CEREBROSPINAL FLUID NORMAL VALUES

Bilirubin	0
Cells	0-5/mm^3, all lymphocytes
Chloride	110-129 mEq/L
Glucose	48-86 mg/dl or ≥60% of serum glucose
pH	7.34-7.43
Pressure	7-20 cm water
Protein, lumbar	15-45 mg/dl
Albumin	58%
α_1-globulins	9%
α_2-globulins	8%
β-globulins	10%
γ-globulins	10 (5-12)%
Protein, cisternal	15-25 mg/dl
Protein, ventricular	5-15 mg/dl

ENDOCRINOLOGIC NORMAL VALUES

HORMONE AND METABOLITE NORMAL VALUES

Adrenocorticotropin (ACTH), serum	15-100 pg/ml	
Aldosterone (mean ± standard deviation)		
Serum		
210 mEq/day sodium diet		
Supine	48 ± 29 pg/ml	
Upright (2 hr)	65 ± 23 pg/ml	
110 mEq/day sodium diet		
Supine	107 ± 45 pg/ml	
Upright (2 hr)	532 ± 228 pg/ml	
Urine	5-19 μg/24 hr	
Calcitonin, serum		
Basal	0.15-0.35 ng/ml	
Stimulated	<06 ng/ml	
Catecholamines, free urinary	<110 μg/24 hr	
Chorionic gonadotropin, serum		
Pregnancy		
First month	10-10.000 mIU/ml	
Second and third months	10,000-100,000 mIU/ml	
Second trimester	10,000-30,000 mIU/ml	
Third trimester	5000-15,000 mIU/ml	
Nonpregnant	<3 mIU/ml	
Cortisol		
Serum		
8 AM	5-25 μg/dl	
8 PM	<10 μg/dl	
Cosyntropin stimulation (30-90 min after 0.25 mg cosyntropin intramuscularly or intravenously)	>10 μg/dl rise over baseline	
Overnight suppression (8 AM serum cortisol after 1 mg dexamethasone orally at 11 PM)	≤5 μg/dl	
Urine	20-70 μg/24 hr	
C-peptide, serum	0.28-0.63 pmol/ml	
11-Deoxycortisol, serum		
Basal	0-1.4 μg/dl	
Metyrapone stimulation (30 mg/kg orally 8 hr prior to level)	>7.5 μg/dl	
Epinephrine, plasma	<35 pg/ml	
Estradiol, serum		
Male	20-50 pg/ml	
Female	25-200 pg/ml	
Estrogens, urine (increased during pregnancy; decreased after menopause)	*Male*	*Female*
Total	4-25 μg/24 hr	5-100 μg/24 hr
Estriol	1-11 μg/24 hr	0-65 μg/24 hr
Estradiol	0-6 μg/24 hr	0-14 μg/24 hr
Estrone	3-8 μg/24 hr	4-31 μg/24 hr
Etiocholanolone, serum	<1.2 μg/dl	
Follicle-stimulating hormone, serum		
Male	2-18 mIU/ml	
Female		
Follicular phase	5-20 mIU/ml	
Peak midcycle	30-50 mIU/ml	
Luteal phase	5-15 mIU/ml	
Postmenopausal	>50 mIU/ml	

Free thyroxine index, serum	1-4 ng/dl
Gastrin, serum (fasting)	30-200 pg/ml
Growth hormone, serum	
Adult, fasting	<5 ng/ml
Glucose load (100 g orally)	<5 ng/ml
Levodopa stimulation (500 mg orally in a fasting state)	>5 ng/ml rise over baseline within 2 hr
17-Hydroxycorticosteroids, urine	
Male	2-12 mg/24 hr
Female	2-8 mg/24 hr
5′-Hydroxyindoleacetic acid (5′-HIAA), urine	2-9 mg/24 hr
Insulin, plasma	
Fasting	6-20 μU/ml
Hypoglycemia (serum glucose < 50 mg/dl)	<5 μU/ml
17-Ketosteroids, urine	
Under 8 years old	0-2 mg/24 hr
Adolescent	0-18 mg/24 hr
Adult	
Male	8-18 mg/24 hr
Female	5-15 mg/24 hr
Luteinizing hormone, serum	
Male adult	2-18 mIU/ml
Female adult	
Basal	5-22 mIU/ml
Ovulation	30-250 mIU/ml
Postmenopausal	>30 mIU/ml
Metanephrines, urine	<1.3 mg/24 hr
Norepinephrine	
Plasma	150-450 pg/ml
Urine	<100 μg/24 hr
Parathyroid hormone, serum	
C-terminal	150-350 pg/ml
N-terminal	230-630 pg/ml
Pregnanediol, urine	
Female	
Follicular phase	<1.5 mg/24 hr
Luteal phase	2.0-4.2 mg/24 hr
Postmenopausal	0.2-1.0 mg/24 hr
Male	<1.5 mg/24 hr
Progesterone, serum	
Female	
Follicular phase	0.02-0.9 ng/ml
Luteal phase	6-30 ng/ml
Male	<2 ng/ml
Prolactin, serum	
Nonpregnant	
Day	5-25 ng/ml
Night	20-40 ng/ml
Pregnant	150-200 ng/ml
Radioactive iodine (^{131}I) uptake (RAIU)	5%-25% at 24 hr (varies with iodine intake)
Renin activity, plasma (mean ± standard deviation)	
Normal diet	
Supine	1.1 ± 0.8 ng/ml/hr
Upright	1.9 ± 1.7 ng/ml/hr
Low-sodium diet	
Supine	2.7 ±1.8 ng/ml/hr
Upright	6.6 ± 2.5 ng/ml/hr
Diuretics and low-sodium diet	10.0 ± 3.7 ng/ml/hr
Testosterone, total plasma	
Bound	
Adolescent male	<100 ng/dl
Adult male	300-1100 ng/dl
Female	25-90 ng/dl
Unbound	
Adult male	3-24 ng/dl
Female	0.09-1.30 ng/dl
Thyroid-stimulating hormone, serum	<10 μU/ml
Thyroxine (T_4), serum	
Total	4-11 μg/dl
Free	0.8-2.4 ng/dl
Thyroxine-binding globulin capacity, serum	15-25 μg T_4/dl
Thyroxine index, free	1-4 ng/dl
Tri-iodothyronine (T_3), serum	70-190 ng/dl
T_3 resin uptake	25%-45%
Vanillylmandelic acid (VMA), urine	1-8 mg/24 hr

ENDOCRINE FUNCTION TESTS

ADRENAL GLAND	
Glucorticoid suppression: overnight dexamethasone suppression test (8 am serum cortisol after 1 mg dexamethasone orally at 11pm)	≤5 µg/dl
Glucocorticoid stimulation; cosyntropin stimulation test (serum cortisol 30-90 min after 0.25 mg cosyntropin intramuscularly or intravenously)	>10 µg/ml more than baseline serum cortisol
Metyrapone test, single dose (8AM serum deoxycortisol after 30 mg/kg metyrapone orally at midnight)	>7.5 µg/dl
Aldosterone suppression: sodium depletion test (urine aldosterone collected on day 3 of 200 mEq day/sodium diet)	<20 µg/24 hr
PANCREAS	
Glucose tolerance test* (serum glucose after 100 g glucose orally)	
60 min after ingestion	<180 mg/dl
90 min after ingestion	<160 mg/dl
120 min after ingestion	<125 mg/dl
PITUITARY GLAND	
Adrenocorticotropic hormone (ACTH) stimulation. See Adrenal gland, Metyrapone test	
Growth hormone stimulation: insulin tolerance test (serum growth hormone after 0.1 U/kg regular insulin intravenously after an overnight fast to induce a 50% fall in serum glucose concentration or symptomatic hypoglycemia)	<5 ng/ml rise over baseline
Levodopa test (serum growth hormone after 0.5 g levodopa orally while fasting)	>5 ng/ml rise over baseline within 2 hr
Growth hormone suppression: glucose tolerance test (serum growth hormone after 100 g glucose orally after 8 hr fast)	<5 ng/ml within 2 hr
Luteinizing hormone (LH) stimulation: gonadotropin-releasing hormone (GnRH) test (serum LH after 100 µg GnRH intravenously or intramuscularly)	4- to 6-fold rise over baseline
Thyroid-stimulating hormone (TSH) stimulation: thyrotropin-releasing hormone (TRH) stimulation test (serum TSH after 400 µg TRH intraveneously)	>2-fold rise over baseline within 2 hr
THYROID GLAND	
Radioactive iodine uptake (RAIU) suppression test (RAIU on day 7 after 25 µg tri-iodothyronine orally 4 times daily)	< 10% to <50% baseline
Thyrotropin-releasing hormone (TRH) stimulation test. See Pituitary gland, Thyroid-stimulating hormone (TSH) stimulation	

*Add 10 mg/dl for each decade over 50 years of age.

PULMONARY FUNCTION TESTS

Abbreviations

P_B	= barometric pressure (mm Hg)
F_IO_2	= inspired oxygen fraction (0.21 = room air)
$PaCO_2$	= partial pressure of carbon dioxide in arterial blood (mm Hg)
P_ACO_2	= partial pressure of carbon dioxide in alveolar gas (mm Hg)
PaO_2	= partial pressure of oxygen in arterial blood (mm Hg)
P_AO_2	= partial pressure of oxygen in alveolar gas (mm Hg)

Alveolar-arterial oxygen gradient (F_IO_2 = 0.21)

$P_{(A-a)}$ in adolescents = <10 mm Hg
adults <40 years = 10 mm Hg
<40 years = 10-15 mm Hg

Alveolar oxygen partial pressure (sea level, F_IO_2 = 0.21)

$P_AO_2 = 150 - (1.2 \times PaCO_2)$

Blood gases (F_IO_2 = 0.21)

	Arterial	*Alveolar*
PO_2	80-105 mm Hg	90-115 mm Hg
PCO_2	38-44 mm Hg	38-44 mm Hg
pH	7.35-7.45	

Spirometric volumes and lung volumes are size-dependent. Typical normal values for adults are provided.

Lung volumes	*Male*	*Female*
Total lung capacity (TLC)	6-7 L	5-6 L
Functional residual capacity (FRC)	2-3 L	2-3 L
Residual values (RV)	1-2 L	1-2 L
Measures of air flow		
Forced vital capacity (FVC)	4.0 L	3.0 L
1 sec forced vital capacity (FEV_1)	>3.0 L	>2.0 L
Pulmonary resistance (RL)	<3.0 cm H_2O/sec/L	
Airway resistance (Raw)	<2.5 H_2O/sec/L	
Other		
Pulmonary compliance (C_L)	0.2 L/cm H_2O	
Diffusing capacity (D_LCO)	25 ml CO/min/mm Hg	

1998

EIGHTH EDITION

Mosby's GenRx™

THE COMPLETE REFERENCE FOR GENERIC AND BRAND DRUGS

Mosby

St. Louis Baltimore Boston Carlsbad Chicago Minneapolis New York Philadelphia Portland
London Milan Sydney Tokyo Toronto

Mosby
Dedicated to Publishing Excellence

A Times Mirror
Company

Vice President: Don E. Ladig
Publisher: L. Suzanne BeDell
Editor: Jabin White
Editorial Systems Manager: Donna L. Hanlon
Database Publishing Editor: Nicole Alexander
Database Publishing Editor: Kerri E. Rabbitt
Database Publishing Editor: Lisa A. Rupe
Project Manager: Linda McKinley
Production Editor: René Spencer
Composition Specialist: Pamela Merritt
Design Coordinator: Renée Duenow
Manufacturing Manager: David R. Graybill
Consulting Editor, International Equivalents: Robert E. Pearson

Mosby's GenR$_x$ accepts no payment for listing; inclusion in the publication of any product, company, or individual does not imply endorsement by the editors or publisher.

The information in this edition was obtained from the FDA, the Health Care Financing Administration, pharmaceutical supplier catalogs, and other publicly available sources. While the publisher has attempted to provide accurate information, it freely admits the possibility of error, and will not accept liability for incorrect information, no matter whether the error was from the FDA, supplier information, or actual information handling by the publisher, including typographical errors. The publisher does not warrant or guarantee any of the products described herein and has not performed any independent analysis in connection with any of the product information contained herein. Users should verify important product information with the appropriate supplier.

Printed in the United States of America
Composition by PageCentre, Inc., and Mosby Electronic Production
Digital photography by Black Dot Group, Ambrosi and Associates, Inc.
Printing/binding by Rand McNally

Mosby–Year Book, Inc.
11830 Westline Industrial Drive
St. Louis, Missouri 63146

ISBN 0-8151-3783-4
ISSN 1094-5768

98 99 00 01 02 / 9 8 7 6 5 4 3 2 1

EDITORIAL REVIEW PANEL

CONTENTS

How to Use, vi
FDA Pregnancy Categories, ix
DEA Schedules of Controlled Substances, ix
Poison Control Centers in the United States and Canada, x
Key Addresses and Phone Numbers, xiii
Oral Solid Dosage Forms That Should Not Be Crushed, xv
Discontinued Products, xix
Manufacturers Listed by NDC Number, xxi
Drug Names that Look Alike and Sound Alike, xxiii
Drug ID Imprint Guide, xxv
Comparative Tables, xl

Section I
KEYWORD INDEX

Alphabetical index of generic and brand names, approved and unlabeled indications, pharmacologic classes and therapeutic uses, pregnancy categories, and FDA approval and patent expiration dates. The page number is given where the entry appears.

DRUG IDENTIFICATION GUIDE

Full-color pictures of capsules and tablets organized alphabetically by generic name. Easy-to-use index that includes generic and brand names. Page location can be found at the end of this section.

Section II
DRUG INFORMATION

Complete manufacturer's package insert supplemented with valuable information, including brand names (U.S. and international), FDA-approved and unlabeled indications, therapeutic use, pharmacologic class, FDA approval date, innovator drug, pregnancy category, top-selling drugs grouped by Top 100 and 200, formulary coverage, benchmark cost of therapy, ICD-9 codes, controlled substance schedule, AWP, HCFA pricing, and FDA-related bioequivalent products.

Section III
SUPPLIER PROFILES

Contains alphabetical listing of suppliers/manufacturers and includes the following key information on each company: NDC number, addresses, telephone and fax numbers, and listing of company representatives.

DIRECTORY OF AIDS DRUG ASSISTANCE PROGRAMS IN THE UNITED STATES, GUAM, AND VIRGIN ISLANDS

Listing of AIDS drug assistance programs listed by U.S. state or territory including Puerto Rico, Guam, and the U.S. Virgin Islands. These are state-funded programs that assist financially depleted patients.

HOW TO USE

The 1998 edition of *Mosby's GenR$_x$* represents a compilation of the most current information on prescription pharmaceuticals and their suppliers available today. The result is a reference that serves the diverse needs of health care professionals. By providing a superior indexing system, thorough prescribing information, and invaluable price listings, *Mosby's GenR$_x$* is the complete, unbiased guide to prescription pharmaceuticals, both branded and generic.

The intention of this book is not to promote the use of generic drugs over brand-name products, or vice versa. Generic drugs are in wide use across the United States. Many state and private health insurance plans promote or mandate generic substitution, and some brand-name pharmaceutical companies have now launched their own generic lines. In short, generic drugs are an integral part of the health care delivery system.

Mosby's GenR$_x$ serves as a guide identifying drugs available as generics, whether there are any therapeutic equivalency problems, and whether there are any significant economic benefits. *Mosby's GenR$_x$* is designed for ease of use. A completely unbiased source of pharmaceutical information, the book is organized in a way that makes sense to both professionals and support staff. It also contains a wealth of information on the pharmaceutical industry, which can be useful for investors, researchers, and marketers.

Prescribing information, as approved by the FDA, is included wherever possible. In some cases, information is not included because it is unavailable. For example, most drugs that predate the FDA approval process (pre-1938) have no official prescribing information. Every effort has been made in these cases to obtain the information; there is no editorial policy against the inclusion of any particular drug or the products of any company. Drugs available without a prescription are not covered in the print version of *Mosby's GenR$_x$*.

Should you have any questions or comments on how to use the book, please call *Mosby's GenR$_x$* hotline at Mosby–Year Book, Inc. (1-800-638-1393).

KEYWORD INDEX

The Keyword Index allows the user to find the correct generic name by looking up any words that might relate to the name.

The many features and advantages of the Keyword Index are enhanced by the fact that they are all found in one place. Each entry within the Keyword Index lists the appropriate page in the Drug Information Section (Section II) where more complete information about the specific drug is located.

FDA-standard names use USP (U.S. Pharmacopeial Convention, Inc.) approved names for single ingredients. For multiple-ingredient drugs, each generic chemical is included in alphabetical order, separated by a semicolon (";") between each entity (*e.g.,* Hydrochlorothiazide; Triamterene). This is not necessarily the same order of ingredients used in product names for multiple-ingredient drugs; however, because suppliers use different formats, this FDA-standard format allows for easy grouping of identical drugs.

Products are also indexed under therapeutic and pharmacologic categories. Most drugs fall into several categories, so this index can be a more powerful way to locate drugs than references that are organized by therapeutic category.

Listings of indications are included among index terms so alternative drug therapies can be identified. Also included are unlabeled indications for some drugs. These unlabeled uses are not described in the FDA prescribing information, but they are included as index categories.

Drugs are also grouped under various categories such as the following:

- Products still under Drug Efficacy Study Implementation (DESI) review that are unapproved for effectiveness but remain on the market legally
- Orphan drugs
- Top-selling drugs grouped by top 200
- Drugs with worldwide sales in U.S. dollars, at the manufacturer's level, more than $1 billion, $500 million, and $100 million
- Drug Enforcement Administration Schedules of Controlled Substances: C-II, C-III, C-IV, C-V
- FDA Pregnancy Categories
- FDA Approval Date
- Patent Expiration Date
- FDA's evaluation of New Molecular Entities:
- Class 1A (Important Therapeutic Advantage)
- Class 1B (Modest Therapeutic Gain)
- Class 1C (Little or No Therapeutic Advantage)
- Class 1P ("Priority Review")
- Class 1S ("Standard Review")

The two categories 1P and 1S are the current FDA designations used for new molecular entities.

Classes 1A, 1B, 1C are no longer assigned.

The Keyword Index also includes a benchmark Cost of Therapy, in parens, for many drugs. Thus different chemicals can be compared in the Keyword Index based on their overall cost of therapy.

DRUG INFORMATION

The purpose of this section is to provide complete information for pharmaceutical decision making, organized alphabetically by generic name, including prescribing information as well as how supplied (equivalency ratings and costs). The core of this information is the FDA-approved labeling for each generic drug. The information is supplemented by data from standard pharmacology texts and peer-reviewed medical journals, as suggested by our editorial panel.

Immediately under the generic name are up to four headings of summary information for that drug: Categories, Brand Names, Formularies, and Cost of Therapy.

CATEGORIES

The list of categories includes FDA-approved and unlabeled indications, pharmacologic class, and therapeutic use. If any unlabeled indications are listed, they are identified by an asterisk and a footnote stating "Indication Not Approved by FDA." This section can be quickly scanned in alphabetical order for the Pregnancy Category, DEA Controlled Substance Schedule, Patent Expiration Date, FDA Class (Evaluations of New Molecular Entities), Top Sales Ranking (Top 200, etc.), and relative worldwide sales volume at the manufacturers level (Sales > $1 Billion, etc.), FDA Approval Date.

BRAND NAMES

Drugs listed under brand names are U.S. brand names, branded generic names, and brand names no longer in use. The primary innovator brand name appears in boldface type. All U.S. brand names listed in this section will be found in the Keyword Index. Also included among the brand names are international brand equivalents used in 137 countries. These names appear in italics and are designated by a footnote.

FORMULARIES

Following the brand names is the formularies section. This section indicates coverage by major, usually national, managed-care drug formularies. Coverage means that the health plans using those formularies typically reimburse their members for use of those drugs. In most cases, all available forms, routes, and strengths are covered, but in some cases they are not. For up-to-date information, please check with your local carrier. This formulary coverage does not indicate the preferred supplier, which is generally the innovator brand when FDA-rated equivalent generics are not available; when they are available, substitution is usually required at the time of drug dispensing. Information on the formulary coverage of drugs was obtained from drug manufacturers who have succeeded in getting their drugs placed on the formularies, from the managed care organization itself, or from government documents and press releases. Included among the formularies is "WHO," indicating inclusion on the World Health Organization's List of Essential Drugs for Developing Countries, intended for use by countries establishing a national drug list for the first time.

COST OF THERAPY

The next section, Cost of Therapy, calculates a net cost based on dosage as in the FDA-approved package insert. The assumptions are provided in the Cost of Therapy section and include primary indication, primary form, starting strength, number of doses per day, and total number of days of therapy required. Cost of Therapy typically uses oral forms only, and the number of days is assumed to be 365 for maintenance drugs. These assumptions are then applied to the prices that appear in the How Supplied section to arrive at a dollar figure. The price used is the lowest supplier price in 100s, which closely approximates the acquisition price of generics.

PRESCRIBING INFORMATION

Next appears complete FDA-approved prescribing information; each monograph is organized into as many as 14 sections:

- Description
- Clinical pharmacology
- Clinical studies
- Indications and usage
- Contraindications
- Adverse reactions
- Warnings
- Precautions
- Drug interactions
- Drug abuse and dependence
- Overdosage
- Dosage and administration
- Animal pharmacology
- References
- Centers for Disease Control dosage information
- Patient information

In addition, some monographs also have a Patient Package Insert when available.

The prescribing information included in this volume is the FDA-approved labeling found in the pharmaceutical suppliers' package inserts. In many cases the monographs in this section are a combination of the prescribing information for different forms, routes, strengths, and indications.

In some of these combination cases, only certain sections of the monograph pertain to all of the products.

HOW SUPPLIED

Equivalency ratings. The breakdown of product listings between "rated equivalent" and "not rated equivalent" is a format that is derived directly from the Food and Drug Administration publication: "Approved Drug Products with Therapeutic Equivalence Evaluations," commonly known as the "Orange Book."

The Orange Book is considered to be the most reliable information source for determining which drug products are therapeutically equivalent.

Most drug labels are required to show the name of the original manufacturer as well as the distributor (if any). If a particular distributor's product is listed as "not rated equivalent," check to see whether the manufacturer is also listed as "not rated equivalent" for the same drug form, strength, and route. Judgment should be based on whether the original manufacturer is listed as "rated therapeutically equivalent." Some original manufacturers are not listed in *Mosby's GenR$_x$* because they do not market their own products and are not registered with the FDA Drug Listing Branch.

There are some products that are available from many sources in one form but only as a branded single source in another. For example, indomethacin is available from many sources as an oral capsule, but only one manufacturer produces the intravenous injection (Indocin I.V., Merck). The injection is "not rated equivalent" because there is no rating in the Orange Book for single-source products.

All single-source products for which there are no other generically available forms, routes, or strengths are listed as "equivalents not available."

Drugs not rated by the Orange Book are listed in the How Supplied section as "equivalents not available." These are (1) drugs that predate the FDA approval process (before 1938) or (2) drug products marketed between 1938 and 1962 that were approved for safety but not effectiveness and are still under the scientific and legal-administrative review procedures of the Drug Efficacy Study Implementation (DESI) process.

Equivalency criteria

Pharmaceutical equivalents: Drug products are considered pharmaceutical equivalents if they contain the same active ingredient(s), are of the same dosage form, and are identical in strength or concentration and route of administration. Pharmaceutically equivalent drug products are formulated to contain the same amount of active ingredient in the same dosage form and to meet the same compendial or other applicable standards (*i.e.*, strength, quality, purity, and identity), but they may differ in characteristics such as shape, scoring configuration, packaging, excipients (including colors, flavors, preservatives), expiration time, and, within certain limits, labeling.

Therapeutic equivalents: Drug products are considered to be therapeutic equivalents only if they are pharmaceutical equivalents and can be expected to have the same clinical effect when administered to patients under the conditions specified in the labeling. The FDA classifies as therapeutically equivalent those products that meet the following general criteria:

1. They are approved as safe and effective, or approved under section 505(j) of the Federal Food, Drug, and Cosmetic Act;
2. They are pharmaceutical equivalents in that they:
   (a) contain identical amounts of the same active drug ingredient in the same dosage form and route of administration, and
   (b) meet compendia or other applicable standards of strength, quality, purity, and identity;
3. They are bioequivalent in that:
   (a) they do not present a known or potential bioequivalence problem, and they meet an applicable in vitro standard, or
   (b) if they do present a known or potential problem, they are shown to meet an appropriate bioequivalence standard;
4. They are adequately labeled;
5. They are manufactured in compliance with Current Good Manufacturing Practice regulations.

The concept of therapeutic equivalence, as used to develop this list, applies only to drug products containing the same active ingredient(s). A single-source drug product in this list repackaged and/or distributed by other than the applicant holder is considered to be therapeutically equivalent to the single-source drug product.

The FDA considers drug products to be therapeutically equivalent if they meet the criteria outlined above, even though they may differ in certain other characteristics such as shape, scoring configuration, packaging, excipients (including colors, flavors, preservatives), expiration time, and minor aspects of labeling (*e.g.,* the presence of pharmacokinetic information). When such differences are important in the care of a particular patient, it may be appropriate for the prescribing physician to require that a particular brand be dispensed as a medical necessity.

Although the therapeutic equivalency information contained in the Orange Book is widely used, product selection is a professional decision that is based on policies at the state level to minimize the cost of drugs to consumers. Health professionals and the states are under no mandate to accept the therapeutic equivalence recommendations in the Orange Book. The FDA takes no official position on state regulation of drug product selection by pharmacists.

If the FDA has rated any products as therapeutic equivalents, they are listed as RATED THERAPEUTICALLY EQUIVALENT. These products are designated with "A" codes by the FDA. Readers may be familiar with the term "A rated," which simply translates as RATED THERAPEUTICALLY EQUIVALENT. Products not rated equivalent are listed as NOT RATED EQUIVALENT, and if no alternative products are available, supplier information is listed as EQUIVALENTS NOT AVAILABLE. Some of these products have received a "B" code by the FDA. These are drug products that the FDA does not at this time consider to be therapeutically equivalent to other pharmaceutically equivalent products. Additionally, some of these products have not been evaluated by the FDA in terms of therapeutic equivalence.

Product listings. Product information is supplied, grouped by Dosage Form and Strength, and sorted by price within package size, giving the product name used by the supplier, the supplier's FDA short name, and the product's official NDC (National Drug Code) number, using 5-4-2 format. The labeler code, assigned by the FDA, is the first five digits of all product NDC numbers listed for this supplier. The rest of the NDC number includes four digits assigned by the supplier to identify their unique drug and two digits to identify the package size.

- Brand names are in all capital letters for easy identification.
- Innovator is listed in bold.
- U.D. indicates Unit Dose packaging.

Prices are AWP (Average Wholesale Price), a benchmark price used for reimbursement. AWP represents the amount a retail pharmacist or a dispensing physician might pay for a product without any special discounts. There are, however, many discounts already in place, so the AWP often approximates the price that a consumer might pay. The prices listed here are not intended to serve as an up-to-date substitute for supplier price lists. The price listings give the reader a good idea of the range between the high and low prices.

In making prescribing decisions and considering generic substitution, physicians can not only determine whether 'equivalent' generic alternatives are available but also evaluate whether the cost differential between brands and generics justifies a possible risk in substitution. Furthermore, decisions about alternative drug entities can also be based partially on their economic impact.

To that end, the H.C.F.A. FFP (the Health Care Finance Administration's Federal Financial Participation "upper limits" price for that package size) for each drug is listed along with the other listings by AWP. This is the price reimbursable by Medicare when reimbursement is available. Many states have also adopted this price for use in their Medicaid programs, and many insurance carriers use this price.

In many states the existence of a H.C.F.A. FFP price means that substitution is mandatory unless the prescribing physician specifies otherwise, and Medicaid reimburses the dispensing pharmacist at the FFP price plus a dispensing fee.

The H.C.F.A. FFP price is a better approximation of actual price for generics; therefore to estimate the difference in price between the generic and brand, the brand should be compared with the FFP, if one is given.

SUPPLIER PROFILES

The Supplier Profiles section can be used to obtain additional information on a particular supplier.

Suppliers in Section II, Drug Information, are listed alphabetically in this section by their FDA short names. Also included are parent companies of listed suppliers and a number of biotechnology companies, research and development organizations, and major foreign manufacturers that do not currently have pharmaceutical products on the market in the United States.

Beneath the FDA short name is the full company name, ownership information (if appropriate), and complete address. To the right of the name is the telephone number (with toll-free 800 numbers where available) for inquiries about the company's products. Fax numbers are also listed, where available.

Opposite the FDA short name are the five-digit NDC (National Drug Code) labeler codes for this supplier. The labeler code, assigned by the FDA, is the first five digits of all product NDC numbers listed for each supplier. Codes that start with the letter "P" designate parent companies; those starting with "A" have no products on the U.S. market.

Also included are estimates of medical product sales volume and total employees. The companies are described as either manufacturers or distributors, if this information is available.

Federal Procurement eligibility, including coverage by the 1990 Medicaid Rebate Law, is also listed. As of April 1, 1991, OBRA-90 will provide Medicaid coverage only for products of those manufacturers that have signed rebate agreements with the federal government.

Ownership of each company is identified by the FDA short name of the owner or the designations *public* and *private*.

A listing of names and titles of key executives in general management, marketing, production, and research follows. The names listed under research (many may appear for larger firms) are listed alphabetically, without respect to position or exact location.

Subsidiaries (each of which has its own separate listing) are listed at the bottom of each supplier profile.

Former names of suppliers and their subsidiaries are cross-referenced within the section.

FDA PREGNANCY CATEGORIES

Pregnancy Category	*Definition*
A	Adequate studies in pregnant women have not demonstrated a risk to the fetus in the first trimester of pregnancy and there is no evidence of risk in later trimesters.
B	Animal studies have not demonstrated a risk to the fetus, but there are no adequate studies in pregnant women **or** Animal studies have shown an adverse effect, but adequate studies in pregnant women have not demonstrated a risk to the fetus during the first trimester of pregnancy, and there is no evidence of risk in later trimesters.
C	Animal studies have shown an adverse effect on the fetus, but there are no adequate studies in humans; the benefits of the drugs in pregnant women may be acceptable despite its potential risks **or** There are no animal reproduction studies and no adequate studies in humans.
D	There is evidence of human fetal risk, but the potential benefits from the use of the drug in pregnant women may be acceptable despite its potential risks.
X	Studies in animals or humans demonstrate fetal abnormalities or adverse reaction reports indicate evidence of fetal risk. The risk of use in a pregnant woman clearly outweighs any possible benefit.

Regardless of the designated Pregnancy Category or presumed safety, no drug should be administered during pregnancy unless it is clearly needed and potential benefits outweigh potential risks.

DRUG ENFORCEMENT ADMINISTRATION SCHEDULES OF CONTROLLED SUBSTANCES

The controlled substances that come under jurisdiction of the Controlled Substances Act are divided into five schedules. Examples of controlled substances and their schedules are as follows:

SCHEDULE I SUBSTANCES

The controlled substances in this schedule are those that have no accepted medical use in the United States and have a high abuse potential. Some examples are heroin, marijuana, LSD, peyote, mescaline, psilocybin, THC, MDA, ketobemidone, acetylmethadol, fenethylline, tilidine, methaqualone, and dihydromorphine.

SCHEDULE II SUBSTANCES

The controlled substances in this schedule have a high abuse potential with severe psychic or physical dependence liability. Schedule II controlled substances consist of certain narcotic, stimulant, and depressant drugs. Some examples of Schedule II controlled narcotic substances are opium, morphine, codeine, hydromorphone, methadone, meperidine, cocaine, oxycodone, anileridine, and oxymorphone. Also in Schedule II are amphetamine, methamphetamine, phenmetrazine, methylphenidate, amobarbital, pentobarbital, secobarbital, fentanyl, etorphine hydrochloride, and phencyclidine.

SCHEDULE III SUBSTANCES

The controlled substances in this schedule have an abuse potential less than those in Schedules I and II and include compounds containing limited quantities of certain narcotic drugs and nonnarcotic drugs such as derivatives of barbituric acid (except those that are listed in another schedule), glutethimide, methyprylon, nalorphine, benzphetamine, chlorphentermine, clortermine, phendimetrazine, and paregoric. Any suppository dosage form containing amobarbital, secobarbital, or pentobarbital is in this schedule.

SCHEDULE IV SUBSTANCES

The controlled substances in this schedule have an abuse potential less than those listed in Schedule III and include drugs such as barbital, phenobarbital, mephobarbital, chloral hydrate, ethchlorvynol, ethinamate, meprobamate, paraldehyde, methohexital, fenfluramine, diethylpropion, phentermine, chlordiazepoxide, diazepam, oxazepam, clorazepate, flurazepam, clonazepam, prazepam, lorazepam, alprazolam, halazepam, triazolam, mebutamate, dextropropoxyphene, and pentazocine.

SCHEDULE V SUBSTANCES

The controlled substances in this schedule have an abuse potential less than those listed in Schedule IV and consist of preparations containing limited quantities of certain narcotic drugs generally for antitussive and antidiarrheal purposes.

POISON CONTROL CENTERS OF THE UNITED STATES AND CANADA

Following are the names and addresses of poison centers in the United States, with emergency telephone numbers.

ALABAMA

Alabama Poison Center, Tuscaloosa
408-A Paul Bryant Drive
Tuscaloosa, AL 35401
Emergency Phone: (800) 462-0800 (AL only); (205) 345-0600
Fax: (205) 759-7994

Regional Poison Control Center
The Children's Hospital of Alabama
1600 – 7th Avenue South
Birmingham, AL 35233-1711
Emergency Phone: (205) 939-9201; (800) 292-6678 (AL only); (205) 933-4050
Fax: (205) 939-9245

ARIZONA

Arizona Poison and Drug Information Center
Arizona Health Sciences Center; Rm. #1156
1501 N. Campbell Avenue
Tucson, AZ 85724
Emergency Phone: (800) 362-0101 (AZ only); (502) 626-6016
Fax: (520) 626-2720

Samaritan Regional Poison Center
Good Samaritan Regional Medical Center
Ancillary-1
1111 E. McDowell Road
Phoenix, AZ 85006
Emergency Phone: (602) 253-3334
Fax: (602) 256-7579

CALIFORNIA

California Poison Control System-Fresno
Valley Children's Hospital
3151 N. Millbrook, IN31
Fresno, CA 93703
Emergency Phone: (800) 346-5922 (Central CA only); (209) 445-1222
Fax: (209) 241-6050

California Poison Control System-San Diego
UCSD Medical Center
200 West Arbor Drive
San Diego, CA 92103-8925
Emergency Phone: (619) 543-6000; (800) 876-4766 (619 area code only)
Fax: (619) 692-1867

California Poison Control System-Sacramento
2315 Stockton Boulevard
Sacramento, CA 95817
Emergency Phone: (916) 734-3692; (800) 342-9293 (Northern California only)
Fax: (916) 734-7796

COLORADO

Rocky Mountain Poison and Drug Center
8802 E. 9th Avenue
Denver, CO 80220-6800
Emergency Phone: (303) 629-1123
Fax: (303) 739-1119

CONNECTICUT

Connecticut Regional Poison Control Center
University of Connecticut Health Center
263 Farmington Avenue
Farmington, CT 06030-5365
Emergency Phone: (800) 343-2722 (CT only); (203) 679-3056
Fax: (203) 679-1623

DISTRICT OF COLUMBIA

National Capital Poison Center
3201 New Mexico Avenue, NW, Suite 310
Washington, DC 20016
Emergency Phone: (202) 625-3333; (202) 362-8563 (TTY)
Fax: (202) 362-8377

FLORIDA

Florida Poison Information Center-Jacksonville
University Medical Center
University of Florida Health Science Center-Jacksonville
655 West 8th Street
Jacksonville, FL 32209
Emergency Phone: (904) 549-4480; (800) 282-3171 (FL only)
Fax: (904) 549-4063

Florida Poison Information Center-Miami
University of Miami, School of Medicine
Department of Pediatrics
P.O. Box 016960 (R-131)
Miami, FL 33101
Emergency Phone: (800) 282-3171 (FL only)
Fax: (305) 242-9762

The Florida Poison Information Center and Toxicology Resource Center
Tampa General Hospital
P.O. Box 1289
Tampa, FL 33601
Emergency Phone: (813) 253-4444 (Tampa); (800) 282-3171 (FL)
Fax: (813) 253-4443

GEORGIA

Georgia Poison Center
Grady Memorial Hospital
80 Butler Street S.E.
P.O. Box 26066
Atlanta, GA 30335-3801
Emergency Phone: (800) 282-5846 (GA only); (404) 616-9000
Fax: (404) 616-6657

HAWAII

Hawaii Poison Control Center
1319 Punahou Street
Honolulu, HI 96826
Emergency Phone: (808) 941-4411; (808) 941-4412; (800) 362-3585

INDIANA

Indiana Poison Center
Methodist Hospital of Indiana
1701 N. Senate Boulevard
P.O. Box 1367
Indianapolis, IN 46206-1367
Emergency Phone: (800) 382-9097 (IN only); (317) 929-2323
Fax: (317) 929-2337

KENTUCKY

Kentucky Regional Poison Center of Kosair Children's Hospital
Medical Towers South, Suite 572
P.O. Box 35070
Louisville, KY 40232-5070
Emergency Phone: (502) 629-7275; (800) 722-5725 (KY only)
Fax: (502) 629-7277

LOUISIANA

Louisiana Drug and Poison Information Center
Northeast Louisiana University
Sugar Hall
Monroe, LA 71209-6430
Emergency Phone: (800) 256-9822 (LA only); (318) 362-5393
Fax: (318) 342-1744

MARYLAND

Maryland Poison Center
20 N. Pine Street
Baltimore, MD 21201
Emergency Phone: (410) 528-7701; (800) 492-2414 (MD only)
Fax: (410) 706-7184

National Capital Poison Center (DC suburbs only)
3201 New Mexico Avenue, NW, Suite 310
Washington, DC 20016
Emergency Phone: (202) 625-3333; (202) 362-8563 (TTY)

MASSACHUSETTS

Massachusetts Poison Control System
300 Longwood Avenue
Boston, MA 02115
Emergency Phone: (617) 232-2120; (800) 682-9211
Fax: (617) 738-0032

MICHIGAN

Poison Control Center
Children's Hospital of Michigan
4160 John Road, Suite 425
Detroit, MI 48201
Emergency Phone: (313) 745-5711
Fax: (313) 745-5493

MINNESOTA

Hennepin Regional Poison Center
Hennepin County Medical Center
701 Park Avenue
Minneapolis, MN 55415
Emergency Phone: (612) 347-3141;
Petline: (612) 337-7387; TDD (612) 337-7474
Fax: (612) 904-4289

Minnesota Regional Poison Center
8100 34th Avenue S.
P.O. Box 1309
Minneapolis, MN 55440-1309
Emergency Phone: (612) 221-2113
Fax: (612) 851-8166

MISSOURI

Cardinal Glennon Children's Hospital Regional Poison Center
1465 S. Grand Boulevard
St. Louis, MO 63104
Emergency Phone: (314) 772-5200; (800) 366-8888
Fax: (314) 577-5355

MONTANA

Rocky Mountain Poison and Drug Center
8801 E. 9th Avenue
Denver, CO 80220
Emergency Phone: (303) 629-1123
Fax: (303) 739-1119

NEBRASKA

The Poison Center
8301 Dodge Street
Omaha, NE 68114
Emergency Phone: (402) 390-5555 (Omaha); (800) 955-9119 (NE and WY)
Fax: (404) 354-3049

NEW JERSEY

New Jersey Poison Information and Education System
201 Lyons Ave.
Newark, NJ 07112
Emergency Phone: (800) 962-1253
Fax: (201) 705-8098

NEW MEXICO

New Mexico Poison and Drug Information Center
University of New Mexico
Health Sciences Library, Room 125
Albuquerque, NM 87131-1076
Emergency Phone: (505) 843-2551, (800) 432-6866 (NM only)
Fax: (505) 277-5892

NEW YORK

Central New York Poison Control Center
SUNY Health Science Center
750 East Adams Street
Syracuse, NY 13210
Emergency Phone: (315) 476-4766; (800) 252-5655 (NY only)
Fax: (315) 464-7077

Finger Lakes Regional Poison Center
601 Elmwood Avenue, Box 321
Room G-3275
Rochester, NY 14642
Emergency Phone: (800) 333-0542; (716) 275-3232
Fax: (716) 244-1677

Hudson Valley Regional Poison Center
Phelps Memorial Hospital Center
701 North Broadway
North Tarrytown, NY 10591
Emergency Phone: (800) 336-6997; (914) 366-3030
Fax: (914) 353-1050

Long Island Regional Poison Control Center
Winthrop University Hospital
259 First Street
Mineola, NY 11501
Emergency Phone: (516) 542-2323, 2324, 2325, 3813
Fax: (516) 739-2070

New York City Poison Control Center
N.Y.C. Department of Health
455 First Avenue, Room 123
New York, NY 10016
Emergency Phone: (212) 340-4494; (212) P-O-I-S-O-N-S; (212) 689-9014 (TDD)
Fax: (212) 447-8223

NORTH CAROLINA

Carolinas Poison Center
1012 S. Kings Drive, Suite 206
P.O. Box 32861
Charlotte, NC 28232-2861
Emergency Phone: (704) 355-4000; (800) 84-TOXIN (800-848-6946)

OHIO

Central Ohio Poison Center
700 Children's Drive
Columbus, OH 43205-2696
Emergency Phone: (614) 228-1323; (800) 682-7625; (614) 228-2272 (TTY); (614) 461-2012
Fax: (614) 221-2672

Cincinnati Drug & Poison Information Center and Regional Poison Control System
P.O. Box 670144
Cincinnati, OH 45267-0144
Emergency Phone: (513) 558-5111; (800) 872-5111 (OH only)
Fax: (513) 558-5301

OREGON

Oregon Poison Center
Oregon Health Sciences University
3181 S.W. Sam Jackson Park Road, CB550
Portland, OR 97201
Emergency Phone: (503) 494-8968, (800) 452-7165 (OR only)
Fax: (503) 494-4980

PENNSYLVANIA

Central Pennsylvania Poison Center
University Hospital
Milton S. Hershey Medical Center
Hershey, PA 17033
Emergency Phone: (800) 521-6110
Fax: (717) 531-6932

The Poison Control Center
3600 Sciences Center, Suite 220
Philadelphia, PA 19104-2641
Emergency Phone: (215) 386-2100
Fax: (215) 590-4419

Pittsburgh Poison Center
3705 Fifth Avenue
Pittsburgh, PA 15213
Emergency Phone: (412) 681-6669
Fax: (412) 692-7497

RHODE ISLAND

Rhode Island Poison Center
593 Eddy Street
Providence, RI 02903
Emergency Phone: (401) 444-5727
Fax: (401) 444-8062

TENNESSEE

Middle Tennessee Poison Center
The Center for Clinical Toxicology
Vanderbilt University Medical Center
1161 21st Avenue South
501 Oxford House
Nashville, TN 37232-4632
Emergency Phone: (615) 936-2034; (800) 288-9999
Fax: (615) 936-2046

TEXAS

Central Texas Poison Center
Scott & White Memorial Hospital
2401 S. 31st Street
Temple, TX 76508
Emergency Phone: (800) 764-7661
Fax: (817) 724-1731

North Texas Poison Center
5201 Harry Hines Boulevard
P.O. Box 35926
Dallas, TX 75235
Emergency Phone: (800) 764-7661; (800) 441-0040 (Texas Watts)
Fax: (214) 590-5008

Southeast Texas Poison Center
The University of Texas Medical Branch
301 University
Galveston, TX 77550-2780
Emergency Phone: (409) 765-1420 (Galveston); (713) 654-1701 (Houston); (800) 764-7661
Fax: (409) 772-3917

UTAH
Utah Poison Control Center
410 Chipeta Way, Suite 230
Salt Lake City, UT 84108
Emergency Phone: (801) 581-2151; (800) 456-7707 (UT only)
Fax: (801) 581-4199

VIRGINIA
Blue Ridge Poison Center
Box 67 Blue Ridge
University of Virginia Medical Center
Charlottesville, VA 22901
Emergency Phone: (804) 924-5543; (800) 451-1428
Fax: (804) 971-8657

National Capital Poison Center (Northern VA only)
3201 New Mexico Avenue, NW, Suite 310
Washington, DC 20016
Emergency Phone: (202) 625-3333, (202) 362-8563 (TTY)

WASHINGTON
Washington Poison Center
155 NE 100th Street
Suite #400
Seattle, WA 98125
Emergency Phone: (206) 526-2121; (206) 517-2394; (800) 732-6985; (800) 572-0638 (TDD)
Fax: (206) 526-8490

WEST VIRGINIA
West Virginia Poison Center
3110 MacCorkle Avenue S.E.
Charleston, WV 25304
Emergency Phone: (800) 642-3625 (WV only); (304) 348-4211
Fax: (304) 348-9560

WYOMING
The Poison Center
8301 Dodge Street
Omaha, NE 68114
Emergency Phone: (402) 390-5555 (Omaha); (800) 955-9119 (NE and WY)
Fax: (404) 354-3049

Following are the names and addresses of poison centers in Canada.

ALBERTA
Poison and Drug Information Service
Foothills Hospital
1403-29th St. N.W.
Calgary, AB T2N 2T9
(800) 332-1414; (403) 670-1414; Fax: (403) 670-1472

BRITISH COLUMBIA
B.C. Drug and Poison Information Centre
St. Paul's Hospital
1081 Burrard St.
Vancouver, BC V6Z 1Y6
(800) 567-8911; (604) 682-5050 (Greater Vancouver & lower mainland); Fax: (604) 631-5262

MANITOBA
Provincial Poison Information Centre
Children's Hospital Helath Sciences Centre
840 Sherbrook St.
Winnipeg, MB R3A 1S1
(204) 787-2591; (204) 787-2444 (general inquiries); Fax: (204) 787-1775

NEW BRUNSWICK
Monoton
Poison Control Centre
The Monoton Hospital
135 McBeath Ave.
Monoton, NB E1C 6Z8
(506) 857-5555; (506) 857-2108 (general inquiries); Fax: (506) 857-5360

Saint John
Emergency Department
Saint John Regional Hospital
P.O. Box 2100
Saint John, NB E2L 4L2
(506) 648-6222; Fax: (506) 867-3259

NEWFOUNDLAND
Emergency Department
The Dr. Charles A. Janeway Child Health Centre
710 Janeway Place
St. John's, NF A1A 1R8
(709) 722-1110 (emergency inquiries); Fax: (709) 926-0830

NORTHWEST TERRITORIES
Emergency Department
Stanton Yellowknife Hospital
P.O. Box 10
Yellowknife, NT X1A 2N1
(403) 669-4100; Fax: (403) 669-4171

NOVA SCOTIA
Poison Control Centre
The Izaak Walton Killam/Grace HealthCare Centre for Children, Women and Families
P.O. Box 3070
Halifax, NS B3J 3G9
(902) 428-8161; (800) 565-8161 (toll-free from P.E.I.); Fax: (902) 428-3213

ONTARIO
Ottawa
Ontario Regional Poison Information Centre
Children's Hospital of Eastern Ontario
401 Smyth Road
Ottawa, ON K1H 8L1
(800) 267-1373; (613) 737-1100; (613) 737-2320 (general inquiries); Fax: (613) 738-4862

Toronto
Ontario Regional Poison Information Centre
The Hospital for Sick Children
555 University Ave.
Toronto, ON M5G 1X8
(800) 268-9017; (416) 813-5900; Fax: (416) 813-7489

PRINCE EDWARD ISLAND
See Nova Scotia listing for address.
(800) 565-8161

QUEBEC
Centre antipoison du Québec
Le Centre Hospitalier de l'Université Laval
2705, boul. Laurier
Sainte-Foy, PQ G1V 4G2
(800) 463-5060; (418) 656-8090; Fax: (418) 654-2747

SASKATCHEWAN
Regina
Emergency Department
Regina General Hospital
1440 14th Ave.
Regina, SK S4P 0W5
(800) 667-4545; (306) 766-4545; Fax: (306) 766-4357

Saskatoon
Emergency Department
Royal University Hospital
Saskatoon, SK S7N 0X8
(800) 363-7474; (306) 655-1010; Fax: (306) 655-1011

YUKON TERRITORY
Emergency Department
Whitehorse General Hospital
5 Hospital Road
Whitehorse, YT Y1A 3H7
(403) 667-8728; Fax: (403) 667-8762

KEY ADDRESSES AND PHONE NUMBERS

Academy of Managed Care Pharmacy
Judith A. Cahill, CEBS
Executive Director
1650 King St. Suite 402
Alexandria, VA 22314
(703) 683-8416; Fax: (703) 683-8417

American Association of Colleges of Pharmacy
Dr. Richard P. Penna
Executive Vice President
1426 Prince St.
Alexandria, VA 22314-2841
(703) 739-2330; Fax: (703) 836-8982

American Association of Pharmaceutical Scientists
John B. Cox
Executive Director
1650 King St.
Alexandria, VA 22314-2747
(703) 548-3000; Fax: (703) 684-7349

American College of Apothecaries
D.C. Huffman, Jr., Ph.D.
Executive Vice President
P.O. Box 341266
Bartlett, TN 38184
(901) 383-8119; Fax: (901) 383-8882

American College of Clinical Pharmacy
Robert Elenbaas, Pharm.D.
Executive Director
3101 Broadway, Suite 380
Kansas City, MO 64111
(816) 531-2177; Fax: (816) 531-4990

American Council on Pharmaceutical Education
Daniel A. Nona
Executive Director
311 W. Superior St., Suite 512
Chicago, IL 60610
(312) 664-3575; Fax: (312) 664-4652

American Foundation for Pharmaceutical Education
Robert M. Bachman
President
One Church St., Suite 202
Rockville, MD 20850
(301) 738-2160; Fax: (301) 738-2161

American Institute of the History of Pharmacy
Gregory J. Higby, Ph.D.
Executive Director
425 North Charter St.
Madison, WI 53706-1508
(608) 262-5378

American Pharmaceutical Association
John A. Gans, Pharm.D.
Executive Vice President
2215 Constitution Ave., NW
Washington, DC 20037
(202) 628-4410; Fax: (202) 783-2351

American Society for Automation in Pharmacy
William A. Lockwood, Jr.
Executive Director
482 Norristown Rd., Suite 112
Blue Bell, PA 19422-2359
(610) 825-7783; Fax: (610) 825-7641

American Society for Pharmacy Law
John A. Cronin, Pharm.D., J.D.
Executive Director
P.O. Box 7163
Auburn, CA 95604-7163
(916) 801-5867; Fax: (916) 823-5259

American Society of Consultant Pharmacists
R. Timothy Webster
Executive Director
1321 Duke St.
Alexandria, VA 22314-3563
(703) 739-1300; Fax: (703) 739-1321

American Society of Health-Systems Pharmacists
Joseph A. Oddis, Sc.D.
Executive Vice President
7272 Wisconsin Ave.
Bethesda, MD 20814
(301) 657-3000; Fax: (301) 657-8278

American Society of Pharmacognosy
Dr. Charles D. Hufford
School of Pharmacy
University of Mississippi
University, MS 38677
(601) 232-7026; Fax: (601) 232-7026

Association of Drug Repackagers, Inc.
439A Causeway Blvd.
Dunedin, FL 34698
(813) 789-2954; Fax: (813) 785-9941

The Drug, Chemical & Allied Trades Association, Inc.
Tara A. Powers
Director, Membership Services
2 Roosevelt Ave., Suite 301
Syosset, NY 11791
(516) 496-3317; Fax: (516) 496-2231

The Food and Drug Law Institute
John C. Villforth
President
1000 Vermont Ave., NW, Suite 200
Washington, DC 20005
(202) 371-1420; Fax: (202) 371-0649

Generic Pharmaceutical Industry Association
Robert A. Waspe
President
1620 "I" St., NW, Suite 800
Washington, DC 20006
(202) 833-9070; Fax: (202) 833-9612

National Association of Boards of Pharmacy
Carmen A. Catizone
Executive Director
700 Busse Highway
Park Ridge, IL 60068-2402
(708) 698-6227; Fax: (708) 698-0124

National Association of Chain Drug Stores, Inc.
Ronald L. Ziegler
President/CEO
413 North Lee St.
Alexandria, VA 22313-1480
(703) 549-3001; Fax: (703) 836-4869

National Assocation of Pharmaceutical Manufacturers
Robert S. Milanese
President
320 Old Country Rd.
Garden City, L.I., NY 11530
New York, NY 10017
(516) 741-3699; Fax: (516) 741-3696

National Community Pharmacists Association
Calvin J. Anthony
Executive Vice President
205 Daingerfield Rd.
Alexandria, VA 22314
(703) 683-8200; Fax: (703) 683-3619

National Council for Prescription Drug Programs
Lee Ann C. Stember
President
4201 N. 24th St., Suite 365
Phoenix, AZ 85016-6268
(602) 957-9105; Fax: (602) 955-0749

National Council of State Pharmaceutical Association Executives
A.H. Mebane, III, R.Ph.
Executive Director
P.O. Box 151
Chapel Hill, NC 27514-0151
(919) 967-2237; Fax: (919) 968-9430

National Council on Patient Information and Education (NCPIE)
William Ray Bullman, MAM
Executive Director
666 11th St., NW, Suite 810
Washington, DC 20001
(202) 347-6711; Fax: (202) 638-0773

National Managed Healthcare Congress
70 Blanchard Rd., Suite 4000
Burlington, MA 01803
(617) 270-6000; Fax: (617) 270-6004

National Pharmaceutical Alliance
Christine Sizemore
Executive Director
421 King St., Suite 222
Alexandria, VA 22314
(703) 836-8816; Fax: (703) 549-4749

National Pharmaceutical Council
John Norris
President
1894 Preston White Drive
Reston, VA 22091
(703) 620-6390; Fax: (703) 476-0904

National Wholesale Druggist's Association
Ronald J. Streck
President
1821 Michael Faraday Dr., Ste. 400
Reston, VA 22090
(703) 787-0000; Fax: (703) 787-6930

Nonprescription Drug Manufacturers Association
James D. Cope
President
1150 Connecticut Ave., NW
Washington, DC 20036
(202) 429-9260; Fax: (202) 223-6835

Parenteral Drug Association, Inc.
Edmund M. Fry
President
7500 Old Georgetown Rd., Suite 620
Bethesda, MD 20814
(301) 986-0293; Fax: (301) 986-0296

Pediatric Pharmacy Advocacy Group, Inc.
Kellie D. McQueen, Pharm.D.
Director
1056 East 19th Ave.
Denver, CO 80110
(303) 861-6835; Fax: (303) 837-2817

Pharmaceutical Care Management Association
Delbert D. Konnor
Executive Vice President
2300 Ninth St. So., Suite 210
Alexandria, VA 22204
(703) 920-8480; Fax: (703) 920-8491

Pharmaceutical Research and Manufacturers of America
Alan F. Holmer
President
1100 15th St., NW
Washington, DC 20005
(202) 835-3400; Fax: (202) 835-3429

The U.S. Pharmacopeial Convention, Inc.
Jerome A. Halperin
Executive Vice President
12601 Twinbrook Pkwy.
Rockville, MD 20852
(301) 881-0666; Fax: (301) 816-8299

U.S. Adopted Names (USAN) Council
Ruta Freimanis, Pharm.D.
Director, Office of Drug Nomenclature
American Medical Association
515 N. State St.
Chicago, IL 60610
(312) 464-4045; Fax: (312) 464-4184

ORAL SOLID DOSAGE FORMS THAT SHOULD NOT BE CRUSHED

John F. Mitchell, PharmD, FASHP
Editor
Medical Education Systems, Inc.
West Bloomfield, Michigan

Note: This listing includes revisions to the article as published in Hospital Pharmacy

Drug Product	Manufacturer	Dosage Forms	Reasons/Comments
Accutane	Roche	Capsule	Mucous membrane irritant
Actifed 12 Hour	Burroughs Wellcome	Capsule	Slow release (#)
Acutrim (various)	Ciba Self-Medication	Tab	Slow release
Aerolate SR, JR, III	Fleming & Co.	Capsule	Slow release (*,#)
Afrinol Repetabs	Schering	Tablet	Slow release
Allerest 12 Hour	Ciba Self-Medication	Capsule	Slow release
Artane Sequels	Lederle	Capsule	Slow release (*,#)
Arthritis Bayer Time Release	Glenbrook	Capsule	Slow release
ASA Enseals	Lilly	Tablet	Enteric-coated
Asbron G Inlay	Sandoz	Tablet	Multiple compressed tablet (#)
Atrohist Plus	Adams	Tablet	Slow release
Atrohist Sprinkle	Adams	Capsule	Slow release (*)
Azulfidine Entabs	Pharmacia Labs	Tablet	Enteric-coated
Baros	Lafayette	Tablet	Effervescent Tab (d)
Bayer Low Adult 81mg Strength	Sterling Health	Tablet	Enteric-coated
Bayer Regular Strength 325mg Caplet	Sterling Health	Tablet	Enteric-coated
Betachron E-R	Inwood	Capsule	Slow release
Betapen-VK	Bristol	Tablet	Taste (c)
Biohist-LA	Wakefield	Tablet	Slow release (g)
Bisacodyl	(various)	Tablet	Enteric-coated (a)
BiscoLax	Raway	Tablet	Enteric-coated (a)
Bontril SR	Carnrick	Capsule	Slow release
Breonesin	Sanofi Winthrop	Capsule	Liquid filled (b)
Brexin LA	Savage	Capsule	Slow release (#)
Bromfed	Muro	Capsule	Slow release (#)
Bromfed PD	Muro	Capsule	Slow release (#)
Calan SR	Searle	Tablet	Slow release (g)
Cama Arthritis Pain Reliever	Sandoz Consumer	Tablet	Multiple compressed tablet
Carbiset-TR	Nutripharm	Tablet	Slow release
Cardizem	Marion-Merrell Dow	Tablet	Slow release
Cardizem CD	Marion-Merrell Dow	Capsule	Slow release (*)
Cardizem SR	Marion-Merrell Dow	Capsule	Slow release (*)
Carter's Little Pills	Carter-Wallace	Tablet	Enteric-coated
Cefal Filmtab	Abbott	Tablet	Enteric-coated
Ceftin	Glaxo	Tablet	Taste **Note:** use suspension for children
Charcoal Plus	Kramer Laboratories	Tablet	Enteric-coated
Chloral Hydrate	(various)	Capsule	**Note:** product is in liquid form within a special capsule (#)
Chlorpheniramine Maleate Time Release	(various)	Capsule	Slow release
Chlor-Trimeton Repetab	Schering	Tablet	Slow release (#)
Choledyl SA	Parke-Davis	Tablet	Slow release (#)
Cipro	Miles	Tablet	Taste (c)
Claritin-D	Schering	Tablet	Slow release
Codimal LA	Central	Capsule	Slow release
Codimal LA Half	Central	Capsule	Slow release
Colace	Mead Johnson	Capsule	Taste (c)
Comhist LA	Norwich Eaton	Capsule	Slow release (*)
Compazine Spansule	SmithKline Beecham	Capsule	Slow release (#)
Congress SR, JR	Fleming & Co.	Capsule	Slow release
Constant T	Geigy	Tablet	Slow release (*)
Contac	SmithKline Beecham	Capsule	Slow release (*)
Cotazym S	Organon	Capsule	Enteric-coated (*)
Covera-HS	Searle	Tablet	Slow release
Creon 10, 20	Solvay	Capsule	Enteric-coated (*)
Cystospaz-M	Schwartz Pharma	Capsule	Slow release
Cytoxan	Bristol-Myers	Tablet	**Note:** drug may be crushed but maker recommends using inj.
Dallergy	Laser	Capsule	Slow release
Dallergy-D	Laser	Capsule	Slow release
Dallergy-JR	Laser	Capsule	Slow release
Deconamine SR	Berlex	Capsule	Slow release (#)
Deconsal II	Adams	Tablet	Slow release
Deconsal Sprinkle	Adams	Capsule	Slow release (*)
Defen-LA	Horizon	Tablet	Slow release (g)
Demazine Repetabs	Schering	Tablet	Slow release (#)
Depakene	Abbott	Capsule	Slow release mucous membrane irritant (#)
Depakote	Abbott	Capsule	Enteric-coated
Desoxyn Gradumets	Abbott	Tablet	Slow release
Desyrel	Mead Johnson	Tablet	Taste (c)
Dexatrim, Max. Strength	Thompson Medical	Tablet	Slow release

Drug Product	Manufacturer	Dosage Forms	Reasons/Comments
Dexedrine Spansule	Smith Kline Beecham	Capsule	Slow release
Diamox Sequels	Lederle	Capsule	Slow release
Dilatrate SR	Reed & Carnrick	Capsule	Slow release
Dimetane Extentab	A.H. Robins	Tablet	Slow release (#)
Disobrom	Geneva	Tablet	Slow release
Disophrol Chronotab	Schering	Tablet	Slow release
Dital	UAD	Capsule	Slow release
Donnatal Extentab	A.H. Robins	Tablet	Slow release (#)
Donnazyme	A.H. Robins	Tablet	Enteric-coated
Drisdol	Sanofi Winthrop	Capsule	Liquid filled (b)
Drixoral	Schering	Tablet	Slow release (#)
Drixoral Sinus	Schering	Tablet	Slow release
Dulcolax	Boehringer Ingelheim	Tablet	Entric-coated (a)
Dynabac	Bock Pharmacal	Tablet	Enteric-coated
Easprin	Parke-Davis	Tablet	Enteric-coated
Ecotrin	SmithKline Beecham	Tablet	Enteric-coated
E.E.S. 400	(various)	Tablet	Enteric-coated (#)
Efidac 24	Ciba Self-Medication	Tablet	Slow release
Efidac 24 chlorpheniramine	Ciba Self-Medication	Tablet	Slow release
Elixophyllin SR	Forest	Capsule	Slow release (*,#)
E-Mycin	Boots	Tablet	Enteric-coated
Endafed	UAD	Capsule	Slow release
Entex LA	Norwich Eaton	Tablet	Slow release (#)
Entozyme	A.H. Robins	Tablet	Enteric-coated
Equanil	Wyeth-Ayerst	Tablet	Taste (c)
Ergostat	Parke-Davis	Tablet	Sublingual form (f)
Eryc	Parke-Davis	Capsule	Enteric-coated (*)
Ery-tab	Abbott	Tablet	Enteric-coated
Erythrocin Stearate	(various)	Tablet	Enteric-coated
Erythromycin Base	(various)	Tablet	Enteric-coated
Eskalith CR	SmithKline Beecham	Tablet	Slow release
Exgest LA	Carnrick	Tablet	Slow release
Fedahist Timecaps	Schwarz Pharma	Capsule	Slow release (#)
Feldene	Pfizer	Capsule	Mucous membrane irritant
Feocyte	Dunhall	Tablet	Slow release
Feosol	SmithKline Beecham	Tablet	Enteric-coated (#)
Feosol Spansule	SmithKline Beecham	Capsule	Slow release (*,#)
Feratab	Upsher-Smith	Tablet	Enteric-coated (#)
Fergon	Sanofi Winthrop	Capsule	Slow release (*)
Fero-Grad 500 mg	Abbott	Tablet	Slow release
Fero-Gradumet	Abbott	Tablet	Slow release
Ferralet SR	Mission	Tablet	Slow release
Festal II	Hoechst-Roussel	Tablet	Enteric-coated

Drug Product	Manufacturer	Dosage Forms	Reasons/Comments
K-Lyte	Mead Johnson	Tablet	Effervescent tablet (d)
K-Lyte CL	Mead Johnson	Tablet	Effervescent tablet (d)
K-Tab	Abbott	Tablet	Slow release (#)
Levsinex Timecaps	Schwarz Pharma	Capsule	Slow release
Lodrane LD	ECR Pharmaceutical	Capsule	Slow release (*)
Mag-Tab	Niche	Tablet	Slow release
Meprospan	Wallace	Capsule	Slow release (*)
Mestinon Timespan	ICN Pharmaceutical	Tablet	Slow release (#)
MI-Cebrin	Dista	Tablet	Enteric-coated
MI-Cebrin T	Dista	Tablet	Enteric-coated
Micro K	A.H. Robins	Capsule	Slow release (*,#)
Motrin	Upjohn	Tablet	Taste (c)
MS Contin	Purdue Frederick	Tablet	Slow release (#)
MSC Triaminic	Sandoz	Tablet	Enteric-coated
Muco-Fen-LA	Wakefield	Tablet	Slow release (g)
Naldecon	Bristol Labs	Tablet	Slow release (#)
Naprelan	Wyeth	Tablet	Slow release
Nasatab LA	ECR Pharmaceutical	Tablet	Slow release (g)
Nico 400	Jones Medical	Capsule	Slow release
Nicobid	Rhone-Poulenc Rorer	Capsule	Slow release
Nitro Bid	Marion-Merrell Dow	Capsule	Slow release (*)
Nitrocine Timecaps	Schwarz Pharma	Capsule	Slow release
Nitroglyn	Kenwood	Capsule	Slow release (*)
Nitrostat	Parke-Davis	Tablet	Sublingual route (f)
Nitro-Time	Time-Cap Labs	Capsule	Slow release
Nitrong	Rhone-Poulenc Rorer	Tablet	Sublingual route (f)
Noctec	Apothecon	Capsule	**Note:** product is in liquid form within a special capsule (#)
Nolamine	Carnrick	Tablet	Slow release
Nolex LA	Carnrick	Tablet	Slow release
Norflex	3M Pharmaceuticals	Tablet	Slow release
Norpace CR	Searle	Capsule	Slow release form within a special capsule
Novafed	Marion-Merrell Dow	Capsule	Slow release
Novafed A	Marion-Merrell Dow	Capsule	Slow release
Ondrox	Unimed	Tablet	Slow release
Optilets 500 Filmtab	Abbott	Tablet	Enteric-coated
Optilets M 500 Filmtab	Abbott	Tablet	Enteric-coated
Oragrafin	Squibb Diagnostics	Capsule	**Note:** product is in liquid form within a special capsule
Oramorph SR	Roxane	Tablet	Slow release (#)
Ornade Spansule	SmithKline Beecham	Capsule	Slow release
Oxycontin	Purdue Pharma	Tablet	Slow release
Pabalate	A.H. Robins	Tablet	Enteric-coated
Pabalate SF	A.H. Robins	Tablet	Enteric-coated
Pancrease	Ortho McNeil	Capsule	Enteric-coated (*)
Pancrease MT	Ortho McNeil	Capsule	Enteric-coated (*)
Panmycin	Upjohn	Capsule	Taste

Feverall Sprinkle Caps	Upsher-Smith	Capsule	Taste (*) **Note:** capsule contents intended to be placed in a teaspoonful of water or soft food
Fumatinic	Laser	Capsule	Slow release
Gastrocrom	Fisons	Capsule	**Note:** contents may be dissolved in water for administration
Geocillin	Roerig	Tablet	Taste
Glucotrol XL	Pratt	Tablet	Slow release
Gris-Peg	Herbert Laboratories	Tablet	**Note:** crushing may result in precipitation as larger particles
Guaifed	Muro	Capsule	Slow release
Guaifed-PD	Muro	Capsule	Slow release
Guaifenex LA	Ethex	Tablet	Slow release (g)
Guaifenex PSE 120	Ethex	Tablet	Slow release (g)
Guaimax-D	Central	Tablet	Slow release
Humabid DM	Adams	Tablet	Slow release
Humabid DM Sprinkle	Adams	Capsule	Slow release (*)
Humabid LA	Adams	Tablet	Slow release
Humabid Sprinkle	Adams	Capsule	Slow release (*)
Hydergine L-C	Sandoz	Capsule	**Note:** product is in liquid form within a special capsule (#)
Hydergine Sublingual	Sandoz	Tablet	Sublingual route (#)
Hytakerol	Sanofi Winthrop	Capsule	Liquid filled (b,#)
Iberet	Abbott	Tablet	Slow release (#)
Iberet 500	Abbott	Tablet	Slow release (#)
ICaps Time Release	LaHaye Labs	Tablet	Slow release
ICaps Plus	LaHaye Labs	Tablet	Slow release
Ilotycin	Dista	Tablet	Enteric-coated
Imdur	Key	Tablet	Slow release (g)
Inderal LA	Wyeth-Ayerst	Capsule	Slow release
Inderide LA	Wyeth-Ayerst	Capsule	Slow release
Indocin SR	MSD	Capsule	Slow release (*,#)
Ionamin	Fisons	Capsule	Slow release
Isoclor Timesule	Fisons	Capsule	Slow release (#)
Isoptin SR	Knoll	Tablet	Slow release
Isordil Sublingual	Wyeth-Ayerst	Tablet	Sublinqual form (f)
Isordil Tembid	Wyeth-Ayerst	Tablet	Slow release
Isosorbide Dinitrate Sublingual	(various)	Tablet	Sublingual form (f)
Isosorbide Dinitrate SR	(various)	Tablet	Slow release
Isuprel Glossets	Sanofi Winthrop	Tablet	Sublingual form (f)
K + 8	Alra	Tablet	Slow release (#)
K + 10	Alra	Tablet	Slow release (#)
Kaon CL 6.7 mEq	Adria	Tablet	Slow release (#)
Kaon CL 10	Adria	Tablet	Slow release (#)
K + Care	Alra	Tablet	Effervescent tablet (d,#)
K-Lease	Adria	Capsule	Slow release (*,#)
Klor-Con	Upsher-Smith	Tablet	Slow release (#)
Klor-Con/EF	Upsher-Smith	Tablet	Effervescent tablet (d,#)
Klorvess	Sandoz	Tablet	Effervescent tablet (d,#)
Klotrix	Mead Johnson	Tablet	Slow release (#)

Papaverine Sustained Action	(various)	Capsule	Slow release
Pathilon Sequels	Lederle	Capsule	Slow release (*)
Pavabid Plateau	Marion-Merrell Dow	Capsule	Slow release (*)
PBZ-SR	Geigy	Tablet	Slow release (#)
Pentasa	Hoescht Marion Roussel	Tablet	Slow release
Perdiem	Rhone-Poulenc Rorer	Granules	Wax coated
Peritrate SA	Parke-Davis	Tablet	Slow release (g)
Permitil Chronotab	Schering	Tablet	Slow release (#)
Phazyme	Reed & Carnrick	Tablet	Slow release
Phazyme 95	Reed & Carnrick	Tablet	Slow release
Phenergan	Wyeth-Ayerst	Tablet	Taste (c,#)
Phyllocontin	Purdue Frederick	Tablet	Slow release
Plendil	Astra Merck	Tablet	Slow release
Polaramine Repetabs	Schering	Tablet	Slow release (#)
Pneumomist	ECR Pharmaceutical	Tablet	Slow release (g)
Prelu-2	Boehringer Ingelheim	Capsule	Slow release
Prevacid	TAP Pharmaceutical	Capsule	Slow release
Prilosec	Astra Merck	Capsule	Slow release
Pro-Banthine	Schiapparelli Searle	Tablet	Taste
Procanbid	Parke-Davis	Tablet	Slow release
Procainmide HCL SR	(various)	Tablet	Slow release
Procan SR	Parke-Davis	Tablet	Slow release
Procardia	Pfizer	Capsule	Delays absorption (e,b)
Procardia XL	Pfizer	Tablet	Slow release **Note:** AUC is unaffected
Profen II	Wakefield	Tablet	Slow release (g)
Profen-LA	Wakefield	Tablet	Slow release (g)
Pronestyl SR	Bristol-Myers Squibb	Tablet	Slow release
Proscar	Merck	Tablet	**Note:** crushed tablets should not be handled by women who are pregnant or who may become pregnant
Proventil Repetabs	Schering	Tablet	Slow release (#)
Prozac	Dista	Capsule	Slow release (*)
Quadra Hist	Schein	Tablet	Slow release
Quibron-T SR	Bristol-Myers Squibb	Tablet	Slow release (#)
Quinaglute Dura Tabs	Berlex	Tablet	Slow release
Quinalan Lanatabs	Lannett	Tablet	Slow release
Quinalan SR	Lannett	Tablet	Slow release
Quinidex Extentabs	A.H. Robins	Tablet	Slow release
Quin-Release	Major	Tablet	Slow release
Respa-1st	Respa	Tablet	Slow release (g)
Respa-DM	Respa	Tablet	Slow release (g)
Respa-GF	Respa	Tablet	Slow release (g)
Respahist	Respa	Capsule	Slow release (*)
Respaire SR	Laser	Capsule	Slow release
Respid	Boehringer Ingelheim	Tablet	Slow release

Drug Product	Manufacturer	Dosage Forms	Reasons/Comments
Ritalin SR	Ciba	Tablet	Slow release
Robimycin Robitab	A.H. Robins	Tablet	Enteric-coated
Rondec TR	Dura	Tablet	Slow release (#)
Roxanol SR	Roxane	Tablet	Slow release (#)
Ru-Tuss	Boots	Tablet	Slow release
Ru-Tuss DE	Boots	Tablet	Slow release
Sinemet CR	DuPont Pharm	Tablet	Slow release
Singlet	Marion-Merrell Dow	Tablet	Slow release
Slo-Bid Gyrocaps	Rhone-Poulenc Rorer	Capsule	Slow release (*)
Slo-Niacin	Upsher Smith	Tablet	Slow release (g)
Slo-Phyllin GG	Rhone-Poulenc Rorer	Capsule	Slow release (#)
Slo-Phyllin Gyrocaps	Rhone-Poulenc Rorer	Capsule	Slow release (*,#)
Slow-FE	Ciba Consumer	Tablet	Slow release (#)
Slow-FE with Folic Acid	Ciba Consumer	Tablet	Slow release
Slow-K	Summit	Tablet	Slow release (#)
Slow-Mag	Searle	Tablet	Slow release
Sorbitrate SA	ICI Pharma	Tablet	Slow release
Sorbitrate Sublingual	ICI Pharma	Tablet	Sublingual route
Sparine	Wyeth-Ayert	Tablet	Taste (c)
S-P-T	Fleming	Capsule	**Note:** liquid gelantin thyroid suspension
Sudafed 12 hour	Burroughs Wellcome	Capsule	Slow release (#)
Sudex	Atley	Tablet	Slow release (g)
Sustaire	Pfizer	Tablet	Slow release (#)
Syn-RX	Adams Lab	Tablet	Slow release
Syn-RX DM	Adams Lab	Tablet	Slow release
Tavist-D	Sandoz	Tablet	Multiple compressed tablet
Tedral SA	Parke-Davis	Tablet	Slow release
Tegretol-XR	Ciba Geigy	Tablet	Slow release
Teldrin	SmithKline Beecham	Capsule	Slow release (*)
Tepanil Ten-Tab	3M Pharmaceutical	Tablet	Slow release
Tessalon Perles	Forest	Capsule	Slow release
Theo-24	Searle	Tablet	Slow release (#)
Theobid	Russ	Capsule	Slow release (*,#)
Theobid Jr.	Russ	Capsule	Slow release (*,#)
Theoclear LA	Central	Capsule	Slow release (#)
Theochron	(various)	Tablet	Slow release
Theo-Dur	Key	Tablet	Slow release (#)
Theo-Dur Sprinkle	Key	Capsule	Slow release (*,#)
Theo-Sav	Savage	Tablet	Slow release (g)
Theo-X	Carnrick	Tablet	Slow release
Theolair SR	3M Pharmaceuticals	Tablet	Slow release (#)
Theovent	Schering	Capsule	Slow release (#)
Theox	Carnrick	Tablet	Slow release
Therapy Bayer	Glenbrook	Caplet	Enteric-coated
Thorazine Spansule	SmithKline Beecham	Capsule	Slow release
Touro A&H	Dartmouth	Capsule	Slow release
Touro DM	Dartmouth	Tablet	Slow release
Touro EX	Dartmouth	Tablet	Slow release
Touro LA	Dartmouth	Tablet	Slow release
T-Phyl	Purdue Frederick	Tablet	Slow release
Trental	Hoechst-Roussel	Tablet	Slow release
Triaminic	Sandoz	Tablet	Enteric-coated (#)
Triaminic 12	Sandoz	Tablet	Slow release (#)
Triaminic TR	Sandoz	Tablet	Multiple compressed tablet (#)
Trilafon Repetabs	Schering	Tablet	Slow release (#)
Tri-Phen-Chlor Time Released	Rugby	Tablet	Slow release
Tri-Phen-Mine SR	Goldline	Tablet	Slow release
Triptone Caplets	Commerce	Tablet	Slow release
Toprol XL	Astra	Tablet	Slow release (g)
Tuss LA	Hyrex	Tablet	Slow release
Tuss Ornade Spansule	Smith Kline Beecham	Capsule	Slow release
Tylenol Extended Relief	McNeil	Capsule	Slow release
Uniphyl	Purdue Frederick	Tablet	Slow release
ULR-LA	Geneva	Tablet	Slow release
Valrelease	Roche	Capsule	Slow release
Verelan	Lederle	Capsule	Slow release (*)
Volmax	Muro	Tablet	Slow release
Wellbutrin	Burroughs Wellcome	Tablet	Anesthetize mucous membrane
Wyamycin S	Wyeth-Ayerst	Tablet	Slow release
Wygesic	Wyeth-Ayerst	Tablet	Taste
ZORprin	Boots	Tablet	Slow release
Zymase	Organon	Capsule	Enteric-coated

(*) Capsule may be opened and the contents taken without crushing or chewing; soft food such as applesauce or pudding may facilitate administration; contents may generally be administered via nasogastric tube using an appropriate fluid provided entire contents are washed down the tube.
(#) Liquid dosage forms of the product are available; however, dose, frequency of administration and manufacturers may differ from that of the solid dosage form.
(a) Antacids and/or milk may prematurely dissolve the coating of the tablet.
(b) Capsule may be opened and the liquid contents removed for administration.
(c) The taste of this product in a liquid form would likely be unacceptable to the patient; administration via nasogastric tube should be acceptable.
(d) Effervescent tablets must be dissolved in the amount of diluent recommended by the manufacturer.
(e) If the liquid capsule is crushed or the contents expressed, the active ingredient will be, in part, absorbed sublingually.
(f) Tablets are made to disintegrate under the tongue.
(g) Tablet is scored and may be broken in half without affecting release characteristics.

DISCONTINUED PRODUCTS

Brand Name	*NDC*
Adenocard	57317-0232-10
Alagesic Tablets	55726-0300-01
Alahist IM Injection	55726-0602-10
Albalon-A Solution	11980-0137-15
Aldactone 25mg 1000	00025-1001-52
Aldomet 500mg Tablet	00006-0516-28
Aldomet 500mg Tablet	00006-0516-78
Aldoril 25 Tablet	00006-0456-28
Alupent Inhalant Solution	00182-6087-92
Alurate Elixir 16 Oz	00004-1000-28
Ambien 10mg 30	00025-5421-30
Ami-Tex PSE Tablets	52152-0130-05
Amicar Tablets 500mg	00005-4665-23
Aminatal Plus Tablets	52152-0022-05
Anaplex Liquid	59010-0125-16
Apresoline-Esidrix	00083-0129-30
Aquamist	12830-0777-01
Aristocort 1mg Tablets	57317-0602-50
Aristocort 8mg Tablets	57317-0603-50
Aristocort A Cream 0.025%	57317-0042-15
Aristocort A Cream 0.025%	57317-0042-60
Aristocort A Cream 0.5%	57317-0062-15
Aristocort A Ointmnt 0.1%	57317-0072-15
Aristocort A Ointmnt 0.1%	57317-0072-60
Aristocort Cream Lp .025%	57317-0082-05
Aristocort Cream Lp .025%	57317-0082-15
Aristocort Cream R 0.1%	57317-0092-05
Aristocort Cream R 0.1%	57317-0092-15
Aristocort Cream R 0.1%	57317-0092-24
Aristocort Cream R 0.1%	57317-0092-60
Aristocort Oint 0.1%	00005-5175-40
Aristocort Oint 0.1%	00005-5175-70
Aristocort Ointment 0.1%	00005-5175-09
Aristocort Ointmnt Hp .5%	57317-0113-15
Aristocort Ointmnt R .1%	57317-0112-15
Aristocort Ointmnt R .1%	57317-0112-24
Artane Sequels 5mg	00005-4438-32
Asbron G Elxir	00078-0201-33
Asbron G Tablets	00078-0202-05
Ativan Tab 0.5mg	00008-0081-07
Ativan Tabs 0.5mg	00008-0081-06
Ativan Tabs 1mg	00008-0064-08
Ativan Tabs 1mg	00008-0064-09
Ativan Tabs 2mg	00008-0065-08
Atrohist Sprinkle	53014-0022-10
Aygestin	00046-0894-50
Azactam	00003-2550-20
B Com C B12 Injection	55726-0123-11
B-Plex	00182-4061-01
Bactrim Tabs	00004-0050-49
Baldex Ointment	00303-9934-38
Baldex Solution	00303-9930-05
Benadryl Capsules	00071-0471-32
Benadryl Elixir	00071-2220-32
Benadryl Kapseals	00071-0373-32
Benemid 0.5gm Tablet	00006-0501-28
Benztropine 2mg	24208-0048-01
Betapen-VK	00015-7506-64
Betapen-VK	00015-7508-60
Betapen-VK	00015-7509-60
Bicnu Injection 100mg	00015-3012-18
Bromatane DC Cough Syrup	00182-1714-40
Bromotuss Cough Syrup	00536-0272-97
Butazolidin	00028-0014-01
Butazolidin	00028-0014-10
Butazolidin	00028-0014-61
Butazolidin	00028-0044-01
Butazolidin	00028-0044-10
Butazolidin	00028-0044-61
Calan 120mg	00025-1861-34
Calan 120mg	00025-1861-51
Calan 80mg	00025-1851-34
Calan SR 240mg	00025-1891-60
Carbodec DM Syrup C	00536-0432-90
Cardene 20mg	00033-2437-53
Cardene 30mg	00033-2438-53
Cardene SR 30mg	00033-2440-53
Cardene SR 45mg	00033-2441-53
Cefadroxil 1000mg Tablets	00182-1282-16
Cefadroxil For Oral Susp	00182-7017-70
Cefadyl Injection 1g	00015-7628-22
Cefadyl Injection 2g	00015-7629-18
Cefizox 2gm/50ml	57317-0221-50
Celontin Kapseals	00071-0537-24
Chlor-Trimeton Injection	00085-0200-06
Chlorofair	24208-0690-06
Chloromycetin Kapseals	00071-0379-09
Choloxin 1mg Tablets	00048-1230-03
Clinoril 150mg Tablet	00006-0941-78
Clinoril 200mg Tablet	00006-0942-28
Col-Probenecid	00182-0478-10
Comtussin HC Syrup	00536-2701-85
Corgard 80mg Tablets	00003-0241-55
Cort D LA Injection	55726-0092-05
Cort K Injection	55726-0204-05
Cort-A Injection	55726-0042-05
Cort-K Injection	55726-0197-05
Cortatrigen	00182-6051-83
CPC B 12 Injection	55726-0991-30
CPC Cort D Injection	55726-0807-05
CPC Optic Suspension	55726-0771-05
CPC Otic Soln	55726-0708-10
CPC Otic Susp	55726-0771-10
Cyanoco	00008-0264-01
Cyanoco	00008-0264-03
Cyanoco	00008-0265-01
Cyclocort Cream 0.1%	57317-0054-15
Cyclocort Cream 0.1%	57317-0054-30
Cyclocort Cream 0.1%	57317-0054-60
Cyclocort Lotion 0.1%	57317-0404-20
Cyclocort Lotion 0.1%	57317-0404-60
Cyclocort Ointment 0.1%	57317-0115-30
Cyclocort Ointment 0.1%	57317-0115-60
Cystospaz	00998-2225-10
Deca Durabolin	00052-0697-71
Decadron 6mg Tablet	00006-0147-50
Decongestabs TD Tab	00349-2315-01
Decongestabs TD Tab	00349-2315-10
Decongestant A-T Elixir	00364-7384-16
Delhistine CS Sugar Free	00536-2904-85
Delhistine DM Syrup	00536-2703-85
Demerol HCl Smartpak	00024-0324-63
Depakene Softgel	00182-1169-01
Depmed 80 Injection	55726-0196-05
Detussin Expectorant Liquid	00364-7258-16
DHE 45 Amp	00078-0041-03
Diabeta 2.5mg Tablets	00039-0051-06
Diamox Tabs 125mg	00005-4398-23
Diamox Tabs 250mg	00005-4469-23
Diamox Tabs 250mg	00005-4469-34
Diapid Nasp	00078-0042-38
Dilex-G Tablets	55726-0100-01
Dilex-T Liquid	55726-1540-16
Diulo 2.5mg 100	00025-0501-31
Diulo 2.5mg 100	00905-0501-31
Diulo 5mg 100	00025-0511-31
Diulo 5mg 100	00905-0511-31
Diupres 500 100 Tablets	00006-0405-68
Diupres 500 1000 Tablets	00006-0405-82
Dolobid 500mg Tablet	00006-0697-28
Doloph 10mg/ml	00054-1218-11
Donnatal No. 2 Tablets	00031-4264-63
Dynapen	00015-7892-30
Dynapen	00015-7893-60
Dyrenium	00108-3806-21
E-Lor	00785-1117-01
Ear Drops Rx	00536-8440-70
Ec-Naprosyn 375mg	18393-0255-11
Ec-Naprosyn 500mg	18393-0256-11
Ees 200	24208-0965-94
Ees 200mg	24208-0965-39
Ees 400mg	24208-0970-39
Ees 400mg	24208-0970-94
Elavil 10mg 100 Tablets	00006-0023-68
Elavil 10mg 1000 Tablets	00006-0023-82
Elavil 10mg/ml Inj 10ml	00006-3286-10
Elavil 25mg 100 Tablets	00006-0045-68
Elavil 25mg 1000 Tablets	00006-0045-82
Elavil 25mg 5000 Tablets	00006-0045-86
Elavil 50mg 100 Tablets	00006-0102-68
Elavil 50mg 1000 Tablets	00006-0102-82
Encron - 10 Caps	00536-5694-01
Estrace	00087-0755-47
Estrace	00087-0756-47
Exna Tablets	00031-5449-63
Ferotrinsic Caps	00536-3804-10
Fioricet Tab	00078-0084-65
Fluorascein/Proparac	24208-0733-60
Gantrisin 0.5g 100 Tablets	00004-0009-01
Gantrisin 0.5g 100 Tablets	00004-0009-49
Gantrisin 0.5g 500 Tablets	00004-0009-14
Gemcor	00245-0670-15
Gemcor	00245-0670-60
Generet 500	00182-1343-26
Gentrasul Soln	00303-9929-05
GerIMal 1mg Sub Tabs	00536-3857-10
Gris-Peg 250mg Tablets	00023-0773-25
Guiatuss Dac	00677-1179-33
Haldol	00045-0240-10
Hem Fe	59310-0105-10
Hemocyte Injection	52747-0400-30
Hi-Tex Pse	55782-0600-01
Hi-Tuss Dm	55782-0100-16
Hydeltra	00006-7572-01
Hydeltra	00006-7572-03
Hydropres 25 1000 Tablets	00006-0053-82
Hyosophen Tabs	00536-3920-50
Ilopan Injection 250mg/ml	00013-2356-95
Inderal Tabs 80mg	00046-0428-99
Indocin 25mg Capsule	00006-0025-28
Indocin 25mg Capsule	00006-0025-78
Infectrol Ointment	00303-9932-38
Infectrol Susp	00303-9927-05
Innovar	50458-0020-02
Innovar	50458-0020-05
Iodinated Glycerol 30mg	00677-1345-01
Iophen C Liq Nat	00839-6756-69
Iophen Elixir	00472-1423-04
Iophen Elixir	00472-1423-16
Isuprel Mistometer	00024-0878-05
Kaon Elixir-Grap	00013-3203-51
Kaon Elixir-Grap	00013-3203-53
Kay Ciel Liquid	00182-1205-40
Keflin	00002-7001-01
Keflin	00002-7001-25
Keflin	00002-7260-25
Keflin	00002-7261-10
Kefzol	00002-7265-01
Kefzol	00002-7265-25
Kenalog-40	00003-0293-20
Kerlone 20mg 100	00025-5201-34
Klonopin 2.0mg Rxp Tabs	00004-0098-45
Klorvess Tab	00078-0206-44
Lanolin Hydrous Topical	00536-2950-98
Lasix Inject 10ml	00039-0069-08
Leucov Cal 15mg Tablets	00005-4501-83
Leucov Cal 15mg Tablets	00005-4501-90
Leucov Cal 5mg Tablets	00005-4536-23
Leucov Cal 5mg Tablets	00005-4536-38
Leucov Cal Inj 100mg	00205-4646-94
Leucov Cal Inj 350mg	00205-4645-77
Leucov Cal Inj 50mg	00205-5330-92
Logen	00182-1047-43
Lypholyte II 200ml	00469-1462-00
Mandelamine Granules	00071-2176-03
Mandol	00002-7068-10
Mandol	00002-7072-16
Mandol	00002-7268-25
Mandol	00002-7269-10
Marax Syrup	00182-6062-40
Margesic No. 3	00682-0806-01
Marpres	00682-1800-01
Med-Hist-Tablets	52349-0200-10
Mellaril 15mg	00078-0008-65
Mepron Tablets 250mg	00173-0126-62
Meprospan-200	00037-1401-01
Meprospan-400	00037-1301-01
Mestinon TIMespan	00187-3010-50
Metandren	00083-0030-30
Metandren	00083-0032-30
Metaprel Sol	00078-0210-26
Methotrx Lpf Sod 250mg	00205-5337-98
Metrogel	55326-0100-21
Mexitil 250mg Capsules	00597-0068-61
Migergot Supp	00839-7283-92
Migrex Capsules	00349-8783-01
Migrex Capsules	00349-8783-05
Migrex Capsules	00349-8914-01
Minoxidil	00182-1280-05
Minoxidil Tabs	00591-5642-01
Minoxidil Tabs	00591-5642-03
Minoxidil Tabs	00591-5643-01
Moban	00056-0072-70
Moban	00056-0076-70
Multi-Ret 500 Tablets	52152-0047-04
Multiple Trace Element	00517-6010-25
Muro 128 2%	00303-9906-15
Muro 128 5%	00303-9905-38
Muro 128 5%	00303-9928-15
Muro 128 5%	00303-9928-30
Murocoll - 2	00303-9903-05
Myphetane DC Cough Syrup	00832-8461-04
N.T.A.	00677-1081-43
Naldelate	00677-0770-33
Naldelate Pediatric Syrup	00472-1007-28
Nasabid	12463-0250-01
Nasahist L A	00588-3888-01
Nelova .5/35 21 Day	00047-0929-11
Nelova 10/11 21 Day	00047-0941-11
Neo-Synalar Crm .025% 15g	00033-2505-13
Neo-Synalar Crm .025% 30g	00033-2505-14
Neo-Synalar Crm .025% 60g	00033-2505-17
Neocidin Opthalmic Solution	00904-5033-10
New-Decongest	00182-1488-05
New-Decongest Pediatric	00182-1495-41
Niacor	00245-0066-11
Nitro-Dur	00085-3305-10
Nitro-Dur	00085-3310-10
Nitro-Dur	00085-3315-10
Nitro-Dur	00085-3320-10
Nitro-Dur	00085-3330-10
Nitrol Ointment 2%	00013-5804-47
Nitrol Ointment 2%	00013-5804-55
Norethin 1/35E-28	00905-0231-06

Brand Name	NDC
Norethin 1/50M-21	00905-0431-06
Norethin 1/50M-28	00905-0441-06
Norethin 1/35E-21	00905-0221-06
Norlestrin	00071-0901-47
Norlestrin	00071-0904-47
Norlestrin Fe	00071-0905-39
Norlestrin Fe	00071-0905-45
Norlestrin Fe	00071-0907-38
Noroxin 400mg Tablet	00006-0705-20
Noroxin 400mg Tablet	00006-0705-28
Norpace 100mg 500	00025-2752-51
Norpace 150mg 1000	00025-2762-52
Norpace 150mg 500	00025-2762-51
Norpace SR Caps	00182-1846-01
Ocutricin	24208-0790-59
Ocutricin HC	24208-0526-61
Ocutricin HC	24208-0785-55
Opcon	00303-9910-15
Opcon A	24208-0781-15
Opcon-A	00303-9911-15
Orflagen	00182-0813-01
Organidin	00037-4224-40
Organidin Tabs	00037-4224-03
Otitricin Otic	24208-0556-61
Otitricin Otic	24208-0556-62
P.E.T.N.	00182-1203-01
Pantopon Amps 20mg 10	00004-1918-06
Para-Hist Hd	00813-0050-16
Paregoric	00364-7043-16
Paregoric	00426-8457-28
Paregoric	00832-8457-16
Paregoric	00832-8457-28
Parlodel 2.5mg	00078-0017-65
Pathocil Cap 250mg	00008-0360-02
Pathocil Cap 500mg	00008-0593-01
Pathocil Sus 62.5mg/5ml	00008-0361-03
Pedia Profen	00045-0469-16
Pedia Profen	00045-0801-16
Pedia Profen	00045-0801-17
Peg-Lyte	51285-0835-40
Pepcid 20mg 4500 Tablets	00006-0963-70
Pepcid 40mg 4500 Tablets	00006-0964-70
Persantine 25mg Tablets	00597-0017-10
Persantine 25mg Tablets	00597-0017-61
Persantine 50mg Tablets	00597-0018-61
Persantine 75mg Tablets	00597-0019-61
Pharmalyte	51079-0718-45
Phen 50 Injection	55726-0258-10
Phen-25 Injection	55726-0259-10
Pilostat 1%	00303-9938-15
Pilostat 1% Twin	00303-9950-30
Pilostat 2%	00303-9939-15
Pilostat 2% Twin	00303-9952-30
Pilostat 4%	00303-9940-15
Pilostat 4% Twin	00303-9953-30
Pilostat 5%	24208-0815-64

Brand Name	NDC
Pipracil 2gm Infusion	00206-3879-47
Plendil 5mg ER Tablets	00006-0451-28
Polargen	00182-1222-01
Poly-Histine Cs Syrup	00563-1633-04
Poly-Histine-D Ped Caps	00563-1658-30
Poly-Vi-Flor Drops	00182-1052-67
Polycillin	00015-7988-40
Polycillin	00015-7988-64
Polycillin	00015-7988-77
Polycillin	00015-7992-41
Polycillin	00015-7992-90
Polycillin	00015-7998-40
Polycillin	00015-7998-50
Polycillin	00015-7998-64
Polycillin	00015-7998-77
Polycillin Injection 125mg	00015-7401-18
Polycillin Pediatric	00015-7884-20
Polycillin Pediatric	00015-7884-40
Polycillin Pediatric	00015-7884-77
Polycillin-N Injection 250mg	00015-7402-18
Polymox	00015-7276-35
Polymox	00015-7277-16
Polymox	00015-7277-35
Polymox	00015-7278-66
Polymox	00015-7279-60
Polymox	00015-7279-66
Polymox	00015-7279-80
Pred Cort 50	55726-0249-10
Predair 0.125%	24208-0705-02
Predsulfair	24208-0645-55
Predsulfair	24208-0775-60
Predsulfair	24208-0775-64
Prenatal Maternal Multi	58177-0217-04
Prilosec 20mg Capsule	00006-0742-28
Prilosec 20mg Capsule	00006-0742-31
Probampacin	00182-0674-68
Proben-C Tabs	00536-4365-10
Prochlorper 10mg/Tubex	00008-0542-02
Prochlorperazine Eds	00364-2231-48
Proloid	00071-0251-24
Proloid	00071-0252-24
Proloid	00071-0253-24
Proloid	00071-0254-24
Proloid	00071-0257-24
Pronestyl	00003-0757-80
Propantheline Br 15mg	00405-4879-01
Prostaphlin	00015-7977-58
Prostaphlin	00015-7982-58
Prostaphlin Injection 250mg	00015-7978-20
Quadra-Hist ER Pediatric	00364-7332-16
Quinidine Gluconate SR	00364-0604-90
Rep Horm 3-20 20mg/ml	00536-1720-70
Rep Horm 3-40 40mg/ml	00536-1741-70
Restoril 15mg	00078-0098-65
Restoril 30mg	00078-0099-65
Robaxisal Tablets	00031-7469-64

Brand Name	NDC
Robinul Tablets	00031-7824-70
Robitussin A-C Syrup	00031-8674-05
Rocephin 1gm 10x100ml	00004-1964-03
Ru-Tuss Tablets	00048-0058-01
Ru-Tuss Tablets	00048-0058-05
Rubex 10mg/Vial Inj	00015-3351-22
Rubramin PC	00003-0519-40
Rufen 400mg Tablets	00048-0039-05
Rufen 600mg Tablets	00048-0062-05
Selsun Rx	00182-0677-37
Serax 10mg-Redipak Capsules	00008-0051-01
Serax 15mg-Redipak Capsules	00008-0006-01
Serax 30mg-Redipak Capsules	00008-0052-01
Serpasil	00083-0035-30
Serpasil	00083-0036-30
Serpasil	00083-0036-40
Serpasil	00083-0036-45
Serpasil	00083-0036-65
Serpasil-Apresoline	00083-0040-30
Serpasil-Apresoline	00083-0104-30
Serpasil-Esidrix	00083-0013-30
Serpasil-Esidrix	00083-0097-30
Sinubid	00071-0177-24
SublIMaze	50458-0030-02
SublIMaze	50458-0030-05
SublIMaze	50458-0030-10
SublIMaze	50458-0030-20
Sucostrin Injection	00003-0719-15
Sudex	59702-0120-01
Sulfacet	00536-2507-70
Sulfair 15%	24208-0665-04
Sulindac 150mg Tabs	00536-5645-05
Sulindac Tabs	00364-2442-06
Sulindac Tabs	00591-5661-01
Sulphrin	00303-9920-05
Sulpred	24208-0915-60
Sulpred	24208-0915-62
Sulten-10	00303-9921-15
Sumycin 250	00003-0655-46
Sumycin 500	00003-0763-46
Surmontil 50mg	00008-4133-04
Symadine	00032-4140-01
Synkayvite 10mg	00004-1924-06
Synkayvite 5mg 100 Tablets	00004-0037-01
Synkyavite Amps 5mg	00004-1923-06
Syntocinon Nasp 2ml	00078-0061-23
Syntocinon Nasp 5ml	00078-0061-25
Taractan Concentrate	00004-1010-28
TB Old Tine Test	00005-2722-34
Tegretol	00028-0027-01
Tegretol	00028-0027-10
Tegretol	00028-0027-61
Theelin Aqueous Susp	00071-4040-10
Theolate Liquid	00472-1540-28
Theomax DF Syrup	00364-0840-16
TIMoptic-Xe 0.25%	00006-3557-91

Brand Name	NDC
TIMoptic-Xe 0.5%	00006-3558-91
Tonocard 600mg Tablet	00006-0709-28
Tornalate MDI Refill	51479-0012-02
TralMcinolone .025%	24208-0650-04
Travase Ointment	00048-1500-52
Tri-Statin 11 Cream	00536-4910-31
Tri-Statin 11 Cream	00536-4910-98
Triavil 4-10 100 Tablets	00006-0934-68
Triavil 4-10 500 Tablets	00006-0934-74
Trimox 250	00003-1738-25
Trimox 500	00003-0109-45
Trimpex 100mg 100 Tablets	00004-0127-49
Triotann-S Pediatric Susp	51285-0713-55
Triphasil-21	00008-2535-02
Triphasil-28	00008-2536-02
Tropicamide 0.5%	24208-0590-59
Tussidin DM Liquid	55370-0309-12
Tussidin DM Liquid	55370-0309-48
Tussidin DM NR Liquid	59743-0032-16
Tussidin NR Liquid	59743-0031-16
Uni Lom	00677-0463-01
Uni Lom	00677-0463-10
Uni-Multihist DM Syrup	00677-1490-33
Uni-Tuss HC Syrup	00677-1491-33
Unipres	00032-1132-01
Urecholine 10mg Tablets	00006-0412-28
Urecholine 25mg Tablets	00006-0457-28
Urex Tablets	00089-0371-50
Uri-Sep SC Blue	00839-7796-16
Urinary Antiseptic No. 2	00349-2345-10
Urised	00998-2183-10
Urised	00998-2183-20
Usept	54979-0145-01
Usept	54979-0145-10
Vascor	00045-0684-10
Vascor	00045-0684-33
Vasodilan	00087-0543-05
Vistaject Injection	55726-0171-10
Vit A Solubilized Capsules	00364-1002-02
Vit B-6 100mg/ml Inj	00536-3350-70
Vit D 50000 Units Capsules	00536-4783-10
Vitamin A 50mu Solu	00677-0469-01
Volmax 4mg	00451-0398-00
Volmax 8mg	00451-0399-00
Vontrol	00007-5442-20
Vosol	00037-3611-30
Wygesic Tab-Redipak	00008-0085-04
Wytensin Tab 4mg	00008-0073-05
Xotic-HC Ear Drops	59630-0130-01
Yovital	49729-0017-10
Zenate Tablets	00032-1146-01
Zephrex LA Tablets	00563-2627-30
Zincvit Caps 60s	00482-0010-01
Zincvit Caps 60s	49729-0010-01
Zyloprim 100mg Tablets	00081-0996-75
Zyloprim 100mg Tablets	00173-0996-75

MANUFACTURERS LISTED BY NDC NUMBER

00002	Eli Lilly
00003	Bristol Myers Squibb
00004	Roche
00005	Lederle Pharm
00006	Merck
00007	SKB Pharm
00008	Wyeth Labs
00009	Pharmacia & Upjohn
00011	Becton Dickinson
00013	Pharmacia & Upjohn
00014	Searle
00015	Mead Johnson
00016	Pharmacia & Upjohn
00019	Mallinckrodt Medcl
00021	Reed & Carnrick
00023	Allergan
00024	Sanofi Winthrop
00025	Searle
00026	Bayer
00028	Novartis
00029	Beecham
00031	AH Robins
00032	Solvay Pharms
00033	Syntex Labs
00034	Purdue Frederick
00037	Wallace Labs
00038	Stuart Pharm
00039	Hoechst Marion Roussel
00041	Oral B Labs
00043	Novartis
00044	Knoll Labs
00045	McNeil Lab
00046	Ayerst
00047	Warner Chilcott
00048	Knoll Pharms
00049	Roerig
00052	Organon
00053	Centeon
00054	Roxane
00056	Dupont Pharma
00058	Ciba Vision
00062	Ortho Pharm
00065	Alcon
00066	Dermik Labs
00068	Hoechst Marion Roussel
00069	Pfizer Labs
00070	Arcola
00071	Parke-Davis
00072	Westwood Squibb
00074	Abbott
00075	Rhone-Poulenc Rorer
00076	Star Pharms FL
00077	Vision Pharms
00078	Novartis
00081	Glaxo Wellcome
00083	Novartis
00085	Schering
00086	Carnrick
00087	Bristol Myers Squibb
00088	Hoechst Marion Roussel
00089	3M Pharms
00091	Schwarz Pharma (US)
00093	Teva
00095	Ecr Pharms
00096	PC
00108	SKB Pharm
00118	Miles Spokane
00122	Rexall
00126	Colgate Oral
00131	Schwarz Pharma (US)
00140	Roche Prod
00143	West Ward Pharm
00144	Superior
00145	Stiefel Labs
00147	Camall
00148	Manufac Chems
00149	Procter Gamble Pharm
00161	Miles Cutter
00168	Fougera
00169	Novo Nordisk Pharm
00172	Zenith Labs
00173	Glaxo Wellcome
00178	Mission Pharma
00182	Goldline Labs
00185	Eon Labs Mfg
00186	Astra Pharm
00187	ICN Pharms
00191	Ortega Pharm
00192	Bayer Pharm
00195	Rhone-Poulenc Rorer
00196	Rachelle Labs
00205	Lederle Parenterals
00206	Lederle Piperacillin
00209	Marsam
00217	Dunhall Pharms
00222	Boyle Pharm
00223	Consolidated Mc
00225	Ascher
00228	Purepac Pharm
00245	Upsher Smith
00249	Geriatric Pharm
00254	Vintage Pharms
00256	Fleming
00258	Inwood Labs
00259	Mayrand Pharms
00261	Drug Industries
00263	Rystan
00264	McGaw
00268	Ctr Labs
00273	Lorvic
00274	Scherer
00277	Laser
00281	Savage Labs
00288	Fluoritab
00298	Vortech Pharms
00299	Galderma
00300	TAP Pharm
00302	Genetco
00303	Bausch & Lomb
00304	Balan
00310	Zeneca Pharms
00314	Hyrex Pharms
00316	Del Ray Lab
00327	Guardian Labs
00332	Teva
00338	Baxter Hlthcare
00339	Caremark
00349	Parmed Pharms
00364	Schein Pharm (US)
00372	Scot Tussin
00374	Lyne Labs
00378	Mylan
00386	Gebauer Chem
00396	Milex Prod
00402	Steris Labs
00405	Aligen Independ
00406	Mallinckrodt
00407	Nycomed
00418	Pasadena
00421	Fielding
00433	Res Inds
00436	Century Pharms
00451	Muro Pharm
00456	Forest Pharms
00463	C O Truxton
00469	Fujisawa USA
00472	Alpharma
00478	Rexar
00482	Bradley Pharms
00485	Edwards Pharms
00486	Beach Pharms
00487	Nephron
00496	Ferndale Labs
00514	Dow Hickam
00516	Glenwood
00517	Am Regent
00524	Boots Pharm
00525	Pam Am Labs
00527	Lannett
00535	Gilbert Labs
00536	Rugby
00539	Amer Urologicals
00548	Intl Med Sys
00555	Barr
00556	HR Cenci
00563	Bock Pharma
00574	Paddock Labs
00575	Baker Norton Pharms
00585	Fisons
00588	Keene Pharms
00590	Du Pont Merck
00597	Boehringer Pharms
00601	Kabi Vitrum
00603	Qualitest Pharms
00615	Vangard Labs
00641	Elkins Sinn
00642	Everett Labs
00659	Circle Pharms
00662	Roerig Pfizer
00663	Pfizer Pharm
00665	Intl Labs
00677	United Res
00682	Marnel Pharceut
00686	Raway
00689	Jones Medical
00703	Gensia Labs
00713	GW Labs
00722	Anabolic
00777	Dista
00781	Geneva Pharms
00785	UAD Labs
00813	Pharmics
00814	IDE-Interstate
00820	Logen Pharm
00832	Rosemont
00834	Saron
00839	HL Moore Drug Exch
00879	Halsey Drug
00884	Pedinol Pharma
00904	Major Pharms
00905	SCS Pharm
00941	Renal Division
00944	Baxter Hyland
00961	Cook-Waite Labs
00998	Alcon-PR
08065	Alcon Surgical
08880	Sherwood-Davis & Geck
10019	Ohmeda Pharm
10023	Alba Pharma
10116	Bartor Pharcal
10267	Contract Pharma
10337	Doak Dermatologics
10360	Dynapedic
10361	E Z Em
10733	Medcl Prods Labs
10760	Minette Pharm
10812	Neutrogena
10892	Lunsco
10952	Recsei Labs
10974	Pegasus Med Svs
11089	McGregor
11584	Intl Ethical
11793	Connaught Labs
11808	Ion
11980	Allergan-Amer
11994	E I Dupont De
12463	Abana Pharms
12496	Reckitt & Colman
12535	Kenyon Drug
12634	Apotheca
12758	Mason Pharms
12830	RA McNeil
12870	Arzol Chem
12939	Marlop Pharms
13143	Melville
14362	Mass Biol Labs
17156	Medi Physics
17224	Calvin Scott
17236	Dixon Shane
17314	Alza
17317	Amend
17478	Akorn
18393	Syntex PR
20254	Concord Labs
23317	NMC Labs
23594	Lemax
28105	Hill Dermac
29294	Pharm Tech
29936	Genderm Corp
30727	Merit Pharms
37000	Procter Gamble Mfg
38130	Embrex Economed
38245	Copley Pharm
39506	Somerset
39769	Solopak Labs
42037	Rose Laboratories
42987	Syntex FP
43567	MD Pharm
44087	Serono Labs
44184	Bajamar Chem
44437	Bolan Pharm
44514	Talbert Phcy
45802	Clay Park Labs
45809	Shionogi USA
46287	Carolina Med
46672	Mikart
46703	H & H Labs
47028	Seneca Pharms
47202	TX Drug Reps
47854	Syosset Labs
48017	Ctr Labs Hermal
48433	Reg Svc
49072	McGuff
49158	Thames Pharma
49230	Fresenius
49281	Connaught Labs
49326	AJ Bart
49483	Time-Caps Labs
49502	Dey Labs
49669	Alpha Therapeutic
49730	Hercon Labs
49884	Par Pharm
49938	Jacobus Pharm
50111	Sidmak Labs
50242	Genentech
50383	Hi Tech Pharma
50419	Berlex Labs
50434	Heran Pharm

50458	Janssen Phar
50467	Challenge Prod
50474	UCB Pharma
50550	Charter Labs
50564	Jerome Stevens
50694	Seres Labs
50732	H N Norton Co.
50752	Geneva Pharms
50914	Iso-Tex Dxs
50930	Parnell Pharm
50962	Xactdose
50991	Poly Pharms
51079	UDL
51081	Nutripharm Labs
51234	Teral Labs
51285	Duramed Pharms
51432	Harber Pharm
51479	Dura
51641	Alra Labs
51801	Nomax
51822	Clincl Formula
51875	Royce
52041	Dayton Labs
52083	Kramer P I
52189	Invamed
52238	Optopics
52268	Braintree
52316	DSC Labs
52349	Med Tek Pharms
52384	Teregen Labs
52446	Qualitest Drugs
52544	Watson Labs
52555	Martec Pharms
52584	General Inj & Vac
52637	AF Hauser
52747	US Pharm
52761	Genderm
52765	Quality Res Pharms
52769	Am Red Cross
52906	Universal Labs
53014	Medeva Pharms
53095	Viratek
53118	Millgood
53124	Lederle-Praxis
53159	Palisades Pharms
53169	Boehringer Mannheim
53191	Bio-Tech Pharm
53258	Voluntary Hosp
53265	Able Labs
53298	ALK
53445	Amer Preferred
53489	Mutual Pharm
53633	PRL Enterpr
53706	Delta Pharma
53746	Interpharm
53862	Labs Atral
53879	Sorter
53905	Chiron Thera
54022	Vitaline
54092	Roberts Labs
54129	Immuno-US
54171	Robar
54198	Liquipharm
54396	BTG Pharms
54482	Sigma-Tau
54627	Valmed
54686	Ethitek Pharms
54696	Baucom Labs
54765	Gynopharma
54799	Ocusoft
54807	RID
54838	Silarx Pharms
54859	Llorens Pharm
54921	IPR
54945	Americal Pharm
54979	Pharmacist Choice
55053	Econolab
55326	Curatek Pharms
55370	Mova Pharms
55372	Stafford Miller
55390	Bedford Labs
55496	TIE Pharm
55505	Kramer
55513	Amgen
55515	Oclassen Pharms
55516	Dynapharm
55566	Ferring Labs
55688	Speywood Pharm
55762	Primus
55782	Highland Pkging
55806	Effcon Labs
55953	Novopharm (US)
55959	OTC Pharm
55982	Macnary
56126	US Trading
56146	Nexstar
57217	Smith & Nephew
57267	Novartis
57294	Smithkline Consumer
57317	Fujisawa Pharm (US)
57480	Medirex
57548	Eveready Drugs
57664	Caraco Pharm
57665	Enzon
57685	Adv Remedies
57706	Storz Ophthalm
57779	Equipharm
57783	Squibb-Mark
57844	Gate Pharms
58063	MGI Pharma
58154	Infinity Pharm
58160	SKB Biols
58173	Bergmar Pharm
58177	Ethex
58178	US Bioscience
58196	Jordan Pharms
58223	Kirkman Sales
58238	Deliz
58281	Medtronic
58298	Elge
58337	Berna Prod
58406	Immunex
58407	Huckaby Pharma
58437	Penn Labs
58441	Insource
58468	Genzyme
58521	Richwood Pharm
58605	Am Pharms
58607	ME Pharm
58634	Am Generics
58768	Ciba Vision
58809	GM Pharms
58869	Dartmouth Pharms
58887	Novartis
58914	Scandipharm
58916	Nutraceutical Labs
58980	Stratus Pharms
59004	Winsor Pharm
59010	Medi-Plex Pharm
59015	Ampharco
59075	Athena
59081	Lafayette Pharms
59148	Otsuka America Pharm
59196	WE Pharm
59197	Topi-Cana
59229	Horus Therapeutics
59310	Wakefield Pharms
59366	Glades Pharms
59390	Altaire Pharm
59417	Lotus Biochem
59426	Cooper Vision Pharm
59528	Nephro-Tech
59582	Tmk Pharm
59591	West Point Pharma
59618	Global Source
59627	Biogen
59630	Horizon Pharm
59676	Ortho Biotech
59702	Atley Pharms
59730	N Am Biologicals
59741	Bio Pharm
59743	Alphagen Labs
59747	Solopak Mdcl
59762	Greenstone
59772	Apothecon
59785	Venture Pharm
59879	Pecos
59911	ESI Lederle
59930	Warrick Pharms
60258	Cypress Pharm
60267	Hope Pharms
60322	Hamilton Pharma
60432	Morton Grove
60505	Apotex
60574	Medimmune
60575	Respa Pharms
60793	King Pharms
60809	Glasgow Pharm
60814	Rexall Rexall
60904	Horizon Pharms
60951	Endo Labs
60976	Flemming Pharms
61113	Astra Merck
61147	Yorpharm
61314	Falcon Ophthalmics
61570	Monarch
61799	Liposome
61958	Gilead Sciences
63010	Agouron Pharm
71114	Circa
99207	Medicis
99999	H.C.F.A. F F P

DRUG NAMES THAT LOOK ALIKE AND SOUND ALIKE

Accupril	Accutane
Acetohexamide	Acetazolamide
Achromycin	Aureomycin
Actinomycin	Achromycin
Actinomycin	Aureomycin
Adenosine (Adenocard)	Adenosine Phosphate
Adriamycin	Aredia
Adriamycin	Idamycin
Albuterol	Atenolol
Allopurinol	Apresoline
Alprazolam	Lorazepam
Altace	Alteplase
Altenol	Atenolol
Ambien	Amen
Amikin	Amicar
Amiloride	Amiodipine
Amiodarone	Amrinone
Amitriptyline	Nortriptyline
Amoxapine	Amoxicillin
Amoxapine	Amoxil
Amoxicillin	Amoxil
Amoxicillin	Atarax
Anfranil	Enalapril
Anusol-HC	Anusol
Arasine	Ara-C
Artane	Altace
Asacol	Ansaid
Asacol	Os-Cal
Asparaginase	Pegaspargase
Atrovent	Alupent
Attenuvax	Meruvax
Bactocil	Pathocil
Belladonna	Belladenal
Benadryl	Benylin
Benadryl Dye-Free	Benadryl
Bentyl	Aventyl
Benylin	Ventolin
Benzac W Wash	Benzac W
Betagan	Betagan
Betagan	Betoptic
Betalin	Benylin
Betoptic 05%	Beloptic S
Bicillin	V-Cillin
Brethine	Banthine
Brevital	Bretylol
Brevital	Brevibloc
Bumex	Buprenex
Butabarbital	Butalbital
Cafergot	Carafate
Calcitriol	Calciferol
Captopril	Capitrol
Carboplatin	Cisplatin
Cardene	Cardizem
Cardene SR	Cardizem SR
Cardizem CD	Cardizem SR
Cardura	Coumadin
Cataflam	Catapres
Catapres	Catarase
Cefaclor	Cephalexin
Cefotan	Ceftin
Cefotaxime	Celtizoxime
Cefprozil	Cefazolin
Cefprozil	Cefuroxime
Ceftazidime	Ceftizoxime
Cefuroxime	Cefotaxime
Cefuroxime	Deferoxamine
Cefzil	Ceftin
Cefzil	Kefzol
Centoxin	Cytoxan
Cephapirin	Cephradine
Chlor-Trimeton	Chlor-Trimeton (Nondrowsy)

Chlorpromazine	Chlorpropamide
Chlorpromazine	Prochlorperazine
Clinoril	Clozaril
Clinoril	Oruvail
Clomipramine	Clomiphene
Clomipramine	Norpramin (Desipramine)
Clonidine	Klonopin (Clonazepam)
Codeine	Iodine
Cordarone	Inocor
Corgard	Cognex
Coumadin	Compazine
Cozaar	Zocor
Cyclobenzaprine	Cyproheptadine
Cyclophosphamide	Cyclosporine
Cyclosporine	Cycloserine
Cytovene	Cytosar
Cytoxan	Cytosar (Cytarabine)
Cytoxan	Cytotec
Dantrium	Danazol
Daunorubicin	Doxorubicin
DDAVP Nasal	DDAVP wl Rhinal Tube
Decadron	Decaderm
Decadron	Percodan
Depo-Estradiol	Depo-Testadiol
Depo-Medrol	Solu-Medrol
DES	E.E.S.
Diabeta	Zebeta
Dialose Plus (Docusate Potassium/ Casanthranol)	Dialose Plus (Docusate Sodium/ Phenolphtalein)
Diazepam	Ditropan
Diflucan	Diprivan
Dilaudid	Demerol
Diphenatol	Diphenidol
Diphenhydramine	Dicyclomine
Diupres	Daypro
Dobutrex	Diamox
Dolobid	Slobid
Dopamine	Dobutamine
Doxepin	Doxcycline
Doxorubicin	Idarubicin
Drisdol	Drysol
Dyazide	Thiacide
Dyclone	Dilone
DynaCirc	Dynacin
Echogen	Epogen
Edecrin	Eulexin
Elavil	Mellaril
Eldepryl	Enalapril
Eludax	Eurax
Enalapril	Ramipril
Enduron	Imuran
Erex	Urex
Estraderm	Testoderm
Estratest	Eskalith
Estratest	Estratab
Estratest	Estratest HS
Ethmozine	Erythrocin
Etidronate	Etretinate
Etornidate	Etidronate
Eurax	Urex
Fam-Pren Forte	Parafon Forte
Feldene	Seldane
Fioricet	Fiorinal
Flumadine	Fludarabine
Fluorouracil	Flucytosine
Folinic Acid	Folic Acid
FUDR	Fludara

Gamimune N	CytoGam
Gamulin Rh	MICRhoGAM
Garamycin	Kanamycin
Gilipizide	Glyburide
Glucophage	Glutofac
Glucotrol	Glyburide
Halfprin	1/2 Halfprin
Halodrin	Haldrone
Halotestin	Haloperidol
Hemoccult	Seracult
Hexadrol	Hexalol
Hycodan	Vicodin
Hydrocodone	Hydrocortisone
Hydromorphone	Meperidine
Hydromorphone	Morphine
Hydroxyzine	Hyralazine
Hytone	Vytone
IMDUR	K-Dur
Imferon	Interferon
Imferon	Roferon-A
Imipenem	Omnipen
Imipramine	Desipramine
Imovax	Imovax I.D.
Imuran	Imferon
Inderal	Adderall
Inderal	Isordil
Inderal LA	IMDUR
Inhibace (Captopril in Israel)	Inhibace (Cilazapril in Switzerland & Japan)
Interleukin 2	Interferon 2
K-Lor	Klor
K-Phos Neutral	Neutra-Phos-K
Klonopin	Clonidine
Lamictal	Lomotil
Lanoxin Lasix	Lomotil
Lenoxin Levoxine	Lanoxin
Leucovorin Leukine	Leukeran
Levbid	Lithobid
Levocabastine	Levobunolol
Levoxyl	Luvox
Levsin	Levoxine
Librium	Librax
Lithobid	Lithotabs
Lithostat	Lithobid
Lodine	Codeine
Lodine	Iodine
Lopid Lorabid	Slo-Bid
Lortab	Cortef
Lortab	Lorabid
Lotensin	Lioresal
Lotensin	Loniten
Lotrimin	Lotrisone
Lotrimin	Otrivin
Lovastalin	Lotensin
Lupron	Lopurin
Luride	Lortab
Luvox	Lasix
Magnesium Sulfate	Magnesium Gluceptate
Materna	Ibuprofen
Mazicon	Mivacron
Medigesic	Medi-Gesic
Medrol ADT	Medrol Dosepak
Mepron (Atovaquone in U.S.)	Mepron (Meprobamate in Australia)
Methyldopa	L-Dopa (Levodopa)
Methylphenidate	Methadone
Methylprednisolone	Medroxyprogesterone
Metolazone	Methotrexate
Metolazone	Metoclopramide

Metoprolol	Misoprostol
Micronase	Micro-K
Monopril	Monoket
Monopril	Minoxidil
Mylanta Gas	Mylicon
Myoflex	Mycelex
Narcan	Norcuron
Nasalide	Nasalcrom
Navoban	Navelbine
Nicobid	Nitro-Bid
Nicoderm	Nitroderm
Nifedipine Nicardipine	Nimodipine
Norflex	Noroxin (Norfloxacin)
Norpramin	Nortriptyline
Norvasc	Navane
Novolin 70/30 Penfill Prefilled	Novolin 70/30
Nuprin	Lupron
Ocu-Mycin	Ocumycin
Ocufen	Ocuflox (Ofloxacin)
Ocufen	Ocupress
Organidin	Organidin NR
Orinase	Ornade
Oruvail	Elavil
Paraplatin	Platinol
Paroxetine	Paciltaxel
Paxil	Paciltaxel
Paxil	Taxol
Pediapred	Pediaprofen
Pediaprofen	Pediazole
Pediaprofen	Prelone
Penicillamine	Penicillin
Pentobarbital	Phenobarbital
Percodan	Percorten
Periactin	Perative
Permax	Bumex
Phenelzine	Phenylzin
Phenergan	Theragran
Phenobarbital	Pentobarbital
Pindolol	Parlodel
Pitocin	Pitressin
Plendil	Pindolol
Plendil	Prinivil
Pondimin	Prednisone
Pravachol	Prevacid
Pravachol	Propranolol
Prednisone	Methylprednisolone
Prednisone	Prednisolone
Premarin	Primaxin
Prepidil	Bepridil
Prilosec	Prednisone
Prilosec	Prozac
Prinivil	Prilosec
Prinivil	Proventil
Proctocream HC	Proctocort
Profen LA Profen II	Profen
Prokine	Proleukin
Proloid	Prolixin
Promethazine	Promethazine with Codeine
Propranolol	Propulsid
Provera	Premarin
Provera	Provir
Prozac Proscar	Prosom
Psorion	Psorcon
Quinidine	Quinine
ReFresh (breath drops)	Refresh (lubricant eye drops)
Reglan	Megace
Regroton	Hygroton
Reno-M-60	Renografin-60
Reserpine	Risperdal (Risperidone)

ReVia	Revex	Sulfasalazine	Sulfisoxazole	Tri-Norinyl	Triphasil	Versed	Vepesid
Ridaura	Cardura	Symmetrel	Synthroid	Triad (Zinc Oxide/ Petrolatum/Mineral Oil)	Triad (Butalbital/ Acetaminophen/ Caffeine)	Vincristine	Vinblastine
Rifampin	Rifabutin	Taxol	Paxil			Virilon	Verelan
Rimantadine Amantadine	Ranitidine	Tedral	Teldrin			Viroptic	Timoptic
Roxanol	Roxicet	Tegretol	Toradol	Triaminic	Triaminicin	Wymox	Tylox
Salagen (Asprin, Buffered) name retired in 1993	Salagen (Pilocarpine) name reissued in 1994	Temaril	Demerol	Tridrate	Trandate	Xanax	Lanoxin
		Terbinatine	Terfenadine	Trifluoperazine	Trihexyphenidyl	Xanax	Tylox
		Tetradecyl Sulfate	Tetracycline	Trimox	Diamox	Xanax	Zantac
Seldane D	Semprex D	Thiamine	Tenormin	Trimox	Tylox	Yocon	Zocor
Serax	Eurax	Thyrar	Thyrolar	Tronothane	Tronolane	Zantac	Xanax
Serax	Xerac	Timoptic	Viroptic	Tussi-Organidin DM	Tussi-Organidin	Zarontin	Zentron
Sinequan	Serentil	Tobrex	Tobradex	Uridon	Vicodin	Zinacef	Zithromax
Sodium Phosphates	Potassium Phosphates	Toradol	Inderal	Urispas	Urised	Zocor	Zoloft
		Toradol	Torecan	Vancenase	Vanceril	Zofran	Zantac
Soma	Soma Compound	Toradol	Tramadol	Vantin	Ventolin	Zonalon	Zone A Forte
Stadol	Haldol	Torsemide	Furosemide	Versed	Vistaril	Zosyn	Zofran

DRUG ID IMPRINT GUIDE

Imprint	Generic Name	Form	Strength	Manufacturer	Color
10 I E 246	Donepezil HCl	Tablet	10mg	Roerig	Yellow
1102 I 60 mg	Fexofenadine HCl	Capsule	60mg	Hoechst Marion Roussel	Pink/White
245	Bumetanide	Tablet	0.5mg	Mylan	Green
3 M I 342	Theophylline	Tablet	125mg	3M	White
3 M I SR 200	Theophylline	Tablet	200mg	3M	White
3 M I SR 250	Theophylline	Tablet	250mg	3M	White
3 M I SR 300	Theophylline	Tablet	300mg	3M	White
3 M I SR 500	Theophylline	Tablet	500mg	3M	White
3 M I THEO LAIR 250	Theophylline	Tablet	250mg	3M	White
317	Cimetidine	Tablet	300mg	Mylan	Lt. Green
370	Bumetanide	Tablet	1mg	Mylan	Yellow
372	Cimetidine	Tablet	400mg	Mylan	Lt. Green
3M I 221	Orphenadrine	Tablet	100mg	3M	White
4	Fluphenazine	Tablet	1mg	Mylan	White
4	Ibuprofen	Tablet	400mg	Luchem	White
40	Verapamil HCl	Tablet	40mg	Knoll	Blue
417	Bumetanide	Tablet	2mg	Mylan	Clay brown
4804	Oxazepam	Capsule	10mg	Zenith	Blue / White
4805	Oxazepam	Capsule	15mg	Zenith	White
5 I E 245	Donepezil HCl	Tablet	5mg	Roerig	White
537	Naproxen Sodium	Tablet	275mg	Geneva	Dove Blue
54 213 54 213	Lithium	Capsule	150mg	Roxane	White
54 339	Prednisone	Tablet	2.5mg	Roxane	White
54 463 54 463	Lithium	Capsule	300mg	Roxane	Shrimp Pink
54 582	Oxycodone	Tablet	5mg	Roxane	White
54 892	Dexamethasone	Tablet	4mg	Roxane	Lt. Green
54 902	Aspirin/Oxycodone HCl/ Oxycodone Terephthalate	Tablet	325/4.5/0.38mg	Roxane	White
54 960	Dexamethasone	Tablet	0.75mg	Roxane	Lt. Blue
54543	Acetaminophen/ Oxycodone HCl	Tablet	325/5mg	Roxane	White
63-7	Desipramine	Tablet	10mg	Hoechst Marion Roussel	Blue
635	Chlorambucil	Tablet	2mg	Glaxo Wellcome	White
74	Fluphenazine	Tablet	5mg	Mylan	Green
742 PRILOSEC 20	Omeprazole	Capsule	20mg	Merck	Purple
751	Cyclobenzaprine HCl	Tablet	10mg	Mylan	Dk. Yellow
879 525 I 879 525	Doxycycline	Capsule	50mg	Halsey	Lt. Blue / White
9	Fluphenazine	Tablet	2.5mg	Mylan	Yellow
93 I 851	Metronidazole	Tablet	250mg	Lemmon	White
93 93 I 852	Metronidazole	Tablet	500mg	Lemmon	White
93350 I 4	Acetaminophen/Codeine	Tablet	300/60mg	Lemmon	White
9350 I 2	Acetaminophen/Codeine	Tablet	300/15mg	Lemmon	White
97	Fluphenazine	Tablet	10mg	Mylan	Peach
A I Adx 1	Anastrozole	Tablet	1mg	Zeneca	White
A MO	Metoprolol Succinate	Tablet	50mg	Astra	White
A MS	Metoprolol Succinate	Tablet	100mg	Astra	White
A MY	Metoprolol Succinate	Tablet	200mg	Astra	White
Abbott logo I CHEW EZ	Erythromycin Ethylsuccinate	Tablet	200mg	Abbott	White

Imprint	Generic Name	Form	Strength	Manufacturer	Color
Abbott logo EC	Erythromycin	Tablet	250mg	Abbott	Pink
Abbott logo ED	Erythromycin	Tablet	500mg	Abbott	Pink
Abbott logo EE	Erythromycin Ethylsuccinate	Tablet	400mg	Abbott	Pink
Abbott logo EH	Erythromycin	Tablet	333mg	Abbott	White
Abbott logo EK	Erythromycin	Tablet	500mg	Abbott	White
Abbott logo ENDURON	Methyclothiazide	Tablet	5mg	Abbott	Salmon
Abbott logo I ES	Erythromycin Stearate	Tablet	250mg	Abbott	Pink
Abbott logo I ET	Erythromycin Stearate	Tablet	500mg	Abbott	Hot Pink
Abbott logo HH	Terazosin HCl	Capsule	1mg	Abbott	Grayish Beige
Abbott logo HK	Terazosin HCl	Capsule	5mg	Abbott	Hot Pink
Abbott logo HN	Terazosin HCl	Capsule	10mg	Abbott	Turquoise
Abbott logo HY	Terazosin HCl	Capsule	2mg	Abbott	Yellow-Green
Abbott logo I K-TAB	Potassium Chloride	Tablet	750mg	Abbott	Bright Yellow
Abbott logo KL	Clarithromycin	Tablet	500mg	Abbott	Neon Yellow
Abbott logo KT	Clarithromycin	Tablet	250mg	Abbott	Neon Yellow
Abbott logo NR	Divalproex	Tablet	250mg	Abbott	Peach
Abbott logo NS	Divalproex	Tablet	500mg	Abbott	Pink
Abbott logo NT	Divalproex	Tablet	125mg	Abbott	Dk. Fuschia
Abbott logo PCE	Erythromycin	Tablet	333mg	Abbott	White w/ Pink specks
Abbott logo TL I T	Clorazepate	Tablet	3.75mg	Abbott	Lt. Blue
Abbott logo TM I T	Clorazepate	Tablet	7.5mg	Abbott	Lt. Peach
Abbott logo UC	Estazolam	Tablet	1mg	Abbott	White
Abbott logo UD	Estazolam	Tablet	2mg	Abbott	Clay Pink
ACTIGALL 300mg White	Ursodiol	Capsule	300mg	Summit	Pale Pink /
ADAMS I 012	Guaifenesin	Tablet	600mg	Adams	Mint Green
ADAMS I 017	Guaifenesin/ Pseudoephedrine HCl	Tablet	600/60mg	Adams	Blue
ADAPIN I 25mg Cream	Doxepin HCl	Capsule	25mg	Lotus	Yellow /
ADRIA MYCOBUTIN	Rifabutin	Capsule	150mg	Adria Labs	Rust
AHR 1 I TENEX	Guanfacine HCl	Tablet	1mg	A. H. Robins	Pale Pink
AHR 10 I REGLAN	Metoclopramide HCl	Tablet	10mg	A. H. Robins	White
AHR 2 I TENEX	Guanfacine HCl	Tablet	2mg	A. H. Robins	Pale Yellow
AHR 4650	Pancreatin	Tablet	500mg	A. H. Robins	Green
AHR 6447	Fenfluramine HCl	Tablet	20mg	A. H. Robins	Orange
AHR DONNATAL EXTENTAB	Atropine/Hyoscyamine/ Phenobarbital/ Scopolamine	Tablet	0.0582/0.3111/ 48.6/0.0195mg	A. H. Robins	Green
AHR MICRO - K 5720	Potassium Chloride	Capsule	600mg	A. H. Robins	Light Peach
AHR MICRO-K 10 5730	Potassium Chloride	Capsule	750mg	A. H. Robins	White/Light Peach
AHR I REGLAN 5	Metoclopramide HCl	Tablet	5mg	A. H. Robins	Lt. Green
AHR I ROBAXIN 750	Methocarbamol	Tablet	750mg	A. H. Robins	Orange
AHR ROBAXISAL	Methocarbamol/Aspirin	Tablet	400/325mg	A. H. Robins	White I Pink
AL	Clorazepate	Tablet	7.5mg	Able	Lt. Blue
ALKERAN A2A	Melphalan	Tablet	2mg	Glaxo Wellcome	Off White
AM	Clorazepate	Tablet	3.75mg	Able	Lt. Peach

Imprint	Generic Name	Form	Strength	Manufacturer	Color
AMB 10 I 5421	Zolpidem	Tablet	10mg	Searle	White
AMB 5 I 5401	Zolpidem	Tablet	5mg	Searle	Clay Peach
AMOXIL I 125	Amoxicillin	Tablet	125mg	SmithKline Beecham	Lt. Pink
AMOXIL I 250	Amoxicillin	Tablet	250mg	SmithKline Beecham	Light Pink
AMOXIL 250 I AMOXIL 250	Amoxicillin	Capsule	250mg	SmithKline Beecham	Dk. Blue / Bright Pink
AMOXIL 500 I AMOXIL 500	Amoxicillin	Capsule	500mg	SmithKline Beecham	Dk. Blue / Bright Pink
ANAFRANIL 25mg	Clomipramine HCl	Capsule	25mg	Basel	Lt. Orange / Yellow
ANAFRANIL 50mg	Clomipramine HCl	Capsule	50mg	Basel	Turquoise / Yellow
ANAFRANIL 75mg	Clomipramine HCl	Capsule	75mg	Basel	Dk. Yellow / Lt. Yellow
ANSAID 100mg	Flurbiprofen	Tablet	100mg	Upjohn	Blue
ANSAID 50mg	Flurbiprofen	Tablet	50mg	Upjohn	White
ANTIVERT I 210 White	Meclizine HCl	Tablet	12.5mg	Roerig	Bright Blue I
ANTIVERT I 211 White	Meclizine HCl	Tablet	25mg	Roerig	Bright YellowI
ANTIVERT I 214 BlueIBright Yellow	Meclizine HCl	Tablet	50mg	Roerig	Bright
ASACOL	Mesalamine	Tablet	400mg	Procter & Gamble	Rust
ATARAX 10	Hydroxyzine HCl	Tablet	10mg	Roerig	Orange
ATARAX 100	Hydroxyzine HCl	Tablet	100mg	Roerig	Purple
ATARAX 50	Hydroxyzine HCl	Tablet	50mg	Roerig	Gold
AUGMENTIN 200 I SB	Amoxicillin/Clavulanate	Tablet	200mg	SmithKline Beecham	Pink
AUGMENTIN I 250/125	Amoxicillin/Clavulanate	Tablet	250/125mg	SmithKline Beecham	White
AUGMENTIN I 500/125	Amoxicillin/Clavulanate	Tablet	500/125mg	SmithKline Beecham	White
AUGMENTIN 875 I SB	Amoxicillin/Clavulanate	Tablet	875/125mg	SmithKline Beecham	White
B I 252	Dipyridamole	Tablet	25mg	Barr	White
B I 285	Dipyridamole	Tablet	50mg	Barr	White
B I 95 ; B I 96 ; B I 97 ; B I11	Ethinyl Estradiol/ Levonorgestrel	Tablet	Inert; 0.03/ 0.125; 0.03/0.05; 0.04/0.075mg	Berlex	Clay ; White ; Gold ; Green
B1 11	Clonidine HCl	Tablet	0.3mg	Boehringer Ingelheim	Lt. Orange
B1 I 19	Dipyridamole	Tablet	75mg	Boehringer Ingelheim	Orange
B1 6	Clonidine HCl	Tablet	0.1mg	Boehringer Ingelheim	Mauve
B1 7	Clonidine HCl	Tablet	0.2mg	Boehringer Ingelheim	Orange
B1 8	Clonidine HCl/ Chlorthalidone	Tablet	0.1/15mg	Boehringer Ingelheim	Pink
B2C	Digoxin	Capsule	0.1mg	Glaxo Wellcome	Transparent Yellow
BARR I 033	Chlordiazepoxide HCl	Capsule	10mg	Barr	Balck / Seafoam Green
BARR I 286	Dipyridamole	Tablet	75mg	Barr	White
BARR I 555 483	Amiloride HCl/Hydrochlorothiazide	Tablet	5/50mg	Barr	Yellow
BEECHAM 185	Penicillin V Potassium	Tablet	250mg	SmithKline Beecham	White
BEECHAM 186	Penicillin V Potassium	Tablet	500mg	SmithKline Beecham	White
BENTYL 10 I BENTYL 10	Dicyclomine HCl	Capsule	10mg	Hoechst Marion Roussel	Blue
BENTYL 20	Dicyclomine HCl	Tablet	20mg	Hoechst Marion Roussel	Lt. Blue
BETAPACE I 160 mg	Sotalol HCl	Tablet	160mg	Berlex	Pale Blue
BETAPACE I 240 mg	Sotalol HCl	Tablet	240mg	Berlex	Pale Blue
BETAPACE I 80 mg	Sotalol HCl	Tablet	80mg	Berlex	Pale Blue
BI 72	Metaproterenol	Tablet	20mg	Boehringer Ingelheim	White

Imprint	Generic Name	Form	Strength	Manufacturer	Color
BOCK	Pheniramine/ Phenylpropanolamine HCl/Phenyltoloxamine/ Pyrilamine	Capsule	16/50/16/16mg	Bock	Red/Clear
BOCK I Z LA	Guaifenesin/ Pseudoephedrine HCl	Tablet	600/120mg	Bock	Orange
BRICANYL 5	Terbutaline	Tablet	5mg	Hoechst Marion Roussel	White
BRISTOL 7278 I BRISTOL 7278	Amoxicillin	Capsule	250mg	Bristol-Myers Squibb	Burgandy / Lt. Pink
BRISTOL 7279 I BRISTOL 7279	Amoxicillin	Capsule	500mg	Bristol-Myers Squibb	Burgandy / Lt. Pink
BRISTOL 7992 I BRISTOL 7992	Ampicillin/Ampicillin Trihydrate	Capsule	250mg	Bristol-Myers Squibb	Dk. Red / Gray
BRISTOL 7993 I BRISTOL 7993	Ampicillin/Ampicillin Trihydrate	Capsule	500mg	Bristol-Myers Squibb	Dk. Red / Gray
BRL 30 I 3101	Diltiazem HCl	Tablet	30mg	Rugby	Light Blue
C I 86120	Acetaminophen/ Dichloralphenazone/ Isometheptene Mucate	Capsule	325/100/65mg	Carnrick	Burgandy/ Fuschia stripe down middle
C I 8673	Phenylpropanolamine HCl/Guaifenesin	Tablet	75/400mg	Carnrick	White w/Blue Dots
C I Clock face	Quinidine Gluconate	Tablet	324mg	Berlex	White
CALAN 120	Verapamil HCl	Tablet	120mg	Searle	Rust
CALAN I 40	Verapamil HCl	Tablet	40mg	Searle	Peach
CALAN I 80	Verapamil HCl	Tablet	80mg	Searle	Pale Peach
CALAN I SR 120	Verapamil HCl	Tablet	120mg	Searle	Pale Purple
CALAN I SR 180	Verapamil HCl	Tablet	180mg	Searle	Pale Pink
CALAN I SR 240	Verapamil HCl	Tablet	240mg	Searle	Greenish-Yellow
CAPOTEN 100	Captopril	Tablet	100mg	Bristol-Myers Squibb	White
CAPOTEN I 12.5	Captopril	Tablet	12.5mg	Bristol-Myers Squibb	White
CAPOTEN 25	Captopril	Tablet	25mg	Bristol-Myers Squibb	White
CAPOTEN 50	Captopril	Tablet	50mg	Bristol-Myers Squibb	White
CAPOZIDE 25/15	Captopril/ Hydrochlorothiazide	Tablet	25/15mg	Bristol-Myers Squibb	White w/ orange specks
CAPOZIDE 50/15	Captopril/ Hydrochlorothiazide	Tablet	50/15mg	Bristol-Myers Squibb	White w/ orange specks
CAPOZIDE 50/25	Captopril/ Hydrochlorothiazide	Tablet	50/25mg	Bristol-Myers Squibb	Peach
CARAFATE I 1712	Sucralfate	Tablet	1g	Hoechst Marion Roussel	Pale Pink
CARDIZEM I 120mg	Diltiazem HCl	Tablet	120mg	Hoechst Marion Roussel	Cream
CARDIZEM I 90mg	Diltiazem HCl	Tablet	90mg	Hoechst Marion Roussel	Lt. Green
CARDURA I 1mg	Doxazosin	Tablet	1mg	Roerig	White
CARDURA I 2mg	Doxazosin	Tablet	2mg	Roerig	Dk. Yellow
CARDURA I 4mg	Doxazosin	Tablet	4mg	Roerig	Peach
CARDURA I 8mg	Doxazosin	Tablet	8mg	Roerig	Lt. Green
CATAFLAM I 50	Diclofenac Potassium	Tablet	50mg	Novartis	Dk. Peach
CB 300	Cimetidine	Tablet	300mg	Pen	Lt. Yellow
CB 800	Cimetidine	Tablet	800mg	Pen	Lt. Yellow
CC 232	Phentermine HCl	Tablet	37.5mg	Camall	White with blue specks
CDX50 I CASODEX	Bicalutamide	Tablet	50mg	Zeneca	White
CEDAX 400	Ceftibuten	Capsule	400mg	Schering	White
CIBA I 110	Maprotiline	Tablet	25mg	Novartis	Bright Orange
CIBA I 135	Maprotiline	Tablet	75mg	Novartis	White

BIOCRAFT 01 I BIOCRAFT 01	Amoxicillin	Capsules	250mg	Biocraft	Brown / Cream
BIOCRAFT 03 I BIOCRAFT 03	Amoxicillin	Capsule	500mg	Biocraft	Cream
BIOCRAFT 05 I BIOCRAFT 05	Ampicillin Sodium	Capsule	250mg	Biocraft	Dk. Red / Gray
BIOCRAFT 115 I BIOCRAFT 115	Cephalexin HCl	Capsule	250mg	Biocraft	Red / Gray
BIOCRAFT 117 I BIOCRAFT 117	Cephalexin HCl	Capsule	500mg	Biocraft	Red
BIOCRAFT 149 I BIOCRAFT 149	Clindamycin HCl	Capsule	150mg	Biocraft	Dk. Red / Royal Blue
BIOCRAFT I 33	Sulfamethoxazole/ Trimethoprim	Tablet	800/160mg	Biocraft	White
BIOCRAFT I 49	Penicillin V Potassium	Tablet	500mg	Biocraft	White
BIOCRAFT I 91	Penicillin V Potassium	Tablet	250mg	Biocraft	White
BL I 130	Albuterol	Tablet	2mg	Biocraft	White
BL I 19	Imipramine HCl	Tablet	10mg	Biocraft	Gold
BL I 20	Imipramine HCl	Tablet	25mg	Biocraft	Rust (Burnt Orange)
BL 207 I CORGARD 40	Nadolol	Tablet	40mg	Bristol-Myers Squibb	Blue
BL 208 I CORGARD 120mg	Nadolol	Tablet	120mg	Bristol-Myers Squibb	Blue
BL I 21	Imipramine HCl	Tablet	50mg	Biocraft	Green
BL 241 I CORGARD 80	Nadolol	Tablet	80mg	Bristol-Myers Squibb	Blue
BL 246 I CORGARD 160mg	Nadolol	Tablet	160mg	Bristol-Myers Squibb	Blue
BL 519	Theophylline	Tablet	300mg	Roberts	White
BL 93	Metoclopramide HCl	Tablet	10mg	Biocraft	White
BL NJ I NALDECON	Chlorpheniramine/ Phenylpropanolamine HCl/Phenylephrine/ Phenytoloxamine	Tablet	5/40/10/15mg	Bristol-Myers Squibb	White w/ Fuschia Specks
BL V1	Penicillin V Potassium	Tablet	250mg	Bristol-Myers Squibb	White
BL V2	Penicillin V Potassium	Tablet	500mg	Bristol-Myers Squibb	White
BM Logo 103 I 10	Torsemide	Tablet	10mg	Boehringer Mannheim	White
BM Logo 104 I 20	Torsemide	Tablet	20mg	Boehringer Mannheim	White
BM Logo 105 I 100	Torsemide	Tablet	100mg	Boehringer Mannheim	White
BMP 140 I BMP 140	Ampicillin Sodium	Capsule	250mg	SmithKline Beecham	Dk. Brown / Orange
BMP 141 I BMP 141	Ampicillin Sodium	Capsule	500mg	SmithKline Beecham	Dk. Brown / Orange
BMP 165 I BMP 165	Dicloxacillin	Capsule	250mg	SmithKline Beecham	Blue/Cream
BMP 166 I BMP 166	Dicloxacillin	Capsule	500mg	SmithKline Beecham	Blue/Cream
BMP 180	Amoxicillin/Clavulanate	Tablet	125/31.25mg	SmithKline Beecham	Brown Speckled
BMP 188	Acetaminophen/ Hydrocodone	Tablet	650/7.5mg	Monarch	Lt. Peach
BMP 190	Amoxicillin/Clavulanate	Tablet	250/62.5mg	SmithKline Beecham	Brown Speckled
BMS 100 I 32	Nefazodone HCl	Tablet	100mg	Bristol-Myers Squibb	White
BMS 150 I 39	Nefazodone HCl	Tablet	150mg	Bristol-Myers Squibb	Peach
BMS 1965 20	Stavudine	Capsule	20mg	Bristol-Myers Squibb	Beige
BMS 1966 30	Stavudine	Capsule	30mg	Bristol-Myers Squibb	Rust/Beige
BMS 1967 40	Stavudine	Capsule	40mg	Bristol-Myers Squibb	Rust
BMS 200 I 33	Nefazodone HCl	Tablet	200mg	Bristol-Myers Squibb	Beige
BMS I 5040	Atenolol	Tablet	50mg	Bristol-Myers Squibb	White
BMS 7720 250	Cefprozil	Tablet	250mg	Bristol-Myers Squibb	Lt. Pink
BMS 7721 500	Cefprozil	Tablet	500mg	Bristol-Myers Squibb	White
CIBA 139 APRESAZIDE 25/25	Hydralazine/ Hydrochlorothiazide	Capsule	25/25mg	Novartis	Blue / White
CIBA 16	Methylphenidate HCl	Tablet	20mg	Novartis	White
CIBA I 22	Hydrochlorothiazide	Tablet	25mg	Novartis	Pink
CIBA I 26	Maprotiline	Tablet	50mg	Novartis	Bright Orange
CIBA I 3	Methylphenidate HCl	Tablet	10mg	Novartis	Mint Green
CIBA I 34	Methylphenidate HCl	Tablet	20mg	Novartis	Pale Yellow
CIBA I 46	Hydrochlorothiazide	Tablet	50mg	Novartis	Yellow
CIBA I 7	Methylphenidate HCl	Tablet	5mg	Novartis	Yellow Green
CIBA I 73	Hydralazine	Tablet	50mg	Novartis	Pale Blue
CIPRO I 250	Ciprofloxacin HCl	Tablet	250mg	Miles	White
CIPRO I 500	Ciprofloxacin HCl	Tablet	500mg	Miles	White
CIPRO I 750	Ciprofloxacin HCl	Tablet	750mg	Miles	White
CL 400	Ergotamine Tartrate/ Caffeine	Tablet	1/100mg	Geneva	Light Mauve
CLARITIN 10 I 458	Loratadine	Tablet	10mg	Schering	White
CLARITIN D	Loratadine/ Pseudoephedrine HCl	Tablet	5/120mg	Schering	White
CLEOCIN 150mg I CLEOCIN 150mg	Clindamycin HCl	Capsule	150mg	Upjohn	Burgandy / Purple
CLEOCIN 300mg I CLEOCIN 300mg	Clindamycin HCl	Capsule	300mg	Upjohn	Burgandy
CLOZARIL I 100	Clozapine	Tablet	100mg	Sandoz	Yellow
CLOZARIL I 25	Clozapine	Tablet	25mg	Sandoz	Lt. Yellow
COGNEX 10	Tacrine HCl	Capsule	10mg	Parke-Davis	Green/Yellow
COGNEX 20	Tacrine HCl	Capsule	20mg	Parke-Davis	Blue/Yellow
COGNEX 30	Tacrine HCl	Capsule	30mg	Parke-Davis	Red/Yellow
COGNEX 40	Tacrine HCl	Capsule	40mg	Parke-Davis	Purple/Yellow
COPLEY I 114	Procainamide HCl	Tablet	750mg	Copley	Beige
COPLEY 169	Diltiazem HCl	Tablet	90mg	Copley	Lt. Blue
COPLEY I 188	Procainamide HCl	Capsule	500mg	Copley	Pink
COPLEY 662	Diltiazem HCl	Tablet	60mg	Copley	White
CORTEF 5	Hydrocortisone	Tablet	5mg	Upjohn	White
CORZIDE 40/5 I PPP 283	Bendroflumethiazide/ Nadolol	Tablet	5/40mg	Bristol-Myers Squibb	White w/ blue specks
CORZIDE 80/5 I PPP 284	Bendroflumethiazide/ Nadolol	Tablet	5/80mg	Bristol-Myers Squibb	White w/ blue specks
COTRIM I 93	Sulfamethoxazole/ Trimethoprim	Tablet	400/80mg	Lemmon	White
COTRIM DS I 93	Sulfamethoxazole/ Trimethoprim	Tablet	800/160mg	Lemmon	White
CY 250	Ganciclovir	Capsule	250mg	Syntex	Green w/ blue bands
Cycrin logo	Medroxyprogesterone	Tablet	2.5mg	ESI	White
Cycrin logo I CYC RIN	Medroxyprogesterone	Tablet	10mg	ESI	Pale Peach
Cycrin logo I CYC RIN	Medroxyprogesterone	Tablet	5mg	ESI	Lavender
DAN 25 I 5542	Thioridazine HCl	Tablet	25mg	Schein Danbury	Beige
DAN I 526	Isoniazid	Tablet	300mg	Schein Danbury	White
DAN 5440 I DAN 5440	Doxycycline	Capsule	100mg	Schein Danbury	Blue
DAN I 5513	Carisoprodol	Tablet	350mg	Schein Danbury	White
DAN I 5538	Quinidine Gluconate	Tablet	324mg	Schein Danbury	White
DAN I 5543	Allopurinol	Tablet	100mg	Schein Danbury	White
DAN I 5544	Allopurinol	Tablet	300mg	Schein Danbury	Dk. Peach
DAN 5560 I DAN 5560	Disopyramide	Capsule	100mg	Schein Danbury	Green / White
DAN I 5590	Tolazamide	Tablet	500mg	Schein Danbury	White
DAN I 5599	Trazodone HCl	Tablet	100mg	Schein Danbury	White
DAN I 5600	Trazodone HCl	Tablet	50mg	Schein Danbury	White
DAN 5605 I 0.5	Haloperidol	Tablet	0.5mg	Schein Danbury	White
DAN 5609 I 0.1	Clonidine HCl	Tablet	0.1mg	Schein Danbury	White

Imprint	Generic Name	Form	Strength	Manufacturer	Color
DAN 5624 | 1	Lorazepam	Tablet	1mg	Schein Danbury	White
DAN 5625 | 0.5	Lorazepam	Tablet	0.5mg	Schein Danbury	White
DAN 5633 | DAN 5633	Doxepin HCl	Capsule	100mg	Schein Danbury	Lt. Green / White
DAN 5636 DAN 5636	Meclofenamate	Capsule	50mg	Schein Danbury	Rust
DAN 5637 DAN 5637	Meclofenamate	Capsule	100mg	Schein Danbury	Rust / White
DAN | 5658	Cyclobenzaprine HCl	Tablet	10mg	Schein Danbury	White
DAN | 5660	Sulindac	Tablet	200mg	Schein Danbury	Yellow-Gold
DAN 5694 MINOCYCLINE 50	Minocycline HCl	Capsule	50mg	Schein Danbury	Yellow
DAN 5695 MINOCYCLINE 100	Minocycline HCl	Capsule	100mg	Schein Danbury	Gray/Yellow
DAN 5696 PRAZOSIN	Prazosin HCl	Capsule	2mg	Schein Danbury	Light Gray
DAN 5730 | 10	Baclofen	Tablet	10mg	Schein Danbury	White
DANTRIUM 100mg | 0149 0033	Dantrolene	Capsule	100mg	Procter & Gamble	Dk. Orange / Peach
DANTRIUM 25mg | 0149 0030	Dantrolene	Capsule	25mg	Procter & Gamble	Dk. Orange / Peach
DANTRIUM 50mg | 0149 0031	Dantrolene	Capsule	50mg	Procter & Gamble	Dk. Orange / Peach
DARAPRIM A3A	Pyrimethamine	Tablet	25mg	Glaxo Wellcome	White
DAYPRO | 13 81	Oxaprozin	Tablet	600mg	Searle	White
DELTASONE 10	Prednisone	Tablet	10mg	Upjohn	White
DELTASONE 2.5	Prednisone	Tablet	2.5mg	Upjohn	Pink
DELTASONE 20	Prednisone	Tablet	20mg	Upjohn	Peach
DELTASONE 5	Prednisone	Tablet	5mg	Upjohn	White
DELTASONE 50	Prednisone	Tablet	50mg	Upjohn	White
DIAMOX D3	Acetazolamide	Capsule	500mg	Storz	Orange transparent
DIPENTUM | 250 mg	Olsalazine Sodium	Capsule	250mg	Pharmacia/Upjohn	Light Brown
DISTA 3104 PROZAC 10mg	Fluoxetine HCl	Capsule	10mg	Dista	Green / White
DISTA 3105 PROZAC 20mg	Fluoxetine HCl	Capsule	20mg	Dista	Green / Cream
DISTA H09 ILOSONE 250mg	Erythromycin Estolate	Capsule	250mg	Dista	Red / Beige
DISTA H69 | KEFLEX 250mg	Cephalexin	Capsule	250mg	Dista	Red / Gray
DISTA H71 | KEFLEX 500mg	Cephalexin	Capsule	500mg	Dista	Red
Dista H77 NALFON	Fenoprofen	Capsule	300mg	Dista	Beige / Yellow
DORAL | 15	Quazepam	Tablet	15mg	Wallace	Peach
DORAL | 75	Quazepam	Tablet	7.5mg	Wallace	Peach
DUPONT | COUMADIN 1	Warfarin Sodium	Tablet	1mg	DuPont	Strawberry Pink
DUPONT | COUMADIN 10	Warfarin Sodium	Tablet	10mg	DuPont	White
DUPONT | COUMADIN 2	Warfarin Sodium	Tablet	2mg	DuPont	Lavender
DUPONT | COUMADIN 2 1/2	Warfarin Sodium	Tablet	2.5mg	DuPont	Lime Green
DUPONT | COUMADIN 4	Warfarin Sodium	Tablet	4mg	DuPont	Robin's Egg Blue
DUPONT | COUMADIN 5	Warfarin Sodium	Tablet	5mg	DuPont	Peach
DUPONT | COUMADIN 7 1/2	Warfarin Sodium	Tablet	7.5mg	DuPont	Yellow
DuPont | NTR	Naltrexone HCl	Tablet	50mg	DuPont	Peach
DUPONT | PERCOCET	Acetaminophen/ Oxycodone HCl	Tablet	325/5mg	DuPont	White

Imprint	Generic Name	Form	Strength	Manufacturer	Color
Forest logo TG	Thyroid	Tablet	180mg	Forest	Beige
Forest logo TH	Thyroid	Tablet	240mg	Forest	Beige
Forest logo TI	Thyroid	Tablet	300mg	Forest	Beige
Forest logo TJ	Thyroid	Tablet	90mg	Forest	Beige
Forest logo YC	Liotrix	Tablet	15mg	Forest	Lavender | White
Forest logo YD	Liotrix	Tablet	30mg	Forest	Lt. Orange | White
Forest logo YE	Liotrix	Tablet	60mg	Forest	Pink | White
Forest logo YF	Liotrix	Tablet	120mg	Forest	Lt. Green | White
Forest logo YH	Liotrix	Tablet	180mg	Forest	Yellow | White
FOSAMAX | MRK 212	Alendronate Sodium	Tablet	40mg	Merck	White
FOSAMAX | MRK 936	Alendronate Sodium	Tablet	10mg	Merck	White
G 0556	Hydrochlorothiazide	Tablet	25mg	Zenith Goldline	Peach
G 0557	Hydrochlorothiazide	Tablet	50mg	Zenith Goldline	Peach
G | 1189 500	Chlorzoxazone	Tablet	500mg	Goldline-Royce	Lt. Green
G 3722	Alprazolam	Tablet	0.25mg	Greenstone	White
G86C879 | 3	Aspirin/Codeine	Tablet	325/30mg	Halsey	White
GEIGY 105	Terbutaline	Tablet	5mg	Novartis	White
GEIGY | 136	Imipramine HCl	Tablet	50mg	Novartis	Rust
GEIGY | 140	Imipramine HCl	Tablet	25mg	Novartis	Rust
GEIGY 20	Imipramine HCl	Capsule	75mg	Novartis	Rust
GEIGY 22	Imipramine HCl	Capsule	150mg	Novartis	Rust
GEIGY | 32	Imipramine HCl	Tablet	10mg	Novartis	Rust
GEIGY 40	Imipramine HCl	Capsule	100mg	Novartis	Gold/Rust
GEIGY | 51 51	Metoprolol Tartrate	Tablet	50mg	Novartis	Pink
GEIGY | 71 71	Metoprolol Tartrate	Tablet	100mg	Novartis	Lt. Blue
GEIGY 72	Terbutaline	Tablet	2.5mg	Novartis	White
GG 101	Methocarbamol	Tablet	750mg	Geneva	White
GG 166	Desipramine	Tablet	75mg	Geneva	White
GG 167	Desipramine	Tablet	100mg	Geneva	White
GG 168	Desipramine	Tablet	150mg	Geneva	White
GG 172	Hydrochlorothiazide/ Triamterene	Tablet	50/75mg	Geneva	Greenish Yellow
GG 190	Methocarbamol	Tablet	500mg	Geneva	White
GG 254	Fenoprofen	Tablet	600mg	Geneva	White
GG 260	Hydroxychloroquine Sulfate	Tablets	200mg	Geneva	White
GG | 30	Thioridazine HCl	Tablet	10mg	Geneva	Orange
GG 417	Naproxen Sodium	Tablet	275mg	Mylan	Yellow
GG 418	Naproxen Sodium	Tablet	550mg	Geneva	White
GG | 42	Imipramine HCl	Tablet	50mg	Geneva	Green
GG 437 | 100	Chlorpromazine	Tablet	100mg	Geneva	Burnt Orange
GG | 47	Imipramine HCl	Tablet	25mg	Geneva	Peach
GG 502 | GG 502	Chlorpheniramine/ Phenylpropanolamine HCl	Capsule	12/75mg	Geneva Blue /	Transparent Transparent Clear
GG 51 | 1	Trifluoperazine	Tablet	1mg	Geneva	Lavender
GG 53 | 2	Trifluoperazine	Tablet	2mg	Geneva	Lavender
GG 536 GG 536	Nitrofurantoin	Capsule	100mg	Geneva	Yellow
GG 541 | GG 541	Diphenhydramine	Capsule	50mg	Geneva	Fuschia Pink
GG 55 | 5	Trifluoperazine	Tablet	5mg	Geneva	Lavender
GG 565 GG 565	Nortriptyline HCl	Capsule	10mg	Geneva	White w/ black and gold letters

DUPONT I PERCODAN	Aspirin/Oxycodone HCl/ Oxycodone Terephthalate	Tablet	325/4.5/0.38mg	DuPont	Yellow
DUPONT I SYMMETREL	Amantadine HCl	Capsule	100mg	DuPont	Red
Duramed logo 301	Methylprednisolone	Tablet	4mg	Duramed	White
DYAZIDE SB	Hydrochlorothiazide/ Triamterene	Capsule	25/37.5mg	SmithKline Beecham	White / Maroon
DYNABAC UC5364	Dirithromycin	Tablet	250mg	Bock	White
E-MYCIN 250	Erythromycin	Tablet	250mg	Knoll	Peach
E-MYCIN 333mg	Erythromycin	Tablet	333mg	Knoll	White
EMCYT KP 132	Estramustine Phosphate	Capsule	140mg	Kabi Pharmacia	White w/ black letters
EMPIRIN 3	Aspirin/Codeine	Tablet	325/30mg	Glaxo Wellcome	White
ENTEX 0146 0412	Phenylephrine/ Phenylpropanolamine HCl/Guaifenesin	Capsule	5/45/200mg	Procter & Gamble	Orange/White
ENTEX LA I 0146 0436	Phenylpropanolamine HCl/Guaifenesin	Tablet	75/400mg	Procter & Gamble	Orange
ENTEX PSE I NE	Guaifenesin/ Pseudoephedrine HCl	Tablet	600/120mg	Procter & Gamble	Yellow
Eon logo 1217	Nitroglycerin	Capsule	9mg	Eon	Gold / Green
ERYC PD 696	Erythromycin	Capsule	250mg	Parke-Davis	Orange / Clear
ETHEX	Potassium Chloride	Capsule	750mg	Ethex	White
FAMVIR I 500	Famciclovir	Tablet	500mg	SmithKline Beecham	White
FLAGYL I 500	Metronidazole	Tablet	500mg	Searle	Blue
FLINT I 100	Levothyroxine	Tablet	0.1mg	Knoll	Yellow
FLINT I 112	Levothyroxine	Tablet	0.112mg	Knoll	Pink
FLINT I 125	Levothyroxine	Tablet	0.125mg	Knoll	Beige
FLINT I 150	Levothyroxine	Tablet	0.15mg	Knoll	Lt. Blue
FLINT I 200	Levothyroxine	Tablet	0.2mg	Knoll	Lt. Pink
FLINT I 25	Levothyroxine	Tablet	0.025mg	Knoll	Peach
FLINT I 300	Levothyroxine	Tablet	0.3mg	Knoll	Lt. Green
FLINT I 50	Levothyroxine	Tablet	0.05mg	Knoll	White
FLINT I 75	Levothyroxine	Tablet	0.075mg	Knoll	Lavender
FLOXIN 200mg	Ofloxacin	Tablet	200mg	Ortho	Cream
FLOXIN 300mg	Ofloxacin	Tablet	300mg	Ortho	White
FLOXIN 400mg	Ofloxacin	Tablet	400mg	Ortho	Lt. Yellow
FOREST I 678	Acetaminophen/ Butalbital/Caffeine	Tablet	500/50/40mg	Forest	White
FOREST I FLUMADINE 100	Rimantadine	Tablet	100mg	Forest	Peach
Forest logo I 100	Levothyroxine	Tablet	0.1mg	Forest	Yellow
Forest logo I 112	Levothyroxine	Tablet	0.112mg	Forest	Pink
Forest logo I 125	Levothyroxine	Tablet	0.125mg	Forest	Lavender
Forest logo I 137	Levothyroxine	Tablet	0.137mg	Forest	Cyan
Forest logo I 150	Levothyroxine	Tablet	0.150mg	Forest	Palest Blue
Forest logo I 200	Levothyroxine	Tablet	0.2mg	Forest	Lt. Pink
Forest logo I 25	Levothyroxine	Tablet	0.025mg	Forest	Peach
Forest logo I 300	Levothyroxine	Tablet	0.3mg	Forest	Lt. Green
Forest logo 3581	Theophylline	Tablet	300mg	Forest	White
Forest logo 3583	Theophylline	Tablet	200mg	Forest	White
Forest logo 3584	Theophylline	Tablet	100mg	Forest	White
Forest logo I 50	Levothyroxine	Tablet	0.05mg	Forest	White
Forest logo I 75	Levothyroxine	Tablet	0.075mg	Forest	Gray
Forest logo I 88	Levothyroxine	Tablet	0.088mg	Forest	Mint Green
Forest logo TC	Thyroid	Tablet	15mg	Forest	Beige
Forest logo TD	Thyroid	Tablet	30mg	Forest	Beige
Forest logo TE	Thyroid	Tablet	60mg	Forest	Beige
Forest logo TF	Thyroid	Tablet	120mg	Forest	Beige

GG 566 GG 566	Nortriptyline HCl	Capsule	25mg	Geneva	White w/ black and gold letter
GG 567 GG 567	Nortriptyline HCl	Capsule	50mg	Geneva	White w/ black and gold letters
GG 568 GG 568	Nortriptyline HCl	Capsule	75mg	Geneva	White w/ Br. Orange letter
GG 573 I GG 573	Doxepin HCl	Capsule	50mg	Geneva	White w/ pink and green stripes
GG 576 I GG 576	Doxepin HCl	Capsule	10mg	Geneva	White w/ red and gold stripes
GG 58 I 10	Trifluoperazine	Tablet	10mg	Geneva	lavender
GG 580	Hydrochlorothiazide/ Triamterene	Capsule	25/50mg	Geneva	Red
GG 591	Propoxyphene HCl	Capsule	65mg	Geneva	Pink
GG 596	Thiothixene	Capsule	2mg	Geneva	White w/ blue and gold bands
GG 597	Thiothixene	Capsule	5mg	Geneva	White w/ orange and brown bands
GG 598	Thiothixene	Capsule	10mg	Geneva	White w/ blue and black bands
GG 606	Hydrochlorothiazide/ Triamterene	Capsule	25/37.5mg	Geneva	White
GG 63	Desipramine	Tablet	10mg	Geneva	White
GG 64	Desipramine	Tablet	25mg	Geneva	White
GG 65	Desipramine	Tablet	50mg	Geneva	White
GG 66	Diazepam	Tablet	2mg	Geneva	White
GG 68	Diazepam	Tablet	10mg	Geneva	Green
GG 725	Naproxen	Tablet	375mg	Geneva	Orange
GG 726	Naproxen	Tablet	500mg	Geneva	Yellow
GG 771	Glipizide	Tablet	5mg	Geneva	White
GG 772	Glipizide	Tablet	10mg	Geneva	White
GG 85	Spironolactone	Tablet	25mg	Geneva	White
GG 95	Spironolactone/ Hydrochlorothiazide	Tablet	25/25mg	Geneva	White
GG L7	Atenolol	Tablet	25mg	Geneva	White
Gilbert logo I 535-11	Acetaminophen/ Butalbital/Caffeine	Tablet	325/50/40mg	Forest	White
GL 500	Metformin HCl	Tablet	500mg	Lipha	White
GL 850	Metformin HCl	Tablet	850mg	Lipha	White
GLAXO I 387	Cefuroxime Axetil	Tablet	500mg	Glaxo Wellcome	Lt. Blue
GLAXO I 394	Cefuroxime Axetil	Tablet	125mg	Glaxo Wellcome	Blue
GLAXO I 395	Cefuroxime Axetil	Tablet	250mg	Glaxo Wellcome	White
GLAXO I 4	Ondansetron HCl	Tablet	4mg	Glaxo Wellcome	White
GLAXO I 8	Ondansetron HCl	Tablet	8mg	Glaxo Wellcome	Mustard Yellow
GLAXO Logo Y9C 100	Zidovudine	Capsule	100mg	Glaxo Wellcome	White w/ blue bands
GLAXO TRANDATE 100	Labetalol HCl	Tablet	100mg	Glaxo Wellcome	Peach
GLAXO I ZANTAC 150	Ranitidine HCl	Tablet	150mg	Glaxo Wellcome	Peach
GLAXO I ZANTAC 150	Ranitidine HCl	Capsule	150mg	Glaxo Wellcome	Beige
GLAXO I ZANTAC 300	Ranitidine HCl	Tablet	300mg	Glaxo Wellcome	Yellow
GLAXO ZANTAC 300	Ranitidine HCl	Capsule	300mg	Glaxo Wellcome	Beige
GLUCOTROL XL 10	Glipizide	Tablet	10mg	Pfizer	White

Imprint	Generic Name	Form	Strength	Manufacturer	Color
GLUCOTROL XL 5	Glipizide	Tablet	5mg	Pfizer	White
Goldline logo 03	Hydralazine	Tablet	25mg	Goldline-Royce	Orange
Goldline Logo 1300	Verapamil HCl	Tablet	80mg	Goldline-Royce	White
Goldline logo 1872	Hydrochlorothiazide/ Triamterene	Tablet	50/75mg	Goldline-Royce	Greenish Yellow
GRISACTIN 250	Griseofulvin	Capsule	250mg	Wyeth-Ayerst	Yellow
HALCION 0.125	Triazolam	Tablet	0.125mg	Upjohn	White
HALCION 0.25	Triazolam	Tablet	0.25mg	Upjohn	Blue
HALOTESTIN 10	Fluoxymesterone	Tablet	10mg	Upjohn	Green
HALOTESTIN 2	Fluoxymesterone	Tablet	2mg	Upjohn	Palest Peach
HALOTESTIN 5	Fluoxymesterone	Tablet	5mg	Upjohn	Pale Green
HD 567	Acetaminophen/ Butalbital/Caffeine	Tablet	325/50/40mg	Halsey	White
HOECHST ALTACE 1.25mg	Ramipril	Capsule	1.25mg	Hoechst Marion Roussel	Yellow
HOECHST ALTACE 10mg	Ramipril	Capsule	10mg	Hoechst Marion Roussel	Blue
HOECHST ALTACE 5 mg	Ramipril	Capsule	5mg	Hoechst Marion Roussel	Red
HOECHST I Dia B	Glyburide	Tablet	1.25mg	Hoechst Marion Roussel	Peach
HOECHST I Dia B	Glyburide	Tablet	2.5mg	Hoechst Marion Roussel	Pink
HOECHST I Dia B	Glyburide	Tablet	5mg	Hoechst Marion Roussel	Green
HOECHST I LASIX	Furosemide	Tablet	20mg	Hoechst Marion Roussel	White
HOECHST I LASIX 40	Furosemide	Tablet	40mg	Hoechst Marion Roussel	White
HOECHST I LASIX 80	Furosemide	Tablet	80mg	Hoechst Marion Roussel	White
Hoechst logo I AMARYL	Glimepiride	Tablet	2mg	Hoechst Marion Roussel	Green
HOECHST I TRENTAL	Pentoxifylline	Tablet	400mg	Hoechst Marion Roussel	Bright Pink
HOEHST ALTACE 2.5 mg	Ramipril	Capsule	2.5mg	Hoechst Marion Roussel	Orange
HYZAAR I MRK 717	Hydrochlorothiazide/ Losartan Potassium	Tablet	12.5/50mg	Merck	Yellow
IBU 600	Ibuprofen	Tablet	600mg	Knoll	White
IBU 800	Ibuprofen	Tablet	800mg	Knoll	White
IM DUR I 60 60	Isosorbide Mononitrate	Tablet	60mg	Schering	Lt. Yellow
IMURAN 50	Azathioprine	Tablet	50mg	Glaxo Wellcome	Lt. Yellow
INDERAL 10 I I	Propranolol HCl	Tablet	10mg	Wyeth-Ayerst	Peach
INDERAL 20 I I	Propranolol HCl	Tablet	20mg	Wyeth-Ayerst	Pale Blue
INDERAL 40 I I	Propranolol HCl	Tablet	40mg	Wyeth-Ayerst	Lt. Green
INDERAL 60 I I	Propranolol HCl	Tablet	60mg	Wyeth-Ayerst	Pink
INDERAL 80 I I	Propranolol HCl	Tablet	80mg	Wyeth-Ayerst	Yellow
INDERAL LA 120	Propranolol HCl	Capsule	120mg	Wyeth-Ayerst	Dk. Blue/ Lt. Blue
INDERAL LA 160	Propranolol HCl	Capsule	160mg	Wyeth-Ayerst	Dark Blue w/ Gray Bands
INDERAL LA 60	Propranolol HCl	Capsule	60mg	Wyeth-Ayerst	Lt. Blue/White
INDERAL LA 80	Propranolol HCl	Capsule	80mg	Wyeth-Ayerst	Lt. Blue w/ Gray Stripes
INDERIDE 40/25 I I	Propranolol HCl/ Hydrochlorothiazide	Tablet	40/25mg	Wyeth-Ayerst	White
INDERIDE LA 120/50	Propranolol HCl/ Hydrochlorothiazide	Capsule	120/50mg	Wyeth-Ayerst	Maroon/Cream w/ beige bands
INDERIDE LA 160/50	Propranolol HCl/ Hydrochlorothiazide	Tablet	160/50mg	Wyeth-Ayerst	Maroon
INDERIDE LA 80/50	Propranolol HCl/ Hydrochlorothiazide	Capsule	80/50mg	Wyeth-Ayerst	Cream w/ beige bands
INV 209	Benztropine Mesylate	Tablet	1mg	Invamed	White
INV 227	Metoclopramide HCl	Tablet	5mg	Invamed	White
INV286	Naproxen Sodium	Tablet	275mg	Invamed	White
INV287	Naproxen Sodium	Tablet	550mg	Invamed	White
Inwood logo 3609	Propranolol HCl	Capsule	60mg	Inwood	Brown/Clear

Imprint	Generic Name	Form	Strength	Manufacturer	Color
KUI	Ergocalciferol	Tablet	1.25mg	Schwarz	Yellow
LEDERLE 1145	Minocycline HCl	Tablet	50mg	Lederle	Beige/Green
LEDERLE 119	Indomethacin	Capsule	25mg	Lederle	Pink/White
LEDERLE 120	Indomethacin	Capsule	50mg	Lederle	Pink/White
LEDERLE A3 250mg	Tetracycline HCl	Capsule	250mg	Lederle	Gold/Purple
LEDERLE A5 500mg	Tetracycline HCl	Capsule	500mg	Lederle	Purple/Gold
Lederle logo I M22	Methyldopa	Tablet	250mg	Lederle	Peach
Lederle logo I P 46	Propranolol HCl	Tablet	40mg	Lederle	Greish Brown
LEDERLE M46 LEDERLE 100mg	Minocycline HCl	Capsule	100mg	Lederle	Light Green/Dark Green
LEDERLE V7 VERELAN 180mg	Verapamil HCl	Capsule	180mg	Lederle	Yellow / Gray
LEDERLE V8 VERELAN 1 20mg	Verapamil HCl	Capsule	120mg	Lederle	Yellow
LEDERLE V9 VERELAN 240mg	Verapamil HCl	Capsule	240mg	Lederle	Blue / Yellow
LILLY 3061 I CECLOR 250 mg	Cefaclor	Capsule	250mg	Lilly	Purple / White
LILLY 3062 I CECLOR 500mg	Cefaclor	Capsule	500mg	Lilly	Purple / Gray
LILLY 3144 AXID 150mg	Nizatidine	Capsule	150mg	Lilly	Gold / Cream
LILLY 3145 AXID 300mg	Nizatidine	Capsule	300mg	Lilly	Clay/Cream
LILLY 3170 LORABID 200 mg	Loracarbef	Capsule	200mg	Lilly	Pale Blue / Gray
LILLY 3171 LORABID	Loracarbef	Capsule	400mg	Lilly	Pale Blue / Peach
LILLY I DARVOCET -N 100	Propoxyphene Napsylate/ Acetaminophen	Tablet	100/650mg	Lilly	Bright Orange
LILLY DARVOCET N 50	Propoxyphene Napsylate/ Acetaminophen	Tablet	50/325mg	Lilly	Bright Orange
LILLY DARVON-N 100	Propoxyphene Napsylate	Tablet	100mg	Lilly	Cream
LILLY V-CILLIN K 125	Penicillin V Potassium	Tablet	125mg	Lilly	White
LILLY V-CILLIN K 250	Penicillin V Potassium	Tablet	250mg	Lilly	White
LILLY V-CILLIN K 500	Penicillin V Potassium	Tablet	500mg	Lilly	White
LIORESAL I 10 10	Baclofen	Tablet	10mg	Novartis	White
LIORESAL I 20 20	Baclofen	Tablet	20mg	Novartis	White
LL 200 I SUPRAX	Cefixime	Tablet	200mg	Lederle	White
LL 400 I SUPRAX	Cefixime	Tablet	400mg	Lederle	White
LL I A 51	Alprazolam	Tablet	0.25mg	Lederle	White
LL I A 52	Alprazolam	Tablet	0.5mg	Lederle	Yellow
LL I A 53	Alprazolam	Tablet	1mg	Lederle	Light Green
LL I B 1	Bisoprolol	Tablet	5mg	Lederle	Pink
LL I B 12	Bisoprolol/ Hydrochlorothiazide	Tablet	2.5/6.25mg	Lederle	Dk. Yellow
LL I B 13	Bisoprolol/ Hydrochlorothiazide	Tablet	5/6.25mg	Lederle	Pink
LL I B 14	Bisoprolol/ Hydrochlorothiazide	Tablet	10/6.25mg	Lederle	White
LL D2 I DIAMOX 250	Acetazolamide	Tablet	250mg	Storz	White
LL DI I DIAMOX 125	Acetazolamide	Tablet	125mg	Storz	White
LL M8 I MAXZIDE	Hydrochlorothiazide/ Triamterene	Tablet	50/75mg	Lederle	Yellow
LL M9 I MAXZIDE	Hydrochlorothiazide/ Triamterene	Tablet	25/37.5mg	Lederle	Green
LL I N 1	Methazolamide	Tablet	50mg	Lederle	Orange
LODINE 200	Etodolac	Capsule	200mg	Wyeth-Ayerst	Gray
LODINE 300	Etodolac	Capsule	300mg	Wyeth-Ayerst	Gray

Inwood logo 3610	Propranolol HCl	Capsule	80mg	Inwood	Blue/Clear
Inwood logo 3611	Propranolol HCl	Capsule	120mg	Inwood	Blue/Clear
Inwood logo 3612	Propranolol HCl	Capsule	160mg	Inwood	Blue/Clear
IONAMIN 15	Phentermine HCl	Capsule	15mg	Fisons	Gray / Yellow
IONAMIN 30	Phentermine HCl	Capsule	30mg	Fisons	Yellow
ISMO 20	Isosorbide Mononitrate	Tablet	20mg	Wyeth-Ayerst	Orange
ISOPTIN SR I 2Triangles	Verapamil HCl	Tablet	240mg	Knoll	Greenish yellow
ISOPTIN SR180mg	Verapamil HCl	Tablet	180mg	Knoll	Pink
JANSSEN I AST 10	Astemizole	Tablet	10mg	Janssen	White
JANSSEN IMODIUM	Loperamide	Capsule	2mg	Janssen	Dk. Green / Lt. Green
JANSSEN I NIZORAL	Ketoconazole	Tablet	200mg	Janssen	White
JANSSEN I P 10	Cisapride	Tablet	10mg	Janssen	White
JANSSEN I P 20	Cisapride	Tablet	20mg	Janssen	Lt. Blue
JANSSEN I R 1	Risperidone	Tablet	1mg	Janssen	White
JANSSEN I R 2	Risperidone	Tablet	2mg	Janssen	Peach
JANSSEN I R 3	Risperidone	Tablet	3mg	Janssen	Yellow
JANSSEN I R 4	Risperidone	Tablet	4mg	Janssen	Green
JANSSEN SPORANOX 100	Itraconazole	Capsule	100mg	Janssen	L. Blue/Pink
JANSSEN I VERMOX	Mebendazole	Tablet	100mg	Janssen	Pale Peach
K-DUR 10	Potassium Chloride	Tablet	750mg	Schering	White Granule
K-DUR 20	Potassium Chloride	Tablet	1500mg	Schering	White Granule
K1	Granisetron HCl	Tablet	1mg	SmithKline Beecham	White
KEFTAB 500	Cephalexin HCl	Tablet	500mg	Dista	Green
KEMADRIN S3A	Procyclidine HCl	Tablet	5mg	Glaxo Wellcome	White
KERLONE 10	Betaxolol HCl	Tablet	10mg	Searle	White
KERLONE 20 I B	Betaxolol HCl	Tablet	20mg	Searle	White
KLONOPIN I 1	Clonazepam	Tablet	1mg	Roche	Blue
KLONOPIN I 1/2	Clonazepam	Tablet	0.5mg	Roche	Orange
KLONOPIN I 2	Clonazepam	Tablet	2mg	Roche	White
KLOR-CON 10	Potassium Chloride	Tablet	750mg	Upsher-Smith	Bright Yellow
KLOR-CON 8	Potassium Chloride	Tablet	600mg	Upsher-Smith	Robin's Egg Blue
KLOTRIX10mEq 770 BL	Potassium Chloride	Tablet	750mg	Bristol-Myers Squibb	Peach
KNOLL I 120 SR	Verapamil HCl	Tablet	120mg	Knoll	Light Pink
KNOLL I ISOPTIN 120	Verapamil HCl	Tablet	120mg	Knoll	White
KNOLL I ISOPTIN 80	Verapamil HCl	Tablet	80mg	Knoll	Bright Yellow
Knoll Logo 150	Propafenone	Tablet	150mg	Knoll	White
Knoll logo I 2	Hydromorphone HCl	Tablet	2mg	Knoll	Orange
Knoll Logo 300	Propafenone	Tablet	300mg	Knoll	White
Knoll logo I 4	Hydromorphone HCl	Tablet	4mg	Knoll	Yellow
Knoll logo I 90	Guaifenesin/ Pseudoephedrine HCl	Tablet	600/120mg	Knoll	Light Blue
KP I 102	Sulfasalazine	Tablet	500mg	Pharmacia/Upjohn	Ochre
KREMERS URBAN I 053	Chlorpheniramine/ Pseudoephedrine HCl	Capsule	10/65mg	Schwarz	Transparent Yellow / Cream
KREMERS URBAN I 055	Chlorpheniramine/ Pseudoephedrine HCl	Capsule	8/120mg	Schwarz	White
KREMERS URBAN 537 Brown	Hyoscyamine Sulfate	Capsule	0.375mg	Schwarz	Clear / Clay
KU I 050	Chlorpheniramine/ Pseudoephedrine HCl	Tablet	4/60mg	Schwarz	Transparent w/ blue and white tiny
KU I 202	Belladonna Alkaloids/ Phenobarbital	Tablet	0.0194/0.1037/ 16.2/0.0065mg	Schwarz	Charcoal Black
KU I 531	Hyoscyamine Sulfate	Tablet	0.125mg	Schwarz	White

LODINE 400	Etodolac	Tablet	400mg	Wyeth-Ayerst	Yellow
logo I CARDIZEM SR 120mg	Diltiazem HCl	Capsule	120mg	Hoechst Marion Roussel	Brown / Lt. Brown
logo I CARDIZEM SR 60mg	Diltiazem HCl	Capsule	60mg	Hoechst Marion Roussel	Brown / Lt. Yellow
logo I CARDIZEM SR 90mg	Diltiazem HCl	Capsule	90mg	Hoechst Marion Roussel	Brown / Dk. Yellow
LORELCO 250	Probucol	Tablet	250mg	Hoechst Marion Roussel	White
LORELCO 500	Probucol	Tablet	500mg	Hoechst Marion Roussel	White
LOTENSIN I 10	Benazepril HCl	Tablet	10mg	Novartis	Golden Yellow
LOTENSIN I 20	Benazepril HCl	Tablet	20mg	Novartis	Lt. Mauve
LOTENSIN I 40	Benazepril HCl	Tablet	40mg	Novartis	Mauve
LOTENSIN I 5	Benazepril HCl	Tablet	5mg	Novartis	Yellow
LOTENSIN HCT I 57 57	Benazepril HCl/ Hydrochlorothiazide	Tablet	5/6.25mg	Novartis	White
LOTENSIN HCT I 72 72	Benazepril HCl/ Hydrochlorothiazide	Tablet	10/12.5mg	Novartis	Lt. Pink
LOTENSIN HCT I 75 75	Benazepril HCl/ Hydrochlorothiazide	Tablet	20/25mg	Novartis	Mauve
LUCHEM I 7 41	Phenylpropanolamine HCl/Guaifenesin	Tablet	75/400mg	Luchem	Blue w/White Dots
M 1	Clonidine HCl/ Chlorthalidone	Tablet	0.1/15mg	Mylan	Yellow
M 11	Penicillin V Potassium	Tablet	250mg	Mylan	White
M 221	Timolol	Tablet	10mg	Mylan	Green
M 27	Clonidine HCl/ Chlorthalidone	Tablet	0.2/15mg	Mylan	Yellow
M 30	Clorazepate	Tablet	3.75mg	Mylan	Lt. Blue
M 32	Metoprolol Tartrate	Tablet	50mg	Mylan	Pink
M 40	Clorazepate	Tablet	7.5mg	Mylan	Peach
M 47	Metoprolol Tartrate	Tablet	100mg	Mylan	Light Blue
M 54	Thioridazine HCl	Tablet	10mg	Mylan	Orange
M 541	Cimetidine	Tablet	800mg	Mylan	Lt. Green
M 55	Timolol	Tablet	5mg	Mylan	Green
M 58	Thioridazine HCl	Tablet	25mg	Mylan	Orange
M 59 I 50	Thioridazine HCl	Tablet	50mg	Mylan	Orange
M 61	Thioridazine HCl	Tablet	100mg	Mylan	Orange
M 715	Timolol	Tablet	20mg	Mylan	Green
M 72	Clonidine HCl/ Chlorthalidone	Tablet	0.3/15mg	Mylan	Yellow
M 98	Penicillin V Potassium	Tablet	500mg	Mylan	White
M400	Erythromycin Ethylsuccinate	Tablet	400mg	Mylan	Light Brown
MACRODANTIN 0149 0009	Nitrofurantoin	Capsule	100mg	Procter & Gamble	Yellow
MACRODANTIN 25mg 0149 0007	Nitrofurantoin	Capsule	25mg	Procter & Gamble	White w/ black letters
MACRODANTIN 50mg 0149 0008	Nitrofurantoin	Capsule	50mg	Procter & Gamble	Yellow / White w/ black letters
MARION I 13 75	Oxybutynin	Tablet	5mg	Hoechst Marion Roussel	Lt. Blue
MARION I 1771	Diltiazem HCl	Tablet	30mg	Hoechst Marion Roussel	Lt. Green
MARION I 1772	Diltiazem HCl	Tablet	60mg	Hoechst Marion Roussel	Lt. Yellow
MARION logo I CARDIZEM CD 120mg	Diltiazem HCl	Capsule	120mg	Hoechst Marion Roussel	Royal Blue / Lt. Blue
MARION logo I CARDIZEM CD 180mg	Diltiazem HCl	Capsule	180mg	Hoechst Marion Roussel	Royal Blue / Lt. Blue
MARION logo I CARDIZEM CD 240mg	Diltiazem HCl	Capsule	240mg	Hoechst Marion Roussel	Royal Blue

Imprint	Generic Name	Form	Strength	Manufacturer	Color
MARION logo I CARDIZEM CD 300mg	Diltiazem HCl	Capsule	300mg	Hoechst Marion Roussel	Royal Blue / Gray
MAXAQUIN 400	Lomefloxacin HCl	Tablet	400mg	Searle	White
MCNEIL I 659	Tramadol HCl	Tablet	50mg	McNeil	White
MCNEIL I HALDOL 1	Haloperidol	Tablet	1mg	McNeil	Bright Yellow w/ hole in the middle
MCNEIL I HALDOL 2	Haloperidol	Tablet	2mg	McNeil	Lavender w/ hole in the middle
MCNEIL I PARAFON FORTE DSC	Chlorzoxazone	Tablet	500mg	McNeil	Lt. Green
MCNEIL TOLECTIN 600	Tolmetin	Tablet	600mg	McNeil	Orange
MCNEIL TOLECTIN DS	Tolmetin	Capsule	400mg	McNeil	Orange w/ Gray bands
MCNEIL I TYLENOL	Acetaminophen/Codeine CODEINE 2	Tablet	300/15mg	McNeil	White
MCNEIL I TYLENOL	Acetaminophen/Codeine CODEINE 3	Tablet	300/30mg	McNeil	White
MCNEIL I TYLENOL CODEINE 4	Acetaminophen/Codeine	Tablet	300/60mg	McNeil	White
MCNEIL TYLOX I MCNEIL TYLOX	Acetaminophen/ Oxycodone HCl	Capsule	500/5mg	McNeil	Dk. Red
MD I 530	Methylphenidate HCl	Tablet	10mg	MD	White
MD I 531	Methylphenidate HCl	Tablet	5mg	MD	Yellow-Green
MD I 532	Methylphenidate HCl	Tablet	20mg	MD	Peach
MD I 535	Diphenoxylate HCl/ Atropine	Tablet	2.5/0.025mg	MD	White
MEDROL 16	Methylprednisolone	Tablet	16mg	Upjohn	White
MEDROL 4	Methylprednisolone	Tablet	4mg	Upjohn	White
MIA 108	Acetaminophen/ Hydrocodone	Tablet	500/5mg	Mikart	White
MICRONASE 1.25	Glyburide	Tablet	1.25mg	Upjohn	White
MICRONASE 2.5	Glyburide	Tablet	2.5mg	Upjohn	Pink
MICRONASE 5	Glyburide	Tablet	5mg	Upjohn	Blue
MILES 095	Clotrimazole	Lozenge	10mg	Miles	White
MILES 30 I 884	Nifedipine	Tablet	30mg	Miles	Clay
MILES 60 I 885	Nifedipine	Tablet	60mg	Miles	Rust
MILES 90 I 886	Nifedipine	Tablet	90mg	Miles	Rust
MJ 021	Estradiol	Tablet	0.5mg	Bristol-Myers Squibb	White
MJ 10 I BUSPAR	Buspirone HCl	Tablet	10mg	Bristol-Myers Squibb	White
MJ 158 I M	Fosinopril	Tablet	10mg	Bristol-Myers Squibb	White
MJ 5 I BUSPAR	Buspirone HCl	Tablet	5mg	Bristol-Myers Squibb	White
MJ 503 I 50	Cyclophosphamide	Tablet	50mg	Bristol-Myers Squibb	White w/ green specks
MJ 609 I M	Fosinopril	Tablet	20mg	Bristol-Myers Squibb	White
MJ 755	Estradiol	Tablet	1mg	Bristol-Myers Squibb	Purple
MJ 756	Estradiol	Tablet	2mg	Bristol-Myers Squibb	Teal Green
MJ 775 DESYREL	Trazodone HCl	Tablet	50mg	Bristol-Myers Squibb	Peach
MJ 776 DESYREL	Trazodone HCl	Tablet	100mg	Bristol-Myers Squibb	White
MJ 778 I 50 50 50	Trazodone HCl	Tablet	150mg	Bristol-Myers Squibb	Peach
MJI850 ; MJI583	Ethinyl Estradiol/ Norethindrone	Tablet	Inert; 0.035/ 0.4mg	Bristol-Myers Squibb	Green ; Pale Peach
MJI850 ; MJI584	Ethinyl Estradiol/ Norethindrone	Tablet	Inert; 0.05/1mg	Bristol-Myers Squibb	Green ; Creamy Yellow
MONODOX 100 I M 259	Doxycycline Monohydrate	Capsule	100mg	Oclassen	Brown / Yellow

Imprint	Generic Name	Form	Strength	Manufacturer	Color
MSD 714 I VASOTEC	Enalapril	Tablet	20mg	Merck	Peach
MSD 72I PROSCAR	Finasteride	Tablet	5mg	Merck	Blue
MSD 720 I VASERTIC	Enalapril/ Hydrochlorothiazide	Tablet	10/25mg	Merck	Mauve
MSD 726 I ZOCOR	Simvastatin	Tablet	5mg	Merck	Pale Yellow
MSD 730 I MEVACOR	Lovastatin	Tablet	10mg	Merck	Peach
MSD 731 I MEVACOR	Lovastatin	Tablet	20mg	Merck	Lt. Blue
MSD 732 I MEVACOR	Lovastatin	Tablet	40mg	Merck	Lt. Green
MSD 735 I ZOCOR	Simvastatin	Tablet	10mg	Merck	Pale Pink
MSD 740 I ZOCOR	Simvastatin	Tablet	20mg	Merck	Pale Peach
MSD 749 I ZOCOR	Simvastatin	Tablet	40mg	Merck	Pink
MSD 917 I M	Amiloride HCl/ Hydrochlorothiazide	Tablet	5/50mg	Merck	Light Peach
MSD 931 I FLEXARIL	Cyclobenzaprine HCl	Tablet	10mg	Merck	Dk. Yellow
MSD 941 I CLINORIL	Sulindac	Tablet	150mg	Merck	Yellow-Gold
MSD 942 I CLINORIL	Sulindac	Tablet	200mg	Merck	Yellow-Gold
MSD 963 I PEPCID	Famotidine	Tablet	20mg	Merck	Beige
MSD 964 I PEPCID	Famotidine	Tablet	40mg	Merck	Brown
MSD 97 I DECADRON	Dexamethasone	Tablet	4mg	Merck	White
MSD INDOCIN SR 693	Indomethacin	Capsule	75mg	Merck	Lt. Blue/Clear
MUTUAL 105 I MUTUAL 105	Doxycycline	Capsule	100mg	Mutual	Blue
MUTUAL 165	Piroxicam	Capsule	10mg	Mutual	Purple / White
MUTUAL 166	Piroxicam	Capsule	20mg	Mutual	Purple
MUTUAL 179	Tolmetin	Capsule	400mg	Mutual	Orange
MYLAN 10 10	Piroxicam	Capsule	10mg	Mylan	Yellow / Green (dull)
MYLAN 101	Tetracycline HCl	Capsule	250mg	Mylan	Gold / Red
MYLAN 106	Erythromycin Stearate	Tablet	250mg	Mylan	Yellow
MYLAN 107	Erythromycin Stearate	Tablet	500mg	Mylan	Yellow
MYLAN 1200	Acebutolol HCl	Capsule	200mg	Mylan	Orange
MYLAN I 130	Acetaminophen/ Propoxyphene HCl	Tablet	650/65mg	Mylan	Orange
MYLAN 1400	Acebutolol HCl	Capsule	400mg	Mylan	Orange
MYLAN 143	Indomethacin	Capsule	25mg	Mylan	Green
MYLAN 148 I MYLAN 148	Doxycycline	Capsule	100mg	Mylan	Blue
MYLAN I 155	Acetaminophen/ Propoxyphene Napsylate	Tablet	650/100mg	Mylan	Fuschia Pink
MYLAN 167	Doxycycline	Tablet	100mg	Mylan	White
MYLAN 2020	Piroxicam	Capsule	20mg	Mylan	Apple Green
MYLAN I 211	Chlordiazepoxide HCl/ Amitriptyline	Tablet	5/12.5mg	Mylan	Neon Green
MYLAN 214	Haloperidol	Tablet	2mg	Mylan	Peach
MYLAN 257	Haloperidol	Tablet	1mg	Mylan	Peach
MYLAN 271	Diazepam	Tablet	2mg	Mylan	White
MYLAN I 277	Chlordiazepoxide HCl/ Amitriptyline	Tablet	10/25mg	Mylan	Cream
MYLAN 3000 MYLAN 3000	Meclofenamate	Capsule	100mg	Mylan	Rust / White
MYLAN 3125 I MYLAN 3125	Doxepin HCl	Capsule	25mg	Mylan	Yellow / White
MYLAN 327	Haloperidol	Tablet	5mg	Mylan	Peach
MYLAN 345	Diazepam	Tablet	5mg	Mylan	Peach
MYLAN 351	Haloperidol	Tablet	0.5mg	Mylan	Peach
MYLAN 4010	Temazepam	Capsule	15mg	Mylan	Gold
MYLAN 4250 I MYLAN 4250	Doxepin HCl	Capsule	50mg	Mylan	Yellow

MONODOX 50 l M 260	Doxycycline Monohydrate	Capsule	50mg	Oclassen	Lt. Yellow / White
MOTRIN 400mg	Ibuprofen	Tablet	400mg	Upjohn	Bright Orange
MOTRIN 600mg	Ibuprofen	Tablet	600mg	Upjohn	Lt. Orange
MOTRIN 800mg	Ibuprofen	Tablet	800mg	Upjohn	Orange
MP 112	Sulindac	Tablet	150mg	Mutual	Yellow-Gold
MP 114	Trazodone HCl	Tablet	100mg	Mutual	White
MP 116	Sulindac	Tablet	200mg	Mutual	Yellow-Gold
MP 118	Trazodone HCl	Tablet	50mg	Mutual	White
MP 142	Benztropine Mesylate	Tablet	2mg	Mutual	White
MP 178	Pindolol	Tablet	5mg	Mutual	White
MP 183	Pindolol	Tablet	10mg	Mutual	White
MP 184	Metoprolol Tartrate	Tablet	50mg	Mutual	Orange
MP 185	Metoprolol Tartrate	Tablet	100mg	Mutual	Bright Yellow
MP 44	Benztropine Mesylate	Tablet	1mg	Mutual	White
MP 50	Tolmetin	Tablet	200mg	Mutual	White
MP 51	Prednisone	Tablet	5mg	Mutual	White
MP 52	Prednisone	Tablet	10mg	Mutual	White
MP 53	Prednisone	Tablet	20mg	Mutual	Peach
MP 71	Allopurinol	Tablet	100mg	Mutual	White
MP 74	Chlorzoxazone	Tablet	500mg	Mutual	Lt. Green
MP 80	Allopurinol	Tablet	300mg	Mutual	Dk. Peach
MP 81	Sulfamethoxazole/ Trimethoprim	Tablet	400/80mg	Mutual	White
MP 85	Sulfamethoxazole/ Trimethoprim	Tablet	800/160mg	Mutual	White
MRK l 951	Losartan Potassium	Tablet	25mg	Merck	Light Green
MRK l 952	Losartan Potassium	Tablet	50mg	Merck	Green
MSD 105 l HYDRODIURIL	Hydrochlorothiazide	Tablet	50mg	Merck	Peach
MSD 106 l PRINIVIL	Lisinopril	Tablet	10mg	Merck	Beige
MSD 136 l BLOCADREN	Timolol	Tablet	10mg	Merck	Light Blue
MSD 14 l VASOTEC	Enalapril	Tablet	2.5mg	Merck	Lt. Yellow
MSD 140 l PRINZIDE	Hydrochlorothiazide/ Lisinopril	Tablet	12.5/20mg	Merck	Beige
MSD 142 l PRINZIDE	Hydrochlorothiazide/ Lisinopril	Tablet	25/20mg	Merck	Peach
MSD 19 l PRINIVIL	Lisinopril	Tablet	5mg	Merck	White
MSD 207 l PRINIVIL	Lisinopril	Tablet	20mg	Merck	Pale Pink
MSD 237 l PRINIVIL	Lisinopril	Tablet	40mg	Merck	Clay Pink
MSD 25 INDOCIN	Indomethacin	Capsule	25mg	Merck	Lt. Blue/White
MSD 401 l ALDOMET	Methyldopa	Tablet	250mg	Merck	Gold
MSD 42 l HYDRODIURIL	Hydrochlorothiazide	Tablet	25mg	Merck	Peach
MSD 452 l PLENDIL	Felodipine	Tablet	10mg	Merck	Clay Pink
MSD 456 l ALDORIL	Hydrochlorothiazide/ Methyldopa	Tablet	25/250mg	Merck	White
MSD 50 INDOCIN	Indomethacin	Capsule	50mg	Merck	Lt. Blue/White
MSD 516 l ALDOMET	Methyldopa	Tablet	500mg	Merck	Gold
MSD 517 l TRIAVIL	Amitriptyline HCl/ Perphenazine	Tablet	50/4mg	Merck	Lt. Peach
MSD 53 l HYDROPRES	Reserpine/ Hydrochlorothiazide	Tablet	0.125/50mg	Merck	Seafoam Green
MSD 60 l COGENTIN	Benztropine Mesylate	Tablet	2mg	Merck	White
MSD 675 l DOLOBID	Diflunisal	Tablet	250mg	Merck	Light Peach
MSD 69 l BLOCADREN	Timolol	Tablet	5mg	Merck	Light Blue
MSD 697 l DOLOBID	Diflunisal	Tablet	500mg	Merck	Orange
MSD 705 l NOROXIN	Norfloxacin	Tablet	400mg	Merck	Salmon
MSD 707 l TONOCARD	Tocainide HCl	Tablet	400mg	Merck	Yellow
MSD 712 l VASOTEC	Enalapril	Tablet	5mg	Merck	White
MSD 713 l VASOTEC	Enalapril	Tablet	10mg	Merck	Mauve

MYLAN 4415	Flurazepam HCl	Capsule	15mg	Mylan	Blue / White
MYLAN l 442	Amitriptyline HCl/ Perphenazine	Tablet	25/2mg	Mylan	Purple
MYLAN 4430	Flurazepam HCl	Capsule	30mg	Mylan	Blue
MYLAN 457	Lorazepam	Tablet	1mg	Mylan	White
MYLAN 477	Diazepam	Tablet	10mg	Mylan	Lt. Green
MYLAN 5050	Temazepam	Capsule	30mg	Mylan	Yellow
MYLAN 512	Verapamil HCl	Tablet	80mg	Mylan	White
MYLAN 5375 l MYLAN 5375	Doxepin HCl	Capsule	75mg	Mylan	Green
MYLAN 6410 l MYLAN 6410	Doxepin HCl	Capsule	100mg	Mylan	Green / White
MYLAN 7250	Cefaclor	Capsule	250mg	Mylan	Pink / White
MYLAN 7500	Cefaclor	Capsule	500mg	Mylan	Pink / Gray
MYLAN 772	Verapamil HCl	Tablet	120mg	Mylan	White
MYLAN 777	Lorazepam	Tablet	2mg	Mylan	White
N/A	Nicotine Polacrilex	Gum	2mg	Hoechst Marion Roussel	Beige Square
N/A	Nitroglycerin	Tablet	0.3mg	Parke-Davis	White
N/A	Nitroglycerin	Tablet	0.4mg	Parke-Davis	White
N/A	Nitroglycerin	Tablet	0.6mg	Parke-Davis	White
N2 l N	Methazolamide	Tablet	25mg	Storz	White
NAPROSYN l 375	Naproxen	Tablet	375mg	Syntex	Clay Pink
NAPROSYN l 500	Naproxen	Tablet	500mg	Syntex	Off White
NAPROXEN l 250	Naproxen	Tablet	250mg	Hamilton	Lime Green
NATURETIN 10 l PPP 618	Bendroflumethiazide	Tablet	10mg	Bristol-Myers Squibb	Lt. Orange
NATURETIN 5 l PPP 606	Bendroflumethiazide	Tablet	5mg	Bristol-Myers Squibb	Lt. Green
NEI 406	Etidronate Disodium	Tablet	400mg	Procter & Gamble	White
NOLVADEX 600	Tamoxifen	Tablet	10mg	Zeneca	White
NORPRAMIN 100	Desipramine	Tablet	100mg	Hoechst Marion Roussel	Lt. Orange
NORPRAMIN 25	Desipramine	Tablet	25mg	Hoechst Marion Roussel	Dk. Yellow
NORPRAMIN 50	Desipramine	Tablet	50mg	Hoechst Marion Roussel	Green
NORPRAMIN 75	Desipramine	Tablet	75mg	Hoechst Marion Roussel	Orange
NORVASC 10	Amlodipine	Tablet	10mg	Pfizer	White
NORVASC l 2.5	Amlodipine	Tablet	2.5mg	Pfizer	White
NORVASC 5	Amlodipine	Tablet	5mg	Pfizer	White
NORWHICH EATON MACROBID	Nitrofurantoin	Capsule	100mg	Procter & Gamble	Black / Yellow
ORINASE 500	Tolbutamide	Tablet	500mg	Upjohn	White
Ortho 1801	Estropipate	Tablet	0.625mg	Ortho	Orange
ORTHO 214	Griseofulvin	Tablet	500mg	Ortho	White
Ortho 535 ; Ortho 135 ; Ortho ; Ortho 75	Ethinyl Estradiol/ Norethindrone	Tablet	Inert; 0.035/0.75; 0.035/0.5; 0.035/1mg	Ortho	White ; Peach ; Green ; Pale Peach
ORTHO ; ORTHO 135	Ethinyl Estradiol/ Norethindrone	Tablet	Inert; 0.035/1mg	Ortho	Green ; Peach
ORUVAIL 200	Ketoprofen	Capsule	200mg	Wyeth-Ayerst	Pink/White
P.D 007	Phenytoin	Tablet	50mg	Parke-Davis	Cream
P.D 362	Phenytoin Sodium	Capsule	100mg	Parke-Davis	White w/ Orange Band
P.D 365	Phenytoin Sodium	Capsule	30mg	Parke-Davis	Cream w/ Pink Band
P&GI402	Etidronate Disodium	Tablet	200mg	Procter & Gamble	White
PAR 028	Hydralazine	Tablet	50mg	Pharm Resources	Orange
PAR l 034	Meclizine HCl	Tablet	12.5mg	Pharm Resources	Bright Blue l White
PAR l 035	Meclizine HCl	Tablet	25mg	Pharm Resources	Bright Yellowl White
PAR 076	Fluphenazine	Tablet	5mg	Pharm Resources	Maroon Pink
PAR 119	Nystatin	Tablet	500,000 units	Pharm Resources	Dk. Brown

Imprint	Generic Name	Form	Strength	Manufacturer	Color
PAR 225	Haloperidol	Tablet	2mg	Pharm Resources	Pink
PAR 226	Haloperidol	Tablet	5mg	Pharm Resources	Green
PAR 227	Haloperidol	Tablet	10mg	Pharm Resources	Mint Green
PAR 240	Temazepam	Capsule	15mg	Pharm Resources	White/Green
PAR 241	Temazepam	Capsule	30mg	Pharm Resources	White
Parke-Davis logo I BENADRYL	Diphenhydramine	Capsule	25mg	Parke-Davis	Pink/ Red / White
PARLODEL 2 1/2	Bromocriptine	Tablet	2.5mg	Sandoz	White
PARNATE SKF	Tranylcypromine	Tablet	10mg	SmithKline Beecham	Burgandy
PAXIL I 10	Paroxetine HCl	Tablet	10mg	SmithKline Beecham	Yellow
PAXIL I 20	Paroxetine HCl	Tablet	20mg	SmithKline Beecham	Pink
PAXIL I 30	Paroxetine HCl	Tablet	30mg	SmithKline Beecham	Blue
PAXIL I 40	Paroxetine HCl	Tablet	40mg	SmithKline Beecham	Green
PD 156 I 20	Atorvastatin Calcium	Tablet	20mg	Parke-Davis	White
PD 205	Procainamide HCl	Tablet	750mg	Parke-Davis	Orange
PD 373 I PD 373	Diphenhydramine	Capsule	50mg	Parke-Davis	Pink / White / Pink
PD 527 I 5	Quinapril HCl	Tablet	5mg	Parke-Davis	Clay Brown
PD 530 I 10	Quinapril HCl	Tablet	10mg	Parke-Davis	Clay Brown
PD 532 I 20	Quinapril HCl	Tablet	20mg	Parke-Davis	Clay Brown
PD 535 I 40	Quinapril HCl	Tablet	40mg	Parke-Davis	Clay Brown
PD 737 I LOPID	Gemfibrozil	Tablet	600mg	Parke-Davis	White w/ blue letters
PFIZER 094 I VIBRA	Doxycycline	Capsule	50mg	Pfizer	Blue / White
PFIZER 095 I VIBRA	Doxycycline	Capsule	100mg	Pfizer	Blue
PFIZER 099 I VIBRATAB	Doxycycline	Tablet	100mg	Pfizer	Peach
PFIZER 261 PROCARDIA 20	Nifedipine	Capsule	20mg	Pfizer	Rust / Orange
PFIZER 260 PROCARDIA	Nifedipine	Capsule	10mg	Pfizer	Orange
PFIZER 305 I PFIZER 305	Azithromycin	Capsule	250mg	Pfizer	Dk. Orange
PFIZER 393	Chlorpropamide	Tablet	100mg	Pfizer	Lt. Blue
PFIZER 394	Chlorpropamide	Tablet	250mg	Pfizer	Lt. Blue
PFIZER 411	Glipizide	Tablet	5mg	Pfizer	White
PFIZER 412	Glipizide	Tablet	10mg	Pfizer	White
PFIZER 430 MINIZIDE	Prazosin HCl/Polythiazide	Capsule	1/0.5mg	Pfizer	Teal Green
PFIZER 431 MINIPRESS	Prazosin HCl	Capsule	1mg	Pfizer	White
PFIZER 432 MINIZIDE	Prazosin HCl/Polythiazide	Capsule	2/0.5mg	Pfizer	Teal/Pink
PFIZER 436 MINIZIDE	Prazosin HCl/Polythiazide	Capsule	5/0.5mg	Pfizer	Teal/Blue
PFIZER 438 MINIPRESS	Prazosin HCl	Capsule	5mg	Pfizer	Blue/White
PFIZER I 551	Cetirizine	Tablet	10mg	Pfizer	White
PFIZER FELDENE 322	Piroxicam	Capsule	10mg	Pfizer	Lt. Blue/ Maroon
PFIZER FELDENE 323	Piroxicam	Capsule	20mg	Pfizer	Maroon
PFIZER MINIPRESS	Prazosin HCl	Capsule	2mg	Pfizer	Pink/White
PFIZER VISTARIL 543	Hydroxyzine Pamoate	Capsule	100mg	Pfizer	Gray / Dk. Green
Pharmacia logo I 101	Sulfasalazine	Tablet	500mg	Pharmacia/Upjohn	Ochre
PLAQUENIL	Hydroxychloroquine Sulfate	Tablet	200mg	Sanofi Winthrop	White
PLENDIL I 451	Felodipine	Tablet	5mg	Merck	Pink
PPP 232 I CORGARD 20	Nadolol	Tablet	20mg	Bristol-Myers Squibb	Blue
PPP 431	Procainamide HCl	Capsule	250mg	Bristol-Myers Squibb	Orange
PPP 434	Procainamide HCl	Tablet	375mg	Bristol-Myers Squibb	Orange
PPP 438	Procainamide HCl	Tablet	500mg	Bristol-Myers Squibb	Orange
PPP 756	Procainamide HCl	Capsule	375mg	Bristol-Myers Squibb	White/Orange
PPP 757	Procainamide HCl	Capsule	500mg	Bristol-Myers Squibb	Yellow/Orange
PPP 784 I DURICEF 500mg	Cefadroxil	Tablet	1g	Bristol-Myers Squibb	Red / White

Imprint	Generic Name	Form	Strength	Manufacturer	Color
ROBERTS 068	Theophylline/Guaifenesin	Capsule	300/180mg	Roberts	White / Yellow
ROBERTS I ETHMOZINE 200	Moricizine HCl	Tablet	200mg	Roberts	Light Green
ROBERTS I ETHMOZINE 250	Moricizine HCl	Tablet	250mg	Roberts	Light Peach
ROBERTS I ETHMOZINE 300	Moricizine HCl	Tablet	300mg	Roberts	Ligth Blue
ROCHE I 0245	Saquinavir	Capsule	200mg	Roche	Light Brown and Green
ROCHE ACCUTANE 10	Isotretinoin	Capsule	10mg	Roche	Lt. Pink
ROCHE ACCUTANE 20	Isotretinoin	Capsule	20mg	Roche	Maroon
ROCHE ACCUTANE 40	Isotretinoin	Capsule	40mg	Roche	Mustard Yellow
ROCHE AZO GANTRISIN	Phenazopyridine HCl/ Sulfisoxazole	Tablet	50/500mg	Roche	Rust
ROCHEI BACTRIM	Sulfamethoxazole/ Trimethoprim	Tablet	400/80mg	Roche	Light Green
ROCHE I BACTRIM-DS	Sulfamethoxazole/ Trimethoprim	Tablet	800/160mg	Roche	White
ROCHE I BUMEX 0.5	Bumetanide	Tablet	0.5mg	Roche	Green
ROCHE I BUMEX 1	Bumetanide	Tablet	1mg	Roche	Yellow
ROCHE I BUMEX 2	Bumetanide	Tablet	2mg	Roche	Mauve
ROCHE DALMANE 15	Flurazepam HCl	Capsule	15mg	Roche	Orange / Yellow
ROCHE DALMANE 30	Flurazepam HCl	Capsule	30mg	Roche	Red / Yellow
ROCHE GANTRISIN	Sulfisoxazole	Tablet	500mg	Roche	White
ROCHE I HIVID 0.375	Zalcitabine	Tablet	0.375mg	Roche	Palest Pink
ROCHE I HIVID 0.750	Zalcitabine	Tablet	0.750mg	Roche	Palest Purple
ROCHE LIBRAX I ROCHE LIBRAX	Chlordiazepoxide HCl/ Clidinium	Capsule	5/2.5mg	Roche	Lt. Green
ROCHE I LIBRITABS 5	Chlordiazepoxide HCl	Tablet	5mg	Roche	Turquoise Green
ROCHE I LIBRIUM 10	Chlordiazepoxide HCl	Capsule	10mg	Roche	Black / Lt. Green
ROCHE I LIBRIUM 25	Chlordiazepoxide HCl	Capsule	25mg	Roche	Lt. Green / White
ROCHE I LIBRIUM 5	Chlordiazepoxide HCl	Capsule	5mg	Roche	Lt. Green / Yellow
ROCHE I LIMBITROL	Chlordiazepoxide HCl/ Amitriptyline	Tablet	5/12.5mg	Roche	Lt. Blue
ROCHE I ROCALTROL 0.25	Calcitriol	Capsule	0.25mcg	Roche	Orange
ROCHE I ROCALTROL 0.5	Calcitriol	Capsule	0.5mcg	Roche	Orange
ROERIG I 143	Carbenicillin Indanyl Sodium	Tablet	382mg	Roerig	Yellow
ROERIG 534 I SINEQUAN	Doxepin HCl	Capsule	10mg	Roerig	Red / Fuschia
ROERIG 535 I SINEQUAN	Doxepin HCl	Capsule	25mg	Roerig	Pink / Blue
ROERIG 536 I SINEQUAN	Doxepin HCl	Capsule	50mg	Roerig	Cream / Pink
ROERIG 537 I SINEQUAN	Doxepin HCl	Capsule	150mg	Roerig	Royal Blue
ROERIG 538 I SINEQUAN	Doxepin HCl	Capsule	100mg	Roerig	Blue / Lt. Pink
ROERIG 571 NAVANE	Thiothixene	Capsule	1mg	Roerig	Orange / Yellow
ROERIG 572 NAVANE	Thiothixene	Capsule	2mg	Roerig	Blue / Yellow
ROERIG 573 NAVANE	Thiothixene	Capsule	5mg	Roerig	White / Orange
ROERIG 574 NAVANE	Thiothixene	Capsule	10mg	Roerig	White / Blue
ROERIG I DIFLUCAN 100	Fluconazole	Tablet	100mg	Roerig	Pink
ROERIG I DIFLUCAN 200	Fluconazole	Tablet	200mg	Roerig	Pink
ROERIG I DIFLUCAN 50	Fluconazole	Tablet	50mg	Roerig	Pink
Royce Logo I 256 20	Baclofen	Tablet	20mg	Royce	White

PPP 785	Cefadroxil	Capsule	500mg	Bristol-Myers Squibb	White
PPP 863	Fluphenazine	Tablet	1mg	Bristol-Myers Squibb	Pink
PPP 864	Fluphenazine	Tablet	2.5mg	Bristol-Myers Squibb	Yellow
PPP 877	Fluphenazine	Tablet	5mg	Bristol-Myers Squibb	Green
PPP 956	Fluphenazine	Tablet	10mg	Bristol-Myers Squibb	Coral
PPP C I 832	Chlorpheniramine/ Phenylpropanolamine HCl/Phenylephrine/ Phenytoloxamine	Tablet	5/40/10/15mg	URL	White w/ Fuschia Specks
PRECOSE I 50	Acarbose	Tablet	50mg	Bayer	Cream
PREMARIN 0.3	Estrogens, Conjugated	Tablet	0.3mg	Wyeth-Ayerst	Dark Green
PREMARIN 0.625	Estrogens, Conjugated	Tablet	0.625mg	Wyeth-Ayerst	Dark Burgandy
PREMARIN 0.625 ; CYC RIN	Estrogens, Conjugated; Medroxyprogesterone	Tablet	0.625/5mg	Wyeth-Ayerst	Dark Burgundy; Light purple
PREMARIN 0.625 ; Wyeth Logo	Estrogens, Conjugated; Medroxyprogesterone	Tablet	0.625/2.5mg	Wyeth-Ayerst	Maroon ; White
PREMARIN 0.9	Estrogens, Conjugated	Tablet	0.9mg	Wyeth-Ayerst	White w/ pink letters
PREMARIN 1.25	Estrogens, Conjugated	Tablet	1.25mg	Wyeth-Ayerst	Yellow w/ black letters
PREMARIN 2.5	Estrogens, Conjugated	Tablet	2.5mg	Wyeth-Ayerst	Purple w/ white letters
PROCARDIA XL 30	Nifedipine	Tablet	30mg	Pfizer	Pink
PROCARDIA XL 60	Nifedipine	Tablet	60mg	Pfizer	Pink
PROCARDIA XL 90	Nifedipine	Tablet	90mg	Pfizer	Pink
PROLOPRIM 09A	Trimethoprim	Tablet	100mg	Glaxo Wellcome	White
PROLOPRIM 200	Trimethoprim	Tablet	200mg	Glaxo Wellcome	Yellow
PROVENTIL 4 I 573 573	Albuterol	Tablet	4mg	Schering	White
PROVERA 10	Medroxyprogesterone	Tablet	10mg	Upjohn	White
PROVERA 2.5	Medroxyprogesterone	Tablet	2.5mg	Upjohn	Peach
PROVERA 5	Medroxyprogesterone	Tablet	5mg	Upjohn	White
PT I GLYNASE 1.5	Glyburide	Tablet	1.5mg	Upjohn	White
PT I GLYNASE 3	Glyburide	Tablet	3mg	Upjohn	Blue
Purepac logo I 023	Aspirin/Butalbital/Caffeine	Tablet	325/50/40mg	Purepac	White
PurePac logo I 026	Phenobarbital	Tablet	15mg	Purepac	White
Purepac logo I 028	Phenobarbital	Tablet	30mg	Purepac	White
Purepac logo I 063	Lorazepam	Tablet	2mg	Purepac	White
Purepac logo I 321	Propranolol HCl	Tablet	60mg	Purepac	Salmon Pink
R I 4250	Atropine/Hyoscyamine/ Phenobarbital/ Scopolamine	Tablet	0.0194/0.1037/ 16.2/0.0065mg	A. H. Robins	White
R I 7	Indapamide	Tablet	1.25mg	Rhone-Poulenc Rorer	Orange
R I 8	Indapamide	Tablet	2.5mg	Rhone-Poulenc Rorer	White
R&C logo 22	Penbutolol	Tablet	20mg	Reed and Carnrick	Yellow
R-500	Prazosin HCl	Capsule	1mg	Purepac	White
RELAFEN I 500	Nabumetone	Tablet	500mg	SmithKline Beecham	White
RELAFEN I 750	Nabumetone	Tablet	750mg	SmithKline Beecham	Clay
RESTORIL 15 mg FOR SLEEP	Temazepam	Capsule	15mg	Sandoz	Maroon/Pink
RESTORIL 30 mg FOR SLEEP	Temazepam	Capsule	30mg	Sandoz	Maroon/Light Blue
RESTORIL 7.5 mg FOR SLEEP	Temazepam	Capsule	7.5mg	Sandoz	Light Blue/Pink
RIDAURA	Auranofin	Capsule	3mg	SmithKline Beecham	Brown / Cream
ROBERTS 067	Theophylline/Guaifenesin	Capsule	150/90mg	Roberts	Yellow

RP 069 I RP 069	Theophylline	Tablet	300mg	Roberts	Cream
RPC I 073	Propantheline Bromide	Tablet	7.5mg	Roberts	White w/ Red letters
RPC I 074	Propantheline Bromide	Tablet	15mg	Roberts	Pale Peach w/ Red Letters
RPR 202	Riluzole	Tablet	50mg	Rhone-Poulenc Rorer	White
RPR I 5100	Enoxacin	Tablet	200mg	Rhone-Poulenc Rorer	Lt. Blue
RPR I 5140	Enoxacin	Tablet	400mg	Rhone-Poulenc Rorer	Blue
RPR DILACOR XR 120	Diltiazem HCl	Capsule	120mg	Rhone-Poulenc Rorer	Lt. Orange / White
RPR DILACOR XR 180	Diltiazem HCl	Capsule	180mg	Rhone-Poulenc Rorer	Orange / White
RPR DILACOR XR 240	Diltiazem HCl	Capsule	240mg	Rhone-Poulenc Rorer	Brown / White
RPR logo I H 20	Chlorthalidone	Tablet	50mg	Rhone-Poulenc Rorer	Lt. Blue
RPR logo I H 22	Chlorthalidone	Tablet	25mg	Rhone-Poulenc Rorer	Peach
RPR Slo-bid 100mg	Theophylline	Capsule	100mg	Rhone-Poulenc Rorer	White w/ red letters
RPR Slo-bid 125mg	Theophylline	Capsule	125mg	Rhone-Poulenc Rorer	White w/ red letters
RPR Slo-bid 200mg	Theophylline	Capsule	200mg	Rhone-Poulenc Rorer	White w/ red letters
RPR Slo-bid 300mg	Theophylline	Capsule	300mg	Rhone-Poulenc Rorer	White w/ red letters
RPR Slo-Bid 75mg	Theophylline	Capsule	75mg	Rhone-Poulenc Rorer	White w/ red letters
RS I 0920	Isosorbide Dinitrate	Capsule	40mg	Schwarz	Lt. Pink/Clear
RUGBY I 0230	Doxycycline	Capsule	100mg	Rugby	Lt. Blue
RUGBY I 0280	Doxycycline	Capsule	50mg	Rugby	Lt. Blue / White
RUGBY 3367 I RUGBY 3367	Dicyclomine HCl	Capsule	10mg	Rugby	Blue
RUGBY I 3372	Benztropine Mesylate	Tablet	2mg	Rugby	White
RUGBY I 3377	Dicyclomine HCl	Tablet	20mg	Rugby	Lt. Blue
RUGBY 3435	Carisoprodol	Tablet	350mg	Rugby	White
RUGBY I 3835	Furosemide	Tablet	80mg	Rugby	Off-White
RUGBY I 3840	Furosemide	Tablet	20mg	Rugby	Off-White
RUGBY I 3841	Furosemide	Tablet	40mg	Rugby	Off-White
RUGBY I 3919	Hydrochlorothiazide	Tablet	50mg	Rugby	Peach
RUGBY I 3922	Hydrochlorothiazide	Tablet	25mg	Rugby	Peach
RUGBY I 3986	Meclizine HCl	Tablet	12.5mg	Rugby	White I Bright Blue
RUGBY I 3988	Meclizine HCl	Tablet	25mg	Rugby	White I Bright Yellow
RUGBY 4094	Nystatin	Tablet	500,000 units	Rugby	Dk. Brown
RUGBY I 4324	Prednisone	Tablet	5mg	Rugby	White
RUGBY I 4325	Prednisone	Tablet	10mg	Rugby	White
RUGBY I 4326	Prednisone	Tablet	20mg	Rugby	Peach
RUGBY I 4328	Prednisone	Tablet	50mg	Rugby	White
RUGBY I 4956	Hydrochlorothiazide/ Triamterene	Tablet	50/75mg	Rugby	Yellow
RUGBY I 5663	Cimetidine	Tablet	400mg	Rugby	White
Rugby logo I 3487	Chlordiazepoxide HCl	Capsule	5mg	Rugby	Yellow / Light Green
S I 5	Selegiline HCl	Tablet	5mg	Somerset	White
S I 770	Isosorbide Dinitrate	Tablet	5mg	Zeneca	Green
S I 773	Isosorbide Dinitrate	Tablet	30mg	Zeneca	White
S I 774	Isosorbide Dinitrate	Tablet	40mg	Zeneca	Lt. Blue
S I 780	Isosorbide Dinitrate	Tablet	10mg	Zeneca	Yellow

Imprint	Generic Name	Form	Strength	Manufacturer	Color
S I 820	Isosorbide Dinitrate	Tablet	20mg	Zeneca	Blue
SANDOZ I CAFERGOT	Ergotamine Tartrate/ Caffeine	Tablet	1/100mg	Sandoz	Light Pink
SANDOZ I FIORNAL	Aspirin/Butalbital/Caffeine	Tablet	325/50/40mg	Sandoz	White
Sandoz logo 20 Lescol	Fluvastatin	Capsule	20mg	Sandoz	Cream / Maroon
Sandoz logo 40 Lescol	Fluvastatin	Capsule	40mg	Sandoz	Gold / Maroon
Sandoz logo 78 240	Cyclosporine	Capsule	25mg	Sandoz	Lt. Mauve
Sandoz logo 78 241	Cyclosporine	Capsule	100mg	Sandoz	Dk. Mauve
Sandoz logo I 782	Thioridazine HCl	Tablet	10mg	Sandoz	Lime Green
Sandoz logo FC I SANDOZ 78 107	Aspirin/Butalbital/ Caffeine/Codeine	Capsule	325/50/40/30mg	Sandoz	Blue / Bright Yellow
Sandoz logo FIORCET I Sandoz logo	Acetaminophen/ Butalbital/Caffeine	Tablet	325/50/40mg	Sandoz	Lt. Blue
Sandoz logo FIORCET WITH CODEINE	Acetaminophen/ Butalbital/Caffeine/ Codeine	Capsule	325/50/40/30mg	Sandoz	Blue / Gray
Sandoz logo I HYDERGINE	Ergoloid Mesylates	Tablet	1mg	Sandoz	White
Sandoz logo I MEL 200	Thioridazine HCl	Tablet	200mg	Sandoz	Hot Pink
Sandoz logo I MELLARRIL 50	Thioridazine HCl	Tablet	50mg	Sandoz	WHITE
Sandoz logo I MELLARRILL 25	Thioridazine HCl	Tablet	25mg	Sandoz	Beige
Sandoz logo I PARLODEL 5 mg	Bromocriptine	Capsule	5mg	Sandoz	Rust / White
SANDOZ PAMELOR 10mg	Nortriptyline HCl	Capsule	10mg	Sandoz	Br. Orange / White
SANDOZ PAMELOR 25mg	Nortriptyline HCl	Capsule	25mg	Sandoz	Br. Orange / White
SANDOZ PAMELOR 50mg	Nortriptyline HCl	Capsule	50mg	Sandoz	White w/ black etters
SANDOZ PAMELOR 75mg	Nortriptyline HCl	Capsule	75mg	Sandoz	Br. Orange w/ Black letters
Sandozlogo 2.5 DynaCirc	Isradipine	Capsule	2.5mg	Sandoz	White
Sandozlogo 5 DynaCirc	Isradipine	Capsule	5mg	Sandoz	Lt. Pink
Sanofi logo I D 35	Meperidine HCl	Tablet	50mg	Sanofi Winthrop	White
Sanofi logo I D 37	Meperidine HCl	Tablet	100mg	Sanofi Winthrop	White
Sanofi logo I T 51	Pentazocine/Naloxone	Tablet	0.05/50mg	Sanofi Winthrop	Yellow
Savage logo I KAON-CL	Potassium Chloride	Tablet	750mg	Savage	White
SB TAGAMET 300	Cimetidine	Tablet	300mg	SmithKline Beecham	Lt. Green
SB TAGAMET 400 I SB TAGAMET 400	Cimetidine	Tablet	400mg	SmithKline Beecham	Lt. Green
SB TAGAMET 800 I SB TAGAMET 800	Cimetidine	Tablet	800mg	SmithKline Beecham	Lt. Green
SCHERING 244 I NORMODYNE 100	Labetalol HCl	Tablet	100mg	Schering	Peach
SCHERING 438 I NORMODYNE 300	Labetalol HCl	Tablet	300mg	Schering	Blue
SCHERING 752 I NORMODYNE 200	Labetalol HCl	Tablet	200mg	Schering	White
Schering logo 431	Albuterol	Tablet	4mg	Schering	White
SCHWARZ I 475	Enzymes/ Hyoscyamine Sulfate/ Phenyltoloxamine	Capsule	30/2/0.0625/ 1200/15/6mg	Schwarz	Green/Cream
SCHWARZ I 522	Pancrelipase	Capsule	30/2/1200/6mg	Schwarz	Yellow/Cream

Imprint	Generic Name	Form	Strength	Manufacturer	Color
SKF ORNADE I SKF ORNADE	Chlorpheniramine/ Phenylpropanolamine HCl	Capsule	12/75mg	SmithKline Beecham	Orange / Transparent Clear
SKF S04	Trifluoperazine	Tablet	2mg	SmithKline Beecham	Blue
SKF T74	Chlorpromazine	Tablet	25mg	SmithKline Beecham	Orange
SKF TAGAMET 200	Cimetidine	Tablet	200mg	SmithKline Beecham	Lt. Green
SL I 07	Hydroxyzine HCl	Tablet	10mg	Sidmak	White
SL I 08	Hydroxyzine HCl	Tablet	25mg	Sidmak	White
SL I 309	Hydroxyzine HCl	Tablet	50mg	Sidmak	White
SL 362	Chlorthalidone	Tablet	25mg	Sidmak	Peach
SL 370	Amitriptyline HCl	Tablet	100mg	Sidmak	Red
SL 373	Chlorpropamide	Tablet	250mg	Sidmak	Lt. Blue
SL 441 I 50 100	Trazodone HCl	Tablet	150mg	Sidmak	White
SL 456	Oxybutynin	Tablet	5mg	Sidmak	Pale Blue
SL 467	Propranolol HCl	Tablet	10mg	Sidmak	Peach
SL 468	Propranolol HCl	Tablet	20mg	Sidmak	Light Blue
SL 469	Propranolol HCl	Tablet	40mg	Rugby	Light Green
SL 471	Propranolol HCl	Tablet	80mg	Rugby	Yellow
SL I 66	Amitriptyline HCl	Tablet	10mg	Sidmak	Dark Pink
SL I 67	Amitriptyline HCl	Tablet	25mg	Sidmak	Green
Slow-K	Potassium Chloride	Tablet	600mg	Summit	Beige
SOLVAY 2808	Prednisone	Tablet	1mg	Solvay	Pink
SOLVAY 4205	Fluvoxamine	Tablet	50mg	Solvay	Yellow
SOLVAY 4210	Fluvoxamine	Tablet	100mg	Solvay	Clay (Pinkish Brown)
SOLVAY 7512	Lithium	Capsule	300mg	Solvay	Shrimp Pink
SOLVAY 7516	Lithium	Tablet	300mg	Solvay	White
SP 15 I 715	Moexipril HCl	Tablet	15mg	Schwarz	Clay Pink
SP 538	Hyoscyamine Sulfate	Tablet	0.375mg	Schwarz	Orange
SP 7.5 I 707	Moexipril HCl	Tablet	7.5mg	Schwarz	Clay Pink
SQUIBB 113 I SQUIBB	Cephradine	Capsule	250mg	Bristol-Myers Squibb	Blue / Orange
SQUIBB 114 I SQUIBB 114	Cephradine	Capsule	500mg	Bristol-Myers Squibb	Blue
SQUIBB 154 I10	Pravastatin	Tablet	10mg	Bristol-Myers Squibb	White
SQUIBB 178 I 20	Pravastatin	Tablet	20mg	Bristol-Myers Squibb	White
SQUIBB 181 I SQUIBB 181	Cephalexin HCl	Capsule	250mg	Bristol-Myers Squibb	Green / White
SQUIBB 194 I 40	Pravastatin	Tablet	40mg	Bristol-Myers Squibb	White
SQUIBB 239 I SQUIBB 239	Cephalexin HCl	Capsule	500mg	Bristol-Myers Squibb	Green / Lt. Green
SQUIBB 580	Nystatin	Tablet	500,000 units	Bristol-Myers Squibb	Brown
SQUIBB 603	Tetracycline HCl	Tablet	500mg	Bristol-Myers Squibb	Hot Pink
SQUIBB 655	Tetracycline HCl	Capsule	250mg	Bristol-Myers Squibb	Fuschia
SQUIBB 663	Tetracycline HCl	Tablet	250mg	Bristol-Myers Squibb	Pink
SQUIBB 763	Tetracycline HCl	Capsule	500mg	Bristol-Myers Squibb	Fuschia/White
STUART 142 I ZESTORETIC	Hydrochlorothiazide/ Lisinopril	Tablet	12.5/20mg	Stuart	White
STUART 145 I ZESTORETIC	Hydrochlorothiazide/ Lisinopril	Tablet	20/25mg	Stuart	Pale Peach
STUART 40 I ELAVIL	Amitriptyline HCl	Tablet	10mg	Stuart	Lt. Blue
STUART 41 I ELAVIL	Amitriptyline HCl	Tablet	50mg	Stuart	Lt. Brown
STUART 42 I ELAVIL	Amitriptyline HCl	Tablet	75mg	Stuart	Lt. Orange
STUART 43 I ELAVIL	Amitriptyline HCl	Tablet	100mg	Stuart	Pink
STUART 45 I ELAVIL	Amitriptyline HCl	Tablet	25mg	Stuart	Dk. Yellow
STUART 47 I ELAVIL	Amitriptyline HCl	Tablet	150mg	Stuart	Lt. Blue

SCHWARZ I 525	Pancrelipase	Capsule	30/80/30 in thousands of units of amylase, lipase, protease	Schwarz	Cream
SCHWARZ I 532	Hyoscyamine Sulfate	Tablet	0.125mg	Schwarz	Mint Blue
SCHWARZ 610 I 10	Isosorbide Mononitrate	Tablet	10mg	Schwarz	White
SCHWARZ 620 I 20	Isosorbide Mononitrate	Tablet	20mg	Schwarz	White
SEARLE 1001 I ALDACTONE 25	Spironolactone	Tablet	25mg	Searle	Yellow
SEARLE 1011 I ALDACTAZIDE 25	Spironolactone/ Hydrochlorothiazide	Tablet	25/25mg	Searle	Beige
SEARLE 1021 I ALDACTAZIDE 50	Spironolactone/ Hydrochlorothiazide	Tablet	50/50mg	Searle	Beige
SEARLE 1031 I ALDACTONE 100	Spironolactone	Tablet	100mg	Searle	Peach
SEARLE 1041 I ALDACTONE 50	Spironolactone	Tablet	50mg	Searle	Peach
SEARLE I 1451	Misoprostol	Tablet	0.1mg	Searle	White
SEARLE 1461 I Searle logo	Misoprostol	Tablet	0.2mg	Searle	White
Searlel151 ; Searlel P	Ethinyl Estradiol/ Ethynodiol Diacetate	Tablet	Inert; 0.035/1mg	Searle	White ; Blue
SEARLE 1831 I FLAGYL 250	Metronidazole	Tablet	250mg	Searle	Blue
SEARLE 2732 I NORPACE 100mg	Disopyramide	Capsule	100mg	Searle	Brown / Orange
SEARLE 2762 I SEARLE 2762	Disopyramide	Capsule	150mg	Searle	Orange
SEARLE I 61	Diphenoxylate HCl/ Atropine	Tablet	2.5/0.025mg	Searle	White
SELDANE	Terfenadine	Tablet	60mg	Hoechst Marion Roussel	White
SELDANE D	Pseudoephedrine HCl/T erfenadine	Tablet	120/60mg	Hoechst Marion Roussel	White
SEPTRA DS 02C	Sulfamethoxazole/ Trimethoprim	Tablet	800/160mg	Glaxo Wellcome	Pink
SEPTRA Y2B	Sulfamethoxazole/ Trimethoprim	Tablet	400/80mg	Glaxo Wellcome	Pink
SGPI1/50 / SGP	Mestranol/Norethindrone	Tablet	Inert; 0.05/1mg	Rugby	White / Peach
SGP / SGP I 0.5/35	Ethinyl Estradiol/ Norethindrone	Tablet	Inert; 0.035/.5	Rugby	Pale Peach / White
SGP / SGP I 1/35	Ethinyl Estradiol/ Norethindrone	Tablet	Inert; 0.035/1	Rugby	Peach / Pale Blue
SINEMET I 647	Carbidopa/Levodopa	Tablet	10/100mg	DuPont	Lt. Blue
SINEMET I 650	Carbidopa/Levodopa	Tablet	25/100mg	DuPont	Yellow
SINEMET I 654	Carbidopa/Levodopa	Tablet	50/200mg	DuPont	Lt. Blue
SINEMET CR I 521	Carbidopa/Levodopa	Tablet	25/250mg	DuPont	Lt. Peach
SKB logo 3346 I 15 mg Black/Transparent	Prochlorperazine	Capsule	15mg	SmithKline Beecham	
SKF C44	Prochlorperazine	Capsule	10mg	SmithKline Beecham	Black/ Transparent
SKF C66	Prochlorperazine	Tablet	5mg	SmithKline Beecham	Yellow
SKF C67	Prochlorperazine	Tablet	10mg	SmithKline Beecham	Yellow
SKF C69	Prochlorperazine	Tablet	25mg	SmithKline Beecham	Yellow-Green
SKF E33 I SKF E33	Phenoxybenzamine HCl	Capsule	10mg	SmithKline Beecham	Red
SKF ESKALITH SKF ESKALITH	Lithium	Capsule	300mg	SmithKline Beecham	Gray / Br. Yellow
SKF J10	Lithium	Tablet	450mg	SmithKline Beecham	Pale Yellow

SYNTEX 2437 CARDENE 20mg	Nicardipine HCl	Capsule	20mg	Syntex	White w/ pink letters, Blue stripe
SYNTEX 2438 CARDENE 30mg	Nicardipine HCl	Capsule	30mg	Syntex	Dk. Blue; Lt. Blue
SYNTEX 2440 CARDENE SR 30mg	Nicardipine HCl	Capsule	30mg	Syntex	Clay
SYNTEX 2441 CARDENE SR 45mg	Nicardipine HCl	Capsule	45mg	Syntex	Lt. Blue
SYNTEX 2442 CARDENE SR 60mg	Nicardipine HCl	Capsule	60mg	Syntex	Blue/White
SYNTEX I 274	Naproxen Sodium	Tablet	275mg	Syntex	Lt. Blue
SYNTEX I ANAPROX 06	Naproxen Sodium	Tablet	550mg	Syntex	Blue
SYNTEX I NAPROSYN 250	Naproxen	Tablet	250mg	Syntex	Beige
SYNTEX I TORADOL	Ketorolac	Tablet	10mg	Syntex	White; Red Letters
T	Benzonatate	Tablet	100mg	Forest	Transparent Yellow
T I 107	Atenolol	Tablet	25mg	Zeneca	White
T 109	Carbamazepine	Tablet	200mg	Teva	White
Tap logo I PREVACID 15	Lansoprazole	Capsule	15mg	Tap Pharm	Pink/Green
Tap logo I PREVACID 30	Lansoprazole	Capsule	30mg	Tap Pharm	Pink/Black
TAVIST 1 I TAVIST 1	Clemastine	Tablet	1.34mg	Sandoz	White
TAVIST I 7872	Clemastine	Tablet	2.68mg	Sandoz	White
TCL 1221	Nitroglycerin	Capsule	2.5mg	Time Caps	Purple / clear
TCL 1222	Nitroglycerin	Capsule	6.5mg	Time Caps	Gold (clear) / Black
TEGRETOL I 27 27	Carbamazepine	Tablet	200mg	Basel	Pink
TEGRETOL I 52 52	Carbamazepine	Tablet	100mg	Basel	White w/ red specks
TENORETIC I 115	Atenolol/Chlorthalidone	Tablet	50/25mg	Zeneca	White
TENORETIC I 117	Atenolol/Chlorthalidone	Tablet	100/25mg	Zeneca	White
TENORMIN I 101	Atenolol	Tablet	100mg	Zeneca	White
TENORMIN I 105	Atenolol	Tablet	50mg	Zeneca	White
TENUATE 75	Diethylpropion	Tablet	75mg	Hoechst Marion Roussel	White
THEODUR 100	Theophylline	Tablet	100mg	Schering	White
THEODUR 200	Theophylline	Tablet	200mg	Schering	White
THEODUR 300	Theophylline	Tablet	300mg	Schering	White
THEODUR 450	Theophylline	Tablet	450mg	Schering	White
THIS END UP I DEPAKOTE SPRINKLE 125mg	Divalproex	Capsule	125mg	Abbott	Lt. Blue / White
TICLID I 250	Ticlopidine HCl	Tablet	250mg	Syntex	White
TIGAN 100mg	Trimethobenzamide HCl	Capsule	100mg	SmithKline Beecham	Blue / White
TIGAN 250mg	Trimethobenzamide HCl	Capsule	250mg	SmithKline Beecham	Blue
TOLINASE 100	Tolazamide	Tablet	100mg	Upjohn	White
TOLINASE 250	Tolazamide	Tablet	250mg	Upjohn	White
TONOCARD I 709	Tocainide HCl	Tablet	600mg	Merck	Yellow
TOP I 25	Topiramate	Tablet	25mg	McNeil	White
TOPAMAX I 100	Topiramate	Tablet	100mg	McNeil	Yellow
TOPAMAX I 200	Topiramate	Tablet	200mg	McNeil	Salmon
TRANDATE 200	Labetalol HCl	Tablet	200mg	Glaxo Wellcome	White
TRINALIN 703	Azatadine/ Pseudoephedrine	Tablet	1/120mg	Schering	Dk. Orange
U 3617	Cefpodoxime	Tablet	100mg	Upjohn	Orange
U 3618	Cefpodoxime	Tablet	200mg	Upjohn	Dk. Orange
U 3772 I U 3772	Estropipate	Tablet	0.625mg	Upjohn	Yellow
U 3773 I U 3773	Estropipate	Tablet	1.25mg	Upjohn	Orange

Imprint	Generic Name	Form	Strength	Manufacturer	Color
U 3774 I U 3774	Estropipate	Tablet	2.5mg	Upjohn	Blue
U 400 I PF	Theophylline	Tablet	400mg	Purdue Frederick	White
UAD I 6350	Acetaminophen/ Hydrocodone	Tablet	650/10mg	Forest	Lt. Blue
URISPAS SKF	Flavoxate HCl	Tablet	100mg	SmithKline Beecham	White
USV I 21	Chlorthalidone	Tablet	100mg	Rhone-Poulenc Rorer	White
USV I R31	Reserpine/Chlorthalidone	Tablet	0.25/50mg	Rhone-Poulenc Rorer	Pink
USV I R32	Reserpine/Chlorthalidone	Tablet	0.125/25mg	Rhone-Poulenc Rorer	White
UU I 201	Acetaminophen/ Hydrocodone	Tablet	650/7.5mg	Forest	White
V 2064 I 3	Acetaminophen/Codeine	Tablet	300/30mg	Vintage	White
V 5013	Phenobarbital	Tablet	60mg	Vintage	White
VALIUM 10	Diazepam	Tablet	10mg	Roche	Lt. Blue
VALIUM 2	Diazepam	Tablet	2mg	Roche	White
VALIUM 5	Diazepam	Tablet	5mg	Roche	Yellow
VALTREX 500 mg	Valacyclovir HCl	Capsule	500mg	Glaxo Wellcome	Blue
VASCOR 300	Bepridil HCl	Tablet	300mg	McNeil	Lt. Blue
VASCOR 400	Bepridil HCl	Tablet	400mg	McNeil	Lt. Blue
VICODIN	Acetaminophen/ Hydrocodone	Tablet	500/5mg	Knoll	White
VICODIN ES	Acetaminophen/ Hydrocodone	Tablet	750/7.5mg	Knoll	White
VIDEX BL I 100	Didanosine	Tablet	100mg	Bristol-Myers Squibb	White
VIDEX BL I 150	Didanosine	Tablet	150mg	Bristol-Myers Squibb	White
VISKEN 10 I V	Pindolol	Tablet	10mg	Sandoz	Off-White
VISKEN 5 I V	Pindolol	Tablet	5mg	Sandoz	White
VISTARIL I 541	Hydroxyzine HCl	Capsule	25mg	Pfizer	Dk. Green / Lt. Green
VISTARIL I 542	Hydroxyzine HCl	Capsule	50mg	Pfizer	White / Dk. Green
VOLTAREN	Diclofenac Sodium	Tablet	25mg	Novartis	Dk. Yellow
VOLTAREN 50	Diclofenac Sodium	Tablet	50mg	Novartis	Dk. Peach
VOLTAREN 75	Diclofenac Sodium	Tablet	75mg	Novartis	Lt. Pink
W 100 I 705	Venlafaxine HCl	Tablet	100mg	Wyeth-Ayerst	Peach
W 25 I 701	Venlafaxine HCl	Tablet	25mg	Wyeth-Ayerst	Peach
W 37.5 I 781	Venlafaxine HCl	Tablet	37.5mg	Wyeth-Ayerst	Peach
W 50 I 703	Venlafaxine HCl	Tablet	50mg	Wyeth-Ayerst	Peach
WI641 ; WI642 ; W643 ; WI650	Ethinyl Estradiol/ Levonorgestrel	Tablet	Inert; 0.03/0.05; 0.03/0.125; 0.04/0.075mg	Wyeth-Ayerst	Clay Pink ; White ; Gold ; Green
W 75 I 704	Venlafaxine HCl	Tablet	75mg	Wyeth-Ayerst	Peach
WALLACE I 0430	Felbamate	Tablet	400mg	Carter-Wallace	Yellow
WALLACE I 0431	Felbamate	Tablet	600mg	Carter-Wallace	Peach
WALLACE 2103 I SOMA C	Aspirin/Carisoprodol	Tablet	325/200mg	Wallace	White / Peach
WALLACE 2403 I SOMA CC	Aspirin/Carisoprodol/ Codeine	Tablet	325/200/16mg	Wallace	White / Yellow
WALLACE 37-2001 I SOMA	Carisoprodol	Tablet	350mg	Wallace	White
WALLACE 521	Dyphylline	Tablet	200mg	Carter-Wallace	White
WALLACE 713	Phenylephrine Tannate/ Chlorpheniramine Tannate/Pyrilamine Tannate	Tablet	25/8/25mg	Wallace	Oat (Creamy Brown)
WALLACE 731	Dyphylline	Tablet	400mg	Carter-Wallace	White
WATSON 302	Furosemide	Tablet	80mg	Watson	White
WATSON 308	Propranolol HCl	Tablet	80mg	Watson	Pale Yellow
WATSON 365 I 15	Clorazepate	Tablet	15mg	Watson	Pink

Imprint	Generic Name	Form	Strength	Manufacturer	Color
WHITBY I 6 12	Guaifenesin/ Pseudoephedrine HCl	Tablet	600/60mg	Whitby	White
WHITBY I 902	Acetaminophen/ Hydrocodone	Tablet	500/5mg	Whitby	White w/ blue specks
WHITBY I 903	Acetaminophen/ Hydrocodone	Tablet	500/7.5mg	Whitby	White w/ green specks
WHR 50mg	Theophylline	Capsule	50mg	Rhone-Poulenc Rorer	White w/ red letters
WINTHROP I T37	Acetaminophen/ Pentazocine	Tablet	650/25mg	Sanofi Winthrop	Lt. Blue
WPPH 157	Indomethacin	Capsule	75mg	West Point	Lt. Blue/Clear
WPPH I 174	Methyldopa	Tablet	125mg	West Point	Gold
WPPH I 176	Methyldopa	Tablet	500mg	West Point	Gold
WYETH 179 I SECTRAL 400	Acebutolol HCl	Capsule	400mg	Wyeth-Ayerst	Brown/Orange
WYETH I 19	Promethazine HCl	Tablet	12.5mg	Wyeth-Ayerst	Light Orange
WYETH I 227	Promethazine HCl	Tablet	50mg	Wyeth-Ayerst	Pale Pink
WYETH 27	Promethazine HCl	Tablet	25mg	Wyeth-Ayerst	White
WYETH 4133	Trimipramine	Capsule	50mg	Wyeth-Ayerst	Blue / Orange
WYETH I 4152	Isosorbide Dinitrate	Tablet	5mg	Wyeth-Ayerst	Lt. Pink
WYETH I 4153	Isosorbide Dinitrate	Tablet	10mg	Wyeth-Ayerst	White
WYETH I 4154	Isosorbide Dinitrate	Tablet	20mg	Wyeth-Ayerst	Green
WYETH 4158	Trimipramine	Capsule	100mg	Wyeth-Ayerst	Blue / White
WYETH 4177 I SECTRAL 200	Acebutolol HCl	Capsule	200mg	Wyeth-Ayerst	Periwinkle / Orange
WYETH 4181 ORUDIS 50	Ketoprofen	Capsule	50mg	Wyeth-Ayerst	Dk. Green/Lt. Green
WYETH 4187 ORUDIS 75	Ketoprofen	Capsule	75mg	Wyeth-Ayerst	Dk. Green/ White
WYETH 4188 I C 200	Amiodarone	Tablet	200mg	Wyeth-Ayerst	Pink
WYETH I 4191	Aspirin/Caffeine/ Dihydrocodeine	Capsule	356.4/30/16mg	Wyeth-Ayerst	Bright Blue / Lt. Gray
WyethI445 ; WyethI56	Ethinyl Estradiol/ Norgestrel	Tablet	Inert; 0.5/0.05	Wyeth-Ayerst	Pink ; White
Wyeth I 486 I Wyeth I 75	Ethinyl Estradiol/ Levonorgestrel	Tablet	Inert; 0.03/ 0.15mg	Wyeth-Ayerst	Pink / Orange
Wyeth I 486 Wyeth I 78	Ethinyl Estradiol/ Norgestrel	Tablet	Inert; 0.3/0.03	Wyeth-Ayerst	Pink / White
WYETH I 559	Amoxicillin	Capsule	250mg	Wyeth-Ayerst	Gray / Lt. Green
WYETH I 560	Amoxicillin	Capsule	500mg	Wyeth-Ayerst	Gray / Lt. Green
WYETH 64	Lorazepam	Tablet	1mg	Wyeth-Ayerst	White
WYETH 65 I 2	Lorazepam	Tablet	2mg	Wyeth-Ayerst	White
WYETH 73 I W	Guanabenz	Tablet	4mg	Wyeth-Ayerst	Peach
WYETH 74 I W 8	Guanabenz	Tablet	8mg	Wyeth-Ayerst	Grayish Purple
WYETH 81	Lorazepam	Tablet	0.5mg	Wyeth-Ayerst	White
WYETH I 85	Acetaminophen/ Propoxyphene HCl	Tablet	650/65mg	Wyeth-Ayerst	Green
Wyeth Logo I MYSOLINE 250	Primidone	Tablet	250mg	Wyeth-Ayerst	Beige
WYETH-51 SERAX 10	Oxazepam	Capsule	10mg	Wyeth-Ayerst	Pink / White
WYETH-6 SERAX 15	Oxazepam	Capsule	15mg	Wyeth-Ayerst	Red / White
XANAX 0.25	Alprazolam	Tablet	0.25mg	Upjohn	White
XANAX 0.5	Alprazolam	Tablet	0.5mg	Upjohn	Peach
XANAX 1.0	Alprazolam	Tablet	1mg	Upjohn	Light Blue
XANAX 2	Alprazolam	Tablet	2mg	Upjohn	White
Z 2978	Tolazamide	Tablet	100mg	Zenith	White

WATSON 387	Acetaminophen/ Hydrocodone	Tablet	750/7.5mg	Watson	White
WC I 084	Gemfibrozil	Tablet	600mg	Warner-Chilcott	White w/ blue letters
WC 242	Carbamazepine	Tablet	100mg	Warner-Chilcott	Pink Speckled
WC 698	Phenobarbital	Tablet	100mg	Warner-Chilcott	White
WC 730 I WC 730	Amoxicillin	Capsule	250mg	Warner-Chilcott	Dk. Pink / Lt. Pink
WC 731 I WC 731	Amoxicillin	Capsule	500mg	Warner-Chilcott	Dk. Pink / Lt. Pink
WD 04 I DANOCRINE 100mg	Danazol	Capsule	100mg	Sanofi Winthrop	Dk. Yellow
WD 05 I DANOCRINE 200mg	Danazol	Capsule	200mg	Sanofi Winthrop	Dk. Orange
WELLBUTRIN 100	Bupropion HCl	Tablet	100mg	Glaxo Wellcome	Dark Burgandy
WELLBUTRIN 75	Bupropion HCl	Tablet	75mg	Glaxo Wellcome	Dk. Yellow
Wellcome logo I SEMPREX D	Acrivastine/ Pseudoephedrine HCl	Capsule	8/60mg	Glaxo Wellcome	Green / White
Wellcome logo I ZOVIRAX 200	Acyclovir	Capsule	200mg	Glaxo Wellcome	Medium Blue
WELLCOME P 7 F	Atovaquone	Tablet	250mg	Glaxo Wellcome	Lt. Yellow
WESTWARD FLURAZEPAM 15	Flurazepam HCl	Capsule	15mg	Westward	White / Blue
WESTWARD FLURAZEPAM 30	Flurazepam HCl	Capsule	30mg	Westward	Blue
WHITBY 2842 THEO-24 200mg	Theophylline	Capsule	200mg	Whitby	Orange / Clear
WHITBY 2852 THEO-24 300mg	Theophylline	Capsule	300mg	Whitby	Red / Clear
Z 2999	Chlorthalidone	Tablet	50mg	Zenith	Lt. Green
Z 3926 I 5	Diazepam	Tablet	5mg	Zenith	Yellow
Z4280 I SR 240	Verapamil HCl	Tablet	240mg	Zenith	White
ZANTAC 150 I 427	Ranitidine HCl	Tablet	150mg	Glaxo Wellcome	Beige
ZAROXOLYN I 21/2	Metolazone	Tablet	2.5mg	Fisons	Purple
ZENECA 10 I 891	Nisoldipine	Tablet	10mg	Zeneca	Oyster
ZENECA 20 I 892	Nisoldipine	Tablet	20mg	Zeneca	Yellow Cream
ZENECA 30 I 893	Nisoldipine	Tablet	30mg	Zeneca	Mustard
ZENECA 40 I 894	Nisoldipine	Tablet	40mg	Zeneca	Burnt Orange
Zeneca logo I 853	Isosorbide Dinitrate	Tablet	2.5mg	Zeneca	White
ZENITH 50mg 2130	Nitrofurantoin	Capsule	50mg	Zenith	Lt. Pink / White
ZESTORETIC I 141	Hydrochlorothiazide/ Lisinopril	Tablet	12.5/10mg	Zeneca	Light Peach
ZESTORETIC I 142	Hydrochlorothiazide/ Lisinopril	Tablet	12.5/20mg	Zeneca	White
ZESTORETIC I 145	Hydrochlorothiazide/ Lisinopril	Tablet	25/20mg	Zeneca	Light Peach
ZESTRIL 10 I 131	Lisinopril	Tablet	10mg	Stuart	Pale Pink
ZESTRIL I 130	Lisinopril	Tablet	5mg	Stuart	Lt. Clay Pink
ZESTRIL 2 1/2 I 135	Lisinopril	Tablet	2.5mg	Zeneca	White
ZESTRIL 20 I 132	Lisinopril	Tablet	20mg	Stuart	Clay Pink
ZESTRIL 40 I 134	Lisinopril	Tablet	40mg	Stuart	Lt. Yellow
ZOLOFT I 100 mg	Sertraline HCl	Tablet	100mg	Roerig	Pale Yellow
ZOLOFT I 50 mg	Sertraline HCl	Tablet	50mg	Roerig	Pale Blue
ZOVIRAX 800	Acyclovir	Tablet	800mg	Glaxo Wellcome	Lt. Blue
ZOVIRAX I Triangle	Acyclovir	Tablet	400mg	Glaxo Wellcome	White
ZYLOPRIM 100	Allopurinol	Tablet	100mg	Glaxo Wellcome	White
ZYLOPRIM 300	Allopurinol	Tablet	300mg	Glaxo Wellcome	Dk. Peach

COMPARATIVE TABLES

The following comparative drug tables were developed by practicing physicians to assist providers in choosing medications of a given therapeutic class. These tables allow clinicians to compare drugs on the basis of important pharmacologic or clinical characteristics. Whenever possible, the information is based on definitive drug data and should help the reader obtain maximal therapeutic effect with minimal adverse effects. When applicable, accepted clinical practice guide lines have been incorporated into the tables.

Analgesics

NONNARCOTIC ANALGESICS

Generic drug name	*Brand name*	*Usual adult dose (mg)*	*Maximum adult daily dose (mg)*	*Oral dose forms (mg)*	*Nonprescription strength (mg)*	*Chemical class*	*Comment*
Acetaminophen	Tylenol	325-650 q4-6h	4000	80, 160, 325, 500, 650	All forms	Aminophenol	Hepatotoxicity if overdosed and in persons with cirrhosis (limit dose to 2000 mg/d in cirrhotics)
SALICYLATES							
Acetylsalicylic acid	Aspirin	325-975 q4h	6000	81, 165, 325, 500, 650, 975	All forms	Salicylate	Antagonizes effect of probenecid; increases effect of sulfonylureas; reduces renal clearance of methotrexate
Choline magnesium trisalicylate	Trilisate	500-1000 q12h	3000	500, 750, 1000	NA	Salicylate	Antagonizes effect of probenecid; increases effect of sulfonylureas; reduces renal clearance of methotrexate
Salsalate	Disalcid	500-1000 q8h 750-1500 q12h	3000	500, 750, 1000	NA	Salicylate	Antagonizes effect of probenecid; increases effect of sulfonylureas; reduces renal clearance of methotrexate
SHORT-ACTING NSAIDS							
Diclofenac	Cataflam	50 tid	200	25, 50	NA	Acetic acid	Formulation is immediate release
Diclofenac	Voltaren	25-75 bid-tid	200	25, 50, 75	NA	Acetic acid	Formulation is delayed release; also available in qd dose form
Fenoprofen	Nalfon	300-600 q6h	3200	200, 300, 600	NA	Propionic acid	Highly protein bound (to albumin); greater renal toxicity
Ibuprofen	Motrin, Rufen	400-600 q6h	3200	200, 300, 400, 600, 800	200	Propionic acid	Also approved for primary dysmenorrhea
Indomethacin	Indocin, Indocin SR	25-50 q8h or 75 q12h (sustained release)	200	25, 50, 75 (sustained release)	NA	Acetic acid	Available in suppository, suspension, and sustained-release forms
Ketoprofen	Orudis Oruvail	50-75 q6-8h	300	12.5, 25, 50, 75; 100, 150 200 (sustained release)	12.5	Propionic acid	High rate of dyspepsia (11%), available in sustained-release form
Ketorolac	Toradol	10 q4-6h	40	10	NA	Acetic acid	100% bioavailable; indicated only as continuation of parenteral ketorolac, short term
Meclofenamate	Meclomen	50-100 q6h	400	50, 100	NA	Anthranilic acid	High rate of diarrhea (10%-33%)
Mefenamic acid	Ponstel	500, then 250 q6h	1000	250	NA	Anthranilic acid	Also approved for primary dysmenorrhea
Tolmetin	Tolectin	400 q6-8h	2000	200, 400, 600	NA	Acetic acid	High rate of nausea (11%)
INTERMEDIATE-ACTING NSAIDS							
Diflunisal	Dolobid	500 q12h	1500	250, 500	NA	Salicylate derivative	Not metabolized to salicylate; increases acetaminophen level by 50% when coadministered
Etodolac	Lodine	200-400 bid-qid	1200	200, 300	NA	Acetic acid	Antacids reduce peak concentration by 20%
Flurbiprofen	Ansaid	50-100 bid-tid	300	50, 100	NA	Phenylalkanoic acid	May cause CNS stimulation

Continued

NONNARCOTIC ANALGESICS—CONT'D

Generic drug name	Brand name	Usual adult dose (mg)	Maximum adult daily dose (mg)	Oral dose forms (mg)	Nonprescription strength (mg)	Chemical class	Comment
INTERMEDIATE-ACTING NSAIDS—CONT'D							
Naproxen	Naprosyn, Napralan	250-500 q8-12h	1250	220, 250, 375, 500	220	Propionic acid	Approved for acute gout; may increase effect of protein-bound drugs such as phenytoin, sulfonylureas, and warfarin; available in qd dose form
Naproxen	Anaprox, Anaprox, DS	275-550 q8-12h	1375	275, 550	220	Propionic acid	Approved for acute gout; may increase effect of protein-bound drugs such as phenytoin, sulfonylureas, and warfarin
Sulindac	Clinoril	150-200 q12h	400	150, 200	NA	Acetic acid	Approved for acute gout; less renal toxicity
LONG-ACTING NSAIDS							
Nabumetone	Relafen	500-750 bid; 1000-1500 qd	1500	500, 750	NA	Nonacidic	High rate of diarrhea (14%); metabolized to active agent
Piroxicam	Feldene	10-20 qd	20	10, 20	NA	Oxicam	High rate of dyspepsia (20%); may increase effect of protein-bound drugs such as phenytoin, sulfonylureas, and warfarin
Oxaprozin	Daypro	1200 qd	1800	600	NA	Proprionic acid	
PARENTERAL NSAID							
Ketorolac	Toradol	30 or 60 initially, then 15-30 q6h (all IM)	150 1st day, then 120 qd	15, 30, 60	NA	Acetic acid	Total duration of treatment should not exceed 5 days; 30 mg equal to 6-12 mg morphine sulfate but 10 times as expensive

NARCOTIC AND NARCOTIC-LIKE ANALGESICS

Generic drug name	Brand name	Usual adult dose (mg) and routes	Parenteral dose (mg) equal to 10 mg morphine sulfate IM	Oral dose (mg) equal to listed parenteral dose	Comment
NARCOTIC-LIKE AGENTS					
Buprenorphine	Buprenex	0.3 q6h IM	0.3	NA	Mixed agonist-antagonist; schedule V controlled substance
Butorphanol	Stadol	1-4 q3-4h IM, Nasal	2-3	NA	Mixed agonist-antagonist; not a controlled substance
Nalbuphine	Nubain	10 q6h IM, IV, or SC	10	NA	Mixed agonist-antagonist; not a controlled substance
Tramadol	Ultram	50-100 q4-6h PO	NA	NA	100 mg equialagesic to 60 mg codeine; long term use may cause dependence and withdrawal syndromes; toxicity includes seizures
NARCOTICS					
Fentanyl	Sublimaze, Duragesic (transdermal)	0.05-0.1 q1-2h IM or IV; 25-100 mcg/h transdermal (base dose on total morphine dose); 0.2-0.4 as lozenge	0.125	NA	Primary use is IV or epidural for perioperative or patient-controlled analgesia; transdermal form available but costly
Oxymorphone	Numorphan	1-1.5 q4-6h IM; 5 q4-6h PR	1	NA	Major use is perioperative
Hydromorphone	Dilaudid	2 q4-6h PO; 1-2 q4-6h IM; 3 q6-8h PR	1.5	7.5	High abuse potential
Levorphanol	Levo-Dromoran	2 q6-8h PO	NA	4	Long acting
Methadone	Dolophine	5-10 q4-6h PO	NA	20	Different $t_{1/2}$ for analgesia and prevention of opiate withdrawal
Morphine sulfate	Roxanol	5-20 q4h IM; 5-20 q6h PR; 10 q4h SL; 10-30 mg q4h PO	10	60 (single dose)	Oral bioavailability poor; sublingual form useful for breakthrough pain
Morphine, sustained release	MS Contin	15-60 q6-12h PO	NA	30 (repeated doses)	Not appropriate for prn use
Oxycodone	Percocet, Percodan, Tylox, Oxycontin	5-10 q4-6h PO	NA	25	Often combined with aspirin (Percodan) or acetaminophen (Percocet, Tylox); available in long-acting form (Oxycontin)
Hydrocodone	Vicodin	5-10 q4-6h PO	NA	30	Only available combined with acetaminophen or aspirin

Continued

NARCOTIC AND NARCOTIC-LIKE ANALGESICS—CONT'D

Generic drug name	*Brand name*	*Usual adult dose (mg) and routes*	*Parenteral dose (mg) equal to 10 mg morphine sulfate IM*	*Oral dose (mg) equal to listed parenteral dose*	*Comment*
NARCOTICS—CONT'D					
Pentazocine	Talwin	30-60 q3-4h IM; 50-100 q4h PO	45	135	Mixed narcotic agonist-antagonist
Meperidine	Demerol	50-125 q3-4h IM; 50-100 q4h PO	75	250	May be used IV; metabolite normeperidine may accumulate with prolonged use causing excitation or seizures
Codeine	Codeine	15-60 q4h PO	130	200	Schedule II unless combined with acetaminophen or aspirin; used as cough suppressant
Propoxyphene	Darvon	32-100 q4h PO	180	360	Less abuse potential than codeine at usual doses

Antibiotics

CEPHALOSPORIN ANTIBIOTICS

Generic drug name (generation in parentheses)	*Brand name*	*Usual adult dose (g)*	*Adjust dose for Renal insufficiency*	*Comment*
ORAL				
Cefadroxil (1)	Duricef	0.5-1.0 q12-24h	Y	
Cephalexin (1)	Keflex	0.25-0.5 q6h	Y	Cheapest in its therapeutic class
Cephradine (1)	Velosef	0.5 q6h	Y	
Cefaclor (2)	Ceclor	0.25-0.5 q8h	N	
Cefpodoxime proxetil (2)	Vantin	0.1-0.4 q12h	Y	
Cefprozil (2)	Cefzil	0.25-0.5 q12h	Y	
Cefuroxime axetil (2)	Ceftin	0.25-0.5 q12h	Y	
Ceftibuten (2)	Cedax	0.4 q24h	Y	
Cefixime (3)	Suprax	0.4 q24h	Y	Single dose therapy for gonococcal genital and pharyngeal infections
PARENTERAL (IV/IM)				
Cefazolin (1)	Ancef, Kefzol	1-2 q6-8h	Y	
Cephalothin (1)	Keflin	1-2 q4-6h	Y	
Cephapirin (1)	Cefadyl	1 q4-6h	Y	
Cefamandole (2)	Mandol	0.5-1.0 q4-8h	Y	
Cefmetazole (2)	Zefazone	2 q6-12h	Y	
Cefonicid (2)	Monocid	1-2 q24h	Y	May be useful in outpatient therapy of endocarditis
Ceforanide (2)	Precef	0.5-1.0 q12h	Y	
Cefotetan (2)	Cefotan	1-2 q12h	Y	Covers GI anaerobes
Cefoxitin (2)	Mefoxin	1-2 q4-6h	Y	Covers GI anaerobes
Cefuroxime (2)	Zinacef	0.75-1.5 q8h	Y	Crosses blood-brain barrier
Cefepime (3)	Maxipime	0.5-2.0 q12h	Y	
Cefoperazone (3)	Cefobid	1-2 q8-12h	N	
Cefotaxime (3)	Claforan	1-2 q4-6h	Y	Crosses blood-brain barrier
Ceftazidine (3)	Fortaz	1-2 q6-8h	Y	
Ceftizoxime (3)	Cefizox	1-2 q6-8h	Y	Crosses blood-brain barrier
Ceftriaxone (3)	Rocephin	1-2 q12-24h	N	May be useful in outpatient therapy of endocarditis; single-dose (250 mg IM) therapy for gonococcal genital and pharyngeal infections; crosses blood-brain barrier

MACROLIDE ANTIBIOTICS

Generic drug name	*Trade name*	*Usual adult dose (mg)*	*Comment*
Azithromycin	Zithromax	500, followed by 250 q24h	Single dose therapy for chlamydial urethritis or cervicitis (1000 mg); antibacterial spectrum includes *Hemophilus influenzae;* indicated to prevent *Mycobacterium avium-intracellulare* infection (1200 mg qwk)
Clarithromycin	Biaxin	250-500 q12h	Antibacterial spectrum includes *H. influenzae;* used to treat *Helicobacter pylori* and to prevent *Mycobacterium avium-intracellulare* infection
Dirithromycin	Dynabac	500 q24h	Antibacterial spectrum includes *H. influenzae*
Erythromycin	Erythromycin	250-500 q6-12h	Available as combination product with sulfisoxazole (extends spectrum to include *H. influenzae*); coating does not decrease GI side effects

PENICILLIN ANTIBIOTICS

Generic drug name	Brand name	Usual adult dose (g)	Comment
ORAL			
Penicillin V	Penicillin VK	0.25-0.5 q6h	
Broad Spectrum Penicillins			
Amoxicillin	Amoxicillin	0.25-0.5 q8h	
Amoxicillin-Clavulanate	Augmentin	One tablet (0.25 or 0.5 amoxicillin/0.125 clavulanate) q8h, or one tablet (0.875 mg amoxicillin/0.125 clavulanate) q12h	Spectrum extended to include beta-lactamase producers such as *Hemophilus influenza, Moraxella catarrhalis, Staphylococcus aureus* (except MRSA), and *Escherichia coli*
Ampicillin	Ampicillin	0.5-1.0 q6h	
Bacampicillin	Spectrobid	0.4-0.8 q12h	Gives higher and more sustained serum levels of ampicillin
Penicillinase Resistant Penicillins			
Cloxacillin	Tegopen	0.25-0.5 q6h	Oral penicillin of choice for *S. aureus* (except MRSA)
Dicloxacillin	Dycill	0.25-0.5 q6h	Oral penicillin of choice for *S. aureus* (except MRSA)
PARENTERAL (IV)			
Penicillin G	Penicillin	1-3 million U q4-6h	Procaine and benzathine forms available for IM use
Broad Spectrum Penicillins			
Ampicillin	Ampicillin	1-2 q4-6h	
Ampicillin-Sulbactam	Unasyn	1-2/0.5-1.0 q6h	Spectrum extended to include beta-lactamase producers such as *H. influenza, M. catarrhalis, S. aureus* (except MRSA), and *E. coli*
Carbenicillin	Geopen	4-5 q4-6h	
Ticarcillin	Ticar	2-3 q4-6h	
Ticarcillin-Clavulanic Acid	Timentin	3.1 (3.0 ticarcillin, 0.1 clavulanate potassium)	Spectrum extended to include beta-lactamase producers such as *S. aureus* (except MRSA), *E. coli, Klebsiella* sp. and *Bacieroldes fragilis*
Azlocillin	Azlin	2-3 q4-6h	Spectrum includes enterococci, *Klebsiella, Enterobacter,* and *Serratia* sp
Mezlocillin	Mezlin	2-4 q4-8h	Spectrum includes enterococci, *Klebsiella, Enterobacter,* and *Serratia* sp
Piperacillin	Pipracil	3-4 q4-6h	Spectrum includes enterococci, *Klebsiella, Enterobacter, Acinetobacter,* and *Serratia* sp
Piperacillin-Tazobactam	Zosyn	3.375 (3.0 piperacillin, 0.375 tazobactam) q4-6h	Spectrum includes enterococci, *Klebsiella, Enterobacter, Acinetobacter,* and *Serratia* sp; extended to include beta-lactamase producers such as *S. aureus* (except MRSA) and *B. fragilis*
Penicillinase Resistant Penicillins			
Methicillin	Methicillin	1-2 q4-6h	Parenteral penicillin of choice for *S. aureus* (except MRSA)
Nafcillin	Nafcillin	0.5-2.0 q4-6h	Parenteral penicillin of choice for *S. aureus* (except MRSA)
Oxacillin	Oxacillin	0.5-2.0 q4-6h	Parenteral penicillin of choice for *S. aureus* (except MRSA)

Note: MRSA = Methicillin resistant *S. aureus.*

QUINOLONE ANTIBIOTICS

Generic drug name	Brand name	Usual adult dose (mg)	Cost (10 days of oral therapy)	Comment
Cinoxacin	Cinobac	PO: 250 q6h or 500 q12h	$36	Approved only to treat UTIs; *Enterococcus, Staphylococcus,* and *Pseudomonas* sp are resistant
Ciprofloxacin	Cipro	PO: 250-750 q12h IV: 200-400 q12h	$56	Available for ophthalmic use; useful in oral therapy of osteomyelitis; approved for *Campylobacter, Salmonella,* and *Shigella* infections; antibacterial spectrum includes *Mycobacterium avium-intracellulare*
Enoxacin	Penetrex	PO: 400 q12h	$57	Approved only to treat UTIs
Levofloxacin	Levaquin	PO: 100 q8h	NA	Levo-form of ofloxacin
Lomefloxacin	Maxaquin	PO: 400 q24h	$61	Not effective for *Pseudomonas aeruginosa* infections outside of the urinary tract
Norfloxacin	Noroxin	PO: 400 q12h	$57	Available for ophthalmic use; approved only to treat UTIs and conjuctivitis
Ofloxacin	Floxin	PO: 200-400 q12h IV: 200-400 q12h	$61	Available for ophthalmic use
Sparfloxacin	Zagam	PO: 100-400 load, then 100-300 q24h	NA	Enhanced activity against gram-positive cocci and anaerobes

SULFONAMIDE ANTIBIOTICS

Generic drug name	Brand name	Usual adult dose	Comment
SYSTEMIC			
Sulfamethoxazole	Gantanol	PO: 500-1000 mg q12h	Primary use is for UTIs
Sulfamethoxazole-trimethoprim	Septra, Septra DS, Bactrim, Bactrim DS, Co-trimoxazole	PO: 800 mg/160 mg q12h IV: 10-20 mg/kg/d based on trimethoprim component divided into q6-12h schedule	First line therapy for *Pneumocystis carinii* pneumonia
Sulfadiazine	Sulfadiazine	PO: 500-1000 mg q6h	Used with pyrimethamine to treat toxoplasmosis
Sulfisoxazole	Gantrisin	PO: 500-1000 mg q6h	Available in combination with erythromycin ethylsuccinate for oral use
TOPICAL			
Silver sulfadiazine	Silvadene	TOP: 1% cream to affected area qd-bid (desired thickness 1-2 mm)	Primary use is for 2nd and 3rd degree burns
Sodium sulfacetamide	Sodium Sulamyd	OPHTH: 10% sol in affected eye q2-4h; 10% oint; 0.5 inch into lower conjunctival sac QID	Primary indication is bacterial conjunctivitis

SYSTEMIC ANTIFUNGAL ANTIBIOTICS

Generic drug name	*Brand name*	*Usual adult dose*	*Common indications*	*Comment*
Amphotericin B	Fungizone	IV: 0.4-0.6 mg/kg/d for 8-10 wk	Histoplasmosis, blastomycosis, candidiasis, cryptococcosis, coccidioidomycosis, aspergillosis, mucormycosis	Used topically in bladder; causes multiple electrolyte abnormalities (hypokalemia, renal tubular acidosis, hypomagnesemia, azotemia); give 1 mg test dose prior to giving full dose
Fluconazole	Diflucan	PO or IV: 100-400 qd	Blastomycosis, histoplasmosis, candidiasis, coccidioidomycosis	Increases serum rifabutin levels and toxicity; increases effect of cyclosporine, terfenadine, astemizole, warfarin, sulfonylureas, and others; single dose oral treatment for vaginal infection
Flucytosine	Ancobon	PO: 12.5-37.5 mg/kg q6h	Cryptococcosis, candidiasis, chromoblastomycosis	Usually used in combination with amphotericin B (allows lower dose); converted to 5-fluorouracil in fungal cell
Griseofulvin	Fulvicin, Gris-PEG	PO: 500 mg qd-bid (microcrystalline) PO: 330 mg qd-bid (ultra microcrystalline)	Dermatophytes	Hepatic mixed function oxidase inducer; absorption enhanced when taken with fatty foods
Itraconazole	Sporanox	PO: 100-200 mg qd-bid	Onychomycosis, blastomycosis, histoplasmosis, candidiasis, coccidioidomycosis, sporotrichosis, cryptococcosis, aspergillosis	Hepatic mixed function oxidase inhibitor (cytochrome P450 3A—affects cyclosporine, terfenadine, astemizole, warfarin, sulfonylureas, and others)
Ketoconazole	Nizoral	PO: 200-400 mg qd-bid	Blastomycosis, histoplasmosis, candidiasis, coccidioidomycosis, dermatophytes	Hepatic mixed function oxidase inhibitor (cytochrome P450 3A—affects cyclosporine, terfenadine, astemizole, warfarin, sulfonylureas, and others); requires acid pH for absorption; reduces testosterone synthesis; available in topical form
Miconazole	Monistat	IV: 200-1200 mg q8h	Coccidioidomycosis, candidiasis, cryptococcosis	Increases warfarin and sulfonylurea effect; used topically for cutaneous and vaginal infections
Terbinafine	Lamisil	PO: 250 mg qd	Onychomycosis	Hepatic clearance increased by rifampin, decreased by cimetidine

TETRACYCLINE ANTIBIOTICS

Generic drug name	*Brand name*	*Usual adult dose (mg)*	*Cost ($) per dose*	*Comment*
Chlortetracycline	Aureomycin	NA	NA	Ophthalmic ointment only
Demeclocycline	Declomycin	300 bid	6.75 (300 mg)	Used to treat diabetes insipidus
Doxycycline	Vibramycin	100 qd-bid	0.12 (100 mg)	
Minocycline	Minocin	100 bid	1.96 (100 mg)	
Oxytetracycline	Terramycin	250-500 qid	0.17 (250 mg)	Available combined with phenazopyridine and sulfamethizole
Tetracycline	Tetracycline	250-500 qid	0.04 (250 mg)	

Antidepressants

SELECTIVE SEROTONIN REUPTAKE INHIBITOR (SSRI) ANTIDEPRESSANTS

Generic drug name	*Brand name*	*Usual adult dose (mg/d)*	*Drug and active metabolite ($t_{1/2}$) (hr)*	*Serotonin reuptake inhibition*	*Anticholinergic effect*	*Drowsiness*	*Degree of cytochrome P450 system inhibition*	*Comment*
Fluoxetine	Prozac	20-40 (starting dose 10 in elderly)	24-72 (acute); 96-144 (chronic); (norfluoxetine: 96-384)	3+	0	0	2-3+	Up to 60 mg/d for obsessive-compulsive disorder
Fluvoxamine	Luvox	50-300	15-26 (no active metabolite)	3+	0	1+	2+	Indicated only for obsessive-compulsive disorder
Paroxetine	Paxil	20-50 (starting dose 10 in elderly)	21 (no active metabolite)	4+	1+	1+	2+	May cause weight gain
Sertraline	Zoloft	50-200 (starting dose 12.5-25 in elderly)	26 (desinethylsertraline: 62-104)	4+	0	0	1+	Metabolite weakly active

TRICYCLIC AND TETRACYCLIC ANTIDEPRESSANTS

Generic drug name	*Brand name*	*Usual adult dose (mg) for acute therapy (maintenance dose is ½-⅔ of this; lower doses recommended for elderly persons)*	*Relative sedation*	*Relative anticholinergic effect*	*Relative delay of cardiac conduction*	*Relative postural hypotension*	*Comment*
TRICYCLIC							
Amitriptyline	Elavil	75-300	3+	2+	3+	3+	Used for chronic pain
Clomipramine	Anafranil	25-250	2+	2+	2+	2+	Primary use is for obsessive-compulsive disorder; may lower seizure threshold; may increase plasma concentration of protein bound drugs (*e.g.,* digoxin, warfarin)
Desipramine	Norpramin	75-300	1+	1+	3+	1+	Used for chronic pain; metabolite of imipramine
Doxepin	Sinequan	75-300	3+	3+	1+	3+	Potent antihistamine
Imipramine	Tofranil	50-300	2+	2+	3+	2+	Used for chronic pain, panic disorder, and headache
Nortriptyline	Pamelor	50-150	1+	1+	2+	2+	Used for chronic pain, panic disorder, and headache; metabolite of amitriptyline
Protriptyline	Vivactil	15-60	0+	2+	2+	1+	
Trimipramine	Surmontil	50-300	2+	2+	3+	2+	
TETRACYCLIC							
Amoxapine	Asendin	200-600	2+	1+	1+	1+	Metabolite has neuroleptic side effect
Maprotiline	Ludiomil	75-300	2+	1+	1+	1+	May lower seizure threshold
HETEROCYCLIC							
Nefazodone	Serzone	200-600	2+	1+	0+	1+	Divided doses on bid schedule; do not administer with terfenadine or astemizole; may increase plasma concentration of protein bound drugs (*e.g.,* digoxin, warfarin)
Trazodone	Desyrel	150-600	3+	1+	0+	2+	Risk of priapism in males and similar phenomenon in females; may increase plasma concentration of protein bound drugs (*e.g.,* digoxin, warfarin); should be given in divided doses

MISCELLANEOUS ANTIDEPRESSANTS, INCLUDING FOODS THAT INTERACT WITH MAOIS

Generic drug name	*Brand name*	*Usual dose (mg/d)*	*Anticholinergic effect*	*Drowsiness*	*Orthostatic hypotension*	*Cardiac dysrhythmias*	*Comment*
Bupropion	Wellbutrin	300-450	0	0	0	1+	Single dose should not exceed 150 mg; inhibits dopamine reuptake; given bid or tid
Mirtazapine	Remeron	15-45	2+	3+	0	0-1+	Do not use with MAOIs
Venlafaxine	Effexor	75-375	1+	1+	0	1+	Inhibits serotonin and norepinephrine reuptake; given bid or tid
Monoamine oxidase inhibitors (MAOIs)							Avoid foods rich in amines (see below) and selected medications while taking MAOI and for 14 days after last dose
Isocarboxazid	Marplan	10-30	2+	2+	3+	1+	May be given as single daily dose
Phenelzine	Nardil	15-90	2+	2+	3+	1+	Given in divided doses
Tranylcypromine	Parnate	30-60	2+	1+	3+	1+	Given in divided doses

Avoid the following foods if taking MAOIs (contain tyramine and other amines, often as a result of aging or fermenting): broad beans; red wines; yeast extracts; beer with yeast; chicken or beef liver; caviar, anchovies, and pickled herring; fermented sausages (bologna, pepperoni, salami, and summer sausage); and aged cheeses (Boursault, Brie, Camembert, cheddar, Emmenthaler, Gruyere, mozzarella, parmesan, romano, Roquefort, and Stilton).

Antihistamines

SYSTEMIC ANTIHISTAMINES

Generic drug name	*Trade name*	*Usual adult dose (mg)*	*Cost per dose ($)*	*Comment*
FIRST GENERATION AGENTS				
Acrivastine	Semprex-D	8 qid	0.47	Available only in combination with pseudoephedrine
Azatadine	Trinalin	1 bid	0.95	Available only in combination with pseudoephedrine
Bromodiphenhydramine	Ambenyl and others	12.5-25.0 qid	0.10	Available only as a syrup and in combination with codeine phosphate
Brompheniramine	Dimetane	4 q4h	0.03	Also available as syrup, extended release capsule, and in combination with decongestants
Carbinoxamine	Rondec and others	4 qid	0.09	Only available in combination with pseudoephedrine; available as syrup and extended release tablet

Continued

SYSTEMIC ANTIHISTAMINES—CONT'D

Generic drug name	Trade name	Usual adult dose (mg)	Cost per dose ($)	Comment
FIRST GENERATION AGENTS—CONT'D				
Chlorpheniramine	Chlor-Trimeton and others	4 qid	0.01	Also available as syrup, extended release capsule, and in combination with decongestants
Clemastine	Tavist and others	1.34 bid	0.31	Also available as syrup and in combination with decongestants
Cyproheptadine	Periactin and others	4 qid	0.02	Also available as syrup
Diphenhydramine	Benadryl and others	25-50 qid	0.02	Also available as syrup
Hydroxyzine	Atarax, Vistaril	10-75 qid	0.03	Also available as syrup
Pheniramine	Triaminic and others	4 qid	0.40	Only available in combination with phenylpropanolamine and pyrilamine; available as syrup and extended release tablet
Pyrilamine	Triaminic and others	4 qid	0.40	Only available in combination with phenylpropanolamine and pheniramine; available as syrup and extended release tablet
Trimeprazine	Temaril and others	2.5 qid	1.05	Also available as syrup and extended release capsule
Tripelennamine	PBZ and others	25-50 qid	0.06	Also available as sustained action tablets
Triprolidine	Actifed and others	2.5 qid	0.03	Also available in combination with pseudoephedrine and as syrup
SECOND GENERATION AGENTS				
Astemizole	Hismanal	10 qd	1.84	Non-sedating agent; prescription required in U.S.; potential drug interaction with macrolides and azole antifungals; potential for QT interval prolongation
Cetirizine	Zyrtec	10 qd	1.61	Less-sedating agent; prescription required in U.S.; no drug interaction with macrolides and azole antifungals; QT interval prolongation not reported
Fexofenadine	Allegra	60 bid	0.86	Non-sedating agent; prescription required in U.S.; potential drug interaction with macrolides and azole antifungals; QT interval prolongation not reported
Loratadine	Claritin	10 qd	1.93	Non-sedating agent; prescription required in U.S.; potential drug interaction with macrolides and azole antifungals; QT interval prolongation not reported; also available in combination with pseudoephedrine
Terfenadine	Seldane	60 bid	0.94	Non-sedating agent; prescription required in U.S.; potential drug interaction with macrolides and azole antifungals; potential for QT interval prolongation; also available in combination with pseudoephedrine;
MISCELLANEOUS AGENTS				
Doxepin	Sinequan	10-50 qd-tid	0.04	Sedating tricyclic antidepressant
Promethazine	Phenergan	12.5 tid-qid	0.06	Phenothiazine derivative; well tolerated by children; available as syrup

Antiretroviral

ANTIRETROVIRAL DRUGS

Generic drug name	Trade name	Usual adult dose (mg)	Dose change in renal insufficiency	Drug interactions	Comment
NUCLEOSIDE REVERSE TRANSCRIPTASE INHIBITORS					
Didanosine (ddI)	Videx	125-200 q12h on empty stomach	Reduce dose if CrCl <60 ml/min	Dapsone, ganciclovir, itraconazole, quinolones; additive neuropathic effect with dapsone, isoniazid, metronidazole, phenytoin, vincristine	Take 2 pills at a time to ensure adequate buffering; available as a powder; penetrates into CSF
Lamivudine (3TC)	Epivir	150 q12h	Reduce dose if CrCl <50 ml/min	Trimethoprim-sulfamethoxazole	Available as oral solution; penetrates into CSF; no proven benefit as monotherapy
Stavudine (d4T)	Zerit	30-40 q12h	Reduce dose if CrCl <50 ml/min	Additive neuropathic effect with dapsone, isoniazid, metronidazole, phenytoin, vincristine	Antagonism with zidovudine; penetrates into CSF; no proven benefit as monotherapy
Zalcitabine (ddC)	Hivid	0.75 q8h	Reduce dose if CrCl <40 ml/min	Antacids, amphotericin, foscarnet, aminoglycosides, probenecid, cimetidine, pentamidine; additive neuropathic effect with dapsone, isoniazid, metronidazole, phenytoin, vincristine	No proven benefit as monotherapy
Zidovudine (AZT)	Retrovir	100-200 q8h or 300 q12h	Reduce dose if CrCl <10 ml/min	Ganciclovir, interferon, probenecid, rifampin, valproic acid	Available as syrup, injection; penetrates into CSF
NON-NUCLEOSIDE REVERSE TRANSCRIPTASE INHIBITORS					
Nevirapine	Viramune	200 qd for 14d, then 200 bid	No	Cimetidine, clarithromycin, dirithromycin, erythromycin, indinavir, ketoconazole, rifabutin, rifampin, ritonavir, saquinavir, troleandomycin, zidovudine	Do not use as monotherapy due to resistance induction

Continued

ANTIRETROVIRAL DRUGS—CONT'D

Generic drug name	*Trade name*	*Usual adult dose (mg)*	*Dose change in renal insufficiency*	*Drug interactions*	*Comment*
PROTEASE INHIBITORS					
Indinavir	Crixivan	800 q8h (400 mg tablets)	No	Astemizole, cisapride, didanosine, ketoconazole, midazolam, nevirapine, rifabutin, rifampin, terfenadine, triazolam	Do not take with large meal; associated with nephrolithiasis; no proven benefit as monotherapy
Ritonavir	Norvir	600 q12h (100 mg tablets)	No	Alprazolam, amiodarone, astemizole, calcium channel blockers, carbamazepine, cisapride, clonazepam, corticosteroids, desipramine, diazepam, encainide, estrogens, fluoxetine, flurazepam, itraconazole, ketoconazole, macrolide antibiotics, midazolam, narcotics, neuroleptics, NSAIDs, omeprazole, phenytoin, quinidine, rifabutin, rifampin, sulfonylureas, terfenadine, theophylline, trazodone, triazolam, warfarin	Take with food; start with 300 mg q12h, increase in 100 mg increments to 600 mg q12h; no proven benefits as monotherapy
Saquinavir	Invirase	600 q8h (200 mg tablets)	No	Astemizole, cisapride, ketoconazole, nevirapine, rifabutin, rifampin, ritonavir, terfenadine	Take with high fat meal to enhance bioavailability; no proven benefit as monotherapy

Hypoglycemic Agents

ORAL HYPOGLYCEMIC AGENTS

Generic drug name	*Brand name*	*Equipotent dose or usual dose range (mg)*	*Usual adult dose schedule*	*Adjust dose in renal insufficiency*	*Cost of dose ($)*	*Comment*
FIRST GENERATION SULFONYLUREA						
Acetohexamide	Dymelor	500	qd-bid	Yes	0.29	Do not use if CrCl <50 ml/min
Chlorpropamide	Diabenese	250	qd	Yes	0.05	Do not use if CrCl <50 ml/min
Tolazamide	Tolinase	250	qd-bid	Yes	0.09	Do not use if CrCl <50 ml/min
Tolbutamide	Orinase	1000	bid-tid	No	0.06	Do not use if CrCl <50 ml/min
SECOND GENERATION SULFONYLUREA						
Glipizide	Glucotrol	10	bid	Yes	0.33	Do not use if CrCl <10 ml/min; available as qd formulation (Glucotrol XL)
Glyburide	Diabeta, Micronase	5	qd-bid	Yes	0.51	Do not use if CrCl <10 ml/min
MISCELLANEOUS						
Acarbose	Precose	25-100	tid	No	0.46 (50 mg)	Take dose at the start of each meal
Metformin	Glucophage	500-850	bid-tid	Yes	0.46 (500 mg)	Do not use if serum creat >1.4 mg/dl (male) or >1.3 mg/dl (female); max daily dose 2550 mg

Lipid Lowering Agents

Generic drug name	*Brand name*	*Usual adult dose*	*Maximum effect on serum lipid levels*	*Cost ($) per dose*
BILE ACID BINDING RESINS			LDL-cholesterol reduced 20%-35%; HDL-cholesterol not changed; triglycerides increased 5%-20%	
Cholestyramine	Questran	8 g bid-tid		1.38 (4 g); available in bulk form
Colestipol	Colestid	10 g bid-tid		1.23 (5 g); available in bulk form
Niacin	Niacin	1-2 g bid-tid	LDL-cholesterol reduced 20%; HDL-cholesterol increased 20%; triglycerides reduced 40%	0.03 (500 mg)
FIBRIC ACID DERIVATIVES			LDL-cholesterol reduced 10%; HDL-cholesterol increased 10%-25%; triglycerides reduced 40%-60%	
Clofibrate	Atromid-S	500 qid		0.13 (500 mg)
Gemfibrozil	Lopid	600 bid		0.75 (600 mg)
HMG CO A REDUCTASE INHIBITORS			LDL-cholesterol reduced 20%-40%; HDL-cholesterol increased 5%-15%; triglycerides reduced 5%-25%	
Fluvastatin	Lescol	20-40 mg qhs		1.28 (40 mg)
Lovastatin	Mevacor	20-40 mg qhs		2.12 (20 mg)
Pravastatin	Pravachol	20-40 mg qhs		1.89 (20 mg)
Simvastatin	Zocor	10-20 mg qhs		1.88 (10 mg)

KEYWORD INDEX

Free To Purchasers Only

International Brand Index

Call 1-800-638-1393 to receive a copy of the International Brand Index. This practical guide allows you to look up international brand name drugs from 137 countries, and their U.S. equivalent generic names. It also lists the name of the country the international product is from. Since many international brands have the same name as U.S. brand name products, this supplement is a valuable tool in avoiding potential mistakes. Call us for your free index!

CATEGORY/BRAND

Generic Name *(cost of therapy)* Page No.

ANTIMALARIAL AGENTS *(cont'd)*
Quinine Sulfate *($82.12)* II-1865

ANTIMANIC AGENTS
Divalproex Sodium *($818.18)* II-724
Lithium Carbonate *($14.17)* II-1312
Lithium Citrate *($33.75)* II-1313

ANTIMETABOLITES
Azathioprine *($54.72)* II-193
Daunorubicin Citrate Liposome *($2,942.65)* II-607
Daunorubicin Hydrochloride *($2,942.65)* II-609
Floxuridine *($490.56)* II-925
Fluorouracil *($564.18)* II-946
Interferon Alfa-2A, Recombinant *($59,200.09)* II-1177
Interferon Alfa-2B, Recombinant *($16,445.33)* II-1181
Mercaptopurine *($5.04)* II-1389
Mitoxantrone Hydrochloride *($87.60)* II-1498
Plicamycin *($51.20)* II-1762
Thioguanine *($97.78)* II-2059

ANTIMICROBIALS
Acetic Acid *($8.73)* II-26
Acyclovir *($129.02)* II-35
Amikacin Sulfate *($123.22)* II-81
Aminosalicylate Sodium *($483.84)* II-94
Aminosalicylic Acid *($2,030.40)* II-95
Amoxicillin *($7.05)* II-112
Amoxicillin; Clavulanate Potassium *($117.36)* II-115
Amphotericin B *($117.36)* II-122
Ampicillin *($3.76)* II-126
Ampicillin Sodium *($3.76)* II-128
Ampicillin Sodium; Sulbactam Sodium *($230.36)* II-130
Ampicillin Trihydrate; Probenecid *($230.36)* II-132
Atovaquone *($538.68)* II-176
Aztreonam *($225.37)* II-201
Bacampicillin Hydrochloride *($225.37)* II-209
Bacitracin *($225.37)* II-210
Belladonna; Phenazo *($225.37)* II-227
Bismuth; Hydrocortisone *($277.14)* II-260
Butabarbital; Hyoscyamine Hydrobromide; Phenazopyridine Hydrochloride *($8.28)* II-301
Butoconazole Nitrate *($8.28)* II-302
Calcium Chloride *($779.85)* II-315
Carbenicillin Indanyl Sodium *($147.16)* II-329
Carbol Fuchsin *($338.35)* II-337
Cefaclor *($117.48)* II-349
Cefadroxil *($60.75)* II-351
Cefamandole Nafate *($60.75)* II-353
Cefazolin Sodium *($60.75)* II-355
Cefepime Hydrochloride *($60.75)* II-358
Cefixime *($63.14)* II-361
Cefonicid Sodium *($63.14)* II-367
Cefoperazone Sodium *($63.14)* II-369
Ceforanide *($63.14)* II-371
Cefotaxime Sodium *($63.14)* II-373
Cefotetan Disodium *($63.14)* II-376
Cefoxitin Sodium *($255.75)* II-379
Ceftazidime *($155.06)* II-388
Ceftazidime (Arginine) *($155.06)* II-392
Ceftibuten *($155.06)* II-395
Ceftizoxime Sodium *($155.06)* II-398
Ceftriaxone Sodium *($4.00)* II-401
Cefuroxime Axetil *($183.30)* II-403
Cefuroxime Sodium *($90.00)* II-407
Cephalexin *($2.83)* II-411
Cephalexin Hydrochloride *($39.34)* II-414
Cephalothin Sodium *($39.34)* II-415
Cephapirin Sodium *($39.34)* II-417
Cephradine *($8.76)* II-418
Chloramphenicol *($20.00)* II-428
Chloramphenicol Sodium Succinate *($20.00)* II-428
Ciclopirox Olamine II-473
Cidofovir II-474
Cilastatin Sodium; Imipenem *($618.00)* II-477
Cinoxacin *($16.78)* II-486
Ciprofloxacin Hydrochloride *($39.20)* II-488
Clavulanate Potassium; Ticarcillin Disodium *($43.47)* II-511
Clindamycin Hydrochloride *($28.17)* II-517
Clindamycin Phosphate *($28.17)* II-519
Clioquinol; Hydrocortisone *($28.17)* II-524
Clofazimine *($28.17)* II-527
Clotrimazole *($5.14)* II-544
Cloxacillin Sodium *($5.14)* II-545
Colistimethate Sodium *($760.95)* II-561
Dapsone *($2,942.65)* II-606
Demeclocycline Hydrochloride *($214.32)* II-616
Dexamethasone *($53.32)* II-626
Dexamethasone; Tobramycin *($53.32)* II-640
Dicloxacillin Sodium *($5.32)* II-668
Doxycycline *($3,775.85)* II-759
Erythromycin *($3.39)* II-806
Erythromycin Estolate *($3.39)* II-808
Erythromycin Ethylsuccinate *($7.46)* II-810
Erythromycin Ethylsuccinate; Sulfisoxazole Acetyl *($7.46)* II-812
Erythromycin Gluceptate *($7.46)* II-814
Erythromycin Lactobionate *($7.46)* II-815
Erythromycin Stearate *($3.60)* II-817
Ethambutol Hydrochloride *($571.50)* II-857
Ethionamide *($642.56)* II-872
Famciclovir *($129.15)* II-890
Flucytosine *($86.84)* II-930
Foscarnet Sodium *($26,632.22)* II-977
Ganciclovir Sodium *($12,702.00)* II-997
Gentamicin Sulfate *($547.50)* II-1009
Griseofulvin, Microcrystalline *($166.00)* II-1042
Griseofulvin, Ultramicrocrystalline *($166.00)* II-1043
Hydroxyzine Hydrochloride *($3.10)* II-1135
Hyoscamine; Methenamine; Methylene Blue; Phenyl Salicylate; Sodium Biphosphate *($30.81)* II-1138
Indinavir Sulfate *($240.79)* II-1162
Interferon Alfa-2A, Recombinant *($59,200.09)* II-1177
Isoniazid *($4.46)* II-1213
Isoniazid; Pyrazinamide; Rifampin *($1,620.00)* II-1215
Isoniazid; Rifampin *($1,019.88)* II-1215
Isosorbide Dinitrate *($19.12)* II-1220
Itraconazole *($970.85)* II-1230
Kanamycin Sulfate *($970.85)* II-1234
Ketoconazole *($18.96)* II-1238
Lamivudine *($324.41)* II-1253

ANTIMICROBIALS *(cont'd)*
Lidocaine; Oxytetracycline Hydrochloride *($60.88)* II-1298
Lincomycin Hydrochloride *($60.88)* II-1300
Meropenem *($5.04)* II-1391
Methenamine Hippurate *($95.81)* II-1415
Methenamine Mandelate *($95.81)* II-1415
Methenamine Mandelate; Sodium Acid Phosphate *($95.81)* II-1416
Methicillin Sodium *($95.81)* II-1417
Methylene Blue *($49.27)* II-1438
Metronidazole *($0.95)* II-1463
Mezlocillin Sodium Monohydratee *($900.30)* II-1470
Miconazole *($20.88)* II-1473
Minocycline Hydrochloride *($39.25)* II-1483
Nafcillin Sodium *($309.04)* II-1536
Nalidixic Acid *($32.48)* II-1540
Neomycin Sulfate *($149.65)* II-1566
Neomycin Sulfate; Polymyxin B Sulfate *($149.65)* II-1567
Netilmicin Sulfate *($149.65)* II-1570
Nitrofurantoin *($1,325.21)* II-1594
Nitrofurantoin, Macrocrystalline *($16.24)* II-1596
Norfloxacin *($16.73)* II-1609
Novobiocin Sodium *($252.29)* II-1614
Nystatin *($252.29)* II-1614
Ofloxacin *($43.09)* II-1620
Oxacillin Sodium *($117.73)* II-1641
Oxytetracycline Hydrochloride *($316.12)* II-1656
Oxytetracycline Hydrochloride; Phenazopyridine Hydrochloride; Sulfamethizole *($316.12)* II-1657
Paromomycin Sulfate *($48.54)* II-1673
Penciclovir *($362.37)* II-1685
Penicillin G Benzathine *($362.37)* II-1689
Penicillin G Benzathine; Penicillin G Procaine *($362.37)* II-1690
Penicillin G Potassium *($362.37)* II-1691
Penicillin G Procaine *($362.37)* II-1694
Penicillin G Procaine; Probenecid *($362.37)* II-1696
Penicillin V Potassium *($3.27)* II-1698
Phenazopyridine Hydrochloride *($110.78)* II-1718
Phenazopyridine Hydrochloride; Sulfisoxazole *($110.78)* II-1719
Piperacillin Sodium *($169.72)* II-1752
Piperacillin Sodium; Tazobactam Sodium *($169.72)* II-1755
Polymyxin B Sulfate *($51.20)* II-1770
Potassium Iodide II-1782
Prednisolone Acetate; Sulfacetamide Sodium *($11.13)* II-1792
Prednisolone Sodium Phosphate *($11.13)* II-1793
Pyrazinamide *($606.85)* II-1851
Ribavirin *($4,124.53)* II-1889
Rifampin *($578.98)* II-1893
Rimantadine Hydrochloride *($578.98)* II-1897
Ritonavir *($2,708.38)* II-1906
Saquinavir Mesylate *($2,708.38)* II-1924
Selenium Sulfide *($1,576.07)* II-1937
Silver Sulfadiazine *($158.60)* II-1941
Sodium Sulfacetamide *($649.99)* II-1954
Spectinomycin Hydrochloride *($1,177.85)* II-1968
Streptomycin Sulfate *($1,441.75)* II-1976
Sulconazole Nitrate *($82.53)* II-1985
Sulfabenzamide; Sulfacetamide; Sulfathiazole *($82.53)* II-1986
Sulfacetamide Sodium *($82.53)* II-1986
Sulfacytine *($82.53)* II-1987
Sulfadiazine *($82.53)* II-1988
Sulfamethizole *($82.53)* II-1989
Sulfamethoxazole *($82.53)* II-1990
Sulfamethoxazole; Trimethoprim *($2.50)* II-1991
Sulfanilamide *($2.50)* II-1995
Sulfasalazine *($156.80)* II-1996
Sulfinpyrazone *($156.80)* II-1997
Sulfisoxazole *($156.80)* II-1998
Terbinafine Hydrochloride *($463.51)* II-2030
Terconazole *($400.33)* II-2032
Tetracycline Hydrochloride *($1.15)* II-2044
Thioridazine Hydrochloride *($8.80)* II-2062
Tobramycin *($203.45)* II-2083
Tobramycin Sulfate *($203.45)* II-2084
Triamcinolone Acetonide *($474.79)* II-2117
Trimethoprim *($71.83)* II-2142
Trimetrexate Glucuronate *($71.83)* II-2143
Troleandomycin *($178.41)* II-2151
Valacyclovir Hydrochloride *($6,363.68)* II-2162
Vancomycin Hydrochloride *($14.00)* II-2173
Vidarabine *($56.72)* II-2190
Zidovudine *($3,488.45)* II-2212

ANTIMIGRAINE/OTHER HEADACHES
Acetaminophen; Butalbital *($401.06)* II-8
Acetaminophen; Butalbital; Caffeine *($401.06)* II-9
Acetaminophen; Dichloralphenazone; Isometheptene Mucate *($6.75)* II-15
Aspirin; Butalbital; Caffeine II-158
Belladonna; Caffeine; Ergotamine; Pentobarbital *($225.37)* II-225
Belladonna; Ergotamine Tartrate; Phenobarbital *($225.37)* II-225
Caffeine; Ergotamine Tartrate *($8.28)* II-307
Dihydroergotamine Mesylate *($27.52)* II-694
Ergoloid Mesylates II-804
Ergotamine Tartrate II-805
Methysergide Maleate *($98.55)* II-1449
Sumatriptan Succinate *($11.96)* II-2003

ANTIMITOTICS
Podofilox *($51.20)* II-1765

ANTIMUSCARINICS/ANTISPASMODICS
Acetaminophen; Atropine; Ethaverine; Salicylic Acid *($401.06)* II-8
Albuterol; Ipratropium Bromide *($35.36)* II-50
Atropine Sulfate *($538.68)* II-181
Atropine; Phenobarbital *($538.68)* II-188
Belladonna *($225.37)* II-223
Belladonna Alkaloids; Phenobarbital *($225.37)* II-223
Belladonna; Butabarbital Sodium *($225.37)* II-225
Belladonna; Enzyme; Phenobarbital *($225.37)* II-225
Belladonna; Ergotamine Tartrate; Phenobarbital *($225.37)* II-225
Benztropine Mesylate *($9.59)* II-236
Chlordiazepoxide Hydrochloride; Clidinium Bromide *($10.65)* II-434
Clidinium Bromide *($43.50)* II-517
Dicyclomine Hydrochloride *($5.32)* II-672
Glycopyrrolate *($107.85)* II-1030

ANTIMUSCARINICS/ANTISPASMODICS *(cont'd)*
Homatropine Hydrobromide *($85.57)* II-1089
Homatropine Methylbromide *($85.57)* II-1090
Hyoscyamine Sulfate *($1,532.63)* II-1138
Hyoscyamine Sulfate; Phenobarbital *($1,532.63)* II-1140
Ipratropium Bromide *($311.27)* II-1203
Mepenzolate Bromide *($618.82)* II-1379
Methantheline Bromide *($95.81)* II-1413
Methscopolamine Bromide *($656.74)* II-1432
Propantheline Bromide *($917.82)* II-1831
Scopolamine *($7.49)* II-1931
Scopolamine Hydrobromide *($7.49)* II-1932
Tridihexethyl Chloride *($3.70)* II-2132

ANTIMYCOBACTERIALS
Aminosalicylate Sodium *($483.84)* II-94
Aminosalicylic Acid *($2,030.40)* II-95
Clofazimine *($28.17)* II-527
Dapsone *($2,942.65)* II-606
Ethambutol Hydrochloride *($571.50)* II-857
Ethionamide *($642.56)* II-872
Isoniazid *($4.46)* II-1213
Isoniazid; Pyrazinamide; Rifampin *($1,620.00)* II-1215
Isoniazid; Rifampin *($1,019.88)* II-1215
Kanamycin Sulfate *($970.85)* II-1234
Pyrazinamide *($606.85)* II-1851
Rifampin *($578.98)* II-1893
Streptomycin Sulfate *($1,441.75)* II-1976

ANTIMYCOTICS
Itraconazole *($970.85)* II-1230
Tioconazole *($203.45)* II-2080

ANTINEOPLASTICS
Aldesleukin *($35.36)* II-51
Altretamine *($6,132.00)* II-74
Amifostine *($123.22)* II-80
Aminophylline *($40.29)* II-91
Anastrozole *($230.36)* II-137
Asparaginase II-154
Bcg Live *($225.37)* II-204
Betamethasone Acetate; Betamethasone Sodium Phosphate *($526.07)* II-244
Bicalutamide *($262.94)* II-257
Bleomycin Sulfate *($41.77)* II-269
Busulfan *($214.27)* II-297
Carboplatin *($2,803.56)* II-337
Carmustine *($2,803.56)* II-342
Chlorambucil *($20.00)* II-426
Chlorotrianisene *($10.65)* II-442
Cisplatin *($4,325.75)* II-498
Cladribine *($4,325.75)* II-503
Cyclophosphamide *($1,020.28)* II-580
Cytarabine *($2,942.65)* II-593
Dacarbazine *($2,942.65)* II-596
Dactinomycin *($2,942.65)* II-597
Daunorubicin Citrate Liposome *($2,942.65)* II-607
Daunorubicin Hydrochloride *($2,942.65)* II-609
Dexrazoxane Hydrochloride *($47.60)* II-648
Diethylstilbestrol *($1,946.41)* II-680
Diethylstilbestrol Diphosphate *($1,946.41)* II-682
Digoxin *($27.52)* II-688
Docetaxel *($7.50)* II-732
Doxorubicin Hydrochloride *($3,775.85)* II-754
Doxorubicin, Liposomal *($3,775.85)* II-756
Estradiol *($73.14)* II-822
Estradiol Cypionate; Testosterone Cypionate *($73.14)* II-828
Estramustine Phosphate Sodium *($73.14)* II-834
Estrogenic Substances *($73.14)* II-835
Estrogens, Conjugated *($107.99)* II-835
Estrogens, Esterified *($107.99)* II-849
Estrogens, Esterified; Methyltestosterone *($107.99)* II-850
Estrone *($107.99)* II-851
Estropipate *($107.99)* II-853
Ethinyl Estradiol *($9.06)* II-861
Etoposide *($1,741.30)* II-884
Floxuridine *($490.56)* II-925
Fludarabine Phosphate *($86.84)* II-931
Fluorouracil *($564.18)* II-946
Fluoxymesterone *($202.08)* II-953
Flutamide *($3,603.42)* II-965
Gallium Nitrate *($1,034.77)* II-996
Gemcitabine Hydrochloride *($12,702.00)* II-1003
Goserelin Acetate *($107.85)* II-1035
Hydroxyprogesterone Caproate *($498.80)* II-1133
Hydroxyurea *($643.75)* II-1133
Idarubicin Hydrochloride *($37.01)* II-1148
Ifosfamide *($37.01)* II-1151
Interferon Alfa-2A, Recombinant *($59,200.09)* II-1177
Interferon Alfa-2B, Recombinant *($16,445.33)* II-1181
Interferon Alfa-N3 *($16,445.33)* II-1190
Interferon Gamma-1B, Recombinant *($13,140.00)* II-1199
Irinotecan Hydrochloride *($311.27)* II-1205
Leucovorin Calcium *($1,346.36)* II-1264
Leuprolide Acetate *($1,346.36)* II-1266
Levamisole Hydrochloride *($1,267.35)* II-1272
Lomustine *($44.87)* II-1319
Masoprocol *($36.79)* II-1348
Mechlorethamine Hydrochloride *($36.79)* II-1357
Medroxyprogesterone Acetate *($231.11)* II-1362
Megestrol Acetate *($231.11)* II-1370
Melphalan *($618.82)* II-1372
Mercaptopurine *($5.04)* II-1389
Mesna *($149.71)* II-1400
Methotrexate Sodium *($656.74)* II-1422
Methylprednisolone *($98.55)* II-1440
Methylprednisolone Acetate *($98.55)* II-1442
Methylprednisolone Sodium Succinate *($98.55)* II-1446
Methyltestosterone *($98.55)* II-1448
Mitomycin *($87.60)* II-1496
Mitotane *($87.60)* II-1497
Mitoxantrone Hydrochloride *($87.60)* II-1498
Nilutamide *($96.46)* II-1589
Paclitaxel *($3,200.13)* II-1660
Pegaspargase *($170.91)* II-1680
Pentostatin *($3.65)* II-1708
Plicamycin *($51.20)* II-1762
Porfimer Sodium *($51.20)* II-1773
Prednisolone *($11.13)* II-1790
Prednisolone Acetate *($11.13)* II-1792
Prednisone *($9.59)* II-1800

AUTONOMIC DRUGS *(cont'd)*
Hyoscyamine Sulfate; Phenobarbital *($1,532.63)* II-1140
Interferon Beta-1A *($16,445.33)* II-1192
Interferon Beta-1B, Recombinant *($13,140.00)* II-1195
Ipratropium Bromide *($311.27)* II-1203
Isoetharine Hydrochloride *($311.27)* II-1211
Isoetharine Mesylate *($204.98)* II-1211
Isoproterenol Hydrochloride *($1,019.88)* II-1216
Isoproterenol Hydrochloride; Phenylephrine Bitartrate *($113.58)* II-1218
Levodopa *($263.38)* II-1277
Mepenzolate Bromide *($618.82)* II-1379
Mephentermine Sulfate *($618.82)* II-1382
Metaproterenol Sulfate *($95.81)* II-1402
Metaraminol Bitartrate *($95.81)* II-1405
Metaxalone *($95.81)* II-1406
Methantheline Bromide *($95.81)* II-1413
Methocarbamol *($146.18)* II-1419
Methoxamine Hydrochloride *($656.74)* II-1428
Methscopolamine Bromide *($656.74)* II-1432
Methylcellulose *($656.74)* II-1435
Methysergide Maleate *($98.55)* II-1449
Metocurine Iodide II-1454
Metyrosine *($0.95)* II-1467
Mivacurium Chloride *($87.60)* II-1500
Neostigmine Bromide *($149.65)* II-1569
Neostigmine Methylsulfate *($149.65)* II-1569
Nicotine *($330.50)* II-1580
Norepinephrine Bitartrate *($57.97)* II-1605
Orphenadrine Citrate *($117.73)* II-1641
Pancuronium Bromide *($3,200.13)* II-1668
Pergolide Mesylate *($559.54)* II-1711
Pheniramine; Phenylpropanolamine; Pyrilamine *($108.64)* II-1722
Phenoxybenzamine Hydrochloride *($0.23)* II-1726
Phentolamine Mesylate *($0.23)* II-1729
Phenylephrine Hydrochloride *($174.65)* II-1732
Phenylephrine Hydrochloride; Phenylpropanolamine; Pseudoephedrine *($174.65)* II-1734
Phenylpropanolamine Hydrochloride *($174.65)* II-1735
Physostigmine Salicylate *($74.46)* II-1739
Physostigmine Sulfate *($74.46)* II-1739
Pipecuronium Bromide *($169.72)* II-1750
Pirbuterol Acetate II-1758
Procyclidine Hydrochloride *($334.63)* II-1819
Propantheline Bromide *($917.82)* II-1831
Pseudoephedrine Hydrochloride *($125.52)* II-1849
Pyridostigmine Bromide *($606.85)* II-1852
Rimantadine Hydrochloride *($578.98)* II-1897
Ritodrine Hydrochloride *($578.98)* II-1904
Rocuronium Bromide *($2,708.38)* II-1909
Salmeterol Xinafoate *($2,708.38)* II-1920
Scopolamine *($7.49)* II-1931
Scopolamine Hydrobromide *($7.49)* II-1932
Selegiline Hydrochloride *($1,576.07)* II-1935
Succinylcholine Chloride *($1,441.75)* II-1979
Sumatriptan Succinate *($11.96)* II-2003
Tacrine Hydrochloride *($11.96)* II-2010
Terbutaline Sulfate *($400.33)* II-2031
Tizanidine Hydrochloride *($203.45)* II-2081
Tridihexethyl Chloride *($3.70)* II-2132
Trihexyphenidyl Hydrochloride *($71.83)* II-2139
Tubocurarine Chloride *($178.41)* II-2153
Vecuronium Bromide *($14.00)* II-2180
Yohimbine Hydrochloride *($112.78)* II-2205

AUTOPLEX T
Anti-Inhibitor Coagulant Complex *($2,438.75)* II-143

AVC
Sulfanilamide *($2.50)* II-1995

AVENTYL HCL
Nortriptyline Hydrochloride *($252.29)* II-1612

AVITENE
Collagen Hemostat *($760.95)* II-562

AVITROL VAGINAL SULFA
Sulfanilamide *($2.50)* II-1995

AVONEX
Interferon Beta-1A *($16,445.33)* II-1192

AXID
Nizatidine *($57.97)* II-1602

AXOTAL
Aspirin; Butalbital II-158

AYGESTIN
Norethindrone Acetate *($57.97)* II-1608

AZACTAM
Aztreonam *($225.37)* II-201

AZALIDES
Azithromycin Dihydrate *($30.50)* II-197

AZALINE
Sulfasalazine *($156.80)* II-1996

AZATADINE MALEATE
Azatadine Maleate *($54.72)* II-191
Azatadine Maleate; Pseudoephedrine Sulfate *($54.72)* II-192

AZATHIOPRINE
Azathioprine *($54.72)* II-193

AZATHIOPRINE SODIUM
Azathioprine *($54.72)* II-193

AZDONE
Aspirin; Hydrocodone Bitartrate II-163

AZELAIC ACID
Azelaic Acid *($54.72)* II-195

AZELASTINE
Azelastine *($54.72)* II-195

AZELEX
Azelaic Acid *($54.72)* II-195

AZITHROMYCIN DIHYDRATE
Azithromycin Dihydrate *($30.50)* II-197

AZMA-AID
Ephedrine Hydrochloride; Phenobarbital; Theophylline Anhydrous *($2.84)* II-789

AZMACORT
Triamcinolone Acetonide *($474.79)* II-2117

AZO-GANTRISIN
Phenazopyridine Hydrochloride; Sulfisoxazole *($110.78)* II-1719

AZO-STANDARD
Phenazopyridine Hydrochloride *($110.78)* II-1718

AZO-SULFISOXAZOLE
Phenazopyridine Hydrochloride; Sulfisoxazole *($110.78)* II-1719

AZO-TRUXAZOLE
Phenazopyridine Hydrochloride; Sulfisoxazole *($110.78)* II-1719

AZOLID
Phenylbutazone *($174.65)* II-1730

AZT
Zidovudine *($3,488.45)* II-2212

AZTREONAM
Aztreonam *($225.37)* II-201

AZULFIDINE
Sulfasalazine *($156.80)* II-1996

B & O
Belladonna; Opium *($225.37)* II-226

B-12-1000
Cyanocobalamin *($155.12)* II-573

B-A-C
Aspirin; Butalbital; Caffeine II-158

B-A-C #3
Aspirin; Butalbital; Caffeine; Codeine Phosphate II-159

B-COMPLEX-100
Vitamin B Complex *($1,272.33)* II-2200

B-FEDRINE
Brompheniramine Maleate; Pseudoephedrine Hydrochloride *($395.91)* II-280

B-FEDRINE PD
Brompheniramine Maleate; Pseudoephedrine Hydrochloride *($395.91)* II-280

B-JECT
Vitamin B Complex *($1,272.33)* II-2200

B-PLEX
Vitamin B Complex *($1,272.33)* II-2200
Vitamin B Complex; Vitamin C *($1,272.33)* II-2200

B-S-P
Betamethasone Sodium Phosphate *($526.07)* II-249

BACAMPICILLIN HYDROCHLORIDE
Bacampicillin Hydrochloride *($225.37)* II-209

BACI-RX
Bacitracin *($225.37)* II-210

BACITRACIN
Bacitracin *($225.37)* II-210
Bacitracin; Hydrocortisone Acetate; Neomycin Sulfate; Polymyxin B Sulfate *($225.37)* II-212

BACITRACIN POLYMYXIN
Bacitracin Zinc; Polymyxin B Sulfate *($225.37)* II-211

BACITRACIN POLYMYXIN B
Bacitracin Zinc; Polymyxin B Sulfate *($225.37)* II-211

BACITRACIN ZINC
Bacitracin Zinc; Neomycin Sulfate; Polymyxin B Sulfate *($225.37)* II-211
Bacitracin Zinc; Polymyxin B Sulfate *($225.37)* II-211

BACK PAIN
Colchicine *($6.64)* II-558

BACLOFEN
Baclofen *($225.37)* II-213

BACTEREMIA
Chloramphenicol Sodium Succinate *($20.00)* II-428
Clavulanate Potassium; Ticarcillin Disodium *($43.47)* II-511
Penicillin G Benzathine; Penicillin G Procaine *($362.37)* II-1690
Penicillin G Procaine *($362.37)* II-1694
Penicillin G Sodium *($362.37)* II-1697
Pneumococcal Vaccine *($51.20)* II-1763
Polymyxin B Sulfate *($51.20)* II-1770
Septomonab *($1,576.07)* II-1937
Streptomycin Sulfate *($1,441.75)* II-1976

BACTERIAL MENINGITIS
Meropenem *($5.04)* II-1391

BACTERIAL SEPSIS
Amikacin Sulfate *($123.22)* II-81
Gentamicin Sulfate *($547.50)* II-1009

BACTERIAL VAGINOSIS
Clindamycin Phosphate *($28.17)* II-519
Metronidazole *($0.95)* II-1463

BACTERIOSTATIC SODIUM CHLORIDE
Sodium Chloride *($649.99)* II-1947

BACTERIOSTATIC WATER
Water For Injection, Sterile *($112.78)* II-2205

BACTICIN
Bacitracin *($225.37)* II-210

BACTICORT
Hydrocortisone; Neomycin Sulfate; Polymyxin B Sulfate *($498.80)* II-1121

BACTOCILL
Oxacillin Sodium *($117.73)* II-1641

BACTRIM
Sulfamethoxazole; Trimethoprim *($2.50)* II-1991

BACTROBAN
Mupirocin *($1,061.16)* II-1522

BALANCED SALT SOLUTION
Balanced Salt Solution *($225.37)* II-217

BALDEX
Dexamethasone Sodium Phosphate *($53.32)* II-631

BALDNESS
Minoxidil *($87.60)* II-1486

BALNADE
Chlorpheniramine Maleate; Phenylpropanolamine Hydrochloride *($4.50)* II-453

BALNADE DMH
Caramiphen; Phenylpropanolamine *($538.37)* II-325

BALNEOL-HC
Hydrocortisone *($29.20)* II-1103

BALSA-DERM
Balsam Peru; Castor Oil; Trypsin *($225.37)* II-218

BALSAM PERU
Balsam Peru; Castor Oil; Trypsin *($225.37)* II-218

BALTANE
Brompheniramine Maleate *($395.91)* II-277

BALTANE DC
Brompheniramine Maleate; Codeine Phosphate; Phenylpropanolamine Hydrochloride *($395.91)* II-278

BALTANE DX
Brompheniramine Maleate; Dextromethorphan Hydrobromide; Pseudoephedrine Hydrochloride *($395.91)* II-279

BALTAPP
Brompheniramine Maleate; Phenylpropanolamine Hydrochloride *($395.91)* II-280

BAN-TUSS HC
Hydrocodone Bitartrate; Phenylephrine Hydrochloride; Phenylpropanolamine Hydrochloride; Pyrilamine *($19.45)* II-1102

BANAN
Cefpodoxime Proxetil *($40.90)* II-383

BANCAP
Acetaminophen; Butalbital *($401.06)* II-8

BANCAP-HC
Acetaminophen; Hydrocodone Bitartrate *($6.75)* II-15

BANEX
Guaifenesin; Phenylephrine Hydrochloride; Phenylpropanolamine Hydrochloride *($521.80)* II-1049

BANEX-LA
Guaifenesin; Phenylpropanolamine Hydrochloride *($521.80)* II-1049

BANFLEX
Orphenadrine Citrate *($117.73)* II-1641

BANOPHEN
Diphenhydramine Hydrochloride *($18.50)* II-706
Diphtheria Antitoxin *($18.50)* II-707
Diphtheria Tetanus Toxoids *($18.50)* II-708

BANQUIN
Hydroquinone *($498.80)* II-1129

BANTHINE
Methantheline Bromide *($95.81)* II-1413

BAR-TEST
Barium Sulfate *($225.37)* II-218

BARBASED
Butabarbital Sodium *($8.28)* II-299

BARBIDONNA
Belladonna Alkaloids; Phenobarbital *($225.37)* II-223

BARBITA
Phenobarbital *($0.23)* II-1722

BARBITURATE ANESTHETICS
Methohexital Sodium *($146.18)* II-1420
Thiopental Sodium *($97.78)* II-2060

BARBITURATE ANTICONVULSANTS
Primidone *($9.59)* II-1806

BARBITURATES
Amobarbital Sodium *($375.00)* II-108
Amobarbital; Secobarbital *($2.13)* II-110
Aprobarbital II-152
Butabarbital Sodium *($8.28)* II-299
Hydroxyzine Hydrochloride *($3.10)* II-1135
Hydroxyzine Pamoate *($30.81)* II-1137
Mephobarbital *($44.90)* II-1383
Methohexital Sodium *($146.18)* II-1420
Pentobarbital Sodium *($3.65)* II-1704
Phenobarbital *($0.23)* II-1722
Phenobarbital; Phenytoin *($0.23)* II-1725
Secobarbital Sodium *($0.14)* II-1933
Sodium Bicarbonate *($649.99)* II-1946
Thiopental Sodium *($97.78)* II-2060

BARICON
Barium Sulfate *($225.37)* II-218

BARIUM SULFATE
Barium Sulfate *($225.37)* II-218

BARO-CAT
Barium Sulfate *($225.37)* II-218

BAROBAG ENEMA KIT
Barium Sulfate *($225.37)* II-218

BAROCYL
Sodium Thiosalicylate *($649.99)* II-1956
Sodium Thiosulfate *($649.99)* II-1956

BAROFLAVE
Barium Sulfate *($225.37)* II-218

BAROPHEN
Belladonna Alkaloids; Phenobarbital *($225.37)* II-223

BETA ADRENERGIC STIMULATORS *(cont'd)*
Terbutaline Sulfate *($400.33)* II-2031

BETA BLOCKERS
Acebutolol Hydrochloride *($401.06)* II-6
Atenolol *($16.93)* II-169
Atenolol; Chlorthalidone *($183.41)* II-172
Bendroflumethiazide; Nadolol *($479.02)* II-231
Betaxolol Hydrochloride *($262.94)* II-252
Betaxolol Hydrochloride; Chlorthalidone *($262.94)* II-256
Bisoprolol Fumarate *($277.14)* II-260
Bisoprolol Fumarate; Hydrochlorothiazide *($277.14)* II-263
Carteolol Hydrochloride *($360.36)* II-344
Carvedilol *($360.36)* II-347
Celiprolol Hydrochloride *($90.00)* II-410
Dilevalol *($27.52)* II-696
Esmolol Hydrochloride *($3.60)* II-818
Hydrochlorothiazide; Metoprolol Tartrate *($340.61)* II-1098
Hydrochlorothiazide; Propranolol Hydrochloride *($44.23)* II-1099
Hydrochlorothiazide; Timolol Maleate *($470.92)* II-1100
Labetalol Hydrochloride *($324.41)* II-1248
Levobunolol Hydrochloride *($103.78)* II-1274
Metipranolol Hydrochloride II-1450
Metoprolol Succinate *($162.89)* II-1458
Metoprolol Tartrate *($43.25)* II-1460
Nadolol *($309.04)* II-1532
Penbutolol Sulfate *($362.37)* II-1683
Pindolol *($169.72)* II-1748
Propranolol Hydrochloride *($14.89)* II-1841
Sotalol Hydrochloride *($1,177.85)* II-1961
Timolol Maleate *($203.45)* II-2076

BETA-2
Isoetharine Hydrochloride *($311.27)* II-1211

BETA-C-PLEX
Vitamin B Complex; Vitamin C *($1,272.33)* II-2200

BETA-CAROTENE
Beta-Carotene *($2,848.96)* II-242

BETA-HC
Hydrocortisone *($29.20)* II-1103

BETA-LACTAM ANTIBIOTICS
Aztreonam *($225.37)* II-201
Cefixime *($63.14)* II-361
Cefoxitin Sodium *($255.75)* II-379
Cilastatin Sodium; Imipenem *($618.00)* II-477
Loracarbef *($176.12)* II-1322
Meropenem *($5.04)* II-1391
Piperacillin Sodium; Tazobactam Sodium *($169.72)* II-1755

BETA-VAL
Betamethasone Valerate *($526.07)* II-251

BETABORO OTIC
Acetic Acid *($8.73)* II-26

BETADERM
Betamethasone *($526.07)* II-243
Betamethasone Valerate *($526.07)* II-251

BETADINE
Povidone-Iodine II-1783

BETAGAN
Levobunolol Hydrochloride *($103.78)* II-1274

BETALIN 12
Cyanocobalamin *($155.12)* II-573

BETALIN S
Thiamine Hydrochloride *($97.78)* II-2057

BETAMETHACOT
Betamethasone Valerate *($526.07)* II-251

BETAMETHASONE
Betamethasone *($526.07)* II-243

BETAMETHASONE ACETATE
Betamethasone Acetate; Betamethasone Sodium Phosphate *($526.07)* II-244

BETAMETHASONE DIPROPIONATE
Betamethasone Dipropionate *($526.07)* II-246
Betamethasone Dipropionate; Clotrimazole *($526.07)* II-248

BETAMETHASONE SODIUM PHOSPHATE
Betamethasone Acetate; Betamethasone Sodium Phosphate *($526.07)* II-244
Betamethasone Sodium Phosphate *($526.07)* II-249

BETAMETHASONE VALERATE
Betamethasone Valerate *($526.07)* II-251

BETANATE
Betamethasone Dipropionate *($526.07)* II-246

BETAPACE
Sotalol Hydrochloride *($1,177.85)* II-1961

BETAPEN-VK
Penicillin V Potassium *($3.27)* II-1698

BETASERON
Interferon Beta-1B, Recombinant *($13,140.00)* II-1195

BETATREX
Betamethasone Valerate *($526.07)* II-251

BETAXOLOL HYDROCHLORIDE
Betaxolol Hydrochloride *($262.94)* II-252
Betaxolol Hydrochloride; Chlorthalidone *($262.94)* II-256

BETHANECHOL CHLORIDE
Bethanechol Chloride *($262.94)* II-256

BETHAPRIM
Sulfamethoxazole; Trimethoprim *($2.50)* II-1991

BETIMOL
Timolol *($8.80)* II-2074

BETOPTIC
Betaxolol Hydrochloride *($262.94)* II-252

BEUZOTHIAZOLE
Riluzole *($578.98)* II-1895

BEXIBEE
Cyanocobalamin; Thiamine Hydrochloride *($155.12)* II-577

BEXOPHENE
Aspirin; Caffeine; Propoxyphene Hydrochloride II-160

BIAMINE
Thiamine Hydrochloride *($97.78)* II-2057

BIAVAX II
Mumps And Rubella Virus Vaccine Live *($1,061.16)* II-1521

BIAXIN
Clarithromycin *($43.47)* II-505

BICALUTAMIDE
Bicalutamide *($262.94)* II-257

BICILLIN C-R
Penicillin G Benzathine; Penicillin G Procaine *($362.37)* II-1690

BICILLIN L-A
Penicillin G Benzathine *($362.37)* II-1689

BICITRA
Citric Acid; Sodium Citrate *($4,325.75)* II-502

BICNU
Carmustine *($2,803.56)* II-342

BIFILM
Lactic Acid; Salicylic Acid *($324.41)* II-1251

BILATERAL TORSION
Testosterone Enanthate *($56.37)* II-2039
Testosterone Propionate *($56.37)* II-2041

BILE ACID SEQUESTRANTS
Colestipol Hydrochloride *($760.95)* II-559

BILE SALTS
Bile Salts; Pancreatin; Pepsin *($262.94)* II-257

BILEZYME
Dehydrocholic Acid; Desoxycholic; Enzymes *($2,942.65)* II-611

BILIARY TRACT INFECTIONS
Cefazolin Sodium *($60.75)* II-355

BILTRICIDE
Praziquantel *($616.08)* II-1786

BIO-GAN
Trimethobenzamide Hydrochloride *($71.83)* II-2141

BIO-K
Potassium *($51.20)* II-1775

BIO-SOL EAR
Acetic Acid *($8.73)* II-26

BIO-SOL HC
Acetic Acid; Hydrocortisone *($8.73)* II-27

BIO-STATIN
Nystatin *($252.29)* II-1614

BIO-SYN
Fluocinolone Acetonide *($564.18)* II-940

BIO-TRIPLE
Gramicidin; Neomycin Sulfate; Polymyxin B Sulfate *($107.85)* II-1039

BIO-TROPIN
Somatropin, Biosynthetic *($13,107.15)* II-1958
Sorbitol *($13,107.15)* II-1960

BIO-TUSS C
Codeine Phosphate; Iodinated Glycerol *($154.83)* II-554

BIO-TUSS DM
Dextromethorphan Hydrobromide; Iodinated Glycerol *($53.87)* II-653

BIO-WELL
Lindane *($60.88)* II-1302

BIOCEF
Cephalexin *($2.83)* II-411

BIOCLATE
Antihemophilic Factor (Human) *($2,438.75)* II-145

BIOCORT
Hydrocortisone; Neomycin Sulfate *($498.80)* II-1121

BIOCOT
Hydrocortisone; Neomycin Sulfate; Polymyxin B Sulfate *($498.80)* II-1121

BIOCYCLINE
Tetracycline Hydrochloride *($1.15)* II-2044

BIODEC
Carbinoxamine Maleate; Pseudoephedrine Hydrochloride *($338.35)* II-337

BIODEC-DM
Carbinoxamine Maleate; Dextromethorphan Hydrobromide; Pseudoephedrine Hydrochloride *($338.35)* II-336

BIOGROTON
Chlorthalidone *($14.23)* II-463

BIOHIST-LA
Carbinoxamine Maleate; Pseudoephedrine Hydrochloride *($338.35)* II-337

BIOLOGICAL RESPONSE MODIFIERS
Filgrastim *($2,132.20)* II-915

BIOLOGICALS
Abciximab II-1
Aldesleukin *($35.36)* II-51
Anistreplase, Anisoylated Psac *($2,438.75)* II-140
Digoxin Immune Fab (Ovine) *($27.52)* II-693
Diphtheria; Haemophilus B; Pertussis; Tetanus *($18.50)* II-708
Diphtheria; Pertussis; Tetanus *($18.50)* II-711
Dornase Alfa *($7.50)* II-740
Glatiramer Acetate *($547.50)* II-1014
Haemophilus B Conjugate Vaccine *($87.52)* II-1061
Haemophilus B; Tetanus Toxoid *($87.52)* II-1066
Hepatitis A Vaccine *($87.52)* II-1080
Hepatitis B Immune Globulin *($87.52)* II-1082
Hepatitis B Vaccine, Recombinant *($85.57)* II-1083
Immune Serum Globulin Human *($93.30)* II-1158
Influenza Virus Vaccine *($23.57)* II-1170

BIOLOGICALS *(cont'd)*
Interferon Alfa-2A, Recombinant *($59,200.09)* II-1177
Interferon Alfa-2B, Recombinant *($16,445.33)* II-1181
Interferon Beta-1A *($16,445.33)* II-1192
Interferon Beta-1B, Recombinant *($13,140.00)* II-1195
Lymphocyte Immune Globulin *($713.30)* II-1340
Measles Virus Vaccine Live *($36.79)* II-1349
Measles And Rubella Virus Vaccine Live *($36.79)* II-1351
Measles, Mumps And Rubella Virus Vaccine Live *($36.79)* II-1353
Mumps Virus Vaccine Live *($1,061.16)* II-1519
Pneumococcal Vaccine *($51.20)* II-1763
Polio Vaccine, Oral Live *($51.20)* II-1768
Respiratory Syncytial Virus Immune Globulin *($12.77)* II-1883
Tetanus Toxoid *($56.37)* II-2042
Typhoid Vaccine *($178.41)* II-2155
Varicella Vaccine *($14.00)* II-2176

BIOMOX
Amoxicillin *($7.05)* II-112

BIONADE C
Caramiphen; Phenylpropanolamine *($538.37)* II-325

BIONATE 50-2
Estradiol Cypionate; Testosterone Cypionate *($73.14)* II-828

BIOPHEN
Iodinated Glycerol *($311.27)* II-1201

BIOPHEN-DM
Dextromethorphan Hydrobromide; Iodinated Glycerol *($53.87)* II-653

BIOTIS
Hydrocortisone; Neomycin Sulfate; Polymyxin B Sulfate *($498.80)* II-1121

BIOTRACE
Minerals; Multivitamins *($20.88)* II-1482

BIOTUSS LA
Guaifenesin; Phenylpropanolamine Hydrochloride *($521.80)* II-1049

BIOTUSSIN AC
Codeine Phosphate; Guaifenesin *($3,744.90)* II-552

BIOTUSSIN DAC
Codeine Phosphate; Guaifenesin; Pseudoephedrine Hydrochloride *($3,744.90)* II-553

BIOZYME-C
Collagenase *($760.95)* II-563

BIPERIDEN HYDROCHLORIDE
Biperiden Hydrochloride *($277.14)* II-257

BIPHETAMINE
Amphetamine Resin Complex; Dextroamphetamine Resin Complex *($117.36)* II-118
Amphetamine Sulfate *($117.36)* II-119

BIPHETAP
Brompheniramine Maleate; Phenylpropanolamine Hydrochloride *($395.91)* II-280

BIPHOSPHONATES
Alendronate Sodium *($35.36)* II-55
Etidronate Disodium *($660.59)* II-877
Pamidronate Disodium *($3,200.13)* II-1663

BIPOLAR DISORDER
Carbamazepine *($147.16)* II-326
Divalproex Sodium *($818.18)* II-724
Lithium Carbonate *($14.17)* II-1312
Lithium Citrate *($33.75)* II-1313
Valproate Sodium *($6,363.68)* II-2164
Valproic Acid *($189.50)* II-2169

BISKAPEC
Bismuth; Kaolin; Paregoric; Pectin *($277.14)* II-260

BISMUTH
Bismuth; Hydrocortisone *($277.14)* II-260
Bismuth; Kaolin; Paregoric; Pectin *($277.14)* II-260

BISMUTH CITRATE
Bismuth Citrate; Ranitidine *($277.14)* II-258

BISOPROLOL FUMARATE
Bisoprolol Fumarate *($277.14)* II-260
Bisoprolol Fumarate; Hydrochlorothiazide *($277.14)* II-263

BISORINE
Isoetharine Hydrochloride *($311.27)* II-1211

BITES
Calcium Gluconate *($779.85)* II-316
Rabies Immune Globulin *($82.12)* II-1866

BITEX
Codeine Phosphate; Guaifenesin *($3,744.90)* II-552

BITOLTEROL MESYLATE
Bitolterol Mesylate *($41.77)* II-266

BLACK WIDOW SPIDER
Calcium Gluconate *($779.85)* II-316

BLADDER CARCINOMA
Bcg Live *($225.37)* II-204
Bcg Vaccine *($225.37)* II-206
Cisplatin *($4,325.75)* II-498
Doxorubicin Hydrochloride *($3,775.85)* II-754
Interferon Alfa-2B, Recombinant *($16,445.33)* II-1181
Thiotepa *($8.80)* II-2065

BLADDER PAIN
Pentosan Polysulfate Sodium *($3.65)* II-1707

BLADDER URINE
Neomycin Sulfate; Polymyxin B Sulfate *($149.65)* II-1567

BLADDER, NEUROGENIC
Methantheline Bromide *($95.81)* II-1413
Oxybutynin Chloride *($316.12)* II-1652

BLASTOMA
Carmustine *($2,803.56)* II-342

ERGO-CAFF
Caffeine; Ergotamine Tartrate *($8.28)* II-307
ERGO-CAFF PB
Belladonna; Caffeine; Ergotamine; Pentobarbital *($225.37)* II-225
ERGOBEL
Belladonna; Ergotamine Tartrate; Phenobarbital *($225.37)* II-225
ERGOCALCIFEROL
Ergocalciferol II-803
ERGOLOID MESYLATES
Ergoloid Mesylates II-804
ERGOMAR
Ergotamine Tartrate II-805
ERGOMETRINE
Ergonovine Maleate II-805
ERGONOVINE MALEATE
Ergonovine Maleate II-805
ERGOSTAT
Ergotamine Tartrate II-805
ERGOT PREPARATIONS
Belladonna; Caffeine; Ergotamine; Pentobarbital *($225.37)* II-225
Caffeine; Ergotamine Tartrate *($8.28)* II-307
Dihydroergotamine Mesylate *($27.52)* II-694
Ergotamine Tartrate II-805
Methylergonovine Maleate *($49.27)* II-1438
Methysergide Maleate *($98.55)* II-1449
ERGOTAMINE
Belladonna; Caffeine; Ergotamine; Pentobarbital *($225.37)* II-225
ERGOTAMINE TARTRATE
Belladonna; Ergotamine Tartrate; Phenobarbital *($225.37)* II-225
Caffeine; Ergotamine Tartrate *($8.28)* II-307
Ergotamine Tartrate II-805
ERGOTRATE MALEATE
Ergonovine Maleate II-805
ERIDIUM
Phenazopyridine Hydrochloride *($110.78)* II-1718
ERYCETTE
Erythromycin *($3.39)* II-806
ERYGEL
Erythromycin *($3.39)* II-806
ERYPAR
Erythromycin Stearate *($3.60)* II-817
ERYPED
Erythromycin Ethylsuccinate *($7.46)* II-810
ERYSIPELAS
Penicillin G Benzathine; Penicillin G Procaine *($362.37)* II-1690
Penicillin G Potassium *($362.37)* II-1691
Penicillin G Procaine *($362.37)* II-1694
Penicillin V Potassium *($3.27)* II-1698
ERYSIPELOID
Penicillin G Procaine *($362.37)* II-1694
Penicillin G Sodium *($362.37)* II-1697
ERYTHEMA MULTIFORME
Betamethasone *($526.07)* II-243
Betamethasone Acetate; Betamethasone Sodium Phosphate *($526.07)* II-244
Betamethasone Sodium Phosphate *($526.07)* II-249
Corticotropin *($760.95)* II-564
Cortisone Acetate *($155.12)* II-565
Dexamethasone *($53.32)* II-626
Dexamethasone Acetate *($53.32)* II-629
Dexamethasone Sodium Phosphate *($53.32)* II-631
Hydrocortisone *($29.20)* II-1103
Hydrocortisone Cypionate *($498.80)* II-1115
Hydrocortisone Sodium Phosphate *($498.80)* II-1116
Hydrocortisone Sodium Succinate *($498.80)* II-1118
Methylprednisolone *($98.55)* II-1440
Methylprednisolone Acetate *($98.55)* II-1442
Methylprednisolone Sodium Succinate *($98.55)* II-1446
Prednisolone *($11.13)* II-1790
Prednisolone Sodium Phosphate *($11.13)* II-1793
Prednisone *($9.59)* II-1800
Triamcinolone *($24.63)* II-2115
Triamcinolone Acetonide *($474.79)* II-2117
ERYTHRASMA
Erythromycin Estolate *($3.39)* II-808
Erythromycin Ethylsuccinate *($7.46)* II-810
Erythromycin Lactobionate *($7.46)* II-815
Erythromycin Stearate *($3.60)* II-817
ERYTHRO
Erythromycin Ethylsuccinate *($7.46)* II-810
ERYTHROBLASTOPENIA
Betamethasone *($526.07)* II-243
Betamethasone Acetate; Betamethasone Sodium Phosphate *($526.07)* II-244
Corticotropin *($760.95)* II-564
Cortisone Acetate *($155.12)* II-565
Dexamethasone Acetate *($53.32)* II-629
Hydrocortisone *($29.20)* II-1103
Hydrocortisone Cypionate *($498.80)* II-1115
Methylprednisolone *($98.55)* II-1440
Prednisolone *($11.13)* II-1790
Prednisone *($9.59)* II-1800
Triamcinolone *($24.63)* II-2115
ERYTHROCIN
Erythromycin Lactobionate *($7.46)* II-815
ERYTHROCIN STEARATE
Erythromycin Stearate *($3.60)* II-817
ERYTHROCOT
Erythromycin Stearate *($3.60)* II-817
ERYTHROMYCIN
Benzoyl Peroxide; Erythromycin *($479.02)* II-234
Erythromycin *($3.39)* II-806
ERYTHROMYCIN BASE
Erythromycin *($3.39)* II-806
ERYTHROMYCIN ESTOLATE
Erythromycin Estolate *($3.39)* II-808
ERYTHROMYCIN ETHYLSUCCINATE
Erythromycin Ethylsuccinate *($7.46)* II-810
Erythromycin Ethylsuccinate; Sulfisoxazole Acetyl *($7.46)* II-812
ERYTHROMYCIN GLUCEPTATE
Erythromycin Gluceptate *($7.46)* II-814
ERYTHROMYCIN LACTOBIONATE
Erythromycin Lactobionate *($7.46)* II-815
ERYTHROMYCIN STEARATE
Erythromycin Stearate *($3.60)* II-817
ERYTHROMYCIN W/SULFISOXAZOLE
Erythromycin Ethylsuccinate; Sulfisoxazole Acetyl *($7.46)* II-812
ERYTHROMYCINS
Azithromycin Dihydrate *($30.50)* II-197
Clarithromycin *($43.47)* II-505
Dirithromycin *($18.50)* II-718
Erythromycin *($3.39)* II-806
Erythromycin Estolate *($3.39)* II-808
Erythromycin Ethylsuccinate *($7.46)* II-810
Erythromycin Ethylsuccinate; Sulfisoxazole Acetyl *($7.46)* II-812
Erythromycin Lactobionate *($7.46)* II-815
Erythromycin Stearate *($3.60)* II-817
ERYTHROPOIETIN
Epoetin Alfa II-793
ERYTHROPOISIS ENHANCERS
Epoetin Alfa II-793
Epoetin Beta II-800
ERYTHROZONE
Erythromycin Estolate *($3.39)* II-808
ERYTRA-DERM
Erythromycin *($3.39)* II-806
ERYTRO
Erythromycin *($3.39)* II-806
ERYZOLE
Erythromycin Ethylsuccinate; Sulfisoxazole Acetyl *($7.46)* II-812
ESDINATE
Estradiol Cypionate *($73.14)* II-827
ESDIVAL
Estradiol Valerate *($73.14)* II-831
ESERDINE
Deserpidine; Methyclothiazide *($128.55)* II-618
ESERINE SALICYLATE
Physostigmine Salicylate *($74.46)* II-1739
ESERINE SULFATE
Physostigmine Sulfate *($74.46)* II-1739
ESGIC
Acetaminophen; Butalbital; Caffeine *($401.06)* II-9
ESGIC-PLUS
Acetaminophen; Butalbital; Caffeine *($401.06)* II-9
ESIDRIX
Hydrochlorothiazide *($3.68)* II-1094
ESIMIL
Guanethidine Monosulfate; Hydrochlorothiazide *($181.29)* II-1059
ESKALITH
Lithium Carbonate *($14.17)* II-1312
ESKALITH-CR
Lithium Carbonate *($14.17)* II-1312
ESMOLOL HYDROCHLORIDE
Esmolol Hydrochloride *($3.60)* II-818
ESOPHAGEAL CANCER
Porfimer Sodium *($51.20)* II-1773
ESOPHAGITIS
Bethanechol Chloride *($262.94)* II-256
Cimetidine *($16.78)* II-482
Famotidine *($83.37)* II-892
Lansoprazole *($1,346.36)* II-1260
Methscopolamine Bromide *($656.74)* II-1432
Nizatidine *($57.97)* II-1602
Omeprazole *($101.64)* II-1631
Ranitidine Hydrochloride *($93.96)* II-1871
ESOPHOTRAST
Barium Sulfate *($225.37)* II-218
ESOTROPIA
Demecarium Bromide *($214.32)* II-615
Echothiophate Iodide *($344.26)* II-1
Isoflurophate *($204.98)* II-1212
ESPASMOTEX
Acetaminophen; Atropine; Ethaverine; Salicylic Acid *($401.06)* II-8
ESTAZOLAM
Estazolam *($6.19)* II-820
ESTERIFIED ESTROGENS
Estrogens, Esterified *($107.99)* II-849
ESTINYL
Ethinyl Estradiol *($9.06)* II-861
ESTONE L.A.-20
Estradiol Valerate *($73.14)* II-831
ESTRA-C
Estradiol Cypionate *($73.14)* II-827
ESTRA-L
Estradiol Valerate *($73.14)* II-831
ESTRA-V
Estradiol Valerate *($73.14)* II-831
ESTRACE
Estradiol *($73.14)* II-822
ESTRADERM
Estradiol *($73.14)* II-822
ESTRADIOL
Estradiol *($73.14)* II-822
ESTRADIOL CYPIONATE
Estradiol Cypionate *($73.14)* II-827
Estradiol Cypionate; Testosterone Cypionate *($73.14)* II-828
ESTRADIOL VALERATE
Estradiol Valerate *($73.14)* II-831
Estradiol Valerate; Testosterone Enanthate *($73.14)* II-833
ESTRAGUARD
Dienestrol *($1,946.41)* II-677
ESTRAMUSTINE PHOSPHATE SODIUM
Estramustine Phosphate Sodium *($73.14)* II-834
ESTRATAB
Estrogens, Esterified *($107.99)* II-849
ESTRATEST
Estrogens, Esterified; Methyltestosterone *($107.99)* II-850
ESTRO-A
Estrone *($107.99)* II-851
ESTRO-CYP
Estradiol Cypionate *($73.14)* II-827
ESTRO-L.A.
Estradiol Cypionate *($73.14)* II-827
ESTRO-SPAN
Estradiol Valerate *($73.14)* II-831
ESTRO-SPAN C
Estradiol Cypionate *($73.14)* II-827
ESTROFEM
Estradiol Cypionate *($73.14)* II-827
ESTROGEN
Estradiol Cypionate *($73.14)* II-827
Estradiol Valerate *($73.14)* II-831
Estrogenic Substances *($73.14)* II-835
ESTROGEN DEFICIENCY
Estropipate *($107.99)* II-853
ESTROGENIC SUBSTANCES
Estrogenic Substances *($73.14)* II-835
ESTROGENS
Diethylstilbestrol *($1,946.41)* II-680
Estradiol *($73.14)* II-822
Estradiol Cypionate *($73.14)* II-827
Estradiol Valerate *($73.14)* II-831
Estrogenic Substances *($73.14)* II-835
Estropipate *($107.99)* II-853
Ethinyl Estradiol *($9.06)* II-861
ESTROGENS, CONJUGATED
Estrogens, Conjugated *($107.99)* II-835
Estrogens, Conjugated; Medroxyprogesterone Acetate *($107.99)* II-840
Estrogens, Conjugated; Meprobamate *($107.99)* II-844
Estrogens, Conjugated; Methyltestosterone *($107.99)* II-846
ESTROGENS, ESTERIFIED
Chlordiazepoxide; Estrogens, Esterified *($10.65)* II-434
Estrogens, Esterified *($107.99)* II-849
Estrogens, Esterified; Methyltestosterone *($107.99)* II-850
ESTROJECT-2
Estrogenic Substances *($73.14)* II-835
ESTROJECT-L.A.
Estradiol Cypionate *($73.14)* II-827
ESTRONE
Estrogenic Substances *($73.14)* II-835
Estrone *($107.99)* II-851
ESTRONOL
Estrone *($107.99)* II-851
ESTRONOL-LA
Estradiol Cypionate *($73.14)* II-827
ESTROPIPATE
Estropipate *($107.99)* II-853
ESTROSTEP 21
Ethinyl Estradiol; Norethindrone Acetate *($146.86)* II-870
ESTROSTEP FE
Ethinyl Estradiol; Ferrous Fumarate; Norethindrone Acetate *($57.57)* II-863
ETHACRYNATE SODIUM
Ethacrynic Acid *($310.68)* II-856
ETHACRYNIC ACID
Ethacrynic Acid *($310.68)* II-856
ETHAMBUTOL HYDROCHLORIDE
Ethambutol Hydrochloride *($571.50)* II-857
ETHAMOLIN
Ethanolamine Oleate *($571.50)* II-859
ETHANOLAMINE OLEATE
Ethanolamine Oleate *($571.50)* II-859
ETHANOLAMINES
Clemastine Fumarate *($43.50)* II-515
Diphenhydramine Hydrochloride *($18.50)* II-706
ETHAQUIN
Ethaverine Hydrochloride *($571.50)* II-860

FEMBUTAL
Acetaminophen; Butalbital; Caffeine *($401.06)* II-9
Aspirin; Butalbital; Caffeine II-158

FEMCET
Acetaminophen; Butalbital; Caffeine *($401.06)* II-9

FEMINATE
Estradiol Valerate *($73.14)* II-831

FEMINONE
Ethinyl Estradiol *($9.06)* II-861

FEMOGEN
Estrogens, Esterified *($107.99)* II-849

FEMSTAT
Butoconazole Nitrate *($8.28)* II-302

FEN-A-COUGH
Carbetapentane Tannate; Chlorpheniramine Tannate; Ephedrine Tannate; Phenylephrine Hydrochloride *($147.16)* II-330

FENACLOR
Chlorpheniramine Maleate; Phenindamine Tartrate; Phenylpropanolamine Hydrochloride *($0.76)* II-450

FENAHISTINE DM
Brompheniramine; Dextromethorphan Hydrobromide; Phenylpropanolamine *($395.91)* II-280

FENATUSS
Carbetapentane Tannate; Chlorpheniramine Tannate; Ephedrine Tannate; Phenylephrine Hydrochloride *($147.16)* II-330

FENESIN
Guaifenesin *($93.44)* II-1044

FENEX DM
Dextromethorphan Hydrobromide; Guaifenesin *($47.60)* II-651

FENEX LA
Guaifenesin *($93.44)* II-1044

FENEX-PSE
Guaifenesin; Pseudoephedrine Hydrochloride *($521.80)* II-1050

FENFLURAMINE HYDROCHLORIDE
Fenfluramine Hydrochloride *($311.63)* II-901

FENOPROFEN CALCIUM
Fenoprofen Calcium *($369.56)* II-902

FENTANYL
Fentanyl *($369.56)* II-904

FENTANYL CITRATE
Droperidol; Fentanyl Citrate *($3,775.85)* II-767
Fentanyl Citrate *($369.56)* II-908

FENTANYL ORALET
Fentanyl Citrate *($369.56)* II-908
Ferric Subsulfate *($369.56)* II-913
Ferrous Gluconate *($369.56)* II-913

FENTANYL W/DROPERIDOL
Droperidol; Fentanyl Citrate *($3,775.85)* II-767

FENTEX
Guaifenesin; Phenylephrine Hydrochloride; Phenylpropanolamine Hydrochloride *($521.80)* II-1049

FENTUSS
Guaifenesin; Hydrocodone Bitartrate *($93.44)* II-1045

FEOSTAT
Iron Dextran *($311.27)* II-1209

FERCON
Cyanocobalamin; Folic Acid; Iron Polysaccharide Complex *($155.12)* II-576

FERLIVIT
Ferrous Sulfate; Liver Extract; Vitamin B Complex *($369.56)* II-913

FERNDEX
Dextroamphetamine Sulfate *($47.60)* II-650

FERNISONE
Prednisone *($9.59)* II-1800

FERO-VITA
Ferrous Sulfate; Vitamin B Complex *($369.56)* II-913

FERRIC SUBSULFATE
Ferric Subsulfate *($369.56)* II-913

FERRO-B
Ferrous Sulfate; Vitamin B Complex *($369.56)* II-913

FERRO-CYTE
Ferrous Sulfate; Liver Extract; Vitamin B Complex *($369.56)* II-913

FERROUS FUMARATE
Cyanocobalamin; Ferrous Fumarate; Vitamin C *($155.12)* II-576
Docusate Sodium; Ferrous Fumarate; Folic Acid; Multivitamins *($7.50)* II-736
Ethinyl Estradiol; Ferrous Fumarate; Norethindrone Acetate *($57.57)* II-863

FERROUS GLUCONATE
Cyanocobalamin; Ferrous Gluconate; Folic Acid *($155.12)* II-576
Ferrous Gluconate *($369.56)* II-913

FERROUS SULFATE
Ferrous Sulfate; Folic Acid; Vitamin C *($369.56)* II-913
Ferrous Sulfate; Liver Extract; Vitamin B Complex *($369.56)* II-913
Ferrous Sulfate; Vitamin B Complex *($369.56)* II-913

FERROUS SULFATE CACODYLATE
Ferrous Sulfate Cacodylate *($369.56)* II-913

FERTILITY AGENTS
Bromocriptine Mesylate *($395.91)* II-274
Clomiphene Citrate *($191.69)* II-530
Menotropins *($618.82)* II-1377
Urofollitropin *($178.41)* II-2157

FESTALAN
Pancrelipase *($3,200.13)* II-1667

FETRIN
Cyanocobalamin; Ferrous Fumarate; Vitamin C *($155.12)* II-576

FEVER
Acetaminophen; Codeine Phosphate *($6.75)* II-12
Acetaminophen; Phenylpropanolamine; Phenyltoloxamine *($6.75)* II-20
Acetaminophen; Propoxyphene Hydrochloride *($6.75)* II-21
Acetaminophen; Propoxyphene Napsylate *($8.73)* II-23
Aspirin; Caffeine; Propoxyphene Hydrochloride II-160
Aspirin; Codeine Phosphate II-162
Azithromycin Dihydrate *($30.50)* II-197
Chlorpheniramine Maleate; Phenylephrine Hydrochloride; Phenylpropanolamine; Pyrilamine *($5.13)* II-452
Choline Magnesium Trisalicylate *($14.23)* II-468
Dantrolene Sodium *($2,942.65)* II-603
Erythromycin Ethylsuccinate *($7.46)* II-810
Erythromycin Stearate *($3.60)* II-817
Ibuprofen *($37.01)* II-1141
Methenamine Mandelate *($95.81)* II-1415
Penicillin G Procaine *($362.37)* II-1694
Penicillin G Sodium *($362.37)* II-1697
Sulfadiazine *($82.53)* II-1988
Thiabendazole *($97.78)* II-2056
Typhoid Vaccine *($178.41)* II-2155

FEVER BLISTERS
Acyclovir *($129.02)* II-35
Famciclovir *($129.15)* II-890
Penciclovir *($362.37)* II-1685
Valacyclovir Hydrochloride *($6,363.68)* II-2162

FEXOFENADINE HYDROCHLORIDE
Fexofenadine Hydrochloride *($369.56)* II-913

FIBRATES
Clofibrate *($191.69)* II-528
Gemfibrozil *($547.50)* II-1006

FIBRILLATION
Amiodarone Hydrochloride *($2,240.73)* II-96
Anisindione *($230.36)* II-139
Bretylium Tosylate *($41.77)* II-272
Dicumarol *($5.32)* II-670
Digitoxin *($425.80)* II-687
Digoxin *($27.52)* II-688
Digoxin Immune Fab (Ovine) *($27.52)* II-693
Diltiazem Hydrochloride *($118.80)* II-696
Dobutamine Hydrochloride *($7.50)* II-730
Esmolol Hydrochloride *($3.60)* II-818
Heparin Sodium *($87.52)* II-1077
Quinidine Gluconate *($125.92)* II-1860
Quinidine Polygalacturonate *($752.63)* II-1863
Quinidine Sulfate *($82.12)* II-1863
Verapamil Hydrochloride *($56.72)* II-2186
Warfarin Sodium *($112.78)* II-2200

FIBRINOGEN
Aminocaproic Acid *($24.38)* II-88
Aprotinin Bovine II-152

FIBRINOLYSIN
Chloramphenicol; Desoxyribonuclease; Fibrinolysin *($20.00)* II-430
Desoxyribonuclease; Fibrinolysin *($266.34)* II-625

FIBRINOLYTIC & PROTEOLYTIC
Aminocaproic Acid *($24.38)* II-88
Aprotinin Bovine II-152
Balsam Peru; Castor Oil; Trypsin *($225.37)* II-218
Chloramphenicol; Desoxyribonuclease; Fibrinolysin *($20.00)* II-430
Desoxyribonuclease; Fibrinolysin *($266.34)* II-625
Papain; Urea *($3,200.13)* II-1670
Sutilains *($11.96)* II-2010
Tranexamic Acid *($177.93)* II-2107

FIBROTICS
Aminobenzoate Potassium *($24.38)* II-87

FILGRASTIM
Filgrastim *($2,132.20)* II-915

FILIBON F.A.
Prenatal Formula *($9.59)* II-1803

FINASTERIDE
Finasteride *($713.42)* II-919

FIOREX
Aspirin; Butalbital; Caffeine II-158

FIORGEN
Aspirin; Butalbital; Caffeine II-158

FIORICET
Acetaminophen; Butalbital; Caffeine *($401.06)* II-9

FIORICET W/CODEINE
Acetaminophen; Butalbital; Caffeine; Codeine Phosphate *($401.06)* II-10

FIORINAL
Aspirin; Butalbital; Caffeine II-158

FIORINAL W CODEINE
Aspirin; Butalbital; Caffeine; Codeine Phosphate II-159

FIORMOR
Aspirin; Butalbital; Caffeine II-158

FIORPAP
Acetaminophen; Butalbital; Caffeine *($401.06)* II-9

FIORTAL
Aspirin; Butalbital; Caffeine II-158

FISH TAPEWORM
Cyanocobalamin *($155.12)* II-573

FK-506
Tacrolimus *($7,971.60)* II-2014

FLAGYL
Metronidazole *($0.95)* II-1463

FLAGYL 375
Metronidazole *($0.95)* II-1463

FLAREX
Fluorometholone Acetate *($564.18)* II-944

FLATULENCE
Amylase; Cellulase; Lipase; Protease *($230.36)* II-135
Dexpanthenol *($47.60)* II-647
Enzymes; Hyoscyamine Sulfate; Phenyltoloxamine Citrate *($2.84)* II-788
Pancrelipase *($3,200.13)* II-1667

FLAVOXATE HYDROCHLORIDE
Flavoxate Hydrochloride *($713.42)* II-921

FLAXEDIL
Gallamine Triethiodide *($1,034.77)* II-996

FLECAINIDE ACETATE
Flecainide Acetate *($490.56)* II-922

FLEROXACIN
Fleroxacin *($490.56)* II-925

FLEXAPHEN
Acetaminophen; Chlorzoxazone *($401.06)* II-12

FLEXERIL
Cyclobenzaprine Hydrochloride *($155.12)* II-577

FLEXIBLE COLLODION
Collodion *($760.95)* II-563

FLEXICORT
Hydrocortisone *($29.20)* II-1103

FLEXOJECT
Orphenadrine Citrate *($117.73)* II-1641

FLEXON
Orphenadrine Citrate *($117.73)* II-1641

FLEXOR
Orphenadrine Citrate *($117.73)* II-1641

FLEXTRA
Acetaminophen; Chlorzoxazone *($401.06)* II-12

FLEXTRA-DS
Acetaminophen; Phenyltoloxamine *($6.75)* II-21

FLOLAN
Epoprostenol Sodium II-800

FLOMAX
Tamsulosin Hydrochloride *($1,036.35)* II-2019

FLONASE
Fluticasone Propionate *($534.03)* II-967

FLONASE AQ
Fluticasone Propionate *($534.03)* II-967

FLORINEF
Fludrocortisone Acetate *($86.84)* II-933

FLOROMET
Fluorometholone *($564.18)* II-943

FLORONE
Diflorasone Diacetate *($1,946.41)* II-684

FLORONE E
Diflorasone Diacetate *($1,946.41)* II-684

FLOROPRYL
Isoflurophate *($204.98)* II-1212

FLOSEQUINAN
Flosequinan *($490.56)* II-925

FLOVENT
Fluticasone Propionate *($534.03)* II-967

FLOXIN
Ofloxacin *($43.09)* II-1620

FLOXURIDINE
Floxuridine *($490.56)* II-925

FLOXYFRAL
Fluvoxamine Maleate *($139.06)* II-972

FLU SHIELD
Influenza Virus Vaccine *($23.57)* II-1170

FLUCONAZOLE
Fluconazole *($86.84)* II-926

FLUCYTOSINE
Flucytosine *($86.84)* II-930

FLUDARA
Fludarabine Phosphate *($86.84)* II-931
Fludeoxyglucose, F-18 *($86.84)* II-933

FLUDARABINE PHOSPHATE
Fludarabine Phosphate *($86.84)* II-931

FLUDEOXYGLUCOSE, F-18
Fludeoxyglucose, F-18 *($86.84)* II-933

FLUDROCORTISONE ACETATE
Fludrocortisone Acetate *($86.84)* II-933

FLUEX
Fluocinonide *($564.18)* II-942

FLUIMMUNE
Influenza Virus Vaccine *($23.57)* II-1170

FLUMADINE
Rimantadine Hydrochloride *($578.98)* II-1897

FLUMAZENIL
Flumazenil *($86.84)* II-934

FLUMEZIDE
Bendroflumethiazide; Rauwolfia Serpentina *($479.02)* II-232

FLUNISOLIDE
Flunisolide *($564.18)* II-937

FLUOCET
Fluocinolone Acetonide *($564.18)* II-940

FLUOCIN
Fluocinonide *($564.18)* II-942

MED-HIST-IM
Brompheniramine Maleate *($395.91)* II-277
MED-HIST-PL
Chlorpheniramine Maleate; Pseudoephedrine Hydrochloride *($4.50)* II-454
MED-JEC-40
Methylprednisolone Acetate *($98.55)* II-1442
MED-PRO
Medroxyprogesterone Acetate *($231.11)* II-1362
MEDASULF
Prednisolone Acetate; Sulfacetamide Sodium *($11.13)* II-1792
MEDATUSSIN PLUS
Chlorpheniramine Maleate; Guaifenesin; Phenylpropanolamine *($0.76)* II-447
MEDE-SCAN
Barium Sulfate *($225.37)* II-218
MEDEBAR M
Barium Sulfate *($225.37)* II-218
MEDENT
Guaifenesin; Pseudoephedrine Hydrochloride *($521.80)* II-1050
MEDEX-LA
Guaifenesin; Phenylpropanolamine Hydrochloride *($521.80)* II-1049
MEDI-TUSS DAC
Codeine Phosphate; Guaifenesin; Pseudoephedrine Hydrochloride *($3,744.90)* II-553
MEDI-TUSS W/CODEINE
Codeine Phosphate; Guaifenesin *($3,744.90)* II-552
MEDICORT 50
Prednisolone Acetate *($11.13)* II-1792
MEDIDEX
Dexamethasone Sodium Phosphate *($53.32)* II-631
MEDIDEX-LA
Dexamethasone Acetate *($53.32)* II-629
MEDIDIOL 10
Estradiol Valerate *($73.14)* II-831
MEDIGESIC
Acetaminophen; Butalbital; Caffeine *($401.06)* II-9
MEDIHALER-ISO
Isoproterenol Hydrochloride *($1,019.88)* II-1216
MEDIPAIN 5
Acetaminophen; Hydrocodone Bitartrate *($6.75)* II-15
MEDIPRED
Methylprednisolone Acetate *($98.55)* II-1442
MEDISOL-SP
Hydrocortisone; Neomycin Sulfate; Polymyxin B Sulfate *($498.80)* II-1121
MEDISPAZ
Hyoscyamine Sulfate *($1,532.63)* II-1138
MEDISPAZ-IM
Dicyclomine Hydrochloride *($5.32)* II-672
MEDITEST
Testosterone Cypionate *($56.37)* II-2038
MEDIVERT
Meclizine Hydrochloride *($36.79)* II-1359
MEDLONE 21
Methylprednisolone *($98.55)* II-1440
MEDRALONE
Methylprednisolone Acetate *($98.55)* II-1442
MEDREX
Methylprednisolone Acetate *($98.55)* II-1442
MEDROL
Methylprednisolone *($98.55)* II-1440
MEDROXYPROGESTERONE ACETATE
Estrogens, Conjugated; Medroxyprogesterone Acetate *($107.99)* II-840
Medroxyprogesterone Acetate *($231.11)* II-1362
MEDRYSONE
Medrysone *($231.11)* II-1367
MEDULLOBLASTOMA
Carmustine *($2,803.56)* II-342
MEFENAMIC ACID
Mefenamic Acid *($231.11)* II-1367
MEFLOQUINE HYDROCHLORIDE
Mefloquine Hydrochloride *($231.11)* II-1368
MEFOXIN
Cefoxitin Sodium *($255.75)* II-379
MEGA C A PLUS
Ascorbic Acid II-154
MEGACE
Megestrol Acetate *($231.11)* II-1370
MEGAGESIC
Acetaminophen; Hydrocodone Bitartrate *($6.75)* II-15
MEGALONE
Fleroxacin *($490.56)* II-925
MEGAMOR
Acetaminophen; Hydrocodone Bitartrate *($6.75)* II-15
MEGAPRIN
Aspirin II-157
MEGATON
Vitamin B Complex; Vitamin C *($1,272.33)* II-2200
MEGESTROL ACETATE
Megestrol Acetate *($231.11)* II-1370
MELANEX
Hydroquinone *($498.80)* II-1129
MELANOL
Hydroquinone *($498.80)* II-1129
MELANOMA
Aldesleukin *($35.36)* II-51
Amifostine *($123.22)* II-80
Dacarbazine *($2,942.65)* II-596
Doxorubicin Hydrochloride *($3,775.85)* II-754
Hydroxyurea *($643.75)* II-1133
Interferon Alfa-2A, Recombinant *($59,200.09)* II-1177
Interferon Alfa-2B, Recombinant *($16,445.33)* II-1181
Melphalan *($618.82)* II-1372
Paclitaxel *($3,200.13)* II-1660
Polyribonucleotide *($51.20)* II-1771
MELATE
Antihemophilic Factor (Human) *($2,438.75)* II-145
MELFIAT
Phendimetrazine Tartrate *($110.78)* II-1719
MELLARIL
Thioridazine Hydrochloride *($8.80)* II-2062
MELLARIL-S
Thioridazine Hydrochloride *($8.80)* II-2062
MELPAQUE HP
Hydroquinone *($498.80)* II-1129
MELPHALAN
Melphalan *($618.82)* II-1372
MELQUIN
Hydroquinone *($498.80)* II-1129
MENADIOL SODIUM DIPHOSPHATE
Menadiol Sodium Diphosphate *($618.82)* II-1374
MENADOL
Ibuprofen *($37.01)* II-1141
MENAVAL
Estradiol Valerate *($73.14)* II-831
MENEST
Estrogens, Esterified *($107.99)* II-849
MENI-D
Meclizine Hydrochloride *($36.79)* II-1359
MENINGITIS
Betamethasone *($526.07)* II-243
Betamethasone Acetate; Betamethasone Sodium Phosphate *($526.07)* II-244
Betamethasone Sodium Phosphate *($526.07)* II-249
Cefotaxime Sodium *($63.14)* II-373
Ceftazidime *($155.06)* II-388
Ceftazidime (Arginine) *($155.06)* II-392
Ceftizoxime Sodium *($155.06)* II-398
Ceftriaxone Sodium *($4.00)* II-401
Cefuroxime Sodium *($90.00)* II-407
Cephalothin Sodium *($39.34)* II-415
Chloramphenicol *($20.00)* II-428
Chloramphenicol Sodium Succinate *($20.00)* II-428
Corticotropin *($760.95)* II-564
Cortisone Acetate *($155.12)* II-565
Dexamethasone *($53.32)* II-626
Dexamethasone Acetate *($53.32)* II-629
Dexamethasone Sodium Phosphate *($53.32)* II-631
Dexamethasone Sodium Phosphate; Lidocaine Hydrochloride *($53.32)* II-636
Fluconazole *($86.84)* II-926
Flucytosine *($86.84)* II-930
Gentamicin Sulfate *($547.50)* II-1009
Hydrocortisone *($29.20)* II-1103
Hydrocortisone Cypionate *($498.80)* II-1115
Hydrocortisone Sodium Phosphate *($498.80)* II-1116
Hydrocortisone Sodium Succinate *($498.80)* II-1118
Itraconazole *($970.85)* II-1230
Methylprednisolone *($98.55)* II-1440
Methylprednisolone Acetate *($98.55)* II-1442
Methylprednisolone Sodium Succinate *($98.55)* II-1446
Metronidazole *($0.95)* II-1463
Miconazole *($20.88)* II-1473
Penicillin G Benzathine; Penicillin G Procaine *($362.37)* II-1690
Penicillin G Potassium *($362.37)* II-1691
Penicillin G Procaine *($362.37)* II-1694
Penicillin G Sodium *($362.37)* II-1697
Phenobarbital *($0.23)* II-1722
Polymyxin B Sulfate *($51.20)* II-1770
Prednisolone *($11.13)* II-1790
Prednisolone Sodium Phosphate *($11.13)* II-1793
Prednisone *($9.59)* II-1800
Sulfadiazine *($82.53)* II-1988
Sulfamethoxazole *($82.53)* II-1990
Sulfisoxazole *($156.80)* II-1998
Tobramycin Sulfate *($203.45)* II-2084
Triamcinolone *($24.63)* II-2115
Triamcinolone Acetonide *($474.79)* II-2117
Triamcinolone Diacetate *($474.79)* II-2125
MENINGITIS VACCINE
Meningitis Vaccine *($618.82)* II-1376
MENOJECT-L.A.
Estradiol Cypionate; Testosterone Cypionate *($73.14)* II-828
MENOMUNE-A C Y W-135
Meningitis Vaccine *($618.82)* II-1376
MENOPAK-E
Estrogens, Conjugated *($107.99)* II-835
MENOPAUSE
Chlordiazepoxide; Estrogens, Esterified *($10.65)* II-434
Chlorotrianisene *($10.65)* II-442
Clonidine Hydrochloride *($17.52)* II-539
Estradiol *($73.14)* II-822
Estradiol Cypionate *($73.14)* II-827
Estradiol Cypionate; Testosterone Cypionate *($73.14)* II-828
Estrogens, Conjugated *($107.99)* II-835
Estrogens, Conjugated; Medroxyprogesterone Acetate *($107.99)* II-840
Estrogens, Conjugated; Meprobamate *($107.99)* II-844
Estrogens, Conjugated; Methyltestosterone *($107.99)* II-846
Estrogens, Esterified *($107.99)* II-849
Estrogens, Esterified; Methyltestosterone *($107.99)* II-850
MENOPAUSE *(cont'd)*
Estrone *($107.99)* II-851
Estropipate *($107.99)* II-853
Ethinyl Estradiol *($9.06)* II-861
MENORRHAGIA
Progesterone *($75.00)* II-1819
MENOTROPINS
Menotropins *($618.82)* II-1377
MENRIUM
Chlordiazepoxide; Estrogens, Esterified *($10.65)* II-434
MENSTRUAL PREPARATIONS
Mefenamic Acid *($231.11)* II-1367
MENTANE
Velnacrine *($14.00)* II-2183
MEPENZOLATE BROMIDE
Mepenzolate Bromide *($618.82)* II-1379
MEPERGAN
Meperidine Hydrochloride; Promethazine Hydrochloride *($618.82)* II-1381
MEPERIDINE HCL
Meperidine Hydrochloride *($618.82)* II-1380
MEPERIDINE HYDROCHLORIDE
Meperidine Hydrochloride *($618.82)* II-1380
Meperidine Hydrochloride; Promethazine Hydrochloride *($618.82)* II-1381
MEPHENTERMINE SULFATE
Mephentermine Sulfate *($618.82)* II-1382
MEPHENYTOIN
Mephenytoin *($618.82)* II-1383
MEPHOBARBITAL
Mephobarbital *($44.90)* II-1383
MEPHYTON
Phytonadione *($74.46)* II-1740
Pilocarpine *($74.46)* II-1741
MEPIVACAINE HYDROCHLORIDE
Mepivacaine Hydrochloride *($44.90)* II-1385
MEPRIAM
Meprobamate *($5.04)* II-1388
MEPROBAMATE
Aspirin; Meprobamate II-164
Benactyzine Hydrochloride; Meprobamate *($225.37)* II-227
Estrogens, Conjugated; Meprobamate *($107.99)* II-844
Meprobamate *($5.04)* II-1388
MEPROBAN-400
Meprobamate *($5.04)* II-1388
MEPROGESIC
Aspirin; Meprobamate II-164
MEPRON
Atovaquone *($538.68)* II-176
MEPROSPAN
Meprobamate *($5.04)* II-1388
MEPROZINE
Meperidine Hydrochloride; Promethazine Hydrochloride *($618.82)* II-1381
MERCAPTOPURINE
Mercaptopurine *($5.04)* II-1389
MEROPENEM
Meropenem *($5.04)* II-1391
MERREM IV
Meropenem *($5.04)* II-1391
MERSALO
Mersalyl Sodium; Theophylline *($5.04)* II-1395
MERSALYL SODIUM
Mersalyl Sodium; Theophylline *($5.04)* II-1395
MERUVAX II
Rubella Virus Vaccine Live *($2,708.38)* II-1917
MESALAMINE
Mesalamine *($149.71)* II-1395
MESANTOIN
Mephenytoin *($618.82)* II-1383
MESCLOR
Chlorpheniramine Maleate; Pseudoephedrine Hydrochloride *($4.50)* II-454
MESERPIDINE
Deserpidine; Methyclothiazide *($128.55)* II-618
MESNA
Mesna *($149.71)* II-1400
MESNEX
Mesna *($149.71)* II-1400
MESORIDAZINE BESYLATE
Mesoridazine Besylate *($921.11)* II-1400
MESTINON
Pyridostigmine Bromide *($606.85)* II-1852
MESTRANOL
Mestranol; Norethindrone *($139.56)* II-1402
METABOLIC ACIDOSIS
Dantrolene Sodium *($2,942.65)* II-603
Potassium Chloride *($51.20)* II-1777
Potassium Gluconate *($51.20)* II-1781
Sodium Bicarbonate *($649.99)* II-1946
Sodium Lactate *($649.99)* II-1951
Tromethamine *($178.41)* II-2151
METAHISTINE D
Pheniramine; Phenylpropanolamine; Pyrilamine *($108.64)* II-1722
METAHYDRIN
Trichlormethiazide *($3.70)* II-2130

PHEOCHROMOCYTOMA
Metyrosine *($0.95)* II-1467
Phenoxybenzamine Hydrochloride *($0.23)* II-1726
Propranolol Hydrochloride *($14.89)* II-1841

PHEOCHROMOCYTOMA TEST
Clonidine Hydrochloride *($17.52)* II-539
Phentolamine Mesylate *($0.23)* II-1729

PHERAZINE
Promethazine Hydrochloride *($0.76)* II-1825

PHERAZINE DM
Dextromethorphan Hydrobromide; Promethazine Hydrochloride *($5.49)* II-654

PHERAZINE VC
Phenylephrine Hydrochloride; Promethazine Hydrochloride *($174.65)* II-1734

PHERAZINE VC W/CODEINE
Codeine Phosphate; Phenylephrine Hydrochloride; Promethazine Hydrochloride *($154.83)* II-555

PHERAZINE W/CODEINE
Codeine Phosphate; Promethazine Hydrochloride *($6.64)* II-555

PHILIP
Epinephrine *($64.18)* II-791
Prednisone *($9.59)* II-1800

PHINATATE
Chlorpheniramine Tannate; Phenylephrine Tannate; Pyrilamine Tannate *($4.50)* II-457

PHISO-SCRUB
Hexachlorophene *($85.57)* II-1087

PHISOHEX
Hexachlorophene *($85.57)* II-1087

PHN-OTIC
Hydrocortisone; Neomycin Sulfate; Polymyxin B Sulfate *($498.80)* II-1121

PHONOPHOBIA
Sumatriptan Succinate *($11.96)* II-2003

PHOS-CAL
Calcium Glycerophosphate *($779.85)* II-317

PHOS-FLUR
Acidulated Phosphate Fluoride *($8.73)* II-33
Sodium Fluoride *($649.99)* II-1949

PHOSLO
Calcium Acetate *($779.85)* II-314
Calcium Chloride *($779.85)* II-315
Calcium Gluceptate *($779.85)* II-315
Calcium Gluconate *($779.85)* II-316

PHOSPHATE FLUORIDE
Sodium Fluoride *($649.99)* II-1949

PHOSPHOLINE IODIDE
Echothiophate Iodide *($344.26)* II-1

PHOSPHORUS PREPARATIONS
Potassium Acid Phosphate; Sodium Acid Phosphate *($51.20)* II-1776
Potassium Phosphate; Sodium Phosphate II-1782

PHOTODAMAGED SKIN
Tretinoin *($13.58)* II-2112

PHOTOFRIN
Porfimer Sodium *($51.20)* II-1773

PHOTOPHOBIA
Hydroxypropyl Cellulose *($498.80)* II-1133

PHOTOSENSITIZER
Methoxsalen *($656.74)* II-1429
Trioxsalen *($178.41)* II-2147

PHRENILIN
Acetaminophen; Butalbital *($401.06)* II-8

PHRENILIN FORTE
Acetaminophen; Butalbital *($401.06)* II-8

PHYLLOCONTIN
Aminophylline *($40.29)* II-91

PHYSIOLYTE
Electrolytes; Multiminerals *($12.37)* II-777

PHYSIOSOL
Electrolytes; Multiminerals *($12.37)* II-777

PHYSOSTIGMINE
Physostigmine *($74.46)* II-1739
Physostigmine; Pilocarpine *($74.46)* II-1740

PHYSOSTIGMINE SALICYLATE
Physostigmine Salicylate *($74.46)* II-1739

PHYSOSTIGMINE SULFATE
Physostigmine Sulfate *($74.46)* II-1739

PHYTOMENADIONE
Phytonadione *($74.46)* II-1740
Pilocarpine *($74.46)* II-1741

PHYTONADIONE
Phytonadione *($74.46)* II-1740

PIERRE'S EAR WAX REMOVER
Carbamide Peroxide *($147.16)* II-329

PIGMENTING AGENTS
Hydroquinone *($498.80)* II-1129
Methoxsalen *($656.74)* II-1429
Trioxsalen *($178.41)* II-2147

PILAGAN
Pilocarpine Nitrate *($97.13)* II-1745

PILOCARPINE
Epinephrine; Pilocarpine *($64.18)* II-793
Physostigmine; Pilocarpine *($74.46)* II-1740
Pilocarpine *($74.46)* II-1741

PILOCARPINE HYDROCHLORIDE
Pilocarpine Hydrochloride *($74.46)* II-1742

PILOCARPINE NITRATE
Pilocarpine Nitrate *($97.13)* II-1745

PILOKAIR
Pilocarpine Hydrochloride *($74.46)* II-1742

PILOPINE HS
Pilocarpine Hydrochloride *($74.46)* II-1742

PILOSOL
Pilocarpine Hydrochloride *($74.46)* II-1742

PILOSTAT
Pilocarpine Hydrochloride *($74.46)* II-1742

PIMA
Potassium Iodide II-1782

PIMOZIDE
Pimozide *($97.13)* II-1745

PINDOLOL
Pindolol *($169.72)* II-1748

PINTA
Penicillin G Benzathine *($362.37)* II-1689
Penicillin G Benzathine; Penicillin G Procaine *($362.37)* II-1690
Penicillin G Procaine *($362.37)* II-1694

PINWORM
Mebendazole *($36.79)* II-1355

PIOTEN
Brompheniramine Maleate; Phenylpropanolamine Hydrochloride *($395.91)* II-280

PIPECURONIUM BROMIDE
Pipecuronium Bromide *($169.72)* II-1750

PIPERACILLIN SODIUM
Piperacillin Sodium *($169.72)* II-1752
Piperacillin Sodium; Tazobactam Sodium *($169.72)* II-1755

PIPERIDINES
Astemizole *($55.49)* II-167
Azatadine Maleate *($54.72)* II-191
Cyproheptadine Hydrochloride *($1.56)* II-589
Terfenadine *($56.37)* II-2033

PIPRACIL
Piperacillin Sodium *($169.72)* II-1752

PIRBUTEROL ACETATE
Pirbuterol Acetate II-1758

PIROSAL
Sodium Thiosalicylate *($649.99)* II-1956
Sodium Thiosulfate *($649.99)* II-1956

PIROXICAM
Piroxicam *($51.20)* II-1760

PITOCIN
Oxytocin *($316.12)* II-1658

PITRESSIN
Vasopressin *($14.00)* II-2180

PITUITARY
Corticotropin *($760.95)* II-564
Desmopressin Acetate *($19.63)* II-621
Gonadorelin Acetate *($107.85)* II-1033
Liothyronine Sodium *($60.88)* II-1303
Somatrem *($13,107.15)* II-1956
Somatropin, Biosynthetic *($13,107.15)* II-1958
Vasopressin *($14.00)* II-2180

PITUITARY FUNCTION
Arginine Hydrochloride II-154
Menotropins *($618.82)* II-1377

PITYRIASIS ROSEA
Liver Derivative Complex *($33.75)* II-1315

PITYRIASIS RUBRA PILARIS
Salicylic Acid *($2,708.38)* II-1919

PLACEBO
Lactose *($324.41)* II-1252

PLACIDYL
Ethchlorvynol *($9.06)* II-860

PLAGUE
Doxycycline *($3,775.85)* II-759
Minocycline Hydrochloride *($39.25)* II-1483
Streptomycin Sulfate *($1,441.75)* II-1976

PLAGUE VACCINE
Plague Vaccine *($51.20)* II-1762

PLAQUENIL
Hydroxychloroquine Sulfate *($498.80)* II-1131

PLASMA FRACTIONS, HUMAN
Immune Serum Globulin Human *($93.30)* II-1158
Varicella-Zoster Immune Globulin (Human) *($14.00)* II-2178

PLASMA-LYTE
Electrolytes; Multiminerals *($12.37)* II-777

PLATELET AGGREGATION INHIBITORS
Ticlopidine Hydrochloride *($8.80)* II-2072

PLATELET DEPLETION
Anagrelide Hydrochloride *($230.36)* II-135
Molgramostim *($87.60)* II-1506

PLATELET INHIBITORS
Dipyridamole *($18.50)* II-715

PLATINOL
Cisplatin *($4,325.75)* II-498

PLEGINE
Phendimetrazine Tartrate *($110.78)* II-1719

PLEGISOL
Cardioplegic Solution *($2,803.56)* II-342

PLENDIL
Felodipine *($311.63)* II-899

PLICAMYCIN
Plicamycin *($51.20)* II-1762

PLURI-B
Vitamin B Complex *($1,272.33)* II-2200

PMB
Estrogens, Conjugated; Meprobamate *($107.99)* II-844

PNEUMAX
Guaifenesin; Phenylephrine Hydrochloride *($521.80)* II-1048

PNEUMOCOCCAL DISEASE
Pneumococcal Vaccine *($51.20)* II-1763

PNEUMOCOCCAL INFECTIONS
Penicillin G Potassium *($362.37)* II-1691
Penicillin G Procaine *($362.37)* II-1694
Penicillin G Sodium *($362.37)* II-1697

PNEUMOCOCCAL VACCINE
Pneumococcal Vaccine *($51.20)* II-1763

PNEUMOCONIOSIS
Betamethasone Acetate; Betamethasone Sodium Phosphate *($526.07)* II-244
Cortisone Acetate *($155.12)* II-565
Dexamethasone *($53.32)* II-626
Dexamethasone Acetate *($53.32)* II-629
Dexamethasone Sodium Phosphate *($53.32)* II-631
Dexamethasone Sodium Phosphate; Lidocaine Hydrochloride *($53.32)* II-636
Hydrocortisone *($29.20)* II-1103
Hydrocortisone Sodium Phosphate *($498.80)* II-1116
Hydrocortisone Sodium Succinate *($498.80)* II-1118
Methylprednisolone *($98.55)* II-1440
Methylprednisolone Acetate *($98.55)* II-1442
Methylprednisolone Sodium Succinate *($98.55)* II-1446
Prednisolone Sodium Phosphate *($11.13)* II-1793
Prednisone *($9.59)* II-1800
Triamcinolone *($24.63)* II-2115
Triamcinolone Acetonide *($474.79)* II-2117
Triamcinolone Diacetate *($474.79)* II-2125

PNEUMOCYSTIS CARINII PNEUMONIA
Atovaquone *($538.68)* II-176
Eflornithine Hydrochloride *($12.37)* II-776
Pentamidine Isethionate *($3.27)* II-1701
Prednisone *($9.59)* II-1800
Sulfamethoxazole; Trimethoprim *($2.50)* II-1991
Trimetrexate Glucuronate *($71.83)* II-2143

PNEUMOMIST
Guaifenesin *($93.44)* II-1044

PNEUMONIA
Atovaquone *($538.68)* II-176
Azithromycin Dihydrate *($30.50)* II-197
Aztreonam *($225.37)* II-201
Bacitracin *($225.37)* II-210
Cefaclor *($117.48)* II-349
Cefamandole Nafate *($60.75)* II-353
Cefmetazole Sodium *($63.14)* II-364
Cefotaxime Sodium *($63.14)* II-373
Cefoxitin Sodium *($255.75)* II-379
Cefpodoxime Proxetil *($40.90)* II-383
Ceftazidime *($155.06)* II-388
Ceftazidime (Arginine) *($155.06)* II-392
Cefuroxime Sodium *($90.00)* II-407
Cephradine *($8.76)* II-418
Clarithromycin *($43.47)* II-505
Clindamycin Phosphate *($28.17)* II-519
Demeclocycline Hydrochloride *($214.32)* II-616
Dexamethasone; Tobramycin *($53.32)* II-640
Dirithromycin *($18.50)* II-718
Doxycycline *($3,775.85)* II-759
Erythromycin *($3.39)* II-806
Erythromycin Estolate *($3.39)* II-808
Erythromycin Ethylsuccinate *($7.46)* II-810
Erythromycin Gluceptate *($7.46)* II-814
Erythromycin Lactobionate *($7.46)* II-815
Erythromycin Stearate *($3.60)* II-817
Fluconazole *($86.84)* II-926
Gentamicin Sulfate *($547.50)* II-1009
Lidocaine; Oxytetracycline Hydrochloride *($60.88)* II-1298
Loracarbef *($176.12)* II-1322
Metronidazole *($0.95)* II-1463
Minocycline Hydrochloride *($39.25)* II-1483
Ofloxacin *($43.09)* II-1620
Oxytetracycline Hydrochloride *($316.12)* II-1656
Penicillin G Benzathine; Penicillin G Procaine *($362.37)* II-1690
Penicillin G Procaine *($362.37)* II-1694
Penicillin G Sodium *($362.37)* II-1697
Piperacillin Sodium; Tazobactam Sodium *($169.72)* II-1755
Pneumococcal Vaccine *($51.20)* II-1763
Streptomycin Sulfate *($1,441.75)* II-1976
Tetracycline Hydrochloride *($1.15)* II-2044
Trimetrexate Glucuronate *($71.83)* II-2143
Troleandomycin *($178.41)* II-2151

PNEUMONITIS
Betamethasone *($526.07)* II-243
Clindamycin Hydrochloride *($28.17)* II-517
Corticotropin *($760.95)* II-564
Cortisone Acetate *($155.12)* II-565
Dexamethasone *($53.32)* II-626
Hydrocortisone *($29.20)* II-1103
Hydrocortisone Cypionate *($498.80)* II-1115
Methylprednisolone *($98.55)* II-1440
Prednisolone *($11.13)* II-1790
Prednisone *($9.59)* II-1800
Ticarcillin Disodium *($8.80)* II-2070
Triamcinolone *($24.63)* II-2115
Triamcinolone Acetonide *($474.79)* II-2117

PNEUMOTUSSIN HC
Guaifenesin; Hydrocodone Bitartrate *($93.44)* II-1045

PNEUMOVAX 23
Pneumococcal Vaccine *($51.20)* II-1763

PNU-IMUNE 23
Pneumococcal Vaccine *($51.20)* II-1763

PODOBEN
Podophyllum Resin *($51.20)* II-1766

PODOCON-25
Podophyllum Resin *($51.20)* II-1766

PODODERM
Podophyllum Resin ($51.20) II-1766
PODOFILOX
Podofilox ($51.20) II-1765
PODOFIN
Podophyllum Resin ($51.20) II-1766
PODOPHYLLUM RESIN
Podophyllum Resin ($51.20) II-1766
POISON IVY
Poison Ivy Extract ($51.20) II-1766
POISON IVY EXTRACT
Poison Ivy Extract ($51.20) II-1766
POISONING
Atropine Sulfate ($538.68) II-181
Edetate Calcium Disodium ($12.37) II-773
Hyoscyamine Sulfate ($1,532.63) II-1138
Sodium Bicarbonate ($649.99) II-1946
POLARAMINE
Dexchlorpheniramine Maleate ($47.60) II-641
Dexchlorpheniramine; Guaifenesin; Pseudoephedrine ($47.60) II-643
POLIO VACCINE, INACTIVATED
Polio Vaccine, Inactivated ($51.20) II-1766
POLIO VACCINE, ORAL LIVE
Polio Vaccine, Oral Live ($51.20) II-1768
POLIOMYELITIS
Polio Vaccine, Inactivated ($51.20) II-1766
Polio Vaccine, Oral Live ($51.20) II-1768
POLIOVAX
Polio Vaccine, Inactivated ($51.20) II-1766
POLOCAINE
Mepivacaine Hydrochloride ($44.90) II-1385
POLY HIST FORTE
Chlorpheniramine Maleate; Phenylephrine Hydrochloride; Phenylpropanolamine; Pyrilamine ($5.13) II-452
POLY OTIC
Hydrocortisone; Neomycin Sulfate; Polymyxin B Sulfate ($498.80) II-1121
POLY TUSSIN
Ammonium Chloride; Hydrocodone ($375.00) II-107
POLY-D
Pheniramine; Phenylpropanolamine; Pyrilamine ($108.64) II-1722
Pheniramine; Phenyltoloxamine; Pyrilamine ($108.64) II-1722
POLY-DEX
Dexamethasone; Neomycin Sulfate; Polymyxin B Sulfate ($53.32) II-640
POLY-DM
Brompheniramine; Dextromethorphan Hydrobromide; Phenylpropanolamine ($395.91) II-280
POLY-FERROUS SULFATE
Folic Acid; Multivitamins; Poly-Ferrous Sulfate ($139.06) II-977
POLY-HISTINE
Pheniramine; Phenyltoloxamine; Pyrilamine ($108.64) II-1722
POLY-HISTINE CS
Brompheniramine Maleate; Codeine Phosphate; Phenylpropanolamine Hydrochloride ($395.91) II-278
POLY-HISTINE-D
Pheniramine; Phenylpropanolamine; Pyrilamine ($108.64) II-1722
POLY-HISTINE-DM
Brompheniramine; Dextromethorphan Hydrobromide; Phenylpropanolamine ($395.91) II-280
POLY-PRED
Neomycin Sulfate; Polymyxin B Sulfate; Prednisolone Acetate ($149.65) II-1568
POLY-RX
Polymyxin B Sulfate ($51.20) II-1770
POLY-TEARS
Dextran ($47.60) II-649
POLY-TUSSIN
Chlorpheniramine Maleate; Hydrocodone; Phenylephrine Hydrochloride ($0.76) II-449
POLY-TUSSIN XP
Guaifenesin; Hydrocodone Bitartrate; Pseudoephedrine Hydrochloride ($93.44) II-1046
POLYCILLIN
Ampicillin ($3.76) II-126
POLYCILLIN-N
Ampicillin Sodium ($3.76) II-128
POLYCILLIN-PRB
Ampicillin Trihydrate; Probenecid ($230.36) II-132
POLYCIN-B
Bacitracin Zinc; Polymyxin B Sulfate ($225.37) II-211
POLYCITRA K
Citric Acid; Potassium Citrate ($4,325.75) II-502
POLYCYSTIC OVARIAN SYNDROME
Urofollitropin ($178.41) II-2157
POLYCYTHEMIA VERA
Mechlorethamine Hydrochloride ($36.79) II-1357
POLYDIPSIA
Desmopressin Acetate ($19.63) II-621
POLYETHYLENE GLYCOL 3350
Polyethylene Glycol 3350; Potassium Chloride; Sodium Bicarbonate; Sodium Chloride; Sodium Sulfate ($51.20) II-1769
POLYGELINE
Urea ($178.41) II-2157
POLYGESIC
Acetaminophen; Hydrocodone Bitartrate ($6.75) II-15
POLYHISTAMINE
Pheniramine; Phenylpropanolamine; Pyrilamine ($108.64) II-1722
POLYHISTAMINE PPA
Pheniramine; Phenylpropanolamine; Pyrilamine ($108.64) II-1722
POLYMOX
Amoxicillin ($7.05) II-112
POLYMYXIN B SULFATE
Bacitracin Zinc; Neomycin Sulfate; Polymyxin B Sulfate ($225.37) II-211
Bacitracin Zinc; Polymyxin B Sulfate ($225.37) II-211
Bacitracin; Hydrocortisone Acetate; Neomycin Sulfate; Polymyxin B Sulfate ($225.37) II-212
Chloramphenicol; Hydrocortisone Acetate; Polymyxin B Sulfate ($20.00) II-430
Dexamethasone; Neomycin Sulfate; Polymyxin B Sulfate ($53.32) II-640
Gramicidin; Neomycin Sulfate; Polymyxin B Sulfate ($107.85) II-1039
Hydrocortisone Acetate; Neomycin Sulfate; Polymyxin B Sulfate ($29.20) II-1110
Hydrocortisone; Neomycin Sulfate; Polymyxin B Sulfate ($498.80) II-1121
Hydrocortisone; Polymyxin B Sulfate ($498.80) II-1123
Neomycin Sulfate; Polymyxin B Sulfate ($149.65) II-1567
Neomycin Sulfate; Polymyxin B Sulfate; Prednisolone Acetate ($149.65) II-1568
Oxytetracycline Hydrochloride; Polymyxin B Sulfate ($316.12) II-1658
Polymyxin B Sulfate ($51.20) II-1770
Polymyxin B Sulfate; Trimethoprim Sulfate ($51.20) II-1771
POLYMYXINS
Colistimethate Sodium ($760.95) II-561
Neomycin Sulfate; Polymyxin B Sulfate ($149.65) II-1567
Oxytetracycline Hydrochloride ($316.12) II-1656
Polymyxin B Sulfate ($51.20) II-1770
POLYRIBONUCLEOTIDE
Polyribonucleotide ($51.20) II-1771
POLYSACCHARIDE-IRON COMPLEX
Cyanocobalamin; Folic Acid; Iron Polysaccharide Complex ($155.12) II-576
Folic Acid; Multivitamins; Poly-Ferrous Sulfate ($139.06) II-977
POLYSPORIN
Bacitracin Zinc; Polymyxin B Sulfate ($225.37) II-211
POLYTHIAZIDE
Polythiazide ($51.20) II-1771
Polythiazide; Prazosin Hydrochloride ($51.20) II-1772
Polythiazide; Reserpine ($51.20) II-1772
POLYTINE CS
Brompheniramine Maleate; Codeine Phosphate; Phenylpropanolamine Hydrochloride ($395.91) II-278
POLYTINE DM
Brompheniramine; Dextromethorphan Hydrobromide; Phenylpropanolamine ($395.91) II-280
POLYTINIC
Ferrous Sulfate; Folic Acid; Vitamin C ($369.56) II-913
POLYTRACIN
Bacitracin Zinc; Polymyxin B Sulfate ($225.37) II-211
POLYTRIM
Polymyxin B Sulfate; Trimethoprim Sulfate ($51.20) II-1771
POLYURIA
Desmopressin Acetate ($19.63) II-621
PONDIMIN
Fenfluramine Hydrochloride ($311.63) II-901
PONSTEL
Mefenamic Acid ($231.11) II-1367
PONTOCAINE
Tetracaine Hydrochloride ($56.37) II-2043
PORFIMER SODIUM
Porfimer Sodium ($51.20) II-1773
PORPHYRIA
Beta-Carotene ($2,848.96) II-242
Chlorpromazine Hydrochloride ($22.10) II-457
PORTALAC
Lactulose ($324.41) II-1252
POSITUSS
Ammonium Chloride; Hydrocodone ($375.00) II-107
POSTURAL HYPOTENSION
Midodrine Hydrochloride ($20.88) II-1477
POTABA
Aminobenzoate Potassium ($24.38) II-87
POTASALAN
Potassium Chloride ($51.20) II-1777
POTASSIUM
Potassium ($51.20) II-1775
Potassium (Gluconate And Citrate) ($51.20) II-1775
POTASSIUM ACETATE
Potassium Acetate ($51.20) II-1775
POTASSIUM ACID PHOSPHATE
Potassium Acid Phosphate ($51.20) II-1776
Potassium Acid Phosphate; Sodium Acid Phosphate ($51.20) II-1776
POTASSIUM BICARBONATE
Potassium ($51.20) II-1775
Potassium Bicarbonate ($51.20) II-1777
POTASSIUM CHLORIDE
Polyethylene Glycol 3350; Potassium Chloride; Sodium Bicarbonate; Sodium Chloride; Sodium Sulfate ($51.20) II-1769
POTASSIUM CHLORIDE (cont'd)
Potassium Chloride ($51.20) II-1777
POTASSIUM CITRATE
Citric Acid; Potassium Citrate ($4,325.75) II-502
Codeine Phosphate; Phenylephrine Hydrochloride; Pheniramine; Potassium Citrate ($154.83) II-554
Hydrocodone; Pheniramine; Potassium Citrate; Pyrilamine; Vitamin C ($19.45) II-1103
Potassium Citrate ($51.20) II-1781
Potassium Citrate; Sodium Citrate ($51.20) II-1781
POTASSIUM GLUCONATE
Potassium Gluconate ($51.20) II-1781
POTASSIUM IODIDE
Aminophylline; Ephedrine; Phenobarbital; Potassium Iodide ($40.29) II-94
Chlorpheniramine Maleate; Codeine Phosphate; Phenylephrine Hydrochloride; Potassium Iodide ($0.76) II-446
Ephedrine Hydrochloride; Potassium Iodide; Phenobarbital; Theophylline ($2.84) II-790
Ephedrine; Potassium Iodide ($2.84) II-791
Potassium Iodide II-1782
Potassium Iodide; Theophylline Anhydrous II-1782
POTASSIUM PERMANGANATE
Potassium Permanganate II-1782
POTASSIUM PHOSPHATE
Potassium Phosphate II-1782
Potassium Phosphate; Sodium Phosphate II-1782
POTASSIUM SALICYLATE
Aminobenzoate Potassium; Potassium Salicylate ($24.38) II-87
POTASSIUM SPARING DIURETICS
Amiloride Hydrochloride ($93.07) II-83
Amiloride Hydrochloride; Hydrochlorothiazide ($24.38) II-85
Hydrochlorothiazide; Spironolactone ($44.23) II-1099
Hydrochlorothiazide; Triamterene ($19.45) II-1100
Spironolactone ($33.06) II-1968
Triamterene ($289.08) II-2127
POTASSIUM SUPPLEMENTS
Potassium ($51.20) II-1775
Potassium (Gluconate And Citrate) ($51.20) II-1775
Potassium Acetate ($51.20) II-1775
Potassium Chloride ($51.20) II-1777
Potassium Gluconate ($51.20) II-1781
POTASSIUM-REMOVING RESINS
Sodium Polystyrene Sulfonate ($649.99) II-1954
POVIDONE-IODINE
Povidone-Iodine II-1783
POXI
Chlordiazepoxide Hydrochloride ($10.65) II-432
PRAMILET-FA
Prenatal Formula ($9.59) II-1803
PRAMOSONE
Hydrocortisone Acetate; Pramoxine Hydrochloride ($29.20) II-1112
PRAMOXINE HYDROCHLORIDE
Chloroxylenol; Hydrocortisone; Pramoxine Hydrochloride ($10.65) II-443
Hydrocortisone Acetate; Pramoxine Hydrochloride ($29.20) II-1112
PRASTERONE
Dehydroepiandrosterone ($2,942.65) II-612
PRAVACHOL
Pravastatin Sodium ($616.08) II-1783
PRAVASTATIN SODIUM
Pravastatin Sodium ($616.08) II-1783
PRAZIQUANTEL
Praziquantel ($616.08) II-1786
PRAZOSIN HYDROCHLORIDE
Polythiazide; Prazosin Hydrochloride ($51.20) II-1772
Prazosin Hydrochloride ($45.55) II-1787
PRE-OP
Hexachlorophene ($85.57) II-1087
PRECARE
Prenatal Formula ($9.59) II-1803
PRECEF
Ceforanide ($63.14) II-371
PRECOCIOUS PUBERTY
Histrelin Acetate ($85.57) II-1088
Leuprolide Acetate ($1,346.36) II-1266
Nafarelin Acetate ($309.04) II-1534
PRECOSE
Acarbose II-4
PRED FORTE
Prednisolone Acetate ($11.13) II-1792
PRED MILD
Prednisolone Acetate ($11.13) II-1792
PRED-G
Gentamicin Sulfate; Prednisolone Acetate ($547.50) II-1013
PRED-IDE
Prednisolone Acetate; Sulfacetamide Sodium ($11.13) II-1792
PREDACORTEN
Methylprednisolone Acetate ($98.55) II-1442
PREDAIR
Prednisolone Sodium Phosphate ($11.13) II-1793
PREDAIR-A
Prednisolone Acetate ($11.13) II-1792
Prednisolone Sodium Phosphate ($11.13) II-1793
PREDAJECT-50
Prednisolone Acetate ($11.13) II-1792

PRURITUS *(cont'd)*
Fluocinolone Acetonide *($564.18)* II-940
Fluocinonide *($564.18)* II-942
Gramicid; Neomycin; Nystatin; Triamcinolone *($107.85)* II-1039
Guaifenesin; Hydrocodone Bitartrate; Pheniramine Maleate; Phenylpropanolamine Hydrochloride *($93.44)* II-1046
Hydrocortisone *($29.20)* II-1103
Hydrocortisone Acetate *($29.20)* II-1106
Hydrocortisone Acetate; Pramoxine Hydrochloride *($29.20)* II-1112
Hydrocortisone Acetate; Urea *($29.20)* II-1113
Hydrocortisone Butyrate *($29.20)* II-1114
Hydrocortisone Valerate *($498.80)* II-1120
Hydrocortisone; Iodoquinol *($498.80)* II-1121
Hydroxyzine Hydrochloride *($3.10)* II-1135
Hydroxyzine Pamoate *($30.81)* II-1137
Lidocaine *($60.88)* II-1290
Lidocaine Hydrochloride *($60.88)* II-1293
Mometasone Furoate *($87.60)* II-1508
Nystatin; Triamcinolone Acetonide *($252.29)* II-1617
Pseudoephedrine Hydrochloride; Terfenadine *($63.54)* II-1850
Terfenadine *($56.37)* II-2033
Triamcinolone Acetonide *($474.79)* II-2117
Trimeprazine Tartrate *($71.83)* II-2140

PSENCLOR-SA
Chlorpheniramine Maleate; Pseudoephedrine Hydrochloride *($4.50)* II-454

PSEUBROM
Brompheniramine Maleate; Pseudoephedrine Hydrochloride *($395.91)* II-280

PSEUBROM-PD
Brompheniramine Maleate; Pseudoephedrine Hydrochloride *($395.91)* II-280

PSEUDO G/PSI
Guaifenesin; Pseudoephedrine Hydrochloride *($521.80)* II-1050

PSEUDO-CAR DM
Carbinoxamine Maleate; Dextromethorphan Hydrobromide; Pseudoephedrine Hydrochloride *($338.35)* II-336

PSEUDO-CHLOR
Chlorpheniramine Maleate; Pseudoephedrine Hydrochloride *($4.50)* II-454

PSEUDO-G/PSI
Guaifenesin; Pseudoephedrine Hydrochloride *($521.80)* II-1050

PSEUDOCOT-C
Chlorpheniramine Maleate; Pseudoephedrine Hydrochloride *($4.50)* II-454

PSEUDOCOT-G
Guaifenesin; Pseudoephedrine Hydrochloride *($521.80)* II-1050

PSEUDOCOT-T
Pseudoephedrine Hydrochloride; Triprolidine Hydrochloride *($63.54)* II-1850
Pyrazinamide *($606.85)* II-1851

PSEUDOEPHEDRINE
Butabarbital; Guaifenesin; Pseudoephedrine; Theophylline *($8.28)* II-301
Chlorpheniramine Maleate; Guaifenesin; Pseudoephedrine *($0.76)* II-448
Chlorpheniramine Maleate; Phenylpropanolamine; Pseudoephedrine *($4.50)* II-454
Dexbrompheniramine; Pseudoephedrine *($53.32)* II-641
Dexchlorpheniramine; Guaifenesin; Pseudoephedrine *($47.60)* II-643
Dextromethorphan Hydrobromide; Guaifenesin; Pseudoephedrine *($47.60)* II-652
Dextromethorphan Hydrobromide; Pseudoephedrine *($5.49)* II-655
Guaifenesin; Pseudoephedrine; Theophylline *($521.80)* II-1052
Hydrocodone; Pseudoephedrine *($19.45)* II-1103
Phenylephrine Hydrochloride; Phenylpropanolamine; Pseudoephedrine *($174.65)* II-1734

PSEUDOEPHEDRINE DX
Brompheniramine Maleate; Dextromethorphan Hydrobromide; Pseudoephedrine Hydrochloride *($395.91)* II-279

PSEUDOEPHEDRINE HYDROCHLORIDE
Acrivastine; Pseudoephedrine Hydrochloride II-33
Brompheniramine Maleate; Dextromethorphan Hydrobromide; Pseudoephedrine Hydrochloride *($395.91)* II-279
Brompheniramine Maleate; Pseudoephedrine Hydrochloride *($395.91)* II-280
Carbinoxamine Maleate; Dextromethorphan Hydrobromide; Pseudoephedrine Hydrochloride *($338.35)* II-336
Carbinoxamine Maleate; Pseudoephedrine Hydrochloride *($338.35)* II-337
Chlorpheniramine Maleate; Codeine Phosphate; Pseudoephedrine Hydrochloride *($0.76)* II-447
Chlorpheniramine Maleate; Dextromethorphan Hydrobromide; Guaifenesin; Phenpropanolamine; Pseudoephedrine Hydrochloride *($0.76)* II-447
Chlorpheniramine Maleate; Hydrocodone Bitartrate; Pseudoephedrine Hydrochloride *($0.76)* II-448
Chlorpheniramine Maleate; Pseudoephedrine Hydrochloride *($4.50)* II-454
Codeine Phosphate; Guaifenesin; Pseudoephedrine Hydrochloride *($3,744.90)* II-553
Codeine Phosphate; Pseudoephedrine Hydrochloride *($6.64)* II-556
Codeine Phosphate; Pseudoephedrine Hydrochloride; Triprolidine Hydrochloride *($6.64)* II-556
Guaifenesin; Hydrocodone Bitartrate; Pseudoephedrine Hydrochloride *($93.44)* II-1046
Guaifenesin; Pseudoephedrine Hydrochloride *($521.80)* II-1050
Pseudoephedrine Hydrochloride *($125.52)* II-1849
Pseudoephedrine Hydrochloride; Terfenadine *($63.54)* II-1850
Pseudoephedrine Hydrochloride; Triprolidine Hydrochloride *($63.54)* II-1850

PSEUDOEPHEDRINE SULFATE
Azatadine Maleate; Pseudoephedrine Sulfate *($54.72)* II-192
Loratadine; Pseudoephedrine Sulfate *($65.43)* II-1326

PSEUDOEPHEDRINE W/CODEINE
Codeine Phosphate; Pseudoephedrine Hydrochloride *($6.64)* II-556

PSEUDOFEN
Guaifenesin; Pseudoephedrine Hydrochloride *($521.80)* II-1050

PSEUDOFEN-PD
Guaifenesin; Pseudoephedrine Hydrochloride *($521.80)* II-1050

PSEUDOGEST
Dextromethorphan Hydrobromide; Guaifenesin; Pseudoephedrine *($47.60)* II-652
Pseudoephedrine Hydrochloride *($125.52)* II-1849

PSEUDOHYPOPARATHYROIDISM
Calcitriol *($779.85)* II-312

PSEUDOPHEDRINE CARBINOXAMINE
Carbinoxamine Maleate; Pseudoephedrine Hydrochloride *($338.35)* II-337

PSEUDOPHEDRINE W/CARBINOXAMINE
Carbinoxamine Maleate; Pseudoephedrine Hydrochloride *($338.35)* II-337

PSITTACOSIS
Demeclocycline Hydrochloride *($214.32)* II-616
Doxycycline *($3,775.85)* II-759
Minocycline Hydrochloride *($39.25)* II-1483
Oxytetracycline Hydrochloride *($316.12)* II-1656

PSORCON
Diflorasone Diacetate *($1,946.41)* II-684

PSORIASIS
Acitretin *($8.73)* II-33
Amcinonide *($123.22)* II-79
Anthralin *($2,438.75)* II-143
Betamethasone *($526.07)* II-243
Betamethasone Acetate; Betamethasone Sodium Phosphate *($526.07)* II-244
Betamethasone Sodium Phosphate *($526.07)* II-249
Calcipotriene *($8.28)* II-309
Clobetasol Propionate *($28.17)* II-524
Coal Tar *($3,744.90)* II-550
Corticotropin *($760.95)* II-564
Cortisone Acetate *($155.12)* II-565
Cyclosporine *($3,863.16)* II-582
Dexamethasone *($53.32)* II-626
Dexamethasone Acetate *($53.32)* II-629
Dexamethasone Sodium Phosphate *($53.32)* II-631
Dexamethasone Sodium Phosphate; Lidocaine Hydrochloride *($53.32)* II-636
Etretinate *($1,741.30)* II-886
Hydrocortisone *($29.20)* II-1103
Hydrocortisone Cypionate *($498.80)* II-1115
Hydrocortisone Sodium Phosphate *($498.80)* II-1116
Hydrocortisone Sodium Succinate *($498.80)* II-1118
Methotrexate Sodium *($656.74)* II-1422
Methoxsalen *($656.74)* II-1429
Methylprednisolone *($98.55)* II-1440
Methylprednisolone Acetate *($98.55)* II-1442
Methylprednisolone Sodium Succinate *($98.55)* II-1446
Prednisolone *($11.13)* II-1790
Prednisolone Sodium Phosphate *($11.13)* II-1793
Prednisone *($9.59)* II-1800
Salicylic Acid *($2,708.38)* II-1919
Triamcinolone *($24.63)* II-2115
Triamcinolone Acetonide *($474.79)* II-2117
Triamcinolone Diacetate *($474.79)* II-2125

PSORION
Betamethasone Dipropionate *($526.07)* II-246

PSYCHOSTIMULANTS
Amphetamine Resin Complex; Dextroamphetamine Resin Complex *($117.36)* II-118
Amphetamine Sulfate *($117.36)* II-119
Amphetamine; Dextroamphetamine *($117.36)* II-120
Benzphetamine Hydrochloride *($479.02)* II-234
Desipramine Hydrochloride *($19.63)* II-618
Dexfenfluramine Hydrochloride *($47.60)* II-644
Dextroamphetamine Sulfate *($47.60)* II-650
Diethylpropion Hydrochloride *($1,946.41)* II-679
Fenfluramine Hydrochloride *($311.63)* II-901
Imipramine Hydrochloride *($4.19)* II-1153
Imipramine Pamoate *($93.30)* II-1156
Mazindol *($36.79)* II-1349
Methamphetamine Hydrochloride *($95.81)* II-1412
Methylphenidate Hydrochloride *($64.36)* II-1439
Pemoline *($170.91)* II-1682
Phendimetrazine Tartrate *($110.78)* II-1719
Phentermine Hydrochloride *($0.23)* II-1727
Phentermine Resin Complex *($0.23)* II-1728

PSYCHOTHERAPEUTIC AGENTS
Amitriptyline Hydrochloride *($2.50)* II-99
Amitriptyline Hydrochloride; Chlordiazepoxide *($69.87)* II-102
Amitriptyline Hydrochloride; Perphenazine *($18.22)* II-102
Amoxapine *($96.19)* II-110
Benactyzine Hydrochloride; Meprobamate *($225.37)* II-227
Bupropion Hydrochloride *($167.85)* II-291
Chlorpromazine Hydrochloride *($22.10)* II-457
Clomipramine Hydrochloride *($54.80)* II-532
Clozapine *($3,744.90)* II-547
Desipramine Hydrochloride *($19.63)* II-618
Doxepin Hydrochloride *($8.03)* II-750
Droperidol *($3,775.85)* II-766
Droperidol; Fentanyl Citrate *($3,775.85)* II-767
Fluoxetine Hydrochloride *($202.08)* II-948
Fluphenazine Decanoate *($202.08)* II-954
Fluphenazine Enanthate *($202.08)* II-955
Fluphenazine Hydrochloride *($81.86)* II-957
Fluvoxamine Maleate *($139.06)* II-972
Haloperidol *($87.52)* II-1070
Haloperidol Decanoate *($87.52)* II-1073
Imipramine Hydrochloride *($4.19)* II-1153
Imipramine Pamoate *($93.30)* II-1156
Lithium Carbonate *($14.17)* II-1312
Lithium Citrate *($33.75)* II-1313

PSYCHOTHERAPEUTIC AGENTS *(cont'd)*
Loxapine Succinate *($713.30)* II-1338
Maprotiline Hydrochloride *($36.79)* II-1346
Mesoridazine Besylate *($921.11)* II-1400
Mirtazapine *($87.60)* II-1491
Molindone Hydrochloride *($87.60)* II-1506
Nefazodone Hydrochloride *($149.65)* II-1559
Nortriptyline Hydrochloride *($252.29)* II-1612
Paroxetine Hydrochloride *($170.91)* II-1673
Perphenazine *($110.78)* II-1714
Phenelzine Sulfate *($108.64)* II-1720
Pimozide *($97.13)* II-1745
Prochlorperazine *($52.11)* II-1816
Promazine Hydrochloride *($75.00)* II-1824
Promethazine Hydrochloride *($0.76)* II-1825
Propiomazine Hydrochloride *($917.82)* II-1832
Protriptyline Hydrochloride *($125.52)* II-1848
Risperidone *($578.98)* II-1900
Sertraline Hydrochloride *($158.60)* II-1937
Thioridazine Hydrochloride *($8.80)* II-2062
Thiothixene *($8.80)* II-2066
Tranylcypromine Sulfate *($123.66)* II-2108
Trazodone Hydrochloride *($13.58)* II-2110
Trifluoperazine Hydrochloride *($16.65)* II-2135
Triflupromazine *($16.65)* II-2137
Trimipramine Maleate *($178.41)* II-2146
Venlafaxine Hydrochloride *($14.00)* II-2183

PSYCHOTIC DISORDERS
Chlorpromazine Hydrochloride *($22.10)* II-457
Doxepin Hydrochloride *($8.03)* II-750
Fluphenazine Decanoate *($202.08)* II-954
Fluphenazine Enanthate *($202.08)* II-955
Fluphenazine Hydrochloride *($81.86)* II-957
Haloperidol *($87.52)* II-1070
Haloperidol Decanoate *($87.52)* II-1073
Loxapine Succinate *($713.30)* II-1338
Mesoridazine Besylate *($921.11)* II-1400
Molindone Hydrochloride *($87.60)* II-1506
Olanzapine *($43.09)* II-1625
Perphenazine *($110.78)* II-1714
Prochlorperazine *($52.11)* II-1816
Promazine Hydrochloride *($75.00)* II-1824
Propranolol Hydrochloride *($14.89)* II-1841
Rauwolfia Serpentina *($562.02)* II-1875
Risperidone *($578.98)* II-1900
Thioridazine Hydrochloride *($8.80)* II-2062
Thiothixene *($8.80)* II-2066
Trifluoperazine Hydrochloride *($16.65)* II-2135
Triflupromazine *($16.65)* II-2137

PT 105
Phendimetrazine Tartrate *($110.78)* II-1719

PUBERTY
Testosterone Enanthate *($56.37)* II-2039
Testosterone Propionate *($56.37)* II-2041

PULMICORT
Budesonide *($395.91)* II-280

PULMO
Theophylline *($97.78)* II-2047

PULMONARY ABSCESS
Cefoxitin Sodium *($255.75)* II-379
Clindamycin Hydrochloride *($28.17)* II-517
Clindamycin Phosphate *($28.17)* II-519
Metronidazole *($0.95)* II-1463
Mezlocillin Sodium Monohydratee *($900.30)* II-1470
Ticarcillin Disodium *($8.80)* II-2070

PULMONARY DISEASE
Albuterol; Ipratropium Bromide *($35.36)* II-50
Azithromycin Dihydrate *($30.50)* II-197
Cilastatin Sodium; Imipenem *($618.00)* II-477
Doxapram Hydrochloride *($459.90)* II-746
Ethambutol Hydrochloride *($571.50)* II-857
Ipratropium Bromide *($311.27)* II-1203
Itraconazole *($970.85)* II-1230

PULMONARY EDEMA
Furosemide *($15.91)* II-988
Oxymorphone Hydrochloride *($316.12)* II-1655

PULMONARY EMBOLISM
Alteplase, Recombinant *($2,750.00)* II-71
Anisindione *($230.36)* II-139
Dalteparin Sodium *($2,942.65)* II-599
Danaparoid Sodium *($2,942.65)* II-600
Dicumarol *($5.32)* II-670
Enoxaparin Sodium *($2.84)* II-787
Heparin Sodium *($87.52)* II-1077
Reteplase *($12.77)* II-1885
Streptokinase *($33.06)* II-1974
Urokinase *($6,363.68)* II-2159
Warfarin Sodium *($112.78)* II-2200

PULMONARY EMPHYSEMA
Ephedrine Hydrochloride; Potassium Iodide; Phenobarbital; Theophylline *($2.84)* II-790
Guaifenesin; Oxtriphylline *($521.80)* II-1047
Iodinated Glycerol *($311.27)* II-1201
Iodinated Glycerol; Theophylline *($311.27)* II-1201
Potassium Iodide II-1782
Potassium Iodide; Theophylline Anhydrous II-1782

PULMONARY HYPERTENSION
Epoprostenol Sodium II-800

PULMONARY INFECTIONS
Flucytosine *($86.84)* II-930

PULMOZYME
Dornase Alfa *($7.50)* II-740

PUPIL DILATION
Hydroxyamphetamine Hydrobromide; Tropicamide *($498.80)* II-1130

PURINETHOL
Mercaptopurine *($5.04)* II-1389

RESPIRATORY & ALLERGY MEDICATIONS *(cont'd)*
Pseudoephedrine Hydrochloride; Triprolidine Hydrochloride *($63.54)* II-1850
Salmeterol Xinafoate *($2,708.38)* II-1920
Terbutaline Sulfate *($400.33)* II-2031
Terfenadine *($56.37)* II-2033
Tetrahydrozoline Hydrochloride *($1.15)* II-2047
Theophylline *($97.78)* II-2047
Triamcinolone Acetonide *($474.79)* II-2117
Trimeprazine Tartrate *($71.83)* II-2140
Tripelennamine Hydrochloride *($178.41)* II-2148
Triprolidine Hydrochloride *($178.41)* II-2149
Zafirlukast *($112.78)* II-2206
Zileuton *($3,488.45)* II-2216

RESPIRATORY DEPRESSION
Atropine Sulfate; Edrophonium Chloride *($538.68)* II-186
Doxapram Hydrochloride *($459.90)* II-746
Edrophonium Chloride *($12.37)* II-775
Epinephrine *($64.18)* II-791
Naloxone Hydrochloride *($32.48)* II-1543
Pyridostigmine Bromide *($606.85)* II-1852

RESPIRATORY DISTRESS
Cetyl Alcohol; Colfosceril Palmitate; Tyloxapol *($20.00)* II-422
Epinephrine *($64.18)* II-791
Indomethacin *($23.57)* II-1165

RESPIRATORY DISTRESS SYNDROME, NEONATAL
Beractant *($2,848.96)* II-240
Cetyl Alcohol; Colfosceril Palmitate; Tyloxapol *($20.00)* II-422

RESPIRATORY INSUFFICIENCY
Doxapram Hydrochloride *($459.90)* II-746

RESPIRATORY MUSCLE RELAXANT
Aminophylline *($40.29)* II-91
Aminophylline; Amobarbital; Ephedrine *($40.29)* II-94
Aminophylline; Ephedrine; Phenobarbital; Potassium Iodide *($40.29)* II-94
Aminophylline; Guaifenesin *($40.29)* II-94
Butabarbital; Ephedrine; Guaifenesin; Theophylline *($8.28)* II-301
Butabarbital; Guaifenesin; Pseudoephedrine; Theophylline *($8.28)* II-301
Dyphylline *($388.36)* II-770
Dyphylline; Ephedrine; Guaifenesin; Phenobarbital *($388.36)* II-771
Dyphylline; Guaifenesin *($284.70)* II-771
Ephedrine Hydrochloride; Phenobarbital; Theophylline Anhydrous *($2.84)* II-789
Ephedrine Hydrochloride; Potassium Iodide; Phenobarbital; Theophylline *($2.84)* II-790
Ephedrine Sulfate; Hydroxyzine Hydrochloride; Theophylline *($2.84)* II-790
Ephedrine; Guaifenesin; Phenobarbital; Theophylline *($2.84)* II-791
Ephedrine; Guaifenesin; Theophylline *($2.84)* II-791
Guaifenesin; Oxtriphylline *($521.80)* II-1047
Guaifenesin; Pseudoephedrine; Theophylline *($521.80)* II-1052
Guaifenesin; Theophylline *($46.86)* II-1052
Hydroxyzine Hydrochloride *($3.10)* II-1135
Iodinated Glycerol; Theophylline *($311.27)* II-1201
Oxtriphylline *($316.12)* II-1650
Potassium Iodide; Theophylline Anhydrous II-1782
Theophylline *($97.78)* II-2047
Zafirlukast *($112.78)* II-2206

RESPIRATORY STIMULANTS
Doxapram Hydrochloride *($459.90)* II-746

RESPIRATORY SYNCYTIAL VIRUS
Ribavirin *($4,124.53)* II-1889

RESPIRATORY SYNCYTIAL VIRUS IMMUNE GLOBULIN
Respiratory Syncytial Virus Immune Globulin *($12.77)* II-1883

RESPIRATORY TRACT INFECTIONS
Acetaminophen; Chlorpheniramine Maleate; Hydrocodone Bitartrate; Phenylephrine Hydrochloride *($401.06)* II-11
Amoxicillin *($7.05)* II-112
Amoxicillin; Clavulanate Potassium *($117.36)* II-115
Ampicillin *($3.76)* II-126
Azithromycin Dihydrate *($30.50)* II-197
Aztreonam *($225.37)* II-201
Bacampicillin Hydrochloride *($225.37)* II-209
Cefaclor *($117.48)* II-349
Cefamandole Nafate *($60.75)* II-353
Cefazolin Sodium *($60.75)* II-355
Cefmetazole Sodium *($63.14)* II-364
Cefonicid Sodium *($63.14)* II-367
Cefoperazone Sodium *($63.14)* II-369
Ceforanide *($63.14)* II-371
Cefotaxime Sodium *($63.14)* II-373
Cefotetan Disodium *($63.14)* II-376
Cefoxitin Sodium *($255.75)* II-379
Cefpodoxime Proxetil *($40.90)* II-383
Cefprozil *($155.06)* II-386
Ceftazidime *($155.06)* II-388
Ceftazidime (Arginine) *($155.06)* II-392
Ceftizoxime Sodium *($155.06)* II-398
Ceftriaxone Sodium *($4.00)* II-401
Cefuroxime Axetil *($183.30)* II-403
Cefuroxime Sodium *($90.00)* II-407
Cephalexin *($2.83)* II-411
Cephalexin Hydrochloride *($39.34)* II-414
Cephalothin Sodium *($39.34)* II-415
Cephapirin Sodium *($39.34)* II-417
Cephradine *($8.76)* II-418
Chlorpheniramine Maleate; Codeine Phosphate; Phenylephrine Hydrochloride; Potassium Iodide *($0.76)* II-446
Cilastatin Sodium; Imipenem *($618.00)* II-477
Ciprofloxacin Hydrochloride *($39.20)* II-488
Clarithromycin *($43.47)* II-505
Clavulanate Potassium; Ticarcillin Disodium *($43.47)* II-511
Clindamycin Hydrochloride *($28.17)* II-517
Clindamycin Phosphate *($28.17)* II-519
Dornase Alfa *($7.50)* II-740
Doxycycline *($3,775.85)* II-759
Erythromycin *($3.39)* II-806
Erythromycin Ethylsuccinate *($7.46)* II-810

RESPIRATORY TRACT INFECTIONS *(cont'd)*
Erythromycin Gluceptate *($7.46)* II-814
Erythromycin Lactobionate *($7.46)* II-815
Ethambutol Hydrochloride *($571.50)* II-857
Gentamicin Sulfate *($547.50)* II-1009
Guaifenesin *($93.44)* II-1044
Lomefloxacin Hydrochloride *($44.87)* II-1316
Loracarbef *($176.12)* II-1322
Metronidazole *($0.95)* II-1463
Mezlocillin Sodium Monohydratee *($900.30)* II-1470
Minocycline Hydrochloride *($39.25)* II-1483
Netilmicin Sulfate *($149.65)* II-1570
Ofloxacin *($43.09)* II-1620
Penicillin G Benzathine *($362.37)* II-1689
Penicillin G Benzathine; Penicillin G Procaine *($362.37)* II-1690
Penicillin G Potassium *($362.37)* II-1691
Penicillin G Procaine *($362.37)* II-1694
Penicillin G Sodium *($362.37)* II-1697
Penicillin V Potassium *($3.27)* II-1698
Piperacillin Sodium *($169.72)* II-1752
Piperacillin Sodium; Tazobactam Sodium *($169.72)* II-1755
Ribavirin *($4,124.53)* II-1889
Sparfloxacin *($1,177.85)* II-1964
Streptomycin Sulfate *($1,441.75)* II-1976
Tetracycline Hydrochloride *($1.15)* II-2044
Ticarcillin Disodium *($8.80)* II-2070
Tobramycin Sulfate *($203.45)* II-2084
Troleandomycin *($178.41)* II-2151
Vancomycin Hydrochloride *($14.00)* II-2173

RESPIRATORY TRACT SECRETIONS
Ribavirin *($4,124.53)* II-1889

RESPIRATORY VACCINE, MIXED
Respiratory Vaccine, Mixed *($12.77)* II-1885

RESPIRATORY/CEREBRAL STIMULANT
Amphetamine Resin Complex; Dextroamphetamine Resin Complex *($117.36)* II-118
Amphetamine Sulfate *($117.36)* II-119
Amphetamine; Dextroamphetamine *($117.36)* II-120
Benzphetamine Hydrochloride *($479.02)* II-234
Caffeine; Sodium Benzoate *($8.28)* II-308
Dexfenfluramine Hydrochloride *($47.60)* II-644
Dextroamphetamine Sulfate *($47.60)* II-650
Diethylpropion Hydrochloride *($1,946.41)* II-679
Doxapram Hydrochloride *($459.90)* II-746
Fenfluramine Hydrochloride *($311.63)* II-901
Mazindol *($36.79)* II-1349
Methamphetamine Hydrochloride *($95.81)* II-1412
Methoxamine Hydrochloride *($656.74)* II-1428
Methylphenidate Hydrochloride *($64.36)* II-1439
Pemoline *($170.91)* II-1682
Phendimetrazine Tartrate *($110.78)* II-1719
Phentermine Hydrochloride *($0.23)* II-1727
Phentermine Resin Complex *($0.23)* II-1728
Phenylpropanolamine Hydrochloride *($174.65)* II-1735

RESPIVIR
Respiratory Syncytial Virus Immune Globulin *($12.77)* II-1883

RESTENOSIS
Abciximab II-1

RESTLESS LEG SYNDROME
Carbamazepine *($147.16)* II-326

RESTORIL
Temazepam *($0.27)* II-2022

RETAVASE
Reteplase *($12.77)* II-1885

RETEPLASE
Reteplase *($12.77)* II-1885

RETICULUM CELL SARCOMA
Bleomycin Sulfate *($41.77)* II-269

RETIN-A
Tretinoin *($13.58)* II-2112

RETINITIS
Cidofovir II-474
Foscarnet Sodium *($26,632.22)* II-977
Ganciclovir Sodium *($12,702.00)* II-997
Molgramostim *($87.60)* II-1506

RETINOCHOROIDITIS
Betamethasone Acetate; Betamethasone Sodium Phosphate *($526.07)* II-244
Cortisone Acetate *($155.12)* II-565
Dexamethasone *($53.32)* II-626
Dexamethasone Acetate *($53.32)* II-629
Dexamethasone Sodium Phosphate *($53.32)* II-631
Dexamethasone Sodium Phosphate; Lidocaine Hydrochloride *($53.32)* II-636
Hydrocortisone *($29.20)* II-1103
Hydrocortisone Sodium Phosphate *($498.80)* II-1116
Hydrocortisone Sodium Succinate *($498.80)* II-1118
Methylprednisolone *($98.55)* II-1440
Methylprednisolone Acetate *($98.55)* II-1442
Methylprednisolone Sodium Succinate *($98.55)* II-1446
Prednisolone Sodium Phosphate *($11.13)* II-1793
Prednisone *($9.59)* II-1800
Triamcinolone *($24.63)* II-2115
Triamcinolone Acetonide *($474.79)* II-2117
Triamcinolone Diacetate *($474.79)* II-2125

RETINOIC ACID
Tretinoin *($13.58)* II-2112

RETROBULBAR ANESTHETICS
Epinephrine Bitartrate; Etidocaine Hydrochloride *($64.18)* II-792
Etidocaine Hydrochloride *($642.56)* II-875

RETROVIR
Zidovudine *($3,488.45)* II-2212

REV-EYES
Dapiprazole Hydrochloride *($2,942.65)* II-605
Dapsone *($2,942.65)* II-606

REVERSOL
Edrophonium Chloride *($12.37)* II-775

REVEX
Nalmefene Hydrochloride *($32.48)* II-1541

REXIGEN FORTE
Phendimetrazine Tartrate *($110.78)* II-1719

REXIN
Benactyzine Hydrochloride; Meprobamate *($225.37)* II-227

REXOLATE
Sodium Thiosalicylate *($649.99)* II-1956
Sodium Thiosulfate *($649.99)* II-1956

REZINE
Hydroxyzine Hydrochloride *($3.10)* II-1135

REZULIN
Troglitazone *($178.41)* II-2149

RHABDOMYOSARCOMA
Dactinomycin *($2,942.65)* II-597
Vincristine Sulfate *($56.72)* II-2195

RHEOMACRODEX
Dextran; Dextrose *($47.60)* II-649
Dextran; Sodium Chloride *($47.60)* II-650

RHEOMACRODEX IN DEXTROSE 5%
Dextran; Dextrose *($47.60)* II-649

RHEOMACRODEX IN DEXTROSE 5PC
Dextran; Dextrose *($47.60)* II-649

RHEOMACRODEX IN NORMAL SALINE
Dextran; Sodium Chloride *($47.60)* II-650

RHESONATIV
Rho (D) Immune Globulin *($12.77)* II-1887

RHEUMATIC FEVER
Azithromycin Dihydrate *($30.50)* II-197
Cefaclor *($117.48)* II-349
Cefadroxil *($60.75)* II-351
Cefazolin Sodium *($60.75)* II-355
Cefixime *($63.14)* II-361
Ceforanide *($63.14)* II-371
Cefpodoxime Proxetil *($40.90)* II-383
Cefprozil *($155.06)* II-386
Cefuroxime Axetil *($183.30)* II-403
Cephalexin *($2.83)* II-411
Cephalexin Hydrochloride *($39.34)* II-414
Cephradine *($8.76)* II-418
Demeclocycline Hydrochloride *($214.32)* II-616
Erythromycin *($3.39)* II-806
Erythromycin Estolate *($3.39)* II-808
Erythromycin Ethylsuccinate *($7.46)* II-810
Erythromycin Gluceptate *($7.46)* II-814
Erythromycin Lactobionate *($7.46)* II-815
Erythromycin Stearate *($3.60)* II-817
Loracarbef *($176.12)* II-1322
Oxytetracycline Hydrochloride *($316.12)* II-1656
Penicillin G Benzathine *($362.37)* II-1689
Penicillin G Benzathine; Penicillin G Procaine *($362.37)* II-1690
Penicillin G Potassium *($362.37)* II-1691
Penicillin G Procaine *($362.37)* II-1694
Penicillin G Sodium *($362.37)* II-1697
Penicillin V Potassium *($3.27)* II-1698
Sulfadiazine *($82.53)* II-1988
Troleandomycin *($178.41)* II-2151

RHEUMATREX
Methotrexate Sodium *($656.74)* II-1422

RHINATATE
Chlorpheniramine Tannate; Phenylephrine Tannate; Pyrilamine Tannate *($4.50)* II-457

RHINDECON
Phenylpropanolamine Hydrochloride *($174.65)* II-1735

RHINITIS
Acetaminophen; Phenylpropanolamine; Phenyltoloxamine *($6.75)* II-20
Acrivastine; Pseudoephedrine Hydrochloride II-33
Astemizole *($55.49)* II-167
Azatadine Maleate *($54.72)* II-191
Azatadine Maleate; Pseudoephedrine Sulfate *($54.72)* II-192
Azelastine *($54.72)* II-195
Beclomethasone Dipropionate *($225.37)* II-219
Betamethasone *($526.07)* II-243
Betamethasone Acetate; Betamethasone Sodium Phosphate *($526.07)* II-244
Betamethasone Sodium Phosphate *($526.07)* II-249
Brompheniramine Maleate; Pseudoephedrine Hydrochloride *($395.91)* II-280
Budesonide *($395.91)* II-280
Carbinoxamine Maleate; Pseudoephedrine Hydrochloride *($338.35)* II-337
Cetirizine Hydrochloride *($8.76)* II-420
Chlorpheniramine Maleate *($0.76)* II-444
Chlorpheniramine Maleate; Codeine Phosphate; Guaifenesin *($0.76)* II-445
Chlorpheniramine Maleate; Codeine Phosphate; Pseudoephedrine Hydrochloride *($0.76)* II-447
Chlorpheniramine Maleate; Phenylephrine Hydrochloride; Phenylpropanolamine Hydrochloride *($0.76)* II-450
Chlorpheniramine Maleate; Phenylephrine Hydrochloride; Phenylpropanolamine; Phenyltoloxamine *($5.13)* II-451
Chlorpheniramine Maleate; Phenylephrine Hydrochloride; Phenylpropanolamine; Pyrilamine *($5.13)* II-452
Chlorpheniramine Maleate; Phenylephrine Hydrochloride; Phenyltoloxamine Citrate *($5.13)* II-452
Chlorpheniramine Maleate; Phenylpropanolamine Hydrochloride *($4.50)* II-453
Chlorpheniramine Maleate; Pseudoephedrine Hydrochloride *($4.50)* II-454
Chlorpheniramine Tannate; Phenylephrine Tannate; Pyrilamine Tannate *($4.50)* II-457
Clemastine Fumarate *($43.50)* II-515
Clemastine Fumarate; Phenylpropanolamine Hydrochloride *($43.50)* II-517
Codeine Phosphate; Guaifenesin; Pseudoephedrine Hydrochloride *($3,744.90)* II-553
Codeine Phosphate; Phenylephrine Hydrochloride; Promethazine Hydrochloride *($154.83)* II-555

TRIAMCINOLONE HEXACETONIDE
Triamcinolone Hexacetonide *($474.79)* II-2125

TRIAMCOT
Triamcinolone Acetonide *($474.79)* II-2117
Triamcinolone Diacetate *($474.79)* II-2125

TRIAMILL
Pheniramine; Phenylpropanolamine; Pyrilamine *($108.64)* II-1722

TRIAMINIC
Pheniramine; Phenylpropanolamine; Pyrilamine *($108.64)* II-1722

TRIAMINIC DH
Guaifenesin; Hydrocodone Bitartrate; Pheniramine Maleate; Phenylpropanolamine Hydrochloride *($93.44)* II-1046

TRIAMINIC EXPECTORANT DH
Guaifenesin; Hydrocodone Bitartrate; Pheniramine Maleate; Phenylpropanolamine Hydrochloride *($93.44)* II-1046

TRIAMINIC W/CODEINE
Codeine Phosphate; Guaifenesin; Phenylpropanolamine *($3,744.90)* II-553

TRIAMOLONE 40
Triamcinolone Diacetate *($474.79)* II-2125

TRIAMONIDE 40
Triamcinolone Acetonide *($474.79)* II-2117

TRIAMTERENE
Hydrochlorothiazide; Triamterene *($19.45)* II-1100
Triamterene *($289.08)* II-2127

TRIANIDE
Triamcinolone Acetonide *($474.79)* II-2117

TRIAPHED
Pseudoephedrine Hydrochloride; Triprolidine Hydrochloride *($63.54)* II-1850
Pyrazinamide *($606.85)* II-1851

TRIAPHED-C
Codeine Phosphate; Pseudoephedrine Hydrochloride; Triprolidine Hydrochloride *($6.64)* II-556

TRIAPRIN
Acetaminophen; Butalbital *($401.06)* II-8

TRIATEX
Triamcinolone Acetonide *($474.79)* II-2117

TRIAVIL
Amitriptyline Hydrochloride; Perphenazine *($18.22)* II-102

TRIAZ
Benzoyl Peroxide *($479.02)* II-233

TRIAZOLAM
Triazolam *($3.70)* II-2128

TRIAZOLE
Sulfamethoxazole; Trimethoprim *($2.50)* II-1991

TRIAZOLES
Fluconazole *($86.84)* II-926

TRIBAN
Trimethobenzamide Hydrochloride *($71.83)* II-2141

TRIBENZAGAN
Trimethobenzamide Hydrochloride *($71.83)* II-2141

TRIBIOTIC
Gramicidin; Neomycin Sulfate; Polymyxin B Sulfate *($107.85)* II-1039

TRICHINOSIS
Corticotropin *($760.95)* II-564
Cortisone Acetate *($155.12)* II-565
Dexamethasone *($53.32)* II-626
Dexamethasone Acetate *($53.32)* II-629
Dexamethasone Sodium Phosphate *($53.32)* II-631
Dexamethasone Sodium Phosphate; Lidocaine Hydrochloride *($53.32)* II-636
Hydrocortisone *($29.20)* II-1103
Hydrocortisone Cypionate *($498.80)* II-1115
Hydrocortisone Sodium Phosphate *($498.80)* II-1116
Hydrocortisone Sodium Succinate *($498.80)* II-1118
Methylprednisolone *($98.55)* II-1440
Methylprednisolone Acetate *($98.55)* II-1442
Methylprednisolone Sodium Succinate *($98.55)* II-1446
Prednisolone *($11.13)* II-1790
Prednisolone Sodium Phosphate *($11.13)* II-1793
Prednisone *($9.59)* II-1800
Thiabendazole *($97.78)* II-2056
Triamcinolone *($24.63)* II-2115
Triamcinolone Acetonide *($474.79)* II-2117
Triamcinolone Diacetate *($474.79)* II-2125

TRICHLOREX
Trichlormethiazide *($3.70)* II-2130

TRICHLORMAS
Trichlormethiazide *($3.70)* II-2130

TRICHLORMETHIAZIDE
Reserpine; Trichlormethiazide *($12.77)* II-1882
Trichlormethiazide *($3.70)* II-2130

TRICHLOROACETIC ACID
Trichloroacetic Acid *($3.70)* II-2132

TRICHLOROMONOFLUOROMETHANE
Dichlorodifluoromethane; Trichloromonofluoromethane *($4.20)* II-663

TRICHOMONAS
Clindamycin Phosphate *($28.17)* II-519
Metronidazole *($0.95)* II-1463

TRICHOMONIASIS
Metronidazole *($0.95)* II-1463

TRICHURIASIS
Thiabendazole *($97.78)* II-2056

TRICHURIS
Mebendazole *($36.79)* II-1355
Thiabendazole *($97.78)* II-2056

TRICOSAL
Choline Magnesium Trisalicylate *($14.23)* II-468

TRICYCLIC ANTIDEPRESSANTS
Amitriptyline Hydrochloride *($2.50)* II-99
Amitriptyline Hydrochloride; Chlordiazepoxide *($69.87)* II-102
Amitriptyline Hydrochloride; Perphenazine *($18.22)* II-102
Amoxapine *($96.19)* II-110
Clomipramine Hydrochloride *($54.80)* II-532
Desipramine Hydrochloride *($19.63)* II-618
Doxepin Hydrochloride *($8.03)* II-750
Imipramine Hydrochloride *($4.19)* II-1153
Imipramine Pamoate *($93.30)* II-1156
Loxapine Succinate *($713.30)* II-1338
Nortriptyline Hydrochloride *($252.29)* II-1612
Protriptyline Hydrochloride *($125.52)* II-1848
Trimipramine Maleate *($178.41)* II-2146

TRICYCLICS
Amitriptyline Hydrochloride *($2.50)* II-99
Amitriptyline Hydrochloride; Perphenazine *($18.22)* II-102
Amoxapine *($96.19)* II-110
Clomipramine Hydrochloride *($54.80)* II-532
Desipramine Hydrochloride *($19.63)* II-618
Doxepin Hydrochloride *($8.03)* II-750
Imipramine Hydrochloride *($4.19)* II-1153
Imipramine Pamoate *($93.30)* II-1156
Loxapine Succinate *($713.30)* II-1338
Nortriptyline Hydrochloride *($252.29)* II-1612
Protriptyline Hydrochloride *($125.52)* II-1848
Trimipramine Maleate *($178.41)* II-2146

TRIDERM
Triamcinolone Acetonide *($474.79)* II-2117

TRIDESILON
Desonide *($266.34)* II-623

TRIDIHEXETHYL CHLORIDE
Tridihexethyl Chloride *($3.70)* II-2132

TRIDIL
Nitroglycerin *($70.62)* II-1599

TRIDIONE
Trimethadione *($71.83)* II-2140

TRIENTINE HYDROCHLORIDE
Trientine Hydrochloride *($3.70)* II-2133

TRIETHANOLAMINE POLYPEPTIDE OLEATE CONDENSATE
Triethanolamine Polypeptide Oleate Condensate *($3.70)* II-2134

TRIETHYLENETHIOPHOSPHORAMIDE
Thiotepa *($8.80)* II-2065

TRIFED
Pseudoephedrine Hydrochloride; Triprolidine Hydrochloride *($63.54)* II-1850
Pyrazinamide *($606.85)* II-1851

TRIFLUOPERAZINE HYDROCHLORIDE
Trifluoperazine Hydrochloride *($16.65)* II-2135

TRIFLUPROMAZINE
Triflupromazine *($16.65)* II-2137

TRIFLURIDINE
Trifluridine *($16.65)* II-2138

TRIGEMINAL NEURALGIA
Carbamazepine *($147.16)* II-326

TRIGONITIS
Atropine Sulfate; Benzoic Acid; Hyoscyamine; Methenamine; Methylene Blue; Phenyl Salicylate *($538.68)* II-183
Hyoscamine; Methenamine; Methylene Blue; Phenyl Salicylate; Sodium Biphosphate *($30.81)* II-1138

TRIHEXANE
Trihexyphenidyl Hydrochloride *($71.83)* II-2139

TRIHEXIDYL
Trihexyphenidyl Hydrochloride *($71.83)* II-2139

TRIHEXY
Trihexyphenidyl Hydrochloride *($71.83)* II-2139

TRIHEXYPHENIDYL HYDROCHLORIDE
Trihexyphenidyl Hydrochloride *($71.83)* II-2139

TRIHIST-CS
Brompheniramine Maleate; Codeine Phosphate; Phenylpropanolamine Hydrochloride *($395.91)* II-278

TRIHIST-D
Pheniramine; Phenylpropanolamine; Pyrilamine *($108.64)* II-1722

TRIHIST-DM
Brompheniramine; Dextromethorphan Hydrobromide; Phenylpropanolamine *($395.91)* II-280

TRIKATES
Potassium *($51.20)* II-1775

TRILAFON
Perphenazine *($110.78)* II-1714

TRILISATE
Choline Magnesium Trisalicylate *($14.23)* II-468

TRILITRON
Pseudoephedrine Hydrochloride; Triprolidine Hydrochloride *($63.54)* II-1850
Pyrazinamide *($606.85)* II-1851

TRILOG
Triamcinolone Acetonide *($474.79)* II-2117

TRILONE
Triamcinolone Diacetate *($474.79)* II-2125

TRIMAZIDE
Trimethobenzamide Hydrochloride *($71.83)* II-2141

TRIMEPRAZINE TARTRATE
Trimeprazine Tartrate *($71.83)* II-2140

TRIMETHADIONE
Trimethadione *($71.83)* II-2140

TRIMETHOBENZAMIDE HYDROCHLORIDE
Trimethobenzamide Hydrochloride *($71.83)* II-2141

TRIMETHOPRIM
Sulfamethoxazole; Trimethoprim *($2.50)* II-1991
Trimethoprim *($71.83)* II-2142

TRIMETHOPRIM SULFATE
Polymyxin B Sulfate; Trimethoprim Sulfate *($51.20)* II-1771

TRIMETREXATE GLUCURONATE
Trimetrexate Glucuronate *($71.83)* II-2143

TRIMIPRAMINE MALEATE
Trimipramine Maleate *($178.41)* II-2146

TRIMOX
Amoxicillin *($7.05)* II-112

TRIMPEX
Trimethoprim *($71.83)* II-2142

TRIMSTAT
Phendimetrazine Tartrate *($110.78)* II-1719

TRIMTABS
Phendimetrazine Tartrate *($110.78)* II-1719

TRIN TUSS
Carbetapentane Tannate; Chlorpheniramine Tannate; Ephedrine Tannate; Phenylephrine Hydrochloride *($147.16)* II-330

TRINALIN
Azatadine Maleate; Pseudoephedrine Sulfate *($54.72)* II-192

TRINIDIN
Iodinated Glycerol *($311.27)* II-1201

TRINPRIN
Aspirin II-157

TRINTEX
Guaifenesin; Phenylephrine Hydrochloride; Phenylpropanolamine Hydrochloride *($521.80)* II-1049
Guaifenesin; Phenylpropanolamine Hydrochloride *($521.80)* II-1049

TRIOSTAT
Liothyronine Sodium *($60.88)* II-1303

TRIOTANN
Chlorpheniramine Tannate; Phenylephrine Tannate; Pyrilamine Tannate *($4.50)* II-457

TRIOTANN-S
Chlorpheniramine Tannate; Phenylephrine Tannate; Pyrilamine Tannate *($4.50)* II-457

TRIOXSALEN
Trioxsalen *($178.41)* II-2147

TRIPEDIA
Diphtheria; Pertussis; Tetanus *($18.50)* II-711

TRIPELENNAMINE HYDROCHLORIDE
Tripelennamine Hydrochloride *($178.41)* II-2148

TRIPHASIL
Ethinyl Estradiol; Levonorgestrel *($255.62)* II-863

TRIPHED
Pseudoephedrine Hydrochloride; Triprolidine Hydrochloride *($63.54)* II-1850
Pyrazinamide *($606.85)* II-1851

TRIPHENYL
Chlorpheniramine Maleate; Phenylpropanolamine Hydrochloride *($4.50)* II-453
Pheniramine; Phenylpropanolamine; Pyrilamine *($108.64)* II-1722

TRIPLE ANTIBIOTIC
Bacitracin Zinc; Neomycin Sulfate; Polymyxin B Sulfate *($225.37)* II-211
Gramicidin; Neomycin Sulfate; Polymyxin B Sulfate *($107.85)* II-1039

TRIPLE ANTIBIOTIC W/HYDROCORTISONE
Bacitracin; Hydrocortisone Acetate; Neomycin Sulfate; Polymyxin B Sulfate *($225.37)* II-212

TRIPLE SULFA
Sulfabenzamide; Sulfacetamide; Sulfathiazole *($82.53)* II-1986

TRIPLE TANNATE-S
Chlorpheniramine Tannate; Phenylephrine Tannate; Pyrilamine Tannate *($4.50)* II-457

TRIPLE-GEN
Hydrocortisone; Neomycin Sulfate; Polymyxin B Sulfate *($498.80)* II-1121

TRIPLEN
Tripelennamine Hydrochloride *($178.41)* II-2148

TRIPOLE-S
Estradiol Cypionate; Testosterone Cypionate *($73.14)* II-828

TRIPROLIDINE HYDROCHLORIDE
Codeine Phosphate; Pseudoephedrine Hydrochloride; Triprolidine Hydrochloride *($6.64)* II-556
Pseudoephedrine Hydrochloride; Triprolidine Hydrochloride *($63.54)* II-1850
Triprolidine Hydrochloride *($178.41)* II-2149

TRIPROLIDINE P-EPHED CODEINE
Codeine Phosphate; Pseudoephedrine Hydrochloride; Triprolidine Hydrochloride *($6.64)* II-556

TRIPROLIDINE W/PSEUDOEPHEDRINE
Pseudoephedrine Hydrochloride; Triprolidine Hydrochloride *($63.54)* II-1850
Pyrazinamide *($606.85)* II-1851

TRISORALEN
Trioxsalen *($178.41)* II-2147

TRISTO-PLEX
Triamcinolone Diacetate *($474.79)* II-2125

TRISTOJECT
Triamcinolone Diacetate *($474.79)* II-2125

NOTES

Keyword Page

NOTES

Keyword Page

NOTES

Keyword **Page**

NOTES

Keyword Page

NOTES

Keyword Page

NOTES

Keyword Page

NOTES

Keyword Page

Mosby's GenRx™

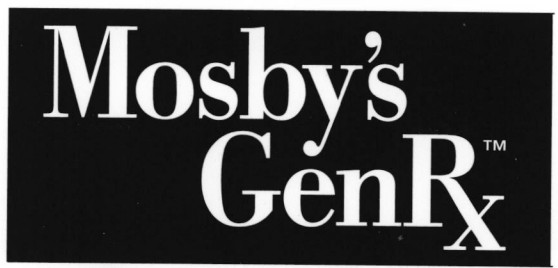

THE COMPLETE REFERENCE
FOR GENERIC AND BRAND DRUGS

DRUG IDENTIFICATION GUIDE

Provides full-color pictures of capsules and tablets.
Products are arranged in alphabetical order by generic name.

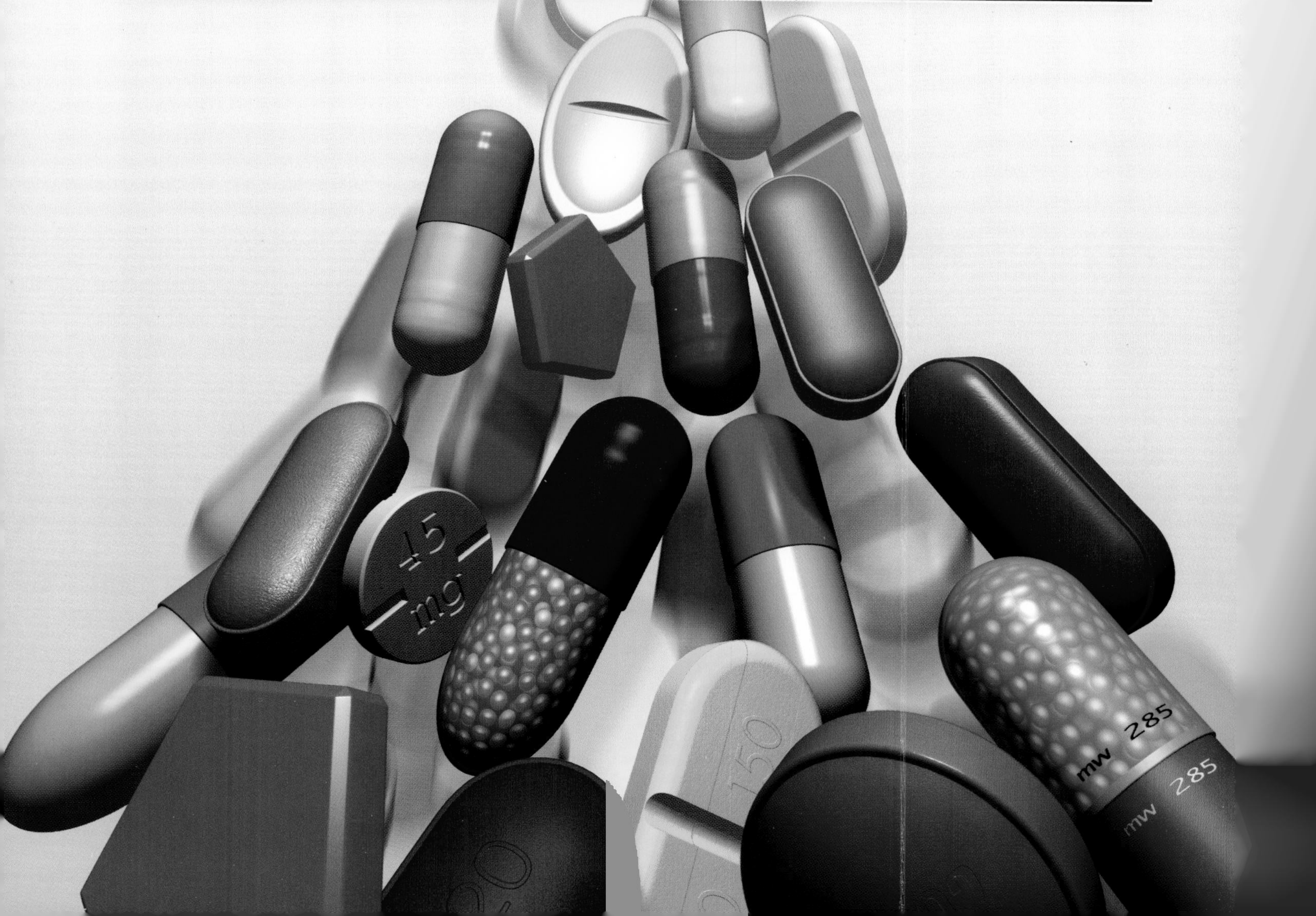

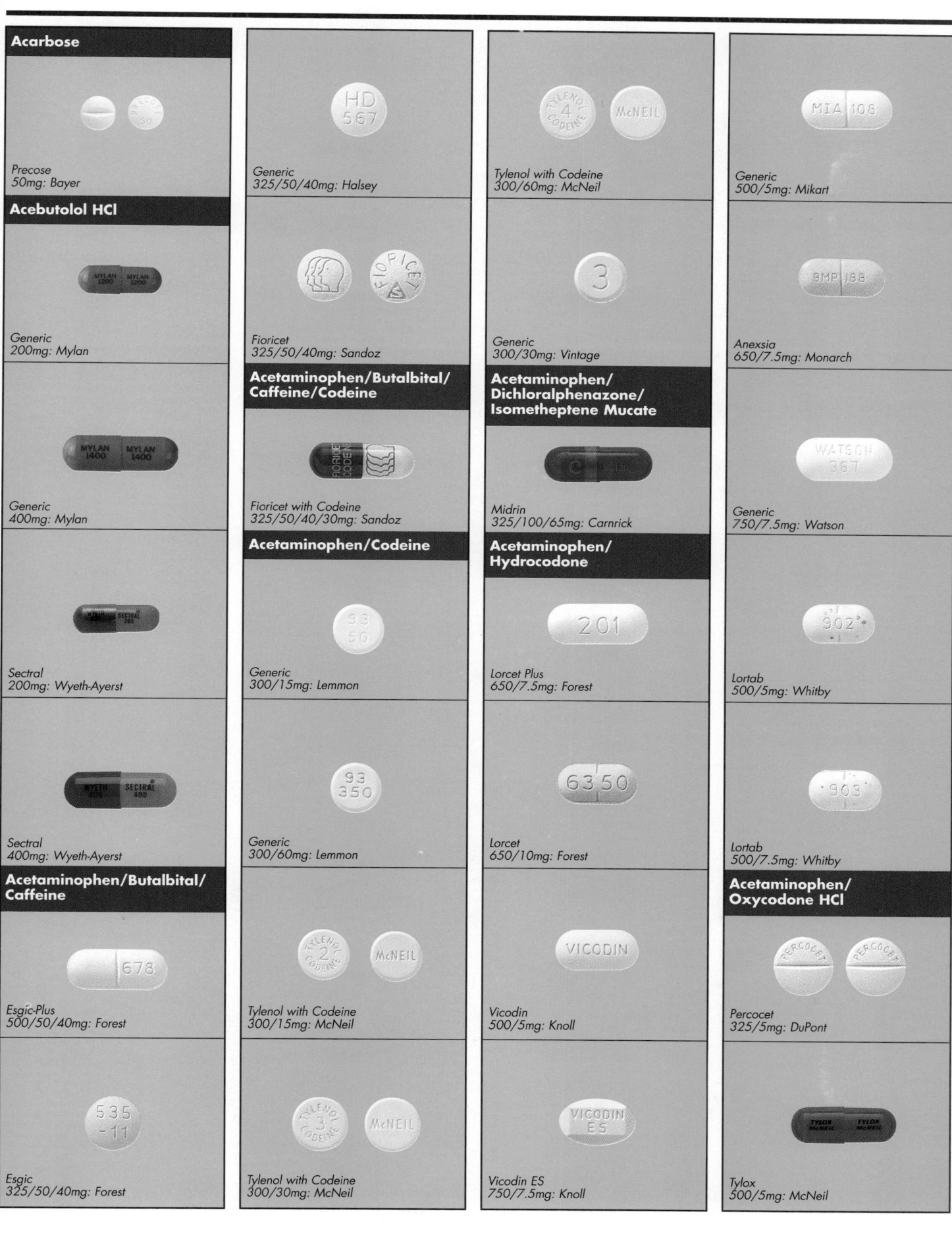

Acarbose

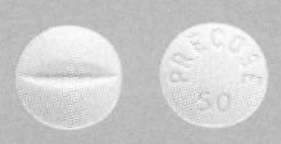

Precose
50mg: Bayer

Acebutolol HCl

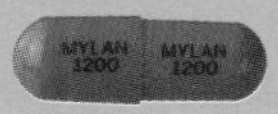

Generic
200mg: Mylan

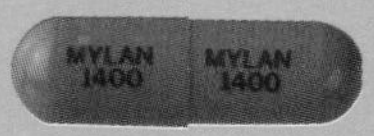

Generic
400mg: Mylan

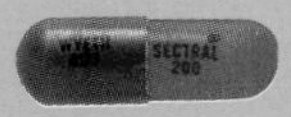

Sectral
200mg: Wyeth-Ayerst

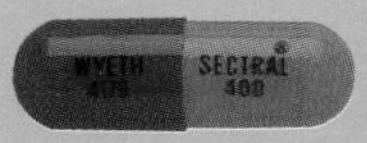

Sectral
400mg: Wyeth-Ayerst

Acetaminophen/Butalbital/Caffeine

Esgic-Plus
500/50/40mg: Forest

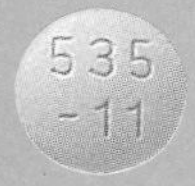

Esgic
325/50/40mg: Forest

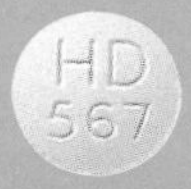

Generic
325/50/40mg: Halsey

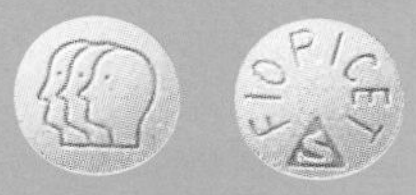

Fioricet
325/50/40mg: Sandoz

Acetaminophen/Butalbital/Caffeine/Codeine

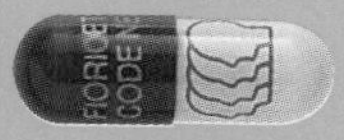

Fioricet with Codeine
325/50/40/30mg: Sandoz

Acetaminophen/Codeine

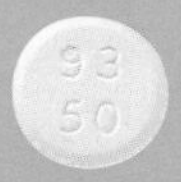

Generic
300/15mg: Lemmon

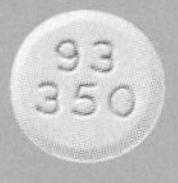

Generic
300/60mg: Lemmon

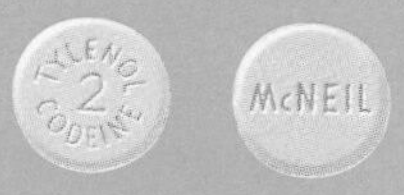

Tylenol with Codeine
300/15mg: McNeil

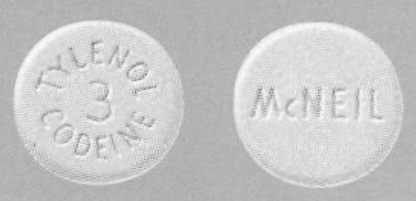

Tylenol with Codeine
300/30mg: McNeil

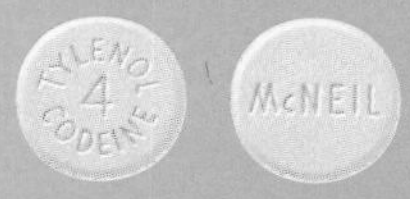

Tylenol with Codeine
300/60mg: McNeil

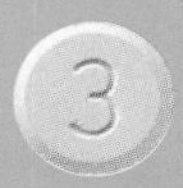

Generic
300/30mg: Vintage

Acetaminophen/Dichloralphenazone/Isometheptene Mucate

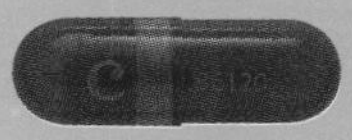

Midrin
325/100/65mg: Carnrick

Acetaminophen/Hydrocodone

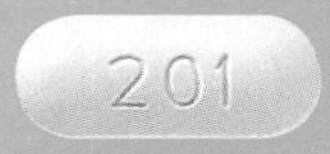

Lorcet Plus
650/7.5mg: Forest

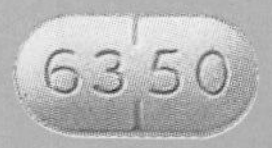

Lorcet
650/10mg: Forest

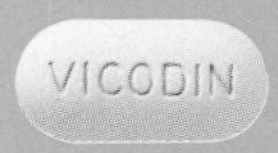

Vicodin
500/5mg: Knoll

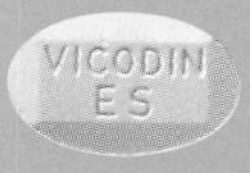

Vicodin ES
750/7.5mg: Knoll

Generic
500/5mg: Mikart

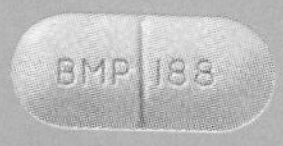

Anexsia
650/7.5mg: Monarch

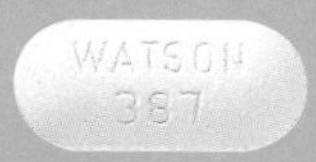

Generic
750/7.5mg: Watson

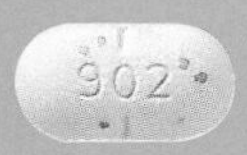

Lortab
500/5mg: Whitby

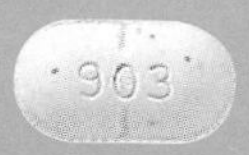

Lortab
500/7.5mg: Whitby

Acetaminophen/Oxycodone HCl

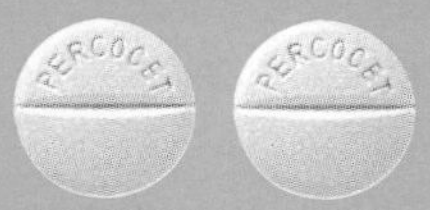

Percocet
325/5mg: DuPont

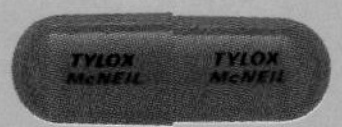

Tylox
500/5mg: McNeil

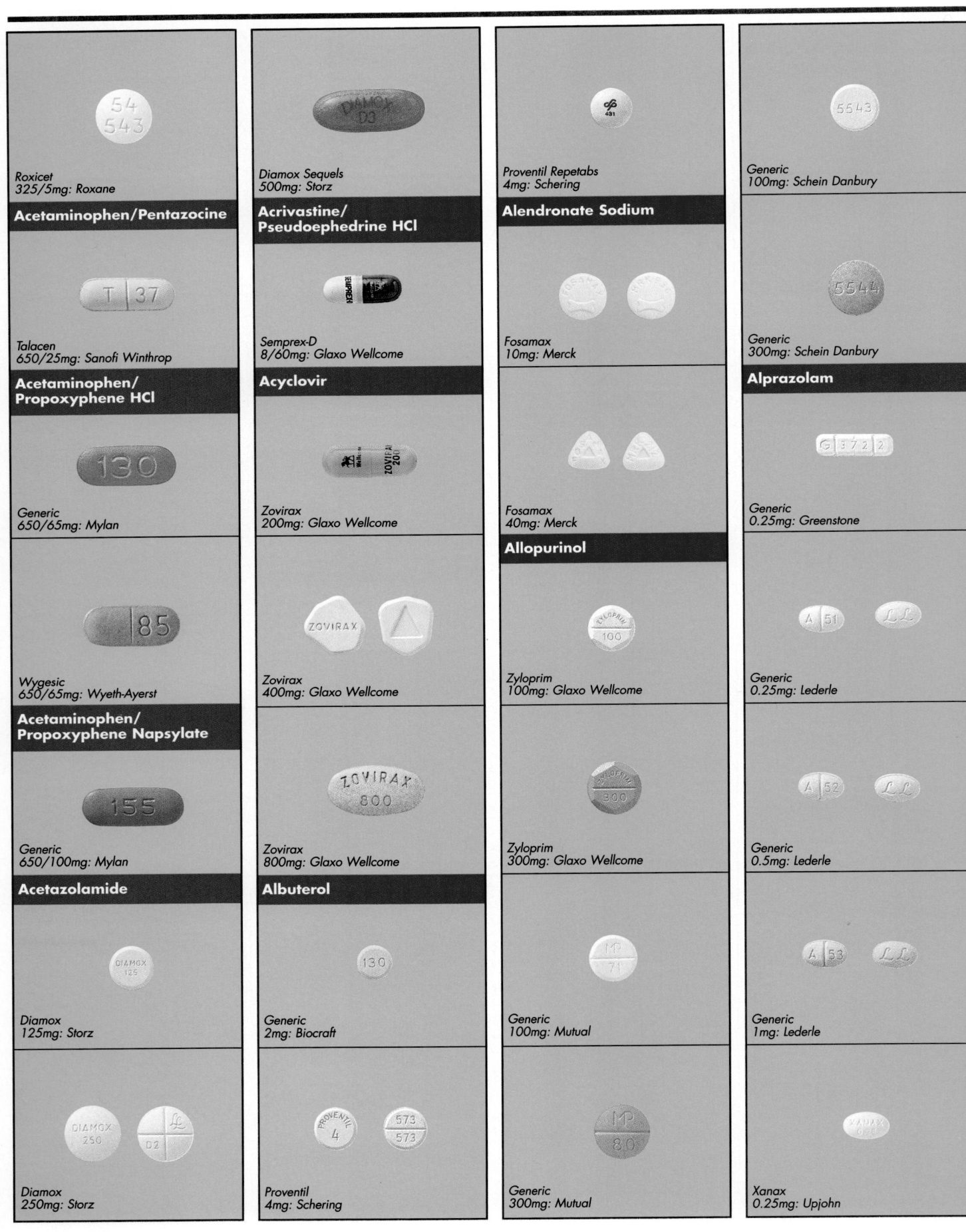

Roxicet
325/5mg: Roxane

Acetaminophen/Pentazocine

Talacen
650/25mg: Sanofi Winthrop

Acetaminophen/ Propoxyphene HCl

Generic
650/65mg: Mylan

Wygesic
650/65mg: Wyeth-Ayerst

Acetaminophen/ Propoxyphene Napsylate

Generic
650/100mg: Mylan

Acetazolamide

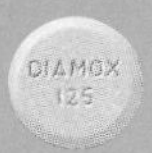

Diamox
125mg: Storz

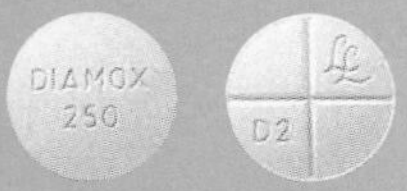

Diamox
250mg: Storz

Diamox Sequels
500mg: Storz

Acrivastine/ Pseudoephedrine HCl

Semprex-D
8/60mg: Glaxo Wellcome

Acyclovir

Zovirax
200mg: Glaxo Wellcome

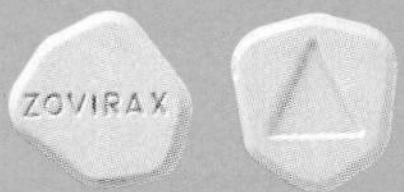

Zovirax
400mg: Glaxo Wellcome

Zovirax
800mg: Glaxo Wellcome

Albuterol

Generic
2mg: Biocraft

Proventil
4mg: Schering

Proventil Repetabs
4mg: Schering

Alendronate Sodium

Fosamax
10mg: Merck

Fosamax
40mg: Merck

Allopurinol

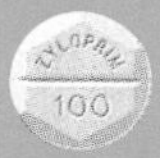

Zyloprim
100mg: Glaxo Wellcome

Zyloprim
300mg: Glaxo Wellcome

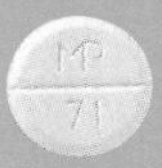

Generic
100mg: Mutual

Generic
300mg: Mutual

Generic
100mg: Schein Danbury

Generic
300mg: Schein Danbury

Alprazolam

Generic
0.25mg: Greenstone

Generic
0.25mg: Lederle

Generic
0.5mg: Lederle

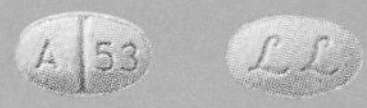

Generic
1mg: Lederle

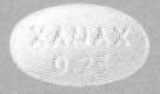

Xanax
0.25mg: Upjohn

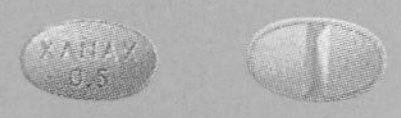

Xanax
0.5mg: Upjohn

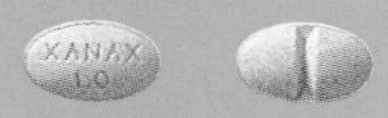

Xanax
1mg: Upjohn

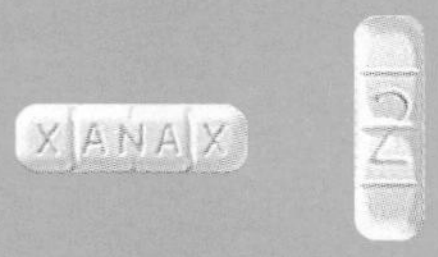

Xanax
2mg: Upjohn

Amantadine HCl

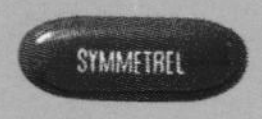

Symmetrel
100mg: DuPont

Amiloride HCl/ Hydrochlorothiazide

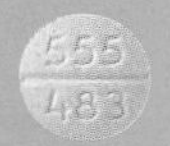

Generic
5/50mg: Barr

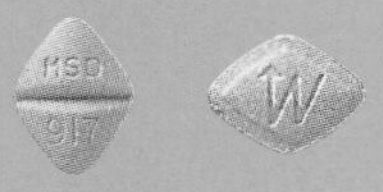

Moduretic
5/50mg: Merck

Amiodarone

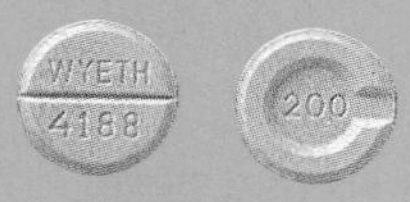

Cordarone
200mg: Wyeth-Ayerst

Amitriptyline HCl

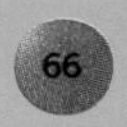

Generic
10mg: Sidmak

Generic
25mg: Sidmak

Generic
100mg: Sidmak

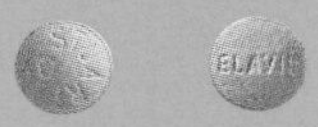

Elavil
10mg: Stuart

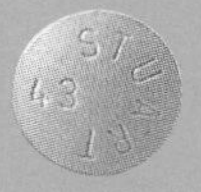

Elavil
25mg: Stuart

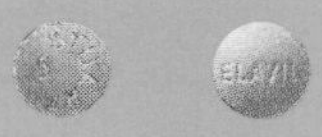

Elavil
50mg: Stuart

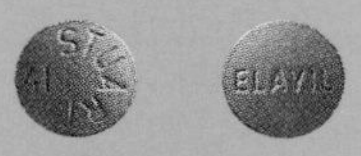

Elavil
75mg: Stuart

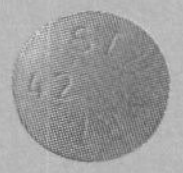
Elavil
100mg: Stuart

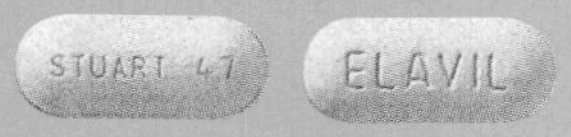

Elavil
150mg: Stuart

Amitriptyline HCl/ Perphenazine

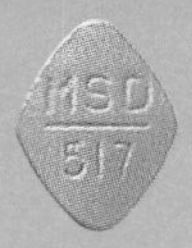

Triavil 4-50
50/4mg: Merck

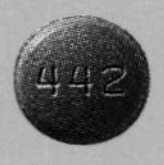

Generic
25/2mg: Mylan

Amlodipine

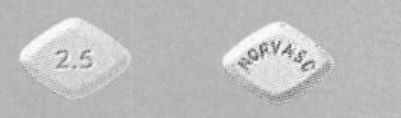

Norvasc
2.5mg: Pfizer

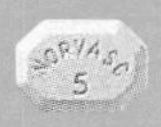

Norvasc
5mg: Pfizer

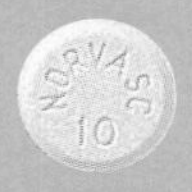

Norvasc
10mg: Pfizer

Amoxicillin

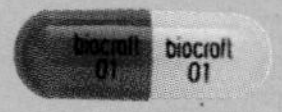

Generic
250mg: Biocraft

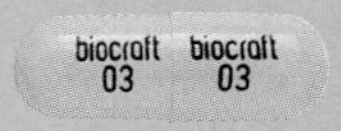

Generic
500mg: Biocraft

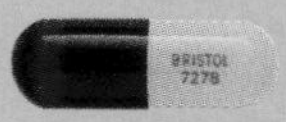
Trimox
250mg: Bristol-Myers Squibb

Trimox
500mg: Bristol-Myers Squibb

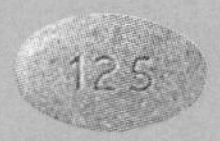

Amoxil
125mg: SmithKline Beecham

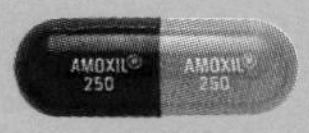
Amoxil
250mg: SmithKline Beecham

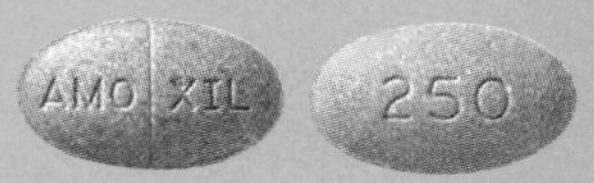

Amoxil
250mg: SmithKline Beecham

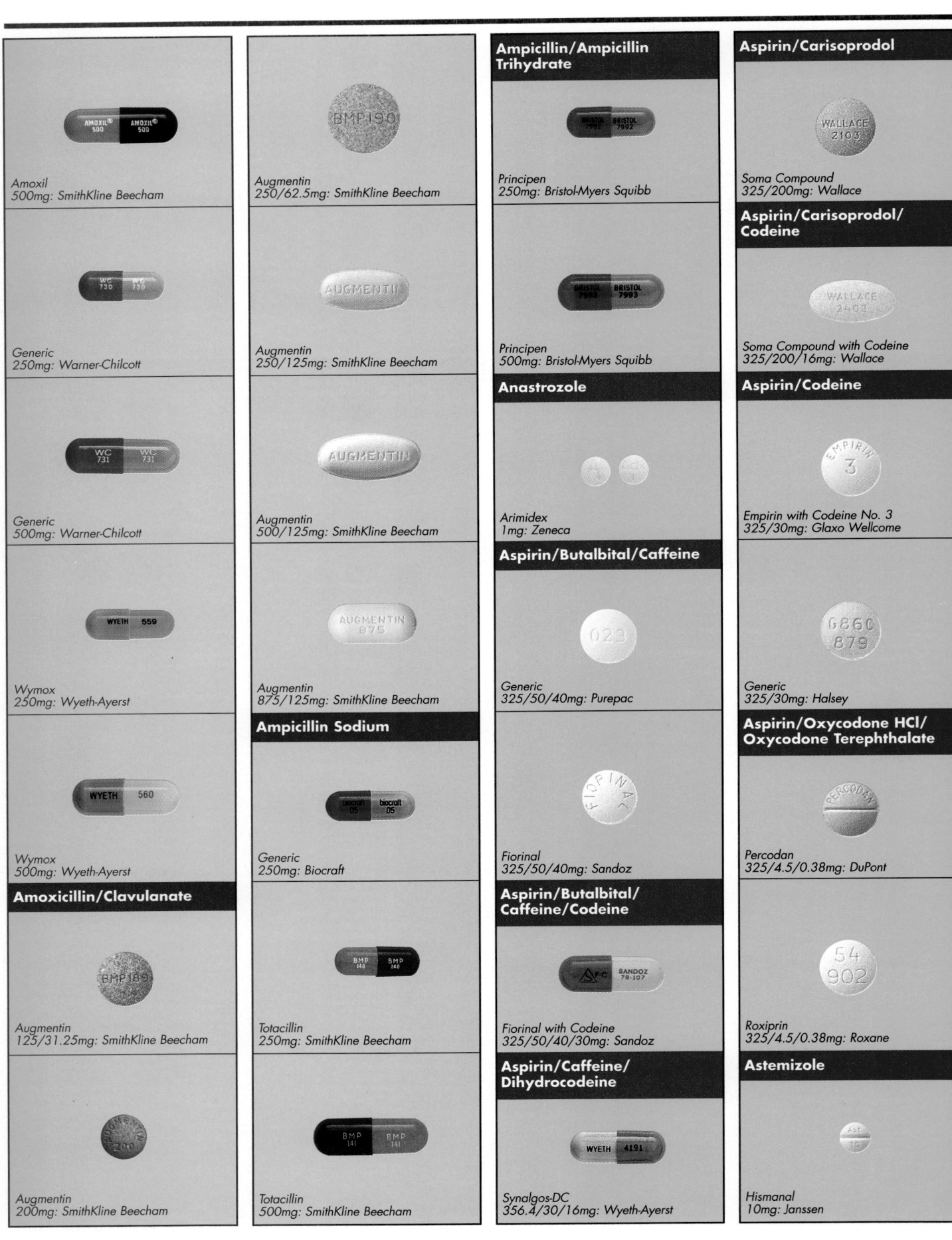

Amoxil
500mg: SmithKline Beecham

Generic
250mg: Warner-Chilcott

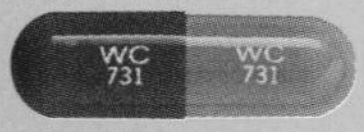

Generic
500mg: Warner-Chilcott

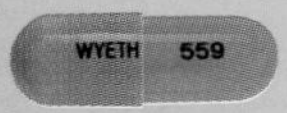

Wymox
250mg: Wyeth-Ayerst

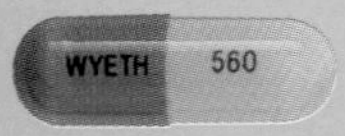

Wymox
500mg: Wyeth-Ayerst

Amoxicillin/Clavulanate

Augmentin
125/31.25mg: SmithKline Beecham

Augmentin
200mg: SmithKline Beecham

Augmentin
250/62.5mg: SmithKline Beecham

Augmentin
250/125mg: SmithKline Beecham

Augmentin
500/125mg: SmithKline Beecham

Augmentin
875/125mg: SmithKline Beecham

Ampicillin Sodium

Generic
250mg: Biocraft

Totacillin
250mg: SmithKline Beecham

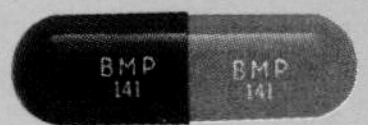

Totacillin
500mg: SmithKline Beecham

Ampicillin/Ampicillin Trihydrate

Principen
250mg: Bristol-Myers Squibb

Principen
500mg: Bristol-Myers Squibb

Anastrozole

Arimidex
1mg: Zeneca

Aspirin/Butalbital/Caffeine

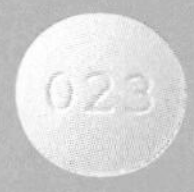

Generic
325/50/40mg: Purepac

Fiorinal
325/50/40mg: Sandoz

Aspirin/Butalbital/Caffeine/Codeine

Fiorinal with Codeine
325/50/40/30mg: Sandoz

Aspirin/Caffeine/Dihydrocodeine

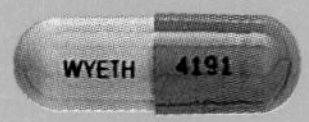

Synalgos-DC
356.4/30/16mg: Wyeth-Ayerst

Aspirin/Carisoprodol

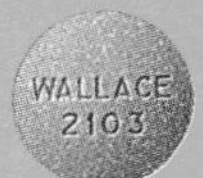

Soma Compound
325/200mg: Wallace

Aspirin/Carisoprodol/Codeine

Soma Compound with Codeine
325/200/16mg: Wallace

Aspirin/Codeine

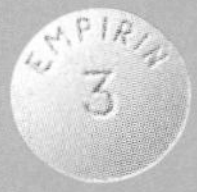

Empirin with Codeine No. 3
325/30mg: Glaxo Wellcome

Generic
325/30mg: Halsey

Aspirin/Oxycodone HCl/Oxycodone Terephthalate

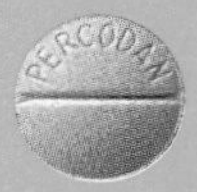

Percodan
325/4.5/0.38mg: DuPont

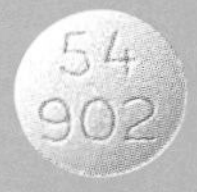

Roxiprin
325/4.5/0.38mg: Roxane

Astemizole

Hismanal
10mg: Janssen

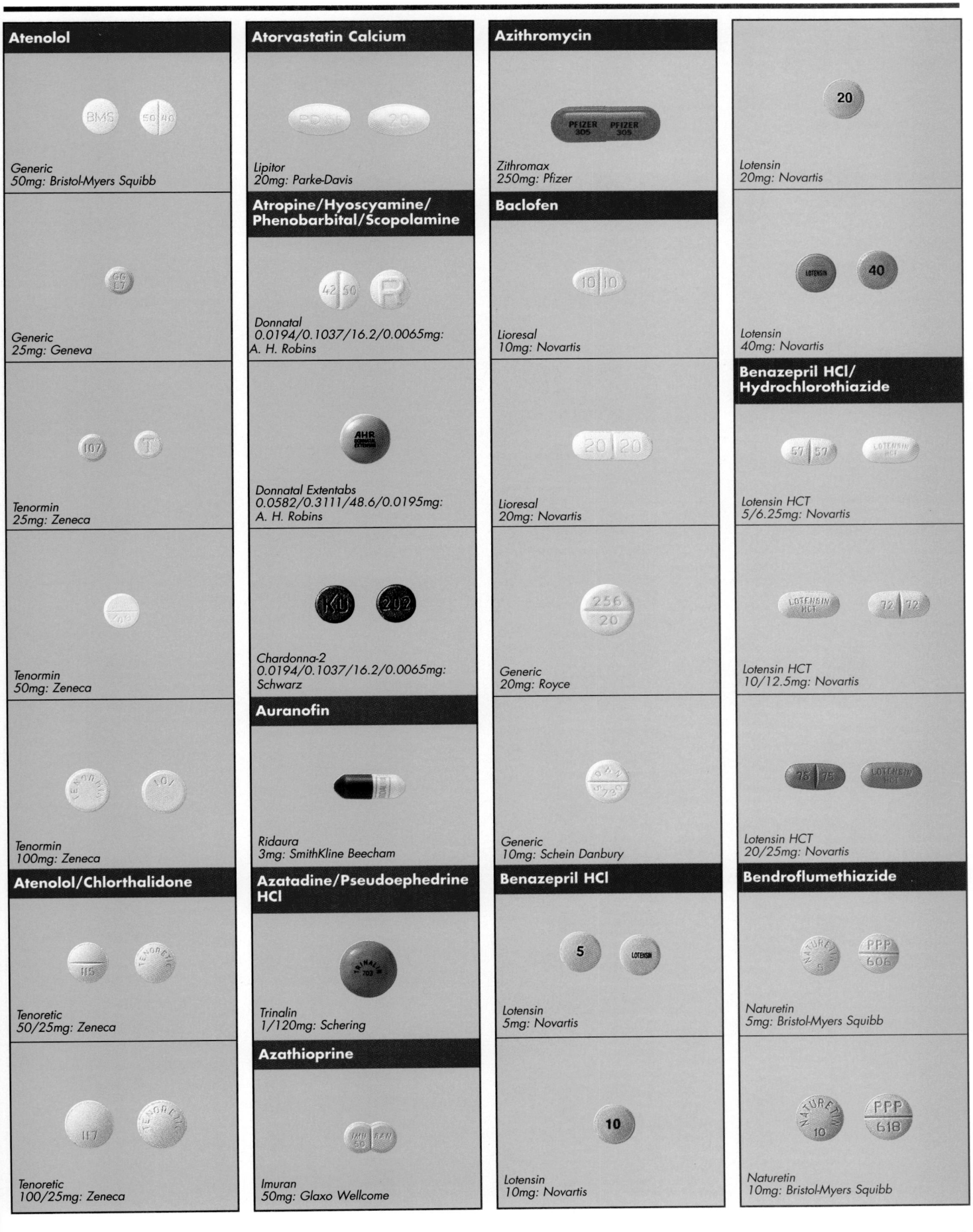

Atenolol

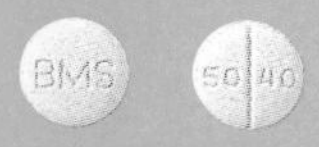

Generic
50mg: Bristol-Myers Squibb

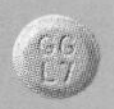

Generic
25mg: Geneva

Tenormin
25mg: Zeneca

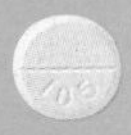

Tenormin
50mg: Zeneca

Tenormin
100mg: Zeneca

Atenolol/Chlorthalidone

Tenoretic
50/25mg: Zeneca

Tenoretic
100/25mg: Zeneca

Atorvastatin Calcium

Lipitor
20mg: Parke-Davis

Atropine/Hyoscyamine/Phenobarbital/Scopolamine

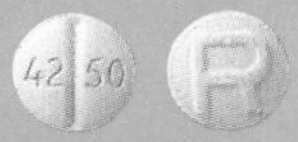

Donnatal
0.0194/0.1037/16.2/0.0065mg: A. H. Robins

Donnatal Extentabs
0.0582/0.3111/48.6/0.0195mg: A. H. Robins

Chardonna-2
0.0194/0.1037/16.2/0.0065mg: Schwarz

Auranofin

Ridaura
3mg: SmithKline Beecham

Azatadine/Pseudoephedrine HCl

Trinalin
1/120mg: Schering

Azathioprine

Imuran
50mg: Glaxo Wellcome

Azithromycin

Zithromax
250mg: Pfizer

Baclofen

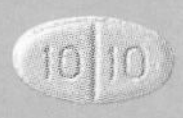

Lioresal
10mg: Novartis

Lioresal
20mg: Novartis

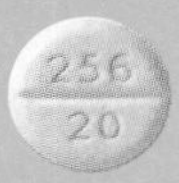

Generic
20mg: Royce

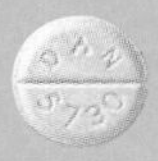

Generic
10mg: Schein Danbury

Benazepril HCl

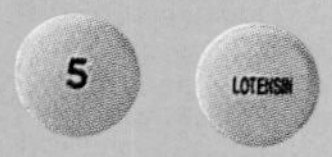

Lotensin
5mg: Novartis

Lotensin
10mg: Novartis

Lotensin
20mg: Novartis

Lotensin
40mg: Novartis

Benazepril HCl/Hydrochlorothiazide

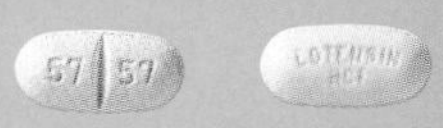

Lotensin HCT
5/6.25mg: Novartis

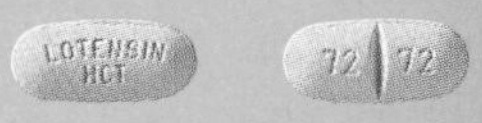

Lotensin HCT
10/12.5mg: Novartis

Lotensin HCT
20/25mg: Novartis

Bendroflumethiazide

Naturetin
5mg: Bristol-Myers Squibb

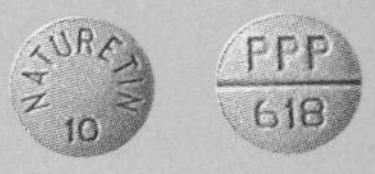

Naturetin
10mg: Bristol-Myers Squibb

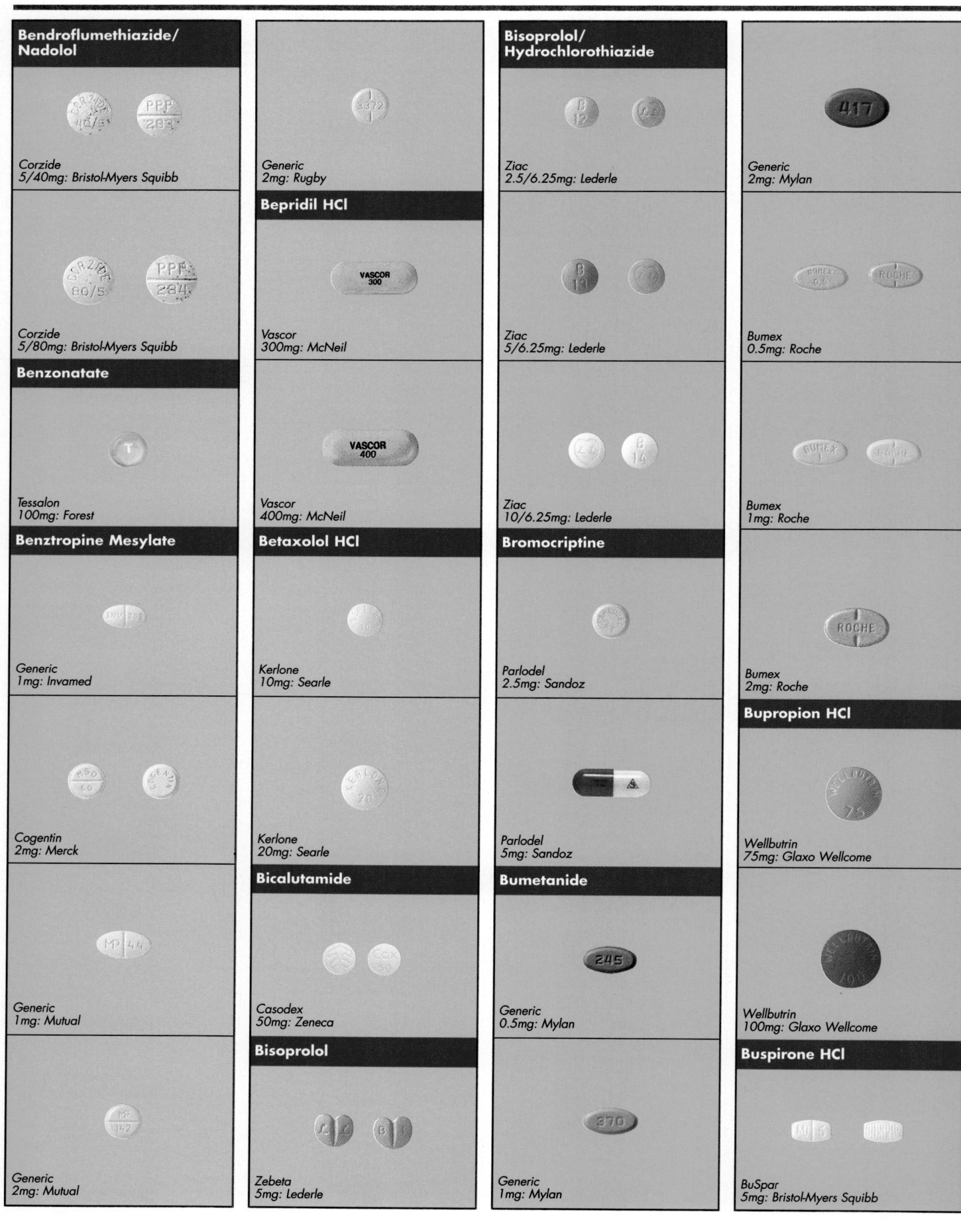

Bendroflumethiazide/ Nadolol

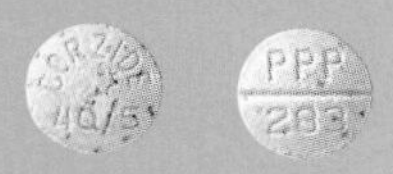

Corzide
5/40mg: Bristol-Myers Squibb

Corzide
5/80mg: Bristol-Myers Squibb

Benzonatate

Tessalon
100mg: Forest

Benztropine Mesylate

Generic
1mg: Invamed

Cogentin
2mg: Merck

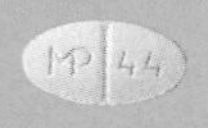

Generic
1mg: Mutual

Generic
2mg: Mutual

Generic
2mg: Rugby

Bepridil HCl

Vascor
300mg: McNeil

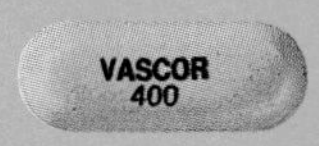

Vascor
400mg: McNeil

Betaxolol HCl

Kerlone
10mg: Searle

Kerlone
20mg: Searle

Bicalutamide

Casodex
50mg: Zeneca

Bisoprolol

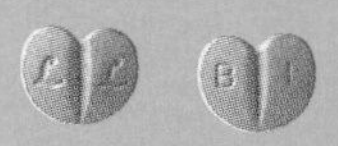

Zebeta
5mg: Lederle

Bisoprolol/ Hydrochlorothiazide

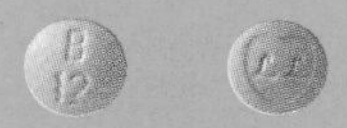

Ziac
2.5/6.25mg: Lederle

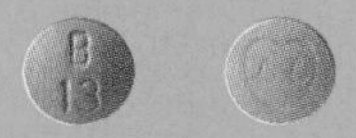

Ziac
5/6.25mg: Lederle

Ziac
10/6.25mg: Lederle

Bromocriptine

Parlodel
2.5mg: Sandoz

Parlodel
5mg: Sandoz

Bumetanide

Generic
0.5mg: Mylan

Generic
1mg: Mylan

Generic
2mg: Mylan

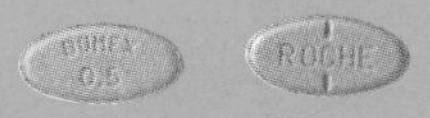

Bumex
0.5mg: Roche

Bumex
1mg: Roche

Bumex
2mg: Roche

Bupropion HCl

Wellbutrin
75mg: Glaxo Wellcome

Wellbutrin
100mg: Glaxo Wellcome

Buspirone HCl

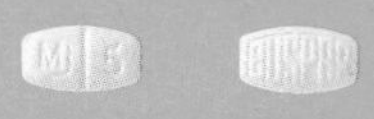

BuSpar
5mg: Bristol-Myers Squibb

BuSpar
10mg: Bristol-Myers Squibb

Calcitriol

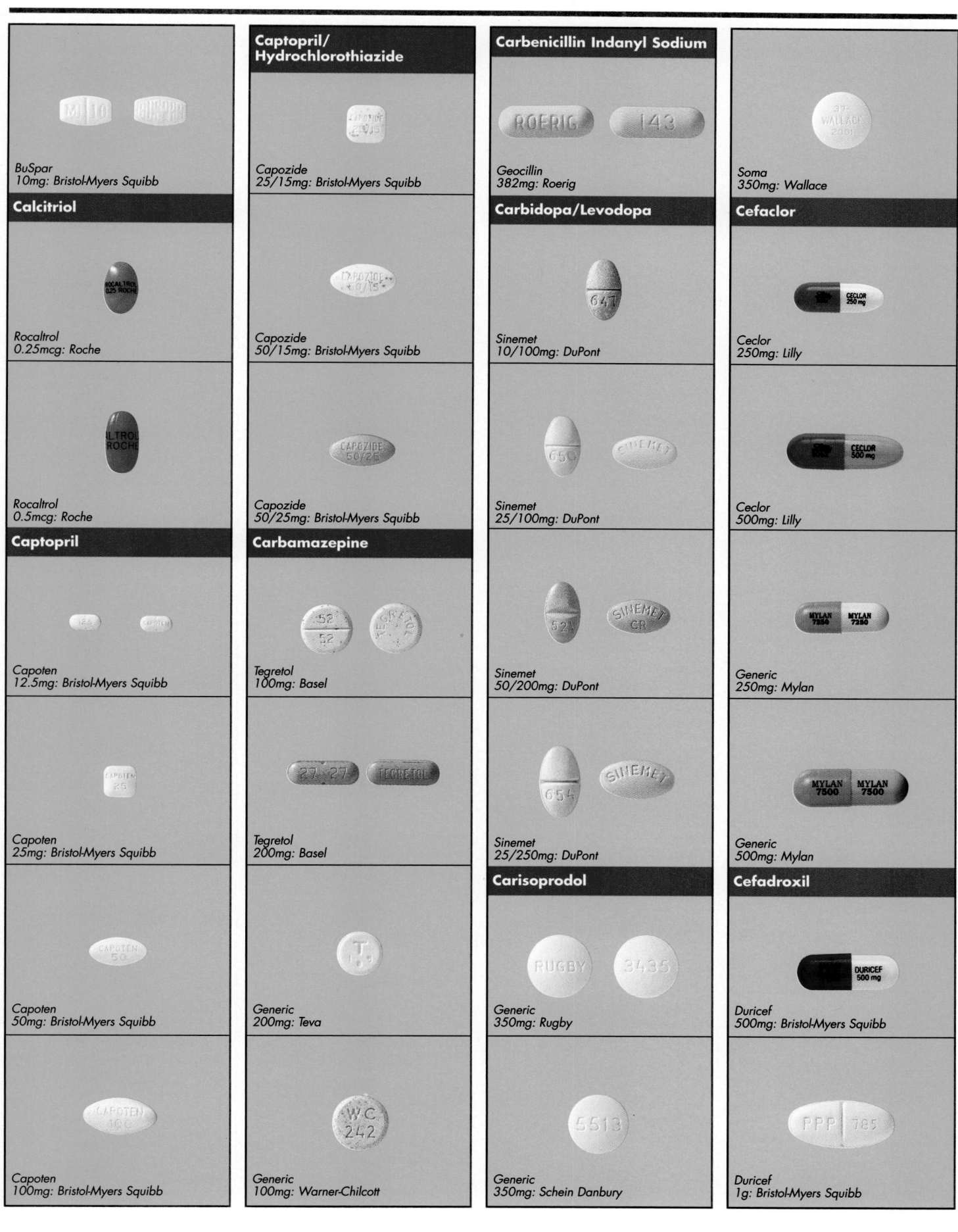

Rocaltrol
0.25mcg: Roche

Rocaltrol
0.5mcg: Roche

Captopril

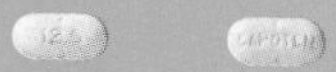
Capoten
12.5mg: Bristol-Myers Squibb

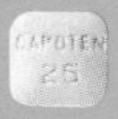

Capoten
25mg: Bristol-Myers Squibb

Capoten
50mg: Bristol-Myers Squibb

Capoten
100mg: Bristol-Myers Squibb

Captopril/ Hydrochlorothiazide

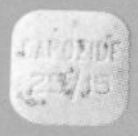
Capozide
25/15mg: Bristol-Myers Squibb

Capozide
50/15mg: Bristol-Myers Squibb

Capozide
50/25mg: Bristol-Myers Squibb

Carbamazepine

Tegretol
100mg: Basel

Tegretol
200mg: Basel

Generic
200mg: Teva

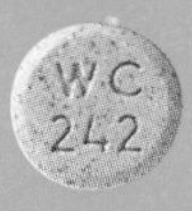

Generic
100mg: Warner-Chilcott

Carbenicillin Indanyl Sodium

Geocillin
382mg: Roerig

Carbidopa/Levodopa

Sinemet
10/100mg: DuPont

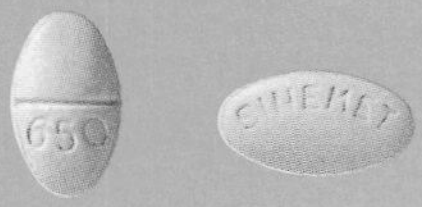

Sinemet
25/100mg: DuPont

Sinemet
50/200mg: DuPont

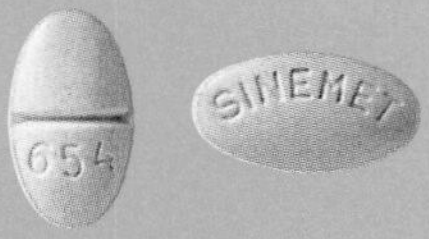

Sinemet
25/250mg: DuPont

Carisoprodol

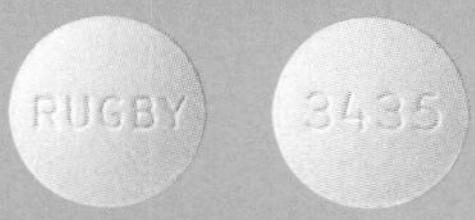

Generic
350mg: Rugby

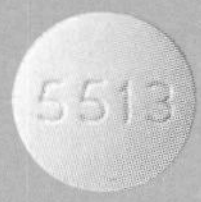

Generic
350mg: Schein Danbury

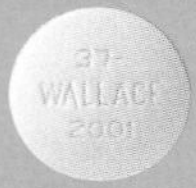

Soma
350mg: Wallace

Cefaclor

Ceclor
250mg: Lilly

Ceclor
500mg: Lilly

Generic
250mg: Mylan

Generic
500mg: Mylan

Cefadroxil

Duricef
500mg: Bristol-Myers Squibb

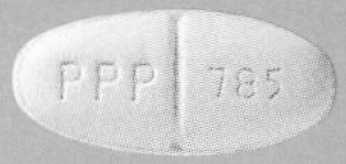

Duricef
1g: Bristol-Myers Squibb

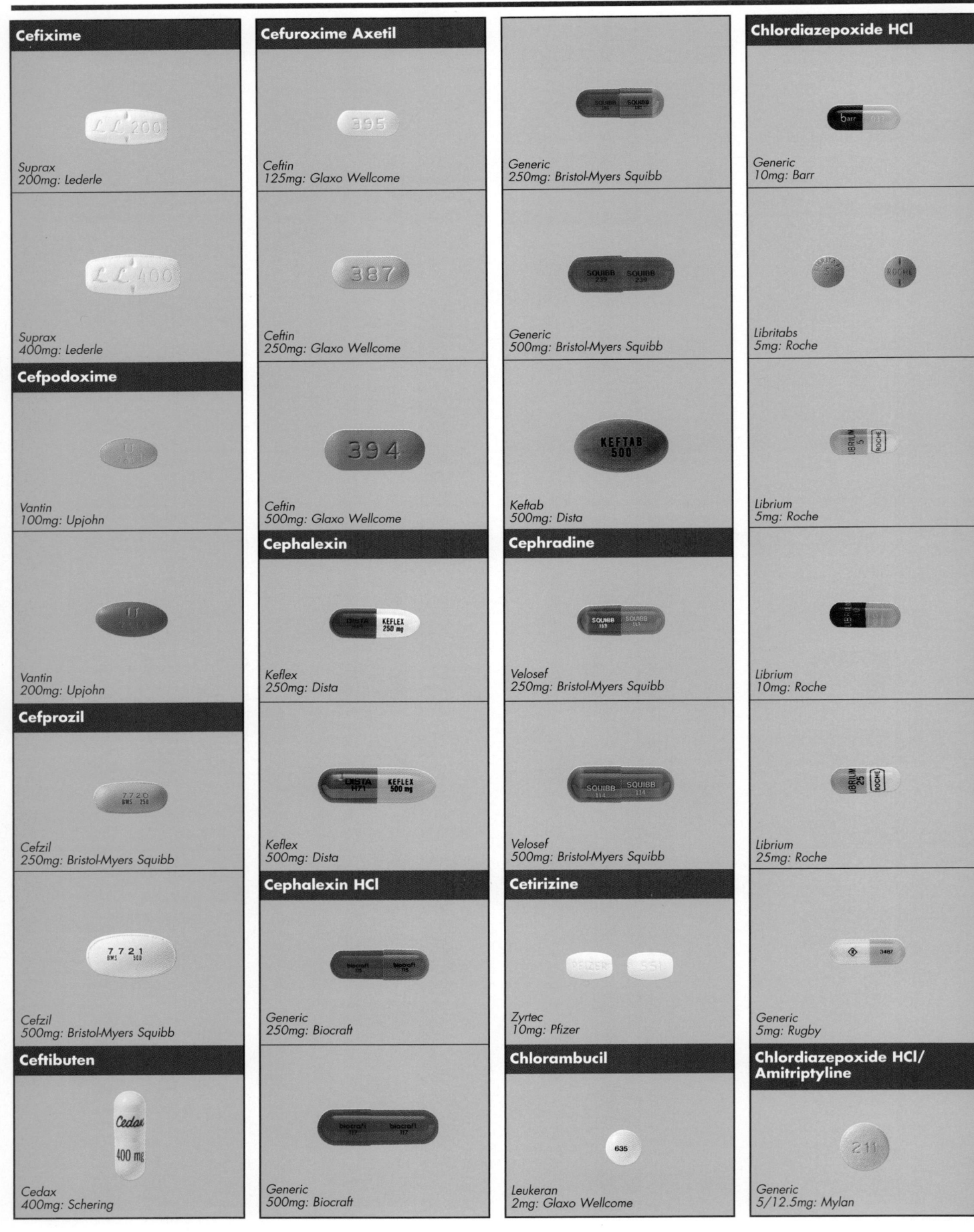

Cefixime

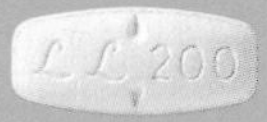

Suprax
200mg: Lederle

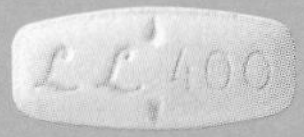

Suprax
400mg: Lederle

Cefpodoxime

Vantin
100mg: Upjohn

Vantin
200mg: Upjohn

Cefprozil

Cefzil
250mg: Bristol-Myers Squibb

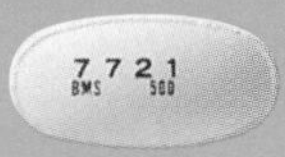

Cefzil
500mg: Bristol-Myers Squibb

Ceftibuten

Cedax
400mg: Schering

Cefuroxime Axetil

Ceftin
125mg: Glaxo Wellcome

Ceftin
250mg: Glaxo Wellcome

Ceftin
500mg: Glaxo Wellcome

Cephalexin

Keflex
250mg: Dista

Keflex
500mg: Dista

Cephalexin HCl

Generic
250mg: Biocraft

Generic
500mg: Biocraft

Generic
250mg: Bristol-Myers Squibb

Generic
500mg: Bristol-Myers Squibb

Keftab
500mg: Dista

Cephradine

Velosef
250mg: Bristol-Myers Squibb

Velosef
500mg: Bristol-Myers Squibb

Cetirizine

Zyrtec
10mg: Pfizer

Chlorambucil

Leukeran
2mg: Glaxo Wellcome

Chlordiazepoxide HCl

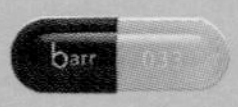

Generic
10mg: Barr

Libritabs
5mg: Roche

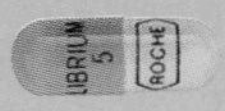

Librium
5mg: Roche

Librium
10mg: Roche

Librium
25mg: Roche

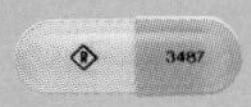

Generic
5mg: Rugby

Chlordiazepoxide HCl/ Amitriptyline

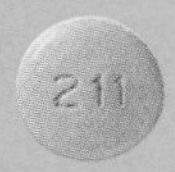

Generic
5/12.5mg: Mylan

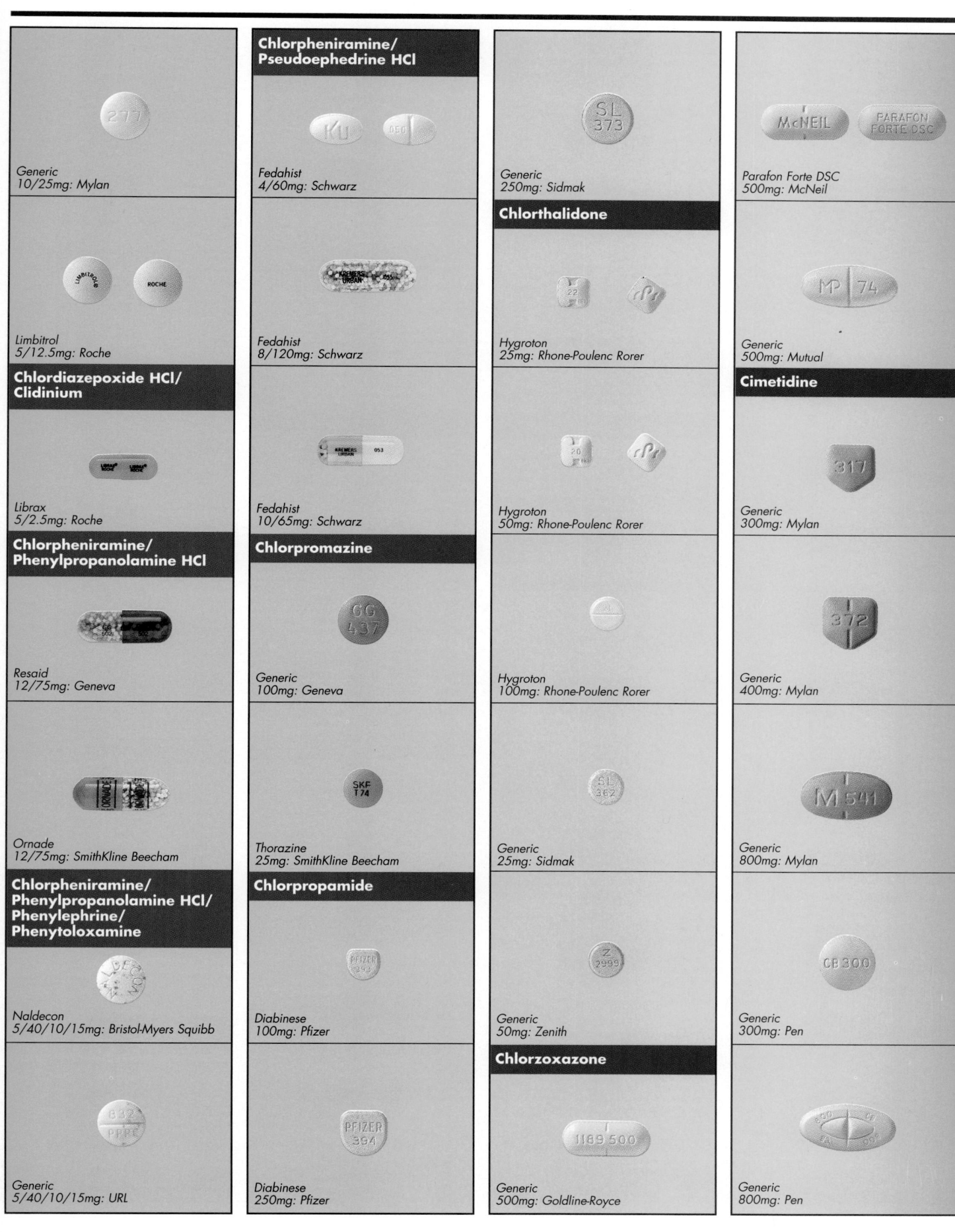

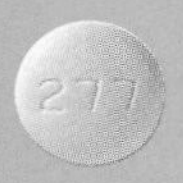

Generic
10/25mg: Mylan

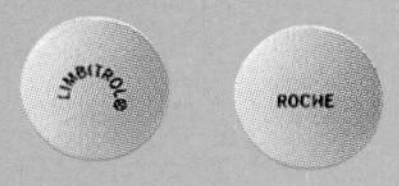

Limbitrol
5/12.5mg: Roche

Chlordiazepoxide HCl/ Clidinium

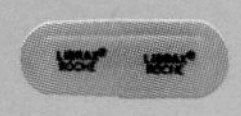

Librax
5/2.5mg: Roche

Chlorpheniramine/ Phenylpropanolamine HCl

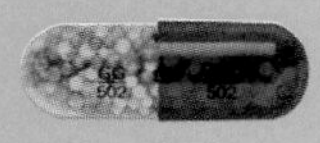

Resaid
12/75mg: Geneva

Ornade
12/75mg: SmithKline Beecham

Chlorpheniramine/ Phenylpropanolamine HCl/ Phenylephrine/ Phenytoloxamine

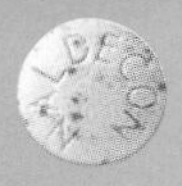

Naldecon
5/40/10/15mg: Bristol-Myers Squibb

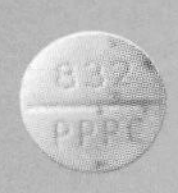

Generic
5/40/10/15mg: URL

Chlorpheniramine/ Pseudoephedrine HCl

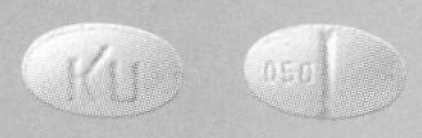

Fedahist
4/60mg: Schwarz

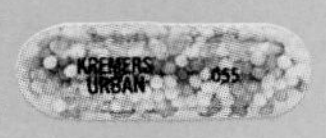

Fedahist
8/120mg: Schwarz

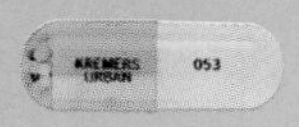

Fedahist
10/65mg: Schwarz

Chlorpromazine

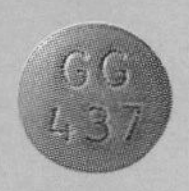

Generic
100mg: Geneva

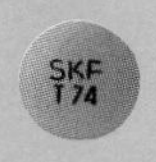

Thorazine
25mg: SmithKline Beecham

Chlorpropamide

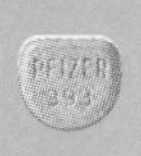

Diabinese
100mg: Pfizer

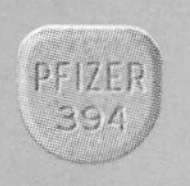

Diabinese
250mg: Pfizer

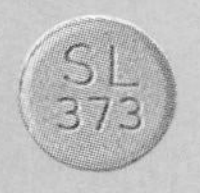

Generic
250mg: Sidmak

Chlorthalidone

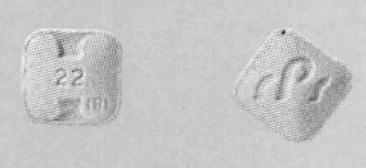

Hygroton
25mg: Rhone-Poulenc Rorer

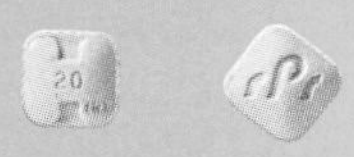

Hygroton
50mg: Rhone-Poulenc Rorer

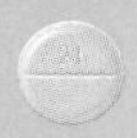

Hygroton
100mg: Rhone-Poulenc Rorer

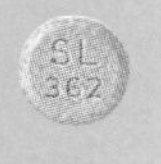

Generic
25mg: Sidmak

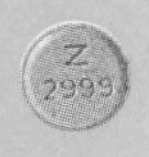

Generic
50mg: Zenith

Chlorzoxazone

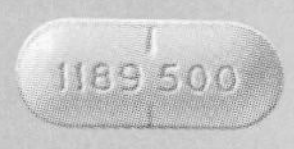

Generic
500mg: Goldline-Royce

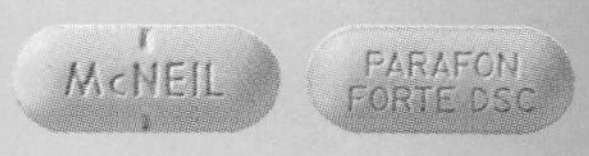

Parafon Forte DSC
500mg: McNeil

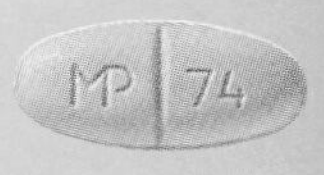

Generic
500mg: Mutual

Cimetidine

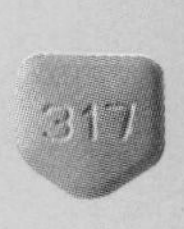

Generic
300mg: Mylan

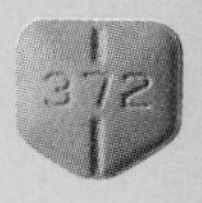

Generic
400mg: Mylan

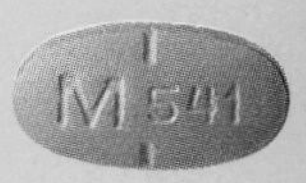

Generic
800mg: Mylan

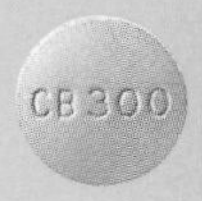

Generic
300mg: Pen

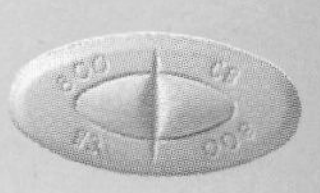

Generic
800mg: Pen

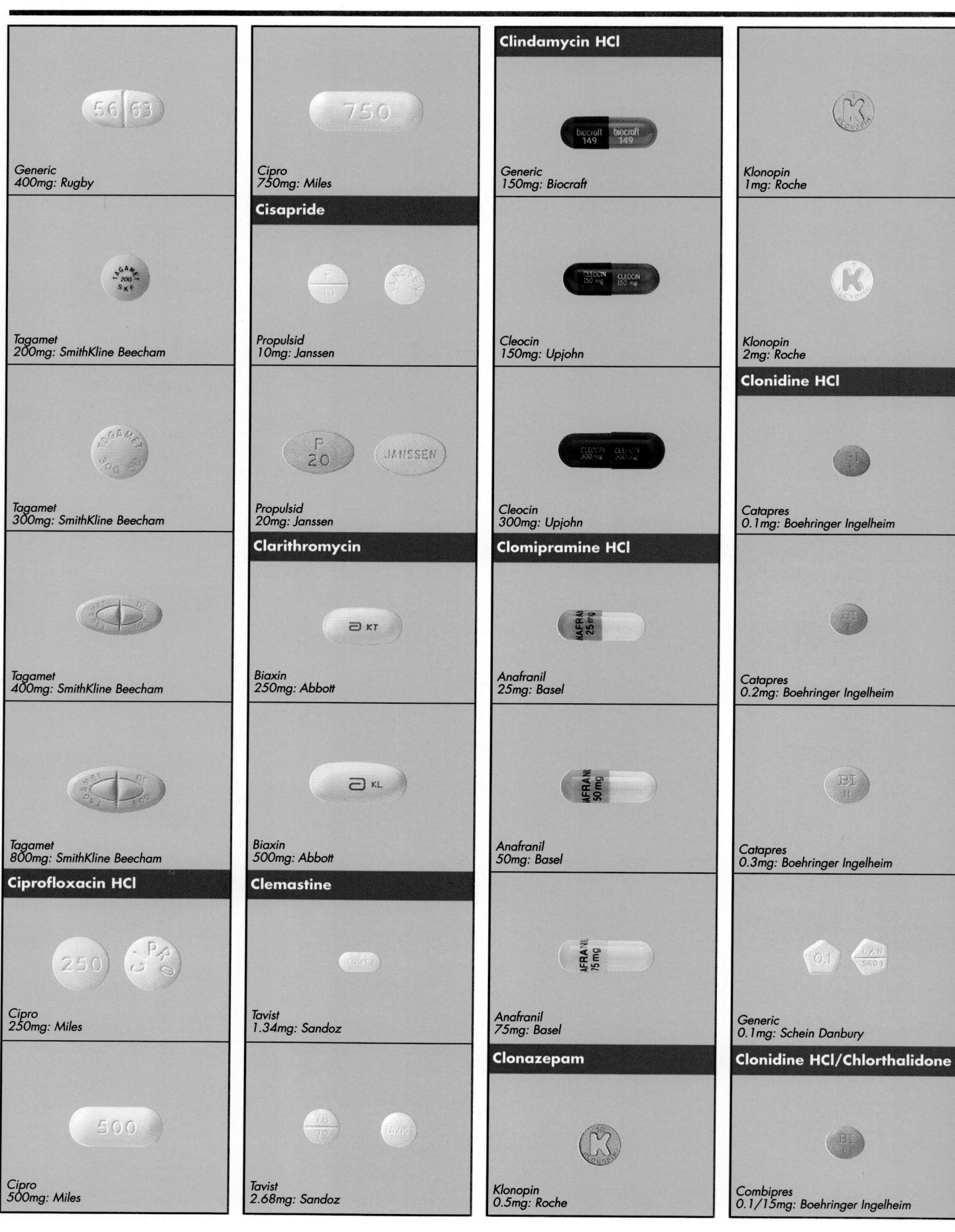

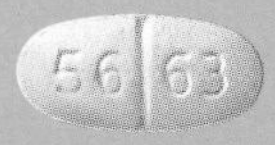

Generic
400mg: Rugby

Tagamet
200mg: SmithKline Beecham

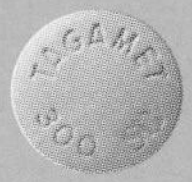

Tagamet
300mg: SmithKline Beecham

Tagamet
400mg: SmithKline Beecham

Tagamet
800mg: SmithKline Beecham

Ciprofloxacin HCl

Cipro
250mg: Miles

Cipro
500mg: Miles

Cipro
750mg: Miles

Cisapride

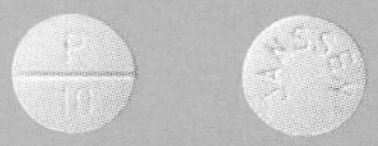

Propulsid
10mg: Janssen

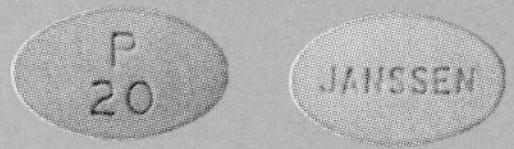

Propulsid
20mg: Janssen

Clarithromycin

Biaxin
250mg: Abbott

Biaxin
500mg: Abbott

Clemastine

Tavist
1.34mg: Sandoz

Tavist
2.68mg: Sandoz

Clindamycin HCl

Generic
150mg: Biocraft

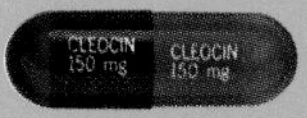

Cleocin
150mg: Upjohn

Cleocin
300mg: Upjohn

Clomipramine HCl

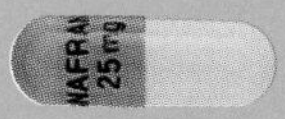

Anafranil
25mg: Basel

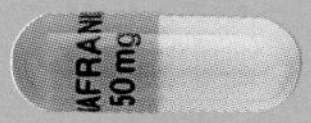

Anafranil
50mg: Basel

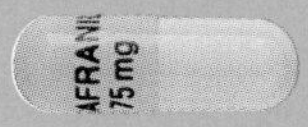

Anafranil
75mg: Basel

Clonazepam

Klonopin
0.5mg: Roche

Klonopin
1mg: Roche

Klonopin
2mg: Roche

Clonidine HCl

Catapres
0.1mg: Boehringer Ingelheim

Catapres
0.2mg: Boehringer Ingelheim

Catapres
0.3mg: Boehringer Ingelheim

Generic
0.1mg: Schein Danbury

Clonidine HCl/Chlorthalidone

Combipres
0.1/15mg: Boehringer Ingelheim

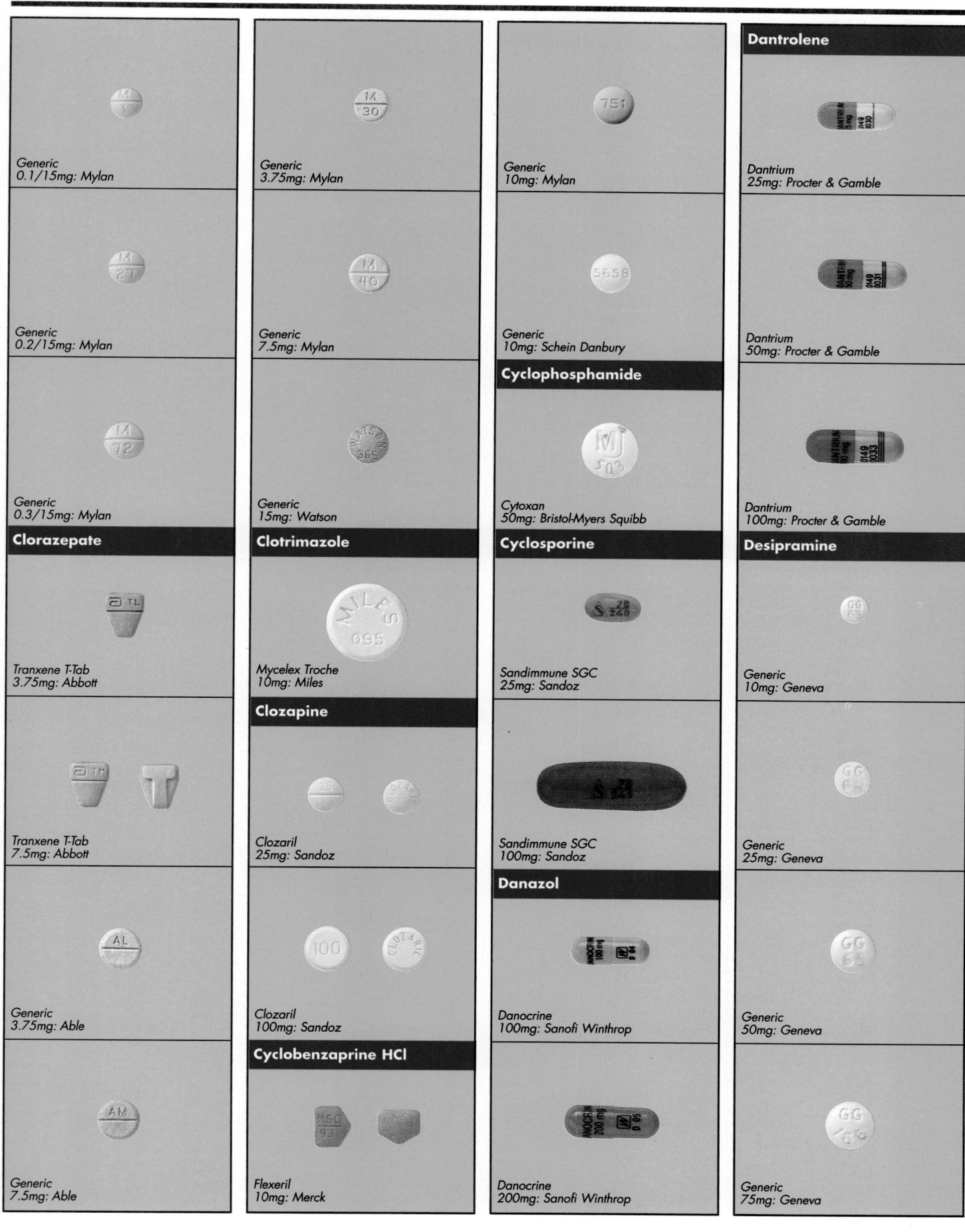

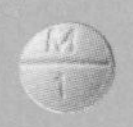

Generic
0.1/15mg: Mylan

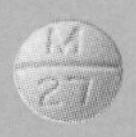

Generic
0.2/15mg: Mylan

Generic
0.3/15mg: Mylan

Clorazepate

Tranxene T-Tab
3.75mg: Abbott

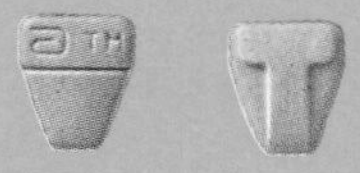

Tranxene T-Tab
7.5mg: Abbott

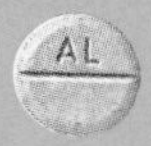

Generic
3.75mg: Able

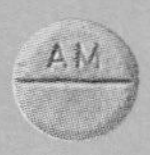

Generic
7.5mg: Able

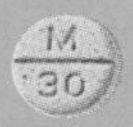

Generic
3.75mg: Mylan

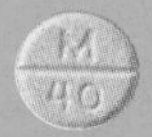

Generic
7.5mg: Mylan

Generic
15mg: Watson

Clotrimazole

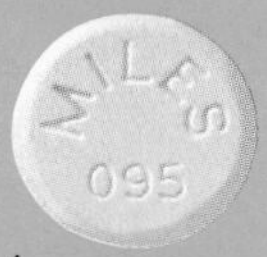

Mycelex Troche
10mg: Miles

Clozapine

Clozaril
25mg: Sandoz

Clozaril
100mg: Sandoz

Cyclobenzaprine HCl

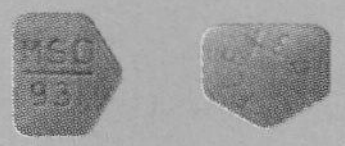

Flexeril
10mg: Merck

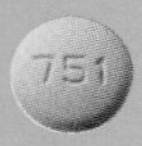

Generic
10mg: Mylan

Generic
10mg: Schein Danbury

Cyclophosphamide

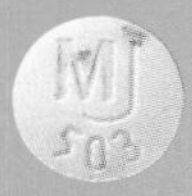

Cytoxan
50mg: Bristol-Myers Squibb

Cyclosporine

Sandimmune SGC
25mg: Sandoz

Sandimmune SGC
100mg: Sandoz

Danazol

Danocrine
100mg: Sanofi Winthrop

Danocrine
200mg: Sanofi Winthrop

Dantrolene

Dantrium
25mg: Procter & Gamble

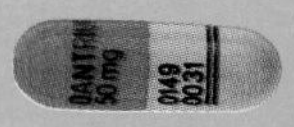

Dantrium
50mg: Procter & Gamble

Dantrium
100mg: Procter & Gamble

Desipramine

Generic
10mg: Geneva

Generic
25mg: Geneva

Generic
50mg: Geneva

Generic
75mg: Geneva

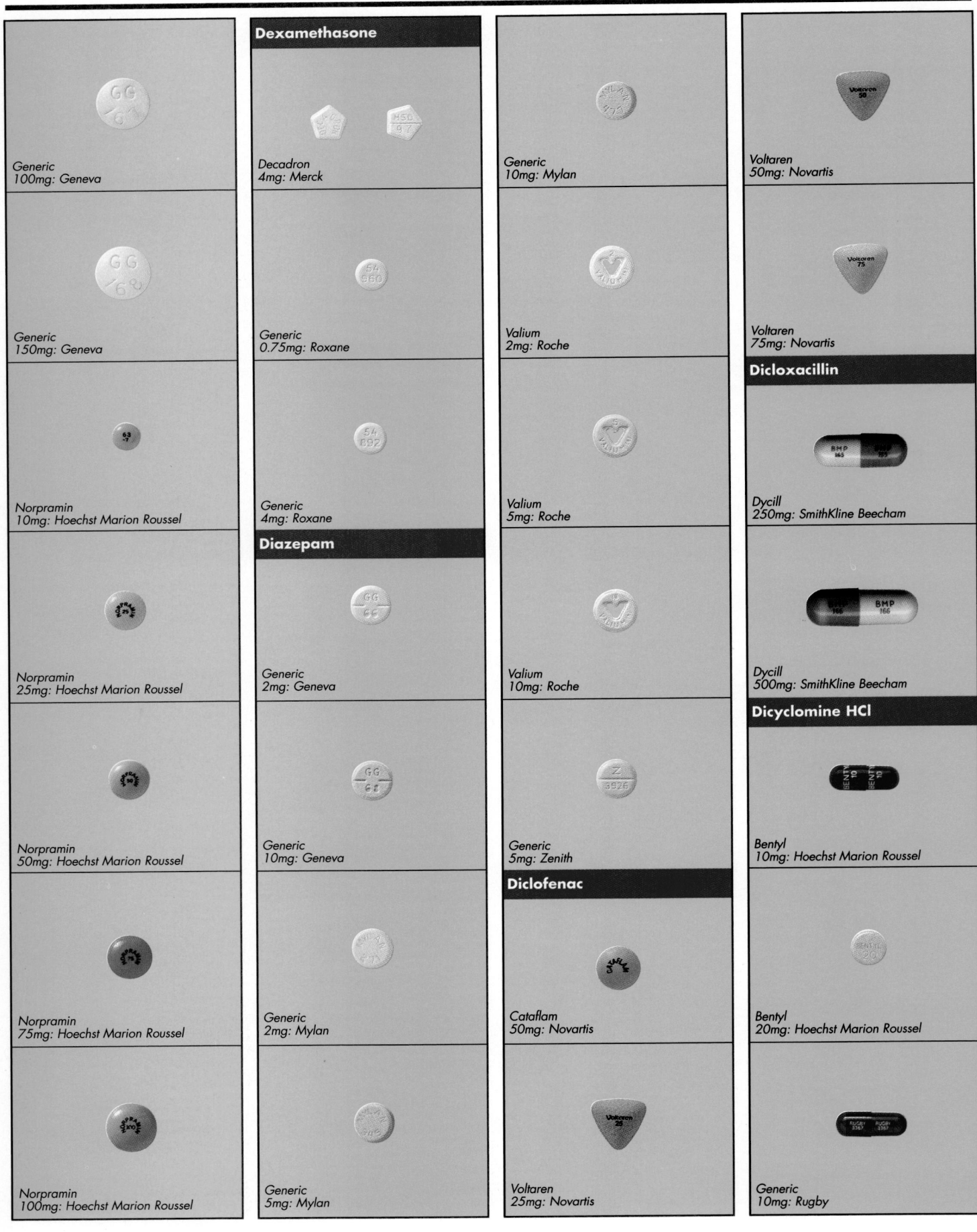

Generic
100mg: Geneva

Generic
150mg: Geneva

Norpramin
10mg: Hoechst Marion Roussel

Norpramin
25mg: Hoechst Marion Roussel

Norpramin
50mg: Hoechst Marion Roussel

Norpramin
75mg: Hoechst Marion Roussel

Norpramin
100mg: Hoechst Marion Roussel

Dexamethasone

Decadron
4mg: Merck

Generic
0.75mg: Roxane

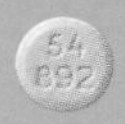

Generic
4mg: Roxane

Diazepam

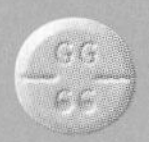

Generic
2mg: Geneva

Generic
10mg: Geneva

Generic
2mg: Mylan

Generic
5mg: Mylan

Generic
10mg: Mylan

Valium
2mg: Roche

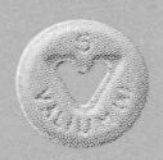

Valium
5mg: Roche

Valium
10mg: Roche

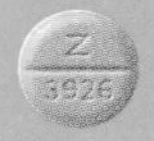

Generic
5mg: Zenith

Diclofenac

Cataflam
50mg: Novartis

Voltaren
25mg: Novartis

Voltaren
50mg: Novartis

Voltaren
75mg: Novartis

Dicloxacillin

Dycill
250mg: SmithKline Beecham

Dycill
500mg: SmithKline Beecham

Dicyclomine HCl

Bentyl
10mg: Hoechst Marion Roussel

Bentyl
20mg: Hoechst Marion Roussel

Generic
10mg: Rugby

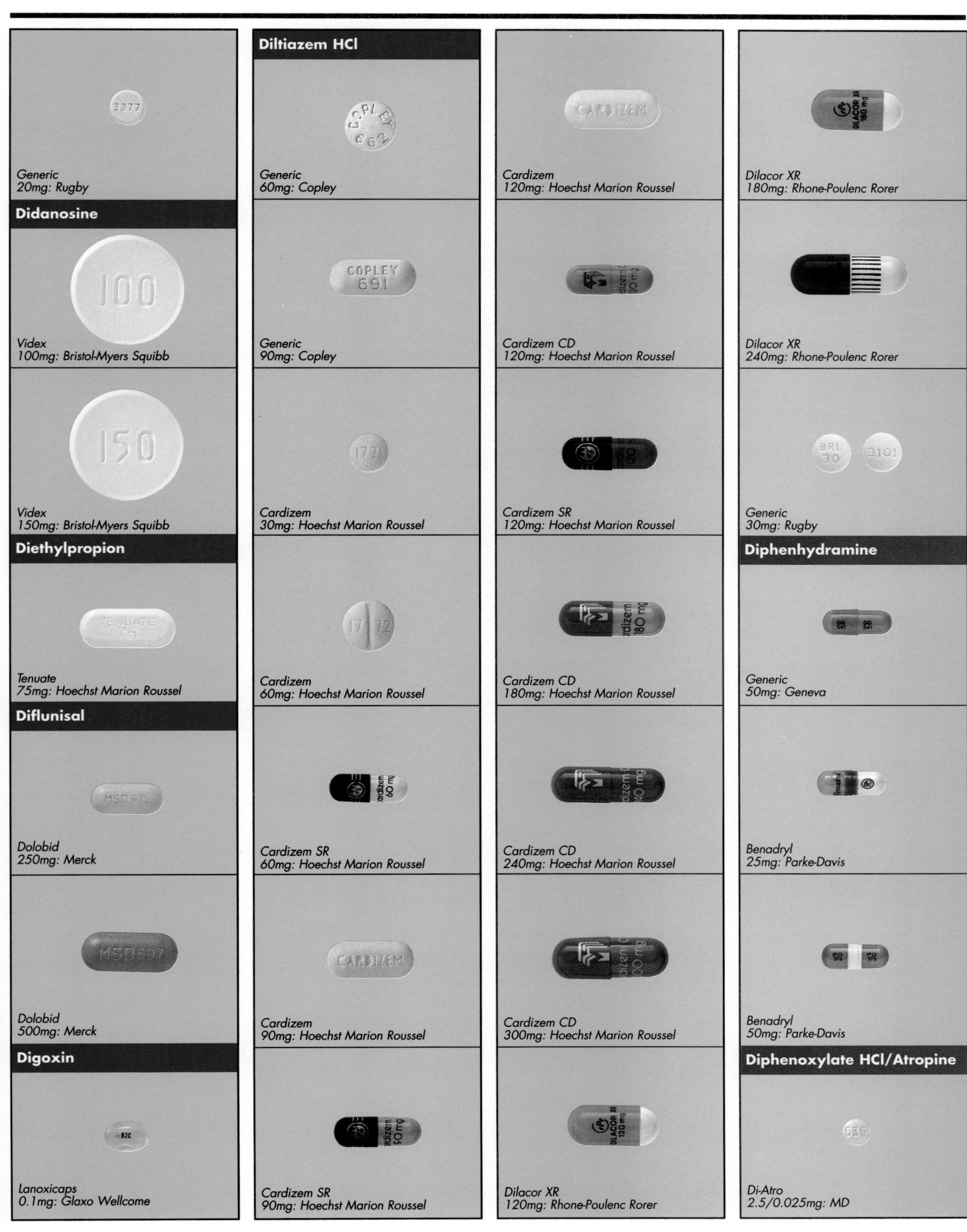

Generic
20mg: Rugby

Didanosine

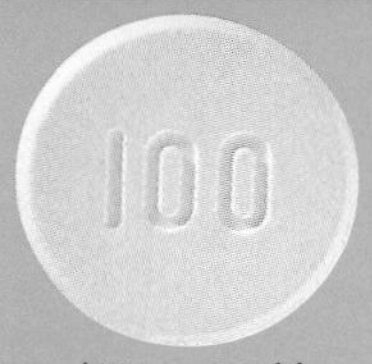

Videx
100mg: Bristol-Myers Squibb

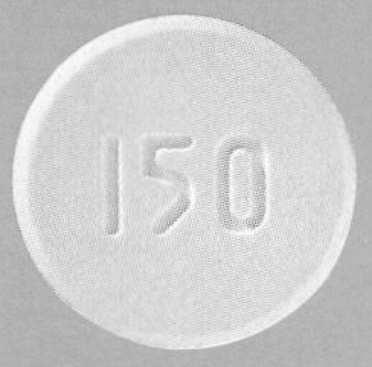

Videx
150mg: Bristol-Myers Squibb

Diethylpropion

Tenuate
75mg: Hoechst Marion Roussel

Diflunisal

Dolobid
250mg: Merck

Dolobid
500mg: Merck

Digoxin

Lanoxicaps
0.1mg: Glaxo Wellcome

Diltiazem HCl

Generic
60mg: Copley

Generic
90mg: Copley

Cardizem
30mg: Hoechst Marion Roussel

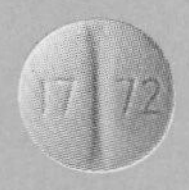

Cardizem
60mg: Hoechst Marion Roussel

Cardizem SR
60mg: Hoechst Marion Roussel

Cardizem
90mg: Hoechst Marion Roussel

Cardizem SR
90mg: Hoechst Marion Roussel

Cardizem
120mg: Hoechst Marion Roussel

Cardizem CD
120mg: Hoechst Marion Roussel

Cardizem SR
120mg: Hoechst Marion Roussel

Cardizem CD
180mg: Hoechst Marion Roussel

Cardizem CD
240mg: Hoechst Marion Roussel

Cardizem CD
300mg: Hoechst Marion Roussel

Dilacor XR
120mg: Rhone-Poulenc Rorer

Dilacor XR
180mg: Rhone-Poulenc Rorer

Dilacor XR
240mg: Rhone-Poulenc Rorer

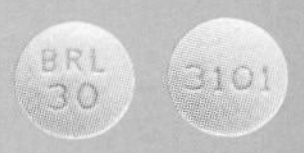

Generic
30mg: Rugby

Diphenhydramine

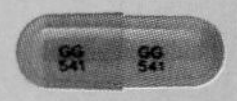

Generic
50mg: Geneva

Benadryl
25mg: Parke-Davis

Benadryl
50mg: Parke-Davis

Diphenoxylate HCl/Atropine

Di-Atro
2.5/0.025mg: MD

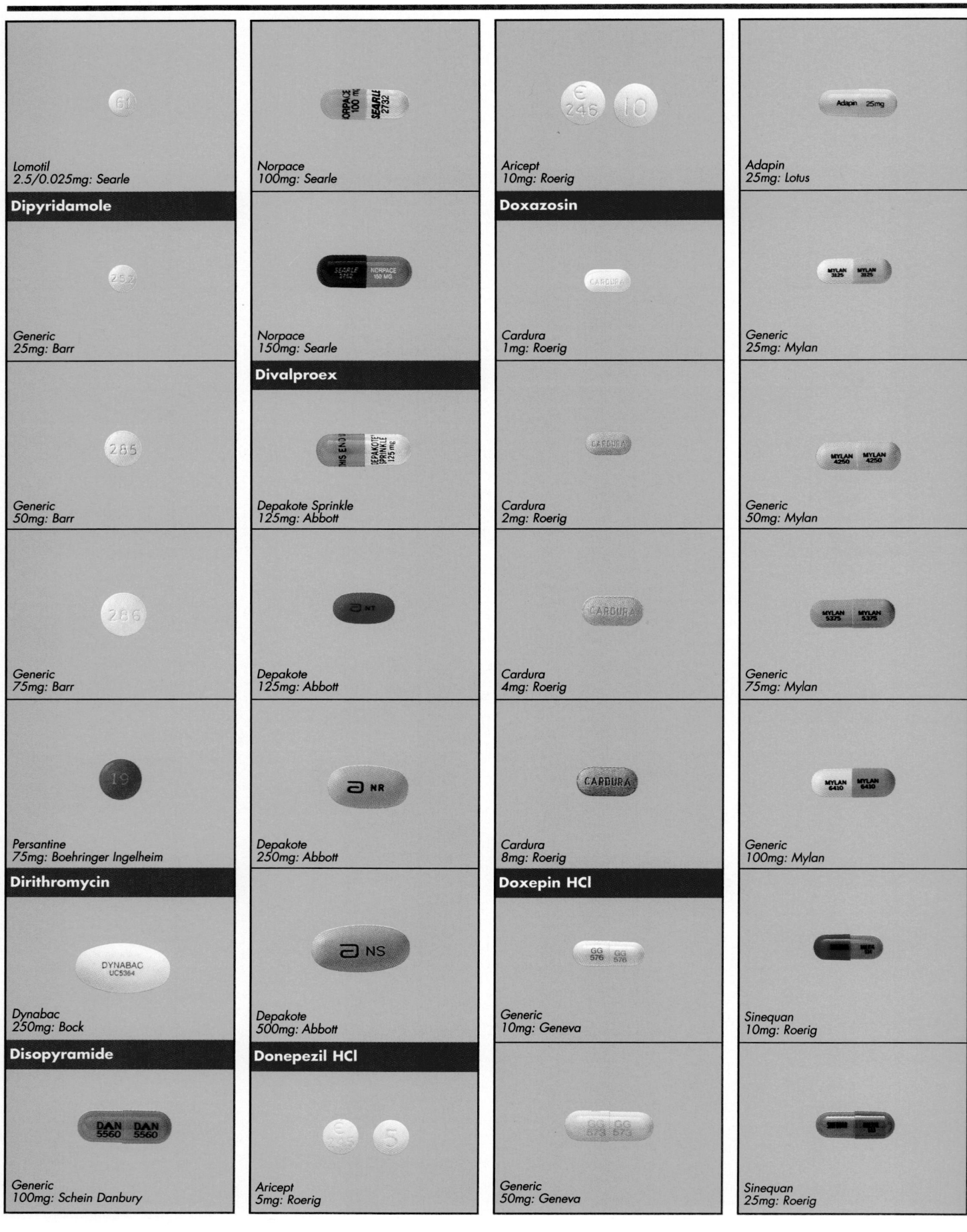

Lomotil
2.5/0.025mg: Searle

Dipyridamole

Generic
25mg: Barr

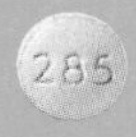

Generic
50mg: Barr

Generic
75mg: Barr

Persantine
75mg: Boehringer Ingelheim

Dirithromycin

Dynabac
250mg: Bock

Disopyramide

Generic
100mg: Schein Danbury

Norpace
100mg: Searle

Norpace
150mg: Searle

Divalproex

Depakote Sprinkle
125mg: Abbott

Depakote
125mg: Abbott

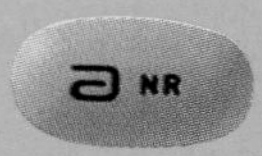

Depakote
250mg: Abbott

Depakote
500mg: Abbott

Donepezil HCl

Aricept
5mg: Roerig

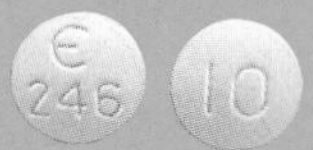

Aricept
10mg: Roerig

Doxazosin

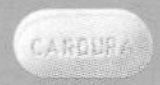

Cardura
1mg: Roerig

Cardura
2mg: Roerig

Cardura
4mg: Roerig

Cardura
8mg: Roerig

Doxepin HCl

Generic
10mg: Geneva

Generic
50mg: Geneva

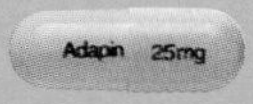

Adapin
25mg: Lotus

Generic
25mg: Mylan

Generic
50mg: Mylan

Generic
75mg: Mylan

Generic
100mg: Mylan

Sinequan
10mg: Roerig

Sinequan
25mg: Roerig

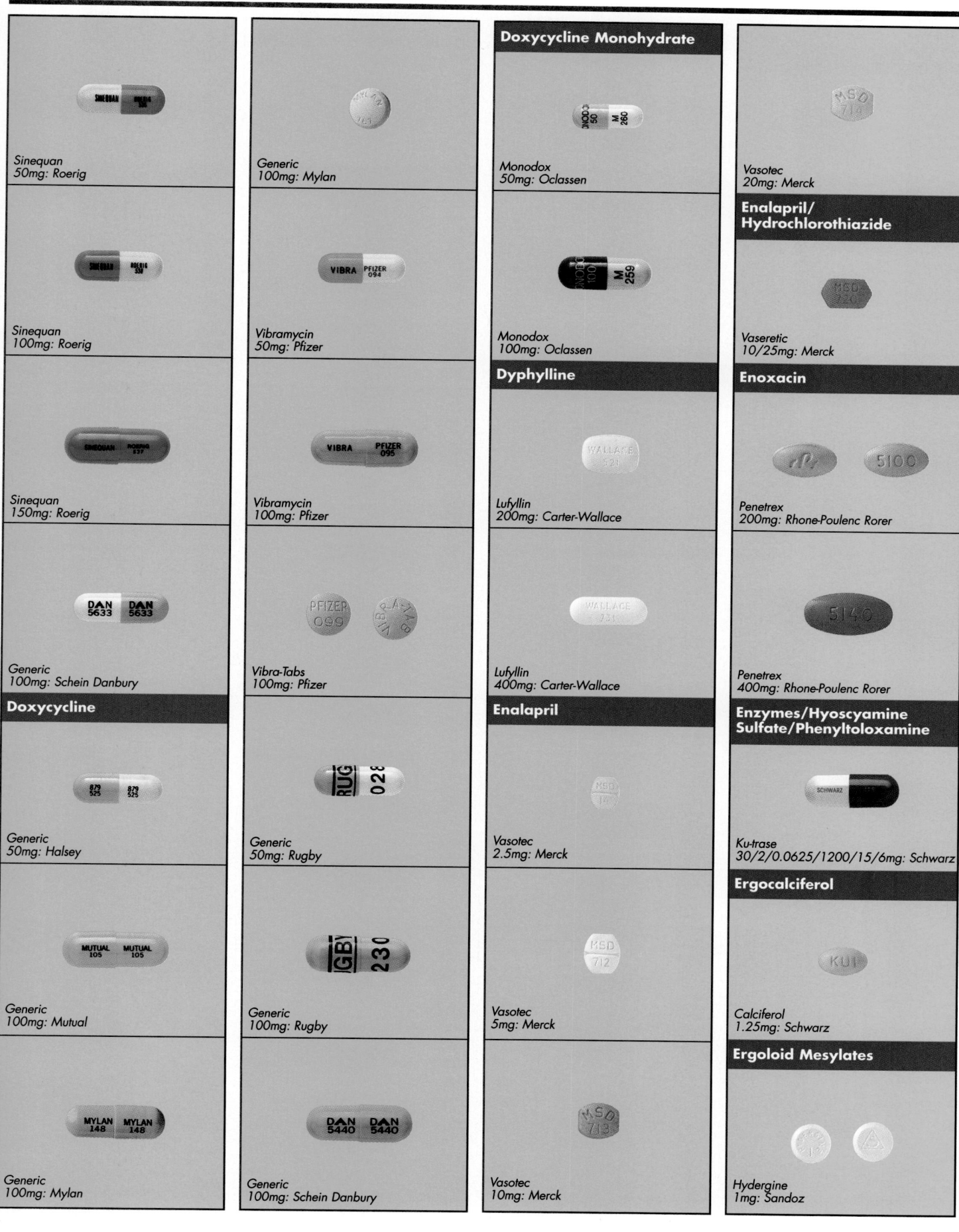

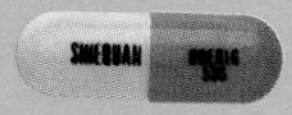

Sinequan
50mg: Roerig

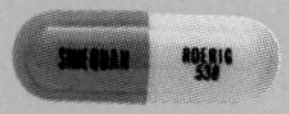

Sinequan
100mg: Roerig

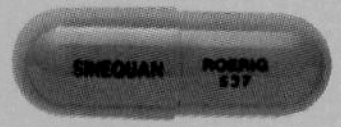

Sinequan
150mg: Roerig

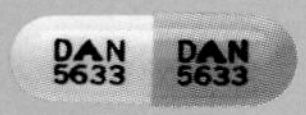

Generic
100mg: Schein Danbury

Doxycycline

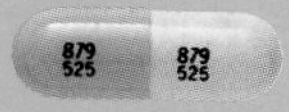

Generic
50mg: Halsey

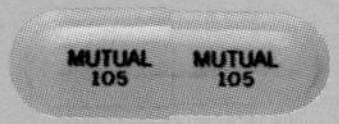

Generic
100mg: Mutual

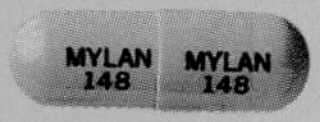

Generic
100mg: Mylan

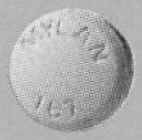

Generic
100mg: Mylan

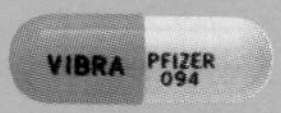

Vibramycin
50mg: Pfizer

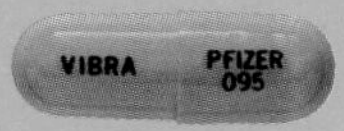

Vibramycin
100mg: Pfizer

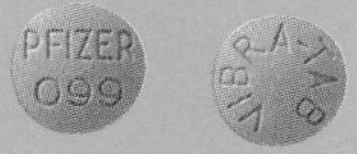

Vibra-Tabs
100mg: Pfizer

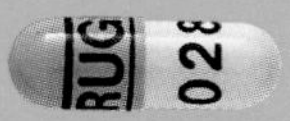

Generic
50mg: Rugby

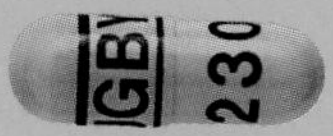

Generic
100mg: Rugby

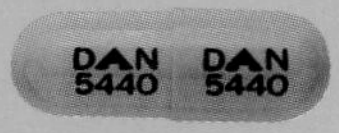

Generic
100mg: Schein Danbury

Doxycycline Monohydrate

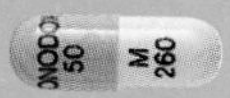

Monodox
50mg: Oclassen

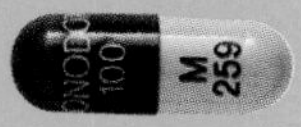

Monodox
100mg: Oclassen

Dyphylline

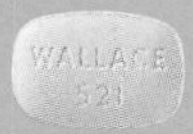

Lufyllin
200mg: Carter-Wallace

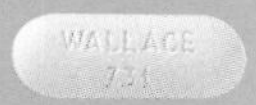

Lufyllin
400mg: Carter-Wallace

Enalapril

Vasotec
2.5mg: Merck

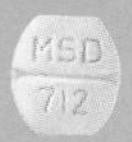

Vasotec
5mg: Merck

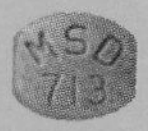

Vasotec
10mg: Merck

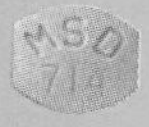

Vasotec
20mg: Merck

Enalapril/ Hydrochlorothiazide

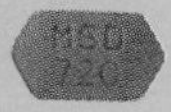

Vaseretic
10/25mg: Merck

Enoxacin

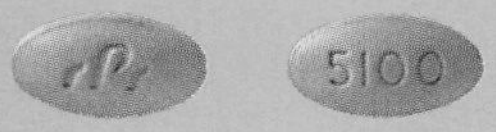

Penetrex
200mg: Rhone-Poulenc Rorer

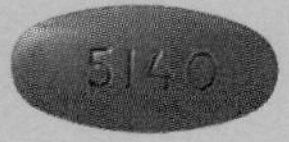

Penetrex
400mg: Rhone-Poulenc Rorer

Enzymes/Hyoscyamine Sulfate/Phenyltoloxamine

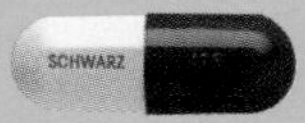

Ku-trase
30/2/0.0625/1200/15/6mg: Schwarz

Ergocalciferol

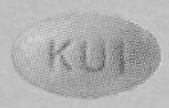

Calciferol
1.25mg: Schwarz

Ergoloid Mesylates

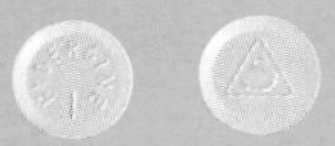

Hydergine
1mg: Sandoz

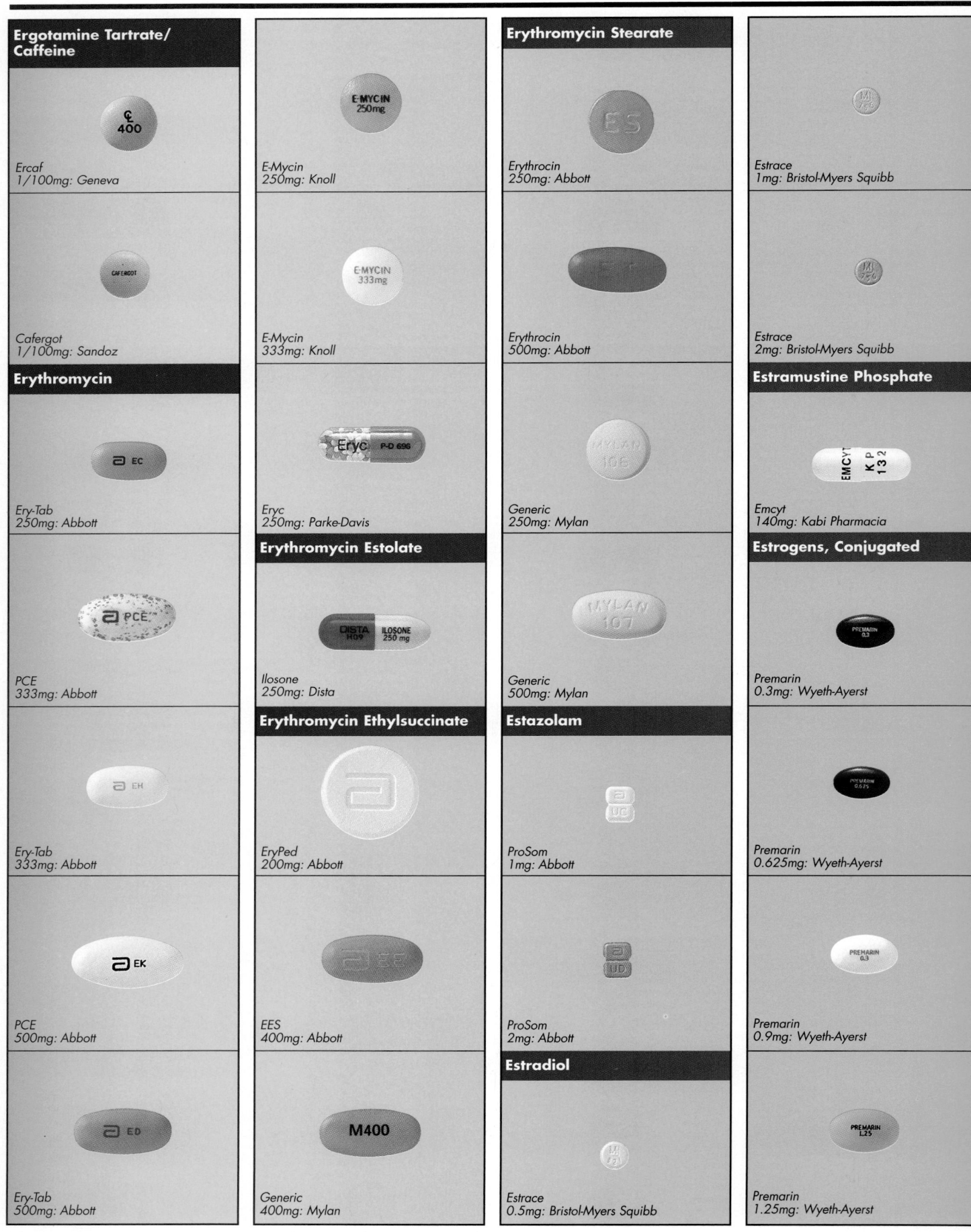

Ergotamine Tartrate/ Caffeine

Ercaf
1/100mg: Geneva

Cafergot
1/100mg: Sandoz

Erythromycin

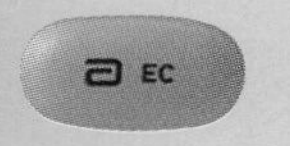

Ery-Tab
250mg: Abbott

PCE
333mg: Abbott

Ery-Tab
333mg: Abbott

PCE
500mg: Abbott

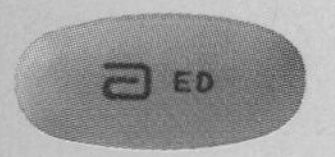

Ery-Tab
500mg: Abbott

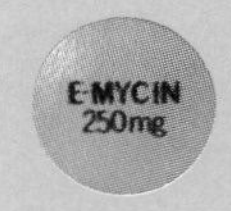

E-Mycin
250mg: Knoll

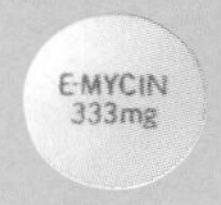

E-Mycin
333mg: Knoll

Eryc
250mg: Parke-Davis

Erythromycin Estolate

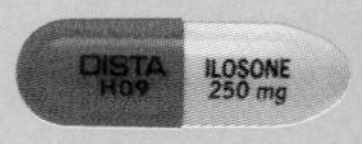

Ilosone
250mg: Dista

Erythromycin Ethylsuccinate

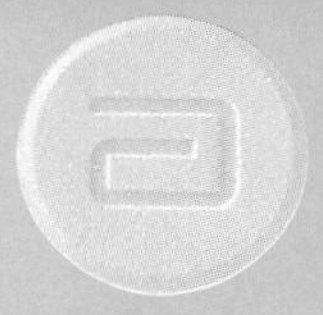

EryPed
200mg: Abbott

EES
400mg: Abbott

Generic
400mg: Mylan

Erythromycin Stearate

Erythrocin
250mg: Abbott

Erythrocin
500mg: Abbott

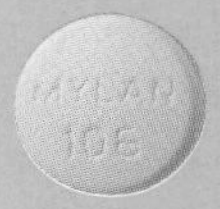

Generic
250mg: Mylan

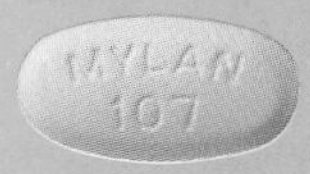

Generic
500mg: Mylan

Estazolam

ProSom
1mg: Abbott

ProSom
2mg: Abbott

Estradiol

Estrace
0.5mg: Bristol-Myers Squibb

Estrace
1mg: Bristol-Myers Squibb

Estrace
2mg: Bristol-Myers Squibb

Estramustine Phosphate

Emcyt
140mg: Kabi Pharmacia

Estrogens, Conjugated

Premarin
0.3mg: Wyeth-Ayerst

Premarin
0.625mg: Wyeth-Ayerst

Premarin
0.9mg: Wyeth-Ayerst

Premarin
1.25mg: Wyeth-Ayerst

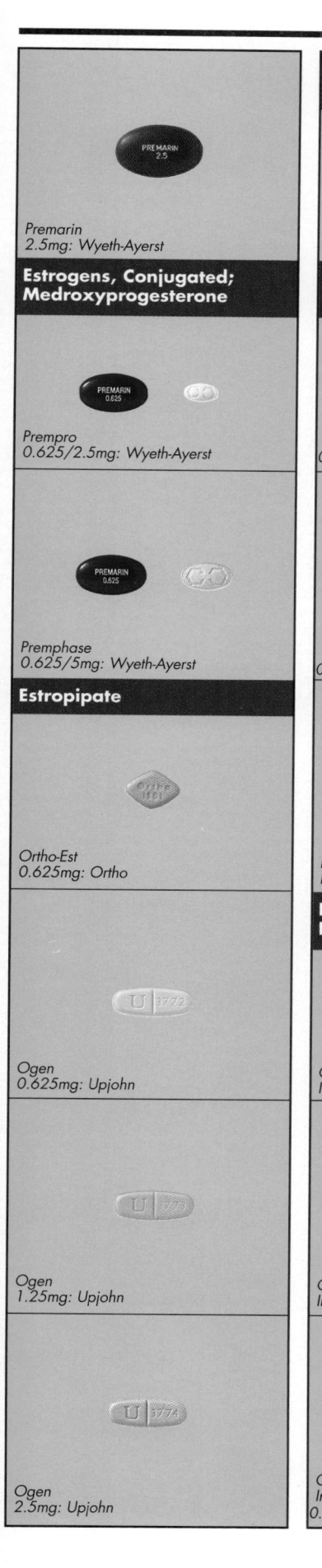

Premarin
2.5mg: Wyeth-Ayerst

Estrogens, Conjugated; Medroxyprogesterone

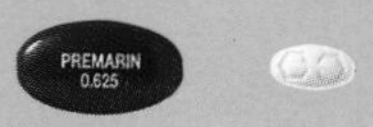

Prempro
0.625/2.5mg: Wyeth-Ayerst

Premphase
0.625/5mg: Wyeth-Ayerst

Estropipate

Ortho-Est
0.625mg: Ortho

Ogen
0.625mg: Upjohn

Ogen
1.25mg: Upjohn

Ogen
2.5mg: Upjohn

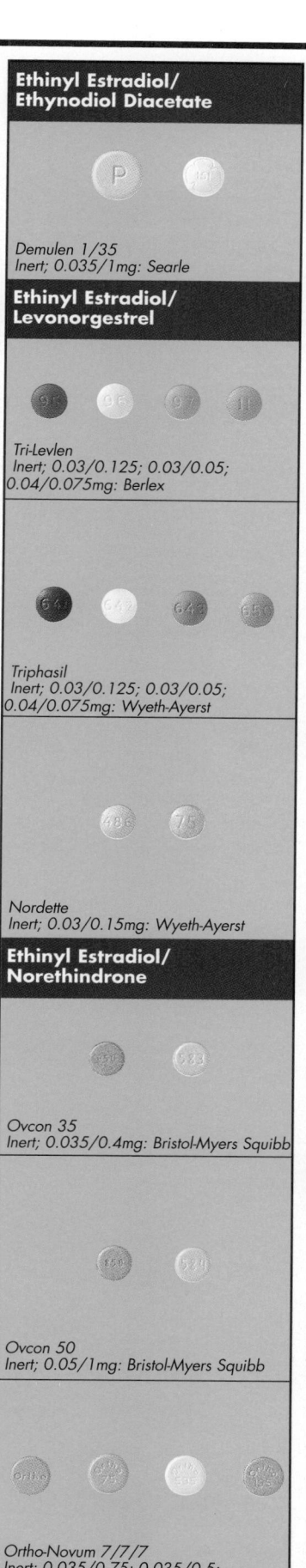

Ethinyl Estradiol/ Ethynodiol Diacetate

Demulen 1/35
Inert; 0.035/1mg: Searle

Ethinyl Estradiol/ Levonorgestrel

Tri-Levlen
Inert; 0.03/0.125; 0.03/0.05; 0.04/0.075mg: Berlex

Triphasil
Inert; 0.03/0.125; 0.03/0.05; 0.04/0.075mg: Wyeth-Ayerst

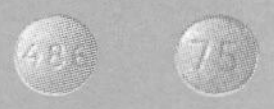

Nordette
Inert; 0.03/0.15mg: Wyeth-Ayerst

Ethinyl Estradiol/ Norethindrone

Ovcon 35
Inert; 0.035/0.4mg: Bristol-Myers Squibb

Ovcon 50
Inert; 0.05/1mg: Bristol-Myers Squibb

Ortho-Novum 7/7/7
Inert; 0.035/0.75; 0.035/0.5; 0.035/1mg: Ortho

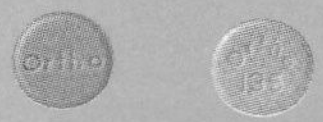

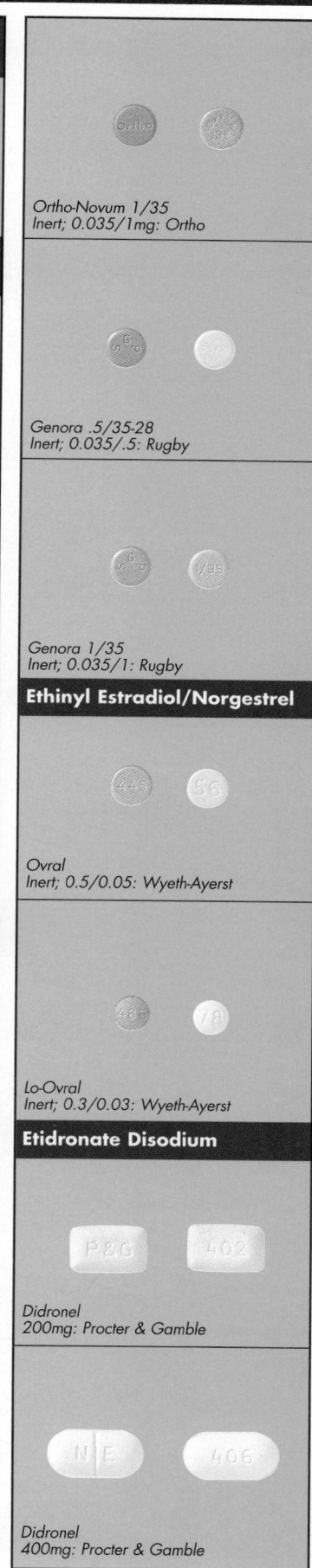

Ortho-Novum 1/35
Inert; 0.035/1mg: Ortho

Genora .5/35-28
Inert; 0.035/.5: Rugby

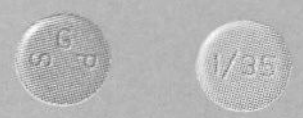

Genora 1/35
Inert; 0.035/1: Rugby

Ethinyl Estradiol/Norgestrel

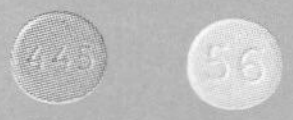

Ovral
Inert; 0.5/0.05: Wyeth-Ayerst

Lo-Ovral
Inert; 0.3/0.03: Wyeth-Ayerst

Etidronate Disodium

Didronel
200mg: Procter & Gamble

Didronel
400mg: Procter & Gamble

Etodolac

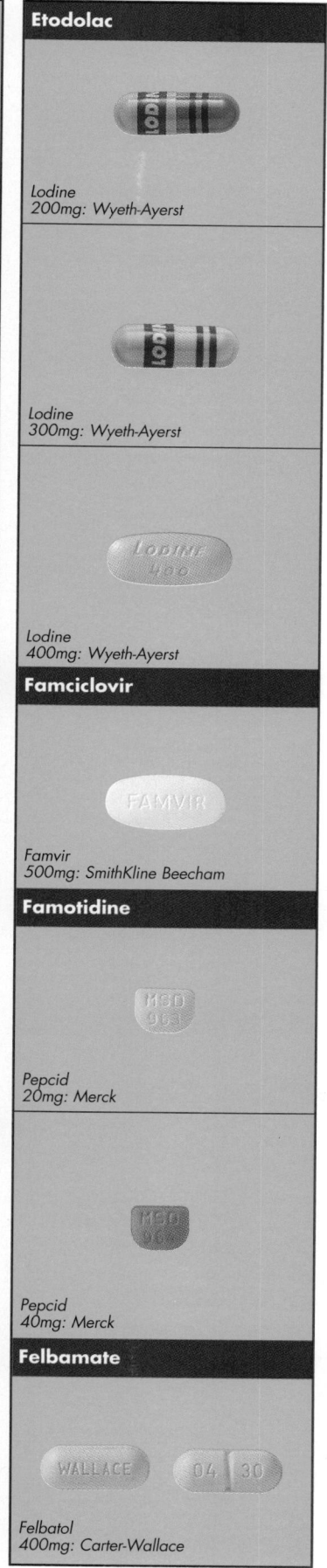

Lodine
200mg: Wyeth-Ayerst

Lodine
300mg: Wyeth-Ayerst

Lodine
400mg: Wyeth-Ayerst

Famciclovir

Famvir
500mg: SmithKline Beecham

Famotidine

Pepcid
20mg: Merck

Pepcid
40mg: Merck

Felbamate

Felbatol
400mg: Carter-Wallace

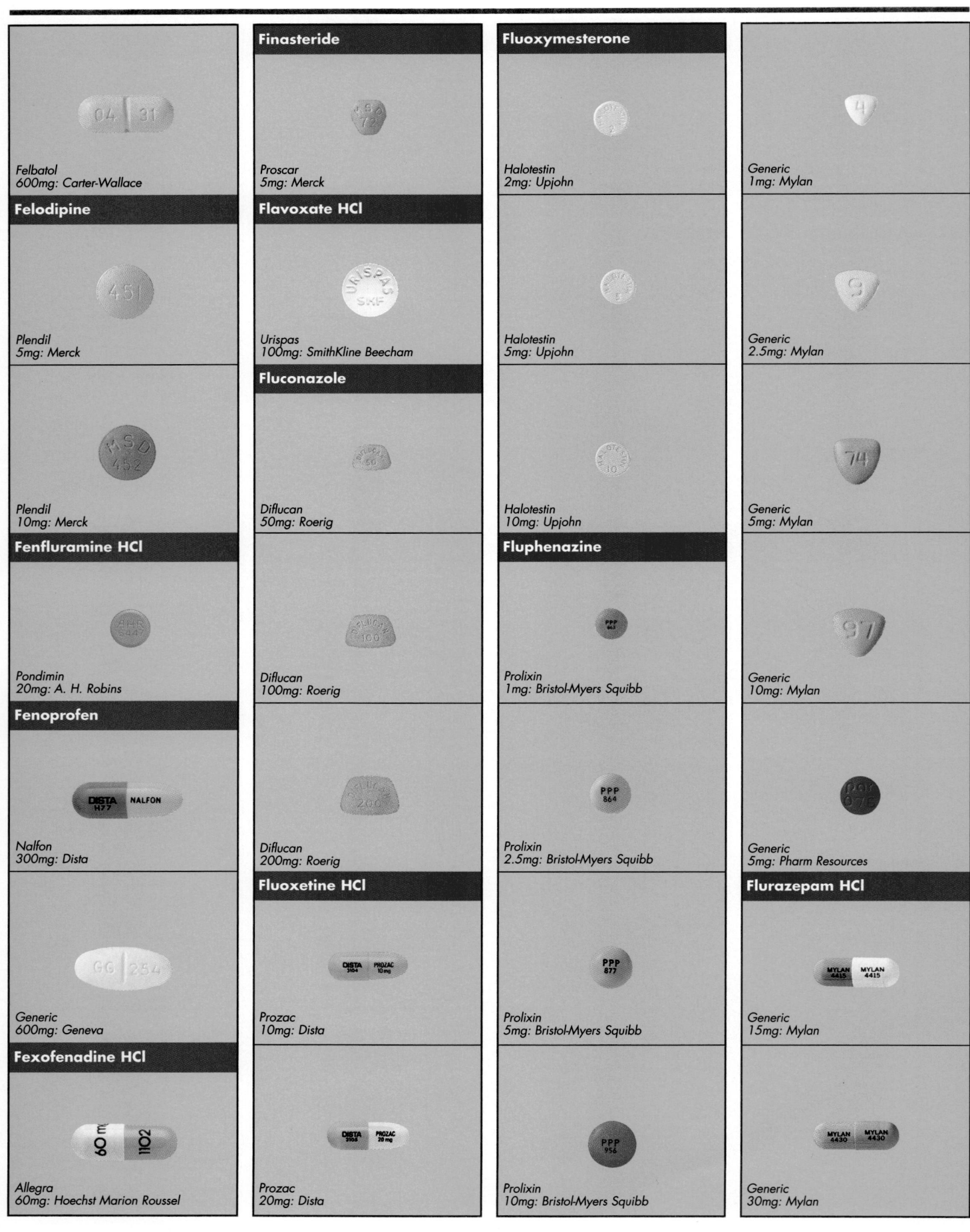

Felbatol
600mg: Carter-Wallace

Felodipine

Plendil
5mg: Merck

Plendil
10mg: Merck

Fenfluramine HCl

Pondimin
20mg: A. H. Robins

Fenoprofen

Nalfon
300mg: Dista

Generic
600mg: Geneva

Fexofenadine HCl

Allegra
60mg: Hoechst Marion Roussel

Finasteride

Proscar
5mg: Merck

Flavoxate HCl

Urispas
100mg: SmithKline Beecham

Fluconazole

Diflucan
50mg: Roerig

Diflucan
100mg: Roerig

Diflucan
200mg: Roerig

Fluoxetine HCl

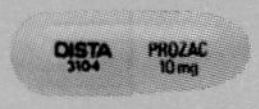

Prozac
10mg: Dista

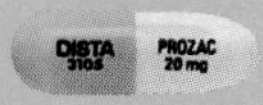

Prozac
20mg: Dista

Fluoxymesterone

Halotestin
2mg: Upjohn

Halotestin
5mg: Upjohn

Halotestin
10mg: Upjohn

Fluphenazine

Prolixin
1mg: Bristol-Myers Squibb

Prolixin
2.5mg: Bristol-Myers Squibb

Prolixin
5mg: Bristol-Myers Squibb

Prolixin
10mg: Bristol-Myers Squibb

Generic
1mg: Mylan

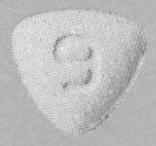

Generic
2.5mg: Mylan

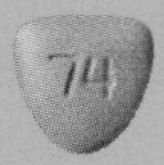

Generic
5mg: Mylan

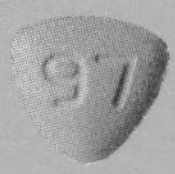

Generic
10mg: Mylan

Generic
5mg: Pharm Resources

Flurazepam HCl

Generic
15mg: Mylan

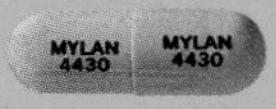

Generic
30mg: Mylan

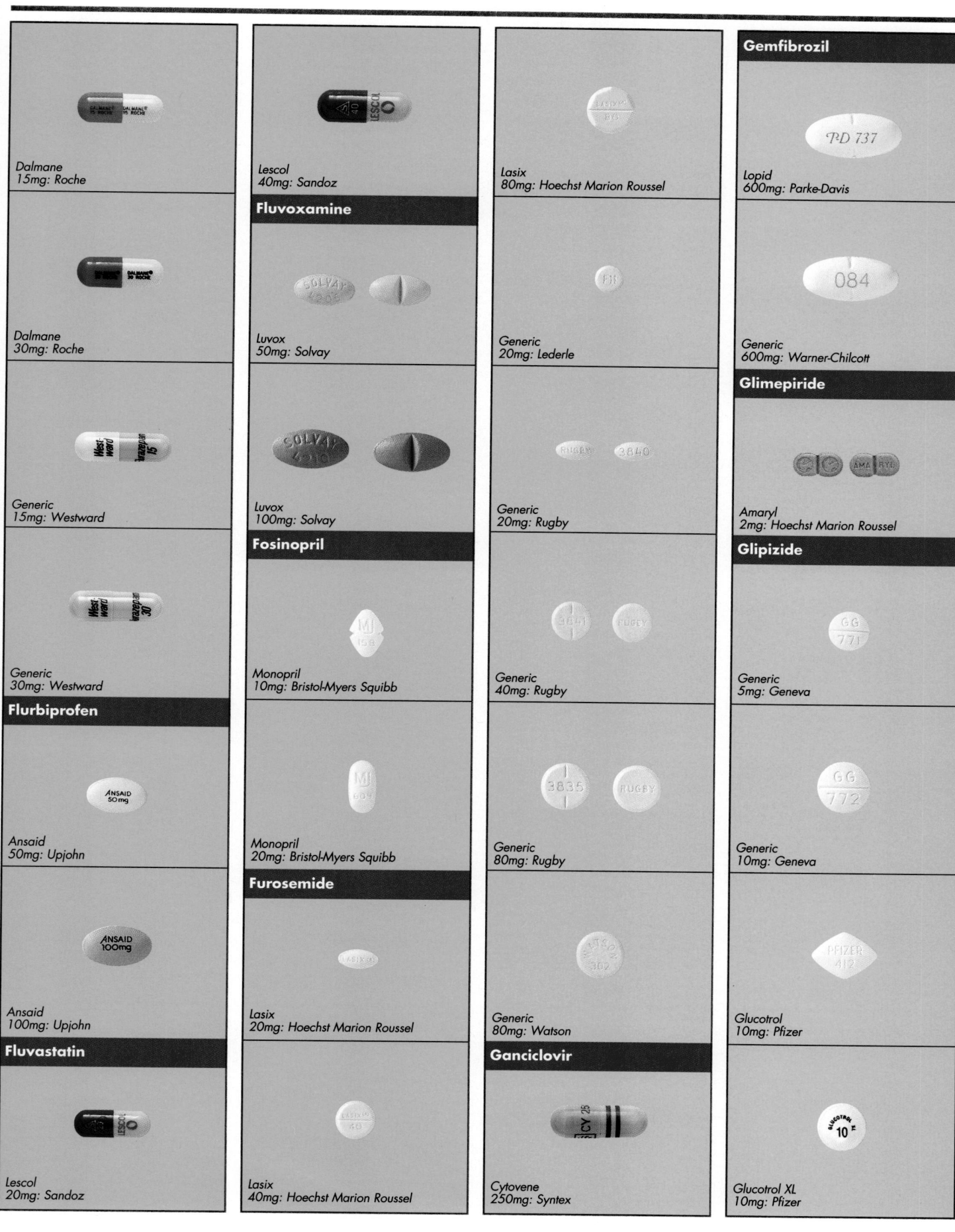

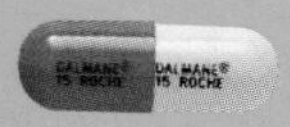

Dalmane
15mg: Roche

Dalmane
30mg: Roche

Generic
15mg: Westward

Generic
30mg: Westward

Flurbiprofen

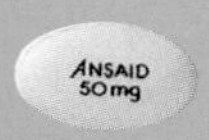

Ansaid
50mg: Upjohn

Ansaid
100mg: Upjohn

Fluvastatin

Lescol
20mg: Sandoz

Lescol
40mg: Sandoz

Fluvoxamine

Luvox
50mg: Solvay

Luvox
100mg: Solvay

Fosinopril

Monopril
10mg: Bristol-Myers Squibb

Monopril
20mg: Bristol-Myers Squibb

Furosemide

Lasix
20mg: Hoechst Marion Roussel

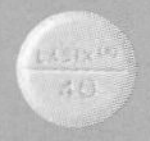

Lasix
40mg: Hoechst Marion Roussel

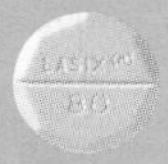

Lasix
80mg: Hoechst Marion Roussel

Generic
20mg: Lederle

Generic
20mg: Rugby

Generic
40mg: Rugby

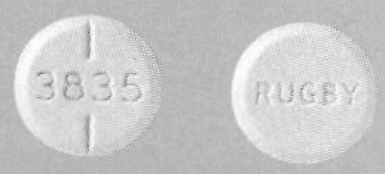

Generic
80mg: Rugby

Generic
80mg: Watson

Ganciclovir

Cytovene
250mg: Syntex

Gemfibrozil

Lopid
600mg: Parke-Davis

Generic
600mg: Warner-Chilcott

Glimepiride

Amaryl
2mg: Hoechst Marion Roussel

Glipizide

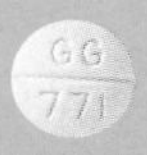

Generic
5mg: Geneva

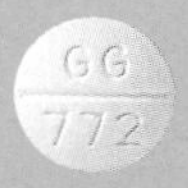

Generic
10mg: Geneva

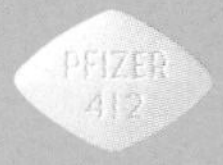

Glucotrol
10mg: Pfizer

Glucotrol XL
10mg: Pfizer

Glucotrol
5mg: Pfizer

Glucotrol XL
5mg: Pfizer

Glyburide

DiaBeta
1.25mg: Hoechst Marion Roussel

DiaBeta
2.5mg: Hoechst Marion Roussel

DiaBeta
5mg: Hoechst Marion Roussel

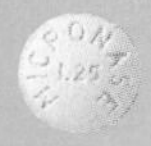

Micronase
1.25mg: Upjohn

Glynase Prestab
1.5mg: Upjohn

Micronase
2.5mg: Upjohn

Glynase Prestab
3mg: Upjohn

Micronase
5mg: Upjohn

Granisetron HCl

Kytril
1mg: SmithKline Beecham

Griseofulvin

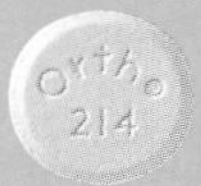

Grifulvin V
500mg: Ortho

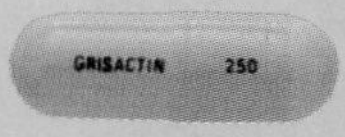

Grisactin
250mg: Wyeth-Ayerst

Guaifenesin

Humibid LA
600mg: Adams

Guaifenesin/ Pseudoephedrine HCl

Deconsal-II
600/60mg: Adams

Zephrex LA
600/120mg: Bock

Ru-Tuss DE
600/120mg: Knoll

Entex PSE
600/120mg: Procter & Gamble

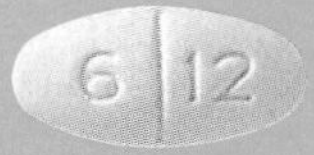

Duratuss
600/60mg: Whitby

Guanabenz

Wytensin
4mg: Wyeth-Ayerst

Wytensin
8mg: Wyeth-Ayerst

Guanfacine HCl

Tenex
1mg: A. H. Robins

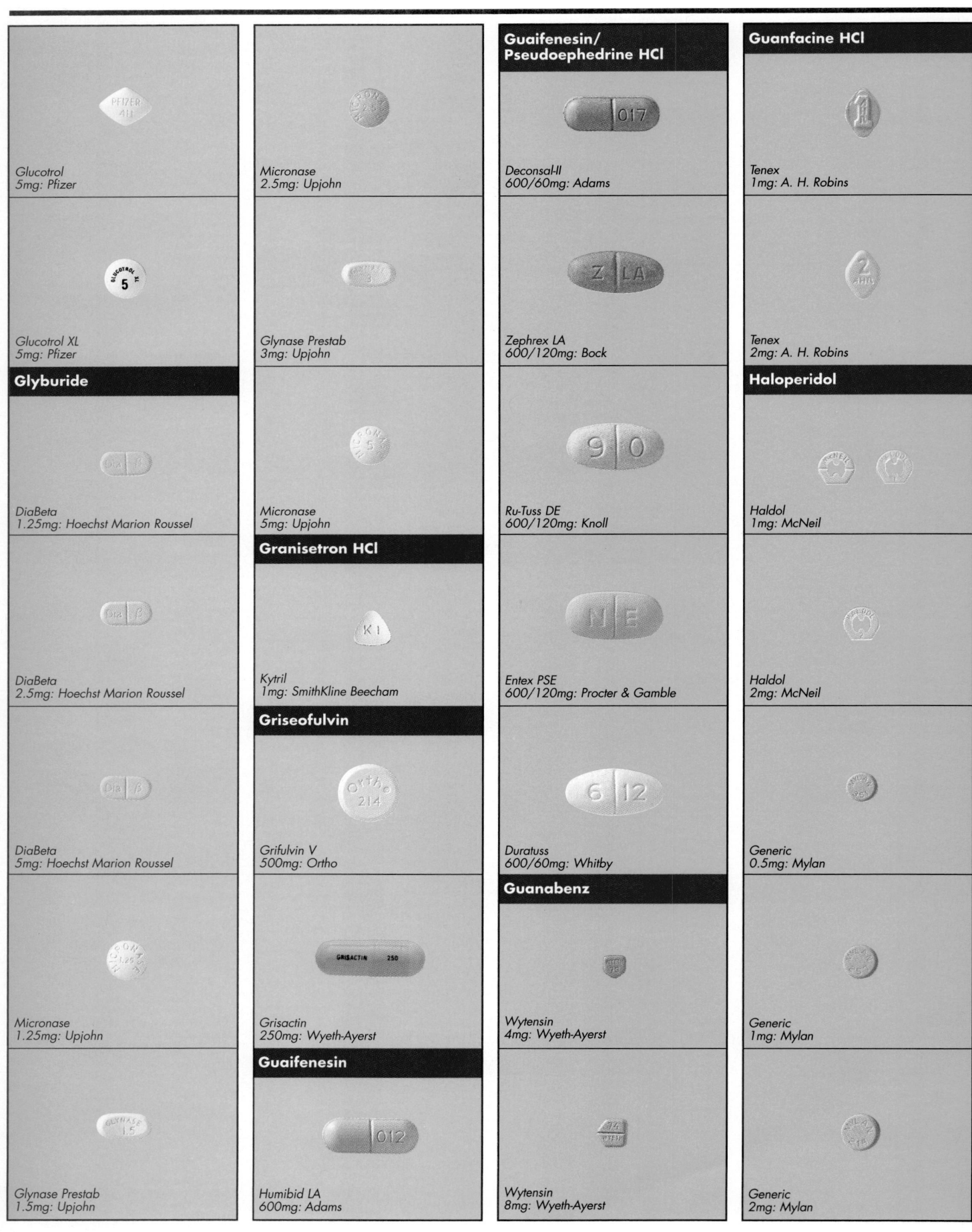

Tenex
2mg: A. H. Robins

Haloperidol

Haldol
1mg: McNeil

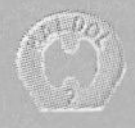

Haldol
2mg: McNeil

Generic
0.5mg: Mylan

Generic
1mg: Mylan

Generic
2mg: Mylan

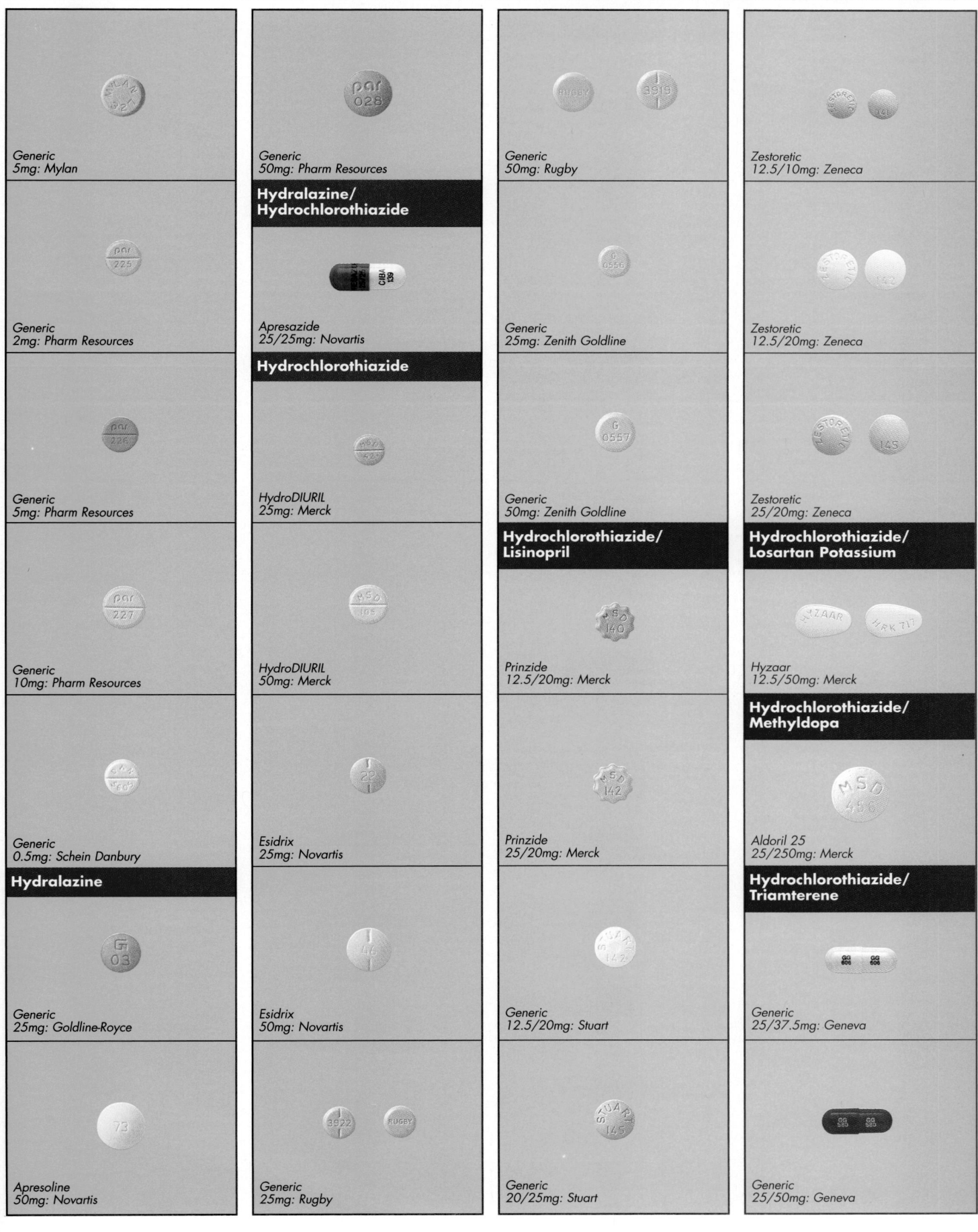

Generic
5mg: Mylan

Generic
2mg: Pharm Resources

Generic
5mg: Pharm Resources

Generic
10mg: Pharm Resources

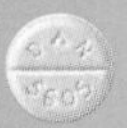

Generic
0.5mg: Schein Danbury

Hydralazine

Generic
25mg: Goldline-Royce

Apresoline
50mg: Novartis

Generic
50mg: Pharm Resources

Hydralazine/ Hydrochlorothiazide

Apresazide
25/25mg: Novartis

Hydrochlorothiazide

HydroDIURIL
25mg: Merck

HydroDIURIL
50mg: Merck

Esidrix
25mg: Novartis

Esidrix
50mg: Novartis

Generic
25mg: Rugby

Generic
50mg: Rugby

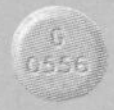

Generic
25mg: Zenith Goldline

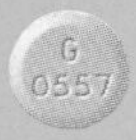

Generic
50mg: Zenith Goldline

Hydrochlorothiazide/ Lisinopril

Prinzide
12.5/20mg: Merck

Prinzide
25/20mg: Merck

Generic
12.5/20mg: Stuart

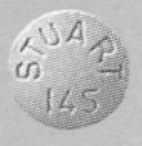

Generic
20/25mg: Stuart

Zestoretic
12.5/10mg: Zeneca

Zestoretic
12.5/20mg: Zeneca

Zestoretic
25/20mg: Zeneca

Hydrochlorothiazide/ Losartan Potassium

Hyzaar
12.5/50mg: Merck

Hydrochlorothiazide/ Methyldopa

Aldoril 25
25/250mg: Merck

Hydrochlorothiazide/ Triamterene

Generic
25/37.5mg: Geneva

Generic
25/50mg: Geneva

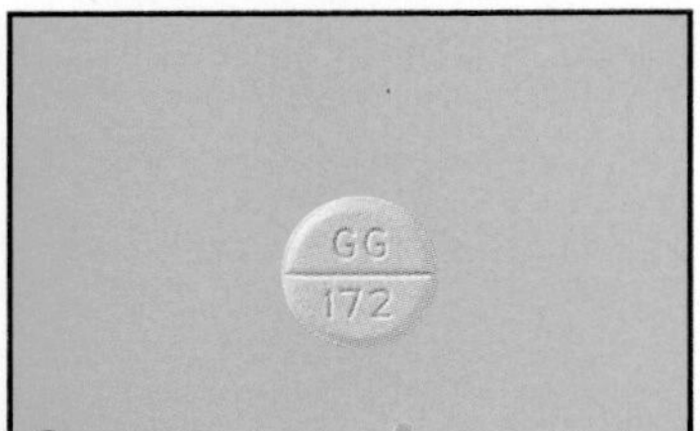

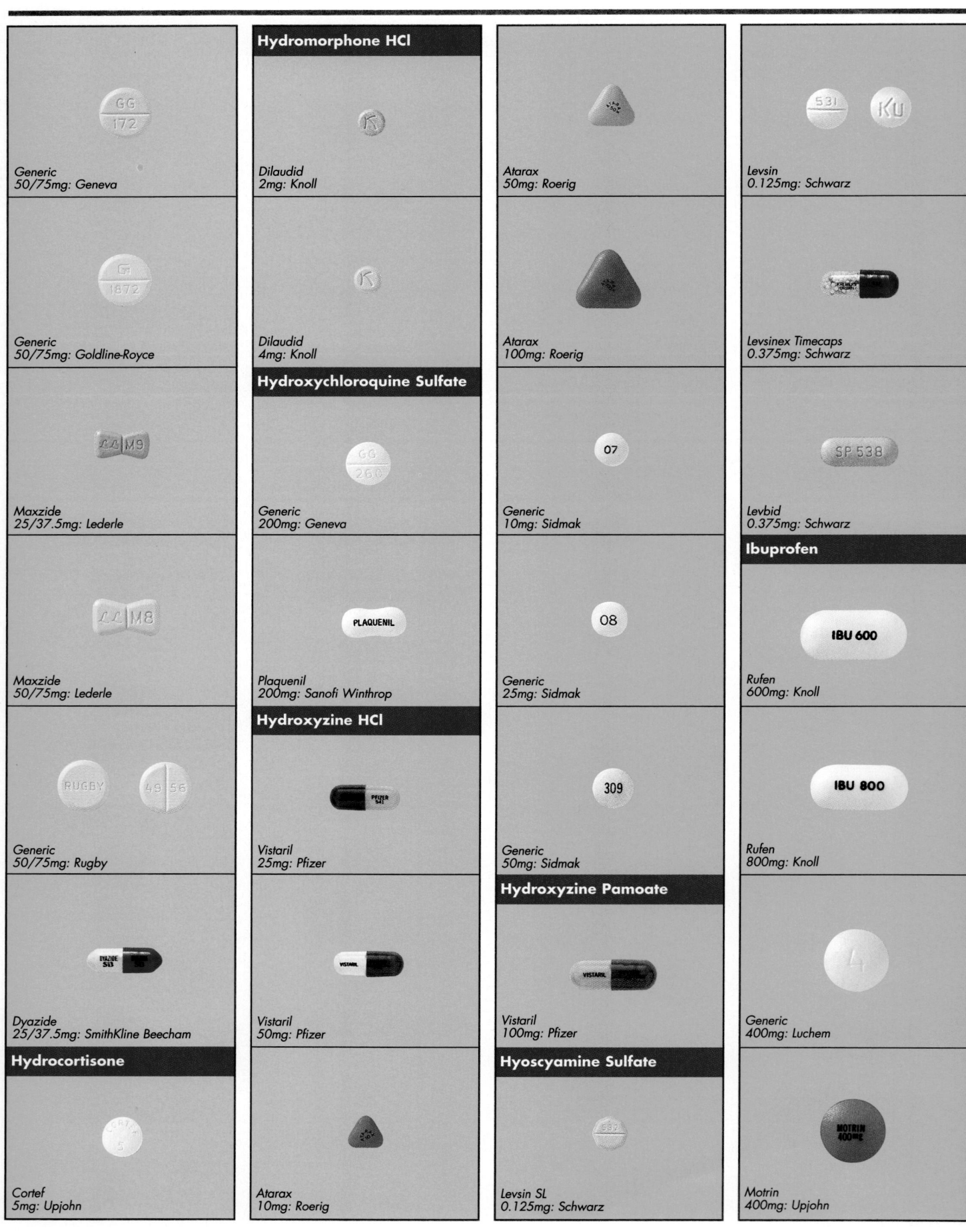

Generic
50/75mg: Geneva

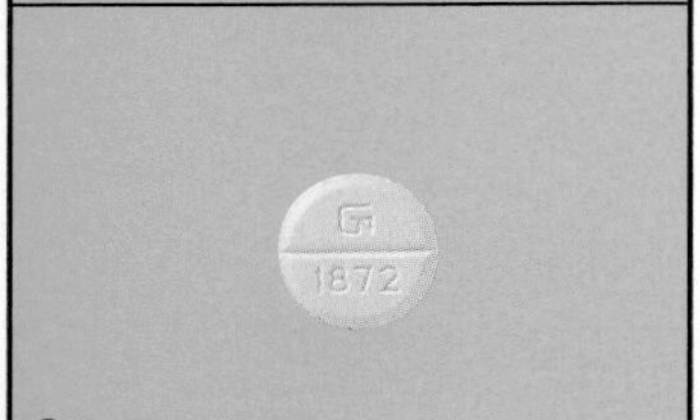

Generic
50/75mg: Goldline-Royce

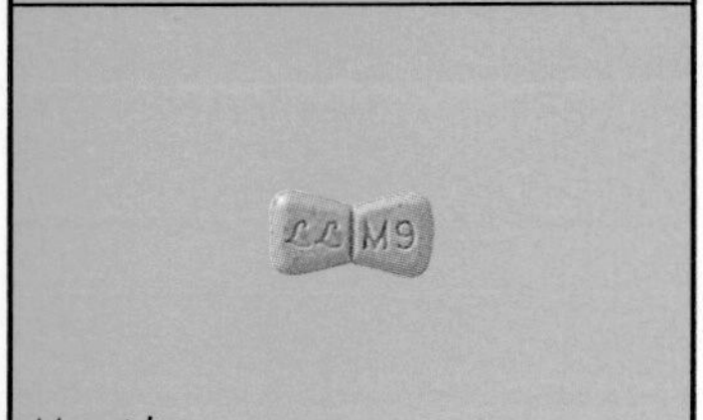

Maxzide
25/37.5mg: Lederle

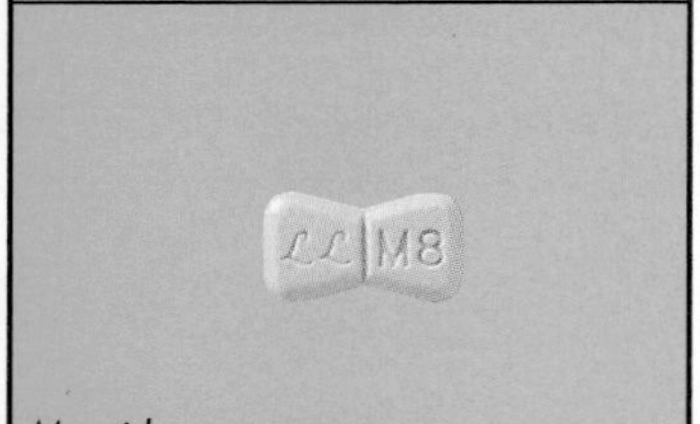

Maxzide
50/75mg: Lederle

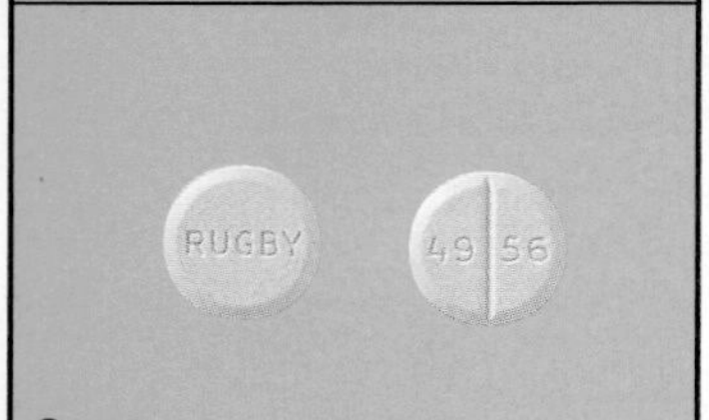

Generic
50/75mg: Rugby

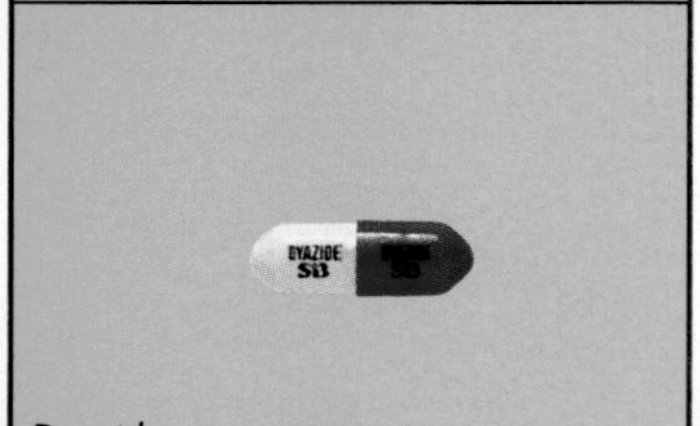

Dyazide
25/37.5mg: SmithKline Beecham

Hydrocortisone

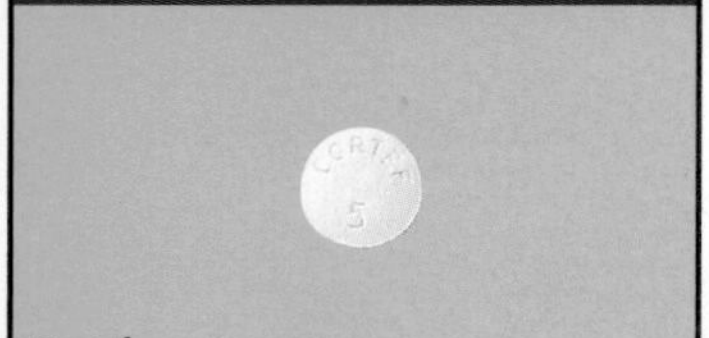

Cortef
5mg: Upjohn

Hydromorphone HCl

Dilaudid
2mg: Knoll

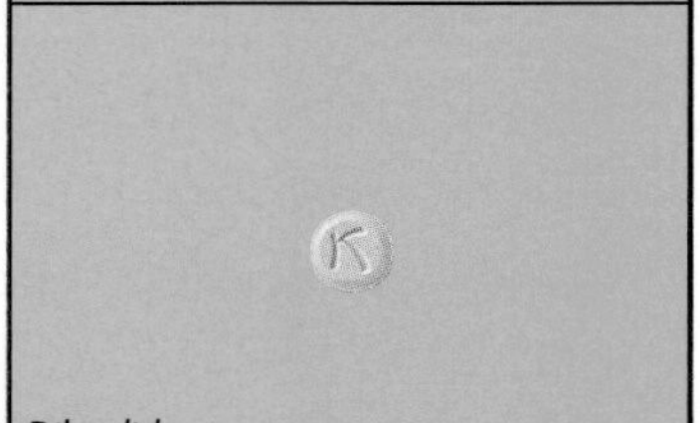

Dilaudid
4mg: Knoll

Hydroxychloroquine Sulfate

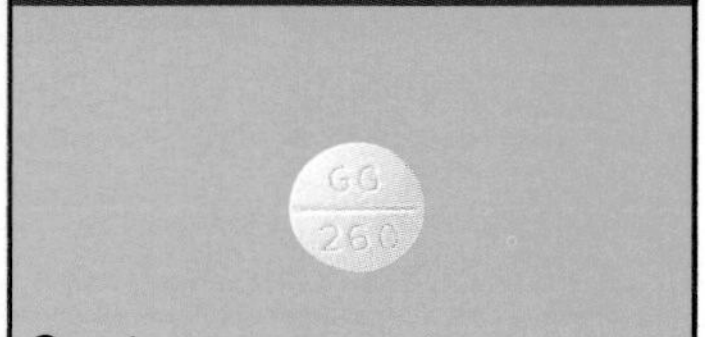

Generic
200mg: Geneva

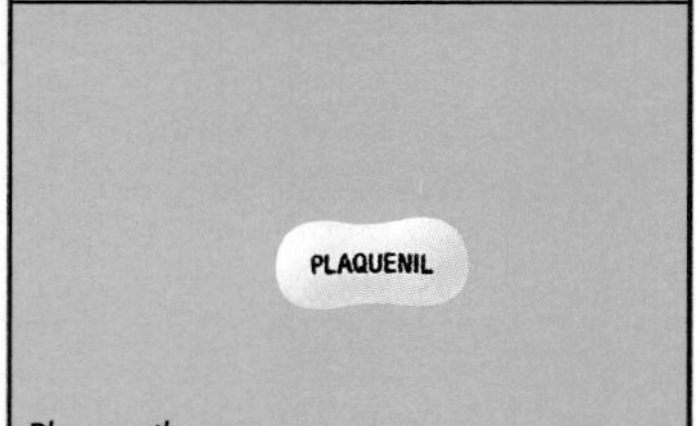

Plaquenil
200mg: Sanofi Winthrop

Hydroxyzine HCl

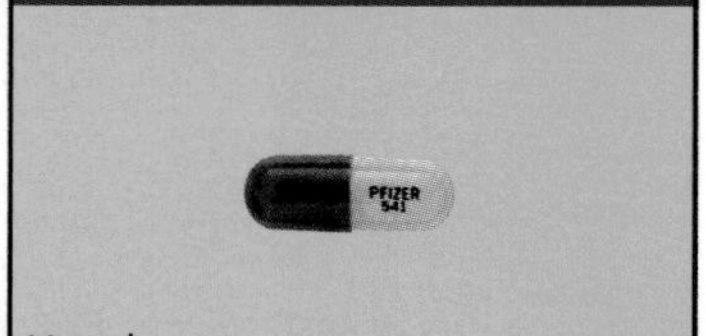

Vistaril
25mg: Pfizer

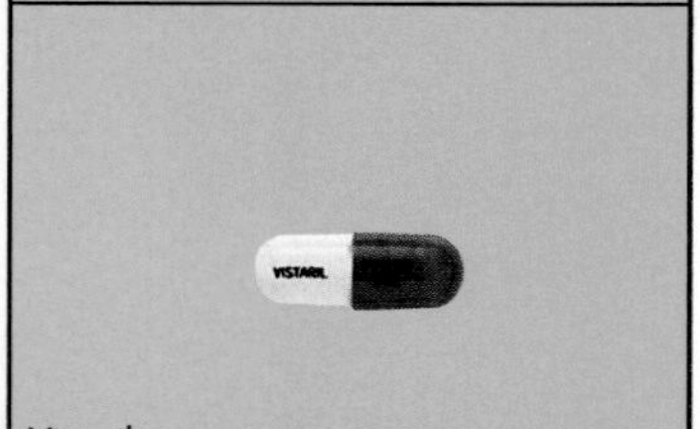

Vistaril
50mg: Pfizer

Atarax
10mg: Roerig

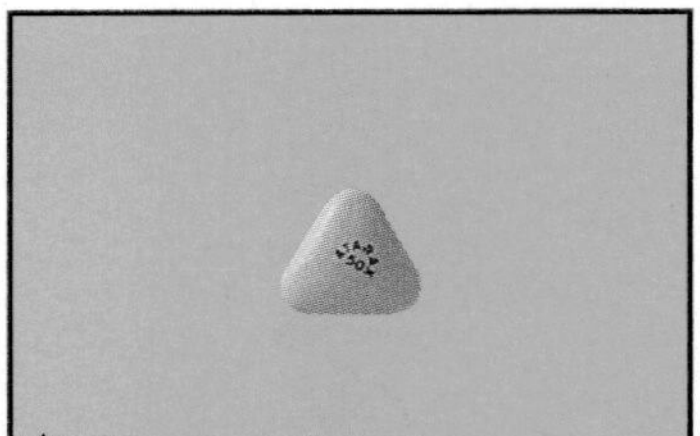

Atarax
50mg: Roerig

Atarax
100mg: Roerig

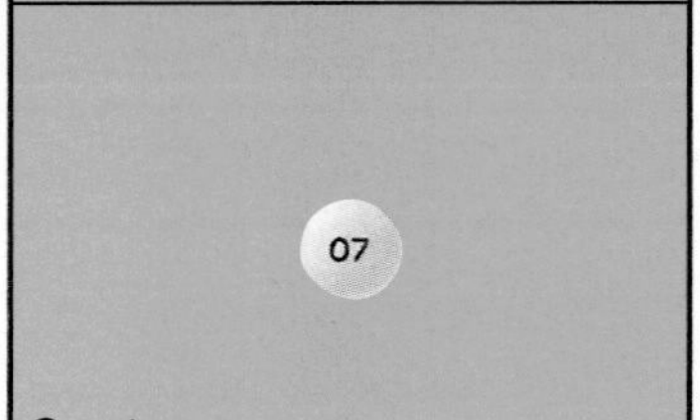

Generic
10mg: Sidmak

Generic
25mg: Sidmak

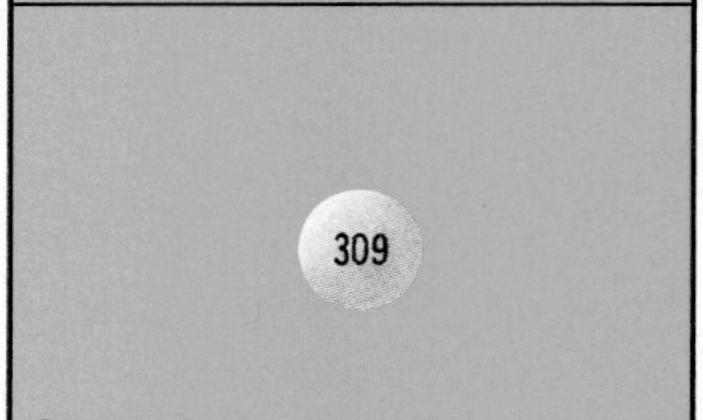

Generic
50mg: Sidmak

Hydroxyzine Pamoate

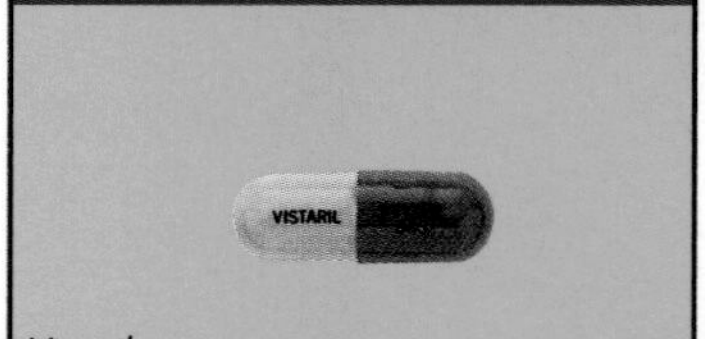

Vistaril
100mg: Pfizer

Hyoscyamine Sulfate

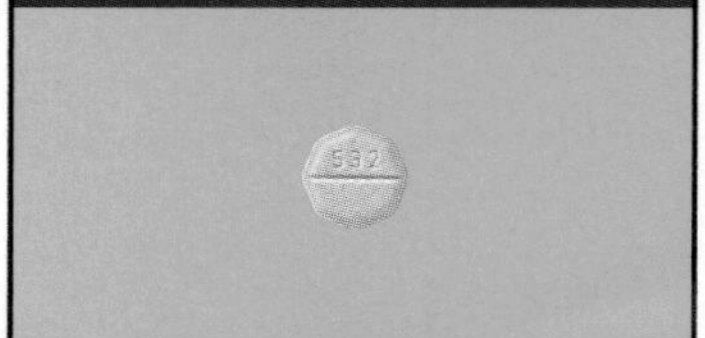

Levsin SL
0.125mg: Schwarz

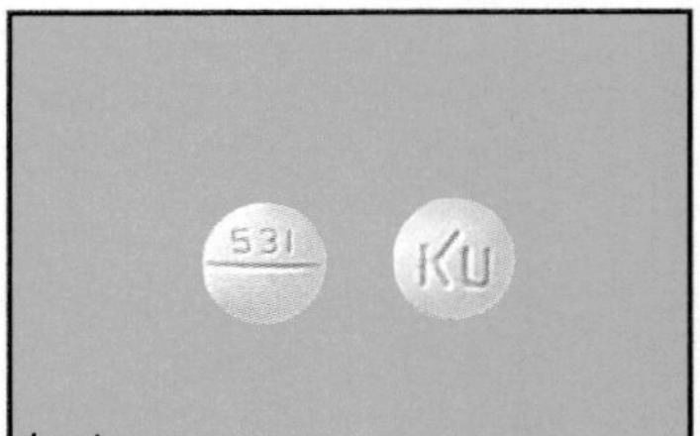

Levsin
0.125mg: Schwarz

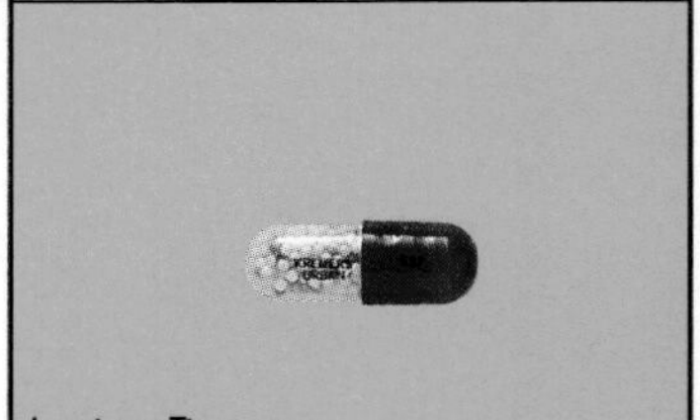

Levsinex Timecaps
0.375mg: Schwarz

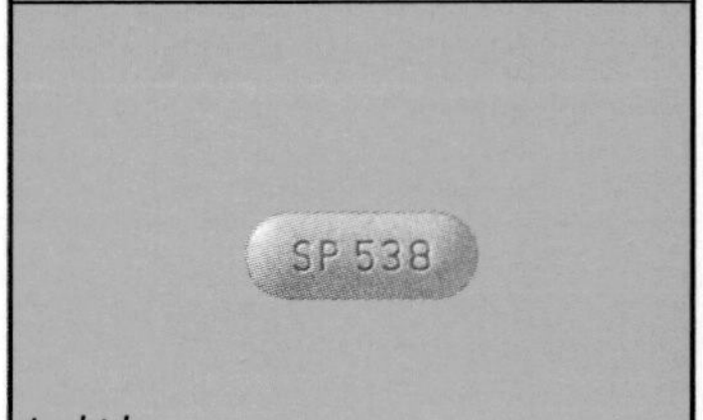

Levbid
0.375mg: Schwarz

Ibuprofen

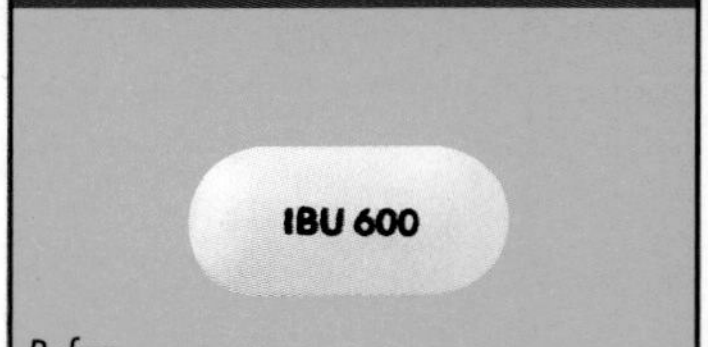

Rufen
600mg: Knoll

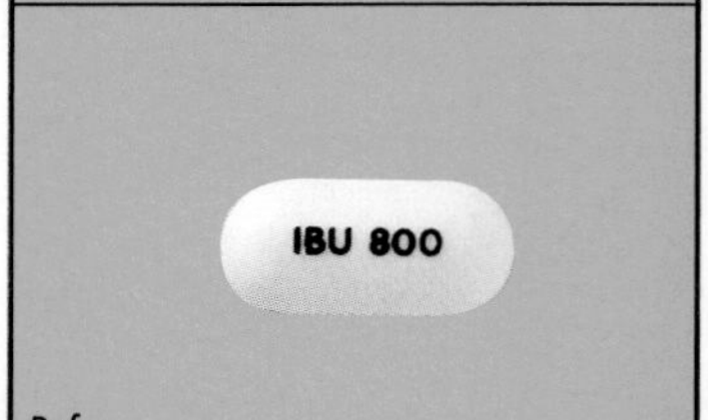

Rufen
800mg: Knoll

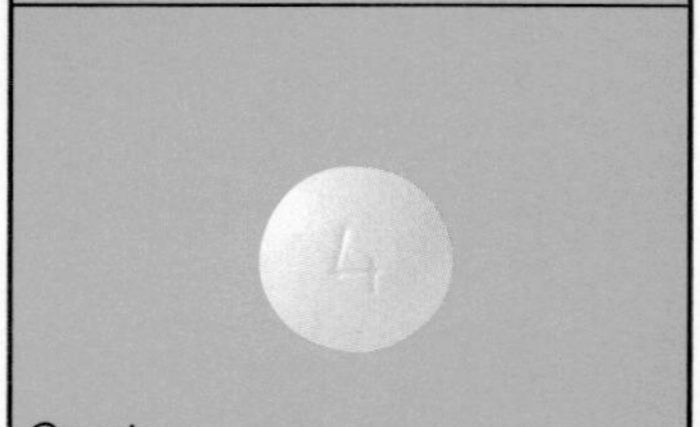

Generic
400mg: Luchem

Motrin
400mg: Upjohn

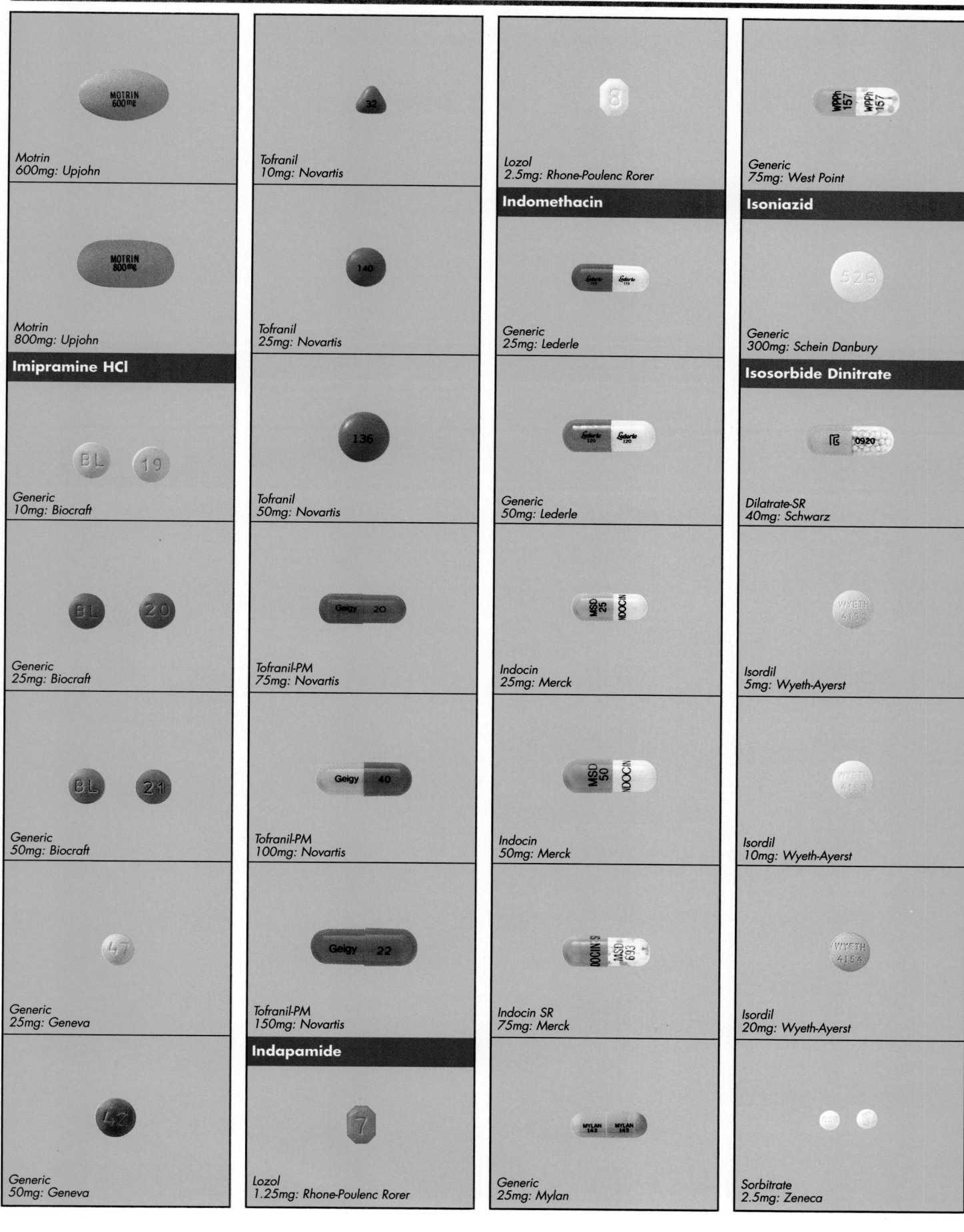

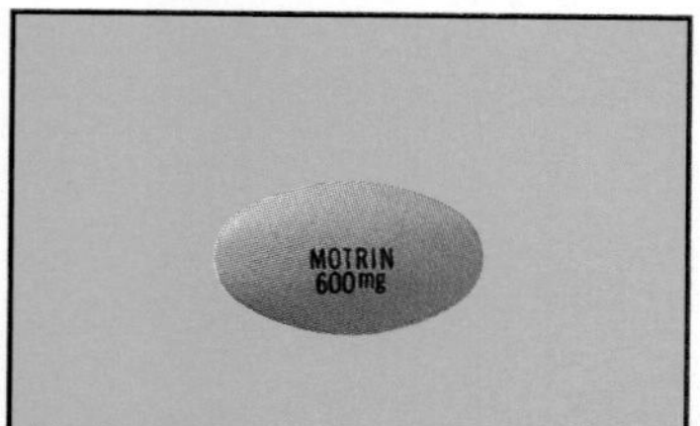

Motrin
600mg: Upjohn

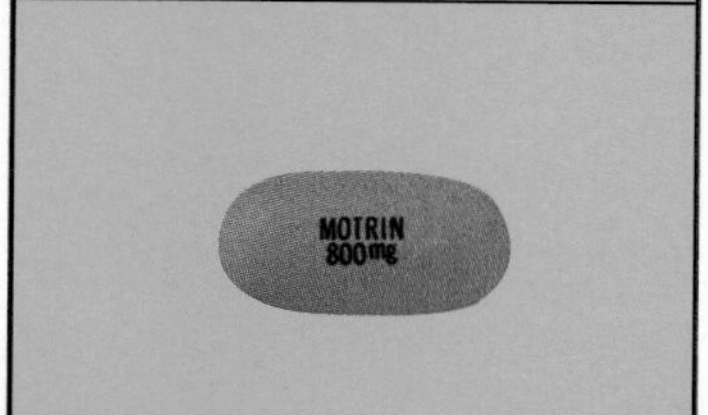

Motrin
800mg: Upjohn

Imipramine HCl

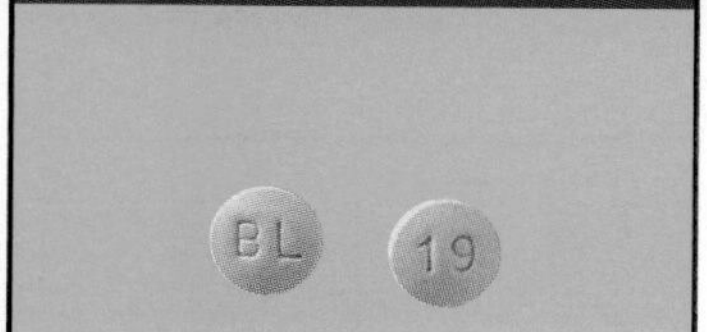

Generic
10mg: Biocraft

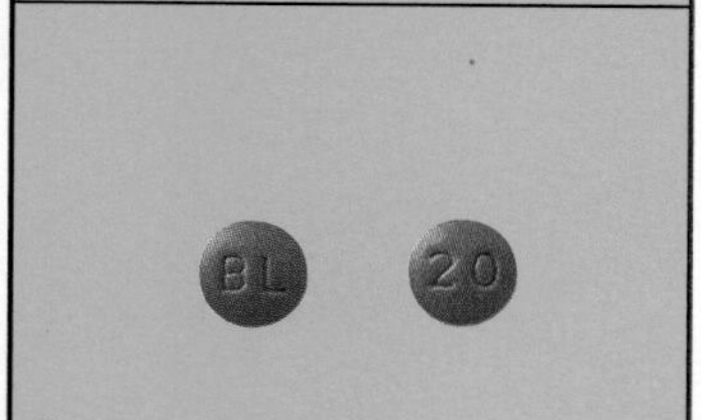

Generic
25mg: Biocraft

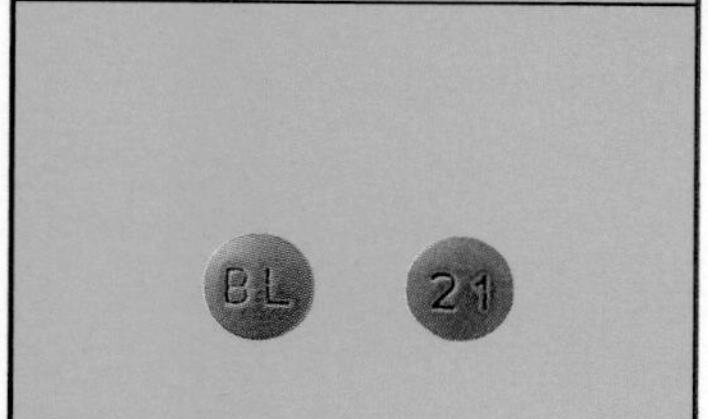

Generic
50mg: Biocraft

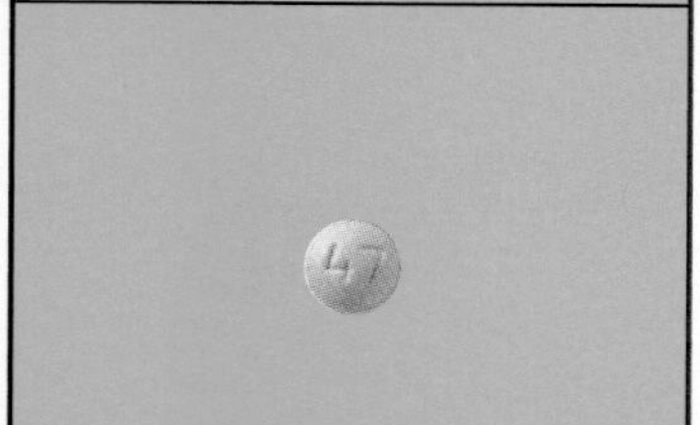

Generic
25mg: Geneva

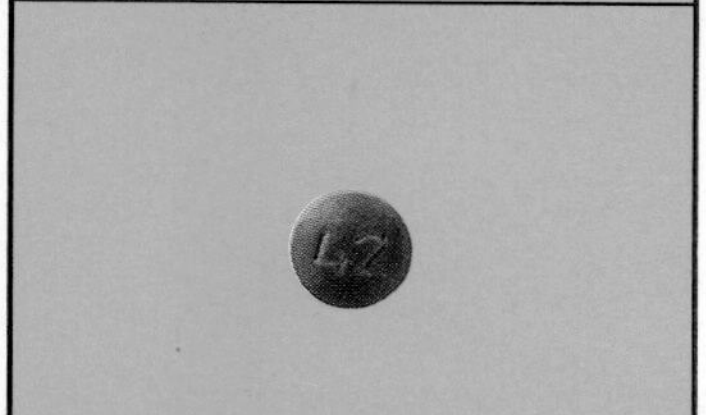

Generic
50mg: Geneva

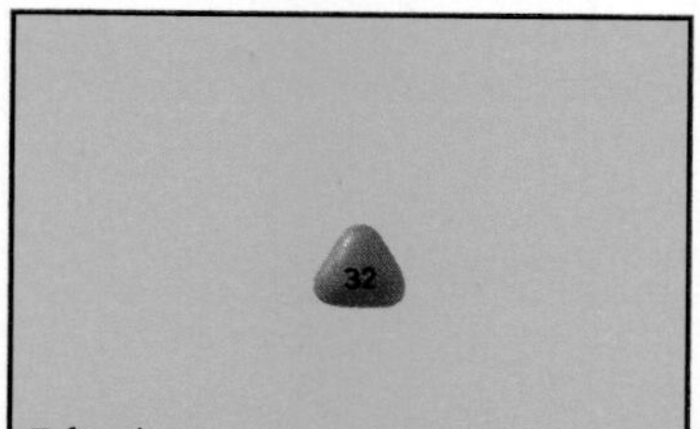

Tofranil
10mg: Novartis

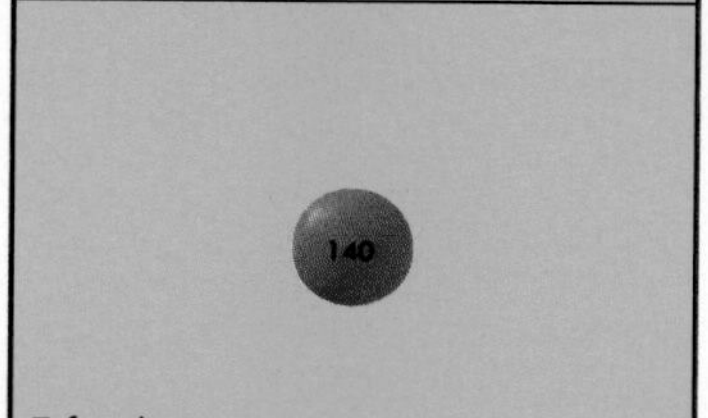

Tofranil
25mg: Novartis

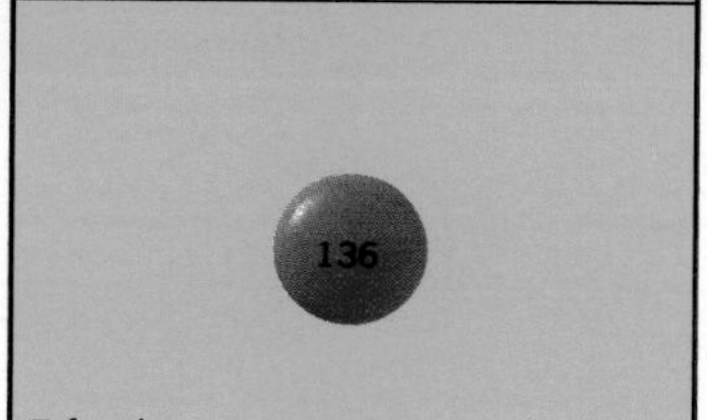

Tofranil
50mg: Novartis

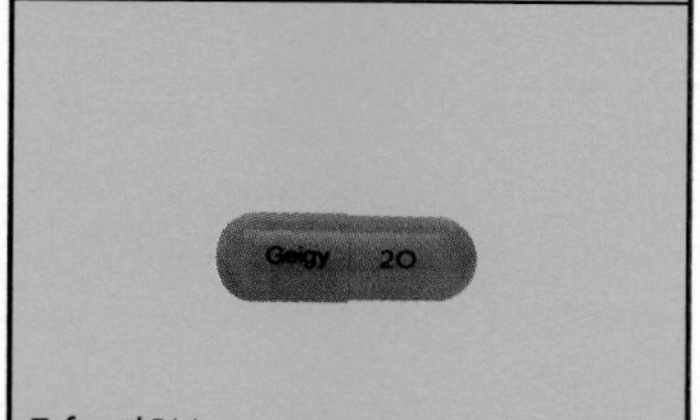

Tofranil-PM
75mg: Novartis

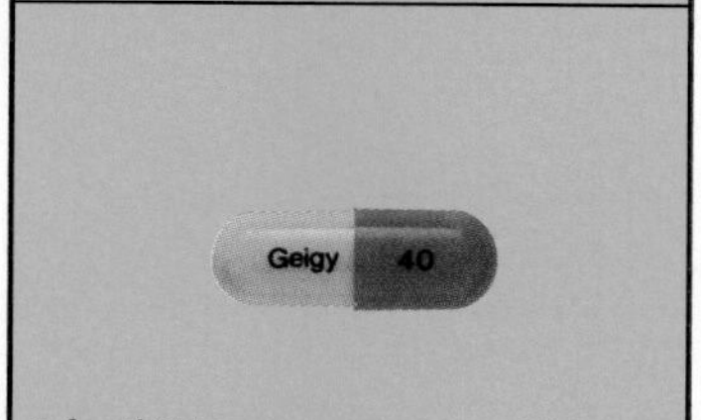

Tofranil-PM
100mg: Novartis

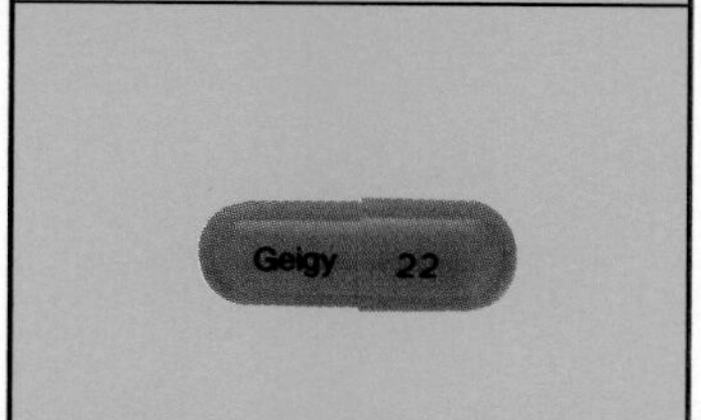

Tofranil-PM
150mg: Novartis

Indapamide

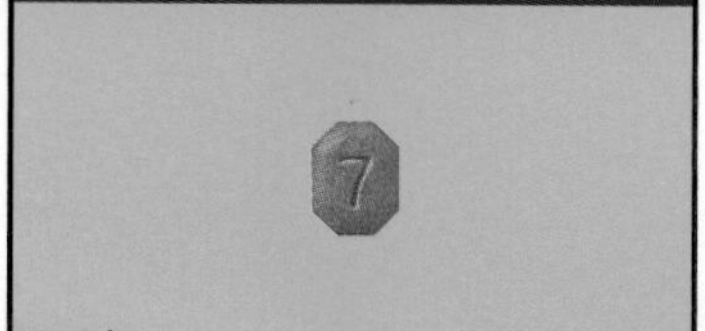

Lozol
1.25mg: Rhone-Poulenc Rorer

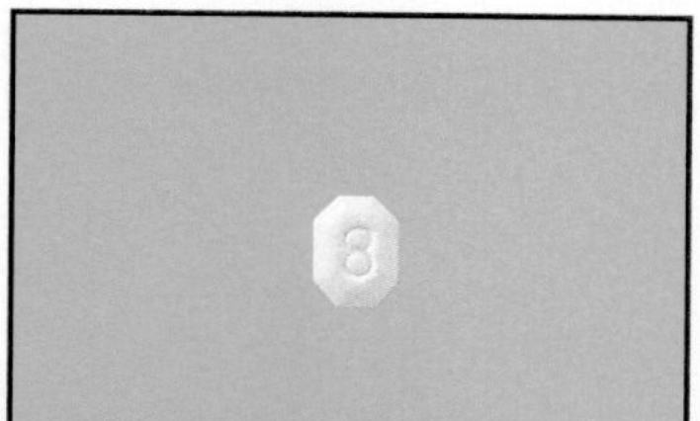

Lozol
2.5mg: Rhone-Poulenc Rorer

Indomethacin

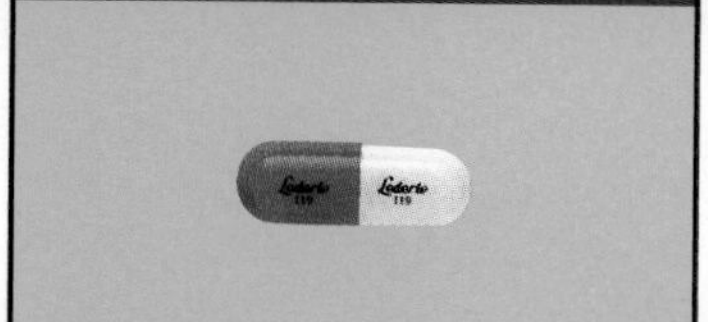

Generic
25mg: Lederle

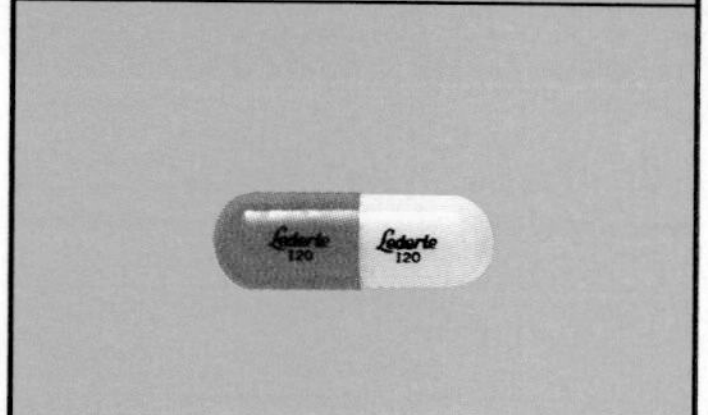

Generic
50mg: Lederle

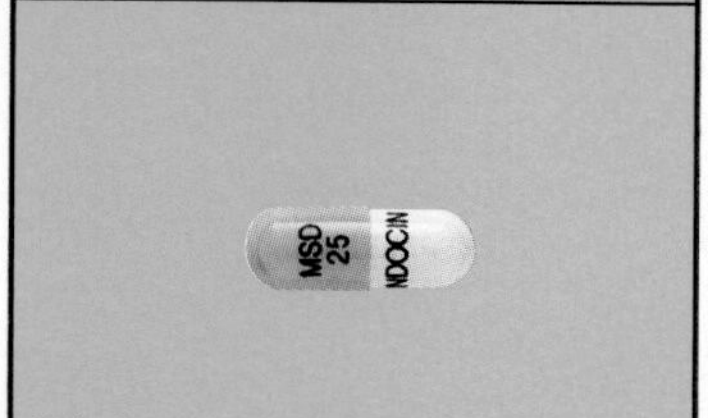

Indocin
25mg: Merck

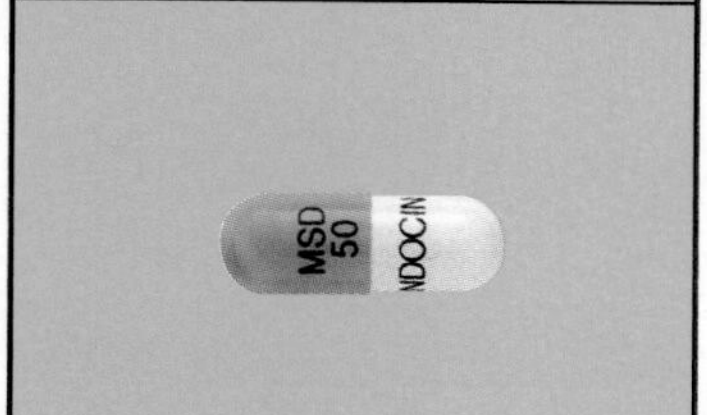

Indocin
50mg: Merck

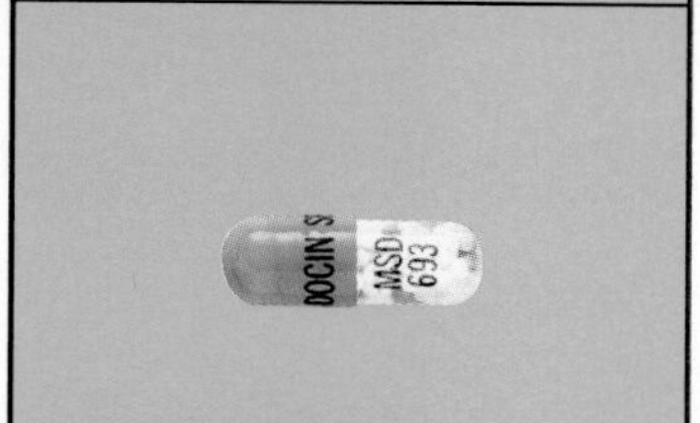

Indocin SR
75mg: Merck

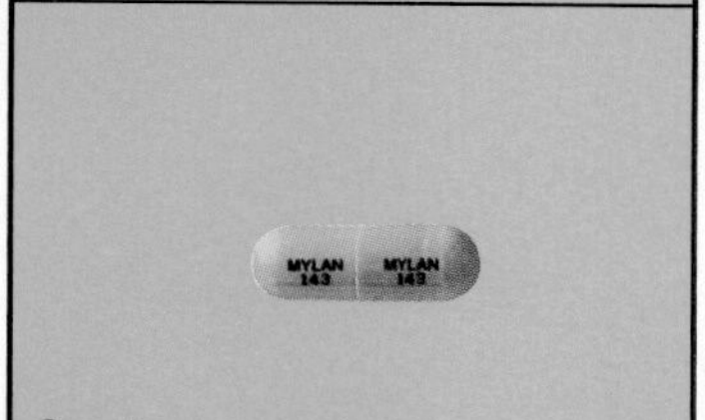

Generic
25mg: Mylan

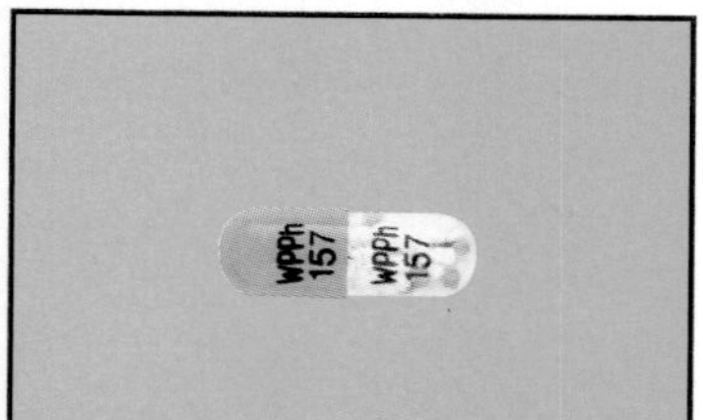

Generic
75mg: West Point

Isoniazid

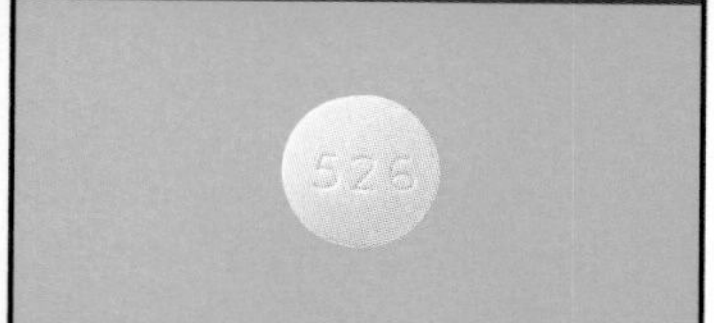

Generic
300mg: Schein Danbury

Isosorbide Dinitrate

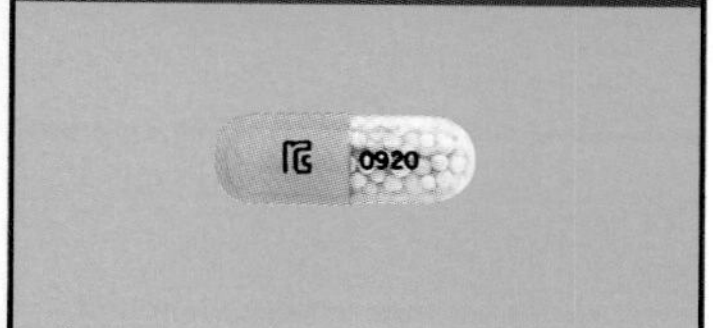

Dilatrate-SR
40mg: Schwarz

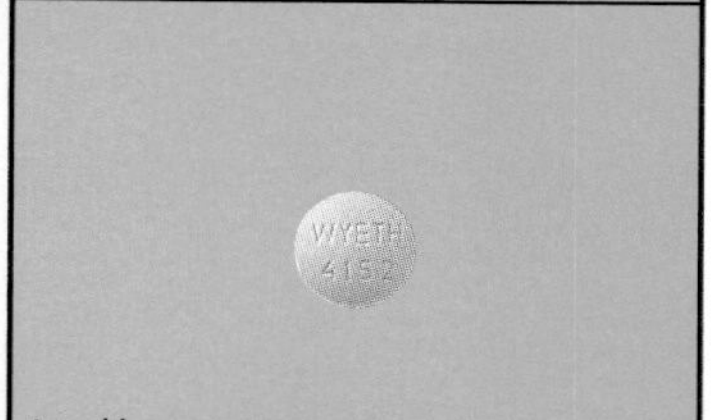

Isordil
5mg: Wyeth-Ayerst

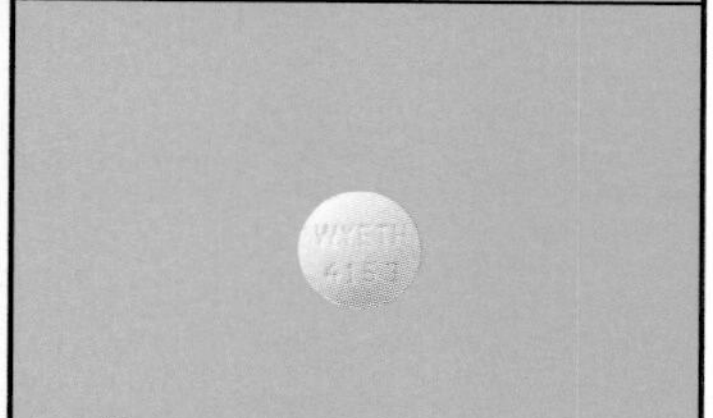

Isordil
10mg: Wyeth-Ayerst

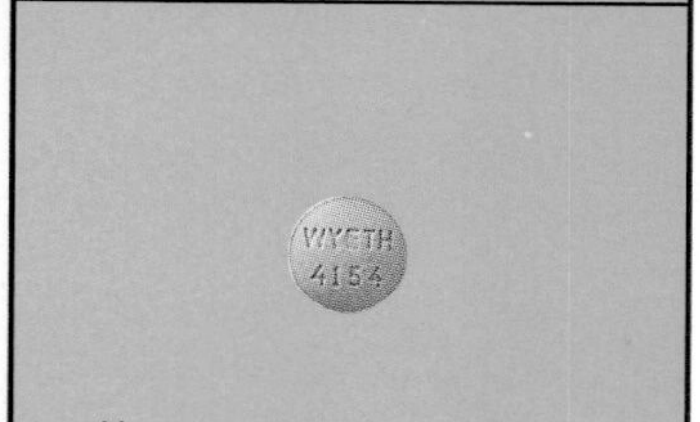

Isordil
20mg: Wyeth-Ayerst

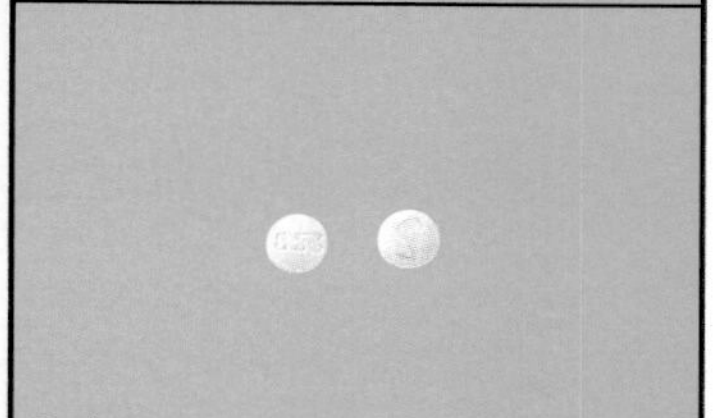

Sorbitrate
2.5mg: Zeneca

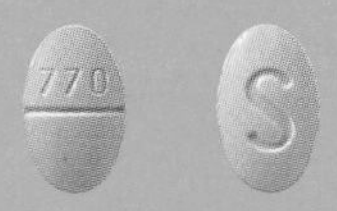

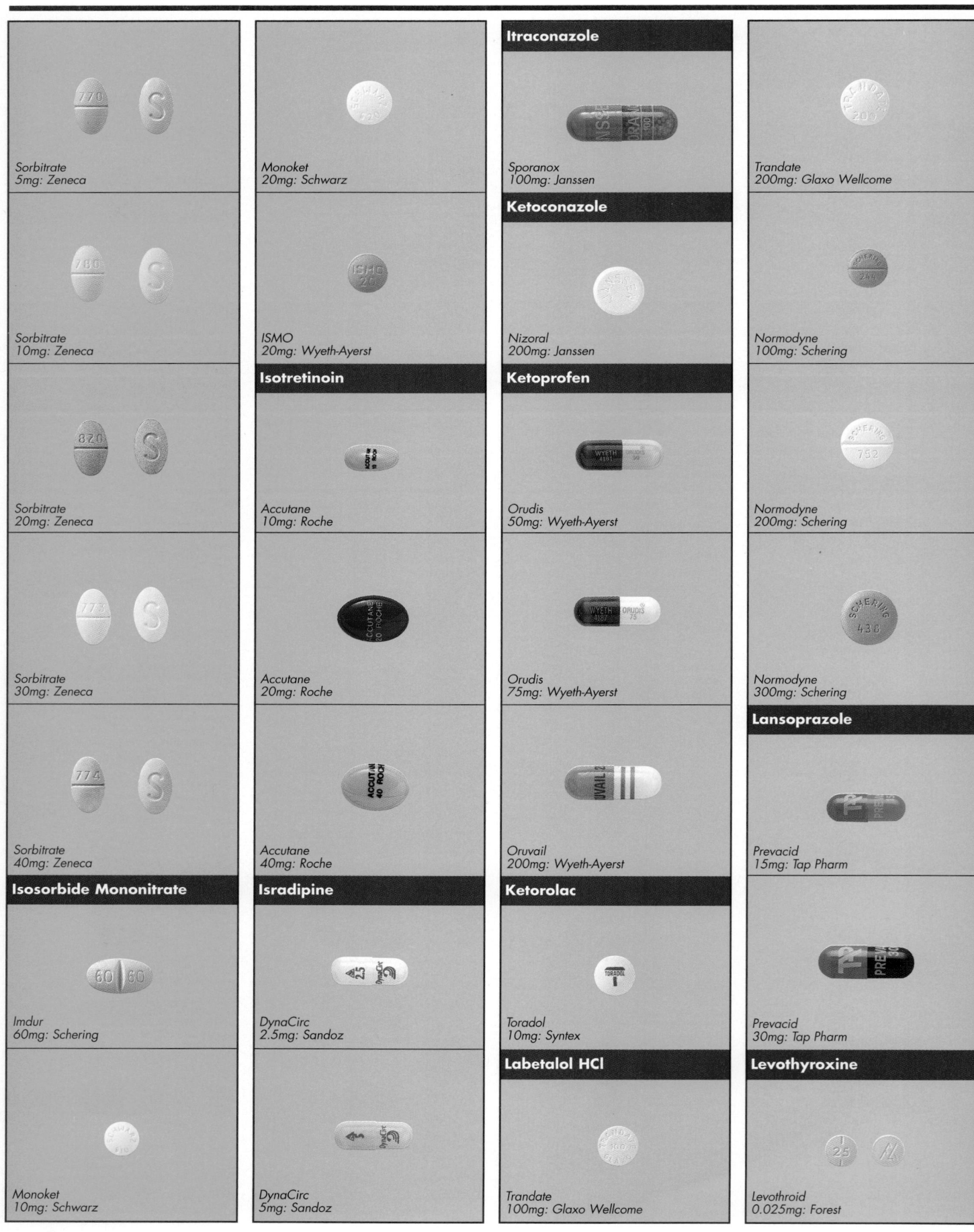

Sorbitrate
5mg: Zeneca

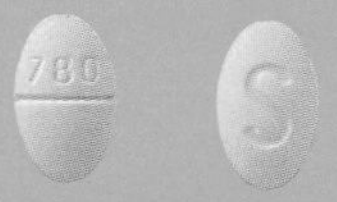

Sorbitrate
10mg: Zeneca

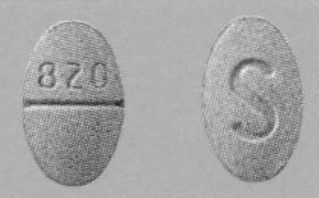

Sorbitrate
20mg: Zeneca

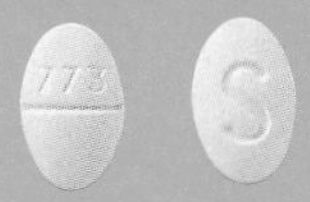

Sorbitrate
30mg: Zeneca

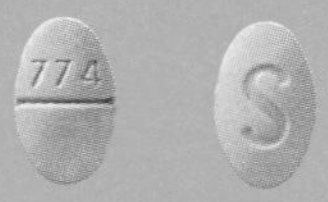

Sorbitrate
40mg: Zeneca

Isosorbide Mononitrate

Imdur
60mg: Schering

Monoket
10mg: Schwarz

Monoket
20mg: Schwarz

ISMO
20mg: Wyeth-Ayerst

Isotretinoin

Accutane
10mg: Roche

Accutane
20mg: Roche

Accutane
40mg: Roche

Isradipine

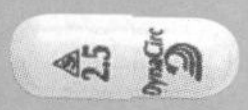

DynaCirc
2.5mg: Sandoz

DynaCirc
5mg: Sandoz

Itraconazole

Sporanox
100mg: Janssen

Ketoconazole

Nizoral
200mg: Janssen

Ketoprofen

Orudis
50mg: Wyeth-Ayerst

Orudis
75mg: Wyeth-Ayerst

Oruvail
200mg: Wyeth-Ayerst

Ketorolac

Toradol
10mg: Syntex

Labetalol HCl

Trandate
100mg: Glaxo Wellcome

Trandate
200mg: Glaxo Wellcome

Normodyne
100mg: Schering

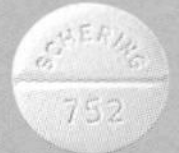

Normodyne
200mg: Schering

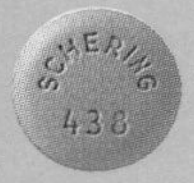

Normodyne
300mg: Schering

Lansoprazole

Prevacid
15mg: Tap Pharm

Prevacid
30mg: Tap Pharm

Levothyroxine

Levothroid
0.025mg: Forest

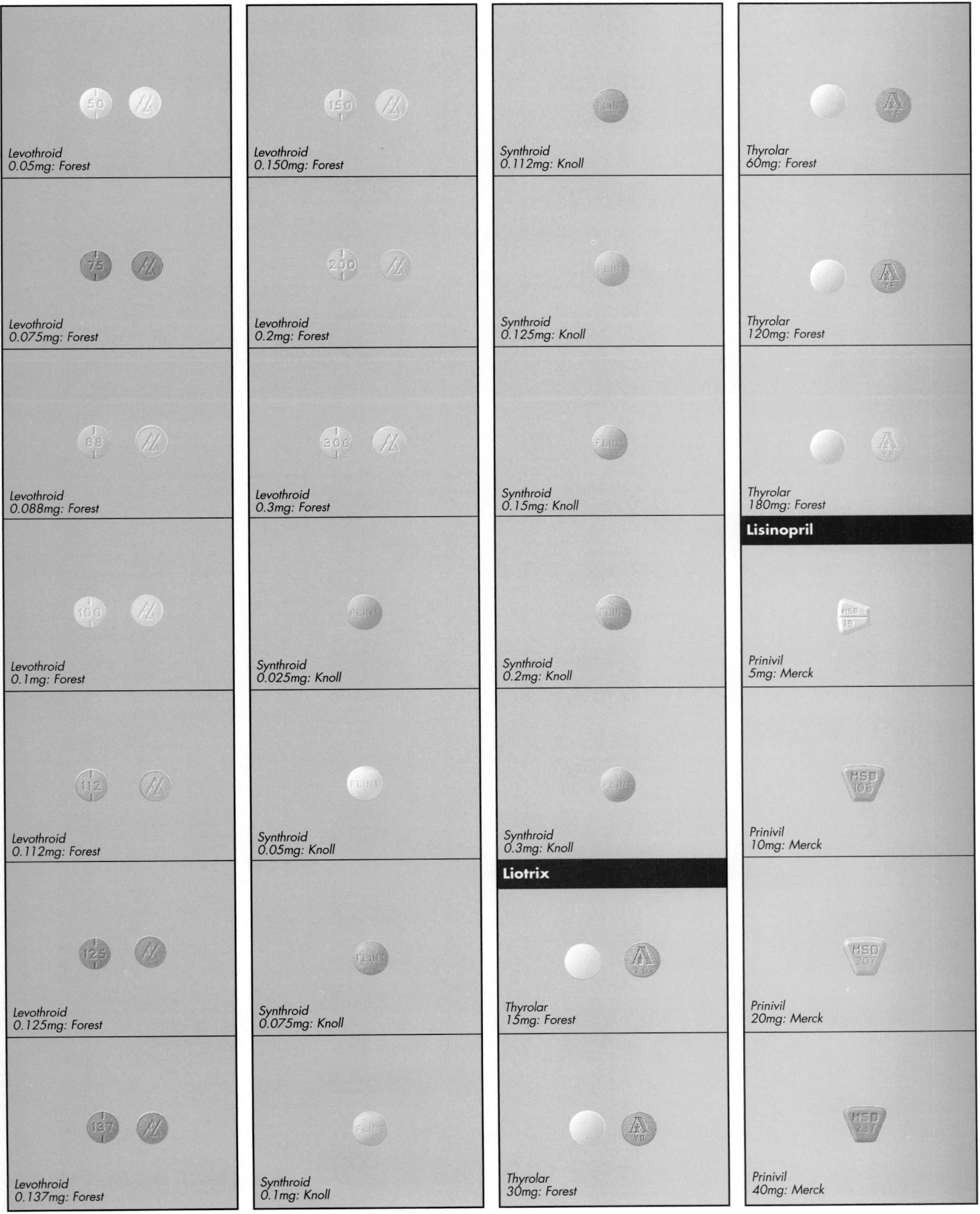

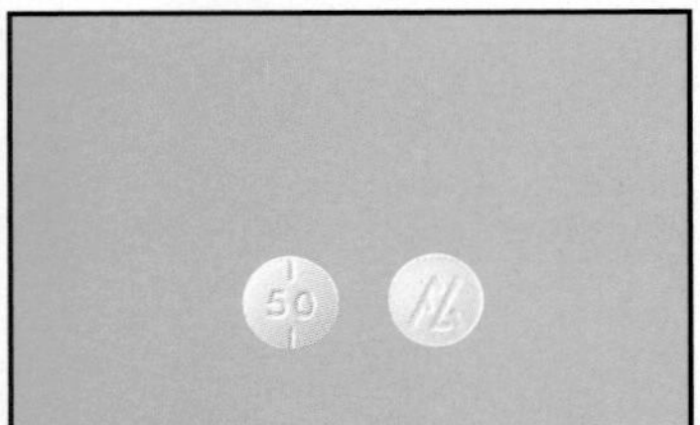

Levothroid
0.05mg: Forest

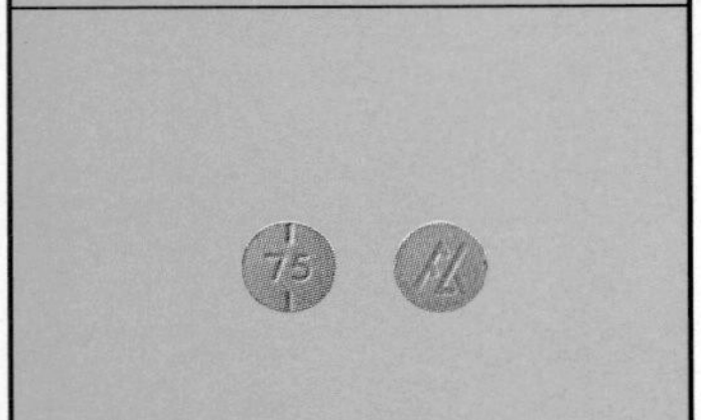

Levothroid
0.075mg: Forest

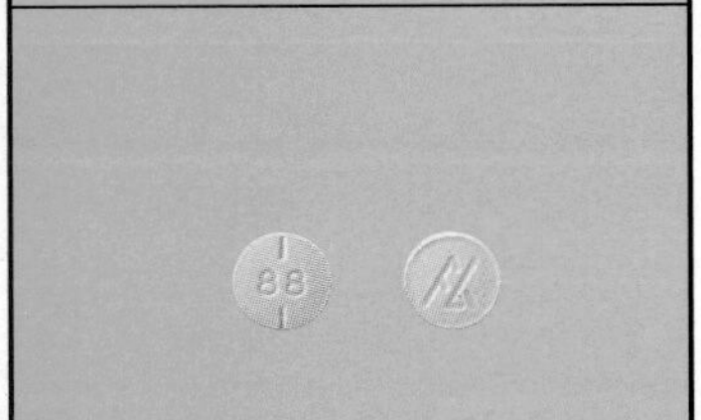

Levothroid
0.088mg: Forest

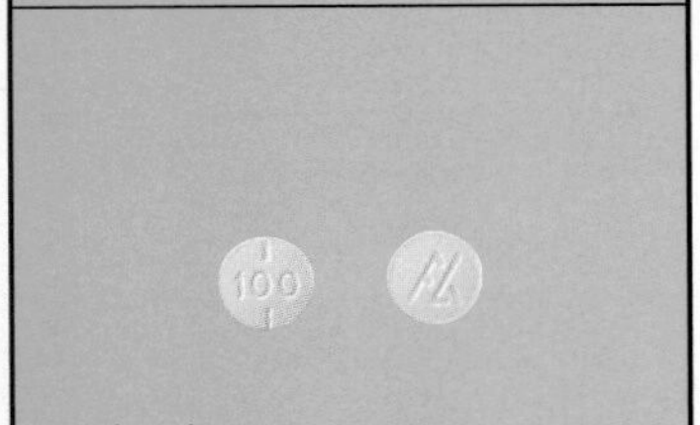

Levothroid
0.1mg: Forest

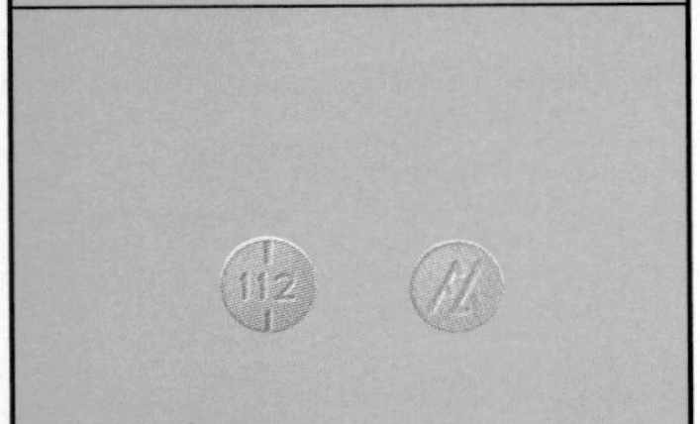

Levothroid
0.112mg: Forest

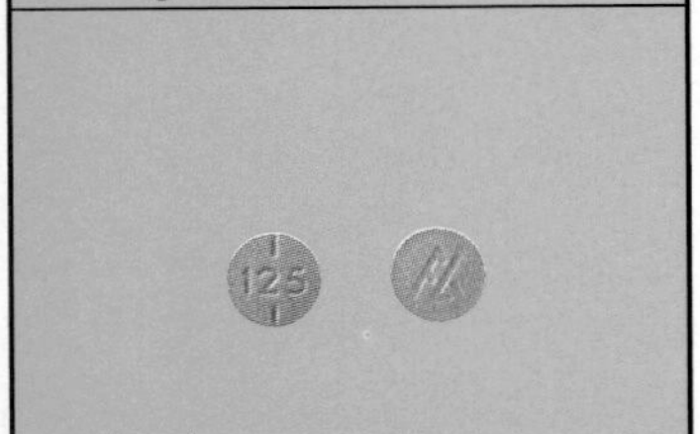

Levothroid
0.125mg: Forest

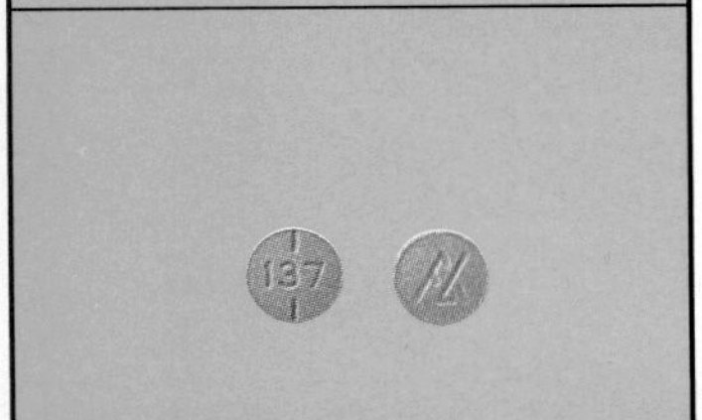

Levothroid
0.137mg: Forest

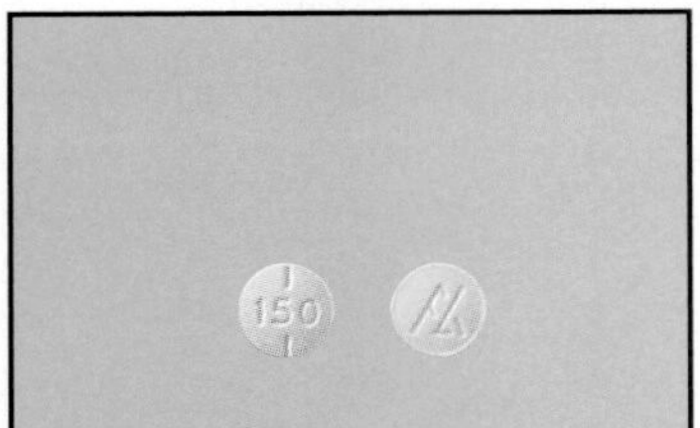

Levothroid
0.150mg: Forest

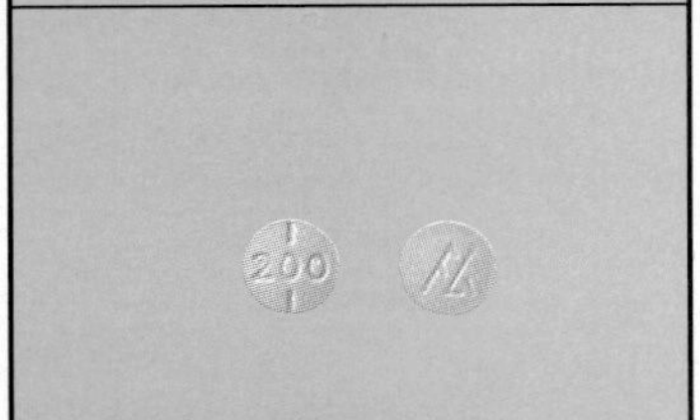

Levothroid
0.2mg: Forest

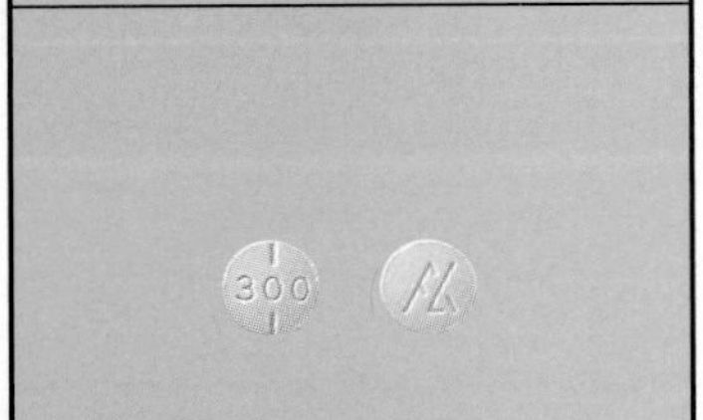

Levothroid
0.3mg: Forest

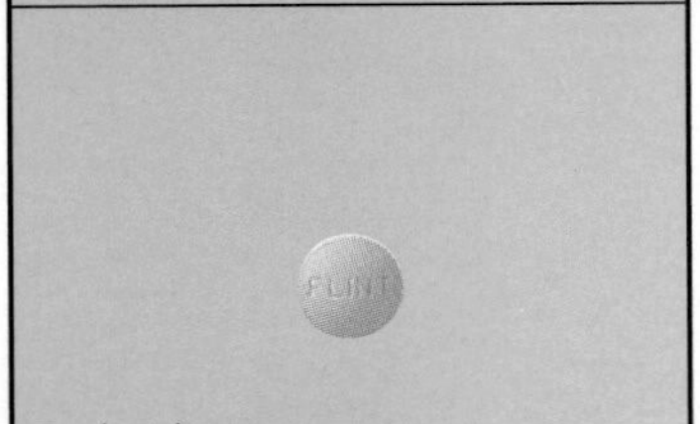

Synthroid
0.025mg: Knoll

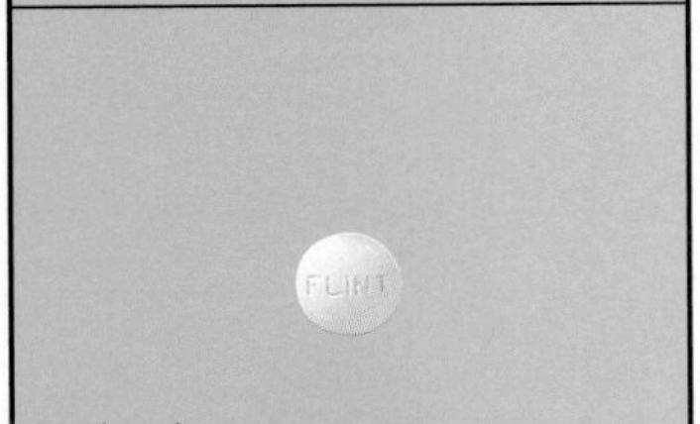

Synthroid
0.05mg: Knoll

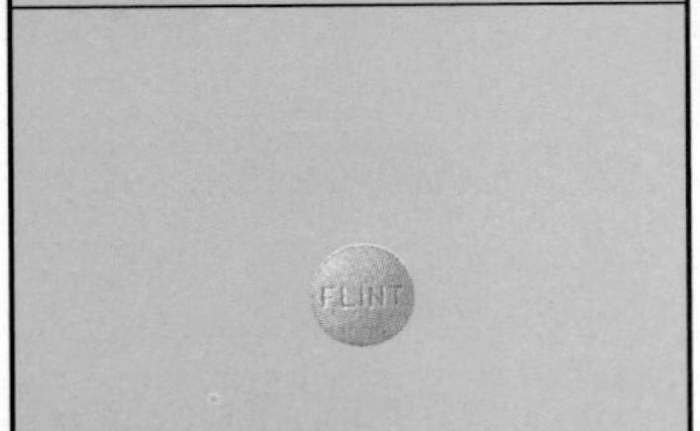

Synthroid
0.075mg: Knoll

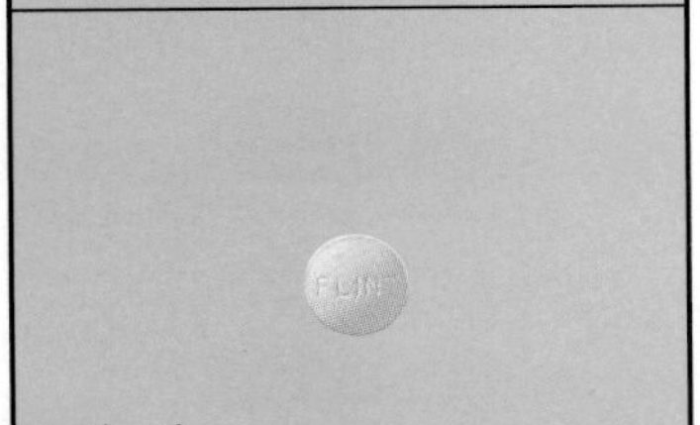

Synthroid
0.1mg: Knoll

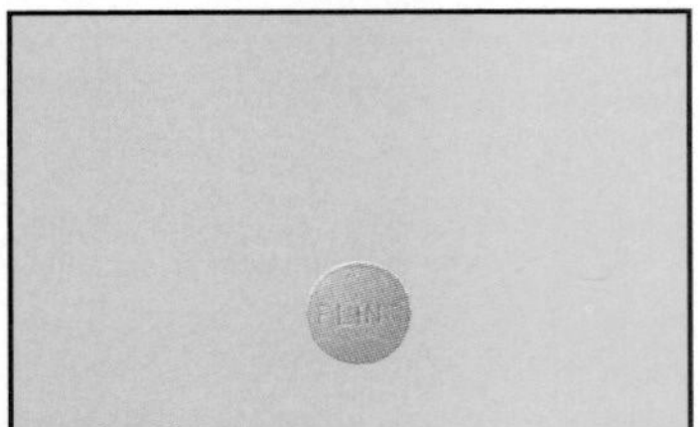

Synthroid
0.112mg: Knoll

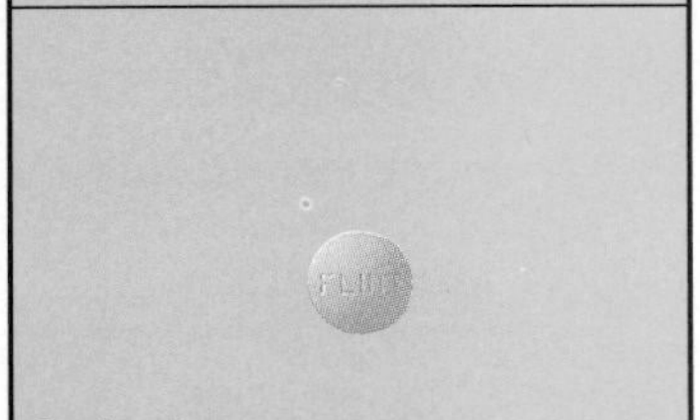

Synthroid
0.125mg: Knoll

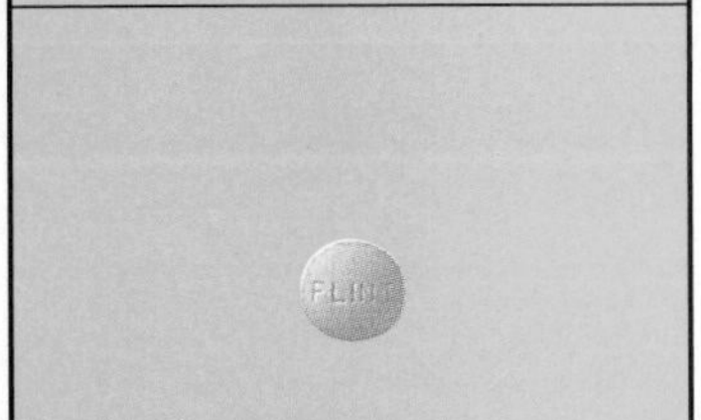

Synthroid
0.15mg: Knoll

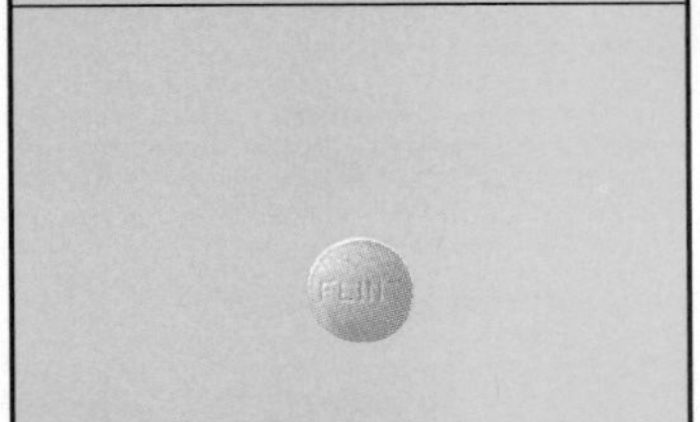

Synthroid
0.2mg: Knoll

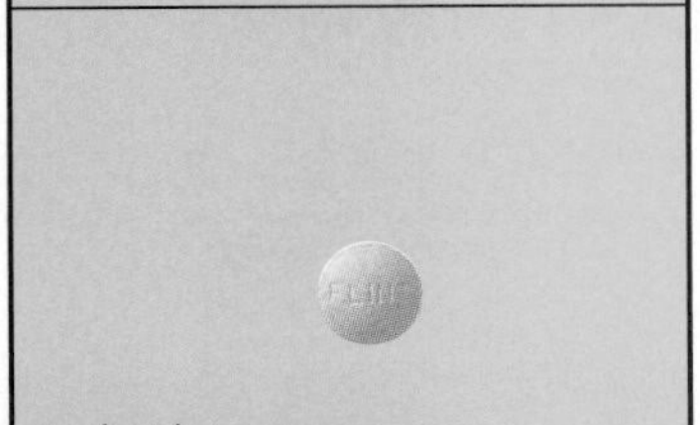

Synthroid
0.3mg: Knoll

Liotrix

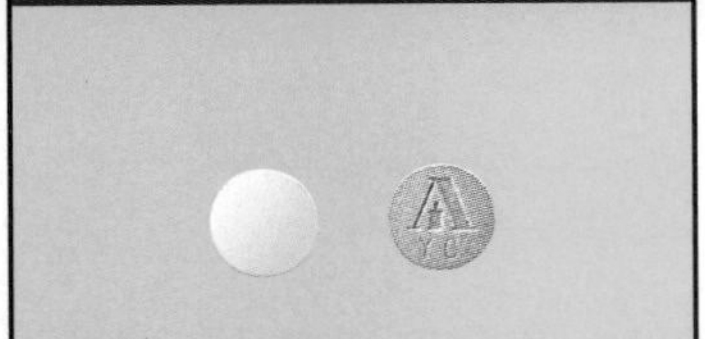

Thyrolar
15mg: Forest

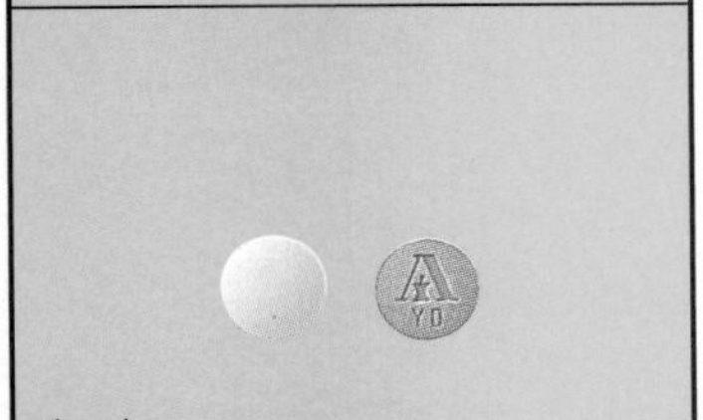

Thyrolar
30mg: Forest

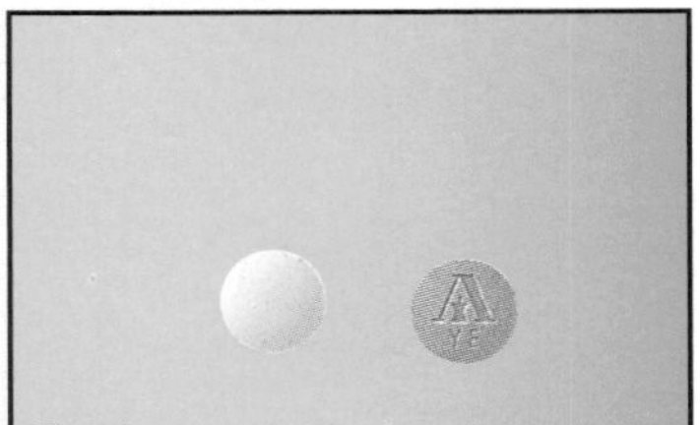

Thyrolar
60mg: Forest

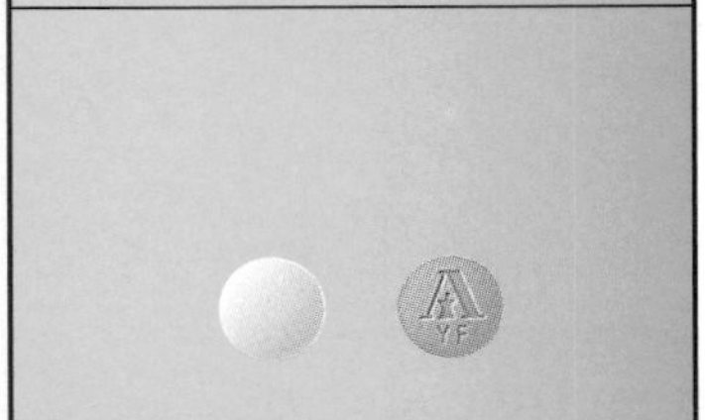

Thyrolar
120mg: Forest

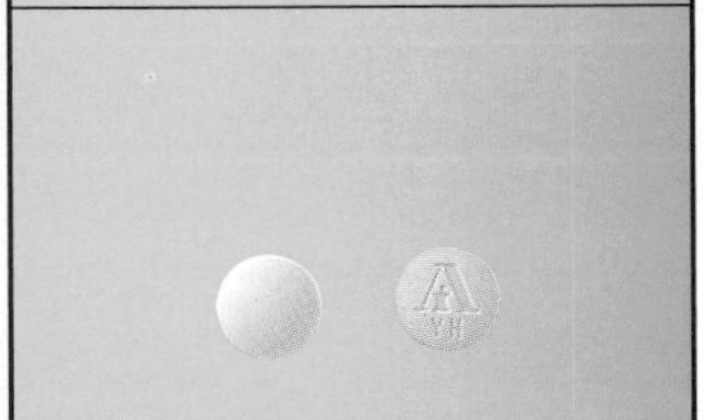

Thyrolar
180mg: Forest

Lisinopril

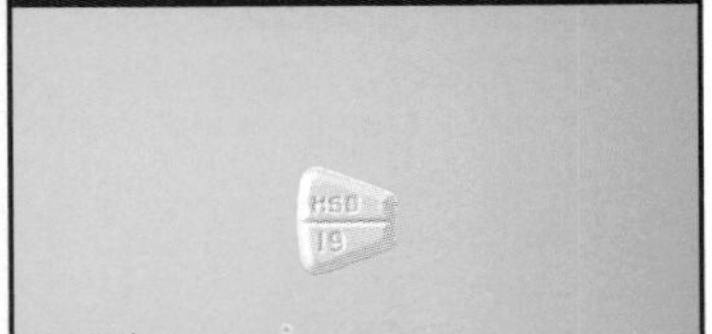

Prinivil
5mg: Merck

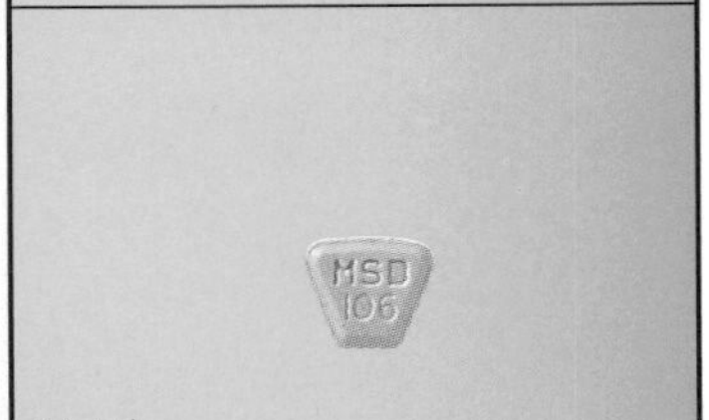

Prinivil
10mg: Merck

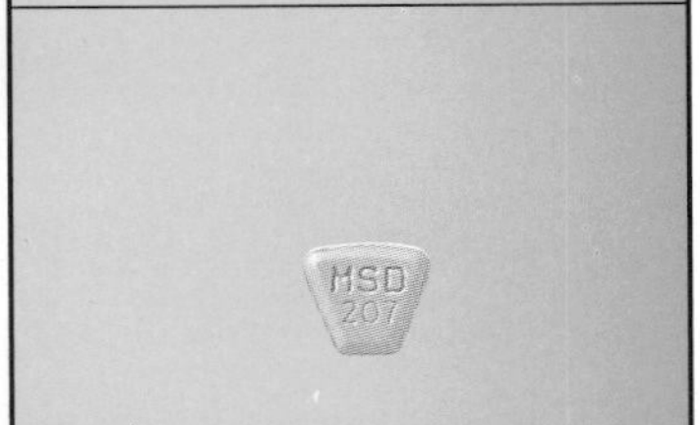

Prinivil
20mg: Merck

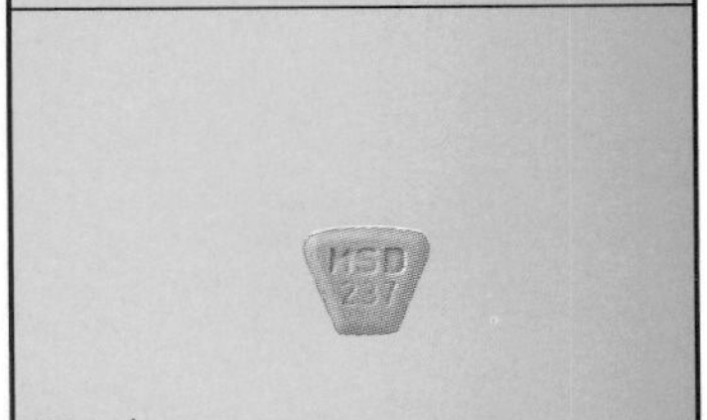

Prinivil
40mg: Merck

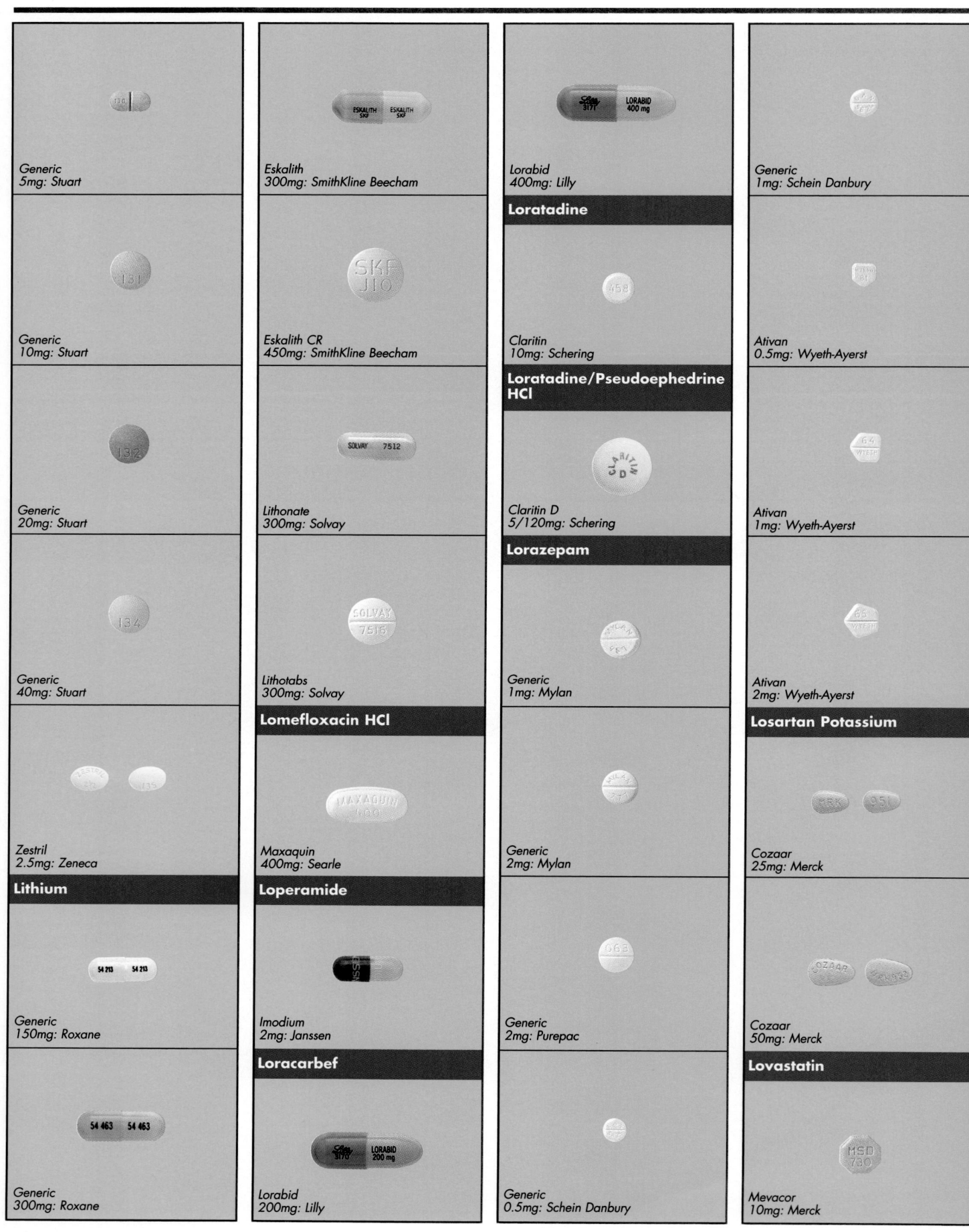

Generic
5mg: Stuart

Generic
10mg: Stuart

Generic
20mg: Stuart

Generic
40mg: Stuart

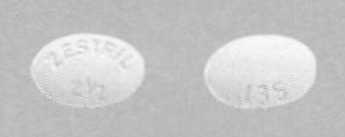

Zestril
2.5mg: Zeneca

Lithium

Generic
150mg: Roxane

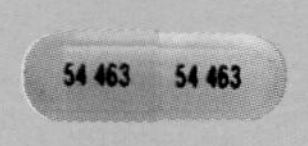

Generic
300mg: Roxane

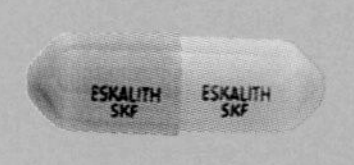

Eskalith
300mg: SmithKline Beecham

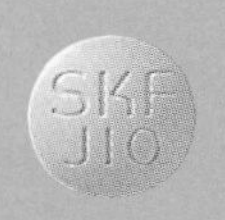

Eskalith CR
450mg: SmithKline Beecham

Lithonate
300mg: Solvay

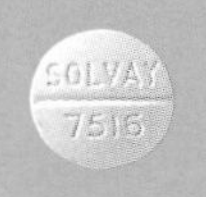

Lithotabs
300mg: Solvay

Lomefloxacin HCl

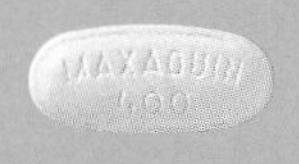

Maxaquin
400mg: Searle

Loperamide

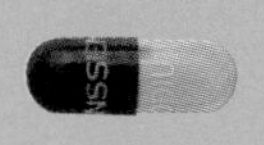

Imodium
2mg: Janssen

Loracarbef

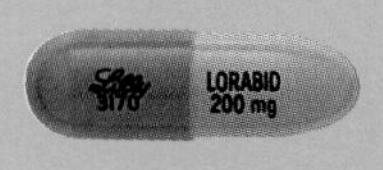

Lorabid
200mg: Lilly

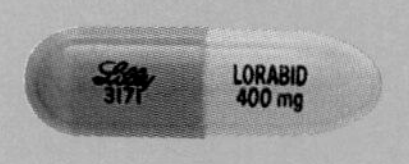

Lorabid
400mg: Lilly

Loratadine

Claritin
10mg: Schering

Loratadine/Pseudoephedrine HCl

Claritin D
5/120mg: Schering

Lorazepam

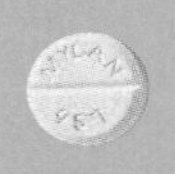

Generic
1mg: Mylan

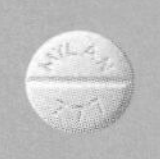

Generic
2mg: Mylan

Generic
2mg: Purepac

Generic
0.5mg: Schein Danbury

Generic
1mg: Schein Danbury

Ativan
0.5mg: Wyeth-Ayerst

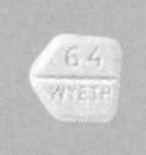

Ativan
1mg: Wyeth-Ayerst

Ativan
2mg: Wyeth-Ayerst

Losartan Potassium

Cozaar
25mg: Merck

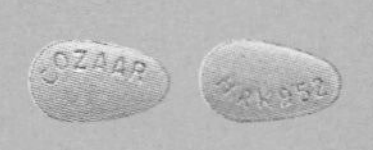

Cozaar
50mg: Merck

Lovastatin

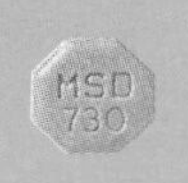

Mevacor
10mg: Merck

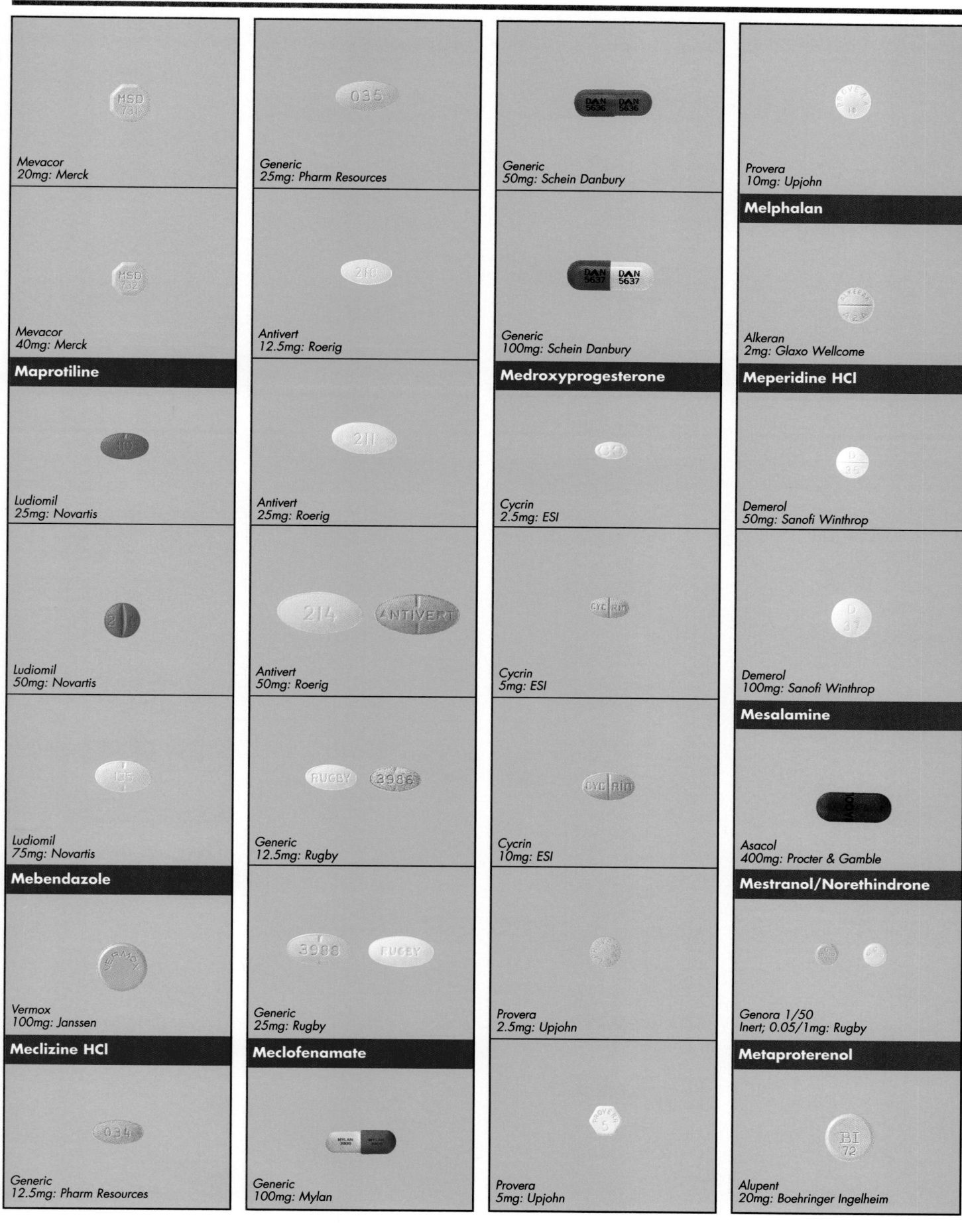

Mevacor
20mg: Merck

Mevacor
40mg: Merck

Maprotiline

Ludiomil
25mg: Novartis

Ludiomil
50mg: Novartis

Ludiomil
75mg: Novartis

Mebendazole

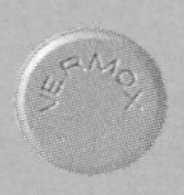

Vermox
100mg: Janssen

Meclizine HCl

Generic
12.5mg: Pharm Resources

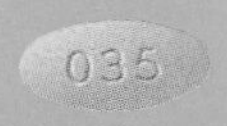

Generic
25mg: Pharm Resources

Antivert
12.5mg: Roerig

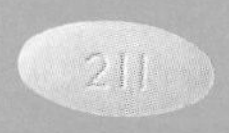

Antivert
25mg: Roerig

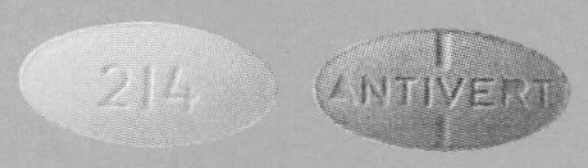

Antivert
50mg: Roerig

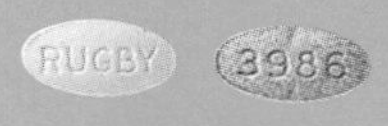

Generic
12.5mg: Rugby

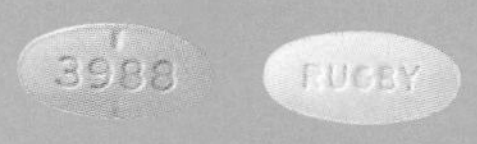

Generic
25mg: Rugby

Meclofenamate

Generic
100mg: Mylan

Generic
50mg: Schein Danbury

Generic
100mg: Schein Danbury

Medroxyprogesterone

Cycrin
2.5mg: ESI

Cycrin
5mg: ESI

Cycrin
10mg: ESI

Provera
2.5mg: Upjohn

Provera
5mg: Upjohn

Provera
10mg: Upjohn

Melphalan

Alkeran
2mg: Glaxo Wellcome

Meperidine HCl

Demerol
50mg: Sanofi Winthrop

Demerol
100mg: Sanofi Winthrop

Mesalamine

Asacol
400mg: Procter & Gamble

Mestranol/Norethindrone

Genora 1/50
Inert; 0.05/1mg: Rugby

Metaproterenol

Alupent
20mg: Boehringer Ingelheim

Metformin HCl

Glucophage
500mg: Lipha

Glucophage
850mg: Lipha

Methazolamide

Generic
50mg: Lederle

Neptazane
25mg: Storz

Methocarbamol

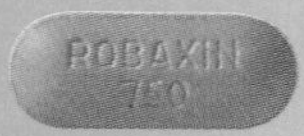

Robaxin
750mg: A. H. Robins

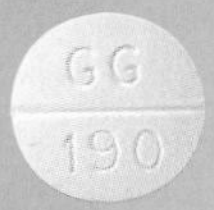

Generic
500mg: Geneva

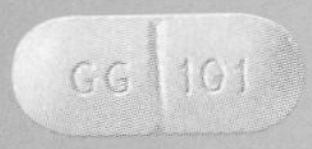

Generic
750mg: Geneva

Methocarbamol/Aspirin

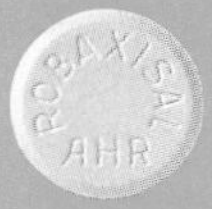

Robaxisal
400/325mg: A. H. Robins

Methyclothiazide

Enduron
5mg: Abbott

Methyldopa

Generic
250mg: Lederle

Aldomet
250mg: Merck

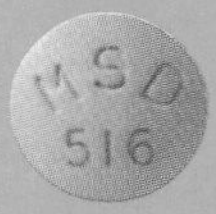

Aldomet
500mg: Merck

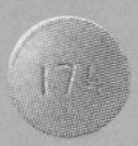

Generic
125mg: West Point

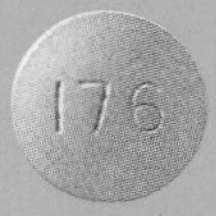

Generic
500mg: West Point

Methylphenidate HCl

Generic
5mg: MD

Generic
10mg: MD

Generic
20mg: MD

Ritalin
5mg: Novartis

Ritalin
10mg: Novartis

Ritalin
20mg: Novartis

Ritalin-SR
20mg: Novartis

Methylprednisolone

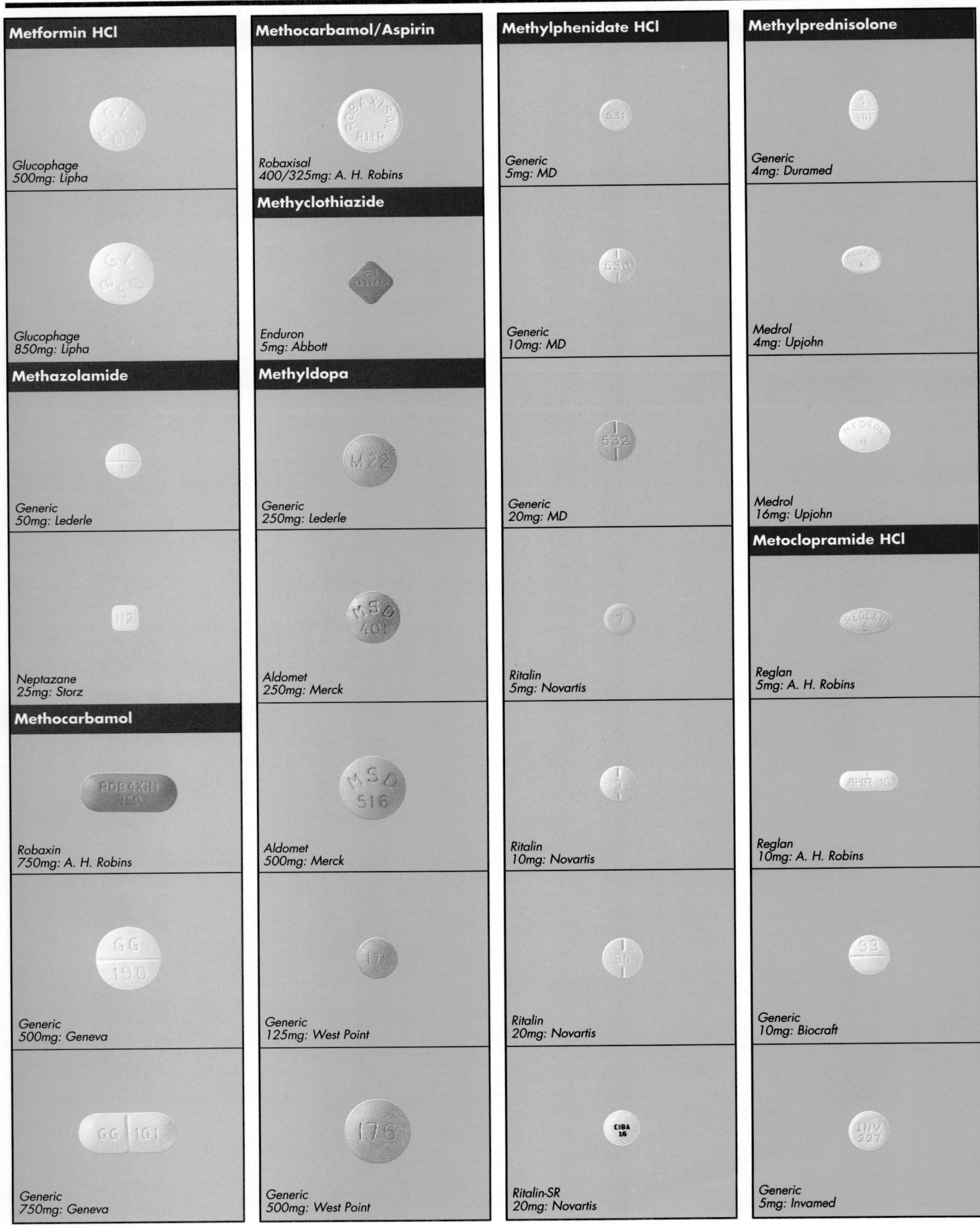

Generic
4mg: Duramed

Medrol
4mg: Upjohn

Medrol
16mg: Upjohn

Metoclopramide HCl

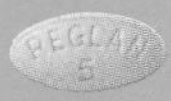

Reglan
5mg: A. H. Robins

Reglan
10mg: A. H. Robins

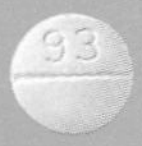

Generic
10mg: Biocraft

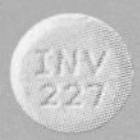

Generic
5mg: Invamed

Metolazone

Zaroxolyn
2.5mg: Fisons

Metoprolol Succinate

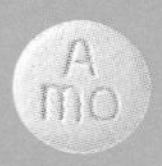

Toprol XL
50mg: Astra

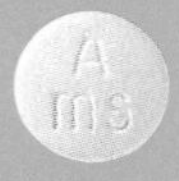

Toprol XL
100mg: Astra

Toprol XL
200mg: Astra

Metoprolol Tartrate

Generic
50mg: Mutual

Generic
100mg: Mutual

Generic
50mg: Mylan

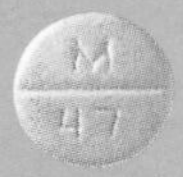

Generic
100mg: Mylan

Lopressor
50mg: Novartis

Lopressor
100mg: Novartis

Metronidazole

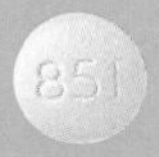

Generic
250mg: Lemmon

Generic
500mg: Lemmon

Flagyl
250mg: Searle

Flagyl
500mg: Searle

Minocycline HCl

Minocin
50mg: Lederle

Minocin
100mg: Lederle

Generic
50mg: Schein Danbury

Generic
100mg: Schein Danbury

Misoprostol

Cytotec
0.1mg: Searle

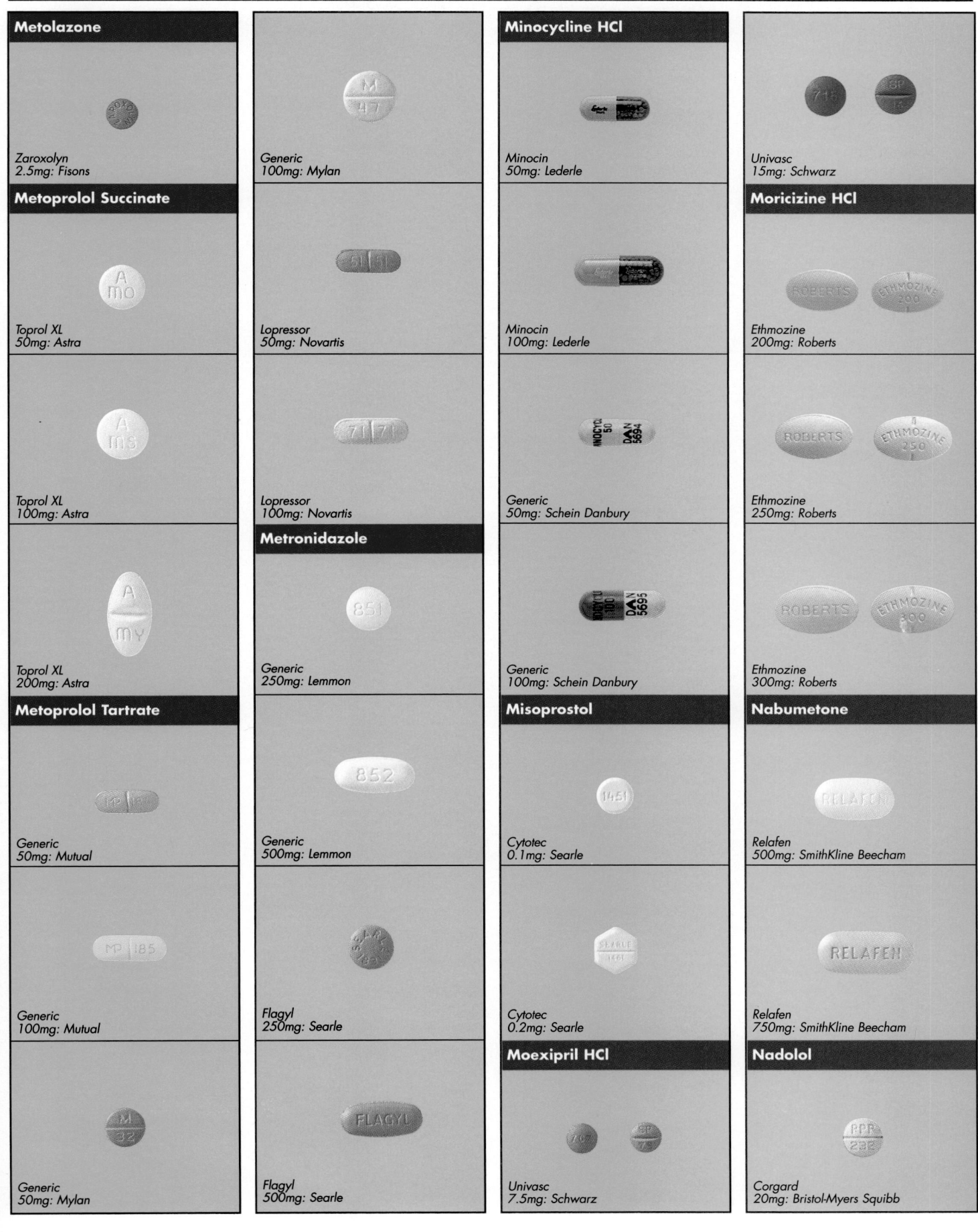

Cytotec
0.2mg: Searle

Moexipril HCl

Univasc
7.5mg: Schwarz

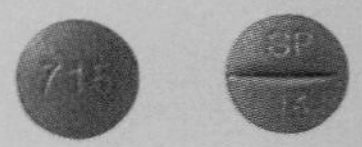

Univasc
15mg: Schwarz

Moricizine HCl

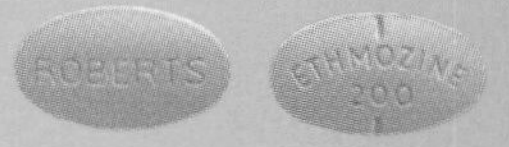

Ethmozine
200mg: Roberts

Ethmozine
250mg: Roberts

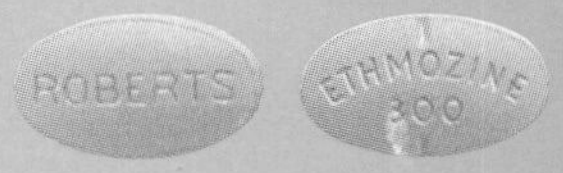

Ethmozine
300mg: Roberts

Nabumetone

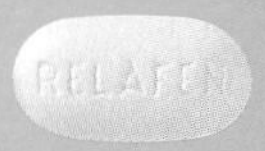

Relafen
500mg: SmithKline Beecham

Relafen
750mg: SmithKline Beecham

Nadolol

Corgard
20mg: Bristol-Myers Squibb

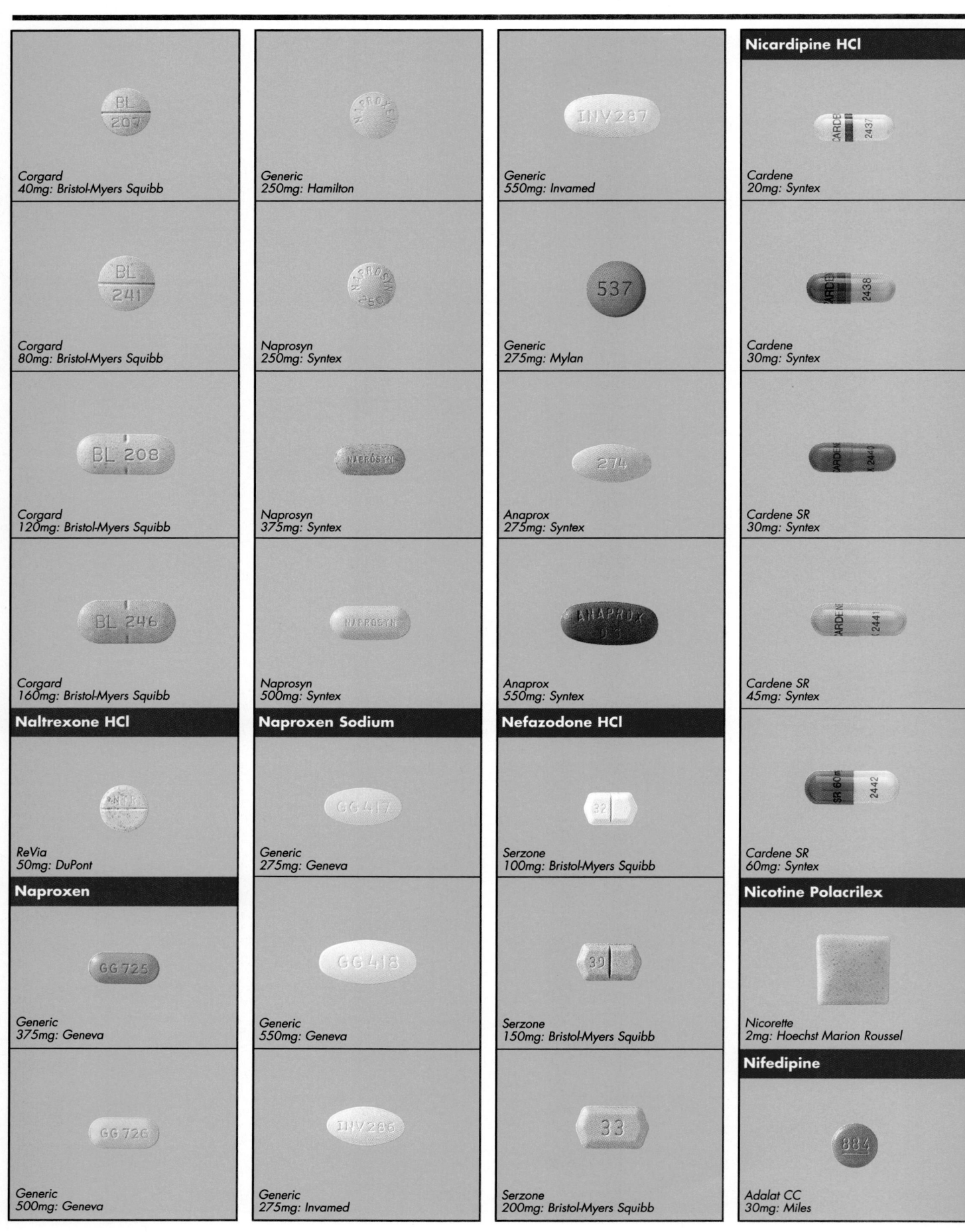

Corgard
40mg: Bristol-Myers Squibb

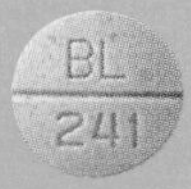

Corgard
80mg: Bristol-Myers Squibb

Corgard
120mg: Bristol-Myers Squibb

Corgard
160mg: Bristol-Myers Squibb

Naltrexone HCl

ReVia
50mg: DuPont

Naproxen

Generic
375mg: Geneva

Generic
500mg: Geneva

Generic
250mg: Hamilton

Naprosyn
250mg: Syntex

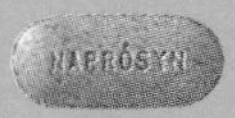

Naprosyn
375mg: Syntex

Naprosyn
500mg: Syntex

Naproxen Sodium

Generic
275mg: Geneva

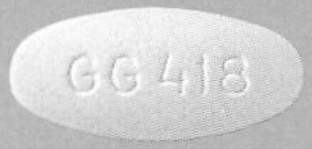

Generic
550mg: Geneva

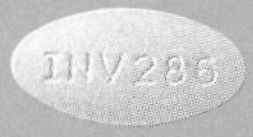

Generic
275mg: Invamed

Generic
550mg: Invamed

Generic
275mg: Mylan

Anaprox
275mg: Syntex

Anaprox
550mg: Syntex

Nefazodone HCl

Serzone
100mg: Bristol-Myers Squibb

Serzone
150mg: Bristol-Myers Squibb

Serzone
200mg: Bristol-Myers Squibb

Nicardipine HCl

Cardene
20mg: Syntex

Cardene
30mg: Syntex

Cardene SR
30mg: Syntex

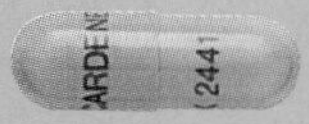

Cardene SR
45mg: Syntex

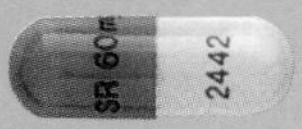

Cardene SR
60mg: Syntex

Nicotine Polacrilex

Nicorette
2mg: Hoechst Marion Roussel

Nifedipine

Adalat CC
30mg: Miles

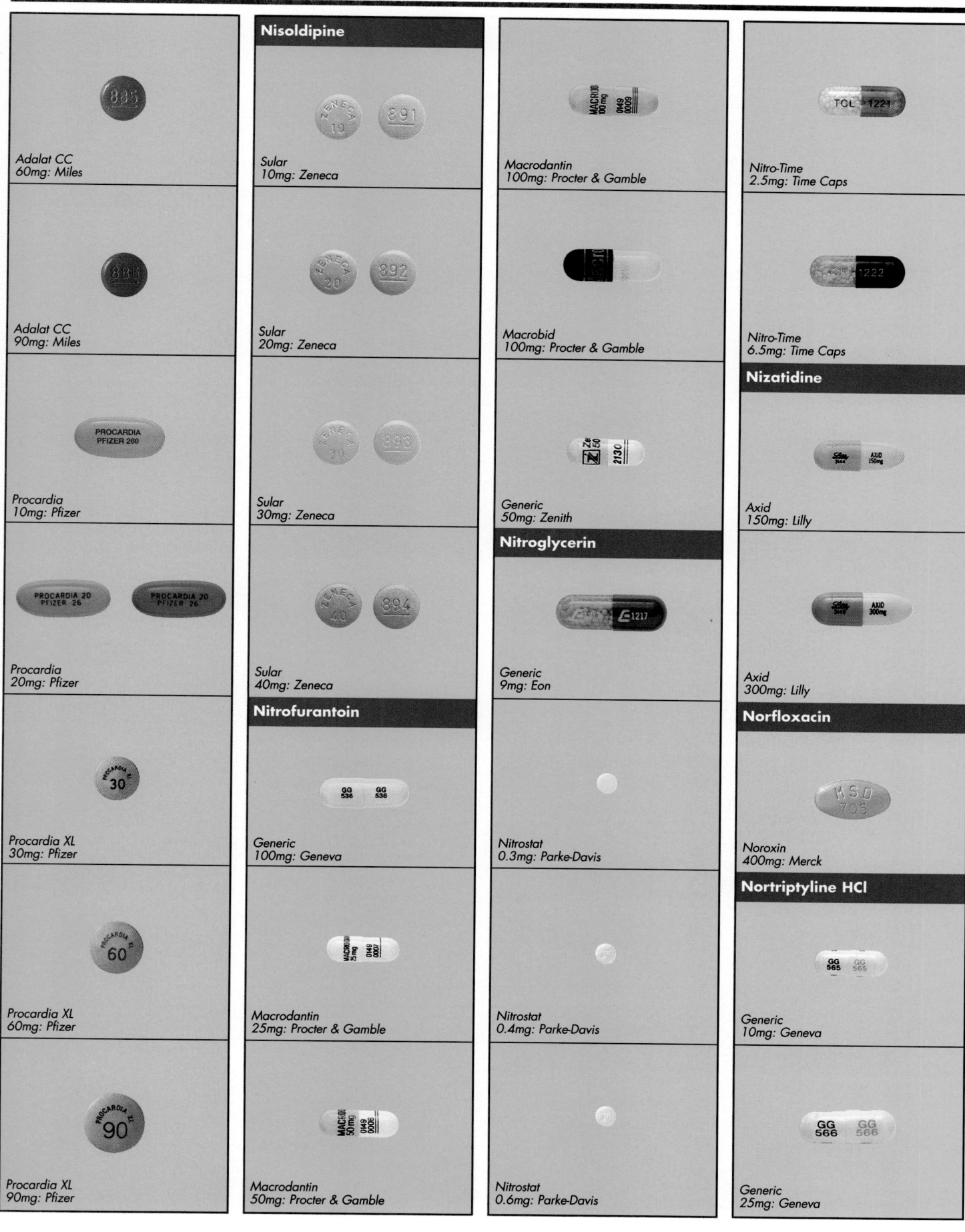

Adalat CC
60mg: Miles

Adalat CC
90mg: Miles

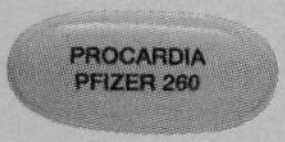

Procardia
10mg: Pfizer

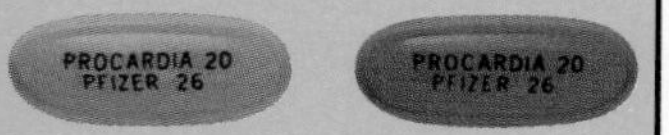

Procardia
20mg: Pfizer

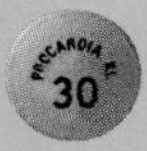

Procardia XL
30mg: Pfizer

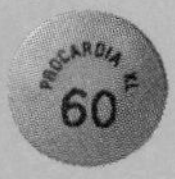

Procardia XL
60mg: Pfizer

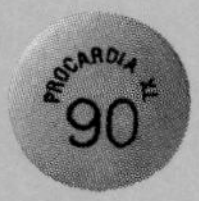

Procardia XL
90mg: Pfizer

Nisoldipine

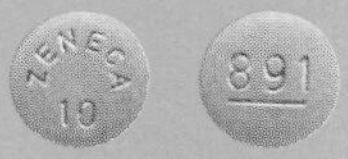

Sular
10mg: Zeneca

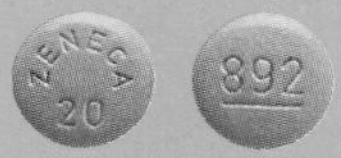

Sular
20mg: Zeneca

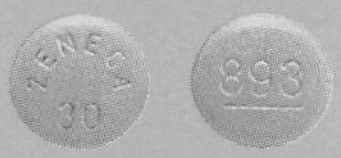

Sular
30mg: Zeneca

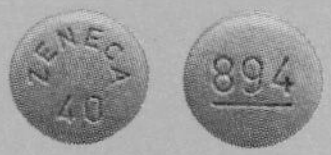

Sular
40mg: Zeneca

Nitrofurantoin

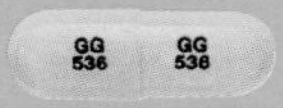

Generic
100mg: Geneva

Macrodantin
25mg: Procter & Gamble

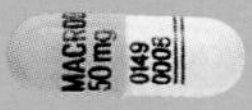

Macrodantin
50mg: Procter & Gamble

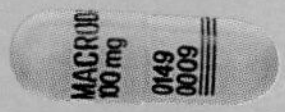

Macrodantin
100mg: Procter & Gamble

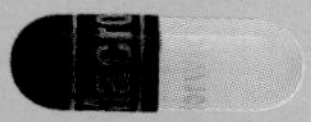

Macrobid
100mg: Procter & Gamble

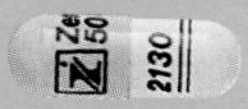

Generic
50mg: Zenith

Nitroglycerin

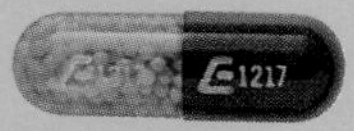

Generic
9mg: Eon

Nitrostat
0.3mg: Parke-Davis

Nitrostat
0.4mg: Parke-Davis

Nitrostat
0.6mg: Parke-Davis

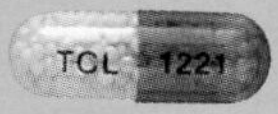

Nitro-Time
2.5mg: Time Caps

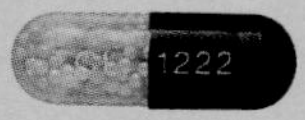

Nitro-Time
6.5mg: Time Caps

Nizatidine

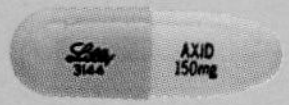

Axid
150mg: Lilly

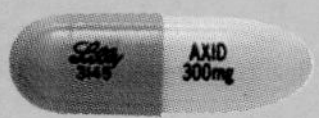

Axid
300mg: Lilly

Norfloxacin

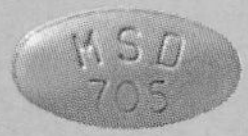

Noroxin
400mg: Merck

Nortriptyline HCl

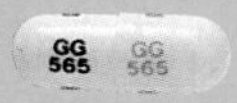

Generic
10mg: Geneva

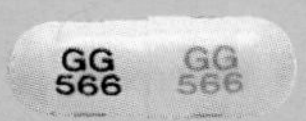

Generic
25mg: Geneva

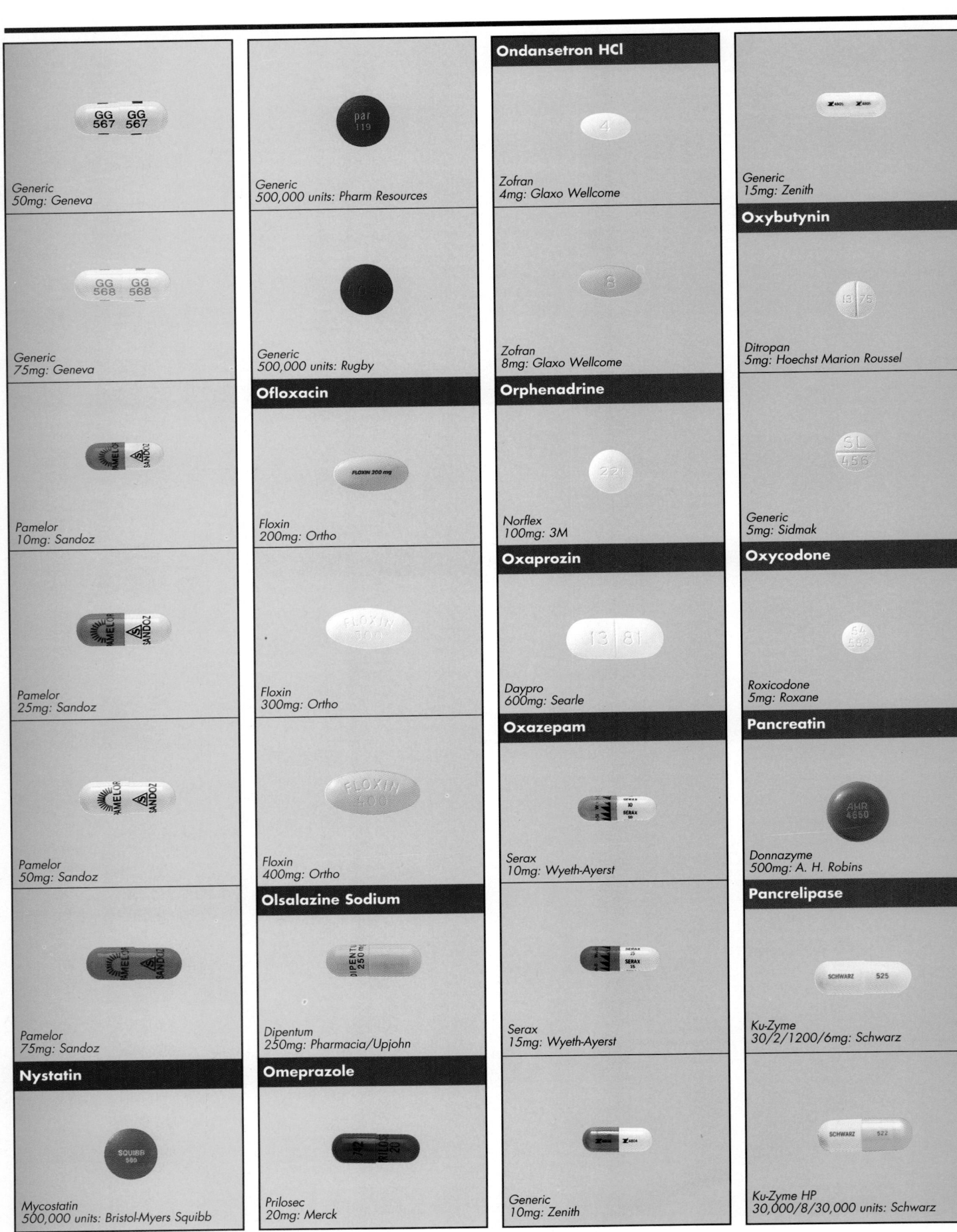

Generic
50mg: Geneva

Generic
75mg: Geneva

Pamelor
10mg: Sandoz

Pamelor
25mg: Sandoz

Pamelor
50mg: Sandoz

Pamelor
75mg: Sandoz

Nystatin

Mycostatin
500,000 units: Bristol-Myers Squibb

Generic
500,000 units: Pharm Resources

Generic
500,000 units: Rugby

Ofloxacin

Floxin
200mg: Ortho

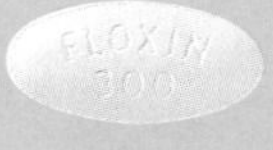

Floxin
300mg: Ortho

Floxin
400mg: Ortho

Olsalazine Sodium

Dipentum
250mg: Pharmacia/Upjohn

Omeprazole

Prilosec
20mg: Merck

Ondansetron HCl

Zofran
4mg: Glaxo Wellcome

Zofran
8mg: Glaxo Wellcome

Orphenadrine

Norflex
100mg: 3M

Oxaprozin

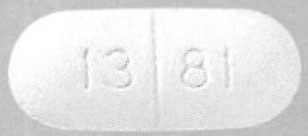

Daypro
600mg: Searle

Oxazepam

Serax
10mg: Wyeth-Ayerst

Serax
15mg: Wyeth-Ayerst

Generic
10mg: Zenith

Generic
15mg: Zenith

Oxybutynin

Ditropan
5mg: Hoechst Marion Roussel

Generic
5mg: Sidmak

Oxycodone

Roxicodone
5mg: Roxane

Pancreatin

Donnazyme
500mg: A. H. Robins

Pancrelipase

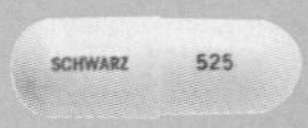

Ku-Zyme
30/2/1200/6mg: Schwarz

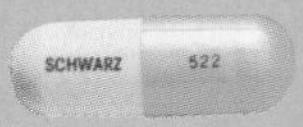

Ku-Zyme HP
30,000/8/30,000 units: Schwarz

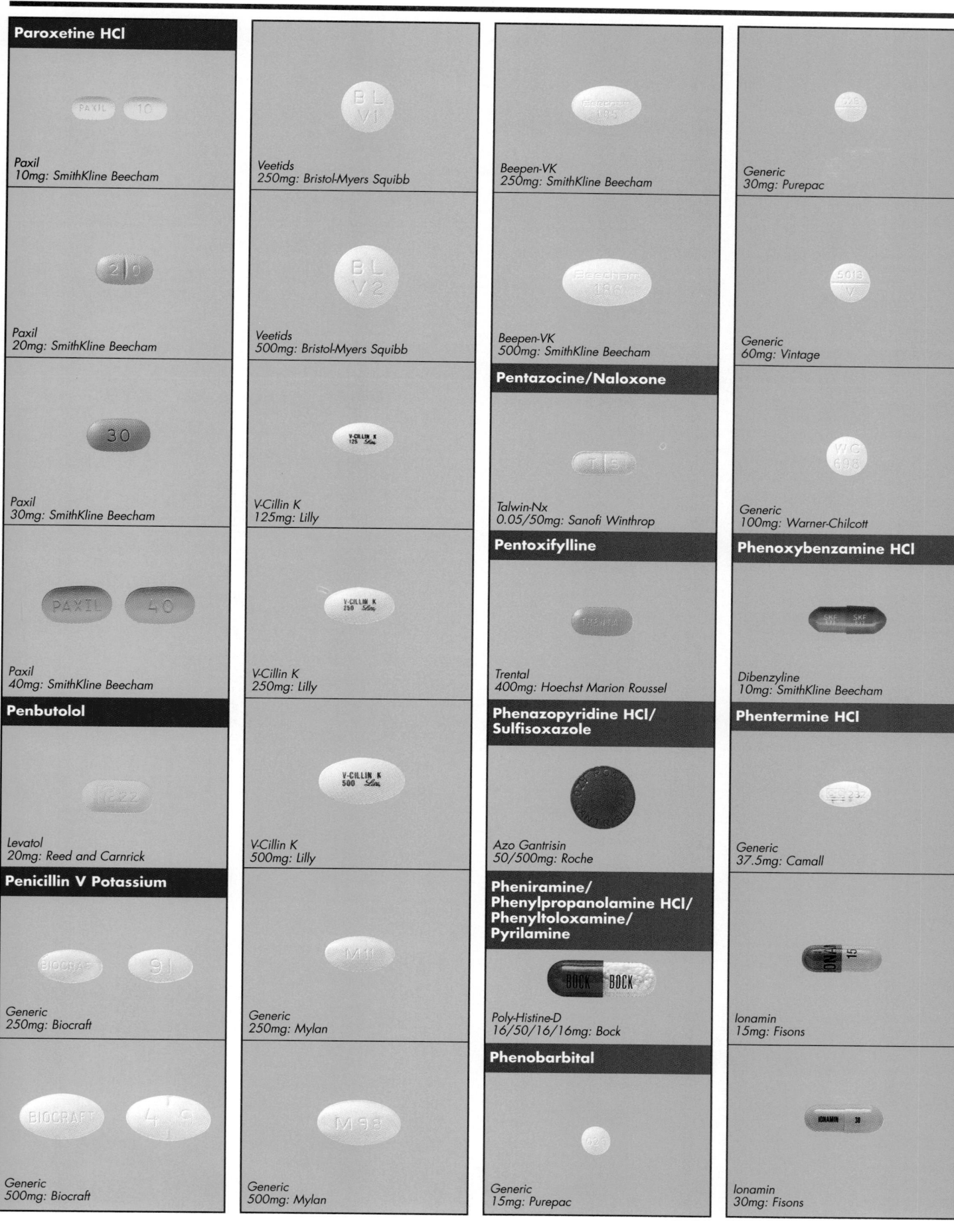

Paroxetine HCl

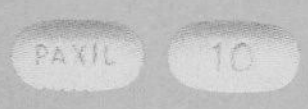

Paxil
10mg: SmithKline Beecham

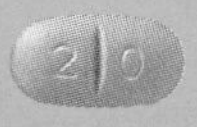

Paxil
20mg: SmithKline Beecham

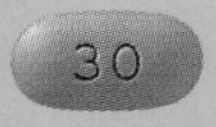

Paxil
30mg: SmithKline Beecham

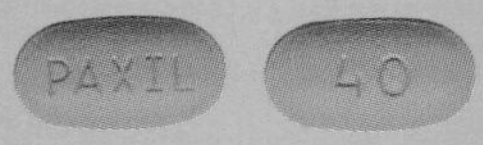

Paxil
40mg: SmithKline Beecham

Penbutolol

Levatol
20mg: Reed and Carnrick

Penicillin V Potassium

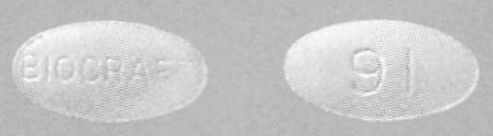

Generic
250mg: Biocraft

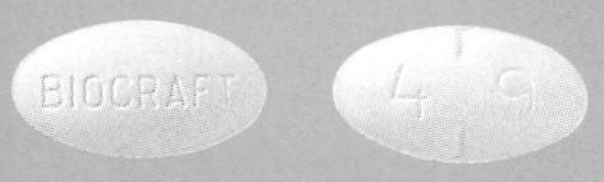

Generic
500mg: Biocraft

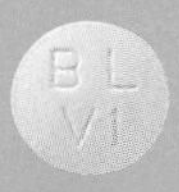

Veetids
250mg: Bristol-Myers Squibb

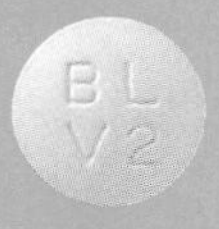

Veetids
500mg: Bristol-Myers Squibb

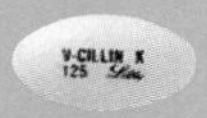

V-Cillin K
125mg: Lilly

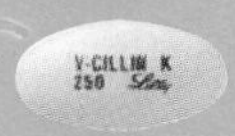

V-Cillin K
250mg: Lilly

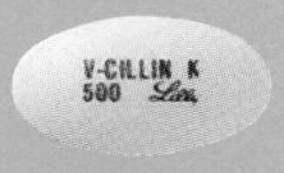

V-Cillin K
500mg: Lilly

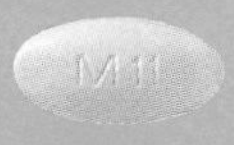

Generic
250mg: Mylan

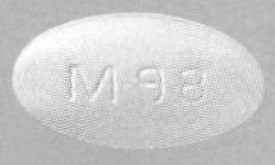

Generic
500mg: Mylan

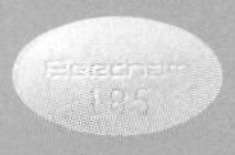

Beepen-VK
250mg: SmithKline Beecham

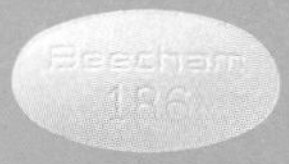

Beepen-VK
500mg: SmithKline Beecham

Pentazocine/Naloxone

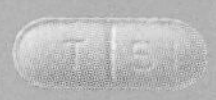

Talwin-Nx
0.05/50mg: Sanofi Winthrop

Pentoxifylline

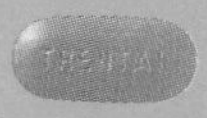

Trental
400mg: Hoechst Marion Roussel

Phenazopyridine HCl/ Sulfisoxazole

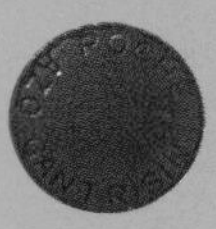

Azo Gantrisin
50/500mg: Roche

Pheniramine/ Phenylpropanolamine HCl/ Phenyltoloxamine/ Pyrilamine

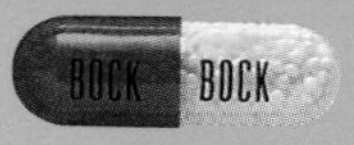

Poly-Histine-D
16/50/16/16mg: Bock

Phenobarbital

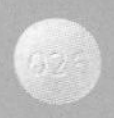

Generic
15mg: Purepac

Generic
30mg: Purepac

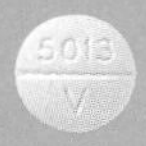

Generic
60mg: Vintage

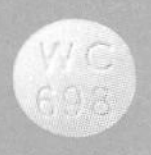

Generic
100mg: Warner-Chilcott

Phenoxybenzamine HCl

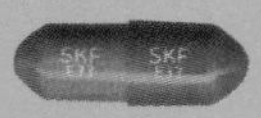

Dibenzyline
10mg: SmithKline Beecham

Phentermine HCl

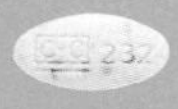

Generic
37.5mg: Camall

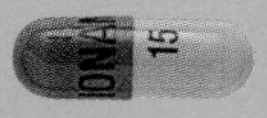

Ionamin
15mg: Fisons

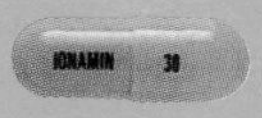

Ionamin
30mg: Fisons

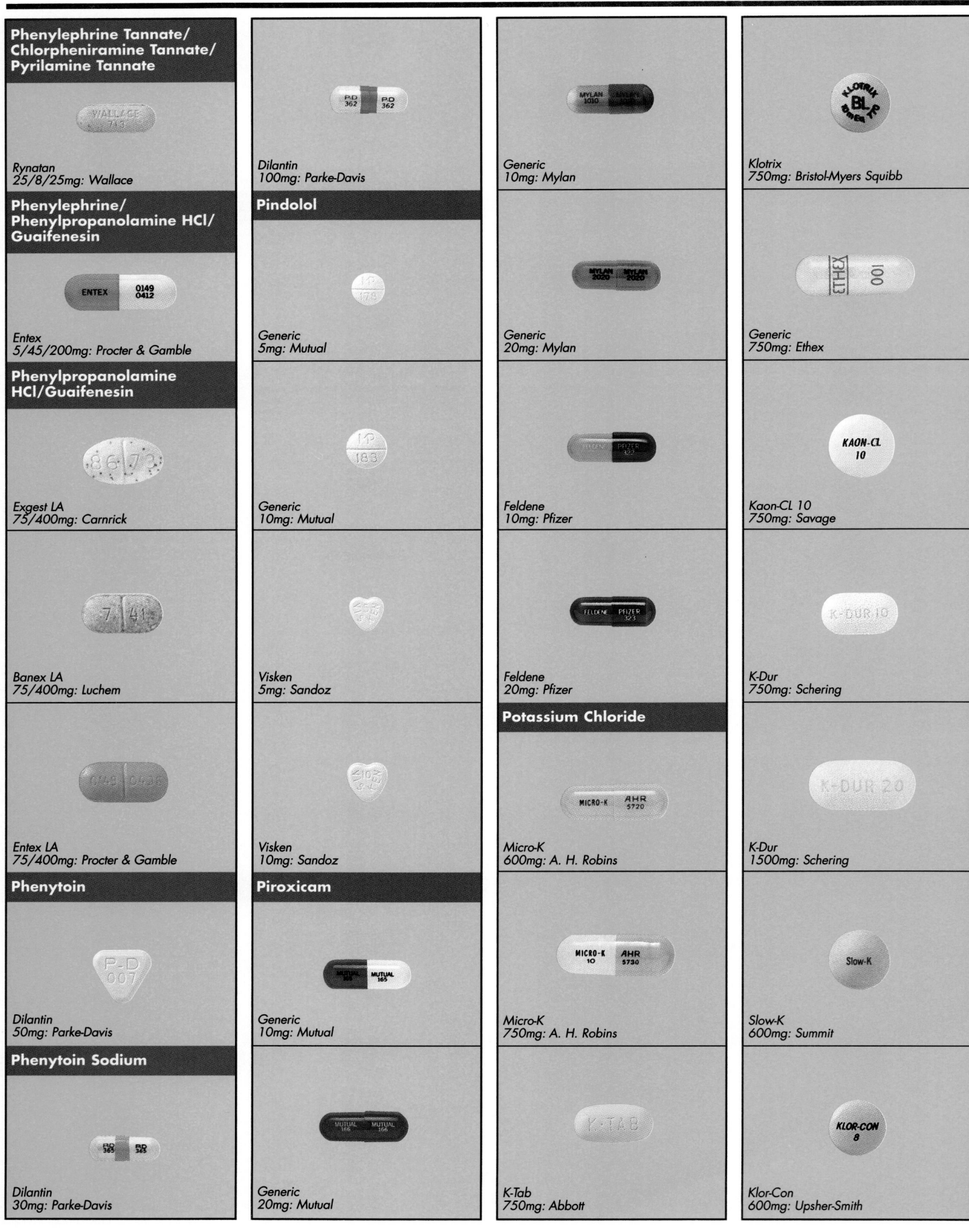

Phenylephrine Tannate/ Chlorpheniramine Tannate/ Pyrilamine Tannate

Rynatan
25/8/25mg: Wallace

Phenylephrine/ Phenylpropanolamine HCl/ Guaifenesin

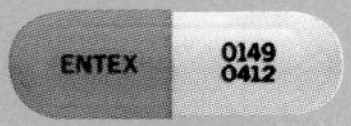

Entex
5/45/200mg: Procter & Gamble

Phenylpropanolamine HCl/Guaifenesin

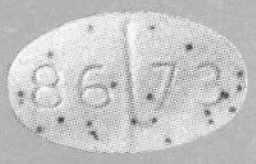

Exgest LA
75/400mg: Carnrick

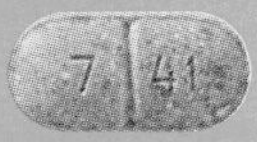

Banex LA
75/400mg: Luchem

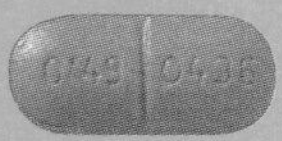

Entex LA
75/400mg: Procter & Gamble

Phenytoin

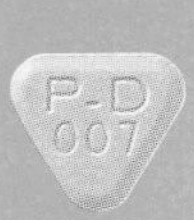

Dilantin
50mg: Parke-Davis

Phenytoin Sodium

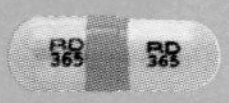

Dilantin
30mg: Parke-Davis

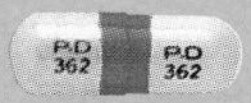

Dilantin
100mg: Parke-Davis

Pindolol

Generic
5mg: Mutual

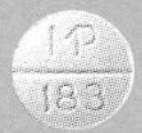

Generic
10mg: Mutual

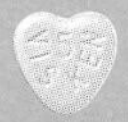

Visken
5mg: Sandoz

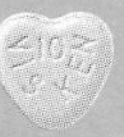

Visken
10mg: Sandoz

Piroxicam

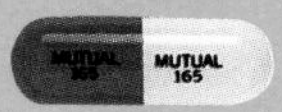

Generic
10mg: Mutual

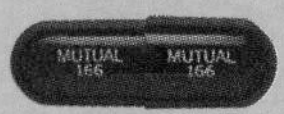

Generic
20mg: Mutual

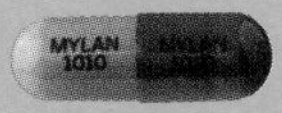

Generic
10mg: Mylan

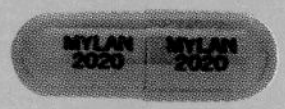

Generic
20mg: Mylan

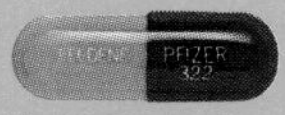

Feldene
10mg: Pfizer

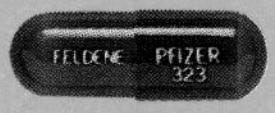

Feldene
20mg: Pfizer

Potassium Chloride

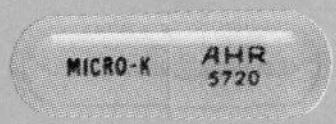

Micro-K
600mg: A. H. Robins

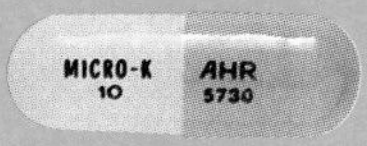

Micro-K
750mg: A. H. Robins

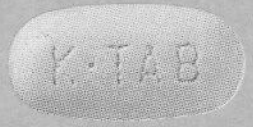

K-Tab
750mg: Abbott

Klotrix
750mg: Bristol-Myers Squibb

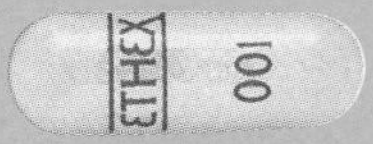

Generic
750mg: Ethex

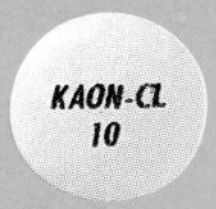

Kaon-CL 10
750mg: Savage

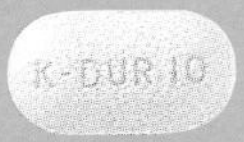

K-Dur
750mg: Schering

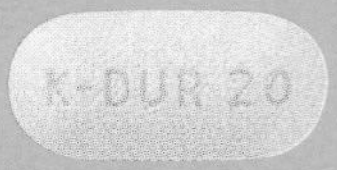

K-Dur
1500mg: Schering

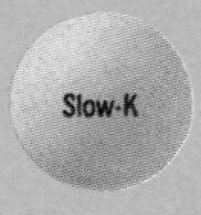

Slow-K
600mg: Summit

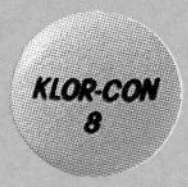

Klor-Con
600mg: Upsher-Smith

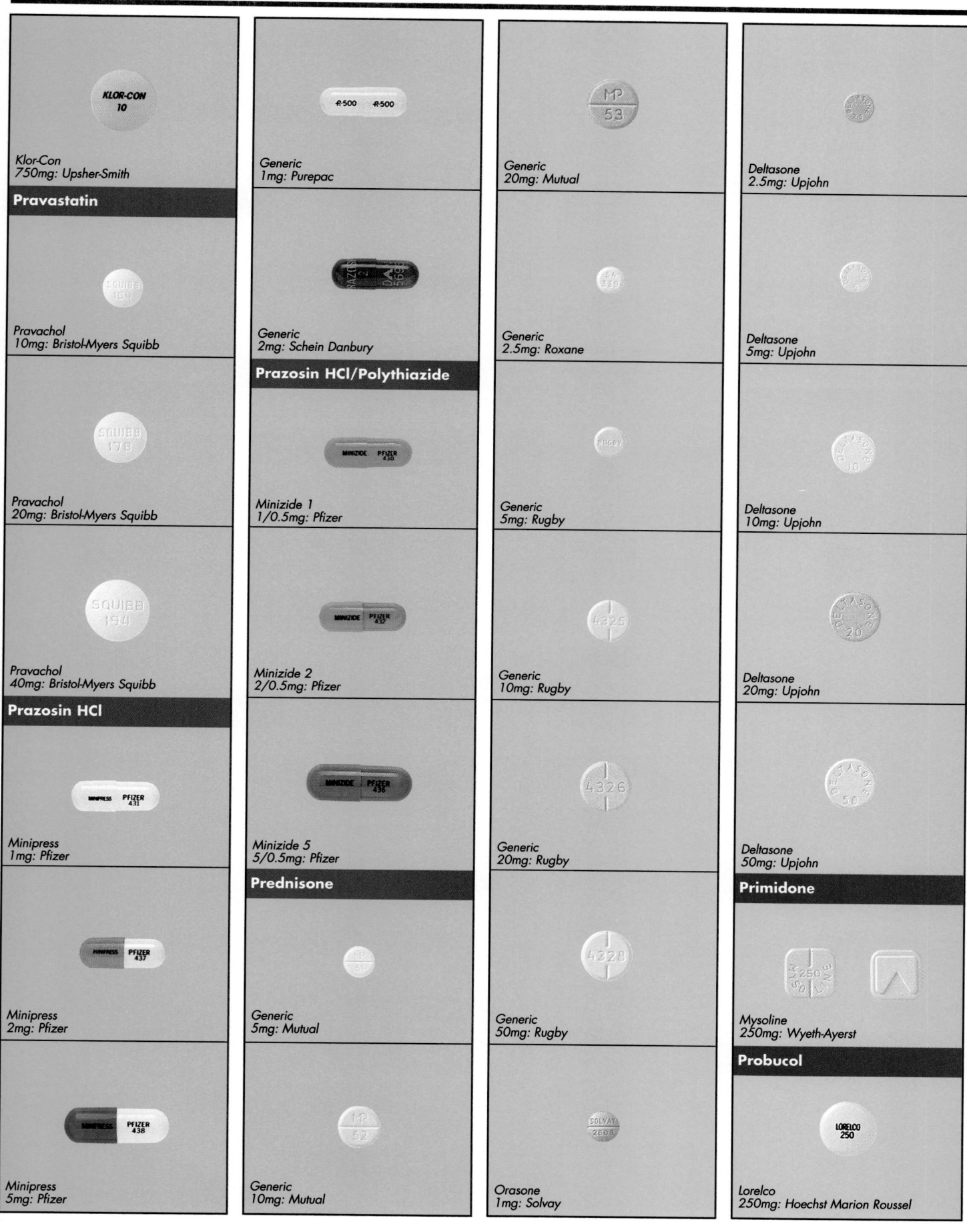

Klor-Con
750mg: Upsher-Smith

Pravastatin

Pravachol
10mg: Bristol-Myers Squibb

Pravachol
20mg: Bristol-Myers Squibb

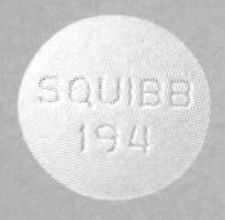

Pravachol
40mg: Bristol-Myers Squibb

Prazosin HCl

Minipress
1mg: Pfizer

Minipress
2mg: Pfizer

Minipress
5mg: Pfizer

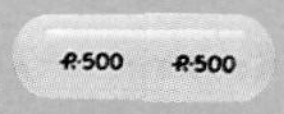

Generic
1mg: Purepac

Generic
2mg: Schein Danbury

Prazosin HCl/Polythiazide

Minizide 1
1/0.5mg: Pfizer

Minizide 2
2/0.5mg: Pfizer

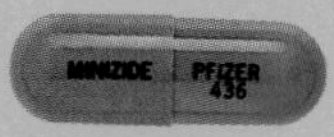

Minizide 5
5/0.5mg: Pfizer

Prednisone

Generic
5mg: Mutual

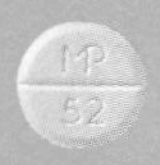

Generic
10mg: Mutual

Generic
20mg: Mutual

Generic
2.5mg: Roxane

Generic
5mg: Rugby

Generic
10mg: Rugby

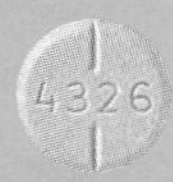

Generic
20mg: Rugby

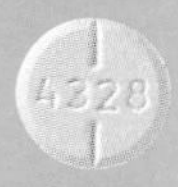

Generic
50mg: Rugby

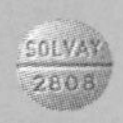

Orasone
1mg: Solvay

Deltasone
2.5mg: Upjohn

Deltasone
5mg: Upjohn

Deltasone
10mg: Upjohn

Deltasone
20mg: Upjohn

Deltasone
50mg: Upjohn

Primidone

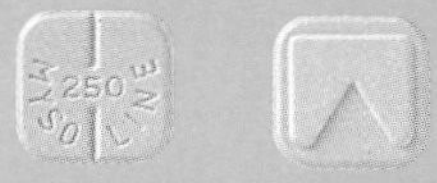

Mysoline
250mg: Wyeth-Ayerst

Probucol

Lorelco
250mg: Hoechst Marion Roussel

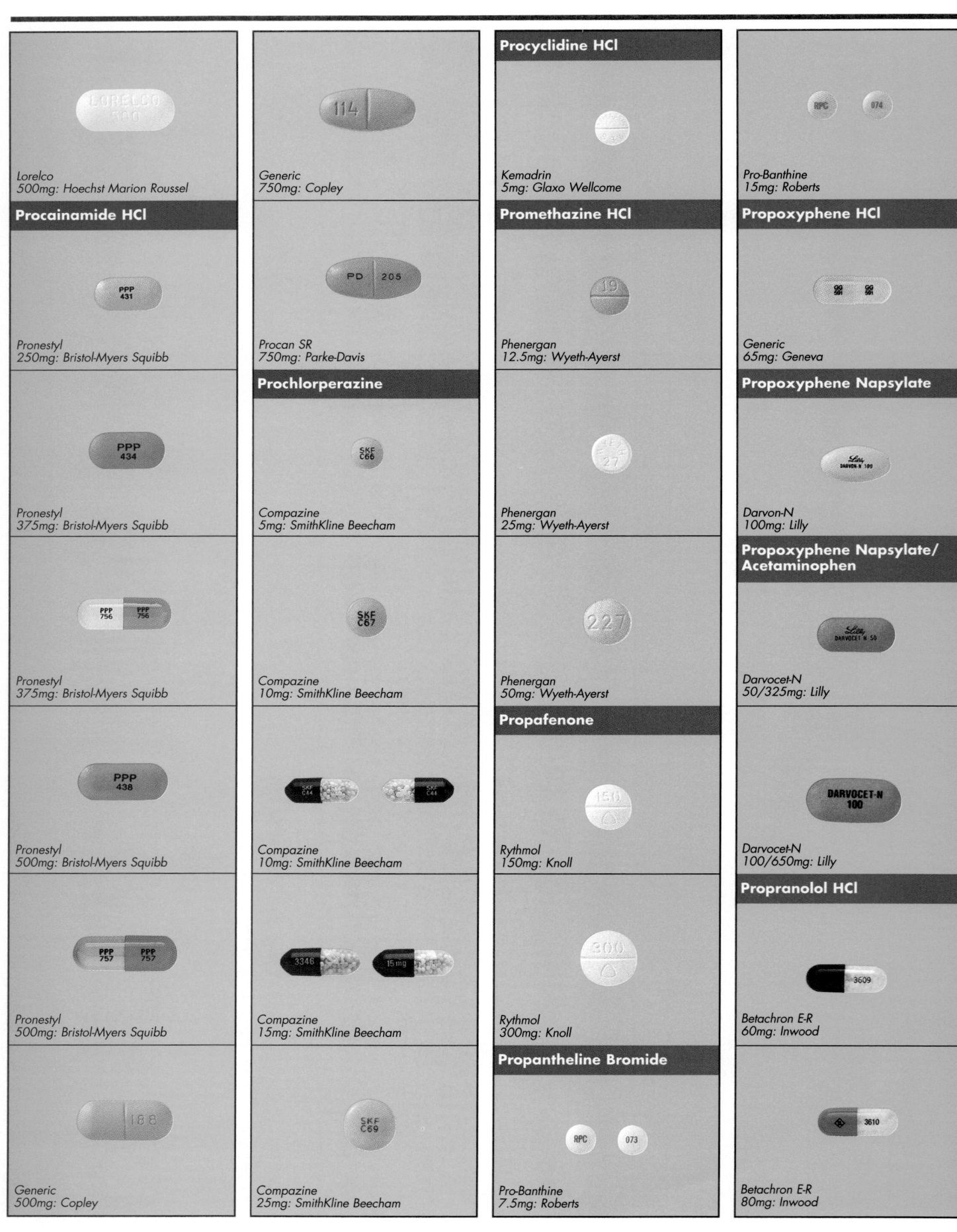

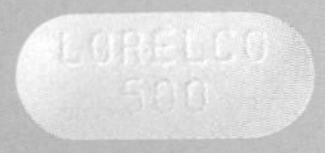

Lorelco
500mg: Hoechst Marion Roussel

Procainamide HCl

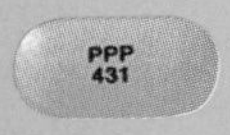

Pronestyl
250mg: Bristol-Myers Squibb

Pronestyl
375mg: Bristol-Myers Squibb

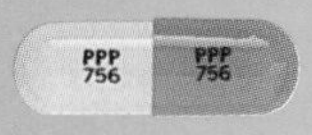

Pronestyl
375mg: Bristol-Myers Squibb

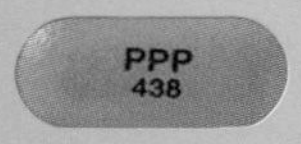

Pronestyl
500mg: Bristol-Myers Squibb

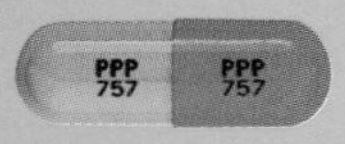

Pronestyl
500mg: Bristol-Myers Squibb

Generic
500mg: Copley

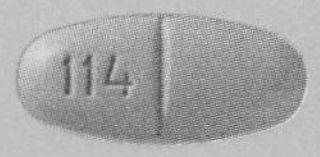

Generic
750mg: Copley

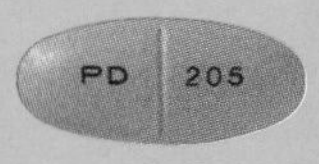

Procan SR
750mg: Parke-Davis

Prochlorperazine

Compazine
5mg: SmithKline Beecham

Compazine
10mg: SmithKline Beecham

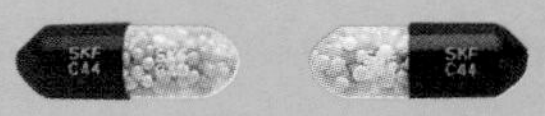

Compazine
10mg: SmithKline Beecham

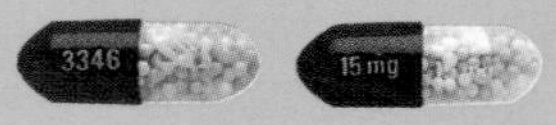

Compazine
15mg: SmithKline Beecham

Compazine
25mg: SmithKline Beecham

Procyclidine HCl

Kemadrin
5mg: Glaxo Wellcome

Promethazine HCl

Phenergan
12.5mg: Wyeth-Ayerst

Phenergan
25mg: Wyeth-Ayerst

Phenergan
50mg: Wyeth-Ayerst

Propafenone

Rythmol
150mg: Knoll

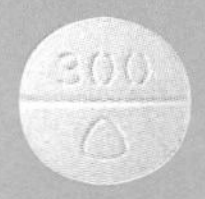

Rythmol
300mg: Knoll

Propantheline Bromide

Pro-Banthine
7.5mg: Roberts

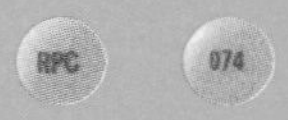

Pro-Banthine
15mg: Roberts

Propoxyphene HCl

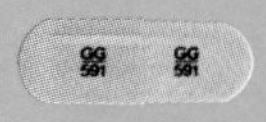

Generic
65mg: Geneva

Propoxyphene Napsylate

Darvon-N
100mg: Lilly

Propoxyphene Napsylate/ Acetaminophen

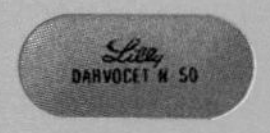

Darvocet-N
50/325mg: Lilly

Darvocet-N
100/650mg: Lilly

Propranolol HCl

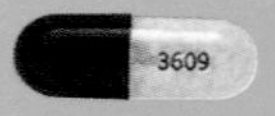

Betachron E-R
60mg: Inwood

Betachron E-R
80mg: Inwood

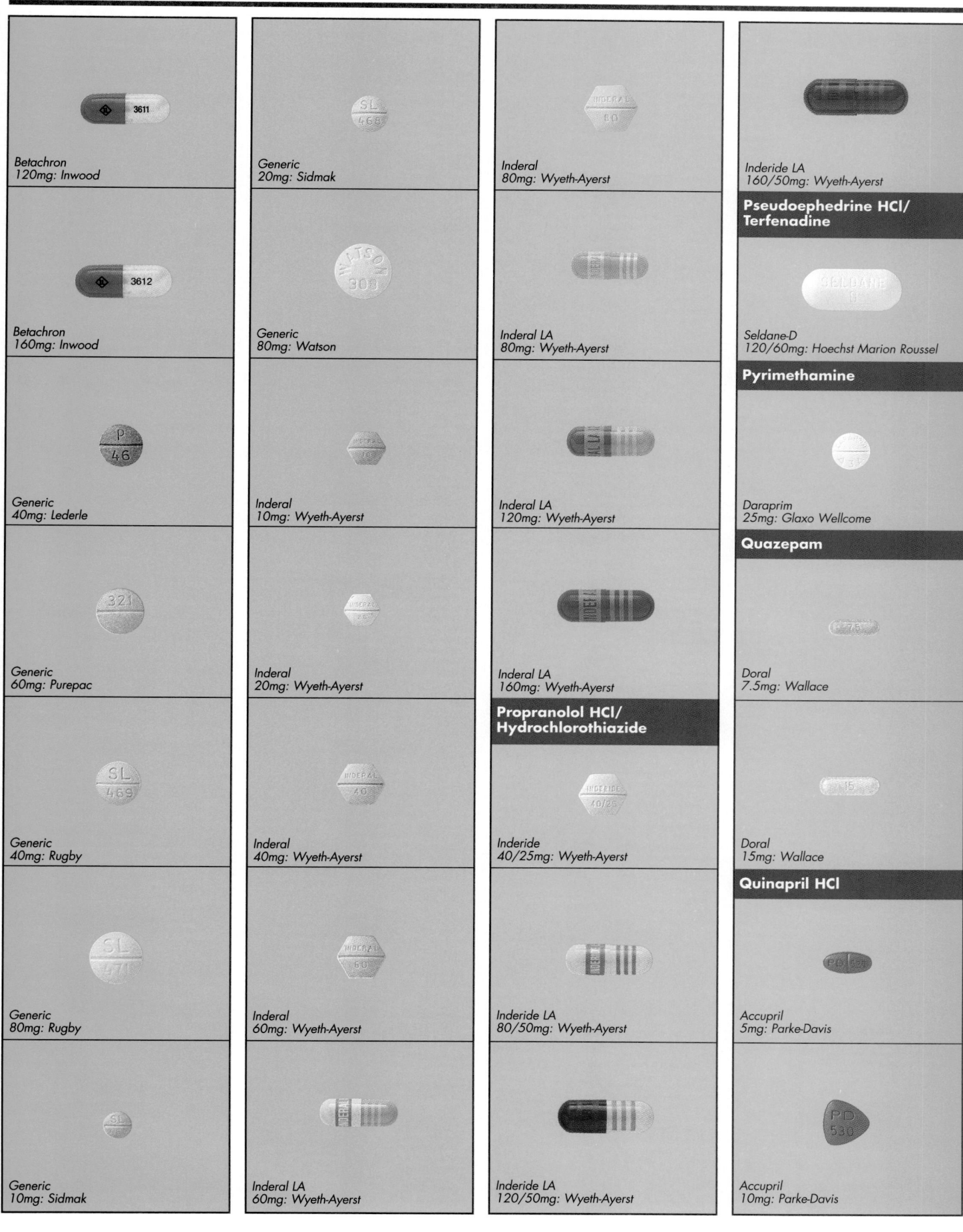

Betachron
120mg: Inwood

Betachron
160mg: Inwood

Generic
40mg: Lederle

Generic
60mg: Purepac

Generic
40mg: Rugby

Generic
80mg: Rugby

Generic
10mg: Sidmak

Generic
20mg: Sidmak

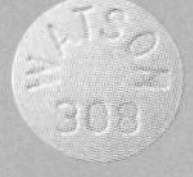

Generic
80mg: Watson

Inderal
10mg: Wyeth-Ayerst

Inderal
20mg: Wyeth-Ayerst

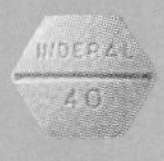

Inderal
40mg: Wyeth-Ayerst

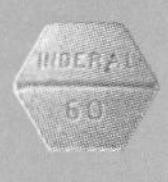

Inderal
60mg: Wyeth-Ayerst

Inderal LA
60mg: Wyeth-Ayerst

Inderal
80mg: Wyeth-Ayerst

Inderal LA
80mg: Wyeth-Ayerst

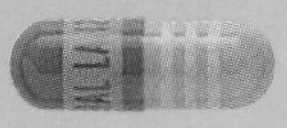

Inderal LA
120mg: Wyeth-Ayerst

Inderal LA
160mg: Wyeth-Ayerst

Propranolol HCl/ Hydrochlorothiazide

Inderide
40/25mg: Wyeth-Ayerst

Inderide LA
80/50mg: Wyeth-Ayerst

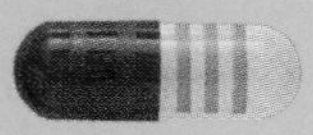

Inderide LA
120/50mg: Wyeth-Ayerst

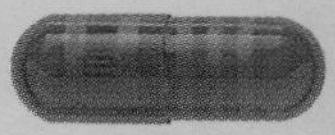

Inderide LA
160/50mg: Wyeth-Ayerst

Pseudoephedrine HCl/ Terfenadine

Seldane-D
120/60mg: Hoechst Marion Roussel

Pyrimethamine

Daraprim
25mg: Glaxo Wellcome

Quazepam

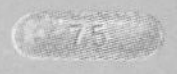

Doral
7.5mg: Wallace

Doral
15mg: Wallace

Quinapril HCl

Accupril
5mg: Parke-Davis

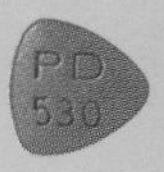

Accupril
10mg: Parke-Davis

Accupril
20mg: Parke-Davis

Accupril
40mg: Parke-Davis

Quinidine Gluconate

Quinaglute Dura-Tabs
324mg: Berlex

Generic
324mg: Schein Danbury

Ramipril

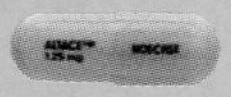

Altace
1.25mg: Hoechst Marion Roussel

Altace
2.5mg: Hoechst Marion Roussel

Altace
5mg: Hoechst Marion Roussel

Altace
10mg: Hoechst Marion Roussel

Ranitidine HCl

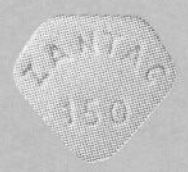

Zantac
150mg: Glaxo Wellcome

Zantac 150 Efferdose
150mg: Glaxo Wellcome

Zantac
150mg: Glaxo Wellcome

Zantac
300mg: Glaxo Wellcome

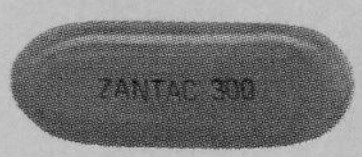

Zantac
300mg: Glaxo Wellcome

Reserpine/Chlorthalidone

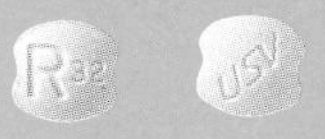

Demi-Regroton
0.125/25mg: Rhone-Poulenc Rorer

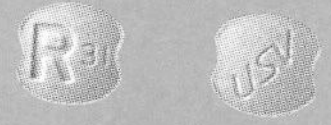

Regroton
0.25/50mg: Rhone-Poulenc Rorer

Reserpine/Hydrochlorothiazide

Hydropres 50
0.125/50mg: Merck

Rifabutin

Mycobutin
150mg: Adria Labs

Riluzole

Rilutek
50mg: Rhone-Poulenc Rorer

Rimantadine

Flumadine
100mg: Forest

Risperidone

Risperdal
1mg: Janssen

Risperdal
2mg: Janssen

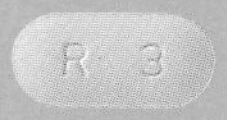

Risperdal
3mg: Janssen

Risperdal
4mg: Janssen

Saquinavir

Invirase
200mg: Roche

Selegiline HCl

Eldepryl
5mg: Somerset

Sertraline HCl

Zoloft
50mg: Roerig

Zoloft
100mg: Roerig

Simvastatin

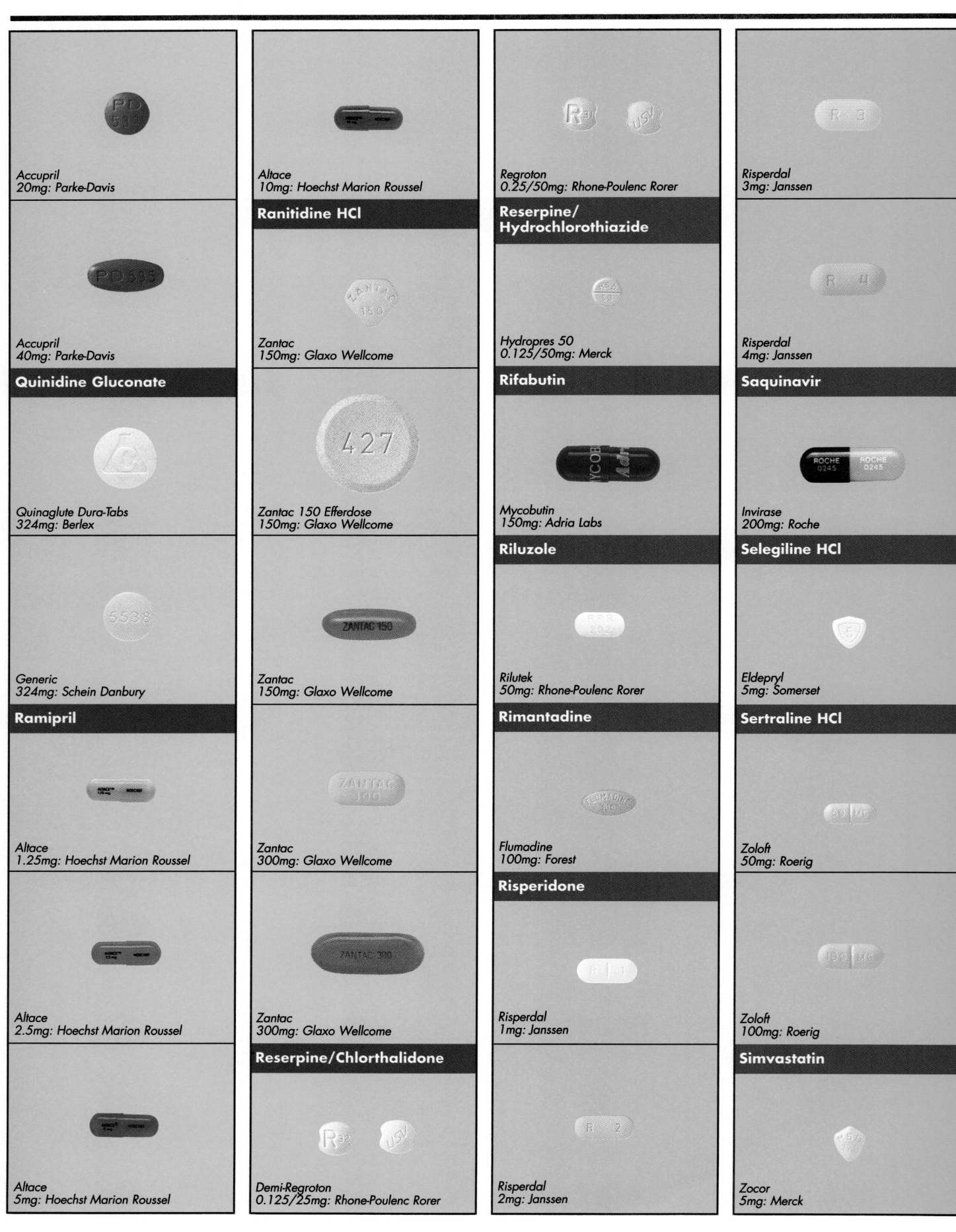

Zocor
5mg: Merck

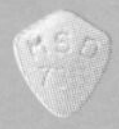

Zocor
10mg: Merck

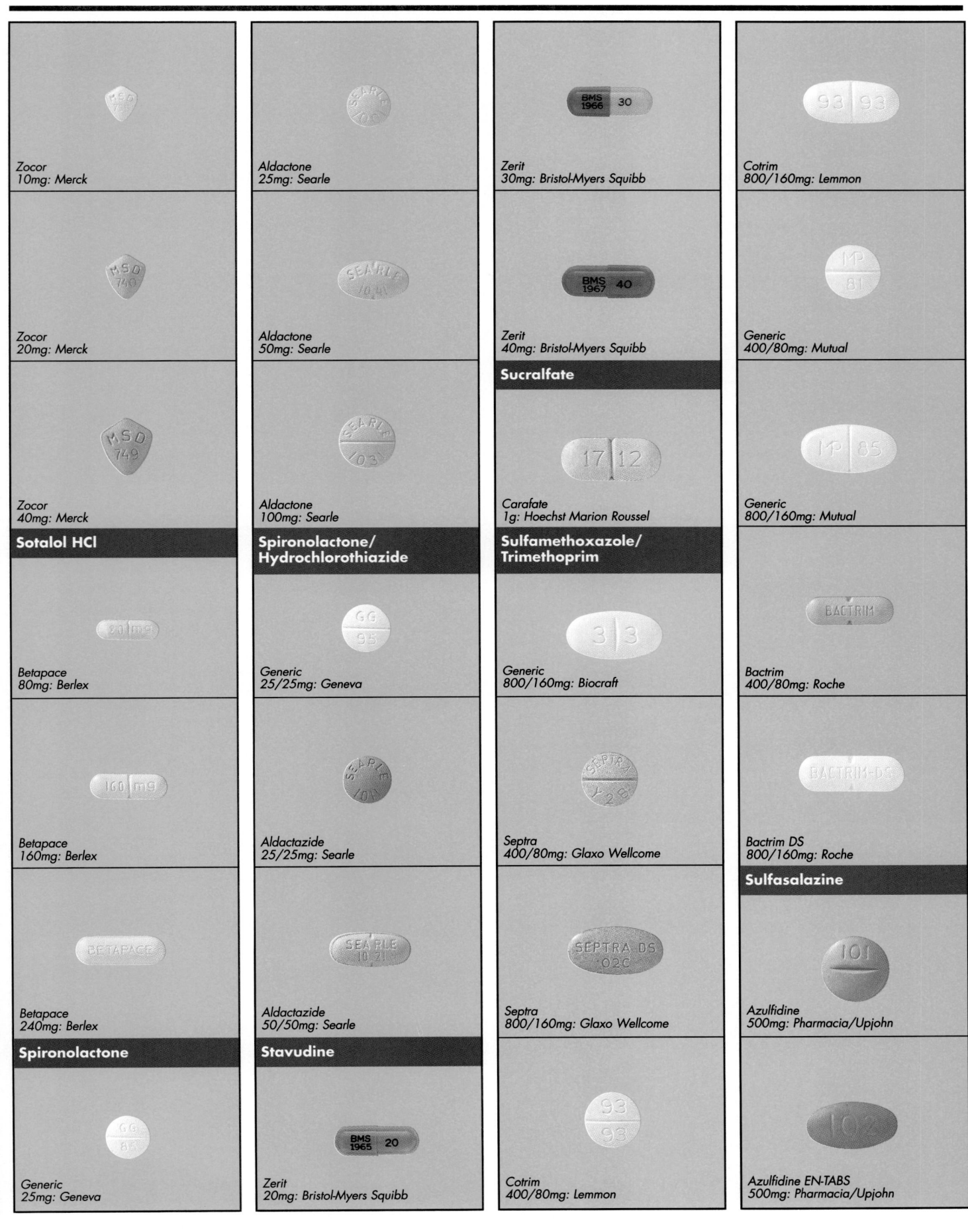

Zocor
20mg: Merck

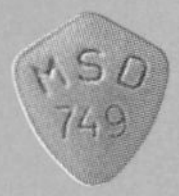

Zocor
40mg: Merck

Sotalol HCl

Betapace
80mg: Berlex

Betapace
160mg: Berlex

Betapace
240mg: Berlex

Spironolactone

Generic
25mg: Geneva

Aldactone
25mg: Searle

Aldactone
50mg: Searle

Aldactone
100mg: Searle

Spironolactone/ Hydrochlorothiazide

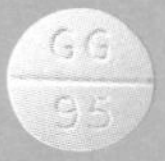

Generic
25/25mg: Geneva

Aldactazide
25/25mg: Searle

Aldactazide
50/50mg: Searle

Stavudine

Zerit
20mg: Bristol-Myers Squibb

Zerit
30mg: Bristol-Myers Squibb

Zerit
40mg: Bristol-Myers Squibb

Sucralfate

Carafate
1g: Hoechst Marion Roussel

Sulfamethoxazole/ Trimethoprim

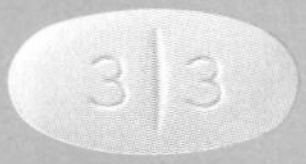

Generic
800/160mg: Biocraft

Septra
400/80mg: Glaxo Wellcome

Septra
800/160mg: Glaxo Wellcome

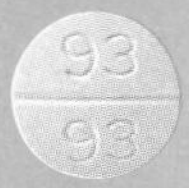

Cotrim
400/80mg: Lemmon

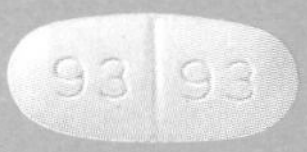

Cotrim
800/160mg: Lemmon

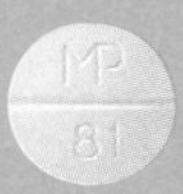

Generic
400/80mg: Mutual

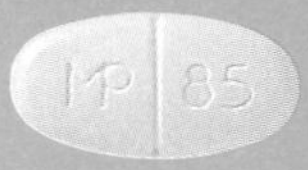

Generic
800/160mg: Mutual

Bactrim
400/80mg: Roche

Bactrim DS
800/160mg: Roche

Sulfasalazine

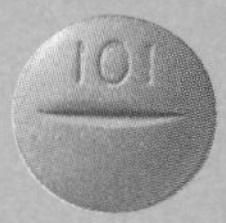

Azulfidine
500mg: Pharmacia/Upjohn

Azulfidine EN-TABS
500mg: Pharmacia/Upjohn

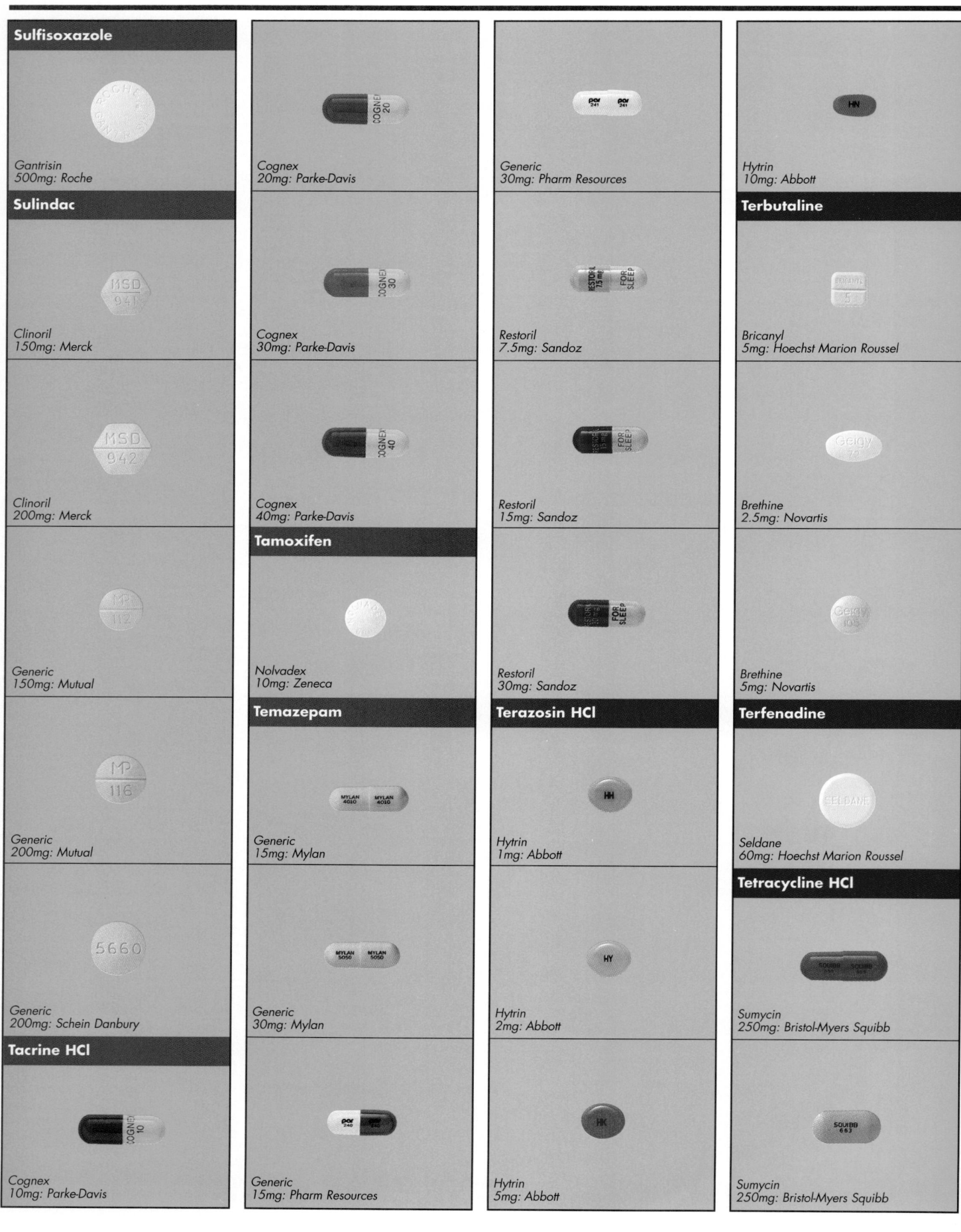

Sulfisoxazole

Gantrisin
500mg: Roche

Sulindac

Clinoril
150mg: Merck

Clinoril
200mg: Merck

Generic
150mg: Mutual

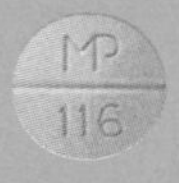

Generic
200mg: Mutual

Generic
200mg: Schein Danbury

Tacrine HCl

Cognex
10mg: Parke-Davis

Cognex
20mg: Parke-Davis

Cognex
30mg: Parke-Davis

Cognex
40mg: Parke-Davis

Tamoxifen

Nolvadex
10mg: Zeneca

Temazepam

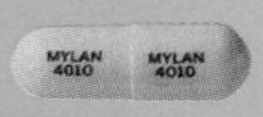

Generic
15mg: Mylan

Generic
30mg: Mylan

Generic
15mg: Pharm Resources

Generic
30mg: Pharm Resources

Restoril
7.5mg: Sandoz

Restoril
15mg: Sandoz

Restoril
30mg: Sandoz

Terazosin HCl

Hytrin
1mg: Abbott

Hytrin
2mg: Abbott

Hytrin
5mg: Abbott

Hytrin
10mg: Abbott

Terbutaline

Bricanyl
5mg: Hoechst Marion Roussel

Brethine
2.5mg: Novartis

Brethine
5mg: Novartis

Terfenadine

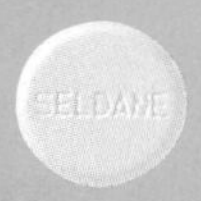

Seldane
60mg: Hoechst Marion Roussel

Tetracycline HCl

Sumycin
250mg: Bristol-Myers Squibb

Sumycin
250mg: Bristol-Myers Squibb

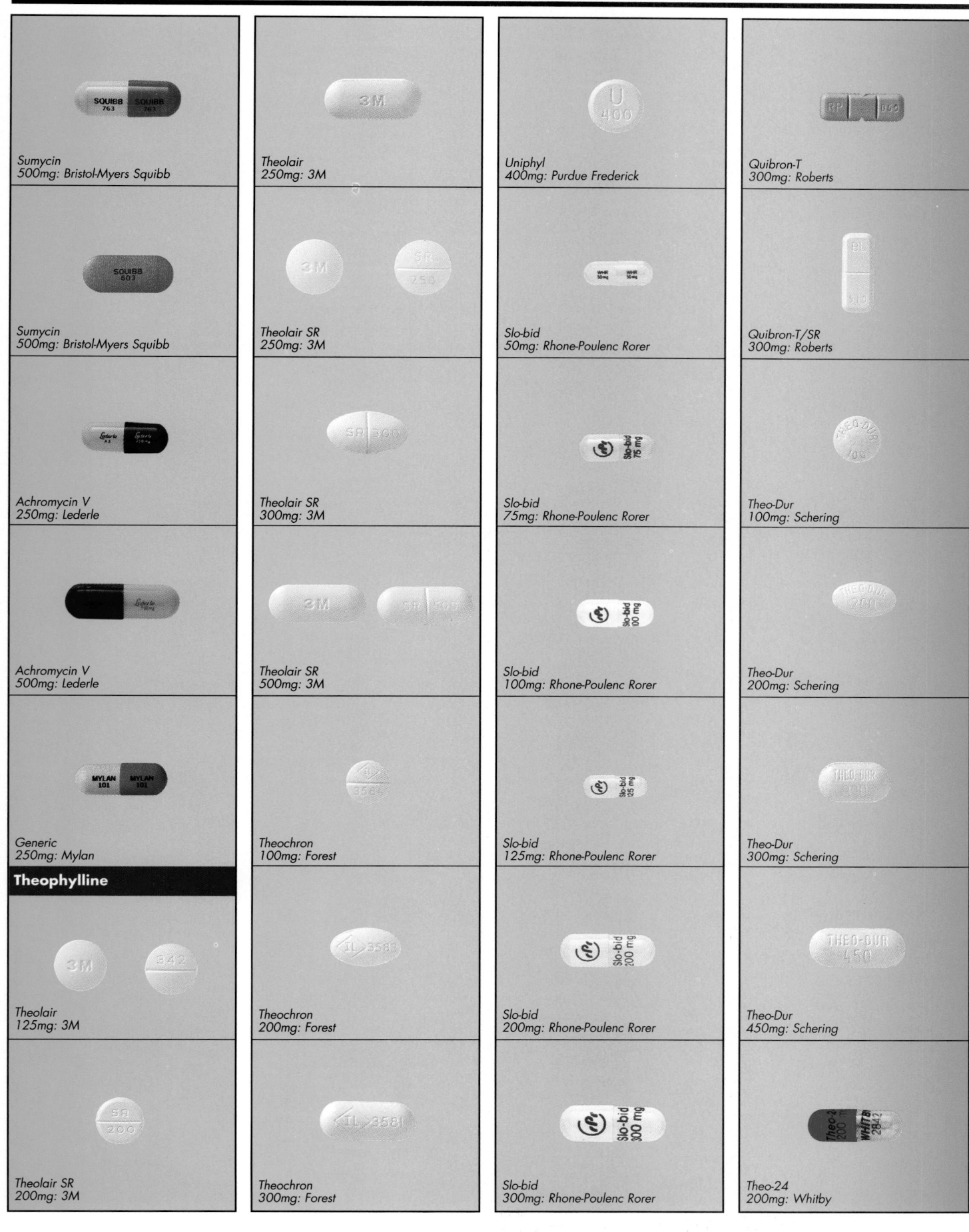

Sumycin
500mg: Bristol-Myers Squibb

Sumycin
500mg: Bristol-Myers Squibb

Achromycin V
250mg: Lederle

Achromycin V
500mg: Lederle

Generic
250mg: Mylan

Theophylline

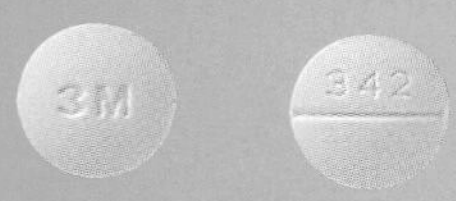

Theolair
125mg: 3M

Theolair SR
200mg: 3M

Theolair
250mg: 3M

Theolair SR
250mg: 3M

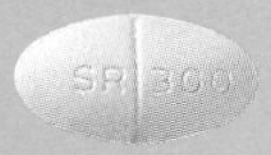

Theolair SR
300mg: 3M

Theolair SR
500mg: 3M

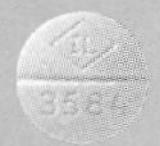

Theochron
100mg: Forest

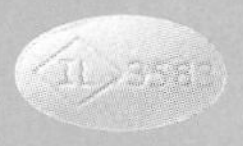

Theochron
200mg: Forest

Theochron
300mg: Forest

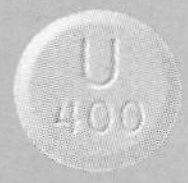

Uniphyl
400mg: Purdue Frederick

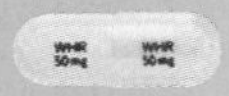

Slo-bid
50mg: Rhone-Poulenc Rorer

Slo-bid
75mg: Rhone-Poulenc Rorer

Slo-bid
100mg: Rhone-Poulenc Rorer

Slo-bid
125mg: Rhone-Poulenc Rorer

Slo-bid
200mg: Rhone-Poulenc Rorer

Slo-bid
300mg: Rhone-Poulenc Rorer

Quibron-T
300mg: Roberts

Quibron-T/SR
300mg: Roberts

Theo-Dur
100mg: Schering

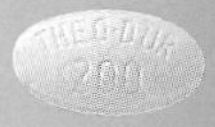

Theo-Dur
200mg: Schering

Theo-Dur
300mg: Schering

Theo-Dur
450mg: Schering

Theo-24
200mg: Whitby

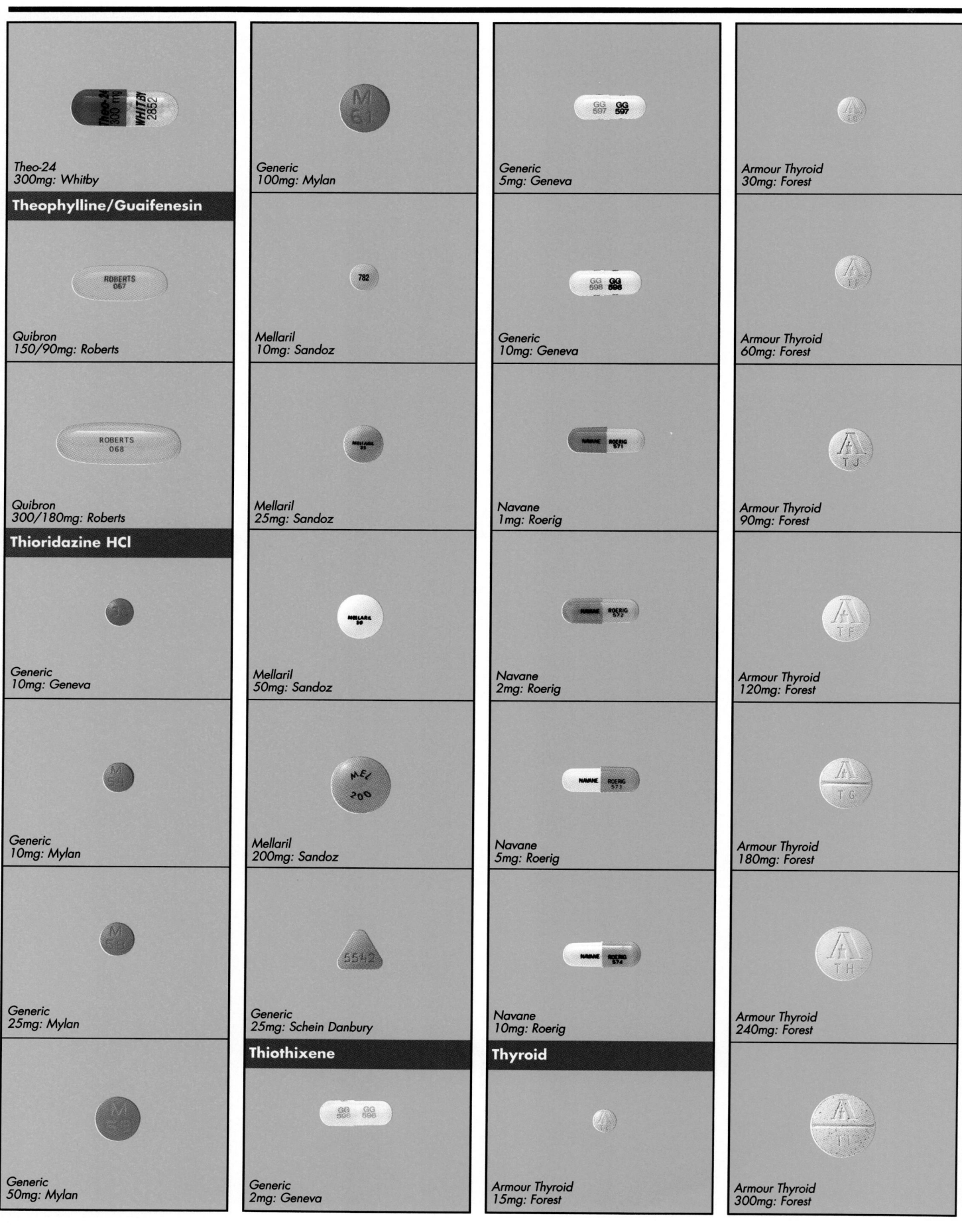

Theo-24
300mg: Whitby

Theophylline/Guaifenesin

Quibron
150/90mg: Roberts

Quibron
300/180mg: Roberts

Thioridazine HCl

Generic
10mg: Geneva

Generic
10mg: Mylan

Generic
25mg: Mylan

Generic
50mg: Mylan

Generic
100mg: Mylan

Mellaril
10mg: Sandoz

Mellaril
25mg: Sandoz

Mellaril
50mg: Sandoz

Mellaril
200mg: Sandoz

Generic
25mg: Schein Danbury

Thiothixene

Generic
2mg: Geneva

Generic
5mg: Geneva

Generic
10mg: Geneva

Navane
1mg: Roerig

Navane
2mg: Roerig

Navane
5mg: Roerig

Navane
10mg: Roerig

Thyroid

Armour Thyroid
15mg: Forest

Armour Thyroid
30mg: Forest

Armour Thyroid
60mg: Forest

Armour Thyroid
90mg: Forest

Armour Thyroid
120mg: Forest

Armour Thyroid
180mg: Forest

Armour Thyroid
240mg: Forest

Armour Thyroid
300mg: Forest

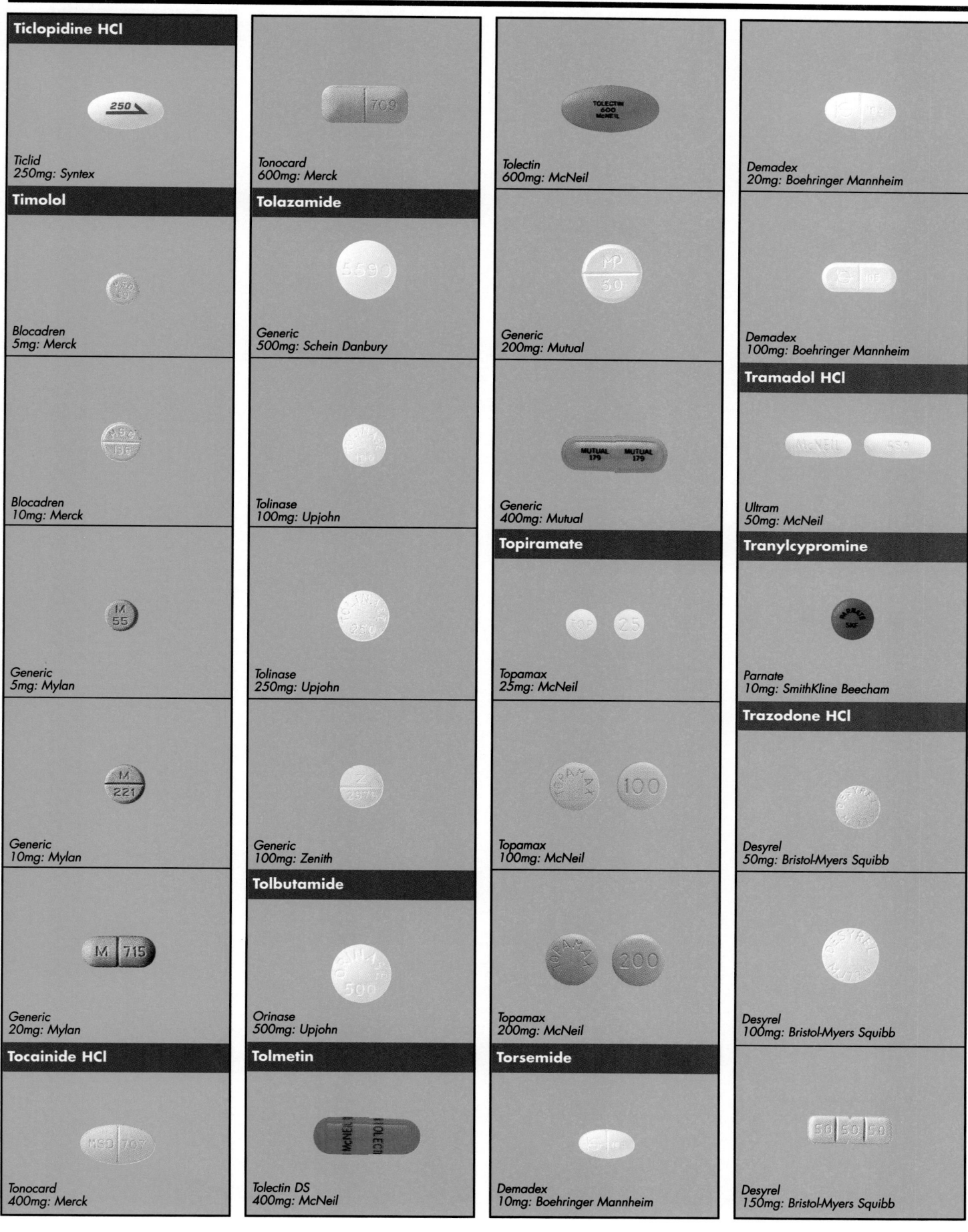

Ticlopidine HCl

Ticlid
250mg: Syntex

Timolol

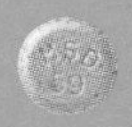

Blocadren
5mg: Merck

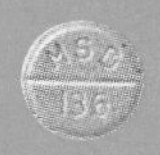

Blocadren
10mg: Merck

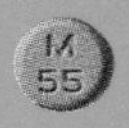

Generic
5mg: Mylan

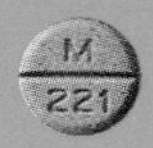

Generic
10mg: Mylan

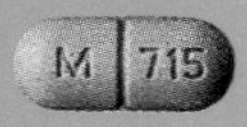

Generic
20mg: Mylan

Tocainide HCl

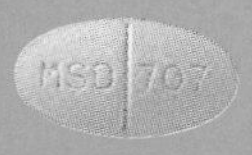

Tonocard
400mg: Merck

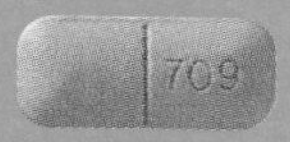

Tonocard
600mg: Merck

Tolazamide

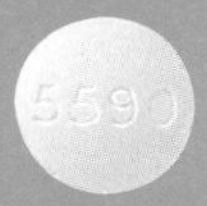

Generic
500mg: Schein Danbury

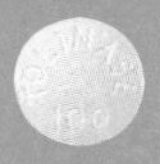

Tolinase
100mg: Upjohn

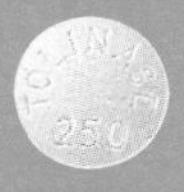

Tolinase
250mg: Upjohn

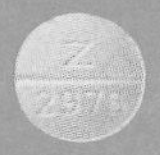

Generic
100mg: Zenith

Tolbutamide

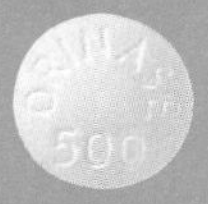

Orinase
500mg: Upjohn

Tolmetin

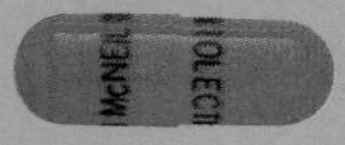

Tolectin DS
400mg: McNeil

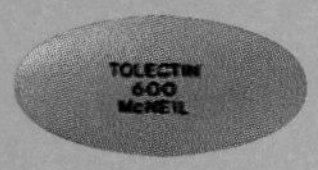

Tolectin
600mg: McNeil

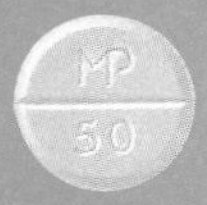

Generic
200mg: Mutual

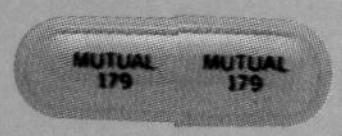

Generic
400mg: Mutual

Topiramate

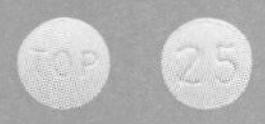

Topamax
25mg: McNeil

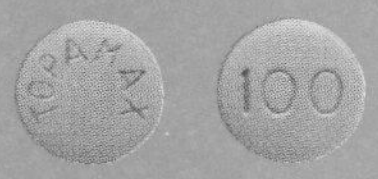

Topamax
100mg: McNeil

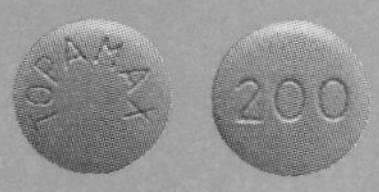

Topamax
200mg: McNeil

Torsemide

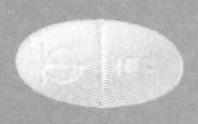

Demadex
10mg: Boehringer Mannheim

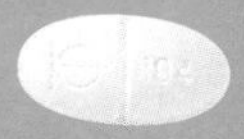

Demadex
20mg: Boehringer Mannheim

Demadex
100mg: Boehringer Mannheim

Tramadol HCl

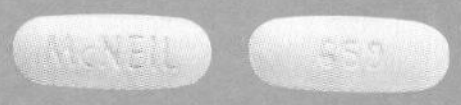

Ultram
50mg: McNeil

Tranylcypromine

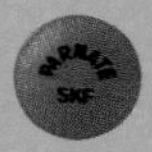

Parnate
10mg: SmithKline Beecham

Trazodone HCl

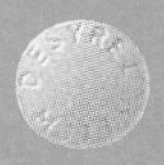

Desyrel
50mg: Bristol-Myers Squibb

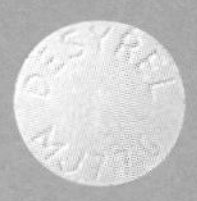

Desyrel
100mg: Bristol-Myers Squibb

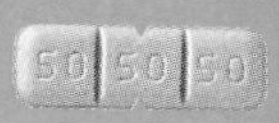

Desyrel
150mg: Bristol-Myers Squibb

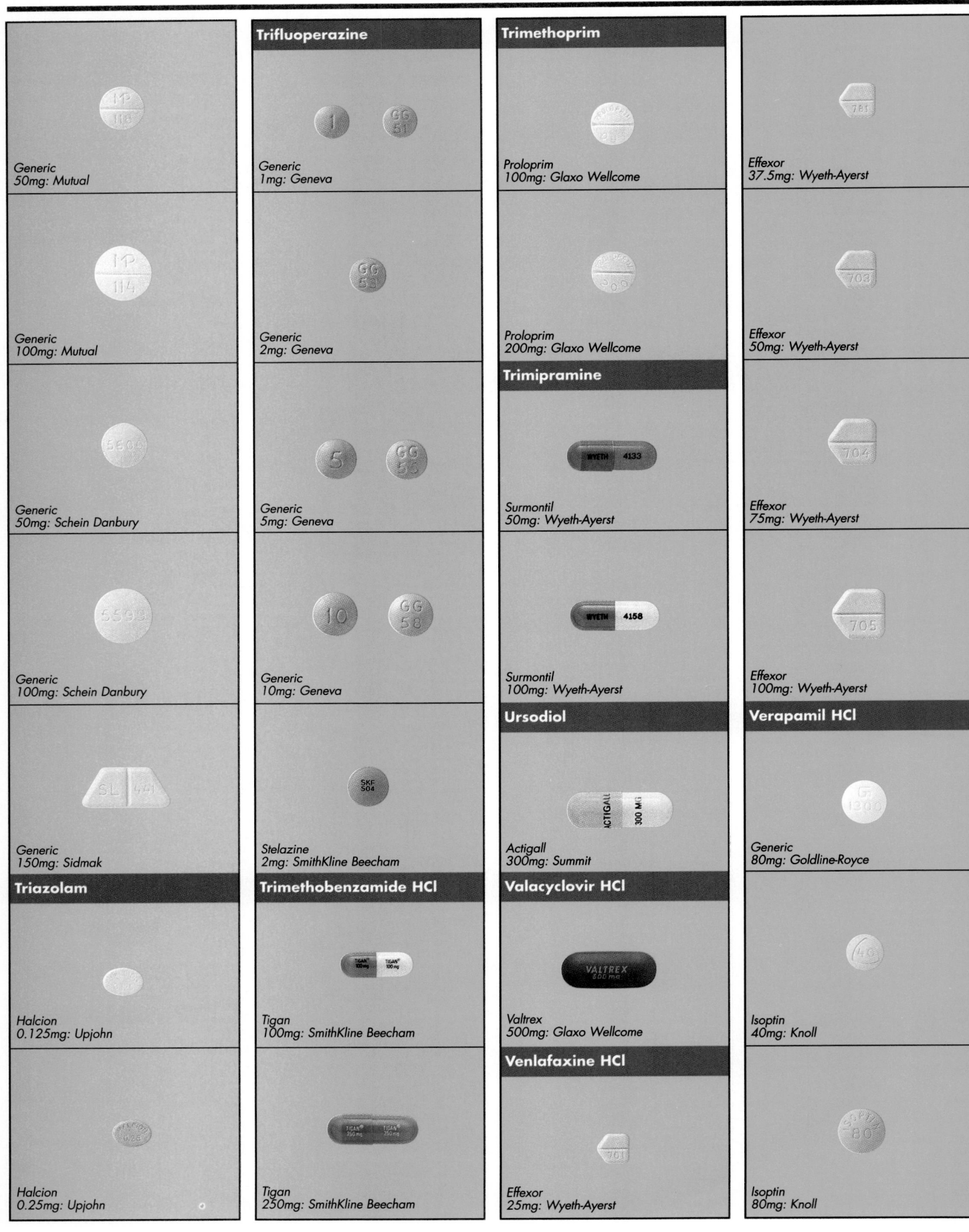

Generic
50mg: Mutual

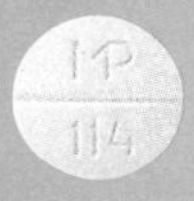

Generic
100mg: Mutual

Generic
50mg: Schein Danbury

Generic
100mg: Schein Danbury

Generic
150mg: Sidmak

Triazolam

Halcion
0.125mg: Upjohn

Halcion
0.25mg: Upjohn

Trifluoperazine

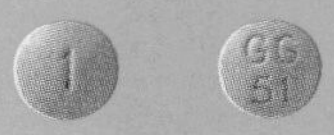

Generic
1mg: Geneva

Generic
2mg: Geneva

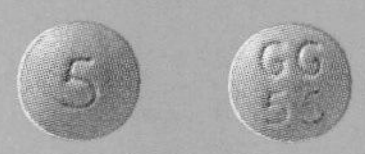

Generic
5mg: Geneva

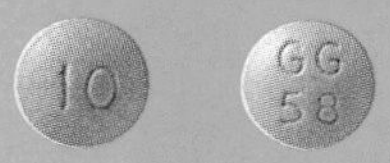

Generic
10mg: Geneva

Stelazine
2mg: SmithKline Beecham

Trimethobenzamide HCl

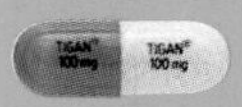

Tigan
100mg: SmithKline Beecham

Tigan
250mg: SmithKline Beecham

Trimethoprim

Proloprim
100mg: Glaxo Wellcome

Proloprim
200mg: Glaxo Wellcome

Trimipramine

Surmontil
50mg: Wyeth-Ayerst

Surmontil
100mg: Wyeth-Ayerst

Ursodiol

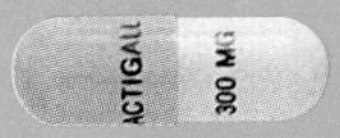

Actigall
300mg: Summit

Valacyclovir HCl

Valtrex
500mg: Glaxo Wellcome

Venlafaxine HCl

Effexor
25mg: Wyeth-Ayerst

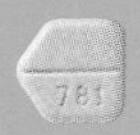

Effexor
37.5mg: Wyeth-Ayerst

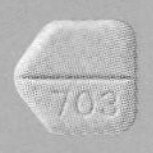

Effexor
50mg: Wyeth-Ayerst

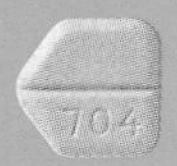

Effexor
75mg: Wyeth-Ayerst

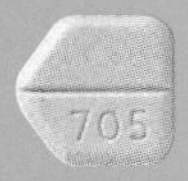

Effexor
100mg: Wyeth-Ayerst

Verapamil HCl

Generic
80mg: Goldline-Royce

Isoptin
40mg: Knoll

Isoptin
80mg: Knoll

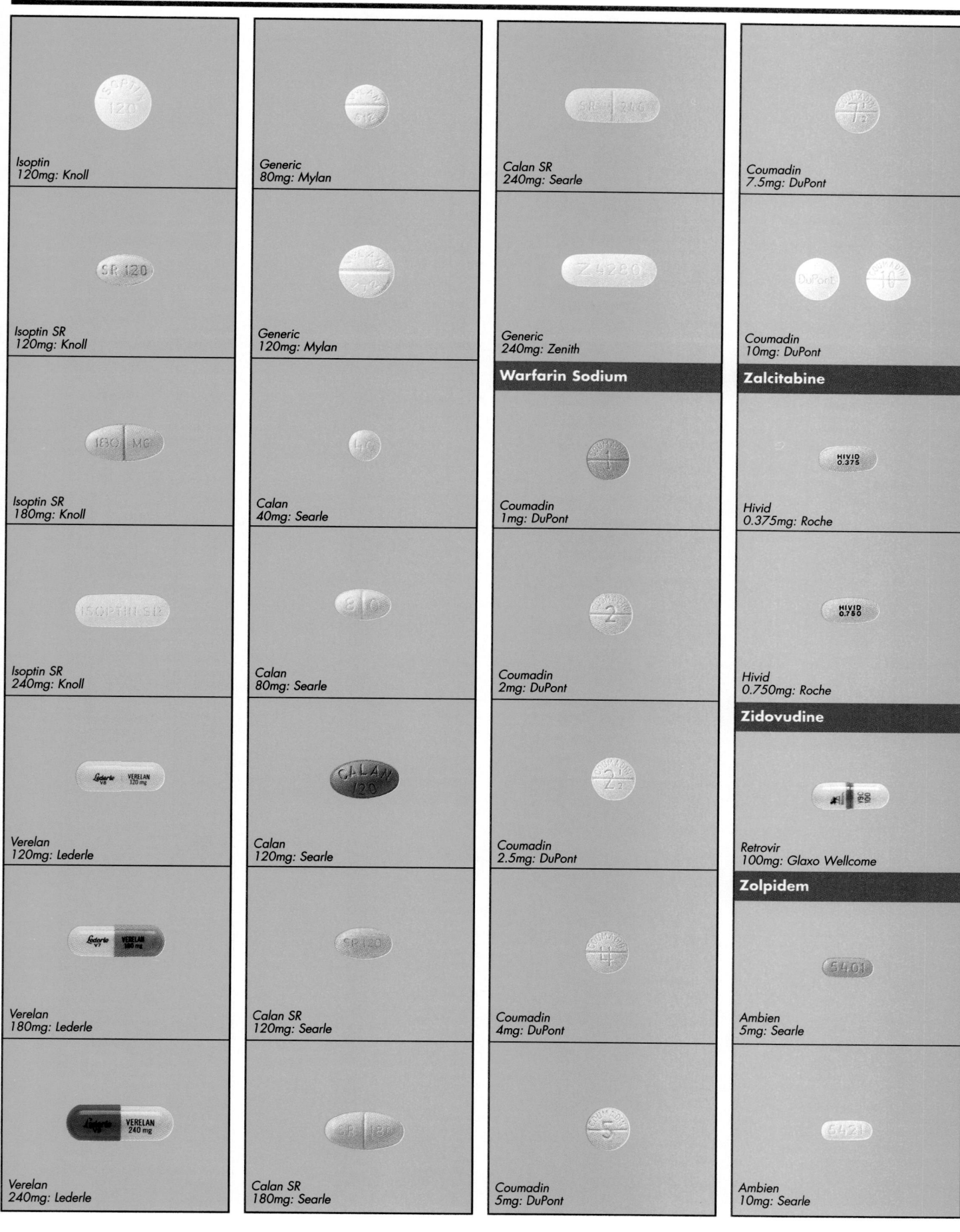

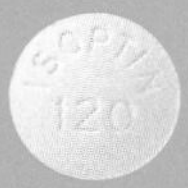

Isoptin
120mg: Knoll

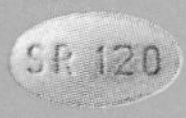

Isoptin SR
120mg: Knoll

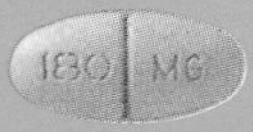

Isoptin SR
180mg: Knoll

Isoptin SR
240mg: Knoll

Verelan
120mg: Lederle

Verelan
180mg: Lederle

Verelan
240mg: Lederle

Generic
80mg: Mylan

Generic
120mg: Mylan

Calan
40mg: Searle

Calan
80mg: Searle

Calan
120mg: Searle

Calan SR
120mg: Searle

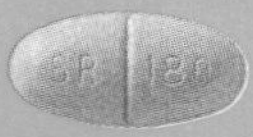

Calan SR
180mg: Searle

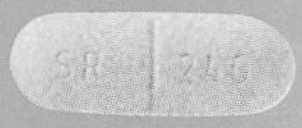

Calan SR
240mg: Searle

Generic
240mg: Zenith

Warfarin Sodium

Coumadin
1mg: DuPont

Coumadin
2mg: DuPont

Coumadin
2.5mg: DuPont

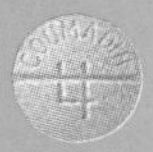

Coumadin
4mg: DuPont

Coumadin
5mg: DuPont

Coumadin
7.5mg: DuPont

Coumadin
10mg: DuPont

Zalcitabine

Hivid
0.375mg: Roche

Hivid
0.750mg: Roche

Zidovudine

Retrovir
100mg: Glaxo Wellcome

Zolpidem

Ambien
5mg: Searle

Ambien
10mg: Searle

INDEX

DRUG INFORMATION

ABCIXIMAB *(003211)*

CATEGORIES: Angina; Angioplasty; Anticoagulants; Anticoagulants/Thrombolytics; Biologicals; Blood Clotting; Blood Formation/Coagulation; Coagulants and Anticoagulants; Coagulopathies; Embolism; Restenosis; Recombinant DNA Origin; FDA Approved 1994 Dec

BRAND NAMES: 7E3; CentoRx; **ReoPro; Reopro**

DESCRIPTION:

Abciximab is the Fab fragment of the chimeric human-murine monoclonal antibody 7E3. Abciximab binds to the glycoprotein IIb/IIIa (GPIIb/IIIa) receptor of human platelets and inhibits platelet aggregation.

The chimeric 7E3 antibody is produced by continuous perfusion in mammalian cell culture. The 47,615 dalton Fab fragment is purified from cell culture supernatant by a series of steps involving specific viral inactivation and removal procedures, digestion with papain and column chromatography.

ReoPro is a clear, colorless, sterile, non-pyrogenic solution for intravenous (IV) use. Each single-use vial contains 2 mg/ml of abciximab in a buffered solution (pH 7.2) of 0.01 M sodium phosphate, 0.15 M sodium chloride and 0.001% polysorbate 80 in Water for Injection. No preservatives are added.

CLINICAL PHARMACOLOGY:

General: Abciximab binds to the intact GPIIb/IIIa receptor, which is a member of the integrin family of adhesion receptors and the major platelet surface receptor involved in platelet aggregation. Abciximab inhibits platelet aggregation by preventing the binding of fibrinogen, von Willebrand factor, and other adhesive molecules to GPIIb/IIIa receptor sites on activated platelets. The mechanism of action is thought to involve steric hindrance and/or conformational effects to block access of large molecules to the receptor rather than interacting directly with the RGD (arginine-glycine-aspartic acid) binding site of GPIIb/IIIa.

Pre-Clinical Experience: Maximal inhibition of platelet aggregation was observed *in vivo* when ≥80% of GPIIb/IIIa receptors were blocked by abciximab. In non-human primates, abciximab bolus doses of 0.25 mg/kg generally achieved a blockade of at least 80% of platelet receptors and fully inhibited platelet aggregation. Inhibition of platelet function was temporary following a bolus dose, but receptor blockade could be sustained at ≥80% by continuous intravenous infusion. The inhibitory effects of abciximab were substantially diminished by the transfusion of platelets in monkeys. The antithrombotic efficacy of prototype antibodies (murine 7E3 Fab and $F(ab')_2$) and abciximab was evaluated in dog, monkey and baboon models of coronary, carotid and femoral artery thrombosis. Doses of the murine version of 7E3 or abciximab sufficient to produce high-grade (≥80%) GPIIb/IIIa receptor blockade prevented acute thrombosis and yielded lower rates of thrombosis compared with aspirin and/or heparin.

Pharmacokinetics: Following intravenous bolus administration, free plasma concentrations of abciximab decrease rapidly with an initial half-life of less than 10 minutes and a second phase half-life of about 30 minutes, probably related to rapid binding to the platelet GPIIb/IIIa receptors. Platelet function generally recovers over the course of 48 hours,[1,2] although abciximab remains in the circulation for up to 10 days in a platelet-bound state. Intravenous administration of a 0.25 mg/kg bolus dose of abciximab followed by continuous infusion of 10 mcg/min produces approximately constant free plasma concentrations throughout the infusion. At the termination of the infusion period, free plasma concentrations fall rapidly for approximately 6 hours then decline at a slower rate.

Pharmacodynamics: Intravenous administration in humans of single bolus doses of abciximab from 0.15 mg/kg to 0.30 mg/kg produced rapid dose-dependent inhibition of platelet function as measured by *ex vivo* platelet aggregation in response to adenosine diphosphate (ADP) or by prolongation of bleeding time. At the two highest doses (0.25 and 0.30 mg/kg) at 2 hours post injection, over 80% of the GPIIb/IIIa receptors were blocked and platelet aggregation in response to 20 μM ADP was almost abolished. The median bleeding time increased to over 30 minutes at both doses compared with a baseline value of approximately 5 minutes.

Intravenous administration in humans of a single bolus dose of 0.25 mg/kg followed by a continuous of 10 mcg/min for periods of 12 to 96 hours produced sustained high-grade GPIIb/IIIa receptor blockade (≥80%) and inhibition of platelet function (*ex vivo* platelet aggregation in response to 5 μM or 20 μM ADP less than 20% of baseline and bleeding time greater than 30 minutes) for the duration of the infusion in most patients. Results in patients who received the 0.25 mg/kg bolus followed by a 5 mcg/min infusion for 24 hours showed a similar initial receptor blockade and inhibition of platelet aggregation, but the response was not maintained throughout the infusion period.

Low levels of GPIIb/IIIa receptor blockade are present for up to 10 days following cessation of the infusion. Bleeding time returned to ≤12 minutes within 12 hours following the end of infusion in 15 to 20 patients (75%), and within 24 hours in 18 of 20 patients (90%). *Ex vivo*

CLINICAL PHARMACOLOGY: *(cont'd)*

platelet aggregation in response to 5 μM ADP returned to ≥50% of baseline within 24 hours following the end of infusion in 11 of 32 patients (34%) and within 48 hours in 23 of 32 patients (72%). In response to 20 μM ADP, *ex vivo* platelet aggregation returned to ≥50% of baseline within 24 hours in 20 of 32 patients (62%) and within 48 hours in 28 of 32 patients (88%).

Clinical Safety and Efficacy Experience: The Evaluation of c7E3 to Prevent Ischemic Complications (EPIC) trial was a multicenter, double-blind, placebo-controlled trial of abciximab in patients undergoing percutaneous transluminal coronary angioplasty or atherectomy (PTCA)[3]. In the EPIC trial, 2099 patients between 26 and 83 years of age who were at high risk for abrupt closure of the treated coronary vessel were randomly allocated to one of three treatments: 1) an abciximab bolus (0.25 mg/kg) followed by an abciximab infusion (10 mcg/min) for twelve hours (bolus plus infusion group); 2) an abciximab bolus (0.25 mg/kg) followed by a placebo infusion (bolus group), or: 3) a placebo bolus followed by a placebo infusion (placebo group). Patients at high risk during or following PTCA were defined as those with unstable angina or a non-Q-wave myocardial infarction (n=489), those with an acute Q-wave myocardial infarction within twelve hours of symptom onset (n=66), and those who were at high risk because of coronary morphology and/or clinical characteristics as defined in INDICATIONS AND USAGE(n=1544). Treatment with study agent in each of the three arms was initiated 10-60 minutes before the onset of PTCA. All patients initially received an intravenous heparin bolus (10,000 to 12,000 units) and boluses of up to 3,000 units thereafter to a maximum of 20,000 units during PTCA. Heparin infusion was continued for twelve hours to maintain a therapeutic elevation of activated partial thromboplastin time (APTT, 1.5-2.5 times normal). Unless contraindicated, aspirin (325 mg) was administered orally two hours prior to the planned procedure and then once daily.

The primary endpoint was the occurrence of any of the following events within 30 days of PTCA: death, myocardial infarction (MI), or the need for urgent intervention for recurrent ischemia (*i.e.,* urgent PTCA, urgent coronary artery bypass graft (CABG) surgery, a coronary stent, or an intra-aortic balloon pump). The 30-day (Kaplan-Meier) primary endpoint event rates for each treatment group by intention-to-treat analysis of all randomized patients are shown in TABLE 1. The 4.5% lower incidence of the primary endpoint in the bolus plus infusion treatment group, compared with the placebo group, was statistically significant, whereas the 1.3% lower incidence in the bolus treatment group was not. A lower incidence of the primary endpoint was observed in the bolus plus infusion treatment arm for all three high-risk subgroups: patients with unstable angina, patients presenting within twelve hours of the onset of symptoms or an acute myocardial infarction, and patients with other high-risk clinical and/or morphologic characteristics as defined in INDICATIONS AND USAGE. The treatment effect was largest in the first two subgroups and smallest in the third subgroup.

TABLE 1 Primary Outcome Events

Event	Placebo (n=696)	Bolus (n=695)	Bolus + Infusion (n=708)
	Number of Patients (%)		
Primary Endpoint*	89 (12.8)	79 (11.5)	59 (8.3)
p-value vs. placebo		0.428	0.008
Components of Primary Endpoint†			
Death	12 (1.7)	9 (1.3)	12 (1.7)
Acute myocardial infarctions in surviving patients.	55 (7.9)	40 (5.8)	31 (4.4)
Urgent interventions in surviving patients without an acute myocardial infarction	22 (3.2)	30 (4.4)	16 (2.2)

*Patients who experienced more than one event in the first 30 days are counted only once.
†Patients are counted only once under the most serious component (death > acute MI > urgent intervention).

Mortality was uncommon and similar rates were observed in all arms. The rate of acute myocardial infarctions was significantly lower in the groups treated with abciximab. While 80% of myocardial infarctions in the study were non-Q-wave infarctions, patients in the bolus plus infusion arm experienced a lower incidence of both Q-wave and non-Q-wave infarctions. Urgent intervention rates were lower in the groups treated with abciximab, mostly because of lower rates of emergency PTCA and, to a lesser extent, emergency CABG surgery. The primary endpoint events in the bolus plus infusion treatment group were reduced mostly in the first 48 hours and this benefit was sustained through 30 days and six months.[3,4] At the 6 months follow-up visit this event rate remained lower in the bolus plus infusion arm (12.3%) than in the placebo arm (17.6%).

INDICATIONS AND USAGE:

Abciximab is indicated as an adjunct to percutaneous transluminal coronary angioplasty or atherectomy (PTCA) for the prevention of acute cardiac ischemic complications in patients at high risk for abrupt closure of the treated coronary vessel.

Patients at high risk for abrupt closure include those undergoing PTCA with at least one of the following conditions:

Unstable angina or a non-Q-wave myocardial infarction

An acute Q-wave myocardial infarction within 12 hours of the onset symptoms

Other high-risk clinical and/or morphologic characteristics (as adapted from the classification of the ACC/AHA (see Footnote):

two type B lesions in the artery to be dilated,

one type B lesion in the artery to be dilated in a woman of at least 65 years of age,

one type B lesion in the artery to be dilated in a patient with diabetes mellitus,

one type C lesion in the artery to be dilated, or

angioplasty of an infarct-related lesion within seven days of myocardial infarction.

Abciximab is intended for use with aspirin and heparin and has been studied only in that setting, as described in CLINICAL PHARMACOLOGY.

FOOTNOTE: Ryan et al., 1988 [7]*Classification of Coronary Lesions According to ACC/AHA Criteria:*

Type A Lesions (High Success, >85%; Low Risk):

Discrete (<10 mm length)	Little or no calcification
Concentric	Less than totally occulsive
Readily accessible	Not ostial in location
Nonangulated segment, <45°	No major branch involvement
Smooth contour	Absence of thrombus

Type B Lesions (Moderate Success, 60 to 85%; Moderate Risk:

Tubular (10 to 20 mm length)	Moderate to heavy calcification
Eccentric	Total occlusions <3 months old
Moderate tortuosity of proximal segment	Ostial in location
Moderately angulated segment >45°, <90°	Some thrombus present
Irregular contour	

Type C Lesions (Low Success, <60%; High Risk):

Diffuse (>2 cm length)	Total occlusion >3 months old
Excessive tortuosity of proximal segment	Inability to protect major side branches
Extremely angulated segments >90°	Degenerated vein grafts with friable lesions

CONTRAINDICATIONS:

Because abciximab increases the risks of bleeding, it is contraindicated in the following clinical situations:

Active internal bleeding

Recent (within six weeks) gastrointestinal (GI) or genitourinary bleeding of clinical significance

History of cerebrovascular accident (CVA) within 2 years, or CVA with a significant residual neurological deficit

Bleeding diathesis

Administration of oral anticoagulants within seven days unless prothrombin time is ≤ 1.2 times control

Thrombocytopenia (< 100,000 cells µl)

Recent (within six weeks) major surgery or trauma

Intracranial neoplasm, arteriovenous malformation, or aneurysm

Severe uncontrolled hypertension

Presumed or documented history of vasculitis

Use of intravenous dextran before PTCA, or intent to use it during PTCA

Abciximab is also contraindicated in patients with known hypersensitivity to any component of this product or to murine proteins.

WARNINGS: ADMINISTRATION OF ABCIXIMAB IS ASSOCIATED WITH AN INCREASED FREQUENCY OF MAJOR BLEEDING COMPLICATIONS INCLUDING RETROPERITONEAL BLEEDING, SPONTANEOUS GASTROINTESTINAL AND GENITOURINARY BLEEDING AND BLEEDING AT THE ARTERIAL ACCESS SITE. THIS RISK IS FURTHER INCREASED IN PATIENTS WHO WEIGH LESS THAN 75 KG. APPROPRIATE MANAGEMENT OF THERAPY AND COMPLICATIONS (as described in PRECAUTIONS, BLEEDING PRECAUTIONS) IS POSSIBLE ONLY WHEN ADEQUATE DIAGNOSIS AND TREATMENT FACILITIES AND QUALIFIED PHYSICIANS ARE READILY AVAILABLE.

Increased Risk of Bleeding (see ADVERSE REACTIONS)

The most common complication encountered during abciximab therapy is bleeding. The types of bleeding associated with abciximab therapy fall into two broad categories:

Bleeding observed at the arterial access site for cardiac catherization.

Internal bleeding involving the gastrointestinal tract, genitourinary tract, or retroperitoneal sites.

In the following conditions, clinical data suggest that the risks of major bleeds due to abciximab therapy may be increased and should be weighed against the anticpated benefits:

Patients who weigh less than 75 kg

Patients >65 years old

Patients with a history of prior GI disease

Patients receiving thrombolytics

The following conditions are also associated with an increased risk of bleeding in the angioplasty setting which may be additive to that of abciximab:

PCTA within 12 hours of the onset of symptoms for acute myocarial infarction

Prolonged PTCA (lasting more than 70 minutes)

Failed PTCA

Heparin anticoagulation may contribute to the risk of bleeding. (See PRECAUTIONS Laboratory Monitoring).

Should serious bleeding occur that is not controllable with pressure, the infusion of abciximab and any concomitant heparin should be stopped (see also PRECAUTIONS Restoration of Platelet Function).

PRECAUTIONS:

Readministration: There are no data concerning readministration of abciximab. Administration of abciximab may result in human anti-chimeric antibody (HACA) formation (see ADVERSE REACTIONS) that can cause allergic or hypersensitivity reactions (including anaphylaxis), thrombocytopenia or diminished benefit upon readministration of abciximab.

Use of Thrombolytics, Anticoagulants and Other Antiplatelet Agents: In the EPIC trial, abciximab was used concomitantly with heparin and aspirin (see CLINICAL PHARMACOLOGY). Because abciximab inhibits platelet aggregation, caution should be employed when it is used with other drugs that affect hemostasis, including thrombolytics, oral anticoagulants, non-steroidal anti-inflammatory drugs, dipyridamole, and ticlopidine.

In the EPIC trial, there was limited experience with the administration of abciximab with low molecular weight dextran. Low molecular weight dextran was usually given for the deployment of a coronary stent, for which oral anticoagulants were also given. In the 11 patients who received low molecular weight dextran with abciximab, 5 had major bleeding events and 4 had minor bleeding events. None of the 5 placebo patients treated with low molecular weight dextran had a major or minor bleeding event. (See CONTRAINDICATIONS.)

There are limited data on the use of abciximab in patients receiving thrombolytic agents. Because of concern about synergistic effects on bleeding, systemic thrombolytic therapy should be used judiciously.

BLEEDING PRECAUTIONS

Therapy with abciximab requires careful attention to all potential bleeding sites (including catheter insertion sites, arterial and venous puncture sites, cut down sites, needle puncture sites, and gastrointestinal, genitourinary, and retroperitoneal sites).

Femoral Artery Access Site: Abciximab is associated with an increase in bleeding rate particularly at the site of arterial access for femoral sheath placement. Care should be taken when attempting vascular access that only the anterior wall of the femoral artery is punctured, avoiding a Seldinger (through and through) technique for obtaining sheath access. Femoral vein sheath placement should be avoided unless needed. While the vascular sheath is in place, patients should be maintained on complete bed rest with the head of the bed ≤30° and the affected limb restrained in a straight position. Heparin should be discontinued at least 4 hours prior to arterial sheath removal. Following sheath removal, pressure should be applied to the femoral artery for at least 30 minutes using either manual compression or a mechanical device for hemostasis. A pressure dressing should be applied following hemostasis. The patient should be maintained on bed rest for 6 to 8 hours following sheath removal or discontinuation of abciximab, whichever is later.

The sheath insertion site and distal pulses of affected leg(s) should be frequently checked while the femoral artery sheath is in place and for 6 hours after femoral artery sheath removal. Any hematoma should be measured and monitored for enlargement.

General Nursing Care: Arterial and venous punctures, intramuscular injections, and use of urinary catheters, nasotracheal intubation, nasogastric tubes and automatic blood pressure cuffs should be minimized. When obtaining intravenous access, non-compressible sites (*e.g.,* subclavian or jugular veins) should be avoided. Saline or heparin locks should be considered for blood drawing. Vascular puncture points should be documented and monitored. Gentle care should be provided when removing dressings.

LABORATORY MONITORING

Before infusion of abciximab, platelet count, prothrombin time and APTT should be measured to identify pre-existing hemostatic abnormalities. During and following abciximab treatment, platelet counts and extent of heparin anticoagulation, as assessed by activated clotting times of APTT, should be monitored closely.

THROMBOCYTOPENIA

Platelet counts should be monitored prior to treatment, 2 to 4 hours following the bolus dose of abciximab and at 24 hours or prior to discharge, whichever is first. If a patient experiences an acute platelet decrease (*e.g.,* a platelet decrease to less than 100,000 cells/mcl or a decrease of at least 25% from pre-treatment value), additional platelet counts should be determined. These platelet counts should be drawn in separate tubes containing ethylenediaminetetraacetic acid (EDTA), citrate or heparin to exclude pseudothrombocytopenia due to *in vitro* anticoagulant interaction. If true thrombocytopenia is verified, abciximab should be immediately discontinued and the condition appropriately monitored and treated. For patients with thrombocytopenia in the EPIC trial, a daily platelet count was obtained until it returned to normal. If a patient's platelet count dropped to 60,000 cells/mcl, heparin and aspirin were discontinued. If a platlet count dropped below 50,000 cells/mcl, platelets were transfused.

Restoration of Platelet Function: In the event of serious uncontrolled bleeding or the need for surgery (especially major procedures within 48-72 hours of treatment with abciximab), an Ivy bleeding time should be determined. Preliminary evidence suggets that platelet function may be restored, at least in part, with platelet transfusions.

ALLERGIC REACTIONS

Anaphylaxis may occur at any time during administration. If it does, administration of abciximab should be immediately stopped and standard appropriate resuscitative measures should be initiated.

PREGNANCY CATEGORY C

Animal reproduction studies have not been conducted with abciximab. It is also not known whether abciximab can cause fetal harm when administered to a pregnant woman or can affect reproduction capacity. Abciximab should be given to a pregnant woman only if clearly needed.

PEDIATRIC USE

Safety and effectiveness in children have not been studied.

CARCINOGENESIS, MUTAGENESIS, AND IMPAIRMENT OF FERTILITY

In vitro and *in vivo* mutagenicity studies have not been demonstrated any mutagenic effect. Long-term studies in animals have not been performed to evaluate the carcinogenic potential or effects on fertility in male or female animals.

NURSING MOTHERS

It is not known whether this drug is excreted in human milk or absorbed systemically after ingestion. Because many drugs are excreted in human milk, caution should be exercised when abciximab is administered to a nursing woman.

ADVERSE REACTIONS:

Bleeding: The most common complication of abciximab therapy is bleeding. In the EPIC trial, abciximab treatment was associated with statistically significant increases in both major and minor bleeding events and in bleeding requiring transfusions (see TABLE 2). Bleeding was classified as major or minor by the criteria of the Thrombolysis in Myocardial Infarction study group[5]. Major bleeding events were defined as either an intracranial hemorrhage or a decrease in hemoglobin greater than 5 g/dl. Minor bleeding events included spontaneous gross hematuria, spontaneous hematemesis, observed blood loss with a hemoglobin decrease of more than 3 g/dl, or a decrease in hemoglobin of at least 4 g/dl without an identified bleeding site. In patients who received transfusions, the number of units of blood lost was estimated through an adaption of the method of Landefeld et al.[6]

ADVERSE REACTIONS: *(cont'd)*

TABLE 2 Bleeding Events and Transfusions

	Placebo (n=696)	Bolus (n=695)	Bolus + Infusion (n=708)
	Number of Patients (%)		
Major Bleeding*	46 (6.6)	77 (11.1)	99 (14.0)
p-value vs. placebo		0.003	<0.001
Minor Bleeding*	68 (9.8)	107 (15.4)	120 (16.9)
p-value vs. placebo		0.002	<0.001
Bleeding requiring transfusions†	52 (7.5)	97 (14.0)	119 (16.8)
p-value vs. placebo		<0.002	<0.001

* For major and minor bleeding, patients are counted only once according to the most severe classification. Numbers include bleeding events associated with CABG surgery.
† Includes transfusions of any type: packed red blood cells, whole blood, platelets, fresh frozen plasma, and cryoprecipitate.

Major bleeding events occurred most commonly in patients treated with the bolus plus infusion regimen. Ten patients who had major bleeding events died; 5 were in the bolus plus infusion treatment group (one of these five patients was randomized, but not treated with abciximab), 3 were in the bolus treatment group, and 2 were in the placebo treatment group. Of the patients with major bleeding who died, 2 patients (1 patient in the bolus plus infusion treatment group and 1 patient in the placebo treatment group) had deaths attributable to bleeding, both had hemorrhagic stroke.

Major bleeding events not associated with CABG surgery occurred in 23 (3.3%) patients in the placebo group, 60 (8.6%) patients in the bolus group and 75 (10.6%) patients in the bolus plus infusion group; the sites of bleeding in these patients are listed in TABLE 3. The incidence if intracranial hemorrhage was similar in all three groups. Approximately 70% of abciximab-treated patients with major bleeding had bleeding at the arterial access site in the groin. Abciximab-treated patients also had a higher incidence of major bleeding events from gastrointestinal, genitourinary, retroperitoneal, and other sites.

Excess spontaneous major organ bleeding occurred primarily in patients weighing 75 kg or less who received abciximab.

Although data are limited, abciximab treatment was not associated with excess major bleeding in patients who underwent CABG surgery. The incidence of CABG surgery-related major blood loss was similar in all 3 groups (3-5%). Some patients with prolonged bleeding times received platelet transfusions to correct the bleeding time prior to surgery.

TABLE 3 Bleeding Locations in Patients with Major Bleeding Events*

	Placebo	Bolus	Bolus + Infusion
Patients with Major bleeding not associated with CABG	23	60	75
Intracranial	2	1	3†
Spontaneous gross hematuria	1	4	4
Other genitourinary	2	5	8
Spontaneous hematemesis	0	5	11
Other gastrointestinal	1	11	11
Retroperitoneal	2	2	12
Femoral artery access site	16	43	50
Other access site	1	1	4
Oral	1	4	4
Other‡	1	9	11
Decrease in Hct/Hgb only	3	7	11

* Indicates the number of patients with major bleeding not associated with CABG surgery; patients may be included for more than one bleeding site.
† Includes one patient randomized but not treated.
‡ Includes hemoptysis, pulmonary bleeding, epistaxis, ocular bleeding, otic bleeding and bleeding associated with procedures and surgery other than CABG surgery.

Thrombocytopenia: In the EPIC study, patients treated with abciximab were more likely than patients treated with placebo to experience decreases in platelet counts and to require platelet transfusions (see TABLE 4).

TABLE 4 Thrombocytopenia and Platelet Transfusions*

	Placebo (n=696)	Bolus + Infusion (n=708)
	Number of Patietns (%)	
Patients with decrease of platelets to <50,000 cells/mcl*	5 (0.7)	11 (1.6)
Patients with decrease of platelets to <100,000 cells/mcl*	24 (3.4)	37 (5.2)
Patients who received platelet transfusions†	18 (2.6)	39 (5.5)

* Patients with a platelet count of <50,000 cells/mcl are also included in the category of patients with a platelet count of <100,000 cells/mcl.
† Includes patients receiving platelet transfusions for thrombocytopenia or any other reason.

Human Anti-Chimeric Antibody Development: HACA may appear in response to the administration of abciximab. In the EPIC trial, positive responses occurred in 6.5% (40/617) of the patients in the bolus plus infusion group versus 0% (0/605) of patients treated with placebo. There was no excess of hypersensitivity or allergic reactions related to abciximab treatment compared with placebo treatment. See also PRECAUTIONSAllergic Reactions.

Other Adverse Reactions: TABLE 5 shows adverse events other than bleeding and thrombocytopenia from the EPIC trial which occurred in patients in the bolus plus infusion arm at an incidence of more than 0.5% higher than in those treated with placebo. Hypotension was often related to bleeding complications associated with abciximab therapy.

The following additional adverse events from the EPIC trial were reported by investigators for patients treated with a bolus plus infusion of abciximab at incidences which were less than 0.5% higher than for patients in the placebo arm:

Cardiovascular System: atrial fibrillation/flutter (3.5%), vascular disorder (1.8%), pulmonary edema (1.5%), complete AV block (1.3%), supraventricular tachycardia (1.0%), weak pulse (1.0%), palpitation (0.7%), intermittent claudication (0.4%), pericardial effusion (0.4%), limb embolism (0.3%), pulmonary embolism (0.3%), ventricular arrhythmia (0.3%);

Gastrointestinal System: diarrhea (0.9%), constipation (0.3%), ileus (0.3%);

Hemic and Lymphatic System: hemolytic anemia (0.3%), petechiae (0.3%);

Nervous System: abnormal thinking (2.1%), dizziness (1.8%), coma (0.4%), brain ischemia (0.3%), insomnia (0.3%);

Musculoskeletal System: myopathy (0.4%), cellulitis (0.3%), myalgia (0.3%);

ADVERSE REACTIONS: *(cont'd)*

TABLE 5 Adverse Events Among Treated Patients in the EPIC Trial

Event	Placebo (n=681)	Bolus + Infusion (n=678)
	Number of Patients (%)	
Cardiovascular System		
Hypotension	82 (12.0)	143 (21.1)
Bradycardia	20 (2.9)	35 (5.2)
Gastrointestinal System		
Nausea	109 (16.0)	125 (18.4)
Vomiting	61 (9.0)	77 (11.4)
Hemic and Lymphatic System		
Anemia	3 (0.4)	8 (1.2)
Leukocytosis	1 (0.1)	7 (1.0)
Nervous System		
Hypesthesia*	2 (0.3)	7 (1.0)
Confusion	0 (0.0)	4 (0.6)
Respiratory System		
Pleural Effusion/Pleurisy	2 (0.2)	9 (1.3)
Pneumonia	3 (0.4)	7 (1.0)
Miscellaneous		
Pain*	8 (2.6)	23 (3.4)
Peripheral Edema	3 (0.4)	11 (1.6)
Abnormal Vision	1 (0.1)	3 (0.7)

* Involving primarily the extremities

Urogenital System: urinary tract infection (1.9%), urinary retention (0.4%), abnormal renal function (0.3%);

Miscellaneous: dysphonia (0.3%), pruritis (0.3%).

OVERDOSAGE:

There has been no experience of overdosage in human clinical trials. It is recommended that infusion be discontinued after 12 hours to avoid effects of prolonged platelet receptor blockade.

DOSAGE AND ADMINISTRATION:

Abciximab is intended for use in patients undergoing PTCA. The safety and efficacy of abciximab have only been investigated with concomitant administration of heparin and aspirin as described in CLINICAL PHARMACOLOGY.

In patients with failed PTCAs the continuous infusion of abciximab should be stopped because there is no evidence for abciximab efficacy in that setting.

In the event of serious bleeding that cannot be controlled by compression, abciximab and heparin should be discontinued immediately (see PRECAUTIONS Restoration of Platelet Function).

Adults: The recommended dosage of abciximab is an intravenous bolus of 0.25 mg/kg administered 10-60 minutes before the start of PTCA, followed by a continuous intravenous infusion of 10 mcg/min for twelve (12) hours.

INSTRUCTIONS FOR ADMINISTRATION

1. Parental drug products should be inspected visually for particulate matter prior to administration. Preparations of abciximab containing visibly opaque particles should NOT be used.

2. Hypersensitivity reactions should be anticipated whenever protein solutions such as abciximab are administered. Epinephrine, dopamine, theophylline, antihistamines and corticosteroids should be available for immediate use. If symptoms of an allergic reaction or anaphylaxis appear, the infusion should be stopped and appropriate treatment given.

3. As with all parental drug products, aseptic procedures should be used during the administration of abciximab.

4. Withdraw the necessary amount of abciximab (2 mg/ml) for bolus injection through a sterile, non-pyrogenic, low protein-binding 0.2 or 0.22 µm filter (Millipore SLGV025LS or equivalent) into a syringe. The bolus should be administered 10-60 minutes before the procedure.

5. Withdraw 4.5 ml of abciximab for the continuous infusion through a sterile, non-pyrogenic, low protein-binding 0.2 or 0.22 µm filter (Millipore SLGV025LS or equivalent) into a syringe. Inject into 250 ml of sterile 0.9% saline or 5% dextrose and infuse at a rate of 17 ml/hour (10 mcg/min) for 12 hours via a continuous infusion pump equipped with an in-line sterile, non-pyrogenic, low protein-binding 0.2 or 0.22 µm filter (Abbott #4524 or equivalent). Discard the unused portion at the end of the 12-hour infusion.

6. Abciximab should be administered in a separate intravenous line; no other medication should be added to the infusion solutions.

7. No incompatibilities have been observed with glass bottles or polyvinyl chloride bags and administration sets.

REFERENCES:

1. Tcheng J, Ellis SG, George BS. Pharmacodynamics of chimeric glycoprotein IIB/IIIa integrin antiplatelet antibody Fab 7E3 in high risk coronary angioplasty. *Circulation*; 1994;**90**:757-1764 **2.** Simoons ML, de Boer MJ, van der Brand MJBM, et al. Randomized trial of a GPIIb/IIIa platelet receptor blocker in refractory unstable angina.*Circulation;*1994;**89**:596-603. **3.** EPIC Investigators. Use of a monoclonal antibody directed against the platelet glycoprotein IIb/IIIa receptor in high-risk coronary angioplasty. *N Engl J Med*1994;**330**:956-961. **4.** Topol EJ, Califf RM, Weisman HF, et al. Randomized trial of coronary intervention with antibody against platelet IIb/IIIa integrin for reduction of clinical restenosis: result six months. *The Lancet*1994:**343**:881-886. **5.** Rao, AK, Pratt C, Berke A, et al. Thrombolysis in Myocardial Infarction (TIMI) Trial - Phase I: Hemorrhagic manifestations and changes in plasma fibrinogen and the fibrinolytic system in patients treated with recombinant tissue plasminogen activator and streptokinase. *J An Coll Cardiol*1988;**11**:1-11. **6.** Landefeld CS, Cook El, Flatley M, et al. Identification and preliminary validation of predictors of major bleeding in hospitalized patients starting anticoagulant therapy. *Am J Med.* 1987;**82**:703-713. **7.** Ryan TJ, Faxon DP, Gunnar RM, et al. Guidelines for percutaneous transluminal coronary angioplasty: A report of the American College of Cardiology/American Heart Association task force on assessment of diagnostic and therapeutic cardiovascular procedures. (Subcommittee on Percutaneous Transluminal Coronary Angioplasty). *J Am Coll Cardiol* 1988;**12**:529-545.

HOW SUPPLIED:

ReoPro 2 mg/ml is supplied in 5 ml vials containing 10 mg.

Vials should be stored at 2 to 8°C (36 to 46°F). Do not freeze. Do not shake. Do not use beyond the expiration date. Discard any unused portion left in the vial.

HOW SUPPLIED - EQUIVALENTS NOT AVAILABLE:

Injection, Solution - Intravenous - 2 mg/ml

5 ml $540.02 REOPRO, Lilly 00002-7140-01

FOOTNOTE: Ryan et al., 1988 [7]
Classification of Coronary Lesions According to ACC/AHA Criteria

Type A Lesions (High Success, >85%; Low Risk)	
·Discrete (<10 mm length)	·Little or no calcification
·Concentric	·Less than totally occulsive
·Readily accessible	·Not ostial in location
·Nonangulated segment, <45°	·No major branch involvement
·Smooth contour	·Absence of thrombus
Type B Lesions (Moderate Success, 60 to 85%; Moderate Risk	
·Tubular (10 to 20 mm length)	·Moderate to heavy calcification
·Eccentric	·Total occlusions <3 months old
·Moderate tortuosity of proximal segment	·Ostial in location
·Irregular contour	·Some thrombus present
Type C Lesions (Low Success, <60%; High Risk)	
·Diffuse (>2 cm length)	·Total occlusion >3 months old
·Excessive tortuosity of proximal segment	·Inability to protect major side branches
·Extremely angulated segments >90°	·Degenerated vein grafts with friable lesions

ACARBOSE *(003262)*

CATEGORIES: Alpha Glucosidase Inhibitors; Antidiabetic Agents; Blood Glucose Regulators; Diabetes; Diabetes Mellitus; Hormones; Hyperglycemia; FDA Class 1S ("Standard Review"); FDA Approved 1995 Sep

BRAND NAMES: Glucobay; *Glumida*; **Precose**; *Prandase*
(International brand names outside U.S. in italics)

FORMULARIES: PCS

DESCRIPTION:

Acarbose tablets are oral alpha-glucosidase inhibitors for use in the management of non-insulin-dependent diabetes mellitus (NIDDM). Acarbose is an oligosaccharide which is obtained from fermentation processes of a microorganism, *Actinoplanes utahensis*, and is chemically known as 0-4,6-dideoxy-4-[[(1S, 4R, 5S,6S)-4,5,6-trihydroxy -3-(hydroxymethyl)-2-cyclohexen-1-yl] amino]-α-D-glucopyranosyl-(1 → 4)-0-α-D-glucopyranosyl -(1 → 4)-D-glucose. It is a white to off-white powder with a molecular weight of 645.6. Acarbose is soluble in water and has a $pK_a$of 5.1. Its empirical formula is $C_{25}H_{43}NO_{18}$.

Precose is available as 50 mg and 100 mg tablets for oral use. The active ingredients are starch, microcrystalline cellulose, magnesium stearate, and colloidal silicon dioxide.

CLINICAL PHARMACOLOGY:

Acarbose is a complex oligosaccharide that delays the digestion of ingested carbohydrates, thereby resulting in a smaller rise in blood glucose concentration following meals. As a consequence of plasma glucose reduction, acarbose reduces levels of glycosylated hemoglobin in patients with Type II (non-insulin dependent) diabetes mellitis. Systemic nonenzymatic protein glycosylation, as reflected by levels of glycosylated hemoglobin, is a function of average blood glucose concentration over time.

MECHANISM OF ACTION

In contrast to sulfonylureas, acarbose does not enhance insulin secretion. The antihyperglycemic action of acarbose results from a competitive, reversible inhibition of pancreatic alpha-amylase and membrane-bound intestinal alpha-glucoside hydrolase enzymes. Pancreatic alph-amylase hydrolyzes complex starches to oligosaccharides in the lumen of the small intestine, while the membrane-bound intestinal alpha-glucosidases hydrolyze oligosaccharides, trisaccharides, and disaccharides to glucose and other monosaccharides in the brush border of the small intestine. In diabetic patients, this enzyme inhibition results in a delayed glucose absorption and a lowering of postprandial hyperglycemia.

Because its mechanism of action is different, the effect of acarbose to enhance glycemic control is additive to that of sulfonylureas when used in combination. In addition, acarbose diminishes the insulinotropic and weight-increasing effects of sulfonylureas.

Acarbose has no inhibitory activity against lactase and consequently would not be expected to induce lactose intolerance.

PHARMACOKINETICS

Absorption: In a study of 6 healthy men, less than 2% of an oral dose of acarbose was absorbed as active drug, while approximately 35% of total radioactivity from a ^{14}C-labeled oral dose was absorbed. An average of 51% of an oral dose was excreted in the feces as unabsorbed drug-related radioactivity within 96 hours of ingestion. Because acarbose acts locally within the gastrointestinal tract, this low systemic bioavailability of parent compound is therapeutically desired. Following oral dosing of healthy volunteers with ^{14}C-labeled acarbose, peak plasma concentrations or radioactivity were attained 14-24 hours after dosing, while peak plasma concentrations of active drug were attained at approximately 1 hour. The delayed absorption of acarbose-related radioactivity reflects the absorption of metabolites that may be formed by either intestinal bacteria or intestinal enzymatic hydrolysis.

Metabolism: Acarbose is metabolized exclusively within the gastrointestinal tract, principally by intestinal bacteria, but also by digestive enzymes. A fraction of these metabolites (approximately 34% of the dose) was absorbed and subsequently excreted in the urine. At least 13 metabolites have been separated chromatographically from urine specimens. The major metabolites have been identified as 4-methylpyrogallol derivatives (*i.e.,* sulfate, methyl, and glucuronides conjugates). One metabolite (formed by cleavage of a glucose molecule from acarbose) also has alpha-glucosidase inhibitory activity. This metabolite, together with the parent compound, recovered from the urine, accounts for less than 2% of the total administered dose.

Excretion: The fraction of acarbose that is absorbed as intact drug is almost completely excreted by the kidneys. When acarbose was given *intravenously*, 89% of the dose was recovered in the urine as active drug within 48 hours. In contrast, less than 2% of an *oral dose* was recovered in the urine as active (*i.e.,* parent compound and active metabolite) drug. This is consistent with the low bioavailability of the parent drug. The plasma elimination half-life of acarbose activity is approximately 2 hours in healthy volunteers. Consequently, drug accumulation does not occur with three times a day (t.i.d.) oral dosing.

Special Populations: The mean steady-state area under the curve (AUC) and maximum concentrations of acarbose were approximately 1.5 times higher in elderly compared to young volunteers; however, these differences were not statistically significant. Patients with severe renal impairment (Cl_{cr}<25 mL/min/1.73m^2) attained about 5 times higher peak plasma concentrations of acarbose and 6 times larger AUCs than volunteers with normal renal function. No studies of acarbose pharmacokinetic parameters according to race have been performed. In U.S. controlled clinical studies of acarbose in patients with NIDDM, reductions in glycosylated hemoglobin levels were similar in whites (n=478) and blacks (n=167) with a trend toward a better response in hispanics (n=132).

CLINICAL STUDIES:

Clinical Experience in Non-Insulin Dependent Diabetes Mellitus (NIDDM) Patients on Dietary Treatment Only: Results from six controlled, fixed—dose, monotherapy studies of acarbose in the treatment of NIDDM, involving 769 acarbose-treated patients, were combined and a weighted average of the difference from placebo in the mean change from baseline in glycosylated hemoglobin (HbA1c) was calculated for each dose level as presented below:

TABLE 1

Mean Change in HbA1c in Fixed-Dose Monotherapy Studies

Dose of Acarbose*	N	Change in HbA1c %	p-Value
25 mg t.i.d.	110	−0.44	0.0307
50 mg t.i.d.	131	−0.77	0.0001
100 mg t.i.d.	244	−0.74	0.0001
200 mg t.i.d. **	231	−0.86	0.0001
300 mg t.i.d. **	53	−1.00	0.0001

* Acarbose was statistically significantly different from placebo at all doses. Although there were no statistically significant differences among mean results for doses ranging from 50 to 300 mg t.i.d., some patients may derive benefit by increasing the dosage from 50 to 100 mg t.i.d.
** Although studies utilized a maximum dose of 200 or 300 mg t.i.d., the maximum recommended dose for patients ≤ 60 kg is 50 mg t.i.d.; the maximum recommended dose for patients > 60 kg is 100 mg t.i.d.

Results from these six, fixed-dose, monotherapy studies were also combined to derive a weighted average of the difference from placebo in mean change from baseline for one-hour postprandial plasma glucose levels.

Clinical Experience in NIDDM Patients Receiving Sulfonylureas: Acarbose was studied as adjunctive therapy to sulfonylurea treatment in two large, placebo-controlled, double-blind, randomized studies conducted in the United States in which 540 patients were included in the efficacy analysis. In addition, acarbose was studied as adjunctive therapy to sulfonylurea treatment in a third study, conducted in Canada, in which patients were stratified according to background therapy. Study 1 (TABLE 2) involved patients under treatment at entry with diet alone who were subsequently randomized to four treatment groups. At the end of the study, patients in the acarbose + tolbutamide group showed a mean treatment effect on glycosylated hemoglobin (HbA1c) of −1.78% and were receiving a significantly lower mean daily dose of tolbutamide than patients in the tolbutamide-group alone. Also, the efficacy in the acarbose + tolbutamide group was significantly better than in the other three treatment groups. Study 2 (TABLE 2) involved patients taking background treatment with maximum daily doses of sulfonylureas. At the end of this study, the mean effect of the addition of acarbose to maximum sulfonylurea therapy was a change in HbA1c of −0.54%. In addition, there was a significantly greater proportion of patients in the acarbose + sulfonylurea group who reduced their sulfonylurea dose as compared to patients in the placebo + sulfonylurea group. In study 3 (TABLE 2), the addition of acarbose to a background treatment of sulfonylurea produced an additional change in mean HbA1c of −0.8%

TABLE 2

Study	Treatment	Mean Baseline*	HbA1c (%) Mean Change from Baseline	Treatment Difference**	p-Value
1	Placebo	9.48	+0.05	-	-
	Acarbose 200‡ mg t.i.d	9.19	−0.71	−0.76	0.0005
	Tolbutamide 250–1000 mg t.i.d. (mean dose 2.4 g/d)	9.28	−1.22	−1.27	0.0001
	Acarbose 200‡ mg t.i.d. + Tolbutamide 250-1000 mg t.i.d. (mean dose 1.9 g/d)	8.99	−1.73	−1.78	0.0001
2	Sulfonylurea + Placebo	9.56	+0.24	-	-
	Sulfonylurea + Acarbose 50-300 ‡ mg t.i.d.	9.64	−0.30	−0.54	0.0096
3	Sulfonylurea + Placebo	8.00	+0.10	-	-
	Sulfonylurea + Acarbose 50-200 ‡ mg t.i.d	8.10	−0.80	−0.90	0.0020

* Normal range : 4-6%
* * The result of subtracting the placebo group average.
‡ Although studies utilized a maximum dose of 200 or 300 mg t.i.d., the maximum recommended dose for patients ≤60 kg is 50 mg t.i.d; the maximum recommended dose for patients > 60 kg is 100 mg t.i.d.

INDICATIONS AND USAGE:

Acarbose, as monotherapy, is indicated as an adjunct to diet to lower blood glucose in patients with non-insulin-depenedent diabetes melitus (NIDDM) whose hyperglycemia cannot be managed on diet alone. Acarbose may also be used in combination with a sulfonylurea when diet plus either acarbose or a sulfonylurea do not result in adequate glycemic control. The effect of acarbose to enhance glycemic control is additive to that of the sulfonylureas when used in combination, presumably because its mechanism of action is different.

In initiating treatment for NIDDM, diet should be emphasized as the primary form of treatment. Caloric restriction and weight loss are essential in the obese diabetic patient. Proper dietary management alone may be effective in controlling blood glucose and symptoms of hyperglycemia. The importance of regular physical activity when appropriate should also be stressed. If this treatment program fails to result in adequate glycemic control, the use of acarbose must be viewed by both the physician and patient as a treatment in addition to diet, and not as a substitute for diet or as a convenient mechanism for avoiding dietary restraint.

CONTRAINDICATIONS:

Acarbose is contraindicated in patients with known hypersensitivity to the drug and in patients with diabetic ketoacidosis, or cirrhosis. Acarbose is also contraindicated in patients with inflammatory bowel disease, colonic ulceration, partial intestinal obstruction, or in patients predisposed to intestinal obstruction. In addition, acarbose is contraindicated in patients who have chronic intestinal diseases associated with marked disorders of digestion or absorption and in patients who have conditions that may deteriorate as a result of increased gas formation in the intestine.

PRECAUTIONS:

GENERAL

Hypoglycemia: Because of its mechanism of action, acarbose when administered alone should not cause hypoglycemia in the fasted or postprandial state. Sulfonylurea agents may cause hypoglycemia. Because acarbose given in combination with a sulfonylurea will cause a further

PRECAUTIONS: *(cont'd)*

lowering of blood glucose, it may increase the hypoglycemic potential of the sulfonylurea. Oral glucose (dextrose), whose absorption is not inhibited by acarbose should be used instead of sucrose (cane sugar) in the treatment of mild to moderate hypoglycemia. Sucrose, whose hydrolysis to glucose and fructose is inhibited by acarbose, is unsuitable for the rapid correction of hypoglycemia. Severe hypoglycemia may require the use of either intravenous glucose infusion or glucagon injection.

Elevated Serum Transaminase Levels: In clinical trials, at doses of 50 mg t.i.d. and 100 mg t.i.d., the incidence of serum transaminase elevations with acarbose was the same with placebo. In long-term studies (up to 12 months, and including acarbose doses up to 300 mg t.i.d.) conducted in the United States, treatment-emergent elevations of serum transaminases (AST and/or ALT) occurred in 15% of acarbose-treated patients as compared to 7% of placebo-treated patients. These serum transaminase elevations appear to be dose related. At doses greater than 100 mg t.i.d., the incidence of serum transaminase elevations greater than three times the upper limit of normal was two to three times higher in the acarbose group than in the placebo group. These elevations were asymptomatic, reversible, more common in females, and, in general, were not associated with other evidence of liver dysfunction.

In international post-marketing experience with acarbose in over 500,000 patients, 19 cases of serum transaminase elevations > 500 IU/L (12 of which were associated with jaundice) have been reported. Fifteen of these 19 cases received treatment with 100 mg t.i.d or greater and 13 of 16 patients for whom weight was reported weighed < 60 kg. In the 18 cases where follow-up was recorded, hepatic abnormalities improved or resolved upon discontinuation of acarbose.

Loss of Control of Blood Glucose: When diabetic patients are exposed to stress such as fever, trauma, infection, or surgery, a temporary loss of control of blood glucose may occur. At such times, temporary insulin therapy may be necessary.

INFORMATION FOR THE PATIENT

Patients should be told to take acarbose orally three times a day at the start (with the first bite) of each main meal. It is important that patients continue to adhere to dietary instructions, a regular exercise program, and regular testing of urine and/or blood glucose.

Acarbose itself does not cause hypoglycemia even when administered to patients in the fasted state. Sulfonylurea drugs and insulin, however, can lower blood sugar levels enough to cause symptoms or sometimes life-threatening hypoglycemia. Because acarbose given in combination with a sulfonylurea or insulin will cause a further lowering of blood sugar, it may increase the hypoglycemic potential of these agents. The risk of hypoglycemia, its symptoms and treatment, and conditions that predispose to its development should be well understood by patients and responsible family members. Because acarbose prevents the breakdown of table sugar, patients should have a readily available source of glucose (dextrose, D-glucose) to treat symptoms of low blood sugar when taking acarbose in combination with a sulfonylurea or insulin.

If side effects occur with acarbose, they usually develop during the first few weeks of therapy. They are most commonly mild-to-moderate gastrointestinal effects, such as flatulence, diarrhea, or abdominal discomfort and generally diminish in frequency and intensity with time.

LABORATORY TESTS

Therapeutic response to acarbose should be monitored by periodic blood glucose tests. Measurement of glycosylated hemoglobin levels is recommended for the monitoring of long-term glycemic control.

Acarbose, particularly at doses in excess of 50 mg t.i.d., may give rise to elevations of serum transaminases and, in rare instances, hyperbilirubinemia. It is recommended that serum transaminase levels be checked every three months during the first year of treatment with acarbose and periodically thereafter. If elevated transaminases are observed, a reduction in dosage or withdrawal of therapy may be indicated, particularly if the elevations persist.

RENAL IMPAIRMENT

Plasma concentrations of acarbose in renally impaired volunteers were proportionally increased relative to the degree of renal dysfunction. Long-term clinical trials in diabetic patients with significant renal dysfunction (serum creatinine > 2.0 mg/dL) have not been conducted. Therefore, treatment of these patients with acarbose is not recommended.

CARCINOGENESIS, MUTAGENESIS, AND IMPAIRMENT OF FERTILITY

Nine chronic toxicity/carcinogenicity studies were conducted in three animal species (rat, hamster, dog) including two rat strains (Sprague-Dawley and Wistar)

In the first rat study, Sprague-Dawley rats received acarbose in feed at high doses (up to approximately 500 mg/kg body weight) for 104 weeks. Acarbose treatment resulted in a significant increase in the incidence of renal tumors (adenomas and adenocarcinomas) and benign Leydig cell tumors. This study was repeated with a similar outcome. Further studies were performed to separate direct carcinogenic effects of acarbose from indirect effects resulting from the carbohydrate malnutrition induced by the large doses of acarbose employed in the studies. In one study using Sprague-Dawley rats, acarbose was mixed with feed but carbohydrate deprivation was prevented by the addition of glucose to the diet. In a 26-month study of Sprague-Dawley rats, acarbose was administered by daily postprandial gavage so as to avoid the pharmacologic effects of the drug. In both of these studies, the increase incidence of renal tumors found in the original studies did not occur. Acarbose was also given in food and by postprandial gavage in two separate studies in Wistar rats. No increased incidence of renal tumors was found in either of these Wistar rat studies. In two feeding studies of hamsters, with and without glucose supplementation, there was no evidence of carcinogenicity.

Acarbose showed no mutagenic activity when tested in six *in vitro* and three *in vivo* assays.

Fertility studies conducted in rats after oral administration produced no untoward effect on fertility or on the overall capability to reproduce.

PREGNANCY, TERATOGENIC EFFECTS, PREGNANCY CATEGORY B

The safety of acarbose in pregnant women has not been established. Reproduction studies have been performed in rats at doses up to 480 mg/kg (corresponding to 9 times the exposure in humans, based on drug blood levels) and have revealed no evidence of impaired fertility or harm to the fetus due to acarbose. In rabbits, reduced maternal body weight gain, probably the result of pharmacodynamic activity of high doses of acarbose in the intestines, may have been responsible for a slight increase in the number of embryonic losses. However, rabbits given 160 mg/kg acarbose (Corresponding to 10 times the dose in man, based on body surface area) showed no evidence of embryotoxicity and there was no evidence of teratogenicity at a dose 32 times the dose in man (based on body surface area). There are, however, no adequate and well-controlled studies of acarbose in pregnant women. Because animal reproduction studies are not always predictive of the human response, this drug should be used during pregnancy only if clearly needed. Because current information strongly suggests that abnormal blood glucose levels during pregnancy are associated with a higher incidence of congenital anomalies as well as increase neonatal morbidity and mortality, most experts recommend that insulin be used during pregnancy to maintain blood glucose levels as close to normal as possible.

NURSING MOTHERS

A small amount of radioactivity has been found in the milk of lactating rats after administration of radiolabled acarbose. It is not known whether this drug is excreted in human milk. Acarbose should not be administered to a nursing woman.

PRECAUTIONS: *(cont'd)*

PEDIATRIC USE

Safety and effectiveness of acarbose in pediatric patients have not been established.

DRUG INTERACTIONS:

Certain drugs tend to produce hyperglycemia and may lead to loss of blood glucose control. These drugs include the thiazides and other diuretics, corticosteroids, phenothiazines, thyroid products, estrogens, oral contraceptives, phenytoin, nicotinic acid, sympathomimetics, calcium channel-blocking drugs, and isoniazid. When such drugs are administered to a patient receiving acarbose, the patient should be closely observed for loss of blood glucose control. When such drugs are withdrawn from patients receiving acarbose in combination with sulfonylureas or insulin, patients should be observed closely for any evidence of hypoglycemia.

Intestinal absorbents (*e.g.,* charcoal) and digestive enzyme preparations containing carbohydrate splitting enzymes (*e.g.,* amylase, pancreatin) may reduce the effect of acarbose and should not be taken concomitantly.

Drug-Drug Interactions: Studies in healthy volunteers have shown that acarbose has no effect on either the pharmacokinetics or pharmacodynamics of digoxin, nifedipine, propranolol, or ranitidine. Acarbose did not interfere with the absorption or disposition of the sulfonylurea glyburide in diabetic patients.

ADVERSE REACTIONS:

Digestive Tract: Gastrointestinal symptoms are the most common reactions to acarbose. In U.S. placebo-controlled trials, the incidences of abdominal pain, diarrhea, and flatulence were 21%, 33%, and 77%, respectively in 1075 patients treated with acarbose 50-300 mg t.i.d. whereas the corresponding incidences were 9%, 12%, and 32% in 818 placebo-treated patients. Abdominal pain and diarrhea tended to return to pretreatment levels over time and the frequency and intensity of flatulence tended to abate with time. The increased gastrointestinal tract symptoms in patients treated with acarbose is a manifestation of the mechanism of action of acarbose and is related to the presence of undigested carbohydrate in the lower GI tract. Rarely, these gastrointestinal events may be severe and might be confused with paralytic ileus.

Elevated Serum Transaminase Levels: See PRECAUTIONS.

Other Abnormal Laboratory Findings: Small reductions in hematocrit occurred more often in acarbose-treated patients than in placebo-treated patients but were not associated with reductions in hemoglobin. Low serum calcium and low plasma vitamin B_6 levels were associated with acarbose therapy but were thought to be either spurious or of no clinical significance.

OVERDOSAGE:

Unlike sulfonylureas or insulin, an overdose of acarbose will not result in hypoglycemia. An overdose may result in transient increases in flatulence, diarrhea, and abdominal discomfort which shortly subside.

DOSAGE AND ADMINISTRATION:

There is no fixed dosage regimen for the management of diabetes mellitus with acarbose or any other pharmacologic agent. Dosage of acarbose must be individualized on the basis of both effectiveness and tolerance while not exceeding the maximum recommended dose of 100 mg t.i.d. acarbose should be taken three times daily at the start (with the first bite) of each main meal. Acarbose should be started at a low dose, with gradual dose escalation as described below, both to reduce gastrointestinal side effects and to permit identification of the minimum dose required for adequate glycemic control of the patient.

During treatment initiation and dose titration (see below), one-hour postprandial plasma glucose should be used to determine the therapeutic response to acarbose and identify the minimum effective dose for the patient. Thereafter, glycosylated hemoglobin should be measured at intervals of approximately three months. The therapeutic goal should be to decrease both postprandial plasma glucose and glycosylated hemoglobin levels to normal or near normal by using the lowest effective dose of acarbose, either as monotherapy or in combination with sulfonylureas.

Initial Dosage: The recommended starting dosage of acarbose is 25 mg (half of a 50-mg tablet), given orally three times daily at the start (with the first bite) of each main meal.

Maintenance Dosage: Dosage of acarbose should be adjusted at 4-8 week intervals based on one-hour postprandial glucose levels and on tolerance. After the initial dosage of 25 mg t.i.d., the dosage can be increased to 50 mg t.i.d. Some patients may benefit from further increasing the dosage to 100 mg t.i.d. The maintenance dose ranges from 50 mg t.i.d. to 100 mg t.i.d. However, since patients with low body weight may be at increased risk for elevated serum transaminases, only patients with body weight > 60 kg should be considered for dose titration above 50 mg t.i.d. (see PRECAUTIONS). If no further reduction in postprandial glucose or glycosylated hemoglobin levels is observed with titration to 100 mg t.i.d., consideration should be given to lowering the dose. Once an effective and tolerated dosage is established, it should be maintained.

Maximum Dosage: The maximum recommended dose for patients ≤ 60 kg is 50 mg t.i.d. The maximum recommended dose for patients > 60 kg is 100 mg t.i.d.

Patients Receiving Sulfonylureas: Sulfonylurea agents may cause hypoglycemia. Acarbose given in combination with a sulfonylurea will cause a further lowering of blood glucose and may increase the hypoglycemic potential of the sulfonylurea. If hypoglycemia occurs, appropriate adjustments in the dosage of these agents should be made.

REFERENCES:

1. Precose TM (acarbose tablets) Package Insert. **2.** American Diabetes Association Implications of the Diabetes Control and Complications Trial. *Diabetes Care.* 1993;16(11):1517-1520. **3.** Coniff RF, Shapiro JA, Robbins D, et al. Reduction of glycosylated hemoglobin and postprandial hyperglycemia by acarbose in patients with NIDDM. *Diabetes Care.* 1993. **4.** Coniff RF, Shapiro JA, Seaton TB, Bray GA. Multicenter, placebo-controlled trial comparing acarbose (BAY g 5421) with placebo, tolbutamide, and tolbutamide-plus-acarbose in non-insulin-dependent diabetes melitus. *Am J Med.* 1995;98:443-451.. **5.** Hanefeld, M. Acarbose efficacy review. *Practical Diabetes Supplement*1993;10(6):S21-S27.

PATIENT INFORMATION:

Acarbose is used with diet or in combination with other medications to lower blood sugar (glucose) in diabetics. Do not use if you have cirrhosis or chronic bowel or intestinal disease. Inform your doctor if pregnant or nursing. Take 3 times daily at the start of each main meal. When acarbose is taken with other blood glucose-lowering medications, it may cause the blood sugar to decrease too much. Acarbose is not a substitute for a good diet, regular exercise and regular urine or blood glucose testing. May cause diarrhea, flatulence, and abdominal discomfort.

HOW SUPPLIED:

Do not store above 25°C (77°F). Protect from moisture. For bottles, keep container tightly closed.

HOW SUPPLIED - EQUIVALENTS NOT AVAILABLE:

Tablet - Oral - 50 mg

100's	$45.61	PRECOSE, Bayer	00026-2861-51
100's	$47.89	PRECOSE, Bayer	00026-2861-48

Tablet - Oral - 100 mg

100's	$58.80	PRECOSE, Bayer	00026-2862-51
100's	$61.74	PRECOSE, Bayer	00026-2862-48

ACEBUTOLOL HYDROCHLORIDE *(000002)*

CATEGORIES: Antihypertensives; Arrhythmia; Beta Adrenergic Blocking Agents; Beta Blockers; Cardiovascular Drugs; Hypertension; Pregnancy Category B; FDA Approved 1984 Dec

BRAND NAMES: *Acecor; Acetanol; Alol; Monitan; Neptal; Prent; Rhodiasectral;* **Sectral**
(International brand names outside U.S. in italics)

FORMULARIES: Aetna; BC-BS; Medi-Cal

COST OF THERAPY: $401.06 (Hypertension; Capsule; 400 mg; 1/day; 365 days)

PRIMARY ICD9: 401.1 (Essential Hypertension, Benign)

DESCRIPTION:

Sectral (acebutolol HCl) is a selective, hydrophilic beta-adrenoreceptor blocking agent with mild intrinsic sympathomimetic activity for use in treating patients with hypertension and ventricular arrhythmias. It is marketed in capsule form for oral administration. Sectral capsules are provided in two dosage strengths which contain 200 or 400 mg of acebutolol as the hydrochloride salt. The inactive ingredients present are D&C Red 22, FD&C Blue 1, FD&C Yellow 6, gelatin, povidone, starch, stearic acid, and titanium dioxide. The 200 mg dosage strength also contains D&C Red 28 and the 400 mg dosage strength also contains FD&C Red 40.

Acebutolol HCl is a white or slightly off-white powder freely soluble in water, and less soluble in alcohol. Chemically it is defined as the hydrochloride salt of Butanamide, N-[3-acetyl-4-[2-hydroxy-3-[(1- methylethyl)amino]propoxy]phenyl]-,(±)- or (±)-3'-Acetyl-4'-[2- hydroxy-3-(isopropylamino)propoxy] butyranilide.

CLINICAL PHARMACOLOGY:

Acebutolol HCl is a cardioselective, β-adrenoreceptor blocking agent, which possesses mild intrinsic sympathomimetic activity (ISA) in its therapeutically effective dose range.

PHARMACODYNAMICS

β_1-cardioselectivity has been demonstrated in experimental animal studies. In anesthetized dogs and cats, acebutolol HCl is more potent in antagonizing isoproterenol-induced tachycardia (β_1) than in antagonizing isoproterenol-induced vasodilatation (β_2). In guinea pigs and cats, it is more potent in antagonizing this tachycardia than in antagonizing isoproterenol-induced bronchodilatation (β_2). ISA of acebutolol HCl has been demonstrated in catecholamine- depleted rats by tachycardia induced by intravenous administration of this agent. A membrane-stabilizing effect has been detected in animals, but only with high concentrations of acebutolol HCl.

Clinical studies have demonstrated β_1-blocking activity at the recommended doses by: a) reduction in the resting heart rate and decrease in exercise-induced tachycardia; b) reduction in cardiac output at rest and after exercise; c) reduction of systolic and diastolic blood pressures at rest and postexercise; d) inhibition of isoproterenol- induced tachycardia.

The β_1-selectivity of acebutolol HCl has also been demonstrated on the basis of the following vascular and bronchial effects:

Vascular Effects: Acebutolol HCl has less antagonistic effects on peripheral vascular β_2-receptors at rest and after epinephrine stimulation than nonselective β-antagonists.

Bronchial Effects: In single-dose studies in asthmatics examining effects of various beta-blockers on pulmonary function, low doses of acebutolol produce less evidence of bronchoconstriction and less reduction of beta$_2$ agonist, bronchodilating effects, than nonselective agents like propranolol but more than atenolol.

ISA has been observed with acebutolol HCl in man, as shown by a slightly smaller (about 3 beats per minute) decrease in resting heart rate when compared to equivalent β-blocking doses of propranolol, metoprolol or atenolol. Chronic therapy with acebutolol HCl induced no significant alteration in the blood lipid profile.

Acebutolol HCl has been shown to delay AV conduction time and to increase the refractoriness of the AV node without significantly affecting sinus node recovery time, atrial refractory period, or the HV conduction time. The membrane-stabilizing effect of acebutolol HCl is not manifest at the doses used clinically.

Significant reductions in resting and exercise heart rates and systolic blood pressures have been observed 1.5 hours after acebutolol HCl administration with maximal effects occurring between 3 and 8 hours postdosing in normal volunteers. Acebutolol HCl has demonstrated a significant effect on exercise-induced tachycardia 24 to 30 hours after drug administration.

There are significant correlations between plasma levels of acebutolol and both the reduction in resting heart rate and the percent of β- blockade of exercise-induced tachycardia.

The antihypertensive effect of acebutolol HCl has been shown in double-blind controlled studies to be superior to placebo and similar to propranolol and hydrochlorothiazide. In addition, patients responding to acebutolol HCl administered twice daily had a similar response whether the dosage regimen was changed to once daily administration or continued on a b.i.d. regimen. Most patients responded to 400 to 800 mg per day in divided doses.

The antiarrhythmic effect of acebutolol HCl was compared with placebo, propranolol, and quinidine. Compared with placebo, acebutolol HCl significantly reduced mean total ventricular ectopic beats (VEB), paired VEB, multiform VEB, R-on-T beats, and ventricular tachycardia (VT). Both acebutolol HCl and propranolol significantly reduced mean total and paired VEB and VT. Acebutolol HCl and quinidine significantly reduced resting total and complex VEB; the antiarrhythmic efficacy of acebutolol HCl was also observed during exercise.

PHARMACOKINETICS AND METABOLISM

Acebutolol HCl is well absorbed from the GI tract. It is subject to extensive first-pass hepatic biotransformation, with an absolute bioavailability of approximately 40% for the parent compound. The major metabolite, an N-acetyl derivative (diacetolol), is pharmacologically active. This metabolite is equipotent to acebutolol HCl and in cats is more cardioselective than acebutolol HCl; therefore, this first-pass phenomenon does not attenuate the therapeutic effect of acebutolol HCl. Food intake does not have a significant effect on the area under the plasma concentration-time curve (AUC) of acebutolol HCl although the rate of absorption and peak concentration decreased slightly.

CLINICAL PHARMACOLOGY: *(cont'd)*

The plasma elimination half-life of acebutolol HCl is approximately 3 to 4 hours, while that of its metabolite, diacetolol, is 8 to 13 hours. The time to reach peak concentration for acebutolol HCl is 2.5 hours and for diacetolol, after oral administration of acebutolol HCl, 3.5 hours.

Within the single oral dose range of 200 to 400 mg, the kinetics are dose proportional. However, this linearity is not seen at higher doses, probably due to saturation of hepatic biotransformation sites. In addition, after multiple dosing the lack of linearity is also seen by AUC increases of approximately 100% as compared to single oral dosing. Elimination via renal excretion is approximately 30% to 40% and by nonrenal mechanisms 50% to 60%, which includes excretion into the bile and direct passage through the intestinal wall.

Acebutolol HCl has a low binding affinity for plasma proteins (about 26%). Acebutolol HCl and its metabolite, diacetolol, are relatively hydrophilic and, therefore, only minimal quantities have been detected in the cerebrospinal fluid (CSF).

Drug interaction studies with tolbutamide and warfarin indicated no influence on the therapeutic effects of these compounds. Digoxin and hydrochlorothiazide plasma levels were not affected by concomitant acebutolol HCl administration. The kinetics of acebutolol HCl were not significantly altered by concomitant administration of hydrochlorothiazide, hydralazine, sulfinpyrazone, or oral contraceptives.

In patients with renal impairment, there is no effect on the elimination half-life of acebutolol HCl, but there is decreased elimination of the metabolite, diacetolol, resulting in a two- to three-fold increase in its half-life. For this reason, the drug should be administered with caution in patients with renal insufficiency (see PRECAUTIONS.) Acebutolol HCl and its major metabolite are dialyzable.

Acebutolol HCl crosses the placental barrier and is secreted in breast milk.

In geriatric patients, the bioavailability of acebutolol HCl and its metabolite is increased, approximately two-fold, probably due to decreases in the first-pass metabolism and renal function in the elderly.

INDICATIONS AND USAGE:

Hypertension: Acebutolol HCl is indicated for the management of hypertension in adults. It may be used alone or in combination with other antihypertensive agents, especially thiazide-type diuretics.

Ventricular Arrhythmias: Acebutolol HCl is indicated in the management of ventricular premature beats; it reduces the total number of premature beats, as well as the number of paired and multiform ventricular ectopic beats, and R-on-T beats.

CONTRAINDICATIONS:

Acebutolol HCl is contraindicated in: 1) persistently severe bradycardia; 2) second- and third-degree heart block; 3) overt cardiac failure; and 4) cardiogenic shock. (See WARNINGS.)

WARNINGS:

CARDIAC FAILURE

Sympathetic stimulation may be essential for support of the circulation in individuals with diminished myocardial contractility, and its inhibition by β-adrenergic receptor blockade may precipitate more severe failure. Although β-blockers should be avoided in overt cardiac failure, acebutolol HCl can be used with caution in patients with a history of heart failure who are controlled with digitalis and/or diuretics. Both digitalis and acebutolol HCl impair AV conduction. If cardiac failure persists, therapy with acebutolol HCl should be withdrawn.

IN PATIENTS WITHOUT A HISTORY OF CARDIAC FAILURE

In patients with aortic or mitral valve disease or compromised left ventricular function, continued depression of the myocardium with β- blocking agents over a period of time may lead to cardiac failure. At the first signs of failure, patients should be digitalized and/or be given a diuretic and the response observed closely. If cardiac failure continues despite adequate digitalization and/or diuretic, acebutolol HCl therapy should be withdrawn.

EXACERBATION OF ISCHEMIC HEART DISEASE FOLLOWING ABRUPT WITHDRAWAL

Following abrupt cessation of therapy with certain β-blocking agents in patients with coronary artery disease, exacerbation of angina pectoris and, in some cases, myocardial infarction and death have been reported. Therefore, such patients should be cautioned against interruption of therapy without a physician's advice. Even in the absence of overt ischemic heart disease, when discontinuation of acebutolol HCl is planned, the patient should be carefully observed, and should be advised to limit physical activity to a minimum while acebutolol HCl is gradually withdrawn over a period of about two weeks. (If therapy with an alternative β-blocker is desired, the patient may be transferred directly to comparable doses of another agent without interruption of β-blocking therapy.) If an exacerbation of angina pectoris occurs, antianginal therapy should be restarted immediately in full doses and the patient hospitalized until his condition stabilizes.

PERIPHERAL VASCULAR DISEASE

Treatment with β-antagonists reduces cardiac output and can precipitate or aggravate the symptoms of arterial insufficiency in patients with peripheral or mesenteric vascular disease. Caution should be exercised with such patients, and they should be observed closely for evidence of progression of arterial obstruction.

BRONCHOSPASTIC DISEASES

Patients with bronchospastic disease should, in general, not receive a β-blocker. Because of its relative β_1-selectivity, however, low doses of acebutolol HCl may be used with caution in patients with bronchospastic disease who do not respond to, or who cannot tolerate, alternative treatment. Since β_1-selectivity is not absolute and is dose-dependent, the lowest possible dose of acebutolol HCl should be used initially, preferably in divided doses to avoid the higher plasma levels associated with the longer dose-interval. A bronchodilator, such as theophylline or a β_2-stimulant, should be made available in advance with instructions concerning its use.

ANESTHESIA AND MAJOR SURGERY

The necessity, or desirability, of withdrawal of a β-blocking therapy prior to major surgery is controversial. β-adrenergic receptor blockade impairs the ability of the heart to respond to β-adrenergically mediated reflex stimuli. While this might be of benefit in preventing arrhythmic response, the risk of excessive myocardial depression during general anesthesia may be enhanced and difficulty in restarting and maintaining the heart beat has been reported with beta- blockers. If treatment is continued, particular care should be taken when using anesthetic agents which depress the myocardium, such as ether, cyclopropane, and trichlorethylene, and it is prudent to use the lowest possible dose of acebutolol HCl. Acebutolol HCl, like other β-blockers, is a competitive inhibitor of β-receptor agonists, and its effect on the heart can be reversed by cautious administration of such agents (*e.g.*, dobutamine or isoproterenol—see OVERDOSAGE).

Manifestations of excessive vagal tone (*e.g.*, profound bradycardia, hypotension) may be corrected with atropine 1 to 3 mg IV in divided doses.

WARNINGS: *(cont'd)*

DIABETES AND HYPOGLYCEMIA

β-blockers may potentiate insulin-induced hypoglycemia and mask some of its manifestations such as tachycardia; however, dizziness and sweating are usually not significantly affected. Diabetic patients should be warned of the possibility of masked hypoglycemia.

THYROTOXICOSIS

β-adrenergic blockade may mask certain clinical signs (tachycardia) of hyperthyroidism. Abrupt withdrawal of β-blockade may precipitate a thyroid storm; therefore, patients suspected of developing thyrotoxicosis from whom acebutolol HCl therapy is to be withdrawn should be monitored closely.

PRECAUTIONS:

IMPAIRED RENAL OR HEPATIC FUNCTION

Studies on the effect of acebutolol in patients with renal insufficiency have not been performed in the U.S. Foreign published experience shows that acebutolol has been used successfully in chronic renal insufficiency. Acebutolol is excreted through the GI tract, but the active metabolite, diacetolol, is eliminated predominantly by the kidney. There is a linear relationship between renal clearance of diacetolol and creatinine clearance. Therefore, the daily dose of acebutolol should be reduced by 50% when the creatinine clearance is less than 50 ml/min and by 75% when it is less than 25 ml/min. Acebutolol HCl should be used cautiously in patients with impaired hepatic function.

Acebutolol HCl has been used successfully and without problems in elderly patients in the U.S. clinical trials without specific adjustment of dosage. However, elderly patients may require lower maintenance doses because the bioavailability of both acebutolol HCl and its metabolite are approximately doubled in this age group.

INFORMATION FOR THE PATIENT

Patients, especially those with evidence of coronary artery disease, should be warned against interruption or discontinuation of acebutolol HCl therapy without a physician's supervision. Although cardiac failure rarely occurs in properly selected patients, those being treated with β-adrenergic blocking agents should be advised to consult a physician if they develop signs or symptoms suggestive of impending CHF, or unexplained respiratory symptoms.

Patients should also be warned of possible severe hypertensive reactions from concomitant use of α-adrenergic stimulants, such as the nasal decongestants commonly used in OTC cold preparations and nasal drops.

CLINICAL LABORATORY FINDINGS

Acebutolol HCl, like other β-blockers, has been associated with the development of antinuclear antibodies (ANA). In prospective clinical trials, patients receiving acebutolol HCl had a dose-dependent increase in the development of positive ANA titers, and the overall incidence was higher than that observed with propranolol. Symptoms (generally persistent arthralgias and myalgias) related to this laboratory abnormality were infrequent (less than 1% with both drugs). Symptoms and ANA titers were reversible upon discontinuation of treatment.

CARCINOGENESIS, MUTAGENESIS, AND IMPAIRMENT OF FERTILITY

Chronic oral toxicity studies in rats and mice, employing dose levels as high as 300 mg/kg/day, which is equivalent to 15 times the maximum recommended (60 kg) human dose, did not indicate a carcinogenic potential for acebutolol HCl. Diacetolol, the major metabolite of acebutolol HCl in man, was without carcinogenic potential in rats when tested at doses as high as 1800 mg/kg/day. Acebutolol HCl and diacetolol were also shown to be devoid of mutagenic potential in the Ames Test. Acebutolol HCl, administered orally to two generations of male and female rats at doses of up to 240 mg/kg/day (equivalent to 12 times the maximum recommended therapeutic dose in a 60- kg human) and diacetolol, administered to two generations of male and female rats at doses of up to 1000 mg/kg/day, had no significant impact on reproductive performance or fertility.

PREGNANCY CATEGORY B

Teratogenic Effects: Reproduction studies have been performed with acebutolol HCl in rats (up to 630 mg/kg/day) and rabbits (up to 135 mg/kg/day). These doses are equivalent to approximately 31.5 and 6.8 times the maximum recommended therapeutic dose in a 60-kg human, respectively. The compound was not teratogenic in either species. In the rabbit, however, doses of 135 mg/kg/day caused slight fetal growth retardation; this effect was considered to be a result of maternal toxicity, as evidenced by reduced food intake, a lowered rate of body weight gain, and mortality. Studies have also been performed in these species with diacetolol (at doses of up to 450 mg/kg/day in rabbits and up to 1800 mg/kg/day in rats). Other than a significant elevation in post- implantation loss with 450 mg/kg/day diacetolol, a level at which food consumption and body weight gain were reduced in rabbit dams and a nonstatistically significant increase in incidence of bilateral cataract in rat fetuses from dams treated with 1800 mg/kg/day diacetolol, there was no evidence of harm to the fetus. There are no adequate and well- controlled trials in pregnant women. Because animal teratology studies are not always predictive of the human response, acebutolol HCl should be used during pregnancy only if the potential benefit justifies the risk to the fetus.

Nonteratogenic Effects: Studies in humans have shown that both acebutolol and diacetolol cross the placenta. Neonates of mothers who have received acebutolol during pregnancy have reduced birth weight, decreased blood pressure, and decreased heart rate. In the newborn the elimination half-life of acebutolol was 6 to 14 hours, while the half-life of diacetolol was 24 to 30 hours for the first 24 hours after birth, followed by a half-life of 12 to 16 hours. Adequate facilities for monitoring these infants at birth should be available.

LABOR AND DELIVERY

The effect of acebutolol HCl on labor and delivery in pregnant women is unknown. Studies in animals have not shown any effect of acebutolol HCl on the usual course of labor and delivery.

NURSING MOTHERS

Acebutolol and diacetolol also appear in breast milk with a milk:plasma ratio of 7.1 and 12.2, respectively. Use in nursing mothers is not recommended.

PEDIATRIC USE

Safety and effectiveness in children have not been established.

DRUG INTERACTIONS:

Catecholamine-depleting drugs, such as reserpine, may have an additive effect when given with β-blocking agents. Patients treated with acebutolol HCl plus catecholamine depletors should, therefore, be observed closely for evidence of marked bradycardia or hypotension which may present as vertigo, syncope/presyncope, or orthostatic changes in blood pressure without compensatory tachycardia. Exaggerated hypertensive responses have been reported from the combined use of β-adrenergic antagonists and α-adrenergic stimulants, including those contained in proprietary cold remedies and vasoconstrictive nasal drops. Patients receiving β-blockers should be warned of this potential hazard.

Blunting of the antihypertensive effect of beta-adrenoceptor blocking agents by nonsteroidal anti-inflammatory drugs has been reported.

No significant interactions with digoxin, hydrochlorothiazide, hydralazine, sulfinpyrazone, oral contraceptives, tolbutamide, or warfarin have been observed.

ADVERSE REACTIONS:

Acebutolol HCl is well tolerated in properly selected patients. Most adverse reactions have been mild, not required discontinuation of therapy, and tended to decrease as duration of treatment increases.

The following table (TABLE 1), shows the frequency of treatment-related side effects derived from controlled clinical trials in patients with hypertension, angina pectoris, and arrhythmia. These patients received acebutolol HCl, propranolol, or hydrochlorothiazide as monotherapy, or placebo.

TABLE 1 Total Volunteered And Elicited (U.S. Studies)

Body System/ Adverse Reaction	Acebutolol HCl (N=1002) %	Propranolol (N=424) %	Hydrochlorothiazide (N=178) %	Placebo (N=314) %
Cardiovascular				
Chest Pain	2	4	4	1
Edema	2	2	4	1
Central Nervous System				
Depression	2	1	3	1
Dizziness	6	7	12	2
Fatigue	11	17	10	4
Headache	6	9	13	4
Insomnia	3	6	5	1
Abnormal dreams	2	3	0	1
Dermatologic				
Rash	2	2	4	1
Gastrointestinal				
Constipation	4	2	7	0
Diarrhea	4	5	5	1
Dyspepsia	4	6	3	1
Flatulence	3	4	7	1
Nausea	4	6	3	0
Genitourinary				
Micturition (frequency)	3	1	9	<1
Musculoskeletal				
Arthralgia	2	1	3	2
Myalgia	2	1	4	0
Respiratory				
Cough	1	1	2	0
Dyspnea	4	6	4	2
Rhinitis	2	1	4	<1
Special Senses				
Abnormal Vision	2	2	3	0

The following selected (potentially important) side effects were seen in up to 2% of acebutolol HCl patients:

Cardiovascular: hypotension, bradycardia, heart failure.

Central Nervous System: anxiety, hyper/hypoesthesia, impotence.

Dermatological: pruritus.

Gastrointestinal: vomiting, abdominal pain.

Genitourinary: dysuria, nocturia.

Liver and Biliary System: A small number of cases of liver abnormalities (increased SGOT, SGPT, LDH) have been reported in association with acebutolol therapy. In some cases increased bilirubin or alkaline phosphatase, fever, malaise, dark urine, anorexia, nausea, headache, and/or other symptoms have been reported. In some of the reported cases, the symptoms and signs were confirmed by rechallenge with acebutolol. The abnormalities were reversible upon cessation of acebutolol therapy.

Musculoskeletal: back pain, joint pain.

Respiratory: pharyngitis, wheezing.

Special Senses: conjunctivitis, dry eye, eye pain.

Autoimmune: In extremely rare instances, systemic lupus erythematosus has been reported.

The incidence of drug-related adverse effects (volunteered and solicited) according to acebutolol HCl dose is shown (TABLE 2). (Data from 266 hypertensive patients treated for 3 months on a constant dose.)

TABLE 2

Body System	400 mg/day (N=132)	800 mg/day (N=63)	1200 mg/day (N=71)
Cardiovascular	5%	2%	1%
Gastrointestinal	3%	3%	7%
Musculoskeletal	2%	3%	4%
Central Nervous System	9%	13%	17%
Respiratory	1%	5%	6%
Skin	1%	2%	1%
Special Senses	2%	2%	6%
Genitourinary	2%	3%	1%

POTENTIAL ADVERSE EFFECTS

In addition, certain adverse effects not listed above have been reported with other β-blocking agents and should also be considered as potential adverse effects of acebutolol HCl.

Central Nervous System: Reversible mental depression progressing to catatonia (an acute syndrome characterized by disorientation for time and place), short-term memory loss, emotional lability, slightly clouded sensorium, and decreased performance (neuropsychometrics).

Cardiovascular: Intensification of AV block (see CONTRAINDICATIONS.)

Allergic: Erythematous rash, fever combined with aching and sore throat, laryngospasm, and respiratory distress.

Hematologic: Agranulocytosis, nonthrombocytopenic, and thrombocytopenic purpura.

Gastrointestinal: Mesenteric arterial thrombosis and ischemic colitis.

Miscellaneous: Reversible alopecia and Peyronie's disease. The oculomucocutaneous syndrome associated with the β-blocker practolol has not been reported with acebutolol HCl during investigational use and extensive foreign clinical experience.

OVERDOSAGE:

No specific information on emergency treatment of overdosage is available for acebutolol HCl. However, overdosage with other β-blocking agents has been accompanied by extreme bradycardia, advanced atrioventricular block, intraventricular conduction defects, hypotension, severe congestive heart failure, seizures, and in susceptible patients, bronchospasm and hypoglycemia. Although specific information on the emergency treatment of acebutolol HCl

OVERDOSAGE: *(cont'd)*

overdose is not available, on the basis of the pharmacological actions and the observations in treating overdoses with other β- blockers, the following general measures should be considered:

1. Empty stomach by emesis or lavage.

2. Bradycardia: IV atropine (1 to 3 mg in divided doses). If antivagal response is inadequate, administer isoproterenol cautiously since larger than usual doses of isoproterenol may be required.

3. Persistent hypotension in spite of correction of bradycardia: Administer vasopressor (*e.g.*, epinephrine, levarterenol, dopamine, or dobutamine) with frequent monitoring of blood pressure and pulse rate.

4. Bronchospasm: A theophylline derivative, such as aminophylline and/or parenteral β_2-stimulant, such as terbutaline.

5. Cardiac failure: Digitalize the patient and/or administer a diuretic. It has been reported that glucagon is useful in this situation.

Acebutolol HCl is dialyzable.

DOSAGE AND ADMINISTRATION:

HYPERTENSION

The initial dosage of acebutolol HCl in uncomplicated mild-to-moderate hypertension is 400 mg. This can be given as a single daily dose, but in occasional patients twice daily dosing may be required for adequate 24- hour blood-pressure control. An optimal response is usually achieved with dosages of 400 to 800 mg per day, although some patients have been maintained on as little as 200 mg per day. Patients with more severe hypertension or who have demonstrated inadequate control may respond to a total of 1200 mg daily (administered b.i.d.), or to the addition of a second antihypertensive agent. Beta-1 selectivity diminishes as dosage is increased.

VENTRICULAR ARRYTHMIA

The usual initial dose of acebutolol HCl is 400 mg daily given as 200 mg b.i.d. Dosage should be increased gradually until an optimal clinical response is obtained, generally at 600 to 1200 mg per day. If treatment is to be discontinued, the dosage should be reduced gradually over a period of about two weeks.

USE IN OLDER PATIENTS

Older patients have an approximately 2-fold increase in bioavailability and may require lower maintenance doses. Doses above 800 mg/day should be avoided in the elderly.

HOW SUPPLIED:

Sectral (acebutolol HCl) is available in the following dosage strengths:

200 mg, opaque purple and orange capsule marked "WYETH 4177" and "Sectral 200"

400 mg, opaque brown and orange capsule marked "WYETH 4179" and "Sectral 400"

Keep tightly closed

Store at room temperature, approx. 25° C (77° F)

Dispense in a tight container

Use carton to protect contents from light

The appearance of these capsules is a trademark of Wyeth-Ayerst Laboratories.

HOW SUPPLIED - RATED THERAPEUTICALLY EQUIVALENT:

Capsule, Gelatin - Oral - 200 mg

100's	$91.30	Acebutolol Hcl, Mylan	00378-1200-01
100's	**$98.18**	**SECTRAL, Wyeth Labs**	**00008-4177-01**
100's	**$105.89**	**SECTRAL, Wyeth Labs**	**00008-4177-04**

Capsule, Gelatin - Oral - 400 mg

100's	$109.88	Acebutolol Hydrochloride, H.C.F.A. F F P	99999-0002-02
100's	$121.40	Acebutolol Hcl, Mylan	00378-1400-01
100's	**$130.53**	**SECTRAL, Wyeth Labs**	**00008-4179-01**

ACETAMINOPHEN *(000005)*

CATEGORIES: Analgesics; Analgesics/Antipyretics; Antipyretics; Central Nervous System Agents; Headache; Pain

BRAND NAMES: APAP; *Abenol* (Canada); *Acamol*; *Acetalgin*; *Acetam*; *Acetamol*; *Acetan*; *Afebrin*; *Algiafin*; *Alvedon*; *Anaflon* (Germany); *Analgiser*, *Anapark*; *Arfen*; *Asidon*; *Ben-U-Ron* (Germany); *Benuron* (Japan); *Biogesic*; *Bodrex*; *Calapol*; *Calip*; *Calpol* (Japan); *Ceetamol*; *Claradol*; *Crocin*; *Custodial*; *Daga*; *Datril* (Mexico); *Depyretin*; *Dhamol*; *Dirox*; *Dolamin*; *Doliprane* (France); *Dolofen*; *Dolomol*; *Dolorol*; *Doltem*; *Drilan*; *Dymadon*; Ed-Apap; *Efferalgan 500*; *Ennagesic*; *Exdol* (Canada); *Fanalgic*; *Focus*; *Fonafor*; *Gelocatil*; *Geluprane 500* (France); *Lemgrip*; *Lotemp*; *Lusadol*; *Malidens*; *Metagesic*; *Mexalen*; *Minopan*; *Napamol*; *NEBS* (Japan); *Nebs*; *Nektol 500*; *Nendol*; *Neodol* (Mexico); *Pacemol*; *Pacimol*; *Pamol*; *Panadol* (Australia, England, France, Canada); *Panamax*; *Panodil*; *Paracet*; *Paracetamol*; *Paralgin*; *Paralief*; *Paramol*; *Paratabs*; *Parmol*; *Pinex*; *Predimol*; *Puernol*; *Pymadon*; *Pyragesic*; *Reliv*; *Remedol*; *Robigesic* (Canada); *Salzone*; *Saridon*; *Setamol*; *Taganopain*; *Tempra* (Canada, Mexico, Japan); *Tempra Drops*; *Tempte*; *Termofren*; *Tinten*; *Turpan*; *Tylenol* (France, Germany, Canada, Japan); *Tynogesic*; *Winadol*; *Winasorb*; *Zolben* *(International brand names outside U.S. in italics)*

FORMULARIES: Aetna; DoD; WHO

Prescribing information not available at time of publication.

HOW SUPPLIED - EQUIVALENTS NOT AVAILABLE:

Solution - Oral - 160 mg/5ml

240 ml	$7.80	ED-APAP, Edwards Pharms	00485-0057-08

ACETAMINOPHEN; ASPIRIN; CAFFEINE; HYDROCODONE *(000288)*

CATEGORIES: Analgesics; Antipyretics; Central Nervous System Agents; Opiate Agonists (Controlled); Pain; DEA Class CIII; FDA Pre 1938 Drugs

BRAND NAMES: Anodynos-Dhc; Dhc Plus

Prescribing information not available at time of publication.

HOW SUPPLIED - EQUIVALENTS NOT AVAILABLE:

Capsule, Gelatin - Oral

100's	$40.82	DHC PLUS, Purdue Frederick	00034-8000-80

ACETAMINOPHEN; ATROPINE; ETHAVERINE; SALICYLIC ACID *(000017)*

CATEGORIES: Analgesics; Anticholinergic Agents; Antimuscarinics/Antispasmodics; Autonomic Drugs; Gastrointestinal Drugs; Pain; Peripheral Vasodilators; FDA Pre 1938 Drugs

BRAND NAMES: Espasmotex

Prescribing information not available at time of publication.

HOW SUPPLIED - EQUIVALENTS NOT AVAILABLE:

Tablet, Uncoated - Oral - 150 mg/0.3 mg/2

20's	$3.00	ESPASMOTEX, Kramer P I	52083-0836-20
60's	$9.00	ESPASMOTEX, Kramer P I	52083-0836-60

ACETAMINOPHEN; BUTALBITAL *(000020)*

CATEGORIES: Analgesics; Analgesics/Antipyretics; Antimigraine/Other Headaches; Antipyretics; Anxiolytics, Sedatives, Hypnotic; Central Nervous System Agents; Headache; Pain; Sedatives/Hypnotics; FDA Approved 1984 Oct

BRAND NAMES: Bancap; Bucet; Bupap; Conten; Greatab; Indogesic; Isopap; Midrinol; **Phrenilin**; Phrenilin Forte; Sedapap; Tencon; Triaprin

DESCRIPTION:

(Warning—May be habit forming)

Phrenilin: Each Phrenilin tablet for oral administration, contains Butalbital*, USP 50 mg * (WARNING—May be habit forming), Acetaminophen, USP 325 mg.

In addition each Phrenilin tablet contains the following inactive ingredients: alginic acid, cornstarch, D&C Red No. 27 - Aluminum Lake, FD&C Blue No. 1 - Aluminum Lake, gelatin, magnesium stearate, microcrystalline cellulose and pregelatinized starch.

Phrenilin Forte: Phrenilin Forte capsule for oral administration contains Butalbital*, USP 50 mg *(WARNING—May be habit forming), Acetaminophen, USP, 650 mg.

In addition, each Phrenilin Forte capsule may also contain the following inactive ingredients: benzyl alcohol, butylparaben, D&C Red No. 28, D&C Red No. 33, edetate calcium disodium, FD&C Blue No. 1, FD&C Red No. 40, gelatin, methylparaben, silicon dioxide, sodium lauryl sulfate, sodium propionate and titanium dioxide.

Butalbital (5-allyl-5-isobutylbarbituric acid), a slightly bitter, white, odorless, crystalline powder, is a short to intermediate-acting barbiturate. It has the following structural formula: $C_{11}H_{16}N_2O_3$. The molecular weight is 224.26.

Acetaminophen (4'-hydroxyacetanalide), a slightly bitter, white, odorless, crystalline powder, is a non-opiate, non-salicylate analgesic and antipyretic. It has the following molecular formula: $C_8H_9NO_2$. It's molecular weight is 151.16.

CLINICAL PHARMACOLOGY:

This combination drug product is intended as a treatment for tension headache.

It consists of a fixed combination of butalbital and acetaminophen. The role each component plays in the relief of the complex of symptoms known as tension headache is incompletely understood.

PHARMACOKINETICS

The behavior of the individual components is described below.

Butalbital: Butalbital is well absorbed from the gastrointestinal tract and is expected to distribute to most tissues in the body. Barbiturates in general may appear in breast milk and readily cross the placental barrier. They are bound to plasma and tissue proteins to a varying degree and binding increases directly as a function of lipid solubility.

Elimination of butalbital is primarily via the kidney (59% to 88% of the dose) as unchanged drug or metabolites. The plasma half-life is about 35 hours. Urinary excretion products include parent drug (about 3.6% of the dose), 5-isobutyl-5-(2,3-dihydroxypropyl) barbituric acid (about 24% of the dose), 5-allyl-5 (3-hydroxy-2-methyl-1-propyl) barbituric acid (about 4.8% of the dose), products with the barbituric acid ring hydrolyzed with excretion of urea (about 14% of the dose), as well as unidentified materials. Of the material excreted in the urine, 32% is conjugated.

See OVERDOSAGE for toxicity information.

ACETAMINOPHEN

Acetaminophen is rapidly absorbed from the gastrointestinal tract and is distributed throughout most body tissues. The plasma half life is 1.25 to 3 hours, but may be increased by liver damage and following overdosage. Elimination of acetaminophen is principally by liver metabolism (conjugation) and subsequent renal excretion of metabolites. Approximately 85% of an oral dose appears in the urine within 24 hours of administration, most as the glucuronide conjugate, with small amounts of other conjugates and unchanged drug.

See OVERDOSAGE for toxicity information.

INDICATIONS AND USAGE:

Acetaminophin; butalbital capsules are indicated for the relief of the symptom complex of tension (or muscle contraction) headache.

Evidence supporting the efficacy and safety of this combination product in the treatment of multiple recurrent headaches is unavailable. Caution in this regard is required because butalbital is habit-forming and potentially abusable.

CONTRAINDICATIONS:

This product is contraindicated under the following conditions:

Hypersensitivity or intolerance to any component of this product.

Patients with porphyria.

WARNINGS:

Butalbital is habit-forming and potentially abusable. Consequently, the extended use of this product is not recommended.

PRECAUTIONS:

GENERAL

Acetaminophin; butalbital should be prescribed with caution in certain special-risk patients, such as the elderly or debilitated, and those with severe impairment of renal or hepatic function, or acute abdominal conditions.

INFORMATION FOR THE PATIENT

This product may impair mental and/or physical abilities required for the performance of potentially hazardous tasks such as driving a car or operating machinery. Such tasks should be avoided while taking this product.

Alcohol; and other CNS depressants may produce an additive CNS depression, when taken with this combination product, and should be avoided.

Butalbital may be habit-forming. Patients should take the drug only for as long as it is prescribed, in the amounts prescribed, and no more frequently than prescribed.

LABORATORY TESTS

In patients with severe hepatic or renal disease, effects of therapy should be monitored with serial liver and/or renal function tests.

DRUG/LABORATORY TEST INTERACTIONS

Acetaminophen may produce false-positive test results for urinary 5-hydroxyindoleacetic acid.

CARCINOGENESIS, MUTAGENESIS, AND IMPAIRMENT OF FERTILITY

No adequate studies have been conducted in animals to determine whether acetaminophen or butalbital have a potential for carcinogenesis, mutagenesis or impairment of fertility.

PREGNANCY CATEGORY C

Teratogenic Effects: Animal reproduction studies have not been conducted with this combination product. It is also not known whether butalbital and acetaminophen can cause fetal harm when administered to a pregnant woman or can affect reproduction capacity. These products should be given to a pregnant woman only when clearly needed.

Nonteratogenic Effects: Withdrawal seizures were reported in a two-day-old male infant whose mother had taken a butalbital-containing drug during the last two months of pregnancy. Butalbital was found in the infant's serum. The infant was given phenobarbital 5 mg/kg, which was tapered without further seizure or other withdrawal symptoms.

NURSING MOTHERS

Barbiturates and acetaminophen are excreted in breast milk in small amounts, but the significance of their effects on nursing infants is not known. Because of potential for serious adverse reactions in nursing infants from butalbital and acetaminophen, a decision should be made whether to discontinue nursing or to discontinue the drug, taking into account the importance of the drug to the mother.

PEDIATRIC USE

Safety and effectiveness in children below the age of 12 have not been established.

DRUG INTERACTIONS:

The CNS effects of butalbital may be enhanced by monoamine oxidase (MAO) inhibitors.

Butalbital and acetaminophen may enhance the effects of: other narcotic analgesics, alcohol, general anesthetics, tranquilizers such as chlordiazepoxide, sedative-hypnotics, or other CNS depressants, causing increased CNS depression.

ADVERSE REACTIONS:

Frequently Observed: The most frequently reported adverse reactions are drowsiness, lightheadedness, dizziness, sedation, shortness of breath, nausea, vomiting, abdominal pain, and intoxicated feeling.

Infrequently Observed: All adverse events tabulated below are classified as infrequent.

Central Nervous: headache, shaky-feeling, tingling, agitation, fainting, fatigue, heavy eyelids, high energy, hot spells, numbness, sluggishness, seizure. Mental confusion, excitement or depression can also occur due to intolerance, particularly in elderly or debilitated patients, or due to overdosage of butalbital

Autonomic Nervous: dry mouth, hyperhidrosis

Gastrointestinal: difficulty swallowing, heartburn, flatulence, constipation

Cardiovascular: tachycardia

Musculoskeletal: leg pain, muscle fatigue

Genitourinary: diuresis

Miscellaneous: pruritus, fever, earache, nasal congestion, tinnitus, euphoria, allergic reactions

Several cases of dermatological reactions, including toxic epidermal necrolysis and erythema multiforme, have been reported.

The following adverse drug events may be borne in mind as potential effects of the components of this product. Potential effects of high dosage are listed in the OVERDOSAGE section.

Acetaminophen: allergic reactions, rash, thrombocytopenia, agranulocytosis

DRUG ABUSE AND DEPENDENCE:

Butalbital: *Barbiturates may be habit-forming.* Tolerance, psychological dependence, and physical dependence may occur especially following prolonged use of high doses of barbiturates. The average daily dose for the barbiturate addict is usually about 1500 mg. As tolerance to barbiturates develops, the amount needed to maintain the same level of intoxication increases; tolerance to a fatal dosage, however, does not increase more than two-fold. As this occurs, the margin between an intoxication dosage and fatal dosage becomes smaller. The lethal dose of a barbiturate is far less if alcohol is also ingested. Major withdrawal symptoms (convulsions and delirium) may occur within 16 hours and last up to 5 days after abrupt cessation of these drugs. Intensity of withdrawal symptoms gradually declines over a period of approximately 15 days. Treatment of barbiturate dependence consists of cautious and gradual withdrawal of the drug. Barbiturate-dependent patients can be withdrawn by using a number of different withdrawal regimens. One method involves initiating treatment at the patient's regular dosage level and gradually decreasing the daily dosage as tolerated by the patient.

OVERDOSAGE:

Following an acute overdosage of butalbital and acetaminophen, toxicity may result from the barbiturate or the acetaminophen.

Signs and Symptoms: Toxicity from barbiturate poisoning include drowsiness, confusion, coma; respiratory depression; hypotension;and hypovolemic shock.

In Acetaminophen Overdosage: dose-dependent, potentially fatal hepatic necrosis is the most serious adverse effect. Renal tubular necroses, hypoglycemic coma and thrombocytopenia may also occur. Early symptoms following a potentially hepatotoxic overdose may include: nausea, vomiting, diaphoresis and general malaise. Clinical and laboratory evidence of hepatic toxicity may not be apparent until 48 to 72 hours post-ingestion. In adults hepatic toxicity has rarely been reported with acute overdoses of less than 10 grams, or fatalities with less than 15 grams.

OVERDOSAGE: *(cont'd)*

Treatment: A single or multiple overdose with these combination products is a potentially lethal polydrug overdose, and consultation with a regional poison control center is recommended.

Immediate treatment includes support of cardiorespiratory function and measures to reduce drug absorption. Vomiting should be induced mechanically, or with syrup of ipecac, if the patient is alert (adequate pharyngeal and laryngeal reflexes). Oral activated charcoal (1 g/kg) should follow gastric emptying. The first dose should be accompanied by an appropriate cathartic. If repeated doses are used, the cathartic might be included with alternate doses as required. Hypotension is usually hypovolemic and should respond to fluids. Pressors should be avoided. A cuffed endotracheal tube should be inserted before gastric lavage of the unconscious patient and, when necessary, to provide assisted respiration. If renal function is normal, forced diuresis may aid in the elimination of the barbiturate. Alkalinization of the urine increases renal excretion of some barbiturates, especially phenobarbital.

Meticulous attention should be given to maintaining adequate pulmonary ventilation. In severe cases of intoxication, peritoneal dialysis, or preferably hemodialysis may be considered. If hypoprothrombinemia occurs due to acetaminophen overdose, vitamin K should be administered intravenously.

If the dose of acetaminophen may have exceeded 140 mg/kg, acetylcysteine should be administered as early as possible. Serum acetaminophen levels should be obtained, since levels four or more hours following ingestion help predict acetaminophen toxicity. Do not await acetaminophen assay results before initiating treatment. Hepatic enzymes should be obtained initially, and repeated at 24-hour intervals.

Methemoglobinemia over 30% should be treated with methylene blue by slow intravenous administration.

TOXIC DOSES FOR ADULTS

(Butalbital 50 mg and acetaminophen 325 mg tablets)

Butalbital: toxic dose 1 g (20 tablets)

Acetaminophen: toxic dose 10 g (30 tablets)

(Butalbital 50 mg and acetaminophen 650 mg capsules)

Butalbital: toxic dose 1 g (20 capsules)

Acetaminophen: toxic dose 10 g (15 capsules)

DOSAGE AND ADMINISTRATION:

Phrenilin: One or two tablets every four hours. Total daily dosage should not exceed 6 tablets.

Phrenilin Forte: One capsule every four hours. Total daily dosage should not exceed 6 capsules.

Extended and repeated use of these products is not recommended because of the potential for physical dependence.

Store at controlled room temperature, 15°-30°C (59°-86°F). Dispense in a tight container.

HOW SUPPLIED - RATED THERAPEUTICALLY EQUIVALENT:

Capsule, Gelatin - Oral - 650 mg/50 mg

100's	$22.20	TENCON, Intl Ethical	11584-1029-01
100's	**$24.70**	**PHRENILIN FORTE, Carnrick**	**00086-0056-10**
100's	$25.49	BUCET, UAD Labs	00785-2307-01
100's	$45.05	AXOCET, Savage Labs	00281-0198-17

Tablet, Uncoated - Oral - 325 mg/50 mg

100's	**$21.05**	**PHRENILIN, Carnrick**	**00086-0050-10**

Tablet, Uncoated - Oral - 650 mg/50 mg

100's	$24.50	BUPAP, Medi-Plex Pharm	59010-0240-01
100's	$28.80	Bupap, ECR Pharms	00095-0240-01
100's	$29.95	Repan-Cf, Everett Labs	00642-0166-10
100's	$33.00	SEDAPAP, Mayrand Pharms	00259-1278-01
100's	$41.60	GREATAB, Am Pharms	58605-0511-01
100's	$45.60	MIDRINOL, Am Pharms	58605-0514-01

HOW SUPPLIED - NOT RATED EQUIVALENT:

Capsule, Gelatin - Oral - 325 mg/50 mg

100's	$18.00	TRIAPRIN, Dunhall Pharms	00217-2811-01
500's	$80.00	TRIAPRIN, Dunhall Pharms	00217-2811-03

ACETAMINOPHEN; BUTALBITAL; CAFFEINE

(000021)

CATEGORIES: Analeptics; Analgesics; Analgesics/Antipyretics; Antimigraine/Other Headaches; Antipyretics; Central Nervous System Agents; Central Pain Syndromes; Headache; Pain; Sedatives/Hypnotics; Anesthesia*; DEA Class CIII; FDA Approved 1984 Nov

* Indication not approved by the FDA

BRAND NAMES: Algesic; Amaphen; Americet; Anolor 300; Anoquan; Apap W/ Caffeine & Butalbital; Butace; Butalbital/Apap/Caffeine; Butaphen; Dolmar; Endolor; Equi-Cet; Esgic; Esgic-Plus; Ezol; Fembutal; Femcet; **Fioricet**; Fiorpap; G-1; Geone; Ide-Cet; Isocet; Isopap; Margesic; Medigesic; Minotal; Mygracet; Pacaps; Pharmagesic; Repan; Rogesic; Tacet; Tencet; Triad; Two-Dyne

FORMULARIES: Aetna; BC-BS; FHP; PCS

DESCRIPTION:

***WARNING: May be habit forming** Each tablet for oral administration contains: butalbital*, USP: 50 mg; acetaminophen, USP: 325 mg; caffeine, USP: 40 mg.

Active Ingredients: Butalbital, USP; acetaminophen, USP; and caffeine, USP.

Fioricet Inactive Ingredients: Crospovidone, FD&C Blue #1, magnesium stearate, microcrystalline cellulose, povidone, pregelatinized starch, and stearic acid.

Butalbital, 5-allyl-5-isobutylbarbituric acid, a white, odorless, crystalline powder having a slightly bitter taste, is a short- to intermediate-acting barbiturate.

$C_{11}H_{16}N_2O_3$, Molecular weight 224.26

Acetaminophen, 4'-hydroxyacetanilide, is a non-opiate, non-salicylate analgesic, and antipyretic which occurs as a white, odorless, crystalline powder possessing a slightly bitter taste.

$C_8H_9NO_2$, Molecular weight 151.16.

Caffeine, 1,3,7-trimethylxanthine, is a central nervous system stimulant which occurs as a white powder or white glistening needles. It also has a bitter taste.

CLINICAL PHARMACOLOGY:

Pharmacologically, this drug combines the analgesic properties of acetaminophen-caffeine with the anxiolytic and muscle relaxant properties of butalbital.

INDICATIONS AND USAGE:

This drug is indicated for the relief of the symptoms complex of tension (or muscle contraction) headache.

CONTRAINDICATIONS:

Hypersensitivity to acetaminophen, caffeine or barbiturates. Patients with porphyria.

PRECAUTIONS:

GENERAL

Barbiturates should be administered with caution, if at all, to patients who are mentally depressed, have suicidal tendencies, or a history of drug abuse.

Elderly or debilitated patients may react to barbiturates with marked excitement, depression, and confusion. In some persons, barbiturates repeatedly produce excitement rather than depression.

INFORMATION FOR THE PATIENT

Practitioners should give the following information and instructions to patients receiving barbiturates:

A. The use of barbiturates carries with it an associated risk of psychological and/or physical dependence. The patient should be warned against increasing the dose of the drug without consulting a physician.

B. Barbiturates may impair mental and/or physical abilities required for the performance of potentially hazardous tasks (*e.g.,* driving, operating machinery, etc.).

C. Alcohol should not be consumed while taking barbiturates. Concurrent use of the barbiturates with other CNS depressants (*e.g.,* alcohol narcotics, tranquilizers, and antihistamines) may result in additional CNS depressant effects.

PREGNANCY

Adequate studies have not been performed in animals to determine whether this drug affects fertility in males or females, has teratogenic potentia,l or has other adverse effects on the fetus. There are no well-controlled studies in pregnant women. Although there is no clearly defined risk, one cannot exclude the possibility of infrequent or subtle damage to the human fetus. This drug should be used in pregnant women only when clearly needed.

NURSING MOTHERS

The effects of this drug on infants of nursing mothers are not known. Barbiturates are excreted in the breast milk of nursing mothers. The serum levels in infants are believed to be significant with therapeutic doses.

PEDIATRIC USE

Safety and effectiveness in children below the age of 12 have not been established.

DRUG INTERACTIONS:

Patients receiving narcotic analgesics, antipsychotics, antianxiety agents, or other CNS depressants (including alcohol) concomitantly with this drug may exhibit additive CNS depressant effects (TABLE 1).

TABLE 1

Drugs	Effect
Butalbital w/coumarin anticoagulants	Decreased effect of anticoagulant because of increased metabolism resulting from enzyme induction.
Butalbital w/tricyclic antidepressants	Decreased blood levels of the antidepressant.

ADVERSE REACTIONS:

The most frequent adverse reactions are drowsiness and dizziness. Less frequent adverse reactions are lightheadedness and gastrointestinal disturbances including nausea, vomiting, and flatulence. Mental confusion or depression can occur due to intolerance or overdosage of butalbital.

DRUG ABUSE AND DEPENDENCE:

Prolonged use of barbiturates can produce drug dependence, characterized by psychic dependence and tolerance. The abuse liability of this drug is similar to that of other barbiturate-containing drug combinations. Caution should be exercised when prescribing medication for patients with a known propensity for taking excessive quantities of drugs, which is not uncommon in patients with chronic tension headache.

OVERDOSAGE:

The toxic effects of acute overdosage of this drug are attributable mainly to its barbiturate component and, to a lesser extent, acetaminophen. Because toxic effects of caffeine occur in very high dosages only, the possibility of significant caffeine toxicity from this drug overdosage is unlikely.

BARBITURATE

Signs and Symptoms

Drowsiness; confusion; coma; respiratory depression; hypotension; shock.

Treatment

1. Maintenance of an adequate airway, with assisted respiration and oxygen administration as necessary.

2. Monitoring of vital signs and fluid balance.

3. If the patient is conscious and has not lost the gag reflex, emesis may be induced with ipecac. Care should be taken to prevent pulmonary aspiration of vomitus. After completion of vomiting, 30 g activated charcoal in a glass of water may be administered.

4. If emesis is contraindicated, gastric lavage may be performed with a cuffed endotracheal tube in place with the patient in the facedown position. Activated charcoal may be left in the emptied stomach and a saline cathartic administered.

5. Fluid therapy and other standard treatment of shock, if needed.

6. If renal function is normal, forced diuresis may aid in the elimination of the barbiturate. Alkalinization of the urine increases renal excretion of some barbiturates, especially phenobarbital.

7. Although not recommended as a routine procedure, hemodialysis may be used in severe barbiturate intoxication or if the patient is anuric or in shock.

ACETAMINOPHEN

Signs and Symptoms: In acute acetaminophen overdosage, dose dependent, potentially fatal hepatic necrosis is the most serious adverse effect. Renal tubular necrosis, hypoglycemic coma, and thrombocytopenia may also occur.

OVERDOSAGE: *(cont'd)*

In adults, hepatic toxicity has rarely been reported with acute overdoses of less than 10 g and fatalities with less than 15 g. Importantly, young children seem to be more resistant than adults to the hepatotoxic effect of an acetaminophen overdose.

Early Symptoms Following A Potentially Hepatotoxic Overdosage May Include: nausea, vomiting, diaphoresis, and general malaise. Clinical and laboratory evidence of hepatic toxicity may not be apparent until 48 to 72 hours postingestion.

Treatment:The stomach should be emptied promptly by lavage or by induction of emesis with syrup of ipecac. Patients' estimates of the quantity of a drug ingested are notoriously unreliable. Therefore, if an acetaminophen overdose is suspected, a serum acetaminophen assay should be obtained as early as possible, but no sooner than four hours following ingestion. Liver function studies should be obtained initially and repeated at 24-hour intervals.

The antidote N-acetylcysteine should be administered as early as possible, preferably within 16 hours of the overdose ingestion for optimal results, but in any case within 24 hours. Following recovery, there are no residual, structural, or functional hepatic abnormalities.

DOSAGE AND ADMINISTRATION:

One or 2 tablets every 4 hours as needed. Do not exceed 6 tablets per day.

Store and Dispense: Store below 86°F; dispense in a tight container.

HOW SUPPLIED - RATED THERAPEUTICALLY EQUIVALENT:

Capsule, Gelatin - Oral - 325 mg/50 mg/40

100's	$11.93	Butalbital/Apap/Caffeine, H.C.F.A. F F P	99999-0021-01
100's	$17.32	TWO-DYNE, Hyrex Pharms	00314-2229-01
100's	$21.10	MARGESIC, Marnel Pharceut	00682-0804-01
100's	$21.75	ALAGESIC, Poly Pharms	50991-0302-01
100's	$23.70	Butalbital/Apap/Caffeine, Qualitest Pharms	00603-2546-21
100's	$23.75	Geone, Alphagen Labs	59743-0004-01
100's	$25.65	MINOTAL, Bolan Pharm	44437-0343-01
100's	$28.08	REPAN, Everett Labs	00642-0164-10
100's	$35.95	TRIAD, UAD Labs	00785-2305-01
100's	$41.88	PACAPS, Lunsco	10892-0116-10
100's	$86.41	ESGIC, Gilbert Labs	00535-0012-01
500's	$59.65	Butalbital/Apap/Caffeine, H.C.F.A. F F P	99999-0021-02
1000's	$119.30	Butalbital/Apap/Caffeine, H.C.F.A. F F P	99999-0021-03

Tablet - Oral - 350/40/25 mg

100's	$14.00	APAP; Butalbital; Caffeine, Duramed Pharms	51285-0849-02
500's	$58.00	APAP; Butalbital; Caffeine, Duramed Pharms	51285-0849-04

Tablet, Uncoated - Oral - 325 mg/50 mg/40

100's	$4.50	Butalbital/Apap/Caffeine, H.C.F.A. F F P	99999-0021-04
100's	$5.40	Butalbital APAP & Caffeine, United Res	00677-1242-01
100's	$10.60	APAP/CAFFEINE/BUTALBITAL, Major Pharms	00904-3280-60
100's	$12.00	Butalbital/APAP/Caffeine, Qualitest Pharms	00603-2547-21
100's	$13.50	Tacet, Baucom Labs	54696-0513-01
100's	$13.75	Butalbital/Apap/Caffeine, Aligen Independ	00405-0026-01
100's	$13.89	Butalbital W/Apap & Caffeine, Parmed Pharms	00349-8793-01
100's	$13.90	Butalbital/Aceta./Caff., Schein Pharm (US)	00364-2297-01
100's	$14.32	Fiorpap, Geneva Pharms	50752-0275-05
100's	$14.40	Butalbital Apap & Caffeine, Halsey Drug	00879-0567-01
100's	$14.80	Isocet, Rugby	00536-5567-01
100's	$15.20	Butalbital/Aceta./Caff., Geneva Pharms	00781-1901-01
100's	$15.25	Butalbital/Apap/Caffeine, Teva	00093-0854-01
100's	$15.25	Butalbital Apap Caffeine, Goldline Labs	00182-1274-01
100's	$15.25	Butalbital Acetaminophen & Caffeine, Mikart	46672-0053-10
100's	$15.92	Butalbital/Apap/Caffeine, HL Moore Drug Exch	00839-7480-06
100's	$15.92	Butalbital CMPD w/ APAP & Caf, HL Moore Drug Exch	00839-7831-06
100's	$16.20	Butalbital/Aceta./Caff., Martec Pharms	52555-0079-01
100's	$17.21	Butalbital/Apap/Caffeine, Major Pharms	00904-3280-61
100's	$21.75	ALGESIC, Poly Pharms	50991-0300-01
100's	$27.04	REPAN, Everett Labs	00642-0162-10
100's	$33.80	EQUI-CET, Equipharm	57779-0111-04
100's	$41.00	AMERICET, Am Pharms	58605-0501-01
100's	**$49.68**	**FIORICET, Novartis**	**00078-0084-05**
100's	**$54.30**	**FIORICET, Novartis**	**00078-0084-06**
100's	$97.39	ESGIC, Forest Pharms	00456-0630-01
500's	$22.50	Butalbital/Apap/Caffeine, H.C.F.A. F F P	99999-0021-05
500's	$26.99	Butalbital/Apap/Caffeine, Balan	00304-1940-05
500's	$38.81	Butalbital/Aceta./Caff., HL Moore Drug Exch	00839-7480-12
500's	$43.95	Butalbital Apap & Caffeine, Halsey Drug	00879-0567-05
500's	$44.62	Butalbital/Apap/Caffeine, Aligen Independ	00405-0026-02
500's	$49.88	Butalbital W/Apap & Caffeine, Parmed Pharms	00349-8793-05
500's	$52.75	Butalbital/Aceta./Caff., Schein Pharm (US)	00364-2297-05
500's	$52.90	APAP/CAFFEINE/BUTALBITAL, Major Pharms	00904-3280-40
500's	$54.41	Butalbital/APAP/Caffeine, Qualitest Pharms	00603-2547-28
500's	$55.95	Isocet, Rugby	00536-5567-05
500's	$71.60	Fiorpap, Geneva Pharms	50752-0275-08
500's	$74.95	Butalbital Apap Caffeine, Goldline Labs	00182-1274-05
500's	$74.95	Butalbital/Aceta./Caff., Mikart	46672-0053-50
500's	$168.00	Equi-Cet, Equipharm	57779-0111-06
500's	**$237.42**	**FIORICET, Novartis**	**00078-0084-08**
500's	$445.15	ESGIC, Forest Pharms	00456-0630-02
1000's	$45.00	Butalbital/Apap/Caffeine, H.C.F.A. F F P	99999-0021-06
1000's	$89.77	Butalbital/Apap/Caffeine, Parmed Pharms	00349-8793-10
1000's	$118.50	Butalbital Apap & Caffeine, Halsey Drug	00879-0567-10

HOW SUPPLIED - NOT RATED EQUIVALENT:

Tablet, Uncoated - Oral - 500 mg/50 mg/40

100's	$73.34	ESGIC-PLUS, Forest Pharms	00456-0678-01
500's	$341.00	ESGIC-PLUS, Forest Pharms	00456-0678-02

ACETAMINOPHEN; BUTALBITAL; CAFFEINE; CODEINE PHOSPHATE *(000022)*

CATEGORIES: Analgesics; Antipyretics; Central Nervous System Agents; Opiate Agonists (Controlled); Pain; DEA Class CIII; FDA Approved 1992 Jul

BRAND NAMES: Amaphen W/Codeine; Ezol IIi; **Fioricet W/Codeine**

Prescribing information not available at time of publication.

HOW SUPPLIED - EQUIVALENTS NOT AVAILABLE:

Capsule, Gelatin - Oral - 30 mg

100's	$104.16	FIORICET WITH CODEINE #3, Novartis	00078-0243-05

ACETAMINOPHEN; CAFFEINE *(000025)*

CATEGORIES: Analgesics; Central Nervous System Agents

BRAND NAMES: *Claradol 500 Cafeine* (France); *Dexamol Plus*; *Head-O*; Migralan; *Oskadon*; *Panadol Extra*; *Paracetamol Plus-Ratiopharm* (Germany); *Picapan* *(International brand names outside U.S. in italics)*

Prescribing information not available at time of publication.

HOW SUPPLIED - EQUIVALENTS NOT AVAILABLE:

Capsule, Gelatin - Oral - 325 mg/100 mg/6

100's	$120.00	MIGRALAM, AJ Bart	49326-0116-90
500's	$504.00	MIGRALAM, AJ Bart	49326-0116-75

ACETAMINOPHEN; CAFFEINE; CODEINE PHOSPHATE; SALICYLIC ACID *(000027)*

CATEGORIES: Analgesics; Antipyretics; Central Nervous System Agents; Opiate Agonists (Controlled); Pain; DEA Class CIII; FDA Pre 1938 Drugs

BRAND NAMES: Codalan

Prescribing information not available at time of publication.

HOW SUPPLIED - EQUIVALENTS NOT AVAILABLE:

Tablet, Uncoated - Oral - 150 mg/30 mg/8

100's	$4.30	CODALAN NO 1, Lannett	00527-0903-01
500's	$13.50	CODALAN NO 1, Lannett	00527-0903-05
1000's	$26.00	CODALAN NO 1, Lannett	00527-0903-10

Tablet, Uncoated - Oral - 150 mg/30 mg/15

100's	$5.10	CODALAN NO 2, Lannett	00527-0904-01
500's	$21.30	CODALAN NO 2, Lannett	00527-0904-05
1000's	$38.00	CODALAN NO 2, Lannett	00527-0904-10

Tablet, Uncoated - Oral - 150 mg/30 mg/30

100's	$8.30	CODALAN NO 3, Lannett	00527-0905-01
500's	$35.50	CODALAN NO 3, Lannett	00527-0905-05
1000's	$71.00	CODALAN NO 3, Lannett	00527-0905-10

ACETAMINOPHEN; CHLORPHENIRAMINE MALEATE; CODEINE PHOSPHATE; PHENYLEPHRINE HYDROCHLORIDE *(000038)*

CATEGORIES: Antipyretics; Antitussives; Central Nervous System Agents; Common Cold; Cough Preparations; Opiate Agonists (Controlled); Respiratory & Allergy Medications; DEA Class CIII; FDA Pre 1938 Drugs

BRAND NAMES: Colrex Compound; Colrex-Compound

Prescribing information not available at time of publication.

ACETAMINOPHEN; CHLORPHENIRAMINE MALEATE; HYDROCODONE BITARTRATE; PHENYLEPHRINE HYDROCHLORIDE *(000036)*

CATEGORIES: Antitussives; Antitussives/Expectorants/Mucolytics; Common Cold; Congestion; Cough Preparations; Nasal Congestion; Respiratory & Allergy Medications; Respiratory Tract Infections; Pregnancy Category C; DEA Class CIII; FDA Pre 1938 Drugs

BRAND NAMES: **Hycomine Compound**

DESCRIPTION:

Hycomine compound tablets contain hydrocodone (dihydrocodeinone) bitartrate, a semi-synthetic centrally-acting narcotic antitussive; chlorpheniramine maleate, an antihistamine; phenylephrine hydrochloride, a sympathomimetic amine decongestant; acetaminophen, an analgesic/antipyretic; and caffeine, a centrally-acting stimulant, for oral administration.

Each hycomine compound tablet contains:

Hydrocodone bitartrate, USP... 5 mg

WARNING: May be habit forming

Chlorpheniramine maleate, USP 2 mg

Phenylephrine hydrochloride, USP 10 mg

Acetaminophen, USP 250 mg

Caffeine, anhydrous 30 mg

Hycomine Compound tablets also contain: cherry flavor, colloidal silicon dioxide, FD&C Red 40, magnesium stearate, microcrystalline cellulose, povidone and starch.

CLINICAL PHARMACOLOGY:

Clinical trials have proven hydrocodone bitartrate to be an effective antitussive agent which is pharmacologically 2 to 8 times as potent as codeine. At equi-effective doses, its sedative action is greater than codeine. The precise mechanism of action of hydrocodone and other opiates is not known, however, hydrocodone is believed to act by directly depressing the cough center. In excessive doses, hydrocodone, like other opium derivatives, will depress respiration. The effects of hydrocodone in therapeutic doses on the cardiovascular system is insignificant. The constipation effects of hydrocodone are much weaker than that of morphine and no stronger than that of codeine. Hydrocodone can produce miosis, euphoria, physical and psychological dependence. At therapeutic antitussive doses, it does exert analgesic effects. Following a 10 mg oral dose of hydrocodone administered to five adult male human subjects, the mean peak concentration was 23.6 ± 5.2 ng/ml. Maximum serum levels were achieved at 1.3 ± 0.3 hours and the half-life was determined to be 3.8 ± 0.3 hours. Hydrocodone exhibits a complex pattern of metabolism including O-demethylation, N-demethylation and 6-keto reduction to the corresponding 6-α-and 6-β-hydroxymetabolites.

Chlorpheniramine maleate is a competitive H_1-receptor histamine blocking drug, thereby counteracting the effects of histamine release associated with allergic manifestations of upper respiratory tract inflammatory disorders. H_1-blocking drugs inhibit the actions of histamine on smooth muscle, capillary permeability, and can both stimulate and depress the central nervous system. Phenylephrine hydrochloride effects its vasoconstrictor activity by releasing noradrenaline from sympathetic nerve endings, and from direct stimulation of α-adrenoreceptors in blood vessels. Acetaminophen is an antipyretic and peripherally acting analgesic. Caffeine is a central nervous system stimulant.

INDICATIONS AND USAGE:

Hycomine compound is indicated for the symptomatic relief of cough, nasal congestion, and discomfort associated with upper respiratory tract infections.

CONTRAINDICATIONS:

Hycomine compound is contraindicated in patients hypersensitive to any component of the drug, and concurrent MAO inhibitor therapy. Patients known to be hypersensitive to other opioids, antihistamines, or sympathomimetic amines may exhibit cross sensitivity with hycomine compound. Phenylephrine is contraindicated in patients with heart disease, hypertension, diabetes or hyperthyroidism. Hydrocodone is contraindicated in the presence of an intracranial lesion associated with increased intracranial pressure and whenever ventilatory function is depressed.

WARNINGS:

May be habit forming. Hydrocodone can produce drug dependence of the morphine type and therefore has the potential for being abused. Psychic dependence and tolerance may develop upon repeated administration of hycomine compound and it should be prescribed and administered with the same degree of caution appropriate to the use of other narcotic drugs. (See DRUG ABUSE AND DEPENDENCE.)

Respiratory Depression: Hycomine compound produces dose-related respiratory depression by directly acting on brain stem respiratory centers. If respiratory depression occurs, it may be antagonized by the use of naloxone HCl and other supportive measures when indicated.

Head Injury and Increased Intracranial Pressure: The respiratory depressant properties of narcotics and their capacity to elevate cerebrospinal fluid pressure may be markedly exaggerated in the presence of head injury, other intracranial lesions or a pre-existing increase in intracranial pressure. Furthermore, narcotics produce adverse reactions which may obscure the clinical course of patients with head injuries.

Acute Abdominal Conditions: The administration of hycomine compound or other narcotics may obscure the diagnosis or clinical course of patients with acute abdominal conditions.

Phenylephrine: Hypertensive crises can occur with concurrent use of phenylephrine and monoamine oxidase (MAO) inhibitors, indomethacin or with beta-blockers and methyldopa.

If a hypertensive crisis occurs these drugs should be discontinued immediately and therapy to lower blood pressure should be instituted immediately. Fever should be managed by means of external cooling.

Chlorpheniramine: Antihistamines may produce drowsiness or excitation, particularly in children and elderly patients.

PRECAUTIONS:

GENERAL

Before prescribing medication to suppress or modify cough, it is important to ascertain that the underlying cause of cough is identified, that modification of cough does not increase the risk of clinical or physiologic complications, and that appropriate therapy for the primary disease is provided.

Usage in Ambulatory Patients : Hydrocodone, like all narcotics, and antihistamines such as chlorpheniramine maleate, may impair the mental and/or physical abilities required for the performance of potentially hazardous tasks such as driving a car or operating machinery; phenylephrine may produce a rapid pulse, dizziness or palpitations; patients should be cautioned accordingly.

CARCINOGENESIS, MUTAGENESIS, AND IMPAIRMENT OF FERTILITY

Carcinogenicity, mutagenicity and reproduction studies have not been conducted with hycomine compound.

PREGNANCY CATEGORY C

Teratogenic Effects: Animal reproduction studies have not been conducted with hycomine compound. It is also not known whether this drug can cause fetal harm when administered to pregnant woman or can affect reproductive capacity. Hycomine compound should be given to a pregnant woman only if clearly needed.

Nonteratogenic Effects: Babies born to mothers who have been taking opioids regularly prior to delivery will be physically dependent.

The withdrawal signs include irritability and excessive crying, tremors, hyperactive reflexes, increased respiratory rate, increased stools, sneezing, yawning, vomiting and fever. The intensity of the syndrome does not always correlate with the duration of maternal opioid use of dose. Chlorpromazine 0.7-1.0 mg/kg q 6 h, phenobarbital 2 mg/kg q 6 h, and paregoric 2-4 drops/kg q 4 h, have been used to treat withdrawal symptoms in infants. The duration of therapy is 4 to 28 days, with the dosages decreased as tolerated.

NURSING MOTHERS

It is not known whether this drug is excreted in human milk. Because many drugs are excreted in human milk and because of the potential for serious adverse reactions in nursing infants from hycomine compound, a decision should be made whether to discontinue nursing or discontinue the drug, taking into account the importance of the drug to the mother.

PEDIATRIC USE

Safety and effectiveness in children below the age of 2 years have not been established.

DRUG INTERACTIONS:

Patients receiving other narcotic analgesics, general anesthetics, phenothiazines, other tranquilizers, sedative-hypnotics or other CNS depressants (including alcohol) concomitantly with hydrocodone may exhibit an additive CNS depression. When such combined therapy is contemplated, the dose of one or both agents should be reduced. The use of phenylephrine with other sympathomimetic amines and MAO inhibitors may produce an additive elevation of blood pressure. MAO inhibitors may prolong the anticholinergic effects of antihistamines (see WARNINGS.)

ADVERSE REACTIONS:

Respiratory System: Hydrocodone produces dose-related respiratory depression by acting directly on the brain stem respiratory centers.

Cardiovascular System: Hypertension, postural hypotension, tachycardia and palpitations.

Genitourinary System: Ureteral spasm, spasm of vesical sphincters and urinary retention have been reported with opiates.

Central Nervous System: Sedation, drowsiness, mental clouding, lethargy, impairment of mental and physical performance, anxiety, fear, dysphoria, dizziness, psychic dependence, mood changes, and blurred vision.

Gastrointestinal System: Nausea and vomiting occur more frequently in ambulatory than in recumbent patients.

DRUG ABUSE AND DEPENDENCE:

Special care should be exercised in prescribing hydrocodone for emotionally unstable patients and for those with a history of drug misuse. Such patients should be closely supervised when long-term therapy is contemplated.

Hycomine compound is a Schedule III narcotic. Psychic dependence, physical dependence, and tolerance may develop upon repeated administration of narcotics; therefore, this drug should always be prescribed and administered with caution. Physical dependence is the condition in which continued administration of the drug is required to prevent the appearance of a withdrawal syndrome.

Patients physically dependent on opioids will develop an abstinence syndrome upon abrupt discontinuation of the opioid following the administration of a narcotic antagonist. The character and severity of the withdrawal symptoms are related to the degree of physical dependence. Manifestations of opioid withdrawal are similar to but milder than that of morphine and include lacrimation, rhinorrhea, yawning, sweating, restlessness, dilated pupils, anorexia, gooseflesh, irritability and tremor. In more severe forms, nausea, vomiting, intestinal spasm and diarrhea, increased heart rate and blood pressure, chills, and pains in bones and muscles of the back and extremities may occur. Peak effects will usually be apparent at 48 to 72 hours.

Treatment of withdrawal is usually managed by providing sufficient quantities of an opioid to suppress severe withdrawal symptoms and then gradually reducing the dose of opioid over a period of several days.

OVERDOSAGE:

The signs and symptoms of overdosage of the individual components of hycomine compound may be modified in varying degrees by the presence of other active ingredients. Overdosage with phenylephrine alone may result in tremor, restlessness, increased motor activity, agitation and hallucinations.

ACETAMINOPHEN

Signs and Symptoms: In acute acetaminophen overdosage, dose-dependent, potentially fatal hepatic necrosis is the most serious adverse effect. Renal tubular necrosis, hypoglycemic coma and thrombocytopenia may also occur.

Acetaminophen in massive overdosage may cause hepatic toxicity in some patients. In cases of suspected overdose, you may wish to call your regional poison center for assistance in diagnosis and for directions in the use of N-acetylcysteine as an antidote.

In adults, hepatic toxicity has rarely been reported with acute overdoses of less than 10 grams and fatalities with less than 15 grams. Importantly, young children seem to be more resistant than adults to the hepatotoxic effect of an acetaminophen overdose. Despite this, the measures outlined below should be initiated in any adult or child suspected of having ingested an acetaminophen overdose.

Early symptoms following a potentially hepatotoxic overdose may include nausea, vomiting, diaphoresis and general malaise. Clinical and laboratory evidence of hepatic toxicity may not be apparent until 48 to 72 hours post-ingestion.

Treatment: The stomach should be emptied promptly by lavage or by induction of emesis with syrup of ipecac. Patient's estimates of the quantity of a drug ingested are notoriously unreliable. Therefore, if an acetaminophen overdose is suspected, a serum acetaminophen assay should be obtained as early as possible, but no sooner than four hours following ingestion. Liver function studies should be obtained initially and repeated at 24-hour intervals.

The antidote N-acetylcysteine should be administered as early as possible, preferably within 16 hours of the overdosage ingestions for optimal results, but in any case, within 24 hours. Following recovery, there are no residual structural or functional hepatic abnormalities.

HYDROCODONE

Signs and Symptoms: Serious overdosage with hydrocodone is characterized by respiratory depression (a decrease in respiratory rate and/or tidal volume, Cheyne-Stokes respiration, cyanosis), extreme somnolence progressing to stupor or coma, skeletal muscle flaccidity, cold and clammy skin, and sometimes bradycardia and hypotension. In severe overdosage apnea, circulatory collapse, cardiac arrest and death may occur.

Treatment: Primary attention should be given to the reestablishment of adequate respiratory exchange through a provision of a patent airway and the institution of assisted or controlled ventilation. The narcotic antagonist naloxone HCl is a specific antidote for respiratory depression which may result from overdosage or unusual sensitivity to narcotics including hydrocodone. Therefore an appropriate dose of naloxone HCl should be administered, preferably by the IV route simultaneously with efforts at respiratory resuscitation. For further information, see full prescribing information of naloxone HCl. An antagonist should not be administered in the absence of clinically significant respiratory depression. Oxygen, IV fluids, vasopressors and other supportive measures should be employed as indicated. Gastric emptying may be useful in removing unabsorbed drug. Activated charcoal may be of benefit.

DOSAGE AND ADMINISTRATION:

Usual dosage, not less than 4 hours apart:

Adults: 1 tablet 4 times a day.

Children: 6 to 12 years: 1/2 tablet 4 times a day.

Store at controlled room temperature (59° - 86°F, 15° - 30°C).

(DuPont Pharma 6015-14/Rev. 8/94)

HOW SUPPLIED - EQUIVALENTS NOT AVAILABLE:

Tablet, Uncoated - Oral - 250 mg/30 mg/2

100's	**$66.60**	**HYCOMINE COMPOUND, Dupont Pharma**	**00056-0048-70**
500's	**$293.70**	**HYCOMINE COMPOUND, Dupont Pharma**	**00056-0048-85**

ACETAMINOPHEN; CHLORPHENIRAMINE MALEATE; PHENYLEPHRINE HYDROCHLORIDE *(000045)*

CATEGORIES: Antihistamines; Antitussives/Expectorants/Mucolytics; Common Cold; Respiratory & Allergy Medications; FDA Pre 1938 Drugs

BRAND NAMES: Aclophen; Decongestant; Oragest-Td; Simplet

Prescribing information not available at time of publication.

HOW SUPPLIED - EQUIVALENTS NOT AVAILABLE:

Tablet, Coated, Sustained Action - Oral - 500 mg/8 mg/40

100's	$13.00	ACLOPHEN, Nutripharm Labs	51081-0831-10

ACETAMINOPHEN; CHLORPHENIRAMINE MALEATE; PHENYLPROPANOLAMINE *(000048)*

CATEGORIES: Allergies; Analgesics; Antihistamines; Common Cold; Cough Preparations; Nasal Congestion; Pain; Respiratory & Allergy Medications; FDA Pre 1938 Drugs

BRAND NAMES: *Acetacol*; Alumadrine; *Beaflu*; *Coldflu*; *Coldrex*; *Contracol*; *Coritab*; *Cortafrin* (Mexico); *Dupagen*; *Febricol*; *Fortaflu*; Histosal; *Neo-Bromexan Forte*; Norel Plus; Phenate; *Procold*; Sinapap; *Sinuzin-D*
(International brand names outside U.S. in italics)

Prescribing information not available at time of publication.

HOW SUPPLIED - EQUIVALENTS NOT AVAILABLE:

Tablet, Coated, Sustained Action - Oral - 325 mg/4 mg/40

100's	$22.00	SINAPAP, Bolan Pharm	44437-0283-01

Tablet, Uncoated - Oral - 500 mg/4 mg/25

100's	$10.50	HISTOSAL, Ferndale Labs	00496-0258-02
100's	$14.00	ALUMADRINE, Fleming	00256-0107-01
1000's	$128.25	ALUMADRINE, Fleming	00256-0107-02

ACETAMINOPHEN; CHLORZOXAZONE *(000050)*

CATEGORIES: Analgesics; Autonomic Drugs; DESI Drugs; Neuromuscular; Pain; Skeletal Muscle Hyperactivity; Skeletal Muscle Relaxants; FDA Pre 1938 Drugs

BRAND NAMES: Cetazone; Chlorofon-F; *Clorxafen*; Chlorzoxacet-F; *Duodil*; Eze-Ds; Flexaphen; Flextra; *Flogodisten*; *Fukiton*; Lobac; Miflex; *Myolgin*; Panflex; *Paraflex Spezial* (Germany); *Parafon*; *Parafon Forte* (Canada, Mexico); Paragen-Forte; *Paras*; Pyregesic Forte; Q-Zon; *Relaxin-P*; Rofon Forte; Saroflex; Skelex; *Solaxit* (Japan); Spasgesic; *Zafor*
(International brand names outside U.S. in italics)

Prescribing information not available at time of publication.

HOW SUPPLIED - EQUIVALENTS NOT AVAILABLE:

Tablet, Uncoated - Oral - 300 mg/250 mg

100's	$18.39	Chlorzoxazone W/Acetaminophen, Voluntary Hosp	53258-0177-13
200's	$19.50	Chlorzoxazone W/Acetaminophen, Voluntary Hosp	53258-0177-14
1000's	$29.38	CHLOROFON-F, Rugby	00536-3450-10

ACETAMINOPHEN; CODEINE PHOSPHATE *(000051)*

CATEGORIES: Analgesics; Antianxiety Drugs; Antipsychotics/Antimanics; Antipyretics; Central Nervous System Agents; Dental; Narcotics, Synthetics & Combinations; Opiate Agonists (Controlled); Pain; Sedatives/Hypnotics; Common Cold*; Fever*; Hay Fever*; Headache*; Influenza*; Migraine*; Pruritus*; Sinus Congestion*; Sinusitis*; Pregnancy Category C; DEA Class CIII; DEA Class CV; Sales > $100 Million; FDA Approval Pre 1982; Top 200 Drugs
* Indication not approved by the FDA

BRAND NAMES: APAP W/Codeine; Acetaminophen W/Codeine; *Algesidal* (France); *Atasol*; *Claradol Codeine* (France); *Codabrol*; *Cod-Acamol Forte*; *Codalgin* (Australia); *Codapane* (Australia); Codaphen; *Codicet*; *Codisal*; *Codisal Forte*; *Codoliprane* (France); *Codral Pain Relief* (Australia); *Cosutone*; *Dafalgan Codeine* (France); *Dolorol Forte*; *Dymadon Co* (Australia); *Dymadon Forte* (Australia); Empracet W/Codeine Phosphate; *Liquigesic Co* (Australia); Margesic; *Maxadol*; *Medocodene*; *Migraleve Yellow*; Myapap And Codeine; *Paceco*; *Panadeine*; *Panadeine Co*; *Panadeine Forte* (Australia); *Panadiene* (Australia, Japan); *Panado-Co*; *Panado-Co Caplets*; *Panamax* (Australia); *Paracod*; *Paracodol*; *Paradine*; *Parake*; Phenaphen W/Codeine; Proval #3; Pyregesic-C; *Rockamol Plus*; *Sunetheton*; *Tricoton*; Ty-Deine; Ty-Pap W/Codeine; Ty-Tab W/Codeine; Tylagesic 3; **Tylenol W Codeine**; *Tylenol W/Codeine No. 4* (Canada); *Tylex CD* (Mexico)
(International brand names outside U.S. in italics)

FORMULARIES: Aetna; BC-BS; CIGNA; DoD; FHP; Humana; Kaiser; Medco; Medi-Cal; PCS; PruCare; United

COST OF THERAPY: $6.75 (Pain; Tablet; 300 mg/30 mg; 4/day; 25 days)

DESCRIPTION:

Acetaminophen, 4'-hydroxyacetanilide, is a non-opiate, non-salicylate analgesic and antipyretic which occurs as a white, odorless, crystalline powder, possessing a slightly bitter taste. It has the following structural formula:

$C_8H_9NO_2$, with a molecular meight of 151.16

Codeine is an alkaloid, obtained from opium or prepared from morphine by methylation. Codeine phosphate occurs as fine, white, needle-shaped crystals, or white, crystalline powder. It is affected by light. Its chemical name is: 7,8-didehydro-4,5α-epoxy-3-methoxy-17-methylmorphinan-6α-ol phosphate (1:1) (salt) hemihydrate. It has the following molecular formula: $C_{18}H_{21}NO_3 \cdot H_3PO_4 \cdot 1/2H_2O$ with a molecular weight of 406.37

TABLETS AND ELIXIR

Each Tylenol with codeine tablet contains:

No. 2 codeine phosphate*... 15 mg

Acetaminophen... 300 mg

No. 3 codeine phosphate*... 30 mg

Acetaminophen... 300 mg

No. 4 codeine phosphate*... 60 mg

Acetaminophen... 300 mg

Each 5 ml of Tylenol with codeine elixir contains:

Codeine phosphate* 12 mg

Acetaminophen 120 mg

Alcohol 7%

* *Warning:* may be habit forming.

DESCRIPTION: *(cont'd)*

Tylenol Inactive Ingredients: tablets–powdered cellulose, magnesium stearate, sodium metabisulfite†, pregelatinized starch, starch (corn); elixir–alcohol, citric acid, propylene glycol, sodium benzoate, saccharin sodium, sucrose, natural and artificial flavors, FD&C Yellow #6.

†See WARNINGS.

CAPSULES

Each Phenaphen w/codeine No. 2 capsule contains:

Acetaminophen, USP... 325 mg

Codeine phosphate, USP... 15 mg

*Warning: may be habit forming.

Phenaphen Inactive Ingredients: Corn starch, FD&C Yellow #10, edible ink, FD&C Blue #1, FD&C Red #40, FD&C Yellow #6, gelatin, magnesium stearate, sodium starch glycolate, stearic acid.

Each Phenaphen w/codeine No. 3 capsule contains:

Acetaminophen, USP... 325 mg

Codeine phosphate, USP... 30 mg

Warning: may be habit forming.

Phenaphen Inactive Ingredients: FD&C Yellow #10, edible ink, FD&C Blue #1, (FD&C Green #3 and Red #40), FD&C Yellow #6, gelatin, magnesium stearate, sodium starch glycolate, stearic acid.

Each Phenaphen w/codeine No. 4 capsule contains:

Acetaminophen, USP... 325 mg

Codeine phosphate, USP... 60 mg

Warning: may be habit forming.

Phenaphen Inactive Ingredients: Corn starch, FD&C Yellow #10, edible ink, FD&C Green #3 or Blue #1, FD&C Yellow #6, gelatin, lactose, magnesium stearate, sodium starch glycolate stearic acid.

CLINICAL PHARMACOLOGY:

Acetaminophen and codeine phosphate tablets, oral solution USP, and capsules, combine the analgesic effects of a centrally acting analgesic, codeine, with a peripherally acting analgesic, acetaminophen.

PHARMACOKINETICS

The behavior of the individual components is described below.

Codeine: Codeine is readily absorbed from the gastrointestinal tract. It is rapidly distribued from the intravascular spaces to the various body tissues, with preferential uptake by parenchymatous organs such as the liver, spleen, and kidney. Codeine crosses the blood-brain barrier, and is found in fetal tissue and breast milk. The plasma concentration does not correlate with brain concentration or relief of pain; however, codeine is not bound to plasma proteins and does not accumulate in body tissues.

The plasma half-life is about 2.9 hours. The elimination of codeine is primarily via the kidneys, and about 90% of an oral dose is excreted by the kidneys within 24 hours of dosing. The urinary secretion products consist of free and glucuronide conjugated codeine (about 70%), free and conjugated norcodeine (about 10%), free and conjugated morphine (about 10%), normorphine (4%), and hydrocodone(1%). The remainder of the dose is excreted in the feces.

At therapeutic doses, the analgesic effect reaches a peak within 2 hours and persists between 4 and 6 hours. (See OVERDOSAGEfor toxicity information.)

Acetaminophen: Acetaminophen is rapidly absorbed from the gastrointestinal tract and is distributed throughout most body tissues. The plasma half-life is 1.5 to 3 hours, but may be increased by liver damage and following overdosage. Elimination of acetaminophen is principally by liver metabolism (conjugation) and subsequent renal excretion of metabolites. Approximately 85% of an oral dose appears in the urine within 24 hours of administration, most as the glucuronide conjugate, with small amounts of other conjugates and unchanged drug. (See OVERDOSAGE for toxicity information.)

INDICATIONS AND USAGE:

Acetaminophen and codeine phosphate tablets and capsules are indicated for the relief of mild to moderately severe pain.

Acetaminophen and codeine phosphate oral solution USP is indicated for the relief of mild to moderate pain.

CONTRAINDICATIONS:

Acetaminophen and codeine phosphate tablets, oral solution USP, or capsules, should not be administered to patients who have previously exhibited hypersensitivity to any component.

WARNINGS:

Acetaminophen and codeine phosphate tablets contain sodium metabisulfite, a sulfite that may cause allergic-type reactions including anaphylactic symptoms and life-threatening or less severe asthmatic episodes in certain susceptible people. The overall prevalence of sulfite sensitivity in the general population is unknown and probably low. Sulfite sensitivity is seen more frequently in asthmatic than in nonasthmatic people.

In the presence of head injury or other intracranial lesions, the respiratory depressant effects of codeine and other narcotics may be markedly enhanced, as well as their capacity for elevating cerebral spinal fluid pressure. Narcotics also produce other CNS depressant effects, such as drowsiness, that may further obscure the clinical course of patients with head injuries.

Codeine or other narcotics may obscure signs on which to judge the diagnosis or clinical course of patients with acute abdominal conditions.

Codeine is habit forming and potentially abusable. Consequently, the extended use of this product is not recommended.

PRECAUTIONS:

GENERAL

Head Injury and Increased Intracranial Pressure: The respiratory depressant effects of narcotics and their capacity to elevate cerebrospinal fluid pressure may be markedly exaggerated in the presence of head injury other intracranial lesions or a pre-existing increase in intracranial pressure. Furthermore, narcotics produce adverse reactions which may obscure the clinical course of patients with head injuries.

Acute Abdominal Conditions: The administration of this product or other narcotics may obscure the diagnosis or clinical course of patients with acute abdominal conditions.

Special Risk Patients: This drug should be given with caution to certain patients such as the elderly or debilitated, and those with severe impairment of hepatic or renal function, hypothyroidism, Addison's disease, and prostatic hypertrophy or urethral stricture.

PRECAUTIONS: *(cont'd)*

INFORMATION FOR THE PATIENT

Codeine may impair the mental and/or physical abilities required for the performance of potentially hazardous tasks such as driving a car or operating machinery. The patient using this drug should be cautioned accordingly.

The patient should understand the single-dose and 24-hour dose limits, and the time interval between doses.

Alcohol and other CNS depressants may produce an additive CNS depression when taken with this combination product and should be avoided.

Codeine may be habit forming. Patients should take the drug only for as long as it is prescribed, in the amounts prescribed, and no more frequently than prescribed.

CARCINOGENESIS, MUTAGENESIS, AND IMPAIRMENT OF FERTILITY

No long-term studies in animals have been performed with acetaminophen or codeine to determine carcinogenic potential or effects on fertility.

Acetaminophen and codeine have been found to have no mutagenic potential using the Ames Salmonella-Microsomal Activation test, the Basc test on Drosophila germ cells, and the Micronucleus test on mouse bone marrow.

PREGNANCY CATEGORY C

Teratogenic Effects: *Codeine:* A study in rats and rabbits reported no teratogenic effect of codeine administered during the period of organogenesis in doses ranging from 5 to 120 mg/kg. In the rat, doses at the 120 mg/kg level, in the toxic range for the adult animal, were associated with an increase in embryo resorption at the time of implantation. In another study a single 100 mg/kg dose of codeine administered to pregnant mice reportedly resulted in delayed ossification in the offspring.

There are no studies in humans, and the significance of these findings to humans, if any, is not known.

Acetaminophen and codeine phosphate tablets, oral solution USP, or capsules, should be used during pregnancy only if the potential benefit justifies the potential risk to the fetus.

Nonteratogenic Effects: Dependence has been reported in newborns whose mothers took opiates regularly during pregnancy. Withdrawal signs include irritability, excessive crying, tremors, hyperreflexia, fever, vomiting, and diarrhea. These signs usually appear during the first few days of life.

LABOR AND DELIVERY

Narcotic analgesics cross the placental barrier. The closer to delivery and the larger the dose used, the greater the possibility of respiratory depression in the newborn. Narcotic analgesics should be avoided during labor if delivery of a premature infant is anticipated. If the mother has received narcotic analgesics during labor, newborn infants should be observed closely for signs of respiratory depression. Resuscitation may be required (see OVERDOSAGE.) The effect of codeine, if any, on the later growth, development, and functional maturation of the child is unknown.

NURSING MOTHERS

Some studies have reported detectable amounts of codeine in breast milk. The levels are probably not clinically significant after usual therapeutic dosage. The possibility of clinically important amounts being excreted in breast milk in individuals abusing codeine should be considered.

PEDIATRIC USE

Safe dosage of acetaminophen and codeine phosphate oral solution USP has not been established in children below the age of three years.

DRUG INTERACTIONS:

Patients receiving other narcotic analgesics, antipsychotics, antianxiety agents, or other CNS depressants (including alcohol) concomitantly with this drug may exhibit an additive CNS depression. When such combined therapy is contemplated, the dose of one or both agents should be reduced.

The concurrent use of anticholinergics with codeine may produce paralytic ileus.

ADVERSE REACTIONS:

The most frequently observed adverse reactions include lightheadedness, dizziness, sedation, shortness of breath, nausea, and vomiting. These effects seem to be more prominent in ambulatory than in non-ambulatory patients, and some of these adverse reactions may be alleviated if the patient lies down. Other adverse reactions include allergic reactions, euphoria, dysphoria, constipation, abdominal pain, and pruritus.

At higher doses, codeine has most of the disadvantages of morphine including respiratory depression.

DRUG ABUSE AND DEPENDENCE:

Acetaminophen and codeine phosphate tablets and capsules are a Schedule III controlled substance.

Acetaminophen with codeine phosphate oral solution USP is a Schedule V controlled substance.

Codeine can produce drug dependence of the morphine type and, therefore, has the potential for being abused. Psychic dependence, physical dependence, and tolerance may develop upon repeated administration of this drug, and it should be prescribed and administered with the same degree of caution appropriate to the use of other oral narcotic-containing medications.

OVERDOSAGE:

ACETAMINOPHEN

Signs and Symptoms: In acute acetaminophen overdosage, dose-dependent, potentially fatal hepatic necrosis is the most serious adverse effect. Renal tubular necrosis, hypoglycemic coma, and thrombocytopenia may also occur.

In adults, hepatic toxicity has rarely been reported with acute overdoses of less than 10 g and fatalities with less than 15 g. Importantly, young children seem to be more resistant than adults to the hepatotoxic effect of an acetaminophen overdose. Despite this, the measures outlined below should be initiated in any adult or child suspected of having ingested an acetaminophen overdose.

Early symptoms following a potentially hepatotoxic overdose may include: nausea, vomiting, diaphoresis, and general malaise. Clinical and laboratory evidence of hepatic toxicity may not be apparent until 48 to 72 hours postingestion.

Treatment: The stomach should be emptied promptly by lavage or by induction of emesis with syrup of ipecac. Patients' estimates of the quantity of a drug ingested are notoriously unreliable. Therefore, if an acetaminophen overdose is suspected, a serum acetaminophen assay should be obtained as early as possible, but no sooner than four hours following ingestion. Liver function studies should be obtained initially and repeated at 24-hour intervals.

The antidote, N-acetylcysteine, should be administered as early as possible, preferably within 16 hours of the overdose ingestion for optimal results, but in any case, within 24 hours. Following recovery, there are no residual, structural or functional hepatic abnormalities.

OVERDOSAGE: *(cont'd)*

CODEINE

Signs and Symptoms: Serious overdose with codeine is characterized by respiratory depression (a decrease in respiratory rate and/or tidal volume, Cheyne-Stokes respiration, cyanosis), extreme somnolence progressing to stupor or coma, skeletal muscle flaccidity, cold and clammy skin, and sometimes bradycardia and hypotension. In severe overdosage, apnea, circulatory collapse, cardiac arrest, and death may occur. Toxicity from codeine poisoning includes the opioid triad of: pinpoint pupils, depression of respiration, and loss of consciousness. Convulsions may occur.

Treatment: Meticulous attention should be given to maintaining adequate pulmonary ventilation. In severe cases of intoxication, peritoneal dialysis, or preferably hemodialysis may be considered. If hypoprothrombinemia occurs due to acetaminophen overdose, vitamin K should be administered intravenously. The narcotic antagonist naloxone is a specific antidote against respiratory depression which may result from overdosage or unusual sensitivity to narcotics, including codeine. Therefore, an appropriate dose of naloxone hydrochloride should be administered, preferably by the intravenous route, and simultaneously with efforts at respiratory resuscitation. Since the duration of action of codeine may exceed that of the antagonist, the patient should be kept under continued surveillance and repeated doses of the antagonist should be administered as needed to maintain adequate respiration.

An antagonist should not be administered in the absence of clinically significant respiratory or cardiovascular depression. Oxygen, intravenous fluids, vasopressors, and other supportive measures should be employed as indicated.

Gastric emptying may be useful in removing unabsorbed drug.

DOSAGE AND ADMINISTRATION:

TABLETS AND CAPSULES

Dosage should be adjusted according to severity of pain and response of the patient. It should be kept in mind, however, that tolerance to codeine can develop with continued use and that the incidence of untoward effects is dose related. Adult doses of codeine higher than 60 mg fail to give commensurate relief of pain but merely prolong analgesia and are associated with an appreciably increased incidence of undesirable side effects. Equivalently high doses in children would have similar effects.

TABLE 1 Usual Adult Dosage

	Single Doses (Range)	Maximum 24 Hour Dose
Codeine Phosphate	15 mg - 60 mg	360 mg
Acetaminophen	300 mg - 1000 mg	4000 mg

Doses may be repeated up to every 4 hours.

The prescriber must determine the number of tablets or capsules per dose and the maximum number of tablets or capsules per 24 hours based upon the above dosage guidance. This information should be conveyed in the prescription.

For children, the single dose of codeine phosphate is 0.5 mg/kg. This dose may be repeated up to every 4 hours.

ELIXIR

Acetaminophen and codeine phosphate oral solution USP contains 120 mg of acetaminophen and 12 mg of codeine phosphate/5 ml and is given orally.

The usual doses are:

Children: *7 to 12 Years:* 10 ml (2 teaspoonfuls) 3 or 4 times daily. *3 to 6 Years:* 5 ml (1 teaspoonful) 3 or 4 times daily. *Under 3 Years:* Safe dosage has not been established.

Adults: 15 ml (1 tablespoonful) every 4 hours as needed.

STORAGE

Tablets, Elixir, and Capsules: Dispense in tight, light-resistant container.

Capsules: Store at controlled room temperature between 15° C and 30° C (59° F and 86° F).

PATIENT INFORMATION:

Acetaminophen with codeine is used for the relief of moderate to severe pain. Inform your physican if you are pregnant or nursing. This medication may cause dizziness, drowsiness, or blurred vision; use caution while driving or operating hazardous machinery. Do not take any other sedating drugs or drink alcohol while taking acetaminophen with codeine. This medication may be habit forming. Withdrawal symptoms may occur after you stop taking it. Inform your physician if shortness of breath or breathing difficulty occur. May cause nausea, vomiting or constipation; notify your physician if these occur. May be taken with food if gastrointestinal upset occurs.

HOW SUPPLIED - RATED THERAPEUTICALLY EQUIVALENT:

Elixir - Oral - 120 mg/12 mg/5m

5 ml x 100	$46.59	Acetaminophen w/Codeine, Roxane	00054-8013-04
12.5 ml x 100	$50.55	Acetaminophen w/Codeine, Roxane	00054-8002-04
15 ml x 100	$53.24	Acetaminophen w/Codeine, Roxane	00054-8017-04
118 ml	$5.30	APAP w/Codeine, Goldline Labs	00182-1078-37
120 ml	$2.25	APAP w/Codeine, Rugby	00536-0082-97
120 ml	$3.74	Acetaminophen W/Codeine, Morton Grove	60432-0245-04
120 ml	$3.80	Acetaminophen w/Codeine, Alpharma	00472-1419-04
120 ml	$3.98	Acetaminophen w/Codeine, HL Moore Drug Exch	00839-6786-65
480 ml	$11.39	Acetaminophen w/Codeine, Balan	00304-2007-98
480 ml	$12.06	Acetaminophen w/Codeine, Qualitest Pharms	00603-1020-58
480 ml	$12.63	Acetaminophen W/Codeine, Mikart	46672-0561-16
480 ml	$12.95	APAP w/Codeine, Schein Pharm (US)	00364-7207-16
480 ml	$12.95	APAP & Codeine, Geneva Pharms	00781-6052-16
480 ml	$13.20	Acetaminophen W/Codeine, Morton Grove	60432-0245-16
480 ml	$13.25	Acetaminophen W/Codeine, Major Pharms	00904-7775-16
480 ml	$13.35	Acetaminophen w/Codeine, HL Moore Drug Exch	00839-6786-69
480 ml	$13.50	APAP w/Codeine, Rugby	00536-0082-85
480 ml	$13.50	APAP w/Codeine, United Res	00677-0996-33
480 ml	$14.00	Acetaminophen w/Codeine, Alpharma	00472-1419-16
480 ml	$14.10	APAP w/Codeine, Goldline Labs	00182-1078-40
480 ml	$14.10	Acetaminophen W/Codeine, Aligen Independ	00405-0012-16
480 ml	$18.75	CAPITAL W/CODEINE, Carnrick	00086-0046-16
480 ml	$47.57	TYLENOL W/CODEINE, McNeil Lab	00045-0508-16
500 ml	$19.13	Acetaminophen w/Codeine, Roxane	00054-3005-63
3840 ml	$67.47	Acetaminophen w/Codeine, Balan	00304-2007-99
3840 ml	$80.76	APAP w/Codeine, Rugby	00536-0082-90
3840 ml	$83.60	Acetaminophen w/Codeine, Alpharma	00472-1419-28
3840 ml	$84.60	TY-PAP W/CODEINE, Major Pharms	00904-0173-28
3840 ml	$84.60	Acetaminophen W/Codeine, Major Pharms	00904-7775-28

Tablet, Uncoated - Oral - 300 mg/15 mg

100's	$4.43	Acetaminophen w/Codeine, H.C.F.A. F F P	99999-0051-01
100's	$6.45	Acetaminophen w/Codeine, Halsey Drug	00879-0051-01
100's	$7.50	Acetaminophen 300, Major Pharms	00904-0571-60
100's	$7.56	Acetaminophen w/Codeine, Qualitest Pharms	00603-2337-21

HOW SUPPLIED - RATED THERAPEUTICALLY EQUIVALENT: *(cont'd)*

100's	$7.85	Acetaminophen W/Codeine, Vintage Pharms	00254-2063-28
100's	$7.95	APAP/Codeine Phosphate 300, Harber Pharm	51432-0476-03
100's	$8.13	APAP w/Codeine, Schein Pharm (US)	00364-0323-01
100's	$8.20	Acetaminophen w/Codeine, Teva	00093-0050-01
100's	$8.20	APAP w/Codeine, Rugby	00536-3228-01
100's	$8.20	Acetaminophen w/Codeine, United Res	00677-0611-01
100's	$8.20	Acetaminophen & Codeine, Mutual Pharm	53489-0159-01
100's	$8.22	Acetaminophen w/Codeine No. 2, HL Moore Drug Exch	00839-6717-06
100's	$9.43	Acetaminophen & Codeine Phosphate, Aligen Independ	00405-0007-01
100's	$27.55	TYLENOL W/CODEINE NO.2, McNeil Lab	00045-0511-60
500's	$22.15	Acetaminophen w/Codeine, H.C.F.A. F F P	99999-0051-02
500's	$29.80	Acetaminophen With Codeine Phosphate, Halsey Drug	00879-0051-05
500's	$32.80	Acetaminophen w/Codeine, United Res	00677-0611-05
500's	$32.80	Acetaminophen & Codeine, Mutual Pharm	53489-0159-05
500's	$138.35	TYLENOL W/CODEINE NO.2, McNeil Lab	00045-0511-72
1000's	$44.30	Acetaminophen w/Codeine, H.C.F.A. F F P	99999-0051-03
1000's	$45.74	Acetaminophen With Codeine Phosphate, Halsey Drug	00879-0051-10
1000's	$55.10	Acetaminophen w/Codeine, Teva	00093-0050-10
1000's	$55.20	Acetaminophen 300, Major Pharms	00904-0571-80
1000's	$57.30	APAP w/Codeine, Rugby	00536-3228-10

Tablet, Uncoated - Oral - 300 mg/30 mg

30's	$6.79	Acetaminophen W/Codeine, Talbert Phcy	44514-0223-18
50's	$11.32	Acetaminophen W/Codeine, Talbert Phcy	44514-0223-33
100's	$6.75	Acetaminophen w/Codeine, H.C.F.A. F F P	99999-0051-04
100's	$7.50	Aceta w/Codeine, Century Pharms	00436-0182-01
100's	$8.00	Acetaminophen w/Codeine, Halsey Drug	00879-0052-01
100's	$8.96	Acetaminophen w/Codeine, Qualitest Pharms	00603-2338-21
100's	$9.00	Acetaminophen & Codeine, Mutual Pharm	53489-0160-01
100's	$9.57	Acetaminophen & Codeine, HL Moore Drug Exch	00839-6245-06
100's	$9.87	Acetaminophen W/Codeine, Amer Preferred	53445-0948-01
100's	$9.90	Acetaminophen W/Codeine, Vintage Pharms	00254-2064-28
100's	$9.90	APAP/Codeine Phosphate 300, Major Pharms	00904-0175-60
100's	$10.00	Acetaminophen w/Codeine, United Res	00677-0612-01
100's	$10.13	Acetaminophen w/Codeine No.3, Purepac Pharm	00228-2001-10
100's	$10.81	Acetaminophen w/Codeine, Geneva Pharms	00781-1752-01
100's	$11.75	Acetaminophen w/Codeine, Geneva Pharms	00781-1752-13
100's	$11.76	APAP/Codeine Phosphate 300, Aligen Independ	00405-0008-01
100's	$12.25	APAP w/Codeine, Rugby	00536-3227-01
100's	$12.60	Acetaminophen w/Codeine, Teva	00093-0150-01
100's	$12.60	APAP w/Codeine, Goldline Labs	00182-0948-01
100's	$12.60	APAP w/Codeine, Schein Pharm (US)	00364-0324-01
100's	$13.35	Acetaminophen & Codeine, Roxane	00054-8022-25
100's	$15.75	Acetaminophen & Codeine, Medirex	57480-0500-01
100's	$16.25	Ty-Tab W/Codeine, Major Pharms	00904-0175-61
100's	$17.80	APAP w/Codeine, Goldline Labs	00182-0948-89
100's	$18.24	Acetaminophen/Codeine #3, Vangard Labs	00615-0430-13
100's	$18.24	Acetaminophen & Codeine #3, Vangard Labs	00615-0430-47
100's	$20.25	Acetaminophen & Codeine, Roxane	00054-8022-24
100's	$29.95	TYLENOL W/CODEINE NO.3, McNeil Lab	00045-0513-60
250's	$35.21	Acetaminophen w/Codeine, Roxane	00054-8022-11
500's	$33.75	Acetaminophen w/Codeine, H.C.F.A. F F P	99999-0051-05
500's	$40.05	Acetaminophen w/Codeine, United Res	00677-0612-05
500's	$40.05	Acetaminophen & Codeine, Mutual Pharm	53489-0160-05
500's	$40.10	Acetaminophen With Codeine Phosphate, Halsey Drug	00879-0052-05
500's	$129.59	TYLENOL W/CODEINE NO.3, McNeil Lab	00045-0513-70
500's	$142.67	TYLENOL W/CODEINE NO.3, McNeil Lab	00045-0513-72
600's	$99.80	Acetaminophen & Codeine, Medirex	57480-0500-06
750's	$124.76	Acetaminophen W/Codeine, Glasgow Pharm	60809-0506-55
750's	$124.76	Acetaminophen W/Codeine, Glasgow Pharm	60809-0506-72
1000's	$10.50	Acetaminophen & Codeine Phosphate, Harber Pharm	51432-0478-03
1000's	$41.95	Tylagesic 3, H & H Labs	46703-0037-10
1000's	$58.80	PYREGESIC-C, C O Truxton	00463-6278-10
1000's	$66.40	APAP/Codeine Phosphate 300, Major Pharms	00904-0175-80
1000's	$66.88	APAP/Codeine Phosphate 300, Aligen Independ	00405-0008-03
1000's	$67.50	Acetaminophen w/Codeine, H.C.F.A. F F P	99999-0051-06
1000's	$70.25	Acetaminophen w/Codeine, Halsey Drug	00879-0052-10
1000's	$70.88	Acetaminophen w/Codeine, Qualitest Pharms	00603-2338-32
1000's	$72.00	Aceta w/Codeine, Century Pharms	00436-0182-10
1000's	$74.40	Acetaminophen W/Codeine, Vintage Pharms	00254-2064-38
1000's	$74.90	Acetaminophen w/Codeine, United Res	00677-0612-10
1000's	$74.90	Acetaminophen & Codeine, Mutual Pharm	53489-0160-10
1000's	$74.99	Acetaminophen & Codeine, HL Moore Drug Exch	00839-6245-16
1000's	$76.54	Acetaminophen w/Codeine No.3, Purepac Pharm	00228-2001-96
1000's	$81.98	Acetaminophen w/Codeine, Geneva Pharms	00781-1752-10
1000's	$89.95	APAP w/Codeine, Rugby	00536-3227-10
1000's	$93.65	Acetaminophen W/Codeine, Amer Preferred	53445-1338-00
1000's	$98.95	Acetaminophen & Codeine, Parmed Pharms	00349-8861-10
1000's	$99.85	Acetaminophen w/Codeine, Teva	00093-0150-10
1000's	$99.85	APAP w/Codeine, Goldline Labs	00182-0948-10
1000's	$99.97	APAP w/Codeine, Schein Pharm (US)	00364-0324-02
1000's	$101.50	Acetaminophen & Codeine Phosphate, Harber Pharm	51432-0478-06
1000's	$107.93	Acetaminophen & Codeine, Roxane	00054-4022-31
1000's	$235.55	TYLENOL W/CODEINE NO.3, McNeil Lab	00045-0513-80

Tablet, Uncoated - Oral - 300 mg/60 mg

100's	$10.43	Acetaminophen w/Codeine, H.C.F.A. F F P	99999-0051-07
100's	$16.40	APAP w/Codeine, Goldline Labs	00182-1338-89
100's	$16.76	Acetaminophen & Codeine Phosphate, Aligen Independ	00405-0009-01
100's	$17.50	Acetaminophen w/Codeine, Mutual Pharm	53489-0161-01
100's	$17.55	Acetaminophen W/Codeine, Vintage Pharms	00254-2065-28
100's	$17.70	Acetaminophen w/Codeine, Qualitest Pharms	00603-2339-21
100's	$17.90	Acetaminophen & Codeine Phosphate, Major Pharms	00904-3916-60
100's	$18.50	Acetaminophen w/Codeine, United Res	00677-0632-01
100's	$19.10	Acetaminophen w/Codeine, Teva	00093-0350-01
100's	$19.10	Acetaminophen, Geneva Pharms	00781-1654-01
100's	$19.14	APAP w/Codeine, Goldline Labs	00182-1338-01
100's	$19.14	Acetaminophen & Codeine No.4, Purepac Pharm	00228-2003-10
100's	$19.15	Acetaminophen w/Codeine, Rugby	00536-3215-01
100's	$19.29	Acetaminophen w/Codeine No 4, HL Moore Drug Exch	00839-6499-06
100's	$21.75	Acetaminophen & Codeine, Parmed Pharms	00349-2324-01
100's	$21.87	APAP w/Codeine, Schein Pharm (US)	00364-0526-01
100's	$52.91	TYLENOL W/CODEINE NO.4, McNeil Lab	00045-0515-60
500's	$52.15	Acetaminophen w/Codeine, H.C.F.A. F F P	99999-0051-08
500's	$60.00	Acetaminophen Codeine Phosphate 60, Halsey Drug	00879-0415-05
500's	$71.70	Acetaminophen w/Codeine, Qualitest Pharms	00603-2339-28
500's	$75.70	Acetaminophen & Codeine Phosphate, Major Pharms	00904-3916-40
500's	$78.80	Acetaminophen W/Codeine, Vintage Pharms	00254-2065-35
500's	$80.65	Acetaminophen w/Codeine, United Res	00677-0632-05
500's	$80.65	Acetaminophen & Codeine, Mutual Pharm	53489-0161-05
500's	$82.51	Acetaminophen, Geneva Pharms	00781-1654-05

HOW SUPPLIED - RATED THERAPEUTICALLY EQUIVALENT:
(cont'd)

500's	$82.95	Acetaminophen W/Codeine, Aligen Independ	00405-0009-02
500's	$84.95	Acetaminophen w/Codeine, Rugby	00536-3215-05
500's	$85.10	Acetaminophen w/Codeine, Teva	00093-0350-05
500's	$85.39	Acetaminophen w/Codeine, HL Moore Drug Exch	00839-6499-12
500's	$85.55	APAP w/Codeine, Goldline Labs	00182-1338-05
500's	$85.55	Acetaminophen & Codeine No.4, Purepac Pharm	00228-2003-50
500's	$228.56	TYLENOL W/CODEINE NO.4, McNeil Lab	00045-0515-70
500's	$254.20	TYLENOL W/CODEINE NO.4, McNeil Lab	00045-0515-72
1000's	$104.30	Acetaminophen w/Codeine, H.C.F.A. F F P	99999-0051-09
1000's	$112.82	Acetaminophen Codeine Phosphate 60, Halsey Drug	00879-0415-10
1000's	$143.30	Acetaminophen & Codeine, Parmed Pharms	00349-2324-10
1000's	$143.50	APAP w/Codeine, Schein Pharm (US)	00364-0526-02
1000's	$153.18	Acetaminophen w/Codeine, Teva	00093-0350-10

HOW SUPPLIED - NOT RATED EQUIVALENT:

Capsule, Gelatin - Oral - 325 mg/15 mg

500's	$57.10	PHENAPHEN W/CODEINE, AH Robins	00031-6242-70

Capsule, Gelatin - Oral - 325 mg/30 mg

100's	$34.23	PHENAPHEN W/CODEINE NO. 3, AH Robins	00031-6257-63
500's	$162.15	PHENAPHEN W/CODEINE NO. 3, AH Robins	00031-6257-70

Capsule, Gelatin - Oral - 325 mg/60 mg

100's	$58.73	PHENAPHEN W/CODEINE NO. 4, AH Robins	00031-6274-63

Elixir - Oral - 120 mg/12 mg/5m

480 ml	$8.95	Acetaminophen W/Codeine, Harber Pharm	51432-0508-20

Tablet, Uncoated - Oral - 300 mg/7.5 mg

100's	$18.40	TYLENOL W/CODEINE NO.1, McNeil Lab	00045-0510-60

Tablet, Uncoated - Oral - 300 mg/15 mg

100's	$6.60	Acetaminophen W/Codeine, Duramed Pharms	51285-0600-02
1000's	$8.20	Acetaminophen & Codeine, Goldline Labs	00182-1268-01

Tablet, Uncoated - Oral - 300 mg/30 mg

100's	$8.45	Acetaminophen W/Codeine, Duramed Pharms	51285-0601-02
1000's	$75.25	Acetaminophen W/Codeine, Duramed Pharms	51285-0601-05

Tablet, Uncoated - Oral - 300 mg/60 mg

100's	$14.75	Acetaminophen W/Codeine, Duramed Pharms	51285-0602-02
500's	$70.35	Acetaminophen W/Codeine, Duramed Pharms	51285-0602-04

ACETAMINOPHEN; DICHLORALPHENAZONE; ISOMETHEPTENE MUCATE *(000064)*

CATEGORIES: Analgesics; Analgesics/Antipyretics; Antimigraine/Other Headaches; Antipyretics; Autonomic Drugs; Central Nervous System Agents; DESI Drugs; Headache; Pain; Sympatholytic Agents; Migraine*; Tension*; FDA Pre 1938 Drugs
* Indication not approved by the FDA

BRAND NAMES: Alidrin; Amidrine; Apap/Isometheptene/Dichlphen; Atarin; Carmid; Drinex; Duradrin; I.D.A.; Iso-Acetazone; Isocom; Isometh/D-Chloralphenaz/Apap; Isopap; Midchlor; **Midrin**; Migain; Migquin; Migraine; Migrapap; Migratine; Migrazone; Migrend; Migrex; Mitride

FORMULARIES: Aetna; BC-BS; DoD; PCS

DESCRIPTION:

Each red Midrin capsule with pink band contains isometheptene mucate 65 mg, dichloralphenazone 100 mg, and acetaminophen 325 mg.

Isometheptene mucate is a white, crystalline powder having a characteristic aromatic odor and bitter taste. It is an unsaturated aliphatic amine with sympathomimetic properties.

Dichloralphenazone is a white, microcrystalline powder, with slight odor and tastes saline at first, becoming acrid. It is a mild sedative.

Acetaminophen, a non-salicylate, occurs as a white, odorless, crystalline powder possessing a slightly bitter taste.

Midrin capsules contain FD&C Yellow #6 as a color additive.

CLINICAL PHARMACOLOGY:

Isometheptene mucate, a sympathomimetic amine, acts by constricting dilated cranial and cerebral arterioles, thus reducing the stimuli that lead to vascular headaches. Dichloralphenazone, a mild sedative, reduces the patient's emotional reaction to the pain of both vascular and tension headaches. Acetaminophen raises the threshold to painful stimuli, thus exerting an analgesic effect against all types of headaches.

INDICATIONS AND USAGE:

For relief of tension and vascular headaches.*

***Based on a review of this drug (isometheptene mucate) by the National Academy of Sciences—National Research Council and/or other information, FDA has classified the other indication as "possibly" effective in the treatment of migraine headache. Final classification of the less-than-effective indication requires further investigation.**

CONTRAINDICATIONS:

This drug is contraindicated in glaucoma and/or severe cases of renal disease, hypertension, organic heart disease, hepatic disease and in those patients who are on monoamine-oxidase (MAO) inhibitor therapy.

PRECAUTIONS:

Caution should be observed in hypertension, peripheral vascular disease and after recent cardiovascular attacks.

ADVERSE REACTIONS:

Transient dizziness and skin rash may appear in hypersensitive patients. This can usually be eliminated by reducing the dose.

DOSAGE AND ADMINISTRATION:

For Relief of Migraine Headache: The usual adult dosage is two capsules at once, followed by one capsule every hour until relieved, up to five capsules within a 12-hour period.

For Relief of Tension Headache: The usual adult dosage is one or two capsules every 4 hours up to 8 capsules a day.

Store at controlled room temperature 15 to 30° C (59 to 86° F) in a dry place.

HOW SUPPLIED - RATED THERAPEUTICALLY EQUIVALENT:

Capsule, Gelatin - Oral - 325 mg/100 mg/6

100's	$17.95	Isometh/Dichloralphenaz/Apap, Mikart	46672-0253-10
250's	$31.75	Isometh/Dichloralphenaz/Apap, Mikart	46672-0253-25

HOW SUPPLIED - NOT RATED EQUIVALENT:

Capsule, Gelatin - Oral - 325 mg/100 mg/6

50's	$8.25	Isocom, Palisades Pharms	53159-0424-05
50's	$9.86	MIGRAZONE, HL Moore Drug Exch	00839-7561-04
50's	**$22.25**	**MIDRIN, Carnrick**	**00086-0120-05**
100's	$16.00	Isocom, Palisades Pharms	53159-0424-01
100's	$16.35	Atarin, Athena	59075-0576-10
100's	$16.49	MIGREX, Balan	00304-1653-01
100's	$16.75	Migrazone, Pharmacist Choice	54979-0144-01
100's	$16.81	MIGRAZONE, HL Moore Drug Exch	00839-7561-06
100's	$16.95	Migraine, Pecos	59879-0106-01
100's	$17.85	Migain, Global Source	59618-0460-15
100's	$19.43	MITRIDE, IDE-Interstate	00814-4860-14
100's	$19.71	Migquin, Vintage Pharms	00254-4270-28
100's	$19.95	DURADRIN, Duramed Pharms	51285-0364-02
100's	$20.00	Isometh/Dichloralphenaz/Apap, Goldline Labs	00182-1234-01
100's	$20.45	Isometh/Dichloralphenaz/Apap, United Res	00677-1125-01
100's	$20.50	MIDCHLOR, Schein Pharm (US)	00364-2342-01
100's	$20.80	Migquin, Qualitest Pharms	00603-4664-21
100's	$21.45	Alidrin, Aligen Independ	00405-4039-01
100's	$22.11	ISO-ACETAZONE, Rugby	00536-3932-01
100's	**$38.85**	**MIDRIN, Carnrick**	**00086-0120-10**
250's	$30.67	Isocom, Palisades Pharms	53159-0424-25
250's	$37.75	Migquin, Vintage Pharms	00254-4270-33
250's	$37.75	Migquin, Qualitest Pharms	00603-4664-24
250's	$46.45	MIGRATINE, Major Pharms	00904-7622-70
500's	$73.83	Apap/Isometheptene/Dichlphen, Jerome Stevens	50564-0508-05
500's	$102.00	Migrazone, Pharmacist Choice	54979-0144-05
500's	$107.75	ISO-ACETAZONE, Rugby	00536-3932-05

ACETAMINOPHEN; HYDROCODONE BITARTRATE *(000070)*

CATEGORIES: Analgesics; Antipyretics; Antitussives; Antitussives/Expectorants/Mucolytics; Central Nervous System Agents; Narcotics, Synthetics & Combinations; Opiate Agonists (Controlled); Pain; Pregnancy Category C; DEA Class CIII; Sales > $100 Million; FDA Approved 1982 May; Top 200 Drugs

BRAND NAMES: Allay; Amacodone; Anexsia; Anolor Dh 5; **Bancap-HC**; Co-Gesic; Dolacet; Dolagesic; Dolphen; Duocet; Gesic 5; Hy-5; Hy-Phen; Hyco-Pap; Hycomed; Hycotab; Hydrocet; Hydrocodone W/Acetaminophen; Hydrogesic; Lorcet; Lorcet 10/650; Lorcide Panseals; Lortab; Margesic; Medipain 5; Megagesic; Megamor; Norcet; Oncet; Panacet; Polygesic; Propain Hc; Ro-Codone; Rogesic #3; Senefen III; Stagesic; Tycolet; Ultragesic; Vanacet; Vapocet; Vendone; Vicodin; Vicodin ES; Zydone

FORMULARIES: Aetna; BC-BS; FHP; PCS

DESCRIPTION:

Each tablet contains: hydrocodone bitartrate* 5 mg and acetaminophen 500 mg.

Other ingredients include colloidal silicon dioxide, corn starch, croscarmelllose sodium, dibasic calcium phosphate, magnesium stearate, microcrystalline cellulose, povidone, and stearic acid.

Each extra strength tablet contains hydrocodone bitartrate* 7.5 mg and acetaminophen 750 mg.

Other ingredients include colloidal silicon dioxide, corn starch, croscarmellose sodium, magnesium stearate, povidone, and stearic acid.

Hydrocodone bitartrate is an opioid analgesic and antitussive and occurs as fine white crystals or as a crystalline powder. It is affected by light. The chemical name is: 4,5α-epoxy-3-methoxy-17-methylmorphinan-6-one tartrate (1:1) hydrate (2:5).

Acetaminophen, 4'-hydroxyacetanilide, is a nonopiate nonsalicylate analgesic and antipyretic which occurs as a white odorless crystalline powder possessing a slightly bitter taste.

*** Warning: May be habit forming**

CLINICAL PHARMACOLOGY:

Hydrocodone is a semisynthetic narcotic analgesic and antitussive with multiple actions qualitatively similar to those of codeine. Most of these involve the central nervous system and smooth muscle. The precise mechanism of action of hydrocodone and other opiates is not known, although it is believed to relate to the existence of opiate receptors in the central nervous system. In addition to analgesia, narcotics may produce drowsiness, changes in mood, and mental clouding.

Radioimmunoassay techniques have recently been developed for the analysis of hydrocodone in human plasma. After a 10 mg oral dose of hydrocodone bitartrate, a mean peak serum drug level of 23.6 ng/ml and an elimination half-life of 3.8 hours were found.

The analgesic action of acetaminophen involves peripheral and central influences, but the specific mechanism is as yet undetermined. Antipyretic activity is mediated through hypothalamic heat regulating centers. Acetaminophen inhibits prostaglandin synthetase. Therapeutic doses of acetaminophen have negligible effects on the cardiovascular or respiratory systems; however, toxic doses may cause circulatory failure and rapid, shallow breathing.

PHARMACOKINETICS

The behavior of the individual components is described below.

Hydrocodone: Following a 10 mg oral dose of hydrocodone administered to five adult male subjects, the mean peak concentration was 23.6 ± 5.2 ng/ml. Maximum serum levels were achieved at 1.3 ± 0.3 hours and the half-life was determined to be 3.8 ± 0.3 hours. Hydrocodone exhibits a complex pattern of metabolism including O-demethylation, N-demethylation, and 6-keto reduction to the corresponding 6-α- and 6-β-hydroxy-metabolites. (See OVERDOSAGE for toxicity information.)

CLINICAL PHARMACOLOGY: *(cont'd)*

Acetaminophen: Acetaminophen is rapidly absorbed from the gastrointestinal tract and is distributed throughout most body tissues. The plasma half-life is 1.25 to 3 hours but may be increased by liver damage and following overdosage. Elimination of acetaminophen is principally by liver metabolism (conjugation) and subsequent renal excretion of metabolites. Approximately 85% of an oral dose appears in the urine within 24 hours of administration, most as the glucuronide conjugate, with small amounts of other conjugates and unchanged drug. (See OVERDOSAGE for toxicity information.)

INDICATIONS AND USAGE:

For the relief of moderate to moderately severe pain.

CONTRAINDICATIONS:

Hypersensitivity to acetaminophen or hydrocodone.

WARNINGS:

Respiratory Depression: At high doses or in sensitive patients, hydrocodone may produce dose-related respiratory depression by acting directly on the brain stem respiratory center. Hydrocodone also affects the center that controls respiratory rhythm and may produce irregular and periodic breathing.

Head Injury and Increased Intracranial Pressure: The respiratory depressant effects of narcotics and their capacity to elevate cerebrospinal fluid pressure may be markedly exaggerated in the presence of head injury, other intracranial lesions, or a pre-existing increase in intracranial pressure. Furthermore, narcotics produce adverse reactions which may obscure the clinical course of patients with head injuries.

Acute Abdominal Conditions: The administration of narcotics may obscure the diagnosis or clinical course of patients with acute abdominal conditions.

PRECAUTIONS:

SPECIAL RISK PATIENTS

As with any narcotic analgesic agent, hydrocodone bitartrate and acetaminophen tablets should be used with caution in elderly or debilitated patients and those with severe impairment of hepatic or renal function, hypothyroidism, Addison's disease, prostatic hypertrophy, or urethral stricture. The usual precautions should be observed and the possibility of respiratory depression should be kept in mind.

INFORMATION FOR THE PATIENT

Hydrocodone bitartrate and acetaminophen tablets, like all narcotics, may impair the mental and/or physical abilities required for the performance of potentially hazardous tasks such as driving a car or operating machinery; patients should be cautioned accordingly.

Alcohol and other CNS depressants may produce an additive CNS depression when taken with this combination product and should be avoided.

Hydrocodone may be habit forming. Patients should take the drug only for as long as it is prescribed, in the amounts prescribed, and no more frequently than prescribed.

LABORATORY TESTS

In patients with severe hepatic or renal disease, effects of therapy should be monitored with serial liver and/or renal function tests.

Drug/Laboratory Test Interactions: Acetaminophen may produce false-positive test results for urinary 5-hydroxyindoleacetic acid.

COUGH REFLEX

Hydrocodone suppresses the cough reflex. As with all narcotics, caution should be exercised when hydrocodone bitartrate and acetaminophen tablets are used postoperatively and in patients with pulmonary disease.

PREGNANCY CATEGORY C

Teratogenic Effects: Hydrocodone has been shown to be teratogenic in hamsters when given in doses 700 times the human dose. There are no adequate and well-controlled studies in pregnant women. Hydrocodone bitartrate and acetaminophen tablets should be used during pregnancy only if the potential benefit justifies the potential risk to the fetus.

Nonteratogenic Effects: Babies born to mothers who have been taking opioids regularly prior to delivery will be physically dependent. The withdrawal signs include irritability and excessive crying, tremors, hyperactive reflexes, increased respiratory rate, increased stools, sneezing, yawning, vomiting, and fever. The intensity of the syndrome does not always correlate with the duration of maternal opioid use or dose. There is no consensus on the best method of managing withdrawal. Chlorpromazine 0.7 to 1 mg/kg every 6 hours, and paregoric 2 to 4 drops/kg every 4 hours, have been used to treat withdrawal symptoms in infants. The duration of therapy is 4 to 28 days, with the dosage decreased as tolerated.

LABOR AND DELIVERY

As with all narcotics, administration of hydrocodone bitartrate and acetaminophen tablets to the mother shortly before delivery may result in some degree of respiratory depression in the newborn, especially if higher doses are used.

NURSING MOTHERS

Acetaminophen is excreted in breast milk in small amounts, but the significance of its effects on nursing infants is not known. It is not known whether hydrocodone is excreted in human milk. Because many drugs are excreted in human milk and because of the potential for serious adverse reactions in nursing infants from hydrocodone bitartrate and acetaminophen tablets, a decision should be made whether to discontinue nursing or to discontinue the drug, taking into account the importance of the drug to the mother.

PEDIATRIC USE

Safety and effectiveness in children have not been established.

DRUG INTERACTIONS:

Patients receiving other narcotic analgesics, antipsychotics, antianxiety agents, or other CNS depressants (including alcohol) concomitantly with hydrocodone and acetaminophen tablets may exhibit an additive CNS depression. When combined therapy is contemplated, the dose of one or both agents should be reduced.

The use of MAO inhibitors or tricyclic antidepressants with hydrocodone preparations may increase the effect of either the antidepressant or hydrocodone.

The concurrent use of anticholinergics with hydrocodone may produce paralytic ileus.

ADVERSE REACTIONS:

The most frequently observed adverse reactions include lightheadedness, dizziness, sedation, nausea, and vomiting. These effects seem to be more prominent in ambulatory than in nonambulatory patients and some of these adverse reactions may be alleviated if the patient lies down.

Other adverse reactions include:

Central Nervous System: Drowsiness, mental clouding, lethargy, impairment of mental and physical performance, anxiety, fear, dysphoria, psychic dependence, mood changes.

ADVERSE REACTIONS: *(cont'd)*

Gastrointestinal System: The antiemetic phenothiazines are useful in suppression of the nausea and vomiting which may occur; however, some phenothiazine derivatives seem to be antianalgesic and to increase the amount of narcotic required to produce pain relief, while other phenothiazines reduce the amount of narcotic required to produce a given level of analgesia. Prolonged administration of hydrocodone bitartrate and acetaminophen tablets may produce constipation.

Genitourinary System: Ureteral spasm, spasm of vesical sphincters, and urinary retention have been reported.

Respiratory Depression: Hydrocodone bitartrate may produce dose-related respiratory depression by acting directly on the brain stem respiratory center. Hydrocodone also affects the center that controls respiratory rhythm and may produce irregular and periodic breathing.

If significant respiratory depression occurs, it may be antagonized by the use of naloxone hydrochloride. Apply other supportive measures when indicated.

Dermatological: Skin rash, pruritus.

DRUG ABUSE AND DEPENDENCE:

Hydrocodone bitartrate and acetaminophen tablets are subject to the Federal Controlled Substance Act (Schedule III).

Psychic dependence, physical dependence, and tolerance may develop upon repeated administration of narcotics; therefore, hydrocodone bitartrate and acetaminophen tablets should be prescribed and administered with caution. However, psychic dependence is unlikely to develop when hydrocodone bitartrate and acetaminophen tablets are used for a short time for the treatment of pain.

Physical dependence, the condition in which continued administration of the drug is required to prevent the appearance of a withdrawal syndrome, assumes clinically significant proportions only after several weeks of continued narcotic use, although some mild degree of physical dependence may develop after a few days of narcotic therapy. Tolerance, in which increasingly large doses are required in order to produce the same degree of analgesia, is manifested initially by a shortened duration of analgesic effect and subsequently by decreases in the intensity of analgesia. The rate of development of tolerance varies among patients.

OVERDOSAGE:

ACETAMINOPHEN

Signs and Symptoms: In acute acetaminophen overdosage, dose-dependent, potentially fatal hepatic necrosis is the most serious adverse effect. Renal tubular necrosis, hypoglycemic coma, and thrombocytopenia may also occur.

In adults, hepatic toxicity has rarely been reported with acute overdoses of less than 10 g and fatalities with less than 15 g. Importantly, young children seem to be more resistant than adults to the hepatotoxic effect of an acetaminophen overdose. Despite this, the measures outlined below should be initiated in any adult or child suspected or having ingested an acetaminophen overdose.

Early symptoms following a potentially hepatotoxic overdose may include: nausea, vomiting, diaphoresis, and general malaise. Clinical and laboratory evidence of hepatic toxicity may not be apparent until 48 to 72 hours postingestion.

Treatment: The stomach should be emptied promptly by lavage or by induction of emesis with syrup of ipecac. Patients' estimates of the quantity of a drug ingested are notoriously unreliable. Therefore, if an acetaminophen overdose is suspected, a serum acetaminophen assay should be obtained as early as possible, but no sooner than four hours following ingestion. Liver function studies should be obtained initially and repeated at 24-hour intervals.

The antidote, N-acetylcysteine, should be administered as early as possible, preferably within 16 hours of the overdose ingestion for optimal results, but in any case, within 24 hours. Following recovery, there are no residual structural or functional hepatic abnormalities.

HYDROCODONE

Signs and Symptoms: Serious overdose with hydrocodone is characterized by respiratory depression (a decrease in respiratory rate and/or tidal volume, Cheyne-Stokes respiration, cyanosis), extreme somnolence progressing to stupor or coma, skeletal muscle flaccidity, cold and clammy skin, and sometimes bradycardia and hypotension. In severe overdose, apnea, circulatory collapse, cardiac arrest and death may occur.

Treatment: Primary attention should be given to the reestablishment of adequate respiratory exchange through provision of a patent airway and the institution of assisted or controlled ventilation. The narcotic antagonist naloxone is a specific antidote against respiratory depression which may result from overdosage or unusual sensitivity to narcotics, including hydrocodone. Therefore, an appropriate dose of naloxone hydrochloride should be administered, preferably by the intravenous route, and simultaneously with efforts at respiratory resuscitation. Since the duration of action of hydrocodone may exceed that of the antagonist, the patient should be kept under continued surveillance and repeated doses of the antagonist should be administered as needed to maintain adequate respiration.

An antagonist should not be administered in the absence of clinically significant respiratory or cardiovascular depression. Oxygen, intravenous fluids, vasopressors, and other supportive measures should be employed as indicated.

Gastric emptying may be useful in removing unabsorbed drug.

DOSAGE AND ADMINISTRATION:

Dosage should be adjusted according to the severity of pain and the response of the patient. However, it should be kept in mind that tolerance to hydrocodone can develop with continued use and that the incidence of untoward effects is dose related.

The usual adult dosage (for the 500 mg/5 mg tablet) is one or two tablets every four to six hours as needed for pain. The total 24 hour dose should not exceed 8 tablets.

The usual adult dosage (for the 650 mg/7.5 mg tablet) is one tablet every four to six hours as needed for pain. The total 24 hour dose should not exceed 5 tablets.

Storage: Store at controlled room temperature 15° to 30° C. (59° to 86° F).

PATIENT INFORMATION:

Acetaminophen with hydrocodone is used for the relief of moderate to severe pain. Inform your physican if you are pregnant or nursing. This medication may cause dizziness, drowsiness, or blurred vision; use caution while driving or operating hazardous machinery. Do not take any other sedating drugs or drink alcohol while taking acetaminophen with hydrocodone. This medication may be habit forming. Withdrawal symptoms may occur after you stop taking acetaminophen with hydrocodone. Inform your physician if shortness of breath or breathing difficulty occur. May cause nausea, vomiting or constipation; notify your physician if these occur. May be taken with food if GI upset occurs.

HOW SUPPLIED - RATED THERAPEUTICALLY EQUIVALENT:

Capsule, Gelatin - Oral - 500 mg/5 mg

100's	$17.63	Hydrocodone w/Acetaminophen, H.C.F.A. F F P	99999-0070-01
100's	$19.50	Vendone, Venture Pharm	59785-0200-10

HOW SUPPLIED - RATED THERAPEUTICALLY EQUIVALENT:
(cont'd)

100's	$22.00	HYDROGESIC, Edwards Pharms	00485-0050-01
100's	$22.70	HYDROCET, Carnrick	00086-0057-10
100's	$23.95	Hydrocodone w/Acetaminophen, Major Pharms	00904-3442-60
100's	$24.00	Medipain 5, Medi-Plex Pharm	59010-0415-01
100's	$24.40	MARGESIC H, Marnel Pharceut	00682-0808-01
100's	$25.15	Hydrocodone 5, H N Norton Co.	50732-0786-01
100's	$26.14	POLYGESIC, Poly Pharms	50991-0005-01
100's	$26.25	STAGESIC, Huckaby Pharma	58407-0091-01
100's	$27.95	Hydrocodone w/APAP, Rugby	00536-3964-01
100's	$28.50	Hycomed, Med Tek Pharms	52349-0300-10
100's	$29.88	HYCO PAP, Lunsco	10892-0113-10
100's	$34.01	LORCET-HD, UAD Labs	00785-1120-01
100's	$34.65	ZYDONE, Dupont Pharma	00056-0091-70
100's	$39.05	Hydrocodone W/Acetaminophen, Goldline Labs	00182-0156-01
100's	$39.05	ALLAY, H N Norton Co.	50732-0128-01
100's	$98.96	BANCAP HC, Forest Pharms	00456-0601-01
500's	$88.15	Hydrocodone w/Acetaminophen, H.C.F.A. F F P	99999-0070-02
500's	$117.37	Hydrocodone 5, H N Norton Co.	50732-0786-05
500's	$417.73	BANCAP HC, Forest Pharms	00456-0601-02

Tablet, Uncoated - Oral - 500 mg/2.5 mg

100's	$30.30	Hydrocodone w/Acetaminophen, Qualitest Pharms	00603-3880-21
100's	$33.14	Hydrocodone w/Acetaminophen, Warner Chilcott	00047-0318-24
100's	$33.35	Hydrocodone w/Acetaminophen, Watson Labs	52544-0388-01
100's	$47.56	LORTAB 2.5/500, UCB Pharma	50474-0925-01

Tablet, Uncoated - Oral - 500 mg/5 mg

30's	$4.34	Hydrocodone W/Acetaminophen, Talbert Phcy	44514-0413-18
50's	$8.00	Hydrocodone W/Acetaminophen, Talbert Phcy	44514-0413-33
100's	$5.46	Hydrocodone w/Acetaminophen, H.C.F.A. F F P	99999-0070-03
100's	$6.53	Hydrocodone & Acetaminophen, United Res	00677-1184-01
100's	$15.05	Hydrocodone Bitartrate/APAP, Halsey Drug	00879-0574-01
100's	$16.50	Hydrocodone & Acetaminophen 5, H N Norton Co.	50732-0785-01
100's	$16.65	Hydrocodone Bitartrate/APAP 5/50, Mikart	46672-0052-10
100's	$16.95	Hydrocodone W/Acetaminophen, Vintage Pharms	00254-3592-28
100's	$17.10	Hydrocodone W/Acetaminophen, King Pharms	60793-0017-01
100's	$18.50	Hydrocodone/Acetaminophen, Major Pharms	00904-3440-60
100's	$19.29	Hydrocodone w/Acetaminophen, HL Moore Drug Exch	00839-7176-06
100's	$19.50	Hydrocodone W/Acetaminophen, Geneva Pharms	50752-0290-05
100's	$19.75	Hydrocodone & Acetaminophen, Watson Labs	52544-0349-01
100's	$20.25	Hydrocodone w/Acetaminophen, Qualitest Pharms	00603-3881-21
100's	$20.76	Hydrocodone w/Acetaminophen, Parmed Pharms	00349-8494-01
100's	$20.84	Hydrocodone W/Acetaminophen, Caremark	00339-4049-12
100's	$21.21	Hydrocodone Bitartrate 5, Aligen Independ	00405-0015-01
100's	$21.90	Hydrocodone w/Acetaminophen, Goldline Labs	00182-1765-01
100's	$21.90	Hydrocodone & Acetaminophen, Martec Pharms	52555-0076-01
100's	$22.62	Hydrocodone W/Acetaminophen, Endo Labs	60951-0639-70
100's	$24.95	VANACET, GM Pharms	58809-0838-01
100's	$25.99	Hydrocodone & Acetaminophen, Geneva Pharms	00781-1606-01
100's	$26.02	Hydrocodone w/Acetaminophen, Schein Pharm (US)	00364-0744-01
100's	$27.00	Panacet, ECR Pharms	00095-0141-01
100's	$27.54	HY-PHEN, Ascher	00225-0450-15
100's	$28.05	Hydrocodone w/Acetaminophen, Warner Chilcott	00047-0448-24
100's	$28.76	Hydrocodone/APAP, Major Pharms	00904-3440-61
100's	$31.50	Hydrocodone w/Acetaminophen, Rugby	00536-3914-01
100's	$31.80	CO-GESIC, Schwarz Pharma (US)	00131-2104-37
100's	$34.09	ANEXSIA, Monarch	61570-0001-01
100's	$37.00	Hydrocodone w/Acetaminophen, Goldline Labs	00182-1765-89
100's	$39.32	VICODIN, Knoll Labs	00044-0727-02
100's	$42.70	LORTAB 5/500, UCB Pharma	50474-0902-60
100's	$46.78	VICODIN, Knoll Labs	00044-0727-41
100's	$47.56	LORTAB 5/500, UCB Pharma	50474-0902-01
500's	$27.30	Hydrocodone w/Acetaminophen, H.C.F.A. F F P	99999-0070-04
500's	$32.65	Hydrocodone w/APAP, United Res	00677-1184-05
500's	$63.21	Hydrocodone Bitartrate/APAP, Halsey Drug	00879-0574-05
500's	$71.48	Hydrocodone W/Acetaminophen, Vintage Pharms	00254-3592-35
500's	$73.90	Hydrocodone/Acetaminophen, Major Pharms	00904-3440-40
500's	$78.85	Hydrocodone W/Acetaminophen, Endo Labs	60951-0639-85
500's	$80.00	Hydrocodone & Acetaminophen 5, H N Norton Co.	50732-0785-05
500's	$80.15	Hydrocodone w/Acetaminophen, Qualitest Pharms	00603-3881-28
500's	$80.50	Hydrocodone W/Acetaminophen, King Pharms	60793-0017-05
500's	$80.75	Hydrocodone Bitartrate/APAP 5/50, Mikart	46672-0052-50
500's	$84.00	Hydrocodone w/Acetaminophen, Schein Pharm (US)	00364-0744-05
500's	$87.10	Hydrocodone w/ APAP, Aligen Independ	00405-0015-02
500's	$87.60	Hydrocodone & Acetaminophen, Martec Pharms	52555-0076-05
500's	$97.50	Hydrocodone W/Acetaminophen, Geneva Pharms	50752-0290-08
500's	$97.55	Hydrocodone w/Acetaminophen, Warner Chilcott	00047-0448-30
500's	$97.75	Hydrocodone w/Acetaminophen, Goldline Labs	00182-1765-05
500's	$97.75	Hydrocodone & Acetaminophen, Watson Labs	52544-0349-05
500's	$97.80	Hydrocodone & Acetaminophen, Geneva Pharms	00781-1606-05
500's	$97.81	Hydrocodone w/Acetaminophen, HL Moore Drug Exch	00839-7176-12
500's	$100.30	Hydrocodone w/Acetaminophen, Parmed Pharms	00349-8494-05
500's	$133.45	Hydrocodone w/Acetaminophen, Rugby	00536-3914-05
500's	$151.73	CO-GESIC, Schwarz Pharma (US)	00131-2104-41
500's	$182.87	VICODIN, Knoll Labs	00044-0727-03
500's	$224.30	LORTAB 5/500, UCB Pharma	50474-0902-50
1000's	$54.60	Hydrocodone w/Acetaminophen, H.C.F.A. F F P	99999-0070-05
1000's	$121.44	Hydrocodone W/Acetaminophen, Vintage Pharms	00254-3592-38
1000's	$165.10	Hydrocodone W/Acetaminophen, Endo Labs	60951-0639-90
1000's	$168.25	Hydrocodone W/Acetaminophen, King Pharms	60793-0017-10
1000's	$169.95	Hydrocodone W/Acetaminophen, Parmed Pharms	00349-8494-10

Tablet, Uncoated - Oral - 500 mg/7.5 mg

30's	$7.35	Hydrocodone w/Acetaminophen, H.C.F.A. F F P	99999-0070-06
100's	$24.53	Hydrocodone w/Acetaminophen, H.C.F.A. F F P	99999-0070-07
100's	$29.95	Hydrocodone W/Acetaminophen, Harber Pharm	51432-0798-03
100's	$33.80	Hydrocodone w/Acetaminophen, Qualitest Pharms	00603-3882-21
100's	$37.05	Hydrocodone W/Acetaminophen, Goldline Labs	00182-0691-01
100's	$37.75	Hydrocodone W/Acetaminophen, Geneva Pharms	50752-0291-05
100's	$37.97	Hydrocodone W/Acetaminophen, Watson Labs	52544-0385-01
100's	$39.29	Hydrocodone W/Acetaminophen, HL Moore Drug Exch	00839-7781-06
100's	$39.75	Hydrocodone w/Acetaminophen, Warner Chilcott	00047-0319-24
100's	$39.75	Hydrocodone w/Acetaminophen, Major Pharms	00904-7631-60
100's	$39.95	Hydrocodone W/Acetaminophen, Geneva Pharms	00781-1513-01
100's	$40.55	Hydrocodone W/Acetaminophen, Aligen Independ	00405-0016-01
100's	$43.05	Hydrocodone/APAP, Rugby	00536-5507-01
100's	$45.12	LORTAB 7.5/500, UCB Pharma	50474-0907-60
100's	$54.71	LORTAB 7.5/500, UCB Pharma	50474-0907-01
500's	$119.75	Hydrocodone W/Acetaminophen, Harber Pharm	51432-0798-05
500's	$122.65	Hydrocodone w/Acetaminophen, H.C.F.A. F F P	99999-0070-08
500's	$146.30	Hydrocodone w/Acetaminophen, Qualitest Pharms	00603-3882-28
500's	$158.80	Hydrocodone W/Acetaminophen, Goldline Labs	00182-0691-05
500's	$162.00	Hydrocodone w/Acetaminophen, Major Pharms	00904-7631-40

HOW SUPPLIED - RATED THERAPEUTICALLY EQUIVALENT:
(cont'd)

500's	$167.25	Hydrocodone W/Acetaminophen, Geneva Pharms	50752-0291-08
500's	$167.73	Hydrocodone w/Acetaminophen, Warner Chilcott	00047-0319-30
500's	$167.73	Hydrocodone w/Acetaminophen, Watson Labs	52544-0385-05
500's	$167.75	Hydrocodone W/Acetaminophen, Geneva Pharms	00781-1513-05
500's	$176.38	Hydrocodone Bitartrate/APAP, HL Moore Drug Exch	00839-7781-12
500's	$176.56	Hydrocodone W/Acetaminophen, Aligen Independ	00405-0016-02
500's	$241.69	LORTAB 7.5/500, UCB Pharma	50474-0907-50

Tablet, Uncoated - Oral - 650 mg/7.5 mg

100's	$34.25	Hydrocodone W/Acetaminophen, Qualitest Pharms	00603-3884-21
100's	$37.94	Hydrocodone W/Acetaminophen, Inwood Labs	00258-3622-01
100's	$38.25	Hydrocodone W/Acetaminophen, Endo Labs	60951-0640-70
100's	$38.34	Hydrocodone W/Acetaminophen, Goldline Labs	00182-0692-01
100's	$38.35	Hydrocodone W/Acetaminophen, Major Pharms	00904-5022-60
100's	$39.50	Hydrocodone W/Acetaminophen, King Pharms	60793-0016-01
100's	$45.00	Hydrocodone W/Acetaminophen, Rugby	00536-5731-01
100's	$47.70	ANEXSIA, Monarch	61570-0002-01
100's	$49.69	LORCET PLUS, UAD Labs	00785-1122-01
100's	$54.25	LORCET PLUS, UAD Labs	00785-1122-63
500's	$154.95	Hydrocodone W/Acetaminophen, Qualitest Pharms	00603-3884-28
500's	$160.79	Hydrocodone W/Acetaminophen, Goldline Labs	00182-0692-05
500's	$164.25	Hydrocodone W/Acetaminophen, Endo Labs	60951-0640-85
500's	$170.00	Hydrocodone W/Acetaminophen, King Pharms	60793-0016-05
500's	$176.64	Hydrocodone W/Acetaminophen, Inwood Labs	00258-3622-05
500's	$207.74	ANEXSIA, Monarch	61570-0002-05
500's	$209.21	LORCET PLUS, UAD Labs	00785-1122-50
1000's	$309.95	Hydrocodone W/Acetaminophen, King Pharms	60793-0016-10

Tablet, Uncoated - Oral - 650 mg/10 mg

100's	$35.14	Hydrocodone W/Acetaminophen, Inwood Labs	00258-3658-01
100's	$50.78	Hydrocodone W/Acetaminophen, Watson Labs	52544-0503-01
100's	$59.74	LORCET, UAD Labs	00785-6350-01
100's	$64.27	LORCET, UAD Labs	00785-6350-63
500's	$170.26	Hydrocodone W/Acetaminophen, Inwood Labs	00258-3658-05
500's	$231.47	Hydrocodone W/Acetaminophen, Watson Labs	52544-0503-05
500's	$277.78	LORCET 10/650, UAD Labs	00785-6350-50

Tablet, Uncoated - Oral - 750 mg/7.5 mg

30's	$6.54	Hydrocodone w/Acetaminophen, H.C.F.A. F F P	99999-0070-09
100's	$21.83	Hydrocodone w/Acetaminophen, H.C.F.A. F F P	99999-0070-10
100's	$30.60	Hydrocodone W/Acetaminophen, United Res	00677-1504-01
100's	$34.40	Hydrocodone w/APAP, Qualitest Pharms	00603-3883-21
100's	$35.35	Hydrocodone W/Acetaminophen, Geneva Pharms	50752-0292-05
100's	$35.44	Hydrocodone W/Acetaminophen, Goldline Labs	00182-0681-01
100's	$35.44	Hydrocodone W/Acetaminophen, Watson Labs	52544-0387-01
100's	$37.21	Hydrocodone W/Acetaminophen, Caremark	00339-4051-12
100's	$37.55	Hydrocodone w/Acetaminophen, Major Pharms	00904-7632-60
100's	$39.00	Hydrocodone w/Acetaminophen, Warner Chilcott	00047-0486-24
100's	$39.00	Hydrocodone W/Acetaminophen, Geneva Pharms	00781-1532-01
100's	$39.21	Hydrocodone W/Acetaminophen, Schein Pharm (US)	00364-2505-01
100's	$40.59	Hydrocodone W/Acetaminophen, HL Moore Drug Exch	00839-7728-06
100's	$41.66	Hydrocodone W/Acetaminophen, Aligen Independ	00405-0017-01
100's	$42.50	Hydrocodone W/Acetaminophen, Rugby	00536-5508-01
100's	$42.50	Hydrocodone W/Acetaminophen, King Pharms	60793-0024-01
100's	$43.36	VICODIN ES, Knoll Labs	00044-0728-02
100's	$51.59	VICODIN ES, Knoll Labs	00044-0728-41
500's	$109.15	Hydrocodone w/Acetaminophen, H.C.F.A. F F P	99999-0070-11
500's	$160.74	Hydrocodone w/APAP, Qualitest Pharms	00603-3883-28
500's	$165.45	Hydrocodone W/Acetaminophen, Geneva Pharms	50752-0292-08
500's	$165.56	Hydrocodone w/Acetaminophen, Warner Chilcott	00047-0486-30
500's	$165.56	Hydrocodone W/Acetaminophen, Goldline Labs	00182-0681-05
500's	$165.56	Hydrocodone w/Acetaminophen, Watson Labs	52544-0387-05
500's	$165.95	Hydrocodone w/Acetaminophen, Major Pharms	00904-7632-40
500's	$166.58	Hydrocodone W/Acetaminophen, HL Moore Drug Exch	00839-7728-12
500's	$174.27	Hydrocodone W/Acetaminophen, Aligen Independ	00405-0017-02
500's	$182.00	Hydrocodone W/Acetaminophen, Rugby	00536-5508-05
500's	$182.00	Hydrocodone W/Acetaminophen, Geneva Pharms	00781-1532-05
500's	$202.57	VICODIN ES, Knoll Labs	00044-0728-03

HOW SUPPLIED - NOT RATED EQUIVALENT:

Elixir - Oral

480 ml	$43.83	ANEXSIA, Monarch	61570-0101-16
480 ml	$53.39	LORTAB ELIXIR, UCB Pharma	50474-0909-16

Tablet, Uncoated - Oral - 556 mg/5 mg

100's	$23.88	Duocet Tablets, Mason Pharms	12758-0067-01

ACETAMINOPHEN; OXYCODONE HYDROCHLORIDE *(000072)*

CATEGORIES: Analgesics; Antipyretics; Central Nervous System Agents; Narcotics, Synthetics & Combinations; Opiate Agonists (Controlled); Pain; Pregnancy Category C; DEA Class CII; Sales > $100 Million; FDA Approval Pre 1982; Top 200 Drugs

BRAND NAMES: Endocet; Oxycet; *Oxycocet* (Canada); Oxycodone W/APAP; Oxycodone W/Acetaminophen; **Percocet**; *Percocet-Demi* (Canada); *Percocet-5* (Canada); Roxicet; Roxilox; Tylox
(International brand names outside U.S. in italics)

FORMULARIES: Aetna; BC-BS; CIGNA; FHP; Humana; Kaiser; Medco; Medi-Cal; PruCare; United; PCS

DESCRIPTION:

Each tablet of oxycodone and acetaminophen contains:

Oxycodone Hydrochloride USP:... 5 mg*

WARNING — May be habit forming.

Acetaminophen USP:... 325 mg

*5 mg Oxycodone HCl is equivalent to 4.4815 mg oxycodone.

Inactive Ingredients: Microcrystalline cellulose, povidone, pregelatinized starch, stearic acid, and other ingredients.

Acetaminophen occurs as a white, odorless, crystalline powder possessing a slightly bitter taste.

The oxycodone component is 14-hydroxydihydrocodeinone, a white, odorless, crystalline powder having a saline, bitter taste. It is derived from the opium alkaloid thebaine.

CLINICAL PHARMACOLOGY:

The principal ingredient, oxycodone, is a semisynthetic narcotic analgesic with multiple actions qualitatively similar to those of morphine; the most prominent of these involve the central nervous system and organs composed of smooth muscle. The principal actions of therapeutic value of the oxycodone in oxycodone w/APAP are analgesia and sedation.

Oxycodone is similar to codeine and methadone in that it retains at least one-half of its analgesic activity when administered orally.

Acetaminophen is a non-opiate, non-salicylate analgesic and antipyretic.

INDICATIONS AND USAGE:

Oxycodone w/APAP is indicated for the relief of moderate to moderately severe pain.

CONTRAINDICATIONS:

Oxycodone w/APAP should not be administered to patients who are hypersensitive to oxycodone or acetaminophen.

WARNINGS:

Contains sodium metabisulfite, a sulfite that may cause allergic-type reactions including anaphylactic symptoms and life-threatening or less severe asthmatic episodes in certain susceptible people. The overall prevalence of sulfite sensitivity in the general population is unknown and probably low. Sulfite sensitivity is seen more frequently in asthmatic than in nonasthmatic people.

Drug Dependence: Oxycodone can produce drug dependence of the morphine type and, therefore, has the potential for being abused. Psychic dependence, physical dependence, and tolerance may develop upon repeated administration of oxycodone w/APAP, and it should be prescribed and administered with the same degree of caution appropriate to the use of other oral narcotic-containing medications. Like other narcotic-containing medications, oxycodone w/APAP is subject to the Federal Controlled Substances Act (Schedule II).

PRECAUTIONS:

GENERAL

Head Injury and Increased Intracranial Pressure: The respiratory depressant effects of narcotics and their capacity to elevate cerebrospinal fluid pressure may be markedly exaggerated in the presence of head injury, other intracranial lesions, or a pre-existing increase in intracranial pressure. Furthermore, narcotics produce adverse reactions which may obscure the clinical course of patients with head injuries.

Acute Abdominal Conditions: The administration of oxycodone w/APAP or other narcotics may obscure the diagnosis or clinical course in patients with acute abdominal conditions.

Special Risk Patients: Oxycodone w/APAP should be given with caution to certain patients such as the elderly or debilitated, and those with severe impairment of hepatic or renal function, hypothyroidism, Addison's disease, and prostatic hypertrophy or urethral stricture.

INFORMATION FOR THE PATIENT

Oxycodone may impair the mental and/or physical abilities required for the performance of potentially hazardous tasks such as driving a car or operating machinery. The patient using oxycodone w/APAP should be cautioned accordingly.

PREGNANCY CATEGORY C

Animal reproductive studies have not been conducted with oxycodone w/APAP. It is also not known whether oxycodone w/APAP can cause fetal harm when administered to a pregnant woman or can affect reproductive capacity. Oxycodone w/APAP should not be given to a pregnant woman unless in the judgment of the physician, the potential benefits outweigh the possible hazards.

Nonteratogenic Effects: Use of narcotics during pregnancy may produce physical dependence in the neonate.

LABOR AND DELIVERY

As with all narcotics, administration of oxycodone w/APAP to the mother shortly before delivery may result in some degree of respiratory depression in the newborn and the mother, especially if higher doses are used.

NURSING MOTHERS

It is not known whether the components of oxycodone w/APAP are excreted in human milk. Because many drugs are excreted in human milk, caution should be exercised when oxycodone w/APAP is administered to a nursing mother.

PEDIATRIC USE

Safety and effectiveness in children have not been established.

DRUG INTERACTIONS:

Patients receiving other narcotic analgesics, general anesthetics, phenothiazines, other tranquilizers, sedative-hypnotics, or other CNS depressants (including alcohol) concomitantly with oxycodone w/APAP may exhibit an additive CNS depression. When such combined therapy is contemplated, the dose of one or both agents should be reduced.

The use of MAO inhibitors or tricyclic antidepressants with oxycodone preparations may increase the effect of either the antidepressant or oxycodone.

The concurrent use of anticholinergics with narcotics may produce paralytic ileus.

ADVERSE REACTIONS:

The most frequently observed adverse reactions include lightheadedness, dizziness, sedation, nausea, and vomiting. These effects seem to be more prominent in ambulatory than in non-ambulatory patients, and some of these adverse reactions may be alleviated if the patient lies down.

Other adverse reactions include euphoria, dysphoria, constipation, skin rash, and pruritus. At higher doses, oxycodone has most of the disadvantages of morphine including respiratory depression.

DRUG ABUSE AND DEPENDENCE:

Oxycodone w/APAP is a Schedule II controlled substance.

Oxycodone can produce drug dependence and has the potential for being abused. See WARNINGS.

OVERDOSAGE:

ACETAMINOPHEN

Signs and Symptoms: In acute acetaminophen overdosage, dose-dependent, potentially fatal hepatic necrosis is the most serious adverse effect. Renal tubular necrosis, hypoglycemic coma, and thrombocytopenia may also occur.

In adults, hepatic toxicity has rarely been reported with acute overdoses of less than 10 g and fatalities with less than 15 g. Importantly, young children seem to be more resistant than adults to the hepatotoxic effect of an acetaminophen overdose.

OVERDOSAGE: *(cont'd)*

Despite this, the measures outlined below should be initiated in any adult or child suspected of having ingested an acetaminophen overdose.

Early symptoms following a potentially hepatotoxic overdose may include: nausea, vomiting, diaphoresis, and general malaise. Clinical and laboratory evidence of hepatic toxicity may not be apparent until 48 to 72 hours postingestion.

Treatment: The stomach should be emptied promptly by lavage or by induction of emesis with syrup of ipecac. Patients' estimates of the quantity of a drug ingested are notoriously unreliable. Therefore, if an acetaminophen overdose is suspected, a serum acetaminophen assay should be obtained as early as possible, but no sooner than four hours following ingestion. Liver function studies should be obtained initially and repeated at 24-hour intervals.

The antidote, N-acetylcysteine, should be administered as early as possible, preferably within 16 hours of the overdose ingestion for optimal results, but in any case, within 24 hours. Following recovery, there are no residual, structural, or functional hepatic abnormalities.

OXYCODONE

Signs and Symptoms: Serious overdosage with oxycodone is characterized by respiratory depression (a decrease in respiratory rate and/or tidal volume, Cheyne-Stokes respiration, cyanosis), extreme somnolence progressing to stupor or coma, skeletal muscle flaccidity, cold and clammy skin, and sometimes bradycardia and hypotension. In severe overdosage apnea, circulatory collapse, cardiac arrest, and death may occur.

Treatment: Primary attention should be given to the reestablishment of adequate respiratory exchange through provision of a patent airway and the institution of assisted or controlled ventilation. The narcotic antagonist naloxone hydrochloride is a specific antidote against respiratory depression which may result from overdosage or unusual sensitivity to narcotics, including oxycodone. Therefore, an appropriate dose of naloxone hydrochloride (usual initial adult dose 0.4 mg to 2 mg) should be administered, preferably by the intravenous route, and simultaneously with efforts at respiratory resuscitation. Since the duration of action of oxycodone may exceed that of the antagonist, the patient should be kept under continued surveillance and repeated doses of the antagonist should be administered as needed to maintain adequate respiration.

An antagonist should not be administered in the absence of clinically significant respiratory or cardiovascular depression. Oxygen, intravenous fluids, vasopressors, and other supportive measures should be employed as indicated.

Gastric emptying may be useful in removing unabsorbed drug.

DOSAGE AND ADMINISTRATION:

Dosage should be adjusted according to the severity of the pain and the response of the patient. It may occasionally be necessary to exceed the usual dosage recommended below in cases of more severe pain or in patients who have become tolerant to the analgesic effect of narcotics.

Oxycodone w/APAP is given orally. The usual adult dosage is one tablet every 6 hours as needed for pain.

Store at controlled room temperature (15°-30° C, 59°-86° F). Protect from moisture.

PATIENT INFORMATION:

Acetaminophen with oxycodone is used for the relief of moderate to severe pain.

Inform your physican if you are pregnant or nursing.

This medication may cause dizziness, drowsiness, or blurred vision; use caution while driving or operating hazardous machinery. Do not take any other sedating drugs or drink alcohol while taking acetaminophen with oxycodone.

This medication may be habit forming. Withdrawal symptoms may occur after you stop taking it.

Inform your physician if shortness of breath or breathing difficulty occur.

May cause nausea, vomiting or constipation; notify your physician if these occur.

May be taken with food if GI upset occurs.

HOW SUPPLIED - RATED THERAPEUTICALLY EQUIVALENT:

Capsule, Gelatin - Oral - 500 mg/5 mg

100's	$29.93	Oxycodone & Acetaminophen, H.C.F.A. F F P	99999-0072-01
100's	$38.94	ROXILOX, Roxane	00054-2795-25
100's	$41.67	Oxycodone w/Acetaminophen, Qualitest Pharms	00603-4997-21
100's	$46.50	Oxycodone w/Acetaminophen, Major Pharms	00904-1973-60
100's	$46.61	Oxycodone W/Acetaminophen, Aligen Independ	00405-0140-01
100's	$48.75	Oxycodone & Acetaminophen, Halsey Drug	00879-0532-01
100's	$49.50	Oxycodone W/Acetaminophen, Duramed Pharms	51285-0644-02
100's	$51.95	Oxycodone & Acetaminophew, Parmed Pharms	00349-8659-01
100's	$54.38	Oxycodone & Acetaminophen, Schein Pharm (US)	00364-2395-01
100's	$54.75	Oxycodone & Acetaminophen 5, Goldline Labs	00182-9175-01
100's	$57.59	Oxycodone w/Acetaminophen, Rugby	00536-3219-01
100's	$71.04	TYLOX, McNeil Lab	00045-0526-60
100's	$93.41	TYLOX, McNeil Lab	00045-0526-79
500's	$149.65	Oxycodone & Acetaminophen, H.C.F.A. F F P	99999-0072-02
500's	$226.65	Oxycodone & Acetaminophen, Halsey Drug	00879-0532-05

Tablet, Uncoated - Oral - 325 mg/5 mg

100's	$13.43	Oxycodone & Acetaminophen, H.C.F.A. F F P	99999-0072-03
100's	$14.50	Oxycodone With Acetaminophen, IDE-Interstate	00814-5600-14
100's	$19.33	Oxycodone w/Acetaminophen, Qualitest Pharms	00603-4998-21
100's	$19.55	Oxycodone w/ APAP, Major Pharms	00904-0465-60
100's	$22.15	Oxycodone W/Acetaminophen, King Pharms	60793-0195-01
100's	$22.27	Oxycodone W/Acetaminophen, Rugby	00536-5670-01
100's	$22.50	Oxycodone & Acetaminophen, Parmed Pharms	00349-8859-01
100's	$22.50	Endocet, Endo Labs	60951-0602-70
100's	$22.55	ROXICET, Roxane	00054-4650-25
100's	$22.95	APAP w/Oxycodone, Goldline Labs	00182-1465-01
100's	$25.69	Oxycodone & Acetaminophen, Schein Pharm (US)	00364-0605-01
100's	$25.97	ROXICET, Roxane	00054-8650-24
100's	$27.90	Oxycodone W/Acetaminophen, Aligen Independ	00405-0139-01
100's	$29.85	Oxycodone W/Acetaminophen, Mallinckrodt	00406-0512-01
100's	**$68.63**	**PERCOCET, Du Pont Merck**	**00590-0127-70**
100's	**$68.63**	**PERCOCET, Du Pont Merck**	**00590-0127-75**
250's	$43.26	Oxycodone w/Acetaminophen, Roxane	00054-8650-11
500's	$64.47	ROXICET, Roxane	00054-4650-29
500's	$67.15	Oxycodone & Acetaminophen, H.C.F.A. F F P	99999-0072-04
500's	$79.45	Oxycodone w/Acetaminophen, Major Pharms	00904-0465-40
500's	$86.75	Oxycodone W/Acetaminophen, Mallinckrodt	00406-0512-05
500's	$91.95	Oxycodone & Acetaminophen, Parmed Pharms	00349-8859-05
500's	$92.33	Oxycodone W/Acetaminophen, Aligen Independ	00405-0139-02
500's	$96.95	Oxycodone W/Acetaminophen, King Pharms	60793-0195-05
500's	$98.45	Endocet, Endo Labs	60951-0602-85
500's	$104.95	Oxycodone W/Acetaminophen, Rugby	00536-5670-05
500's	$105.66	Oxycodone & Acetaminophen, Schein Pharm (US)	00364-0605-05

HOW SUPPLIED - RATED THERAPEUTICALLY EQUIVALENT: *(cont'd)*

500's	$108.00	APAP w/Oxycodone, Goldline Labs	00182-1465-05
500's	**$325.00**	**PERCOCET, Du Pont Merck**	**00590-0127-85**

HOW SUPPLIED - NOT RATED EQUIVALENT:

Solution - Oral - 325 mg/5 mg

5 ml x 40	$43.25	ROXICET, Roxane	00054-8648-16
500 ml	$36.28	ROXICET, Roxane	00054-3686-63

Tablet, Uncoated - Oral - 500 mg/5 mg

100's	$51.31	ROXICET 5/500 CAPLETS, Roxane	00054-8784-24
100's	$52.26	ROXICET 5/500 CAPLETS, Roxane	00054-4784-25

ACETAMINOPHEN; PENTAZOCINE HYDROCHLORIDE *(000074)*

CATEGORIES: Analgesics; Antipyretics; Central Nervous System Agents; Narcotic Agonist-Antagonist; Opiate Partial Agonists; Pain; Pregnancy Category C; DEA Class CIV; FDA Approved 1982 Sep

BRAND NAMES: **Talacen**

DESCRIPTION:

Talacen is a combination of pentazocine hydrochloride, USP, equivalent to 25 mg base and acetaminophen, USP, 650 mg.

Pentazocine is a member of the benzazocine series (also known as the benzomorphan series). Chemically, pentazocine is 1,2,3,4,5,6-hexahydro -6,11 -dimethyl-3-(3-methyl-2-butenyl)-2, 6-methano-3-benzazocin-8-ol, a white, crystalline substance soluble in acidic aqueous solutions.

Chemically, acetaminophen is Acetamide, *N*-(4-hydroxyphenyl).

Pentazocine is an analgesic and acetaminophen is an analgesic and antipyretic.

Talacen is a pale blue, scored caplet for oral administration.

Talacen Inactive Ingredients: Colloidal Silicon Dioxide, FD&C Blue #1, Gelatin, Microcrystalline Cellulose, Potassium Sorbate, Pregelatinized Starch, Sodium Lauryl Sulfate, Sodium Metabisulfite, Sodium Starch Glycolate, Stearic Acid.

CLINICAL PHARMACOLOGY:

Pentazocine HCl/APAP is an analgesic possessing antipyretic actions.

Pentazocine is an analgesic with agonist/antagonist action which when administered orally is approximately equivalent on a mg for mg basis in analgesic effect to codeine.

Acetaminophen is an analgesic and antipyretic.

Onset of significant analgesia with pentazocine usually occurs between 15 and 30 minutes after oral administration, and duration of action is usually three hours or longer. Onset and duration of action and the degree of pain relief are related both to dose and the severity of pretreatment pain. Pentazocine weakly antagonizes the analgesic effects of morphine, meperidine, and phenazocine; in addition, it produces incomplete reversal of cardiovascular, respiratory, and behavioral depression induced by morphine and meperidine. Pentazocine has about 1/50 the antagonistic activity of nalorphine. It also has sedative activity.

Pentazocine is well absorbed from the gastrointestinal tract. Plasma levels closely correspond to the onset, duration, and intensity of analgesia. The mean peak concentration in 24 normal volunteers was 1.7 hours (range 0.5 to 4.0 hours) after oral administration and the mean plasma elimination half-life was 3.6 hours (range 1.5 to 10 hours).

The action of pentazocine is terminated for the most part by biotransformation in the liver with some free pentazocine excreted in the urine. The products of the oxidation of the terminal methyl groups and glucuronide conjugates are excreted by the kidney. Elimination of approximately 60% of the total dose occurs within 24 hours. Pentazocine passes the placental barrier.

Onset of significant analgesic and antipyretic activity of acetaminophen when administered orally occurs within 30 minutes and is maximal at approximately 2 1/2 hours. The pharmacological mode of action of acetaminophen is unknown at this time.

Acetaminophen is rapidly and almost completely absorbed from the gastrointestinal tract. In 24 normal volunteers the mean peak plasma concentration was 1 hour (range 0.25 to 3 hours) after oral administration and the mean plasma elimination half-life was 2.8 hours (range 2 to 4 hours).

The effect of pentazocine on acetaminophen plasma protein binding or vice versa has not been established. For acetaminophen there is little or no plasma protein binding at normal therapeutic doses. When toxic doses of acetaminophen are ingested and drug plasma levels exceed 90 mcg/ml, plasma binding may vary from 8% to 43%.

Acetaminophen is conjugated in the liver with glucuronic acid and to a lesser extent with sulfuric acid. Approximately 80% of acetaminophen is excreted in the urine after conjugation and about 3% is excreted unchanged. The drug is also conjugated to a lesser extent with cysteine and additionally metabolized by hydroxylation.

If pentazocine HCl/APAP is taken every 4 hours over an extended period of time, accumulation of pentazocine and to a lesser extent, acetaminophen, may occur.

INDICATIONS AND USAGE:

Pentazocine HCl/APAP is indicated for the relief of mild to moderate pain.

CONTRAINDICATIONS:

Pentazocine HCl/APAP should not be administered to patients who are hypersensitive to either pentazocine or acetaminophen.

WARNINGS:

Contains sodium metabisulfite, a sulfite that may cause allergic-type reactions including anaphylactic symptoms and life-threatening or less severe asthmatic episodes in certain susceptible people. The overall prevalence of sulfite sensitivity in the general population is unknown and probably low. Sulfite sensitivity is seen more frequently in asthmatic than in nonasthmatic people.

Head Injury and Increased Intracranial Pressure: As in the case of other potent analgesics, the potential of pentazocine for elevating cerebrospinal fluid pressure may be attributed to CO_2retention due to the respiratory depressant effects of the drug. These effects may be markedly exaggerated in the presence of head injury, other intracranial lesions, or a preexisting increase in intracranial pressure. Furthermore, pentazocine can produce effects which may obscure the climcal course of patients with head injuries. In such patients, Pentazocine HCl/APAP must be used with extreme caution and only if its use is deemed essential.

WARNINGS: *(cont'd)*

Acute CNS Manifestations: Patients receiving therapeutic doses of pentazocine have experienced hallucinations (usually visual), disorientation, and confusion which have cleared spontaneously within a period of hours. The mechanism of this reaction is not known. Such patients should be closely observed and vital signs checked. If the drug is reinstituted, it should be done with caution since these acute CNS manifestations may recur.

There have been instances of psychological and physical dependence on parenteral pentazocine in patients with a history of drug abuse, and rarely, in patients without such a history. (See DRUG ABUSE AND DEPENDENCE.))

Due to the potential for increased CNS depressant effects, alcohol should be used with caution in patients who are currently receiving pentazocine.

Pentazocine may precipitate opioid abstinence symptoms in patients receiving courses of opiates for pain relief.

PRECAUTIONS:

In prescribing pentazocine HCl/APAP for chronic use, the physician should take precautions to avoid increases in dose by the patient.

GENERAL

Myocardial Infarction: As with all drugs, pentazocine HCl/APAP should be used with caution in patients with myocardial infarction who have nausea or vomiting.

Certain Respiratory Conditions: Although respiratory depression has rarely been reported after oral administration of pentazocine, the drug should be administered with caution to patients with respiratory depression from any cause, severely limited respiratory reserve, severe bronchial asthma and other obstructive respiratory conditions, or cyanosis.

Impaired Renal or Hepatic Function: Decreased metabolism of the drug by the liver in extensive live disease may predispose to accentuation of side effects. Although laboratory tests have not indicated that pentazocine causes or increases renal or hepatic impairment, the drug should be administered with caution to patients with such impairment.

Since acetaminophen is metabolized by the liver, the question of the safety of its use in the presence of liver disease should be considered.

Biliary Surgery: Narcotic drug products are generally considered to elevate biliary tract pressure for varying periods following their administration. Some evidence suggests that pentazocine may differ from other marketed narcotics in this respect (*i.e.,* it causes little or no elevation in biliary tract pressures). The clinical significance of these findings, however, is not yet known.

CNS Effect: Caution should be used when pentazocine HCl/APAP is administered to patients prone to seizures; seizures have occurred in a few such patients in association with the use of pentazocine although no cause and effect relationship has been established.

INFORMATION FOR THE PATIENT

Since sedation, dizziness, and occasional euphoria have been noted, ambulatory patients should be warned not to operate machinery, drive cars, or unnecessarily expose themselves to hazards. Pentazocine may cause physical and psychological dependence when taken alone and may have additive CNS depressant properties when taken in combination with alcohol or other CNS depressants.

CARCINOGENESIS, MUTAGENESIS, AND IMPAIRMENT OF FERTILITY

Carcinogenesis, mutagenesis, and impairment of fertility studies have not been done with this combination product.

Pentazocine, when administered orally or parenterally, had no adverse effect on either the reproductive capabilities or the course of pregnancy in rabbits and rats. Embryotoxic effects on the fetuses were not shown.

The daily administration of 4 mg/kg to 20 mg/kg pentazocine subcutaneously to female rats during a 14 day pre-mating period and until the 13th day of pregnancy did not have any adverse effects on the fertility rate.

There is no evidence in long-term animal studies to demonstrate that pentazocine is carcinogenic.

PREGNANCY CATEGORY C

Teratogenic Effects: Animal reproduction studies have not been conducted with pentazocine HCl/APAP. It is also not known whether pentazocine HCl/APAP can cause fetal harm when administered to pregnant women or can affect reproduction capacity. Pentazocine HCl/APAP should be given to pregnant women only if clearly needed. However, animal reproduction studies with pentazocine have not demonstrated teratogenic or embryotoxic effects.

Nonteratogenic Effects: There has been no experience in this regard with the combination pentazocine and acetaminophen. However, there have been rare reports of possible abstinence syndromes in newborns after prolonged use of pentazocine during pregnancy.

LABOR AND DELIVERY

Patients receiving pentazocine during labor have experienced no adverse effects other than those that occur with commonly used analgesics. Pentazocine HCl/APAP should be used with caution in women delivering premature infants. The effect of pentazocine HCl/APAP on the mother and fetus, the duration of labor or delivery, the possibility that forceps delivery or other intervention or resuscitation of the newborn may be necessary, or the effect of pentazocine HCl/APAP, on the later growth, development, and functional maturation of the child are unknown at the present time.

NURSING MOTHERS

It is not known whether this drug is excreted in human milk. Because many drugs are excreted in human milk, caution should be exercised when pentazocine HCl/APAP is administered to a nursing woman.

PEDIATRIC USE

Safety and effectiveness in children below the age of 12 have not been established.

DRUG INTERACTIONS:

Pentazocine is a mild narcotic antagonist. Some patients previously given narcotics, including methadone for the daily treatment of narcotic dependence, have experienced withdrawal symptoms after receiving pentazocine.

ADVERSE REACTIONS:

Clinical experience with pentazocine HCl/APAP has been insufficient to define all possible adverse reactions with this combination. However, reactions reported after oral administration of pentazocine hydrochloride in 50 mg dosage include:

Gastrointestinal: nausea, vomiting, infrequently constipation; and rarely abdominal distress, anorexia, diarrhea.

CNS effects: dizziness, lightheadedness, hallucinations, sedation, euphoria, headache, confusion, disorientation; infrequently weakness, disturbed dreams, insomnia, syncope, visual blurring and focusing difficulty, depression; and rarely tremor, irritability, excitement, tinnitus.

Autonomic: sweating; infrequently flushing; and rarely chills.

Allergic: infrequently rash; and rarely urticaria, edema of the face.

ADVERSE REACTIONS: *(cont'd)*

Cardiovascular: infrequently decrease in blood pressure, tachycardia.

Hematologic: rarely depression of white blood cells (especially granulocytes), which is usually reversible, moderate transient eosinophilia.

Other: rarely respiratory depression, urinary retention, paresthesia, toxic epidermal necrolysis, and in one instance, an apparent anaphylactic reaction has been reported.

Numerous clinical studies have shown that acetaminophen, when taken in recommended doses, is relatively free of adverse effects in most age groups, even in the presence of a variety of disease states.

A few cases of hypersensitivity to acetaminophen have been reported, as manifested by skin rashes, thrombocytopenic purpura, rarely hemolytic anemia and agranulocytosis. Occasional individuals respond to ordinary doses with nausea and vomiting and diarrhea.

DRUG ABUSE AND DEPENDENCE:

Controlled Substance: Pentazocine HCl/APAP is a Schedule IV controlled substance.

Abuse and Dependence: There have been some reports of dependence and of withdrawal symptoms with orally administered pentazocine. There have been recorded instances of psychological and physical dependence in patients using parenteral pentazocine. Abrupt discontinuance following the extended use of parenteral pentazocine has resulted in withdrawal symptoms. Patients with a history of drug dependence should be under close supervision while receiving pentazocine HCl/APAP. There have been rare reports of possible abstinence syndromes in newborns after prolonged use of pentazocine during pregnancy.

Some tolerance to the analgesic and subjective effects of pentazocine develops with frequent and repeated use.

Drug addicts who are given closely spaced doses of pentazocine (*e.g.,* 60 mg to 90 mg every 4 hours) develop physical dependence which is demonstrated by abrupt withdrawal or by administration of naloxone. The withdrawal symptoms exhibited after chronic doses of more than 500 mg of pentazocine per day have similar characteristics, but to a lesser degree, of opioid withdrawal and may be associated with drug seeking behavior.

OVERDOSAGE:

Manifestations: Clinical experience with pentazocine HCl/APAP has been insufficient to define the signs of overdosage with this product. It may be assumed that signs and symptoms of pentazocine HCl/APAP overdose would be a combination of those observed with pentazocine overdose and acetaminophen overdose.

For pentazocine alone in single doses above 60 mg there have been reports of the occurrence of nalorphine-like psychotomimetic effects such as anxiety, nightmares, strange thoughts, and hallucinations. Marked respiratory depression associated with increased blood pressure and tachycardia have also resulted from excessive doses as have dizziness, nausea, vomiting, lethargy, and paresthesias. The respiratory depression is antagonized by naloxone (see Treatment.)

In acute acetaminophen overdose, dose-dependent, potentially fatal hepatic necrosis is the most serious adverse effect. Renal tubular necrosis, hypoglycemic coma, and thrombocytopenia may also occur.

In adults, a single dose of 10 g to 15 g (200 mg/kg to 250 mg/kg) of acetaminophen may cause hepatotoxicity. A dose of 25 g or more is potentially fatal. The potential seriousness of the intoxication may not be evident during the first two days of acute acetaminophen poisoning. During the first 24 hours, nausea, vomiting, anorexia, and abdominal pain occur. These may persist for a week or more. Liver injury may become evident the second day, initial signs being elevation of serum transaminase and lactic dehydrogenase activity, increased serum bilirubin concentration, and prolongation of prothrombin time. Serum albumin concentration and alkaline phosphatase activity may remain normal. The hepatotoxicity may lead to encephalopathy, coma, and death. Transient azotemia is evident in a majority of patients and acute renal failure occurs in some.

There have been reports of glycosuria and impaired glucose tolerance, but hypoglycemia may also occur. Metabolic acidosis and metabolic alkalosis have been reported. Cerebral edema and nonspecific myocardial depression have also been noted. Biopsy reveals centrolobular necrosis with sparing of the periportal area. The hepatic lesions are reversible over a period of weeks or months in nonfatal cases.

The severity of the liver injury can be determined by measurement of the plasma halftime of acetaminophen during the first day of acute poisoning. If the halftime exceeds 4 hours, hepatic necrosis is likely and if the halftime is greater than 12 hours, hepatic coma will probably occur. Only minimal liver damage has developed when the serum concentration was below 120 mcg/ml at 12 hours after ingestion of the drug. If serum bilirubin concentration is greater than 4 mg/100 ml during the first 5 days, encephalopathy may occur.

The seven day oral LD_{50} value for pentazocine HCl/APAP in mice is 3,570 mg/kg.

Treatment: Oxygen, intravenous fluids, vasopressors, and other supportive measures should be employed as indicated. Assisted or controlled ventilation should also be considered. For respiratory depression due to overdosage or unusual sensitivity to Talacen, parenteral naloxone is a specific and effective antagonist.

The toxic effects of acetaminophen may be prevented or minimized by antidotal therapy with N-acetylcysteine. In order to obtain the best possible results, N-acetylcysteine should be administered within approximately 16 hours of ingestion of the overdose.

Vigorous supportive therapy is required in severe intoxication. Procedures to limit the continuing absorption of the drug must be readily performed since the hepatic injury is dose dependent and occurs early in the course of intoxication. Induction of vomiting or gastric lavage, followed by oral administration of activated charcoal should be done in all cases.

If hemodialysis can be initiated within the first 12 hours, it is advocated for patients with a plasma acetaminophen concentration exceeding 120 mcg/ml at 4 hours after ingestion of the drug.

DOSAGE AND ADMINISTRATION:

Adult: The usual adult dose is 1 tablet every 4 hours as needed for pain relief, up to a maximum of 6 tablets per day.

The usual duration of therapy is dependent upon the condition being treated but in any case should be reviewed regularly by the physician. The effect of meals on the rate and extent of bioavailability of both pentazocine and acetaminophen has not been documented.

HOW SUPPLIED - EQUIVALENTS NOT AVAILABLE:

Tablet, Uncoated - Oral - 25 mg/650 mg

100's	$71.91	TALACEN, Sanofi Winthrop	00024-1937-04
250's	$198.07	TALACEN, Sanofi Winthrop	00024-1937-14

ACETAMINOPHEN; PHENYLPROPANOLAMINE; PHENYLTOLOXAMINE *(000078)*

CATEGORIES: Allergies; Autonomic Drugs; Common Cold; Congestion; Cough Preparations; Fever; Nasal Congestion; Pain; Respiratory & Allergy Medications; Rhinitis; Sinusitis; Sympathomimetic Agents; FDA Pre 1938 Drugs

BRAND NAMES: Sinubid; *Sinutab*; *Sinutab SA* (Canada)
(International brand names outside U.S. in italics)

DESCRIPTION:

Sinubid is an analgesic/decongestant/antihistamine combination product for oral administration. Each two layer sustained-release tablet contains:

600 mg acetaminophen

100 mg phenylpropanolamine hydrochloride

66 mg phenyltoloxamine citrate

Also contains calcium sulfate, NF; carnauba wax; confectioners sugar, NF; D and C red No. 30 lake; ethylcellulose, NF, 45 cps; FD and C blue No. 2 lake; FD and C yellow No. 6 lake; hydrogenated vegetable oil; hydroxypropyl methylcellulose, USP, 2910; lactose, USP; locust bean gum; magnesium stearate, NF; stearic acid, NF; syloid 244 silica gel; talc, USP; titanium dioxide, USP.

CLINICAL PHARMACOLOGY:

This drug is designed to provide symptomatic relief of coryza and nasal congestion when given twice a day (every 12 hours). This drug can provide symptomatic relief of headache, fever, and other symptoms associated with mucosal congestion (nasopharyngeal), general malaise, and irritability associated with the common cold, allergic and vasomotor disorders, sinusitis, and rhinitis.

This drug contains an analgesic-antipyretic (acetaminophen) to relieve the pain of sinus headache and nasal congestion. This analgesic-antipyretic is rapidly absorbed and as effective as aspirin in raising the pain threshold, but has the advantage of causing little or no gastric irritation. This drug, because it contains no salicylates, can be used by patients who are allergic to aspirin.

Decongestion of the nasopharyngeal mucosa is provided by phenylpropanolamine hydrochloride, a sympathomimetic amine which provides symptomatic relief. Because its vasoconstrictor activity is similar to that of ephedrine, but less likely to cause CNS stimulation, this drug may eliminate the need for topical decongestants.

Phenyltoloxamine citrate is a mild antihistamine which may provide symptomatic relief of seasonal and perennial allergic rhinitis, vasomotor rhinitis, nasal and sinus symptoms of sinusitis, and adjunctive therapy for bacterial sinusitis in uncomplicated upper respiratory infections.

INDICATIONS AND USAGE:

This drug is indicated for the rapid, prolonged, symptomatic relief of nasal congestion in sinus or other frontal headache; allergic and vasomotor manifestations of upper respiratory disorders such as sinusitis, allergic rhinitis, vasomotor rhinitis, coryza; facial pain and "pressure" of acute and chronic sinusitis; and for the relief of accompanying fever. This drug is indicated only for intermittent treatment of the above noted acute symptoms.

CONTRAINDICATIONS:

This compound should not be used in patients whose oversensitivity to small doses of sympathomimetic amines produces sleeplessness, dizziness, light-headedness, weakness, tremulousness, or cardiac arrhythmias. The drug is contraindicated in any patient hypersensitive to any of the ingredients of the formulation.

WARNINGS:

Instruct patients not to drive or operate machinery if drowsiness occurs. Individuals should not ingest alcoholic beverages, monoamine oxidase inhibitors, or barbiturates while taking this medication.

PRECAUTIONS:

GENERAL

Individuals with high blood pressure, heart disease, diabetes mellitus, chronic renal disease, or thyroid disease should use only as directed by a physician.

INFORMATION FOR THE PATIENT

Patients taking this medication should be instructed not to operate heavy machinery, drive an auto or ingest alcoholic beverages, sedatives or monoamine oxidase inhibitors.

CARCINOGENESIS, MUTAGENESIS, AND IMPAIRMENT OF FERTILITY

No long-term studies have been conducted with this drug.

PREGNANCY CATEGORY C

Animal reproduction studies have not been conducted with this drug. It is also not known whether this drug can cause fetal harm when administered to a pregnant woman or can affect reproduction capacity. This drug should be given to a pregnant woman only if clearly needed.

NURSING MOTHERS

This drug should not be used in nursing mothers.

DRUG INTERACTIONS:

See WARNINGS.

ADVERSE REACTIONS:

The following adverse reactions have been reported for each of the individual or combinations of ingredients:

Acetaminophen: urticaria, epigastric distress, dizziness, and palpitation.

Phenylpropanolamine HCl: anxiety, restlessness, tension, insomnia, tremor, weakness, headache, vertigo, sweating, arrhythmia, nausea, and vomiting. Phenyltoloxamine Citrate—urticaria, drowsiness, disturbed coordination, inability to concentrate, dizziness, insomnia, tremors, nervousness, palpitation, convulsions, muscular weakness, gastric distress, diarrhea, intestinal cramps, blurred vision, hypotension, urinary retention, dryness of mouth, throat and nose.

OVERDOSAGE:

Antihistamine overdosage reactions may vary from CNS depression to stimulation. There is no specific therapy for acute overdosage with antihistamines. The latent period from ingestion to appearance of toxic effects is short (1.5 - 2 hours). General symptomatic and supportive measures should be instituted and maintained for as long as necessary.

DOSAGE AND ADMINISTRATION:

Adults: One tablet twice daily (every 12 hours).
Children: 6-12 years of age: One half tablet twice daily (every 12 hours).
Not to be given to children under the age of 12.
Tablets should not be chewed.
Store between 15-30°C (59-86°F).

ACETAMINOPHEN; PHENYLTOLOXAMINE *(000079)*

CATEGORIES: Analgesics; Analgesics/Antipyretics; Central Nervous System Agents

BRAND NAMES: Dologesic; Flextra-Ds; Relagesic

Prescribing information not available at time of publication.

HOW SUPPLIED - EQUIVALENTS NOT AVAILABLE:

Liquid - Oral

180 ml	$9.99	DOLOGESIC, Llorens Pharm	54859-0512-06

Tablet, Uncoated - Oral - 500 mg/30 mg

50's	$8.30	DOLOGESIC, Llorens Pharm	54859-0101-50

Tablet, Uncoated - Oral - 500 mg/50 mg

100's	$43.69	FLEXTRA-DS, Poly Pharms	50991-0830-01

Tablet, Uncoated - Oral - 650 mg/50 mg

100's	$32.95	RELAGESIC, Intl Ethical	11584-0476-01

ACETAMINOPHEN; PROPOXYPHENE HYDROCHLORIDE *(000081)*

CATEGORIES: Analgesics; Antipyretics; Central Nervous System Agents; Fever; Narcotics, Synthetics & Combinations; Opiate Agonists (Controlled); Pain; DEA Class CIV; FDA Approval Pre 1982

BRAND NAMES: *Corbutyl*; *Cosalgesic*; *Distalgesic*; Dolene Ap-65; E-Lor; Genagesic; Propoxyphene HCl w/APAP; Propoxyphene HCl APAP; **Wygesic**
(International brand names outside U.S. in italics)

FORMULARIES: Aetna; FHP

DESCRIPTION:

Acetaminophen with propoxyphene HCl tablets contain 65 mg propoxyphene HCl and 650 mg acetaminophen. The inactive ingredients present are cellulose, D&C Yellow 10, FD&C Blue 1, FD&C Yellow 6, hydrogenated vegetable oil, hydroxypropyl methylcellulose, methylcellulose, polacrilin potassium, polyethylene glycol, and titanium dioxide.

Propoxyphene hydrochloride is an odorless white crystalline powder with a bitter taste. It is freely soluble in water. Chemically, it is (S-(R*, S*))-α-(2-(dimethylamino) -1-methylethyl)-α-phenylbenzeneethanol, propanoate (ester), hydrochloride.

Acetaminophen is a white, crystalline powder, possessing a slightly bitter taste. It is soluble in boiling water and freely soluble in alcohol. Chemically, it is N-Acetyl-p- aminophenol.

CLINICAL PHARMACOLOGY:

Acetaminophen with propoxyphene HCl is a centrally acting narcotic analgesic agent.

Equimolar doses of propoxyphene hydrochloride provide similar plasma concentrations. Following administration of 65, 130, or 195 mg of propoxyphene hydrochloride, the bioavailability of propoxyphene is equivalent to that of 100, 200, or 300 mg respectively of propoxyphene napsylate. Peak plasma concentrations of propoxyphene are reached in 2 to 2-1/2 hours. After a 65 mg oral dose of propoxyphene hydrochloride, peak plasma levels of 0.05 to 0.1 mcg/ml are achieved.

Repeated doses of propoxyphene at 6-hour intervals lead to increasing plasma concentrations, with a plateau after the ninth dose at 48 hours.

Propoxyphene is metabolized in the liver to yield norpropoxyphene. Propoxyphene has a half-life of 6 to 12 hours, whereas that of norpropoxyphene is 30 to 36 hours.

Norpropoxyphene has substantially less central nervous system depressant effect than propoxyphene, but a greater local anesthetic effect, which is similar to that of amitriptyline and antiarrhythmic agents, such as lidocaine and quinidine.

In animal studies in which propoxyphene and norpropoxyphene were continuously infused in large amounts, intracardiac conduction time (P-R and QRS intervals) was prolonged. Any intracardiac conduction delay attributable to high concentrations of norpropoxyphene may be of relatively long duration.

MECHANISM OF ACTION

Propoxyphene is a mild narcotic analgesic structurally related to methadone. The potency of propoxyphene hydrochloride is from two-thirds to equal that of codeine.

Propoxyphene hydrochloride and acetaminophen provide the analgesic activity of propoxyphene napsylate and the antipyretic-analgesic activity of acetaminophen.

The combination of propoxyphene and acetaminophen produces greater analgesia than that produced by either propoxyphene or acetaminophen alone.

INDICATIONS AND USAGE:

Acetaminophen with propoxyphene HCl is indicated for the relief of mild-to-moderate pain, either when pain is present alone or when it is accompanied by fever.

CONTRAINDICATIONS:

Hypersensitivity to propoxyphene or to acetaminophen.

WARNINGS:

DO NOT PRESCRIBE PROPOXYPHENE FOR PATIENTS WHO ARE SUICIDAL OR ADDICTION PRONE.
PRESCRIBE PROPOXYPHENE WITH CAUTION FOR PATIENTS TAKING TRANQUILIZERS OR ANTIDEPRESSANT DRUGS AND PATIENTS WHO USE ALCOHOL IN EXCESS.
TELL YOUR PATIENTS NOT TO EXCEED THE RECOMMENDED DOSE AND TO LIMIT THIER INTAKE OF ALCOHOL.
Propoxyphene products in excessive doses, either alone or in combination with other CNS depressants, including alcohol, are a major cause of drug-related deaths. Fatalities within the first hour of overdosage are not uncommon. In a survey of deaths due to overdosage conducted in 1975, in approximately 20% of the fatal cases, death occurred within the first hour (5% occurred within 15 minutes). Propoxyphene should not be taken in doses higher than those recommended by the physician. The judicious prescribing of propoxyphene is essential to the safe use of this drug. With patients who are depressed or suicidal, consideration should be given to the use of nonnarcotic analgesics. Patients should be cautioned about the concomitant use of propoxyphene products and alcohol because of potentially serious CNS-additive effects of these agents. Because of its added depressant effects, propoxyphene should be prescribed with caution for those patients whose medical condition requires the concomitant administration of sedatives, tranquilizers, muscle relaxants, antidepressants, or other CNS-depressant drugs. Patients should be advised of the additive depressant effects of these combinations.
Many of the propoxyphene-related deaths have occurred in patients with previous histories of emotional disturbances or suicidal ideation or attempts as well as histories of misuse of tranquilizers, alcohol, and other CNS-active drugs. Some deaths have occurred as a consequence of the accidental ingestion of excessive quantities of propoxyphene alone or in combination with other drugs. Patients taking propoxyphene should be warned not to exceed the dosage recommended by the physician.

PRECAUTIONS:

GENERAL

Propoxyphene should be administered with caution to patients with hepatic or renal impairment since higher serum concentrations or delayed elimination may occur.

PREGNANCY

Safe use in pregnancy has not been established relative to possible adverse effects on fetal development. Instances of withdrawal symptoms in the neonate have been reported following usage during pregnancy. Therefore, propoxyphene should not be used in pregnant women unless, in the judgment of the physician, the potential benefits outweigh the possible hazards.

NURSING MOTHERS

Low levels of propoxyphene have been detected in human milk. In postpartum studies involving nursing mothers who were given propoxyphene, no adverse effects were noted in infants receiving mother's milk.

PEDIATRIC USE

Propoxyphene is not recommended for use in children, because documented clinical experience has been insufficient to establish safety and a suitable dosage regimen in the pediatric age group.

A patient Information Sheet is available for this product. See PATIENT PACKAGE INSERT.

DRUG INTERACTIONS:

The CNS-depressant effect of propoxyphene is additive with that of other CNS depressants, including alcohol.

As is the case with many medicinal agents, propoxyphene may slow the metabolism of a concomitantly administered drug. Should this occur, the higher serum concentrations of that drug may result in increased pharmacologic or adverse effects of that drug. Such occurrences have been reported when propoxyphene was administered to patients on antidepressants, anticonvulsants, or warfarin-like drugs.

ADVERSE REACTIONS:

In a survey conducted in hospitalized patients, less than 1% of patients taking propoxyphene hydrochloride at recommended doses experienced side effects. The most frequently reported have been dizziness, sedation, nausea, and vomiting. Some of these adverse reactions may be alleviated if the patient lies down.

Other adverse reactions include constipation, abdominal pain, skin rashes, light headedness, headache, weakness, euphoria, dysphoria, and minor visual disturbances.

Liver dysfunction has been reported in association with both active components of propoxyphene and acetaminophen tablets.

Propoxyphene therapy has been associated with abnormal liver-function tests and, more rarely, with instances of reversible jaundice.

Hepatic necrosis may result from acute overdoses of acetaminophen (see OVERDOSAGE). In chronic ethanol abusers, this has been reported rarely with short-term use of acetaminophen doses of 2.5 to 10 g/day. Fatalities have occurred.

DRUG ABUSE AND DEPENDENCE:

Propoxyphene, when taken in higher-than-recommended doses over long periods of time, can produce drug dependence characterized by psychic dependence and, less frequently, physical dependence and tolerance. Propoxyphene will only partially suppress the withdrawal syndrome in individuals physically dependent on morphine or other narcotics. The abuse liability of propoxyphene is qualitatively similar to that of codeine although quantitatively less, and propoxyphene should be prescribed with the same degree of caution appropriate to the use of codeine.

USAGE IN AMBULATORY PATIENTS

Propoxyphene may impair the mental and/or physical abilities required for the performance of potentially hazardous tasks, such as driving a car or operating machinery. The patient should be cautioned accordingly.

OVERDOSAGE:

In all cases of suspected overdosage, call your regional Poison Control Center to obtain the most up-to-date information about the treatment of overdosage. This recommendation is made because, in general, information regarding the treatment of overdosage may change more rapidly than do package inserts.

Initial consideration should be given to the management of the CNS effects of propoxyphene overdosage. Resuscitative measures should be initiated promptly.

SYMPTOMS OF PROPOXYPHENE OVERDOSAGE

The manifestations of acute overdosage with propoxyphene are those of narcotic overdosage. The patient is usually somnolent, but may be stuporous or comatose and convulsing. Respiratory depression is characteristic. The ventilatory rate and/or tidal volume is decreased, which results in cyanosis and hypoxia. Pupils, initially pinpoint, may become dilated as hypoxia increases. Cheyne-Stokes respiration and apnea may occur. Blood pressure and heart rate are usually normal initially, but blood pressure falls and cardiac performance deteriorates, which ultimately results in pulmonary edema and circulatory collapse unless the

OVERDOSAGE: *(cont'd)*

respiratory depression is corrected and adequate ventilation is restored promptly. Cardiac arrhythmias and conduction delay may be present. A combined respiratory-metabolic acidosis occurs, owing to retained CO_2 (hypercapnia) and to lactic acid formed during anaerobic glycolysis. Acidosis may be severe if large amounts of salicylates have also been ingested. Death may occur.

TREATMENT OF PROPOXYPHENE OVERDOSAGE

Attention should be directed first to establishing a patent airway and to restoring ventilation. Mechanically assisted ventilation, with or without oxygen, may be required, and positive-pressure respiration may be desirable if pulmonary edema is present.

The narcotic antagonist naloxone hydrochloride will markedly reduce the degree of respiratory depression, and 0.4 to 2 mg should be administered promptly, preferably intravenously. If the desired degree of counteraction with improvement in respiratory functions is not obtained, naloxone should be repeated at 2- to 3-minute intervals. The duration of action of the antagonist may be brief. If no response is observed after 10 mg of naloxone have been administered, the diagnosis of propoxyphene toxicity should be questioned. Naloxone hydrochloride may also be administered by continuous intravenous infusion.

TREATMENT OF PROPOXYPHENE OVERDOSAGE IN CHILDREN

The usual initial dose of naloxone in children is 0.01 mg/kg body weight given intravenously. If this dose does not result in the desired degree of clinical improvement, a subsequent increased dose of 0.1 mg/kg body weight may be administered. If an IV route of administration is not available, naloxone may be administered IM or subcutaneously in divided doses. If necessary, naloxone can be diluted with sterile water for injection.

Blood gases, pH, and electrolytes should be monitored in order that acidosis and any electrolyte disturbance present may be corrected promptly. Acidosis, hypoxia, and generalized CNS depression predispose to the development of cardiac arrhythmias. Ventricular fibrillation or cardiac arrest may occur and necessitate the full complement of cardiopulmonary resuscitation (CPR) measures. Respiratory acidosis rapidly subsides as ventilation is restored and hypercapnia eliminated, but lactic acidosis may require intravenous bicarbonate for prompt correction.

Electrocardiographic monitoring is essential. Prompt correction of hypoxia, acidosis, and electrolyte disturbance (when present) will help prevent these cardiac complications and will increase the effectiveness of agents administered to restore normal cardiac function.

In addition to the use of a narcotic antagonist, the patient may require careful titration with an anticonvulsant to control convulsions. Analeptic drugs (for example, caffeine or amphetamine) should not be used because of their tendency to precipitate convulsions.

General supportive measures, in addition to oxygen, include, when necessary, intravenous fluids, vasopressor-inotropic compounds, and, when infection is likely, anti-infective agents. Gastric lavage may be useful, and activated charcoal can adsorb a significant amount of ingested propoxyphene. Dialysis is of little value in poisoning due to propoxyphene. Efforts should be made to determine whether other agents, such as alcohol, barbiturates, tranquilizers, or other CNS depressants, were also ingested, since these increase CNS depression as well as cause specific toxic effects.

SYMPTOMS OF ACETAMINOPHEN OVERDOSAGE

Shortly after oral ingestion of an overdosage of acetaminophen and for the next 24 hours, anorexia, nausea, vomiting, and abdominal pain have been noted. The patient may then present no symptoms, but evidence of liver dysfunction may be apparent during the next 24 to 48 hours, with elevated serum transaminase and lactic dehydrogenase levels, an increase in serum bilirubin concentrations, and a prolonged prothrombin time. Death from hepatic failure may result 3 to 7 days after overdosage.

Acute renal failure may accompany the hepatic dysfunction and has been noted in patients who do not exhibit signs of fulminant hepatic failure. Typically, renal impairment is more apparent 6 to 9 days after ingestion of the overdose.

TREATMENT OF ACETAMINOPHEN OVERDOSAGE

Acetaminophen in massive overdosage may cause hepatic toxicity in some patients. In all cases of suspected overdose, you may wish to call your regional poison center for assistance in diagnosis and for directions in the use of N-acetylcysteine as an antidote.

In adults, hepatic toxicity has rarely been reported with acute overdoses of less than 10 g and fatalities with less than 15 g. Importantly, young children seem to be more resistant than adults to the hepatotoxic effect of an acetaminophen overdose. Despite this, the measures outlined below should be initiated in any adult or child suspected of having ingested an acetaminophen overdose. Clinical and laboratory evidence of hepatic toxicity may not be apparent until 48 to 72 hours postingestion. Early symptoms following a potentially hepatotoxic overdose may include: nausea, vomiting, diaphoresis, and general malaise.

The stomach should be emptied promptly by lavage or by induction of emesis with syrup of ipecac. Patients' estimates of the quantity of a drug ingested are notoriously unreliable. Therefore, if an acetaminophen overdose is suspected, a serum acetaminophen assay should be obtained as early as possible, but no sooner than four hours following ingestion. Liver-function studies should be obtained initially and repeated at 24-hour intervals.

The antidote, N-acetylcysteine, should be administered as early as possible, preferably within 16 hours of the overdose ingestion for optimal results, but in any case, within 24 hours. Following recovery, there are no residual, structural or functional hepatic abnormalities.

DOSAGE AND ADMINISTRATION:

This product is given orally. The usual dose is 65 mg propoxyphene HCl and 650 mg acetaminophen every 4 hours as needed for pain. The maximum recommended dose of propoxyphene HCl is 390 mg per day.

Consideration should be given to a reduced total daily dosage in patients with hepatic or renal impairment.

Store at controlled room temperature, 15°-30° C (59°-86° F).

Dispense in a tight, light-resistant container as defined in the USP.

ANIMAL PHARMACOLOGY:

The acute lethal doses of the hydrochloride and napsylate salts of propoxyphene were determined in 4 species. The results shown in TABLE 1 indicate that on a molar basis, the napsylate salt is less toxic than the hydrochloride. This may be due to the relative insolubility and retarded absorption of propoxyphene napsylate.

Some indication of the relative insolubility and retarded absorption of propoxyphene napsylate was obtained by measuring plasma propoxyphene levels in 2 groups of 4 dogs following oral administration of equimolar doses of the 2 salts.

Although none of the animals in this experiment died, 3 of the 4 dogs given propoxyphene hydrochloride exhibited convulsive seizures during the time interval corresponding to the peak plasma levels. The 4 animals receiving the napsylate salt were ataxic but not acutely ill.

TABLE 1 Acute Oral Toxicity Of Propoxyphene

Species	LD50 (mg/kg) = SE LD50 (mMole/kg) Propoxyphene Hydrochloride	Propoxyphene Napsylate
Mouse	282 ± 39 0.75	915 ± 163 1.62
Rat	230 ± 44 0.61	647 ± 95 1.14
Rabbit	ca. 82 0.22	>183 > 0.32
Dog	ca. 100 0.27	>183 > 0.32

PATIENT PACKAGE INSERT:

SUMMARY

Products containing propoxyphene are used to relieve pain.

LIMIT YOUR INTAKE OF ALCOHOL WHILE TAKING THIS DRUG. Make sure your doctor knows if you are taking tranquilizers, sleep aids, antidepressants, antihistamines, or any other drugs that make you sleepy. Combining propoxyphene with alcohol or these drugs in excessive doses is dangerous.

Use care while driving a car or using machines until you see how the drug affects you, because propoxyphene can make you sleepy. Do not take more of the drug than your doctor prescribed. Dependence has occurred when patients have taken propoxyphene for a long period of time at doses greater than recommended.

The rest of this monograph gives you more information about propoxyphene. Please read it and keep it for further use.

Uses for Propoxyphene: Products containing propoxyphene are used for the relief of mild to moderate pain. Products which contain propoxyphene plus acetaminophen are prescribed for the relief of pain or pain associated with fever.

Before Taking Propoxyphene: Make sure your doctor knows if you have ever had an allergic reaction to propoxyphene or acetaminophen.

The effect of propoxyphene in children under 12 has not been studies. Therefore, use of the drug in this age group is not recommended.

How To Take Propoxyphene: Follow your doctor's directions exactly. Do not increase the amount you take without your doctor's approval. If you miss a dose of the drug, do not take twice as much the next time.

Pregnancy: Do not take propoxyphene during pregnancy unless your doctor knows you are pregnant and specifically recommends its use. Cases of temporary dependence in the newborn have occurred when the mother has taken propoxyphene consistently in the weeks before delivery. As a general principle, no drug should be taken during pregnancy unless it is clearly necessary.

General Caution: Heavy use of alcohol with propoxyphene is hazardous and may lead to overdosage symptoms (see OVERDOSAGE); THEREFORE, LIMIT YOUR INTAKE OF ALCOHOL WHILE TAKING PROPOXYPHENE.

Combinations of excessive doses of propoxyphene, alcohol, and tranquilizers are dangerous. Make sure your doctor knows if you are taking tranquilizers, sleep aids, antidepressant drugs, antihistamines, or any other drugs that make you sleepy. The use of these drugs with propoxyphene increases their sedative effects and may lead to overdosage symptoms, including death (see OVERDOSAGE.)

Propoxyphene may cause drowsiness or impair your mental and/or physical abilities; therefore, use caution when driving a vehicle or operating dangerous machinery. DO NOT perform any hazardous task until you have seen your response to this drug.

Propoxyphene may increase the concentration in the body of medications such as anticoagulants ("blood thinners"), antidepressants, or drugs used for epilepsy. The result may be excessive or adverse effects of these medications. Make sure your doctor knows if you are taking any of these medications.

Dependence: You can become dependent on propoxyphene if you take it in higher than recommended doses over a long period of time. Dependence is a feeling of need for the drug and a feeling that you cannot perform normally without it.

Overdosage: An overdosage of propoxyphene, alone or in combination with other drugs, including alcohol, may cause weakness, difficulty in breathing, confusion, anxiety, and more severe drowsiness and dizziness. Extreme overdosage may lead to unconsciousness and death.

If the propoxyphene product contains acetaminophen, the overdosage symptoms include nausea, vomiting, lack of appetite, and abdominal pain. Liver damage may occur.

In any suspected overdosage situation, contact your doctor or nearest hospital emergency room. GET EMERGENCY HELP IMMEDIATELY. KEEP THIS AND ALL DRUGS OUT OF THE REACH OF CHILDREN.

Possible Side Effects: When propoxyphene is taken as directed, side effects are infrequent. Among those reported are drowsiness, dizziness, nausea, and vomiting. If these effects occur, it may help if you lie down and rest.

Less frequently reported side effects are constipation, abdominal pain, skin rashes, light-headedness, headache, weakness, minor visual disturbances, and feelings of elation or discomfort.

If side effects occur and concern you, contact your doctor.

Other Information: The safe and effective use of propoxyphene depends on your taking it exactly as directed. This drug has been prescribed specifically for you and your present condition. Do not give this drug to others who may have similar symptoms. Do not use it for any other reason.

If you would like more information about propoxyphene, ask your doctor or pharmacist. They have a more technical leaflet (professional labeling) you may read.

HOW SUPPLIED - RATED THERAPEUTICALLY EQUIVALENT:

Tablet, Coated - Oral - 650 mg/65 mg

100's	$12.46	DOLENE AP-65, Lederle Pharm	00005-4643-23
100's	$14.93	Propoxyphene HCl w/Apap, H.C.F.A. F F P	99999-0081-01
100's	$18.95	Propoxyphene Hcl W/Apap, Harber Pharm	51432-0392-03
100's	$19.40	Propoxyphene Hcl w/Apap, Qualitest Pharms	00603-5463-21
100's	$21.50	Propoxyphene HCl & Acetaminophen, Geneva Pharms	00781-1378-01
100's	$22.50	Propoxyphene Apap, IDE-Interstate	00814-6464-14
100's	$26.35	Propoxyphene Hcl & APAP, Mylan	00378-0130-01
100's	$31.30	Propoxyphene Hcl w/Apap, Geneva Pharms	00781-1378-13
100's	**$47.36**	**WYGESIC, Wyeth Labs**	**00008-0085-01**
500's	$74.65	Propoxyphene HCl w/Apap, H.C.F.A. F F P	99999-0081-02
500's	$78.75	Propoxyphene Hcl W/Apap, Harber Pharm	51432-0392-05
500's	$94.60	Propoxyphene Hcl w/Apap, Qualitest Pharms	00603-5463-28
500's	$98.62	Propoxyphene HCl & Acetaminophen, Geneva Pharms	00781-1378-05
500's	$98.62	Propoxyphene Hcl w/Apap, HL Moore Drug Exch	00839-1566-12
500's	$106.95	Propoxyphene Apap, IDE-Interstate	00814-6464-28

HOW SUPPLIED - RATED THERAPEUTICALLY EQUIVALENT: *(cont'd)*

500's	$125.15	Propoxyphene Hcl & APAP, Mylan	00378-0130-05
500's	**$221.21**	**WYGESIC, Wyeth Labs**	**00008-0085-02**

ACETAMINOPHEN; PROPOXYPHENE NAPSYLATE *(000082)*

CATEGORIES: Analgesics; Antipyretics; Central Nervous System Agents; Fever; Opiate Agonists (Controlled); Pain; DEA Class CIV; Sales > $100 Million; FDA Approval Pre 1982; Top 200 Drugs

BRAND NAMES: **Darvocet-N**; *Distalgesic*; *Dologesic*; *Dologesic-32*; *Dolostop*; Doxapap-N; Propacet; Propoxyphene Napsylate W/APAP; Ro-Cet-N 100
(International brand names outside U.S. in italics)

FORMULARIES: Aetna; BC-BS; FHP; PCS

COST OF THERAPY: $8.73 (Pain; Tablet; 650 mg/100 mg; 4/day; 25 days)

DESCRIPTION:

Propoxyphene napsylate, USP is an odorless, white, crystalline powder with a bitter taste. It is very slightly soluble in water and soluble in methanol, ethanol, chloroform, and acetone. Chemically, it is (αS,1R)-α-[2-(Dimethylamino)-1-methylethyl]-α-phenylphenethyl propionate compound with 2-naphthalenesulfonic acid (1:1) monohydrate. Its molecular weight is 565.72.

Propoxyphene napsylate differs from propoxyphene hydrochloride in that it allows more stable liquid dosage forms and tablet formulations. Because of differences in molecular weight, a dose of 100 mg (176.8 μmol) of propoxyphene napsylate is required to supply an amount of propoxyphene equivalent to that present in 65 mg (172.9 μmol) of propoxyphene hydrochloride.

Each Darvocet-N 50 tablet contains 50 mg (88.4 μmol) propoxyphene napsylate and 325 mg (2,150 μmol) acetaminophen.

Each Darvocet-N 100 tablet contains 100 mg (176.8 μmol) propoxyphene napsylate and 650 mg (4,300 μmol) acetaminophen.

Each tablet also contains amberlite, cellulose, FD&C Yellow #6, magnesium stearate, stearic acid, titanium dioxide, and other inactive ingredients.

CLINICAL PHARMACOLOGY:

Propoxyphene is a centrally acting narcotic analgesic agent. Equimolar doses of propoxyphene hydrochloride or napsylate provide similar plasma concentrations. Following administration of 65, 130, or 195 mg of propoxyphene hydrochloride, the bioavailability of propoxyphene is equivalent to that of 100, 200, or 300 mg respectively of propoxyphene napsylate. Peak plasma concentrations of propoxyphene are reached in 2 to 2 ½ hours. After a 100-mg oral dose of propoxyphene napsylate, peak plasma levels of 0.05 to 0.1 mcg/ml are achieved. The napsylate salt tends to be absorbed more slowly than the hydrochloride. At or near therapeutic doses, this absorption difference is small when compared with that among subjects and among doses (for graphic illustration please see manufacturer's original package insert).

Because of this several hundredfold difference in solubility, the absorption rate of very large doses of the napsylate salt is significantly lower than that of equimolar doses of the hydrochloride.

Repeated doses of propoxyphene at 6-hour intervals lead to increasing plasma concentrations with a plateau after the ninth dose at 48 hours.

Propoxyphene is metabolized in the liver to yield norpropoxyphene. Propoxyphene has a half-life of 6 to 12 hours, whereas that of norpropoxyphene is 30 to 36 hours.

Norpropoxyphene has substantially less central-nervous-system-depressant effect than propoxyphene but a greater local anesthetic effect, which is similar to that of amitriptyline and antiarrhythmic agents, such as lidocaine and quinidine.

In animal studies in which propoxyphene and norpropoxyphene were continuously infused in large amounts, intracardiac conduction time (PR and QRS intervals) was prolonged. Any intracardiac conduction delay attributable to high concentrations of norpropoxyphene may be of relatively long duration.

Propoxyphene is a mild narcotic analgesic structurally related to methadone. The potency of propoxyphene napsylate is from two thirds to equal that of codeine.

Propoxyphene napsylate and acetaminophen tablets provide the analgesic activity of propoxyphene napsylate and the antipyretic-analgesic activity of acetaminophen.

The combination of propoxyphene and acetaminophen produces greater analgesia than that produced by either propoxyphene or acetaminophen administered alone.

INDICATIONS AND USAGE:

These products are indicated for the relief of mild to moderate pain, either when pain is present alone or when it is accompanied by fever.

CONTRAINDICATIONS:

Hypersensitivity to propoxyphene or acetaminophen.

WARNINGS:

Do not prescribe propoxyphene for patients who are suicidal or addiction-prone.
Prescribe propoxyphene with caution for patients taking tranquilizers or antidepressant drugs and patients who use alcohol in excess.
Tell your patients not to exceed the recommended dose and to limit their intake of alcohol.
Propoxyphene products in excessive doses, either alone or in combination with other CNS depressants, including alcohol, are a major cause of drug-related deaths. Fatalities within the first hour of overdosage are not uncommon. In a survey of deaths due to overdosage conducted in 1975, death occurred within the first hour in approximately 20% of the fatal cases (5% occurred within 15 minutes). Propoxyphene should not be taken in doses higher than those recommended by the physician. The judicious prescribing of propoxyphene is essential to the safe use of this drug. With patients who are depressed or suicidal, consideration should be given to the use of non-narcotic analgesics. Patients should be cautioned about the concomitant use of propoxyphene products and alcohol because of potentially serious CNS-additive effects of these agents. Because of its added depressant effects, propoxyphene should be prescribed with caution for patients whose medical condition requires the concomitant administration of sedatives, tranquilizers, muscle relaxants, antidepressants, or other CNS-depressant drugs. Patients should be advised of the additive depressant effects of these combinations. Many of the propoxyphene-related deaths have occurred in patients with previous histories of emotional disturbances or suicidal ideation or attempts as well as histories of misuse of tranquilizers, alcohol, and other CNS-active drugs. Some deaths have occurred as a consequence of the accidental ingestion of excessive quantities of propoxyphene alone or in combination with other drugs. Patients taking propoxyphene should be warned not to exceed the dosage recommended by the physician.

Usage in Ambulatory Patients: Propoxyphene may impair the mental and/or physical abilities required for the performance of potentially hazardous tasks, such as driving a car or operating machinery. The patient should be cautioned accordingly.

PRECAUTIONS:

General: Propoxyphene should be administered with caution to patients with hepatic or renal impairment since higher serum concentrations or delayed elimination may occur.

Pregnancy: Safe use in pregnancy has not been established relative to possible adverse effects on fetal development. Instances of withdrawal symptoms in the neonate have been reported following usage during pregnancy. Therefore, propoxyphene should not be used in pregnant women unless, in the judgment of the physician, the potential benefits outweigh the possible hazards.

Nursing Mothers: Low levels of propoxyphene have been detected in human milk. In postpartum studies involving nursing mothers who were given propoxyphene, no adverse effects were noted in infants receiving mother's milk.

Pediatric Use: Propoxyphene is not recommended for use in children, because documented clinical experience has been insufficient to establish safety and a suitable dosage regimen in the pediatric age group.

Geriatric Use: The rate of propoxyphene metabolism may be reduced in some patients. Increased dosing interval should be considered.

A patient information sheet is available for this product. (See PATIENT PACKAGE INSERT.)

DRUG INTERACTIONS:

The CNS-depressant effect of propoxyphene is additive with that of other CNS depressants, including alcohol.

As is the case with many medicinal agents, propoxyphene may slow the metabolism of a concomitantly administered drug. Should this occur, the higher serum concentrations of that drug may result in increased pharmacologic or adverse effects of that drug. Such occurrences have been reported when propoxyphene was administered to patients taking antidepressants, anticonvulsants, or warfarin-like drugs. Severe neurologic signs, including coma, have occurred with concurrent use of carbamazepine.

ADVERSE REACTIONS:

In a survey conducted in hospitalized patients, less than 1% of patients taking propoxyphene hydrochloride at recommended doses experienced side effects. The most frequently reported were dizziness, sedation, nausea, and vomiting. Some of these adverse reactions may be alleviated if the patient lies down.

Other adverse reactions include constipation, abdominal pain, skin rashes, lightheadedness, headache, weakness, euphoria, dysphoria, hallucinations, and minor visual disturbances.

Liver dysfunction has been reported in association with both active components of propoxyphene napsylate and acetaminophen tablets, USP. Propoxyphene therapy has been associated with abnormal liver function tests and more rarely with instances of reversible jaundice (including cholestatic jaundice). Hepatic necrosis may result from acute overdose of acetaminophen (see OVERDOSAGE). In chronic ethanol abusers, this has been reported rarely with short-term use of acetaminophen dosages of 2.5 to 10 g/day. Fatalities have occurred.

Renal papillary necrosis may result from chronic acetaminophen use, particularly when the dosage is greater than recommended and when combined with aspirin.

Subacute painful myopathy has occurred following chronic propoxyphene overdosage.

DRUG ABUSE AND DEPENDENCE:

Propoxyphene, when taken in higher-than-recommended doses over long periods of time, can produce drug dependence characterized by psychic dependence and, less frequently, physical dependence and tolerance. Propoxyphene will only partially suppress the withdrawal syndrome in individuals physically dependent on morphine or other narcotics. The abuse liability of propoxyphene is qualitatively similar to that of codeine although quantitatively less. Propoxyphene should be prescribed with the same degree of caution appropriate to the use of codeine.

OVERDOSAGE:

Management of Overdosage: In all cases of suspected overdosage, call your regional Poison Control Center to obtain the most up-to-date information about the treatment of overdose. Telephone numbers of certified poison control centers are listed at the beginning of Physicians GenRx. This recommendation is made because, in general, information regarding the treatment of overdosage may change more rapidly than do package inserts.

Initial consideration should be given to the management of the CNS effects of propoxyphene overdosage. Resuscitative measures should be initiated promptly.

Symptoms of Propoxyphene Overdosage: The manifestations of acute overdosage with propoxyphene are those of narcotic overdosage. The patient is usually somnolent but may be stuporous or comatose and convulsing. Respiratory depression is characteristic. The ventilatory rate and/or tidal volume is decreased, which results in cyanosis and hypoxia. Pupils, initially pinpoint, may become dilated as hypoxia increases. Cheyne-Stokes respiration and apnea may occur. Blood pressure and heart rate are usually normal initially, but blood pressure falls and cardiac performance deteriorates, which ultimately results in pulmonary edema and circulatory collapse, unless the respiratory depression is corrected and adequate ventilation is restored promptly. Cardiac arrhythmias and conduction delay may be present. A combined respiratory- metabolic acidosis occurs owing to retained CO_2 (hypercapnia) and to lactic acid formed during anaerobic glycolysis. Acidosis may be severe if large amounts of salicylates have also been ingested. Death may occur.

Treatment of Propoxyphene Overdosage: Attention should be directed first to establishing a patent airway and to restoring ventilation. Mechanically assisted ventilation, with or without oxygen, may be required, and positive pressure respiration may be desirable if pulmonary edema is present. The narcotic antagonist naloxone will markedly reduce the degree of respiratory depression, and 0.4 to 2 mg should be administered promptly, preferably intravenously. If the desired degree of counteraction with improvement in respiratory functions is not obtained, naloxone should be repeated at 2- to 3-minute intervals. The duration of action

OVERDOSAGE: *(cont'd)*

of the antagonist may be brief. If no response is observed after 10 mg of naloxone have been administered, the diagnosis of propoxyphene toxicity should be questioned. Naloxone may also be administered by continuous intravenous infusion.

Treatment of Propoxyphene Overdosage in Children: The usual initial dose of naloxone in children is 0.01 mg/kg body weight given intravenously. If this dose does not result in the desired degree of clinical improvement, a subsequent increased dose of 0.1 mg/kg body weight may be administered. If an IV route of administration is not available, naloxone may be administered IM or subcutaneously in divided doses. If necessary, naloxone can be diluted with sterile water for injection.

Blood gases, pH, and electrolytes should be monitored in order that acidosis and any electrolyte disturbance present may be corrected promptly. Acidosis, hypoxia, and generalized CNS depression predispose to the development of cardiac arrhythmias. Ventricular fibrillation or cardiac arrest may occur and necessitate the full complement of cardiopulmonary resuscitation (CPR) measures. Respiratory acidosis rapidly subsides as ventilation is restored and hypercapnia eliminated, but lactic acidosis may require intravenous bicarbonate for prompt correction.

Electrocardiographic monitoring is essential. Prompt correction of hypoxia, acidosis, and electrolyte disturbance (when present) will help prevent these cardiac complications and will increase the effectiveness of agents administered to restore normal cardiac function.

In addition to the use of a narcotic antagonist, the patient may require careful titration with an anticonvulsant to control convulsions. Analeptic drugs (*e.g.,* caffeine or amphetamine) should not be used because of their tendency to precipitate convulsions.

General supportive measures in addition to oxygen include when necessary: intravenous fluids, vasopressor-inotropic compounds, and when infection is likely anti-infective agents. Gastric lavage may be useful, and activated charcoal can adsorb a significant amount of ingested propoxyphene. Dialysis is of little value in poisoning due to propoxyphene. Efforts should be made to determine whether other agents, such as alcohol, barbiturates, tranquilizers, or other CNS depressants, were also ingested, since these increase CNS depression as well as cause specific toxic effects.

Symptoms of Acetaminophen Overdosage: Shortly after oral ingestion of an overdose of acetaminophen and for the next 24 hours anorexia, nausea, vomiting, diaphoresis, general malaise, and abdominal pain have been noted. The patient may then present no symptoms, but evidence of liver dysfunction may become apparent up to 72 hours after ingestion with elevated serum transaminase and lactic dehydrogenase levels, an increase in serum bilirubin concentrations, and a prolonged prothrombin time. Death from hepatic failure may result 3 to 7 days after overdosage.

Acute renal failure may accompany the hepatic dysfunction and has been noted in patients who do not exhibit signs of fulminant hepatic failure. Typically, renal impairment is more apparent 6 to 9 days after ingestion of the overdose.

Treatment of Acetaminophen Overdosage: Acetaminophen in massive overdosage may cause hepatic toxicity in some patients. *In all cases of suspected overdose, immediately call your regional poison center* for assistance in diagnosis and for directions in the use of N-acetylcysteine as an antidote.

In adults, hepatic toxicity has rarely been reported with acute overdoses of less than 10 g and fatalities with less than 15 g. Importantly, young children seem to be more resistant than adults to the hepatotoxic effect of an acetaminophen overdose. Despite this, the measures outlined below should be initiated in any adult or child suspected of having ingested an acetaminophen overdose.

Because clinical and laboratory evidence of hepatic toxicity may not be apparent until 48 to 72 hours postingestion, liver function studies should be obtained initially and repeated at 24-hour intervals. Early symptoms following a potentially hepatotoxic overdose may include: nausea, vomiting, disphoresis, and general malaise.

The stomach should be emptied promptly by lavage or by induction of emesis with syrup of ipecac. Patients' estimates of the quantity of a drug ingested are notoriously unreliable. Therefore, if an acetaminophen overdose is suspected, a serum acetaminophen assay should be obtained as early as possible, but no sooner than 4 hours following ingestion. The antidote, N-acetylcysteine, should be administered as early as possible, and within 16 hours of the overdose ingestion for optimal results. Following recovery, there are no residual, structural, or functional hepatic abnormalities.

DOSAGE AND ADMINISTRATION:

These products are given orally. The usual dosage is 100 mg propoxyphene napsylate and 650 mg acetaminophen every 4 hours as needed for pain. The maximum recommended dose of propoxyphene napsylate is 600 mg per day.

Consideration should be given to a reduced total daily dosage in patients with hepatic or renal impairment.

Store at controlled room temperature, 59° to 86°F (15° to 30°C).

ANIMAL PHARMACOLOGY:

Animal Toxicology: The acute lethal doses of the hydrochloride and napsylate salts of propoxyphene were determined in 4 species. The results shown in TABLE 1 indicate that on a molar basis the napsylate salt is less toxic than the hydrochloride. This may be due to the relative insolubility and retarded absorption of propoxyphene napsylate.

TABLE 1 Acute Oral Toxicity Of Propoxyphene

Species	LD50(mg/kg) ± SE / LD50(mmol/kg): Propoxyphene Hydrochloride	Propoxyphene Napsylate
Mouse	282 ± 39 / 0.75	915 ± 163 / 1.62
Rat	230 ± 44 / 0.61	647 ± 95 / 1.14
Rabbit	ca. 82 / 0.22	>183 / >0.32
Dog	ca. 100 / 0.27	>183 / >0.32

Some indication of the relative insolubility and retarded absorption of propoxyphene napsylate was obtained by measuring plasma propoxyphene levels in 2 groups of 4 dogs following oral administration of equimolar doses of the 2 salts. The peak plasma concentration observed with propoxyphene hydrochloride was much higher than that obtained after administration of the napsylate salt.

Although none of the animals in this experiment died, 3 of the 4 dogs given propoxyphene hydrochloride exhibited convulsive seizures during the time interval corresponding to the peak plasma levels. The 4 animals receiving the napsylate salt were mildly ataxic but not acutely ill. (For graphic illustration please see manufacturer's original package insert).

PATIENT PACKAGE INSERT:

YOUR PRESCRIPTION FOR A PROPOXYPHENE PRODUCT

Summary: Products containing propoxyphene are used to relieve pain.

LIMIT YOUR INTAKE OF ALCOHOL WHILE TAKING THIS DRUG. Make sure your doctor knows if you are taking tranquilizers, sleep aids, antidepressants, antihistamines, or any other drugs that make you sleepy. Combining propoxyphene with alcohol or these drugs in excessive doses is dangerous.

Use care while driving a car or using machines until you see how the drug affects you because propoxyphene can make you sleepy. Do not take more of the drug than your doctor prescribed. Dependence has occurred when patients have taken propoxyphene for a long period of time at doses greater than recommended.

The rest of this leaflet gives you more information about propoxyphene. Please read it and keep it for future use.

Uses of Propoxyphene: Products containing propoxyphene are used for the relief of mild to moderate pain. Products that contain propoxyphene plus aspirin or acetaminophen are prescribed for the relief of pain or pain associated with fever.

Before Taking Propoxyphene: Make sure your doctor knows if you have ever had an allergic reaction to propoxyphene, aspirin, or acetaminophen. Some forms of propoxyphene products contain aspirin to help relieve the pain. Your doctor should be advised if you have a history of ulcers or if you are taking an anticoagulant ("blood thinner"). The aspirin may irritate the stomach lining and may cause bleeding, particularly if an ulcer is present. Also, bleeding may occur if you are taking an anticoagulant. In a small group of people, aspirin may cause an asthma attack. If you are one of these people, be sure your drug does not contain aspirin.

The effect of propoxyphene in children under 12 has not been studied. Therefore, use of the drug in this age group is not recommended.

Also, due to the possible association between aspirin and Reye Syndrome, those propoxyphene products containing aspirin should not be given to children, including teenagers, with chicken pox or flu unless prescribed by a physician. The following propoxyphene product contains aspirin: propoxyphene hydrochloride, aspirin, and caffeine, USP.

How to Take Propoxyphene: Follow your doctor's directions exactly. Do not increase the amount you take without your doctor's approval. If you miss a dose of the drug, do not take twice as much the next time.

Pregnancy: Do no take propoxyphene during pregnancy unless your doctor knows you are pregnant and specifically recommends its use. Cases of temporary dependence in the newborn have occurred when the mother has taken propoxyphene consistently in the weeks before delivery. As a general principle, no drug should be taken during pregnancy unless it is clearly necessary.

General Cautions: Heavy use of alcohol with propoxyphene is hazardous and may lead to overdosage symptoms (see OVERDOSAGE.) THEREFORE, LIMIT YOUR INTAKE OF ALCOHOL WHILE TAKING PROPOXYPHENE.

Combinations of excessive doses of propoxyphene, alcohol, and tranquilizers are dangerous. Make sure your doctor knows if you are taking tranquilizers, sleep aids, antidepressant drugs, antihistamines, or any other drugs that make you sleepy. The use of these drugs with propoxyphene increases their sedative effects and may lead to overdosage symptoms including death (see OVERDOSAGE).

Propoxyphene may cause drowsiness or impair your mental and/or physical abilities; therefore, use caution when driving a vehicle or operating dangerous machinery. DO NOT perform any hazardous task until you have seen your response to this drug.

Propoxyphene may increase the concentration in the body of medications, such as anticoagulants ("blood thinners"), antidepressants, or drugs used for epilepsy. The result may be excessive or adverse effects of these medications. Make sure your doctor knows if you are taking any of these medications.

Dependence: You can become dependent on propoxyphene if you take it in higher than recommended doses over a long period of time. Dependence is a feeling of need for the drug and a feeling that you cannot perform normally without it.

Overdose: An overdose of propoxyphene, alone or in combination with other drugs, including alcohol, may cause weakness, difficulty in breathing, confusion, anxiety, and more severe drowsiness and dizziness. Extreme overdosage may lead to unconsciousness and death.

If the propoxyphene product contains acetaminophen, the overdosage symptoms include nausea, vomiting, lack of appetite, and abdominal pain. Liver damage may occur even after symptoms disappear. Death can occur days later.

When the propoxyphene product contains aspirin, symptoms of taking too much of the drug are headache, dizziness, ringing in the ears, difficulty in hearing, dim vision, confusion, drowsiness, sweating, thirst, rapid breathing, nausea, vomiting, and, occasionally, diarrhea.

In any suspected overdosage situation, contact your doctor or nearest hospital emergency room. GET EMERGENCY HELP IMMEDIATELY. KEEP THIS DRUG AND ALL DRUGS OUT OF THE REACH OF CHILDREN.

Possible Side Effects: When propoxyphene is taken as directed, side effects are infrequent. Among those reported are drowsiness, dizziness, nausea, and vomiting. If these effects occur, it may help if you lie down and rest.

Less frequently reported side effects are constipation, abdominal pain, skin rashes, lightheadedness, headache, weakness, hallucinations, minor visual disturbances, and feelings of elation or discomfort.

If side effects occur and concern you, contact your doctor.

Other Information: The safe and effective use of propoxyphene depends on your taking it exactly as directed. This drug has been prescribed specifically for you and your present condition. Do not give this drug to others who may have similar symptoms. Do not use it for any other reason.

If you would like more information about propoxyphene, ask your doctor or pharmacist. They have a more technical leaflet (professional labeling) you may read.

HOW SUPPLIED - RATED THERAPEUTICALLY EQUIVALENT:

Tablet, Coated - Oral - 325 mg/50 mg

100's	$19.00	Propoxyphene Nap w/APAP, Major Pharms	00904-7622-60
100's	**$29.24**	**DARVOCET-N, Lilly**	**00002-0351-02**
500's	**$120.54**	**DARVOCET-N, Lilly**	**00002-0351-03**

Tablet, Coated - Oral - 650 mg/100 mg

30's	$2.61	Propoxyphene Nap w/Aceta, H.C.F.A. F F P	99999-0082-01
30's	$6.56	Propoxyphene Napsylatew/Apap, Talbert Phcy	44514-0750-18
50's	$10.93	Propoxyphene Napsylate W/Apap, Talbert Phcy	44514-0750-33
100's	$8.73	Propoxyphene Nap w/Aceta, United Res	00677-1034-01
100's	$8.73	Propoxyphene Nap w/Aceta, H.C.F.A. F F P	99999-0082-02
100's	$13.05	Propoxyphene-N-100 (White), IDE-Interstate	00814-6454-14
100's	$22.75	Propoxyphene Napsylate w/APAP, United Res	00677-1467-01
100's	$22.77	Propoxyphene Nap w/APAP, Voluntary Hosp	53258-0614-01
100's	$22.95	Propoxyphene Nap w/Aceta, HL Moore Drug Exch	00839-7123-06
100's	$23.30	Propoxyphene Nap w/Aceta, Goldline Labs	00182-1266-01
100's	$23.50	Propoxyphene Nap w/Aceta, Halsey Drug	00879-0630-01

HOW SUPPLIED - RATED THERAPEUTICALLY EQUIVALENT: *(cont'd)*

100's	$23.50	Propoxyphene Nap w/Aceta, Halsey Drug	00879-0711-01
100's	$23.95	Propoxyphene Nap w/APAP, Harber Pharm	51432-0391-03
100's	$24.53	Propoxyphene Nap w/Aceta, Aligen Independ	00405-0178-01
100's	$26.55	PROPACET 100, Teva	00093-0590-01
100's	$26.55	Propoxyphene Nap w/Aceta, Teva	00093-0890-01
100's	$28.44	Propoxyphene Nap w/APAP, Voluntary Hosp	53258-0614-13
100's	$29.06	Propoxyphene Nap w/Aceta, Goldline Labs	00182-0317-01
100's	$29.06	Propoxyphene Nap w/Aceta, Purepac Pharm	00228-2085-10
100's	$29.95	Propoxyphene Nap w/Aceta, Rugby	00536-4361-01
100's	$30.00	Propoxyphene Nap w/Aceta, Zenith Labs	00172-3981-60
100's	$33.49	Propoxyphene Nap w/Aceta, Geneva Pharms	00781-1720-01
100's	$33.75	Propoxyphene Nap w/APAP, Schein Pharm (US)	00364-0767-01
100's	$33.75	Propoxyphene Napsylate & APAP, Mylan	00378-0155-01
100's	$33.75	Propoxyphene Napsylate W/Apap, HL Moore Drug Exch	00839-7330-06
100's	$34.00	Propoxyphene Nap w/Aceta, Goldline Labs	00182-0317-89
100's	$34.08	Propoxyphene Nap w/Aceta, Vangard Labs	00615-0455-13
100's	$34.08	Propoxyphene Nap w/Aceta, Vangard Labs	00615-0455-47
100's	$34.20	Propoxyphene Nap w/Aceta, Medirex	57480-0507-01
100's	$38.20	Propoxyphene Nap w/Aceta, Geneva Pharms	00781-1720-13
100's	**$55.16**	**DARVOCET-N 100, Lilly**	**00002-0363-02**
100's	**$59.54**	**DARVOCET-N 100, Lilly**	**00002-0363-33**
500's	$35.75	Propoxyphene Napsylate W/Apap, H & H Labs	46703-0100-05
500's	$43.65	Propoxyphene Nap w/Aceta, United Res	00677-1034-05
500's	$43.65	Propoxyphene Nap w/Aceta, H.C.F.A. F F P	99999-0082-03
500's	$49.95	Propoxyphene Nap w/Aceta, Balan	00304-1580-05
500's	$59.25	Propoxyphene-N-100 (White), IDE-Interstate	00814-6454-28
500's	$81.33	Propoxyphene Nap w/Aceta, Martec Pharms	52555-0212-05
500's	$103.50	Propoxyphene Nap w/Aceta, Halsey Drug	00879-0630-05
500's	$103.50	Propoxyphene Nap w/Aceta, Halsey Drug	00879-0711-05
500's	$108.00	Propoxyphene Napsylate w/APAP, United Res	00677-1467-05
500's	$108.30	Propoxyphene Napsylate W/Apap, Major Pharms	00904-2281-40
500's	$108.30	Propoxyphene Napsylate W/Apap, Major Pharms	00904-7702-40
500's	$108.30	Propoxyphene Napsylate W/Apap, Major Pharms	00904-7703-40
500's	$109.34	Propoxyphene Nap w/Aceta, Goldline Labs	00182-1266-05
500's	$118.41	Propoxyphene Nap w/APAP, Voluntary Hosp	53258-0614-05
500's	$118.75	Propoxyphene Nap w/APAP, Qualitest Pharms	00603-5466-28
500's	$119.75	Propoxyphene Nap w/Aceta, Aligen Independ	00405-0178-02
500's	$119.75	Propoxyphene Napsylate W/Apap, Harber Pharm	51432-0391-05
500's	$124.86	Propoxyphene Nap w/Aceta, Goldline Labs	00182-0317-05
500's	$124.86	Propoxyphene Nap w/Aceta, Purepac Pharm	00228-2085-50
500's	$125.00	Propoxyphene Nap w/APAP, Amer Preferred	53445-0317-05
500's	$130.90	Propoxyphene Nap w/Aceta, Teva	00093-0490-05
500's	$130.90	PROPACET 100, Teva	00093-0590-05
500's	$130.90	Propoxyphene Nap w/Aceta, Teva	00093-0890-05
500's	$130.95	Propoxyphene Nap w/Aceta, HL Moore Drug Exch	00839-7123-12
500's	$142.85	Propoxyphene Nap w/Aceta, Zenith Labs	00172-3981-70
500's	$150.93	Propoxyphene Nap w/APAP, HL Moore Drug Exch	00839-7330-12
500's	$159.08	Propoxyphene Nap w/Aceta, Geneva Pharms	00781-1720-05
500's	$159.50	Propoxyphene Napsylate & APAP, Mylan	00378-0155-05
500's	$159.50	Propoxyphene Napsylate & APAP, Mylan	00378-1155-05
500's	$159.51	Propoxyphene Nap w/APAP, Schein Pharm (US)	00364-0767-05
500's	$159.51	Propoxyphene Nap w/Aceta, Rugby	00536-4361-05
500's	**$262.00**	**DARVOCET-N 100, Lilly**	**00002-0363-03**
500's	**$280.79**	**DARVOCET-N 100, Lilly**	**00002-0363-43**
500's	**$289.87**	**DARVOCET-N 100, Lilly**	**00002-0363-46**
600's	$226.00	Propoxyphene Nap w/Aceta, Medirex	57480-0507-06
750's	$259.99	Propoxyphene Napsylate W/Apap, Glasgow Pharm	60809-0500-55
750's	$259.99	Propoxyphene Napsylate W/Apap, Glasgow Pharm	60809-0500-72
1000's	$169.00	Propoxyphene/Acetaminophen, Halsey Drug	00879-0630-10
1000's	$169.00	Propoxyphene/Acetaminophen, Halsey Drug	00879-0711-10

ACETAMINOPHEN; SALICYLAMIDE *(000084)*

CATEGORIES: Analgesics; Antipyretics; Central Nervous System Agents; Pain; FDA Pre 1938 Drugs

BRAND NAMES: Duoprin-S; Panritis Forte

Prescribing information not available at time of publication.

HOW SUPPLIED - EQUIVALENTS NOT AVAILABLE:

Tablet, Uncoated - Oral - 250 mg/600 mg

100's	$23.95	PANRITIS FORTE CT, Pam Am Labs	00525-0803-01

ACETAZOLAMIDE *(000086)*

CATEGORIES: Anticonvulsants; Antiglaucomatous Agents; Carbonic Anhydrase Inhibitors; Diuretics; EENT Drugs; Eye, Ear, Nose, & Throat Preparations; Edema; Epilepsy; Glaucoma; Intraocular Pressure; Mountain Sickness; Ophthalmics; Renal Drugs; Seizures; Tonic-Clonic Seizures; FDA Approval Pre 1982

BRAND NAMES: *Acetamide*; *Acetazolam* (Canada); Acetazolamide Sodium; Ak-Zol; *Albox* (Japan); *Apo-Acetazolamide*; *Azol*; *Carbinib*; *Defiltran* (Germany); *Dehydratin*; **Diamox**; Diamox Sequels; Diamox Sodium; *Diamox Sustets*; *Diuramid* (Germany); *Edemox*; *Ederen*; *Glaucomed*; *Glaucomide*; *Glauconox*; *Glaupax* (Japan); *Glaupax Retard*; *Inidrase*; *Ledimox* (Japan); *Lediamox*; *Nephramid*; Ocu-Zolamide; *Oratrol*; Storzolamide

(International brand names outside U.S. in italics)

FORMULARIES: Aetna; BC-BS; CIGNA; FHP; Humana; Kaiser; Medco; Medi-Cal; PCS; PruCare; United; WHO

DESCRIPTION:

Acetazolamide, an inhibitor of the enzyme carbonic anhydrase is a white to faintly yellowish white crystalline, odorless powder, weakly acidic, very slightly soluble in water and slightly soluble in alcohol. The chemical name is *N*-(5-Sulfa-moyl-1,3,4-thiadiazol-2yl)-acetamide.

Acetazolamide is available as oral tablets containing 125 mg and 250 mg of acetazolamide respectively and the following inactive ingredients: Corn Starch, Dibasic Calcium Phosphate, Magnesium Stearate, Povidone, and Sodium Starch Glycolate.

Acetazolamide sustained-release capsules, for oral administration, each containing 500 mg of acetazolamide and the following inactive ingredients: Benzoin, Ethylcellulose, Ethyl Vanillin, FD&C Blue No. 1, FD&C Yellow No.6, Gelatin, Glycerin, Magnesium Stearate, Methylparaben, Mineral Oil, Mono- and Diglycerides, Propylene Glycol, Propylparaben, Silicon Dioxide, Sucrose, Talc, Terpene Resin, Vanillin, and White Wax.

DESCRIPTION: *(cont'd)*

Acetazolamide is also available for intravenous use, and is supplied as a sterile powder requiring reconstitution. Each vial contains an amount of acetazolamide sodium equivalent to 500 mg of acetazolamide. The bulk solution is adjusted to pH 9.2 using sodium hydroxide and, if necessary, hydrochloric acid prior to lyophilization.

CLINICAL PHARMACOLOGY:

Acetazolamide is a potent carbonic anhydrase inhibitor, effective in the control of fluid secretion (*e.g.,* some types of glaucoma), in the treatment of certain convulsive disorders (*e.g.,* epilepsy) and in the promotion of diuresis in instances of abnormal fluid retention (*e.g.,* cardiac edema).

Acetazolamide is not a mercurial diuretic. Rather, it is a nonbacteriostatic sulfonamide possessing a chemical structure and pharmacological activity distinctly different from the bacteriostatic sulfonamides.

Acetazolamide is an enzyme inhibitor that acts specifically on carbonic anhydrase, the enzyme that catalyzes the reversible reaction involving the hydration of carbon dioxide and the dehydration of carbonic acid. In the eye, this inhibitory action of acetazolamide decreases the secretion of aqueous humor and results in a drop in intraocular pressure, a reaction considered desirable in cases of glaucoma and even in certain nonglaucomatous conditions. Evidence seems to indicate that acetazolamide has utility as an adjuvant in the treatment of certain dysfunctions of the central nervous system (*e.g.,* epilepsy). Inhibition of carbonic anhydrase in this area appears to retard abnormal, paroxysmal, excessive discharge from central nervous system neurons. The diuretic effect of acetazolamide is due to its action in the kidney on the reversible reaction involving hydration of carbon dioxide and dehydration of carbonic acid. The result is renal loss of HCO_3ion, which carries out sodium, water, and potassium. Alkalinization of the urine and promotion of diuresis is thus effected. Alteration in ammonia metabolism occurs due to increased reabsorption of ammonia by the renal tubules as a result of urinary alkalinization.

Placebo-controlled clinical trials have shown that prophylactic administration of Acetazolamide at a dose of 250 mg every eight to 12 hours (or a 500 mg controlled-release capsule once daily) before and during rapid ascent to altitude results in fewer and/or less severe symptoms (such as headache, nausea, shortness of breath, dizziness, drowsiness, and fatigue) of acute mountain sickness (AMS). Pulmonary function (*e.g.,* minute ventilation, expired vital capacity, and peak flow) is greater in the Acetazolamide treated group, both in subjects with AMS and asymptomatic subjects. The acetazolamide treated climbers also had less difficulty in sleeping.

INDICATIONS AND USAGE:

For adjunctive treatment of: edema due to congestive heart failure; drug-induced edema; centrencephalic epilepsies (petit mal, unlocalized seizures); chronic simple (open-angel) glaucoma, secondary glaucoma, and preoperatively in acute angle-closure glaucoma where delay of surgery is desired in order to lower intraocular pressure. Acetazolamide is also indicated for the prevention of amelioration of symptoms associated with acute mountain sickness in climbers attempting rapid ascent and in those who are very susceptible to acute mountain sickness despite gradual ascent.

CONTRAINDICATIONS:

Acetazolamide therapy is contraindicated in situations in which sodium and/or potassium blood serum levels are depressed, in cases of marked kidney and liver disease or dysfunction, in suprarenal gland failure, and in hyperchloremic acidosis. It is contraindicated in patients with cirrhosis because of the risk of development of hepatic encephalopathy.

Long-term administration of acetazolamide is contraindicated in patients with chronic non-congestive angle-closure glaucoma since it may permit organic closure of the angle to occur while the worsening glaucoma is masked by lowered intraocular pressure.

WARNINGS:

Fatalities have occurred, although rarely, due to severe reactions to sulfonamides including Stevens-Johnson syndrome, toxic epidermal necrolysis, fulminant hepatic necrosis, agranulocytosis, aplastic anemia, and other blood dyscrasias. Sensitizations may recur when a sulfonamide is readministered irrespective of the route of administration. If signs of hypersensitivity or other serious reactions occur, discontinue use of this drug.

Caution is advised for patients receiving concomitant high-dose aspirin and acetazolamide, as anorexia, tachypnea, lethargy, coma and death have been reported.

PRECAUTIONS:

GENERAL

Increasing the dose does not increase the diuresis and may increase the incidence of drowsiness and/or paresthesia. Increasing the dose often results in a decrease in diuresis. Under certain circumstances, however, very large doses have been given in conjunction with other diuretics in order to secure diuresis in complete refractory failure.

INFORMATION FOR THE PATIENT

Adverse reactions common to all sulfonamide derivatives may occur: anaphylaxis, fever, rash (including erythema multiforme, Stevens-Johnson syndrome, toxic epidermal necrolysis), crystalluria, renal calculus, bone marrow depression, thrombocytopenic purpura, hemolytic anemia, leukopenia, pancytopenia and agranulocytosis. Precaution is advised for early detection of such reactions and the drug should be discontinued and appropriate therapy instituted.

In patients with pulmonary obstruction or emphysema where alveolar ventilation may be impaired, acetazolamide which may precipitate or aggravate acidosis, should be used with caution.

Gradual ascent is desirable to try to avoid acute mountain sickness. If rapid ascent is undertaken and acetazolamide is used, it should be noted that such use does not obviate the need for prompt descent if severe forms of high altitude sickness occur, i.e., high altitude pulmonary edema (HAPE) or high-altitude cerebral edema.

Caution is advised for patients receiving concomitant high-dose aspirin and acetazolamide, as anorexia, tachypnea, lethargy, coma and death have been reported (see WARNINGS.)

LABORATORY TESTS

To monitor for hematologic reactions common to all sulfonamides, it is recommended that a baseline CBC and platelet count be obtained on patients prior to initiating acetazolamide therapy and at regular intervals during therapy. If significant changes occur, early discontinuance and institution of appropriate therapy are important. Periodic monitoring of serum electrolytes is recommended.

CARCINOGENESIS, MUTAGENESIS, AND IMPAIRMENT OF FERTILITY

Long-term studies in animal to evaluate the carcinogenic potential of acetazolamide have not been conducted. In a bacterial mutagenicity assay, acetazolamide was not mutagenic when evaluated with and without metabolic activation. The drug had no effect on fertility when administered in the diet to male and female rats at a daily intake of up to 4 times the recommended human dose of 100 mg in a 50 kg individual.

PRECAUTIONS: *(cont'd)*

PREGNANCY CATEGORY C

Acetazolamide, administered orally or parenterally, has been shown to be teratogenic (defects of the limbs) in mice, rats, hamsters and rabbits. There are no adequate and well-controlled studies in pregnant women. Acetazolamide should be used in pregnancy only if the potential benefit justifies the potential risk to the fetus.

NURSING MOTHERS

Because of the potential for serious adverse reaction in nursing infants from acetazolamide, a decision should be made whether to discontinue nursing or to discontinue the drug taking into account the importance of the drug to the mother.

PEDIATRIC USE

The safety and effectiveness of acetazolamide in children have not been established.

ADVERSE REACTIONS:

Adverse reactions, occurring most often early in therapy, include: paresthesias, particularly a "tingling" feeling in the extremities, hearing dysfunction or tinnitus, loss of appetite, taste alteration and gastrointestinal disturbances such as nausea, vomiting and diarrhea, polyuria, and occasional instances of drowsiness and confusion.

Metabolic acidosis and electrolyte imbalance may occur.

Transient myopia has been reported. This condition invariably subsides upon diminution or discontinuance of the medication.

Other occasional adverse reactions include urticaria, melena, hematuria, glycosuria, hepatic insufficiency, flaccid paralysis, photosensitivity and convulsions. Also see PRECAUTIONS, Information for the Patient for possible reactions common to sulfonamide derivatives. Fatalities have occurred although rarely, due to severe reactions to sulfonamides including Stevens-Johnson syndrome, toxic epidermal necrolysis, fulminant hepatic necrosis, agranulocytosis, aplastic anemia and other blood dyscrasias (see WARNINGS.)

OVERDOSAGE:

No data are available regarding acetazolamide overdosage in humans as no cases of acute poisoning with this drug have been reported. Animal data suggest that acetazolamide is remarkably nontoxic. No specific antidote is known. Treatment should be symptomatic and supportive.

Electrolyte imbalance, development of an acidotic state, and central nervous effects might be expected to occur. Serum electrolyte levels (particularly potassium) and blood pH levels should be monitored.

Supportive measures are required to restore electrolyte and pH balance. The acidotic state can usually be corrected by the administration of bicarbonate.

Despite its high intraerythrocytic distribution and plasma protein binding properties, Acetazolamide may be dialyzable. This may be particularly important in the management of acetazolamide overdosage when complicated by the presence of renal failure.

DOSAGE AND ADMINISTRATION:

Preparation and Storage of Parenteral Solution: Each 500 mg vial containing sterile acetazolamide sodium parenteral should be reconstituted with at least 5 ml of Sterile Water for injection prior to use. Reconstituted solutions retain potency for one week if refrigerated. Since this product contains no preservative, use within 24 hours of reconstitution is strongly recommended. The direct intravenous route of administration is preferred. Intramuscular administration is not recommended.

TABLETS

Glaucoma Acetazolamide should be used as an adjunct to the usual therapy. The dosage employed in the treatment of *chronic simple (open-angle) glaucoma* ranges from 250 mg to 1 g of acetazolamide per 24 hours, usually in divided doses for amounts over 250 mg. It has usually been found that a dosage in excess of 1 g per 24 hours does not produce an increased effect. In all cases, the dosage should be adjusted with careful individual attention both to symptomatology and ocular tension. Continuous supervision by a physician is advisable.

In treatment of secondary glaucoma and in the preoperative treatment of some cases of *acute congestive (closed-angle) glaucoma*, the preferred dosage is 250 mg every four hours, although some cases have responded to 250 mg twice daily on short-term therapy. In some acute cases, it may be more satisfactory to administer an initial dose of 500 mg followed by 125 mg every four hours depending on the individual case. Intravenous therapy may be used for rapid relief to ocular tension in acute cases. A complementary effect has been noted when acetazolamide has been used in conjunction with miotics or mydriatics as the case demanded.

SUSTAINED-RELEASE CAPSULES

The recommended dosage is 1 capsules (500 mg) two times a day. Usually 1 capsule is administered in the morning and 1 capsule in the evening. It may be necessary to adjust the dose, but it has usually been found that dosage in excess of 2 capsules (1 g) does not produce an increased effect. The dosage should be adjusted with careful individual attention both to symptomatology and intraocular tension. In all cases, continuous supervision by a physician is advisable.

In those unusual instances where adequate control is not obtained by twice-a-day administration of acetazolamide sustained-release capsules the desired control may be established by means of acetazolamide tablets or parenteral. Use tablets or parenteral in accordance with the more frequent dosage schedules recommended for these dosage forms, such as 250 mg every four hours, or an initial dose of 500 mg followed by 250 mg or 125 mg every four hours, depending on the case in question.

Epilepsy: It is not clearly shown whether the beneficial effects observed in epilepsy are due to direct inhibition of carbonic anhydrase in the central nervous system or whether they are due to the slight degree of acidosis produced by the divided dosage. The best results to date have been seen in petit mal in children. Good results, however, have been seen in patients, both children and adult, in other types of seizures such as grand mal, mixed seizure patterns, myoclonic jerk patterns, etc. The suggested total daily dose is 8 to 30 mg per kg in divided doses. Although some patients respond to a low dose, the optimum range appears to be from 375 to 1000 mg daily. However, some investigators feel that daily doses in excess of 1 g do not produce any better results than a 1 g dose. When acetazolamide is given in combination with other anticonvulsants, it is suggested that the starting dose should be 250 mg once daily in addition to the existing medications. This can be increased to levels as indicated above.

The change from other medications to acetazolamide should be gradual and in accordance with usual practice in epilepsy therapy.

Congestive Heart Failure: For diuresis in congestive heart failure, the starting dose in usually 250 to 375 mg once daily in the morning (5 mg/kg). If, after an initial response, the patient fails to continue to lose edema fluid, do not increase the dose but allow for kidney recovery by skipping medication for a day. Acetazolamide yields best diuretic results when given on alternate days, or for two days alternating with a day of rest.

Failures in therapy may be due to overdosage or too frequent dosage. The use of acetazolamide does not eliminate the need for other therapy such as digitalis, bed rest, and salt restriction.

DOSAGE AND ADMINISTRATION: *(cont'd)*

Drug-Induced Edema: Recommended dosage is 250 to 375 mg of acetazolamide once a day for one or two days, alternating with a day of rest.

Acute Mountain Sickness: Dosage is 500 mg to 1000 mg daily, in divided doses using tablets or sustained-release capsules as appropriate. In circumstances of rapid ascent, such as in rescue or military operations, the higher dose level of 1000 mg is recommended. It is preferable to initiate dosing 24 to 48 hours before ascent and to continue for 48 hours while at high altitude, or longer as necessary to control symptoms.

Note: The dosage recommendations for glaucoma and epilepsy differ considerably from those for congestive heart failure, since the first two conditions are not dependent upon carbonic anhydrase inhibition in the kidney which requires intermittent dosage if it is to recover from the inhibitory effect of the therapeutic agent.

Parenteral drug products should be inspected visually for particulate matter and discoloration prior to administration, whenever solution and container permit.

STORAGE

Store at Controlled Room Temperature 15-30°C (59-86°F).

(Tablets and Injection: Storz, 11/93, 31916-93); (Capsules: Storz, 3/94, 40713-94)

HOW SUPPLIED - RATED THERAPEUTICALLY EQUIVALENT:

Injection, Lyphl-Soln - Intravenous - 500 mg/5ml

1's	$31.20	Acetazolamide Sodium, Bedford Labs	55390-0460-01
5 ml	**$36.59**	**DIAMOX, Storz Ophthalm**	**57706-0762-96**

Tablet, Uncoated - Oral - 125 mg

100's	$6.70	Acetazolamide, Mutual Pharm	53489-0166-01
100's	$8.39	Acetazolamide, United Res	00677-1248-01
100's	$9.05	Acetazolamide, HL Moore Drug Exch	00839-7687-06
100's	**$30.06**	**DIAMOX, Storz Ophthalm**	**57706-0754-23**
500's	$27.00	Acetazolamide, Mutual Pharm	53489-0166-05
1000's	$51.00	Acetazolamide, Mutual Pharm	53489-0166-10

Tablet, Uncoated - Oral - 250 mg

100's	$5.95	Acetazolamide, Raway	00686-0042-10
100's	$7.26	Acetazolamide, US Trading	56126-0203-11
100's	$8.95	Acetazolamide, Consolidated Midland	00223-0039-01
100's	$9.00	Acetazolamide, Goldline Labs	00182-0818-01
100's	$9.00	Acetazolamide, Major Pharms	00904-0350-60
100's	$9.17	Acetazolamide, HL Moore Drug Exch	00839-5953-06
100's	$9.85	Acetazolamide, Mutual Pharm	53489-0167-01
100's	$12.00	Acetazolamide, IDE-Interstate	00814-0265-14
100's	$13.80	Acetazolamide, Aligen Independ	00405-4019-01
100's	$15.00	Acetazolamide, Raway	00686-0052-20
100's	$28.00	Acetazolamide, Schein Pharm (US)	00364-0400-01
100's	**$38.78**	**DIAMOX, Storz Ophthalm**	**57706-0755-23**
100's	**$44.89**	**DIAMOX, Storz Ophthalm**	**57706-0755-60**
500's	$38.75	Acetazolamide, Mutual Pharm	53489-0167-05
500's	$42.35	Acetazolamide, United Res	00677-0577-05
1000's	$49.00	Acetazolamide, Raway	00686-0042-14
1000's	$72.00	Acetazolamide, Mutual Pharm	53489-0167-10
1000's	$77.80	Acetazolamide, Major Pharms	00904-0350-80
1000's	$80.99	Acetazolamide, HL Moore Drug Exch	00839-5953-16
1000's	$85.00	Acetazolamide, Consolidated Midland	00223-0039-02
1000's	$90.55	Acetazolamide, Aligen Independ	00405-4019-03
1000's	**$368.23**	**DIAMOX, Storz Ophthalm**	**57706-0755-34**

HOW SUPPLIED - NOT RATED EQUIVALENT:

Capsule, Gelatin, Sustained Action - Oral - 500 mg

100's	**$96.30**	**DIAMOX SEQUELS, Storz Ophthalm**	**57706-0753-23**

ACETIC ACID *(000087)*

CATEGORIES: Anti-Infectives; Antibacterials; Antimicrobials; Dermatitis; Dermatologicals; EENT Drugs; Electrolytic, Caloric-Water Balance; Eye, Ear, Nose, & Throat Preparations; Infections; Irrigating Solutions; Otic Preparations; Otologic; Pharmaceutical Aids; Wet Dressings; Diaper Rash*; Insect Bites*; FDA Approval Pre 1982

* Indication not approved by the FDA

BRAND NAMES: Aa-Sol; Acetasol; Acetic Acid, Glacial; Acetic Acid Otic; Acetic Acid Aluminum; Acetic Aluminum; *Aquaear;* Betaboro Otic; Bio-Sol Ear; Borofair; Burotic; Burow's Solution; Burrow's Otic; Domeboro; Orlex; Vaolate; **Vosol**
(International brand names outside U.S. in italics)

FORMULARIES: Aetna; BC-BS; FHP; Medi-Cal; PCS

DESCRIPTION:

Vosol (acetic acid otic solution, USP) is a solution of acetic acid (2%), in a propylene glycol vehicle containing propylene glycol diacetate (3%), benzethonium chloride (0.02%), and sodium acetate (0.015%). The empirical formula for acetic acid is CH_3COOH, with a molecular weight of 60.05.

Acetic acid is available as a nonaqueous otic solution buffered at pH 3 for use in the external ear canal.

CLINICAL PHARMACOLOGY:

Acetic acid is anti-bacterial and anti-fungal; propylene glycol is hydrophilic and provides a low surface tension; benzethonium chloride is a surface active agent that promotes contact of the solution with tissues.

INDICATIONS AND USAGE:

For the treatment of superficial infections of the external auditory canal caused by organisms susceptible to the action of the antimicrobial.

CONTRAINDICATIONS:

Hypersensitivity to acetic acid or any of the ingredients. Perforated tympanic membrane is frequently considered a contraindication to the use of any medication in the external ear canal.

WARNINGS:

Discontinue promptly it sensitization or irritation occurs.

PRECAUTIONS:

Transient stinging or burning may be noted occasionally when the solution is first instilled into the acutely inflamed ear.

ADVERSE REACTIONS:

Stinging or burning may be noted occasionally; local irritation has occurred very rarely.

DOSAGE AND ADMINISTRATION:

Carefully remove all cerumen and debris to allow acetic acid to contact infected surfaces directly. To promote continuous contact, insert a wick saturated with acetic acid into the ear canal; the wick may also be saturated after insertion. Instruct the patient to keep the wick in for at least 24 hours and to keep it most by adding 3 to 5 drops of acetic acid every 4 to 6 hours. The wick may be removed after 24 hours but the patient should continue to instill 5 drops of acetic acid 3 or 4 times daily thereafter, for as long as indicated.

Store at room temperature; avoid excessive heat. Keep container tightly closed.

HOW SUPPLIED - RATED THERAPEUTICALLY EQUIVALENT:

Solution - Irrigation - 0.25 %

250 ml	$18.53	Acetic Acid, Abbott	00074-6143-02
500 ml x 12	$18.31	Acetic Acid, McGaw	00264-2304-10
1000 ml	$20.70	Acetic Acid, Baxter Hlthcare	00338-0656-04
1000 ml	$21.73	Acetic Acid, Abbott	00074-6143-09
1000 ml x 12	$21.43	Acetic Acid, McGaw	00264-2304-00
2000 ml x 6	$17.44	Acetic Acid, McGaw	00264-2304-50

Solution - Oral - 2 %

15 ml	$3.75	VASOTATE, Major Pharms	00904-0315-35

Solution - Otic - 2 %

15 ml	$2.60	Acetic Acid Otic, Thames Pharma	49158-0195-42
15 ml	$3.32	Acetic Acid Otic, Qualitest Pharms	00603-7035-41
15 ml	$3.48	Acetic Acid Otic, UDL	51079-0262-15
15 ml	$3.50	Acetic Acid Otic, Goldline Labs	00182-1775-64
15 ml	$3.63	ACETASOL, HL Moore Drug Exch	00839-6644-61
15 ml	$3.65	ACETIC ACID OTIC, Harber Pharm	51432-0499-10
15 ml	$3.78	Acetic Acid Otic, Schein Pharm (US)	00364-0732-72
15 ml	$5.25	Acetic Acid Otic, Rugby	00536-2102-72
15 ml	$10.00	ACETASOL, Alpharma	00472-0880-99
15 ml	**$99.88**	**VOSOL, Wallace Labs**	**00037-3611-10**
60 ml	$7.09	BOROFAIR OTIC, HL Moore Drug Exch	00839-7383-64
60 ml	$7.77	Acetic Acid/Aluminum, Aligen Independ	00405-2126-56
60 ml	$10.30	BOROFAIR, Major Pharms	00904-3524-03
60 ml	$10.80	BURROW'S OTIC, Rugby	00536-0252-96
60 ml	$16.00	DOMEBORO, Bayer	00026-4312-02

Solution/Drops - Otic - 2 %

15 ml	$1.87	Acetic Acid, H.C.F.A. F F P	99999-0087-01

HOW SUPPLIED - NOT RATED EQUIVALENT:

Solution - Otic - 2 %

15 ml	$3.95	Acetasol, Raway	00686-0880-09

ACETIC ACID; HYDROCORTISONE *(000088)*

CATEGORIES: Anti-Infectives; Anti-Inflammatory Agents; Antibacterials; Dermatologicals; EENT Drugs; Eye, Ear, Nose, & Throat Preparations; Infections; Inflammation; Otic Hydrocortisones; Otic Preparations; Otologic; Steroids; FDA Approval Pre 1982

BRAND NAMES: Acetasol HC; Acetic Acid W/HC; Bio-Sol HC; Orlex HC; Otobalm HC; Otomycet-HC; Otosol-HC; Vasolate HC; **Vosol HC**; *Vosol HC* (Canada)

(International brand names outside U.S. in italics)

FORMULARIES: Aetna; BC-BS; Medi-Cal; PCS

DESCRIPTION:

Hydrocortisone and acetic acid otic solution is a solution containing hydrocortisone (1%) and acetic acid (2%) in a propylene glycol vehicle containing propylene glycol diacetate (3%), benzethonium chloride (0.02%), sodium acetate (0.015%) and citric acid (0.2%). The empirical formulas for acetic acid and hydrocortisone are CH_3COOH and $C_{21}H_{30}O_5$, with a molecular weight of 60.05 and 326.46, respectively.

Chemically, hydrocortisone is Pregn-4-ene-3,20-dione, 11, 17, 21- trihydroxy-11β)-.

Acetic acid/hydrocortisone is available as a nonaqueous otic solution buffered at pH 3 for use in the external ear canal.

CLINICAL PHARMACOLOGY:

Acetic acid is antibacterial and antifungal; hydrocortisone is anti-inflammatory, anti-allergic and anti-pruritic; propylene glycol is hydrophilic and provides low surface tension; benzethonium chloride is a surface active agent that promotes contact of the solution with tissues.

INDICATIONS AND USAGE:

For the treatment of superficial infections caused by organisms susceptible to the action of the antimicrobial, complicated by inflammation.

CONTRAINDICATIONS:

Hypersensitivity to hydrocortisone and acetic acid otic solution or any of the ingredients; herpes simplex, varicella. Perforated tympanic membrane is frequently considered a contraindication to the use of any medication in the external ear canal.

WARNINGS:

Discontinue promptly if sensitization or irritation occurs.

PRECAUTIONS:

Transient stinging or burning may be noted occasionally when the solution is first instilled into the acutely inflamed ear.

ADVERSE REACTIONS:

Stinging or burning may be noted occasionally; local irritation has occurred very rarely.

DOSAGE AND ADMINISTRATION:

Carefully remove all cerumen and debris to allow acetic acid/hydrocortisone to contact infected surfaces directly. To promote continuous contact, insert a wick saturated with this solution into the ear canal; the wick may also be saturated after insertion. Instruct the patient to keep the wick in for at least 24 hours and to keep it moist by adding 3 to 5 drops of hydrocortisone and acetic acid otic solution every 4 to 6 six hours. The wick may be removed after 24 hours but the patient should continue to instill 5 drops of the solution 3 or 4 times daily thereafter, for as long as indicated.

Storage: Store at room temperature; avoid excessive heat. Keep container tightly closed.

HOW SUPPLIED - RATED THERAPEUTICALLY EQUIVALENT:

Solution - Otic - 2 %/1 %

10 ml	$3.98	Acetic Acid Hydrocortisone, Thames Pharma	49158-0197-43
10 ml	$4.50	OTICOT HC, C O Truxton	00463-8054-10
10 ml	$5.26	Acetic Acid HC, Qualitest Pharms	00603-7036-39
10 ml	$5.30	ACETASOL HC, Goldline Labs	00182-1776-63
10 ml	$6.15	VASOTATE-HC OTIC, Major Pharms	00904-0316-10
10 ml	$7.15	Acetic Acid Hydrocortisone, Schein Pharm (US)	00364-0751-54
10 ml	$7.95	Acetic Acid W/Hydrocortisone, Rugby	00536-2110-70
10 ml	$10.63	Acetic Acid Hydrocortisone, Geneva Pharms	00781-6311-70
10 ml	$12.00	ACETASOL HC, Alpharma	00472-0882-82
10 ml	$12.00	ACETASOL HC, HL Moore Drug Exch	00839-6645-90
10 ml	$23.90	OTOSOL-HC, Universal Labs	52906-1005-00
10 ml	**$121.33**	**VOSOL HC, Wallace Labs**	**00037-3811-12**

HOW SUPPLIED - NOT RATED EQUIVALENT:

Solution - Otic - 2 %/1 %

10 ml	$2.25	Acetasol Hc, Raway	00686-0882-82
10 ml	$5.65	Acetic Acid Hc, Harber Pharm	51432-0501-09

ACETIC ACID; OXYQUINOLINE SULFATE *(000091)*

CATEGORIES: Anti-Infectives; Skin/Mucous Membrane Agents; Vaginal Preparations; Pregnancy Category C; FDA Pre 1938 Drugs

BRAND NAMES: Aci-Jel

DESCRIPTION:

Aci-Jel Vaginal Jelly is a bland, non-irritating, water-dispersible, buffered acid jelly for intravaginal use. Aci-Jel is classified as a Vaginal Therapeutic Jelly.

Aci-Jel contains 0.921% glacial acetic acid ($C_2H_4O_2$), 0.025% oxyquinoline sulfate ($C_{18}H_{16}N_2O_6S$), 0.7% ricinoleic acid ($C_{18}H_{34}O_3$), and 5% glycerin ($C_3H_8O_3$) compounded with tragacanth, acacia, propylparaben, potassium hydroxide, stannous chloride, egg albumin, potassium bitartrate, perfume and purified water. Aci-Jel is formulated to pH 3.9-4.1

CLINICAL PHARMACOLOGY:

Acetic acid and oxyquinoline sulfate acts to restore and maintain normal vaginal acidity through its buffer action.

INDICATIONS AND USAGE:

Acetic acid and oxyquinoline sulfate is indicated as adjunctive therapy in those case where restoration and maintenance of vaginal acidity is desirable.

CONTRAINDICATIONS:

None known.

WARNINGS:

No serious adverse reactions or potential safety hazards have been reported with the use of acetic acid and oxyquinoline sulfate.

PRECAUTIONS:

General: No special care is required for the safe and effective use of acetic acid and oxyquinoline sulfate.

Laboratory Tests: The monitoring of vaginal acidity (pH) may be helpful in following the patients response. (The normal vaginal pH has been shown to be in the range of 4.0 to 5.0)

Carcinogenesis: No long-term studies in animals have been performed to evaluate carcinogenic potential.

Pregnancy Category C: Animal reproduction studies have not been conducted with acetic acid and oxyquinoline sulfate. It is also not known whether acetic acid and oxyquinoline sulfate can cause fetal harm when administered to a pregnant woman or can affect reproduction capacity. Acetic acid and oxyquinoline sulfate should be given to a pregnant woman only if clearly needed.

Nursing Mothers: It is not known whether this drug is excreted in human milk. Because many drugs are excreted in human milk, caution should be exercised when acetic acid and oxyquinoline sulfate is administered to a nursing woman.

DRUG INTERACTIONS:

No incidence of drug interactions have been reported with concomitant use of acetic acid and oxyquinoline sulfate and any other medications.

ADVERSE REACTIONS:

Occasional cases of local stinging and burning have been reported.

DOSAGE AND ADMINISTRATION:

The usual dose is one applicatorful, administered intravaginally, morning and evening. Duration of treatment may be determined by the patients response to therapy.

DIRECTIONS FOR PUNCTURING TUBE END AND USING ORTHO* VAGINAL APPLICATOR

1. Puncturing the tube end: Remove cap from tube. Reverse cap and place puncture tip onto tube. Push cap firmly until tube end is punctured.

2. Filling the applicator: Screw applicator onto tube. Squeeze tube forcing contents into barrel until it is full. Then remove applicator from the tube.

Lie on your back with knees drawn up. Hold filled applicator into the vagina as far as it will go comfortably. Press plunger and deposit material. While keeping the plunger depressed, remove the applicator from vagina.

3. Care of the applicator: After each use, pull applicator apart and wash with soap and warm water.

To reassemble, gently push plunger back into barrel as far as it will go.

Note: Store at controlled room temperature. See end flap for lot number and expiration date.

PATIENT INFORMATION:

The vagina is normally moist and contains several different kinds of bacteria (small, one-celled plantlike organisms). The vaginal fluid is also normally somewhat acidic. Acidity is measured on a scale called pH; the lower the pH value, the more acid the fluid. Normal vaginal pH is in a range from 3.8 to 4.2.

The acidic vaginal fluid is the result of bacterial growth and metabolism. Like the acidity if the stomach, the vaginal acidity may be a means by which the body "defends" itself, by killing off harmful bacteria and other organisms which are "foreign" (not normal) to it.

Certain factors tend to lessen the vaginal acidity.

Examples would be mucus from the cervix (mouth of the womb), blood, or cellular material from vaginal tissues after a surgical procedure. Your health professional may recommend certain hygienic steps, such as douching, to reduce such factors.

The vaginal acidity may be promoted or maintained by the use of a vaginal jelly, or gel, such as acetic acid and oxyquinoline sulfate* therapeutic vaginal jelly, which is itself acidic. Such a preparation may be recommended by your health professional in conjunction with the treatment of vaginal infections or to help prevent the recurrence of vaginal infections.

HOW SUPPLIED - EQUIVALENTS NOT AVAILABLE:

Jelly - Vaginal - 0.921 %/5 %/0.0

85 gm $25.02 ACI-JEL, Ortho Pharm 00062-5421-01

ACETOHEXAMIDE *(000092)*

CATEGORIES: Antidiabetic Agents; Blood Glucose Regulators; Diabetes; Diabetes Mellitus; Hormones; Hyperglycemia; Sulfonylureas; FDA Approval Pre 1982

BRAND NAMES: *Dimelin* (Japan); *Dimelor* (Canada); **Dymelor**; *Gamadiabet*; *Ordimel*; *Toyobexin* (Japan)
(International brand names outside U.S. in italics)

FORMULARIES: Aetna; Medi-Cal

DESCRIPTION:

Acetohexamide is an oral blood-glucose lowering drug of the sulfonylurea class. Acetohexamide is a white to off-white, crystalline, practically odorless powder. It is practically insoluble in water and ether, soluble in pyridine and dilute solutions of alkali hydroxides, and slightly soluble in alcohol and chloroform. Chemically, it is benzenesulfonamide, 4-acetyl-*N*-[[cyclohexylamino]carbonyl]- or 1-[(*p*-acetylphenyl)sulfonyl]-3-cyclohexylurea. The empirical formula for acetohexamide is $C_{15}H_2ON_2O_4S$. Its molecular weight is 324.39.

Acetohexamide is supplied in 250-mg (770 µmol) and 500-mg (1,540 µmol) tablets. The tablets contain corn starch, magnesium stearate, polacrillin potassium, and talc. The 500 mg tablet also contains D&C Yellow #10 and FD&C Yellow #6.

CLINICAL PHARMACOLOGY:

Acetohexamide appears to lower the blood glucose acutely by stimulating the release of insulin from the pancreas, an effect that is dependent on functioning β cells in the pancreatic islets. The mechanism by which acetohexamide lowers blood glucose during long-term administration has not been clearly established.

Acetohexamide is rapidly absorbed from the gastrointestinal tract, and maximum hypoglycemic activity is observed about 3 hours after ingestion. The total duration of action is 12 to 24 hours. Much of the activity is ascribable to a metabolite, hydroxyhexamide, which has a plasma half-life of approximately 6 hours; the parent compound, acetohexamide, has a plasma half-life of 1.3 hours. In persons with normal renal and hepatic function, more than 80% is excreted, largely as metabolites, in 24 hours.

INDICATIONS AND USAGE:

Acetohexamide is indicated as an adjunct to diet for lowering the blood glucose in patients with non-insulin-dependent diabetes mellitus (type II) whose hyperglycemia cannot be controlled by diet alone.

In initiating treatment for non-insulin-dependent diabetes, diet should be emphasized as the primary form of treatment. Caloric restriction and weight loss are essential in the obese diabetic patient. Proper dietary management alone may be effective in controlling the blood glucose and symptoms of hyperglycemia. The importance of regular physical activity should also be stressed, and cardiovascular risk factors should be identified and corrective measures taken when possible.

If this treatment program fails to reduce symptoms and/or blood glucose, the use of an oral sulfonylurea or insulin should be considered. The use of acetohexamide must be viewed by both the physician and patient as a treatment in addition to diet, and not as a substitute for diet or as a convenient mechanism for avoiding dietary restraint. Furthermore, loss of blood glucose control with diet alone may be transient, thus requiring only short-term administration of acetohexamide.

During maintenance programs, acetohexamide should be discontinued if satisfactory lowering of blood glucose is no longer achieved. Judgements should be based on regular clinical and laboratory evaluations.

In considering the use of acetohexamide in asymptomatic patients, it should be recognized that controlling the blood glucose in non-insulin-dependent diabetes has not been definitely established as being effective in preventing the long-term cardiovascular or neural complications of diabetes.

CONTRAINDICATIONS:

Acetohexamide is contraindicated in patients with:

1. Known hypersensitivity to the drug

2. Diabetic ketoacidoses, with or without coma. This condition should be treated with insulin.

3. Insulin-dependent (type I) diabetes mellitus, as sole therapy.

4. Diabetes when complicated by pregnancy (see PRECAUTIONS, Pregnancy).

WARNINGS:

SPECIAL WARNING ON INCREASED RISK OF CARDIOVASCULAR MORTALITY

The administration of oral hypoglycemic drugs has been reported to be associated with increased cardiovascular mortality as compared to treatment with diet alone or diet plus insulin. This warning is based on the study conducted by the University Group Diabetes Program (UGDP), a long-term prospective clinical trial designed to evaluate the effectiveness of glucose-lowering drugs in preventing or delaying vascular complications in patients with non-insulin-dependent diabetes. The study involved 823 patients who were randomly assigned to 1 of 4 treatment groups (*Diabetes* 1970;19 [suppl 2]:747-830).

WARNINGS: *(cont'd)*

UGDP reported that patients treated for 5 to 8 years with diet plus a fixed dose of tolbutamide (1.5 g/day) had a rate of cardiovascular mortality approximately 2 1/2 times that of patients treated with diet alone. A significant increase in total mortality was not observed, but the use of tolbutamide was discontinued based on the increase in cardiovascular mortality, thus limiting the opportunity for the study to show an increase in overall mortality. Despite controversy regarding the interpretation of these results, the findings of the UGDP study provide an adequate basis for this warning. The patient should be informed of the potential risks and advantages of acetohexamide and of alternative modes of therapy.

Although only 1 drug in the sulfonylurea class (tolbutamide) was included in this study, it is prudent from a safety standpoint to consider that this warning may also apply to other oral hypoglycemic drugs in this class, in view of their close similarities in mode of action and chemical structure.

PRECAUTIONS:

GENERAL

Hypoglycemia: All sulfonylurea drugs are capable of producing severe hypoglycemia. Proper patient selection, dosage, and instructions are important for avoiding hypoglycemic episodes. Renal or hepatic insufficiency may cause elevated blood levels of acetohexamide, and the latter may also diminish gluconeogenic capacity, both of which increase the risk of serious hypoglycemic reactions. Elderly, debilitated or malnourished patients, and those with adrenal or pituitary insufficiency are particularly susceptible to the hypoglycemic action of glucose-lowering drugs. Hypoglycemia may be difficult to recognize in the elderly and in people who are taking β-adrenergic blocking drugs.

Hypoglycemia is more likely to occur when caloric intake is deficient, after severe or prolonged exercise, when alcohol is ingested, or when more than 1 glucose-lowering drug is used.

Loss of Control of Blood Glucose: When a patient stabilized on any diabetic regimen is exposed to stress, such as fever, trauma, infection, or surgery, a loss of control may occur. At such times, it may be necessary to discontinue acetohexamide and administer insulin.

The effectiveness of any oral hypoglycemic drug, including acetohexamide, in lowering blood glucose to a desired level decreases in many patients over a period of time; this decrease in effectiveness may be due to progression of the severity of the diabetes or to diminished responsiveness to the drug. This phenomenon is known as secondary failure, to distinguish it from primary failure in which the drug is ineffective in an individual patient when first given.

LABORATORY TESTS

Blood and urine glucose should be monitored periodically. Measurement of glycosylated hemoglobin may be useful.

CARCINOGENESIS, MUTAGENESIS, AND IMPAIRMENT OF FERTILITY

Long-term studies in rats and mice revealed no evidence of carcinogenicity of acetohexamide. A sister chromatid exchange study performed with acetohexamide showed no evidence of mutagenicity. No animal studies have been conducted to determine whether acetohexamide has the potential to impair fertility.

PREGNANCY CATEGORY C

Teratogenic Effects: Acetohexamide has been shown to be teratogenic in animals. However, teratogenesis in animals has been observed following administration of high doses of the sulfonylurea agents. There are no adequate and well-controlled studies in pregnant women. Therefore, acetohexamide is not recommended for the management of diabetes when complicated by pregnancy.

Because recent information suggests that abnormal blood glucose levels during pregnancy are associated with a higher incidence of congenital abnormalities, many experts recommend that insulin be used during pregnancy to maintain blood glucose levels as close to normal as possible.

Nonteratogenic Effects Prolonged severe hypoglycemia (4 to 10 days) has been reported in neonates born to mothers who were receiving a sulfonylurea drug at the time of delivery. This has been reported more frequently with the use of agents with prolonged half-lives. The use of acetohexamide is not recommended for the management of diabetes when complicated by pregnancy.

NURSING MOTHERS

It is not known whether this drug is excreted in human milk. Because some sulfonylurea drugs are excreted in human milk and because of the potential for serious adverse reactions in nursing infants from acetohexamide, a decision should be made whether to discontinue nursing or to discontinue the drug, taking into account the importance of the drug to the mother.

DRUG INTERACTIONS:

The hypoglycemic action of sulfonylurea agents may be potentiated by certain drugs, including nonsteroidal anti-inflammatory agents and other drugs that are highly protein bound, salicylates, sulfonamides, chloramphenicol, probenecid, coumarins, monoamine oxidase inhibitors, and β-adrenergic blocking agents. When such drugs are administered to a patient receiving acetohexamide, the patient should be observed closely for hypoglycemia. When such drugs are withdrawn from a patient receiving acetohexamide, the patient should be observed closely for loss of control.

Certain drugs tend to produce hyperglycemia and may lead to loss of control. These drugs include the thiazides and other diuretics, corticosteroids, phenothiazines, thyroid products, estrogens, oral contraceptives, phenytoin, nicotinic acid, sympathomimetics, calcium channel blocking drugs, and isoniazid. When such drugs are administered to a patient receiving acetohexamide, the patient should be closely observed for loss of control. When such drugs are withdrawn from a patient receiving acetohexamide, the patient should be observed closely for hypoglycemia.

A potential interaction between oral miconazole and oral hypoglycemic agents leading to severe hypoglycemia has been reported. Whether this interaction also occurs with the intravenous, topical, or vaginal preparations of miconazole is not known.

ADVERSE REACTIONS:

Hypoglycemia: See PRECAUTIONSand OVERDOSAGE.

Gastrointestinal Reactions: Cholestatic jaundice may occur rarely; acetohexamide should be discontinued if this occurs. Gastrointestinal disturbances, eg, nausea, epigastric fullness, and heartburn, are the most common reactions and occur in 1 to 40 patients. These reactions tend to be dose related and may disappear when dosage is reduced.

Dermatologic Reactions: Allergic skin reactions, eg, pruritus, erythema, urticaria, and morbilliform or maculopapular eruptions, occur in less than 1 in 100 patients. These may be transient and may disappear despite continued use of acetohexamide; if skin reactions persist, the drug should be discontinued.

Porphyria cutanea tarda and photosensitivity reactions have been reported with this and other sulfonylurea agents.

ADVERSE REACTIONS: *(cont'd)*

Endocrine Reactions: Cases of hyponatremia and the syndrome of inappropriate antidiuretic hormone (SIADH) secretion have been reported with this and other sulfonylurea agents.

Hematologic Reactions: Leukopenia, agranulocytosis, thrombocytopenia, hemolytic anemia, aplastic anemia, and pancytopenia have been reported with sulfonylurea agents.

Metabolic Reactions: Hepatic porphyria and disulfiram-like reactions have been reported with sulfonylurea agents.

OVERDOSAGE:

Signs and Symptoms: Hypoglycemia is the predominant finding in cases of sulfonylurea overdose (including overdose with acetohexamide), but this condition may be preceded by nausea, vomiting, and mild epigastric pain. Symptoms of hypoglycemia may include headache, weakness, confusion, dizziness, lethargy, convulsions, coma and death. Patients may be especially susceptible hypoglycemia if they are elderly, if they have had restricted carbohydrate intake (especially during periods of exercise), or if they have kidney or liver dysfunction.

Treatment: To obtain up-to-date information about the treatment of overdose, a good resource is your certified Regional Poison Control Center. Telephone numbers of certified poison control centers are listed in *Physicians GenRx*. In managing overdosage, consider the possibility of multiple drug overdoses, interaction among drugs, and unusual drug kinetics in your patient.

Overdosage of sulfonylureas, including acetohexamide, can produce hypoglycemia. Mild hypoglycemic symptoms without loss of consciousness or neurologic findings should be treated aggressively with oral glucose and adjustments in drug dosage and/or meal patterns. Close monitoring should continue until the physician is assured that the patient is out of danger. Severe hypoglycemic reactions with coma, seizure, or other neurologic impairment occur infrequently but constitute medical emergencies requiring immediate hospitalization. If hypoglycemic coma is diagnosed or suspected, the patient should be given a rapid intravenous injection of concentrated (50%) glucose solution. This should be followed by a continuous infusion of a more dilute (10%) glucose solution at a rate that will maintain the blood glucose at a level of about 100 mg/dl. Patients should be closely monitored for a minimum of 24 to 48 hours, since hypoglycemia may recur after apparent clinical recovery.

Monitor the patient's vital signs, blood gases, glucose, serum electrolytes, etc. Absorption of drugs from the gastrointestinal tract may be decreased by giving activated charcoal, which, in many cases, is more effective than emesis or lavage; consider charcoal instead of or in addition to gastric emptying. Repeated doses of charcoal over time may hasten elimination of some drugs that have been absorbed. Safeguard the patient's airway when employing gastric emptying or charcoal.

DOSAGE AND ADMINISTRATION:

There is no fixed dosage regimen for the management of diabetes mellitus with acetohexamide or any other hypoglycemic agent. In addition to the usual monitoring of urinary glucose, the patient's blood glucose must also be monitored periodically to determine the minimum effective dose for a patient; to detect primary failure, i.e., inadequate lowering of blood glucose with the recommended dose of medication; and to detect secondary failure; i.e., loss of an adequate blood-glucose lowering response after an initial period of effectiveness. Glycosylated hemoglobin levels may also be of value in monitoring the patient's response to therapy.

Short-term administration of acetohexamide may be sufficient during periods of transient loss of control in patients usually well controlled on diet.

Daily oral dosage of acetohexamide may range between 250 mg and 1.5 g.

No loading dose is required. Patients who do not respond to 1.5 g daily usually will not respond to a higher dose. For this reason, doses in excess of 1.5 g daily are not recommended.

The majority of patients receiving 1 g or less/day can be controlled on a convenient once-daily dosage. Patients who need 1.5 g/day usually benefit from twice-daily dosage, given before the morning and evening meals.

Various measures have been employed to establish patients on acetohexamide, and the following procedures are suggested.

PATIENTS NOT PREVIOUSLY RECEIVING INSULIN OR DRUG THERAPY

In mild, stable diabetes (after dietary regulation), therapy may be initiated with 250 mg daily before breakfast; subsequent adjustment of the dosage may be made by increments of 250 to 500 mg every 5 to 7 days as necessary. The 250-mg or 500-mg tablet (scored and easily broken in half) may be used.

Because of reports of hyperresponsiveness to acetohexamide of some elderly patients with diabetes, patients in this group should be started with a single dose of 250 mg before breakfast, and their blood and urine sugars should be checked during the first 24 hours of therapy. If control appears to be satisfactory, this dose may be continued on a daily basis or, if necessary, gradually increased. If, however, there appears to be a tendency toward hypoglycemia, this dose should be reduced or the drug should be discontinued.

PATIENTS RECEIVING OTHER ORAL AGENTS

When transfer is made from tolbutamide, the initial dose of acetohexamide should be about half the tolbutamide dose (eg., 250 mg of acetohexamide in place of 500 mg of tolbutamide), up to a maximum of 1.5 g of acetohexamide.

When transfer is made from chlorpropamide, the initial dose of acetohexamide should be about double the chlorpropamide dose (eg, 500 mg of acetohexamide in place of 250 mg of chlorpropamide).

A transition period usually is required because of the long half-life of chlorpropamide. Subsequent adjustment of dosage should be made according to clinical response. The maximum recommended dose of acetohexamide is 1.5 g.

Clinical reports on the efficacy of once-daily dosage of acetohexamide indicate that its effect on the blood sugar is better sustained than that of tolbutamide. However, patients requiring more than 1 g of acetohexamide daily should be treated with divided doses.

PATIENTS RECEIVING INSULIN

In general, patients who were previously maintained on insulin in small dosage (eg., up to 20 units/day) may be placed on acetohexamide directly and their insulin administration abruptly discontinued. Patients receiving larger doses of insulin, such as 20 to 40 units or more/day, should have an initial reduction of insulin dosage by 25% to 30% daily or every other day and subsequent further reduction depending on the response to acetohexamide. An initial dose of 250 mg of acetohexamide can be used, with readjustment depending on response to therapy. Because of the potential hazards of hypoglycemia in the elderly, patients in this age group should be carefully observed during the transition from insulin to acetohexamide.

During the period of insulin withdrawal, the patient should test his/her blood or urine for sugar and urine for acetone at least 3 times a day and report the results frequently to his/her physician so that appropriate adjustments of therapy may be made. In some cases, it may be advisable to consider hospitalization during the transition period from insulin to acetohexamide.

DOSAGE AND ADMINISTRATION: *(cont'd)*

It should be noted that, as with other sulfonylureas, primary and secondary failures may occur with acetohexamide.

In elderly, debilitated or malnourished patients, and patients with impaired renal or hepatic function, the initial and maintenance doses should be conservative to avoid hypoglycemic reactions (see PRECAUTIONS).

Store at controlled room temperature, 59° to 86°F (15° to 30°C).

PATIENT INFORMATION:

Patients should be informed of the potential risks and advantages of acetohexamide and of alternative modes of therapy. They should also be informed about the importance of adherence to dietary instructions, of a regular exercise program, and of regular testing of urine and/or blood glucose.

The risks of hypoglycemia, its symptoms and treatment, and conditions that predispose to its development should be explained to patients and responsible family members. Primary and secondary failure should also be explained.

HOW SUPPLIED - RATED THERAPEUTICALLY EQUIVALENT:

Tablet, Uncoated - Oral - 250 mg

50's	**$12.86**	**DYMELOR, Lilly**	**00002-2103-50**
100's	$15.75	Acetohexamide, Major Pharms	00904-1990-60
100's	$18.48	Acetohexamide, HL Moore Drug Exch	00839-7386-06
100's	$23.63	Acetohexamide, H.C.F.A. F F P	99999-0092-01
100's	$26.38	Acetohexamide, Barr	00555-0442-02
100's	$26.42	Acetohexamide, Schein Pharm (US)	00364-2232-01
100's	$27.60	Acetohexamide 250, Aligen Independ	00405-4024-01
200's	$47.26	Acetohexamide, H.C.F.A. F F P	99999-0092-02
200's	**$47.89**	**DYMELOR, Lilly**	**00002-2103-22**
500's	**$114.70**	**DYMELOR, Lilly**	**00002-2103-03**

Tablet, Uncoated - Oral - 500 mg

50's	$16.12	Acetohexamide, H.C.F.A. F F P	99999-0092-03
50's	**$22.53**	**DYMELOR, Lilly**	**00002-2107-50**
100's	$29.03	Acetohexamide, HL Moore Drug Exch	00839-7387-06
100's	$29.95	Acetohexamide, Major Pharms	00904-1991-60
100's	$32.25	Acetohexamide, H.C.F.A. F F P	99999-0092-04
100's	**$37.03**	**DYMELOR, Lilly**	**00002-2107-33**
100's	$37.48	Acetohexamide, Barr	00555-0443-02
100's	$37.69	Acetohexamide, Schein Pharm (US)	00364-2233-01
100's	$48.20	Acetohexamide 500, Aligen Independ	00405-4025-01
200's	$64.50	Acetohexamide, H.C.F.A. F F P	99999-0092-05
200's	**$86.52**	**DYMELOR, Lilly**	**00002-2107-22**
500's	**$213.47**	**DYMELOR, Lilly**	**00002-2107-03**

ACETOHYDROXAMIC ACID *(000093)*

CATEGORIES: Ammonia Detoxicants; Antagonists and Antidotes; Antidotes; Electrolytic, Caloric-Water Balance; Urinary Tract Infections; Pregnancy Category X; FDA Approved 1983 May

BRAND NAMES: A.H.A.; **Lithostat**; *Uronefrex* (France)
(International brand names outside U.S. in italics)

DESCRIPTION:

Acetohydroxamic acid is a stable, synthetic compound derived from hydroxylamine and ethyl acetate. Its molecular structure is similar to urea.

Acetohydroxamic acid is weakly acidic, highly soluble in water, and chelates metals - notably iron. The molecular weight is 75.068. Acetohydroxamic acid has a pKa of 9.32 and a melting point of 89-91°C. Acetohydroxamic acid is a urease inhibitor. Available as 250 mg tablets.

CLINICAL PHARMACOLOGY:

Acetohydroxamic acid reversibly inhibits the bacterial enzyme urease, thereby inhibiting the hydrolysis of urea & production of ammonia in urine infected with urea-splitting organisms. The reduced ammonia levels and decreased pH enhance the effectiveness of antimicrobial agents and allow an increased cure rate of these infections.

Acetohydroxamic acid is well absorbed from the gastrointestinal tract after oral administration; peak blood levels occur from 0.25 to 1 hour after dosing. The compound is distributed throughout body water, and there is no known binding to any tissue. Acetohydroxamic acid chelates with dietary iron without the gut. This reaction may interfere with absorption of acetohydroxamic acid and with iron. Concomitant hypochromic anemia should be treated with intramuscular iron.

In rodents, the metabolic fate of acetohydroxamic acid is well known; 55% is excreted unchanged in urine, 25% is excreted as acetamide or acetate and 7% is excreted by the lungs as carbon dioxide. Less than 1% is excreted in the feces. Approximately 5% of the administered dose is unaccounted for. In rodents, acetohydroxamic acid shows a dose-related change in pharmacokinetics; with increasing dose, there is an increase in the half-life and an increase in the percent of the administered dose recovered in urine as unchanged acetohydroxamic acid.

Pharmacokinetics in man are generally similar to rodents including the dose-related increase in half-life, but they are not as well characterized as in the rodent. Thirty-six to sixty-five percent (36 - 65%) of the oral dosage is excreted unchanged in the urine. It is unaltered acetohydroxamic acid in the urine that provides the therapeutic effect, but the precise concentration of acetohydroxamic acid in urine that is necessary to inhibit urease is incompletely delineated.

Therapeutic benefit may be obtained from concentrations as low as 8 mcg/ml; higher concentrations (*i.e.,* 30 mcg/ml) are expected to provide more complete inhibition of urease. The plasma half-life of acetohydroxamic acid is approximately 5-10 hours in subjects with normal renal function and is prolonged in patients with reduced renal function.

Acetohydroxamic acid has been evaluated clinically in patients with urea-splitting urinary infections, often accompanied by struvite stone disease, that were recalcitrant to other forms of medical and surgical management. In these clinical trials, acetohydroxamic acid reduced the pathologically elevated urinary ammonia and pH levels that result from the hydrolysis of urea by the enzyme, urease.

Acetohydroxamic acid does not acidify urine directly nor does it have a direct anti-bacterial effect. The usefulness of reducing ammonia levels and decreasing urinary pH is suggested by single (not yet replicated) clinical trials in which urease inhibition:

1) allowed successful antibiotic treatment of urea-splitting Proteus infections after surgical removal of struvite stones in patients not cured by 3 months of antibacterial treatment alone, and 2) reduced the rate of stone growth in patients who were not candidates for surgical removal of stones.

INDICATIONS AND USAGE:

Acetohydroxamic acid is indicated as adjunctive therapy in patients with chronic urea-splitting urinary infection. Acetohydroxamic acid is intended to decrease urinary ammonia and alkalinity, but it should not be used in lieu of curative surgical treatment (for patients with stones) or antimicrobial treatment. Long-term treatment with acetohydroxamic acid may be warranted to maintain urease inhibition as long as urea-splitting infection is present. Experience with acetohydroxamic acid does not go beyond 7 years. A patient package insert should be distributed to each patient who receives acetohydroxamic acid.

CONTRAINDICATIONS:

Acetohydroxamic acid should not be used in:

a. Patients whose physical state and disease are amenable to definitive surgery and appropriate antimicrobial agents

b. Patients whose urine is infected by non-urease producing organisms

c. Patients whose urinary infections can be controlled by culture-specific oral antimicrobial agents

d. Patients whose renal function is poor (*i.e.,* serum creatinine more than 2.5 mg/dl and/or creatinine clearance less than 20 ml/min)

e. Female patients who do not evidence a satisfactory method of contraception

f. Patients who are pregnant

Acetohydroxamic acid may cause fetal harm when administered to a pregnant woman. Acetohydroxamic acid was teratogenic (retarded and/or clubbed rear leg at 750 mg/kg and above and exencephaly and encephalocele at 1,500 mg/kg) when given intraperitoneally to rats. Acetohydroxamic acid is contraindicated in women who are or may become pregnant. If this drug is used during pregnancy, or if the patient becomes pregnant while taking this drug, the patient should be informed of the potential hazard to the fetus.

WARNINGS:

A Coombs negative hemolytic anemia has occurred in patients receiving acetohydroxamic acid. Gastrointestinal upset characterized by nausea, vomiting, anorexia and generalized malaise have accompanied the most severe forms of hemolytic anemia. Approximately 15% of patients receiving acetohydroxamic acid have had only laboratory findings of an anemia. However, most patients developed a mild reticulocytosis. The untoward reactions have reverted to normal following cessation of treatment. A complete blood count, including a reticulocyte count, is recommended after two weeks of treatment. If the reticulocyte count exceeds 6%, a reduced dosage should be entertained. A CBC and reticulocyte count are recommended at 3-month intervals for the duration of treatment.

PRECAUTIONS:

GENERAL

Hematologic Effects: Bone marrow depression (leukopenia, anemia, and thrombocytopenia) has occurred in experimental animals receiving large doses of acetohydroxamic acid, but has not been seen in man to date. Acetohydroxamic acid is a known inhibitor of DNA synthesis and also chelates metals - notably iron. Its bone marrow suppressant effect is probably related to its ability to inhibit DNA synthesis, but anemia could also be related to depletion of iron stores. To date, the only clinical effect noted has been hemolysis, with a decrease in the circulating red blood cells, hemoglobin and hematocrit. Abnormalities in platelet or white blood cell count have not been noted. However, clinical monitoring of the platelet and white cell count is recommended.

Monitoring Liver Function: Abnormalities of liver function have not been reported to date. However, a chloro-benzene derivative of acetohydroxamic acid caused significant liver dysfunction in an unrelated study. Therefore, close monitoring of liver function is recommended. (See Carcinogenesis, Mutagenesis, Impairment Of Fertility for discussion of possible hepatic carcinogenesis.)

Use In Patients With Renal Impairment: Since acetohydroxamic acid is eliminated primarily by the kidneys, patients with significantly impaired renal function should be closely monitored, and a reduction of daily dose may be needed to avoid excessive drug accumulation. (See DOSAGE AND ADMINISTRATION.)

CARCINOGENESIS, MUTAGENESIS, IMPAIRMENT OF FERTILITY

Well controlled, long-term animal studies that identify the carcinogenic potential of acetohydroxamic acid treatment have not been conducted. Acetamide, a metabolite of acetohydroxamic acid, has been shown to cause hepatocellular carcinoma in rats at oral doses 1,500 times the human dose. Acetohydroxamic acid is cytotoxic and was positive for mutagenicity in the Ames test.

PREGNANCY CATEGORY X

(See CONTRAINDICATIONS.)

NURSING MOTHERS

It is not known whether acetohydroxamic acid is secreted in human milk. Because many drugs are excreted in human milk, and because of the potential for serious adverse reactions in nursing infants from acetohydroxamic acid, a decision should be made to discontinue nursing or the drug, taking into account the significance of the drug to the mother's well being.

PEDIATRIC USE

Children with chronic, recalcitrant, urea-splitting urinary infection may benefit from treatment with acetohydroxamic acid. However, detailed studies involving dosage and dose intervals in children have not been established. Children have tolerated a dose of 10 mg/kg/day, taken in two or three divided doses, satisfactorily for periods up to one year. Close monitoring of such patients is mandatory.

DRUG INTERACTIONS:

Acetohydroxamic acid has been used concomitantly with insulin, oral and parenteral antibiotics, and progestational agents. No clinically significant interactions have been noted, but until wider clinical experience is obtained, acetohydroxamic acid should be used with caution in patients receiving other therapeutic agents. Acetohydroxamic acid taken in association with alcoholic beverages has resulted in a rash. (See ADVERSE REACTIONS.)

Acetohydroxamic acid chelates heavy metals - notably iron. The absorption of iron and acetohydroxamic acid from the intestinal lumen may be reduced when both drugs are taken concomitantly. When iron administration is indicated, intramuscular iron is probably the product of choice.

ADVERSE REACTIONS:

Experience with acetohydroxamic acid is limited. About 150 patients have been treated, most for periods of more than a year.

Adverse reactions have occurred in up to thirty percent (30%) of the patients receiving acetohydroxamic acid. In some instances the reactions were symptomatic; in others only changes in laboratory parameters were noted. Adverse reactions seem to be more prevalent in patients with preexisting thrombophlebitis or phlebothrombosis and/or in patients with advanced degrees of renal insufficiency. The risk of adverse reactions is highest during the first year of treatment. Chronic treatment does not seem to increase the risk nor the severity of adverse reactions.

The following reactions have been reported:

Neurological: Mild headaches are commonly reported (about 30%) during the first 48 hours of treatment. These headaches are mild, responsive to oral salicylate-type analgesics, and usually disappear spontaneously. The headaches have not been associated with vertigo, tinnitus, or visual or auditory abnormalities. Tremulousness and nervousness have also been reported.

Gastrointestinal: Gastrointestinal symptoms, nausea, vomiting, anorexia, and malaise have occurred in 20-25% of patients. In most patients the symptoms were mild, transitory, and did not result in interruption of treatment. Approximately 3% of patients developed a hemolytic anemia of sufficient magnitude to warrant interruption in treatment; several of these patients also had symptoms of gastrointestinal upset.

Hematological: Approximately 15% of patients have had laboratory findings characteristic of a hemolytic anemia. A mild reticulocytosis (5 - 6%) without anemia, is even more prevalent. The laboratory findings are occasionally accompanied by systemic symptoms such as malaise, lethargy and fatigue, and gastrointestinal symptoms. Symptoms and laboratory findings have invariably improved following cessation of treatment with acetohydroxamic acid. The hematological abnormalities are more prevalent in patients with advanced renal failure.

Dermatological: A nonpruritic, macular skin rash has occurred in the upper extremities and on the face of several patients taking acetohydroxamic acid on a long-term basis, usually when acetohydroxamic acid has been taken concomitantly with alcoholic beverages, but in a few patients in the absence of alcohol consumption. The rash commonly appears 30 - 45 minutes after ingestion of alcoholic beverages; it characteristically disappears spontaneously in 30 - 60 minutes. The rash may be associated with a general sensation of warmth. In some patients the rash is sufficiently severe to warrant discontinuation of treatment, but most patients have continued treatment, avoiding alcohol or using smaller quantities of it. Alopecia has also been reported in patients taking acetohydroxamic acid.

Cardiovascular: Superficial phlebitis involving the lower extremities has occurred in several patients on acetohydroxamic acid during the early (Phase II) clinical trials. Several of the affected patients had phlebitic episodes prior to treatment. One patient developed deep vein thrombosis of the lower extremities. The patient with phlebothrombosis had an associated traumatic injury to the groin. It is unclear whether the phlebitis was related to or exacerbated by treatment with acetohydroxamic acid. No patient in the three (3) year controlled (Phase III) clinical trial developed phlebitis. In all instances these vascular abnormalities returned to normal following appropriate medical therapy. Embolic phenomena have been reported in three patients taking acetohydroxamic acid in the Phase II trial. The phlebitis and emboli resolved following discontinuation of acetohydroxamic acid and implementation of appropriate medical therapy. Several patients have resumed treatment with acetohydroxamic acid without ill effect. Palpitations have also been reported in patients taking acetohydroxamic acid.

Respiratory: No symptoms have been reported. Radiographic evidence of small pulmonary emboli has been seen in three patients with phlebitis in their lower legs.

Psychiatric: Depression, anxiety, nervousness, and tremulousness have been observed in approximately 20% of patients taking acetohydroxamic acid. In most patients the symptoms were mild and transitory, but in about 6% of patients the symptoms were sufficiently distressing to warrant interruption or discontinuation of treatment.

OVERDOSAGE:

Acute deliberate overdosage in man has not occurred, but would be expected to induce the following symptoms: anorexia, malaise, lethargy, diminished sense of well being, tremulousness, anxiety, nausea and vomiting. Laboratory findings are likely to include an elevated reticulocyte count and a severe hemolytic reaction requiring hospitalization, symptomatic treatment, and possibly blood transfusions. Concomitant reduction in platelets and/or white blood cells should be anticipated.

Milder overdosages resulting in hemolysis have occurred in an occasional patient with reduced renal function after several weeks or months of continuous treatment.

The acute LD 50 of acetohydroxamic acid in animals (rats) is 4.8 g/kg.

Recommended treatment for an overdosage reaction consists of 1) cessation of treatment, 2) close monitoring of hematologic status, 3) symptomatic treatment, and 4) blood transfusions as required by the clinical circumstances. The drug is probably dialyzable, but this property has not been tested clinically.

DOSAGE AND ADMINISTRATION:

Acetohydroxamic acid should be administered orally, one tablet 3-4 times a day in a total daily dose of 10-15 mg/kg/day. The recommended starting dose is 12 mg/kg/day, administered at 6-8 hour intervals at a time when the stomach is empty. The maximum daily dose should be no more than 1.5 grams, regardless of body weight.

The dosage should be reduced in patients with reduced renal function. Patients whose serum creatinine is greater than 1.8 mg/dl should take no more than 1.0 g/day; such patients should be dosed at q-12-h intervals. Further reductions in dosage to prevent the accumulation of toxic concentrations in the blood may also be desirable. Insufficient data exists to accurately characterize the optimum dose and/or dose interval in patients with moderate degrees of renal insufficiency.

Patients with advanced renal insufficiency (*i.e.,* serum creatinine more than 2.5 mg/dl) should not be treated with acetohydroxamic acid. The risk of accumulation of toxic blood levels of acetohydroxamic acid seems to be greater than the chances for a beneficial effect in such patients.

In children an initial dose of 10 mg/kg/day is recommended. Close monitoring of the patient's clinical condition and hematologic status is recommended. Titration of the dose to higher or lower levels may be required to obtain an optimum therapeutic effect and/or to reduce the risk of side effects.

Storage: Acetohydroxamic acid should be stored in a dry place at room temperature, 15°-30°C (59°-86°F). Container should be closed tightly.

HOW SUPPLIED - EQUIVALENTS NOT AVAILABLE:

Tablet, Uncoated - Oral - 250 mg

100's	$82.50	LITHOSTAT, Mission Pharma	00178-0500-01

ACETYLCARBROMAL *(000099)*

CATEGORIES: Anxiolytics, Sedatives, Hypnotic; Central Nervous System Agents; Sedatives/Hypnotics; FDA Pre 1938 Drugs

BRAND NAMES: Paxarel

Prescribing information not available at time of publication.

HOW SUPPLIED - EQUIVALENTS NOT AVAILABLE:

Tablet, Coated - Oral - 250 mg

100's	$5.50	PAXAREL, Circle Pharms	00659-3241-01

ACETYLCHOLINE CHLORIDE *(000100)*

CATEGORIES: Antiglaucomatous Agents; EENT Drugs; Eye, Ear, Nose, & Throat Preparations; Intraocular Miotic; Iridectomy; Miosis; Miotics; Ophthalmics; Parasympathomimetic Agents; Surgical Aid, Ophthalmic; Cataract*; FDA Approval Pre 1982

* Indication not approved by the FDA

BRAND NAMES: **Miochol**; Miochol-E

DESCRIPTION:

Acetylcholine chloride is a parasympathomimetic preparation for intraocular use packaged in a vial of two compartments; the lower chamber containing acetylcholine chloride 20 mg and mannitol 60 mg; the upper chamber containing sterile water for injection 2 ml.

The reconstituted liquid will be a sterile isotonic solution containing 20 mg acetylcholine chloride (1:100 solution) and 3% mannitol. Mannitol is used in the process of lyophilizing acetylcholine chloride, and is not considered an active ingredient.

The chemical name for acetylcholine chloride, $C_7H_{16}ClNO_2$, is 2-acetoxyethyltrimethylammonium chloride.

CLINICAL PHARMACOLOGY:

Acetylcholine is a naturally occurring neurohormone which mediates nerve impulse transmission at all cholinergic sites involving somatic and autonomic nerves. After release from the nerve ending, acetylcholine is rapidly inactivated by the enzyme acetylcholinesterase by hydrolysis to acetic acid and choline.

Direct application of acetylcholine to the iris will cause rapid miosis of short duration. Topical ocular instillation of acetylcholine to the intact eye causes no discernible response as cholinesterase destroys the molecule more rapidly than it can penetrate the cornea.

INDICATIONS AND USAGE:

To obtain complete miosis of the iris in seconds after delivery of the lens in cataract surgery, in penetrating keratoplasty, iridectomy and other anterior segment surgery where rapid, complete miosis may be required.

CONTRAINDICATIONS:

There are presently no known contraindications to the use of acetylcholine intraocular.

WARNINGS:

If blister or peelable backing is damaged or broken, sterility of the enclosed bottle cannot be assured. Open under aseptic conditions only.

WARNING: DO NOT GAS STERILIZE

PRECAUTIONS:

General: In the reconstitution of the solution, as described under Directions for Using Univial, if the center rubber plug seal in the univial does not go down or is down, do not use the vial.

If miosis is to be obtained quickly and completely with acetylcholine, obstructions to miosis, such as anterior or posterior synechiae, may require surgery prior to administration of acetylcholine. In cataract surgery, use acetylcholine only after delivery of the lens. **NOTE:** Aqueous solutions of acetylcholine chloride are unstable. Prepare solution immediately before use. Do not use solution which is not clear and colorless. Discard any solution that has not been used.

Pediatric Use: Safety and effectiveness in children have not been established.

DRUG INTERACTIONS:

Although clinical studies with acetylcholine chloride and animal studies with acetylcholine or carbachol revealed no interference, and there is no known pharmacological basis for an interaction, there have been reports that acetylcholine chloride and carbachol have been ineffective when used in patients treated with topical nonsteroidal anti-inflammatory agents.

ADVERSE REACTIONS:

Infrequent cases of corneal edema, corneal clouding, and corneal decompensation have been reported with the use of acetylcholine.

Adverse reactions have been reported rarely which are indicative of systemic absorption. These include bradycardia, hypotension, flushing, breathing difficulties and sweating.

OVERDOSAGE:

Atropine sulfate (0.5 to 1 mg) should be given intramuscularly or intravenously and should be readily available to counteract possible overdosage. Epinephrine (0.1 to 1 mg subcutaneously) is also of value in overcoming severe cardiovascular or bronchoconstrictor responses.

DOSAGE AND ADMINISTRATION:

With a new needle of sturdy gauge, 18-20, draw all of the solution into a dry, sterile syringe. Replace needle with a suitable atraumatic cannula for intraocular irrigation.

The acetylcholine solution is instilled into the anterior chamber before or after securing one or more sutures. Instillation should be gentle and parallel to the iris face and tangential to pupil border.

If there are no mechanical hindrances, the pupil is rapidly constricted and the peripheral iris drawn away from the angle of the anterior chamber. Any anatomical hindrance to miosis may require surgery to permit the desired effect of the drug. In most cases, 1/2 to 2 ml produces satisfactory miosis. The acetylcholine solution need not be flushed from the chamber after miosis occurs. Since the action of acetylcholine is of short duration, pilocarpine may be applied topically before dressing to maintain miosis.

DOSAGE AND ADMINISTRATION: *(cont'd)*

In cataract surgery, use acetylcholine only after delivery of the lens.

NOTE: Aqueous solutions of acetylcholine chloride are unstable. Prepare solution immediately before use. Do not use solution which is not clear and colorless. Discard any solution that has not been used.

DIRECTIONS FOR USING THE UNIVIAL: STERILE UNLESS PACKAGE OPEN OR BROKEN

1. Inspect univial while inside unopened blister. Diluent must be in upper chamber. **2.**Peel open blister. **3.** Aseptically transfer univial to sterile field. Maintain sterility of outer container during preparation of solution. **4.** Immediately before use, give plunger-stopper a quarter turn and press to force diluent and center plug into lower chamber. **5.** Shake gently to dissolve drug. **6.**Discard univial and any unused solution.

Keep From Freezing: Store at 15°-30°C (59°-86°F).

HOW SUPPLIED - EQUIVALENTS NOT AVAILABLE:

Injection, Conc, W/Buf - Intraocular; Ir - 1 %

2 ml	$34.74	MIOCHOL, SYSTEM PAK/IOCARE BSALT, Ciba Vision	00058-2764-54

Kit - Ophthalmic - 1 %

1's	$24.18	MIOCHOL-E, Ciba Vision	00058-2775-53

Solution - Ophthalmic - 1 %

2 ml	$22.02	MIOCHOL-E, Ciba Vision	00058-2772-52

ACETYLCYSTEINE *(000101)*

CATEGORIES: Acetaminophen Overdose; Amyloidosis; Anesthesia; Antidotes; Antitussives/Expectorants/Mucolytics; Atelectasis; Brochopulmonary Disease; Bronchial Studies; Bronchiectasis; Bronchitis; Cough Preparations; Cystic Fibrosis; Diagnostic Agents; Emphysema; Mucolytic Agents; Respiratory & Allergy Medications; Tracheostomy Care; Tuberculosis; Hypercholesterolemia*; FDA Approval Pre 1982

* Indication not approved by the FDA

BRAND NAMES: *Acetyst*; *Agisolvan*; *Airbron* (Canada); *Alveolex*; *Alveolux*; *Bromuc*; *Ecomucyl*; *Encore*; *Exomuc* (France); *Fabrol* (England); *Fluimicil* (Germany); *Fluimucil* (France); *Mucofillin* (Japan); *Mucolid*; *Mucolitico*; *Mucomiste*; Mucomyst; Mucosil; Mucosol; *Mukolit*; *Mukosil*; *Respaire*; *Siran 200*

(International brand names outside U.S. in italics)

FORMULARIES: BC-BS; Medi-Cal

DESCRIPTION:

Acetylcysteine is for inhalation (mucolytic agent) or oral administration (acetaminophen antidote), and available as sterile, unpreserved solutions (not for injection). The solutions contain 20% or 10% acetylcysteine, with disodium edetate in purified water. Sodium hydroxide is added to adjust pH to 7. Acetylcystine is the N-acetyl derivative of the N-acetyl derivative of the naturally occurring amino acid, cysteine. The compound is a white crystalline powder with the molecular formula $C_5H_9NO_3S$, a molecular weight of 163.2, and chemical name of N-acetyl-L-cysteine.

This product contains the following inactive ingredients: disodium edetate, sodium hydroxide, and purified water.

CLINICAL PHARMACOLOGY:

The viscosity of pulmonary mucous secretions depends on the concentrations of mucoprotein and to a lesser extent deoxyribonucleic acid (DNA). The latter increases with increasing purulence owing to cellular debris. The mucolytic action of acetylcysteine is related to the sulfhydryl group in the molecule. This group probably "opens" disulfide linkages in mucous thereby lowering the viscosity. The mucolytic activity of acetylcysteine is unaltered by the presence of DNA, and increases with increasing pH. Significant mucolysis occurs between pH 7 and 9.

Acetylcysteine undergoes rapid deacetylation *in vivo* to yield cysteine or oxidation to yield diacetylcystine.

Occasionally, patients exposed to the inhalation of an acetylcysteine aerosol respond with the development of increased airways obstruction of varying and unpredictable severity. Those patients who are reactors cannot be identified *a priori* from a random patient population. Even when patients are known to have reacted previously to the inhalation of an acetylcysteine aerosol, they may not react during a subsequent treatment. The converse is also true; patients who have had inhalation treatments of acetylcysteine without incident may still react to a subsequent inhalation with increased airways obstruction. Most patients with bronchospasm are quickly relieved by the use of a bronchodilator given by nebulization. If bronchospasm progresses, the medication should be discontinued immediately.

AS AN ANTIDOTE FOR ACETAMINOPHEN OVERDOSE

(Antidotal) Acetaminophen is rapidly absorbed from the upper gastrointestinal tract with peak plasma levels occurring between 30 and 60 minutes after therapeutic doses and usually within 4 hours following an overdose. The parent compound, which is nontoxic, is extensively metabolized in the liver to form principally the sulfate and glucuronide conjugates which are also nontoxic and are rapidly excreted in the urine. A small fraction of an ingested dose is metabolized in the liver by the cytochrome P-450 mixed function oxidase enzyme system to form a reactive, potentially toxic, intermediate metabolite which preferentially conjugates with hepatic glutathione to form the nontoxic cysteine and mercapturic acid derivatives which are then excreted by the kidney. Therapeutic doses of acetaminophen do not saturate the glucuronide and sulfate conjugation pathways and do not result in the formation of sufficient reactive metabolic to deplete glutathione stores. However, following ingestation of a large overdose (150 mg/kg or greater) the glucuronide and sulfate conjugation pathways are saturated resulting in a larger fraction of the drug being metabolized via the P-450 pathway. The increased formation of reactive metabolite may deplete the hepatic stores of glutathione with subsequent binding of the metabolite to protein molecules within the hepatocyte resulting in cellular necrosis. Acetylcysteine has been shown to reduce the extent of liver injury following acetaminophen overdose. Its effectiveness depends on early administration, with benefit seen principally in patients treated within 16 hours of the overdose. Acetylcysteine probably the liver by maintaining or restoring the glutathione levels, or by acting as an alternate substrate for conjugation with, and thus detoxification of, the reactive metabolite.

INDICATIONS AND USAGE:

Acetylcysteine is indicated as adjuvant therapy for patients with abnormal, viscid, or inspissated mucous secretions in such conditions as:

Chronic bronchopulmonary disease (chronic emphysema, emphysema with bronchitis, chronic asthmatic bronchitis, tuberculosis, bronchiectasis and primary amyloidosis of the lung)

Acute bronchopulmonary disease (pneumonia, bronchitis, tracheobronchitis)

INDICATIONS AND USAGE: *(cont'd)*

Pulmonary complications of cystic fibrosis

Tracheostomy care

Pulmonary complications associated with surgery

Use during anesthesia

Post-traumatic chest conditions

Atelectasis due to mucous obstruction

Diagnostic bronchial studies (bronchograms, bronchospirometry and bronchial wedge catheterization)

ACETYLCYSTEINE AS AN ANTIDOTE FOR ACETAMINOPHEN OVERDOSE

Acetylcysteine, administered orally, is indicated as an antidote to prevent or lessen hepatic injury which may occur following the ingestion of a potentially hepatotoxic quantity of acetaminophen.

It is essential to initiate treatment as soon as possible after the overdose and, in any case, within 24 hours of ingestion.

CONTRAINDICATIONS:

Acetylcysteine is contraindicated in those patients who are sensitive to it.

ACETYLCYSTEINE AS AN ANTIDOTE FOR ACETAMINOPHEN OVERDOSE

There are no contraindications to oral administration of acetylcysteine in the treatment of acetaminophen overdose.

WARNINGS:

After proper administration of acetylcysteine, an increased volume of liquefied bronchial secretions may occur. When cough is inadequate, the open airway must be maintained by mechanical suction if necessary. When there is a large mechanical block due to foreign body or local accumulation, the airway should be cleared by endotracheal aspiration, with or without bronchoscopy. Asthmatics under treatment with acetylcysteine should be watched carefully. If bronchospasm progresses, the medication should be discontinued immediately.

AS AN ANTIDOTE FOR ACETAMINOPHEN OVERDOSE

Generalized urticaria has been observed rarely in patients receiving oral acetylcysteine for acetaminophen overdose. If this occurs or other allergic symptoms appear, treatment with acetylcysteine should be discontinued unless it is deemed essential and the allergic symptoms can be otherwise controlled.

If encephalopathy due to hepatic failure becomes evident, acetylcysteine treatment should be discontinued to avoid further administration of nitrogenous substances. There are no data indicating that acetylcysteine adversely influences hepatic failure, but this remains a theoretical possibility.

PRECAUTIONS:

With the administration of acetylcysteine, the patient may initially notice a slight disagreeable odor which soon is not noticeable. With a face mask there may be a stickiness on the face after nebulization which is easily removed by washing with water.

Under certain conditions, a color change may take place in the solution of acetylcysteine in the opened bottle. The light purple color is the result of a chemical reaction which does not significantly impair the safety or mucolytic effectiveness of acetylcysteine.

Continued nebulization of an acetylcysteine solution with a dry gas will result in an increased concentration of the drug in the nebulizer because of evaporation of the solvent. Extreme concentration may impede nebulization and efficient delivery of the drug. Dilution of the nebulizing solutions with Sterile Water for Injection, USP, as concentration occurs, will obviate this problem.

AS AN ANTIDOTE FOR ACETAMINOPHEN OVERDOSE

Occasionally severe and persistent vomiting occurs as a symptom of acute acetaminophen overdose. Treatment with oral acetylcysteine may aggravate the vomiting. Patients at risk of gastric hemorrhage (*e.g.,* esophageal varices, peptic ulcers, etc.) should be evaluated concerning the risk of upper gastrointestinal hemorrhage versus the risk of developing hepatic toxicity, and treatment with acetylcysteine given accordingly.

Dilution of the acetylcysteine minimizes the propensity of oral acetylcysteine to aggravate vomiting.

CARCINOGENESIS, MUTAGENESIS, AND IMPAIRMENT OF FERTILITY

Carcinogenesis: Carcinogenicity studies in laboratory animals have not been performed with acetylcysteine in combination with isoproterenol.

Long-term oral studies of acetylcysteine alone in rats (12 months of treatment followed by 6 months of observation) at doses up to 1000 mg/kg/day (5.2 times the human dose) provided no evidence of oncogenic activity.

Mutagenesis: Published data* indicate that acetylcysteine is not mutagenic in the Ames test, both with and without metabolic activation.

Impairment of Fertility: A reproductive toxicity test to assess potential impairment of fertility was performed with acetylcysteine (10%) combined with isoproterenol (0.05%) and administered as an aerosol into a chamber of 12.43 cubic meters. The combination was administered for 25, 30, or 35 twice a day for 68 days before mating, to 200 male and 150 female rats; no adverse effects were noted in dams or pups. Females after mating were continued on treatment for the next 42 days.

Reproductive toxicity studies of acetylcysteine in the rat given oral doses of acetylcysteine up to 1,000 mg/kg (2.6 or 5.2 times the human dose) in the Segment 1 Study.

PREGNANCY CATEGORY B

Reproduction studies of acetylcysteine with isoproterenol have been performed in rats and of acetylcysteine alone in rabbits at doses up to 2.6 times the human dose. These have revealed no evidence of impaired fertility or harm to the fetus due to acetylcysteine. There are, however, no adequate and well-controlled studies in pregnant women. Because animal reproduction studies may not always be predictiveness of responses, this drug should be used during pregnancy only if clearly needed.

Teratogenic Effects: In a teratology study of acetylcysteine in the rabbit, oral doses of 500 mg/kg/day (2.6 times the human dose) were administered to pregnant does by intubation on days 6 through 16 of gestation. Acetylcysteine was found to be nonteratogenic under the conditions of study.

In the rabbit, two groups (one of 14 and one of 16 pregnant females) were exposed to an aerosol of 10% acetylcysteine and 0.05% isoproterenol hydrochloride for 30 or 35 minutes twice a day from the 6th through the 18th day of pregnancy. No teratogenic effects were observed among the offspring.

Teratology and a perinatal and postnatal toxicity study in rats were performed with a combination of acetylcysteine and isoproterenol administered by the inhalation route. In the rat, two groups of 25 pregnant females each were exposed to the aerosol for 30 and 35 minutes, respectively, twice a day from the 6th through the 15th day of gestation. No teratogenic effects were observed among the offspring.

PRECAUTIONS: *(cont'd)*

In the pregnant rat (30 rats per group), twice-daily exposure to an aerosol of acetylcysteine and isoproterenol for 30 or 35 minutes from the 15th day of gestation through the 21st day postpartum was without adverse effect on dams or newborns.

NURSING MOTHERS

It is not known whether this drug is excreted in human milk. Because many drugs are excreted in human milk, caution should be exercised when acetylcysteine is administered to a pregnant woman.

ADVERSE REACTIONS:

Adverse effects have included stomatitis, nausea, vomiting, fever, rhinorrhea, drowsiness, clamminess, chest tightness, and bronchoconstriction. Clinically overt acetylasthmatics bronchospasm occurs infrequently and unpredictably even in patients with asthmatic bronchitis or bronchitis complicating bronchial asthma. Acquired sensitization to acetylcysteine has been reported rarely. Reports of sensitization in patients have not been confirmed by patch testing. Sensitization has been confirmed in several inhalation therapists who reported a history of dermal eruptions after frequent and extended exposure to acetylcysteine. Reports of irritation to the tracheal and bronchial tracts have been received and although hemoptysis has occurred in patients receiving acetylcysteine such findings are not uncommon in patients with bronchopulmonary disease and a causal relationship has not been established.

AS AN ANTIDOTE FOR ACETAMINOPHEN OVERDOSE

Oral administration of acetylcysteine, especially in the large doses needed to treat acetaminophen overdose, may result in nausea, vomiting and other gastrointestinal symptoms. Rash with or without mild fever has been observed rarely.

DOSAGE AND ADMINISTRATION:

Acetylcysteine Solution 10% and 20%, is available in glass vials containing 4 ml or 30 ml. The 20% solution may be diluted to a lesser concentration with either Sodium Chloride Inhalation Solution, USP, Sodium Chloride Injection, USP, or Sterile Water for Injection, USP. The 10% solution may be used undiluted.

Acetylcysteine does not contain an antimicrobial agent, and care must be taken to minimize contamination of the sterile solution. If only a portion of the solution in a vial is used, store the remainder in a refrigerator and use within 96 hours.

Nebulization—face mask, mouth piece, tracheostomy: When nebulized into a face mask, mouth piece or tracheostomy, 1 to 10 ml of the 20% solution or 2 to 20 ml of the 10% solution may be given every 2 to 6 hours; the recommended dose for most patients is 3 to 5 ml of the 20% solution or 6 to 10ml of the 10% solution 3 to 4 times a day.

Nebulization Tent, Croupette: In special circumstances it may be necessary to nebulize into a tent or Croupette, and this method of use must be individualized to take into account the available equipment and the patient's particular needs. This form of administration requires very large volumes of the solution, occasionally as much as 300 ml during a single treatment period. If a tent or Croupette must be used, the recommended dose is the volume of solution (using 10% or 20% acetylcysteine) that will maintain a very heavy mist in the tent or Croupette for the desired period. Administration for intermittent or continuous prolonged periods, including overnight, may be desirable.

Direct Installation: When used by direct instillation, 1 to 2 ml of the 10% or 20% solution may then be given as often as every hour.

When used for the routine nursing care of patients with tracheostomy, 1 to 2 ml of the 10% to 20% solution may be given every 1 to 4 hours by instillation into the tracheostomy.

Acetylcysteine may be introduced directly into a particular segment of the bronchopulmonary tree by inserting (under local anesthesia and direct vision) a small plastic catheter into the trachea. Two to 5 ml of the 20% solution may then be instilled by means of a syringe connected to the catheter.

Acetylcysteine may also be given through a percutaneous intratracheal catheter. One to 2 ml of the 20% or 2 to 4 ml of the 10% solution every 1 to 4 hours may then be given by a syringe attached to the catheter.

Diagnostic Bronchograms: For diagnostic bronchial studies, 2 or 3 administrations of 1 to 2 ml of the 20% solution or 2 to 4 ml of the 10% solution should be given by nebulization or by instillation intratracheally, prior to the procedure.

ADMINISTRATION OF AEROSOL

Materials: Acetylcysteine may be administered using conventional nebulizers made of plastic or glass. Certain materials used in nebulization equipment react with acetylcysteine. The most reactive of these are certain metals (notably iron and copper) and rubber. Where material may come into contact with acetylcysteine solution, parts made of the following acceptable materials should be used: glass, plastic, aluminum, anodized aluminum, chromed metal, tantalum, sterling silver, or stainless steel. Silver may become tarnished after exposure, but this is not harmful to the drug action or to the patient.

NEBULIZING GASES

Compressed tank gas (air) on an air compressor should be used to provide pressure for nebulizing the solution. Oxygen may also be used but should be used with usual caution in patients with severe respiratory disease and CO_2 retention.

Apparatus: Acetylcysteine is usually administered as fine nebulae for its local effect, and the nebulizer used should be capable of providing optimal quantities of a suitable range of particle sizes.

Commercially available nebulizers will produce nebulae of acetylcysteine satisfactory for retention in the respiratory tract. Most of the nebulizers tested will supply a high proportion of the drug solution as particles of less than 10 microns in diameter. Mitchell[a] has shown that particles less than 10 microns should be retained in the respiratory tract satisfactorily.

Units that nebulized acetylcysteine with a satisfactory efficiency were the Maxi-Myst Nebulizer (Mead Johnson Pharmaceuticals, Evansville, Indiana), Hand-E-Vent intermittent positive pressure breathing device (Ohio Medical Products, 3030 Airco Drive, Madison, Wisconsin), and various other intermittent positive pressure breathing devices, No. 40 De Vilbiss (The De Vilbiss Co., Somerset, Pennsylvania), Bennett Twin-Jet Nebulizer (Puritan Bennett Corp., Oak at 13th., Kansas City, Missouri).

The nebulized solution may be inhaled directly from the nebulizer. Nebulizers may also be attached to plastic face masks or plastic mouthpieces. Suitable nebulizers may also be fitted for use with the various intermittent positive pressure breathing (IPPB) machines. The nebulizing equipment should be cleaned immediately after use because the residues may clog the smaller orifices or corrode metal parts.

Hand bulbs are not recommended for routine use for nebulizing acetylcysteine because their output is generally too small. Some hand-operated nebulizers deliver particles that are larger than optimum for inhalation therapy.

Acetylcysteine should not be placed directly into the chamber of a heated (hot pot) nebulizer. A heated nebulizer may be part of the nebulization assembly to provide a warm saturated atmosphere if the acetylcysteine aerosol is introduced by means of a separate unheated nebulizer. Usual precautions for administration of warm saturated nebulae should be observed.

DOSAGE AND ADMINISTRATION: *(cont'd)*

The nebulized solution may be breathed directly from the nebulizer. Nebulizers may also be attached to plastic face masks, plastic face tents, plastic mouth pieces, conventional plastic oxygen tents, or head tents. Suitable nebulizers may also be fitted for use with the various intermittent positive pressure breathing (IPPB) machine.

The nebulizing equipment should be cleaned immediately after use; the residues may occlude the fine orifices or corrode metal parts.

Prolonged Nebulization: When three fourths of the initial volume of acetylcysteine solution has been nebulized, a quantity of Sterile Water for Injection, USP (approximately equal to the volume of solution remaining) should be added to the nebulizer. This obviates any concentration of the agent in the residual solvent remaining after prolonged nebulization.

COMPATIBILITY

The physical and chemical compatibility of acetylcysteine solutions with other drugs commonly administered by nebulization, direct instillation, or topical application, has been studied.

Acetylcysteine should not be mixed with all antibiotics. For example, the antibiotics tetracycline hydrochloride, oxytetracycline hydrochloride, and erythromycin lactobionate were found to be incompatible when mixed in the same solution. These agents may be administered from separate solutions if administration of these agents is desirable.

If it is deemed advisable to prepare an admixture, it should be administered as soon as possible after preparation. Do not store unused mixtures.

AS AN ANTIDOTE FOR ACETAMINOPHEN OVERDOSE

Regardless of the quantity of acetaminophen reported to have been ingested, administer acetylcysteine immediately if 24 hours or less have elapsed from the reported time of ingestion of an overdose of acetaminophen. Do not await results of assays for acetaminophen level before initiating treatment with acetylcysteine. The following procedures are recommended:

1. The stomach should be emptied promptly by lavage or by inducing emesis with syrup of ipecac. Syrup of ipecac should be given in a dose of 15 ml for children up to age 12, and 30 ml for adolescents and adults followed immediately by copious quantities of water. The dose should be repeated if emesis does not occur in 20 minutes.

2. In the case of a mixed drug overdose activated charcoal may be indicated. However, if activated charcoal has been administered, lavage before administering acetylcysteine treatment. Activated charcoal adsorbs acetylcysteine *in vitro* and may do so in patients and thereby may reduce in effectiveness.

3. Draw blood for acetaminophen plasma assay and for baseline SGOT, SGPT, bilirubin, prothrombin time, creatinine, BUN, blood sugar and electrolytes. The acetaminophen assay provides a basis for determining the need for continuing with the maintenance doses of acetylcysteine treatment. If an assay cannot be obtained or if the acetaminophen level is clearly in the toxic range (above the dashed line of the nomogram) dosing with acetylcysteine should be continued for the full course of therapy. The laboratory measurements are used to monitor hepatic and renal function and electrolyte and fluid balance.

4. Administer the loading dose of acetylcysteine, 140 mg per kg of body weight. (Prepare acetylcysteine for oral administration as described in the Dosage Guide and Preparation table).

5. Four hours after the loading dose administer the first maintenance dose (70 mg of acetylcysteine per kg of body weight). The maintenance dose is then repeated at 4 hour intervals for a total of 17 doses unless the acetaminophen assay reveals a nontoxic level as discussed below.

6. If the patient vomits the loading dose or any maintenance dose within one hour of administration, repeat the dose.

7. In the occasional instances where the patient is persistently unable to retain the orally administered acetylcysteine, the antidote may be administered by duodenal intubation.

8. Repeat SGOT, SGPY, bilirubin, prothrombin time, creatinine, BUN, blood sugar and electrolytes daily if the acetaminophen plasma level is in the potentially toxic range as discussed below.

Table 1 Dosage Guide And Preparation

Body Weight (kg)	Body Weight (lb)	Acetylcysteine grams	Acetylcysteine ml of 20%	Diluent ml	5% Solution Total ml
Loading Dose of Acetylcysteine**					
100-109	220-240	15	75	225	300
90-99	198-218	14	70	210	280
80-89	176-196	13	65	195	260
70-79	154-174	11	55	165	220
60-69	132-152	10	50	150	200
50-59	110-130	8	40	120	160
40-49	88-108	7	35	105	140
30-39	66-86	6	30	90	120
20-29	44-64	4	20	60	80
Maintenance Dose**					
100-109	220-240	7.5	37	113	150
90-99	198-218	7	35	105	140
80-89	176-196	6.5	33	97	130
70-79	154-174	5.5	28	82	110
60-69	132-152	5	25	75	100
50-59	110-130	4	20	60	80
40-49	88-108	3.5	18	52	70
30-39	66-86	3	15	45	60
20-29	44-64	2	10	30	40

Doses in relation to body weight are as shown above.

** If patient weighs less than 20 kg (usually patients younger than 6 years), calculate the doses of acetylcysteine solution. Each ml of 20% acetylcysteine solution, contains 200 mg of acetylcysteine. The loading dose is 140 mg per kilogram of body weight. The maintenance dose is 70 mg/kg. Three (3) ml of diluent are added to each ml of 20% acetylcysteine solution. Do not decrease the proportion of diluent.

PREPARATION OF ACETYLCYSTEINE FOR ORAL ADMINISTRATION

Oral administration requires dilution of the 20% solution with cola drinks, Fresca or other soft drinks, to a final concentration of 5% (see Dosage Guide and Preparation table). If administered via gastric tube or Miller-Abbott tube, water may be used as the diluent. The dilutions should be freshly prepared and utilized within one hour. Remaining undiluted solutions in opened vials can be stored in the refrigerator up to 96 hours. **ACETYLCYSTEINE IS NOT APPROVED FOR PARENTERAL INJECTION.**

ACETAMINOPHEN ASSAYS - INTERPRETATION AND METHODOLOGY

The acute ingestion of acetaminophen in quantities of 150 mg/kg or greater may result in hepatic toxicity. However, the reported history of the quantity of a drug ingested as an overdose is often inaccurate and is not a reliable guide to therapy of the overdose. **THEREFORE, PLASMA OR SERUM ACETAMINOPHEN CONCENTRATIONS, DETERMINED AS EARLY AS POSSIBLE, BUT NO SOONER THAN FOUR HOURS FOLLOWING ACUTE OVERDOSE, ARE ESSENTIAL IN ASSESSING THE POTENTIAL RISK OF HEPATOTOXICITY. IF AN ASSAY FOR ACETAMINOPHEN CANNOT BE OBTAINED, IT IS NECESSARY TO ASSUME THAT THE OVERDOSE IS POTENTIALLY TOXIC.**

INTERPRETATION OF ACETAMINOPHEN ASSAYS

1. When results of the plasma acetaminophen assay are available refer to the nomogram above to determine if plasma concentration is in the potentially toxic range. Values above the solid line connecting 200 mcg/ml at 4 hours with 50 mcg/ml at 12 hours are associated with a possibility of hepatic toxicity if an antidote is not administered. (Do not wait for assay results to begin acetylcysteine treatment.)

2. If the plasma level is above the broken line continue with maintenance doses of acetylcysteine. It is better to err on the safe side and thus the broken line is plotted 25% below the solid line which defines possible toxicity.

3. If the initial plasma level is below the broken line described above, there is minimal risk of hepatic toxicity and acetylcysteine treatment can be discontinued.

ACETAMINOPHEN ASSAY METHODOLOGY

Assay procedures most suitable for determining acetaminophen concentrations utilize high pressure liquid chromatography (HPLC) or gas liquid chromatography (GLC). The assay should measure only parent acetaminophen and not conjugated. The assay procedures listed below fulfill this requirement:

SELECTED TECHNIQUES (NONINCLUSIVE)

HPLC:

1. Blair, D and Rumack, BH, Clin Chem 23(4):743-745 (April) 1977.

2. Howie, D, Andriaenssens, PI and Prescott, LF, Journ Pharm and Pharmacol 29(4)235-237 (April) 1977.

GLC:

3. Prescott, LF, Journ Pharm and Pharmacol 23 (10):807-808 (October) 1971.

Colorimetric

4. Glynn, JP and Kendal, SE, The Lancet 1:1147-1148 (May 17) 1975.

SUPPORTIVE TREATMENT OF ACETAMINOPHEN OVERDOSE

1. Maintain fluid and electrolyte balance based on clinical evaluation of state of hydration and serum electrolytes.

2. Treat as necessary for hypoglycemia.

3. Administer vitamin K_1if prothrombin time ratio exceeds 1.5 or fresh frozen plasma if the prothrombin time ratio exceeds 3.0. 4. Diuretics and forced diuresis should be avoided (See TABLE 1.)

HOW SUPPLIED - RATED THERAPEUTICALLY EQUIVALENT:

Solution - Inhalation; Ora - 10 %

4 ml x 12	$30.74	Acetylcysteine, Roxane	00054-8059-05
4 ml x 12	$67.80	Acetylcysteine, Dey Labs	49502-0181-04
4 ml x 12	$103.21	MUCOMYST-10, Bristol Myers Squibb	00087-0572-03
10 ml x 3	$19.56	Acetylcysteine, Roxane	00054-3027-02
10 ml x 3	$40.26	Acetylcysteine, Dey Labs	49502-0181-10
10 ml x 3	$62.02	MUCOMYST-10, Bristol Myers Squibb	00087-0572-01
30 ml x 3	$34.94	Acetylcysteine, Roxane	00054-3025-02
30 ml x 3	$110.48	Acetylcysteine, Dey Labs	49502-0181-30
30 ml x 3	$168.24	MUCOMYST-10, Bristol Myers Squibb	00087-0572-02

Solution - Inhalation; Ora - 20 %

4 ml x 12	$33.54	Acetylcysteine, Roxane	00054-8060-05
4 ml x 12	$81.36	Acetylcysteine, Dey Labs	49502-0182-04
4 ml x 12	$123.89	MUCOMYST, Bristol Myers Squibb	00087-0570-07
10 ml x 3	$24.45	Acetylcysteine, Roxane	00054-3028-02
10 ml x 3	$48.66	Acetylcysteine, Dey Labs	49502-0182-10
10 ml x 3	$74.17	MUCOMYST, Bristol Myers Squibb	00087-0570-03
30 ml x 3	$39.13	Acetylcysteine, Roxane	00054-3026-02
30 ml x 3	$133.43	Acetylcysteine, Dey Labs	49502-0182-30
30 ml x 3	$203.22	MUCOMYST, Bristol Myers Squibb	00087-0570-09
100 ml	$92.21	Acetylcysteine, Dey Labs	49502-0182-00

HOW SUPPLIED - NOT RATED EQUIVALENT:

Solution - Inhalation; Ora - 10 %

30 ml x 10	$93.75	Acetylcysteine, Jordan Pharms	58196-0200-73

ACIDULATED PHOSPHATE FLUORIDE *(000104)*

CATEGORIES: Dental; Dental Caries; Homeostatic & Nutrient; Vitamins; FDA Pre 1938 Drugs

BRAND NAMES: Fluorinse; Gel II; Liquiflur; Nafrinse; *Orofluor Solution*; **Phos-Flur**
(International brand names outside U.S. in italics)

Prescribing information not available at time of publication.

HOW SUPPLIED - EQUIVALENTS NOT AVAILABLE:

Solution - Oral - 2.2 mg/5ml

500 ml	$7.55	LIQUI-FLUR, CHERRY FLAVORED, Liquipharm	54198-0108-16
500 ml	$7.55	LIQUI-FLUR, CINNAMON FLAVORED, Liquipharm	54198-0109-16
500 ml	$7.55	LIQUI-FLUR, LIME FLAVORED, Liquipharm	54198-0110-16
500 ml	$7.55	LIQUI-FLUR, ORANGE FLAVORED, Liquipharm	54198-0111-16

ACITRETIN *(003200)*

CATEGORIES: Dermatologicals; Psoriasis; Skin/Mucous Membrane Agents; Pregnancy Category X; FDA Unapproved

BRAND NAMES: *Neotigason* (England, Germany); **Soriatane**
(International brand names outside U.S. in italics)

Prescribing information not available at time of publication.

ACRIVASTINE; PSEUDOEPHEDRINE HYDROCHLORIDE *(003163)*

CATEGORIES: Allergies; Antihistamines; Respiratory & Allergy Medications; Rhinitis; Rhinorrhea; Sneezing; FDA Class 1S ("Standard Review"); FDA Approved 1994 Mar

BRAND NAMES: Duact; **Semprex-D**

FORMULARIES: Medi-Cal

COST OF THERAPY: (Rhinitis; Capsule; 8 mg/60 mg; 4/day; 30 days)

PRIMARY ICD9: 477.9 (Allergic Rhinitis, Cause Unspecified)

DESCRIPTION:

Semprex-D Capsules (acrivastine and pseudoephedrine HCl), are a fixed combination product formulation for oral administration. Acrivastine is an antihistamine and pseudoephedrine is a decongestant. Each capsule contains 8 mg acrivastine and 60 mg pseudoephedrine HCl and the inactive ingredients: lactose, magnesium stearate and sodium starch glycolate. The green and white capsule shell consists of gelatin, D&C Yellow No. 10, FD&C Green No. 3, and titanium dioxide.The yellow band around the capsule consists of gelatin and D&C Yellow No. 10. The capsules may contain one or more parabens and are printed with edible black and white inks.

The chemical name of acrivastine is (*E,E*),-3-[6-[1-(4-methylphenyl)-3-(1-pyrrolidinyl)-1-propenyl]-2-propenoic acid; the molecular formula is $C_{22}H_{24}N_2O_2$. As an analog of triprolidine hydrochloride, acrivastine is classified as an alkylamine antihistamine. Acrivastine is an odorless, white to pale cream crystalline powder that is soluble in chloroform and alcohol and slightly soluble in water.

The chemical name of pseudoephedrine hydrochloride is [*S*-(R*,R*)]-α-[1-(methylamino) ethyl]benzenemethanol hydrochloride; the molecular formula is $C_{10}H_{15}NO{\cdot}HCl$. Pseudoephedrine is one of the naturally occurring dextrorotatory diastereoisomers of ephedrine and is classified as an indirect sympathomimetic amine. Pseudoephedrine hydrochloride occurs as odorless, fine white to off-white crystals or powder; the drug is soluble in water, alcohol and chloroform.

CLINICAL PHARMACOLOGY:

Acrivastine a structural analog of triprolidine hydrochloride, exhibits H_1-antihistamine activity in isolated tissues, animals, and humans, and has sedative effects in humans (see PRECAUTIONS.) The propionic acid derivative of acrivastine is a metabolite in several animal species (as well as in man) and also exhibits H_1-antihistamine activity.

Pseudoephedrine hydrochloride is an indirect sympathomimetic agent; that is, it releases norepinephrine from adrenergic nerves.

In vitro tests and *in vivo* studies in animals of acrivastine and pseudoephedrine in combination failed to demonstrate evidence of any beneficial or deleterious pharmacologic interaction between the two agents.

PHARMACOKINETICS AND METABOLISM

Acrivastine was absorbed rapidly from combination capsule following oral administration and was bioavailable as a solution of acrivastine. After administration of acrivastine and pseudoephedrine hydrochloride capsules, maximum plasma acrivastine concentrations were achieved at 1.14 ± 0.23 hour. A mass balance study in 7 healthy volunteers showed that acrivastine is primarily eliminated by the kidneys. Over a 72-hour collection period, about 84% of the administered total radioactivity was recovered in urine and about 13% in feces, for a combined recovery of about 97%. Further, 67% of the administered radioactive dose was recovered in urine and the unchanged drug, 11% as the propionic acid metabolite, and 6% as other unknown metabolites.

Acrivastine exhibits linear kinetics over dosages ranging from 2 to 32 mg t.i.d. The mean ± SD terminal half-life for acrivastine was 1.9 ± 0.3 hours following single oral doses and increased to 3.5 ± 1.9 hours at steady state. The terminal half-life for the propionic acid metabolite was 3.8 ± 1.4 hours. Because of the short half lives of both acrivastine and its metabolites, accumulation in the plasma following multiple dosing is not expected.

The steady-state maximum acrivastine plasma concentration was 227 ± 47 ng/ml. The oral clearance and apparent volume of distribution were 2.9 ± 0.7 ml/min/kg and 0.46 ± 0.05 l/kg, respectively, following a single oral dose; oral clearance did not change at steady state (2.86 ± 0.75 ml/min/kg). The apparent volume of distribution increased to 0.82 ± 0.6 l/kg to parallel the increase in the elimination half-life of the drug.

Acrivastine binding to human plasma proteins was 50 ± 2.0% and was concentration-independent over the range of 5 to 1000 ng/ml. The main binding protein was serum albumin although the drug was slightly bound to α 1-acid glycoprotein. No displacement interaction was observed between acrivastine and either phenytoin or theophylline. The binding of acrivastine was not affected by the presence of pseudoephedrine.

Pseudoephedrine hydrochloride was also rapidly absorbed from the combination capsule, and the capsule was as bioavailable as a solution of pseudoephedrine. Steady state maximum plasma concentration for pseudoephedrine was 498 ± 129 ng/ml. The terminal half-life, oral clearance and apparent volume of distribution were 6.2 ± 1.8 hours, 5.9 ± 1.7 ml/min/kg, and 3.0 ± 0.4 l/kg, respectively. Elimination of pseudoephedrine is primarily through the renal route as 55 to 75% of an administered dose appears unchanged in the urine. Pseudoephedrine elimination, however, is highly dependent upon urine pH; the plasma half-life decreased to about 4 hours at pH 5 and increased to 13 hours at pH 8.

Pseudoephedrine did not bind to human plasma proteins over the concentration range of 50 to 2000 ng/ml.

Acrivastine and pseudoephedrine do not influence the pharmacokinetics of the other drug when administered concomitantly.

SPECIAL POPULATIONS

A single dose pharmacokinetic study showed that the elimination half-lives of acrivastine, the propionic acid metabolite of acrivastine, and pseudoephedrine were prolonged in patients with chronic renal insufficiency. Compared to normal volunteers, the elimination half-life of acrivastine was about 50% increased in patients with mild renal insufficiency (creatinine clearance = 26 to 48 ml/min) and was increased by about 130% in patients with moderate (creatinine clearance = 12 to 17 ml/min) or severe (creatinine clearance 6 to 10 ml/min) renal insufficiency. Oral clearance of acrivastine was diminished by the same magnitude as the half-life was prolonged in each of the three renally impaired groups. The elimination half-life of the propionic acid metabolite of acrivastine was about 140% increased in patients with mild renal insufficiency and about 5 times increased in patients with moderate or severe renal insufficiency.

Compared to normal volunteers, the elimination half-life of pseudoephedrine was about 3 times increased in patients with mild renal insufficiency, about 7 times increased in patients with moderate renal insufficiency, and about 10 times increased in patients with severe renal insufficiency. Oral clearance of pseudoephedrine was diminished by about the same magnitude as the half-life was prolonged in each of the three renally impaired groups (see PRECAUTIONS, Impaired Renal Function.)

The total body load removed by dialysis is approximately 20%, 27%, and 38% for acrivastine, the propionic acid metabolite of acrivastine, and pseudoephedrine, respectively, and therefore, a supplemental dose after a dialysis session is not required.

Based on a multiple dose cross study comparison, the apparent volume of distribution for acrivastine was 44% lower in elderly (n=36, 65-75 yr) than in young volunteers (n=16, 19-33yr). This difference could be attributed to the decrease in total body water that occurs with aging. Despite this difference, no appreciable differences in plasma acrivastine concentrations were seen in the elderly compared to the young, and no appreciable accumulation of acrivastine occurred in plasma at steady-state. The elimination half-life for pseudoephedrine was 18% longer in elderly (7.9 hours) than in younger subjects (6.7 hours), presumably due to the deadline in average renal function that occurs with aging. Despite the difference, clearance of pseudoephedrine was not appreciably different in elderly and younger subjects. Elderly patients should therefore be given the same dosage as younger patients. Acrivastine and pseudoephedrine hydrochloride capsules are not recommended, however, in patients with renal impairment (see PRECAUTIONS, Impaired Renal Function.)

The effect of age and sex on the pharmacokinetics parameters of acrivastine and pseudoephedrine was determined in 93 healthy volunteers who participated in various studies. All of the 93 volunteers were Caucasian (81 males and 12 females); 57 were between the ages of 18 and 38 years and 36 were between the ages of 65 and 75 years. There were no age- or sex-related differences in the pharmacokinetic parameters of either acrivastine or pseudoephedrine.

The effect of race on acrivastine and pseudoephedrine pharmacokinetics was examined by screening data obtained from 1035 patients, age 12 to 71 years, who participate in the 8 safety and efficacy studies. No race-related differences were observed in the pharmacokinetics of either acrivastine or pseudoephedrine.

CLINICAL STUDIES:

In healthy volunteers, histamine-induced wheal and flare areas were significantly reduced relative to placebo at 30 minutes after administration of a single dose of acrivastine 8 mg. Maximum reductions of wheal and flare occurred by 1 to 2 hours and significant reductions relative to placebo persisted for up to 6 hours a single oral dose of acrivastine 8 mg. No additional reductions of wheal and flare were observed following single doses of acrivastine up to 24 mg. The exact correlation between responses on skin testing and clinical efficacy is not established.

Five randomized, placebo- and or active-controlled trials compared acrivastine and pseudoephedrine hydrochloride with its acrivastine and pseudoephedrine components for the symptomatic relief of seasonal allergic rhinitis. In these studies, 696 patients received four daily doses of acrivastine 8 mg plus pseudoephedrine hydrochloride 60 mg (*i.e.,* acrivastine and pseudoephedrine hydrochloride capsules or bioequivalent formulations administered concurrently) or the same doses of the components for 14 days. The combination reduced the intensity of sneezing, rhinorrhea, pruritus, and lacrimation more than pseudoephedrine and reduced the intensity of nasal congestion more than acrivastine, demonstrating a contribution of each of the components. The onset of antihistaminic and nasal decongestant actions occurred within one or two hours after the first dose of acrivastine and pseudoephedrine hydrochloride capsules. Somnolence occurred in about 12% of patients given acrivastine and pseudoephedrine hydrochloride compared with about 6% on placebo.

INDICATIONS AND USAGE:

Acrivastine and pseudoephedrine hydrochloride capsules are indicated for relief of symptoms associated with seasonal allergic rhinitis such as sneezing, rhinorrhea, pruritus, lacrimation, and nasal congestion. Acrivastine and pseudoephedrine hydrochloride capsules should be administered when both antihistaminic activity of acrivastine and the nasal decongestant activity of pseudoephedrine are desired (see CLINICAL PHARMACOLOGY.) The efficacy of acrivastine and pseudoephedrine hydrochloride capsules beyond 14 days of continuous treatment in patients with seasonal allergic rhinitis has not been adequately investigated in clinical trials.

Acrivastine and pseudoephedrine hydrochloride capsules have not been adequately studied for effectiveness in relieving the symptoms of the common cold.

CONTRAINDICATIONS:

Acrivastine and pseudoephedrine hydrochloride capsules are contraindicated in patients with a known sensitivity to acrivastine, other alkylamine antihistamines (*e.g.,* triprolidine), pseudoephedrine, other sympathomimetic amines (*e.g.,* phenylpropanolamine), or to any other components of the formulation. Acrivastine and pseudoephedrine hydrochloride capsules are contraindicated in patients with severe hypertension or severe coronary artery disease. Acrivastine and pseudoephedrine hydrochloride capsules are contraindicated in patients taking monoamine oxidase (MAO) inhibitors and for two weeks after stopping use of an MAO inhibitor (see DRUG INTERACTIONS.)

WARNINGS:

Acrivastine and pseudoephedrine hydrochloride capsules should be used with caution in patients with hypertension, diabetes mellitus, ischemic heart disease, increased intraocular pressure, hyperthyroidism, prostatic hypertrophy, stenosing peptic ulcer, or pyloroduodenal obstruction. Overdose of sympathomimetic amines may produce CNS stimulation with convulsions or cardiovascular collapse with accompanying hypotension. The elderly are more likely to have adverse reactions to sympathomimetic amines.

PRECAUTIONS:

GENERAL

Acrivastine is sedating in some patients. In controlled clinical trials, somnolence (*i.e.,* drowsiness, sedation, sleepiness) was more common with acrivastine and pseudoephedrine hydrochloride capsules (by an average of 6%) than with placebo (see ADVERSE REACTIONS.)

Patients should be advised to assess their individual responses to acrivastine and pseudoephedrine hydrochloride capsules before engaging in any activity requiring mental alertness, such as driving a motor vehicle or operating machinery. Concurrent use of acrivastine and pseudoephedrine hydrochloride capsules with alcohol or other CNS depressants may cause additional reductions in alertness and impairment of CNS performance and should be avoided (see DRUG INTERACTIONS.)

IMPAIRED RENAL FUNCTION

Acrivastine and pseudoephedrine are excreted primarily through the kidneys. Both compounds therefore accumulate in patients with impaired renal function. Due to the differential effects of renal failure on the serum half-life and clearance of acrivastine and pseudoephedrine, use of acrivastine and pseudoephedrine hydrochloride capsules, a fixed combination product, in patients with renal impairment (creatinine clearance ≤ 48 ml/min) is not recommended (see OVERDOSAGE and CLINICAL PHARMACOLOGY).

GERIATRIC USE (APPROXIMATELY 60 YEARS OR OLDER)

Elderly patients who participate in clinical trials did not differ in effectiveness or adverse effects from younger patients. Antihistamines, however, as a pharmaceutical class, are more likely to cause dizziness, sedation, bladder-neck obstruction, and hypotension in elderly patients. The elderly are also more likely to have adverse reactions to sympathomimetics such as pseudoephedrine (see CLINICAL PHARMACOLOGY and WARNINGS).

INFORMATION FOR THE PATIENT

Patients taking acrivastine and pseudoephedrine hydrochloride capsules should receive the following information. acrivastine and pseudoephedrine hydrochloride capsules are prescribed to reduce symptoms associated with seasonal allergic rhinitis. Patients should be instructed to take acrivastine and pseudoephedrine hydrochloride capsules only as prescribed and not to

PRECAUTIONS: *(cont'd)*

exceed the prescribed dose. Patients should be advised against the concurrent use of acrivastine and pseudoephedrine hydrochloride with over-the-counter antihistamines and decongestants. Patients who are or may become pregnant should be told that this product should be used in pregnancy or during lactation only if the potential benefit justifies the potential risks to the fetus or nursing infant. Due to the risk of hypertensive crisis, patients should be instructed not to take acrivastine and pseudoephedrine hydrochloride capsules if they are presently taking a monoamine oxidase inhibitor or for two weeks after stopping use of MAO inhibitor. Patients should be advised to assess their individual responses to acrivastine and pseudoephedrine hydrochloride capsules before engaging in any activity requiring mental alertness, such as driving a car or operating machinery. Patients should be advised that the concurrent use of acrivastine and pseudoephedrine hydrochloride capsules with alcohol and other CNS depressants may lead to additional reductions in alertness and impairment of CNS performance and should be avoided.

CARCINOGENESIS, MUTAGENESIS, AND IMPAIRMENT OF FERTILITY

Carcinogenicity studies with the combination of acrivastine and pseudoephedrine have not been performed. Oral doses of acrivastine alone at levels up to 40 mg/kg/day (236 mg/m^2/day or 10 times the recommended human daily dose) for 20 to 22 months in rats and up to 250 mg/kg/day (750 mg/m^2/day or 32 times the recommended human daily dose) for 20 to 24 months in mice revealed no evidence of carcinogenic potential. No evidence of mutagenicity (with or without metabolic activation) was observed in the Ames Salmonella mutagenicity assay or in the L5178Y/tk$^{+/-}$ lymphoma assay. In an *in vitro* cytogenetic study performed in cultured human lymphocytes, acrivastine induced structural chromosomal abnormalities in the absence of metabolic activation, but not in its presence. In an *in vivo* cytogenic study in rats given single oral doses of acrivastine up to 1000 mg/kg (5900 mg/m^2 or 249 times the recommended human daily dose) there were no structural chromosomal alterations.

Reproduction-fertility studies in rats given acrivastine alone at levels up to 200 mg/kg/day (1180 mg/m^2/day 50 times the recommended human daily dose) had no effect on male or female fertility. Similarly, no effect on fertility was seen in male rats given acrivastine 20 mg/kg/day and pseudoephedrine 100 mg/kg/day (118 and 590 mg/m^2/day or 5 and 3 times the recommended human daily dose, respectively) or in female rats given acrivastine 4 mg/kg/day and pseudoephedrine 20 mg/kg/day (23.6 and 118 mg/m^2/day or 1 and 0.7 times the recommended human daily doses, respectively).

PREGNANCY CATEGORY B

Teratogenic Effects: No evidence of teratogenicity was seen in rats and rabbits given acrivastine 1000 and 400 mg/kg/day, respectively (5900 and 4720 mg/m^2/day or 249 and 200 times the recommended human daily dose). No evidence of teratogenicity was seen in rats given a combination of acrivastine 30 mg/kg/day and pseudoephedrine 150 mg/kg/day (177 and 885 mg/m^2/day or 8 and 5 times the recommended human daily dose respectively). Similarly, no evidence of teratogenicity was observed in rabbits given acrivastine 20 mg/kg/day and pseudoephedrine 100 mg/kg/day (236 and 1180 mg/m^2/day or 10 and 7 times the recommended human daily doses, respectively). There are, however, no adequate and well-controlled studies in pregnant women. Because animal teratology studies are not always predictive of human responses, acrivastine and pseudoephedrine hydrochloride capsules should be used during pregnancy only if the potential benefit justifies the potential risks to the fetus.

Nonteratogenic Effects: In a perinatal-postnatal study in rats, acrivastine given alone at levels up to 500 mg/kg/day (2950 mg/m^2/day or 124 times the recommended human daily dose) was associated with maternal and neonatal morality at the maximum dose level. Neonatal survival was decreased in rats given a combination of acrivastine 20 mg/kg/day and pseudoephedrine 100 mg/kg/day (118 and 590 mg/m^{2}5 and 3 times the human dose, respectively).

NURSING MOTHERS

It is not know whether acrivastine is excreted in human milk. Acrivastine and pseudoephedrine hydrochloride capsules should only be used in nursing mothers when the potential benefit justifies the potential risks to the nursing infant.

PEDIATRIC USE

Safety and effectiveness of acrivastine and pseudoephedrine hydrochloride capsules in children under the age of 12 years have not been established.

DRUG INTERACTIONS:

MAO inhibitors and beta-adrenergic agonists increase the effects of sympathomimetic amines. Concomitant use of sympathomimetic amines with MAO inhibitors can result in a hypertensive crisis (see CONTRAINDICATIONS.) Because MAO inhibitors are long-acting, acrivastine and pseudoephedrine hydrochloride capsules should not be taken with MAO inhibitors or for two weeks after stopping use of a MAO inhibitor.

Because of their pseudoephedrine content, acrivastine and pseudoephedrine hydrochloride capsules may reduce the antihypertensive effects of drugs that interfere with sympathetic activity. Care should be taken in the administration of acrivastine and pseudoephedrine hydrochloride capsules concomitantly with other sympathomimetic amines because the combined effects on the cardiovascular system may be harmful to the patient.

Concomitant administration of acrivastine and pseudoephedrine hydrochloride capsules with alcohol and other CNS depressants may result in additional reductions in alertness and impairment of CNS performance and should be avoided.

No formal drug interaction studies between acrivastine and pseudoephedrine hydrochloride capsules and other possible co-administered drugs have been performed.

ADVERSE REACTIONS:

Information on the incident of adverse events in clinical investigations conducted in the U.S. was obtained from 33 controlled and 15 uncontrolled clinical studies in which 2499 patients received acrivastine and 2631 patients received acrivastine plus pseudoephedrine hydrochloride for treatment periods ranging from one day to one year. The majority of patients in clinical trials were exposed to acrivastine or acrivastine plus pseudoephedrine for less than 90 days. Acrivastine dosages ranged from 3 to 96 mg/day; 1336 patients received dosages equal to or greater than acrivastine 24 mg/day. Acrivastine plus pseudoephedrine hydrochloride dosages ranged from acrivastine 8 to 48 mg/day plus pseudoephedrine hydrochloride 60 to 240 mg/day. A total of 2335 patients received three of four daily doses of acrivastine 8 mg plus pseudoephedrine hydrochloride 60 mg.

In controlled clinical trials, only 12 spontaneously elicited adverse events were reported with frequencies greater than 1% in the acrivastine plus pseudoephedrine hydrochloride treatment group (see TABLE 1.)

The nature and overall frequency of adverse events from international clinical trials (35 studies involving approximately 1600 patients) were similar to the results obtained in the U.S. studies.

Post-marketing clinical experience reports with acrivastine and acrivastine plus pseudoephedrine have included rare serious hypersensitivity reactions manifested by anaphylaxis, angioedema, bronchospasm, and erythema multiforme. No deaths associated with use of acrivastine or acrivastine plus pseudoephedrine have been reported.

Pseudoephedrine may cause ephedrine-like reactions such as tachycardia, palpitations, headache, dizziness, or nausea (see WARNINGS and OVERDOSAGE).

TABLE 1 Adverse Event Reported in Clinical Trials* (Percent of Patients Reporting)†

	Controlled Studies			
	Placebo (N=1767)	Acrivastine (N=1935)	Pseudoephedrine (N=887)	Acrivastine plus Pseudoephedrine (N=1650)
CNS				
Somnolence‡	6	12	8	12
Headache	18	19	19	19
Dizziness	2	3	3	3
Nervousness‡	1	2	4	3
Insomnia‡	1	1	6	4
Miscellaneous				
Nausea	2	3	3	2
Dry Mouth‡	2	3	5	7
Asthenia	2	3	2	2
Dyspepsia	1	1	2	2
Pharyngitis	2	1	1	3
Cough Increase	1	2	1	2
Dysmenorrhea	1	2	3	2

* Includes all events regardless of causal relationship to treatment.
† Includes all adverse events with reported frequency of >1% for the acrivastine plus pseudoephedrine treatment group.
‡ Semprex-D demonstrates a statistically higher frequency of events than placebo, $p \leq 0.05$.

OVERDOSAGE:

There have been no reports of overdosage with acrivastine and pseudoephedrine hydrochloride capsules. In the clinical trial program and in international post-marketing experience, there have been two reported overdoses with acrivastine. Doses were 72 mg and 322 mg. Both patients recovered without sequelae. Adverse events included trembling, stridor loss of consciousness and possible convulsions in the first patient and somnolence in the second.

Since acrivastine and pseudoephedrine have pharmacologically different actions, it is difficult to predict how an individual will respond to overdosage with acrivastine and pseudoephedrine hydrochloride capsules. However, acute overdosage with acrivastine and pseudoephedrine hydrochloride capsules may produce clinical signs of either CNS stimulation or depression. Overdosage of sympathomimetics has been associated with the following events: fear, anxiety, tenseness, restlessness, tremor, weakness, pallor, respiratory difficulty, dysuria, insomnia, hallucinations, convulsions, CNS depression, arrhythmias, and cardiovascular collapse with hypotension. Treatment for overdosage with acrivastine and pseudoephedrine hydrochloride capsules should follow general symptomatic and supportive principles.

In a placebo-controlled, double-blind clinical trial in 18 healthy male subjects, single doses of acrivastine up to 400 mg (50 times the recommended antihistamine dose) produced only a weak vagolytic effect, manifested as an increase in heart rate, and did not cause cardiac repolarization delays (*i.e.,* increased QTc). Daily doses of acrivastine up to 2400 mg (75 times the recommended antihistamine dose) in an uncontrolled study in 38 cancer patients produced a 15 beats per minute increase in mean heart rate and occasional episodes of nausea and vomiting. The effects of acrivastine plus pseudoephedrine at single or multiple doses higher than the recommended daily dose of acrivastine and pseudoephedrine hydrochloride capsules (*i.e.,* 32 mg acrivastine plus 240 mg pseudoephedrine) on heart rate and cardiac repolarization have not been investigated in clinical trials.

The mean LD_{50} (single, oral dose) of acrivastine is greater than 4000 mg/kg (23600 mg/m^2 or 1000 times the recommended human daily dose) in rats and greater than 1200 mg/kg (3600 mg/m^2 or 153 times the recommended human daily dose) in mice. The mean LD_{50} (single, oral dose) of pseudoephedrine hydrochloride is 2206 mg/kg (13015 mg/m^{2}or 73 times the recommended human daily dose in rats 726 mg/kg (2178 mg/m^2 12 times the recommended human daily dose) in mice. The toxic and lethal concentrations of acrivastine and pseudoephedrine in human biologic fluids are not known. Based upon pharmacokinetic screening data from clinical trials, the maximum plasma acrivastine concentration after dosing with acrivastine 8 mg was 393 ng/ml and the maximum plasma pseudoephedrine concentration after dosing with pseudoephedrine hydrochloride 60 mg was 1308 ng/ml.

DOSAGE AND ADMINISTRATION:

The recommended dosage for adults and children 12 years and older is one capsule administered orally, every 4 to 6 hours four times a day.

HOW SUPPLIED:

Semprex-D Capsules (dark green opaque cap and white opaque body with a yellow band) contain acrivastine 8 mg and pseudoephedrine hydrochloride 60 mg. The cap is printed with "Wellcome" and the unicorn logo in white ink, and the body is printed with "Semprex-D" in black ink.

The capsules should be stored at 15° to 25°C (59° to 77°F) in a dry place and protected from light.

For How Supplied Information, Contact Burroughs Wellcome (NDA# NULL)

ACYCLOVIR *(000105)*

CATEGORIES: Anti-Infectives; Antimicrobials; Antivirals; Chickenpox; Dermatologicals; Encephalitis; Fever Blisters; Herpes; Herpes Genitalis; Herpes Simplex; Herpes Simplex Encephalitis; Herpes Zoster; Infections; Lesions; Sexually Transmitted Diseases; Skin/Mucous Membrane Agents; Topical; Varicella; Varicella, Community-Acquired; Varicella Zoster; Viral Agents; Pregnancy Category C; Sales > $1 Billion; FDA Approved 1982 Mar; Patent Expiration 1997 Apr; Top 200 Drugs

BRAND NAMES: *Acic Creme* (Germany); *Acicloftal*; *Aciclor*; *Aciclosina*; *Aclovir*; *Acyclo-V* (Australia); *Acyvir*; *Azovir*; *Cicloferon* (Mexico); *Cicloviral*; *Clinovir*; *Clovix*; *Cusiviral*; *Cyclivex*; *Cyclovir*; *Deherp*; *Eduvir*; *Herpefug* (Germany); *Herpex*; *Herpoviric Rp Creme* (Germany); *Hexidol*; *Inmerax*; *Lisovyr*; *Maynor*; *Norum*; *Oppvir*; *Poviral*; *Quavir*; *Supraviran Creme* (Germany); *Vacrovir*; *Vicorax*; *Virogon*; *Virex*; *Virless*; *Zevin*; *Zoter*; *Zovir*; **Zovirax**; Zovirax Ointment 5%; Zovirax Sterile Powder; *Zyclir* (Australia)
(International brand names outside U.S. in italics)

FORMULARIES: Aetna; BC-BS; DoD; Medi-Cal; PCS

COST OF THERAPY: $129.02 (Herpes Zoster; Tablet; 800 mg; 5/day; 7 days)

DESCRIPTION:

IV Infusion: Zovirax is the brand name for acyclovir, an antiviral drug active against herpesviruses. Zovirax Sterile Powder is a formulation for intravenous administration. Each 5.49 mg of sterile lyophilized acyclovir sodium is equivalent to 5 mg acyclovir.

The chemical name of acyclovir sodium is 9-[(2-hydroxyethoxy)methyl] guanine sodium.

Acyclovir sodium is a white, crystalline powder with a molecular weight of 247 daltons, and a solubility in water exceeding 100 mg/ml. Each 500 mg or 1000 mg vial of acyclovir sterile powder when reconstituted with 10 ml or 20 ml, respectively, sterile diluent yields 50 mg/ml acyclovir (pH approximately 11). Further dilution in any appropriate intravenous solution must be performed before infusion (see Method of Preparation). At physiologic pH, acyclovir exists as the un-ionized form with a molecular weight of 225 daltons and a maximum solubility of 2.5 mg/ml at 37°C.

Oral Forms: Zovirax Capsules, Tablets, and Suspension are formulations for oral administration. Each capsule contains 200 mg of acyclovir and the inactive ingredients corn starch, lactose, magnesium stearate, and sodium lauryl sulfate. The capsule shell consists of gelatin, FD&C Blue No.2, and titanium dioxide. May contain one or more parabens. Printed with edible black ink.

Each 800 mg tablet of Zovirax contains 800 mg of acyclovir and the inactive ingredients FD&C Blue No.2, magnesium stearate, microcrystalline cellulose, povidone, and sodium starch glycolate.

Each 400 mg tablet of Zovirax contains 400 mg of acyclovir and the inactive ingredients magnesium stearate, microcrystalline cellulose, povidone, and sodium starch glycolate.

Each teaspoonful (5 ml) of Zovirax Suspension contains 200 mg of acyclovir and the inactive ingredients methylparaben 0.1% and propylparaben 0.02% (added as a preservative), carbomethylcellulose sodium, flavor, glycerin, microcrystalline cellulose, and sorbitol.

The chemical name of acyclovir sodium is 9-[(2- hydroxyethoxy)methyl]guanine.

Ointment: Zovirax is an antiviral drug effective against herpes viruses. Zovirax Ointment 5% is a formulation for topical administration. Each gram of Zovirax Ointment 5% contains 50 mg of acyclovir in a polyethylene glycol (PEG) base.

The chemical name of acyclovir is 2-amino-1,9-dihydro-9-[(2-hydroxyethoxy)methyl] guanine.

Acyclovir is a white, crystalline powder with a molecular weight of 225 daltons, and a maximum solubility in water of 1.3 mg/ml.

CLINICAL PHARMACOLOGY:

MECHANISM OF ANTIVIRAL EFFECTS

Acyclovir is a synthetic purine nucleoside analogue with *in vitro* and *in vivo* inhibitory activity against human herpes viruses including herpes simplex types 1 (HSV-1) and 2 (HSV-2), varicella-zoster virus (VZV), Epstein-Barr virus (EBV) and cytomegalovirus (CMV). In cell cultures, acyclovir has the highest antiviral activity against HSV-1, followed in decreasing order of potency against HSV-2, VZV, EBV and CMV.[1]

The inhibitory activity of acyclovir for HSV-1, HSV-2, VZV and EBV is highly selective. The enzyme thymidine kinase (TK) of normal uninfected cells does not effectively use acyclovir as a substrate. However, TK encoded by HSV, VZV and EBV[2] converts acyclovir into acyclovir monophosphate, a nucleotide analogue. The monophosphate is further converted into diphosphate by cellular guanylate kinase and into triphosphate by a number of cellular enzymes.[3] Acyclovir triphosphate interferes with Herpes simplex virus DNA polymerase and inhibits viral DNA replication. Acyclovir triphosphate also inhibits cellular α-DNA polymerase but to a lesser degree. *In vitro*, acyclovir triphosphate can be incorporated into growing chains of DNA by viral DNA polymerase and to a much smaller extent by cellular α-DNA polymerase.[4]When incorporation occurs, the DNA chain is terminated.[5,6]Acyclovir is preferentially taken up and selectively converted to the active triphosphate form by herpesvirus-infected cells. Thus, acyclovir is much less toxic *in vitro* for normal uninfected cells because: 1) less is taken up; 2) less is converted to the active form 3) cellular α-DNA polymerase is less sensitive to effects to the active form. The mode of acyclovir phosphorylation in cytomegalovirus-infected cells is not clearly established but may involve virally induced cell kinases or an unidentified viral enzyme. Acyclovir is not efficiently activated in cytomegalovirus infected cells, which may account for the reduced susceptibility of cytomegalovirus to acyclovir *in vitro*.

MICROBIOLOGY

The quantitative relationship between the *in vitro* susceptibility of herpes simplex virus to acyclovir and the clinical response to therapy has not been established in man, and virus sensitivity testing has not been standardized. Sensitivity testing results, expressed as the concentration of drug required to inhibit by 50% the growth of virus in cell culture (ID_{50}), vary greatly depending upon the particular assay used,[7]the cell type employed,[8] and the laboratory performing the test.[1] The ID_{50} of acyclovir against HSV-1 isolates may range from 0.02 mcg/ml (plaque reduction in Vero cells) to 5.9-13.5 mcg/ml (plaque reduction in green monkey kidney (GMK) cells).[1] The ID_{50} against HSV-2 ranges from 0.01 mcg/ml to 9.9 mcg/ml (plaque reduction in Vero and GMK cells, respectively).[1]

Using a dye-uptake method in Vero cells,[9]which gives ID_{50} values approximately 5- to 10-fold higher than plaque reduction assays, 1417 isolates (553 HSV-1 AND 864 HSV-2) from approximately 500 patients were examined over a 5-year period.[10]. These assays found that 90% of HSV-1 isolates were sensitive to ≤0.9 mcg/ml acyclovir and 50% of all isolates were sensitive ot ≤0.2 mcg/ml acyclovir. For HSV-2 isolates, 90% were sensitive to ≤2.2 mcg/ml and 50% of all isolates were sensitive to ≤0.7 mcg/ml of acyclovir. Isolates with significantly diminished sensitivity were found in 44 patients. It must be emphasized that neither the patients nor the isolates were randomly selected and, therefore, do not represent the general population.

Most of the less sensitive HSV clinical isolates have been relatively deficient in the viral TK.[11-19] Strains with alterations in viral TK[20] or viral DNA polymerase[21] have also been reported. Prolonged exposure to low concentrations (0.1 mcg/ml) of acyclovir in cell culture has resulted in the emergence of a variety of acyclovir-resistant strains.[22]

The ID_{50} against VZV ranges from 0.17-1.53 mcg/ml (yield reduction, human foreskin fibroblasts) to 1.85-3.98 mcg/ml [foci reduction, human embryo fibroblasts (HEF)]. Reproduction of EBV genome is suppressed by 50% in superinfected Raji cells or P3HR-1 lymphoblastoid cells by 1.5 mcg/ml acyclovir. CMV is relatively resistant to acyclovir with ID_{50}values ranging from 2.3-17.6 mcg/ml (plaque reduction, HEF cells) to 1.82-56.8 mcg/ml (DNA hybridization, HEF cells). The latent state of the genome of any of the human herpesviruses is not known to be sensitive to acyclovir.[1]

PHARMACOKINETICS

IV Injection: The pharmacokinetics of acyclovir has been evaluated in 95 patients (9 studies). Results were obtained in adult patients with normal renal function during Phase I/II studies after single doses ranging from 0.5 to 15 mg/kg and after multiple doses ranging from 2.5 to 15 mg/kg every 8 hours. Pharmacokinetics was also determined in pediatric patients with normal renal function ranging in age from 1 to 17 years at doses of 250 mg/m^2 or 500 mg/m^{2}every 8 hours. In these studies, dose-independent pharmacokinetics is observed in the range of 0.5 to 15 mg/kg. Proportionality between dose and plasma levels is seen after single doses or at steady state after multiple dosing.[23] When acyclovir was administered to adults at 5 mg/kg (approximately 250 mg/m^2) by 1-hr infusions every 8 hours, mean steady-state peak and trough concentrations of 9.8 mcg/ml (5.5 to 13.8 mcg/ml) and 0.7 mcg/ml (0.2 to 1.0 mcg/ml), respectively, were achieved. Similar concentrations are achieved in children over 1 year of age when doses of 250 mg/m^2 are given by 1-hr infusions every 8 hours. At a dose of 10 mg/kg given by 1-hr infusion every 8 hours, mean steady-state peak and trough concentrations were 22.9 μ/ml (14.1 to 44.1μ /ml) and 1.9 mcg/ml (0.5 to 2.9 μ/ml). Similar concentrations were achieved in children dosed at 500 mg/m^2 given by 1-hr infusion every 8 hours. Concentrations achieved in the cerebrospinal fluid are approximately 50% of plasma values. Plasma protein binding is relatively low (9% to 33%) and drug interactions involving binding site displacement are not anticipated.[23]

Renal excretion of unchanged drug by glomerular filtration and tubular secretion is the major route of acyclovir elimination accounting for 62 to 91% of the dose as determined by ^{14}C-labelled drug. The only major urinary metabolite detected in 9-carboxymethoxymethylguanine. This may account for up to 14.1% of the dose in patients with normal renal function. An insignificant amount of drug is recovered in feces and expired CO^2 and there is no evidence to suggest tissue retention.[23] However, postmortem examinations have shown that acyclovir is widely distributed in tissues and body fluids including brain, kidney, lung, liver, muscle, spleen, uterus, vaginal mucosa, vaginal secretions, cerebrospinal fluid and herpetic vesicular fluid.

The half-life and total body clearance of acyclovir is dependent on renal function as shown below (TABLE 1):[23]

TABLE 1 Half-Life

Creatinine Clearance (ml/min/1.73m^2)	Half-Life (hr)	Total Body Clearance (ml/min/1.73m^2)
>80	2.5	327
50-80	3.0	248
15-50	3.5	190
0 (Anuric)	19.5	29

Acyclovir was administered at a dose of 2.5 mg/kg to 6 adult patients with severe renal failure. The peak and trough plasma levels during the 47 hours preceding hemodialysis were 8.5 mcg/ml and 0.7 mcg/ml, respectively.[24,25]

Consult DOSAGE AND ADMINISTRATION section for recommended adjustment in dosing based upon creatinine clearance. The half-life and total body clearance of acyclovir in pediatric patients over 1 year of age is similar to those in adults with normal renal function (see DOSAGE AND ADMINISTRATION).

Oral Forms: The pharmacokinetics of acyclovir after oral administration have been evaluated in 6 clinical studies involving 110 adult patients. In one uncontrolled study of 35 immunosuppressed patients with herpes simplex or varicella-zoster infection, acyclovir capsules were administered in doses of 200 to 1000 mg every 4 hours, 6 times daily for 5 days, and steady-state plasma levels were reached by the second day of dosing. Mean steady-state peak and trough concentrations following the final 200 mg dose were 0.49 mcg/ml (0.47 to 0.54 mcg/ml) and 0.31 mcg/ml (0.18 to 0.41 mcg/ml) respectively, and following the final 800 mg dose were 2.8 mcg/ml (2.3 to 3.1 mcg/ml) and 1.8 mcg/ml (1.3 to 2.5 mcg/ml), respectively. In another uncontrolled study of 20 younger immunocompetent patients with recurring genital herpes simplex infections, acyclovir capsules were administered in doses of 800 mg every 6 hours, 4 times daily for 5 days; the mean steady-state peak and trough complications were 1.4 mcg/ml (0.66 to 1.8 mcg/ml) and 0.55 mcg/ml (0.14 to 1.1 mcg/ml), respectively.

In general, the pharmacokinetics of acyclovir in children is similar to adults. Mean half-life after oral doses of 300 mg/m^{2}and 600 mg/m^2, in children ages 7 months to 7 years, was 2.6 hours. (range 1.59 to 3.74 hours).

A single oral dose bioavailability study in 23 normal volunteers showed that acyclovir capsules 200 mg are bioequivalent to 200 mg acyclovir in aqueous solution; and in a separate study in 20 volunteers, it was shown that acyclovir suspension is bioequivalent to acyclovir capsules. In a different single-dose bioavailability/bioequivalence study in 24 volunteers, one acyclovir 800 mg tablet was demonstrated to be bioequivalent to four Zovirax 200 mg capsules.

In a multiple-dose crossover study where 23 volunteers received acyclovir as one 200 mg capsule, one 400 mg tablet, and one 800 mg tablet 6 times daily, absorption decreased with increasing dose and the estimated bioavailabilities of acyclovir were 20%, 15%, and 10%, respectively. The decrease in bioavailability is believed to be a function of the dose and not the dosage farm. It was demonstrated that acyclovir is not proportional over the dosing range 200 mg to 800 mg. In this study, steady-state peak and trough concentrations of acyclovir were 0.83 and 0.46 mcg/ml, 1.21 and 0.63 mcg/ml, and 1.61 and 0.83 mcg/ml for the 200, 400, and 800 mg dosing regimens, respectively. In another study in 6 volunteers, the influence of food on the absorption of acyclovir was not apparent.

Following oral administration, the mean plasma half-life of acyclovir in volunteers and patients with normal renal function ranged from 2.5 to 3.3 hours. The mean renal excretion of unchanged drug accounts for 14.4% (8.6% to 19.8%) of the orally administered dose. The only urinary metabolite (identified by high performance liquid chromatography) is 9- [(carboxymethoxy)methyl]guanine. The half-life and total body clearance of acyclovir are dependent on renal function. A dosage adjustment is recommended for patients with reduced renal function (see DOSAGE AND ADMINISTRATION).

Orally administered acyclovir in children less than 2 years of age has not yet been fully studied.

OINTMENT

Acyclovir is a synthetic acyclic purine nucleoside analogue with *in vitro* inhibitory activity against Herpes simplex types 1 and 2 (HSV-1 and HSV-2), varicella-zoster, Epstein-Barr and cytomegalovirus. In cell cultures, the inhibitory activity of acyclovir for Herpes simplex virus is highly selective. Cellular thymidine kinase does not effectively utilize acyclovir as a substrate. Herpes simplex virus-coded thymidine kinase, however, converts acyclovir into acyclovir monophosphate, a nucleotide. The monophosphate is further converted into diphosphate by cellular guanylate kinase and into triphosphate by a number of cellular enzymes. Acyclovir triphosphate interferes with Herpes simplex virus DNA polymerase and inhibits viral DNA replication. Acyclovir triphosphate also inhibits cellular α-DNA polymerase but to a lesser degree. *In vitro*, acyclovir triphosphate can be incorporated into growing chains of DNA by viral DNA polymerase and to a much smaller extent by cellular α-DNA polymerase. When incorporation occurs, the DNA chain is terminated. Acyclovir is preferentially taken up and selectively converted to the active triphosphate form by herpesvirus-infected cells. Thus, acyclovir is much less toxic *in vitro* for normal uninfected cells because: 1) less is taken up; 2) less is converted to the active form; 3) cellular α-DNA polymerase is less sensitive to the effects of the active form.

The relationship between *in vitro* susceptibility of Herpes simplex virus to antiviral drugs and clinical response has not been established. The techniques and cell culture types used for determining *in vitro* susceptibility may influence the results obtained. Using a quantitative assay to determine the acyclovir concentration producing 50% inhibition of viral cytopathic effect (ID_{50}), 28 HSV-1 clinical isolates has a mean ID_{50} of 0.17 mcg/ml and 32 HSV-2 clinical isolates had a mean $ID_{50}$of 0.46 mcg/ml. Results from other studies using different assays have yielded mean ID_{50} values for clinical HSV-1 isolates of 0.018, 0.03 and 0.043 mcg/ml and for clinical HSV-2 isolates of 0.0027, 0.36 and 0.03 mcg/ml, respectively.

CLINICAL PHARMACOLOGY: *(cont'd)*

Two clinical pharmacology studies were performed with acyclovir ointment 5% in adult immunocompromised patients, at risk of developing mucocutaneous Herpes simplex virus infections or with localized varicella-zoster infections. These studies were designed to evaluate the dermal tolerance, systemic toxicity and percutaneous absorption of acyclovir.

In one of these studies, which included 16 inpatients, the complete ointment or its vehicle were randomly administered in a dose of 1 cm strips (25 mg acyclovir) four times a day for seven days to an intact skin surface area of 4.5 square inches. No local intolerance, systemic toxicity or contact dermatitis were observed. In addition, no drug was detected in blood and urine by radioimmunoassay (sensitivity, 0.01 mcg/ml).

The other study included eleven patients with localized varicella-zoster. In this uncontrolled study, acyclovir was detected in the blood of 9 patients and in the urine of all patients tested. Acyclovir levels in plasma ranged from <0.01 to 0.28 mcg/ml in eight patients with normal renal function, and from <0.01 to 0.78 mcg/ml in one patient with impaired renal function. Acyclovir excreted in the urine ranged <0.02 to 9.4 percent of the daily dose. Therefore systemic absorption of acyclovir after topical application is minimal.

INDICATIONS AND USAGE:

IV INFUSION

Acyclovir sterile powder is indicated for the treatment of initial and recurrent mucosal and cutaneous Herpes simplex (HSV-1 and HSV-2) and varicella-zoster (shingles) infections in immunocompromised patients. It is also indicated for herpes simplex encephalitis in patients over 6 months of age and for severe initial clinical episodes of herpes genitalis in patients who are not immunocompromised.

Herpes Simplex Infections in Immunocompromised Patients: A multicenter trial of acyclovir sterile powder at a dose of 250 mg/m^2 every 8 hours (750 mg/m^2/day) for 7 days was conducted in 98 immunocompromised patients (73 adults and 25 children) with oro-facial, esophageal, genital and other localized infections (52 treated with acyclovir and 46 with placebo). Acyclovir significantly decreased virus excretion, reduced pain, and promoted scabbing and rapid healing of lesions.[14,26,27,28]

Initial Episodes of Herpes Genitalis: In placebo-controlled trials, 58 patients with initial genital herpes were treated with intravenous acyclovir 5 mg/kg or placebo (27 patients treated with acyclovir and 31 treated with placebo) every eight hours for 5 days. Acyclovir decreased the duration of viral excretion, new lesion formation, and duration of vesicles and promoted healing of lesions.[28,29,30]

Herpes Simplex Encephalitis: Sixty-two patients ages 6 months to 79 years with brain biopsy-proven herpes simplex encephalitis were randomized to receive either acyclovir (30 mg/kg/day) or adenine arabinoside (Vira-A) (15 mg/kg/day) for 10 days (28 were treated with acyclovir and 34 with Vira-A).[31] Overall mortality for acyclovir recipients at 6 months was 18% compared to 59% for Vira-A treated patients (p = 0.003). The proportion of acyclovir recipients functioning normally or with only mild sequelae (*e.g.,* decreased attention span) was 39% compared to 9% of Vira-A treated patients (p = 0.01). The remaining patients in both groups had moderate (*e.g.,* hemiparesis, speech impediment or seizure) or severe (continuous supportive care required) neurologic sequelae.

After 12 months of follow-up, two additional acyclovir recipients had died, resulting in an overall mortality of 25% compared to 59% for Vira-A treated patients (p = 0.02). Morbidity assessments at that time indicated that 32% of acyclovir recipients were functioning normally, or with only mild sequelae compared to 12% Vira-A patients (p = 0.06). Moderate to severe impairment was noted in all remaining patients in both groups who were available for evaluation. Patients less than 30 years of age and those who had the least severe neurologic involvement at time of entry into study had the best outcome with acyclovir treatment. An additional controlled study performed in Europe[32] demonstrated similar findings. The superiority of acyclovir over Vira-A for neonatal herpes encephalitis has not been demonstrated.

Varicella-Zoster Infections in Immunocompromised Patients: A multicenter trial of acyclovir sterile powder at a dose of 500 mg/m^2 every 8 hours for 7 days was conducted in immunocompromised patients with zoster infections (shingles). Ninety-four (94) patients were evaluated (52 patients were treated with acyclovir and 42 with placebo). Acyclovir halted progression of infection as determined by significant reductions in cutaneous dissemination, visceral dissemination, or the proportion of patients deemed treatment failures.[28,33]

A comparative trial of acyclovir and vidarabine was conducted in 22 severely immunocompromised patients with zoster infections. Acyclovir was shown to be superior to vidarabine as demonstrated by significant differences in the time of new lesion formation, the time to pain reduction, the time lesion crusting, the time to complete healing, the incidence of fever and the duration of positive viral cultures. In addition, cutaneous dissemination occurred in none of the 10 acyclovir recipients compared to 5 to the 10 vidarabine recipients who presented with localized dermatomal disease.[34]

Diagnosis: Diagnosis is confirmed by virus isolation. Accelerated viral culture assays or immunocytology allow more rapid diagnosis than standard viral culture. In initial episodes of genital herpes, appropriate examinations should be performed to rule out other sexually transmitted diseases. Whereas cutaneous lesions associated with Herpes simplex and varicella-zoster infections are often characteristic, the finding of multinucleated giant cells in smears prepared from lesion exudate or scrapings may assist in the diagnosis.[35]

The Tzanck smear does not distinguish varicella-zoster from herpes simplex infections. Culture of varicella-zoster is not widely available.

Herpes encephalitis should be confirmed by brain biopsy to obtain tissue examination and viral culture and to exclude other causes of neurologic disease. A presumptive diagnosis of herpes encephalitis may be made on the basis of focal changes in the temporal lobe visualized with various diagnostic methods including magnetic resonance imaging, computerized tomography, radionuclide scans or electroencephalography. Culture of the cerebrospinal fluid for herpes simplex virus is unreliable.

ORAL FORMS

Acyclovir capsules and suspension are indicated for the treatment of initial episodes and the management of recurrent episodes of genital herpes in certain patients.

Acyclovir capsules, tablets, and suspension are indicated for the acute treatment of herpes zoster (shingles) and chickenpox (varicella).

Genital Herpes Infections: The severity of disease is variable depending upon the immune status of the patient, the frequency and duration of episodes, and the degree of cutaneous or systemic involvement. These factors should determine patient management, which may include symptomatic support and counseling only, or the institution of specific therapy. The physical, emotional and psycho-social difficulties posed by herpes infections as well as the degree of debilitation, particularly in immunocompromised patients, are unique for each patient, and the physician should determine therapeutic alternatives based on his or her understanding of the individuals patient's needs. Thus orally administered acyclovir is not appropriate in treating all genital herpes infections. The following guidelines may be useful in weighing the benefit/risk considerations in specific disease categories:

First Episodes (primary and nonprimary infections—commonly known as initial genital herpes): Double-blind, placebo-controlled studies have demonstrated that orally administered acyclovir significantly reduced the duration of acute infection (detection of virus in lesions by tissue culture) and lesion healing. The duration of pain and new lesion formation was decreased in

INDICATIONS AND USAGE: *(cont'd)*

some patient groups. The promptness of initiation of therapy and/or the patient's prior exposure to herpes simplex virus may influence the degree of benefit from therapy. Patients with mild disease may derive less benefit than those with more severe episodes. In patients with extremely severe episodes, in which prostration, central nervous system involvement, urinary retention or inability to take oral medication require hospitalization and more aggressive management, therapy may be best initiated with intravenous acyclovir.

Recurrent Episodes: Double-blind, placebo-controlled studies in patients with frequent recurrences (6 or more episodes per year) have shown that orally administered acyclovir given daily for 4 months to 3 years prevented or reduced the frequency and/or severity of recurrences in greater than 95% of patients.

In a study of 283 patients who received 400 mg (two 200mg capsules) twice daily for three years, 45%, 52% and 63% of patients remained free of recurrences in the first, second and third years, respectively. Serial analyses of the 3 month recurrence rates for the 283 patients showed that 71% to 87% were recurrence-free in each quarter, indicating that the effects are constant over time.

The frequency and severity of episodes of untreated genital herpes may change over time. After 1 year of therapy, the frequency and severity of the patient's genital herpes infection should be re-evaluated to assess the need for continuation of acyclovir therapy. Re-evaluation will usually require a trial off acyclovir to assess the need for reinstitution of suppressive therapy. Some patients, such as those with very frequent or severe episodes before treatment, may warrant uninterrupted suppression for more than a year.

Chronic suppressive therapy is most appropriate when, in the judgment of the physician, the benefits of such a regimen outweigh known or potential adverse effects. In general, orally administered acyclovir should not be used for the suppression of recurrent disease in mildly affected patients. Unanswered questions concerning the relevance to humans of *in vitro* mutagenicity studies and reproductive toxicity studies and reproductive toxicity studies in animals given high parenteral doses of acyclovir for short periods (See PRECAUTIONS, Carcinogenesis, Mutagenesis, and Impairment of Fertility) should be borne in mind when designing long-term management for individual patients. Discussion of these issues with patients will provide them the opportunity to weigh the potential for toxicity against the severity of their disease. Thus, this regimen should be considered only for appropriate patients with annual re-evaluation.

Limited studies have shown that there are certain patients for whom intermittent short-term treatment of recurrent episodes is effective. This approach may be more appropriate than a suppressive regimen in patients with infrequent recurrences.

Immunocompromised patients with recurrent herpes infection can be treated with either intermittent or chronic suppressive therapy. Clinically significant resistance, although rare, is more likely to be seen with prolonged or repeated therapy in severely immunocompromised patients with active lesions.

Herpes Zoster Infections: In a double-blind, placebo-controlled study of 187 normal patients with localized cutaneous zoster infection (93 randomized to acyclovir and 94 to placebo), acyclovir (800 mg 5 times daily for 10 days) shortened the times to lesion scabbing, healing and complete cessation of pain, and reduced the duration or viral shedding and the duration of new lesion formation.

In a similar double-blind, placebo-controlled study in 83 normal patients with herpes zoster (40 randomized to acyclovir and 43 to placebo), acyclovir (800 mg 5 times daily for 7 days) shortened the times to complete lesion scabbing, healing and cessation of pain, reduced the duration of new lesion formulation, and reduced the prevalence of localized zoster-associated neurologic symptoms (paresthesia, dysesthesia, or hyperesthesia).

Chickenpox: In a double blind-placebo-controlled efficacy study in 110 normal patients, ages 5 to 16 years, who presented **within 24 hours**of the onset of a typical chickenpox rash, acyclovir was administered orally 4 times daily for 5 to 7 days at doses of 10, 15, or 20 mg/kg depending on the age group. Acyclovir treatment reduced the maximum number of lesions (336 vs. greater than 500; lesions beyond 500 were not counted). Acyclovir treatment also shortened the mean time to 50% healing (7.1 days vs. 8.7 days), reduced the number of vesicular lesions by the second day of treatment (49 vs. 113), and decreased the proportion of patients with fever (temperature greater than 100°F) by the second day (19% vs. 57%). Acyclovir treatment did not effect the antibody response to varicella-zoster virus measured one month and one year following treatment.

In two concurrent double-blind, placebo-controlled studies, a total of 883 normal patients, ages 2 to 18 years were enrolled **within 24 hours** of the onset of a typical chickenpox rash, and acyclovir was administered at 20 mg/kg orally up to 800 mg 4 times daily for 5 days. In the larger study of 815 children ages 2 to 12 years, acyclovir treatment reduced the median maximum number of lesions (277 vs. 386), reduced the median number of vesicular lesions by the second day of treatment (26 vs. 40), and reduced the proportion of patients with moderate to severe itching by the third day of treatment (15% vs. 34%). In addition, in both studies (883 patients ages 2 to 18 years), acyclovir treatment also decreased the proportion of patients with fever (temperature greater than 100°F), anorexia, and lethargy by the second day of treatment, and decreased the mean number of residual lesions on Day 28. There were no substantial differences in VZV-specific humoral or cellular immune responses measured at one month following treatment in patients receiving acyclovir compared to patients receiving placebo.

Diagnosis: Diagnosis is confirmed by virus isolation. Accelerated viral culture assays or immunocytology allow more rapid diagnosis than standard viral culture. For patients with initial episodes of genital herpes, appropriate examinations should be performed to rule-out other sexually transmitted diseases. While cutaneous lesions associated with herpes simplex and varicella-zoster infections are often characteristic, the finding of multinucleated giant cells in smears prepared from lesion exudate or scrapings may provide additional support to the clinical diagnosis.

Multinucleated giant cells in smears do not distinguish varicella-zoster from herpes simplex infections.

OINTMENT

Acyclovir ointment 5% is indicated in the management of initial herpes genitalis and in limited non-life threatening mucocutaneous Herpes simplex virus infections in immunocompromised patients. In clinical trials of initial herpes genitalis. Acyclovir Ointment 5% has shown a decrease in healing time and in some cases a decrease in duration of viral shedding and duration of pain. In studies in immunocompromised patients with mainly herpes labialis, there was a decrease in duration of viral shedding and a slight decrease in duration of pain.

By contrast, in studies of recurrent herpes genitalis and of herpes labialis in nonimmunocompromised patients, there was no evidence of clinical benefit, there was some decrease in duration of viral shedding and a slight decrease in the duration of pain.

Diagnosis: Whereas cutaneous lesions associated with Herpes simplex infections are often characteristic, the finding of multinucleated giant cells in smears prepared from lesion exudate or scrapings may assist in the diagnosis. Positive cultures for herpes simplex virus offer a reliable means for confirmations of the diagnosis. In genital herpes, appropriate examinations should be performed to rule out other sexually transmitted diseases.

CONTRAINDICATIONS:

Acyclovir is contraindicated for patients who develop hypersensitivity or chemical intolerance to the drug or components of the formulation.

WARNINGS:

IV Infusion: Acyclovir sterile powder is intended for intravenous infusion only, and should not be administered topically, intramuscularly, orally, subcutaneously, or in the eye. Intravenous infusions must be given over a period of at least 1 (one) hour to reduce the risk of renal tubular damage (see PRECAUTIONS and DOSAGE AND ADMINISTRATION).

Oral Forms: Acyclovir capsules, tablets, and suspension are for oral ingestion only.

Ointment: Acyclovir ointment is intended for cutaneous use only and should not be used in the eye.

PRECAUTIONS:

GENERAL

IV Infusion: The recommended dosage, frequency of applications, and length of treatment should not be exceeded (see DOSAGE AND ADMINISTRATION).

Although the aqueous solubility of acyclovir sodium (for infusion) is >100 mg/ml, precipitation of acyclovir crystals in renal tubules can occur if the maximum solubility of free acyclovir (2.5 mg/ml at 37°C in water) is exceeded or if the drug is administered by bolus injection. This complication causes a rise in serum creatinine and blood urea nitrogen (BUN), and a decrease in renal creatinine clearance. Ensuing renal tubular damage can produce acute renal failure.

Abnormal renal function (decreased creatinine clearance) can occur as a result of acyclovir administration and depends on the state of the patients' hydration, other treatments, and the rate of drug administration. Bolus administration of the drug leads to a 10% incidence of renal dysfunction, while in controlled studies, infusion of 5 mg/kg (250/m^2) and 10 mg/kg (500 mg/m^2) over an hour was associated with a lower frequency—3.8%. Concomitant use of other nephrotoxic drugs, pre-existing renal disease, and dehydration make further renal impairment with acyclovir more likely. In most instances, alterations of renal function were transient and resolved spontaneously or with improvement of water and electrolyte balance, drug dosage adjustment or discontinuation of drug administration. However, in some instances, these changes may progress to acute renal failure.

Administration of acyclovir by intravenous infusion must be accompanied by adequate hydration. Since maximum urine concentration occurs within the first 2 hours following infusion, particular attention should be given to establishing sufficient urine flow during that period in order to prevent precipitation in renal tubules. Recommended urine output is ≥ 500 ml per gram of drug infused. In patients with encephalitis, the recommended hydration should be balanced by the risk of cerebral edema.

When dosage adjustment are required they should be based on estimated creatinine clearance (see DOSAGE AND ADMINISTRATION).

Approximately 1% of patients receiving intravenous acyclovir have manifested encephalopathic changes characterized by either lethargy, obtundation, tremors, confusion, hallucinations, agitation, seizures or coma. Acyclovir should be used with caution in those patients who have underlying neurologic abnormalities and those with serious renal, hepatic, or electrolyte abnormalities or significant hypoxia. It should also be used with caution in patients who have manifested prior neurologic reactions to cytotoxic drugs or those receiving concomitant intrathecal methotrexate or interferon.

Exposure of HSV isolates to acyclovir *in vitro* can lead to the emergence of less sensitive viruses. These viruses usually are deficient in thymidine kinase (required for acyclovir activation) and are less pathogenic in animals. Similar isolates have been observed in severely immunocompromised patients during the course of controlled and uncontrolled studies of intravenously administered acyclovir. These occurred in patients with severe combined immunodeficiencies or following bone marrow transplantation. The presence of these viruses was not associated with a worsening of clinical illness and, in some instances, the virus disappeared spontaneously. The possibility of the appearance of less sensitive viruses must be recognized when treating such patients.[11-19] The relationship between the *in vitro* sensitivity of herpes simplex or varicella-zoster virus to acyclovir and clinical response to therapy has not been established.

Oral Forms: Acyclovir has caused decreased spermatogenesis at high parenteral doses in some animals and mutagenesis in some acute studies of this drug at high concentrations of drug (see PRECAUTIONS, Carcinogenesis, Mutagenesis, and Impairment of Fertility). The recommended dosage should not be exceeded (see DOSAGE AND ADMINISTRATION).

Exposure of herpes simplex and varicella-zoster isolates to acyclovir *in vitro* can lead to the emergence of less sensitive viruses. The possibility of the appearance of less sensitive viruses in humans must be borne in mind when treating patients. The relationship between the *in vitro* sensitivity of herpes simplex or varicella-zoster virus to acyclovir clinical response to therapy has yet to be established (see CLINICAL PHARMACOLOGY, Microbiology).

Because of the possibility that less sensitive virus may be selected in patients who are receiving acyclovir, all patients should be advised to take particular care to avoid potential transmission virus if active lesions are present while they are on therapy. In severely immunocompromised patients, the physician should be aware that prolonged or repeated courses of acyclovir may result in selection of resistant viruses which may not fully respond to continued acyclovir therapy.

Caution should be exercised when administering acyclovir to patients receiving potentially nephrotoxic agents since this may increase the risk of renal dysfunction.

Ointment: The recommended dosage, frequency of applications, and length of treatment should not be exceeded (see DOSAGE AND ADMINISTRATION). There exist no data which demonstrate that the use of acyclovir ointment 5% will either prevent transmission of infection to other persons or prevent recurrent infections when applied in the absence of signs and symptoms. Acyclovir ointment 5% should not be used for the prevention of recurrent HSV infections. Although clinically significant viral resistance associated with the use of acyclovir ointment 5% has not been observed, this possibility exists.

INFORMATION FOR THE PATIENT

Oral Forms: Patients are instructed to consult with their physician if they experience severe or troublesome adverse reactions, they become pregnant or intend to become pregnant, they intend to breast feed while taking orally administered acyclovir, or they have any other questions.

GENITAL HERPES INFECTIONS

Oral Forms: Genital herpes is a sexually transmitted disease and patients should avoid intercourse when visible lesions are present because of the risk of infecting intimate partners. Acyclovir capsules, tablets and suspension are for oral ingestion only. Medication should not be shared with others. The prescribed dosage should not be exceeded. Acyclovir does not eliminate latent viruses. Patients are instructed to consult with their physician if they do not receive sufficient relief in the frequency and severity of their genital herpes recurrences.

There are still unanswered questions concerning reproductive/gonadal toxicity and mutagenesis; long term studies are continuing. decreased sperm production has been seen at high doses in some animals; a placebo-controlled clinical study using 400 mg or 1000 mg of acyclovir per day for 6 months in humans did not show similar findings. Chromosomal breaks were

PRECAUTIONS: *(cont'd)*

seen *in vitro* after brief exposure to high concentrations. Some other currently marketed medications also cause chromosomal breaks, and the significance of this finding is unknown. A placebo-controlled clinical study using 800 mg of acyclovir per day for 1 year in humans did not show any abnormalities in structure or number of chromosomes.

HERPES ZOSTER INFECTIONS

Oral Forms: Adults age 50 or older tend to have more severe shingles, and treatment with acyclovir showed more significant benefit for older patients. Treatment was begun within 72 hours of rash onset in these studies, and was more useful if started within the first 48 hours.

CHICKENPOX

Oral Forms: Although chickenpox in otherwise healthy children is usually a self-limited disease of mild to moderate severity, adolescents and adults tend to have more severe disease. Treatment was initiated within 24 hours of the typical chickenpox rash in the controlled studies, and there is no information regarding the effects of treatment begun later in the disease course. It is unknown whether the treatment of chickenpox in childhood has any effect on long-term immunity. However, there is no evidence to indicate that acyclovir treatment on chickenpox would have any effect on either decreasing or increasing the incidence or severity of subsequent recurrences of herpes zoster (shingles) later in life. Intravenous acyclovir is indicated for the treatment of varicella-zoster infections in immunocompromised patients.

CARCINOGENESIS, MUTAGENESIS, AND IMPAIRMENT OF FERTILITY

IV Infusion and Oral Forms: The data presented below include references to peak steady state plasma acyclovir concentrations observed in humans treated with 800 mg given orally 6 times a day (dosing appropriate for treatment of herpes zoster or herpes encephalitis), or 200 mg given orally 6 times a day (dosing appropriate for treatment of primary genital herpes or herpes simplex infections in immunocompromised patients). Plasma drug concentrations in animal studies are expressed as multiples of human exposure to acyclovir at the higher and lower dosing schedules (see CLINICAL PHARMACOLOGY, Pharmacokinetics).

Acyclovir was tested in lifetime bioassays in rats and mice at single daily doses of up to 450 mg/kg administered by gavage. There was no statistically significant difference in the incidence of tumors between treated and control animals, nor did acyclovir shorten the latency of tumors. At 450 mg/kg/day, plasma concentrations in both the mouse and rat bioassay were lower than concentrations in humans.

Acyclovir was tested in two *in vitro* cell transformation assays. Positive results were observed at the highest concentration tested (31 to 63 times human levels) in one system and the resulting morphologically transformed cells formed tumors when inoculated into immunosuppressed, syngeneic, weanling mice. Acyclovir was negative (40 to 80 times human levels) in the other, possibly less sensitive, transformation assay.

In acute cytogenetic studies, there was an increase, though not statistically significant, in the incidence of chromosomal damage of maximum tolerated parenteral doses of acyclovir (100 mg/kg) in rats (62 to 125 times human levels) but not in Chinese hamster; higher doses of 500 and 1000 mg/kg were clastogenic in Chinese hamsters (380 to 760 times human levels). In addition, to activity was found after 5 days dosing in a dominant lethal study in mice (36 to 73 times human levels). In all 4 microbial assays, no evidence of mutagenicity was observed. Positive results were obtained in 2 of 7 genetic toxicity assays using mammalian cells *in vitro*. In human lymphocytes, a positive response for chromosomal damage was seen at concentrations 150 to 300 times the acyclovir plasma levels achieved in man. At one locus in mouse lymphoma cells, mutagenicity was observed at concentrations 250 to 500 times human plasma levels. Results in the other five mammalian cell loci follow: at 3 loci in a Chinese hamster ovary cell line, the results were inconclusive at concentrations at least 1850 times human levels; at 2 other loci in mouse lymphoma cells, no evidence of mutagenicity was observed at concentrations at least 1500 times human levels.

Acyclovir has not been shown to impair fertility or reproduction in mice (450 mg/kg/day, p.o.) or in rats (25 mg/kg/day, SC). In the mouse study plasma levels were 9 to 18 times human levels, while in the rat study they were 8 to 15 times human levels. At 50 mg/kg/day, SC in the rat (1 to 2 times human levels), there was a statistically significant increase in post-implantation loss, but no concomitant decrease in littler size. In female rabbits treated subcutaneously with acyclovir subsequent to mating, there was a statistically significant decrease in implantation efficiency but no concomitant decrease in litter size at a dose of 50 mg/kg/day (1 to 3 times human levels). No effect upon implantation efficiency was observed when the same dose was administered intravenously (4 to 9 times human levels). In a rat peri- and postnatal study at 50 mg/kg/day, SC (1 to 2 times human levels), there was a statistically significant decrease in the group mean numbers of corpora lutea, total implantation sites and live fetuses in the F^1 generation. Although not statistically significant, there was also a dose-related decrease in group mean numbers of live fetuses and implantation sites at 12.5 mg/kg/day and 25 mg/kg/day, SC. The intravenous administration of 100 mg/kg/day, a dose known to cause obstructive nephropathy in rabbits, caused a significant increase in fetal resorptions and a corresponding decrease in litter size (plasma levels were not measured). However, at a maximum tolerated intravenous dose of 50 mg/kg/day in rabbits (4 to 9 times human levels), no drug-related reproductive effects were observed.

Intraperitoneal doses of 80 or 320 mg/kg/day acyclovir given to rats for 6 and 1 months, respectively, caused testicular atrophy. Plasma levels were not measured in the one-month study and were 2 to 4 times human levels in the six-month study. Testicular atrophy was persistent through the 4-week postdose recovery phase after 320 mg/kg/day; some evidence of recovery of sperm production was evident 30 days postdose. Intravenous dose of 100 and 200 mg/kg/day acyclovir given to dogs for 31 days caused aspermatogenesis. At 100 mg/kg/day plasma levels were 4 to 8 times human levels, while at 200 mg/kg/day they were 13 to 25 times human levels. No testicular abnormalities were seen in dogs given 50 mg/kg/day IV for one month (2 to 3 times human levels) and in dogs given 60 mg/kg/day orally for one year (the same as human levels).

Ointment: Acyclovir was tested in lifetime bioassays in rats and mice at single daily doses of 50, 150 and 450 mg/kg/day given by gavage. These studies showed no statistically significant difference in the incidence of benign and malignant tumors produced in drug-treated as compared to control animals, nor did acyclovir induce the occurrence of tumors earlier in drug-treated animals as compared to control. In two *in vitro* cell transformation assays, used to provide preliminary assessment of potential oncogenicity in advance of these more definitive lifetime bioassays in rodents, conflicting results were obtained. Acyclovir was positive at the highest dose used in one system and the resulting morphologically transformed cells formed tumors when inoculated into immunosuppressed, syngeneic, weanling mice. Acyclovir was negative in another transformation system.

No chromosome damage was observed at maximum tolerated parenteral doses of 100 mg/kg acyclovir in rats or Chinese hamsters; higher doses of 500 and 1000 mg/kg were clastogenic in Chinese hamsters. In addition, no activity was found in a dominant lethal study in mice. In 9 of 11 microbial and mammalian cell assays, no evidence of mutagenicity was observed. In two mammalian cell assays (human lymphocytes and L5178Y mouse lymphoma cells *in vitro*), positive response for mutagenicity and chromosomal damage occurred, but only at concentrations at least 1000 times the plasma levels achieved in humans following topical application.

PRECAUTIONS: *(cont'd)*

Acyclovir does not impair fertility or reproduction in mice at oral doses up to 450 mg/kg/day or in rats at subcutaneous doses up to 25 mg/kg/day. In rabbits given a high dose of acyclovir (50 mg/kg/day SC), there was a statistically significant decrease in implantation efficiency.

PREGNANCY CATEGORY C

IV Infusion and Oral Forms

Teratogenic Effects: Acyclovir was not teratogenic in the mouse (450 mg/kg/day, p.o.), rabbit (50 mg/kg/day, SC and IV) or in standard tests in the rat (50 mg/kg/day, SC). These exposures resulted in plasma levels the same as, 4 and 9, and 1 and 2 times, respectively, human levels. In a non-standard test in rats there were fetal abnormalities, such as head and tail anomalies, and maternal toxicity.[37] In this test, rats were given 3 SC doses of 100 mg/kg acyclovir on gestation day 10, resulting in plasma levels 5 and 10 times human levels. There are no adequate and well-controlled studies in pregnant women. Acyclovir should not be used during pregnancy unless the potential benefit justifies the potential risk to the fetus. Although acyclovir was not teratogenic in standard animal studies, the drug's potential for causing chromosome breaks at high concentration should be taken into consideration in making this determination.

Pregnancy Exposure Registry: To monitor maternal fetal outcomes of pregnant women exposed to systemic acyclovir, Glaxo Wellcome Co. maintains an Acyclovir Pregnancy Registry. Physicians are encouraged to register patients by calling (800) 722-9292 ext. 8465.

Ointment

Teratogenic Effects: Acyclovir was not teratogenic in the mouse (450,g/kg/day, P.O.), rabbit (50 mg/kg/day, S.C. and I.V.), or in standard tests in the rat (50 mg/kg/day S.C.). In a non-standard test in rats, fetal abnormalities, such as head and tail anomalies, were observed following subcutaneous administration of acyclovir at very high doses associated with toxicity to the maternal rat. The clinical relevance of these findings is uncertain. There are no adequate and well-controlled studies in pregnant women. Acyclovir should not be used during pregnancy unless the potential benefit justifies the potential risk to the fetus.

NURSING MOTHERS

Acyclovir concentrations have been documented in breast milk in two women following oral administration of acyclovir and ranged from 0.6 to 4.1 times corresponding plasma levels.[38,39] These concentrations would potentially expose the nursing infant to a dose acyclovir up to 0.3 mg/kg/day. Caution should be exercised when acyclovir is administered to a nursing woman.

Ointment: It is not known whether topically applied acyclovir is excreted in breast milk. After oral administration of acyclovir, concentrations have been documented in breast milk in two women and ranged from 0.6 to 4.1 times the corresponding plasma levels. Caution should be exercised when acyclovir ointment is administered to a nursing woman.

PEDIATRIC USE

Oral Forms: Safety and effectiveness in children less than 2 years of age have not been established.

Ointment: Safety and effectiveness in children have not been established.

DRUG INTERACTIONS:

IV Infusion, Oral Forms: Co-administration of probenecid with acyclovir has been shown to increase the mean half-life and the area under the concentration-time curve. Urinary excretion and renal clearance were correspondingly reduced.[36] The clinical effects of this combination have not been studied.

Ointment: Clinical experience has identified no interactions resulting from topical or systemic administration of other drugs concomitantly with acyclovir ointment 5%.

ADVERSE REACTIONS:

IV INFUSION

The adverse reactions listed below have been observed in controlled and uncontrolled clinical trials in approximately 700 patients who received acyclovir at ≈5 mg/kg (250 mg/m²) three times daily, and approximately 300 patients who received ≈10 mg/kg (500 mg/m²) three times daily.

The most frequent adverse reactions reported during acyclovir administration were inflammation or phlebitis at the injection site in approximately 9% of the patients, and transient elevations of serum creatinine of BUN in 5% to 10% (the higher incidence occurred usually following rapid (less than 10 minutes) intravenous infusion). Nausea and/or vomiting occurred in approximately 7% of the patients (the majority occurring in nonhospitalized patients who received 10 mg/kg). Itching, rash or hives occurred in approximately 2% of patients. Elevation of transaminases occurred in 1-2% of patients.

Approximately 1% of patients receiving intravenous acyclovir have manifested encephalopathic changes characterized by either lethargy, obtundation, tremors, confusion, hallucinations, agitation, seizures or coma see PRECAUTIONS.

Adverse reactions which occurred at a frequency of less than 1% and which were probably or possibly related to intravenous acyclovir administration were: anemia, anuria, hematuria, hypotension, edema, anorexia, lightheadedness, thirst, headache, diaphoresis, fever, neutropenia, thrombocytopenia, abnormal urinalysis (characterized by an increase in formed elements in urine sediment) and pain on urination.

Other reactions have been reported with a frequency of less than 1% in patients receiving acyclovir, but a causal relationship between acyclovir and the reaction could not be determined. These include pulmonary edema with cardiac tamponade, abdominal pain, chest pain, thrombocytosis, leukocytosis, neutrophilia, ischemia of digits, hypokalemia, purpura fulminans, pressure on urination, hemoglobinemia and rigors.

Observed During Clinical Practice: Based on clinical practice experience in patients treated with acyclovir sterile powder in the U.S., spontaneously reported adverse events are uncommon. Data are insufficient to support an estimate of their incidence or to establish causation. These events may also occur as part of underlaying disease process. Voluntary reports of adverse events which have been received since market introduction include:

General: fever, pain, and rarely, anaphylaxis

Digestive: elevated liver function tests, nausea

Hemic and Lymphatic: leukopenia

Nervous: agitation, coma, confusion, convulsions, hallucinations, obtundation, psychosis

Skin: rash

Urogenital: elevated blood urea nitrogen, elevated creatinine, renal failure

ORAL FORMS

Herpes Simplex

Short-Term Administration: The most frequent adverse events reported during clinical trials of treatment of genital herpes with orally administered acyclovir were nausea and/or vomiting in 8 of 298 patient treatments (2.7%) and headache in 2 of 298 (0.6%). Nausea and/or vomiting occurred in 2 of 287 (0.7%) of patients who received placebo.

Less frequent adverse events, each of which occurred in 1 of 298 patient treatments with orally administered acyclovir (0.3%), included diarrhea, dizziness, anorexia, fatigue, edema, skin rash, leg pain, inguinal adenopathy, medication taste, and sore throat.

ADVERSE REACTIONS: *(cont'd)*

Long-Term Administration: The most frequent adverse events reported in a clinical trial for the prevention of recurrences with continuous administration of 400 mg (two 200 mg capsules) 2 times daily for 1 year in 586 patients treated with acyclovir were: nausea (4.8%), diarrhea (2.4%), headache (1.9%), and rash (1.7%). The 589 control patients receiving intermittent treatment of recurrences with acyclovir for 1 year reported diarrhea (2.7%), nausea (2.4%), headache (2.2%), and rash (1.5%).

The most frequent adverse effects reported during the second year by 390 patients who elected to continue daily administration of 400 mg (two 200 mg capsules) 2 times daily for 2 years were headache (1.5%), rash (1.3%), and paresthesia (0.8%). Adverse events reported by 329 patients during the third year include asthenia (1.2%), paresthesia (1.2%), and headache (0.9%).

Herpes Zoster

The most frequent adverse effects reported during three clinical trials of treatment of herpes zoster (shingles) with 800 mg of acyclovir 5 times daily for 7 to 10 days in 323 patients were: malaise (11.5%), nausea (8.0%), headache (5.9%), vomiting (2.5%), diarrhea (1.5%), and constipation (0.9%). The 323 placebo recipients reported malaise (11.1%), nausea (11.5%), headache (11.1%), vomiting (2.5%), diarrhea (0.3%), and constipation (2.4%).

Chickenpox

The most frequent adverse events reported during three clinical trials of treatment with chickenpox with oral acyclovir in 495 patients were: diarrhea (3.2%), abdominal pain (0.6%), rash (0.6%), vomiting (0.6%), and flatulence (0.4%). The 498 patients receiving placebo reported: diarrhea (2.2%), flatulence (0.8%), and insomnia (0.4%).

Observed During Clinical Practice

Based on clinical practice experience in patients treated with oral acyclovir in the U.S., spontaneously reported adverse events are uncommon. Data are insufficient to support an estimate of their incidence or to establish causation. These events may also occur as part of the underlying disease process. Voluntary reports of adverse events which have been received since market introduction include:

General: fever, headache, pain, peripheral edema, and rarely, anaphylaxis

Nervous: confusion, dizziness, hallucinations, paresthesia, somnolence (These symptoms may be marked, especially in older adults.)

Digestive: diarrhea, elevated liver function tests, gastrointestinal distress, nausea

Hemic and Lymphatic: leukopenia, lymphadenopathy

Musculoskeletal: myalgia

Skin: alopecia, pruritus, rash, urticaria

Special Senses: visual abnormalities

Urogenital: elevated creatinine

OINTMENT

Because ulcerated genital lesions are characteristically tender and sensitive to any contact or manipulation, patients may experience discomfort upon application of ointment. In the controlled trials, mild pain (including transient burning and stinging) was reported by 103 (28.3%) of 364 patients treated with acyclovir and by 115 (31.1%) of 370 patients treated with placebo; treatment was discontinued in 2 of these patients. Other local reactions among acyclovir-treated patients included pruritus in 15 (4.1%), rash in 1 (0.3%) and vulvitis in 1 (0.3%). Among the placebo-treated patients, pruritus was reported by 17 (4.6%) and rash by 1 (0.3%).

In all studies, there was no significant difference between the drug and placebo group in the rate or type of reported adverse reactions nor were there any differences in abnormal clinical laboratory findings.

Observed During Clinical Practice: Based on clinical practice experience in patients treated with acyclovir ointment in the U.S., spontaneously reported adverse reactions are uncommon. Data are insufficient to support an estimate of their incidence or to establish causation. These events may also occur as part of the underlying disease process. Voluntary reports of adverse events which have been received since market introduction include:

General: edema and/or pain at the application site

Skin: pruritus, rash

OVERDOSAGE:

IV Infusion: Overdosage has been reported following administration of bolus injections, or inappropriately high doses, and in patients whose fluid and electrolyte balance was not properly monitored. This has resulted in elevations in BUN, serum creatinine and subsequent renal failure. Lethargy, convulsions and coma have been reported rarely.

Precipitation of acyclovir in renal tubules may occur when the solubility (2.5 mg/ml) in the intratubular fluid is exceeded (see PRECAUTIONS). Renal lesions related to obstruction of renal tubules by precipitated drug crystals occurred in the following species: rats treated with IV and IP doses of 20 mg/kg/day for 21 and 31 days, respectively, and at SC doses of 100 mg/kg/day for 10 days; rabbits at SC and IV doses of 50 mg/kg/day for 13 days; and dogs at IV doses of 100 mg/kg/day for 31 days. In the event of overdosage, sufficient urine flow must be maintained to prevent precipitation of drug in renal tubules. Recommended urine output is ≥500 ml per gram of drug infused. A six-hour hemodialysis results in a 60% decrease in plasma acyclovir concentration. Data concerning peritoneal dialysis are incomplete but indicate that this method may be significantly less efficient in removing acyclovir from the blood. In the event of acute renal failure and anuria, the patient may benefit from hemodialysis until renal function is restored (see DOSAGE AND ADMINISTRATION).

Oral Forms: Patients have ingested intentional overdoses of up to 100 capsules (20 g) of acyclovir, with no unexpected adverse effects.

Precipitation of acyclovir in renal tubules may occur when the solubility (2.5 mg/ml) in the intratubular fluid is exceeded. Renal lesions considered to be related to obstruction of renal tubules by precipitated drug crystals occurred in the following species: rats treated with IV and IP doses of 20 mg/kg/day for 21 and 31 days, respectively, and at SC doses of 100 mg/kg/day for 10 days; rabbits and SC and IV doses of 50 mg/kg/day for 13 days; and dogs at IV doses of 100 mg/kg/day for 31 days. A 6-hour hemodialysis results in a 60% decrease in plasma acyclovir concentration. Data concerning peritoneal dialysis are incomplete but indicate that this method may be significantly less efficient in removing acyclovir from blood. In the event of acute renal failure and anuria, the patient may benefit from hemodialysis until renal function is restored(see DOSAGE AND ADMINISTRATION).

Ointment: Overdosage by topical application of acyclovir ointment 5% is unlikely because of limited transcutaneous absorption (see CLINICAL PHARMACOLOGY).

DOSAGE AND ADMINISTRATION:

IV INFUSION

CAUTION—RAPID OR BOLUS INTRAVENOUS AND INTRAMUSCULAR OR SUBCUTANEOUS INJECTION MUST BE AVOIDED. Therapy should be initiated as early as possible following onset of signs and symptoms. For diagnosis—see INDICATIONS AND USAGE.

DOSAGE AND ADMINISTRATION: *(cont'd)*

Dosage

Herpes Simplex Infections: *Mucosal and Cutaneous Herpes Simplex (HSV-1 and HSV-2) Infections in immunocompromised Patients:* 5 mg/kg infused at a constant rate over 1 hour, every 8 hours (15 mg/kg/day) for 7 days in adult patients with normal renal function. In children under 12 years of age, more accurate dosing can be attained by infusing 250 mg/m^2 at a constant rate over 1 hour, every 8 hours (750 mg/m^2/day) for 7 days.

Severe Initial Clinial Episodes of Herpes Genitalis: The same dose given above—administered for 5 days.

Herpes Simplex Encephalitis: 10 mg/kg infused at a constant rate over at least 1 hour, every 8 hours for 10 days. In children between 6 months and 12 years of age, more accurate dosing is achieved by infusing 500 mg/m^2, at a constant rate over at least one hour, every 8 hours for 10 days.

Varicella Zoster Infections

Zoster in Immunocompromised Patients: 10 mg/kg infused at a constant rate over 1 hour, every 8 hours for 7 days in adult patients with normal renal function. In children under 12 years of age, equivalent plasma concentrations are attained by infusing 500 mg/m^2at a constant rate over at least 1 hour, every 8 hours for 7 days. Obese patients should be dosed at 10 mg/kg (Ideal Body Weight). A maximum dose equivalent to 500 mg/m^2 every 8 hours should be exceeded for any patient.

Patients with Acute or Chronic Renal Impairment: Refer to DOSAGE AND ADMINISTRATION section for recommended doses, and adjust the dosing interval as indicated in TABLE 2.

TABLE 2 Dosage for Renally Impaired Patients

Creatinine Clearance ($ml/min/1.73m^2$)	Percent of Recommended Dose	Dosing Interval (hours)
>50	100%	8
25-50	100%	12
10-25	100%	24
0-10	50%	24

Hemodialysis: For patients who require dialysis, the mean plasma half-life of acyclovir during hemodialysis is approximately 5 hours. This results in a 60% decrease in plasma concentrations following a six-hour dialysis period. Therefore, the patient's dosing schedule should be adjusted so that an additional dose is administered after each dialysis.[24,25]

Peritoneal Dialysis: No supplemental dose appears to be necessary after adjustment of the dosing interval.[40,41]

Method of Preparation: Each 10 ml vial contains acyclovir sodium equivalent to 500 mg of acyclovir. Each 20 ml vial contains acyclovir sodium equivalent to 1000 mg of acyclovir. The contents of the vial should be dissolved in Sterile Water for Injection as shown in TABLE 3.

TABLE 3

Contents of Vial	Amount of Diluent
500 mg	10 ml
1000 mg	20 ml

The resulting solution in each case contains 50 mg acyclovir per ml (pH approximately 11). Shake the vial well to assure complete dissolution before measuring and transferring each individual dose. DO NOT USE BACTERIOSTATIC WATER FOR INJECTION CONTAINING BENZYL ALCOHOL OR PARABENS.

Administration: The calculated dose should then be removed and added to any appropriate intravenous solution at a volume selected for administration during each 1 hour infusion. Infusion concentrations of approximately 7 mg/ml or lower are recommended. In clinical studies, the average 70 kg adult received between 60 and 150 ml of fluid per dose. Higher concentrations (*e.g.,*10 mg/ml) may produce phlebitis or inflammation at the injection site upon inadvertent extravasation. Standard, commercially available electrolyte and glucose solutions are suitable for intravenous administration; biologic or colloidal fluids (*e.g.,* blood products, protein solutions, etc.) are not recommended.

Once in solution in the vial at a concentration of 50 mg/ml, the drug should be used within 12 hours. Once diluted for administration, each dose should be used within 24 hours. Refrigeration of reconstituted solutions may result in formation of a precipitate which will redissolve at room temperature.

ORAL FORMS

Treatment of Initial Genital Herpes

200 mg (one 200 mg capsules or one teaspoonful [5 ml] suspension) every 4 hours, 5 times daily for 10 days.

Chronic Suppressive Therapy for Recurrent Disease

400 mg (two 200 mg capsules, one 400 mg tablet, or two teaspoonfuls [10 ml] suspension) 2 times daily for up to 12 months, followed by re-evaluation. See INDICATIONS AND USAGE and PRECAUTIONSfor considerations on continuation of suppressive therapy beyond twelve months. Alternative regimens have included doses ranging from 200 mg 3 times daily to 200 mg 5 times daily.

Intermittent Therapy: 200 mg (one 200 mg capsule or one teaspoonful [5 ml] suspension) every 4 hours, 5 times daily for 5 days. Therapy should be initiated at the earliest sign or symptom (prodrome) of recurrence.

Acute Treatment of Herpes Zoster: 800 mg (four 200 mg capsules, two 400 mg tablets, one 800 mg tablet, or four teaspoonfuls [20 ml] suspension) every 4 hours orally 5 times daily for 7 to 10 days.

Treatment of Chickenpox: 20 mg/kg (not to exceed 80 mg) orally, 4 times daily for 5 days. Therapy should be initiated at the earliest sign or symptom. Children over 40 kg should receive the adult dose for chicken pox.

Patients with Acute or Chronic Renal Impairment: Comprehensive pharmacokinetic studies have been completed following IV acyclovir infusions in patients with renal impairment. Based on these studies, dosage adjustments are recommended in the following chart (TABLE 4), for genital herpes and herpes zoster indications:

TABLE 4

Normal Dosage Regimen	Creatine Clearance ($ml/min/1.73\ m^3$)	Adjusted Dosage Regimen Dose (mg)	Dosing Intervals
200 mg every 4 hrs	> 10	200	every 4 hrs, 5x/day
	0-10	200	every 12 hrs
400 mg every 12 hrs	> 10	400	every 12 hrs
	0-10	200	every 12 hrs
800 mg every 4 hours	> 25	800	every 4 hrs, 5x/day
	10-25	800	every 8 hrs
	0-10	800	every 12 hrs

DOSAGE AND ADMINISTRATION: *(cont'd)*

Hemodialysis: For Patients who require hemodialysis, the mean plasma half-life of acyclovir during hemodialysis is approximately 5 hours. This results in a 60% decrease in plasma concentrations following a 6-hour dialysis period. Therefore, the patient's dosing schedule should be adjusted so that an additional dose is administered after each dialysis.

Peritoneal Dialysis: No Supplemental dose appears to be necessary after adjustment of the dosing interval.

OINTMENT

Apply sufficient quantity to adequately cover all lesions every 3 hours 6 times per day for 7 days. The dose size per application will vary depending upon the total lesion area but should approximate a one-half inch ribbon of ointment per 4 square inches of surface area. A finger cot or rubber glove should be used when applying acyclovir to prevent other body sites and transmission of infection to other persons. **Therapy should be initiated as early as possible following onset of signs and symptoms.**

ANIMAL PHARMACOLOGY:

Topical treatment of guinea pigs with 10% acyclovir in polyethylene glycol ointment for three weeks did not result in cutaneous irritation or systemic toxicity. Also, a wide variety of animal tests by parenteral routes demonstrated that acyclovir has a low order of toxicity.

REFERENCES:

(*References are from Zovirax IV Infusion labeling*). **1.** O'Brien JJ, Campoli-Richards DM. Acyclovir — an updated review of its antiviral activity, pharmacokinetic properties and therapeutic efficacy. *Drugs.* 1989;37:233-309. **2.** Littler E, Zeuthen J, McBride AA, et al. Identification of an Epstein-Barr virus- coded thymidine kinase. The *EMBO Journal.*1986;5(8):1959-1966. **3.** Miller WH, Miller RL. Phosphorylation of acyclovir (acycloguanosine) monophosphate by GMP kinase. *J Biol Chem.*1980;255:7204-7207. **4.** Furman PA, St Clair MH, Fyfe JA, et al. Inhibition of herpes simplex virus-induced DNA polymerase activity and viral DNA replication by 9-(2-hydroxyethoxymethyl)guanine and its triphosphate. *J Virol.* 1979;32:72-77. **5.** Derse D, Cheng YC, Furman PA, et al. Inhibition of purified human and herpes simplex virus-induced DNA polymerases by 9-(2- hydroxyethoxymethyl)guanine triphosphate: Effects on primer-template function. *J Biol Chem.*1981;256: 11447-11451. **6.** McGuirt PV, Shaw JE, Elion GB, et al. Identification of small DNA fragments synthesized in herpes simplex virus-infected cells in the presence of acyclovir. *Antimicrob Agents Chemother.*1984;25:507-509. **7.** Barry DW, Blum MR. Antiviral drugs: acyclovir In: Turner P, Shand DG eds. *Recent Advances in Clinical Pharmacology.* ed 3. New York: Churchill Livingstone, 1983: chap 4. **8.** DeClercq E. Comparative efficacy of antiherpes drugs in different cell lines. *Antimicrob Agents Chemother.*1982;21:661-663. **9.** McLaren C, Ellis MN, Hunter GA. A colorimetric assay for the measurement of the sensitivity of herpes simplex viruses to antiviral agents. *Antiviral Res.* 1983;3:223- 234. **10.** Barry DW, Nusinoff-Lehrman S. Viral resistance in clinical practice: summary of five years experience with acyclovir. In: Kono R, Nakajima A eds. *Herpes Viruses and Virus Chemotherapy (Ex Med IntCongr Ser 667).* New York: *Excerpta Medica,*1985:269-270. **11.** Dekker C, Ellis MN, McLaren C, et al. Virus resistance in clinical practice. *J Antimicrob Chemother.*1983;12(suppl B):137-152 **12.** Sibrack CD, Gutman LT, Wilfert CM, et al. Pathogenicity of acyclovir-resistant herpes simplex virus type 1 from an immunodeficient child. *J Infect Dis.* 1982;146:673-682. **13.** Crumpacker CS, Schnipper LE, Marlowe SI, et al. Resistance to antiviral drugs of herpes simplex virus isolated from a patient treated with acyclovir. *N Engl J Med.*1982;306:343-346. **14.** Wade JC, Newton B, McLaren C, et al. Intravenous acyclovir to treat mucocutaneous herpes simplex virus infection after marrow transplantation: a double-blind trial. *Ann Intern Med.*1982;96:265-269. **15.** Burns WH, Saral R, Santos GW, et al. Isolation and characterization of resistant herpes simplex virus after acyclovir therapy. *Lancet.* 1982;1:421-423. **16.** Straus SE, Takiff HE, Seidlin M. et al. Suppression of frequently recurring genital herpes: a placebo-controlled double-blind trial of oral acyclovir. *N Engl J Med* 1984;310:1545-1550. **17.** Collins P. Viral sensitivity following the introduction of acyclovir. *Am J Med.*1988;85 (2A):129-134. **18.** Erlich KS, Mills J, Chatis P, et al. Acyclovir-resistant herpes simplex virus infections in patients with the acquired immunodeficiency syndrome. *N Engl J Med.*1989;320(5):293-296. **19.** Hill EL, Ellis MN, Barry DW. In: 28th*Intersci Conf on Antimicrob Agents Chemother. Los Angeles,*1988, Abst. No 0840:260. **20.** Ellis MN, Keller PM, Fyfe JA, et al. Clinical isolates of herpes simplex virus type 2 that induces a thymidine kinase with altered substrate specificity.*Antimicrob Agents Chemother.*1987;31(7): 1117-1125. **21.** Collins P, Larder BA, Oliver NM, et al. Characterization of a DNA polymerase mutant of herpes simplex virus from a severely immunocompromised patient receiving acyclovir. *J gen Virol.*1989;(70):375-382. **22.** Field HJ, Darby G, Wildy P. Isolation and characterization of acyclovir-resistant mutants of herpes simplex virus.*J gen Virol.*1980;49:115-124. **23.** Blum MR, Liao SH, deMiranda P. Overview of acyclovir pharmacokinetic disposition in adults and children. *Am J Med.*1982;73:186-192. **24.** Laskin OL, Longstreth JA, Whelton A, et al. Effect of renal failure on the pharmacokinetics of acyclovir. *Am J Med.*1982;73:197-201. **25.** Krasny HC, Liao SH, deMiranda P, et al. Influence of hemodialysis on acyclovir pharmacokinetic in patients with chronic renal failure *Am. J Med.* 1982;73:202-204. **26.** Mitchell CD, Bean B, Gentry SR, et al. Acyclovir therapy for mucocutaneous herpes simplex infections in immunocompromised patients. *Lancet.*1981;1:1389-1392. **27.** Meyers JD, Wade JC, Mitchell CD, et al. Multicenter collaborative trial of intravenous acyclovir for treatment of mucocutaneous herpes simplex virus infection in the immunocompromised host. *Am J Med.* 1982;73:229-235. **28.** Data on file, Burroughs Wellcome Co. **29.** Corey L, Fife KH, Benedetti JK, et al. Intravenous acyclovir for the treatment of primary genital herpes.*Ann Intern Med.* 1983;98(6):914- 921. **30.** Mindel A, Adler MW, Sutherland S, et al. Intravenous acyclovir treatment for primary genital herpes. *Lancet.*1982;1:697-700. **31.** Whitley RJ, Alford CA, Hirsch MS, et al. Vidarabine versus acyclovir therapy in herpes simplex encephalitis. *N Engl J Med.* 1986;314(3): 144-149. **32.** Skoldenberg B, Forsgren M, Alestig K, et al. Acyclovir versus vidarabine in herpes simplex encephalitis: randomized multicenter study in consecutive Swedish patients. *Lancet.* 1984;2(8405):707-711. **33.** Balfour HH Jr, Bean B, Laskin OL, et al. Acyclovir halts progression of herpes zoster in immunocompromised patients. *N Engl J Med.* 1983;308(24):1448-1453. **34.** Shepp DH, Danliker PS, Meyers JD. Treatment of varicella-zoster virus infection in severely immunocompromised patients. *N Engl J Med.* 1986;314:208- 212. **35.** Naib ZM, Nahmias AJ, Josey WE, et al. Relation of cytohistopathology of genital herpesvirus infection to cervical anaplasia. *Cancer Res.* 1973;33:1452-1463. **36.** Laskin OL, deMiranda P, King DH, et al. Effects of probenecid on the pharmacokinetics and elimination of acyclovir in humans.*Antimicrob Agents Chemother.* 1982;21:804-807. **37.** Stahlmann R, Klug S, Lewandowski C, et al. Teratogenicity of acyclovir in rats. *Infection.*1987; 15:261-262. **38.** Lau RJ, Emery MG, Galinsky RE, et al. Unexpected accumulation of acyclovir in breast milk with estimate of infant exposure. *ObstetGynecol.*1987;69(3):468-471. **39.** Meyer LJ, deMiranda P, Sheth N, et al. Acyclovir in human breast milk. *Am J Obstet Gynecol.*1988;158(3):586-588. **40.** Boelart J, Schurgers M, Daneels R, et al. Multiple dose pharmacokinetics of intravenous acyclovir in patients on continuous ambulatory peritoneal dialysis. *J Antimicrob Chemother.* 1987;20:69- 76. **41.** Shah GM, Winer RL, Krasny HC. Acyclovir pharmacokinetics in a patient on continuous ambulatory peritoneal dialysis. *Am J Kidney Dis.* 1986;507-510.

PATIENT INFORMATION:

Acyclovir is used for the treatment of genital herpes, varicella-zoster (shingles) and chickenpox. It is not a cure. Inform your physician if you are pregnant or nursing. Inform your physician if you have kidney disease. Drink six to eight glasses of water each day while receiving an intravenous infusion of acyclovir or while taking the oral form of acyclovir. Acyclovir may be taken with or without food. Do not use the topical ointment in the eyes. Shake the suspension well before each use.

HOW SUPPLIED:

IV Infusion: Store at 15° to 25°C (59° to 77°F).

Capsules: Zovirax Capsules (blue, opaque cap and body) containing 200 mg acyclovir and printed with "Wellcome ZOVIRAX 200"—Bottle of 100, and unit dose pack of 100. Store at 15° to 25°C (59° to 77°F) and protect from light and moisture.

Tablets: Zovirax Tablets are light blue, oval, and contain 800 mg acyclovir, engraved with "ZOVIRAX 800". Store at 15° to 25°C (59° to 77°F) and protect from light and moisture.

Zovirax Tablets are white, shield-shaped, containing 400 mg acyclovir and engraved with "ZOVIRAX" on one side and a triangle on the other side. Store at 15° to 25°C (59° to 77°F) and protect from light and moisture.

Suspension: Zovirax Suspension is off-white, banana-flavored, containing 200 mg acyclovir in each teaspoonful (5 ml). Store at 15° to 25°C (59° to 77°F).

Ointment: Zovirax Ointment 5% is supplied in 15 g tubes. Each gram contains 50 mg acyclovir in a polyethylene glycol base. Store at 15° to 25°C (59° to 77°F) in a dry place.

HOW SUPPLIED - RATED THERAPEUTICALLY EQUIVALENT:

Capsule - Oral - 200 mg

100's	$97.70	Acyclovir, Schein Pharm (US)	00364-2692-01

Capsule, Gelatin - Oral - 200 mg

100's	**$108.56**	**ZOVIRAX, Glaxo Wellcome**	**00173-0991-55**
100's	**$123.65**	**ZOVIRAX, Glaxo Wellcome**	**00173-0991-56**

HOW SUPPLIED - RATED THERAPEUTICALLY EQUIVALENT: *(cont'd)*

Tablet - Oral - 400 mg

100's	$189.60	Acyclovir, Schein Pharm (US)	00364-2689-01
500's	$900.60	Acyclovir, Schein Pharm (US)	00364-2689-05

Tablet - Oral - 800 mg

100's	$368.65	Acyclovir, Schein Pharm (US)	00364-2690-01

Tablet, Uncoated - Oral - 400 mg

100's	**$210.68**	**ZOVIRAX, Glaxo Wellcome**	**00173-0949-55**

Tablet, Uncoated - Oral - 800 mg

100's	**$409.67**	**ZOVIRAX, Glaxo Wellcome**	**00173-0945-55**
100's UD	**$417.85**	**ZOVIRAX, Glaxo Wellcome**	**00173-0945-56**

HOW SUPPLIED - NOT RATED EQUIVALENT:

Injection, Lyphl-Susp - Intravenous - 500 mg/10ml

10 ml x 10	**$566.03**	**ZOVIRAX, Glaxo Wellcome**	**00173-0995-01**
20 ml x 10	**$943.37**	**ZOVIRAX, Glaxo Wellcome**	**00173-0952-01**

Ointment - Topical - 5%

3 gm	**$17.18**	**ZOVIRAX, Glaxo Wellcome**	**00173-0993-41**
15 gm	**$39.73**	**ZOVIRAX, Glaxo Wellcome**	**00173-0993-94**

Suspension - Oral - 200 mg/5ml

480 ml	**$93.55**	**ZOVIRAX, Glaxo Wellcome**	**00173-0953-96**

ADAPALENE *(003292)*

CATEGORIES: Acne; Acne Vulgaris; Dermatologicals; Skin/Mucous Membrane Agents; Topical; Pregnancy Category C

BRAND NAMES: **Differin**; *Differin Gel* (Germany); *Differine* (France)
(International brand names outside U.S. in italics)

DESCRIPTION:

Adapalene gel is used for the topical treatment of acne vulgaris. Each gram of adapalene gel contains adapalene 0.1% (1 mg) in a vehicle consisting of propylene glycol, carbomer 940, poloxamer 182, edelate disodium, methylparaben, sodium hydroxide, and purified water. May contain hydrochloric acid to adjust pH.

The chemical name of adapalene is 6–[3–(1–adamantyl)-4–methoxyphenyl] -2–nephthoic acid. Adapalene is a white to off-white powder which is soulable in tetrahydrofuran, sparingly soluable in ethanol, and practically insoluable in water. The molecular formula is $C_{28}H_{28}O_3$ and the molecular weight is 412.52.

CLINICAL PHARMACOLOGY:

Adapalene is a chemically stable, retinoid-like compound. Biochemical and pharmacological profile studies have demonstrated that adapalene is a modulator of cellular differentiation, keratinization, and inflammatory processes all of which represent important features in the pathology of acne vulgaris.

Mechanistically, adalapene binds to specific retinoic acid nuclear receptors but does not bind to the cytosolic receptor protein. Although the exact mode of action of adapalene is unknown, it is suggested that topical adalapene may normalize the differentiation of follicular epithelial cells resulting in decreased microcomadone formation.

PHARMACOKINETICS

Absorption of adapalene through human skin is low. Only trace amounts (<0.25 ng/mL) of parent substance have been found in the plasma of acne patients following chronic topical application of adalapene in controlled clinical trials. Excretion appears to be primarily by the biliary route.

INDICATIONS AND USAGE:

Adapalene gel is indicated for the topical treatment of acne vulgaris.

CONTRAINDICATIONS:

Adapalene gel should not be administered to individuals who are hypersensitive to adapalene or any of the components in the vehicle gel.

WARNINGS:

Use of adapalene gel should be discontinued if hypersensitivity to any of the ingredients is noted. Patients with sunburn should be advised not to use this product until fully recovered.

PRECAUTIONS:

GENERAL

If a reaction suggesting sensitivity or chemical irritation occurs, use of the medication should be discontinued. Exposure to sunlight, including sunlamps, should be minimized during the use of adapalene. Patients who normally experience high levels of sun exposure, and those with inherent sensitivity to the sun should be warned to exercise caution. Use of sunscreen products and protective clothing over treated areas is recommended when exposure cannot be avoided. Weather extremes, such as wind or cold, also may be irritating to patients under treatment with adapalene.

Avoid contact with eyes, lips, angles of the nose, and mucous membranes. The product should not be applied to cuts, abrasions, eczemelous skin, or sunburned skin.

Certain cutaneous signs and symptoms such as erythema, dryness, scaling, burning, or pruritus may be experienced during treatment. These are most likely to occur during the first two to four weeks and will usually lessen with continued use of the medication. Depending upon the severity of adverse events, patients should be instructed to reduce the frequency of application or discontinue use.

CARCINOGENESIS, MUTAGENESIS, AND IMPAIRMENT OF FERTILITY

Carcinogenicity studies have been conducted in mice at topical doses of 0.3, 0.9, and 2.6 mg/kg/day and in rats at oral doses of 0.15. 0.5, and 1.5 mg/kg/day, approximately 4-75 times the maximal daily human topical dose. In the oral study, positive linear trends were observed in the incidence of follicular cell adenomas and carcinomas in the thyroid glands of female rats, and in the incidence of benign and malignant pheochromocytomas in the adrenal medullas of male rats.

No photocarcinogenicity studies were conducted. Animal studies have shown an increased tumorigenic risk with the use of pharmacologically similar drugs (*e.g.,* retinoids) when exposed to UV irridation in the laboratory, or to sunlight. Although the significance of these studies to human use is not clear, patients should be advised to avoid or minimize exposure to either sunlight or artificial UV irridation sources.

In a series of *in vivo* and *in vitro* studies, adapalene did not exhibit mutagenic or genotoxic activities.

PRECAUTIONS: *(cont'd)*

PREGNANCY, TERATOGENIC EFFECTS, PREGNANCY CATEGORY C

No teratogenic effects were seen in rats at oral doses of adapalene 0.15 to 5.0 mg/kg/day, up to 120 times the maximal daily human topical dose. Cutaneous route teratology studies conducted in rats and rabbits at doses of 0.6, 2.0, and 6.0 mg/kg/day up to 150 times the maximal daily human topical dose exhibited no fetotoxicity and only minimal increases in supernumerary ribs in rats. There are no adequate and well-controlled studies in pregnant women. Adapalene should be used during pregnancy only if the potential benefit justifies the potential risk to the fetus.

NURSING MOTHERS

It is not known whether this drug is excreted in human milk. Because many drugs are excreted in human milk, caution should be exercised when adapalene gel is administered to a nursing woman.

PEDIATRIC USE

Safety and effectiveness in pediatric patients below the age of 12 have not been established.

DRUG INTERACTIONS:

As adapalene gel has the potential to produce local irritation in some patients, concomitant use of other potentially irritating topical products (medicated or abrasive soaps and cleansers, soaps and cosmetics that have a strong drying effect, and products with high concentrations of alcohol, astringents, spices, or lime) should be approached with caution. Particular caution should be exercised in using preparations containing sulfur, resorcinol, or salicylic acid in combination with adapalene gel. If these preparations have been used, it is advisable not to start therapy with adapalene gel until the effects of such preparations in the skin have been subsided.

ADVERSE REACTIONS:

Some adverse effects such as erythema, scaling, dryness, pruritus, and burning will occur in 10 - 40% of patients. Pruritus or burning immediately after application also occurs in approximately 20% of patients. The following adverse experiences were reported in approximately 1% or less of patients: skin irritation, burning/stinging, erythema, sunburn, and acne flares. These are most commonly seen during the first month of therapy and decrease in frequency and severity thereafter. All adverse effects with use of adapalene gel during clinical trials were reversible upon discontinuation of therapy.

OVERDOSAGE:

Adapalene gel is intended for cutaneous use only. If the medication is applied excessively, no more rapid or better results will be obtained and marked redness, peeling, or discomfort may occur. The acute oral toxicity of adapalene gel in mice and rats is greater than 10 mL/kg. Chronic ingestion of the drug may lead to the same side effects as those associated with excessive oral intake of Vitamin A.

DOSAGE AND ADMINISTRATION:

Adapalene gel should be applied once a day to affected areas after washing in the evening before retiring. A thin film of the gel should be applied, avoiding eyes, lips, and mucous membranes.

During the early weeks of therapy, an apparent exacerbation of acne may occur. This is due to the action of the medication on previously unseen lesions and should not be considered a reason to discontinue therapy. Therapeutic results should be noticed after eight to twelve weeks of treatment.

HOW SUPPLIED:

Adapalene gel, 0.1% is supplied in the following sizes: 15 g laminate tube; 45 g laminate tube.

Storage: Store at controlled room temperature 20° - 25 C°(68° - 77°F).

Caution: Federal law prohibits dispensing without prescription.

HOW SUPPLIED - EQUIVALENTS NOT AVAILABLE:

Gel - Topical - 0.1%

15 g	$22.08	DIFFERIN, Galderma	00299-5910-15
45 g	$52.14	DIFFERIN, Galderma	00299-5910-45

ADENOSINE *(000107)*

CATEGORIES: Antiarrhythmic Agents; Atrial Fibrillation; Cardiovascular Drugs; Homeostatic & Nutrient; Myocardial Perfusion; Nutrition, Enteral/Parenteral; Stress Test; Tachycardia; Vasodilating Agents; Vitamins; Pregnancy Category C; FDA Approved 1989 Oct

BRAND NAMES: Adenic; Adeno-Jec; Adenocar; **Adenocard**; *Adenocor*, Adenoscan; Adenosine Phosphate; *Adrekar* (Germany); Atp
(International brand names outside U.S. in italics)

DESCRIPTION:

INTRAMUSCULAR INJECTION

Adenosine Phosphate Injection is a sterile solution of adenosine-5-monophosphate available for intramuscular use. Adenosine phosphate (AMP) has the molecular formula $C_{10}H_{14}N_5O_7$ with a molecular wight of 347.22. It is Adenosine-5-Monophosphoric Acid and occurs as white crystals with a melting point of 196° - 200°C. It is readily soluble in boiling water.

Each ml contains: Adenosine-5-Monophosphate 25 mg, Benzyl alcohol 1.5% as a preservative, in water for Injection q.s. Sodium Hydroxide is added to adjust pH and convert Adenosine-5-Monophosphate to the sodium salt.

INTRAVENOUS INJECTION

Adenosine is an endogenous nucleoside occurring in all cells of the body. It is chemically 6-amino-9-β-D-ribofuranosyl-9-H-purine.

$C_{10}H_{13}N_5O_4$ M.W. = 267.24

Adenosine is a white crystalline powder. It is soluble in water and practically insoluble in alcohol. Solubility increases by warming and lowering the pH. Adenosine is not chemically related to other antiarrhythmic drugs. Adenosine is a sterile solution for rapid bolus intravenous injection and is available in 6 mg/2 ml vials. Each ml contains 3 mg adenosine and 9 mg sodium chloride in Water for Injection. The pH of the solution is between 5.5 and 7.5.

CLINICAL PHARMACOLOGY:

INTRAMUSCULAR INJECTION

It is not yet understood by what exact mechanism adenosine phosphate provides certain therapeutic benefits. Perhaps correction of deficiencies or underlying biochemical imbalances at the cellular level provides this clinical benefit. However, the rationale for the therapeutic use of adenosine phosphate must rely essentially upon clinical evidence until more is known about cellular biochemistry and its relation to normal and disturbed physiological processes.

CLINICAL PHARMACOLOGY: *(cont'd)*

INTRAVENOUS INJECTION

Mechanism of Action: Adenosine slows conduction time through the A-V node, can interrupt the reentry pathways through the A-V-node, and can restore normal sinus rhythm in patients with paroxysmal supraventricular tachycardia (PSVT), including PSVT associated with Wolff-Parkinson-White Syndrome.

Adenosine is antagonized competitively by methylxanthines such as caffeine and theophylline, and potentiated by blockers of nucleoside transport such as dipyridamole. Adenosine is not blocked by atropine.

Hemodynamics: The usual intravenous bolus dose of 6 or 12 mg adenosine will have no systemic hemodynamic effects. When larger doses are given by infusion, adenosine decreases blood pressure by decreasing peripheral resistance.

Pharmacokinetics: Intravenously administered adenosine is removed from the circulation very rapidly. Following an intravenous bolus, adenosine is taken up by erythrocytes and vascular endothelial cells. The half-life of intravenous adenosine is estimated to be less than 10 seconds. Adenosine enters the body pool and is primarily metabolized to inosine and adenosine monophosphate (AMP).

Hepatic and Renal Failure: Hepatic and renal failure should have no effect on the activity of a bolus adenosine injection. Since adenosine has a direct action, hepatic and renal function are not required for the activity or the metabolism of a bolus adenosine injection.

CLINICAL STUDIES:

In controlled studies in the United States, bolus doses of 3, 6, 9, and 12 mg were studied. A cumulative 60% of patients with paroxysmal supraventricular tachycardia had converted to normal sinus rhythm within one minute after an intravenous bolus dose of 6 mg adenosine (some converted on 3 mg and failures were given 6 mg), and a cumulative 92% converted after a bolus dose of 12 mg. Seven to sixteen percent of patients converted after 1–4 placebo bolus injections. Similar responses were seen in a variety of patient subsets, including those using or not using digoxin, those with Wolff-Parkinson-White Syndrome, males, females, blacks, caucasians, and hispanics.

Adenosine is not effective in converting rhythms other than PSVT, such as atrial flutter, atrial fibrillation, or ventricular tachycardia, to normal sinus rhythm. To date, such patients have not had adverse consequences following administration of adenosine.

INDICATIONS AND USAGE:

INTRAMUSCULAR INJECTION

The symptomatic relief of varicose vein complications with stasis dermatitis.

INTRAVENOUS INJECTION

Intravenous Adenosine is indicated for the following:

Conversion to sinus rhythm of paroxysmal supraventricular tachycardia (PSVT), including that associated with accessory bypass tracts (Wolff-Parkinson-White Syndrome). When clinically advisable, appropriate vagal maneuvers (*e.g.*, Valsalva maneuver), should be attempted prior to adenosine administration.

It is important to be sure the adenosine solution actually reaches the systemic circulation see DOSAGE AND ADMINISTRATION.

Adenosine does not convert atrial flutter, atrial fibrillation, or ventricular tachycardia to normal sinus rhythm. In the presence of atrial flutter or atrial fibrillation, a transient modest slowing of ventricular response may occur immediately following adenosine administration.

CONTRAINDICATIONS:

INTRAMUSCULAR INJECTION

Adenosine Phosphate Injection is contraindicated in patients with a history of myocardial infarction; cerebral hemorrhage.

INTRAVENOUS INJECTION

Intravenous adenosine is contraindicated in:

1. Second- or third-degree A-V block (except in patients with a functioning artificial pacemaker).

2. Sick sinus syndrome (except in patients with a functioning artificial pacemaker).

3. Known hypersensitivity to adenosine.

WARNINGS:

INTRAMUSCULAR INJECTION

Adenosine phosphate and adenosine adenosine are not interchangeable drugs. Therefore, extreme care should be utilized to avoid possible inadvertent interchange, since use could result in serious toxicity and/or therapeutic failure, which may be potentially fatal.

Anaphylactoid reactions following administration of Adenosine phosphate injection have been reported. If patient complains of dyspnea and tightness in the chest following an injection, further injections should not be made. Prompt treatment for the allergic reaction should be immediately instituted when and if they occur.

Usage in Pregnancy: Safe use of adenosine phosphate has not been established with respect to adverse effects upon fetal development. Therefore, this drug should not be used in women of child-bearing potential and particularly during early pregnancy unless in the judgment of the physician the benefits outweigh the potential hazards.

Usage in Children: Adenosine phosphate is not recommended for use in children because documented clinical experience has been insufficient to establish safety and a suitable dosage regimen in the pediatric age group.

INTRAVENOUS INJECTION

Heart Block: Adenosine exerts its effect by decreasing conduction through the A-V node and may produce a short lasting first-, second- or third-degree heart block. In extreme cases, transient asystole may result (one case has been reported in a patient with atrial flutter who was receiving carbamazepine). Appropriate therapy should be instituted as needed. Patients who develop high-level block on one dose of adenosine should not be given additional doses. Because of the very short half-life of adenosine, these effects are generally self-limiting.

Rarely, ventricular fibrillation has been reported following adenosine administration, including both resuscitated and fatal events. In most instances, these cases were associated with the concomitant use of digoxin. Although no causal relationship or drug-drug interaction has been established, adenosine should be used with caution in patients receiving digoxin. Appropriate resuscitative measures should be available.

Arrhythmias at Time of Conversion: At the time of conversion to normal sinus rhythm, a variety of new rhythms may appear on the electrocardiogram. They generally last only a few seconds without intervention, and may take the form of premature ventricular contractions, atrial premature contractions, sinus bradycardia, sinus tachycardia, skipped beats, and varying degrees of A-V nodal block. Such findings were seen in 55% of patients.

PRECAUTIONS:

GENERAL

Intramuscular Injection: Do not inject intravenously.

Intravenous Injection: *Asthma:* Most patients with asthma who have received intravenous adenosine have not experienced exacerbation of their asthma. Cases of bronchospasm have been reported rarely in both asthmatic and nonasthmatic patients. Inhaled adenosine has been reported to induce bronchoconstriction in asthmatic patients, but not in normal individuals.

CARCINOGENESIS, MUTAGENESIS, AND IMPAIRMENT OF FERTILITY

Studies in animals have not been performed to evaluate the carcinogenic potential of adenosine. Adenosine was negative for genotoxic potential in the Salmonella (Ames Test) and Mammalian Microsome Assay.

Adenosine, however, like other nucleosides at millimolar concentrations present for several doubling times of cells in culture, is known to produce a variety of chromosomal alterations. In rats and mice, adenosine administered intraperitoneally once a day for 5 days at 50, 100, and 150 mg/kg [10–30 (rats) and 5–15 (mice) times human dosage on a mg/M^2 basis] caused decreased spermatogenesis and increased numbers of abnormal sperm, a reflection of the ability of adenosine to produce chromosomal damage.

PREGNANCY CATEGORY C

Animal reproduction studies have not been conducted with adenosine; nor have studies been performed in pregnant women. As adenosine is a naturally occurring material, widely dispersed throughout the body, no fetal effects would be anticipated. However, since it is not known whether adenosine can cause fetal harm when administered to pregnant women, adenosine should be used during pregnancy only if clearly needed.

PEDIATRIC USE

No controlled studies have been conducted in pediatric patients.

DRUG INTERACTIONS:

INTRAVENOUS INJECTION

Intravenous adenosine has been effectively administered in the presence of other cardioactive drugs, such as digitalis, quinidine, beta-adrenergic blocking agents, calcium channel blocking agents, and angiotensin converting enzyme inhibitors, without any change in the adverse reaction profile. The use of adenosine in patients receiving digitalis may be rarely associated with ventricular fibrillation (see WARNINGS).

The effects of adenosine are antagonized by methylxanthines such as caffeine and theophylline. In the presence of these methylxanthines, larger doses of adenosine may be required or adenosine may not be effective.

Adenosine effects are potentiated by dipyridamole. Thus, smaller doses of adenosine may be effective in the presence of dipyridamole. Carbamazepine has been reported to increase the degree of heart block produced by other agents. As the primary effect of adenosine is to decrease conduction through the A-V node, higher degrees of heart block may be produced in the presence of carbamazepine.

ADVERSE REACTIONS:

INTRAMUSCULAR INJECTION

Flushing, dizziness, and palpitation may occur. Hypotension, dyspnea, epigastric discomfort, and nausea. Occasional local rash and diuresis. Increase in symptoms of bursitis and tendinitis.

INTRAVENOUS INJECTION

The following reactions were reported with intravenous adenosine used in controlled U.S. clinical trials. The placebo group has a less than 1% rate of all of these reactions.

Cardiovascular: Facial flushing (18%), headache (2%), sweating, palpitations, chest pain, hypotension (less than 1%).

Respiratory: Shortness of breath/dyspnea (12%), chest pressure (7%), hyperventilation, head pressure (less than 1%).

Central Nervous System: Lightheadedness (2%), dizziness, tingling in arms, numbness (1%), apprehension, blurred vision, burning sensation, heaviness in arms, neck and back pain (less than 1%).

Gastrointestinal: Nausea (3%), metallic taste, tightness in throat, pressure in groin (less than 1%).

In post-market clinical experience with adenosine, cases of prolonged asystole, ventricular tachycardia, ventricular fibrillation, transient increase in blood pressure, and bronchospasm, in association with adenosine use, have been reported.

OVERDOSAGE:

The half-life of adenosine is less than 10 seconds. Thus, adverse effects are generally rapidly self-limiting. Treatment of any prolonged adverse effects should be individualized and be directed toward the specific effect. Methylxanthines, such as caffeine and theophylline, are competitive antagonists of adenosine.

DOSAGE AND ADMINISTRATION:

INTRAMUSCULAR INJECTION

For Intramuscular Use Only.

Adults: Usually 1 ml (25 mg) once or twice daily until relief is obtained and then 1 ml (25 mg) two or three times weekly for maintenance.

Parenteral drug products should be inspected visually for particulate matter and discoloration prior to administration, whenever the solution and container permit.

Store at controlled room temperature 15-30°C (59-86°F).

INTRAVENOUS INJECTION

For rapid bolus intravenous use only.

Adenosine injection should be given as a rapid bolus by the peripheral intravenous route. To be certain the solution reaches the systemic circulation, it should be administered either directly into a vein or, if given into an IV line, it should be given as close to the patient as possible and followed by a rapid saline flush.

The dose recommendation is based on clinical studies with peripheral venous bolus dosing. Central venous (CVP or other) administration of adenosine has not been systematically studied.

The recommended intravenous doses for adults are as follows:

Initial dose: 6 mg given as a rapid intravenous bolus (administered over a 1-2 second period).

Repeat administration: If the first dose does not result in elimination of the supraventricular tachycardia within 1-2 minutes, 12 mg should be given as a rapid intravenous bolus. This 12 mg dose may be repeated a second time if required.

Doses greater than 12 mg are not recommended.

NOTE: Parenteral drug products should be inspected visually for particulate matter and discoloration prior to administration.

DOSAGE AND ADMINISTRATION: *(cont'd)*

Store at controlled room temperature 15 - 30°C (59 - 86°F).

DO NOT REFRIGERATE as crystallization may occur. If crystallization has occurred, dissolve crystals by warming to room temperature. The solution must be clear at the time of use.

Contains no preservatives. Discard unused portion.

(IM Injection, Steris Labs, 910308A1)

HOW SUPPLIED - EQUIVALENTS NOT AVAILABLE:

Injection, Solution - Intramuscular - 25 mg/ml

10 ml	$5.60	Adenosine Phosphate, McGuff	49072-0011-10
10 ml	$7.20	Adenosine Phosphate, Steris Labs	00402-0087-10
10 ml	$8.50	Adenosine Phosphate, Pasadena	00418-6420-10
10 ml	$11.95	Adenosine Phosphate, Consolidated Midland	00223-7717-10
10 ml	$18.50	ADENIC, Intl Ethical	11584-1006-01

Injection, Solution - Intravenous - 3 mg/ml

2 ml	**$30.43**	**ADENOCARD, Fujisawa USA**	**00469-7234-12**
2 ml x 10	**$263.63**	**ADENOCARD IV, Fujisawa USA**	**00469-0871-02**
5 ml	**$59.60**	**ADENOCARD, Fujisawa USA**	**00469-7234-14**
30 ml	**$223.75**	**ADENOSCAN, Fujisawa USA**	**00469-0871-30**

ALBENDAZOLE *(003225)*

CATEGORIES: Anthelmintics; Anti-Infectives; Antiparasitics; Helminths; Infections; Parasiticidal; FDA Approved 1996 Jul

BRAND NAMES: *ABZ; Adazol; Albatel; Albenzol; Albezole; Alminth; Altoo; Alzental; Alzol; Bendex; Emanthal; Eskazole* (Germany, England, Mexico, Japan); *Fintel; Gascop* (Mexico); *Helben; Helmindazol; Helminzol; Loveral* (Mexico); *Rotopar*; **Valbazen**; *Vermin Plus* (Mexico); *Zeben; Zentel* (France, Mexico)
(International brand names outside U.S. in italics)

FORMULARIES: WHO

DESCRIPTION:

Albendazole is an orally administered broad-spectrum anthelmintic. Chemically it is Methyl 5-(propyl-thio)-2-benzimidazolecarbamate. Its molecular formula is $C_{12}H_{15}N_3O_2S$.

Albendazole is a white to off-white powder. It is soluble in dimthylsulfoxide, strong acids and strong bases. It is slightly soluble in methanol, chloroform, ethyl acetate and acetonitrile. Albendazole is practically insoluble in water. Each white to off-white film-coated Albenza tablet contains 200 mg of albendazole.

Albenza inactive ingredients contain: carnauba wax, hydroxypropyl methylcellulose, lactose monohydrate, magnesium stearate, microcrystalline cellulose, povidone, sodium lauryl sulfate, sodium saccharin, sodium starch glycolate, and starch.

CLINICAL PHARMACOLOGY:

PHARMACOKINETICS

Absorption and Metabolism: Albendazole is poorly absorbed from the gastrointestinal tract due to its low aqueous solubility. Albendazole concentrations are negligible or undectable in plasma as it is rapidly converted to the sulfoxide metabolite prior to reaching the systemic circulation. The systemic anthelmintic activity has been attributed to the primary metabolite, albendazole sulfoxide. Oral bioavailability appears to be enhanced when albendazole is coadministered with a fatty meal (estimated fat content 40 g) as evidenced by higher (up to 5-fold on average) plasma concentrations of albendazole sulfoxide as compared to the fasted state.

Maximal plasma concentrations of albendazole sulfoxide are typically achieved 2 to 5 hours after dosing and are on average 1.31 mcg/ml (range 0.46 to 1.58 mcg/ml) following oral doses of albendazole (400 mg) in siz hydatid disease patients, when administered with a fatty meal. Plasma concentrations of albendazole sulfoxide increase in a dose-proportional manner over the therapeutic dose range following ingestion of a fatty meal (fat content 43.1 g). The mean apparent terminal elimination half-life of albendazole sulfoxide typically ranges from 8 to 12 hours in twenty-five normal subjects, as well as in fourteen hydatid and eight neurocysticercosis patients.

Following 4 weeks of treatment with albendazole (200 mg three times daily), twelve patients' plasma concentrations of albendazole sulfoxide were approximately 20% lower than those observed during the first half of the treatment period, suggesting that albendazole may include its own metabolism.

DISTRIBUTION

Albendazole sulfoxide is 70% bound to plasma protein and is widely distributed throughout the body; it has been detected in urine, bile, liver, cyst wall, cyst fluid, cerebral spinal fluid (CSF). Concentrations in plasma were 3- to 10-fold and 2- to 4-fold higher than those simultaneously determined in cyst fluid and CSF, respectively. Limited *in vitro* and clinical data suggest that albendazole sulfoxide may be eliminated from cysts at a slower rate than observed in plasma.

METABOLISM AND EXCRETION

Albendazole is rapidly converted in the liver to the primary metabolite, albendazole sulfoxide, which is further metabolized to albendazole sulfone and other primary oxidative metabolites that have been identified in human urine. Following oral administration, albendazole has not been detected in human urine. Urinary excretion of albendazole sulfoxide is a minor elimination pathway with less than 1% of the dose recovered in the urine. Biliary elimination presumably accounts for a portion of the elimination as evidenced by biliary concentrations of albendazole sulfoxide similar to those achieved in plasma.

SPECIAL POPULATIONS

Patients with Impaired Renal Function: The pharmacokinetics of albendazole in patients with impaired renal function have not been studied. However, since renal elimination of albendazole and its primary metabolite, albendazole sulfoxide, is negligible, it is unlikely that clearance of these compounds would be altered in these patients.

Biliary Effects: In patients with evidence of extrahepatic obstruction (n=5), the systemic availability of albendazole sulfoxide was increased, as indicated by a 2-fold increase in maximum serum concentration and a 7-fold increase in area under the curve. The rate of absorption/conversion and elimination of albendazole sulfoxide appeared to be prolonged with mean T_{max} and serum elimination half-life values of 10 hours and 31.7 hours, respectively. Plasma concentrations of aprent albendazole were measurable in only one of five patients.

Pediatrics: Following single-dose administration of 200 mg to 300 mg (approximately 10 mg/kg) albendazole to three fasted and two fed pediatric patients with hydatid cyst disease (age range 6 to 13 years), albendazole sulfoxide pharmacokinetics were similar to those observed in fed adults.

CLINICAL PHARMACOLOGY: *(cont'd)*

Elderly Patients: Although no studies have investigated the effect of age on albendazole sulfoxide pharmacokinetics, data in twenty-six hydatid cyst patients (up to 79 years) suggest pharmacokinetics similar to those in young healthy subjects.

MICROBIOLOGY

The prinicpal mode of action for albendazole is by its inhibitory effect on tublin polymerization which results in the loss of cytoplasmic microtubules.

In the specified treatment indications albendazole appears to be active against the larval forms of the following organisms: *Echinococcus granulosus* and *Taenia solium*.

INDICATIONS AND USAGE:

Albendazole is indicated for the treatment of the following infections:

Neurocysticercosis: Albendazole is indicated for the treatment of parenchymal neurocysticercosis due to active lesions caused by larval forms of the pork tapeworm, *Taenia solium*.

Lesions considered responsive to albendazole therapy appear as nonenhancing cysts with no surrounding edema on contrast-enhanced computerized tomography. Clinical studies in patients with lesions of this type demonstrate a 74% to 88% reduction in number of cysts; 40% to 70% of albendazole-treated patients showed resolution of all active cysts.

Hydatid Disease: Albendazole is indicated for the treatment of cystic hydatid disease of the liver, lung, and peritoneum, caused by the larval form of the dog tapeworm, *Echinococcus granulosus*.

This indication is based on combined clinical studies which demonstrated non-infectious cyst contents in approximately 80-90% of patients given albendazole for 3 cycles of therapy of 28 days each (see DOSAGE AND ADMINISTRATION.) Clinical cure (disappearance of cysts) was seen in approximately 30% of these patients, and improvement (reduction in cyst diameter of ≥25%) was seen in a additional 40%.

Note: When medically feasible, surgery is considered the treatment of choice for hydatid disease. When administering albendazole in the pre- or post-surgical setting, optimal killing of cyst contents is achieved when three courses of therapy have been given.

Note: The efficacy of albendazole in the therapy of alveolar hydatid disease caused by *Echinococcus multiocularis* has not been clearly demonstrated in clinical studies.

CONTRAINDICATIONS:

Albendazole is contraindicated in patients with known hypersensitivity to the benzimidazole class of compounds or any components of albendazole.

WARNINGS:

Rare fatalities associated with the use of albendazole have been reported due to granulocytopenia or pancytopenia. (See PRECAUTIONS.) Blood counts should be monitored at the beginning of each 28-day cycle of therapy, and every 2 weeks while on therapy with albendazole. Albendazole may be continued if the total white blood cell count and absolute neutrophil count decrease appear modest and do not progress.

Albandazole should not be used in pregnant women except in clinical circumstances where no alternative management is appropriate. Patients should not become pregnant for at least 1 month following cessation of albendazole therapy. If a patient becomes pregnant while taking this drug, albendazole should be discontinued immediately. If pregancy occurs while taking this drug, the patient should be apprised of the potential hazard to the fetus.

PRECAUTIONS:

GENERAL

Patients being treated for neurocysticercosis should receive appropriate steroid and anticonvulsant therapy as required. Oral or intravenous corticosteroids should be considered to prevent cerebral hypertensive episodes during the first week of anticysticeral therapy.

Cysticercosis may, in rare cases, involve the retina. Before initiating therapy for neurocysticercosis, the patient should be examined for the pressence of retinal lesions. If such lesions are visualized, the need for anticysticeral therapy should be weighed against the possibility of retinal damage caused by albendazole-induced changes to the retinal lesion.

INFORMATION FOR THE PATIENT

Patients should be advised that:

Albendazole may cause fetal harm, therefore, women of childbearing age should begin treatment after a negative pregnancy test.

Women of childbearing age should be cautioned against becoming pregnant while on albendazole or within 1 month of completing treatment.

During albendazole therapy, because of the possibility of harm to the liver or bone marrow, routine (every 2 weeks) monitoring of blood counts and liver function tests should take place.

Albendazole should be taken with food.

LABORATORY TESTS

White Blood Cell Count: Albendazole has been shown to cause occasional (less than 1% of treated patients) reversible reductions in total white blood cell count. Rarely, more significant reductions may be encountered including granulocytopenia, agranulocytosis, or pancytopenia. Blood counts should be performed at the start of each 28-day treatment cycle and every 2 weeks during each 28-day cycle. Albedazole may be continued if the total white blood cell count decrease appears modest and does not progress.

Liver Function: In clinical trials, treatment with albendazole has been associated with mild to moderate elevations of hepatic enzymes in approximately 16% of patients. These have returned to normal upon discontinuation of therapy. Liver function tests (transaminases) should be performed before the start of each treatment cycle and at least every 2 weeks during treatment. If enzymes are significantly increased, albendazole therapy should be discontinued. Therapy can be reinstituted when liver enzymes have returned to pretreatment levels, but laboratory tests should be performed frequently during repeat therapy.

Patients with abnormal liver function test results prior to commencing albendazole therapy should be carefully evaluated, since the drug is metabolized by the liver and has been associated with hepatoxicity in a few patients.

Theophylline: Although single doses of albendazole have been shown not to inhibit theophylline metabolism (see DRUG INTERACTIONS), albendazole does induce cytochrome P450 1A in human hepatoma cells. Therefore, it is recommended that plasma concentrations of theophylline be monitored during and after treatment with albendazole.

CARCINOGENESIS, MUTAGENESIS, AND IMPAIRMENT OF FERTILITY

Long-term carcinogeicity studies were conducted in mice and rats. In the mouse study, albendazole was administered in the diet at doses of 25, 100, and 400 mg/kg/day (0.1, 0.5, and 2 times the recommended human dose based on body surface area in mg/m^2, respectively) for 108 weeks. In the rat study, albendazole was administered in the diet at doses of 3.5, 7, and 20 mg/kg/day (0.4, 0.8, and 0.21 times the recommended human dose based on body surface area in mg/m^2, respectively) for 117 weeks. There was no evidence of increased incidence of tumors in the treated mice and rats when compared to the control group.

PRECAUTIONS: *(cont'd)*

In genotoxicity tests, albendazole was found negative in an Ames Salmonella/Microsome Plate mutation assay with and without metabolic activation or with and without pre-incubation, cell-mediated Chines Hamster Ovary chromosomal aberration test and *in vivo* mouse micronucleus test. In the *in vitro* BALB/3T3 cells transformation assay, albendazole produced weak activity in the presence of metabolic activation while no activity was found in the absence of metabolic activation.

Albendazole did not adversely affect male or female fertility in the rat at an oral dose of 30 mg/kg/day (0.32 times the recommended human dose based on body surface are in mg/m^2).

PREGNANCY, TERATOGENIC EFFECTS, PREGNANCY CATEGORY C

Albendazole has been shown to be teratogenic (to cause embryotoxicity and skeletal malformations) in pregnant rats and rabbits. The teratogenic response in the rat was shown at oral doses of 10 and 30 mg/kg/day (0.10 times and 0.32 times the recommended human dose based on body surface area in mg/m^2, respectively) during gestation days 6 to 15 and in pregnant rabbits at oral doses of 30 mg/kg/day (0.6 times the recommended human dose based on body surface area in mg/m^2) administered during gestation days 7 to 19. In the rabbit study, maternal toxicity (33% mortality) was noted at 30 mg/kg/day. In mice, no teratogenic effects were observed at oral doses up to 30 mg/kg/day (0.16 times the recommended human dose based on body surface area in mg/m^2), administered during gestation days 6 to 15.

There are no adequate and well-controlled studies of albendazole administration in prenant women. Albendazole should be used during pregnancy only if the potential benefit justifies the potential risk to the fetus. (See WARNINGS.)

NURSING MOTHERS

Albendazole is excreted in animal milk. It is not known whether it is excreted in human milk. Because many drugs are excreted in human milk, caution should be exercised when albendazole is administered to a nursing woman.

PEDIATRIC USE

Experience in children under the age of 6 years is limited. In hydatid disease, infection in infants and young children in uncommon, but no problems have been encountered in those who have been treated. In neurocysticercosis, infection is more frequently encountered. In five published studies involving pediatric patients as young as 1 year, no significant problems were encountered, and the efficacy appeared similar to the adult population.

GERIATRIC USE

Experience in patients 65 years of age or older is limited. The number of patients treated for either hydatid disease or neurocysticercosis is limited, but no problems associated with an older population have been observed.

DRUG INTERACTIONS:

Dexamethasone: Steady-state trough concentrations of albendazole sulfoxide were about 56% higher when 8 mg dexamethasone was coadministered with each dose of albendazole (15 mg/kg/day) in eight neurocysticercosis patients.

Praziquantel: In the fed state, praziquantel (40 mg/kg) increased mean maximum plasma concentration and area under the curve of albendazole sulfoxide by about 50% in healthy subjects (n=10) compared with a separate group of subjects (n=6) given albendazole alone. Mean T_{max} and mean plasma elimination half-life of albendazole sulfoxide were unchanged. The pharmacokinetics of praziquantel were unchanged following coadministration with albendazole (400 mg).

Cimetidine: Albendazole sulfoxide concentrations in bile and cystic fluid were increased (about 2-fold) in hydatid cyst patients treated with cimetidine (10 mg/kg/day) (n=7) compared with albendazole (20 mg/kg/day) alone (n=12). Albendazole sulfoxide plasma concentrations were unchanged 4 hours after dosing.

Theophylline: The pharmacokinetics of theophylline (amino-phylline 5.8 mg/kg infused over 20 minutes) were unchanged following a single oral dose of albendazole (400 mg) in 6 healthy subjects.

ADVERSE REACTIONS:

The adverse event profile of albendazole differs between hydatid disease and neurocysticercosis. Adverse events occurring with a frequency of ≥1% in either disease are described in TABLE 1.

These symptoms were usually mild and resolved without treatment. Treatment discontinuations were predominantly due to leukopenia (0.7%) or hepatic abnormalities (3.8% in hydatid disease). The following incidence reflects events that were reported by investigators to be at least possibly or probably related to albendazole.

TABLE 1 Adverse Event Incidence ≥1% in Hydatid Disease and Neurocysticercosis

Adverse Event	Hydatid Disease	Neurocysticercosis
Abnormal Liver Function Tests	15.6	<1.0
Abdominal Pain	6.0	0
Nausea / Vomiting	3.7	6.2
Headache	1.3	11.0
Dizziness / Vertigo	1.2	<1.0
Raised Intracranial Pressure	0	1.5
Meningeal Signs	0	1.0
Reversible Alopecia	1.6	<1.0
Fever	1.0	0

The following adverse events were observed at an incidence of <1%:

Hematologic: Leukopenia. There have been rare reports of granulocytopenia, pancytopenia, agranulocytosis, or thrombocytopenia (see WARNINGS.)

Dermatologic: Rash, urticaria.

Hypersensitivity: Allergic reactions.

Renal: Acute renal failure related to albendazole therapy has been observed.

OVERDOSAGE:

Significant toxicity and mortality were shown in male and female mice at doses exceeding 5,000 mg/kg; in rats, at estimated doses between 1,300 and 2,400 mg/kg; in hamsters, at doses exceeding 10,000 mg/kg; and in rabbits, at estimated doses between 500 and 1,250 mg/kg. In the animals, symptoms were demonstrated in a dose-response relationship and included diarrhea, vomiting, tachycardia, and respiratory distress.

One overdosage has been reported with albendazole in a patient who took at least 16 grams over 12 hours. No untoward effects were reported. In case of overdosage, symptomatic therapy (*e.g.,* gastric lavage and activated charcoal) and general supportive measures are recommended.

DOSAGE AND ADMINISTRATION:

Dosing of albendazole will vary, depending upon which parasitic infection is being treated. See TABLE 2

DOSAGE AND ADMINISTRATION: *(cont'd)*

TABLE 2

Indication: Hydatid Disease		
Patient Weight	60 kg or greater	Less than 60 kg
Dose	400 mg twice a day, w/ meals	15 mg/kg/day given in divided doses twice a day, w/ meals (maximum total dose 800 mg)
Duration	28 day cycle followed by a 14 day albendazole free, interval for the total of 3 cycles	
NOTE: When administered albendazole in the pre- or post-surgical setting, optimal killing of cyst contents is achieved when three courses of therapy have been given.		
Indication: Neurocysticercosis		
Patient Weight	60 kg or greater	Less than 60 kg
Dose	400 mg b.i.d, with meals	15 mg/kg/day given in divided doses b.i.d. with meals (maximum total daily dose 800 mg)
Duration	8-30 days	

Patients being treated for neurocysticercosis should receive appropriate steroid and anticonvulsant therapy as required. oral or intravenous corticosteroids should be considered to prevent cerebral hypertensive episodes during the first week of reatment.

PATIENT INFORMATION:

This drug is uded in the treatment of infestations due to pork tapeworm and dog tapeworm. This drug may cause fetal harm; do not take during pregnancy.

Because of possible harm to the liver or bone marrow, blood counts and liver function tests should be performed every two weeks.

This medicine can affect the dosage of other drugs; inform your physician of any other medications you are taking.

Albendazole may cause abnormal liver function tests, stomach pain, nausea/vomiting, headache, dizziness, vertigo, hair loss or fever. Inform your doctor or physician if these occur.

Take this drug with food.

HOW SUPPLIED:

Albenza (albendazole) is supplied as 200 mg, white to off-white, circular, biconvex, beveledged, film-coated Tiltab tablets in bottles of 112.

Storage: Store between 20° and 25°C (68° and 77°F).

For How Supplied Information, Contact SKB Pharms (NDA# 020666)

ALBUTEROL *(000115)*

CATEGORIES: Airway Obstruction; Antiasthmatics/Bronchodilators; Asthma; Autonomic Drugs; Beta Adrenergic Stimulators; Bronchial Dilators; Bronchospasm; Respiratory & Allergy Medications; Sympathomimetic Agents; Sympathomimetics, Beta Agonist; Pregnancy Category C; Sales > $1 Billion; FDA Approval Pre 1982

BRAND NAMES: *Aerolin*; Airet; *Airomir*; Albuterol Sulfate; *Almotex*; *Anebron*; Arm-A-Med; *Asmadil*; *Asmalin*; *Asmanil*; *Asmasal*; *Asmatol*; *Asmaven* (England); *Asmidon* (Japan); *Asmol*; *Asmol Uni-Dose*; *Asthalin*; *Broncho-Spray* (Germany); *Broncovaleas*; *Bronter*; *Bugonol*; *Butamol*; *Buto-Asma*; *Butotal*; *Cobutolin* (England); *Dilatamol*; *Farcolin*; *Grafalin*; *Libretin*; *Medolin*; *Mozal*; *Novosalmol* (Canada); *Parasma*; Proventil; Proventil Inhaler; Proventil Solutions; Proventil Syrup; *Respax* (Australia); *Respolin* (Australia); *Sabutal*; *Salbetol*; *Salbron*; *Salbulin* (England); *Salbusian*; *Salbutalan* (Mexico); *Salbutamol*; *Salbutan*; *Salbutol*; *Salbuven*; *Salbuvent*; *Salmaplon*; *Salomol*; *Sedalin*; *Sultanol* (Germany, Japan); *Suprasma*; *Theosal*; *Tobybron*; *Vencronyl*; *Venetlin* (Japan); *Ventilan*; **Ventolin**; *Ventoline* (France); Ventolin Rotacaps; Volmax
(International brand names outside U.S. in italics)

FORMULARIES: Aetna; BC-BS; CIGNA; DoD; FHP; Foundation; Humana; Kaiser; Medco; Medi-Cal; PCS; PruCare; United; WHO

COST OF THERAPY: $35.36 (Asthma; Tablet; 2 mg; 3/day; 365 days)

PRIMARY ICD9: 493.90 (Asthma, Unspecified, Without Mention of Status Asthmaticus)

DESCRIPTION:

The World Health Organization recommended name for albuterol base is salbutamol.

Oral Forms: Albuterol sulfate, USP is the racemic form of albuterol and a relatively selective beta$_2$-adrenergic bronchodilator. Albuterol sulfate has the chemical name (±) α'-[(*tert*-butylamino) methyl]-4- hydroxy-*m*-xylene-α,α'-diol sulfate (2:1) (salt).

Albuterol sulfate has a molecular weight of 576.7, and the empirical formula is $(C_{13}H_{21}NO_3)_2 \cdot H_2SO_4$. Albuterol sulfate is a white crystalline powder, soluble in water and slightly soluble in ethanol.

Inhalation Forms: Albuterol, USP, is racemic (α'-[(*tert*-butylamino) methyl]-4-hydroxy-*m*-xylene-α, α'-diol) and a relatively selective beta$_2$-adrenergic bronchodilator.

The molecular weight of albuterol is 239.3, and the empirical formula is $C_{13}H_{21}NO_3$. Albuterol is a white to off-white crystalline solid. It is soluble in ethanol, sparingly soluble in water, and very soluble in chloroform.

Ventolin Tablets: Each Ventolin tablet contains 2 or 4 mg of albuterol as 2.4 or 4.8 mg, respectively, of albuterol sulfate. Each tablet also contains the inactive ingredients corn starch, lactose, and magnesium stearate.

Proventil Repetabs: Each Proventil Repetab extended-release tablet contains a total of 4 mg (2 mg in the coating for immediate release and 2 mg in the core for release after several hours) of albuterol as 4.8 mg of albuterol sulfate. The inactive ingredients for albuterol extended-release tablets include: acacia, butylparaben, calcium phosphate, calcium sulfate, carnauba wax, corn starch, lactose, magnesium stearate, neutral soap, oleic acid, rosin, sugar, talc, titanium dioxide, white wax, and zein.

Ventolin Syrup: Ventolin syrup contains 2 mg of albuterol as 2.4 mg of albuterol sulfate in each teaspoonful (5 ml). The inactive ingredients for albuterol syrup include: citric acid, FD&C Yellow No. 6, flavor, hydroxypropyl methylcellulose, saccharin, sodium benzoate, sodium citrate, and water.

Ventolin Inhalation Aerosol: Ventolin Inhalation Aerosol is a metered-dose aerosol unit for oral inhalation. It contains a microcrystalline (95% ≤10 µm) suspension of albuterol in propellants (trichloromonofluoromethane and dichlorodifluoromethane) with oleic acid. Each actuation delivers from the mouthpiece 90 mcg of albuterol. Each 6.8-g canister provides at least 80 inhalations and each 17-g canister provides at least 200 inhalations.

DESCRIPTION: *(cont'd)*

Ventolin Inhalation Solution, 0.5%: Ventolin inhalation solution, 0.5% is in concentrated form. Dilute 0.5 ml of the solution with 2.5 ml of sterile normal saline solution before administration. Each milliliter of Ventolin inhalation solution contains 5 mg of albuterol (as 6 mg of albuterol sulfate) in an aqueous solution containing benzalkonium chloride; sulfuric acid is used to adjust the pH to between 3 and 5. Ventolin inhalation solution contains no sulfiting agents. Ventolin inhalation solution is a clear, colorless to light yellow solution.

Ventolin Nebules Inhalation Solution, 0.083%: Ventolin Nebules inhalation solution requires no dilution before administration. Each milliliter of Ventolin Nebules inhalation solution contains 0.83 mg of albuterol (as 1 mg of albuterol sulfate) in an isotonic, sterile, aqueous solution containing sodium chloride; sulfuric acid is used to adjust the pH to between 3 and 5. Ventolin Nebules inhalation solution contains no sulfiting agents or preservatives. Ventolin Nebules inhalation solution is a clear, colorless solution.

Ventolin Rotacaps: Ventolin Rotacaps are capsules for inhalation contain a dry powder presentation of albuterol sulfate intended for oral inhalation only. Each light blue and clear, hard gelatin capsule contains a mixture of 200 mcg of microfine (95% ≤10 µm) albuterol (as the sulfate) with 25 mg of lactose. The contents of each capsule are inhaled using a specially designed plastic device for inhaling powder called the Rotahaler. When turned, this device opens the capsule and facilitates dispersion of the albuterol sulfate into the airstream created when the patient inhales through the mouthpiece. Ventolin Rotacaps for inhalation are an alternative inhalation form of albuterol to the metered-dose pressurized inhaler.

CLINICAL PHARMACOLOGY:

ORAL FORMS

Albuterol is longer acting than isoproterenol in most patients by any route of administration because it is not a substrate for the cellular uptake processes for catecholamines nor for catechol-*O*-methyl transferase.

Animal studies show that albuterol does not pass the blood-brain barrier.

Tablets and Extended-Release Tablets: *In vitro* studies and *in vivo*pharmacologic studies have demonstrated that albuterol has a preferential effect on $beta_2$-adrenergic receptors compared with isoproterenol. While it is recognized that $beta_2$-adrenergic receptors are the predominant receptors in bronchial smooth muscle, recent data indicate that there is a population of $beta_2$-receptors in the human heart, existing in a concentration between 10% and 50%. The precise function of these receptors, however, is not yet established.

The pharmacologic effects of beta-adrenergic agonist drugs, including albuterol, are at least in part attributable to stimulation through beta-adrenergic receptors of intracellular adenyl cyclase, the enzyme that catalyzes the conversion of adenosine triphosphate (ATP) to cyclic-3', 5'-adenosine monophosphate (cyclic AMP). Increased cyclic AMP levels are associated with relaxation of bronchial smooth muscle and inhibition of release of mediators of immediate hypersensitivity from cells, especially from mast cells.

Albuterol has been shown in most controlled clinical trials to have more effect on the respiratory tract, in the form of bronchial smooth muscle relaxation, than isoproterenol at comparable doses while producing fewer cardiovascular effects. Controlled clinical studies and other clinical experience have shown that inhaled albuterol, like other beta-adrenergic agonist drugs, can produce a significant cardiovascular effect in some patients, as measured by pulse rate, blood pressure, symptoms, and/or electrocardiographic changes.

Albuterol is rapidly and well absorbed following oral administration. In studies involving normal volunteers, the mean steady-state peak and trough plasma levels of albuterol were 6.7 and 3.8 ng/ml, respectively, following dosing with a 2 mg albuterol tablet every 6 hours and 14.8 and 8.6 ng/ml, respectively, following dosing with a 4 mg albuterol tablet every 6 hours. Maximum albuterol plasma levels are usually obtained between 2 and 3 hours after dosing and the elimination half-life is 5 to 6 hours. These data indicate that albuterol, administered orally, is dose proportional and exhibits dose independent pharmacokinetics.

Albuterol extended-release tablets have been formulated to provide a duration of action of up to 12 hours. In studies conducted in normal volunteers, the mean steady-state peak and trough plasma levels of albuterol were 6.5 and 3.0 ng/ml, respectively, following dosing with a 4 mg albuterol extended-release tablet every 12 hours. In addition, it has been shown that administration of a 4 mg albuterol extended-release tablet every 12 hours is bioequivalent to administration of a 2 mg albuterol tablet every 6 hours.

Recent studies in laboratory animals (minipigs, rodents, and dogs) recorded the occurrence of cardiac arrhythmias and sudden death (with histologic evidence of myocardial necrosis) when beta-agonists and methylxanthines were administered concurrently. The significance of these findings when applied to humans is currently unknown.

In other studies, the analysis of urine samples of subjects given titrated albuterol (4-10 mg) orally showed that 65% to 90% of the dose was excreted over 3 days, with the majority of the dose being excreted within the first 24 hours. Sixty percent of this radioactivity was shown to be the metabolite of albuterol. Feces collected over this period contained 4% of the administered dose.

In controlled clinical trials in patients with asthma, the onset of improvement in pulmonary function, as measured by maximal midexpiratory flow rate, MMEF, was noted within 30 minutes after a dose of albuterol tablets with peak improvement occurring between 2 and 3 hours. In controlled clinical trials, in which measurements were conducted for 6 hours, significant clinical improvement in pulmonary function (defined as maintaining a 15% or more increase in FEV_1, and a 20% or more increase in MMEF over baseline values) was observed in 60% of patients at 4 hours and in 40% at 6 hours. In other single-dose, controlled clinical trials, clinically significant improvement was observed in at least 40% of the patients at 8 hours with the 4 mg albuterol tablet. No decrease in the effectiveness of albuterol tablets has been reported in patients who received long-term treatment with the drug in uncontrolled studies of periods up to 6 months.

In another controlled clinical study in asthmatic patients, it has been demonstrated that the initiation of therapy with either the 4 mg albuterol extended-release tablet dosed every 12 hours, or the 2 mg albuterol tablet dosed every 6 hours, achieve therapeutically equivalent effects.

Syrup: The prime action of beta-adrenergic drugs is to stimulate adenyl cyclase, the enzyme that catalyzes the formation of-3',5'-adenosine monophosphate (cyclic AMP) from adenosine triphosphate (ATP). The cyclic AMP thus formed mediates the cellular responses. Based on pharmacologic studies in animals, albuterol appears to exert direct and preferential action on $beta_2$-adrenoceptors, including those of the bronchial tree and uterus, and may have less cardiac stimulant effect than isoproterenol when given in the usual recommended dose.

After oral administration of 10 ml of albuterol syrup (4 mg of albuterol) in normal volunteers, albuterol is rapidly absorbed. Maximum plasma albuterol concentrations of about 18 ng/ml are achieved within 2 hours, and the drug is eliminated with a half-life of about 5 hours. In other studies, the analysis of urine samples of patients given 8 mg of titrated albuterol orally showed that 76% of the dose was excreted over 3 days, with the majority of the dose being excreted within the first 24 hours. Sixty percent of this radioactivity was shown to be the metabolite. Feces collected over this period contained 4% of the administered dose.

CLINICAL PHARMACOLOGY: *(cont'd)*

INHALATION FORMS

In vitro studies and *in vivo* pharmacologic studies have demonstrated that albuterol has a preferential effect on $beta_2$-adrenergic receptors compared with isoproterenol. While it is recognized that $beta_2$-adrenergic receptors are the predominant receptors in bronchial smooth muscle, recent data indicate that there is a population of $beta_2$-receptors in the human heart existing in a concentration between 10% and 50%. The precise function of these, however, is not yet established (see WARNINGS.)

The pharmacologic effects of beta-adrenergic agonist drugs, including albuterol, are at least in part attributable to stimulation through beta-adrenergic receptors of intracellular adenyl cyclase, the enzyme that catalyzes the conversion of adenosine triphosphate (ATP) to cyclic-3', 5'-adenosine monophosphate (cyclic AMP). Increased cyclic AMP levels are associated with relaxation of bronchial smooth muscle and inhibition of release of mediators of immediate hypersensitivity from cells, especially from mast cells.

Albuterol has been shown in most controlled clinical trials to have more effect on the respiratory tract, in the form of bronchial smooth muscle relaxation, than isoproterenol at comparable doses while producing fewer cardiovascular effects. Controlled clinical studies and other clinical experience have shown that inhaled albuterol, like other beta-adrenergic agonist drugs, can produce a significant cardiovascular effect in some patients, as measured by pulse rate, blood pressure, symptoms, and/or electrocardiographic changes.

Albuterol is longer acting than isoproterenol in most patients by any route of administration because it is not a substrate for the cellular uptake processes for catecholamines nor for catechol-*O*-methyl transferase.

Inhalation Aerosol: Because of its gradual absorption from the bronchi, systemic levels of albuterol are low after inhalation of recommended doses. Studies undertaken with four subjects administered tritiated albuterol resulted in maximum plasma concentrations occurring within 2 to 4 hours. Due to the sensitivity of the assay method, the metabolic rate and half-life of elimination of albuterol in plasma could not be determined. However, urinary excretion provided data indicating that albuterol has an elimination half-life of 3.8 hours. Approximately 72% of the inhaled dose is excreted within 24 hours in the urine, and consists of 28% as unchanged drug and 44% as metabolite.

Animal studies show that albuterol does not pass the blood-brain barrier.

Recent studies in laboratory animals (minipigs, rodents, and dogs) recorded the occurrence of cardiac arrhythmias and sudden death (with histologic evidence of myocardial necrosis) when beta-agonists and methylxanthines were administered concurrently. The significance of these findings when applied to humans is currently unknown.

The effects of rising doses of albuterol and isoproterenol aerosols were studied in volunteers and asthmatic patients. Results in normal volunteers indicated that albuterol is one half to one quarter as active as isoproterenol in producing increases in heart rate. In asthmatic patients similar cardiovascular differentiation between the two drugs was also seen.

In controlled clinical trials involving adults with asthma, the onset of improvement in pulmonary function was within 15 minutes, as determined by both MMEF (maximum midexpiratory flow rate) and FEV_1(forced expiratory volume in 1 second). MMEF measurements also showed that near maximum improvement in pulmonary function generally occurs within 60 to 90 minutes following two inhalations of albuterol and that clinically significant improvement generally continues for 3 to 4 hours in most patients. Some patients showed a therapeutic response (defined by maintaining FEV_1values 15% or more above baseline) that was still apparent at 6 hours. Continued effectiveness of albuterol was demonstrated over a 13-week period in these same trials.

In controlled clinical trials involving children 4 to 12 years of age, FEV_1 measurements showed that maximum improvement in pulmonary function occurs within 30 to 60 minutes. The onset of clinically significant (≥15%) improvement in FEV_1 was observed as soon as 5 minutes following 180 mcg of albuterol in 18 of 30 (60%) children in a controlled dose-ranging study. Clinically significant improvement in FEV_1 continued in the majority of patients for 2 hours and in 33% to 47% for 4 hours among 56 patients receiving inhalation aerosol in one pediatric study. In a second study among 48 patients receiving inhalation aerosol, clinically significant improvement continued in the majority for up to 1 hour and in 23% to 40% for 4 hours. In addition, at least 50% of the patients in both studies achieved an improvement in $FEF_{25\%-75\%}$ (forced expiratory flow rate between 25% and 75% of the forced vital capacity) of at least 20% for 2 to 5 hours. Continued effectiveness of albuterol was demonstrated over the 12-week study period.

In other clinical studies in adults and children, two inhalations of albuterol inhalation aerosol taken approximately 15 minutes before exercise prevented exercise-induced bronchospasm, as demonstrated by the maintenance of FEV_1 within 80% of baseline values in the majority of patients. One study in adults also evaluated the duration of the prophylactic effect to repeated exercise challenges, which was evident at 4 hours in the majority of patients and at 6 hours in approximately one third of the patients.

Inhalation Solution: Studies in asthmatic patients have shown that less than 20% of a single albuterol dose was absorbed following either intermittent positive- pressure breathing (IPPB) or nebulizer administration; the remaining amount was recovered from the nebulizer and apparatus and expired air. Most of the absorbed dose was recovered in the urine 24 hours after drug administration. Following a 3-mg dose of nebulized albuterol, the maximal albuterol plasma levels at 0.5 hours were 2.1 ng/ml (range, 1.4 to 3.2 ng/ml). There was a significant dose-related response in FEV_1(forced expiratory volume in 1 second) and peak flow rate. It has been demonstrated that following oral administration of 4 mg of albuterol, the elimination half-life was 5 to 6 hours.

Animal studies show that albuterol does not pass the blood-brain barrier. Recent studies in laboratory animals (minipigs, rodents, and dogs) recorded the occurrence of cardiac arrhythmias and sudden death (with histologic evidence of myocardial necrosis) when beta-agonists and methylxanthines were administered concurrently. The significance of these findings when applied to humans is currently unknown.

In controlled clinical trials, most patients exhibited an onset of improvement in pulmonary function within 5 minutes as determined by FEV_1. FEV_1 measurements also showed that the maximum average improvement in pulmonary function usually occurred at approximately 1 hour following inhalation of 2.5 mg of albuterol by compressor-nebulizer and remained close to peak for 2 hours. Clinically significant improvement in pulmonary function (defined as maintenance of a 15% or more increase in FEV_1 over baseline values) continued for 3 to 4 hours in most patients, with some patients continuing up to 6 hours.

In repetitive dose studies, continued effectiveness was demonstrated throughout the 3-month period of treatment in some patients.

Capsules for Inhalation: Studies undertaken with four subjects administered tritiated albuterol from a metered-dose aerosol inhaler resulted in maximum plasma concentrations occurring within 2 to 4 hours. Due to the sensitivity of the assay method, the metabolic rate and half-life of elimination of albuterol in plasma could not be determined. However, urinary excretion provided data indicating that albuterol has an elimination half-life of 3.8 hours. Approximately 72% of the inhaled dose is excreted within 24 hours in the urine, and consists of 28% as unchanged drug and 44% as metabolite.

Animal studies show that albuterol does not pass the blood-brain barrier.

CLINICAL PHARMACOLOGY: *(cont'd)*

Recent studies in laboratory animals (minipigs, rodents, and dogs) recorded the occurrence of cardiac arrhythmias and sudden death (with histologic evidence of myocardial necrosis) when beta-agonists and methylxanthines were administered concurrently. The significance of these findings when applied to humans is currently unknown.

In single, dose-range, crossover trials with albuterol capsules for inhalation in patients 12 years of age and older, the onset of improvement in pulmonary function was within 5 minutes as determined by a 15% increase in FEV_1 (forced expiratory volume in 1 second) following administration of either a 200- or 400-mcg dose. Maximum increases in FEV_1 occurred within 60 minutes following inhalation of either dose. The duration of effect (defined as an increase in $FEV_1$of 15% or greater in a single-dose study) was 1 to 2 hours after the 200-mcg dose and 3 to 4 hours after the 400-mcg dose. In a single-dose study, an increase in $FEF_{25\%-75\%}$ (forced expiratory flow rate between 25% and 75% of the forced vital capacity) of 20% or greater continued for 3 to 4 hours after the 200-mcg dose and for 3 to 6 hours following the 400-mcg dose. A therapeutic response continued for 4 hours in the majority of patients and for 6 hours in 38% of the patients following the 400-mcg dose. Twenty-two percent of the patients receiving the 200-mcg dose had a duration of effect of 8 hours.

In 12-week, double-blind, comparative evaluations in patients 12 years of age and older of one 200-mcg albuterol capsule for inhalation versus two inhalations of albuterol inhalation aerosol, the two dosage regimens were found to be equivalent. Based on a 15% or more increase in FEV_1 determinations, both provided a therapeutic response that persisted for 2 or 3 hours in 50% of 231 patients aged 12 years and older. Similar results were found in two controlled, 12-week clinical trials involving 204 children aged 4 to 11 years. Both formulations produced a therapeutic response (defined as maintenance of mean increase over baseline of at least 15% in FEV_1, or 20% in $FEF_{25\%-75\%}$). Therapeutic improvement of $FEF_{25\%-75\%}$ persisted for 3 to 5 hours in over 50% of the children throughout the study. Continued effectiveness and safety of albuterol capsules for inhalation were demonstrated over the 12-week study periods in both adults and children.

In other clinical studies in adults and children, one 200-mcg albuterol capsule for inhalation taken approximately 15 minutes before exercise prevented exercise-induced bronchospasm, as demonstrated by the maintenance of FEV_1 within 80% of baseline values in the majority of patients. One study in adults also evaluated the duration of the prophylactic effect to repeated exercise challenges, which was evident at 4 hours in the majority of patients and at 6 hours in approximately one third of the patients.

INDICATIONS AND USAGE:

ORAL FORMS

Albuterol tablets and extended-release tablets are indicated for the relief of bronchospasm in patients with reversible obstructive airway disease.

Albuterol syrup is indicated for the relief of bronchospasm in adults and in children 2 years of age and older with reversible obstructive airway disease.

In controlled clinical trials in patients with asthma, the onset of improvement in pulmonary function, as measured by maximum midexpiratory flow rate (MMEF) and forced expiratory volume in 1 second (FEV_1), was within 30 minutes after a dose of albuterol syrup. Peak improvement of pulmonary function occurred between 2 and 3 hours.

In controlled clinical trials, in which measurements were conducted for 6 hours, significant clinical improvement in pulmonary function (defined as maintaining a 15% or more increase in FEV_1, and a 20% or more increase in MMEF over baseline values) was observed in 60% of patients at 4 hours and in 40% at 6 hours. In other single-dose, controlled clinical trials, clinically significant improvement was observed in at least 40% of the patients at 8 hours with the 4 mg albuterol tablet. No decrease in the effectiveness of albuterol tablets has been reported in patients who received long-term treatment with the drug in uncontrolled studies of periods up to 6 months.

In a controlled clinical trial involving 55 children, clinically significant improvement (defined as maintenance of mean values over baseline of 15% or 20% or more in the FEV_1 and MMEF, respectively) continued to be recorded up to 6 hours. No decrease in the effectiveness was reported in one uncontrolled study of 32 children who took albuterol syrup for a 3-month period.

INHALATION FORMS

Inhalation Aerosol: Albuterol inhalation aerosol is indicated for the prevention and relief of bronchospasm in patients 4 years of age and older with reversible obstructive airway disease and for the prevention of exercise-induced bronchospasm in patients 4 years of age and older.

Albuterol inhalation aerosol can be used with or without concomitant steroid therapy.

Inhalation Solutions: Albuterol inhalation solution is indicated for the relief of bronchospasm in patients with reversible obstructive airway disease and acute attacks of bronchospasm.

Capsules for Inhalation: Albuterol capsules for inhalation are indicated for the prevention and relief of bronchospasm in patients 4 years of age and older with reversible obstructive airway disease and for the prevention of exercise-induced bronchospasm in patients 4 years of age and older. The capsules for inhalation formulation is particularly useful in patients who are unable to properly use the pressurized aerosol form of albuterol or who prefer an alternative formulation. Albuterol capsules for inhalation can be used with or without concomitant steroid therapy.

CONTRAINDICATIONS:

Albuterol is contraindicated in patients with a history of hypersensitivity to any of its components.

WARNINGS:

ORAL FORMS

Immediate hypersensitivity reactions may occur after administration of albuterol, as demonstrated by rare cases of urticaria, angioedema, anaphylaxis, rash, bronchospasm, and oropharyngeal edema.

Albuterol, like other beta-adrenergic agonists, can produce a significant cardiovascular effect in some patients, as measured by pulse rate, blood pressure, symptoms, and/or electrocardiographic changes.

Rarely, erythema multiforme and Stevens-Johnson syndrome have been associated with the administration of albuterol sulfate syrup in children.

INHALATION FORMS

As with other inhaled beta-adrenergic agonists, albuterol inhalation solution can produce paradoxical bronchospasm that can be life-threatening. If it occurs, the preparation should be discontinued immediately and alternative therapy instituted.

Fatalities have been reported in association with excessive use of inhaled sympathomimetic drugs and with the home use of nebulizers.The exact cause of death is unknown, but cardiac arrest following the unexpected development of a severe acute asthmatic crisis and subsequent hypoxia is suspected. It is therefore essential that the physician instruct the patient in the need for further evaluation if his/her asthma becomes worse. In individual patients, any $beta^2$-adrenergic agonist, including albuterol inhalation solution, may have a clinically significant cardiac effect.

WARNINGS: *(cont'd)*

Immediate hypersensitivity reactions may occur after administration of albuterol, as demonstrated by rare cases of urticaria, angioedema, rash, bronchospasm, and oropharyngeal edema.

Inhalation Aerosol: The contents of albuterol inhalation aerosol are under pressure. Do not puncture. Do not use or store near heat or open flame. Exposure to temperatures above 120°F may cause bursting. Never throw container into fire or incinerator. Keep out of reach of children.

Capsules for Inhalation: Inhalation of albuterol capsule particles may result if damage to the capsule has occurred from handling by the patient.

PRECAUTIONS:

GENERAL

Since albuterol is a sympathomimetic amine, it should be used with caution in patients with cardiovascular disorders, including ischemic heart disease, hypertension, or cardiac arrhythmias, in patients with hyperthyroidism or diabetes mellitus, and in patients who are unusually responsive to sympathomimetic amines or who have convulsive disorders. Significant changes in systolic and diastolic blood pressure could be expected to occur in some patients after use of any beta adrenergic bronchodilator.

Large doses of intravenous albuterol have been reported to aggravate preexisting diabetes mellitus and ketoacidosis. Additionally, albuterol and other beta agonists, when given intravenously or inhaled, may cause a decrease in serum potassium, possibly through intracellular shunting. The decrease is usually transient, not requiring supplementation. The relevance of these observations to the use of albuterol tablets and extended-release tablets is unknown.

Inhalation Aerosol and Solution: Albuterol, as with all sympathomimetic amines, should be used with caution in patients with cardiovascular disorders, especially coronary insufficiency, cardiac arrhythmias, and hypertension; in patients with convulsive disorders, hyperthyroidism, or diabetes mellitus; and in patients who are unusually responsive to sympathomimetic amines.

Large doses of intravenous albuterol have been reported to aggravate pre-existing diabetes mellitus and ketoacidosis. As with other beta-agonists, inhaled and intravenous albuterol may produce significant hypokalemia in some patients, possibly through intracellular shunting, which has the potential to produce adverse cardiovascular effects. The decrease is usually transient, not requiring supplementation.

Aerosol and Capsules for Inhalation: Although there have been no reports concerning the use of albuterol inhalation during labor and delivery, it has been reported that high doses of albuterol administered intravenously inhibit uterine contractions. Although this effect is extremely unlikely as a consequence of use, it should be kept in mind.

Capsules for Inhalation: Although no effect on the cardiovascular system is usually seen after the administration of inhaled albuterol at recommended doses, cardiovascular and central nervous system (CNS) effects seen with all sympathomimetic drugs can occur after use of inhaled albuterol and may require discontinuation of the drug. As with all sympathomimetic amines, albuterol should be used with caution in patients with cardiovascular disorders, including coronary insufficiency, hypertension, and cardiac arrhythmia; in patients with hyperthyroidism or diabetes mellitus; in patients who are unusually responsive to sympathomimetic amines; and in patients with convulsive disorders. Clinically significant changes in systolic and diastolic blood pressure have been seen in individual patients and could be expected to occur in some patients after use of any beta-adrenergic bronchodilator. As with other beta-agonists, inhaled and intravenous albuterol may produce significant hypokalemia in some patients, possibly through intracellular shunting, which has the potential to produce adverse cardiovascular effects. The decrease is usually transient, not requiring supplementation.

INFORMATION FOR THE PATIENT

Tablets and Extended-Release Tablets: Patients being treated with albuterol tablets or extended-release tablets should receive the following information and instructions. This information is intended to aid in the safe and effective use of this medication. It is not a disclosure of all possible adverse or intended effects.

Albuterol tablets and extended-release tablets should not be taken more frequently than recommended. Do not increase the dose or frequency of medication, or add other medications to your therapy without medical consultation. If symptoms get worse, medical consultation should be sought promptly. If pregnant or nursing, consult your physician.

Syrup: The action of albuterol syrup may last up to 6 hours and therefore it should not be taken more frequently than recommended. Do not increase the dose or frequency of medication without medical consultation. If symptoms get worse, medical consultation should be sought promptly. If pregnant or nursing, consult with your physician.

Inhalation Forms: The action of albuterol inhalation aerosol may last up to 6 hours, and therefore it should not be used more frequently than recommended. Do not increase the number or frequency of doses without medical consultation. If recommended dosage does not provide relief of symptoms or symptoms become worse, seek immediate medical attention. While taking albuterol inhalation, other inhaled antiasmatic drugs should not be used unless prescribed.

Children should use albuterol inhalation aerosol or capsules under adult supervision, as instructed by the patient's physician.

Inhalation Aerosol: In general, the technique for administering albuterol inhalation aerosol to children is similar to that for adults, since children's smaller ventilatory exchange capacity automatically provides proportionally smaller aerosol intake.

Inhalation Solutions: Drug compatibility (physical and chemical), efficacy, and safety of albuterol inhalation solution when mixed with other drugs in a nebulizer have not been established.

CARCINOGENESIS, MUTAGENESIS, AND IMPAIRMENT OF FERTILITY

Oral Forms: Albuterol sulfate, like other agents in its class, caused a significant dose-related increase in the incidence of benign leiomyomas of the mesovarium in a 2-year study in the rat, at doses corresponding to 3, 16, and 78 times the maximum human oral dose [or in syrup study 2, 9, and 46 times the maximum human (child weighing 21 kg) oral dose]. In another study this effect was blocked by the coadministration of propranolol. The relevance of these findings to humans is not known. An 18-month study in mice and a lifetime study in hamsters revealed no evidence of tumorigenicity. Studies with albuterol revealed no evidence of mutagenesis. Reproduction studies in rats revealed no evidence of impaired fertility.

Inhalations Forms: Albuterol sulfate caused a significant dose-related increase in the incidence of benign leiomyomas of the mesovarium in a 2-year study in the rat at oral doses of 2, 10, and 50 mg/kg, corresponding to 93, 463, and 2315 [10, 50, and 250 (solution)] [42, 208, and 1042 (capsules)] times, respectively, the maximum inhalational dose for a 50-kg human. In another study this effect was blocked by the coadministration of propranolol. The relevance of these findings to humans is not known. An 18-month study in mice [at doses corresponding to 10,417 times the human inhalational dose (capsules)] and a lifetime study in hamsters [at doses corresponding to 1,042 times the human inhalational dose (capsules)] revealed no evidence of tumorigenicity. Studies with albuterol revealed no evidence of mutagenesis. Reproduction studies in rats revealed no evidence of impaired fertility.

PRECAUTIONS: *(cont'd)*

PREGNANCY, TERATOGENIC EFFECTS, PREGNANCY CATEGORY C

Tablets and Extended-Release Tablets: Albuterol has been shown to be teratogenic in mice when given subcutaneously in doses corresponding to 0.4 times the maximum human oral dose [in syrup study 0.2 times the maximum human (child weighing 21 kg) oral dose]. There are no adequate and well-controlled studies in pregnant women. Albuterol should be used during pregnancy only if the potential benefit justifies the potential risk to the fetus. A reproduction study in CD-1 mice with albuterol showed cleft palate formation in 5 of 111 (4.5%) fetuses at 0.25 mg/kg and in 10 of 108 (9.3%) fetuses at 2.5 mg/kg; none were observed at 0.025 mg/kg. Cleft palate also occurred in 22 of 72 (30.5%) fetuses treated with 2.5 mg/kg isoproterenol (positive control). A reproduction study in Stride Dutch rabbits revealed cranioschisis in 7 of 19 (37%) fetuses at 50 mg/kg, corresponding to 78 times the maximum human oral dose of albuterol.

During marketing, various congenital anomalies, including cleft palate and limb defects, have been reported in the offspring of patients being treated with albuterol. Some of the mothers were taking multiple medications during their pregnancies. Because no consistent pattern of defects can be discerned, a relationship between albuterol use and congenital anomalies cannot be established.

Inhalation Forms: Albuterol has been shown to be teratogenic in mice when given in doses corresponding to 14 [1.25 (solution)] [5 (capsules)] times the human dose. There are no adequate and well-controlled studies in pregnant women. Albuterol should be used during pregnancy only if the potential benefit justifies the potential risk to the fetus. A reproduction study in CD-1 mice given albuterol subcutaneously (0.025, 0.25, and 2.5 mg/kg, corresponding to 1.15, 11.5, and 115 [0.125, 1.25, and 12.5 (solution)] [0.52, 5.2, and 52 (capsules)] times, respectively, the maximum inhalational dose for a 50-kg human) showed cleft palate formation in 5 of 111 (4.5%) fetuses at 0.25 mg/kg and in 10 of 108 (9.3%) fetuses at 2.5 mg/kg. None was observed at 0.025 mg/kg. Cleft palate also occurred in 22 of 72 (30.5%) fetuses treated with 2.5 mg/kg of isoproterenol (positive control). A reproduction study with oral albuterol in Stride Dutch rabbits revealed cranioschisis in 7 of 19 (37%) fetuses at 50 mg/kg, corresponding to 2315 [250 (solution)] [1042 (capsules)] times the maximum inhalational dose for a 50-kg human.

During worldwide marketing experience, various congenital anomalies, including cleft palate and limb defects, have been rarely reported in the offspring of patients being treated with albuterol. Some of the mothers were taking multiple medications during their pregnancies. No consistent pattern of defects can be discerned, and a relationship between albuterol use and congenital anomalies has not been established.

LABOR AND DELIVERY

Oral albuterol has been shown to delay preterm labor in some reports. There are presently no well-controlled studies that demonstrate that it will stop preterm labor or prevent labor at term. Therefore, cautious use of albuterol is required in pregnant patients when given for relief of bronchospasm so as to avoid interference with uterine contractility. Use in such patients should be restricted to those patients in whom the benefits clearly outweigh the risks.

Use in such patients should be restricted to those patients in whom the benefits clearly outweigh the risks.

NURSING MOTHERS

It is not known whether this drug is excreted in human milk. Because of the potential for tumorigenicity shown for albuterol in animal studies, a decision should be made whether to discontinue nursing or to discontinue the drug, taking into account the importance of the drug to the mother.

PEDIATRIC USE

Tablets and Extended-Release Tablets: Safety and effectiveness in children below the age of 6 years for albuterol tablets, and below the age of 12 years for albuterol extended-release tablets have not been established.

Syrup: Safety and effectiveness in children below the age of 2 years have not yet been adequately demonstrated.

Inhalation Aerosol and Capsules for Inhalation: Safety and effectiveness in children below 4 years of age have not been established.

Inhalation Solutions: Safety and effectiveness in children below 12 years of age have not been established.

DRUG INTERACTIONS:

ORAL FORMS

The concomitant use of albuterol and other oral sympathomimetic agents is not recommended since such combined use may lead to deleterious cardiovascular effects. This recommendation does not preclude the judicious use of an aerosol bronchodilator of the adrenergic stimulant type in patients receiving albuterol tablets or syrup. Such concomitant use, however, should be individualized and not given on a routine basis. If regular coadministration is required, then alternative therapy should be considered.

Albuterol should be administered with extreme caution to patients being treated with monoamine oxidase inhibitors or tricyclic antidepressants, since the action of albuterol on the vascular system may be potentiated.

Beta-receptor blocking agents and albuterol inhibit the effect of each other.

Since albuterol may lower serum potassium, care should be taken in patients also using other drugs which lower serum potassium as the effects may be additive.

After single-dose administration of albuterol to normal volunteers who had received digoxin for 10 days, a 16% to 22% decrease in serum digoxin levels was demonstrated. The clinical significance of these findings for patients with obstructive airway disease who are receiving albuterol and digoxin on a chronic basis is unclear. Nevertheless, it would be prudent to carefully evaluate the serum digoxin levels in patients who are concurrently receiving digoxin and albuterol.

ADVERSE REACTIONS:

ORAL FORMS

In addition to the reactions listed separately below, albuterol, like other sympathomimetic agents, can cause adverse reactions such as hypertension, angina, vomiting, vertigo, CNS stimulation, unusual taste, and drying or irritation of the oropharynx.

The reactions are generally transient in nature, and it is usually not necessary to discontinue treatment with albuterol extended-release tablets or albuterol tablets. In selected cases, however, dosage may be reduced temporarily; after the reaction has subsided, dosage should be increased in small increments to the optimal dosage.

Tablets and Extended-Release Tablets: The adverse reactions to albuterol are similar in nature to those of other sympathomimetic agents. The most frequent adverse reactions to albuterol tablets were nervousness and tremor, with each occurring in approximately 20 of 100 patients (20%). Other reported reactions were headache, 7 of 100 patients (7%); tachycardia and palpitations, 5 of 100 patients (5%); muscle cramps, 3 of 100 patients (3%); insomnia, nausea, weakness, and dizziness, each occurred in 2 of 100 patients (2%). Drowsiness, flushing, restlessness, irritability, chest discomfort, and difficulty in micturition each occurred in fewer than 1 of 100 patients (less than 1%).

ADVERSE REACTIONS: *(cont'd)*

In a clinical study of 1 week duration comparing a 4 mg albuterol extended-release tablet administered every 12 hours to a 2 mg albuterol tablet administered every 6 hours, the following adverse reactions considered to be possibly or probably treatment related were reported: nervousness in 1 of 50 (2%) and 3 of 50 patients (6%) for albuterol extended-release and albuterol tablets, respectively; nausea in 2 of 50 (4%) for both; vomiting in 1 of 50 (2%) and 2 of 50 (4%) for albuterol extended-release and albuterol tablets, respectively; somnolence in 1 of 50 (2%) for both. The following adverse reactions were reported for albuterol tablets only: tremor in 3 of 50 patients (6%), tinnitus, dyspepsia, and rash each occurred in 1 of 50 patients (2%).

Rare cases of urticaria, angioedema, rash, bronchospasm, and oropharyngeal edema have been reported after the use of albuterol.

Although not reported for albuterol extended-release tablets in the above study, there have been reports of tremor in other trials. When all clinical experience is considered, the incidence of tremor is approximately the same as that seen with albuterol tablets.

In addition to those adverse reactions reported above, albuterol, like other sympathomimetic agents, can cause adverse reactions such as hypertension, angina, vomiting, vertigo, central nervous system stimulation, unusual taste, and drying or irritation of the oropharynx.

Syrup: The adverse reactions to albuterol are similar in nature to those to other sympathomimetic agents. The most frequent adverse reactions to albuterol syrup in adults and older children were tremor, 10 of 100 patients; nervousness and shakiness, each 9 of 100 patients. Other reported adverse reactions were headache, 4 of 100 patients; dizziness and increased appetite, each 3 of 100 patients; hyperactivity and excitement, each 2 of 100 patients; tachycardia, epistaxis, irritable behavior, and sleeplessness, each 1 of 100 patients. The following adverse effects occurred in less than 1 of 100 patients each: muscle spasm, disturbed sleep, epigastric pain, cough, palpitations, stomachache, irritable behavior, dilated pupils, sweating, chest pain, weakness.

In young children 2 to 6 years of age, some adverse reactions were noted more frequently than in adults and older children. Excitement was noted in approximately 20% of patients and nervousness in 15%. Hyperkinesia occurred in 4% of patients, insomnia, tachycardia, and gastrointestinal symptoms in 2% each. Anorexia, emotional lability, pallor, fatigue, and conjunctivitis were seen in 1%.

INHALATION FORMS

Inhalation Aerosol

The adverse reactions to albuterol are similar in nature to reactions to other sympathomimetic agents, although the incidence of certain cardiovascular effects is lower with albuterol.

A 13-week, double-blind study compared albuterol and isoproterenol aerosols in 147 asthmatic patients aged 12 years and older. The results of this study showed that the incidence of cardiovascular effects was: palpitations, fewer than 10 per 100 with albuterol and fewer than 15 per 100 with isoproterenol; tachycardia, 10 per 100 with both albuterol and isoproterenol; and increased blood pressure, fewer than 5 per 100 with both albuterol and isoproterenol. In the same study, both drugs caused tremor or nausea in fewer than 15 patients per 100, and dizziness or heartburn in fewer than 5 per 100 patients. Nervousness occurred in fewer than 10 per 100 patients receiving albuterol and in fewer than 15 per 100 patients receiving isoproterenol.

Twelve-week, double-blind studies involving the use of albuterol inhalation aerosol 180 mcg q.i.d. by 104 asthmatic children aged 4 to 11 years showed the following side effects:

Central Nervous System: Headache, 3 of 104 patients (3%); nervousness, lightheadedness, agitation, nightmares, hyperactivity, and aggressive behavior, each in 1%.

Gastrointestinal: Nausea and/or vomiting, 6 of 104 (6%); stomachache, 3 of 104 (3%); diarrhea in 1%.

Oropharyngeal: Throat irritation, 6 of 104 (6%); discoloration of teeth in 1%.

Respiratory: Epistaxis, 3 of 104 (3%); coughing, 2 of 104 (2%).

Musculoskeletal: Tremor and muscle cramp, each in 1%.

Rare cases of urticaria, angioedema, rash, bronchospasm, hoarseness, and oropharyngeal edema have been reported after the use of inhaled albuterol.

In addition, albuterol, like other sympathomimetic agents, can cause adverse reactions such as hypertension, angina, vertigo, central nervous system stimulation, insomnia, and unusual taste.

Inhalation Solutions

The results of clinical trials with albuterol inhalation solution, 0.5% in 135 patients showed the following side effects that were considered probably or possibly drug related:

Central Nervous System: Tremors (20%), dizziness (7%), nervousness (4%), headache (3%), insomnia (1%).

Gastrointestinal: Nausea (4%), dyspepsia (1%).

Ear, Nose and Throat: Pharyngitis (<1%), nasal congestion (1%).

Cardiovascular: Tachycardia (1%), hypertension (1%).

Respiratory: Bronchospasm (8%), cough (4%), bronchitis (4%), wheezing (1%).

No clinically relevant laboratory abnormalities related to albuterol inhalation solution administration were determined in these studies.

In comparing the adverse reactions reported for patients treated with albuterol inhalation solution with those of patients treated with isoproterenol during clinical trials of 3 months, the following moderate to severe reactions, as judged by the investigators, were reported. TABLE 1 does not include mild reactions.

Rare cases of urticaria, angioedema, rash, bronchospasm, and oropharyngeal edema have been reported after the use of inhaled albuterol.

Capsules for Inhalation

The adverse reactions to albuterol are similar in nature to reactions to other sympathomimetic agents, although the incidence of certain cardiovascular effects is lower with albuterol. Results of clinical trials with albuterol capsules for inhalation 200 mcg in 172 patients aged 12 years and older (adults) and 129 patients aged 4 to 12 years (children) showed the following side effects:

CNS: *Adults:*Headache in 4 of 172 patients (2%); nervousness in 2 of 172 (1%); dizziness, insomnia, lightheadedness, each in <1%. *Children:*Headache in 6 of 129 (5%); dizziness and hyperactivity, each in <1%.

Gastrointestinal: *Adults:*Burning in stomach in <1%. *Children:*Nausea and/or vomiting in 5 of 129 (4%), stomachache in 2 of 129 (2%), diarrhea in <1%.

Oropharyngeal: *Adults:*Throat irritation in 3 of 172 (2%); dry mouth and voice changes, each in <1%. *Children:*Throat irritation in 3 of 129 (2%); unusual taste in 2 of 129 (2%).

Respiratory: *Adults:*Cough in 8 of 172 (5%), bronchospasm in 2 of 172 (1%). *Children:*Cough and nasal congestion, each in 3 of 129 (2%); hoarseness and epistaxis, each in 2 of 129 (2%).

Musculoskeletal: *Adults:*Tremor in 2 of 172 (1%). *Children:*None reported.

Rare cases of urticaria, angioedema, rash, hoarseness, and oropharyngeal edema have been reported after the use of inhaled albuterol.

ADVERSE REACTIONS: *(cont'd)*

TABLE 1 Percent Incidence of Moderate To Severe Adverse Reactions
Inhalation Solutions

Reaction	Albuterol n=65	Isoproterenol n=65
Central Nervous System		
Tremor	10.7%	13.8%
Headache	3.1%	1.5%
Insomnia	3.1%	1.5%
Cardiovascular		
Hypertension	3.1%	3.1%
Arrhythmias	0%	3.0%
Palpitation*	0%	22.0%
Respiratory		
Bronchospasm†	15.4%	18.0%
Cough	3.1%	5.0%
Bronchitis	1.5%	5.0%
Wheezing	1.5%	1.5%
Sputum Increase	1.5%	1.5%
Dyspnea	1.5%	1.5%
Gastrointestinal		
Nausea	3.1%	0%
Dyspepsia	1.5%	0%
Systemic		
Malaise	1.5%	0%

* The finding of no arrhythmias and no palpitations after albuterol administration in this clinical study should not be interpreted as indicating that these adverse effects cannot occur after the administration of inhaled albuterol.
† In most cases of bronchospasm, this term was generally used to describe exacerbations in the underlying pulmonary disease.

In addition, albuterol, like other sympathomimetic agents, can cause adverse reactions such as hypertension, angina, vertigo, and CNS stimulation.

OVERDOSAGE:

The expected symptoms with overdosage are those of excessive beta-stimulation and/or occurrence or exaggeration of any of the symptoms listed under ADVERSE REACTIONS (*e.g.,* seizures, angina, hypertension or hypotension, tachycardia with rates up to 200 beats per minute, arrhythmias, nervousness, headache, tremor, dry mouth, palpitation, nausea, dizziness, fatigue, malaise, and insomnia). Hypokalemia may also occur.

Treatment consists of discontinuation of albuterol together with appropriate symptomatic therapy.

The oral LD_{50} in male and female rats and mice was greater than 2000 mg/kg.

There is insufficient evidence to determine if dialysis is beneficial for overdosage of albuterol tablets. Dialysis is not appropriate treatment for overdosage of albuterol syrup.

INHALATION FORMS

The expected symptoms with overdosage are those of excessive beta-stimulation and/or occurrence or exaggeration of any of the symptoms listed under ADVERSE REACTIONS, e.g., seizures, angina, hypertension or hypotension, tachycardia with rates up to 200 beats per minute, arrhythmias, nervousness, headache, tremor, dry mouth, palpitation, nausea, dizziness, fatigue, malaise, and insomnia. Hypokalemia may also occur.

The oral LD_{50} in male and female rats and mice was greater than 2000 mg/kg. The inhalational LD_{50}could not be determined.

As with all sympathomimetic aerosol medications, cardiac arrest and even death may be associated with abuse.

Treatment consists of discontinuation of albuterol solution together with appropriate symptomatic therapy.

Inhalation Aerosol: Dialysis is not appropriate treatment for overdosage of albuterol inhalation aerosol. The judicious use of a cardioselective beta-receptor blocker, such as metoprolol tartrate, is suggested, bearing in mind the danger of inducing an asthmatic attack.

Inhalation Solutions: There is insufficient evidence to determine if dialysis is beneficial for overdosage of albuterol inhalation solution.

Capsules for Inhalation: Dialysis is not appropriate treatment for overdosage of albuterol capsules for inhalation.

DOSAGE AND ADMINISTRATION:

ORAL FORMS

Tablets

The following dosages of albuterol tablets and extended-release tablets are expressed in terms of albuterol base.

Extended-Release Tablets

Usual Dose: The usual starting dosage of albuterol extended-release tablets for adults and children 12 years and over is 4 or 8 mg (one or two tablets) every 12 hours.

Dosage Adjustment: Doses of albuterol extended-release tablets above 8 mg twice a day should be used only when the patient fails to respond to lower doses. The dose should be increased cautiously stepwise up to a maximum of 16 mg twice a day if a favorable response does not occur with the 4 mg initial dose.

The total daily dose should not exceed 32 mg in adults and children 12 years and over.

Switching to Albuterol Extended-Release Tablets: Patients currently maintained on albuterol tablets can be switched to albuterol extended-release tablets. For example, the administration of a 4 mg albuterol extended-release tablet every 12 hours is equivalent to one 2 mg albuterol tablet every 6 hours. Multiples of this regimen up to the maximum recommended daily dose also apply.

Tablets

Usual Dosage: The usual starting dosage for children 6 to 12 years of age is 2 mg three or four times a day.

The usual starting dosage for adults and children 12 years and over is 2 mg or 4 mg three or four times a day.

Dosage Adjustment: For children from 6 to 12 years of age who fail to respond to the initial starting dosage of 2 mg four times a day, the dosage may be cautiously increased stepwise, but not to exceed 24 mg per day (given in divided doses).

For adults and children 12 years and over, a dosage above 4 mg four times a day should be used only when the patient fails to respond to lower doses. The dose should be increased cautiously stepwise up to a maximum of 8 mg four times a day as tolerated if a favorable response does not occur with the 4 mg initial dose.

DOSAGE AND ADMINISTRATION: *(cont'd)*

Elderly Patients and Those Sensitive to Beta-Adrenergic Stimulators: An initial dosage of 2 mg three or four times a day is recommended for elderly patients and for those with a history of unusual sensitivity to beta-adrenergic stimulators. If adequate bronchodilation is not obtained, dosage may be increased gradually to as much as 8 mg three or four times a day.

The total daily dose should not exceed 32 mg in adults and children 12 years and over.

Syrup

The following dosages of albuterol syrup are expressed in terms of albuterol base.

Usual Dosage: The usual starting dosage for adults and children over 14 years of age is 2 mg (1 teaspoonful) or 4 mg (2 teaspoonfuls) three or four times a day.

The usual starting dosage for children 6 to 14 years of age is 2 mg (1 teaspoonful) three or four times a day.

For children 2 to 6 years of age, dosing should be initiated at 0.1 mg/kg of body weight three times a day. This starting dosage should not exceed 2 mg (1 teaspoonful) three times a day.

Dosage Adjustment: For adults and children over age 14, a dosage above 4 mg four times a day should be used *only* when the patient fails to respond. If a favorable response does not occur, the dosage may be cautiously increased stepwise, but the dosage should not exceed 8 mg four times a day.

For children from 6 to 14 years of age who fail to respond to the initial starting dosage of 2 mg four times a day, the dosage may be cautiously increased stepwise, but not to exceed 24 mg per day (given in divided doses).

For children 2 to 6 years of age who do not respond satisfactorily to the initial dosage, the dosage may be increased stepwise to 0.2 mg/kg of body weight three times a day, but not to exceed a maximum of 4 mg (2 teaspoonfuls) given three times a day.

For elderly patients and those sensitive to beta-adrenergic stimulation, the initial dosage should be restricted to 2 mg three or four times a day and individually adjusted thereafter.

INHALATION FORMS

The use of albuterol inhalation can be continued as medically indicated to control recurring bouts of bronchospasm. During this time most patients gain optimal benefit from regular use. Safe usage for periods extending over several years has been documented.

If a previously effective dosage regimen fails to provide the usual relief, medical advice should be sought immediately as this is often a sign of seriously worsening asthma which would require reassessment of therapy.

Drug compatibility (physical and chemical), efficacy, and safety of albuterol inhalation solution when mixed with other drugs in a nebulizer have not been established.

Inhalation Aerosol

For treatment of acute episodes of bronchospasm or prevention of asthmatic symptoms, the usual dosage for adults and children 4 years of age and older is two inhalations repeated every 4 to 6 hours; in some patients, one inhalation every 4 hours may be sufficient. More frequent administration or a larger number of inhalations are not recommended.

Exercise-Induced Bronchospasm Prevention: The usual dosage for adults and children 4 years and older is two inhalations 15 minutes before exercise.

Inhalation Solution, 0.5%

To avoid cross contamination, proper aseptic technique should be used.

The usual dosage for adults and children 12 years and older is 2.5 mg of albuterol administered three to four times daily by nebulization. More frequent administration or higher doses are not recommended. To administer 2.5 mg of albuterol, dilute 0.5 ml of the 0.5% inhalation solution with 2.5 ml of sterile normal saline solution. The flow rate is regulated to suit the particular nebulizer so that the albuterol inhalation solution will be delivered over approximately 5 to 15 minutes.

Inhalation Solution, 0.083%

The usual dosage for adults and children 12 years and older is 2.5 mg of albuterol administered three to four times daily by nebulization. More frequent administration or higher doses are not recommended. To administer 2.5 mg of albuterol, administer the contents of one sterile unit dose nebule (3 ml of 0.083% inhalation solution) by nebulization. The flow rate is regulated to suit the particular nebulizer so that albuterol inhalation solution will be delivered over approximately 5 to 15 minutes.

Capsules for Inhalation

The usual dosage of capsules for inhalation for adults and children 4 years of age and older is the contents of one 200-mcg capsule inhaled every 4 to 6 hours using a Rotahaler inhalation device. In some patients, the contents of two 200-mcg capsules inhaled every 4 to 6 hours may be required. Larger doses or more frequent administration is not recommended.

Exercise-Induced Bronchospasm Prevention: The usual dosage of albuterol capsules for inhalation for adults and children 4 years of age and older is the contents of one 200-mcg capsule inhaled using a Rotahaler 15 minutes before exercise.

PATIENT PACKAGE INSERT:

VENTOLIN INHALATION AEROSOL

Before using your Ventolin inhalation aerosol, read complete instructions carefully. Children should use Ventolin inhalation aerosol under adult supervision, as instructed by the patient's doctor. The refill canister is to be used only with the blue inhalation aerosol adapter.

1. **Shake The Inhaler Well** immediately before each use. **Then remove the cap from the mouthpiece;** the strap on the cap will stay attached to the actuator. If the strap is removed from the actuator and lost, the inhaler mouthpiece should be inspected for the presence of foreign objects before each use. Make sure the cannister is fully and firmly inserted into the actuator.

2. **BREATHE OUT FULLY THROUGH THE MOUTH,** expelling as much air from your lungs as possible. Place the mouthpiece fully into the mouth, holding the inhaler in its upright position and closing the lips around it.

3. **WHILE BREATHING IN DEEPLY AND SLOWLY THROUGH THE MOUTH. FULLY DEPRESS THE TOP OF THE METAL CANISTER** with your index finger.

4. **HOLD YOUR BREATH AS LONG AS POSSIBLE.** Before breathing out, remove the inhaler from your mouth and release your finger from the canister.

5. Wait one minute and **SHAKE** the inhaler again. Repeat steps 2 through 4 for each inhalation prescribed by your doctor.

6. **CLEANSE THE INHALER THOROUGHLY AND FREQUENTLY.** Remove the metal canister and cleanse the plastic case and cap by rinsing thoroughly in warm, running water at least once a day. After thoroughly drying the plastic case and cap, gently replace the canister into the case with a twisting motion and put the cap back on the mouthpiece.

7. As with all aerosol medications, it is recommended to "test spray" into the air before using for the first time and in cases where the aerosol has not been used for a prolonged period of time.

8. **DISCARD THE CANISTER AFTER YOU HAVE USED THE LABELED NUMBER OF INHALATIONS.** The correct amount of medication in each inhalation cannot be assured after this point.

The refill canister is to be used only with the blue Ventolin inhalation adapter.

PATIENT PACKAGE INSERT: *(cont'd)*

Dosage: Use only as directed by your doctor.
Warnings: The action of Ventolin inhalation aerosol may last up to 6 hours, and therefore it should not be used more frequently than recommended. Do not increase the number or frequency of doses without consulting your doctor. If recommended dosage does not provide relief of symptoms or symptoms become worse, seek immediate medical attention. While taking Ventolin inhalation aerosol, other inhaled medicines should be used only as prescribed by your doctor.
Contents Under Pressure: Do not puncture. Do not use or store near heat or open flame. Exposure to temperatures above 120°F may cause bursting. Never throw container into fire or incinerator. Keep out of reach of children.
Store between 15° and 30°C (59° and 86°F). As with most inhaled medications in aerosol canisters, the therapeutic effect of this medication may decrease when the canister is cold. Shake well before using.

VENTOLIN INHALATION SOLUTION, 0.5%

Patient's Instructions for Use. *Potency expressed as albuterol. Read complete instructions carefully before using.

1. Draw 0.5 ml of Ventolin inhalation solution into the specially marked dropper that comes with each multidose bottle.

2. Squeeze the solution into the nebulizer reservoir through the appropriate opening.

3. Add 2.5 ml of sterile normal saline solution, as your doctor has directed.

4. Gently swirl the nebulizer to mix the contents and connect it with the mouthpiece or face mask.

5. Connect the nebulizer to the compressor.

6. Sit in a comfortable, upright position; place the mouthpiece in your mouth (or put on the face mask); and turn on the compressor.

7. Breathe as calmly, deeply, and evenly as possible until no more mist is formed in the nebulizer chamber (about 5 to 15 minutes). At this point, the treatment is finished.

8. Clean the nebulizer (see manufacturer's instructions).

Note: Use only as directed by your doctor. More frequent administration or higher doses are not recommended.

Drug compatibility (physical and chemical), efficacy, and safety of Ventolin inhalation solution when mixed with other drugs in a nebulizer have not been established.

Store between 2° and 25°C (36° and 77°F).

VANTOLIN NEBULES INHALATION SOLUTION, 0.083%

Patient's Instructions for Use. *Potency expressed as albuterol. Read complete instructions carefully before using.

1. Twist open the top of one Nebule unit-of-use dose container and squeeze the contents into the nebulizer reservoir.

2. Connect the nebulizer reservoir to the mouthpiece or face mask.

3. Connect the nebulizer to the compressor.

4. Sit in a comfortable, upright position; place the mouthpiece in your mouth (or put on the face mask); and turn on the compressor.

5. Breathe as calmly, deeply, and evenly as possible until no more mist is formed in the nebulizer chamber (about 5 to 15 minutes). At this point, the treatment is finished.

6. Clean the nebulizer (see manufacturer's instructions).

Note: Use only as directed by your doctor. More frequent administration or higher doses are not recommended.

Drug compatibility (physical and chemical), efficacy, and safety of Ventolin inhalation solution when mixed with other drugs in a nebulizer have not been established.

Protect from light. Store in a refrigerator between 2° and 8°C (36° and 46°F). Inhalation solution may be held at room temperature for up to 2 weeks before use. (Nebules must be used within 2 weeks of removal from refrigerator; record date the nebules are removed from the refrigerator in the space provided on the product carton.) Discard if solution becomes discolored. (Note: Inhalation solution is colorless.)

VENTOLIN ROTACAPS CAPSULES FOR INHALATION

Patient's Instructions for Use. Instructions for Administration of Ventolin Rotacaps with the Rotahaler Inhalation Device

Note: Ventolin Rotacaps should be stored in a dry place and not exposed to temperature extremes. Ventolin Rotacaps should be stored below 86°F. Do not remove Ventolin Rotacaps from the original packaging until you are ready to use the Rotahaler inhalation device.

Bottle Packs: Store Ventolin Rotacaps in the original bottle. You may transfer a daily supply of capsules to the smaller, reusable bottle that fits into the carrying case. Do not remove capsules from the bottle until you are ready to use the Rotahaler inhalation device.

Hospital Unit Dose Pack: To remove a capsule from a unit dose blister pack, tear off one section of the paper backing starting at the corner marked "PEEL."

The Ventolin Rotacaps for inhalation capsule appears partially filled; the partial filling of dry powder facilitates the delivery of the medication.

Children should use Ventolin Rotacaps under adult supervision, as instructed by the patient's doctor.

Preparing the Rotahaler For Use:

1. Remove the Rotahaler from its container and check to be sure it is clean and dry. Inspect the mouthpiece for the presence of foreign objects before each use.

2. Keeping the Rotahaler upright (vertical), hold the darker colored end in one hand and turn the lighter colored end as far as it will go in either direction.

3. Take a Ventolin Nebule from its pack and insert the clear (thinner) end into the raised octagonal hole located in the lighter colored end of the Rotahaler inhalation device. This will force the previously used capsule shell into the Rotahaler chamber. Push the new capsule in until it is level with the top of the hole. (**Note:** When first using or after washing the Rotahaler, the raised octagonal hole will be empty).

4. Hold the Rotahaler level (horizontally) with the white dot uppermost and turn the lighter colored end (the end where the capsule was inserted) as far as it will go in the opposite direction. This will open the capsule.

YOUR ROTAHALER IS NOW READY FOR USE. KEEP LEVEL.

Using the Rotahaler:

5. Keep the Rotahaler level. Breathe out fully. Raise the Rotahaler to your mouth and gently place the mouthpiece (darker colored end) between your teeth and lips.

6. Breathe in through your mouth as quickly and as deeply as you can.

7. Hold your breath briefly; then remove the Rotahaler from your mouth and exhale.

PATIENT PACKAGE INSERT: *(cont'd)*

8. If a dose of two capsules is recommended by your doctor, repeat steps 2 through 7.

After Using the Rotahaler:

1. After each use, pull the two halves of the Rotahaler apart and throw away the loose capsule shells.

2. Reassemble the Rotahaler and replace it in its container.

Care of Your Rotahaler: Keep the Rotahaler clean and dry at all times. Once every 2 weeks wash the two halves of your Rotahaler in warm water. Make sure that the empty capsule shell is removed from the raised octagonal hole before washing your inhaler.

Dry your Rotahaler thoroughly before reassembling it. Avoid excessive heat.

Dosage: Use only as directed by your doctor.

Warnings: The action of Ventolin Rotacaps may last for 6 hours or longer, and therefore they should not be used more frequently than recommended. Do not increase the frequency of doses without consulting your doctor. If recommended dosage does not provide relief of symptoms or symptoms become worse, seek immediate medical attention. While taking Ventolin Rotacaps, other inhaled bronchodilators should be used only as prescribed by your doctor.

HOW SUPPLIED:

Ventolin: 4 mg tablets are white, round, compressed tablets impressed with "VENTOLIN 4" on one side and "GLAXO" on both sides. *Storage:* Store between 2 and 25°C (36 and 77°F)

Proventil Repetabs: 4 mg extended-release tablets are white, round, coated tablets branded in red on one side with the Schering trademark and the number 431. *Storage:* Store between 2 and 30°C (3 and 86°F).

Ventolin Syrup: Syrup is a clear, orange-yellow liquid with a strawberry flavor. *Storage:* Store between 2 and 30°C (36 and 86°F).

Ventolin Inhalation Aerosol: Store between 15° and 30°C (59° and 86°F). As with most inhaled medications in aerosol canisters, the therapeutic effect of this medication may decrease when the canister is cold. Shake well before using.

Ventolin Inhalation Solution, 0.5%: Store between 2° and 25°C (36° and 77°F).

Ventolin Nebules Inhalation Solution, 0.083%: Protect from light. Store in a refrigerator between 2° and 8°C (36° and 46°F). Inhalation solution may be held at room temperature for up to 2 weeks before use. (Nebules must be used within 2 weeks of removal from refrigerator; record date the nebules are removed from the refrigerator in the space provided on the product carton.) Discard if solution becomes discolored. (Note: Inhalation solution is colorless.)

Ventolin Rotacaps Capsules for Inhalation: The 200 mcg capsule is light blue and clear with "VENTOLIN" printed on the blue cap and "GLAXO" printed on the clear cap. Store between 2° and 30°C (36° and 86°F). Replace cap securely after each opening.

HOW SUPPLIED - RATED THERAPEUTICALLY EQUIVALENT:

Aerosol, Metered - Inhalation - 0.09 mg/inh

6.8 gm	**$14.57**	**Ventolin, Glaxo Wellcome**	**00173-0463-00**
17 gm, 200 inh	**$24.43**	**VENTOLIN, REFILL, Glaxo Wellcome**	**00173-0321-98**
17 gm, 200 inh	**$26.50**	**VENTOLIN, INHALER, Glaxo Wellcome**	**00173-0321-88**

Solution - Inhalation - 0.083 %

3 ml	$25.37	Albuterol, Astra USA	00186-1491-04
3 ml x 25	$30.00	Albuterol, Copley Pharm	38245-0669-17
3 ml x 25	$30.25	Albuterol, Goldline Labs	00182-8010-24
3 ml x 25	$30.25	Albuterol, Dey Labs	49502-0697-03
3 ml x 25	$30.25	Albuterol, Warrick Pharms	59930-1500-08
3 ml x 25	$30.42	Albuterol Sulfate, Qualitest Pharms	00603-1005-40
3 ml x 25	$30.50	Albuterol Sulfate, HL Moore Drug Exch	00839-7860-18
3 ml x 25	$30.50	Albuterol, Major Pharms	00904-7731-17
3 ml x 25	$32.00	Albuterol Sulfate, United Res	00677-1522-72
3 ml x 25	$32.20	Albuterol Sulfate, Aligen Independ	00405-2131-25
3 ml x 25	$32.50	Albuterol Sulfate, Rugby	00536-2677-04
3 ml x 25	$32.50	Albuterol Sulfate, Geneva Pharms	00781-9150-93
3 ml x 25	**$35.65**	**VENTOLIN, NEBULIZER, Glaxo Wellcome**	**00173-0419-00**
3 ml x 25	$36.98	PROVENTIL, Schering	00085-0209-01
3 ml x 25	$49.48	AIRET, Medeva Pharms	53014-0075-25
3 ml x 30	$36.30	Albuterol, Dey Labs	49502-0697-33
3 ml x 60	$60.22	Arm-A-Med (Albuterol Sulfate), Astra USA	00186-1491-17
3 ml x 60	$72.50	Albuterol Sulfate, United Res	00677-1522-73
3 ml x 60	$72.60	Albuterol, Dey Labs	49502-0697-60
3 ml x 60	$72.60	Albuterol, Warrick Pharms	59930-1500-06
3 ml x 60	$73.17	Albuterol Sulfate, HL Moore Drug Exch	00839-7860-35
3 ml x 60	$106.88	AIRET, Medeva Pharms	53014-0075-60

Solution - Inhalation - 0.5 %

20 ml	$11.25	Albuterol, Astra USA	00186-1490-01
20 ml	$12.45	Albuterol, United Res	00677-1521-22
20 ml	$12.50	Albuterol, Qualitest Pharms	00603-1006-43
20 ml	$12.50	Albuterol, Copley Pharm	38245-0640-09
20 ml	$13.91	Albuterol Sulfate, Schein Pharm (US)	00364-2530-55
20 ml	$13.95	Albuterol, Goldline Labs	00182-6014-65
20 ml	$13.95	Albuterol, Rugby	00536-2675-73
20 ml	$13.95	Albuterol, Geneva Pharms	00781-7535-80
20 ml	$14.50	Albuterol, Harber Pharm	51432-0745-11
20 ml	$14.65	Albuterol, Aligen Independ	00405-2130-52
20 ml	$14.65	Albuterol, Major Pharms	00904-7658-55
20 ml	$14.99	Albuterol, Warrick Pharms	59930-1515-04
20 ml	$15.86	Albuterol Sulfate, HL Moore Drug Exch	00839-7861-97
20 ml	$16.23	PROVENTIL, Schering	00085-0208-02
20 ml	**$17.09**	**VENTOLIN, Glaxo Wellcome**	**00173-0385-58**

Syrup - Oral - 2 mg/5ml

16 oz	**$32.08**	**VENTOLIN, Glaxo Wellcome**	**00173-0351-54**
100's	$119.56	Albuterol Sulfate Syrup 2, Xactdose	50962-0402-05
473 ml	$11.73	Albuterol Sulfate, H.C.F.A. F F P	99999-0115-02
473 ml	$26.73	Albuterol Sulfate, Par Pharm	49884-0411-33
473 ml	$26.85	Albuterol Sulfate, Duramed Pharms	51285-0720-57
480 ml	$7.44	Albuterol Sulfate, H.C.F.A. F F P	99999-0115-01
480 ml	$9.36	Albuterol Sulfate, United Res	00677-1505-33
480 ml	$24.75	Albuterol Sulfate, Aligen Independ	00405-2135-16
480 ml	$24.75	Albuterol Sulfate, Qualitest Pharms	00603-1007-58
480 ml	$24.75	Albuterol Sulfate, Warrick Pharms	59930-1510-05
480 ml	$25.95	Albuterol Sulfate, Harber Pharm	51432-0340-20
480 ml	$26.00	Albuterol Sulfate, Goldline Labs	00182-6015-40
480 ml	$26.00	Albuterol Sulfate, Schein Pharm (US)	00364-2522-16
480 ml	$26.00	Albuterol Sulfate, Rugby	00536-0415-85
480 ml	$26.23	Albuterol Sulfate, Mova Pharms	55370-0315-48
480 ml	$26.26	Albuterol Sulfate, HL Moore Drug Exch	00839-7746-69
480 ml	$26.26	Albuterol Sulfate, HL Moore Drug Exch	00839-7859-69
480 ml	$26.38	Albuterol Sulfate, Watson Labs	52544-0419-16
480 ml	$27.23	Albuterol Sulfate, Dupont Pharma	00056-0197-16

HOW SUPPLIED - RATED THERAPEUTICALLY EQUIVALENT:
(cont'd)

480 ml	$27.90	Albuterol Sulfate, Major Pharms	00904-7681-16
480 ml	$27.92	Albuterol Sulfate, Teva	00093-0661-16
480 ml	$27.92	Albuterol Sulfate, Geneva Pharms	00781-6067-16
480 ml	$27.92	Albuterol Sulfate, Dey Labs	49502-0795-16
480 ml	$33.88	PROVENTIL SYRUP, Schering	00085-0315-02

Tablet, Uncoated - Oral - 2 mg

100's	$3.23	Albuterol Sulfate, United Res	00677-1359-01
100's	$3.23	Albuterol Sulfate, H.C.F.A. F F P	99999-0115-03
100's	$8.00	Albuterol Sulfate, Raway	00686-0656-20
100's	$9.75	Albuterol Sulfate, Harber Pharm	51432-0381-03
100's	$20.44	Albuterol Sulfate, Squibb-Mark	57783-6891-01
100's	$22.57	Albuterol Sulfate, Vangard Labs	00615-3517-13
100's	$23.07	Albuterol Sulfate, HL Moore Drug Exch	00839-7867-06
100's	$23.50	Albuterol Sulfate, Mova Pharms	55370-0111-07
100's	$23.50	Albuterol, Novopharm (US)	55953-0480-40
100's	$23.60	Albuterol Sulfate, Qualitest Pharms	00603-2093-21
100's	$23.64	Albuterol Sulfate, Mutual Pharm	53489-0176-01
100's	$23.65	Albuterol Sulfate, Warrick Pharms	59930-1520-01
100's	$24.00	Albuterol Sulfate 2, Aligen Independ	00405-4030-01
100's	$24.00	Albuterol Sulfate, Martec Pharms	52555-0581-01
100's	$24.50	Albuterol Sulfate, HL Moore Drug Exch	00839-7611-06
100's	$24.75	Albuterol Sulfate, Rugby	00536-3008-01
100's	$24.90	Albuterol Sulfate, Parmed Pharms	00349-8994-01
100's	$24.90	Albuterol Sulfate Tablets, Major Pharms	00904-2876-60
100's	$25.00	Albuterol Sulfate, Goldline Labs	00182-1011-01
100's	$25.00	Albuterol, Teva	00332-2226-09
100's	$25.00	Albuterol Sulfate, Copley Pharm	38245-0132-10
100's	$25.38	Albuterol Sulfate, Major Pharms	00904-2876-61
100's	$25.50	Albuterol Sulfate 2, Lederle Pharm	00005-3062-43
100's	$25.50	Albuterol Sulfate, Sidmak Labs	50111-0491-01
100's	$26.00	Albuterol Sulfate, Schein Pharm (US)	00364-2438-01
100's	$26.21	Albuterol Sulfate, MD Pharm	43567-0563-07
100's	$27.29	Albuterol Sulfate, Parmed Pharms	00349-8713-01
100's	$28.05	Albuterol Sulfate, Teva	00093-0665-01
100's	$28.05	Albuterol Sulfate 2 Mg, Geneva Pharms	00781-1671-01
100's	$28.06	Albuterol Sulfate, Dupont Pharma	00056-0198-70
100's	$28.25	Albuterol Sulfate, Warner Chilcott	00047-0956-24
100's	$28.25	Albuterol Sulfate, Mylan	00378-0255-01
100's	**$35.77**	**VENTOLIN, Glaxo Wellcome**	**00173-0341-43**
100's	$37.80	PROVENTIL, Schering	00085-0252-02
250's	$8.07	Albuterol Sulfate, H.C.F.A. F F P	99999-0115-04
250's	$63.12	Albuterol Sulfate, Parmed Pharms	00349-8713-25
500's	$16.15	Albuterol Sulfate, United Res	00677-1359-05
500's	$16.15	Albuterol Sulfate, H.C.F.A. F F P	99999-0115-05
500's	$48.75	Albuterol Sulfate, Harber Pharm	51432-0381-05
500's	$96.85	Albuterol Sulfate, Qualitest Pharms	00603-2093-28
500's	$97.08	Albuterol Sulfate, Squibb-Mark	57783-6891-02
500's	$100.52	Albuterol Sulfate, Martec Pharms	52555-0581-05
500's	$112.00	Albuterol Sulfate, Mova Pharms	55370-0111-08
500's	$112.00	Albuterol, Novopharm (US)	55953-0480-70
500's	$112.22	Albuterol Sulfate, Mutual Pharm	53489-0176-05
500's	$112.25	Albuterol Sulfate, Warrick Pharms	59930-1520-02
500's	$112.90	Albuterol Sulfate Tablets, Major Pharms	00904-2876-40
500's	$117.59	Albuterol Sulfate, HL Moore Drug Exch	00839-7611-12
500's	$119.95	Albuterol Sulfate, Rugby	00536-3008-05
500's	$120.00	Albuterol, Teva	00332-2226-13
500's	$120.00	Albuterol Sulfate, Copley Pharm	38245-0132-50
500's	$121.12	Albuterol Sulfate 2, Lederle Pharm	00005-3062-31
500's	$122.00	Albuterol Sulfate, Parmed Pharms	00349-8994-05
500's	$122.00	Albuterol Sulfate, Sidmak Labs	50111-0491-02
500's	$122.66	Albuterol Sulfate, MD Pharm	43567-0563-11
500's	$126.32	Albuterol Sulfate 2 Mg Tablets, Aligen Independ	00405-4030-02
500's	$134.19	Albuterol Sulfate, Teva	00093-0665-05
500's	$134.20	Albuterol Sulfate, Dupont Pharma	00056-0198-85
500's	$134.40	Albuterol Sulfate, Mylan	00378-0255-05
500's	**$169.84**	**VENTOLIN, Glaxo Wellcome**	**00173-0341-44**
500's	$179.43	PROVENTIL, Schering	00085-0252-03

Tablet, Uncoated - Oral - 4 mg

100's	$5.40	Albuterol Sulfate, United Res	00677-1360-01
100's	$5.40	Albuterol Sulfate, H.C.F.A. F F P	99999-0115-06
100's	$24.95	Albuterol Sulfate, Raway	00686-0658-20
100's	$34.66	Albuterol Sulfate, Vangard Labs	00615-3518-13
100's	$35.00	Albuterol Sulfate, Mova Pharms	55370-0112-07
100's	$35.00	Albuterol, Novopharm (US)	55953-0499-40
100's	$35.16	Albuterol Sulfate, Qualitest Pharms	00603-2094-21
100's	$35.18	Albuterol Sulfate, Mutual Pharm	53489-0177-01
100's	$35.20	Albuterol Sulfate, Warrick Pharms	59930-1530-01
100's	$35.25	Albuterol Sulfate, Martec Pharms	52555-0582-01
100's	$35.30	Albuterol Sulfate Tablets 4 Mg, Major Pharms	00904-2877-60
100's	$35.51	Albuterol Sulfate, HL Moore Drug Exch	00839-7612-06
100's	$36.38	Albuterol Sulfate, Major Pharms	00904-2877-61
100's	$36.95	Albuterol Sulfate, MD Pharm	43567-0564-07
100's	$37.50	Albuterol Sulfate, Goldline Labs	00182-1012-01
100's	$37.50	Albuterol, Teva	00332-2228-09
100's	$37.50	Albuterol Sulfate, Copley Pharm	38245-0134-10
100's	$37.60	Albuterol Sulfate, Schein Pharm (US)	00364-2439-01
100's	$38.00	Albuterol Sulfate, Sidmak Labs	50111-0492-01
100's	$38.05	Albuterol Sulfate 4, Aligen Independ	00405-4031-01
100's	$39.46	Albuterol Sulfate 4, Lederle Pharm	00005-3063-43
100's	$39.55	Albuterol Sulfate, Teva	00093-0666-01
100's	$39.95	Albuterol Sulfate, Rugby	00536-3009-01
100's	$41.00	Albuterol Sulfate, Dupont Pharma	00056-0199-70
100's	$41.30	Albuterol Sulfate, Parmed Pharms	00349-8714-01
100's	$41.30	Albuterol Sulfate, Parmed Pharms	00349-8995-01
100's	$41.30	Albuterol Sulfate 4 Mg, Geneva Pharms	00781-1672-01
100's	$41.50	Albuterol Sulfate, Warner Chilcott	00047-0957-24
100's	$41.50	Albuterol Sulfate, Mylan	00378-0572-01
100's	**$53.35**	**VENTOLIN, Glaxo Wellcome**	**00173-0342-43**
100's	$56.38	PROVENTIL, Schering	00085-0573-02
250's	$13.50	Albuterol Sulfate, H.C.F.A. F F P	99999-0115-07
250's	$93.89	Albuterol Sulfate, Parmed Pharms	00349-8714-25
500's	$27.00	Albuterol Sulfate, United Res	00677-1360-05
500's	$27.00	Albuterol Sulfate, H.C.F.A. F F P	99999-0115-08
500's	$87.50	Albuterol Sulfate, Harber Pharm	51432-0382-05
500's	$132.68	Albuterol Sulfate, Martec Pharms	52555-0582-05
500's	$144.00	Albuterol Sulfate, Qualitest Pharms	00603-2094-28
500's	$164.60	Albuterol Sulfate Tablets 4 Mg, Major Pharms	00904-2877-40
500's	$168.00	Albuterol Sulfate, Mova Pharms	55370-0112-08
500's	$168.00	Albuterol, Novopharm (US)	55953-0499-70
500's	$168.01	Albuterol Sulfate, HL Moore Drug Exch	00839-7612-12
500's	$168.25	Albuterol Sulfate, Warrick Pharms	59930-1530-02

HOW SUPPLIED - RATED THERAPEUTICALLY EQUIVALENT:
(cont'd)

500's	$168.32	Albuterol Sulfate, Mutual Pharm	53489-0177-05
500's	$176.75	Albuterol Sulfate, MD Pharm	43567-0564-11
500's	$180.00	Albuterol, Teva	00332-2228-13
500's	$180.00	Albuterol Sulfate, Copley Pharm	38245-0134-50
500's	$182.00	Albuterol Sulfate, Parmed Pharms	00349-8995-05
500's	$182.00	Albuterol Sulfate, Sidmak Labs	50111-0492-02
500's	$186.69	Albuterol Sulfate 4, Lederle Pharm	00005-3063-31
500's	$187.00	Albuterol Sulfate, Rugby	00536-3009-05
500's	$189.47	Albuterol Sulfate, Aligen Independ	00405-4031-02
500's	$197.00	Albuterol Sulfate, Teva	00093-0666-05
500's	$200.20	Albuterol Sulfate, Dupont Pharma	00056-0199-85
500's	$200.50	Albuterol Sulfate, Mylan	00378-0572-05
500's	**$253.62**	**VENTOLIN, Glaxo Wellcome**	**00173-0342-44**
500's	$267.93	PROVENTIL, Schering	00085-0573-03

HOW SUPPLIED - NOT RATED EQUIVALENT:

Aerosol, Metered - Inhalation - 0.09 mg/inh

17 gm	$22.20	PROVENTIL, Schering	00085-0614-03
17 gm	$24.09	PROVENTIL, Schering	00085-0614-02

Capsule, Gelatin - Inhalation - 200 mcg

24's UD	**$21.48**	**VENTOLIN ROTACAPS, Glaxo Wellcome**	**00173-0389-03**
100's	**$26.51**	**VENTOLIN, ROTACAPS, REFILL, Glaxo Wellcome**	**00173-0389-02**
100's	**$31.28**	**VENTOLIN, ROTACAPS, Glaxo Wellcome**	**00173-0389-01**

Powder

25 gm	$52.50	Albuterol, Paddock Labs	00574-0512-25
100 gm	$135.00	Albuterol Sulfate, Elge	58298-0509-01
100 gm	$187.50	Albuterol, Paddock Labs	00574-0512-01

Tablet, Coated, Sustained Action - Oral - 4 mg

100's	$63.24	VOLMAX, Muro Pharm	00451-0398-50
100's	$63.31	PROVENTIL REPETABS, Schering	00085-0431-02
100's	$79.28	PROVENTIL REPETABS, Schering	00085-0431-04
500's	$307.10	PROVENTIL, Schering	00085-0431-03

Tablet, Coated, Sustained Action - Oral - 8 mg

100's	$117.42	VOLMAX, Muro Pharm	00451-0399-50

ALBUTEROL; IPRATROPIUM BROMIDE
(003214)

CATEGORIES: Antiasthmatics/Bronchodilators; Anticholinergic Agents; Antimuscarinics/Antispasmodics; Autonomic Drugs; Bronchial Dilators; Bronchospasm; Pulmonary Disease; Respiratory & Allergy Medications; Sympathomimetic Agents; FDA Unapproved

BRAND NAMES: *Albugenol TR*; **Combivent**; *Combivent Aerosol*
(International brand names outside U.S. in italics)

Prescribing information not available at time of publication.

HOW SUPPLIED - EQUIVALENTS NOT AVAILABLE:

Aerosol - Inhalation - 0.103mg-0.018mg

14.7 gm	$35.52	COMBIVENT, Boehringer Pharms	00597-0013-14

ALCLOMETASONE DIPROPIONATE *(000116)*

CATEGORIES: Anti-Inflammatory Agents; Dermatologicals; Dermatoses; Inflammation; Pruritus; Skin/Mucous Membrane Agents; Steroids; Pregnancy Category C; FDA Approved 1982 Dec

BRAND NAMES: *Acloderm*; *Aclosone* (France); **Aclovate**; *Alderm*; *Almeta* (Japan); *Delonal* (Germany); *Demiderm*; *Legederm*; *Logoderm* (Australia, Mexico); *Lomesone*; *Miloderme*; *Modraderm*; *Modrasone* (England); *Perderm*
(International brand names outside U.S. in italics)

FORMULARIES: Aetna; BC-BS; Medi-Cal

For Dermatologic Use Only—Not for Ophthalmic Use.

DESCRIPTION:

Aclovate Cream and Ointment contain alclometasone dipropionate (7α-chloro-11β, 17,21-trihydroxy-16α-methylpregna-1,4-diene-3,20-dione 17,21-dipropionate), a synthetic corticosteroid for topical dermatologic use. The corticosteroids constitute a class of primarily synthetic steroids used topically as anti-inflammatory and antipruritic agents.

Chemically, alclometasone dipropionate is $C_{28}H_{37}ClO_7$.

Alclometasone dipropionate has the molecular weight of 521. It is a white powder, insoluble in water, slightly soluble in propylene glycol, and moderately soluble in hexylene glycol.

Each gram of alclometasone dipropionate cream contains 0.5 mg of alclometasone dipropionate in a hydrophilic, emollient cream base of propylene glycol, white petrolatum, cetearyl alcohol, glyceryl stearate, PEG 100 stearate, Ceteth-20, monobasic sodium phosphate, chlorocresol, phosphoric acid, and purified water.

Each gram of alclometasone dipropionate ointment contains 0.5 mg of alclometasone dipropionate in an ointment base of hexylene glycol, white wax, propylene glycol stearate, and white petrolatum.

CLINICAL PHARMACOLOGY:

Like other topical corticosteroids, alclomestasone dipropionate has anti-inflammatory, antipruritic, and vasoconstrictive properties. The mechanism of the anti-inflammatory activity of the topical steroids, in general, is unclear. However, corticosteroids are thought to act by the induction of phospholipase A_2 inhibitory proteins, collectively called lipocortins. It is postulated that these proteins control the biosynthesis of potent mediators of inflammation such as prostaglandins and leukotienes by inhibiting the release of their common precursor, arachidonic acid. Arachidonic acid is released from membrane phospholipids by phospholipase A_2.

PHARMACOKINETICS

The extent of percutaneous absorption of topical corticosteroids, including alclometasone dipropionate, is determined by many factors, including the vehicle and the integrity of the epidermal barrier. Occlusive dressings with hydrocortisone for up to 24 hours have not been demonstrated to increase penetration; however, occlusion of hydrocortisone for 96 hours markedly enhances penetration. Topical corticosteroids can be absorbed from normal intact skin. Inflammation and/or other disease processes in the skin may increase percutaneous

CLINICAL PHARMACOLOGY: *(cont'd)*

absorption. A study utilizing a radiolabeled alclometasone dipropionate ointment formulation was performed to measure systemic absorption and excretion. Results indicated that approximately 3% of the steroid was absorbed during 8 hours of contact with intact skin of normal volunteers.

Studies performed with alclometasone dipropionate cream and ointment indicate that these products are in the low to medium range of potency as compared with other topical corticosteroids.

INDICATIONS AND USAGE:

Alclometasone dipropionate cream and ointment are low to medium potency corticosteroids indicated for the relief of the inflammatory and pruitic manifestations of corticosteroid-responsive dermatoses. Alclometasone dipropionate cream and ointment may be used in pediatric patients 1 year of age or older, although the safety and efficacy of drug use for longer than 3 weeks have not been established (see PRECAUTIONS, Pediatric Use.) Since the safety and efficacy of alclometasone dipropionate cream and ointment have not been established in pediatric patients below 1 year of age, their use in this age-group is not recommended.

CONTRAINDICATIONS:

Alclometasone dipropionate cream and ointment are contraindicated in those patients with a history of hypersensitivity to any of the components in these preparations.

PRECAUTIONS:

GENERAL

Systemic absorption of topical corticosteroids can produce reversible hypothalmic-pituitary-adrenal (HPA) axis suppression with the potential for glucocorticosteroid insufficiency after withdrawal of treatment. Manifestations of Cushing's syndrome, hyperglycemia, and glucosuria can also be produced in some patients by systemic absorption of topical corticosteroids while on treatment.

Patients applying a topical steroid to a large surface area or to areas under occlusion should be evaluated periodically for evidence of HPA axis suppression. This may be done by using the ACTH stimulation, A.M. plasma cortisol, and urinary free cortisol tests.

The effects of alclometasone dipropionate cream and ointment on the HPA axis have been evaluated. In one study, alclometasone dipropionate cream and ointment were applied to 30% of the body twice daily for 7 days, and occlusive dressings were used in selected patients either 12 hours or 24 hours daily. In another study, alclometasone dipropionate cream was applied to 80% of the body surface of normal subjects twice daily for 21 days with daily 12–hour periods of whole body occlusion. Average plasma and urinary free cortisol levels and urinary levels of 17–hydroxysteroids were decreased (about 10%), suggesting suppression of the HPA axis under these conditions. Plasma cortisol levels have also been demonstrated to decrease in pediatric patients treated twice daily for 3 weeks without occlusion.

If HPA axis suppression is noted, an attempt should be made to withdraw the drug, to reduce the frequency of application, or to substitute a less potent corticosteroid. Recovery of HPA axis function is generally prompt upon discontinuation of topical coricosteroids. Infrequently, signs and symptoms of glucocorticosteroid insufficiency may occur, requiring supplemental systemic corticosteroids. For information on systemic supplementation, see prescribing information for those products.

Pediatric patients may be more susceptible to systemic toxicity from equivalent doses due to their larger skin surface area to body mass ratios (see PRECAUTIONS, Pediatric Use.)

If irritation develops, alclometasone dipropionate cream and ointment should be discontinued and appropriate therapy instituted. Allergic contact dermatitis with corticosteroids is usually diagnosed by observing a *failure to heal* rather than noting a clinical exacerbation, as with most topical products not containing corticosteroids. Such an observation should be corroborated with appropriate diagnostic patch testing.

If concomitant skin infections are present or develop, an appropriate antifungal or antibacterial agent should be used. If a favorable response does not occur promptly, use of alclometasone dipropionate cream and ointment should be discontinued until the infection has been adequately controlled.

INFORMATION FOR THE PATIENT:

Patients using topical corticosteroids should receive the following information and instructions:

1. This medication is to be used as directed by the physician. It is for external use only. Avoid contact with the eyes.

2. This medication should not be used for any disorder other than that for which it was prescribed.

3. The treated skin area should not be bandaged, otherwise covered or wrapped so as to be occlusive, unless directed by the physician.

4. Patients should report to their physician any signs of local adverse reactions.

5. Parents of pediatric patients should be advised not to use alclometasone dipropionate cream and ointment in the treatment of diaper dermatitis. Alclometasone dipropionate cream and ointment should not be applied in the diaper area as diapers or plastic pants may constitute occlusive dressing (see DOSAGE AND ADMINISTRATION.)

6. This medication should not be used on the face, underarms, or groin areas unless directed by the physician.

7. As with other corticosteroids, therapy should be discontinued when control is achieved. If no improvement is seen within 2 weeks, contact the physician.

LABORATORY TESTS

The following tests may be helpful in evaluating patients for HPA axis suppression:

ACTH stimulation test

A.M. plasma cortisol test

Urinary free cortisol test

CARCINOGENESIS, MUTAGENESIS, AND IMPAIRMENT OF FERTILITY

Long-term animal studies have not been performed to evaluate the carcinogenic potential or the effect on fertility of topical corticosteroids.

PREGNANCY CATEGORY C

Teratogenic Effects: Corticosteroids have been shown to be teratogenic in laboratory animals when administered systemically at relatively low dosage levels. Some corticosteroids have been shown to be teratogenic after dermal application in laboratory animals. There are no adequate and well-controlled studies in pregnant women. Alclometasone dipropionate cream and ointment should be used during pregnancy only if the potential benefit justifies the potential risk to the fetus.

NURSING MOTHERS

Systemically administered corticosteroids appear in human milk and could suppress growth, interfere with endogenous corticosteroid production, or cause other untoward effects. It is not known whether topical administration of topical corticosteroids could result in sufficient

PRECAUTIONS: *(cont'd)*

systemic absorption to produce detectable quantities in human milk, caution should be exercised when alclometasone dipropionate cream and ointment is administered to a nursing woman.

PEDIATRIC USE

Alclometasone dipropionate cream and ointment may be used with caution in pediatric patients 1 year of age or older, although the safety and efficacy of drug use for longer than 3 weeks have not been established. Use of alclometasone dipropionate cream and ointment is supported by results from adequate and well-controlled studies in pediatric patients with corticosteroid-responsive dermatoses. Since the safety and efficacy of alclometasone dipropionate cream and ointment have not been established in pediatric patients below 1 year of age, its use in this age-group is not recommended. Because of a higher ratio of skin surface area to body mass, pediatric patients are at a greater risk than adults of HPA axis suppression and Cushing's syndrome when they are treated with topical corticosteroids. They are therefore also at greater risk of adrenal insufficiency during and/or after withdrawal of treatment. Adverse effects, including striae, have been reported with use of topical corticosteroids in infants and children. Pediatric patients applying alclometasone dipropionate cream and ointment to >20% of the body surface area are at higher risk for HPA axis suppression.

HPA axis suppression, Cushing's syndrome, linear growth retardation, delayed weight gain, and intracranial hypertension have been reported in pediatric patients receiving topical corticosteroids. Manifestations of adrenal suppression in pediatric patients include low plasma cortisol levels and absence of response to ACTH stimulation. Manifestations of intracranial hypertension include bulging fontanelles, headaches, and bilateral papilledema.

Alclometasone dipropionate cream and ointment should not be used in the treatment of diaper dermatitis.

ADVERSE REACTIONS:

The following local adverse reactions have been reported with alclometasone dipropionate cream in approximately 2% of patients: itching and burning, erythema, dryness, irritation, and papular rashes.

The following local adverse reactions have been reported with alclometasone dipropionate ointment in approximately 1% of patients: itching, burning, and erythema.

The following additional local adverse reactions have been reported infrequently with topical corticosteroids, but may occur more frequently with the use of occlusive dressings. These reactions are listed in an approximately decreasing order of occurrence: folliculitis, acneiform eruptions, hypopigmentation, perioral dermatitis, allergic contact dermatitis, secondary infection, skin atrophy, striae, and miliaria.

OVERDOSAGE:

Topically applied alclometasone dipropionate cream and ointment can be absorbed in sufficient amounts to produce systemic effects (see PRECAUTIONS.)

DOSAGE AND ADMINISTRATION:

Apply a thin film of alclometasone dipropionate cream or ointment to the affected skin areas two or three times daily; massage gently until the medication disappears.

Alclometasone dipropionate cream and ointment may be used in pediatric patients 1 year of age or older. Safety and effectiveness of alclometasone dipropionate cream and ointment in pediatric patients for more than 3 weeks of use have not been established. Use in pediatric patients under 1 year of age is not recommended.

As with other corticosteroids, therapy should be discontinued when control is achieved. If no improvement is seen within 2 weeks, reassessment of diagnosis may be necessary.

Alclometasone dipropionate cream and ointment should not be used with occlusive dressings unless directed by a physician. Alclometasone dipropionate cream and ointment should not be applied in the diaper area if the child still requires diapers or plastic pants as these garments may constitute occlusive dressing.

PATIENT INFORMATION:

Patients using alclometasone dipropionate cream and ointment should receive the following information and instructions.

1. This medication is to be used as directed by the physician. It is for external use only. Avoid contact with the eyes.

2. This medication should not be used for any disorder other than that for which it was prescribed.

3. The treated skin area should not be bandaged or otherwise covered or wrapped as to be occlusive unless directed by the physician.

4. Patients should report any signs of local adverse reactions, especially under occlusive dressings, to the physician.

5. Parents of pediatric patients should be advised not to use tight-fitting diapers or plastic pants on a child being treated in the diaper area, as these garments may constitute occlusive dressings.

HOW SUPPLIED:

Aclovate Cream, 0.5% and Aclovate Ointment 0.5% are supplied in 15, 45, and 60 gram tubes.

Store between 2° and 30°C (36° and 86°F).

HOW SUPPLIED - EQUIVALENTS NOT AVAILABLE:

Cream - Topical - 0.05 %

15 gm	**$11.20**	**ACLOVATE, Glaxo Wellcome**	**00173-0401-00**
45 gm	**$23.34**	**ACLOVATE, Glaxo Wellcome**	**00173-0401-01**
60 gm	**$29.56**	**ACLOVATE, Glaxo Wellcome**	**00173-0401-06**

Ointment - Topical - 0.05 %

15 gm	**$11.20**	**ACLOVATE, Glaxo Wellcome**	**00173-0402-00**
45 gm	**$23.34**	**ACLOVATE, Glaxo Wellcome**	**00173-0402-01**
60 gm	**$29.56**	**ACLOVATE, Glaxo Wellcome**	**00173-0402-06**

ALDESLEUKIN *(003125)*

CATEGORIES: Antineoplastics; Biologicals; Cancer; Oncologic Drugs; Renal Carcinoma; Renal Cell Carcinoma; AIDS Related Complex*; Melanoma*; Recombinant DNA Origin; FDA Approved 1992 May

* Indication not approved by the FDA

BRAND NAMES: Interleukin-2; **Proleukin**

FORMULARIES: Medi-Cal

WARNING:
Aldesleukin for injection should be administered only in a hospital setting under the supervision of a qualified physician experienced in the use of anti-cancer agents. An intensive care facility and specialists skilled in cardiopulmonary or intensive care medicine must be available.
Aldesleukin administration has been associated with capillary leak syndrome (CLS). CLS results in hypotension and reduced organ perfusion which may be severe and can result in death.
Therapy with aldesleukin should be restricted to patients with normal cardiac and pulmonary functions as defined by thallium stress testing and formal pulmonary function testing. Extreme caution should be used in patients with normal thallium stress tests and pulmonary function tests who have a history of prior cardiac or pulmonary disease.
Aldesleukin administration should be held in patients developing moderate to severe lethargy or somnolence; continued administration may result in coma.

DESCRIPTION:

Aldesleukin for injection, a human recombinant interleukin-2 product, is a highly purified protein with a molecular weight of approximately 15,300 daltons. The chemical name is desalanyl-1, serine-125 human interleukin-2. Aldesleukin, a lymphokine, is produced by recombinant DNA technology using a genetically engineered *E. coli* strain containing an analog of the human interleukin-2 gene. Genetic engineering techniques were used to modify the human IL-2 gene, and the resulting expression clone encodes a modified human interleukin-2. This recombinant form differs from native interleukin-2 in the following ways: a) aldesleukin is not glycosylated because it is derived from *E. coli*; b) The molecule has no N-terminal alanine; the codon for this amino acid was deleted during the genetic engineering procedure; c) The molecule has serine substituted for cysteine at amino acid position 125; this was accomplished by site specific manipulation during the genetic engineering procedure; and d) the aggregation state of aldesleukin is likely to be different from that of native interleukin-2.

Biological activities tested *in vitro*for the native non-recombinant molecule have been reproduced with aldesleukin.[1,2]

Aldesleukin is supplied as a sterile, white to off-white, lyophilized cake in single-use vials intended for intravenous (IV) administration. When reconstituted with 1.2 ml Sterile Water for Injection, USP, each ml contains 18 million IU (1.1 mg) aldesleukin, 50 mg mannitol, and 0.18 mg sodium dodecyl sulfate, buffered with approximately 0.17 mg monobasic and 0.89 mg dibasic sodium phosphate to a pH of 7.5 (range 7.2 to 7.8). The manufacturing process for aldesleukin involves fermentation in a defined medium constraining tetracycline hydrochloride. The presence of the antibiotic is not detectable in the final product. Aldesleukin contains no preservatives in the final product.

Aldesleukin biological potency is determined by a lymphocyte proliferation bioassay and is expressed in International Units (IU) as established by the World Health Organization 1st International Standard for interleukin-2 (human). The relationship between potency and protein mass is as follows:

18 million (18 x 10^6) IU aldesleukin = 1.1 mg protein

CLINICAL PHARMACOLOGY:

Aldesleukin has been shown to possess the biological activity of human native interleukin-2.[1,2] *In vitro* studies performed on human cell lines demonstrate the immunoregulatory properties of aldesleukin, including: a) enhancement of lymphocyte mitogenesis and stimulation of long-term growth of human Interleukin-2 dependent cell lines; b) enhancement of lymphocyte cytotoxicity; c) induction of killer cell [lymphokine-activated (LAK) and natural (NK)] activity; and d) induction of interferon-gamma production.

The *in vivo* administration of aldesleukin in select murine tumor models and in the clinic produces multiple immunological effects in a dose dependent manner. These effects include activation of cellular immunity with profound lymphocytosis, eosinophilia, and thrombocytopenia, and the production of cytokines including tumor necrosis factor, IL-1 and gamma interferon.[3] *In vivo* experiments in murine tumor models have shown inhibition of tumor growth.[4] The exact mechanism by which aldesleukin mediates its antitumor activity in animals and humans is unknown.

PHARMACOKINETICS

aldesleukin exists as biologically active, non-covalently bound microaggregates with an average size of 27 recombinant interleukin-2 molecules. The solubilizing agent, sodium dodecyl sulfate, may have an effect on the kinetic properties of this product. The pharmacokinetic profile of aldesleukin is characterized by high plasma concentrations following a short IV infusion, rapid distribution to extravascular, extracellular space and elimination from the body by metabolism in the kidneys with little or no bioactive protein excreted in the urine.

Studies of IV aldesleukin in sheep and humans indicate that approximately 30% of the administered dose initially distributes to the plasma.

This is consistent with studies in rats that demonstrate a rapid (<1 minute) and preferential uptake of approximately 70% of an administered dose into the liver, kidney and lung.

The serum half-life (T 1/2) curves of aldesleukin remaining in the plasma are derived from studies done in 52 cancer patients following a 5-minute IV infusion.[5] These patients were shown to have a distribution and elimination T 1/2 of 13 and 85 minutes, respectively.

The relatively rapid clearance rate of aldesleukin has led to dosage schedules characterized by frequent, short infusions. Observed serum levels are proportional to the dose of aldesleukin.

Following the initial rapid organ distribution described above, the primary route of clearance of circulating aldesleukin is the kidney. In humans and animals, aldesleukin is cleared from the circulation by both glomerular filtration and peritubular extraction in the kidney.[6-8]This dual mechanism for delivery of aldesleukin to the proximal tubule may account for the preservation of clearance in patients with rising serum creatinine values. Greater than 80% of the amount of aldesleukin distributed to plasma, cleared from the circulation and presented to the kidney is metabolized to amino acids in the cells lining the proximal convoluted tubules. In humans, the mean clearance rate in cancer patients is 268 ml/min.

IMMUNOGENICITY

Fifty-seven of 77 renal cancer patients (74%) treated with the every 8 hour aldesleukin regimen developed low titers of non-neutralizing anti-interleukin-2 antibodies. Neutralizing antibodies were not detected in this group of patients, but have been detected in 1/106 (<1%) patients treated with IV aldesleukin using a wide variety of schedules and doses. The clinical significance of anti-interleukin-2 antibodies is unknown.

CLINICAL EXPERIENCE

Two hundred and fifty-five patients with metastatic renal cell cancer were treated with single agent aldesleukin. Treatment was given by the every 8-hour regimen in 7 clinical studies conducted at 21 institutions. To be eligible for study, patients were required to have bidimensionally measurable disease; Eastern Cooperative Oncology Group (ECOG) Performance Status (PS) of 0 or 1 (see TABLE 2); and normal organ function, including normal

CLINICAL PHARMACOLOGY: *(cont'd)*

cardiac stress test and pulmonary function tests. Patients with brain metastases, active infections, organ allografts, and diseases requiring steroid treatment were excluded. In addition, it was noted that 218 of the 255 (85%) patients had undergone nephrectomy prior to treatment with aldesleukin.

aldesleukin was given by 15 minute IV infusion every 8 hours for up to 5 days (maximum of 14 doses). No treatment was given on days 6 to 14 and then dosing was repeated for up to 5 days on days 15 to 19 (maximum of 14 doses). These 2 cycles constituted 1 course of therapy. All patients were treated with 28 doses or until dose-limiting toxicity occurred requiring ICU-level support. Patients received a median of 20 of 28 scheduled doses of aldesleukin. Doses were held for specific toxicities (See DOSAGE AND ADMINISTRATION, Dose Modification.) A variety of serious adverse events were encountered including: hypotension; oliguria/anuria; mental status changes including coma; pulmonary congestion and dyspnea; GI bleeding; respiratory failure leading to intubation; ventricular arrhythmias; myocardial ischemia and/or infarction; ileus or intestinal perforation; renal failure requiring dialysis; gangrene; seizures; sepsis and death (See ADVERSE REACTIONS.)

Due to the toxicities encountered during the clinical trials, investigators used the following concomitant medications. Acetaminophen and indomethacin were started immediately prior to aldesleukin to reduce fever. Renal function was particularly monitored because indomethacin may cause synergistic nephrotoxicity. Meperidine was added to control the rigors associated with fever. Ranitidine or cimetidine were given for prophylaxis of gastrointestinal irritation and bleeding. Antiemetics and antidiarrheals were used as needed to treat other gastrointestinal side effects. These medications were discontinued 12 hours after the last dose of aldesleukin. Hydroxyzine or diphenhydramine was used to control symptoms from pruritic rashes and continued until resolution of pruritus.**NOTE: Prior to the use of any product mentioned in this paragraph, the physician should refer to the package insert for the respective product.**

For the 255 patients in the aldesleukin database, objective response was seen in 15% or 37 patients with nine (4%) complete and 28 (11%) partial responders. The 95% confidence interval for response was 11 to 20%. Onset of tumor regression has been observed as early as 4 weeks after completion of the first course of treatment and tumor regression may continue for up to 12 months after the start of treatment. Durable responses were achieved with a median duration of objective (partial or complete) response by Kaplan-Meier projection of 23.2 months (1 to 50 months). The median duration of objective partial response was 18.8 months. The proportion of responding patients who will have response durations of 12 months or greater is projected to be 85% for all responders and 79% for patients with partial responses (Kaplan-Meier) (TABLE 1).

TABLE 1

Complete Responders	Partial Responders	Response Rate	Onset of Response	Median Duration of Response
9 (4%)	28 (11%)	15%	1 to 12 mos.	23.2 months (range 1-50)

Response was observed in both lung and non-lung sites (*e.g.,* liver, lymph node, renal bed recurrences, soft tissue). Patients with individual bulky lesions (>5 x 5 cm) as well as large cumulative tumor burden (>25 cm^2 tumor area) achieved durable responses.

An analysis of prognostic factors showed that performance status as defined by the ECOG (see TABLE 2) was a significant predictor of response. PS 0 patients had an 18% overall rate or objective response, which included all 9 complete response patients and 21 of 28 partial response patients. PS 1 patients had a lower rate of response (9%), all of which were partial responses. In this group it was notable that 6 of the 7 responders had resolution of tumor related symptoms and improved performance status to PS O. All seven patients were fully functional and 4 of the 7 returned to work, suggesting that responses among the PS 1 patients were clinically meaningful as well (see TABLE 3.)

In addition, the frequency of toxicity was related to the performance status. As a group, PS 0 patients, when compared with PS 1 patients, had lower rates of adverse events with fewer on-study deaths (4% vs. 6%), less frequent intubations (8% vs. 25%), gangrene (0% vs. 6%), coma (1% vs. 6%), GI bleeding (4% vs. 8%), and sepsis (6% vs. 18%). These differences in toxicity are reflected in the shorter mean time to hospital discharge for PS 0 patients (2 vs. 3 days) as well as the smaller percentage of PS 0 patients experiencing a delayed (>7 days) discharge from the hospital (8% vs. 19%).

TABLE 2 Performance Status Scale

Performance Status Equivalent ECOG*	Karnofsky	Performance Status Definitions
0	100	Asymptomatic
1	80-90	Symptomatic; fully ambulatory
2	60-70	Symptomatic; in bed less than 50% of day
3	40-50	Symptomatic; in bed more than 50% of day
4	20-30	Bedridden

* Eastern Cooperative Oncology Group
Zubrod, CG, et al. J Chron Dis 11:7-33, 1960

TABLE 3 Aldesleukin Response Analyzed By Ecog* Performance Status (PS)

Pre-Treatment ECOG PS	No. of Patients Treated (n=255)	Response CR	Response PR	Patients Responding	On-Study Death Rate
0	166	9	21	18%	4%
1	80	0	7	9%	6%
≥2	9	0	0	0%	0%

* Eastern Cooperative Oncology Group

INDICATIONS AND USAGE:

Aldesleukin is indicated for the treatment of adults (≥ 18 years of age) with metastatic renal cell carcinoma.

Careful patient selection is mandatory prior to the administration of aldesleukin. (See CONTRAINDICATIONS, WARNINGS and PRECAUTIONS regarding patient screening, including recommended cardiac and pulmonary function tests and laboratory tests.)

Evaluation of clinical studies to date reveals that patients with more favorable ECOG performance status (ECOG PS O) at treatment initiation respond better to aldesleukin, with a higher response rate and lower toxicity (See CLINICAL PHARMACOLOGY, Clinical Experience.) Therefore, selection of patients for treatment should include assessment of performance status, as described in TABLE 2.

Experience in patients with PS > 1 is extremely limited.

CONTRAINDICATIONS:

Aldesleukin is contraindicated in patients with a known history of hypersensitivity to interleukin-2 or any component of the aldesleukin formulation.

CONTRAINDICATIONS: *(cont'd)*

Patients with an abnormal thallium stress test or pulmonary function tests are excluded from treatment with aldesleukin. Patients with organ allografts should be excluded as well. In addition, retreatment with aldesleukin is contraindicated in patients who experienced the following toxicities while receiving an earlier course of therapy:

Sustained ventricular tachycardia (≥5 beats)

Cardiac rhythm disturbances not controlled or unresponsive to management

Recurrent chest pain with ECG changes, consistent with angina or myocardial infarction

Intubation required > 72 hours

Pericardial tamponade

Renal dysfunction requiring dialysis > 72 hours

Coma or toxic psychosis lasting > 48 hours

Repetitive or difficult to control seizures

Bowel ischemia/perforation

GI bleeding requiring surgery

WARNINGS:

(See BOXED WARNING)

Aldesleukin administration has been associated with capillary leak syndrome (CLS) which results from extravasation of plasma proteins and fluid into the extravascular space and loss of vascular tone. CLS results in hypotension and reduced organ perfusion which may be severe and can result in death. The CLS may be associated with cardiac arrhythmias (supraventricular and ventricular), angina, myocardial infarction, respiratory insufficiency requiring intubation, gastrointestinal bleeding or infarction, renal insufficiency, and mental status changes.

Because of the severe adverse events which generally accompany aldesleukin therapy at the recommended dosages, thorough clinical evaluation should be performed to exclude from treatment patients with significant cardiac, pulmonary, renal, hepatic, or CNS impairment.

Should adverse events occur, which require dose modification, dosage should be withheld rather than reduced (See DOSAGE AND ADMINISTRATION, Dose Modification.)

Aldesleukin may exacerbate pre-existing autoimmune disease. Because not all patients who develop interleukin-2-associated autoimmune phenomena have a pre-existing history of autoimmune disease, awareness and close monitoring for thyroid abnormalities or other potentially autoimmune phenomena is warranted. Two patients with quiescent Crohn's disease had activation of their disease following treatment with aldesleukin, and both required surgical intervention.

Aldesleukin may exacerbate disease symptoms in patients with clinically unrecognized or untreated CNS metastases. All patients should have thorough evaluation and treatment of CNS metastases prior to receiving aldesleukin therapy. They should be neurologically stable with a negative CT scan. In addition, extreme caution should be exercised in treating patients with a history of seizure disorder because aldesleukin may cause seizures.

Intensive aldesleukin treatment is associated with impaired neutrophil function (reduced chemotaxis) and with an increased risk of disseminated infection, including sepsis and bacterial endocarditis, in treated patients. Consequently, pre-existing bacterial infections should be adequately treated prior to initiation of aldesleukin therapy. Additionally, all patients with indwelling central lines should receive antibiotic prophylaxis effective against *S. aureus*.[9-11] Antibiotic prophylaxis which has been associated with a reduced incidence of staphylococcal infections in aldesleukin studies includes the use of oxacillin, nafcillin, ciprofloxacin, or vancomycin. Disseminated infections acquired in the course of aldesleukin treatment are a major contributor to treatment morbidity and use of antibiotic prophylaxis and aggressive treatment of suspected and documented infections may reduce the morbidity of aldesleukin treatment. **NOTE: Prior to the use of any product mentioned in this paragraph, the physician should refer to the package insert for the respective product.**

PRECAUTIONS:

GENERAL

Patients should have normal cardiac, pulmonary, hepatic, and CNS function at the start of therapy. Patients who have had a nephrectomy are still eligible for treatment if they have serum creatinine levels ≤ 1.5 mg/dl.

Adverse events are frequent, often serious, and sometimes fatal.

Capillary leak syndrome (CLS) begins immediately after aldesleukin treatment starts and is marked by increased capillary permeability to protein and fluids and reduced vascular tone. In most patients, this results in a concomitant drop in mean arterial blood pressure within 2 to 12 hours after the start of treatment. With continued therapy, clinically significant hypotension (defined as systolic blood pressure below 90 mm Hg or a 20 mm Hg drop from baseline systolic pressure) and hypoperfusion will occur. In addition, extravasation of protein and fluids into the extravascular space will lead to edema formation and creation of effusions.

Medical management of CLS begins with careful monitoring of the patient's fluid and organ perfusion status. This is achieved by frequent determination of blood pressure and pulse, and by monitoring organ function, which includes assessment of mental status and urine output. Hypovolemia is assessed by catheterization and central pressure monitoring.

Flexibility in fluid and pressor management is essential for maintaining organ perfusion and blood pressure. Consequently, extreme caution should be used in treating patients with fixed requirements for large volumes of fluid (*e.g.,* patients with hypercalcemia).

Patients with hypovolemia are managed by administering IV fluids, either colloids or crystalloids. IV fluids are usually given when the central venous pressure (CVP) is below 3 to 4 mm H_2O. Correction of hypovolemia may require large volumes of IV fluids but caution is required because unrestrained fluid administration may exacerbate problems associated with edema formation or effusions.

With extravascular fluid accumulation, edema is common and some patients may develop ascites or pleural effusions. Management of these events depends on a careful balancing of the effects of fluid shifts so that neither the consequences of hypovolemia (*e.g.,* impaired organ perfusion) nor the consequences of fluid accumulations (*e.g.,* pulmonary edema) exceeds the patient's tolerance.

Clinical experience has shown that early administration of dopamine (1 to 5 mcg/kg/min) to patients manifesting capillary leak syndrome, before the onset of hypotension, can help to maintain organ perfusion particularly to the kidney and thus preserve urine output. Weight and urine output should be carefully monitored. If organ perfusion and blood pressure are not sustained by dopamine therapy, clinical investigators have increased the dose of dopamine to 6 to 10 mcg/kg/min or have added phenylephrine hydrochloride (1 to 5 mcg/kg/min) to low dose dopamine(See CLINICAL PHARMACOLOGY, Clinical Experience.) Prolonged use of pressors, either in combination or as individual agents, at relatively high doses, may be associated with cardiac rhythm disturbances. **NOTE: Prior to the use of any product mentioned in this paragraph, the physician should refer to the package insert for the respective product.**

PRECAUTIONS: *(cont'd)*

Failure to maintain organ perfusion, demonstrated by altered mental status, reduced urine output, a fall in the systolic blood pressure below 90 mm Hg or onset of cardiac arrhythmias, should lead to holding the subsequent doses until recovery of organ perfusion and a return of systolic blood pressure above 90 mm Hg are observed (See DOSAGE AND ADMINISTRATION, Dose Modification.)

Recovery from CLS begins soon after cessation of aldesleukin therapy. Usually, within a few hours, the blood pressure rises, organ perfusion is restored and resorption of extravasated fluid and protein begins. If there has been excessive weight gain or edema formation, particularly if associated with shortness of breath from pulmonary congestion, use of diuretics, once blood pressure has normalized, has been shown to hasten recovery.

Oxygen is given to the patient if pulmonary function monitoring confirms that P_aO_2 is decreased.

Aldesleukin administration may cause anemia and/or thrombocytopenia. Packed red blood cell transfusions have been given both for relief of anemia and to insure maximal oxygen carrying capacity. Platelet transfusions have been given to resolve absolute thrombocytopenia and to reduce the risk of GI bleeding. In addition, leukopenia and neutropenia are observed.

Aldesleukin administration results in fever, chills, rigors, pruritus, and gastrointestinal side effects in most patients treated at recommended doses. These side effects have been aggressively managed as described in the CLINICAL PHARMACOLOGY, Clinical Experience.

Renal and hepatic function are impaired during aldesleukin treatment. Use of concomitant medications known to be nephrotoxic or hepatotoxic may further increase toxicity to the kidney or liver. In addition, reduced kidney and liver function secondary to aldesleukin treatment may delay elimination of concomitant medications and increase the risk of adverse events from those drugs.

Patients may experience mental status changes including irritability, confusion, or depression while receiving aldesleukin. These mental status changes may be indicators of bacteremia or early bacterial sepsis. Mental status changes due solely to aldesleukin are generally reversible when drug administration is discontinued. However, alterations in mental status may progress for several days before recovery begins.

Impairment of thyroid function has been reported following aldesleukin treatment. A small number of these patients required thyroid replacement therapy. This impairment of thyroid function may be a manifestation of autoimmunity.

Aldesleukin enhancement of cellular immune function may increase the risk of allograft rejection in transplant patients.

LABORATORY TESTS

The following clinical evaluations are recommended for all patients, prior to beginning treatment and then daily during drug administration.

Standard hematologic tests—including CBC, differential and platelet counts

Blood chemistries—including electrolytes, renal and hepatic function tests

Chest x-rays

All patients should have baseline pulmonary function tests with arterial blood gases. Adequate pulmonary function should be documented (FEV_1 >2 liters or ≥ 75% of predicted for height and age) prior to initiating therapy. All patients should be screened with a stress thallium study. Normal ejection fraction and unimpaired wall motion should be documented. If a thallium stress test suggests minor wall motion abnormalities of questionable significance, a stress echocardiogram to document normal wall motion may be useful to exclude significant coronary artery disease.

Daily monitoring during therapy with aldesleukin should include vital signs (temperature, pulse, blood pressure, and respiration rate) and weight. In a patient with a decreased blood pressure, especially less than 90 mm Hg, constant cardiac monitoring for rhythm should be conducted. If an abnormal complex or rhythm is seen, an ECG should be performed. Vital signs in these hypotensive patients should be taken hourly and central venous pressure (CVP) checked.

During treatment, pulmonary function should be monitored on a regular basis by clinical examination, assessment of vital signs and pulse oximetry. Patients with dyspnea or clinical signs of respiratory impairment (tachypnea or rales) should be further assessed with arterial blood gas determination. These tests are to be repeated as often as clinically indicated.

Cardiac function is assessed daily by clinical examination and assessment of vital signs. Patients with signs or symptoms of chest pain, murmurs, gallops, irregular rhythm or palpitations should be further assessed with an ECG examination and CPK evaluation. If there is evidence of cardiac ischemia or congestive heart failure, a repeat thallium study should be done.

CARCINOGENESIS, MUTAGENESIS, AND IMPAIRMENT OF FERTILITY

There have been no studies conducted assessing the carcinogenic or mutagenic potential of aldesleukin.

There have been no studies conducted assessing the effect of aldesleukin on fertility. It is recommended that this drug not be administered to fertile persons of either sex not practicing contraception.

PREGNANCY CATEGORY C

Animal reproduction studies have not been conducted with aldesleukin. It is also not known whether aldesleukin can cause fetal harm when administered to a pregnant woman or can affect reproduction capacity. In view of the known adverse effects of aldesleukin, it should only be given to a pregnant woman with extreme caution, weighing the potential benefit with the risks associated with therapy.

NURSING MOTHERS

It is not known whether this drug is excreted in human milk. Because many drugs are excreted in human milk and because of the potential for serious reactions in nursing infants from aldesleukin, a decision should be made whether to discontinue nursing or to discontinue the drug, taking into account the importance of the drug to the mother.

PEDIATRIC USE

Safety and effectiveness in children under 18 years of age have not been established.

DRUG INTERACTIONS:

Aldesleukin may affect central nervous function. Therefore, interactions could occur following concomitant administration of psychotropic drugs (*e.g.,* narcotics, analgesics, antiemetics, sedatives, tranquilizers).

Concurrent administration of drugs possessing nephrotoxic (*e.g.,* aminoglycosides, indomethacin), myelotoxic (*e.g.,* cytotoxic chemotherapy), cardiotoxic (*e.g.,* doxorubicin) or hepatotoxic (*e.g.,* methotrexate, asparaginase) effects with aldesleukin may increase toxicity in these organ systems. The safety and efficacy of aldesleukin in combination with chemotherapies have not been established.

Although glucocorticoids have been shown to reduce aldesleukin-induced side effects including fever, renal insufficiency, hyperbilirubinemia, confusion, and dyspnea,[12] concomitant administration of these agents with aldesleukin may reduce the antitumor effectiveness of aldesleukin and thus should be avoided.

DRUG INTERACTIONS: *(cont'd)*

Beta-blockers and other antihypertensives may potentiate the hypotension seen with aldesleukin.

Delayed adverse reactions to iodinated contrast media: A review of the literature revealed that 12.6% (range 11-28%) of 501 patients treated with various interleukin-2-containing regimens who were subsequently administered radiographic iodinated contrast media experienced acute, atypical adverse reactions. The onset of symptoms usually occurred within hours (most commonly 1 to 4 hours) following the administration of contrast media. These reactions include fever, chills, nausea, vomiting, pruritus, rash, diarrhea, hypotension, edema, and oliguria. Some clinicians have noted that these reactions resemble the immediate side effects caused by interleukin-2 administration, however the cause of contrast reactions after interleukin-2 therapy is unknown. Most events reported to occur when contrast media was given within 4 weeks after the last dose of interleukin-2. These events were also reported to occur when contrast media was given several months after interleukin-2 treatment.[13]

ADVERSE REACTIONS:

The rate of drug-related deaths in the 255 metastatic renal cell carcinoma patients on study who received single-agent aldesleukin was 4% (11/255).

Frequency and severity of adverse reactions to aldesleukin have generally been shown to be dose-related and schedule-dependent. Most adverse reactions are self-limiting and are usually, but not invariably, reversible within 2 or 3 days of discontinuation of therapy.

Examples of adverse reactions with permanent sequelae include: myocardial infarction, bowel perforation/infarction, and gangrene.

The most frequently reported serious adverse reactions include hypotension, renal dysfunction with oliguria/anuria, dyspepsia or pulmonary congestion, and mental status changes (*i.e.,* lethargy, somnolence, confusion, and agitation). Other serious toxicities have included myocardial ischemia, myocarditis, gangrene, respiratory failure leading to intubation, GI bleeding requiring surgery, intestinal perforation/ileus, coma, seizure, sepsis, and renal impairment requiring dialysis. The incidence of these events has been higher in PS 1 patients than in PS 0 patients (See CLINICAL PHARMACOLOGY, Clinical Experience.)

The following data on adverse reactions are based on 373 patients (255 with renal cell cancer and 118 with other tumors) treated with the recommended every 8-hour 15-minute infusion dosing regimen. These patients had metastatic or recurrent carcinoma and were enrolled in investigational trials in the United States.

Organ systems in which reactions occurred in a significant number of the patients treated are found in Table 4 below:

Other serious adverse events were derived from trials involving more than 1,800 patients treated with aldesleukin-based regimens using a variety of doses and schedules. These events each occurred with a frequency of <1% and included: liver or renal failure resulting in death; duodenal ulceration; fatal intestinal perforation; bowel necrosis; fatal cardiac arrest, myocarditis, and supraventricular tachycardia; permanent or transient blindness secondary to optic neuritis; fatal malignant hyperthermia; pulmonary edema resulting in death; respiratory arrest; fatal respiratory failure; fatal stroke; transient ischemic attack; meningitis; cerebral edema; pericarditis; allergic interstitial nephritis; tracheo-esophageal fistula; fatal pulmonary emboli; severe depression leading to suicide.

Exacerbation of pre-existing autoimmune disease (Crohn's Disease and Thyroid Disease, (see WARNINGS) and delayed adverse reactions to iodinated contrast media (see PRECAUTIONS) have also been reported. In clinical investigations, persistent but non-progressive vitiligo has been observed in malignant melanoma patients treated with interleukin-2.

OVERDOSAGE:

Side effects following the use of aldesleukin are dose-related. Administration of more than the recommended dose has been associated with a more rapid onset of expected dose-limiting toxicities. Adverse reactions generally will reverse when the drug is stopped, particularly because its serum half-life is short (see CLINICAL PHARMACOLOGY, Pharmacokinetics.) Any continuing symptoms should be treated supportively. Life-threatening toxicities have been ameliorated by the intravenous administration of dexamethasone,[12] which may result in loss of therapeutic effect from aldesleukin. **NOTE: Prior to the use of dexamethasone, the physician should refer to the package insert for this product.**

DOSAGE AND ADMINISTRATION:

Aldesleukin) for injection should be administered by a 15-minute IV infusion every 8 hours. Before initiating treatment, carefully review INDICATIONS AND USAGE, CONTRAINDICATIONS, WARNINGS, PRECAUTIONS, and ADVERSE REACTIONS, particularly regarding patient selection, possible serious adverse events, patient monitoring and withholding dosage.

The following schedule has been used to treat adult patients with metastatic renal cell carcinoma. Each course of treatment consists of two 5-day treatment cycles separated by a rest period.

600,000 IU/kg (0.037 mg/kg) dose administered every 8 hours by a 15-minute IV infusion for a total of 14 doses. Following 9 days of rest, the schedule is repeated for another 14 doses, for a maximum of 28 doses per course.

During clinical trials, doses were frequently held for toxicity (see Dose Modification.) Patients treated with this schedule received a median of 20 of the 28 doses during the first course of therapy.

Retreatment: Patients should be evaluated for response approximately 4 weeks after completion of a course of therapy and again immediately prior to the scheduled start of the next treatment course. Additional courses of treatment may be given to patients only if there is some tumor shrinkage following the last course and retreatment is not contraindicated (see CONTRAINDICATIONS.) Each treatment course should be separated by a rest period of at least 7 weeks from the date of hospital discharge. Tumors have continued to regress up to 12 months following the initiation of aldesleukin therapy.

Dose Modification: Dose modification for toxicity should be accomplished by holding or interrupting a dose rather than reducing the dose to be given. Decisions to stop, hold, or restart aldesleukin therapy must be made after a global assessment of the patient. With this in mind, the following guidelines should be used: Treatment with aldesleukin should be permanently discontinued for (TABLE 5):

Reconstitution and Dilution Directions: Reconstitution and dilution procedures other than those recommended may alter the delivery and/or pharmacology of aldesleukin and thus should be avoided.

1. Aldesleukin is a sterile, white to off-white, preservative-free, lyophilized powder suitable for IV infusion upon reconstitution and dilution. **EACH VIAL CONTAINS 22 MILLION IU (1.3 MG) OF ALDESLEUKIN AND SHOULD BE RECONSTITUTED ASEPTICALLY WITH 1.2 ML OF STERILE WATER FOR INJECTION, USP. WHEN RECONSTITUTED AS DIRECTED, EACH ML CONTAINS 18 MILLION IU (1.1 MG) OF ALDESLEUKIN.** The resulting solution should be a clear, colorless to slightly yellow liquid. The vial is for single-use only and any unused portion should be discarded.

2. During reconstitution, the Sterile Water for Injection, USP should be directed at the side of the vial and the contents gently swirled to avoid excess foaming. **DO NOT SHAKE.**

DOSAGE AND ADMINISTRATION: *(cont'd)*

TABLE 4 Incidence of Adverse Events

Events by Body System	% of Patients	Events by Body System	% of Patients
Cardiovascular		Gastrointestinal	
Hypotension	85	Nausea and Vomiting	87
(requiring pressors)	71	Diarrhea	76
Sinus Tachycardia	70	Stomatitis	32
Arrhythmias	22	Anorexia	27
Atrial	8	GI Bleeding	13
Supraventricular	5	— requiring surgery	2
Ventricular	3	Dyspepsia	7
Junctional	1	Constipation	5
Bradycardia	7	Intestinal Perforation/Ileus	2
Premature Ventricular Contractions	5	Pancreatitis	<1
Premature Atrial Contractions	4	Neurologic	
Myocardial Ischemia	3	Mental Status Changes	73
Myocardial Infarction	2	Dizziness	17
Cardiac Arrest	2	Sensory Dysfunction	10
Congestive Heart Failure	1	Special Sensory Disorders (vision, speech, taste)	7
Myocarditis	1	Syncope	3
Stroke	1	Motor Dysfunction	2
Gangrene	1	Coma	1
Pericardial Effusion	1	Seizure (grand mal)	1
Endocarditis	1	Renal	
Thrombosis	1	Oliguria/Anuria	76
Pulmonary		BUN Elevation	63
Pulmonary Congestion	54	Serum Creatinine Elevation	61
Dyspnea	52	Proteinuria	12
Pulmonary Edema	10	Hematuria	9
Respiratory Failure (leading to intubation)	9	Dysuria	3
Tachypnea	8	Renal Impairment Requiring Dialysis	2
Pleural Effusion	7	Urinary Retention	1
Wheezing	6	Urinary Frequency	1
Apnea	1	Dermatologic	
Pneumothorax	1	Pruritus	48
Hemoptysis	1	Erythema	41
Hepatic		Rash	26
Elevated Bilirubin	64	Dry Skin	15
Elevated Transaminase	56	Exfoliative Dermatitis	14
Elevated Alkaline Phosphatase	56	Purpura/Petechiae	4
Jaundice	11	Urticaria	2
Hepatomegaly	1	Musculoskeletal	
Hematologic		Arthralgia	6
Anemia	77	Myalgia	6
Thrombocytopenia	64	Arthritis	1
Leukopenia	34	Muscle Spasm	1
Coagulation Disorders	10	Endocrine	
Leukocytosis	9	Hypothyroidism	<1
Eosinophilia	6	General	
Abnormal Laboratory Findings		Fever and/or Chills	89
Hypomagnesemia	16	Pain (all sites)	54
Acidosis	16	Abdominal	15
Hypocalcemia	15	Chest	12
Hypophosphatemia	11	Back	9
Hypokalemia	9	Fatigue/Weakness/Malaise	53
Hyperuricemia	9	Edema	47
Hypoalbuminemia	8	Infection (including urinary tract, injection site, catheter tip, phlebitis, sepsis)	23
Hypoproteinemia	7	Weight Gain (≥ 10%)	23
Hyponatremia	4	Headache	12
Hyperkalemia	4	Weight Loss (≥ 10%)	5
Alkalosis	4	Conjunctivitis	4
Hypoglycemia	2	Injection Site Reactions	3
Hyperglycemia	2	Allergic Reactions (non-anaphylactic)	1
Hypocholesterolemia	1		
Hypercalcemia	1		
Hypernatremia	1		
Hyperphosphatemia	1		

TABLE 5

Organ System	Permanently discontinue treatment for the following toxicities
Cardiovascular	Sustained ventricular tachycardia (≥5 beats) Cardiac rhythm disturbances not controlled or unresponsive to management Recurrent chest pain with ECG changes, documented angina or myocardial infarction Pericardial tamponade
Pulmonary	Intubation required >72 hours
Renal	Renal dysfunction requiring dialysis >72 hours
Central Nervous System	Coma or toxic psychosis lasting >48 hours Repetitive or difficult to control seizures
Gastrointestinal	Bowel ischemia/perforation/GI bleeding requiring surgery

3. The dose of aldesleukin, reconstituted in Sterile Water for Injection, USP (without preservative) should be diluted aseptically in 50 ml of 5% Dextrose Injection, USP and infused over a 15-minute period. Although glass bottles and plastic (polyvinyl chloride) bags have been used in clinical trials with comparable results, it is recommended that plastic bags be used as the dilution container since experimental studies suggest that use of plastic containers results in more consistent drug delivery. In-line filters should not be used when administering aldesleukin.

DOSAGE AND ADMINISTRATION: *(cont'd)*

Doses should be held and restarted according to the following:

Organ System	Hold dose for	Subsequent doses may be given if
Cardiovascular	Atrial fibrillation, supraventricular tachycardia, or bradycardia that requires treatment or is recurrent or persistent	Patient is asymptomatic with full recovery to normal sinus rhythm
	Systolic bp <90 mm Hg with increasing requirements for pressors	Systolic bp ≥90 mm Hg and stable or improving requirements for pressors
	Any ECG change consistent with MI or ischemia with or without chest pain; suspicion of cardiac ischemia	Patient is asymptomatic, MI has been ruled out, clinical suspicion of angina is low
Pulmonary	O_2 saturation <94% on room air or <90% with 2 liters O_2 nasal prongs	O_2 saturation ≥94% on room air or ≥90% with 2 liters O_2 by nasal prongs
Central Nervous System	Mental status changes, including moderate confusion or agitation	Mental status changes completely resolved
Systemic	Sepsis syndrome, patient is clinically unstable	Sepsis syndrome has resolved, patient is clinically stable, infection is under treatment
Renal	Serum creatinine ≥4.5 mg/dl or a serum creatinine of 4 mg/dl in the presence of severe volume overload, acidosis, or hyperkalemia	Serum creatinine <4 mg/dl and fluid and electrolyte status is stable
	Persistent oliguria, urine output of ≤10 ml/hour for 16 to 24 hours with rising serum creatinine	Urine output >10 ml/hour with a decrease of serum creatinine ≥1.5 mg/dl or normalization of serum creatinine
Hepatic	Signs of hepatic failure including encephalopathy, increasing ascites, liver pain, hypoglycemia	All signs of hepatic failure have resolved*
Gastrointestinal	Stool guaiac repeatedly >3-4+	Stool guaiac negative
Skin	Bullous dermatitis or marked worsening of pre-existing skin condition (avoid topical steroid therapy)	Resolution of all signs of bullous dermatitis

* Discontinue all further treatment for that course. Consider starting a new course of treatment of least 7 weeks after cessation of adverse event and hospital discharge.

4. Before and after reconstitution and dilution, store in a refrigerator at 2° to 8°C (36° to 46°F). Do not freeze. Administer aldesleukin within 48 hours of reconstitution. The solution should be brought to room temperature prior to infusion in the patient.

5. Reconstitution or dilution with Bacteriostatic Water for Injection, USP, or 0.9% Sodium Chloride Injection, USP should be avoided because of increased aggregation. Animal studies have shown that dilution with albumin can alter the pharmacology of aldesleukin. Aldesleukin should not be mixed with other drugs.

6. Parenteral drug products should be inspected visually for particulate matter and discoloration prior to administration, whenever solution and container permit.

REFERENCES:

1. Doyle MV, Lee MT, Fong S. Comparison of the biological activities of human recombinant interleukin-2$_{125}$and native interleukin-2. *J Biol Response Mod*1985;4:96-109. **2.** Ralph P, Nakoinz I, Doyle M, et al. Human B and T lymphocyte stimulating properties of interleukin-2 (IL-2) muteins. In: *Immune Regulation by Characterized Polypeptides.* Alan R. Liss, Inc. 1987:453-62. **3.** Winkelhake JL and Gauny SS. Human recombinant interleukin-2 as an experimental therapeutic.*Pharmacol Rev*1990; 42:1-28. **4.** Rosenberg SA, Mule JJ, Spiess PJ, et al. Regression of established pulmonary metastases and subcutaneous tumor mediated by the systemic administration of high-dose recombinant interleukin-2. *J Exp Med* 1985;161:1169-88. **5.** Konrad MW, Hemstreet G, Hersh EM, et al. Pharmacokinetics of recombinant interleukin-2 in humans. *Cancer Res* 1990; 50:2009-17. **6.** Donohue JH and Rosenberg SA. The fate of interleukin-2 after *in vivo* administration. *J Immunol* 1983; 130:2203-8. **7.** Koths K, Halenbeck R. Pharmacokinetic studies on 35S-labeled recombinant interleukin-2 in mice. In: Sorg C and Schimpl A, eds. *Cellular and Molecular Biology of Lymphokines.* Academic Press: Orlando, Fl, 1985:779. **8.** Moyer BR, Young JD, Bauer RJ, et al. Renal mechanisms for the clearance of recombinant human IL-2 in the rat. *Pharmaceutical Res* 1990; 7:S284 (abstract). **9.** Bock SN, Lee RE, Fisher B, et al. A prospective randomized trial evaluating prophylactic antibiotics to prevent triple-lumen catheter-related sepsis in patients treated with immunotherapy. *J Clin Oncol* 1990;8:161-69. **10.** Hartman LC, Urba, WJ, Steis RG, et al. Use of prophylactic antibiotics for prevention of intravascular catheter-related infections in interleukin-2-treated patients. *J Natl Cancer Inst* 1989; 81:1190-93. **11.** Snydman DR, Sullivan B, Gill M, et al. Nosocomial sepsis associated with interleukin-2. *Ann Intern Med* 1990; 112:102-07. **12.** Mier JW, Vachino G, Klempner MS, et al. Inhibition of interleukin-2-induced tumor necrosis factor release by dexamethasone: Prevention of an acquired neutrophil chemotaxis defect and differential suppression of interleukin-2-associated side effects. *Blood 1990;*76:1933-40. **13.** Choyke PL, Miller DL, Lotze MT, et al. Delayed reactions to contrast media after interleukin-2 immunotherapy.*Radiology* 1992; 183:111-114.

HOW SUPPLIED:

Proleukin for injection is supplied in individually-boxed single-use vials. Each contains 22 x 10^6 IU of Proleukin. Discard unused portion.

Store vials of lyophilized aldesleukin in a refrigerator at 2° to 8°C (36° to 46°F).

Reconstituted or diluted aldesleukin is stable for up to 48 hours at refrigerated and room temperatures, 2° to 25°C (36° to 77°F). However, since this product contains no preservative, the reconstituted and diluted solutions should be stored in the refrigerator.

Do not use beyond the expiration date printed on the vial. **Note:**This product contains no preservative.

HOW SUPPLIED - EQUIVALENTS NOT AVAILABLE:

Injection, Lyophilized-Powder - 22 million IU

1's	$395.00	**PROLEUKIN, Chiron Thera**	**53905-0991-01**

ALENDRONATE SODIUM *(003232)*

CATEGORIES: Biphosphonates; Bone Metabolism Regulators; Homeostatic & Nutrient; Osteoporosis; Paget's Disease; FDA Class 1P ("Priority Review"); FDA Approved 1995 Sep; Top 200 Drugs; Top 200 Drugs

BRAND NAMES: *Fosalan*; **Fosamax**
(International brand names outside U.S. in italics)

FORMULARIES: PCS

DESCRIPTION:

Fosamax is an aminobisphosphonate that acts as a specific inhibitor of osteoclast-mediated bone resorption. Bisphosphonates are synthetic analogs of pyrophosphate that bind to the hydroxyapatite found in bone.

Alendronate sodium is chemically described as (4-amino-1- hydroxybutylidene) bisphosphonic acid monosodium salt trihydrate.

DESCRIPTION: *(cont'd)*

The empirical formula of alendronate sodium is $C_4H_{12}NNaO_7P_2{\cdot}3H_2O$ and its formula weight is 325.12.

Alendronate sodium is a white, crystalline, nonhygroscopic powder. It is soluble in water, very slightly soluble in alcohol, and practically insoluble in chloroform.

Tablets alendronate sodium for oral administration contain either 13.05 mg or 52.21 mg of alendronate monosodium salt trihydrate, which is the molar equivalent of 10.0 mg and 40.0 mg, respectively, of free acid, and the following inactive ingredients: microcrystalline cellulose, anhydrous lactose, croscarmellose sodium, and magnesium stearate.

CLINICAL PHARMACOLOGY:

MECHANISM OF ACTION

Animal studies have indicated the following mode of action. At the cellular level, alendronate shows preferential localization to sites of bone resorption, specifically under osteoclasts. The osteoclasts adhere normally to the bone surface but lack the ruffled border that is indicative of active resorption. Alendronate does not interfere with osteoclast recruitment or attachment, but it does inhibit osteoclast activity. Studies in mice on the localization of radioactive [^{3}H]alendronate in bone showed about 10-fold higher uptake on osteoclast surfaces than on osteoblast surfaces. Bones examined 6 and 49 days after [^{3}H]alendronate administration in rats and mice, respectively, showed that normal bone was formed on top of the alendronate, which was incorporated inside the matrix. While incorporated in bone matrix, alendronate is not pharmacologically active. Thus, alendronate must be continuously administered to suppress osteoclasts on newly formed resorption surfaces. Histomorphometry in baboons and rats showed that alendronate treatment reduces bone turnover (*i.e.,* the number of sites at which bone is remodeled). In addition, bone formation exceeds bone resorption at these remodeling sites, leading to progressive gains in bone mass.

PHARMACOKINETICS

Absorption: Relative to an intravenous (IV) reference dose, the mean oral bioavailability of alendronate in women was 0.7% for doses ranging from 5 to 40 mg when administered after an overnight fast and two hours before a standardized breakfast. Oral bioavailability of the 10 mg tablet in men (0.59%) was similar to that in women (0.78%) when administered after an overnight fast and 2 hours before breakfast.

A study examining the effect of timing of a meal on the bioavailability of alendronate was performed in 49 postmenopausal women. Bioavailability was decreased (by approximately 40%) when 10 mg alendronate was administered either 0.5 or 1 hour before a standardized breakfast, when compared to dosing 2 hours before eating. Bioavailability was negligible whether alendronate was administered with or up to two hours after a standardized breakfast. Concomitant administration of alendronate with coffee or orange juice reduced bioavailability by approximately 60%.

In a trial in elderly patients given 5 mg of alendronate (n = 86) 30 minutes before breakfast, similar bone mineral density changes were noted when compared to the pivotal trials, in which one of the treatment arms was 5 mg alendronate administered 60 minutes before breakfast.

Distribution: Preclinical studies (in male rats) show that alendronate transiently distributes to soft tissues following 1 mg/kg IV administration but is then rapidly redistributed to bone or excreted in the urine. The mean steady-state volume of distribution, exclusive of bone, is at least 28:1 in humans. Concentrations of drug in plasma following therapeutic oral doses are too low (less than 5 ng/ml) for analytical detection. Protein binding in human plasma is approximately 78%.

Metabolism: There is no evidence that alendronate is metabolized in animals or humans.

Excretion: Following a single IV dose of [^{14}C]alendronate, approximately 50% of the radioactivity was excreted in the urine within 72 hours and little or no radioactivity was recovered in the feces. Following a single 10 mg IV dose, the renal clearance of alendronate was 71 ml/min, and systemic clearance did not exceed 200 ml/min. Plasma concentrations fell by more than 95% within 6 hours following IV administration. The terminal half-life in humans is estimated to exceed 10 years, probably reflecting release of alendronate from the skeleton. Based on the above, it is estimated that after 10 years of oral treatment with alendronate sodium (10 mg daily) the amount of alendronate released daily from the skeleton is approximately 25% of that absorbed from the gastrointestinal tract.

SPECIAL POPULATIONS

Pediatric: Alendronate pharmacokinetics have not been investigated in patients <18 years of age.

Gender: Bioavailability and the fraction of an IV dose excreted in urine were similar in men and women.

Geriatric: Bioavailability and disposition (urinary excretion) were similar in elderly (≥65 years of age) and younger patients. No dosage adjustment is necessary (see DOSAGE AND ADMINISTRATION).

Race: Pharmacokinetic differences due to race have not been studied.

Renal Insufficiency: Preclinical studies show that, in rats with kidney failure, increasing amounts of drug are present in plasma, kidney, spleen, and tibia. In healthy controls, drug that is not deposited in bone is rapidly excreted in the urine. No evidence of saturation of bone uptake was found after 3 weeks dosing with cumulative IV doses of 35 mg/kg in young male rats. Although no clinical information is available, it is likely that, as in animals, elimination of alendronate via the kidney will be reduced in patients with impaired renal function. Therefore, somewhat greater accumulation of alendronate in bone might be expected in patients with impaired renal function.

No dosage adjustment is necessary for patients with mild-to-moderate renal insufficiency (creatinine clearance 35 to 60 ml/min). **Alendronate sodium is not recommended for patients with more severe renal insufficiency (creatinine clearance <35 ml/min) due to lack of experience.**

Hepatic Insufficiency: As there is evidence that alendronate is not metabolized or excreted in the bile, no studies were conducted in patients with hepatic insufficiency. No dosage adjustment is necessary.

PHARMACODYNAMICS

Osteoporosis In Postmenopausal Women: Osteoporosis is characterized by low bone mass that leads to an increased risk of fracture. The diagnosis can be confirmed by the finding of low bone mass, evidence of fracture on x-ray, a history of osteoporotic fracture, or height loss or kyphosis, indicative of vertebral fracture. Osteoporosis occurs in both males and females but is most common among women following the menopause, when bone turnover increases and the rate of bone resorption exceeds that of bone formation. These changes result in progressive bone loss and lead to osteoporosis in a significant proportion of women over age 50. Fractures, usually of the spine, hip, and wrist, are the common consequences. From age 50 to age 90, the risk of hip fracture in white women increases 50-fold and the risk of vertebral fracture 15- to 30-fold. It is estimated that approximately 40% of 50-year-old women will sustain one or more osteoporosis-related fractures of the spine, hip, or wrist during their remaining lifetimes. Hip fractures, in particular, are associated with substantial morbidity, disability, and mortality.

Alendronate is an aminobisphosphonate that binds to bone hydroxyapatite and specifically inhibits the activity of osteoclasts, the bone-resorbing cells. Alendronate reduces bone resorption with no direct effect on bone formation, although the latter process is ultimately reduced

CLINICAL PHARMACOLOGY: *(cont'd)*

because bone resorption and formation are coupled during bone turnover. Alendronate thus reduces the elevated rate of bone turnover observed in postmenopausal women to approximate more closely that in premenopausal women.

Daily oral doses of alendronate (5, 20, and 40 mg for six weeks) in postmenopausal women produced biochemical changes indicative of dose-dependent inhibition of bone resorption, including decreases in urinary calcium and urinary markers of bone collagen degradation (such as deoxypyridinoline and cross-linked N-telopeptides of type I collagen). These biochemical changes tended to return toward baseline values as early as 3 weeks following the discontinuation of therapy with alendronate and did not differ from placebo after 7 months.

In long-term (two- or three-year) studies, alendronate sodium 10 mg/day reduced urinary excretion of markers of bone resorption, including deoxypyridinoline and cross-linked N-telopeptides of type I collagen, by approximately 50-60% to reach levels similar to those seen in healthy premenopausal women. The decrease in the rate of bone resorption indicated by these markers was evident as early as one month and at three to six months reached a plateau that was maintained for the entire duration of treatment with alendronate sodium. In addition, the markers of bone formation, serum osteocalcin and alkaline phosphatase, were also reduced by approximately 50% and 25 to 30%, respectively, to a plateau after 6 to 12 months. These data indicate that the rate of bone turnover reached a new steady-state, despite the progressive increase in the total amount of alendronate deposited within bone.

As a result of inhibition of bone resorption, asymptomatic reductions in serum calcium and phosphate concentrations were also observed following treatment with alendronate sodium. In the long-term studies, reductions from baseline in serum calcium (approximately 2%) and phosphate (approximately 4 to 6%) were evident the first month after the initiation of alendronate sodium 10 mg, but no further decreases were observed for the three-year duration of the studies. The reduction in serum phosphate may reflect not only the positive bone mineral balance due to alendronate sodium but also a decrease in renal phosphate reabsorption.

Paget's disease: Paget's disease of bone is a chronic, focal skeletal disorder characterized by greatly increased and disorderly bone remodeling. Excessive osteoclastic bone resorption is followed by osteoblastic new bone formation, leading to the replacement of the normal bone architecture by disorganized, enlarged, and weakened bone structure.

Clinical manifestations of Paget's disease range from no symptoms to severe morbidity due to bone pain, bone deformity, pathological fractures, and neurological and other complications. Serum alkaline phosphatase, the most frequently used biochemical index of disease activity, provides an objective measure of disease severity and response to therapy.

Alendronate sodium decreases the rate of bone resorption directly, which leads to an indirect decrease in bone formation. In clinical trials, alendronate sodium 40 mg once daily for six months produced highly significant decreases in serum alkaline phosphatase as well as in urinary markers of bone collagen degradation. As a result of the inhibition of bone resorption, alendronate sodium induced generally mild, transient, and asymptomatic decreases in serum calcium phosphate.

CLINICAL STUDIES:

Osteoporosis in postmenopausal women: The efficacy of alendronate sodium 10 mg once daily in postmenopausal women, 44 to 84 years of age, with osteoporosis (lumbar spine bone mineral density [BMD] of at least 2 standard deviations below the premenopausal mean) was demonstrated in four double-blind, placebo-controlled clinical studies of two or three years' duration. These included two large three-year, multicenter studies of virtually identical design, one performed in the United States (U.S.) and the other in 15 different countries (Multinational), which enrolled 478 and 516 patients, respectively.

Highly significant increases in BMD, relative both to baseline and placebo, were seen at each measurement site in each study in patients who received alendronate sodium 10 mg/day. Total body BMD also increased significantly in each study, suggesting that the increases in bone mass of the spine and hip did not occur at the expense of other skeletal sites. Increases in BMD were evident as early as three months and continued throughout the three years of treatment. Thus, alendronate sodium appears to reverse the progression of osteoporosis. Alendronate sodium was similarly effective regardless of age, race, baseline rate of bone turnover, and baseline BMD in the range studied (at least 2 standard deviations below the premenopausal mean).

To assess the effects of alendronate sodium on vertebral fracture incidence, the U.S. and Multinational studies were combined in an analysis that compared placebo to the pooled dosage groups of alendronate sodium (5 or 10 mg for three years or 20 mg for two years followed by 5 mg for one year). There was a significant 48% reduction in the proportion of patients treated with alendronate sodium experiencing one or more new vertebral fractures relative to those treated with placebo (3.2% vs. 6.2%). A reduction in the total number of new vertebral fractures (4.2 vs. 11.3 per 100 patients) was also observed. In the pooled analysis, patients who received alendronate sodium had a statistically significant smaller loss in stature than those who received placebo (-3.0 mm vs. -4.6 mm). Furthermore, of patients who sustained any vertebral fracture, those treated with alendronate sodium experienced less height loss (5.9 mm vs. 23.3 mm) due to a reduction in both the number and severity of fractures.

The effects of treatment withdrawal were assessed in a study that included patients treated with alendronate sodium for one or two years. Following discontinuation, neither further increases in bone mass nor accelerated rate of bone loss was noted. These data indicate that continuous daily treatment with alendronate sodium is required to maintain the effect of the drug.

Bone histology in 270 postmenopausal patients with osteoporosis treated with alendronate sodium at doses ranging from 1 to 20 mg/day for one, two, or three years revealed normal mineralization and structure, as well as the expected decrease in bone turnover relative to placebo. These data, together with the normal bone histology and increased bone strength observed in rats and baboons exposed to long-term alendronate treatment, support the conclusion that bone formed during therapy with alendronate sodium is of normal quality.

Paget's disease: The efficacy of alendronate sodium 40 mg once daily for six months was demonstrated in two double-blind clinical studies of male and female patients with moderate to severe Paget's disease (alkaline phosphatase at least twice the upper limit of normal): a placebo-controlled multinational study and a U.S. comparative study with etidronate disodium 400 mg/day.

At six months the suppression in alkaline phosphatase in patients treated with alendronate sodium was significantly greater than that achieved with etidronate and contrasted with the complete lack of response in placebo-treated patients. Response (defined as either normalization of serum alkaline phosphatase or decrease from baseline ≥60%) occurred in approximately 85% of patients treated with alendronate sodium in the combined studies vs. 30% in the etidronate group and 0% in the placebo group. Alendronate sodium was similarly effective irrespective of age, gender, race, prior use of other bisphosphonates, or baseline alkaline phosphatase within the range studied (at least twice the upper limit of normal).

Bone histology was evaluated in 33 patients with Paget's disease treated with alendronate sodium 40 mg/day for 6 months. As in patients treated for osteoporosis (see CLINICAL STUDIES, Osteoporosis In Postmenopausal Women), alendronate sodium did not impair mineralization, and the expected decrease in the rate of bone turnover was observed. Normal

CLINICAL STUDIES: *(cont'd)*

lamellar bone was produced during treatment with alendronate sodium, even where preexisting bone was woven and disorganized. Overall, bone histology data support the conclusion that bone formed during treatment with alendronate sodium is of normal quality.

INDICATIONS AND USAGE:

Alendronate sodium is indicated for the treatment of:

Osteoporosis in postmenopausal women. Osteoporosis may be confirmed by the finding of low bone mass (for example, at least 2 standard deviations below the premenopausal mean) or by the presence or history of osteoporotic fracture. (See CLINICAL PHARMACOLOGY, Pharmacodynamics.)

Paget's disease of bone. Treatment is indicated in patients with Paget's disease of bone having alkaline phosphatase at least two times the upper limit of normal, or those who are symptomatic, or those at risk for future complications from their disease.

CONTRAINDICATIONS:

Abnormalities of the esophagus which delay emptying such as stricture or achalasia.

Inability to stand or sit upright for at least 30 minutes.

Hypersensitivity to any component of this product.

Hypocalcemia (see PRECAUTIONS, General.)

WARNINGS:

Alendronate sodium, like other biophosphonates, may cause local irritation of the upper gastrointestinal mucosa.

Esophageal adverse experiences, such as esophagitis, esophageal ulcers and esophageal erosions have been reported in patients receiving treatment with alendronate sodium. In some cases these have been severe and required hospitalization. Physicians should therefore be alert to any signs of symptoms signaling a possible esophageal reaction and patients should discontinue alendronate sodium and seek medical attention if they develope dysphagia, odynophagia or retrosternal pain.

The risk of severe esophageal adverse experiences appears to be greater in patients who lie down after taking alendronate sodium and/or who fail to swallow it with a full glass of water, and/or continue to take alendronate sodium after developing symptoms suggestive of esophageal irritation. Therefore, it is very important that the full dosing instructions are provided to, and understood by, the patient (see DOSAGE AND ADMINISTRATION).

Because of possible irritant effects of alendronate sodium on the upper gastrointestinal mucosa, caution should be used when alendronate sodium is given to patients with active upper gastrointestinal problems, such as dysphagia, esophageal diseases, gastritis, duodenitis, or ulcers.

PRECAUTIONS:

General: Alendronate sodium is not recommended for patients with renal insufficiency (creatinine clearance <35 ml/min). (See DOSAGE AND ADMINISTRATION.)

Causes of osteoporosis other than estrogen deficiency and aging should be considered.

Hypocalcemia must be corrected before initiating therapy with alendronate sodium (see CONTRAINDICATIONS). Other disturbances of mineral metabolism (such as vitamin D deficiency) should also be effectively treated. Presumably due to the effects of alendronate sodium on increasing bone mineral, small, asymptomatic decreases in serum calcium and phosphate may occur, especially in patients with Paget's disease, in whom the pretreatment rate of bone turnover may be greatly elevated. Adequate calcium and vitamin D intake should be ensured to provide for these enhanced needs.

Information for the Patient: Patients should be instructed that the expected benefits of alendronate sodium may only be obtained when each tablet is taken with plain water the first thing in the morning at least 30 minutes before the first food, beverage, or medication of the day. Even dosing with orange juice or coffee has been shown to markedly reduce the absorption of alendronate sodium (see CLINICAL PHARMACOLOGY, Absorption).

To facilitate delivery to the stomach and thus reduce the potential for esophageal irritation patients should be instructed to swallow alendronate sodium with a full glass of water (6–8 oz) and not to lie down for at least 30 minutes and until after their first food of the day. Patients should not chew or suck on the tablet. Patients should be specifically instructed not to take alendronate sodium at bedtime or before arising for the day. Patients should be informed that failure to follow these instructions may increase their risk of esophageal problems. Patients should be instructed that if they develop symptoms of esophageal disease (such as difficulty or pain upon swallowing, retrosternal pain or new or worsening heartburn) they should stop taking alendronate sodium and consult their physician.

Patients should be instructed to take supplemental calcium and vitamin D, if daily dietary intake is inadequate. Weight-bearing exercise should be considered along with the modification of certain behavioral factors, such as excessive cigarette smoking, and/or alcohol consumption, if these factors exist.

Physicians should instruct their patients to read the patient package insert before starting therapy with alendronate sodium and to reread it each time the prescription is renewed.

Carcinogenesis, Mutagenesis, and Impairment of Fertility: Harderian gland (a retroorbital gland not present in human) adenomas were increased in high-dose female mice (p=0.003) in a 92-week carcinogenicity study at doses of alendronate of 1, 3, and 10 mg/kg/day (males) or 1, 2, and 5 mg/kg/day (females). These doses are equivalent to 0.5 to 4 times the 10 mg human dose based on surface area, mg/m^2.

Parafollicular cell (thyroid) adenomas were increased in high-dose male rats (p=0.003) in a 2-year carcinogenicity study at doses of 1 and 3.75 mg/kg body weight. These doses are equivalent to 1 and 3 times the 10 mg human dose based on body surface area.

Alendronate was not genotoxic in the *in vitro* microbial mutagenesis assay with and without metabolic activation, in an *in vitro* mammalian cell mutagenesis assay, in an *in vitro* alkaline elution assay in rat hepatocytes, and in an *in vivo* chromosomal aberration assay in mice. In an *in vitro* chromosomal aberration assay in Chinese hamster ovary cells, however, alendronate was weakly positive at concentrations ≥5 mM in the presence of cytotoxicity.

Alendronate had no effect on fertility (male or female) in rats at oral doses up to 5 mg/kg/day (four times the 10 mg human dose based on surface area).

Pregnancy Category C: Reproduction studies in rats showed decreased postimplantation survival at 2 mg/kg/day and decreased body weight gain in normal pups at 1 mg/kg/day. Sites of incomplete fetal ossification were statistically significantly increased in rats beginning at 10 mg/kg/day in vertebral (cervical, thoracic, and lumbar), skull, and sternebral bones. The above doses ranged from 1 times (1 mg/kg) to 9 times (10 mg/kg) the 10 mg human dose based on surface area, mg/m^2. No similar fetal effects were seen when pregnant rabbits were treated at doses up to 35 mg/kg/day (50 times the 10 mg human dose based on surface area, mg/m^2).

Both total and ionized calcium decreased in pregnant rats at 15 mg/kg/day (13 times the 10 mg human dose based on surface area) resulting in delays and failures of delivery. Protracted parturition due to maternal hypocalcemia occurred in rats at doses as low as 0.5 mg/kg/day (0.5 times the recommended human dose), when rats were treated from before mating

PRECAUTIONS: *(cont'd)*

through gestation. Maternotoxicity (late pregnancy deaths) occurred in the female rats treated with 15 mg/kg/day for varying periods of time ranging from treatment only during pre-mating to treatment only during early, middle, or late gestation; these deaths were lessened but not eliminated by cessation of treatment. Calcium supplementation either in the drinking water or by minipump could not ameliorate the hypocalcemia or prevent maternal and neonatal deaths due to delays in delivery; calcium supplementation IV prevented maternal, but not fetal deaths.

There are no studies in pregnant women. Alendronate sodium should be used during pregnancy only if the potential benefit justifies the potential risk to the mother and fetus.

Nursing Mothers: Alendronate was secreted in the milk of rats after an IV dose. It is not known whether alendronate is excreted in human milk. Alendronate sodium has not been studied in nursing women and should not be given to them.

Pediatric Use: Safety and effectiveness in pediatric patients have not been established.

Geriatric Use: Of the patients receiving alendronate sodium in the two large osteoporosis studies and Paget's disease studies (see CLINICAL STUDIES), 45% and 70%, respectively, were 65 years of age or over. No overall differences in efficacy or safety were observed between these patients and younger patients but greater sensitivity of some older individuals cannot be ruled out.

Use in Men: Safety and effectiveness in male osteoporosis have not been established.

DRUG INTERACTIONS:

Intravenous ranitidine was shown to double the bioavailability of oral alendronate. The clinical significance of this increased bioavailability and whether similar increases will occur in patients given oral H_2-antagonists is unknown; no other specific drug interaction studies were performed.

Products containing calcium and other multivalent cations likely will interfere with absorption of alendronate (TABLE 1).

TABLE 1 Summary of Pharmacokinetic Parameters in the Normal Population

Absolute bioavailability of tablet taken 2 hours before first meal of the day	Mean	90% Confidence Interval
10 mg tablet	0.78% (females)	(0.61, 1.04)
	0.59% (males)	(0.43, 0.81)
40 mg tablet	0.60% (females)	(0.46, 0.78)
Renal Clearance (ml/min) (n=6)	71	(64, 78)

(See CLINICAL PHARMACOLOGY, Pharmacokinetics.)

Estrogen: A small number of postmenopausal women in the osteoporosis trials received estrogen (intravaginal, transdermal, or oral) while taking alendronate sodium. No adverse experiences attributable to their concomitant use were identified.

Concomitant use of hormone replacement therapy and alendronate sodium in the treatment of osteoporosis in postmenopausal women is not recommended because of lack of clinical experience.

Calcium Supplements/Antacids: It is unlikely that calcium supplements, antacids, and some oral medications will interfere with absorption of alendronate sodium. Therefore, patients must wait at least one-half hour after taking alendronate sodium before taking any other drug.

NSAIDS/Aspirin: The risk of upper gastrointestinal adverse events associated with NSAIDS does not appear to be greater with concomitant treatment with alendronate sodium 10 mg/day. However, in patients receiving concomitant therapy with doses of alendronate sodium greater than 10 mg/day and aspirin-containing compounds, the incidence of upper gastrointestinal adverse events was increased.

Other: Although specific interaction studies were not performed, alendronate sodium 10 mg/day was used in postmenopausal osteoporosis studies with a wide range of commonly prescribed drugs without evidence of clinical adverse interactions. These included antacids, anticholinergics, aspirin-containing compounds, benzodiazepines, beta-blockers, calcium channel blockers, diuretics, gastric acid secretion inhibitors, glucocorticoids, nonsteroidal anti-inflammatory drugs (NSAIDS), sedative hypnotics, thiazides, thyroid hormones, vasoconstrictors, and vasodilators.

ADVERSE REACTIONS:

Adverse experiences associated with alendronate sodium usually have been mild, and generally have not required discontinuation of therapy.

Osteoporosis In Postmenopausal Women: Alendronate sodium has been evaluated for safety in clinical studies in more than 1800 postmenopausal patients. In two large, three-year, placebo-controlled, double-blind, multicenter studies (United States and Multinational), discontinuation of therapy due to any clinical adverse experience occurred in 4.1% of 196 patients treated with alendronate sodium 10 mg/day and 6.0% of 397 patients treated with placebo. Adverse experiences reported by the investigators as possibly, probably, or definitely drug related in ≥1% of patients treated with either alendronate sodium 10 mg/day or placebo are presented in the following table (TABLE 2).

Rarely, rash and erythema have occurred.

One patient treated with alendronate sodium (10 mg/day), who had a history of peptic ulcer disease and gastrectomy and who was taking concomitant aspirin developed an anastomotic ulcer with mild hemorrhage, which was considered drug related. Aspirin and alendronate sodium were discontinued and the patient recovered.

The adverse experience profile was similar for the 401 patients treated with either 5 or 20 mg doses of alendronate sodium in the United States and Multinational studies.

Paget's Disease: In clinical studies (osteoporosis and Paget's disease), adverse experiences reported in 175 patients taking alendronate sodium 40 mg/day for 3-12 months were similar to those in postmenopausal women treated with alendronate sodium 10 mg/day. However, there was an apparent increased incidence of upper gastrointestinal adverse experiences in patients taking alendronate sodium 40 mg/day (17.7% alendronate sodium vs. 10.2% placebo). One case of esophagitis and two cases of gastritis resulted in discontinuation of treatment.

Additionally, musculoskeletal pain, which has been described in patients with Paget's disease treated with other bisphosphonates, was reported by the investigators as possibly, probably, or definitely drug related in approximately 6% of patients treated with alendronate sodium 40 mg/day versus approximately 1% of patients treated with placebo, but rarely resulted in discontinuation of therapy. Discontinuation of therapy due to any clinical adverse experience occurred in 6.4% of patients with Paget's disease treated with alendronate sodium 40 mg/day and 2.4% of patients treated with placebo.

Laboratory Test Findings: In double-blind, multicenter, controlled studies, asymptomatic, mild, and transient decreases in serum calcium and phosphate were observed in approximately 18% and 10%, respectively, of patients taking alendronate sodium versus approximately 12% and 3% of those taking placebo. However, the incidences of decreases in serum calcium to <8.0 mg/dl (2.0 mM) and serum phosphate to ≤2.0 mg/dl (0.65 mM) were similar in both treatment groups.

ADVERSE REACTIONS: *(cont'd)*

TABLE 2 Drug-Related Adverse Experiences Reported in ≥1% of Patients**

	10 mg/day Alendronate Na % (n = 196)	Placebo % (n = 397)
Gastrointestinal		
abdominal pain	6.6	4.8
nausea	3.6	4.0
dyspepsia	3.6	3.5
constipation	3.1	1.8
diarrhea	3.1	1.8
flatulence	2.6	0.5
acid regurgitation	2.0	4.3
esophageal ulcer	1.5	0.0
vomiting	1.0	1.5
dysphagia	1.0	0.0
abdominal distention	1.0	0.8
gastritis	0.5	1.3
Musculoskeletal		
musculoskeletal pain	4.1	2.5
muscle cramp	0.0	1.0
Nervous System/Psychiatric		
headache	2.6	1.5
dizziness	0.0	1.0
Special Senses		
taste perversion	0.5	1.0

** Considered possibly, probably, or definitively drug related as assessed by the investigators

Post-Marketing Experience: The following adverse reactions have been reported in post-marketing use: esophagitis, esophageal erosions and esophageal ulcers (see WARNINGS and DOSAGE AND ADMINISTRATION).

OVERDOSAGE:

Significant lethality after single oral doses was seen in female rats and mice at 552 mg/kg (3256 mg/m²) and 966 mg/kg (2898 mg/m²), respectively. In males, these values were slightly higher, 626 and 1280 mg/kg, respectively. There was no lethality in dogs at oral doses up to 200 mg/kg (4000 mg/m²).

No specific information is available on the treatment of overdosage with alendronate sodium. Hypocalcemia, hypophosphatemia, and upper gastrointestinal adverse events, such as upset stomach, heartburn, esophagitis, gastritis, or ulcer, may result from oral overdosage. Milk or antacids ahould be given to blind alendronate. Due to risk of esophageal irritation, vomiting should not be induced and the patient should remain fully upright.

Dialysis would not be beneficial.

DOSAGE AND ADMINISTRATION:

Alendronate sodium must be taken *at least* one-half hour before the first food, beverage, or medication of the day with plain water only (see PRECAUTIONS, Information for the Patient). Other beverages (including mineral water), food, and some medications are likely to reduce the absorption of alendronate sodium (see DRUG INTERACTIONS). Waiting longer than 30 minutes before eating will improve the absorption of alendronate sodium. Waiting less than 30 minutes, or taking alendronate sodium with food, beverages (other than plain water) or other medications will lessen the effect of alendronate sodium by decreasing its absorption into the body. To facilitate delivery to the stomach, alendronate sodium should be taken with a full glass of water (6-8 oz.) and patients should avoid lying down for at least 30 minutes thereafter (see PRECAUTIONS, Information for the Patient).

Patients with osteoporosis or Paget's disease should receive supplemental calcium and vitamin D, if dietary intake is inadequate (see PRECAUTIONS, General).

No dosage adjustment is necessary for the elderly or for patients with mild-to-moderate renal insufficiency (creatinine clearance 35 to 60 ml/min). Alendronate sodium is not recommended for patients with more severe renal insufficiency (creatinine clearance <35 ml/min) due to lack of experience.

Osteoporosis In Postmenopausal Women: The recommended dosage is 10 mg once a day. Safety of treatment with alendronate sodium for longer than four years has not been studied; extension studies are ongoing.

Paget's Disease Of Bone: The recommended treatment regimen is 40 mg once a day for six months.

Retreatment Of Paget's Disease: In clinical studies in which patients were followed every six months, relapses during the 12 months following therapy occurred in 9% (3 out of 32) of patients who responded to treatment with alendronate sodium. Specific retreatment data are not available, although responses to alendronate sodium were similar in patients who had received prior bisphosphonate therapy and those who had not. Retreatment with alendronate sodium may be considered, following a six-month post-treatment evaluation period in patients who have relapsed, based on increases in serum alkaline phosphatase, which should be measured periodically. Retreatment may also be considered in those who failed to normalize their serum alkaline phosphatase.

ANIMAL PHARMACOLOGY:

The relative inhibitory activities on bone resorption and mineralization of alendronate and etidronate were compared in the Schenk assay, which is based on histological examination of the epiphyses of growing rats. In this assay, the lowest dose of alendronate that interfered with bone mineralization (leading to osteomalacia) was 6000-fold the antiresorptive dose. The corresponding ratio for etidronate was one to one. These data suggest that alendronate administered in therapeutic doses is highly unlikely to induce osteomalacia.

PATIENT INFORMATION:

Alendronate sodium is used to treat osteoporosis and Paget's disease, both diseases which weaken bones. Alendronate sodium is effective in decreasing bone loss but does require you to understand exactly how to take this medication. You may have also been prescribed Vitamin D and/or exercises both which should be followed as prescribed in order to get the greatest benefit. This drug should not be taken if you have a low calcium level that is not being corrected with calcium supplementation. Alendronate sodium will irritate the esophagus and stomach. It is very important to take this medication the first thing in the morning with a FULL glass of water and to not lie down for at least 30 minutes after taking the medication. Food should not be eaten or other medications taken for 30 minutes. Drinking juice or coffee with alendronate sodium decreases the absorption and may lessen the benefit you receive. If you experience any signs of difficult swallowing, painful swallowing or upper

PATIENT INFORMATION: *(cont'd)*

chest pain report these to your physician immediately. You should receive patient information on this drug each time you get a refill. Because taking this correctly is very important, read this information to refresh your memory.

HOW SUPPLIED:

Tablets Fosamax, 10 mg, are white, round, uncoated tablets with a bone image and code MRK 936 on one side and a bone image and Fosamax on the other.

Tablets Fosamax, 40 mg, are white triangular-shaped, uncoated tablets with code MRK 212 on one side and Fosamax on the other.

Storage: Store in a well-closed container at controlled room temperature 15-30°C (59-86°F).

HOW SUPPLIED - EQUIVALENTS NOT AVAILABLE:

Tablet, Uncoated - Oral - 10 mg

30's	$50.04	FOSAMAX, Merck	00006-0936-31
100's	$166.80	FOSAMAX, Merck	00006-0936-28
100's	$166.80	FOSAMAX, Merck	00006-0936-58

Tablet, Uncoated - Oral - 40 mg

30's	$126.00	FOSAMAX, Merck	00006-0212-31

ALFENTANIL HYDROCHLORIDE *(000122)*

CATEGORIES: Analgesics; Anesthesia; Antipyretics; Central Nervous System Agents; Endotracheal Intubation; Intubation; Narcotic Analgesics; Narcotics, Synthetics & Combinations; Opiate Agonists (Controlled); Pregnancy Category C; DEA Class CII; FDA Approved 1986 Dec

BRAND NAMES: **Alfenta**; *Rapifen* (Europe, Mexico)
(International brand names outside U.S. in italics)

DESCRIPTION:

Alfentanil hydrochloride injection is an opioid analgesic chemically designated as N-[1-[2-(4-ethyl-4,5-dihydro-5-oxo-1H-tetrazol-1-yl)ethyl]-4-(methoxymethyl)-4-piperidinyl]-N-phenylpropanamide monohydrochloride (1:1) with a molecular weight of 452.98.

Alfenta is a sterile, non-pyrogenic, preservative free aqueous solution containing alfentanil hydrochloride equivalent to 500 mcg per ml of alfentanil base for intravenous injection. The solution, which contains sodium chloride for isotonicity, has a pH range of 4.0-6.0.

CLINICAL PHARMACOLOGY:

Alfentanil hydrochloride is an opioid analgesic with a rapid onset of action.

At doses of 8-40 mcg/kg for surgical procedures lasting up to 30 minutes, alfentanil provides analgesic protection against hemodynamic responses to surgical stress with recovery times generally comparable to those seen with equipotent fentanyl dosages.

For longer procedures, doses of up to 75 mcg/kg attenuate hemodynamic responses to laryngoscopy, intubation and incision, with recovery time comparable to fentanyl. At doses of 50-75 mcg/kg followed by a continuous infusion of 0.5-3.0 mcg/kg/min, alfentanil attenuates the catecholamine response with more rapid recovery and reduced need for postoperative analgesics as compared to patients administered enflurane. At doses of 5 mcg/kg, alfentanil provides analgesia for the conscious but sedated patient. Based on patient response, doses higher than 5 mcg/kg may be needed. Elderly or debilitated patients may require lower doses. High intrasubject and intersubject variability in the pharmacokinetic disposition of alfentanil has been reported.

The pharmacokinetics of alfentanil can be described as a three-compartment model with sequential distribution half-lives of 1 and 14 minutes; and a terminal elimination half-life of 90-111 minutes (as compared to a terminal elimination half-life of approximately 475 minutes for fentanyl and approximately 265 minutes for sufentanil at doses of 250 mcg). The liver is the major site of biotransformation.

Alfentanil has an apparent volume of distribution of 0.4-1 L/kg, which is approximately one-fourth to one-tenth that of fentanyl, with an average plasma clearance of 5 ml/kg/min as compared to approximately 8 ml/kg/min for fentanyl.

Only 1.0% of the dose is excreted as unchanged drug; urinary excretion is the major route of elimination of metabolites. Plasma protein binding of alfentanil is approximately 92%.

In one study involving 15 patients administered alfentanil with nitrous oxide/oxygen, a narrow range of plasma alfentanil concentrations, approximately 310-340 ng/ml, was shown to provide adequate anesthesia for intra-abdominal surgery, while lower concentrations, approximately 190 ng/ml, blocked responses to skin closure. Plasma concentrations between 100-200 ng/ml provided adequate anesthesia for superficial surgery.

Alfentanil has an immediate onset of action. At dosages of approximately 105 mcg/kg, alfentanil produces hypnosis as determined by EEG patterns; an aesthetic ED_{90} of 182 mcg/kg for alfentanil in unpremedicated patients has been determined, based upon the ability to block response to placement of a nasopharyngeal airway. Based on clinical trials, induction dosage requirements range from 130-245 mcg/kg. For procedures lasting 30-60 minutes, loading dosages of up to 50 mcg/kg produce the hemodynamic responses to endotracheal intubation and skin incision comparable to those from fentanyl. A pre-intubation loading dose of 50-75 mcg/kg prior to a continuous infusion attenuates the response to laryngoscopy, intubation and incision. Subsequent administration of alfentanil infusion administered at a rate of 0.5-3 mcg/kg/min with nitrous oxide/oxygen attenuates sympathetic responses to surgical stress with more rapid recovery than enflurane.

Requirements for volatile inhalation anesthetics were reduce by 30 to 50%during the first 60 minutes of maintenance in patients administered anesthetic doses (above 130 mcg/kg) of alfentanil as compared to patients given doses of 4-5 mg/kg thiopental for anesthetic induction. At anesthetic induction dosages, alfentanil provides a deep level of anesthesia during the first hour of anesthetic maintenance and provides attenuation of the hemodynamic response during intubation and incision.

Following an anesthetic dose of alfentanil, requirements for alfentanil infusion are reduced by 30 to 50% for the first hour of maintenance.

Patients with compromised liver function and those over 65 years of age have been found to have reduced plasma clearance and extended terminal elimination of alfentanil, which may prolong postoperative recovery.

Repeated or continuous administration of alfentanil produces increasing plasma concentrations and an accumulation of the drug, particularly in patients with reduced plasma clearance.

Bradycardia may be seen in patients administered alfentanil. The incidence and degree of bradycardia may be more pronounced when alfentanil is administered in conjunction with non-vagolytic neuromuscular blocking agents or in the absence of anticholinergic agents such as atropine.

CLINICAL PHARMACOLOGY: *(cont'd)*

Administration of intravenous diazepam immediately prior to or following high doses of alfentanil has been shown to produce decreases in blood pressure that may be secondary to vasodilation; recovery may also be prolonged.

Patients administered doses up to 200 mcg/kg of alfentanil have shown no significant increase in histamine levels and no clinical evidence of histamine release.

Skeletal muscle rigidity is related to the dose and speed of administration of alfentanil. Muscular rigidity will occur with an immediate onset following anesthetic induction dosages. Preventative measures (see WARNINGS) may reduce the rate and severity.

The duration and degree of respiratory depression and increased airway resistance usually increase with dose, but have also been observed at lower doses. Although higher doses may produce apnea and a longer duration of respiratory depression, apnea may also occur at low doses.

During monitored anesthesia care (MAC), attention must be given to the respiratory effects of alfentanil injection. Decreased oxygen saturation, apnea, decreased respiratory rate, and upper airway obstruction can occur. (See WARNINGS)

INDICATIONS AND USAGE:

Alfentanil hydrochloride is indicated:

as an analgesic adjunct given in incremental doses in the maintenance of anesthesia with barbiturate/nitrous oxide/oxygen.

as an analgesic administered by continuous infusion with nitrous oxide/oxygen in the maintenance of general anesthesia.

as a primary anesthetic agent for the induction of anesthesia in patients undergoing general surgery in which endotracheal intubation and mechanical ventilation are required.

as the analgesic component for monitored anesthesia care (MAC).

SEE TABLE 1 FOR MORE COMPLETE INFORMATION ON THE USE OF ALFENTANIL.

CONTRAINDICATIONS:

Alfentanil hydrochloride is contraindicated in patients with known hypersensitivity to the drug.

WARNINGS:

ALFENTANIL SHOULD BE ADMINISTERED ONLY BY PERSONS SPECIFICALLY TRAINED IN THE USE OF INTRAVENOUS AND GENERAL ANESTHETIC AGENTS AND IN THE MANAGEMENT OF RESPIRATORY EFFECTS OF POTENT OPIOIDS.

AN OPIOID ANTAGONIST, RESUSCITATIVE AND INTUBATION EQUIPMENT AND OXYGEN SHOULD BE READILY AVAILABLE.

BECAUSE OF THE POSSIBILITY OF DELAYED RESPIRATORY DEPRESSION, MONITORING OF THE PATIENT MUST CONTINUE WELL AFTER SURGERY.

Alfentanil hydrochloride administered in initial dosages up to 20 mcg/kg may cause skeletal muscle rigidity, particularly of the truncal muscles. The incidence and severity of muscle rigidity is usually dose- related. Administration of alfentanil at anesthetic induction dosages (above 130 mcg/kg) will consistently produce muscular rigidity with an immediate onset. The onset of muscular rigidity occurs earlier than with other opioids. Alfentanil may produce muscular rigidity that involves all skeletal muscles, including those of the neck and extremities. The incidence may be reduced by: 1) routine methods of administration of neuromuscular blocking agents for balanced opioid anesthesia; 2) administration of up to 1/4 of the full paralyzing dose of a neuromuscular blocking agent just prior to administration of alfentanil at dosages up to 130 mcg/kg; following loss of consciousness, a full paralyzing dose of a neuromuscular blocking agent should be administered; or 3) simultaneous administration of alfentanil and a full paralyzing dose of a neuromuscular blocking agent when alfentanil is used in rapidly administered anesthetic dosages (above 130 mcg/kg).

The neuromuscular blocking agent used should be appropriate for the patient's cardiovascular status. Adequate facilities should be available for postoperative monitoring and ventilation of patients administered alfentanil. It is essential that these facilities be fully equipped to handle all degrees of respiratory depression.

PATIENTS RECEIVING MONITORED ANESTHESIA CARE (MAC) SHOULD BE CONTINUOUSLY MONITORED BY PERSONS NOT INVOLVED IN THE CONDUCT OF THE SURGICAL OR DIAGNOSTIC PROCEDURE; OXYGEN SUPPLEMENTATION SHOULD BE IMMEDIATELY AVAILABLE AND PROVIDED WHERE CLINICALLY INDICATED; OXYGEN SATURATION SHOULD BE CONTINUOUSLY MONITORED; THE PATIENT SHOULD BE OBSERVED FOR EARLY SIGNS OF HYPOTENSION, APNEA, UPPER AIRWAY OBSTRUCTION AND/OR OXYGEN DESATURATION.

Severe and unpredictable potentiation of monoamine oxidase (MAO) inhibitors has been reported for other opioid analgesics, and rarely with alfentanil. Therefore when alfentanil is administered to patients who have received MAO inhibitors within 14 days, appropriate monitoring and ready availability of vasodilators and beta-blockers for the treatment of hypertension is recommended.

PRECAUTIONS:

DELAYED RESPIRATORY DEPRESSION, RESPIRATORY ARREST, BRADYCARDIA, ASYSTOLE, ARRHYTHMIAS AND HYPOTENSION HAVE ALSO BEEN REPORTED. THEREFORE, VITAL SIGNS MUST BE MONITORED CONTINUOUSLY.

General: The initial dose of alfentanil should be appropriately reduced in elderly and debilitated patients. The effect of the initial dose should be considered in determining supplemental doses. In obese patients (more then 20% above ideal total body weight), the dosage of alfentanil should be determined on the basis of lean body weight. In one clinical trial, the dose of alfentanil required to produce anesthesia, as determined by appearance of delta waves in EEG, was 40% lower in geriatric patients than that needed in healthy young patients.

In patients with compromised liver function and in geriatric patients, the plasma clearance of alfentanil may be reduced and postoperative recovery may be prolonged.

Induction doses of alfentanil should be administered slowly (over three minutes). Administration may produce loss of vascular tone and hypotension. Consideration should be given to fluid replacement prior to induction.

Diazepam administered immediately prior to or in conjunction with high doses of alfentanil may produce vasodilation, hypotension and result in delayed recovery.

Bradycardia produced by alfentanil may be treated with atropine. Severe bradycardia and asystole have been successfully treated with atropine and conventional resuscitative methods.

The hemodynamic effects of a particular muscle relaxant and the degree of skeletal muscle relaxation required should be considered in the selection of a neuromuscular blocking agent.

Following an anesthetic induction dose of alfentanil, requirements for volatile inhalation anesthetics of alfentanil infusion are reduced by 30 to 50% for the first hour of maintenance.

PRECAUTIONS: *(cont'd)*

Alfentanil infusions should be discontinued at least 10-15 minutes prior to the end of surgery during general anesthesia. During administration of alfentanil for Monitored Anesthesia Care (MAC), infusions may be continued to the end of the procedure.

Respiratory depression caused by opioid analgesics can be reversed by opioid antagonists such as naloxone. Because the duration of respiratory depression produced by alfentanil may last longer than the duration of the opioid antagonist action, appropriate surveillance should be maintained. As with all potent opioids, profound analgesia is accompanied by respiratory depression and diminished sensitivity to CO_2 stimulation which may persist into or recur in the postoperative period.

Intraoperative hyperventilation may further after postoperative response to CO_2. Appropriate postoperative monitoring should be employed, particularly after infusions and large doses of alfentanil, to ensure that adequate spontaneous breathing is established and maintained in the absence of stimulation prior to discharging the patient from the recovery area.

Head Injuries: Alfentanil may obscure the clinical course of patients with head injuries.

Impaired Respiration: Alfentanil should be used with caution in patients with pulmonary disease, decreased respiratory reserve or potentially compromised respiration. In such patients, opioids may additionally decrease respiratory drive and increase airway resistance. During anesthesia, this can be managed by assisted or controlled respiration.

Impaired Hepatic or Renal Function: In patients with liver or kidney dysfunction, alfentanil should be administered with caution due to the importance of these organs in the metabolism and excretion of alfentanil.

Carcinogenesis, Mutagenesis and Impairment of Fertility: No long-term animal studies of alfentanil have been performed to evaluate carcinogenic potential. No structural chromosome mutations were produced in the *in vivo* micronucleus test in female rats at single intravenous doses of alfentanil as high as 20 mg/kg body weight (approximately 40 times the upper human dose), equivalent to a dose of 103 mg/m^2 body surface area. No dominant lethal mutations were produced in the *in vivo* dominant lethal test in male and female mice at the maximum intravenous dose of 20 mg/kg (60 mg/m^2). No mutagenic activity was revealed in the *in vitro* Ames*Salmonella typhimurium* test, with and without metabolic activation.

Pregnancy Category C: Alfentanil has been shown to have an embryocidal effect in rats and rabbits when given in doses 2.5 times the upper human dose for a period of 10 days to over 30 days. These effects could have been due to maternal toxicity (decreased food consumption with increased mortality) following prolonged administration of the drug.

No evidence of teratogenic effects has been observed after administration for alfentanil in rats or rabbits.

There are no adequate and well-controlled studies in pregnant women. Alfentanil should be used during pregnancy only if the potential benefit justifies the potential risk to the fetus.

Labor and Delivery: There are insufficient data to support the use of alfentanil in labor and delivery. Placental transfer of the drug has been reported: therefore, use in labor and delivery is not recommended.

Nursing Mothers: In one study of nine women undergoing postpartum tubal ligation, significant levels of alfentanil were detected in colostrum four hours after administration of 60 mcg/kg of alfentanil, with no detectable levels present after 28 hours. Caution should be exercised when alfentanil is administered to a nursing woman.

Pediatric Use: Adequate data to support the use of alfentanil in children under 12 years of age are not presently available.

DRUG INTERACTIONS:

Both the magnitude and duration of central nervous system and cardiovascular effects may be enhanced when alfentanil is administered in combination with other CNS depressants such as barbiturates, tranquilizers, opioids, or inhalation general anesthetics. Postoperative respiratory depression may be enhanced or prolonged by these agents. In such cases of combined treatment, the dose of one or both agents should be reduced. Limited clinical experience indicates that requirements for volatile inhalation anesthetics are reduced by 30 to 50% for the first sixty (60) minutes following alfentanil induction.

The concomitant use of erythromycin with alfentanil can significantly inhibit alfentanil clearance and may increase the risk of prolonged or delayed respiratory depression. Cimetidine reduces the clearance of alfentanil. Therefore smaller alfentanil doses will be required with prolonged administration and the duration of action of alfentanil may be extended.

Perioperative administration of drugs affecting hepatic blood flow or enzyme function may reduce plasma clearance and prolong recovery.

ADVERSE REACTIONS:

The most common adverse reactions of opioids are respiratory depression and skeletal muscle rigidity, particularly of the truncal muscles. Alfentanil may produce muscular rigidity that involves the skeletal muscles of the neck and extremities. (See CLINICAL PHARMACOLOGY, WARNINGS, and PRECAUTIONS) on the management of respiratory depression and skeletal muscle rigidity.

The adverse experience profile from 696 patients receiving alfentanil for Monitored Anesthesia Care (MAC) is similar to the profile established with alfentanil during general anesthesia. Respiratory events reported during MAC included hypoxia, apnea, and bradypnea. Other adverse events reported by patients receiving alfentanil for MAC, in order of decreasing frequency, were nausea, hypotension, vomiting, pruritus, confusion, somnolence and agitation.

The following adverse reaction information is derived from controlled and open clinical trials in 785 patients who received intravenous alfentanil during induction and maintenance of general anesthesia. The controlled trial included treatment comparisons with fentanyl, thiopental sodium, enflurane, saline placebo and halothane. The incidence of certain side effects is influenced by the type of use (*e.g.,* chest wall rigidity has a higher reported incidence in clinical trials of alfentanil induction) and by the type of surgery, (*e.g.,* nausea and vomiting have a higher reported incidence in patients undergoing gynecologic surgery). The overall reports of nausea and vomiting with alfentanil were comparable to fentanyl.

Incidence Greater than 1% - Probably Causally Related (Derived from clinical trials)

Gastrointestinal: nausea (28%); vomiting (18%)

Cardiovascular: arrhythmia, bradycardia (14%); hypertension (18%); hypotension (10%); tachycardia (12%)

Musculoskeletal: chest wall rigidity (17%); skeletal muscle movements*

Respiratory: apnea*, postoperative respiratory depression

Central Nervous System: blurred vision, dizziness*, sleepiness/postoperative sedation

* Incidence 3% to 9%

All others 1% to 3%

Incidence Less than 1% - Probably Causally Related(Derived from clinical trials)

Adverse events reported in post-marketing surveillance, not seen in clinical trials, are *italicized.*

Central Nervous System: headache*, *myoclonic movements,* postoperative confusion*, postoperative euphoria*, shivering*

ADVERSE REACTIONS: *(cont'd)*

Dermatological: itching*, urticaria*

Injection Site: pain*

Musculoskeletal: *skeletal muscle rigidity of neck and extremities*

Respiratory: bronchospasm, hypercarbia*, laryngospasm*

* Incidence 0.3% to 1%

DRUG ABUSE AND DEPENDENCE:

Alfentanil hydrochloride is a Schedule II controlled drug substance that can produce drug dependence of the morphine type and therefore has the potential for being abused.

Opioid analgesics have been associated with abuse and dependence in health care providers and others with ready access to such drugs. Alfentanil should be handled accordingly.

OVERDOSAGE:

Overdosage would be manifested by extension of the pharmacological actions of alfentanil hydrochloride (see CLINICAL PHARMACOLOGY) as with other potent opioid analgesics. No experience of overdosage with alfentanil was reported during clinical trials. The intravenous LD_{50} of alfentanil is 43-51 mg/kg in rats, 72-74 mg/kg in mice, 72-82 mg/kg in guinea pigs and 60-88 mg/kg in dogs. Intravenous administration of an opioid antagonist such as naloxone should be employed as a specific antidote to manage respiratory depression.

The duration of respiratory depression following overdosage with alfentanil may be longer than the duration of action of the opioid antagonist. Administration of an opioid antagonist should not preclude immediate establishment of a patent airway, administration of oxygen, and assisted or controlled ventilation as indicated for hypoventilation or apnea. If respiratory depression is associated with muscular rigidity, a neuromuscular blocking agent may be required to facilitate assisted or controlled ventilation. Intravenous fluids and vasoactive agents may be required to manage hemodynamic instability.

DOSAGE AND ADMINISTRATION:

The dosage of alfentanil hydrochloride should be individualized in each patient according to body weight, physical status, underlying pathological condition, use of other drugs, and type and duration of surgical procedure and anesthesia. In obese patients (more than 20% above ideal total body weight), the dosage of alfentanil should be determined on the basis of lean body weight. The dose of alfentanil should be reduced in elderly or debilitated patients (see PRECAUTIONS).

Vital signs should be monitored routinely.

See Dosage Guidelines for the use of alfentanil: 1) by incremental injection as an analgesic adjunct to anesthesia with barbiturate/nitrous oxide/oxygen for short surgical procedures (expected duration of less than one hour); 2) by continuous infusion as a maintenance analgesic with nitrous oxide/oxygen for general surgical procedures; and 3) by intravenous injection in anesthetic doses for the induction of anesthesia for general surgical procedures with a minimum expected duration of 45 minutes; and 4) by intravenous injection as the analgesic component for monitored anesthesia care (MAC).

TABLE 1 Dosage Guidelines
Dosage Should Be Individualized And Titrated For Use During General Anesthesia

SPONTANEOUS BREATHING/ASSISTED VENTILATION	
Induction of Analgesia: 8-20 mcg/kg	
Maintenance of Analgesia: 3-5 mcg/kg q 5-20 min or 0.5 to 1 mcg/kg/min	
Total dose: 8-40 mcg/kg	
ASSISTED OR CONTROLLED VENTILATION	
Incremental Injection (To attenuate response to laryngoscopy and intubation)	Induction of Analgesia: 20-50 mcg/kg Maintenance of Analgesia: 5-15 mcg/kg q 5-20 min Total dose: Up to 75 mcg/kg
Continuous Infusion (To provide attenuation of response to intubation and incision)	Infusion rates are variable and should be titrated to the desired clinical effect. SEE INFUSION DOSAGE GUIDELINES BELOW. Induction of Analgesia: 50-75 mcg/kg Maintenance of Analgesia: 0.5 to 3 mcg/kg/min (Average rate 1 to 1.5 mcg/kg/min) Total dose: Dependent on duration of procedure
Anesthetic Induction	Induction of Anesthesia: 130-245 mcg/kg Maintenance of Anesthesia: 0.5 to 1.5 mcg/kg/min or general anesthetic Total dose: Dependent on duration of procedure At these doses, truncal rigidity should be expected and a muscle relaxant should be utilized. Administer slowly (over 3 minutes). Concentration of inhalation agents reduced by 30-50% for initial hour.
MONITORED ANESTHESIA CARE (MAC) (For sedated and responsive, spontaneously breathing patients)	Induction of MAC: 3-8 mcg/kg Maintenance of MAC: 3-5 mcg/kg q 5-20 min or 0.25 to 1 mcg/kg/min Total dose: 3-40 mcg/kg

INFUSION DOSAGE

Continuous Infusion: 0.5-3.0 mcg/kg/min administered with nitrous oxide/oxygen in patients undergoing general surgery. Following an anesthetic induction dose of alfentanil, infusion rate requirements are reduced by 30-50% for the first hour of maintenance.

Changes in vital signs that indicate a response to surgical stress or lightening of anesthesia may be controlled by increasing the rate up to a maximum of 4.0 mcg/kg/min and/or administration of bolus doses of 7 mcg/kg. If changes are not controlled after three bolus doses given over a five minute period, a barbiturate, vasodilator, and/or inhalation agent should be used. Infusion rates should always be adjusted downward in the absence of these signs until there is some response to surgical stimulation.

Rather than an increase in infusion rate, 7 mcg/kg bolus doses of alfentanil or a potent inhalation agent should be administered in response to signs of lightening of anesthesia within the last 15 minutes of surgery. Administration of alfentanil infusion should be discontinued at least 10-15 minutes prior to the end of surgery.

Usage In Children: Clinical data to support the use of alfentanil in patients under 12 years of age are not presently available. Therefore, such use is not recommended.

Premedication: The selection of preanesthetic medications should be based upon the needs of the individual patient.

Neuromuscular Blocking Agents: The neuromuscular blocking agent selected should be compatible with the patient's condition, taking into account the hemodynamic effects of a particular muscle relaxant and the degree of skeletal muscle relaxation required (see CLINICAL PHARMACOLOGY, WARNINGS, and PRECAUTIONS).

DOSAGE AND ADMINISTRATION: *(cont'd)*

In patients administered anesthetic (induction) dosages of alfentanil, it is essential that qualified personnel and adequate facilities are available for the management of intraoperative and postoperative respiratory depression.

Also see WARNINGS and PRECAUTIONS.

For purposes of administering small volumes of alfentanil accurately, the use of a tuberculin syringe or equivalent is recommended.

The physical and chemical compatibility of alfentanil have been demonstrated in solution with normal saline, 5% dextrose in normal saline, 5% dextrose in water and Lactated Ringers. Clinical studies of alfentanil infusion have been conducted with alfentanil diluted to a concentration range of 25 mcg/ml to 80 mcg/ml.

As an example of the preparation of alfentanil for infusion, 20 ml of alfentanil added to 230 ml of diluent provides a 40 mcg/ml solution of alfentanil.

Parenteral drug products should be inspected visually for particulate matter and discoloration prior to administration, whenever solution and container permit.

SAFETY AND HANDLING

Alfentanil hydrochloride is supplied in individually sealed dosage forms which pose no known risk to health-care providers having incidental contact. Accidental dermal exposure to alfentanil should be treated by rinsing the affected area with water.

Protect from light. Store at room temperature 15°-30°C (59°-86°F).

HOW SUPPLIED:

Each ml of Alfenta (alfentanil hydrochloride) Injection for intravenous use contains alfentanil hydrochloride equivalent to 500 mcg of alfentanil base.

(Janssen, 2/94), 7614601)

HOW SUPPLIED - EQUIVALENTS NOT AVAILABLE:

Injection, Solution - Intravenous - 500 mcg/ml

2 ml x 10	$74.98	ALFENTA, Janssen Phar	50458-0060-02
5 ml x 10	$134.39	ALFENTA, Janssen Phar	50458-0060-05
10 ml x 5	$108.50	ALFENTA, Janssen Phar	50458-0060-10
20 ml x 5	$189.90	ALFENTA, Janssen Phar	50458-0060-20

ALGLUCERASE *(003042)*

CATEGORIES: Enzymes; Gaucher's Disease; Orphan Drugs; Thrombocytopenia; Pregnancy Category C; FDA Class 1A ("Important Therapeutic Advantage"); Sales > $100 Million; FDA Approved 1991 Apr

BRAND NAMES: **Ceredase**

COST OF THERAPY: $140,452.00 (Gaucher's Disease; Injection; 80 unit/ml; 1.3/day; 365 days)

PRIMARY ICD9: 272.7 (Lipidoses)

DESCRIPTION:

Alglucerase is a modified form of the enzyme, β-glucocerebrosidase (β-D-glucosyl-N-acyl-sphingosine glucohydrolase, EC 3.2.1.45). Alglucerase is a monomeric glycoprotein of 497 amino acids with carbohydrates making up approximately 6% of the molecule (M_r = 59,300 as determined by SDS-PAGE). The unmodified enzyme (b-glucocerebrosidase) also contains 497 amino acids and contains approximately 12% carbohydrate (M_r= 67,000). The carbohydrates on the unmodified enzyme consist of N-linked carbohydrate chains of the complex and high mannose type. Glucocerebrosidase and alglucerase catalyze the hydrolysis of the glycolipid, glucocerebroside, within the lysosomes of the reticuloendothelial system.

Alglucerase is prepared by modification of the oligosaccharide chains of human β-glucocerebrosidase. The modification alters the sugar residues at the non-reducing ends of the oligosaccharide chains of the glycoprotein so that they are predominantly terminated with mannose residues which specifically recognized by carbohydrate receptors on macrophage cells. Alglucerase is supplied as a clear sterile non-pyrogenic solution of alglucerase in a citrate buffered solution (53 mM citrate, 143 mM sodium) containing 1% albumin human USP. The enzyme is supplied as 400 international units per bottle (80 units/ml) and 50 units per bottle (10 units/ml) with a fill volume 5 ml per bottle. An enzyme unit (U) is defined as the amount of enzyme required to hydrolyze one minute one micromole of the synthetic substrate, 4-methylumbelliferyl-β-glucoside.

Alglucerase is purified from a large pool of human placental tissue collected from selected donors. Steps have been introduced into the manufacturing process to reduce further the risk of viral contamination. However, no procedure has been shown to be totally effective in removing viral infectivity. (See PRECAUTIONS.) Each lot of product has been tested and found negative for hepatitis B surface antigen (HBsAg) and for human immunodeficiency virus (HIV-1) and antibody (HIV-1/2).

Human chorionic gonadotropin (hCG), a naturally occurring hormone in human placenta, has been detected in alglucerase. Although it is likely the hCG is partially deglycosylated, *in vitro* studies demonstrate biological activity of approximately 3 units of hCG activity per unit of alglucerase. Preliminary studies suggest that the deglycosylated hCG in alglucerase is rapidly cleared at a rate which is approximately forty times greater than that of native hCG.

Therefore, *in vivo* biological activity and clearance of the material may be different to the naturally occurring hormone and is currently under investigation.

CLINICAL PHARMACOLOGY:

Alglucerase catalyzes the hydrolysis of the glycolipid, glucocerebroside, to glucose and ceramide as part of the normal degradation pathway for membrane lipids. Glucocerebroside is primarily derived from hematologic cell turnover. Gaucher disease is characterized by a functional deficiency in β-glucocerebrosidase enzymatic activity and the resultant accumulation of lipid glucocerebroside in tissue macrophages which become engorged and are termed Gaucher cells. Gaucher cells are typically found in liver, spleen and bone marrow and occasionally, as well, in lung, kidney and intestine. Secondary hematologic sequelae include severe anemia and thrombocytopenia in addition to the characteristic progressive hepatosplenomegaly. Skeletal complications, including osteonecrosis and osteopenia with secondary pathological fractures, are a common feature of Gaucher disease.

Pharmacokinetics Following an intravenous infusion of different doses (between 0.6 and 234 unit/kg) of alglucerase over a 4-hour period, steady-state enzymatic activity was achieved by 60 minutes. Individual steady-state activity and area under the curve of the activity increased linearly with the infused dose (0.6 to 121 units/kg). Following infusion termination, plasma enzymatic activity declined rapidly with elimination of half-life ranging between 3.6 and 10.4 minutes. Plasma clearance of alglucerase, calculated from its plasma enzymatic activity, was variable and ranged between 6.34 and 25.39 ml/min/kg, whereas the volume of distribution ranged from 49.4 to 282.1 ml/kg. Within the dosage range of 0.6 and 121 units/kg, elimination half-life, plasma clearance, and volume of distribution values appear to be independent of the infused dose.

CLINICAL PHARMACOLOGY: *(cont'd)*

Pharmacologic Actions: Chronic administration of alglucerase in 13 patients with Type 1 Gaucher disease induced the following effects:

1. Splenomegaly and hepatomegaly were significantly reduced, presumably by disruption of the lysosomal storage sites and metabolism of glucocerebroside in Gaucher cells. This effect was demonstrated within 6 months of initiation of therapy.

2. Hematologic deficiencies in hemoglobin, hematocrit, erythrocyte and platelet counts were significantly improved. In most patients a change in hemoglobin was the first observable effect. In some patients hemoglobin levels were normalized after 6 months of therapy.

3. Improved mineralization of bone, as revealed by plain radiographs of long bones, occurred in three patients after prolonged treatment as a result of a reduction in the osteolytic actions of lipid-laden Gaucher cells in the marrow.

4. Cachexia and wasting in children were reduced.

INDICATIONS AND USAGE:

Alglucerase is indicated for use as long-term enzyme replacement therapy for patients with a confirmed diagnosis of Type 1 Gaucher disease who exhibit signs and symptoms that are severe enough to result in one or more of the following conditions:

a) moderate-to-severe anemia;

b) thrombocytopenia with bleeding tendency;

c) bone disease;

d) significant hepatomegaly or splenomegaly.

CONTRAINDICATIONS:

There are no known contraindications to the use of alglucerase.

WARNINGS:

Approximately 14% of 538 patients treated clinically and tested to date have developed IgG antibody to alglucerase during the first year of therapy. It appears that patients who will develop IgG antibody are most likely to do so within 6 months of treatment and will rarely develop antibodies to alglucerase after 12 months of therapy. **Approximately 25% of patients with detectable IgG antibodies experienced symptoms of hypersensitivity.**

Thus, patients with antibody to alglucerase have a higher risk of hypersensitivity reaction. Conversely, not all patients with symptoms of hypersensitivity have detectable antibody and further evaluation of their antibody isotypes and mechanisms is continuing. It is suggested that patients be monitored periodically for IgG antibody formation.

At present, should a patient experience a reaction with symptoms suggestive of hypersensitivity, it is recommended that a serum sample for tryptase levels and complement activation be drawn within two hours of the event after appropriate treatment of the symptoms. Subsequent serum for testing antibody to alglucerase would be helpful. Decreased efficacy has been noted in less than 0.5% of treated patients due to antibodies to alglucerase.

PRECAUTIONS:

General: Therapy with alglucerase should be directed by physicians knowledgeable in the management of patients with Gaucher disease. Treatment with alglucerase should be approached with caution in patients who have exhibited symptoms of hypersensitivity to the product. Pre-treatment with antihistamines has allowed continued use of alglucerase in some patients. (See ADVERSE REACTIONS.) As hCG has been detected in alglucerase physicians should be alert for signs of early virilization in males under the age of ten, although no cases of precocious puberty have been reported to date. Alglucerase should also be used with caution in patients with androgen sensitive malignancies, *e.g.*, prostate cancer and patients with known prior allergies to hCG.

Alglucerase is prepared from pooled human placental tissue that may contain the causative agents of some viral diseases. Manufacturing steps have been designed to reduce the risk of transmitting viral infectious agents. These steps have demonstrated *in vitro* inactivation of a panel of model viruses, including human immunodeficiency virus (HIV-1). The risk of contamination from slowly acting or latent viruses, including the Creutzfeldt-Jacob disease agent, is believed to be remote but has not been tested. Accordingly, the benefits and the risks of treatment with this product should be assessed prior to use.

Carcinogenesis, Mutagenesis, and Impairment of Fertility: Studies have not been conducted to assess the potential effects of alglucerase on carcinogenesis, mutagenesis, or impairment of fertility in animals or man.

Pregnancy Category C: Animal reproductive studies have not been conducted with alglucerase. It is also not know whether alglucerase can cause fetal harm when administered to a pregnant woman, or can affect reproductive capacity. Alglucerase should be given to a pregnant woman only if clearly needed.

Nursing Mothers: Since alglucerase may be excreted in human milk caution should be exercised when alglucerase is administered to a nursing woman.

ADVERSE REACTIONS:

Experience in over 1000 patients treated with alglucerase has revealed a small number of adverse events. Some of these events were related to the route of administration including discomfort, pruritus, burning and swelling or sterile abscess at the site of venipuncture. The remaining experiences consisted of slight fever, chills, abdominal discomfort, nausea or vomiting. None of these events were judged to require medical intervention.

Symptoms suggestive of hypersensitivity have been noted in a limited number of patients. Onset of such symptoms has occurred during or shortly after infusions; these symptoms have included pruritus, flushing, urticaria/angioedema (a small number of patients have had upper airway involvement), chest discomfort, respiratory symptoms, nausea and abdominal cramping. Hypotension was reported to occur during one of these events. (See WARNINGS.)

Pre-treatment with antihistamines and reduced rate of infusion has allowed continued use of alglucerase in most patients. Additional adverse symptoms which have been reported include: fatigue, vasomotor irritability or hot flash, weakness, headache, light headedness, dysosmia, oral ulcerations, backache and transient peripheral edema, menstrual abnormalities and diarrhea.

Because it contains human chorionic gonadotropin, alglucerase may cause a false positive pregnancy test.

OVERDOSAGE:

No obvious toxicity was detected after single doses of up to 234 units/kg. There is no experience with larger doses.

DOSAGE AND ADMINISTRATION:

Alglucerase is administered by intravenous infusion over 1-2 hours. Dosage should be individualized for each patient. Initial dosage may be as little as 2.5 units/kg of body weight 3 times a week up to as much as 60 units/kg administered as frequently as once a week or as infrequently as every 4 weeks. 60 units/kg every 2 weeks is the dose for which the most data is available. Disease severity may dictate that drug be initiated with relatively high doses or

DOSAGE AND ADMINISTRATION: *(cont'd)*

relatively frequent administration. After patient response is well-established, a reduction in dosage may be attempted for maintenance therapy. Progressive reductions can be made at intervals of 3-6 months while carefully monitoring response parameters.

Alglucerase should not be shaken. Each bottle should be inspected visually for particulate matter and discoloration before use. Any bottles exhibiting particulate matter or discoloration should not be used. DO NOT USE alglucerase after the expiration date on the bottle.

On the day of use, the appropriate amount of alglucerase for each patient is diluted with 0.9% sodium chloride IV solution to a final volume not to exceed 200 ml. Aseptic techniques should be used when diluting the dose.

Alglucerase, when diluted to 100 to 200 ml, has been shown to be stable for up to 18 hours when stored at 2-8°C. The use of an in-line particulate filter is recommended for the infusion apparatus. Since alglucerase does not contain any preservative, after opening, bottles should not be stored for subsequent use.

Relatively low toxicity, combined with the extended time course of response, allows small dosage adjustments to be made occasionally to avoid discarding partially used bottle. Thus, the dosage administered in individual infusions may be slightly increased or decreased to utilize fully each bottle as long as the monthly administered dosage remains substantially unaltered.

HOW SUPPLIED:

Ceredase is supplied as a clear sterile citrate buffered solution (53 mM citrate, 143 mM sodium) containing 1% albumin human USP. Store at 2-8°C.

(Genzyme Corporation, 10/94 1811/REV 5)

HOW SUPPLIED - EQUIVALENTS NOT AVAILABLE:

Injection, Solution - Intravenous - 10 unit/ml

5 ml $185.00 CEREDASE, Genzyme 58468-1781-01

Injection, Solution - Intravenous - 80 unit/ml

5 ml $1480.00 CEREDASE, Genzyme 58468-1060-01

ALLOPURINOL *(000133)*

CATEGORIES: Antigout; Arthritis; Calcium Oxalate Stone Preventative; Cancer; Electrolytic, Caloric-Water Balance; Gout; Kidney Stones; Leukemia; Lithiasis; Lymphoma; Pain; Uricosuric Agents; Xanthine Oxidase Inhibitors; Pregnancy Category C; FDA Approval Pre 1982

BRAND NAMES: *Abburic*; *Adenock* (Japan); *Aipico*; *Alinol*; *Allo 300* (Germany); *Allo-Basan*; *Allo-Puren* (Germany); *Allopin*; *Allopur*; *Allopurinol*; *Alloremed*; *Alloril*; *Allorin*; *Alloscan*; *Allozym* (Japan); *Allurase*; *Allurit*; *Alonol*; *Alopron*; *Aloral*; *Alositol* (Japan); *Alpurin*; *Alunlan*; *Aluline*; *Aluprin*; *Aluron*; *Anoprolin* (Japan); *Anzief* (Japan); *Apo-Allopurinol* (Canada); *Aprinol* (Japan); *Apulonga* (Germany); *Apurin*; *Apurol*; *Atisuril* (Mexico); *Bleminol* (Germany); *Caplenal* (England); *Capurate*; *Cellidrin* (Germany); *Clint*; *Cosuric*; *Dabrosan* (Germany); *Embarin* (Germany); *Epidropal* (Germany); *Epuric*; *Foligan* (Germany); *Geapur*; *Gichtex*; *Hamarin* (England); *Isanol*; *Isoric*; *Ketanrift* (Japan); *Ketobun-A* (Japan); *Litinol*; *Llanol*; *Lo-Uric*; Lopurin; *Lysuron*; *Lysuron 300*; *Masaton* (Japan); *Medoric*; *Mefanol*; *Mephanol*; *Milurit*; *Miniplanor* (Japan); *Neufan* (Japan); *Nipurol*; *No-Uric*; *Novopurol* (Canada); *Progout* (Australia); *Puricemia*; *Puricos*; *Purinase*; *Purinol* (Canada); *Purinox*; *Remid* (Germany); *Riball* (Japan); *Salterprim*; *Suspendol* (Germany); *Takanarumin* (Japan); *Tonnic*; *Unizuric*; *Unizuric 300* (Mexico); *Uracuad*; *Urapurin*; *Uric* (Japan); *Uricad*; *Uricemil*; *Uriconorm*; *Uriconorm-E*; *Urinol*; *Uripurinol* (Germany); *Urocuad*; *Urogquad*; *Uroquad*; *Urosin* (Germany); *Xanturic* (France); *Xylonol*; *Zylapour*; *Zylol*; **Zyloprim**; *Zyloric* (Europe)
(International brand names outside U.S. in italics)

FORMULARIES: Aetna; BC-BS; CIGNA; DoD; FHP; Humana; Kaiser; Medco; Medi-Cal; PCS; PruCare; United; WHO

DESCRIPTION:

Allopurinol is known chemically as 1,5-dihydro-4*H*-pyrazolo [3,4-*d*]pyrimidin-4-one. It is a xanthine oxidase inhibitor which is administered orally. Each scored white tablet contains 100 mg allopurinol and the inactive ingredients lactose, magnesium stearate, potato starch, and povidone. Each scored peach tablet contains 300 mg allopurinol and the inactive ingredients corn starch, FD&C Yellow No. 6 Lake, lactose, magnesium stearate, and povidone. Its solubility in water at 37°C is 80.0 mg/dl and is greater in an alkaline solution.

CLINICAL PHARMACOLOGY:

Allopurinol acts on purine catabolism, without disrupting the biosynthesis of purines. It reduces the production of uric acid by inhibiting the biochemical reactions immediately preceding its formation.

Allopurinol is a structural analogue of the natural purine base, hypoxanthine. It is an inhibitor of xanthine oxidase, the enzyme responsible for the conversion of hypoxanthine to xanthine and of xanthine to uric acid, the end product of purine metabolism in man. Allopurinol is metabolized to the corresponding xanthine analogue, oxipurinol (alloxanthine), which also is an inhibitor of xanthine oxidase.

It has been shown that reutilization of both hypoxanthine and xanthine for nucleotide and nucleic acid synthesis is markedly enhanced when their oxidations are inhibited by allopurinol and oxipurinol. This reutilization does not disrupt normal nucleic acid anabolism, however, because feedback inhibition is an integral part of purine biosynthesis. As a result of xanthine oxidase inhibition, the serum concentration of hypoxanthine plus xanthine in patients receiving allopurinol for treatment of hyperuricemia is usually in the range of 0.3 to 0.4 mg/dl compared to a normal level of approximately 0.15 mg/dl. A maximum of 0.9 mg/dl of these oxypurines has been reported when the serum urate was lowered to less than 2 mg/dl by high doses of allopurinol. These values are far below the saturation levels at which point their precipitation would be expected to occur (above 7 mg/dl).

The renal clearance of hypoxanthine and xanthine is at least 10 times greater than that of uric acid. The increased xanthine and hypoxanthine in the urine have not been accompanied by problems of nephrolithiasis. Xanthine crystalluria has been reported in only three patients. Two of the patients had Lesch-Nyhan syndrome, which is characterized by excessive uric acid production combined with a deficiency of the enzyme, hypoxanthine-guanine phosphoribosyltransferase (HGPRTase). This enzyme is required for the conversion of hypoxanthine, xanthine, and guanine to their respective nucleotides. The third patient had lymphosarcoma and produced an extremely large amount of uric acid because of rapid cell lysis during chemotherapy.

CLINICAL PHARMACOLOGY: *(cont'd)*

Allopurinol is approximately 90% absorbed from the gastrointestinal tract. Peak plasma levels generally occur at 1.5 hours and 4.5 hours for allopurinol and oxipurinol respectively, and after a single oral dose of 300 mg allopurinol, maximum plasma levels of about 3 mcg/ml of allopurinol and 6.5 mcg/ml of oxipurinol are produced.

Approximately 20% of the ingested allopurinol is excreted in the feces. Because of its rapid oxidation to oxipurinol and a renal clearance rate approximately that of glomerular filtration rate, allopurinol has a plasma half-life of about 1-2 hours. Oxipurinol, however, has a longer plasma half-life (approximately 15.0 hours) and therefore effective xanthine oxidase inhibition is maintained over a 24-hour period with single daily doses of allopurinol. Whereas allopurinol is cleared essentially by glomerular filtration, oxipurinol is reabsorbed in the kidney tubules in a manner similar to the reabsorption of uric acid.

The clearance of oxipurinol is increased by uricosuric drugs, and as a consequence, the addition of a uricosuric agent reduces to some degree the inhibition of xanthine oxidase by oxipurinol and increases to some degree the urinary excretion of uric acid. In practice, the net effect of such combined therapy may be useful in some patients in achieving minimum serum uric acid levels provided the total urinary uric acid load does not exceed the competence of the patient's renal function.

Hyperuricemia may be primary, as in gout, or secondary to diseases such as acute and chronic leukemia, polycythemia vera, multiple myeloma, and psoriasis. It may occur with the use of diuretic agents, during renal dialysis, in the presence of renal damage, during starvation or reducing diets and in the treatment of neoplastic disease where rapid resolution of tissue masses may occur. Asymptomatic hyperuricemia is not an indication for allopurinol treatment (see INDICATIONS AND USAGE).

Gout is a metabolic disorder which is characterized by hyperuricemia and resultant deposition of monosodium urate in the tissues, particularly the joints and kidneys. The etiology of this hyperuricemia is the overproduction of uric acid in relation to the patient's ability to excrete it. If progressive deposition of urates is to be arrested or reversed, it is necessary to reduce the serum uric acid level below the saturation point to suppress urate precipitation.

Administration of allopurinol generally results in a fall in both serum and urinary uric acid within two to three days. The degree of this decrease can be manipulated almost at will since it is dose-dependent. A week or more of treatment with allopurinol may be required before its full effects are manifested; likewise, uric acid may return to pretreatment levels slowly (usually after a period of seven to ten days following cessation of therapy). This reflects primarily the accumulation and slow clearance of oxipurinol. In some patients a dramatic fall in urinary uric acid excretion may not occur, particularly in those with severe tophaceous gout. It has been postulated that this may be due to the mobilization of urate from tissue deposits as the serum uric acid level begins to fall.

Allopurinol's action differs from that of uricosuric agents, which lower the serum uric acid level by increasing urinary excretion of uric acid. Allopurinol reduces both the serum and urinary uric acid levels by inhibiting the formation of uric acid. The use of allopurinol to block the formation of urates avoids the hazard of increased renal excretion of uric acid posed by uricosuric drugs.

Allopurinol can substantially reduce serum and urinary uric acid levels in previously refractory patients even in the presence of renal damage serious enough to render uricosuric drugs virtually ineffective. Salicylates may be given conjointly for their antirheumatic effect without compromising the action of allopurinol. This is in contrast to the nullifying effect of salicylates on uricosuric drugs.

Allopurinol also inhibits the enzymatic oxidation of mercaptopurine, the sulfur-containing analogue of hypoxanthine, to 6-thiouric acid. This oxidation, which is catalyzed by xanthine oxidase, inactivates mercaptopurine. Hence, the inhibition of such oxidation by allopurinol may result in as much as a 75% reduction in the therapeutic dose requirement of mercaptopurine when the two compounds are given together.

INDICATIONS AND USAGE:

THIS IS NOT AN INNOCUOUS DRUG. IT IS NOT RECOMMENDED FOR THE TREATMENT OF ASYMPTOMATIC HYPERURICEMIA.

Allopurinol reduces serum and urinary uric acid concentrations. Its use should be individualized for each patient and requires an understanding of its mode of action and pharmacokinetics (see CLINICAL PHARMACOLOGY, CONTRAINDICATIONS, WARNINGS and PRECAUTIONS).

Allopurinol is indicated in:

(1) the management of patients with signs and symptoms of primary or secondary gout (acute attacks, tophi, joint destruction, uric acid lithiasis and/or nephropathy).

(2) the management of patients with leukemia, lymphoma and malignancies who are receiving cancer therapy which causes elevations of serum and urinary uric acid levels. Allopurinol treatment should be discontinued when the potential for overproduction of uric acid is no longer present.

(3) the management of patients with recurrent calcium oxalate calculi whose daily uric acid excretion exceeds 800 mg/day in male patients and 750 mg/day in female patients. Therapy in such patients should be carefully assessed initially and reassessed periodically to determine in each case that treatment is beneficial and that the benefits outweigh the risks.

CONTRAINDICATIONS:

Patients who have developed a severe reaction to allopurinol should not be restarted on the drug.

WARNINGS:

ALLOPURINOL SHOULD BE DISCONTINUED AT THE FIRST APPEARANCE OF SKIN RASH OR OTHER SIGNS WHICH MAY INDICATE AN ALLERGIC REACTION. In some instances a skin rash may be followed by more severe hypersensitivity reactions such as exfoliative, urticarial and purpuric lesions as well as Stevens-Johnson syndrome (erythema multiforme exudativum), and/or generalized vasculitis, irreversible hepatotoxicity and on rare occasions death.

In patients receiving mercaptopurine (Purinethol) or azathioprine (Imuran), the concomitant administration of 300-600 mg of allopurinol per day will require a reduction in dose to approximately one-third to one-fourth of the usual dose of mercaptopurine or azathioprine. Subsequent adjustment of doses of mercaptopurine or azathioprine should be made on the basis of therapeutic response and the appearance of toxic effects (see CLINICAL PHARMACOLOGY).

A few cases of reversible clinical hepatotoxicity have been noted in patients taking allopurinol, and in some patients asymptomatic rises in serum alkaline phosphatase or serum transaminase have been observed. If anorexia, weight loss or pruritus develop in patients on allopurinol, evaluation of liver function should be part of their diagnostic workup. In patients with pre-existing liver disease, periodic liver function tests are recommended during the early stages of therapy.

Due to the occasional occurrence of drowsiness, patients should be alerted to the need for due precaution when engaging in activities where alertness is mandatory.

WARNINGS: *(cont'd)*

The occurrence of hypersensitivity reactions to allopurinol may be increased in patients with decreased renal function receiving thiazides and allopurinol concurrently. For this reason, in this clinical setting, such combinations should be administered with caution and patients should be observed closely.

PRECAUTIONS:

General: An increase in acute attacks of gout has been reported during the early stages of allopurinol administration, even when normal or subnormal serum uric acid levels have been attained. Accordingly, maintenance doses of colchicine generally should be given prophylactically when allopurinol is begun. In addition, it is recommended that the patient start with a low dose of allopurinol (100 mg daily) and increase at weekly intervals by 100 mg until a serum uric acid level of 6 mg/dl or less is attained but without exceeding the maximum recommended dose (800 mg per day). The use of colchicine or anti-inflammatory agents may be required to suppress gouty attacks in some cases. The attacks usually become shorter and less severe after several months of therapy. The mobilization of urates from tissue deposits which cause fluctuations in the serum uric acid levels may be a possible explanation for these episodes. Even with adequate allopurinol therapy, it may require several months to deplete the uric acid pool sufficiently to achieve control of the acute attacks.

A fluid intake sufficient to yield a daily urinary output of at least two liters and the maintenance of a neutral or, preferably, slightly alkaline urine are desirable to (1) avoid the theoretical possibility of formation of xanthine calculi under the influence of allopurinol therapy and (2) help prevent renal precipitation of urates in patients receiving concomitant uricosuric agents.

Some patients with pre-existing renal disease or poor urate clearance have shown a rise in BUN during allopurinol administration. Although the mechanism responsible for this has not been established, patients with impaired renal function should be carefully observed during the early stages of allopurinol administration and dosage decreased or the drug withdrawn if increased abnormalities in renal function appear and persist.

Renal failure in association with allopurinol administration has been observed among patients with hyperuricemia secondary to neoplastic diseases. Concurrent conditions such as multiple myeloma and congestive myocardial disease were present among those patients whose renal dysfunction increased after allopurinol was begun. Renal failure is also frequently associated with gouty nephropathy and rarely with allopurinol-associated hypersensitivity reactions. Albuminuria has been observed among patients who developed clinical gout following chronic glomerulonephritis and chronic pyelonephritis.

Patients with decreased renal function require lower doses of allopurinol than those with normal renal function. Lower than recommended doses should be used to initiate therapy in any patients with decreased renal function and they should be observed closely during the early stages of allopurinol administration. In patients with severely impaired renal function or decreased urate clearance, the half-life of oxipurinol in the plasma is greatly prolonged. Therefore, a dose of 100 mg per day or 300 mg twice a week, or perhaps less, may be sufficient to maintain adequate xanthine oxidase inhibition to reduce serum urate levels.

Bone marrow depression has been reported in patients receiving allopurinol, most of whom received concomitant drugs with the potential for causing this reaction. This has occurred as early as six weeks to as long as six years after the initiation of allopurinol therapy. Rarely a patient may develop varying degrees of bone marrow depression, affecting one or more cell lines, while receiving allopurinol alone.

Information for the Patient: Patients should be informed of the following:

(1) They should be cautioned to discontinue allopurinol and to consult their physician immediately at the first sign of a skin rash, painful urination, blood in the urine, irritation of the eyes, or swelling of the lips or mouth. (2) They should be reminded to continue drug therapy prescribed for gouty attacks since optimal benefit of allopurinol may be delayed for two to six weeks. (3) They should be encouraged to increase fluid intake during therapy to prevent renal stones. (4) If a single dose of allopurinol is occasionally forgotten, there is no need to double the dose at the next scheduled time. (5) There may be certain risks associated with the concomitant use of allopurinol and dicumarol, sulfinpyrazone, mercaptopurine, azathioprine, ampicillin, amoxicillin and thiazide diuretics, and they should follow the instructions of their physician. (6) Due to the occasional occurrence of drowsiness, patients should take precautions when engaging in activities where alertness is mandatory. (7) Patients may wish to take allopurinol after meals to minimize gastric irritation.

Laboratory Tests: The correct dosage and schedule for maintaining the serum uric acid within the normal range is best determined by using the serum uric acid as an index.

In patients with pre-existing liver disease, periodic liver function tests are recommended during the early stages of therapy (see WARNINGS.)

Allopurinol and its primary active metabolite oxipurinol are eliminated by the kidneys; therefore, changes in renal function have a profound effect on dosage. In patients with decreased renal function or who have concurrent illnesses which can affect renal function such as hypertension and diabetes mellitus, periodic laboratory parameters of renal function, particularly BUN and serum creatinine or creatinine clearance, should be performed and the patient's allopurinol dosage reassessed.

The prothrombin time should be reassessed periodically in the patients receiving dicumarol who are given allopurinol.

Drug/Laboratory Test Interactions: Allopurinol is not known to alter the accuracy of laboratory tests.

Pregnancy, Teratogenic Effects, Pregnancy Category C: Reproductive studies have been performed in rats and rabbits at doses up to twenty times the usual human dose (5 mg/kg/day), and it was concluded that there was no impaired fertility or harm to the fetus due to allopurinol. There is a published report of a study in pregnant mice given 50 or 100 mg/kg allopurinol intraperitoneally on gestation days 10 or 13. There were increased numbers of dead fetuses in dams given 100 mg/kg allopurinol but not in those given 50 mg/kg. There were increased numbers of external malformations in fetuses at both doses of allopurinol on gestation day 10 and increased numbers of skeletal malformations in fetuses at both doses on gestation day 13. It cannot be determined whether this represented a fetal effect or an effect secondary to maternal toxicity. There are, however, no adequate or well-controlled studies in pregnant women. Because animal reproduction studies are not always predictive of human response, this drug should be used during pregnancy only if clearly needed.

Experience with allopurinol during human pregnancy has been limited partly because women of reproductive age rarely require treatment with allopurinol. There are two unpublished reports and one published paper of women giving birth to normal offspring after receiving allopurinol during pregnancy.

Nursing Mothers: Allopurinol and oxipurinol have been found in the milk of a mother who was receiving allopurinol. Since the effect of allopurinol on the nursing infant is unknown, caution should be exercised when allopurinol is administered to a nursing woman.

Pediatric Use: Allopurinol is rarely indicated for use in children with the exception of those with hyperuricemia secondary to malignancy or to certain rare inborn errors of purine metabolism (see INDICATIONS AND USAGE and DOSAGE AND ADMINISTRATION).

DRUG INTERACTIONS:

In patients receiving mercaptopurine (Purinethol) or azathioprine (Imuran), the concomitant administration of 300-600 mg of allopurinol per day will require a reduction in dose to approximately one-third to one-fourth of the usual dose of mercaptopurine or azathioprine. Subsequent adjustment of doses of mercaptopurine or azathioprine should be made on the basis of therapeutic response and the appearance of toxic effects (see CLINICAL PHARMACOLOGY).

It has been reported that allopurinol prolongs the half-life of the anticoagulant, dicumarol. The clinical basis of this drug interaction has not been established but should be noted when allopurinol is given to patients already on dicumarol therapy.

Since the excretion of oxipurinol is similar to that of urate, uricosuric agents, which increase the excretion of urate, are also likely to increase the excretion of oxipurinol and thus lower the degree of inhibition of xanthine oxidase. The concomitant administration of uricosuric agents and allopurinol has been associated with a decrease in the excretion of oxypurines (hypoxanthine and xanthine) and an increase in urinary uric acid excretion compared with that observed with allopurinol alone. Although clinical evidence to date has not demonstrated renal precipitation of oxypurines in patients either on allopurinol alone or in combination with uricosuric agents, the possibility should be kept in mind.

The reports that the concomitant use of allopurinol and thiazide diuretics may contribute to the enhancement of allopurinol toxicity in some patients have been reviewed in an attempt to establish a cause-and-effect relationship and a mechanism of causation. Review of these case reports indicates that the patients were mainly receiving thiazide diuretics for hypertension and that tests to rule out decreased renal function secondary to hypertensive nephropathy were not often performed. In those patients in whom renal insufficiency was documented, however, the recommendation to lower the dose of allopurinol was not followed. Although a causal mechanism and a cause-and-effect relationship have not been established, current evidence suggests that renal function should be monitored in patients on thiazide diuretics and allopurinol even in the absence of renal failure, and dosage levels should be even more conservatively adjusted in those patients on such combined therapy if diminished renal function is detected.

An increase in the frequency of skin rash has been reported among patients receiving ampicillin or amoxicillin concurrently with allopurinol compared to patients who are not receiving both drugs. The cause of the reported association has not been established.

Enhanced bone marrow suppression by cyclophosphamide and other cytotoxic agents has been reported among patients with neoplastic disease, except leukemia, in the presence of allopurinol. However, in a well-controlled study of patients with lymphoma on combination therapy, allopurinol did not increase the marrow toxicity of patients treated with cyclophosphamide, doxorubicin, bleomycin, procarbazine and/or mechlorethamine.

Tolbutamide's conversion to inactive metabolites has been shown to be catalyzed by xanthine oxidase from rat liver. The clinical significance, if any, of these observations is unknown.

Chlorpropamide's plasma half-life may be prolonged by allopurinol, since allopurinol and chlorpropamide may compete for excretion in the renal tubule. The risk of hypoglycemia secondary to this mechanism may be increased if allopurinol and chlorpropamide are given concomitantly in the presence of renal insufficiency.

ADVERSE REACTIONS:

Data upon which the following estimates of incidence of adverse reactions are made are derived from experiences reported in the literature, unpublished clinical trials and voluntary reports since marketing of allopurinol began. Past experience suggested that the most frequent event following the initiation of allopurinol treatment was an increase in acute attacks of gout (average 6% in early studies). An analysis of current usage suggests that the incidence of acute gouty attacks has diminished to less than 1%. The explanation for this decrease has not been determined but may be due in part to initiating therapy more gradually (see PRECAUTIONS and DOSAGE AND ADMINISTRATION.

The most frequent adverse reaction to allopurinol is skin rash. Skin reactions can be severe and sometimes fatal. Therefore, treatment with allopurinol should be discontinued immediately if a rash develops (see WARNINGS.) Some patients with the most severe reaction also had fever, chills, arthralgias, cholestatic, jaundice, eosinophilia and mild leukocytosis or leukopenia. Among 55 patients with gout treated with allopurinol for 3 to 34 months (average greater than 1 year) and followed prospectively, Rundles observed that 3% of patients developed a type of drug reaction which was predominantly a pruritic maculopapular skin eruption, sometimes scaly or exfoliative. However, with current usage, skin reactions have been observed less frequently than 1%. The explanation for this decrease is not obvious. The incidence of skin rash may be increased in the presence of renal insufficiency. The frequency of skin rash among patients receiving ampicillin or amoxicillin concurrently with allopurinol has been reported to be increased (see PRECAUTIONS.)

Most Common Reactions* Probably Causally Related

Gastrointestinal: diarrhea, nausea, alkaline phosphatase increase, SGOT/SGPT increase

Metabolic and Nutritional: acute attacks of gout

Skin and Appendages: rash, maculopapular rash

*Early clinical studies and incidence rates from early clinical experience with allopurinol suggested that these adverse reactions were found to occur at a rate of greater than 1%. The most frequent event observed was acute attacks of gout following the initiation of therapy. Analyses of current usage suggest that the incidence of these adverse reactions is now less than 1%. The explanation for this decrease has not been determined, but it may be due to following recommended usage (see ADVERSE REACTIONS introduction,INDICATIONS AND USAGE,PRECAUTIONS and DOSAGE AND ADMINISTRATION).

Incidence Less Than 1% Probably Causally Related

Body as a whole: ecchymosis, fever, headache

Cardiovascular: necrotizing angiitis, vasculitis

Gastrointestinal: hepatic necrosis, granulomatous hepatitis, hepatomegaly, hyperbilirubinemia, cholestatic jaundice, vomiting, intermittent abdominal pain, gastritis, dyspepsia

Hemic and Lymphatic: thrombocytopenia, eosinophilia, leukocytosis, leukopenia

Musculoskeletal: myopathy, arthralgias

Nervous: peripheral neuropathy, neuritis, paresthesia, somnolence

Respiratory: epistaxis

Skin and Appendages: erythema multiforme exudativum (Stevens-Johnson syndrome), toxic epidermal necrolysis (Lyell's syndrome), hypersensitivity vasculitis, purpura, vesicular bullous dermatitis, exfoliative dermatitis, eczematoid dermatitis, pruritus, urticaria, alopecia, onycholysis, lichen planus

Special Senses: taste loss/perversion

Urogenital: renal failure, uremia (see PRECAUTIONS)

Incidence Less Than 1% Causal Relationship Unknown

Body as a whole: malaise

Cardiovascular: pericarditis, peripheral vascular disease, thrombophlebitis, bradycardia, vasodilation

Endocrine: infertility (male), hypercalcemia, gynecomastia (male)

ADVERSE REACTIONS: *(cont'd)*

Gastrointestinal: hemorrhagic pancreatitis, gastrointestinal bleeding, stomatitis, salivary gland swelling, hyperlipidemia, tongue edema, anorexia

Hemic and Lymphatic: aplastic anemia, agranulocytosis, eosinophilic fibrohistiocytic lesion of bone marrow, pancytopenia, prothrombin decrease, anemia, hemolytic anemia, reticulocytosis, lymphadenopathy, lymphocytosis

Musculoskeletal: myalgia

Nervous: optic neuritis, confusion, dizziness, vertigo, foot drop, decrease in libido, depression, amnesia, tinnitus, asthenia, insomnia

Respiratory: bronchospasm, asthma, pharyngitis, rhinitis

Skin and Appendages: furunculosis, facial edema, sweating, skin edema

Special Senses: cataracts, macular retinitis, iritis, conjunctivitis, amblyopia

Urogenital: nephritis, impotence, primary hematuria, albuminuria

OVERDOSAGE:

Massive overdosing or acute poisoning by allopurinol has not been reported.

In mice the 50% lethal dose (LD_{50}) is 160 mg/kg given intraperitoneally (i.p.) with deaths delayed up to five days and 700 mg/kg orally (p.o.) (approximately 140 times the usual human dose) with deaths delayed up to three days. In rats the acute LD_{50} is 750 mg/kg i.p. and 6000 mg/kg p.o. (approximately 1200 times the human dose).

In the management of overdosage there is no specific antidote for allopurinol. There has been no clinical experience in the management of a patient who has taken massive amounts of allopurinol.

Both allopurinol and oxipurinol are dialyzable; however, the usefulness of hemodialysis or peritoneal dialysis in the management of a allopurinol overdose is unknown.

DOSAGE AND ADMINISTRATION:

The dosage of allopurinol to accomplish full control of gout and to lower serum uric acid to normal or near-normal levels varies with the severity of the disease. The average is 200 to 300 mg per day for patients with mild gout and 400 to 600 mg per day for those with moderately severe tophaceous gout. The appropriate dosage may be administered in divided doses or as a single equivalent dose with the 300 mg tablet. Dosage requirements in excess of 300 mg should be administered in divided doses. The minimal effective dosage is 100 to 200 mg daily and the maximal recommended dosage is 800 mg daily. To reduce the possibility of flare-up of acute gouty attacks, it is recommended that the patient start with a low dose of allopurinol (100 mg daily) and increase at weekly intervals by 100 mg until a serum uric acid level of 6 mg/dl or less is attained but without exceeding the maximal recommended dosage.

Normal serum urate levels are usually achieved in one to three weeks. The upper limit of normal is about 7 mg/dl for men and postmenopausal women and 6 mg/dl for premenopausal women. Too much reliance should not be placed on a single serum uric acid determination since, for technical reasons, estimation of uric acid may be difficult. By selecting the appropriate dosage and, in certain patients, using uricosuric agents concurrently, it is possible to reduce serum uric acid to normal or, if desired, to as low as 2 to 3 mg/dl and keep it there indefinitely.

While adjusting the dosage of allopurinol in patients who are being treated with colchicine and/or anti-inflammatory agents, it is wise to continue the latter therapy until serum uric acid has been normalized and there has been freedom from acute gouty attacks for several months.

In transferring a patient from a uricosuric agent to allopurinol, the dose of the uricosuric agent should be gradually reduced over a period of several weeks and the dose of allopurinol gradually increased to the required dose needed to maintain a normal serum uric acid level.

It should also be noted that allopurinol is generally better tolerated if taken following meals. A fluid intake sufficient to yield a daily urinary output of at least two liters and the maintenance of a neutral or, preferably, slightly alkaline urine are desirable.

Since allopurinol and its metabolites are primarily eliminated only by the kidney, accumulation of the drug can occur in renal failure, and the dose of allopurinol should consequently be reduced. With a creatinine clearance of 10 to 20 ml/min, a daily dosage of 200 mg of allopurinol is suitable. When the creatinine clearance is less than 10 ml/min the daily dosage should not exceed 100 mg. With extreme renal impairment (creatinine clearance less than 3 ml/min) the interval between doses may also need to be lengthened.

The correct size and frequency of dosage for maintaining the serum uric acid just within the normal range is best determined by using the serum uric acid level as an index.

For the prevention of uric acid nephropathy during the vigorous therapy of neoplastic disease, treatment with 600 to 800 mg daily for two or three days is advisable together with a high fluid intake. Otherwise similar considerations to the above recommendations for treating patients with gout govern the regulation of dosage for maintenance purposes in secondary hyperuricemia.

The dose of allopurinol recommended for management of recurrent calcium oxalate stones in hyperuricosuric patients is 200 to 300 mg/day in divided doses or as the single equivalent. This dose may be adjusted up or down depending upon the resultant control of the hyperuricosuria based upon subsequent 24 hour urinary urate determinations. Clinical experience suggests that patients with recurrent calcium oxalate stones may also benefit from dietary changes such as the reduction of animal protein, sodium, refined sugars, oxalate-rich foods, and excessive calcium intake as well as an increase in oral fluids and dietary fiber.

Children, 6 to 10 years of age, with secondary hyperuricemia associated with malignancies may be given 300 mg allopurinol daily while those under 6 years are generally given 150 mg daily. The response is evaluated after approximately 48 hours of therapy and a dosage adjustment is made if necessary.

Store at 15° to 25°C (59° to 77°F) in a dry place and protect from light.

HOW SUPPLIED - RATED THERAPEUTICALLY EQUIVALENT:

Tablet, Uncoated - Oral - 100 mg

100's	$3.23	Allopurinol, United Res	00677-0870-01
100's	$3.23	Allopurinol, Geneva Pharms	00781-1080-01
100's	$3.23	Allopurinol, H.C.F.A. F F P	99999-0133-01
100's	$5.33	Allopurinol, IDE-Interstate	00814-0510-14
100's	$7.75	Allopurinol, Mova Pharms	55370-0527-07
100's	$8.03	Allopurinol, Bristol Myers Squibb	00003-0845-50
100's	$8.07	Allopurinol, Qualitest Pharms	00603-2117-21
100's	$8.10	Allopurinol, Voluntary Hosp	53258-0101-01
100's	$8.81	Allopurinol, Boots Pharm	00524-0405-01
100's	$8.95	Allopurinol, Goldline Labs	00182-1481-01
100's	$8.95	Allopurinol, Par Pharm	49884-0104-01
100's	$8.95	Allopurinol, Mutual Pharm	53489-0156-01
100's	$9.20	Allopurinol, Aligen Independ	00405-4036-01
100's	$9.25	Zyolprim, Rugby	00536-3027-01
100's	$9.25	Allopurinol, HL Moore Drug Exch	00839-7064-06
100's	$9.25	Allopurinol, Major Pharms	00904-2613-60
100's	$9.69	Allopurinol, Parmed Pharms	00349-2332-01
100's	$9.69	Allopurinol, Parmed Pharms	00349-8911-01

HOW SUPPLIED - RATED THERAPEUTICALLY EQUIVALENT: *(cont'd)*

100's	$9.79	Allopurinol, HL Moore Drug Exch	00839-7713-06
100's	$9.80	Allopurinol, Schein Pharm (US)	00364-0632-01
100's	$11.01	Allopurinol, Voluntary Hosp	53258-0101-13
100's	$12.23	Allopurinol, Amer Preferred	53445-1481-01
100's	$12.40	Allopurinol, Geneva Pharms	00781-1080-13
100's	$12.45	Allopurinol USP, Medirex	57480-0800-01
100's	$13.21	Allopurinol, Schein Pharm (US)	00364-0632-90
100's	$14.40	Allopurinol, Goldline Labs	00182-1481-89
100's	$15.30	Allopurinol, Major Pharms	00904-2613-61
100's	$15.75	Allopurinol, Vangard Labs	00615-1592-13
100's	$18.36	Allopurinol, Mylan	00378-0137-01
100's	**$21.40**	**ZYLOPRIM, Glaxo Wellcome**	**00173-0996-55**
100's	$66.83	Allopurinol, Boots Pharm	00524-0405-10
360's	$27.02	Allopurinol, Rugby	00536-3027-07
500's	$16.15	Allopurinol, Geneva Pharms	00781-1080-05
500's	$16.15	Allopurinol, H.C.F.A. F F P	99999-0133-03
500's	$34.00	Allopurinol, Goldline Labs	00182-1481-05
500's	$36.00	Allopurinol, Mutual Pharm	53489-0156-05
500's	$37.49	Allopurinol, Bristol Myers Squibb	00003-0845-60
500's	$43.41	Allopurinol, Par Pharm	49884-0104-05
600's	$80.40	Allopurinol USP, Medirex	57480-0800-06
750's	$101.18	Allopurinol, Glasgow Pharm	60809-0106-55
750's	$101.18	Allopurinol, Glasgow Pharm	60809-0106-72
775's	$104.55	Allopurinol, Glasgow Pharm	60809-0106-66
775's	$104.55	Allopurinol, Glasgow Pharm	60809-0106-88
1000's	$32.30	Allopurinol, United Res	00677-0870-10
1000's	$32.30	Allopurinol, H.C.F.A. F F P	99999-0133-02
1000's	$42.75	Allopurinol, IDE-Interstate	00814-0510-30
1000's	$61.82	Allopurinol, HL Moore Drug Exch	00839-7064-16
1000's	$67.70	Allopurinol, Major Pharms	00904-2613-80
1000's	$68.77	Allopurinol, Qualitest Pharms	00603-2117-32
1000's	$70.00	Allopurinol, Mutual Pharm	53489-0156-10
1000's	$72.20	Allopurinol, Aligen Independ	00405-4036-03
1000's	$83.48	Allopurinol, Parmed Pharms	00349-2332-10
1000's	$89.20	Allopurinol, Parmed Pharms	00349-8911-10
1000's	$89.50	Allopurinol, Goldline Labs	00182-1481-10
1000's	$89.50	Allopurinol, Schein Pharm (US)	00364-0632-02
1000's	$89.50	Allopurinol, Rugby	00536-3027-10
1000's	$89.50	Allopurinol, Par Pharm	49884-0104-10
1000's	$93.96	Allopurinol, HL Moore Drug Exch	00839-7713-16
1000's	$94.25	Allopurinol, Mylan	00378-0137-10
1000's	$104.12	LOPURIN, Knoll Pharms	00048-0051-10
1080's	$55.44	Allopurinol, Rugby	00536-3027-11

Tablet, Uncoated - Oral - 300 mg

100's	$7.43	Allopurinol, United Res	00677-0871-01
100's	$7.43	Allopurinol, Geneva Pharms	00781-1082-01
100's	$7.43	Allopurinol, H.C.F.A. F F P	99999-0133-04
100's	$13.05	Allopurinol, IDE-Interstate	00814-0511-14
100's	$18.10	Allopurinol, Mova Pharms	55370-0529-07
100's	$20.15	Allopurinol, Bristol Myers Squibb	00003-0288-50
100's	$20.94	Allopurinol, Qualitest Pharms	00603-2118-21
100's	$21.20	Allopurinol 300, Major Pharms	00904-2614-60
100's	$21.80	Allopurinol, Boots Pharm	00524-0410-01
100's	$22.30	Allopurinol, Aligen Independ	00405-4037-01
100's	$22.50	Allopurinol, Rugby	00536-3028-01
100's	$22.60	Allopurinol, Goldline Labs	00182-1482-01
100's	$22.60	Allopurinol, Par Pharm	49884-0105-01
100's	$22.80	Allopurinol, Voluntary Hosp	53258-0102-01
100's	$22.94	Allopurinol, Parmed Pharms	00349-8912-01
100's	$23.00	Allopurinol, Mutual Pharm	53489-0157-01
100's	$23.69	Allopurinol, HL Moore Drug Exch	00839-7714-06
100's	$25.94	Allopurinol, Parmed Pharms	00349-2331-01
100's	$26.15	Allopurinol, Schein Pharm (US)	00364-0633-01
100's	$30.37	Allopurinol, Geneva Pharms	00781-1082-13
100's	$30.50	Allopurinol USP, Medirex	57480-0801-01
100's	$31.56	Allopurinol, Voluntary Hosp	53258-0102-13
100's	$33.50	Allopurinol, Schein Pharm (US)	00364-0633-90
100's	$33.70	Allopurinol, Goldline Labs	00182-1482-89
100's	$35.75	Allopurinol, Vangard Labs	00615-1593-13
100's	$38.82	Allopurinol, Major Pharms	00904-2614-61
100's	$50.29	Allopurinol, Mylan	00378-0181-01
100's	**$58.62**	**ZYLOPRIM, Glaxo Wellcome**	**00173-0998-55**
100's	$161.20	Allopurinol 300, Boots Pharm	00524-0410-10
500's	$37.15	Allopurinol, United Res	00677-0871-05
500's	$37.15	Allopurinol, Geneva Pharms	00781-1082-05
500's	$37.15	Allopurinol, H.C.F.A. F F P	99999-0133-06
500's	$60.83	Allopurinol, IDE-Interstate	00814-0511-28
500's	$78.35	Allopurinol, Major Pharms	00904-2614-40
500's	$80.68	Allopurinol, Aligen Independ	00405-4037-02
500's	$85.50	Allopurinol, Qualitest Pharms	00603-2118-28
500's	$85.94	Allopurinol, Rugby	00536-3028-05
500's	$86.55	Allopurinol, Mova Pharms	55370-0529-08
500's	$88.20	Allopurinol, Knoll Labs	00044-0410-05
500's	$95.00	Allopurinol, Mutual Pharm	53489-0157-05
500's	$109.60	Allopurinol, Par Pharm	49884-0105-05
500's	$112.50	Allopurinol, Goldline Labs	00182-1482-05
500's	$112.95	Allopurinol, Schein Pharm (US)	00364-0633-05
500's	$113.00	Allopurinol 300, Purepac Pharm	00228-2103-50
500's	$116.86	Allopurinol, Parmed Pharms	00349-2331-05
500's	$116.86	Allopurinol, Parmed Pharms	00349-8912-05
500's	$117.25	Allopurinol, Mylan	00378-0181-05
500's	**$288.32**	**ZYLOPRIM, Glaxo Wellcome**	**00173-0998-70**
600's	$200.60	Allopurinol USP, Medirex	57480-0801-06
1000's	$74.30	Allopurinol, United Res	00677-0871-10
1000's	$74.30	Allopurinol, Mutual Pharm	53489-0157-10
1000's	$74.30	Allopurinol, H.C.F.A. F F P	99999-0133-05
1000's	$149.07	Zyloprim, Rugby	00536-3028-10
1000's	$219.22	Allopurinol, Goldline Labs	00182-1482-10
1000's	$219.22	Allopurinol, Par Pharm	49884-0105-10
1000's	$228.73	Allopurinol, Parmed Pharms	00349-2331-10
1000's	$228.73	Allopurinol, Parmed Pharms	00349-8912-10
1000's	$230.18	Allopurinol, HL Moore Drug Exch	00839-7714-16
1080's	$133.61	Allopurinol, Rugby	00536-3028-11

ALPRAZOLAM *(000140)*

CATEGORIES: Antianxiety Drugs; Anxiety; Anxiolytics, Sedatives, Hypnotic; Benzodiazepines; Central Nervous System Agents; Depression; Nausea; Pain; Panic Disorder; Tension; Tinnitus*; Pregnancy Category D; DEA Class CIV; Sales > $500 Million; FDA Approval Pre 1982; Patent Expiration 1993 Sep; Top 200 Drugs
* Indication not approved by the FDA

BRAND NAMES: *Alcelam* ; *Algad*; *Alpaz*; *Alplax*; *Alpram*; *Alprax*; Alprazolam Intensol; *Alprox*; *Alzam*; *Alzolam*; *Anpress*; *Ansiopax*; *Azor*; *Cassadan* (Germany); *Constan* (Japan); *Frontal*; *Kalma* (Australia); *Panix*; *Pharnax*; *Prinox*; *Ralozam* (Australia); *Relaxol*; *Restyl*; *Solanax* (Japan); *Tafil* (Germany, Mexico); *Tensivan*; *Trankimazin*; *Tranquinal*; *Tricalma*; *Valeans*; *Xanagis*; **Xanax**; *Xanor*; *Zacetin*; *Zanapam*; *Zenax*; *Zolarem*; *Zoldac*; *Zoldax*; *Zotran*
(International brand names outside U.S. in italics)

FORMULARIES: Aetna; BC-BS

COST OF THERAPY: $18.10 (Anxiety; Tablet; 0.25 mg; 3/day; 120 days)

DESCRIPTION:

Alprazolam Tablets contain alprazolam which is a triazolo analog of the 1, 4 benzodiazepine class of central nervous system-active compounds.

The chemical name of alprazolam is 8-Chloro-1-methyl-6-phenyl-4H-s-triazolo (4,3-α)(1,4) benzodiazepine.

Alprazolam is a white crystalline powder, which is soluble in methanol or ethanol but which has no appreciable solubility in water at physiological pH.

Each alprazolam Tablet, for oral administration, contains 0.25, 0.5, 1 or 2 mg of alprazolam.

Inactive ingredients: Cellulose, corn starch, docusate sodium, lactose, magnesium stearate, silicon dioxide and sodium benzoate. In addition, the 0.5 mg tablet contains FD&C Yellow No. 6 and the 1 mg tablet contains FD&C Blue No. 2.

CLINICAL PHARMACOLOGY:

CNS agents of the 1,4 benzodiazepine class presumably exert their effects by binding at stereo specific receptors at several sites within the central nervous system. Their exact mechanism of action is unknown. Clinically, all benzodiazepines cause a dose-related central nervous system depressant activity varying from mild impairment of task performance to hypnosis.

Following oral administration, alprazolam is readily absorbed. Peak concentrations in the plasma occur in one to two hours following administration. Plasma levels are proportionate to the dose given; over the dose range of 0.5 to 3.0 mg, peak levels of 8.0 to 37 ng/ml were observed. Using a specific assay methodology, the mean plasma elimination half-life of alprazolam has been found to be about 11.2 hours (range: 6.3-26.0 hours) in healthy adults.

The predominant metabolites are α-hydroxy-alprazolam and a benzophenone derived from alprazolam. The biological activity of α-hydroxy-alprazolam is approximately one-half that of alprazolam. The benzophenone metabolite is essentially inactive. Plasma levels of these metabolites are extremely low, thus precluding precise pharmacokinetic description. However, their half-lives appear to be of the same order of magnitude as that of alprazolam. Alprazolam and its metabolites are excreted primarily in the urine.

The ability of alprazolam to induce human hepatic enzyme systems has not yet been determined. However, this is not a property of benzodiazepines in general. Further, alprazolam did not affect the prothrombin or plasma warfarin levels in male volunteers administered sodium warfarin orally.

In vitro, alprazolam is bound (80%) to human serum protein.

Changes in the absorption, distribution, metabolism and excretion of benzodiazepines have been reported in a variety of disease states including alcoholism, impaired hepatic function and impaired renal function. Changes have also been demonstrated in geriatric patients. A mean half-life of alprazolam of 16.3 hours has been observed in healthy elderly subjects (range: 9.0-26.9 hours, n = 16) compared to 11.0 hours (range: 6.3-15.8 hours, n = 16) in healthy adult subjects. The co-administration of oral contraceptives to healthy women increased the half-life of alprazolam as compared to that in healthy control women (mean: 12.4 hours, n = 11 versus 9.6 hours, n = 9). There was a prolongation in the mean half-life of alprazolam from 12.4 hours (range: 7.2-18.4 hours, n = 9) to 16.6 hours (range: 10.0-24.3 hours, n = 9) by the co-administration of cimetidine to the same healthy adults. In patients with alcoholic liver disease the half-life of alprazolam ranged between 5.8 and 65.3 hours (mean: 19.7 hours, n = 17) as compared to between 6.3 and 26.9 hours (mean = 11.4 hours, n = 17) in healthy subjects. In an obese group of subjects the half-life of alprazolam ranged between 9.9 and 40.4 hours (mean = 21.8 hours, n = 12) as compared to between 6.3 and 15.8 hours (mean = 10.6 hours, n = 12) in healthy subjects.

Because of its similarity to other benzodiazepines, it is assumed that alprazolam undergoes transplacental passage and that it is excreted in human milk.

CLINICAL STUDIES:

ANXIETY DISORDERS

AlprazolamTablets were compared to placebo in double blind clinical studies (doses up to 4 mg/day) in patients with a diagnosis of anxiety or anxiety with associated depressive symptomatology. Alprazolam was significantly better than placebo at each of the evaluation periods of these four week studies as judged by the following psychometric instruments: Physician's Global Impressions, Hamilton Anxiety Rating Scale, Target Symptoms, Patient's Global Impressions and Self-Rating Symptom Scale.

PANIC DISORDER

Support for the effectiveness of alprazolam in the treatment of panic disorder came from three short-term, placebo controlled studies (up to 10 weeks) in patients with diagnoses closely corresponding to DSM-III-R criteria for panic disorder.

The average dose of alprazolam was 5-6 mg/day in two of the studies, and the doses of alprazolam were fixed at 2 and 6 mg/day in the third study. In all three studies, alprazolam was superior to placebo on a variable defined as "the number of patients with zero panic attacks" (range, 37-83% met this criterion), as well as on a global improvement score. In two of the three studies, alprazolam was superior to placebo on a variable defined as "change from baseline on the number of panic attacks per week" (range, 3.3-5.2), and also on a phobia rating scale. A subgroup of patients who were improved on alprazolam during short-term treatment in one of these trials was continued on an open basis up to eight months, without apparent loss of benefit.

INDICATIONS AND USAGE:

Alprazolam is indicated for the management of anxiety disorder (a condition corresponding most closely to the APA Diagnostic and Statistical Manual (DSM-III-R) diagnosis of generalized anxiety disorder) or the short-term relief of symptoms of anxiety. Anxiety or tension associated with the stress of everyday life usually does not require treatment with an anxiolytic.

INDICATIONS AND USAGE: *(cont'd)*

Generalized anxiety disorder is characterized by unrealistic or excessive anxiety and worry (apprehensive expectation) about two or more life circumstances, for a period of six months or longer, during which the person has been bothered more days than not by these concerns. At least 6 of the following 18 symptoms are often present in these patients:*Motor Tension* (trembling, twitching, or feeling shaky; muscle tension, aches, or soreness; restlessness; easy fatigability);*Autonomic Hyperactivity* (shortness of breath or smothering sensations; palpitations or accelerated heart rate; sweating, or cold clammy hands; dry mouth; dizziness or lightheadedness; nausea, diarrhea, or other abdominal distress; flushes or chills; frequent urination; trouble swallowing or 'lump in throat'); *Vigilance and Scanning* (feeling keyed up or on edge; exaggerated startle response; difficulty concentrating or 'mind going blank' because of anxiety; trouble falling or staying asleep; irritability). These symptoms must not be secondary to another psychiatric disorder or caused by some organic factor.

Anxiety associated with depression is responsive to alprazolam.

Alprazolam is also indicated for the treatment of panic disorder, with or without agoraphobia.

Studies supporting this claim were conducted in patients whose diagnoses corresponded closely to the DSM-III-R criteria for panic disorder (See CLINICAL STUDIES.)

Panic disorder is an illness characterized by recurrent panic attacks. The panic attacks, at least initially, are unexpected. Later in the course of this disturbance certain situations, *e.g.*, driving a car or being in a crowded place, may become associated with having a panic attack. These panic attacks are not triggered by situations in which the person is the focus of others attention (as in social phobia). The diagnosis requires four such attacks within a four-week period, or one or more attacks followed by at least a month of persistent fear of having another attack. The panic attacks must be characterized by at least four of the following symptoms: dyspnea or smothering sensations; dizziness, unsteady feelings, or faintness; palpitations or tachycardia; trembling or shaking; sweating; choking; nausea or abdominal distress; depersonalization or derealization; paresthesias; hot flashes or chills; chest pain or discomfort; fear of dying; fear of going crazy or of doing something uncontrolled. At least some of the panic attack symptoms must develop suddenly, and the panic attack symptoms must not be attributable to some known organic factors. Panic disorder is frequently associated with some symptoms of agoraphobia.

Demonstrations of the effectiveness of alprazolam by systematic clinical study are limited to four months duration for anxiety disorder and four to ten weeks duration for panic disorder; however, patients with panic disorder have been treated on an open basis for up to eight months without apparent loss of benefit. The physician should periodically reassess the usefulness of the drug for the individual patient.

CONTRAINDICATIONS:

Alprazolam Tablets are contraindicated in patients with known sensitivity to this drug or other benzodiazepines. Alprazolam may be used in patients with open angle glaucoma who are receiving appropriate therapy, but is contraindicated in patients with acute narrow angle glaucoma.

WARNINGS:

DEPENDENCE AND WITHDRAWAL REACTIONS, INCLUDING SEIZURES

Certain adverse clinical events, some life-threatening, are a direct consequence of physical dependence to alprazolam. These include a spectrum of withdrawal symptoms; the most important is seizure (see DRUG ABUSE AND DEPENDENCE.) Even after relatively short-term use at the doses recommended for the treatment of transient anxiety and anxiety disorder (*i.e.*, 0.75 to 4.0 mg per day), there is some risk of dependence. Postmarketing surveillance data suggest that the risk of dependence and its severity appear to be greater in patients treated with relatively high doses (above 4 mg per day) and for long periods (more than 8-12 weeks).

THE IMPORTANCE OF DOSE AND THE RISKS OF ALPRAZOLAM AS A TREATMENT FOR PANIC DISORDER

Because the management of panic disorder often requires the use of average daily doses of alprazolam above 4 mg, the risk of dependence among panic disorder patients may be higher than that among those treated for less severe anxiety. Experience in randomized placebo-controlled discontinuation studies of patients with panic disorder showed a high rate of rebound and withdrawal symptoms in patients treated with alprazolam compared to placebo treated patients.

Relapse or return of illness was defined as a return of symptoms characteristic of panic disorder (primarily panic attacks) to levels approximately equal to those seen at baseline before active treatment was initiated. Rebound refers to a return of symptoms of panic disorder to a level substantially greater in frequency, or more severe in intensity than seen at baseline. Withdrawal symptoms were identified as those which baseline. Withdrawal symptoms were identified as those which were generally not characteristic of panic disorder and which occurred for the first time more frequently during discontinuation than at baseline.

In a controlled clinical trial in which 63 patients were randomized to alprazolam and where withdrawal symptoms were specifically sought, the following were identified as symptoms of withdrawal: heightened sensory perception, impaired concentration, dysosmia, clouded sensorium, paresthesias, muscle cramps, muscle twitch, diarrhea, blurred vision, appetite decrease and weight loss. Other symptoms, such as anxiety and insomnia, were frequently seen during discontinuation, but it could not be determined if they were due to return of illness, rebound or withdrawal.

In a larger database comprised of both controlled and uncontrolled studies in which 641 patients received alprazolam, discontinuation-emergent symptoms which occurred at a rate of over 5% in patients treated with alprazolam and at a greater rate than the placebo treated group were as follows.

Discontinuation-Emergent Symptom Incidence: Percentage of 641 Alprazolam-Treated Panic Disorder Patients Reporting Events.

Neurologic	
Insomnia (29.5)	Muscular twitching (6.9)
Lightheadedness (19.3)	Impaired Coordination (6.6)
Abnormal involuntary movement (17.3)	Muscle tone disorders (5.9)
Headache (17.0)	Weakness (5.8)
Psychiatric	
Anxiety (19.2)	Memory impairment (5.5)
Fatigue and Tiredness (18.4)	Depression (5.1)
Irritability (10.5)	Confusional state (5.0)
Cognitive disorder (10.3)	
Gastrointestinal	
Diarrhea (13.6)	Decreased salivation (10.6)
Nausea/Vomiting (16.5)	
Metabolic-Nutritional	
Weight loss (13.3)	Decreased appetite (12.8)
Dermatological	
Sweating (14.4)	

WARNINGS: *(cont'd)*

Cardiovascular

Tachycardia (12.2)

Special Senses

Blurred vision (10.0)

From the studies cited, it has not been determined whether these symptoms are clearly related to the dose and duration of therapy with alprazolam in patients with panic disorder.

In two controlled trials of six to eight weeks duration where the ability of patients to discontinue medication was measured, 71%-93% of alprazolam treated patients tapered completely off therapy compared to 89%-96% of placebo treated patients. The ability of patients to completely discontinue therapy with alprazolam after long-term therapy has not been reliably determined.

Seizures attributable to alprazolam were seen after drug discontinuance or dose reduction in 8 of 1980 patients with panic disorder or in patients participating in clinical trials where alprazolam doses of greater than 4 mg daily for over 3 months were permitted. Five of these cases clearly occurred during abrupt dose reduction, or discontinuation from daily doses of 2 to 10 mg. Three cases occurred in situations where there was not a clear relationship to abrupt dose reduction or discontinuation. In one instance, seizure occurred after discontinuation from a single dose of 1 mg after tapering at a rate of 1 mg every three days from 6 mg daily. In two other instances, the relationship to taper is indeterminate; in both of these cases the patients had been receiving doses of 3 mg daily prior to seizure. The duration of use in the above 8 cases ranged from 4 to 22 weeks. There have been occasional voluntary reports of patients developing seizures while apparently tapering gradually from alprazolam. The risk of seizure seems to be greatest 24-72 hours after discontinuation (see DOSAGE AND ADMINISTRATION for recommended tapering and discontinuation schedule).

STATUS EPILEPTICUS AND ITS TREATMENT

The medical event voluntary reporting system shows that withdrawal seizures have been reported in association with the discontinuation of alprazolam. In most cases, only a single seizure was reported; however, multiple seizures and status epilepticus were reported as well. Ordinarily, the treatment of status epilepticus of any etiology involves use of intravenous benzodiazepines plus phenytoin or barbiturates, maintenance of a patent airway and adequate hydration. For additional details regarding therapy, consultation with an appropriate specialist may be considered.

INTERDOSE SYMPTOMS

Early morning anxiety and emergence of anxiety symptoms between doses of alprazolam (alprazolam) have been reported in patients with panic disorder taking prescribed maintenance doses of alprazolam. These symptoms may reflect the development of tolerance or a time interval between doses which is longer than the duration of clinical action of the administered dose. In either case, it is presumed that the prescribed dose is not sufficient to maintain plasma levels above those needed to prevent relapse, rebound or withdrawal symptoms over the entire course of the interdosing interval. In these situation, it is recommended that the same total daily dose be given divided as more frequent administrations (see DOSAGE AND ADMINISTRATION.)

RISK OF DOSE REDUCTION

Withdrawal reactions may occur when dosage reduction occurs for any reason. This includes purposeful tapering, but also inadvertent reduction of dose (*e.g.,* the patient forgets, the patient is admitted to a hospital, etc.). Therefore, the dosage of alprazolam should be reduced or discontinued gradually (see DOSAGE AND ADMINISTRATION.)

Alprazolam Tablets are not of value in the treatment of psychotic patients and should not be employed in lieu of appropriate treatment for psychosis. Because of its CNS depressant effects, patients receiving alprazolam should be cautioned against engaging in hazardous occupations or activities requiring complete mental alertness such as operating machinery or driving a motor vehicle. For the same reason, patients should be cautioned about the simultaneous ingestion of alcohol and other CNS depressant drugs during treatment with alprazolam.

Benzodiazepines can potentially cause fetal harm when administered to pregnant women. If alprazolam is used during pregnancy, or if the patient becomes pregnant while taking this drug, the patient should be apprised of the potential hazard to the fetus. Because of experience with other members of the benzodiazepine class, alprazolam is assumed to be capable of causing an increased risk of congenital abnormalities when administered to a pregnant woman during the first trimester. Because use of these drugs is rarely a matter of urgency, their use during the first trimester should almost always be avoided. The possibility that a woman of childbearing potential may be pregnant at the time of institution of therapy should be considered. Patients should be advised that if they become pregnant during therapy or intend to become pregnant they should communicate with their physicians about the desirability of discontinuing the drug.

PRECAUTIONS:

GENERAL

If alprazolam tablets are to be combined with other psychotropic agents or anticonvulsant drugs, careful consideration should be given to the pharmacology of the agents to be employed, particularly with compounds which might potentiate the action of benzodiazepines (see DRUG INTERACTIONS.)

As with other psychotropic medications, the usual precautions with respect to administration of the drug and size of the prescription are indicated for severely depressed patients or those in whom there is reason to expect concealed suicidal ideation or plans.

It is recommended that the dosage be limited to the smallest effective dose to preclude the development of ataxia or oversedation which may be a particular problem in elderly or debilitated patients. (See DOSAGE AND ADMINISTRATION.) The usual precautions in treating patients with impaired renal, hepatic or pulmonary function should be observed. There have been rare reports of death in patients with severe pulmonary disease shortly after the initiation of treatment with alprazolam (alprazolam). A decreased systemic alprazolam elimination rate (*e.g.,* increased plasma half-life) has been observed in both alcoholic liver disease patients and obese patients receiving alprazolam (See CLINICAL PHARMACOLOGY.)

Episodes of hypomania and mania have been reported in association with the use of alprazolam in patients with depression.

Alprazolam has a weak uricosuric effect. Although other medications with weak uricosuric effect have been reported to cause acute renal failure, there have been no reported instances of acute renal failure attributable to therapy with alprazolam.

INFORMATION FOR PATIENTS

For All Users Of Alprazolam

To assure safe and effective use of benzodiazepines, all patients prescribed alprazolam should be provided with the following guidance. In addition, panic disorder patients, for whom higher doses are typically prescribed, should be advised about the risks associated with the use of higher doses.

1. Inform your physician about any alcohol consumption and medicine you are taking now, including medication you may buy without a prescription. Alcohol should generally not be used during treatment with benzodiazepines.

PRECAUTIONS: *(cont'd)*

2. Not recommended for use in pregnancy. Therefore, inform your physician if you are pregnant, if you are planning to have a child, or if you become pregnant while you are taking this medication.

3. Inform your physician if you are nursing.

4. Until you experience how this medication affects you, do not drive a car or operate potentially dangerous machinery, etc.

5. Do not increase the dose even if you think the medication "does not work anymore" without consulting your physician. Benzodiazepines, even when used as recommended, may produce emotional and/or physical dependence.

6. Do not stop taking this medication abruptly or decrease the dose without consulting your physician, since withdrawal symptoms can occur.

Additional Advice For Panic Disorder Patients

The use of alprazolam at the high doses (above 4 mg per day), often necessary to treat panic disorder, is accompanied by risks that you need to carefully consider. When used at high doses for long intervals, which may or may not be required for your treatment, alprazolam has the potential to cause severe emotional and physical dependence in some patients and these patients may find it exceedingly difficult to terminate treatment. In two controlled trials of six to eight weeks duration where the ability of patients to discontinue medication was measured, 7 to 29% of alprazolam treated patients did not completely taper off therapy. The ability of patients to completely discontinue therapy with alprazolam after long-term therapy has not been reliably determined. In all cases, it is important that your physician help you discontinue this medication in a careful and safe manner to avoid overly extended use of alprazolam.

In addition, the extended use at high doses appears to increase the incidence and severity of withdrawal reactions when alprazolam is discontinued. These are generally minor but seizure can occur, especially if you reduce the dose too rapidly or discontinue the medication abruptly. Seizure can be life-threatening.

LABORATORY TESTS

Laboratory tests are not ordinarily required in otherwise healthy patients.

DRUG/LABORATORY TEST INTERACTIONS

Although interactions between benzodiazepines and commonly employed clinical laboratory tests have occasionally been reported, there is no consistent pattern for a specific drug or specific test.

CARCINOGENESIS, MUTAGENESIS, AND IMPAIRMENT OF FERTILITY

No evidence of carcinogenic potential was observed during 2-year bioassay studies of alprazolam in rats at doses up to 30 mg/kg/day (150 times the maximum recommended daily human dose of 10 mg/day) and in mice at doses up to 10 mg/kg/day (50 times the maximum recommended daily human dose).

Alprazolam was not mutagenic in the rat micronucleus test at doses up to 100 mg/kg, which is 500 times the maximum recommended daily human dose of 10 mg/day. Alprazolam also was not mutagenic in vitro in the DNA Damage/Alkaline Elution Assay or the Ames Assay.

Alprazolam produced no impairment of fertility in rats at doses up to 5 mg/kg/day, which is 25 times the maximum recommended daily human dose of 10 mg/day.

PREGNANCY CATEGORY D

Teratogenic Effects: See WARNINGS.

Nonteratogenic Effects: It should be considered that the child born of a mother who is receiving benzodiazepines may be at some risk for withdrawal symptoms from the drug during the postnatal period. Also, neonatal flaccidity and respiratory problems have been reported in children born of mothers who have been receiving benzodiazepines.

LABOR AND DELIVERY

Alprazolam has no established use in labor or delivery.

NURSING MOTHERS

Benzodiazepines are known to be excreted in human milk. It should be assumed that alprazolam is as well. Chronic administration of diazepam to nursing mothers has been reported to cause their infants to become lethargic and to lose weight. As a general rule nursing should not be under taken by mothers who must use alprazolam.

PEDIATRIC USE

Safety and effectiveness in children below the age of 18 years have not been established.

DRUG INTERACTIONS:

The benzodiazepines, including alprazolam, produce additive CNS depressant effects when co-administered with other psychotropic medications, anticonvulsants, antihistaminics, ethanol and other drugs which themselves produce CNS depression.

The steady state plasma concentrations of imipramine and desipramine have been reported to be increased an average of 31% and 20%, respectively, by the concomitant administration of alprazolam tablets in doses up to 4 mg/day. The clinical significance of these changes is unknown.

Pharmacokinetic interactions of benzodiazepines with other drugs have been reported. For example, the clearance of alprazolam and certain other benzodiazepines can be delayed by the co-administration of cimetidine. The clearance of alprazolam can also be delayed by the co-administration of oral contraceptives (See CLINICAL PHARMACOLOGY.) The clinical significance of these interactions is unclear.

ADVERSE REACTIONS:

Side effects of alprazolam tablets, if they occur, are generally observed at the beginning of therapy and usually disappear upon continued medication. In the usual patient, the most frequent side effects are likely to be an extension of the pharmacological activity of alprazolam, e.g. drowsiness or lightheadedness.

The data cited in the two tables below (TABLE 1 and TABLE 2) are estimates of untoward clinical event incidence among patients who participated under the following clinical conditions: relatively short duration (*i.e.,* four weeks) placebo-controlled clinical studies with dosages up to 4 mg/day of alprazolam (for the management of anxiety disorders or for the short-term relief of the symptoms of anxiety) and short-term (up to ten weeks) placebo-controlled clinical studies with dosages up to 10 mg/day of alprazolam in patients with panic disorder, with or without agoraphobia.

These data cannot be used to predict precisely the incidence of untoward events in the course of usual medical practice where patient characteristics, and other factors often differ from those in clinical trials. These figures cannot be compared with those obtained from other clinical studies involving related drug products and placebo as each group of drug trials are conducted under a different set of conditions.

Comparison of the cited figures, however, can provide the prescriber with some basis for estimating the relative contributions of drug and non-drug factors to the untoward event incidence in the population studied. Even this use must be approached cautiously, as a drug may relieve a symptom in one patient but induce it in others. (For example, an anxiolytic drug may relieve dry mouth (a symptom of anxiety) in some subjects but induce it (an untoward event) in others.)

ADVERSE REACTIONS: *(cont'd)*

Additionally, for anxiety disorders the cited figures can provide the prescriber with an indication as to the frequency with which physician intervention (*e.g.*, increased surveillance, decreased dosage or discontinuation of drug therapy) may be necessary because of the untoward clinical event (TABLE 1).

TABLE 1 Anxiety Disorders

	Treatment-Emergent Symptom Incidence ‡		Incidence of intervention Because of Symptom
	Alprazolam	Placebo	Alprazolam
Number of Patients	565	505	565
	% of Patients Reporting		
Central Nervous System			
Drowsiness	41.0	21.6	15.1
Light-headedness	20.8	19.3	1.2
Depression	13.9	18.1	2.4
Headache	12.9	19.6	1.1
Confusion	9.9	10.0	0.9
Insomnia	8.9	18.4	1.3
Nervousness	4.1	10.3	1.1
Syncope	3.1	4.0	*
Dizziness	1.8	0.8	2.5
Akathisia	1.6	1.2	*
Tiredness/Sleepiness	*	*	1.8
Gastrointestinal			
Dry Mouth	14.7	13.3	0.7
Constipation	10.4	11.4	0.9
Diarrhea	10.1	10.3	1.2
Nausea/Vomiting	9.6	12.8	1.7
Increased Salivation	4.2	2.4	*
Cardiovascular			
Tachycardia/Palpitations	7.7	15.6	0.4
Hypotension	4.7	2.2	*
Sensory			
Blurred Vision	6.2	6.2	0.4
Musculoskeletal			
Rigidity	4.2	5.3	*
Tremor	4.0	8.8	0.4
Cutaneous			
Dermatitis/Allergy	3.8	3.1	0.6
Other			
Nasal Congestion	7.3	9.3	*
Weight Gain	2.7	2.7	*
Weight Loss	2.3	3.0	*

* None reported.
† Events reported by 1% or more of alprazolam patients are included.

In addition to the relatively common (*i.e.,* greater than 1%) untoward events enumerated in the table above, the following adverse events have been reported in association with the use of benzodiazepines: dystonia, irritability, concentration difficulties, anorexia, transient amnesia or memory impairment, loss of coordination, fatigue, seizures, sedation, slurred speech, jaundice, musculoskeletal weakness, pruritus, diplopia, dysarthria, changes in libido, menstrual irregularities, incontinence and urinary retention. See TABLE 2

In addition to the relatively common (*i.e.,* greater than 1%) untoward events enumerated in the table above, the following adverse events have been reported in association with the use of alprazolam: seizures, hallucinations, depersonalization, taste alterations, diplopia, elevated bilirubin, elevated hepatic enzymes, and jaundice.

There have also been reports of withdrawal seizures upon rapid decrease or abrupt discontinuation of alprazolam tablets (See WARNINGS.)

To discontinue treatment in patients taking alprazolam, the dosage should be reduced slowly in keeping with good medical practice. It is suggested that the daily dosage of alprazolam be decreased by no more than 0.5 mg every three days (See DOSAGE AND ADMINISTRATION.) Some patients may require an even slower dosage reduction.

Panic disorder has been associated with primary and secondary major depressive disorders and increased reports of suicide among untreated patients. Therefore, the same precaution must be exercised when using the higher doses of alprazolam in treating patients with panic disorders as is exercised with the use of any psychotropic drug in treating depressed patients or those in whom there is reason to expect concealed suicidal ideation or plans.

As with all benzodiazepines, paradoxical reactions such as stimulation, agitation, increased muscle spasticity, sleep disturbances, hallucinations and other adverse behavioral effects such as agitation, rage, irritability, and aggressive or hostile behavior have been reported rarely. In many of the spontaneous case reports of adverse behavioral effects, patients were receiving other CNS drugs concomitantly and/or were described as having underlying psychiatric conditions. Should any of the above events occur, alprazolam should be discontinued. Isolated published reports involving small numbers of patients have suggested that patients who have borderline personality disorder, a prior history of violent or aggressive behavior, or alcohol or substance abuse may be at risk for such evens. Instances of irritability, hostility, and intrusive thoughts have been reported during discontinuation of alprazolam in patients with posttraumatic stress disorder.

Laboratory analyses were performed on patients participating in the clinical program for alprazolam. The following incidences of abnormalities shown in TABLE 3 were observed in patients receiving alprazolam and in patients in the corresponding placebo group. Few of these abnormalities were considered to be of physiological significance.

When treatment with alprazolam is protracted, periodic blood counts, urinalysis and blood chemistry analyses are advisable.

Minor changes in EEG patterns, usually low-voltage fast activity have been observed in patients during therapy with alprazolam and are of no known significance.

POST INTRODUCTION REPORTS

Various adverse drug reactions have been reported in association with the use of alprazolam since market introduction. The majority of these reactions were reported through the medical event voluntary reporting system. Because of the spontaneous nature of the reporting of medical events and the lack of controls, a causal relationship to the use of alprazolam cannot be readily determined. Reported events include: liver enzyme elevations, gynecomastia and galactorrhea.

DRUG ABUSE AND DEPENDENCE:

Physical and Psychological Dependence: Withdrawal symptoms similar, in character to those noted with sedative/hypnotics and alcohol have occurred following discontinuance of benzodiazepines, including alprazolam. The symptoms can range from mild dysphoria and insomnia to a major syndrome that may include abdominal and muscle cramps, vomiting, sweating, tremors and convulsions. Distinguishing between withdrawal emergent signs and

DRUG ABUSE AND DEPENDENCE: *(cont'd)*

TABLE 2 Panic Disorders

	Treatment-Emergent Symptom Incidence*	
	Alprazolam	Placebo
Number of Patients	1388	1231
	% of Patients Reporting	
Central Nervous System		
Drowsiness	76.8	42.7
Fatigue and Tiredness	48.6	42.3
Impaired Coordination	40.1	17.9
Irritability	33.1	30.1
Memory Impairment	33.1	22.1
Lightheadedness/Dizziness	29.8	36.9
Insomnia	29.4	41.8
Headache	29.2	35.6
Cognitive Disorder	28.8	20.5
Dysarthria	23.3	6.3
Anxiety	16.6	24.9
Abnormal Involuntary Movement	14.8	21.0
Decreased Libido	14.4	8.0
Depression	13.8	14.0
Confusional State	10.4	8.2
Muscular Twitching	7.9	11.8
Increased Libido	7.7	4.1
Change in Libido (Not Specified)	7.1	5.6
Weakness	7.1	8.4
Muscle Tone Disorders	6.3	7.5
Syncope	3.8	4.8
Akathisia	3.0	4.3
Agitation	2.9	2.6
Disinhibition	2.7	1.5
Paresthesia	2.4	3.2
Talkativeness	2.2	1.0
Vasomotor Disturbances	2.0	2.6
Derealization	1.9	1.2
Dream Abnormalities	1.8	1.5
Fear	1.4	1.0
Feeling Warm	1.3	0.5
Gastrointestinal		
Decreased Salivation	32.8	34.2
Constipation	26.2	15.4
Nausea/Vomiting	22.0	31.8
Diarrhea	20.6	22.8
Abdominal Distress	18.3	21.5
Increased Salivation	5.6	4.4
Cardiorespiratory		
Nasal Congestion	17.4	16.5
Tachycardia	15.4	26.8
Chest Pain	10.6	18.1
Hyperventilation	9.7	14.5
Upper Respiratory Infection	4.3	3.7
Sensory		
Blurred Vision	21.0	21.4
Tinnitus	6.6	10.4
Musculoskeletal		
Muscular Cramps	2.4	2.4
Muscle Stiffness	2.2	3.3
Cutaneous		
Sweating	15.1	23.5
Rash	10.8	8.1
Other		
Increased Appetite	32.7	22.8
Decreased Appetite	27.8	24.1
Weight Gain	27.2	17.9
Weight Loss	22.6	16.5
Micturition Difficulties	12.2	8.6
Menstrual Disorders	10.4	8.7
Sexual Dysfunction	7.4	3.7
Edema	4.9	5.6
Incontinence	1.5	0.6
Infection	1.3	1.7

* Events reported by 1% or more of alprazolam patients are included.

TABLE 3

	Alprazolam		Placebo	
	Low	High	Low	High
Hematology				
Hematocrit	*	*	*	*
Hemoglobin	*	*	*	*
Total WBC Count	1.4	2.3	1.0	2.0
Neutrophil Count	2.3	3.0	4.2	1.7
Lymphocyte Count	5.5	7.4	5.4	9.5
Monocyte Count	5.3	2.8	6.4	*
Eosinophil Count	3.2	9.5	3.3	7.2
Basophil Count	*	*	*	*
Urinalysis				
Albumin	-	*	-	*
Sugar	-	*	-	*
RBC/HPF	-	3.4	-	5.0
WBC/HPF	-	25.7	-	25.9
Blood Chemistry				
Creatinine	2.2	1.9	3.5	1.0
Bilirubin	*	1.6	*	*
SGOT	*	3.2	1.0	1.8
Alkaline Phosphatase	*	1.7	*	1.8

* Less than 1%

symptoms and the recurrence of illness is often difficult in patients undergoing dose reduction. The long term strategy for treatment of these phenomena will vary with their cause and the therapeutic goal. When necessary, immediate management of withdrawal symptoms requires re-institution of treatment at doses of alprazolam sufficient to suppress symptoms. There have been reports of failure of other benzodiazepines to fully suppress these withdrawal symptoms. These failures have been attributed to incomplete cross-tolerance but may also reflect the use of an inadequate dosing regimen of the substituted benzodiazepine or the effects of concomitant medications.

While it is difficult to distinguish withdrawal and recurrence for certain patients, the time course and the nature of the symptoms may be helpful. A withdrawal syndrome typically includes the occurrence of new symptoms, tends to appear toward the end of taper or shortly

DRUG ABUSE AND DEPENDENCE: *(cont'd)*

after discontinuation, and will decrease with time. In recurring panic disorder, symptoms similar to those observed before treatment may recur either early or late, and they will persist.

While the severity and incidence of withdrawal phenomena appear to be related to dose and duration of treatment, withdrawal symptoms, including seizures, have been reported after only brief therapy with alprazolam at doses within the recommended range for the treatment of anxiety (*e.g.,* 0.75 to 4 mg/day). Signs and symptoms of withdrawal are often more prominent after rapid decrease of dosage or abrupt discontinuance. The risk of withdrawal seizures may be increased at doses above 4 mg/day (See WARNINGS.)

Patients, especially individuals with a history of seizures or epilepsy, should not be abruptly discontinued from any CNS depressant agent, including alprazolam. It is recommended that all patients on alprazolam who require a dosage reduction be gradually tapered under close supervision (See WARNINGS and DOSAGE AND ADMINISTRATION).

Psychological dependence is a risk with all benzodiazepines, including alprazolam. The risk of psychological dependence may also be increased at higher doses and with longer term use, and this risk is further increased in patients with a history of alcohol or drug abuse. Some patients have experienced considerable difficulty in tapering and discontinuing from alprazolam, especially those receiving higher doses for extended periods. Addiction-prone individuals should be under careful surveillance when receiving alprazolam. As with all anxiolytics, repeat prescriptions should be limited to those who are under medical supervision.

CONTROLLED SUBSTANCE CLASS

Alprazolam is a controlled substance under the Controlled Substance Act by the Drug Enforcement Administration and AlprazolamTablets have been assigned to Schedule IV.

OVERDOSAGE:

Manifestations of alprazolam overdosage include somnolence, confusion, impaired coordination, diminished reflexes and coma. Death has been reported in association with overdoses of alprazolam by itself, as it has with other benzodiazepines. In addition, fatalities have been reported in patients who have overdosed with a combination of a single benzodiazepine, including alprazolam, and alcohol; alcohol levels seen in some of these patients have been lower than those usually associated with alcohol-induced fatality.

The acute oral LD_{50} in rats is 331-2171 mg/kg. Other experiments in animals have indicated that cardiopulmonary collapse can occur following massive intravenous doses of alprazolam (over 195 mg/kg; 975 times the maximum recommended daily human dose of 10 mg/day). Animals could be resuscitated with positive mechanical ventilation and the intravenous infusion of norepinephrine bitartrate.

Animal experiments have suggested that forced diuresis or hemodialysis are probably of little value in treating overdosage.

GENERAL TREATMENT OF OVERDOSE

Overdosage reports with alprazolam (alprazolam) tablets are limited. As in all cases of drug overdosage, respiration, pulse rate, and blood pressure should be monitored. General supportive measures should be employed, along with immediate gastric lavage. Intravenous fluids should be administered and an adequate airway maintained. If hypotension occurs, it may be combated by the use of vasopressors. Dialysis is of limited value. As with the management of intentional overdosing with any drug, it should be borne in mind that multiple agents may have been ingested.

Flumazenil (Mazicon), a specific benzodiazepine receptor antagonist, is indicated for the complete or partial reversal of the sedative effects of benzodiazepines and may be used in situations when an overdose with a benzodiazepine is known or suspected. Prior to the administration of flumazenil, necessary measures should be instituted to secure airway, ventilation, and intravenous access. Flumazenil is intended as an adjunct to, not as a substitute for, proper management of benzodiazepine overdose. Patients treated with flumazenil should be monitored for re- sedation, respiratory depression, and other residual benzodiazepine effects for an appropriate period after treatment. **The prescriber should be aware of a risk of seizure in association with flumazenil treatment, particularly in long-term benzodiazepine users and in cyclic antidepressant overdose.** The complete flumazenil prescribing information including CONTRAINDICATIONS, WARNINGS, and PRECAUTIONS should be consulted prior to use.

DOSAGE AND ADMINISTRATION:

Dosage should be individualized for maximum beneficial effect. While the usual daily dosages given below will meet the needs of most patients, there will be some who require higher doses. In such cases, dosage should be increased cautiously to avoid adverse effects.

ANXIETY DISORDERS AND TRANSIENT SYMPTOMS OF ANXIETY

Treatment for patients with anxiety should be initiated with a dose of 0.25 to 0.5 mg given three times daily. The dose may be increased to achieve a maximum therapeutic effect, at intervals of 3 to 4 days, to a maximum daily dose of 4 mg, given in divided doses. The lowest possible effective dose should be employed and the need for continued treatment reassessed frequently. The risk of dependence may increase with dose and duration of treatment.

In elderly patients, in patients with advanced liver disease or in patients with debilitating disease, the usual starting dose is 0.25 mg, given two or three times daily. This may be gradually increased if needed and tolerated. The elderly may be especially sensitive to the effects of benzodiazepines.

If side effects occur at the recommended starting dose, the dose may be lowered.

In all patients, dosage should be reduced gradually when discontinuing therapy or when decreasing the daily dosage. Although there are no systematically collected data to support a specific discontinuation schedule, it is suggested that the daily dosage be decreased by no more than 0.5 mg every three days. Some patients may require an even slower dosage reduction.

PANIC DISORDER

The successful treatment of many panic disorder patients has required the use of alprazolam at doses greater than 4 mg daily. In controlled trials conducted to establish the efficacy of alprazolam in panic disorder, doses in the range of 1 to 10 mg daily were used. The mean dosage employed was approximately 5 to 6 mg daily. Among the approximately 1700 patients participating in a the panic disorder development program, about 300 received maximum alprazolam dosages of greater than 7 mg/day, including approximately 100 patients who received maximum dosages of greater than 9 mg/day. Occasional patients required as much as 10 mg a day to achieve a successful response.

However, in the absence of systematic studies evaluating the dose response relationship, the dosing regimen for the administration of alprazolam to patients with panic disorder must be based on generic principles. Generally, therapy should be initiated at a low dose to minimize the risk of adverse responses in patients especially sensitive to the drug. Thereafter, the dose can be increased at intervals equal to at least 5 times the elimination half-life (about 11 hours in young patients, about 16 hours in elderly patients). Longer titration intervals should probably be used because the maximum therapeutic response may not occur until after the

DOSAGE AND ADMINISTRATION: *(cont'd)*

plasma levels achieve steady state. Dose should be advanced until an acceptable therapeutic response (*i.e.,* a substantial reduction in or total elimination of panic attacks) is achieved, intolerance occurs, or the maximum recommended dose is attained. Because of the danger of withdrawal, abrupt discontinuation of treatment should be avoided. (See WARNINGS, PRECAUTIONS, and DRUG ABUSE AND DEPENDENCE.)

THE FOLLOWING REGIMEN IS ONE THAT FOLLOWS THE PRINCIPLES OUTLINED

Treatment may be initiated with a dose of 0.5 mg three times daily. Depending on the response, the dose may be increased at intervals of 3 to 4 days in increments of no more than 1 mg per day. Slower titration to the higher dose levels may be advisable to allow full expression of the pharmacodynamic effect of alprazolam. To lessen the possibility of interdose symptoms, the times of administration should be distributed as evenly as possible throughout the waking hours, that is, on a three or four times per day schedule.

The necessary duration of treatment for panic disorder patients responding to alprazolam is unknown. After a period of extended freedom from attacks, a carefully supervised tapered discontinuation may be attempted, but there is evidence that this may often be difficult to accomplish without recurrence of symptoms and/or the manifestation of withdrawal phenomena.

In any case, reduction of dose must be undertaken under close supervision and must be gradual. If significant withdrawal symptoms develop, the previous dosing schedule should be reinstituted and, only after stabilization, should a less rapid schedule of discontinuation be attempted. Although no experimental studies have been conducted to assess the comparative benefits of various discontinuation regimens, a possible approach is to reduce the dose by no more than 0.5 mg every three days, with the understanding that some patients may require an even more gradual discontinuation. Some patients may prove resistant to all discontinuation regimens.

Store at controlled room temperature 15-30°C (59-86°F).

ANIMAL PHARMACOLOGY:

When rats were treated with alprazolam at 3, 10, and 30 mg/kg/day (15 to 150 times the maximum recommended human dose) orally for 2 years, a tendency for a dose related increase in the number of cataracts was observed in females and a tendency for a dose related increase in corneal vascularization was observed in males. These lesions did not appear until after 11 months of treatment.

(Upjohn, 4/93, 811 557 722, 691157)

PATIENT INFORMATION:

Alprazolam is used for the treatment of anxiety, panic disorder, and insomnia. Inform your physican if you are pregnant or nursing. Alprazolam may cause dizziness and drowsiness; use caution while driving or operating hazardous machinery. Do not take any other sedating drugs or drink alcohol while taking this medication. Alprazolam may be habit forming. Withdrawal symptoms may occur after you stop taking it. Alprazolam may be taken with or without food.

HOW SUPPLIED - RATED THERAPEUTICALLY EQUIVALENT:

Tablet, Plain Coated - Oral - 0.25 mg

30's	$1.50	Alprazolam, H.C.F.A. F F P	99999-0140-05
100's	$5.03	Alprazolam, H.C.F.A. F F P	99999-0140-06
100's	$5.07	Alprazolam, United Res	00677-1496-01
100's	$46.40	Alprazolam, Major Pharms	00904-7791-60
100's	$46.40	Alprazolam, Major Pharms	00904-7918-60
100's	$48.23	Alprazolam, West Point Pharma	59591-0051-68
100's	$48.23	Alprazolam, Greenstone	59762-3719-01
100's	$50.55	Alprazolam, Qualitest Pharms	00603-2346-21
100's	$51.00	Alprazolam, Roxane	00054-4104-25
100's	$51.95	Alprazolam, Novopharm (US)	55953-0126-40
100's	$51.95	Alprazolam, Novopharm (US)	55953-0868-40
100's	$52.00	Alprazolam, Zenith Labs	00172-4835-60
100's	$52.06	Alprazolam, Aligen Independ	00405-4043-01
100's	$52.22	Alprazolam, Purepac Pharm	00228-2027-10
100's	$52.50	Alprazolam, Par Pharm	49884-0448-01
100's	$52.50	Alprazolam, Martec Pharms	52555-0589-01
100's	$52.80	Alprazolam, Lederle Pharm	00005-3340-43
100's	$52.80	Alprazolam, Goldline Labs	00182-0027-01
100's	$52.95	Alprazolam, Rugby	00536-3235-01
100's	$53.00	Alprazolam, Roxane	00054-8104-25
100's	$53.51	Alprazolam, Schein Pharm (US)	00364-2582-01
100's	$53.55	Alprazolam, Geneva Pharms	00781-1326-01
100's	$55.00	Alprazolam, Vangard Labs	00615-0426-13
100's	$55.08	Alprazolam, HL Moore Drug Exch	00839-7851-06
100's	$55.90	Alprazolam, Mylan	00378-4001-01
100's	$57.00	Alprazolam, Roxane	00054-8104-24
100's	**$59.45**	**XANAX, Pharmacia & Upjohn**	**00009-0029-01**
100's	$62.50	Alprazolam, Goldline Labs	00182-0027-89
100's	$62.50	Alprazolam, Geneva Pharms	00781-1326-13
100's	**$65.80**	**XANAX, Pharmacia & Upjohn**	**00009-0029-46**
500's	$25.15	Alprazolam, H.C.F.A. F F P	99999-0140-07
500's	$25.35	Alprazolam, United Res	00677-1496-05
500's	$224.90	Alprazolam, Major Pharms	00904-7791-40
500's	$224.90	Alprazolam, Major Pharms	00904-7918-40
500's	$233.89	Alprazolam, Greenstone	59762-3719-03
500's	$248.00	Alprazolam, Roxane	00054-4104-29
500's	$249.60	Alprazolam, Qualitest Pharms	00603-2346-28
500's	$252.80	Alprazolam, Novopharm (US)	55953-0126-70
500's	$252.80	Alprazolam, Novopharm (US)	55953-0868-70
500's	$253.20	Alprazolam, Purepac Pharm	00228-2027-50
500's	$253.50	Alprazolam, Zenith Labs	00172-4835-70
500's	$254.20	Alprazolam, Aligen Independ	00405-4043-02
500's	$254.62	Alprazolam, Par Pharm	49884-0448-05
500's	$256.13	Alprazolam, Lederle Pharm	00005-3340-31
500's	$256.13	Alprazolam, Goldline Labs	00182-0027-05
500's	$256.90	Alprazolam, Martec Pharms	52555-0503-05
500's	$256.90	Alprazolam, Martec Pharms	52555-0589-05
500's	$259.25	Alprazolam, Schein Pharm (US)	00364-2582-05
500's	$259.35	Alprazolam, Geneva Pharms	00781-1326-05
500's	$259.90	Xanax, Rugby	00536-3235-05
500's	$267.37	Alprazolam, HL Moore Drug Exch	00839-7851-12
500's	$271.15	Alprazolam, Mylan	00378-4001-05
500's	**$288.32**	**XANAX, Pharmacia & Upjohn**	**00009-0029-02**
1000's	$50.30	Alprazolam, H.C.F.A. F F P	99999-0140-08
1000's	$457.67	Alprazolam, Greenstone	59762-3719-04
1000's	$480.35	Alprazolam, Novopharm (US)	55953-0126-80
1000's	$494.24	Alprazolam, Purepac Pharm	00228-2027-96
1000's	$496.85	Alprazolam, Zenith Labs	00172-4835-80

HOW SUPPLIED - RATED THERAPEUTICALLY EQUIVALENT:
(cont'd)

1000's	$507.39	Alprazolam, Geneva Pharms	00781-1326-10
1000's	**$564.16**	**XANAX, Pharmacia & Upjohn**	**00009-0029-14**

Tablet, Plain Coated - Oral - 0.5 mg

30's	$1.77	Alprazolam, H.C.F.A. F F P	99999-0140-01
100's	$5.93	Alprazolam, H.C.F.A. F F P	99999-0140-02
100's	$6.38	Alprazolam, United Res	00677-1497-01
100's	$57.75	Alprazolam, Major Pharms	00904-7792-60
100's	$57.75	Alprazolam, Major Pharms	00904-7919-60
100's	$60.08	Alprazolam, West Point Pharma	59591-0052-68
100's	$60.08	Alprazolam, Greenstone	59762-3720-01
100's	$63.00	Alprazolam, Roxane	00054-4105-25
100's	$63.50	Alprazolam, Qualitest Pharms	00603-2347-21
100's	$64.88	Alprazolam, Novopharm (US)	55953-0127-40
100's	$64.88	Alprazolam, Novopharm (US)	55953-0880-40
100's	$65.00	Alprazolam, Zenith Labs	00172-4836-60
100's	$65.07	Alprazolam, Purepac Pharm	00228-2029-10
100's	$65.21	Alprazolam, Aligen Independ	00405-4044-01
100's	$65.25	Alprazolam, Par Pharm	49884-0449-01
100's	$65.80	Alprazolam, Martec Pharms	52555-0590-01
100's	$65.81	Alprazolam, Lederle Pharm	00005-3341-43
100's	$65.81	Alprazolam, Goldline Labs	00182-0028-01
100's	$66.00	Alprazolam, Roxane	00054-8105-25
100's	$66.25	Xanax, Rugby	00536-3236-01
100's	$66.63	Alprazolam, Schein Pharm (US)	00364-2583-01
100's	$66.65	Alprazolam, Geneva Pharms	00781-1327-01
100's	$67.32	Alprazolam, Vangard Labs	00615-0401-13
100's	$68.51	Alprazolam, HL Moore Drug Exch	00839-7852-06
100's	$69.65	Alprazolam, Mylan	00378-4003-01
100's	$70.00	Alprazolam, Roxane	00054-8105-24
100's	**$74.06**	**XANAX, Pharmacia & Upjohn**	**00009-0055-01**
100's	$74.25	Alprazolam, Goldline Labs	00182-0028-89
100's	$74.25	Alprazolam, Geneva Pharms	00781-1327-13
100's	**$80.18**	**XANAX, Pharmacia & Upjohn**	**00009-0055-46**
500's	$29.65	Alprazolam, H.C.F.A. F F P	99999-0140-03
500's	$31.90	Alprazolam, United Res	00677-1497-05
500's	$279.95	Alprazolam, Major Pharms	00904-7792-40
500's	$279.95	Alprazolam, Major Pharms	00904-7919-40
500's	$291.16	Alprazolam, Greenstone	59762-3720-03
500's	$308.50	Alprazolam, Qualitest Pharms	00603-2347-28
500's	$310.00	Alprazolam, Roxane	00054-4105-29
500's	$315.32	Alprazolam, Purepac Pharm	00228-2029-50
500's	$316.46	Alprazolam, Par Pharm	49884-0449-05
500's	$316.82	Alprazolam, Aligen Independ	00405-4044-02
500's	$316.88	Alprazolam, Zenith Labs	00172-4836-70
500's	$318.83	Alprazolam, Lederle Pharm	00005-3341-31
500's	$318.83	Alprazolam, Goldline Labs	00182-0028-05
500's	$319.55	Alprazolam, Martec Pharms	52555-0507-05
500's	$319.55	Alprazolam, Martec Pharms	52555-0590-05
500's	$322.75	Xanax, Rugby	00536-3236-05
500's	$322.89	Alprazolam, Geneva Pharms	00781-1327-05
500's	$323.50	Alprazolam, Schein Pharm (US)	00364-2583-05
500's	$332.24	Alprazolam, HL Moore Drug Exch	00839-7852-12
500's	$337.54	Alprazolam, Mylan	00378-4003-05
500's	$345.09	Alprazolam, Novopharm (US)	55953-0127-70
500's	$345.09	Alprazolam, Novopharm (US)	55953-0880-70
500's	**$358.91**	**XANAX, Pharmacia & Upjohn**	**00009-0055-03**
750's	$139.85	Alprazolam, Glasgow Pharm	60809-0502-55
750's	$139.85	Alprazolam, Glasgow Pharm	60809-0502-72
1000's	$59.30	Alprazolam, H.C.F.A. F F P	99999-0140-04
1000's	$570.11	Alprazolam, Greenstone	59762-3720-04
1000's	$615.40	Alprazolam, Purepac Pharm	00228-2029-96
1000's	$621.00	Alprazolam, Zenith Labs	00172-4836-80
1000's	$632.05	Alprazolam, Geneva Pharms	00781-1327-10
1000's	$655.70	Alprazolam, Novopharm (US)	55953-0127-80
1000's	**$702.76**	**XANAX, Pharmacia & Upjohn**	**00009-0055-15**

Tablet, Plain Coated - Oral - 1 mg

30's	$2.43	Alprazolam, H.C.F.A. F F P	99999-0140-09
100's	$8.10	Alprazolam, H.C.F.A. F F P	99999-0140-10
100's	$8.48	Alprazolam, United Res	00677-1498-01
100's	$77.05	Alprazolam, Major Pharms	00904-7793-60
100's	$77.05	Alprazolam, Major Pharms	00904-7920-60
100's	$80.13	Alprazolam, West Point Pharma	59591-0053-68
100's	$80.16	Alprazolam, Greenstone	59762-3721-01
100's	$84.00	Alprazolam, Roxane	00054-4107-25
100's	$85.12	Alprazolam, Qualitest Pharms	00603-2348-21
100's	$85.69	Xanax, Rugby	00536-3237-01
100's	$86.80	Alprazolam, Purepac Pharm	00228-2031-10
100's	$87.00	Alprazolam, Zenith Labs	00172-4837-60
100's	$87.63	Alprazolam, Aligen Independ	00405-4045-01
100's	$87.66	Alprazolam, Novopharm (US)	55953-0131-40
100's	$87.66	Alprazolam, Novopharm (US)	55953-0891-40
100's	$87.76	Alprazolam, Lederle Pharm	00005-3342-43
100's	$87.80	Alprazolam, Par Pharm	49884-0450-01
100's	$88.00	Alprazolam, Roxane	00054-8107-25
100's	$88.40	Alprazolam, Goldline Labs	00182-0029-01
100's	$88.40	Alprazolam, Martec Pharms	52555-0591-01
100's	$88.60	Alprazolam, Schein Pharm (US)	00364-2584-01
100's	$88.95	Alprazolam, Geneva Pharms	00781-1328-01
100's	$89.76	Alprazolam, Vangard Labs	00615-0403-13
100's	$92.00	Alprazolam, Roxane	00054-8107-24
100's	$92.19	Alprazolam, HL Moore Drug Exch	00839-7853-06
100's	$92.50	Alprazolam, Goldline Labs	00182-0029-89
100's	$92.92	Alprazolam, Mylan	00378-4005-01
100's	$96.00	Alprazolam, Geneva Pharms	00781-1328-13
100's	**$98.80**	**XANAX, Pharmacia & Upjohn**	**00009-0090-01**
100's	**$104.08**	**XANAX, Pharmacia & Upjohn**	**00009-0090-46**
100's	**$113.00**	**XANAX, Pharmacia & Upjohn**	**00009-0090-17**
500's	$40.50	Alprazolam, H.C.F.A. F F P	99999-0140-11
500's	$373.75	Alprazolam, Major Pharms	00904-7793-40
500's	$373.75	Alprazolam, Major Pharms	00904-7920-40
500's	$388.71	Alprazolam, Greenstone	59762-3721-03
500's	$411.88	Alprazolam, Qualitest Pharms	00603-2348-28
500's	$414.00	Alprazolam, Roxane	00054-4107-29
500's	$415.29	Xanax, Rugby	00536-3237-05
500's	$420.20	Alprazolam, Novopharm (US)	55953-0131-70
500's	$420.20	Alprazolam, Novopharm (US)	55953-0891-70
500's	$420.96	Alprazolam, Purepac Pharm	00228-2031-50
500's	$424.13	Alprazolam, Zenith Labs	00172-4837-70
500's	$425.66	Alprazolam, Lederle Pharm	00005-3342-31
500's	$425.66	Alprazolam, Goldline Labs	00182-0029-05

HOW SUPPLIED - RATED THERAPEUTICALLY EQUIVALENT:
(cont'd)

500's	$425.83	Alprazolam, Par Pharm	49884-0450-05
500's	$426.65	Alprazolam, Martec Pharms	52555-0508-05
500's	$426.65	Alprazolam, Martec Pharms	52555-0591-05
500's	$431.01	Alprazolam, Schein Pharm (US)	00364-2584-05
500's	$431.05	Alprazolam, Geneva Pharms	00781-1328-05
500's	$434.63	Alprazolam, Aligen Independ	00405-4045-02
500's	$447.12	Alprazolam, HL Moore Drug Exch	00839-7853-12
500's	$450.61	Alprazolam, Mylan	00378-4005-05
500's	**$479.15**	**XANAX, Pharmacia & Upjohn**	**00009-0090-04**
1000's	$81.00	Alprazolam, H.C.F.A. F F P	99999-0140-12
1000's	$760.67	Alprazolam, Greenstone	59762-3721-04
1000's	$798.40	Alprazolam, Novopharm (US)	55953-0131-80
1000's	$821.43	Alprazolam, Purepac Pharm	00228-2031-96
1000's	$831.30	Alprazolam, Zenith Labs	00172-4837-80
1000's	$843.25	Alprazolam, Geneva Pharms	00781-1328-10
1000's	**$937.66**	**XANAX, Pharmacia & Upjohn**	**00009-0090-13**

Tablet, Plain Coated - Oral - 2 mg

100's	$20.66	Alprazolam, H.C.F.A. F F P	99999-0140-13
100's	$136.28	Alprazolam, West Point Pharma	59591-0054-68
100's	$136.28	Alprazolam, Greenstone	59762-3722-01
100's	$145.65	Xanax, Rugby	00536-3238-01
100's	$147.00	Alprazolam, Zenith Labs	00172-4845-60
100's	$147.59	Alprazolam, Purepac Pharm	00228-2039-10
100's	$149.24	Alprazolam, Lederle Pharm	00005-3346-43
100's	$149.24	Alprazolam, Goldline Labs	00182-0030-01
100's	$151.15	Alprazolam, Geneva Pharms	00781-1329-01
100's	$157.98	Alprazolam, Mylan	00378-4007-01
100's	**$167.98**	**XANAX, Pharmacia & Upjohn**	**00009-0094-01**
500's	$103.30	Alprazolam, H.C.F.A. F F P	99999-0140-14
500's	$660.98	Alprazolam, Greenstone	59762-3722-03
500's	$715.83	Alprazolam, Purepac Pharm	00228-2039-50
500's	$716.63	Alprazolam, Zenith Labs	00172-4845-70
500's	$732.55	Alprazolam, Geneva Pharms	00781-1329-05
500's	**$814.78**	**XANAX, Pharmacia & Upjohn**	**00009-0094-03**

HOW SUPPLIED - NOT RATED EQUIVALENT:

Concentrate - Oral - 0.5 mg/5ml

500 ml	$51.75	ALPRAZOLAM, Roxane	00054-3067-63

Concentrate - Oral - 1 mg/ml

30 ml	$37.50	ALPRAZOLAM INTENSOL, Roxane	00054-3068-44

ALPROSTADIL *(000141)*

CATEGORIES: Atresia; Cardiovascular Drugs; Coronary Vasodilators; Impotence; Prostaglandins; Stenosis; Vasodilating Agents; FDA Approval Pre 1982

BRAND NAMES: Caverject; *Edex* (France); *Eglandin*; *Lyple* (Japan); *Minprog* (Germany); *Palux* (Japan); *Promostan*; *Prostandin*; *Prostavasin*; **Prostin VR**; *Prostine VR* (France); *Prostivas*
(International brand names outside U.S. in italics)

WARNING:
Apnea is experienced by about 10 to 12% of neonates with congenital heart defects treated with Prostin VR Pediatric Sterile Solution. Apnea is most often seen in neonates weighing less than 2 kg at birth and usually appears during the first hour of drug infusion. Therefore, respiratory status should be monitored throughout treatment, and Prostin VR Pediatric should be used where ventilatory assistance is immediately available.

DESCRIPTION:

PROSTIN VR PEDIATRIC STERILE SOLUTION

Prostin VR Pediatric Sterile Solution for intravascular infusion contains 500 micrograms alprostadil, more commonly known as prostaglandin E_1, in 1.0 ml dehydrated alcohol.

The chemical name for alprostadil is (11α, 13E, 15S)-11,15dihydroxy-9-oxoprost-13-en-1-oic acid, and the molecular weight is 354.49.

Alprostadil is a white to off-white crystalline powder with a melting point between 110° and 116° C. Its solubility at 35°C is 8000 micrograms per 100 ml double distilled water.

CAVERJECT

For Intracavernosal Use

Caverject Sterile Powder contains alprostadil as the naturally occurring form of prostaglandin E_1 (PGE_1) and designated chemically as (11α, 13E, 15S)-11,15-dihydroxy-9-oxoprost-13-en-1-oic acid. The molecular weight is 354.49.

Alprostadil is a white to off-white crystalline powder with a melting point between 115° and 116°C. Its solubility at 35°C is 8000 micrograms per 100 milliliter double distilled water. Alprostadil is available as a ste freeze-dried powder for intracavernosal use in two sizes: 10-microgram vial—When reconstituted as directed with 1 milliliter of bacteriostatic water for injection or sterile water, both preserved with benzyl alcohol 0.945% w/v, gives 1.13 milliliters of reconstituted solution. Each milliliter contains 10.5 micrograms alprostadil, 172 milligrams lactose, 47 micrograms sodium citrate, and 8.4 milligrams benzyl alcohol. The deliverable amount of alprostadil in each milliliter is 10 micrograms because approximately 0.5 microgram is lost due to adsorption to the vial and syringe; 20-microgram vial—When reconstituted as directed with 1 milliliter of bacteriostatic water for injection or sterile water, both preserved with benzyl alcohol 0.945% w/v, gives 1.13 milliliter of reconstituted solution. Each milliliter contains 20.5 micrograms alprostadil, 172 milligrams lactose, 47 micrograms sodium citrate, and 8.4 milligrams benzyl alcohol. The deliverable amount of alprostadil in

DESCRIPTION: *(cont'd)*

each milliliter is 20 micrograms because approximately 0.5 microgram is lost due to adsorption to the vial and syringe. When necessary, the pH of alprostadil for injection was adjusted with hydrochloric acid and/or sodium hydroxide before lyophilization.

CLINICAL PHARMACOLOGY:

PROSTIN VR PEDIATRIC STERILE SOLUTION

Alprostadil (prostaglandin E_1) is one of a family of naturally occurring acidic lipids with various pharmacologic effects. Vasodilation, inhibition of platelet aggregation, and stimulation of intestinal and uterine smooth muscle are among the most notable of these effects. Intravenous doses of 1 to 10 micrograms of alprostadil per kilogram of body weight lower the blood pressure in mammals by decreasing peripheral resistance. Reflex increases in cardiac output and rate accompany the reduction in blood pressure.

Smooth muscle of the ductus arteriosus is especially sensitive to alprostadil, and strips of lamb ductus markedly relax in the presence of the drug. In addition, administration of alprostadil reopened the closing ductus of new-born rats, rabbits, and lambs. These observations led to the investigation of alprostadil in infants who had congenital defects which restricted the pulmonary or systemic blood flow and who depended on a patent ductus arteriosus for adequate blood oxygenation and lower body perfusion.

In Infants with restricted pulmonary blood flow, about 50% responded to alprostadil infusion with at least a 10 torr increase in blood pO_2 (mean increase about 14 torr and mean increase in oxygen saturation about 23%). In general, patients who responded best had low pretreatment blood pO_2 and were 4 days old or less.

In infants with restricted systemic blood flow, alprostadil often increased pH in those having acidosis, increased systemic blood pressure, and decreased the ratio of pulmonary artery pressure to aortic pressure.

Alprostadil must be infused continuously because it is very rapidly metabolized. As much as 80% of the circulating alprostadil may be metabolized in one pass through the lungs, primarily by β- and ω-oxidation. The metabolites are excreted primarily by the kidney, and excretion is essentially complete within 24 hours after administration. No unchanged alprostadil has been found in the urine, and there is no evidence of tissue retention of alprostadil or its metabolites.

CAVERJECT

Alprostadil has a wide variety of pharmacological actions; vasodilation and inhibition of platelet aggregation are among the most notable of these effects. In most animal species tested, alprostadil relaxed retractor penis and corpus cavernosum urethrae *in vitro*. Alprostadil also relaxed isolated preparations of human corpus cavernosum and spongiosum, as well as cavernous arterial segments contracted by either noradrenaline or $PGF_{2\alpha}$ *in vitro*. In pigtail monkeys *(Macaca nemestrina)*, alprostadil increased cavernous arterial blood flow *in vivo*. The degree and duration of cavernous smooth muscle relaxation in this animal model was dose-dependent.

Alprostadil induces erection by relaxation of trabecular smooth muscle and by dilation of cavernosal arteries. This leads to expansion of lacunar spaces and entrapment of blood by compressing the venules against the tunica albuginea, a process referred to as the corporal veno-occlusive mechanism.

Pharmacokinetics

Absorption: For treatment of erectile dysfunction, alprostadil is administered by injection into the corpora cavernosa. The absolute bioavailability of alprostadil has not been determined.

Distribution: Following intracavernosal injection of 20 micrograms alprostadil, mean peripheral plasma concentrations of alprostadil at 30 and 60 minutes after injection (89 and 102 picograms/milliliter, respectively) were not significantly greater than baseline levels of endogenous alprostadil (96 picograms/milliliter). Alprostadil is bound in plasma primarily to albumin (81% bound) and to a lesser extent α-globulin IV-4 fraction (55% bound). No significant binding to erythrocytes or white blood cells was observed.

Metabolism: Alprostadil is rapidly converted to compounds which are further metabolized prior to excretion. Following intravenous administration, approximately 80% of circulating alprostadil is metabolized in one pass through the lungs, primarily by *beta-* and *omega*-oxidation. Hence, any alprostadil entering the systemic circulation following intracavernosal injection is very rapidly metabolized. Following intracavernosal injection of 20 micrograms alprostadil, peripheral levels of the major circulating metabolite, 13,14-dihydro-15-oxo-PGE_1, increased to reach a peak 30 minutes after injection and returned to pre-dose levels by 60 minutes after injection.

Excretion: The metabolites of alprostadil are excreted primarily by the kidney, with almost 90% of an administered intravenous dose excreted in urine within 24 hour post-dose. The remainder of the dose is excreted in the feces. There is no evidence of this tissue retention of alprostadil or its metabolites following intravenous administration.

Pharmacokinetics in Special Populations

Geriatric: The potential effect of age on the pharmacokinetics of alprostadil has not been formally evaluated. In patients with acute respiratory distress syndrome (ARDS), the mean (± SD) pulmonary extraction of alprostadil was 72% ± 15% in 11 elderly patients aged 65 years or older (mean 71 ± 6 years) and 65% ± 20% in 6 young patients aged 35 years or younger (mean, 28 ± 5 years).

Pediatric: Alprostadil plasma concentrations were measured in 10 neonates (gestational age of 34 weeks in 2 infants and 38 to 40 weeks in 8 infants) receiving steady-state intravenous infusions of alprostadil to treat underlying cardiac malformations. Infusion rates of alprostadil ranged from 5 to 50 (median, 45) nanograms/kilogram/minute, resulting in alprostadil plasma concentrations ranging between 22 and 530 (median, 56) picograms/milliliter. The wide range of alprostadil plasma concentrations in neonates reflects high variability in individual clearances of alprostadil in this patient population.

Gender: The potential influence of gender on the pharmacokinetics of alprostadil has not been formally studied in healthy subjects. Two studies determined the pulmonary extraction of alprostadil following intravascular administration in 23 patients with ARDS. The mean (± SD) pulmonary extraction was 66% ± 20% in 17 male patients and 69% ± 18% in 6 female patients, suggesting that the pharmacokinetics of alprostadil are not influenced by gender.

Race: The potential influence of race on the pharmacokinetics of alprostadil has not been formally evaluated.

Renal and Hepatic Insufficiency: Pulmonary first-pass metabolism is the primary factor influencing the systemic clearance of alprostadil. Although the pharmacokinetics of alprostadil have not been formally examined in patients with renal or hepatic insufficiency, alterations in renal or hepatic function would not be expected to have a major influence on the pharmacokinetics of alprostadil.

Pulmonary Disease: The pulmonary extraction of alprostadil following intravascular administration was reduced by 15% (66 ± 32% vs 78 ± 2.4%) in patients with ARDS compared with a control group of patients with normal respiratory function who were undergoing cardiopulmonary bypass surgery. Pulmonary clearance was found to vary as a function of cardiac output and pulmonary intrinsic clearance in a group of 14 patients with ARDS or at a risk of developing ARDS following trauma or sepsis. In this study, the extraction efficiency of alprostadil ranged from subnormal (11%) to normal (90%), with overall mean of 67%.

INDICATIONS AND USAGE:

PROSTIN VR PEDIATRIC STERILE SOLUTION

Prostin VR Pediatric Sterile Solution is indicated for palliative, not definitive, therapy to temporarily maintain the patency of the ductus arteriosus until corrective or palliative surgery can be performed in neonates who have congenital heart defects and who depend upon the patent ductus for survival. Such congenital heart defects include pulmonary atresia, pulmonary stenosis, tricuspid atresia, tetralogy of Fallot, interruption of the aortic arch, coarctation of the aorta, or transposition of the great vessels with or without other defects.

In infants with restricted pulmonary blood flow, the increase in blood oxygenation is inversely proportional to pretreatment pO_2values; that is, patients with low pO_2 values respond best, and patients with pO_2 values of 40 torr or more usually have little response.

Prostin VR Pediatric should be administered only by trained personnel in facilities that provide pediatric intensive care.

CAVERJECT

Caverject is indicated for the treatment of erectile dysfunction due to neurogenic, vasculogenic, psychogenic, or mixed etiology.

Intracavernosal Caverject may be a useful adjunct to other diagnostic tests in the diagnosis of erectile dysfunction.

CONTRAINDICATIONS:

PROSTIN VR PEDIATRIC STERILE SOLUTION

None.

CAVERJECT

Alprostadil should not be used in patients who have a known hypersensitivity to the drug, in patients who have conditions that might predispose them to priapism, such as sickle cell anemia or trait, multiple myeloma, or leukemia, or in patients with anatomical deformation of the penis, such as angulation, cavernosal fibrosis, or Peyronie's disease. Patients with penile implants should not be treated with Alprostadil.

Alprostadil should not be used in women or children and is not for use in newborns.

Alprostadil should not be used in men for whom sexual activity is inadvisable or contraindicated.

WARNINGS:

PROSTIN VR PEDIATRIC STERILE SOLUTION

See BOXED WARNING.

NOTE: Prostin VR Pediatric Sterile Solution must be diluted before it is administered. See DOSAGE AND ADMINISTRATION, Dilution Instructions.

The administration of Prostin VR Pediatric to neonates may result in gastric outlet obstruction secondary to antral hyperplasia. This effect appears to be related to duration of therapy and cumulative dose of the drug. Neonates receiving Prostin VR Pediatric ar recommended doses for more than 120 hours should be closely monitored for evidence of antral hyperplasia and gastric outlet obstruction.

Prostin VR Pediatric should be infused for the shortest time and at the lowest dose that will produce the desired effects. The risks of long-term infusion of Prostin VR Pediatric should be weighed against the possible benefits that critically ill infants may derive from its administration.

PRECAUTIONS:

PROSTIN VR PEDIATRIC STERILE SOLUTION

General: Cortical proliferation of the long bones, first observed in dogs, has also been observed in infants during long-term infusions of alprostadil. The cortical proliferation in infants regressed after withdrawal of the drug.

In infants treated with Prostin VR Pediatric at the usual doses for 10 hours to 12 days and who died of causes unrelated to ductus structural weakness, tissue sections of the ductus and pulmonary arteries have shown intimal lacerations, a decrease in medial muscularity and disruption of the medial and internal elastic lamina. Localized and aneurysmal dilatations and vessel wall edema also were seen compared to a series of pathological specimens from infants not treated with Prostin VR Pediatric. The incidence of such structural alterations has not been defined.

Because alprostadil inhibits platelet aggregation, use Prostin VR Pediatric cautiously in neonates with bleeding tendencies.

Prostin VR Pediatric should not be used in neonates with respiratory distress syndrome. A differential diagnosis should be made between respiratory distress syndrome (hyaline membrane disease) and cyanotic heart disease (restricted pulmonary blood flow). If full diagnostic facilities are not immediately available, cyanosis (pO_2 less than 40 torr) and restricted pulmonary blood flow apparent on an X-ray are appropriate indicators of congenital heart defects.

Necessary Monitoring: In all neonates, arterial pressure should be monitored intermittently by umbilical artery catheter, auscultation, or with a Doppler transducer. *Should arterial pressure fall significantly, decrease the rate of infusion immediately.*

In infants with restricted pulmonary blood flow, measure efficacy of Prostin VR Pediatric by monitoring improvement in blood oxygenation. In infants with restricted systemic blood flow, measure efficacy by monitoring improvement of systemic blood pressure and blood pH.

Carcinogenesis, Mutagenesis, and Impairment of Fertility: Long-term carcinogenicity studies and fertility studies have not been done. The Ames and Alkaline Elution assays reveal no potential for mutagenesis.

CAVERJECT

General: Priapism (erection lasting over 6 hours) is known to occur following intracavernosal administration of vasoactive substances, including alprostadil. The patient should be instructed to immediately report to his physician or, if unavailable, to seek immediate medial assistance for any erection that persists for longer than 6 hours. Treatment of priapism should be according to established medical practice.

The overall incidence of penile fibrosis, including Peyronie's disease, reported in clinical studies with alprostadil was 3%. In one self-injection clinical study where duration of use was up to 18 months, the incidence of fibrosis was 7.8%. Regular follow-up of patients, with careful examination of the penis, is strongly recommended to detect signs of penile fibrosis. Treatment with alprostadil should be discontinued in patients who develop penile angulation, cavernosal fibrosis, or Peyronie's disease.

Patients on anticoagulants, such as warfarin or heparin, may have increased propensity for bleeding after intracavernosal injection.

Underlying treatable medical causes of erectile dysfunction should be diagnosed and treated prior to initiation of therapy with alprostadil.

The safety and efficacy of combinations of alprostadil and other vasoactive agents have not been systematically studied. Therefore, the use of such combinations is not recommended.

The patient should be instructed not to re-use or to share needles or syringes. As with all prescription medicines, the patient should not allow anyone else to use this medicine.

PRECAUTIONS: *(cont'd)*

Information for the Patient: To ensure safe and effective use of alprostadil, the patient should be thoroughly instructed and trained in the self-injection technique before he begins intracavernosal treatment with alprostadil at home. The desirable dose should be established in the physician's office. The instructions for preparation of the solution of alprostadil should be carefully followed. Vials with precipitates or discoloration should be discarded. The reconstituted vial is designed for one use only and should be discarded after withdrawal or proper volume if the solution. The content of the reconstituted vial is design for one use only and should be discarded after withdrawal of proper volume of the solution. The content of the reconstituted vial should not be shaken. The needle must be properly discarded after use; it must not be re-used or shared with other persons. Patient instructions for administration are included in each package of alprostadil.

The dose of alprostadil that is established in the physician's office should not be changed by the patient without consulting the physician. The patient may expect an erection to occur within 5 to 20 minutes. A standard treatment goal is to produce an erection lasting no longer than 1 hour. Generally, alprostadil should be used no more than 3 times per week, with at least 24 hours between each use.

Patients should be aware of possible side effects of therapy with alprostadil; the most frequently occurring is penile pain after injection, usually mild to moderate in severity. A potentially serious adverse reaction with intracavernosal therapy is priapism. Accordingly, the patient should be instructed to contact the physician's office immediately or, if unavailable, to seek immediate medical assistance if an erection persists for longer than 6 hours.

The patient should report any penile pain that was not present before or that increased in intensity, as well as the occurrence of nodules or hard tissue in the penis to his physician as soon as possible. As with any intravenous injection, an infection is a possibility. Patients should be instructed to report to the physician any penile redness, swelling, tenderness or curvature of the erect penis. The patient must visit the physician's office for regular checkups for assessment of the therapeutic benefit and safety of treatment with alprostadil.

Note: Use of intracavernosal offers no protection from the transmission of sexually transmitted diseases. Individuals who use alprostadil should be counseled about the protective measures that are necessary to guard against the spread of sexually transmitted diseases, including the human immunodeficiency virus (HIV).

The injection of alprostadil can induce a small amount of bleeding at the site of injection (see ADVERSE REACTIONS, Hematoma, Ecchymosis, Hemorrhage At The Site Of Injection). In patients infected with blood-borne diseases, this could increase the risk of transmission of blood- borne diseases between partners.

In clinical trials, concomitant use of agents such as antihypertensive drugs, diuretics, antidiabetic agents (including insulin), or non-steroidal anti-inflammatory drugs had no effect on the efficacy or safety of alprostadil.

Carcinogenesis, Mutagenesis, and Impairment of Fertility: Long-term carcinogenicity studies have not been conducted. Rat reproductive studies indicate that alprostadil at doses of up to 0.2 milligram/kilogram/day does not adversely affect or alter rat spermatogenesis, providing a 200-fold margin of safety compared with the usual human doses. The following battery of mutagenicity assays revealed no potential for mutagenesis: bacterial mutation (Ames), alkaline elution, rat micronucleus, sister chromatid exchange, CHO/HGPRT mammalian cell forward gene mutation, and unscheduled DNA synthesis (UDS).

A 1 year irritancy study was conducted in three groups of 5 male Cynomolgus monkeys injected intracavernosally twice weekly with either vehicle or 3 or 8.25 micrograms of alprostadil per injection. An additional two groups of 6 monkeys each were injected with vehicle or with 8.25 micrograms/injection twice weekly as described previously plus they received multiple doses during weeks 44, 48, and 52. Three monkeys from each group were retained for a 4-week recovery period. There was no evidence of drug-related penile irritancy or nonpenile tissue lesions, which could be directly related to alprostadil. The irritancy which was noted for control and treated monkeys was considered to be a result of the injection procedure itself, and any lesions noted were shown to be reversible. At the end of 4-week recovery period, the histological changes in the penis had regressed.

Pregnancy, Nursing Mothers, and Pediatric Use: Alprostadil is not indicated for use in newborns, children, or women.

DRUG INTERACTIONS:

PROSTIN VR PEDIATRIC STERILE SOLUTION

No drug interactions have been reported between Prostin VR Pediatric and the therapy standard in neonates with restricted pulmonary or systemic blood flow. Standard therapy includes antibiotics, such as penicillin and gentamicin; vasopressors, such as dopamine and isoproterenol; cardiac glycosides; and diuretics, such as furosemide.

CAVERJECT

The potential for pharmacokinetic drug-drug interactions between alprostadil and other agents has not been formally studied.

ADVERSE REACTIONS:

PROSTIN VR PEDIATRIC STERILE SOLUTION

Central Nervous System Apnea has been reported in about 12% of the neonates treated. (See BOXED WARNING.) Other common adverse reactions reported have been fever in about 14% of the patients treated and seizures in about 4%. The following reactions have been reported in less than 1% of the patients: cerebral bleeding, hyperextension of the neck, hyperirritability, hypothermia, jitteriness, lethargy, and stiffness.

Cardiovascular System: The most common adverse reactions reported have been flushing in about 10% of patients (more common after intraarterial dosing), bradycardia in about 7%, hypotension in about 4%, tachycardia in about 3%, cardiac arrest in about 1%, and edema in about 1%. The following reactions have been reported in less than 1% of the patients: congestive heart failure, hyperemia, second degree heart block, shock, spasm of the right ventricle infundibulum, supraventricular tachycardia, and ventricular fibrillation.

Respiratory System: The following reactions have been reported in less than 1% of the patients: bradypnea, bronchial wheezing, hypercapnia, respiratory depression, respiratory distress, and tachypnea.

Gastrointestinal System: See WARNINGS. The most common adverse reaction reported has been diarrhea in about 2% of the patients. The following reactions have been reported in less than 1% of the patients: gastric regurgitation, and hyperbilirubinemia.

Hematologic System: The most common hematologic event reported has been disseminated intravascular coagulation in about 1% of the patients. The following events have been reported in less than 1% of the patients: anemia, bleeding, and thrombocytopenia.

Excretory System: Anuria and hematuria have been reported in less than 1% of the patients.

Skeletal System: Cortical proliferation of the long bones has been reported. See PRECAUTIONS.

Miscellaneous: Sepsis has been reported in about 2% of the patients. Peritonitis has been reported in less than 1% of the patients. Hypokalemia has been reported in about 1% and hypoglycemia and hyperkalemia have been reported in less than 1% of the patients.

ADVERSE REACTIONS: *(cont'd)*

CAVERJECT

Local Adverse Reactions: The following local adverse reaction information was derived from controlled and uncontrolled studies, including an uncontrolled 18-month safety study. (TABLE 1)

TABLE 1 Local Adverse Reactions Reported by ≥ 1% of Patients Treated with Alprostadil for up to 18 Months*

Event	Alprostadil N = 1861
Penile pain	37%
Prolonged erection	4%
Penile fibrosis**	3%
Injection site hematoma	3%
Penis disorder***	3%
Injection site ecchymosis	2%
Penile rash	1%
Penile edema	1%

* Expected for penile pain (2%), no significant local adverse reactions were reported by 294 patients who received 1 to 3 injections of placebo.
** See General Precautions.
*** Included numbness, yeast infection, irritation, sensitivity, phimosis, pruritus, erythema, venous leak, penile skin tear, strange feeling of penis, discoloration of penile head, itch at tip of penis.

Penile Pain: Penile pain after intracavernosal administration of Caverject was reported at least once by 37% of patients in clinical studies of up to 18 months in duration. In the majority of the cases, penile pain was rated mild or moderate in intensity. Three percent of patients discontinued treatment because of penile pain. The frequency of penile pain was 2% in 294 patients who received 1 to 3 injections of placebo.

Prolonged Erection/Priapism: In clinical trials, prolonged erection was defined as an erection that lasted for 4 to 6 hours; priapism was defined as erection that lasted 6 hours or longer. The frequency of prolonged erection after intracavernosal administration of Caverject was 4%, while the frequency of priapism was 0.4%. In the majority of cases, spontaneous detumescence occurred. To minimize the chances of prolonged erection or priapism. Caverject should be titrated slowly to the lowest effective dose (see DOSAGE AND ADMINISTRATION). The patient must be instructed to immediately report to his physician or, if unavailable, to seek immediate medical assistance for any erection that persists for longer than 6 hours. If priapism is not treated immediately, penile tissue damage and permanent loss of potency may result.

Hematoma/Ecchymosis: The frequency of hematoma and ecchymosis was 3% and 2%, respectively. In most cases, hematoma/ecchymosis was judged to be a complication of a faulty injection technique. Accordingly, proper instruction of the patient in self-injection is of importance to minimize the potential of hematoma/ecchymosis (see DOSAGE AND ADMINISTRATION).

The following local adverse reactions were reported by fewer than 1% of patients after injection of Caverject: balanitis, injection site hemorrhage, injection site-inflammation, injection site itching, injection site swelling, injection site edema, urethral bleeding, penile warmth, numbness, yeast infection, irritation, sensitivity, phimosis, pruritus, erythema, venous leak, painful erection, and abnormal ejaculation.

Systemic Adverse Events: The following systemic adverse event information was derived from controlled and uncontrolled studies, including an uncontrolled 18-month safety study. (TABLE 2)

TABLE 2 Systemic Adverse Events Reported by ≥ 1% of Patients Treated with Caverject for up to 18 Months*

Body System/Reaction	Alprostadil N=1861
Cardiovascular System	
Hypertension	2%
Central Nervous System	
Headache	2%
Dizziness	1%
Musculoskeletal System	
Back pain	1%
Respiratory System	
Upper respiratory infection	4%
Flu syndrome	2%
Sinusitis	2%
Nasal congestion	1%
Cough	1%
Urogenital System	
Prostatic Disorder**	2%
Miscellaneous	
Localized pain***	2%
Trauma****	2%

* No significant adverse events were more reported 294 patients who received 1 to 3 injections of placebo.
** prostatitis, pain, hypertrophy, enlargement
*** pain in various anatomical structures other than injection site
**** injuries, fractures, abrasions, lacerations, dislocations

The following systemic events, which were reported for < 1% of patients in clinical studies, were judged by investigators to be possibly related to use of alprostadil: testicular pain, scrotal disorder, scrotal edema, hematuria, testicular disorder, impaired urination, urinary frequency, urinary urgency, pelvic pain, hypotension, vasodilation, peripheral vascular disorder, supraventricular extrasystoles, vasovagal reactions, hypesthesia, non-generalized weakness, diaphoresis, rash, non-application site pruritus, skin neoplasm, nausea, dry mouth, increased serum creatinine, leg cramps, and mydriasis.

Hemodynamic changes, manifested as decreases in blood pressure and increases in pulse rate, were observed during clinical studies, principally at doses above 20 micrograms and above 30 micrograms of alprostadil, respectively, and appeared to be dose-dependent. However, these changes were usually clinically unimportant; only three patients discontinued the treatment because of symptomatic hypotension.

Caverject had no clinically important effect on serum or urine laboratory tests.

OVERDOSAGE:

PROSTIN VR PEDIATRIC STERILE SOLUTION

Apnea, bradycardia, pyrexia, hypotension, and flushing may be signs of drug overdosage. If apnea or bradycardia occurs, discontinue the infusion, and provide appropriate medical treatment. Caution should be used in restarting the infusion. If pyrexia or hypotension occurs, reduce the infusion rate until these symptoms subside. Flushing is usually a result of incorrect intraarterial catheter placement, and the catheter should be repositioned.

OVERDOSAGE: *(cont'd)*

CAVERJECT

Overdosage was not observed in clinical trials with alprostadil. If intracavernous overdose of alprostadil occurs, the patient should be under medical supervision until any systemic effects have resolved and/or until penile detumescence has occurred. Symptomatic treatment of any systemic symptoms would appropriate.

DOSAGE AND ADMINISTRATION:

PROSTIN VR PEDIATRIC STERILE SOLUTION

The preferred route of administration for Prostin VR Pediatric Sterile Solution is continuous intravenous infusion into a large vein. Alternatively, Prostin VR Pediatric may be administered through an umbilical artery catheter placed at the ductal opening. Increases in blood pO_2have been the same in neonates who received the drug by either route of administration.

Begin infusion with 0.05 to 0.1 micrograms alprostadil per kilogram of body weight per minute. A starting dose of 0.1 micrograms per kilogram of body weight per minute is the recommended starting dose based on clinical studies; however, adequate clinical response has been reported using a starting dose of 0.05 micrograms per kilogram of body weight per minute. After a therapeutic response is achieved (increased pO_2 in infants with restricted pulmonary blood flow or increased systemic blood pressure and blood pH in infants with restricted systemic blood flow), reduce the infusion rate to provide the lowest possible dosage that maintains the response. This may be accomplished by reducing the dosage from 0.1 to 0.05 to 0.025 to 0.01 micrograms per kilogram of body weight per minute. If response to 0.05 micrograms per kilogram of body weight per minute is inadequate, dosage can be increased up to 0.4 micrograms per kilogram of body weight per minute although, in general, higher infusion rates do not produce greater effects.

Dilution Instructions: To prepare infusion solutions, dilute 1 ml of Prostin VR Pediatric Sterile Solution with Sodium Chloride Injection USP or Dextrose Injection USP. Undiluted Prostin VR Pediatric Sterile Solution may interact with the plastic sidewalls of volumetric infusion chambers causing a change in the appearance of the chamber and creating a hazy solution. Should this occur, the solution and the volumetric infusion chamber should be replaced.

When using a volumetric infusion chamber, the appropriate amount of intravenous infusion solution, avoiding direct contact of the undiluted solution with the walls of the volumetric infusion chamber.

Dilute to volumes appropriate for the pump delivery system available. Prepare fresh infusion solutions every 24 hours. *Discard any solution more than 24 hours old* (TABLE 3).

TABLE 3 Sample Dilutions and Infusion Rates to Provide a Dosage of 0.1 Micrograms per Kilogram of Body Weight per Minute

Add 1 ampoule (500 micrograms) alprostadil to:	Approximate Concentration of resulting solution (micrograms/ml)	Infusion rate (ml/min per kg of body weight)
250 ml	2	0.05
100 ml	5	0.02
50 ml	10	0.01
25 ml	20	0.005

Example: To provide 0.1 micrograms/kilogram of body weight per minute to an infant weighing 2.8 kilograms using a solution of 1 ampoule

Prostin VR Pediatric in 100 ml of saline or dextrose: INFUSION RATE =0.02 ml/min per kg X 2.8 kg = 0.056 ml/min or 3.36 ml/hr.

CAVERJECT

The dose of alprostadil should be individualized for each patient by careful titration under supervision by the physician. In clinical studies, patients were treated with alprostadil in doses ranging from 0.2 to 140 micrograms; however, since 99% of patients received doses of 60 micrograms or less are not recommended. In general, the lowest possible effective dose should always be employed. In clinical studies, over 80% of patients experienced an erection sufficient for sexual intercourse after intracavernosal injection of alprostadil. A 1/2 inch, 27- to 30-gauge needle is generally recommended.

Initial Titration in Physician's Office: *Erectile Dysfunction of Vasculogenic, Psychogenic, or Mixed Etiology.* Dosage titration should be initiated at 2.5 micrograms of alprostadil. If there is a partial response, the dose may be increased by 2.5 micrograms, depending upon erectile response, until the dose that produces an erection suitable for intercourse and not exceeding a duration of 1 hour is reached. If there is no response to the initial 2.5-microgram dose, the second dose may be increased to 7.5 micrograms, followed by increments of 5 to 10 micrograms. The patient must stay in the physician's office until complete detumescence occurs. If there is no response, then the next higher dose should be given within 1 hour. If there is a response, then there should be at least a 1-day interval before the next dose is given.

Erectile Dysfunction of Pure Neurogenic Etiology (Spinal Cord Injury): Dosage titration should initiated at 1.25 micrograms of alprostadil. The dose may be increased by 1.25 micrograms to a dose of 2.5 micrograms, followed by an increment of 2.5 micrograms to a dose of 5 micrograms, and then in 5-microgram increments until the dose that produces an erection suitable for intercourse and not exceeding a duration of 1 hour is reached. The patient must stay in the physician's office until complete detumescence occurs. If there is no response, then the next higher dose may be given within 1 hour. If there is a response, then there should be at least a 1-day interval before the next dose is given.

The majority of patients (56%) in one clinical study involving 579 patients were titrated to doses of greater than 5 micrograms but less than or equal to 20 micrograms. The mean dose at the end of the titration phase was 17.8 micrograms of alprostadil.

Maintenance Therapy: The first injections of alprostadil must be done at the physician's office by medically trained personnel. Self-injection therapy by the patient can be started only after the patient is properly instructed and well trained in the self-injection technique. The physician should make a careful assessment of the patient's skills and competence with this procedure. This intracavernosal injection must be done under sterile conditions. The site of injection is usually along the dorso-lateral aspect of the proximal third of the penis. Visible veins should be avoided. The side of the penis that is injected and the site of the injection must be alternated; the injection site must be cleansed with an alcohol swab.

The dose of alprostadil that is selected for self-injection treatment should provide the patient with an erection that is satisfactory for sexual intercourse and that is maintained for no longer than 1 hour. If the duration of the erection is longer than 1 hour, the dose of alprostadil should be reduced. Self-injection therapy for use at home should be initiated at the dose that was determined in the physician's office; however, dose adjustment, if required (up to 57% of patients in one clinical study), should be made only after consultation with the physician. The dose should be adjusted in accordance with the titration guidelines described above. The effectiveness of alprostadil for long-term use of up to 6 months has been documented in an uncontrolled, self-injection study. The mean dose of alprostadil at the end of 6 months was 20.7 micrograms in this study.

DOSAGE AND ADMINISTRATION: *(cont'd)*

Careful and continuous follow-up of the patient while in the self-injection program must be exercised. This is especially true for the initial self-injections, since adjustments in the dose of alprostadil may be needed. This recommended frequency of injection is no more than 3 times weekly, with at least 24 hours between each dose. The reconstituted vial of alprostadil is intended for single use only and should be discarded after use. The user should be instructed in the proper disposal of the syringe, needle, and vial.

While on self-injection treatment, it is recommended that the patient visit the prescribing physician's office every 3 months. At that time, the efficacy and safety of the therapy should be assessed, and the dose of alprostadil should be adjusted, if needed.

Caverject as an Adjunct to the Diagnosis of Erectile Dysfunction: On the simplest diagnostic test for erectile dysfunction (pharmacologic testing), patients are monitored for the occurrence of an erection after an intracavernosal injection of alprostadil. Extensions of this testing are the use of alprostadil as an adjunct to laboratory investigations, such as duplex or Doppler imaging. ^{133}Xenon washout tests, radioisotope penogram, and penile arteriography, to allow visualization and assessment of penile vasculature. For any less of these tests, a single dose of alprostadil that induces an erection with firm rigidity should be used.

General Procedure for Solution Preparation: Alprostadil is packaged in a 5-milliliter glass vial. Bacteriostatic water for injection or sterile water, both preserved with benzyl alcohol 0.945% w/v, must be used as the diluent for reconstitution. After reconstitution with 1 milliliter of diluent, the volume of the resulting solution is 1.13 milliliters. One milliliter of this solution will contain either 10.5 or 20.5 micrograms of alprostadil depending on vial strength, 172 milligrams of lactose, and 47 micrograms of sodium citrate. The deliverable amount of alprostadil is either 10 or 20 micrograms per milliliter because approximately 0.5 microgram is lost due to adsorption to the vial and syringe. After reconstitution, the solution of alprostadil should be used immediately and not stored or frozen. Parenteral drug products should be inspected visually for particulate matter and discoloration prior to administration whenever the solution and container permit.

HOW SUPPLIED:

PROSTIN VR PEDIATRIC STERILE SOLUTION

Prostin VR Pediatric Sterile Solution is available in packages of 5–1 ml ampoules. Each ml contains 500 micrograms alprostadil in dehydrated alcohol.

Store Prostin VR Pediatric Sterile Solution in a refrigerator at 2-8°C (36-46°F).

CAVERJECT

Alprostadil is a dry lyophilized powder and is supplied in vials containing 11.9 micrograms or 23.2 micrograms of alprostadil for intracavernosal administration. Store at 2° to 8°C (36° to 46°F) until dispensed. After dispensing, alprostadil may be stored up to 3 months at or below 25°C (77°F). When reconstituted and used as directed, the deliverable amount of alprostadil is 10 and 20 micrograms, respectively. The reconstituted solution should be used immediately and not stored or frozen. Only the accompanying diluent or bacteriostatic water for injection with benzyl alcohol should be used when reconstituting alprostadil.

Caverject is available in the following packages:

6-10 microgram vial with diluent syringe

6-20 microgram vial with diluent syringe

HOW SUPPLIED - EQUIVALENTS NOT AVAILABLE:

Injection, Solution - Intravenous - 500 mcg/ml

1 ml x 5	$893.21	PROSTIN VR PEDIATRIC, Pharmacia & Upjohn	00009-3169-06

Kit - Intravenous - 10 mcg

6's	$104.33	CAVERJECT, Pharmacia & Upjohn	00009-3778-08
6's	$104.33	CAVERJECT, Pharmacia & Upjohn	00009-3778-13

Kit - Intravenous - 20 mcg

6's	$134.36	CAVERJECT, Pharmacia & Upjohn	00009-3701-01
6's	$134.36	CAVERJECT, Pharmacia & Upjohn	00009-3701-13

ALTEPLASE, RECOMBINANT *(000143)*

CATEGORIES: Anticoagulants/Thrombolytics; Blood Formation/Coagulation; Cardiovascular Drugs; Embolism; Heart Failure; Myocardial Infarction; Pulmonary Embolism; Recombinant DNA Origin; Thrombolytic Agents; Thrombosis; Congestive Heart Failure*; Pregnancy Category C; Sales > $100 Million; FDA Approved 1987 Nov; Patent Expiration 2000 Dec

* Indication not approved by the FDA

BRAND NAMES: *Actilyse* (Australia, Asia, England, France, Germany, Mexico); *Activacin* (Japan); **Activase**; TPA

(International brand names outside U.S. in italics)

FORMULARIES: Kaiser

COST OF THERAPY: $2,750.00 (Myocardial Infarction; Injection; 1 mg/ml; 100/day; 1 days)

DESCRIPTION:

Alteplase is a tissue plasminogen activator produced by recombinant DNA technology. It is a sterile, purified glycoprotein of 527 amino acids. It is synthesized using the complementary DNA (cDNA) for natural human tissue-type plasminogen activator obtained from a human melanoma cell line. The manufacturing process involves the secretion of the enzyme alteplase into the culture medium by an established mammalian cell line (Chinese Hamster Ovary cells) into which the cDNA for alteplase has been genetically inserted.

Phosphoric acid and/or sodium hydroxide may be used prior to lyophilization for pH adjustment.

Activase is a sterile, white to off-white, lyophilized powder for intravenous administration after reconstitution with Sterile Water for Injection, USP.

TABLE 1 Quantitative Composition of the Lyophilized Product

	100 mg Vial	50 mg Vial	20 mg Vial
Alteplase	100 mg (58 million IU)	50 mg (29 million IU)	20 mg (11.6 million IU)
L-Arginine	3.5 g	1.7 g	0.7 g
Phosphoric Acid	1 g	0.5 g	0.2 g
Polysorbate 80	less than or equal to 11 mg	less than or equal to 4 mg	less than or equal to 1.6 mg
Vacuum	No	Yes	Yes

Biological potency is determined by an *in vitro* clot lysis assay and is expressed in International Units as tested against the WHO standard. The specific activity of alteplase is 580,000 IU/mg.

CLINICAL PHARMACOLOGY:

Alteplase is an enzyme (serine protease) which has the property of fibrin-enhanced conversion of plasminogen to plasmin. It produces limited conversion of plasminogen in the absence of fibrin. When introduced into the systemic circulation at pharmacologic concentration, alteplase binds to fibrin in a thrombus and converts the entrapped plasminogen to plasmin. This initiates local fibrinolysis with limited systemic proteolysis. Following administration of 100 mg alteplase there is a decrease (16%-36%) in circulating fibrinogen.[1,2] In a controlled trial, 8 of 73 patients (11%) receiving alteplase (1.25 mg/kg body weight over 3 hours) experienced a decrease in fibrinogen to below 100 mg/dl.[2]

The clearance of alteplase in AMI patients has shown that it is rapidly cleared from the plasma with an initial half-life of less than 5 minutes. There is no difference in the dominant initial plasma half-life between the 3-Hour and accelerated regimens for AMI. The plasma clearance of alteplase is 380-570 ml/min.[3,4] The clearance is mediated primarily by the liver. The initial volume of distribution approximates plasma volume.

Acute Myocardial Infarction (AMI) Patients: Coronary occlusion due to a thrombus is present in the infarct-related coronary artery in approximately 80% of patients experiencing a transmural myocardial infarction evaluated within 4 hours of onset of symptoms.[5,6]

Two alteplase dose regimens have been studied in patients experiencing acute myocardial infarction. (Please see DOSAGE AND ADMINISTRATION.) The comparative efficacy of these two regimens has not been evaluated.

Accelerated Infusion in AMI Patients: Accelerated infusion of alteplase was studied in an international, multi-center trial (GUSTO) that randomized 41,021 patients with acute myocardial infarction to four thrombolytic regimens. Entry criteria included onset of chest pain within 6 hours of treatment and ST segment elevation of ECG. The regimens included accelerated infusion of alteplase (≤100 mg over 90 minutes, see DOSAGE AND ADMINISTRATION) plus intravenous (IV) heparin (accelerated infusion of alteplase, n=10,396), or the Kabikinase brand of Streptokinase (1.5 million units over 60 minutes) plus IV heparin (SK [IV], n=10,410), or Streptokinase (as above) plus subcutaneous (SQ) heparin (SK [SQ], n=9841). A fourth regimen combined alteplase and Streptokinase. Aspirin and heparin use was directed by the GUSTO study protocol as follows: All patients were to receive 160 mg chewable aspirin administered as soon as possible, followed by 160-325 mg daily. IV heparin was directed to be a 5000 U IV bolus initiated as soon as possible, followed by a 1000 U/hour continuous IV infusion for at least 48 hours; subsequent heparin therapy was at the discretion of the attending physician. SQ heparin was directed to be 12,500 U administered 4 hours after initiation of SK therapy, followed by 12,500 U twice daily for 7 days or until discharge, whichever came first. Many of the patients randomized to receive SQ heparin received some IV heparin, usually in response to recurrent chest pain and/or the need for a medical procedure. Some received IV heparin on arrival to the emergency room prior to enrollment and randomization.

Results for the primary endpoint of the study, 30-day mortality, are shown in TABLE 2. The incidence of 30-day mortality for accelerated infusion of alteplase was 1.0% lower than for SK (IV) and 1.0% lower than for SK (SQ). The secondary endpoints of combined 30-day mortality or nonfatal stroke, and 24-hour mortality, as well as the safety endpoints of total stroke and intracerebral hemorrhage (ICH) are also shown in TABLE 2. The incidence of combined 30-day mortality or nonfatal stroke for the alteplase accelerated infusion was 1.0% lower than for SK (IV) and 0.8% lower than for SK (SQ).

TABLE 2A

Event	Accelerated Activase	SK (IV)	p-value[1]
30-Day Mortality	6.3%	7.3%	0.003
30-Day Mortality or Nonfatal Stroke	7.2%	8.2%	0.006
24-Hour Mortality	2.4%	2.9%	0.009
Any Stroke	1.6%	1.4%	0.32
Intracerebral Hemorrhage	0.7%	0.6%	0.22

1 Two-tailed p-value is for comparison of accelerated infusion of Activase, Alteplase, recombinant to the respective SK control arm.

TABLE 2B

Event	SK (SQ)	p-value[1]
30-Day Mortality	7.3%	0.007
30-Day Mortality or Nonfatal Stroke	8.0%	0.036
24-Hour Mortality	2.8%	0.029
Any Stroke	1.2%	0.03
Intracerebral Hemorrhage	0.5%	0.02

1 Two-tailed p-value is for comparison of accelerated infusion of Activase, Alteplase, recombinant to the respective SK control arm.

Subgroup analysis of patients by age, infarct location, time from symptom onset to thrombolytic treatment, and treatment in the U.S. or elsewhere showed consistently lower 30-day mortality for the alteplase accelerated infusion group. For patients who were over 75 years of age, a predefined subgroup consisting of 12% of patients enrolled, the incidence of stroke was 4.0% for the alteplase accelerated infusion group, 2.8% for SK (IV), and 3.2% for SK (SQ); the incidence of combined 30-day mortality or nonfatal stroke was 20.6% for accelerated infusion of alteplase, 21.5% for SK (IV), and 22.0% for SK (SQ).

An angiographic substudy of the GUSTO trial provided data on infarct-related artery patency. TABLE 3 presents 90-minute, 180-minute, 24 hour, and 5-7 day patency values by TIMI flow grade for the three treatment regimens. Reocclusion rates were similar for all three treatment regimens.

TABLE 3A

Patency (TIMI 2 or 3)	Accelerated Activase	SK(IV)	p-value
90-Minute	n=272 81.3%	n=261 59.0%	<0.0001
180-Minute	n=80 76.3%	n=76 72.4%	0.58
24-Hour	n=81 88.9%	n=72 87.5%	0.24
5-7 Day	n=72 83.3%	n=77 90.9%	0.47

The safety and efficacy of the accelerated infusion of alteplase have not been evaluated using antithrombotic or antiplatelet regimens other than those used in the GUSTO trial.

3-Hour Infusion in AMI Patients: In patients studied in a controlled trial with coronary angiography at 90 and 120 minutes following infusion of alteplase infarct artery patency was observed in 71% and 85% of patients (n=85), respectively.[2] In a second study, where patients

CLINICAL PHARMACOLOGY: *(cont'd)*

TABLE 3B

Patency (TIMI 2 or 3)	SK (SQ)	p-value
90-Minute	n=260 53.5%	<0.0001
180-Minute	n=95 71.6%	0.48
24-Hour	n=67 82.1%	0.79
5-7 Day	n=75 78.7%	0.17

received coronary angiography prior to and following infusion of alteplase within 6 hours of the onset of symptoms, reperfusion of the obstructed vessel occurred within 90 minutes after the commencement of therapy, in 71% of 83 patients.[1]

In a double-blind, randomized trial (138 patients) comparing alteplase to placebo, patients infused with alteplase within 4 hours of onset of symptoms experienced improved left ventricular function at day 10 compared to the placebo group, when ejection fraction was measured by gated blood pool scan (53.2% vs 46.4%, p=0.018). Relative to baseline (day 1) values, the net changes in ejection fraction were +3.6% and -4.7% for the treated and placebo groups, respectively (p=0.0001). Also documented was a reduced incidence of clinical congestive heart failure in the treated group (14%) compared to the placebo group (33%) (p=0.009).[7]

In a second double-blind, randomized trial (145 patients) comparing alteplase, recombinant to placebo, patients infused with alteplase within 2.5 hours of onset of symptoms experienced improved left ventricular function at a mean of 21 days compared to the placebo group, when ejection fraction was measured by gated blood pool scan (52% vs 48%, p=0.08) and by contrast ventriculogram (61% vs 54%, p=0.006). Although the contribution of alteplase alone is unclear, the incidence of nonischemic cardiac complications when taken as a group (*i.e.,* congestive heart failure, pericarditis, atrial fibrillation, and conduction disturbance) was reduced when compared to those patients treated with placebo (p<0.01).[8]

In a double-blind, randomized trial (5013 patients) comparing alteplase to placebo (ASSET study), patients infused with alteplase within 5 hours of the onset of symptoms of acute myocardial infarction experienced improved 30-day survival compared to those treated with placebo. At 1 month, the overall mortality rates were 7.2% for the alteplase -treated group and 9.8% for the placebo-treated group (p=0.001).[9,10] This benefit was maintained at 6 months for alteplase -treated patients (10.4%) compared to those treated with placebo (13.1%, p=0.008).[10]

In a second double-blind, randomized trial (721 patients) comparing alteplase to placebo, patients infused with alteplase within 5 hours of the onset of symptoms experienced improved ventricular function 10-22 days after treatment compared to the placebo group, when global ejection fraction was measured by contrast ventriculography (50.7% vs 48.5%, p=0.01). Patients treated with alteplase had a 19% reduction in infarct size, as measured by cumulative release of HBDH (α-hydroxybutyrate dehydrogenase) activity compared to placebo-treated patients (p=0.001). Patients treated with alteplase had significantly fewer episodes of cardiogenic shock (p=0.02), ventricular fibrillation (p<0.04) and pericarditis (p=0.01) compared to patients treated with placebo. Mortality at 21 days in alteplase -treated patients was reduced to 3.7% compared to 6.3% in placebo-treated patients (1p=0.05).[11] Although these data do not demonstrate unequivocally a significant reduction in mortality for this study, they do indicate a trend that is supported by the results of the ASSET study.

Pulmonary Embolism Patients: In a comparative randomized trial (n=45),[12] 59% of patients (n=22) treated with alteplase (100 mg over 2 hours) experienced moderate or marked lysis of pulmonary emboli when assessed by pulmonary angiography 2 hours after treatment initiation. Alteplase, recombinant-treated patients also experienced a significant reduction in pulmonary embolism-induced pulmonary hypertension within 2 hours of treatment (p=0.003). Pulmonary perfusion at 24 hours, as assessed by radionuclide scan, was significantly improved (p=0.002).

INDICATIONS AND USAGE:

Acute Myocardial Infarction: Alteplase is indicated for use in the management of acute myocardial infarction in adults for the improvement of ventricular function following AMI, the reduction of the incidence of congestive heart failure, and the reduction of mortality associated with AMI. Treatment should be initiated as soon as possible after the onset of AMI symptoms (see CLINICAL PHARMACOLOGY.)

Pulmonary Embolism: Alteplase is indicated in the management of acute massive pulmonary embolism (PE) in adults:

for the lysis of acute pulmonary emboli, defined as obstruction of blood flow to a lobe or multiple segments of the lungs, and

for the lysis of pulmonary emboli accompanied by unstable hemodynamics, e.g., failure to maintain blood pressure without supportive measures.

The diagnosis should be confirmed by objective means, such as pulmonary angiography or noninvasive procedures such as lung scanning.

CONTRAINDICATIONS:

Because thrombolytic therapy increases the risk of bleeding, Alteplase is contraindicated in the following situations:

Active internal bleeding

History of cerebrovascular accident

Recent (within 2 months) intracranial or intraspinal surgery or trauma (see WARNINGS.)

Intracranial neoplasm, arteriovenous malformation, or aneurysm

Known bleeding diathesis

Severe uncontrolled hypertension

WARNINGS:

Bleeding: The most common complication encountered during alteplase, recombinant therapy is bleeding. The type of bleeding associated with thrombolytic therapy can be divided into two broad categories:

Internal bleeding, involving intracranial and retroperitoneal sites, or the gastrointestinal, genitourinary, or respiratory tracts.

uperficial or surface bleeding, observed mainly at invaded or disturbed sites (*e.g.,* venous cutdowns, arterial punctures, sites of recent surgical intervention).

The concomitant use of heparin anticoagulation may contribute to bleeding. Some of the hemorrhagic episodes occurred 1 or more days after the effects of alteplase had dissipated, but while heparin therapy was continuing.

As fibrin is lysed during alteplase therapy, bleeding from recent puncture sites may occur. Therefore, thrombolytic therapy requires careful attention to all potential bleeding sites (including catheter insertion sites, arterial and venous puncture sites, cutdown sites, and needle puncture sites).

WARNINGS: *(cont'd)*

Intramuscular injections and nonessential handling of the patient should be avoided during treatment with alteplase. Venipunctures should be performed carefully and only as required.

Should an arterial puncture be necessary during an infusion of alteplase, it is preferable to use an upper extremity vessel that is accessible to manual compression. Pressure should be applied for at least 30 minutes, a pressure dressing applied, and the puncture site checked frequently for evidence of bleeding.

Should serious bleeding (not controllable by local pressure) occur, the infusion of alteplase and any concomitant heparin should be terminated immediately.

Each patient being considered for therapy with alteplase, recombinant should be carefully evaluated and anticipated benefits weighed against potential risks associated with therapy.

In the following conditions, the risks of alteplase therapy may be increased and should be weighed against the anticipated benefits.

Recent (within 10 days) major surgery, e.g., coronary artery bypass graft, obstetrical delivery, organ biopsy, previous puncture of noncompressible vessels

Cerebrovascular disease

Recent gastrointestinal or genitourinary bleeding (within 10 days)

Recent trauma (within 10 days)

Hypertension: systolic BP ≥ 180 mm Hg and/or diastolic BP ≥ 110 mm Hg

High likelihood of left heart thrombus, e.g., mitral stenosis with atrial fibrillation

Acute pericarditis

Subacute bacterial endocarditis

Hemostatic defects including those secondary to severe hepatic or renal disease

Significant liver dysfunction

Pregnancy

Diabetic hemorrhagic retinopathy, or other hemorrhagic ophthalmic conditions

Septic thrombophlebitis or occluded AV cannula at seriously infected site

Advanced age, *i.e.*, over 75 years old

Patients currently receiving oral anticoagulants, e.g., warfarin sodium

Any other condition in which bleeding constitutes a significant hazard or would be particularly difficult to manage because of its location

Arrhythmias: Coronary thrombolysis may result in arrhythmias associated with reperfusion. These arrhythmias (such as sinus bradycardia, accelerated idioventricular rhythm, ventricular premature depolarizations, ventricular tachycardia) are not different from those often seen in the ordinary course of acute myocardial infarction and may be managed with standard antiarrhythmic measures. It is recommended that antiarrhythmic therapy for bradycardia and/or ventricular irritability be available when infusions of alteplase, recombinant are administered.

Pulmonary Embolism: It should be recognized that the treatment of pulmonary embolism with alteplase has not been shown to constitute adequate clinical treatment of underlying deep vein thrombosis. Furthermore, the possible risk of reembolization due to the lysis of underlying deep venous thrombi should be considered.

PRECAUTIONS:

General: Standard management of myocardial infarction or pulmonary embolism should be implemented concomitantly with alteplase treatment. Noncompressible arterial puncture must be avoided (*i.e.*, internal jugular and subclavian punctures should be avoided to minimize bleeding from noncompressible sites). Arterial and venous punctures should be minimized. In the event of serious bleeding, alteplase and heparin should be discontinued immediately. Heparin effects can be reversed by protamine.

Readministration: There is no experience with readministration of alteplase. If an anaphylactoid reaction occurs, the infusion should be discontinued immediately and appropriate therapy initiated.

Although sustained antibody formation in patients receiving one dose of alteplase has not been documented, readministration should be undertaken with caution. Detectable levels of antibody (a single point measurement) were reported in one patient, but subsequent antibody test results were negative.

Laboratory Tests: During alteplase therapy, if coagulation tests and/or measures of fibrinolytic activity are performed, the results may be unreliable unless specific precautions are taken to prevent *in vitro* artifacts. Alteplase is an enzyme that when present in blood in pharmacologic concentrations remains active under *in vitro* conditions. This can lead to degradation of fibrinogen in blood samples removed for analysis. Collection of blood samples in the presence of aprotinin (150-200 units/ml) can to some extent mitigate this phenomenon.

Use of Antithrombotics: Aspirin and heparin have been administered concomitantly with and following infusions of alteplase. Because heparin, aspirin, or alteplase may cause bleeding complications, careful monitoring for bleeding is advised, especially at arterial puncture sites.

Pregnancy (Category C): Animal reproduction studies have not been conducted with alteplase. It is also not known whether alteplase can cause fetal harm when administered to a pregnant woman or can affect reproduction capacity. Alteplase should be given to a pregnant woman only if clearly needed.

Pediatric Use: Safety and effectiveness of alteplase in pediatric patients have not been established.

Carcinogenesis, Mutagenesis, and Impairment of Fertility: Long-term studies in animals have not been performed to evaluate the carcinogenic potential or the effect on fertility. Short-term studies, which evaluated tumorigenicity of alteplase and effect on tumor metastases in rodents, were negative.

Studies to determine mutagenicity (Ames test) and chromosomal aberration assays in human lymphocytes were negative at all concentrations tested. Cytotoxicity, as reflected by a decrease in mitotic index, was evidenced only after prolonged exposure and only at the highest concentrations tested.

Nursing Mothers: It is not known whether alteplase, recombinant is excreted in human milk. Because many drugs are excreted in human milk, caution should be exercised when alteplase is administered to a nursing woman.

DRUG INTERACTIONS:

The interaction of alteplase, recombinant with other cardioactive drugs has not been studied. In addition to bleeding associated with heparin and vitamin K antagonists, drugs that alter platelet function (such as acetylsalicylic acid, dipyridamole) may increase the risk of bleeding if administered prior to, during, or after alteplase therapy.

ADVERSE REACTIONS:

Bleeding: The most frequent adverse reaction associated with alteplase is bleeding.[13,14] The type of bleeding associated with thrombolytic therapy can be divided into two broad categories:

Internal bleeding, involving the following locations:

ADVERSE REACTIONS: *(cont'd)*

Intracranial and retroperitoneal sites

Gastrointestinal, genitourinary, or respiratory tracts.

Superficial or surface bleeding, observed mainly at invaded or disturbed sites (*e.g.*, venous cutdowns, arterial punctures, sites of recent surgical intervention).

The incidence of all strokes for the alteplase accelerated infusion regimen in the GUSTO trial was 1.6% while the incidence of nonfatal stroke was 0.9%. The incidence of hemorrhagic stroke was 0.7%, not all of which were fatal. The incidence of all strokes, as well as that for hemorrhagic stroke, increased with increasing age (see CLINICAL PHARMACOLOGY), Accelerated Infusion in AMI Patients. Data from previous trials utilizing a 3-hour infusion of ≤100 mg indicated that the incidence of total stroke in six randomized double-blind placebo controlled trials [2,7-11,15] was 1.2% (37/3161) in alteplase-treated patients compared with 0.9% (27/3092) in placebo-treated patients.

The incidence of significant internal bleeding (estimated as >250 cc blood loss) has been reported in studies in over 800 patients. These data do not include patients treated with the alteplase accelerated infusion:

TABLE 4

	Total Dose ≤100 mg	Total Dose >100 mg
gastrointestinal	5%	5%
genitourinary	4%	4%
ecchymosis	1%	<1%
retroperitoneal	<1%	<1%
epistaxis	<1%	<1%
gingival	<1%	<1%

The incidence of intracranial bleeding (ICB) in patients treated with alteplase is as follows:

TABLE 5

Dose	Number of Patients	ICB (%)
100 mg, 3-hours	3272	0.4
≤100 mg, accelerated	10,396	0.7
150 mg	1779	1.3
1-1.4 mg/kg	237	0.4

These data indicate that a dose of 150 mg of alteplase, recombinant should not be used because it has been associated with an increase in intracranial bleeding.[16]

Should serious bleeding in a critical location (intracranial, gastrointestinal, retroperitoneal, pericardial) occur, alteplase therapy should be discontinued immediately, along with any concomitant therapy with heparin. Death and permanent disability are not uncommonly reported in patients that have experienced stroke (including intracranial bleeding) and other serious bleeding episodes.

Fibrin which is part of the hemostatic plug formed at needle puncture sites will be lysed during alteplase therapy. Therefore, alteplase therapy requires careful attention to potential bleeding sites, e.g., catheter insertion sites, and arterial puncture sites.

Allergic Reactions: Allergic-type reactions, e.g., anaphylactoid reaction, laryngeal edema, rash, and urticaria have been reported very rarely (<0.02%). A cause and effect relationship to alteplase therapy has not been established. When such reactions occur, they usually respond to conventional therapy.

Other Adverse Reactions: Cholesterol embolization (CE) has been reported rarely in patients treated with thrombolytic therapy; the true incidence is unknown. This serious condition, which can be lethal, is also known to be associated with invasive vascular procedures (*e.g.*, cardiac catheterization, angiography, vascular surgery) and/or anticoagulant therapy. Clinical features of CE include livedo reticularis, "purple toe" syndrome, acute renal failure, gangrenous digits, hypertension, pancreatitis, myocardial infarction, cerebral infarction, spinal cord infarction, retinal artery occlusion, bowel infarction, and rhabdomyolysis.

Patients with myocardial infarction or pulmonary embolism can experience disease-related events such as cardiogenic shock, arrhythmias, pulmonary edema, heart failure, cardiac arrest, recurrent ischemia, reinfarction, myocardial rupture, mitral regurgitation, pericardial effusion, pericarditis, cardiac tamponade, venous thrombosis and embolism, and electromechanical dissociation. These events can be life-threatening and may lead to death. Other adverse reactions have been reported, principally nausea and/or vomiting, hypotension, and fever. These reactions are frequent sequelae of myocardial infarction and may or may not be attributable to alteplase therapy.

DOSAGE AND ADMINISTRATION:

Alteplase, recombinant is for intravenous administration only.

Extravasation of alteplase infusion can cause ecchymosis and/or inflammation. Management consists of terminating the infusion at that IV site and application of local therapy.

ACUTE MYOCARDIAL INFARCTION

Administer alteplase as soon as possible after the onset of symptoms.

There are two alteplase dose regimens for use in the management of acute myocardial infarction; controlled studies to compare clinical outcomes with these regimens have not been conducted.

Accelerated Infusion: The recommended total dose is based upon patient weight, not to exceed 100 mg. For patients weighing >67 kg, the recommended dose administered is 100 mg as a 15 mg intravenous bolus, followed by 50 mg infused over the next 30 minutes, and then 35 mg infused over the next 60 minutes.

For patients weighing ≤67 kg, the recommended dose is administered as a 15 mg intravenous bolus, followed by 0.75 mg/kg infused over the next 30 minutes not to exceed 50 mg, and then 0.50 mg/kg over the next 60 minutes not to exceed 35 mg.

The safety and efficacy of this accelerated infusion of alteplase regimen has only been investigated with concomitant administration of heparin and aspirin as described in CLINICAL PHARMACOLOGY.

a. The bolus dose may be prepared in one of the following ways:

1. By removing 15 ml from the vial of reconstituted (1 mg/ml) alteplase using a syringe and needle. If this method is used with the 20 mg or 50 mg vials, the syringe should not be printed with air and the needle should be inserted into the alteplase vial stopper. If the 100 mg vial is used, the needle should be inserted away from the puncture mark made by the transfer device.

2. By removing 15 ml from a port (second injection site) on the infusion line after the infusion set is primed.

3. By programming an infusion pump to deliver a 15 ml (1 mg/ml) bolus at the initiation of the infusion.

b. The remainder of the alteplase, recombinant dose may be administered as follows:

20 mg, 50 mg vials: administer using either a polyvinyl chloride bag or glass vial and infusion set

DOSAGE AND ADMINISTRATION: *(cont'd)*

100 mg vials: insert the spike end of an infusion set through the same puncture site created by the transfer device in the stopper of the vial of reconstituted alteplase. Hang the alteplase vial from the plastic molded capping attached to the bottom of the vial.

PULMONARY EMBOLISM

The recommended dose is 100 mg administered by intravenous infusion over 2 hours. Heparin therapy should be instituted or reinstituted near the end of or immediately following the alteplase infusion when the partial thromboplastin time or thrombin time returns to twice normal or less.

The alteplase dose may be administered as follows:

20 mg, 50 mg vials: administer using either a polyvinyl chloride bag or glass vial and infusion set

100 mg vials: insert the spike end of an infusion set through the same puncture site created by the transfer device in the stopper of the vial of reconstituted alteplase. Hang the alteplase vial from the plastic molded capping attached to the bottom of the vial.

A DOSE OF 150 MG OF ALTEPLASE SHOULD NOT BE USED BECAUSE IT HAS BEEN ASSOCIATED WITH AN INCREASE IN INTRACRANIAL BLEEDING.

RECONSTITUTION AND DILUTION

Alteplase should be reconstituted by aseptically adding the appropriate volume of the accompanying Sterile Water for Injection, USP to the vial. It is important that alteplase be reconstituted only with Sterile Water for Injection, USP, without preservatives. Do not use Bacteriostatic Water for Injection, USP. The reconstituted preparation results in a colorless to pale yellow transparent solution containing alteplase 1 mg/ml at approximately pH 7.3. The osmolality of this solution is approximately 215 mOsm/kg.

Because alteplase contains no antibacterial preservatives, it should be reconstituted immediately before use. The solution may be used for intravenous administration within 8 hours following reconstitution when stored between 2-30°C (36-86°F). Before further dilution or administration, the product should be visually inspected for particulate matter and discoloration prior to administration whenever solution and container permit.

Alteplase, recombinant may be administered as reconstituted at 1 mg/ml. As an alternative, the reconstituted solution may be diluted further immediately before administration in an equal volume of 0.9% Sodium Chloride Injection, USP or 5% Dextrose Injection, USP to yield a concentration of 0.5 mg/ml. Either polyvinyl chloride bags or glass vials are acceptable. Alteplase is stable for up to 8 hours in these solutions at room temperature. Exposure to light has no effect on the stability of these solutions. Excessive agitation during dilution should be avoided; mixing should be accomplished with gentle swirling and/or slow inversion. Do not use other infusion solutions, e.g., Sterile Water for Injection, USP or preservative-containing solutions for further dilution.

20 mg and 50 mg vials: Reconstitution should be carried out using a large bore needle (*e.g.,* 18 gauge) and a syringe, directing the stream of Sterile Water for Injection, USP into the lyophilized cake. **DO NOT USE IF VACUUM IS NOT PRESENT.** Slight foaming upon reconstitution is not unusual; standing undisturbed for several minutes is usually sufficient to allow dissipation of any large bubbles.

No other medication should be added to infusion solutions containing alteplase. Any unused infusion solution should be discarded.

100 mg vials: Reconstitution should be carried out using the transfer device provided, adding the contents of the accompanying 100 ml vial of Sterile Water for Injection, USP to the contents of the 100 mg vial of alteplase powder. Slight foaming upon reconstitution is not unusual; standing undisturbed for several minutes is usually sufficient to allow dissipation of any large bubbles. Please refer to the accompanying Instructions for Reconstitution and Administration. **100 mg VIALS DO NOT CONTAIN VACUUM.**

100 mg Vial Reconstitution

1. Use aseptic technique throughout.

2. Remove the protective flip-caps from one vial of alteplase and one vial of Sterile Water for Injection, USP (SWFI).

3. Open the package containing the transfer device by peeling the paper label off the package.

4. Remove the protective cap from one end of the transfer device and keeping the vial of SWFI upright, insert the piercing pin vertically into the center of the stopper of the vial of SWFI.

5. Remove the protective cap from the other end of the transfer device. **DO NOT INVERT THE VIAL OF SWFI.**

6. Holding the vial of alteplase, recombinant upside-down, position it so that the center of the stopper is directly over the exposed piercing pin of the transfer device.

7. Push the vial of alteplase down so that the piercing pin is inserted through the center of the alteplase vial stopper.

8. Invert the two vials so that the vial of alteplase is on the bottom (upright) and the vial of SWFI is upside-down, allowing the SWFI to flow down through the transfer device. Allow the entire contents of the vial of SWFI to flow into the alteplase vial (approximately 0.5 cc of SWFI will remain in the diluent vial). Approximately 2 minutes are required for this procedure.

9. Remove the transfer device and the empty SWFI vial from the alteplase vial. Safely discard both the transfer device and the empty diluent vial according to institutional procedures.

10. Swirl gently to dissolve the alteplase powder. **DO NOT SHAKE.**

No other medication should be added to infusion solutions containing alteplase. Any unused infusion solution should be discarded.

REFERENCES:

1. Mueller H, Rao AK, Forman SA, *et al.*Thrombolysis in myocardial infarction (TIMI): comparative studies of coronary reperfusion and systemic fibrinogenolysis with two forms of recombinant tissue-type plasminogen activator. *J Am Coll Cardiol.*1987;10:479-490. **2.** Topol EJ, Morriss DC, Smalling RW, *et al.* A multicenter, randomized, placebo-controlled trial of a new form of intravenous recombinant tissue-type plasminogen activator (Activase) in acute myocardial infarction. *J Am Coll Cardiol.*1987;9:1205-13. **3.** Seifried E, Tanswell P, Ellbruck D, *et al.*Pharmacokinetics and haemostatic status during consecutive infusions of recombinant tissue-type plasminogen activator in patients with acute myocardial infarction, *Thromb Haemostas.* 1989;61:497-501. **4.** Tanswell P, Tebbe U, Neuhaus K-L, *et al.*Pharmacokinetics and fibrin specificity of Alteplase during accelerated infusions in acute myocardial infarction. *J Am Coll Cardiol.*1992;19:1071-5. **5.** De Wood MA, Spores J, Notske R, *et al.*Prevalence of total coronary occlusion during the early hours of transmural myocardial infarction. *New Engl J Med.*1980;303:897-902. **6.** Chesebro JH, Knatterud G, Roberts R, *et al.* Thrombolysis in myocardial infarction (TIMI) trial, Phase I: a comparison between intravenous tissue plasminogen activator and intravenous streptokinase. *Circulation.* 1987;76(1):142-154. **7.** Guerci AD, Gerstenblith G, Brinker JA, *et al.* A randomized trial of intravenous tissue plasminogen activator for acute myocardial infarction with subsequent randomization to elective coronary angioplasty. *New Engl J Med.* 1987;317:1613-18. **8.** O'Rourke M, Baron D, Keogh A, *et al.*Limitation of myocardial infarction by early infusion of recombinant tissue-plasminogen activator.*Circulation.* 1988;77:1311-15. **9.** Wilcox RG, von der Lippe G, Olsson CG, *et al.* Trial of tissue plasminogen activator for mortality reduction in acute myocardial infarction: ASSET.*Lancet.*1988;2:525-30. **10.** Hampton JR, The University of Nottingham. Personal communication. **11.** Van de Werf F, Arnold AER, *et al.*Effect of intravenous tissue-plasminogen activator on infarct size, left ventricular function and survival in patients with acute myocardial infarction. *Br Med J.* 1988;297:1374-9. **12.** Goldhaber SZ, Kessler CM, Heit J, *et al.* A randomized controlled trial of recombinant tissue plasminogen activator versus urokinase in the treatment of acute pulmonary embolism. *Lancet.*1988;2:293-8. **13.** Califf RM, Topol EJ, George BS, *et al.*Hemorrhagic complications associated with the use of intravenous tissue plasminogen activator in treatment of acute myocardial infarction. *Am J Med.* 1988;85:353-9. **14.** Bovill EG, Terrin ML, Stump DC,*et al.*Hemorrhagic events during therapy with recombinant tissue- type plasminogen activator, heparin, and aspirin for acute myocardial infarction: results from the thrombolysis in myocardial infarction (TIMI), Phase II trial. *Ann Int Med.* 1991;115(4):256-65. **15.** National Heart Foundation of Australia Coronary Thrombolysis Group. Coronary thrombolysis and myocardial infarction

REFERENCES: *(cont'd)*

salvage by tissue plasminogen activator given up to 4 hours after onset of myocardial infarction. *Lancet.* 1988;1: 203-7. **16.** Gore JM, Sloan M, Price TR, *et al.* and the TIMI Investigators. Intracerebral hemorrhage, cerebral infarction, and subdural hematoma after acute myocardial infarction and thrombolytic therapy in the thrombolysis in myocardial infarction study. *Circulation.* 1991;83:448-59.

HOW SUPPLIED:

Activase is supplied as a sterile, lyophilized powder in 20 mg and 50 mg vials containing vacuum and in 100 mg vials without vacuum.

Each 20 mg Activase vial (11.6 million IU) is packaged with diluent for reconstitution (20 ml Sterile Water for Injection, USP): NDC 50242-044-12.

Each 50 mg Activase vial (29 million IU) is packaged with diluent for reconstitution (50 ml Sterile Water for Injection, USP): NDC 50242-044- 13.

Each 100 mg Activase vial (58 million IU) is packaged with diluent for reconstitution (100 ml Sterile Water for Injection, USP), and one transfer device: NDC 50242-085-27.

Storage Store lyophilized Activase at controlled room temperature not to exceed 30°C (86°F), or under refrigeration (2-8°C/36-46°F). Protect the lyophilized material during extended storage from excessive exposure to light.

Do not use beyond the expiration date stamped on the vial.

HOW SUPPLIED - EQUIVALENTS NOT AVAILABLE:

Injection, Lyphl-Soln - Intravenous - 1 mg/ml

20 mg	**$550.00**	**ACTIVASE, VIAL + DILUENT, Genentech**	**50242-0044-12**
50 mg	**$1375.00**	**ACTIVASE, VIAL + DILUENT, Genentech**	**50242-0044-13**
100 mg	**$2750.00**	**ACTIVASE, Genentech**	**50242-0085-27**

ALTRETAMINE *(003001)*

CATEGORIES: Antineoplastics; Cancer; Chemoprotective Agents; Chemotherapy; Ovarian Carcinoma; Pregnancy Category D; FDA Class 1A ("Important Therapeutic Advantage"); FDA Approved 1990 Dec

BRAND NAMES: **Hexalen**; *Hexamethylmelamin* (Germany); Hexamethylmelamine; *Hexastat* (France, Canada); *Hexinawas*
(International brand names outside U.S. in italics)

FORMULARIES: Aetna; Medi-Cal

COST OF THERAPY: $6,132.00 (Ovarian Carcinoma; Capsule; 50 mg; 4/day; 365 days)

WARNING:

1. Hexalen should only be given under the supervision of a physician experienced in the use of antineoplastic agents.
2. Peripheral blood counts should be monitored at least monthly, prior to the initiation of each course of altretamine, and as clinically indicated (see ADVERSE REACTIONS.)
3. Because of the possibility of altretamine-related neurotoxicity, neurologic examination should be performed regularly during altretamine administration (see ADVERSE REACTIONS.)

DESCRIPTION:

Altretamine, is a synthetic cytotoxic antineoplastic s-triazine derivative. Altretamine capsules contain 50 mg of altretamine for oral administration. Inert ingredients include lactose, anhydrous and calcium stearate. Altretamine is known chemically as N, N,N', N',N", N"-hexamethyl-1,3,5-triazine-2,4,6-triamine.

Its empirical formula is $C_9H_{18}N_6$ with a molecular weight of 210.28. Altretamine is a white crystalline powder, melting at 172° ± 1°C. Altretamine is practically insoluble in water but is increasingly soluble at pH3 and below.

CLINICAL PHARMACOLOGY:

The precise mechanism by which altretamine exerts its cytotoxic effect is unknown, although a number of theoretical possibilities have been studied. Structurally, altretamine resembles the alkylating agent triethylenemelamine, yet *in vitro* tests for alkylating activity of altretamine and its metabolites have been negative. Altretamine has demonstrated to be efficacious for certain ovarian tumors resistant to classical alkylating agents. Metabolism of altretamine is a requirement for cytotoxicity. Synthetic monohydroxymethylmelamines, and products of altretamine metabolism, *in vitro* and *in vivo*, can form covalent adducts with tissue macromolecules including DNA, but the relevance of these reactions to antitumor activity is unknown.

Altretamine is well-absorbed following oral administration in humans, but undergoes rapid and extensive demethylation in the liver, producing variation in altretamine plasma levels. The principal metabolites are pentamethylmelamine and tetramethylmelamine.

Pharmacokinetic studies were performed in a limited number of patients and should be considered preliminary. After oral administration of altretamine to 11 patients with advanced ovarian cancer in doses of 120-300 mg/m², peak plasma levels (as measured by gas-chromatographic assay) were reached between 0.5 and 3 hours, varying from 0.2 to 20.8 mg/L.Half-life of the β-phase of elimination ranged from 4.7 to 10.2 hours. Altretamine and metabolites show binding to plasma proteins. The free fractions of altretamine, pentamethylmelamine and tetramethylmelamine are 6%, 25% and 50%, respectively.

Following oral administration of ^{14}C-ring-labeled altretamine (4 mg/kg), urinary recovery of radioactivity was 61% at 24 hours and 90% at 72 hours. Human urinary metabolites were N-demethylated homologues of altretamine with <1% unmetabolized altretamine excreted at 24 hours.

After intraperitoneal administration of ^{14}C-ring-labeled altretamine to mice, tissue distribution was rapid in all organs, reaching a maximum at 30 minutes. The excretory organs (liver and kidney) and the small intestine showed high concentrations of radioactivity, whereas relatively low concentrations were found in other organs, including the brain.

There have been no formal pharmacokinetic studies in patients with compromised hepatic and/or renal function, though altretamine has been administered both concurrently and following nephrotoxic drugs such as cisplatin.

Altretamine has been administered in 4 divided doses, with meals and at bedtime, though there is no pharmacokinetic data on this schedule nor information from formal interaction studies about the effect of food on its bioavailability or pharmacokinetics.

In two studies in patients with persistent or recurrent ovarian cancer following first-line treatment with cisplatin and/or alkylating agent- based combinations, altretamine was administered as a single agent for 14 or 21 days of a 28 day cycle. In the 51 patients with measurable or evaluable disease, there were 6 clinical complete responses, 1 pathologic

CLINICAL PHARMACOLOGY: *(cont'd)*

complete response, and 2 partial responses for an overall response rate of 18%. The duration of these responses ranged from 2 months in a patient with a palpable pelvic mass to 36 months in a patient who achieved a pathologic complete response. In some patients, tumor regression was associated with improvement in symptoms and performance status.

INDICATIONS AND USAGE:

Altretamine is indicated for use as a single agent in the palliative treatment of patients with persistent or recurrent ovarian cancer following first-line therapy with a cisplatin and/or alkylating agent-based combination.

CONTRAINDICATIONS:

Altretamine is contraindicated in patients who have shown hypersensitivity to it. Altretamine should not be employed in patients with preexisting severe bone marrow depression or severe neurologic toxicity. Altretamine has been administered safely, however, to patients heavily pretreated with cisplatin and/or alkylating agents, including patients with preexisting cisplatin neuropathies. Careful monitoring of neurologic function in these patients is essential.

WARNINGS:

(See BOXED WARNING.)

Concurrent administration of altretamine and antidepressants of the monoamine oxidase (MAO) inhibitor class may cause severe orthostatic hypotension. Four patients, all over 60 years of age, were reported to have experienced symptomatic hypotension after 4 to 7 days of concomitant therapy with altretamine and MAO inhibitors.

Altretamine causes mild to moderate myelosuppression and neurotoxicity. Blood counts and a neurologic examination should be performed prior to the initiation of each course of therapy and the dose of altretamine adjusted as clinically indicated (see DOSAGE AND ADMINISTRATION.)

PREGNANCY CATEGORY D

Altretamine has been shown to be embryotoxic and teratogenic in rats and rabbits when given at doses 2 and 10 times the human dose. Altretamine may cause fetal damage when administered to a pregnant woman. If altretamine is used during pregnancy, or if the patient becomes pregnant while taking the drug, the patient should be apprised of the potential hazard to the fetus. Women of childbearing potential should be advised to avoid becoming pregnant.

PRECAUTIONS:

General: Neurologic examination should be performed regularly (see ADVERSE REACTIONS.)

Laboratory Tests: Peripheral blood counts should be monitored at least monthly, prior to the initiation of each course of altretamine, and as clinically indicated (see ADVERSE REACTIONS.)

Carcinogenesis, Mutagenesis, and Impairment of Fertility: The carcinogenic potential of altretamine has not been studied in animals, but drugs with similar mechanisms of action have been shown to be carcinogenic. Altretamine was weakly mutagenic when tested in strain TA100 of *Salmonella typhimurium.* Altretamine administered to female rats 14 days prior to breeding through the gestation period had no adverse effect on fertility, but decreased post-natal survival at 120 mg/m²/day and was embryocidal at 240 mg/m²/day. Administration of 120 mg/m²/day altretamine to male rats for 60 days prior to mating resulted in testicular atrophy, reduced fertility and a possible dominant lethal mutagenic effect. Male rats treated with altretamine at 450 mg/m²/day for 10 days had decreased spermatogenesis, atrophy of testes, seminal vesicles and ventral prostate.

Pregnancy Category D: (see WARNINGS)

Nursing Mothers: It is not known whether altretamine is excreted in human milk. Because there is a possibility of toxicity in nursing infants secondary to altretamine treatment of the mother, it is recommended that breast feeding be discontinued if the mother is treated with altretamine.

Pediatric Use: The safety and effectiveness of altretamine in children have not been established.

DRUG INTERACTIONS:

Concurrent administration of altretamine and antidepressants of the MAO inhibitor class may cause severe orthostatic hypotension (see WARNINGS.) Cimetidine, and inhibitor of microsomal drug metabolism, increased altretamine's half-life and toxicity in a rat model.

Data from a randomized trial of altretamine and cisplatin plus or minus pyridoxine in ovarian cancer indicated that pyridoxine significantly reduced neurotoxicity; however, it adversely affected response duration suggesting that pyridoxine should not be administered with altretamine and/or cisplatin (1).

ADVERSE REACTIONS:

Gastrointestinal: With continuous high-dose daily altretamine, nausea and vomiting of gradual onset occur frequently. Although in most instances these symptoms are controllable with anti-emetics, at times the severity requires altretamine dose reduction or, rarely, discontinuation of altretamine therapy. In some instances, a tolerance of these symptoms develops after several seeks of therapy. The incidence and severity of nausea and vomiting are reduced with moderate-dose administration of altretamine. In 2 clinical studies of single-agent altretamine utilizing a moderate, intermittent dose and schedule, only 1 patient (1%) discontinued altretamine due to severe nausea and vomiting.

Neurotoxicity: Peripheral neuropathy and central nervous system symptoms (mood disorders, disorders of consciousness, ataxia, dizziness, vertigo) have been reported. They are more likely to occur in patients receiving continuous high-dose daily altretamine (altretamine) than moderate-dose altretamine administered on an intermittent schedule. Neurologic toxicity has been reported to be reversible when therapy is discontinued. Data from a randomized trial of altretamine and cisplatin plus or minus pyridoxine in ovarian cancer indicated that pyridoxine significantly reduced neurotoxicity; however, it adversely affected response duration suggesting that pyridoxine should not be administered with altretamine and/or cisplatin [1].

Hematologic: Altretamine causes mild to moderate dose-related myelosuppression. Leukopenia below 3000 WBC/mm³ occurred in <15% of patients on a variety of intermittent or continuous dose regimens. Less than 1% had leukopenia below 1000 WBC/mm³. Thrombocytopenia below 50,000 platelets/mm³ was seen in <10% of patients. When given in doses of 8-12 mg/kg/day over a 21 day course, nadirs of leukocyte and platelet counts were reached by 3-4 weeks, and normal counts were regained by 6 weeks. With continuous administration at doses of 6-8 mg/kg/day, nadirs are reached in 6-8 weeks (median).

Data in TABLE 1 are based on the experience of 76 patients with ovarian cancer previously treated with a cisplatin-based combination regimen who received single-agent altretamine. In one study, altretamine, 260 mg/m²/day, was administered for 14 days of a 28 day cycle. In another study, altretamine, 6-8 mg/kg/day, was administered for 21 days of a 28 day cycle.

ADVERSE REACTIONS: *(cont'd)*

TABLE 1 Adverse Experiences in 76 Previously Treated Ovarian Cancer Patients Receiving Single-Agent Altretamine

Adverse Event	%
Gastrointestinal	
Nausea and Vomiting	33
Mild to moderate	32
Severe	1
Increased Alkaline Phosphatase	9
Neurologic	
Peripheral Sensory Neuropathy	31
Mild	22
Moderate to Severe	9
Anorexia and Fatigue	1
Seizures	1
Hematologic	
Leukopenia	5
WBC 2000-2999/mm³	4
WBC <2000/mm³	1
Thrombocytopenia	9
Platelets 75,000-99,000/mm³	6
Platelets <75,000/mm³	3
Anemia	33
Mild	20
Moderate to Severe	13
Renal	
Serum Creatinine 1.6-3.75 mg/dl	7
BUN	9
25-40 mg%	5
41-60 mg%	3
>60 mg%	1

Additional adverse reaction information is available from 13 single-agent altretamine studies (total of 1014 patients) conducted under the auspices of the National Cancer Institute. The treated patients had a variety of tumors and many were heavily pretreated with other chemotherapies; most of these trials utilized high, continuous daily doses of altretamine (6- 12 mg/kg/day). In general, adverse reaction experiences were similar in the two trials described above. Additional toxicities, not reported in the above table, included hepatic toxicity, skin rash, pruritus and alopecia, each occurring in <1% of patients.

OVERDOSAGE:

No case of acute overdosage in humans has been described. The oral LD_{50} dose in rats was 1050 mg/kg and 437 mg/kg in mice.

DOSAGE AND ADMINISTRATION:

Altretamine is administered orally. Doses are calculated on the basis of body surface area.

Altretamine may be administered either for 14 or 21 consecutive days in a 28 day cycle at a dose of 260 mg/m²/day. The total daily dose should be given as 4 divided oral doses after meals and at bedtime. There is no pharmacokinetic information supporting this dosing regimen and the effect of food on altretamine bioavailability or pharmacokinetics has not been evaluated.

Altretamine should be temporarily discontinued (for 14 days or longer) and subsequently restarted at 200 mg/m²/day for any of the following situations:

1) Gastrointestinal intolerance unresponsive to symptomatic measures;

2) White blood count <2000/mm³ or granulocyte count <1000/mm³;

3) Platelet count <75,000/mm³;

4) Progressive neurotoxicity.

If neurologic symptoms fail to stabilize on the reduced dose schedule, altretamine should be discontinued indefinitely.

Procedures for proper handling and disposal of anticancer drugs should be considered. Several guidelines on this subject have been published (2-8). There is no general agreement that all of the procedures recommended in the guidelines are necessary or appropriate.

HOW SUPPLIED:

Hexalen (altretamine) is available in 50 mg clear, hard gelatin capsules. The capsules are imprinted with the following description: USB001 Hexalen 50mg.

Store at controlled room temperature 15-30°C (59- 86°F)

REFERENCES:

1. Wiernik PH, et al. Hexamethylmelamine and Low or Moderate Dose Cisplatin With or Without Pyridoxine for Treatment of Advanced Ovarian Carcinoma: A Study of the Eastern Cooperative Oncology Group.*Cancer Investigation* 10(1): 1-9, 1992. **2.** Recommendations for the Safe Handling of Parenteral Antineoplastic Drugs. NIH Publication No. 83- 2621. For sale by the Superintendent of Documents, U.S. Government Printing Office, Washington, D.C. 20402. **3.** AMA Council Report. Guidelines for Handling Parenteral Antineoplastics. *Journal of the American Medical Association* March 15, 1985. **4.** National Study Commission on Cytotoxic Exposure - Recommendations for Handling Cytotoxic Agents. Available from Louis P. Jeffrey, Sc.D., Director of Pharmacy Services, Rhode Island Hospital, 593 Eddy Street, Providence, Rhode Island 02902. **5.** Clinical Oncological Society of Australia: Guidelines and Recommendations for Safe Handling of Antineoplastic Agents. *Medical Journal of Australia* 1:426-428, 1983. **6.** Jones RB, et al. Safe Handling of Chemotherapeutic Agents: A Report from the Mount Sinai Medical Center. *CA - A Cancer Journal for Clinicians* Sept/Oct, 258-263, 1983. **7.** American Society of Hospital Pharmacists Technical Assistance Bulletin on Handling Cytotoxic Drugs in Hospitals. *American Journal of Hospital Pharmacy* 42:131-137, 1985. **8.** OSHA Work Practice Guidelines for Personnel Dealing with Cytotoxic (Antineoplastic) Drugs. *American Journal of Hospital Pharmacy* 43:1193-1204, 1986.

HOW SUPPLIED - EQUIVALENTS NOT AVAILABLE:

Capsule, Gelatin - Oral - 50 mg

100's $420.00 HEXALEN 50, US Bioscience — 58178-0001-70

Tablet, Film-coated - Oral - 5 mg

60's $251.99 ZYPREXA, Lilly — 00002-4115-60

Tablet, Film-coated - Oral - 7.5 mg

60's $251.99 ZYPREXA, Lilly — 00002-4116-60

Tablet, Film-coated - Oral - 10 mg

60's $367.27 ZYPREXA, Lilly — 00002-4117-60

ALUMINUM ACETATE; PHENOL; RESCORCINOL *(000145)*

CATEGORIES: Antipruritics/Local Anesthetics; Antiseptics/Disinfectants; Dermatologicals; Skin/Mucous Membrane Agents; FDA Pre 1938 Drugs

Prescribing information not available at time of publication.

HOW SUPPLIED - EQUIVALENTS NOT AVAILABLE:

Gel - Topical - 3 %/10 %

1 oz	$6.30	DERMA CAS GEL, Hill Dermac	28105-0198-01
6 oz	$36.00	DERMA CAS GEL, Hill Dermac	28105-0198-06

ALUMINUM CHLORIDE HEXAHYDRATE *(000154)*

CATEGORIES: Acidifying Agents; Acne; Anti-Infectives; Antiperspirants; Deodorants; Dermatologicals; Histomoniasis; Hyperhidrosis; Local Infections; Mucous Membrane Agents; Skin/Mucous Membrane Agents; Topical; FDA Pre 1938 Drugs

BRAND NAMES: *Anhydrol Forte* (England); *Driclor* (England); **Drysol**; *Etiaxil*; *Hidrosol*; Lumicaine; *Prespir* (Mexico); *Sinol*; Xerac Ac
(International brand names outside U.S. in italics)

DESCRIPTION:

Xerac AC: A solution of aluminum chloride (hexahydrate) 6.25% (w/v) in anhydrous ethyl alcohol (s.d. alcohol 40) 96% (v/v).

Drysol: A solution of aluminum chloride (hexahydrate) 20% w/v in anhydrous ethyl alcohol (s.d. alcohol 40) 93% v/v.

INDICATIONS AND USAGE:

Xerac AC: For topical application as an antiperspirant (anhidrotic).

Drysol: An aid in the management of hyperhidrosis.

WARNINGS:

ANTIPERSPIRANT

For External Use Only. Some users of this product will experience skin irritation. If this occurs, discontinue use. Avoid contact with the eyes. This product may be harmful to certain fabrics. Keep the container tightly closed when not in use to prevent evaporation. Keep this and all medication out of reach of children.

HYPERHIDROSIS

For external use only. Keep out of the reach of children. Avoid contact with the eyes. If irritation or sensitization occurs, discontinue use or consult with a physician. Aluminum chloride hexahydrate may be harmful to certain metals and fabrics. Do not use near open flame.

ADVERSE REACTIONS:

ANTIPERSPIRANT

Transient stinging or itching may occur. It is not evidence of contact sensitivity and may be prevented or reduced by applying this drug only to skin which is completely dry or by removing the solution with soap and water.

HYPERHIDROSIS

Aluminum chloride hexahydrate will probably produce a burning or prickling sensation. Keep can tightly closed when not in use to prevent evaporation.

DOSAGE AND ADMINISTRATION:

ANTIPERSPIRANT

Apply this product to the axillae at bedtime or as directed by a physician. Application is facilitated by the special swab applicator head of the dispenser. To help prevent irritation, the area should be completely dry prior to application. Do not apply aluminum chloride to broken or irritated skin. Keep container tightly closed.

Assembly Instructions: Remove and discard original cap. Push special Dab-O-Matic applicator into bottle opening using the white cap as holder. Screw cap down to seat applicator.

HYPERHIDROSIS

Apply aluminum chloride hexahydrate to the affected area once a day, only at bedtime. To help prevent irritation, the area should be completely dry prior to application. Do not apply aluminum chloride hexahydrate to broken, irritated or recently shaved skin.

For Maximum Effect: Your doctor may instruct you to cover the treated area with saran wrap held in place by a snug fitting "T" or body shirt, mitten or sock. (Never hold saran wrap in place with tape). Wash the treated area the following morning. Excessive sweating may be stopped after two or more treatments. Thereafter, apply aluminum chloride hexahydrate once or twice weekly or as needed.

Assembly Instructions: Remove and discard original cap. Push special Dab-O-Matic applicator into bottle opening using the white cap as a holder. Screw cap down to seat applicator.

HOW SUPPLIED:

Xerac AC: Plastic bottle with special applicator, 35 cc and 60 cc

HOW SUPPLIED - EQUIVALENTS NOT AVAILABLE:

Solution - Topical - 6.25 %

35 ml	$5.78	XERAC AC, Person and Covey	00096-0709-35
60 ml	$7.72	XERAC AC, Person and Covey	00096-0709-60
60 ml	$7.82	Lumicaine, HL Moore Drug Exch	00839-0092-92
60 ml	$7.82	Lumicaine, HL Moore Drug Exch	00839-6286-64

Solution - Topical - 20 %

35 ml	**$6.75**	**DRYSOL, Person and Covey**	**00096-0707-35**
37.5 ml	**$6.25**	**DRYSOL, Person and Covey**	**00096-0707-37**
60 ml	**$9.10**	**DRYSOL DAB-O-MATIC, Person and Covey**	**00096-0707-60**

AMANTADINE HYDROCHLORIDE *(000174)*

CATEGORIES: Anticholinergic Agents; Antiparkinson Agents; Antivirals; Autonomic Drugs; Extrapyramidal Movement Disorders; Influenza; Neuromuscular; Parkinsonism; Skeletal Muscle Hyperactivity; Viral Agents; Pregnancy Category C; FDA Approval Pre 1982

BRAND NAMES: *Aldinam*; *Amanda*; Amantadine Hcl; *Amantan*; *Amantix*; *Amantrel*; *Amazolon* (Japan); *Amixx* (Germany); *Antadine*; *Atarin*; *Boidan* (Japan); *Contenton*; *Enzil*; *Grippin-Merz* (Germany); *Hofcomant*; *Mantadan*; *Mantadix* (France); *Mantandan*; *Padiken* (Mexico); *Parkintrel*; *Paritrel*; *PK-Merz* (Germany); *Prayanol*; *Protexin*; *Shikitan*; Symadine; **Symmetrel**; *Topharmin*; *Tregor* (Germany); *Virofral*; *Virosol*
(International brand names outside U.S. in italics)

FORMULARIES: Aetna; BC-BS; CIGNA; FHP; Humana; Kaiser; Medco; Medi-Cal; PCS; PruCare; United

COST OF THERAPY: $123.22 (Parkinsonism; Capsule; 100 mg; 2/day; 365 days)

DESCRIPTION:

This drug is designated generically as amantadine hydrochloride (amantadine HCl) and chemically as 1-adamantanamine hydrochloride.

Amantadine HCl is a stable white or nearly white crystalline powder, freely soluble in water and soluble in alcohol and in chloroform.

Amantadine HCl has pharmacological actions as both an anti-Parkinson and an antiviral drug.

Amantadine HCl is available in capsules and syrup.

Symmetrel Capsules Contain: FD&C Red 40, gelatin, glycerin, hydrogenated vegetable oil, lecithin, methylparaben, propylparaben, soybean oil, titanium dioxide, vegetable shortening, white printing ink, and yellow wax.

Symmetrel Syrup Contains: artificial raspberry flavor, citric acid, methylparaben, propylparaben, and sorbitol sodium.

CLINICAL PHARMACOLOGY:

Mechanism of Action: Parkinson's Disease The mechanism of action of amantadine in the treatment of Parkinson's disease and drug-induced extrapyramidal reactions is not known. It has been shown to cause an increase in dopamine release in the animal brain. The drug does not possess anticholinergic activity in dogs at doses of 31.5 mg/kg, equivalent to an approximate human dose of 15.8 mg/kg (based on body surface area conversions).

Mechanism of Activity: Antiviral The mechanism by which amantadine exerts its antiviral activity is not clearly understood. It appears to mainly prevent the release of infectious viral nucleic acid into the host cell by interfering with the function of the transmembrane domain of the viral M2 protein. In certain cases, amantadine is also known to prevent virus assembly during virus replication. It does not appear to interfere with the immunogenicity of inactivated influenza A virus vaccine.

Antiviral Activity: Amantadine inhibits the replication of influenza A virus isolates from each of the subtypes, i.e., H1N1, H2N2 and H3N2. It has very little or no activity against influenza B virus isolates. A quantitative relationship between the *in vitro* susceptibility of influenza A virus to amantadine and the clinical response to therapy has not been established in man. Sensitivity test results, expressed as the concentration of amantadine required to inhibit by 50% the growth of virus (ED_{50}) in tissue culture vary greatly (from 0.1 mcg/ml to 25.0 mcg/ml) depending upon the assay protocol used, size of virus inoculum, isolates of influenza A virus strains tested, and the cell type used. Host cells in tissue culture readily tolerated amantadine up to a concentration of 100 mcg/ml.

Drug Resistance: Influenza A variants with reduced *in vitro* sensitivity to amantadine have been isolated from epidemic strains in areas where adamantine derivatives are being used. Influenza viruses with reduced *in vitro* sensitivity have been shown to be transmissible and to cause typical influenza illness. The quantitative relationship between the *in vitro* sensitivity of influenza A variants to amantadine and the clinical response to therapy has not been established.

Pharmacokinetics: Amantadine is well absorbed orally. Maximum plasma concentrations are directly related to dose for doses up to 200 mg/day. Doses above 200 mg/day may result in a greater than proportional increase in maximum plasma concentrations. It is primarily excreted unchanged in the urine by glomerular filtration and tubular secretion. Eight metabolites of amantadine have been identified in human urine. One metabolite, an N-acetylated compound, was quantified in human urine and accounted for 5-15% of the administered dose. Plasma acetylamantadine accounted for up to 80% of the concurrent amantadine plasma concentration in 5 of 12 healthy volunteers following the ingestion of a 200 mg dose of amantadine. Acetylamantadine was not detected in the plasma of the seven volunteers. The contribution of this metabolite to efficacy or toxicity is not known.

There appears to be a relationship between plasma amantadine concentrations and toxicity. As concentration increases toxicity seems to be more prevalent, however absolute values of amantadine concentrations associated with adverse effects have not been fully defined.

Amantadine pharmacokinetics were determined in 24 normal adult male volunteers after the oral administration of a single amantadine 100 mg capsule. The mean ± SD maximum plasma concentration was 0.22 ± 0.03 mcg/ml (range 0.18 to 0.32 mcg/ml). The time to peak concentration was 3.3 ± 1.5 hours (range: 1.5 to 8.0 hours). The apparent oral clearance was 0.28 ± 0.11 L/hr/kg (range: 0.14 to 0.62 L/hr/kg). The half-life was 17 ± 4 hours (range: 10 to 25 hours). Across other studies, amantadine plasma half-life has averaged 16 ± 6 hours (range: 9 to 31 hours) in 19 healthy volunteers.

After oral administration of a single dose of 100 mg amantadine syrup to five healthy volunteers, the mean ± SD maximum plasma concentration C_{max} was 0.24 ± 0.04 mcg/ml and ranged from 0.18 to 0.28 mcg/ml. After 15 days of amantadine 100 mg b.i.d., the C_{max} was 0.47 ± 0.11 mcg/ml in four of the five volunteers. The administration of amantadine tablets as a 200 mg single dose to 6 healthy subjects resulted in a C_{max} of 0.51 ± 0.14 mcg/ml. Across studies, the time to C_{max} (T_{max}) averaged about 2 to 4 hours.

Plasma amantadine clearance ranged from 0.2 to 0.3 L/hr/kg after the administration of 5 mg to 25 mg intravenous doses of amantadine to 15 healthy volunteers.

In six healthy volunteers, the ratio of amantadine renal clearance to apparent oral plasma clearance was 0.79 ± 0.17 (mean ± SD).

The volume of distribution determined after the intravenous administration of amantadine to 15 healthy subjects was 3 to 8 L/kg, suggesting tissue binding. Amantadine, after single oral 200 mg doses to 6 healthy young subjects and to 6 healthy elderly subjects has been found in nasal mucus at mean ± SD concentrations of 0.15 ± 0.16, 0.28 ± 0.26, and 0.39 ± 0.34 mcg/g at 1, 4, and 8 hours after dosing, respectively. These concentrations represented 31 ± 33%, 59 ± 61%, and 95 ± 86% of the corresponding plasma amantadine concentrations. Amantadine is approximately 67% bound to plasma proteins over a concentration range of 0.1 to 2.0 mcg/ml. Following the administration of amantadine 100 mg as a single dose, the mean ± SD red blood cell to plasma ratio ranged from 2.7 ± 0.5 in six healthy subjects to 1.4 ± 0.2 in 8 patients with renal insufficiency.

The apparent oral plasma clearance of amantadine is reduced and the plasma half-life and plasma concentrations are increased in healthy elderly individuals age 60 and older. After single dose administration of 25 to 75 mg to 7 healthy, elderly male volunteers, the apparent plasma clearance of amantadine was 0.10 ± 0.04 L/hr/kg (range 0.06 to 0.17 L/hr/kg) and the half-life was 29 ± 7 hours (range 20 to 41 hours). Whether these changes are due to decline in renal function or other age related factors is not known.

CLINICAL PHARMACOLOGY: *(cont'd)*

Compared with otherwise healthy adult individuals, the clearance of amantadine is significantly reduced in adult patients with renal insufficiency. The elimination half-life increases two to three fold or greater when creatinine clearance is less than 40 ml/min/1.73m^{2}and averages eight days in patients on chronic maintenance hemodialysis. Amantadine is removed in negligible amounts by hemodialysis.

The pH of the urine has been reported to influence the excretion rate of amantadine. Since the excretion rate of amantadine increases rapidly when the urine is acidic, the administration of urine acidifying drugs may increase the elimination of the drug from the body.

INDICATIONS AND USAGE:

Amantadine HCl is indicated for the prophylaxis and treatment of signs and symptoms of infection caused by various strains of influenza A virus. Amantadine HCl is also indicated in the treatment of parkinsonism and drug-induced extrapyramidal reactions.

Influenza A Prophylaxis: Amantadine HCl is indicated for chemoprophylaxis against signs and symptoms of influenza A virus infection when early vaccination is not feasible or when the vaccine is contraindicated or not available. In the prophylaxis of influenza, early vaccination on an annual basis as recommended by the Centers for Disease Control's Immunization Practices Advisory Committee is the method of choice. Because amantadine does not completely prevent the host immune response to influenza A infection, individuals who take this drug may still develop immune responses to natural disease or vaccination and may be protected when later exposed to antigenically related viruses. Following vaccination during an influenza A outbreak, amantadine prophylaxis should be considered for the 2 to 4 week time period required to develop an antibody response.

Influenza A Treatment: Amantadine HCl is also indicated in the treatment of uncomplicated respiratory tract illness caused by influenza A virus strains especially when administered early in the course of illness. There are no well-controlled clinical studies demonstrating that treatment with amantadine will avoid the development of influenza A virus pneumonitis or other complications in high risk patients.

There is no clinical evidence indicating that amantadine is effective in the prophylaxis or treatment of viral respiratory tract illnesses other than those caused by influenza A strains.

Parkinson's Disease/Syndrome: Amantadine HCl is indicated in the treatment of idiopathic Parkinson's disease (Paralysis Agitans), postencephalitic parkinsonism, and symptomatic parkinsonism which may follow injury to the nervous system by carbon monoxide intoxication. It is indicated in those elderly patients believed to develop parkinsonism in association with cerebral arteriosclerosis. In the treatment of Parkinson's disease, amantadine is less effective than levodopa, (-)-3- (3,4-dihydroxyphenl)-L-alanine, and its efficacy in comparison with the anticholinergic antiparkinson drugs has not yet been established.

Drug-Induced Extrapyramidal Reactions: Amantadine HCl is indicated in the treatment of drug-induced extrapyramidal reactions. Although anticholinergic-type side effects have been noted with amantadine HCl when used in patients with drug-induced extrapyramidal reactions, there is a lower incidence of these side effects than that observed with anticholinergic antiparkinson drugs.

CONTRAINDICATIONS:

Amantadine HCl is contraindicated in patients with known hypersensitivity to the drug.

WARNINGS:

Deaths: Deaths have been reported from overdose with amantadine HCl. The lowest reported acute lethal dose was 2 grams. Acute toxicity may be attributable to the anticholinergic effects of amantadine. Drug overdose has resulted in cardiac, respiratory, renal or central nervous system toxicity. Cardiac dysfunction includes arrhythmia, tachycardia and hypertension (see OVERDOSAGE.)

Suicide Attempts: Suicide attempts, some of which have been fatal, have been reported in patients treated with amantadine HCl, many of whom received short courses for influenza treatment or prophylaxis. The incidence of suicide attempts is not known and the pathophysiologic mechanism is not understood. Suicide attempts and suicidal ideation have been reported in patients with and without prior history of psychiatric illness. Amantadine HCl can exacerbate mental problems in patients with a history of psychiatric disorders or substance abuse. Patients who attempt suicide may exhibit abnormal mental states which include disorientation, confusion, depression, personality changes, agitation, aggressive behavior, hallucinations, paranoia, other psychotic reactions, and somnolence or insomnia. Because of the possibility of serious adverse effects, caution should be observed when prescribing amantadine HCl to patients being treated with drugs having CNS effects, or for whom the potential risks outweigh the benefit of treatment. Because some patients have attempted suicide by overdosing with amantadine, prescriptions should be written for the smallest quantity consistent with good patient management.

CNS Effects: Patients with a history of epilepsy or other "seizures" should be observed closely for possible increased seizure activity.

Patients receiving amantadine HCl who note central nervous system effects or blurring of vision should be cautioned against driving or working in situations where alertness and adequate motor coordination are important.

Other: Patients with a history of congestive heart failure or peripheral edema should be followed closely as there are patients who developed congestive heart failure while receiving amantadine HCl.

Patients with Parkinson's disease improving on amantadine HCl should resume normal activities gradually and cautiously, consistent with other medical considerations, such as the presence of osteoporosis or phlebothrombosis.

PRECAUTIONS:

Amantadine HCl should not be discontinued abruptly in patients with Parkinson's disease since a few have experienced a parkinsonian crisis, i.e., a sudden marked clinical deterioration, when this medication was suddenly stopped. The dose of anticholinergic drug or of amantadine HCl should be reduced if atropine-like effects appear when these drugs are used concurrently.

Neuroleptic Malignant Syndrome (NMS): Sporadic cases of possible Neuroleptic Malignant Syndrome (NMS) have been reported in association with dose reduction or withdrawal of amantadine HCl therapy.

NMS is an uncommon but life-threatening syndrome characterized by fever or hyperthermia; neurologic findings include muscle rigidity, involuntary movements, altered consciousness; other disturbances such as autonomic dysfunction, tachycardia, tachypnea, hyper- or hypotension; laboratory findings such as creatine phosphokinase elevation, leukocytosis and increased serum myoglobin.

The early diagnosis of this condition is important for the appropriate management of these patients. Considering NMS as a possible diagnosis and ruling out other acute illnesses (*e.g.,* pneumonia, systemic infection, etc.) is essential. This may be especially complex if the clinical presentation includes both serious medical illness and untreated or inadequately treated extrapyramidal signs and symptoms (EPS). Other important considerations in the differential diagnosis include central anticholinergic toxicity, heat stroke, drug fever and primary central nervous system (CNS) pathology.

The management of NMS should include: 1) intensive symptomatic treatment and medical monitoring, and 2) treatment of any concomitant serious medical problems for which specific treatments are available. Dopamine agonists, such as bromocriptine, and muscle relaxants, such as dantrolene are often used in the treatment of NMS, however, their effectiveness has not been demonstrated in controlled studies.

Other: Because amantadine HCl is mainly excreted in the urine, it accumulates in the plasma and in the body when renal function declines. Thus, the dose of amantadine HCl should be reduced in patients with renal impairment and in individuals who are 65 years of age or older. The dose of amantadine HCL may need careful adjustment in patients with congestive heart failure, peripheral edema, or orthostatic hypotension.

Care should be exercised when administering amantadine HCl to patients with liver disease, a history of recurrent eczematoid rash, or to patients with psychosis or severe psychoneurosis not controlled by chemotherapeutic agents. Rare instances of reversible elevation of liver enzymes have been reported in patients receiving amantadine HCl, though a specific relationship between the drug and such changes has not been established.

Carcinogenesis and Mutagenesis: Long-term *in vivo* animal studies designed to evaluate the carcinogenic potential of amantadine HCl have not been performed. In several *in vitro* assays for gene mutation, amantadine HCl did not increase the number of spontaneously observed mutations in four strains of *Salmonella typhimurium* (Ames Test) or in a mammalian cell line (Chinese Hamster Ovary cells) when incubations were performed either with or without a liver metabolic activation extract. Further, there was no evidence of chromosome damage observed in an *in vitro* test using freshly derived and stimulated human peripheral blood lymphocytes (with and without metabolic activation) or in an *in vivo* mouse bone marrow micronucleus test (140-550 mg/kg; estimated human equivalent doses of 11.7-45.8 mg/kg based on body surface area conversion).

Impairment of Fertility: In a three litter reproduction study in rats, amantadine at a dose of 32 mg/kg/day (estimated human equivalent dose of 4.5 mg/kg/day, based on body surface area conversions) administered to both males and females slightly impaired fertility. There were no effects on fertility at a dose level of 10 mg/kg/day (estimated human equivalent dose of 1.4 mg/kg/day); intermediate doses were not tested.

Pregnancy Category C: Amantadine HCl has been shown to be embryotoxic and teratogenic in rats at 50 mg/kg/day (estimated human equivalent dose of 7.1 mg/kg/day based on body surface area conversion), while a dose of 37 mg/kg/day (estimated human equivalent dose of 5.3 mg/kg/day) was without effect. Embryotoxic and teratogenic drug effects were not seen in rabbits that received 32 mg/kg/day (estimated human equivalent dose of 9.6 mg/kg/day, based on body surface area conversion). There are no adequate and well-controlled studies in pregnant women. Amantadine HCl should be used during pregnancy only if the potential benefit justifies the potential risk to the embryo or the fetus.

Nursing Mothers: Amantadine HCl is excreted in human milk. Use is not recommended in nursing mothers.

Pediatric Use: The safety and efficacy of amantadine HCl in newborn infants and infants below the age of 1 year have not been established.

Geriatric Use: Because amantadine HCl is primarily excreted in the urine, it accumulates in the plasma and in the body when renal function declines. Thus, the dose of amantadine HCl should be reduced in patients with renal impairment and in individuals who are 65 years of age or older. The dose of amantadine HCl may need reduction in patients with congestive heart failure, peripheral edema, or orthostatic hypotension (see DOSAGE AND ADMINISTRATION.)

DRUG INTERACTIONS:

Careful observation is required when amantadine HCl is administered concurrently with central nervous system stimulants.

Coadministration of thioridazine has been reported to worsen the tremor in elderly patients with Parkinson's disease, however, it is not known if other phenothiazines produce a similar response.

Coadministration of Dyazide (triamterene/hydrochlorothiazide) resulted in a higher plasma amantadine concentration in a 61 year old man receiving amantadine HCl 100 mg TID for Parkinson's disease. It is not known which of the components of Dyazide contributed to the observation or if related drugs produce a similar response.

ADVERSE REACTIONS:

The adverse reactions reported most frequently at the recommended dose of amantadine HCl (5-10%) are: nausea, dizziness (lightheadedness), and insomnia.

Less frequently (1-5%) reported adverse reactions are: depression, anxiety and irritability, hallucinations, confusion, anorexia, dry mouth, constipation, ataxia, livedo reticularis, peripheral edema, orthostatic hypotension, headache, somnolence, nervousness, dream abnormality, agitation, dry nose, diarrhea and fatigue.

Infrequently (0-1.1%) occurring adverse reactions are: congestive heart failure, psychosis, urinary retention, dyspnea, fatigue, skin rash, vomiting, weakness, slurred speech, euphoria, confusion, thinking abnormality, amnesia, hyperkinesia, hypertension, decreased libido, and visual disturbance, including punctuate subepithelial or other corneal opacity, corneal edema, decreased visual acuity, sensitivity to light, and optic nerve palsy.

Rare (less than 0.1%) occurring adverse reactions are: instances of convulsion, leukopenia, neutropenia, eczematoid dermatitis, oculogyric episodes, suicidal attempt, suicide, and suicidal ideation (see WARNINGS.)

OVERDOSAGE:

Deaths have been reported from overdose with amantadine HCl. The lowest reported acute lethal dose was 2 grams. Acute toxicity may be attributable to the anticholinergic effects of amantadine. Drug overdose has resulted in cardiac, respiratory, renal or central nervous system toxicity. Cardiac dysfunction includes arrhythmia, tachycardia and hypertension. Pulmonary edema and respiratory distress (including adult respiratory distress syndrome - ARDS) have been reported; renal dysfunction including increased BUN, decreased creatinine clearance and renal insufficiency can occur. Central nervous system effects that have been reported include insomnia, anxiety, aggressive behavior, hypertonia, hyperkinesia, tremor, confusion, disorientation, depersonalization, fear, delirium, hallucinations, psychotic reactions, lethargy, somnolence and coma. Seizures may be exacerbated in patients with prior history of seizure disorders. Hyperthermia has also been observed in cases where a drug overdose has occurred.

There is no specific antidote for an overdose of amantadine HCl. However, slowly administered intravenous physostigmine in 1 and 2 mg doses in an adult[2] at 1 to 2 hour intervals and 0.5 mg doses in a child[3] at 5 to 10 minute intervals up to a maximum of 2 mg/hour have been reported to be effective in the control of central nervous system toxicity caused by amantadine HCl. For acute overdosing, supportive measures should be employed along with immediate gastric lavage or induction of emesis. Fluids should be forces, and if necessary,

OVERDOSAGE: *(cont'd)*

given intravenously. The pH of the urine has been reported to influence the excretion rate of amantadine HCl. Since the excretion rate of amantadine HCl increases rapidly when the urine is acidic, the administration of urine acidifying drugs may increase in the elimination of the drug from the body. The blood pressure, pulse, respiration and temperature should be monitored. The patient should be observed for hyperactivity and convulsions; if required, sedation, and anticonvulsant therapy should be administered. The patient should be observed for the possible development of arrhythmias and hypotension; if required, appropriate antiarrhythmic and antihypotensive therapy should be given. The blood electrolytes, urine pH and urinary output should be monitored. If there is no record to recent voiding, catheterization should be done.

DOSAGE AND ADMINISTRATION:

The dose of amantadine HCl may need reduction in patients with congestive heart failure, peripheral edema, orthostatic hypotension, or impaired renal function (see Dosage for Impaired Renal Function).

DOSAGE FOR PROPHYLAXIS AND TREATMENT OF UNCOMPLICATED INFLUENZA A VIRUS ILLNESS

Adult: The adult daily dosage of amantadine is 200 mg; two 100 mg capsules (or four teaspoonfuls of syrup) as a single daily dose. The daily dosage may be split into one capsule of 100 mg (or two teaspoonfuls of syrup) twice a day. If central nervous system effects develop in once-a-day dosage, a split dosage schedule may reduce such complaints. In persons 65 years of age or older, the daily dosage of amantadine HCl is 100 mg.

A 100 mg daily dose has also been shown in experimental challenge studies to be effective as prophylaxis in healthy adults who are not at high risk for influenza-related complications. However, it has not been demonstrated that a 100 mg daily dose is as effective as a 200 mg daily dose for prophylaxis, nor has the 100 mg daily dose been studied in the treatment of acute influenza illness. In recent clinical trials, the incidence of central nervous system (CNS) side effects associated with the 100 mg daily dose was at or near the level of placebo. The 100 mg dose is recommended for persons who have demonstrated intolerance to 200 mg of amantadine daily because of CNS or other toxicities.

Children 1 yr.-9 yrs. of age: The total daily dose should be calculated on the basis of 2 to 4 mg/lb/day (4.4 to 8.8 mg/kg/day), but not to exceed 150 mg per day.

Children 9 yrs.-12 yrs. of age: The total daily dose is 200 mg given as one capsule of 100 mg (or two teaspoonfuls of syrup) twice a day. The 100 mg daily dose has not been studied in children. Therefore, there are no data which demonstrate that this dose is as effective as or safer than the 200 mg daily dose in this patient population.

Prophylactic dosing should be started in anticipation of an influenza A outbreak and before or after contact with individuals with influenza A virus respiratory tract illness.

Amantadine HCl should be continued daily for at least 10 days following a known exposure. If amantadine HCl is used chemoprophylactically in conjunction with inactivated influenza A virus vaccine until protective antibody responses develop, then it should be administered for 2 to 4 weeks after the vaccine has been given. When inactivated influenza A virus vaccine is unavailable or contraindicated, amantadine HCl should be administered for the duration of known influenza A in the community because of repeated and unknown exposure.

Treatment of influenza A virus illness should be started as soon as possible, preferably within 24 to 48 hours after onset of signs and symptoms, and should be continued for 24 to 48 hours after the disappearance of signs and symptoms.

DOSAGE FOR PARKINSONISM

Adult: The usual dose of amantadine HCl is 100 mg twice a day when used alone. Amantadine HCl has an onset of action usually within 48 hours.

The initial dose of amantadine HCl is 100 mg daily for patients with serious associated medical illness or who are receiving high doses of other antiparkinson drugs. After one to several weeks at 100 mg once daily, the dose may be increased to 100 mg twice daily, if necessary.

Occasionally, patients whose responses are not optimal with amantadine HCl at 200 mg daily may benefit from an increase up to 400 mg daily in divided doses. However, such patients should be supervised closely by their physicians.

Patients initially deriving benefit from amantadine HCl not uncommonly experience a fall-off of effectiveness after a few months. Benefit may be regained by increasing the dose to 300 mg daily. Alternatively, temporary discontinuation of amantadine HCl for several weeks, followed by reinitiation of the drug, may result in regaining benefit in some patients. A decision to use other antiparkinson drugs may be necessary.

Dosage for Concomitant Therapy: Some patients who do not respond to anticholinergic antiparkinson drugs may respond to amantadine HCl. When amantadine HCl or anticholinergic antiparkinson drugs are each used with marginal benefit, concomitant use may produce additional benefit.

When amantadine HCl and levodopa are initiated concurrently, the patient can exhibit rapid therapeutic benefits. Amantadine HCl should be held constant at 100 mg daily or twice daily while the daily dose of levodopa is gradually increased to optimal benefit.

When amantadine HCl is added to optimal well-tolerate doses of levodopa, additional benefit may result, including smoothing out the fluctuations in improvement which sometimes occur in patients on levodopa alone. Patients who require a reduction in their usual dose of levodopa because of development of side effects may possibly regain lost benefit with the addition of amantadine HCl.

DOSAGE FOR DRUG-INDUCED EXTRAPYRAMIDAL REACTIONS

Adult: The usual dose of amantadine HCl is 100 mg twice a day. Occasionally, patients whose responses are not optimal with amantadine HCl at 200 mg daily may benefit from an increase up to 300 mg daily in divided doses.

Dosage for Impaired Renal Function: Depending upon creatinine clearance, the following dosage adjustments are recommended.

TABLE 1

Creatinine Clearance ml/min/1.73m²	Amantadine HCl Dosage
30-50	200 mg 1st day and 100 mg each day thereafter
15-29	200 mg 1st day followed by 100 mg on alternate days
<15	200 mg every 7 days

The recommended dosage for patients on hemodialysis is 200 mg every 7 days.

Store at controlled room temperature (59°-86°F, 15°-30°C).

REFERENCES:

1. W.W. Wilson and A.H. Rajput, Amantadine-Dyazide Interaction, Can Med Assoc J. 129:974-975, 1983. **2.** D.F. Casey, N Engl. J. Med. 298:516, 1978. **3.** C.D. Berkowitz, J. Pediatr. 95:144, 1979. **4.** V.W. Horadam, et. al., Ann. Intern. Med. 94:454, 1981.

HOW SUPPLIED - RATED THERAPEUTICALLY EQUIVALENT:

Capsule, Elastic - Oral - 100 mg

30's	$5.06	Amantadine HCl, H.C.F.A. F F P	99999-0174-01
100's	$16.88	Amantadine HCl, H.C.F.A. F F P	99999-0174-02
100's	$19.13	Amantadine Hcl, United Res	00677-1128-01
100's	$19.13	Amantadine Hcl, United Res	00677-1346-01
100's	$19.13	Amantadine, United Res	00677-1452-01
100's	$19.13	Amantadine Hcl, Martec Pharms	52555-0122-01
100's	$20.46	Amantadine Hcl, US Trading	56126-0364-11
100's	$27.75	Amantadine Hcl, Solvay Pharms	00032-4140-06
100's	$29.50	Amantadine Hcl, Raway	00686-0481-20
100's	$30.59	Amantadine Hcl, Qualitest Pharms	00603-2163-21
100's	$30.59	Amantadine Hcl, Qualitest Pharms	00603-2164-21
100's	$31.05	Amantadine, HL Moore Drug Exch	00839-7250-06
100's	$31.50	Amantadine, Goldline Labs	00182-1258-01
100's	$31.50	Amantadine Hcl, Parmed Pharms	00349-8613-01
100's	$31.50	Amantadine Hcl, Rosemont	00832-1015-00
100's	$31.50	Amantadine Hcl, Major Pharms	00904-3430-60
100's	$31.50	Amantadine Hcl, Major Pharms	00904-3431-60
100's	$32.95	Amantadine Hcl, Geneva Pharms	00781-2106-01
100's	$33.50	Symmetrel, Rugby	00536-3090-01
100's	$34.75	Amantadine, Intl Labs	00665-4140-06
100's	$35.71	Amantadine Hcl, HL Moore Drug Exch	00839-7471-06
100's	$36.20	Amantadine Hcl, Aligen Independ	00405-4042-01
100's	$36.58	Amantadine Hcl, Duramed Pharms	51285-0839-02
100's	$37.93	Amantadine HCl, Schein Pharm (US)	00364-2146-01
100's	$43.22	Amantadine HCl, Warner Chilcott	00047-0853-24
100's	$62.73	Amantadine Hcl, Major Pharms	00904-3430-61
100's	**$84.72**	**SYMMETREL, Dupont Pharma**	**00056-0105-70**
500's	$84.40	Amantadine HCl, H.C.F.A. F F P	99999-0174-03
500's	$119.65	Amantadine Hcl, Major Pharms	00904-3430-40
500's	$119.65	Amantadine Hcl, Major Pharms	00904-3431-40
500's	$122.30	Amantadine Hcl, Parmed Pharms	00349-8613-05
500's	$122.30	Amantadine Hcl, Rosemont	00832-1015-50
500's	$129.53	Amantadine Hcl, HL Moore Drug Exch	00839-7250-12
500's	$130.78	Amantadine Hcl, Qualitest Pharms	00603-2163-28
500's	$130.78	Amantadine Hcl, Qualitest Pharms	00603-2164-28
500's	$177.95	Amantadine Hcl, Duramed Pharms	51285-0839-04
500's	$181.00	Amantadine Hydrochloride Capsules 100 Mg, Aligen Independ	00405-4042-02
500's	**$411.84**	**SYMMETREL, Dupont Pharma**	**00056-0105-85**

Syrup - Oral - 50 mg/5ml

480 ml	$31.48	Amantadine HCl, H.C.F.A. F F P	99999-0174-04
480 ml	$40.00	Amantadine Hcl, Raway	00686-0190-07
480 ml	$57.50	Symmetrel, Rugby	00536-2665-85
480 ml	$59.95	Amantadine Hcl, Qualitest Pharms	00603-1010-58
480 ml	$59.95	Amantadine Hcl, Copley Pharm	38245-0180-07
480 ml	$59.95	Amantadine Hcl, Mikart	46672-0606-16
480 ml	$61.51	Amantadine HCl, Alpharma	00472-0833-16
480 ml	$62.15	Amantadine Hcl, Endo Labs	60951-0656-16
480 ml	$63.00	Amantadine Hcl, Goldline Labs	00182-6016-40
480 ml	$63.11	Amantadine Hcl, Aligen Independ	00405-2140-16
480 ml	$64.00	Amantadine Hcl, Hi Tech Pharma	50383-0807-16
480 ml	$64.95	Amantadine Hcl, Harber Pharm	51432-0729-20
480 ml	$68.04	Amantadine Hcl, King Pharms	60793-0113-12
480 ml	$70.70	Amantadine Hcl, Major Pharms	00904-3432-16
480 ml	$70.86	Amantadine Hcl, HL Moore Drug Exch	00839-7667-69
480 ml	**$72.45**	**SYMMETREL, Dupont Pharma**	**00056-0205-16**

AMBENONIUM CHLORIDE *(000175)*

CATEGORIES: Autonomic Drugs; Cholinesterase Inhibitors; Myasthenia Gravis; Neuromuscular; Parasympathomimetic Agents; FDA Approval Pre 1982

BRAND NAMES: **Mytelase**

FORMULARIES: Aetna; Medi-Cal

DESCRIPTION:

Ambenonium chloride is a white crystalline powder soluble in water to 20 percent weight/volume.

CLINICAL PHARMACOLOGY:

A cholinesterase inhibitor with all the pharmacologic actions of acetylcholine, both of muscarinic & nicotinic types. Cholinesterase inactivates acetylcholine. Myasthenia gravis is a pathologic exhaustion of voluntary muscles, resulting in a state resembling paralysis, due either to an underproduction of acetylcholine or to an overproduction and activity of cholinesterase at the myoneural junction. Like neostigmine, ambenonium suppresses cholinesterase but it has the advantage of a longer duration of action and fewer side effects on the gastro-intestinal tract. Because its action is longer, administration of ambenonium is necessary only every three or four hours, depending upon the clinical response. Usually medication is not required throughout the night so that the patient can sleep uninterruptedly.

INDICATIONS AND USAGE:

Myasthenia gravis.

CONTRAINDICATIONS:

Since belladonna derivatives (atropine, etc.) may suppress the parasympathomimetic (muscarinic) symptoms of excessive gastrointestinal stimulation, leaving only the more serious symptoms of fasciculation and paralysis of voluntary muscle as signs of overdosage, routine administration of atropine with Ambenonium is contraindicated.

Because ambenonium has a more prolonged action than other antimyasthenic drugs, simultaneous administration with other cholinergics is contraindicated except under strict medical supervision. The overlap in duration of action of several drugs complicates dosage schedules. Thus, when transferring to Ambenonium chloride all other cholinergics should be suspended until the patient has been stabilized. In most instances the myasthenic symptoms are effectively controlled by Ambenonium alone.

Ambenonium should be used with caution in patients with asthma or in patients with mechanical intestinal or urinary obstruction.

OVERDOSAGE:

Overstimulation with Ambenonium has a clinical picture of increasing parasympathomimetic action which is more or less characteristic when not masked by the use of atropine. Signs and symptoms of overdosage, including up to cholinergic crises, vary considerably. They are usually manifested by increasing gastrointestinal stimulation with epigastric distress, abdominal cramps, diarrhea and vomiting, excessive salivation, pallor, cold sweating, urinary urgency, blurring of vision and eventually fasciculation and paralysis of voluntary muscles

OVERDOSAGE: *(cont'd)*

including those of the tongue (thick tongue and difficulty in swallowing), shoulder, neck and arms. Miosis, increase in blood pressure with or without bradycardia, and finally subjective sensations of internal trembling and often severe anxiety and panic may complete the picture. A cholinergic crisis is usually differentiated from the weakness and paralysis of myasthenia gravis insufficiently treated by cholinergic drugs by the fact that myasthenic weakness is not accompanied by any of the above signs and symptoms except the last two subjective ones (of anxiety and panic).

Since the warning of overdosage is minimal, the existence of a narrow margin between the first appearance of side effects and serious toxic effects must be borne in mind constantly. If signs of overdosage occur with ambenonium (excessive gastrointestinal stimulation, excessive salivation, miosis and more serious fasciculations of voluntary muscles) discontinue temporarily all cholinergic medication and administer from 0.5 to 1 mg. (1/120 to 1/60 grain) atropine intravenously. Give other supportive treatment as indicated (artificial respiration, tracheotomy, oxygen, etc.).

CAUTION: Since belladonna derivatives (atropine) may suppress symptoms of excessive gastrointestinal stimulation, leaving only the more serious symptoms of fasciculation of voluntary muscle as a sign of overdosage, routine administration of atropine with ambenonium is contraindicated.

DOSAGE AND ADMINISTRATION:

The oral dose must be individualized according to the patient's response because the disease varies widely in its severity in different patients, and patients vary in their sensitivity to cholinergic drugs. There is a highly critical point of maximum therapeutic effectiveness with optimum muscle strength and no gastrointestinal disturbances requiring close supervision of a physician familiar with the disease.

Since the warning of overdosage is minimal and the requirements of patients vary tremendously, great care and supervision are required. That a narrow margin exists between the first appearance of side effects and serious toxic effects must be borne in mind constantly. Caution in increasing dosage is essential.

For the moderately severe myasthenic patient from 5 to 25 mg Ambenonium chloride three or four times daily is an effective dose. Some patients do well with as little as 5 mg per dose, while others require as much as from 50 to 75 mg per dose. The physician should start with a 5 mg dose, carefully observing the effect of the drug in each patient. The dosage may be gradually increased to determine the effective and safe dose for each patient. In addition to individual variations in dosage requirements, the amount of cholinergic medication necessary to control symptoms may fluctuate in each patient, depending upon his activity and the current status of the disease, including spontaneous remission. A few patients have required greater doses for adequate control of the myasthenic symptoms, but increasing the dosage above 200 mg daily requires exacting supervision of a physician well aware of the signs and treatment of overdosage with cholinergic medication.

HOW SUPPLIED - EQUIVALENTS NOT AVAILABLE:

Tablet, Uncoated - Oral - 10 mg

100's $81.56 MYTELASE, Sanofi Winthrop 00024-1287-04

AMCINONIDE *(000176)*

CATEGORIES: Anti-Inflammatory Agents; Dermatitis; Dermatologicals; Dermatoses; Glucocorticoids; Hormones; Pruritus; Psoriasis; Skin/Mucous Membrane Agents; Steroids; Topical; Pregnancy Category C; FDA Approval Pre 1982

BRAND NAMES: *Amciderm* (Germany); *Amcinil*; *Amicla*; **Cyclocort**; *Cycloderm*; *Penticort* (France); *Visderm* (Japan); *Visderm H* (Mexico)
(International brand names outside U.S. in italics)

FORMULARIES: Aetna; BC-BS

DESCRIPTION:

The topical corticosteroids constitute a class of primarily synthetic steroids used as anti-inflammatory and antipruritic agents.

Topical Lotion 0.1%: Each gram of Cyclocort (amcinonide) topical Lotion contains 1 mg of the active steroid amcinonide in Aquatain,* a white, smooth, homogeneous, opaque emulsion composed of Benzyl Alcohol 1% (wt/wt) as preservative, Emulsifying Wax, Glycerin, Isopropyl Palmitate, Lactic Acid, Purified Water, and Sorbitol Solution. In addition, contains Polyethylene Glycol 400.

Sodium hydroxide may be used to adjust pH to approximately 4.4 during manufacture.

Topical Cream 0.1%: Each gram Cyclocort (amcinonide) topical cream contains 1 mg of the active steroid amcinonide in Aquatain,* a white smooth, homogeneous, opaque emulsion composed of Benzyl Alcohol 2% (wt/wt) as preservative, Emulsifying Wax, Glycerin, Isopropyl Palmitate, Lactic Acid, Purified Water, and Sorbitol Solution.

*Aquatain is non-staining, water-washable, paraben-free, spermaceti-free, and has a light texture and consistency.

Topical Ointment 0.1%: Each gram of Cyclocort (amcinonide) topical Ointment contains 1 mg of the active steroid amcinonide in a specially formulated base composed of Benzyl Alcohol 2% (wt/wt) as preservative, White Petrolatum, Emulsifying Wax, and Tenox II (Butylated Hydroxyanisole, Propyl Gallate, Citric Acid, Propylene Glycol).

Molecular Weight 502.58 $C_{28}H_{35}FO_7$ Pregna-1,4-diene-3,20-dione, 21-(acetyloxy)-16,17-(cyclopentyl-idenebis(oxy))-9-fluoro-11-hydroxy-, (11β,16α).

CLINICAL PHARMACOLOGY:

Topical corticosteroids have anti-inflammatory, antipruritic, and vasoconstrictive actions.

The mechanism of anti-inflammatory activity of the topical corticosteroids is unclear. Various laboratory methods, including vasoconstrictor assays, are used to compare and predict potencies and/or clinical efficacies of the topical corticosteroids. There is some evidence to suggest that a recognizable correlation exists between vasoconstrictor potency and therapeutic efficacy in man.

PHARMACOKINETICS

The extent of percutaneous absorption of topical corticosteroids is determined by many factors, including the vehicle, the integrity of the epidermal barrier, and the use of occlusive dressings.

Topical corticosteroids can be absorbed from normal intact skin. Inflammation and/or other disease processes in the skin increase percutaneous absorption. Occlusive dressings substantially increase the percutaneous absorption of topical corticosteroids (see DOSAGE AND ADMINISTRATION.)

Once absorbed through the skin, topical corticosteroids are handled through pharmacokinetic pathways similar to systemically-administered corticosteroids. Corticosteroids are bound to plasma proteins in varying degrees.

CLINICAL PHARMACOLOGY: *(cont'd)*

Corticosteroids are metabolized primarily in the liver and are then excreted by the kidneys. Some of the topical corticosteroids and their metabolites are also excreted into the bile.

INDICATIONS AND USAGE:

Topical corticosteroids are indicated for the relief of the inflammatory and pruritic manifestations of corticosteroid-responsive dermatoses.

CONTRAINDICATIONS:

Topical corticosteroids are contraindicated in those patients with a history of hypersensitivity to any of the components of the preparation.

PRECAUTIONS:

GENERAL

Systemic absorption of topical corticosteroids has produced reversible hypothalamic-pituitary-adrenal (HPA) axis suppression, manifestations of Cushing's syndrome, hyperglycemia, and glucosuria in some patients.

Conditions that augment system absorption include the application of the more potent steroids, use over large surface areas, prolonged use, and the addition of occlusive dressings. Therefore, patients receiving a large dose of a potent topical steroid applied to a large surface area or under an occlusive dressing should be evaluated periodically for evidence of HPA-axis suppression by using the urinary free-cortisol and ACTH stimulation tests. If HPA-axis suppression is noted, an attempt should be made to withdraw the drug, to reduce the frequency of application, or to substitute with a less potent steroid.

Recovery of HPA-axis function is generally prompt and complete upon discontinuation of the drug.

Infrequently, signs and symptoms of steroid withdrawal may occur, requiring supplemental systemic corticosteroids.

Children may absorb proportionally larger amounts of topical corticosteroids and thus be more susceptible to systemic toxicity (see PRECAUTIONS, Pediatric Use.)

If irritation develops, topical corticosteroids should be discontinued and appropriate therapy instituted.

In the presence of dermatological infections, the use of an appropriate antifungal or antibacterial agent should be instituted. If a favorable response does not occur promptly the corticosteroid should be discontinued until the infection has been adequately controlled.

The products are not for ophthalmic use.

INFORMATION FOR THE PATIENT

Patients using topical corticosteroids should receive the following information and instructions.

1. This medication is to be used as directed by the physician. It is for external use only. Avoid contact with the eyes.

2. Patients should be advised not to use this medication for any disorder other than for which it was prescribed.

3. The treated skin area should not be bandaged or otherwise covered or wrapped, as to be occlusive, unless directed by the physician.

4. Patients should report any signs of local adverse reactions, especially those that occur under occlusive dressings.

5. Parents of pediatric patients should be advised not to use tight-fitting diapers or plastic pants on a child being treated in the diaper area, as these garments may constitute occlusive dressings.

LABORATORY TESTS

The following tests may be helpful in evaluating the HPA-axis suppression.

Urinary free-cortisol test

ACTH stimulation test

CARCINOGENESIS, MUTAGENESIS, AND IMPAIRMENT OF FERTILITY

Long-term animal studies have not been performed to evaluate the carcinogenic potential of topical corticosteroids or their effect on fertility.

Studies to determine mutagenicity with prednisolone and hydrocortisone have revealed negative results.

PREGNANCY CATEGORY C

Corticosteroids are generally teratogenic in laboratory animals when administered systemically at relatively low dosage levels. The more potent corticosteroids have been shown to be teratogenic after dermal application in laboratory animals. There are no adequate and well-controlled studies in pregnant women on teratogenic effects from topically-applied corticosteroids. Therefore, topical corticosteroids should be used during pregnancy only if the potential benefit justifies the potential risk to the fetus. Drugs of this class should not be used extensively on pregnant patients, in large amounts, or for prolonged periods of time.

NURSING MOTHERS

It is not known whether topical administration of corticosteroids could result in sufficient systemic absorption to produce detectable quantities in breast milk. Systemically-administered corticosteroids are secreted into breast milk in quantities not likely to have a deleterious effect on the infant. Nevertheless, a decision should be made whether to discontinue nursing or to discontinue the drug, taking into account the importance of the drug to the mother.

PEDIATRIC USE

Pediatric patients may demonstrate greater susceptibility to topical corticosteroid-included HPA-axis suppression and Cushing's syndrome than mature patients because of a higher ratio of skin surface area to body weight.

Hypothalamic-pituitary-adrenal (HPA) axis suppression, Cushing's syndrome, and intracranial hypertension have been reported in children receiving topical corticosteroids. Manifestations of adrenal suppression in children include linear growth retardation, delayed weight gain, low plasma cortisol levels, and absence of response to ACTH stimulation. Manifestations of intracranial hypertension include bulging fontanelles, headaches, and bilateral papilledema.

Administration of topical corticosteroids to children should be limited to the least amount compatible with an effective therapeutic regimen. Chronic corticosteroid therapy may interfere with the growth and development of children.

ADVERSE REACTIONS:

In the clinical trials with Cyclocort Lotion, the investigators reported a 4.7% incidence of side effects. In a weekly acceptability evaluation, approximately 20% of the patients treated with Cyclocort Lotion or placebo reported itching, stinging, soreness, or burning at one or more of the visits.

The following local adverse reactions are reported infrequently with topical corticosteroids, but may occur more frequently with the use of occlusive dressings. These reactions are listed in an approximate decreasing order of occurrence.

ADVERSE REACTIONS: *(cont'd)*

Burning, itching, irritation, dryness, folliculitis, hypertrichosis, acneiform eruptions, hypopigmentation, perioral dermatitis, allergic contact dermatitis, maceration of the skin, secondary infection, skin atrophy, striae, miliaria

OVERDOSAGE:

Topically-applied corticosteroids can be absorbed in sufficient amounts to produce systemic effects (see PRECAUTIONS.)

DOSAGE AND ADMINISTRATION:

Topical corticosteroids are generally applied to the affected area as a thin film from two to three times daily depending on the severity of the condition.

The lotion may be applied topically to the specified lesions, particularly to those in hairy areas, two times per day. The lotion should be rubbed into the affected area completely, and the area should be protected from washing, clothing, rubbing, etc. until the lotion has dried.

Occlusive dressings may be a valuable therapeutic adjunct for the management of psoriasis or recalcitrant conditions.

If an infection develops, the use of occlusive dressings should be discontinued and appropriate antimicrobial therapy instituted.

Store at controlled room temperature 15-30°C (59-86°F). DO NOT FREEZE.

HOW SUPPLIED - EQUIVALENTS NOT AVAILABLE:

Cream - Topical - 0.1 %

15 gm	**$15.98**	**CYCLOCORT, Fujisawa USA**	**00469-7054-15**
30 gm	**$23.79**	**CYCLOCORT, Fujisawa USA**	**00469-7054-30**
60 gm	**$39.98**	**CYCLOCORT, Fujisawa USA**	**00469-7054-60**

Lotion - Topical - 0.1 %

60 ml	**$36.54**	**CYCLOCORT, Fujisawa USA**	**00469-7404-60**

Ointment - Topical - 0.1 %

15 gm	**$15.34**	**CYCLOCORT, Fujisawa Pharm (US)**	**57317-0115-15**
30 gm	**$23.79**	**CYCLOCORT, Fujisawa USA**	**00469-7115-30**
60 gm	**$39.98**	**CYCLOCORT, Fujisawa USA**	**00469-7115-60**

AMIFOSTINE *(003071)*

CATEGORIES: Antineoplastics; Chemoprotective Agents; Melanoma; Orphan Drugs; Ovarian Carcinoma; FDA Approved 1995 Dec

BRAND NAMES: **Ethyol**; *Ethyol 500*
(International brand names outside U.S. in italics)

DESCRIPTION:

Ethyol(amifostine) is an organic thiophosphate cytoprotective agent known chemically as ethanethiol, 2-[(3-aminopropyl)amino]-, dihydrogen phosphate (ester) and has the following structural formula: $H_2N(CH_2)_3NH(CH_2)_2S\text{-}PO_3H_2$.

Amifostine is a white crystalline powder which is freely soluble in water. Its empirical formula is $C_5H_{15}N_2O_3PS$ and it has a molecular weight of 214.22.

Amifostine is supplied as a sterile lyophilized powder mixture with mannitol requiring reconstitution for intravenous infusion. Each single-use 10 mL vial contains 500 mg of amifostine (anhydrous basis) and 500 mg of mannitol.

CLINICAL PHARMACOLOGY:

Amifostine is a pro drug that is dephosphorylated by alkaline phosphatase in tissues to a pharmacologically active free thiol metabolite that can reduce the toxic effects of cisplatin. The ability to differentially protect normal tissues is attributed to the higher capillary alkaline phosphatase activity, higher pH and better vascularity of normal tissues relative to tumor tissue, which results in a more rapid generation of the active thiol metabolite as well as a higher rate constant for uptake. The higher concentration of free thiol in normal tissues is available to bind to, and thereby detoxify, reactive metabolites of cisplatin; and also can act as a scavenger of free radicals that may be generated in tissues exposed to cisplatin. Several preclinical studies in mice and rats have demonstrated that pretreatment with amifostine results in protection from nephrotoxicity following administration of single and multiple doses of cisplatin.

Pharmacokinetics: Clinical pharmacokinetic studies show that amifostine is rapidly cleared from the plasma with a distribution half-life of < 1 minute and an elimination half-life of approximately 8 minutes. Less than 10% of amifostine remains in the plasma 6 minutes after drug administration. Amifostine is rapidly metabolized to an active free thiol metabolite. A disulfide metabolite is produced subsequently and is less active than the free thiol. After a 10-second bolus dose of 150 mg/m^2 of amifostine, renal excretion of the parent drug and its two metabolites was low during the hour following drug administration, averaging 0.69%, 2.64% and 2.22% of the administered dose for the parent, thiol and disulfide, respectively. Measurable levels of the free thiol metabolite have been found in bone marrow cells 5-8 minutes after intravenous infusion of amifostine. Pretreatment with dexamethasone or metoclopramide has no effect on amifostine pharmacokinetics.

CLINICAL STUDIES:

A randomized controlled trial compared six cycles of cyclophosphamide 1000 mg/m^2, and cisplatin 100 mg/m^2 with or without amifostine pretreatment at 910 mg/m^2, in two successive cohorts of 121 patients with advanced ovarian cancer. In both cohorts, after multiple cycles of chemotherapy, pretreatment with amifostine significantly reduced the cumulative renal toxicity associated with cisplatin as assessed by the proportion of patients who had ≥40% decrease in creatinine clearance from pretreatment values, protracted elevations in serum creatinine (>1.5 mg/dL), or severe hypomagnesemia. Subgroup analyses suggested that the effect of amifostine was present in patients who had received nephrotoxic antibiotics, or who had preexisting diabetes or hypertension (and thus may have been at increased risk for significant nephrotoxicity), as well as in patients who lacked these risks. Selected analyses of the effects of amifostine in reducing the cumulative renal toxicity of cisplatin in the randomized ovarian cancer study are provided in TABLES 1 and 2, below.

TABLE 1 Proportion of Patients with ≥40% Reduction in Calculated Creatinine Clearance*

	Amifostine + CP	**CP**	**p-value 2-sided**
All Patients	16/122 (13%)	36/120 (30%)	0.001
First Cohort	10/63	20/58	0.018
Second Cohort	6/59	16/62	0.026

* Creatinine clearance values were calculated using the Cockcroft-Gault formula.**Nephron** 1976; 16:31-41.

CLINICAL STUDIES: *(cont'd)*

TABLE 2 NCI Toxicity Grades of Serum Magnesium Levels for Each Patient's Last Cycle of Therapy

NCI-CTC Grade: (mEq/L)	**0 >1.4**	**1 ≤1.4-<1.1**	**2 ≤1.1->0.8**	**3 ≤0.8->0.5**	**4 ≤0.5**	**p-value***
All Patients						
Amifostine + CP	92	13	3	0	0	
CP	73	18	7	5	1	0.001
First Cohort						
Amifostine + CP	49	10	3	0	0	
CP	35	8	6	3	1	0.017
Second Cohort						
Amifostine + CP	43	3	0	0	0	
CP	38	10	1	2	0	0.012

*Based on 2-sided Mantel-Haenszel Chi-Square statistic.

In the randomized ovarian cancer study, amifostine had no detectable effect on the antitumor efficacy of cisplatin-cyclophosphamide chemotherapy. Objective response rates (including pathologically confirmed complete remission rates), time to progression, and survival duration were all similar in the amifostine and control study groups. TABLE 3 below summarizes the principal efficacy findings of the randomized ovarian cancer study.

TABLE 3

	Amifostine + CP	**CP**
Complete pathologic tumor response rate	21.3%	15.8%
Time to progression (months)		
Median (± 95% Cl)	15.8 (13.2, 25.1)	18.1 (12.5, 20.4)
Mean (± Std error)	19.8 (± 1.04)	19.1 (± 1.58)
Hazard Ratio (95% Confidence Interval)	0.98 (0.64, 1.4)	
Survival (months)		
Median (± 95% Cl)	31.3 (28.3, 38.2)	31.8 (26.3, 39.8)
Mean (± Std error)	33.7 (± 2.03)	34.3 (± 2.04)
Hazard Ratio (95% Confidence Interval)	0.97 (0.69, 1.32)	

A Phase II trial of amifostine, 740-910 mg/m^2, and cisplatin, 120 mg/m^2, administered on day 1 and vinblastine, 5 mg/m^2, administered on days 1, 8, 15 and 22 of each monthly cycle was conducted in 25 patients with Stage IV non-small cell lung cancer. This regimen was repeated until disease progression or unacceptable toxicity occurred, or a maximum of six cycles had been administered. Among 13 patients who received 4 or more cycles of this intensive cisplatin regimen, 1 had a ≥40% reduction in creatinine clearance. These results are consistent with the randomized ovarian cancer trial. Sixteen of the 25 patients treated demonstrated a partial response to chemotherapy. With a median follow-up of 19 months, the median survival was 17 months. At one year, 64% of the patients were alive. These results indicate that amifostine may not adversely affect the efficacy of this chemotherapy for non-small cell lung cancer..

INDICATIONS AND USAGE:

Amifostine is indicated to reduce the cumulative renal toxicity associated with repeated administration of cisplatin in patients with advanced ovarian cancer or non-small cell lung cancer. In these settings, the clinical data do not suggest that the effectiveness of cisplatin based chemotherapy regimens is altered by amifostine. There are at present only limited data on the effects of amifostine on the efficacy of chemotherapy in other settings; therefore amifostine should not be administered to patients in other settings where chemotherapy can produce a significant survival benefit or cure (*e.g.,* certain malignancies of germ cell origin), except in the context of a clinical study.

CONTRAINDICATIONS:

Amifostine is contraindicated in patients with known sensitivity to aminothiol compounds or mannitol.

WARNINGS:

1. Effectiveness of the Cytotoxic Regimen: Limited data are currently available regarding the preservation of antitumor efficacy when amifostine is administered prior to cisplatin therapy in settings other than advanced ovarian cancer or non-small cell lung cancer. Although some animal data suggest interference is possible, in most tumor models the antitumor effects of chemotherapy are not altered by amifostine. The possibility of interference with the efficacy of cancer treatment would be of particular concern in those settings where chemotherapy can produce a significant survival benefit or cure. Amifostine should therefore not be used in patients receiving chemotherapy for other malignancies in which chemotherapy can produce a significant survival benefit or cure (*e.g.,* certain malignancies of germ cell origin), except in the context of a clinical study.

2. Hypotension: Patients who are hypotensive or in a state of dehydration should not receive amifostine. Patients receiving antihypertensive therapy that cannot be stopped for 24 hours preceding amifostine treatment also should not receive amifostine. Patients should be adequately hydrated prior to amifostine infusion and kept in a supine position during the infusion. Blood pressure should be monitored every 5 minutes during the infusion. It is important that the duration of the infusion be 15 minutes, as administration of amifostine as a longer infusion is associated with a higher incidence of side effects. If hypotension requiring interruption of therapy occurs, patients should be placed in the Trendelenburg position and be given an infusion of normal saline using a separate i.v. line. Guidelines for interrupting and restarting amifostine infusion if a decrease in systolic blood pressure should occur are provided in the DOSAGE AND ADMINISTRATIONsection.

3. Nausea and Vomiting: Antiemetic medication should be administered prior to and in conjunction with amifostine (see DOSAGE AND ADMINISTRATION). When amifostine is administered with highly emetogenic chemotherapy, the fluid balance of the patient should be carefully monitored.

4. Hypocalcemia: Reports of clinically relevant hypocalcemia are rare, but serum calcium levels should be monitored in patients at risk of hypocalcemia, such as those with nephrotic syndrome. If necessary, calcium supplements can be administered.

PRECAUTIONS:

General: Patients should be adequately hydrated prior to the infusion and blood pressure should be monitored during the infusion. Amifostine should be administered as a 15-minute infusion (see DOSAGE AND ADMINISTRATION).

The safety of amifostine administration has not been established in elderly patients, or patients with preexisting cardiovascular or cerebrovascular conditions such as ischemic heart disease, arrhythmias, congestive heart failure, or history of stroke or transient ischemic

PRECAUTIONS: *(cont'd)*

attacks. Amifostine should be used with particular care in these and other patients in whom the common amifostine adverse effects of nausea/vomiting and hypotension may be more likely to have serious consequences.

Carcinogenesis, Mutagenesis and Impairment of Fertility: No long-term animal studies have been performed to evaluate the carcinogenic potential of amifostine. Amifostine was negative in the Ames test and in the mouse micronucleus test. The free thiol metabolite, however, was positive in the Ames test with S9 microsomal fraction in the TA1535 Salmonella typhimurium strain and at the TK locus in the mouse L5178Y cell assay. The metabolite was negative in the mouse micronucleus test and negative for clastogenicity in human lymphocytes.

Pregnancy Category C: Amifostine has been shown to be embryotoxic in rabbits at doses of 50 mg/kg, approximately sixty percent of the recommended dose in humans on a body surface area basis. There are no adequate and well-controlled studies in pregnant women. Amifostine should be used during pregnancy only if the potential benefit justifies the potential risk to the fetus.

Nursing Mothers: No information is available on the excretion of amifostine or its metabolites into human milk. Because many drugs are excreted in human milk and because of the potential for adverse reactions in nursing infants, it is recommended that breast feeding be discontinued if the mother is treated with amifostine.

DRUG INTERACTIONS:

There are no known drug interactions with amifostine. However, special consideration should be given to the administration of amifostine in patients receiving antihypertensive medications or other drugs that could potentiate hypotension.

ADVERSE REACTIONS:

Amifostine produced a transient reduction in blood pressure in 62% of patients treated. The mean time of onset was 14 minutes into the 15-minute period of amifostine infusion, and the mean duration was 6 minutes. In some cases, the infusion had to be prematurely terminated due to a more pronounced drop in systolic blood pressure. In general, the blood pressure returned to normal within 5-15 minutes. Fewer than 3% of patients discontinued amifostine due to blood pressure reductions. Short term, reversible loss of consciousness has been reported rarely. Blood pressure reductions during amifostine administration have not been reported to cause long-term CNS, cardiovascular or renal sequelae, but clinical studies performed to date have not evaluated the safety of amifostine in elderly patients or patients with preexisting cardiovascular or cerebrovascular conditions.

Hypotension that requires interruption of the amifostine infusion should be treated with fluid infusion and postural management of the patient (supine or Trendelenburg position). If the blood pressure returns to normal within 5 minutes and the patient is asymptomatic, the infusion may be restarted, so that the full dose of amifostine can be administered.

Nausea and/or vomiting occur frequently after amifostine infusion and may be severe. In the ovarian cancer randomized study, the incidence of severe nausea/vomiting on day 1 of cyclophosphamide-cisplatin chemotherapy was 10% in patients who did not receive amifostine, and 19% in patients who did receive amifostine. Other effects which have been described during or following amifostine infusion are flushing/feeling of warmth, chills/feeling of coldness, dizziness, somnolence, hiccups and sneezing. These effects have not generally precluded the completion of chemotherapy.

Decrease in serum calcium concentrations is a known pharmacological effect of amifostine. At the recommended doses, clinically significant hypocalcemia has occurred rarely (<1%).

Allergic reactions, ranging from mild skin rashes to rigors, have occurred rarely (<1%). There has been no reported occurrence of anaphylaxis with amifostine.

OVERDOSAGE:

In clinical trials, the maximum single dose of amifostine was 1300 mg/m^2. No information is available on single doses higher than this in adults. In the setting of a clinical trial, children have received single amifostine doses of up to 2700 mg/m^2 with no unexpected effects. Multiple infusions (up to three) of 740-910 mg/m^{2}doses of amifostine have been administered within a 24-hour period under study conditions without unexpected effects. Administration of amifostine at 2 and 4 hours after the initial dose has not led to increased or cumulative side effects, such as increased nausea and vomiting or hypotension. The most likely symptom of overdosage is hypotension, which should be managed by infusion of normal saline and other supportive measures, as clinically indicated.

DOSAGE AND ADMINISTRATION:

In adults, the recommended starting dose of amifostine is 910 mg/m^2 administered once daily as a 15-minute i.v. infusion, starting within 30 minutes prior to chemotherapy. The 15-minute infusion is better tolerated than more extended infusions. Further reductions in infusion times have not been systematically investigated. The infusion of amifostine should be interrupted if the systolic blood pressure decreases significantly from the baseline value as listed in the guideline (TABLE 4) below:

TABLE 4 Guideline for Interrupting Amifostine Infusion Due to Decrease in Systolic Blood Pressure

	Baseline Systolic Blood Pressure (mm Hg)				
	<100	100-119	120-139	140-179	≥180
Decrease in systolic blood pressure during infusion of Ethyol (mm Hg)	20	25	30	40	50

If the blood pressure returns to normal within 5 minutes and the patient is asymptomatic, the infusion may be restarted so that the full dose of amifostine may be administered. If the full dose of amifostine cannot be administered, the dose of amifostine for subsequent cycles should be 740 mg/m^2.

Only limited experience is available for the usage of amifostine in children or elderly patients (more than 70 years of age).

It is recommended that antiemetic medication, including dexamethasone 20 mg i.v. and a serotonin $5HT_3$ receptor antagonist, be administered prior to and in conjunction with amifostine. Additional antiemetics may be required based on the chemotherapy drugs administered.

RECONSTITUTION

Amifostine for Injection is supplied as a sterile lyophilized powder mixture requiring reconstitution for intravenous infusion. Each single-use vial contains 500 mg of amifostine (anhydrous basis) and 500 mg of mannitol.

Prior to intravenous injection, amifostine for Injection is reconstituted with 9.5 mL of sterile Sodium Chloride Injection, USP 0.9%. The reconstituted solution (500 mg amifostine/10 mL) is chemically stable for up to 5 hours at room temperature (approximately 25°C) or up to 24 hours under refrigeration (2°C to 8°C).

DOSAGE AND ADMINISTRATION: *(cont'd)*

Amifostine prepared in polyvinylchloride (PVC) bags at concentrations ranging from 5 mg/mL to 40 mg/mL is chemically stable for up to 5 hours when stored at room temperature (25°C) or up to 24 hours when stored under refrigeration (2°C to 8°C).

CAUTION: Parenteral products should be inspected visually for particulate matter and discoloration prior to administration whenever solution and container permit. Do not use if cloudiness or precipitate is observed.

INCOMPATIBILITIES

The compatibility of amifostine with solutions other than 0.9% Sodium Chloride for Injection, or Sodium Chloride solutions with other additives, has not been examined. The use of other solutions is not recommended.

HOW SUPPLIED:

Ethyol for Injection is supplied as a sterile lyophilized powder in 10 mL single-use vials. Each single-use vial contains 500 mg of amifostine (anhydrous basis) and 500 mg of mannitol.

Store the lyophilized dosage form in a refrigerator (2°C to 8°C).

HOW SUPPLIED - EQUIVALENTS NOT AVAILABLE:

Injection - Intravenous - 500 mg

1's	$312.00	ETHYOL, Alza	17314-3123-01
3's	$936.00	ETHYOL, Alza	17314-3123-03

AMIKACIN SULFATE *(000178)*

CATEGORIES: Aminoglycosides; Anti-Infectives; Antibiotics; Antimicrobials; Bacterial Sepsis; Burns; Infections; Intra-Abdominal Infections; Septicemia; Tuberculosis*; Pregnancy Category D; FDA Approval Pre 1982

* Indication not approved by the FDA

BRAND NAMES: *Acemycin*; *Akacin*; *Akicin*; *Akim*; *Alostil*; *Amicacina*; *Amicasil*; *Amicin*; *Amikafur* (Mexico); *Amikan*; *Amikayect* (Mexico); **Amikin**; *Amiklin* (France); *Amiktam*; *Amukin*; *Biklin* (Germany); *Briklin*; *Chemacin*; *Gamikal* (Mexico); *Glukamin*; *Kacinth-A*; *Kanbine*; *Lanomycin*; *Likacin*; *Lukadin*; *Miacin*; *Migacin*; *Orlobin*; *Pediakin*; *Pierami*; *Savox*; *Selaxa*; *Tybikin*; *Yectamid* (Mexico)
(International brand names outside U.S. in italics)

WARNING:

Patients treated with parenteral aminoglycosides should be under close clinical observation because of the potential ototoxicity and nephrotoxicity associated with their use. Safety for treatment periods which are longer than 14 days has not been established.

Neurotoxicity, manifested as vestibular and permanent bilateral auditory ototoxicity can occur in patients with preexisting renal damage and in patients with normal renal function treated at higher doses and/or for periods longer than those recommended. The risk of aminoglycoside-induced ototoxicity is greater in patients with renal damage. High frequency deafness usually occurs first and can be detected only by audiometric testing. Vertigo may occur and may be evidence of vestibular injury. Other manifestations of neurotoxicity may include numbness, skin tingling, muscle twitching, and convulsions. The risk of hearing loss due to aminoglycosides increases with the degree of exposure to either high peak or high trough serum concentrations. Patients developing cochlear damage may not have symptoms during therapy to warn them of developing eighth-nerve toxicity, and total or partial irreversible bilateral deafness may occur after the drug has been discontinued. Aminoglycoside-induced ototoxicity is usually irreversible.

Aminoglycosides are potentially nephrotoxic. The risk of nephrotoxicity is greater in patients with impaired renal function and in those who receive high doses or prolonged therapy.

Neuromuscular blockade and respiratory paralysis have been reported following parenteral injection, topical instillation (as in orthopedic and abdominal irritation or in local treatment of empyema), and following oral use of aminoglycosides. The possibility of these phenomena should be considered if aminoglycosides are administered by any route, especially in patients receiving anesthetics, neuromuscular blocking agents such as tubocurarine, succinylcholine, decamethonium, or in patients receiving massive transfusions of citrate-anticoagulated blood. If blockade occurs, calcium salts may reverse these phenomena, but mechanical respiratory assistance may be necessary. Renal and eight-nerve function should be closely monitored especially in patients with known or suspected renal impairment at the onset of therapy and also in those whose renal function is initially normal but who develop signs of renal dysfunction during therapy. Serum concentrations of amikacin should be monitored when feasible to assure adequate levels and to avoid potentially toxic levels and prolonged peak concentrations above micrograms per ml. Urine should be examined for decreased specific gravity, increased excretion of proteins, and the presence of cells or casts. Blood urea nitrogen, serum creatinine, or creatinine clearance should be measured periodically. Serial audiograms should be obtained where feasible in patients old enough to be tested, particularly high risk patients. Evidence of ototoxicity (dizziness, vertigo, tinnitus, roaring in the ears, and hearing loss) or nephrotoxicity requires discontinuation of the drug or dosage adjustment. Concurrent and/or sequential systemic, oral, or topical use of other neurotoxic or nephrotoxic products, particularly bacitracin, cisplatin, amphotericin B, cephaloridine, paromomycin, viomycin, polymyxin B, colistin, vancomycin, or other aminoglycosides should be avoided. Other factors that may increase risk of toxicity are advanced age and dehydration.

The concurrent use of Amikin with potent diuretics (ethacrynic acid, or furosemide) should be avoided since diuretics by themselves may cause ototoxicity. In addition, when administered intravenously, diuretics may enhance aminoglycoside toxicity by altering antibiotic concentrations in serum and tissue.

DESCRIPTION:

Amikacin sulfate is a semi-synthetic aminoglycoside antibiotic derived from kanamycin. It is $C_{22}H_{43}N_5O_{13}$·$2H_2SO_4$. D-Streptamine, O-3-amino-3-deoxy-α-D -glucopyranosyl - (1→6)-O-(6-amino- 6-deoxy-α-D- glucopyranosyl- (1→4))-N[1]-(4-amino-2-hydroxyl-1 -oxobutyl)-2 -deoxy-, (S)-,sulfate (1:2) (salt).

The dosage form is supplied as a sterile, colorless to light straw colored solution. The 100 mg per 2 ml vial contains, in addition to amikacin sulfate, 0.13% sodium bisulfite and 0.5% sodium citrate with pH adjusted to 4.5 with sulfuric acid. The 500 mg per 2 ml vial and the 1 gram per 4 ml vial contain 0.66% sodium bisulfite and 2.5% sodium citrate with pH adjusted to 4.5 with sulfuric acid.

Vial headspace contains nitrogen.

CLINICAL PHARMACOLOGY:

Intramuscular Administration: Amikin is rapidly absorbed after intramuscular administration. In normal adult volunteers, average peak serum concentrations of about 12, 16, and 21 mcg/ml are obtained 1 hour after intramuscular administration of 250-mg (3.7 mg/kg), 375-mg (5 mg/kg), 500-mg (7.5 mg/kg), single doses, respectively. At 10 hours, serum levels are about 0.3 mcg/ml, 1.2 mcg/ml, and 2.1 mcg/ml, respectively.

Tolerance studies in normal volunteers reveal that amikacin is well tolerated locally following repeated intramuscular dosing, and when given at maximally recommended doses, no ototoxicity or nephrotoxicity has been reported. There is no evidence of drug accumulation with repeated dosing for 10 days when administered according to recommended doses.

With normal renal function, about 91.9% of an intramuscular dose is excreted unchanged in the urine in the first 8 hours, and 98.2% within 24 hours. Mean urine concentrations for 6 hours are 563 mcg/ml following a 250-mg dose. 697 mcg/ml following a 375-mg dose, and 832 mcg/ml following a 500-mg dose.

Preliminary intramuscular studies in newborns of different weights (less than 1.5 kg, 1.5 to 2.0 kg, over 2.0 kg) at a dose of 7.5 mg/kg revealed that, like other aminoglycosides, serum half-life values were correlated inversely with post-natal age and renal clearances of amikacin. The volume of distribution indicates that amikacin, like other aminoglycosides, remains primarily in the extracellular fluid space of neonates. Repeated dosing every 12 hours in all the above groups did not demonstrate accumulation after 5 days.

Intravenous Administration: Single doses of 500 mg (7.5 mg/kg) administered to normal adults as an infusion over a period of 30 minutes produced a mean peak serum concentration of 38 mcg/ml at the end of the infusion, and levels of 24 mcg/ml, 18 mcg/ml, and 0.75 mcg/ml at 30 minutes, 1 hour, and 10 hours post-infusion, respectively. Eighty-four percent of the administered dose was excreted in the urine in 9 hours and about 94% within 24 hours.

Repeat infusions of 7.5 mg/kg every 12 hours in normal adults were well tolerated and caused no drug accumulation.

General: Pharmacokinetic studies in normal adult subjects reveal the mean serum half-life to be slightly over 2 hours with a mean total apparent volume of distribution of 24 liters (28% of the body weight). By the ultrafiltration technique, reports of serum protein binding range from 0 to 11%. The mean serum clearance rate is about 100 ml/min and the renal clearance rate is 94 ml/min in subjects with normal renal function.

Amikacin is excreted primarily by glomerular filtration. Patients with impaired renal function or diminished glomerular filtration pressure excrete the drug much more slowly (effectively prolonging the serum half-life). Therefore, renal function should be monitored carefully and dosage adjusted accordingly see suggested dosage schedule under DOSAGE AND ADMINISTRATION.

Following administration at the recommended dose, therapeutic levels are found in bone, heart, gallbladder, and lung tissue in addition to significant concentrations in urine, bile, sputum, bronchial secretions, interstitial, pleural, and synovial fluids.

Spinal fluid levels in normal infants are approximately 10% to 20% of the serum concentrations and may reach 50% when the meninges are inflamed. Amikin has been demonstrated to cross the placental barrier and yield significant concentrations in amniotic fluid. The peak fetal serum concentration is about 16% of the peak maternal serum concentration and maternal and fetal serum half-life values are about 2 and 3.7 hours, respectively.

MICROBIOLOGY

Gram-negative: Amikacin is active *in vitro* against*Pseudomonas* species, *Escherichia coli*, *Proteus* species (indole-positive and indole-negative), *Providencia* species,*Klebsiella-Enterobacter-Serratia* species, *Acinetobacter* (formerly *Mima-Herellea*) species, and *Citrobacter freundii*.

When strains of the above organisms are found to be resistant to other aminoglycosides, including gentamicin, tobramycin and kanamycin, many are susceptible to amikacin *in vitro*.

Gram-positive: Amikacin is active *in vitro* against penicillinase and nonpenicillinase-producing *Staphylococcus* species including methicillin-resistant strains. However, aminoglycosides in general have a low order of activity against other Gram-positive organisms; viz, *Streptococcus pyogenes*, enterococci, and *Streptococcus pneumoniae* (formerly *Diplococcus pneumoniae*).

Amikacin resists degradation by most aminoglycoside inactivating enzymes known to affect gentamicin, tobramycin, and kanamycin.

In vitro studies have shown that Amikin combined with a beta-lactam antibiotic acts synergistically against many clinically significant Gram-negative organisms.

Disc Susceptibility Tests: Quantitative methods that require measurement of zone diameters give the most precise estimates of antibiotic susceptibility. One such procedure* has been recommended for use with discs to test susceptibility to amikacin. Interpretation involves correlation of the diameters obtained in the disc test with MIC values for amikacin. When the causative organism is tested by the Kirby-Bauer method of disc susceptibility, a 30-mcg amikacin disc should give a zone of 17 mm or greater to indicate susceptibility. Zone sizes of 14 mm or less indicate resistance. Zone sizes of 15 to 16 mm indicate intermediate susceptibility. With this procedure, a report from the laboratory of "susceptible" indicates that the infecting organism is likely to respond to therapy. A report of "resistant" indicates that the infecting organism is not likely to respond to therapy. A report of "intermediate susceptibility" suggests that the organism would be susceptible if the infection is confined to tissues and fluids (*e.g.,* urine) in which high antibiotic levels are attained.

INDICATIONS AND USAGE:

Amikin is indicated in the short-term treatment of serious infections due to susceptible strains of Gram-negative bacteria, including*Pseudomonas* species, *Escherichia coli*, species of indole-positive and indole-negative *Proteus*, *Providencia* species,*Klebsiella-Enterobacter-Serratia* species, and *Acinetobacter (Mima-Herellea)* species.

Clinical studies have shown Amikin to be effective in bacterial septicemia (including neonatal sepsis); in serious infections of the respiratory tract, bones and joints, central nervous system (including meningitis) and skin and soft tissue intra-abdominal infections (including peritonitis); and in burns and postoperative infections (including postvascular surgery). Clinical studies have shown Amikin also to be effective in serious complicated and recurrent urinary tract infections due to these organisms. Aminoglycosides, including Amikin injectable, are not indicated in uncomplicated initial episodes of urinary tract infections unless the causative organisms are not susceptible to antibiotics having less potential toxicity.

INDICATIONS AND USAGE: *(cont'd)*

Bacteriologic studies should be performed to identify causative organisms and their susceptibilities to amikacin. Amikin may be considered as initial therapy in suspected Gram-negative infections and therapy may be instituted before obtaining the results of susceptibility testing. Clinical trials demonstrated that Amikin was ineffective in infections caused by gentamicin and/or tobramycin-resistant strains of Gram-negative organisms, particularly *Proteus rettgeri, Providencia stuartii, Serratia marcescens,* and *Pseudomonas aeruginosa.* The decision to continue therapy with the drug should be based on results of the susceptibility tests, the severity of the infection, the response of the patient and the important additional considerations contained in the WARNINGSbox above.

Amikin has also been shown to be effective in staphylococcal infections and may be considered as initial therapy under certain conditions in the treatment of known or suspected staphylococcal disease such as, severe infections where the causative organism may be either a Gram-negative bacterium or a staphylococcus, infections due to susceptible strains of staphylococci in patients allergic to other antibiotics, and in mixed staphylococcal/Gram-negative infections.

In certain severe infections such as neonatal sepsis, concomitant therapy with a penicillin-type drug may be indicated because of the possibility of infections due to Gram-positive organisms such as streptococci or pneumococci.

CONTRAINDICATIONS:

A history of hypersensitivity to amikacin is a contraindication for its use. A history of hypersensitivity or serious toxic reactions to aminoglycosides may contraindicate the use of any other aminoglycosides because of the known cross-sensitivities of patients to drugs in this class.

WARNINGS:

See BOXED WARNING.

Aminoglycosides can cause fetal harm when administered to a pregnant woman. Aminoglycosides cross the placenta and there have been several reports of total irreversible, bilateral congenital deafness in children whose mothers received streptomycin during pregnancy. Although serious side effects to the fetus or newborns have not been reported in the treatment of pregnant women with other aminoglycosides, the potential for harm exists. Reproduction studies of amikacin have been performed in rats and mice and revealed no evidence of impaired fertility or harm to the fetus due to amikacin. There are no well controlled studies in pregnant women, but investigational experience does not include any positive evidence of adverse effects to the fetus. If this drug is used during pregnancy, or if the patient becomes pregnant while taking this drug, the patient should be apprised of the potential hazard to the fetus.

Contains sodium bisulfite, a sulfite that may cause allergic-type reactions including anaphylactic symptoms and life-threatening or less severe asthmatic episodes in certain susceptible people. The overall prevalence of sulfite sensitivity in the general population is unknown and probably low. Sulfite sensitivity is seen more frequently in asthmatic than nonasthmatic people.

PRECAUTIONS:

Aminoglycosides are quickly and almost totally absorbed when they are applied topically, except to the urinary bladder, in association with surgical procedures. Irreversible deafness, renal failure, and death due to neuromuscular blockade have been reported following irritation of both small and large surgical fields with an aminoglycoside preparation.

Amikin is potentially nephrotoxic, ototoxic and neurotoxic. The concurrent or serial use of other ototoxic or nephrotoxic agents should be avoided either systemically or topically because of the potential for additive effects. Increased nephrotoxicity has been reported following concomitant parenteral administration of aminoglycoside antibiotics and cephalosporins. Concomitant cephalosporins may spuriously elevate creatinine determinations.

Since Amikin is present in high concentrations in the renal excretory system, patients should be well hydrated to minimize chemical irritation of the renal tubules. Kidney function should be assessed by the usual methods prior to starting therapy and daily during the course of treatment.

It signs or renal irritation appear (casts, white or red cells, or albumin), hydration should be increased. A reduction in dosage (see DOSAGE AND ADMINISTRATION) may be desirable if other evidence of renal dysfunction occurs such as decreased creatinine clearance; decreased urine specific gravity; increased BUN, creatinine, or oliguria increases or if a progressive decrease in urinary output occurs, treatment should be stopped.

Note: When patients are well hydrated and kidney function is normal the risk of nephrotoxic reactions with amikacin is low if the dosage recommendations (see DOSAGE AND ADMINISTRATION) are not exceeded.

Elderly patients may have reduced renal function which may not be evident in routine screening tests such as BUN or serum creatinine. A creatinine clearance determination may be more useful. Monitoring of renal function during treatment with aminoglycosides is particularly important.

Aminoglycosides should be used with caution in patients with muscular disorders such as myasthenia gravis or parkinsonism since these drugs may aggravate muscle weakness because of their potential curare-like effect on the neuromuscular junction.

In vitro mixing of aminoglycosides with beta-lactam antibiotics (penicillin or cephalosporins) may result in a significant mutual inactivation. A reduction in serum half-life or serum level may occur when an aminoglycoside or penicillin-type drug is administered by separate routes. Inactivation of the aminoglycosides is clinically significant only in patients with severely impaired renal function. Inactivation may continue in specimens of body fluids collected for assay, resulting in inaccurate aminoglycosides readings. Such specimens should be properly handled (assayed promptly, frozen, or treated with beta-lactamase).

Cross-allergenicity among aminoglycosides has been demonstrated.

As with other antibiotics, the use of amikacin may result in overgrowth of nonsusceptible organisms. If this occurs, appropriate therapy should be instituted.

Aminoglycosides should not be given concurrently with potent diuretics (See BOXED WARNING.)

Carcinogenesis, Mutagenesis, and Impairment of Fertility: Long term studies in animals to evaluate carcinogenic potential have not been performed, and mutagenicity has not been studied. Amikin administered subcutaneously to rats at doses up to 4 times the human daily dose did not impair male or female fertility.

Pregnancy Category D: (See WARNINGS.)

Nursing Mothers: It is not known whether Amikin is excreted in human milk. Because many drugs are excreted in human milk and because of the potential for serious adverse reactions in nursing infants from Amikin, a decision should be made whether to discontinue the drug, taking into account the importance of the drug to the mother.

Pediatric Use: Aminoglycosides should be used with caution in premature and neonatal infants because of the renal immaturity of these patients and the resulting prolongation of serum half-life of these drugs.

ADVERSE REACTIONS:

All aminoglycosides have the potential to induce auditory, vestibular, and renal toxicity and neuromuscular blockade (see BOXED WARNING.) They occur more frequently in patients with present or past history of renal impairment, of treatment with other ototoxic or nephrotoxic drugs, and in patients treated for longer periods and/or with higher doses than recommended.

Neurotoxicity-Ototoxicity: Toxic effects on the eighth cranial nerve can result in hearing loss, loss of balance, or both. Amikacin primarily affects auditory function. Cochlear damage includes high frequency deafness and usually occurs before clinical hearing loss can be detected.

Neurotoxicity-Neuromuscular Blockage: Acute muscular paralysis and apnea can occur following treatment with aminoglycosides drugs.

Nephrotoxicity: Elevation of serum creatinine, albuminuria, presence of red and white cells, casts, azotemia, and oliguria have been reported. Renal function changes are usually reversible when the drug is discontinued.

Other: In addition to those described above, other adverse reactions which have been reported on rare occasions are skin rash, drug fever. headache, paresthesia, tremor, nausea and vomiting, eosinophilia, arthralgia, and hypotension.

Overdosage: In the event of overdosage or toxic reaction, peritoneal dialysis or hemodialysis will aid in the removal of amikacin from the blood. In the newborn infant, exchange transfusion may also be considered.

DOSAGE AND ADMINISTRATION:

The patient's pretreatment body weight should be obtained for calculation of correct dosage. Amikin may be given intramuscularly or intravenously.

The status of renal function should be estimated by measurement of the serum creatinine concentration or calculation of the endogenous creatinine clearance rate. The blood urea nitrogen (BUN) is much less reliable for this purpose. Reassessment of renal function should be made periodically during therapy.

Whenever possible, amikacin concentrations in serum should be measured to assure adequate but not excessive levels. It is desirable to measure both peak and tough serum concentrations intermittently during therapy. Peak concentrations (30 to 90 minutes after injection) above 35 mcg per ml and trough concentrations (just prior to the next dose) above 10 mcg per ml should be avoided. Dosage should be adjusted as indicated.

Intramuscular Administration for Patients with Normal Renal Function: The recommended dosage for adults, children and older infants (see BOXED WARNING) with normal renal function is 15 mg/kg/day divided into 2 or 3 equal doses administered at equally-divided intervals i.e., 7.5 mg/kg q.12h or 5 mg/kg q.8h. Treatment of patients in the heavier weight classes should not exceed 1.5 g/day.

When amikacin is indicated is newborns (see BOXED WARNING), it is recommended that a loading dose of 10 mg/kg be administered initially to be followed with 7.5 mg/kg every 12 hours.

The usual duration of treatment is 7 to 10 days. It is desirable to limit the duration of treatment to short term whenever feasible. The total daily dose by all routes of administration should not exceed 15 mg/kg/day. In difficult and complicated infections where treatment beyond 10 days is considered, the use of Amikin should be reevaluated. It continued, amikacin serum levels, and renal, auditory, and vestibular functions should be monitored. At the recommended dosage level, uncomplicated infections due to amikacin-sensitive organisms should respond in 24 to 48 hours, If definite clinical response does not occur within 3 to 5 days, therapy should be stopped and the antibiotic susceptibility patterns of the invading organism should be rechecked. Failure of the infection to respond may be due to resistance of the organism or to the presence of septic foci requiring surgical drainage.

When Amikin is indicated in uncomplicated urinary tract infections, a dose of 250 mg twice daily may be used (TABLE 1):

TABLE 1 Dosage Guidelines: Adult And Children With Normal Renal Function

Patient Weight		Dosage	
lbs	kg	7.5 mg/kg q. 12h OR	5 mg/kg q. 8h
99	45	337.5 mg	225 mg
110	50	375 mg	250 mg
121	55	412.5 mg	275 mg
132	60	450 mg	300 mg
143	65	487.5 mg	325 mg
154	70	525 mg	350 mg
165	75	562.6 mg	375 mg
176	80	600 mg	400 mg
187	85	637.5 mg	425 mg
198	90	675 mg	450 mg
209	95	712.5 mg	475 mg
220	100	750 mg	500 mg

Available as: 100 mg/2 ml vial, 500 mg/2 ml vial, 1 g/4 ml vial, 500 mg/2 ml Disposable Syringe

Intramuscular Administration for Patients with Impaired Renal Function: Whenever possible, serum amikacin concentrations should be monitored by appropriate assay procedures. Doses may be adjusted in patients with impaired renal function either by administering normal doses at prolonged intervals or by administering reduced doses at a fixed interval.

Both methods are based on the patient's creatinine clearance or serum creatinine values since these have been found to correlate with aminoglycoside half-lives in patients with diminished renal function. These dosage schedules must be used in conjunction with careful clinical and laboratory observations of the patient and should be modified as necessary. Neither method should be used when dialysis is being performed.

Normal Dosage at Prolonged Intervals: If the creatinine clearance rate is not available and the patient's condition is stable, a dosage interval in hours for the normal dose can be calculated by multiplying the patient's serum creatinine by 9, e.g., if the serum creatinine concentration is 2 mg/100 ml, the recommended single dose (7.5 mg/kg) should be administered every 18 hours.

Reduced Dosage at Fixed Time Intervals: When renal function is impaired and it is desirable to administer Amikin at a fixed time interval, dosage must be reduced. In these patients, serum Amikin concentrations should be measured to assure accurate administration of Amikin and to avoid concentrations above 35 mcg/ml. If serum assay determinations are not available and the patient's condition is stable, serum creatinine and creatinine clearance values are the most readily available indicators of the degree of renal impairment to use as a guide for dosage.

First, initiate therapy by administering a normal dose, 7.5 mg/kg, as a loading dose. This loading dose is the same as the normally recommended dose which would be calculated for a patient with normal renal function as described above.

DOSAGE AND ADMINISTRATION: *(cont'd)*

To determine the size of maintenance doses administered every 12 hours, the loading dose should be reduced in proportion to the reduction in the patient's creatinine clearance rate (TABLE 2):

TABLE 2

Maintenance Dose Every 12 Hours = [(observed CC in ml/min) ÷ (normal CC in ml/min)] × calculated loading dose in mg
(CC - creatinine clearance rate)

An alternate rough guide for determining reduced dosage at 12-hours intervals (for patients whose steady state serum creatinine values are known) is to divide the normally recommended dose by the patient's serum creatinine.

The above dosage schedules are not intended to be rigid recommendations but are provided as guides to dosage when the measurement of amikacin serum levels is not feasible.

Intravenous Administration: The individual dose, the total daily dose, and the total cumulative dose of Amikin are identical to the dose recommended for intramuscular administration. The solution of intravenous use is prepared by adding the contents of a 500 mg vial to 100 or 200 ml of sterile diluent such as Normal Saline or 5% Dextrose in Water or any of the compatible solutions listed below.

The solution is administered to adults over a 30 to 60 minute period. The total daily dose should not exceed 15 mg/kg/day and may be divided into either 2 or 3 equally-divided doses at equally-divided intervals.

In pediatric patients the amount of fluid used will depend on the amount of Amikin ordered for the patient. It should be a sufficient amount to infuse the Amikin over a 30 to 60 minute period. Infants should receive a 1 to 2 hour infusion.

Stability in IV Fluids: Amikin is stable for 24 hours at room temperature at concentrations of 0.25 and 5.0 mg/ml in the following solutions:

5% Dextrose Injection, USP

5% Dextrose and 0.2% Sodium Chloride Injection, USP

5% Dextrose and 0.45% Sodium Chloride Injection, USP

0.9% Sodium Chloride Injection, USP

Lactated Ringer's Injection, USP

NormosolM in 5% Dextrose Injection, USP (or Plasma-Lyte 56 Injection in 5% Dextrose in Water)

NormosolR in 5% Dextrose Injection, USP (or Plasma-Lyte 148 Injection in 5% Dextrose in Water)

In the above solutions with Amikin concentrations of 0.25 and 5.0 mg/ml, solutions aged for 60 days at 4° C and then stored at 25° C had utility times of 24 hours.

At the same concentrations, solutions frozen and aged for 30 days at -15° C, thawed, and stored at 25° C had utility times of 24 hours.

Parenteral drug products should be inspected visually for particulate matter and discoloration prior to administration whenever the solution and container permit.

Aminoglycosides administered by any of the above routes should not be physically premixed with other drugs but should be administered separately.

Because of the potential toxicity of aminoglycosides, "fixed dosage" recommendations which are not based upon body weight are not advised. Rather, it is essential to calculate the dosage to fit the needs of each patient.

REFERENCES:

* Bauer, A.W., Kirby, W.M.M., Sherris, J.C., and Turck, M.: Antibiotic Testing by a Standardized Single Disc Method, Am. J. Clin. Pathol., 45:493, 1966; Standardized Disc Susceptibility Test, FEDERAL REGISTER, 37: 20527-29, 1972.

HOW SUPPLIED:

Amikin (sterile amikacin sulfate infection) is supplied in vials as a colorless solution which requires no refrigeration. It is stable at room temperature for 2 years. At times the solution may become a very pale yellow; this does not indicate a decrease in potency.

HOW SUPPLIED - RATED THERAPEUTICALLY EQUIVALENT:

Injection, Solution - Intramuscular; - 50 mg/ml

2 ml	**$35.25**	**AMIKIN, Mead Johnson**	**00015-3015-20**
2 ml	$81.94	AMIKACIN SULFATE, Abbott	00074-1955-01
2 ml x 10	$325.00	Amikacin Sulfate, Bedford Labs	55390-0225-02
2 ml x 10	$369.96	Amikacin Sulfate, Gensia Labs	00703-9022-03
2 ml x 10	$400.00	Amikacin Sulfate, Jordan Pharms	58196-0240-38

Injection, Solution - Intramuscular; - 250 mg/ml

2 ml	**$47.00**	**AMIKIN, Mead Johnson**	**00015-3020-20**
2 ml	**$47.00**	**AMIKIN, Mead Johnson**	**00015-3020-97**
2 ml	**$68.56**	**AMIKIN, SYRINGE, Mead Johnson**	**00015-3020-21**
2 ml	$99.75	AMIKACIN SULFATE, Abbott	00074-1956-01
2 ml	$110.44	AMIKACIN SULFATE, Abbott	00074-1958-01
2 ml x 10	$437.50	Amikacin Sulfate, Bedford Labs	55390-0226-02
2 ml x 10	$626.88	Amikacin Sulfate, Gensia Labs	00703-9032-03
2 ml x 10	$637.50	Amikacin Sulfate, Elkins Sinn	00641-0123-23
4 ml	**$92.87**	**AMIKIN, Mead Johnson**	**00015-3023-20**
4 ml	$203.06	AMIKACIN SULFATE, Abbott	00074-1957-01
4 ml x 10	$875.00	Amikacin Sulfate, Bedford Labs	55390-0226-04
4 ml x 10	$1200.00	Amikacin Sulfate, Elkins Sinn	00641-2357-43
4 ml x 10	$1269.24	Amikacin Sulfate, Gensia Labs	00703-9040-03
50 ml	$1015.31	AMIKACIN SULFATE, Abbott	00074-3212-02

HOW SUPPLIED - NOT RATED EQUIVALENT:

Injection, Solution - Intravenous - 62.5 mg/ml

8 ml	$103.31	AMIKACIN SULFATE, Abbott	00074-2434-03

AMILORIDE HYDROCHLORIDE *(000179)*

CATEGORIES: Antihypertensives; Congestive Heart Failure; Diuretics; Electrolyte Solutions; Homeostatic & Nutrient; Hypertension; Hypokalemia; Potassium Sparing Diuretics; Renal Drugs; Pregnancy Category B; FDA Approval Pre 1982

BRAND NAMES: *Amilo*; *Amikal*; *Amilospare*; *Arumil*; *Kaluril*; *Medamor*; **Midamor**; *Midoride*; *Modamide* (France); *Nirulid*; *Pandiuren*; *Puritrid*; *Ride*
(International brand names outside U.S. in italics)

FORMULARIES: Aetna; WHO

COST OF THERAPY: $93.07 (Hypertension; Tablet; 5 mg; 1/day; 365 days)

PRIMARY ICD9: 401.1 (Essential Hypertension, Benign)

DESCRIPTION:

Amiloride HCl, an antikaliuretic-diuretic agent, is a pyrazine-carbonyl-guanidine that is unrelated chemically to other known antikaliuretic or diuretic agents. It is the salt of a moderately strong base (pKa 8.7). It is designated chemically as 3,5-diamino-6-chloro-*N*-(diaminomethylene)pyrazinecarboxamide monohydrochloride, dihydrate and has a molecular weight of 302.14. Its empirical formula is $C_6H_8ClN_7O{\cdot}HCl{\cdot}2H_2O$.

Amiloride HCl is available for oral use as tablets containing 5 mg of anhydrous amiloride HCl. Each tablet contains the following inactive ingredients: calcium phosphate, D&C Yellow 10, iron oxide, lactose, magnesium stearate and starch.

CLINICAL PHARMACOLOGY:

Amiloride HCl is a potassium-conserving (antikaliuretic) drug that possesses weak (compared with thiazide diuretics) natriuretic, diuretic, and antihypertensive activity. These effects have been partially additive to the effects of thiazide diuretics in some clinical studies. When administered with a thiazide or loop diuretic, amiloride HCl has been shown to decrease the enhanced urinary excretion of magnesium which occurs when a thiazide or loop diuretic is used alone. Amiloride HCl has potassium-conserving activity in patients receiving kaliuretic-diuretic agents.

Amiloride HCl is not an aldosterone antagonist and its effects are seen even in the absence of aldosterone.

Amiloride HCl exerts its potassium sparing effect through the inhibition of sodium reabsorption at the distal convoluted tubule, cortical collecting tubule and collecting duct; this decreases the net negative potential of the tubular lumen and reduces both potassium and hydrogen secretion and their subsequent excretion. This mechanism accounts in large part for the potassium sparing action of amiloride.

Amiloride HCl usually begins to act within 2 hours after an oral dose. Its effect on electrolyte excretion reaches a peak between 6 and 10 hours and lasts about 24 hours. Peak plasma levels are obtained in 3 to 4 hours and the plasma half-life varies from 6 to 9 hours. Effects on electrolytes increase with single doses of amiloride HCl up to approximately 15 mg.

Amiloride HCl is not metabolized by the liver but is excreted unchanged by the kidneys. About 50 percent of a 20 mg dose of amiloride HCl is excreted in the urine and 40 percent in the stool within 72 hours. Amiloride HCl has little effect on glomerular filtration rate or renal blood flow. Because amiloride HCl is not metabolized by the liver, drug accumulation is not anticipated in patients with hepatic dysfunction, but accumulation can occur if the hepatorenal syndrome develops.

INDICATIONS AND USAGE:

Amiloride HCl is indicated as adjunctive treatment with thiazide diuretics or other kaliuretic-diuretic agents in congestive heart failure or hypertension to:

a. help restore normal serum potassium levels in patients who develop hypokalemia on the kaliuretic diuretic

b. prevent development of hypokalemia in patients who would be exposed to particular risk if hypokalemia were to develop, e.g., digitalized patients or patients with significant cardiac arrhythmias.

The use of potassium-conserving agents is often unnecessary in patients receiving diuretics for uncomplicated essential hypertension when such patients have a normal diet. Amiloride HCl has little additive diuretic or antihypertensive effect when added to a thiazide diuretic.

Amiloride HCl should rarely be used alone. It has weak (compared with thiazides) diuretic and antihypertensive effects. Used as single agents, potassium sparing diuretics, including amiloride HCl, result in an increased risk of hyperkalemia (approximately 10% with amiloride). Amiloride HCl should be used alone only when persistent hypokalemia has been documented and only with careful titration of the dose and close monitoring of serum electrolytes.

CONTRAINDICATIONS:

Hyperkalemia: Amiloride HCl should not be used in the presence of elevated serum potassium levels (greater than 5.5 mEq per liter).

Antikaliuretic Therapy or Potassium Supplementation: Amiloride HCl should not be given to patients receiving other potassium-conserving agents, such as spironolactone or triamterene. Potassium supplementation in the form of medication, potassium-containing salt substitutes or a potassium-rich diet should not be used with amiloride HCl except in severe and/or refractory cases of hypokalemia. Such concomitant therapy can be associated with rapid increases in serum potassium levels. If potassium supplementation is used, careful monitoring of the serum potassium level is necessary.

Impaired Renal Function: Anuria, acute or chronic renal insufficiency, and evidence of diabetic nephropathy are contraindications to the use of amiloride HCl. Patients with evidence of renal functional impairment (blood urea nitrogen (BUN) levels over 30 mg per 100 ml or serum creatinine levels over 1.5 mg per 100 ml) or diabetes mellitus should not receive the drug without careful, frequent and continuing monitoring of serum electrolytes, creatinine, and BUN levels. Potassium retention associated with the use of an antikaliuretic agent is accentuated in the presence of renal impairment and may result in the rapid development of hyperkalemia.

Hypersensitivity: Amiloride HCl is contraindicated in patients who are hypersensitive to this product.

WARNINGS:

HYPERKALEMIA

Like other potassium-conserving agents, amiloride may cause hyperkalemia (serum potassium levels greater than 5.5 mEq per liter) which, if uncorrected, is potentially fatal. Hyperkalemia occurs commonly (about 10%) when amiloride is used without a kaliuretic diuretic. This incidence is greater in patients with renal impairment, diabetes mellitus (with or without recognized renal insufficiency), and in the elderly. When amiloride HCl is used concomitantly with a thiazide diuretic in patients without these complications, the risk of hyperkalemia is reduced to about 1-2 percent. It is thus essential to monitor serum potassium levels carefully in any patient receiving amiloride, particularly when it is first introduced, at the time of diuretic dosage adjustments, and during any illness that could affect renal function.

The risk of hyperkalemia may be increased when potassium-conserving agents, including amiloride HCl, are administered concomitantly with an angiotensin-converting enzyme inhibitor. See DRUG INTERACTIONS. Warning signs or symptoms of hyperkalemia include paresthesias, muscular weakness, fatigue, flaccid paralysis of the extremities, bradycardia, shock, and ECG abnormalities. Monitoring of the serum potassium level is essential because mild hyperkalemia is not usually associated with an abnormal ECG.

WARNINGS: *(cont'd)*

When abnormal, the ECG in hyperkalemia is characterized primarily by tall, peaked T waves or elevations from previous tracings. There may also be lowering of the R wave and increased depth of the S wave, widening and even disappearance of the P wave, progressive widening of the QRS complex, prolongation of the PR interval, and ST depression.

Treatment of Hyperkalemia: If hyperkalemia occurs in patients taking amiloride HCl, the drug should be discontinued immediately. If the serum potassium level exceeds 6.5 mEq per liter, active measures should be taken to reduce it. Such measures include the intravenous administration of sodium bicarbonate solution or oral or parenteral glucose with a rapid-acting insulin preparation. If needed, a cation exchange resin such as sodium polystyrene sulfonate may be given orally or by enema. Patients with persistent hyperkalemia may require dialysis.

DIABETES MELLITUS

In diabetic patients, hyperkalemia has been reported with the use of all potassium-conserving diuretics, including amiloride HCl, even in patients without evidence of diabetic nephropathy. Therefore, amiloride HCl should be avoided, if possible, in diabetic patients and, if it is used, serum electrolytes and renal function must be monitored frequently.

Amiloride HCl should be discontinued at least three days before glucose tolerance testing.

METABOLIC OR RESPIRATORY ACIDOSIS

Antikaliuretic therapy should be instituted only with caution in severely ill patients in whom respiratory or metabolic acidosis may occur, such as patients with cardiopulmonary disease or poorly controlled diabetes. If amiloride HCl is given to these patients, frequent monitoring of acid-base balance is necessary. Shifts in acid-base balance alter the ratio of extracellular/intracellular potassium, and the development of acidosis may be associated with rapid increases in serum potassium levels.

PRECAUTIONS:

GENERAL

Electrolyte Imbalance and BUN Increases: Hyponatremia and hypochloremia may occur when amiloride HCl is used with other diuretics and increases in BUN levels have been reported. These increases usually have accompanied vigorous fluid elimination, especially when diuretic therapy was used in seriously ill patients, such as those who had hepatic cirrhosis with ascites and metabolic alkalosis, or those with resistant edema. Therefore, when amiloride HCl is given with other diuretics to such patients, careful monitoring of serum electrolytes and BUN levels is important. In patients with pre-existing severe liver disease, hepatic encephalopathy, manifested by tremors, confusion, and coma, and increased jaundice, have been reported in association with diuretics, including amiloride HCl.

CARCINOGENICITY, MUTAGENICITY, IMPAIRMENT OF FERTILITY

There was no evidence of a tumorigenic effect when amiloride HCl was administered for 92 weeks to mice at doses up to 10 mg/kg/day (25 times the maximum daily human dose). Amiloride HCl has also been administered for 104 weeks to male and female rats at doses up to 6 and 8 mg/kg/day (15 and 20 times the maximum daily dose for humans, respectively) and showed no evidence of carcinogenicity.

Amiloride HCl was devoid of mutagenic activity in various strains of *Salmonella typhimurium* with or without a mammalian liver microsomal activation system (Ames test).

PREGNANCY CATEGORY B

Teratogenicity studies with amiloride HCl in rabbits and mice given 20 and 25 times the maximum human dose, respectively, revealed no evidence of harm to the fetus, although studies showed that the drug crossed the placenta in modest amounts. Reproduction studies in rats at 20 times the expected maximum daily dose for humans showed no evidence of impaired fertility. At approximately 5 or more times the expected maximum daily dose for humans, some toxicity was seen in adult rats and rabbits and a decrease in rat pup growth and survival occurred.

There are, however, no adequate and well-controlled studies in pregnant women. Because animal reproduction studies are not always predictive of human response, this drug should be used during pregnancy only if clearly needed.

NURSING MOTHERS

Studies in rats have shown that amiloride is excreted in milk in concentrations higher than that found in blood, but it is not known whether amiloride HCl is excreted in human milk. Because many drugs are excreted in human milk and because of the potential for serious adverse reactions in nursing infants from amiloride HCl, a decision should be made whether to discontinue nursing or to discontinue the drug, taking into account the importance of the drug to the mother.

PEDIATRIC USE

Safety and effectiveness in children have not been established.

DRUG INTERACTIONS:

When amiloride HCl is administered concomitantly with an angiotensin-converting enzyme inhibitor, the risk of hyperkalemia may be increased. Therefore, if concomitant use of these agents is indicated because of demonstrated hypokalemia, they should be used with caution and with frequent monitoring of serum potassium. (See WARNINGS.)

Lithium generally should not be given with diuretics because they reduce its renal clearance and add a high risk of lithium toxicity. Read circulars for lithium preparations before use of such concomitant therapy.

In some patients, the administration of a non-steroidal anti-inflammatory agent can reduce the diuretic, natriuretic, and antihypertensive effects of loop, potassium-sparing and thiazide diuretics. Therefore, when amiloride HCl and non-steroidal anti-inflammatory agents are used concomitantly, the patient should be observed closely to determine if the desired effect of the diuretic is obtained. Since indomethacin and potassium-sparing diuretics, including amiloride HCl, each may be associated with increased serum potassium levels, the potential effects on potassium kinetics and renal function should be considered when these agents are administered concurrently.

ADVERSE REACTIONS:

Amiloride HCl is usually well tolerated and, except for hyperkalemia (serum potassium levels greater than 5.5 mEq per liter (see WARNINGS), significant adverse effects have been reported infrequently. Minor adverse reactions were reported relatively frequently (about 20%) but the relationship of many of the reports to amiloride HCl is uncertain and the overall frequency was similar in hydrochlorothiazide treated groups. Nausea/anorexia, abdominal pain, flatulence, and mild skin rash have been reported and probably are related to amiloride. Other adverse experiences that have been reported with amiloride are generally those known to be associated with diuresis, or with the underlying disease being treated.

The adverse reactions for amiloride HCl listed in TABLE 1 have been arranged into two groups: (1) incidence greater than one percent; and (2) incidence one percent or less. The incidence for group (1) was determined from clinical studies conducted in the United States (837 patients treated with amiloride HCl). The adverse effects listed in group (2) include reports from the same clinical studies and voluntary reports since marketing. The probability of a causal relationship exists between amiloride HCl and these adverse reactions, some of which have been reported only rarely.

ADVERSE REACTIONS: *(cont'd)*

TABLE 1

	Incidence >1%	Incidence ≤ 1%
Body As A Whole	Headache* Weakness Fatigability	Back pain Chest pain Neck/shoulder ache Pain, extremities
Cardiovascular	None	Angina pectoris Orthostatic hypotension Arrhythmia Palpitation
Digestive	Nausea/anorexia* Diarrhea* Vomiting* Abdominal pain Gas pain Appetite changes Constipation	Jaundice GI bleeding Abdominal fullness GI disturbance Thirst Heartburn Flatulence Dyspepsia
Metabolic	Elevated serum potassium levels (>5.5 mEq per liter)†	None
Integumentary	None	Skin rash Itching Dryness of mouth Pruritus Alopecia
Musculoskeletal	Muscle cramps	Joint pain Leg ache
Nervous	Dizziness Encephalopathy	Paresthesia Tremors Vertigo
Psychiatric	None	Nervousness Mental confusion Insomnia Decreased libido Depression Somnolence
Respiratory	Cough Dyspnea	Shortness of breath
Special Senses	None	Visual disturbances Nasal congestion Tinnitus Increased intraocular pressure
Urogenital	Impotence	Polyuria Dysuria Urinary frequency Bladder spasms

* Reactions occurring in 3% to 8% of patients treated with Amiloride HCl. (Those reactions occurring in less than 3% of the patients are unmarked.)
† See WARNINGS.

CAUSAL RELATIONSHIP UNKNOWN

Other reactions have been reported but occurred under circumstances where a causal relationship could not be established. However, in these rarely reported events, that possibility cannot be excluded. Therefore, these observations are listed to serve as alerting information to physicians.

Activation of probable pre-existing peptic ulcer

Aplastic anemia

Neutropenia

Abnormal liver function

OVERDOSAGE:

No data are available in regard to overdosage in humans.

The oral LD_{50} of amiloride hydrochloride (calculated as the base) is 56 mg/kg in mice and 36 to 85 mg/kg in rats, depending on the strain.

It is not known whether the drug is dialyzable.

The most likely signs and symptoms to be expected with overdosage are dehydration and electrolyte imbalance. These can be treated by established procedures. Therapy with amiloride HCl should be discontinued and the patient observed closely. There is no specific antidote. Emesis should be induced or gastric lavage performed. Treatment is symptomatic and supportive. If hyperkalemia occurs, active measures should be taken to reduce the serum potassium levels.

DOSAGE AND ADMINISTRATION:

Amiloride HCl should be administered with food.

Amiloride HCl, one 5 mg tablet daily, should be added to the usual antihypertensive or diuretic dosage of a kaliuretic diuretic. The dosage may be increased to 10 mg per day, if necessary. More than two 5 mg tablets of amiloride HCl daily usually are not needed, and there is little controlled experience with such doses. If persistent hypokalemia is documented with 10 mg, the dose can be increased to 15 mg, then 20 mg, with careful monitoring of electrolytes.

In treating patients with congestive heart failure after an initial diuresis has been achieved, potassium loss may also decrease and the need for amiloride HCl should be re-evaluated. Dosage adjustment may be necessary. Maintenance therapy may be on an intermittent basis.

If it is necessary to use amiloride HCl alone (see INDICATIONS AND USAGE), the starting dosage should be one 5 mg tablet daily. This dosage may be increased to 10 mg per day, if necessary. More than two 5 mg tablets usually are not needed, and there is little controlled experience with such doses. If persistent hypokalemia is documented with 10 mg, the dose can be increased to 15 mg, then 20 mg, with careful monitoring of electrolytes.

STORAGE

Protect from moisture, freezing and excessive heat.

HOW SUPPLIED - RATED THERAPEUTICALLY EQUIVALENT:

Tablet, Uncoated - Oral - 5 mg

100's	$25.50	Amiloride Hcl, IDE-Interstate	00814-4060-14
100's	$25.64	Amiloride Hcl, HL Moore Drug Exch	00839-7181-06
100's	$27.35	Amiloride Hcl, Aligen Independ	00405-4047-01
100's	$29.50	Amiloride Hcl, Harber Pharm	51432-0710-03
100's	$37.07	Amiloride Hcl, Par Pharm	49884-0117-01
100's	**$46.08**	**MIDAMOR, Merck**	**00006-0092-68**
500's	$175.09	Amiloride Hcl, Par Pharm	49884-0117-05
1000's	$276.29	Amiloride Hcl, Par Pharm	49884-0117-10

AMILORIDE HYDROCHLORIDE; HYDROCHLOROTHIAZIDE *(000180)*

CATEGORIES: Antihypertensives; Cardiovascular Drugs; Congestive Heart Failure; Diuretics; Electrolyte Solutions; Electrolytic, Caloric-Water Balance; Hypertension; Potassium Sparing Diuretics; Renal Drugs; Thiazides; Pregnancy Category B; Sales > $100 Million; FDA Approval Pre 1982

BRAND NAMES: *Adco-Retic*; *Add-Acten*; *Ameide*; *Ameride*; *Amil-Co* (England); *Amilco*; *Amilco Mite*; *Amilide*; *Amiloretic*; Amiloride Hcl W/Hctz; *Amiloscan*; *Amithiazide*; *Amitrid*; *Amitrid Mite*; *Amizide* (Australia); *Betaretic*; Hydro-Ride; *Hydrozide*; *Hyperetic*; *Kaluril*; *Lorinid*; *Lorinid Mite*; *Lorizide*; *Miduret*; *Modizide*; *Moduret* (Canada); **Moduretic**; *Moduretic Mite*; *Nirulid*; *Pandiuren*; *Rhefluin* (Mexico); *Scandiuret*; *Tiaden*; *Uniretic*
(International brand names outside U.S. in italics)

FORMULARIES: Aetna

COST OF THERAPY: $24.38 (Hypertension; Tablet; 5 mg/50 mg; 1/day; 365 days) vs. Potential Cost of $24,027.04 (Coronary Bypass)

PRIMARY ICD9: 401.1 (Essential Hypertension, Benign)

DESCRIPTION:

Amiloride hydrochloride with hydrochlorothiazide (miloride w/ HCTZ) combines the potassium-conserving action of amiloride HCl with the natriuretic action of hydrochlorothiazide.

FOR COMPLETE PRESCRIBING INFORMATION, REFER TO THE INDIVIDUAL DRUG MONOGRAPHS (AMILORIDE HYDROCHLORIDE; HYDROCHLOROTHIAZIDE).

INDICATIONS AND USAGE:

Amiloride HCl w/ HCTZ is indicated in those patients with hypertension or with congestive heart failure who develop hypokalemia when thiazides or other kaliuretic diuretics are used alone, or in whom maintenance of normal serum potassium levels is considered to be clinically important, e.g., digitalized patients, or patients with significant cardiac arrhythmias.

The use of potassium-conserving agents is often unnecessary in patients receiving diuretics for uncomplicated essential hypertension when such patients have a normal diet.

Amiloride HCl w/ HCTZ may be used alone or as an adjunct to other antihypertensive drugs, such as methyldopa or beta blockers. Since amiloride HCl w/ HCTZ enhances the action of these agents, dosage adjustments may be necessary to avoid an excessive fall in blood pressure and other unwanted side effects.

This fixed combination drug is not indicated for the initial therapy of edema or hypertension except in individuals in whom the development of hypokalemia cannot be risked.

DOSAGE AND ADMINISTRATION:

Amiloride HCl w/ HCTZ should be administered with food.

The usual starting dosage is 1 tablet a day. The dosage may be increased to 2 tablets a day, if necessary. More than 2 tablets of amiloride HCl w/ HCTZ daily usually are not needed and there is no controlled experience with such doses. The daily dose is usually given as a single dose but may be given in divided doses. Once an initial diuresis has been achieved, dosage adjustment may be necessary. Maintenance therapy may be on an intermittent basis.

Storage: Keep container tightly closed. Protect from light, moisture, freezing, -20°C (-4°F) and store at room temperature, 15-30°C (59-86°F).

HOW SUPPLIED - RATED THERAPEUTICALLY EQUIVALENT:

Tablet - Oral - 5 mg/ 50 mg

100's	$38.95	Amiloride HCl & HCTZ, Mylan	00378-0577-01

Tablet - Oral - 5/50 mg

100's	$38.50	Amiloride Hcl; HCTZ, Duramed Pharms	51285-0885-02
1000's	$368.00	Amiloride Hcl; HCTZ, Duramed Pharms	51285-0885-05

Tablet, Uncoated - Oral - 5 mg/50 mg

100's	$6.68	Amiloride HCL w/HCTZ, United Res	00677-1223-01
100's	$7.08	Amiloride HCL w/HCTZ, H.C.F.A. F F P	99999-0180-01
100's	$28.81	Amiloride HCL w/HCTZ, Barr	00555-0483-02
100's	$28.90	Amiloride HCL w/HCTZ, Teva	00332-2205-09
100's	$32.45	Amiloride HCL w/HCTZ, Schein Pharm (US)	00364-2260-01
100's	$32.55	Amiloride Hcl & Hydrochlorothiazide, Major Pharms	00904-2113-60
100's	$32.55	Amiloride Hcl W/Hctz, Major Pharms	00904-2114-60
100's	$32.75	Amiloride Hcl W/Hctz, West Point Pharma	59591-0162-68
100's	$32.75	Amiloride Hcl W/Hctz, Endo Labs	60951-0764-70
100's	$33.34	Amiloride Hcl W/Hctz, Qualitest Pharms	00603-2188-21
100's	$33.90	Amiloride Hcl & Hydrochlorothiazi, Aligen Independ	00405-4053-01
100's	$34.75	Moduretic, Rugby	00536-5699-01
100's	$34.97	Amiloride HCL w/HCTZ, Vangard Labs	00615-3516-13
100's	$36.30	Amiloride HCL w/HCTZ, Major Pharms	00904-2113-61
100's	$37.95	Amiloride Hcl W/Hctz, Martec Pharms	52555-0338-01
100's	$38.00	Amiloride HCL w/HCTZ, Goldline Labs	00182-1877-01
100's	$38.00	Amiloride Hcl W/Hctz, Royce	51875-0358-01
100's	$38.50	Amiloride HCL w/HCTZ, Geneva Pharms	00781-1119-01
100's	$40.00	Amiloride Hcl W/Hctz, Raway	00686-0421-20
100's	**$46.06**	**MODURETIC, Merck**	**00006-0917-54**
100's	**$52.08**	**MODURETIC 5-50, Merck**	**00006-0917-68**
100's	**$56.38**	**MODURETIC 5-50, Merck**	**00006-0917-28**
100's	$242.33	Amiloride HCL w/HCTZ, HL Moore Drug Exch	00839-7446-16
500's	$35.40	Amiloride HCL w/HCTZ, H.C.F.A. F F P	99999-0180-03
1000's	$30.44	Amiloride HCL w/HCTZ, HL Moore Drug Exch	00839-7446-06
1000's	$70.80	Amiloride HCL w/HCTZ, H.C.F.A. F F P	99999-0180-02
1000's	$255.00	Amiloride HCL w/HCTZ, Teva	00332-2205-15
1000's	$255.60	Amiloride Hcl W/Hctz, Martec Pharms	52555-0338-10
1000's	$272.10	Amiloride Hcl & Hydrochlorothiazide, Major Pharms	00904-2113-80
1000's	$272.10	Amiloride Hcl W/Hctz, Major Pharms	00904-2114-80
1000's	$273.69	Amiloride HCL w/HCTZ, Barr	00555-0483-05
1000's	$279.50	Amiloride HCL w/HCTZ, Schein Pharm (US)	00364-2260-02
1000's	$280.00	Amiloride Hcl W/Hctz, United Res	00677-1223-10
1000's	$280.08	Moduretic, Rugby	00536-5699-10
1000's	$313.58	Amiloride Hcl W/Hctz, Qualitest Pharms	00603-2188-32
1000's	$360.00	Amiloride Hcl W/Hctz, Royce	51875-0358-04

AMINO ACETATE; DEXTROSE; ELECTROLYTES *(000183)*

CATEGORIES: Caloric Agents; Electrolytic, Caloric-Water Balance; Homeostatic & Nutrient; Nutrition, Enteral/Parenteral; FDA Pre 1938 Drugs

BRAND NAMES: *Aminomel 10 G-E* (Germany); *Aminomel 6 G-E* (Germany); *Aminomel 8 G-E* (Germany); *Aminosol*; Aminosyn; Freamine IIi; *Laev-Amin 2.5%*; *Laev-Amin 10%*; Parenteral Nutrition Kit; *Plasamin*; *Synthamin 8% with Dextrose 50%*; *Synthamin 10% with Dextrose 50%*; Travasol; *Vamin*; *Vamin 9*; *Vamin 9 glucose* (England); *Vamin glucose*; *Vamin Glucose*; *Vamin glukos*; *Vamina Mit glucose*
(International brand names outside U.S. in italics)

Prescribing information not available at time of publication.

HOW SUPPLIED - EQUIVALENTS NOT AVAILABLE:

Injection, Solution - Intravenous

1's	$77.66	PARENTERAL NUTRITION KIT, Baxter Hlthcare	00338-0783-98
1's	$84.56	PARENTERAL NUTRITION KIT, Baxter Hlthcare	00338-0785-98
1's	$100.87	PARENTERAL NUTRITION KIT, Baxter Hlthcare	00338-0787-98
1's	$107.81	PARENTERAL NUTRITION KIT, Baxter Hlthcare	00338-0789-98

Injection, Solution - Intravenous - 8.5 %

3 kits	$102.78	FREAMINE III - HYPERALIMENTATION KIT, McGaw	00264-1167-90

AMINO ACIDS *(000185)*

CATEGORIES: Caloric Agents; Electrolytic, Caloric-Water Balance; Homeostatic & Nutrient; Nutrition, Enteral/Parenteral; Vitamins; FDA Approval Pre 1982

BRAND NAMES: Aminess; Aminess 5.2% Essential Amino Acids W/ Histadine; Aminosyn 10%; Aminosyn 10% (Ph6); Aminosyn 3.5%; Aminosyn 5%; Aminosyn 7%; Aminosyn 7% (Ph6); Aminosyn 8.5%; Aminosyn 8.5% (Ph6); Aminosyn II 10%; Aminosyn II 3.5%; Aminosyn II 3.5%/Dextrose 25%; Aminosyn II 3.5%/Dextrose 5%; Aminosyn II 4.25%/Dextrose 10%; Aminosyn II 4.25%/Dextrose 20%; Aminosyn II 4.25%/Dextrose 25%; Aminosyn II 5%; Aminosyn II 7%; Aminosyn II 8.5%; Aminosyn II In Dextrose; Aminosyn W/25% Dextrose; Aminosyn W/5Pc Dextrose; Aminosyn-Hbc 7%; Aminosyn-Pf 10%; Aminosyn-Pf 7%; Aminosyn-Rf 5.2%; Branchamin; Branchamin 4%; Freamine Hbc 6.9%; Freamine IIi; Freamine IIi 10%; Freamine IIi 8.5%; Hepatamine 8%; L-Histidine Monohydrochloride; Nephramine 5.4%; Novamine; Novamine 11.4%; Novamine 15%; Novamine 8.5%; Parenteral Nutrition Kit; Renamin; Renamin W/O Electrolytes; Travasol; Travasol 10%; Travasol 10% W/O Electrolytes; Travasol 5.5% W/O Electrolytes; Travasol 8.5% W/O Electrolytes; Travasol W/Dextrose; Trophamine; Trophamine 10%

Prescribing information not available at time of publication.

HOW SUPPLIED - EQUIVALENTS NOT AVAILABLE:

Injection, Solution - Intravenous - 4.25 %

1000 ml	$102.60	AMINOSYN II 4.25% IN 10% DEXTROSE, Abbott	00074-7751-29
1000 ml	$103.52	AMINOSYN II/ELECTROLYTES IN DEXTROSE, Abbott	00074-7752-29

Injection, Solution - Intravenous

250 ml	$75.00	RENAMIN, Baxter Hlthcare	00338-0471-02
400 ml	$107.35	AMINESS, Baxter Hlthcare	00338-0488-17
500 ml	$45.77	TRAVASOL, Baxter Hlthcare	00338-0623-03
500 ml	$73.09	TRAVASOL, Baxter Hlthcare	00338-0625-03
500 ml	$83.44	TRAVASOL, Baxter Hlthcare	00338-0629-03
500 ml	$93.60	BRANCHAMIN, Baxter Hlthcare	00338-0477-03
500 ml	$150.00	RENAMIN, Baxter Hlthcare	00338-0471-03
1000 ml	$61.76	AMINOSYN W/5PC DEXTROSE, Abbott	00074-7674-09
1000 ml	$68.87	AMINOSYN W/25% DEXTROSE, Abbott	00074-7673-09
1000 ml	$69.32	TRAVASOL, Baxter Hlthcare	00338-0833-04
1000 ml	$71.45	AMINOSYN W/25% DEXTROSE, Abbott	00074-7675-09
1000 ml	$91.54	TRAVASOL, Baxter Hlthcare	00338-0623-04
1000 ml	$146.22	TRAVASOL, Baxter Hlthcare	00338-0625-04
1000 ml	$166.80	TRAVASOL, Baxter Hlthcare	00338-0629-04
2000 ml	$57.36	TRAVASOL, Baxter Hlthcare	00338-0821-04
2000 ml	$59.63	TRAVASOL, Baxter Hlthcare	00338-0823-04
2000 ml	$64.49	TRAVASOL, Baxter Hlthcare	00338-0829-04
2000 ml	$67.04	TRAVASOL, Baxter Hlthcare	00338-0831-04
2000 ml	$74.17	TRAVASOL, Baxter Hlthcare	00338-0839-04
2000 ml	$112.00	TRAVASOL, Baxter Hlthcare	00338-0623-06
2000 ml	$148.26	TRAVASOL, Baxter Hlthcare	00338-0625-06
2000 ml	$152.66	AMINOSYN II 3.5% IN 5% DEXTROSE, Abbott	00074-7701-27
2000 ml	$170.26	AMINOSYN II 3.5%/DEXTROSE 25%, Abbott	00074-7700-27
2000 ml	$173.74	AMINOSYN II 4.25%/DEXTROSE 10%, Abbott	00074-7751-27
2000 ml	$175.34	AMINOSYN II 4.25%/DEXTROSE 20%, Abbott	00074-7752-27
2000 ml	$176.62	AMINOSYN II 4.25% IN 25% DEXTROSE, Abbott	00074-7702-27
2000 ml	$333.60	TRAVASOL, Baxter Hlthcare	00338-0629-06
2000 ml	$333.60	TRAVASOL, Baxter Hlthcare	00338-0644-06

AMINO ACIDS; ELECTROLYTES *(000189)*

CATEGORIES: Caloric Agents; Electrolyte Solutions; Electrolytic, Caloric-Water Balance; Homeostatic & Nutrient; Nutrition, Enteral/Parenteral; FDA Pre 1938 Drugs

BRAND NAMES: *Aminomel 6E* (Germany); *Aminomel 8E* (Germany); *Aminomel 10E* (Germany); *Aminomel 12.5E* (Germany); *Aminoplasmal-L 5%*; *Aminoplasmal L5*; *Aminoplasmal L10*; *Aminoplasmal 5%*; *Aminoplasmal 7%*; *Aminoplasmal 10%*; *Aminoplasmal 12.5%*; *Aminoplasmol 5%*; *Aminoplasmol 10%*; *Aminoplasmol 12.5%*; Aminosyn; Branchamin; *Cletamin*; *Eloamin 7%*; *Eloamin 10%*; Freamine; *Green Hepa*; Hepatamine; *Intrafusin 10%*; *Levamin Normo Con Electrolitos* (Mexico); *Neozamin*; Nephramine; Novamine; Procalamine; *Rectisol*; Renamin; *Serepamine*; *Synthamin with Electrolytes*; *Synthamin 9 with Electrolytes*; *Synthamin 13 with Electrolytes*; *Synthamin 17 with Electrolytes*; *Synthamin 5.5% with Electrolytes*; *Synthamin 8% with Electrolytes*; *Synthamin 10% with Electrolytes*; Travasol; Trophamine; *Vamin 9* (England); *Vamin 14* (England); *Vamin 14 g n 1*
(International brand names outside U.S. in italics)

Prescribing information not available at time of publication.

HOW SUPPLIED - EQUIVALENTS NOT AVAILABLE:

Injection, Solution - Intravenous - 3 %

1000 ml	$44.76	PROCALAMINE, McGaw	00264-1915-07
1000 ml x 6	$59.55	3% FREAMINE 111, McGaw	00264-1904-00
1000 ml x 10	$48.90	PROCALAMINE, McGaw	00264-1915-00

Injection, Solution - Intravenous - 3.5 %

1000 ml	$58.67	AMINOSYN 3.5%, Abbott	00074-2989-05
1000 ml	$61.40	AMINOSYN 3.5% M, Abbott	00074-4154-05
1000 ml	$90.13	AMINOSYN II 3.5% IN 5% DEXTROSE, Abbott	00074-7701-29
1000 ml	$94.64	AMINOSYN II 3.5% M IN 5% DEXTROSE, Abbott	00074-7740-29
1000 ml	$100.52	AMINOSYN II 3.5% IN 25% DEXTROSE, Abbott	00074-7700-29
1000 ml	$104.79	AMINOSYN II 3.5%, Abbott	00074-1083-05
1000 ml	$109.21	AMINOSYN II W/ELEC IN DEX W/CA, Abbott	00074-7756-29

Injection, Solution - Intravenous - 4.25 %

1000 ml	$104.27	AMINOSYN II 4.25% IN 25% DEXTROSE, Abbott	00074-7702-29
1000 ml	$107.51	AMINOSYN II 4.25% M IN 10% DEXTROSE, Abbott	00074-7742-29
1000 ml	$109.83	AMINOSYN II/LYTE/CA/D20W, Abbott	00074-7753-29
1000 ml	$113.20	AMINOSYN II W/ELEC IN DEX W/CA, Abbott	00074-7757-29

Injection, Solution - Intravenous - 5 %

500 ml	$53.56	AMINOSYN, Abbott	00074-2990-03
1000 ml	$104.79	AMINOSYN, Abbott	00074-2990-05
1000 ml	$118.99	AMINOSYN II 5% IN 25% DEXTROSE, Abbott	00074-7744-29

Injection, Solution - Intravenous - 5.2 %

300 ml	$93.92	AMINOSYN-RF 5.2%, Abbott	00074-4072-02

Injection, Solution - Intravenous - 6 %

500 ml x 12	$73.16	TROPHAMINE, McGaw	00264-1936-10

Injection, Solution - Intravenous - 6.9 %

750 ml fill 100	$84.61	6.9 % FREAMINE HBC, McGaw	00264-1935-04

Injection, Solution - Intravenous - 7 %

250 ml	$55.06	AMINOSYN-PF 7%, Abbott	00074-1616-02
500 ml	$72.40	AMINOSYN II 7%, Abbott	00074-1086-03
500 ml	$72.40	AMINOSYN 7%, Abbott	00074-2992-03
500 ml	$73.46	AMINOSYN-PF 7%, Abbott	00074-1616-03
500 ml	$76.01	AMINOSYN-HBC 7%, Abbott	00074-1108-03
500 ml	$76.23	AMINOSYN 7% WITH ELECTROLYTES, Abbott	00074-5852-03
500 ml	$100.88	AMINOSYN, Abbott	00074-2996-01
500 ml	$105.47	AMINOSYN W/ELECTROLYTES, Abbott	00074-4343-01
1000 ml	$152.08	AMINOSYN-HBC 7%, Abbott	00074-1108-05

Injection, Solution - Intravenous - 8 %

500 ml x 6	$102.00	HEPATAMINE, McGaw	00264-1937-10

Injection, Solution - Intravenous - 8.5 %

500 ml	$76.00	AMINOSYN II 8.5 % WITH ELECTROLYTES, Abbott	00074-1089-03
500 ml	$76.74	AMINOSYN II 8.5%, Abbott	00074-1088-03
500 ml	$76.74	AMINOSYN 8.5%, Abbott	00074-5855-03
500 ml	$80.58	AMINOSYN 8.5% WITH ELECTROLYTES, Abbott	00074-5856-03
500 ml	$106.00	AMINOSYN, Abbott	00074-4041-01
500 ml	$113.19	AMINOSYN W/ELECTROLYTES, Abbott	00074-4183-01
500 ml glass bo	$78.02	8.5% FREAMINE III WITH ELECTROLYTES, McGaw	00264-1931-10
500 ml x 12	$74.38	FREAMINE III, McGaw	00264-1903-10
1000 ml	$153.52	AMINOSYN II 8.5%, Abbott	00074-1088-05
1000 ml	$153.52	AMINOSYN 8.5%, Abbott	00074-5855-05
1000 ml	$161.14	Aminosyn 8.5%/Electrolytes Injection, Abbott	00074-5856-05
1000 ml glass b	$137.96	8.5% FREAMINE III WITH ELECTROLYTES, McGaw	00264-1931-00
1000 ml x 6	$148.88	FREAMINE III, McGaw	00264-1903-00

Injection, Solution - Intravenous - 10 %

500 ml	$87.60	AMINOSYN II 10%, Abbott	00074-1090-03
500 ml	$87.60	AMINOSYN 10%, Abbott	00074-2991-03
500 ml	$102.29	TROPHAMINE, McGaw	00264-1934-10
500 ml x 12	$84.82	10% FREAMINE III AMINO ACID, McGaw	00264-1901-10
1000 ml	$153.18	AMINOSYN 10%, Abbott	00074-4360-05
1000 ml	$173.76	AMINOSYN-PF 10%, Abbott	00074-1617-05
1000 ml	$175.12	AMINOSYN II 10%, Abbott	00074-1090-05
1000 ml	$175.12	AMINOSYN 10%, Abbott	00074-2991-05
1000 ml x 6	$162.98	10% FREAMINE III AMINO ACID, McGaw	00264-1901-00
2000 ml	$2101.44	AMINOSYN II, Abbott	00074-7121-07

Injection, Solution - Intravenous - 15 %

2000 ml	$495.00	NOVAMINE, Baxter Hlthcare	00338-0498-06
2000 ml	$3152.04	AMINOSYN II, Abbott	00074-7122-07

Injection, Solution - Intravenous

250 ml	$25.12	AMINOSYN, Abbott	00074-2990-02
500 ml	$30.24	TRAVASOL, Baxter Hlthcare	00338-0624-03
500 ml	$33.47	3.5 % TRAVASOL M WITH ELECTROLYTE 45, Baxter Hlthcare	00338-0627-03
500 ml	$48.46	TRAVASOL, Baxter Hlthcare	00338-0457-03
500 ml	$49.21	AMINOSYN, Abbott	00074-4358-03
500 ml	$52.17	AMINOSYN 8.5%, Abbott	00074-4359-03
500 ml	$59.54	AMINOSYN 10%, Abbott	00074-4360-03
500 ml	$76.77	TRAVASOL, Baxter Hlthcare	00338-0459-03
500 ml	$79.72	TRAVASOL, Baxter Hlthcare	00338-0626-03
500 ml	$83.99	TRAVASOL, Baxter Hlthcare	00338-0644-03
500 ml	$91.44	AMINOSYN, Abbott	00074-4019-01
500 ml	$95.14	NOVAMINE, Baxter Hlthcare	00338-0489-03
500 ml	$112.32	NOVAMINE, Baxter Hlthcare	00338-0494-03
500 ml x 12	$38.33	FREAMINE II 8.5% AMINO ACID, McGaw	00264-1906-10
1000 ml	$55.88	3.5 % TRAVASOL M WITH ELECTROLYTE 45, Baxter Hlthcare	00338-0627-04
1000 ml	$72.31	AMINOSYN II/ELECTROLYTES IN 25% DEX, Abbott	00074-7741-29
1000 ml	$75.02	AMINOSYN II/ELECTROLYTES IN 25% DE, Abbott	00074-7743-29
1000 ml	$96.92	TRAVASOL, Baxter Hlthcare	00338-0457-04
1000 ml	$104.33	AMINOSYN, Abbott	00074-4359-05
1000 ml	$126.20	AMINOSYN-PF 10%, Abbott	00074-1146-05
1000 ml	$154.77	TRAVASOL, Baxter Hlthcare	00338-0459-04
1000 ml	$182.66	NOVAMINE, Baxter Hlthcare	00338-0489-04
1000 ml	$234.17	NOVAMINE, Baxter Hlthcare	00338-0494-04
2000 ml	$118.58	TRAVASOL, Baxter Hlthcare	00338-0457-06
2000 ml	$156.50	TRAVASOL, Baxter Hlthcare	00338-0459-06
2000 ml	$160.30	AMINOSYN II 3.5% M IN 5% DEXTROSE, Abbott	00074-7740-27
2000 ml	$184.98	AMINOSYN II W/LYTE/CA/D25W, Abbott	00074-7756-27
2000 ml	$186.02	AMINOSYN II/LYTE/CA/D20W, Abbott	00074-7753-27
2000 ml	$191.72	AMINOSYN II W/LYTE/CA/D25W, Abbott	00074-7757-27

HOW SUPPLIED - EQUIVALENTS NOT AVAILABLE: *(cont'd)*

2000 ml	$201.56	AMINOSYN II 5% IN 25% DEXTROSE, Abbott	00074-7744-27
2000 ml	$216.24	AMINOSYN II W/LYTE/CA/D25W, Abbott	00074-7754-27

AMINOBENZOATE POTASSIUM *(000199)*

CATEGORIES: DESI Drugs; Fibrotics; Pemphigus; Scleroderma; Vitamin B Complex; Vitamins; FDA Pre 1938 Drugs

BRAND NAMES: *Fibroderm*; **Potaba**; *Potabex* (Mexico)
(International brand names outside U.S. in italics)

DESCRIPTION:

Potaba is chemically pure potassium p-aminobenzoate, KPAB.

Advantages: Potaba offers a means of treatment of serious and often chronic entities involving fibrosis and nonsuppurative inflammation.

CLINICAL PHARMACOLOGY:

P-Aminobenzoate is considered a member of the vitamin B complex. Small amounts are found in cereal, eggs, milk & meats. Detectable amounts are normally present in human blood, spinal fluid, urine, and sweat. PABA is a component of several biologically important systems, and it participates in a number of fundamental biological processes.

It has been suggested that the antifibrosis action of Potaba is due to its medication of increased oxygen uptake at the tissue level. Fibrosis is believed to occur from either too much serotonin or too little monoamine oxidase activity over a period of time. Monoamine oxidase requires an adequate supply of oxygen to function properly. By increasing oxygen supply at the tissue level Potaba may enhance MAO activity and prevent or bring about regression of fibrosis.[3]

Clinical Uses: PEYRONIE'S DISEASE: 21 patients with Peyronie's disease were placed on Potaba therapy for periods ranging from 3 months to 2 years. Pain disappeared from 16 to 16 cases in which it has been present. There was objective improvement in penile deformity in 10 of 17 patients, and decrease in plaque size in 16 of 21. The authors suggest that this medication offers no hazard of further local injury as may result from other therapy. There were no significant untoward effects encountered in long term Potaba therapy.[5, 10]

Scleroderma: Of 135 patients with diffuse systemic sclerosis treated with Potaba every patient but one has shown softening of the involved skin if treatment has been continued for 3 months or longer. The responses have been reported in a number of publications.[9] The treatment program consists of systemic antifibrosis therapy with Potaba, physical therapy, including deep breathing exercises and dynamic traction splints where indicated, and bethanechol chloride (MYOTONACHOL, Glenwood) for relief of dysphagia as well as all doses of reserpine for amelioration of Raynaud's phenomena.[1,3]

Dermatomyositis: Five patients with scleroderma and 2 with dermatomyositis were treated with Potaba. There was striking clinical improvement in each patient. Doses of 15-20 grams per day were well tolerated, and patients were easily able to take these doses.[6]

Morphea and Linear Scleroderma: All 14 patients with localized forms of scleroderma placed on long-term Potaba treatment showed softening of the sclerotic component of their disorder. Treatment is particularly indicated in patients where persistent compressive sclerosis may contribute even greater disfigurement of functional embarrassment from secondary pressure atrophy.[8,9]

CONTRAINDICATIONS:

Potaba should not be administered to patients taking sulfonamides.

INDICATIONS AND USAGE:

Based on a review of this drug by the National Academy of Sciences-National Research Council and/or other information, FDA has classified the indications as follows:

"Possibly" effective: Potassium aminobenzoate is possibly effective in the treatment of scleroderma, dermatomyositis, morphea, linear scleroderma, pemphigus, and Peyronie's disease.

Final classification of the less-than-effective indications requires further investigation.

PRECAUTIONS:

Should anorexia or nausea occur, therapy is interrupted until the patient is eating normally again. This permits prompt subsidence of symptoms and also avoids the possible development of hypoglycemia. Give cautiously to patients with renal disease. If a hypersensitivity reaction should occur, Potaba should be stopped.

Usage In Pregnancy: Safety for use in pregnancy or during lactation has not been established.

ADVERSE REACTIONS:

Anorexia, nausea, fever and rash have occurred infrequently and subside with omission of the drug. Desensitization can be accomplished and treatment resumed.

DOSAGE AND ADMINISTRATION:

The average adult daily dose of Potaba is 12 grams, usually given in four to six divided doses. Tablets and capsules 0.5 gram are given at the rate of 4 tablets or capsules 6 times daily, or 6 given four times daily, usually with meals and at bed-time with a snack. Tablets must be taken with an adequate amount of liquid to prevent gastrointestinal upset.

Potaba Envules contain 2 grams pure drug each. 6 Envules are given for a total of 12 grams Potaba daily.

Potaba Powder is used to prepare solutions, which are kept refrigerated, but for no longer than one week. 100 grams Potaba powder make 1 quart of 10% solution when dissolved in potable tap water. Children are given 1 gram Potaba daily in divided doses for each 10 lbs. of body weight.

REFERENCES:

1. From: Inflammation and Diseases of Connective Tissue, Edited by Drs. Lewis C. Mills and John H. Moyer, Published by W.B. Saunders Company, Phila. 1961. **3.** Zarafonetis, Chris J.D.: Treatment of Scleroderma, Annals of Int. Med. 50:343-365 (1959). **5.** Zarafonetis, C.J.D., and Horrax, T.M.: Treatment of Peyronie's Disease with Potaba, Journ. of Urology 81:770-772 (June 1959). **6.** Grace, William J., Kennedy, Richard J., Formato, Anthony: Therapy of Scleroderma and Dermatomyositis, N.Y. State J. of Med. 63:140-144, 1963. **8.** Zarafonetis, C. J.D.: Treatment of Localized Forms of Scleroderma, Am. J. Med Sci. 243:147-158. **9.** Zarafonetis, Chris J. D.: Antifibrotic Therapy With Potaba, Amer. Jrnl. of Med. Sci. 248: No. 5/551-561 (nov. 1964). **10.** Horrax, Trudeau M.: Peyronie's Disease, Scientific Exhibit, AMer. Urological Assn. Annl. Meet., New Orleans, May 1965.

HOW SUPPLIED:

Potaba capsules 0.5 gm.:
NDC-0516-0051-25 bottle of 250
NDC-0516-0051-10 bottle of 1000.
Potaba Powder 2.0 Envules:
NDC-0516-0052-50 box of 50 X 2.0 gm.

HOW SUPPLIED: *(cont'd)*

NDC-0516-0053-01 bottle of 100 gm. bulk
NDC-0516-0053-16 bottle of 1 lb. bulk
Potaba Tablets 0.5 gm.:
NDC-0516-0054-01 bottle OF 100
NDC-0516-0054-10 bottle of 1000.

HOW SUPPLIED - EQUIVALENTS NOT AVAILABLE:

Capsule - Oral - 0.5 gm

250's	$56.92	POTABA, Glenwood	00516-0051-25
1000's	$211.11	POTABA, Glenwood	00516-0051-10

Powder - Oral - 2 gm/envule

50's	$42.64	POTABA, Glenwood	00516-0052-50

Powder - Oral

100 gm	$44.62	POTABA, Glenwood	00516-0053-01

Tablet, Uncoated - Oral - 0.5 gm

100's	$24.08	POTABA, Glenwood	00516-0054-01
1000's	$202.28	POTABA, Glenwood	00516-0054-10

AMINOBENZOATE POTASSIUM; POTASSIUM SALICYLATE *(000200)*

CATEGORIES: Analgesics; Antiarthritics; Antipyretics; Arthritis; Central Nervous System Agents; Congestive Heart Failure; Glomerulonephritis; Heart Failure; Hypertension; Nonsteroidal Anti-Inflammatory; Pain; Salicylates; Pregnancy Category C; FDA Pre 1938 Drugs

BRAND NAMES: **Pabalate-SF**

DESCRIPTION:

These tablets are intended for oral administration.

Each enteric-coated tablet contains:
Potassium Salicylate..................... 0.3 g
Potassium Aminobenzoate.................. 0.3 g
Potassium content per tablet: 131.5 mg (3.4 mEq)

Pabalate-SF Inactive Ingredients: Acacia, Acetylated Monoglycerides, Calcium Carbonate, Calcium Sulfate, Carnauba Wax, Cellulose Acetate Phthalate, Diethyl Phthalate, Docusate Sodium, Edible Ink, FD&C Blue 1 Aluminum Lake, FD&C Blue 2 Aluminum Lake, FD&C Red 3 Aluminum Lake, Gelatin, Magnesium Stearate, Polysorbates, Shellac, Stearic Acid, Sucrose, Talc, Titanium Dioxide, Wheat Flour, White Wax. May contain FD&C Red 40 and Yellow 6 Aluminum Lakes.

Analgesic Drug Product

CLINICAL PHARMACOLOGY:

Potassium salicylate is a mild analgesic with anti-inflammatory and antipyretic activity. Compared to aspirin, potassium salicylate has substantially less effect on platelet adhesiveness. In large doses, however, it has a hypoprothrombinemic effect. Potassium salicylate in conventional dosage form dissolves in the stomach and is absorbed as unionized salicylic acid. However, in aminobenzoate potassium - potassium salicylate, the enteric coating delays release of the salicylate until the tablet reaches the alkaline medium of the intestine. After absorption, salicylic acid is extensively bound to plasma protein, and the bound portion is in equilibrium with the free salicylate in the plasma. The action of potassium aminobenzoate in this formulation has not been established.

INDICATIONS AND USAGE:

Aminobenzoate potassium/potassium salicylate tablets are indicated for the temporary relief of mild to moderate pain complicated by conditions in which the restriction of sodium intake may be desirable, such as: congestive heart failure, essential hypertension and glomerulonephritis.

CONTRAINDICATIONS:

Hypersensitivity to any of the ingredients. Presence of an active ulcer, hypoprothrombinemia, Vitamin K deficiency, severe hepatic or renal damage, hemophilia, or hyperkalemia. Do not administer to patients who are receiving a potassium-sparing diuretic.

WARNINGS:

Salicylates have been reported to be associated with the development of Reye syndrome in children and teenagers with chicken pox, influenza, and influenza-like infections. There have been several reports, published and unpublished, concerning non-specific small bowel lesions consisting of stenosis with or without ulceration, associated with the administration of enteric-coated thiazides with potassium salts. These lesions may occur with enteric-coated potassium tablets alone or when they are used with nonenteric-coated thiazides, or certain other oral diuretics. These small bowel lesions have caused obstruction, hemorrhage, and perforation. Surgery was frequently required and deaths have occurred.

Based on a large survey of physicians and hospitals, both American and foreign, the incidence of these lesions is low, and a causal relationship in man has not been definitely established.

Available information tends to implicate enteric-coated potassium salts although lesions of this type also occur spontaneously. Therefore, coated potassium-containing formulations should be administered only when indicated, and should be discontinued immediately if abdominal pain, distension, nausea, vomiting, or gastrointestinal bleeding occur.

When prescribing aminobenzoate potassium - potassium salicylate for patients who are receiving concurrent potassium supplementation (*e.g.*, to replace potassium excreted during thiazide therapy), it should be kept in mind that each tablet contains 131.5 mg (3.4 mEq) of potassium. A decrease in supplemental potassium dosage should be considered in order to The use of potassium salts in patients with chronic renal disease, or any other condition which impairs potassium excretion, requires particularly careful monitoring of the serum potassium concentration and appropriate dosage adjustment.

PRECAUTIONS:

General: Treatment with salicylates may interfere with blood clotting; therefore, salicylate therapy should be stopped at least one week prior to surgery.

Carcinogenesis, Mutagenesis: Long-term studies in animals have not been performed to evaluate carcinogenic potential.

Pregnancy Category C: Animal reproduction studies have not been conducted with aminobenzoate potassium - potassium salicylate.

PRECAUTIONS: *(cont'd)*

Safe use of this drug has not been established with regard to possible adverse effects upon fetal development. Therefore, the drug should not be used in women who are or may become pregnant and particularly during early pregnancy unless in the judgment of the physician the potential benefits outweigh the possible hazards.

Nursing Mothers: Salicylates appear in human milk in moderate amounts. They can produce a bleeding tendency by decreasing the amount of prothrombin in the infant's blood. As a general rule, nursing should not be undertaken while a patient is on this drug.

Pediatric Use: Safety and effectiveness in children below the age of 12 have not been established.

DRUG INTERACTIONS:

This product contains aminobenzoic acid which inhibits the bacteriostatic action of sulfonamides when the two are administered concurrently.

ADVERSE REACTIONS:

Hyperkalemia is a potential adverse effect (see CONTRAINDICATIONS and WARNINGS). The most frequent adverse reactions to products such as aminobenzoate potassium - potassium salicylate which contain potassium and/or salicylates are nausea and gastrointestinal upset. Fine rash with or without pruritus and urticaria occur less frequently. The occasional occurrence of mild salicylism may require adjustment in dosage.

OVERDOSAGE:

Overdose may cause symptoms of hyperkalemia and/or salicylate intoxication. Mild chronic overdosage, termed salicylism, may cause symptoms such as tinnitus, nausea, headache, hyperventilation, dizziness, drowsiness, mental confusion, dimness of vision, sweating, thirst, and occasionally diarrhea. Withdrawal of salicylates and supportive therapy may be sufficient treatment.

A more severe degree of salicylate intoxication may occur with acute massive overdosage or the chronic administration of more moderate overdoses, especially in infants and children. CNS effects are more pronounced and may progress to delirium, hallucinations, generalized convulsions and coma.

A variety of cutaneous lesions may be observed. A most important feature of salicylate intoxication is a disturbance of acid-base balance and plasma electrolytes. Careful monitoring of these laboratory parameters along with plasma glucose concentration is essential. The type and quantity of repair solutions used will depend upon interpretation of the laboratory data. Bicarbonate solution should be administered IV in order to produce alkaline diuresis. Correction of hypoglycemia and ketosis by the administration of glucose is essential.

Since hyperthermia and dehydration are immediate threats to life, external sponging and the administration of adequate quantities of IV fluids are important first steps to correct these conditions and maintain adequate renal function. If hemorrhagic phenomena *(petechiae, thrombocytopenia)* occur, whole blood transfusions and vitamin K may be necessary.

The gastrointestinal tract should be emptied either by emesis or purging to remove undissolved tablets in cases of acute ingestion of a large single dose. Since enteric-coated tablets do not disintegrate in the stomach, they cannot be removed by lavage. Rapid and immediate removal of salicylate from the body by alkaline diuresis is essential. In more severe cases, extrarenal measures such as peritoneal dialysis, hemodialysis, hemoperfusion or exchange transfusion may be required.

DOSAGE AND ADMINISTRATION:

The average adult dose is two tablets every 4 hours. Due to the enteric coating, tablets should not be taken within one hour of ingesting milk or antacids. For Chicken Pox or Flu, (see WARNINGS.)

HOW SUPPLIED - EQUIVALENTS NOT AVAILABLE:

Tablet, Enteric Coated - Oral

100's	$7.50	PABALATE-SF, AH Robins	00031-5883-63
500's	$34.35	PABALATE-SF, AH Robins	00031-5883-70

AMINOCAPROIC ACID *(000202)*

CATEGORIES: Antiheparin Agents; Bleeding; Blood Formation/Coagulation; Coagulants and Anticoagulants; Fibrinogen; Fibrinolytic & Proteolytic; Hemostatics; Shock; FDA Approval Pre 1982

BRAND NAMES: **Amicar**; *Amiplong*; *Capracid*; *Capramol* (France); *Caproamin*; *Caprolisin*; *Epsicaprom*; *Epsikapron*; *Epsilonaminocapronsav*; *Hemocaprol*; *Hemocid*; *Ipron*; *Ipsilon* (Japan); *Resplamin* (Japan)
(International brand names outside U.S. in italics)

FORMULARIES: BC-BS

DESCRIPTION:

Aminocaproic acid, USP is 6-aminohexanoic acid, which acts as an inhibitor of fibrinolysis.

Aminocaproic acid is soluble in water, acids, and alkalies; it is sparingly soluble in methanol and practically insoluble in chloroform.

Aminocaproic acid Injection, USP, for intravenous administration, is a sterile pyrogen free solution containing 250 mg/ml of Aminocaproic Acid with Benzyl Alcohol 0.9% as preservative and Water for Injection qs 100%. Hydrochloric acid may be added to adjust pH to approximately 6.8 during manufacture.

Aminocaproic acid Syrup, USP 25%, for oral administration, contains 250 mg/ml of Aminocaproic Acid with Potassium Sorbate 0.2% and Sodium Benzoate 0.1% as preservatives and the following inactive ingredients: Citric Acid, Flavorings, Sodium Saccharin and Sorbitol.

Each aminocaproic acid Tablet, USP, for oral administration, contains 500 mg of Aminocaproic Acid and the following inactive ingredients: Magnesium Stearate, Stearic Acid and Povidone.

CLINICAL PHARMACOLOGY:

The fibrinolysis-inhibitory effects of aminocaproic acid appear to be exerted principally via inhibition of plasminogen activators & to a lesser degree through antiplasmin activity.

In adults, oral absorption appears to be a zero-order process with an absorption rate of 5.2 g/hr. The mean lag time in absorption is 10 minutes. After a single oral dose of 5 g, absorption was complete (F=1). Mean ± SD peak plasma concentrations (164 ± 28 mcg/ml) were reached within 1.2 ± 0.45 hours.

CLINICAL PHARMACOLOGY: *(cont'd)*

After oral administration, the apparent volume of distribution was estimated to be 23.1 ± 6.6 l (mean ± SD). Correspondingly, the volume of distribution after intravenous administration has been reported to be 30.0 ± 8.2 l. After prolonged administration, aminocaproic acid has been found to distribute throughout extravascular and intravascular compartments of the body, penetrating human red blood cells as well as other tissue cells.

Renal excretion is the primary route of elimination, whether aminocaproic acid is administered orally or intravenously. Sixty-five percent of the dose is recovered in the urine as unchanged drug and 11% of the dose appears as the metabolite adipic acid. Renal clearance (116 ml/min) approximates endogenous creatinine clearance. The total body clearance is 169 ml/min. The terminal elimination half-life for aminocaproic acid is approximately 2 hours.

INDICATIONS AND USAGE:

Aminocaproic acid is useful in enhancing hemostasis when fibrinolysis contributes to bleeding. In life-threatening situations, fresh whole blood transfusions, fibrinogen infusions, and other emergency measures may be required.

Fibrinolytic bleeding may frequently be associated with surgical complications following heart surgery (with or without cardiac bypass procedures) and portacaval shunt; hematological disorders such as aplastic anemia; abruptio placentae; hepatic cirrhosis; neoplastic disease such as carcinoma of the prostate, lung, stomach, and cervix.

Urinary fibrinolysis, usually a normal physiological phenomenon, may frequently be associated with life-threatening complications following severe trauma, anoxia, and shock. Symptomatic of such complications is surgical hematuria (following prostatectomy and nephrectomy) or nonsurgical hematuria (accompanying polycystic or neoplastic diseases of the genitourinary system). (See WARNINGS.)

CONTRAINDICATIONS:

Aminocaproic acid should not be used when there is evidence of an active intravascular clotting process.

When there is uncertainty as to whether the cause of bleeding is primary fibrinolysis or disseminated intravascular coagulation (DIC), this distinction must be made before administering aminocaproic acid.

The following tests can be applied to differentiate the two conditions:

Platelet count is usually decreased in DIC but normal in primary fibrinolysis.

Protamine paracoagulation test is positive in DIC; a precipitate forms when protamine sulphate is dropped into citrated plasma. The test is negative in the presence of primary fibrinolysis.

The euglobulin clot lysis test is abnormal in primary fibrinolysis but normal in DIC. Aminocaproic acid must not be used in the presence of DIC without concomitant heparin.

WARNINGS:

In patients with upper urinary tract bleeding, aminocaproic acid administration has been known to cause intrarenal obstruction in the form of glomerular capillary thrombosis or clots in the renal pelvis and ureters. For this reason, aminocaproic acid should not be used in hematuria of upper urinary tract origin, unless the possible benefits outweigh the risk.

Subendocardial hemorrhages have been observed in dogs given intravenous infusions of 0.2 times the maximum human therapeutic dose of aminocaproic acid and in monkeys given 8 times the maximum human therapeutic dose of aminocaproic acid.

Fatty degeneration of the myocardium has been reported in dogs given intravenous doses of aminocaproic acid at 0.8 to 3.3 times the maximum human therapeutic dose and in monkeys given intravenous doses of aminocaproic acid at 6 times the maximum human therapeutic dose.

Rarely, skeletal muscle weakness with necrosis of muscle fibers has been reported following prolonged administration. Clinical presentation may range from mild myalgias with weakness and fatigue to a severe proximal myopathy with rhabdomyolysis, myoglobinuria, and acute renal failure. Muscle enzymes, especially creatine phosphokinase (CPK) are elevated. CPK levels should be monitored in patients on long-term therapy. Aminocaproic acid administration should be stopped if a rise in CPK is noted. Resolution follows discontinuation of aminocaproic acid; however, the syndrome may recur if aminocaproic acid is restarted.

The possibility of cardiac muscle damage should also be considered when skeletal myopathy occurs. One case of *cardiac* and *hepatic lesions* observed in man has been reported. The patient received 2 g of aminocaproic acid every 6 hours for a total dose of 26 g. Death was due to continued cerebrovascular hemorrhage. Necrotic changes in the heart and liver were noted at autopsy.

PRECAUTIONS:

GENERAL

Aminocaproic acid inhibits both the action of plasminogen activators and to a lesser degree, plasmin activity. The drug should NOT be administered without a definite diagnosis and/or laboratory finding indicative of hyperfibrinolysis (hyperplasminemia).*

Rapid intravenous administration of the drug should be avoided since this may induce hypotension, bradycardia, and/or arrhythmia.

Inhibition of fibrinolysis by aminocaproic acid may theoretically result in clotting or thrombosis. However, there is no definite evidence that administration of aminocaproic acid has been responsible for the few reported cases of intravascular clotting which followed this treatment. Rather, it appears that such *intravascular clotting* was most likely due to the patient's preexisting clinical condition (*e.g.*, the presence of DIC). It has been postulated that *extravascular clots* formed *in vivo*may not undergo spontaneous lysis as do normal clots.

Reports have appeared in the literature of an increased incidence of certain neurological deficits such as hydrocephalus, cerebral ischemia, or cerebral vasospasm associated with the use of antifibrinolytic agents in the treatment of subarachnoid hemorrhage (SAH). All of these events have also been described as part of the natural course of SAH, or as a consequence of diagnostic procedures such as angiography. Drug relatedness remains unclear.

Thrombophlebitis, a possibility with all intravenous therapy, should be guarded against by strict attention to the proper insertion of the needle and the fixing of its position.

LABORATORY TESTS

The use of aminocaproic acid should be accompanied by tests designed to determine the amount of fibrinolysis present. There are presently available (a) general tests such as those for the determination of the lysis of a clot of blood or plasma and (b) more specific tests for the study of various phases of fibrinolytic mechanisms. These latter tests include both semiquantitative and quantitative techniques for the determination of profibrinolysin, fibrinolysin, and antifibrinolysin.

DRUG LABORATORY TEST INTERACTIONS

Prolongation of the template bleeding time has been reported during continuous intravenous infusion of aminocaproic acid at dosages exceeding 24 g/day. Platelet function studies in these patients have not demonstrated any significant platelet dysfunction. However, *in vitro* studies have shown that at high concentrations (7.4 mMol/l or 0.97 mg/ml and greater) EACA inhibits ADP and collagen-induced platelet aggregation, the release of ATP and

PRECAUTIONS: *(cont'd)*

serotonin, and the binding of fibrinogen to the platelets in a concentration-response manner. Following a 10 g bolus of aminocaproic acid, transient peak plasma concentrations of 4.6 mMol/l or 0.60 mg/ml have been obtained. The concentration of aminocaproic acid necessary to maintain inhibition of fibrinolysis is 0.99 mMol/l or 0.13 mg/ml. Administration of a 5 g bolus followed by 1 to 1.25 g/hr., should achieve and sustain plasma levels of 0.13 mg/ml. Thus, concentrations which have been obtained *in vivo* clinically in patients with normal renal function are considerably lower than the *in vitro* concentrations found to induce abnormalities in platelet function tests. However, higher plasma concentrations of aminocaproic acid may occur in patients with severe renal failure.

CARCINOGENESIS, MUTAGENESIS, AND IMPAIRMENT OF FERTILITY

Long-term studies in animals to evaluate the carcinogenic potential of aminocaproic acid and studies to evaluate its mutagenic potential have not been conducted. Dietary administration of an equivalent of the maximum human therapeutic dose of aminocaproic acid to rats of both sexes impaired fertility as evidenced by decreased implantations, litter sizes and number of pups born.

PREGNANCY CATEGORY C

Animal teratological studies have not been conducted with aminocaproic acid. It is also not known whether aminocaproic acid can cause fetal harm when administered to a pregnant woman or can affect reproduction capacity. Aminocaproic acid should be given to a pregnant woman only if clearly needed.

NURSING MOTHERS

It is not known whether this drug is excreted in human milk. Because many drugs are excreted in human milk, caution should be exercised when aminocaproic acid is administered to a nursing woman.

PEDIATRIC USE

Safety and effectiveness in children have not been established.

ADVERSE REACTIONS:

Occasionally nausea, cramps, diarrhea, hypotension, dizziness, tinnitus, malaise, conjunctival suffusion, nasal stuffiness, headache, and skin rash have been reported as results of the administration of aminocaproic acid. Only rarely has it been necessary to discontinue or reduce medication because of one or more of these effects. Myopathy (see WARNINGS) may be accompanied by general weakness, fatigue, and elevated serum enzymes. Rarely, rhabdomyolysis with myoglobinuria and renal failure may occur.

There have also been some reports of dry ejaculation during the period of aminocaproic acid treatment. These have been reported to date only in hemophilia patients who received the drug after undergoing dental surgical procedures. However, this symptom resolved in all patients within 24 to 48 hours of completion of therapy.

Two cases of convulsions have been reported to occur following intravenous administration of aminocaproic acid.

OVERDOSAGE:

Signs, symptoms, laboratory findings, and complications have not been reported in association with acute overdosage of aminocaproic acid. Concentrations of aminocaproic acid in biologic fluids related to toxicity and/or death in humans are not known. Further, the single dose of aminocaproic acid causing symptoms of overdosage or considered to be life-threatening is unknown.

The intravenous and oral LD_{50} of aminocaproic acid were 3.0 and 12.0 g/kg respectively in the mouse and 3.2 and 16.4 g/kg respectively in the rat. An intravenous infusion dose of 2.3 g/kg was lethal in the dog. On intravenous administration, tonic-clonic convulsions were observed in dogs and mice.

No treatment for overdosage is known, although evidence exists that aminocaproic acid is removed by hemodialysis and may be removed by peritoneal dialysis.

DOSAGE AND ADMINISTRATION:

Intravenous: Aminocaproic acid Injection is administered by infusion, utilizing the usual compatible intravenous vehicles (*e.g.,* Sterile Water for Injection, Sodium Chloride for Injection, 5% Dextrose or Ringer's Injection). Although Sterile Water for Injection is compatible for intravenous injection the resultant solution is hypo-osmolar. RAPID INJECTION OF AMINOCAPROIC ACID INJECTION UNDILUTED INTO A VEIN IS NOT RECOMMENDED.

For the treatment of *acute* bleeding syndromes due to elevated fibrinolytic activity, it is suggested that 16 to 20 ml (4 to 5 g) of aminocaproic acid Injection in 250 ml of diluent be administered by infusion during the first hour of treatment, followed by a continuing infusion at the rate of 4 ml (1 g) per hour in 50 ml of diluent. This method of treatment would ordinarily be continued for about 8 hours or until the bleeding situation has been controlled.

Parenteral drug products should be inspected visually for particulate matter and discoloration prior to administration, whenever solution and container permit.

Oral Therapy: If the patient is able to take medication by mouth, an identical dosage regimen may be followed by administering aminocaproic acid Tablets or aminocaproic acid Syrup 25% as follows: For the treatment of acute bleeding syndromes due to elevated fibrinolytic activity, it is suggested that 10 tablets (5 g) or 4 teaspoonfuls of syrup (5 g) of aminocaproic acid be administered during the first hour of treatment, followed by a continuing rate of 2 tablets (1 g) or 1 teaspoonful of syrup (1.25 g) per hour. This method of treatment would ordinarily be continued for about 8 hours or until the bleeding situation has been controlled.

Injection: Store at Controlled Room Temperature 15-30°C (59-86°F). DO NOT FREEZE.

Syrup: Store at Controlled Room Temperature 15-30°C (59-86°F). Dispense in tight containers. DO NOT FREEZE.

Tablets: Store at Controlled Room Temperature 15-30°C (59-86°F). Dispense in tight containers.

REFERENCES:

* Stefanini M, Dameshek W: The Hemorrhagic Disorders, Ed. 2, New York, Grune and Stratton. 1962; pp. 510-514.

HOW SUPPLIED - RATED THERAPEUTICALLY EQUIVALENT:

Injection, Solution - Intravenous - 250 mg/ml

20 ml	$7.01	Aminocaproic Acid, Abbott	00074-4346-73
20 ml	$7.27	Aminocaproic Acid, Abbott	00074-3443-05
20 ml	**$16.24**	**AMICAR, Lederle Parenterals**	**00205-4668-37**
20 ml	$17.50	Aminocaproic Acid, Consolidated Midland	00223-7126-20
20 ml x 5	$13.44	Aminocaproic Acid, Am Regent	00517-9120-05
20 ml x 10	$100.25	Aminocaproic Acid, Elkins Sinn	00641-2235-43
20 ml x 25	$377.50	Aminocaproic Acid, Fujisawa USA	00469-1720-40
96 ml	$65.58	Aminocaproic Acid, Fujisawa USA	00469-1721-00
96 ml	**$74.04**	**AMICAR, Lederle Parenterals**	**00205-4668-73**

HOW SUPPLIED - NOT RATED EQUIVALENT:

Syrup - Oral - 1.25 gm/5ml

473 ml	**$344.32**	**AMICAR, Immunex**	**58406-0611-90**

Tablet, Uncoated - Oral - 500 mg

100's	**$137.94**	**AMICAR, Immunex**	**58406-0612-61**

AMINOGLUTETHIMIDE *(000203)*

CATEGORIES: ACTH; Adrenal Corticosteroid Inhibitors; Adrenal Function; Adrenal Hyperplasia; Cancer; Cushing's Syndrome; Hormones; Tumors; Adenoma*; Pregnancy Category D; FDA Approval Pre 1982

* Indication not approved by the FDA

BRAND NAMES: **Cytadren**; *Orimeten* (England, Germany); *Orimetene* (France); *Rodazol* (Germany)

(International brand names outside U.S. in italics)

DESCRIPTION:

Aminoglutethimide is an inhibitor of adrenocortical steroid synthesis. Its chemical name is 3-(4-aminophenyl)-3-ethyl-2,6-piperidinedione.

Aminoglutethimide USP is a fine, white or creamy white, crystalline powder. It is very slightly soluble in water, and readily soluble in most organic solvents. It forms water-soluble salts with strong acids. Its molecular weight is 232.28.

Cytadren is available as 250-mg tablets for oral administration.

Cytadren Inactive Ingredients: Cellulose compounds, colloidal silicon dioxide, starch, stearic acid, and talc.

CLINICAL PHARMACOLOGY:

Aminogluthethimide inhibits the enzymatic conversion of cholesterol to Δ^5-pregnenolone, resulting in a decrease in the production of adrenal glucocorticoids, mineralocorticoids, estrogens, & androgens.

Aminogluthethimide blocks several other steps in steroid synthesis, including the C-11, C-18, and C-21 hydroxylations and the hydroxylations required for the aromatization of androgens to estrogens, mediated through the binding of aminogluthethimide to cytochrome P-450 complexes.

A decrease in adrenal secretion of cortisol is followed by an increased secretion of pituitary adrenocorticotropic hormone (ACTH), which will overcome the blockade of adrenocortical steroid synthesis by aminogluthethimide. The compensatory increase in ACTH secretion can be suppressed by the simultaneous administration of hydrocortisone. Since aminogluthethimide increases the rate of metabolism of dexamethasone but not that of hydrocortisone, the latter is preferred as the adrenal glucocorticoid replacement.

Although aminogluthethimide inhibits the synthesis of thyroxine by the thyroid gland, the compensatory increase in thyroid-stimulating hormone (TSH) is frequently of sufficient magnitude to overcome the inhibition of thyroid synthesis due to aminogluthethimide. In spite of an increase in TSH, aminogluthethimide has not been associated with increased prolactin secretion.

Note: aminogluthethimide was marketed previously as an anticonvulsant but was withdrawn from marketing for that indication in 1966 because of the effects on the adrenal gland.

PHARMACOKINETICS

Aminogluthethimide is rapidly and completely absorbed after oral administration. In 6 healthy male volunteers, maximum plasma levels of aminogluthethimide averaged 5.9 mcg/ml at a median of 1.5 hours after ingestion of two 250-mg tablets. The bioavailability of tablets is equivalent to equal doses given as a solution. After ingestion of a single oral dose, 34-54% is excreted in the urine as unchanged drug during the first 48 hours, and an additional fraction as the N-acetyl derivative.

The half-life of aminogluthethimide in normal volunteers given single oral doses averaged 12.5 ± 1.6 hours.

Upon withdrawal of therapy with aminogluthethimide, the ability of the adrenal glands to synthesize steroid returns, usually within 72 hours.

CLINICAL STUDIES:

Clinical investigations included 9 patients aged 2 1/2 to 16 years; 4 of these were aged 10 or less. Seven of the patients received other therapies (drugs or irradiation) either with aminogluthethimide or within a short period before initiation of therapy with aminogluthethimide. Diagnoses included 5 patients with adrenal carcinoma, 3 with adrenal hyperplasia, and 1 with ectopic ACTH-producing tumor. Duration of treatment ranged from 3 days to 6 1/2 months. Dosages ranged from 0.375 g to 1.5 g daily. In general, smaller doses were used for younger patients; for example, a 2 1/2-year-old received 0.5-0.75 g daily, a 3 1/2-year-old received 0.5 g daily, and all others over 10 years of age received 0.75-1.5 g daily. Results are difficult to evaluate because of the concomitant therapy, duration of therapy, or inadequate laboratory documentation. Most patients did show decreases in plasma or urinary steroids at some time during treatment, but these may have been due to other therapeutic modalities or their combinations.

INDICATIONS AND USAGE:

Aminogluthethimide is indicated for the suppression of adrenal function in selected patients with Cushing's syndrome. Morning levels of plasma cortisol in patients with adrenal carcinoma and ectopic ACTH-producing tumors were reduced on the average to about one half of the pretreatment levels, and in patients with adrenal hyperplasia to about two thirds of the pretreatment levels, during 1-3 months of therapy with aminogluthethimide. Data available from the few patients with adrenal adenoma suggest similar reductions in plasma cortisol levels. Measurements of plasma cortisol showed reductions to at least 50% of baseline or to normal levels in one third or more of the patients studied, depending on diagnostic groups and time of measurement.

Because aminogluthethimide does not affect the underlying disease process, it is used primarily as an interim measure until more definitive therapy such as surgery can be undertaken or in cases where such therapy is not appropriate. Only small numbers of patients have been treated for longer than 3 months. A decreased effect or "escape phenomenon" seems to occur more frequently in patients with pituitary-dependent Cushing's syndrome, probably because of increasing ACTH levels in response to decreasing glucocorticoid levels.

Aminogluthethimide should be used only in those patients who are responsive to treatment.

CONTRAINDICATIONS:

Aminogluthethimide is contraindicated in those patients with serious forms, and/or more severe manifestations, of hypersensitivity to glutethimide or aminoglutethimide.

WARNINGS:

Aminogluthethimide may cause adrenocortical hypofunction, especially under conditions of stress, such as surgery, trauma, or acute illness. Patients should be carefully monitored and given hydrocortisone and mineralocorticoid supplements as indicated. Dexamethasone should not be (see DRUG INTERACTIONS.)

Aminogluthethimide also may suppress aldosterone production by the adrenal cortex and may cause orthostatic or persistent hypotension. The blood pressure should be monitored in all patients at appropriate intervals. Patients should be advised of the possible occurrence of weakness and dizziness as symptoms of hypotension, and of measures to be taken should they occur.

The effects of aminogluthethimide may be potentiated if it is taken in combination with alcohol.

Aminogluthethimide can cause fetal harm when administered to a pregnant woman. In the earlier experience with the drug in about 5000 patients, two cases of pseudohermaphroditism were reported in female infants whose mothers were treated with aminogluthethimide and concomitant anticonvulsants. Normal pregnancies have also occurred in patients treated with aminogluthethimide.

When administered to rats at doses 1/2 and 1 1/4 times the maximum daily human dose, aminogluthethimide caused a decrease in fetal implantation, an increase in fetal deaths, and a variety of teratogenic effects. The compound also caused pseudohermaphroditism in rats treated with approximately 3 times the maximum daily human dose. If this drug must be used during pregnancy, or if the patient becomes pregnant while taking the drug, the patient should be apprised of the potential hazard to the fetus.

PRECAUTIONS:

General: This drug should be administered only by physicians familiar with its use and hazards. Therapy should be initiated in a hospital. (See DOSAGE AND ADMINISTRATION.)

Information for the Patient: Patients should be warned that drowsiness may occur and that they should not drive, operate potentially dangerous machinery, or engage in other activities that may become hazardous because of decreased alertness.

Patients should also be warned of the possibility of hypotension and its symptoms (see WARNINGS.)

Laboratory Tests: Hypothyroidism may occur in association with aminogluthethimide; hence, appropriate clinical observations should be made and laboratory studies of thyroid function performed as indicated. Supplementary thyroid hormone may be required.

Hematologic abnormalities in patients receiving aminogluthethimide have been reported (see ADVERSE REACTIONS.) Therefore, baseline hematologic studies should be performed, followed by periodic hematologic evaluation.

Since elevations in SGOT, alkaline phosphatase, and bilirubin have been reported, appropriate clinical observations and regular laboratory studies should be performed before and during therapy.

Serum electrolyte levels should be determined periodically.

Carcinogenesis, Mutagenesis, and Impairment of Fertility: Long-term carcinogenicity studies in animals and mutagenicity studies have not been performed with aminogluthethimide.

Aminogluthethimide affects fertility in female rats (see WARNINGS.) The relevance of these findings to humans is not known.

Pregnancy Category D: See WARNINGS.

Nursing Mothers: It is not known whether this drug is excreted in human milk. Because many drugs are excreted in human milk and because of the potential for serious adverse reactions in nursing infants from aminogluthethimide, a decision should be made whether to discontinue nursing or to discontinue the drug, taking into account the importance of the drug to the mother.

Pediatric Use: Safety and effectiveness in children have not been established (see CLINICAL STUDIES) in children.

DRUG INTERACTIONS:

Aminogluthethimide accelerates the metabolism of dexamethasone; therefore, if glucocorticoid replacement is needed, hydrocortisone should be prescribed.

Aminoglutethimide diminishes the effect of coumarin and warfarin.

ADVERSE REACTIONS:

Untoward effects have been reported in about 2 out of 3 patients with Cushing's syndrome who were treated for 4 or more weeks with aminogluthethimide as the only adrenocortical suppressant.

The most frequent and reversible side effects were drowsiness (approximately 1 in 3 patients), morbilliform skin rash (1 in 6 patients), nausea and anorexia (each approximately 1 in 8 patients), and dizziness (about 1 in 20 patients). The dizziness was possibly caused by lowered vascular resistance or orthostasis. These reactions often disappear spontaneously with continued therapy.

OTHER EFFECTS OBSERVED

Hematologic: Single instances of neutropenia, leukopenia (patient received concomitant o,p'-DDD), pancytopenia (patient received concomitant 5-fluorouracil), and agranulocytosis occurred in 4 of 27 patients with Cushing's syndrome caused by adrenal carcinoma who were treated for at least 4 weeks. In 1 patient with adrenal hyperplasia, hemoglobin levels and hematocrit decreased during the course of treatment with aminogluthethimide. From the earlier experience with the drug used as an anticonvulsant in 1,214 patients, transient leukopenia was the only hematologic effect and was reported once; Coombs'-negative hemolytic anemia also occurred once. In approximately 300 patients with nonadrenal malignancy, 1 in 25 showed some degree of anemia, and 1 in 150 developed pancytopenia during treatment with aminogluthethimide.

Endocrine: Adrenal insufficiency occurred in about 1 in 30 patients with Cushing's syndrome who were treated with aminogluthethimide for 4 or more weeks. This insufficiency tended to involve glucocorticoids as well as mineralocorticoids. Hypothyroidism is occasionally associated with thyroid enlargement and may be detected or confirmed by measuring plasma levels of the thyroid hormone. Masculinization and hirsutism have occasionally occurred in females, as has precocious sexual development in males.

Central Nervous System: Headache was reported in about 1 in 20 patients.

Cardiovascular: Hypotension, occasionally orthostatic, occurred in 1 in 30 patients receiving aminogluthethimide. Tachycardia occurred in 1 in 40 patients.

Gastrointestinal and Liver: Vomiting occurred in 1 in 30 patients. Isolated instances of abnormal findings on liver function tests were reported. Suspected hepatotoxicity occurred in less than 1 in 1000 patients.

Skin: In addition to rash (1 in 6 patients, and often reversible with continued therapy), pruritus was reported in 1 in 20 patients. These may be allergic or hypersensitive reactions. Urticaria has occurred rarely.

ADVERSE REACTIONS: *(cont'd)*

Miscellaneous: Fever was reported in several patients who were treated with aminogluthethimide for less than 4 weeks; some of these patients also received other drugs. Myalgia occurred in 1 in 30 patients.

OVERDOSAGE:

ACUTE TOXICITY

No deaths due to overdosage with aminogluthethimide have been reported.

The highest known doses that have been survived are 7 g (33-year-old woman) and 7.5-10.0 g (16-year-old girl).

Oral LD_{50}'s (mg/kg): rats, 1800; dogs, >100. Intravenous LD_{50}'s (mg/kg): rats, 156; dogs >100.

SIGNS AND SYMPTOMS

An acute overdose with aminogluthethimide may reduce the production of steroids in the adrenal cortex to a degree that is clinically relevant. The following manifestations may be expected:

Respiratory Function: Respiratory depression, hyperventilation.

Cardiovascular System: Hypotension, hypovolemic shock due to dehydration.

Central Nervous System Muscles: Somnolence, lethargy, coma, ataxia, dizziness, fatigue. (Extreme weakness has been reported with divided doses of 3 g daily.)

Gastrointestinal System: Nausea, vomiting.

Renal Function: Loss of sodium and water.

Laboratory Findings: Hyponatremia, hypochloremia, hyperkalemia, hypoglycemia.

The signs and symptoms of acute overdosage with aminogluthethimide may be aggravated or modified if alcohol, hypnotics, tranquilizers, or tricyclic antidepressants have been taken at the same time.

TREATMENT

Symptomatic treatment of overdosage is recommended.

Since aminoglutethimide and glutethimide are chemically related, measures that have been used in successfully removing glutethimide from the body might be useful in removing aminoglutethimide.

Gastric lavage and unspecified supportive treatment have been employed. Full consciousness following deep coma was regained 40 hours or less after ingestion of 3 or 4 g without lavage. No evidence of hematologic, renal, or hepatic effects was subsequently found.

Close monitoring should be provided, and appropriate measures taken to support vital functions, if necessary.

If deficiency of circulating glucocorticoid develops, an intravenous infusion of a soluble hydrocortisone preparation (100 mg of hydrocortisone sodium succinate in 500 ml of isotonic sodium chloride solution) and 50 ml of 40% glucose solution should be given within 3 hours. After the initial infusion is completed, an intravenous administration of hydrocortisone, 10 mg per hour, should be continued until the patient is able to take oral cortisone.

If hypovolemia or hypotension occurs, an intravenous administration of norepinephrine, 10 mg, in 500 ml of isotonic sodium chloride should be administered according to the patient's needs and response. After rehydration, 500 ml of plasma or blood should be given for maintenance of sufficient circulatory volume.

Dialysis may be considered in severe intoxication.

DOSAGE AND ADMINISTRATION:

ADULTS

Treatment should be instituted in a hospital until a stable dosage regimen is achieved. Therapy should be initiated with 250 mg orally four times daily, preferably at 6-hour intervals. Adrenocortical response should be followed by careful monitoring of plasma cortisol levels until the desired level of suppression is achieved. If the level of cortisol suppression is inadequate, the dosage may be increased in increments of 250 mg daily at intervals of 1-2 weeks to a total daily dose of 2 g. Dose reduction or temporary discontinuation of therapy may be required in the event of adverse effects, including extreme drowsiness, severe skin rash, or excessively low cortisol levels. If a skin rash persists for longer than 5-8 days or becomes severe, the drug should be discontinued. It may be possible to reinstate therapy at a lower dosage following the disappearance of a mild or moderate rash. Mineralocorticoid replacement (*e.g.,* fludrocortisone) may be necessary. If glucocorticoid replacement therapy is needed, 20-30 mg of hydrocortisone orally in the morning will replace endogenous secretion.

HOW SUPPLIED - EQUIVALENTS NOT AVAILABLE:

Tablet, Uncoated - Oral - 250 mg

100's	$104.35	CYTADREN, Novartis	00083-0024-30

AMINOHIPPURATE SODIUM *(000204)*

CATEGORIES: Diagnostic Agents; Kidney Function; Renal Function; Pregnancy Category C; FDA Approval Pre 1982

DESCRIPTION:

Aminohippurate sodium is an agent to measure effective renal plasma flow (ERPF). It is the sodium salt of para-aminohippuric acid, commonly abbreviated "PAH". It is water soluble, lipid-insoluble and has a pKa of 3.83. The empirical formula of the anhydrous salt is $C_9H_9N_2NaO_3$.

It is provided as a sterile, non-preserved 20 percent aqueous solution for injection, with a pH of 6.7 to 7.6. Each 10 ml contains: Aminohippurate sodium 2 g. Inactive ingredients: Sodium hydroxide to adjust pH, water for injection, q.s.

CLINICAL PHARMACOLOGY:

PAH is filtered by the glomeruli and is actively secreted by the proximal tubules. At low plasma concentrations (1.0 to 2.0 mg/100 ml), an average of 90 percent of PAH is cleared by the kidneys from the renal bloodstream in a single circulation. It is ideally suited for measurement of ERPF since it has a high clearance, is essentially nontoxic at the plasma concentrations reached with recommended doses and its analytical determination is relatively simple and accurate.

PAH is also used to measure the functional capacity of the renal tubular secretory mechanism or transport maximum (Tm_{PAH}). This is accomplished by elevating the plasma concentration to levels (40-60 mg/100 ml) sufficient to saturate the maximal capacity of the tubular cells to secrete PAH.

Inulin clearance is generally measured during Tm_{PAH} determinations since glomerular filtration rate (GFR) must be known before calculations of secretory Tm measurements can be done (see DOSAGE AND ADMINISTRATION.)

INDICATIONS AND USAGE:

Estimation of effective renal plasma flow.

Measurement of the functional capacity of the renal tubular secretory mechanism.

CONTRAINDICATIONS:

Hypersensitivity to this product or to its components.

PRECAUTIONS:

General: Intravenous solutions must be given with caution to patients with low cardiac reserve, since a rapid increase in plasma volume can precipitate congestive heart failure.

For measurement of ERPF, small doses of PAH are used. However, in research procedures to measure Tm_{PAH}, high plasma levels are required to saturate the capacity of the tubular cells. During these procedures the intravenous administration of PAH solutions should be carried out slowly and with caution. The patient should be continuously observed for any adverse reactions.

Carcinogenesis, Mutagenesis, and Impairment of Fertility: Long-term studies in animals have not been done to evaluate any effects upon fertility or carcinogenic potential of PAH.

Pregnancy Category C: Animal reproduction studies have not been done with PAH. It is also not known whether or not PAH can cause fetal harm when given to a pregnant woman or can effect reproduction capacity. PAH should be given to a pregnant woman only if clearly needed.

Nursing Mothers: It is not known whether this drug is excreted in human milk. Because many drugs are excreted in human milk, caution should be exercised when PAH is administered to a nursing woman.

Pediatric Use: Safety and effectiveness in children have not been established.

DRUG INTERACTIONS:

Renal clearance measurements of PAH cannot be made with any sufficient accuracy in patients receiving sulfonamides, procaine, or thiazolesulfone. These compounds interfere with chemical color development essential to the analytical procedures.

Probenecid depresses tubular secretion of certain weak acids such as PAH. Therefore, patients receiving probenecid will have erroneously low ERPF and Tm_{PAH} values.

ADVERSE REACTIONS:

Vasomotor disturbances, flushing, tingling, nausea, vomiting, and cramps may occur.

Patients may have a sensation of warmth or the desire to defecate or urinate during or shortly following initiation of infusion.

OVERDOSAGE:

The intravenous LD_{50} in female mice is 7.22 g/kg.

DOSAGE AND ADMINISTRATION:

For intravenous use only

Clearance measurements using single injection technics are generally inaccurate, particularly in the measurement of ERPF. For this reason, intravenous infusions at fixed rates are used to sustain the plasma PAH concentration at the desired level.

To measure ERPF, the concentration of PAH in the plasma should be maintained at 2 mg per 100 ml, which can be achieved with a priming dose of 6 to 10 mg/kg and an infusion dose of 10 to 24 mg/min.

As a research procedure for the measurement of Tm_{PAH}, the plasma level of PAH must be sufficient to saturate the capacity of the tubular secretory cells. Concentrations of from 40 to 60 mg per 100 ml are usually necessary.

Technical details in these tests may be found in Smith[1]; Wesson[2]; Bauer[3]; Pitts[4]; and Schnurr[5].

Parenteral drug products shouls be inspected visually for particulate matter and discoloration prior to use, whenever solution and container permit. NOTE: The normal color range for this product is a colorless to yellow/brown solution. The efficacy is not affected by changes within this color range.

CALCULATIONS

Effective Renal Plasma Flow (ERPF): The clearance of PAH, which is extracted almost completely from the plasma during its passage the renal circulation, constitutes a measure of ERPF hence (TABLE 1):

TABLE 1

$ERPF = U_{PAH} V \div P_{PAH}$
Where U_{PAH} = concentration of PAH (mg/ml) in the urine
V = rate of urine excretion (ml-min), and
P_{PAH} = plasma concentration of PAH (mg/ml)
Example: U_{PAH} = 8.0 mg/ml
V = 1.5 ml/min
P_{PAH} = 0.02 mg/ml
$ERPF = 8.0 \times 1.5 \div 0.02 = 600$ ml/min

Based on PAH clearance studies, the normal values for ERPF are:

men 675 ± 150 ml/min

women 595 ± 125 ml/min

Maximum Tubular Secretory (Tm_{PAH})Mechanism

The quantity of PAH secreted by the tubules (Tm_{PAH}) is given by the difference between the total rate of excretion ($U_{PAH}V$) and the quantity filtered by the glomeruli (GFR x P_{PAH}).

$Tm_{PAH} = U_{PAH}V$ - (GFR x P_{PAH} x 0.83)

The factor, 0.83, corrects for that portion of PAH which is bound to plasma protein and hence is unfilterable.

Example: U_{PAH} = 9.55 mg/ml
V = 16.68 ml/min
GFR = 120 ml/min
P_{PAH} = 0.60 mg/ml
Then Tm_{PAH} = 9.55 x 16.68 - (120 x 6.60 x 0.83) = 100 mg/min

Average normal values of Tm_{PAH} are 80-90 mg/min.

The value of the expression $U_{PAH}V$, used in calculations of ERPF and Tm_{PAH}, may be found by determining the amount of PAH in a measured volume of urine excreted within a specific period of time.

These calculations are based on a body surface area of 1.73 m^2. Corrections for variations in surface area are made by multiplying the values obtained for ERPF and Tm_{PAH} by 1.73/A, where A is the subject surface area.

Storage: Avoid storage at temperatures below -20°C (-4°F) and above 40°C (104°F).

REFERENCES:

1. Smith, H.W.: Lectures on the kidney, University Extension Division, University of Kansas, Lawrence, Kansas, 1943 **2.** Wesson, L.G., Jr: "Physiology of the Human Kidney," New York, Grune & Stratton, 1969, pp.632-655. **3.** Bauer, J.D.; Ackerman, P.G.; Toro, G.: "Brays Clinical Laboratory Methods," ed. 7, St. Louis, Mosby, 1968. **4.** Pitts, R.F.: "Physiology of the Kidney and Body Fluids," ed. 2, Chicago, Year Book Medical Publishers, 1968. **5.** Schnurr, E., Lahme, W., Kuppers, H.: Measurement of renal clearance of inulin and PAH in the steady state without urine collection; Clinical Nephrology, *13* (1); (26-29), 1980.

HOW SUPPLIED - EQUIVALENTS NOT AVAILABLE:

Injection, Solution - Intravenous - 20 %

10 ml $5.69 Sodium Aminohippurate, Merck 00006-3395-11

AMINOPHYLLINE *(000207)*

CATEGORIES: Airway Obstruction; Antiasthmatics/Bronchodilators; Asthma; Bronchial Dilators; Bronchitis; Bronchospasm; Chronic Bronchitis; Emphysema; Respiratory & Allergy Medications; Respiratory Muscle Relaxant; Smooth Muscle Relaxants; Xanthine Derivatives; Antineoplastics*; Pregnancy Category C; FDA Approval Pre 1982

* Indication not approved by the FDA

BRAND NAMES: *Aminofilina*; *Aminomal*; **Aminophyllin**; *Aminophyllinum*; *Anephyllin* (Japan); *Asiphylline*; *Asthcontin*; *Bufasma*; *Cardophyllin*; *Corophyllin* (Canada); *Diaphyllin*; *Elixophyllin*; *Eufilin*; *Eufilina*; *Eufilina Mite*; *Euphyllin* (Germany); *Euphyllin Retard*; *Inophyline*; *Kyophyllin* (Japan); *Neophyllin*; Norphyl; *Novphyllin*; *Palaron* (Canada); *Peterphyllin*; Phyllocontin; *Phyllotemp* (Germany); *Planphylline* (France); *Somophylin*; Somophyllin; *Synthophyllin*; *Tefamin*; *Teofylamin*; *Theourin*; Truphylline

(International brand names outside U.S. in italics)

FORMULARIES: Aetna; FHP; Medi-Cal; WHO

COST OF THERAPY: $40.29 (Asthma; Tablet; 200 mg; 3/day; 365 days)

PRIMARY ICD9: 493.90 (Asthma, Unspecified, Without Mention of Status Asthmaticus)

DESCRIPTION:

This monograph contains full prescribing information where noted for the Tablet and Oral Solution form and for the Injection form.

Tablets and Oral Solution: Aminophylline, a xanthine bronchodilator, is a 2:1 complex of theophylline and ethylenediamine. Aminophylline dihydrate contains approximately 79% of anhydrous theophylline, whereas aminophylline anhydrous contains approximately 86% anhydrous theophylline. Aminophylline occurs as white or slightly yellowish granules or powder, having a slight ammoniacal odor and a bitter taste. *Inactive Ingredients:* The oral solution contains ethylenediamine, flavoring, FD&C Yellow No. 6, glycerin, methylparaben, propylparaben, saccharin sodium, sorbitol, and water.

The tablets contain colloidal silicon dioxide, calcium phosphate dibasic, magnesium stearate, and sodium starch glycolate.

Injection: Aminophylline Injection is a sterile solution of theophylline in water for injection. Aminophylline (dihydrate) is approximately 79% of anhydrous theophylline by weight. Aminophylline Injection is administered by intravenous infusion.

Each milliliter contains aminophylline (calculated as the dihydrate) 25 mg (equivalent to 19.7 mg anhydrous theophylline) prepared with the aid of ethylenediamine. The solution may contain an excess of ethylenediamine for pH adjustment. pH is 8.8 (8.6 to 9.0). The osmolar concentration is 0.17 mOsmol/ml (calc.). Headspace nitrogen gassed.

The solution contains no bacteriostat or antimicrobial agent and is intended for use only as a single-dose injection. When smaller doses are required the unused portion should be discarded.

Aminophylline, a xanthine bronchodilator, is a 2:1 complex of theophylline and ethylenediamine and has the chemical name 1H-Purine- 2,6,-dione,3,7-dihydro-1,3-dimethyl-,compounded with 1,2-ethanediamine (2:1).

CLINICAL PHARMACOLOGY:

AMINOPHYLLINE SHOULD BE CONSIDERED AS A MIXTURE OF THEOPHYLLINE AND BASE. ITS ACTIVITY IS THAT OF THEOPHYLLINE ALONE.

Theophylline directly relaxes the smooth muscle of the bronchial airway and pulmonary blood vessels, thus acting mainly as a bronchodilator and smooth muscle relaxant. It has also been demonstrated that aminophylline has a potent effect on diaphragmatic contractility in normal persons and may then be capable of reducing fatigability and therapy improve contractility in patients with chronic obstructive airway disease. The exact mode of action remains unsettled. Although theophylline does cause inhibition of phosphodiesterase with a resultant increase in intracellular cyclic AMP, other agents similarly inhibit the enzyme producing a rise of cyclic AMP but are unassociated with any demonstrable bronchodilation. Other mechanisms proposed include an effect on translocation of intracellular calcium; prostaglandin antagonism; stimulation of catecholamines endogenously; inhibition of cyclic guanosine monophosphate metabolism and adenosine receptor antagonism. None of these mechanisms has been proved, however.

In vitro, theophylline has been shown to act synergistically with beta agonists and there are now available data which demonstrate an additive effect *in vivo*with combined use.

Pharmacokinetics: The half-life of theophylline is influenced by a number of known variables. It may be prolonged in chronic alcoholics, particularly those with liver disease (cirrhosis or alcoholic liver disease), in patients with congestive heart failure, and in those patients taking certain other drugs (see DRUG INTERACTIONS.) Newborns and neonates have extremely slow clearance rates compared to older infants and children, i.e., those over 1 year. Older children have rapid clearance rates while most non-smoking adults have clearance rates between these two extremes. In premature neonates the decreased clearance is related to oxidative pathways that have yet to be established (TABLE 1):

TABLE 1 Theophylline Elimination Characteristics

	Half-Life (in hours) Range	Mean
Children	1-9	3.7
Adults	3-15	7.7

In cigarette smokers (1-2 packs/day) the mean half-life is 4-5 hours, much shorter than in non-smokers. The increase in clearance associated with smoking is presumably due to stimulation of the hepatic metabolic pathway by components of cigarette smoke. The duration of this effect after cessation of smoking is unknown but may require 6 months to 2 years before the rate approaches that of the non-smoker.

INDICATIONS AND USAGE:

For relief and/or prevention of symptoms from asthma and reversible bronchospasm associated with chronic bronchitis and emphysema.

CONTRAINDICATIONS:

This product is contraindicated in individuals who have shown hypersensitivity to its components, including ethylenediamine.

It is also contraindicated in patients with active peptic ulcer disease, and in individuals with underlying seizure disorders (unless receiving appropriate anticonvulsant medications).

WARNINGS:

Serum levels above 20 mcg/ml are rarely found after appropriate administration of the recommended doses. However, in individuals in whom theophylline plasma clearance in reduced *for any reason,* even conventional doses may result in increased serum levels and potential toxicity. Reduced theophylline clearance has been documented in the following readily identifiable groups: 1) patients with impaired liver function; 2) patients over 55 years of age, particularly males and those with chronic lung disease; 3) those with cardiac failure from any cause; 4) patients with sustained high fever; 5) neonates and infants under 1 year of age; and 6) those patients taking certain drugs (see DRUG INTERACTIONS.) Frequently, such patients have markedly prolonged theophylline serum levels following discontinuation of the drug.

Reduction of dosage and laboratory monitoring is especially appropriate in the above individuals.

Serious side effects such as ventricular arrhythmias, convulsions or even death may appear as the first sign of toxicity without any previous warning. Less serious signs of theophylline toxicity (*i.e.,* nausea and restlessness) may occur frequently when initiating therapy, but are usually transient; when such signs are persistent during maintenance therapy, they are often associated with serum concentrations above 20 mcg/ml. Stated differently;*serious toxicity is not reliable preceded by less severe side effects.*A serum concentration measurement is the only reliable method of predicting potentially life-threatening toxicity.

Many patients who require theophylline exhibit tachycardia due to their underlying disease process so that the cause/effect relationship to elevated serum theophylline concentrations may not be appreciated.

Theophylline products may cause or worsen arrhythmias and any significant change in rate and/or rhythm warrants monitoring and further investigation.

Studies is laboratory animals (minipigs, rodents, and dogs) recorded the occurrence of cardiac arrhythmias and sudden death (with histologic evidence of myocardial necrosis) when beta-agonists and methylxanthines were administered concurrently. The significance of these findings when applied to humans is currently unknown.

PRECAUTIONS:

General: On the average, theophylline half-life is shorter in cigarette and marijuana smokers than in non-smokers, but smokers can have half-lives as long as non-smokers. Theophylline should not be administered concurrently with other xanthines. Use with caution in patients with hypoxemia, hypertension, or those with a history of peptic ulcer. Theophylline may occasionally act as a local irritant to G.I. tract (when administered orally), although gastrointestinal symptoms are more commonly centrally mediated and associated with serum drug concentrations over 20 mcg/ml.

Laboratory Tests: Serum levels should be monitored periodically to determine the theophylline level associated with observed clinical response and as the method of predicting toxicity. For such measurements, the serum sample should be obtained at the time of peak concentration, 1 or 2 hours after administration for immediate release products. It is important that the patient will not have missed or taken additional doses during the previous 48 hours and that dosing intervals will have been reasonably equally spaced. DOSAGE ADJUSTMENT BASED ON SERUM THEOPHYLLINE MEASUREMENTS WHEN THESE INSTRUCTIONS HAVE NOT BEEN FOLLOWED MAY RESULT IN RECOMMENDATIONS THAT PRESENT RISK OF TOXICITY TO THE PATIENT.

Drug/Laboratory Test Interactions: Currently available analytical methods, including high pressure liquid chromatography and immunoassay techniques, for measuring serum theophylline levels are specific. Metabolites and other drugs generally do not affect the results. Other new analytic methods are also now in use. The physician should be aware of the laboratory method used and whether other drugs will interfere with the assay for theophylline.

Carcinogenesis, Mutagenesis, and Impairment of Fertility: Long-term carcinogenicity studies have been performed with theophylline.

Chromosome-breaking activity was detected in human cell cultures at concentrations of theophylline up to 50 times the therapeutic serum concentrations in humans. Theophylline was not mutagenic in the dominant lethal assay in male mice given theophylline intraperitoneally in doses up to 30 times the maximum daily human oral dose.

Studies to determine the effect on fertility have not been performed with theophylline.

Pregnancy Category C: Animal reproduction studies have not been conducted with theophylline. It is also not known whether theophylline can cause fetal harm when administered to a pregnant woman or can affect reproduction capacity. Xanthines should be given to a pregnant woman only if clearly needed.

Nursing Mothers: Theophylline is distributed into breast milk and may cause irritability or other sings of toxicity in nursing infants. Because of the potential for serious adverse reactions in nursing infants from theophylline, a decision should be made whether to discontinue nursing or to discontinue the drug, taking into account the importance of the drug to the mother.

Pediatric Use: Sufficient numbers of infants under the age of 1 year have not been studied in clinical trials to support use in this age group; however, there is evidence recorded that the use of dosage recommendations for older infants and young children (16 mg/kg/24 hours) may result in the development of toxic serum levels. Such findings very probably reflect differences in the metabolic handling of the drug related to absent or undeveloped enzyme systems. Consequently, the use of the drug in this age group should carefully consider the associated benefits and risks. If used, the maintenance dose must be conservative and in accord with the following guidelines:

Laboratory Tests: *Tablets and Oral Solution:* The importance of taking only the prescribed dose and time interval between doses should be reinforced. *Injection:* Serum levels should be monitored periodically to determine the theophylline level associated with observed clinical response and as the method of predicting toxicity.

DRUG INTERACTIONS:

Tablets and Oral Solution: Toxic synergism with ephedrine has been documented any may occur with other sympathomimetic bronchodilators. In addition, the following drug interactions have been demonstrated (TABLE 2):

TABLE 2 Aminophylline, Drug Interactions

Theophylline with:	
Allopurinol (high-dose)	Increased serum theophylline levels
Cimetidine	Increased serum theophylline levels
Ciprofloxacin	Increased serum theophylline levels
Erythromycin, Troleandomycin	Increased serum theophylline levels
Lithium carbonate	Increased renal excretion of lithium
Oral Contraceptives	Increased serum theophylline levels
Phenytoin	Decreased theophylline and phenytoin serum levels
Propranolol	Increased serum theophylline levels
Rifampin	Decreased serum theophylline levels

ADVERSE REACTIONS:

The following adverse reactions have been observed, but there has not been enough systematic collection of data to support an estimate of their frequency. The most consistent adverse reactions are usually due to overdosage.

1. Gastrointestinal: Nausea, vomiting, epigastric pain, hematemesis, diarrhea.

2. Central nervous system: Headaches, irritability, restlessness, insomnia, reflex hyperexcitability, muscle twitching, clonic and tonic generalized convulsions.

3. Cardiovascular: Palpitation, tachycardia, extrasystoles, flushing, hypotension, circulatory failure, ventricular arrhythmias.

4. Respiratory: Tachypnea.

5. Renal: Potentiation of diuresis.

6. Others: Alopecia, hyperglycemia and inappropriate ADH syndrome, rash (consider ethylenediamine).

OVERDOSAGE:

TABLETS

Management: It is suggested that the management principles (consistent with the clinical status of the patient when first seen) outlined below be instituted and that simultaneous contact with a Regional Poison Control Center be established. In this way both updated information and individualization regarding required therapy may be provided.

1. When potential oral overdose is established and seizure has not occurred:

a) If patient is alert and seen within the early hours after ingestion, induction of emesis may be of value. Gastric lavage has been demonstrated to be of no value in influencing outcome in patients who present more than 1 hour after ingestion.

b) Administer a cathartic. Sorbitol solution is reported to be of value.

c) Administer repeated doses of activated charcoal and monitor theophylline serum levels.

d) Prophylactic administration of phenobarbital has been shown to increase the seizure threshold in laboratory animals, and administration of this drug can be considered.

2. If patient presents with a seizure:

a) Establish in airway.

b) Administer oxygen.

c) Treat the seizure with intravenous diazepam, 0.1 to 0.3 mg/kg up to 10 mg. If seizures cannot be controlled, the use of general anesthetic should be considered.

d) Monitor vital signs, maintain blood pressure and provide adequate hydration.

3. If post-seizure coma is present:

a) Maintain airway and oxygenation.

b) If a result of oral mediation, follow above recommendations to prevent absorption of the drug, but intubation and lavage will have to be performed instead of inducing emesis, and the cathartic and charcoal will need to be introduced via a large bore gastric lavage tube.

c) Continue to provide full supportive care and adequate hydration until the drug is metabolized. In general, drug metabolism is sufficiently rapid so as not to warrant dialysis. If repeated oral activated charcoal is ineffective (as noted by stable or rising serum levels) charcoal hemoperfusion may be indicated.

Injection: Management of Toxic Symptoms:

1. Discontinue drug immediately.

2. There is no known specific antidote.

3. Treatment is supportive and symptomatic.

4. Avoid administration of sympathomimetic drugs.

5. Administer intravenous fluids, oxygen and other supportive measures to prevent hypotension; correct dehydration and acid-base imbalance.

6. For hyperthermia, use a cooling blanket or give sponge baths as necessary.

7. Maintain patient airway and use artificial respiration in case of respiratory depression.

8. Control convulsions with intravenous diazepam (0.1 to 0.3 mg/kg up to 10 mg). If seizures cannot be controlled, the use of general anesthesia should be considered.

9. Monitor serum theophylline levels until below 20 mcg/ml.

DOSAGE AND ADMINISTRATION:

Effective use of theophylline (*e.g.,* the concentration of drug in the serum associated with optimal benefit and minimal risk of toxicity) is considered to occur when the theophylline concentration is maintained from 10 to 20 mcg/ml. The early studies from which these levels were derived were carried out in patients immediately or shortly after recovery from acute exacerbations of their disease (some hospitalized with status asthmaticus).

Although the 20 mcg/ml level remains appropriate as a critical value (above which toxicity in more likely to occur) for safety purposes, additional data are now available which indicate that the serum theophylline concentrations required to produce maximum physiologic benefit may, in fact, fluctuate with the degree of bronchospasm present and are variable. Therefore, the physician should individualize the range appropriate to the patient's requirements, based of both symptomatic response and improvement in pulmonary function. It should be stressed that serum theophylline concentrations maintained at the upper level of the 10 to 20 mcg/ml range may be associated with potential toxicity when factors known to reduce theophylline clearance are operative. (See WARNINGS.)

Theophylline does not distribute into fatty tissue. Dosage should be calculated on the basis of lean (ideal) body weight where mg/kg doses are presented.

Caution should be exercised for younger children who cannot complain of minor side effects. Older adults, those with cor pulmonale, congestive heart failure, and/or liver disease may have usually low dosage requirements and thus may experience toxicity at the maximal dosage recommended below.

DOSAGE AND ADMINISTRATION: *(cont'd)*

Tablets and Oral Solution: If it is not possible to obtain serum level determinations, restriction of the daily dose (in otherwise healthy adults) to greater than 13 mg/kg/day, to a maximum of 900 mg, in divided doses will result in relatively few patients exceeding serum levels of 20 mcg/ml and the resultant greater risk of toxicity.

Frequency of Dosing: When immediate release products with rapid absorption are used, to maintain serum levels generally requires administration every 6 hours. This is particularly true in children, but dosing intervals up to 8 hours may be satisfactory in adults since they eliminate the drug at a slower rate. Some children, and adults requiring higher than average doses (those having rapid rates of clearance, e.g., half-lives of under 6 hours) may benefit and be more effectively controlled during chronic therapy when given products with sustained-release characteristics since these provide longer dosing intervals and/or less fluctuation in serum concentration between dosing.

Dosage guidelines are approximately only and the wide range of theophylline clearance between individuals (particularly those with concomitant disease) makes indiscriminate usage hazardous.

Dosage Guidelines: *All dosages expressed in terms of Theophylline. For conversion to mg Aminophylline, the following equivalents apply:

1 mg Theophylline equivalent to:

a) 1.16 mg Aminophylline Anhydrous

b) 1.27 Aminophylline Dihydrate (as contained in the tablets)

ACUTE SYMPTOMS OF BRONCHOSPASM REQUIRING RAPID ATTAINMENT OF THEOPHYLLINE SERUM LEVELS FOR BRONCHODILATION

Note: Status asthmaticus should be considered a medical emergency and is defined as that degree of bronchospasm which is not rapidly responsive to usual doses of conventional bronchodilators. Optimal therapy for such patients frequently requires with *additional medication,* parenterally administered, and *close monitoring,*preferably in an intensive care setting.

Patients not currently receiving theophylline products TABLE 3:

TABLE 3

	Theophylline Oral Loading	Dosage Maintenance
Children age 1 to under 9 years	5 mg/kg	4 mg/kg q 6 hrs
Children age 9 to under 16 years; and Smokers	5 mg/kg	3 mg/kg q 6 hrs
Otherwise healthy non-smoking adults	5 mg/kg	3 mg/kg q 8 hrs
Older patients and patients with cor pulmonale	5 mg/kg	2 mg/kg q 8 hrs
Patients with congestive heart failure	5 mg/kg	1-2 mg/kg q 12 hrs

Patients currently receiving theophylline products: Determine, where possible, the time, amount, dosage form, and route of administration of the last dose the patient received. The loading dose for theophylline is based on the principle that each 0.5 mg/kg of theophylline administered as a loading dose will result in a 1.0 mcg/ml increase in serum theophylline concentration. Ideally, the loading dose should be deferred if a serum theophylline concentration can be obtained rapidly. If this is not possible, the clinician must exercise judgement in selecting a dose based on the potential for benefit and risk. When there is sufficient respiratory distress to warrant a small risk, then 2.5 mg/kg or theophylline administered in rapidly absorbed form is likely to increase serum concentration by approximately 5 mcg/ml. If the patient is not experiencing theophylline toxicity, this is unlikely to result in dangerous adverse effects. Subsequent to the decision regarding use of a loading dose for this group to patients, the maintenance dosage recommendations are the same as those described above.

CHRONIC THERAPY

Theophylline is a treatment for the management of reversible bronchospasm (asthma, chronic bronchitis and emphysema) to prevent symptoms and maintain patent airways. A dosage form which allows small incremental doses is desirable for initiating therapy. A liquid preparation should be considered for children to permit both greater ease of and more accurate dosage adjustment. Slow clinical titration is generally preferred to assure acceptance and safety of the medication, and to allow the patient to develop tolerance transient caffeine-like side effects.

Initial Dose: 16 mg/kg/24 hours or 400 mg/24 hours (whichever is less) of theophylline in divided doses at 6 to 8 hour intervals.

Increasing Dose: The above dosage may be increased in approximately 25 percent increments at 3 day intervals so long as the drug is tolerated; until clinical response is satisfactory or the maximum dose as indicated in section III (below) is reached. The serum concentration may be checked at these intervals, but at a minimum, should be determined at the end of this adjustment period. It is important that no patient be maintained on any dosage that is not tolerated. When instructing patients to increase dosage according to the schedule above, they should be told not to take a subsequent dose if apparent side effects occur and to resume therapy at a lower dose once adverse effects have disappeared.

MAXIMUM DOSE OF THEOPHYLLINE WHERE THE SERUM CONCENTRATION IS NOT MEASURED

WARNING: DO NOT ATTEMPT TO MAINTAIN ANY DOSE THAT IS NOT TOLERATED. Not to exceeded the following: (or 900 mg, whichever is less) (TABLE 4):

TABLE 4

Age 1 to under 9 years	24 mg/kg/day
Age 9 to under 12 years	20 mg/kg/day
Age 12 to under 16 years	18 mg/kg/day
Age 16 years and older	13 mg/kg/day

MEASUREMENT OF SERUM THEOPHYLLINE CONCENTRATIONS DURING CHRONIC THERAPY:

If the above maximum doses are to be maintained or exceeded, serum theophylline measurement is essential. See PRECAUTIONS, Laboratory Tests for guidance.

FINAL ADJUSTMENT OF DOSAGE

Dosage adjustment after serum theophylline measurement (TABLE 5):

The serum concentration may be rechecked at appropriate intervals, but at least at the end of any adjustment period. When the patient's condition is otherwise clinically stable and none of the recognized factors which alter elimination are present, measurement of serum levels need be repeated only every 6 to 12 months.

Injection: Acute symptoms of bronchospasm requiring rapid attainment of theophylline serum levels for bronchodilation.

NOTE: Status asthmaticus should be considered a medical emergency and defined as that degree of bronchospasm which is not rapidly responsive to usual doses of conventional bronchodilators. Optimal therapy for such patients frequently requires both *additional medication,*parenterally administered, and *close monitoring,* preferably in an intensive care setting.

Patients not currently receiving theophylline products (* = equivalent dosage of theophylline) (TABLE 6):

DOSAGE AND ADMINISTRATION: *(cont'd)*

TABLE 5

If serum theophylline is:	Directions:
Within desired range	Maintain dosage if tolerated
Too high 20 to 25 mcg/ml	Decrease doses by about 10% and recheck serum level after 3 days:
20 to 30 mcg/ml	Skip the next dose and decrease subsequent doses by about 25%. Recheck serum level after 3 days.
Over 30 mcg/ml	Skip next 2 doses and decrease subsequent doses by 50%. Recheck serum level after 3 days.
Too Low	Increase dosage by 25% at 3 day intervals until either the desired serum concentration and/or clinical response is achieved. The total daily dose may need to be administered at more frequent intervals if symptoms occur repeatedly at the end of a dosing interval.

TABLE 6

	Aminophylline Dosage Loading	Maintenance
Children age 1 to 9 years	6.3 mg/kg *(5.0)	1.0 mg/kg/hr *(0.79)
Children age 9 to 16 years and smokers	6.3 mg/kg *(5.0)	0.8 mg/kg hr *(0.63)
Otherwise healthy non-smoking adults	6.3 mg/kg *(5.0)	0.5 mg/kg hr *(0.40)
Older patients and patients with cor pulmonale	6.3 mg/kg *(5.0)	0.3 mg/kg hr *(0.24)
Patients with congestive heart failure	6.3 mg/kg *(5.0)	0.1-0.2 mg/kg/hr *(0.08-0.16)

Patients Currently Receiving Theophylline Products

Determine, where possible, the time, amount, dosage form, and route of administration of the last dose the patient received. The loading dose for theophylline is based on the principle that each 0.5 mg/kg of theophylline administered as a loading dose will result in a 1 mcg/ml increase in serum theophylline concentration. Ideally, the loading dose should be deferred if a serum theophylline concentration can be obtained rapidly. If this is not possible, the clinician must exercise judgement in selecting a dose based on the potential for benefit and risk. When there is sufficient respiratory distress to warrant a small risk, then 2.5 mg/kg or theophylline administered in rapidly absorbed form is likely to increase the serum concentration by approximately 5 mcg/ml. If the patient is not experiencing theophylline toxicity, this is unlikely to result in dangerous adverse effects. Subsequent to the decision regarding use of a loading dose for this group to patients, the maintenance dosage recommendations are the same as those described above.

Principles of IV Therapy: The loading dose of aminophylline can be given by very slow IV push, or more conveniently, may be infused in a small quantity (usually 100 to 200 ml) of 5% dextrose injection or 0.9% Sodium Chloride Injection, USP. Do not exceed the rate of 25 mg/min. Thereafter, maintenance therapy can be administered by a large volume infusion to deliver the desired amount of drug each hour. Aminophylline is compatible with the most commonly use IV solutions. Oral therapy should be substituted for IV aminophylline as soon as adequate improvement is achieved.

Intravenous Admixture Incompatibility: Although there have been reports of aminophylline precipitating in acidic media, these reports do not apply to the dilute solutions found in IV infusions. Aminophylline Injection should not be mixed in a syringe with other drugs but should be added separately to the IV solution. When an IV solution containing Aminophyllin is given "piggyback", the IV system already in place should be turned off while the aminophylline is infused if there is a potential problem with admixture incompatibility. Because of the alkalinity of Aminophylline containing solutions, drugs known to be alkali labile should be avoided in admixtures. These included epinephrine HCl, norepinephrine bitartrate, isoproterenol HCl and penicillin G potassium. It is suggested that specialized literature be consulted before preparing admixtures with Aminophylline and other drugs.Parenteral drug products should be inspected visually for particulate matter discoloration prior to administration, whenever solution and container permit. Do not administer unless solution is clear and container is undamaged. Discard unused portion. Do not use if crystals have separated from solution.

INITIAL MAINTENANCE DOSAGE

(of anhydrous theophylline) 1 mg theophylline anhydrous-1.3 mg aminophylline dihydrate.

Premature Infants

Up to 24 days postnatal age: 1.0 mg/kg q 12h

Beyond 24 days postnatal age: 1.5 mg/kg q 12h

Infants 6 to 52 Weeks

[(0.2 x age in weeks) + 5.0] x kg body wt : 24 hour dose in mg.

Up to 26 weeks , divide into q8h dosing intervals.

From 26-52 weeks , divide into q6h dosing intervals.

Final Dosage should be guided by serum concentrations after a steady state (no further accumulation of drug) has been achieved.

PROTECT FROM LIGHT. Keep syringes and vials in carton until time of use.

SINGLE DOSE CONTAINER: Discard unused portion.

Store at controlled room temperature 15- 30°C (59-86°F).

(Tablets and Oral Solution: Roxane Laboratories, 7/94) (Injection: Abbott Laboratories: 6/93)

HOW SUPPLIED - RATED THERAPEUTICALLY EQUIVALENT:

Injection, Solution - Intravenous - 25 mg/ml

10 ml	$2.14	Aminophylline, Abbott	00074-7385-01
10 ml	$2.40	Aminophylline, Abbott	00074-5921-01
10 ml	$15.54	AMINOPHYLLINE, Abbott	00074-4909-18
10 ml x 10	$95.88	Aminophylline, Fujisawa USA	00469-9314-87
10 ml x 25	$19.69	Aminophylline, Am Regent	00517-3810-25
10 ml x 100	$86.00	Aminophylline, Raway	00686-3810-25
20 ml	$2.68	Aminophylline, Abbott	00074-7386-01
20 ml	$3.33	Aminophylline, Abbott	00074-5922-01
20 ml	$16.49	AMINOPHYLLINE, Abbott	00074-4906-19
20 ml	$21.72	Aminophylline, Fujisawa USA	00469-8000-40
20 ml x 25	$22.19	Aminophylline, Am Regent	00517-3820-25
20 ml x 25	$22.81	Aminophylline, Fujisawa USA	00469-0005-25

Solution - Oral - 105 mg/5ml

10 ml x 40	$21.33	Aminophylline, Roxane	00054-8049-16
15 ml cups x 40	$22.28	Aminophylline, Roxane	00054-8050-16

HOW SUPPLIED - RATED THERAPEUTICALLY EQUIVALENT:
(cont'd)

237 ml	$11.55	Aminophylline Dye Free Liquid 105, Schein Pharm (US)	00364-7342-76
237 ml	$12.32	Aminophylline - Dye Free, Alpharma	00472-0873-08
240 ml	$4.00	Aminophylline, Raway	00686-0873-08
240 ml	$11.20	Aminophylline, Harber Pharm	51432-0505-19
240 ml	$12.13	Somophyllin DF, Rugby	00536-0202-59
500 ml	$16.67	Aminophylline, Roxane	00054-3045-63

Tablet, Uncoated - Oral - 100 mg

100's	$2.47	Aminophylline, West Ward Pharm	00143-1020-01
100's	$3.25	Aminophylline, Consolidated Midland	00223-0100-01
100's	$3.44	Aminophylline, H.C.F.A. F F P	99999-0207-01
100's	$3.45	Aminophylline, Schein Pharm (US)	00364-0004-01
100's	$3.45	Aminophylline, United Res	00677-0003-01
100's	$3.45	Aminophylline, Geneva Pharms	00781-1214-01
100's	$3.50	Aminophylline, Roxane	00054-4025-25
100's	$3.90	Aminophyllin, Rugby	00536-3046-01
100's	$4.20	Aminophylline, Major Pharms	00904-2273-60
100's	$4.55	Aminophylline, Aligen Independ	00405-4060-01
100's	$8.26	Aminophylline, Roxane	00054-8025-25
1000's	**$11.32**	**Aminophylline, West Ward Pharm**	**00143-1020-10**
1000's	$13.00	Aminophylline, C O Truxton	00463-6001-10
1000's	$16.50	Aminophylline, Goldline Labs	00182-0109-10
1000's	$18.00	Aminophylline, Roxane	00054-4025-31
1000's	$19.95	Aminophylline, Major Pharms	00904-2273-80
1000's	$20.30	Aminophylline, United Res	00677-0003-10
1000's	$20.32	Aminophylline, Aligen Independ	00405-4060-03
1000's	$21.50	Aminophylline, Consolidated Midland	00223-0100-02
1000's	$22.55	Aminophylline, HL Moore Drug Exch	00839-5053-16
1000's	$30.95	Aminophylline, Rugby	00536-3046-10
1000's	$34.40	Aminophylline, H.C.F.A. F F P	99999-0207-02

Tablet, Uncoated - Oral - 200 mg

100's	$3.68	Aminophylline, West Ward Pharm	00143-1025-01
100's	$3.72	Aminophylline, Roxane	00054-4026-25
100's	$4.50	Aminophylline, Consolidated Midland	00223-0102-01
100's	$4.90	Aminophylline, HL Moore Drug Exch	00839-1011-06
100's	$5.38	Aminophylline, United Res	00677-0007-01
100's	$5.39	Aminophylline, H.C.F.A. F F P	99999-0207-03
100's	$5.64	Aminophylline, Aligen Independ	00405-4061-01
100's	$5.68	Aminophyllin, Rugby	00536-3060-01
100's	$5.99	Aminophylline, Schein Pharm (US)	00364-0005-01
100's	$6.00	Aminophylline, Major Pharms	00904-2283-60
100's	$8.96	Aminophylline, Roxane	00054-8026-25
1000's	$16.99	Aminophylline, West Ward Pharm	00143-1025-10
1000's	$22.00	Aminophylline, C O Truxton	00463-6003-10
1000's	$24.47	Aminophylline, Roxane	00054-4026-31
1000's	$29.50	Aminophylline, Consolidated Midland	00223-0102-02
1000's	$33.00	Aminophylline, Goldline Labs	00182-0110-10
1000's	$33.30	Aminophylline, United Res	00677-0007-10
1000's	$33.40	Aminophylline, Major Pharms	00904-2283-80
1000's	$39.79	Aminophylline, Aligen Independ	00405-4061-03
1000's	$40.97	Aminophylline, HL Moore Drug Exch	00839-1011-16
1000's	$53.90	Aminophylline, H.C.F.A. F F P	99999-0207-04

HOW SUPPLIED - NOT RATED EQUIVALENT:

Injection, Solution - Intravenous - 1 mg/ml

500 ml	$8.62	Aminophylline, Abbott	00074-6466-03
1000 ml	$10.23	Aminophylline, Abbott	00074-6466-05

Injection, Solution - Intravenous - 2 mg/ml

500 ml	$10.24	Aminophylline, Abbott	00074-6467-03

Injection, Solution - Intravenous - 25 mg/ml

10 ml x 10	$51.60	Aminophylline, Voluntary Hosp	53258-9314-08
10 ml x 25	$18.00	Aminophylline, Gensia Labs	00703-5104-04
10 ml x 25	$18.44	Aminophylline, Fujisawa USA	00469-0051-25
10 ml x 25	$30.00	Aminophylline, Consolidated Midland	00223-7130-10
10 ml x 100	$44.37	Aminophylline, Am Regent	00517-0232-70
10 ml x 100	$110.00	Aminophylline, Consolidated Midland	00223-7130-00
20 ml x 25	$22.50	Aminophylline, Gensia Labs	00703-5115-04
20 ml x 25	$40.00	Aminophylline, Consolidated Midland	00223-7136-20

Suppository - Rectal - 250 mg

10's	$8.75	Aminophylline, GW Labs	00713-0125-09
10's	$14.34	Aminophyllin, Rugby	00536-1301-19
10's	$14.50	Aminophylline, Consolidated Midland	00223-5010-10
25's	$4.81	Aminophyllin, Rugby	00536-1301-04
25's	$17.50	Aminophylline, GW Labs	00713-0125-25
25's	$24.00	Aminophylline, Consolidated Midland	00223-5010-25

Suppository - Rectal - 500 mg

10's	$9.94	Aminophylline, GW Labs	00713-0103-09
10's	$16.08	Aminophylline, Qualitest Pharms	00603-8022-10
10's	$16.47	Aminophyllin, Rugby	00536-1310-19
10's	$17.00	Aminophylline, Consolidated Midland	00223-5012-10
25's	$19.88	Aminophylline, GW Labs	00713-0103-25
25's	$29.50	Aminophylline, Consolidated Midland	00223-5012-25
50's	$31.81	Aminophylline, GW Labs	00713-0103-50
50's	$49.50	Aminophylline, Consolidated Midland	00223-5012-50

Tablet, Uncoated - Oral - 100 mg

100's	$3.45	Aminophylline, Goldline Labs	00182-0109-01

Tablet, Uncoated - Oral - 200 mg

100's	$5.40	Aminophylline, Goldline Labs	00182-0110-01

Tablet, Uncoated, Sustained Action - Oral - 225 mg

100's	$35.55	PHYLLOCONTIN, Purdue Frederick	00034-0225-80

AMINOPHYLLINE; AMOBARBITAL; EPHEDRINE *(000208)*

CATEGORIES: DESI Drugs; Respiratory Muscle Relaxant; Smooth Muscle Relaxants; FDA Pre 1938 Drugs

BRAND NAMES: Asthmacon

Prescribing information not available at time of publication.

HOW SUPPLIED - EQUIVALENTS NOT AVAILABLE:

Capsule, Gelatin - Oral

100's	$4.50	Asthmacon, Consolidated Midland	00223-0160-01
1000's	$40.00	Asthmacon, Consolidated Midland	00223-0160-02

AMINOPHYLLINE; EPHEDRINE; PHENOBARBITAL; POTASSIUM IODIDE *(000205)*

CATEGORIES: Antiasthmatics/Bronchodilators; DESI Drugs; Iodide Salts; Respiratory & Allergy Medications; Respiratory Muscle Relaxant; Smooth Muscle Relaxants; FDA Pre 1938 Drugs

BRAND NAMES: Mudrane

Prescribing information not available at time of publication.

HOW SUPPLIED - EQUIVALENTS NOT AVAILABLE:

Tablet, Uncoated - Oral - 130 mg/16 mg/8

100's	$24.48	MUDRANE, ECR Pharms	00095-0050-01

AMINOPHYLLINE; GUAIFENESIN *(000206)*

CATEGORIES: Antiasthmatics/Bronchodilators; Respiratory & Allergy Medications; Respiratory Muscle Relaxant; Smooth Muscle Relaxants; FDA Pre 1938 Drugs

BRAND NAMES: **Mudrane Gg-2**

Prescribing information not available at time of publication.

HOW SUPPLIED - EQUIVALENTS NOT AVAILABLE:

Tablet, Uncoated - Oral - 130 mg/100 mg

100's	**$21.00**	**MUDRANE GG-2, ECR Pharms**	**00095-0033-01**

AMINOSALICYLATE SODIUM *(000211)*

CATEGORIES: Anti-Infectives; Antimicrobials; Antimycobacterials; Antituberculosis Agents; Tuberculosis; FDA Approval Pre 1982

BRAND NAMES: 5-Aminosalicylic Acid; *Aminox*; *Eupasal*; *Nemasol*; **PAS Sodium**; Sodium Aminosalicylate; Sodium P.A.S.; Teebacin
(International brand names outside U.S. in italics)

COST OF THERAPY: $483.84 (Tuberculosis; Tablet; 0.5 gm; 28/day; 180 days)

PRIMARY ICD9: 011.93 (Pulmonary Tuberculosis, Unspecified, Tubercle Bacilli Found)

DESCRIPTION:

Sodium Aminosalicylate, USP is a white to cream colored crystalline powder. It is practically odorless and has a sweet, saline taste. Its solutions decompose slowly and darken in color. One gram dissolves in about 2 ml. of water. It is sparingly soluble in alcohol and very slightly soluble in ether and in chloroform. A 2% solution has pH of 6.5 to 8.5. Therapeutic class: Antitubercular.

$C_7H_6NNaO_3 \cdot 2H_2O$

Molecular Weight: 211.2

CLINICAL PHARMACOLOGY:

Sodium aminosalicylate is bacteriostatic against *Mycobacterium tuberculosis.* It inhibits the onset of bacterial resistance to streptomycin & isoniazid.

INDICATIONS AND USAGE:

Treatment of tuberculosis, always in combination with streptomycin, isoniazid, or both, when due to susceptible strains of tubercle bacilli.

CONTRAINDICATIONS:

Sever hypersensitivity to sodium aminosalicylate and its congeners.

PRECAUTIONS:

All drugs should be stopped at the first sign suggesting a hypersensitive reaction. They may be restarted one at a time, in very small but gradually increasing doses to determine whether the manifestations are drug induced and, if so, which drug is responsible. Oral hyposensitization to sodium aminosalicylate products can only occasionally be accomplished.

Should be used with caution in patients with impaired renal or hepatic functions, and with gastric ulcer.

Patients receiving anticoagulants may require adjustments of their dosage.

Crystalluria may be prevented by the maintenance of urine at a neutral or an alkaline pH.

Sodium aminosalicylate should be used with caution in patients with known or impending congestive hear failure and in other situations in which excess sodium is potentially harmful, such as severe liver disease.

ADVERSE REACTIONS:

The most common side effect is gastrointestinal intolerance manifested by nausea, vomiting, diarrhea, and abdominal pain.

Hypersensitivity Reactions: Fever, skin eruptions of various types, infectious mononucleosis-like syndrome, leukopenia, agranulocytosis, thrombocytopenia, hemolytic anemia, jaundice, hepatitis, encephalopathy, Loeffler's syndrome and vasculitis.

Endocrine Reactions: Goiter with or without myxedema.

DOSAGE AND ADMINISTRATION:

Sodium aminosalicylate should be administered with isoniazid, streptomycin, or both.

Adults: 14 to 16 g/day sodium aminosalicylate in two to three divided doses orally.

Children: 275 to 420 mg/kg/day in 3 to 4 divided doses daily.

Caution: Sodium aminosalicylate deteriorates rapidly in contact with water, heat and sunlight. A brownish or purplish color of the powder or tablets, and especially of a solution made with them, is indicative of such deterioration. If deterioration is evident, the drug should be discarded.

DOSAGE AND ADMINISTRATION: *(cont'd)*
Dispense tablets in tight, light-resistant containers as defined in the USP.

HOW SUPPLIED - EQUIVALENTS NOT AVAILABLE:

Powder

100 gm	$49.05	5-Aminosalicylic Acid, Paddock Labs	00574-0515-01

Tablet, Coated - Oral - 0.5 gm

100's	$9.60	Sodium P.A.S., Lannett	00527-1149-01
500's	$41.80	Sodium P.A.S., Lannett	00527-1149-05
500's	$102.18	Sodium P.A.S., Palisades Pharms	53159-0014-05

AMINOSALICYLIC ACID *(003227)*

CATEGORIES: Anti-Infectives; Antibiotics; Antimicrobials; Antimycobacterials; Antituberculosis Agents; Tuberculosis; FDA Approved 1994 Jun

BRAND NAMES: *Eupasal Sodico*; *Nemasol Sodium* (Canada); **Paser** *(International brand names outside U.S. in italics)*

COST OF THERAPY: $2,030.40 (Tuberculosis; Granules; 4 gm; 3/day; 180 days)

PRIMARY ICD9: 011.93 (Pulmonary Tuberculosis, Unspecified, Tubercle Bacilli Found)

DESCRIPTION:

Paser granules are a delayed release granule preparation of aminosalicylic acid (p-aminosalicylic acid; 4-aminosalicylic acid) for use with other anti-tuberculosis drugs for the treatment of all forms of active tuberculosis due to susceptible strains of tubercle bacilli. The granules are designed for gradual release to avoid high peak levels not useful (and perhaps toxic) with bacteriostatic drugs. Aminosalicylic acid is rapidly degraded in acid media; the protective acid-resistant outer coating is rapidly dissolved in neutral media so a mildly acidic food such as orange, apple or tomato juice, yogurt or apple sauce should be used.

Aminosalicylic acid (p-aminosalicylic acid) is 4-Amino-2-hydroxybenzoic acid. Paser granules are the free base of aminosalicylic acid and do NOT contain sodium or a sugar. The molecular formula is $C_7H_7NO_3$ with a molecular weight of 153.14. With heat p-aminosalicylic acid is decarboxylated to produce CO_2 and m-aminophenol. If the airtight packets are swollen, storage has been improper. DO NOT USE if packets are swollen or the granules have lost their tan color and are dark brown or purple.

Paser granules are supplied as off-white tan colored granules with an average diameter of 1.5 mm and an average content of 60% aminosalicylic acid by weight. The acid resistant outer coating will be completely removed by a few minutes at a neutral pH. The inert ingredients are: colloidal silicon dioxide, dibutyl sebacate, hydroxypropyl methyl cellulose, methacrylic acid copolymer, microcrystalline cellulose, talc. The packets contain 4 grams of aminosalicylic acid for oral administration three times a day by sprinkling on apple sauce or yogurt to be eaten without chewing. Suspension in an acidic fruit drink such as orange juice or tomato juice will protect the coating for at least 2 hours. Swirling the juice in the glass will help resuspend the granules if they sink.

CLINICAL PHARMACOLOGY:

Mechanism of Action: Aminosalicylic acid is bacteriostatic against Mycobacterium tuberculosis. It inhibits the onset of bacterial resistance to streptomycin and isoniazid. The mechanism of action has been postulated to be inhibition of folic acid synthesis (but without potentiation with antifolic compounds) and/or inhibition of synthesis of the cell wall component, mycobactin, thus reducing iron uptake by M. tuberculosis.

Characteristics: The two major considerations in the clinical pharmacology of aminosalicylic acid are the prompt production of a toxic inactive metabolite under acid conditions and the short serum half life of one hour for the free drug. Both are discussed below.

After two hours in simulated gastric fluid, 10% of unprotected aminosalicylic acid is decarboxylated to form meta-aminophenol, a known hepatotoxin. The acid-resistant coating of the Paser granules protects against degradation in the stomach. The small granules are designed to escape the usual restriction on gastric emptying of large particles. Under neutral conditions such as are found in the small intestine or in neutral foods, the acid-resistant coating is dissolved within one minute. Care must be taken in the administration of these granules to protect the acid-resistant coating by maintaining the granules in an acidic food during dosage administration. Patients who have neutralized gastric acid with antacids will not need to protect the acid resistant coating with an acidic food since no acid is present to spoil the drug. Antacids may influence the absorption of other medications and are not necessary for Paser consumed with an acidic food.

Because Paser granules are protected by an enteric coating absorption does not commence until they leave the stomach; the soft skeletons of the granules remain and may be seen in the stool.

Absorption And Excretion: In a single 4 gram pharmacokinetic study with food in normal volunteers the initial time to a 2 mcg/ml serum level of aminosalicylic acid was 2 hours with a range of 45 minutes to 24 hours; the median time to peak was 6 hours with a range of 1.5 to 24 hours; the mean peak level was 20 mcg/ml with a range of 9 to 35 mcg/ml; a level of 2 mcg/ml was maintained for an average of 7.9 hours with a range of 5 to 9; a level of 1 mcg/ml was maintained for an average of 8.8 hours with a range of 6 to 11.5 hours. The recommended schedule is 4 grams every 8 hours.

80% of aminosalicylic acid is excreted in the urine, with 50% or more of the dosage excreted in acetylated form. The acetylation process is not genetically determined as is the case for isoniazid. Aminosalicylic acid is excreted by glomerular filtration; although previously reported otherwise, probenecid, a tubular blocking agent, does not enhance plasma concentration. In a 1954 study thyroxine synthesis but not iodide uptake was reported reduced about 40% when the sodium salt (not Paser granules) of aminosalicylic acid was administered one hour before radio-iodine; the sodium salt typically produces a serum level over 120 mcg/ml at one hour lasting one hour. Occasional goiter development can be prevented by the administration of thyroxine but not iodide.

Penetration into the cerebrospinal fluid occurs only if the meninges are inflamed.

Approximately 50-60% of aminosalicylic acid is protein bound; binding is reported to be reduced 50% in kwashiorkor.

Microbiology: The aminosalicylic acid MIC for M. tuberculosis in 7H11 agar was less than 1.0 mcg/ml for nine strains including three multidrug resistant strains, but 4 and 8 mcg/ml for two other multidrug resistant strains. The 90% inhibition in 7H12 broth (Bactec) showed little dose response but was interpreted as being less than or equal to 0.12-0.25 mcg/ml for eight strains of which three were multi-resistant, 0.50 mcg/ml for one resistant strain, questionable for four non-resistant strains and greater than 1 mcg/ml for one non-resistant and three resistant strains. Aminosalicylic acid is not active *in vitro* against M. avium.

INDICATIONS AND USAGE:

Paser is indicated for the treatment of tuberculosis in combination with other active agents. It is most commonly used in patients with Multi-drug Resistant TB (MDR-TB) or in situations when therapy with isoniazid and rifampin is not possible due to a combination of resistance and/or intolerance. When Paser is added to the treatment regimen in patients with proven or suspected drug resistance, it should be accompanied by at least one and preferably two other new agents to which the patient's organism is known or expected to be susceptible.

CONTRAINDICATIONS:

Hypersensitivity to any component of this medication.

Severe renal disease.

Patients with severe renal disease will accumulate aminosalicylic acid and its acetyl metabolite but will continue to acetylate, thus leading exclusively to the inactive acetylated form; deacetylation, if any, is not significant.

The half life of free aminosalicylic acid in renal disease is 30.8 minutes in comparison to 26.4 minutes in normal volunteers, but the half life of the inactive metabolite is 309 minutes in uremic patients in comparison to 51 minutes in normal volunteers. Although aminosalicylic acid passes dialysis membranes, the frequency of dialysis usually is not comparable to the half-life of 50 minutes for the free acid. Patients with end stage renal disease should not receive aminosalicylic acid.

WARNINGS:

Liver Function In retrospective study of 7492 patients on rapidly absorbed aminosalicylic acid preparations, drug-induced hepatitis occurred in 38 patients (0.5%); in these 38 the first symptom usually appeared within three months of the start of therapy with a rash as the most common event followed by fever and much less frequently by GI disturbances of anorexia, nausea or diarrhea. Only one patient was diagnosed on routine biochemistry.

Premonitory symptoms in 90% of these 38 patients preceded jaundice by afew days to several weeks with the mean time of onset 33 days with a range of 7-90 days. Half of the adverse reactions occurred during the third, fourth or fifth weeks. When aminosalicylic acid-induced hepatitis was diagnosed, hepatomegaly was invariably present with lymphadenopathy in 46%, leucocytosis in 79%, and eosinophilia in 55%. Prompt recognition with discontinuation led to the recovery of all 38 patients. If recognized in the premonitory stage, the reaction is reported to "settle" in 24 hours and no jaundice ensues. From other reported studies failure to recognize the reaction can result in a mortality of up to 21%. The patient must be monitored carefully during the first three months of therapy and treatment must be discontinued immediately at the first sign of a rash, fever or other premonitory signs of intolerance.

PRECAUTIONS:

General: All drugs should be stopped at the first sign suggesting a hypersensitivity reaction. They may be restarted one at a time in very small but gradually increasing doses to determine whether the manifestations are drug-induced and, if so, which drug is responsible.

Desensitization has been accomplished successfully in 15 of 17 patients starting with 10 mg aminosalicylic acid given as a single dose. The dosage is doubled every 2 days until reaching a total of 1 gram after which the dosage is divided to follow the regular schedule of administration. If a mild temperature rise or skin reaction develops, the increment is to be dropped back one level or the progression held for one cycle. Reactions are rare after a total dosage of 1.5 grams.

Patients with hepatic disease may not tolerate aminosalicylic acid as well as normal patients, even though the metabolism in patients with hepatic disease has been reported to be comparable to that in normal volunteers.

Information for the Patient: The patient should be advised that the first signs of hypersensitivity include a rash, often followed by fever, and much less frequently, GI disturbances of anorexia, nausea or diarrhea. If such symptoms develop the patient should immediately cease taking the medication and arrange for a prompt clinical visit.

Patients should be advised that poor compliance in taking anti-TB medication often lead to treatment failure, and, not infrequently, to the development of resistance of the organisms in the individual patient.

Patients should be advised that the skeleton of the granules may be seen in the stool.

The coating to protect the Paser granules dissolves promptly under neutral conditions; the granules therefore should be administered by sprinkling on acidic foods such as apple sauce or yogurt or by suspension in a fruit drink which will protect the coating, but the granules sink and will have to be swirled. The coating will last at least 2 hours in either system. All juices tested to date have been satisfactory; tested are: tomato, orange, grapefruit, grape, cranberry, apple, "fruit punch".

Patients should be advised NOT to use if the packets are swollen or the granules have lost their tan color and are dark brown or purple. The patient should inform the pharmacist or physician immediately and return the medication.

Laboratory Tests: Aminosalicylic acid has been reported to interfere technically with the serum determinations of albumin by dye-binding, SGOT by the azoene dye method and with qualitative urine test for ketones, bilirubin, urobilinogen or porphobilinogen.

Carcinogenesis, Mutagenesis, and Impairment of Fertility: Sodium aminosalicylate produced an occipital bone defect, probably with a dose response, when administered to ten pregnant Wistar rats at five doses from 3.85 to 385 mg/kg from days 6 to 14. There were no significant changes from controls in any group in corpora lutea, early resorptions, total resorptions, fetal death, litter size, or hematomas. For all except the 77 mg/kg group, fetal weights were significantly greater than controls. Chinchilla rabbits on 5 mg/kg from days 7 to 14 did not show any significant differences as compared to controls for the same parameters studied.

Sodium aminosalicylic acid was not mutagenic in Ames tester strain TA 100. In human lymphocyte cultures *in vitro* clastogenic effects of achromatic, chromatid, isochromatic breaks or chromatid translocations were not seen at 153 or 600 mcg/ml. At 1500 and 3000 mcg/ml there was a dose related increase in chromatid aberrations.

Patients on isoniazid and aminosalicylic acid have been reported to have an increased number of chromosomal aberrations as compared to controls.

Pregnancy Category C: Aminosalicylic acid has been reported to produce occipital malformations in rats when given at doses within the human dose range. Although there probably is a dose response, the frequency of abnormalities was comparable to controls at the highest level tested (two times the human dosage). When administered to rabbits at 5 mg/kg, throughout all three trimesters, no teratologic or embryocidal effects were seen. Literature reports on aminosalicylic acid in pregnant women always report coadministration of other medications. Because there are no adequate and well controlled studies of aminosalicylic acid in humans, Paser granules should be given to a pregnant woman only if clearly needed.

Nursing Mothers: After administration of a different preparation of aminosalicylic acid to one patient, the maximum concentration in the milk was 1 mcg/ml at 3 hours with a half-life of 2.5 hours; the maximum maternal plasma concentration was 70 mcg/ml at two hours.

DRUG INTERACTIONS:

Aminosalicylic acid at a dosage of 12 grams in a rapidly available form has been reported to produce a 20 percent reduction in the acetylation of isoniazid, especially in patients who are rapid acetylators; INH serum levels, half lives and excretions in fast acetylators still remain half of the levels seen in slow acetylators with or without p-aminosalicylic acid. The effect is dose related and, while it has not been studied with the current delayed release preparation, the lower serum levels with this preparation will result in a reduced effect on the acetylation of INH.

Aminosalicylic acid has previously been reported to block the absorption of rifampin. A subsequent report has shown that this blockade was due to an excipient not included in Paser granules. Oral administration of a solution containing both aminosalicylic acid and rifampin showed full absorption of each product.

As a result of competition, Vitamin B_{12} absorption has been reduced 55% by 5 grams of aminosalicylic acid with clinically significant erythrocyte abnormalities developing after depletion; patients on therapy of more than one month should be considered for maintenance B_{12}.

A malabsorption syndrome can develop in patients on aminosalicylic acid but is usually not complete. The complete syndrome includes steatorrhea, an abnormal small bowel pattern on x-ray, villus atrophy, depressed cholesterol, reduced D-xylose and iron absorption. Triglyceride absorption always is normal.

In one literature report 8 hours after the last dosage of aminosalicylic acid at 2 gm qid serum digoxin levels were reduced 40% in two of ten patients but not changed in the remaining eight.

ADVERSE REACTIONS:

The most common side effect is gastrointestinal intolerance manifested by nausea, vomiting, diarrhea, and abdominal pain.

Hypersensitivity Reactions: Fever, skin eruptions of various types, including exfoliative dermatitis, infectious mononucleosis-like, or lymphoma-like syndrome, leucopenia, agranulocytosis, thrombocytopenia, Coombs' positive hemolytic anemia, jaundice, hepatitis, pericarditis, hypoglycemia, optic neuritis, encephalopathy, Leoffler's syndrome, vasculitis and a reduction in prothrombin.

Crystalluria may be prevented by the maintenance of urine at a neutral or an alkaline pH.

OVERDOSAGE:

Overdosage has not been reported.

DOSAGE AND ADMINISTRATION:

Paser granules should be administered with other drugs to which the organism is known or expected to be susceptible. It is most commonly administered to patients with Multi-drug Resistant TB (MDR-TB) or in other situations in which therapy with isoniazid or rifampin is not possible due to a combination of resistance and/or intolerance. The adult dosage of four grams (one packet) three times per day or correspondingly smaller doses in children should be given by sprinkling on apple sauce or yogurt or by swirling in the glass to suspend the granules in an acidic drink such as tomato or orange juice.

DO NOT USE if the packet is swollen or the granules have lost their tan color, turning dark brown or purple.

HOW SUPPLIED:

Carton of 30 Paser packets.

Each packet contains four grams aminosalicylic acid.

Paser granules are supplied in packets containing 4 grams of aminosalicylic acid for administration three times a day by suspension in an acidic drink or food with a pH less than 5. Examples include apple sauce, yogurt, tomato or orange juice.

Store below 77°F (25°C). AVOID EXCESSIVE HEAT. DO NOT USE if packet is swollen or the granules have lost their tan color, turning dark brown or purple.

(Jacobus Pharmaceutical Co. Inc. 07/94)

HOW SUPPLIED - EQUIVALENTS NOT AVAILABLE:

Granule - Oral - 4 gm

30's UD	$112.80	PASER, Jacobus Pharm	49938-0107-04

AMIODARONE HYDROCHLORIDE *(000212)*

CATEGORIES: Antiarrhythmic Agents; Arrhythmia; Cardiovascular Drugs; Fibrillation; Orphan Drugs; Renal Drugs; Tachycardia; Pregnancy Category D; FDA Approved 1985 Dec

BRAND NAMES: *Aldarin*; *Aldarone*; *Amidodacore*; *Amiorit*; *Amiodarona*; *Amiorone*; *Ancaron* (Japan); *Angoron*; *Aratac* (Australia); *Atlansil*; *Braxan* (Mexico); *Cardarone*; *Cardiorona* (Mexico); *Corbionax* (France); *Cordarex* (Germany); *Cordaron*; **Cordarone**; Cordarone I.V.; *Cordarone X* (Australia, England); *Coronovo*; *Kendaron*; *Myodura*; *Procor*; *Rythmarone*; *Sedacoron*; *Tachydaron* (Germany); *Tiaryt*; *Trangorex*
(International brand names outside U.S. in italics)

FORMULARIES: Aetna; BC-BS; Medi-Cal; PCS

COST OF THERAPY: $2,240.73 (Arrhythmia; Tablet; 200 mg; 2/day; 365 days)

DESCRIPTION:

Cordarone is a member of a new class of antiarrhythmic drugs with predominantly Class III (Vaughan Williams' classification) effects, available for oral administration as pink, scored tablets containing 200 mg of amiodarone hydrochloride. The inactive ingredients present are colloidal silicon dioxide, lactose, magnesium stearate, povidone, starch, and FD&C Red 40. Cordarone is a benzofuran derivative: 2-butyl-3- benzofuranyl 4-(2-(diethylamino)-ethoxy)-3,5-diiodophenyl ketone, hydrochloride. It is not chemically related to any other available antiarrhythmic drug.

Amiodarone HCl is a white to cream-colored crystalline powder. It is slightly soluble in water, soluble in alcohol, and freely soluble in chloroform. It contains 37.3% iodine by weight.

CLINICAL PHARMACOLOGY:

ELECTRYPHOPHYSIOLOGY/ MESCHANISMS OF ACTION

In animals, amiodarone is effective in the prevention or suppression of experimentally induced arrhythmias. The antiarrhythmic effect of amiodarone may be due to at least two major properties: 1) a prolongation of the myocardial cell-action potential duration and refractory period and 2) noncompetitive alpha-and beta-adrenergic inhibition.

CLINICAL PHARMACOLOGY: *(cont'd)*

Amiodarone prolongs the duration of the action potential of all cardiac fibers while causing minimal reduction of dV/dt (maximal upstroke velocity of the action potential). The refractory period is prolonged in all cardiac tissues.

Amiodarone increases the cardiac refractory period without influencing resting membrane potential, except in automatic cells where the slope of the prepotential is reduced, generally reducing automaticity. These electrophysiologic effects are reflected in a decreased sinus rate of 15 to 20%, increased PR and QT intervals of about 10%, the development of U-waves, and changes in T-wave contour. These changes should not require discontinuation of amiodarone as they are evidence of its pharmacological action, although amiodarone can cause marked sinus bradycardia or sinus arrest and heart block. On rare occasions, QT prolongation has been associated with worsening of arrhythmia (see WARNINGS.)

HEMODYNAMICS

In animal studies and after intravenous administration in man, amiodarone relaxes vascular smooth muscle, reduces peripheral vascular resistance (afterload), and slightly increases cardiac index. After oral dosing, however, amiodarone produces no significant change in left ventricular ejection fraction (LVEF), even in patients with depressed LVEF. After acute intravenous dosing in man, amiodarone may have a mild negative inotropic effect.

PHARMACOKINETICS

Following oral administration in man, amiodarone is slowly and variably absorbed. The bioavailability of amiodarone is approximately 50%, but has varied between 35 and 65% in various studies. Maximum plasma concentrations are attained 3 to 7 hours after a single dose. Despite this, the onset of action may occur in 2 to 3 days, but more commonly takes 1 to 3 weeks, even with loading doses. Plasma concentrations with chronic dosing at 100 to 600 mg/day are approximately dose proportional, with a mean 0.5 mg/L increase for each 100 mg/day. These means, however, include considerable individual variability.

Amiodarone has a very large but variable volume of distribution, averaging about 60 L/kg, because of extensive accumulation in various sites, especially adipose tissue and highly perfused organs, such as the liver, lung, and spleen. One major metabolite of amiodarone, desethylamiodarone, has been identified in man; it accumulates to an even greater extent in almost all tissues. The pharmacological activity of this metabolite, however, is not known. During chronic treatment, the plasma ratio of metabolite to parent compound is approximately one.

The main route of elimination is via hepatic excretion into bile, and some enterohepatic recirculation may occur. However, its kinetics in patients with hepatic insufficiency have not been elucidated. Amiodarone has a very low plasma clearance with negligible renal excretion, so that it does not appear necessary to modify the dose in patients with renal failure. In patients with renal impairment, the plasma concentration of amiodarone is not elevated. Neither amiodarone nor its metabolite is dialyzable.

In patients, following discontinuation of chronic oral therapy, amiodarone has been shown to have a biphasic elimination with an initial one-half reduction of plasma levels after 2.5 to 10 days. A much slower terminal plasma-elimination phase shows a half-life of the parent compound ranging from 26 to 107 days, with a mean of approximately 53 days and most patients in the 40- to 55-day range. In the absence of a loading-dose period, steady-state plasma concentrations, at constant oral dosing, would therefore be reached between 130 and 535 days, with an average of 265 days. For the metabolite, the mean plasma-elimination half-life was approximately 61 days. These data probably reflect an initial elimination of drug from well-perfused tissue (the 2.5- to 10-day half-life phase), followed by a terminal phase representing extremely slow elimination from poorly perfused tissue compartments such as fat.

The considerable intersubject variation in both phases of elimination, as well as uncertainty as to what compartment is critical to drug effect, requires attention to individual responses once arrhythmia control is achieved with loading doses because the correct maintenance dose is determined, in part, by the elimination rates. Daily maintenance doses of amiodarone should be based on individual patient requirements (see DOSAGE AND ADMINISTRATION.)

Amiodarone and its metabolite have a limited transplacental transfer of approximately 10 to 50%. The parent drug and its metabolite have been detected in breast milk.

Amiodarone is highly protein-bound (approximately 96%).

Although electrophysiologic effects, such as prolongation of QTc, can be seen within hours after a parenteral dose of amiodarone, effects on abnormal rhythms are not seen before 2 to 3 days and usually require 1 to 3 weeks, even when a loading dose is used. There may be a continued increase in effect for longer periods still. There is evidence that the time to effect is shorter when a loading-dose regimen is used.

Consistent with the slow rate of elimination, antiarrhythmic effects persist for weeks or months after amiodarone is discontinued, but the time of recurrence is variable and unpredictable. In general, when the drug is resumed after recurrence of the arrhythmia, control is established relatively rapidly compared to the initial response, presumably because tissue stores were not wholly depleted at the time of recurrence.

PHARMACODYNAMICS

There is no well-established relationship of plasma concentration to effectiveness, but it does appear that concentrations much below 1 mg/L are often ineffective and that levels above 2.5 mg/L are generally not needed. Within individuals dose reductions and ensuing decreased plasma concentrations can result in loss of arrhythmia control. Plasma-concentration measurements can be used to identify patients whose levels are unusually low, and who might benefit from a dose increase, or unusually high, and who might have dosage reduction in the hope of minimizing side effects. Some observations have suggested a plasma concentration, dose, or dose/duration relationship for side effects such as pulmonary fibrosis, liver-enzyme elevations, corneal deposits and facial pigmentation, peripheral neuropathy, gastrointestinal and central nervous system effects.

MONITORING EFFECTIVENESS

Predicting the effectiveness of any antiarrhythmic agent in long-term prevention of recurrent ventricular tachycardia and ventricular fibrillation is difficult and controversial, with highly qualified investigators recommending use of ambulatory monitoring, programmed electrical stimulation with various stimulation regimens, or a combination of these, to assess response. There is no present consensus on many aspects of how best to assess effectiveness, but there is a reasonable consensus on some aspects:

1. If a patient with a history of cardiac arrest does not manifest a hemodynamically unstable arrhythmia during electrocardiographic monitoring prior to treatment, assessment of the effectiveness of amiodarone requires some provocative approach, either exercise or programmed electrical stimulation (PES).

2. Whether provocation is also needed in patients who do manifest their life-threatening arrhythmia spontaneously is not settled, but there are reasons to consider PES or other provocation in such patients. In the fraction of patients whose PES-inducible arrhythmia can be made noninducible by amiodarone (a fraction that has varied widely in various series from less than 10% to almost 40%, perhaps due to different stimulation criteria), the prognosis has been almost uniformly excellent, with very low recurrence (ventricular tachycardia or sudden death) rates. More controversial is the meaning of continued inducibility. There has been an impression that continued inducibility in amiodarone patients may not

CLINICAL PHARMACOLOGY: *(cont'd)*

foretell a poor prognosis but, in fact, many observers have found greater recurrence rates in patients who remain inducible than in those who do not. A number of criteria have been proposed, however, for identifying patients who remain inducible but who seem likely nonetheless to do well on amiodarone. These criteria include increased difficulty of induction (more stimuli or more rapid stimuli), which has been reported to predict a lower rate of recurrence, and ability to tolerate the induced ventricular tachycardia without severe symptoms, a finding that has been reported to correlate with better survival but not with lower recurrence rates. While these criteria require confirmation and further study in general, *easier* inducibility or *poorer* tolerance of the induced arrhythmia should suggest consideration of a need to revise treatment.

Several predictors of success not based on PES have also been suggested, including complete elimination of all nonsustained ventricular tachycardia on ambulatory monitoring and very low premature ventricular-beat rates (less than 1 VPB/1,000 normal beats).

While these issues remain unsettled for amiodarone, as for other agents, the prescriber of amiodarone should have access to (direct or through referral), and familiarity with, the full range of evaluatory procedures used in the care of patients with life-threatening arrhythmias.

It is difficult to describe the effectiveness rates of amiodarone, as these depend on the specific arrhythmia treated, the success criteria used, the underlying cardiac disease of the patient, the number of drugs tried before resorting to amiodarone, the duration of follow-up, the dose of amiodarone, the use of additional antiarrhythmic agents, and many other factors. As amiodarone has been studied principally in patients with refractory life-threatening ventricular arrhythmias, in whom drug therapy must be selected on the basis of response and cannot be assigned arbitrarily, randomized comparisons with other agents or placebo have not been possible. Reports of series of treated patients with a history of cardiac arrest and mean follow-up of one year or more have given mortality (due to arrhythmia) rates that were highly variable, ranging from less than 5% to over 30%, with most series in the range of 10 to 15%. Overall arrhythmia-recurrence rates (fatal and nonfatal) also were highly variable (and, as noted above, depended on response to PES and other measures), and depend on whether patients who do not seem to respond initially are included. In most cases, considering only patients who seemed to respond well enough to be placed on long-term treatment, recurrence rates have ranged from 20 to 40% in series with a mean follow-up of a year or more.

INDICATIONS AND USAGE:

Because of its life-threatening side effects and the substantial management difficulties associated with its use (see WARNINGS), amiodarone is indicated only for the treatment of the following documented, life-threatening recurrent ventricular arrhythmias when these have not responded to documented adequate doses of other available antiarrhythmics or when alternative agents could not be tolerated.

1. Recurrent ventricular fibrillation.
2. Recurrent hemodynamically unstable ventricular tachycardia.

As is the case for other antiarrhythmic agents, there is no evidence from controlled trials that the use of amiodarone favorably affects survival.

Amiodarone should be used only by physicians familiar with and with access to (directly or through referral) the use of all available modalities for treating recurrent life-threatening ventricular arrhythmias, and who have access to appropriate monitoring facilities, including in-hospital and ambulatory continuous electrocardiographic monitoring and electrophysiologic techniques. Because of the life-threatening nature of the arrhythmias treated, potential interactions with prior therapy, and potential exacerbation of the arrhythmia, initiation of therapy with amiodarone should be carried out in the hospital.

CONTRAINDICATIONS:

Amiodarone is contraindicated in severe sinus-node dysfunction, causing marked sinus bradycardia; second- and third-degree atrioventricular block; and when episodes of bradycardia have caused syncope (except when used in conjunction with a pacemaker).

Amiodarone is contraindicated in patients with a known hypersensitivity to the drug.

WARNINGS:

Amiodarone is intended for use only in patients with the indicated life-threatening arrhythmias because its use is accompanied by substantial toxicity.

Amiodarone has several potentially fatal toxicities, the most important of which is pulmonary toxicity (hypersensitivity pneumonitis or interstitial/alveolar pneumonitis) that has resulted in clinically manifest disease at rates as high as 10 to 17% in some series of patients with ventricular arrhythmias given doses around 400 mg/day, and as abnormal diffusion capacity without symptoms in a much higher percentage of patients. Pulmonary toxicity has been fatal about 10% of the time. Liver injury is common with amiodarone, but is usually mild and evidenced only by abnormal liver enzymes. Overt liver disease can occur, however, and has been fatal in a few cases. Like other antiarrhythmics, amiodarone can exacerbate the arrhythmia, e.g., by making the arrhythmia less well tolerated or more difficult to reverse. This has occurred in 2 to 5% of patients in various series, and significant heart block or sinus bradycardia has been seen in 2 to 5%. All of these events should be manageable in the proper clinical setting in most cases. Although the frequency of such proarrhythmic events does not appear greater with amiodarone than with many other agents used in this population, the effects are prolonged when they occur. Even in patients at high risk of arrhythmic death, in whom the toxicity of amiodarone is an acceptable risk, amiodarone poses major management problems that could be life-threatening in a population at risk of sudden death, so that every effort should be made to utilize alternative agents first.

The difficulty of using amiodarone effectively and safely itself poses a significant risk to patients. Patients with the indicated arrhythmias must be hospitalized while the loading dose of amiodarone is given, and a response generally requires at least one week, usually two or more. Because absorption and elimination are variable, maintenance-dose selection is difficult, and it is not unusual to require dosage decrease or discontinuation of treatment. In a retrospective survey of 192 patients with ventricular tachyarrhythmias, 84 required dose reduction and 18 required at least temporary discontinuation because of adverse effects, and several series have reported 15 to 20% overall frequencies of discontinuation due to adverse reactions. The time at which a previously controlled life-threatening arrhythmia will recur after discontinuation or dose adjustment is unpredictable, ranging from weeks to months. The patient is obviously at great risk during this time and may need prolonged hospitalization. Attempts to substitute other antiarrhythmic agents when amiodarone must be stopped

WARNINGS: *(cont'd)*

will be made difficult by the gradually, but unpredictably, changing amiodarone body burden. A similar problem exists when amiodarone is not effective; it still poses the risk of an interaction with whatever subsequent treatment is tried.

PULMONARY TOXICITY

Amiodarone may cause a clinical syndrome of cough and progressive dyspnea accompanied by functional, radiographic, gallium-scan, and pathological data consistent with pulmonary toxicity, the frequency of which varies from 2 to 7% in most published reports, but is as high as 10 to 17% in some reports. Therefore, when amiodarone therapy is initiated, a baseline chest X-ray and pulmonary-function tests, including diffusion capacity, should be performed. The patient should return for a history, physical exam, and chest X-ray every 3 to 6 months.

Preexisting pulmonary disease does not appear to increase the risk of developing pulmonary toxicity; however, these patients have a poorer prognosis if pulmonary toxicity does develop.

Pulmonary toxicity secondary to amiodarone seems to result from either indirect or direct toxicity as represented by hypersensitivity pneumonitis or interstitial/alveolar pneumonitis, respectively.

Hypersensitivity pneumonitis usually appears earlier in the course of therapy, and rechallenging these patients with amiodarone results in a more rapid recurrence of greater severity. Bronchoalveolar lavage is the procedure of choice to confirm this diagnosis, which can be made when a T suppressor/cytotoxic (CD8-positive) lymphocytosis is noted. Steroid therapy should be instituted and amiodarone therapy discontinued in these patients.

Interstitial/alveolar pneumonitis may result from the release of oxygen radicals and/or phospholipidosis and is characterized by findings of diffuse alveolar damage, interstitial pneumonitis or fibrosis in lung biopsy specimens. Phospholipidosis (foamy cells, foamy macrophages), due to inhibition of phospholipase, will be present in most cases of amiodarone-induced pulmonary toxicity; however, these changes also are present in approximately 50% of all patients on amiodarone therapy. These cells should be used as markers of therapy, but not as evidence of toxicity. A diagnosis of amiodarone-induced interstitial/alveolar pneumonitis should lead, at a minimum, to dose reduction or, preferably, to withdrawal of the amiodarone to establish reversibility, especially if other acceptable antiarrhythmic therapies are available. Where these measures have been instituted, a reduction in symptoms of amiodarone-induced pulmonary toxicity was usually noted within the first week, and a clinical improvement was greatest in the first two to three weeks. Chest X-ray changes usually resolve within two to four months. According to some experts, steroids may prove beneficial. Prednisone in doses of 40 to 60 mg/day or equivalent doses of other steroids have been given and tapered over the course of several weeks depending upon the condition of the patient. In some cases rechallenge with amiodarone at a lower dose has not resulted in return of toxicity. Recent reports suggest that the use of lower loading and maintenance doses of amiodarone are associated with a decreased incidence of amiodarone-induced pulmonary toxicity.

In a patient receiving amiodarone, any new respiratory symptoms should suggest the possibility of pulmonary toxicity, and the history, physical exam, chest X-ray, and pulmonary-function tests (with diffusion capacity) should be repeated and evaluated. A 15% decrease in diffusion capacity has a high sensitivity but only a moderate specificity for pulmonary toxicity; as the decrease in diffusion capacity approaches 30%, the sensitivity decreases but the specificity increases. A gallium scan also may be performed as part of the diagnostic workup.

Fatalities, secondary to pulmonary toxicity, have occurred in approximately 10% of cases. However, in patients with life-threatening arrhythmias, discontinuation of amiodarone therapy due to suspected drug-induced pulmonary toxicity should be undertaken with caution, as the most common cause of death in these patients is sudden cardiac death. Therefore, every effort should be made to rule out other causes of respiratory impairment (*i.e.*, congestive heart failure with Swan-Ganz catheterization if necessary, respiratory infection, pulmonary embolism, malignancy, etc.) before discontinuing amiodarone in these patients. In addition, bronchoalveolar lavage, transbronchial lung biopsy, and/or open lung biopsy may be necessary to confirm the diagnosis, especially in those cases where no acceptable alternative therapy is available.

If a diagnosis of amiodarone-induced hypersensitivity pneumonitis is made, amiodarone should be discontinued, and treatment with steroids should be instituted. If a diagnosis of amiodarone-induced interstitial/alveolar pneumonitis is made, steroid therapy should be instituted and, preferably, amiodarone discontinued or, at a minimum, reduced in dosage. Some cases of amiodarone-induced interstitial/alveolar pneumonitis may resolve following a reduction in amiodarone dosage in conjunction with the administration of steroids. In some patients, rechallenge at a lower dose has not resulted in return of interstitial/alveolar pneumonitis; however, in some patients (perhaps because of severe alveolar damage) the pulmonary lesions have not been reversible.

WORSENED ARRHYTHMIA

Amiodarone, like other antiarrhythmics, can cause serious exacerbation of the presenting arrhythmia, a risk that may be enhanced by the presence of concomitant antiarrhythmics. Exacerbation has been reported in about 2 to 5% in most series, and has included new ventricular fibrillation, incessant ventricular tachycardia, increased resistance to cardioversion, and polymorphic ventricular tachycardia associated with QT prolongation (Torsade de Pointes).

In addition, amiodarone has caused symptomatic bradycardia or sinus arrest with suppression of escape foci in 2 to 4% of patients.

LIVER DYSFUNCTION

Elevations of hepatic enzyme levels are seen frequently in patients exposed to amiodarone and in most cases are asymptomatic. If the increase exceeds three times normal, or doubles in a patient with an elevated baseline, discontinuation of amiodarone or dosage reduction should be considered. In a few cases in which biopsy has been done, the histology has resembled that of alcoholic hepatitis or cirrhosis. Hepatic failure has been a rare cause of death in patients treated with amiodarone.

PREGNANCY CATEGORY D

Amiodarone has been shown to be embryotoxic (increased fetal resorption and growth retardation) in the rat when given orally at a dose of 200 mg/kg/day (18 times the maximum recommended maintenance dose). Similar findings have been noted in one strain of mice at a dose of 5 mg/kg/day (approximately 1/2 the maximum recommended maintenance dose) and higher, but not in a second strain nor in the rabbit at doses up to 100 mg/kg/day (9 times the maximum recommended maintenance dose).

NEONATAL HYPO- OR HYPERTHYROIDISM

Amiodarone can cause fetal harm when administered to a pregnant woman. Although amiodarone use during pregnancy is uncommon, there have been a small number of published reports of congenital goiter/hypothyroidism and hyperthyroidism. If amiodarone is used during pregnancy, or if the patient becomes pregnant while taking amiodarone, the patient should be apprised of the potential hazard to the fetus.

In general, amiodarone should be used during pregnancy only if the potential benefit to the mother justifies the unknown risk to the fetus.

PRECAUTIONS:

CORNEAL MICRODEPOSITS; IMPAIRMENT OF VISION

Corneal microdeposits appear in the majority of adults treated with amiodarone. They are usually discernible only by slit-lamp examination, but give rise to symptoms such as visual halos or blurred vision in as many as 10% of patients. Corneal microdeposits are reversible upon reduction of dose or termination of treatment. Asymptomatic microdeposits are not a reason to reduce dose or discontinue treatment.

PHOTOSENSITIVITY

Amiodarone has induced photosensitization in about 10% of patients; some protection may be afforded by the use of sun-barrier creams or protective clothing. During long-term treatment, a blue-gray discoloration of the exposed skin may occur. The risk may be increased in patients of fair complexion or those with excessive sun exposure, and may be related to cumulative dose and duration of therapy.

THYROID ABNORMALITIES

Amiodarone inhibits peripheral conversion of thyroxine (T_4) to triiodothyronine (T_3) and may cause increased thyroxine levels, decreased T_3 levels, and increased levels of inactive reverse T_3 (rT_3) in clinically euthyroid patients. It is also a potential source of large amounts of inorganic iodine. Because of its release of inorganic iodine, or perhaps for other reasons, amiodarone can cause either hypothyroidism or hyperthyroidism. Thyroid function should be monitored prior to treatment and periodically thereafter, particularly in elderly patients, and in any patient with a history of thyroid nodules, goiter, or other thyroid dysfunction. Because of the slow elimination of amiodarone and its metabolites, high plasma iodide levels, altered thyroid function, and abnormal thyroid-function tests may persist for several weeks or even months following amiodarone withdrawal.

Hypothyroidism has been reported in 2 to 4% of patients in most series, but in 8 to 10% in some series. This condition may be identified by relevant clinical symptoms and particularly by elevated serum TSH levels. In some clinically hypothyroid amiodarone-treated patients, free thyroxine index values may be normal. Hypothyroidism is best managed by amiodarone dose reduction and/or thyroid hormone supplement. However, therapy must be individualized, and it may be necessary to discontinue amiodarone in some patients. Hyperthyroidism occurs in about 2% of patients receiving amiodarone, but the incidence may be higher among patients with prior inadequate dietary iodine intake. Amiodarone-induced hyperthyroidism usually poses a greater hazard to the patient than hypothyroidism because of the possibility of arrhythmia break-through or aggravation. In fact, IF ANY NEW SIGNS OF ARRHYTHMIA APPEAR, THE POSSIBILITY OF HYPERTHYROIDISM SHOULD BE CONSIDERED. Hyperthyroidism is best identified by relevant clinical symptoms and signs, accompanied usually by abnormally elevated levels of serum T_3 RIA, and further elevations of serum T_4, and a subnormal serum TSH level (using a sufficiently sensitive TSH assay). The finding of a flat TSH response to TRH is confirmatory of hyperthyroidism and may be sought in equivocal cases. Since arrhythmia breakthroughs may accompany amiodarone-induced hyperthyroidism, aggressive medical treatment is indicated, including, if possible, dose reduction or withdrawal of amiodarone. The institution of antithyroid drugs, beta-adrenergic blockers and/or temporary corticosteroid therapy may be necessary. The action of antithyroid drugs may be especially delayed in amiodarone-induced thyrotoxicosis because of substantial quantities of preformed thyroid hormones stored in the gland. Radioactive iodine therapy is contraindicated because of the low radioiodine uptake associated with amiodarone-induced hyperthyroidism. Experience with thyroid surgery in this setting is extremely limited, and this form of therapy runs the theoretical risk of inducing thyroid storm. Amiodarone-induced hyperthyroidism may be followed by a transient period of hypothyroidism.

SURGERY

Hypotension Postbypass: Rare occurrences of hypotension upon discontinuation of cardiopulmonary bypass during open-heart surgery in patients receiving amiodarone have been reported. The relationship of this event to amiodarone therapy is unknown.

Adult Respiratory Distress Syndrome (ARDS): Postoperatively, rare occurrences of ARDS have been reported in patients receiving amiodarone therapy who have undergone either cardiac or noncardiac surgery. Although patients usually respond well to vigorous respiratory therapy, in rare instances the outcome has been fatal. One possible mechanism of this deleterious effect may be the generation of superoxide radicals during oxygenation; therefore, the operative FiO_2 should be kept as close to room air as possible.

LABORATORY TEST

Elevations in liver enzymes (SGOT and SGPT) can occur. Liver enzymes in patients on relatively high maintenance doses should be monitored on a regular basis. Persistent significant elevations in the liver enzymes or hepatomegaly should alert the physician to consider reducing the maintenance dose of amiodarone or discontinuing therapy.

Amiodarone alters the results of thyroid-function tests, causing an increase in serum T_4 and serum reverse T_3, and a decline in serum T_3 levels. Despite these biochemical changes, most patients remain clinically euthyroid.

ELECTROLYTE DISTURBANCES

Since antiarrhythmic drugs may be ineffective or may be arrhythmogenic in patients with hypokalemia, any potassium of magnesium deficiency should be corrected before instituting amiodarone therapy.

CARCINOGENESIS, MUTAGENESIS, AND IMPAIRMENT OF FERTILITY

Amiodarone reduced fertility of male and female rats at a dose level of 90 mg/kg/day (8 x highest recommended human maintenance dose). Amiodarone caused a statistically significant, dose-related increase in the incidence of thyroid tumors (follicular adenoma and/or carcinoma) in rats. The incidence of thyroid tumors was greater than control even at the lowest dose level of amiodarone tested, i.e., 5 mg/kg/day or approximately equal to 1/2 the highest recommended human maintenance dose. Mutagenicity studies (Ames, micronucleus, and lysogenic tests) with amiodarone were negative.

PREGNANCY CATEGORY D

See WARNINGS.

LABOR AND DELIVERY

It is not known whether the use of amiodarone during labor or delivery has any immediate or delayed adverse effects. Preclinical studies in rodents have not shown any effect of amiodarone on the duration of gestation or on parturition.

NURSING MOTHERS

Amiodarone is excreted in human milk, suggesting that breast-feeding could expose the nursing infant to a significant dose of the drug. Nursing offspring of lactating rats administered amiodarone have been shown to be less viable and have reduced body-weight gains. Therefore, when amiodarone therapy is indicated, the mother should be advised to discontinue nursing.

PEDIATRIC USE

The safety and effectiveness of amiodarone in children have not been established.

DRUG INTERACTIONS:

Although only a small number of drug-drug interactions with amiodarone have been explored formally, most of these have shown such an interaction. The potential for other interactions should be anticipated, particularly for drugs with potentially serious toxicity, such as other antiarrhythmics. If such drugs are needed, their dose should be reassessed and, where appropriate, plasma concentration measured.

In view of the long and variable half-life of amiodarone, potential for drug interactions exists not only with concomitant medication but also with drugs administered after discontinuation of amiodarone.

DIGITALIS

Administration of amiodarone to patients receiving digoxin therapy regularly results in an increase in the serum digoxin concentration that may reach toxic levels with resultant clinical toxicity. **On initiation of amiodarone, the need for digitalis therapy should be reviewed and the dose reduced by approximately 50% or discontinued.** If digitalis treatment is continued, serum levels should be closely monitored and patients observed for clinical evidence of toxicity. These precautions probably should apply to digitoxin administration as well.

ANTICOAGULANTS

Potentiation of warfarin-type anticoagulant response is almost always seen in patients receiving amiodarone and can result in serious or fatal bleeding. **The dose of the anticoagulant should be reduced by one-third to one-half, and prothrombin times should be monitored closely.**

ANTIARRHYTHMIC AGENTS

Other antiarrhythmic drugs, such as quinidine, procainamide, disopyramide, and phenytoin, have been used concurrently with amiodarone.

There have been case reports of increased steady-state levels of quinidine, procainamide, and phenytoin during concomitant therapy with amiodarone. In general, any added antiarrhythmic drug should be initiated at a lower than usual dose with careful monitoring.

In general, combination of amiodarone with other antiarrhythmic therapy should be reserved for patients with life-threatening ventricular arrhythmias who are incompletely responsive to a single agent or incompletely responsive to amiodarone. During transfer to amiodarone the dose levels of previously administered agents should be reduced by 30 to 50% several days after the addition of amiodarone, when arrhythmia suppression should be beginning. The continued need for the other antiarrhythmic agent should be reviewed after the effects of amiodarone have been established, and discontinuation ordinarily should be attempted. If the treatment is continued, these patients should be particularly carefully monitored for adverse effects, especially conduction disturbances and exacerbation of tachyarrhythmias, as amiodarone is continued. In amiodarone-treated patients who require additional antiarrhythmic therapy, the initial dose of such agents should be approximately half of the usual recommended dose.

Amiodarone should be used with caution in patients receiving beta-blocking agents or calcium antagonists because of the possible potentiation of bradycardia, sinus arrest, and AV block; if necessary, amiodarone can continue to be used after insertion of a pacemaker in patients with severe bradycardia or sinus arrest (TABLE 1):

TABLE 1 Summary Of Drug Interaction With Amiodarone

Concomitant Drug	Interaction: Onset (days)	Interaction: Magnitude	Recommended Dose Reduction of Concomitant Drug
Warfarin	3 to 4	Increases prothrombin time by 100%	↓ 1/3 to 1/2
Digoxin	1	Increases serum concentration by 70%	↓ 1/2
Quinidine	2	Increases serum concentration by 33%	↓ 1/3 to 1/2 (or discontinue)
Procainamide	<7	Increases plasma concentration by 55%; NAPA* concentration by 33%	↓ 1/3 (or discontinue)

* NAPA = n-acetyl procainamide.

ADVERSE REACTIONS:

Adverse reactions have been very common in virtually all series of patients treated with amiodarone for ventricular arrhythmias, with relatively large doses of drug (400 mg/day and above) occurring in about three-fourths of all patients and causing discontinuation in 7 to 18%. The most serious reactions are pulmonary toxicity, exacerbation of arrhythmia, and rare serious liver injury (see WARNINGS), but other adverse effects constitute important problems. They are often reversible with dose reduction and virtually always reversible with cessation of amiodarone treatment. Most of the adverse effects appear to become more frequent with continued treatment beyond six months, although rates appear to remain relatively constant beyond one year. The time and dose relationships of adverse effects are under continued study. Neurologic problems are extremely common, occurring in 20 to 40% of patients and including malaise and fatigue, tremor and involuntary movements, poor coordination and gait, and peripheral neuropathy; they are rarely a reason to stop therapy and may respond to dose reductions.

Gastrointestinal complaints, most commonly nausea, vomiting, constipation, and anorexia, occur in about 25% of patients but rarely require discontinuation of drug. These commonly occur during high-dose administration (*i.e.,* loading dose) and usually respond to dose reduction or divided doses.

Asymptomatic corneal microdeposits are present in virtually all adult patients who have been on drug for more than 6 months. Some patients develop eye symptoms of halos, photophobia, and dry eyes. Vision is rarely affected and drug discontinuation is rarely needed.

Dermatological adverse reactions occur in about 15% of patients, with photosensitivity being most common (about 10%). Sunscreen and protection from sun exposure may be helpful, and drug discontinuation is not usually necessary. Prolonged exposure to amiodarone occasionally results in a blue-gray pigmentation. This is slowly and occasionally incompletely reversible on discontinuation of drug but is of cosmetic importance only.

Cardiovascular adverse reactions, other than exacerbation of the arrhythmias, include the uncommon occurrence of congestive heart failure (3%) and bradycardia. Bradycardia usually responds to dosage reduction but may require a pacemaker for control. CHF rarely requires drug discontinuation. Cardiac conduction abnormalities occur infrequently and are reversible on discontinuation of drug.

The following side-effect rates are based on a retrospective study of 241 patients treated for 2 to 1,515 days (mean 441.3 days).

The following side effects were each reported in 10 to 33% of patients:

Gastrointestinal: Nausea and vomiting.

The following side effects were each reported in 4 to 9% of patients:

Dermatologic: Solar dermatitis/photosensitivity.

Neurologic: Malaise and fatigue, tremor/abnormal involuntary movements, lack of coordination, abnormal gait/ataxia, dizziness, paresthesias.

ADVERSE REACTIONS: *(cont'd)*

Gastrointestinal: Constipation, anorexia.

Ophthalmologic: Visual disturbances.

Hepatic: Abnormal liver-function tests.

Respiratory: Pulmonary inflammation or fibrosis.

The following side effects were each reported in 1 to 3% of patients:

Thyroid: Hypothyroidism, hyperthyroidism.

Neurologic: Decreased libido, insomnia, headache, sleep disturbances.

Cardiovascular: Congestive heart failure, cardiac arrhythmias, SA node dysfunction.

Gastrointestinal: Abdominal pain.

Hepatic: Nonspecific hepatic disorders.

Other: Flushing, abnormal taste and smell, edema, abnormal salivation, coagulation abnormalities.

The following side effects were each reported in less than 1% of patients:

Blue skin discoloration, rash, spontaneous ecchymosis, alopecia, hypotension, and cardiac conduction abnormalities.

Rare occurrences of hepatitis, cholestatic hepatitis, cirrhosis, optic neuritis, epididymitis, vasculitis, pseudotumor cerebri, and thrombocytopenia have been reported in patients receiving amiodarone.

In surveys of almost 5,000 patients treated in open U.S. studies and in published reports of treatment with amiodarone, the adverse reactions most frequently requiring discontinuation of amiodarone included pulmonary infiltrates or fibrosis, paroxysmal ventricular tachycardia, congestive heart failure, and elevation of liver enzymes. Other symptoms causing discontinuations less often included visual disturbances, solar dermatitis, blue skin discoloration, hyperthyroidism, and hypothyroidism.

OVERDOSAGE:

There have been a few reported cases of amiodarone overdose in which 3 to 8 grams were taken. There were no deaths or permanent sequelae. Animal studies indicate that amiodarone has a high oral LD_{50}(>3,000 mg/kg).

In addition to general supportive measures, the patient's cardiac rhythm and blood pressure should be monitored, and if bradycardia ensues, a β-adrenergic agonist or a pacemaker may be used. Hypotension with inadequate tissue perfusion should be treated with positive inotropic and/or vasopressor agents. Neither amiodarone nor its metabolite is dialyzable.

DOSAGE AND ADMINISTRATION:

BECAUSE OF THE UNIQUE PHARMACOKINETIC PROPERTIES, DIFFICULT DOSING SCHEDULE, AND SEVERITY OF THE SIDE EFFECTS IF PATIENTS ARE IMPROPERLY MONITORED, AMIODARONESHOULD BE ADMINISTERED ONLY BY PHYSICIANS WHO ARE EXPERIENCED IN THE TREATMENT OF LIFE-THREATENING ARRHYTHMIAS WHO ARE THOROUGHLY FAMILIAR WITH THE RISKS AND BENEFITS OF AMIODARONE THERAPY, AND WHO HAVE ACCESS TO LABORATORY FACILITIES CAPABLE OF ADEQUATELY MONITORING THE EFFECTIVENESS AND SIDE EFFECTS OF TREATMENT.

In order to insure that an antiarrhythmic effect will be observed without waiting several months, loading doses are required. A uniform, optimal dosage schedule for administration of amiodarone has not been determined. Individual patient titration is suggested according to the following guidelines.

For life-threatening ventricular arrhythmias, such as ventricular fibrillation or hemodynamically unstable ventricular tachycardia: Close monitoring of the patients is indicated during the loading phase, particularly until risk of recurrent ventricular tachycardia or fibrillation has abated. Because of the serious nature of the arrhythmia and the lack of predictable time course of effect, loading should be performed in a hospital setting. Loading doses of 800 to 1,600 mg/day are required for 1 to 3 weeks (occasionally longer) until initial therapeutic response occurs. (Administration of amiodarone in divided doses with meals is suggested for total daily doses of 1,000 mg or higher, or when gastrointestinal intolerance occurs.) If side effects become excessive, the dose should be reduced. Elimination of recurrence of ventricular fibrillation and tachycardia usually occurs within 1 to 3 weeks, along with reduction in complex and total ventricular ectopic beats.

Upon starting amiodarone therapy, an attempt should be made to gradually discontinue prior antiarrhythmic drugs (see DRUG INTERACTIONS.) When adequate arrhythmia control is achieved, or if side effects become prominent, amiodarone dose should be reduced to 600 to 800 mg/day for one month and then to the maintenance dose, usually 400 mg/day (see CLINICAL PHARMACOLOGY, Monitoring Effectiveness.) Some patients may require larger maintenance doses, up to 600 mg/day, and some can be controlled on lower doses. Amiodarone may be administered as a single daily dose, or in patients with severe gastrointestinal intolerance, as a b.i.d. dose. In each patient, the chronic maintenance dose should be determined according to antiarrhythmic effect as assessed by symptoms, Holter recordings, and/or programmed electrical stimulation and by patient tolerance. Plasma concentrations may be helpful in evaluating nonresponsiveness or unexpectedly severe toxicity (see CLINICAL PHARMACOLOGY.)

The lowest effective dose should be used to prevent the occurrence of side effects. In all instances, the physician must be guided by the severity of the individual patient's arrhythmia and response to therapy.

When dosage adjustments are necessary, the patient should be closely monitored for an extended period of time because of the long and variable half-life of amiodarone and the difficulty in predicting the time required to attain a new steady-state level of drug. Dosage suggestions are summarized in TABLE 2:

TABLE 2

	Loading Dose (Daily)	Adjustment and Maintenance Dose (Daily)	
Ventricular Arrhythmias	1 to 3 weeks	~1 month	Usual maintenance
	800 to 1,600 mg	600 to 800 mg	400 mg

Store at Room Temperature, Approx. 25°C (77°F).

HOW SUPPLIED - EQUIVALENTS NOT AVAILABLE:

Injection, Solution - Intravenous - 50 mg/ml

3 ml x 10	$687.50	CORDARONE I.V., Wyeth Labs	00008-0814-01

Tablet, Uncoated - Oral - 200 mg

60's	$182.72	CORDARONE, Wyeth Labs	00008-4188-04
100's	$306.95	CORDARONE, Wyeth Labs	00008-4188-06

AMITRIPTYLINE HYDROCHLORIDE *(000213)*

CATEGORIES: Antianxiety Drugs; Antidepressants; Central Nervous System Agents; Depression; Sedatives; Psychotherapeutic Agents; Tricyclics; Tricyclic Antidepressants; Migraine*; FDA Approval Pre 1982
* Indication not approved by the FDA

BRAND NAMES: *Adepril*; *Amicen*; *Amilent*; *Amilit*; *Amineurin* (Germany); *Amiplin*; *Amiprin* (Japan); Amitid; Amitril; *Amitrip*; *Amyline*; *Amyzol*; *Anapsique* (Mexico); *Apo-Amitriptyline* (Canada); *Domical* (England); *Elatrol*; *Elatrolet*; **Elavil**; Emitrip; *Enafon*; *Endep* (Australia); Enovil; *Etravil* ; *Lantron* (Japan); *Laroxyl* (France, Germany); *Larozyl*; *Lentizol* (England); *Levate* (Canada); *Miketorin* (Japan); *Novoprotect* (Germany); *Novotriptyn* (Canada); *Pinsanu*; *Pinsaun*; *Quietal*; *Redomex*; *Saroten Retard*; *Saroten* (Germany); *Sarotena*; *Sarotex*; *Syneudon* (Germany); *Teperin*; *Trepiline*; *Tridep*; *Tripta*; *Triptizol*; *Trynol*; *Tryptal*; *Tryptanol* (Australia, Mexico, Japan); *Tryptine* (Australia); *Tryptizol* (England); *Trytomer*; *Uxen*; Vanatrip *(International brand names outside U.S. in italics)*

FORMULARIES: Aetna; BC-BS; CIGNA; FHP; Foundation; Humana; Kaiser; Medco; Medi-Cal; PCS; PruCare; United; WHO

COST OF THERAPY: $2.50 (Depression; Tablet; 50 mg; 1/day; 90 days)

PRIMARY ICD9: 311 (Depressive Disorder, Not Elsewhere Classified)

DESCRIPTION:

Amitriptyline HCl is 3-(10,11-dihydro-5*H*-dibenzo [*a,d*] cycloheptene-5-ylidene)-*N,N*-dimethyl-1-propanamine hydrochloride. Its empirical formula is $C_{20}H_{23}N \cdot HCl$.

Amitriptyline HCl, a dibenzocycloheptadiene derivative, has a molecular weight of 313.87. It is a white, odorless, crystalline compound which is freely soluble in water.

Amitriptyline HCl is supplied as 10 mg, 25 mg, 50 mg, 75 mg, 100 mg, and 150 mg tablets and as a sterile solution for intramuscular use. Inactive ingredients of the tablets are calcium phosphate, cellulose, colloidal silicon dioxide, hydroxypropyl cellulose, hydroxypropyl methylcellulose, lactose, magnesium stearate, starch, stearic acid, talc, and titanium dioxide. 10 mg amitriptyline HCl tablets also contain FD&C Blue 1. 25 mg amitriptyline HCl tablets also contain D&C Yellow 10, FD&C Blue 1, and FD&C Yellow 6. 50 mg amitriptyline HCl tablets also contain D&C Yellow 10, FD&C Yellow 6 and iron oxide. 75 mg amitriptyline HCl tablets also contain FD&C Yellow 6. 100 mg amitriptyline HCl tablets also contain FD&C Blue 2 and FD&C Red 40. 150 mg amitriptyline HCl tablets also contain FD&C Blue 2 and FD&C Yellow 6.

Each milliliter of the sterile solution contains: Amitriptyline hydrochloride: 10 mg; Dextrose: 44 mg; Water for Injection, q.s.: 1 ml

Added as preservatives: Methylparaben: 1.5 mg; Propylparaben: 0.2 mg

CLINICAL PHARMACOLOGY:

Amitriptyline HCl is an antidepressant with sedative effects. Its mechanism of action in man is not known. It is not a monoamine oxidase inhibitor and it does not act primarily by stimulation of the central nervous system.

Amitriptyline inhibits the membrane pump mechanism responsible for uptake of norepinephrine and serotonin in adrenergic and serotonergic neurons. Pharmacologically this action may potentiate or prolong neuronal activity since reuptake of these biogenic amines is important physiologically in terminating transmitting activity. This interference with the reuptake of norepinephrine and/or serotonin is believed by some to underlie the antidepressant activity of amitriptyline.

METABOLISM

Studies in man following oral administration of ^{14}C-labeled drug indicated that amitriptyline is rapidly absorbed and metabolized. Radioactivity of the plasma was practically negligible, although significant amounts of radioactivity appeared in the urine by 4 to 6 hours and one-half to one-third of the drug was excreted within 24 hours.

Amitriptyline is metabolized by N-demethylation and bridge hydroxylation in man, rabbit, and rat. Virtually the entire dose is excreted as glucuronide or sulfate conjugate of metabolites, with little unchanged drug appearing in the urine. Other metabolic pathways may be involved.

INDICATIONS AND USAGE:

For the relief of symptoms of depression. Endogenous depression is more likely to be alleviated than are other depressive states.

CONTRAINDICATIONS:

Amitriptyline HCl is contraindicated in patients who have shown prior hypersensitivity to it.

It should not be given concomitantly with monoamine oxidase inhibitors. Hyperpyretic crises, severe convulsions, and deaths have occurred in patients receiving tricyclic antidepressant and monoamine oxidase inhibiting drugs simultaneously. When it is desired to replace a monoamine oxidase inhibitor with amitriptyline HCl, a minimum of 14 days should be allowed to elapse after the former is discontinued. Amitriptyline HCl should then be initiated cautiously with gradual increase in dosage until optimum response is achieved.

This drug is not recommended for use during the acute recovery phase following myocardial infarction.

WARNINGS:

Amitriptyline HCl may block the antihypertensive action of guanethidine or similarly acting compounds.

It should be used with caution in patients with a history of seizures and, because of its atropine-like action, in patients with a history of urinary retention, angle-closure glaucoma or increased intraocular pressure. In patients with angle-closure glaucoma, even average doses may precipitate an attack.

Patients with cardiovascular disorders should be watched closely. Tricyclic antidepressant drugs, including amitriptyline HCl, particularly when given in high doses, have been reported to produce arrhythmias, sinus tachycardia, and prolongation of the conduction time. Myocardial infarction and stroke have been reported with drugs of this class.

Close supervision is required when amitriptyline HCl is given to hyperthyroid patients or those receiving thyroid medication.

Amitriptyline HCl may enhance the response to alcohol and the effects of barbiturates and other CNS depressants. In patients who may use alcohol excessively, it should be borne in mind that the potentiation may increase the danger inherent in any suicide attempt or overdosage. Delirium has been reported with concurrent administration of amitriptyline and disulfiram.

Usage in Pregnancy: Teratogenic effects were not observed in mice, rats, or rabbits when amitriptyline was given orally at doses of 2 to 40 mg/kg/day (up to 13 times the maximum recommended human dose**). Studies in literature have shown amitriptyline to be tera-

WARNINGS: *(cont'd)*

togenic in mice and hamsters when given by various routes of administration at doses of 28 to 100 mg/kg/day (9 to 33 times the maximum recommended human dose), producing multiple malformations. Another study in the rat reported that an oral dose of 25 mg/kg/day (8 times the maximum recommended human dose) produced delays in ossification of fetal vertebral bodies without other signs of embryotoxicity. In rabbits, an oral dose of 60 mg/kg/day (20 times the maximum recommended human dose) was reported to cause incomplete ossification of the cranial bones.

Amitriptyline has been shown to cross the placenta. Although a causal relationship has not been established, there have been a few reports of adverse events, including CNS effects, limb deformities, or developmental delay, in infants whose mothers had taken amitriptyline during pregnancy.

There are no adequate and well-controlled studies in pregnant women. Amitriptyline HCl should be used during pregnancy only if the potential benefit to the mother justifies the potential risk to the fetus.

Nursing Mothers: Amitriptyline is excreted into breast milk. In one report in which a patient received amitriptyline 100 mg/day while nursing her infant, levels of 83 - 141 ng/ml were detected in the mother's serum. Levels of 135-151 ng/ml were found in the breast milk, but no trace of the drug could be detected in the infant's serum.

Because of the potential for serious adverse reactions in nursing infants from amitriptyline, a decision should be made whether to discontinue nursing or to discontinue the drug, taking into account the importance of the drug to the mother.

Usage in Children: In view of the lack of experience with the use of this drug in children, it is not recommended at the present time for patients under 12 years of age.

PRECAUTIONS:

Schizophrenic patients may develop increased symptoms of psychosis; patients with paranoid symptomatology may have an exaggeration of such symptoms. Depressed patients, particularly those with known manic-depressive illness, may experience a shift to mania or hypomania. In these circumstances the dose of amitriptyline may be reduced or a major tranquilizer such as perphenazine may be administered concurrently.

The possibility of suicide in depressed patients remains until significant remission occurs. Potentially suicidal patients should not have access to large quantities of this drug. Prescriptions should be written for the smallest amount feasible.

Concurrent administration of amitriptyline HCl and electroshock therapy may increase the hazards associated with such therapy. Such treatment should be limited to patients for whom it is essential.

When possible, the drug should be discontinued several days before elective surgery.

Both elevation and lowering of blood sugar levels have been reported.

Amitriptyline HCl should be used with caution in patients with impaired liver function.

Information for the Patient: While on therapy with amitriptyline HCl, patients should be advised as to the possible impairment of mental and/or physical abilities required for performance of hazardous tasks, such as operating machinery or driving a motor vehicle.

DRUG INTERACTIONS:

Drugs Metabolized by P450 2D6 — The biochemical activity of the drug metabolizing isozyme cytochrome P450 2D6 (debrisoquin hydroxylase) is reduced in a subset of the caucasian population (about 7-10% of caucasians are so called "poor metabolizers"); reliable estimates of the prevalence of reduced P450 2D6 isozyme activity among Asian, African and other populations are not yet available. Poor metabolizers have higher than expected plasma concentrations of tricyclic antidepressants (TCAs) when given usual doses. Depending on the fraction of drug metabolized by P450 2D6, the increase in plasma concentration may be small, or quite large (8-fold increase in plasma AUC of the TCA).

In addition, certain drugs inhibit the activity of this isozyme and make normal metabolizers resemble poor metabolizers. An individual who is stable on a given dose of TCA may become abruptly toxic when given one of these inhibiting drugs as concomitant therapy. The drugs that inhibit cytochrome P450 2D6 include some that are not metabolized by the enzyme (quinidine; cimetidine) and many that are substrates for P450 2D6 (many other antidepressants, phenothiazines, and the Type 1C antiarrhythmics propafenone and flecainide). While all the selective serotonin reuptake inhibitors (SSRIs), e.g., fluoxetine, sertraline, and paroxetine, inhibit P450 2D6, they may vary in the extent of inhibition. The extent to which SSRI-TCA interactions may pose clinical problems will depend on the degree of inhibition and the pharmacokinetics of the SSRI involved. Nevertheless, caution is indicated in the coadministration of TCAs with any of the SSRIs and also in switching from one class to the other. Of particular importance, sufficient time must elapse before initiating TCA treatment in a patient being withdrawn from fluoxetine, given the long half-life of the parent and active metabolite (at least 5 weeks may be necessary).

Concomitant use of tricyclic antidepressants with drugs that can inhibit cytochrome P450 2D6 may require lower doses than usually prescribed for either the tricyclic antidepressant or the other drug. Furthermore, whenever one of these other drugs is withdrawn from co-therapy, an increased dose of tricyclic antidepressant may be required. It is desirable to monitor TCA plasma levels whenever a TCA is going to be coadministered with another drug known to be an inhibitor of P450 2D6.

Monoamine Oxidase Inhibitors: (See CONTRAINDICATIONS.) Guanethidine or similarly acting compounds; thyroid medication; alcohol, barbiturates and other CNS depressants; and disulfiram (see WARNINGS.)

When amitriptyline HCl is given with anticholinergic agents or sympathomimetic drugs, including epinephrine combined with local anesthetics, close supervision and careful adjustment of dosages are required.

Hyperpyrexia has been reported when amitriptyline HCl is administered with anticholinergic agents or with neuroleptic drugs, particularly during hot weather.

Paralytic ileus may occur in patients taking tricyclic antidepressants in combination with anticholinergic-type drugs.

Cimetidine is reported to reduce hepatic metabolism of certain tricyclic antidepressants, thereby delaying elimination and increasing steady-state concentrations of these drugs. Clinically significant effects have been reported with the tricyclic antidepressants when used concomitantly with cimetidine. Increases in plasma levels of tricyclic antidepressants, and in the frequency and severity of side effects, particularly anticholinergic, have been reported when cimetidine was added to the drug regimen. Discontinuation of cimetidine in well-controlled patients receiving tricyclic antidepressants and cimetidine may decrease the plasma levels and efficacy of the antidepressants.

Caution is advised if patients receive large doses of ethchlorvynol concurrently. Transient delirium has been reported in patients who were treated with one gram of ethchlorvynol and 75 - 150 mg of amitriptyline HCl.

ADVERSE REACTIONS:

Within each category the following adverse reactions are listed in order of decreasing severity. Included in the listing are a few adverse reactions which have not been reported with this specific drug. However, pharmacological similarities among the tricyclic antidepressant drugs require that each of the reactions be considered when amitriptyline is administered.

Cardiovascular: Myocardial infarction; stroke; nonspecific ECG changes and changes in AV conduction; heart block; arrhythmias; hypotension, particularly orthostatic hypotension; syncope; hypertension; tachycardia; palpitation.

CNS and Neuromuscular: Coma; seizures; hallucinations; delusions; confusional states; disorientation; incoordination; ataxia; tremors; peripheral neuropathy; numbness, tingling, and paresthesias of the extremities; extrapyramidal symptoms including abnormal involuntary movements and tardive dyskinesia; dysarthria; disturbed concentration; excitement; anxiety; insomnia; restlessness; nightmares; drowsiness; dizziness; weakness; fatigue; headache; syndrome of inappropriate ADH (antidiuretic hormone) secretion; tinnitus; alteration in EEG patterns.

Anticholinergic: Paralytic ileus; hyperpyrexia; urinary retention; dilatation of the urinary tract; constipation; blurred vision, disturbance of accommodation, increased ocular pressure, mydriasis; dry mouth.

Allergic: Skin rash; urticaria; photosensitization; edema of face and tongue.

Hematologic: Bone marrow depression including agranulocytosis, leukopenia, thrombocytopenia; purpura; eosinophilia.

Gastrointestinal: Rarely hepatitis (including altered liver function and jaundice); nausea; epigastric distress; vomiting; anorexia; stomatitis; peculiar taste; diarrhea; parotid swelling; black tongue.

Endocrine: Testicular swelling and gynecomastia in the male; breast enlargement and galactorrhea in the female; increased or decreased libido; impotence; elevation and lowering of blood sugar levels.

Other: Alopecia; edema; weight gain or loss; urinary frequency; increased perspiration.

Withdrawal Symptoms: After prolonged administration, abrupt cessation of treatment may produce nausea, headache, and malaise. Gradual dosage reduction has been reported to produce, within two weeks, transient symptoms including irritability, restlessness, and dream and sleep disturbance.

These symptoms are not indicative of addiction. Rare instances have been reported of mania or hypomania occurring within 2-7 days following cessation of chronic therapy with tricyclic antidepressants.

Causal Relationship Unknown: Other reactions, reported under circumstances where a causal relationship could not be established, are listed to serve as alerting information to physicians:

Body as a Whole: Lupus-like syndrome (migratory arthritis, positive ANA and rheumatoid factor).

Digestive: Hepatic failure, ageusia.

OVERDOSAGE:

Manifestations: High doses may cause temporary confusion, disturbed concentration, or transient visual hallucinations. Overdosage may cause drowsiness; hypothermia; tachycardia and other arrhythmic abnormalities, such as bundle branch block; ECG evidence of impaired conduction; congestive heart failure; dilated pupils; disorders or ocular motility; convulsions; severe hypotension; stupor; coma; and, polyradiculoneuropathy. Other symptoms may be agitation, hyperactive reflexes, muscle rigidity, vomiting, hyperpyrexia, or any of those listed under ADVERSE REACTIONS.

There has been a report of fatal dysrhythmia occurring as late as 56 hours after amitriptyline overdose.

All patients suspected of having taken an overdosage should be admitted to a hospital as soon as possible. Treatment is symptomatic and supportive. Empty the stomach as quickly as possible by emesis followed by gastric lavage upon arrival at the hospital. Following gastric lavage, activated charcoal may be administered. Twenty to 30 g of activated charcoal may be given every four to six hours during the first 24 to 48 hours after ingestion. An ECG should be taken and close monitoring of cardiac function instituted if there is any sign of abnormality. Maintain an open airway and adequate fluid intake; regulate body temperature.

The intravenous administration of 1-3 mg of physostigmine salicylate is reported to reverse the symptoms of tricyclic antidepressant poisoning. Because physostigmine is rapidly metabolized, the dosage of physostigmine should be repeated as required particularly if life threatening signs such as arrhythmias, convulsions, and deep coma recur or persist after the initial dosage of physostigmine. Because physostigmine itself may be toxic, it is not recommended for routine use.

Standard measures should be used to manage circulatory shock and metabolic acidosis. Cardiac arrhythmias may be treated with neostigmine, pyridostigmine, or propranolol. Should cardiac failure occur, the use of digitalis should be considered. Close monitoring of cardiac function for not less than five days is advisable.

Anticonvulsants may be given to control convulsions. Amitriptyline increases the CNS depressant action but not the anticonvulsant action of barbiturates; therefore, an inhalation anesthetic, diazepam, or paraldehyde is recommended for control of convulsions.

Dialysis is of no value because of low plasma concentrations of the drug.

Since overdosage is often deliberate, patients may attempt suicide by other means during the recovery phase.

Deaths by deliberate or accidental overdosage have occurred with this class of drugs.

DOSAGE AND ADMINISTRATION:

Oral Dosage: Dosage should be initiated at a low level and increased gradually, noting carefully the clinical response and any evidence of intolerance.

Initial Dosage for Adults: For outpatients 75 mg of amitriptyline HCl a day in divided doses is usually satisfactory. If necessary, this may be increased to a total of 150 mg per day. Increases are made preferably in the late afternoon and/or bedtime doses. A sedative effect may be apparent before the antidepressant effect is noted, but an adequate therapeutic effect may take as long as 30 days to develop.

An alternate method of initiating therapy in outpatients is to begin with 50 to 100 mg amitriptyline HCl at bedtime. This may be increased by 25 or 50 mg as necessary in the bedtime dose to a total of 150 mg per day.

Hospitalized patients may require 100 mg a day initially. This can be increased gradually to 200 mg a day if necessary. A small number of hospitalized patients may need as much as 300 mg a day.

Adolescent and Elderly Patients: In general, lower dosages are recommended for these patients. Ten mg 3 times a day with 20 mg at bedtime may be satisfactory in adolescent and elderly patients who do not tolerate higher dosages.

Maintenance: The usual maintenance dosage of amitriptyline HCl is 50 to 100 mg per day. In some patients 40 mg per day is sufficient. For maintenance therapy the total daily dosage may be given in a single dose preferably at bedtime. When satisfactory improvement has

DOSAGE AND ADMINISTRATION: *(cont'd)*

been reached, dosage should be reduced to the lowest amount that will maintain relief of symptoms. It is appropriate to continue maintenance therapy 3 months or longer to lessen the possibility of relapse.

Intramuscular Dosage: Initially, 20 to 30 mg (2 to 3 ml) four times a day.

When amitriptyline HCl injection is administered intramuscularly, the effects may appear more rapidly than with oral administration.

When amitriptyline HCl injection is used for initial therapy in patients unable or unwilling to take amitriptyline HCl tablets, the tablets should replace the injection as soon as possible.

Usage in Children: In view of the lack of experience with the use of this drug in children, it is not recommended at the present time for patients under 12 years of age.

Plasma Levels: Because of the wide variation in the absorption and distribution of tricyclic antidepressants in body fluids, it is difficult to directly correlate plasma levels and therapeutic effect. However, determination of plasma levels may be useful in identifying patients who appear to have toxic effects and may have excessively high levels, or those in whom lack of absorption or noncompliance is suspected. Adjustments in dosage should be made according to the patient's clinical response and not on the basis of plasma levels.***

REFERENCES:

1. Ayd FJ Jr: Amitriptyline therapy for depressive reactions. Psychosomatics 1960;1:320-325. **2.** Diamond S: Human metabolizer of amitriptyline tagged with carbon 14. Curr Ther Res, Mar 1965, pp 170-175. **3.** Dorfman W: Clinical experiences with amitriptyline: A preliminary report. Psychosomatics 1960;1:153-155. **4.** Fallette JM, Stasney CR, Mintz AA: Amitriptyline poisoning treated with physostigmine. South Med J 1970;63:1492-1493. **5.** Hollister LE, Overall JE, Johnson M, et al: Controlled comparison of amitriptyline, imipramine and placebo in hospitalized depressed patients. J Nerv Ment Dis 1964;139:370-375. **6.** Hordern A, Burt CG, Holt NF: Depressive states: A pharmacotherapeutic study, Springfield study. Springfield, III, Charles C. Thomas, 1965. **7.** Klerman GL, Cole JO: Clinical pharmacology of imipramine and related antidepressant compounds. Int J Psychiatry 1976;3:267-304. **8.** McConaghy N, Joffe AD, Kingston WR, et al: Correlation of clinical features of depressed outpatients with response to amitriptyline and protriptyline. Br J Psychiatry 1968;114:103-106. **9.** McDonald IM, Perkins M, Marjerrison G, et al: A controlled comparison of amitriptyline and electroconvulsive therapy in the treatment of depression. Am J Psychiatry 1966;122:1427-1431. **10.** Slovis T, Ott J, Teitelbaum, et al: Physostigmine therapy in acute tricyclic antidepressant poisoning. Clin Toxicol 1971;4:451-459. **11.** Symposium on depression with special studies of a new antidepressant, amitriptyline. Dis Nerv Syst, (Sect 2) May 1961, pp 5-56.

* Registered trademark of Zeneca Inc.

** Based on a maximum recommended amitriptyline dose of 150 mg/day or 3 mg/kg/day for a 50 kg patient.

*** Hollister LE: JAMA 1979;241:2350-2533.

HOW SUPPLIED:

Tablets: Elavil, 10 mg, are blue, round, film coated tablets, identified with "40" debossed on one side and "Elavil" on the other side. Elavil, 25 mg, are yellow, round, film coated tablets, identified with "45" debossed on one side and "Elavil" on the other side. Elavil, 50 mg, are beige, round, film coated tablets, identified with "41" debossed on one side and "Elavil" on the other side. Elavil, 75 mg, are orange, round, film coated tablets, identified with "42" debossed on one side and "Elavil" on the other side. Elavil, 100 mg, are mauve, round, film coated tablets, identified with "43" debossed on one side and "Elavil" on the other side. Elavil, 150 mg, are blue, capsule shaped, film coated tablets, identified with "47" debossed on one side and "Elavil" on the other side.

Injection: Elavil, 10 mg/ml, is a clear, colorless solution, and is supplied in 10 ml vials:

Storage: Store amitriptyline HCl tablets in a well-closed container. Avoid storage at temperatures above 30°C (86°F). In addition, amitriptyline HCl tablets 10 mg must be protected from light and stored in a well-closed, light-resistant container.

Protect amitriptyline HCl injection from freezing and avoid storage above 30°C (86°F).

HOW SUPPLIED - RATED THERAPEUTICALLY EQUIVALENT:

Injection, Solution - Intramuscular - 10 mg/ml

10 ml	$4.00	Amitriptyline Hcl, Consolidated Midland	00223-7180-10
10 ml	**$8.88**	**ELAVIL, Stuart Pharm**	**00038-0049-10**

Tablet, Coated - Oral - 10 mg

100's	$1.73	Amitriptyline HCl, H.C.F.A. F F P	99999-0213-01
100's	$3.55	Amitriptyline Hcl, Major Pharms	00904-0200-60
100's	$3.74	Amitriptyline HCl, Teva	00332-2120-09
100's	$3.89	Amitriptyline Hcl, Roxane	00054-4041-25
100's	$4.00	Amitriptyline Hcl, Mutual Pharm	53489-0104-01
100's	$4.20	Amitriptyline Hcl, Sidmak Labs	50111-0366-01
100's	$4.28	Amitriptyline Hcl, United Res	00677-0475-01
100's	$4.40	Amitriptyline Hcl, Parmed Pharms	00349-1040-01
100's	$4.50	Elavil, Rugby	00536-3071-01
100's	$4.50	Amitriptyline Hcl, Qualitest Pharms	00603-2212-21
100's	$4.50	Amitriptyline Hcl, Martec Pharms	52555-0975-01
100's	$4.53	Amitriptyline Hcl, Purepac Pharm	00228-2131-10
100's	$4.62	Amitriptyline Hcl, MD Pharm	43567-0538-07
100's	$4.65	Amitriptyline Hcl, Geneva Pharms	00781-1486-01
100's	$4.68	Amitriptyline HCl 10, Aligen Independ	00405-4066-01
100's	$4.95	Amitriptyline Hcl, Goldline Labs	00182-1018-01
100's	$5.40	Amitriptyline HCl., Schein Pharm (US)	00364-0573-01
100's	$5.40	Amitriptyline Hcl, HL Moore Drug Exch	00839-6191-06
100's	$5.95	Amitriptyline Hcl, Mylan	00378-2610-01
100's	$8.50	Amitriptyline Hcl, Medirex	57480-0301-01
100's	$8.53	Amitriptyline Hcl, Roxane	00054-8041-25
100's	$12.80	Amitriptyline Hcl, Goldline Labs	00182-1018-89
100's	$13.99	Amitriptyline HCl, Geneva Pharms	00781-1486-13
100's	$14.03	Amitriptyline HCl, Vangard Labs	00615-0828-13
100's	$15.18	Amitriptyline Hcl, Major Pharms	00904-0200-61
100's	$15.71	ENDEP, Roche Prod	00140-0106-01
100's	**$18.59**	**ELAVIL, Stuart Pharm**	**00038-0040-10**
600's	$89.00	Amitriptyline Hcl, Medirex	57480-0301-06
1000's	$17.30	Amitriptyline HCl, H.C.F.A. F F P	99999-0213-02
1000's	$26.50	Amitriptyline Hcl, Major Pharms	00904-0200-80
1000's	$29.75	Amitriptyline Hcl, Mutual Pharm	53489-0104-10
1000's	$31.00	Elavil, Rugby	00536-3071-10
1000's	$31.70	Amitriptyline Hcl, United Res	00677-0475-10
1000's	$31.72	Amitriptyline Hcl, Purepac Pharm	00228-2131-96
1000's	$33.85	Amitriptyline HCl 10, Aligen Independ	00405-4066-03
1000's	$35.66	Amitriptyline HCl, Teva	00332-2120-15
1000's	$37.67	Amitriptyline Hcl, HL Moore Drug Exch	00839-6191-16
1000's	$38.00	Amitriptyline Hcl, Sidmak Labs	50111-0366-03
1000's	$40.60	Amitriptyline Hcl, Parmed Pharms	00349-1040-10
1000's	$40.85	Amitriptyline Hcl, Qualitest Pharms	00603-2212-32
1000's	$40.89	Amitriptyline Hcl, MD Pharm	43567-0538-12
1000's	$44.55	Amitriptyline Hcl, Goldline Labs	00182-1018-10
1000's	$44.70	Amitriptyline HCl, Geneva Pharms	00781-1486-10
1000's	$45.00	Amitriptyline HCl., Schein Pharm (US)	00364-0573-02
1000's	$53.55	Amitriptyline Hcl, Mylan	00378-2610-10
1000's	**$177.13**	**ELAVIL, Stuart Pharm**	**00038-0040-34**

HOW SUPPLIED - RATED THERAPEUTICALLY EQUIVALENT: *(cont'd)*

Tablet, Coated - Oral - 25 mg

30's	$.60	Amitriptyline HCl, H.C.F.A. F F P	99999-0213-03
30's	$1.85	Amitriptyline Hydrochloride, Major Pharms	00904-0201-46
60's	$1.21	Amitriptyline HCl, H.C.F.A. F F P	99999-0213-04
60's	$2.30	Amitriptyline Hcl, Major Pharms	00904-0201-52
100's	$2.03	Amitriptyline HCl, H.C.F.A. F F P	99999-0213-05
100's	$4.94	Amitriptyline HCl 25, Aligen Independ	00405-4067-01
100's	$5.25	Amitriptyline Hcl, Major Pharms	00904-0201-60
100's	$5.70	Amitriptyline Hcl, United Res	00677-0476-01
100's	$5.70	Amitriptyline Hcl, Mutual Pharm	53489-0105-01
100's	$6.00	Amitriptyline HCl, Teva	00332-2122-09
100's	$6.25	Elavil, Rugby	00536-3072-01
100's	$6.75	Amitriptyline Hcl, Qualitest Pharms	00603-2213-21
100's	$6.96	Amitriptyline Hcl, MD Pharm	43567-0539-07
100's	$7.11	Amitriptyline Hcl, Purepac Pharm	00228-2132-10
100's	$7.20	Amitriptyline Hcl, Sidmak Labs	50111-0367-01
100's	$7.82	Amitriptyline Hcl, Roxane	00054-4042-25
100's	$8.25	Amitriptyline Hcl, Parmed Pharms	00349-1041-01
100's	$8.75	Amitriptyline Hcl, Martec Pharms	52555-0976-01
100's	$9.20	Amitriptyline Hcl, Medirex	57480-0302-01
100's	$9.50	Amitriptyline Hcl, Goldline Labs	00182-1019-01
100's	$10.01	Amitriptyline HCl, Schein Pharm (US)	00364-0574-01
100's	$10.46	Amitriptyline Hcl, HL Moore Drug Exch	00839-6192-06
100's	$10.50	Amitriptyline HCl, Geneva Pharms	00781-1487-01
100's	$10.95	Amitriptyline Hcl, Mylan	00378-2625-01
100's	$13.12	Amitriptyline Hcl, Roxane	00054-8042-25
100's	$14.90	Amitriptyline Hcl, Geneva Pharms	00781-1487-13
100's	$15.00	Amitriptyline Hcl, Goldline Labs	00182-1019-89
100's	$16.17	Amitriptyline HCl, Vangard Labs	00615-0829-13
100's	$17.41	Amitriptyline Hcl, Major Pharms	00904-0201-61
100's	$31.05	ENDEP, Roche Prod	00140-0107-01
100's	**$37.26**	**ELAVIL, Stuart Pharm**	**00038-0045-10**
100's	**$40.88**	**ELAVIL, Stuart Pharm**	**00038-0045-39**
600's	$145.80	Amitriptyline Hcl, Medirex	57480-0302-06
1000's	$20.30	Amitriptyline HCl, H.C.F.A. F F P	99999-0213-06
1000's	$29.50	Amitriptyline Hcl, Major Pharms	00904-0201-80
1000's	$35.30	Amitriptyline Hcl, United Res	00677-0476-10
1000's	$35.30	Amitriptyline Hcl, Mutual Pharm	53489-0105-10
1000's	$36.62	Amitriptyline HCl 25, Aligen Independ	00405-4067-03
1000's	$46.49	Amitriptyline Hcl, Purepac Pharm	00228-2132-96
1000's	$47.05	Amitriptyline Hcl, HL Moore Drug Exch	00839-6192-16
1000's	$49.95	Elavil, Rugby	00536-3072-10
1000's	$55.85	Amitriptyline HCl, Schein Pharm (US)	00364-0574-02
1000's	$57.04	Amitriptyline HCl, Teva	00332-2122-15
1000's	$57.20	Amitriptyline Hcl, Qualitest Pharms	00603-2213-32
1000's	$58.10	Amitriptyline Hcl, Sidmak Labs	50111-0367-03
1000's	$59.85	Amitriptyline Hcl, Martec Pharms	52555-0976-10
1000's	$61.00	Amitriptyline Hcl, Parmed Pharms	00349-1041-10
1000's	$61.95	Amitriptyline Hcl, MD Pharm	43567-0539-12
1000's	$66.16	Amitriptyline Hcl, Roxane	00054-4042-31
1000's	$78.75	Amitriptyline Hcl, Geneva Pharms	00781-1487-10
1000's	$85.50	Amitriptyline Hcl, Goldline Labs	00182-1019-10
1000's	$98.55	Amitriptyline Hcl, Mylan	00378-2625-10
1000's	**$354.18**	**ELAVIL, Stuart Pharm**	**00038-0045-34**
5000's	$101.50	Amitriptyline HCl, H.C.F.A. F F P	99999-0213-07
5000's	**$1726.70**	**ELAVIL, Stuart Pharm**	**00038-0045-50**

Tablet, Coated - Oral - 50 mg

30's	$.83	Amitriptyline HCl, H.C.F.A. F F P	99999-0213-08
30's	$2.10	Amitriptyline Hcl, Major Pharms	00904-0202-46
100's	$2.78	Amitriptyline HCl, H.C.F.A. F F P	99999-0213-09
100's	$6.85	Amitriptyline HCl 50, Aligen Independ	00405-4068-01
100's	$8.35	Amitriptyline Hcl, United Res	00677-0477-01
100's	$8.50	Amitriptyline Hcl, Mutual Pharm	53489-0106-01
100's	$8.60	Amitriptyline Hcl, Major Pharms	00904-0202-60
100's	$9.30	Amitriptyline Hcl, MD Pharm	43567-0540-07
100's	$9.93	Amitriptyline Hcl, Roxane	00054-4043-25
100's	$10.68	Amitriptyline HCl, Teva	00332-2124-09
100's	$10.95	Elavil, Rugby	00536-3073-01
100's	$11.19	Amitriptyline Hcl, HL Moore Drug Exch	00839-6193-06
100's	$11.20	Amitriptyline HCl., Schein Pharm (US)	00364-0575-01
100's	$11.20	Amitriptyline Hcl, Qualitest Pharms	00603-2214-21
100's	$11.20	Amitriptyline Hcl, Sidmak Labs	50111-0368-01
100's	$11.33	Amitriptyline Hcl, Purepac Pharm	00228-2133-10
100's	$11.40	Amitriptyline Hcl, Martec Pharms	52555-0977-01
100's	$11.44	Amitriptyline Hcl, Medirex	57480-0303-01
100's	$11.75	Amitriptyline Hcl, Parmed Pharms	00349-1042-01
100's	$12.25	Amitriptyline Hcl, Goldline Labs	00182-1020-01
100's	$12.40	Amitriptyline HCl, Geneva Pharms	00781-1488-01
100's	$12.95	Amitriptyline Hcl, Mylan	00378-2650-01
100's	$19.20	Amitriptyline Hcl, Goldline Labs	00182-1020-89
100's	$20.07	Amitriptyline Hcl, Major Pharms	00904-0202-61
100's	$20.66	Amitriptyline HCl, Vangard Labs	00615-0830-13
100's	$22.70	Amitriptyline Hcl, Roxane	00054-8043-25
100's	$24.49	Amitriptyline HCl, Geneva Pharms	00781-1488-13
100's	**$66.28**	**ELAVIL, Stuart Pharm**	**00038-0041-10**
100's	**$68.99**	**ELAVIL, Stuart Pharm**	**00038-0041-39**
250's	$6.95	Amitriptyline HCl, H.C.F.A. F F P	99999-0213-10
250's	$15.20	Amitriptyline Hcl, MD Pharm	43567-0540-10
500's	$13.90	Amitriptyline HCl, H.C.F.A. F F P	99999-0213-11
500's	$37.95	Elavil, Rugby	00536-3073-05
600's	$236.60	Amitriptyline Hcl, Medirex	57480-0303-06
1000's	$27.80	Amitriptyline HCl, H.C.F.A. F F P	99999-0213-12
1000's	$41.80	Amitriptyline Hcl, Major Pharms	00904-0202-80
1000's	$49.30	Amitriptyline Hcl, United Res	00677-0477-10
1000's	$49.30	Amitriptyline Hcl, Mutual Pharm	53489-0106-10
1000's	$54.29	Amitriptyline HCl 50, Aligen Independ	00405-4068-03
1000's	$60.20	Amitriptyline Hcl, Sidmak Labs	50111-0368-03
1000's	$64.95	Elavil, Rugby	00536-3073-10
1000's	$65.75	Amitriptyline Hcl, HL Moore Drug Exch	00839-6193-16
1000's	$74.49	Amitriptyline Hcl, Purepac Pharm	00228-2133-96
1000's	$74.95	Amitriptyline Hcl, Parmed Pharms	00349-1042-10
1000's	$80.24	Amitriptyline HCl., Schein Pharm (US)	00364-0575-02
1000's	$81.84	Amitriptyline Hcl, MD Pharm	43567-0540-12
1000's	$89.47	Amitriptyline Hcl, Roxane	00054-4043-31
1000's	$101.33	Amitriptyline HCl, Teva	00332-2124-15
1000's	$101.50	Amitriptyline Hcl, Qualitest Pharms	00603-2214-32
1000's	$103.50	Amitriptyline Hcl, Martec Pharms	52555-0977-10
1000's	$110.25	Amitriptyline Hcl, Goldline Labs	00182-1020-10
1000's	$110.50	Amitriptyline HCl, Geneva Pharms	00781-1488-10
1000's	$116.55	Amitriptyline Hcl, Mylan	00378-2650-10
1000's	**$629.16**	**ELAVIL, Stuart Pharm**	**00038-0041-34**

HOW SUPPLIED - RATED THERAPEUTICALLY EQUIVALENT: *(cont'd)*

Tablet, Coated - Oral - 75 mg

100's	$3.53	Amitriptyline HCl, H.C.F.A. F F P	99999-0213-13
100's	$8.94	Amitriptyline HCl 75, Aligen Independ	00405-4069-01
100's	$9.00	Amitriptyline Hcl, Major Pharms	00904-0203-60
100's	$9.13	Amitriptyline Hcl, Purepac Pharm	00228-2134-10
100's	$9.75	Amitriptyline Hcl, Mutual Pharm	53489-0107-01
100's	$10.20	Amitriptyline Hcl, United Res	00677-0478-01
100's	$11.50	Elavil, Rugby	00536-3074-01
100's	$13.70	Amitriptyline Hcl, HL Moore Drug Exch	00839-6194-06
100's	$13.86	Amitriptyline Hcl, MD Pharm	43567-0541-07
100's	$13.95	Amitriptyline Hcl, Parmed Pharms	00349-1043-01
100's	$14.60	Amitriptyline Hcl, Qualitest Pharms	00603-2215-21
100's	$14.62	Amitriptyline HCl, Teva	00332-2126-09
100's	$15.08	Amitriptyline Hcl, Roxane	00054-4045-25
100's	$15.15	Amitriptyline Hcl, Sidmak Labs	50111-0369-01
100's	$15.15	Amitriptyline Hcl, Martec Pharms	52555-0978-01
100's	$15.50	Amitriptyline Hcl, Goldline Labs	00182-1021-01
100's	$16.28	Amitriptyline HCl, Geneva Pharms	00781-1489-01
100's	$16.29	Amitriptyline HCl., Schein Pharm (US)	00364-0576-01
100's	$16.30	Amitriptyline Hcl, Mylan	00378-2675-01
100's	$17.90	Amitriptyline Hcl, Medirex	57480-0304-01
100's	$23.30	Amitriptyline Hcl, Goldline Labs	00182-1021-89
100's	$24.36	Amitriptyline Hcl, Major Pharms	00904-0203-61
100's	$25.81	Amitriptyline HCl, Vangard Labs	00615-0831-13
100's	$25.87	Amitriptyline HCl 75, Geneva Pharms	00781-1489-13
100's	$38.98	Amitriptyline Hcl, Roxane	00054-8045-25
100's	$76.20	ENDEP, Roche Prod	00140-0114-01
100's	**$90.76**	**ELAVIL, Stuart Pharm**	**00038-0042-10**
500's	$17.65	Amitriptyline HCl, H.C.F.A. F F P	99999-0213-14
500's	$36.00	Amitriptyline Hcl, Mutual Pharm	53489-0107-05
1000's	$35.30	Amitriptyline HCl, H.C.F.A. F F P	99999-0213-15
1000's	$64.00	Amitriptyline Hcl, Sidmak Labs	50111-0369-03
1000's	$181.58	Amytriptyline HCl, HL Moore Drug Exch	00839-6194-16

Tablet, Coated - Oral - 100 mg

100's	$4.28	Amitriptyline HCl, H.C.F.A. F F P	99999-0213-16
100's	$9.42	Amitriptyline HCl 100, Aligen Independ	00405-4070-01
100's	$9.50	Amitriptyline Hcl, Major Pharms	00904-0204-60
100's	$11.58	Amitriptyline Hcl, Purepac Pharm	00228-2135-10
100's	$11.90	Amitriptyline Hcl, Mutual Pharm	53489-0108-01
100's	$11.95	Elavil, Rugby	00536-3075-01
100's	$12.05	Amitriptyline Hcl, United Res	00677-0568-01
100's	$16.97	Amitriptyline Hcl, MD Pharm	43567-0542-07
100's	$17.92	Amitriptyline Hcl, Roxane	00054-4046-25
100's	$18.48	Amitriptyline HCl, Teva	00332-2128-09
100's	$18.88	Amitriptyline Hcl, Qualitest Pharms	00603-2216-21
100's	$18.95	Amitriptyline Hcl, Parmed Pharms	00349-1044-01
100's	$19.25	Amitriptyline Hcl, Sidmak Labs	50111-0370-01
100's	$19.25	Amitriptyline Hcl, Martec Pharms	52555-0979-01
100's	$19.30	Amitriptyline HCl., Schein Pharm (US)	00364-0577-01
100's	$19.50	Amitriptyline Hcl, Goldline Labs	00182-1063-01
100's	$19.70	Amitriptyline Hcl, HL Moore Drug Exch	00839-6223-06
100's	$19.90	Amitriptyline HCl, Geneva Pharms	00781-1490-01
100's	$19.95	Amitriptyline Hcl, Mylan	00378-2685-01
100's	$24.50	Amitriptyline Hcl, Medirex	57480-0424-01
100's	$29.15	Amitriptyline Hcl, Major Pharms	00904-0204-61
100's	$38.00	Amitriptyline Hcl, Goldline Labs	00182-1063-89
100's	$40.19	Amitriptyline HCl, Geneva Pharms	00781-1490-13
100's	$40.21	Amitriptyline HCl, Vangard Labs	00615-0832-13
100's	$47.69	Amitriptyline Hcl, Roxane	00054-8046-25
100's	**$114.76**	**ELAVIL, Stuart Pharm**	**00038-0043-10**
500's	$21.40	Amitriptyline HCl, H.C.F.A. F F P	99999-0213-17
500's	$47.75	Elavil, Rugby	00536-3075-05
600's	$147.00	Amitriptyline Hcl, Medirex	57480-0424-06

Tablet, Coated - Oral - 150 mg

30's	$2.09	Amitriptyline HCl, H.C.F.A. F F P	99999-0213-18
30's	**$49.91**	**ELAVIL, Stuart Pharm**	**00038-0047-30**
100's	$6.98	Amitriptyline HCl, H.C.F.A. F F P	99999-0213-19
100's	$14.18	Elavil, Rugby	00536-3076-01
100's	$14.85	Amitriptyline Hcl, Sidmak Labs	50111-0371-01
100's	$15.20	Amitriptyline Hcl, Mutual Pharm	53489-0109-01
100's	$16.20	Amitriptyline Hcl, United Res	00677-0645-01
100's	$16.25	Amitriptyline Hcl, Qualitest Pharms	00603-2217-21
100's	$17.19	Amitriptyline HCl 150, Aligen Independ	00405-4071-01
100's	$21.50	Amitriptyline HCl, Goldline Labs	00182-1486-01
100's	$22.13	Amitriptyline Hcl, HL Moore Drug Exch	00839-6401-06
100's	$26.62	Amitriptyline HCl, Schein Pharm (US)	00364-0578-01
100's	$26.62	Amitriptyline HCl, Geneva Pharms	00781-1491-01
100's	$26.62	Amitriptyline Hcl, Major Pharms	00904-0205-60
100's	$26.62	Amitriptyline Hcl, MD Pharm	43567-0543-07
100's	$26.75	Amitriptyline Hcl, Mylan	00378-2695-01
100's	$37.80	Amitriptyline HCl, Geneva Pharms	00781-1491-13
100's	$147.86	ENDEP, Roche Prod	00140-0124-01
100's	**$163.28**	**ELAVIL, Stuart Pharm**	**00038-0047-10**
600's	$228.60	Amitriptyline Hcl, Medirex	57480-0425-06

HOW SUPPLIED - NOT RATED EQUIVALENT:

Tablet, Coated - Oral - 10 mg

100's	$2.43	Amitriptyline Hcl, Voluntary Hosp	53258-0185-01
100's	$3.08	Amitriptyline Hcl, IDE-Interstate	00814-0635-14
100's	$3.21	Amitriptyline Hcl, US Trading	56126-0133-11
100's	$6.12	Amitriptyline Hcl, Voluntary Hosp	53258-0185-13
100's	$8.35	Amitriptyline Hcl, TIE Pharm	55496-1001-09

Tablet, Coated - Oral - 25 mg

100's	$2.85	Amitriptyline Hcl, Voluntary Hosp	53258-0186-01
100's	$8.01	Amitriptyline Hcl, Voluntary Hosp	53258-0186-13
100's	$12.64	Amitriptyline Hcl, TIE Pharm	55496-1002-09

Tablet, Coated - Oral - 50 mg

100's	$3.84	Amitriptyline Hcl, Voluntary Hosp	53258-0187-01
100's	$4.11	Amitriptyline Hcl, US Trading	56126-0135-11
100's	$9.15	Amitriptyline Hcl, Raway	00686-2226-13
100's	$9.18	Amitriptyline Hcl, Voluntary Hosp	53258-0187-13
100's	$21.86	Amitriptyline Hcl, TIE Pharm	55496-1003-09
100's	$59.08	VANATRIP, GM Pharms	58809-0717-01

Tablet, Coated - Oral - 75 mg

100's	$5.55	Amitriptyline Hcl, Voluntary Hosp	53258-0188-01
100's	$12.60	Amitriptyline Hcl, Voluntary Hosp	53258-0188-13
100's	$13.90	Amitriptyline Hcl, Raway	00686-2231-13
100's	$37.59	Amitriptyline Hcl, TIE Pharm	55496-1004-09
500's	$33.95	Amitriptyline Hcl, Halsey Drug	00879-0491-05

HOW SUPPLIED - NOT RATED EQUIVALENT: *(cont'd)*

Tablet, Coated - Oral - 100 mg

100's	$6.60	Amitriptyline Hcl, US Trading	56126-0137-11
100's	$8.55	Amitriptyline Hcl, Voluntary Hosp	53258-0189-01
100's	$14.85	Amitriptyline Hcl, Voluntary Hosp	53258-0189-13
100's	$18.50	Amitriptyline Hcl, Raway	00686-2233-13
500's	$52.95	Amitriptyline Hcl, Halsey Drug	00879-0492-05

AMITRIPTYLINE HYDROCHLORIDE; CHLORDIAZEPOXIDE *(000214)*

CATEGORIES: Anorexia; Antianxiety Drugs; Antidepressants; Anxiety; Benzodiazepines; Central Nervous System Agents; Depression; Insomnia; Psychotherapeutic Agents; Sedatives; Tricyclic Antidepressants; Tranquilizers; DEA Class CIV; FDA Approval Pre 1982

BRAND NAMES: *Amitrol*; *Amitrol D.S.*; Lamitrip; **Limbitrol**; *Limbitrol F*; *Limbitryl* *(International brand names outside U.S. in italics)*

COST OF THERAPY: $69.87 (Depression; Tablet; 25 mg/10 mg; 3/day; 90 days)

PRIMARY ICD9: 311 (Depressive Disorder, Not Elsewhere Classified)

DESCRIPTION:

FOR COMPLETE PRESCRIBING INFORMATION, REFER TO THE INDIVIDUAL DRUG MONOGRAPHS (AMITRIPTYLINE HYDROCHLORIDE; CHLORDIAZEPOXIDE).

INDICATIONS AND USAGE:

Amitriptyline HCl-chlordiazepoxide is indicated for the treatment of patients with moderate to severe depression associated with moderate to severe anxiety.

The therapeutic response to amitriptyline HCl-chlordiazepoxide occurs earlier and with fewer treatment failures than when either amitriptyline or chlordiazepoxide is used alone.

Symptoms likely to respond in the first week of treatment include: insomnia, feelings of guilt or worthlessness, agitation, psychic and somatic anxiety, suicidal ideation and anorexia.

DOSAGE AND ADMINISTRATION:

Optimum dosage varies with the severity of the symptoms and the response of the individual patient. When a satisfactory response is obtained, dosage should be reduced to the smallest amount needed to maintain the remission. The larger portion of the total daily dose may be taken at bedtime. In some patients, a single dose at bedtime may be sufficient. In general, lower dosages are recommended for elderly patients.

Amitriptyline HCl-chlordiazepoxide double strength tablets are recommended in an initial dosage of three or four tablets daily in divided doses; this may be increased to six tablets daily as required. Some patients respond to smaller doses and can be maintained on two tablets daily.

Amitriptyline HCl-chlordiazepoxide tablets in an initial dosage of three or four tablets daily in divided doses may be satisfactory in patients who do not tolerate higher doses.

HOW SUPPLIED:

Amitrol DS (double strength) Tablets contain 10 mg chlordiazepoxide and 25 mg amitriptyline (as the hydrochloride salt).

Amitrol Tablets contain 5 mg chlordiazepoxide and 12.5 mg amitriptyline (as the hydrochloride salt).

HOW SUPPLIED - RATED THERAPEUTICALLY EQUIVALENT:

Tablet, Plain Coated - Oral - 12.5 mg/5 mg

50's	**$28.32**	**LIMBITROL, Roche Prod**	**00140-0070-02**
100's	$19.43	Amitriptyline/Chlordiazepoxide, H.C.F.A. F F P	99999-0214-01
100's	$21.62	Amitriptyline/Chlordiazepoxide, Rugby	00536-3475-01
100's	$27.75	Chlordiazepoxide & Amitriptyline Hcl, Geneva Pharms	00781-1982-01
100's	$32.44	Amitriptyline/Chlordiazepoxide, Aligen Independ	00405-0037-01
100's	$39.49	Chlordiazepoxide & Amitriptyline, HL Moore Drug Exch	00839-7279-06
100's	$42.70	Amitriptyline/Chlordiazepoxide, Qualitest Pharms	00603-2690-21
100's	$42.75	Chlordiazepoxide & Amitriptyline Hcl, Mylan	00378-0211-01
100's	**$65.86**	**LIMBITROL, Roche Prod**	**00140-0070-01**
100's	**$67.94**	**LIMBITROL, Roche Prod**	**00140-0070-49**
500's	$97.15	Amitriptyline/Chlordiazepoxide, H.C.F.A. F F P	99999-0214-02
500's	$176.85	Chlordiazepoxide & Amitriptyline, HL Moore Drug Exch	00839-7279-12
500's	$198.25	Chlordiazepoxide & Amitriptyline Hcl, Mylan	00378-0211-05
500's	$198.25	Amitriptyline/Chlordiazepoxide, Qualitest Pharms	00603-2690-28
500's	**$328.14**	**LIMBITROL, Roche Prod**	**00140-0070-14**

Tablet, Plain Coated - Oral - 25 mg/10 mg

50's	**$39.91**	**LIMBITROL, Roche Prod**	**00140-0071-02**
100's	$25.88	Amitriptyline/Chlordiazepoxide, H.C.F.A. F F P	99999-0214-03
100's	$34.08	Chlordiazepoxide/Amitriptyline, Geneva Pharms	00781-1983-01
100's	$40.28	Chlordiazepoxide/Amitriptyline, Rugby	00536-3492-01
100's	$41.80	Amitriptyline/Chlordiazepoxide, Aligen Independ	00405-0038-01
100's	$59.33	Chlordiazepoxide & Amitriptyline, HL Moore Drug Exch	00839-7280-06
100's	$62.49	Amitriptyline/Chlordiazepoxide, Qualitest Pharms	00603-2691-21
100's	$62.50	Chlordiazepoxide & Amitriptyline Hcl, Mylan	00378-0277-01
100's	**$92.97**	**LIMBITROL, Roche Prod**	**00140-0071-01**
100's	**$95.07**	**LIMBITROL, Roche Prod**	**00140-0071-49**
500's	$129.40	Amitriptyline/Chlordiazepoxide, H.C.F.A. F F P	99999-0214-04
500's	$265.68	Chlordiazepoxide & Amitriptyline, HL Moore Drug Exch	00839-7280-12
500's	$296.60	Amitriptyline/Chlordiazepoxide, Qualitest Pharms	00603-2691-28
500's	$296.65	Chlordiazepoxide & Amitriptyline Hcl, Mylan	00378-0277-05
500's	**$463.76**	**LIMBITROL, Roche Prod**	**00140-0071-14**

AMITRIPTYLINE HYDROCHLORIDE; PERPHENAZINE *(000215)*

CATEGORIES: Antianxiety Drugs; Antidepressants; Antipsychotics/Antimanics; Anxiety; Central Nervous System Agents; Depression; Neuroleptics; Phenothiazines; Psychotherapeutic Agents; Schizophrenia; Tranquilizers; Tricyclics; Tricyclic Antidepressants; FDA Approval Pre 1982; Top 200 Drugs

BRAND NAMES: *Anxipress-D; Deprelio; Elavil; Elavil Plus* (Canada); Etrafon; *Longopax* (Germany); *Minitran; Mutabase; Mutabon; Mutabon-A; Mutabon-D; Mutabon-F; Mutabon-M; Mutabon A* (Mexico); *Mutabon D* (Mexico); *Mutabon F; Mutabon M; Neuragon-A; Neuragon-B;* Per-Trip; *Pertriptyl; Proavil;* Talazil; **Triavil**; *Triptafen* (England); *Triptafen M* (England)
(International brand names outside U.S. in italics)

FORMULARIES: BC-BS; Medi-Cal

COST OF THERAPY: $18.22 (Depression; Tablet; 25 mg/2 mg; 3/day; 90 days)

PRIMARY ICD9: 311 (Depressive Disorder, Not Elsewhere Classified)

DESCRIPTION:

Perphenazine and amitriptyline hydrochloride tablets are available in multiple strengths to afford dosage flexibility for optimum management. They are available as perphenazine and amitriptyline hydrochloride 2-10 tablets, 2 mg perphenazine and 10 mg amitriptyline hydrochloride; perphenazine and amitriptyline hydrochloride tablets, 2 mg perphenazine and 25 mg amitriptyline hydrochloride; perphenazine and amitriptyline hydrochloride tablets, 4 mg perphenazine and 25 mg amitriptyline hydrochloride.

FOR COMPLETE PRESCRIBING INFORMATION, REFER TO THE INDIVIDUAL DRUG MONOGRAPHS (AMITRIPTYLINE HYDROCHLORIDE; PERPHENAZINE).

INDICATIONS AND USAGE:

Perphenazine and amitriptyline hydrochloride tablets are indicated for the treatment of patients with moderate to severe anxiety and/or agitation and depressed mood; patients with depression in whom anxiety and/or agitation are moderate or severe; patients with anxiety and depression associated with chronic physical disease; patients in whom depression and anxiety cannot be clearly differentiated.

Schizophrenic patients who have associated symptoms of depression should be considered for therapy with perphenazine and amitriptyline hydrochloride.

DOSAGE AND ADMINISTRATION:

Initial Dosage: In psychoneurotic patients whose anxiety and depression warrant combined therapy, one perphenazine and amitriptyline hydrochloride tablet (2-25) or one perphenazine and amitriptyline hydrochloride tablet (4-25) three or four times a day is recommended.

In elderly patients and adolescents, a lower initial dosage may be needed. The dosage may then be adjusted cautiously to produce an adequate response.

In more severely ill patients with schizophrenia, two perphenazine and amitriptyline hydrochloride tablets (4-25) three times a day are recommended as the initial dosage. If necessary, a fourth dose may be given at bedtime. The total daily dosage should not exceed eight tablets of any strength.

Maintenance Dosage: Depending on the condition being treated, the onset of therapeutic response may vary from a few days to a few weeks or even longer. After a satisfactory response is noted, dosage should be reduced to the smallest dose which is effective for relief of the symptoms for which perphenazine and amitriptyline hydrochloride tablets are being administered. A useful maintenance dosage is one perphenazine and amitriptyline hydrochloride tablet (2-25) or one perphenazine and amitriptyline hydrochloride tablet (4-25) two to four times a day. In some patients, maintenance dosage is required for many months.

Perphenazine and amitriptyline hydrochloride 2-10 tablets (2-10) can be used to increase flexibility in adjusting maintenance dosage to the lowest amount consistent with relief of symptoms.

Storage: Perphenazine and amitriptyline hydrochloride 2-10, 2-25, 4-25 tablets between 2°C and 25°C (36° and 77°F). In addition, protect unit-dose packages from excessive moisture.

PATIENT INFORMATION:

Amitriptyline; perphenazine is used for the treatment of anxiety and depression. Inform your physician if you are pregnant or nursing. This medication may cause drowsiness or dizziness; use caution while driving or operating hazardous machinery. Do not take any other sedating drugs or drink alcohol while taking this medication. Do not take this medication with monoamine oxidase inhibitors. Amitriptyline; perphenazine may increase susceptibility to heat stroke; avoid becoming overheated. Some patients may develop tardive dyskinesia (muscle spasms, uncontrolled twitching in the face and body, and uncontrolled tongue or jaw movement) during long-term therapy. Talk with your physician regarding this possible side effect. Amitriptyline; perphenazine may be habit forming. Withdrawal symptoms may occur after you stop taking it. This medication may be taken with food if GI upset occurs.

HOW SUPPLIED - RATED THERAPEUTICALLY EQUIVALENT:

Tablet - Oral - 2/10 mg

100's	$24.75	Amitriptyline Hcl; Perphenazine, Duramed Pharms	51285-0887-02
500's	$117.12	Amitriptyline Hcl; Perphenazine, Duramed Pharms	51285-0887-04

Tablet - Oral - 10/4 mg

100's	$28.20	Amitriptyline Hcl; Perphenazine, Duramed Pharms	51285-0888-02
500's	$87.00	Amitriptyline Hcl; Perphenazine, Duramed Pharms	51285-0888-04

Tablet - Oral - 25/2 mg

500's	$131.00	Amitriptyline Hcl; Perphenazine, Duramed Pharms	51285-0889-04

Tablet - Oral - 25/4 mg

100's	$31.09	Amitriptyline Hcl; Perphenazine, Duramed Pharms	51285-0889-02
500's	$142.72	Amitriptyline Hcl; Perphenazine, Duramed Pharms	51285-0890-04

Tablet, Plain Coated - Oral - 10 mg/2 mg

100's	$5.33	Amitriptyline W/Perphenazine, H.C.F.A. F F P	99999-0215-01
100's	$5.40	Perphenazine & Amitripryline Hcl, United Res	00677-1120-01
100's	$15.00	Perphenazine w/ Amitriptyline Hcl, Aligen Independ	00405-4787-01
100's	$17.00	Perphenazine & Amitriptyline Hcl, Goldline Labs	00182-1235-01
100's	$17.68	Amitriptyline W/Perphenazine, Qualitest Pharms	00603-5115-21
100's	$18.40	Perphenazine & Amitriptyline Hcl, Major Pharms	00904-1820-60
100's	$18.95	Amitriptyline W/Perphenazine, Royce	51875-0247-01
100's	$19.30	Amitriptyline W/Perphenazine, Martec Pharms	52555-0460-01
100's	$21.25	Perphenazine & Amitriptyline HCl, Rugby	00536-3077-01
100's	$24.30	Perphenazine & Amitriptyline Hcl, HL Moore Drug Exch	00839-6225-06
100's	$24.85	Perphenazine & Amitriptyline HCl, Geneva Pharms	00781-1265-01
100's	$24.95	Perphenazine & Amitriptyline Hcl, Mylan	00378-0330-01
100's	$35.00	Perphenazine/Amitriptyline, Geneva Pharms	00781-1265-13
100's	$38.84	Amitriptyline W/Perphenazine, Major Pharms	00904-7636-61
500's	$26.65	Amitriptyline W/Perphenazine, H.C.F.A. F F P	99999-0215-02
500's	$75.51	Amitriptyline/Perphenazine, Qualitest Pharms	00603-5115-28
500's	$79.95	Perphenazine & Amitriptyline Hcl, Rugby	00536-3077-05
500's	$80.00	Perphenazine & Amitriptyline Hcl, Goldline Labs	00182-1235-05
500's	$86.40	Perphenazine & Amitriptyline Hcl, Major Pharms	00904-1820-40
500's	$89.10	Amitriptyline W/Perphenazine, Royce	51875-0247-02
500's	$90.80	Amitriptyline W/Perphenazine, Martec Pharms	52555-0460-05

HOW SUPPLIED - RATED THERAPEUTICALLY EQUIVALENT:

(cont'd)

500's	$91.13	Perphenazine & Amitriptyline Hcl, HL Moore Drug Exch	00839-6225-12
500's	$117.29	Perphenazine & Amitriptyline HCl, Geneva Pharms	00781-1265-05
500's	$117.35	Perphenazine & Amitriptyline Hcl, Mylan	00378-0330-05

Tablet, Plain Coated - Oral - 10 mg/4 mg

100's	$6.23	Amitriptyline W/Perphenazine, H.C.F.A. F F P	99999-0215-03
100's	$19.00	Perphenazine & Amitriptyline Hcl, Goldline Labs	00182-1237-01
100's	$19.00	Perphenazine & Amitriptyline Hcl, Aligen Independ	00405-4789-01
100's	$19.54	Amitriptyline W/Perphenazine, Qualitest Pharms	00603-5117-21
100's	$20.30	Perphenazine & Amitriptyline Hcl, Major Pharms	00904-1840-60
100's	$20.95	Perphenazine & Amitriptyline HCl, Rugby	00536-3078-01
100's	$21.20	Amitriptyline W/Perphenazine, Royce	51875-0249-01
100's	$21.60	Amitriptyline W/Perphenazine, Martec Pharms	52555-0462-01
100's	$24.30	Perphenazine & Amitriptyline Hcl, HL Moore Drug Exch	00839-6226-06
100's	$28.50	Perphenazine & Amitriptyline Hcl, Mylan	00378-0042-01
100's	$28.50	Perphenazine/Amitriptyline HCl, Geneva Pharms	00781-1266-01
100's	$52.88	Amitriptyline W/Perphenazine, Major Pharms	00904-7638-61
500's	$31.15	Amitriptyline W/Perphenazine, H.C.F.A. F F P	99999-0215-04
500's	$83.87	Amitriptyline W/Perphenazine, Qualitest Pharms	00603-5117-28
500's	$96.85	Amitriptyline W/Perphenazine, Royce	51875-0249-02

Tablet, Plain Coated - Oral - 25 mg/2 mg

100's	$6.75	Amitriptyline W/Perphenazine, H.C.F.A. F F P	99999-0215-05
100's	$7.13	Perphenazine & Amitriptyline Hcl, United Res	00677-1121-01
100's	$19.50	Perphenazine W/ Amitriptyline Hcl, Aligen Independ	00405-4788-01
100's	$22.61	Amitriptyline W/Perphenazine, Qualitest Pharms	00603-5116-21
100's	$23.40	Perphenazine & Amitriptyline Hcl, Major Pharms	00904-1825-60
100's	$24.15	Amitriptyline W/Perphenazine, Royce	51875-0248-01
100's	$24.50	Perphenazine/Amitriptyline, HL Moore Drug Exch	00839-6217-06
100's	$24.65	Perphenazine & Amitriptyline Hcl, Goldline Labs	00182-1236-01
100's	$24.65	Amitriptyline W/Perphenazine, Martec Pharms	52555-0461-01
100's	$24.95	Perphenazine/Amitriptyline HCl, Rugby	00536-3082-01
100's	$28.89	Perphenazine/Amitriptyline HCl, Geneva Pharms	00781-1273-01
100's	$28.95	Perphenazine & Amitriptyline Hcl, Mylan	00378-0442-01
100's	$43.00	Perphenazine/Amitriptyline, Geneva Pharms	00781-1273-13
100's	$44.85	Amitriptyline W/Perphenazine, Major Pharms	00904-7637-61
500's	$33.75	Amitriptyline W/Perphenazine, H.C.F.A. F F P	99999-0215-06
500's	$92.40	Amitriptyline/Perphenazine, Qualitest Pharms	00603-5116-28
500's	$109.75	Perphenazine & Amitriptyline Hcl, Major Pharms	00904-1825-40
500's	$109.95	Amitriptyline W/Perphenazine, Rugby	00536-3082-05
500's	$112.60	Amitriptyline W/Perphenazine, Royce	51875-0248-02
500's	$112.95	Perphenazine & Amitriptyline Hcl, Goldline Labs	00182-1236-05
500's	$114.85	Amitriptyline W/Perphenazine, Martec Pharms	52555-0461-05
500's	$116.10	Perphenazine & Amitriptyline Hcl, HL Moore Drug Exch	00839-6217-12
500's	$131.29	Perphenazine/Amitriptyline HCl, Geneva Pharms	00781-1273-05
500's	$131.95	Perphenazine & Amitriptyline Hcl, Mylan	00378-0442-05

Tablet, Plain Coated - Oral - 25 mg/4 mg

100's	$8.13	Amitriptyline W/Perphenazine, H.C.F.A. F F P	99999-0215-07
100's	$8.48	Perphenazine & Amitriptyline Hcl, United Res	00677-1123-01
100's	$21.00	Perphenazine & Amitriptyline Hcl, Aligen Independ	00405-4790-01
100's	$24.00	Perphenazine & Amitriptyline Hcl, Goldline Labs	00182-1238-01
100's	$25.11	Amitriptyline W/Perphenazine, Qualitest Pharms	00603-5118-21
100's	$25.80	Perphenazine & Amitriptyline Hcl, Major Pharms	00904-1845-60
100's	$25.85	Perphenazine & Amitriptyline HCl, Rugby	00536-3083-01
100's	$26.25	Amitriptyline W/Perphenazine, Royce	51875-0250-01
100's	$26.78	Amitriptyline W/Perphenazine, Martec Pharms	52555-0464-01
100's	$26.99	Perphenazine & Amitriptyline Hcl 4, HL Moore Drug Exch	00839-6227-06
100's	$31.30	Perphenazine & Amitriptyline Hcl, Mylan	00378-0574-01
500's	$40.65	Amitriptyline W/Perphenazine, H.C.F.A. F F P	99999-0215-08
500's	$104.86	Amitriptyline/Perphenazine, Qualitest Pharms	00603-5118-28
500's	$115.25	Perphenazine & Amitriptyline Hcl, Rugby	00536-3083-05
500's	$120.95	Perphenazine & Amitriptyline Hcl, Major Pharms	00904-1845-40
500's	$122.50	Perphenazine & Amitriptyline Hcl, Goldline Labs	00182-1238-05
500's	$124.30	Amitriptyline W/Perphenazine, Royce	51875-0250-02
500's	$126.78	Amitriptyline W/Perphenazine, Martec Pharms	52555-0464-05
500's	$127.56	Perphenazine & Amitriptyline Hcl 4, HL Moore Drug Exch	00839-6227-12
500's	$143.05	Perphenazine & Amitriptyline Hcl, Mylan	00378-0574-05

Tablet, Plain Coated - Oral - 50 mg/4 mg

60's	$10.75	Amitriptyline W/Perphenazine, H.C.F.A. F F P	99999-0215-09
60's	**$78.01**	**TRIAVIL 4-50, Merck**	**00006-0517-60**
100's	$13.80	Amitriptyline W/Perphenazine, US Trading	56126-0185-11
100's	$17.93	Amitriptyline W/Perphenazine, H.C.F.A. F F P	99999-0215-10
100's	$33.00	Perphenazine/Amitriptyline, Aligen Independ	00405-4791-01
100's	$37.78	Amitriptyline W/Perphenazine, Qualitest Pharms	00603-5119-21
100's	$43.27	Perphenazine & Amitriptyline Hcl, HL Moore Drug Exch	00839-7233-06
100's	$54.25	Perphenazine & Amitriptyline Hcl, Mylan	00378-0073-01
100's	$54.25	Perphenazine/Amitriptyline HcL, Geneva Pharms	00781-1268-01
100's	**$127.83**	**TRIAVIL 4-50, Merck**	**00006-0517-68**

HOW SUPPLIED - NOT RATED EQUIVALENT:

Tablet, Plain Coated - Oral - 10 mg/2 mg

100's	$15.63	Amitriptyline W/Perphenazine, Bristol Myers Squibb	00003-0193-50
100's	$16.25	Amitriptyline W/Perphenazine, Lederle Pharm	00005-3372-23
100's	$20.85	Perphenazine & Amitriptyline Hcl, Parmed Pharms	00349-8882-01
100's	$34.60	Amitriptyline W/Perphenzine, Amer Preferred	53445-0818-01
100's	$67.16	ETRAFON 2-10, Schering	00085-0287-04
100's	$70.82	ETRAFON 2-10, Schering	00085-0287-08
500's	$75.00	Amitriptyline W/Perphenazine, Bristol Myers Squibb	00003-0193-60
500's	$92.29	Perphenazine & Amitriptyline Hcl, Parmed Pharms	00349-8882-05

Tablet, Plain Coated - Oral - 10 mg/4 mg

100's	$6.23	Amitriptyline W/Perphenazine, United Res	00677-1122-01
100's	$10.20	Amitriptyline W/Perphenazine, US Trading	56126-0183-11
100's	$17.50	Amitriptyline W/Perphenazine, Bristol Myers Squibb	00003-0267-50
100's	$36.48	Amitriptyline W/Perphenzine, Amer Preferred	53445-0820-01
100's	$62.68	ETRAFON A, Schering	00085-0119-04
100's	$66.18	ETRAFON A, Schering	00085-0119-08
500's	$85.00	Amitriptyline W/Perphenazine, Bristol Myers Squibb	00003-0267-60

Tablet, Plain Coated - Oral - 25 mg/2 mg

100's	$13.28	Amitriptyline W/Perphenazine, IDE-Interstate	00814-5956-14
100's	$13.56	Amitriptyline W/Perphenazine, US Trading	56126-0182-11
100's	$20.00	Amitriptyline W/Perphenazine, Bristol Myers Squibb	00003-0259-50
100's	$24.08	Perphenazine & Amitriptyline Hcl, Parmed Pharms	00349-8883-01
100's	$39.63	Perphenazine & Amitriptyline Hcl, Amer Preferred	53445-0819-01
100's	$85.40	ETRAFON, Schering	00085-0598-04
100's	$89.00	ETRAFON, Schering	00085-0598-08

HOW SUPPLIED - NOT RATED EQUIVALENT: *(cont'd)*

500's	$96.88	Amitriptyline W/Perphenazine, Bristol Myers Squibb	00003-0259-60
500's	$113.37	Perphenazine & Amitriptyline Hcl, Parmed Pharms	00349-8883-05

Tablet, Plain Coated - Oral - 25 mg/4 mg

100's	$14.70	Amitriptyline W/Pherphenazine, US Trading	56126-0184-11
100's	$21.88	Amitriptyline W/Perphenazine, Bristol Myers Squibb	00003-0271-50
100's	$28.00	Perphenazine & Amitriptyline Hcl, Parmed Pharms	00349-8885-01
100's	$40.87	Amitriptyline W/Perphenzine, Amer Preferred	53445-0821-01
100's	$92.76	ETRAFON FORTE, Schering	00085-0720-04
100's	$96.41	ETRAFON FORTE, Schering	00085-0720-08
500's	$105.00	Amitriptyline W/Perphenazine, Bristol Myers Squibb	00003-0271-60
500's	$137.30	Perphenazine & Amitriptyline Hcl, Parmed Pharms	00349-8885-05

AMLEXANOX *(003316)*

CATEGORIES: Anti-Inflammatory Agents; Aphthous Ulcer; Antihistamines; Leukotriene Inhibitor; Mouth and Throat; Topical; FDA Approved 1996 Dec

BRAND NAMES: **Aphthasol**; *Elics* (Japan)
(International brand names outside U.S. in italics)

DESCRIPTION:

For Oral Cavity Use Only
Not for Ophthalmic Use

Aphthasol contains 5% amlexanox in an adhesive oral paste. Chemically, amlexanox is 2-amino-7- isopropyl-5-oxo-5H-[1]benzopyrano[2,3-b]pyridine-3-carboxylic acid. It has a molecular formula of $C_{16}H_{14}N_2O_4$ and has molecular weight of 298.30. Amlexanox is odorless, white to yellowish-white crystalline powder.

Each gram of Aphthasol beige colored oral paste contains 50 mg of amlexanox in an adhesive oral paste base consisting of benzyl alcohol, gelatin, glyceryl monostearate, mineral oil, pectin, petrolatum, and sodium carboxymethylcellulose.

CLINICAL PHARMACOLOGY:

MECHANISM OF ACTION

The mechanism of action by which amlexanox accelerates healing of aphthous ulcers is unknown. *In vitro* studies have demonstrated amlexanox to be a potent inhibitor of the formation and/or release of inflammatory mediators (histamine and leukotrienes) from mast cells, neutrophils and mononuclear cells. Given orally to animals, amlexanox has demonstrated anti-allergic and anti-inflammatory activities and has been shown to suppress both immediate and delayed type hypersensitivity reactions. The relevance of these activities of amlexanox to its effects on aphthous ulcers has not been established.

PHARMACOKINETICS AND METABOLISM

After a single oral application of 100 mg of paste (5 mg amlexanox), maximal serum levels of approximately 120 ng/ml are observed at 2.4 hours. Most of the systemic absorption of amlexanox is via the gastrointestinal tract, and the amount absorbed directly through the active ulcer is not a significant portion of the applied dose. The half-life for elimination was 3.5 ± 1.1 hours in healthy individuals. Approximately 17% of the dose is eliminated into the urine as unchanged amlexanox, a hydroxylated metabolite, and their conjugates. With multiple applications 4 times daily, steady state levels were reached within one week, and no accumulation was observed with up to four weeks of usage.

CLINICAL STUDIES:

The safety of amlexanox oral paste, 5%, was established in a study in which 100 patients with aphthous ulcers applied the medication 4 times daily for 28 days with no significant topical or systemic adverse effects.

The effectiveness was demonstrated in three controlled clinical studies of patients with mild to moderate aphthous ulcers which evaluated 464 patients receiving amlexanox oral paste, 5%, 465 patients receiving a placebo paste, and 195 patients receiving no treatment. Amlexanox oral paste, 5%, was shown to accelerate healing of aphthous ulcers in a statistically significant manner as compared to both vehicle and no treatment.

Amlexanox Oral Paste, 5%, Versus No Treatment: In the combined database of the two studies including a no treatment group, there was a significant difference in the rate of ulcer healing which translated to a reduction of 1.6 days in the median time to complete healing and reduction of 1.3 days in the median time to complete pain relief. After 3 days of treatment there was a significant difference in both percent of patients with complete healing of ulcers (21% vs. 8%) and percent of patients with complete resolution of pain (44% vs. 20%).

Amlexanox Oral Paste, 5%, Versus Vehicle: In the combined database of the three studies, there was a significant difference in the rate of ulcer healing which translated into a reduction of 0.7 days in the median time to complete healing, and a reduction of 0.7 days in the median time to complete pain relief. After 4 days of treatment there was a significant difference in both percent of patients with complete healing of ulcers (37% vs. 27%) and percent of patients with complete resolution of pain (60% vs. 49%).

Pain relief occurred in conjunction with healing of the ulcers, Amlexanox oral paste, 5%, by itself, was not shown to be an analgesic medication.

The safety and effectiveness of the product in immunocomprimised individuals has not been assessed.

INDICATIONS AND USAGE:

Amlexanox oral paste, 5%, is indicated for the treatment of aphthous ulcers in people with normal immune systems.

CONTRAINDICATIONS:

Amlexanox oral paste, 5%, is contraindicated in patients with known hypersensitivity to amlexanox or other ingredients in the formulation.

PRECAUTIONS:

GENERAL

Wash hands immediately after applying amlexanox oral paste, 5%, directly to ulcers with the finger tips. In the event that a rash or contact mucositis occurs, discontinue use.

Information for Patients

1. Apply the paste as soon as possible after noticing the symptoms of an aphthous ulcer. Continue to use the paste 4 times daily, preferably following oral hygiene after breakfast, lunch, dinner and at bedtime.

2. Squeeze a dab of paste approximately ¼ inch (0.5 cm) onto a finger tip. Dab the paste onto each ulcer in the mouth using gentle pressure.

3. Wash hands immediately after applying amlexanox oral paste, 5%.

4. Wash eyes promptly if they should come in contact with paste.

PRECAUTIONS: *(cont'd)*

5. Use the paste until the ulcer heals. If significant healing or pain reduction has not occurred in 10 days, consult your dentist or physician.

6. Keep out of the reach of children.

CARCINOGENESIS, MUTAGENESIS, AND IMPAIRMENT OF FERTILITY

Amlexanox was not carcinogenic when administered orally to rats for two years and to mice for 18 months. *In vitro* (Ames) and *in vivo* (mouse micronucleus) mutagenicity tests amlexanox were negative. Amlexanox at doses up to two hundred times the projected human daily dose, on a mg/m^2 basis, did not significantly affect fertility or general reproductive performance in rats.

Pregnancy Category B: Teratology studies were performed with rats and rabbits at doses up to two hundred and six hundred times, respectively, the projected human daily dose, on a mg/m^2 basis. No adverse fetal effects were observed. At doses up to two hundred times the projected human daily dose, on a mg/m^2 basis, amlenanox did not have significant effect on peri- and postnatal development of rat fetuses. There are no adequate and well-controlled studies in pregnant women. Because animal reproduction studies are not always predictive of human response, this drug should be used during pregnancy only if clearly needed.

NURSING MOTHERS

Amlexanox was found in the milk of lactating rats; therefore, caution should be exercised when administering amlexanox oral paste, 5%, to a nursing woman.

PEDIATRIC USE

Safety and effectiveness of amlexanox oral paste, 5%, in pediatric patients have not been established.

ADVERSE REACTIONS:

Adverse reactions considered related or possibly related to amlexanox oral paste, 5%, were not reported by more than 5% of patients. Adverse reactions reported by 1-2% of patients were transient pain, stinging and/or burning at the site of application. Infrequent (<1%) adverse reactions in the clinical studies were contact mucositis, nausea, and diarrhea.

OVERDOSAGE:

There are no reports of human ingestion overdosage. Ingestion of a full tube of 5 grams of paste would result in systemic exposure well below the maximum nontoxic dose of amlexanox in animals. Gastrointestinal upset such as diarrhea and vomiting could result from an overdose.

DOSAGE AND ADMINISTRATION:

The paste should be applied as soon as possible after noticing the symptoms of an aphthous ulcer and should be used 4 times daily, preferably following oral hygiene after breakfast, lunch, dinner, and at bedtime. Squeeze a dab of paste approximately ¼ inch (0.5 cm) onto a finger tip. With gentle pressure, dab the paste onto each ulcer in the mouth. Use of the medication should be continued until the ulcer heals. If significant healing or pain reduction has not occurred in 10 days, consult your dentist or physician.

PATIENT INFORMATION:

Amelexanox is an oral paste used for the treatment of aphthous ulcers. Inform your physician if you are pregnant or nursing. May cause pain, stinging or burning of the mouth. If rash or contact mucositis occurs, discontinue use. Apply paste as soon as ulcer symptoms are noticed. Use 4 times daily after meals and at bedtime. Wash hands after use. Keep out of eyes. If healing or pain reduction has not occurred in 10 days, consult your physician or dentist.

HOW SUPPLIED:

Amlexanox oral paste, 5%, is supplied in 5 gm tubes. Amlexanox oral paste, 5%, should be stored at controlled room temperature, 15°-30°C (59°-86°F).

AMLODIPINE BESYLATE *(003072)*

CATEGORIES: Angina; Antihypertensives; Calcium Channel Blockers; Cardiovascular Drugs; Hypertension; Renal Drugs; Vasospastic Angina; Heart Failure*; Pregnancy Category C; FDA Class 1S ("Standard Review"); Sales > $1 Billion; FDA Approved 1992 Jul; Top 200 Drugs
* Indication not approved by the FDA

BRAND NAMES: *Amcard*; *Amdepin*; *Amdipin*; *Amlodin* (Japan); *Amlogard*; *Amlopin*; *Amlor* (France); *Amlosyn*; *Istin* (England); *Norvas* (Mexico); **Norvasc**; *Norvask*; *Tensivask*
(International brand names outside U.S. in italics)

FORMULARIES: Aetna; BC-BS; CIGNA; FHP; Humana; Kaiser; Medco; WellPoint; PCS

COST OF THERAPY: $375.00 (Hypertension; Tablet; 5 mg; 1/day; 365 days)

PRIMARY ICD9: 401.1 (Essential Hypertension, Benign)

DESCRIPTION:

Amlodipine besylate is a long-acting calcium channel blocker.

Amlodipine besylate is chemically described as (R.S.) 3-ethyl-5-methyl-2-(2-aminoethoxymethyl)-4-(2-chlorophenyl)-1,4-dihydro-6-methyl-3,5-pyridinedicarboxylate benzenesulphonate. Its empirical formula is: $C_{20}H_{25}ClN_2O_5 \cdot C_6H_6O_3S$.

Amlodipine besylate is a white crystalline powder with a molecular weight of 567.1. It is slightly soluble in water and sparingly soluble in ethanol. Amlodipine besylate tablets are formulated as white tablets equivalent to 2.5, 5 and 10 mg of amlodipine for oral administration. In addition to the active ingredient, amlodipine besylate, each tablet contains the following inactive ingredients: microcrystalline cellulose, dibasic calcium phosphate anhydrous, sodium starch glycolate, and magnesium stearate.

CLINICAL PHARMACOLOGY:

MECHANISM OF ACTION

Amlodipine besylate is a dihydropyridine calcium antagonist (calcium ion antagonist or slow channel blocker) that inhibits the transmembrane influx of calcium ions into vascular smooth muscle and cardiac muscle. Experimental data suggest that amlodipine besylate binds to both dihydropyridine and nondihydropyridine binding sites. The contractile processes of cardiac muscle and vascular smooth muscle are dependent upon the movement of extracellular calcium ions into these cells through specific ion channels. Amlodipine besylate inhibits calcium ion influx across cell membranes selectively, with a greater effect on vascular smooth muscle cells than on cardiac muscle cells. Negative inotropic effects can be detected *in vitro* but such effects have not been seen in intact animals at therapeutic doses. Serum calcium concentration is not affected by amlodipine besylate. Within the physiologic pH range,

CLINICAL PHARMACOLOGY: *(cont'd)*

amlodipine besylate is an ionized compound (pKa=8.6), and its kinetic interaction with the calcium channel receptor is characterized by a gradual rate of association and dissociation with the receptor binding site, resulting in a gradual onset of effect.

Amlodipine besylate is a peripheral arterial vasodilator that acts directly on vascular smooth muscle to cause a reduction in peripheral vascular resistance and reduction in blood pressure.

The precise mechanisms by which amlodipine besylate relieves angina have not been fully delineated, but are thought to include the following:

Exertional Angina: In patients with exertional angina, amlodipine besylate reduces the total peripheral resistance (after-load) against which the heart works and reduces the rate pressure product, and thus myocardial oxygen demand, at any given level of exercise.

Vasospastic Angina: Amlodipine besylate has been demonstrated to block constriction and restore blood flow in coronary arteries and arterioles in response to calcium, potassium epinephrine, serotonin, and thromboxane A_2 analog in experimental animal models and in human coronary vessels *in vitro*. This inhibition of coronary spasm is responsible for the effectiveness of amlodipine besylate in vasospastic (Prinzmetal's or variant) angina.

PHARMACOKINETICS AND METABOLISM

After oral administration of therapeutic doses of amlodipine besylate, absorption produces peak plasma concentrations between 6 and 12 hours. Absolute bioavailability has been estimated to be between 64 and 90%. The bioavailability of amlodipine besylate is not altered by the presence of food.

Amlodipine besylate is extensively (about 90%) converted to inactive metabolites via hepatic metabolism with 10% of the parent compound and 60% of the metabolites excreted in the urine. *Ex vivo* studies have shown that approximately 93% of the circulating drug is bound to plasma proteins in hypertensive patients. Elimination from the plasma is biphasic with a terminal elimination half-life of about 30-50 hours. Steady state plasma levels of amlodipine besylate are reached after 7 to 8 days of consecutive daily dosing.

The pharmacokinetics of amlodipine besylate are not significantly influenced by renal impairment. Patients with renal failure may therefore receive the usual initial dose.

Elderly patients and patients with hepatic insufficiency have decreased clearance of amlodipine with a resulting increase in AUC of approximately 40-60%, and a lower initial dose may be required.

PHARMACODYNAMICS

Hemodynamics: Following administration of therapeutic doses to patients with hypertension, amlodipine besylate produces vasodilation resulting in a reduction of supine and standing blood pressures. These decreases in blood pressure are not accompanied by a significant change in heart rate or plasma catecholamine levels with chronic dosing. Although the acute intravenous administration of amlodipine decreases arterial blood pressure and increases heart rate in hemodynamic studies of patients with chronic stable angina, chronic administration of oral amlodipine in clinical trials did not lead to clinically significant changes in heart rate or blood pressures in normotensive patients with angina.

With chronic once daily oral administration, antihypertensive effectiveness is maintained for at least 24 hours. Plasma concentrations correlate with effect in both young and elderly patients. The magnitude of reduction in blood pressure with amlodipine besylate is also correlated with the height of pretreatment elevation; thus, individuals with moderate hypertension (diastolic pressure 105-114 mmHg) had about a 50% greater response than patients with mild hypertension (diastolic pressure 90-104 mmHg). Normotensive subjects experienced no clinically significant change in blood pressures (+1/-2 mmHg).

As with other calcium channel blockers, hemodynamic measurements of cardiac function at rest and during exercise (or pacing) in patients with normal ventricular function treated with amlodipine besylate have generally demonstrated a small increase in cardiac index without significant influence on dP/dt or on left ventricular end diastolic pressure or volume. In hemodynamic studies, amlodipine besylate has not been associated with a negative inotropic effect when administered in the therapeutic dose range to intact animals and man, even when co-administered with beta-blockers to man. Similar findings, however, have been observed in normals or well-compensated patients with heart failure with agents possessing significant negative inotropic effects.

In a double-blind, placebo-controlled clinical trial involving 118 patients with well compensated heart failure (NYHA Class II and Class III), treatment with amlodipine besylate did not lead to worsened heart failure, based on measures of exercise tolerance, left ventricular ejection fraction and clinical symptomatology. Studies in patients with NYHA Class IV heart failure have not been performed and, in general, all calcium channel blockers should be used with caution in any patient with heart failure.

In hypertensive patients with normal renal function, therapeutic doses of amlodipine besylate resulted in a decrease in renal vascular resistance and an increase in glomerular filtration rate and effective renal plasma flow without change in filtration fraction or proteinuria.

ELECTROPHYSIOLOGIC EFFECTS

Amlodipine besylate does not change sinoatrial nodal function or atrioventricular conduction in intact animals or man. In patients with chronic stable angina, intravenous administration of 10 mg did not significantly alter A-H and H-V conduction and sinus node recovery time after pacing. Similar results were obtained in patients receiving amlodipine besylate and concomitant beta blockers. In clinical studies in which amlodipine besylate was administered in combination with beta-blockers to patients with either hypertension or angina, no adverse effects on electrocardiographic parameters were observed. In clinical trials with angina patients alone, amlodipine besylate therapy did not alter electrocardiographic intervals or produce higher degrees of AV blocks.

EFFECTS IN HYPERTENSION

The antihypertensive efficacy of amlodipine besylate has been demonstrated in a total of 15 double-blind, placebo-controlled, randomized studies involving 800 patients on amlodipine besylate and 538 on placebo. Once daily administration produced statistically significant placebo-corrected reductions in supine and standing blood pressures at 24 hours postdose, averaging about 12/6 mmHg in the standing position and 13/7 mmHg in the supine position in patients with mild to moderate hypertension. Maintenance of the blood pressure effect over the 24 hour dosing interval was observed, with little difference in peak and trough effect. Tolerance was not demonstrated in patients studied for up to 1 year. The 3 parallel, fixed dose, dose response studies showed that the reduction in supine and standing blood pressures was dose-related within the recommended dosing range. Effects on diastolic pressure were similar in young and older patients. The effect on systolic pressure was greater in older patients, perhaps because of greater baseline systolic pressure. Effects were similar in black and white patients.

EFFECTS IN CHRONIC STABLE ANGINA

The effectiveness of 5-10 mg/day of amlodipine besylate in exercise-induced angina has been evaluated in 8 placebo-controlled, double-blind clinical trials of up to 6 weeks duration involving 1038 patients (648 amlodipine besylate, 354 placebo) with chronic stable angina. In 5 of the 8 studies significant increases in exercise time (bicycle or treadmill) were seen with the 10 mg dose. Increases in symptom-limited exercise time averaged 12.8% (63 sec) for amlodipine besylate 10 mg, and averaged 7.9% (38 sec) for amlodipine besylate 5 mg. Amlodipine besylate 10 mg also increased time to 1 mm ST segment deviation in several studies and decreased angina attack rate. The sustained efficacy of amlodipine besylate in

CLINICAL PHARMACOLOGY: *(cont'd)*

angina patients has been demonstrated over long-term dosing. In patients with angina there were no clinically significant reductions in blood pressures (4/1 mmHg) or changes in heart rate (+0.3 bpm).

EFFECTS IN VASOSPASTIC ANGINA

In a double-blind, placebo-controlled clinical trial of 4 weeks duration in 50 patients, amlodipine besylate therapy decreased attacks by approximately 4/week compared with a placebo decrease of approximately 1/week (p<0.01). Two of 23 amlodipine besylate and 7 of 27 placebo patients discontinued from the study due to lack of clinical improvement.

INDICATIONS AND USAGE:

1. Hypertension: Amlodipine besylate is indicated for the treatment of hypertension. It may be used alone or in combination with other antihypertensive agents.

2. Chronic Stable Angina: Amlodipine besylate is indicated for the treatment of chronic stable angina. amlodipine besylate may be used alone or in combination with other antianginal agents.

3. Vasospastic Angina (Prinzmetal's or Variant Angina): Amlodipine besylate is indicated for the treatment of confirmed or suspected vasospastic angina. Amlodipine besylate may be used as monotherapy or in combination with other antianginal drugs.

CONTRAINDICATIONS:

Amlodipine besylate is contraindicated in patients with known sensitivity to amlodipine.

WARNINGS:

Increased Angina and/or Myocardial Infarction: Rarely, patients, particularly those with severe obstructive coronary artery disease, have developed documented increased frequency, duration and/or severity of angina or acute myocardial infarction on starting calcium channel blocker therapy or at the time of dosage increase. The mechanism of this effect has not been elucidated.

PRECAUTIONS:

General: Since the vasodilation induced by amlodipine besylate is gradual in onset, acute hypotension has rarely been reported after oral administration of amlodipine besylate. Nonetheless, caution should be exercised when administering amlodipine besylate as with any other peripheral vasodilator particularly in patients with severe aortic stenosis.

Use in Patients with Congestive Heart Failure: Although hemodynamic studies and a controlled trial in NYHA Class II-III heart failure patients have shown that amlodipine besylate did not lead to clinical deterioration as measured by exercise tolerance, left ventricular ejection fraction, and clinical symptomatology, studies have not been performed in patients with NYHA Class IV heart failure. In general, all calcium channel blockers should be used with caution in patients with heart failure.

Beta-Blocker Withdrawal: Amlodipine besylate is not a beta-blocker and therefore gives no protection against the dangers of abrupt beta-blocker withdrawal; any such withdrawal should be by gradual reduction of the dose of beta-blocker.

Patients with Hepatic Failure: Since amlodipine besylate is extensively metabolized by the liver and the plasma elimination half-life (t 1/2) is 56 hours in patients with impaired hepatic function, caution should be exercised when administering amlodipine besylate to patients with severe hepatic impairment.

Drug/Laboratory Test Interactions: None known.

Carcinogenesis, Mutagenesis, and Impairment of Fertility: Rats and mice treated with amlodipine in the diet for two years, at concentrations calculated to provide daily dosage levels of 0.5, 1.25, and 2.5 mg/kg/day showed no evidence carcinogenicity. The highest dose (for mice, similar to, and for rats twice* the maximum recommended clinical dose of 10 mg on a mg/m^2 basis), was close to the maximum tolerated dose for mice but not for rats.

Mutagenicity studies revealed no drug related effects at either the gene or chromosome levels.

There was no effect on the fertility of rats treated with amlodipine (males for 64 days and females 14 days prior to mating) at doses up to 10 mg/kg/day (8 times* the maximum recommended human dose of 10 mg on a mg/m^2 basis).

Pregnancy Category C: No evidence of teratogenicity or other embryo/fetal toxicity was found when pregnant rats or rabbits were treated orally with up to 10 mg/kg amlodipine (respectively 8 times* and 23 times* the maximum recommended human dose of 10 mg on a mg/m^2 basis) during their respective periods of major organogenesis. However, litter size was significantly decreased (by about 50%) and the number of intrauterine deaths was significantly increased (about 5-fold) in rats administered 10 mg/kg amlodipine for 14 days before mating and throughout mating and gestation. Amlodipine has been shown to prolong both the gestation period and the duration of labor in rats at this dose. There are no adequate and well-controlled studies in pregnant women. Amlodipine should be used during pregnancy only if the potential benefit justifies the potential risk to the fetus.

Nursing Mothers: It is not known whether amlodipine is excreted in human milk. In the absence of this information, it is recommended that nursing be discontinued while amlodipine besylate is administered.

Pediatric Use: Safety and effectiveness of amlodipine besylate in children have not been established.

DRUG INTERACTIONS:

In vitro data in human plasma indicate that amlodipine besylate has no effect on the protein binding of drugs tested (digoxin, phenytoin, warfarin, and indomethacin). Special studies have indicated that the co-administration of amlodipine besylate with digoxin did not change serum digoxin levels or digoxin renal clearance in normal volunteers; that co-administration with cimetidine did not alter the pharmacokinetics of amlodipine; and that co-administration with warfarin did not change the warfarin prothrombin response time.

In clinical trials, amlodipine besylate has been safely administered with thiazide diuretics, beta-blockers, angiotensin converting enzyme inhibitors, long-acting nitrates, sublingual nitroglycerin, digoxin, warfarin, non-steroidal anti-inflammatory drugs, antibiotics, and oral hypoglycemic drugs.

ADVERSE REACTIONS:

Amlodipine besylate has been evaluated for safety in more than 11,000 patients in U.S. and foreign clinical trials. In general, treatment with amlodipine besylate was well-tolerated at doses up to 10 mg daily. Most adverse reactions reported during therapy with amlodipine besylate were of mild or moderate severity. In controlled clinical trials directly comparing amlodipine besylate (N=1730) in doses up to 10 mg to placebo (N=1250), discontinuation of amlodipine besylate due to adverse reactions was required in only about 1.5% of patients and was not significantly different from placebo (about 1%). The most common side effects are headache and edema. The incidence (%) of side effects which occurred in a dose related manner are as follows (TABLE 1):

Other adverse experiences which were not clearly dose related but which were reported with an incidence greater than 1.0% in placebo-controlled clinical trials include TABLE 2:

ADVERSE REACTIONS: *(cont'd)*

TABLE 1

Adverse Event	2.5 mg N=275	5.0 mg N=296	10.0 mg N=268	Placebo N=520
Edema	1.8	3.0	10.8	0.6
Dizziness	1.1	3.4	3.4	1.5
Flushing	0.7	1.4	2.6	0.0
Palpitation	0.7	1.4	4.5	0.6

TABLE 2 Placebo Controlled Studies

Adverse Event	Norvasc (%) (N=1730)	Placebo (%) (N=1250)
Headache	7.3	7.8
Fatigue	4.5	2.8
Nausea	2.9	1.9
Abdominal Pain	1.6	0.3
Somnolence	1.4	0.6

For several adverse experiences that appear to be drug and dose related, there was a greater incidence in women than men associated with amlodipine treatment as shown in the TABLE 3:

TABLE 3

ADR	Amlodipine Besylate M=% (N=1218)	Amlodipine Besylate F=% (N=512)	Placebo M=% (N=914)	Placebo F=% (N=336)
Edema	5.6	14.6	1.4	5.1
Flushing	1.5	4.5	0.3	0.9
Palpitations	1.4	3.3	0.9	0.9
Somnolence	1.3	1.6	0.8	0.3

The following events occurred in ≤1% but >0.1% of patients in controlled clinical trials or under conditions of open trials or marketing experience where a casual relationship is uncertain; they are listed to alert the physician to a possible relationship:

Cardiovascular: arrhythmia (including ventricular tachycardia and atrial fibrillation), bradycardia, chest pain, hypotension, peripheral ischemia, syncope, tachycardia, postural dizziness, postural hypotension.

Central and Peripheral Nervous System: hypoesthesia, paresthesia, tremor, vertigo.

Gastrointestinal: anorexia, constipation, dyspepsia,** dysphagia, diarrhea, flatulence, vomiting, gingival hyperplasia.

General: asthenia,** back pain, hot flushes, malaise, pain, rigors, weight gain.

Musculo-skeletal System: arthralgia, arthrosis, muscle cramps,** myalgia.

Psychiatric: sexual dysfunction (male** and female), insomnia, nervousness, depression, abnormal dreams, anxiety, depersonalization.

Respiratory System: dyspnea,** epistaxis.

Skin and Appendages: pruritus,** rash,** rash erythematous, rash maculopapular.

*Based on patient weight of 50 kg.

**These events occurred in less than 1% in placebo controlled trials, but the incidence of these side effects was between 1% and 2% in all multiple dose studies.

Special Senses: abnormal vision, conjunctivitis, diplopia, eye pain, tinnitus.

Urinary System: micturition frequency, micturition disorder, nocturia.

Autonomic Nervous System: dry mouth, increased sweating.

Metabolic and Nutritional: thirst.

Hemopoietic: purpura.

The Following Events Occurred In ≤0.1% Of Patients: Cardiac failure, pulse irregularity, extrasystoles, skin discoloration, urticaria, skin dryness, alopecia, dermatitis, muscle weakness, twitching, ataxia, hypertonia, migraine, cold and clammy skin, apathy, agitation, amnesia, gastritis, increased appetite, loose stools, coughing, rhinitis, dysuria, polyuria, parosmia, taste perversion, abnormal visual accommodation, and xerophthalmia.

Other reactions occurred sporadically and cannot be distinguished from medications or concurrent disease states such as myocardial infarction and angina.

Amlodipine besylate therapy has not been associated with clinically significant changes in routine laboratory tests. No clinically relevant changes were noted in serum potassium, serum glucose, total triglycerides, total cholesterol, HDL cholesterol, uric acid, blood urea nitrogen, creatinine or liver function tests.

Amlodipine besylate has been used safely in patients with chronic obstructive pulmonary disease, well compensated congestive heart failure, peripheral vascular disease, diabetes mellitus, and abnormal lipid profiles.

OVERDOSAGE:

Single oral doses of 40 mg/kg and 100 mg/kg in mice and rats, respectively, caused deaths. A single oral dose of 4 mg/kg or higher in dogs caused a marked peripheral vasodilation and hypotension.

Overdosage might be expected to cause excessive peripheral vasodilation with marked hypotension and possibly a reflex tachycardia. In humans, experience with intentional overdosage of amlodipine besylate is limited. Reports of intentional overdosage include a patient who ingested 250 mg and was asymptomatic and was not hospitalized; another (120 mg) was hospitalized, underwent gastric lavage and remained normotensive; the third (105 mg) was hospitalized and had hypotension (90/50 mmHg) which normalized following plasma expansion. A patient who took 70 mg amlodipine and an unknown quantity of benzodiazepine in a suicide attempt, developed shock which was refractory to treatment and died the following day with abnormally high benzodiazepine plasma concentration. A case of accidental drug overdose has been documented in a 19 month old male who ingested 30 mg amlodipine (about 2 mg/kg). During the emergency room presentation, vital signs were stable with no evidence of hypotension, but as heart rate of 180 bpm. Ipecac was administered 3.5 hours after ingestion and on subsequent observation (overnight) no sequelae were noted.

If massive overdose should occur, active cardiac and respiratory monitoring should be instituted. Frequent blood pressure measurements are essential. Should hypotension occur, cardiovascular support including elevation of the extremities and the judicious administration of fluids should be initiated. If hypotension remains unresponsive to these conservative measures, administration of vasopressors (such as phenylephrine), should be considered with attention to circulating volume and urine output. Intravenous calcium gluconate may help to reverse the effects of calcium entry blockade. As amlodipine besylate is highly protein bound, hemodialysis is not likely to be of benefit.

DOSAGE AND ADMINISTRATION:

The usual initial antihypertensive oral dose of amlodipine besylate is 5 mg once daily with a maximum dose of 10 mg once daily. Small, fragile, or elderly individuals, or patients with hepatic insufficiency may be started on 2.5 mg once daily and this dose may be used when adding amlodipine besylate to other antihypertensive therapy.

Dosage should be adjusted according to each patient's need. In general, titration should proceed over 7 to 14 days so that the physician can fully assess the patient's response to each dose level. Titration may proceed more rapidly, however, if clinically warranted, provided the patient is assessed frequently.

The recommended dose for chronic stable or vasospastic angina is 5-10 mg, with the lower dose suggested in the elderly and in patients with hepatic insufficiency. Most patients will require 10 mg for adequate effect. See ADVERSE REACTIONS for information related to dosage and side effects.

Co-administration with Other Antihypertensive and/or Antianginal Drugs: amlodipine besylate has been safely administered with thiazides, ACE inhibitors, beta-blockers, long-acting nitrates, and/or sublingual nitroglycerin.

PATIENT INFORMATION:

Amlodipine besylate is ued to treat high blood pressure and a heart condition called angina. It is referred to as a calcium-channel blocker. The most common side effects include headache and swelling (edema). If you experience difficulty breathing, contact your doctor immediately. Rarely, in patients with severe disease, more frequent and more sever chest pain has been reported. If this occurs, contact your doctor immediately. There have been no significant drug interactions reported to date. Dizziness and lightheadedness can result when the mediation is first started. If this persists longer than one week, contact your physician. Your blood pressure should be checked regularly to assure adequate control.

HOW SUPPLIED:

Norvasc 2.5 mg tablets (amlodipine besylate equivalent to 2.5 mg of amlodipine per tablet) are supplied as white, diamond, flat-faced, beveled edged engraved with "NORVASC" on one side and "2.5" on the other side.

Norvasc 5 mg tablets (amlodipine besylate equivalent to 5 mg of amlodipine per tablet) are white, elongated octagon, flat-faced, beveled edged engraved with both "NORVASC" and "5" on one side and plain on the other side.

Norvasc 10 mg tablets (amlodipine besylate equivalent to 10 mg of amlodipine per tablet) are white, round, flat-faced, beveled edged engraved with both "NORVASC" and "10" on one side and plain on the other side.

Store bottles at controlled room temperature, 59° to 86°F (15° to 30°C) and dispense in tight, light-resistant containers (USP).

HOW SUPPLIED - EQUIVALENTS NOT AVAILABLE:

Tablet, Uncoated - Oral - 2.5 mg

100's $102.74 NORVASC, Pfizer Labs 00069-1520-66

Tablet, Uncoated - Oral - 5 mg

100's $102.74 NORVASC, Pfizer Labs 00069-1530-41
100's $102.74 NORVASC, Pfizer Labs 00069-1530-66
300's $302.06 NORVASC, Pfizer Labs 00069-1530-72

Tablet, Uncoated - Oral - 10 mg

100's $177.78 NORVASC, Pfizer Labs 00069-1540-41
100's $177.78 NORVASC, Pfizer Labs 00069-1540-66

AMLODIPINE BESYLATE; BENAZEPRIL HYDROCHLORIDE *(003212)*

CATEGORIES: ACE Inhibitors; Angina; Angiotensin Converting Enzyme Inhibitors; Antihypertensives; Calcium Channel Blockers; Cardiovascular Drugs; Hypertension; FDA Class 4S ("Standard Review"); FDA Approved 1995 Mar

BRAND NAMES: **Lotrel**

DESCRIPTION:

Lotrel is a combination of amlodipine besylate and benazepril hydrochloride. The capsules are formulated for oral administration with a combination of amlodipine besylate equivalent to 2.5 mg or 5 mg of amlodipine and 10 mg or 20 mg of benazepril hydrochloride. The inactive ingredients of the capsules are calcium phosphate, cellulose compounds, colloidal silicon dioxide, crospovidone, gelatin, hydrogenated castor oil, iron oxides, lactose, magnesium stearate, polysorbate 80, silicon dioxide, sodium lauryl sulfate, sodium starch glycolate, starch, talc, and titanium dioxide.

FOR COMPLETE PRESCRIBING INFORMATION REFER TO THE INDIVIDUAL DRUG MONOGRAPHS (AMLODIPINE BESYLATE; BENAZEPRIL HYDROCHLORIDE).

INDICATIONS AND USAGE:

Amlodipine besylate; benazepril HCl in indicated for the treatment of hypertension.

This fixed combination drug is not indicated for the initial therapy of hypertension. (See DOSAGE AND ADMINISTRATION.)

In using amlodipine besylate; benazepril HCl, consideration should be given to the fact that an ACE inhibitor, captopril, has caused agranulocytosis, particularly in patients with renal impairment or collagen-vascular disease. Available data are insufficient to show that benazepril does not have a similar risk.

DOSAGE AND ADMINISTRATION:

Amlodipine is an effective treatment of hypertension in once-daily doses of 2.5-10 mg while benazepril is effective in doses of 10-80 mg. In clinical trials of amlodipine/benazepril combination therapy using amlodipine doses of 2.5-5 mg and benazepril doses of 10-20 mg, the antihypertensive effects increased with increasing dose of amlodipine in all patient groups, and the effects increased with increasing dose of benazepril in nonblack groups. All patient groups benefited from the reduction in amlodipine-induced edema.

The hazards of benazepril are generally independent of dose; those of amlodipine are a mixture of dose-dependent phenomena (primarily peripheral edema) and dose-independent phenomena, the former much more common than the latter. When benazepril is added to a regimen of amlodipine, the incidence of edema is substantially reduced. Therapy with any combination of amlodipine and benazepril will thus be associated with both sets of dose-independent hazards, but the incidence of edema will generally be less than that seen with similar (or higher) doses of amlodipine monotherapy.

DOSAGE AND ADMINISTRATION: *(cont'd)*

Rarely, the dose-independent hazards of benazepril are serious. To minimize dose-independent hazards, it is usually appropriate to begin therapy with amlodipine besylate; benazepril HCl only after a patient has either (a) failed to achieve the desired antihypertensive effect with one or the other monotherapy, or (b) demonstrated inability to achieve adequate antihypertensives effect with amlodipine therapy without developing edema.

Dose Titration Guided by Clinical Effect: A patient whose blood pressure is not adequately controlled with amlodipine (or another dihydropyridine) alone or with benazepril (or another ACE inhibitor) alone may be switched to combination therapy with amlodipine besylate;benazepril HCl. The addition of benazepril to a regimen of amlodipine should not be expected to provide additional antihypertensive effect in African-Americans. However, all patient groups benefit from the reduction in amlodipine-induced edema. Dosage must be guided by clinical response; steady-state levels of benazepril and amlodipine will be reached after approximately 2 and 7 days of dosing, respectively.

In patients whose blood pressures are adequately controlled with amlodipine but who experience unacceptable edema, combination therapy may achieve similar (or better) blood-pressure control without edema. Especially in nonblacks, it may be prudent to minimize the risk of excessive response by reducing the dose of amlodipine as benazepril is added to the regimen.

Replacement Therapy: For convenience, patients receiving amlodipine and benazepril from separate tablets may instead wish to receive capsules of amlodipine besylate; benazepril HCl containing the same component doses.

Use in Patients With Metabolic Impairments: Regimens of therapy with Lotrel need not take account of renal function as long as the patient's creatinine clearance is >30 ml/min/1.73m^2 (serum creatinine roughly ≤3 mg/dl or 265 μmol/l). In patients with more severe renal impairment, the recommended initial dose of benazepril is 5 mg. Amlodipine besylate; benazepril HCl is not recommended in these patients.

In small, elderly, frail, or hepatically impaired patients, the recommended initial dose of amlodipine, as monotherapy or as a component of combination therapy, is 2.5 mg.

HOW SUPPLIED:

Lotrel is available as capsules containing amlodipine/benazepril HCl 2.5/10 mg, 5/10 mg, and 5/20 mg.

Capsules are imprinted with "Lotrel" and a portion of the NDC code. Samples, when available, are identified by the word *SAMPLE* appearing on each capsule.

Storage: Do not store above 86°F (30°C). Protect from moisture and light.

Dispense in tight, light-resistant container (USP).

HOW SUPPLIED - EQUIVALENTS NOT AVAILABLE:

Capsule, Gelatin - Oral - 10 mg/2.5 mg

100's	$129.67	LOTREL, Novartis	00083-2255-30

Capsule, Gelatin - Oral - 10 mg/5 mg

100's	$129.67	LOTREL, Novartis	00083-2260-30

Capsule, Gelatin - Oral - 20 mg/5 mg

100's	$136.15	LOTREL, Novartis	00083-2265-30

AMMONIUM CHLORIDE *(000219)*

CATEGORIES: Acidifying Agents; Alkalosis; Antagonists and Antidotes; Antidotes; Electrolyte, Caloric-Water Balance; Hyperchloremia; Urinary Acidifiers; Pregnancy Category C; FDA Approval Pre 1982

DESCRIPTION:

Ammonium chloride injection, USP, 100 mEq, is a sterile, nonpyrogenic solution of ammonium chloride (NH_4Cl) in water for injection administered (after dilution) by the intravenous route. Each mL contains 267.5 mg of ammonium chloride (5 mEq of ammonium and 5 mEq of chloride) and 2.0 mg of edetate disodium (anhydrous) added as a stabilizer. Approximate ph 5.0, adjusted with hydrochloric acid. 10 mOsm/mL (calc). It is intended to be used only after dilution in a larger volume of isotonic (0.9%) sodium chloride injection.

The solution contains no bacteriostat, antimicrobial agent or added buffer (except for ph adjustment) and is intended only for dilution as a single-dose additive. When smaller doses are required the unused portion should be discarded with the entire additive unit.

Ammonium chloride injection, USP is an electrolyte replenisher and systemic acidifier.

Ammonium chloride, USP is chemically designated NH_4Cl, colorless crystals or white granular powder freely soluble in water.

CLINICAL PHARMACOLOGY:

The ammonium ion (NH_4+) in the body plays an important role in the maintenance of acid-base balance. The kidney uses ammonium (NH_4+) in place of sodium (Na+) to combine with fixed anions in maintaining acid-base balance, especially as a homeostatic compensatory mechanism in metabolic acidosis.

When a loss of hydrogen ions (H+) occurs and serum chloride (Cl-) decreases, sodium is made available for combination with bicarbonate ($HC0_3$-). This creates an excess of sodium bicarbonate ($NaHC0_3$) which leads to a rise in blood ph and a state of metabolic alkalosis.

The therapeutic effects of ammonium chloride depend upon the ability of the kidney to utilize ammonia in the excretion of an excess of fixed anions and the conversion of ammonia to urea by the liver, thereby liberating hydrogen (H+) and chloride (Cl-) ions into the extracellular fluid.

INDICATIONS AND USAGE:

Ammonium chloride injection, USP, after dilution in isotonic sodium chloride injection, may be indicated in the treatment of patients with (1) hypochloremic states and (2) metabolic alkalosis.

CONTRAINDICATIONS:

Ammonium chloride is contraindicated in patients with severe impairment of renal or hepatic function.

Ammonium chloride should not be administered when metabolic alkalosis due to vomiting of hydrochloric acid is accompanied by loss of sodium (excretion of sodium bicarbonate in the urine).

PRECAUTIONS:

Do not administer unless the solution is clear and seal is intact. Discard unused portion.

Patients receiving ammonium chloride should be constantly observed for symptoms of ammonia toxicity (pallor, sweating, retching, irregular breathing, bradycardia, cardiac arrhythmias, local and general twitching, tonic convulsions and coma).

PRECAUTIONS: *(cont'd)*

It should be used with caution in patients with high total CO_2 and buffer base secondary to primary respiratory acidosis.

Intravenous administration should be slow to avoid local irritation and toxic effects.

When exposed to low temperatures, concentrated solutions of ammonium chloride may crystallize. If crystals are observed, the vial should be warmed to room temperature in a water bath prior to use.

Pregancy Category C: Animal reproduction studies have not been conducted with ammonium chloride. It is also not known whether ammonium chloride can cause fetal harm when administered to a pregnant woman or can affect reproduction capacity. Ammonium chloride should be given to a pregnant woman only if clearly needed.

ADVERSE REACTIONS:

Rapid intravenous administration of ammonium chloride may be accompanied by pain or irritation at the site of injection or along the venous route.

Reactions which may occur because of the solution or the technique of administration include febrile response, infection at the site of injection, venous thrombosis or phlebitis extending from the site of injection, extravasation and hypervolemia (from large volume diluent).

If an adverse reaction does occur, discontinue the infusion, evaluate the patient, institute appropriate therapeutic countermeasures and save the remainder of the fluid for examination if deemed necessary.

OVERDOSAGE:

Overdosage of ammonium chloride has resulted in a serious degree of metabolic acidosis, disorientation, confusion and coma. Should metabolic acidosis occur following overdosage, the administration of an alkalinizing solution such as sodium bicarbonate or sodium lactate will serve to correct the acidosis.

DOSAGE AND ADMINISTRATION:

Ammonium chloride injection, USP, is administered intravenously and must be diluted before use. Solutions for intravenous infusion should not exceed a concentration of 1% to 2% of ammonium chloride.

Dosage is dependent upon the condition and tolerance of the patient. It is recommended that the contents of one to two vials (100 to 200 mEq) be added to 500 or 1000 mL of isotonic (0.9%) sodium chloride injection. The rate of intravenous infusion should not exceed 5 mL per minute in adults (approximately 3 hours for infusion of 1000 mL). Dosage should be monitored by repeated serum bicarbonate determinations.

Parenteral drug products should be inspected visually for particulate matter and discoloration prior to administration, whenever solution and container permit. (See PRECAUTIONS.)

Protect from freezing and extreme heat.

HOW SUPPLIED - RATED THERAPEUTICALLY EQUIVALENT:

Injection, Conc-Soln - Intravenous - 5.35 gm/20ml

500 ml x 12	$14.71	Ammonium Chloride, McGaw	00264-1493-10

HOW SUPPLIED - NOT RATED EQUIVALENT:

Injection, Conc-Soln - Intravenous - 5.35 gm/20ml

20 ml	$4.87	Ammonium Chloride, Abbott	00074-6043-01

AMMONIUM CHLORIDE; HYDROCODONE *(000166)*

CATEGORIES: Antitussives; Antitussives/Expectorants/Mucolytics; Common Cold; Cough Preparations; DESI Drugs; Expectorants; Respiratory & Allergy Medications; DEA Class CIII; FDA Pre 1938 Drugs

BRAND NAMES: Hexatussin; Hyfed; N-Tussin; **P-V-Tussin**; Poly Tussin; Posituss; Q-V Tussin; Tusset

Prescribing information not available at time of publication.

HOW SUPPLIED - EQUIVALENTS NOT AVAILABLE:

Syrup - Oral

120 ml	$6.62	HYFED, H N Norton Co.	50732-0812-04
480 ml	$14.84	Hexatussin, HL Moore Drug Exch	00839-7483-69
480 ml	$24.07	HYFED SYRUP, H N Norton Co.	50732-0812-16

AMMONIUM LACTATE *(000223)*

CATEGORIES: Dermatologicals; Emollients; Ichthyosis; Moisturizers; Pruritus; Skin/Mucous Membrane Agents; Xerosis; Pregnancy Category C; FDA Approved 1985 Apr

BRAND NAMES: **Lac-Hydrin**

DESCRIPTION:

Ammonium Lactate, specially formulates 12% lactic acid neutralized with ammonium hydroxide, as ammonium lactate to provide a lotion pH of 4.5-5.5. Ammonium Lactate also contains light mineral oil, glyceryl stearate, PEG-100 stearate, propylene glycol, polyoxyl 40 stearate, glycerin, magnesium aluminum silicate, laureth-4, cetyl alcohol methyl and propylparabens, methylcellulose, fragrance, quaternium-15 and water. Lactic acid is a racemic mixture of 2-hydroxypropanoic acid.

CLINICAL PHARMACOLOGY:

It is generally accepted that the water content of the stratum corneum is a controlling factor in maintaining skin flexibility. When the stratum corneum contains more than 10% water it remain soft and pliable; however, when the water content drops below 10% the stratum corneum becomes less flexible and rough, and may exhibit scaling and cracking and the underlying skin may become irritated.[1,2]

Symptomatic relief of dry skin is provided by skin protectants containing hygroscopic substances (humectants) which increase skin moisture. Lactic acid, an α-hydroxy acid, is reported to be one of the most effective naturally occurring humectants in the skin.[3] The α-hydroxy acids (and their salts), in addition to having beneficial effects on dry skin, have also been shown to reduce excessive epidermal keratinization in patients with hyperkeratotic conditions (*e.g.,* ichthyosis).[4]

PHARMACOKINETICS

The mechanism of action of topically applied neutralized lactic acid is not yet known.

INDICATIONS AND USAGE:

Ammonium lactate is indicated for the treatment of dry, scaly skin (xerosis) and ichthyosis vulgaris and for temporary relief of itching associated with these conditions.

CONTRAINDICATIONS:

Known hypersensitivity to any of the label ingredients.

PRECAUTIONS:

GENERAL For external use only. Avoid contact with eyes, lips or mucous membranes. Caution is advised when used on the face of fair-skinned individuals since irritation may occur. A mild, transient stinging may occur on application to abraded or inflamed areas or in individuals with sensitive skin.

Carcinogenesis, Mutagenesis, and Impairment of Fertility Ammonium lactate was non-mutagenic in the Ames/Salmonella/Microsome Plate Assay. Reproductive studies in rats given lactic acid orally showed no effect on the sex ratio of the offspring.[5]

Pregnancy Category C Animal reproduction studies have not been conducted with Ammonium Lactate. It is also not known whether Ammonium Lactate can cause fetal harm when administered to a pregnant woman or can affect reproduction capacity. Ammonium Lactate should be given to a pregnant women only if clearly needed.

Nursing Mothers Although lactic acid is a normal constituent of blood and tissues, it is not known to what extent this drug affects normal lactic acid levels in human milk. Because many drugs are excreted in human milk, caution should be exercised when Ammonium Lactate is administered to a nursing woman.

Pediatric Use Safety and effectiveness of Ammonium Lactate have been demonstrated in infants and children. No unusual toxic effects were reported.

ADVERSE REACTIONS:

The most frequent adverse experiences in patients with xerosis are transient stinging (1 in 30 patients), burning (1 in 30 patients), erythema (1 in 50 patients) and peeling (1 in 60 patients). Other adverse reactions which occur less frequently are irritation, eczema, petechiae, dryness and hyperpigmentation.

Due to the more severe initial skin conditions associated with ichthyosis, there was a higher incidence of transient stinging, burning and erythema (each occurring in 1 in 10 patients).

OVERDOSAGE:

The oral administration of Ammonium Lactate to rats and mice showed this drug to be practically non-toxic (LD_{50}>15 ml/kg).

DOSAGE AND ADMINISTRATION:

Shake well, Apply to the affected areas and rub in thoroughly. Use twice daily or as directed by a physician.

REFERENCES:

1. Blank IH: Further observation on factors which influence the water content of the stratum corneum. *J Invest Dermatol 21:* 259-271, 1953. **2.** Blank IH: Factors which influence the water content of the stratum corneum. *J Invest Dermatol 18:* 433-440, 1952. **3.** Middleton JD: Sodium lactate as a moisturizer. *Cosmetics andToiletries 93:* 85-86, 1978. **4.** Van Scott EJ and Yu RJ: Modulations of keratinization with α-hydroxy acids and related compounds. In: *Recent Advances in Dermatopharmacology,* P. Frost, E.E. Gomez and N. Zaias (eds) Spectrum Publications, Inc. NY, 211-217, 1977. **5.** D'Amour FE: Effects of feeding Sodium bicarbonate or lactic acid upon the sex ration in rats. Science 79: 61-62, 1934.

HOW SUPPLIED - EQUIVALENTS NOT AVAILABLE:

Lotion - Topical - 12 %

225 gm	$23.18	LAC-HYDRIN, Westwood Squibb	00072-5708-01
225 gm	$23.18	LAC-HYDRIN, Westwood Squibb	00072-5712-08
400 gm	$36.51	LAC-HYDRIN, Westwood Squibb	00072-5712-14
400 gm	$36.51	LAC-HYDRIN, Westwood Squibb	00072-5714-01

AMOBARBITAL SODIUM *(000227)*

CATEGORIES: Anxiolytics, Sedatives, Hypnotic; Barbiturates; Central Nervous System Agents; Sedatives/Hypnotics; DEA Class CII; FDA Pre 1938 Drugs

BRAND NAMES: **Amytal Sodium**

WARNING:
MAY BE HABIT-FORMING
CAUTION: These products are to be under the direction of a physician.
The intravenous administration of Amytal Sodium (Amobarbital Sodium) carries with it the potential dangers inherent in the intravenous use of any potent hypnotic.
The barbiturates are nonselective central nervous system (CNS) depressants that are primarily used as sedative hypnotics. In subhypnotic doses, they are also used as anticonvulsants. The barbiturates and their sodium salts are subject to control under Federal Controlled Substances Act.

DESCRIPTION:

Amobarbital sodium is a white, friable, granular powder that is odorless, has a bitter taste, and is hygroscopic. It is very soluble in water, soluble in alcohol, and practically insoluble in ether and chloroform. Amobarbital sodium is sodium 5-ethyl-5-isopentylbarbiturate and has the empirical formula $C_{11}H_{17}N_2NaO_3$. Its molecular weight 248.26.

Amobarbital sodium is a substituted pyrimidine derivative in which the basic structure is barbituric acid, a substance that has no CNS activity.

Vials Amobarbital sodium are for parenteral administration. The vials contain 250 mg (1 mmol) or 500 mg (2 mmol) sterile amobarbital sodium.

CLINICAL PHARMACOLOGY:

Barbiturates are capable of producing all levels of CNS mood alteration, from excitation to mild sedation, hypnosis, and deep coma. Overdosage can produce death. In high enough therapeutic doses, barbiturates induce anesthesia.

Barbiturates depress the sensory cortex, decrease motor activity, alter cerebellar function, and produce drowsiness, sedation, and hypnosis.

Barbiturate-induced sleep differs from physiologic sleep. Sleep laboratory studies have demonstrated that barbiturates reduce the amount of time spent in the rapid eye movement (REM) phase of sleep or the dreaming stage. Also, Stages III and IV sleep are decreased. Following abrupt cessation of barbiturates used regularly, patients may experience markedly increased dreaming, nightmares, and/or insomnia. Therefore, withdrawal of a single therapeutic dose over 5 to 6 days has been recommended to lessen the REM rebound and disturbed sleep that contribute to the drug withdrawal syndrome (for example, the dose should be decreased from 3 to 2 doses/day for 1 week).

In studies, secobarbital sodium and pentobarbital sodium have been found to lose most of their effectiveness for both inducing and maintaining sleep by the end of 2 weeks of continued drug administration, even with the use of multiple doses. As with secobarbital sodium and pentobarbital sodium, other barbiturates (including amobarbital) might be expected to lose most of their effectiveness for inducing and maintaining sleep after about 2 weeks. The short-, immediate-, and to a lesser degree, long-acting barbiturates have been widely prescribed for treating insomnia. Although the clinical literature abounds with claims that the short-acting barbiturates are superior for producing sleep whereas the intermediate-acting compounds are more effective in maintaining sleep, controlled studies have failed to demonstrate these differential effects. Therefore, as sleep medications, the barbiturates are of limited value beyond short-term use.

Barbiturates have little analgesic action at subanesthetic doses. Rather, in subanesthetic doses, these drugs may increase the reaction to painful stimuli. All barbiturates exhibit anticonvulsant activity in anesthetic doses. However, of the drugs in this class, only phenobarbital, mephobarbital, and metharbital are effective as oral anticonvulsants in subhypnotic doses.

Barbiturates are respiratory depressants, and the degree of respiratory depression is dependent upon the dose. With hypnotic doses, respiratory depression produced by barbiturates is similar to that which occurs during physiologic sleep and is accompanied by a slight decrease in blood pressure and heart rate.

Studies in laboratory animals have shown that barbiturates cause reduction in the tone and contractility of the uterus, ureters, and urinary bladder. However, concentrations of the drugs required to produce this effect in humans are not reached with sedative-hypnotic doses.

Barbiturates do not impair normal hepatic function but have been shown to induce liver microsomal enzymes, thus increasing and/or altering the metabolism of barbiturates and other drugs (see DRUG INTERACTIONS).

PHARMACOKINETICS

Barbiturates are absorbed in varying degrees following oral or parenteral administration. The salts are more rapidly absorbed than are the acids. The rate of absorption is increased if the sodium salt in ingested as a dilute solution or taken on an empty stomach.

The onset of action for oral administration of barbiturates varies from 20 to 60 minutes. For intramuscular (IM) administration, the onset of action is slightly faster. Following intravenous (IV) administration, the onset of action ranges from almost immediately for pentobarbital sodium to 5 minutes for phenobarbital sodium. Maximal CNS depression may not occur until 15 minutes or more after IV administration for phenobarbital sodium. Duration of action, which is not related to the rate at which the barbiturates are redistributed throughout the body, varies among persons and in the same person from time to time. Amobarbital sodium, an intermediate-acting barbiturate, is a CNS depressant. For the oral form, the onset of sedative and hypnotic action is 3/4 to 1 hour, with a duration of action ranging from 6 to 8 hours. These values should serve as a guide but not be used to predict exact duration of effect. No studies have demonstrated that the different routes of administration are equivalent with respect to bioavailability.

Barbiturates are weak acids that are absorbed and rapidly distributed to all tissues and fluids, with high concentrations in the brain, liver, and kidneys. Lipid solubility of the barbiturates is the dominant factor in their distribution within the body. The more lipid soluble the barbiturate, the more rapidly it penetrates all tissues of the body. Barbiturates are bound to plasma and tissue proteins to a varying degree, with the degree of binding increasing directly as a function of lipid solubility.

Phenobarbital has the lowest lipid solubility, lowest plasma binding, lowest brain protein binding, the longest delay in onset of activity, and the longest duration of action. At the opposite extreme is secobarbital, which has the highest lipid solubility, highest plasma protein binding, highest brain protein binding, the shortest delay in onset of activity, and the shortest duration of action. Amobarbital sodium is classified as an intermediate barbiturate. The plasma half-life for amobarbital sodium in adults ranges between 16 and 40 hours, with a mean of 25 hours.

Barbiturates are metabolized primarily by the hepatic microsomal enzyme system, and the metabolic products are excreted in the urine and, less commonly in the feces. Only a negligible amount of amobarbital sodium is eliminated unchanged in the urine.

INDICATIONS AND USAGE:

A. Sedative

B. Hypnotic, for the short-term treatment of insomnia, since it appears to lose its effectiveness for sleep induction and sleep maintenance after 2 weeks (see CLINICAL PHARMACOLOGY).

C. Preanesthetic

CONTRAINDICATIONS:

Amobarbital sodium is contraindicated in patients who are hypersensitive to barbiturates, in patients with a history of manifest or latent porphyria, and in patients with marked impairment of liver function or respiratory disease in which dyspnea or obstruction is evident.

WARNINGS:

1. Habit Forming: Amobarbital sodium may be habit forming. Tolerance, psychological and physical dependence may occur with continued use (see DRUG ABUSE AND DEPENDENCE and CLINICAL PHARMACOLOGY, Pharmacokinetics). Patients who have psychological dependence on barbiturates may increase the dosage or decrease the dosage interval without consulting a physician and may subsequently develop a physical dependence on barbiturates. In order to minimize the possibility of overdosage or the development of dependence, the prescribing and dispensing of sedative-hypnotic barbiturates should be limited to the amount required for the interval until the next appointment. Abrupt cessation after prolonged use in a person who is dependent on the drug may result in withdrawal symptoms, including delirium, convulsions, and possibly death. Barbiturates should be withdrawn gradually from any patient known to be taking excessive doses over long periods of time (see DRUG ABUSE AND DEPENDENCE).

2. Intravenous Administration: Too rapid administration may cause respiratory depression, apnea, laryngospasm, or vasodilation with fall in blood pressure.

3. Acute or Chronic Pain: Caution should be exercised when barbiturates are administered to patients with acute or chronic pain, because paradoxical excitement could be induced or important symptoms could be masked. However, the use of barbiturates as sedatives in the postoperative surgical period and as adjuncts to cancer chemotherapy is well established.

4. Usage in Pregnancy: Barbiturates can cause fetal damage when administered to a pregnant women. Retrospective, case-controlled studies have suggested a connection between the maternal consumption of barbiturates and a higher than expected incidence of fetal abnor-

WARNINGS: *(cont'd)*

malities. Barbiturates readily cross the placental barrier and are distributed throughout fetal tissues; the highest concentrations are found in the placenta fetal liver and brain. Fetal blood levels approach maternal blood levels following parenteral administration.

Withdrawal symptoms occur in infants born to women who receive barbiturates throughout the last trimester of pregnancy (see DRUG ABUSE AND DEPENDENCE).

If amobarbital sodium is used during pregnancy or if the patient becomes pregnant while taking this drug, the patient should be apprised of the potential hazard to the fetus.

5. Synergistic Effects: The concomitant use of alcohol or other CNS depressants may produce additive CNS-depressant effects.

PRECAUTIONS:

GENERAL

Barbiturates may be habit forming. Tolerance and psychological and physical dependence may occur with continuing use (see DRUG ABUSE AND DEPENDENCE).

Barbiturates should be administered with caution, if at all, to patients who are mentally depressed, have suicidal tendencies, or have a history of drug abuse. Particular caution is also indicated before administering barbiturates to patients who have abused other classes of drugs (see WARNINGS).

Elderly or debilitated patients may react to barbiturates with marked excitement, depression, or confusion. In some persons, especially children, barbiturates, repeatedly produce excitement rather than depression.

In patients with hepatic damage, barbiturates should be administered with caution and initially in reduced doses. Barbiturates should not be administered to patients showing the premonitory signs of hepatic coma.

Parenteral solutions of barbiturates are highly alkaline. Therefore, extreme care should be taken to avoid perivascular extravasation or intra-arterial injection. Extravascular injection may cause local tissue damage with subsequent necrosis; consequences of intra-arterial injection may vary from transient pain to gangrene of the limb. Any complaint of pain in the limb warrant stopping injection.

The systemic effects of exogenous and endogenous corticosteroids may be diminished by amobarbital sodium. Thus, this product should be administered with caution to patients with borderline hypoadrenal function, regardless of whether it is of pituitary or of primary adrenal origin.

INFORMATION FOR THE PATIENT

The following information should be given to patients receiving barbiturates.

1. The use of barbiturates carries with it an associated risk of psychological and/or physical dependence.

2. Barbiturates may impair the mental and/or physical abilities required for the performance of potentially hazardous tasks, such as driving a car or operating machinery. The patient should be cautioned accordingly.

3. Alcohol should not be consumed while taking barbiturates. The concurrent use of the barbiturates with other CNS depressants (*e.g.,* alcohol, narcotics, tranquilizers, and antihistamines) may result in additional CNS-depressant effects.

LABORATORY TESTS

Prolonged therapy with barbiturates should be accompanied by periodic evaluation of organ systems, including hematopoietic, renal, and hepatic systems (see PRECAUTIONS, General and ADVERSE REACTIONS).

CARCINOGENESIS

1. Animal Data: Phenobarbital sodium is carcinogenic in mice and rats after lifetime administration. In mice, it produced benign and malignant liver cell tumors. In rats, benign liver cell tumors were observed very late in life.

2. Human Data: In a 29-year epidemiologic study of 9,136 patients who were treated on an anticonvulsant protocol that included phenobarbital, results indicated a higher than normal incidence of hepatic carcinoma. Previously, some of these patients had been treated with thorotrast, a drug that is known to produce hepatic carcinomas. Thus, this study did not provide sufficient evidence that phenobarbital sodium is carcinogenic on humans.

A retrospective study of 84 children with brain tumors matched to 73 normal controls and 78 cancer controls (malignant disease other than brain tumors) suggested an association between exposure to barbiturates prenatally and an increased incidence of brain tumors.

PREGNANCY CATEGORY D

See WARNINGS, Usage in Pregnancy.

Nonteratogenic Effects: Reports of infants suffering from long-term barbiturate exposure *in utero* included the acute withdrawal syndrome of seizures and hyperirritability from birth to a delayed onset of up to 14 days (see DRUG ABUSE AND DEPENDENCE).

LABOR AND DELIVERY

Hypnotic doses of barbiturates do not appear to impair uterine activity significantly during labor. Full anesthetic doses of barbiturates decrease the force and frequency of uterine contractions. Administration of sedative-hypnotic barbiturates to the mother during labor may result in respiratory depression in the newborn. Premature infants are particularly susceptible to the depressant effects of barbiturates. If barbiturates are used during labor and delivery, resuscitation equipment should be available.

Data are not available to evaluate the effect of barbiturates when forceps delivery or other intervention is necessary or to determine the effect of barbiturates on the later growth, development, and functional maturation of the child.

NURSING MOTHERS

Caution should be exercised when amobarbital sodium is administered to a nursing woman because small amounts of barbiturates are excreted in the milk.

USAGE IN CHILDREN

Safety and effectiveness have not been established in children below the age of 6 years.

DRUG INTERACTIONS:

Most reports of clinically significant drug interactions occurring with the barbiturates have involved phenobarbital. However, the application of these data to other barbiturates appears valid and warrants serial blood level determinations of the relevant drugs when there are multiple therapies.

Anticoagulants: Phenobarbital lowers the plasma levels of dicumarol and cause decrease in anticoagulant activity as measured by the prothrombin time. Barbiturates can induce hepatic microsomal enzymes, resulting in increased metabolism and decreased anticoagulant response of oral anticoagulants (*e.g.,* warfarin, acenocoumarol, dicumarol, and phenprocoumon). Patients stabilized on anticoagulant therapy may require dosage adjustments if barbiturates are added to or withdrawn from their dosage regimen.

Corticosteroids: Barbiturates appear to enhance the metabolism of exogenous corticosteroids, probably through the induction of hepatic microsomal enzymes. Patients stabilized on corticosteroid therapy may require dosage adjustments if barbiturates are added to or withdrawn from their dosage regimen.

DRUG INTERACTIONS: *(cont'd)*

Griseofulvin: Phenobarbital appears to interfere with the absorption of orally administered griseofulvin, thus decreasing its blood level. The effect of the resultant decreased blood levels of griseofulvin on therapeutic response has not been established. However, it would be preferable to avoid concomitant administration of these drugs.

Doxycycline: Phenobarbital has been shown to shorten the half-live of doxycycline for as long as 2 weeks after barbiturate therapy is discontinued.

This mechanism is probably through the induction of hepatic microsomal enzymes that metabolize the antibiotic. If amobarbital sodium and doxycycline are administered concurrently, the clinical response to doxycycline should be monitored closely.

Phenytoin, Sodium Valproate, Valproic Acid: The effect of barbiturates on the metabolism of phenytoin appears to be variable. Some investigators report an accelerating effect, whereas others report no effect. Because the effect of barbiturates on the metabolism of phenytoin is not predictable, phenytoin and barbiturate blood levels should be monitored more frequently if these drugs are given concurrently. Sodium valproate and valproic acid appear to increase the amobarbital sodium serum levels; therefore, amobarbital sodium blood levels should be closely monitored and appropriate dosage adjustments made as clinically indicated.

CNS Depressants: The concomitant use of other CNS depressants, including other sedatives or hypnotics, antihistamines, tranquilizers, or alcohol, may produce additive depressant effects.

Monoamine Oxidase Inhibitors (MAOIs): MAOIs prolong the effects of barbiturates, probably because metabolism of the barbiturate is inhibited.

Estradiol, Estrone, Progesterone, and Other Steroidal Hormones: Pretreatment with or concurrent administration of phenobarbital may decrease the effect of estradiol by increasing its metabolism. There have been reports of patients treated with antiepileptic drugs (*e.g.,* phenobarbital) who become pregnant while taking oral contraceptives. An alternative contraceptive method might be suggested to women taking barbiturates.

ADVERSE REACTIONS:

The following adverse reactions and their incidence were compiled from surveillance of thousands of hospitalized patients who received barbiturates. Because such patients may be less aware of certain of the the milder adverse effects of barbiturates, the incidence of these reactions may be somewhat higher in fully ambulatory patients.

MORE THAN 1 IN 100 PATIENTS

The most common adverse reaction, estimated to occur at a rate of 1 to 3 patients per 100, is the following:

Nervous System: Somnolence

LESS THAN 1 IN 100 PATIENTS

Adverse reactions estimated to occur at a rate of less than 1 in 100 patients are listed below, grouped by organ system and by decreasing order of occurrence:

Nervous System: Agitation, confusion, hyperkinesia, ataxia, CNS depression, nightmares, nervousness, psychiatric disturbance, hallucinations, insomnia, anxiety, dizziness, abnormality in thinking

Respiratory System: Hypoventilation, apnea, postoperative atelectasis

Cardiovascular System: Bradycardia, hypotension, syncope

Digestive System: Nausea, vomiting, constipation

Other Reported Reactions: Headache, injection site reactions, hypersensitivity reactions (angioedema, skin rashes, exfoliative dermatitis), fever, liver damage, megaloblastic anemia following chronic phenobarbital use.

DRUG ABUSE AND DEPENDENCE:

Controlled Substance: Amobarbital sodium is a Schedule II drug.

Dependence: Barbiturates may be habit-forming. Tolerance, psychological dependence, and physical dependence may occur, especially following prolonged use of high doses of barbiturates. Daily administration in excess of 400 mg of pentobarbital or secobarbital for approximately 90 days is likely to produce some degree of physical dependence. A dosage of 600 to 800 mg for at least 35 days is sufficient to produce withdrawal seizures. The average daily dose for the barbiturate addict is usually about 1.5 g. As tolerance to barbiturates develops, the amount needed to maintain the same level of intoxication increases; tolerance to a fatal dosage, however, does not increase more than twofold. As this occurs, the margin between intoxicating dosage and fatal dosage becomes smaller.

Symptoms of acute intoxication with barbiturates include unsteady gait, slurred speech, and sustained nystagmus. Mental signs of chronic intoxication include confusion, poor judgement, irritability, insomnia, and somatic complaints.

Symptoms of barbiturate dependence are similar to those of chronic alcoholism. If an individual appears to be intoxicated with alcohol to a degree that is radically disproportionate to the amount of alcohol in his or her blood, the use of barbiturates should be suspected. The lethal dose of a barbiturate is far less if alcohol is also ingested.

The symptoms of barbiturate withdrawal can be severe and may cause death. Minor withdrawal symptoms may appear 8 to 12 hours after the last dose of a barbiturate. These symptoms usually appear in the following order: anxiety, muscle twitching, tremor of hands and fingers, progressive weakness, dizziness, distortion in visual perception, nausea, vomiting, insomnia, and orthostatic hypotension. Major withdrawal symptoms (convulsions and delirium) may occur within 16 hours and last up to 5 days after abrupt cessation of barbiturates. The intensity of withdrawal symptoms gradually declines over a period of approximately 15 days. Individuals susceptible to barbiturate abuse and dependence include alcoholics and opiate abusers, as well as other sedative-hypnotic and amphetamine abusers.

Drug dependence on barbiturates arises from repeated administration on a continuous basis, generally in amounts exceeding therapeutic dose levels. The characteristics of drug dependence on barbiturates include: (a) a strong desire or need to continue taking the drug; (b) a tendency to increase the dose; (c) a psychic dependence on the effects of the drug related to subjective and individual appreciation of those effects; and (d) a physical dependence on the effects of the drug, requiring its presence for maintenance of homeostasis and resulting in a definite, characteristic, and self-limited abstinence syndrome when the drug is withdrawn.

Treatment of barbiturate dependence consists of cautious and gradual withdrawal of the drug. Barbiturate-dependent patients can be withdrawn by using a number of different withdrawal regimens. In all cases, withdrawal requires an extended period of time. One method involves substituting a 30-mg dose of phenobarbital for each 100- to 200-mg dose of barbiturate that the patient has been taking. The total daily amount of phenobarbital is then administered in 3 or 4 divided doses, not to exceed 600 mg daily. If signs of withdrawal occur on the first day of treatment, a loading dose of 100 to 200 mg of phenobarbital may be administered IM in addition to the oral dose. After stabilization on phenobarbital, the total daily dose is decreased by 30 mg/day as long as withdrawal is proceeding smoothly. A modification of this regimen involves initiating treatment at the patient's regular dosage level and decreasing the daily dosage by 10% if tolerated by the patient.

DRUG ABUSE AND DEPENDENCE: *(cont'd)*

Infants that are physically dependent on barbiturates may be given phenobarbital, 3 to 10 mg/kg/day. After withdrawal symptoms (hyperactivity, disturbed sleep, tremors, and hyperreflexia) are relieved, the dosage of phenobarbital should be gradually decreased and completely withdrawn over a 2-week period.

OVERDOSAGE:

The toxic dose of barbiturates varies considerably. In general, an oral dose of 1 g of most barbiturates produces serious poisoning in an adult. Toxic effects and fatalities have occurred following overdoses of amobarbital sodium alone and in combination with other CNS depressants. Death commonly occurs after 2 to 10 g of ingested barbiturate. The sedated, therapeutic blood levels of amobarbital range between 2 to 10 mcg/ml; the usual lethal blood level ranges from 40 to 80 mcg/ml. Barbiturate intoxication may be confused with alcoholism, bromide intoxication, and various neurologic disorders. Potential tolerance must be considered when evaluating significance of dose and plasma concentration.

Signs and Symptoms: Symptoms of oral overdose may occur within 15 minutes beginning with CNS depression, absent or sluggish reflexes, underventilation, hypotension, and hypothermia and may progress to pulmonary edema and death. Hemorrhagic blisters may develop, especially at pressure points.

In extreme overdose, all electrical activity in the brain may cease, in which case a "flat" EEG normally equated with clinical death cannot be accepted. This effect is fully reversible unless hypoxic damage occurs. Consideration should be given to the possibility of barbiturate intoxication even in situations that appear to involve trauma.

Complications such as pneumonia, pulmonary edema, cardiac arrhythmias, congestive heart failure, and renal heart failure may occur. Uremia may increase CNS sensitivity to barbiturates if renal function is impaired. Differential diagnosis should include hypoglycemia, head trauma, cerebrovascular accidents, convulsive states, and diabetic coma.

Treatment: To obtain up-to-date information about the treatment of overdose, a good resource is your certified Regional Poison Control Center. Telephone numbers of certified poison control centers are listed in *Physicians' GenRx*. In managing overdosage, consider the possibility of multiple drug overdoses, interaction among drugs, and unusual drug kinetics in your patient.

Protect the patient's airway and support ventilation and perfusion. Meticulously monitor and maintain, within acceptable limits, the patient's vital signs, blood gases, serum electrolytes, etc. Absorption of drugs from which, in many cases, is more effective than emesis or lavage; consider charcoal instead of or in addition to gastric emptying. Repeated doses of charcoal over time may hasten elimination of some drugs that have been absorbed. Safeguard the patient's airway when employing gastric emptying or charcoal.

Diuresis and peritoneal dialysis are of little value; hemodialysis and hemoperfusion enhance drug clearance and should be considered in serious poisoning. If the patient has chronically abused sedatives withdrawal reactions may be manifest following acute overdose.

Preparation of Solution: Solutions of amobarbital sodium should be made up aseptically with Sterile Water for Injection. The accompanying table will aid in preparing solutions of various concentrations. Ordinarily, a 10% solution is used. After Sterile Water for Injection is added, the vial should be rotated to facilitate solution of the powder. **Do not shake the vial.**

Several minutes may be required for the drug to dissolve completely, but under no circumstances should a solution be injected if it has not become absolutely clear within 5 minutes. Also, a solution that forms a precipitate after clearing should not be used. Amobarbital sodium hydrolyzes in solution or on exposure to air. Not more than 30 minutes should elapse from the time the vial is opened until its contents are injected. Prior to administration, parenteral drug products should be inspected visually for particulate matter and discoloration whenever solution containers permit. (See TABLE 1.)

TABLE 1 Quantity of Sterile Water for Injection Required to Dilute the Contents of a Given Vial of Amobarbital Sodium to Obtain the Percentages Listed. Solutions Derived Will Be in Weight/Volume

Amobarbital Sodium Vial Number	Content in Weight	1%	2.5%	5%	10%	20%
386	250 mg	25 ml	10 ml	5 ml	2.5 ml	1.25 ml
387	0.5 g	50 ml	20 ml	10 ml	5 ml	2.5 ml

DOSAGE AND ADMINISTRATION:

The dose of amobarbital sodium must be individualized with full knowledge of its particular characteristics and recommended rate of administration. Factors of consideration are the patient's age, weight, and condition. The maximum single dose for an adult is 1 g.

Intramuscular Use: Intramuscular injection of the sodium salts of barbiturates should be made deeply into a large muscle. The average intramuscular dose ranges from 65 mg to 0.5 g. A volume of 5 ml (irrespective of concentration) should not be exceeded at any one site because of possible tissue irritation. Twenty percent solutions may be used so that a small volume can contain a large dose. After IM injection of a hypnotic dose, the patient's vital signs should be monitored. Superficial intramuscular or subcutaneous injections may be painful and may produce sterile abscesses or sloughs.

Intravenous Use: Intravenous injection is restricted to conditions in which other routes are not feasible, either because the patient is unconscious (as in cerebral hemorrhage, eclampsia, or status epilepticus), because the patient resists (as in delirium), or because prompt action is imperative. Slow IV injection is essential, and patients should be carefully observed during administration. This requires that blood pressure, respiration, and cardiac function be maintained, vital signs be recorded and equipment for resuscitation and artificial ventilation be available. The rate of IV injection for adults should be exceed 50 mg/min to prevent sleep or sudden respiratory depression. The final dosage is determined to a great extent by the patient's reaction to the slow administration of the drug.

ADULTS

a. Sedative: 30 to 50 mg given 2 or 3 times daily.

b. Hypnotic: 65 to 200 mg at bedtime.

Special Patient Population: Dosage should be reduced in the elderly or debilitated because these patients may be more sensitive to barbiturates. Dosage should be reduced for patients with impaired renal function or hepatic disease. Ordinarily, an intravenous dose of 65 mg to 0.5 g may be given to a child 6 to 12 years of age.

HOW SUPPLIED - EQUIVALENTS NOT AVAILABLE:

Capsule, Gelatin - Oral - 200 mg

100's $22.53 AMYTAL SODIUM, Lilly 00002-0633-02

Injection, Lyphl-Soln - Intramuscular; - 0.5 gm/vial

10 ml x 10 $82.49 AMYTAL SODIUM, Lilly 00002-7215-10
10 ml x 25 $189.01 AMYTAL SODIUM, Lilly 00002-7215-25

HOW SUPPLIED - EQUIVALENTS NOT AVAILABLE: *(cont'd)*

Injection, Solution - Intravenous - 250 mg

10's $47.01 AMYTAL SODIUM, Lilly 00002-7214-10

Powder

30 gm $9.50 Amobarbital Sodium, Lannett 00527-0603-31

AMOBARBITAL; EPHEDRINE *(000228)*

CATEGORIES: Antiasthmatics/Bronchodilators; Autonomic Drugs; Respiratory & Allergy Medications; Sympathomimetic Agents; DEA Class CIII; FDA Pre 1938 Drugs

BRAND NAMES: **Amytal W/Ephedrine**

Prescribing information not available at time of publication.

HOW SUPPLIED - EQUIVALENTS NOT AVAILABLE:

Capsule, Gelatin - Oral

100's $10.99 EPHEDRINE & AMYTAL, Lilly 00002-0614-02

AMOBARBITAL; SECOBARBITAL *(000229)*

CATEGORIES: Anesthesia; Anxiolytics, Sedatives, Hypnotic; Barbiturates; Central Nervous System Agents; Insomnia; Sedatives/Hypnotics; DEA Class CII; FDA Pre 1938 Drugs

BRAND NAMES: **Tuinal**

COST OF THERAPY: $2.13 (Insomnia; Capsule; 100 mg/100 mg; 1/day; 7 days) vs. Potential Cost of $3,628.44 (Psychoses)

DESCRIPTION:

Chemically, Secobarbital Sodium is sodium 5-allyl-5-(1-methylbutyl) barbiturate, with the empirical formula $C_{12}H_{17}N_2NaO_3$. Its molecular weight is 260.27.

Amytal Sodium is sodium 5-ethyl-5-isopentylbarbiturate with the empirical formula $C_{11}H_{17}N_2NaO_3$. Its molecular weight is 248.26.

FOR COMPLETE PRESCRIBING INFORMATION REFER TO THE INDIVIDUAL DRUG MONOGRAPHS (AMOBARBITAL; SECOBARBITAL).

INDICATIONS AND USAGE:

A. Hypnotic, for the short-term treatment of insomnia, since it appears to lose its effectiveness for sleep induction and sleep maintenance after 2 weeks.

B. Preanesthetic.

DOSAGE AND ADMINISTRATION:

The dose of Amobarbital/Secobarbital must be individualized with full knowledge of its particular characteristics and recommended rate of administration. Factors of consideration are the patient's age, weight, and condition.

Adults: 100 mg (50 mg each of secobarbital sodium and amobarbital sodium) to 200 mg (100 mg each of secobarbital sodium and amobarbital sodium) at bedtime or 1 hour preoperatively.

Special Patient Population: Dosage should be reduced in the elderly or debilitated because these patients may be more sensitive to barbiturates. Dosage should be reduced for patients with impaired renal function or hepatic disease.

Store at controlled room temperature, 59 to 86°F (15° to 30°C) Dispense in a tight container.

HOW SUPPLIED - EQUIVALENTS NOT AVAILABLE:

Capsule, Gelatin - Oral - 50 mg/50 mg

100's $22.87 TUINAL, Lilly 00002-0665-02

Capsule, Gelatin - Oral - 100 mg/100 mg

100's $30.52 TUINAL, Lilly 00002-0666-02
1000's $232.28 TUINAL, Lilly 00002-0666-04

AMOXAPINE *(000230)*

CATEGORIES: Antidepressants; Anxiety; Central Nervous System Agents; Depression; Psychotherapeutic Agents; Tricyclics; Tricyclic Antidepressants; Pregnancy Category C; FDA Approval Pre 1982

BRAND NAMES: *Amoxan* (Japan); **Asendin**; *Asendis* (England); *Defanyl* (France); *Demolox* (Mexico)
(International brand names outside U.S. in italics)

COST OF THERAPY: $96.19 (Depression; Tablet; 50 mg; 2/day; 90 days)

PRIMARY ICD9: 311 (Depressive Disorder, Not Elsewhere Classified)

DESCRIPTION:

Amoxapine is an antidepressant of the dibenzoxazepine class, chemically distinct from the dibenzazepines, dibenzocycloheptenes, and dibenzoxepines.

It is designated chemically as 2-chloro-11-(1-piperazinyl) dibenz-(*b,f*)(1,4)oxazepine. The molecular weight is 313.8. The molecular formula is $C_{17}H_{16}ClN_3O$.

Amoxapine is supplied for oral administration as 25 mg, 50 mg, 100 mg, and 150 mg tablets.

Asendin Inactive Ingredients: All tablets contain lactose, microcrystalline cellulose, magnesium stearate, and croscarmellose sodium. In addition, 50 mg tablets contain D & C Red No. 30 and D & C Yellow No. 10, 100 mg tablets contain FD & C Blue No. 1 and 150 mg tablets contain D & C Red No. 30 and D & C Yellow No. 10.

CLINICAL PHARMACOLOGY:

Amoxapine is an antidepressant with a mild sedative component to its action. The mechanism of its clinical action in man is not well understood. In animals, amoxapine reduced the uptake of norepinephrine and serotonin and blocked the response of dopamine receptors to dopamine. Amoxapine is not a monoamine oxidase inhibitor.

Amoxapine is absorbed rapidly and reaches peak blood levels approximately 90 minutes after ingestion. It is almost completely metabolized. The main route of excretion is the kidney. *In vitro* tests show that amoxapine binding to human serum is approximately 90%.

CLINICAL PHARMACOLOGY: *(cont'd)*

In man, amoxapine serum concentration declines with a half-life of eight hours. However, the major metabolite, 8-hydroxyamoxapine, has a biologic half-life of 30 hours. Metabolites are excreted in the urine in conjugated form as glucuronides.

Clinical studies have demonstrated that amoxapine has a more rapid onset of action than either amitriptyline or imipramine. The initial clinical effect may occur within four to seven days and occurs within two weeks in over 80% of responders.

INDICATIONS AND USAGE:

Amoxapine is indicated for the relief of symptoms of depression in patients with neurotic or reactive depressive disorders as well as endogenous and psychotic depressions. It is indicated for depression accompanied by anxiety or agitation.

CONTRAINDICATIONS:

Amoxapine is contraindicated in patients who have shown prior hypersensitivity to dibenzoxazepine compounds. It should not be given concomitantly with monoamine oxidase inhibitors. Hyperpyretic crises, severe convulsions and deaths have occurred in patients receiving tricyclic antidepressants and monoamine oxidase inhibitors simultaneously. When it is desired to replace a monoamine oxidase inhibitor with amoxapine, a minimum of 14 days should be allowed to elapse after the former is discontinued. Amoxapine should then be initiated cautiously with gradual increase in dosage until optimum response is achieved. The drug is not recommended for use during the acute recovery phase following myocardial infarction.

WARNINGS:

TARDIVE DYSKINESIA

Tardive dyskinesia, a syndrome consisting of potentially irreversible, involuntary, dyskinetic movements may develop in patients treated with neuroleptic (*i.e.,* antipsychotics) drugs. (Amoxapine is not an antipsychotic, but it has substantive neuroleptic activity.) Although the prevalence of the syndrome appears to be highest among the elderly, especially elderly women, it is impossible to rely upon prevalence estimates to predict, at the inception of neuroleptic treatment, which patients are likely to develop the syndrome. Whether neuroleptic drug products differ in their potential to cause tardive dyskinesia is unknown.

Both the risk of developing the syndrome and the likelihood that it will become irreversible are believed to increase as the duration of treatment and the total cumulative dose of neuroleptic drugs administered to the patient increase. However, the syndrome can develop, although much less commonly, after relatively brief treatment periods at low doses.

There is no known treatment for established cases of tardive dyskinesia, although the syndrome may remit, partially or completely, if neuroleptic treatment is withdrawn. Neuroleptic treatment itself, however, may suppress (or partially suppress) the signs and symptoms of the syndrome and thereby may possibly mask the underlying disease process. The effect that symptomatic suppression has upon the long-term course of the syndrome is unknown.

Given these considerations, neuroleptics should be prescribed in a manner that is most likely to minimize the occurrence of tardive dyskinesia. Chronic neuroleptic treatment should generally be reserved for patients who suffer from a chronic illness that, 1) is known to respond to neuroleptic drugs, and 2) for whom alternative, equally effective, but potentially less harmful treatments are not available or appropriate. In patients who do require chronic treatment, the smallest dose and the shortest duration of treatment producing a satisfactory clinical response should be sought. The need for continued treatment should be reassessed periodically.

If signs and symptoms of tardive dyskinesia appear in a patient on neuroleptics, drug discontinuation should be considered. However, some patients may require treatment despite the presence of the syndrome.

(For further information about the description of tardive dyskinesia and its clinical detection, please refer to the sections on Information for Patients and ADVERSE REACTIONS.)

NEUROLEPTIC MALIGNANT SYNDROME (NMS)

A potentially fatal symptom complex sometimes referred to as Neuroleptic Malignant Syndrome (NMS) has been reported in association with antipsychotic drugs and with amoxapine. Clinical manifestations of NMS are hyperpyrexia, muscle rigidity, altered mental status and evidence of autonomic instability (irregular pulse or blood pressure, tachycardia, diaphoresis, and cardiac dysrhythmias).

The diagnostic evaluation of patients with this syndrome is complicated. In arriving at a diagnosis, it is important to identify cases where the clinical presentation includes both serious medical illness (*e.g.,* pneumonia, systemic infection, etc.) and untreated or inadequately treated extrapyramidal signs and symptoms (EPS). Other important considerations in the differential diagnosis include central anticholinergic toxicity, heat stroke, drug fever and primary central nervous system (CNS) pathology.

The management of NMS should include 1) immediate discontinuation of antipsychotic drugs and other drugs not essential to concurrent therapy, 2) intensive symptomatic treatment and medical monitoring, and 3) treatment of any concomitant serious medical problems for which specific treatments are available. There is no general agreement about specific pharmacological treatment regimens for uncomplicated NMS.

If a patient requires antipsychotic drug treatment after recovery from NMS, the potential reintroduction of drug therapy should be carefully considered. The patient should be carefully monitored since recurrences of NMS have been reported.

Amoxapine should be used with caution in patients with a history of urinary retention, angle-closure glaucoma or increased intraocular pressure. Patients with cardiovascular disorders should be watched closely. Tricyclic antidepressant drugs, particularly when given in high doses, can induce sinus tachycardia, changes in conduction time, and arrhythmias. Myocardial infarction and stroke have been reported with drugs of this class.

Extreme caution should be used in treating patients with a history of convulsive disorder or those with overt or latent seizure disorders.

PRECAUTIONS:

GENERAL

In prescribing the drug it should be borne in mind that the possibility of suicide is inherent in any severe depression, and persists until a significant remission occurs; the drug should be dispensed in the smallest suitable amount. Manic depressive patients may experience a shift to the manic phase. Schizophrenic patients may develop increased symptoms of psychosis; patients with paranoid symptomatology may have an exaggeration of such symptoms. This may require reduction of dosage or the addition of a major tranquilizer to the therapeutic regimen. Antidepressant drugs can cause skin rashes and/or "drug fever" in susceptible individuals. These allergic reactions may, in rare cases, be severe. They are more likely to occur during the first few days of treatment, but may also occur later. Amoxapine should be discontinued if rash and/or fever develop. Amoxapine possesses a degree of dopamine-blocking activity which may cause extrapyramidal symptoms in <1% of patients. Rarely, symptoms indicative of tardive dyskinesia have been reported.

PRECAUTIONS: *(cont'd)*

INFORMATION FOR THE PATIENT

Given the likelihood that some patients exposed chronically to neuroleptics will develop tardive dyskinesia, it is advised that all patients in whom chronic use is contemplated be given, if possible, full information about this risk. The decision to inform patients and/or their guardians must obviously take into account the clinical circumstances and the competency of the patient to understand the information provided.

Patients should be warned of the possibility of drowsiness that may impair performance of potentially hazardous tasks such as driving an automobile or operating machinery.

THERAPEUTIC INTERACTIONS

Concurrent administration with electroshock therapy may increase the hazards associated with such therapy.

CARCINOGENESIS, MUTAGENESIS, AND IMPAIRMENT OF FERTILITY

In a 21-month toxicity study at three dose levels in rats, pancreatic islet cell hyperplasia occurred with slightly increased incidence at doses 5-10 times the human dose. Pancreatic adenocarcinoma was detected in low incidence in the mid-dose group only, and may possibly have resulted from endocrinemediated organ hyperfunction. The significance of these findings to man is not known.

Treatment of male rats with 5-10 times the human dose resulted in a slight decrease in the number of fertile matings. Female rats receiving oral doses within the therapeutic range displayed a reversible increase in estrous cycle length.

PREGNANCY:PREGNANCY CATEGORY C

Studies performed in mice, rats, and rabbits have demonstrated no evidence of teratogenic effect due to amoxapine. Embryotoxicity was seen in rats and rabbits given oral doses approximating the human dose. Fetotoxic effects (intrauterine death, stillbirth, decreased birth weight) were seen in animals studied at oral doses 3-10 times the human dose. Decreased postnatal survival (between days 0-4) was demonstrated in the offspring of rats at 5-10 times the human dose. There are no adequate and well-controlled studies in pregnant women. Amoxapine should be used during pregnancy only if the potential benefit justifies the potential risk to the fetus.

NURSING MOTHERS

Amoxapine, like many other systemic drugs, is excreted in human milk. Because effects of the drug on infants are unknown, caution should be exercised when amoxapine is administered to nursing women.

PEDIATRIC USE

Safety and effectiveness in children below the age of 16 have not been established.

DRUG INTERACTIONS:

(See CONTRAINDICATIONS) about concurrent usage of tricyclic antidepressants and monoamine oxidase inhibitors. Paralytic ileus may occur in patients taking tricyclic antidepressants in combination with anticholinergic drugs. Amoxapine may enhance the response to alcohol and the effects of barbiturates and other CNS depressants. Serum levels of several tricyclic antidepressants have been reported to be significantly increased when cimetidine is administered concurrently. Although such an interaction has not been reported to date with amoxapine, specific interaction studies have not been done, and the possibility should be considered.

ADVERSE REACTIONS:

Adverse reactions reported in controlled studies in the United States are categorized with respect to incidence below. Following this is a listing of reactions known to occur with other antidepressant drugs of this class but not reported to date with amoxapine tablets.

INCIDENCE GREATER THAN 1%

The most frequent types of adverse reactions occurring with amoxapine tablets in controlled clinical trials were sedative and anticholinergic: these included drowsiness (14%), dry mouth (14%), constipation (12%), and blurred vision (7%).

Less frequently reported reactions are:

CNS and Neuromuscular: anxiety, insomnia, restlessness, nervousness, palpitations, tremors, confusion, excitement, nightmares, ataxia, alterations in EEG patterns

Allergic: edema, skin rash

Endocrine: elevation of prolactin levels

Gastrointestinal: nausea

Other: dizziness, headache, fatigue, weakness, excessive appetite, increased perspiration

INCIDENCE LESS THAN 1%

Anticholinergic: disturbances of accommodation, mydriasis, delayed micturition, urinary retention, nasal stuffiness

Cardiovascular: hypotension, hypertension, syncope, tachycardia

Allergic: drug fever, urticaria, photosensitization, pruritus, rarely vasculitis, hepatitis

CNS and Neuromuscular: tingling, paresthesias of the extremities, tinnitus, disorientation, seizures, hypomania, numbness, incoordination, disturbed concentration, hyperthermia, extrapyramidal symptoms, including, rarely, tardive dyskinesia. Neuroleptic malignant syndrome has been reported (See WARNINGS.)

Hematologic: leukopenia, agranulocytosis

Gastrointestinal: epigastric distress, vomiting, flatulence, abdominal pain, peculiar taste, diarrhea

Endocrine: increased or decreased libido, impotence, menstrual irregularity, breast enlargement and galactorrhea in the female, syndrome of inappropriate antidiuretic hormone secretion

Other: lacrimation, weight gain or loss, altered liver function, painful ejaculation

DRUG RELATIONSHIP UNKNOWN

The following reactions have been reported very rarely, and occurred under uncontrolled circumstances where a drug relationship was difficult to assess. These observations are listed to serve as alerting information to physicians.

Anticholinergic: paralytic ileus

Cardiovascular: atrial arrhythmias (including atrial fibrillation), myocardial infarction, stroke, heart block

CNS and Neuromuscular: hallucinations

Hematologic: thrombocytopenia, eosinophilia, purpura, petechiae

Gastrointestinal: parotid swelling

Endocrine: change in blood glucose levels

Other: pancreatitis, hepatitis, jaundice, urinary frequency, testicular swelling, anorexia, alopecia

ADDITIONAL ADVERSE REACTIONS

The following reactions have been reported with other antidepressant drugs, but not with amoxapine tablets.

ADVERSE REACTIONS: *(cont'd)*

Anticholinergic: sublingual adenitis, dilation of the urinary tract
CNS and Neuromuscular: delusions
Gastrointestinal: stomatitis, black tongue
Endocrine: gynecomastia

OVERDOSAGE:

SIGNS AND SYMPTOMS

Toxic manifestations of amoxapine overdosage differ significantly from those of other tricyclic antidepressants. Serious cardiovascular effects are seldom if ever observed. However, CNS effects -particularly grand mal convulsions-occur frequently, and treatment should be directed primarily toward prevention or control of seizures. Status epilepticus may develop and constitutes a neurologic emergency. Coma and acidosis are other serious complications of substantial amoxapine overdosage in some cases.

Renal failure may develop two to five days after toxic overdosage in patients who may appear otherwise recovered. Acute tubular necrosis with rhabdomyolysis and myoglobinuria is the most common renal complication in such cases. This reaction probably occurs in less than 5% of overdose cases, and typically in those who have experienced multiple seizures.

TREATMENT

Treatment of amoxapine overdosage should be symptomatic and supportive, but with special attention to prevention or control of seizures. If the patient is conscious, induced emesis followed by gastric lavage with appropriate precautions to prevent pulmonary aspiration should be accomplished as soon as possible. Following lavage, activated charcoal may be administered to reduce absorption, and repeated administrations may facilitate drug elimination. An adequate airway should be established in comatose patients and assisted ventilation instituted if necessary. Seizures may respond to standard anticonvulsant therapy such as intravenous diazepam and/or phenytoin. The value of physostigmine appears less certain. Status epilepticus, should it develop, requires vigorous treatment such as that described by Delgado- Escueta et al (*N Engl J Med* 1982; 306:1337-1340).

Convulsions, when they occur, typically begin within 12 hours after ingestion. Because seizures may occur precipitously in some overdosage patients who appear otherwise relatively asymptomatic, the treating physician may wish to consider prophylactic administration of anticonvulsant medication during this period.

Treatment of renal impairment, should it occur, is the same as that for nondrug-induced renal dysfunction.

Serious cardiovascular effects are remarkably rare following amoxapine overdosage, and the ECG typically remains within normal limits except for sinus tachycardia. Hence, prolongation of the QRS interval beyond 100 milliseconds within the first 24 hours is *not* a useful guide to the severity of overdosage with this drug.

Fatalities and, rarely, neurologic sequelae have resulted from prolonged status epilepticus in amoxapine overdosage patients. While the lethal dose appears higher than that of other tricyclic antidepressants (80% of lethal amoxapine overdosages have involved ingestion of 3 grams or more), many factors other than amount ingested are important in assessing probability of survival. These include age and physical condition of the patient, concomitant ingestion of other drugs, and especially the interval between drug ingestion and initiation of emergency treatment.

DOSAGE AND ADMINISTRATION:

Effective dosage of amoxapine tablets may vary from one patient to another. Usual effective dosage is 200 to 300 mg daily. Three weeks constitutes an adequate period of trial providing dosage has reached 300 mg daily (or lower level of tolerance) for at least two weeks. If no response is seen at 300 mg, dosage may be increased, depending upon tolerance, up to 400 mg daily. Hospitalized patients who have been refractory to antidepressant therapy and who have no history of convulsive seizures may have dosage raised cautiously up to 600 mg daily in divided doses.

Amoxapine tablets may be given in a single daily dose, not to exceed 300 mg, preferably at bedtime. If the total daily dose exceeds 300 mg, it should be given in divided doses.

INITIAL DOSAGE FOR ADULTS

Usual starting dosage is 50 mg two or three times daily. Depending upon tolerance, dosage may be increased to 100 mg two or three times daily by the end of the first week. (Initial dosage of 300 mg daily may be given, but notable sedation may occur in some patients during the first few days of therapy at this level.) Increases above 300 mg daily should be made only if 300 mg daily has been ineffective during a trial period of at least two weeks. When effective dosage is established, the drug may be given in a single dose (not to exceed 300 mg) at bedtime.

ELDERLY PATIENTS

In general, lower dosages are recommended for these patients. Recommended starting dosage of amoxapine tablets is 25 mg two or three times daily. If no intolerance is observed, dosage may be increased by the end of the first week to 50 mg two or three times daily. Although 100-150 mg daily may be adequate for many elderly patients, some may require higher dosage. Careful increases up to 300 mg daily are indicated in such cases.

Once an effective dosage is established, amoxapine tablets may conveniently be given in a single bedtime dose, not to exceed 300 mg.

MAINTENANCE

Recommended maintenance dosage of amoxapine tablets is the lowest dose that will maintain remission. If symptoms reappear, dosage should be increased to the earlier level until they are controlled.

For maintenance therapy at dosages of 300 mg or less, a single dose at bedtime is recommended.

Store at controlled room temperature, 15 - 30° C (59 - 86° F). Dispense in a tight container.

HOW SUPPLIED - RATED THERAPEUTICALLY EQUIVALENT:

Tablet, Uncoated - Oral - 25 mg

100's	$32.87	Amoxapine, Harber Pharm	51432-0511-03
100's	$40.95	Amoxapine, H.C.F.A. F F P	99999-0230-01
100's	$41.03	Amoxapine, United Res	00677-1432-01
100's	$46.70	Amoxapine, HL Moore Drug Exch	00839-7604-06
100's	$49.20	Amoxapine, Qualitest Pharms	00603-2240-21
100's	$49.56	Amoxapine, Major Pharms	00904-3994-61
100's	$51.95	Amoxapine, Parmed Pharms	00349-8702-01
100's	$52.87	Amoxapine, Martec Pharms	52555-0539-01
100's	$52.95	Amoxapine, Schein Pharm (US)	00364-2432-01
100's	$52.95	Amoxapine, Major Pharms	00904-3994-60
100's	$52.97	Asendin, Rugby	00536-3003-01
100's	$61.45	Amoxapine, Geneva Pharms	00781-1844-01
100's	$61.48	Amoxapine 25, Goldline Labs	00182-1043-01
100's	$61.48	Amoxapine, Watson Labs	52544-0379-01
100's	$64.72	Amoxapine, Aligen Independ	00405-4076-01
100's	**$72.33**	**ASENDIN, Lederle Pharm**	**00005-5389-23**

HOW SUPPLIED - RATED THERAPEUTICALLY EQUIVALENT: *(cont'd)*

Tablet, Uncoated - Oral - 50 mg

10's	**$133.53**	**ASENDIN, Lederle Pharm**	**00005-5390-60**
100's	$53.44	Amoxapine, Harber Pharm	51432-0513-03
100's	$63.23	Amoxapine, United Res	00677-1378-01
100's	$63.23	Amoxapine, H.C.F.A. F F P	99999-0230-02
100's	$76.48	Amoxapine, HL Moore Drug Exch	00839-7605-06
100's	$78.54	Amoxapine, Major Pharms	00904-3995-61
100's	$82.95	Amoxapine, Parmed Pharms	00349-8703-01
100's	$83.85	Asendin, Rugby	00536-3004-01
100's	$84.20	Amoxapine, Major Pharms	00904-3995-60
100's	$85.41	Amoxapine, Qualitest Pharms	00603-2241-21
100's	$85.55	Amoxapine, Schein Pharm (US)	00364-2433-01
100's	$86.85	Amoxapine, Martec Pharms	52555-0540-01
100's	$99.90	Amoxapine, Geneva Pharms	00781-1845-01
100's	$99.95	Amoxapine 50, Goldline Labs	00182-1044-01
100's	$99.95	Amoxapine, Aligen Independ	00405-4077-01
100's	$99.95	Amoxapine, Watson Labs	52544-0380-01
100's	**$121.29**	**ASENDIN, Lederle Pharm**	**00005-5390-23**
500's	$285.00	Amoxapine, Bristol Myers Squibb	00003-3688-82
500's	$316.15	Amoxapine, H.C.F.A. F F P	99999-0230-03
500's	$474.34	Amoxapine, Watson Labs	52544-0380-05
500's	**$576.14**	**ASENDIN, Lederle Pharm**	**00005-5390-31**

Tablet, Uncoated - Oral - 100 mg

10's	**$208.38**	**ASENDIN, Lederle Pharm**	**00005-5391-60**
100's	$89.16	Amoxapine, Harber Pharm	51432-0518-03
100's	$110.70	Amoxapine, United Res	00677-1379-01
100's	$110.70	Amoxapine, H.C.F.A. F F P	99999-0230-04
100's	$128.99	Amoxapine, HL Moore Drug Exch	00839-7606-06
100's	$134.80	Amoxapine, Qualitest Pharms	00603-2242-21
100's	$135.70	Amoxapine, Major Pharms	00904-3996-60
100's	$138.77	Asendin, Rugby	00536-3005-01
100's	$139.95	Amoxapine, Parmed Pharms	00349-8709-01
100's	$143.47	Amoxapine, Martec Pharms	52555-0541-01
100's	$144.50	Amoxapine, Schein Pharm (US)	00364-2434-01
100's	$166.80	Amoxapine, Geneva Pharms	00781-1846-01
100's	$166.83	Amoxapine 100, Goldline Labs	00182-1045-01
100's	$166.83	Amoxapine, Aligen Independ	00405-4078-01
100's	$166.83	Amoxapine, Watson Labs	52544-0381-01
100's	**$196.27**	**ASENDIN, Lederle Pharm**	**00005-5391-23**

Tablet, Uncoated - Oral - 150 mg

30's	$42.16	Amoxapine, Harber Pharm	51432-0519-30
30's	$50.55	Amoxapine, United Res	00677-1380-07
30's	$50.55	Amoxapine, H.C.F.A. F F P	99999-0230-05
30's	$60.95	Amoxapine, HL Moore Drug Exch	00839-7607-19
30's	$62.95	Amoxapine, Major Pharms	00904-3997-46
30's	$63.15	Amoxapine, Qualitest Pharms	00603-2243-16
30's	$66.86	Asendin, Rugby	00536-3006-07
30's	$67.51	Amoxapine, Schein Pharm (US)	00364-2435-30
30's	$67.85	Amoxapine, Martec Pharms	52555-0542-30
30's	$70.00	Amoxapine, Geneva Pharms	00781-1847-31
30's	$78.90	Amoxapine 150, Goldline Labs	00182-1046-17
30's	$78.90	Amoxapine, Aligen Independ	00405-4079-30
30's	$78.90	Amoxapine, Watson Labs	52544-0382-30
30's	**$92.82**	**ASENDIN, Lederle Pharm**	**00005-5392-38**
100's	$43.87	Amoxapine, Rugby	00536-3006-01
100's	$168.50	Amoxapine, H.C.F.A. F F P	99999-0230-06
100's	$249.85	Amoxapine, Watson Labs	52544-0382-01

AMOXICILLIN *(000231)*

CATEGORIES: Anti-Infectives; Antibacterials; Antibiotics; Antimicrobials; Gonorrhea; Infections; Influenza; Neuromuscular; Penicillins; Respiratory Tract Infections; Sexually Transmitted Diseases; H. Pylori*; Lyme Disease*; Otitis Media*; Peptic Ulcer*; Skeletal Muscle Hyperactivity*; Ulcer*; Pregnancy Category B; Sales > $500 Million; FDA Approval Pre 1982; Top 200 Drugs
* Indication not approved by the FDA

BRAND NAMES: *Abdimox*; A-Cillin; *Acimox* (Mexico); *Actimoxi*; *Adbiotin*; *Agerpen*; *A-Gram* (France); *Alfamox*; *Almodan* (England); *Aloxyn* (Germany); *Alphamox* (Australia); *AM 73*; *Amagesen Solutab* (Germany); *Amcill*; *Amoclen*; *Amodex* (France); *Amo-flamsian*; *Amoflux*; *Amolin* (Japan); *Amosine*; *Amox*; *Amoxa*; *Amoxal*; *Amoxapen*; *Amoxaren*; *Amoxcillin*; *Amoxi*; *Amoxi-basan* (Germany); *Amoxibiotic*; *Amoxicilina*; Amoxicillin Trihydrate; *Amoxidal*; *Amoxiden*; *Amoxidin*; *Amoxihexal* (Germany); **Amoxil**; *Amoxillin*; *Amoxin*; *Amoxipen*; *Amoxipenil*; *Amoxisol* (Mexico); *Amoxivan*; *Amoxivet* (Mexico); *Amoxtrex*; *Amoxy*; *Amoxybid*; *Amoxycillin*; *Amoxy-diolan* (Germany); *Amoxypen* (Germany); *Ampidroxyl*; *Anemol*; *Apitart*; *Apo-Amoxi*; *Ardine*; *Aspenil*; *Audumic*; *Azillin*; *Bactamox*; *Bimox*; *Bintamox*; Biomox; *Bioxidona*; *Bioxyllin*; *Bridopen*; *Bristamox* (France); *Cabermox*; *Cilamox* (Australia); *Clamox*; *Clamoxyl* (Australia, France, Germany, Japan); *Clavoxilin*; *Coamoxin*; Colmox; Comox; *Comoxyl*; *Damoxicil*; *Delacillin*; *Deniren*; *Draximox*; *Efpinex* (Japan); Entamox; *Eupen*; *Excillin*; *Farconcil*; *Fisamox* (Australia); *Flemoxin*; *Fullcilina*; *Gemox*; *Gimalxina* (Mexico); *Gomcillin*; *Grinsul*; *Grunamox*; *Hiconcil* (France); *Hidramox* (Mexico); *Hipen*; *Hosboral*; *Ibiamox*; *Ikamoxil*; *Imacillin*; *Imaxilin*; *Imox*; *Imoxil*; *Intermox*; *Isimoxin*; *Izoltil*; *Jerramcil*; *Kamoxin*; *Kymoxin*; *Lamoxy*; *Larocilin*; Larotid; *Limox*; *Majorpen*; *Matasedrin*; *Maxcil*; *Medimox*; *Meixil*; *Mopen*; *Morgenxil*; *Mox*; *Moxacin* (Australia); *Moxaline*; *Moxarin*; *Moxcil*; *Moxilen*; *Moxlin*; *Moxylin*; *Moxypen*; *Moxyvit*; *Novabritine*; *Novamoxin* (Canada); *Novenzymin*; *Optium*; *Ospamox*; *Pamocil*; *Pamoxin*; *Pamoxicillin*; *Pasetocin* (Japan); *Penamox* (Mexico); *Penbiosyn*; *Penmox*; *Pensyn*; *Piramox*; Polymox; *Posmox*; *Protexillin*; *Rancil*; *Ranmoxy*; *Ranoxyl*; *Reloxyl*; *Respimox*; *Rhamoxilina*; *Robamox*; *Rocillin*; Romoxil; *Saltermox*; *Samosillin*; *Samthongcillin*; *Sawacillin* (Japan); *Sawamezin* (Japan); Senox; *Servamox*; *Sia-mox*; *Sigmopen*; *Sil-A-mox*; *Simoxil*; *Simplamox*; *Specillin*; *Supercillin*; *Superpeni*; *Supramox*; *Suprapen*; *Teramoxyl*; *Tolodina*; *Triafamox*; *Triamoxil*; *Trilaxin*; Trimox; *Twicyl*; *Unicillin*; Utimox; *Velamox*; *Virgoxillin*; *Widecillin*; *Winmox*; Wymox; *Yisulon*; *Zamocillin*; *Zamox*; *Zamoxil*; *Zerrsox*; *Zimox*
(International brand names outside U.S. in italics)

FORMULARIES: Aetna; BC-BS; CIGNA; DoD; FHP; Foundation; Humana; Kaiser; Medco; Medi-Cal; PCS; PruCare; United; WHO

COST OF THERAPY: $7.05 (Respiratory Infections; Capsule; 500 mg; 3/day; 14 days)

WARNING:
SERIOUS AND OCCASIONALLY FATAL HYPERSENSITIVITY (ANAPHYLACTIC) REACTIONS HAVE BEEN REPORTED IN PATIENTS ON PENICILLIN THERAPY. ALTHOUGH ANAPHYLAXIS IS MORE FREQUENT FOLLOWING PARENTERAL THERAPY, IT HAS OCCURRED IN PATIENTS ON ORAL PENICILLINS. THESE REACTIONS ARE MORE LIKELY TO OCCUR IN INDIVIDUALS WITH A HISTORY OF PENICILLIN HYPERSENSITIVITY AND OR A HISTORY OF SENSITIVITY TO MULTIPLE ALLERGENS. THERE HAVE BEEN REPORTS OF INDIVIDUALS WITH A HISTORY OF PENICILLIN HYPERSENSITIVITY WHO HAVE EXPERIENCED SEVERE REACTIONS WHEN TREATED WITH CEPHALOSPORINS. BEFORE INITIATING THERAPY WITH AMOXICILLIN, CAREFUL INQUIRY SHOULD BE MADE CONCERNING PREVIOUS HYPERSENSITIVITY REACTIONS TO PENICILLINS, CEPHALOSPORINS, OR OTHER ALLERGENS. IF AN ALLERGIC REACTION OCCURS, AMOXICILLIN SHOULD BE DISCONTINUED AND APPROPRIATE THERAPY INSTITUTED. SERIOUS ANAPHYLACTIC REACTIONS REQUIRE IMMEDIATE EMERGENCY TREATMENT WITH EPINEPHRINE. OXYGEN, INTRAVENOUS STEROIDS, AND AIRWAY MANAGEMENT, INCLUDING INTUBATION, SHOULD ALSO BE ADMINISTERED AS INDICATED.

DESCRIPTION:

Amoxicillin is a semisynthetic penicillin, an analog of ampicillin, with a broad spectrum of bactericidal activity against many gram-positive and gram-negative microorganisms. Chemically it is D-(-)-α-amino-p-hydroxybenzyl penicillin trihydrate.

Amoxicillin capsules, tablets and powder for oral suspension are intended for oral administration.

Amoxil Capsules: Each capsule, with royal blue opaque cap and pink opaque body, contains 250 mg or 500 mg amoxicillin as the trihydrate. Inactive ingredients: D&C Red No. 28, FD&C Blue No. 1, FD&C Red No. 40, gelatin, magnesium stearate, magnesium sulfate and titanium dioxide.

Amoxil Tablets: Each oval, pink, cherry-banana-peppermint-flavored tablet contains 125 mg or 250 mg amoxicillin as the trihydrate. The tablets are imprinted with the product name AMOXIL on one side and 125 or 250 on the other side. Inactive ingredients: citric acid, corn starch, FD&C Red No. 40, flavorings, glycine, mannitol, magnesium stearate, saccharin sodium, silica gel and sucrose.

Amoxil Oral Suspension: Each 5 ml of reconstituted suspension contains 125 mg or 250 mg amoxicillin as the trihydrate. The oral suspension 125 mg/5 ml (reconstituted) is a strawberry-flavored pink suspension; the 250 mg/5 ml or 50 mg/ml is a bubble-gum flavored pink suspension. Inactive ingredients: FD&C Red No. 3, flavorings, silica gel, sodium benzoate, sodium citrate, sucrose and xanthan gum.

Pediatric Drops for Oral Suspension: Each ml of reconstituted suspension contains 50 mg amoxicillin as the trihydrate.

CLINICAL PHARMACOLOGY:

Amoxicillin is stable in the presence of gastric acid and is well absorbed from the gastrointestinal tract and may be given without regard to meals. It is rapidly absorbed after oral administration. It diffuses readily into most body tissues and fluids, with the exception of brain and spinal fluid, except when meninges are inflamed. The half-life of amoxicillin is 61.3 minutes. Most of the amoxicillin is excreted unchanged in the urine; its excretion can be delayed by concurrent administration of probenecid. Amoxicillin is not highly protein-bound. In blood serum, amoxicillin is approximately 20% protein-bound as compared to 60% for penicillin G.

Orally administered doses of 250 mg and 500 mg amoxicillin capsules result in average peak blood levels one to two hours after administration in the range of 3.5 mcg/ml to 5.0 mcg/ml and 5.5 mcg/ml to 7.5 mcg/ml respectively.

Orally administered doses of amoxicillin suspension 125 mg/5 ml and 250 mg/5 ml result in average peak blood levels one to two hours after administration in the range of 1.5 mcg/ml to 3.0 mcg/ml and 3.5 mcg/ml to 5.0 mcg/ml respectively. Amoxicillin chewable tablets, 125 mg and 250 mg, produced blood levels similar to those achieved with the corresponding doses of amoxicillin oral suspensions.

Detectable serum levels are observed up to 8 hours after an orally administered dose of amoxicillin. Following a 1 g dose and utilizing a special skin window technique to determine levels of the antibiotic, it was noted that therapeutic levels were found in the interstitial fluid. Approximately 60 percent of an orally administered dose of amoxicillin is excreted in the urine within 6 to 8 hours.

MICROBIOLOGY

Amoxicillin is similar to ampicillin in its bactericidal action against susceptible organisms during the stage of active multiplication. It acts through the inhibition of biosynthesis of cell wall mucopeptide. While *in vitro* studies have demonstrated the susceptibility of most strains of the following gram-positive bacteria:

alpha-and beta-hemolytic streptococci

Diplococcus pneumoniae

nonpenicillinase-producing staphylococci

Streptococcus faecalis

Clinical efficacy for infections other than those indicated in INDICATIONS AND USAGE has not been documented. It is active *in vitro* against many strains of *Haemophilus influenzae, Neisseria gonorrhoeae, Escherichia coli* and *Proteus mirabilis.* Because it does not resist destruction by penicillinase, it is not effective against penicillinase-producing bacteria, particularly resistant staphylococci. All strains of *Pseudomonas* and most strains of *Klebsiella* and *Enterobacter* are resistant.

CLINICAL STUDIES:

Disk Susceptibility Tests: Quantitative methods that require measurement of zone diameters give the most precise estimates of antibiotic susceptibility. One such procedure[1] has been recommended for use with disks for testing susceptibility to ampicillin-class antibiotics. Interpretations correlate diameters of the disk test with MIC values for amoxicillin. With this procedure, a report from the laboratory of "susceptible" indicates that the infecting organism is likely to respond to therapy. A report of "resistant" indicates that the infecting organism is not likely to respond to therapy. A report of "intermediate susceptibility" suggests that the organism would be susceptible if high dosage is used, or if the infection is confined to tissues and fluids (*e.g.,* urine), in which high antibiotic levels are attained.

INDICATIONS AND USAGE:

Amoxicillin is indicated in the treatment of infections due to susceptible strains of the following:

Gram-negative organisms: *H. influenzae, E. coli, P. mirabilis* and *N. gonorrhoea*

Gram-positive organisms: Streptococci (including *Streptococcus faecalis*), *D. pneumoniae* and nonpenicillinase-producing staphylococci.

Therapy may be instituted prior to obtaining results from bacteriological and susceptibility studies to determine the causative organisms and their susceptibility to amoxicillin.

Indicated surgical procedures should be performed.

CONTRAINDICATIONS:

A history of allergic reaction to any of the penicillins is a contraindication.

WARNINGS:

Pseudomembranous colitis has been reported with nearly all antibacterial agents, including amoxicillin, and may range in severity from mild to life-threatening. Therefore, it is important to consider this diagnosis in patients who present with diarrhea subsequent to the administration of antibacterial agents.

Treatment with antibacterial agents alters the normal flora of the colon and may permit overgrowth of clostridia. Studies indicate that a toxin produced by *Clostridium difficile* is a primary cause of "antibiotic-associated colitis."

After the diagnosis of pseudomembranous colitis has been established, therapeutic measures should be initiated. Mild cases of pseudomembranous colitis usually respond to drug discontinuation alone. In moderate to severe cases, consideration should be given to management with fluids and electrolytes, protein supplementation and treatment with an antibacterial drug clinically effective against *C. difficile* colitis.

Usage In Pregnancy: Safety for use in pregnancy has not been established.

PRECAUTIONS:

General: The possibility of superinfections with mycotic organisms or bacterial pathogens should be kept in mind during therapy. In such cases, (usually involving *Enterobacter, Pseudomonas* or *Candida*), discontinue the drug and substitute appropriate treatment.

Laboratory Tests: As with any potent drug, periodic assessment of renal, hepatic and hematopoietic function should be made during prolonged therapy.

Cases of gonorrhea with a suspected lesion of syphilis should have darkfield examinations before receiving amoxilcillin, and monthly serological tests for a minimum of four months

Carcinogenesis, Mutagenesis, and Impairment of Fertility: Long term studies in animals have not been performed with these drugs.

Pregnancy Category B: Reproduction studies have been performed in mice and rats at doses up to ten (10) times the maximum human dose and have revealed no evidence of impaired fertility or harm to the fetus due to amoxicillin. There are however, no adequate and well-controlled studies in pregnant women. Because animal reproductive studies are not always predictive of human response, this drug should be used during pregnancy only if clearly needed.

Labor and Delivery: Oral ampicillin-class antibiotics are poorly absorbed during labor. Studies in guinea pigs showed that intravenous administration of ampicillin slightly decreased the uterine tone and frequency of contractions, but moderately increased the height and duration of the contractions. However, it is not known whether the use of these drugs in humans during labor or delivery has immediate or delayed adverse effects on the fetus, prolongs the duration of labor, or increases the likelihood that forceps delivery or other obstetrical intervention or resuscitation of the newborn will be necessary.

Nursing Mothers: Amoxicillin is excreted in human milk in very small amounts. Therefore, caution should be exercised when amoxicillin is administered to a nursing woman.

Pediatric Use: Guidelines for administration of amoxicillin to pediatric patients are presented in DOSAGE AND ADMINISTRATION.

ADVERSE REACTIONS:

As with other penicillins, it may be expected that untoward reactions will be essentially limited to sensitivity phenomena. They are more likely to occur in individuals who have previously demonstrated hypersensitivity to penicillins and in those with a history of allergy, asthma, hay fever or urticaria. The following adverse reactions have been reported as associated with the use of penicillin:

Gastrointestinal: Glossitis, stomatitis, black "hairy" tongue, nausea, vomiting and diarrhea (these reactions are usually associated with oral dosage forms).

Hypersensitivity Reactions: Erythematous maculopapular rashes, erythema multiforme, Stevens-Johnson Syndrome, toxic epidermal necrolysis and urticaria have been reported. *NOTE:* These hypersensitivity reactions may be controlled with antihistamines and, if necessary, systemic corticosteroids. Whenever such reactions occur, amoxicillin should be discontinued unless, in the opinion of the physician, the condition being treated is life-threatening and amenable only to penicillin therapy. Serious anaphylactic reactions require the immediate use of epinephrine, oxygen, and intravenous steroids.

Liver: A moderate rise in serum glutamic oxaloacetic transaminase (SGOT) has been noted, but the significance of this finding is unknown.

Hemic and Lymphatic Systems: Anemia, thrombocytopenia, thrombocytopenic purpura, eosinophilia, leukopenia and agranulocytosis have been reported during therapy with penicillins. These reactions are usually reversible on discontinuation of therapy and are believed to be hypersensitivity phenomena.

Central Nervous System: Reversible hyperactivity, agitation, anxiety, insomnia, confusion, behavioral changes, and/or dizziness have been reported rarely.

DOSAGE AND ADMINISTRATION:

Infections of the ear, nose and throat due to streptococci, pneumococci, nonpenicillinase-producing staphylococci and *H. influenzae.*

Infections of the genitourinary tract due to *E. coli, Proteus mirabilis* and *Streptococcus faecalis.*

Infections of the skin and soft-tissues due to streptococci, susceptible staphylococci and *E. coli:*

TABLE 1 Usual Dosage for Infections of the Skin and Soft-Tissues

Adults:	250 mg every 8 hours
Children:	20 mg/kg/day in divided doses every 8 hours

Children weighing 20 kg or more should be dosed according to the adult recommendations.

In severe infections or those caused by less susceptible organisms:

500 mg every 8 hours for adults and 40 mg/kg/day in divided doses every 8 hours for children may be needed.

DOSAGE AND ADMINISTRATION: *(cont'd)*

Infections of the lower respiratory tract due to streptococci, pneumococci, nonpenicillinase-producing staphylococci and *H. influenzae:*

TABLE 2 Usual Dosage for Infections of the Lower Respiratory Tract

Adults:	500 mg every 8 hours
Children:	40 mg/kg/day in divided doses every 8 hours

Children weighing 20 kg or more should be dosed according to the adult recommendations.

Gonorrhea, Acute Uncomplicated: Ano-genital and urethral infections due to *N. gonorrhoeae* (males and females):

TABLE 3 Usual Dosage for Gonorrhea, Acute Uncomplicated

Adults:	3 grams as a single oral dose
Prepubertal children:	50 mg/kg amoxicillin combined with 25 mg/kg probenecid as a single dose

Note: Since probenecid is contraindicated in children under 2 years, this regimen should not be used in these cases.

LARGER DOSES MAY BE REQUIRED FOR STUBBORN OR SEVERE INFECTIONS.

THE CHILDREN'S DOSAGE IS INTENDED FOR INDIVIDUALS WHOSE WEIGHT WILL NOT CAUSE A DOSAGE TO BE CALCULATED GREATER THAN THAT RECOMMENDED FOR ADULTS.

IT SHOULD BE RECOGNIZED THAT IN THE TREATMENT OF CHRONIC URINARY TRACT INFECTIONS, FREQUENT BACTERIOLOGICAL AND CLINICAL APPRAISALS ARE NECESSARY. SMALLER DOSES THAN THOSE RECOMMENDED ABOVE SHOULD NOT BE USED. EVEN HIGHER DOSES MAY BE NEEDED AT TIMES. IN STUBBORN INFECTIONS, THERAPY MAY BE REQUIRED FOR SEVERAL WEEKS. IT MAY BE NECESSARY TO CONTINUE CLINICAL AND/OR BACTERIOLOGICAL FOLLOW-UP FOR SEVERAL MONTHS AFTER CESSATION OF THERAPY. EXCEPT FOR GONORRHEA, TREATMENT SHOULD BE CONTINUED FOR A MINIMUM OF 48 TO 72 HOURS BEYOND THE TIME THAT THE PATIENT BECOMES ASYMPTOMATIC OR EVIDENCE OF BACTERIAL ERADICATION HAS BEEN OBTAINED. IT IS RECOMMENDED THAT THERE BE AT LEAST 10 DAYS' TREATMENT FOR ANY INFECTION CAUSED BY HEMOLYTIC STREPTOCOCCI TO PREVENT THE OCCURRENCE OF ACUTE RHEUMATIC FEVER OR GLOMERULONEPHRITIS.

DOSAGE AND ADMINISTRATION OF PEDIATRIC DROPS: Usual dosage for all indications except infections of the lower respiratory tract:

TABLE 4 Dosage and Administration of Pediatric Drops

Under 6 kg (13 lbs):	0.75 ml every 8 hours
6 to 7 kg (13 to 15 lbs):	1.0 ml every 8 hours
8 kg (16 to 18 lbs):	1.25 ml every 8 hours

TABLE 5 Infections Of The Lower Respiratory Tract

Under 6 kg (13 lbs):	1.25 ml every 8 hours
6 to 7 kg (13 to 15 lbs):	1.75 ml every 8 hours
8 kg (16 to 18 lbs):	2.25 ml every 8 hours

Children weighing more than 8 kg (18 lbs) should receive the appropriate dose of the oral suspension 125 mg or 250 mg/5 ml.

After reconstitution, the required amount of suspension should be placed directly on the child's tongue for swallowing. Alternate means of administration are to add the required amount of suspension to formula, milk, fruit juice, water, ginger ale or cold drinks. These preparations should then be taken immediately. To be certain the child is receiving full dosage, such preparations should be consumed in entirety.

Directions For Mixing Oral Suspension: Prepare suspension at time of dispensing as follows: Tap bottle until all powder flows freely. Add approximately 1/3 of the total amount of water for reconstitution (see TABLE 6) and shake vigorously to wet powder. Add remainder of the water and again shake vigorously.

TABLE 6

	Amount of Water Required for Reconstitution	
Bottle Size	**125 mg per 5 ml**	**250 mg per 5 ml**
80 ml	62 ml*	59 ml†
100 ml	78 ml*	74 ml†
150 ml	116 ml*	111 ml†
125 mg unit dose	5 ml	–
250 mg unit dose	–	5 ml

* Each teaspoonful (5 ml) will contain 125 mg amoxicillin.
† Each teaspoonful (5 ml) will contain 250 mg amoxicillin.

Directions For Mixing Pediatric Drops: Prepare pediatric drops at time of dispensing as follows: Add the required amount of water (see TABLE 7) to the bottle and shake vigorously. Each ml of suspension will then contain amoxicillin trihydrate equivalent to 50 mg amoxicillin.

TABLE 7

Bottle Size	**Amount of Water Required for Reconstitution**
15 ml	12 ml
30 ml	23 ml

NOTE: SHAKE BOTH ORAL SUSPENSION AND PEDIATRIC DROPS WELL BEFORE USING. Keep bottle tightly closed. Any unused portion of the reconstituted suspension must be discarded after 14 days. Refrigeration preferable, but not required.

REFERENCES:

1. Bauer, A. W., Kirby, W. M. M., Sherris, J. C., and Turck, M.: Antibiotic Testing by a Standardized Single Disc Method, Am. J. Clin. Pathol., 45:493, 1966. Standardized Disc Susceptibility Test, Federal Register 37: 20527-29, 1972.

PATIENT INFORMATION:

Amoxicillin is an antibiotic for treatment of infection.

Take at regular intervals, around the clock. Always finish course of therapy.

Take with or without meals.

PATIENT INFORMATION: *(cont'd)*

May cause serious allergic reactions in those with penicillin allergy.

May cause nausea, vomiting and diarrhea; notify your doctor or pharmacist if these occur.

HOW SUPPLIED - RATED THERAPEUTICALLY EQUIVALENT:

Capsule, Gelatin - Oral - 250 mg

30's	$2.31	Amoxicillin, H.C.F.A. F F P	99999-0231-01
30's	$5.87	Amoxicillin, Novopharm (US)	55953-0724-27
30's	$7.00	Amoxicillin, Teva	00332-3107-04
30's	$7.14	Amoxicillin, Talbert Phcy	44514-0076-18
100's	$7.73	Amoxicillin, H.C.F.A. F F P	99999-0231-02
100's	$9.00	MOXILIN, Intl Ethical	11584-0391-00
100's	$10.88	Amoxicillin, IDE-Interstate	00814-0690-14
100's	$12.25	Amoxicillin, Raway	00686-0600-20
100's	$12.40	Amoxicillin, Novopharm (US)	55953-0724-40
100's	$12.49	POLYMOX, Mead Johnson	00015-7278-58
100's	$15.29	Amoxicillin, Novopharm (US)	55953-0724-01
100's	$15.95	Amoxicillin, Major Pharms	00904-2617-60
100's	$16.50	Amoxicillin, Teva	00093-0613-01
100's	$16.73	Amoxicillin, HL Moore Drug Exch	00839-6037-06
100's	$19.50	Amoxicillin, Martec Pharms	52555-0148-01
100's	$19.80	Amoxicillin, Geneva Pharms	00781-2020-01
100's	$19.95	Senox, Seneca Pharms	47028-0053-01
100's	$20.25	Amoxicillin, Schein Pharm (US)	00364-2040-01
100's	$20.43	Amoxil, Rugby	00536-0070-01
100's	$20.95	Amoxicillin, Goldline Labs	00182-1070-01
100's	$20.95	Amoxicillin, Teva	00332-3107-09
100's	$21.05	WYMOX, Wyeth Labs	00008-0559-01
100's	**$21.60**	**AMOXIL, Beecham**	**00029-6006-30**
100's	**$21.60**	**AMOXIL, Beecham**	**00029-6006-31**
100's	$21.67	Amoxicillin, United Res	00677-0660-01
100's	$21.72	Amoxicillin, Lederle Pharm	00005-3144-23
100's	$21.79	Amoxicillin, Dupont Pharma	00056-0153-70
100's	$22.05	Amoxicillin, Aligen Independ	00405-4083-01
100's	$23.95	Amoxicillin, Major Pharms	00904-2617-61
100's	$24.76	Amoxicillin, Warner Chilcott	00047-0730-24
100's	$24.89	TRIMOX, Bristol Myers Squibb	00003-0101-50
100's	$24.89	TRIMOX, Bristol Myers Squibb	00003-0101-51
100's	$24.95	TRIMOX 250, Bristol Myers Squibb	00003-0230-51
100's	$24.97	Amoxicillin, Qualitest Pharms	00603-2266-21
100's	$25.10	Amoxicillin Trihydrate, Mylan	00378-0204-01
100's	$26.50	Amoxicillin, Goldline Labs	00182-1070-89
500's	$38.65	Amoxicillin, H.C.F.A. F F P	99999-0231-03
500's	$46.05	Amoxicillin, IDE-Interstate	00814-0690-28
500's	$56.83	Amoxicillin, Novopharm (US)	55953-0724-70
500's	$61.25	Amoxicillin, Major Pharms	00904-2617-40
500's	$62.48	POLYMOX, Mead Johnson	00015-7278-86
500's	$73.67	Amoxicillin, Labs Atral	53862-0100-02
500's	$75.00	Amoxicillin, Teva	00093-0613-05
500's	$75.50	Amoxicillin, United Res	00677-0660-05
500's	$77.69	Amoxicillin, HL Moore Drug Exch	00839-6037-12
500's	$82.00	Amoxicillin, Geneva Pharms	00781-2020-05
500's	$89.00	Amoxicillin, Martec Pharms	52555-0148-05
500's	$91.00	Amoxicillin, Schein Pharm (US)	00364-2040-05
500's	$94.50	WYMOX, Wyeth Labs	00008-0559-02
500's	$99.85	Amoxicillin, Goldline Labs	00182-1070-05
500's	$99.85	Amoxicillin, Teva	00332-3107-13
500's	$99.90	Amoxil, Rugby	00536-0070-05
500's	$101.95	Amoxicillin, Dupont Pharma	00056-0153-85
500's	**$102.90**	**AMOXIL, Beecham**	**00029-6006-32**
500's	$103.44	Amoxicillin, Lederle Pharm	00005-3144-31
500's	$107.75	Amoxicillin, Parmed Pharms	00349-0190-05
500's	$110.12	Amoxicillin, Aligen Independ	00405-4083-02
500's	$117.09	Amoxicillin, Amer Preferred	53445-1070-05
500's	$118.53	TRIMOX, Bristol Myers Squibb	00003-0101-60
500's	$118.82	Amoxicillin, Warner Chilcott	00047-0730-30
500's	$118.95	Amoxicillin, Mylan	00378-0204-05
500's	$118.95	Amoxicillin, Qualitest Pharms	00603-2266-28
1000's	$77.30	Amoxicillin, H.C.F.A. F F P	99999-0231-04
1000's	$107.98	Amoxicillin, Novopharm (US)	55953-0724-80
1000's	$133.80	Amoxicillin, Parmed Pharms	00349-0190-10

Capsule, Gelatin - Oral - 500 mg

30's	$6.65	Amoxicillin, Talbert Phcy	44514-0077-18
30's	$6.88	Amoxicillin, H.C.F.A. F F P	99999-0231-05
30's	$8.85	Amoxicillin, Novopharm (US)	55953-0716-27
30's	$13.75	Amoxicillin, Teva	00332-3109-04
50's	$10.88	Amoxicillin, IDE-Interstate	00814-0692-08
50's	$11.47	Amoxicillin, H.C.F.A. F F P	99999-0231-06
50's	$12.40	Amoxicillin, Novopharm (US)	55953-0716-33
50's	$15.75	Amoxicillin, Teva	00093-0615-53
50's	$16.19	Amoxicillin, HL Moore Drug Exch	00839-6038-04
50's	$16.95	Amoxicillin, Major Pharms	00904-2618-51
50's	$19.60	Amoxicillin, Martec Pharms	52555-0149-00
50's	$19.70	WYMOX, Wyeth Labs	00008-0560-01
50's	$20.25	Amoxicillin, United Res	00677-0661-02
50's	$20.31	Amoxicillin, Lederle Pharm	00005-3145-18
50's	$21.60	Amoxicillin, Schein Pharm (US)	00364-2041-50
50's	$23.00	Amoxil, Rugby	00536-0080-06
50's	$23.35	Amoxicillin, Goldline Labs	00182-1071-19
50's	$23.35	Amoxicillin, Teva	00332-3109-07
50's	$23.35	Amoxicillin, Aligen Independ	00405-4084-50
50's	$23.35	Amoxicillin, Qualitest Pharms	00603-2267-19
50's	$23.50	Amoxicillin, Mylan	00378-0205-89
100's	$16.80	MOXILIN, Intl Ethical	11584-0401-00
100's	$17.95	Amoxicillin, Raway	00686-0601-20
100's	$22.94	Amoxicillin, H.C.F.A. F F P	99999-0231-07
100's	$23.27	Amoxicillin, Novopharm (US)	55953-0716-40
100's	$24.74	POLYMOX, Mead Johnson	00015-7279-58
100's	$24.95	Amoxicillin, Warner Chilcott	00047-0731-24
100's	$26.15	Amoxicillin, Novopharm (US)	55953-0716-01
100's	$39.00	Amoxicillin, United Res	00677-0661-01
100's	$39.00	Amoxicillin, Geneva Pharms	00781-2613-01
100's	$39.95	Amoxicillin, Dupont Pharma	00056-0154-70
100's	**$40.40**	**AMOXIL, Beecham**	**00029-6007-30**
100's	**$41.10**	**AMOXIL, Beecham**	**00029-6007-31**
100's	$43.41	Trimox, Bristol Myers Squibb	00003-0109-55
100's	$45.50	Amoxicillin, Goldline Labs	00182-1071-89
100's	$46.53	TRIMOX 500, Bristol Myers Squibb	00003-0109-51
250's	$57.35	Amoxicillin, H.C.F.A. F F P	99999-0231-08
250's	$96.20	Amoxil, Rugby	00536-0080-02
500's	$81.60	MOXILIN, Intl Ethical	11584-0405-00
500's	$83.78	Amoxicillin, IDE-Interstate	00814-0692-28
500's	$110.77	Amoxicillin, Novopharm (US)	55953-0716-70

HOW SUPPLIED - RATED THERAPEUTICALLY EQUIVALENT: *(cont'd)*

500's	$114.70	Amoxicillin, H.C.F.A. F F P	99999-0231-09
500's	$117.50	Amoxicillin, Aligen Independ	00405-4084-02
500's	$123.97	POLYMOX, Mead Johnson	00015-7279-86
500's	$136.00	Amoxicillin, Teva	00093-0615-05
500's	$145.10	Amoxicillin, Major Pharms	00904-2618-40
500's	$145.93	Amoxicillin, Labs Atral	53862-0200-03
500's	$148.49	Amoxicillin, HL Moore Drug Exch	00839-6038-12
500's	$157.00	Amoxicillin, Martec Pharms	52555-0149-05
500's	$170.91	Amoxil, Rugby	00536-0080-05
500's	$172.88	Amoxicillin, Qualitest Pharms	00603-2267-28
500's	$174.98	Amoxicillin, United Res	00677-0661-05
500's	$175.00	Amoxicillin, Geneva Pharms	00781-2613-05
500's	$175.50	WYMOX, Wyeth Labs	00008-0560-02
500's	$177.19	Amoxicillin, Schein Pharm (US)	00364-2041-05
500's	$184.48	Amoxicillin, Warner Chilcott	00047-0731-30
500's	$184.48	Amoxicillin, Goldline Labs	00182-1071-05
500's	$184.48	Amoxicillin, Teva	00332-3109-13
500's	$189.00	Amoxicillin, Parmed Pharms	00349-0999-05
500's	$189.09	Amoxicillin, Amer Preferred	53445-1071-05
500's	**$189.90**	**AMOXIL, Beecham**	**00029-6007-32**
500's	$190.31	TRIMOX, Bristol Myers Squibb	00003-0109-60
500's	$190.94	Amoxicillin, Lederle Pharm	00005-3145-31
500's	$194.50	Amoxicillin, Dupont Pharma	00056-0154-85
500's	$196.95	Amoxicillin, Mylan	00378-0205-05
1000's	$210.46	Amoxicillin, Novopharm (US)	55953-0716-80
1000's	$229.00	Amoxicillin, Parmed Pharms	00349-0999-10
1000's	$229.40	Amoxicillin, H.C.F.A. F F P	99999-0231-10

Powder, Reconstitution - Oral - 125 mg/5ml

5 ml x 10	**$1.00**	**AMOXIL, Beecham**	**00029-6008-18**
5 ml x 100	$108.50	TRIMOX 125, Bristol Myers Squibb	00003-1737-25
80 ml	$1.95	Amoxicillin, IDE-Interstate	00814-0700-52
80 ml	$2.24	Amoxicillin, H.C.F.A. F F P	99999-0231-11
80 ml	$2.50	Amoxicillin, Harber Pharm	51432-0691-13
80 ml	$2.69	Amoxicillin, HL Moore Drug Exch	00839-6115-71
80 ml	$2.72	Amoxicillin, Lederle Pharm	00005-3146-43
80 ml	$2.80	Amoxil, Rugby	00536-0090-81
80 ml	$2.90	Amoxicillin, Schein Pharm (US)	00364-7215-60
80 ml	$2.98	Amoxicillin, Dupont Pharma	00056-0249-34
80 ml	$3.08	Amoxicillin, Novopharm (US)	55953-0149-38
80 ml	$3.10	TRIMOX 125, Bristol Myers Squibb	00003-1737-30
80 ml	$3.12	Amoxicillin, Warner Chilcott	00047-2500-16
80 ml	$3.12	Amoxicillin, Teva	00332-4150-30
80 ml	$3.22	Amoxicillin, Aligen Independ	00405-2225-58
80 ml o/s	$1.72	POLYMOX, Mead Johnson	00015-7276-70
80 ml x 6	**$2.70**	**AMOXIL, Beecham**	**00029-6008-21**
100 ml	$1.73	Amoxicillin, H.C.F.A. F F P	99999-0231-12
100 ml	$2.10	Amoxicillin, IDE-Interstate	00814-0700-54
100 ml	$2.82	Amoxicillin, HL Moore Drug Exch	00839-6115-73
100 ml	$2.95	Amoxicillin, Major Pharms	00904-2619-04
100 ml	$3.00	WYMOX, Wyeth Labs	00008-0557-02
100 ml	$3.12	Amoxicillin, Lederle Pharm	00005-3146-46
100 ml	$3.25	Amoxicillin, Harber Pharm	51432-0691-14
100 ml	$3.29	Amoxicillin, Dupont Pharma	00056-0249-36
100 ml	$3.37	Amoxicillin, Novopharm (US)	55953-0149-40
100 ml	$3.40	Amoxil, Rugby	00536-0090-82
100 ml	$3.47	Amoxicillin, Martec Pharms	52555-0141-01
100 ml	$3.55	Amoxicillin, United Res	00677-0452-27
100 ml	$3.56	TRIMOX 125, Bristol Myers Squibb	00003-1737-40
100 ml	$3.59	Amoxicillin, Warner Chilcott	00047-2500-17
100 ml	$3.59	Amoxicillin, Goldline Labs	00182-1072-70
100 ml	$3.59	Amoxicillin, Teva	00332-4150-32
100 ml	$3.59	Amoxicillin, Aligen Independ	00405-2225-60
100 ml	$3.59	Amoxicillin, Qualitest Pharms	00603-6500-64
100 ml	$3.73	Amoxicillin, Schein Pharm (US)	00364-7215-61
100 ml	$3.76	Amoxicillin, Mylan	00378-0206-02
100 ml o/s	$2.12	POLYMOX, Mead Johnson	00015-7276-72
100 ml x 6	**$3.10**	**AMOXIL, Beecham**	**00029-6008-23**
150 ml	$1.93	Amoxicillin, H.C.F.A. F F P	99999-0231-13
150 ml	$2.63	Amoxicillin, IDE-Interstate	00814-0700-58
150 ml	$3.47	WYMOX, Wyeth Labs	00008-0557-03
150 ml	$3.59	Amoxicillin, Lederle Pharm	00005-3146-49
150 ml	$3.70	Amoxicillin, Major Pharms	00904-2619-07
150 ml	$3.71	Amoxicillin, HL Moore Drug Exch	00839-6115-75
150 ml	$4.10	Amoxicillin, United Res	00677-0452-28
150 ml	$4.11	TRIMOX 125, Bristol Myers Squibb	00003-1737-45
150 ml	$4.14	Amoxicillin, Goldline Labs	00182-1072-72
150 ml	$4.14	Amoxicillin, Teva	00332-4150-34
150 ml	$4.14	Amoxicillin, Qualitest Pharms	00603-6500-66
150 ml	$4.20	Amoxil, Rugby	00536-0090-74
150 ml	$4.25	Amoxicillin, Harber Pharm	51432-0691-15
150 ml	$4.26	Amoxicillin, Schein Pharm (US)	00364-7215-62
150 ml	$4.71	Amoxicillin, Aligen Independ	00405-2225-78
150 ml	$4.71	Amoxicillin, Novopharm (US)	55953-0149-47
150 ml	$4.72	Amoxicillin, Warner Chilcott	00047-2500-18
150 ml	$4.72	Amoxicillin, Mylan	00378-0206-06
150 ml	$4.72	Amoxicillin, Martec Pharms	52555-0141-07
150 ml	$4.79	Amoxicillin, Dupont Pharma	00056-0249-38
150 ml o/s	$3.24	POLYMOX, Mead Johnson	00015-7276-73
150 ml x 6	**$3.55**	**AMOXIL, Beecham**	**00029-6008-22**
200 ml	$3.46	Amoxicillin, H.C.F.A. F F P	99999-0231-14
200 ml	$8.75	Amoxicillin, Warner Chilcott	00047-2500-20

Powder, Reconstitution - Oral - 250 mg/5ml

5 ml x 10	**$1.05**	**AMOXIL, Beecham**	**00029-6009-18**
15 ml	**$1.80**	**AMOXIL PEDIATRIC DROPS, Beecham**	**00029-6035-20**
30 ml	**$3.45**	**AMOXIL PEDIATRIC DROPS, Beecham**	**00029-6038-39**
50 ml	$2.34	POLYMOX, Mead Johnson	00015-7277-17
80 ml	$3.00	Amoxicillin, IDE-Interstate	00814-0701-52
80 ml	$3.75	Amoxicillin, Harber Pharm	51432-0692-13
80 ml	$3.75	Amoxicillin, Novopharm (US)	55953-0130-38
80 ml	$3.78	Amoxicillin, Schein Pharm (US)	00364-7216-60
80 ml	$3.95	Amoxicillin, Major Pharms	00904-2620-06
80 ml	$4.31	Amoxicillin, HL Moore Drug Exch	00839-6116-71
80 ml	$4.32	Amoxicillin, H.C.F.A. F F P	99999-0231-15
80 ml	$4.64	Amoxicillin, Lederle Pharm	00005-3147-43
80 ml	$4.72	Amoxil, Rugby	00536-0105-81
80 ml	$4.98	Amoxicillin, Dupont Pharma	00056-0250-34
80 ml	$5.31	TRIMOX 250, Bristol Myers Squibb	00003-1738-30
80 ml	$5.35	Amoxicillin, Warner Chilcott	00047-2501-16
80 ml	$5.35	Amoxicillin, Teva	00332-4155-30
80 ml	$5.38	Amoxicillin, Aligen Independ	00405-2250-58
80 ml o/s	$2.78	POLYMOX, Mead Johnson	00015-7277-70

HOW SUPPLIED - RATED THERAPEUTICALLY EQUIVALENT: *(cont'd)*

80 ml x 6	**$4.60**	**AMOXIL, Beecham**	**00029-6009-21**
100 ml	$2.55	Amoxicillin, H.C.F.A. F F P	99999-0231-16
100 ml	$3.30	Amoxicillin, IDE-Interstate	00814-0701-54
100 ml	$3.59	Amoxicillin, Teva	00332-4155-32
100 ml	$4.42	Amoxicillin, Novopharm (US)	55953-0130-40
100 ml	$4.80	Amoxicillin, Major Pharms	00904-2620-04
100 ml	$4.85	Amoxicillin, HL Moore Drug Exch	00839-6116-73
100 ml	$5.12	Amoxicillin, Mylan	00378-0207-02
100 ml	$5.15	WYMOX, Wyeth Labs	00008-0558-02
100 ml	$5.15	Amoxicillin, Martec Pharms	52555-0142-01
100 ml	$5.20	Amoxicillin, Schein Pharm (US)	00364-7216-61
100 ml	$5.30	AmoxicilliN, United Res	00677-0453-27
100 ml	$5.49	Amoxicillin, Lederle Pharm	00005-3147-46
100 ml	$5.95	Amoxil, Rugby	00536-0105-82
100 ml	$6.09	TRIMOX 250, Bristol Myers Squibb	00003-1738-40
100 ml	$6.13	Amoxicillin, Warner Chilcott	00047-2501-17
100 ml	$6.13	Amoxicillin, Goldline Labs	00182-1073-70
100 ml	$6.13	Amoxicillin, Aligen Independ	00405-2250-60
100 ml	$6.13	Amoxicillin, Qualitest Pharms	00603-6501-64
100 ml	$6.19	Amoxicillin, Dupont Pharma	00056-0250-36
100 ml o/s	$3.47	POLYMOX, Mead Johnson	00015-7277-72
100 ml x 6	**$5.30**	**AMOXIL, Beecham**	**00029-6009-23**
150 ml	$2.77	Amoxicillin, H.C.F.A. F F P	99999-0231-17
150 ml	$3.90	Amoxicillin, IDE-Interstate	00814-0701-58
150 ml	$4.14	Amoxicillin, Teva	00332-4155-34
150 ml	$5.85	Amoxicillin, Major Pharms	00904-2620-07
150 ml	$5.96	WYMOX, Wyeth Labs	00008-0558-03
150 ml	$6.06	Amoxicillin, HL Moore Drug Exch	00839-6116-75
150 ml	$6.15	Amoxicillin, Novopharm (US)	55953-0130-47
150 ml	$6.35	Amoxicillin, Lederle Pharm	00005-3147-49
150 ml	$6.35	Amoxicillin, Martec Pharms	52555-0142-07
150 ml	$6.75	Amoxil, Rugby	00536-0105-74
150 ml	$6.90	Amoxicillin, United Res	00677-0453-28
150 ml	$6.96	Amoxicillin, Mylan	00378-0207-06
150 ml	$7.06	TRIMOX 250, Bristol Myers Squibb	00003-1738-45
150 ml	$7.11	Amoxicillin, Warner Chilcott	00047-2501-18
150 ml	$7.11	Amoxicillin, Goldline Labs	00182-1073-72
150 ml	$7.11	Amoxicillin, Aligen Independ	00405-2250-78
150 ml	$7.11	Amoxicillin, Qualitest Pharms	00603-6501-66
150 ml	$7.12	Amoxicillin, Schein Pharm (US)	00364-7216-62
150 ml	$7.49	Amoxicillin, Dupont Pharma	00056-0250-38
150 ml o/s	$5.23	POLYMOX, Mead Johnson	00015-7277-73
150 ml x 6	**$6.10**	**AMOXIL, Beecham**	**00029-6009-22**
200 ml	$5.10	Amoxicillin, H.C.F.A. F F P	99999-0231-18
200 ml	$12.23	Amoxicillin, Warner Chilcott	00047-2501-20

Suspension - Oral - 125 mg/5 ml

200 ml	$3.46	Amoxicillin, H.C.F.A. F F P	99999-0231-19
200 ml	$5.87	Amoxicillin, Novopharm (US)	55953-0149-53

Suspension - Oral - 250 mg/5ml

15 ml	$3.74	TRIMOX, Bristol Myers Squibb	00003-1738-15
100 ml	$2.46	MOXILIN, Intl Ethical	11584-0381-00
150 ml	$2.82	MOXILIN, Intl Ethical	11584-0381-05
200 ml	$5.10	Amoxicillin, H.C.F.A. F F P	99999-0231-20
200 ml	$7.69	Amoxicillin, Novopharm (US)	55953-0130-53

Tablet, Chewable - Oral - 125 mg

60's	**$8.85**	**AMOXIL, Beecham**	**00029-6004-39**

Tablet, Chewable - Oral - 250 mg

30's	$7.40	Amoxicillin, Teva	00332-2268-04
30's	**$7.60**	**AMOXIL, Beecham**	**00029-6005-13**
100's	$22.82	Amoxicillin, Goldline Labs	00182-1962-01
100's	$22.82	Amoxicillin, Teva	00332-2268-09
100's	$22.82	Amoxicillin, Qualitest Pharms	00603-2274-21
100's	$22.85	Amoxicillin, HL Moore Drug Exch	00839-7776-06
100's	$22.85	Amoxicillin, Major Pharms	00904-7713-60
100's	$22.95	Amoxicillin, Warner Chilcott	00047-0038-24
100's	$23.02	Amoxicillin, Aligen Independ	00405-4086-01
100's	$23.07	Amoxicillin, Geneva Pharms	00781-1098-01
100's	$23.50	Amoxicillin, Harber Pharm	51432-0785-03
100's	**$25.35**	**AMOXIL, Beecham**	**00029-6005-30**
100's	$25.52	Amoxicillin Chewable, Schein Pharm (US)	00364-2569-01
500's	$101.00	Amoxicillin, Teva	00332-2268-13
500's	$106.32	Amoxicillin, Aligen Independ	00405-4086-02
500's	$114.75	Amoxicillin, Major Pharms	00904-7713-40
500's	$124.59	AMOXICILLIN, HL Moore Drug Exch	00839-7776-12
500's	$135.00	Amoxicillin, Goldline Labs	00182-1962-05

AMOXICILLIN; CLAVULANATE POTASSIUM

(000232)

CATEGORIES: Anti-Infectives; Antibiotics; Antimicrobials; Hemophilus; Infections; Otitis Media; Penicillins; Respiratory Tract Infections; Skin Infections; Sinusitis; Urinary Tract Infections; Pregnancy Category B; Sales > $1 Billion; FDA Approved 1984 Aug; Patent Expiration 2000 Dec; Top 200 Drugs

BRAND NAMES: *Amocla*; *Amonate*; *Amoxsiklav*; *Ancla*; *Augmentan* (Germany); **Augmentin**; *Augmentine*; *Auspilic*; *Clamobit*; *Clamoxyl*; *Clavinex*; *Clavoxilin Plus*; *Clavulin* (Canada); *Clavamox* (Germany); *Clavumox*; *Viaclav*; *Xiclav*
(International brand names outside U.S. in italics)

FORMULARIES: Aetna; BC-BS; Foundation; Medi-Cal; PCS

COST OF THERAPY: $117.36 (Respiratory Infections; Tablet; 500 mg/125 mg; 3/day; 14 days)

DESCRIPTION:

Augmentin is an oral antibacterial combination consisting of the semisynthetic antibiotic amoxicillin and the β-lactamase inhibitor, clavulanate potassium (the potassium salt of clavulanic acid). Amoxicillin is an analog of ampicillin, derived from the basic penicillin nucleus, 6-aminopenicillanic acid. The amoxicillin molecular formula is $C_{16}H_{19}N_3O_5S \cdot 3H_2O$ and the molecular weight is 419.45. Chemically, amoxicillin is *(2S,5R,6R)*-6-[(*R*)-(-)-2-Amino-2-(*p*- hydroxyphenyl)acetamido]-3,3-dimethyl-7-oxo-4-thia-1-azabicyclo [3.2.0]heptane-2-carboxylic acid trihydrate.

Clavulanic acid is produced by the fermentation of *Streptomyces clavuligerus*. It is a β-lactam structurally related to the penicillins and possesses the ability to inactivate a wide variety of β-lactamases by blocking the active sites of these enzymes. Clavulanic acid is particularly

DESCRIPTION: *(cont'd)*

active against the clinically important plasmid mediated β-lactamases frequently responsible for transferred drug resistance to penicillins and cephalosporins. The clavulanate potassium molecular formula is $C_8H_8KNO_5$ and the molecular weight is 237.25. Chemically clavulanate potassium is potassium Z-(3R, 5R)-2-(β-hydroxyethylidene) clavam-3-carboxylate.

Inactive Ingredients: *Tablets:* Colloidal silicon dioxide, ethyl cellulose, hydroxypropyl cellulose, hydroxypropyl methylcellulose, magnesium stearate, microcrystalline cellulose, sodium starch glycolate and titanium dioxide. *Powder for Oral Suspension:* Colloidal silicon dioxide, flavorings, mannitol, silica gel, sodium saccharin, succinic acid and xanthan gum. *Chewable Tablets:* Colloidal silicon dioxide, D&C Yellow No. 10, glycine, magnesium stearate, mannitol and sodium saccharin.

Augmentin is available in 250 mg and 500 mg white filmcoated tablets, 125 mg and 250 mg lemon-lime-flavored chewable tablets, and 125 mg/5 ml banana-flavored and 250 mg/5 ml orange-flavored oral suspensions. Each Augmentin 250 mg and 500 mg tablet contains 250 mg and 500 mg amoxicillin as the trihydrate, respectively, together with 125 mg clavulanic acid as the potassium salt. Each 125 mg chewable tablet and each teaspoonful (5 ml) of reconstituted Augmentin 125 mg/5 ml oral suspension contain 125 mg amoxicillin and 31.25 mg clavulanic acid as the potassium salt while each 250 mg chewable tablet and each 5 ml of reconstituted Augmentin 250 mg/5 ml oral suspension contain 250 mg amoxicillin and 62.5 mg clavulanic acid as the potassium salt.

Each Augmentin tablet contains 0.63 mEq potassium. Each 125 mg chewable tablet and each 5 ml of reconstituted Augmentin 125 mg/5 ml oral suspension contain 0.16 mEq potassium. Each 250 mg chewable tablet and each 5 ml of reconstituted Augmentin 250 mg/5 ml oral suspension contain 0.32 mEq potassium.

CLINICAL PHARMACOLOGY:

Amoxicillin and clavulanate potassium are well absorbed from the gastrointestinal tract after oral administration of Augmentin. Augmentin is stable in the presence of gastric acid and may be given without regard to meals.

Oral administration of 1 amoxicillin; clavulanate potassium 250 mg or amoxicillin; clavulanate potassium 500 mg tablet provides average peak serum concentrations 1 to 2 hours after dosing of 4.4 mcg/ml and 7.6 mcg/ml, respectively, for amoxicillin and 2.3 mcg/ml for clavulanic acid. The areas under the serum concentration curves obtained during the first 6 hours after dosing were 11.4 mcg/ml.hr. and 20.2 mcg/ml.hr. for amoxicillin, respectively, when 1 amoxicillin; clavulanate potassium 250 mg or 500 mg tablet was administered to adult volunteers. The corresponding area under the serum concentration curve for clavulanic acid was 5 mcg/ml.hr. Oral administration of 5 ml of amoxicillin; clavulanate potassium 250 mg/5 ml suspension or the equivalent dose of 10 ml amoxicillin; clavulanate potassium 125 mg/5 ml suspension provides average peak serum concentrations approximately 1 hour after dosing of 6.9 mcg/ml for amoxicillin and 1.6 mcg/ml for clavulanic acid. The areas under the serum concentration curves obtained during the first 6 hours after dosing were 12.6 mcg/ml.hr. for amoxicillin and 2.9 mcg/ml.hr. for clavulanic acid when 5 ml of amoxicillin; clavulanate potassium 250 mg/5 ml suspension or equivalent dose of 10 ml of amoxicillin; clavulanate potassium 125 mg/5 ml suspension was administered to adult volunteers. One amoxicillin; clavulanate potassium 250 mg chewable tablet or 2 amoxicillin; clavulanate potassium 125 mg chewable tablets are equivalent to 5 ml of amoxicillin; clavulanate potassium 250 mg/5 ml suspension and provide similar serum levels of amoxicillin and clavulanic acid.

Amoxicillin serum concentrations achieved with amoxicillin; clavulanate potassium are similar to those produced by the oral administration of equivalent doses of amoxicillin alone. The half-life of amoxicillin after the oral administration of amoxicillin; clavulanate potassium is 1.3 hours and that of clavulanic acid is 1.0 hour.

Approximately 50% to 70% of the amoxicillin and approximately 25% to 40% of the clavulanic acid are excreted unchanged in urine during the first 6 hours after administration of a single amoxicillin; clavulanate potassium 250 mg or 500 mg tablet or 10 ml of amoxicillin; clavulanate potassium 250 mg/5 ml suspension.

Concurrent administration of probenecid delays amoxicillin excretion but does not delay renal excretion of clavulanic acid.

Neither component in amoxicillin; clavulanate potassium is highly protein-bound; clavulanic acid has been found to be approximately 30% bound to human serum and amoxicillin approximately 20% bound.

Amoxicillin diffuses readily into most body tissues and fluids with the exception of the brain and spinal fluids. The results of experiments involving the administration of clavulanic acid to animals suggest that this compound, like amoxicillin, is well distributed in body tissues.

Two hours after oral administration of a single 35 mg/kg dose of amoxicillin; clavulanate potassium suspension to fasting children, average concentrations of 3.0 mcg/ml of amoxicillin and 0.5 mcg/ml of clavulanic acid were detected in middle ear effusions.

Microbiology: Amoxicillin is a semisynthetic antibiotic with a broad spectrum of bactericidal activity against many gram-positive and gram-negative microorganisms. Amoxicillin is, however, susceptible to degradation by β-lactamases and therefore the spectrum of activity does not include organisms which produce these enzymes. Clavulanic acid is a β-lactam, structurally related to the penicillins, which possesses the ability to inactivate a wide range of β-lactamase enzymes commonly found in microorganisms resistant to penicillins and cephalosporins. In particular, it has good activity against the clinically important plasmid mediated β-lactamases frequently responsible for transferred drug resistance.

The formulation of amoxicillin with clavulanic acid in amoxicillin; clavulanate potassium protects amoxicillin from degradation by β-lactamase enzymes and effectively extends the antibiotic spectrum of amoxicillin to include many bacteria normally resistant to amoxicillin and other β-lactam antibiotics. Thus amoxicillin; clavulanate potassium possesses the distinctive properties of a broad-spectrum antibiotic and a β-lactamase inhibitor.

While *in vitro* studies have demonstrated the susceptibility of most strains of the following organisms, clinical efficacy for infections other than those included in the INDICATIONS AND USAGE section has not been documented:

Gram-Positive Bacteria: *Staphylococcus aureus* (β-lactamase and non-β-lactamase producing), *Staphylococcus epidermidis* (β-lactamase and non-β-lactamase producing),*Staphylococcus saprophyticus* (β-lactamase and non-β-lactamase producing), *Streptococcus faecalis** (*Enterococcus*), *Streptococcus pneumoniae** (*D. pneumoniae*), *Streptococcus pyogenes**, *Streptococcus viridans**

Anaerobes: *Clostridium species**, *Peptococcus species**, *Peptostreptococcus species**

*These are non-B-lactamase-producing strains and therefore are susceptible to amoxicillin alone.

Gram-Negative Bacteria: *Hemophilus influenzae* (β-lactamase and non-β-lactamase producing), *Moraxella* (*Branhamella*) *catarrhalis* (β-lactamase and non-β- lactamase producing); *Escherichia coli* (β-lactamase and non- β-lactamase producing), *Klebsiella species* (All known strains are β-lactamase producing), *Enterobacter species* (Although most strains of *Enterobacter* species are resistant *in vitro*, clinical efficacy has been demonstrated with amoxicillin; clavulanate potassium in urinary tract infections caused by these organisms.), *Proteus mirabilis* (β-lactamase and non-β-lactamase producing),*Proteus vulgaris* (β-lactamase and non-β-lactamase producing), *Neisseria gonorrhoeae* (β-lactamase and non-β-lactamase producing), *Legionella species* (β-lactamase and non-β-lactamase producing).

Anaaerobes: *Bacteroides species*, including *B. fragilis* (β-lactamase and non-β-lactamase producing).

SUSCEPTIBILITY TESTING

Diffusion Technique: For Kirby-Bauer method of susceptibility testing, a 30 mcg amoxicillin; clavulanate potassium (20 mcg amoxicillin + 10 mcg clavulanic acid) diffusion disk should be used. With this procedure, a report from the laboratory of "Susceptible" indicates that the infecting organism is likely to respond to amoxicillin; clavulanate potassium therapy and a report of "Resistant" indicates that the infecting organism is not likely to respond to therapy. An "intermediate susceptibility" report suggests that the infecting organism would be susceptible to amoxicillin; clavulanate potassium if the higher dosage is used or if the infection is confined to tissues or fluids (*e.g.,* urine) in which high antibiotic levels are attained.

Dilution Techniques: Broth or agar dilution methods may be used to determine the minimal inhibitory concentration (MIC) value for susceptibility of bacterial isolates to Augmentin. Tubes should be inoculated to contain 10^4 to 10^5organisms/ml or plates "spotted" with $10^3$to 10^4 organisms.

The recommended dilution method employs a constant amoxicillin/clavulanic acid ratio of 2 to 1 in all tubes with increasing concentrations of amoxicillin. MICs are reported in terms of amoxicillin concentration in the presence of clavulanic acid at a constant 2 parts amoxicillin to 1 part clavulanic acid. (TABLE 1)

TABLE 1 Recommended Augmentin Susceptibility Ranges [1,2]

ORGANISMS	Resistant	Intermediate	Susceptible	MIC[3] Correlates mcg/ml R	S
Gram-Negative Enteric-Bacteria	≤13 mm	14 to 17 mm	≥18 mm	≥32/16	≤8/4
Staphylococcus[4] and *Hemophilus* spp.	≤19 mm	-	≥20 mm	-	≤4/2 ≤4/2

1 The non-β-lactamase-producing organisms which are normally susceptible to ampicillin, such as streptococci, will have similar zone sizes as for ampicillin disks.
2 The quality control cultures should have the following assigned daily ranges for Augmentin: (TABLE 2)
3 Expressed as concentration of amoxicillin/clavulanic acid.
4 Organisms which show susceptibility to Augmentin but are resistant to methicillin/oxacillin should be considered resistant.

TABLE 2

		Disks	MIC Range (mcg/ml)
E. coli	(ATCC 25922)	19 to 25 mm	2/1 to 8/4
S. aureus	(ATCC 25923)	28 to 36 mm	0.25/0.12 to 0.5/0.25
E. coli	(ATCC 35218)	18 to 22 mm	4/2 to 16/8

INDICATIONS AND USAGE:

Amoxicillin; clavulanate potassium is indicated in the treatment of infections caused by susceptible strains of the designated organisms in the conditions listed below:

Lower Respiratory Tract Infections: caused by β-lactamase-producing strains of *Hemophilus influenzae* and *Moraxella* (*Branhamella*) *catarrhalis.*

Otitis Media: caused by β-lactamase-producing strains of *Hemophilus influenzae* and *Moraxella* (*Branhamella*) *catarrhalis.*

Sinusitis: caused by β-lactamase-producing strains of *Hemophilus influenzae* and *Moraxella* (*Branhamella*) *catarrhalis.*

Skin and Skin Structure Infections: caused by β-lactamase-producing strains of *Staphylococcus aureus*, *Escherichia coli* and *Klebsiella* spp.

Urinary Tract Infections: caused by β-lactamase-producing strains of *Escherichia coli*, *Klebsiella* spp. and *Enterobacter* spp.

While amoxicillin; clavulanate potassium is indicated only for the conditions listed above, infections caused by ampicillin-susceptible organisms are also amenable to Augmentin treatment due to its amoxicillin content. Therefore, mixed infections caused by ampicillin-susceptible organisms and β-lactamase-producing organisms susceptible to amoxicillin; clavulanate potassium should not require the addition of another antibiotic.

Bacteriological studies, to determine the causative organisms and their susceptibility to amoxicillin; clavulanate potassium, should be performed together with any indicated surgical procedures.

Therapy may be instituted prior to obtaining the results from bacteriological and susceptibility studies to determine the causative organisms and their susceptibility to amoxicillin; clavulanate potassium when there is reason to believe the infection may involve any of the β-lactamase-producing organisms listed above. Once the results are known, therapy should be adjusted, if appropriate.

CONTRAINDICATIONS:

Amoxicillin; clavulanate potassium is contraindicated in patients with a history of allergic reactions to any penicillin. It is also contraindicated in patients with a previous history of amoxicillin; clavulanate potassium-associated cholestatic jaundice/hepatic dysfunction.

WARNINGS:

SERIOUS AND OCCASIONALLY FATAL HYPERSENSITIVITY (ANAPHYLACTIC) REACTIONS HAVE BEEN REPORTED IN PATIENTS ON PENICILLIN THERAPY. THESE REACTIONS ARE MORE LIKELY TO OCCUR IN INDIVIDUALS WITH A HISTORY OF PENICILLIN HYPERSENSITIVITY AND/OR A HISTORY OF SENSITIVITY TO MULTIPLE ALLERGENS. THERE HAVE BEEN REPORTS OF INDIVIDUALS WITH A HISTORY OF PENICILLIN HYPERSENSITIVITY WHO HAVE EXPERIENCED SEVERE REACTIONS WHEN TREATED WITH CEPHALOSPORINS. BEFORE INITIATING THERAPY WITH AUGMENTIN, CAREFUL INQUIRY SHOULD BE MADE CONCERNING PREVIOUS HYPERSENSITIVITY REACTIONS TO PENICILLINS, CEPHALOSPORINS OR OTHER ALLERGENS. IF AN ALLERGIC REACTION OCCURS, AUGMENTIN SHOULD BE DISCONTINUED AND THE APPROPRIATE THERAPY INSTITUTED. **SERIOUS ANAPHYLACTIC REACTIONS REQUIRE IMMEDIATE EMERGENCY TREATMENT WITH EPINEPHRINE. OXYGEN, INTRAVENOUS STEROIDS AND AIRWAY MANAGEMENT, INCLUDING INTUBATION, SHOULD ALSO BE ADMINISTERED AS INDICATED.**

WARNINGS: *(cont'd)*

Pseudomembranous colitis has been reported with nearly all antibacterial agents, including amoxicillin; clavulanate potassium, and has ranged in severity from mild to life-threatening. Therefore, it is important to consider this diagnosis in patients who present with diarrhea subsequent to the administration of antibacterial agents.

Treatment with antibacterial agents alters the normal flora of the colon and may permit overgrowth of clostridia. Studies indicate that a toxin produced by *Clostridium difficile* is one primary cause of "antibiotic associated colitis."

After the diagnosis of pseudomembranous colitis has been established, appropriate therapeutic measures should be initiated. Mild cases of pseudomembranous colitis usually respond to drug discontinuation alone. In moderate to severe cases, consideration should be given to management with fluids and electrolytes, protein supplementation and treatment with an antibacterial drug clinically effective against *Clostridium difficile* colitis.

Amoxicillin; clavulanate potassium should be used with caution in patients with evidence of hepatic dysfunction. Hepatic toxicity associated with the use of amoxicillin; clavulanate potassium is usually reversible. On rare occasions, deaths have been reported (less than 1 death reported per estimated 4 million prescriptions worldwide). These have generally been cases associated with serious underlying diseases or concomitant medications (see CONTRAINDICATIONS and ADVERSE REACTIONS, Liver.

PRECAUTIONS:

GENERAL

While amoxicillin; clavulanate potassium possesses the characteristic low toxicity of the penicillin group of antibiotics, periodic assessment of organ system functions, including renal, hepatic and hematopoietic function, is advisable during prolonged therapy.

A high percentage of patients with mononucleosis who receive ampicillin develop a skin rash. Thus, ampicillin class antibiotics should not be administered to patients with mononucleosis. The possibility of superinfections with mycotic or bacterial pathogens should be kept in mind during therapy. If superinfections occur (usually involving *Pseudomonas* or *Candida*), the drug should be discontinued and/or appropriate therapy instituted.

DRUG/LABORATORY TEST INTERACTIONS

Oral administration of amoxicillin; clavulanate potassium will result in high urine concentrations of amoxicillin. High urine concentrations of ampicillin may result in false-positive reactions when testing for the presence of glucose in urine using Clinitest, Benedict's Solution or Fehling's Solution. Since this effect may also occur with amoxicillin and therefore amoxicillin; clavulanate potassium, it is recommended that glucose tests based on enzymatic glucose oxidase reactions (such as Clinistix or Tes-Tape) be used.

Following administration of ampicillin to pregnant women a transient decrease in plasma concentration of total conjugated estriol, estriol-glucuronide, conjugated estrone and estradiol has been noted. This effect may also occur with amoxicillin and therefore amoxicillin; clavulanate potassium.

CARCINOGENESIS, MUTAGENESIS, AND IMPAIRMENT OF FERTILITY

Long-term studies in animals have not been performed to evaluate carcinogenic or mutagenic potential.

PREGNANCY CATEGORY B

Reproduction studies have been performed in mice and rats at doses up to ten (10) times the human dose and have revealed no evidence of impaired fertility or harm to the fetus due to amoxicillin; clavulanate potassium. There are, however, no adequate and well-controlled studies in pregnant women. Because animal reproduction studies are not always predictive of human response, this drug should be used during pregnancy only if clearly needed.

LABOR AND DELIVERY

Oral ampicillin class antibiotics are generally poorly absorbed during labor. Studies in guinea pigs have shown that intravenous administration of ampicillin decreased the uterine tone, frequency of contractions, height of contractions and duration of contractions. However, it is not known whether the use of amoxicillin; clavulanate potassium in humans during labor or delivery has immediate or delayed adverse effects on the fetus, prolongs the duration of labor, or increases the likelihood that forceps delivery or other obstetrical intervention or resuscitation of the newborn will be necessary.

NURSING MOTHERS

Ampicillin class antibiotics are excreted in the milk; therefore, caution should be exercised when amoxicillin; clavulanate potassium is administered to a nursing woman.

DRUG INTERACTIONS:

Probenecid decreases the renal tubular secretion of amoxicillin. Concurrent use with amoxicillin; clavulanate potassium may result in increased and prolonged blood levels of amoxicillin.

The concurrent administration of allopurinol and ampicillin increases substantially the incidence of rashes in patients receiving both drugs as compared to patients receiving ampicillin alone. It is not known whether this potentiation of ampicillin rashes is due to allopurinol or the hyperuricemia present in these patients. There are no data with amoxicillin; clavulanate potassium and allopurinol administered concurrently.

Amoxicillin; clavulanate potassium should not be co-administered with Antabuse (disulfiram).

ADVERSE REACTIONS:

Amoxicillin; clavulanate potassium is generally well tolerated. The majority of side effects observed in clinical trials were of a mild and transient nature and less than 3% of patients discontinued therapy because of drug-related side effects. The most frequently reported adverse effects were diarrhea/loose stools (9%), nausea (3%), skin rashes and urticaria (3%), vomiting (1%) and vaginitis (1%). The overall incidence of side effects, and in particular diarrhea, increased with the higher recommended dose. Other less frequently reported reactions include: abdominal discomfort, flatulence and headache.

The following adverse reactions have been reported for ampicillin class antibiotics:

Gastrointestinal: Diarrhea, nausea, vomiting, indigestion, gastritis, stomatitis, glossitis, black "hairy" tongue, enterocolitis, mucocutaneous candidiasis, and pseudomembranous colitis. Onset of pseudomembranous colitis symptoms may occur during or after antibiotic treatment (see WARNINGS.)

Hypersensitivity Reactions: Skin rashes, pruritus, urticaria, angioedema, serum sickness-like reactions (urticaria or skin rash accompanied by arthritis, arthralgia, myalgia and frequently fever), erythema multiforme (rarely Stevens-Johnson Syndrome) and an occasional case of exfoliative dermatitis (including toxic epidermal necrolysis) have been reported. These reactions may be controlled with antihistamines and, if necessary, systemic corticosteroids. Whenever such reactions occur, the drug should be discontinued, unless the opinion of the physician dictates otherwise. Serious and occasional fatal hypersensitivity (anaphylactic) reactions can occur with oral penicillin (See WARNINGS.)

Liver: A moderate rise in AST (SGOT) and/or ALT (SGPT) has been noted in patients treated with ampicillin class antibiotics but the significance of these findings is unknown. Hepatic dysfunction, including increases in serum transaminases (AST and/or ALT), serum bilirubin and/or alkaline phosphatase, has been infrequently reported with Augmentin. The

ADVERSE REACTIONS: *(cont'd)*

histologic findings on liver biopsy have consisted of predominantly cholestatic, hepatocellular, or mixed cholestatic-hepatocellular changes. The onset of signs/symptoms of hepatic dysfunction may occur during or several weeks after therapy has been discontinued. The hepatic dysfunction, which may be severe, is usually reversible. On rare occasions, deaths have been reported (less than 1 death reported per estimated 4 million prescriptions worldwide). These have generally been cases associated with serious underlying diseases or concomitant medications.

Renal: Interstitial nephritis and hematuria have been reported rarely.

Hemic and Lymphatic Systems: Anemia, thrombocytopenia, thrombocytopenic purpura, eosinophilia, leukopenia and agranulocytosis have been reported during therapy with penicillins. These reactions are usually reversible on discontinuation of therapy and are believed to be hypersensitivity phenomena. A slight thrombocytosis was noted in less than 1% of the patients treated with amoxicillin; clavulanate potassium.

Central Nervous System: Reversible hyperactivity, agitation, anxiety, insomnia, confusion, behavioral changes, and/or dizziness have been reported rarely.

OVERDOSAGE:

Amoxicillin may be removed from circulation by hemodialysis.

The molecular weight, degree of protein binding and pharmacokinetic profile of clavulanic acid together with information from a single patient with renal insufficiency all suggest that this compound may also be removed by hemodialysis.

DOSAGE AND ADMINISTRATION:

The amoxicillin; clavulanate potassium 250 mg tablet and the 250 mg chewable tablet do *not* contain the same amount of clavulanic acid (as the potassium salt). The amoxicillin; clavulanate potassium 250 mg tablet contains 125 mg clavulanic acid, whereas the 250 mg chewable tablet contains 62.5 mg of clavulanic acid. Therefore, the amoxicillin; clavulanate potassium 250 mg tablet and the 250 mg chewable tablet should *not* be substituted for each other, as they are not interchangeable.

Since both the amoxicillin; clavulanate potassium 250 mg and 500 mg tablets contain the same amount of clavulanic acid (125 mg, as the potassium salt), 2 amoxicillin; clavulanate potassium 250 mg tablets are not equivalent to 1 amoxicillin; clavulanate potassium 500 mg tablet. Therefore, 2 amoxicillin; clavulanate potassium 250 mg tablets should not be substituted for 1 amoxicillin; clavulanate potassium 500 mg tablet for treatment of more severe infections.

DOSAGE

Adults: The usual adult dose is 1 amoxicillin; clavulanate potassium 250 mg tablet every 8 hours. For more severe infections and infections of the respiratory tract, the dose should be 1 amoxicillin; clavulanate potassium 500 mg tablet every 8 hours.

Children: The usual dose is 20 mg/kg/day, based on amoxicillin component, in divided doses every 8 hours. For otitis media, sinusitis and lower respiratory tract infections, the dose should be 40 mg/kg/day, based on the amoxicillin component, in divided doses every 8 hours. Severe infections should be treated with the higher recommended dose.

Children weighing 40 kg and more: should be dosed according to the adult recommendations.

Due to the different amoxicillin to clavulanic acid ratios in the amoxicillin; clavulanate potassium 250 mg tablet (250/125) versus the amoxicillin; clavulanate potassium 250 mg chewable tablet (250/62.5), the amoxicillin; clavulanate potassium 250 mg tablet should not be used until the child weighs at least 40 kg and more.

Directions For Mixing Oral Suspension: Prepare a suspension at time of dispensing as follows: Tap bottle until all the powder flows freely. Add approximately 2/3 of the total amount of water for reconstitution (see TABLE 3 and TABLE 4) and shake vigorously to suspend powder. Add remainder of the water and again shake vigorously.

TABLE 3 Amoxicillin; clavulanate potassium 125 mg/5 ml Suspension

Bottle Size	Amount of Water Required for Reconstitution
75 ml	67 ml
100 ml	90 ml
150 ml	134 ml

Each teaspoonful (5 ml) will contain 125 mg amoxicillin and 31.25 mg of clavulanic acid as the potassium salt.

TABLE 4 Amoxicillin; clavulanate potassium 250 mg/5 ml Suspension

Bottle Size	Amount of Water Required for Reconstitution
75 ml	65 ml
100 ml	87 ml
150 ml	130 ml

Each teaspoonful (5 ml) will contain 250 mg amoxicillin and 62.5 mg of clavulanic acid as the potassium salt.

NOTE: SHAKE ORAL SUSPENSION WELL BEFORE USING.

RECONSTITUTED SUSPENSION MUST BE STORED UNDER REFRIGERATION AND DISCARDED AFTER 10 DAYS.

Administration: The absorption of amoxicillin; clavulanate potassium is unaffected by food. Therefore, amoxicillin; clavulanate potassium may be administered without regard to meals.

CDC GUIDELINES FOR TREATMENT OF SEXUALLY TRANSMITTED DISEASES

Chancroid (Hemophilus ducreyi infection)[1]: One '500' tablet 3 times daily for 7 days as an alternative to erythromycin or ceftriaxone (not evaluated in the U.S.).

Disseminated gonococcal infection[1] : Following appropriate parenteral therapy with ceftriaxone, ceftizoxime or cefotaxime, reliable patients with uncomplicated disease may be discharged from the hospital 24 to 48 hours after all symptoms resolve and may complete the therapy (for a total of 1 week of antibiotic therapy) with an oral regimen of one '500' tablet 3 times a day.

[1]CDC 1989 Sexually Transmitted Diseases Treatment Guidelines. *Morbidity and Mortality Weekly Report*1989 Sept. 1;38(No.S-8):1–43.

PATIENT INFORMATION:

Amoxicillin Clavulanate is an antibiotic for the treatment of infection. Take at regular intervals and complete the entire course of therapy. Do not take this medication if you are allergic to any type of penicillin. Notify your physician if you are pregnant or nursing. This antibiotic may decrease the effectiveness of birth control pills; use another form of birth control while taking this medication. Shake the suspension well before each use and store it in the refrigerator. May cause nausea, vomiting, or diarrhea; notify your physician if these occur. Amoxicillin Clavulanate may be taken with or without food.

HOW SUPPLIED:

Augmentin 250 mg Tablets: Each white oval filmcoated tablet, debossed with Augmentin on 1 side and 250/125 on the other side, contains 250 mg amoxicillin as the trihydrate and 125 mg clavulanic acid as the potassium salt.

Augmentin 500 mg Tablets: Each white oval filmcoated tablet, debossed with Augmentin on 1 side and 500/125 on the other side, contains 500 mg amoxicillin as the trihydrate and 125 mg clavulanic acid as the potassium salt.

Augmentin 125 mg/5 ml For Oral Suspension: Each 5 ml of reconstituted banana-flavored suspension contains 125 mg amoxicillin and 31.25 mg clavulanic acid as the potassium salt.

Augmentin 250 mg/5 ml For Oral Suspension: Each 5 ml of reconstituted orange-flavored suspension contains 250 mg amoxicillin and 62.5 mg clavulanic acid as the potassium salt.

Augmentin 125 mg Chewable Tablets: Each yellow mottled round tablet, debossed with BMP 189, contains 125 mg amoxicillin as the trihydrate and 31.25 mg clavulanic acid as the potassium salt.

Augmentin 250 mg Chewable Tablets: Each yellow mottled round tablet, debossed with BMP 190, contains 250 mg amoxicillin as the trihydrate and 62.5 mg clavulanic acid as the potassium salt.

Store tablets and dry powder at or below 25°C (77°F). Dispense in tightly closed, moisture-proof containers. Store reconstituted suspension under refrigeration. Discard unused suspension after 10 days.

HOW SUPPLIED - EQUIVALENTS NOT AVAILABLE:

Powder, Reconstitution - Oral - 125 mg/31.25 mg

75 ml x 6	$14.00	AUGMENTIN 125, Beecham	00029-6085-39
100 ml	$18.65	AUGMENTIN, Beecham	00029-6085-23
150 ml x 6	$27.40	AUGMENTIN 125, Beecham	00029-6085-22

Powder, Reconstitution - Oral - 250 mg/62.5 mg/

75 ml x 6	$26.65	AUGMENTIN 250, Beecham	00029-6090-39
100 ml	$35.55	AUGMENTIN, Beecham	00029-6090-23
150 ml x 6	$52.20	AUGMENTIN 250, Beecham	00029-6090-22

Tablet, Chewable - Oral - 125 mg/31.25 mg

30's	$27.40	AUGMENTIN, Beecham	00029-6073-47

Tablet, Chewable - Oral - 250 mg/62.5 mg

30's	$52.20	AUGMENTIN, Beecham	00029-6074-47

Tablet, Uncoated - Oral - 250 mg/125 mg

30's	$57.65	AUGMENTIN, Beecham	00029-6075-27
100's	$197.05	AUGMENTIN, Beecham	00029-6075-31

Tablet, Uncoated - Oral - 500 mg/125 mg

30's	$81.80	AUGMENTIN 500, Beecham	00029-6080-27
100's	$279.45	AUGMENTIN 500, Beecham	00029-6080-31

AMPHETAMINE RESIN COMPLEX; DEXTROAMPHETAMINE RESIN COMPLEX

(000233)

CATEGORIES: Amphetamines; Anorexients/CNS Stimulants; Attention Deficit Disorders; Behavior Problems; Central Nervous System Agents; Obesity; Psychostimulants; Respiratory/Cerebral Stimulant; Stimulants; DEA Class CII; FDA Approval Pre 1982

BRAND NAMES: **Biphetamine**; Obetrol; Saccamine

FORMULARIES: Aetna

WARNING:
AMPHETAMINES HAVE A HIGH POTENTIAL FOR ABUSE. THEY SHOULD THUS BE TRIED ONLY IN WEIGHT REDUCTION PROGRAMS FOR PATIENTS IN WHOM ALTERNATIVE THERAPY HAS BEEN INEFFECTIVE. ADMINISTRATION OF d- AND dl-AMPHETAMINE FOR PROLONGED PERIODS OF TIME IN OBESITY MAY LEAD TO DRUG DEPENDENCE AND MUST BE AVOIDED. PARTICULAR ATTENTION SHOULD BE PAID TO THE POSSIBILITY OF SUBJECTS OBTAINING d- AND dl-AMPHETAMINE FOR NON-THERAPEUTIC USE OR DISTRIBUTION TO OTHERS, AND THE DRUG SHOULD BE PRESCRIBED OR DISPENSED SPARINGLY.

DESCRIPTION:

BIPHETAMINE 12 1/2

Each capsule contains cationic exchange resin complexes equivalent to:

Amphetamine: 6.25 mg

Dextroamphetamine: 6.25 mg

BIPHETAMINE 20

Each capsule contains cationic exchange resin complexes equivalent to:

Amphetamine: 10 mg

Dextroamphetamine 10 mg

Other ingredients in Biphetamine: dibasic calcium phosphate, FD&C Blue No. 1, FD&C Red No. 40, FD&C Yellow No. 6, gelatin, lactose, magnesium stearate, titanium dioxide and other ingredients in trace quantities.

CLINICAL PHARMACOLOGY:

Amphetamine is a sympathomimetic amine with CNS stimulant activity. Peripheral actions include elevation of systolic and diastolic blood pressures and weak bronchodilator and respiratory stimulant action.

Behavioral Effects in Children: There is neither specific evidence which clearly establishes the mechanism whereby amphetamine produces its mental and behavioral effects in children, nor conclusive evidence regarding how these effects relate to the condition of the central nervous system.

Anorectic: Drugs of this class used in obesity are commonly known as "anorectics" or "anorexigenics". It has not been established, however, that the action of such drugs in treating obesity is primarily one of appetite suppression. For example, other central nervous system actions or metabolic effects may be involved.

Adult obese subjects instructed in dietary management and treated with anorectic drugs lose more weight, on the average, than those treated with placebo and diet, as determined in relatively short-term clinical trials.

CLINICAL PHARMACOLOGY: *(cont'd)*

The magnitude of increased weight loss of drug-treated patients over placebo-treated patients is, on the average, only a fraction of a pound a week. However, some patients lose more weight than this and some lose less. The rate of weight loss is greatest in the first weeks of therapy for both drug and placebo subjects and tends to decrease in succeeding weeks. The origins of the increased weight loss due to the various possible drug effects are not established. The amount of weight loss associated with the use of an "anorectic" drug varies from trial to trial, and may be related in part to variables other than the drug prescribed, such as the physician-investigator, the population treated, and the diet prescribed. Studies do not permit conclusions as to the relative importance of the drug and non-drug factors on weight loss.

The natural history of obesity is measured in years, whereas most studies cited are restricted to a few weeks duration; thus, the total impact of drug-induced weight loss over that of diet alone must be considered clinically limited.

Blood levels of amphetamine were determined in human subjects following the administration of Biphetamine Capsules and amphetamine phosphate capsules. Efficiency of absorption was the same for the resinate as for the soluble salt. The average absorption rate was slower and less variable for the resinate. Blood levels with the resinate reached a slightly lower, later, and flatter peak and a slightly higher blood level was maintained over a period of 16 hours. The clinical significance of these differences is not known. In efficiency studies a single dose of Biphetamine was given early in the day and the results obtained were comparable to those which have been reported for multiple daily doses of a soluble salt.

INDICATIONS AND USAGE:

Behavioral Syndrome in Children: Biphetamine is indicated as an integral part of a total treatment program which typically includes other remedial measures (psychological, educational, social) for a stabilizing effect in children with a behavioral syndrome characterized by the following group of developmentally inappropriate symptoms: moderate to serve distractibility, short attention span, hyperactivity, emotional lability, and impulsivity. The diagnosis of this syndrome should not be made with finality when these symptoms are only of comparatively recent origin. Nonlocalizing (soft) neurological signs, learning disability, and abnormal EEG may not be present, and a diagnosis of central nervous system dysfunction may or may not be warranted.

Exogenous Obesity: As a short-term (a few weeks) adjunct in a regimen of weight reduction based on caloric restriction for patients refractory to alternative therapy (*e.g.* repeated diets, group programs and other drugs). The limited usefulness of amphetamine (see CLINICAL PHARMACOLOGY) should be weighed against possible risks inherent in use of the drug, such as those described below.

CONTRAINDICATIONS:

Advanced arteriosclerosis

Symptomatic cardiovascular disease

Moderate to severe hypertension

Hyperthyroidism

Known hypersensitivity or idiosyncrasy to the sympathomimetic amines

Glaucoma

Agitated states.

Patients with a history of drug abuse.

During or within 14 days following the administration of monoamine oxidase inhibitors (hypertensive crises may result).

WARNINGS:

When tolerance to the "anorectic" effect develops, the recommended dose should not be exceeded in an attempt to increase the effect; rather the drug should be discontinued.

Amphetamine may impair the ability of the patient to engage in potentially hazardous activities such as operating machinery or driving a motor vehicle; the patient should therefore be cautioned accordingly.

Drug Dependence: Amphetamine has been extensively abused. Tolerance, extreme psychological dependence, and severe social disability have occurred. There are reports of patients who have increased the dosage to many times that recommended. Abrupt cessation following prolonged high dosage administration results in extreme fatigue and mental depression; changes are also noted on the sleep EEG. Manifestations of chronic intoxication with amphetamine include severe dermatoses, marked insomnia, irritability, hyperactivity, and personality changes. The most severe manifestation of chronic intoxication is psychosis, often clinically indistinguishable from schizophrenia.

Usage in Pregnancy: Safe use in pregnancy has not been established. Reproduction studies in mammals at high multiples of the human dose have suggested both an embryotoxic and a teratogenic potential. Use of amphetamine by women who are or who may become pregnant, and especially by those in the first trimester of pregnancy, requires that the potential benefit be weighed against the possible hazard to mother and infant.

Usage in Children: Amphetamine is not recommended for use as an anorectic agent in children under 12 years of age or for behavior syndrome in children under 3 years of age.

Clinical experience suggests that in psychotic children, administration of amphetamine may exacerbate symptoms of behavior disturbance and thought disorder.

Data are inadequate to determine whether chronic administration of amphetamine may be associated with growth inhibition; therefore, growth should be monitored during treatment.

PRECAUTIONS:

Caution is to be exercised in prescribing amphetamine for patients with mild hypertension.

Insulin requirements in diabetes mellitus may be altered in association with the use of amphetamine and the concomitant dietary regimen.

Amphetamine may decrease the hypotensive effect of guanethidine.

The least amount feasible should be prescribed or dispensed at one time in order to minimize the possibility of overdosage.

Drug treatment is not indicated in all cases of this behavioral syndrome and should be considered only in light of the complete history and evaluation of the child. The decision to prescribe Biphetamine (amphetamine) should depend on the physician's assessment of the chronicity and severity of the child's symptoms and their appropriateness for his/her age. Prescription should not depend solely on the presence of one or more of the behavioral characteristics.

When these symptoms are associated with acute stress reactions, treatment with Biphetamine is usually not indicated.

Usage in Nursing Mothers: Amphetamines are excreted in human milk. Mothers taking amphetamines should be advised to refrain from nursing.

Long-term effects of Biphetamine in children have not been well-established.

ADVERSE REACTIONS:

Cardiovascular: Palpitation, tachycardia, elevation of blood pressure. There have been isolated reports of cardiomyopathy associated with chronic amphetamine use.

Central nervous system: Overstimulation, restlessness, dizziness, insomnia, euphoria, dysphoria, tremor, headache; rarely psychotic episodes at recommended doses.

Gastrointestinal: Dryness of the mouth, unpleasant taste, diarrhea, constipation, other gastrointestinal disturbances.

Allergic: Urticaria.

Endocrine: Impotence, changes in Libido.

OVERDOSAGE:

Manifestations of acute overdosage with amphetamine include restlessness, tremor, hyperreflexia, rapid respiration, confusion, assaultiveness, hallucinations, panic states. Fatigue and depression usually follow the central stimulation.

Cardiovascular effects include arrhythmias, hypertension or hypotension and circulatory collapse. Gastrointestinal symptoms include nausea, vomiting, diarrhea, and abdominal cramps. Fatal poisoning usually terminates in convulsions and coma.

While not reported to date with Biphetamine, hyperpyrexia and rhabdomyolysis can occur with amphetamine overdosage.

Management of acute amphetamine intoxication is largely symptomatic and includes lavage and sedation with a barbiturate. Experience with hemodialysis or peritoneal dialysis is inadequate to permit recommendation in this regard. Acidification of the urine increases amphetamine excretion. Intravenous phentolamine (Regitine) has been suggested or pharmacological grounds for possible acute, severe hypertension, if this complicates amphetamine overdosage.

DOSAGE AND ADMINISTRATION:

Biphetamine should be administered at the lowest effective dosage and dosage should be individually adjusted. Late evening medication should be avoided because of possible insomnia.

Biphetamine capsules should be swallowed whole.

BEHAVIORAL SYNDROME

Amphetamine is not recommended for children under 3 years of age.

Recommended regimen for establishment of optimal response with short acting dextroamphetamine product:

In children from 3 to 5 years of age, start with 2.5 mg daily; daily dosage may be raised in increments of 2.5 mg at weekly intervals until optimal response is obtained.

In children 6 years of age and older, start with 5 mg once or twice daily; daily dosage may be raised in increments of 5 mg at weekly intervals until optimal response is obtained. Only in rare cases will it be necessary to exceed a total of 40 milligrams per day.

Once the optimal response dosage level for amphetamine has been established, Biphetamine capsules may be used for once-a-day dosage wherever appropriate for reasons of convenience.

Biphetamine 12 1/2 and 20 capsules are approximately equivalent to 10 mg and 15 mg, respectively, of dextroamphetamine administered as a single dose.

Where possible, drug administration should be interrupted occasionally to determine if there is a recurrence of behavioral symptoms sufficient to require continued therapy.

OBESITY

One capsule daily, 10-14 hours before retiring; capsule strength may be adjusted to individual requirements.

HOW SUPPLIED - EQUIVALENTS NOT AVAILABLE:

Tablet, Uncoated - Oral - 5 mg/5 mg

100's	$52.43	OBETROL 10, Rexar	00478-5432-01
500's	$357.50	OBETROL 10, Rexar	00478-5432-05
1000's	$471.90	OBETROL 10, Rexar	00478-5432-10

Tablet, Uncoated - Oral - 10 mg/10 mg

100's	$76.26	OBETROL 20, Rexar	00478-5433-01
500's	$357.50	OBETROL 20, Rexar	00478-5433-05
1000's	$686.40	OBETROL 20, Rexar	00478-5433-10

AMPHETAMINE SULFATE *(000234)*

CATEGORIES: Amphetamines; Anorexients/CNS Stimulants; Attention Deficit Disorders; Behavior Problems; Central Nervous System Agents; Narcolepsy; Obesity; Psychostimulants; Respiratory/Cerebral Stimulant; Stimulants; Pregnancy Category C; DEA Class CII; FDA Approved 1984 Aug

BRAND NAMES: *Amfetamin*; *Centramina*; *Simpatina*
(International brand names outside U.S. in italics)

> WARNING:
> AMPHETAMINES HAVE A HIGH POTENTIAL FOR ABUSE. THEY SHOULD BE TRIED ONLY IN WEIGHT REDUCTION PROGRAMS FOR PATIENTS IN WHOM ALTERNATIVE THERAPY HAS BEEN INEFFECTIVE. ADMINISTRATION OF AMPHETAMINES FOR PROLONGED PERIODS OF TIME IN OBESITY MAY LEAD TO DRUG DEPENDENCE AND MUST BE AVOIDED. PARTICULAR ATTENTION SHOULD BE PAID TO THE POSSIBILITY OF SUBJECTS OBTAINING AMPHETAMINES FOR NON-THERAPEUTIC USE OR DISTRIBUTION TO OTHERS, AND THE DRUGS SHOULD BE PRESCRIBED OR DISPENSED SPARINGLY.

DESCRIPTION:

Amphetamine sulfate is a white odorless crystalline powder. It has a slightly bitter taste. Its solutions are acid to litmus, having a pH of 5 to 6. It is freely soluble in water, slightly soluble in alcohol and practically insoluble in ether. Dextroamphetamine sulfate is the dextrorotary isomer of amphetamine sulfate. The chemical name is (+)-alpha-methylphenethylamine Sulfate (2:1)

CLINICAL PHARMACOLOGY:

Amphetamines are non-catecholamine, sympathomimetic amines with CNS stimulant activity. Peripheral actions include elevations of systolic and diastolic blood pressure, wand weak bronchodilator, and respiratory stimulant action.

CLINICAL PHARMACOLOGY: *(cont'd)*

Amphetamine, as the racemic form, differs from dextroamphetamine in a number of ways. The l isomer is more potent than the d isomer in cardiovascular activity, but much less potent in causing CNS excitatory effects. The racemic mixture also is less effective as an appetite suppressant when compared to dextroamphetamine.

There is neither specific evidence which clearly establishes the mechanism whereby amphetamines produce mental and behavioral effects in children, nor conclusive evidence regarding how these effects relate to the condition of the central nervous system.

Drugs of this class used in obesity are commonly known as "anorectics" or "anorexigenics." It has not been established, however, that the action of such drugs in treating obesity is primarily one of appetite suppression. Other central nervous system actions/ or metabolic effects, may be involved, for example. Adult obese subjects instructed in dietary and treated with "anorectic" drugs lose more weight on the average than those treated with placebo and diet, as determined in relatively short- term clinical trials.

The magnitude of increased weight loss of drug-treated patients over placebo-treated patients is only a fraction of a pound a week. The rate of weight loss is greatest in the first weeks of therapy for both drug and placebo subjects and tends to decrease in succeeding weeks. The origins of the increased weight loss due to the various possible drug effects are not established. The amount of weight loss associated with the use of an "anorectic" drug varies from trial to trial, and the increased weight loss appears to be related in part to variables other than the drug prescribed, such as the physician-investigator, the population treated, and the diet prescribed. Studies do not permit conclusions as to the relative importance of the drug and nondrug factors, or weight loss.

The natural history of obesity is measured in years, whereas the studies cited are restricted to few week's duration; thus, the total impact of drug-induced weight loss over that of diet alone must be considered clinically limited.

INDICATIONS AND USAGE:

Amphetamine sulfate is indicated:

1. In Narcolepsy

2. In Attention Deficit Disorder with Hyperactivity: as an integral part of a total treatment program which typically includes other remedial measures (psychological, educational, social) for a stabilizing effect in children with a behavioral syndrome characterized by the following group of developmentally inappropriate symptoms: moderate to severe distractibility, short attention span, hyperactivity, emotional lability, and impulsivity. The diagnosis of this syndrome should not be made with finality when these symptoms are only of comparatively recent origin. Nonlocalizing (soft) neurological signs, learning disability, and abnormal EEG may or may not be present, and a diagnosis of central nervous system dysfunction may or may not be warranted.

3. In Exogenous Obesity: as a short-term (a few weeks) adjunct in a regimen of weight reduction based on caloric restriction, for patients refractory to alternative therapy, e.g., repeated diets, group programs; and other drugs. The limited usefulness of amphetamines (see CLINICAL PHARMACOLOGY) should be weighed against possible risks inherent in the use of the drug, such as those described below.

Clinical experience suggests that in psychotic children, administration of amphetamines may exacerbate symptoms of behavior disturbance and thought disorder.

Amphetamines have been reported to exacerbate motor and phonic tics and Tourette's syndrome. Therefore, clinical evaluation for tics and Tourette's syndrome in children and their families should precede use of stimulant medications.

Data is inadequate to determine whether chronic administration of amphetamines may be associated with growth inhibition; therefore, growth should be monitored during treatment.

Drug treatment is not indicated in all cases of Attention Deficit Disorder with Hyperactivity and should be considered only in light of the complete history and evaluation of the child.

The decision to prescribe amphetamines should depend on the physician's assessment of the chronically and severity of the child's symptoms and their appropriateness for his/her age. Prescription should not depend solely on the presence of one or more of the behavioral characteristics.

When these symptoms are associated with acute stress reactions, treatment with amphetamines is usually not indicated.

CONTRAINDICATIONS:

Advanced arteriosclerosis, symptomatic cardiovascular disease, moderate to severe hypertension, hyperthyroidism, known hypersensitivity or idiosyncrasy to the sympathomimetic amines, glaucoma. Agitated states.

Patients with a history of drug abuse.

During within 14 days following the administration of monoamine oxidase inhibitors (hypertensive rises may result).

WARNINGS:

When tolerance to the "anorectic" effect develops, the recommended dose should not be exceeded in an attempt to increase the effect, rather, the drug should be discontinued.

PRECAUTIONS:

GENERAL

Caution is to be exercised in prescribing amphetamines for patients with even mild hypertension. The least amount feasible should be prescribed or dispensed at one time in order to minimize the possibility of overdosage.

INFORMATION FOR THE PATIENT

Amphetamines may impair the ability of the patient to engage in potentially hazardous activities such as operating machinery or vehicles: the patient should therefore be cautioned accordingly.

DRUG/LABORATORY TEST INTERACTIONS

Amphetamines can cause a significant elevation in plasma corticosteroid levels. This increase is greatest in the evening.

Amphetamines may interfere with urinary steroid determinations.

CARCINOGENESIS, MUTAGENESIS, AND IMPAIRMENT OF FERTILITY

Mutagenicity studies and long-term studies in animals to determine the carcinogenic potential of dextroamphetamine sulfate have not been performed.

PREGNANCY, TERATOGENIC EFFECTS, PREGNANCY CATEGORY C

Amphetamine sulfate has been shown to have embryotoxic and teratogenic effects when administered to A/Jax mice and C57BL mice in doses approximately 41 times the maximum human dose. Embryotoxic effects were not seen in New Zealand white rabbits given the drug in doses 7 times the human dose. There are no adequate and well-controlled studies in pregnant women. Amphetamine sulfate should be used during pregnancy only if the potential benefit justifies the potential risk to the fetus.

PRECAUTIONS: *(cont'd)*

Nonteratogenic Effects: Infants born to mother dependent on amphetamines have an increased risk if premature delivery and low birth weight. Also, these infants may experience symptoms of withdrawal as demonstrated by dysphoria, including agitation, and significant lassitude.

NURSING MOTHERS

It is not known whether this drug is excreted in breast milk; efforts to measure amphetamines in breast milk have been unsuccessful. Because many drugs are excreted in human milk, caution should be exercised when amphetamine sulfate is administered to a nursing woman.

PEDIATRIC USE

Long term effects of amphetamines in children have not been well established.

Amphetamines are not recommended for use as anorectic agents in children under 12 years of age.

DRUG INTERACTIONS:

Acidifying Agents: Gastrointestinal acidifying agents (guanethidine, reserpine, glutamic acid HCl, ascorbic acid, fruit juices, etc.) lower absorption of amphetamines. Urinary acidifying agents (ammonium chloride, sodium acid phosphate, etc.) increase the concentration of the ionized species of the amphetamine molecule, thereby increasing urinary excretion. Both groups of agents lower blood levels and efficacy of amphetamines.

Adrenergic Blockers: Adrenergic blockers are inhibited by amphetamines.

Alkalinizing agents, Gastrointestinal alkalinizing agents (sodium bicarbonate, etc.): increase absorption of amphetamines. Urinary alkalinizing agents (acetazolamide, some thiazides) increase the concentration of the non-ionized species of the amphetamine molecules, thereby decreasing urinary excretion. Both groups of agents increase blood levels and therefore potentiate the action of amphetamines.

Antidepressants, Tricyclic: Amphetamines may enhance the activity of tricyclic or sympathomimetic agents; d-amphetamine with desipramine or protriptyline and possibly other tricyclics cause striking and sustained increases in the concentration of d- amphetamine in the brain; cardiovascular effects can be potentiated.

MAO Inhibitors: MAO antidepressants, as well as a metabolite of furazolidone, slow amphetamine metabolism. This slowing potentiates amphetamines, increasing their effect on the release of norepinephrine and other monoamines from adrenergic nerve endings; this can cause headaches and other signs of hypertensive crisis. A variety of neurological toxic effects and malignant hyperpyrexia can occur, sometimes with fatal results.

Antihypertensives: Amphetamines may antagonize the hypotensive effects of antihypertensives.

Chlorpromazine: Chlorpromazine blocks a dopamine and norepinephrine reuptake, thus inhibiting the central stimulant affects of amphetamines, and can be used to treat amphetamine poisoning.

Ethosuximide: Amphetamines may delay intestinal absorption of ethosuximide.

Haloperidol: Haloperidol blocks dopamine and norepinephrine reuptake, thus inhibiting the central stimulant affects of amphetamines.

Lithium Carbonate: The antiobesity and stimulatory effects of amphetamines may be inhibited by lithium carbonate.

Meperidine: Amphetamines potentiate the analgesic effect of meperidine.

Methenamine therapy: Urinary excretion of amphetamines is increased, and efficacy is reduced by acidifying agents used in methenamine therapy.

Norepinephrine: Amphetamines enhance the adrenergic effect of norepinephrine.

Phenobarbital: Amphetamines may delay the intestinal absorption of phenobarbital. Co-administration of phenobarbital may produce a synergistic anticonvulsant action.

Phenytoin: Amphetamines may delay intestinal absorption of phenytoin. Co-administration of phenytoin may produce a synergistic anticonvulsant action.

Propoxyphene: In cases of propoxyphene overdosage, amphetamine CNS stimulation is potentiated and fatal convulsions can occur.

Veratrum Alkaloids: Amphetamines inhibit the hypotensive effect of veratrum alkaloids.

ADVERSE REACTIONS:

Cardiovascular: Palpitations, tachycardia, elevation of blood pressure.

Central Nervous System: Psychotic episodes at recommended doses (rare), overstimulation, restlessness, dizziness, insomnia, euphoria, dyskinesia, dysphoria, tremor, headaches, exacerbation of motor and phonic tics and Tourette's syndrome.

Gastrointestinal: Dryness of the mouth, unpleasant taste, diarrhea, constipation and other gastrointestinal disturbances. Anorexia and weight loss may occur as undesirable effects when amphetamines are used for other than the anorectic effect.

Allergic: Urticaria.

Endocrine: Impotence, changes in libido.

DRUG ABUSE AND DEPENDENCE:

Amphetamine sulfate is a Schedule II controlled substance. Amphetamines have been extensively abused. Tolerance, extreme psychological dependence, and severe social disability have occurred. There are reports of patients who have increased the dosage to many times that recommended. Abrupt cessation following prolonged high dosage administration results in extreme fatigue and mental depression; changes are also noted in the sleep EEG.

Manifestations of chronic intoxication with amphetamines include severe dermatosis, marked insomnia, irritability, hyperactivity and personality changed. The most severe manifestation of chronic intoxication is psychosis, often clinically indistinguishable from schizophrenia. This is rare with oral amphetamine.

OVERDOSAGE:

Individual patient response to amphetamine varies widely. While toxic symptoms occasionally occur as an idiosyncrasy at doses as low as 2 mg, they are rare with doses of less than 15 mg. 30 mg can produce severe reactions, yet doses of 400 to 500 mg are not necessarily fatal.

In rats, the oral LD_{50} of dextroamphetamine sulfate is 96.8 mg/kg.

SYMPTOMS

Manifestations of acute overdosage with amphetamines include restlessness, tremor, hyperreflexia, rapid respiration, confusion, assaultiveness, hallucinations, panic states. Fatigue and depression usually follow the central stimulation. Cardiovascular effects include arrhythmias, hypertension, or hypotension and circulatory collapse. Gastrointestinal symptoms include nausea, vomiting, diarrhea, and abdominal cramps. Fatal poisoning us usually proceeded by convulsions and coma.

TREATMENT

Management of acute amphetamine intoxication is largely symptomatic and includes gastric lavage and sedation with a barbiturate. Experience with hemodialysis or peritoneal dialysis is inadequate to permit recommendation in this regard. Acidification of the urine increases

OVERDOSAGE: *(cont'd)*

amphetamine excretion. If acute, severe hypertension complicates amphetamine overdosage, administration of intravenous phentolamine has been suggested. However, a gradual drop in pressure will usually result when sufficient sedation has been achieved.

Chlorpromazine antagonizes the central stimulant effects of amphetamines and can be used to treat amphetamine intoxication.

DOSAGE AND ADMINISTRATION:

NARCOLEPSY

Narcolepsy seldom occurs in children under 12 years of age, however, when it does, amphetamine sulfate may be used. The Suggested initial dose for patients aged 6 to 12 is 5 mg daily; daily dose may be raised in increments of 5 mg at weekly intervals until optimal response is obtained. If bothersome adverse reactions appear (*e.g.,* insomnia or anorexia), dosage should be reduced.

ATTENTION DEFICIT DISORDER WITH HYPERACTIVITY

Not recommended for children under 3 years of age.

In children from 3 to 5 years of age, start with 2.5 mg daily; daily dosage may be raised in increments if 2,5 at weekly intervals until optimal response is obtained.

In children 6 years of age or older, start with 5 mg, once or twice daily: daily dosage may be raised in increments of 5 mg at weekly intervals until optimal response is obtained. Only in rare cases will it be necessary to exceed a total of 40 milligrams per day.

With tablets give first dose on awakening; additional doses (1 or 2) at intervals of 4 to 6 hours. Where possible, drug administration should be interrupted occasionally to determine if there is a recurrence of behavioral symptoms sufficient to require continued therapy.

EXOGENOUS OBESITY

Usual adult dose is 5 to 30 milligrams per day in divided doses.

HOW SUPPLIED - EQUIVALENTS NOT AVAILABLE:

Tablet, Plain Coated - Oral - 5 mg

1000's $40.27 Amphetamine Sulfate, Lannett 00527-1138-10

Tablet, Plain Coated - Oral - 10 mg

1000's $55.16 Amphetamine Sulfate, Lannett 00527-1139-10

AMPHETAMINE; DEXTROAMPHETAMINE

(003289)

CATEGORIES: Amphetamines; Anorexients/CNS Stimulants; Attention Deficit Disorders; Behavior Problems; Central Nervous System Agents; Obesity; Psychostimulants; Respiratory/Cerebral Stimulant; Stimulants; DEA Class CII; FDA Approved 1996 Feb

BRAND NAMES: **Adderall**

PRIMARY ICD9: 347 (Narcolepsy)

> WARNING:
> AMPHETAMINES HAVE A HIGH POTENTIAL FOR ABUSE. THEY SHOULD THUS BE TRIED ONLY IN WEIGHT REDUCTION PROGRAMS FOR PATIENTS IN WHOM ALTERNATIVE THERAPY HAS BEEN INEFFECTIVE. ADMINISTRATION OF AMPHETAMINES FOR PROLONGED PERIODS OF TIME IN OBESITY MAY LEAD TO DRUG DEPENDENCE AND MUST BE AVOIDED. PARTICULAR ATTENTION SHOULD BE PAID TO THE POSSIBILITY OF SUBJECTS OBTAINING AMPHETAMINES FOR NON-THERAPEUTIC USE OR DISTRIBUTION TO OTHERS, AND THE DRUGS SHOULD BE PRESCRIBED OR DISPENSED SPARINGLY.

DESCRIPTION:

A single entity amphetamine product combining the neutral salts of dextroamphetamine and amphetamine, with the dextro isomer of amphetamine saccharate and d, l-amphetamine asperate.

TABLE 1

	10 mg	20 mg
Dextroamphetamine Saccharate	2.5 mg	5 mg
Amphetamine Aspartate	2.5 mg	5 mg
Dextroamphetamine Sulfate USP	2.5 mg	5 mg
Amphetamine Sulfate USP	2.5 mg	5 mg
Total amphetamine base equivalence	6.3 mg	12.6 mg

Inactive ingredients: sucrose, lactose, corn starch, acacia and magnesium stearate.

Colors: *Adderall 10 mg:* contains FD & C Blue #1. *Aderall 20 mg:* contains FD & C Yellow #6 as a color additive.

CLINICAL PHARMACOLOGY:

MECHANISM OF ACTION

Amphetamines are non-catecholamine sympathomimetic amines with CNS stimulant activity. Peripheral actions include elevation of systolic and diastolic blood pressures and weak bronchodilator and respiratory stimulant action. Drugs of this class used in obesity are commonly known as "anorectics" or "anorexigenics". It has not been established, however, that the action of such drugs in treating obesity is primarily one of appetite suppression. For example, other central nervous system actions or metabolic effects may be involved.

There is neither specific evidence which clearly establishes the mechanism whereby amphetamine produces meental and behavioral effects in children, nor conclusive evidence regarding how these effects relate to the condition of the central nervous system dysfunction may or may not be warranted.

CLINICAL STUDIES:

Adult obese subjects instructed in dietary management and treated with "anorectic" drugs, lose more weight on the average than those treated with placebo and diet, as determined in relatively short-term clinical trials.

The magnitude of increased weight loss of drug-treated patients over placebo-treated patients is only a fraction of a pound a week. The rate of weight loss is greater in the first weeks of therapy for both drug and placebo subjects and tends to decrease in succeeding weeks. The origins of the increased weight loss due to the various possible drug effects are not estab-

CLINICAL STUDIES: *(cont'd)*

lished. The amount of weight loss associated with the use of an "anorectic" drug varies from trial to trial, and the increased weight loss appears to be related in part to variables other than the drug prescribed, such as the physician-investigator, the population treated, and the diet prescribed. Studies do not permit conclusions as to the relative importance of the drug and non-drug factors on weight loss.

The natural history of obesity is measured in years, whereas the studies cited are restricted to a few weeks duration, thus, the total impact of drug-induced weight loss over that of diet alone must be considered clinically limited.

INDICATIONS AND USAGE:

ATTENTION DEFICIT DISORDER WITH HYPERACTIVITY

Amphetamines are indicated as an integral part of a total treatment program which typically includes other remedial measures (psychological, educational, social) for a stabilizing effect in children with a behavioral syndrome characterized by the following group of developmentally inappropriate symptoms:

moderate to serve distractibility
short attention span
hyperactivity
emotional lability
impulsivity

The diagnosis of this syndrome should not be made with finality when these symptoms are only of comparatively recent origin. Nonlocalizing (soft) neurological signs, learning disability, and abnormal EEG may not be present, and a diagnosis of central nervous system dysfunction may or may not be warranted.

IN NARCOLEPSY

Exogenous obesity: As a short-term (a few weeks) adjunct in a regimen of weight reduction based on caloric restriction for patients refractory to alternative therapy (*e.g.*, repeated diets, group programs and other drugs). The limited usefulness of amphetamine (see Mechanism of Action) should be weighed against possible risks inherent in use of the drug, such as those described below.

CONTRAINDICATIONS:

Advanced arteriosclerosis, symptomatic cardiovascular disease, moderate to severe hypertension, hyperthyroidism, known hypersensitivity or idiosyncrasy to the sympathomimetic amines, glaucoma, agitated states, and patients with a history of drug abuse.

During or within 14 days following the administration of monoamine oxidase inhibitors (hypertensive crises may result).

WARNINGS:

When tolerance to the "anorectic" effect develops, the recommended dose should not be exceeded in an attempt to increase the effect; rather the drug should be discontinued. Clinical experience suggests that in psychotic children, administration of amphetamine may exacerbate symptoms of behavior disturbance and thought disorder. Data are inadequate to determined whether chronic administration of amphetamine may be associated with growth inhibition; therefore, growth should be monitored during treatment.

Usage in Nursing Mothers: Amphetamines are excreted in human milk. Mothers taking amphetamines should be advised to refrain from nursing.

PRECAUTIONS:

GENERAL

Caution is to be exercised in prescribing amphetamine for patients with mild hypertension.

The least amount feasible should be prescribed or dispensed at one time in order to minimize the possibility of overdosage.

INFORMATION FOR THE PATIENT

Amphetamines may impair the ability of the patient to engage in potentially hazardous activities such as operating machinery or vehicles; the patient should therefore be cautioned accordingly.

DRUG/LABORATORY TEST INTERACTIONS

Amphetamines can cause a significant elevation in plasma corticosteroid levels. This increase is greatest in the evening.

Amphetamines may interfere with urinary steroid determinations.

Carcinogenesis, Mutagenesis, and Impairment of Fertility: Mutagenicity studies and long-term studies in animals to determine the carcinogenic potential of Amphetamine, have not been performed.

Pregnancy, Teratogenic Effects, Pregnancy Category C: Amphetamine has been shown to have embryotoxic and teratogenic effects when administered to A/Jax mice and C57BL mice in doses approximately 41 times the maximum human dose. Embryotoxic effects were not seen in New Zealand white rabbits given the drug in doses 7 times the human dose nor in rats given 12.5 times the maximum human dose. There are no adequate and well-controlled studies in pregnant women. Amphetamines should be used during pregnancy only if the potential benefit justifies the potential risk to the fetus.

Nonteratogenic Effects: Infants born to mothers dependent on amphetamines have an increased risk of premature delivery and low birth weight. Also, these infants may experience symptoms of withdrawal as demonstrated by dysphoria, including agitation, and significant lassitude.

Pediatric Use: Long-term effects of amphetamines in children have not been well established. Amphetamines are not recommended for use as anorectic agents in children under 12 years of age, or in children 3 years of age with Attention Deficit Disorder with Hyperactivity described under INDICATIONS AND USAGE.

Amphetamines have been reported to exacerbate motor and phonic tics and Tourette's syndrome. Therefore, clinical evaluation for tics and Tourette's syndrome in children and their families should precede use of stimulant medications.

Drug treatment is not indicated in all cases of Attention Deficit Disorder with Hyperactivity and should be considered only in light of the complete history and evaluation of the child. The decision to prescribe amphetamines should depend on the physician's assessment of the chronicity and severity of the child's symptoms and their appropriateness for his/her age. Prescription should not depend solely on the presence of one or more of the behavioral characteristics. When these symptoms are associated with acute stress reactions, treatment with amphetamines is usually not indicated.

DRUG INTERACTIONS:

Acidifying agents: Gastrointestinal acidifying agents (guanethidine, reserpine, glutamic acid HCl, ascorbic acid, fruit juices, etc.) lower absorption of amphetamines.

Urinary acidifying agents: (ammonium chloride, sodium acid phosphate, etc.) increase the concentration of the ionized species of the amphetamine molecule, thereby increasing urinary excretion. Both groups of agents lower blood levels and efficacy of amphetamines.

DRUG INTERACTIONS: *(cont'd)*

Adrenergic blockers: Adrenergic blockers are inhibited by amphetamines.

Alkalinizing agents: Gastrointestinal alkalinizing agents (sodium bicarbonate, etc.) increase absorption of amphetamines. Urinary alkalinizing agents (acetazolamide, some thiazides) increase the concentration of the non-ionized species of the amphetamine molecule, thereby decreasing urinary excretion. Both groups of agents increase blood levels and therefore potentiate the actions of amphetamines.

Antidepressants, tricyclic: Amphetamines may enhance the activity of tricyclic or sympathomimetic agents; d-amphetamine with desipramine or protriptyline and possibly other tricyclics cause striking and sustained increases in the concentration of d=amphetamine in the brain; cardiovascular effects can be potentiated.

MAO inhibitors: MAOI antidepressants, as well as a metabolite of furazolidone, slow amphetamine metabolism. This slowing potentiates amphetamines, increasing their effect on the release of norepinephrine and other monoamines from adrenergic nerve endings; this can cause headaches and other signs of hypertensive crisis. A variety of neurological toxic effects and malignant hyperpyrexia can occur, sometimes with fatal results.

Antihistamines: Amphetamines may counteract the sedative effect of antihistamines.

Antihypertensives: Amphetamines may antagonize the hypotensive effects of antihypertensives.

Chlorpromazine: Chlorpromazine blocks dopamine and norepinephrine reuptake, thus inhibiting the central stimulant effects of amphetamines, and can be used to treat amphetamine poisoning.

Ethosuximide: Amphetamines may delay intestinal absorption of ethosuximide.

Haloperidol: Haloperidol blocks dopamine and norepinephrine reuptake, thus inhibiting the central stimulant effects of amphetamines.

Lithium carbonate: The antiobesity and stimulatory effects of amphetamines may be inhibited by lithiium carbonate.

Meperidine: Amphetamines potentiate the analgesic effect of meperidine.

Methenamine therapy: Urinary excretion of amphetamines is increased, and efficacy is reduced, by acidifying agents used in methenamine therapy.

Norepinephrine: Amphetamines enhance the adrenergic effect of norepinephrine.

Phenobarbital: Amphetamines may delay intestinal absorption of phenobarbital; co-administration of phenobarbital may product a synergistic anticonvulsant action.

Phenytoin: Amphetamines may delay intestinal absorption of phenytoin; co-administration of phenytoin may produce a synergistic anticonvulsant action.

Propoxyphene: In most cases of propoxyphene overdosage, amphetamine CNS stimulation is potential and fatal convulsions can occur.

Veratrum alkaloids: Amphetamines inhibit the hypertensive effect of veratrum alkaloids.

ADVERSE REACTIONS:

Cardiovascular: Palpitation, tachycardia, elevation of blood pressure. There have been isolated reports of cardiomyopathy associated with chronic amphetamine use.

Central nervous system: Overstimulation, restlessness, dizziness, insomnia, euphoria, dysphoria, tremor, headache; rarely psychotic episodes at recommended doses.

Gastrointestinal: Dryness of the mouth, unpleasant taste, diarrhea, constipation, other gastrointestinal disturbances.

Allergic: Urticaria.

Endocrine: Impotence, changes in Libido.

DRUG ABUSE AND DEPENDENCE:

Dextroamphetamine sulfate is a Schedule II controlled substance.

Amphetamines have been extensively abused. Tolerance, extreme psychological dependence, and severe social disability have occurred. There are reports of patients who have increased the dosage to many times that recommended. Abrupt cessation following prolonged high dosage administration results in extreme fatigue and mental depression; changes are also noted on the sleep EEG. Manifestations of chronic intoxication with amphetamines include severe dermatoses, marked insomnia, irritability, hyperactivity, and personality changes. The most severe manifestation of chronic intoxication is psychosis, often clinically indistinguishable from schizophrenia. This is rare with oral amphetamines.

OVERDOSAGE:

Individual patient response to amphetamines varies widely. While toxic symptoms occasionally occur as an idosyncrasy at doses as low as 2 mg, they are rare with doses of less than 15 mg; 30 mg can produce severe reactions, yet doses of 400 to 500 mg are not necessarily fatal.

In rats, the oral LD50 of dextroamphetamine sulfate is 96.8 mg/kg.

SYMPTOMS

Manifestations of acute overdosage with amphetamines include restlessness, tremor, hyperreflexia, rapid respiration, confusion, assaultiveness, hallucinations, panic states, hyperpyrexia and rhabdomolysis.

Fatigue and depression usually follow the central stimulation.

Cardiovascular effects include arrhythmias, hypertension or hypotension and circulatory collapse.

Gastrointestinal symptoms include nausea, vomiting, diarrhea, and abdominal cramps. Fatal poisoning is usally preceded by convulsions and coma.

TREATMENT

Consult with a Certified Poison Control Center for up to date guidance and advice. Management of acute amphetamine intoxication is largely symptomatic and includes gastric lavage, administration of activated charcoal, administration of a cathartic and sedation. Experience with hemodialysis or peritoneal dialysis is inadequate to permit recommendation in this regard. Acidification of the urine increases amphetamine excretion, but is believed to increase risk of acute renal failure if myoglobinuria is present. If acute, severe hypertension complicates amphetamine overdosage, administration of intravenous phentolamine (Regitine, CIBA) has been suggested. However, a gradual drop in blood pressure will usually result when sufficient sedation has been achieved. Chlorpromazine antagonizes the central stimulant effects of amphetamines and can be used to treat amphetamine intoxication.

DOSAGE AND ADMINISTRATION:

Regardless of indication, amphetamines should be administered at the lowest effective dosage and dosage should be individually adjusted. Late evening doses should be avoided because of the resulting insomnia.

Attention Deficit Disorder with Hyperactivity: Not recommended for children under 3 years of age. In children from 3 to 5 years of age, start with 2.5 mg daily; daily dosage may be raised in increments of 2.5 mg at weekly intervals until optimal response is obtained.

DOSAGE AND ADMINISTRATION: *(cont'd)*

In children 6 years of age and older, start with 5 mg once or twice daily; daily dosage may be raised in increments of 5 mg at weekly intervals until optimal response is obtained. Only in rare cases will it be necessary to exceed a total of 40 mg per day. Give first dose on awakening; additional doses (1 or 2) at intervals of 4 to 6 hours.

Where possible, drug administration should be interrupted occasionally to determine if there is a recurrence of behavioral symptoms sufficient to require continued therapy.

NARCOLEPSY

Usual dose 5 mg to 60 mg per day in divided doses, depending on the individual patient response.

Narcolepsy seldom occurs in children under 12 years of age; however, when it does, dextroamphetamine sulfate, may be used. The suggested initial dose for patients aged 6–12 is 5 mg daily; daily dose may be raised in increments of 5 mg at weekly intervals until optimal response is obtained. In patients 12 years of age and older, start with 10 mg daily; daily dosage may be raised in increments of 10 mg at weekly intervals until optimal response is obtained. If bothersome adverse reactions appear (*e.g.*, insomnia or anorexia), dosage should be reduced. Give first dose on awakening; additional doses (1 or 2) at intervals of 4 to 6 hours.

EXOGENOUS OBESITY

Usual adult dose is 5 mg to 30 mg per day in divided doses, taken 30 to 60 minutes before meals. Not recommended for use in children under 12 years of age.

PATIENT INFORMATION:

Amphetamines are used for narcolepsy, attention deficit disorder and obesity.

Do not take if you have hypertension. Inform your doctor if you are pregnant or nursing. To avoid insomnia, do not take this drug in the evening. May impair ability to perform hazardous tasks; patients should use caution while driving or operating machinery.

May cause insomnia, dizziness, overstimulation and GI upset. Inform your doctor or pharmacist if these effects occur.

HOW SUPPLIED:

Dispense in a tight, light-resistant container.

Storage: Store in controlled room temperature 15°-30°C (59°-86°F).

HOW SUPPLIED - EQUIVALENTS NOT AVAILABLE:

Tablet - Oral - 10 mg

10 mg x 100	$49.95	ADDERALL, Richwood Pharm	58521-0032-01

Tablet - Oral - 20 mg

20 mg x 100	$74.90	ADDERALL, Richwood Pharm	58521-0033-01

AMPHOTERICIN B *(000235)*

CATEGORIES: Anti-Infectives; Antibiotics; Antifungals; Antimicrobials; Aspergillosis; Blastomycosis; Candidiasis; Coccidioidomycosis; Cryptococcosis; Histoplasmosis; Infections; Mucormycosis; Skin/Mucous Membrane Agents; Sporotrichosis; Zygomycosis; FDA Approval Pre 1982

BRAND NAMES: Amphocin; *Ampho-Moronal* (Germany); *Fungilin*; **Fungizone IV**; *Fungizone* (France); **Fungizone Topical**
(International brand names outside U.S. in italics)

FORMULARIES: Medi-Cal; WHO

> **WARNING:**
> **Intravenous Injection:** This drug should be used primarily for treatment of patients with progressive and potentially life-threatening fungal infections; it should not be used to treat noninvasive forms of fungal disease such as oral thrush, vaginal candidiasis and esophageal candidiasis in patients with normal neutrophil counts.

DESCRIPTION:

INJECTION

Amphotericin B is an antifungal polyene antibiotic obtained from a strain of *Streptomyces nodosus.* Amphotericin B is designated chemically as (1R-(1R*,3S*,5R*,6R*,9R*,11R*,15S*,16R*,17R*,18S*,19E,21E,23E,25E,27E,29E,31E,33R*,35S*-,36R*,37S*))-33-((3-Amino-3,6-dideoxy-β-D-mannopyranosyl)-oxy)-1,3,5,6,9,11,17,37-octahydroxy-15,16,18-trimethyl-1 3-oxo-14,39-dioxabicyclo(33.3.1)nonatriaconta-19,21,23,25,29,31-heptaene-36- carboxylic acid.

Each vial of Fungizone contains a sterile, nonpyrogenic, lyophilized cake (which may partially reduce to powder following manufacture) providing 50 mg amphotericin B and 41 mg sodium desoxycholate with 20.2 mg sodium phosphates as a buffer.

Crystalline amphotericin B is insoluble in water; therefore, the antibiotic is solubilized by the addition of sodium desoxycholate to form a mixture which provides a colloidal dispersion for intravenous infusion following reconstitution.

At the time of manufacture the air in the vial is replaced by nitrogen.

TOPICAL

Lotion: Amphotericin B lotion contains the antifungal antibiotic amphotericin B at a concentration of 3% (30 mg/ml) in a tinted, unscented aqueous lotion vehicle with thimerosal, titanium dioxide, guar gum, propylene glycol, cetyl alcohol, Stearyl alcohol, sorbitan monopalmitate, polysorbate 20, glyceryl monostearate, polyethylene glycol monostearate, simethicone, sorbic acid, sodium citrate, methylparaben, and propylparaben.

Ointment: Amphotericin B ointment contains the antifungal antibiotic Amphotericin B U.S.P. at a concentration of 3 % (30 mg/g) in a tinted form of Plastibase (Plasticized Hydrocarbon Gel), a polyethylene and mineral oil gel base with titanium dioxide.

CLINICAL PHARMACOLOGY:

INJECTION

Microbiology: Amphotericin B shows a high order of *in vitro* activity against many species of fungi. *Histoplasma capsulatum, Coccidioides immitis, Candida* species, *Blastomyces dermatitidis, Rhodotorula, Cryptococcus neoformans, Sporothrix schenckii, Mucor mucedo,* and *Aspergillus fumigatus* are all inhibited by concentrations of amphotericin B ranging from 0.03 to 1.0 mcg/ml *in vitro.* While *Candida albicans* is generally quite susceptible to amphotericin B, non-*albicans* species may be less susceptible. *Pseudallescheria boydii* and *Fusarium* sp. are often resistant to amphotericin B. The antibiotic is without effect on bacteria, rickettsiae and viruses.

CLINICAL PHARMACOLOGY: *(cont'd)*

Susceptibility Testing: Standardized techniques for susceptibility testing for antifungal agents have not been established and results of susceptibility studies have not been correlated with clinical outcomes.

Pharmacokinetics: Amphotericin B is fungistatic or fungicidal depending on the concentration obtained in body fluids and the susceptibility of the fungus. The drug acts by binding to sterols in the cell membrane of susceptible fungi with a resultant change in membrane permeability allowing leakage of intercellular components. Mammalian cell membranes also contain sterols and it has been suggested that the damage to human cells and fungal cells may share common mechanisms.

An initial intravenous infusion of 1 to 5 infusion of 1 to 5 mg of amphotericin B per day, gradually increased to 0.4 to 0.6 mg/kg daily, produces peak plasma concentrations ranging from approximately 0.5 to 2 mcg/ml. Following a rapid initial fall, plasma concentrations plateau at about 0.5 mcg/ml. An elimination half-life of approximately 15 days follows an initial plasma half-life of about 24 hours. Amphotericin B circulating in plasma is highly (>90%) to plasma proteins and is poorly dialyzable. Approximately two thirds of concurrent plasma concentrations have been detected in fluids from inflamed pleura, peritoneum, synovium, and aqueous humor. Concentrations in the cerebrospinal fluid seldom exceed 2.5 percent of those in the plasma. Little amphotericin B penetrates into vitreous humor or normal amniotic fluid. Complete details of tissue distribution are not known.

Amphotericin B is excreted very slowly (over weeks to months) by the kidneys with two to five percent of a given dose being excreted in the biologically active form. Details of possible metabolic pathways are not know. After treatment is discontinued, the drug can be detected in the urine for at least seven weeks due to the slow disappearance of the drug. The cumulative urinary output over a seven day period amounts to approximately 40 percent of the amount of drug infused.

TOPICAL

Amphotericin B is an antibiotic with antifungal activity produced by a strain of *Streptomyces nodosus.* It has been shown to exhibit greater *in vitro* activity than nystatin against *Candida (Monilia) albicans.* In clinical studies involving cutaneous and mucocutaneous candidal infections, results with topical preparations of amphotericin B were comparable to those obtained with nystatin in similar formulations.

Although amphotericin B exhibits some *in vitro* activity against the superficial dermatophytes (ringworm organisms), it has not demonstrated an effectiveness *in vivo* on topical application. Amphotericin B has no significant effect either *in vitro* or clinically against gram-positive or gram-negative bacteria, or viruses.

INDICATIONS AND USAGE:

Injection: Amphotericin B for injection should be administered primarily to patients with progressive, potentially-life-threatening fungal infections. This potent drug should not be used to threat noninvasive fungal infections, such as oral thrush, vaginal candidiasis and esophageal candidiasis in patients with normal neutrophil counts.

Amphotericin B for injection is specifically intended to treat potentially life-threatening fungal infection: aspergillosis, cryptococcosis (torulosis). North American blastomycosis, systemic candidiasis, coccidioidomycosis, histoplasmosis, zygomycosis including mucormycosis due to susceptible species of the genera *Absidia, Mucor* and *Rhizopus*, and infections due to related susceptible species of *Conidiobolus* and *Basidiobolus,* and sporotrichosis.

Amphotericin B may be useful in the treatment of American mucocutaneous leishmaniasis, but it is not drug of choice as primary therapy.

Topical: Amphotericin B lotion and ointment are indicated in the treatment of cutaneous and mucocutaneous mycotic infections caused by *Candida (Monilia)* species.

CONTRAINDICATIONS:

INJECTION

This product is contraindicated in those patients who have shown hypersensitivity to amphotericin B or any other component in the formulation unless, in the opinion of the physician, the condition requiring treatment is life-threatening and amenable only to amphotericin B therapy.

TOPICAL

The preparations are contraindicated in patients with a history of hypersensitivity to any of its components.

WARNINGS:

Injection: Amphotericin B is frequently the only effective treatment available for potentially life-threatening fungal disease. In each case, its possible life-saving benefit must be balanced against its untoward and dangerous side effects.

PRECAUTIONS:

INJECTION

General

Amphotericin B should be administered intravenously under close clinical observation by medically trained personnel. It should be reserved for treatment of patients with progressive, potentially life-threatening fungal infections due to susceptible organisms (see INDICATIONS AND USAGE.)

Acute reactions including fever, shaking chills, hypotension, anorexia, nausea, vomiting headache, and tachypnea are common 1 to 3 hours after starting an intravenous infusion. These reactions are usually more severe with the first few doses of amphotericin B and usually diminish with subsequent doses.

Rapid Intravenous Infusion: has been associated with hypotension, hypokalemia, arrhythmias, and shock and should, therefore, be avoided (see DOSAGE AND ADMINISTRATION.)

Amphotericin B should be used with care in patients with reduced renal function; frequent monitoring of renal function is recommended (see PRECAUTIONS, Laboratory Tests) and ADVERSE REACTIONS). In some patients hydration and sodium repletion prior to amphotericin B administration may reduce the risk of developing nephrotoxicity. Supplemental alkali medication may decrease renal tubular acidosis complications.

Since acute pulmonary reactions have been reported in patients given amphotericin B during or shortly after leukocyte transfusion, it is advisable to temporally separate these infusions as far as possible and to monitor pulmonary function (See DRUG INTERACTIONS.)

Leukoencephalopathy has been reported following use of amphotericin B. Literature reports have suggested that total body irradiation may be a predisposition.

Whenever medication is interrupted for a period longer than seven days, therapy should be resumed by starting with the lowest dosage level e.g. 0.25 mg/kg of body weight, and increased gradually as outlined under DOSAGE AND ADMINISTRATION.

PRECAUTIONS: *(cont'd)*

Laboratory Tests

Renal function should be monitored frequently during amphotericin B therapy (see ADVERSE REACTIONS). It is also advisable to monitor on a regular basis liver function, serum electrolytes (particularly magnesium and potassium), blood counts, and hemoglobin concentrations. Laboratory test results should be used as a guide to subsequent dosage adjustments.

Carcinogenesis, Mutagenesis, and Impairment of Fertility

No long-term studies in animals have been performed to evaluate carcinogenic potential. There also have been no studies to determine mutagenicity or whether this medication affects fertility in males or females.

Pregnancy, Teratogenic Effects, Pregnancy Category B

Reproduction studies in animals have revealed no evidence of harm to the fetus due to amphotericin B for injection. Systemic fungal infections have been successfully treated in pregnant women with amphotericin B for injection without obvious effects to the fetus, but the number of cases reported has been small. Because animal reproduction studies are not always predictive of human response, and adequate and well-controlled studies have not been conducted in pregnant women, this drug should be used during pregnancy only if clearly indicated.

Nursing Mothers

It is not known whether amphotericin B is excreted in human milk. Because many drugs are excreted in human milk and considering the potential toxicity of amphotericin B, it is prudent to advise a nursing mother to discontinue nursing.

Pediatric Use

Safety and effectiveness in pediatric patients have not been established through adequate and well-controlled studies. Systemic fungal infections have been successfully treated in pediatric patients without reports of unusual side effects. Amphotericin B for Injection when administered to pediatric patient should be limited to the smallest dose compatible with an effective therapeutic regimen.

TOPICAL

Should a reaction of hypersensitivity occur the drug should be immediately withdrawn and appropriate measures taken.

The lotion preparation is not for ophthalmic use.

DRUG INTERACTIONS:

INJECTION

When administered concurrently, the following drugs may interact with amphotericin B:

Antineoplastic Agents: may enhance the potential for renal toxicity, bronchospasm and hypotension. Antineoplastic agents (*e.g.* nitrogen mustard, etc.) should be given concomitantly only with great caution.

Corticosteroids and Corticotropin (ACTH): may potentiate amphotericin B-induced hypokalemia which may predispose the patient to cardiac dysfunction. Avoid concomitant use unless necessary to control side effects of amphotericin B. If used concomitantly, closely monitor serum electrolytes and cardiac function (see ADVERSE REACTIONS).

Digitalis Glycosides: Amphotericin B-induced hypokalemia may potentiate digitalis toxicity. Serum potassium levels and cardiac function should be closely monitored and any deficit promptly corrected.

Flucytosine: While a synergistic relationship with amphotericin B has been reported, concomitant use may increase the toxicity of flucytosine by possible increasing its cellular uptake and/or impairing its renal excretion.

Imidazoles (*e.g.* ketoconazole, miconazole, clotrimazole, fluconazole, etc.): *In vitro* and animal studies with the combination of amphotericin B and imidazoles suggest that imidazoles may induce fungal resistance to amphotericin B. Combination therapy should be administered with caution, especially in immunocompromised patients.

Other Nephrotoxic Medications: Agents such as aminoglycosides, cyclosporine, and pentamidine may enhance the potential for drug-induced renal toxicity, and should be used concomitantly only with great caution. Intensive monitoring of renal function is recommended in patients requiring any combination of nephrotoxic medications (see PRECAUTIONS, Laboratory Tests.)

Skeletal Muscle Relaxants: Amphotericin B-induced hypokalemia may enhance the curariform effect of skeletal muscle relaxants (*e.g.,* tubocurarine). Serum potassium levels should be monitored and deficiencies corrected.

Leukocyte Transfusions: Acute pulmonary toxicity has been reported in patients receiving intravenous amphotericin B and leukocyte transfusions (see PRECAUTIONS, General.)

ADVERSE REACTIONS:

INJECTION

Although some patients may tolerate full intravenous doses of amphotericin B without difficulty, most will exhibit some intolerance, often at less than the full therapeutic dose.

Tolerance may be improved by treatment with aspirin, antipyretics (*e.g.,* acetaminophen), antihistamines, or antiemetics. Meperidine (25 to 50 mg IV) has been shown in some patients to decrease the duration of shaking chills and fever that may accompany the infusion of amphotericin B.

Administration of amphotericin B on alternate days may decrease anorexia and phlebitis.

Intravenous administration of small doses of adrenal corticosteroids just prior to or during the amphotericin B infusion may help decrease febrile reactions. Dosage and duration of such corticosteroid therapy should be kept to a minimum (see DRUG INTERACTIONS).

Addition of heparin (1000 units per infusion), and the use of a pediatric scalp-vein needle may lessen the incidence of thrombophlebitis. Extravasation may cause chemical irritation.

The adverse reactions most commonly observed are:

General (body as a whole): fever (sometimes accompanied by shaking chills usually occurring within 15 to 20 minutes after initiation of treatment); malaise; weight loss.

Cardiopulmonary: hypotension; tachypnea.

Gastrointestinal: anorexia, nausea; vomiting; diarrhea; dyspepsia; cramping epigastric pain.

Hematologic: normochromic, normocytic anemia.

Local: pain at the injection site with or without phlebitis or thrombophlebitis.

Musculoskeletal: generalized pain, including muscle and joint pains.

Neurologic: headache.

Renal: decreased renal function and renal function abnormalities including: azotemia, hypokalemia, hyposthenuria, renal tubular acidosis; and nephrocalcinosis. These usually improve with interruption of therapy. However, some permanent impairment often occurs, especially in those patients receiving large amounts (over 5 g) of amphotericin B or receiving other nephrotoxic agents. In some patients hydration and sodium repletion prior to amphotericin B administration may reduce the risk of developing nephrotoxicity. Supplemental alkali medication may decrease renal tubular acidosis.

ADVERSE REACTIONS: *(cont'd)*

The following adverse reactions have also been reported:

General (body as a whole): flushing

Allergic: anaphylactoid and other allergic reactions; bronchospasm; wheezing

Cardiopulmonary: cardiac arrest; shock; cardiac failure; pulmonary edema; hypersensitivity pneumonitis; arrhythmias, including ventricular fibrillation; dyspnea; hypertension

Dermatologic: rash, in particular maculopapular; pruritus

Gastrointestinal: acute liver failure; hepatitis; jaundice; hemorrhagic gastroenteritis; melena

Hematologic: agranulocytosis; coagulation defects; thrombocytopenia; leukopenia; eosinophilia; leukocytosis

Neurologic: convulsions; hearing loss; tinnitus; transient vertigo; visual impairment; diplopia; peripheral neuropathy; other neurologic symptoms

Renal: acute renal failure, anuria; oliguria

Altered Laboratory Findings

Serum Electrolytes: Hypomagnesemia; hypo-and hyperkalemia; hypocalcemia.

Liver function Tests: Elevations of AST, ALT, GGT, bilirubin, and alkaline phosphatase.

Renal Function Tests: Elevations of BUN and serum creatinine.

TOPICAL

No evidence of any systemic toxicity or side effects has been observed during or following even prolonged, intensive and extensive application of amphotericin B lotion or ointment.

Lotion: The preparation is extremely well tolerated by all age groups, including infants, even when therapy must be continued for many months. It is not a primary irritant and apparently has only a slight sensitizing potential. Local intolerance, which seldom occurs, has included increased pruritus with or without other subjective or objective evidence of local irritation, or exacerbation of preexisting candidal lesions. Allergic contact dermatitis is rare.

Ointment: The preparation is usually well tolerated by all age groups. It is not a primary irritant and apparently has only a slight sensitizing potential. However, it is well to remember that any oleaginous ointment vehicle may occasionally irritate when applied to moist, intertriginous areas.

OVERDOSAGE:

Injection: Amphotericin B overdoses can results in cardio-respiratory arrest. If an overdose is suspected discontinue therapy and monitor the patient's clinical status (*e.g.* cardio-respiratory, renal, and liver function, hematologic status, serum electrolytes) and administer supportive therapy, as required. Amphotericin B is not hemodialyzable.

Prior to reinstituting therapy, the patient's condition should be stabilized (including correction of electrolyte deficiencies, etc.)

DOSAGE AND ADMINISTRATION:

INJECTION

CAUTION: Under no circumstances should a total daily dose of 1.5 mg/kg be exceeded. Amphotericin B overdoses can result in cardio-respiratory arrest (see OVERDOSAGE).

Amphotericin B intravenous injection should be administered by *slow* intervenous infusion. Intravenous infusion should be given over a period of approximately 2 to 6 hours (depending on the dose) observing the usual precautions for intravenous therapy (see PRECAUTIONS, General). The recommended concentration for intravenous infusion is 0.1 mg/ml (1 mg/10 ml).

Since patient tolerance varies greatly, the dosage of amphotericin B must be individualized and adjusted according to the patient's clinical status (*e.g.,* site and severity of infection, etiologic agent, cardio-renal function, etc.).

A single intravenous **test dose** (1 mg in 20 ml of 5% dextrose solution) administered over 20-30 minutes may be preferred. The patient's temperature, pulse, respiration and blood pressure should be recorded every 30 minutes for 2 to 4 hours.

In patients with **good cardio-renal function** and a **well tolerated test dose**, therapy is usually initiated with a daily dose of 0.25 mg/kg of body weight. However, in those patients having **severe and rapidly progressive fungal infection**, therapy may be initiated with a daily dose of 0.3 mg/kg of body weight. In patients with**impaired cardio-renal function** or a **severe reaction to the test dose**, therapy should be initiated with smaller daily doses (*i.e.* 5 to 10 mg).

Depending on the patient's cardio-renal status (see PRECAUTIONS, Laboratory Tests) doses may gradually be increased by 5 to 10 mg per day to final daily dosage of 0.5 to 0.7 mg/kg.

There is sufficient data presently available to define total dosage requirements and duration of treatment necessary for eradication of specific mycoses. The optimal dose is unknown. Total daily dosage may range up to 1.0 mg/kg per day or up to 1.5 mg/kg when given on alternate days.

Sporotrichosis: Therapy with intravenous amphotericin B for sporotrichosis has ranged up to nine months with a total dose up to 2.5 g.

Aspergillosis: Aspergillosis has been treated with amphotericin B intravenously for a period up to 11 months with a total dose up to 3.6 g.

Rhinocerebral Phycomycosis: This fulminating disease, generally occurs in association with diabetic ketoacidosis. It is, therefore, imperative that diabetic control be restored in order for treatment with amphotericin B intravenous injection to be successful. In contradistinction, pulmonary phycomycosis, which is more common in association with hematologic malignancies, is often an incidental finding at autopsy. A cumulative dose of at least 3 g of amphotericin is recommended to treat rhinocerebral phycomycosis. Although a total dose of 3 to 4 will infrequently cause lasting renal impairment, this would seem a reasonable minimum where there is clinical evidence of invasion of deep tissue. Since rhinocerebral phycomycosis usually follows a rapidly fatal course, the therapeutic approach must necessarily be more aggressive than that used in more indolent mycoses.

Preparation of Solutions

Reconstitute as Follows: An initial concentrate of 5 mg amphotericin B per ml is first prepared by rapidly expressing 10 ml Sterile Water for Injection USP *without a bacteriostatic* agent directly into the lyophilized cake, using a sterile needle (minimum diameter: 20 gauge) and syringe. Shake the vial immediately until the colloidal solution is clear. The infusion solution, providing 0.1 mg amphotericin B per ml, is then obtained by further dilution (1:50) with 5% Dextrose Injection USP*of pH above 4.2.* The pH of each container of Dextrose Injection should be ascertained before use. Commercial Dextrose Injection usually has a pH above 4.2; however, if it is below 4.2., then 1 or 2 ml of buffer should be added to the Dextrose Injection before it is used to dilute the concentrated solution of amphotericin B. The recommended buffer has the following composition:

Dibasic sodium phosphate (anhydrous): 1.59 g

Monobasic sodium phosphate (anhydrous): 0.96 g

Water for Injection USP: qs 100. ml

The buffer should be sterilized before it is added to the Dextrose Injection, either by filtration through a bacterial retentive stone, mat, or membrane, or by autoclaving for 30 minutes at 15 lb pressure (121°C).

DOSAGE AND ADMINISTRATION: *(cont'd)*

CAUTION: Aseptic technique must be strictly observed in all handling, since no preservative or bacteriostatic agent is present in the antibiotic or in the materials used to prepare it for administration. **All entries into the vial or into the diluents must be made with a sterile needle. Do not reconstitute with saline solutions. The use of any diluent other than the ones recommended or the presence of a bacteriostatic agent (*e.g.* benzyl alcohol) in the diluent may cause precipitation of the antibiotic. Do not use the initial concentrate or the infusion solution if there is any evidence of precipitation or foreign matter in either one.**

An in-line membrane filter may be used for intravenous infusion of amphotericin B; **however, the mean pore diameter of the filter should not be less than 1.0 micron in order to assure passage of the antibiotic dispersion.**

TOPICAL

Amphotericin B lotion or ointment should be applied liberally to the candidal lesions two to four times daily. Duration of therapy depends on individual patient response. Intertriginous lesions usually respond within a few days, and treatment may be completed in one to three weeks. Similarly, candidiasis of the diaper area, perleche, and glabrous skin lesions usually clear in one to two weeks. Interdigital (erosio) lesions may require two to four weeks of intensive therapy, paronychias also require relatively prolonged therapy, and those onychomycoses which respond may require several months or more of treatment. (Relapses are frequently encountered in the last three clinical conditions.)

Note: The preparation does not stain the skin when thoroughly rubbed into the lesion, although nail lesions may be stained.

The patient should be informed that any discoloration of fabrics is readily removed with soap and warm water or a standard cleaning fluid.

HOW SUPPLIED:

INJECTION

Fungizone Intravenous: Available as single vials providing 50 mg amphotericin B as a yellow to orange lyophilized cake (which may partially reduce to powder following manufacture). *Storage:* Prior to reconstitution Fungizone Intravenous should be stored in the refrigerator, protected against exposure to light. The concentrate (5 mg amphotericin B per ml after reconstitution with 10 ml Sterile Water for Injection USP) may be stored in the dark, at room temperature for 24 hours, or at refrigerator temperatures for one week with minimal loss of potency and clarity. Any unused material should then be discarded. Solutions prepared for intravenous infusion (0.1 mg or less amphotericin B per ml) should be used promptly after preparation and should be protected from light during administration.

Fungizone Lotion: in 30 ml plastic squeeze bottles providing 30 mg amphotericin B per ml.

Fungizone Ointment: is supplied in tubes providing 3% Amphotericin B U.S.P. (30 mg/g).

Storage: Store at room temperature, avoid freezing.

(Lotion: Apothecon, 6/92, J4-453A)

(Ointment: E.R. Squibb & Sons, Inc., 9/72, J2-151D)

HOW SUPPLIED - RATED THERAPEUTICALLY EQUIVALENT:

Injection, Lyphl-Soln - Intravenous - 50 mg/15ml vial

1's	**$21.61**	**FUNGIZONE IV, Bristol Myers Squibb**	**00003-0437-30**
1's	**$21.61**	**FUNGIZONE IV, Bristol Myers Squibb**	**00003-0437-32**
1's	$31.20	AMPHOTERICIN B, Gensia Labs	00703-9785-01
1's	$34.54	Amphocin, Pharmacia & Upjohn	00013-1405-44
1's	**$42.30**	**FUNGIZONE, TISSUE CULTURE, Bristol Myers Squibb**	**00003-0437-60**

HOW SUPPLIED - NOT RATED EQUIVALENT:

Cream - Topical - 3 %

20 gm	$30.43	FUNGIZONE, Bristol Myers Squibb	00003-0411-20

Lotion - Topical - 3 %

30 ml	$41.74	FUNGIZONE, Bristol Myers Squibb	00003-0412-30

Ointment - Topical - 3 %

20 gm	$29.25	FUNGIZONE, Bristol Myers Squibb	00003-0426-20

AMPHOTERICIN B LIPID COMPLEX *(003277)*

CATEGORIES: Anti-Infectives; Antifungals; Aspergillosis; Infections; FDA Approved 1995 Nov

BRAND NAMES: **Abelcet**; ABLC; *Ambisome*
(International brand names outside U.S. in italics)

DESCRIPTION:

Amphotericin B Lipid Complex (ABLC) is a sterile, pyrogen-free suspension for intravenous infusion. ABLC consists of amphotericin B complexed with two phospholipids in a 1:1 drug-to-lipid molar ratio. The two phospholipids, L-α-dimyristoylphosphatidylcholine (DMPC) and L-α-dimyristoylphosphatidylglycerol (DMPG), are present in a 7:3 molar ratio. ABLC is yellow and opaque in appearance, with a pH of 5.5–6.0.

NOTE: Liposomal encapsulation or incorporation in a lipid complex can substantially affect a drug's functional properties relative to those of the unencapsulated or nonlipid-associated drug. In addition, different liposomal or lipid-complexed products with a common active ingredient may vary from one to another in the chemical composition and physical form of the lipid component. Such differences may affect functional properties of these drug products.

Amphotericin B is a polygene, antifungal antibiotic produced from a strain of *Streptomyces nodsus*. Amphotericin B is designated chemically as [1R-(1R*, 3S*, 5R*, 6R*, 9R*, 11R*, 15S*, 16R*, 17R*, 18S*, 19E, 21E, 23E, 25E, 27E, 29E, 31E, 33R*, 35S*, 36R*, 37S*)]-33-[(3-Amino-3, 6-dideoxy -β-D-mannopyranosyl) oxy]-1, 3, 5, 6, 9, 11, 17, 37-octahydroxy-15, 16, 18- trimethyl -13-oxo-14, 39-dioxabicyclo[33.3.1]nonatriacontra-19, 21, 23, 25, 27, 29, 31-heptaene-36-carboxylic acid.

It has a molecular weight of 924.09 and a molecular formula of $C_{47}H_{73}NO_{17}$.

ABLC is provided as a sterile, opaque suspension in 20 ml glass, single-use vials. Each vial of ABLC contains 100 mg of amphotericin B (see DOSAGE AND ADMINISTRATION), and each ml of ABLC contains:

Amphotericin B USP: 5.0 mg

L-α-Dimyristoylphosphatidylcholine (DMPC): 3.4 mg

L-α-Dimyristoylphosphatidylglycerol (DMPG): 1.5 mg

Sodium Chloride USP: 9.0 mg

Water for Injection USP: q.s. 1.0 ml

CLINICAL PHARMACOLOGY:

MECHANISM OF ACTION

The active component of ABLC, amphotericin B, acts by binding to sterols in the cell membrane of susceptible fungi, with a resultant change in the permeability of the membrane. Mammalian cell membranes also contain sterols, and damage to human cells is believed to occur through the same mechanism of action.

ACTIVITY *IN VITRO* AND *IN VIVO*

ABLC shows *in vitro* activity against *Aspergillus* sp. (n=3) and *Candida* (n=10), with MICs generally <1 mcg/ml. Depending upon the species and strain of *Aspergillus* and *Candida* tested, significant *in vitro* differences in susceptibility to amphotericin B have been reported (MICs ranging from 0.1 to >10mcg/ml). However, standardized techniques for susceptibility testing for antifungal agents have not been established, and results of susceptibility studies do not necessarily correlate with clinical outcome.

ABLC is active in animal models against *Aspergillus fumigatus, Candida albicans. C. guillermondi, C. stellatoideae, and C. tropicalis*, in which end-points were prolonged survival of infected animals and clearance of microorganisms from target organ(s).

DRUG RESISTANCE

Mutants with decreased susceptibility to amphotericin B have been isolated from several fungal species after serial passage in culture media containing the drug, and from some patients receiving prolonged therapy. However, the clinical relevance of drug resistance to clinical outcome has not been established.

PHARMACOKINETICS

The assay used to measure amphotericin B in the blood after the administration of ABLC does not distinguish amphotericin B that is complexed with the phospholipids of ABLC from amphotericin B that is uncomplexed.

The pharmacokinetics of amphotericin B after the administration of ABLC are nonlinear. Volume of distribution and clearance from blood increase with increasing dose of ABLC, resulting in less than proportional increase in blood concentrations of amphotericin B over a dose range of 0.6-5.0 mg/kg/day. The pharmacokinetics of amphotericin B in whole blood after the administration of ABLC and amphotericin B desoxycholate are in TABLE 1.

TABLE 1 Pharmacokinetic Parameters of Amphotericin B in Whole Blood in Patients Administered Multiple Doses of ABLC or Amphotericin B Desoxycholate

Pharmacokinetic Parameter	ABC 5 mg/kg/day for 5-7 days Mean ± SD	Amphotericin B 0.6 mg/kg/day for 42 days[a] Mean ± SD
Peak Concentration (mcg/ml)	1.7 ± 0.8 (n=10)[b]	1.1 ± 0.2 (n=5)
Concentration at End of Dosing Interval (mcg/ml)	0.6 ± 0.3 (n=10)[b]	0.4 ± 0.2 (n=5)
Area Under Blood Concentration-Time Curve (AUC_{0-24h}) (mcg·h/ml)	14 ± 7 (n=14)[b,c]	1701 ± 5 (n=5)
Clearance (ml/h/kg)	436 ± 188.5 (n=14)[b,c]	38 ± 15 (n=5)
Apparent Volume of Distribution (Vd_{area}) (l/kg)	131 ± 57.7 (n=8)[c]	5 ± 2.8 (n=5)
Terminal elimination Half-Life (h)	173.4 ± 78 (n=8)[c]	91.1 ± 40.9 (n=5)
Amount Excreted in Urine Over 24h After Last Dose (% of dose)[d]	0.9 ± 0.4 (n=8)[c]	9.6 ± 2.5 (n=8)

a Data from patients with Mucocutaneous Leishmaniasis. Inusion rate was 0.25 mg/kg/h.
b Data from studies in patients with cytologically proven cancer being treated with chemotherapy or neutropenic patients with presumed or proven fungal infection. Infusion rate was 2.5 mg/kg/h.
c Data from patients with Mucocutaneous Leishmaniasis. Infusion rate was 4.0 mg/kg/h.
d Percentage of dose excreted in 24 hours after last dose.

The large volume of distribution and high clearance value from the blood of amphotericin B after the administration of ABLC probably reflect uptake by tissues. The long terminal elimination half-life probably reflects a slow redistribution from tissues. Although amphotericin B is excreted slowly, there is little accumulation in the blood after repeated dosing. AUC of amphotericin B increased approximately 34% from day 1 after the administration of ABLC 5 mg/kg/day for 7 days. The effect of gender or ethnicity on the pharmacokinetics of ABLC has not been studied.

Tissue concentrations of amphotericin B have been obtained at autopsy from one heart transplant patient who received three doses of ABLC at 5.3 mg/kg/day (see TABLE 2).

TABLE 2

Organ	Amphotericin B Tissue Concentration (mcg/g)
Spleen	290.0
Lung	222.0
Liver	196.0
Lymph Node	7.6
Kidney	6.9
Heart	5.0
Brain	1.6

This pattern of distribution is consistent with that observed in preclinical studies in dogs in which greatest concentrations of amphotericin B after ABLC administration were observed in the liver, spleen, and lung; however, the relationship of tissue concentrations of amphotericin B to its biological activity when administered as ABLC is unknown.

Metabolism: The metabolic pathways of ABLC are not known. The effect of hepatic impairment on the disposition of ABLC is not known.

Renal Impairment: The effect of renal impairment on the disposition of ABLC is not known. The effect of dialysis on the elimination of ABLC has not been studied; however, amphotericin B is not removed by hemodialysis when administered as amphotericin B desoxycholate.

CLINICAL STUDIES:

Aspergillosis: Data were pooled from two emergency-use studies and one small, prospective, single-arm study in which ABLC was provided for the treatment of patients with aspergillosis. Most patients enrolled in these studies were judged by the physicians to be clinically refactory to conventional amphotericin B treatment (n=101) or to have developed nephrotoxicity while receiving conventional amphotericin B therapy (n=47). Smaller numbers of patients were entered because they had acute toxicity that contraindicated further conventional amphotericin B therapy (n=13), had preexisting renal insufficiency from other causes that contraindicated conventional amphotericin B therapy (n=11), or were refactory to itraconazole (n=6).

CLINICAL STUDIES: *(cont'd)*

Patients were defined by their individual physician as being refractory to or "failing" conventional amphotericin B therapy based on overall clinical judgment after receiving a minimum total dose of 500 mg of amphotericin B. Nephrotoxicity was defined as a serum creatinine that had increased to >2.5 mg/dL in adults or a creatinine clearance of <25 ml/min while receiving conventional amphotericin B therapy.

TABLE 3 Demographic Characteristics: Patients with Definite or Probable Aspergillosis

Parameter	N=178
Age (y)	
Median	39
Range	1/82
Gender (M/F)	120/58
Race	
Caucasian	137 (77%)
African-American	18 (10%)
Hispanic	15 (8%)
Asian	4 (2%)
Other	4 (2%)
Baseline Neutrophils (PMN/mm³)	
Median	3,719
<500/mm³	45 (25%)
Underlying Disease, n(%)	
Leukemia	77 (43%)
Lymphoma	14 (8%)
AIDS	11 (6%)
Solid Organ Cancer	11 (6%)
Other[a]	65 (37%)
Site of Infection	
Pulmonary	116 (65%)
Sinus	27 (15%)
CNS	6 (3%)
Other[b]	29 (16%)
Prior Dose of Amphotericin B for Patients Who Were Refractory to Amphotericin B (N=101)	
<7.5 mg/kg	10 (10%)
7.5-15 mg/kg	30 (30%)
>15 mg/kg	59 (58%)
Unknown	2 (2%)

a Myelodysplasia (10), transplant (9), congenital immunodeficiency (6), end-stage disease (5), diabetes mellitus (3), cardiovascular disease (3), intravenous drug users (2), cystic fibrosis (1), liver cirrhosis (1), sarcoidosis (1), and unknown (24).
b Skin (7), pleural fluid (4), ear (3), spine (3), heart valve (2), orbit (2), kidneys (1), lip/face (1), liver (1), penis (1), perianal abscess (1), prostate/urine (1), retroperitoneal abscess (1), and tonsil (1).

A retrospective response analysis was conducted based in the definitions previously developed by the Mycoses Study Group.[1] A "complete response" was defined as resolution of all attributable symptoms, signs, and radiologic and/or bronchoscopic abnormalities present at enrollment; a "partial response" was defined as major improvement of the above-mentioned parameters. The total number of responders was the sum of the number of "complete" and "partial" responses.

Of the 178 patients, 111 were considered evaluable for response. Sixty-seven were excluded on the basis of unconfirmed diagnostics, confounding factors, failure of other drugs, or receiving ≤4 doses of ABLC. All 178 patients were included in the safety analysis.

TABLE 4

Patient Group (n)	Complete Response	Partial Response	Total Responders
Amphotericin B refactory/failure (65)	17%	11%	28%
Nephrotoxicity (37)[a]	22%	30%	51%
Others (9)[b]	22%	44%	67%
Combined	19%	20%	39%

a Including 30 patients with due to amphotericin B, 7 due to preexisting renal disease.
b Including acute toxicity to conventional amphotericin B therapy.

There is no direct comparable control group for the patients described in the above table to be certain how similar patients would have responded had controventional amphotericin B therapy been continued. A retrospective historical control study of patients treated from January 1990 to December 1993 at four medical centers (University of Pittsburgh, H. Lee Moffitt Cancer Center and Research Institute, M.D. Anderson Cancer Center, Fred Hutchinson Cancer Research Center) who developed aspergillosis infection and were treated with conventional amphotericin B at first-line treatment was analyzed using the Mycoses Study Group classification of diagnosis and response. In 60 evaluable patients who had survived at least longer than 4 days after the diagnosis, the response rate was 23%. It should be cautioned that the results are not directly comparable to those of the ABLC group.

Renal Function: Patients with aspergillosis who initiated treatment with ABLC when serum creatinine was above 2.5 mg/dl experienced a decline in serum creatinine during treatment. Serum creatinine levels were also lower during treatment with ABLC when compared to the serum creatinine levels in patients treated with conventional amphotericin B in historical control group cited above, although meaningful statistical testing of the differences between these two groups is precluded since these data were obtained from two separate studies.

In a randomized study of ABLC for the treatment of invasive candidiasis, it was demonstrated in patients with normal baseline renal function that the incidence of nephrotoxicity was significantly less for ABLC at a dose of 5 mg/kg/day than for conventional amphotericin B at a dose of 0.7 mg/kg/day.

Despite generally less nephrotoxicity of ABLC observed at a dose of 5 mg/kg/day compared with conventional amphotericin B therapy at a dose range of 0.6-1.0 mg/kg/day, dose-limiting renal toxicity may still be observed with ABLC. Renal toxicity of doses greater than 5 mg/kg/ day of ABLC has not been formally studied.

INDICATIONS AND USAGE:

ABLC is indicated for the treatment of aspergillosis in patients who are refractory to or intolerant of conventional amphotericin B therapy. This indication is based on results obtained primarily from emergency-use studies of ABLC for the treatment of aspergillosis (see CLINICAL STUDIES).

CONTRAINDICATIONS:

ABLC is contraindicated in patients who have shown hypersensitivity to amphotericin B or any other component in the formulation.

WARNINGS:

Anaphylaxis has been reported with amphotericin B desoxycholate and other amphotericin B-containing drugs. One case of anaphylaxis has been reported with ABLC. Facilities for cardiopulmonary resuscitation should be available during administration due to the possibility of anaphylactoid reaction. If severe respiratory distress occurs, the infusion should be immediately discontinued. The patient should not receive further infusions of ABLC.

PRECAUTIONS:

General: As with any amphotericin B-containing product, during the initial dosing of ABLC, the drug should be administered intravenously under close clinical observation by medically trained personnel.

Acute reactions including fever and chills may occur 1 to 2 hours after starting an intravenous infusion of ABLC. These reactions are usually more common with the first few doses of ABLC and generally diminish with subsequent doses. Infusion has been rarely associated with hypertension, brochospasm, arrhythmias, and shock.

Laboratory Tests: Serum creatinine should be monitored frequently during ABLC therapy (see ADVERSE REACTIONS). It is also advisable to regularly monitor liver function, serum electrolytes (particularly magnesium and potassium), and complete blood counts.

Carcinogenesis, Mutagenesis, and Impairment of Fertility: No long-term studies in animals have been performed to evaluate the carcinogenic potential of ABLC. The following *in vitro* (with and without metabolic activation) and *in vivo* studies to assess ABLC for mutagenic potential were conducted: bacterial reverse mutation assay, mouse lymphoma forward mutation assay, chromosomal aberration assay in CHO cells, and *in vivo* mouse micronucleus assay. ABLC was found to be without mutagenic effects in all assay systems. Studies demonstrated that ABLC had no impact on fertility in male and female rats at doses up to 0.32 times the recommended human dose (based on body surface area considerations).

Pregnancy, Teratogenic Effects, Pregnancy Category B: Reproductive studies in rats and rabbits at doses of ABLC up to 0.64 times the human dose revealed no harm to the fetus. There are no reports of pregnant women having been treated with ABLC. Because animal reproductive studies are not always predictive of human response, and adequate and well-controlled studies have not been conducted in pregnant women, ABLC should be used during pregnancy only after taking into account the importance of the drug to the mother.

Pediatric Use: A small number of children, age 16 and under, with aspergillosis (n=40), have been treated with ABLC. No serious, unexpected adverse events have been reported.

Nursing Mothers: It is not known whether ABLC is excreted in human milk. Because many drugs are excreted in human milk, and because of the potential for serious adverse reactions in nursing infants from ABLC, taking into account the importance of the drug to the mother, a decision should be made whether to discontinue nursing or to discontinue the drug.

DRUG INTERACTIONS:

No formal clinical studies of drug interactions have been conducted with ABLC. However, when administered concomitantly, the following drugs are known to interact with amphotericin B; therefore, the following drugs may interact with ABLC:

Antineoplastic agents: Concurrent use of antineoplastic agents and amphotericin B may enhance the potential for renal toxicity, bronchospasm, and hypotension. Antineoplastic agents should be given concomitantly with ABLC with great caution.

Corticosteroids and Corticotropin (ACTH): Concurrent use of corticosteroids and corticotropin (ACTH) with amphotericin B may potentiate hypokalemia which could predispose the patient to cardiac dysfunction. If used concomitantly with ABLC, serum electrolytes and cardiac function should be closely monitored.

Cyclosporin A: Data from a prospective study of prophylactic ABLC in 22 patients undergoing bone marrow transplantation suggested that concurrent initiation of cyclosporin A and ABLC within several days of bone marrow ablation may be associated with increased nephrotoxicity.

Digitalis glycosides: Concurrent use of amphotericin B may induce hypokalemia and may potentiate digitalis toxicity. When administered concomitantly with ABLC, serum potassium levels should be closely monitored.

Flucytosine: Concurrent use of flucytosine with amphotericin B-containing preparations may increase the toxicity of flucytosine by possibly increasing its cellular uptake and/or impairing its renal excretion. Flucytosine should be given concomitantly with ABLC with caution.

Imidazoles (*e.g.,* ketoconazole, miconazole, clotrimazole, fluconazole, etc.): Antagonism between amphotericin B and imidazole derivatives such as miconazole and ketoconazole, which inhibit ergosterol synthesis, has been reported in both *in vitro* and *in vivo* animal studies. The clinical significance of these findings has not been determined.

Leukocyte transfusions: Acute pulmonary toxicity has been reported in patients receiving intravenous amphotericin B and leukocyte transfusions. Leukocyte transfusions and ABLC should not be given concurrently.

Other nephrotoxic medications: Concurrent use of amphotericin B and agents such as aminoglycosides, cyclosporine, and pentamidine may enhance the potential for drug-induced renal toxicity. Aminoglycosides, cyclosporine, and pentamidine should be used concomitantly with ABLC only with great caution. Intensive monitoring of renal function is recommend in patients requiring any combination of nephrotoxic medications.

Skeletal muscle relaxants: Amphotericin B-induced hypokalemia may enhance the curariform effect of skeletal muscle relaxants (*e.g.,* tubocurarine) due to hypokalemia. When administered concomitantly with ABLC, serum potassium levels should be closely monitored.

Zidovudine: Increased myelotoxicity and nephrotoxicity were observed in dogs when either ABLC (at doses 0.16 or 0.5 times the recommended human dose) or amphotericin B desoxycholate (at 0.5 times the recommended human dose) were administered concomitantly with zidovudine for 30 days. If zidovudine is used concomitantly with ABLC, renal and hematologic function should be closely monitored.

ADVERSE REACTIONS:

The total safety data base is composed of 813 patients treated with ABLC, of whom 667 were treated with 5.0 mg/kg/day. Of these 667 patients, 194 patients were treated in four comparative studies, 418 patients were treated in emergency-use studies, and 55 patients were treated in open-label, non-comparative studies. Most had underlying hematologic neoplasms, and many were receiving multiple concomitant medications. In the emergence-use studies, the median duration of therapy was 22 days for ABLC-treated patients. Nine percent of ABLC patients discontinued treatment due to adverse events, regardless of presumed relationship to drug. In general, the adverse events most commonly reported with ABLC were transient chills and fever during infusion of the drug. TABLE 5 shows all reported adverse events that occurred with an incidence of ≥3% in the emergency-use studies and the corresponding incidence for patients with documented or suspected aspergillosis.

The following adverse events have also been reported with ABLC:

Body as a whole: malaise, weight loss, injection site reaction including inflammation

Allergic: bronchospasm, wheezing, asthma, anaphylactoid and other allergic reactions

ADVERSE REACTIONS: *(cont'd)*

TABLE 5

Adverse Event	All Fungal Infection n=418 %	Aspergillosis n=218 %
Body as a Whole		
Chills	16	15
Fever	12	15
Multiple Organ Failure	10	9
Sepsis	7	9
Headache	4	7
Infection	4	6
Pain	4	4
Abdominal Pain	3	5
Cardiovascular System		
Hypotension	7	6
Cardic Arrest	5	5
Digestive System		
Nausea	8	6
Vomiting	6	6
Diarrhea	5	10
Gastrointestinal Hemorrhage	3	3
Hemic and Lymphatic System		
Thrombocytopenia	5	4
Leukopenia	4	4
Anemia	4	4
Metabolic and Nutritional Disorders		
Increased Serum Creatinine	11	12
Bilirubinemia	4	5
Hypokalemia	4	6
Acidosis	3	3
Respiratory System		
Respiratory Failure	9	10
Dyspnea	5	8
Respiratory Disorder	4	3
Pneumonia	3	5
Skin and Appendages		
Rash	3	5
Urogenital System		
Kidney Failure	5	4

Cardiopulmonary: cardiac failure, pulmonary edema, shock, myocardial infarct, hemoptysis, arrhythmias including ventricular fibrillation, hypertension, tachypnea, thrombrophlebtis, pulmonary embolus, cardiomyopathy

Dermatological: maculopapular rash, pruritus, exfoliative dermatitis, erythema multiforme

Gastrointestinal: acute liver failure, hepatitis, jaundice, melena, anorexia, dyspepsia, cramping, epigastic pain, veno-occlusive liver disease

Hematologic: coagulation defects, blood dyscrasias including eosinophilia, leukocytosis

Musculoskeletal: myasthenia, generalized pain, including bone, muscle, and joint pains

Neurologic: convulsions, tinnitus, visual impairment, hearing loss, peripheral neuropathy, transient vertigo, diplopia, encephalopathy, extrapyramidal syndrome and other neurologic symptoms

Urogenital: acute renal failure, oliguria, decreased renal function, anuria, renal tubular acidosis, impotence

Altered Laboratory Findings

Serum electrolyte abnormalities: hypomagnesemia, hyperkalemia, hypocalcemia

Liver function test abnormalities: increased AST, ALT, alkaline phosphatase

Renal function test abnormalities: increased BUN

Other test abnormalities: acidosis, hyperamylasemia, hypoglycemia, hyperglycemia

OVERDOSAGE:

Amphotericin B descoxycholate overdose has been reported to result in cardio-respiratory arrest. Ten patients have been reported who have received one or more doses of ABLC between 7–13 mg/kg. None of these patients had a serious acute reaction to ABLC. If an overdose is suspected, discontinue therapy, monitor the patient's clinical status, and administer supportive therapy as required. ABLC is not hemodialyzable.

DOSAGE AND ADMINISTRATION:

The recommended daily dosage for adults and children is 5.0 mg/kg given as a single infusion. ABLC should be administered by intravenous infusion at a rate of 2.5 mg/kg/hr. If the infusion time exceeds 2 hours, mix the contents by shaking the infusion bag every 2 hours. Facilities for cardiopulmonary resuscitation should be available due to the possibility of anaphylactiod reaction.

Renal toxicity of ABLC, as measured by serum creatinine levels, has been shown to be dose dependent. There are no firm guidelines for dose adjustment based on laboratory test results, and decisions about dose adjustments should be made only after taking into account the overall clinical condition of the patient.

Preparation of Admixture for Infusion: Shake the vial gently until there is no evidence of any yellow sediment at the bottom. Withdraw the appropriate dose of ABLC from the required number of vials into one or more sterile 20 ml syringes using an 18–gauge needle. Remove the needle from each syringe filled with ABLC and replace with the 5–micron filter needle supplied with each vial. Each filter needle must be used to filter the content of only one vial; a new filter needle should be used for each subsequent syringe. Insert the filter needle of the syringe into an IV bag containing 5.0% Dextrose Injection USP, and empty the contents of the syringe into the bag. The infusion concentration should be 1 mg/ml. For pediatric patients and patients with cardiovascular disease the drug may be diluted with 5.0% Dextrose Injection to a final infusion concentration of 2 mg/ml. Do not use the admixture after dilution with 5.0% Dextrose Injection if there is any evidence of foreign matter. Vials are for single use. Unused material should be discarded. Aseptic technique must be strictly observed throughout handling of ABLC since no bacteriostatic agent of preservative is present.

DO NOT DILUTE WITH SALINE SOLUTIONS OR MIX WITH OTHER DRUGS OR ELECTROLYTES as the compatibility of ABLC with these materials has not been established. An existing intravenous line should be flushed with 5.0% Dextrose Injection before infusion of ABLC, or a separate infusion line should be used. *Do not use an in-line filter less than 5 microns with ABLC.*

The diluted ready-for-use admixture is stable for up to 15 hours at 2° to 8°C (36° to 46°F) and an additional 6 hours at room temperature.

REFERENCES:

1. Denning DW, Lee JY, Hostetler JS, et al. NIAID Mycoses Study Group multicenter trial of oral itraconazole therapy for invasive aspergillosis. *AM J Med.* 97:135–144, 1994.

HOW SUPPLIED:

Each vial contains 100 mg of Abelcet in 20 ml of suspension. Single-use vials along with single-use filter needles are individually packaged.

Storage: Prior to admixture, ABLC should be stored at 2° to 8°C (36° to 46°F) and protected from exposure to light. Do not freeze. ABLC should be retained in the carton until time of use.

The admixed ABLC and 5.0% Dextrose Injection may be stored for 15 hours at 2° to 8°C (36° to 46°F) and an additional 6 hours at room temperature. Do not freeze. Any unused material should be discarded

HOW SUPPLIED - EQUIVALENTS NOT AVAILABLE:

Suspension - Intravenous - 100 mg

vial	$130.00	ABELCET, Liposome	61799-0101-41

AMPHOTERICIN; TETRACYCLINE *(000236)*

CATEGORIES: Anti-Infectives; Antibiotics; Tetracyclines

BRAND NAMES: Mysteclin-F

Prescribing information not available at time of publication.

HOW SUPPLIED - EQUIVALENTS NOT AVAILABLE:

Capsule, Gelatin - Oral - 250 mg/50 mg

16's	$14.05	MYSTECLIN-F, Bristol Myers Squibb	00003-0779-16
100's	$83.75	MYSTECLIN-F, Bristol Myers Squibb	00003-0779-50
100's	$83.75	MYSTECLIN-F, Bristol Myers Squibb	00003-0779-53

Syrup - Oral

240 ml	$32.97	MYSTECLIN-F, Bristol Myers Squibb	00003-0464-30

AMPICILLIN *(000239)*

CATEGORIES: Anti-Infectives; Antibacterials; Antibiotics; Antimicrobials; Gonorrhea; Infections; Penicillins; Respiratory Tract Infections; Pregnancy Category B; FDA Approval Pre 1982; Top 200 Drugs

BRAND NAMES: *Acupillin*; *Adumic*; *Aimelin*; *Aldribid*; *Aletmicina*; *Alphacin* (Australia); *Amblosin*; Amcap; Amcill; *Amcillin*; Amficot; *Amfipen* (England); *Amipenix* (Japan); *Ampat*; *Ampecu*; *Ampen*; *Ampesid*; *Ampex*; *Ampexin*; *Ampibel*; *Ampibex*; *Ampiblan*; *Ampicher*; *Ampicilina*; Ampicillin; *Ampicin*; *Ampiclox*; *Ampicyn*; *Ampidar*; *Ampifen*; *Ampikel*; *Ampil*; *Ampilag*; *Ampilin*; *Ampillin*; *Ampipen*; *Ampisol*; *Ampivral*; *Ampliblan*; *Amplibin*; Amplin; *Ampolin*; *Anglopen* (Mexico); *Apo-Ampi* (Canada); *Austrapen*; *Bacipen*; *Binotal* (Germany, Mexico); *Bionacillin*; *Bremcillin*; *Bridopen*; *Britapen*; *Broacil*; *Camicil*; *Cimexillin*; *Cinpillin*; *Citicil*; *Coampi*; *Copharcilin*; *Cryocil*; D-Amp; *Deripen*; *Dexypen*; *Dhacillin*; *Dibacilina* (Mexico); *Doktacillin*; *Doltirol*; *Dotirol*; *Duacillin*; *Eracillin*; *Eskaycillin*; *Eurotrexil*; *Excillin*; *Extrapen*; *Fortapen*; *Herpen*; *Hostes*; *Ificillin*; *Ikacillin*; *Ingacillin*; *Intramed*; *Isocillin*; *Iwacillin* (Japan); *Jenampin* (Germany); *Lampicin* (Mexico); *Magnapen*; Marcillin; *Marticil*; *Maxipen*; *Nelpicil*; *Novo-Ampicillin* (Canada); *Nuvapen*; *Omnipen* (Mexico); *Pamecil*; *Pelitin*; Penamp; *Penbritin* (Canada, Mexico, England); *Penbrex*; *Penibrin*; *Penodil*; *Penstabil* (Germany); *Pentrex*; *Pentrexyl* (England, Mexico); *Petercillin*; *Pilitin*; Polycillin; Pfizerpen A; *Primapen*; **Principen**; *Protexillin*; *Radiocillina*; *Resan*; *Rimacillin*; *Rophabiotic*; *Rosampline*; *Roscillin*; *Semicillin*; *Servicillin*; *Standacillin*; *Statcillin*; *Supicillin*; *Synthocilin*; *Tampicillin*; *Tokiocillin*; *Tolimal*; Totacillin; *Totapen* (France); *Trifalicina*; *Trifarcin*; *Trihypen*; *Trilaxan*; *Trilaxin*; *Ukapen*; *Vacillin*; *Vialicina*; *Viccillin*; *Vidopen* (England); *Virgoxillin*; *Virucil*; *Vitapen*; *Winpicillin*

(International brand names outside U.S. in italics)

FORMULARIES: Aetna; BC-BS; CIGNA; FHP; Humana; Kaiser; Medco; Medi-Cal; PruCare; United

COST OF THERAPY: $3.76 (Urinary Tract Infections; Capsule; 500 mg; 4/day; 7 days)

DESCRIPTION:

Ampicillin is a semisynthetic penicillin derived from the basic penicillin nucleus, 6-amino-penicillanic acid.

Ampicillin capsules contain 250 mg or 500 mg ampicillin. The inactive ingredients are magnesium stearate and FD&C Yellow No. 6.

Ampicillin for oral suspension is a powder that; when reconstituted as directed, yields a suspension of 125 mg or 250 mg ampicillin per 5 ml. The inactive ingredients are FD&C Red 3, flavoring, silica gel, sodium benzoate, sodium citrate, sucrose, and xanthan gum.

CLINICAL PHARMACOLOGY:

MICROBIOLOGY

Ampicillin is similar to benzyl penicillin in its bactericidal action against sensitive organisms during the stage of active multiplication. It acts through the inhibition of biosynthesis of cell wall mucopeptide. Ampicillin differs *in vitro* spectrum. It exerts high *in vitro* activity against many strains of *Haemophilus influenzae, Neisseria gonorrhoeae, Neisseria meningitidis, Neisseria catarrhalis, Escherichia coli, Proteus mirabilis, Bacteroides funduliformis, and Salmonella and Shigella* organisms.

In vitro studies have also demonstrated the sensitivity of many strains of the following gram-positive bacteria: alpha-hemolytic streptococci, *Diplococcus pneumoniae*, nonpenicillinase-producing staphylococci, *Bacillus anthracis*, and most strains of enterococci and clostridia. Ampicillin generally provides less *in vitro* activity than penicillin G does against gram-positive bacteria. Because it does not resist destruction by penicillinase, it is not effective against penicillin-producing bacteria, particularly resistant staphylococci. All strains of *Pseudomonas* and most strains of *Klebsiella* and *Aerobacter* organisms are resistant.

PHARMACOKINETICS

Ampicillin is acid stable and therefore well absorbed. Food, however, retards absorption. Blood serum levels of approximately 2 mcg/ml are attained within 1 to 2 hours following a 250-mg oral dose given to fasting adults. Detectable amounts persist for about 6 hours.

Ampicillin diffuses readily into all body tissues and fluids with the exception of brain and spinal fluid except when meninges are inflamed. Higher serum levels are obtained following IM injection. Most of the ampicillin is excreted unchanged in the urine; and this excretion can be delayed by concurrent administration of probenecid. The active form appears in the

CLINICAL PHARMACOLOGY: *(cont'd)*

bile in higher concentrations than those found in the serum. Ampicillin is one of the least serum bound of all the penicillins; averaging about 20% compared to approximately 60% to 90% for other penicillins.

INDICATIONS AND USAGE:

Ampicillin is indicated primarily in the treatment of infections due to susceptible strains of the following:

Gram-Negative Organisms: *Shigella, Salmonella* (including *S. typhosa*), *H. influenzae, E. coli, P. mirabilis, N. gonorrhoeae,* and *N. meningitidis.*

Gram-Positive Organisms: Streptococci, *D. pneumoniae,* and nonpenicillinase-producing staphylococci.

Because of its wide spectrum and bactericidal action, ampicillin may be useful in instituting therapy; however, bacteriologic studies to determine the causative organisms and their sensitivity to Ampicillin should be performed.

CONTRAINDICATIONS:

A history of an allergic reaction to any of the penicillins is a contraindication.

WARNINGS:

SERIOUS AND OCCASIONALLY FATAL HYPERSENSITIVITY (ANAPHYLACTOID) REACTIONS HAVE BEEN REPORTED IN PATIENTS ON PENICILLIN THERAPY. ALTHOUGH ANAPHYLAXIS IS MORE FREQUENT FOLLOWING PARENTERAL THERAPY, IT HAS OCCURRED IN PATIENTS ON ORAL PENICILLINS. THESE REACTIONS ARE MORE APT TO OCCUR IN INDIVIDUALS WITH A HISTORY OF SENSITIVITY TO MULTIPLE ALLERGENS. THERE HAVE BEEN REPORTS OF INDIVIDUALS WITH A HISTORY OF PENICILLIN HYPERSENSITIVITY WHO EXPERIENCED SEVERE REACTIONS WHEN TREATED WITH CEPHALOSPORINS. BEFORE THERAPY WITH A PENICILLIN, CAREFUL INQUIRY SHOULD BE MADE CONCERNING PREVIOUS HYPERSENSITIVITY REACTIONS TO PENICILLINS, CEPHALOSPORINS, AND OTHER ALLERGENS. IF AN ALLERGIC REACTION OCCURS, THE DRUG SHOULD BE DISCONTINUED AND THE APPROPRIATE THERAPY SHOULD BE INSTITUTED. SERIOUS ANAPHYLACTOID REACTIONS REQUIRE IMMEDIATE EMERGENCY TREATMENT WITH EPINEPHRINE. OXYGEN, INTRAVENOUS STEROIDS, AND AIRWAY MANAGEMENT, INCLUDING INTUBATION, SHOULD ALSO BE ADMINISTERED AS INDICATED.

USAGE IN PREGNANCY

Safety for use in pregnancy has not been established.

PRECAUTIONS:

As with any antibiotic preparation, constant observation for signs of overgrowth of nonsusceptible organisms, including fungi, is essential. If superinfection should occur (usually involving *Aerobacter, Pseudomonas,* or *Candida* organisms), the drug should be discontinued and/or appropriate therapy instituted. As with any potent agent, it is advisable to check periodically for organ system dysfunction during prolonged therapy; this includes renal, hepatic, and hematopoietic systems. This is particularly important in premature infants, neonates, and other infants.

ADVERSE REACTIONS:

As with other penicillins, it may be expected that untoward reactions will be essentially limited to sensitivity phenomena. These reactions are more likely to occur in individuals who have previously demonstrated hypersensitivity to penicillins and in those with a history of allergy, asthma, hay fever, or urticaria. The following adverse reactions have been reported as associated with the use of ampicillin:

Gastrointestinal: Glossitis, stomatitis, black "hairy" tongue, nausea, vomiting, enterocolitis, pseudomembranous colitis, and diarrhea. (These reactions are usually associated with oral dosage forms.)

Hypersensitivity Reactions: An erythematous maculopapular rash has been reported fairly frequently. Urticaria and erythema multiforme have been reported occasionally. A few cases of exfoliative dermatitis have been reported. Anaphylaxis is the most serious reaction experienced and has usually been associated with the parenteral dosage form.

Liver: A moderate rise in serum glutamic-oxaloacetic transaminase (SGOT) has been noted, particularly in infants, but the significance of this finding is unknown.

Hemic and Lymphatic Systems: Anemia, thrombocytopenia, thrombocytopenic purpura, eosinophilia, leukopenia, and agranulocytosis have been reported during therapy with the penicillins. These reactions are usually reversible on discontinuation of therapy and are believed to be sensitivity reactions.

Note: Urticaria, other skin rashes, and serum sickness-like reactions may be controlled with antihistamines and, if necessary, systemic corticosteroids. Whenever such reactions occur, ampicillin should be discontinued unless, in the opinion of the physician, the condition being treated is life-threatening and amenable only to ampicillin therapy.

DOSAGE AND ADMINISTRATION:

INFECTIONS OF THE EAR, NOSE, AND THROAT

Infections of the ear, nose, throat, and lower respiratory tract due to streptococci, pneumococci, and nonpenicillinase-producing staphylococci and also those infections of the upper and lower respiratory tract due to *H. influenzae*.

Adults: 250 mg every 6 hours.

Children: 50 mg/kg/day in divided doses every 6 or 8 hours.

INFECTIONS OF THE GENITOURINARY TRACT CAUSED BY SENSITIVE GRAM-NEGATIVE AND GRAM-POSITIVE BACTERIA

Adults: 500 mg every 6 hours.

Larger doses may be required for severe infections.

Children: 100 mg/kg/day in divided doses every 6 hours.

UNCOMPLICATED URETHRITIS DUE TO N. GONORRHOEAE

Adult Males and Females: 3.5-g single oral dose administered simultaneously with 1 g of probenecid.

Cases of gonorrhea with a suspected lesion of syphilis should have dark-field examinations before receiving ampicillin and monthly serologic tests for a minimum of 4 months.

INFECTIONS OF THE GASTROINTESTINAL TRACT

Adults: 500 mg every 6 hours.

Children: 100 mg/kg/day in divided doses every 6 hours.

Larger doses may be required for stubborn or severe infections. The children's dosage is intended for individuals whose weight will not cause a dosage to be calculated greater than that recommended for adults. Children weighing more than 20 kg should be dosed according to the adult recommendations.

DOSAGE AND ADMINISTRATION: *(cont'd)*

It should be recognized that in the treatment of chronic urinary tract and intestinal infections, frequent bacteriologic follow-up is required for several months after cessation of therapy.

Treatment should be continued for a minimum of 48 to 72 hours beyond the time that the patient becomes asymptomatic or evidence of bacterial eradication has been obtained. It is recommended that there be at least 10 days of treatment for any infection caused by hemolytic streptococci to help prevent the occurrence of acute rheumatic fever to glomerulonephritis.

DIRECTIONS FOR MIXING ORAL SUSPENSION

Prepare suspension at time of dispensing as follows: Tap bottle until all powder flows freely. Add approximately $\frac{1}{2}$ of the total amount of water for reconstitution (TABLE 1), and shake vigorously to wet powder. Add the remainder of the water and again shake vigorously.

TABLE 1

Bottle Size (ml)	Amount of Water Required for Reconstitution (ml)
125 mg per 5 ml*	
100	78
200	155
250 mg per 5 ml†	
100	74
200	148

* Each teaspoonful (5 ml) will contain 125 mg ampicillin.
† Each teaspoonful (5 ml) will contain 250 mg ampicillin.

SHAKE WELL BEFORE USING. Keep bottle tightly closed. Any unused portion of the reconstituted suspension must be discarded after 14 days under refrigeration.

PATIENT INFORMATION:

Ampicillin is an antibiotic for the treatment of infection.

Take at regular intervals and complete the entire course of therapy.

Do not take this medication if you are allergic to any type of penicillin.

Notify your physician if you are pregnant or nursing.

This antibiotic may decrease the effectiveness of birth control pills; use another form of birth control while taking this medication.

Shake the suspension well before each use and store it in the refrigerator.

May cause nausea, vomiting, or diarrhea; notify your physician if these occur.

Ampicillin should be taken on an empty stomach, one hour before or two hours after meals with a full glass of water.

HOW SUPPLIED - RATED THERAPEUTICALLY EQUIVALENT:

Capsule, Gelatin - Oral - 250 mg

40's	$2.94	Ampicillin, H.C.F.A. F F P	99999-0239-01
40's	$7.25	Ampicillin, Teva	00332-3111-06
100's	$6.59	Ampicillin, Mead Johnson	00015-7992-58
100's	$7.37	Ampicillin, H.C.F.A. F F P	99999-0239-02
100's	$8.55	Ampicillin, Lederle Pharm	00005-3586-23
100's	$9.30	AMFICOT, C O Truxton	00463-5011-01
100's	$10.00	Ampicillin, Raway	00686-0602-20
100's	$10.05	Ampicillin, IDE-Interstate	00814-0720-14
100's	$11.00	Ampicillin, HL Moore Drug Exch	00839-5087-06
100's	$11.20	Ampicillin, Schein Pharm (US)	00364-2001-01
100's	$11.50	Ampicillin, Rugby	00536-0010-01
100's	$11.65	Ampicillin, United Res	00677-0010-01
100's	**$11.73**	**PRINCIPEN 250, Bristol Myers Squibb**	**00003-0122-50**
100's	**$11.73**	**PRINCIPEN 250, Bristol Myers Squibb**	**00003-0122-51**
100's	$11.75	Ampicillin, Major Pharms	00904-2017-60
100's	$11.76	Ampicillin, Geneva Pharms	00781-2555-01
100's	$11.93	Ampicillin, Goldline Labs	00182-0163-01
100's	$11.93	Ampicillin, Teva	00332-3111-09
100's	$11.93	Ampicillin, Qualitest Pharms	00603-2290-21
100's	$12.11	Ampicillin, Aligen Independ	00405-4089-01
100's	$14.86	Ampicillin, Warner Chilcott	00047-0402-24
100's	$15.10	Ampicillin, Mylan	00378-0115-01
100's	$18.85	Ampicillin, Goldline Labs	00182-0163-89
500's	$32.99	Ampicillin, Mead Johnson	00015-7992-85
500's	$36.60	Ampicillin, IDE-Interstate	00814-0720-28
500's	$36.85	Ampicillin, H.C.F.A. F F P	99999-0239-03
500's	$40.76	Ampicillin, Lederle Pharm	00005-3586-31
500's	**$41.54**	**PRINCIPEN 250, Bristol Myers Squibb**	**00003-0122-60**
500's	$41.55	Ampicillin, Geneva Pharms	00781-2555-05
500's	$44.67	Ampicillin, HL Moore Drug Exch	00839-5087-12
500's	$45.30	Ampicillin, Schein Pharm (US)	00364-2001-05
500's	$46.40	Ampicillin, Major Pharms	00904-2017-40
500's	$47.95	Ampicillin, Rugby	00536-0010-05
500's	$50.57	Ampicillin, United Res	00677-0010-05
500's	$52.25	TOTACILLIN, Beecham	00029-6615-32
500's	$57.51	Ampicillin, Goldline Labs	00182-0163-05
500's	$57.51	Ampicillin, Teva	00332-3111-13
500's	$57.51	Ampicillin, Qualitest Pharms	00603-2290-28
500's	$59.32	Ampicillin, Aligen Independ	00405-4089-02
500's	$62.71	OMNIPEN, Wyeth Labs	00008-0053-05
500's	$71.62	Ampicillin, Warner Chilcott	00047-0402-30
500's	$71.65	Ampicillin, Mylan	00378-0115-05
1000's	$73.70	Ampicillin, Teva	00332-3111-15
1000's	$73.70	Ampicillin, H.C.F.A. F F P	99999-0239-04
1000's	$87.00	Ampicillin, Schein Pharm (US)	00364-2001-02
1000's	$88.05	Ampicillin, Rugby	00536-0010-10

Capsule, Gelatin - Oral - 500 mg

40's	$5.37	Ampicillin, H.C.F.A. F F P	99999-0239-05
40's	$13.65	Ampicillin, Teva	00332-3113-06
100's	$13.43	Ampicillin, H.C.F.A. F F P	99999-0239-06
100's	$13.50	Ampicillin, Mead Johnson	00015-7993-58
100's	$15.85	Ampicillin, Lederle Pharm	00005-3587-23
100's	$17.55	Ampicillin, Raway	00686-0603-20
100's	**$17.70**	**PRINCIPEN, Bristol Myers Squibb**	**00003-0134-50**
100's	**$17.70**	**PRINCIPEN, UNIMATIC, Bristol Myers Squibb**	**00003-0134-51**
100's	$17.85	Ampicillin, IDE-Interstate	00814-0722-14
100's	$19.44	Ampicillin, HL Moore Drug Exch	00839-5130-06
100's	$19.95	Ampicillin, Major Pharms	00904-2073-60
100's	$20.00	Ampicillin, Schein Pharm (US)	00364-2002-01
100's	$20.20	Ampicillin, Rugby	00536-0016-01
100's	$20.80	Ampicillin, Geneva Pharms	00781-2999-01
100's	$21.00	Ampicillin, Goldline Labs	00182-0641-01

HOW SUPPLIED - RATED THERAPEUTICALLY EQUIVALENT: *(cont'd)*

100's	$21.25	Ampicillin, United Res	00677-0011-01
100's	$21.29	Ampicillin, Teva	00332-3113-09
100's	$21.29	Ampicillin, Qualitest Pharms	00603-2291-21
100's	$21.60	MARCILLIN, Marnel Pharceut	00682-9113-01
100's	$22.00	Ampicillin, Mylan	00378-0116-01
100's	$24.19	Ampicillin, Aligen Independ	00405-4090-01
100's	$25.70	OMNIPEN, Wyeth Labs	00008-0309-03
100's	$26.51	Ampicillin, Warner Chilcott	00047-0404-24
100's	$32.00	Ampicillin, Goldline Labs	00182-0641-89
500's	$67.15	Ampicillin, Teva	00332-3113-13
500's	$67.15	Ampicillin, H.C.F.A. F F P	99999-0239-07
500's	$67.61	Ampicillin, Mead Johnson	00015-7993-85
500's	**$75.81**	**PRINCIPEN, Bristol Myers Squibb**	**00003-0134-60**
500's	$75.83	Ampicillin, Lederle Pharm	00005-3587-31
500's	$77.25	Ampicillin, IDE-Interstate	00814-0722-28
500's	$83.50	Ampicillin, Geneva Pharms	00781-2999-05
500's	$86.50	Ampicillin, Major Pharms	00904-2073-40
500's	$88.68	Ampicillin, HL Moore Drug Exch	00839-5130-12
500's	$94.05	Ampicillin, Schein Pharm (US)	00364-2002-05
500's	$95.50	Ampicillin, Rugby	00536-0016-05
500's	$101.00	Ampicillin, United Res	00677-0011-05
500's	$102.70	Ampicillin, Goldline Labs	00182-0641-05
500's	$102.70	Ampicillin, Qualitest Pharms	00603-2291-28
500's	$104.55	TOTACILLIN, Beecham	00029-6620-32
500's	$117.20	Ampicillin, Aligen Independ	00405-4090-02
500's	$120.94	OMNIPEN, Wyeth Labs	00008-0309-06
500's	$127.90	Ampicillin, Warner Chilcott	00047-0404-30
500's	$127.95	Ampicillin, Mylan	00378-0116-05

Powder, Reconstitution - Oral - 100 mg/ml

20 ml	$3.04	Ampicillin, Mead Johnson	00015-7884-21

Powder, Reconstitution - Oral - 125 mg/5ml

5 ml x 100	**$28.13**	**PRINCIPEN 125, Bristol Myers Squibb**	**00003-0969-15**
80 ml	$3.06	POLYCILLIN, Mead Johnson	00015-7988-35
100 ml	$1.50	TOTACILLIN, Beecham	00029-6625-23
100 ml	$1.52	Ampicillin, Mead Johnson	00015-7988-62
100 ml	$2.10	Ampicillin, Schein Pharm (US)	00364-2003-61
100 ml	$2.11	Ampicillin, Lederle Pharm	00005-3588-46
100 ml	$2.24	OMNIPEN, Wyeth Labs	00008-0054-03
100 ml	$2.25	Ampicillin, Harber Pharm	51432-0689-14
100 ml	$2.25	Ampicillin, H.C.F.A. F F P	99999-0239-08
100 ml	**$2.30**	**PRINCIPEN 125, Bristol Myers Squibb**	**00003-0969-09**
100 ml	$2.35	Ampicillin, Major Pharms	00904-4010-04
100 ml	$2.87	Ampicillin, Warner Chilcott	00047-2301-17
100 ml	$2.87	AMPICILLIN, Goldline Labs	00182-0274-70
100 ml	$2.90	Ampicillin, Balan	00304-0584-63
100 ml	$34.50	AMFICOT, C O Truxton	00463-5013-01
150 ml	$2.31	Ampicillin, Mead Johnson	00015-7988-51
150 ml	$3.15	OMNIPEN, Wyeth Labs	00008-0054-02
150 ml	**$3.21**	**PRINCIPEN 125, Bristol Myers Squibb**	**00003-0969-52**
150 ml	$3.37	Ampicillin, H.C.F.A. F F P	99999-0239-09
200 ml	$2.95	TOTACILLIN, Beecham	00029-6625-24
200 ml	$3.08	Ampicillin, Mead Johnson	00015-7988-63
200 ml	$3.19	Ampicillin, Lederle Pharm	00005-3588-60
200 ml	$3.52	Ampicillin, H.C.F.A. F F P	99999-0239-10
200 ml	$3.86	OMNIPEN, Wyeth Labs	00008-0054-04
200 ml	$3.95	Ampicillin, Major Pharms	00904-4010-08
200 ml	**$3.99**	**PRINCIPEN 125, Bristol Myers Squibb**	**00003-0969-61**
200 ml	$4.50	Ampicillin, Balan	00304-0584-65
200 ml	$4.50	Ampicillin, HL Moore Drug Exch	00839-5144-78
200 ml	$4.62	AMPICILLIN, Warner Chilcott	00047-2301-20
200 ml	$4.62	Ampicillin, Mylan	00378-0117-04
200 ml	$4.64	Ampicillin, Goldline Labs	00182-0274-73

Powder, Reconstitution - Oral - 250 mg/5ml

80 ml	$4.26	POLYCILLIN, Mead Johnson	00015-7998-35
100 ml	$2.10	TOTACILLIN, Beecham	00029-6630-23
100 ml	$2.20	Ampicillin, Mead Johnson	00015-7998-62
100 ml	$2.90	Ampicillin, Lederle Pharm	00005-3589-46
100 ml	$3.15	Ampicillin, H.C.F.A. F F P	99999-0239-11
100 ml	$3.31	OMNIPEN, Wyeth Labs	00008-0055-03
100 ml	$3.35	AMPICILLIN, C O Truxton	00463-5014-01
100 ml	**$3.43**	**PRINCIPEN 250, Bristol Myers Squibb**	**00003-0972-52**
100 ml	$3.88	Ampicillin, Warner Chilcott	00047-2302-17
100 ml	$3.90	Ampicillin, Goldline Labs	00182-0275-70
100 ml	$3.90	Ampicillin, Major Pharms	00904-4014-04
100 ml	$4.18	Ampicillin, Balan	00304-0585-63
150 ml	$3.28	Ampicillin, Mead Johnson	00015-7998-51
150 ml	$4.72	Ampicillin, H.C.F.A. F F P	99999-0239-12
150 ml	$4.95	OMNIPEN, Wyeth Labs	00008-0055-02
200 ml	$2.70	MARCILLIN, Marnel Pharceut	00682-9116-01
200 ml	$4.20	TOTACILLIN, Beecham	00029-6630-24
200 ml	$4.37	Ampicillin, Mead Johnson	00015-7998-63
200 ml	$4.94	Ampicillin, Lederle Pharm	00005-3589-60
200 ml	$5.10	Ampicillin, H.C.F.A. F F P	99999-0239-13
200 ml	$5.92	OMNIPEN, Wyeth Labs	00008-0055-04
200 ml	**$6.12**	**PRINCIPEN 250, Bristol Myers Squibb**	**00003-0972-61**
200 ml	$6.30	Ampicillin, HL Moore Drug Exch	00839-6445-78
200 ml	$6.50	Ampicillin, Major Pharms	00904-4014-08
200 ml	$6.58	Ampicillin, Balan	00304-0585-65
200 ml	$6.67	Ampicillin, Warner Chilcott	00047-2302-20
200 ml	$6.69	Ampicillin, Goldline Labs	00182-0275-73

AMPICILLIN SODIUM *(000237)*

CATEGORIES: Anti-Infectives; Antibacterials; Antibiotics; Antimicrobials; Influenza; Ocular Infections; Ophthalmics; Penicillins; Salmonella Typhi; FDA Approval Pre 1982

BRAND NAMES: Omnipen-N; Penbritin-S; Polycillin-N; Totacillin-N

DESCRIPTION:

Ampicillin Sodium is derived from the penicillin nucleus, 6-aminopenicillanic acid (6-APA), isolated by Beecham. Chemically it is D (-) α-aminobenzyl penicillin sodium salt.

CLINICAL PHARMACOLOGY:

MICROBIOLOGY

Ampicillin Sodium is similar to benzyl penicillin in its bactericidal action against sensitive organisms during the stage of active multiplication. It acts through the inhibition of biosynthesis of cell wall mucopeptide. Ampicillin Sodium differs in *in vitro* spectrum from benzyl

CLINICAL PHARMACOLOGY: *(cont'd)*

penicillin in the Gram-negative spectrum. It exerts high *in vitro* activity against many strains of *Haemophilus influenzae, Neisseria gonorrhoeae, Neisseria meningitidis, Neisseria catarrhalis, Escherichia coli, Proteus mirabilis, Bacteroides funduliformis, Salmonellae* and *Shigellae.*

In vitro studies have also demonstrated the sensitivity of many strains of the following Gram-positive bacteria: alpha- and beta-hemolytic streptococci, *Diplococcus pneumoniae* , nonpenicillinase-producing staphylococci, *Bacillus anthracis,* and most strains of enterococci and clostridia. Ampicillin generally provides less *in vitro* activity than penicillin G against Gram-positive bacteria. Because it does not resist destruction by penicillinase, it is not effective against penicillinase-producing bacteria, particularly resistant staphylococci. All strains of Pseudomonas and most strains of Klebsiella and Aerobacter are resistant.

PHARMACOKINETICS

Ampicillin Sodium diffuses readily into all body tissues and fluids with the exception of brain and spinal fluid except when meninges are inflamed. It produces high and persistent blood levels. Most of the Ampicillin is excreted unchanged in the urine and this excretion can be delayed by concurrent administration of probenecid. The active form appears in the bile in higher concentrations than found in the serum. Ampicillin Sodium is one of the least serum bound of all the penicillins, averaging about 20% compared to approximately 60%-90% for other penicillins.

INDICATIONS AND USAGE:

Ampicillin Sodium is indicated in the treatment of infections due to susceptible strains of the following:

Gram-negative Organisms: *Shigellae, Salmonellae* (including *S. typhosa*), *H. influenzae, E. coli, P. mirabilis, N. gonorrhoeae,* and *N. meningitidis.*

Gram-positive Organisms: Streptococci, *D. pneumoniae,* and nonpenicillinase-producing staphylococci.

Because of its wide spectrum and bactericidal action, it may be useful in instituting therapy; however, bacteriological studies to determine the causative organisms and their sensitivity to Ampicillin should be performed.

Indicated surgical procedures should be performed.

CONTRAINDICATIONS:

A history of allergic reaction to any of the penicillins is a contraindication.

WARNINGS:

SERIOUS AND OCCASIONALLY FATAL HYPERSENSITIVITY (ANAPHYLACTOID) REACTIONS HAVE BEEN REPORTED IN PATIENTS ON PENICILLIN THERAPY. ALTHOUGH ANAPHYLAXIS IS MORE FREQUENT FOLLOWING PARENTERAL THERAPY, IT HAS OCCURRED IN PATIENTS ON ORAL PENICILLINS. THESE REACTIONS ARE MORE APT TO OCCUR IN INDIVIDUALS WITH A HISTORY OF PENICILLIN HYPERSENSITIVITY AND/OR HYPERSENSITIVITY REACTIONS TO MULTIPLE ALLERGENS. THERE HAVE BEEN REPORTS OF INDIVIDUALS WITH A HISTORY OF PENICILLIN HYPERSENSITIVITY WHO HAVE EXPERIENCED SEVERE REACTIONS WHEN TREATED WITH CEPHALOSPORINS. BEFORE THERAPY WITH A PENICILLIN, CAREFUL INQUIRY SHOULD BE MADE CONCERNING PREVIOUS HYPERSENSITIVITY REACTIONS TO PENICILLINS, CEPHALOSPORINS, AND OTHER ALLERGENS. IF AN ALLERGIC REACTION OCCURS, THE DRUG SHOULD BE DISCONTINUED AND THE APPROPRIATE THERAPY INSTITUTED. **SERIOUS ANAPHYLACTOID REACTIONS REQUIRE IMMEDIATE EMERGENCY TREATMENT WITH EPINEPHRINE. OXYGEN, INTRAVENOUS STEROIDS, AND AIRWAY MANAGEMENT, INCLUDING INTUBATION, SHOULD ALSO BE ADMINISTERED AS INDICATED.**

USAGE IN PREGNANCY: SAFETY FOR USE IN PREGNANCY HAS NOT BEEN ESTABLISHED.

PRECAUTIONS:

As with any antibiotic preparation, constant observation for signs of overgrowth of non-susceptible organisms, including fungi, is essential. Should superinfection occur (usually involving Aerobacter, Pseudomonas, or Candida), the drug should be discontinued and/or appropriate therapy instituted. As with any potent agent, it is advisable to check periodically for organ system dysfunction during prolonged therapy; this includes renal, hepatic, and hematopoietic systems. This is particularly important in premature, neonates and other infants.

ADVERSE REACTIONS:

As with other penicillins, it may be expected that untoward reactions will be essentially limited to sensitivity phenomena. They are more likely to occur in individuals who have previously demonstrated hypersensitivity to penicillins and in those with a history of allergy, asthma, hay fever, or urticaria.

The following adverse reactions have been reported as associated with the use of Ampicillin:

Gastrointestinal: Glossitis, stomatitis, black "hairy" tongue, nausea, vomiting, and diarrhea. (These reactions are usually associated with oral dosage forms.)

Hypersensitivity Reactions: An erythematous maculopapular rash has been reported fairly frequently. Urticaria and erythema multiforme have been reported occasionally. A few cases of exfoliative dermatitis have been reported. Anaphylaxis is the most serious reaction experienced and has usually been associated with the parenteral dosage form.

Note: Urticaria, other skin rashes, and serum sicknesslike reactions may be controlled with antihistamines and, if necessary, systemic corticosteroids. Whenever such reactions occur, Ampicillin should be discontinued unless, in the opinion of the physician, the condition being treated is life-threatening and amenable only to Ampicillin therapy.

Liver: A moderate rise in serum glutamic oxaloacetic transaminase (SGOT) has been noted, particularly in infants, but the significance of this finding is unknown.

Hemic and Lymphatic Systems: Anemia, thrombocytopenia, thrombocytopenic purpura, eosinophilia, leukopenia, and agranulocytosis have been reported during therapy with the penicillins. These reactions are usually reversible on discontinuation of therapy and are believed to be sensitivity reactions.

DOSAGE AND ADMINISTRATION:

Infections of the ear, nose, throat, and lower respiratory tract due to streptococci, pneumococci, and nonpenicillinase-producing staphylococci, and also those infections of **the upper and lower respiratory tract** due to *H. influenzae:Adults:* 250-500 mg every 6 hours. *Children:* 12.5 mg/kg every 6 hours.

Infection of the genitourinary tract caused by sensitive Gram-negative and Gram-positive bacteria: *Adults:* 500 mg every 6 hours. *Children:* 12.5 mg/kg every 6 hours.

Urethritis due to *N. gonorrhoeae* in adult males: 500 mg every 12 hours for 1 day. Treatment may be repeated if necessary.

DOSAGE AND ADMINISTRATION: *(cont'd)*

Cases of gonorrhea with a suspected lesion of syphilis should have dark-field examinations before receiving Ampicillin, and monthly serological tests for a minimum of 4 months.

Infections of the gastrointestinal tract: *Adults:* 500 mg every 6 hours. *Children:* 12.5 mg/kg every 6 hours.

Larger doses may be required for stubborn or severe infections. The children's dosage is intended for individuals whose weight will not cause a dosage to be calculated greater than that recommended for adults. Children weighing more than 20 kg should be dosed according to the adult recommendations.

It should be recognized that in the treatment of chronic urinary tract and intestinal infections, frequent bacteriological and clinical appraisals are necessary. Smaller doses than those recommended above should not be used. Even higher doses may be needed at times. In stubborn infections, therapy may be required for several weeks. It may be necessary to continue clinical and/or bacteriological follow-up for several months after cessation of therapy.

Treatment should be continued for a minimum of 48 to 72 hours beyond the time that the patient becomes asymptomatic or evidence of bacterial eradication has been obtained. It is recommended that there be at least 10 days' treatment for any infection caused by hemolytic streptococci to help prevent the occurrence of acute rheumatic fever or glomerulonephritis.

Bacterial meningitis: Children with bacterial meningitis caused by *N. meningitidis* or *H. influenzae* have been successfully treated with doses of 150-200 mg/kg/day. A few adults have been successfully treated for bacterial meningitis with doses ranging from 8 to 14 gm daily. Treatment was initiated with intravenous drip therapy for at least 3 days, and continued with frequent (every 3 to 4 hours) intramuscular therapy.

Septicemia: For adults, a dosage of 8 to 14 gm daily is recommended, starting with IV administration for at least 3 days and continuing with the IM route every 3 to 4 hours. For children, a dosage of 150-200 mg/kg/day is recommended, starting with IV administration for at least 3 days and continuing with the IM route every 3 to 4 hours.

As with other parenteral drugs, Ampicillin Sodium should be inspected visually for particulate matter and discoloration.

DIRECTIONS FOR USE-INTRAMUSCULAR ADMINISTRATION

250 mg, 500 mg, 1 gm and 2 gm Standard Vials

(Concentrations of approximately 125 mg/ml and 250 mg/ml). For initial reconstitution, use Sterile Water for Injection, U.S.P.

TABLE 1

Vial Size	Amount of Diluent to be Added	Volume After Reconstitution	Concentration
250 mg	0.9 ml	1.0 ml	250 mg/ml
	1.9 ml	2.0 ml	125 mg/ml
500 mg	1.7 ml	2.0 ml	250 mg/ml
1 gm	3.4 ml	4.0 ml	250 mg/ml
	7.4 ml	8.0 ml	125 mg/ml
2 gm	6.8 ml	8.0 ml	250 mg/ml

Add the required amount of Sterile Water for Injection, U.S.P. and shake vigorously to reconstitute. As with all intramuscular preparations, Ampicillin Sodium should be injected well within the body of a relatively large muscle using usual techniques and precautions.

Stability: Use solutions within one hour after reconstitution. Stability studies demonstrate that Ampicillin Sodium at 125 mg/ml and 250 mg/ml concentrations maintain their potencies up to 1 hour.

Intravenous Therapy: Intravenous therapy is recommended in serious infections when prompt, effective levels of the antibiotic must reach the site of the infection. Such infections include meningitis, subacute bacterial endocarditis, peritonitis, septicemia, severe forms of chronic bronchitis, osteomyelitis, pneumonia and pyelonephritis due to susceptible organisms.

The 1 gm and 2 gm in the Standard Vials and the Piggyback Bottles may be given either intravenous drip or by direct intravenous injection. For direct intravenous injection, dissolve 1 gm or 2 gm in at least 7.4 ml Sterile Water for Injection, U.S.P. and administer slowly over 10 to 15 minutes.

CAUTION: More rapid administration may result in convulsive seizures.

Direct Intravenous Injection: (Concentrations of 50 mg/ml and 100 mg/ml).

Reconstitute 250 mg or 500 mg in 5 ml of Sterile Water for Injection, U.S.P. Administer every six hours by slow injection (3 to 4 minutes).

Stability: The resulting solutions must be used within 2 hours at room temperature (70°-75°F) or within 4 hours if kept under refrigeration (40°F).

Continuous Intravenous Infusion: (Concentration of ≤ 30 mg/ml.)

Reconstitute as directed under Intramuscular Administration (as described above), withdraw the entire contents, then further dilute to a concentration of ≤ 30 mg/ml.

Stability: For IV solutions, see Stability Period section below.

500 mg, 1 gm and 2 gm Piggyback Bottles

For initial reconstitution, use Sterile Water for Injection, U.S.P., Sodium Chloride Injection, U.S.P. or 5% Dextrose in Water*.

Intravenous Drip Infusion: (Concentrations of approximately 5 mg/ml to 20 mg/ml).

500 mg Piggyback Bottle: Reconstitute with a minimum of 50 ml of Sterile Water for Injection, U.S.P., Sodium Chloride Injection, U.S.P., or 5% Dextrose in Water* and shake well.

TABLE 2

Amount of Diluent to be Added	Concentration
50 ml	10 mg/ml
100 ml	5 mg/ml

1 gm Piggyback Bottle: Reconstitute with a minimum of 49 ml of sterile Water for Injection, U.S.P., Sodium Chloride Injection, U.S.P., or 5% Dextrose in Water* and shake well.

TABLE 3

Amount of Diluent to be Added	Concentration
49 ml	20 mg/ml
99 ml	10 mg/ml

2 gm Piggyback Bottle: Reconstitute with 99 ml of Sterile Water for Injection, U.S.P., Sodium Chloride Injection, U.S.P., 5% Dextrose in Water* and shake well.

Stability: For IV solutions, see Stability Period section below.

DOSAGE AND ADMINISTRATION: *(cont'd)*

TABLE 4

Amount of Diluent to be Added	Concentration
99 ml	20 mg/ml

*If the piggyback bottle is reconstituted using 5% Dextrose in Water to a concentration of ≤ 20 mg/ml, the resulting solution is stable for 2 hours at room temperature (70°-75°F) or 3 hours under refrigeration (40°F).

TABLE 5 Stability Period

Intravenous Solution	Concentration	Room Temperature (70-75°F)	Refrigeration (40°F)
Sterile Water for Injection, U.S.P.	≤ 30 mg/ml	8 hours	48 hours
	≤ 20 mg/ml	8 hours	72 hours
Sodium Chloride Injection, U.S.P.	≤ 30 mg/ml	8 hours	48 hours
	≤ 20 mg/ml	8 hours	72 hours
5% Dextrose in Water	≤ 20 mg/ml	2 hours	3 hours
5% Dextrose in 0.45% Sodium Chloride Solution	≤ 10 mg/ml	2 hours	3 hours
Lactated Ringer's Solution	≤ 30 mg/ml	8 hours	24 hours

Unused portions of any solution must be discarded after the time periods listed above.

Store dry powder at room temperature (70°-75°F) or below.

CDC GUIDELINES FOR TREATMENT OF SEXUALLY TRANSMITTED DISEASES

Gonococcal infections:[1] Disseminated gonococcal infection (hospitalization recommended): When the infecting organism is proven to be penicillin-sensitive, parenteral treatment may be switched to ampicillin 1 g every 6 hours (or equivalent).

Rape victims (prophylaxis of infection): Alternative regimen for pregnant women or when tetracycline is contraindicated: 3.5 g orally with 1 g probenecid.

[1]CDC 1989 Sexually Transmitted Diseases Treatment Guidelines. *Morbidity and Mortality Weekly Report* 1989 Sept. 1;38(No.S-8):1–43.

HOW SUPPLIED - RATED THERAPEUTICALLY EQUIVALENT:

Injection, Dry-Soln - Intramuscular; - 1 gm/vial

1's	$1.84	TOTACILLIN-N, Beecham	00029-6610-25
1's	$1.85	TOTACILLIN-N, ADD-VANTAGE, Beecham	00029-6610-40
1's	$2.17	POLYCILLIN-N, Mead Johnson	00015-7404-20
1's	$2.20	Totacillin-N, Beecham	00029-6610-07
1's	$2.34	POLYCILLIN-N, ADD-VANTAGE, Mead Johnson	00015-7404-18
1's	$2.79	TOTACILLIN-N, PIGGYBACK, Beecham	00029-6610-21
1's	$3.49	POLYCILLIN-N, PIGGYBACK, Mead Johnson	00015-7404-36
10's	$23.82	Ampicillin Sodium, Marsam	00209-0250-22
10's	$26.50	Ampicillin Sodium, Bristol Myers Squibb	00003-2919-10
10's	$28.68	Ampicillin Sodium, Gensia Labs	00703-8138-03
10's	$34.80	Ampicillin Sodium, Gensia Labs	00703-8139-03
10's	$37.98	Ampicillin Sodium, Elkins Sinn	00641-2254-43
10's	$43.70	Ampicillin Sodium, Piggyback, Marsam	00209-0300-42
10's	$46.71	Ampicillin Sodium, Elkins Sinn	00641-2255-43
10's	$48.60	Ampicillin Sodium, Bristol Myers Squibb	00003-2919-20

Injection, Dry-Soln - Intramuscular; - 2 gm/vial

1's	$3.38	Totacillin-N, Beecham	00029-6612-07
2 gm	$3.36	POLYCILLIN-N, Mead Johnson	00015-7405-20
2 gm	$3.52	POLYCILLIN-N, Mead Johnson	00015-7405-18
2 gm	$4.94	POLYCILLIN-N, Mead Johnson	00015-7405-28
2 gm x 10	$46.80	Sterile Ampicillin Sodium, Bristol Myers Squibb	00003-2920-10
2 gm x 10	$66.99	Ampicillin Sodium, Elkins Sinn	00641-2256-43
2 gm x 10	$76.09	Ampicillin Sodium, Elkins Sinn	00641-2257-43
10's	$50.40	Ampicillin Sodium, Gensia Labs	00703-8148-03
10's	$57.48	Ampicillin Sodium, Gensia Labs	00703-8149-03
10's	$69.00	Ampicillin Sodium, Bristol Myers Squibb	00003-2920-20
20 ml x 10	$3.03	TOTACILLIN-N, Beecham	00029-6612-22
20 ml x 10	$42.08	Ampicillin Sodium, Vial, Marsam	00209-0350-22
21 ml x 10	$2.85	TOTACILLIN-N ADD-VANTAGE, Beecham	00029-6612-40
100 ml x 10	$3.62	TOTACILLIN-N, Beecham	00029-6612-21
100 ml x 10	$62.04	Ampicillin Sodium, Piggyback, Marsam	00209-0400-42

Injection, Dry-Soln - Intramuscular; - 10 gm/vial

10 gm	$18.32	POLYCILLIN-N, Mead Johnson	00015-7100-28
10 gm x 10	$254.90	Sterile Ampicillin Sodium 10, Bristol Myers Squibb	00003-2921-20
10 gm x 10	$373.35	Ampicillin Sodium, Elkins Sinn	00641-2259-43
10's	$280.80	Ampicillin Sodium, Gensia Labs	00703-8158-03
100 ml x 10	$16.33	TOTACILLIN-N, Beecham	00029-6613-21
100 ml x 10	$229.32	Ampicillin Sodium, Bulk, Marsam	00209-0450-52

Injection, Dry-Soln - Intramuscular; - 125 mg/vial

1 gm x 10	$42.46	OMNIPEN-N, Wyeth Labs	00008-0315-40
1gm x 10	$47.61	OMNIPEN-N, Wyeth Labs	00008-0315-24
2 gm x 10	$68.20	OMNIPEN-N, Wyeth Labs	00008-0315-10
2 gm x 10	$71.95	OMNIPEN-N, Wyeth Labs	00008-0315-42
2gm x 10	$77.40	OMNIPEN-N, Wyeth Labs	00008-0315-26
6 ml x 10	$12.13	Ampicillin Sodium, Vial, Marsam	00209-0050-22
10 gm x 10	$379.75	OMNIPEN-N, Wyeth Labs	00008-0315-43
10's	$14.28	Ampicillin Sodium, Gensia Labs	00703-8108-03
125 mg	$0.97	POLYCILLIN-N, Mead Johnson	00015-7401-20
125 mg x 10	$13.50	Sterile Ampicillin Sodium 125, Bristol Myers Squibb	00003-2916-10
125 mg x 10	$19.68	OMNIPEN-N, Wyeth Labs	00008-0315-07
250 mg x 10	$23.19	OMNIPEN-N, Wyeth Labs	00008-0315-05
500 mg x 10	$30.33	OMNIPEN-N, Wyeth Labs	00008-0315-06
500 mg x 10	$34.08	OMNIPEN-N, Wyeth Labs	00008-0315-38

Injection, Dry-Soln - Intramuscular; - 250 mg/vial

6 ml x 10	$1.01	TOTACILLIN-N, Beecham	00029-6600-24
6 ml x 10	$14.20	Ampicillin Sodium, Vial, Marsam	00209-0100-22
10's	$17.40	Ampicillin Sodium, Gensia Labs	00703-8118-03
250 mg	$1.14	POLYCILLIN-N, Mead Johnson	00015-7402-20
250 mg x 10	$15.80	Sterile Ampicillin Sodium 250, Bristol Myers Squibb	00003-2917-10
250 mg x 10	$22.74	Ampicillin Sodium, Elkins Sinn	00641-2251-43

Injection, Dry-Soln - Intramuscular; - 500 mg/vial

6 ml x 10	$1.31	TOTACILLIN-N, Beecham	00029-6605-24
6 ml x 10	$18.61	Ampicillin Sodium, Vial, Marsam	00209-0150-22
10's	$22.68	Ampicillin Sodium, Gensia Labs	00703-8128-03
10's	$31.08	Ampicillin Sodium, Gensia Labs	00703-8129-03
100 ml x 10	$38.75	Ampicillin Sodium, Piggyback, Marsam	00209-0200-42
500 mg	$1.49	POLYCILLIN-N, Mead Johnson	00015-7403-20

HOW SUPPLIED - RATED THERAPEUTICALLY EQUIVALENT: *(cont'd)*

500 mg	$3.10	POLYCILLIN-N, Mead Johnson	00015-7403-31
500 mg x 10	$20.70	Sterile Ampicillin Sodium 500, Bristol Myers Squibb	00003-2918-10
500 mg x 10	$29.75	Ampicillin Sodium, Elkins Sinn	00641-2252-43
500 mg x 10	$40.93	Ampicillin Sodium, Elkins Sinn	00641-2253-43
500 mg x 10	$43.10	Sterile Ampicillin Sodium 500, Bristol Myers Squibb	00003-2918-20

AMPICILLIN SODIUM; SULBACTAM SODIUM

(000238)

CATEGORIES: Anti-Infectives; Antibiotics; Antimicrobials; Gynecologic Infections; Infections; Intra-Abdominal Infections; Penicillins; Skin Infections; Pregnancy Category B; Sales > $100 Million; FDA Approved 1986 Dec; Patent Expiration 1999 Dec

BRAND NAMES: *Betamp*; *Sulbacin*; *Unacid* (Germany); *Unacim* (France); **Unasyn**; *Unasyna* (Mexico)
(International brand names outside U.S. in italics)

COST OF THERAPY: $230.36 (Infections; Injection; 1.5 gm; 4/day; 10 days)

PRIMARY ICD9: 136.9 (Unspecified Infections and Parasitic Diseases)

DESCRIPTION:

Unasyn is an injectable antibacterial combination consisting of the semisynthetic antibiotic ampicillin sodium and the beta-lactamase inhibitor sulbactam sodium for intravenous and intramuscular administration.

Ampicillin sodium is derived from the penicillin nucleus, 6-aminopenicillanic acid. Chemically, it is monosodium (2S, 5R, 6R)-6-[(R)-2-amino-2-phenylacetamido]-3, 3-dimethyl-7-oxo-4-thia-1-aza-bicyclo(3.2.0)heptane-2-carboxylate and has a molecular weight of 371.39. Its chemical formula is $C_{16}H_{18}N_3NaO_4S$.

Sulbactam sodium is a derivative of the basic penicillin nucleus. Chemically, sulbactam sodium is sodium penicillinate sulfone; sodium (2S,5R)-3,3-dimethyl-7-oxo-4-thia-1-azabicyclo (3.2.0)heptane-2-carboxylate 4, 4-dioxide. Its chemical formula is $C_8H_{10}NNaO_5S$ with a molecular weight of 255.22.

Ampicillin sodium;sulbactam sodium parenteral combination, is available as a white to off-white dry powder for reconstitution. Ampicillin sodium;sulbactam sodium dry powder is freely soluble in aqueous diluents to yield pale yellow to yellow solutions containing ampicillin sodium and sulbactam sodium equivalent to 250 mg ampicillin per ml and 125 mg sulbactam per ml. The pH of the solutions is between 8.0 and 10.0.

Dilute solutions (up to 30 mg ampicillin and 15 mg sulbactam per ml) are essentially colorless to pale yellow. The pH of dilute solutions remains the same.

1.5 g of Unasyn (1 g ampicillin as the sodium salt plus 0.5 g sulbactam as the sodium salt) parenteral contains approximately 115 mg (5 mEq) of sodium.

3 g of Unasyn (2 g ampicillin as the sodium salt plus 1 g sulbactam as the sodium salt) parenteral contains approximately 230 mg (10 mEq) of sodium.

Ampicillin sodium;sulbactam sodium pharmacy bulk package is a vial containing a sterile preparation of ampicillin sodium and sulbactam sodium for parenteral use that contains many single doses. The pharmacy bulk package is for use in pharmacy admixture setting; it provides many single doses of ampicillin sodium;sulbactam sodium for addition to suitable parenteral fluids in preparation of admixtures for intravenous infusion.

CLINICAL PHARMACOLOGY:

GENERAL

Immediately after completion of a 15-minute intravenous infusion of ampicillin sodium;sulbactam sodium, peak serum concentrations of ampicillin and sulbactam are attained. Ampicillin serum levels are similar to those produced by the administration of equivalent amounts of ampicillin alone. Peak ampicillin serum levels ranging from 109 to 150 mcg/ml are attained after administration of 2000 mg of ampicillin plus 1000 mg sulbactam and 40 to 71 mcg/ml after administration of 1000 mg ampicillin plus 500 mg sulbactam. The corresponding mean peak serum levels for sulbactam range from 48 to 88 mcg/ml and 21 to 40 mcg/ml, respectively. After an intramuscular injection of 1000 mg ampicillin plus 500 mg sulbactam, peak ampicillin serum levels ranging from 8 to 37 mcg/ml and peak sulbactam serum levels ranging from 6 to 24 mcg/ml are attained.

The mean serum half-life of both drugs is approximately 1 hour in healthy volunteers.

Approximately 75% to 85% of both ampicillin and sulbactam is excreted unchanged in the urine during the first 8 hours after administration of ampicillin sodium;sulbactam sodium to individuals with normal renal function. Somewhat higher and more prolonged serum levels of ampicillin and sulbactam can be achieved with the concurrent administration of probenecid.

In patients with impaired renal function, the elimination kinetics of ampicillin and sulbactam are similarly affected; hence the ratio of one to the other will remain constant whatever the renal function. The dose of ampicillin sodium;sulbactam sodium in such patients should be administered less frequently in accordance with the usual practice for ampicillin (see DOSAGE AND ADMINISTRATION).

Ampicillin has been found to be approximately 28% reversibly bound to human serum protein and sulbactam approximately 38% reversibly bound.

The average levels (TABLE 1) of ampicillin and sulbactam were measured in the tissues and fluids listed.

TABLE 1 Concentration of Unasyn in Various Body Tissues and Fluids

Fluid or Tissue	Dose (g) Ampicillin;Sulbactam	Concentration (mcg/ml or mcg/g) Ampicillin;Sulbactam
Peritoneal fluid	0.5/0.5 IV	7/14
Blister fluid (cantharides)	0.5/0.5 IV	8/20
Tissue fluid	1/0.5 IV	8/4
Intestinal mucosa	0.5/0.5 IV	11/18
Appendix	2/1 IV	3/40

Penetration of both ampicillin and sulbactam into cerebrospinal fluid in the presence of inflamed meninges has been demonstrated after IV administration of Unasyn.

MICROBIOLOGY

Ampicillin is similar to benzyl penicillin in its bactericidal action against susceptible organisms during the stage of active multiplication. It acts through the inhibition of cell wall mucopeptide biosynthesis. Ampicillin has a broad spectrum of bactericidal activity against many gram-positive and gram-negative aerobic and anaerobic bacteria. (Ampicillin is, however, degraded by beta-lactamases; and therefore the spectrum of activity does not normally include organisms that produce these enzymes.)

CLINICAL PHARMACOLOGY: *(cont'd)*

A wide range of beta-lactamases found in microorganisms resistant to penicillins and cephalosporins have been shown in biochemical studies with cell free bacterial systems to be irreversibly inhibited by sulbactam. Although sulbactam alone possesses little useful antibacterial activity except against *Neisseriaceae* organisms; whole organism studies have shown that sulbactam restores ampicillin activity against beta-lactamase–producing strains. In particular, sulbactam has good inhibitory activity against the clinically important plasmid-mediated beta-lactamases most frequently responsible for transferred drug resistance. Sulbactam has no effect on the activity of ampicillin against ampicillin susceptible strains.

The presence of sulbactam in the ampicillin sodium; sulbatcam sodium formulation effectively extends the antibiotic spectrum of ampicillin to include many bacteria normally resistant to it and to other beta-lactam antibiotics. Thus ampicillin sodium; sulbatcam sodium possesses the properties of a broad-spectrum antibiotic and a beta-lactamase inhibitor.

While *in vitro* studies have demonstrated the susceptibility of most strains of the following organisms, clinical efficacy for infections other than those included in the INDICATIONS AND USAGE section has not been documented.

Gram-Positive Bacteria: *Staphylococcus aureus* (beta-lactamase and non–beta-lactamase producing), *Staphylococcus epidermidis* (beta-lactamase and non–beta-lactamase producing),*Staphylococcus saprophyticus* (beta-lactamase and non–beta-lactamase producing), *Streptococcus faecalis* (Enterococcus), Streptococcus pneumoniae** (formerly *D. pneumoniae*), *Streptococcus pyogenes*†, *Streptococcus viridans.**

Gram-Negative Bacteria: *Haemophilus influenzae* (beta-lactamase and non–beta-lactamase producing), *Moraxella catarrhalis* (beta-lactamase and non–beta-lactamase producing), *Escherichia coli* (beta-lactamase and non–beta-lactamase producing), *Klebsiella* species (all known strains are beta-lactamase producing), *Proteus mirabilis* (beta-lactamase and non–beta-lactamase producing), *Proteus vulgaris, Providencia rettgeri, Providencia stuartii, Morganella morganii*, and *Neisseria gonorrhoeae* (beta-lactamase and non–beta-lactamase producing).

Anaerobes: *Clostridium* spp.,* *Peptococcus* spp.,* *Peptostreptococcus* spp., *Bacteroides* spp., including *B. fragilis.*

*These are not beta-lactamase producing strains and therefore are susceptible to ampicillin alone.

SUSCEPTIBILITY TESTING

Diffusion Technique: For the Kirby-Bauer method of susceptibility testing, a 20 mcg (10 mcg ampicillin + 10 mcg sulbactam) diffusion disk should be used. The method is one outlined in the NCCLS publication M 2-A 3*. With this procedure, a report from the laboratory of "Susceptible" indicates that the infecting organism is likely to respond to ampicillin sodium; sulbatcam sodium therapy; and a report of "Resistant" indicates that the infecting organism is not likely to respond to therapy. An "Intermediate" susceptibility report suggests that the infecting organism would be susceptible to ampicillin sodium; sulbatcam sodium if a higher dosage is used or if the infection is confined to tissues or fluids (*e.g.,* urine) in which high antibiotic levels are attained.

Dilution Techniques: Broth or agar dilution methods may be used to determine the minimal inhibitory concentration (MIC) value for susceptibility of bacterial isolates to ampicillin;sulbactam. The method used is one outlined in the NCCLS publication M 7-A.** Tubes should be inoculated to contain 10^5 to 10^6organisms/ml or plates "spotted" with 10^4 organisms.

The recommended dilution method employs a constant ampicillin/sulbactam ratio of 2:1 in all tubes with increasing concentrations of ampicillin. MICs are reported in terms of ampicillin concentration in the presence of sulbactam at a constant 2 parts ampicillin to 1 part sulbactam (TABLE 2)

TABLE 2 Recommended Ampicillin;Sulbactam, Susceptibility Ranges *, †, ‡

	Resistant (mm)	Intermediate (mm)	Susceptible (mm)
Gram(-) and Staphylococcus			
Kirby-Bauer Zone sizes	≤11 mm	12-13 mm	≥14 mm
MIC (mcg of ampicillin/ml)	≥32	16	≤8
Haemophilus influenzae			
Bauer/Kirby Zones sizes	≤19	—	≥20
MIC (mcg of ampicillin/ml)	≥4	—	≤2

*The non-beta-lactamase producing organisms that are normally susceptible to ampicillin, such as streptococci, will have similar zone sizes as for ampicillin disks.
†staphylococci resistant to methicillin, oxacillin, or nafcillin must be considered resistant to Unasyn.
‡The quality-control cultures should have the assigned daily ranges for ampicillin;sulbactam: (TABLE 3)

TABLE 3

	Disks (mm)	Mode MIC (mcg/ml ampicillin;mcg/ml sulbactam)
E. coli	(ATCC 25922) 20-24	2/1
S. aureus	(ATCC 25923) 29-37	0.12/0.06
E. coli	(ATCC 35218) 13-19	8/4

INDICATIONS AND USAGE:

Ampicillin sodium;sulbactam sodium is indicated for the treatment of infections due to susceptible strains of the designated microorganisms in the conditions listed.

Skin and Skin Structure Infections: Caused by beta-lactamase producing strains of *Staphylococcus aureus, Escherichia coli,*† *Klebsiella* spp.† (including *K. pneumoniae*†), *Proteus mirabilis,*† *Bacteroides fragilis*†, *Enterobacter* spp.,† and *Acinetobacter calcoaceticus.*†

Intra-abdominal Infections: Caused by beta-lactamase producing strains of *Escherichia coli, Klebsiella* spp. (including *K. pneumoniae*†), *Bacteroides* spp. (including *B. fragilis*), and *Enterobacter* spp.†

Gynecologic Infections: Caused by beta-lactamase producing strains of *Escherichia coli,*† and *Bacteroides* spp.† (including *B. fragilis*†).

†Efficacy for this organism in this organ system was studied in fewer than 10 infections.

While ampicillin sodium;sulbactam sodium is indicated only for the conditions listed, infections caused by ampicillin-susceptible organisms are also amenable to treatment with ampicillin sodium; sulbatctam sodium due to its ampicillin content. Therefore mixed infections

INDICATIONS AND USAGE: *(cont'd)*

caused by ampicillin-susceptible organisms and beta-lactamase producing organisms susceptible to ampicillin sodium/sulbactam sodium should not require the addition of another antibiotic.

Appropriate culture and susceptibility tests should be performed before treatment in order to isolate and identify the organisms causing infection and to determine their susceptibility to ampicillin sodium;sulbactam sodium.

When there is reason to believe the infection may involve any of the beta-lactamase producing organisms listed in the indicated organ systems; therapy may be instituted prior to obtaining the results from bacteriologic and susceptibility studies. Once the results are known, therapy should be adjusted if appropriate.

CONTRAINDICATIONS:

The use of ampicillin sodium/sulbactam sodium is contraindicated in individuals with a history of hypersensitivity reactions to any of the penicillins.

WARNINGS:

SERIOUS AND OCCASIONALLY FATAL HYPERSENSITIVITY (ANAPHYLACTIC) REACTIONS HAVE BEEN REPORTED IN PATIENTS ON PENICILLIN THERAPY. THESE REACTIONS ARE MORE APT TO OCCUR IN INDIVIDUALS WITH A HISTORY OF PENICILLIN HYPERSENSITIVITY AND/OR HYPERSENSITIVITY REACTIONS TO MULTIPLE ALLERGENS. THERE HAVE BEEN REPORTS OF INDIVIDUALS WITH A HISTORY OF PENICILLIN HYPERSENSITIVITY WHO HAVE EXPERIENCED SEVERE REACTIONS WHEN TREATED WITH CEPHALOSPORINS. BEFORE THERAPY WITH A PENICILLIN, CAREFUL INQUIRY SHOULD BE MADE CONCERNING PREVIOUS HYPERSENSITIVITY REACTIONS TO PENICILLINS, CEPHALOSPORINS, AND OTHER ALLERGENS. IF AN ALLERGIC REACTION OCCURS, AMPICILLIN SODIUM; SULBATCTAM SODIUM SHOULD BE DISCONTINUED AND THE APPROPRIATE THERAPY INSTITUTED.

Pseudomembranous colitis has been reported with nearly all antibacterial agents, including ampicillin sodium;sulbactam sodium and has ranged in severity from mild to life threatening. Therefore it is important to consider this diagnosis in patients who present with diarrhea subsequent to the administration of antibacterial agents.

Treatment with antibacterial agents alters the normal flora of the colon and may permit overgrowth of clostridia. Studies indicate that toxin produced by *Clostridium difficile* is one primary cause of "antibiotic-associated colitis."

Mild cases of pseudomembranous colitis usually respond to drug discontinuation alone. In moderate to severe cases, consideration should be given to management with fluids and electrolytes, protein supplementation; and treatment with an antibacterial drug clinically effective against *C. difficile* colitis.

SERIOUS ANAPHYLACTOID REACTIONS REQUIRE IMMEDIATE EMERGENCY TREATMENT WITH EPINEPHRINE. OXYGEN, INTRAVENOUS STEROIDS, AND AIRWAY MANAGEMENT, INCLUDING INTUBATION, SHOULD ALSO BE ADMINISTERED AS INDICATED.

PRECAUTIONS:

General: A high percentage of patients with mononucleosis who receive ampicillin develop a skin rash. Thus ampicillin-class antibiotics should not be administered to patients with mononucleosis. In patients treated with ampicillin sodium;sulbactam sodium the possibility of superinfections with mycotic or bacterial pathogens should be kept in mind during therapy. If superinfections occur (usually involving *Pseudomonas* or*Candida* organisms), the drug should be discontinued and/or appropriate therapy instituted.

Drug/Laboratory Test Interactions: Administration of ampicillin sodium;sulbactam sodium will result in high urine concentration of ampicillin. High urine concentrations of ampicillin may result in false-positive reactions in testing for the presence of glucose in urine using Clinitest, Benedict's solution or Fehling's solution. It is recommended that glucose tests based on enzymatic glucose oxidase reactions (such as Clinistix or Tes-Tape) be used. Following administration of ampicillin to pregnant women, a transient decrease in plasma concentration of total conjugated estriol, estriol-glucuronide, and conjugated estrone and estradiol has been noted. This effect may also occur with ampicillin sodium;sulbactam sodium.

Carcinogenesis, Mutagenesis, and Impairment of Fertility: Long-term studies in animals have not been performed to evaluate carcinogenic or mutagenic potential.

PREGNANCY CATEGORY B: Reproduction studies have been performed in mice, rats, and rabbits at doses up to ten (10) times the human dose and have revealed no evidence of impaired fertility or harm to the fetus due to ampicillin sodium;sulbactam sodium. There are, however, no adequate and well-controlled studies in pregnant women. Because animal reproduction studies are not always predictive of human response, this drug should be used during pregnancy only if clearly needed. (See PRECAUTIONS, Drug/Laboratory Test Interactions)

Labor and Delivery: Studies in guinea pigs have shown that intravenous administration of ampicillin decreased the uterine tone, frequency of contractions, height of contractions, and duration of contractions. However, it is not known whether the use of ampicillin sodium;sulbactam sodium in humans during labor or delivery has immediate or delayed adverse effects on the fetus, prolongs the duration of labor, or increases the likelihood that forceps delivery or other obstetric intervention or resuscitation of the newborn will be necessary.

Nursing Mothers: Low concentrations of ampicillin and sulbactam are excreted in the milk; therefore caution should be exercised when ampicillin sodium;sulbatctam sodium is administered to a nursing woman.

Pediatric Use: The efficacy and safety of ampicillin sodium;sulbactam sodium have not been established in infants and children under the age of 12.

DRUG INTERACTIONS:

Probenecid decreases the renal tubular secretion of ampicillin and sulbactam. Concurrent use of probenecid and ampicillin sodium/sulbactam sodium may result in increased and prolonged blood levels of ampicillin and sulbactam. The concurrent administration of allopurinol and ampicillin substantially increases the incidence of rashes in patients receiving both drugs as compared to patients receiving ampicillin alone. It is not known whether this potentiation of ampicillin rashes is due to allopurinol or the hyperuricemia present in these patients. There are no data with ampicillin sodium;sulbactam sodium and allopurinol administered concurrently. Ampicillin sodium;sulbactam sodium and aminoglycosides should not be reconstituted together due to the *in vitro* inactivation of aminoglycosides by the ampicillin component of ampicillin sodium;sulbactam sodium.

ADVERSE REACTIONS:

Ampicillin sodium;sulbactam sodium is generally well tolerated. These adverse reactions have been reported.

ADVERSE REACTIONS: *(cont'd)*

LOCAL ADVERSE REACTIONS

Pain at IM injection site: 16%

Pain at IV injection site: 3%

Thrombophlebitis: 3%

SYSTEMIC ADVERSE REACTIONS

The most frequently reported adverse reactions were diarrhea in 3% of the patients and rash in less than 2% of the patients.

Additional systemic reactions reported in less than 1% of the patients were: itching, nausea, vomiting, candidiasis, fatigue, malaise, headache, chest pain, flatulence, abdominal distention, glossitis, urine retention, dysuria, edema, facial swelling, erythema, chills, tightness in throat, substernal pain, epistaxis, and mucosal bleeding.

ADVERSE LABORATORY CHANGES

Adverse laboratory changes without regard to drug relationship that were reported during clinical trials were:

Hepatic: Increased AST (SGOT), ALT (SGPT), alkaline phosphatase, and LDH.

Hematologic: Decreased hemoglobin, hematocrit, RBC, WBC, neutrophils, lymphocytes, platelets and increased lymphocytes, monocytes, basophils, eosinophils, and platelets.

Blood Chemistry: Decreased serum albumin and total proteins.

Renal: Increased BUN and creatinine.

Urinalysis: Presence of RBCs and hyaline casts in urine.

These adverse reactions have been reported with ampicillin-class antibiotics and can also occur with ampicillin sodium;sulbactam sodium.

Gastrointestinal: Gastritis, stomatitis, black "hairy" tongue, and enterocolitis. Onset of post-membranous colitis symptoms may occur during or after antibiotic treatment. (See WARNINGS.)

Hypersensitivity Reactions: Urticaria, erythema multiforme, and an occasional case of exfoliative dermatitis have been reported. These reactions may be controlled with antihistamines and, if necessary, systemic corticosteroids. Whenever such reactions occur, the drug should be discontinued, unless the opinion of the physician dictates otherwise. Serious and occasionally fatal hypersensitivity (anaphylactic) reactions can occur with a penicillin. (See WARNINGS.)

Hematologic: In addition to the adverse laboratory changes listed above for ampicillin sodium;sulbactam sodium, agranulocytosis has been reported during therapy with penicillins. All of these reactions are usually reversible on discontinuation of therapy and are believed to be hypersensitivity phenomena. Some individuals have developed a positive direct Coombs' test during treatment with ampicillin sodium;sulbactam sodium, as with other beta-lactam antibiotics.

OVERDOSAGE:

Neurologic adverse reactions, including convulsions, may occur with the attainment of high CSF levels of beta-lactams. Ampicillin may be removed from circulation by hemodialysis. The molecular weight, degree of protein binding, and pharmacokinetics profile of sulbactam suggest that this compound may also be removed by hemodialysis.

DOSAGE AND ADMINISTRATION:

Ampicillin sodium;sulbactam sodium may be administered by either the IV or IM routes. The intent of the pharmacy bulk package is for preparation of solutions for IV infusion only.

For IV administration, the dose can be given by slow IV injection over at least 10 to 15 minutes or can also be delivered, in greater dilutions, with 50 to 100 ml of a compatible diluent as an IV infusion over 15 to 30 minutes.

Ampicillin sodium;sulbactam sodium may be administered by deep IM injection. See DOSAGE AND ADMINISTRATION, Preparation For Intramuscular Injection.

The recommended adult dosage of ampicillin sodium;sulbactam sodium is 1.5 g (1 g ampicillin as the sodium salt plus 0.5 g sulbactam as the sodium salt) to 3 g (2 g ampicillin as the sodium salt plus 1 g sulbactam as the sodium salt) every 6 hours. This 1.5- to 3-g range represents the total of ampicillin content plus the sulbactam content of ampicillin sodium;sulbactam sodium, and corresponds to a range of 1 g ampicillin/0.5 g sulbactam to 2 g ampicillin/1 g sulbactam. The total dose of sulbactam should not exceed 4 g per day.

IMPAIRED RENAL FUNCTION

In patients with impairment of renal function, the elimination kinetics of ampicillin and sulbactam are similarly affected, hence the ration of one to the other will remain constant whatever the renal function. The dose of ampicillin sodium;sulbactam sodium in such patients should be administered less frequently in accordance with the usual practice for ampicillin and according to the recommendations found in TABLE 4.

TABLE 4 Dosage Guide for Patients With Renal Impairment

Creatinine Clearance (ml/min/1.73m^2)	Ampicillin/Sulbactam Half-Life (Hr)	Recommended Unasyn Dosage
≥30	1	1.5-3.0 g q6h-q8h
15-29	5	1.5-3.0 g q12h
5-14	9	1.5-3.0 g q24h

When only serum creatinine is available, a specific formula (based on sex, weight, and age of the patient) (TABLE 5) may be used to convert this value into creatinine clearance. The serum creatinine should represent a steady state of renal function.

TABLE 5

Males: [Weight (kg) × (140 - Age)] ÷ [72 × Serum creatinine]
Females 0.85 × Above value

COMPATIBILITY, RECONSTITUTION, AND STABILITY

Ampicillin sodium;sulbactam sodium sterile powder is to be stored at or below 30° C (86° F) prior to reconstitution.

When concomitant therapy with aminoglycosides is indicated, ampicillin sodium;sulbactam sodium and aminoglycosides should be reconstituted and administered separately, due to the *in vitro* inactivation of aminoglycosides by any of the aminopenicillins.

DIRECTIONS FOR USE

General Dissolution Procedures: Ampicillin sodium;sulbactam sodium sterile powder for intravenous and intramuscular use may be reconstituted with any of the compatible diluents described in this insert. Solutions should be allowed to stand after dissolution to allow any foaming to dissipate in order to permit visual inspection for complete solubilization.

Preparation for Intravenous Use

1.5-g and 3.0-g Bottles: Ampicillin sodium;sulbactam sodium sterile powder in piggyback units may be reconstituted directly to the desired concentrations using any of the following parenteral diluents. Reconstitution of ampicillin sodium;sulbactam sodium, at the specified

DOSAGE AND ADMINISTRATION: *(cont'd)*

concentrations, with these diluents provide stable solutions for the time periods are indicated in TABLE 6. (After the indicated time periods, any unused portions of solutions should be discarded.)

TABLE 6

Diluent	Maximum Concentrations (mg/ml) Ampicillin/Sulbactam	Use Periods
Sterile Water for Injection	45 (30/15)	8 hr @ 25°C
	45 (30/15)	48 hr @ 4°C
	30 (20/10)	72 hr @ 4°C
0.9% Sodium Chloride Injection	45 (30/15)	8 hr @ 25°C
	45 (30/15)	48 hr @ 4°C
	30 (20/10)	72 hr @ 4°C
5% Dextrose Injection	30 (20/10)	2 hr @ 25°C
	30 (20/10)	4 hr @ 4°C
	3 (2/1)	4 hr @ 25°C
Lacated Ringer's Injection	45 (30/15)	8 hr @ 25°C
	45 (30/15)	24 hr @ 4°C
M/6 Sodium Lactate Injection	45 (30/15)	8 hr @ 25°C
	45 (30/15)	8 hr @ 4°C
5% Dextrose in 0.45% Saline	3 (2/1)	4 hr @ 25°C
	15 (10/5)	4 hr @ 4°C
10% Invert Sugar	3 (2/1)	4 hr @ 25°C
	30 (20/10)	3 hr @ 4°C

If piggyback bottles are unavailable, standard vials of ampicillin sodium;sulbactam sodium sterile powder may be used. Initially, the vials may be reconstituted with Sterile Water for Injection to yield solutions containing 375 mg ampicillin sodium;sulbactam sodium per ml (250 mg ampicillin/125 mg sulbactam per ml). An appropriate volume should then be immediately diluted with a suitable parenteral diluent to yield solutions containing 3 to 45 mg ampicillin sodium; sulbatctam sodium per ml (2 to 30 mg ampicillin/1 to 15 mg sulbactam/per ml).

1.5 g ADD-Vantage Vials: ampicillin sodium; sulbatctam sodium in the ADD-Vantage system is intended as a single dose for intravenous administration after dilution with the ADD-Vantage Flexible Diluent Container containing 50 ml, 100 ml, or 250 ml of 0.9% Sodium Chloride Injection, USP.

3 g ADD-Vantage Vials: ampicillin sodium; sulbatctam sodium in the ADD-Vantage system is intended as a single dose for intravenous administration after dilution with the ADD-Vantage Flexible Diluent Container containing 100 ml or 250 ml of 0.9% Sodium Chloride Injection, USP.

ampicillin sodium; sulbatctam sodium in the ADD-Vantage system is to be reconstituted with 0.9% Sodium Chloride Injection, USP, only. Reconstitution of ampicillin sodium; sulbatctam sodium, at the specified concentration, with 0.9% Sodium Chloride Injection, USP, provides stable solutions for the time period indicated below:

Diluent: 0.9% Sodium Chloride Injection

Maximum Concentration (mg/ml) Unasyn (Ampicillin;Sulbactam): 30 (20/10)

Use Period: 8 hours @ 25°C

In 0.9% Sodium Chloride Injection, USP

The final diluted solution of ampicillin sodium;sulbactam sodium should be completely administered *within 8 hours* in order to assure proper potency.

Preparation for Intramuscular Injection

1.5 and 3.0 g Standard Vials: Vials for intramuscular use may be reconstituted with Sterile Water for Injection, USP; 05% Lidocaine Hydrochloride Injection, USP; or 2% Lidocaine Hydrochloride Injection, USP. Consult TABLE 7 for recommended volumes to be added to obtain solutions containing 375 mg ampicillin sodium; sulbatctam sodium per ml (250 mg ampicillin/125 mg sulbactam per ml). Note: *Use only freshly prepared solutions and administer within 1 hour after preparation.*

Directions for Proper Use of Pharmacy Bulk Package

The 15-g vial may be reconstituted with either 92 ml Sterile Water for injection or 0.9% Sodium Chloride Injection. The diluent should be added in two seperate aliquots in a suitable work area, such as a laminar flow hood. Add 50 ml of solution; shake to dissolve. Then add an additional 42 ml and shake. The solution should be allowed to stand after dissolution to allow any foaming to dissipate in order to permit visual inspection for complete solubilization. The resultant solution will have a final concentration of approximately 100 mg/ml ampicillin and 50 mg/ml sulbactam. The closure may be penetrated only one time after reconstitution, if needed, using a suitable sterile transfer device or dispensing set that allows for measured dispensing of the contents.

After reconstitution, use within 2 hours (if stored at room temperature) or within 4 hours (if stored under refrigeration).

TABLE 7

Unasyn Vial Size(g)	Volume of Diluent to be Added (ml)	Withdrawal Volume (ml)*
1.5	3.2	4.0
3.0	6.4	8.0

* There is sufficient excess present to allow withdrawal and administration of the stated volumes.

ANIMAL PHARMACOLOGY:

While reversible glycogenosis was observed in laboratory animals, this phenomenon was dose- and time-dependent and is not expected to develop at the therapeutic doses and corresponding plasma levels attained during the relatively short periods of combined ampicillin/sulbactam therapy in man.

HOW SUPPLIED:

Unasyn is supplied as a sterile off-white dry powder in glass vials and piggyback bottles.

Storage: Ampicillin sodium; sulbactam sodium sterile powder is to be stored at or below 30° C (86° F) prior to reconstitution.

HOW SUPPLIED - EQUIVALENTS NOT AVAILABLE:

Injection, Dry-Soln - Intramuscular; - 1.5 gm

10's	$57.59	UNASYN, VIAL, Roerig	00049-0013-83
10's	$61.11	UNASYN, VIAL, Roerig	00049-0031-83
10's	$66.74	UNASYN, PIGGYBACK, Roerig	00049-0022-83

HOW SUPPLIED - EQUIVALENTS NOT AVAILABLE: *(cont'd)*

Injection, Dry-Soln - Intramuscular; - 3 gm

10's	$108.71	UNASYN, VIAL, Roerig	00049-0014-83
10's	$112.21	UNASYN, Roerig	00049-0032-83
10's	$118.40	UNASYN, PIGGYBACK, Roerig	00049-0023-83

Injection, Solution - Intravenous - 15 gm

1's	$54.86	UNASYN, Roerig	00049-0024-28

AMPICILLIN TRIHYDRATE; PROBENECID

(000240)

CATEGORIES: Anti-Infectives; Antibacterials; Antibiotics; Antimicrobials; Central Nervous System Agents; Gonorrhea; Infections; Penicillins; Sedatives/Hypnotics; Urethritis; Pregnancy Category C; FDA Approval Pre 1982

BRAND NAMES: *Ampicin-PRB* (Canada); *Blenox*; Polycillin-Prb; **Principen W Probenecid**; Probampacin; Probencillin; *Prototapen* (France)
(International brand names outside U.S. in italics)

FORMULARIES: Medi-Cal

DESCRIPTION:

Ampicillin trihydrate is semisynthetic penicillin derived the basic penicillin nucleus, 6-aminopenicillanic acid. Probenecid is a uricosuric and renal tubular blocking agent. Principen with probenecid is provided in single dose bottles containing nine capsules; each capsule contains ampicillin trihydrate equivalent to 389 mg, ampicillin, and 111 mg, probenecid (9 capsules contain ampicillin trihydrate equivalent to 3.5 g, ampicillin, and 1 g probenecid.

CLINICAL PHARMACOLOGY:

Ampicillin is stable in the presence of gastric acid and is well absorbed from the gastrointestinal tract. It diffuses readily into most body tissues and fluids; however, penetration into the cerebrospinal fluid and brain occurs only with meningeal inflammation. Ampicillin is excreted largely unchanged in the urine; its excretion is delayed by concurrent administration of probenecid which inhibits the renal tubular secretion of ampicillin. In blood serum, ampicillin is the least bound of all the penicillins; an average of about 20 percent of the drug is bound to the plasma as compared to 60-90 percent for the other penicillins. Probenecid inhibits the tubular reabsorption of urate, thus increasing serum acid levels. It also inhibits the tubular secretion of penicillin and usually increases penicillin plasma levels by any route the antibiotic is given. A two-fold to four-fold elevation has been demonstrated for various penicillins.

Ampicillin is inactivated by penicillinase and therefore is ineffective against penicillinase-producing organisms.

INDICATIONS AND USAGE:

Ampicillin-Probenecid Capsules are indicated for the treatment of uncomplicated infection (urethral, endocervical or rectal) caused by *N. gonorrhoeae* in men and women.

Urethritis and the presence of gram-negative diplococci in urethral smears is strong presumptive evidence of gonorrhea. Culture or fluorescent antibody studies will confirm the diagnosis.

Susceptibility studies should be performed with recurrent infections or when resistant strains are encountered. Therapy may be instituted prior to obtaining results of susceptibility testing.

CONTRAINDICATIONS:

A history of a previous hypersensitivity reaction to any of the penicillins or to probenecid is a contraindication.

Probenecid is not recommended in persons with known blood dyscrasias or uric acid kidney stones or during an acute attack of gout. It is not recommended in conjunction with ampicillin in the presence of known renal impairment.

WARNINGS:

Serious and occasional fatal hypersensitivity (anaphylactoid) reactions have been reported in patients on penicillin therapy. Although anaphylaxis is more frequent following parenteral administration, it has occurred in patients on oral penicillins. These reactions are more apt to occur in individuals with a history of sensitivity to multiple allergens.

There have been well-documented reports of individuals with a history of penicillin hypersensitivity who have experienced severe hypersensitivity reactions when treated with cephalosporins. Before therapy with a penicillin, careful inquiry should be made concerning previous hypersensitivity reactions to penicillins, cephalosporins, and other allergens. If an allergic reaction occurs, the patient should be treated with the usual agents, e.g. pressor amines, antihistamines, and corticosteroids. **Serious anaphylactoid reactions require immediate emergency treatment with epinephrine. Oxygen, IV steroids and airway management, including intubation, should also be administered as indicated.**

USAGE IN PREGNANCY

The safety of these drugs for use in pregnancy has not yet been established.

PRECAUTIONS:

Cases of gonococcal infection with a suspected lesion of syphilis should have darkfield examinations ruling out syphilis before receiving ampicillin. Patients who do not have suspected lesions of syphilis and are treated with ampicillin should have a follow-up serologic test for syphilis that may have been masked by treatment for gonorrhea. Patients with gonorrhea who also have syphilis should be given additional appropriate parenteral penicillin treatment.

ADVERSE REACTIONS:

AMPICILLIN

As with other penicillins, it may be expected that untoward reactions will be essentially limited to sensitivity phenomena. They are more likely to occur in individuals who have previously demonstrated hypersensitivity to penicillin and in those with a history of allergy, asthma, hay fever, or urticaria.

The following adverse reactions have been reported as associated with ampicillin:

GASTROINTESTINAL

Glossitis, stomatitis, nausea, vomiting, and diarrhea. These reactions are usually associated with oral dosage forms of the drug.

HYPERSENSITIVITY REACTIONS

An erythematous, mildly pruritic maculopapular skin rash has been reported fairly frequently. The rash, which actually does not develop within the first week of therapy, may cover the entire body including the soles, palms, and oral mucosa. The eruption usually disappears in three to seven days. Other hypersensitivity reactions that have been reported are: skin rash,

ADVERSE REACTIONS: *(cont'd)*

pruritus, urticaria, erythema multiforme, and an occasional case of exfoliative dermatitis. Anaphylaxis is the most serious reaction experienced and has usually been associated with the parenteral dosage forms of the drug.

Note: Urticaria, other skin rashes, and serum sickness-like reactions may be controlled by antihistamines, and if necessary, systemic corticosteroids. Serious anaphylactoid reactions require emergency measures (see WARNINGS).

LIVER

Moderate elevation in serum glutamic oxaloacetic transaminase (SGOT) has been noted, but the significance of this finding is unknown.

HEMIC AND LYMPHATIC SYSTEMS

Anemia, thrombocytopenia, thrombocytopenic purpura, eosinophilia, leukopenia, agranulocytosis have been reported during therapy with penicillins. These reactions are usually reversible on discontinuation of therapy and are believed to be hypersensitivity phenomena.

PROBENECID

The following are the principal adverse reactions which have generally been reported as associated with the use of probenecid, generally with more prolonged or repeated administration: hypersensitivity reactions (including anaphylaxis), nephrotic syndrome, hepatic necrosis, aplastic anemia; also other anemias, including hemolytic anemia related to genetic deficiency of glucose-6-phosphate dehydrogenase.

DOSAGE AND ADMINISTRATION:

For the treatment of gonorrhea in both men and women - 3.5 g ampicillin and 1 g probenecid (9 capsules) is administered as a single dose.

Physicians are cautioned to use no less than the above recommended dosage.

Follow-up cultures should be obtained from the original sites(s) of infection 7 to 14 days after therapy. In women it is also desirable to obtain culture test-of-cure from both the endocervical and anal canals.

HOW SUPPLIED - RATED THERAPEUTICALLY EQUIVALENT:

Powder, Reconstitution - Oral - 3.5 gm/1 gm

60 ml	$3.60	Ampicillin W/Probenecid, Raway	00686-4140-20
60 ml	$9.50	Ampicillin W/Probenicid, Harber Pharm	51432-0697-17

HOW SUPPLIED - NOT RATED EQUIVALENT:

Capsule, Gelatin - Oral - 3.5 gm/1 gm

9's	**$9.39**	**PRINCIPEN W/PROBENECID, Bristol Myers Squibb**	**00003-1616-10**

AMRINONE LACTATE *(000241)*

CATEGORIES: Cardiovascular Drugs; Congestive Heart Failure; Coronary Vasodilators; Heart Failure; Inotropic Agents; Pregnancy Category C; FDA Approved 1984 Jul; Patent Expiration 1995 Feb

BRAND NAMES: *Amcoral* (Japan); *Cartonic* (Japan); **Inocor**; *Vesistol*
(International brand names outside U.S. in italics)

DESCRIPTION:

Inocor lactate injection, brand of amrinone lactate, represents a new class of cardiac inotropic agents distinct from digitalis glycosides or catecholamines. Amrinone lactate is designated chemically as 5-Amino [3,4'-bipyridin]-6(1*H*)-one 2-hydroxypropanate.

Amrinone is a pale yellow crystalline compound with a molecular weight of 187.2 and an empirical formula of $C_{10}H_9N_3O$. Each mole of lactic acid has a molecular weight of 90.08 and an empirical formula of $C_3H_6O_3$. The solubilities of amrinone at pH's 4.1, 6.0, and 8.0 are 25, 0.9, and 0.7 mg/ml, respectively.

Amrinone lactate is available as a sterile solution in 20 ml ampuls for intravenous administration. Each ml contains Inocor lactate equivalent to 5 mg of base and 0.25 mg of sodium metabisulfite added as a preservative in Water for Injection. All dosages expressed in the package insert are expressed in terms of the base, amrinone. The pH is adjusted to between 3.2 to 4.0 with lactic acid or sodium hydroxide. The total concentration of lactic acid can vary between 5.0 mg/ml and 7.5 mg/ml.

CLINICAL PHARMACOLOGY:

Amrinone Lactate is a positive inotropic agent with vasodilator activity, different in structure and mode of action from either digitalis glycosides or catecholamines.

The mechanism of its inotropic and vasodilator effects has not been fully elucidated.

With respect to its inotropic effect, experimental evidence indicates that it is not a beta-adrenergic agonist. It inhibits myocardial cyclic adenosine monophosphate (c-AMP) phosphodiesterase activity and increases cellular levels of c-AMP. Unlike, digitalis, it does not inhibit sodium-potassium adenosine triphosphatase activity.

With respect to its vasodilatory activity, amrinone lactate reduces afterload and preload by its direct relaxant effect on vascular smooth muscle.

PHARMACOKINETICS

Following intravenous bolus (1 to 2 minutes) injection of 0.68 mg/kg to 1.2 mg/kg to normal volunteers, amrinone lactate had a volume of distribution of 1.2 liters/kg, and following a distributive phase half-life of about 4.6 minutes in plasma, had a mean apparent first-order terminal elimination half-life of about 3.6 hours. In patients with congestive heart failure receiving infusions of Inocor the mean apparent first-order terminal elimination half-life was about 5.8 hours.

Amrinone has been shown in one study to be 10% to 22% bound to human plasma protein by ultrafiltration *in vitro*, and in another study 35% to 49% bound by either ultrafiltration or equilibrium dialysis.

The primary route of excretion in man is *via* the urine as both amrinone and several metabolites (N-glycolyl, N-acetate, O-glucuronide and N-glucuronide). In normal volunteers, approximately 63% of an oral dose of ^{14}C-labelled amrinone was excreted in the urine over a 96-hour period. In the first 8 hours, 51% of the radioactivity in the urine was amrinone with 5% as the N-acetate, 8% as the N-glycolate, and less than 5% for each glucuronide. Approximately 18% of the administered dose was excreted in the feces in 72 hours.

In a 24-hour nonradioactive intravenous study, 10% to 40% of the dose was excreted in urine as unchanged amrinone with the N-acetyl metabolite representing less than 2% of the dose.

In congestive heart failure patients, after a loading bolus dose, steady-state plasma levels of about 2.4 mcg/ml were able to be maintained by an infusion 5 mcg/kg/min to 10 mcg/mg/min. In some congestive heart failure patients, with associated compromised renal and hepatic perfusion, it is possible that plasma levels of amrinone may rise during the infusion period; therefore, in these patients, it may be necessary to monitor the hemodynamic response and/or drug level. The principal measures of patient response include cardiac index, pulmonary capillary wedge pressure, central venous pressure, and their relationship to plasma concentrations. Additionally, measurements of blood pressure, urine output, and body weight may prove useful, as may such clinical symptoms as orthopnea, dyspnea, and fatigue.

PHARMACODYNAMICS

In patients with depressed myocardial function, amrinone lactate produces a prompt increase in cardiac output due to its inotropic and vasodilator actions.

Following a single intravenous bolus dose of amrinone lactate of 0.75 mg/kg to 3 mg/kg in patients with congestive heart failure, dose-related maximum increases in cardiac output occur (of about 28% at 0.75 mg/kg to about 61% at 3 mg/kg). The peak effect occurs within 10 minutes at all doses. The duration of effect depends upon dose, lasting about 1/2 hour at 0.75 mg/kg and approximately 2 hours at 3 mg/kg.

Over the same range of doses, pulmonary capillary wedge pressure and total peripheral resistance show dose-related decreases (mean maximum decreases of 29% in pulmonary capillary wedge pressure and 29% in systemic vascular resistance). At doses up to 3.0 mg/kg dose-related decreases in diastolic pressure (up to 13%) have been observed. Mean arterial pressure decreases (9.7%) at a dose of 3.0 mg/kg. The heart rate is generally unchanged.

The changes in hemodynamic parameters are maintained during continuous intravenous infusion and for several hours thereafter.

Amrinone lactate is effective in fully digitalized patients without causing signs of cardiac glycoside toxicity. Its inotropic effects are additive to those of digitalis. In cases of atrial flutter/fibrillation, it is possible that amrinone lactate may increase ventricular response rate because of its slight enhancement of A/V conduction. In these cases, prior treatment with digitalis is recommended.

Improvement in left ventricular function and relief of congestive heart failure in patients with ischemic heart disease have been observed. The improvement has occurred without inducing symptoms or electrocardiographic signs of myocardial ischemia.

At constant heart rate and blood pressure, increases in cardiac output occur without measurable increases in myocardial oxygen consumption or changes in arteriovenous oxygen difference.

Inotropic activity is maintained following repeated intravenous doses of amrinone lactate. Amrinone lactate administration produces hemodynamic and symptomatic benefits to patients not satisfactorily controlled by conventional therapy with diuretics and cardiac glycosides.

INDICATIONS AND USAGE:

Amrinone lactate is indicated for the short-term management of congestive heart failure. Because of limited experience and potential for serious adverse effects (see ADVERSE REACTIONS), amrinone lactate should be used only in patients who can be closely monitored and who have not responded adequately to digitalis, diuretics, and/or vasodilators. Although most patients have been studied hemodynamically for periods only up to 24 hours, some patients were studied for longer periods and demonstrated consistent hemodynamic and clinical effects. The duration of therapy should depend on patient responsiveness.

CONTRAINDICATIONS:

Amrinone lactate is contraindicated in patients who are hypersensitive to it.

It is also contraindicated in those patients known to be hypersensitive to bisulfites.

WARNINGS:

Amrinone lactate contains sodium metabisulfite, a sulfite that may cause allergic-type reactions including anaphylactic symptoms and life-threatening or less severe asthmatic episodes in certain susceptible people. The overall prevalence of sulfite sensitivity in the general population is unknown and probably low. Sulfite sensitivity is seen more frequently in asthmatic than in nonasthmatic people.

PRECAUTIONS:

GENERAL

Amrinone Lactate should not be used in patients with severe aortic or pulmonic valvular disease in lieu of surgical relief of the obstruction. Like other inotropic agents, it may aggravate outflow obstruction in hypertrophic subaortic stenosis.

During intravenous therapy with amrinone lactate injection, blood pressure and heart rate should be monitored and the rate of infusion slowed or stopped in patients showing excessive decreases in blood pressure.

Patients who have received vigorous diuretic therapy may have insufficient cardiac filling pressure to respond adequately to Inocor lactate injection, in which case cautious liberalization of fluid and electrolyte intake may be indicated.

Supraventricular and ventricular arrhythmias have been observed in the very high risk population treated. While amrinone per se has not been shown to be arrhythmogenic, the potential for arrhythmia, present in congestive heart failure itself, may be increased by any drug or combination of drugs.

Thrombocytopenia and hepatotoxicity have been noted (see ADVERSE REACTIONS.)

USE IN ACUTE MYOCARDIAL INFARCTION

No clinical trials have been carried out in patients in the acute phase of postmyocardial infarction. Therefore, amrinone lactate is not recommended in these cases.

LABORATORY TESTS FLUID AND ELECTROLYTES

Fluid and electrolyte changes and renal function should be carefully monitored during amrinone lactate therapy. Improvement in cardiac output with resultant diuresis may necessitate a reduction in the dose of diuretic. Potassium loss due to excessive diuresis may predispose digitalized patients to arrhythmias. Therefore, hypokalemia should be corrected by potassium supplementation in advance of or during amrinone use.

CARCINOGENESIS, MUTAGENESIS, AND IMPAIRMENT OF FERTILITY

There was no suggestion of a carcinogenic potential with amrinone when administered orally for up to two years to rats and mice at dose levels up to the maximally tolerated dose of 80 mg/kg/day.

The mouse micronucleus test (at 7.5 to 10 times the maximum human dose) and the Chinese hamster ovary chromosome aberration assay were positive indicating both clastogenic potential and suppression of the number of polychromatic erythrocytes. However, the Ames Salmonella assay, mouse lymphoma study, and cultured human lymphocyte metaphase analysis were all negative. The clastogenic effects are in contrast to negative results obtained in the rat male and female fertility studies, and a three-generation study in rats, both with oral dosing.

Slight prolongation of the rat gestation period was seen in these studies at dose levels of 50 mg/kg/day and 100 mg/kg/day. Dystocia occurred in dams receiving 100 mg/kg/day resulting in increased numbers of stillbirths, decreased litter size, and poor pup survival.

PRECAUTIONS: *(cont'd)*

PREGNANCY CATEGORY C

In New Zealand white rabbits, amrinone has been shown to produce fetal skeletal and gross external malformations at oral doses of 16 mg/kg and 50 mg/kg which were toxic for the rabbit. Studies in French Hy/Cr rabbits using oral doses up to 32 mg/kg/day did not confirm this finding. No malformations were seen in rats receiving amrinone intravenously at the maximum dose used, 15 mg/kg/day (approximately the recommended daily intravenous dose for patients with congestive heart failure). There are no adequate and well-controlled studies in pregnant women. Amrinone should be used during pregnancy only if the potential benefit justifies the potential risk to the fetus.

NURSING MOTHERS

Caution should be exercised when amrinone is administered to nursing women since it is not known whether it is excreted in human milk.

PEDIATRIC USE

Safety and effectiveness in children have not been established.

DRUG INTERACTIONS:

In a relatively limited experience, no untoward clinical manifestations have been observed in patients in which amrinone lactate was used concurrently with the following drugs; digitalis glycosides; lidocaine, quinidine; metoprolol, propranolol; hydralazine, prazosin; isosorbide dinitrate, nitroglycerine; chlorthalidone, ethacrynic acid, furosemide, hydrochlorothiazide, spironolactone; captopril; heparin, warfarin; potassium supplements; insulin; diazepam.

One case report of excessive hypotension has been reported when amrinone was used concurrently with disopyramide.

Until additional experience is available, concurrent administration with Norpace (disopyramide) should be undertaken with caution.

Chemical Interactions: A chemical interaction occurs slowly over a 24-hour period when the intravenous solution of Amrinone Lactate is mixed directly with dextrose (glucose)-containing solutions.**THEREFORE, AMRINONE LACTATE SHOULD NOT BE DILUTED WITH SOLUTIONS THAT CONTAIN DEXTROSE (GLUCOSE) PRIOR TO INJECTION.**

A chemical interaction occurs immediately, which is evidenced by the formation of a precipitate when furosemide is injected into an intravenous line of an infusion of amrinone. Therefore, furosemide should not be administered in intravenous lines containing amrinone.

ADVERSE REACTIONS:

Thrombocytopenia: Intravenous amrinone lactate resulted in platelet count reductions to below 100,000/mm^3 or normal limits in 2.4 percent of the patients.

It is more common in patients receiving prolonged therapy. To date, in closely-monitored clinical trials, in patients whose platelet counts were not allowed to remain depressed, no bleeding phenomena have been observed.

Platelet reduction is dose dependent and appears due to a decrease in platelet survival time. Several patients who developed thrombocytopenia while receiving amrinone had bone marrow examinations which were normal. There is no evidence relating platelet reduction to immune response or to a platelet activating factor.

Gastrointestinal Effects: Gastrointestinal adverse reactions reported with Inocor lactate injection during clinical use included nausea (1.7%), vomiting (0.9%), abdominal pain (0.4%) and anorexia (0.4%).

Cardiovascular Effects: Cardiovascular adverse reactions reported with Inocor lactate injection include arrhythmia (3%) and hypotension (1.3%).

Hepatic Toxicity: In dogs, at IV doses between 9 mg/kg/day and 32 mg/kg/day amrinone showed dose-related hepatotoxicity manifested either as enzyme elevation or hepatic cell necrosis or both. Hepatotoxicity has been observed in man following long-term oral dosing and has been observed, in a limited experience (0.2%), following intravenous administration of amrinone. There have also been rare reports of enzyme and bilirubin elevation and jaundice.

Hypersensitivity: There have been reports of several apparent hypersensitivity reactions in patients treated with oral amrinone for about two weeks. Signs and symptoms were variable but included pericarditis, pleuritis and ascites (1 case), myositis with interstitial shadowing on chest x-ray and elevated sedimentation rate (1 case) and vasculitis with nodular pulmonary densities, hypoxemia, and jaundice (1 case). The first patient died, not necessarily of the possible reaction, while the last two resolved with discontinuation of therapy. None of the cases were rechallenged so that attribution to amrinone is not certain, but possible hypersensitivity reactions should be considered in any patient maintained for a prolonged period on amrinone.

General: Additional adverse reactions observed in intravenous amrinone clinical studies include fever (0.9%), chest pain (0.2%), and burning at the site of injection (0.2%).

Management of Adverse Reactions Platelet Count Reductions: Asymptomatic platelet count reduction (to <150,000/mm^3) may be reversed within one week of a decrease in drug dosage. Further, with no change in drug dosage, the count may stabilize at lower than pre-drug level without any clinical sequelae. Pre-drug platelet counts and frequent platelet counts during therapy are recommended to assist in decisions regarding dosage modifications.

Should a platelet count less than 150,000/mm^3 occur, the following actions may be considered:

Maintain total daily dose unchanged, since in some cases counts have either stabilized or returned to pretreatment levels.

Decrease total daily dose.

Discontinue amrinone if, in the clinical judgment of the physician, risk exceeds the potential benefit.

Gastrointestinal Side Effects: While gastrointestinal side effects were seen infrequently with intravenous therapy, should severe or debilitating ones occur, the physician may wish to reduce dosage or discontinue the drug based on the usual benefit-to-risk considerations.

Hepatic Toxicity: In clinical experience to date with intravenous administration, hepatotoxicity has been observed rarely. If acute marked alterations in liver enzymes occur together with clinical symptoms suggesting an idiosyncratic hypersensitivity reaction, amrinone therapy should be promptly discontinued.

If less than marked enzyme alterations occur without clinical symptoms, these nonspecific changes should be evaluated on an individual basis. The clinician may wish to continue amrinone, reduce dosage, or discontinue the drug based on the usual benefit/risk considerations.

OVERDOSAGE:

A death has been reported with a massive accidental overdose (840 mg over three hours by initial bolus and infusion) of amrinone, although causal relation is uncertain. Diligence should be exercised during product preparation and administration.

Doses of Inocor lactate injection may produce hypotension because of its vasodilator effect. If this occurs, amrinone administration should be reduced or discontinued. No specific antidote is known, but general measures for circulatory support should be taken.

OVERDOSAGE: *(cont'd)*

In rats, the LD_{50} of amrinone, as the lactate salt, was 102 mg/kg or 130 mg/kg intravenously in two different studies and 132 mg/kg orally (intragastrically); as a suspension in aqueous gum tragacanth the oral LD_{50} was 239 mg/kg.

DOSAGE AND ADMINISTRATION:

Loading doses of amrinone lactate should be administered as supplied (undiluted). Infusions of Amrinone Lactate may be administered in normal, or half normal saline solution to a concentration of 1 mg/ml to 3 mg/ml. Diluted solutions should be used within 24 hours.

Amrinone Lactate may be injected into running dextrose (glucose) infusions through a Y-Connector or directly into the tubing where preferable.

Chemical Interactions: A chemical interaction occurs slowly over a 24-hour period when the intravenous solution of Inocor lactate injection is mixed directly with dextrose (glucose)-containing solutions.**THEREFORE, AMRINONE LACTATE SHOULD NOT BE DILUTED WITH SOLUTIONS THAT CONTAIN DEXTROSE (GLUCOSE) PRIOR TO INJECTION.**

A chemical interaction occurs immediately, which is evidenced by the formation of a precipitate when furosemide is injected into an intravenous line of an infusion of amrinone. Therefore, furosemide should not be administered in intravenous lines containing amrinone.

The following procedure is recommended for the administration of Amrinone Lactate:

1. Initiate therapy with a 0.75 mg/kg loading dose given slowly over 2 to 3 minutes (TABLE 1):

2. Continue therapy with a maintenance infusion between 5 mcg/min and 10 mcg/kg/min.

3. Based on clinical response, an additional loading dose of 0.75 mg/kg may be given 30 minutes after the initiation of therapy.

4. The rate of infusion usually ranges from 5 mcg/kg/min to 10 mcg/kg/min such that the recommended total daily dose (including loading doses) does not exceed 10 mg/kg. A limited number of patients studied at higher doses support a dosage regimen up to 18 mg/kg/day for shortened durations of therapy.

5. The rate of administration and the duration of therapy should be adjusted according to the response of the patient. The physician may wish to reduce or titrate the infusion downward based on clinical responsiveness or untoward effects.

TABLE 1 Loading Dose Determination 0.75 mg/kg (Undiluted)

Patient Wt in kg	30	40	50	60	70	80	90	100	110	120
ml of undiluted Amrinone Lactate	4.5	6.0	7.5	9.0	10.5	12.0	13.5	15.0	16.5	18.0

The following infusion rate chart may be used to assure that the calculations are made correctly.

To utilize the chart, the concentration of amrinone infusion solution used must be 2.5 mg/ml (2500 mcg/ml). This concentration is prepared by mixing the amrinone solution with an equal volume of diluent (normal or half normal saline;)(See TABLE 2):

TABLE 2 Amrinone Lactate Infusion Rate (Ml/Hr) Chart Using 2.5 Mg/Ml Infusion Concentration*

Patient Weight in kg	30	40	50	60	70	80	90	100	110	120
Dosage: 5.0 mcg/kg/min	4	5	6	7	8	10	11	12	13	14
7.5 mcg/kg/min	5	7	9	11	13	14	16	18	20	22
10.0 mcg/kg/min	7	10	12	14	17	19	22	24	26	29

Example: A 70 kg patient would require a loading dose of 10.5 ml of undiluted Inocor. If the physician selects a dose of 7.5 mcg/kg/min for the infusion, the flow rate would be 13 ml/hr at the 2.5 mg/ml concentration of Inocor.

Dilution: To prepare the 2.5 mg/ml concentration recommended for infusion mix Inocor with an equal volume of diluent. For example, mix three 20 ml ampuls of Inocor (3x20 ml= 60 ml) with 60 ml of diluent for a total volume of 120 ml of the final 2.5 mg/ml solution of Inocor.

The above dosing regimens can be expected to place most patients' plasma concentration of amrinone at approximately 3 mcg/ml. Increases in cardiac index show a linear relationship to plasma concentration of a range of 0.5 mcg/ml to 7 mcg/ml. No observations have been made at greater plasma concentrations.

Patient improvement may be reflected by increases in cardiac output, reduction in pulmonary capillary wedge pressure, and such clinical responses as a lessening of dyspnea and an improvement in other symptoms of heart failure, such as orthopnea and fatigue.

Monitoring central venous pressure (CVP) may be valuable in the assessment of hypotension and fluid balance management. Prior correction or adjustment of fluid/electrolytes is essential to obtain satisfactory response with amrinone.

Parenteral drug products should be inspected visually and should not be used if particulate matter or discoloration is observed.

Protect amrinone lactate ampuls from light. Ampul packaging is light resistant for protection during storage.

Storage: Store at room temperature.

HOW SUPPLIED - EQUIVALENTS NOT AVAILABLE:

Injection, Solution - Intravenous - 5 mg/ml

20 ml x 25 $1506.60 INOCOR, Sanofi Winthrop 00024-0888-20

AMYL NITRITE *(000243)*

CATEGORIES: Angina; Antianginals; Cardiovascular Drugs; Coronary Artery Disease; Vasodilating Agents; Pregnancy Category C; FDA Pre 1938 Drugs

BRAND NAMES: Amyl Nitrate; *Amyl Nitrite* (Canada); *Nitrit*
(International brand names outside U.S. in italics)

DESCRIPTION:

Amyl Nitrite is a systemic vasodilator taken by inhalation. It is available in 0.3 ml crushable glass capsules. Amyl nitrite is a clear yellow liquid that volatilizes readily at room temperature with a pungent fruity aroma. It is stabilized with Epoxol 9-5 2%.

Amyl nitrite is a mixture of 2-methylbutyl nitrite and 3-methylbutyl nitrite.

The structural formulas are:

$(CH_3)_2CHCH_2CH_2ONO$ +

$CH_3CH_2CH(CH_3)CH_2ONO$

CLINICAL PHARMACOLOGY:

Nitrites, including amyl nitrite, relax smooth muscles, most prominently in the blood vessels. Administration of nitrites results in prompt dilation of the large coronary blood vessels, decreased systemic vascular resistance, decreased venous return to the heart, and reduced left ventricular energy expenditure. In patients with angina pectoris myocardial ischemia is thereby relieved, resulting in abatement of chest pain. The vapors of amyl nitrite are absorbed rapidly through the pulmonary alveoli, exerting therapeutic effects within one minute of their inhalation. The drug is metabolized rapidly, probably by hydrolytic denitration. Approximately one-third of the inhaled dose is excreted in the urine.

INDICATIONS AND USAGE:

Amyl Nitrite is indicated for the rapid relief of angina pectoris due to coronary artery disease.

CONTRAINDICATIONS:

The use of nitrites is contraindicated in the presence of cerebral hemorrhage or recent head trauma, and in patients who are hypersensitive to such drugs.

PRECAUTIONS:

General Tolerance to nitrites may develop with repeated use. Transient dizziness, weakness, or other signs of cerebral hypoperfusion from postural hypotension may develop following inhalation of amyl nitrite. Brief syncope can also occur, especially if the patient is standing when hypotension develops. Measures that facilitate venous return may be used to hasten recovery: the head-low position, deep breathing and elevation of the extremities. High doses of nitrites may produce methemoglobinemia, especially in individuals with methemoglobin reductase deficiency or other metabolic abnormality that interferes with the normal conversion of methemoglobin back to hemoglobin.

Information for the Patient This drug should be inhaled while the patient is seated or lying down. Taking it after drinking alcohol may worsen its side effects.

Caution: Amyl nitrite is very flammable. Do not use where it may be ignited.

Carcinogenesis, Mutagenesis, and Impairment of Fertility Adequate long-term studies to evaluate the carcinogenic potential of this drug have not been reported.

Pregnancy, Teratogenic Effects, Pregnancy Category C: . Animal reproduction studies have not been conducted with amyl nitrite. It is also not known whether amyl nitrite can cause fetal harm when administered to a pregnant woman or can affect reproduction capacity. Amyl nitrite should be given to a pregnant woman only if clearly needed.

Nursing Mothers: It is not known whether this drug is excreted in human milk. Because many drugs are excreted in human milk, caution should be exercised when amyl nitrite is administered to a nursing woman.

Pediatric Use: Safety and effectiveness in children have not been established.

DRUG INTERACTIONS:

Postural hypotension from nitrites appears to be exacerbated by ingestion of alcohol before treatment.

ADVERSE REACTIONS:

Headache, usually transient and mild, dizziness, and flushing of the face are common reactions to nitrites. Other reactions that have occurred include: syncope, involuntary passage of urine and feces, hypotension, pallor, cold sweat, tachycardia, restlessness, weakness, vomiting and nausea.

DRUG ABUSE AND DEPENDENCE:

Abuse: Volatile nitrites are abused for sexual stimulation, with headache as a common side effect.

Dependence: Tolerance to nitrites can develop, but the conditions required and its duration have not been established.

OVERDOSAGE:

The acute effects of inhalation of large doses of amyl nitrite in animals include signs and symptoms of hypotension, see PRECAUTIONS section for treatment of postural hypotension.

High doses of nitrites may produce methemoglobinemia, especially in individuals with methemoglobin reductase deficiency. Methemoglobinemia should be treated with high-flow oxygen and methylene blue administered slowly at a dose of 0.2 ml/kg (1 to 2 mg/kg) IV. The dose of methylene blue may need to be repeated once in severe cases but treatment with additional doses (*i.e.,* greater than 4 mg/kg) may cause clinical deterioration since large amounts of methylene blue will itself produce methemoglobinemia. Methylene blue is contraindicated in cases of iatrogenic methemoglobinemia caused by the use of nitrites in the treatment of cyanide poisoning.

Information on serious overdosage or the lethal dose in man is not available.

DOSAGE AND ADMINISTRATION:

With the patient seated or recumbent, a capsule of Amyl Nitrite is crushed with the fingers and held to the nostrils for inhalation of the vapors. Two to six inhalations of the vapors from one capsule are usually sufficient to produce therapeutic effects promptly. This dose may be repeated in 3 to 5 minutes if necessary.

The contents of the capsules are flammable. Store in a cool place 8 - 15°C (46° - 59°F) and protect from light.

HOW SUPPLIED - EQUIVALENTS NOT AVAILABLE:

Solution - Inhalation - 5 drop/ampul

0.18 ml x 12	$21.40	Amyl Nitrite, Lilly	00002-2404-12
0.3 ml x 12	$6.60	Amyl Nitrite, Consolidated Midland	00223-7002-12
0.3 ml x 144	$41.76	Amyl Nitrate, Raway	00686-0221-01
12's	$33.15	Amyl Nitrite, Lilly	00002-2405-12

AMYLASE; CELLULASE; LIPASE; PROTEASE

(000244)

CATEGORIES: Abdominal Distention; Diarrhea; Digestants; Dyspepsia; Enzymes & Digestants; Flatulence; Gastrointestinal Drugs; Pregnancy Category C; FDA Pre 1938 Drugs

BRAND NAMES: **Ku-Zyme**

FORMULARIES: Aetna; BC-BS; FHP; Humana; Kaiser; PruCare

DESCRIPTION:

Ku-Zyme Capsules contain four standardized enzymes: lipase, amylase, protease and cellulase. They are derived from fungal, plant and animal sources and are designed for oral digestive enzyme supplement therapy. Each capsule contains:

Lipase: 1,200 USP Units

Amylase: 30 mg

Protease: 6 mg

Cellulase: 2 mg

Inactive Ingredients: D&C Yellow #10, FD&C Yellow #6, gelatin, lactose, magnesium stearate, synthetic red iron oxide, titanium dioxide, and vanillin.

CLINICAL PHARMACOLOGY:

Diminution of secretions from exocrine glands is often a result of the normal aging process. Amylase;Cellulase;Lipase;Protease provides a balanced combination of natural proteolytic, amylolytic, cellulolytic and lipolytic enzymes to enhance digestion of proteins, starch and fat in the gastrointestinal tract. These enzymes do not exert any systemic pharmacologic effects. Amylase;Cellulase;Lipase;Protease should be considered an enzyme supplement and not an enzyme replacement therapy. Enzymes in Amylase;Cellulase;Lipase;Protease are basically derived from fungal and plant sources and possess a broad spectrum of Ph activity. Enzymes are promptly released from the capsules and are bioavailable for digestion of food in the stomach and intestines.

INDICATIONS AND USAGE:

For the relief of functional indigestion when due to enzyme deficiency or imbalance. Amylase;Cellulase;Lipase;Protease relieves symptoms due to faulty digestion including the sensation of fullness after meals, dyspepsia, flatulence, abdominal distention and intolerance to certain foods.

CONTRAINDICATIONS:

There are not known contraindications to the administration of digestive enzymes. These enzymes do not attack living tissues and do not present any danger to the patient with ulceration or inflammation in the digestive tract.

WARNINGS:

Do not administer to patients who are allergic to pork products.

PRECAUTIONS:

Information for the Patient: If capsules are opened, avoid inhalation of the powder. Sensitive individuals may experience allergic reactions.

Carcinogenesis, Mutagenesis, and Impairment of Fertility: Long-term studies in animals have not been performed to evaluate the carcinogenic, mutagenic or impairment of fertility potential of Amylase;Cellulase;Lipase;Protease.

Pregnancy Category C: Animal reproduction studies have not been conducted with Amylase;Cellulase;Lipase;Protease. It is also not known whether Amylase;Cellulase;Lipase;Protease can cause fetal harm when administered to a pregnant woman or can affect reproduction capacity. Amylase;Cellulase;Lipase;Protease should be given to a pregnant woman only if clearly needed.

Nursing Mothers: It is not known whether Amylase;Cellulase;Lipase;Protease is excreted in human milk. Because many drugs are excreted in human milk, caution should be exercised when Amylase;Cellulase;Lipase;Protease is administered to a nursing woman.

ADVERSE REACTIONS:

Virtually unknown. Occasionally a slight looseness of stools may be noticed. If so, dosage should be reduced. Finely powdered pancreatic enzyme may be irritating to the mucous membranes and respiratory tract. Inhalation of the airborne powder may precipitate an asthma attack in sensitive individuals.

OVERDOSAGE:

No systemic toxicity occurs. Excessive dosage may, however, produce a laxative effect.

DOSAGE AND ADMINISTRATION:

1 or 2 capsules taken with each meal or snack. Dosage may be adjusted depending on individual requirements for relief of symptoms due to digestive enzyme deficiency. In patients who experience difficulty in swallowing the capsule, it may be opened and the contents sprinkled on the food. When opening the capsules, avoid inhalation of the powder (see PRECAUTIONS and ADVERSE REACTIONS).

Storage: Store at controlled room temperature 15-30°C (59-86°F).

Protect from high humidity.

(Schwarz/Kremers 2/94)

HOW SUPPLIED - EQUIVALENTS NOT AVAILABLE:

Capsule, Gelatin - Oral - 30 mg/2 mg/75 m

100's	$35.87	KU-ZYME, Schwarz Pharma (US)	00091-3522-01

ANAGRELIDE HYDROCHLORIDE *(003327)*

CATEGORIES: Platelet Depletion; Thrombocythemia; Pregnancy Category C; FDA Approved 1997 Jan

BRAND NAMES: **Agrylin**

DESCRIPTION:

Name: Anagrelide HCl capsules

Dosage Form: 0.5 mg and 1 mg capsules for oral administration

Active Ingredient: Agrylin capsules contain either 0.5 mg or 1 mg of anagrelide base (as anagrelide hydrochloride).

DESCRIPTION: *(cont'd)*

Inactive Ingredients: povidone USP, anhydrous lactose NF, lactose monohydrate NF, microcrystalline cellulose NF, crospovidone NF, magnesium stearate NF.

Pharmacological Classification: Platelet-reducing agent.

Chemical Name: 6,7-dichloro-1, 5-dihydroimidazo(2,1-b)quinazolin-2(3H)-one monohydrochloride monohydrate.

Molecular formula: $C_{10}H_7Cl_2N_3O{\cdot}HCl{\cdot}H_2O$

Molecular weight: 310.55

Appearance: Off-white powder

Solubility: Anagrelide HCl is very slightly soluble in water, sparingly soluble in dimethyl sulfoxide and sparingly soluble in dimethylformamide.

CLINICAL PHARMACOLOGY:

The mechanism by which anagrelide reduces blood platelet count is still under investigation. Studies in patients support a hypothesis of dose-related reduction in platelet production resulting from a decrease in megakaryocyte hypermaturation. In blood withdrawn from normal volunteers treated with anagrelide, a disruption was found in the postmitotic phase of megakaryocyte development and a reduction in megakaryocyte size and plaidy. At therapeutic doses, anagrelide does not produce significant changes in white cell counts or coagulation parameters, and may have a small, but clinically insignificant effect on red cell parameters. Platelet aggregation is inhibited in people at doses higher than those required to reduce platelet count. Anagrelide inhibits cyclic AMP phosphodiesterase, as well as ADP- and collagen-induced platelet aggregation.

Following oral administration of ^{14}C-anagrelide in people, more than 70% of radioactivity was recovered in urine. Based on limited data, there appears to be a trend toward dose linearity between doses of 0.5 mg and 2.0 mg. At fasting and at a dose of 0.5 mg of anagrelide, the plasma half-life is 1.3 hours. The available plasma concentration time data at steady state in patients showed that anagrelide does not accumulate in plasma after repeated administration. The drug is extensively metabolized; less than 1% is recovered in the urine as anagrelide.

When a 0.5 mg dose of anagrelide was taken after food, its bioavailability (based on AUC values) was modestly reduced by an average of 13.8% and its plasma half-life slightly increased (to 1.8 hours), when compared with drug administered to the same subjects in the fasted state. The peak plasma level was lowered by an average of 45% and delayed by 2 hours.

CLINICAL STUDIES:

A total of 551 patients with Essential Thrombocythemia (ET) were treated with anagrelide in three clinical trials. Patients with ET were diagnosed based on the following criteria:

Platelet count ≥ 900,000/mcl on two determinations

Profound megakaryocytic hyperplasia in bone marrow

Absence of Philadelphia chromosome

Normal red cell mass

Normal serum iron and ferritin, and normal marrow in iron stores.

The mean duration of anagrelide therapy for study patients was 65 weeks; 23% of patients received treatment for 2 years. In one unbinded, historically-controlled study, 276 ET patients were treated with anagrelide starting at doses of 0.5-2.0 mg every 6 hours. The dose was increased if the platelet count was still high, but to no more than 12 mg each day. Efficacy was defined as reduction of platelet count to or near physiologic levels (150,000-400,000/mcl). The criteria for defining subjects as "responders" were reduction in platelets for at least 4 weeks to ≤600,000/mcl or by at least 50% from baseline value. Subjects treated for less than 4 weeks were not considered evaluable.

TABLE 1

		Time on Treatment						
		Weeks				Years		
	Baseline	4	12	24	48	2	3	4
Mean*	1045	627	537	506	508	501	474	464
N	274†	265	245	206	179	139	78	11

* x 10^3/mcl
† 276 ET subjects were enrolled in this study. There is no anagrelide information available for two of those subjects. Therefore, 274 subjects represent the intent-to-treat population who received anagrelide hydrochloride.

A second historically-controlled, unblinded study in 35 patients with ET treated with anagrelide showed similar decreases in platelet count over time. For 139 patients who had baseline symptoms thought to be secondary to thrombocytopenia (*e.g.,* headache, dizziness, neurological or visual symptoms) and who were treated for at least one year with anagrelide, there was a significant reduction in frequency of symptoms at one year compared with the first month of treatment.

INDICATIONS AND USAGE:

Anagrelide HCl capsules are indicated for the treatment of patients with Essential Thrombocythemia to reduce the elevated platelet count and the risk of thrombosis and to ameliorate associated symptoms (see CLINICAL STUDIESand DOSAGE AND ADMINISTRATION).

WARNINGS:

Cardiovascular: Anagrelide should be used with caution in patients with known or suspected heart disease, and only if the potential benefits of therapy outweigh the potential risks. Because of the positive inotropic effects and side-effects of anagrelide, a pre-treatment cardiovascular examination is recommended along with careful monitoring during treatment in humans, therapeutic doses of anagrelide may cause cardiovascular effects, including vasodilation, tachycardia, palpitations, and congestive heart failure.

Renal: It is recommended that patients with renal insufficiency (creatinine ≥2 mg/dl) receive anagrelide when, in the physician's judgment, the potential benefits of therapy outweigh the potential risks. These patients should be monitored closely for signs of renal toxicity while receiving anagrelide (see ADVERSE REACTIONS, Urogenital System).

Hepatic: It is recommended that patients with evidence of hepatic dysfunction (bilirubin, SGOT, or measures of liver function >1.5 times the upper limit of normal) receive anagrelide when, in the physician's judgment, the potential benefits of therapy outweigh the potential risks. These patients should be monitored closely for signs of hepatic toxicity while receiving anagrelide (see ADVERSE REACTIONS, Hepatic System).

PRECAUTIONS:

LABORATORY TESTS

Anagrelide therapy requires close clinical supervision of the patient. While the platelet count is being lowered (usually during the first two weeks of treatment), blood counts (hemoglobin, white blood cells), liver function (SGOT, SGPT) and renal function (serum creatinine, BUN) should be monitored.

PRECAUTIONS: *(cont'd)*

In 9 subjects receiving a single 5 mg dose of anagrelide, standing blood pressure fell an average of 22/15 mm Hg, usually accompanied by dizziness. Only minimal changes in blood pressure were observed following a dose of 2 mg.

CESSATION OF ANAGRELIDE HCL TREATMENT

In general, interruption of anagrelide treatment is followed by an increase in platelet count. After sudden stoppage of anagrelide therapy, the increase in platelet count can be observed within four days.

CARCINOGENESIS, MUTAGENESIS, AND IMPAIRMENT OF FERTILITY

No long-term studies in animals have been performed to evaluate carcinogenic potential of anagrelide hydrochloride. Anagrelide hydrochloride was not genotoxic in the Ames test, the mouse lymphoma cell (L5178Y, TK) forward mutation test, the human lymphocyte chromosome aberration test, or the mouse micronucleus test. Anagrelide hydrochloride at oral doses up to 240 mg/kg/day (1440 mg/m^2 /day, 195 times the recommended maximum human dose based on body surface area) was found to have no effect on fertility and reproductive performance of male rats. However, in female rats, at oral doses of 60 mg/kg/day (360 mg/m^2/day, 49 times the recommended maximum human dose based on body surface area) or higher, it disrupted implantation when administered in early pregnancy and retarded or blocked parturition when administered in late pregnancy.

PREGNANCY CATEGORY C

Pregnancy, Teratogenic Effects: Teratology studies have been performed in pregnant rats at oral doses up to 900 mg/kg/day (5400 mg/m^2/day, 730 times the recommended maximum human dose based on body surface area) and in pregnant rabbits at oral doses up to 20 mg/kg/day (240 mg/m^2/day, 32 times the recommended maximum human dose based on body surface area) and have revealed no evidence of impaired fertility or harm to the fetus due to anagrelide hydrochloride.

Pregnancy, Nonteratogenic Effects: A fertility and reproductive performance study performed in female rats revealed that anagrelide hydrochloride at oral doses of 60 mg/kg/day (360 mg/m^2/day, 49 times the recommended maximum human dose based on body surface area) or higher disrupted implantation and exerted adverse effect on embryo/fetal survival.

A perinatal and postnatal study performed in female rats revealed that anagrelide hydrochloride at oral doses of 60 mg/kg/day (360 mg/m^2/day, 49 times the recommended maximum human dose based on body surface area) or higher produced delay or blockage of parturition, deaths of nondelivering pregnant dams and their fully developed fetuses, and increased mortality in the pups born.

Five women became pregnant while on anagrelide treatment at doses of 1 to 4 mg/day. Treatment was stopped as soon as it was realized that they were pregnant. All delivered normal, healthy babies. There are no adequate and well-controlled studies in pregnant women. Anagrelide hydrochloride should be used during pregnancy only if the potential benefit justifies the potential risk to the fetus.

Anagrelide is not recommended in women who are or may become pregnant. If this drug is used during pregnancy, or if the patient becomes pregnant while taking this drug, the patient should be apprised of the potential harm to the fetus. Women of child-bearing potential should be instructed that they must not be pregnant and that they should use contraception while taking anagrelide. Anagrelide may cause fetal harm when administered to a pregnant woman.

NURSING MOTHERS

It is not know whether this drug is excreted in human milk. Because many drugs are excreted in human milk and because of the potential or serious adverse reaction in nursing infants from anagrelide hydrochloride a decision should be made whether to discontinue nursing or discontinue the drug, taking into account the importance of the drug to the mother.

PEDIATRIC USE

The safety and efficacy of anagrelide in patients under the age of 16 years have not been established. Anagrelide has been used successfully in eight pediatric patients (age range 8 to 17 years), including three patients with essential thrombocythemia who were treated at a dose of 1 to 4 mg/day.

DRUG INTERACTIONS:

Bioavailability studies evaluating possible interactions between anagrelide and other drugs have not been conducted. The most common medications used concomitantly with anagrelide have been aspirin, acetaminophen, furosemide, iron, ranitidine, hydroxyurea, and allopurinol. The most frequently used concomitant cardiac medication has been digoxin. Although drug-to-drug interaction studies have not been conducted, there is no clinical evidence to suggest that anagrelide interacts with any of these compounds.

There is a single report which suggests that sucralfate may interfere with anagrelide absorption.

Food has no clinically significant effect on the bioavailability of anagrelide.

ADVERSE REACTIONS:

While most reported adverse events during anagrelide therapy have been mild in intensity and have decreased in frequency with continued therapy, serious adverse events reported in patients with ET and/or in patients with thrombocythemia of other etiologies include: congestive heart failure, myocardial infarction, cardiomyopathy, cardiomegaly, complete heart block, atrial fibrillation, cerebrovascular accident, pericarditis, pulmonary infiltrates, pulmonary fibrosis, pulmonary hypertension, pancreatitis, gastric/duodenal.

Of the 551 ET patients treated with anagrelide for a mean duration of 65 weeks, 82 (15%) were discontinued from the study because of adverse events or abnormal laboratory test results. The most common adverse events for treatment discontinuation were headache, diarrhea, edema, palpitation, and abdominal pain. Overall, the occurrence rate of all adverse events was 17.9 per 1000 treatment days. The occurrence rate of adverse events increased at higher doses of anagrelide.

Adverse events with an incidence of 1% to <5% included:

Body as a Whole System: Fever, flu symptoms, chills, neck pain, photosensitivity.

Cardiovascular System: Arrhythmia, hemorrhage, cardiovascular disease, cerebrovascular accident, angina pectoris, heart failure, postural hypotension, vasodilatation, migraine, syncope.

Digestive System: Constipation, GI distress, GI hemorrhage, gastritis, melena, aphthous stomatitis, eructation, nausea, vomiting.

Hemic and Lymphatic System: Anemia, thrombocytopenia, ecchymosis, lymphadenoma. Platelet counts below 1000,000/mcl occurred in 35 patients and reduction below 50,000/mcl occurred in 7 of the 551 ET patients while on anagrelide therapy. Thrombocythemia promptly recovered upon discontinuation of anagrelide.

Hepatic System: Elevated liver enzymes were observed in 2 of 551 patients during therapy.

Musculoskeletal System: Arthralgia, myalgia, leg cramps.

Nervous System: Depression, somnolence, confusion, insomnia, hypertension, nervousness, amnesia.

Nutritional Disorders: Dehydration

ADVERSE REACTIONS: *(cont'd)*

TABLE 2 Most Frequently Reported Adverse Reactions To Anagrelide (in 5% or greater of 551 patients with ET) in clinical trials

Headache	44.5%
Palpitations	27.2%
Diarrhea	24.3%
Asthenia	22.1%
Edema, other	19.8%
Abdominal pain	17.4%
Nausea	15.1%
Pain, other	14.7%
Dizziness	14.5%
Dyspnea	10.5%
Flatulence	10.5%
Chest pain	7.8%
Rash, including urticaria	7.8%
Vomiting	7.4%
Paresthesia	7.3%
Tachycardia	7.3%
Peripheral edema	7.1%
Dyspepsia	6.4%
Back pain	6.4%
Anorexia	5.8%
Malaise	5.8%

Respiratory System: Rhinitis, epistaxis, respiratory disease, sinusitis, pneumonia, bronchitis, asthma.

Skin and Appendages System: Pruritus, skin disease, alopecia.

Special Senses: Amblyopia, abnormal vision, tinnitus, visual field abnormality, diplopia.

Urogenital System: Dysuria, hematuria.

Of the 551 ET patients, 10 were found to have renal abnormalities. Six of the 10 experienced renal failure (approximately 1%) while on anagrelide treatment. In two, the renal failure was considered to be possibly related to anagrelide treatment.. The remaining 4 were found to have pre-existing renal impairment and were successfully treated with anagrelide. Doses ranged from 1.5-6.0 mg/day with exposure periods of 2 to 12 months. Serum creatinine remained within normal limits and no dose adjustment was required because of renal insufficiency.

OVERDOSAGE:

Acute Toxicity and Symptoms: Single oral doses of anagrelide hydrochloride of 2500, 1500 and 200 mg/kg in mice, rats and monkeys, respectively, were not lethal. Symptoms of acute toxicity were: decreased motor activity in mice and rats and softened stools and decreased appetite in monkeys. There are no reports of overdosage with anagrelide hydrochloride. Platelet reduction from anagrelide therapy is dose-related: theratore, thrombocythemia which can potentially cause bleeding, is expected from overdosage. Should overdosage occur, cardiac, and central nervous system toxicity can also be expected.

Management and Treatment: In case of overdosage, close clinical supervision of the patient is required: this especially includes monitoring of the platelet could for thrombocythemia. Dosage should be decreased or stopped, as appropriate, until the platelet count returns to within the normal range.

DOSAGE AND ADMINISTRATION:

Treatment with anagrelide HCl capsules should be initiated under close medical supervision. The recommended starting dosage of anagrelide HCl is 0.5 mg 4 times daily or 1 mg twice daily, which should be maintained for at least one week. Dosage should then be adjusted to the lowest effective dosage required to reduce and maintain platelet count below 600,000/mcl and ideally to the normal range. The dosage should be increased by not more than 0.5 mg/day in any one week. Dosage should not exceed 10 mg/day or 2.5 mg in a single dose (see PRECAUTIONS). The decision to treat asymptomatic young adults with essential for thrombocythemia should be individualized.

To monitor the effect of anagrelide and prevent the occurrence of thrombocytopenia, platelet counts should be performed every two days during the first week of treatment and at least weekly thereafter until the maintenance dosage is reached.

Typically, platelet count begins to respond with 7 to 14 days at the proper dosage. Most patients will experience an adequate response at a dose of 1.5 to 3.0 mg/day. Patients with known or suspected heart disease, renal insufficiency, or hepatic dysfunction should be monitored closely.

PATIENT INFORMATION:

Anagrelide is used to reduce elevated platelet counts and reduce the risk of thrombosis.

Inform your physician if you have any kidney, liver or heart conditions.

Inform your doctor if you are pregnant or nursing.

Inform your doctor if you are taking any other medications.

May cause headache, palpitations, diarrhea, weakness or water retention.

May be taken with or without food.

HOW SUPPLIED:

Agrylin is available as 0.5 mg, opaque white capsules imprinted "ROBERTS 063" in black ink. 1 mg, opaque, gray capsules imprinted "ROBERTS 064" in black ink.

Store from 15° to 25°C (59° to 77°F), in a light-resistant container.

ANASTROZOLE *(003272)*

CATEGORIES: Antineoplastics; Breast Carcinoma; Cancer; Chemotherapy; Oncologic Drugs; Tumors

BRAND NAMES: **Arimidex**

DESCRIPTION:

Anastrozole tablets for oral administration contain 1 mg of anastrozole, a non-steroidal aromatase inhibitor. It is chemically described as 1,3-Benzenediacentonitrile, α, α, α', α'-tetramethyl -5-(1H-1,2,4-triazol -1-ylmethyl). Its molecular formula is $C_{17}H_{19}N_5$.

Anastrozole is an off-white powder with a molecular weight of 293.4. Anastrozole has moderate aqueous solubility (0.5 mg/mL at 25°C), solubility is independent of pH in the physiological range. Anastrozole is freely soluble in methanol, acetone, ethanol, and tetrahydrofuran, and very soluble in acetonitrite.

Inactive Ingredients: lactose, magnesium stearate, hydroxypropylmethylcellulose, polyethylene glycol, povidone, sodium starch glycolate, and titanium dioxide.

CLINICAL PHARMACOLOGY:

MECHANISM OF ACTION

Many breast cancers have estrogen receptors and growth of these tumors can be stimulated by estrogens. In post-menopausal women, the principle source of circulating estrogen (primarily estradiol) is conversion of adrenally-generated androstenedione to estrone by aromatase in peripheral tissues, such as adipose tissue, with further conversion of estrone to estradiol. Many breast cancers also contain aromatase; the importance of tumor-generated estrogens is uncertain.

Treatment of breast cancer has included efforts to decrease estrogen levels by ovariectomy premenopausally and by use of anti-estrogens and progestational agents both pre- and post-menopausally, these interventions lead to decreased tumor mass or delayed progression of tumor growth in some women.

Anastrozole is a potent and selective non-steroidal aromatase inhibitor. It significantly lowers serum estradiol concentrations and has no detectable effect on formation of adrenal corticosteroids or aldosterone.

PHARMACOKINETICS

Inhibition of aromatase activity is primarily due to anastrozole, the parent drug. Studies with radiolabeled drug have demonstrated that orally administered anastrozole is well absorbed into the systemic circulation with 83 to 85% of the radiolabel recovered in the urine and feces. Food does affect the extent of absorption. elimination of anastrazole is primarily via hepatic metabolism (approximately 85% and to a lesser extent, renal excretion (approximately 11%), and anastrozole has a mean terminal elimination half-life of approximately 50 hours in post menopausal women. The major circulating metabolite of anastrozole, triazole, lacks pharmacologic activity. The pharmacokinetic parameters are similar in patients and in healthy post-menopausal volunteers. The pharmacokinetics of anastrozole are linear over the dose range of 1 to 20 mg and do not change with repeated dosing. Consistent with the approximately 2-day terminal elimination half-life, plasma concentrations approach steady-state levels at about 7 days of once daily dosing and steady-state levels are approximately three-to-four-fold higher than levels observed after a single dose of anastrozole. Anastrozole is 40% bound to plasma proteins in the therapeutic range.

Metabolism and Excretion: Studies in post-menopausal women demonstrated that anastrozole is extensively metabolized with about 10% of the dose excreted in the urine as unchanged drug within 72 hours of dosing, and the remainder (about 60% of the dose) excreted in the urine as metabolites. Metabolism of anastrozole occurs by N-dealkylation, hydroxylation and glucuronidation. Three metabolites of anastrozole have been identified in human plasma and urine. The known metabolites are triazole, a glucuronide conjugate of hydroxy-anastrozole, and a glucuronide of anastrozole itself. Several minor (less than 5% of the radioactive dose) metabolites have not been identified.

Because renal elimination is not a significant pathway of elimination, total body clearance of anastrozole is unchanged even in severe (creatinine clearance less then 30 mL/min/1.73m²) renal impairment; dosing adjustment in patients with renal dsyfunction is not necessary (see Special Populations and DOSAGE AND ADMINISTRATION sections). Dosage adjustment is also unnecessary in patients with stable hepatic cirrhosis (see Special Populations and DOSAGE AND ADMINISTRATION sections).

SPECIAL POPULATIONS

Geriatric: Anastrozole pharmacokinetics have been investigated in post-menopausal female volunteers and patients with breast cancer. No age related effects were seen over the range <50 to >80 years.

Race: Anastrozole pharmacokinetic differences due to race have not been studied.

Renal insufficiency: Anastrozole pharmacokinetics have been investigated in subjects with renal insufficiency. Anastrozole renal clearance decreased proportionally with creatinine clearance and was approximately 50% lower in volunteers with severe renal impairment (creatinine clearance less than 30 mL/min/1.73m²) compared to controls. Since only about 10% of anastrozole is excreted unchanged in the urine, the reduction in renal clearance did not influence the total body clearance (see DOSAGE AND ADMINISTRATION).

Hepatic insufficiency: Hepatic metabolism accounts for approximately 85% of anastrozole elimination. Anastrozole pharmacokinetics have been investigated in subjects with hepatic cirrhosis related to alcohol abuse. The apparent oral clearance (CL/F) of anastrozole was approximately 30% lower in subjects with stable hepatic cirrhosis than in control subjects with normal liver function. However plasma anastrozole concentrations in the subjects with hepatic cirrhosis were within the range of concentrations seen in normal subjects across all clinical trials (see DOSAGE AND ADMINISTRATION), so that no dosage adjustment is needed.

PHARMACODYNAMICS

Effect on Estradiol: Mean serum concentrations of estradiol were evaluated in multiple daily dosing trials with 0.5, 1, 3, 5 and 10 mg of anastrozole in post-menopausal women with advanced breast cancer. Clinically significant suppression of serum estradiol was seen with all doses. Doses of 1 mg and higher resulted in suppression of the mean serum concentrations of estradiol to the lower limit of detection (3.7 pmol/L). The recommended daily dose, 1 mg, reduced estradiol by approximately 70% within 24 hours and by approximately 80% after 14 days of daily dosing. Suppression of serum estradiol was maintained for up to 6 days after cessation of daily dosing with 1 mg of anastrozole.

Effect on Corticosteroids: In multiple daily dosing trials with 3, 5, and 10 mg, the selectivity of anastrozole was assessed by examining effects on corticosteroid synthesis. For all doses, anastrozole did not effect cortisol or aldosterone secretion at baseline or in response to ACTH. No glucocorticoid or mineralicorticoid replacement therapy is necessary with anastrozole.

Other Endocrine Effects: In multiple daily dosing trials with 5 and 10 mg, thyroid stimulation hormone (TSH) was measured; there was no increase in TSH during the administration of anastrozole. Anastrozole does not possess direct progestogenic, androgenic, or estrogenic activity in animals, but does perturb the circulating levels of progesterone, androgens, and estrogens

CLINICAL STUDIES:

Anastrozole was studied in two well-controlled clinical trials (0004, a North American study; 0005, a predominantly European study) in post-menopausal women with advanced breast cancer who had disease progression following tamoxifen therapy for either advanced or early breast cancer. Some of the patients had also received previous cytotoxic treatment. Most patients were ER positive; a small fraction were either ER unknown or ER negative (the ER negative patients were eligible only if they had had a positive response to tamoxifen). Eligible patients with measurable and non-measurable disease were randomized to receive either a single daily dose of 1 mg or 10 mg of anastrozole or megestrol acetate 40 mg four times a day. The studies were double-blinded with respect to anastrozole. Time to progression and objective response (only patients with measurable disease could be considered partial responders) rates were the primary efficacy variables. Objective response rates were calculated based on the Union Internationale Contre le Cancer (UICC) criteria. The rate of prolonged (more than 24 weeks) stable disease, the rate of progression, and survival were also calculated.

CLINICAL STUDIES: *(cont'd)*

Both trials included over 375 patients; demographics and other baseline characteristics were similar for the three treatment groups in each trial. Patients in the 0005 trial had responded better to prior tamoxifen treatment. Of the patients who entered who had prior tamoxifen therapy for advanced disease (58 % in Trial 0004; 57 % in Trial 0005), 18% of these patients in Trial 0004 and 42% in Trial 0005 were reported by the primary investigator to have responded. In Trial 0004, 81% of patients were ER positive, 13% were ER unknown, and 6% were ER negative. In Trial 0005, 58% of patients were ER positive, 37% were ER unknown, and 5% were ER negative. In Trial 0004, 60% of patients had measurable disease compared to 80% in Trial 0005. The sites of metastatic disease were similar among treatment groups for each trails. On average, 40% of the patients had soft tissue metastases, 60% had bone metastases, and 40% had visceral (15% liver) metastases.

As shown in TABLE 1, similar results were observed among treatment groups and between the two trials. None of the within-trial differences were statistically significant.

TABLE 1

	Anastrozole 1 mg	Anastrozole 10 mg	Megestrol Acetate 160 mg
Trial 0004 (N. America)	(n=128)	(n=130)	(n=128)
Median Follow-up (days)	179	182	176
Time to Progression (days)	170	143	151
Objective Response (all patients) (%)	10.2	5.4	5.5
Stable Disease for >24 weeks (%)	26.6	23.8	29.7
Progression (%)	48.4	50.0	51.6
Trial 0005 (Europe, Australia, S. Africa)	(n=135)	(n=118)	(n=125)
Median Follow-up (days)	192	185	182
Time to Progression (days)	132	156	120
Objective Response (all patients) (%)	10.4	12.7	10.4
Stable Disease for >24 weeks (%)	23.7	21.2	22.4
Progression (%)	58.5	50.8	56.0

Approximately 1/3 of the patients in each treatment group in both studies had either an objective response or stabilization of their disease for greater than 24 weeks. Among the 263 patients who received anastrozole 1 mg, there were 6 complete responders and 21 partial responders. In patients who had an objective response, over 60% of the patients responded for greater than 6 months and over 15% responded for greater than 12 months.

To compare the three treatments, hazard ratios for the time to progression (ratio of the likelihood of progression for two treatments over the period of study) and odds ratios for response rates, together with their confidence intervals, were calculated for the pooled studies. These show that in general the three treatments were similar in efficacy, but that confidence intervals were fairly wide. There is, in these data, no indication that anastrozole 10 mg is superior to anastrozole 1 mg. For time to progression for the anastrozole 1 mg comparison to megestrol acetate, the hazard ratio (anastrozole/megestrol acetate) was 0.97 [0.75, 1.24] (p=0.76); for anastrozole 10 mg compared to megestrol acetate, the hazard ratio was 0.93 [0.71, 1.19] (p=0.47). The odds ratio and confidence intervals of the comparison between each dose of anastrozole and megestrol acetate for objective response rate demonstrate that both anastrozole 1 mg and anastrozole 10 mg were similar in efficacy to the comparator. For the anastrozole 1 mg comparison to megestrol acetate, the odds ratio (anastrozole/megestrol acetate) was 1.32 [0.66, 2.65] (p=0.37); for the anastrozole 10 mg comparison to megestrol acetate, the odds ratio was 1.15 [0.55, 2.36] (p=0.68). There were too few deaths occurring across treatment groups of both trials to draw conclusions on overall survival differences.

There were no differences in response seen between women over or under 65. There were too few non-white patients studied to draw conclusions about racial difference in response rates.

INDICATIONS AND USAGE:

Anastrozole is indicated for the treatment of advanced breast cancer in post-menopausal women with disease progression following tamoxifen therapy.

Patients with ER-negative disease and patients who did not respond to previous tamoxifen therapy rarely responded to anastrozole.

CONTRAINDICATIONS:

None known.

WARNINGS:

Anastrozole can cause fetal harm when administered to a pregnant woman. Anastrozole has been found to cross the placenta following oral administration of 0.1 mg/kg in rats and rabbits (about 3/4 and 1.5 times the recommended human dose, respectively, on a mg/m^2 basis). Studies in both rats and rabbits at doses equal to or greater than 0.1 and 0.02 mg/kg/day, respectively (about 3/4 and 1/3, respectively, the recommended human dose on a mg/m^{2}basis), administered during a period of organogenesis showed that anastrozole increased pregnancy loss (increased pre- and/or post-implatation loss, increased resorption, and decreased numbers of live fetuses); effects were dose related in rats. Placental weights were significantly increased in rats at doses of 0.1 mg/kg/day or more.

Evidence of fetotoxicity, including delayed fetal development (i.e. incomplete ossification and depressed fetal body weights), was observed in rats administered doses of 1 mg/kg/day (which produced plasma anastrozole $C_{SSMAX}$and $AUC_{0\text{-}24\ hr}$that were 19 times and 9 times higher than the respective values found in healthy post-menopausal humans at the recommended dose). There was no evidence of teratogenicity in rats administered doses up to 1.0 mg/kg/day. In rabbits, anastrozole caused pregnancy failure at doses equal to or greater than 1.0 mg/kg/day (about 16 times the recommended human dose on a mg/m^2 basis); there was no evidence of teratogenicity in rabbits administered 0.2 mg/kg/day (about 3 times the recommended human dose on a mg/m^2 basis).

There are no adequate and well-controlled studies in pregnant women using anastrozole. If anastrozole is used during pregnancy or if the patient becomes pregnant while receiving this drug, the patient should be apprised of the potential hazard to the fetus or potential risk for loss of the pregnancy.

PRECAUTIONS:

GENERAL

Before starting treatment with anastrozole, pregnancy must be excluded (see WARNINGS).

Anastrozole should be administered under the supervision of a qualified physician experienced in the use of anticancer agents.

LABORATORY TESTS

Three-fold elevations of mean serum gamma glutamyl transferase (GT) levels have been observed among patients with liver metastases receiving anastrozole or megestrol acetate. These changes were likely related to the progression of liver metastases in these patients, although other contributing factors could not be ruled out.

CARCINOGENESIS

No long term studies have been conducted to assess the carcinogenic potential of anastrozole.

PRECAUTIONS: *(cont'd)*

MUTAGENESIS

Anastrozole has not been shown to be mutagenic in *in vitro* tests (Ames and E. coli bacterial tests, CHO-K1 gene mutation assay) or clastogenic either *in vivo* (chromosome aberrations in human lymphocytes) or in *in vitro* (micronucleus test in rats).

IMPAIRMENT OF FERTILITY

Studies to investigate the effect of anastrozole on fertility have not been conducted; however, chronic studies indicated hypertrophy of the ovaries and the presence of follicular cysts in rats administered doses equal to or greater than 1 mg/kg/day (which produced plasma anastrozole $C_{SSMAX}$and $AUC_{0\text{-}24\ hr}$that were 19 and 9 times higher than the respective values found in post-menopausal humans at the recommended dose). In addition, hyperplastic uteri were observed in chronic studies of female dogs administered doses equal to or greater than 1 mg/kg/day (which produced plasma anastrozole $C_{SSMAX}$and $AUC_{0\text{-}24\ hr}$ that were 22 times and 16 times higher than the respective values found in post-menopausal humans at the recommended dose). It is not known whether these effects on the reproductive organs of animals are associated with impaired fertility in humans.

Pregnancy Category D: (see WARNINGS).

Nursing Mothers It is not known if anastrozole is excreted in human milk. Because many drugs are excreted in human milk, caution should be exercised when anastrozole is administered to a nursing woman (see WARNINGS and PRECAUTIONS).

Pediatric Use The safety and efficacy of anastrozole in pediatric patients have not been established.

Geriatric Use Fifty percent of patients in studies 0004 and 0005 were 65 or older. Response rates and time to progression were similar for the over 65 and younger patients.

DRUG INTERACTIONS:

Anastrozole inhibited reactions catalyzed by cytochrome P450 1A2, 2C8/9, and 3A4 *in vitro* with Ki values which were approximately 30 times higher than the mean steady-state C_{max} values observed following a 1-mg daily dose. Anastrozole had no inhibitory effect on reactions catalyzed by cytochome P450 2A6 or 2D6 *in vitro.* Administration of a single 30mg/kg or multiple 10 mg/kg doses of anastrozole to subjects had no effect on the clearance of antipyrine or urinary recovery of antipyrine metabolites. Based on these *in vitro* and *in vivo* results, it is unlikely that co-administration of anastrozole 1 mg with other drugs will result in clinically significant inhibition of cytochrome P450 mediated metabolism.

Anastrozole inhibited *in vitro* metabolic reactions catalyzed by cytochromes P450 1A2, 2C8/9, and 3A4 but only at relatively high concentrations. Anastrozole did not inhibit P450 2A6 or the polymorphic P450 2D6 in human liver microsomes. Anastrozole did not alter the pharmacokinetics of antipyrine. Although there have been no formal interaction studies other than with antipyrine, based on these *in vivo* and *in vitro* studies, it is unlikely that co-administration of a 1-mg dose of anastrozole with other drugs will result in clinically significant drug inhibition of cytochrome P450-mediated metabolism of the other drugs.

DRUG/LABORATORY TEST INTERACTIONS

No clinically significant changes in the results of clinical laboratory tests have been observed.

ADVERSE REACTIONS:

Anastrozole was generally well tolerated in two well-controlled clinical trials (*i.e.,* Trials 0004 and 0005), with less than 3.3% of the anastrozole-treated patients and 4.0% of the megestrol acetate-treated patients withdrawing due to adverse event.

The principle adverse event more common with anastrozole than megestrol acetate was diarrhea. Adverse events reported in greater than 5% of the patients in any of the treatment groups in these two well-controlled clinical trials, regardless of causality, are presented in TABLE 2.

TABLE 2 Number (n) and Percentage of Patients with Adverse Event ‡

	Anastrozole 1 mg (n=262)		Anastrozole 10 mg (n=246)		Megestrol Acetate 160 mg (n=253)	
Adverse Event	n	%	n	%	n	%
Asthenia	42	(16.0)	33	(13.4)	47	(18.6)
Nausea	41	(15.6)	48	(19.5)	28	(11.1)
Headache	34	(13.0)	44	(17.9)	24	(9.5)
Hot Flushes	32	(12.2)	29	(10.6)	21	(8.3)
Pain	28	(10.7)	38	(15.4)	29	(11.5)
Back Pain	28	(10.7)	26	(10.6)	19	(7.5)
Dyspnea	24	(9.2)	27	(11.0)	53	(20.9)
Vomiting	24	(9.2)	26	(10.6)	16	(6.3)
Cough Increased	22	(8.4)	18	(7.3)	19	(7.5)
Diarrhea	22	(8.4)	18	(7.3)	7	(2.8)
Constipation	18	(6.9)	18	(7.3)	21	(8.3)
Abdominal Pain	18	(6.9)	14	(5.7)	18	(7.1)
Anorexia	18	(6.9)	19	(7.7)	11	(4.3)
Bone Pain	17	(6.5)	26	(11.8)	19	(7.5)
Pharyngitis	16	(6.1)	23	(9.3)	15	(5.9)
Dizziness	16	(6.1)	12	(4.9)	15	(5.9)
Rash	15	(5.7)	15	(6.1)	19	(7.5)
Dry Mouth	15	(5.7)	11	(4.5)	13	(5.1)
Peripheral Edema	14	(5.3)	21	(8.5)	28	(11.1)
Pelvic Pain	14	(5.3)	17	(6.9)	13	(5.1)
Depression	14	(5.3)	6	(2.4)	5	(2.0)
Chest Pain	13	(5.0)	18	(7.3)	13	(5.1)
Paresthesia	12	(4.6)	15	(6.1)	9	(3.6)
Vaginal Hemorrhage	6	(2.3)	4	(1.6)	13	(5.1)
Weight Gain	4	(1.5)	9	(3.7)	30	(11.9)
Sweating	4	(1.5)	3	(1.2)	16	(6.3)
Increased Appetite	0	(0)	1	(0.4)	13	(5.1)

‡ A patient may have more than one adverse event.

Other less frequent (2% to 5%) adverse experiences reported in patients receiving anastrozole 1 mg in either Trial 0004 or Trial 0005 are listed below. These adverse experiences are listed by body system and are in order of decreasing frequency within each body system regardless of assessed causality.

Body as a Whole: Flu syndrome; fever; neck pain; malaise; accidental injury; infection

Cardiovascular: Hypertension; thrombophlebitis

Hepatic: Gamma GT increased; SGOT increased; SGPT increased

Hematologic: Anemia; leukopenia

Metabolic and Nutritional: Alkaline phosphatase increased; weight loss; Mean serum total cholesterol levels increased by 0.5 mmol/L among patients receiving anastrozole. Increases in LDL cholesterol have been shown to contribute to these changes.

Musculoskeletal: Myalgia; arthralgia; pathological fracture

Nervous: Somnolence; confusion; insomnia; anxiety; nervousness

ADVERSE REACTIONS: *(cont'd)*

Respiratory: Sinusitis; bronchitis; rhinitis

Skin and Appendages: Hair thinning; pruritus

Urogenital: Urinary tract infection; breast pain

The incidences of the following adverse event groups, potentially causally related to one or both of the therapies because of their pharmacology, were statistically analyzed: weight gain, edema, thromboembolic disease, gastrointestinal disturbance, hot flushes, and vaginal dryness. These six groups, and the adverse events captured in the groups, were prospectively defined. The results are shown in TABLE 3.

TABLE 3 Number (n) and Percentage of Patients

Adverse Event Group	Anastrazole 1 mg (n=262) n	%	Anastrazole 10 mg (n=246) n	%	Megestrol Acetate 160 mg (n=253) n	%
Gastrointestinal Disturbance	77	(29.4)	81	(32.9)	54	(21.3)
Hot Flushes	33	(12.6)	29	(11.8)	35	(13.8)
Edema	19	(7.3)	28	(11.4)	35	(13.8)
Thromboembolic Disease	9	(3.4)	4	(1.6)	12	(4.7)
Vaginal Dryness	5	(1.9)	3	(1.2)	2	(0.8)
Weight Gain	4	(1.5)	10	(4.1)	30	(11.9)

More patients treated with megestrol acetate reported weight gain as an adverse event compared to patients treated with anastrozole 1 mg ($p<0.0001$). Other differences were not statistically significant.

An examination of the magnitude of change in weight in all patients was also conducted. Thirty-four percent (87/253) of the patients treated with megestrol acetate experienced weight gain of 5% or more and 11% (27/253) of the patients treated with megestrol acetate experienced weight gain of 10% or more. Among patients treated with anastrozole 1 mg, 13% (33/262) experienced weight gain of 5% or more and 3% (6/262) experienced weight gain of 10% or more. On average, this 5 to 10% weight gain represented between 6 and 12 pounds.

No patients receiving anastrozole or megestrol acetate discontinued treatment due to drug-related weight gain.

OVERDOSAGE:

Clinical trial have been conducted with anastrozole, up to 60 mg in a single dose given to healthy male volunteers and up to 10 mg daily given to post-menopausal women with advanced breast cancer; these dosages were well tolerated. A single dose of anastrozole that results in life threatening symptoms has not been established. In rats, lethality was observed after single oral doses that were greater than 100 mg/kg (about 800 times the recommended human dose on a mg/m^2 basis) and was associated with severe irritation to the stomach (necrosis, gastritis, ulceration, and hemorrhage).

There is no specific antidote to overdosage and treatment must by symptomatic. In the management of an overdose, consider that multiple agents may haven been taken. Vomiting may be induced if patient is alert. Dialysis may be helpful because anastrozole is not highly protein bound. General supportive care, including frequent monitoring of vital signs and close observation of the patient, is indicated.

DOSAGE AND ADMINISTRATION:

The dose of anastrozole is one 1 mg tablet taken once a day.

Patients treated with anastrozole do not require glucocorticoid or mineralocorticoid replacement therapy.

Patients with Hepatic Impairment: (See CLINICAL PHARMACOLOGY) Hepatic metabolism accounts for approximately 85% of anastrozole elimination. Although clearance of anastrozole was decreased in patients with cirrhosis due to alcohol abuse, plasma anastrozole concentraions stayed in the usual range seen in patients without liver disease. Therefore, no changes in dose are recommended for patients with mild-to-moderate hepatic impairment, although patients should be monitored for side effects. Anastrozole has not been studied in patients with severe hepatic impairment.

Patients with Renal Impairment: No changes in dose are necessary for patients with renal impairment.

PATIENT INFORMATION:

Anastrozole is used for the treatment of advanced breast cancer. Do not use if you are pregnant. Inform your doctor if you are nursing. Take once daily on an empty stomach. May cause weakness, nausea and stomach upset, headache, hot flashes, and back pain. Inform your doctor or pharmacist if these effects occur.

HOW SUPPLIED:

ARIMIDEX

White, biconvex, film coated tablets containing 1 mg of anastrozole. The tablets are impressed on one side with a logo consisting of a letter"A" (upper case) with an arrowhead attached to the foot of the extended right leg of the "A" and on the reverse with the tablet strength marking "Adx 1".

Store at controlled room temperature, 20°-25°C (68°-77°F)

HOW SUPPLIED - EQUIVALENTS NOT AVAILABLE:

Tablet, Coated - Oral - 1 mg

30's $180.00 ARIMIDEX, Zeneca Pharms 00310-0201-30

ANISINDIONE *(000249)*

CATEGORIES: Anticoagulants; Anticoagulants/Thrombolytics; Atrial Fibrillation; Blood Formation/Coagulation; Coagulants and Anticoagulants; Coronary Occlusion; Embolism; Fibrillation; Pulmonary Embolism; Thrombosis; Pregnancy Category X; FDA Approval Pre 1982

BRAND NAMES: **Miradon**

DESCRIPTION:

Miradon Tablets contain a synthetic anticoagulant, anisindione, an indanedione derivative. Each tablet contains 50 mg anisindione.

They also contain: corn starch, FD&C Red No. 3, gelatin, lactose and hydrogenated vegetable oil.

CLINICAL PHARMACOLOGY:

Like phenindione, to which it is related chemically, anisindione exercises its therapeutic action by reducing the prothrombin activity of the blood.

INDICATIONS AND USAGE:

Anisindione is indicated for the prophylaxis & treatment of venous thrombosis and its extension, the treatment of atrial fibrillation with embolization, the prophylaxis and treatment of pulmonary embolism, and as an adjunct in the treatment of coronary occlusion.

CONTRAINDICATIONS:

All contraindications to oral anticoagulant therapy are relative rather than absolute. Contraindications should be evaluated for each patient, giving consideration to the need for and the benefits to be achieved by anticoagulant therapy, the potential dangers of hemorrhage, the expected duration of therapy, and the quality of patient monitoring and compliance.

Hemorrhagic Tendencies or Blood Dyscrasias: In general, oral anticoagulants are contraindicated in patients who are bleeding or who have hemorrhagic blood dyscrasias or hemorrhagic tendencies (*e.g.,* hemophilia, polycythemia vera, purpura, leukemia) or a history of bleeding diathesis. They are contraindicated in patients with recent cerebral hemorrhage, active ulceration of the gastrointestinal tract, including ulcerative colitis, or open ulcerative, traumatic, or surgical wounds. Oral anticoagulants may be contraindicated in patients with recent or contemplated brain, eye, or spinal cord surgery or prostatectomy, and in those undergoing regional or lumbar block anesthesia or continuous tube drainage of the small intestine. Oral anticoagulants may be contraindicated in patients who have severe renal or hepatic disease, subacute bacterial endocarditis, pericarditis, polyarthritis, diverticulitis, visceral carcinoma, or aneurysm. Other conditions in which the oral anticoagulants may be contraindicated include severe or malignant hypertension, eclampsia or preeclampsia, threatened abortion, emaciation, malnutrition, and vitamin C or K deficiencies. Since a high degree of patient cooperation is required for the outpatient use of oral anticoagulants, a lack of such cooperation is a relative contraindication to their use.

Pregnancy: Anisindione is contraindicated in pregnancy because the drug crosses the placental barrier. Oral anticoagulants may cause fetal damage when administered to pregnant women. Fetal or neonatal hemorrhage and intrauterine fetal death have occurred even when maternal prothrombin times were within the therapeutically accepted range. Maternal use of warfarin and anisindione during the first trimester of pregnancy has been reported to cause hypoplastic nasal structures, or other signs of the Conradi-Hunermann syndrome in the offspring. These patients received other drugs in addition to anticoagulants and a positive causal relationship has not been established. If oral anticoagulants must be used during pregnancy, or if the patient becomes pregnant while taking one of these drugs, the patient should be apprised of the potential hazard to the fetus. The possibility of termination of the pregnancy should be considered in light of these risks.

As an alternative to the use of oral anticoagulants in pregnant patients, the use of heparin, which does not cross the placenta, should be considered.

WARNINGS:

Anisindione should be reserved for patients who cannot tolerate the coumarins.

Oral anticoagulants are potent drugs with prolonged and cumulative effects. Treatment must be individualized according to patient response, and the benefit expected from anticoagulant therapy should be weighed against the possible hazards associated with the use of these drugs.

Oral anticoagulants should not be used in the treatment of acute completed strokes due to the risk of fatal cerebral hemorrhage (See INDICATIONS AND USAGE.)

Because agranulocytosis and hepatitis have been associated with the use of anisindione, liver function and blood studies should be performed periodically. Patients should be instructed to report to the physician symptoms such as marked fatigue, chills, fever, or sore throat; the drug should be discontinued promptly since these symptoms may signal the onset of severe toxicity. If leukopenia or evidence of hypersensitivity occurs, the drug should be discontinued. Because of the possibility of renal damage associated with the use of phenindione, the urine should be tested periodically for albumin whenever phenindione or any indanedione anticoagulant is used.

Relatively minor bleeding episodes and hemorrhage occur in 2 to 10% of patients treated with oral anticoagulants. Bleeding will vary in intensity, and may be related to the quality of patient monitoring, compliance on the part of the patient, the incidence of potentially hemorrhagic lesions or the extent of anticoagulation induced. Severe and moderate hypertension, severe to moderate hepatic and renal insufficiency, and infectious diseases or disturbances of intestinal flora as in sprue, or with antibiotic therapy may increase the risks associated with anticoagulant therapy.

Occasionally, fatal hemorrhages can occur. Massive hemorrhage from organ systems may involve cerebral, pericardial, pulmonary, adrenal, hepatic, spinal, gastrointestinal, or genitourinary sites. Gastrointestinal hemorrhage may be secondary to peptic ulceration or silent neoplasm and is responsible for 25% of all deaths due to oral anticoagulant therapy. Bleeding complications in the genitourinary tract may range in severity from microscopic hematuria to gross hematuria to extensive uterine hemorrhage.

Hemorrhagic necrosis and/or gangrene of the skin and subcutaneous tissue, petechial and purpuric hemorrhage, ecchymosis, epistaxis, hematemesis, or hemoptysis, may also occur. Hemorrhage and necrosis have in some cases been reported to result in death or permanent disability. Necrosis appears to be associated with local thrombosis and usually appears within a few days of the start of anticoagulant therapy. In severe cases of necrosis, treatment through debridement or amputation of the affected tissue, limb, breast or penis has been reported. Careful diagnosis is required to determine whether necrosis is caused by an underlying disease. Miradon therapy should be discontinued when anisindione is suspected to be the cause of developing necrosis and heparin therapy may be considered for anticoagulation. Although various treatments have been attempted, no treatment for necrosis has been considered uniformly effective. The risks of anticoagulant therapy may be increased in patients with known or suspected hereditary, familial or clinical deficiency in protein C. This condition, which should be suspected if there is a history of recurrent episodes of thromboembolic disorders in the patient or in the family, has been associated with an increased risk of developing necrosis following warfarin administration, and may be expected following anisindione therapy. Skin necrosis may occur in the absence of protein C deficiency. It has been reported that initiation of anticoagulation therapy with heparin for 4 to 5 days before initiation of therapy with anisindione may minimize the incidence of this reaction. Miradon therapy should be discontinued when it is suspected to be the cause of developing necrosis and heparin therapy may be considered for anticoagulation.

Concurrent use of anticoagulants with streptokinase, urokinase, or alteplase (recombinant) is not recommended and may be hazardous.

(Consult the product information accompanying those preparations).

Abrupt cessation of anticoagulant therapy is not generally recommended; if possible, taper the dose gradually over 3 to 4 weeks.

PRECAUTIONS:

General: Periodic determination of prothrombin time or other suitable coagulation test is essential. The availability of suitable laboratory facilities to monitor therapy accurately with oral anticoagulants is mandatory, both to assure adequate anticoagulation and to avoid toxicity due to overdosage. The dosage of oral anticoagulants depends on the clinical response as monitored by prothrombin time determinations (see DOSAGE AND ADMINISTRATION.) Since heparin prolongs the one-stage prothrombin time, a period of at least 5 hours should elapse after the last intravenous dose and after the last subcutaneous dose of heparin before drawing blood to determine the prothrombin time when heparin and anisindione have been given together. In addition to adequate laboratory facilities, a supply of oral or parenteral phytonadione (vitamin K_1) and a source of whole blood or plasma should be available when emergency treatment of acute overdosage is required (see OVERDOSAGE.)

A number of factors including environmental, mental, medical and nutritional states may affect an individual's response to anticoagulant therapy. Factors which increase sensitivity to the drug and lengthen prothrombin time include: initial hypoprothrombinemia, increased age, poor nutritional status, vitamin K deficiency or malabsorption, congestive heart failure, or vascular damage, hepatic disorders including hepatitis or obstructive jaundice, biliary fistula, febrile states, hyperthyroidism, preparatory bowel sterilization, recent surgery, and x-ray therapy.

Factors which may decrease the response to oral anticoagulants and shorten the prothrombin time include: pregnancy, diabetes mellitus, hyperlipidemia, hypothyroidism, hypercholesterolemia, and hereditary or acquired resistance.

Information for the Patient: The physician should instruct patients to:

Follow carefully the physician's directions for taking this drug and not to alter these directions without his authorization.

Follow carefully the physician's directions for the periodic blood test (prothrombin time) required to assure that the correct dose of the drug is being used.

Discuss with the physician any other medication (prescription or non-prescription) to be used.

Report to the physician any abnormal bleeding, such as blood in the urine, blood in the stool (a black, tarry appearance), bleeding from the gums or nose, patches of discoloration or bruises on the arms, legs, or toes, or excessive bleeding following minor cuts (*e.g.,* while shaving).

Discuss with the physician any plan to become pregnant or to report any pregnancy promptly.

Laboratory Tests: The need for careful control of the degree of anticoagulation, as determined by changes in prothrombin activity, cannot be overemphasized. It should be noted, however, that bleeding during anticoagulant therapy may not always correlate with prothrombin activity.

In long-term therapy with anticoagulants, periodic laboratory evaluation of organ systems, including hematopoietic, renal, and hepatic studies, should be performed (See WARNINGS.)

Drug/Laboratory Test Interferences: Dicumarol and indanedione anticoagulants, including anisindione, or their metabolites may color alkaline urine red-orange, which may interfere with spectrophotometrically determined urinary laboratory tests. The color reverses when the test sample is acidified *in vitro* to a pH below 4.

Carcinogenesis, Mutagenesis, and Impairment of Fertility: Long-term dosing studies to determine the carcinogenic potential of oral anticoagulants, including anisindione, have not been done. Information on mutagenesis is unknown.

Pregnancy, Teratogenic Effects, Pregnancy Category X: (see CONTRAINDICATIONS.)

Labor and Delivery: Anisindione is contraindicated in pregnancy. If oral anticoagulants are used in pregnant women, they should not be administered during the first trimester, and should be discontinued prior to labor and delivery.

Some clinicians suggest the replacement of oral anticoagulants with heparin therapy before term. Heparin is withheld during early labor and reinstituted 6 hours postpartum. After 5 to 7 days, therapy with oral anticoagulants, may be resumed if indicated.

See CONTRAINDICATIONS for the use of oral anticoagulants in pregnancy.

Nursing Mothers: Oral anticoagulants or their metabolites are excreted in the milk of nursing mothers, possibly in amounts sufficient to cause a prothrombopenic state and bleeding in the newborn. As a general rule, nursing should not be undertaken while a patient is receiving an oral anticoagulant.

Pediatric Use: The use of oral anticoagulants in children is not well documented. However, they may be beneficial in children with rare thromboembolic disorder secondary to other disease states such as the nephrotic syndrome or congenital heart lesions. Heparin is probably the initial anticoagulant of choice because of its immediate onset of action.

DRUG INTERACTIONS:

Addition or deletion of any drug from the therapeutic regimen of patients receiving oral anticoagulants may affect patient response to the anticoagulant. Frequent determination of prothrombin time and close monitoring of the patient is essential to ascertain when adjustment of dosage of anticoagulant may be needed.

Because of the variability of individual patient response, multiple interacting mechanisms with some drugs, the dependency of the extent of the interaction on the dosage and duration of therapy and the possible administration of several interacting drugs simultaneously, it is difficult to predict the direction and degree of the ultimate effect of concomitant medications on anticoagulant response. For example, since cholestyramine may reduce the gastrointestinal absorption of both the oral anticoagulants and vitamin K, the net effects are unpredictable. Chloral hydrate may cause an increased prothrombin response by displacing the anticoagulant from protein binding sites or a diminished prothrombin response through increased metabolism of the unbound drug by hepatic enzyme induction, thus leading to inter-patient variation in ultimate prothrombin effect. An interacting drug which leads to a decrease in prothrombin time necessitating an increased dose of oral anticoagulant to maintain an adequate degree of anticoagulation may, if abruptly discontinued, increase the risk of subsequent bleeding.

Drugs that have been reported to diminish oral anticoagulant response, i.e., decreased prothrombin time response, in man significantly include: adrenocortical steroids; alcohol*; antacids; antihistamines; barbiturates; carbamazepine; chloral hydrate*; chlordiazepoxide; cholestyramine; diet high in vitamin K; diuretics*; ethchlorvynol; glutethimide; griseofulvin; haloperidol; meprobamate; oral contraceptives; paraldehyde; primidone; ranitidine*, rifampin; unreliable prothrombin time determinations; vitamin C; warfarin sodium underdosage.

Drugs that reportedly may increase oral anticoagulant response, i.e., increased prothrombin response, in man include: alcohol*; allopurinol; aminosalicylic acid; amiodarone; anabolic steroids; antibiotics; bromelains; chloral hydrate*; chlorpropamide; chymotrypsin; cimetidine; cinchophen; clofibrate; dextran; dextrothyroxine; diazoxide; dietary deficiencies; diflunisal; diuretics*; disulfiram; drugs affecting blood elements; ethacrynic acid; fenoprofen; glucagon; hepatotoxic drugs; ibuprofen; indomethacin; influenza virus vaccine; inhalation anesthetics; mefenamic acid; methyldopa; methylphenidate; metronidazole; miconazole; monoamine oxidase inhibitors; nalidixic acid; naproxen; oxolinic acid; oxyphenbutazone; pentoxifylline; phenylbutazone; phenyramidol; phenytoin; prolonged hot weather; prolonged narcotics; pyrazolones; quinidine; quinine; ranitidine*; salicylates; sulfinpyrazone; sulfonamides, long acting; sulindac; thyroid drugs; tolbutamide; triclofos sodium; trimethoprim/sulfamethoxazole; unreliable prothrombin time determinations; warfarin sodium overdosage.

Oral anticoagulants may potentiate the hypoglycemic action of hypoglycemic agents, e.g., tolbutamide and chlorpropamide, by inhibiting their metabolism in the liver. Because oral anticoagulants may interfere with the hepatic metabolism of phenytoin, toxic levels of the anticonvulsant may occur when an oral anticoagulant and phenytoin are administered concurrently.

Drugs that reduce the number of blood platelets by causing bone marrow depression (such as antineoplastic agents) or drugs which inhibit platelet function (*e.g.,* aspirin and other nonsteroidal anti-inflammatory drugs, dipyridamole, hydrochloroquine, clofibrate, dextran) may increase the bleeding tendency produced by anticoagulants without altering prothrombin time determinations. The beneficial effects on arterial thrombus formation from combined therapy with anti-platelet and anticoagulant medication must be weighed against an increased risk of inducing hemorrhage.

* Increased and decreased prothrombin time responses have been reported.

ADVERSE REACTIONS:

Multisystem adverse reactions have been reported, and some may be serious enough to warrant hospital admission. In general, they may be divided into 2 categories: those which involve abnormal bleeding and other effects which do not. Hemorrhage and/or necrosis are among the hazards of treatment with any anticoagulant and are the main serious complications of therapy. For additional discussion of possible hemorrhagic complications following oral anticoagulant therapy see WARNINGS. Although most of the adverse reactions for oral anticoagulant drugs have been reported for warfarin, dicumarol, and phenindione, all the drugs within this class have similar pharmacologic and clinical properties, and require the same degree of caution in monitoring adverse reactions regardless of the drug administered.

Some indanediones (phenindione) have been associated with undesirable reactions which have not been reported with the coumarins and are not counterbalanced by advantages, thus perhaps favoring the use of the coumarin-type anticoagulants. Changing from one chemical type of oral anticoagulant to the other may eliminate an adverse reaction, such as rash or diarrhea.

Dermatitis is the only untoward reaction consistently associated with anisindione therapy.

Adverse reactions reported following therapy with either coumarin or indanedione anticoagulants include: nausea, diarrhea, pyrexia, dermatitis or exfoliative dermatitis, urticaria, alopecia, and sore mouth or mouth ulcers.

Side effects which have additionally been reported for coumarin derivatives include: vomiting, abdominal cramps, anorexia, priapism, erythemia, and necrosis of the skin and other tissues, manifesting as purple toes and cutaneous gangrene. There is no reason to expect that some or all of these adverse reactions might not occur in patients receiving anisindione.

Additional side effects attributed to the indanedione anticoagulants include: headache, sore throat, blurred vision, paralysis of accommodation, steatorrhea, hepatitis, jaundice, liver damage, renal tubular necrosis, albuminuria, anuria, myeloid immaturity, agranulocytosis, leukocyte agglutinins, red cell aplasia, atypical mononuclear cells, leukopenia, leukocytosis, anemia, thrombocytopenia, and eosinophilia.

Phenprocoumon-induced delayed callus formation following bone fracture have recently been reported.

OVERDOSAGE:

Vitamin K_1 is a specific antidote for anticoagulants, such as anisindione, which reduce prothrombin activity in the blood. Vitamin K_1 may be administered orally or by injection, if the patient is not bleeding or if bleeding is slight. A few hours after administration of vitamin K_1 preparations, such as phytonadione, prothrombin activity increases and clotting time decreases. In the presence of more active hemorrhage, however, transfusions of whole blood or plasma are required until the desired level of prothrombin activity is achieved. Treatment with vitamin K_1 preparations is only adjunctive in such cases.

DOSAGE AND ADMINISTRATION:

InitialDosage: Miradon Tablets, 300 mg the first day, 200 mg the second day, and 100 mg the third day. With initiation of treatment, prothrombin activity decreases rapidly to 50 percent of baseline values within six hours; thereafter, it decreases slowly until it reaches 15 to 30 percent of baseline values in 48 to 72 hours. *Maintenance Dosage:* is established from daily prothrombin-time determinations for each patient, although with Miradon Tablets, the uniform, predictable action of the drug makes it possible to reduce the frequency of prothrombin-time determinations in some cases. Maintenance dosage will vary between 25 to 250 mg a day and should be set to keep the prothrombin time two to two and one-half times the normal value. The dose may be repeated for many days; anisindione does not accumulate in the body.

Prothrombin activity returns to normal within 24 to 72 hours after treatment with the drug is discontinued. Some studies suggest that gradual reduction of dosage over a two-week period may decrease the frequency of recurrence of thromboembolic disease by preventing a rapid rise in prothrombin activity.

HOW SUPPLIED:

Miradon Tablets, 50 mg, pink, scored, compressed tablets are impressed with the Schering trademark and product identification letters, ANK, or numbers 795.

HOW SUPPLIED - EQUIVALENTS NOT AVAILABLE:

Tablet, Uncoated - Oral - 50 mg

100's $39.87 MIRADON, Schering 00085-0795-05

ANISTREPLASE, ANISOYLATED PSAC *(000252)*

CATEGORIES: Biologicals; Blood Formation/Coagulation; Blood Derivatives; Cardiovascular Drugs; Myocardial Infarction; Myocardial Infarction Prophylaxis; Thrombolytic Agents; Thrombosis; Pregnancy Category C; FDA Approved 1990 Jun

BRAND NAMES: **Eminase**; *Iminase*
(International brand names outside U.S. in italics)

COST OF THERAPY: $2,438.75 (Myocardial Infarction; Injection; 30 unit; 1/day; 1 days)

DESCRIPTION:

Eminase (anistreplase) is the p-anisoylated derivative of the Lys-Plasminogen- Streptokinase activator complex prepared *in vitro* by acylating human plasma-derived, purified, heat-treated, Lys-Plasminogen and purified Streptokinase from group C β-hemolytic streptococci.

DESCRIPTION: *(cont'd)*

Anistreplase, Anisoylated Psac has a molecular weight of about 131,000. Each vial of Anistreplase, Anisoylated Psac is supplied as a sterile, lyophilized, white to off-white powder containing 30 units of Anistreplase, <3 mg dimethylsulfoxide, <0.2 mg sodium hydroxide and the following buffers and stabilizers: 150 mcg p-amidinophenyl-p'-anisate (acylating agent), 100 mg mannitol, 46 mg L-lysine, 30 mg Albumin (Human), <2 mg glycerol, and 1.3 mg epsilon-aminocaproic acid. Anistreplase, Anisoylated Psac is intended only for intravenous (IV) injection after reconstitution with Sterile Water for Injection, USP. The preparation contains no preservatives and is intended to be used as a single dose. Potency is expressed in units of Anistreplase by using a reference standard which is specific for Anistreplase, Anisoylated Psac and is not comparable with units used for other fibrinolytics.

The Lys-Plasminogen and the Streptokinase used in the manufacture of Eminase are prepared under U.S. license by Oesterreichisches Institute fuer Haemoderivate GmbH and Behringwerke AG, respectively, under shared manufacturing arrangements.

CLINICAL PHARMACOLOGY:

Anistreplase, Anisoylated Psac is an inactive derivative of a fibrinolytic enzyme with the catalytic center of the activator complex temporarily blocked by an anisoyl group. The anisoyl group does not decrease the high fibrin-binding ability of the complex. Anistreplase, Anisoylated Psac is made *in vitro* from Lys-Plasminogen and Streptokinase. Anistreplase, Anisoylated Psac differs from the complex initially formed *in vivo* upon administration of Streptokinase; the latter complex contains predominately gluplasminogen. Activation of Eminase occurs with release of the anisoyl group by deacylation, a non-enzymatic first-order process with a half-life *in vitro* in human blood of about 2 hours. In solution, deacylation of Anistreplase, Anisoylated Psac starts immediately and the enzymatically active Lys-Plasminogen-Streptokinase activator complex is progressively formed. The production of plasmin from plasminogen by deacylated Anistreplase, Anisoylated Psac can take place in the bloodstream or within the thrombus; the latter process is catalytically more efficient but both may contribute to thrombolysis. The half-life of fibrinolytic activity of the circulating Anistreplase, Anisoylated Psac is 70 to 120 minutes (mean 94 minutes).

A number of controlled clinical studies have been performed with Anistreplase, Anisoylated Psac to demonstrate benefit. Heparin anticoagulation was administered to all patients routinely following (about 4 to 6 hours) dosing with Anistreplase, Anisoylated Psac.

Randomized, controlled studies have demonstrated that Anistreplase, Anisoylated Psac reduces mortality when administered within 6 hours of the onset of the symptoms of acute myocardial infarction (AMI). The benefit of mortality reduction occurs acutely and is maintained for at least one year.

In a study of 1258 patients (AIMS trial), mortality at 30 days postinfarction was decreased (47.2%, p = 0.0001) in patients receiving Anistreplase, Anisoylated Psac as compared with placebo. At one year, the reduction in mortality was maintained (38%, p = 0.001). The incidence of heart failure was less in patients treated with Anistreplase, Anisoylated Psac (17.9%) compared with patients who received placebo (23.3%).[1,2] Similar mortality results were obtained from a smaller, randomized, controlled trial.[1,3]

In a double-blind, randomized trial of Anistreplase, Anisoylated Psac compared with heparin bolus, left ventricular function was improved and infarction size reduced. There was significantly (p <0.01, two sample t-test) higher left ventricular ejection fraction (LVEF) for the Eminase treatment group (53%) compared with the heparin treatment group (47.5%) when measured 4 days after treatment (intent-to-treat analysis). This difference was maintained when patients were reexamined by radionuclide ventriculography at day 19, even when patients who experienced successful angioplasty were excluded from the analysis (p = 0.04). About 3 weeks after treatment, mean infarct size was 24% lower in the patients treated with Anistreplase, Anisoylated Psac compared with those treated with heparin (n = 188, p = 0.02).[1,4] Similarly, if those patients who experienced successful angioplasty were excluded from the analysis, the mean infarct size in patients treated with Anistreplase, Anisoylated Psac was significantly less than that of heparin-treated patients (p <0.01).

In randomized, comparative studies reperfusion rates of between 50% and 68% have been reported in patients receiving Anistreplase, Anisoylated Psac within 6 hours of symptom onset. However, for maximum rates of reperfusion, treatment should be initiated as soon as possible after onset of symptoms.

In two studies,[1,5,6] Anistreplase, Anisoylated Psac and intracoronary (IC) Streptokinase were compared in patients with angiographically proven coronary artery occlusion. Reperfusion occurred about 45 minutes after the start of therapy for both treatment groups. When therapy was initiated within 4 hours of onset of AMI symptoms reperfusion rates of 59% (n = 87) and 68% (n = 41) were observed for Anistreplase, Anisoylated Psac compared with 59% (n = 85) and 70% (n = 43) for IC Streptokinase. Of those patients who had coronary artery reperfusion, angiographically demonstrated reocclusion occurred within 24 hours in 3% to 4% of those treated with Anistreplase, Anisoylated Psac and in 7% to 12% of those treated with Streptokinase.[1,5,6]

In a well-controlled, randomized study, a patency rate of 72% was obtained with Anistreplase, Anisoylated Psac compared with 53% for IV Streptokinase. Patency for the 107 patients was determined by posttreatment angiography.[1,7]

Anistreplase, Anisoylated Psac was also found to have a favorable risk/benefit profile in elderly patients (>65 years, n = 940) who participated in clinical trials. Use of Anistreplase, Anisoylated Psac in patients over 75 years old has not been adequately studied.

INDICATIONS AND USAGE:

Anistreplase, Anisoylated Psac is indicated for use in the management of acute myocardial infarction (AMI) in adults, for the lysis of thrombi obstructing coronary arteries, the reduction of infarct size, the improvement of ventricular function following AMI, and the reduction of mortality associated with AMI. Treatment should be initiated as soon as possible after the onset of AMI symptoms (see CLINICAL PHARMACOLOGY.)

CONTRAINDICATIONS:

Because thrombolytic therapy increases the risk of bleeding, Anistreplase, Anisoylated Psac is contraindicated in the following situations:

active internal bleeding

history of cerebrovascular accident

recent (within 2 months) intracranial or intraspinal surgery or trauma (see WARNINGS)

intracranial neoplasm, arteriovenous malformation, or aneurysm

known bleeding diathesis

severe, uncontrolled hypertension

Anistreplase, Anisoylated Psac should not be administered to patients having experienced severe allergic reactions to either this product or Streptokinase.

WARNINGS:

Bleeding: See ADVERSE REACTIONS. The most common complication associated with Anistreplase, Anisoylated Psac therapy is bleeding. The types of bleeding associated with thrombolytic therapy can be divided into two broad categories:

WARNINGS: *(cont'd)*

1. Internal bleeding involving the gastrointestinal tract, genitourinary tract, retroperitoneal, ocular, or intracranial sites.

2. Superficial or surface bleeding, observed mainly at invaded or disturbed sites (*e.g.,* venous cutdowns, arterial punctures, sites of recent surgical intervention).

The concomitant use of heparin anticoagulation may contribute to the bleeding. Some of the hemorrhagic episodes occurred one or more days after the effects of Anistreplase, Anisoylated Psac had dissipated, but while heparin therapy was continuing.

As fibrin is lysed during Anistreplase, Anisoylated Psac therapy, bleeding from recent puncture sites may occur. Therefore, thrombolytic therapy requires careful attention to all potential bleeding sites (including catheter insertion sites, arterial and venous puncture sites, cutdown sites, and needle puncture sites).

Intramuscular injections and nonessential handling of the patient should be avoided during treatment with Anistreplase, Anisoylated Psac. Venipunctures should be performed carefully and only as required.

Should an arterial puncture be necessary following administration of Anistreplase, Anisoylated Psac, it is preferable to use an upper-extremity vessel that is accessible to manual compression. A pressure dressing should be applied, and the puncture site should be checked frequently for evidence of bleeding.

Each patient being considered for therapy with Anistreplase, Anisoylated Psac should be carefully evaluated and anticipated benefits should be weighed against potential risks associated with therapy.

In the following conditions, the risks of Anistreplase, Anisoylated Psac therapy may be increased and should be weighed against the anticipated benefits:

recent (within 10 days) major surgery (*e.g.,* coronary artery bypass graft, obstetrical delivery, organ biopsy, previous puncture of noncompressible vessels)

cerebrovascular disease

recent gastrointestinal or genitourinary bleeding (within 10 days)

recent trauma (within 10 days) including cardiopulmonary resuscitation

hypertension: systolic BP ≥ 180 mmHg and/or diastolic BP ≥ 110 mmHg

high likelihood of left heart thrombus (*e.g.,* mitral stenosis with atrial fibrillation)

subacute bacterial endocarditis

acute pericarditis

hemostatic defects including those secondary to severe hepatic or renal disease

pregnancy

age > 75 years (Use of Anistreplase, Anisoylated Psac in patients over 75 years old has not been adequately studied.)

diabetic hemorrhagic retinopathy or other hemorrhagic ophthalmic conditions

septic thrombophlebitis or occluded AV cannula at seriously infected site

patients currently receiving oral anticoagulants (*e.g.,* warfarin sodium)

any other condition in which bleeding constitutes a significant hazard or would be particularly difficult to manage because of its location

ARRHYTHMIAS

Coronary thrombolysis may result in arrhythmias associated with reperfusion. These arrhythmias (such as sinus bradycardia, accelerated idioventricular rhythm, ventricular premature depolarizations, ventricular tachycardia) are not different from those often seen in the ordinary course of acute myocardial infarction and may be managed with standard antiarrhythmic measures. It is recommended that antiarrhythmic therapy for bradycardia and/or ventricular irritability be available when injections of Anistreplase, Anisoylated Psa are administered.

HYPOTENSION

Hypotension, sometimes severe, not secondary to bleeding or anaphylaxis, has occasionally been observed soon after intravenous Anistreplase, Anisoylated Psac administration. Patients should be monitored closely and, should symptomatic or alarming hypotension occur, appropriate symptomatic treatment should be administered.

PRECAUTIONS:

GENERAL

Standard management of myocardial infarction should be implemented concomitantly with Anistreplase, Anisoylated Psac treatment. Invasive procedures should be minimized (see WARNINGS.) Anaphylactoid reactions have rarely been reported in patients who received Anistreplase, Anisoylated Psac. Accordingly, adequate treatment provisions such as epinephrine should be available for immediate use.

READMINISTRATION

Because of the increased likelihood of resistance due to antistreptokinase antibody, Anistreplase, Anisoylated Psac may not be effective if administered more than 5 days after prior Anistreplase, Anisoylated Psac or Streptokinase therapy, particularly between 5 days and 12 months. Increased antistreptokinase antibody levels after Anistreplase, Anisoylated Psac or Streptokinase may also increase the risk of allergic reactions following readministration.

Repeated administration of Anistreplase, Anisoylated Psac within one week of the initial dose has occurred in a small number of patients treated for AMI and non-AMI conditions. The incidence of hematomas/bruising was somewhat greater in those patients who received repeat doses of Anistreplase, Anisoylated Psac but otherwise the adverse event profile was similar to those who received one dose.

LABORATORY TESTS

Intravenous administration of Anistreplase, Anisoylated Psac will cause marked decreases in plasminogen and fibrinogen and increases in thrombin time (TT), activated partial thromboplastin time (APTT), and prothrombin time (PT).

Results of coagulation tests and/or measures of fibrinolytic activity performed during Anistreplase, Anisoylated Psac therapy may be unreliable unless specific precautions are taken to prevent *in vitro* artifacts. Anistreplase, Anisoylated Psac, when present in blood in pharmacologic concentrations, remains active under *in vitro* conditions. This can lead to degradation of fibrinogen in blood samples removed for analysis. Collection of blood samples in the presence of aprotinin (2000 to 3000 KIU/ml) can, to some extent, mitigate this phenomenon.

CARCINOGENESIS, MUTAGENESIS, AND IMPAIRMENT OF FERTILITY

Long-term studies in animals have not been performed to evaluate the carcinogenic potential or the effect on fertility. Studies to determine mutagenicity and chromosomal aberration assays in human lymphocytes were negative at all concentrations tested.

PREGNANCY CATEGORY C

Animal reproduction studies have not been conducted with Anistreplase, Anisoylated Psac. It is also not known whether Anistreplase, Anisoylated Psac can cause fetal harm when administered to a pregnant woman or can affect reproduction capacity. Anistreplase, Anisoylated Psac should be given to a pregnant woman only if clearly needed.

PRECAUTIONS: *(cont'd)*

NURSING MOTHERS

It is not known whether Anistreplase, Anisoylated Psac is excreted in human milk. Because many drugs are excreted in human milk, the physician should decide whether the patient should discontinue nursing or not receive Anistreplase, Anisoylated Psac.

PEDIATRIC USE

Safety and effectiveness of Anistreplase, Anisoylated Psac in children have not been established.

DRUG INTERACTIONS:

The interaction of Anistreplase, Anisoylated Psac with other cardioactive drugs has not been studied. In addition to bleeding associated with heparin and vitamin K antagonists, drugs that alter platelet function (such as aspirin and dipyridamole) may increase the risk of bleeding if administered prior to Anistreplase, Anisoylated Psac therapy.

USE OF ANTICOAGULANTS

Anistreplase, Anisoylated Psac alone or in combination with antiplatelet agents and anticoagulants may cause bleeding complications. Therefore, careful monitoring is advised, especially at arterial puncture sites. In clinical studies, a majority of patients treated received anticoagulant therapy postdosing with Anistreplase, Anisoylated Psac during their hospital stay and a minority received heparin pretreatment with Anistreplase, Anisoylated. The use of antiplatelet agents increased the incidence of bleeding events similarly in patients treated with Anistreplase, Anisoylated Psac or non-thrombolytic therapy. There was no evidence of a synergistic effect of combined Anistreplase, Anisoylated Psac and antiplatelet agents on bleeding events. In addition, there was no difference in the incidence of hemorrhagic CVAs in Anistreplase, Anisoylated Psac-treated patients who did or did not receive aspirin.

ADVERSE REACTIONS:

BLEEDING

The incidence of bleeding (major or minor) varied widely from study to study and may depend on the use of arterial catheterization and other invasive procedures, patient population, and/or concomitant therapy. The overall incidence of bleeding in patients treated with Anistreplase, Anisoylated Psac in clinical trials (n = 5275) was 14.6%, with nonpuncture-site bleeding occurring in 10.2%, and puncture-site bleeding occurring in 5.7%, of these patients. Bleeding at the puncture site occurred more frequently in clinical trials in which the patients underwent immediate coronary catheterization (13.3%, n = 637) compared with those who did not (3.0%, n= 2023). The incidence of presumed intracranial bleeding within 7 days postdosing with Anistreplase, Anisoylated Psac was 0.57% (n = 5275; 0.34% etiology confirmed hemorrhagic; 0.23% etiology not confirmed) compared to 0.16% (n = 1249) after nonthrombolytic therapy.

In the AIMS trial the overall incidence of bleeding in patients treated with Anistreplase, Anisoylated Psac was 14.8% compared with 3.8% for placebo. The incidence of specific bleeding events can be seen in TABLE 1.

TABLE 1 Anistreplase; Anisoylated, Adverse Reactions

Type of Bleeding	Anistreplase, Anisoylated Psac (n = 500)	Placebo (n = 501)
Puncture site	4.6%	<1%
Nonpuncture site hematoma	2.8%	<1%
Hematuria/Genitourinary	2.4%	<1%
Hemoptysis	2.2%	<1%
Gastrointestinal hemorrhage	2.0%	1.4%
Intracranial	1.0%	<1%
Gum/Mouth hemorrhage	1.0%	0
Epistaxis	<1%	<1%
Anemia	<1%	<1%
Eye hemorrhage	<1%	<1%
Hemorrhage (unspecified)	<1%	0

In this study there was no difference between Anistreplase, Anisoylated Psac and placebo in the incidence of major bleeding events.

Should serious bleeding (not controlled by local pressure) occur in a critical location (intracranial, gastrointestinal, retroperitoneal, pericardial), any concomitant heparin should be terminated immediately and the administration of protamine to reverse heparinization should be considered. If necessary, the bleeding tendency can be reversed with appropriate replacement therapy.

Minor bleeding can be anticipated mainly at invaded or disturbed sites. If such bleeding occurs, local measures should be taken to control the bleeding (see WARNINGS).

Cardiovascular: The most frequently reported adverse experiences in Anistreplase, Anisoylated Psac clinical trials (n = 5275) were arrhythmia/conduction disorders which were reported in 38% of patients treated with Anistreplase, Anisoylated Psac and 46% of nonthrombolytic control patients. Hypotension occurred in 10.4% of patients treated with Anistreplase, Anisoylated Psac compared to 7.9% for patients who received nonthrombolytic treatment (see WARNINGS).

Allergic-type Reactions: Anaphylactic and anaphylactoid reactions have been observed rarely (0.2%) in patients treated with Anistreplase, Anisoylated Psac and are similar in incidence to Streptokinase (0.1% anaphylactic shock in one study). These included symptoms such as bronchospasm or angioedema.

Other milder or delayed effects such as urticaria, itching, flushing, rashes and eosinophilia have been occasionally observed. A delayed purpuric rash appearing one to two weeks after treatment has been reported in 0.3% of patients. The rash may also be associated with arthralgia, ankle edema, gastrointestinal symptoms, mild hematuria and mild proteinuria. This syndrome was self-limiting and without long-term sequelae.

Risk of Viral Transmission: Six batches of Anistreplase, Anisoylated Psac (five different batches of Lys-Plasminogen) were used in clinical trials designed specifically to monitor possible hepatitis non-A, non-B transmission. No case of hepatitis was diagnosed in patients receiving Anistreplase, Anisoylated Psac. Lys-Plasminogen is derived from human plasma obtained from FDA approved sources and tested for absence of viral contamination, including human immunodeficiency virus type-1 (HIV-1) and hepatitis B surface antigen. The manufacturing process includes a vapor-heat treatment step for inactivation of viruses. The entire manufacturing process has also been validated to yield a cumulative reduction of $\geq 10^{21}$ fold HIV-1 infectious particles, i.e., $\geq 10^{6}$ infectious particles removed by vapor-heat treatment and a cumulative total of $\geq 10^{15}$ infectious particles removed by the various steps in the purification process.

Causal Relationship Unknown: Since the following experiences may also be associated with AMI or other therapy, the causal relationship to Anistreplase, Anisoylated Psac administration is unknown. The following adverse experiences were infrequently (<10%) reported in clinical trials:

Body as a Whole: chills, fever, headache, shock;

Cardiovascular: cardiac rupture, chest pain, emboli;

ADVERSE REACTIONS: *(cont'd)*

Dermatology: purpura, sweating;

Gastrointestinal: nausea and/or vomiting;

Hemic and Lymphatic: thrombocytopenia;

Metabolic and Nutritional: elevated transaminase levels;

Musculoskeletal: arthralgia;

Nervous: agitation, dizziness, paresthesia, tremor, vertigo;

Respiratory: dyspnea, lung edema.

DOSAGE AND ADMINISTRATION:

Administer Anistreplase, Anisoylated Psac as soon as possible after the onset of symptoms. The recommended dose is 30 units of Anistreplase, Anisoylated Psac administered only by intravenous injection over 2 to 5 minutes into an intravenous line or vein.

RECONSTITUTION

1. Slowly add 5 ml of Sterile Water for Injection, USP, by directing the stream of fluid against the side of the vial.
2. Gently roll the vial, mixing the dry powder and fluid. Do not shake. Try to minimize foaming.
3. The reconstituted preparation is a colorless to pale yellow transparent solution. Before administration, the product should be visually inspected for particulate matter and discoloration.
4. Withdraw the entire contents of the vial.
5. The reconstituted solution should not be further diluted before administration or added to any infusion fluids. No other medications should be added to the vial or syringe containing Anistreplase, Anisoylated Psac.
6. If Anistreplase, Anisoylated Psac is not administered within 30 minutes of reconstitution, it should be discarded.

REFERENCES:

1. Data on File. SmithKline Beecham Pharmaceuticals, Philadelphia. 2. AIMS Trial Study Group. Effect of intravenous APSAC on mortality after acute myocardial infarction: preliminary report of a placebo-controlled clinical trial. Lancet 1988: 1:545-9. 3. Meinertz T, Kasper W. Schumacher M, Just H for the APSAC multicenter trial group. The German multicenter trial of anisoylated plasminogen streptokinase activator complex versus heparin for acute myocardial infarction. Am J Cardiol 1988; 62:347-51. 4. Bassand JP, Machecourt J, Cassagnes J, et al. Multicenter trial of intravenous anisoylated plasminogen streptokinase activator complex (APSAC) in acute myocardial infarction: effects on infarct size and left ventricular function. J Am Coll Cardiol 1989; 13:988-97. 5. Anderson JL, Rothbard RL, Hackworthy RA, et al. Multicenter reperfusion trial of intravenous anisoylated plasminogen Streptokinase activator complex (APSAC) in acute myocardial infarction: controlled comparison with intracoronary streptokinase. J Am Coll Cardiol 1988; 11:1153-63. 6. Bonnier HJRM, Visser RF, Klomps HC, Hoffmann HJML and the Dutch Invasive Reperfusion Study Group. Comparison of intravenous anisoylated plasminogen streptokinase activator complex and intracoronary streptokinase in acute myocardial infarction. Am J Cardiol 1988; 62:25-30. 7. Brochie ML, Quilliet L, Kulbertus H, et al. Intravenous anisoylated plasminogen streptokinase activator complex versus intravenous streptokinase in evolving myocardial infarction: preliminary data from a randomized multicentre study. Drugs 1987, 33(Suppl 3):140-5.

HOW SUPPLIED:

Anistreplase, Anisoylated Psac is supplied as a sterile, lyophilized powder in 30-unit vials.

Storage: Store lyophilized Anistreplase, Anisoylated Psac between 2°-8°C (36°-46°F).

Do not use beyond the expiration date printed on the vial.

(SmithKline Beecham, 8/92, 21:95032)

HOW SUPPLIED - EQUIVALENTS NOT AVAILABLE:

Injection, Solution - Intravenous - 30 unit

1's $2438.75 EMINASE, Roberts Labs **57294-0030-20**

ANTAZOLINE PHOSPHATE; NAPHAZOLINE HYDROCHLORIDE *(000254)*

CATEGORIES: Allergies; Antihistamines; Conjunctivitis; EENT Drugs; Eye, Ear, Nose, & Throat Preparations; Ophthalmic Decongestants; Ophthalmics; Respiratory & Allergy Medications; Vasoconstrictors; Pregnancy Category C; FDA Approved 1990 Apr

BRAND NAMES: Ak-Vaso-A; Albalon-A; *Albalon-A Liquifilm* (Australia); *Alergoftal*; Allersol-A; Antazoline-V; *Midazol Ofteno*; *Oftalirio*; Storz-Naf-A; **Vasocon-A**
(International brand names outside U.S. in italics)

FORMULARIES: Aetna; BC-BS

DESCRIPTION:

Vasocon-A (antazoline phosphate/naphazoline hydrochloride) is a combination of an antihistamine and a vasoconstrictor prepared as a sterile solution for ophthalmic administration having the following composition:

Antazoline Phosphate: 5 mg/ml

Naphazoline Hydrochloride: 0.5 mg/ml

in a solution containing polyethylene glycol 8000, sodium chloride, polyvinyl alcohol, edetate disodium and purified water, preserved with benzalkonium chloride (0.1 mg/ml). Sodium hydroxide and/or hydrochloric acid added to adjust pH when necessary. It has a pH of 5.5-6.3 and a tonicity of 280-350 mOsm/kg.

The chemical name for naphazoline hydrochloride is 1 H-imidazole,4,5-dihydro-2-(1-naphthalenyl-methyl)-, monohydrochloride.

The chemical name for antazoline phosphate is 1 H-imidazole-2- methanamine,4,5-dihydro-N-phenyl-N-(phenylmethyl)-, phosphate(1:1).

CLINICAL PHARMACOLOGY:

Antazoline Phosphate;Naphazoline Hydrochloride combines the effects of the antihistamine, antazoline, and the vasoconstrictor, naphazoline. Naphazoline hydrochloride is an alpha-sympathetic receptor agonist (sympathomimetic) producing vasoconstriction. Antazoline phosphate is an H_1-receptor antagonist producing antihistaminic effects.

INDICATIONS AND USAGE:

Antazoline Phosphate;Naphazoline Hydrochloride Ophthalmic Solution is indicated for relief of signs and symptoms of allergic conjunctivitis.

CONTRAINDICATIONS:

Contraindicated in the presence of an anatomically narrow angle or in narrow angle glaucoma or in persons hypersensitive to one or more of the components of this preparation. Antazoline Phosphate;Naphazoline Hydrochloride is contraindicated while soft contact lenses are being worn.

WARNINGS:

Patients under therapy with monoamine oxidase (MAO) inhibitors may experience a severe hypertensive crisis if given a sympathomimetic drug. (See PRECAUTIONS.) Use of drugs in this pharmacologic class may cause CNS depression leading to unconsciousness and/or coma. Marked reduction in body temperature may occur in children, especially infants. Patients are advised not to wear contact lenses during treatment with Antazoline Phosphate;Naphazoline Hydrochloride.

PRECAUTIONS:

GENERAL

Use with caution in the presence of hypertension, cardiovascular abnormalities, hyperglycemia (diabetes), hyperthyroidism, ocular infection or injury and when other medications are being used.

INFORMATION FOR THE PATIENT

For topical use only. To prevent contaminating the dropper tip and solution, care should be taken not to touch the eyelids or surrounding areas with the dropper tip of the bottle. Keep bottle tightly closed when not in use. Protect from light. Do not use if the solution has darkened.

Patients should be advised to discontinue the drug and consult a physician if relief is not obtained within 48 hours of therapy; if irritation, blurring or redness persists or increases; or if symptoms of systemic absorption occur, i.e., dizziness, headache, nausea, decrease in body temperature or drowsiness.

Overuse of this product may produce increased redness/irritation of the eyes.

CARCINOGENESIS, MUTAGENESIS, AND IMPAIRMENT OF FERTILITY

There have been no long-term studies done using naphazoline and/or antazoline in animals to evaluate carcinogenic or mutagenic potential.

PREGNANCY CATEGORY C

Animal reproduction studies have not been conducted with naphazoline and/or antazoline. It is also not known whether naphazoline and/or antazoline can cause fetal harm when administered to a pregnant woman or can affect reproduction capacity. Antazoline Phosphate;Naphazoline Hydrochloride Ophthalmic Solution should be given to a pregnant woman only if clearly needed. There are no available data on the effect of the drug on later growth, development, and functional maturation of the child.

NURSING MOTHERS

It is not known whether naphazoline and/or antazoline are excreted in human milk. Because many drugs are excreted in human milk, caution should be exercised when these drugs are administered to a nursing woman.

PEDIATRIC USE

Safety and effectiveness in children have not been established. See WARNINGS.

DRUG INTERACTIONS:

Concurrent use of maprotiline or tricyclic antidepressants and naphazoline may potentiate the pressor effect of naphazoline. Patients under therapy with MAO inhibitors may experience a severe hypertensive crisis if given a sympathomimetic drug. See WARNINGS.

ADVERSE REACTIONS:

Ocular: The most frequent complaint with the use of Antazoline Phosphate;Naphazoline Hydrochloride Ophthalmic Solution is that of mild transient stinging/burning. Other adverse experiences that have been reported with naphazoline and/or antazoline include mydriasis, increased redness, irritation, blurring, punctate keratitis, lacrimation, increased intraocular pressure.

Systemic: Dizziness, headache, nausea, sweating, nervousness, drowsiness, weakness, hypertension, cardiac irregularities and hyperglycemia.

DOSAGE AND ADMINISTRATION:

Instill one to two drops in the conjunctival sac(s) every two hours as needed, but not to exceed four times per day.

HOW SUPPLIED:

Vasocon-A Ophthalmic Solution:

3 ml and 15 ml plastic dropper tip squeeze bottles.

Do not store above 25°C (77°F).

Keep bottle tightly closed when not in use. protect from light.

HOW SUPPLIED - EQUIVALENTS NOT AVAILABLE:

Solution - Ophthalmic; Top - 0.5 %/0.05 %

15 ml	$4.44	Naphazoline Hcl W/Antazoline, HL Moore Drug Exch	00839-7563-31
15 ml	$7.12	Naphazoline/Antazoline Phosphate, Geneva Pharms	00781-6221-85

ANTHRALIN *(000255)*

CATEGORIES: Dermatologicals; Keratolytic Agents; Pharmaceutical Adjuvants; Psoriasis; Skin/Mucous Membrane Agents; Topical; Pregnancy Category C; FDA Pre 1938 Drugs

BRAND NAMES: *Amitase*; **Anthra-Derm**; Anthra-Tex; *Anthraderm*; *Anthraforte*; *Anthraforte 1* (Canada); *Anthramed*; *Anthranol* (England, France, Mexico); *Anthranol 0.1* (Canada); *Anthranol 0.2* (Canada); *Anthranol 0.4* (Canada); *Anthrascalp* (Canada); *Antralina*; *Desmoline*; Dithranol; *Dithranol-Hermal* (Germany); *Dithrasis* (France); *Dithrocream* (England); *Ditrastick*; Dritho-Scalp; Drithocreme; *Filorose*; Lasan; *Psoradexan*; *Psoralon* (Germany)
(International brand names outside U.S. in italics)

FORMULARIES: Aetna; BC-BS; Medi-Cal; PCS; WHO

DESCRIPTION:

Each gram of Anthralin ointment 0.1%, 0.25%, 0.5% and 1.0% contains 1 mg, 2.5 mg, 5 mg and 10 mg, respectively, of anthralin in a base consisting of mineral oil and white petrolatum. Anthralin is an anti-psoriatic agent with cytostatic, irritant and weak antimicrobial properties.

CLINICAL PHARMACOLOGY:

Although the exact mechanism of Anthralin's activity is unknown, there is experimental evidence that Anthralin binds DNA, inhibiting synthesis of nucleic protein, and thus reduces mitotic activity.

Absorption in man has not been determined. However, based on a study in piglets, it would appear to be quite low.

INDICATIONS AND USAGE:

For the topical treatment of psoriasis.

CONTRAINDICATIONS:

Anthralin ointment is contraindicated in patients with acute psoriasis of where inflammation is present, and in those patients with a history of hypersensitivity to any of the ingredients.

WARNINGS:

Although no renal, hepatic or hematologic abnormalities have been reported as a result of topical application of Anthralin ointment caution is advised in patients with renal disease. Patients with renal disease and those having extensive and prolonged applications should have periodic urine tests for albuminuria. Discontinue use if sensitivity reactions occur.

PRECAUTIONS:

GENERAL

When redness is observed on adjacent normal skin, reduce frequency of application. For external use only. Do not apply to face, genitalia or intertriginous areas. Wash hands thoroughly and carefully after using. anthralin may stain skin, hair and fabric. Keep out of the reach of children. Anthralin is a tumor-promoting agent in two-stage carcinogenesis on mouse skin. However, there have not been any reports of such effects in humans at the usual dosages.

PREGNANCY

Category C Animal reproduction studies have not been conducted with Anthralin ointment. It is also not known whether Anthralin ointment can cause fetal harm when administered to a pregnant woman or can affect reproduction capacity. Anthralin should be given to a pregnant woman only if clearly needed.

NURSING MOTHERS

It is not known whether this drug is excreted in human milk. Because many drugs are excreted in milk and because of the potential for tumorigenicity shown for anthralin in animal studies, a decision should be made whether to discontinue nursing or to discontinue the drug, taking into account the importance of the drug to the mother.

PEDIATRIC USE

Safety and effectiveness in children have not been established.

ADVERSE REACTIONS:

Irritation of normal skin is the most frequently reported adverse reaction.

DOSAGE AND ADMINISTRATION:

The usual dosage regimen begins with the lowest concentration (0.1%) and is gradually increased until the desired effect is obtained. Apply in a thin layer to affected areas once or twice daily, or as directed by a physician.

HOW SUPPLIED - EQUIVALENTS NOT AVAILABLE:

Cream - Topical - 0.1 %

50 gm	$20.79	DRITHOCREME, Dermik Labs	00066-7200-50

Cream - Topical - 0.25 %

50 gm	$22.39	DRITHOCREME, Dermik Labs	00066-7201-50
50 gm	$23.19	DRITHO-SCALP, Dermik Labs	00066-7204-50

Cream - Topical - 0.5 %

50 gm	$25.01	DRITHOCREME, Dermik Labs	00066-7202-50
50 gm	$25.70	DRITHO-SCALP, Dermik Labs	00066-7205-50

Cream - Topical - 1 %

50 gm	$29.36	DRITHOCREME HP, Dermik Labs	00066-7203-50

Ointment - Topical - 0.1 %

45 gm	**$23.12**	**ANTHRA-DERM, Dermik Labs**	**00066-0010-15**

Ointment - Topical - 0.25 %

45 gm	**$23.12**	**ANTHRA-DERM, Dermik Labs**	**00066-0025-15**

Ointment - Topical - 0.5 %

45 gm	**$24.52**	**ANTHRA-DERM, Dermik Labs**	**00066-0050-15**

Ointment - Topical - 1 %

45 gm	**$24.95**	**ANTHRA-DERM, Dermik Labs**	**00066-0100-15**

Ointment - Topical - 4 %

60 gm	$12.94	LASAN, Stiefel Labs	00145-0950-04

Powder

25 gm	$45.50	Anthralin, Millgood	53118-0700-25
25 gm	$79.50	Anthralin, Paddock Labs	00574-0525-25

ANTI-INHIBITOR COAGULANT COMPLEX *(000258)*

CATEGORIES: Antihemophilic Factor; Bleeding; Blood Derivatives; Blood Formation/Coagulation; Coagulants and Anticoagulants; Factor VIII Deficiency; Hemophilia; Hemostatics; Pregnancy Category C; FDA Pre 1938 Drugs

BRAND NAMES: *Autoplex* (Japan); *Autoplex -T*; **Autoplex T**; *Feiba Inumno Tim 4*; *Feiba Tim 4*; Feiba-Vh
(International brand names outside U.S. in italics)

> **WARNING:**
> THIS PRODUCT IS TO BE USED ONLY IN PATIENTS WITH INHIBITORS TO FACTOR VIII.
> THIS IS A POTENT DRUG WITH POTENTIAL HAZARDS. FOR MAXIMAL SAFETY AND EFFICACY, CAREFULLY READ AND FOLLOW DIRECTIONS BELOW.

DESCRIPTION:

Anti-Inhibitor Coagulant Complex, Heat Treated, is a sterile product prepared from pooled human plasma with subsequent alcohol fractionation to Cohn Fraction IV1. It contains, in concentrated form, variable amounts of activated and precursor vitamin-K- dependent clotting factors. Factors of the kinin generating system are also present. The product is standardized by its ability to correct the clotting time of Factor VIII deficient plasma or Factor VIII deficient plasma which contains inhibitors to Factor VIII.

DESCRIPTION: *(cont'd)*

When reconstituted, this product contains a maximum of 2 units per ml of heparin and a residual amount of polyethylene glycol (2 mg per ml. maximum). It also contains 0.02 M sodium citrate and the sodium content is 177 ± 15 milliequivalents per liter.

Laboratory testing of several lots of Anti-Inhibitor Coagulant Complex, Heat treated, has shown the presence of Factor VIII coagulant antigen (VIII:Cag). Although anamnestic response to this antigen following administration of the product was not observed during the clinical trials, the possibility of such a response does exist.

Each lot of Anti-Inhibitor Coagulant Complex, Heat Treated, is assayed and labeled for units of Hyland Factor VIII correctional activity. Factor VIII correctional activity may not be exclusively related to the efficacious component(s). See CLINICAL PHARMACOLOGY.

During the manufacturing process, this product was heated for 6 days at 60°C. This heating step is designed to reduce the risk of transmission of hepatitis and other viral diseases. However, no procedure has been shown to be totally effective in removing hepatitis infectivity from Anti-Inhibitor Coagulant Complex.

Anti-Inhibitor Coagulant Complex, Heat Treated, MUST be administered intravenously.

CLINICAL PHARMACOLOGY:

The Factor VIII correctional activity of Anti-Inhibitor Coagulant complex, Heat treated, is thought to be, in part, related to the factor Xa content of the product. It is additionally hypothesized that the elevated Factor VII-VIIa content of this product is also a contributing factor in the *in vivo* reestablishment of normal hemostasis by way of Factor X activation in conjunction with tissue factor, phospholipid and ionic calcium.

Control of thrombin formation is regulated by (1) the presence of antithrombin III and other serine protease inhibitors which neutralize Factors IXa and Xa, (2) the short biological half-lives of factors VII and VIIa and (3) the presence of circulating Factor VIII inhibitor which additionally controls overactivation of the intrinsic coagulation system.

In work with human immunodeficiency virus (HIV), substantial reduction in viral content has been reported in a recent study of the effects of ethanol fractionation, the process by which Anti- Inhibitor Coagulant Complex, Heat Treated, is manufactured. Wells et al, report 1 to 4 log reduction in each fractionation step they examined.

The effectiveness of the 6-day heating step in reducing viral infectivity was assessed by *in vitro* viral inactivation studies, using as markers, viruses not commonly found in plasma. When known quantities of these viruses were added to the product, the heat treatment employed inactivated the following quantities of virus:

TABLE 1 Anti-Inhibitor Coagulant Complex, Clinical Pharmacology

Sindbis	10.0 Log10	(1.68 Log10/day)
Vesicular stomatitis	5.0 Log10	(0.84 Log10/day)
Herpes simplex	1.6 Log10	(0.26 Log10/day)
HIV	4.5 Log10	(2.00 Log10/day)

In separate experiments, HIV was also studied and these data are reported in TABLE 1.

A retrospective study conducted with patients receiving unheated Anti-Inhibitor Coagulant Complex, supports the effectiveness of the purification process in reducing viral burden in the product. In the study, none of the patients who received that product exclusively seroconverted for HIV antibodies, while 56% of those patients who received other treatment modalities seroconverted during the three year study.

INDICATIONS AND USAGE:

Anti-Inhibitor Coagulant Complex, Heat Treated, is indicated for use in patients with Factor VIII inhibitors who are bleeding or who are to undergo surgery. The intravenous administration of this preparation is intended to control bleeding episodes in such patients.

Approximately 10% of individuals with hemophilia A (classical hemophilia) have laboratory-measurable inhibitors to Factor VIII. For these patients, the treatment of choice depends upon the following factors: the severity of the bleeding episode, the existing level of inhibitor and whether the patient responds to infusion of Factor VIII with increasing antibody titers (anamnestic rise of Factor VIII antibody).

The following table is presented as a guide in determining the preferred therapy with respect to the use of Anti-Inhibitor Coagulant Complex or Antihemophilic Factor (Human) in patients with Factor VIII inhibitors. Inhibitor level categories are given along with the corresponding recommended product or products.

Other regimens have been proposed.

TABLE 2 Anti-Inhibitor Coagulant Complex

Historical Maximum Level of Factor VII Inhibitor	Present Level of Factor VIII Inhibitor		
	< 2 B.U.	2-10 B.U.	> 10 B.U.
< 2 B.U.	AHF	AICC or AHF	AICC
2 - 10 B.U.	AICC or AHF	AICC or AHF	AICC
> 10 B.U.	AICC	AICC	AICC

B.U. designates Bethesda Units.
AHF designates Antihemophilic Factor (Human).
AICC designates Anti-Inhibitor Coagulant Complex

Patients whose present Factor VIII inhibitor levels are greater than 10 Bethesda Units, as well as patients whose inhibitor levels are historically known to rise to greater than 10 Bethesda Units following treatment with Antihemophilic Factor (Human), should be treated with Anti-Inhibitor Coagulant Complex.

Patients whose present Factor VIII inhibitor levels are between 2 and 10 Bethesda Units and whose inhibitor levels are historically known to remain in this range following treatment with Antihemophilic Factor (Human) may be treated with either Antihemophilic Factor (Human) or Anti-Inhibitor Coagulant Complex, depending on the patient's clinical history and the severity of the bleeding episode.

Patients with Factor VIII inhibitor levels of less than 2 Bethesda Units and whose inhibitor levels are historically known to remain at 2 Bethesda Units or less following treatment with Antihemophilic Factor (Human) may be treated with appropriate doses of Antihemophilic Factor (Human).

For patients who have low levels of Factor VIII inhibitor and whose history does not include adequate laboratory indications of an anamnestic response to Antihemophilic Factor (human), the treatment of choice should be based on clinical judgement. In such patients who are having noncritical or minor bleeding episodes, the use of Anti-inhibitor Coagulant Complex, Heat Treated, will maintain the inhibitor at a low level and allow the use of other coagulant therapeutic agents in subsequent major emergencies.

CONTRAINDICATIONS:

The use of Anti-Inhibitor Coagulant Complex, Heat Treated, is contraindicated in patients with signs of fibrinolysis and in patients with disseminated intravascular coagulation (DIC).

WARNINGS:

This product is prepared from pooled units of human plasma which have been individually tested and found nonreactive for hepatitis B surface antigen and antibody to human immunodeficiency virus (HIV) by FDA approved tests. Other screening procedures are used to reduce the risk of transmitting viral infection. However, testing methods presently available are not sensitive enough to detect all units of potentially infectious plasma and treatment methods have not been shown to be totally effective in eliminating viral infectivity from this product.

Individuals who have not received multiple infusions of blood or plasma products are very likely to develop signs and/or symptoms of certain viral infections, especially non A, non B hepatitis as shown by recent data.

If the infusion of the concentrate occurs more than 1 hour following reconstitution, there may be increased prekallikrein activator (PKA) with consequent hypotension.

PRECAUTIONS:

GENERAL

IDENTIFICATION OF THE CLOTTING DEFICIENCY AS THAT CAUSED BY THE PRESENCE OF FACTOR VIII INHIBITORS IS ESSENTIAL BEFORE THE ADMINISTRATION OF ANTI-INHIBITOR COAGULANT COMPLEX, HEAT TREATED, IS INITIATED.

Signs and/or symptoms of hypotension may occur with this product. In these cases, stopping the infusion allows the symptoms to disappear. With all but the most reactive individuals, the infusion may be resumed at a slower rate.

If signs of intravascular coagulation occur, the infusion should be stopped and the patient monitored for DIC by the appropriate laboratory tests. Symptoms of DIC include changes in blood pressure and pulse rate, respiratory distress, chest pain and cough. Laboratory indications of DIC include prolonged thrombin time, prothrombin time and partial thromboplastin time tests. Other indications of DIC are decreased fibrinogen concentration, decreased platelet count and/or the presence of fibrin split products.

Special caution should be taken in the use of this concentrate in newborns, where a high morbidity and mortality may be associated with hepatitis, and in individuals with preexisting liver disease.

LABORATORY TESTS

In some cases, laboratory tests such as the activated partial thromboplastin time test may not correlate with clinical response, in that the appearance of hemostatic improvement may occur without a reduction of partial thromboplastin time. However, the prothrombin time would be expected to be shortened.

In children, fibrinogen levels should be determined prior to the initial infusion and monitored during the course of the treatment.

PREGNANCY CATEGORY C

Animal Reproduction studies have not been conducted with Anti-Inhibitor Coagulant Complex, Heat Treated. It is also not known whether Anti-Inhibitor Coagulant Complex, Heat Treated, can cause fetal harm when administered to a pregnant woman or can affect reproduction capacity. Anti-Inhibitor Coagulant Complex, Heat Treated, should be given to a pregnant woman only if clearly needed.

DRUG INTERACTIONS:

Since only limited data are available on the administration of highly activated prothrombin complex products together with antifibrinolytic agents such as epsilonaminocaproic acid (EACA) or tranexamic acid, the concomitant use of Anti-Inhibitor Coagulant Complex, Heat Treated, with such agents is not recommended.

ADVERSE REACTIONS:

As with other plasma preparations, reactions manifested by fever, chills, or indications of protein sensitivity may be observed with the administration of Anti-Inhibitor Coagulant Complex, Heat Treated. Signs and/or symptoms of high prekallikrein activity, such as changes in blood pressure or pulse rate may also be observed. It is advisable that appropriate medications be available for the treatment of acute allergic reactions or acute vasoactive reactions, should they occur.

A rate of infusion that is too rapid may cause headache, flushing, and changes in pulse rate and blood pressure. In such instances, stopping the infusion allows the symptoms to disappear promptly. With all but the most reactive individuals, infusion may be resumed at a slower rate.

DOSAGE AND ADMINISTRATION:

Each bottle of Anti-Inhibitor Coagulant Complex, Heat Treated, is labeled with number of Hyland Factor VIII Correctional Units that it contains. One Hyland Factor VIII Correctional Unit is that quantity of activated prothrombin complex which upon addition to an equal volume of Factor VIII deficient or inhibitor plasma, will correct the clotting time (ellagic acid-activated partial thromboplastin time) to 35 seconds (normal).

The recommended dosage range is 25 to 100 Hyland Factor VIII Correctional Units per kg of body weight, depending upon the severity of hemorrhage. If no hemostatic improvement is observed approximately 6 hours following the initial administration, the dosage should be repeated.

Subsequent dosage and administration intervals should be adjusted according to the patients clinical response. (See PRECAUTIONS, Laboratory Tests.)

RECONSTITUTION: USE ASEPTIC TECHNIQUE

1. Bring Anti-Inhibitor Coagulant Complex, Heat Treated, (dry concentrate) and Sterile Water for Injection, USP, (diluent) to room temperature.

2. Remove caps from concentrate and diluent bottles to expose central portions of rubber stoppers.

3. Cleanse stoppers with germicidal solution.

4. Remove protective covering from one end of the double-ended needle and insert exposed needle through DILUENT stopper.

5. Remove protective covering from other end of the double-ended needle. Invert diluent bottle over the upright concentrate bottle, the RAPIDLY insert free end of the needle through the concentrate bottle stopper at its center. Vacuum in the concentrate bottle will draw in diluent.

6. Disconnect the two bottles by removing needle from the diluent bottle, then remove needle from concentrate bottle stopper.

Swirl or rotate the concentrate bottle until all material is dissolved.

Parenteral drug products should be inspected visually for particulate matter and discoloration prior to administration, whenever solution and container permit.

DOSAGE AND ADMINISTRATION: *(cont'd)*

NOTE: DO NOT REFRIGERATE AFTER RECONSTITUTION.

RATE OF ADMINISTRATION

It is recommended that Anti-Inhibitor Coagulant Complex, Heat Treated, be infused initially at a rate of 2 ml/min. If infusion at this rate is well tolerated the administration rate may be gradually increased to 10 ml/min.

Administration: Use Aseptic Technique When reconstitution of Anti-Inhibitor Coagulant Complex, is complete, its infusion should commence as soon as practical; however, must be completed within 1 hour.

The reconstituted solution should be at room temperature during infusion.

A. Intravenous Drip Infusion: When a Hyland administration set is used, follow directions for use printed on the administration set container. When an administration set from another source is used, follow directions accompanying that set where necessary. The use of a Hyland administration set is recommended as it contains a suitable filter.

B. Intravenous Syringe Injection:

1. Attach filter needle to syringe and draw back plunger to admit air into the syringe.

2. Insert needle into the reconstituted Anti-Inhibitor Coagulant Complex, Heat Treated.

3. Inject air into bottle and withdraw the reconstituted material into the syringe.

4. Remove and discard the filter needle from the syringe; attach a suitable needle and inject intravenously as instructed under RATE OF ADMINISTRATION.

5. If patient is to receive more than one bottle of concentrate, the contents of two bottles may be drawn into the same syringe by drawing up each bottle through a separate unused filter needle. This practice lessens the loss of concentrate. Please note, filter needles are intended to filter the contents of a single bottle of Anti-Inhibitor Coagulant Complex only.

Storage: Anti-Inhibitor Coagulant Complex, Heat Treated, should be stored under ordinary refrigeration (2° to 8°C, 36° to 46°F). Avoid freezing to prevent damage to the diluent bottle.

HOW SUPPLIED - EQUIVALENTS NOT AVAILABLE:

Injection, Solution - Intravenous - 400 mg/800 unit

1's $1.30 FEIBA VH IMMUNO, Immuno-US 54129-0222-04

ANTIHEMOPHILIC FACTOR (HUMAN) *(000260)*

CATEGORIES: Blood Components/Substitutes; Blood Formation/Coagulation; Blood Derivatives; Coagulants and Anticoagulants; Hemophilia; Hemostatics; Pregnancy Category C; Sales >$100 Million; FDA Pre—1938 Drugs

BRAND NAMES: Alphanate; *Bayer Koate-HP*; *Beriate*; *Beriate hs*; *Beriate HS* (Germany); *Beriate-p*; Bioclate; *Cutter Koate-HP*; Factor VIII; *Haemate*; *Haemate HS* (Germany); *Haemate-P*; *Haemate P*; *Haemosolvate Factor VIII*; Helixate; Hemofil-M; *Hemofil M* (Germany); Humate-P; Hyate:C; Koate; *Koate-hp*; *Koate-HP*; **Koate-Hp**; *Koate HP* (Mexico); *Koate hs*; Kogenate; *Kryobulin*; *Kryobulin S-TIM3 Immuno*; *Kryobulin TIM 3*; Melate; *Monoclate-p*; *Monoclate-P*; *Nordiocto*; Nybcen; *Octa-VI*; *Octa V.I. 500*; *Octonativ-M*; Profilate; *Profilate OSD*; *Profilate SD*; *Ristofact* (Germany)
(International brand names outside U.S. in italics)

FORMULARIES: WHO

DESCRIPTION:

Antihemophilic factor (human), pasteurized (described here as AHF [Human]), is a stable, purified, sterile, lyophilized concentrate of AHF (human) (factor VIII, AHF) to be administered by the intravenous route in the treatment of patients with classic hemophilia (hemophilia A).

AHF (human) is purified from the cold insoluble fraction of pooled human fresh-frozen plasma and contains highly purified and concentrated antihemophilic factor (human). AHF (human) has a high degree of purity with a low amount of non–factor VIII proteins and contains no fibrinogen (as detected by the Clauss method). AHF (human) has a higher AHF potency than cryoprecipitate preparations. Each bottle of AHF (Human) contains the labeled amount of antihemophilic activity in international units. The Unit (IU) is defined by an international standard established by the World Health Organization: one AHF international unit is approximately equal to the level of AHF found in 1.0 ml of fresh-pooled human plasma.

Each 100 IU of AHF (human) contains 60 to 100 mg of glycine, 14 to 28 mg of sodium citrate, 8 to 16 mg of sodium chloride, 16 to 24 mg of albumin (human), 4 to 20 mg of other proteins, and 20 to 44 mg of total proteins.

This product is prepared from pooled human plasma collected in the United States. AHF (human) may also be prepared from source material supplied by other U.S. licensed manufacturers.

AHF (human), pasteurized, is pasteurized by a new procedure: heating to 60° C for 10 hours in aqueous solution form.[1] This procedure has been shown to inactivate several DNA viruses (cytomegalovirus, herpes, and hepatitis B) and RNA viruses (rubella, mumps, measles, and poliomyelitis). However, no procedure has been shown to be totally effective in removing hepatitis infectivity from antihemophilic factor (human). (SeeCLINICAL PHARMACOLOGYand WARNINGS).

AHF (human) contains anti-A and anti-B blood group isoagglutinins. (See PRECAUTIONS).

CLINICAL PHARMACOLOGY:

After IV injection in humans, there is a rapid increase in plasma AHF followed by a rapid decrease in activity (time of equilibration with the extravascular compartment) and a subsequent slower rate of decrease in activity (biological half-life). Studies with AHF (human) in hemophilic patients have demonstrated a mean initial half-disappearance time of 8 hours and a mean half-life of 12 hours.

Tests of infectivity on chimpanzees have confirmed the reliability of this pasteurization method in eliminating the risk of transmission of hepatitis B virus. Two chimpanzee studies were used to evaluate the efficacy of the pasteurization process in inactivating hepatitis B virus. In studies of 6 and 9 months' duration, cryoprecipitate was infected with hepatitis B virus to give a concentration of 3000 infectious units/ml. All chimpanzees injected with either cryoprecipitate or nonpasteurized AHF (human) developed hepatitis B markers (HBsAg, anti-Hbs, anti-Hbc). All chimpanzees injected with the pasteurized AHF (human) product consistently remained serologically negative.

The pasteurization process used in the manufacture of this product has demonstrated *in vitro* inactivation of a number of infectious agents, including HIV, Epstein-Barr virus, cytomegalovirus, herpes simplex virus, rubella virus, measles virus, mumps virus, and poliomyelitis virus. *In vivo* experiments have demonstrated inactivation of hepatitis B virus and at least one type of non-A, non-B hepatitis virus. Furthermore, clinical studies using this product have indicated an absence of transmission of HIV, hepatitis B virus, and non-A, non-B hepatitis.

CLINICAL PHARMACOLOGY: *(cont'd)*

Clinical evidence confirms the hepatitis B safety of the pasteurization procedure. Of the 34 patients who had serologic follow-up for hepatitis B markers, none had developed seroconversion of the antibodies, anti-Hbs or anti-Hbc caused by the administration of AHF (human), pasteurized[2].

A total of 24 lots of AHF (human) were administered to a cohort of 16 patients who had not previously received any blood products. The study showed no elevation in ALT levels over observation periods ranging from 2 months to 12 months.

In a retrospective study of 56 patients, all have remained negative for the presence of HIV-1 antibody for time periods ranging from 2 months to 5 years from initial administration of product.

INDICATIONS AND USAGE:

The usage of AHF (human) is indicated in hemophilia A (classic hemophilia) for the prevention and control of hemorrhagic episodes. AHF (human) is not indicated in von Willebrand's disease.

CONTRAINDICATIONS:

None known.

WARNINGS:

This product is prepared from pooled human plasma, which may contain the causative agents of hepatitis and other viral diseases. Prescribed manufacturing procedures utilized at the plasma collection centers, plasma testing laboratories, and fractionation facilities are designed to reduce the risk of transmitting viral infection. However, the risk of viral infectivity from this product cannot be totally eliminated. Accordingly, the benefits and risks of treatment with this concentrate should be carefully assessed prior to use.

Individuals who receive infusions of blood or plasma products may develop signs and/or symptoms of some viral infections, particularly non-A, non-B hepatitis.

PRECAUTIONS:

It is important to determine that the coagulation disorder is caused by factor VIII deficiency, since no benefit in treating other deficiencies can be expected.

This AHF (human), pasteurized, preparation contains blood group isoagglutinins (anti-A and anti-B). When large or frequently repeated doses are needed, as when inhibitors are present or when presurgical and postsurgical care is involved, patients of blood groups A, B, and AB should be monitored for signs of intravascular hemolysis and decreasing hematocrit values. In the event of severe hemolysis, type-specific cryoprecipitate can be given instead. Hemolytic anemia, when present, may be corrected by the administration of compatible group O red blood cells (human).

Other precautions are as follows:

The filter needle should be used only to transfer solution from the preparation vial to a syringe or infusion bottle or bag. The filter needle must not be used for injection.

The administration equipment and any unused AHF (human), pasteurized, should be discarded.

PREGNANCY CATEGORY C

Animal reproduction studies have not been conducted with AHF (human). It is also not known whether AHF (human) can cause fetal harm when administered to a pregnant woman or can affect reproduction capacity. AHF (human) should be given to a pregnant woman only if clearly needed.

ADVERSE REACTIONS:

AHF (human), pasteurized, is usually tolerated without reaction. Rare cases of allergic reaction and rise in temperature have been observed.

DOSAGE AND ADMINISTRATION:

AHF (human) is for intravenous administration only. Although dosage must be individualized according to the needs of the patient (weight, severity of hemorrhage, presence of inhibitors), the following general dosages are suggested:

1. Overt Bleeding: Initially 15 units per kg of body weight followed by 8 units per kg every 8 hours for the first 24 hours and the same dose every 12 hours for 3 or 4 days.

2. Muscle Hemorrhages:

a. Minor hemorrhages in extremities or nonvital areas: 8 units per kg once a day for 2 or 3 days.

b. Massive hemorrhages in nonvital areas: 8 units per kg by infusion at 12-hour intervals for 2 days and then one a day for 2 more days.

c. Hemorrhages near vital organs (neck, throat, subperitoneal): 15 units per kg initially, then 8 units per kg every 8 hours. After 2 days the dose may be reduced by one-half.

3. Joint Hemorrhages: The usual dose is 8 units per kg every 8 hours for 1 day; then every 12 hours for 1 or 2 days. However, recent experience suggests that a substantially lower dose, 5 to 8 units per kg given once, may be sufficient for most hemorrhages. If aspiration is carried out, 8 units per kg are given just prior to aspiration, 8 hours later, and again on the following day.

4. Surgery: Dosages of 26 to 30 units per kg body weight prior to surgery are recommended. After surgery, 15 units per kg every 8 hours should be administered. Close laboratory control to maintain the blood AHF at the level deemed appropriate for the surgical procedure is recommended for at least 10 days postoperatively. As a general rule, 1 unit of AHF activity per kg will increase the circulating AHF level by 2%. Adequacy of treatment must be judged by the clinical effects—thus the dosage may vary with individual cases.

RECONSTITUTION

1. Warm both diluent and AHF (human), pasteurized, in unopened vials to room temperature (not above 37° C [98° F]).

2. Remove caps from both vials to expose central portions of the rubber stoppers.

3. Treat surface of rubber stoppers with antiseptic solution and allow to dry.

4. Using aseptic technique, pierce the double needle of the blue transfer set into the diluent vial. Remove the protective cap and insert the exposed (longer) needle into the upright AHF (human), pasteurized, vial. The diluent will be transferred into the AHF (human) by vacuum.

5. Remove the diluent vial, then the transfer set, from the AH factor (human) vial.

6. Gently rotate the vial. DO NOT SHAKE VIAL. Vigorous shaking will prolong the reconstitution time. Continue swirling until the powder is dissolved and the solution is ready for administration. To ensure product sterility, AHF (human) should be administered within 3 hours after reconstitution.

7. Parenteral drug products should be inspected visually for particulate matter and discoloration prior to administration whenever solution and container permit.

DOSAGE AND ADMINISTRATION: *(cont'd)*

ADMINISTRATION

Intravenous Injection: Plastic disposable syringes are recommended with AHF (human), pasteurized, solution. The ground-glass surface of all-glass syringes tends to stick with solutions of this type.

1. Open the package containing the disposable filter. Attach the filter to a sterile disposable syringe and take the filter out of the package.

2. Remove the protective cap and—without touching the tip of the filter—insert the disposable filter into the stopper of the AHF (human) vial; inject air.

3. Draw up the solution slowly (when using several syringes, leave the filter in the vial). Discard the filter.

4. Slowly inject the solution (maximally 4 ml/min) intravenously with an infusion kit or with a suitable injection needle. Aspiration of blood into the filled syringe must be avoided.

REFERENCES:

1. Heimburger N, Schwinn H, Gratz P, et al: Factor VIII Concentrate—highly purified and heated in solution. Arzneim Forsch 31(1):619-22, 1981. **2.** Experimental and clinical studies of a new pasteurized antihemophilic factor concentrate. In press. **3.** Abildgaard CF, Simone JV, Corrigan JJ, et al: Treatment of hemophilia with glycine-precipitated factor VIII. New Engl J Med 275:471-475, 1966. **4.** Hilgartner MW: Current Therapy, in Hilgartner MW (ed): Hemophilia in children. Littelton, MA, Publishing Sciences Group Inc., 1976, p 158. **5.** Schimpf K, Rothman P, Zimmermann K: Factor VIII doses in prophylaxis of hemophilia A; A further controlled study, Proc XIth Cong W.F.H. Tokyo, Academia Press, 1976, p 363.

HOW SUPPLIED:

Storage: When stored at refrigerator temperature, 2°to 8° C (36°to 46° F), AHF (human), pasteurized, is stable for the period indicated by the expiration date on its label. Within this period, AHF (human) may be stored at room temperature not to exceed 30° C (86° F), for up to 6 months.

Avoid freezing, which may damage container for the diluent.

HOW SUPPLIED - EQUIVALENTS NOT AVAILABLE:

Injection, Lyphl-Soln - Intravenous

1's	$0.70	PROFILATE HP SOLVENT SUSP, Alpha Therapeutic	49669-4200-01
1's	$0.70	PROFILATE HP SOLVENT SUSP, Alpha Therapeutic	49669-4200-02

Injection, Lyphl-Soln - Intravenous - 250 ahfunit

1's	**$0.90**	**KOATE-HP, Bayer Pharm**	**00192-0664-20**
1's	$1.10	MELATE, Melville	13143-0321-54
1's	$1.18	HELIXATE, Centeon	00053-8120-01
1's	$1.18	KOGENATE, Bayer Pharm	00192-0670-20
10 ml	$0.84	KOATE-HS, Miles	00161-0660-20
250 unt	$1.30	HUMATE-P, Centeon	00053-7605-01

Injection, Lyphl-Soln - Intravenous - 325 ahfunit

1's	$0.90	PROFILATE SD SOLVENT DETERGENT, Alpha Therapeutic	49669-4100-01
1's	$0.90	PROFILATE OSD, Alpha Therapeutic	49669-4300-01

Injection, Lyphl-Soln - Intravenous - 500 ahfunit

1's	**$0.90**	**KOATE-HP, Bayer Pharm**	**00192-0664-30**
1's	$1.10	MELATE, Melville	13143-0321-55
1's	$1.18	HELIXATE, Centeon	00053-8120-02
1's	$1.18	KOGENATE, Bayer Pharm	00192-0670-30
20 ml	$0.84	KOATE-HS, Miles	00161-0660-30
500 unt	$1.30	HUMATE-P, Centeon	00053-7605-02

Injection, Lyphl-Soln - Intravenous - 1000 ahfunit

1's	**$0.90**	**KOATE-HP, Bayer Pharm**	**00192-0664-50**
1's	$1.10	MELATE, Melville	13143-0321-56
1's	$1.18	HELIXATE, Centeon	00053-8120-04
1's	$1.18	KOGENATE, Bayer Pharm	00192-0670-50
40 ml	$0.84	KOATE-HS, Miles	00161-0660-50
1000 unt	$1.30	HUMATE-P, Centeon	00053-7605-04

Injection, Lyphl-Soln - Intravenous - 1325 ahfunit

1's	$0.90	PROFILATE SD SOLVENT DETERGENT, Alpha Therapeutic	49669-4100-02
1's	$0.90	PROFILATE OSD, Alpha Therapeutic	49669-4300-02

Injection, Solution - Intravenous - 310 ahfunit

1's	$1.18	BIOCLATE, Centeon	00053-8110-01

Injection, Solution - Intravenous - 450 ahfunit

1's	$1.10	NYBCEN, Melville	13143-0321-52

Injection, Solution - Intravenous - 550 ahfunit

1's	$1.61	HYATE:C, Speywood Pharm	55688-0106-02

Injection, Solution - Intravenous - 600 ahfunit

1's	$1.18	BIOCLATE, Centeon	00053-8110-02

Injection, Solution - Intravenous - 850 ahfunit

1's	$0.90	HEMOFIL-M, Baxter Hyland	00944-2935-01

Injection, Solution - Intravenous - 900 ahfunit

1's	$1.10	NYBCEN, Melville	13143-0321-53

Injection, Solution - Intravenous - 950 ahfunit

1's	$0.70	ALPHANATE, Alpha Therapeutic	49669-4500-01

Injection, Solution - Intravenous - 1020 ahfunit

1's	$1.18	BIOCLATE, Centeon	00053-8110-03
1's	$1.18	BIOCLATE, Centeon	00053-8110-04

Injection, Solution - Intravenous - 1500 ahfunit

1's	$0.84	KOATE-HS, Miles	00161-0660-60
1's	**$0.90**	**KOATE-HP, Bayer Pharm**	**00192-0664-60**

ANTIHEMOPHILIC FACTOR VIII COMPLEX (HUMAN, MONOCLONAL) *(000259)*

CATEGORIES: Antihemophilic Factor; Blood Formation/Coagulation; Blood Derivatives; Coagulants and Anticoagulants; Factor VIII Deficiency; Hemophilia; Hemostatics; Pregnancy Category C; Recombinant DNA Origin; Sales >$100 Million; FDA Approval Pre–1982

BRAND NAMES: *Antihemophilic Factor (Recombinant)*; Factor VIII; *Kogenate*; KoGENate; **Monoclate Factor VIII:C**; Recombinate
(International brand names outside U.S. in italics)

DESCRIPTION:

Antihemophilic factor (human), Monoclate-P, Factor VIII:C Pasteurized, Monoclonal Antibody Purified is a sterile, stable, lyophilized concentrate of Factor VIII:C with reduced amounts of von Willebrand factor antigen (vWf:Ag) and purified of extraneous plasma-derived protein by use of affinity chromatography. A murine monoclonal antibody to vWf:Ag is used as an affinity ligand to first isolate the factor VIII complex. Factor VIII:C is then dissociated from vWf:Ag, recovered, formulated, and provided as a sterile lyophilized powder.[1-3]The concentrate as formulated contains albumin (human) as a stabilizer, resulting in a concentrate with a specific activity between 5 and 10 U/mg of total protein. In the absence of this added albumin (human) stabilizer, specific activity has been determined to exceed 3000 U/mg of protein.[4] Monoclate-P has been prepared from pooled human plasma and is intended for use in therapy of classic hemophilia (hemophilia A).

This concentrate has been pasteurized by heating at 60° C for 10 hours in aqueous solution form during its manufacture in order to further reduce the risk of viral transmission.[5] However, no procedure has been shown to be totally effective in removing viral infectivity from coagulant factor concentrates. (See CLINICAL PHARMACOLOGYand WARNINGS.)

Monoclate-P is a highly purified preparation of Factor VIII:C. When stored as directed, it will maintain its labeled potency for the period indicated on the container and package labels.[8,9]

Upon reconstitution, a clear, colorless solution is obtained, containing 50 to 150 times as much Factor VIII:C as does an equal volume of plasma.

Each vial contains the labeled amount of antihemophilic factor (AHF) activity as expressed in terms of international units of antihemophilic activity. One unit of antihemophilic activity is equivalent to that quantity of AHF present in 1 ml of normal human plasma. When reconstituted as recommended, the resulting solution contains approximately 300 to 450 millimoles of sodium ions per liter and has 2 to 3 times the tonicity of saline. It contains approximately 2 to 5 millimoles of calcium ions per liter, contributed as calcium chloride, approximately 1% to 2% albumin (human), 0.8% mannitol, and 1.2 mm histidine. The pH is adjusted with hydrochloric acid and/or sodium hydroxide. Monoclate-P also contains trace amounts (≤50 ng per 100 IU of AHF) of the murine monoclonal antibody used in its purification (see CLINICAL PHARMACOLOGY).

Monoclate-P is to be administered only intravenously.

CLINICAL PHARMACOLOGY:

Factor VIII:C is the coagulant portion of the factor VIII complex circulating in plasma. It is noncovalently associated with the von Willebrand protein responsible for von Willebrand factor activity. These two proteins have distinct biochemical and immunologic properties and are under separate genetic control. Factor VIII:C acts as a cofactor for factor IX to activate factor X in the intrinsic pathway of blood coagulation.[6] Hemophilia A, a hereditary disorder of blood coagulation due to decreased levels of Factor VIII:C, results in profuse bleeding into joints, muscles, or internal organs as a result of a trauma. AHF (human), Monoclate-P, Factor VIII:C Pasteurized provides an increase in plasma levels of AHF, thereby enabling temporary correction of hemophilia A bleeding.

Clinical evaluation of Monoclate-P, Factor VIII:C Pasteurized, Monoclonal Antibody Purified concentrate for its half-life characteristics in hemophilic patients showed it to be comparable to other commercially available AHF (human) concentrates. The mean half-life obtained from six patients was 17.5 hours with a mean recovery of 1.9 U/dl rise/U/kg.

The pasteurization process used in the manufacture of this concentrate has demonstrated *in vitro* inactivation of human immunodeficiency virus (HIV) and several model viruses. In two separate studies, HIV was reduced by $\geq 7.0 \log_{10}$ to an undetectable level and by $10.5 \log_{10}$, respectively. In addition to HIV, studies were also performed using three lipid-containing model viruses and one nonlipid encapsulated model virus. Vesicular stomatitis (VSV) was reduced by $\geq 6.79 \log_{10}$ to undetectable levels. Sindbis was reduced by $\geq 6.48 \log_{10}$ to undetectable and Vaccinia was reduced by $\geq 5.36 \log_{10}$ to undetectable. Murine encephalomyocarditis (EMC), a nonlipid encapsulated model virus, was reduced by $\geq 7.1 \log_{10}$ to undetectable levels.

Evidence of the capability of the purification and preparative steps used in the production of antihemophilic factor (human), Monoclate-P, Factor VIII:C Pasteurized, Monoclonal Antibody Purified to reduce viral bioburden was obtained in studies involving the addition of known quantities of virus to cryoprecipitate. These studies were conducted using an earlier form of the concentrate that had not undergone liquid pasteurization (AHF (human), Monoclate, Monoclonal Antibody Purified, Factor VIII:C, Heat-Treated). These studies provide evidence of the viral removal potential of the purification and preparative steps of the manufacturing process (exclusive of heat treatment) that are common to both concentrates. In one study the viruses used were HIV, sindbis virus, vesicular stomatitis virus (VSV), and pseudorabies virus (PsRV). A comparison of the cumulative mean reductions for all viruses tested with the individual values obtained in each experiment indicates that the combined effects of the manufacturing steps, which purify the Factor VIII:C and prepare the concentrate in a final sterile container as a lyophilized powder, contribute viral reduction capabilities of approximately 5 to 6 logs. In a separate study, aluminum hydroxide treatment followed by antibody affinity chromatography reduced vaccinia virus infectivity by 4.81 logs. These studies indicate that the purification and preparative steps of the manufacturing process are capable of providing a nonspecific viral reduction of approximately 5 to 6 logs, independent of the pasteurization process.

Monoclate-P contains trace amounts of mouse protein[7](≤50 ng per 100 IU of AHF). In a study using an earlier form of the concentrate, which had not undergone pasteurization (Monoclate), a number of patients seronegative for anti-HIV-1 were monitored to determine whether they would develop antibody or experience adverse reactions as a result of repeated exposure. These patients were treated on multiple occasions. Prestudy serum measurements of 27 patients for human anti-mouse lgG showed that, prior to treatment, 6 of them had either detectable antibody to mouse proteins or cross-reactive proteins. These patients continued to demonstrate similar or lower antibody levels during the study. Of the remaining 21 patients, 6 were shown to have low antibody levels on one or more occasions. In no case was observance of low antibody level associated with an anamnestic response or any clinical adverse reaction. Patients were observed for periods ranging from 2 to 30 months.

INDICATIONS AND USAGE:

AHF (human), Monoclate-P, Factor VIII:C Pasteurized is indicated for treatment of classic hemophilia (hemophilia A). Affected individuals frequently require therapy following minor accidents. Surgery, when required in such individuals, must be preceded by temporary correction of the clotting abnormality. Presurgical correction of severe AHF deficiency can be accomplished with a small volume of Monoclate-P.

Monoclate-P is not effective in controlling the bleeding of patients with von Willebrand's disease.

CONTRAINDICATIONS:

Known hypersensitivity to mouse protein is a contraindication to AHF (human), Monoclate-P, Factor VIII:C Pasteurized, Monoclonal Antibody Purified.

WARNINGS:

This product is prepared from pooled human plasma, which may contain the causative agents of hepatitis and other viral diseases. Prescribed manufacturing procedures utilized at the plasma collection centers, plasma testing laboratories, and fractionation facilities are designed to reduce the risk of transmitting viral infection. However, the risk of viral infectivity from this product cannot be totally eliminated. Accordingly, the benefits and risks of treatment with this concentrate should be carefully assessed prior to use.

Individuals who receive infusions of blood or plasma products may develop signs and/or symptoms of some viral infections, particularly non-A, non-B hepatitis.

PRECAUTIONS:

GENERAL

Most AHF (human) concentrates contain naturally occurring blood group–specific antibodies. However, the processing of Monoclate-P significantly reduces the presence of blood group specific antibodies in the final product. Nevertheless, when large or frequently repeated doses of product are needed, patients should be monitored by means of hematocrit and direct Coombs' test for signs of progressive anemia.

FORMATION OF ANTIBODIES TO MOUSE PROTEIN

Although no hypersensitivity reactions have been observed, because Monoclate-P contains trace amounts of mouse protein (≤50 ng per 100 IU of AHF), the possibility exists that patients treated with Monoclate-P may develop hypersensitivity to the mouse proteins.

INFORMATION FOR THE PATIENT

Patients should be informed of the early signs of hypersensitivity reactions, including hives, generalized urticaria, tightness of the chest, wheezing, hypotension, and anaphylaxis and should be advised to discontinue use of the concentrate and contact their physician if these symptoms occur.

PREGNANCY CATEGORY C

Animal reproduction studies have not been conducted with AHF (human), Monoclate-P, Factor VIII:C Pasteurized. It is also not known whether Monoclate-P can cause fetal harm when administered to a pregnant woman or affect reproduction capacity. Monoclate-P should be given to a pregnant woman only if clearly needed.

ADVERSE REACTIONS:

Products of this type are known to cause allergic reactions, mild chills, nausea, or stinging at the infusion site.

DOSAGE AND ADMINISTRATION:

AHF (human), Monoclate-P, Factor VIII:C Pasteurized, Monoclonal Antibody Purified is for intravenous administration only. As a general rule, 1 unit of AHF activity per kg will increase the circulating AHF level by 2%.[10] The following formula provides a guide of dosage calculations: See TABLE 1.

TABLE 1

$$\text{Number of AHF} = \frac{\text{Body weight} \times \text{Desired factor VIII} \times 0.5^{10}}{\text{IU required (in kg) increase (\% normal)}}$$

Although dosage must be individualized according to the needs of the patient (weight, severity of hemorrhage, presence of inhibitors), the following general dosages are suggested.[11]

1. Mild Hemorrhages: Minor hemorrhagic episodes will generally subside with a single infusion if a level of 30% or more is attained.

2. Moderate Hemorrhage and Minor Surgery: For more serious hemorrhages and minor surgical procedures, the patient's factor VIII level should be raised to 30%-50% of normal, which usually requires an initial dose of 15 to 25 IU per kg. If further therapy is required, a maintenance dose of 10 to 15 IU per kg every 8 to 12 hours is given.

3. Severe Hemorrhage: In hemorrhages near vital organs (neck, throat, subperitoneal), it may be desirable to raise the factor VIII level to 80%-100% of normal, which can be achieved with an initial dose of 40 to 50 IU per kg and a maintenance dose of 20 to 25 IU per kg every 8 to 12 hours.

4. Major Surgery: For surgical procedures a dose of AHF sufficient to achieve a level 80%-100% of normal should be given an hour prior to surgery. A second dose, half the size of the priming dose, should be given 5 hours after the first dose. Factor VIII levels should be maintained at a daily minimum of 30% for a period of 10 to 14 days postoperatively. Close laboratory control to maintain AHF plasma levels deemed appropriate to maintain hemostasis is recommended.

RECONSTITUTION

1. Warm both the diluent and AHF (human), Monoclate-P, Factor VIII:C Pasteurized, Monoclonal Antibody Purified in unopened vials to room temperature [not above 37° C (98° F)].

2. Remove the caps from both vials to expose the central portions of the rubber stoppers.

3. Treat the surface of the rubber stoppers with antiseptic solution and allow them to dry.

4. Using aseptic technique, insert one end of the double-end needle into the rubber stopper of the diluent vial. Invert the diluent vial, and insert the other end of the double-end needle into the rubber stopper of the Monoclate-P vial. Direct the diluent, which will be drawn in by vacuum, over the entire surface of the Monoclate-P cake. (In order to ensure transfer of all the diluent, adjust the position of the tip of the needle in the diluent vial to the inside edge of the diluent stopper.) Rotate the vial to ensure complete wetting of the cake during the transfer process.

5. Remove the diluent vial to release the vacuum. Then remove the double-end needle from the Monoclate-P vial.

6. Gently swirl the vial until the powder is dissolved and the solution is ready for administration. The concentrate routinely and easily reconstitutes within 1 minute. To ensure sterility, Monoclate-P should be administered within 3 hours after reconstitution.

7. Parenteral drug preparations should be inspected visually for particulate matter and discoloration prior to administration, whenever solution and container permit.

ADMINISTRATION

Caution:This kit contains two devices, a stainless steel 5- micron filter needle, individually labeled as a 5-micron filter needle and contained in a separate blister pack, and an all plastic 5-micron vented filter spike, which is supplied with the four-item administration components blister pack, either of which may be used to withdraw the reconstituted product for administration. The withdrawal directions specific for each of these alternate devices must be followed exactly for whichever device is chosen for use as described below. Product loss or inability to withdraw product will result if the improper instructions are followed.

A. Administration Using the Stainless Steel Filter Needle for Withdrawal (This item is individually packaged in a separate labeled blister pack.)

Intravenous Injection Plastic disposable syringes are recommended with antihemophilic factor (human), Monoclate-P, Factor VIII:C Pasteurized, Monoclonal Antibody Purified, solution. The ground-glass surface of all glass syringes tends to stick with solutions of this type.

DOSAGE AND ADMINISTRATION: *(cont'd)*

1. Using aseptic technique, attach the filter needle to a sterile disposable syringe.

2. Draw air into the syringe equal to or greater than the contents of the vial.

3. Insert the filter needle into the stopper of the Monoclate-P vial, invert the vial, position the filter needle above the level of the liquid, and inject all of the air into the vial.

4. Pull the filter needle back down below the level of the liquid until the tip is at the inside edge of the stopper.

5. Withdraw the reconstituted solution into the syringe, being careful to always keep the tip of the needle below the level of the liquid.*CAUTION:*Failure to inject air into the vial, or allowing air to pass through the filter needle while filling the syringe with reconstituted solution, may cause the needle to clog.

6. Discard the filter needle. Perform venipuncture using the enclosed winged needle with microbore tubing. Attach the syringe to the luer end of the tubing.

7. Administer solution intravenously at a rate (approximately 2 ml/min) comfortable to the patient.

Caution: Use of other winged needles without microbore tubing, although compatible with the concentrate, will result in a larger retention of solution within the winged infusion set.

B. Administration Using the All-Plastic VENTED FILTER SPIKE FOR WITHDRAWAL (THIS SPIKE IS SUPPLIED IN THE FOUR-ITEM ADMINISTRATION COMPONENTS PACK.)

Intravenous Injection: Plastic disposable syringes are recommended with AHF (human), Monoclate-P, Factor VII:C Pasteurized, Monoclonal Antibody Purified solution. The ground-glass surface of all glass syringes tends to stick with solutions of this type.

1. Using aseptic technique, attach the vented filter spike to a sterile disposable syringe.

Caution: DO NOT INJECT AIR INTO THE MONOCLATE-P VIAL. The self-venting feature of the vented filter spike precludes the need to inject air in order to facilitate withdrawal of the reconstituted solution. The injection of air could cause partial product loss through the vent filter.

Caution: The use of other nonvented filter needles or spikes without proper procedure may result in an air lock and prevent the complete transfer of the concentrate.

2. Insert the vented filter spike into the stopper of the Monoclate-P vial, invert the vial, and position the filter spike so that the orifice is at the inside edge of the stopper.

3. Withdraw the reconstituted solution into the syringe.

4. Discard the filter spike. Perform venipuncture using the enclosed winged needle with microbore tubing. Attach the syringe to the luer end of the tubing.

Caution: Use of the other winged needles without microbore tubing, although compatible with the concentrate, will result in a larger retention of solution within the winged infusion set.

5. Administer solution intravenously at a rate (approximately 2 ml/min) comfortable to the patient.

REFERENCES:

1. W. Terry, A. Schreiber, C. Tarr, M. Hrinda, W. Curry, and F. Feldman, "Human Factor VIII:C Produced Using Monoclonal Antibodies," in*Research in Clinic and Laboratory,* Vol. XVI, (#1), 202 (1986) from the XVIIth International Congress of the World Federation of Hemophilia. **2.** A.B. Schreiber, "The Preclinical Characterization of Monoclate Factor VIII C Antihemophilic Factor Human," *Semin Hematol* 25 (2 Suppl. 1), 1988, pp. 27-32. **3.** E. Berntorp and I.M. Nilsson, "Biochemical Properties of Human Factor VIII C Monoclate Purified Using Monoclonal Antibody to VWF," *Thromb Res* O (Suppl. 7), 1987, p. 60, from the Satellite Symposia of the XIth International Congress on Thrombosis and Haemostasis, Brussels, Belgium, July 11, 1987. **4.** S. Chandra, C.C. Huang, R.L. Weeks, K. Beatty and F. Feldman, "Purity of a Factor VIII:C Preparation (Monoclate) Manufactured by Monoclonal Immunoaffinity Chromatography Technique," from the XVIII International Congress of the World Federation of Hemophilia, May 1988. **5.** B. Spire, D. Dormont, F. Barre-Sinousii, L. Montagnier, and J.C. Chermann, "Inactivation of Lymphadenopathy Associated Virus by Heat, Gamma Rays, and Ultraviolet Light," *Lancet,* Jan. 26. 1985, p. 188. **6.** L.W. Hoyer, "The Factor VIII Complex: Structure and Function,"*Blood* 58 (1981), p. 1. **7.** F. Feldman, S. Chandra, R. Kleszynski, C.C. Huang and R.L. Weeks, "Measurement of Murine Protein Levels in Monoclonal Antibody Purified Coagulation Factor," from the XVIII International Congress of the World Federation of Hemophilia, May 1988. **8.** F. Feldman, R. Kleszynski, L. Ho, R. Kling, S. Chandra and C.C. Huang, "Validation of Coagulation Test Methods for Evaluation of Monoclate (Factor VIII:C) Potencies," from the XVIII International Congress of the World Federation of Hemophilia, May 1988. **9.** S. Chandra, C.C. Huang, L. Ho, R. Kling, R.L. Weeks and F. Feldman, "Studies on the Stability of Factor VIII:C (Monoclate) in Lyophilized and Solution Form," from the XVIII International Congress of the World Federation of Hemophilia, May 1988. **10.** C.F. Abilgaard, J.V. Simone, J.J. Corrigan, et al., "Treatment of Hemophilia with Glycine—Precipitated Factor VIII," *New Eng J Med,* 275 (1966), p. 471. **11.** C.K. Kasper, "Hematologic Care," *Comprehensive Management of Hemophilia,* ed. Boone, D.C., Philadelphia, F.A. Davis Co., (1976) pp. 2-20. **Bibliography:** Hershman, R.J., Naconti, S.B., and Shulman, N.R. "Prophylactic Treatment of Factor VIII Deficiency." *Blood* 35 (1970), p. 189.Kasper, C.K., Dietrich, S.I. and Rapaport, S.K. "Hemophilia Prophylaxis in Factor VIII Concentrate." *Arch. Int. Med.*125 (1970), p. 1004.Biggs, R., ed. "The Treatment of Hemophilia A and B and von Willebrands Disease." Oxford: Blackwell, 1978.Fulcher, C.A., Zimmerman, T.S., "Characterization of the Human Factor VIII Procoagulant Protein With a Heterologous Precipitating Antibody."*Proc. Natl. Acad. Sci.* 79 (1982), pp. 1648-1652.Levine, P.H., "Factor VIII C Purified from Plasma Via Monoclonal Antibodies Human Studies." *Semin Hematol* 25 (2 Suppl. 1). 1988, pp. 38-41.

HOW SUPPLIED:

Storage: When stored at refrigerator temperature, 2° to 8°C (36° to 46°F), AHF (human), Monoclate-P, Factor VIII:C Pasteurized, Monoclonal Antibody Purified is stable for the period indicated by the expiration date on its label. Within this period, Monoclate-P may be stored at room temperature, not to exceed 30° C (86° F), for up to 6 months.

Avoid freezing, which may damage the container for the diluent.

HOW SUPPLIED - EQUIVALENTS NOT AVAILABLE:

Injection, Lyphl-Soln - Intravenous - 250 ahfunit/via

1 unit	$0.90	MONOCLATE-P, Centeon	00053-7656-01

Injection, Lyphl-Soln - Intravenous - 310 ahfunit/via

1 unit	$1.18	RECOMBINATE, Baxter Hyland	00944-2938-01

Injection, Lyphl-Soln - Intravenous - 407 ahfunit/via

1 unit	$1.18	RECOMBINATE, Baxter Hyland	00944-2938-03

Injection, Lyphl-Soln - Intravenous - 500 ahfunit/via

1 unit	$0.90	MONOCLATE-P, Centeon	00053-7656-02

Injection, Lyphl-Soln - Intravenous - 600 ahfunit/via

1 unit	$1.18	RECOMBINATE, Baxter Hyland	00944-2938-02

Injection, Lyphl-Soln - Intravenous - 1000 ahfunit/vi

1 unit	$0.90	MONOCLATE-P, Centeon	00053-7656-04

ANTIPYRINE; BENZOCAINE *(000263)*

CATEGORIES: Analgesics; EENT Drugs; Eye, Ear, Nose, & Throat Preparations; Ear Wax; Inflammation; Local Anesthetics; Otic Preparations; Otitis Media; Otologic; Pain; Pregnancy Category C; FDA Pre 1938 Drugs

BRAND NAMES: A B Otic; Allergen; Antipyrine W/Benzocaine; Aurafair; **Auralgan**; *Auralgan (non-prescription)*; *Auralgan Otic*; *Auralgicin*; *Auraltone*; *Auralyt* (Mexico); Aurodex; Auromid; Auroto; Benzotic; Dec-Agesic A.B.; Decon Otic;

Dolotic; Ear Drops; Ear Drops Rx; Earocol; Lanaurine; Otipyrin; *Otised*; Oto; Otocalm; *Ototrisol*
(International brand names outside U.S. in italics)

FORMULARIES: Aetna; BC-BS; FHP; Medi-Cal; PCS

DESCRIPTION:

Each ml Contains:

Antipyrine : 54.0 mg

Benzocaine: 14.0 mg

Glycerin dehydrated q.s. to 1.0 ml

Contains not more than 0.6% moisture (also contains oxyquinoline sulfate).

TOPICAL DECONGESTANT AND ANALGESIC

Antipyrine w/ Benzocaine is an otic solution containing antipyrine, benzocaine, and dehydrated glycerin. The solution congeals at 0° C (32° F) but returns to normal consistency, unchanged, at room temperature.

CLINICAL PHARMACOLOGY:

Antipyrine w/ Benzocaine combines the hygroscopic property of dehydrated glycerin with the analgesic action of antipyrine and benzocaine to relieve pressure, reduce inflammation and congestion, and alleviate pain and discomfort in acute otitis media.

Antipyrine w/ Benzocaine does not blanch the tympanic membrane or mask the landmarks and, therefore, does not distort the otoscopic picture.

INDICATIONS AND USAGE:

ACUTE OTITIS MEDIA OF VARIOUS ETIOLOGIES

Prompt relief of pain and reduction of inflammation in the congestive and serous stages

Adjuvant therapy during systemic antibiotic administration for resolution of the infection

Because of the close anatomical relationship of the eustachian tube to the nasal cavity, otitis media is a frequent problem, especially in children in whom the tube is shorter, wider, and more horizontal than in adults.

REMOVAL OF CERUMEN

Facilitates the removal of excessive or impacted cerumen.

CONTRAINDICATIONS:

Hypersensitivity to any of the components or substances related to them.

Perforated tympanic membrane is considered a contraindication to the use of any medication in the external ear canal.

WARNINGS:

Discontinue promptly if sensitization or irritation occurs.

PRECAUTIONS:

CARCINOGENESIS, MUTAGENESIS, AND IMPAIRMENT OF FERTILITY

No long-term studies in animals or humans have been conducted.

PREGNANCY CATEGORY C

Animal reproduction studies have not been conducted with Antipyrine w/ Benzocaine. It is also not known whether Antipyrine w/ Benzocaine can cause fetal harm when administered to a pregnant woman, or can affect reproduction capacity. Antipyrine w/ Benzocaine should be given to a pregnant woman only if clearly needed.

NURSING MOTHERS

It is not known whether this drug is excreted in human milk. Because many drugs are excreted in human milk, caution should be exercised when Antipyrine w/ Benzocaine is administered to a nursing woman.

DOSAGE AND ADMINISTRATION:

ACUTE OTITIS MEDIA

Instill Antipyrine w/ Benzocaine permitting the solution to run along the wall of the canal until it is filled. Avoid touching the ear with dropper. Then moisten a cotton pledget with Antipyrine w/ Benzocaine and insert into meatus. Repeat every one to two hours until pain and congestion are relieved.

REMOVAL OF CERUMEN

Before: Instill Antipyrine w/ Benzocaine three times daily for two or three days to help detach cerumen from wall of canal and facilitate removal.

After: Antipyrine w/ Benzocaine is useful for drying out the canal or relieving discomfort.

Before and after removal of cerumen, a cotton pledget moistened with Antipyrine w/ Benzocaine should be inserted into the meatus following instillation.

NOTE: Do not rinse dropper after use. Replace dropper in bottle after each use. Hold dropper assembly by screw cap and, without compressing the rubber bulb, insert into drug container and screw down tightly.

Protect the solution from light and heat, and do not use if it is brown or contains a precipitate.

DISCARD THIS PRODUCT SIX MONTHS AFTER DROPPER IS FIRST PLACED IN THE DRUG SOLUTION.

Storage: Store at room temperature (approximately 25° C).

HOW SUPPLIED - RATED THERAPEUTICALLY EQUIVALENT:

Solution - Otic - 54 mg/14 mg

10 ml	$1.51	A/B Otic, Clay Park Labs	45802-0311-68
15 ml	$1.94	A/B OTIC DROPS, Clay Park Labs	45802-0311-56

HOW SUPPLIED - NOT RATED EQUIVALENT:

Solution - Otic - 54 mg/14 mg

10 ml	$1.47	EAR DROPS, HL Moore Drug Exch	00839-6342-30
10 ml	$1.82	Antipyrine/Benzocaine #2, Schein Pharm (US)	00364-7260-54
10 ml	$2.04	Antipyrine W/Benzocaine, Aligen Independ	00405-2025-51
10 ml	**$13.35**	**AURALGAN, Ayerst**	**00046-1000-10**
15 ml	$1.73	EAR DROPS, HL Moore Drug Exch	00839-6342-61
15 ml	$1.88	EAR DROPS ANALGESIC, Rugby	00536-8440-94
15 ml	$1.90	RX OTIC DROPS, Thames Pharma	49158-0178-30
15 ml	$2.18	Antipyrine W/Benzocaine, IDE-Interstate	00814-0790-42
15 ml	$2.50	Antipyrine and Benzocaine, United Res	00677-1406-30
15 ml	$2.65	AURODEX, Major Pharms	00904-0793-35
15 ml	$2.75	Auroto, Consolidated Midland	00223-6416-01
15 ml	$2.91	Ear Drops Rx, Rugby	00536-8440-72
15 ml	$3.00	ALLERGEN, Goldline Labs	00182-1175-33
15 ml	$3.08	AUROTO, Alpharma	00472-0016-99
15 ml	$3.08	A/B Otic, Qualitest Pharms	00603-7020-73

HOW SUPPLIED - NOT RATED EQUIVALENT: *(cont'd)*

15 ml	$4.00	Decon Otic, Norega Labs	51724-0016-15
15 ml	$12.20	BENZOTIC, Alba Pharma	10023-0127-15

ANTIPYRINE; BENZOCAINE; PHENYLEPHRINE HYDROCHLORIDE *(000264)*

CATEGORIES: Analgesics; Anesthesia; EENT Drugs; Eye, Ear, Nose, & Throat Preparations; Local Anesthetics; Otic Preparations; Otitis; Otitis Media; Otologic; Pain; Topical; Pregnancy Category C; FDA Pre 1938 Drugs

BRAND NAMES: Auroto; Otogesic; **Tympagesic**

DESCRIPTION:

Antipyrine/benzocaine/phenylephrine HCl Otic Solution, analgesic-decongestant ear drops, contains phenylephrine hydrochloride USP 0.25%, antipyrine USP 5% and benzocaine USP 5% in propylene glycol USP.

Phenylephrine hydrochloride is a sympathomimetic amine with local vasoconstriction or decongestant action. It is chemically (1) Benzenemethanol, 3- hydroxy-alpha-((methylamino) methyl)-, hydrochloride (R) (2) (-)-m-Hydroxy -alpha- (methylamino)methyl)benzyl alcohol hydrochloride CAS 61-76-7

It occurs as white crystals, has a bitter taste and is freely soluble in water and alcohol. Antipyrine is an analgesic with local anesthetic action. It is chemically 2,3-dimethyl-1-phenyl-3- pyrazolin-5-one. CAS 60-80-0.

Antipyrine appears as colorless crystals or white powder, has a slightly bitter taste and is soluble in water and alcohol. Benzocaine is a local anesthetic. It is chemically ethyl P-aminobenzoate CAS 04-09-7.

It occurs as white crystals or white crystalline powder and is slightly soluble in water and soluble in organic solvents.

CLINICAL PHARMACOLOGY:

Topical application of phenylephrine produces vasoconstriction mainly by a direct effect on alpha-adrenergic receptors. The effects of phenylephrine are similar to those of epinephrine. However, phenylephrine is considered less CNS and cardiostimulatory than epinephrine. Phenylephrine, after its absorption, is metabolized in the liver and the intestine by the enzyme monoamine oxidase (MAO). The type, route and rate of excretion of metabolites have not been defined.

Like other local anesthetics, benzocaine acts by blocking nerve conduction first in autonomic, then in sensory and finally in motor nerve fibers. Its effect appears to be due to decreased nerve cell membrane permeability to sodium ions or competition with calcium ions for membrane binding sites. A vasoconstrictor, such as phenylephrine, is added to decrease the rate of absorption and prolong the duration of action of the anesthetic. Ester-type anesthetics, which include benzocaine, after absorption are comparatively rapidly degraded by esterases mainly in the liver and excreted in the urine as metabolites and in small amounts as the unchanged drug.

Antipyrine is believed to have analgesic and local anesthetic effects on the nerve endings. After absorption, it is slowly metabolized in the liver by oxidation and conjugation with glucuronic acid and is excreted in the urine mainly in the conjugated form.

INDICATIONS AND USAGE:

Antipyrine/benzocaine/phenylephrine HCl otic solution may be used as a topical anesthetic in the external auditory canal to relieve ear pain. It may be used concomitantly with systemic antibiotics as in the treatment of acute otitis media.

CONTRAINDICATIONS:

Antipyrine/benzocaine/phenylephrine otic solution or any medication for use in the external ear canal is contraindicated in the presence of a perforated tympanic membrane or ear discharge and in individuals with a history of hypersensitivity to any of its ingredients.

WARNINGS:

As with all drugs containing a sympathomimetic or an anesthetic, systemic reactions may occur after local application. Phenylephrine may cause blanching and a feeling of coolness in the skin. Allergic and idiosyncratic reactions to local anesthetics have been observed infrequently. Such reactions are unlikely because absorption from the skin of the ear drum or the external ear canal is minimal.

Discontinue promptly if sensitization or irritation occurs.

Cross-sensitivity reactions between members of the Caine group of local anesthetics have been reported.

Contains Sodium Metabisulfite, a sulfite that may cause allergic-type reactions including anaphylactic symptoms and life-threatening or less severe asthmatic episodes in certain susceptible people. The overall prevalence of sulfite sensitivity in the general population is unknown and probably low. Sulfite sensitivity is seen more frequently in asthmatic than in nonasthmatic people.

PRECAUTIONS:

GENERAL

Drugs containing a sympathomimetic should be used with caution in the elderly and in patients with hypertension, increased intraocular pressure, diabetes mellitus, ischemic heart disease, hyperthyroidism and prostatic hypertrophy.

High plasma levels of benzocaine and antipyrine may cause CNS stimulation with nausea and vomiting. Such levels, however, are unlikely to be attained following local application in the external ear.

CARCINOGENESIS, MUTAGENESIS, AND IMPAIRMENT OF FERTILITY

There have been no studies in animals or humans to evaluate the carcinogenesis, mutagenesis or impairment of fertility for this drug.

PREGNANCY CATEGORY C

Animal reproduction studies have not been conducted with antipyrine/benzocaine/phenylephrine HCl otic solution. It is also not known whether this drug can cause fetal harm when administered to a pregnant woman or can effect reproduction capacity. This drug should be given to a pregnant woman only if clearly needed.

NURSING MOTHERS

It is not known whether this drug is excreted in human milk. Because many drugs are excreted in human milk, caution should be exercised when antipyrine/benzocaine/phenylephrine HCl is administered to a nursing woman.

PEDIATRIC USE

Safety and effectiveness in children below the age of 12 has not been established.

DRUG INTERACTIONS:

MAO inhibitors and beta-adrenergic blockers enhance the effects of sympathomimetics. Benzocaine is hydrolyzed in the body to p-aminobenzoic acid which competes with the antibacterial action of sulfonamides. However, these are unlikely to occur because of the limited absorption from the external ear canal.

ADVERSE REACTIONS:

Following its absorption, phenylephrine may produce a pressor response or cause restlessness, anxiety, nervousness, weakness, pallor, headache and dizziness. Absorption of benzocaine and antipyrine in the plasma may cause chills, nausea, vomiting, tinnitus and agranulocytosis. Such reactions are unlikely following application of this solution on the external ear canal. Benzocaine can cause a hypersensitivity reaction consisting of rash, urticaria and edema. Individuals frequently exposed to ester-type local anesthetics can develop contact dermatitis characterized by erythema and pruritus which may progress to vesiculation and oozing.

OVERDOSAGE:

It is more likely to be associated with accidental or deliberate ingestion rather than cutaneous absorption. Phenylephrine present in a bottle (13 ml) or antipyrine/benzocaine/phenylephrine HCl otic solution, if absorbed, may cause hypertension, headache, vomiting and palpitations. Effects of benzocaine overdosage may include yawning, restlessness, excitement, nausea and vomiting. Antipyrine overdosage may cause giddiness, tremor, sweating and skin eruptions.

Treatment is symptomatic. If ingestion of the contents of a bottle or more of antipyrine/benzocaine/phenylephrine HCl otic solution recent or food is present in the stomach, induction of emesis with ipecac syrup, gastric emptying and lavage and introduction of activated charcoal may be recommended.

DOSAGE AND ADMINISTRATION:

Using the dropper, instill antipyrine/benzocaine/phenylephrine HCl otic solution in the external ear canal allowing the solution to run into the canal until filled. Insert a cotton pledget into the meatus after moistening with the otic solution. Repeat every 2 to 4 hours, if necessary, until pain is relieved. Replace dropper in bottle without rinsing.

HOW SUPPLIED - EQUIVALENTS NOT AVAILABLE:

Solution - Otic - 5 %/5 %/0.25 %

13 ml	**$11.84**	**TYMPAGESIC, Savage Labs**	**00281-7363-39**
15 ml	$11.25	Otogesic, Teral Labs	51234-0163-15

ANTITHROMBIN III (HUMAN) *(000268)*

CATEGORIES: Antithrombin III Deficiency; Blood Derivatives; Blood Formation/Coagulation; Coagulants and Anticoagulants; Orphan Drugs; Thromboembolism; Thrombosis; Pregnancy Category C; FDA Approved 1990 Jun

BRAND NAMES: *Anthrobin P* (Japan); *Antithrombin III*; *Antithrombin III Immuno*; *Atenativ* (Germany); *Atenativ 500*; *Athimbin HS 500*; **Atnativ**; *Neuart* (Japan); Thrombate III; Thrombate Iii

(International brand names outside U.S. in italics)

DESCRIPTION:

Antithrombin III (Human), is produced from human plasma. Antithrombin III is a glycoprotein of molecular weight 58,000 (14) and consists of 425 amino acids in a single polypeptide chain crosslinked by three disulfide bridges. Antithrombin III is identical with heparin cofactor I, a factor in plasma necessary for heparin to exert its anticoagulant effect.

Antithrombin III, a sterile white powder, is intended for intravenous administration after reconstitution with Sterile Water for Injection, USP, and contains no preservative.

Antithrombin III (Human) has been heat-treated in solution at 60 ±0.5 °C for not less than 10 hours. Antithrombin III is supplied with 10 ml Sterile Water for Injection, USP. After reconstitution it contains 50 IU Antithrombin III (Human) per ml and has a pH of 6.5 to 7.5. The quantity of antithrombin III in 1 ml of normal pooled human plasma is conventionally taken as one unit. The potency assignment has been determined with a standard calibrated against a World Health Organization (WHO) Antithrombin III Reference Preparation.

TABLE 1 Antithrombin III (Human), Description

Composition of the product:	
I. Antithrombin III (Human)	500 IU
Sodium chloride	90 mg
Albumin (Human)	100 mg
II. Sterile Water for Injection, USP	10 ml

CLINICAL PHARMACOLOGY:

Antithrombin III is a major coagulation inhibitor in blood. It inactivates thrombin and the activated forms of Factors IX, X, XI and XII, i.e., all coagulation enzymes except Factor VIIa and XIIIa (17). The concentration of antithrombin III in normal plasma has been estimated from 0.1 to 0.2 g/L (3, 13). Antithrombin III levels are usually expressed as a percentage of a reference plasma.

In subjects with hereditary antithrombin III deficiency the levels of antithrombin III are found to be about 50% of the level in normal human plasma. (1, 4, 5, 11, 15, 20, 23). These subjects have a high risk of thromboembolic disease even at an early age. Surgery and pregnancy are significant factors precipitating venous thrombosis in antithrombin III deficient patients. Antithrombin III (Human) is given as replacement treatment to patients with hereditary antithrombin III deficiency in connection with surgical or obstetrical procedures or when they suffer from thromboembolism.

Pharmacokinetic studies of Antithrombin III (Human) have been performed (22). The mean biological half-life in three patients with hereditary antithrombin III deficiency and one healthy subject was found to be 3.0 days. The half-life of antithrombin III is decreased by concurrent heparin treatment (3).

In clinical studies thirty-nine patients with hereditary antithrombin III deficiency were treated with Antithrombin III (Human) on sixty separate occasions. In each case antithrombin III was given prophylactically or therapeutically. In 68% of the treatments the doses were between 30 and 50 IU per kg body weight per day and the duration of therapy was two to eight days (range one day to twenty weeks).

Twenty women were given forty-seven prophylactic treatments during delivery and postpartum. Twelve had previous thromboembolic complications. Further, seven women were treated during abortion, all of which had at least two previous incidences of thromboembolism. In all cases treated with antithrombin there was no incidence of thrombosis. The same results were obtained when nine surgical patients were treated (thirteen operations). There was no thrombosis in connection with treatment, although seven patients had previous

CLINICAL PHARMACOLOGY: *(cont'd)*

thrombosis. Additionally, eleven patients were treated for acute thrombosis. Five patients were treated with heparin alone without disappearance of soreness, swelling, and pain. Addition of Antithrombin III (Human) to the regimen reduced the thrombotic signs. The remaining six patients were treated with Antithrombin III (Human) in combination with oral anticoagulants and/or heparin. In all cases but one, the clinical signs of acute thrombosis were reduced or eliminated after the combined treatment.

A test for presence of depressor substance was performed on cats according to the procedure described in the United States Pharmacopeia XX, p. 890. Intravenous injection of Antithrombin III did not affect the blood pressure, heart rate, or respiration in any of the experiments performed (16).

During clinical investigations of Antithrombin III (Human), patients with hereditary deficiency were evaluated for evidence of hepatitis by clinical examination or laboratory tests. Patients with acquired antithrombin III deficiency and patients receiving multiple blood components were considered non-evaluable for the study. None of the evaluable patients demonstrated evidence of hepatitis.

Antithrombin III is heat-treated at 60 °C ±0.5 °C for not less than 10 hours. This heat-treatment process is similar to that reported to inactivate hepatitis B virus in a preparation of Antithrombin III (Human), as judged by inoculation of chimpanzees (21). Model viruses were used to assess the efficacy of the heat-treatment process. For herpes simplex virus type 1, Sindbis virus and vesicular stomatitis virus, this heat treatment procedure completely inactivated virus titers of 10^4-10^6 plaque forming units per ml (PFU/ml) (10). The same heat-treatment process has been shown to completely inactivate at least 10^4 ID_{50}-units of HIV, which was intentionally added to Antithrombin III (Human) (24).

No studies on overdose have been done. However, antithrombin III levels of 150-210% have been found in a few patients, and no signs or symptoms of complications have been identified.

INDICATIONS AND USAGE:

Antithrombin III (Human) is indicated for treatment of patients with hereditary antithrombin III deficiency in connection with surgical or obstetrical procedures or when they suffer from thromboembolism. Dosage should be determined so that the antithrombin III level in plasma is maintained higher than 80% (see PRECAUTIONS and DOSAGE AND ADMINISTRATION.)

Subjects with antithrombin III deficiency should be informed about the risk of thrombosis in connection with pregnancy and surgery and about the inheritance of the disease.

The diagnosis of hereditary antithrombin III deficiency should be based on a clear family history of venous thrombosis as well as decreased plasma antithrombin III levels, and the exclusion of acquired deficiency.

Antithrombin III in plasma may be measured with amidolytic assays by using synthetic chromogenic substrates, or with clotting assays, or with immunoassays. The latter does not detect all congenital antithrombin III deficiencies (19).

The antithrombin III level in neonates of parents with hereditary antithrombin III deficiency should be measured immediately after birth. (Fatal neonatal thromboembolism, such as aortic thrombi in children of women with hereditary antithrombin III deficiency, has been reported [2].) It is recommended that testing and treatment with Antithrombin III (Human) of such neonates be discussed with an expert on coagulation. (7).

CONTRAINDICATIONS:

None known.

WARNINGS:

This product is prepared from pooled units of human plasma which may contain the causative agents of hepatis and other viral diseases. Prescribed manufacturing procedures utilized at the plasma collection centers, plasma testing laboratories and the fractionation facilities are designed to reduce the risk of transmitting viral infection. However, the risk of viral infectivity from this product cannot be totally eliminated.

Individuals who receive infusions of blood or plasma products may develop signs and/or symptoms of some viral infections, particularly non A, non B hepatitis.

The anticoagulant effect of heparin is enhanced by concurrent treatment with Antithrombin III (Human) in patients with hereditary antithrombin III deficiency. Thus, in order to avoid bleeding, reduced dosage of heparin is recommended during treatment with Antithrombin III (Human).

PRECAUTIONS:

Recommended rate of infusion is 50 IU per minute (*i.e.,* 1 ml/min) and should not exceed 100 IU per minute (*i.e.,* 2 ml/min). One healthy subject became dyspneic after a rapid intravenous injection (1500 IU of Antithrombin III [Human] in 5 minutes) and his blood pressure increased.

The diagnosis of hereditary antithrombin III deficiency should be based on a clear family history of venous thrombosis as well as decreased plasma antithrombin III levels, and the exclusion of acquired deficiency.

It is recommended that antithrombin III plasma levels are monitored during the treatment period.

PREGNANCY CATEGORY C

Animal reproduction studies have not been conducted with Antithrombin III (Human). It is also not known whether Antithrombin III (Human) can cause fetal harm when administered to a pregnant woman or can affect reproduction capacity. Antithrombin III (Human) should be given to a pregnant woman only if clearly needed. However, studies in pregnant women have not shown that Antithrombin III (Human) increases the risk of fetal abnormalities if administered during the third trimester of pregnancy (7,18).

Thus far, antithrombin III concentrates have been used in twenty-three full-term pregnancies. All resulted in deliveries with no neonatal complications and with healthy children.

USE IN CHILDREN

Only a few neonates and children have so far been treated with Antithrombin III (Human). Safety and effectiveness in children have not yet been established.

ADVERSE REACTIONS:

No adverse reactions were reported in conjunction with clinical trials in hereditary antithrombin III deficient patients. However, two patients with acquired antithrombin III deficiency with severe disseminated intravascular coagulation, out of sixty-five studied, exhibited diuretic and vasodilatory effects. In one case, the recorded decrease in arterial systolic blood pressure was 25 mm Hg. The other decrease was not recorded.

DOSAGE AND ADMINISTRATION:

Each bottle of Antithrombin III (Human) is labeled with antithrombin III (AT-III) content expressed in international units (IU). The quantity of antithrombin III in 1 ml of normal pooled human plasma is conventionally taken as one unit. The potency assignment has been determined with a standard calibrated against a World Health Organization (WHO) Antithrombin III Reference Preparation.

The amount of Antithrombin III (Human) required to restore the recipient to a normal level varies with the circumstances and the patient. The dose must be individualized according to the needs of the patient and is dependent upon the weight of the patient, the degree of the deficiency and the desired level of antithrombin III to be achieved. It should be based on the medical judgement of the physician and on laboratory control values.

After the first dose the antithrombin III level should increase to about 120% of normal. Thereafter, it should be maintained at levels higher than 80%. In general, this may be achieved by administration of maintenance doses of Antithrombin III once every 24 hours. Initially and until the patient is stabilized the antithrombin III level should be measured at least twice a day, thereafter once a day, and always immediately before the next infusion.

The administration of one International Unit (IU) per kilogram body weight raises the level of antithrombin III (AT-III) by 1.0 to 2.1 percent depending on the condition of the patient. Thus, an initial loading dose of Antithrombin III may be calculated from the following formula (assuming a plasma volume of 40 ml/kg body weight):

Dosage Units = [Desired: AT-III: Level: (%): –: Baseline: AT-II: (%): x: Body: Weight: (kg)] ÷ [1.0%: (IU/kg)]

Thus, if a 70 kg individual has a baseline AT-III level of 57%, the initial Antithrombin III dose would be (120% - 57%) x 70/1.0 = 4410 IU.

Plasma AT-III levels should be measured preceding and 30 minutes after the dose, and the *in vivo* recovery calculated (9). If the recovery differs from an anticipated rise of 1% for each IU/kg administered, the formula should be modified accordingly. For example, if in the above example, the plasma level measured 30 minutes after the infusion is 147%, then the increases in AT-III measured per each 1IU/kg administered is [147% - 57%] x 70 kg/4410 units = 1.43% rise for each IU/kg administered. This would become the new recovery used in the above formula for subsequent infusions.

The above recommendations for dosing are provided only as a general guideline for therapy. The exact loading and maintenance dosages and dosing intervals should be individualized for each subject, based on the individual clinical conditions, response to therapy, and actual plasma AT-III levels achieved. Laboratory tests should be performed to assure that the desired levels are achieved.

When an infusion of Antithrombin III (Human) is indicated for a patient with hereditary deficiency to control an acute thrombotic episode or to prevent thrombosis following surgical or obstetrical procedures, it is desirable to raise the antithrombin III level to normal and maintain this level for 2 to 8 days depending on the indication for treatment, type and extensiveness of surgery, the patient's medical condition, past history and the physician's judgement. Concomitant administration of heparin in each of these situations should be based on the medical judgement of the physician.

Antithrombin III (Human) should be reconstituted by dissolving the powder in 10 ml Sterile Water for Injection, USP. Gently swirl the vial to dissolve the powder. Do not shake. The solution should be brought to room temperature and administered within 3 hours following reconstitution. Antithrombin III may be infused over 5 - 10 minutes. Antithrombin III (Human) should be administered intravenously.

Alternatively, Antithrombin III may be reconstituted with 0.9% Sodium Chloride Injection, USP or 5% Dextrose Injection, USP. After reconstitution Antithrombin III may be further diluted with the same diluent (8).

Parenteral drug products should be inspected visually for particulate matter and discoloration prior to administration whenever solution and container permit.

REFERENCES:

1. BICK R L. Clinical relevance of Antithrombin III. *Semin Thromb Hemostas* 1982, 8, 276. **2.** BJARKE B, HERIN P, BLOMBACK M. Neonatal aortic thrombosis. A possible clinical manifestation of congenital Antithrombin III deficiency. *Acta Paediatr Scand*1974, 63, 297-301. **3.** COLLEN D, SCHETZ J, DE COCK F, HOLMER E, VERSTRAETE M. Metabolism of antithrombin III (heparin cofactor) in man; effects of venous thrombosis and heparin administration. *Eur J Clin Invest*1977, 7, 27-35. **4.** COSGRIFF T M, BISHOP D T, HERSHGOLD E J, SKOLNICK M H, MARTIN B A, BATY B J, CARLSON K S. Familiar antithrombin III deficiency: Its natural history, genetics, diagnosis and treatment. *Medicine* 1983, 62, 209-220. **5.** EGEBERG O. Inherited antithrombin deficiency causing thrombophilia. *Thromb Diath Haemorrh* 1965, 3, 516-530. **6.** HEDNER U & ABILDGAARD U. Repair on the joint meeting of the task forces on nomenclature and standards of inhibitors of coagulation and fibrinolysis. *Thromb Haemost* (Stuttg) 1978, 39, 524-525. **7.** HELLGREN M, TENGBORN L, ABILDGAARD U. Pregnancy in women with congenital antithrombin III deficiency: Experience of treatment with heparin and antithrombin.*Gynecol Obstet Invest* 1982, 14, 127-141. **8.** HOGLUND U. Compatibility test performed on antithrombin, heat treated, added to sodium chloride and glucose infusion solutions. Data on file, Kabi Pharmacia AB. **9.** JAVELIN L. Antithrombin, heat treated - recovery *in vivo*. Data on file, Kabi Pharmacia AB. **10.** Lieu M. Inactivation of model viruses in heat-treated, Antithrombin III. Data on file, Kabi Pharmacia AB. **11.** MARCINIAK E, FARLEY C, H, DESIMONE P A. Familial thrombosis due to antithrombin III deficiency.*Blood* 1974, 43, 219-231. **12.** McDOUGAL S J, MARTIN L S, CORT S P, MOZEN M, HELDEBRANT C M, EVATT B. Thermal inactivation of the acquired immunodeficiency syndrome Virus, Human T Lymphotropic Virus III/Lymph-adenopathy-associated Virus, with Special Reference to Antihemophilic Factor. *J Clin Invest Inc*1985, 76, 875-877. **13.** MURANO G, WILLIAMS L, MILLER-ANDERSON M, ARONSON D L, KING C. Some properties of antithrombin-III and its concentration in human plasma. *Thromb Res* 1980, 18, 259-262. **14.** NORDENMAN B, NYSTROM C, BJORK I. The size and shape of human and bovine antithrombin III. *Eur J Biochem*1977, 78, 195-203. **15.** PENNER J A, HASSOUNA M J, HUNTER M J, CHOCKELY M. A clinical silent antithrombin III defect in an Ann Arbor family. *Clin Res* 1979, 27, 303. **16.** PIHL B. Antithrombin III - test for depressor substances on a heat-treated preparation. Data on file, Kabi Pharmacia AB. **17.** ROSENBERG R D. Actions and interactions of antithrombin and heparin.*N Eng J Med* 1975, 292, 146-151. **18.** SAMSON D, STIRLING Y, WOOLF L, HOWARTH D, SEGHATCHIAN M J, DE CHAZAL R. Management of planned pregnancy in a patient with congenital antithrombin III deficiency. *Br J Haematol* 1984, 56, 243-249. **19.** SAS G, BLASKO G, BANHEGYI D, JAKO J, PALOS L A. Abnormal antithrombin III (Antithrombin III "Budapest") as a cause of a familial thrombophilia.*Thromp Diath Haemorrh* (Stuttg) 1974, 32, 105-115. **20.** SCHAFER A I. Hypercoagulable states. *Annals of Internal Medicine*1985, 102, 814-828. **21.** TABOR E, MURANO G, SNOY P, GERETY R J. Inactivation of hepatitis B virus by heat in antithrombin III stabilized with citrate. *Thromb Res* 1981, 22, 233-238. **22.** TENGBORN L, FROHM B, NILSSON L-E. Catabolism and coagulation properties of heat treated antithrombin III concentrate. *Thromb Res* 1987, 48, 701- 711. **23.** WINTER J H & DOUGLASS A S. Familiar venous thrombosis.*Postgrad Med J* 1983, 59, 677-689. **24.** EINARSSON M, ET AL. Heat inactivation of human immunodeficiency virus in solutions of antithrombin III. *Transfusion* 1989, 29, 148-152.

HOW SUPPLIED:

Antithrombin III (Human) is supplied as a lyophilized powder in 50 ml infusion bottles containing 500 IU of Antithrombin III. Each bottle of Antithrombin III is accompanied by 10 ml Sterile Water for Injection, USP.

Storage: Antithrombin III should be stored at 2 to 8 °C.

HOW SUPPLIED - EQUIVALENTS NOT AVAILABLE:

Injection, Solution - Intravenous - 500 unit

1's	$1.25	**ATNATIV, Baxter Hyland**	**00944-0996-01**
500 unit	$1.25	**ATNATIV 500 UNT, Kabi Vitrum**	**00601-0130-50**

Injection, Solution - Intravenous - 580 unit

1's	$0.86	THROMBATE III, Bayer Pharm	00192-0603-20

Injection, Solution - Intravenous - 1125 unit

1's	$0.86	THROMBATE III, Bayer Pharm	00192-0603-30

APRACLONIDINE HYDROCHLORIDE *(000276)*

CATEGORIES: Alpha Adrenergic Agonists; EENT Drugs; Eye, Ear, Nose, & Throat Preparations; Miotics; Ocular Hypertension; Ophthalmics; Surgical Aid, Ophthalmic; Pregnancy Category C; FDA Approved 1987 Dec

BRAND NAMES: **Iopidine**

DESCRIPTION:

This monograph contains prescribing information for both Iopidine Ophthalmic Solution and Iopidine 0.5% Ophthalmic Solution.

BOTH FORMS

Iopidine Ophthalmic Solution and Iopidine 0.5% Ophthalmic Solution contain apraclonidine hydrochloride, an alpha adrenergic agonist, in a sterile isotonic solution for topical application to the eye. Apraclonidine hydrochloride is a white to off-white powder and is highly soluble in water. Its chemical name is 2-[(4- amino-2,6 dichlorophenyl)imino]imidazolidine monohydrochloride with an empirical formula of $C_9H_{11}Cl_3N_4$.

IOPIDINE OPHTHALMIC SOLUTION

The molecular weight is 281.60. Its ingredients are: Active: Apraclonidine hydrochloride 11.5 mg equivalent to apraclonidine base 10 mg. Preservative: Benzalkonium chloride 0.01%. Inactive: Sodium chloride, sodium acetate, sodium hydroxide and/or hydrochloric acid (pH 4.4-7.8) and purified water.

IOPIDINE 0.5% OPHTHALMIC SOLUTION

The molecular weight is 281.57. Its ingredients are: Active: Apraclonidine hydrochloride 5.73 mg equivalent to apraclonidine base 5 mg. Preservative: Benzalkonium chloride 0.01%. Inactive: Sodium chloride, sodium acetate, sodium hydroxide and/or hydrochloric acid (pH 4.4-7.8) and purified water.

CLINICAL PHARMACOLOGY:

APRACLONIDINE HCL OPHTHALMIC SOLUTION

Apraclonidine HCl is a relatively selective alpha adrenergic agonist and does not have significant membrane stabilizing (local anesthetic) activity. When instilled into the eye, apraclonidine hydrochloride Ophthalmic Solution has the action of reducing intraocular pressure. Ophthalmic apraclonidine has minimal effect on cardiovascular parameters.

Optic nerve head damage and visual field loss may result from an acute elevation in intraocular pressure that can occur after argon or Nd:YAG laser surgical procedures. Elevated intraocular pressure, whether acute or chronic in duration, is a major risk factor in the pathogenesis of visual field loss. The higher the peak or spike of intraocular pressure, the greater the likelihood of visual field loss and optic nerve damage especially in patients with previously compromised nerve optic nerves. The onset of action with Apraclonidine Ophthalmic Solution can usually be noted within one hour and the maximum intraocular pressure reduction usually occurs three to five hours after application of a single dose. The precise mechanism of the ocular hypotensive action of Apraclonidine Ophthalmic Solution is not completely established at this time. Aqueous fluorophotometry studies in man suggest that its predominant action may be related to a reduction of aqueous formation. Controlled clinical studies of patients requiring argon laser trabeculoplasty, argon laster iridotomy or Nd:YAG posterior capsulotomy showed that Apraclonidine Ophthalmic Solution controlled or prevented the postsurgical intraocular pressure rise typically observed in patients after undergoing those procedures. After surgery, the mean intraocular pressure was 1.2 to 4.0 mmHg below the corresponding presurgical baseline pressure before Apraclonidine Ophthalmic Solution treatment. With placebo treatment, postsurgical pressures were 2.5 to 8.4 mmHg higher than their corresponding presurgical baselines. Overall, only 2% of patients treated with Apraclonidine pressure elevations (spike ≥ 10 mmHg) during the first three hours after laser surgery, whereas 22% of placebo-treated patients responded with severe pressure spikes (see TABLE 1.) Of the patients that experienced a pressure spike after surgery, the peak intraocular pressure was above 30 mmHg in seven patients (see TABLE 2) and was above 50 mmHg in seven placebo-treated patients and one Apraclonidine HCl Ophthalmic Solution treated patient.

TABLE 1 Incidence of Intraocular Pressure Spikes ≥ 10 mmHg

			Treatment			
			Apraclonidine HCl		Placebo	
Study	Laser Procedure	P-value	[a]N	(%)	[a]N	(%)
1	Trabeculoplasty	<0.05	0/40	(0%)	6/35	(17%)
2	Trabeculoplasty	-0.06	2/41	(5%)	8/42	(19%)
1	Iridotomy	<0.05	0/11	(0%)	4/10	(40%)
2	Iridotomy	-0.05	0/17	(0%)	4/19	(21%)
1	Nd:YAG Capsulotomy	<0.05	3/80	(4%)	19/83	(23%)
2	Nd:YAG Capsulotomy	<0.05	0/83	(0%)	22/81	(27%)

a N - Number Spikes/Number Eyes.

TABLE 2 Magnitude of Postsurgical Intraocular Pressure in Trabeculoplasty, Iridotomy and Nd:YAG Capsulotomy Patients With Severe Pressure Spikes ≥ 10 mmHg

		Maximum Postsurgical Intraocular Pressure (mmHg)			
Treatment	Total Spikes	20-29 mmHg	30-39 mmHg	40-49 mmHg	>50 mmHg
Apraclonidine	8	1	4	2	1
Placebo	78	16	47	8	7

APRACLONIDINE HCL 0.5% OPHTHALMIC SOLUTION

Apraclonidine hydrochloride is a relatively selective alpha-2-adrenergic agonist. When instilled in the eye, Apraclonidine 0.5% Ophthalmic Solution, has the action of reducing elevated as well as normal intraocular pressure (IOP), whether or not accompanied by glaucoma. Ophthalmic apraclonidine has minimal effect on cardiovascular parameters.

Elevated IOP presents a major risk factor in glaucomatous field loss. The higher the level of IOP the greater the likelihood of optic nerve damage and visual field loss. Apraclonidine HCl 0.5% Ophthalmic Solution has the action of reducing IOP. The onset of action of apraclonidine can usually be noted within one hour, and maximum IOP reduction occurs about three hours after installation. Aqueous flurophotometry studies demonstrate that Apraclonidine's predominant mechanism of action is reduction of aqueous flow via stimulation of the alpha-adrenergic system.

Repeated dose response and comparative studies (0.125% -1.0% apraclonidine) demonstrate that 0.5% apraclonidine is at the top of the dose/response IOP reduction curve.

The clinical utility of Apraclonidine HCl 0.5% Ophthalmic Solution is most apparent for those glaucoma patients on maximally tolerated medical therapy. Patients on maximally tolerated medical therapy with uncontrolled IOP and scheduled to undergo laster

CLINICAL PHARMACOLOGY: *(cont'd)*

trabeculoplasty or trabeculetomy surgery were enrolled into a double-masked, placebo- controlled, multi-center clinical trial to determine if Apraclonidine HCl 0.5% Ophthalmic Solution, dosed three times daily (TID), could delay the need for surgery for up to three months.

All patients enrolled into this trial had advanced glaucoma and were undergoing maximally tolerated medical therapy, i.e., patients were using combinations of a topical beta blocker, sympathomimetics, parasympathomimetics and oral carbonic anhydrase inhibitors. Patients were considered to be treatment failures in this study if, in the opinion of the investigators, their IOP was uncontrolled by the masked study medication or there was evidence of further optic nerve damage or visual field loss, and surgery was indicated. Of 171 patients receiving masked medication, 84 were treated with Apraclonidine HCl 0.5% Ophthalmic Solution and 87 were treated with placebo (Apraclonidine vehicle).

Apraclonidine HCl treatment resulted in a significantly greater percentage of treatment successes compared to patients treated with placebo. In this placebo controlled maximum therapy trial, 14.3% of patients treated with Apraclonidine HCl 0.5% Ophthalmic Solution were discontinued due to adverse events, primarily allergic-like reactions (12.9%).

The IOP lowering efficacy of Apraclonidine HCl 0.5% Ophthalmic Solution diminishes over time in some patients. This loss of effect, or tachyphylaxis, appears to be an individual occurrence with a variable time of onset and should be closely monitored.

An unpredictable decrease of IOP control in some patients and incidence of ocular allergic responses and systemic side effects may limit the utility of Apraclonidine HCl 0.5% Ophthalmic Solution. However, patients on maximally tolerated medical therapy may still benefit from the additional IOP reduction provided by the short-term use of Apraclonidine HCl 0.5% Ophthalmic Solution.

Topical use of Apraclonidine HCl 0.5% Ophthalmic Solution leads to systemic absorption. Studies of Apraclonidine HCl 0.5% Ophthalmic Solution dosed one drop three times a day in both eyes for 10 days in normal volunteers yielded mean peak and trough concentrations of 0.9 ng/ml and 0.5 ng/ml, respectively. The half-life of Apraclonidine HCl 0.5% Ophthalmic Solution was calculated to be 8 hours.

Apraclonidine HCl 0.5% Ophthalmic Solution, because of its alpha adrenergic activity, is a vasoconstrictor. Single dose ocular blood flow studies in monkeys, using the microsphere technique, demonstrated a reduced blood flow for the anterior segment; however, no reduction in blood flow was observed in the posterior segment of the eye after a topical dose of Apraclonidine HCl 0.5% Ophthalmic Solution. Ocular blood flow studies have not been conducted in humans.

INDICATIONS AND USAGE:

APRACLONIDINE OPHTHALMIC SOLUTION

Apraclonidine hydrochloride Ophthalmic Solution is indicated to control or prevent postsurgical elevations in intraocular pressure that occur in patients after argon laser trabeculoplasty, argon laser, iridotomy or Nd:YAG posterior capsulotomy.

APRACLONIDINE 0.5% OPHTHALMIC SOLUTION

Apraclonidine HCl 0.5% Ophthalmic Solution is indicated for short-term adjunctive therapy in patients on maximally tolerated medical therapy who require additional IOP reduction. Patients on maximally tolerated medical therapy who are treated with Apraclonidine HCl 0.5% Ophthalmic Solution to delay surgery should have frequent followup examinations and treatment should be discontinued if the intraocular pressure rises significantly.

The addition of Apraclonidine HCl 0.5% Ophthalmic Solution to patients already using two aqueous suppressing drugs (*i.e.*, beta-blocker plus carbonic anhydrase inhibitor) as part of their maximally tolerated medical therapy may not provide additional benefit. This is because Apraclonidine HCl 0.5% Ophthalmic Solution is an aqueous suppressant may not significantly reduce IOP.

The IOP lowering efficacy of Apraclonidine HCl 0.5% Ophthalmic Solution diminishes over time in some patients. This loss of effect, or tachyphylaxis, appears to be an individual occurrence with a variable time of onset and should be closely monitored. The benefit for most patients is less than one month.

CONTRAINDICATIONS:

BOTH FORMS

Apraclonidine HCl Ophthalmic Solution and Apraclonidine HCl 0.5% Ophthalmic Solution are contraindicated in patients receiving monoamine oxidase inhibitor therapy and for patients with hypersensitivity to any component of this medication or to clonidine.

WARNINGS:

APRACLONIDINE HCL 0.5% OPHTHALMIC SOLUTION

Not for injection or oral ingestion. Topical ophthalmic use only.

PRECAUTIONS:

GENERAL

Apraclonidine HCl Ophthalmic Solution: Since Apraclonidine HCl Ophthalmic Solution is a potent depressor of intraocular pressure, patients who develop exaggerated reductions in intraocular pressure should be closely monitored.

Although the acute administration of two drops of Apraclonidine HCl Ophthalmic Solution has minimal effect on heart rate or blood pressure in clinical studies evaluating patients undergoing anterior segment laser surgery, the preclinical pharmacologic profile of this drug suggests that caution should be observed in treating patients with severe cardiovascular disease including hypertension.

The possibility of a vasovagal attack occurring during laser surgery should be considered and caution used in patients with history of such episodes.

No adverse ocular effects were observed in cynomolgus monkeys treated with two drops of 1.5% Apraclonidine HCl Ophthalmic Solution applied three times daily for three months. No corneal changes were observed in 320 humans given at least one dose of 1.0% Apraclonidine HCl Ophthalmic Solution.

Apraclonidine HCl 0.5% Ophthalmic Solution: Glaucoma patients on maximally tolerated medical therapy who are treated with Apraclonidine HCl 0.5% Ophthalmic Solution to delay surgery should have their visual fields monitored periodically.

Although the topical use of Apraclonidine HCl 0.5% Ophthalmic Solution has not been studied in renal failure patients, structurally related clonidine undergoes a significant increase in half-life in patients with severe reanl impairment. Close montioring of cardiovascualr parameters in patients with impaired renal function is advised if they are candidates for topical Apraclonidine HCl therapy. Close monitoring of cardiovascular parameters in patients with impaired liver function is also advised as the systemic dosage form of clonidine is partly metabolized in the liver.

While the topical administration of Apraclonidine HCl 0.5% Ophthalmic Solution had minimal effect on heart rate or blood pressure in clinical studies evaluating glaucoma patients, the preclinical pharmacology profile of this drug suggest that caution should be observed in treating patients with severe, uncontrolled cardiovascular disease, including hypertension.

PRECAUTIONS: *(cont'd)*

Apraclonidine HCl 0.5% Ophthalmic Solution should be used with caution in patients with coronary insufficiency, recent myocardial infarction, cerebrovascular disease, chronic renal failure, Raynaud's disease, or thromboangiitis obliterans. Caution and monitoring of depressed patients are advised since Apraclonidine has been infrequently associated with depression. Apraclonidine HCl can cause dizziness and somnolence. Patients who engage in hazardous activities requiring mental alertness should be warned of the potential for a decrease in mental alertness while using Apraclonidine.

Use of Apraclonidine HCl 0.5% Ophthalmic Solution can lead to allergic-like reaction characterized wholly or in part by the symptoms of hyperemia, pruritus, discomfort, tearing, foreign body sensation, and edema of the lids and conjunctiva. If ocular allergic-like symptoms occur, Apraclonidine HCl 0.5% Ophthalmic Solution therapy should be discontinued.

Both Forms: Topical ocular administration of two drops of 0.5%, 1.0% and 1.5% Apraclonidine HCl Ophthalmic Solution to New Zealand Albino rabbits three times daily for one month resulted in sporadic and transient instances of minimal corneal cloudiness in the 1.5% group only; no histopathological changes were noted in those eyes.

CARCINOGENESIS, MUTAGENESIS, AND IMPAIRMENT OF FERTILITY

Apraclonidine HCl Ophthalmic Solution: In a variety of *in vitro* cell assays, apraclonidine was nonmutagenic. Studies addressing carcinogenesis and the impairment of fertility have not been conducted.

Apraclonidine HCl 0.5% Ophthalmic Solution: No significant change in tumor incidence or type was observed following two years of oral administration of apraclonidine HCl to rats and mice at dosages of 1.0 and 0.6 mg/kg, up to 20 and 12 times, respectively, the maximum dose recommended for human topical ocular use.

Apraclonidine HCl was not a mutagenic in a series of *in vitro* mutagenicity tests, including the Ames test, a mouse lymphoma forward mutation assay, a chromosome aberration assay in cultured Chinese hamster ovary (CHO) cells, a sister chromatid exchange assay in (CHO) cells, and a cell transformation assay. An *in vivo* mouse micronucleus assay conducted with apraclonidine HCl also provided no evidence of mutagenicity.

Reproduction and fertility studies in rats showed no adverse effects on male or female fertility at a dose of 0.5 mg/kg (5 to 10 times the maximum recommended human dose).

PREGNANCY CATEGORY C

Apraclonidine HCl Ophthalmic Solution: There are no adequate and well controlled studies of Apraclonidine HCl Ophthalmic Solution in pregnant women. Animal reproduction studies have not been conducted with apraclonidine hydrochloride. This medication should be used in pregnancy only if the potential benefit to the mother justifies the potential risk to the fetus.

Apraclonidine HCl 0.5% Ophthalmic Solution: Apraclonidine HCl has been shown to have an embryocidal effect in rabbits when given in an oral dose of 3.0 mg/kg (60 times the maximum recommedned human dose). Dose related maternal toxicity was observed in pregnant rats at 0.3 mg/kg (6 times the maximum recommended human dose). There are no adequate and well controlled studies in pregnant women. Apraclonidine HCl 0.5% Ophthalmic Solution should be used during pregnancy only if the potential benefit justifies the potential risk to the fetus.

NURSING MOTHERS

Apraclonidine HCl Solution: It is not known if topically applied Apraclonidine Ophthalmic Solution is excreted in human milk. A decision should be considered to discontinue nursing temporarily for the one day on which Apraclonidine HCl Ophthalmic Solution is used.

Apraclonidine HCl 0.5% Ophthalmic Solution: It is not known whether this drug is excreted in human milk. Because many drugs are excreted in human milk, caution should be exercised when Apraclonidine HCl 0.5% Ophthalmic Solution is administered to a nursing woman.

PEDIATRIC USE

Both Forms: Safety and effectiveness in pediatric patients have not been established.

PATIENT INFORMATION

Apraclonidine HCl 0.5% Ophthalmic Solution: Do not touch dropper tip to any surface as this may contaminate the contents.

ADVERSE REACTIONS:

APRACLONIDINE HCL OPHTHALMIC SOLUTION

The following adverse events were reported in association with the use of Apraclonidine HCl Opthalmic Solution in laser surgery: ocular injection (1.8%), upper lid elevation (1.3%), irregular heart rate (0.7%), ocular inflammation (0.45%), nasal decongestion (0.45%) conjunctival blanching (0.4%) and mydriasis (0.4%).

The following adverse events were observed in investigational studies dosing Apraclonidine HCl Opthalmic Solution once or twice daily for up to 28 days in nonlaser studies:

Ocular: Conjunctival blanching, upper lid elevation, mydriasis, burning, discomfort, foreign body sensation, dryness, itching, hypotony, blurred or dimmed vision, allergic response, Conjunctival microhemorrhage.

Gastrointestinal: Abdominal pain, diarrhea, stomach discomfort, emesis.

Cardiovascular: Bradycardia, vasovagal attack, palpitations, orthostatic episode.

Central Nervous System: Insomnia, dream disturbances, irritability, decreased libido.

Other: Taste abnormalities, dry mouth, nasal burning or dryness, headache, head cold sensation, chest heaviness or burning, clammy or sweaty palms, body heat sensation, shortness of breath, increased pharyngeal secretion, extremity pain or numbness, fatigue, paresthesia, pruritus not associated with rash.

APRACLONIDINE HCL 0.5% OPHTHALMIC SOLUTION

Use of Apraclonidine HCl 0.5% Ophthalmic Solution can lead to an allergic-like reaction characterized wholly or in part by the symptoms of hyperemia, pruritus, discomfort, tearing, foreign body sensation, and edema of the lids and conjunctiva. If ocular allergic-like symptoms occur, Apraclonidine HCl 0.5% Ophthalmic Solution therapy should be discontinued.

In clinical studies the overall discontinuation rate related to Apraclonidine HCl 0.5% Ophthalmic Solution was 15%. The most commonly reported events leading to discontinuation included (in decreasing order of frequency) hyperemia, pruritus, tearing, discomfort, lid edema, dry mouth, and foreign body sensation. The following adverse reactions (incidences) were reported in clinical studies of Apraclonidine HCl 0.5% (Apraclonidine HCl Ophthalmic Solution) as being possibly, probably, or definitely related to therapy:

Ocular: Hyperemia (13%), pruritus (10%), discomfort (6%), tearing (4%). The following adverse reactions were reported in less than 3% of the patients: lid edema, blurred vision, foreign body sensation, dry eye, conjunctivitis, discharge, blanching. The following adverse reactions were reported in less than 1% of the patients: lid margin crusting, conjunctival follicles, conjunctival edema, edema, abnormal vision, pain, lid disorder, keratitis, blepharitis, photophobia, corneal staining, lid erythema, blepharoconjunctivitis, irritation, corneal erosion, corneal infiltrate, keratopathy, lid scales, lid retraction.

Nonocular Body as a Whole: The following adverse reactions were reported in less than 3% of the patients: headache, asthenia. The following adverse reactions (incidences) were reported in less than 1% of the patients: chest pain, abnormal coordination, malaise, facial edema.

ADVERSE REACTIONS: *(cont'd)*

Cardiovascular: The following adverse reactions were reported in less than 1% of the patients: peripheral edema, arrhythmia. Although no reports of bradycardia related to Apraclonidine HCl 0.5% Ophthalmic Solution were available from clinical studies, the possibility of its occurrence based on Apraclonidine's alpha-2-agonist effect should be considered (see CLINICAL PHARMACOLOGY.)

Central Nervous System: The following adverse reactions were reported in less than 1% of the patients: somnolence, dizziness, nervousness, depression, insomnia, paresthesia.

Digestive System: Dry mouth (10%). The following adverse reactions were reported in less than 1% of the patients: constipation, nausea.

Musculoskeletal: Myalgia (0.2%).

Respiratory System: Dry nose (2%). The following adverse reactions were reported in less than 1% of the patients: rhinitis, dyspnea, pharyngitis, asthma.

Skin: The following adverse reactions were reported in less than 1% of the patients: contact dermatitis, dermatitis.

Special Senses: Taste perversion (3%), parosmia (0.2%).

OVERDOSAGE:

BOTH FORMS

While no instances of accidental or intentional ingestion of ophthalmic apraclonidine are known, overdose with the oral form of clonidine has been reported to cause hypotension, transient hypertension, asthenia, vomiting, irritability, diminished or absent reflexes, lethargy, somnolence, sedation, or coma, pallor, hypothermia, bradycardia, conduction defects, arrhythmias, dryness of the mouth, miosis, apnea, respiratory depression, hypoventilation, and seizure. Treatment of an oral overdose includes supportive and symptomatic therapy, a patent airway should be maintained. Hemodialysis is of limited value since a maximum of 5% of circulating drug is removed.

DOSAGE AND ADMINISTRATION:

APRACLONIDINE HCL OPHTHALMIC SOLUTION

One drop of Apraclonidine HCl Ophthalmic Solution should be instilled in the scheduled operative eye one hour before initiating anterior segment laser surgery and a second drop should be instilled to the same eye immediately upon completion of the laser surgical procedure. Use a separate container for each single- drop dose and discard each container after use.

APRACLONIDINE HCL 0.5% OPHTHALMIC SOLUTION

One to two drops of Apraclonidine HCl 0.5% Ophthalmic Solution should be instilled in the affected eye(s); three times daily. Since Apraclonidine HCl 0.5% Ophthalmic Solution will be used with other ocular glaucoma therapies, an approximate 5 minute interval between instillation of each medication should be practiced to prevent washout of the previous dose.

NOT FOR INJECTION INTO THE EYE.

NOT FOR ORAL INGESTION.

HOW SUPPLIED:

IOPIDINE OPHTHALMIC SOLUTION

Apraclonidine hydrochloride Ophthalmic Solution 1% as base is a sterile, isotonic, aqueous solution containing apraclonidine hydrochloride.

Supplied as follows: 0.1 ml in plastic ophthlamic dispensers, packaged two per pouch. These dispensers are enclosed in a foil over-wrap as an added barrier to evaporation.

Storage: Store at room temperature: Protect from light.

IOPIDINE 0.5% OPHTHALMIC SOLUTION

Iopidine 0.5% Ophthalmic Solution as base in a sterile, isotonic, aqueous solution containing apraclonidine hydrochloride.

Supplied in plastic in ophthalmic DROP-CONTAINER dispenser as follows:

Storage: Store between 2-27°C (36-80°F).

Protect from freezing and light.

(Both forms: Alcon Laboratories, 1/95)

HOW SUPPLIED - EQUIVALENTS NOT AVAILABLE:

Solution - Ophthalmic - 0.5 %

5 ml	$35.31	IOPIDINE, Alcon	00065-0665-05
10 ml	$65.50	IOPIDINE, Alcon	00065-0665-10

Solution - Ophthalmic - 1 %

0.2 ml x 12	$142.50	IOPIDINE, Alcon	00065-0660-10

APROBARBITAL *(000277)*

CATEGORIES: Anxiolytics, Sedatives, Hypnotic; Barbiturates; Central Nervous System Agents; Hypnotics; Insomnia; Sedatives; Sedatives/Hypnotics; Pregnancy Category D; DEA Class CIII; FDA Pre 1938 Drugs

BRAND NAMES: **Alurate**

Prescribing information not available at time of publication.

For How Supplied Information, Contact Roche

APROTININ BOVINE *(003183)*

CATEGORIES: Antiheparin Agents; Bleeding; Blood Formation/Coagulation; Coagulants and Anticoagulants; Fibrinogen; Fibrinolytic & Proteolytic; Hemostatics; Orphan Drugs; FDA Class 1P ("Priority Review"); FDA Approved 1993 Dec

BRAND NAMES: *Antagosan* (France); *Aprotimbin*; *Fase*; *Iniprol* (France); *Midran*; *Pantinol*; *Protosol*; **Trasylol**; *Trazinine*
(International brand names outside U.S. in italics)

DESCRIPTION:

Trasylol (aprotinin injection), $C_{284}H_{432}N_{84}O_{79}S_7$, is a natural proteinase inhibitor obtained from bovine lung. Aprotinin (molecular weight of 6512 daltons) consists of 58 amino acid residues that are arranged in a single polypeptide chain, cross-linked by three disulfide bridges. It is supplied as a clear, colorless, sterile isotonic solution for intravenous administration. Each milliliter contains 10,000 KIU (Kallikrein Inhibitor Units) (1.4 mg/ml) and 9 mg sodium chloride in water for injection. Hydrochloric acid and/or sodium hydroxide is used to adjust the pH to 4.5-6.5.

CLINICAL PHARMACOLOGY:

MECHANISM OF ACTION

Aprotinin is a protease inhibitor with a variety of effects on the coagulation system. It inhibits plasmin and kallikrein, thus directly affecting fibrinolysis. It also inhibits the contact phase activation of coagulation which both initiates coagulation and promotes fibrinolysis. In addition to these effects on the clotting and lysis cascades in blood, aprotinin preserves the adhesive glycoproteins in the platelet membrane making them resistant to damage from the increased plasmin levels and mechanical injury that occur during cardiopulmonary bypass (CPB). The net effect is to inhibit both fibrinolysis and turnover of coagulation factors, and to decrease bleeding, although the precise mechanism of this effect is unclear.

Patients undergoing cardiac surgery with extracorporeal circulation by a heart-lung machine (cardiopulmonary bypass; CPB) develop adverse changes of their blood components, blood cells and specific coagulation proteins. These changes cause a transient hemostatic defect during the intraoperative and immediate postoperative period which may result in diffuse bleeding despite correct surgical technique. At times, this blood loss is severe enough to require multiple blood transfusions and even surgical re-exploration.

PHARMACOKINETICS

The studies comparing the pharmacokinetics of aprotinin in healthy volunteers, cardiac patients undergoing surgery with cardiopulmonary bypass, and women undergoing hysterectomy suggest linear pharmacokinetics over the dose range of 50,000 KIU to 2 million KIU. After intravenous (IV) injection, rapid distribution of aprotinin occurs into the total extracellular space, leading to a rapid initial decrease in plasma aprotinin concentration. Following this distribution phase, a plasma half-life of about 150 minutes is observed. At later time points, (*i.e.*, beyond 5 hours after dosing) there is a terminal elimination phase with a half-life of about 10 hours.

Average steady state intraoperative plasma concentrations were 137 KIU/ml (n=10) after administration of the following dosage regimen: 1 million KIU IV loading dose, 1 million KIU IV loading dose, 1 million KIU into the pump prime volume, 250,000 KIU per hour of operation as continuous intravenous infusion (Regimen B). Average steady state intraoperative plasma concentrations were 250 KIU/ml in patients (n=20) treated with aprotinin during cardiac surgery by administration of Regimen A (exactly double Regimen B): 2 million KIU IV loading dose, 2 million KIU into the pump prime volume, 500,000 KIU per hour of operation as continuous intravenous infusion.

Following a single IV dose of radiolabelled aprotinin, approximately 25-40% of the radioactivity is excreted in the urine over 48 hours. After a 30 minute infusion of 1 million KIU, about 2% is excreted as unchanged drugs. After a larger dose of 2 million KIU infused over 30 minutes, urinary excretion of unchanged aprotinin accounts for approximately 9% of the dose. Animal studies have shown that aprotinin is accumulated primarily in the kidney. Aprotinin, after being filtered by the glomeruli, is active reabsorbed by the proximal tubules in which it is stored in phagolysosomes. Aprotinin is slowly degraded by lysosomal enzymes. The physiological renal handling of aprotinin is similar to that of other small proteins, e.g. insulin.

CLINICAL STUDIES:

Two placebo-controlled, double-blind studies of Aprotinin were conducted in the United States involving 523 patients undergoing repeat coronary artery bypass graft (CABG) surgery, of whom 463 were valid for efficacy analysis. The following treatments were used in the studies: Aprotinin Regimen A (2 million KIU IV loading dose, 2 million KIU into the pump prime volume, 500,000 KIU IV per hour of surgery as a continuous intravenous infusion); Aprotinin Regimen B (1 million KIU IV loading dose, 1 million KIU into the pump prime volume, 250,000 KIU per hour of surgery as a continuous intravenous infusion); a pump prime regimen (2 million KIU into the pump prime volume only); and a placebo regimen (normal saline). In the three studies fewer patients receiving either regimen of Aprotinin (either Regimen A or Regimen B) required any donor blood in comparison to the placebo regimen (TABLE 1)

TABLE 1 Repeat Cabg Patients Who Required Donor Blood

	PLACEBO REGIMEN	APROTININ PUMP PRIME REGIMEN	APROTININ REGIMEN B	APROTININ REGIMEN A
Study 1	40/52 (77%)	Not Studied	23/49 (47%)*	22/53 (42%)*
Study 2	23/32 (72%)	Not Studied	Not Studied	7/23 (30%)*
Study 3	49/65 (75%)	49/68 (72%)	28/60 (47%)*	33/61 (54%)*

* $p \leq 0.0072$ compared to placebo

The number of units of donor blood required by patients was also reduced by Aprotinin Regimens A and B when compared to the placebo regimen:

TABLE 2 UNITS OF DONOR BLOOD REQUIRED BY REPEAT CABG PATIENTS

Study 1

	PLACEBO REGIMEN	APROTINEN REGIMEN B	APROTINEN REGIMEN A
MEAN ± SE	3.5 ± 0.6*	2.0 ± 0.6**	1.8 ± 0.6*
RANGE	0-34	0-18	0-24
MEDIAN	2	0	0

* $p \leq 0.001$ compared to placebo, ANOVA on ranks
** p=0.005 compared to placebo, ANOVA on ranks

Study 2

	PLACEBO REGIMEN	APROTINEN REGIMEN A
MEAN ± SE	3.3 ± 0.7*	0.4 ± 0.8*
RANGE	0-20	0-5
MEDIAN	4	0

* p=0.0001 compare to placebo, ANOVA on ranks

Study 3

	PLACEBO REGIMEN	APROTININ PUMP PRIME REGIMEN	APROTININ REGIMEN B	APROTININ REGIMEN A
MEAN ± SE	3.4 ± 0.5	2.5 ± 0.3	2.3 ± 0.8*	1.6 ± 0.2*
RANGE	0-17	0-13	0-46	0-6
MEDIAN	3.0	2.0	0.0	1.0

* $p \leq 0.0001$ compared to placebo (ANOVA on ranks)

CLINICAL STUDIES: *(cont'd)*

Study 2 also included 151 patients undergoing primary CABG surgery; 74 of the patients receiving Aprotinin and 67 of the patients receiving placebo were valid for efficacy analysis. Fewer patients receiving Aprotinin required any donor blood:

TABLE 3 PRIMARY CABG PATIENTS WHO REQUIRED DONOR BLOOD

	Study 2
PLACEBO REGIMEN	**APROTININ REGIMEN A**
35/67 (52%)	28/74 (38%)
* p=052 compared to placebo	

TABLE 4 UNITS OF DONOR BLOOD REQUIRED BY PRIMARY CABG PATIENTS

	Study 2	
	PLACEBO REGIMEN	**APROTININ REGIMEN A**
MEAN ± SE	2.1 ± 0.3*	1.1 ± 0.3*
RANGE	0-15	0-10
MEDIAN	1	0
* p=0.0246 compared to placebo, ANOVA on ranks		

In these three studies there was no diminution of benefit with age. Male and female patients received benefits from Aprotinin in terms of a reduction in the average number of units of donor blood transfused. Male patients did better than female patients in terms of the percentage of patients who required any donor blood transfusions. However, the number of female patients studied was small.

A double-blind, randomized, Canadian study compared Aprotinin Regimen A (n=28) and placebo (n=23) in primary cardiac surgery patients (mainly CABG) requiring cardiopulmonary bypass who were treated with aspirin within 48 hours of surgery. The mean total blood loss (1209.7 ml vs. 2532.3 ml) and the mean number of units of packed red blood cells transfused (1.6 units vs. 4.3 units) were significantly less ($p<0.008$) in the Aprotinin group compared to the placebo group.

In a U.S. randomized placebo controlled study of Aprotinin Regimen A and Regimen B versus placebo in 212 patients undergoing primary aortic and/or mitral valve replacement or repair, no benefit was found for Aprotinin in terms of the need for transfusion or the number of units of blood required.

INDICATIONS AND USAGE:

Aprotinin is indicated for prophylactic use to reduce perioperative blood loss and the need for blood transfusion in patients undergoing cardiopulmonary bypass in the course of repeat coronary artery bypass graft surgery. Aprotinin is also indicated in selected cases of primary coronary artery bypass graft surgery where the risk of bleeding is especially high (impaired hemostasis, e.g., presence of aspirin or coagulopathy of other origin) or where transfusion is unavailable or unacceptable. This selected use of Aprotinin in primary CABG patients is based on the risk of renal dysfunction and on the risk of anaphylaxis (should a second procedure be needed).

CONTRAINDICATIONS:

Hypersensitivity to aprotinin.

WARNINGS:

Anaphylactic reactions have been reported in less than 0.5% of patients receiving Aprotinin (including first time and re-exposures). Since Aprotinin is a foreign protein, the incidence of hypersensitivity reactions, including anaphylaxis, is considerably higher upon re- exposure. The symptoms of hypersensitivity-type reactions can range from skin eruptions, itching, dyspnea, nausea and tachycardia to fatal anaphylactic shock with circulatory failure. If hypersensitivity reactions occur during injection or infusion, administration should be stopped immediately. Emergency treatment should be initiated.

PRECAUTIONS:

GENERAL

Test Dose and Use of H_1 Antihistamine: All patients treated with Aprotinin should first receive a test dose to assess the potential for allergic reactions. The test dose of 1 ml Aprotinin should be administered intravenously at least 10 minutes prior to the loading dose. Particular caution is necessary when administering Aprotinin (even test doses) to patients who have received aprotinin in the past because of the risk of anaphylaxis. In re-exposure cases, intravenous administration of an H_1 antihistamine antagonist (antihistamine) is recommended shortly before the loading dose of Aprotinin.

Loading Dose: The loading dose of Aprotinin should be given intravenously to patients in the supine position over a 20-30 minute period. Rapid intravenous administration of Aprotinin can cause a transient fall in blood pressure. (See DOSAGE AND ADMINISTRATION.)

Allergic Reactions: Patients who experience any allergic reaction to the test dose of aprotinin should not receive further administration of the drug. Even after the uneventful administration of the 1 ml test dose, or without previous exposure to aprotinin, the full therapeutic dose may cause anaphylaxis. If this happens, the infusion should be stopped immediately and emergency treatment for anaphylaxis should be applied. Patients with a history of allergic reactions to drugs or other agents may be at greater risk of developing an allergic reaction.

Use Of Aprotinin In Patients Undergoing Deep Hypothermic Circulatory Arrest: An increase in both renal failure and mortality compared to age matched historical controls has been reported in patients receiving Aprotinin while undergoing deep hypothermic circulatory arrest in connection with surgery of the aortic arch. The strength of this association is uncertain because there are no data from randomized studies to confirm or refute these findings.

CARCINOGENESIS, MUTAGENESIS, AND IMPAIRMENT OF FERTILITY

Long- term animal studies to evaluate the carcinogenic potential of Aprotinin or studies to determine the effect of Aprotinin on fertility have not been performed.

Results of microbial *in vitro* tests using *Salmonella typhimurium* and *Bacillus subtilis* indicate that Aprotinin is not a mutagen.

PREGNANCY, TERATOGENIC EFFECTS, PREGNANCY CATEGORY B

Reproduction studies have performed in rats at intravenous doses up to 200,000 KIU/kg/day for 11 days, and in rabbits at intravenous doses up to 100,000 KIU/kg/day for 13 days, 2.4 and 1.2 times the human dose on a mg/kg basis and 0.37 and 0.36 times the human mg/m^2 dose. They have revealed no evidence of impaired fertility or harm to the fetus due to Trasylol. There are, however, no adequate and well-controlled studies in pregnant women. Because animal reproduction studies are not always predictive of human response, this drug should be used during pregnancy only if clearly needed.

NURSING MOTHERS

Not applicable.

PRECAUTIONS: *(cont'd)*

PEDIATRIC USE

Safety and effectiveness in children have not been established.

LABORATORY MONITORING OF ANTICOAGULATION DURING CARDIOPULMONARY BYPASS

Aprotinin prolongs whole blood clotting time of heparinized blood as determined by a celite surface activation method. The kaolin activated clotting time appears to be much less affected. In the event of prolonged extracorporeal circulation, patients may require additional heparin, even in the presence of activated clotting time (ACT) levels that appear to represent adequate anticoagulation. Therefore, in patients on cardiopulmonary bypass (CPB) who are receiving Aprotinin, the standard system of monitoring heparinization during CPB, by keeping the celite ACT above 400-450 seconds, may lead to inadequate anticoagulation. In patients undergoing cardiopulmonary bypass with Aprotinin therapy, standard loading doses of heparin should be employed. However, additional heparin should be administered either in a fixed-dose regimen based on patient weight and duration of CPB, or on the basis of heparin levels measured by a method unaffected by Aprotinin (such as protamine titration).

DRUG INTERACTIONS:

Aprotinin is known to have antifibrinolytic activity and, therefore, may inhibit the effects of fibrinolytic agents.

In a study of nine patients with untreated hypertension, Aprotinin infused intravenously in a dose of 2 million KIU over two hours blocked the acute hypotensive effect of 100 mg of captopril.

Aprotinin in the presence of heparin, has been found to prolong the activated clotting time (ACT) as measured by a celite surface activation method. The kaolin activated clotting time appears to be much less affected. However, Aprotinin should not be viewed as a heparin sparing agent. (See PRECAUTIONS, Laboratory Monitoring of Anticoagulation During Cardiopulmonary Bypass.)

ADVERSE REACTIONS:

Studies analyzed to date indicate that Aprotinin is generally well tolerated. The adverse events reported are frequent sequelae of cardiac surgery and are not necessarily attributable to Aprotinin therapy. Adverse events reported, up to the time of discharge from the hospital, from four double-blind, placebo-controlled studies conducted in the United States involving 886 patients undergoing cardiac surgery with cardiopulmonary bypass (Study 1 - repeat CABG; Study 2 - repeat and primary CABG; Study 3 - repeat CABG; Study 4 - primary cardiac valve replacement or repair) are listed in the following table. The table lists only those events which occurred in 2% or more of the patients treated with Aprotinin without regard to causal relationship. (TABLE 5)

TABLE 5

	Percentage of Patients Treated with Aprotinin (N=579)	Percentage Patients Treated with Placebo (N=307)
BODY AS A WHOLE		
Any Event	76	73
Fever	12	8
Infection	6	5
Sepsis	3	2
CARDIOVASCULAR		
Atrial fibrillation	24	22
Myocardial infarction	11	8
Heart failure	10	5
Atrial flutter	8	5
Hypotension	6	6
Ventricular tachycardia	6	4
Pericarditis	5	4
Ventricular extrasystoles	5	4
Arrhythmia	4	5
Supraventricular tachycardia	4	3
Heart arrest	3	2
Congestive Heart Failure	3	1
Peripheral edema	3	1
Ventricular fibrillation	2	5
Hypertension	2	4
Atrial arrhythmia	2	3
Tachycardia	2	5
Surgery*	2	1
DIGESTIVE		
Liver function tests abnormal	5	2
Nausea	3	3
Diarrhea	2	1
Vomiting	2	1
Hemic and Lymphatic		
Leukocytosis	3	2
Thrombocytopenia	2	2
Metabolic and Nutritional		
Creatine phosphokinase increased	5	3
Hyperglycemia	3	2
Nervous		
Confusion	4	3
Respiratory		
Lung disorder	7	7
Pleural effusion	5	6
Pneumonia	4	4
Apnea	3	1
Dyspnea	3	1
Respiratory disorder	3	3
Pneumothorax	3	4
Asthma	3	2
Urogenital		
Kidney function abnormal	5	3
Urinary tract infection	3	4
Kidney Failure	2	1

*These surgical procedures included: rethoracotomy, pacemaker implantation, mitral valve repair, vena cava filter placement, femoral thrombectomy and chest drainage in Aprotinin group and pacemaker placement or revision in the placebo group.

In the pooled analysis of the four U.S. placebo-controlled studies, in patients undergoing cardiopulmonary bypass there was a trend toward an increased incidence of myocardial infarction in patients given Aprotinin (11% vs 8%, p=0.145). Because of the trend seen the earlier U.S. studies (Studies 1 and 2), this issue was addressed prospectively in Study 3 (repeat CABG). In this study, the incidence rates of myocardial infarction as reported by investigators were 16%, 13%, and 7% in Aprotinin Regimen A, Regimen B, and pump prime regimens, respectively, versus 10% in the placebo regimen group. When the data were

ADVERSE REACTIONS: *(cont'd)*

analyzed by a blinded consultant, the incidence rates for definite myocardial infarction were 12%, 15%, and 9% in the Aprotinin Regimen A, Regimen B, and pump prime regimens, respectively, versus 12% in the placebo group. The differences in the incidence rates in both analyses were not statistically significant.

In study of patients undergoing primary or repeat CABG (Study 2), in which graft patency was evaluated by ultrafast computerized tomography (CT), a trend was seen toward an increased incidence of saphenous vein graft closure in patients who received Aprotinin Regimen A versus the placebo regimen.

Less frequent adverse events of concern, without regard to drug relationship, in cardiac surgery patients treated with Aprotinin in U.S. clinical trials were: shock (1.7%), lung edema (1.2%), phlebitis (1.0%), kidney tubular necrosis (0.9%), cerebral embolism (0.5%), liver damage (0.5%), acute kidney failure (0.5%), cerebrovascular accident (0.5%), hemolysis (0.3%), allergic reaction (0.3%).

In comparison to the placebo group, no increase in mortality in patients treated with Aprotinin was observed.

Hypersensitivity and Anaphylaxis: see WARNINGS

Laboratory Findings Serum Creatinine: Pooled data from the four U.S. placebo-controlled studies showed a statistically significant increase in the incidence of post-operative renal dysfunction in the Aprotinin-treated group. The incidence of serum creatinine elevations ≥0.5 mg/dl above baseline was 21 percent in Regimen A, 18 percent in Regimen B compared to 14 percent in the placebo group (p=0.015 and p=0.495, respectively). In patients undergoing coronary artery bypass graft procedures only (Study 1,2,3) the rates were 19 percent and 20 percent in the Aprotinin Regimen A and Regimen B groups and 15 percent in the placebo group (p≥0.345, versus placebo). Postoperative renal dysfunction was observed somewhat more frequently in association with primary cardiac valve procedures (30% for Aprotinin Regimen A, and 14% for Regimen B versus 8% for placebo). In the majority of instances the renal dysfunction was not severe and was reversible. A total of 4 percent of Aprotinin Regimens A and B and 2 percent of the placebo group had a serum creatinine increase of ≥2 mg/dl above the preoperative value.

Patients with baseline elevations in serum creatinine were not at increased risk of developing postoperative renal dysfunction following Aprotinin treatment although there were mean increases in creatine of 0.11 mg/dl after the high dose regimen (A), and of 0.09 mg/dl after the low dose regimen (B), each of which was statistically significant compared to placebo.

Serum Glucose: In the hours after cardiopulmonary bypass surgery, the serum glucose was increased; however, the average serum glucose increase in patients treated with the high dose regimen (61 mg/dl) was less than in the placebo treated group (78 mg/dl).

Serum Transaminases: In U.S. controlled studies, a significantly greater incidence of treatment emergent abnormal liver function tests was reported in all Aprotinin treated (Regimen A, Regimen B and the pump prime regimen) patients (5%) compared to patients treated with placebo regimen (2%). The percent of primary CABG patients developing an elevation of ALT (alanine amino transferase; formerly SGPT, serum glutamic pyruvic transaminase) greater than 1.8 times the upper limit of normal was not higher in the Aprotinin treated group compared to the placebo group. Among the repeat CABG patients, the percent of subjects developing an elevation of ALT of this magnitude was significantly higher in the Aprotinin treated group. This suggests an indirect effect possibly related to the risk of repeated surgery and attendant myocardial dysfunction rather than a primary drug effect. There were no differences between the Aprotinin treated and placebo groups in the incidence of elevated ALT values greater than 3.0 times the upper limit of normal.

Serum Creatine Kinase (CK): There was a trend toward an increased incidence of elevated serum creatine kinase (CK) with increased MB fractions in Aprotinin treated patients.

Partial Thromboplastin Time (PTT) and Active Clotting Time (ACT): Significant elevations in the partial thromboplastin time (PTT) and activated clotting time (ACT) in Aprotinin treated patients are expected in the hours after surgery due to circulating concentrations of Aprotinin which are known to inhibit activation of the intrinsic clotting system by contact with a foreign surface, a method used in these tests. (See PRECAUTIONS, Laboratory Monitoring of Anticoagulation During Cardiopulmonary Bypass.)

OVERDOSAGE:

The maximum amount of Aprotinin that can be safely administered in single or multiple doses has not been determined. Doses up to 17.5 million KIU have been within 24 hour period without any apparent toxicity. There is one poorly documented case, however, of a patient who received a large, but not well determined, amount of Trasylol (in excess of 15 million KIU) in 24 hours. The patient, who had pre- existing liver dysfunction, developed hepatic and renal failure postoperatively and died. Autopsy showed hepatic necrosis and extensive renal tubular and glomerular necrosis. The relationship of these findings to Aprotinin therapy is unclear.

DOSAGE AND ADMINISTRATION:

Aprotinin given prophylactically in both dose Regimen A and Regimen B (half Regimen A) to patients undergoing repeat CABG surgery significantly reduced the donor blood transfusion requirement relative to placebo treatment. In patients given aspirin preoperatively, while there was no difference in the number of patients requiring transfusion whether assigned to Regimen A or B, fewer units of blood and/or blood products were required by patients administered Regimen A. In high risk primary CABG surgery patients, only Regimen A was studied.

Aprotinin is supplied as a solution containing 10,000 KIU/ml, which was equal to 1.4 mg/ml. All intravenous doses of Aprotinin should be administered through a central line. **DO NOT ADMINISTER ANY OTHER DRUG USING THE SAME LINE.** Both regimens include a 1 ml test dose, a loading dose, a dose to be added to the priming fluid of the cardiopulmonary bypass circuit ("pump prime" dose), and a constant infusion dose.

Regimens A and B (both incorporating a 1 ml test dose) are described in the table below (TABLE 6A and 6B):

TABLE 6A

	TEST DOSE	LOADING DOSE
Aprotinin Regimen A	1 ml (1.4 mg, or 10,000 KIU)	200 ml (280 mg, or 2.0 million KIU)
Aprotinin Regimen B	1 ml (1.4 mg, or 10,000 KIU)	100 ml (140 mg, or 1.0 million KIU)

The 1 ml test dose should be administered intravenously at least 10 minutes before the loading dose. With the patient in a supine position, the loading dose is given slowly over 20-30 minutes, after induction of anesthesia but prior to sternotomy. When the loading dose is complete, it is followed by the constant infusion dose, which is continued until surgery is complete and the patient leaves the operating room. The "pump prime" dose is added to the

DOSAGE AND ADMINISTRATION: *(cont'd)*

TABLE 6B

	"PUMP PRIME" DOSE	CONSTANT INFUSION DOSE
Aprotinin Regimen A	200 ml (280 mg, or 2.0 million KIU)	50 ml/hr (70 mg/hr or 500,000 KIU/hr)
Aprotinin Regimen B	100 ml (140 mg, or 1.0 million KIU)	25 ml/hr (35 mg/hr, or 250,000 KIU/hr)

priming fluid of the cardiopulmonary bypass circuit, by replacement of an aliquot of the priming fluid, prior to the institution of cardiopulmonary bypass. Total doses of more than 7 million KIU have not been studied in controlled trials.

Parenteral drug products should be inspected visually for particulate matter and discoloration prior to administration whenever solution and container permit. Discard any unused portion.

Renal and Hepatic Impairment: No formal studies of the pharmacokinetics of aprotinin in patients with preexisting renal insufficiency have been conducted. However, in the placebo-controlled clinical trials conducted in the United States, patients with mildly elevated pretreatment serum creatinine levels did not have a notably higher incidence of clinically significant post-treatment elevations in serum creatinine following Aprotinin Regimen A or Regimen B compared to administration of the placebo regimen. Changes on aprotinin pharmacokinetics with age or impaired renal function are not great enough to require any dose adjustment. No pharmacokinetic data from patients with pre-existing hepatic disease treated with Trasylol are available.

Compatibility: Aprotinin is incompatible *in vitro* with corticosteroids, heparin, tetracyclines, and nutrient solutions containing amino acids or fat emulsion. If Aprotinin is to be given concomitantly with another drug, each drug should be administered separately through different venous lines or catheters.

HOW SUPPLIED:

Storage: Aprotinin should be stored between 2° and 25°C (36° - 77°F).
Protect from freezing.

HOW SUPPLIED - EQUIVALENTS NOT AVAILABLE:

Injection, Solution - Intravenous - 10000 unit/ml

100 ml x 6	**$1080.00**	**TRASYLOL, Bayer**	**00026-8196-36**
200 ml x 6	**$2160.00**	**TRASYLOL, Bayer**	**00026-8197-63**

ARGININE HYDROCHLORIDE *(000278)*

CATEGORIES: Caloric Agents; Diagnostic Agents; Electrolytic, Caloric-Water Balance; Pituitary Function; FDA Approval Pre 1982

BRAND NAMES: R-Gene 10

Prescribing information not available at time of publication.

HOW SUPPLIED - EQUIVALENTS NOT AVAILABLE:

Injection, Solution - Intravenous - 10 %

300 ml	$106.25	R-GENE 10, Pharmacia & Upjohn	00016-0436-24

ASCORBIC ACID *(000290)*

CATEGORIES: Homeostatic & Nutrient; Pharmaceutical Adjuvants; Vitamin C; Vitamins; FDA Pre 1938 Drugs

BRAND NAMES: *Acidylina*; *Agrumina*; *Ascorbin*; *Askorbin*; *C500*; C-Tym; *C-Vimin*; Cebid; *Cebion* (Germany); *Cecap*; *Cecon*; *Cecon Drops*; *Celin*; *Cenol*; Cecore 500; Cee-500; Cetane; *Cetebe* (Germany); *Cetrinets*; **Cevalin**; *Ce-Vi-Sol* (Mexico); *Cewin*; *Citravite*; *Dancimin C*; *Dayvital*; *Flavettes*; *Ikacee*; *Laroscorbine* (France); *Leder C*; *Leder-C*; *Limcee*; Mega C A Plus; *Multiperla-C*; *Oranvital*; *Potent C*; *Pro-C*; *Redoxon* (Australia); *Redoxon C*; *Redoxon Forte* (Mexico); *Scorbex*; *SLC*; *Take-C*; *Tanvimil-C*; *Upsa-C*; *Upsa C*; *Vi-C 500*; *Vicef*; *Vita-Cedol Orange*; *Vitac*; *Vitacemil* (France); Vitamin C; *Vitascarbol 500*; *Vorange*; *Xon-ce*
(International brand names outside U.S. in italics)

FORMULARIES: Aetna; WHO

Prescribing information not available at time of publication.

HOW SUPPLIED - EQUIVALENTS NOT AVAILABLE:

Injection, Solution - Intramuscular; - 250 mg/ml

2 ml x 25	$36.80	Ascorbic Acid, Steris Labs	00402-0457-82
2 ml x 25	$39.00	Ascorbid Acid, Pasadena	00418-0457-82
2 ml x 25	$46.00	Ascorbic Acid, Schein Pharm (US)	00364-2361-42
30 ml	$4.20	Ascorbic Acid, Steris Labs	00402-0080-30
30 ml	$4.77	Ascorbic Acid, Schein Pharm (US)	00364-6635-56
30 ml	$6.80	Ascorbic Acid, Hyrex Pharms	00314-0085-30

Injection, Solution - Intramuscular; - 500 mg/ml

1 ml ampoule x	**$50.70**	**CEVALIN, Lilly**	**00002-1677-25**
2 ml x 25	$60.00	Ascorbic Acid, Consolidated Midland	00223-8875-02
50 ml	$3.80	Ascorbic Acid, McGuff	49072-0037-50
50 ml	$5.30	Ascorbic Acid, Steris Labs	00402-0709-50
50 ml	$5.30	Ascorbic Acid, Steris Labs	00402-1083-50
50 ml	$7.50	Ascorbic Acid, Consolidated Midland	00223-7186-50
50 ml	$12.75	MEGA-C-ACID PLUS 500, Merit Pharms	30727-0339-90
50 ml x 1	$4.38	Ascorbic Acid, Am Regent	00517-5050-01

Syrup - Oral - 500 mg/5ml

480 ml	$13.50	VITAMIN C, Hi Tech Pharma	50383-0167-16

ASPARAGINASE *(000297)*

CATEGORIES: Acute Lymphoblastic Leukemia; Antineoplastics; Chemotherapy; Leukemia; Oncologic Drugs; Pregnancy Category C; FDA Pre 1938 Drugs

BRAND NAMES: Crasnitin (Germany); *Crasnitine*; *Crastinin*; **Elspar**; *Erwinase*; *Kidrolase* (France, Canada); L-Asparaginase; *Laspar*; *Leucogen*; *Leunase* (Australia, Asia, Mexico)
(International brand names outside U.S. in italics)

FORMULARIES: BC-BS; Medi-Cal; WHO

WARNING:
IT IS RECOMMENDED THAT ASPARAGINASE BE ADMINISTERED TO PATIENTS ONLY IN A HOSPITAL SETTING UNDER THE SUPERVISION OF A PHYSICIAN WHO IS QUALIFIED BY TRAINING AND EXPERIENCE TO ADMINISTER CANCER CHEMOTHERAPEUTIC AGENTS, BECAUSE OF THE POSSIBILITY OF SEVERE REACTIONS, INCLUDING ANAPHYLAXIS AND SUDDEN DEATH. THE PHYSICIAN MUST BE PREPARED TO TREAT ANAPHYLAXIS AT EACH ADMINISTRATION OF THE DRUG.
IN THE TREATMENT OF EACH PATIENT THE PHYSICIAN MUST WEIGH CAREFULLY THE POSSIBILITY OF ACHIEVING THERAPEUTIC BENEFIT VERSUS THE RISK OF TOXICITY. THE FOLLOWING DATA SHOULD BE THOROUGHLY REVIEWED BEFORE ADMINISTERING THE COMPOUND.

DESCRIPTION:

Elspar contains the enzyme L-asparagine amidohydrolase, type EC-2, derived from *Escherichia coli*. It is a white crystalline powder that is freely soluble in water and practically insoluble in methanol, acetone and chloroform. Its activity is expressed in terms of International Units (I.U.) according to the recommendation of the International Union of Biochemistry. The specific activity of Asparaginase is at least 225 I.U. per milligram of protein and each vial contains 10,000 I.U. of asparaginase and 80 mg of mannitol, an inactive ingredient, as a sterile, white lyophilized plug or powder for intravenous or intramuscular injection after reconstitution.

CLINICAL PHARMACOLOGY:

MECHANISM OF ACTION

In a significant number of patients with acute leukemia, particularly lymphocytic, the malignant cells are dependent on an exogenous source of asparagine for survival. Normal cells, however, are able to synthesize asparagine and thus are affected less by the rapid depletion produced by treatment with the enzyme asparaginase. This is a unique approach to therapy based on a metabolic defect in asparagine synthesis of some malignant cells. Asparaginase, derived from *Escherichia coli*, is effective in inducing remissions in some patients with acute lymphocytic leukemia.

ASPARAGINE DEPENDENCE TEST

An asparagine dependence test has been utilized during the investigational studies. In this test leukemic cells obtained from some marrow cultures could be shown to require asparagine *in vitro*, suggesting sensitivity to asparaginase therapy *in vivo*. However, present data indicate that the correlation between asparaginase dependence in such tests and the final response to therapy is sufficiently poor that the test is not recommended as a basis for selection of patients for treatment.

PHARMACOKINETICS AND METABOLISM

In a study[1] in patients with metastatic cancer and leukemia, initial plasma levels of L-asparaginase following intravenous administration were correlated to dose. Daily administration resulted in a cumulative increase in plasma levels. Plasma half-life varied from 8 to 30 hours; it did not appear to influenced by dosage, either single or repetitive, and could not be correlated with age, sex, surface area, renal or hepatic function, diagnosis or extent of disease. Apparent volume of distribution was approximately 70-80% of estimated plasma volume. There was some slow movement of asparaginase from vascular to extravascular, extracellular space, L-asparaginase was detected in the lymph. Cerebrospinal fluid levels were less than 1% of concurrent plasma levels. Only trace amounts appeared in the urine.

In a study[2] in which patients with leukemia and metastatic cancer received intra-muscular L-asparaginase, peak plasma levels of asparaginase were reached 14 to 24 hours after dosing. Plasma half-life was 39 to 49 hours. No asparaginase was detected in the urine.

INDICATIONS AND USAGE:

Asparaginase is indicated in the therapy of patients with acute lymphocytic leukemia. This agent is useful primarily in combination with other chemotherapeutic agents in the induction of remissions of the disease in children.[3,4] Asparaginase should not be used as the sole induction agent unless combination therapy is deemed inappropriate. Asparaginase is not recommended for maintenance therapy.

CONTRAINDICATIONS:

Asparaginase is contraindicated in patients with pancreatitis or a history of pancreatitis. Acute hemorrhagic pancreatitis, in some instances fatal, has been reported following asparaginase administration.[4-7] Asparaginase is also contraindicated in patients who have had previous anaphylactic reactions to it.

WARNINGS:

Allergic reactions to asparaginase are frequent and may occur during the primary course of therapy. They are not completely predictable on the basis of the intradermal skin test. Anaphylaxis and death have occurred in a hospital setting with experienced observers.

Once a patient has received asparaginase as part of a treatment regimen, retreatment with this agent at a later time is associated with increased risk of hypersensitivity reactions. In patients found by skin testing to be hypersensitive to asparaginase, and in any patient who has received a previous course of therapy with asparaginase, therapy with this agent should be instituted or reinstituted only after the successful desensitization, and then only if in the judgement of the physician the possible benefit is greater than the increased risk. Desensitization itself may be hazardous. (See DOSAGE AND ADMINISTRATION.)

In view of the unpredictability of the adverse reactions to asparaginase, it is recommended that this product be used in a hospital setting. Asparaginase has an adverse effect on liver function in the majority of patients. Therapy with asparaginase may increase preexisting liver impairment caused by prior therapy or the underlying disease. Because of this there is a possibility that asparaginase may increase the toxicity of other medications.[3,7]

The administration of Asparaginase *intravenously concurrently with or immediately before* a course of vincristine and prednisone may be associated with increased toxicity.[3] (See DOSAGE AND ADMINISTRATION, Recommended Induction Regimens.)

PRECAUTIONS:

GENERAL

This drug may be a contact irritant and both powder and solution must be handled and administered with care. Inhalation of dust or vapors and contact with skin or mucous membranes, especially those of the eyes, must be avoided. In case of contact, wash with copious amounts of water for at least 15 minutes.

PRECAUTIONS: *(cont'd)*

Asparaginase has been reported to have immunosuppressive activity in animal experiments. Accordingly, the possibility that use of the drug in man may predispose to infection should be considered.

Asparaginase toxicity is reported to be greater in adults than in children.[7]

LABORATORY TESTS

The fall in circulating lymphoblasts often is quite marked; normal or below normal leukocyte counts are noted frequently within the first several days after initiating therapy. This may be accompanied by a marked raise in serum uric acid. The possible development of uric acid nephropathy should be borne in mind. Appropriate preventative measures should be taken, e.g., allopurinol, increased fluid intake, alkalization of urine.[8,9]

Frequent serum amylase determinations should be obtained to detect early evidence of pancreatitis. If pancreatitis occurs, therapy should be stopped and not reinstituted.

Blood sugar should be monitored during therapy with asparaginase because hypoglycemia may occur.[4,6,7,10-13]

DRUG/LABORATORY INTERACTIONS

L-asparaginase has been reported to interfere with the interpretation of thyroid function tests by producing a rapid and marked reduction in serum concentrations of thyroxine-binding globulin within two days after the first dose. Serum concentrations of thyroxine-binding globulin returned to pretreatment values within four weeks of the last dose of L- asparaginase.[15]

ANIMAL TOXICOLOGY

A one-month intravenous toxicity study of asparaginase in dogs at doses of 250, 1000, and 2000 I.U./kg/day revealed reduced serum total protein and albumin with loss of body weight at the highest dose level and anorexia, emesis, and diarrhea at all dosage levels. A similar study in monkeys at doses of 100, 300, and 1000 I.U./kg/day also revealed reduction of serum total protein and albumin and body weight loss at all dosage levels. Bromsulphalein retention and fatty changes in the liver were noted in monkeys that were given 300 and 100 kg/day. The rabbit was unusually sensitive to Asparaginase since a single intravenous dose of 1000 I.U./kg caused hypocalcemia associated with necrosis of the parathyroid cells, convulsions, and death in about one third of the animals. Some rabbits that died showed small thymic and lymph node hemorrhages and necrosis of the germinal centers in their lymph nodes and spleen. The intravenous administration of calcium gluconate alleviated or prevented the adverse effects.

Changes in the pancreatic islets (not pancreatitis) ranging from edema to necrosis were observed in the rabbits in the acute intravenous toxicity studies (doses of 12,500 to 50,000 I.U./kg) but not in rabbits that received 100 I.U./kg. The anatomical changes and the hypocalcemia found in the rabbits were not observed in the subacute intravenous studies in the dogs and monkeys.

CARCINOGENESIS, MUTAGENESIS, AND IMPAIRMENT OF FERTILITY

The intraperitoneal injection of 2500 I.U./kg/day for 4 days in newborn Swiss mice resulted in a small increase in pulmonary adenomas; lymphatic leukemia was not increased.

L-asparaginase at concentrations of 152-909 I.U./plate was not mutagenic in the Ames microbial mutagen test with or without metabolic activation.

There are no adequate studies on the effects of asparaginase on fertility.

PREGNANCY CATEGORY C

In mice and rats asparaginase has been shown to retard the weight gain of mothers and fetuses when given in doses of more than 1000 I.U./kg (the recommended human dose). Resorptions, gross abnormalities and skeletal abnormalities were observed. The intravenous administration of 50 or 100 I.U./kg (one-twentieth or one-tenth of the human dose) to pregnant rabbits on Day 8 and 9 of gestation resulted in dose dependent embryotoxicity and gross abnormalities. There are no adequate and well- controlled studies in pregnant women. asparaginase should be used during pregnancy only if the potential benefit outweighs the potential risk to the fetus.

NURSING MOTHERS

It is not known whether this drug is secreted in human milk. Because many drugs are secreted in human milk and because of the potential for serious adverse reactions in nursing infants from asparaginase, a decision should be made whether to discontinue nursing or to discontinue the drug, taking into account the importance of the drug to the mother.

DRUG INTERACTIONS:

Tissue culture and animal studies indicate the asparaginase can diminish or abolish the effect of methotrexate on malignant cells.[14] This effect on methotrexate activity persists as long as plasma asparagine levels are suppressed. These results would seem to dictate against the clinical use of methotrexate with asparaginase, or during the period following asparaginase therapy when asparagine levels are below normal.

ADVERSE REACTIONS:

Allergic reactions, including skin rashes, urticaria, arthralgia, respiratory distress and acute anaphylaxis have been reported. (See WARNINGS.) Acute reactions have occurred in the absence of a positive skin test and during continued maintenance of therapeutic serum levels of asparaginase.

In children with advanced leukemia, a lower incidence of anaphylaxis has been reported with intramuscular administration, although there was a higher incidence of milder hypersensitivity reactions than with intravenous administration.[16]

Fatal hyperthermia has been reported.

Pancreatitis, sometimes fulminant and fatal, has occurred during of following therapy with asparaginase.[4-7,17]

Hyperglycemia with glucosuria and polyuria has been reported in low incidence. Serum and urine acetone usually have been absent or negligible in these patients; this syndrome thus resembles hyperosmolar, nonketotic, hyperglycemia induced by a variety of other agents. This complication usually responds to discontinuance of asparaginase, judicious use of intravenous fluid, and insulin, but may be fatal on occasion.

In addition to hypofibrinogenemia, depression of various other clotting factors has been reported. Most marked has been a decrease in plasma levels of factors V and VIII with a variable decrease in factors VII and IX. A decrease in circulating platelets has occurred in low incidence which, together with the increased levels of fibrin degradation products in the serum, may indicate the development of a consumption coagulopathy. Bleeding has been a problem in a minority of patients with demonstrable coagulopathy. However, intracranial hemorrhage and fatal bleeding associated with low fibrinogen levels have been reported.[6,7,18] Increased fibrinolytic activity, apparently compensatory in nature, also has occurred.

Some patients have shown central nervous effects consisting of depression, somnolence, fatigue, coma, confusion, agitation, and hallucinations varying from mild to severe.[6,7,10,12,13] Rarely, a Parkinson-like syndrome has occurred, with tremor and a progressive increase in muscular tone. These side effects usually have reversed spontaneously after treatment was stopped. Therapy with asparaginase is associated with an increase in blood ammonia during the conversion of asparagine to asparatic acid by the enzyme. No clear correlation exists

ADVERSE REACTIONS: *(cont'd)*

between the degree of elevation of blood ammonia levels and the appearance of CNS changes. Chills, fever, nausea, vomiting, anorexia, abdominal cramps, weight loss, headache, and irritability may occur and usually are mild.

Azotemia, usually pre-renal, occurs frequently. Acute renal shut down and fatal renal insufficiency have been reported during treatment.[5] Proteinuria has occurred infrequently.

A variety of liver function abnormalities have been reported, including elevations of SGOT, SGPT, alkaline phosphatase, bilirubin (direct and indirect), and depression of serum albumin, cholesterol (total and esters), and plasma fibrinogen. Increases and decreases of total lipids have occurred.[19] Marked hypoalbuminemia associated with peripheral edema has been reported.[10] However, these abnormalities usually are reversible on discontinuance of therapy and some reversal may occur during the course of therapy. Fatty changes in the liver have been documented by biopsy. Malabsorption syndrome has been reported.[12]

Rarely, transient bone marrow depression has been observed, as evidenced by a delay in return of hemoglobin or hematocrit levels to normal in patients undergoing hematologic remission of leukemia. Marked leukopenia has been reported.[20]

OVERDOSAGE:

The acute intravenous LD_{50} of asparaginase for mice was about 500,000 I.U./kg and for rabbits about 22,000 I.U./kg.

DOSAGE AND ADMINISTRATION:

As a component of selected multiple agent induction regimens, asparaginase may be administered by either the intravenous or the intramuscular route. When administered intravenously this enzyme should be given over a period of not less than thirty minutes through the side arm of an already running infusion of Sodium Chloride Injection or Dextrose Injection 5% (D_5W). Asparaginase has little tendency to cause phlebitis when given intravenously. Anaphylactic reactions require the immediate use of epinephrine, oxygen, and intravenous steroids.

When administering asparaginase intramuscularly, the volume at a single injection site should be limited to 2 ml. If a volume greater than 2 ml is to be administered, two injection sites should be used.

Unfavorable interactions of asparaginase with some antitumor agents have been demonstrated. It is recommended therefore, that asparaginase be used in combination regimens only by physicians familiar with the benefits and risks of a given regimen. During the period of its inhibition of protein synthesis and cell replication asparaginase may interfere with the action of drugs such as methotrexate which require cell replication for their lethal effect. Asparaginase may interfere with the enzymatic detoxification of other drugs, particularly in the liver.

RECOMMENDED INDUCTION REGIMENS

When using chemotherapeutic agents in combination for the induction of remissions in patients with acute lymphocytic leukemia, regimens are sought which provide maximum chance of success while avoiding excessive cumulative toxicity or negative drug interactions.

One of the following combination regimens incorporating asparaginase is recommended for acute lymphocytic leukemia in children: (In the regimens below, Day 1 is considered to be the first day of therapy.)

Regimen I [3]:

Prednisone: 40 mg/square meter of body surface area per day orally in three divided doses for 15 days, followed by tapering of the dosage as follows: 20 mg/square meter for 2 days, 10 mg/square meter for 2 days, 5 mg/square meter for 2 days, 2.5 mg/square meter for 2 days and then discontinue.

Vincristine Sulfate: 2 mg/square meter of body surface area intravenously once weekly on Days 1,8, and 15 of the treatment period. The maximum single dose should not exceed 2.0 mg.

Asparaginase: 1,000 I.U./kg/day intravenously for ten successive days beginning on Day 22 of the treatment period.

Regimen II [4]:

Prednisone: 40 mg/square meter of body surface area per day orally in three divided doses for 28 days (the total daily dose should be to the nearest 2.5 mg), following which the dosage of prednisone should be discontinued gradually over a 14 day period.

Vincristine Sulfate: 1.5 mg/square meter of body surface area intravenously weekly for four doses, on Days 1,8,15, and 22 of the treatment period. The maximum single dose should not exceed 2.0 mg.

Asparaginase: 6,000 I.U./square meter of body surface area intramuscularly on Days 4,7,10,13,16,19,22,25, and 28 of the treatment period.

When a remission is obtained with either of the above regimens, appropriate maintenance therapy must be instituted. Asparaginase should not be used as part of a maintenance regimen. The above regimens do not preclude a need for special therapy directed toward the prevention of central nervous system leukemia.

It should be noted that asparaginase has been used in combination regimens other than those recommended above. It is important to keep in mind that asparaginase administered intravenously concurrently with or immediately before a course of vincristine and prednisone may be associated with increased toxicity. Physicians using a given regimen should be thoroughly familiar with its benefits and risks. Clinical data are insufficient for a recommendation concerning the use of combination regimens in adults. Asparaginase toxicity is reported to be greater in adults than in children.

Use of asparaginase as the sole induction agent should be undertaken only in an unusual situation when a combined regimen is inappropriate because of toxicity or other specific patient-related factors, or in cases refractory to other therapy. When asparaginase is to be used as the sole induction agent for children or adults the recommended dosage regimen is 200 I.U./kg/day intravenously for 28 days.[5,7,21,22] When complete remissions were obtained with this regimen, they were of short duration, 1 or 3 months. Asparaginase has been used as the sole induction agent in other regimens.[6,21,24] Physicians using a given regimen should be thoroughly familiar with its benefits and risks.

Patients undergoing induction therapy must be carefully monitored and the therapeutic regimen adjusted according to response and toxicity.

Such adjustments should always involve decreasing dosages of one or more agents of discontinuation depending on the degree of toxicity. Patients who have received a course of asparaginase, if retreated, have an increased risk of hypersensitivity reactions. Therefore, retreatment should be undertaken only when the benefit of such therapy is weighed against the increased risk.

INTRADERMAL SKIN TEST

Because of the occurrence of allergic reactions, an intradermal skin test should be performed prior to the initial administration of asparaginase and when asparaginase is given after an interval of a week or more has elapsed between doses. The skin test solution may be prepared as follows: Reconstitute the contents of a 10,000 I.U. vial with 5.0 ml of diluent. From this solution (2,000 I.U./ml) withdraw 0.1 ml and inject it into another vial containing 9.9 ml of diluent, yielding a skin test solution of approximately 20.01 I.U./ml. Use 0.1 ml of this

DOSAGE AND ADMINISTRATION: *(cont'd)*

solution (about 2.0 I.U.) for the intradermal skin test. The skin test site should be observed for at least one hour for the appearance of a wheal or erythema either of which indicates a positive reaction. An allergic reaction even to the skin test dose in certain sensitized individuals may rarely occur. A negative skin test reaction does not preclude the possibility of the development of an allergic reaction.

DESENSITIZATION

Desensitization should be performed before administering the first dose of asparaginase on initiation of therapy in positive reactors, and on retreatment of any patient in whom such therapy is deemed necessary after carefully weighing the increased risk of hypersensitivity reactions. Rapid desensitization of the patient may be attempted with progressively increasing amounts of intravenously administered asparaginase provided adequate precautions are taken to treat an allergic reaction should it occur. One reported schedule[21,22] begins with a total of 1 I.U. given intravenously and doubles the dose every 10 minutes, provided no reaction has occurred, until the accumulated total amount given the planned doses for that day.

For convenience TABLE 1 is included to calculate the number of doses necessary to reach the patient's total dose that day.

TABLE 1 Asparaginase, DOSAGE AND ADMINISTRATION

Injection Number	Asparaginase Dose in I.U.	Accumulated Total Dose
1	1	1
2	2	3
3	4	7
4	8	15
5	16	31
6	32	63
7	64	127
8	128	255
9	256	511
10	512	1023
11	1024	2047
12	2048	4095
13	4096	8191
14	8192	16383
15	16384	32767
16	32768	65535
17	65536	131071
18	131072	262143

For example: A patient weighing 20 kg who is to receive 200 I.U./kg (total dose 4000 I.U.) would receive injections 1 through 12 during desensitization.

DIRECTIONS FOR RECONSTITUTION

Parenteral drug products should be inspected visually for particulate matter and discoloration prior to administration whenever solution and container permit. When reconstituted, asparaginase should be a clear, colorless solution. If the solution becomes cloudy, discard.

FOR INTRAVENOUS USE

Reconstitute with Sterile Water for Injection or with Sodium Chloride Injection. The volume recommended for reconstitution is 5 ml for the 10,000 unit vials. Ordinary shaking during reconstitution does not inactivate the enzyme. This solution may be used for direct intravenous administration within an eight hour period following restoration. For administration by infusion, solutions should be diluted with the isotonic solutions, Sodium Chloride or Dextrose Injection 5%. These solutions should be infused within eight hours and only if clear.

Occasionally, a very small number of gelatinous fiber-like particles may develop on standing. Filtration through a 5.0 micron filter during administration will remove the particles with no resultant loss in potency. Some loss of potency has been observed with the use of a 0.2 micron filter.

FOR INTRAMUSCULAR USE

When asparaginase is administered intramuscularly according to the schedule cited in the induction regimen, reconstitution is carried out by adding 2 ml Sodium Chloride Injection to the 10,000 unit vial. The resulting solution should be used within eight hours and only if clear.

STORAGE

Store at 2-8°C (36-46°F). Asparaginase does not contain a preservative. Unused, reconstituted solution should be stored at 2 to 8°C (36-46°F) and discarded after eight hours, or sooner if it becomes cloudy.

REFERENCES:

1. Ho, D.H.W.; Thetford, B.S.; Carter, C.J.K.; Frei, E.,III: Clinical pharmacologic studies of L-asparaginase, Clin. Pharmacol. Ther. *11:* 408-417, May-June 1970. **2.** Ho, D.H.W.; Yap, H.Y.; Brown, N.; Benjamin, R.S.; Friereich, E.J.; Blumenschein, G.R.; Bodey, G.P.; Clinical Pharmacology of intramuscularly administered L-asparaginase, J. Clin. Pharmacol.*21:* 72-78, Feb.-Mar. 1981. **3.** Jones, B., et al: Blood *42:*1015, Dec. 1973 (Abstract: Optimal Use of Asparaginase in Acute Lymphocytic Leukemia of Childhood). **4.** Ortega, J.A.; Nesbit, M.E.; Donaldson, M.H.; Hittle, R.E.; Weiner, J.; Karon, M.; Hammond, D.: L-asparaginase, vincristine and prednisone for induction of first remission in acute lymphocytic leukemia, Cancer Research *37:* 535-540, Feb. 1977. **5.** Haskell, C.M.; Canellos, G.P.; Leventhal, B.G.; Carbone, P.P.; Block, J.B.; Serpick, A.A.; Selawry, O.S.: L-asparaginase: Therapeutic and toxic effects in patients with neoplastic disease, New Engl. J. Med. *281:* 1028-1034, 1969. **6.** Ohnuma, T., et al: Treatment of adult leukemia with L-asparaginase (NCS-109229), Cancer Chemo. Reports Part I *55* (3):269-275, June 1971. **7.** Zubrod, C.G.: The clinical toxicities of L-asparaginase in the treatment of leukemia and lymphoma, Pediat.*45:*555-559, Apr.1970. **8.** Holland, J.F.; Gildewell, O.J.: Oncologists' Reply: Survival Expectancy in Acute Lymphocytic Leukemia, New Engl. J. Med., Vol.*287:*769-777, 1972. **9.** Wintrobe, M.M.: 'Clinical Hematology,' ed. 6, Philadelphia, Lea & Febiger, 1969, 1044. **10.** Oettgen, H.F.; Stephenson, P.A.; Schwartz, M.K.; Leeper, R.D.; Tallal, L.; Tan, C.C.; Clarkson, B.D.; Golbey, R.B.; Krakoff, I.H.; Karnofsky, D.A..; Murphy, M.L.; Burchenal, J.H.: The toxicity of E. coli L-asparaginase in man, Cancer Research Vol.*30:* 2297-2305, 1970. **11.** Khan, A.; Adachi, M.; Hill, J.M.; Diabetogenic effect of L-asparaginase, J. Clin. Endocrinol. & Metab. *29:* 1373-1376, Oct.1969. **12.** Ohnuma, T.; Holland, J.F.; Freeman, A.; Sinks, L.F.: Biochemical and Pharmacological Studies with Asparaginase in Man, Cancer Research Vol. *30:* 2297-2305, 1970. **13.** Whitecar, J.P., Jr.; Bodey, G.P.; Harris, J.E.; Freireich, E.J.: L- asparaginase, New Engl. J. Med. *282:* 732-734, Mar. 26, 1970 (in Current Concepts). **14.** Capizzi, R.L.: Schedule-dependent synergism and antagonism between methotrexate and asparaginase, Biochem. Pharmacol. *23:* 151-161, 1974. **15.** Garnick, M.B.; Larsen, P.R.: Acute deficiency of thyroxine-binding globulin during L-asparaginase therapy, New Engl. J. Med. *301:* 252-253, Aug. 2, 1979. **16.** Nesbit, M.; Chard, R.; Evans, A.; Karon, M.: Evaluation of intramuscular versus intravenous administration of L-asparaginase in childhood leukemia, Am. J. Ped. Hematology/Oncology *1:* 9-13, Spring 1979. **17.** McLean, R.; Martin, S.; Lam-Po-Tang, P.R.L.: Fatal case L- asparaginase induced pancreatitis, Lancet *2:* 1401-1402, Dec. 18, 1982. **18.** Lederman, G.S.: Stroke due to treatment with L-asparaginase in an adult, N. Engl. J. Med. *307* (26): 1643, Dec. 23, 1982. **19.** Storti, E.; Quaglino, D.: Dysmetabolic and neurologic complications in leukemic patients treated with L-asparaginase, in 'Experimental and Clinical Effects of L-asparaginase,' E. Grundman & H.F. Oettgen (ed.), New York, Springer-Verlag, 1970, pp. 344-349. **20.** Oehlers, M.J.; Fetawadjieff, W.; Woodliff, H.J.: Profound leukopenia following asparaginase treatment in a patient with acute lympho- blastic leukemia, Med. J. Aust. *2:* 907-909, Nov. 1, 1969. **21.** Clarkson, B.; Krakoff, I.; Burchenal, J.; Karnofsky, D.; Golbey, R.; Dowling, M.; Oettgen, H.; Lipton, A.: Chemical results of treatment with E. coli L-asparaginase in adults with leukemia, lymphoma, and solid tumors, Cancer. *25:* 279-305, Feb.1970. **22.** Tallal, L.; Tan, C.; Oetgen, H.; Wollner, N.; McCarthy, M.; Helson, L.; Burchenal, J.; Karnofsky, D.; Murphy, M.L.: E. coli L-asparaginase in the treatment of leukemia and tumors in 131 children, Cancer. *25:* 306-320, Feb. 1970. **23.** Pratt, C.B.; Johnson, W.W.: Duration and severity of fatty metamorphosis of the liver following L-asparaginase therapy, Cancer *28:* 361-364, Aug. 1971. **24.** Pratt, C.B.; Simone, J.V.; Zee, P.; Aur, R.J.; Johnson, W.W.: Comparison of daily versus weekly L-asparaginase for the treatment of childhood acute leukemia, J. Pediat. *77:* 474-483, Sept.1970.

HOW SUPPLIED - EQUIVALENTS NOT AVAILABLE:

Injection, Lyphl-Soln - Intramuscular; - 10,000 unit

10 ml	$54.68	ELSPAR, Merck	00006-4612-00

ASPIRIN *(000299)*

CATEGORIES: Analgesics; Antiarthritics; Antipyretics; Antithrombotics; Arthritis; Cardiovascular Drugs; Central Nervous System Agents; Inflammation; Inflammatory Conditions; Nonsteroidal Anti-Inflammatory; Osteoarthritis; Pain; Salicylates; Angina*; Colon Carcinoma*; Myocardial Infarction*; Stroke Prevention*; Pregnancy Category D; FDA Pre 1938 Drugs
* Indication not approved by the FDA

BRAND NAMES: *AAS*; *ASS* (Germany); *Acesal*; *Acetard*; *Acetosal*; Acetylsalicylic Acid; *Actispirine* (France); *Adiro* (Mexico); *Albyl-E*; Amiprine; *Anacin*; *Anasprin*; *Asalic*; *Asapor*; *ASA500* (Mexico); *Asart*; *Asawin* (Mexico); *Ascriptin*; *Aspec*; *Aspent*; *Aspex*; *Aspilets*; *Aspirem*; *Aspirin*; *Aspirin Bayer*; *Aspirina*; *Aspro* (Australia, Germany, England); *Aspro Clear*; *Bayaspirina*; *Bayer Aspirin*; *Bex*; *Buffered Aspirin*; *Bufferin*; *Cafenol*; *Caprin* (England); *Ceto*; *Claragine* (France); *Colfarit* (Germany); Dasprin; *Dispril*; *Disprin* (Australia, England); *Dusil*; Easprin; *Ecotrin* (Australia); Entaprin; *Eskotrin*; *Globentyl*; *Idotyl*; Megaprin; *Mejoral*; *Melabon* (Germany); *Nu-Seals*; Or-Prin; *Plewin*; *Rhonal* (France); *Ronal*; Salicylic Acid; Sloprin; *Solprin*; *Spren*; *Supirin*; *Tapal*; Trinprin; *Winsprin*; **Zorprin**
(International brand names outside U.S. in italics)

FORMULARIES: Aetna; BC-BS; Medi-Cal; WHO

DESCRIPTION:

Aspirin Delayed-Release Tablets, USP enteric coated tablets contain 15 grains (975 mg) aspirin for oral administration. Also contain: candelilla wax; colloidal silicon dioxide, NF; corn starch 1500; dusty rose Opaspray; hydroxypropyl methylcellulose, USP (15 cps); methylparaben, NF; microcrystalline cellulose, NF; mistron spray talc; polyethylene glycol 3350, NF; propylparaben, NF; stearic acid powder; vanillin, NF; zinc stearate, USP. The enteric coating is designed to prevent the release of aspirin in the stomach and thereby reduce gastric irritation and total occult blood loss. The pharmacologic effects of aspirin include analgesia, antipyresis, antiinflammatory activity, and antirheumatic activity.

CLINICAL PHARMACOLOGY:

Aspirin is a salicylate that has demonstrated antiinflammatory, analgesic, antipyretic, and antirheumatic activity.

Aspirin's mode of action as an antiinflammatory and antirheumatic agent may be due to inhibition of synthesis and release of prostaglandins.

Aspirin appears to produce analgesia by virtue of both a peripheral and CNS effect.

Peripherally, aspirin acts by inhibiting the synthesis and release of prostaglandins. Acting centrally, it would appear to produce analgesia at a hypothalamic site in the brain, although the mode of action is not known.

Aspirin also acts on the hypothalamus to produce antipyresis; heat dissipation is increased as a result of vasodilation and increased peripheral blood flow. Aspirin's antipyretic activity may also be related to inhibition of synthesis and release of prostaglandins.

In a crossover study, aspirin at a dose of one tablet (15 grains) three times a day produced an average fecal blood loss of 1.54 ml per day. Uncoated aspirin at a dosage of three 5-grain tablets given three times a day caused an average fecal blood loss of 4.33 ml per day.

Aspirin tablets are enteric coated. This coating acts to prevent the release of aspirin in the stomach but permits the tablet to dissolve with resultant absorption in the upper portion of the small intestine. This reduces any gastric irritation that may occur with uncoated aspirin but does delay the onset of action. Aspirin is rapidly hydrolyzed primarily in the liver to salicylic acid, which is conjugated with glycine (forming salicyluric acid) and glucuronic acid and excreted largely in the urine. As a result of the rapid hydrolysis, plasma concentrations of aspirin are always low and rarely exceed 20 mcg/ml at ordinary therapeutic doses. The peak salicylate level for uncoated aspirin occurs in about 2 hours; however with enteric coated aspirin tablets this is delayed. A direct correlation between salicylate plasma levels and clinical analgesic effectiveness has not been definitely established, but effective analgesia is usually achieved at plasma levels of 15 to 30 mg per 100 ml. Effective antiinflammatory activity is usually achieved at salicylate plasma levels of 20 to 30 mg per 100 ml. There is also poor correlation between toxic symptoms and plasma salicylate concentrations, but most patients exhibit symptoms of salicylism at plasma salicylate levels of 35 mg per 100 ml. The plasma half-life for aspirin is approximately 15 minutes; that for salicylate lengthens as the dose increases: Doses of 300 to 650 mg have a half-life of 3.1 to 3.2 hours; with doses of 1 gram, the half-life is increased to 5 hours and with 2 grams it is increased to about 9 hours.

Salicylates are excreted mainly by the kidney. Studies in man indicate that salicylate is excreted in the urine as free salicylic acid (10%), salicyluric acid (75%), salicylic phenolic (10%) and acyl (5%) glucuronides and gentisic acid (<1%).

INDICATIONS AND USAGE:

Aspirin, delayed-release, enteric coated tablets, are indicated in patients who need the higher 15 grain dose of aspirin in the long-term palliative treatment of mild to moderate pain and inflammation of arthritic and other inflammatory conditions.

CONTRAINDICATIONS:

Aspirin should not be used in patients who have previously exhibited hypersensitivity to aspirin and/or nonsteroidal antiinflammatory agents.

Aspirin should not be given to patients with a recent history of gastrointestinal bleeding or in patients with bleeding disorders (*e.g.*, hemophilia).

WARNINGS:

Aspirin tablets should be used with caution when anticoagulants are prescribed concurrently, for aspirin may depress the concentration of prothrombin in plasma and thereby increase bleeding time. Large doses of salicylates have a hypoglycemic action and may enhance the effect of the oral hypoglycemics. Consequently, they should not be given concomitantly; if however, this is necessary, the dosage of the hypoglycemic agent must be reduced while the salicylate is given. This hypoglycemic action may also affect the insulin requirements of diabetics.

Although salicylates in large doses are uricosuric agents, smaller amounts may decrease the uricosuric effects of probenecid, sulfinpyrazone, and phenylbutazone.

PRECAUTIONS:

GENERAL

Aspirin tablets should be administered with caution to patients with asthma, nasal polyps, or nasal allergies.

PRECAUTIONS: *(cont'd)*

Consult a physician before giving this medicine to children, including teenagers, with chicken pox or flu.

In patients receiving large doses of aspirin and/or prolonged therapy, mild salicylate intoxication (salicylism) may develop that may be reversed by reduction in dosage.

Although the fecal blood loss with enteric-coated aspirin is less than that with uncoated aspirin tablets, enteric-coated aspirin tablets should be administered with caution to patients with a history of gastric distress, ulcer, or bleeding problems. Occult gastrointestinal bleeding occurs in many patients but is not correlated with gastric distress. The amount of blood lost is usually insignificant clinically, but with prolonged administration, it may result in iron deficiency anemia.

Sodium excretion produced by spironolactone may be decreased in the presence of salicylates.

Salicylates can produce changes in thyroid function tests.

Salicylates should be used with caution in patients with severe hepatic damage, pre-existing hypoprothrombinemia, or Vitamin K deficiency, and in those undergoing surgery.

USAGE IN PREGNANCY

It has been reported that adverse effects were increased in the mother and fetus following chronic ingestion of aspirin. Prolonged pregnancy and labor with increased bleeding before and after delivery, as well as decreased birth weight and increased rate of stillbirth were correlated with high blood salicylate levels. Because of possible adverse effects on the neonate and the potential for increased maternal blood loss, aspirin should be avoided during the last three months of pregnancy.

DRUG INTERACTIONS:

Anticoagulants: See WARNINGS section.

Hypoglycemic Agents: See WARNINGS section.

Uricosuric Agents: Aspirin may decrease the effects of probenecid, sulfinpyrazone, and phenylbutazone.

Spironolactone: See PRECAUTIONS section.

Alcohol: Has a synergistic effect with aspirin in causing gastrointestinal bleeding.

Corticosteroids: Concomitant administration with aspirin may increase the risk of gastrointestinal ulceration and may reduce serum salicylate levels.

Pyrazolone Derivatives (phenylbutazone, oxyphenbutazone, and possibly dipyrone): Concomitant administration with aspirin may increase the risk of gastrointestinal ulceration.

Nonsteroidal Antiinflammatory Agents: Aspirin is contraindicated in patients who are hypersensitive to nonsteroidal antiinflammatory agents.

Urinary Alkalinizers: Decrease aspirin effectiveness by increasing the rate of salicylate renal excretion.

Phenobarbital: Decreases aspirin effectiveness by enzyme induction.

Phenytoin: Serum phenytoin levels may be increased by aspirin.

Propranolol: May decrease aspirin's antiinflammatory action by competing for the same receptors.

Antacids: Enteric-coated aspirin should not be given concurrently with antacids, since an increase in the pH of the stomach may effect the enteric coating of the tablets.

ADVERSE REACTIONS:

Gastrointestinal: Dyspepsia, thirst, nausea, vomiting, diarrhea, acute reversible hepatotoxicity, gastrointestinal bleeding, and/or ulceration.

Special Senses: Tinnitus, vertigo, reversible hearing loss, and dimness of vision.

Hematologic: Prolongation of bleeding time, leukopenia, thrombocytopenia, purpura, decreased plasma iron concentration and shortened erythrocyte survival time.

Dermatologic and Hypersensitivity: Urticaria, angioedema, pruritus, sweating, various skin eruptions, asthma, and anaphylaxis.

Neurologic: Mental confusion, drowsiness, and dizziness.

Body as a Whole: Headache and fever.

OVERDOSAGE:

Overdosage of 200 to 500 mg/kg is in the fatal range. Early symptoms are CNS stimulation with vomiting, hyperpnea, hyperactivity, and possibly convulsions. This progresses quickly to depression, coma, respiratory failure, and collapse. These symptoms are accompanied by severe electrolyte disturbances.

In the treatment of salicylate overdosage, intensive supportive therapy should be instituted immediately. Plasma salicylate levels should be measured in order to determine the severity of the poisoning and to provide a guide for therapy. Emptying of the stomach should be accomplished as soon as possible with ipecac syrup unless the patient is depressed. In depressed patients use airway protected gastric lavage. Delay absorption with activated charcoal and give a saline cathartic. Proceed according to Standard Reference Procedures for Salicylate Intoxication.

DOSAGE AND ADMINISTRATION:

Usual Adult Dosage: One tablet 3 to 4 times daily.

Patients who have displayed no significant adverse effects on a long term qid regimen and who receive a total daily dosage of aspirin no greater than 3.9 grams may be considered for a bid regimen (2 tablets of enteric-coated aspirin twice daily). Patients on the bid enteric-coated aspirin regimen should be closely monitored for serum salicylate levels, increased incidence of CNS-related adverse effects, increased fecal blood loss, or any other signs or symptoms suggestive of significant blood loss.

If necessary, dosage may be increased until relief is obtained, but dosage should be maintained slightly below that which produces tinnitus. Plasma salicylate levels may also be helpful in determining proper dosage (see CLINICAL PHARMACOLOGY) section).

Storage: Store at controlled room temperature 15 to 30°C (59 to 86°F).

HOW SUPPLIED - EQUIVALENTS NOT AVAILABLE:

Tablet, Enteric Coated, Sustained Action - Oral - 800 mg

100's	$9.00	Aspirin, Aligen Independ	00405-4100-01
100's	$9.00	SLOPRIN, Econolab	55053-0514-01
100's	$9.79	Aspirin Controlled Release, Parmed Pharms	00349-8784-01
100's	$11.12	Aspirin Timed Release, Rugby	00536-3320-01
100's	$11.25	Aspirin, United Res	00677-1172-01
100's	$12.85	Aspirin, Major Pharms	00904-0585-60
100's	**$32.80**	**ZORPRIN, Knoll Labs**	**00044-0057-01**

Tablet, Enteric Coated, Sustained Action - Oral - 975 mg

100's	$11.48	Aspirin Delayed-Release, HL Moore Drug Exch	00839-7404-06
100's	$11.55	Aspirin Delayed-Release, Rugby	00536-3321-01
100's	$12.50	Aspirin Delayed-Release, United Res	00677-1347-01
100's	$13.20	Aspirin Delayed-Release, Goldline Labs	00182-1065-01

HOW SUPPLIED - EQUIVALENTS NOT AVAILABLE: *(cont'd)*

100's	$14.50	Aspirin Delayed-Release, Major Pharms	00904-0582-60
100's	$36.64	EASPRIN, Parke-Davis	00071-0490-24

ASPIRIN; BUTALBITAL *(000303)*

CATEGORIES: Analgesics; Antipyretics; Central Nervous System Agents; Nonsteroidal Anti-Inflammatory; Pain; Sedatives/Hypnotics; FDA Approved 1983 Oct

BRAND NAMES: Aspirtal; **Axotal**

Prescribing information not available at time of publication.

HOW SUPPLIED - EQUIVALENTS NOT AVAILABLE:

Tablet, Uncoated - Oral - 650 mg/50 mg

100's	**$49.55**	**AXOTAL, Savage Labs**	**00281-1301-17**

ASPIRIN; BUTALBITAL; CAFFEINE *(000304)*

CATEGORIES: Analgesics; Antimigraine/Other Headaches; Antipyretics; Central Nervous System Agents; Headache; Narcotics, Synthetics & Combinations; Nonsteroidal Anti-Inflammatory; Pain; Sedatives/Hypnotics; Migraine*; Pharyngitis*; Sciatica*; Tonsillitis*; DEA Class CIII; FDA Approved 1983 Aug
* Indication not approved by the FDA

BRAND NAMES: B-A-C; Butal Compound; Butalbital Compound; Butalgen; Farbital; Fembutal; Fiorex; Fiorgen; **Fiorinal**; Fiormor; Fiortal; Fortabs; Idenal; Isobutal; Isolin; Isollyl; Laniroif; Lanorinal; Marnal; Vibutal

FORMULARIES: Aetna; DoD; PCS

DESCRIPTION:

This combination of aspirin, butalbital and caffeine will be abbreviated here as: "butalbital compound."

Each butalbital compound tablet or capsule for oral administration contains: butalbital, USP, 50 mg (Warning: May be habit forming); aspirin, USP, 325 mg; caffeine, USP, 40 mg.

Butalbital, 5-allyl-5-isobutyl-barbituric acid, a white, odorless crystalline powder; is a short- to intermediate-acting barbiturate.

Fiorinal Tablets: *Active Ingredients:* aspirin, USP; butalbital, USP; and caffeine, USP. *Inactive Ingredients:* alginic acid, lactose, microcrystalline cellulose, povidone, stearic acid, and another ingredient.

Fiorinal Capsules: *Active Ingredients:* aspirin, USP; butalbital, USP; and caffeine, USP. *Inactive Ingredients:* D&C Yellow #10, gelatin, microcrystalline cellulose, sodium lauryl sulfate, starch, and talc. *May Also Include:* benzyl alcohol, butylparaben, color additives including FD&C Blue #1, FD&C Green #3, FD&C Yellow #6, edetate calcium disodium, methylparaben, propylparaben, silicon dioxide, sodium propionate.

CLINICAL PHARMACOLOGY:

Pharmacologically, butalbital compound combines the analgesic properties of aspirin with the anxiolytic and muscle relaxant properties of butalbital.

The clinical effectiveness of butalbital compound in tension headache has been established in double-blind, placebo-controlled, multiclinic trials. A factorial design study compared butalbital compound with each of its major components. This study demonstrated that each component contributes to the efficacy of butalbital compound in the treatment of the target symptoms of tension headache (headache pain, psychic tension, and muscle contraction in the head, neck, and shoulder region). For each symptom and the symptom complex as a whole, butalbital compound was shown to have significantly superior clinical effects to either component alone.

INDICATIONS AND USAGE:

Butalbital compound is indicated for the relief of the symptom complex of tension (or muscle contraction) headache.

CONTRAINDICATIONS:

Hypersensitivity to aspirin, caffeine, or barbiturates. Patients with porphyria.

WARNINGS:

Drug Dependency: Prolonged use of barbiturates can produce drug dependence, characterized by psychic dependence, and, less frequently, physical dependence and tolerance. The abuse liability of butalbital compound is similar to that of other barbiturate-containing drug combinations. Caution should be exercised when prescribing medication for patients with a known propensity for taking excessive quantities of drugs, which is not uncommon in patients with chronic tension headache.

Use in Ambulatory Patients: Butalbital compound may impair the mental and/or physical abilities required for the performance of potentially hazardous tasks, such as driving a car or operating machinery. The patient should be cautioned accordingly. Central nervous system (CNS) depressant effects of butalbital may be additive with those of other CNS depressants.

Use in Pregnancy: Adequate studies have not been performed in animals to determine whether this drug affects fertility in males or females, has teratogenic potential, or has other adverse effects on the fetus. While there are no well-controlled studies in pregnant women, over twenty years of marketing and clinical experience does not include any positive evidence of adverse effects on the fetus. Although there is no clearly defined risk, such experience cannot exclude the possibility of infrequent or subtle damage to the human fetus. Butalbital compound should be used in pregnant women only when clearly needed.

Nursing Mothers: The effects of butalbital compound on infants of nursing mothers are not known. Salicylates and barbiturates are excreted in the breast milk of nursing mothers. The serum levels in infants are believed to be insignificant with therapeutic doses.

PRECAUTIONS:

Salicylates should be used with extreme caution in the presence of peptic ulcer or coagulation abnormalities.

Pediatric Use: Safety and effectiveness has not been established in children younger than 12 years of age.

DRUG INTERACTIONS:

Concurrent use with other sedative-hypnotics or alcohol should be avoided. When such combined therapy is necessary, the dose of one or more agents may need to be reduced.

ADVERSE REACTIONS:

The most frequent adverse reactions are drowsiness and dizziness. Less frequent adverse reactions are light-headedness and gastrointestinal disturbances including nausea, vomiting, and flatulence. A single incidence of bone marrow suppression has been reported with the use of butalbital compound. Several cases of dermatological reactions, including toxic epidermal necrolysis and erythema multiforme, have been reported.

OVERDOSAGE:

SIGNS AND SYMPTOMS

The toxic effects of acute overdosage of butalbital compound are attributable mainly to its barbiturate component, and, to a lesser extent, to aspirin. Because toxic effects of caffeine occur in very high dosages only, the possibility of significant caffeine toxicity from butalbital compound overdosage is unlikely.

Acute Barbiturate Poisoning: Symptoms include drowsiness, confusion, and coma; respiratory depression; hypotension; shock.

Acute Aspirin Poisoning: Symptoms include hyperpnea; acid-base disturbances with development of metabolic acidosis; vomiting and abdominal pain; tinnitus; hyperthermia; hypoprothrombinemia; restlessness; delirium; convulsions.

Acute Caffeine Poisoning: May cause insomnia, restlessness, tremor, and delirium; tachycardia and extrasystoles.

TREATMENT

Treatment consists primarily of management of barbiturate intoxication and the correction of the acid-base imbalance due to salicylism. Vomiting should be induced mechanically or with emetics in the conscious patient. Gastric lavage may be used if the pharyngeal and laryngeal reflexes are present and if less than 4 hours have elapsed since ingestion. A cuffed endotracheal tube should be inserted before gastric lavage of the unconscious patient and when necessary to provide assisted respiration. Diuresis, alkalinization of the urine, and correction of electrolyte disturbances should be accomplished through administration of intravenous fluids such as 1% sodium bicarbonate in 5% dextrose in water. Meticulous attention should be given to maintaining adequate pulmonary ventilation. Correction of hypotension may require the administration of levarterenol bitartrate or phenylephrine hydrochloride by intravenous infusion. In severe cases of intoxication, peritoneal dialysis, hemodialysis, or exchange transfusion may be lifesaving. Hypoprothrombinemia should be treated with vitamin K, intravenously.

DOSAGE AND ADMINISTRATION:

One or 2 tablets or capsules every 4 hours. Total daily dose should not exceed 6 tablets or capsules.

HOW SUPPLIED:

Fiorinal Capsules: Color is bright kelly green and lime green, imprinted "FIORINAL 78-103" on each half of capsule. Packages of 100. Also available in ControlPak package, 25 capsules (continuous reverse-numbered roll of sealed blisters).

Fiorinal Tablets: White compressed tablet, engraved "FIORINAL" on one side, "SANDOZ" on other side. Packages of 100. Also available in SandoPak (unit-dose) package of 100 tablets individually blister-sealed.

Store and Dispense: Below 77° F (25° C), tight container.

HOW SUPPLIED - RATED THERAPEUTICALLY EQUIVALENT:

Capsule, Gelatin - Oral - 325 mg/50 mg/40

25's	$8.60	Butalbital Compound, H.C.F.A. F F P	99999-0304-01
25's	**$17.94**	**FIORINAL, Novartis**	**00078-0103-13**
100's	$20.00	Butalbital Compound, Equipharm	57779-0103-04
100's	$33.75	LANORINAL, Lannett	00527-1552-01
100's	$34.43	Butalbital Compound, United Res	00677-1439-01
100's	$34.43	Butalbital Compound, H.C.F.A. F F P	99999-0304-02
100's	$36.70	Butalbital Compound, Qualitest Pharms	00603-2550-21
100's	$37.00	Butalbital Compound, Goldline Labs	00182-0140-01
100's	$37.10	ISOLLYL, Rugby	00536-3933-01
100's	$37.13	Fiormor, HL Moore Drug Exch	00839-7047-06
100's	$37.35	Butalbital/Aspirin/Caffeine, Major Pharms	00904-3934-60
100's	$38.90	Fiortal, Geneva Pharms	50752-0278-05
100's	$39.70	Butalbital Compound, Aligen Independ	00405-0029-01
100's	**$49.68**	**FIORINAL, Novartis**	**00078-0103-05**
500's	$172.15	Butalbital Compound, H.C.F.A. F F P	99999-0304-03
500's	**$237.42**	**FIORINAL, Novartis**	**00078-0103-08**
1000's	$38.20	LANORINAL, Lannett	00527-1552-10
1000's	$249.50	Butalbital Compound, Harber Pharm	51432-0838-06

Tablet, Uncoated - Oral - 325 mg/50 mg/40

30's	$1.07	Butalbital Compound, Talbert Phcy	44514-0088-18
100's	$3.90	FORTABS, United Res	00677-0827-01
100's	$3.90	BUTALBITAL COMPOUND, Geneva Pharms	00781-1435-01
100's	$3.90	Butalbital Compound, H.C.F.A. F F P	99999-0304-04
100's	$4.08	Butalbital Aspirin & Caffeine, Halsey Drug	00879-0566-01
100's	$4.35	Butalbital, Aspirin & Caffeine, West Ward Pharm	00143-1785-01
100's	$4.50	FARBITAL, Major Pharms	00904-3892-60
100's	$4.58	Butalbital Compound, Aligen Independ	00405-0028-01
100's	$5.40	IDENAL, IDE-Interstate	00814-3822-14
100's	$5.76	Butalbital Compound, Caremark	00339-4063-12
100's	$5.95	Butal Compound, Parmed Pharms	00349-8299-01
100's	$5.95	Butalbital Compound, Schein Pharm (US)	00364-0677-01
100's	$6.45	Butalbital Compound, Qualitest Pharms	00603-2548-21
100's	$6.95	FIORMOR, HL Moore Drug Exch	00839-6733-06
100's	$7.10	Fiortal, Geneva Pharms	50752-0277-05
100's	$7.27	FIORGEN PF, Goldline Labs	00182-1631-01
100's	$7.27	Butalbital Compound, Purepac Pharm	00228-2023-10
100's	$7.95	ISOLLYL, Rugby	00536-3937-01
100's	$16.28	Butalbital Compound, Caremark	00339-5843-12
100's	$24.87	Butalbital Compound, Voluntary Hosp	53258-0600-01
100's	$29.64	Butalbital Compound, Voluntary Hosp	53258-0600-13
100's	**$49.68**	**FIORINAL, Novartis**	**00078-0104-05**
100's	**$54.30**	**FIORINAL, Novartis**	**00078-0104-06**
500's	$19.50	Butalbital Compound, H.C.F.A. F F P	99999-0304-05
640's	**$277.68**	**FIORINAL, Novartis**	**00078-0104-65**
1000's	$14.90	LANORINAL, Lannett	00527-1043-10
1000's	$25.00	FARBITAL, Major Pharms	00904-3892-80
1000's	$25.20	LANIROIF, C O Truxton	00463-6110-10
1000's	$26.15	Butalbital, Aspirin & Caffeine, West Ward Pharm	00143-1785-10
1000's	$32.64	Butalbital Aspirin & Caffeine, Halsey Drug	00879-0566-10
1000's	$33.25	BUTALBITAL COMPOUND, Geneva Pharms	00781-1435-10
1000's	$33.75	IDENAL, IDE-Interstate	00814-3822-30
1000's	$36.00	Butalbital Compound, Schein Pharm (US)	00364-0677-02
1000's	$39.00	FORTABS, United Res	00677-0827-10
1000's	$39.00	Butalbital Compound, H.C.F.A. F F P	99999-0304-06
1000's	$42.75	ISOLLYL, Rugby	00536-3937-10
1000's	$50.96	FIORMOR, HL Moore Drug Exch	00839-6733-16

HOW SUPPLIED - RATED THERAPEUTICALLY EQUIVALENT: *(cont'd)*

1000's	$54.59	Fiortal, Geneva Pharms	50752-0277-09
1000's	$56.60	Butalbital Compound, Qualitest Pharms	00603-2548-32
1000's	$56.67	FIORGEN PF, Goldline Labs	00182-1631-10
1000's	$56.67	Butalbital, Aspirin, & Caffeine, Purepac Pharm	00228-2023-96
1000's	$159.95	Fembutal, Quality Res Pharms	52765-1376-00
1000's	**$464.22**	**FIORINAL, Novartis**	**00078-0104-09**

ASPIRIN; BUTALBITAL; CAFFEINE; CODEINE PHOSPHATE *(000302)*

CATEGORIES: Analgesics; Antipyretics; Central Nervous System Agents; Opiate Agonists (Controlled); Pain; Sedatives/Hypnotics; DEA Class CIII; FDA Approved 1990 Oct

BRAND NAMES: Ascomp W/Codeine; B-A-C #3; **Fiorinal W Codeine**; *Fiorinal-C 1 4* (Canada); *Fiorinal-C 1 2* (Canada); Idenal; Isobutal
(International brand names outside U.S. in italics)

FORMULARIES: Aetna; BC-BS; FHP

Prescribing information not available at time of publication.

HOW SUPPLIED - RATED THERAPEUTICALLY EQUIVALENT:

Capsule, Gelatin - Oral - 325 mg/50 mg/40

25's	**$32.70**	**FIORINAL WITH CODEINE NO 3, Novartis**	**00078-0107-13**
100's	**$104.16**	**FIORINAL WITH CODEINE NO 3, Novartis**	**00078-0107-05**
640's	**$592.92**	**FIORINAL W/CODEINE #3, Novartis**	**00078-0107-65**

ASPIRIN; CAFFEINE; CHLORPHENIRAMINE *(000282)*

CATEGORIES: Allergies; Antihistamines; Common Cold; Respiratory & Allergy Medications; FDA Pre 1938 Drugs

BRAND NAMES: Histaphen H.S.; Korigesic; Minagest; S.A.C. W/Chlorpheniramine

Prescribing information not available at time of publication.

HOW SUPPLIED - EQUIVALENTS NOT AVAILABLE:

Tablet, Uncoated - Oral

100's	$12.00	MINAGEST, Minette Pharm	10760-3022-01

ASPIRIN; CAFFEINE; DIHYDROCODEINE BITARTRATE *(000306)*

CATEGORIES: Analgesics; Antipyretics; Central Nervous System Agents; Narcotics, Synthetics & Combinations; Opiate Agonists (Controlled); Pain; DEA Class CIII; FDA Approved 1983 Sep

BRAND NAMES: Dihydrocodeine Compound; Synalgos-Dc

FORMULARIES: Aetna

DESCRIPTION:

Each light aqua and bluish-green capsule contains Dihydrocodeine Bitartrate 16 mg. **(Warning: may be habit forming.)** The empirical formula is $C_{18}H_{23}NO_3 \cdot C_4H_6O_6$and the molecular weight is 451.46. The chemical name is 6-hydroxy-3-methoxy-N- methyl-4,5-epoxy-morphinan Bitartrate.

Acetaminophen 356.4 mg. The empirical formula is $C_8H_9NO_2$ and the molecular weight is 151.16. The chemical name is N-(4-Hydroxyphenyl) acetamide.

Caffeine 30 mg. The empirical formula is $C_8H_{10}N_4O_2$ (anhydrous) and the molecular weight is 194.19. The chemical name is 3,7-Dihydro-1,3,7-trimethyl-1H-purine-2,6-dione.

Dihydrocodeine Compound Capsules also contain the following inactive ingredients: Croscarmellose sodium, FD&C Blue No. 1, FD&C Green No. 3, Gelatin, Silica gel, Silicon dioxide, Sodium lauryl sulfate, Corn starch, Titanium dioxide and Zinc stearate.

CLINICAL PHARMACOLOGY:

Dihydrocodeine Compound Capsules contain dihydrocodeine which is semi-synthetic narcotic analgesic, related to codeine, with multiple actions qualitatively similar to those of codeine; the most prominent of these involve the central nervous system and organs with smooth-muscle components. The principal action of therapeutic value is analgesia.

Dihydrocodeine Compound Capsules also contain acetaminophen, a non-opiate, non-salicylate analgesic, and antipyretic.

Dihydrocodeine Compound Capsules contain caffeine as an analgesic adjuvant. Caffeine is also a CNS and cardiovascular stimulant.

INDICATIONS AND USAGE:

Dihydrocodeine Compound Capsules are indicated for the relief of moderate to moderately severe pain.

CONTRAINDICATIONS:

Hypersensitivity to dihydrocodeine, codeine, acetaminophen, caffeine, or the other components noted above.

WARNINGS:

Dihydrocodeine may impair the mental and/or physical abilities required for the performance of potentially hazardous tasks such as driving a car or operating machinery.

PRECAUTIONS:

GENERAL

Dihydrocodeine Compound Capsules should be given with caution to certain patients such as the elderly or debilitated.

Acetaminophen is relatively non-toxic at therapeutic doses, but it should be used with caution in patients with severe renal or hepatic disease.

Caffeine in high doses may produce CNS and cardiovascular stimulation and GI irritation.

PRECAUTIONS: *(cont'd)*

INFORMATION FOR THE PATIENT

Dihydrocodeine may impair the mental and/or physical abilities required for the performance of potentially hazardous tasks such as driving a car or operating machinery. The patient using Dihydrocodeine Compound Capsules should be cautioned accordingly.

PREGNANCY, TERATOGENIC EFFECTS, PREGNANCY CATEGORY C

Animal reproduction studies have not been conducted with Dihydrocodeine Compound Capsules. It is also not known whether Dihydrocodeine Compound Capsules can cause fetal harm when administered to pregnant women or can affect reproduction capacity in males and females. Dihydrocodeine Compound Capsules should be given to a pregnant woman only if clearly needed.

NURSING MOTHERS

Because of the potential for serious adverse reactions in nursing infants from Dihydrocodeine Compound Capsules, a decision should be made whether to discontinue nursing or to discontinue the drug, taking into account the importance of the drug to the mother.

PEDIATRIC USE

Since there is no experience in children who have received this drug, safety and efficacy in children have not been established.

DRUG INTERACTIONS:

Dihydrocodeine: Patients receiving other narcotic analgesics, general anesthetics, tranquilizers, sedative-hypnotics, or other CNS depressants (including alcohol) concomitantly with Dihydrocodeine Compound Capsules may exhibit an additive CNS depression. When such combined therapy is contemplated, the dose of one or both agents should be reduced.

Caffeine: Caffeine may enhance the cardiac inotropic effects of beta-adrenergic stimulating agents. Co-administration of caffeine and disulfiram may lead to a substantial decrease in caffeine clearance. Caffeine may increase the metabolism of other drugs such as phenobarbital and aspirin. Caffeine accumulation may occur when products or foods containing caffeine are consumed concomitantly with quinolones such as ciprofloxacin.

ADVERSE REACTIONS:

The most frequently observed reactions include light-headedness, dizziness, drowsiness, sedation, nausea, vomiting, constipation, pruritus, and skin reactions.

DRUG ABUSE AND DEPENDENCE:

Dihydrocodeine Compound Capsules are subject to the provisions of the Controlled Substance Act, and has been placed in Schedule III.

Dihydrocodeine can produce drug dependence of the codeine type and therefore has the potential of being abused. Psychic dependence, physical dependence, and tolerance may develop upon repeated administration of dihydrocodeine, and it should be prescribed and administered with the same degree of caution appropriate to the use of other oral narcotic-containing medications.

Prolonged, high intake of caffeine may produce tolerance and habituation. Physical signs of withdrawal, such as headaches, irritation, nervousness, anxiety, dizziness may occur upon abrupt discontinuation.

OVERDOSAGE:

Following an acute overdosage with Dihydrocodeine Compound Capsules, toxicity may result from the dihydrocodeine, acetaminophen, or, less likely, caffeine component. An overdose is a potentially lethal polydrug overdose situation, and consultation with a regional poison control center is recommended. A listing of the poison control centers can be found in *Physicians GenRx*.

SIGNS AND SYMPTOMS

Laboratory Findings: Toxicity from*dihydrocodeine* is typical of opiates and includes pinpoint pupils, respiratory depression, and loss of consciousness. Convulsions, cardiovascular collapse, and death may occur.

Acetaminophen: Dose-dependent hepatic necrosis, hypoglycemic coma, and thrombocytopenia may occur. Early symptoms of hepatotoxicity include nausea, vomiting, diaphoresis, and general malaise. Clinical and laboratory evidence of hepatic toxicity may not be apparent until 48 to 72 hours post-ingestion. In adults, hepatic toxicity has rarely been reported with acute overdoses of less than 10 grams or fatalities with less than 15 grams. Acute*caffeine* poisoning may cause insomnia, restlessness, tremor, delirium, tachycardia, extrasystoles, and seizures.

Because overdose information on Dihydrocodeine Compound Capsules is limited, it is unclear which of the signs and symptoms of toxicity would manifest in any particular overdose situation.

TREATMENT

Immediate treatment includes support of cardiorespiratory function and measures to reduce drug absorption. Vomiting should be induced with syrup of ipecac, if the patient is alert and has adequate laryngeal reflexes. Oral activated charcoal should follow. The first dose should be accompanied by an appropriate cathartic. Gastric lavage may be necessary. Hypotension is usually hypovolemic and should be treated with fluids. Endotracheal intubation and artificial respiration may be necessary. Peritoneal or hemodialysis may be necessary. If hypoprothrombinemia occurs, Vitamin K should be administered.

The pure opioid antagonist, naloxone, is a specific antidote against respiratory depression which results from opioid overdose. Naloxone hydrochloride (usually C.4 to 2.0 mg) should be administered intravenously; however, because its duration of action is relatively short, the patient must be carefully monitored until spontaneous respiration is reliably re-established. Re-administration may be necessary. Naloxone should not be given in the absence of clinically significant respiratory or circulatory depression secondary to opioid overdose.

In adults and adolescents, regardless of the quantity of acetaminophen reported to have been ingested, administer acetylcysteine immediately if 24 hours or less have elapsed from the reported time since ingestion. Do not await the plasma concentration determination of acetaminophen before administering acetylcysteine. Serum liver enzyme levels should be quantitated. Therapy in children involves a similar treatment scheme; however, a regional Poison Control Center should be contacted.

No specific antidote is available for caffeine. In addition to the supportive measures above, administration of demulcents such as aluminum hydroxide gel may diminish GI irritation. Seizures may be treated with intravenous diazepam or a barbiturate.

DOSAGE AND ADMINISTRATION:

The usual adult dose is two (2) DHCplus Capsules orally every four (4) hours. Dosage should be adjusted according to the severity of the pain and the response of the patient. No more than twelve (12) capsules should be taken in a 24-hour period.

Store at controlled room temperature, 15°-30°C (59°-86°F). Protect from moisture.

Dispense in a tight, light-resistant containers as defined in the U.S.P.

HOW SUPPLIED - EQUIVALENTS NOT AVAILABLE:

Capsule, Gelatin - Oral - 356.4 mg/30 mg/

100's	$80.39	SYNALGOS-DC, Wyeth Labs	00008-4191-01
500's	$382.29	SYNALGOS-DC, Wyeth Labs	00008-4191-02

ASPIRIN; CAFFEINE; ORPHENADRINE CITRATE *(000310)*

CATEGORIES: Analgesics; Anticholinergic Agents; Antiparkinson Agents; Autonomic Drugs; Neuromuscular; Pain; Skeletal Muscle Hyperactivity; Skeletal Muscle Relaxants; FDA Approved 1982 Oct

BRAND NAMES: N3 Gesic; *Norflex Compuesto*; **Norgesic**; *Norgesic Forte* (Canada); Orphengesic
(International brand names outside U.S. in italics)

DESCRIPTION:

Norgesic (Aspirin; Caffeine; Orphenadrine Citrate) tablets can be identified by their three layers colored light green, white and yellow. Each round tablet contains Orphenadrine citrate (2-dimethylaminoethyl 2-methyl-benzhydral ether citrate) 25 mg aspirin, 385 mg, and caffeine 30 mg.

Norgesic Forte Tablets are exactly twice the strength of Norgesic. They are identified by their scored capsule shape and by their three layers colored light green, white, and yellow. Each capsule shaped tablet contains orphenadrine citrate 50 mg, aspirin 770 mg, and caffeine 60 mg.

Norgesic and Norgesic Forte also contain: lactose, polyethylene, glycol, povidone, starch, sucrose, zinc stearate, D&C yellow #10, and FD&C blue #1.

CLINICAL PHARMACOLOGY:

Orphenadrine citrate is a centrally acting (brain stem) compound which in animals selectively blocks facilitatory functions of the reticular formation. Orphenadrine does not produce myoneural block, nor does it affect crossed extensor reflexes. Orphenadrine prevents nicotine-induced convulsions but not those produced by strychnine.

Chronic administration of aspirin;caffeine;orphenadrine citrate to dogs and rats has revealed no drug-related toxicity. No blood or urine changes were observed, nor were there any macroscopic or microscopic pathological changes detected. Extensive experience with combinations containing aspirin and caffeine has established them as safe agents. The addition of orphenadrine citrate does not alter the toxicity of aspirin and caffeine.

The mode of therapeutic action of orphenadrine has not been clearly identified, but may be related to its analgesic properties. Orphenadrine citrate also possesses anticholinergic actions.

INDICATIONS AND USAGE:

1. Symptomatic relief of mild to moderate pain of acute musculo-skeletal disorders.

2. The orphenadrine component is indicated as an adjunct to rest, physical therapy, and other measures for the relief of discomfort associated with acute painful musculo-skeletal conditions.

The mode of action of orphenadrine has not been clearly identified, but may be related to its analgesic properties. Aspirin;Caffeine;Orphenadrine Citrate does not directly relax tense skeletal muscles in man.

CONTRAINDICATIONS:

Because of the mild anticholinergic effect of orphenadrine, aspirin;caffeine;orphenadrine citrate should not be used in patients with glaucoma, pyloric or duodenal obstruction, achalasia, prostatic hypertrophy or obstructions at the bladder neck. Aspirin;caffeine;orphenadrine citrate is also contraindicated in patients with myasthenia gravis and in patients known to be sensitive to aspirin or caffeine.

The drug is contraindicated in patients who have demonstrated a previous hypersensitivity to the drug.

WARNINGS:

Reye Syndrome may develop in individuals who have chicken pox, influenza, or flu symptoms. Some studies suggest a possible association between the development of Reye Syndrome and the use of medicines containing salicylate of aspirin. Aspirin;caffeine;orphenadrine citrate contains aspirin and therefore is not recommended for use in patients with chicken pox, influenza, or flu symptoms.

Aspirin;caffeine;orphenadrine citrate may impair the ability of the patient to engage in potentially hazardous activities such as operating machinery or driving a motor vehicle; ambulatory patients should therefore be cautioned accordingly.

Aspirin should be used with extreme caution in the presence of peptic ulcers and coagulation abnormalities.

USAGE IN PREGNANCY

Since safety of the use of this preparation in pregnancy, during lactation, or in the childbearing age has not been established, use of the drug in such patients requires that the potential benefits of the drug be weighed against its possible hazard to the mother and child.

USAGE IN CHILDREN

The safe and effective use of this drug in children has not been established. Usage of this drug in children under 12 years of age is not recommended.

PRECAUTIONS:

Confusion, anxiety and tremors have been reported in few patients receiving propoxyphene and orphenadrine concomitantly. As these symptoms may be simply due to an additive effect, reduction of dosage and/or discontinuation of one or both agents is recommended in such cases.

Safety of continuous long term therapy with Aspirin;caffeine;orphenadrine citrate has not been established; therefore, if Aspirin;caffeine;orphenadrine citrate is prescribed for prolonged use, periodic monitoring of blood, urine and liver function values is recommended.

ADVERSE REACTIONS:

Side effects of Aspirin;caffeine;orphenadrine citrate are those seen with aspirin and caffeine or those usually associated with mild anticholinergic agents. These may include tachycardia, palpitation, urinary hesitancy or retention, dry mouth, blurred vision, dilation of the pupil, increased intraocular tension, weakness, nausea, vomiting, headache, dizziness, constipation, drowsiness, and rarely, urticaria and other dermatoses. Infrequently, an elderly patient may experience some degree of confusion. Mild central excitation and occasional hallucinations may be observed. These mild side effects can usually be eliminated by reduction in dosage. One case of aplastic anemia associated with the use of Aspirin;caffeine;orphenadrine citrate has been reported. No causal relationship has been established. Rare G.I. hemorrhage due to

ADVERSE REACTIONS: *(cont'd)*

aspirin content may be associated with the administration of Aspirin;caffeine;orphenadrine citrate. Some patients may experience transient episodes of lightheadedness, dizziness or syncope.

DOSAGE AND ADMINISTRATION:

Norgesic: Adults 1 to 2 tablets 3 to 4 time daily.

Norgesic Forte: Adults 1/2 to 1 tablet 3 to 4 times daily.

Store below 30°C (86°F).

HOW SUPPLIED - RATED THERAPEUTICALLY EQUIVALENT:

Tablet, Uncoated - Oral - 385 mg/30 mg/25

100's	$74.82	NORGESIC, 3M Pharms	00089-0231-16
100's	$84.18	NORGESIC, 3M Pharms	00089-0231-10
500's	$399.36	NORGESIC, 3M Pharms	00089-0231-50

Tablet, Uncoated - Oral - 770 mg/60 mg/50

100's	$103.44	NORGESIC FORTE, 3M Pharms	00089-0233-16
100's	$122.16	NORGESIC FORTE, 3M Pharms	00089-0233-10
500's	$579.66	NORGESIC FORTE, 3M Pharms	00089-0233-50

ASPIRIN; CAFFEINE; PROPOXYPHENE HYDROCHLORIDE *(000311)*

CATEGORIES: Analgesics; Antipyretics; Central Nervous System Agents; Fever; Narcotics, Synthetics & Combinations; Opiate Agonists (Controlled); Pain; DEA Class CIV; FDA Approved 1983 Mar

BRAND NAMES: Bexophene; Cotanal-65; **Darvon Compound**; *Dibagesic*; *Doloxene Compound*; Doxaphene Compound; Margesic Compound; Propoxyphene Hcl Compound
(International brand names outside U.S. in italics)

FORMULARIES: Aetna; BC-BS

DESCRIPTION:

Darvon (Propoxyphene Hydrochloride, USP, Lilly) is an odorless, white crystalline powder with a bitter taste. It is freely soluble in water. Chemically, it is (2*S*,3*R*)-(+) -4-(Dimethylamino)-3-methyl-1,2-diphenyl-2- butanol propionate (ester) hydrochloride.

Its molecular weight is 375.94.

Each Pulvule contains 65 mg (172.9 μmol) propoxyphene hydrochloride, 389 mg (2,159 μmol) aspirin, and 32.4 mg (166.8 μmol) caffeine.

It also contains F D & C Red No. 3, F D & C Yellow No. 6, gelatin, glutamic acid hydrochloride, iron oxide, kaolin, silicone, titanium dioxide, and other inactive ingredients.

CLINICAL PHARMACOLOGY:

Propoxyphene is a centrally acting narcotic analgesic agent. Equimolar doses of propoxyphene hydrochloride or napsylate provide similar plasma concentrations. Following administration of 65, 130, or 195 mg of propoxyphene hydrochloride, the bioavailability of propoxyphene is equivalent to that of 100, 200, or 300 mg respectively of propoxyphene napsylate. Peak plasma concentrations of propoxyphene are reached in 2 to 2 1/2 hours. After a 65-mg oral dose of propoxyphene hydrochloride, peak plasma levels of 0.05 to 0.1 mcg/ml are achieved.

Repeated doses of propoxyphene at 6-hour intervals lead to increasing plasma concentrations, with a plateau after the ninth dose at 48 hours.

Propoxyphene is metabolized in the liver to yield norpropoxyphene. Propoxyphene has a half-life of 6 to 12 hours, whereas that of norpropoxyphene is 30 to 36 hours.

Norpropoxyphene has substantially less central-nervous-system-depressant effect than propoxyphene but a greater local anesthetic effect, which is similar to that of amitriptyline and antiarrhythmic agents, such as lidocaine and quinidine.

In animal studies in which propoxyphene and norpropoxyphene were continuously infused in large amounts, intracardiac conduction time (PR and QRS intervals) was prolonged. Any intracardiac conduction delay attributable to high concentrations of norpropoxyphene may be of relatively long duration.

Propoxyphene is a mild narcotic analgesic structurally related to methadone. The potency of propoxyphene hydrochloride is from two thirds to equal that of codeine.

The combination of propoxyphene with a mixture of aspirin and caffeine produces greater analgesia than that produced by either propoxyphene or aspirin and caffeine administered alone.

INDICATIONS AND USAGE:

This product is indicated for the relief of mild to moderate pain, either when pain is present alone or when it is accompanied by fever.

CONTRAINDICATIONS:

Hypersensitivity to propoxyphene, aspirin, or caffeine.

WARNINGS:

WARNINGS:
Do not prescribe propoxyphene for patients who are suicidal or addiction-prone.
Prescribe propoxyphene with caution for patients taking tranquilizers or antidepressant drugs and patients who use alcohol in excess.
Tell your patients not to exceed the recommended dose and to limit their intake of alcohol.
Propoxyphene products in excessive doses, either alone or in combination with other CNS depressants, including alcohol, are a major cause of drug-related deaths. Fatalities within the first hour of overdosage are not uncommon. In a survey of deaths due to overdosage conducted in 1975, in approximately 20% of the fatal cases, death occurred within the first hour (5% occurred within 15 minutes). Propoxyphene should not be taken in doses higher than those recommended by the physician. The judicious prescribing of propoxyphene is essential to the safe use of this drug. With patients who are depressed or suicidal, consideration should be given to the use of non-narcotic analgesics. Patients should be cautioned about the concomitant use of propoxyphene products and alcohol because of potentially serious CNS-additive effects of these agents. Because of its added depressant effects, propoxyphene should be prescribed with caution for

WARNINGS: *(cont'd)*

those patients whose medical condition requires the concomitant administration of sedatives, tranquilizers, muscle relaxants, antidepressants, or other CNS-depressant drugs. Patients should be advised of the additive depressant effects of these combinations.

Many of the propoxyphene-related deaths have occurred in patients with previous histories of emotional disturbances or suicidal ideation or attempts as well as histories of misuse of tranquilizers, alcohol, and other CNS-active drugs. Some deaths have occurred as a consequence of the accidental ingestion of excessive quantities of propoxyphene alone or in combination with other drugs. Patients taking propoxyphene should be warned not to exceed the dosage recommended by the physician.

Drug Dependence: Propoxyphene, when taken in higher-than-recommended doses over long periods of time, can produce drug dependence characterized by psychic dependence and, less frequently, physical dependence and tolerance. Propoxyphene will only partially suppress the withdrawal syndrome in individuals physically dependent on morphine or other narcotics. The abuse liability of propoxyphene is qualitatively similar to that of codeine although quantitatively less, and propoxyphene should be prescribed with the same degree of caution appropriate to the use of codeine.

Usage in Ambulatory Patients: Propoxyphene may impair the mental and/or physical abilities required for the performance of potentially hazardous tasks, such as driving a car or operating machinery. The patients should be cautioned accordingly.

Warning: Reye Syndrome is a rare but serious disease which can follow flu or chicken pox in children and teenagers. While the cause of Reye Syndrome is unknown, some reports claim aspirin (or salicylates) may increase the risk of developing this disease.

PRECAUTIONS:

GENERAL

Salicylates should be used with extreme caution in the presence of peptic ulcer or coagulation abnormalities.

Propoxyphene should be administered with caution to patients with hepatic or renal impairment since higher serum concentrations or delayed elimination may occur.

USAGE IN PREGNANCY

Safe use in pregnancy has not been established relative to possible adverse effects on fetal development. Instances of withdrawal symptoms in the neonate have been reported following usage during pregnancy. Therefore, propoxyphene should not be used in pregnant women unless, in the judgment of the physician, the potential benefits outweigh the possible hazards. Aspirin does not appear to have teratogenic effects. However, prolonged pregnancy and labor with increased bleeding before and after delivery, decreased birth weight, and increased rate of stillbirth were reported with high blood salicylate levels. Because of possible adverse effects on the neonate and the potential for increased maternal blood loss, aspirin should be avoided during the last 3 months of pregnancy.

USAGE IN NURSING MOTHERS

Low levels of propoxyphene have been detected in human milk. In postpartum studies involving nursing mothers who were given propoxyphene, no adverse effects were noted in infants receiving mother's milk.

USAGE IN CHILDREN

Propoxyphene is not recommended for use in children, because documented clinical experience has been insufficient to establish safety and a suitable dosage regimen in the pediatric age group.

GERIATRIC USE

The rate of propoxyphene metabolism may be reduced in some patients. Increased dosing interval should be considered.

DRUG INTERACTIONS:

The CNS-depressant effect of propoxyphene is additive with that of other CNS depressants, including alcohol.

Salicylates may enhance the effect of anticoagulants and inhibit the uricosuric effect of uricosuric agents.

As is the case with medicinal agents, propoxyphene may slow the metabolism of a concomitantly administered drug. Should this occur, the higher serum concentrations of that drug may result in increased pharmacologic or adverse effect of that drug. Such occurrences have been reported when propoxyphene was administered to patients on antidepressants, anticonvulsants, or warfarin-like drugs. Severe neurologic signs, including coma, have occurred with concurrent use of carbamazepine.

ADVERSE REACTIONS:

In a survey conducted in hospitalized patients, less than 1% of patients taking propoxyphene hydrochloride at recommended doses experienced side effects. The most frequently reported were dizziness, sedation, nausea, and vomiting. Some of these adverse reactions may be alleviated if the patient lies down.

Other adverse reactions include constipation, abdominal pain, skin rashes, lightheadedness, headache, weakness, euphoria, dysphoria, hallucinations, and minor visual disturbances.

Propoxyphene therapy has been associated with abnormal liver function tests and, more rarely, with instances of reversible jaundice (including cholestatic jaundice).

Renal papillary necrosis may result from chronic aspirin use, particularly when the dosage is greater than recommended and when combined with acetaminophen.

Subacute painful myopathy has occurred following chronic propoxyphene overdosage.

OVERDOSAGE:

In all cases of suspected overdosage, call your regional Poison Control Center to obtain the most up-to-date information about the treatment of overdose. Telephone numbers of certified poison control centers are listed in *Physicians GenRx*. This recommendation is made because, in general, information regarding the treatment of overdosage may change more rapidly than do package inserts.

Initial consideration should be given to the management of the CNS effects of propoxyphene overdosage. Resuscitative measures should be initiated promptly.

SIGNS AND SYMPTOMS

The manifestations of acute overdosage with propoxyphene are those of narcotic overdosage. The patient is usually somnolent but may be stuporous or comatose and convulsing. Respiratory depression is characteristic. The ventilatory rate and/or tidal volume is decreased, which results in cyanosis and hypoxia. Pupils, initially pinpoint, may become dilated as hypoxia increases. Cheyne-Stokes respiration and apnea may occur. Blood pressure and heart rate are usually normal initially, but blood pressure falls and cardiac performance deteriorates, which ultimately results in pulmonary edema and circulatory collapse, unless the respiratory depression is corrected and adequate ventilation is restored promptly. Cardiac

OVERDOSAGE: *(cont'd)*

arrhythmias and conduction delay may be present. A combined respiratory-metabolic acidosis occurs owing to retained CO_2(hypercapnia) and to lactic acid formed during anaerobic glycolysis. Acidosis may be severe if large amounts of salicylates have also been ingested. Death may occur.

TREATMENT

Treatment of Propoxyphene Overdosage in Adults: Attention should be directed first to establishing a patient airway and to restoring ventilation. Mechanically assisted ventilation, with or without oxygen, may be required, and positive pressure respiration may be desirable if pulmonary edema is present. The narcotic antagonist naloxone will markedly reduce the degree of respiratory depression, and 0.4 to 2 mg should be administered promptly, preferably intravenously. If the desired degree of counteraction with improvement in respiratory functions is not obtained, naloxone should be repeated at 2- to 3- minute intervals. The duration of action of the antagonist may be brief. If no response is observed after 10 mg of naloxone have been administered, the diagnosis of propoxyphene toxicity should be questioned. Naloxone may also be administered by continuous intravenous infusion.

Treatment of Propoxyphene Overdosage in Children: The usual initial dose of naloxone in children is 0.01 mg/kg body weight given intravenously. If this dose does not result in the desired degree of clinical improvement, a subsequent increased dose of 0.1 mg/kg body weight may be administered. If an IV route of administration is not available, naloxone may be administered IM or subcutaneously in divided doses. If necessary, naloxone can be diluted with Sterile Water for Injection.

Blood gases, pH, and electrolytes should be monitored in order that acidosis and any electrolyte disturbance present may be corrected promptly. Acidosis, hypoxia, and generalized CNS depression predispose to the development of cardiac arrhythmias. Ventricular fibrillation or cardiac arrest may occur and necessitate the full complement of cardiopulmonary resuscitation (CPR) measures. Respiratory acidosis rapidly subsides as ventilation is restored and hypercapnia eliminated, but lactic acidosis may require intravenous bicarbonate for prompt correction.

Electrocardiographic monitoring is essential. Prompt correction of hypoxia, acidosis, and electrolyte disturbance (when present) will help prevent these cardiac complications and will increase the effectiveness of agents administered to restore normal cardiac function.

In addition to the use of a narcotic antagonist, the patient may require careful titration with an anticonvulsant to control convulsions. Analeptic drugs (for example, caffeine or amphetamine) should not be used because of their tendency to precipitate convulsions.

General supportive measures, in addition to oxygen, include, when necessary, intravenous fluids, vasopressor-inotropic compounds, and, when infection is likely, anti-infective agents. Gastric lavage may be useful and activated charcoal can adsorb a significant amount of ingested propoxyphene. Dialysis is of little value in poisoning due to propoxyphene. Efforts should be made to determine whether other agents, such as alcohol, barbiturates, tranquilizers, or other CNS depressants, were also ingested, since these increase CNS depression as well as cause specific toxic effects.

SIGNS AND SYMPTOMS OF SALICYLATE OVERDOSAGE

Such symptoms include central nausea and vomiting, tinnitus and deafness, vertigo and headaches, mental dullness and confusion, diaphoresis, rapid pulse, and increased respiration and respiratory alkalosis.

TREATMENT OF SALICYLATE OVERDOSAGE

When Darvon Compound-65 has been ingested, the clinical picture may be complicated by salicylism.

The treatment of acute salicylate intoxication includes minimizing drug absorption, promoting elimination through the kidneys, and correcting metabolic derangements affecting body temperature, hydration, acid-base balance, and electrolyte balance. The technique to be employed for eliminating salicylate from the bloodstream depends on the degree of drug intoxication.

If the patient is seen within 4 hours of ingestion, the stomach should be emptied by inducing vomiting or by gastric lavage as soon as possible.

The nomogram of Done is a useful prognostic guide in which the expected severity of salicylate intoxication is based on serum salicylate levels and the time interval between ingestion and taking the blood sample.

Exchange transfusion is most feasible for a small infant. Intermittent peritoneal dialysis is useful for cases of moderate severity in adults. Intravenous fluids alkalinized by the addition of sodium bicarbonate or potassium citrate are helpful. Hemodialysis with the artificial kidney is the most effective means of removing salicylate and is indicated for the very severe cases of salicylate intoxication.

DOSAGE AND ADMINISTRATION:

This product is given orally. The usual dosage is 65 mg propoxyphene hydrochloride, 389 mg aspirin, and 32.4 mg caffeine every 4 hours as needed for pain.

The maximum recommended dose of propoxyphene hydrochloride is 390 mg/day.

Consideration should be given to a reduced total daily dosage in patients with hepatic or renal impairment.

Store at controlled room temperature, 59° to 86°F (15° to 30°C).

PATIENT PACKAGE INSERT:

YOUR PRESCRIPTION FOR A PROPOXYPHENE PRODUCT

Summary: Products containing Propoxyphene are used to relieve pain.

LIMIT YOUR INTAKE OF ALCOHOL WHILE TAKING THIS DRUG.

Make sure your doctor knows if you are taking tranquilizers, sleep aids, antidepressants, antihistamines, or any other drugs that make you sleepy. Combining propoxyphene with alcohol or these drugs in excessive doses is dangerous.

Use care while driving a car or using machines until you see how the drug affects you because propoxyphene can make you sleepy. Do not take more of the drug than your doctor prescribed. Dependence has occurred when patients have taken propoxyphene for a long period of time at doses greater than recommended.

The rest of this leaflet gives you more information about propoxyphene.

Please read it and keep it for future use.

Uses of Propoxyphene: Products containing Darvon are used for the relief of mild to moderate pain. Products that contain Darvon plus aspirin or acetaminophen are prescribed for the relief of pain associated with fever.

Before Taking Propxyphene: Make sure your doctor knows if you have ever had an allergic reaction to propoxyphene, aspirin, or acetaminophen. Some forms of propoxyphene products contain aspirin to help relieve the pain. Your doctor should be advised if you have a history of ulcers or if you are taking an anticoagulant ("blood thinner"). The aspirin may irritate the stomach lining and may cause bleeding, particularly if an ulcer is present. Also, bleeding may occur if you are taking an anticoagulant. In a small group of people, aspirin may cause an asthma attack. If you are one of these people, be sure your drug does not contain aspirin.

PATIENT PACKAGE INSERT: *(cont'd)*

The effect of propoxyphene in children under 12 has not been studied. Therefore, use of the drug in this age group is not recommended.

Also, due to the possible association between aspirin and Reye Syndrome, those propoxyphene products containing aspirin should not be given to children, including teenagers, with chicken pox or flu unless prescribed by a physician. The following propoxyphene product contains: Darvon Compound-65 (Propoxyphene Hydrochloride, Aspirin, and Caffeine, USP, Lilly)

How to Take Propoxyphene: Follow your doctor's directions exactly. Do not increase the amount you take without your doctor's approval. If you miss a dose of the drug, do not take twice as much the next time.

Pregnancy: Do not take propoxyphene during pregnancy unless your doctor knows you are pregnant and specifically recommends its use. Cases of temporary dependence in the newborn have occurred when the mother has taken propoxyphene consistently in the weeks before delivery. **IT IS ESPECIALLY IMPORTANT NOT TO USE DARVON COMPOUND-65 DURING THE LAST 3 MONTHS OF PREGNANCY UNLESS SPECIFICALLY DIRECTED TO DO SO BY A DOCTOR BECAUSE ASPIRIN MAY CAUSE PROBLEMS IN THE UNBORN CHILD OR COMPLICATIONS DURING DELIVERY.** As a general principle, no drug should be taken during pregnancy unless it is clearly necessary.

General Cautions: Heavy use of alcohol with propoxyphene is hazardous and may lead to overdosage symptoms (see OVERDOSAGE.) THEREFORE, LIMIT YOUR INTAKE OF ALCOHOL WHILE TAKING PROPOXYPHENE.

Combinations of excessive doses of propoxyphene, alcohol, and tranquilizers are dangerous. Make sure your doctor knows if you are taking tranquilizers, sleep aids, antidepressant drugs, antihistamines, or any other drugs that make you sleepy. The use of these drugs with propoxyphene increases their sedative effects and may lead to overdosage symptoms, including death (see OVERDOSAGE.)

Propoxyphene may cause drowsiness or impair your mental and/or physical abilities; therefore, use caution when driving a vehicle or operating dangerous machinery. DO NOT perform any hazardous task until you have seen your response to this drug.

Propoxyphene may increase the concentration in the body of medications such as anticoagulants ("blood thinners"), antidepressants, or drugs used for epilepsy. The result may be excessive or adverse effects of these medications. Make sure your doctor knows if you are taking any of these medications.

Dependence: You can become dependent on propoxyphene if you take it in higher than recommended doses over a long period of time. Dependence is a feeling of need for the drug and a feeling that you cannot perform normally without it.

Overdose: An overdose of propoxyphene, alone or in combination with other drugs, including alcohol, may cause weakness, difficulty in breathing, confusion, anxiety, and more severe drowsiness and dizziness. Extreme overdosage may lead to unconsciousness and death.

If the propoxyphene product contains acetaminophen, the overdosage symptoms include nausea, vomiting, lack of appetite, and abdominal pain. Liver damage may occur.

When the propoxyphene product contains aspirin, symptoms of taking too much of the drug are headache, dizziness, ringing in the ears, difficulty in hearing, dim vision, confusion, drowsiness, sweating, thirst, rapid breathing, nausea, vomiting, and, occasionally, diarrhea.

In any suspected overdosage situation, contact your doctor or nearest hospital emergency room. GET EMERGENCY HELP IMMEDIATELY. KEEP THIS DRUG AND ALL DRUGS OUT OF THE REACH OF CHILDREN.

Possible Side Effects: When propoxyphene is taken as directed, side effects are infrequent. Among those reported are drowsiness, dizziness, nausea, and vomiting. If these effects occur, it may help if you lie down and rest.

Less frequently reported side effects are constipation, abdominal pain, skin rashes, lightheadedness, headache, weakness, hallucinations, minor visual disturbances, and feelings of elation or discomfort.

If side effects occur and concern you, contact your doctor.

Other Information: The safe and effective use of propoxyphene depends on your taking it exactly as directed. This drug has been prescribed specifically for you and your present condition. Do not give this drug to others who may have similar symptoms. Do not use it for any other reason.

If you would like more information about propoxyphene, ask your doctor or pharmacist. They may have a more technical leaflet (professional labeling) you may read.

HOW SUPPLIED - RATED THERAPEUTICALLY EQUIVALENT:

Capsule, Gelatin - Oral - 389 mg/32.4 mg/

100's	$10.95	Propoxyphene Hcl Compound, Harber Pharm	51432-0390-03
100's	$16.89	Propoxyphene Compound, United Res	00677-0828-01
100's	$16.89	Propoxyphene HCl Compound, H.C.F.A. F F P	99999-0311-01
100's	$22.25	Propoxyphene Compound, Geneva Pharms	00781-2367-13
100's	$22.88	PROPOXYPHENE COMPOUND 65, IDE-Interstate	00814-6460-14
100's	$23.10	Propoxyphene HCl Compound, Qualitest Pharms	00603-5460-21
100's	$23.20	Propoxyphene Hcl Compound, Major Pharms	00904-7701-60
100's	$23.27	Propoxyphene Compound 65, HL Moore Drug Exch	00839-1561-06
100's	$24.50	Propoxyphene Compound, Teva	00093-0686-01
100's	$24.50	Propoxyphene Compound 65, Goldline Labs	00182-1673-01
100's	$25.00	Propoxyphene Compound 65, Schein Pharm (US)	00364-0668-01
100's	$25.79	Propoxyphene Compound, Aligen Independ	00405-0173-01
100's	$32.95	Propoxyphene w/Aspirin & Caffeine, Rugby	00536-4374-01
100's	$33.50	Propoxyphene Compound-65, Mylan	00378-0131-01
100's	**$36.00**	**DARVON COMPOUND-65, Lilly**	**00002-3111-02**
500's	$39.50	Propoxyphene Compound 65, Harber Pharm	51432-0390-05
500's	$59.25	Propoxyphene Hcl Compound, IDE-Interstate	00814-6460-28
500's	$79.15	Propoxyphene Hcl Compound, Major Pharms	00904-7701-40
500's	$84.45	Propoxyphene HCl Compound, H.C.F.A. F F P	99999-0311-02
500's	$90.78	Propoxyphene Compound, Aligen Independ	00405-0173-02
500's	$110.10	Propoxyphene HCl Compound, Qualitest Pharms	00603-5460-28
500's	$113.00	Propoxyphene w/Aspirin & Caffeine, Rugby	00536-4374-05
500's	$116.45	Propoxyphene Compound, Teva	00093-0686-05
500's	$116.45	Propoxyphene Compound 65, Goldline Labs	00182-1673-05
500's	$116.95	Propoxyphene Compound-65, Mylan	00378-0131-05
500's	**$171.17**	**DARVON COMPOUND-65, Lilly**	**00002-3111-03**
1000's	$63.25	Propoxyphene Hcl Compound, H & H Labs	46703-0009-10
1000's	$86.24	Propoxyphene Compound, Teva	00093-0686-10
1000's	$168.90	Propoxyphene HCl Compound, H.C.F.A. F F P	99999-0311-03

ASPIRIN; CARISOPRODOL *(000314)*

CATEGORIES: Analgesics; Autonomic Drugs; Muscle Relaxants; Neuromuscular; Pain; Skeletal Muscle Hyperactivity; Skeletal Muscle Relaxants; Pregnancy Category C; FDA Approved 1983 Jul

BRAND NAMES: *Carisoprodol and Aspirin* (England); Carisoprodol Compound; **Soma Compound**; Sopridol Compound
(International brand names outside U.S. in italics)

FORMULARIES: Aetna; BC-BS

Prescribing information not available at time of publication.

HOW SUPPLIED - RATED THERAPEUTICALLY EQUIVALENT:

Tablet, Uncoated - Oral - 325 mg/200 mg

100's	$32.50	Carisoprodol Compound, Consolidated Midland	00223-0658-01
100's	$50.25	Carisoprodol Compound, H.C.F.A. F F P	99999-0314-01
100's	$62.93	Carisoprodol Compound, United Res	00677-1068-01
100's	$71.74	Carisoprodol Compound, Amer Preferred	53445-1821-01
100's	$72.50	Carisoprodol Compound, Qualitest Pharms	00603-2583-21
100's	$73.20	SODOL COMPOUND, Major Pharms	00904-0356-60
100's	$75.76	Carisoprodol Compound, Aligen Independ	00405-0032-01
100's	$92.88	Carisoprodol Compound, HL Moore Drug Exch	00839-7162-06
100's	$95.00	Carisoprodol Compound, Goldline Labs	00182-1821-01
100's	$95.95	Carisoprodol Compound, Parmed Pharms	00349-8475-01
100's	$125.98	Carisoprodol & Aspirin, Schein Pharm (US)	00364-2524-01
100's	$127.74	Carisoprodol Compound, Ethex	58177-0236-04
100's	$130.51	Carisoprodol & Aspirin, Par Pharm	49884-0246-01
100's	$141.80	Carisoprodol Compound, Rugby	00536-3429-01
100's	**$166.86**	**SOMA COMPOUND, Wallace Labs**	**00037-2103-01**
500's	$150.00	Carisoprodol Compound, Consolidated Midland	00223-0658-05
500's	**$167.99**	**SOMA COMPOUND, Wallace Labs**	**00037-2103-85**
500's	$251.25	Carisoprodol Compound, H.C.F.A. F F P	99999-0314-02
500's	$338.80	SODOL COMPOUND, Major Pharms	00904-0356-40
500's	$405.50	Carisoprodol Compound, Rugby	00536-3429-05
500's	$456.89	Carisoprodol Compound, Parmed Pharms	00349-8475-05
500's	$460.00	Carisoprodol Compound, Goldline Labs	00182-1821-05
500's	$578.43	Carisoprodol & Aspirin, Par Pharm	49884-0246-05
500's	$578.46	Carisoprodol Compound, HL Moore Drug Exch	00839-7162-12
500's	**$823.08**	**SOMA COMPOUND, Wallace Labs**	**00037-2103-03**
1000's	$275.00	Carisoprodol Compound, Consolidated Midland	00223-0658-03

ASPIRIN; CARISOPRODOL; CODEINE PHOSPHATE *(000315)*

CATEGORIES: Analgesics; Autonomic Drugs; Pain; Skeletal Muscle Relaxants; DEA Class CIII; FDA Approved 1983 Jul

BRAND NAMES: **Soma Compound W/Codeine**

Prescribing information not available at time of publication.

HOW SUPPLIED - RATED THERAPEUTICALLY EQUIVALENT:

Tablet, Uncoated - Oral - 325 mg/200 mg/1

100's	$172.72	SOMA COMPOUND WITH CODEINE, Wallace Labs	00037-2403-01

ASPIRIN; CODEINE PHOSPHATE *(000317)*

CATEGORIES: Analgesics; Antipyretics; Arthritis; Central Nervous System Agents; Fever; Headache; Influenza; Opiate Agonists (Controlled); Pain; Salicylates; Pregnancy Category C; DEA Class CIII; FDA Pre 1938 Drugs

BRAND NAMES: *Analgin Forte*; *Aspalgin*; Aspirin W/Codeine; *Codiphen*; *Codis*; *Codral*; *Codral Forte* (Australia); *Decrin Powders*; *Disprin Forte*; *Dolviron*; Emcodeine; **Empirin W Codeine**; *Rokanite*; *Solcode*
(International brand names outside U.S. in italics)

FORMULARIES: Aetna; BC-BS; FHP; Medi-Cal

DESCRIPTION:

Aspirin with codeine has analgesic antipyretic and anti-inflammatory effects.

The components of aspirin with codeine have the following chemical names and structural formulae:

a. Aspirin (acetylsalicylic acid): 2-(acetyloxy) benzoic acid

b. Codeine phosphate U.S.P.: 7,8-didehydro-4, 5α-epoxy-3-methoxy-17-methylmorphinan- 6α-ol phosphate(1:1) (salt) hemihydrate

FOR COMPLETE PRESCRIBING INFORMATION, REFER TO THE INDIVIDUAL DRUG MONOGRAPHS (ASPIRIN; CODEINE PHOSPHATE).

INDICATIONS AND USAGE:

Aspirin with codeine is indicated for the relief of mild, moderate, and moderate to severe pain.

DOSAGE AND ADMINISTRATION:

Dosage is adjusted according to the severity of pain and the response to the patient. It may occasionally be necessary to exceed the usual dosage recommended below when pain is sever or the patient has become tolerant to the analgesic effect of codeine. Aspirin with codeine is given orally. The usual adult dose for aspirin with codeine No. 3 is one or two tablets every four hours as required. The usual dose for aspirin with codeine No. 4 is one tablet ever four hours as required.

Aspirin with codeine should be taken with food or a full glass of milk or water to lessen gastric irritation.

Storage: Store at 15° to 25°C (59° to 77°F) in a dry place and protect from light.

HOW SUPPLIED - EQUIVALENTS NOT AVAILABLE:

Tablet, Uncoated - Oral - 325 mg/15 mg

100's	$8.95	Aspirin With Codeine Phosphate, Parmed Pharms	00349-8655-01
1000's	$52.10	Aspirin 325, Halsey Drug	00879-0441-10

Tablet, Uncoated - Oral - 325 mg/30 mg

100's	$9.40	EMCODEINE #3, Major Pharms	00904-3900-60
100's	$9.71	Aspirin With Codeine Phosphate No 3, HL Moore Drug Exch	00839-6435-06

HOW SUPPLIED - EQUIVALENTS NOT AVAILABLE: *(cont'd)*

100's	$10.55	Aspirin W/Codeine, Qualitest Pharms	00603-2361-21
100's	$10.60	Aspirin With Codeine 30, Rugby	00536-3328-01
100's	$10.85	Aspirin With Codeine Phosphate 30, Zenith Labs	00172-3984-60
100's	$10.85	Aspirin With Codeine 30, Goldline Labs	00182-1225-01
100's	$10.95	Aspirin 325, Halsey Drug	00879-0442-01
100's	$10.95	Aspirin W/Codeine, Martec Pharms	52555-0333-01
100's	$11.23	Aspirin, United Res	00677-0647-01
100's	$11.97	Aspirin W/Codeine Phosphate, Schein Pharm (US)	00364-0540-01
100's	$12.95	Aspirin With Codeine Phosphate No. 3, Parmed Pharms	00349-4082-01
100's	$13.10	Aspirin W/Codeine, HL Moore Drug Exch	00839-7857-06
100's	$13.44	Aspirin W/Codeine, Aligen Independ	00405-0021-01
100's	$36.73	EMPIRIN WITH CODEINE NO.3, Glaxo Wellcome	00173-0220-55
500's	$36.50	Aspirin 325, Halsey Drug	00879-0442-05
500's	$180.12	EMPIRIN WITH CODEINE NO.3, Glaxo Wellcome	00173-0220-70
1000's	$74.80	Aspirin 325, Halsey Drug	00879-0442-10
1000's	$78.38	Aspirin With Codeine 30, Rugby	00536-3328-10
1000's	$81.66	Aspirin With Codeine Phosphate No 3, HL Moore Drug Exch	00839-6435-16
1000's	$93.50	Aspirin W/Codeine, Qualitest Pharms	00603-2361-32
1000's	$93.55	Aspirin With Codeine Phosphate 30, Zenith Labs	00172-3984-80
1000's	$93.80	Aspirin W/Codeine, Martec Pharms	52555-0333-10
1000's	$109.95	Aspirin With Codeine Phosphate No. 3, Parmed Pharms	00349-4082-10

Tablet, Uncoated - Oral - 325 mg/60 mg

100's	$12.00	Aspirin With Codeine Phosphate No 4, HL Moore Drug Exch	00839-6776-06
100's	$14.65	EMCODEINE # 4, Major Pharms	00904-3907-60
100's	$15.75	Aspirin W/Codeine, Rugby	00536-3329-01
100's	$17.75	Aspirin 325, Halsey Drug	00879-0443-01
100's	$18.35	Aspirin With Codeine, #4, United Res	00677-0676-01
100's	$18.40	Aspirin With Codeine, Zenith Labs	00172-3985-60
100's	$18.40	Aspirin With Codeine Phosphate, Goldline Labs	00182-1226-01
100's	$18.40	Aspirin W/Codeine, Qualitest Pharms	00603-2362-21
100's	$18.97	Aspirin W/Codeine, Martec Pharms	52555-0334-01
100's	$19.10	Aspirin W/Codeine, HL Moore Drug Exch	00839-7858-06
100's	$19.53	Aspirin With Codeine Phosphate, Parmed Pharms	00349-8337-01
100's	$20.29	Aspirin W/Codeine Phosphate, Schein Pharm (US)	00364-0541-01
100's	$20.67	Aspirin 325, Aligen Independ	00405-0022-01
100's	$24.25	Aspirin W/Codeine, Geneva Pharms	00781-1875-13
100's	$85.80	EMPIRIN WITH CODEINE NO. 4, Glaxo Wellcome	00173-0225-55
500's	$74.93	Aspirin W/Codeine, Rugby	00536-3329-05
500's	$83.75	Aspirin 325, Halsey Drug	00879-0443-05
500's	$86.25	Aspirin With Codeine, Zenith Labs	00172-3985-70
500's	$427.87	EMPIRIN WITH CODEINE NO. 4, Glaxo Wellcome	00173-0225-70
1000's	$129.95	Aspirin 325, Halsey Drug	00879-0443-10
1000's	$171.10	Aspirin With Codeine Phosphate, Parmed Pharms	00349-8337-10

ASPIRIN; HYDROCODONE BITARTRATE

(000319)

CATEGORIES: Analgesics; Antipyretics; Central Nervous System Agents; Narcotics, Synthetics & Combinations; Opiate Agonists (Controlled); Pain; Pregnancy Category C; DEA Class CIII; FDA Approved 1988 Jan

BRAND NAMES: Alor; **Azdone**; Damason-P; Lortab Asa; Panasal

FORMULARIES: Aetna

DESCRIPTION:

Each tablet contains:

Hydrocodone Bitartrate: 5 mg

Aspirin: 500 mg

(WARNING: May be habit forming)

Hydrocodone bitartrate is an opioid analgesic and antitussive and occurs as fine, white crystals or as a crystalline powder. It is affected by light. The chemical name is: 4,5 α-epoxy-3-methoxy-17-methylmorphinan-6-one tartrate (1:1) hydrate (2:5).

Aspirin, salicylic acid acetate, is a non-opiate, salicylate analgesic, anti-inflammatory, and antipyretic which occurs as a white, crystalline tabular or needle-like powder and is odorless or has a faint odor.

Inactive Ingredients: Corn Starch, D&C Red #7 (Calcium Lake), Sodium Starch Glycolate, and Stearic Acid.

CLINICAL PHARMACOLOGY:

Hydrocodone: Hydrocodone is a semisynthetic narcotic analgesic and antitussive with multiple actions qualitatively similar to those of codeine. Most of these involve the central nervous system and smooth muscle. The precise mechanism of action of hydrocodone and other opiates, is not known, although it is believed to relate to the existence of opiate receptors in the central nervous system. In addition to analgesia, narcotics may produce drowsiness, changes in mood and mental clouding.

Radioimmunoassay techniques have recently been developed for the analysis of hydrocodone in human plasma. After a 10 mg oral dose of hydrocodone bitartrate, a mean peak serum drug level of 23.6 ng/ml and an elimination half-life of 3.8 hours were found.

Aspirin: The analgesic, anti-inflammatory and antipyretic effects of aspirin are believed to result from inhibition of the synthesis of certain prostaglandins. Aspirin interferes with clotting mechanisms primarily by diminishing platelet aggregation; at high doses prothrombin synthesis can be inhibited.

Aspirin in solution is rapidly absorbed from the stomach and from the upper small intestine. About 50 percent of an oral dose is absorbed in 30 minutes and peak plasma concentrations are reached in about 40 minutes. Higher than normal stomach pH or the presence of food slightly delays absorption.

Once absorbed, aspirin is mainly hydrolyzed to salicylic acid and distributed to all body tissues and fluids, including fetal tissue, breast milk and the central nervous system (CNS). Highest concentrations are found in plasma, liver, renal cortex, heart and lung.

From 50 to 80 percent of salicylic acid and its metabolites in plasma are loosely bound to protein. The plasma half-life of total salicylate is about 3.0 hours, with a 650 mg dose. Higher doses of aspirin cause increaseS in plasma salicylate half-life.

Almost all of a therapeutic dose of aspirin is excreted through the kidneys either as salicylic acid or its metabolites. Renal clearance of salicylate is greatly augmented by an alkaline urine, as is produced by concurrent administration of sodium bicarbonate or potassium citrate.

CLINICAL PHARMACOLOGY: *(cont'd)*

Toxic salicylate blood levels are usually above 30 mg/100 ml. The single lethal dose of aspirin in normal adults is approximately 25-30 g, but patients have recovered from much larger doses with appropriate treatment.

INDICATIONS AND USAGE:

For the relief of moderate to moderately severe pain.

CONTRAINDICATIONS:

Hydrocodone Bitartrate and Aspirin Tablets are contraindicated under the following conditions:

(1) Hypersensitivity or intolerance to hydrocodone or aspirin.

(2) Severe bleeding, disorders of coagulation or primary hemostasis including hemophilia, hypoprothrombinemia, von Willebrand's disease, thrombocytopenias, thrombasthenia and other ill-defined hereditary platelet dysfunctions, severe vitamin K deficiency and severe liver damage.

(3) Anticoagulant therapy.

(4) Peptic ulcer, or other serious gastrointestinal lesions.

WARNINGS:

HYDROCODONE

Respiratory Depression: At high doses or in sensitive patients, hydrocodone may produce dose-related respiratory depression by acting directly on the brain stem respiratory center. Hydrocodone also affects the center that controls respiratory rhythm, and may produce irregular and periodic breathing.

Head Injury and Increased Intracranial Pressure: The respiratory depressant effects of narcotics and their capacity to elevate cerebrospinal fluid pressure may be markedly exaggerated in the presence of head injury, other intracranial lesions or a pre-existing increase in intracranial pressure. Furthermore, narcotics produce adverse reactions which may obscure the clinical course of patients with head injuries.

Acute Abdominal Conditions: The administration of narcotics may obscure the diagnosis or clinical course of patients with acute abdominal conditions.

ASPIRIN

Allergic Reactions: Therapeutic doses of aspirin can cause anaphylactic shock and other severe allergic reactions. A history of allergy is often lacking.

Bleeding: Significant bleeding can result from aspirin therapy in patients with peptic ulcer or other gastrointestinal lesions, and in patients with bleeding disorders. Aspirin administered preoperatively may prolong the bleeding time.

PRECAUTIONS:

SPECIAL RISK PATIENTS

As with any narcotic analgesic agent, Hydrocodone Bitartrate and Aspirin Tablets should be used with caution in elderly or debilitated patients and those with severe impairment of hepatic or renal function, gallbladder disease or gallstones, respiratory impairment, cardiac arrhythmias, inflammatory disorders of the gastrointestinal tract, hypothyroidism, Addison's disease, prostatic hypertrophy or urethral stricture, coagulation disorders, head injuries or acute abdominal conditions. The usual precautions should be observed and the possibility of respiratory depression should not be overlooked.

Precautions should be taken when administering salicylates to persons with known allergies. Hypersensitivity to aspirin is particularly likely in patients with nasal polyps, and relatively common with asthma.

INFORMATION FOR THE PATIENT

Hydrocodone Bitartrate and Aspirin Tablets, like all narcotics, may impair the mental and/or physical abilities required for the performance of potentially hazardous tasks such as driving a car or operating machinery; patients should be cautioned accordingly.

COUGH REFLEX

Hydrocodone suppresses the cough reflex; as with all narcotics, caution should be exercised when Hydrocodone Bitartrate and Aspirin Tablets are used postoperatively and in patients with pulmonary disease.

LABORATORY TESTS

Hypersensitivity to aspirin cannot be detected by skin testing or radioimmunoassay procedures.

DRUG/LABORATORY TEST INTERACTIONS

Aspirin: Aspirin may interfere with the following laboratory determinations.

In Blood: Serum amylase, fasting blood glucose, carbon dioxide, cholesterol, protein, protein bound iodine, uric acid, prothrombin time, bleeding time, and spectrophotometric detection of barbiturates.

In Urine: Glucose, 5-hydroxyindoleacetic acid, Gerhardt ketone, vanillylmandelic acid (VMA), protein, uric acid, and diacetic acid.

PREGNANCY, TERATOGENIC EFFECTS, PREGNANCY CATEGORY C

Hydrocodone: Hydrocodone has been shown to be teratogenic in hamsters when given in doses 700 times the human dose. There are no adequate and well-controlled studies in pregnant women. Hydrocodone Bitartrate and Aspirin Tablets should be used during pregnancy only if the potential benefit justifies the potential risk to the fetus.

Aspirin: Reproductive studies in rats and mice have shown aspirin to be teratogenic and embryocidal at four to six times the human therapeutic dose. Studies in pregnant women however, have not shown that aspirin increases the risk of abnormalities when administered during the first trimester of pregnancy. In controlled studies involving 41,337 pregnant women and their offspring, there was no evidence that aspirin taken during pregnancy caused stillbirth, neonatal death or reduced birthweight. In controlled studies of 50,282 pregnant women and their offspring, aspirin administration in moderate and heavy doses during the first four months of pregnancy showed no teratogenic effect.

NONTERATOGENIC EFFECTS

Hydrocodone: Babies born to mothers who have been taking opioids regularly prior to delivery will be physically dependent. The withdrawal signs include irritability and excessive crying, tremors, hyperactive reflexes, increased respiratory rate, increased stools, sneezing, yawning, vomiting, and fever. The intensity of the syndrome does not always correlate with the duration of maternal opioid use of dose. There is no consensus on the best method of managing withdrawal. Chlorpromazine 0.7 to 1 mg/kg every 6 hours, and paregoric 2 to 4 drops/kg every 4 hours, have been used to treat withdrawal symptoms in infants. The duration of therapy is 4 to 28 days, with the dosage decreased as tolerated.

Aspirin: Therapeutic doses of aspirin in pregnant women close to term may cause bleeding in the mother, fetus, or neonate. During the last six months of pregnancy, regular use of aspirin in high doses may prolong pregnancy and delivery.

PRECAUTIONS: *(cont'd)*

LABOR AND DELIVERY

As with all narcotics, administration of Hydrocodone Bitartrate and Aspirin Tablets to the mother shortly before delivery may result in some degree of respiratory depression in the newborn, especially if higher doses are used. Ingestion of aspirin prior to delivery may prolong delivery or lead to bleeding in the mother or neonate.

NURSING MOTHERS

Aspirin is excreted in human milk in a small amount; the significance of its effect on nursing infants is not known. It is not known whether hydrocodone is excreted in human milk. Because many drugs are excreted in human milk and because of the potential for serious adverse reactions in nursing infants, a decision should be made whether to discontinue nursing or to discontune the drug, taking into account the importance of the drug to the mother.

PEDIATRIC USE

Safety and effectiveness in children have not been established.

DRUG INTERACTIONS:

Hydrocodone: Patients receiving other narcotic analgesics, antipsychotics, antianxiety agents, or other CNS depressants (including alcohol) concomitantly with Hydrocodone Bitartrate and Aspirin Tablets may exhibit additive CNS depression. When combined therapy is contemplated, the dose of one or both agents should be reduced.

The use of MAO inhibitors or tricyclic antidepressants with hydrocodone preparations may increase the effect of either the antidepressant or hydrocodone.

The concurrent use of anticholinergics with hydrocodone, as with all narcotics, may produce paralytic ileus.

Aspirin: Aspirin may **enhance** the effects of:

(1) oral anticoagulants, causing bleeding by inhibiting prothrombin formation in the liver and displacing anticoagulants from plasma protein binding sites.

(2) oral antidiabetic agents and insulin, causing hypoglycemia by contributing an additive effect, and by displacing the oral antidiabetic agent from secondary binding sites.

(3) 6-mercaptopurine and methotrexate, causing bone morrow toxicity and blood dyscrasias by displacing these drugs from secondary binding sites.

(4) non-steroidal anti-inflammatory agents, increasing the risk of peptic ulceration and bleeding by contributing additive effects.

(5) corticosteroids, potentiating anti-inflammatory effects by displacing steroids from protein binding sites. Aspirin intoxication may occur with corticosteroid withdrawal because steroids promote renal clearance of salicylates.

Aspirin may **diminish** the effects of uricosuric agents, such as probenecid and sulfinpyrazone, in the treatment of gout by competing for protein binding sites.

ADVERSE REACTIONS:

The most frequently observed adverse reactions include lightheadedness, dizziness, sedation, nausea and vomiting. These effects seem to be more prominent in ambulatory than in nonambulatory patients and some of these adverse reactions may be alleviated if the patient lies down.Others adverse reactions include:

CENTRAL NERVOUS SYSTEM

Hydrocodone: Drowsiness, mental clouding, lethargy, impairment of mental and physical performance, anxiety, fear, dysphoria, psychic dependence and mood changes.

Aspirin: Headache, drowsiness, and mental confusion can occur in response to chronic use of large doses.

GASTROINTESTINAL SYSTEM

Hydrocodone: The antiemetic phenothiazines are useful in suppressing the nausea and vomiting which may occur; however, some phenothiazine derivatives seem to be antianalgesic and to increase the amount of narcotic required to produce pain relief, while other phenothiazines reduce the amount of narcotic required to produce a given level of analgesia. Prolonged administration of Hydrocodone Bitartrate and Aspirin Tablets may produce constipation.

Aspirin: Some patients are unable to take aspirin or other salicylates without developing nausea or vomiting. Occasional patients respond to aspirin (usually large doses) with dyspepsia or heartburn, which may be accompanied by occult bleeding. Excessive bruising or bleeding is sometimes seen in patients with mild disorders of primary hemostasis who regularly use low doses of aspirin. Prolonged use of aspirin can cause painless erosion of gastric mucosa, occult bleeding, and, infrequently, iron-deficiency anemia. High doses of aspirin can exacerbate symptoms of peptic ulcer and, occasionally, cause extensive bleeding. Excessive bleeding can follow injury or surgery in patients with or without known bleeding disorders who have taken therapeutic doses of aspirin within the preceding 10 days. Hepatotoxicity has been reported in association with prolonged use of large doses of aspirin in patients with lupus erythematosus, rheumatoid arthritis and rheumatic disease.

HEMATOLOGIC

Aspirin: Bone marrow depression, manifested by weakness, fatigue or abnormal bruising or bleeding, has occasionally been reported with aspirin. In patients with glucose-6-phosphate dehydrogenase deficiency, aspirin can cause a mild degree of hemolytic anemia.

RESPIRATORY

Hydrocodone: Hydrocodone bitartrate may produce dose-related respiratory depression by acting directly on the brain stem respiratory center. Hydrocodone also affects the center that controls respiratory rhythm, and may produce irregular and periodic breathing. If significant respiratory depression occurs, it may be antagonized by the use of naloxone hydrochloride. Apply other supportive measures when indicated.

Aspirin: Hyperpnea and hyperventilation can occur in response to chronic use of large doses.

CARDIOVASCULAR

Aspirin: Tachycardia can occur in response to chronic use of large doses of aspirin.

GENITOURINARY

Hydrocodone: Ureteral spasm, spasm of vesical sphincters and urinary retention have been reported.

METABOLIC

Aspirin: In hyperuricemic persons, low doses of aspirin may reduce the effectiveness of uricosuric therapy or precipitate an attack of gout.

ALLERGIC

Aspirin: Therapeutic doses of aspirin can induce mild or severe allergic reactions manifested by skin rashes, urticaria, angioedema, rhinorrhea, asthma, abdominal pain, nausea, vomiting, or anaphylactic shock. A history of allergy is often lacking, and allergic reactions may occur even in patients who have previously taken aspirin without any ill effects. Allergic reactions to aspirin are most likely to occur in patients with a history of allergic disease, especially in patients with nasal polyps or asthma.

OTHER

Aspirin: Sweating and thirst can occur in response to chronic use of large doses of aspirin.

DRUG ABUSE AND DEPENDENCE:

Hydrocodone Bitartrate and Aspirin Tablets are subject to the Federal Controlled Substance Act (Schedule CIII).

Psychic dependence, physical dependence, and tolerance may develop upon repeated administration of narcotics; therefore, Hydrocodone Bitartrate and Aspirin Tablets should be prescribed and administered with caution. However, psychic dependence is unlikely to develop when Hydrocodone Bitartrate and Aspirin Tablets are used for a short time for the treatment of pain.

Physical dependence, the condition in which continued administration of the drug is required to prevent the appearance of a withdrawal syndrome, assumes clinically significant proportions only after several weeks of continued oral narcotic use, although some mild degree of physical dependence may develop after a few days of narcotic therapy. Tolerance, in which increasingly large doses are required in order to produce the same degree of analgesia, is manifested initially by shortened duration of analgesic effect, and subsequently by decreases in the intensity of analgesia. The rate of development of tolerance varies among patients.

OVERDOSAGE:

HYDROCODONE

Signs and Symptoms: Serious overdose with hydrocodone is characterized by respiratory depression (a decrease in respiratory rate and/or tidal volume, Cheyne-Stokes respiration, cyanosis), extreme somnolence progressing to stupor or coma, skeletal muscle flaccidity, cold and clammy skin, and sometimes bradycardia and hypotension. In severe overdosage apnea, circulatory collapse, cardiac arrest and death may occur.

Treatment: Primary attention should be given to the reestablishment of adequate respiratory exchange through provision of a patent airway and institution of assisted or controlled ventilation. If significant respiratory depression occurs, it may be antagonized by the use of naloxone hydrochloride, preferably intravenously. Naloxone promptly reverses the effects of morphine-like opioid antagonists such as hydrocodone. In patients who are physically dependent, small doses of naloxone may be sufficient not only to antagonize respiratory depression, but also to precipitate withdrawal phenomena. The dose of naloxone should therefore be adjusted accordingly in such patients. Since the duration of action of hydrocodone may exceed that of the antagonist, the patient should be kept under continued surveillance and repeated doses of the antagonist should be administered as needed to maintain adequate respiration.

A narcotic antagonist should not be administered in the absence of clinically significant respiratory or cardiovascular depression. Oxygen, intravenous fluids, vasopressors and other supportive measures should be employed as indicated.

Gastric emptying may be useful in removing unabsorbed drug.

ASPIRIN

Signs and Symptoms: The most severe manifestations from aspirin result from cardiovascular and respiratory insufficiency secondary to acid-base and electrolyte disturbances, complicated by hyperthermia and dehydration.

Respiratory alkalosis is characteristic of the early phase of intoxication with aspirin while hyperventilation is occurring, but is quickly followed by metabolic acidosis in most people with severe intoxication.

Concentrations of aspirin in plasma above 30 mg/100 ml are associated with toxicity (See CLINICAL PHARMACOLOGY). The single lethal dose of aspirin in adults is probably about 25-30 g, but is not known with certainty.

Hemodialysis and peritoneal dialysis can be performed to reduce the body aspirin content.

Treatment: Treatment consists primarily of supporting vital functions, increasing salicylate elimination, and correcting the acid-base imbalance due primarily to salicylism.

Gastric emptying (Syrup of Ipecac) and/or lavage is recommended as soon as possible after ingestion, even if the patient has vomited spontaneously. Administration of activated charcoal as a slurry is beneficial after lavage and/or emesis, if less than three hours have passed since ingestion. Charcoal adsorption should **not** be employed prior to emesis or lavage.

Severity of aspirin intoxication is determined by measuring the blood salicylate level. Acid-base status should be closely followed with serial blood gas and serum pH measurements. Fluid and electrolyte balance should also be regularly monitored.

In severe cases, hyperthermia and hypovolemia are the major immediate threats to life. Children should be sponged with tepid water. Replacement fluid should be administered intravenously and augmented with sufficient bicarbonate to correct acidosis, with monitoring of plasma electrolytes and pH, to promote alkaline diuresis of salicylate if renal function is normal.Complete control may also require infusion of glucose to control hypoglycemia.

In patients with renal insufficiency or in cases of life-threatening intoxication, dialysis is usually required. Peritoneal dialysis or exchange transfusion is indicated in infants and young children and hemodialysis in older patients.

DOSAGE AND ADMINISTRATION:

Dosage should be adjusted according to the severity of the pain and the response of the patient. However, tolerance to hydrocodone can develop with continued use and the incidence of untoward effects is dose related.

The usual adult dosage is one or two tablets every four to six hours as needed for pain. The total 24 hour dose should not exceed 8 tablets.

Hydrocodone Bitartrate and Aspirin Tablets should be taken with food or a full glass of milk or water to lessen gastric irritation.

Storage: Store at controlled room temperature 15-30°C (59-86°F). Protect from moisture.

Dispense in a tight, light-resistant container as defined in the USP/NF with a child-resistant closure.

HOW SUPPLIED - EQUIVALENTS NOT AVAILABLE:

Tablet, Uncoated - Oral - 500 mg/5 mg

100's	$26.88	Alor, Atley Pharms	59702-0550-01
100's	$27.00	Panasal, ECR Pharms	00095-0131-01
100's	**$31.50**	**AZDONE, Schwarz Pharma (US)**	**00131-2821-37**
100's	$37.68	DAMASON-P REFORMULATED, Mason Pharms	12758-0057-01
100's	$59.79	LORTAB ASA, UCB Pharma	50474-0500-01
500's	$162.18	Damason-P Reformulated Tablets, Mason Pharms	12758-0057-05
1000's	**$271.00**	**AZDONE, Schwarz Pharma (US)**	**00131-2821-43**
1000's	$316.81	DAMASON-P REFORMULATED, Mason Pharms	12758-0057-10

ASPIRIN; MEPROBAMATE *(000320)*

CATEGORIES: Analgesics; Antipyretics; Anxiety; Central Nervous System Agents; Neuromuscular; Nonsteroidal Anti-Inflammatory; Pain; Skeletal Muscle Hyperactivity; Tension; DEA Class CIV; FDA Approval Pre 1982

BRAND NAMES: Epromate-M; **Equagesic**; Equazine-M; Heptogesic; Meprogesic; Micrainin

FORMULARIES: Aetna

DESCRIPTION:

FOR COMPLETE PRESCRIBING INFORMATION, REFER TO THE INDIVIDUAL DRUG MONOGRAPHS (ASPIRIN; MEPROBAMATE).

INDICATIONS AND USAGE:

As an adjunct in the short-term treatment of pain accompanied by tension and/or anxiety in patients with musculoskeletal disease. Clinical trials have demonstrated that in these situations relief of pain is somewhat greater than with aspirin alone.

The effectiveness of Meprobamate w/ Aspirin in long-term use, that is, more than 4 months, has not been assessed by systematic clinical studies. The physician should periodically reassess the usefulness of the drug for the individual patient.

DOSAGE AND ADMINISTRATION:

The usual dosage of Meprobamate w/ Aspirin is one or two tablets, each tablet containing meprobamate, 200 mg, and aspirin, 325 mg, orally 3 to 4 times daily as needed for the relief of pain when tension or anxiety is present.

Meprobamate w/ Aspirin is not recommended for patients 12 years of age and under.

Keep tightly closed.

Protect from light.

Dispense in light-resistant, tight container.

HOW SUPPLIED - RATED THERAPEUTICALLY EQUIVALENT:

Tablet, Uncoated - Oral - 325 mg/200 mg

100's	$20.90	EPROMATE-M, Major Pharms	00904-0671-60
100's	$24.90	Meprobamate W/Aspirin, Qualitest Drugs	52446-0582-21
100's	$32.79	Meprobamate W/Aspirin, Major Pharms	00904-0671-61
100's	**$74.94**	**EQUAGESIC, Wyeth Labs**	**00008-0091-02**
100's	$124.93	MICRAININ, Wallace Labs	00037-0120-01
500's	$98.05	EPROMATE-M, Major Pharms	00904-0671-40
1000's	$166.70	Meprobamate W/Aspirin, Major Pharms	00904-0671-80

ASPIRIN; METHOCARBAMOL *(000321)*

CATEGORIES: Analgesics; Autonomic Drugs; Muscle Relaxants; Neuromuscular; Pain; Skeletal Muscle Hyperactivity; Skeletal Muscle Relaxants; FDA Approval Pre 1982

BRAND NAMES: *Ortoton Plus* (Germany); Robamol W/Aspirin; **Robaxisal**; *Robaxisal Forte* (England)
(International brand names outside U.S. in italics)

FORMULARIES: Aetna; BC-BS

DESCRIPTION:

For oral administration, Aspirin with methocarbamol is available as a pink and white laminated tablet containing:

Methocarbamol, USP: 400 mg

Aspirin, USP: 325 mg

Inactive Ingredients: Corn Starch, FD&C Red 3, Magnesium Stearate, Povidone, Sodium Lauryl Sulfate, Sodium Starch Glycolate, Stearic Acid.

3-(2-Methoxyphenoxy)-1,2-propanediol 1-Carbamate

CLINICAL PHARMACOLOGY:

Aspirin with methocarbamol provides a double approach to the management of discomforts associated with musculoskeletal disorders.

Methocarbamol: The mechanism of action of methocarbamol in humans has not been established, but may be due to general central nervous system depression. It has no direct action on the contractile mechanism of striated muscle, the motor end plate or the nerve fiber.

Aspirin: Aspirin is a mild analgesic with anti-inflammatory and antipyretic activity.

INDICATIONS AND USAGE:

Aspirin with methocarbamol is indicated as an adjunct to rest, physical therapy, and other measures for the relief of discomfort associated with acute, painful musculoskeletal conditions. The mode of action of methocarbamol has not been clearly identified but may be related to its sedative properties. Methocarbamol does not directly relax tense skeletal muscles in man.

CONTRAINDICATIONS:

Hypersensitivity to methocarbamol or aspirin.

WARNINGS:

Since methocarbamol may possess a general central nervous system depressant effect, patients receiving Aspirin with methocarbamol should be cautioned about combined effects with alcohol and other CNS depressants.

PRECAUTIONS:

Products containing aspirin should be administered with caution to patients with gastritis or peptic ulceration, or those receiving hypoprothrombinemic anticoagulants.

Methocarbamol may cause a color interference in certain screening tests for 5-hydroxyindoleacetic acid (5-HIAA) and vanilmandelic acid (VMA).

PREGNANCY

Safe use of Aspirin with methocarbamol has not been established with regard to possible adverse effects upon fetal development. Therefore, Aspirin with methocarbamol should not be used in women who are or may become pregnant and particularly during early pregnancy unless in the judgment of the physician the potential benefits outweigh the possible hazards.

NURSING MOTHERS

It is not known whether methocarbamol is secreted in human milk; however, aspirin does appear in human milk in moderate amounts. It can produce a bleeding tendency either by interfering with the function of the infant's platelets or by decreasing the amount of prothrombin in the blood. The risk is minimal if the mother takes the aspirin just after nursing and if the infant has an adequate store of vitamin K. As a general rule, nursing should not be undertaken while a patient is on a drug.

PEDIATRIC USE

Safety and effectiveness in children 12 years of age and below have not been established.

PRECAUTIONS: *(cont'd)*

USE IN ACTIVITIES REQUIRING MENTAL ALERTNESS

Aspirin with methocarbamol may rarely cause drowsiness. Until the patient's response has been determined, he should be cautioned against the operation of motor vehicles or dangerous machinery.

ADVERSE REACTIONS:

The most frequent adverse reaction to methocarbamol is dizziness or lightheadedness and nausea. This occurs in about one in 20-25 patients. Less frequent reactions are drowsiness, blurred vision, headache, fever, allergic manifestations such as urticaria, pruritus, and rash.

Adverse reactions that have been associated with the use of aspirin include: nausea and other gastrointestinal discomfort, gastritis, gastric erosion, vomiting, constipation, diarrhea, angioedema, asthma, rash, pruritus, urticaria.

Gastrointestinal discomfort may be minimized by taking Aspirin with methocarbamol with food.

OVERDOSAGE:

Toxicity due to overdosage of methocarbamol is unlikely; however, acute overdosage of aspirin may cause symptoms of salicylate intoxication.

Treatment: Supportive therapy for 24 hours, as methocarbamol is excreted within that time. If salicylate intoxication occurs, especially in children, the hyperpnea may be controlled with sodium bicarbonate. Judicious use of 5% CO_2 with 95% O_2may be of benefit. Abnormal electrolyte patterns should be corrected with appropriate fluid therapy.

DOSAGE AND ADMINISTRATION:

Adults and Children Over 12 Years of Age: Two tablets four times daily. Three tablets four times daily may be used in severe conditions for one to three days in patients who are able to tolerate salicylates. These dosage recommendations provide respectively 3.2 and 4.8 grams of methocarbamol per day.

Storage: Store at controlled room temperature, between 15°C and 30C (59°F and 86F).

HOW SUPPLIED - RATED THERAPEUTICALLY EQUIVALENT:

Tablet, Uncoated - Oral - 325 mg/400 mg

48's	$7.27	Methocarbamol & Aspirin, H.C.F.A. F F P	99999-0321-01
100's	$15.15	Methocarbamol & Aspirin, H.C.F.A. F F P	99999-0321-02
100's	$19.24	Methocarbamol W/Aspirin, HL Moore Drug Exch	00839-6284-06
100's	$22.29	Methocarbamol & Aspirin, Rugby	00536-4028-01
100's	$23.25	Methocarbamol & Aspirin, Major Pharms	00904-0227-60
100's	$23.62	Methocarbamol W/Aspirin, Caremark	00339-5823-12
100's	$23.95	Methocarbamol & Aspirin, United Res	00677-0579-01
100's	$24.30	Methocarbamol With Aspirin, Zenith Labs	00172-2813-60
100's	$24.30	Methocarbamol & Aspirin, Goldline Labs	00182-1911-01
100's	$24.85	Methocarbamol & Aspirin, Par Pharm	49884-0249-01
100's	$25.11	Methocarbamol W/Aspirin, Qualitest Pharms	00603-4489-21
100's	$25.29	Methocarbamol & Aspirin, Aligen Independ	00405-4641-01
100's	**$52.79**	**ROBAXISAL, AH Robins**	**00031-7469-63**
500's	$75.75	Methocarbamol & Aspirin, H.C.F.A. F F P	99999-0321-03
500's	$105.50	Robamol W/Aspirin, Major Pharms	00904-0227-40
500's	$114.55	Methocarbamol With Aspirin, Zenith Labs	00172-2813-70
500's	$115.50	Methocarbamol & Aspirin, Par Pharm	49884-0249-05
500's	**$245.75**	**ROBAXISAL, AH Robins**	**00031-7469-70**

ASPIRIN; OXYCODONE HYDROCHLORIDE; OXYCODONE TEREPHTHALATE *(000322)*

CATEGORIES: Analgesics; Antipyretics; Central Nervous System Agents; Narcotics, Synthetics & Combinations; Opiate Agonists (Controlled); Pain; DEA Class CII; FDA Approval Pre 1982

BRAND NAMES: Codoxy; Endodan; *Oxycodan* (Canada); Oxycodone W/Aspirin; **Percodan**; *Percodan-Demi* (Canada); Roxiprin
(International brand names outside U.S. in italics)

FORMULARIES: Aetna; BC-BS; CIGNA; FHP; Humana; Kaiser; Medco; Medi-Cal; PruCare; United

DESCRIPTION:

Note: This monograph pertains to both Percodan and Percodan-Demi. (The innovator brand name has been left in so as to avoid confusion).

Each tablet of Percodan contains:

Oxycodone hydrochloride: 4.50 mg* (WARNING: May be habit forming)

Oxycodone terephthalate: 0.38 mg** (WARNING: May be habit forming)

Aspirin, USP: 325 mg

*4.50 mg oxycodone HCl is equivalent to 4.0338 mg of oxycodone.

**0.38 mg oxycodone terephthalate is equivalent to 0.3008 mg of oxycodone.

Percodan Tablets also contain: D&C Yellow 10, FD&C Yellow 6, microcrystalline cellulose and starch.

The oxycodone component is 14-hydroxydihydrocodeinone, a white odorless crystalline powder which is derived from the opium alkaloid, thebaine.

Each tablet of Percodan-Demi contains:

Oxycodone hydrochloride: 2.25 mg* (WARNING: May be habit forming)

Oxycodone terephthalate: 0.19 mg** (WARNING: May be habit forming)

Aspirin, USP: 325 mg

*2.25 mg oxycodone HCl is equivalent to 2.0169 mg of oxycodone.

**0.19 mg oxycodone terephthalate is equivalent to 0.1504 mg of oxycodone.

Percodan-Demi Tablets also contain: microcrystalline cellulose and starch.

The oxycodone component is 14-hydroxydihydrocodeinone, a white odorless crystalline powder which is derived from the opium alkaloid, thebaine.

CLINICAL PHARMACOLOGY:

The principal ingredient, oxycodone, is a semisynthetic narcotic analgesic with multiple actions qualitatively similar to those of morphine; the most prominent of these involve the central nervous system and organs composed of smooth muscle. The principle actions of therapeutic value of the oxycodone in Percodan are analgesia and sedation.

Oxycodone is similar to codeine and methadone in that it retains at least one half of its analgesic activity when administered orally.

Percodan also contains the non-narcotic antipyretic-analgesic, aspirin.

INDICATIONS AND USAGE:

For the relief of moderate to moderately severe pain.

CONTRAINDICATIONS:

Hypersensitivity to oxycodone or aspirin.

WARNINGS:

DRUG DEPENDENCE

Oxycodone can produce drug dependence of the morphine type and, therefore, has the potential for being abused. Psychic dependence, physical dependence and tolerance may develop upon repeated administration of Percodan, and it should be prescribed and administered with the same degree of caution appropriate to the use of other oral narcotic-containing medications. Like other narcotic-containing medications, Percodan is subject to the Federal Controlled Substances Act.

USAGE IN AMBULATORY PATIENTS

Oxycodone may impair the mental and/or physical abilities required for the performance of potentially hazardous tasks such as driving a car or operating machinery. The patient using Percodan should be cautioned accordingly.

Interaction with Other Central Nervous System Depressants

Patients receiving other narcotic analgesics, general anesthetics, phenothiazines, other tranquilizers, sedative-hypnotics or other CNS depressants (including alcohol) concomitantly with Percodan may exhibit an additive CNS depression. When such combined therapy is contemplated, the dose of one or both agents should be reduced.

USAGE IN PREGNANCY

Safe use in pregnancy has not been established relative to possible adverse effects on fetal development. Therefore, Percodan should not be used in pregnant women unless, in the judgment of the physician, the potential benefits outweigh the possible hazards.

USAGE IN CHILDREN

Percodan should not be administered to children. Percodan-Demi, containing half the amount of oxycodone, can be considered.)

REYE SYNDROME

Reye Syndrome is a rare but serious disease which can follow flu or chicken pox in children and teenagers. While the cause of Reye Syndrome is unknown, some reports claim aspirin (or salicylates) may increase the risk of developing this disease.

Salicylates should be used with caution in the presence of peptic ulcer or coagulation abnormalities.

PRECAUTIONS:

Head Injury and Increased Intracranial Pressure: The respiratory depressant effects of narcotics and their capacity to elevate cerebrospinal fluid pressure may be markedly exaggerated in the presence of head injury, other intracranial lesions or a pre-existing increase in intracranial pressure. Furthermore, narcotics produce adverse reactions which may obscure the clinical course of patients with head injuries.

Acute Abdominal Conditions: The administration of Percodan or other narcotics may obscure the diagnosis or clinical course in patients with acute abdominal conditions.

Special Risk Patients: Percodan should be given with caution to certain patients such as the elderly or debilitated, and those with severe impairment of hepatic or renal function, hypothyroidism, Addison's disease, and prostatic hypertrophy or urethral stricture.

DRUG INTERACTIONS:

The CNS depressant effects of Percodan may be additive with that of other CNS depressants. (See WARNINGS.)

Aspirin may enhance the effect of anticoagulants and inhibit the uricosuric effects of uricosuric agents.

ADVERSE REACTIONS:

The most frequently observed adverse reactions include lightheadedness, dizziness, sedation, nausea and vomiting. These effects seem to be more prominent in ambulatory than in nonambulatory patients, and some of these adverse reactions may be alleviated if the patient lies down.

Other adverse reactions include euphoria, dysphoria, constipation and pruritus.

DRUG ABUSE AND DEPENDENCE:

Percodan tablets are a Schedule II controlled substance. Oxycodone can produce drug dependence and has the potential for being abused. (See WARNINGS.)

OVERDOSAGE:

Signs and Symptoms: Serious overdose with Percodan is characterized by respiratory depression (a decrease in respiratory rate and/or tidal volume, Cheyne-Stokes respiration, cyanosis), extreme somnolence progressing to stupor or coma, skeletal muscle flaccidity, cold and clammy skin, and sometimes bradycardia and hypotension. In severe overdosage, apnea, circulatory collapse, cardiac arrest and death may occur. The ingestion of very large amounts of Percodan may, in addition, result in acute salicylate intoxication.

Treatment: Primary attention should be given to the reestablishment of adequate respiratory exchange through provision of a patent airway and the institution of assisted or controlled ventilation. The narcotic antagonist naloxone hydrochloride (NARCAN) is a specific antidote against respiratory depression which may result from overdosage or unusual sensitivity to narcotics including oxycodone. Therefore, an appropriate dose of naloxone hydrochloride should be administered (usual initial adult dose: 0.4 mg-2 mg) preferably by the intravenous route, simultaneously with efforts at respiratory resuscitation. Since the duration of action of oxycodone may exceed that of the antagonist, the patient should be kept under continued surveillance and repeated doses of the antagonist should be administered as needed to maintain adequate respiration.

Oxygen, intravenous fluids, vasopressors and other supportive measures should be employed as indicated.

Gastric emptying may be useful in removing unabsorbed drug.

DOSAGE AND ADMINISTRATION:

Dosage should be adjusted according to the severity of the pain and the response of the patient. It may occasionally be necessary to exceed the usual dosage recommended below in cases of more severe pain or in those patients who have become tolerant to the analgesic effect of narcotics.

Percodan is given orally. The usual adult dose is one tablet every 6 hours as needed for pain.

Percodan-Demi is given orally.

Adults: One or two tablets every six hours.

Children 12 Years and Older: One-half tablet every six hours.

DOSAGE AND ADMINISTRATION: *(cont'd)*

Children 6 to 12 Years: One quarter tablet every six hours.

Percodan-Demi is not indicated for children under 6 years of age.

(DuPont Pharmaceuticals, 6/93, 6190-2, 6234-2)

HOW SUPPLIED - RATED THERAPEUTICALLY EQUIVALENT:

Tablet, Uncoated - Oral - 325 mg/2.25 mg/

100's	**$54.06**	**PERCODAN DEMI, Du Pont Merck**	**00590-0166-70**

Tablet, Uncoated - Oral - 325 mg/4.5 mg/0

100's	$17.63	Oxycodone W/Aspirin, H.C.F.A. F F P	99999-0322-01
100's	$18.43	Oxycodone W/Aspirin, Aligen Independ	00405-0143-01
100's	$18.95	Oxycodone & Aspirin, Parmed Pharms	00349-8831-01
100's	$19.55	Oxycodone/Aspirin, Major Pharms	00904-0464-60
100's	$20.23	Oxycodone W/Aspirin, Caremark	00339-4071-12
100's	$21.63	ROXIPRIN, Roxane	00054-4653-25
100's	$22.91	Oxycodone W/Aspirin, King Pharms	60793-0194-01
100's	$22.95	Aspirin & Oxycodone, Goldline Labs	00182-1508-01
100's	$22.95	Oxycodone W/Aspirin, Rugby	00536-5671-01
100's	$23.00	Endodan, Endo Labs	60951-0610-70
100's	$32.12	ROXIPRIN, Roxane	00054-8653-24
100's	**$70.75**	**PERCODAN, Du Pont Merck**	**00590-0135-70**
250's	**$185.63**	**PERCODAN, Du Pont Merck**	**00590-0135-65**
500's	$54.00	Oxycodone/Aspirin, Major Pharms	00904-0464-40
500's	$61.24	CODOXY, Halsey Drug	00879-0464-05
500's	$88.15	Oxycodone W/Aspirin, H.C.F.A. F F P	99999-0322-02
500's	$93.95	Oxycodone & Aspirin, Parmed Pharms	00349-8831-05
500's	$103.50	Endodan, Endo Labs	60951-0610-85
500's	$105.55	Oxycodone W/Aspirin, Rugby	00536-5671-05
500's	$108.00	Aspirin & Oxycodone, Goldline Labs	00182-1508-05
500's	**$343.63**	**PERCODAN, Du Pont Merck**	**00590-0135-85**
1000's	$176.30	Oxycodone W/Aspirin, H.C.F.A. F F P	99999-0322-03
1000's	$209.84	ROXIPRIN, Roxane	00054-4653-31
1000's	**$669.87**	**PERCODAN, Du Pont Merck**	**00590-0135-90**

ASPIRIN; PENTAZOCINE HYDROCHLORIDE

(000323)

CATEGORIES: Analgesics; Anesthesia; Antipyretics; Central Nervous System Agents; Narcotic Agonist-Antagonist; Narcotics, Synthetics & Combinations; Opiate Partial Agonists; Pain; DEA Class CIV; FDA Approval Pre 1982

BRAND NAMES: **Talwin Compound**

DESCRIPTION:

Talwin Compound is a combination of pentazocine hydrochloride, USP, equivalent to 12.5 mg base and aspirin, USP, 325 mg.

Pentazocine is a member of the benzazocine series (also known as the benzomorphan series). Chemically, pentazocine is 1,2,3,4,5,6-hexahydro-6, 11-dimethyl-3-(3-methyl-2-butenyl)-2, 6-methano-3-benzazocin-8-ol, a white, crystalline substance soluble in acidic aqueous solutions.

Chemically, aspirin is Benzoic acid, 2-(acetyloxy).

Inactive Ingredients: Magnesium Stearate, Microcrystalline Cellulose, Sodium Lauryl Sulfate, Starch.

CLINICAL PHARMACOLOGY:

Pentazocine is a potent analgesic which when administered orally is approximately equivalent, on a mg for mg basis, in analgesic effect to codeine. Two Caplets of Talwin Compound when administered orally have the additive analgesic effect equivalent to 25 mg of Talwin plus 650 mg of aspirin. Aspirin;Pentazocine Hydrochloride provides the analgesic effects of pentazocine and the analgesic, anti-inflammatory, and antipyretic actions of aspirin.

Onset of significant analgesia usually occurs between 15 and 30 minutes after oral administration, and duration of action is usually three hours or longer. Onset and duration of action and the degree of pain relief are related both to dose and the severity of pretreatment pain. Pentazocine weakly antagonizes the analgesic effects of morphine, meperidine, and phenazocine; in addition, it produces incomplete reversal of cardiovascular, respiratory, and behavioral depression induced by morphine and meperidine. Pentazocine has about 1/50 the antagonistic activity of nalorphine. It also has sedative activity.

INDICATIONS AND USAGE:

For the relief of moderate pain.

CONTRAINDICATIONS:

Aspirin;Pentazocine HCl should not be administered to patients who are hypersensitive to either pentazocine or salicylates, or in any situation where aspirin is contraindicated.

WARNINGS:

DRUG DEPENDENCE

There have been instances of psychological and physical dependence on parenteral pentazocine in patients with a history of drug abuse, and rarely, in patients without such a history. Abrupt discontinuance following the extended use of parenteral pentazocine has resulted in withdrawal symptoms. There have been a few reports of dependence and of withdrawal symptoms with orally administered pentazocine. Patients with a history of drug dependence should be under close supervision while receiving Aspirin;Pentazocine HCl orally. There have been rare reports of possible abstinence syndromes in newborns after prolonged use of pentazocine during pregnancy.

In prescribing Aspirin;Pentazocine HCl for chronic use, the physician should take precautions to avoid increases in dose by the patient and to prevent the use of the drug in anticipation of pain rather than for the relief of pain.

HEAD INJURY AND INCREASED INTRACRANIAL PRESSURE

The respiratory depressant effect of pentazocine and its potential for elevating cerebrospinal fluid pressure may be markedly exaggerated in the presence of preexisting increase in intracranial pressure. Furthermore, pentazocine can produce effects which may obscure the clinical course of patients with head injuries. In such patients, Aspirin;Pentazocine HCl must be used with extreme caution and only if its use is deemed essential.

USAGE IN PREGNANCY

Safe use of pentazocine during pregnancy (other than labor) has not been established. Animal reproduction studies have not demonstrated teratogenic or embryotoxic effects. However, Aspirin;Pentazocine HCl should be administered to pregnant patients (other than labor) only when, in the judgment of the physician, the potential benefits outweigh the possible hazards.

WARNINGS: *(cont'd)*

Patients receiving pentazocine during labor have experienced no adverse effects other than those that occur with commonly used analgesics. Aspirin;Pentazocine HCl should be used with caution in women delivering premature infants.

ACUTE CNS MANIFESTATIONS

Patients receiving therapeutic doses of pentazocine have experienced hallucinations (usually visual), disorientation, and confusion which have cleared spontaneously within a period of hours. The mechanism of this reaction is not known. Such patients should be closely observed and vital signs checked. If the drug is reinstituted it should be done with caution since these acute CNS manifestations may recur.

Due to the potential for increased CNS depressant effects, alcohol should be used with caution in patients who are currently receiving pentazocine.

USAGE IN CHILDREN

Because clinical experience in children under 12 years of age is limited, administration of Aspirin;Pentazocine HCl in this age group is not recommended.

AMBULATORY PATIENTS

Since sedation, dizziness, and occasional euphoria have been noted, ambulatory patients should be warned not to operate machinery, drive cars, or unnecessarily expose themselves to hazards.

OTHER

Because of its aspirin content, Aspirin;Pentazocine HCl should be used with caution in the presence of peptic ulcer, in conjunction with anticoagulant therapy, or in any situation where the effects of aspirin may be deleterious.

PRECAUTIONS:

Certain Respiratory Conditions: Although respiratory depression has rarely been reported after oral administration of pentazocine, Aspirin;Pentazocine HCl should be administered with caution to patients with respiratory depression from any cause, severely limited respiratory reserve, severe bronchial asthma and other obstructive respiratory conditions, or cyanosis.

Impaired Renal or Hepatic Function: Decreased metabolism of the drug by the liver in extensive liver disease may predispose to accentuation of side effects. Although laboratory tests have not indicated that pentazocine causes or increases renal or hepatic impairment, Aspirin;Pentazocine HCl should be administered with caution to patients with such impairment.

Myocardial Infarction: As with all drugs, Aspirin;Pentazocine HCl should be used with caution in patients with myocardial infarction who have nausea or vomiting.

Biliary Surgery: Narcotic drug products are generally considered to elevate biliary tract pressure for varying periods following administration. Some evidence suggests that pentazocine may differ in this respect (*i.e.,* it causes little or no elevation in biliary tract pressures). The clinical significance of these findings, however, is not yet known.

Patients Receiving Narcotics: Pentazocine is a mild narcotic antagonist. Some patients previously given narcotics, including methadone for the daily treatment of narcotic dependence, have experienced withdrawal symptoms after receiving pentazocine.

CNS Effect: Caution should be used when pentazocine is administered to patients prone to seizures. Seizures have occurred in a few such patients in association with the use of pentazocine although no cause and effect relationship has been established.

ADVERSE REACTIONS:

Reactions reported after oral administration of pentazocine or Aspirin;Pentazocine HCl include:

Gastrointestinal: nausea, vomiting; infrequently constipation; and rarely abdominal distress, anorexia, diarrhea.

CNS Effects: dizziness, lightheadedness, hallucinations, sedation, euphoria, headache, confusion, disorientation; infrequently weakness, disturbed dreams, insomnia, syncope, visual blurring and focusing difficulty, depression; and rarely tremor, irritability, excitement, tinnitus.

Autonomic: sweating infrequently flushing; and rarely chills. Allergic: infrequently rash; and rarely urticaria, edema of the face, and angioneurotic edema.

Cardiovascular: infrequently decrease in blood pressure, tachycardia.

Hematologic: rarely depression of white blood cells (especially granulocytes), which is usually reversible, moderate transient eosinophilia.

Other: rarely respiratory depression, urinary retention, paresthesia, toxic epidermal necrolysis, and angioneurotic edema.

OVERDOSAGE:

SIGNS AND SYMPTOMS

Clinical experience with pentazocine overdosage has been insufficient to define the signs of this condition. Signs of salicylate overdosage include headache, dizziness, confusion, tinnitus, diaphoresis, thirst, nausea, vomiting, diarrhea, tachycardia, tachypnea, Kussmaul breathing, convulsions, and coma. Death is usually from respiratory failure.

TREATMENT

Treatment for overdosage of Aspirin;Pentazocine HCl should include treatment for salicylate poisoning as outlined in standard references.

Oxygen, intravenous fluids, vasopressors, and other supportive measures should be employed as indicated. Assisted or controlled ventilation should also be considered. For respiratory depression due to overdosage or unusual sensitivity to pentazocine, parenteral naloxone is a specific and effective antagonist.

DOSAGE AND ADMINISTRATION:

Adults: The usual adult dose is 2 Caplets three or four times a day.

Children Under 12 years of Age: Since clinical experience in children under 12 years of age is limited, administration of Talwin Compound in this age group is not recommended.

Duration of Therapy: Patients with chronic pain who receive pentazocine orally for prolonged periods have only rarely been reported to experience withdrawal symptoms when administration was abruptly discontinued ([Ss]ee WARNINGS). Tolerance to the analgesic effect of pentazocine has also been reported only rarely. Significant abnormalities of liver and kidney function tests have not been reported, even after prolonged administration of pentazocine.

HOW SUPPLIED - EQUIVALENTS NOT AVAILABLE:

Tablet, Uncoated - Oral - 12.5 mg/325 mg

100's	$83.08	TALWIN COMPOUND, Sanofi Winthrop	00024-1927-04

ASTEMIZOLE *(000332)*

CATEGORIES: Allergies; Antihistamines; Non-Sedating Antihistamines; Piperidines; Respiratory & Allergy Medications; Rhinitis; Urticaria; Pregnancy Category C; Sales > $100 Million; FDA Approved 1988 Dec; Patent Expiration 1999 Dec

BRAND NAMES: Adistan (Mexico); *Alestol*; *Anminlin*; *Asemin*; *Astelong*; *Astem*; *Astemina* (Mexico); *Astemizol*; *Astin*; *Astimal*; *Astizol*; *Cilergil* (Mexico); *Eumine*; **Hismanal**; *Hisnot*; *Hispral*; *Histalong*; *Histamen*; *Histaminos*; *Histamizol*; *Histazole*; *Irene*; *Metodik*; *Mildugen*; *Pollon*; *Pollon-Eze* (England); *Retolen*; *Scantihis*; *Simprox*; *Sines*; *Sisnal*; *Stemiz*; *Tenon*
(International brand names outside U.S. in italics)

FORMULARIES: Aetna; BC-BS

COST OF THERAPY: $55.49 (Rhinitis; Tablet; 10 mg; 1/day; 30 days)

PRIMARY ICD9: 477.9 (Allergic Rhinitis, Cause Unspecified)

DESCRIPTION:

Astemizole is a histamine H_1-receptor antagonist available in scored white tablets for oral use. Each Hismanal tablet contains 10 mg of astemizole and, as inactive ingredients; lactose, cornstarch, microcrystalline cellulose, pregelatinized starch, povidone K90, magnesium stearate, colloidal silicon dioxide, and sodium lauryl sulfate. Astemizole is chemically designated as 1-[(4-fluorophenyl) -methyl] -N-[1-[2-(4-methoxyphenyl) ethyl]-4-piperidinyl]-1H-benzimidazol-2-amine, with a molecular weight of 458.58. The empirical formula is $C_{28}H_{31}FN_4O$.

Astemizole is a white to slightly off-white powder; it is insoluble in water, slightly soluble in ethanol, and soluble in chloroform and methanol.

CLINICAL PHARMACOLOGY:

Astemizole is a long-acting, selective histamine H_1-receptor antagonist. Receptor binding studies in animals demonstrated that at pharmacological doses, Hismanal occupies peripheral H_1-receptors but does not reach H_1-receptors in the brain. Whole body autoradiographic studies in rats, radiolabel tissue distribution studies in dogs, and radioligand binding studies of guinea pig brain H_1-receptors have shown that astemizole does not readily cross the blood-brain barrier. Screening studies in rats at effective antihistaminic doses showed no anticholinergic effects. Studies in humans using the recommended dosage regimens have not been performed to determine whether astemizole is associated with a different frequency of anticholinergic effects than therapeutic doses of other antihistamines.

The absorption of astemizole is reduced by 60% when taken with meals. In single oral dose studies, astemizole was rapidly absorbed from the gastrointestinal tract; peak plasma concentrations of unchanged astemizole were reached within 1 hour. Due to extensive first-pass metabolism and significant tissue distribution, plasma concentrations of unchanged drug were low. Elimination of unchanged astemizole occurred with a half-life of approximately 1 day. Elimination of astemizole plus hydroxylated metabolites, considered together to represent the pharmacologically active fraction in plasma, was biphasic with half-lives of 20 hours for the distribution phase and 7 to 11 days for the elimination phase. The pharmacokinetics of astemizole plus hydroxylated metabolites are dose proportional following single doses of 10 to 30 mg.

Following chronic administration, steady-state plasma concentrations of astemizole plus hydroxylated metabolites (mainly desmethylastemizole) were reached within 4 to 8 weeks; concentrations of the metabolites are substantially higher than those of unchanged astemizole. Astemizole plus hydroxylated metabolites decayed biphasically with an initial half-life of 7 to 9 days, with plasma concentrations being reduced by 75% within this phase, and with a terminal half-life of about 19 days. The initial phase ($t_{1/2}$= 7-9 days) appears to determine the time to reach steady-state plasma concentrations of astemizole plus hydroxylated metabolites. Steady-state plasma concentrations of unchanged astemizole were reached by 6 days (with a range of 6-9 days); unchanged astemizole was eliminated from plasma with a half-life of approximately 2 days (with a range of 1-2.5 days).

Excretion and metabolism studies with ^{14}C-labeled astemizole in volunteers demonstrated that the drug is almost completely metabolized in the liver and primarily excreted in the feces.

Interpatient variability in pharmacokinetic parameters may be greater in patients with liver disease as compared to normal subjects. Systemic evaluation of the pharmacokinetics in patients with hepatic or renal dysfunction has not been performed.

The *in vitro* plasma protein binding of unchanged astemizole (100 ng/ml) was 96.7% with 2.3% being found as free drug in the plasma water. In human blood with an astemizole concentration of 100 ng/ml, 61.5% of astemizole was bound to the plasma proteins, with 36.2% being distributed to the blood cell fraction. The concentration of astemizole found in the blood was the same as that found in the plasma fraction of the blood. Binding studies for the astemizole metabolite(s), which achieve much higher concentrations than astemizole under chronic dosing conditions, have not been conducted.

INDICATIONS AND USAGE:

Astemizole tablets are indicated for the relief of symptoms associated with seasonal allergic rhinitis and chronic idiopathic urticaria. Astemizole should not be used as a prn product for immediate relief of symptoms. Patients should be advised not to increase the dose in an attempt to accelerate the onset of action.

Clinical studies have not been conducted to evaluate the effectiveness of astemizole in the common cold.

CONTRAINDICATIONS:

Concomitant administration of astemizole with erythromycin is contraindicated because erythromycin is known to impair the cytochrome P450 enzyme system, which also influences astemizole metabolism. There have been two reports to date of syncope with torsades de pointes, requiring hospitalization, in patients taking combinations of astemizole 10 mg daily with erythromycin. In each case the QT intervals were prolonged beyond 650 milliseconds the time of the event; one patient also received ketoconazole, and the other patient also had hypokalemia.

Concomitant administration of astemizole with ketoconazole tablets is contraindicated because available human pharmacokinetic data indicate that oral ketoconazole significantly inhibits the metabolism of astemizole, resulting in elevated plasma levels of astemizole and desmethylastemizole. Data suggest that cardiovascular events are associated with elevation of astemizole and/or astemizole metabolite levels resulting in electrocardiographic QT prolongation.

Concomitant administration with itraconazole is also contraindicated based on the chemical resemblance of itraconazole and ketoconazole. *In vitro* data suggest that itraconazole has a less pronounced effect on the biotransformation system responsible for the metabolism of astemizole compared to ketoconazole.

CONTRAINDICATIONS: *(cont'd)*

(See WARNINGS and DRUG INTERACTIONS.)

Astemizole is contraindicated in patients with known hypersensitivity to astemizole or any of the inactive ingredients.

WARNINGS:

QT Prolongation/Ventricular Arrhythmias: RARE CASES OF SERIOUS CARDIOVASCULAR ADVERSE EVENTS; INCLUDING DEATH, CARDIAC ARREST, QT PROLONGATION, TORSADES DE POINTES, AND OTHER VENTRICULAR ARRHYTHMIAS; HAVE BEEN OBSERVED IN PATIENTS EXCEEDING RECOMMENDED DOSES OF ASTEMIZOLE. WHILE THE MAJORITY OF SUCH EVENTS HAVE OCCURRED FOLLOWING SUBSTANTIAL OVERDOSES OF ASTEMIZOLE, TORSADES DE POINTES (ARRHYTHMIAS) HAVE VERY RARELY OCCURRED AT REPORTED DOSES AS LOW AS 20 TO 30 MG DAILY (2-3 TIMES THE RECOMMENDED DAILY DOSE). DATA SUGGEST THAT THESE EVENTS ARE ASSOCIATED WITH ELEVATION OF ASTEMIZOLE AND/OR ASTEMIZOLE METABOLITE LEVELS, RESULTING IN ELECTROCARDIOGRAPHIC QT PROLONGATION.

THESE EVENTS HAVE ALSO OCCURRED AT 10 MG DAILY IN A FEW PATIENTS WITH POSSIBLE AUGMENTING CIRCUMSTANCES (SEE CONTRAINDICATIONSand WARNINGS). IN VIEW OF THE POTENTIAL FOR CARDIAC ARRHYTHMIAS, ADHERENCE TO THE RECOMMENDED DOSE SHOULD BE EMPHASIZED.

DO NOT EXCEED THE RECOMMENDED DOSE OF 10 MG (1 TABLET) DAILY.

SOME PATIENTS APPEAR TO INCREASE THE DOSE OF HISMANAL IN AN ATTEMPT TO ACCELERATE THE ONSET OF ACTION. PATIENTS SHOULD BE ADVISED NOT TO DO THIS AND NOT TO USE HISMANAL AS A PRN PRODUCT FOR IMMEDIATE RELIEF OF SYMPTOMS.

CONCOMITANT ADMINISTRATION OF ASTEMIZOLE WITH KETOCONAZOLE TABLETS, ITRACONAZOLE, OR ERYTHROMYCIN IS CONTRAINDICATED. (SEE CONTRAINDICATIONSand DRUG INTERACTIONS.)

SINCE ASTEMIZOLE IS EXTENSIVELY METABOLIZED BY THE LIVER, THE USE OF ASTEMIZOLE IN PATIENTS WITH SIGNIFICANT HEPATIC DYSFUNCTION SHOULD GENERALLY BE AVOIDED.

IN SOME CASES, SEVERE ARRHYTHMIAS HAVE BEEN PRECEDED BY EPISODES OF SYNCOPE. SYNCOPE IN PATIENTS RECEIVING ASTEMIZOLE SHOULD LEAD TO IMMEDIATE DISCONTINUATION OF TREATMENT AND APPROPRIATE CLINICAL EVALUATION, INCLUDING ELECTROCARDIOGRAPHIC TESTING (LOOKING FOR QT PROLONGATION AND VENTRICULAR ARRHYTHMIA).

(SEE CLINICAL PHARMACOLOGY, CONTRAINDICATIONS, WARNINGS ANDPRECAUTIONS, AND DOSAGE AND ADMINISTRATION.)

Patients known to have conditions leading to QT prolongation may experience QT prolongation and/or ventricular arrhythmias with astemizole at recommended doses. The effect of astemizole in patients who are receiving agents that alter the QT interval is unknown. However, in view of astemizole's known potential for QT prolongation, it is advisable to avoid its use in patients who are taking medications that are reported to prolong QT intervals (including probucol, certain antiarrhythmics, certain tricyclic antidepressants, certain phenothiazines, certain calcium channel blockers such as bepridil, and terfenadine), patients with electrolyte abnormalities such as hypokalemia or hypomagnesemia, or those taking diuretics with potential for inducing electrolyte abnormalities.

Rare cases of cardiovascular events have been observed in patients with hepatic dysfunction. Systematic evaluation of the pharmacokinetics of astemizole in patients with hepatic dysfunction has not been performed. Since astemizole is extensively metabolized by the liver, the use of astemizole in patients with significant hepatic dysfunction should generally be avoided.

PRECAUTIONS:

General: Caution should be given to potential anticholinergic (drying) effects in patients with lower airway diseases.

Caution should be used in patients with cirrhosis or other liver diseases (see CLINICAL PHARMACOLOGY).

Astemizole does not appear to be dialyzable. Caution should also be used when treating patients with renal impairment.

Information for the Patient: Patients taking astemizole should receive the following information and instructions. Antihistamines are prescribed to reduce allergic symptoms. Patients taking astemizole should be advised: (1) to adhere to the recommended dose, and (2) that the use of excessive doses may lead to serious cardiovascular events. DO NOT EXCEED THE RECOMMENDED DOSE. Some patients appear to increase the dose of astemizole in an attempt to accelerate the onset of action. PATIENTS SHOULD BE ADVISED **NOT** TO DO THIS and not to use astemizole as a prn product for immediate relief of symptoms. Patients should be questioned about use of another prescription or over-the-counter medication and should be cautioned regarding the potential for life-threatening arrhythmias with concurrent use of ketoconazole, itraconazole, or erythromycin. Patients should be questioned about pregnancy or lactation before starting astemizole therapy, since the drug should be used in pregnancy or lactation only if the potential benefit justifies the potential risk to fetus or infant. (see Pregnancy). In addition, patients should be instructed to take astemizole on an empty stomach (*e.g.,* at least 2 hours after a meal). No additional food should be taken for at least 1 hour after dosing. Patients should also be instructed to store this medication in a tightly closed container in a cool, dry place, away from heat or direct sunlight, and away from children.

Carcinogenesis, Mutagenesis, and Impairment of Fertility: Carcinogenic potential has not been revealed in rats given 260 times the recommended human dose of astemizole for 24 months or in mice given 400 times the recommended human dose for 18 months. Micronucleus, dominant lethal, sister chromatid exchange and Ames tests of astemizole have not revealed mutagenic activity.

Impairment of fertility was not observed in male or female rats given 200 times the recommended human dose.

PRECAUTIONS: *(cont'd)*

Pregnancy, Teratogenic Effects, Pregnancy Category C: Teratogenic effects were not observed in rats administered 200 times the recommended human dose or in rabbits given 200 times the recommended human dose. Maternal toxicity was seen in rabbits administered 200 times the recommended human dose. Embryocidal effects accompanied by maternal toxicity were observed at 100 times the recommended human dose in rats. Embryotoxicity or maternal toxicity was not observed in rats or rabbits administered 50 times the recommended human dose. There are no adequate and well controlled studies in pregnant women. Hismanal should be used during pregnancy only if the potential benefit justifies the potential risk to the fetus. Metabolites may remain in the body for as long as 4 months after the end of dosing, calculated on the basis of 6 times the terminal half-life. (See CLINICAL PHARMACOLOGY.)

Nursing Mothers: It is not known whether this drug is excreted in human milk.

Because certain drugs are known to be excreted in human milk, caution should be exercised when Hismanal is administered to a nursing woman. Astemizole is excreted in the milk of dogs.

Pediatric Use: Safety and efficacy in children younger than 12 years of age has not been demonstrated.

DRUG INTERACTIONS:

See CONTRAINDICATIONS and WARNINGSfor discussion of information regarding potential drug interactions.

Ketoconazole/Itraconazole: Concomitant administration of ketoconazole tablets or itraconazole with astemizole is contraindicated. (See CONTRAINDICATIONS and WARNINGS.)

Due to the chemical similarity of fluconazole, metronidazole, and miconazole IV to ketoconazole, concomitant use of these products is not recommended.

Macrolides (Including Erythromycin): Concomitant administration of erythromycin with astemizole is contraindicated. (See CONTRAINDICATIONSand WARNINGS.) Concomitant administration of astemizole with other macrolide antibiotics, including troleandomycin, azithromycin, and clarithromycin, is not recommended.

ADVERSE REACTIONS:

For information regarding cardiovascular adverse events (*e.g.,* cardiac arrest, ventricular arrhythmias), see CONTRAINDICATIONSand WARNINGS. In some cases, recognition of severe arrhythmias has been preceded by episodes of syncope. Similarly, rare cases of hypotension, palpitations, and dizziness have also been reported with astemizole use, which may reflect undetected ventricular arrhythmia.

The reported incidences of adverse reactions listed in TABLE 1 are derived from controlled clinical studies in adults. In these studies the usual maintenance dose of astemizole was 10 mg once daily.

TABLE 1 Percent of Patients Reporting Controlled Studies*

Adverse Event	Astemizole (N = 1630) %	Placebo (N = 1109) %	Classic** (N = 304) %
Central Nervous System			
Drowsiness	7.1	6.4	22.0
Headache	6.7	9.2	3.3
Fatigue	4.2	1.6	11.8
Appetite increase	3.9	1.4	0.0
Weight increase	3.6	0.7	1.0
Nervousness	2.1	1.2	0.3
Dizzy	2.0	1.8	1.0
Gastrointestinal System			
Nausea	2.5	2.9	1.3
Diarrhea	1.8	2.0	0.7
Abdominal pain	1.4	1.2	0.7
Eye, Ear, Nose, and Throat			
Mouth dry	5.2	3.8	7.9
Pharyngitis	1.7	2.3	0.3
Conjunctivitis	1.2	1.2	0.7
Other			
Arthralgia	1.2	1.6	0.0

* Duration of treatment in controlled studies ranged from 7 to 182 days

** Classic Drugs: clemastine (N = 137); chlorpheniramine (N = 100); pheniramine maleate (N = 47); d-chlorpheniramine (N = 20)

Adverse reaction information has been obtained from more than 7500 patients in all clinical trials. Weight gain has been reported in 3.6% of astemizole-treated patients involved in controlled studies, with an average treatment duration of 53 days. In 46 of the 59 patients for whom actual weight gain data was available, the average weight gain was 3.2 kg.

Less frequently occurring adverse experiences reported in clinical trials or spontaneously from marketing experience with astemizole include angioedema, asymptomatic liver enzyme elevations, bronchospasm, depression, edema, epistaxis, myalgia, palpitation, paresthesia, photosensitivity, pruritus, and rash.

Marketing experiences include isolated cases of convulsions. A causal relationship with astemizole has not been established.

OVERDOSAGE:

In the event of overdosage, supportive measures; including gastric lavage and emesis should be employed. Substantial overdoses of astemizole can cause death, cardiac arrest, QT prolongation, cardiac arrest, torsades de pointes, and other ventricular arrhythmias. These events can also occur, although rarely, at doses (20-30 mg) close to the recommended dose (10 mg/daily). (See WARNINGS and DOSAGE AND ADMINISTRATION.)

Seizures and syncope have also been reported with overdose and may be associated with a cardiac event.

Overdose patients should be carefully monitored as long as the QT interval is prolonged or arrhythmias are present. In some cases, this has been up to 6 days. In overdose cases in which ventricular arrhythmias are associated with significant QT prolongation, treatment with antiarrhythmics known to prolong QT intervals is not recommended.

Astemizole does not appear to be dialyzable.

Oral LD_{50} values for astemizole were 2052 mg/kg in mice and 3154 mg/kg in rats. In neonatal rats, the oral LD_{50} was 905 mg/kg in males and 1235 mg/kg in females.

DOSAGE AND ADMINISTRATION:

The recommended dosage for adults and children 12 years of age and older is 10 mg (1 tablet) once daily.

Patients should be advised **not** to increase the dose of astemizole in an attempt to accelerate the onset of action. (See WARNINGS.)

DOSAGE AND ADMINISTRATION: *(cont'd)*

Use of astemizole in patients taking ketoconazole, itraconazole, or erythromycin is contraindicated. (See CONTRAINDICATIONS, WARNINGS, and DRUG INTERACTIONS.)

Studies evaluating the need for dosage adjustments for patients with hepatic or renal dysfunction have not been performed. Since astemizole is extensively metabolized by the liver, use of astemizole in patients with significant hepatic dysfunction should generally be avoided.

Astemizole should be taken on an empty stomach, (*e.g.,* at least two hours after a meal). There should be no additional food intake for at least 1 hour post dosing.

HOW SUPPLIED:

Astemizole is available as white scored tablets containing 10 mg of astemizole debossed "JANSSEN" and on the reverse side debossed "AST/10."

Storage: Store tablets at room temperature (59°-86°) (15°- 30°C). Protect from moisture.

HOW SUPPLIED - EQUIVALENTS NOT AVAILABLE:

Tablet, Uncoated - Oral - 10 mg

30's	**$221.99**	**HISMANAL, Janssen Phar**	**50458-0510-13**
100's	**$184.99**	**HISMANAL, Janssen Phar**	**50458-0510-10**

ATENOLOL *(000333)*

CATEGORIES: Angina; Antianginals; Antihypertensives; Atherosclerosis; Beta Adrenergic Blocking Agents; Beta Blockers; Cardiovascular Drugs; Hypertension; Myocardial Infarction; Ischemia*; Migraine*; Pregnancy Category C; Sales >$500 Million; FDA Approval Pre 1982; Patent Expiration 1991 Sep; Top 200 Drugs

* Indication not approved by the FDA

BRAND NAMES: *Aircrit*; *Alinor*; *Altol*; *Anselol*; *Antipressan* (England); *Apo-Atenolol*; *Atcardil*; *Atecard*; *AteHexal* (Germany); *Atenblock*; *Atendol* (Germany); *Atenet*; *Ateni*; *Atenil*; *Atenol*; *Atenolin*; *Atenomel*; *Atereal* (Germany); *Aterol*; *Betablok*; *Betacard*; *Blokium*; *Catenol*; *Coratol*; *Corotenol*; *Evitocor* (Germany); *Farnormin*; *Felo-Bits*; *Hypoten*; *Hipres*; *Internolol*; *Lo-ten*; *Loten*; *Lotenal*; *Myocord*; *Normalol*; *Normiten*; *Noten* (Australia); *Oraday*; *Premorine*; *Prenolol*; *Seles*; *Serten*; *Stermin*; *Tenidon*; *Tenoblock*; *Tenolol*; *Tenoprin*; **Tenormin**; *Tenormine* (France); *Tensimin*; *Tredol*; *Urosin*; *Vascoten*; *Vericordin*; *Wesipin*

(International brand names outside U.S. in italics)

FORMULARIES: Aetna; BC-BS; CIGNA; FHP; Humana; Kaiser; Medco; Medi-Cal; PCS; PruCare; United; WHO

COST OF THERAPY: $16.93 (Hypertension; Tablet; 50 mg; 1/day; 365 days)

PRIMARY ICD9: 401.1 (Essential Hypertension, Benign)

DESCRIPTION:

Atenolol, a synthetic, beta$_1$-selective (cardioselective) adrenoreceptor blocking agent, may be chemically described as benzeneacetamide, 4 -[2'-hydroxy-3'-[(1- methylethyl) amino] propoxy]-.

Atenolol (free base) has a molecular weight of 266. It is a relatively polar hydrophilic compound with a water solubility of 26.5 mg/ml at 37°C and a log partition coefficient (octanol/water) of 0.23. It is freely soluble in 1N HCl (300 mg/ml at 25°C) and less soluble in chloroform (3 mg/ml at 25°C).

TABLETS

Atenolol is available as 25, 50 and 100 mg tablets for oral administration.

Tenormin Inactive Ingredients: Magnesium stearate, microcrystalline cellulose, povidone, sodium starch glycolate.

IV INJECTION

Atenolol for parenteral administration contains 5 mg atenolol in 10 ml sterile, isotonic, citrate-buffered, aqueous solution. The pH of the solution is 5.5-6.5.

Tenormin Inactive Ingredients: Sodium chloride for isotonicity and citric acid and sodium hydroxide to adjust pH.

CLINICAL PHARMACOLOGY:

Atenolol is a beta$_1$-selective (cardioselective) beta-adrenergic receptor blocking agent without membrane stabilizing or intrinsic sympathomimetic (partial agonist) activities. This preferential effect is not absolute, however, and at higher doses, atenolol inhibits beta$_2$-adrenoreceptors, chiefly located in the bronchial and vascular musculature.

PHARMACOKINETICS AND METABOLISM

In humans, absorption of an oral dose is rapid and consistent but incomplete. Approximately 50% of an oral dose is absorbed from the gastrointestinal tract, the remainder being excreted unchanged in the feces. Peak blood levels are reached between two (2) and four (4) hours after ingestion. Unlike propranolol or metoprolol, but like nadolol, atenolol undergoes little or no metabolism by the liver, and the absorbed portion is eliminated primarily by renal excretion. Over 85% of an intravenous dose is excreted in urine within 24 hours compared with approximately 50% for an oral dose. Atenolol also differs from propranolol in that only a small amount (6%-16%) is bound to proteins in the plasma. This kinetic profile results in relatively consistent plasma drug levels with about a fourfold interpatient variation.

The elimination half-life of oral atenolol is approximately 6 to 7 hours, and there is no alteration of the kinetic profile of the drug by chronic administration. Following intravenous administration, peak plasma levels are reached within 5 minutes. Declines from peak levels are rapid (5- to 10-fold) during the first 7 hours; thereafter, plasma levels decay with a half-life similar to that of orally administered drug. Following oral doses of 50 mg or 100 mg, both beta-blocking and antihypertensive effects persist for at least 24 hours. When renal function is impaired, elimination of atenolol is closely related to the glomerular filtration rate; significant accumulation occurs when the creatinine clearance falls below 35 ml/min/1.73m^2 (See DOSAGE AND ADMINISTRATION).

PHARMACODYNAMICS

In standard animal or human pharmacological tests, beta-adrenoreceptor blocking activity of atenolol has been demonstrated by:

(1) reduction in resting and exercise heart rate and cardiac output,

(2) reduction of systolic and diastolic blood pressure at rest and on exercise,

(3) inhibition of isoproterenol induced tachycardia, and

(4) reduction in reflex orthostatic tachycardia.

A significant beta-blocking effect of atenolol, as measured by reduction of exercise tachycardia, is apparent within one hour following oral administration of a single dose. This effect is maximal at about 2 to 4 hours, and persists for at least 24 hours. Maximum reduction in exercise tachycardia occurs within 5 minutes of an intravenous dose. For both orally and

CLINICAL PHARMACOLOGY: *(cont'd)*

intravenously administered drug, the duration of action is dose related and also bears a linear relationship to the logarithm of plasma atenolol concentration. The effect on exercise tachycardia of a single 10 mg intravenous dose is largely dissipated by 12 hours, whereas beta-blocking activity of single oral doses of 50 mg and 100 mg is still evident beyond 24 hours following administration. However, as has been shown for all beta-blocking agents, the antihypertensive effect does not appear to be related to plasma level.

In normal subjects, the beta$_1$ selectivity of atenolol has been shown by its reduced ability to reverse the beta$_2$-mediated vasodilating effect of isoproterenol as compared to equivalent beta-blocking doses of propranolol. In asthmatic patients, a dose of atenolol producing a greater effect on resting heart rate than propranolol resulted in much less increase in airway resistance. In a placebo controlled comparison of approximately equipotent oral doses of several beta blockers, atenolol produced a significantly smaller decrease of FEV$_1$ than nonselective beta blockers such as propranolol and, unlike those agents, did not inhibit bronchodilation in response to isoproterenol.

Consistent with its negative chronotropic effect due to beta blockade of the SA node, atenolol increases sinus cycle length and sinus node recovery time. Conduction in the AV node is also prolonged. Atenolol is devoid of membrane stabilizing activity, and increasing the dose well beyond that producing beta blockade does not further depress myocardial contractility. Several studies have demonstrated a moderate (approximately 10%) increase in stroke volume at rest and during exercise.

In controlled clinical trials, atenolol, given as a single daily oral dose, was an effective antihypertensive agent providing 24-hour reduction of blood pressure. Atenolol has been studied in combination with thiazide-type diuretics, and the blood pressure effects of the combination are approximately additive. Atenolol is also compatible with methyldopa, hydralazine, and prazosin, each combination resulting in a larger fall in blood pressure than with the single agents. The dose range of atenolol is narrow and increasing the dose beyond 100 mg once daily is not associated with increased antihypertensive effect. The mechanisms of the antihypertensive effects of beta-blocking agents have not been established. Several possible mechanisms have been proposed and include:

(1) competitive antagonism of catecholamines at peripheral (especially cardiac) adrenergic neuron sites, leading to decreased cardiac output,

(2) a central effect leading to reduced sympathetic outflow to the periphery, and

(3) suppression of renin activity.

The results from long-term studies have not shown any diminution of the antihypertensive efficacy of atenolol with prolonged use.

By blocking the positive chronotropic and inotropic effects of catecholamines and by decreasing blood pressure, atenolol generally reduces the oxygen requirements of the heart at any given level of effort, making it useful for many patients in the long-term management of angina pectoris. On the other hand, atenolol can increase oxygen requirements by increasing left ventricular fiber length and end diastolic pressure, particularly in patients with heart failure.

In a multicenter clinical trial (ISIS-1) conducted in 16,027 patients with suspected myocardial infarction, patients presenting within 12 hours (mean = 5 hours) after the onset of pain were randomized to either conventional therapy plus atenolol (n = 8,037), or conventional therapy alone (n = 7,990). Patients with a heart rate of < 50 bpm or systolic blood pressure < 100 mm Hg, or with other contraindications to beta blockade were excluded. Thirty-eight percent of each group were treated within 4 hours of onset of pain. The mean time from onset of pain to entry was 5.0 ± 2.7 hours in both groups. Patients in the atenolol group were to receive atenolol IV injection 5-10 mg given over 5 minutes plus atenolol tablets 50 mg every 12 hours orally on the first study day (the first oral dose administered about 15 minutes after the IV dose) followed by either atenolol tablets 100 mg once daily or atenolol tablets 50 mg twice daily on days 2-7. The groups were similar in demographic and medical history characteristics and in electrocardiographic evidence of myocardial infarction, bundle branch block, and first degree atrioventricular block at entry.

During the treatment period (days 0-7), the vascular mortality rates were 3.89% in the atenolol group (313 deaths) and 4.57% in the control group (365 deaths). This absolute difference in rates, 0.68%, is statistically significant at the $P < 0.05$ level. The absolute difference translates into a proportional reduction of 15% (3.89-4.57/4.57 = -0.15). The 95% confidence limits are 1%-27%. Most of the difference was attributed to mortality in days 0-1 (atenolol -121 deaths; control - 171 deaths).

Despite the large size of the ISIS-1 trial, it is not possible to identify clearly subgroups of patients most likely or least likely to benefit from early treatment with atenolol. Good clinical judgment suggests, however, that patients who are dependent on sympathetic stimulation for maintenance of adequate cardiac output and blood pressure are not good candidates for beta blockade. Indeed, the trial protocol reflected that judgment by excluding patients with blood pressure consistently below 100 mm Hg systolic. The overall results of the study are compatible with the possibility that patients with borderline blood pressure (less than 120 mm Hg systolic), especially if over 60 years of age, are less likely to benefit.

The mechanism through which atenolol improves survival in patients with definite or suspected acute myocardial infarction is unknown, as is the case for other beta blockers in the postinfarction setting. Atenolol, in addition to its effects on survival, has shown other clinical benefits including reduced frequency of ventricular premature beats, reduced chest pain, and reduced enzyme elevation.

INDICATIONS AND USAGE:

Acute Myocardial Infarction: Atenolol is indicated in the management of hemodynamically stable patients with definite or suspected acute myocardial infarction to reduce cardiovascular mortality. Treatment can be initiated as soon as the patient's clinical condition allows. (See DOSAGE AND ADMINISTRATION, CONTRAINDICATIONS, and WARNINGS.) In general, there is no basis for treating patients like those who were excluded from the ISIS-1 trial (blood pressure less than 100 mm Hg systolic, heart rate less than 50 bpm) or have other reasons to avoid beta blockade. As noted above, some subgroups (*e.g.,* elderly patients with systolic blood pressure below 120 mm Hg) seemed less likely to benefit.

TABLETS

Hypertension: Atenolol is indicated in the management of hypertension. It may be used alone or concomitantly with other antihypertensive agents, particularly with a thiazide-type diuretic.

Angina Pectoris Due to Coronary Atherosclerosis: Atenolol is indicated for the long-term management of patients with angina pectoris.

CONTRAINDICATIONS:

Atenolol is contraindicated in sinus bradycardia, heart block greater than first degree, cardiogenic shock, and overt cardiac failure (See WARNINGS).

WARNINGS:

Cardiac Failure: Sympathetic stimulation is necessary in supporting circulatory function in congestive heart failure, and beta blockade carries the potential hazard of further depressing myocardial contractility and precipitating more severe failure. In patients who have congestive heart failure controlled by digitalis and/or diuretics, atenolol should be administered cautiously. Both digitalis and atenolol slow AV conduction.

In patients with acute myocardial infarction, cardiac failure which is not promptly and effectively controlled by 80 mg of intravenous furosemide or equivalent therapy is a contraindication to beta-blocker treatment.

In Patients Without a History of Cardiac Failure: Continued depression of the myocardium with beta-blocking agents over a period of time can, in some cases, lead to cardiac failure. At the first sign or symptom of impending cardiac failure, patients should be fully digitalized and/or be given a diuretic and the response observed closely. If cardiac failure continues despite adequate digitalization and diuresis, atenolol should be withdrawn. (See DOSAGE AND ADMINISTRATION.)

Cessation of Therapy With Atenolol: Patients with coronary artery disease, who are being treated with atenolol, should be advised against abrupt discontinuation of therapy. Severe exacerbation of angina and the occurrence of myocardial infarction and ventricular arrhythmias have been reported in angina patients following the abrupt discontinuation of therapy with beta blockers. The last two complications may occur with or without preceding exacerbation of the angina pectoris. As with other beta blockers, when discontinuation of atenolol is planned, the patients should be carefully observed and advised to limit physical activity to a minimum. If the angina worsens or acute coronary insufficiency develops, it is recommended that atenolol be promptly reinstituted, at least temporarily. Because coronary artery disease is common and may be unrecognized, it may be prudent not to discontinue atenolol therapy abruptly even in patients treated only for hypertension (see DOSAGE AND ADMINISTRATION).

Concomitant Use of Calcium Channel Blockers: When calcium channel blockers are coadministered with beta-blockers, bradycardia and heart block can occur and the left ventricular end diastolic pressure can rise. Patients with pre-existing conduction abnormalities or left ventricular dysfunction are particularly susceptible (see PRECAUTIONS).

Bronchospastic Diseases: PATIENTS WITH BRONCHOSPASTIC DISEASE SHOULD, IN GENERAL, NOT RECEIVE BETA BLOCKERS. Because of its relative $beta_1$ selectivity, however, atenolol may be used with caution in patients with bronchospastic disease who do not respond to, or cannot tolerate, other antihypertensive treatment. Since $beta_1$selectivity is not absolute, the lowest possible dose of atenolol should be used with therapy initiated at 50 mg and a $beta_2$-stimulating agent (bronchodilator) should be made available. If dosage must be increased, dividing the dose should be considered in order to achieve lower peak blood levels.

Anesthesia and Major Surgery: It is not advisable to withdraw beta-adrenoreceptor blocking drugs prior to surgery in the majority of patients. However, care should be taken when using anesthetic agents such as those which may depress the myocardium. Vagal dominance, if it occurs, may be corrected with atropine (1-2 mg IV).

Atenolol, like other beta blockers, is a competitive inhibitor of beta-receptor agonists and its effects on the heart can be reversed by administration of such agents: eg, dobutamine or isoproterenol with caution (see OVERDOSAGE).

Diabetes and Hypoglycemia: Atenolol should be used with caution in diabetic patients if a beta-blocking agent is required. Beta blockers may mask tachycardia occurring with hypoglycemia, but other manifestations such as dizziness and sweating may not be significantly affected. At recommended doses atenolol does not potentiate insulin-induced hypoglycemia and, unlike nonselective beta blockers, does not delay recovery of blood glucose to normal levels.

Thyrotoxicosis: Beta-adrenergic blockade may mask certain clinical signs (*e.g.,* tachycardia) of hyperthyroidism. Abrupt withdrawal of beta blockade might precipitate a thyroid storm; therefore, patients suspected of developing thyrotoxicosis from whom atenolol therapy is to be withdrawn should be monitored closely (see DOSAGE AND ADMINISTRATION).

Pregnancy and Fetal Injury: Atenolol can cause fetal harm when administered to a pregnant woman. Atenolol crosses the placental barrier and appears in cord blood. Administration of atenolol, starting in the second trimester of pregnancy, has been associated with the birth of infants that are small for gestational age. No studies have been performed on the use of atenolol in the first trimester and the possibility of fetal injury cannot be excluded. If this drug is used during pregnancy, or if the patient becomes pregnant while taking this drug, the patient should be apprised of the potential hazard to the fetus.

Atenolol has been shown to produce a dose-related increase in embryo/fetal resorptions in rats at doses equal to or greater than 50 mg/kg/day or 25 or more times when maximum recommended human antihypertensive dose*. Although similar effects were not seen in rabbits, the compound was not evaluated in rabbits at doses above 25 mg/kg/day or 12.5 times the maximum recommended human antihypertensive dose*.

*Based on the maximum dose of 100 mg/day in a 50 kg patient.

PRECAUTIONS:

General: *Tablets and IV Injection:* Patients already on a beta blocker must be evaluated carefully before atenolol is administered. Initial and subsequent atenolol dosages can be adjusted downward depending on clinical observations including pulse and blood pressure. Atenolol may aggravate peripheral arterial circulatory disorders.

Impaired Renal Function: The drug should be used with caution in patients with impaired renal function (see DOSAGE AND ADMINISTRATION).

Carcinogenesis, Mutagenesis, and Impairment of Fertility: Two long-term (maximum dosing duration of 18 or 24 months) rat studies and one long-term (maximum dosing duration of 18 months) mouse study, each employing dose levels as high as 300 mg/kg/day or 150 times the maximum recommended human antihypertensive dose,* did not indicate a carcinogenic potential of atenolol. A third (24 month) rat study, employing doses of 500 and 1,500 mg/kg/day (250 and 750 times the maximum recommended human antihypertensive dose*) resulted in increased incidences of benign adrenal medullary tumors in males and females, mammary fibroadenomas in females, and anterior pituitary adenomas and thyroid parafollicular cell carcinomas in males. No evidence of a mutagenic potential of atenolol was uncovered in the dominant lethal test (mouse), in vivo cytogenetics test (Chinese hamster) or Ames test (*S typhimurium*).

Fertility of male or female rats (evaluated at dose levels as high as 200 mg/kg/day or 100 times the maximum recommended human dose*) was unaffected by atenolol administration.

Usage in Pregnancy: Pregnancy Category D: See WARNINGS, Pregnancy and Fetal Injury.

PRECAUTIONS: *(cont'd)*

Nursing Mothers: Atenolol is excreted in human breast milk at a ratio of 1.5 to 6.8 when compared to the concentration in plasma. Caution should be exercised when atenolol is administered to a nursing woman. Clinically significant bradycardia has been reported in breast fed infants. Premature infants, or infants with impaired renal function, may be more likely to develop adverse effects.

Pediatric Use: Safety and effectiveness in children have not been established.

DRUG INTERACTIONS:

Catecholamine-Depleting Drugs (*e.g.,* Reserpine): may have an additive effect when given with beta-blocking agents. Patients treated with atenolol plus a catecholamine depletor should therefore be closely observed for evidence of hypotension and/or marked bradycardia which may produce vertigo, syncope, or postural hypotension.

Calcium Channel Blockers: may also have an additive effect when given with atenolol (See WARNINGS.)

Beta Blockers: may exacerbate the rebound hypertension which can follow the withdrawal of clonidine. If the two drugs are coadministered, the beta blocker should be withdrawn several days before the gradual withdraw of clonidine. If replacing clonidine by beta-blocker therapy, the introduction of beta blockers should be delayed for several days after clonidine administration has stopped.

Information on concurrent usage of atenolol and aspirin is limited. Data from several studies, i.e., TIMI-II, ISIS-2, currently do not suggest any clinical interaction between aspirin and beta blockers in the acute myocardial infarction setting.

While taking beta blockers, patients with a history of anaphylactic reaction to a variety of allergens may have a more severe reaction on repeated challenge, either accidental, diagnostic or therapeutic. Such patients may be unresponsive to the usual doses of epinephrine used to treat the allergic reaction.

Additional Information for the IV Injection: Caution should be exercised with atenolol IV when given in close proximity with drugs that may also have depressant effect on myocardial contractility. On rare occasions, concomitant use of IV beta blockers and IV verapamil has resulted in serious adverse reactions, especially in patients with severe cardiomyopathy, congestive heart failure, or recent myocardial infarction.

ADVERSE REACTIONS:

Most adverse effects have been mild and transient.

The frequency estimates in TABLE 1 were derived from controlled studies in hypertensive patients in which adverse reactions were either volunteered by the patient (US studies) or elicited, e.g., by checklist (foreign studies). The reported frequency of elicited adverse effects was higher for both atenolol and placebo-treated patients than when these reactions were volunteered. Where frequency of adverse effects of atenolol and placebo is similar, causal relationship to atenolol is uncertain.

TABLE 1 Adverse Effects

	Volunteered (US Studies)		Total - Volunteered and Elicited (Foreign + US Studies)	
	Atenolol (n = 164) %	Placebo (n = 206) %	Atenolol (n = 399) %	Placebo (n = 407) %
Cardiovascular				
Bradycardia	3	0	3	0
Cold Extremities	0	0.5	12	5
Postural Hypotension	2	1	4	5
Leg Pain	0	0.5	3	1
Central Nervous System/Neuromuscular				
Dizziness	4	1	13	6
Vertigo	2	0.5	2	0.2
Light-headedness	1	0	3	0.7
Tiredness	0.6	0.5	26	13
Fatigue	3	1	6	5
Lethargy	1	0	3	0.7
Drowsiness	0.6	0	2	0.5
Depression	0.6	0.5	12	9
Dreaming	0	0	3	1
Gastrointestinal				
Diarrhea	2	0	3	2
Nausea	4	1	3	1
Respiratory (see WARNINGS)				
Wheeziness	0	0	3	3
Dyspnea	0.6	1	6	4

Acute Myocardial Infarction: In a series of investigations in the treatment of acute myocardial infarction, bradycardia and hypotension occurred more commonly, as expected for any beta blocker, in atenolol-treated patients than in control patients. However, these usually responded to atropine and/or to withholding further dosage of atenolol. The incidence of heart failure was not increased by atenolol. Inotropic agents were infrequently used. The reported frequency of these and other events occurring during these investigations is given in TABLE 2.

In a study of 477 patients, the following adverse events were reported during either intravenous and/or oral atenolol administration (TABLE 2):

In the subsequent International Study of Infarct Survival (ISIS-1) including over 16,000 patients of whom 8037 were randomized to receive atenolol treatment, the dosage of intravenous and subsequent oral atenolol was either discontinued or reduced for the following reasons (TABLE 3):

During postmarketing experience with atenolol, the following have been reported in temporal relationship to the use of the drug: elevated liver enzymes and/or bilirubin, hallucinations, headache, impotence, Peyronie's disease, postural hypotension which may be associated with syncope, psoriasiform rash or exacerbation of psoriasis, psychoses, purpura, reversible alopecia, thrombocytopenia and visual disturbances. Atenolol, like other beta blockers, has been associated with the development of antinuclear antibodies (ANA), and lupus syndrome.

POTENTIAL ADVERSE EFFECTS

In addition, a variety of adverse effects have been reported with other beta-adrenergic blocking agents, and may be considered potential adverse effects of atenolol:

Hematologic: Agranulocytosis.

Allergic: Fever, combined with aching and sore throat, laryngospasm, and respiratory distress.

Central Nervous System: Reversible mental depression progressing to catatonia; an acute reversible syndrome characterized by disorientation of time and place; short-term memory loss; emotional lability with slightly clouded sensorium; and, decreased performance on neuropsychometrics.

Gastrointestinal: Mesenteric arterial thrombosis, ischemic colitis.

ADVERSE REACTIONS: *(cont'd)*

TABLE 2 Adverse Effects

	Conventional Therapy Plus Atenolol (n=244)	Conventional Therapy Alone (n=233)
Bradycardia	43 (18%)	24 (10%)
Hypotension	60 (25%)	34 (15%)
Bronchospasm	3 (1.2%)	2 (0.9%)
Heart Failure	46 (19%)	56 (24%)
Heart Block	11 (4.5%)	10 (4.3%)
BBB + Major Axis Deviation	16 (6.6%)	28 (12%)
Supraventricular Tachycardia	28 (11.5%)	45 (19%)
Atrial Fibrillation	12 (5%)	29 (11%)
Atrial Flutter	4 (1.6%)	7 (3%)
Ventricular Tachycardia	39 (16%)	52 (22%)
Cardiac Reinfarction	0 (0%)	6 (2.6%)
Total Cardiac Arrests	4 (1.6%)	16 (6.9%)
Nonfatal Cardiac Arrests	4 (1.6%)	12 (5.1%)
Deaths	7 (2.9%)	16 (6.9%)
Cardiogenic Shock	1 (0.4%)	4 (1.7%)
Development of Ventricular Septal Defect	0 (0%)	2 (0.9%)
Development of Mitral Regurgitation	0 (0%)	2 (0.9%)
Renal Failure	1 (0.4%)	0 (0%)
Pulmonary Emboli	3 (1.2%)	0 (0%)

TABLE 3 Reasons For Reduced Dosage

	IV Atenolol Reduced Dose (< 5 mg)*		Oral Partial Dose	
Hypotension/Bradycardia	105	(1.3%)	1168	(14.5%)
Cardiogenic Shock	4	(.04%)	35	(.44%)
Reinfarction	0	(0%)	5	(.06%)
Cardiac Arrest	5	(.06%)	28	(.34%)
Heart Block (> first degree)	5	(.06%)	143	(1.7%)
Cardiac Failure	1	(.01%)	233	(2.9%)
Arrhythmias	3	(.04%)	22	(.27%)
Bronchospasm	1	(.01%)	50	(.62%)

* Full dosage was 10 mg and some patients received less than 10 mg but more than 5 mg.

Other: Erythematous rash, Raynaud's Phenomenon.

Miscellaneous: There have been reports of skin rashes and/or dry eyes associated with the use of beta-adrenergic blocking drugs. The reported incidence is small, and in most cases, the symptoms have cleared when treatment was withdrawn. Discontinuance of the drug should be considered if any such reaction is not otherwise explicable. Patients should be closely monitored following cessation of therapy. (See DOSAGE AND ADMINISTRATION.)

The oculomucocutaneous syndrome associated with the beta blocker practolol has not been reported with atenolol. Furthermore, a number of patients who had previously demonstrated established practolol reactions were transferred to atenolol therapy with subsequent resolution or quiescence of the reaction.

OVERDOSAGE:

Overdosage with atenolol has been reported with patients surviving acute doses as high as 5 g. One death was reported in a man who may have taken as much as 10 g acutely.

The predominant symptoms reported following atenolol overdose are lethargy, disorder of respiratory drive, wheezing, sinus pause and bradycardia. Additionally, common effects associated with overdosage of any beta-adrenergic blocking agent and which might also be expected in atenolol overdose are congestive heart failure, hypotension, bronchospasm and/or hypoglycemia.

Treatment of overdose should be directed to the removal of any unabsorbed drug by induced emesis, gastric lavage, or administration of activated charcoal. Atenolol can be removed from the general circulation by hemodialysis. Other treatment modalities should be employed at the physician's discretion and may include:

Bradycardia: Atropine intravenously. If there is no response to vagal blockade, give isoproterenol cautiously. In refractory cases, a transvenous cardiac pacemaker may be indicated.

Heart Block (Second or Third Degree): Isoproterenol or transvenous cardiac pacemaker.

Cardiac Failure: Digitalize the patient and administer a diuretic. Glucagon has been reported to be useful.

Hypotension: Vasopressors such as dopamine or norepinephrine (levarterenol). Monitor blood pressure continuously.

Bronchospasm: A $beta_2$stimulant such as isoproterenol or terbutaline and/or aminophylline.

Hypoglycemia: Intravenous glucose.

Based on the severity of symptoms, management may require intensive support care and facilities for applying cardiac and respiratory support.

DOSAGE AND ADMINISTRATION:

TABLETS

Hypertension: The initial dose of atenolol is 50 mg given as one tablet a day either alone or added to diuretic therapy. The full effect of this dose will usually be seen within one to two weeks. If an optimal response is not achieved, the dosage should be increased to atenolol 100 mg given as one tablet a day. Increasing the dosage beyond 100 mg a day is unlikely to produce any further benefit.

Atenolol may be used alone or concomitantly with other antihypertensive agents including thiazide type diuretics, hydralazine, prazosin, and alpha-methyldopa.

Angina Pectoris: The initial dose of atenolol is 50 mg given as one tablet a day. If an optimal response is not achieved within one week, the dosage should be increased to atenolol 100 mg given as one tablet a day. Some patients may require a dosage of 200 mg once a day for optimal effect.

Twenty-four hour control with once daily dosing is achieved by giving doses larger than necessary to achieve an immediate maximum effect. The maximum early effect on exercise tolerance occurs with doses of 50 to 100 mg, but at these doses the effect at 24 hours is attenuated, averaging about 50% to 75% of that observed with once a day oral doses of 200 mg.

DOSAGE AND ADMINISTRATION: *(cont'd)*

Elderly Patients or Patients with Renal Impairment: Atenolol is excreted by the kidneys; consequently dosage should be adjusted in cases of severe impairment of renal function. Some reduction in dosage may also be appropriate for the elderly, since decreased kidney function is a physiologic consequence of aging. Atenolol excretion would be expected to decrease with advancing age.

No significant accumulation of atenolol occurs until creatinine clearance falls below 35 ml/min/1.73m^2. Accumulation of atenolol and prolongation of its half-life were studied in subjects with creatinine clearance between 5 and 105 ml/min. Peak plasma levels were significantly increased in subjects with creatinine clearances below 30 ml/min.

The following maximum oral dosages are recommended for elderly, renally-impaired patients and for patients with renal impairment due to other causes. See TABLE 4.

TABLE 4 Dosage And Renal Impairment

Creatinine Clearance (ml/min/1.73m^2)	Atenolol Elimination Half-Life (h)	Maximum Dosage
15 - 35	16 - 27	50 mg daily
< 15	> 27	25 mg daily

Some renally-impaired or elderly patients being treated for hypertension may require a lower starting dose of atenolol: 25 mg given as one tablet a day. If this 25 mg dose is used, assessment of efficacy must be made carefully. This should include measurement of blood pressure just prior to the next dose ("trough" blood pressure) to ensure that the treatment effect is present for a full 24 hours.

Although a similar dosage reduction may be considered for elderly and/or renally-impaired patients being treated for indications other than hypertension, data are not available for these patient populations.

Patients on hemodialysis should be given 25 mg or 50 mg after each dialysis; this should be done under hospital supervision as marked falls in blood pressure can occur.

Cessation of Therapy In Patients with Angina Pectoris: If withdrawal of atenolol therapy is planned, it should be achieved gradually and patients should be carefully observed and advised to limit physical activity to a minimum.

TABLETS AND IV INJECTION

Acute Myocardial Infarction: In patients with definite or suspected acute myocardial infarction, treatment with atenolol IV injection should be initiated as soon as possible after the patient's arrival in the hospital and after eligibility is established. Such treatment should be initiated in a coronary care or similar unit immediately after the patient's hemodynamic condition has stabilized. Treatment should begin with the intravenous administration of 5 mg atenolol over 5 minutes followed by another 5 mg intravenous injection 10 minutes later. Atenolol IV Injection should be administered under carefully controlled conditions including monitoring of blood pressure, heart rate, and electrocardiogram. Dilutions of atenolol IV injection in Dextrose Injection USP, Sodium Chloride Injection USP, or Sodium Chloride and Dextrose Injection may be used. These admixtures are stable for 48 hours if they are not used immediately.

In patients who tolerate the full intravenous dose (10 mg), atenolol tablets 50 mg should be initiated 10 minutes after the last intravenous dose followed by another 50 mg oral dose 12 hours later. Thereafter, atenolol can be given orally either 100 mg once daily or 50 mg twice a day for a further 6-9 days or until discharge from the hospital. If bradycardia or hypotension requiring treatment or any other untoward effects occur, atenolol should be discontinued.

Data from other beta blocker trials suggest that if there is any question concerning the use of IV beta blocker or clinical estimate that there is a contraindication, the IV beta blocker may be eliminated and patients fulfilling the safety criteria may be given atenolol tablets 50 mg twice daily or 100 mg once a day for at least seven days (if the IV dosing is excluded).

Although the demonstration of efficacy of atenolol is based entirely on data from the first seven postinfarction days, data from other beta blocker trials suggest that treatment with beta blockers that are effective in the postinfarction setting may be continued for one to three years if there are no contraindications.

Atenolol is an additional treatment to standard coronary care unit therapy.

ANIMAL PHARMACOLOGY:

Animal Toxicology: Chronic studies employing oral atenolol performed in animals have revealed the occurrence of vacuolation of epithelial cells of Brunner's glands in the duodenum of both male and female dogs at all tested dose levels of atenolol (starting at 15 mg/kg/day or 7.5 times the maximum recommended human antihypertensive dose*) and increased incidence of atrial degeneration of hearts of male rats at 300 but not 150 mg atenolol/kg/day (150 and 75 times the maximum recommended human antihypertensive dose,* respectively).

*Based on the maximum dose of 100 mg/day in a 50 kg patient.

PATIENT INFORMATION:

Atenolol is a beta blocker used for the treatment of high blood pressure, angina (chest pain), and myocardial infarction (heart attack). This medication should be taken even if you feel fine because high blood pressure may not produce physical symptoms. Do not discontinue this medication suddenly without consulting with your physician. Inform your physician if you are pregnant or nursing. This medication may cause dizziness, drowsiness, or blurred vision; use caution while driving or operating hazardous machinery. Do not take other medications which may contain alpha-adrenergic stimulants (nasal decongestants, over-the-counter cold preparations) without consulting your physician or pharmacist. Notify your physician if you experience difficulty breathing, slow pulse rate, or swelling of legs or ankles. Atenolol may alter blood sugar levels or cover up symptoms of very low blood sugar (hypoglycemia) in patients with diabetes. Atenolol may be taken with or without food.

HOW SUPPLIED:

Tablets: Tablets of 25 mg Tenormin, (round, flat, uncoated white tablets identified with "T" debossed on one side and "107" debossed on the other side) are supplied in bottles of 100 tablets.

Tablets of 50 mg atenolol, (round, flat, uncoated white tablets identified with with "TENORMIN" debossed on one side and "107" debossed on the other side, bisected) are supplied in bottles of 100 tablets and 1000 tablets, and unit dose packages of 100 tablets.

Tablets of 100 mg atenolol, (round, flat, uncoated white tablets identified with "TENORMIN" debossed on one side and "101" debossed on the other side) are supplied in bottles of 100 tablets, and in unit dose packages of 100 tablets.

STORAGE

Tablets: Store at controlled room temperature, 15-30°C (59-36°F). Dispense in well-closed, light resistant containers.

IV Injection: Protect from light. Keep ampules in outer packaging until time of use. Store at room temperature.

HOW SUPPLIED: *(cont'd)*

Parenteral drug products should be inspected visually for particulate matter and discoloration prior to administration, whenever solution and container permit.

HOW SUPPLIED - RATED THERAPEUTICALLY EQUIVALENT:

Tablet, Uncoated - Oral - 25 mg

100's	$9.09	Atenolol, H.C.F.A. F F P	99999-0333-01
100's	$23.50	Atenolol, Harber Pharm	51432-0449-03
100's	$60.00	Atenolol, Rugby	00536-3325-01
100's	$65.31	Atenolol, Invamed	52189-0259-24
100's	$67.00	Atenolol, Lederle Pharm	00005-3218-43
100's	$67.00	Atenolol, Goldline Labs	00182-1001-01
100's	$68.00	Atenolol, Goldline Labs	00182-1001-89
100's	$68.57	Atenolol, HL Moore Drug Exch	00839-7951-06
100's	$70.25	Atenolol, Geneva Pharms	00781-1078-01
100's	$70.25	Atenolol, West Point Pharma	59591-0007-68
100's	$70.55	Atenolol, Aligen Independ	00405-4106-01
100's	**$88.40**	**TENORMIN, Zeneca Pharms**	**00310-0107-10**
500's	$45.45	Atenolol, H.C.F.A. F F P	99999-0333-02
500's	$295.00	Atenolol, Rugby	00536-3325-05
500's	$325.30	Atenolol, Invamed	52189-0259-29
1000's	$90.90	Atenolol, H.C.F.A. F F P	99999-0333-03
1000's	$619.75	Atenolol, Lederle Pharm	00005-3218-34
1000's	$650.10	Atenolol, Invamed	52189-0259-30

Tablet, Uncoated - Oral - 50 mg

30's	$1.39	Atenolol, H.C.F.A. F F P	99999-0333-04
30's	$18.37	Atenolol, Talbert Phcy	44514-0876-18
100's	$4.64	Atenolol, H.C.F.A. F F P	99999-0333-05
100's	$4.91	Atenolol, United Res	00677-1478-01
100's	$24.95	SENORMIN, Seneca Pharms	47028-0054-01
100's	$61.25	Atenolol, Qualitest Pharms	00603-2371-21
100's	$61.25	Atenolol, Mova Pharms	55370-0122-07
100's	$61.25	Atenolol, Novopharm (US)	55953-0039-40
100's	$61.50	Atenolol, Aligen Independ	00405-4107-01
100's	$64.16	Atenolol, Schein Pharm (US)	00364-2513-90
100's	$65.00	Atenolol, Major Pharms	00904-7634-60
100's	$65.38	Atenolol, Duramed Pharms	51285-0837-02
100's	$65.38	Atenolol, Invamed	52189-0256-24
100's	$65.40	Atenolol, Martec Pharms	52555-0531-01
100's	$65.55	Atenolol, Rugby	00536-3330-01
100's	$67.49	Atenolol, HL Moore Drug Exch	00839-7723-06
100's	$67.49	Atenolol, HL Moore Drug Exch	00839-7741-06
100's	$67.50	Atenolol, Martec Pharms	52555-0006-01
100's	$67.53	Atenolol, Schein Pharm (US)	00364-2513-01
100's	$68.10	Atenolol, Rexall Rexall	60814-0710-01
100's	$68.26	Atenolol, Lederle Pharm	00005-3219-43
100's	$68.26	Atenolol, Goldline Labs	00182-1004-01
100's	$69.00	Atenolol, Goldline Labs	00182-1004-89
100's	$69.69	Atenolol, Bristol Myers Squibb	00003-5040-50
100's	$70.00	Atenolol, Mutual Pharm	53489-0529-01
100's	$70.38	Atenolol, Vangard Labs	00615-3532-13
100's	$71.75	Atenolol, West Point Pharma	59591-0263-68
100's	$72.75	Atenolol, Teva	00093-0752-01
100's	$73.92	Atenolol, Par Pharm	49884-0456-01
100's	$73.97	Atenolol, Geneva Pharms	00781-1506-01
100's	$75.99	Atenolol, Geneva Pharms	00781-1506-13
100's	$78.16	Atenolol, Major Pharms	00904-7634-61
100's	$84.40	Atenolol, Mylan	00378-0231-01
100's	**$90.20**	**TENORMIN, Zeneca Pharms**	**00310-0105-10**
100's	**$90.20**	**TENORMIN, Zeneca Pharms**	**00310-0105-39**
500's	$23.20	Atenolol, H.C.F.A. F F P	99999-0333-06
500's	$325.65	Atenolol, Invamed	52189-0256-29
500's	$345.50	Atenolol, Major Pharms	00904-7634-40
750's	$448.23	Atenolol, Glasgow Pharm	60809-0102-55
750's	$448.23	Atenolol, Glasgow Pharm	60809-0102-72
1000's	$46.40	Atenolol, H.C.F.A. F F P	99999-0333-07
1000's	$49.10	Atenolol, United Res	00677-1478-10
1000's	$555.00	Atenolol, Rugby	00536-3330-10
1000's	$567.38	Atenolol, Qualitest Pharms	00603-2371-32
1000's	$567.38	Atenolol, Mova Pharms	55370-0122-09
1000's	$567.38	Atenolol, Novopharm (US)	55953-0039-80
1000's	$590.00	Atenolol, Major Pharms	00904-7634-80
1000's	$593.99	Atenolol, HL Moore Drug Exch	00839-7741-16
1000's	$595.50	Atenolol, Martec Pharms	52555-0531-10
1000's	$597.24	Atenolol, Aligen Independ	00405-4107-03
1000's	$598.20	Atenolol, Rexall Rexall	60814-0710-10
1000's	$612.48	Atenolol, Duramed Pharms	51285-0837-05
1000's	$612.48	Atenolol, Invamed	52189-0256-30
1000's	$623.00	Atenolol, Mutual Pharm	53489-0529-10
1000's	$624.40	Atenolol, Martec Pharms	52555-0006-10
1000's	$625.00	Atenolol, Bristol Myers Squibb	00003-5040-75
1000's	$631.42	Atenolol, Lederle Pharm	00005-3219-34
1000's	$631.42	Atenolol, Goldline Labs	00182-1004-10
1000's	$632.00	Atenolol, Schein Pharm (US)	00364-2513-02
1000's	$633.94	Atenolol, SCS Pharm	00905-5711-52
1000's	$635.99	Atenolol, HL Moore Drug Exch	00839-7723-16
1000's	$637.50	Atenolol, Teva	00093-0752-10
1000's	$638.09	Atenolol, Par Pharm	49884-0456-10
1000's	$684.99	Atenolol, Geneva Pharms	00781-1506-10
1000's	$805.90	Atenolol, Mylan	00378-0231-10
1000's	**$891.36**	**TENORMIN, Zeneca Pharms**	**00310-0105-34**

Tablet, Uncoated - Oral - 100 mg

30's	$2.83	Atenolol, H.C.F.A. F F P	99999-0333-08
30's	$26.90	Atenolol, Talbert Phcy	44514-0885-18
100's	$9.45	Atenolol, United Res	00677-1479-01
100's	$9.45	Atenolol, H.C.F.A. F F P	99999-0333-09
100's	$89.85	Atenolol, Rugby	00536-3331-01
100's	$91.85	Atenolol, Qualitest Pharms	00603-2372-21
100's	$91.85	Atenolol, Mova Pharms	55370-0124-07
100's	$91.85	Albuterol, Novopharm (US)	55953-0401-40
100's	$94.50	Atenolol, Major Pharms	00904-7635-60
100's	$94.50	Atenolol, Martec Pharms	52555-0534-01
100's	$95.45	Atenolol, Rexall Rexall	60814-0711-01
100's	$96.23	Atenolol, SCS Pharm	00905-5721-31
100's	$96.50	Atenolol, Mutual Pharm	53489-0530-01
100's	$96.80	Atenolol, Aligen Independ	00405-4108-01
100's	$96.95	Atenolol, Duramed Pharms	51285-0838-02
100's	$96.95	Atenolol, Invamed	52189-0257-24
100's	$97.65	Atenolol, West Point Pharma	59591-0265-68
100's	$98.55	Atenolol, Schein Pharm (US)	00364-2514-01
100's	$98.60	Atenolol, Martec Pharms	52555-0007-01
100's	$99.95	Atenolol, Lederle Pharm	00005-3220-43
100's	$99.95	Atenolol, Goldline Labs	00182-1005-01

HOW SUPPLIED - RATED THERAPEUTICALLY EQUIVALENT: *(cont'd)*

100's	$99.95	Atenolol, Goldline Labs	00182-1005-89
100's	$100.25	Atenolol, Bristol Myers Squibb	00003-5240-50
100's	$100.43	Atenolol, Vangard Labs	00615-3533-13
100's	$101.24	Atenolol, HL Moore Drug Exch	00839-7724-06
100's	$101.24	Atenolol, HL Moore Drug Exch	00839-7742-06
100's	$102.50	Atenolol, Teva	00093-0753-01
100's	$103.05	Atenolol, Par Pharm	49884-0457-01
100's	$103.90	Atenolol, Geneva Pharms	00781-1507-01
100's	$105.00	Atenolol, Major Pharms	00904-7635-61
100's	$105.99	Atenolol, Geneva Pharms	00781-1507-13
100's	**$135.31**	**TENORMIN, Zeneca Pharms**	**00310-0101-10**
100's	**$135.31**	**TENORMIN, Zeneca Pharms**	**00310-0101-39**
100's	$137.50	Atenolol, Mylan	00378-0757-01
100's UD	$97.92	Atenolol, Schein Pharm (US)	00364-2514-90
500's	$47.25	Atenolol, H.C.F.A. F F P	99999-0333-10
500's	$483.50	Atenolol, Invamed	52189-0257-29
1000's	$94.50	Atenolol, United Res	00677-1479-10
1000's	$94.50	Atenolol, H.C.F.A. F F P	99999-0333-11
1000's	$896.00	Atenolol, Mutual Pharm	53489-0530-10
1000's	$924.53	Atenolol, Lederle Pharm	00005-3220-34
1000's	$925.10	Atenolol, Par Pharm	49884-0457-10
1000's	$966.50	Atenolol, Invamed	52189-0257-30
1000's	$1000.12	Atenolol, Rexall Rexall	60814-0711-10

HOW SUPPLIED - NOT RATED EQUIVALENT:

Injection, Solution - Intravenous; Bu - 5 mg/10 ml

10 ml x 6	**$18.42**	**TENORMIN I.V., Zeneca Pharms**	**00310-0108-10**

ATENOLOL; CHLORTHALIDONE *(000334)*

CATEGORIES: Antihypertensives; Beta Adrenergic Blocking Agents; Beta Blockers; Cardiovascular Drugs; Diuretics; Hypertension; Renal Drugs; Pregnancy Category C; FDA Approved 1984 Jun; Patent Expiration 1993 Jan

BRAND NAMES: *Atecard-D*; *Atenigron*; *Ateno-Basan*; Atenolol W/Chlorthalidone; *Blokium D*; *Blokium-Diu*; *Diluxen DC*; *Lo-Ten C*; *Target*; *Teneretic* (Germany); *Tenoclor 25*; *Tenoclor 50*; *Tenoclor 100*; *Tenolone*; *Tenoret* (England); *Tenoret 50*; **Tenoretic**; *Tenoric*; *Tenormin*
(International brand names outside U.S. in italics)

FORMULARIES: BC-BS

COST OF THERAPY: $183.41 (Hypertension; Tablet; 50 mg/25 mg; 1/day; 365 days)

PRIMARY ICD9: 401.1 (Essential Hypertension, Benign)

DESCRIPTION:

Atenolol with chlorthalidone is for the treatment of hypertension. It combines the antihypertensive activity of two agents: a beta$_1$-selective (cardioselective) hydrophilic blocking agent (atenolol) and a monosulfonamyl diuretic (chlorthalidone). Atenolol is Benzeneacetamide, 4-(2'-hydroxy-3'-((1-methylethyl) amino) propoxy)-.

FOR COMPLETE PRESCRIBING INFORMATION REFER TO THE INDIVIDUAL DRUG MONOGRAPHS (ATENOLOL; CHLORTHALIDONE).

INDICATIONS AND USAGE:

Atenolol w/ chlorthalidone is indicated in the treatment of hypertension. This fixed dose combination drug is not indicated for initial therapy of hypertension. If the fixed dose combination represents the dose appropriate to the individual patient's needs, it may be more convenient than the separate components.

DOSAGE AND ADMINISTRATION:

DOSAGE MUST BE INDIVIDUALIZED (see INDICATIONS AND USAGE).

Chlorthalidone is usually given at a dose of 25 mg daily; the usual initial dose of atenolol is 50 mg daily. Therefore, the initial dose should be one atenolol w/ chlorthalidone 50 tablet given once a day. If an optimal response is not achieved, the dosage should be increased to one atenolol w/ chlorthalidone 100 tablet given once a day.

When necessary, another antihypertensive agent may be added gradually beginning with 50 percent of the usual recommended starting dose to avoid an excessive fall in blood pressure.

Since atenolol is excreted via the kidneys, dosage should be adjusted in cases of severe impairment of renal function. No significant accumulation of atenolol occurs until creatinine clearance falls below 35 ml/min/1.73m^2 (normal range is 100-150 ml/min/1.73m^2); therefore, the following maximum dosages (TABLE 1) are recommended for patients with renal impairment.

TABLE 1 DOSAGE AND RENAL IMPAIRMENT

Creatinine Clearance (ml/min/1.73m^2)	Atenolol Elimination Half-life (hrs)	Maximum Dosage
15-35	16-27	50 mg daily
< 15	> 27	50 mg every other day

Storage: Store at controlled room temperature, 15-30°C (59-86°F). Dispense in well-closed, light-resistant containers.

HOW SUPPLIED - RATED THERAPEUTICALLY EQUIVALENT:

Tablet, Uncoated - Oral - 50 mg/25 mg

100's	$50.25	Atenolol W/Chlorthalidone, H.C.F.A. F F P	99999-0334-01
100's	$58.43	Atenolol/Chlorthalidone, United Res	00677-1480-01
100's	$79.40	Atenolol W/Chlorthalidone, Goldline Labs	00182-1942-01
100's	$79.80	Atenolol W/Chlorthalidone, Qualitest Pharms	00603-2374-21
100's	$80.00	Atenolol/Chlorthalidone, Mutual Pharm	53489-0531-01
100's	$80.12	Atenolol 50 Mg/Chlorthalidone 25 Mg Tabl, IPR	54921-0115-10
100's	$80.57	Atenolol W/Chlorthalidone, HL Moore Drug Exch	00839-7807-06
100's	$83.80	Atenolol W/Chlorthalidone, Martec Pharms	52555-0547-01
100's	$84.44	Atenolol W/Chlorthalidone, Caremark	00339-5839-12
100's	$85.65	Atenolol W/Chlorthalidone, Major Pharms	00904-7881-60
100's	$85.90	Atenolol/Chlorthalidone, Rugby	00536-3332-01
100's	$92.14	Atenolol W/Chlorthalidone, Aligen Independ	00405-4103-01
100's	$92.50	Atenolol W/Chlorthalidone, Schein Pharm (US)	00364-2527-01
100's	$92.58	Atenolol W/Chlorthalidone, Geneva Pharms	00781-1315-01
100's	$96.38	Atenolol W/Chlorthalidone, Mylan	00378-2063-01
100's	**$102.98**	**TENORETIC, Zeneca Pharms**	**00310-0115-10**

HOW SUPPLIED - RATED THERAPEUTICALLY EQUIVALENT: *(cont'd)*

Tablet, Uncoated - Oral - 100 mg/25 mg

100's	$72.75	Atenolol W/Chlorthalidone, H.C.F.A. F F P	99999-0334-02
100's	$86.25	Atenolol/Chlorthalidone, United Res	00677-1481-01
100's	$111.45	Atenolol W/Chlorthalidone, Qualitest Pharms	00603-2375-21
100's	$112.00	Atenolol/Chlorthalidone, Mutual Pharm	53489-0532-01
100's	$112.45	Atenolol 100 Mg/Chlorthalidone 25 Mg Tab, IPR	54921-0117-10
100's	$113.09	Atenolol W/Chlorthalidone, HL Moore Drug Exch	00839-7808-06
100's	$113.95	Atenolol W/Chlorthalidone, Goldline Labs	00182-1943-01
100's	$116.90	Atenolol W/Chlorthalidone, Martec Pharms	52555-0548-01
100's	$118.95	Atenolol W/Chlorthalidone, Caremark	00339-5841-12
100's	$120.25	Atenolol W/Chlorthalidone, Major Pharms	00904-7882-60
100's	$129.03	Atenolol w/ Chlorthalidone, Aligen Independ	00405-4104-01
100's	$129.94	Atenolol W/Chlorthalidone, Geneva Pharms	00781-1316-01
100's	$129.95	Atenolol W/Chlorthalidone, Schein Pharm (US)	00364-2528-01
100's	$135.90	Atenolol W/Chlorthalidone, Mylan	00378-2064-01
100's	**$144.60**	**TENORETIC, Zeneca Pharms**	**00310-0117-10**

ATORVASTATIN CALCIUM *(003318)*

CATEGORIES: Antilipemic Agents; Cardiovascular Drugs; Cholesterol; FDA Approved 1996 Dec; HMG-COA Reductase Inhibitors; Heart Disease; Hypercholesterolemia; Hyperlipidemia; Hyperlipoproteinemia; Hypolipidemics; Pregnancy Category X; Vascular Disease

BRAND NAMES: **Lipitor**

DESCRIPTION:

Atorvastatin calcium is a synthetic lipid-lowering agent. Atorvastatin is an inhibitor of 3 hydroxy-3-methylglutaryl-coenzyme A (HMG-CoA) reductase. This enzyme catalyzes the conversion of HMG-CoA to mevalonate, an early and rate-limiting step in cholesterol biosynthesis.

Atorvastatin calcium is [R-(R*,R*)]-2-(4-fluorophenyl)-β, σ-dihydroxy-5-(1-methylethyl)-3-phenyl-4 [(phenylamino)carbonyl]-lH-pyrrole-1-heptanoic acid, calcium salt (2:1) trihydrate. The empirical formula of atorvastatin calcium is $(C_{33}H_{34}FN_2O_5)_2Ca{\cdot}3H_2O$ and its molecular weight is 1209.42.

Atorvastatin calcium is a white to off-white crystalline powder that is insoluble in aqueous solutions of pH 4 and below. Atorvastatin calcium is very slightly soluble in distilled water, pH 7.4 phosphate buffer, and acetonitrile, slightly soluble in ethanol, and freely soluble in methanol.

Lipitor tablets for oral administration contain 10, 20, or 40 mg atorvastatin and the following inactive ingredients: calcium carbonate, USP; candelilla wax, FCC; croscarmellose sodium, NF; hydroxypropyl cellulose, NF; lactose monohydrate, NF; magnesium stearate, NF; microcrystalline cellulose; NF, Opadry White YS-1-7040 (hydroxypropylmethylcellulose, polyethylene glycol, talc, titanium dioxide); polysorbate 80, NF; simethicone emulsion.

CLINICAL PHARMACOLOGY:

MECHANISM OF ACTION

Atorvastatin is a selective, competitive inhibitor of HMG-CoA reductase, the rate-limiting enzyme that converts 3-hydroxy-3-methyl-glutaryl-coenzyme A to mevalonate, a precursor of sterols, including cholesterol. Cholesterol and triglycerides circulate in the bloodstream as part of lipoprotein complexes. With ultracentrifugation, these complexes separate into HDL (high-density lipoprotein), IDL (intermediate-density lipoprotein), LDL (low-density lipoprotein), and VLDL (very-low-density lipoprotein) fractions. Triglycerides (TG) and cholesterol in the liver are incorporated into VLDL and released into the plasma for delivery to peripheral tissues. LDL is formed from VLDL and is catabolized primarily through the high-affinity LDL receptor. Clinical and pathologic studies show that elevated plasma levels of total cholesterol (total-C), LDL-cholesterol (LDL-C), and apolipoprotein B (apo B) promote human atherosclerosis and are risk factors for developing cardiovascular disease, while increased levels of HDL-C are associated with a decreased cardiovascular risk.

In animal models, atorvastatin lowers plasma cholesterol and lipoprotein levels by inhibiting HMG-CoA reductase and cholesterol synthesis in the liver and by increasing the number of hepatic LDL receptors on the cell-surface to enhance uptake and catabolism of LDL; atorvastatin also reduces LDL production and the number of LDL particles. Atorvastatin reduces LDL-C in some patients with homozygous familial hypercholesterolemia (FH), a population that rarely responds to other lipid-lowering medication(s).

A variety of clinical studies have demonstrated that elevated levels of total-C, LDL-C, and apo B (a membrane complex for LDL-C) promote human atherosclerosis. Similarly, decreased levels of HDL-C (and its transport complex, apo A) are associated with the development of atherosclerosis. Epidemiologic investigations have established that cardiovascular morbidity and mortality vary directly with the level of total-C and LDL-C, and inversely with the level of HDL-C.

Atorvastatin reduces total-C, LDL-C, and apo B in patients with homozygous and heterozygous FH, nonfamilial forms of hypercholesterolemia, and mixed dyslipidemia. Atorvastatin also reduces VLDL-C and TG and produces variable increases in HDL-C and apolipoprotein A-1. The effect of atorvastatin on cardiovascular morbidity and mortality has not been determined.

PHARMACODYNAMICS

Atorvastatin as well as some of its metabolites are pharmacologically active in humans. The liver is the primary site of action and the principal site of cholesterol synthesis and LDL clearance. Drug dosage rather than systemic drug concentration correlates better with LDL-C reduction. Individualization of drug dosage should be based on therapeutic response (see DOSAGE AND ADMINISTRATION).

PHARMACOKINETICS AND DRUG METABOLISM

Absorption: Atorvastatin is rapidly absorbed after oral administration; maximum plasma concentrations occur within 1 to 2 hours. Extent of absorption increases in proportion to atorvastatin dose. The absolute bioavailability of atorvastatin (parent drug) is approximately 12% and the systemic availability of HMG-CoA reductase inhibitory activity is approximately 30%. The low systemic availability is attributed to presystemic clearance in gastrointestinal mucosa and/or hepatic first-pass metabolism. Although food decreases the rate and extent of drug absorption by approximately 25% and 9%, respectively, as assessed by C_{max} and AUC, LDL-C reduction is similar whether atorvastatin is given with or without food. Plasma atorvastatin concentrations are lower (approximately 30% for C_{max} and AUC) following evening drug administration compared with morning. However, LDL-C reduction is the same regardless of the time of day of drug administration (see DOSAGE AND ADMINISTRATION).

CLINICAL PHARMACOLOGY: *(cont'd)*

Distribution: Mean volume of distribution of atorvastatin is approximately 565 liters. Atorvastatin is ≥98% bound to plasma proteins. A blood/plasma ratio of approximately 0.25 indicates poor drug penetration into red blood cells. Based on observations in rats, atorvastatin is likely to be secreted in human milk (see CONTRAINDICATIONS, Pregnancy and Lactation and PRECAUTIONS, Nursing Mothers).

Metabolism: Atorvastatin is extensively metabolized to ortho- and parahydroxylated derivatives and various beta-oxidation products. *In vitro* inhibition of HMG-CoA reductase by ortho- and parahydroxylated metabolites is equivalent to that of atorvastatin. Approximately 70% of circulating inhibitory activity for HMG-CoA reductase is attributed to active metabolites. *In vitro* studies suggest the importance of atorvastatin metabolism by cytochrome P450 3A4, consistent with increased plasma concentrations of atorvastatin in humans following coadministration with erythromycin, a known inhibitor of this isozyme (see DRUG INTERACTIONS). In animals, the ortho-hydroxy metabolite undergoes further glucuronidation.

Excretion: Atorvastatin and its metabolites are eliminated primarily in bile following hepatic and/or extra hepatic metabolism: however, the drug does not appear to undergo enterohepatic recirculation. Mean plasma elimination half-life of atorvastatin in humans is approximately 14 hours, but the half-life of inhibitory activity for HMG-CoA reductase is 20 to 30 hours due to the contribution of active metabolites. Less than 2% of a dose of atorvastatin is recovered in urine following oral administration.

SPECIAL POPULATIONS

Geriatric: Plasma concentrations of atorvastatin are higher (approximately 40% for C_{max} and 30% for AUC) in healthy elderly subjects (age ≥65 years) than in young adults. LDL-C reduction is comparable to that seen in younger patient populations given equal doses of atorvastatin.

Pediatric: Pharmacokinetic data in the pediatric population are not available.

Gender: Plasma concentrations of atorvastatin in women differ from those in men (approximately 20% higher for C_{max} and 10% lower for AUC); however, there is no clinically significant difference in LDL-C reduction with atorvastatin between men and women.

Renal Insufficiency: Renal disease has no influence on the plasma concentrations or LDL-C reduction of atorvastatin; thus, dose adjustment in patients with renal dysfunction is not necessary (see DOSAGE AND ADMINISTRATION).

Hemodialysis: While studies have not been conducted in patients with end-stage renal disease, hemodialysis is not expected to significantly enhance clearance of atorvastatin since the drug is extensively bound to plasma proteins.

Hepatic Insufficiency: In patients with chronic alcoholic liver disease, plasma concentrations of atorvastatin are markedly increased. C_{max} and AUC are each 4-fold greater in patients with Childs-Pugh A disease. C_{max} and AUC are approximately 16-fold and 11-fold increased, respectively, in patients with Childs-Pugh B disease (see CONTRAINDICATIONS).

CLINICAL STUDIES:

HYPERCHOLESTEROLEMIA (HETEROZYGOUS FAMILIAL AND NONFAMILIAL) AND MIXED DYSLIPIDEMIA (*FREDRICKSON* TYPES IIA AND IIB)

Atorvastatin reduces total-C, LDL-C, VLDL-C, apo B, and TG, and increases HDL-C in patients with hypercholesterolemia and mixed dyslipidemia. Therapeutic response is seen within 2 weeks, and maximum response is usually achieved within 4 weeks and maintained during chronic therapy.

Atorvastatin is effective in a wide variety of patient populations with hypercholesterolemia, with and without hypertriglyceridemia, in men and women, and in the elderly. Experience in pediatric patients has been limited to patients with homozygous FH.

In two multicenter, placebo-controlled, dose-response studies in patients with hypercholesterolemia, atorvastatin given as a single dose over 6 weeks significantly reduced total-C, LDL-C, apo B, and TG (Pooled results are provided in TABLE 1A and TABLE 1B).

TABLE 1A Dose-Response in Patients With Primary Hypercholesterolemia (Adjusted Mean % Change From Baseline)*

Dose	N	TC	LDL-C	Apo B
Placebo	21	4	4	3
10	22	-29	-39	-32
20	20	-33	-43	-35
40	21	-37	-50	-42
80	23	-45	-60	-50

* Results are pooled from 2 dose-response studies

TABLE 1B Dose-Response in Patients With Primary Hypercholesterolemia (Adjusted Mean % Change From Baseline)*

Dose	TG	HDL-C	Non-HDL-C/HDL-C
Placebo	10	-3	7
10	-19	6	-34
20	-26	9	-41
40	-29	6	-45
80	-37	5	-53

* Results are pooled from 2 dose-response studies

In three multicenter, double-blind studies in patients with hypercholesterolemia, atorvastatin was compared to other HMG-CoA reductase inhibitors. After randomization, patients were treated for 16 weeks with either atorvastatin 10 mg per day or a fixed dose of the comparative agent (TABLE 2A and TABLE 2B).

The impact on clinical outcomes of the differences in lipid-altering effects between treatments shown in TABLE 2A and TABLE 2B is not known. TABLE 2A and TABLE 2B do not contain data comparing the effects of atorvastatin 10 mg and higher doses of lovastatin, pravastatin, and simvastatin. The drugs compared in the studies summarized in the tables are not necessarily interchangeable.

In a large clinical study, the number of patients meeting their National Cholesterol Education Program Adult Treatment Panel (NCEP-ATP) II target LDL-C levels on 10 mg of atorvastatin daily was assessed. After 16 weeks,156/167 (93%) of patients with less than 2 risk factors for CHD and baseline LDL-C ≥190 mg/dl reached a target of ≤160 mg/dl; 141/218 (65%) of patients with 2 or more risk factors for CHD and LDL-C ≥160 mg/dl achieved a level of ≤130 mg/dl LDL-C, and 21/113 (19%) of patients with CHD and LDL-C 2 130 mg/dl reached a target level of ≤100 mg/dl LDL-C.

HOMOZYGOUS FAMILIAL HYPERCHOLESTEROLEMIA

In a study without a concurrent control group, 29 patients ages 6 to 37 years with homozygous FH received maximum daily doses of 20 to 80 mg of atorvastatin. The mean LDL-C reduction in this study was 18%. Twenty five patients with a reduction in LDL-C had a mean response of 20% (range of 7% to 53%, median of 24%); the remaining 4 patients had

CLINICAL STUDIES: *(cont'd)*

TABLE 2A Mean Percent Change From Baseline at End Point (Double-Blind, Randomized, Active-Controlled Trials)

Treatment (Daily Dose)	N	Total-C	LDL-C	Apo B
Study 1				
Atorvastatin 10 mg	707	-27*	-36*	-28*
Lovastatin 20 mg	191	-19	-27	-20
95% CI for Diff[1]		-9.2, -6.5	-10.7, -7.1	-10.0, -6.5
Study 2				
Atorvastatin 10 mg	222	-25†	-35†	-27†
Pravastatin 20 mg	77	-17	-23	-17
95% CI for Diff[1]		-10.8, -6.1	-14.5, -8.2	-13.4, -7.4
Study 3				
Atorvastatin 10 mg	132	-29‡	-37‡	-34‡
Simvastatin 10 mg	45	-24	-30	-30
95% CI for Diff[1]		-8.7, -2.7	-10.1, -2.6	-8.0, -1.1

1 A negative value for the 95% CI for the difference between treatments favors atorvastatin for all except HDL-C, for which a positive value favors atorvastatin. If the range does not include 0, this indicates a statistically significant difference.
* Significantly different from lovastatin, p ≤0.05
† Significantly different from pravastatin, p ≤0.05
‡ Significantly different from simvastatin, p ≤0.05

TABLE 2B Mean Percent Change From Baseline at End Point (Double-Blind, Randomized, Active-Controlled Trials)

Treatment (Daily Dose)	TG	HDL-C	Non-HDL-C/HDL-C
Study 1			
Atorvastatin 10 mg	-17*	+7	-37*
Lovastatin 20 mg	-6	+7	-28
95% CI for Diff[1]	-15.2, -7.1	-1.7, 2.0	-11.7, -7.1
Study 2			
Atorvastatin 10 mg	-17†	+6	-36†
Pravastatin 20 mg	-9	+8	-28
95% CI for Diff[1]	-14.1, -0.7	-4.9, 1.6	-11.5, -4.1
Study 3			
Atorvastatin 10 mg	-23‡	+7	-39‡
Simvastatin 10 mg	-15	+7	-33
95% CI for Diff[1]	-15.1, -0.7	-4.3, 3.9	-9.6, -1.9

1 A negative value for the 95% CI for the difference between treatments favors atorvastatin for all except HDL-C, for which a positive value favors atorvastatin. If the range does not include 0, this indicates a statistically significant difference.
* Significantly different from lovastatin, p ≤0.05
† Significantly different from pravastatin, p ≤0.05
‡ Significantly different from simvastatin, p ≤0.05

7% to 24% increases in LDL-C. Five of the 29 patients had absent LDL-receptor function. Of these, 2 patients also had a portacaval shunt and had no significant reduction in LDL-C. The remaining 3 receptor-negative patients had a mean LDL-C reduction of 22%.

INDICATIONS AND USAGE:

Atorvastatin is indicated as an adjunct to diet to reduce elevated total-C, LDL-C, apo B, and TG levels in patients with primary hypercholesterolemia (heterozygous familial and nonfamilial) and mixed dyslipidemia (*Fredrickson* Types IIa and IIb).

Atorvastatin is also indicated to reduce total-C and LDL-C in patients with homozygous familial hypercholesterolemia as an adjunct to other lipid-lowering treatments (*e.g.*, LDL apheresis) or if such treatments are unavailable.

Therapy with lipid-altering agents should be a component of multiple-risk-factor intervention in individuals at increased risk for atherosclerotic vascular disease due to hypercholesterolemia. Lipid-altering agents should be used in addition to a diet restricted in saturated fat and cholesterol only when the response to diet and other nonpharmacological measures has been inadequate (see *National Cholesterol Education Program (NCEP) Guidelines*, summarized in TABLE 3).

TABLE 3 NCEP Guidelines for Lipid Management

Definite Atherosclerotic Disease*	Two or More Other Risk Factors†	LDL-Cholesterol mg/dl (mmol/L) Initiation Level	LDL-Cholesterol mg/dl (mmol/L) Minimum Goal
No	No	≥190 (≥4.9)	<160 (<4.1)
No	Yes	≥160 (≥4.1)	<130 (<3.4)
Yes	Yes or No	≥130‡ (≥3.4)	≤100 (≤2.6)

* Coronary heart disease or peripheral vascular disease (including symptomatic carotid artery disease).
† Other risk factors for coronary heart disease (CHD) include: age (males: ≥45 years; females: ≥55 years or premature menopause without estrogen replacement therapy); family history of premature CHD; current cigarette smoking; hypertension; confirmed HDL-C <35 mg/dl (<0.91 mmol/L); and diabetes mellitus. Subtract 1 risk factor if HDL-C is ≥60 mg/dl (≥1.6 mmol/L).
‡ In CHD patients with LDL-C levels 100 to 129 mg/dl, the physician should exercise clinical judgment in deciding whether to initiate drug treatment.

At the time of hospitalization for an acute coronary event, consideration can be given to initiating drug therapy at discharge if the LDL-C level is ≥130 mg/dl (NCEP-ATP II).

Prior to initiating therapy with atorvastatin, secondary causes for hypercholesterolemia (*e.g.*, poorly controlled diabetes mellitus, hypothyroidism, nephrotic syndrome, dysproteinemias, obstructive liver disease, other drug therapy, and alcoholism) should be excluded, and a lipid profile performed to measure total-C, LDL-C, HDL-C, and TG. For patients with TG <400 mg/dl (<4.5 mmol/L), LDL-C can be estimated using the following equation: LDL-C = total-C - (0.20 x [TG] + HDL-C). For TG levels >400 mg/dl (>4.5 mmol/L), this equation is less accurate and LDL-C concentrations should be determined by ultracentrifugation.

CONTRAINDICATIONS:

Active liver disease or unexplained persistent elevations of serum transaminases.

Hypersensitivity to any component of this medication.

CONTRAINDICATIONS: *(cont'd)*

PREGNANCY AND LACTATION

Atherosclerosis is a chronic process and discontinuation of lipid-lowering drugs during pregnancy should have little impact on the outcome of long-term therapy of primary hypercholesterolemia. Cholesterol and other products of cholesterol biosynthesis are essential components for fetal development lincluding synthesis of steroids and cell membranes). Since HMG-CoA reductase inhibitors decrease cholesterol synthesis and possibly the synthesis of other biologically active substances derived from cholesterol, they may cause fetal harm when administered to pregnant women. Therefore, HMG-CoA reductase inhibitors are contraindicated during pregnancy and in nursing mothers. ATORVASTATIN SHOULD BE ADMINISTERED TO WOMEN OF CHILDBEARING AGE ONLY WHEN SUCH PATIENTS ARE HIGHLY UNLIKELY TO CONCEIVE AND HAVE BEEN INFORMED OF THE POTENTIAL HAZARDS. If the patient becomes pregnant while taking this drug, therapy should be discontinued and the patient apprised of the potential hazard to the fetus.

WARNINGS:

LIVER DYSFUNCTION

HMG-CoA reductase inhibitors, like some other lipid-lowering therapies, have been associated with biochemical abnormalities of liver function. **Persistent elevations (>3 times the upper limit of normal [ULN] occurring on 2 or more occasions) in serum transaminases occurred in 0.7% of patients who received atorvastatin in clinical trials. The incidence of these abnormalities was 0.2%, 0.6%, 0.6%, and 2.3% for 10, 20, 40, and 80 mg, respectively.**

One patient in clinical trials developed jaundice. Increases in liver function tests (LFT) in other patients were not associated with jaundice or other clinical signs or symptoms. Upon dose reduction, drug interruption, or discontinuation, transaminase levels returned to or near pretreatment levels without sequelae. Eighteen of 30 patients with persistent LFT elevations continued treatment with a reduced dose of atorvastatin.

It is recommended that liver function tests be performed before the initiation of treatment, at 6 and 12 weeks after initiation of therapy or elevation in dose, and periodically (*e.g.*, semiannually) thereafter. Liver enzyme changes generally occur in the first 3 months of treatment with atorvastatin. Patients who develop increased transaminase levels should be monitored until the abnormalities resolve. Should an increase in ALT or AST of >3 times ULN persist, reduction of dose or withdrawal of atorvastatin is recommended.

Atorvastatin should be used with caution in patients who consume substantial quantities of alcohol and/or have a history of liver disease. Active liver disease or unexplained persistent transaminase elevations are contraindications to the use of atorvastatin (see CONTRAINDICATIONS).

SKELETAL MUSCLE

Rhabdomyolysis with acute renal failure secondary to myoglobinuria has been reported with other drugs in this class.

Uncomplicated myalgia has been reported in atorvastatin-treated patients (see ADVERSE REACTIONS). Myopathy, defined as muscle aches or muscle weakness in conjunction with increases in creatine phos phokinase (CPK) values >10 times ULN, should be considered in any patient wlth diffuse myalgias, muscle tenderness or weakness, and/or marked elevation of CPK. Patients should be advised to report promptly unexplained muscle pain, tenderness or weakness, particularly if accompanied by malaise or fever. Atorvastatin therapy should be discontinued if markedly elevated CPK levels occur or myopathy is diagnosed or suspected.

The risk of myopathy during treatment with other drugs in this class is increased with concurrent administration of cyclosporine, fibric acid derivatives, erythromycin, niacin, or azole antifungals. Physicians considering combined therapy with atorvastatin and fibric acid derivatives, erythromycin, immunosuppressive drugs, azole antifungals, or lipid-lowering doses of niacin should carefully weigh the potential benefits and risks and should carefully monitor patients for any signs or symptoms of muscle pain, tenderness, or weakness, particularly during the initial months of therapy and during any periods of upward dosage titration of either drug. Periodic creatine phosphokinase (CPK) determinations may be considered in such situations, but there is no assurance that such monitoring will prevent the occurence of severe myopathy.

Atorvastatin therapy should be temporarily withheld or discontinued in any patient with an acute, serious condition suggestive of a myopathy or having a risk factor predisposing to the development of renal failure secondary to rhabdomyolysis (*e.g.*, severe acute infection, hypotension, major surgery, trauma, severe metabolic, endocrine and electrolyte disorders, and uncontrolled seizures).

PRECAUTIONS:

GENERAL

Before instituting therapy with atorvastatin, an attempt should be made to control hypercholesterolemia with appropriate diet, exercise, and weight reduction in obese patients, and to treat other underlying medical problems (see INDICATIONS AND USAGE).

INFORMATION FOR PATIENTS

Patients should be advised to report promptly unexplained muscle pain, tenderness, or weakness, particularly if accompanied by malaise or fever.

CARCINOGENESIS, MUTAGENESIS, IMPAIRMENT OF FERTILITY

In a 2-year carcinogenicity study in rats at dose levels of 10, 30, and 100 mg/kg/day, 2 rare tumors were found in muscle in high-dose females: in one, there was a rhabdomyosarcoma and, in another, there was a fibrosarcoma. This dose represents a plasma AUC (0-24) value of approximately 16 times the mean human plasma drug exposure after an 80 mg oral dose.

A 2-year carcinogenicity study in mice given 100, 200, or 400 mg/kg/day resulted in a significant increase in liver adenomas in high-dose males and liver carcinomas in high-dose females. These findings occurred at a plasma AUC (0-24) values of approximately 6 times the mean human plasma drug exposure after an 80 mg oral dose.

In vitro, atorvastatin was not mutagenic or clastogenic in the following tests with and without metabolic activation: the Ames test with *Salmonella typhimurium* and *Escherichia coli*, the HGPRT forward mutation assay in Chinese hamster lung cells, and the chromosomal aberration assay in Chinese hamster lung cells. Atorvastatin was negative in the *in vivo* mouse micronucleus test.

Studies in rats performed at doses up to 175 mg/kg (15 times the human exposure) produced no changes in fertility. There was aplasia and aspermia in the epididymis of 2 of 10 rats treated with 100 mg/kg/day of atorvastatin for 3 months (16 times the human AUC at the 80 mg dose); testis weights were significantly lower at 30 and 100 mg/kg and epididymal weight was lower at 100 mg/kg. Male rats given 100 mg/kg/day for 11 weeks prior to mating had decreased sperm motility, spermatid head concentration, and increased abnormal sperm. Atorvastatin caused no adverse effects on semen parameters, or reproductive organ histopathology in dogs given doses of 10, 40, or 120 mg/kg for two years.

PREGNANCY, TERATOGENIC EFFECTS, PREGNANCY CATEGORY X

See CONTRAINDICATIONS.

PRECAUTIONS: *(cont'd)*

Safety in pregnant women has not been established. Atorvastatin crosses the rat placenta and reaches a level in fetal liver equivalent to that of maternal plasma. Atorvastatin was not teratogenic in rats at doses up to 300 mg/kg/day or in rabbits at doses up to 100 mg/kg/day. These doses resulted in multiples of about 30 times (rat) or 20 times (rabbit) the human exposure based on surface area (mg/m^2).

In a study in rats given 20, 100, or 225 mg/kg/day, from gestation day 7 through to lactation day 21 (weaning), there was decreased pup survival at birth, neonate, weaning, and maturity in pups of mothers dosed with 225 mg/kg/day. Body weight was decreased on days 4 and 21 in pups of mothers dosed at 100 mg/kg/day; pup body weight was decreased at birth and at days 4, 21, and 91 at 225 mg/kg/day. Pup development was delayed (rotorod performance at 100 mg/kg/day and acoustic startle at 225 mg/kg/day; pinnae detachment and eye opening at 225 mg/kg/day). These doses correspond to 6 times 1100 mg/kg) and 22 times 1225 mg/kg) the human AUC at 80 mg/day.

Rare reports of congenital anomalies have been received following intrauterine exposure to HMG-CoA reductase inhibitors. There has been one report of severe congenital bony deformity, tracheo-esophageal fistula, and anal atresia (VATER association) in a baby born to a woman who took lovastatin with dextroamphetamine sulfate during the first trimester of pregnancy. Atorvastatin should be administered to women of child-bearing potential only when such patients are highly unlikely to conceive and have been informed of the potential hazards. If the woman becomes pregnant while taking atorvastatin, it should be dis continued and the patient advised again as to the potential hazards to the fetus.

NURSING MOTHERS

Nursing rat pups had plasma and liver drug levels of 50% and 40%, respectively, of that in their mother's milk. Because of the potential for adverse reactions in nursing infants, women taking atorvastatin should not breast-feed (see CONTRAINDICATIONS).

PEDIATRIC USE

Treatment experience in a pediatric population is limited to doses of atorvastatin up to 80 mg/day for 1 year in 8 patients with homozygous FH. No clinical or biochemical abnormalities were reported in these patients. None of these patients was below 9 years of age.

GERIATRIC USE

Treatment experience in adults age ≥70 years with doses of atorvastatin up to 80 mg/day has been evaluated in 221 patients. The safety and efficacy of atorvastatin in this population were similar to those of patients <70 years of age.

DRUG INTERACTIONS:

The risk of myopathy during treatment with other drugs of this class is increased with concurrent administration of cyclosporine, fibric acid derivatives, niacin (nicotinic acid), erythromycin, azole antifungals (see WARNINGS, Skeletal Muscle).

Antacid: When atorvastatin and Maalox TC suspension were coadministered, plasma concentrations of atorvastatin decreased approximately 35%. However, LDL-C reduction was not altered.

Antipyrine: Because atorvastatin does not affect the pharmacokinetics of antipyrine, interactions with other drugs metabolized via the same cytochrome isozymes are not expected.

Colestipol: Plasma concentrations of atorvastatin decreased approximately 25% when colestipol and atorvastatin were coadministered. However, LDL-C reduction was greater when atorvastatin and colestipol were coadministered than when either drug was given alone.

Cimetidine: Atorvastatin plasma concentrations and LDL-C reduction were not altered by coadministration of cimetidine.

Digoxin: When multiple doses of atorvastatin and digoxin were coadministered, steady-state plasma digoxin concentrations increased by approximately 20%. Patients taking digoxin should be monitored appropriately.

Erythromycin: In healthy individuals, plasma concentrations of atorvastatin increased approximately 40% with coadministratlon of atorvastatin and erythromycin, a known inhibitor of cytochrome P450 3A4 (see WARNINGS, Skeletal Muscle).

Oral Contraceptives: Coadministration of atorvastatin and an oral contraceptive increased AUC values for norethindrone and ethinyl estradiol by approximately 30% and 20%. These increases should be considered when selecting an oral contraceptive for a woman taking atorvastatin.

Warfarin: Atorvastatin had no clinically significant effect on prothrombin time when administered to patients receiving chronic warfarin treatment.

Other Concomitant Therapy: In clinical studies, atorvastatin was used concomitantly with antihypertensive agents and estrogen replacement therapy without evidence of clinically significant adverse interactions. Interaction studies with specific agents have not been conducted.

ENDOCRINE FUNCTION

HMG-CoA reductase inhibitors interfere with cholesterol synthesis and theoretically might blunt adrenal and/or gonadal steroid production. Clinical studies have shown that atorvastatin does not reduce basal plasma cortisol concentration or impair adrenal reserve. The effects of HMG-CoA reductase inhibitors on male fertility have not been studied in adequate numbers of patients. The effects, if any, on the pituitary gonadal axis in premenopausal women are unknown. Caution should be exercised if an HMG-CoA reductase inhibitor is administered concomitantly with drugs that may decrease the levels or activity of endogenous steroid hormones, such as ketoconazole, spironolactone, and cimetidine.

CNS TOXICITY

Brain hemorrhage was seen in a female dog treated for 3 months at 120 mg/kg/day. Brain hemorrhage and optic nerve vacuolation were seen in another female dog that was sacrificed in moribund condition after 11 weeks of escalating doses up to 280 mg/kg/day. The 120 mg/kg dose resulted in a systemic exposure approximately 16 times the human plasma area-under-the curve (AUC, 0-24 hours) based on the maximum human dose of 80 mg/day. A single tonic convulsion was seen in each of 2 male dogs (one treated at 10 mg/kg/day and one at 120 mg/kg/day) in a 2-year study. No CNS lesions have been observed in mice after chronic treatment for up to 2 years at doses up to 400 mg/kg/day or in rats at doses up to 100 mg/kg/day. These doses were 6 to 11 times (mouse) and 8 to 16 times (rat) the human AUC (0-24) based on the maximum recommended human dose of 80 mg/day.

CNS vascular lesions, characterized by perivascular hemorrhages, edema, and mononuclear cell infiltration of perivascular spaces, have been observed in dogs treated with other members of this class. A chemically similar drug in this class produced optic nerve degeneration (Wallerian degeneration of retino geniculate fibers) in clinically normal dogs in a dose-dependent fashion at a dose that produced plasma drug levels about 30 times higher than the mean drug level in humans taking the highest recommended dose.

ADVERSE REACTIONS:

Atorvastatin is generally well-tolerated. Adverse reactions have usually been mild and transient. In controlled clinical studies of 2502 patients, <2% of patients were discontinued due to adverse experiences attributable to atorvastatin. The most frequent adverse events thought to be related to atorvastatin were constipation, flatulence, dyspepsia, and abdominal pain.

ADVERSE REACTIONS: *(cont'd)*

Clinical Adverse Experiences: Adverse experiences reported in ≥2% of patients in placebo-controlled clinical studies of atorvastatin, regardless of causality assessment, are shown in TABLE 4.

TABLE 4 Adverse Events in Placebo-Controlled Studies (% of Patients)

Body System/Adverse Event	Placebo N=270	Atorvastatin 10 mg N=863	Atorvastatin 20 mg N=36	Atorvastatin 40 mg N=79	Atorvastatin 80 mg
Body as a Whole					
Infection	10.0	10.3	2.8	10.1	7.4
Headache	7.0	5.4	16.7	2.5	6.4
Accidental Injury	3.7	4.2	0.0	1.3	3.2
Flu Syndrome	1.9	2.2	0.0	2.5	3.2
Abdominal Pain	0.7	2.8	0.0	3.8	2.1
Back Pain	3.0	2.8	0.0	3.8	1.1
Allergic Reaction	2.6	0.9	2.8	1.3	0.0
Asthenia	1.9	2.2	0.0	3.8	0.0
Digestive System					
Constipation	1.8	2.1	0.0	2.5	1.1
Diarrhea	1.5	2.7	0.0	3.8	5.3
Dyspepsia	4.1	2.3	2.8	1.3	2.1
Flatulence	3.3	2.1	2.8	1.3	1.1
Respiratory System					
Sinusitis	2.6	2.8	0.0	2.5	6.4
Pharyngitis	1.5	2.5	0.0	1.3	2.1
Skin And Appendages					
Rash	0.7	3.9	2.8	3.8	1.1
Musculoskeletal System					
Arthralgia	1.5	2.0	0.0	5.1	0.0
Myalgia	1.1	3.2	5.6	1.3	0.0

The following adverse events were reported, regardless of causality assessment, in <2% of patients treated with atorvastatin in clinical trials.

Body as a Whole: Face edema, fever, neck rigidity, malaise, photosensitivity reaction, generalized edema.

Digestive System: Gastroenteritis, liver function tests abnormal, colitis, vomiting, gastritis, dry mouth, rectal hemorrhage, esophagitis. eructation, glossitis, mouth ulceration, anorexia, increased appetite, stomatitis, biliary pain, cheilitis, duodenal ulcer, dysphagia, enteritis, melena, gum hemorrhage, stomach ulcer tenesmus, ulcerative stomatitis, hepatitis, pancreatitis, cholestatic jaundice.

Respiratory System: Pneumonia, dyspnea, asthma, epistaxis.

Nervous System: Paresthesia, somnolence, amnesia, abnormal dreams, libido decreased, emotional lability, incoordination, peripheral neuropathy, torticollis, facial paralysis, hyperkinesia.

Musculoskeletal System: Leg cramps, bursitis, tenosynovitis, myasthenia, tendinous contracture, myositis.

Skin and Appendages: Pruritus, contact dermatitis, alopecia, dry skin, sweating, acne, urticaria, eczema, seborrhea, skin ulcer.

Urogenital System: Urinary frequency, cystitis, hematuria, impotence, dysuria, kidney calculus, nocturia, epididymitis, fibrocystic breast, vaginal hemorrhage, albuminuria, breast enlargement, metrorrhagia, nephritis, urinary incontinence, urinary retention, urinary urgency, abnormal ejaculation, uterine hemorrhage.

Special Senses: Amblyopia, tinnitus, dry eyes, refraction disorder, eye hemorrhage, deafness, glaucoma, parosmia, taste loss, taste perversion.

Cardiovascular System: Palpitation, vasodilatation, syncope, migraine, postural hypotension, phlebitis, arrhythmia.

Metabolic and Nutrtional Disorders: Hyperglycemia, creatine phosphokinase increased, gout, weight gain, hypoglycemia.

Hemic and Lymphatic System: Ecchymosis, anemia, lymphadenopathy, thrombocytopenia, petechia.

OVERDOSAGE:

There is no specific treatment for atorvastatin overdosage. In the event of an overdose, the patient should be treated symptomatically, and supportive measures instituted as required. Due to extensive drug binding to plasma proteins, hemodialysis is not expected to significantly enhance atorvastatin clearance.

DOSAGE AND ADMINISTRATION:

The patient should be placed on a standard cholesterol-lowering diet before receiving atorvastatin and should continue on this diet during treatment with atorvastatin.

HYPERCHOLESTEROLEMIA (HETEROZYGOUS FAMILIAL AND NONFAMILIAL) AND MIXED DYSLIPIDEMIA (*FREDRICKSON* TYPES LLA AND IIB)

The recommended starting dose of atorvastatin is 10 mg once daily. The dosage range is 10 to 80 mg once daily. Atorvastatin can be administered as a single dose at any time of the day, with or without food. Therapy should be individualized according to goal of therapy and response (see **NCEP Guidelines**, summarized in TABLE 3). After initiation and/or upon titration of atorvastatin, lipid levels should be analyzed within 2 to 4 weeks and dosage adjusted accordingly.

Since the goal of treatment is to lower LDL-C, the NCEP recommends that LDL-C levels be used to initiate and assess treatment response. Only if LDL-C levels are not available, should total-C be used to monitor therapy.

HOMOZYGOUS FAMILIAL HYPERCHOLESTEROLEMIA

The dosage of atorvastatin in patients with homozygous FH is 10 to 80 mg daily. Atorvastatin should be used as an adjunct to other lipid-lowering treatments (*e.g.,* LDL apheresis) in these patients or if such treatments are unavailable.

CONCOMITANT THERAPY

Atorvastatin may be used in combination with a bile acid binding resin for additive effect. The combination of HMG-CoA reductase inhibitors and fibrates should generally be avoided (see WARNINGS, Skeletal Muscleand DRUG INTERACTIONS for other drug-drug interactions).

DOSAGE IN PATIENTS WITH RENAL INSUFFICIENCY

Renal disease does not affect the plasma concentrations nor LDL-C reduction of atorvastatin; thus, dosage adjustment in patients with renal dysfunction is not necessary (see CLINICAL PHARMACOLOGY, Pharmacokinetics).

PATIENT INFORMATION:

Atorvastatin calcium is used for the treatment of elevated cholesterol.

Inform physician if you are pregnant or nursing.

PATIENT INFORMATION: *(cont'd)*

Inform physician if you have liver disease. Liver function tests should be performed before starting therapy and periodically thereafter.

Inform physician if you are taking any other medication including over-the-counter drugs.

Inform physician if you experience muscle pain, tenderness or weakness, particularly if accompanied by lethargy or fever.

May cause constipation, flatulence, dyspepsia and abdominal pain.

May be taken at any time of day without regard to meals.

HOW SUPPLIED:

Lipitor is supplied as white, elliptical, film-coated tablets of atorvastatin calcium containing 10, 20, and 40 mg atorvastatin. *10 mg tablets:* coded "PD 155" on one side and "10" on the other. *20 mg tablets:* coded "PD 156" on one side and "20" on the other. *40 mg tablets:* coded "PD 157" on one side and "40" on the other.

Storage: Store at controlled room temperature 20°C to 25°C (68°F to 77°F).

Caution: Federal law prohibits dispensing without prescription.

HOW SUPPLIED - EQUIVALENTS NOT AVAILABLE:

Tablet - Oral - 10 mg

10 mg x 90 $164.16 LIPITOR, Parke-Davis 00071-0155-23

Tablet - Oral - 20 mg

20 mg x 90 $253.80 LIPITOR, Parke-Davis 00071-0156-23

Tablet - Oral - 40 mg

40 mg x 90 $305.64 LIPITOR, Parke-Davis 00071-0157-23

ATOVAQUONE *(003136)*

CATEGORIES: AIDS Related Complex; Anti-Infectives; Antibacterials; Antimicrobials; Antiprotozoals; Antivirals; Pneumocystis Carinii Pneumonia; Pneumonia; Pregnancy Category C; FDA Class 1P ("Priority Review"); FDA Approved 1992 Nov

BRAND NAMES: Mepron (Caribbean); *Wellvone* (Germany)
(International brand names outside U.S. in italics)

FORMULARIES: Medi-Cal; PCS

COST OF THERAPY: $538.68 (PCP; Suspension; 750 mg/5ml; 10/day; 21 days)

DESCRIPTION:

Mepron (atovaquone) is an antiprotozoal agent. The chemical name of atovaquone is *trans*-2 (4-(4-chlorophenyl) cyclohexyl)-3 - hydroxy - 1,4-naphthalenedione. Atovaquone is a yellow crystalline solid that is practically insoluble in water. It has a molecular weight of 366.84 and the molecular formula of $C_{22}H_{19}ClO_3$.

Mepron suspension is a formulation of micro-fine particles of atovaquone. The Atovaquone particles, which were reduced in size to facilitate absoprtion, are significantly smaller than those in the previously marketed tablet formulation. Mepron suspension is for oral administratioin and is bright yellow with a citrus flavor. Each teaspoonful (5 ml) contains 750 mg of atovaquone and the inactive ingredients benzyl alcohol, flavor, poloxamer 188, purified water, saccharin sodium, and xantham gum.

CLINICAL PHARMACOLOGY:

MECHANISM OF ACTION

Atovaquone is a hydroxy-1,4- naphthoquinone, an analog of ubiquinone, with anti-pneumocystis activity. The mechanism of action against *P. Carinii* has not been fully elucidated. In *Plasmodium* species, the site of action appears to be the cytochrome bc_1complex (Complex III). Several metabolic enzymes are linked to the mitochondrial electron transport chain via ubiquinone. Inhibition of electron transport by atovaquone will result in indirect inhibition of these enzymes. The ultimate metabolic effects of such blockade may include inhibition of nucleic acid and ATP synthesis.

MICROBIOLOGY

Pneumocystis carinii: Several laboratories, using different *in vivo* methodologies, have shown the IC_{50} (50% Inhibitory Concentration) of atovaquone against rat*P. carinii* to be in the range of 0.1 to 3.0 mcg/ml.

PHARMACOKINETICS

Absorption: Atovaquone is a highly lipophilic compound with a low aqueous solubility. The bioavailability of atovaquone is highly dependent on formulation and diet. The suspension formulation provides an approximately two-fold increase in atovaquone bioavailability in the fasting or fed state compared to the previously marketed tablet formulation. The absolute bioavailability of a 750 mg dose of atovaquone suspension administered under fed conditions in nine HIV-infected (CD4>100 cells/mm^3) volunteers was 47% ± 15%. In the same study, the bioavailability of a 750 mg dose of the previously marketed tablet formulation was 23% ± 11%.

Administering atovaquone with food enhances its absorption by approximately two-fold. In one study, 15 healthy volunteers received a single dose of 750 mg atovaquone suspension after an overnight fast and following a standard breakfast (23 g fat; 610 kCal). The mean (±SD) area under the concentration-time curve (AUC) values were 324 ± 115 and 801 ± 320 hr·mcg/ml under fasting and fed conditions, respectively, representing a 2.5 ± 1.0 fold increase. The effect of food (23 g fat; 400 kCal) on plasma atovaquone concentrations was also evaluated in a multiple-dose, randomized, crossover study in 19 HIV-infected volunteers (CD4 <200 cells/mm^3) receiving daily doses of 500 mg atovaquone suspension. AUC was 280 ± 114 hr·mcg/ml when atovaquone was administered with food as compared to 169 ± 77 hr·mcg/ml under fasting conditions. Maximum plasma atovaquone concentration (C_{max}) was 15.1 ± 6.1 and 8.8 ± 3.7 mcg/ml when atovaquone was administered with food and under fasting conditions, respectively.

Dose Proportionality: Plasma atovaquone concentrations do not increase proportionally with dose. When atovaquone suspension was administered with food at dosage regimens of 500 mg once daily, 750 mg once daily, average staedy-state plasma atovaquone concentrations were 11.7±4.8, 12.5±5.8, and 13.5±5.1 mcg/ml, respectively. The corresponding C_{max} concentrations were 15.1±6.1, 15.3±7.6, and 15.8±6.4 mcg/ml. When atovaquone suspension was administered to five HIV-infected volunteers at a dose 750 mg twice daily, the average steady-state plasma atovaquone concentration was 21.0±4.9 mcg/ml. The minimum plasma atovaquone concentration (C_{min}) associated with the 750 mg twice daily regimen was 16.7±4.6 mcg/ml.

Distribution: Following the intravenous administration of atovaquone, the volume of distribution at steady-state (Vd_{SS}) was 0.60±0.17 L/kg (n=9). Atovaquone is extensively bound to plasma proteins (99.9%) over the concentration range of 1 to 90 mcg/ml. In three HIV-infected children who received 750 mg of atovaquone as the tablet formulation four times daily for 2 weeks, the cerbrospinal fluid concentrations of atovaquone were 0.04 mcg/ml, and 0.25 mcg/ml, representing less than 1% of the plasma concentration.

Elimination: The plamsa clearance of atovaquone following intravenous administration in nine HIV-infected volunteers was 10.4±5.5 ml/min (0.15±0.09 ml/min/kg). The half-life of atovaquone was 52.5±35.3 hours after I.V. administration and ranged from 67.0±33.4 to 77.5±23.1 hours across studies following administration of atovaquone suspension. The half-life of atpvaquone is long due to presumed enteropathic cycling and eventual fecal elimination. In a study where ^{14}C-labelled atovaquone was administered to healthy volunteers, greater than 94% of the dose was recovered as unchanged atovaquone in the feces over 21 days. Therre was little or no excretion of atovaquone in the urine (less than 0.5%). There is indirect evidence that atovaquone may undergo limited metabolism; however, a specific metabolite has not been identified.

Special Populations

Pediatrics: Preliminary analysis of an ongoing study of atovaquone suspension in 15 HIV-infected, asympotmatic infants and children between 1 month and 13 years of age suggests that the pharmacokinetics of atovaquone is age dependent. Those between 2 and 13 years of age achieved average steady-state plasma atovaquone concentrations of 16.8 ± 6.4 mcg/ml and 37.1 ± 10.9 mcg/ml when given doses of 10 amd 30 mg/kg, respectively. Those between 3 and 24 months of age achieved average steady-state plasma atovaquone concentrations of 5.7±5.1 mcg/ml and 8.9±3.1 mcg/ml when given doses of 10 and 30 mg/kg, respectively.

Hepatic/Renal Impairment: The pharmacokinetics of atovaquone has not been studied in patients with hepatic or renal impairment.

CLINICAL STUDIES:

Relationship Between Plasma Atovaquone Concentration and Clinical Outcome: In a comparative study of atovaquone tablets with trimethoprim-sulfamethoxazole (TMP-SMX) for oral treatment of mild to moderate *Pneumocystis Carinii* pneumonia (PCP) (see INDICATIONS AND USAGE) where AIDS patients received 750 mg atovaquone tablets tree times daily for 21 days, the mean steady-state atovaquone concentration was 13.9±5.9 mcg/ml (n=133). Analysis of these data established a relationship between plasma atovaquone concentration and successful treatment. This is shown in TABLE 1.

TABLE 1 Relationship Between Plasma Atovaquone Concentration and Successful Treatment

Steady-State Plasma Atovaquone Concentrations (mcg/ml)	Successful Treatment* (No. Successes/No. in Group) (%)			
	Observed		Predicted†	
0 to <5	0/6	(0%)	1.5/6	(25%)
5 to <10	18/26	(69%)	14.7/26	(57%)
10 to <15	30/3	(79%)	31.9/3	(84%)
15 to < 20	18/1	(95%)	18.1/1	(95%)
20 to <25	18/1	(100%)	17.8/1	(99%)
25+	5/5	(100%)	5/5	(100%)

* Successful treatment was defined as improvement in clinical and respiratory measures persisting at least 4 weeks after cessation of therapy. This was based on data from patients for which both outcome and steady-state plasma atovaquone concentration data are available.
† Based on logistic regression analysis

A dosing regimen of atovaquone suspension for the treatment of mild to moderate PCP has been selected to achieve average plasma atovaquone concentrations of approximately 20 mcg/ml, because this plasma concentration was previously shown to be well tolerated and associated with the highest treatment success rates (TABLE 1). In an open-label PCP treatment study with atovaquone suspension, dosing regimens of 1000 mg once daily, 750 mg twice daily, 1500 mg once daily, and 1000 mg twice daily were explored. The average steady-state plasma atovaquone concentration achieved at the 750 mg twice daily dose given with meals was 22.0±10.1 mcg.ml (n=18).

INDICATIONS AND USAGE:

Atovaquone is indicated for the acute oral treatment of mild to moderate*Pneumocystis Carinii* in pneumonia in patients who are intolerant to trimethoprim-sulfamethoxazole (TMP-SMX).

This indication is based on the results of comparative pharmacokinetic studies of the suspension and tablet formulations (see CLINICAL PHARMACOLOGY) and clinical efficacy studies of the tablet formulation which established a relationship between plasma atovaquone concentration and successful treatment. The results of a randomized, double-blind trial comparing atovaquone to TMP-SMX in AIDS patients with mild to moderate PCP (defined in the study protocol as an alveolar-atrial oxygen diffusion gradient [(A-a)DO_2]^1 ≤45 mmHg and PaO_2 ≥50 mmHg on room air) and a randomized trial comparing atovaquone to intravenous pentamide isethionate in patients with mild to moderate PCP intolerant to trimethoprim or sulfa-antimicrobials are summarized below:

TMP-SMX Comparative Study: This double-blind, randomized trial initiated in 1990 was designed to compare the safety and efficacy of atovaquone to that of TMP-SMX for the treatment of AIDS in patients with histologically confirmed PCP. Only patients with mild to moderate PCP were eligible for enrollment.

A total of 408 patients were enrolled into the trial at 37 study centers. Eighty-six patients without histologic confirmation of PCP were excluded from efficacy analyses. Of the 322 patients with histologically confirmed PCP. 160 were randomized to receive Mepron and 162 to TMP-SMX.

Study participants randomized to atovaquone treatment were to receive 750 mg (three 250 mg tablets) three times daily for 21 days and those randomized to TMP-SMX were to receive 320 mg TMP plus 1600 mg SMX three times daily for 21 days.

Therapy success was defined as improvement in clinical and respiratory measures persisting at least four weeks after cessation of therapy. Therapy failures included lack of response, treatment discontinuation due to an adverse experience, and unevaluable.

There was a significant difference (P= 0.03) in mortality rates between the treatment groups. Among the 322 patients with confirmed PCP, 13 of 160 (8%) patients treated with atovaquone and four of 162 (2.5%) patients receiving TMP-SMX died during the 21-day treatment course or 8- week follow-up period. In the intent-to-treat analysis for all 408 randomized patients, there were 16 (8%) deaths in the atovaquone arm and seven (3.4%) deaths in the TMP-SMX arm (P = 0.051). Of the 13 patients treated with atovaquone who died, 4 died of PCP and 5 died with a combination of bacterial infections and PCP; bacterial infections did not appear to be a factor in any of the 4 deaths among TMP-SMX-treated patients.

INDICATIONS AND USAGE: *(cont'd)*

A correlation between plasma atovaquone concentrations and death was demonstrated; in general, patients with lower plasma concentrations were more likely to die. For those patients for whom day 4 atovaquone plasma concentration data are available, 5 (63%) of the 8 patients with concentrations < 5 mcg/ml died during participation in the study. However, only 1 (2.0%) of the 49 patients with day 4 plasma concentrations ≥ 5 mcg/ml died.

Sixty-two percent of patients on atovaquone and 64% of patients on TMP-SMX were classified as protocol-defined therapy successes (TABLE 2).

TABLE 2 Outcome of Treatment for PCP-Positive Patients Enrolled in the TMP-SMX Comparative Study

Outcome of Therapy*	No. of Patients Atovaquone (n=160)	TMP-SMX (n=162)	(% of Total) P-value
Therapy Success	99 (62%)	103 (64%)	0.75
Therapy Failure			
Lack of Response	28 (17%)	10 (%6)	< 0.01
Adverse Experience	11 (7%)	33 (20%)	< 0.01
Unevaluable	22 (14%)	16 (%10)	0.28
Required Alternate PCP Therapy During Study	55 (34%)	55 (34%)	0.95

* As defined by the protocol and described in study description above.

The failure rate due to lack of response was significantly larger for atovaquone patients while the failure rate due to adverse experiences was significantly larger for TMP-SMX patients.

There were no significant differences in the effect of either treatment on additional indicators of response (*i.e.,* arterial blood gas measurements, vital signs, serum LDH levels, clinical symptoms, and chest radiographs).

Pentamidine Comparative Study: This unblinded, randomized trial initiated in 1991 was designed to compare the safety and efficacy of atovaquone to that of pentamidine for the treatment of histologically confirmed mild or moderate PCP in AIDS patients. Approximately 80% of the patients had a history of intolerance to trimethoprim or sulfa- antimicrobials (the primary therapy group) or were experiencing intolerance to TMP-SMX with treatment of an episode of PCP at the time of enrollment in the study (the salvage treatment group).

Patients randomized to atovaquone were to receive 750 mg atovaquone (three 250 mg tablets) three times daily for 21 days and those randomized to pentamidine isethionate were to receive a 3 to 4 mg/kg single intravenous infusion daily for 21 days.

A total of 174 patients were enrolled into the trial at 22 study centers. Thirty-nine patients without histologic confirmation of PCP were excluded from the efficacy analyses. Of the 135 patients with histologically confirmed PCP, 70 were randomized to receive atovaquone and 65 to pentamidine. One hundred and ten (110) of these were in the primary therapy group and 25 were in the salvage therapy group. One patient in the primary therapy group randomized to receive pentamidine did not receive study medication.

There was no difference in mortality rates between the treatment groups. Among the 135 patients with confirmed PCP, 10 of 70 (14%) patients randomized to atovaquone and nine of 65 (14%) patients randomized to pentamidine died during the 21-day treatment course or 8-week follow-up period. In the intent-to-treat analysis for all randomized patients, there were 11 (12.5%) deaths in the atovaquone arm and 12 (14%) deaths in the pentamidine arm. For those patients for whom day 4 atovaquone plasma concentration are available, 3 of 5 (60%) patients with concentrations < 5 mcg/ml died during participation in the study. However, only 2 of 21 (9%) patients with day 4 plasma concentrations ≥ 5 mcg/ml died.

The therapeutic outcomes for the 134 patients who received study medication in this trial are presented in TABLE 3.

TABLE 3 Outcome of Treatment for PCP-Positive Patients Enrolled in the Pentamidine Comparative Study

Outcome of Therapy	Primary Treatment Mepron (n=56)	Primary Treatment Pentamidine (n=53)	P-value	Salvage Treatment Mepron (n=14)	Salvage Treatment Pentamidine (n=11)	P-value
Therapy Success	32 (57%)	21 (40%)	0.09	13 (93%)	7 (64%)	0.14
Therapy Failure						
Lack of Response	16 (29%)	9 (17%)	0.18	0	0	—
Adverse Experience	2 (3.6%)	19 (36%)	<0.01	0	3 (27%)	0.07
Unevaluable	6 (11%)	4 (8%)	0.75	1 (7%)	1 (9%)	1.00
Required Alternate PCP Therapy During Study	19 (34%)	29 (55%)	0.04	0	4 (36%)	0.03

Data on Chronic Use: Atovaquone has not been systematically evaluated as a chronic suppressive agent to prevent the development of PCP in patients at high risk for *Pneumocystis carinii* disease.

CONTRAINDICATIONS:

Atovaquone suspension is contraindicated for patients who develop or have a history of potentially life-threatening allergic reactions to any of the components of the formulation.

WARNINGS:

Clinical experience with atovaquone had been limited to patients with mild to moderate PCP [(A-a)DO_2 ≤ 45 mmHg]. Treatment of more severe episodes of PCP has not been systematically studied with this agent. Also, the efficacy of atovaquone in patients who are failing therapy with TMP-SMX has not been systematically studied. Atovaquone has not been evaluated as an agent for PCP prophylaxis.

PRECAUTIONS:

General: Absorption of orally administered atovaquone is limited but can be significantly increased when the drug is taken with food. Atovaquone plasma concentrations have been shown to correlate with the likelihood of successful treatment and survival. Therefore, parenteral therapy with other agents should be considered for patients who have difficulty taking Mepron with food (see CLINICAL PHARMACOLOGY). Gastrointestinal disorders may limit absorption of orally administered drugs. Patients with these disorders also may also not achieve plasma concentrations of atovaquone associated with response to therapy in controlled trials.

Based upon the spectrum of *in vitro* antimicrobial activity, atovaquone is not effective therapy for concurrent pulmonary conditions such as bacterial, viral or fungal pneumonia or mycobacterial diseases. Clinical deterioration in patients may be due to infections with other

PRECAUTIONS: *(cont'd)*

pathogens, as well as progressive PCP. All patients with acute PCP should be carefully evaluated for other possible causes of pulmonary disease and treated with additional agents as appropriate.

Information for the Patient: The importance of taking the prescribed dose of atovaquone should be stressed. Patients should be instructed to take their daily dose of atovaquone with meals as the presence of food will significantly improve the absorption of the drug.

Drug/Laboratory Test Interactions: It is not known if atovaquone interferes with clinical laboratory test or assay results.

Carcinogenesis, Mutagenesis, and Impairment of Fertility: Carcinogenicity studies in rats and mice have not been completed. Atovaquone was negative with or without metabolic activation in the Ames*Salmonella* mutagenicity assay, the Mouse Lymphoma mutagenesis assay, and the Cultured Human Lymphocyte cytogenetic assay. No evidence of genotoxicity was observed in the *in vivo* Mouse Micronucleus assay.

Pregnancy Category C: Atovaquone was not teratogenic and did not cause reproductive toxicity in rats at plasma concentrations up to 5 times the estimated human exposure. Atovaquone caused maternal toxicity in rabbits at plasma concentrations that were approximately equal to the estimated human exposure. Mean fetal body lengths and weights were decreased and there were higher numbers of early resorption and post-implantation loss per diem. It is not clear whether these effects were caused by atovaquone or were secondary to maternal toxicity. Concentrations of atovaquone in rabbit fetuses averaged 30% of the concurrent maternal plasma concentrations. In a separate study in rats given a single ^{14}C-radiolabeled dose, concentrations of radiocarbon in rat fetuses were 18% (middle gestation) and 60% (late gestation) of concurrent maternal plasma concentrations. There are no adequate and well-controlled studies in pregnant women. Atovaquone should be used during pregnancy only the potential benefit justifies the potential risk to the fetus.

Nursing Mothers: It is not known whether atovaquone is excreted into human milk. Because many drugs are excreted into human milk, caution should be exercised when atovaquone is administered to a nursing woman. In a rat study, atovaquone concentrations in the milk were 30% of the concurrent atovaquone concentrations in the maternal plasma.

Pediatric Use: There are no efficacy studies in children. Clinical experience with atovaquone in the pediatric population is limited to a pharmacokinetic and safety study. No children under 4 months of age participated in the phase I trial.

Geriatric Use: Atovaquone has not been systematically evaluated in patients greater than 65 years of age. Caution should be exercised when treating elderly patients reflecting the greater frequency of decreased hepatic, renal and cardiac function in this population.

DRUG INTERACTIONS:

Rifampin: In a study with 13 HIV- infected volunteers, the oral administration of rifampin 600 mg every 24 hours with atovaquone suspension 750 mg every 12 hours resulted in a 52% ± 13% decrease in the average steady-state plasma atovaquone concentration and a 37% ± 42% increase in the average steady-state plasma rifampin concentration. The half-life of atovaquone decreased from 82 ± 35 hours when administered without rifampin.

Rifabutin, another rifamycin is structurally similar to rifampin and may possibly have some of the same drug interactions as rifampin. No interaction trials have been conducted with atovaquone suspension and rifampin.

Trimethoprim/Sulfamethoxazole (TMP-SMX): The possible interaction between atovaquone and TMP-SMX was evaluated in six HIV-infected adult volunteers as part of a larger mulitple-dose, dose escalation, and chronic dosing study of atovaquone suspension. In this cross-over study, atovaquone suspension 500 mg once daily, or Septra® DS Tablets (150 mg trimethoprim and 800 mg sulfamethoxazole) twice daily, or the combination were administered with food to achieve steady-state. No difference was observed in the average steady-state plasma atovaquone concentration after co-administration with TMP-SMX. Co-administration of atovaquone with TMP-SMX resulted in a 17% and 8% decrease in average steady-state concentration of trimethoprim and sulfamethoxazole in plasma, respectively. This effect is minor and would not be expected to produce clinically significant events.

Zidovudine: Data from 14 HIV-infected volunteers who were given atovaquone tablets 750 mg every 12 hours with zidovudine 200 mg every 6 hours showed a 24% ± 12% decrease in zidovudine apparent oral clearance, leading to a 35% ± 23% increase in plasma zidovudine AUC. The glucuronide metabolite : parent ratio decreased from a mean of 4.5 when zidovudine was administered alone to 3.1 when zidovudine was administered with atovaquone tablets. This effect is minor and would not be expected to produce clinically significant events. Zidovudine had no effect on atovaquone pharmacokinetics.

Atovaquone is highly bound to plasma protein (>99.9%). Therefore, caution should be used when administering atovaquone concurrently with other highly plasma protein-bound drugs with narrow therapeutic indices, as competition for binding sites may occur. The extent of plasma protein binding of atovaquone in human plasma is not affected by the presence of therapeutic concentrations of phenytoin (15 mcg/ml), nor is the binding of phenytoin affected by the presence of atovaquone.

ADVERSE REACTIONS:

Because many patients who participated in clinical trials with atovaquone had complications of advanced HIV disease, it was often difficult to distinguish adverse events caused by atovaquone suspension from those caused by the underlying medical conditions. There were no life-threatening or fatal adverse experiences caused by atovaquone.

TABLE 4 summarizes all the clinical adverse experiences reported by ≥ 5% of the study population during the TMP-SMX comparative study of atovaquone (n=408), regardless of attribution.

Although an equal percentage of patients receiving atovaquone and TMP-SMX reported at least one adverse experience, more patients receiving TMP-SMX required discontinuation of therapy due to an adverse event. Nine percent of patients receiving atovaquone were prematurely discontinued from therapy due an adverse event versus 24% of patients receiving TMP-SMX. Four percent of patients receiving atovaquone had therapy discontinued due to development of rash. The majority of cases of rash among patients receiving atovaquone were mild and did not require the discontinuation of dosing. The only other clinical adverse experience that led to premature discontinuation of atovaquone dosing by more than one patient was the development of vomiting (<1%). Twenty-four percent of patients receiving TMP-SMX were prematurely discontinued from therapy due to an adverse experience versus 9% of patients receiving atovaquone. The most common adverse experience requiring discontinuation of dosing in the TMP-SMX group was rash (8%).

Laboratory test abnormalities reported for ≥ 5% of the study population during the treatment period are summarized in TABLE 5. Two percent of patients treated with atovaquone and 7% of patients treated with TMP-SMX had therapy prematurely discontinued due to elevations in ALT/AST. In general, patients treated with atovaquone developed fewer abnormalities in measures of hepatocellular function (ALT, AST, alkaline phosphatase) or amylase values than patients treated with TMP-SMX.

TABLE 6 summarizes the clinical adverse experiences reported by ≥ 5% of the primary therapy study population (n=144) during the comparative trial of atovaquone and intravenous pentamidine, regardless of attribution. A slightly lower percentage of patients who

ADVERSE REACTIONS: *(cont'd)*

TABLE 4 Treatment-Emergent Adverse Experiences in the TMP-SMX Comparative PCP Treatment Study

Treatment-Emergent Adverse-Experience	Number of Patients w/ Treatment-Emergent Adverse Experience (% ot Total) Atovaquone (n=203)	TMP-SMX (n=205)
Rash (including maculopapular)	47 (23%)	69 (34%)*
Nausea	43 (21%)	90 (44%)
Diarrhea	39 (19%)	15 (7%)
Headache	33 (16%)	44 (22%)
Vomiting	29 (14%)	72 (35%)
Fever	28 (14%)	52 (25%)
Insomnia	20 (10%)	18 (9%)
Asthenia	17 (8%)	16 (8%)
Pruritus	11 (5%)	18 (9%)
Monilia, Oral	11 (5%)	21 (10%)
Abdominal Pain	9 (4%)	15 (7%)
Constipation	7 (3%)	35 (17%)
Dizziness	7 (3%)	17 (8%)
No. Patients Discontinuing Therapy due to an Adverse Experience	19 (9%)	50 (24%)
No. Patients Reporting at least one Adverse Experience	127 (63%)	134 (65%)

* $P \leq 0.05$

TABLE 5 Treatment-Emergent Laboratory Test Abnormalities in the TMP-SMX Comparative PCP Treatment Study

Laboratory Test Abnormality	Patients Developing a Laboratory Test Abnormality (% of Total) Atovaquone	TMP-SMX
Anemia (Hgb < 8.0 gm/dl)	6%	7%
Neutropenia (ANC < 750 c/mm^3)	3%	9%
Elevated ALT (> 5 x ULN)	6%	16%
Elevated AST (> 5 x ULN)	4%	14%
Elevated Alkaline Phosphatase (> 2.5 x ULN)	8%	6%
Elevated Amylase (> 1.5 x ULN)	7%	12%
Hyponatremia (< 0.96 x LLN)	7%	26%

ULN = upper limit of normal range
LLN = lower limit of normal range

received atovaquone reported occurrence of adverse events than did those who received pentamidine (63% vs 72%). However, only 7% of patients discontinued treatment with atovaquone due to adverse events while 41% of patients who received pentamidine discontinued treatment for this reason ($P < 0.001$). Of the five patients who discontinued therapy with atovaquone, three reported rash (4%). Rash was not severe in any patient. No other reason for discontinuation of Mepron was cited more than once. The most frequently cited reasons for discontinuation of pentamidine therapy were hypoglycemia (11%) and vomiting (9%).

TABLE 6 Treatment-Emergent Adverse Experiences in the Pentamidine Comparative PCP Treatment Study (Primary Therapy Group)

Treatment-Emergent Adverse-Experience	No. of Patients w/ Treatment-Emergent Adverse Experience (% of Total) Atovaquone (n=73)	Pentamidine (n=71)
Fever	29 (40%)	18 (25%)
Nausea	16 (22%)	26 (37%)
Rash	16 (22%)	9 (13%)
Diarrhea	15 (21%)	22 (31%)
Insomnia	14 (19%)	10 (14%)
Headache	13 (18%)	20 (28%)
Vomiting	10 (14%)	12 (17%)
Cough	10 (14%)*	1 (1%)
Abdominal Pain	7 (10%)	8 (11%)
Pain	7 (10%)	7 (10%)
Sweat	7 (10%)	2 (3%)
Monilia, Oral	7 (10%)	2 (3%)
Asthenia	6 (8%)	10 (14%)
Dizziness	6 (8%)	10 (14%)
Anxiety	5 (7%)	7 (10%)
Anorexia	5 (7%)	7 (10%)
Sinusitis	5 (7%)	4 (6%)
Dyspepsia	4 (5%)	7 (10%)
Rhinitis	4 (5%)	5 (7%)
Taste Perversion	2 (3%)	9 (13%)*
Hypoglycemia	1 (1%)	11 (15%)*
Hypotension	1 (1%)	7 (10%)*
No. Patients Discontinuing Therapy due to an Adverse Experience	5 (7%)	29 (41%)†
No. Patients Reporting at least one Adverse Experience	46 (63%)	51 (72%)

* $P \leq 0.05$
† †$P \leq 0.001$

Laboratory test abnormalities reported in ≥ 5% of patients in the pentamidine comparative study are presented in TABLE 7. Laboratory abnormality was reported as the reason for discontinuation of treatment in two of 73 patients who received atovaquone. One patient (1%) had elevated creatinine and BUN levels and one patient (1%) had elevated amylase levels. Laboratory abnormalities were the sole or contributing factor in 14 patients who prematurely discontinued pentamidine therapy. In the 71 patients who received pentamidine, laboratory parameters most frequently reported as reasons for discontinuation were hypoglycemia (11%), elevated creatinine levels (6%), and leukopenia (4%).

OVERDOSAGE:

There have been no reports of overdosage from the oral administration of atovaquone.

DOSAGE AND ADMINISTRATION:

The recommended oral dose is 750 mg (5 ml) administered with meals twice daily for 21 days (total daily dose 1500 mg). Failure to administer Mepron Suspension with meals may result in lower plasma atovaquone concentrations and may limit response to therapy (see CLINICAL PHARMACOLOGYand PRECAUTIONS).

TABLE 7 Treatment-Emergent Laboratory Test Abnormalities in the Pentamidine Comparative PCP Treatment Study

Laboratory Test Abnormality	Patients Developing a Laboratory Test Abnormality (% of Total) Atovaquone	Pentamidine
Anemia (Hgb < 8.0 gm/dl)	4%	9%
Neutropenia (ANC < 750 cells/mm^3)	5%	9%
Hyponatremia (< 0.96 x LLN)	10%	10%
Hyperkalemia (> 1.18 x ULN)	0%	5%
Alkaline Phosphatase (> 2.5 x ULN)	5%	2%
Hyperglycemia (>1.8 x ULN)	9%	13%
Elevated AST (> 5 x ULN)	0%	5%
Elevated Amylase (> 1.5 x ULN)	8%	4%
Elevated Creatinine (> 1.5 x ULN)	0%	7%

ULN = upper limit of normal range
LLN = lower limit of normal range

HOW SUPPLIED:

Mepron Suspension (bright yellow, citrus flavored) containing 750 mg atovaquone in each teaspoonful (5 ml).

Storage: Store at 15° to 25°C (59° to 77°F). **Do Not Freeze.** Dispense in tight container as defined in USP.

HOW SUPPLIED - EQUIVALENTS NOT AVAILABLE:

Suspension - Oral - 750 mg/5ml

210 ml $538.69 MEPRON, Glaxo Wellcome 00173-0665-18

ATRACURIUM BESYLATE *(000335)*

CATEGORIES: Analeptics; Anesthesia; Autonomic Drugs; Endotracheal Intubation; Muscle Relaxants; Neuromuscular Blocking Agents; Non-Depolarizing Muscle Relaxants; Skeletal Muscle Relaxants; Pregnancy Category C; Sales > $100 Million; FDA Approved 1983 Nov; Patent Expiration 1996 Dec

BRAND NAMES: **Tracrium**

DESCRIPTION:

This drug should be used only by adequately trained individuals familiar with its actions, characteristics, and hazards.

Atracurium besylate is an intermediate-duration, nondepolarizing, skeletal muscle relaxant for intravenous administration. Atracurium besylate is designated as 2,2'-[1,5-pentanediylbis[oxy (3-oxo- 3,1-propanediyl)]] bis[1-[(3, 4-dimethoxyphenyl)methyl]-1,2,3,4-tetrahydro- 6,7-dimethoxy-2- methylisoquinolinium] dibenzenesulfonate. It has a molecular weight of 1243.49, and its molecular formula is $C_{65}H_{82}N_2O_{18}S_2$.

Atracurium besylate is a complex molecule containing four sites at which different stereochemical configurations can occur. The symmetry of the molecule, however, results in only ten, instead of sixteen, possible different isomers. The manufacture of atracurium besylate results in these isomers being produced in unequal amounts but with a consistent ratio. Those molecules in which the methyl group attached to the quaternary nitrogen projects on the opposite side to the adjacent substituted-benzyl moiety predominate by approximately 3:1.

Atracurium besylate is a sterile, non-pyrogenic aqueous solution. Each ml contains 10 mg atracurium besylate. The pH is adjusted to 3.25 to 3.65 with benzenesulfonic acid. The multiple dose vial contains 0.9% benzyl alcohol added as a preservative. Atracurium besylate slowly loses potency with time at the rate of approximately 6% per *year* under refrigeration (5°C). Atracurium besylate should be refrigerated at 2° to 8°C (36° to 46°F) to preserve potency. Rate of loss in potency increases to approximately 5% per *month* at 25°C (77°F). Upon removal from refrigeration to room temperature storage conditions (25°C/77°F), use atracurium besylate within 14 days even if rerefrigerated.

CLINICAL PHARMACOLOGY:

Atracurium besylate is a nondepolarizing skeletal muscle relaxant. Nondepolarizing agents antagonize the neurotransmitter action of acetylcholine by binding competitively with cholinergic receptor sites on the motor end-plate. This antagonism is inhibited, and neuromuscular block reversed, by acetylcholinesterase inhibitors such as neostigmine, edrophonium, and pyridostigmine.

Atracurium besylate can be used most advantageously if muscle twitch response to peripheral nerve stimulation is monitored to assess degree of muscle relaxation.

The duration of neuromuscular block produced by atracurium besylate is approximately one-third to one-half the duration of block by d-tubocurarine, metocurine, and pancuronium at initially equipotent doses. As with other nondepolarizing neuromuscular blockers, the time to onset of paralysis decreases and the duration of maximum effect increases with increasing doses of atracurium besylate.

The ED_{95} (dose required to produce 95% suppression of the muscle twitch response with balanced anesthesia) has averaged 0.23 mg/kg (0.11 to 0.26 mg/kg in various studies). An initial dose of atracurium besylate of 0.4 to 0.5 mg/kg generally produces maximum neuromuscular block within 3 to 5 minutes of injection, with good or excellent intubation conditions within 2 to 2.5 minutes in most patients. Recovery from neuromuscular block (under balanced anesthesia) can be expected to begin approximately 20 to 35 minutes after injection. Under balanced anesthesia, recovery to 25% of control is achieved approximately 35 to 45 minutes after injection, and recovery is usually 95% complete approximately 60 to 70 minutes after injection. The neuromuscular blocking action of atracurium besylate is enhanced in the presence of potent inhalation anesthetics. Isoflurane and enflurane increase the potency of atracurium besylate and prolong neuromuscular block by approximately 35%; however, halothane's potentiating effect (approximately 20%) is marginal (see DOSAGE AND ADMINISTRATION).

Repeated administration of maintenance doses of atracurium besylate has no cumulative effect on the duration of neuromuscular block if recovery is allowed to begin prior to repeat dosing. Moreover, the time needed to recover from repeat doses does not change with additional doses. Repeat doses can therefore be administered at relatively regular intervals with predictable results. After an initial dose of 0.4 to 0.5 mg/kg under balanced anesthesia, the first maintenance dose (suggested maintenance dose is 0.08 to 0.10 mg/kg) is generally required within 20 to 45 minutes, and subsequent maintenance doses are usually required at approximately 15 to 25 minute intervals.

Once recovery from the neuromuscular blocking effects of atracurium besylate begins, it proceeds more rapidly than recovery from d-tubocurarine, metocurine, and pancuronium. Regardless of the dose of atracurium besylate, the time from start of recovery (from complete block) to complete (95%) recovery is approximately 30 minutes under balanced anesthesia, and approximately 40 minutes under halothane, enflurane or isoflurane. Repeated doses have no cumulative effect on recovery rate.

CLINICAL PHARMACOLOGY: *(cont'd)*

Reversal of neuromuscular block produced by atracurium besylate can be achieved with an anticholinesterase agent such as neostigmine, edrophonium, or pyridostigmine, in conjunction with an anticholinergic agent such as atropine or glycopyrrolate. Under balanced anesthesia, reversal can usually be attempted approximately 20 to 35 minutes after an initial atracurium besylate dose of 0.4 to 0.5 mg/kg, or approximately 10 to 30 minutes after a 0.08 to 0.10 mg/kg maintenance dose, when recovery of muscle twitch has started. Complete reversal is usually attained within 8 to 10 minutes of the administration of reversing agents. Rare instances of breathing difficulties, possibly related to incomplete reversal, have been reported following attempted pharmacologic antagonism of atracurium besylate-induced neuromuscular block. As with other agents in this class, the tendency for residual neuromuscular block is increased if reversal is attempted at deep levels of block or if inadequate doses of reversal agents are employed.

The pharmacokinetics of atracurium besylate in man are essentially linear within the 0.3 to 0.6 mg/kg dose range. The elimination half-life is approximately 20 minutes. THE DURATION OF NEUROMUSCULAR BLOCK PRODUCED BY TRACRIUM DOES NOT CORRELATE WITH PLASMA PSEUDOCHOLINESTERASE LEVELS AND IS NOT ALTERED BY THE ABSENCE OF RENAL FUNCTION. This is consistent with the results of *in vitro* studies which have shown that atracurium besylate is inactivated in plasma via two nonoxidative pathways: ester hydrolysis, catalyzed by nonspecific esterases; and Hofmann elimination, a nonenzymatic chemical process which occurs at physiological pH. Some placental transfer occurs in humans.

Radiolabel studies demonstrated that atracurium besylate undergoes extensive degradation in cats, and that neither kidney nor liver plays a major role in its elimination. Biliary and urinary excretion were the major routes of excretion of radioactivity (totaling >90% of the labeled dose within 7 hours of dosing), of which atracurium besylate represented only a minor fraction. The metabolites in bile and urine were similar, including products of Hofmann elimination and ester hydrolysis.

Elderly patients may have slightly altered pharmacokinetic parameters compared to younger patients, with a slightly decreased total plasma clearance which is offset by a corresponding increase in volume of distribution. The net effect is that there has been no significant difference in clinical duration and recovery from neuromuscular block observed between elderly and younger patients receiving atracurium besylate.

Tracrium is a less potent histamine releaser than d-tubocurarine or metocurine. Histamine release is minimal with initial atracurium besylate doses up to 0.5 mg/kg, and hemodynamic changes are minimal within the recommended dose range. A moderate histamine release and significant falls in blood pressure have been seen following 0.6 mg/kg of atracurium besylate. The histamine and hemodynamic responses were poorly correlated. The effects were generally short-lived and manageable, but the possibility of substantial histamine release in sensitive individuals or in patients in whom substantial histamine release would be especially hazardous (*e.g.,*patients with significant cardiovascular disease) must be considered.

It is not known whether the prior use of other nondepolarizing neuromuscular blocking agents has any effect on the activity of atracurium besylate. The prior use of succinylcholine decreases by approximately 2 to 3 minutes the time to maximum block induced by atracurium besylate, and may increase the depth of block. Atracurium besylate should be administered only after a patient recovers from succinylcholine-induced neuromuscular block.

INDICATIONS AND USAGE:

Atracurium besylate is indicated, as an adjunct to general anesthesia, to facilitate endotracheal intubation and to provide skeletal muscle relaxation during surgery or mechanical ventilation.

CONTRAINDICATIONS:

Atracurium besylate is contraindicated in patients known to have a hypersensitivity to it.

WARNINGS:

ATRACURIUM BESYLATE SHOULD BE USED ONLY BY THOSE SKILLED IN AIRWAY MANAGEMENT AND RESPIRATORY SUPPORT. EQUIPMENT AND PERSONNEL MUST BE IMMEDIATELY AVAILABLE FOR ENDOTRACHEAL INTUBATION AND SUPPORT OF VENTILATION, INCLUDING ADMINISTRATION OF POSITIVE PRESSURE OXYGEN. ADEQUACY OF RESPIRATION MUST BE ASSURED THROUGH ASSISTED OR CONTROLLED VENTILATION. ANTICHOLINESTERASE REVERSAL AGENTS SHOULD BE IMMEDIATELY AVAILABLE.
DO NOT GIVE ATRACURIUM BESYLATE BY INTRAMUSCULAR ADMINISTRATION.

Atracurium besylate has no known effect on consciousness, pain threshold, or cerebration. It should be used only with adequate anesthesia.

Atracurium besylate, which has an acid pH, should not be mixed with alkaline solutions (*e.g.,* barbiturate solutions) in the same syringe or administered simultaneously during intravenous infusion through the same needle. Depending on the resultant pH of such mixtures, atracurium besylate may be inactivated and a free acid may be precipitated.

Atracurium besylate 10 ml multiple dose vials contain benzyl alcohol. In newborn infants, benzyl alcohol has been associated with an increased incidence of neurological and other complications which are sometimes fatal. Atracurium besylate 5 ml single use vials do not contain benzyl alcohol.

PRECAUTIONS:

General: Although atracurium besylate is a less potent histamine releaser than d-tubocurarine or metocurine, the possibility of substantial histamine release in sensitive individuals must be considered. Special caution should be exercised in administering atracurium besylate to patients in whom substantial histamine release would be especially hazardous (*e.g.,*patients with clinically significant cardiovascular disease) and in patients with any history (*e.g.,* severe anaphylactoid reactions or asthma) suggesting a greater risk of histamine release. In these patients, the recommended initial atracurium besylate dose is lower (0.3 to 0.4 mg/kg) than for other patients and should be administered slowly or in divided doses over one minute.

Since atracurium besylate has no clinically significant effects on heart rate in the recommended dosage range, it will not counteract the bradycardia produced by many anesthetic agents or vagal stimulation. As a result, bradycardia during anesthesia may be more common with atracurium besylate than with other muscle relaxants.

Atracurium besylate may have profound effects in patients with myasthenia gravis, Eaton-Lambert syndrome, or other neuromuscular diseases in which potentiation of nondepolarizing agents has been noted. The use of a peripheral nerve stimulator is especially important for assessing neuromuscular block in these patients. Similar precautions should be taken in patients with severe electrolyte disorders or carcinomatosis.

PRECAUTIONS: *(cont'd)*

Multiple factors in anesthesia practice are suspected of triggering malignant hyperthermia (MH), a potentially fatal hypermetabolic state of skeletal muscle. Halogenated anesthetic agents and succinylcholine are recognized as the principal pharmacologic triggering agents in MH-susceptible patients; however, since MH can develop in the absence of established triggering agents, the clinician should be prepared to recognize and treat MH in any patient scheduled for general anesthesia. Reports of MH have been rare in cases in which atracurium besylate has been used. In studies of MH-susceptible animals (swine) and in a clinical study of MH-susceptible patients, atracurium besylate did not trigger this syndrome.

Resistance to nondepolarizing neuromuscular blocking agents may develop in burn patients. Increased doses of nondepolarizing muscle relaxants may be required in burn patients and are dependent on the time elapsed since the burn injury and the size of the burn.

The safety of atracurium besylate has not been established in patients with bronchial asthma.

Long-Term Use in Intensive Care Unit (ICU): When there is a need for long-term mechanical ventilation, the benefits-to-risk ratio of neuromuscular block must be considered. The long-term (1 to 10 days) infusion of atracurium besylate during mechanical ventilation in the ICU has been evaluated in several studies. Average infusion rates of 11 to 13 mcg/kg/min (range: 4.5 to 29.5) were required to achieve adequate neuromuscular block. These data suggest that there is wide interpatient variability in dosage requirements. In addition, these studies have shown that dosage requirements may decrease or increase with time. Following discontinuation of infusion of atracurium besylate in these ICU studies, spontaneous recovery of four twitches in a train-of-four occurred in an average of approximately 30 minutes (range: 15 to 75 min) and spontaneous recovery to a train-of-four ratio >75% (the ratio of the height of the fourth to the first twitch in a train-of-four) occurred in an average of approximately 60 minutes (ranges: 32 to 108 min).

Little information is available on the plasma levels and clinical consequences of atracurium metabolites that may accumulate during days to weeks of atracurium administration in ICU patients. Laudanosine, a major biologically active metabolite of atracurium without neuromuscular blocking activity, produces transient hypotension and, in higher doses, cerebral excitatory effects (generalized muscle twitching and seizures) when administered to several species of animals. There have been rare spontaneous reports of seizures in ICU patients who have received atracurium or other agents. These patients usually had predisposing causes (such as head trauma, cerebral edema, hypoxic encephalopathy, viral encephalitis, uremia). There are insufficient data to determine whether or not laudanosine contributes to seizures in ICU patients.

WHETHER THE USE OF ATRACURIUM BESYLATE OR ANY NEUROMUSCULAR BLOCKING AGENT IS CONTEMPLATED IN THE ICU, IT IS RECOMMENDED THAT NEUROMUSCULAR TRANSMISSION BE MONITORED CONTINUOUSLY DURING ADMINISTRATION WITH THE HELP OF A NERVE STIMULATOR. ADDITIONAL DOSES OF TRACRIUM OR ANY OTHER NEUROMUSCULAR BLOCKING AGENT SHOULD NOT BE GIVEN BEFORE THERE IS A DEFINITE RESPONSE TO T_1 OR TO THE FIRST TWITCH. IF NO RESPONSE IS ELICITED, INFUSION ADMINISTRATION SHOULD BE DISCONTINUED UNTIL A RESPONSE RETURNS.

Hemofiltration has a minimal effect on plasma levels of atracurium and its metabolites, including laudanosine. The effects of hemodialysis and hemoperfusion on plasma levels of atracurium and its metabolites are unknown.

Carcinogenesis, Mutagenesis, and Impairment of Fertility: Carcinogenesis and fertility studies have not been performed. Atracurium was evaluated in a battery of three short-term mutagenicity tests. It was non-mutagenic in both the Ames Salmonella assay at concentrations up to 1000 mcg/plate, and in a rat bone marrow cytogenicity assay at up to paralyzing doses. A positive response was observed in the mouse lymphoma assay under conditions (80 and 100 mcg/ml, in the absence of metabolic activation) which killed over 80% of the treated cells; there was no mutagenicity at 60 mcg/ml and lower, concentrations which killed up to half of the treated cells. A far weaker response was observed in the presence of metabolic activation at concentrations (1200 mcg/ml and higher) which also killed over 80% of the treated cells.

Mutagenicity testing is intended to simulate chronic (years to lifetime) exposure in an effort to determine potential carcinogenicity. Thus, a single positive mutagenicity response for a drug used infrequently and/or briefly is of questionable clinical relevance.

Pregnancy, Teratogenic Effects, Pregnancy Category C: Atracurium besylate has been shown to be potentially teratogenic in rabbits when given in doses up to approximately one-half the human dose. There are no adequate and well-controlled studies in pregnant women. Atracurium besylate should be used during pregnancy only if the potential benefit justifies the potential risk to the fetus.

Atracurium besylate was administered subcutaneously on days 6 through 18 of gestation to non-ventilated Dutch rabbits. Treatment groups were given either 0.15 mg/kg once daily or 0.10 mg/kg twice daily. Lethal respiratory distress occurred in two 0.15 mg/kg animals and in one 0.10 mg/kg animal, with transient respiratory distress or other evidence of neuromuscular block occurring in 10 of 19 and in 4 of 20 of the 0.15 mg/kg and 0.10 mg/kg animals, respectively. There was an increased incidence of certain spontaneously occurring visceral and skeletal anomalies or variations in one or both treated groups when compared to non-treated controls. The percentage of male fetuses was lower (41% vs. 51%) and the post-implantation losses were increased (15% vs. 8%) in the group given 0.15 mg/kg once daily when compared to the controls; the mean numbers of implants (6.5 vs. 4.4) and normal live fetuses (5.4 vs. 3.8) were greater in this group when compared to the control group.

Labor and Delivery: It is not known whether muscle relaxants administered during vaginal delivery have immediate or delayed adverse effects on the fetus or increase the likelihood that resuscitation of the newborn will be necessary. The possibility that forceps delivery will be necessary may increase.

Atracurium besylate (0.3 mg/kg) has been administered to 26 pregnant women during delivery by cesarean section. No harmful effects were attributable to atracurium besylate in any of the newborn infants, although small amounts of atracurium besylate were shown to cross the placental barrier. The possibility of respiratory depression in the newborn infant should always be considered following cesarean section during which a neuromuscular blocking agent has been administered. In patients receiving magnesium sulfate, the reversal of neuromuscular block may be unsatisfactory and the dose of atracurium besylate should be lowered as indicated.

Nursing Mothers: It is not known whether this drug is excreted in human milk. Because many drugs are excreted in human milk, caution should be exercised when atracurium besylate is administered to a nursing woman.

Pediatric Use: Safety and effectiveness in children below the age of 1 month have not been established.

Pediatric Use: Since marketing in 1983, uncontrolled clinical experience and limited data from controlled trials have not identified differences in effectiveness, safety, or dosage requirements between healthy elderly and younger patients (see CLINICAL PHARMACOLOGY); however, as with other neuromuscular blocking agents, the use of a peripheral nerve stimulator to monitor neuromuscular function is suggested (see DOSAGE AND ADMINISTRATION).

DRUG INTERACTIONS:

Drugs which may enhance the neuromuscular blocking action of atracurium besylate include: enflurane; isoflurane; halothane; certain antibiotics, especially the aminoglycosides and polymyxins; lithium; magnesium salts; procainamide; and quinidine.

If other muscle relaxants are used during the same procedure, the possibility of a synergistic or antagonist effect should be considered.

The prior administration of succinylcholine does not enhance the duration, but quickens the onset and may increase the depth, of neuromuscular block induced by atracurium besylate. Atracurium besylate should not be administered until a patient has recovered from succinylcholine-induced neuromuscular block.

ADVERSE REACTIONS:

Observed in Controlled Clinical Studies: Atracurium besylate was well tolerated and produced few adverse reactions during extensive clinical trials. Most adverse reactions were suggestive of histamine release. In studies including 875 patients, atracurium besylate was discontinued in only one patient (who required treatment for bronchial secretions), and six other patients required treatment for adverse reactions attributable to atracurium besylate (wheezing in one, hypotension in five). Of the five patients who required treatment for hypotension, three had a history of significant cardiovascular disease. The overall incidence rate for clinically important adverse reactions, therefore, was 7/875 or 0.8%. The table below (TABLE 1) includes all adverse reactions reported attributable to atracurium besylate during clinical trials with 875 patients.

TABLE 1 Percent of Patients Reporting Adverse Reactions

Adverse Reaction	Initial Atracurium Besylate Dose(mg/kg) 0.00-0.30 (n = 485)	0.31-0.50* (n = 366)	≥ 0.60 (n = 24)	Total (n = 875)
Skin Flush	1.0%	8.7%	29.2%	5.0%
Erythema	0.6%	0.5%	0%	0.6%
Itching	0.4%	0%	0%	0.2%
Wheezing/Bronchial Secretions	0.2%	0.3%	0%	0.2%
Hives	0.2%	0%	0%	0.1%

* Includes the recommended initial dosage range for most patients.

Most adverse reactions were of little clinical significance unless they were associated with significant hemodynamic changes. The table below (TABLE 2) summarizes the incidences of substantial vital sign changes noted during Tracrium clinical trials with 530 patients, without cardiovascular disease, in whom these parameters were assessed.

TABLE 2 Percent Of Patients Showing ≥ 30% Vital Sign Changes Following Administration Of Atracurium Besylate

Vital Sign Change	Initial Atracurium besylate Dose (mg/kg) 0.00-0.30 (n = 365)	0.31-0.50* (n = 144)	≥ 0.60 (n = 21)	Total (n = 530)
Mean Arterial Pressure				
Increase	1.9%	2.8%	0%	2.1%
Decrease	1.1%	2.1%	14.3%	1.9%
Heart Rate				
Increase	1.6%	2.8%	4.8%	2.1%
Decrease	0.8%	0%	0%	0.6%

* Includes the recommended initial dosage range for most patients.

Observed in Clinical Practice: Based on initial clinical practice experience in approximately 3 million patients who received atracurium besylate in the U.S. and in the United Kingdom, spontaneously reported adverse reactions were uncommon (approximately 0.01% to 0.02%). The following adverse reactions are among the most frequently reported, but there are insufficient data to support an estimate of their incidence:

General: allergic reactions (anaphylactic or anaphylactoid responses) which, in rare instances, were severe (*e.g.,* cardiac arrest)

Musculoskeletal: inadequate block, prolonged block

Cardiovascular: hypotension, vasodilatation (flushing), tachycardia, bradycardia

Respiratory: dyspnea, bronchospasm, laryngospasm

Integumentary: rash, urticaria, reaction at injection site

There have been rare spontaneous reports of seizures in ICU patients following long-term infusion of atracurium to support mechanical ventilation. There are insufficient data to define the contribution, if any, of atracurium and/or its metabolite laudanosine. (See PRECAUTIONS, Long, Term Use in Intensive Care Unit [ICU]).

OVERDOSAGE:

There has been limited experience with overdosage of atracurium besylate. The possibility of iatrogenic overdosage can be minimized by carefully monitoring muscle twitch response to peripheral nerve stimulation. Excessive doses of atracurium besylate can be expected to produce enhanced pharmacological effects. Overdosage may increase the risk of histamine release and cardiovascular effects, especially hypotension. If cardiovascular support is necessary, this should include proper positioning, fluid administration, and the use of vasopressor agents if necessary. The patient's airway should be assured, with manual or mechanical ventilation maintained as necessary. A longer duration of neuromuscular block may result from overdosage and a peripheral nerve stimulator should be used to monitor recovery. Recovery may be facilitated by administration of an anticholinesterase reversing agent such as neostigmine, edrophonium, or pyridostigmine, in conjunction with an anticholinergic agent such as atropine or glycopyrrolate. The appropriate package inserts should be consulted for prescribing information.

Three pediatric patients (3 weeks, 4 and 5 months of age) unintentionally received doses of 0.8 mg/kg to 1.0 mg/kg of atracurium besylate. The time to 25% recovery (50 to 55 minutes) following these doses, which were 5 to 6 times the ED_{95} dose, was moderately longer than the corresponding time observed following doses 2.0 to 2.5 times the Tracrium ED_{95}dose in infants (22 to 36 minutes). Cardiovascular changes were minimal. Nonetheless the possibility of cardiovascular changes must be considered in the case of overdose.

An adult patient (17 years of age) unintentionally received an initial dose of 1.3 mg/kg of atracurium besylate. The time from injection to 25% recovery (83 minutes) was approximately twice that observed following maximum recommended doses in adults (35 to 45 minutes). The patient experienced moderate hemodynamic changes (13% increase in mean arterial pressure and 27% increase in heart rate) which persisted for 40 minutes and did not require treatment.

OVERDOSAGE: *(cont'd)*

The intravenous LD_{50}s determined in non-ventilated male and female albino mice and male Wistar rats were 1.9, 2.01 and 1.31 mg/kg, respectively. Deaths occurred within 2 minutes and were caused by respiratory paralysis. The subcutaneous LD_{50} determined in non-ventilated male Wistar rats was 282.8 mg/kg. Tremors, ptosis, loss of reflexes and respiratory failure preceded death which occurred 45 to 120 minutes after injection.

DOSAGE AND ADMINISTRATION:

To avoid distress to the patient, atracurium besylate should not be administered before unconsciousness has been induced. Atracurium besylate should not be mixed in the same syringe, or administered simultaneously through the same needle, with alkaline solutions (*e.g.,* barbiturate solutions).

Atracurium besylate should be administered intravenously. DO NOT GIVE ATRACURIUM BESYLATE BY INTRAMUSCULAR ADMINISTRATION. Intramuscular administration of atracurium besylate may result in tissue irritation and there are no clinical data to support this route of administration.

As with other neuromuscular blocking agents, the use of a peripheral nerve stimulator will permit the most advantageous use of atracurium besylate, minimizing the possibility of overdosage or underdosage, and assist in the evaluation of recovery.

Parenteral drug products should be inspected visually for particulate matter and discoloration prior to administration, whenever solution and container permit.

BOLUS DOSES FOR INTUBATION AND MAINTENANCE OF NEUROMUSCULAR BLOCK

Adults: A dose of atracurium besylate of 0.4 to 0.5 mg/kg (1.7 to 2.2 times the ED_{95}), given as an intravenous bolus injection, is the recommended initial dose for most patients. With this dose, good or excellent conditions for nonemergency intubation can be expected in 2 to 2.5 minutes in most patients, with maximum neuromuscular block achieved approximately 3 to 5 minutes after injection. Clinically required neuromuscular block generally lasts 20 to 35 minutes under balanced anesthesia. Under balanced anesthesia, recovery to 25% of control is achieved approximately 35 to 45 minutes after injection, and recovery is usually 95% complete approximately 60 minutes after injection.

Atracurium besylate is potentiated by isoflurane or enflurane anesthesia. The same initial dose of atracurium besylate of 0.4 to 0.5 mg/kg may be used for intubation prior to administration of these inhalation agents; however, if atracurium besylate is first administered under steady state of isoflurane or enflurane, the initial dose of atracurium besylate should be reduced by approximately one-third, i.e., to 0.25 to 0.35 mg/kg, to adjust for the potentiating effects of these anesthetic agents. With halothane, which has only a marginal (approximately 20%) potentiating effect on atracurium besylate, smaller dosage reductions may be considered.

Doses of atracurium besylate of 0.08 to 0.10 mg/kg are recommended for maintenance of neuromuscular block during prolonged surgical procedures. The first maintenance dose will generally be required 20 to 45 minutes after the initial dose of atracurium besylate, but the need for maintenance doses should be determined by clinical criteria. Because atracurium besylate lacks cumulative effects, maintenance doses may be administered at relatively regular intervals for each patient, ranging approximately from 15 to 25 minutes under balanced anesthesia, slightly longer under isoflurane or enflurane. Higher doses of atracurium besylate (up to 0.2 mg/kg) permit maintenance dosing at longer intervals.

Children and Infants: No atracurium besylate dosage adjustments are required for pediatric patients two years of age or older. A dose of atracurium besylate of 0.3 to 0.4 mg/kg is recommended as the initial dose for infants (1 month to 2 years of age) under halothane anesthesia. Maintenance doses may be required with slightly greater frequency in infants and children than in adults.

Special Considerations: An initial dose of atracurium besylate of 0.3 to 0.4 mg/kg, given slowly or in divided doses over one minute, is recommended for adults, children, or infants with significant cardiovascular disease and for adults, children, or infants with any history (*e.g.,* severe anaphylactoid reactions or asthma) suggesting a greater risk of histamine release.

Dosage reductions must be considered also in patients with neuromuscular disease, severe electrolyte disorders, or carcinomatosis in which potentiation of neuromuscular block or difficulties with reversal have been demonstrated. There has been no clinical experience with atracurium besylate in these patients, and no specific dosage adjustments can be recommended. No atracurium besylate dosage adjustments are required for patients with renal disease.

An initial dose of atracurium besylate of 0.3 to 0.4 mg/kg is recommended for adults following the use of succinylcholine for intubation under balanced anesthesia. Further reductions may be desirable with the use of potent inhalation anesthetics. The patient should be permitted to recover from the effects of succinylcholine prior to administration of atracurium besylate. Insufficient data are available for recommendation of a specific initial dose of atracurium besylate for administration following the use of succinylcholine in children and infants.

USE BY CONTINUOUS INFUSION

Infusion in the Operating Room (OR): After administration of a recommended initial bolus dose of atracurium besylate (0.3 to 0.5 mg/kg), a diluted solution of atracurium besylate can be administered by continuous infusion to adults and children aged 2 or more years for maintenance of neuromuscular block during extended surgical procedures.

Infusion of atracurium besylate should be individualized for each patient. The rate of administration should be adjusted according to the patient's response as determined by peripheral nerve stimulation. Accurate dosing is best achieved using a precision infusion device.

Infusion of atracurium besylate should be initiated only after early evidence of spontaneous recovery from the bolus dose. An initial infusion rate of 9 to 10 mcg/kg/min may be required to rapidly counteract the spontaneous recovery of neuromuscular function. Thereafter, a rate of 5 to 9 mcg/kg/min should be adequate to maintain continuous neuromuscular block in the range of 89% to 99% in most pediatric and adult patients under balanced anesthesia. Occasional patients may require infusion rates as low as 2 mcg/kg/min or as high as 15 mcg/kg/min.

The neuromuscular blocking effect of atracurium besylate administered by infusion is potentiated by enflurane or isoflurane and, to a lesser extent, by halothane. Reduction in the infusion rate of atracurium besylate should, therefore, be considered for patients receiving inhalation anesthesia. The rate of atracurium besylate infusion should be reduced by approximately one-third in the presence of steady-state enflurane or isoflurane anesthesia; smaller reductions should be considered in the presence of halothane.

In patients undergoing cardiopulmonary bypass with induced hypothermia, the rate of infusion of atracurium besylate required to maintain adequate surgical relaxation during hypothermia (25° to 28°C) has been shown to be approximately half the rate required during normothermia.

Spontaneous recovery from neuromuscular block following discontinuation of atracurium besylate infusion may be expected to proceed at a rate comparable to that following administration of a single bolus dose.

DOSAGE AND ADMINISTRATION: *(cont'd)*

Infusion in the Intensive Care Unit (ICU): The principles for infusion of atracurium besylate in the OR are also applicable to use in the ICU.

An infusion rate of 11 to 13 mcg/kg/min (range: 4.5 to 29.5) should provide adequate neuromuscular block in adult patients in an ICU. Limited information suggests that infusion rates required for pediatric patients in the ICU may be higher than in adult patients. There may be wide interpatient variability in dosage requirements and these requirements may increase or decrease with time (see PRECAUTIONS, Long, Term Use in Intensive Care Unit [ICU]). Following recovery from neuromuscular block, readministration of a bolus dose may be necessary to quickly re-establish neuromuscular block prior to reinstitution of the infusion.

Infusion Rate Tables: The amount of infusion solution required per minute will depend upon the concentration of atracurium besylate in the infusion solution, the desired dose of atracurium besylate, and the patient's weight. The following tables (TABLE 3 and TABLE 4) provide guidelines for delivery, in ml/hr (equivalent to microdrops/min when 60 microdrops = 1 ml), of atracurium besylate solutions in concentrations of 0.2 mg/ml (20 mg in 100 ml) or 0.5 mg/ml (50 mg in 100 ml) with an infusion pump or a gravity flow device.

TABLE 3 Atracurium Besylate Infusion Rates for a Concentration of 0.2 mg/ml

Patient Weight (Kg)	Drug Delivery Rate (mcg/kg/min)								
	5	6	7	8	9	10	11	12	13
	Infusion Delivery Rate (ml/hr)								
30	45	54	63	72	81	90	99	108	117
35	53	63	74	84	95	105	116	126	137
40	60	72	84	96	108	120	132	144	156
45	68	81	95	108	122	135	149	162	176
50	75	90	105	120	135	150	165	180	195
55	83	99	116	132	149	165	182	198	215
60	90	108	126	144	162	180	198	216	234
65	98	117	137	156	176	195	215	234	254
70	105	126	147	168	189	210	231	252	273
75	113	135	158	180	203	225	248	270	293
80	120	144	168	192	216	240	264	288	312
90	135	162	189	216	243	270	297	324	351
100	150	180	210	240	270	300	330	360	390

TABLE 4 Atracurium Besylate Infusion Rates for a Concentration of 0.5 mg/ml

Patient Weight (Kg)	Drug Delivery Rate (mcg/kg/min)								
	5	6	7	8	9	10	11	12	13
	Infusion Delivery Rate (ml/hr)								
30	18	22	25	29	32	36	40	43	47
35	21	25	29	34	38	42	46	50	55
40	24	29	34	38	43	48	53	58	62
45	27	32	38	43	49	54	59	65	70
50	30	36	42	48	54	60	66	72	78
55	33	40	46	53	59	66	73	79	86
60	36	43	50	58	65	72	79	86	94
65	39	47	55	62	70	78	86	94	101
70	42	50	59	67	76	84	92	101	109
75	45	54	63	72	81	90	99	108	117
80	48	58	67	77	86	96	106	115	125
90	54	65	76	86	97	108	119	130	140
100	60	72	84	96	108	120	132	144	156

Compatibility and Admixtures: Atracurium besylate Infusion solutions may be prepared by admixing atracurium besylate with an appropriate diluent such as 5% Dextrose Injection USP, 0.9% Sodium Chloride Injection USP, or 5% Dextrose and 0.9% Sodium Chloride Injection USP. Infusion solutions should be used with 24 hours of preparation. Unused solutions should be discarded. Solutions containing 0.2 mg/ml or 0.5 mg/ml atracurium besylate in the above diluents may be stored either under refrigeration or at room temperature for 24 hours without significant loss of potency. Care should be taken during admixture to prevent inadvertent contamination. Visually inspect prior to administration.

Spontaneous degradation of atracurium besylate has been demonstrated to occur more rapidly in lactated Ringer's solution than in 0.9% sodium chloride solution. Therefore, it is recommended that Lactated Ringer's Injection USP not be used as a diluent in preparing solutions of Tracrium for infusion.

HOW SUPPLIED:

Tracrium, 10 mg atracurium besylate in each ml. 5 ml Single Use Vial (50 mg atracurium besylate per vial). Tray of 10. 10 ml Multiple Dose Vial (100 mg atracurium besylate per vial). Contains benzyl alcohol (see WARNINGS).

Storage: Atracurium besylate should be refrigerated at 2° to 8°C (36° to 46°F) to preserve potency. DO NOT FREEZE. Upon removal from refrigeration to room temperature storage conditions (25°C/77°F), use atracurium besylate within 14 days even if rerefrigerated.

HOW SUPPLIED - EQUIVALENTS NOT AVAILABLE:

Injection, Solution - Intravenous - 10 mg

5 ml x 10	$283.37	TRACRIUM, Glaxo Wellcome	00173-0940-44
10 ml x 10	$527.51	TRACRIUM, Glaxo Wellcome	00173-0940-95

ATROPINE SULFATE *(000336)*

CATEGORIES: Analeptics; Anesthesia; Antiarrhythmic Agents; Anticholinergic Agents; Anticholinesterase; Antimuscarinics/Antispasmodics; Autonomic Drugs; Bradycardia; Conjunctivitis; Corneal Ulcer; Cycloplegics/Mydriatics; EENT Drugs; Eye, Ear, Nose, & Throat Preparations; Gastrointestinal Drugs; Heart Block; Inflammatory Conditions; Mushroom Poisoning; Mydriasis; Mydriatics; Mydriatics & Cycloplegics; Ophthalmics; Poisoning; Refraction; Renal Drugs; Syncope; FDA Approval Pre 1982

BRAND NAMES: *Atro Ofteno; Atro Ofteno AL 1%;* Atropair; Atropen; *Atropin* (Germany); *Atropin "Dak"; Atropin Dispersa; Atropin Minims; Atropina; Atropina Llorens; Atropine; Atropine Dispersa; Atropine Martinet* (France); *Atropine Sulfate; Atropine Sulfate Tablets* (England); *Atropini Sulfas; Atropinol;* Atropisol; *Atropt* (Australia); *Atrospan; Bellpino-Artin; Borotropin; Cendo Tropine; Chibro-Atropine* (France); *Ciba Vision Atropine; Dispersa-Atropine; Dispersa Atropine; Dosatropine;* I-Tropine; *Isopto* (England); *Isopto Atropin; Isopto Atropina;* **Isopto Atropine**; *Liotropina; Minims-Atropine; Minims Atropine Sulfaat; Minims Atropine Sulfate* (England); Ocu-Tropine; Sal-Tropine; *Skiatropine;* Spectro-Atropine; *Vitatropine* (France); *Ximex Optidrop*

(International brand names outside U.S. in italics)

FORMULARIES: Aetna; BC-BS; FHP; Medi-Cal; PCS; WHO

DESCRIPTION:

Note: This monograph contains complete prescribing information for the Injection and the Ophthalmic Solution of Atropine Sulfate.

INJECTION

Adult: 0.1 mg/ml

Pediatric: 0.05 mg/ml

Atropine sulfate injection, USP is a sterile, nonpyrogenic isotonic solution of atropine sulfate monohydrate in water for injection with sodium chloride sufficient to render the solution isotonic. It is administered parenterally by subcutaneous, intramuscular or intravenous injection.

Each ml contains Atropine sulfate, monohydrate 0.1 mg (adult strength) or 0.05 mg (pediatric strength), and sodium chloride, 9 mg. May contain sodium hydroxide and/or sulfuric acid for pH adjustment 0.308 mOsmol/ml. pH 4.2 (3.0 to 6.5).

The solution contains no bacteriostat, antimicrobial agent or added buffer (except for pH adjustment) and is intended for use only as a single-dose injection. When smaller doses are required the unused portion should be discarded.

Atropine sulfate is a parenteral anticholinergic agent and muscarinic antagonist.

Atropine sulfate, USP is chemically designated 1α H, 5α H-Tropan-3- α ol (±)-tropate (ester), sulfate (2:1) (salt) monohydrate $(C_{17}H_{23}NO_3)_2 \cdot H_2SO_4 \cdot H_2O$, colorless crystals or white crystalline powder very soluble in water.

Atropine, a naturally occurring belladonna alkaloid is a racemic mixture of equal parts of d- and l-hyoscyamine, whose activity is due almost entirely to the levo isomer of the drug.

Sodium chloride, USP is chemically designated NaCl, a white crystalline powder freely soluble in water.

OPHTHALMIC SOLUTION

Atropine sulfate sterile ophthalmic solution is a topical anticholinergic for ophthalmic use.

Chemical name: Benzeneacetic acid, α-(hydroxymethyl)-,8-methyl-8-azabicyclo-(3,2,1) oct-3-yl ester, endo-(±)-, sulfate (2:1)(salt), monohydate.

Atropine sulfate sterile ophthalmic solution contains:Atropine sulfate 1% with chlorobutanol (chloral deriv.) 0.5%; boric acid; sodium citrate; hydrochloric acid and/or sodium hydroxide to adjust the pH; and purified water.

CLINICAL PHARMACOLOGY:

INJECTION

Atropine sulfate is commonly classified as an anticholinergic or antiparasympathetic (parasympatholytic) drug. More precisely, however, it is termed an antimuscarinic agent since it antagonizes the muscarine-like actions of acetyl-choline and other choline esters.

Atropine inhibits the muscarinic actions of acetylcholine on structures innervated by postganglionic cholinergic nerves, and on smooth muscles which respond to endogenous acetylcholine but not so innervated. As with other antimuscarinic agents, the major action atropine is a competitive or surmountable antagonism which can be overcome by increasing the concentration of acetylcholine at receptor sites at the effector organ (*e.g.,* by using anticholinesterase agents which inhibit the enzymatic destruction of acetylcholine). The receptors antagonized by atropine are the peripheral structure that are stimulated or inhibited by muscarine (*i.e.,* exocrine glands and smooth and cardiac muscle). Responses to postganglionic cholinergic nerve stimulation also may be inhibited by atropine but this occurs less readily than with responses to injected (exogenous) choline esters.

Atropine-induced parasympathetic inhibition may be preceded by a transient phase of stimulation, especially on the heart where small doses first slow the rate before characteristic tachycardia develops due to paralysis of vagal control. Atropine exerts a more potent and prolonged effect on heart, intestine and bronchial muscle than scopolamine, but its action on the iris, ciliary body and certain secretory glands is weaker than that of scopolamine. Unlike the latter, atropine in clinical doses not depress the central nervous system but may stimulate the medulla and higher cerebral centers. Although mild vagal excitation occurs, the increased respiratory rate and (sometimes) increased depth of desperation produced by atropine are more probably the result of bronchiolar dilatation. Accordingly, atropine is an unreliable respiratory stimulant and large or repeated doses may depress respiration.

Adequate doses of atropine abolish various types of reflex vagal cardiac slowing or asystole. The drug also prevents or abolishes bradycardia or asystole produced by injection of choline esters, anticholinesterase agents or other parasympathomimetic drugs, and cardiac arrest produced by stimulation of the vagus. Atropine also may lessen the degree of partial heart block when vagal activity is an etiologic factor. In some patients with complete heart block, the idioventricular rate may be accelerated by atropine; in others, the rate is stabilized. Occasionally a large dose may cause atrioventricular (A-V) block and nodal rhythm.

Atropine sulfate injection, USP in clinical doses counteracts the peripheral dilatation and abrupt decrease in blood pressure produced by choline esters. However, when given by itself, atropine does not exert a striking or uniform effect on blood vessels or blood pressure. Systemic doses slightly raise systolic and lower diastolic pressures and can produce significant postural hypotension. Such doses also slightly increase cardiac output and decrease central venous pressure. Occasionally, therapeutic doses dilate cutaneous blood vessels, particularly in the "blush" area (atropine flush), and may cause atropine "fever" due to suppression of sweat gland activity in infants and small children.

Atropine disappears rapidly from the blood following injection and is distributed throughout the body. Much of the drug is destroyed by enzymatic hydrolysis, particularly in the liver; from 13 to 50% is excreted unchanged in the urine. Traces are found in various secretions, including milk. Atropine readily crosses the placental barrier and enters the fetal circulation.

Sodium chloride added to render the solution isotonic for injection of the active ingredient is present in amounts insufficient to affect serum electrolyte balance of sodium (Na^+) and chloride (Cl^-) ions.

OPHTHALMIC SOLUTION

Anticholinergics act directly on the smooth muscles and secretory glands innervated by postganglionic cholinergic nerves. They act by blocking the parasympathomimetic (muscarinic) effects of acetylcholine and parasympathomimetic drugs at these sites.

INDICATIONS AND USAGE:

INJECTION

Atropine sulfate injection, USP is indicated:

(1) as antisialagogue for preanesthetic medication to prevent or reduce secretions of the respiratory tract,

(2) to restore cardiac rate and arterial pressure during anesthesia when vagal stimulation produced by intra-abdominal surgical traction causes a sudden decrease in pulse rate and cardiac action,

INDICATIONS AND USAGE: *(cont'd)*

(3) to lessen the degree of atrioventricular (A-V) heart block when increased vagal tone is a major factor in conduction defect as in some cases due to digitalis,

(4) to overcome severe bradycardia and syncope due to hyperactive carotid sinus reflex,

(5) as an antidote (with external cardiac massage) for cardiovascular collapse from the injudicious use of choline ester (cholinergic) drug,

(6) in the treatment of anticholinesterase poisoning from organophosphorus insecticides, and

(7) as an antidote for the "rapid" type of mushroom poisoning due to the presence of the alkaloid, muscarine, in certain species of fungus such as *Amanita muscaria.*

OPHTHALMIC SOLUTION

Atropine sulfate is used to produce mydriasis and cycloplegia for refraction, or for iris dilation and relaxation of the ciliary muscle desirable in acute inflammatory conditions of the anterior uveal tract.

CONTRAINDICATIONS:

Injection: Atropine generally is contraindicated in patients with glaucoma, pyloric stenosis or prostatic hypertrophy, except in doses ordinarily used for preanesthetic medication.

Ophthalmic Solution: Should not be used in patients with glaucoma or predisposition to narrow-angle glaucoma. Should not be used in children who have previously had a severe systemic reaction to atropine.

WARNINGS:

Injection: Atropine is a highly potent drug and due care is essential to avoid overdosage, especially with intravenous administration. Children are more susceptible than adults to the toxic effects of anticholinergic agents.

Ophthalmic Solution: Excessive use in children and certain susceptible individuals may produce general toxic symptoms. If this occurs, discontinue medication and use appropriate therapy as outlined in the "OVERDOSAGE" section.

PRECAUTIONS:

GENERAL

Injection: Do not administer unless solution is clear and seal is intact. Discard unused portion.

Atropine sulfate injection, USP should be used with caution in all individuals over 40 years of age. Conventional systemic doses may precipitate acute glaucoma in susceptible patients, convert partial organic pyloric stenosis into complete urinary retention in patients with prostatic hypertrophy or cause inspiration of bronchial secretions and formation of dangerous viscid plugs in patients with chronic lung disease.

INFORMATION FOR THE PATIENT

Keep out of reach of children.

CARCINOGENESIS, MUTAGENESIS, AND IMPAIRMENT OF FERTILITY

No studies have been conducted in animals or in humans to evaluate the potential of these effects.

PREGNANCY CATEGORY C

Injection: Animal reproduction studies have not been conducted with atropine. It also is not known whether atropine can cause fetal harm when given to a pregnant woman or can affect reproduction capacity. Atropine should be given to a pregnant woman only if clearly needed.

Ophthalmic Solution: See information above for Atropine Sulfate Injection.

PEDIATRIC USE

See CONTRAINDICATIONS and WARNINGS.

ADVERSE REACTIONS:

Injection: Most of the side effects of atropine are directly related to its antimuscarinic action. Dryness of the mouth, blurred vision, photophobia and tachycardia commonly occur with chronic administration of therapeutic doses. Anhidrosis also may occur and produce heat intolerance or impair temperature regulation in persons living in a hot environment. Constipation and difficulty in micturition may occur in elderly patients. Occasional hypersensitivity reactions have been observed, especially skin rashes which in some instances progressed to exfoliation.

Adverse effects following single or repeated injections of atropine are most often the result of excessive dosage. These include palpitation, dilated pupils, difficulty in swallowing, hot dry skin, thirst, dizziness, restlessness, tremor, fatigue and ataxia. Toxic doses lead to marked palpitation, restlessness and excitement, hallucinations, delirium and coma. Depression and circulatory collapse occur with severe intoxication. In such cases, blood pressure declines and death due to respiratory failure may ensue following paralysis and coma.

Ophthalmic Solution: Prolonged use may cause general systemic reactions, allergic lid reactions, local irritation, hyperemia, edema, follicular, conjunctivitis or dermatitis.

OVERDOSAGE:

INJECTION

In the event of toxic overdosage (See ADVERSE REACTIONS), a short acting barbiturate or diazepam may be given as needed as needed to control marked excitement and convulsions. Large doses for sedation should be avoided because central depressant action may coincide with the depression occurring late in atropine poisoning. Central stimulants are not recommended. Physostigmine, given as an atropine antidote by slow intravenous injection of 1 to 4 mg (0.5 to 1.0 mg in children), rapidly abolishes delirium and coma caused by large doses of atropine. Since physostigmine is rapidly destroyed, the patient may be again lapse into coma after one or two hours, and repeated doses may be required. Artificial respiration with oxygen may be necessary. Icy bags and alcohol sponges help to reduce fever, especially in children.

The fatal dose of atropine is not known; 200 mg doses have been used and doses as high as 1000 mg have been given.

In children, 10 mg or less may be fatal. With a dose as low as 0.5 mg, undesirable minimal symptoms or responses of overdosage may occur. These increase in severity and extent with larger doses of the drug (excitement, hallucinations, delirium and coma with a dose of 10 mg or more).

OPHTHALMIC SOLUTION

General signs and symptoms of atropine toxicity include dryness of mouth and skin, fever, irritability or delirium, tachycardia, and flushing of the face. Should overdosage in the eye(s) occur, flush the eye(s) with water or normal saline. Use of a topical miotic may be required.

If accidentally ingested, induce emesis or gastric lavage with 4% tannic acid. 5 mg of pilocarpine should be administered orally at repeated intervals until the mouth is moist. General supportive measures should be used if needed as listed below:

Respiratory depression: oxygen and artificial respiration

Urinary retention: catheterization

Fever: alcohol sponge baths

OVERDOSAGE: *(cont'd)*

Use extreme caution when employing short-acting barbiturates to control excitement.

DOSAGE AND ADMINISTRATION:

INJECTION

Atropine sulfate injection, USP may be administered subcutaneously, intramuscularly, or intravenously. The average adult dose is 0.5 mg (5 ml of a 0.1 mg/ml solution), range 0.4 to 0.6 mg (4 to 6 ml). As an antisialagogue it is usually injected intramuscularly prior to induction of anesthesia. This produces only minimal blocking of vagal activity, In children, the dosage ranges from 0.1 mg (2 ml of a 0.05 mg solution) in the newborn to 0.6 mg (6 ml of a 0.1 mg/ml solution) in a child age 12 years, injected subcutaneously 30 minutes before surgery. During surgery, the drug is given intravenously when reduction in pulse rate and cessation of cardiac action are due to increased vagal activity; however, if the anesthetic is cyclopropane, doses less than 0.4 mg should be used and should be given slowly to avoid the possible production of ventricular arrhythmia. Usual doses are used to reduce severe bradycardia and syncope associated with hyperactive carotid sinus reflex. For bradyarrhythmias the usual intravenous adult dosage ranges from 0.4 to 1 mg (4 to 10 ml of a 0.1 mg/ml solution) every one to two hours as needed; larger doses up to a maximum of 2 mg may be required. In children, intravenous dosage ranges from 0.01 to 0.33 mg (0.2 to 0.6 ml of a 0.05 mg/ml solution) per kg of body weight. Atropine is also a specific antidote for cardiovascular collapse resulting from injudicious administration of choline ester. When cardiac arrest has occurred, external cardiac massage or other method of resuscitation is required to distribute the drug after intravenous injection.

In anticholinesterase poisoning from exposure to insecticides, large doses of at least 2 to 3 mg (20 to 30 ml of a 0.1 mg/ml solution) should be administered parenterally and repeated until signs of atropine intoxication appear. In the "rapid" type of mushroom poisoning, atropine should be given in doses sufficient to control parasympathomimetic signs before coma and cardiovascular collapse supervene.

Parenteral drug products should be inspected visually for particulate matter and discoloration prior to administration, whenever solution and container permit. See PRECAUTIONS.

Store injection at controlled room temperature 15 to 30°C (59 to 86°F).

OPHTHALMIC SOLUTION

1 or 2 drops in the eyes three times a day or as directed by physician.

(Ophthalmic solution, Allergan PR7340 N-30-4/M)(Injection, Abbott, 06-4740-R10)

HOW SUPPLIED - RATED THERAPEUTICALLY EQUIVALENT:

Injection, Solution - Intramuscular; - 0.4 mg/ml

2 ml x 25	$12.60	Atropine Sulfate, Gensia Labs	00703-2501-04
20 ml	$4.78	Atropine Sulfate, Lilly	00002-1675-01
20 ml x 10	$7.56	Atropine Sulfate, Gensia Labs	00703-2525-03

Injection, Solution - Intramuscular; - 1 mg/ml

2 ml x 25	$12.30	Atropine Sulfate 1, Gensia Labs	00703-2511-04

HOW SUPPLIED - NOT RATED EQUIVALENT:

Injection, Solution - Intramuscular; - 0.1 mg/ml

5 ml	$4.93	Atropine Sulfate, Intl Medication	00548-1038-00
5 ml	$12.22	Atropine Sulfate, Abbott	00074-4910-15
5 ml	$13.03	Atropine Sulfate, Abbott	00074-4910-23
5 ml	$13.55	Atropine Sulfate, Abbott	00074-4910-34
5 ml x 10	$33.30	Atropine Sulfate, Voluntary Hosp	53258-9410-08
5 ml x 10	$64.91	Atropine Sulfate, Astra USA	00186-0648-01
5 ml x 10	$72.63	Atropine Sulfate, Fujisawa USA	00469-9410-87
10 ml	$4.93	Atropine Sulfate, Intl Medication	00548-1039-00
10 ml	$5.30	Atropine Sulfate, Intl Medication	00548-2039-00
10 ml	$12.61	Atropine Sulfate, Abbott	00074-4911-18
10 ml	$13.41	Atropine Sulfate, Abbott	00074-4911-23
10 ml	$13.70	Atropine Sulfate, Intl Medication	00548-3039-00
10 ml	$13.94	Atropine Sulfate, Abbott	00074-4911-34
10 ml x 10	$70.88	Atropine Sulfate, Astra USA	00186-0649-01
10 ml x 10	$75.25	Atropine Sulfate, Fujisawa USA	00469-9411-87

Injection, Solution - Intramuscular; - 0.4 mg/.5ml

0.5 ml x 25	$12.19	Atropine Sulfate, Am Regent	00517-0805-25
0.5 ml x 100	$48.75	Atropine Sulfate, Am Regent	00517-1058-69

Injection, Solution - Intramuscular; - 0.4 mg/ml

0.5 ml x 25	$13.75	Atropine Sulfate, Consolidated Midland	00223-7203-05
1 ml x 25	$8.89	Atropine Sulfate, Elkins Sinn	00641-1380-35
1 ml x 25	$9.23	Atropine Sulfate, Elkins Sinn	00641-0320-25
1 ml x 25	$10.94	Atropine Sulfate, Am Regent	00517-0401-25
1 ml x 25	$15.00	Atropine Sulfate, Consolidated Midland	00223-7192-00
1 ml x 25	$16.25	Atropine Sulfate, Consolidated Midland	00223-7200-01
1 ml x 25	$20.00	Atropine Sulfate, Fujisawa USA	00469-1234-25
1 ml x 100	$34.38	Atropine Sulfate, Am Regent	00517-1057-71
20 ml	$17.50	Atropine Sulfate, Consolidated Midland	00223-7195-20
20 ml x 10	$8.36	Atropine Sulfate, Elkins Sinn	00641-2210-43
20 ml x 25	$37.50	Atropine Sulfate, Fujisawa USA	00469-0234-25

Injection, Solution - Intramuscular; - 0.5 mg/ml

1 ml x 25	$23.13	Atropine Sulfate, Fujisawa USA	00469-0243-25

Injection, Solution - Intramuscular; - 1 mg/ml

1 ml x 25	$9.23	Atropine Sulfate, Elkins Sinn	00641-0330-25
1 ml x 25	$20.00	Atropine Sulfate, Fujisawa USA	00469-0246-25
1 ml x 100	$48.75	Atropine Sulfate, Am Regent	00517-1065-71

Injection, Solution - Intravenous - 0.05 mg/ml

5 ml	$9.65	Atropine Sulfate, Abbott	00074-7897-15

Injection, Solution - Intravenous - 1 mg/ml

1 ml x 25	$12.19	Atropine Sulfate, Am Regent	00517-0101-25
1 ml x 25	$12.19	Atropine Sulfate, Am Regent	00517-1010-25
1 ml x 25	$16.25	Atropine Sulfate, Consolidated Midland	00223-7206-01

Ointment - Ophthalmic - 1 %

3.5 gm	$2.42	Atropine Sulfate, Aligen Independ	00405-0500-08
3.5 gm	$2.45	Atropine Sulfate Ophth, Harber Pharm	51432-0702-30
3.5 gm	$2.75	Atropine Sulfate, Consolidated Midland	00223-4105-03
3.5 gm	$2.88	Atropine Sulfate, Fougera	00168-0065-38
3.5 gm	$3.02	Atropine Sulfate, Schein Pharm (US)	00364-7142-70
3.5 gm	$3.30	Atropine Sulfate, Qualitest Pharms	00603-7071-70
3.5 gm	$3.31	Atropine Sulfate, HL Moore Drug Exch	00839-5492-43
3.5 gm	$4.79	Atropine Sulfate, Lilly	00002-1851-17
3.5 gm x 12	$2.78	Atropine Sulfate, Rugby	00536-6100-91

Powder

30 gm	$64.25	Atropine Sulfate, Mallinckrodt	00406-3692-34
125 gm	$222.86	Atropine Sulfate, Mallinckrodt	00406-3692-37

HOW SUPPLIED - NOT RATED EQUIVALENT: *(cont'd)*

Solution - Ophthalmic - 0.5 %

5 ml	**$10.00**	**ISOPTO ATROPINE, Alcon-PR**	**00998-0302-05**

Solution - Ophthalmic - 1 %

1 ml x 12	$25.80	ATROPISOL OPHTHALMIC, Ciba Vision	00058-0770-12
2 ml	$2.20	Atropine Sulfate, Optopics	52238-0502-02
2 ml	$2.20	Atropine Sulfate, Apotex	60505-7484-01
2 ml	$2.98	Atropine Sulfate, Martec Pharms	52555-0992-01
2 ml	$3.31	ATROPINE CARE, Akorn	17478-0214-20
2 ml	$51.00	Atropine Sulfate, Alcon	00065-0702-12
5 ml	$2.52	Atropine Sulfate, Apotex	60505-7484-02
5 ml	$2.55	Atropine Sulfate, Optopics	52238-0502-05
5 ml	$2.95	Atropine Sulfate, Raway	00686-0750-60
5 ml	$3.10	Atropine Sulfate, Adv Remedies	57685-0050-07
5 ml	$3.16	Atropine Sulfate, Martec Pharms	52555-0992-05
5 ml	$3.48	Atropine Sulfate, Aligen Independ	00405-6010-05
5 ml	$4.06	ATROPINE CARE, Akorn	17478-0214-10
5 ml	$7.20	ATROPISOL OPHTHALMIC, Ciba Vision	00058-0705-05
5 ml	**$10.63**	**ISOPTO ATROPINE, Alcon-PR**	**00998-0303-05**
15 ml	$2.50	Atropine Sulfate Ophthalmic, Goldline Labs	00182-7064-64
15 ml	$2.78	Atropine Sulfate, Rugby	00536-0101-72
15 ml	$2.95	Atropine Sulfate, Apotex	60505-7484-05
15 ml	$3.25	Atropine Sulfate, Qualitest Pharms	00603-7072-41
15 ml	$3.28	Atropine Sulfate, Martec Pharms	52555-0992-10
15 ml	$3.35	Atropine Sulfate, Fougera	00168-0172-15
15 ml	$3.66	Atropine Sulfate, Steris Labs	00402-0796-15
15 ml	$3.84	Atropine Sulfate 1%, Schein Pharm (US)	00364-7128-72
15 ml	$4.00	Atropine Sulfate, Major Pharms	00904-0824-35
15 ml	$4.21	Atropine Sulfate, Aligen Independ	00405-6010-15
15 ml	$4.94	ATROPINE CARE, Akorn	17478-0214-12
15 ml	$8.54	Atropine Sulfate 1% Ophthalmic, Allergan-Amer	11980-0002-15
15 ml	$11.90	Atropine Sulfate, Optopics	52238-0502-15
15 ml	**$14.37**	**ISOPTO ATROPINE, Alcon-PR**	**00998-0303-15**

Solution - Ophthalmic - 3 %

5 ml	**$10.00**	**ISOPTO ATROPINE, Alcon-PR**	**00998-0305-05**

Tablet, Uncoated - Oral - 0.4 mg

100's	$26.95	SAL-TROPINE, Hope Pharms	60267-0742-30

ATROPINE SULFATE; BENZOIC ACID; HYOSCYAMINE; METHENAMINE; METHYLENE BLUE; PHENYL SALICYLATE *(000340)*

CATEGORIES: Analgesics; Anti-Infectives; Antibacterials; Antipyretics; Antiseptics, Urinary Tract; Antispasmodics; Cystitis; Inflammation; Relaxants/Stimulants, Urinary Tract; Renal Drugs; Trigonitis; Urethritis; Urinary Anti-Infectives; Urinary Antibacterial; Urinary Tract Infections; Pregnancy Category C; FDA Pre 1938 Drugs

BRAND NAMES: Atrosept; Cystemms-V; Dolsed; Hexalol; Lanased; Ro-Sed; Trac-2X; Uaa; Urapine; Uretron; Uri-Sep Sc Blue; Uridon; Urimar T; Urimed; Urin D.S.; Urinary Antiseptic; **Urised**; Urisep; Uriseptic; Uritabs; Uritan Purple; Uritin; Urivin; Uro-Ves; Urstat; Usept

FORMULARIES: Aetna; BC-BS

DESCRIPTION:

Atropine Sulfate 0.03 mg, Hyoscyamine 0.03 mg, Methenamine 40.8 mg, Methylene Blue 5.4 mg, Phenyl Salicylate 18.1 mg, Benzoic Acid 4.5 mg

TABLE 1

Established Name	Chemical Name
Methenamine	Hexamethylenetetramine
Phenyl Salicylate	2-Hydroxybenzoic acid phenyl ester
Methylene Blue	Methylthionine chloride
Benzoic acid	Benzenecarboxylic acid
Atropine sulfate	d/ tropyl tropate
Hyoscyamine	Methylthionine chloride,/- tropyl tropate

Urised is a purple, round, sugar coated tablet for oral administration. It is a combination of antiseptics (Methenamine, Methylene Blue, Phenyl Salicylate, Benzoic Acid) and parasympatholytics (Atropine Sulfate, Hyoscyamine).

Each Urised Tablet-Contains: Methenamine - 40.8 mg; Phenyl Salicylate - 18.1 mg; Methylene Blue - 5.4 mg; Benzoic Acid - 4.5 mg; Atropine Sulfate - 0.03 mg; Hyoscyamine Sulfate - 0.03 mg

CLINICAL PHARMACOLOGY:

Methenamine itself does not have antiseptic, irritant, or toxic properties in the urine. Methenamine, in an acid urine (pH 6 or below), hydrolyzes into formaldehyde within the urinary tract providing mild antiseptic activity. When given as directed and the daily urine volume is 1000 to 1500 ml, a daily dose of 2 grams will yield a urinary concentration of 18-60 mcg/ml of free formaldehyde in the urine. This is more than the minimal inhibitory dose of formaldehyde which must be available for most urinary tract pathogens. Methenamine is readily absorbed from the gastrointestinal tract and is rapidly excreted almost entirely in the urine. Methylene blue and benzoic acid are mild but effective antiseptics which contribute to the antiseptic properties of methenamine. Phenyl salicylate is mild analgesic and antipyretic with weak antiseptic activity. All of these compounds are readily absorbed from the gastrointestinal tract and excreted in the urine. Through parasympatholytic action, atropine sulfate and hyoscyamine sulfate relax smooth muscle spasms resulting from parasympathetic stimulation.[2]

INDICATIONS AND USAGE:

Urinary Antiseptic Tablets are indicated for the relief of discomfort of the lower urinary tract caused by hypermotility resulting from inflammation or diagnostic procedures and in the treatment of cystitis, urethritis, and trigonitis when caused by organisms which maintain or produce an acid urine and are susceptible to formaldehyde.

CONTRAINDICATIONS:

Glaucoma, urinary bladder neck obstruction, pyloric or duodenal obstruction, or cardiospasm. Hypersensitivity to any of the ingredients.

WARNINGS:

Do not exceed recommended dose. Methenamine may combine with sulfonamides in the urine to give mutual antagonism and should not be used with sulfonamides.

PRECAUTIONS:

Administer with caution to persons with known idiosyncrasy to atropine-like compounds and to patients suffering from cardiac disease. Bacteriological studies of the urine may be helpful in following the patient response. Methylene blue interferes with the analysis for some urinary components such as free formaldehyde. Drugs and/or foods which produce an alkaline urine should be restricted.[3] Patient should be advised that the urine may become blue to blue-green and the feces may be discolored as a result of excretion of methylene blue. Methenamine preparations should not be given to patients taking sulfonamides since insoluble precipitates may form with formaldehyde in the urine. No known long-term animal studies have been performed to evaluate carcinogenic potential. The precautions related to drug interaction, diagnostic interference, medical problems and side effects to use of belladonna alkaloids, should be observed.

Pregnancy Category C: Animal reproduction studies have not been conducted with Urinary Antiseptic Tablets. It is also not known whether this product can cause fetal harm when administered to pregnant women or can affect reproduction capacity. This product should be given to a pregnant woman only if clearly needed.

Nursing Mothers: It is not known whether this drug is excreted in human milk. Because many drugs are excreted in human milk, caution should be exercised when Urinary Antiseptic Tablets are administered to a nursing women.

Prolonged Use: There have been no studies to establish the safety of prolonged use in humans.

ADVERSE REACTIONS:

Prolonged use may result in generalized skin rash, pronounced dryness of the mouth, flushing, difficulty in initiating micturition, rapid pulse, dizziness or blurring of vision. If any of these reactions occur, discontinue use immediately. Acute urinary retention may be precipitated in prostatic. See OVERDOSAGE.

DRUG ABUSE AND DEPENDENCE:

A dependence on the use of Urised has not been reported and due to the nature of its ingredients, abuse is not expected.

OVERDOSAGE:

By exceeding the recommended dosage of Urinary Antiseptic Tablets, symptomology related to the overdose of its individual active ingredients may be expected as follows:

Atropine Sulfate, Hyoscyamine Sulfate: Symptoms associated with an overdosage of this product will not probably be manifested in the symptoms related to overdosage of the alkaloids atropine sulfate and hyoscyamine sulfate. Such symptoms as dryness of mucous membranes; dilation of pupils; hot, dry, flushed skin; hyperpyrexia; tachycardia, palpitations; elevated blood pressure; coma; circulatory collapse and death from respiratory failure can occur due to overdosage of these alkaloids.

Methenamine: If large amounts of the drug (2-8 gm daily) are used over extended periods, (3-4 weeks), bladder and gastrointestinal irritation, painful and frequent micturition, albuminuria and gross hematuria may be expected.

Methylene Blue: Symptoms of methylene blue overdosage associated with the overdosage of this product is not expected to be discernible from those associated with the other active ingredients in this product.

Benzoic Acid: Symptoms of benzoic acid overdosage associated with the overdosage of this product is not expected to be discernible from those associated with the other active ingredients in this product.

Phenyl Salicylate: Symptoms of phenyl salicylate overdosage include burning pain in throat and mouth, white necrotic lesions in the mouth, abdominal pain, vomiting, bloody diarrhea, pallor, sweating, weakness, headache, dizziness and tinnitus. The symptoms however, are not expected to be discernible from those associated with the other active ingredients in this product.

REFERENCES:

1. Gollamudi, R., Straughn, A.B., and Meyer, M.C., *"Urinary Excretion of Methenamine and Formaldehyde: Evaluation of 10 Methenamine Products in Humans,"* J. Pharm. Sci, 70, 596, 1981. **2.** Goodman, L.S. and Gilman, G., *The Pharmacological Basis of Therapeutics,* Sixth Edition, Macmillan Pub Co. 121, 971, 980, 1119 (1980). **3.** *AMA Drug Evaluation,* Fifth Edition, 1745 (1983).

DOSAGE AND ADMINISTRATION:

Adults: Two tablets four times daily. See PRECAUTIONS.

Usual Pediatric dosage: *Children (up to 6 years of age):* Use is not recommended. *Children (6 years of age and older):* Dosage must be individualized by physician.

Storage: Dispense in a tight, light-resistant container as defined in the USP. Store at controlled room temperature 15 - 30°C (59 - 86°F). Protect from moisture.

HOW SUPPLIED - EQUIVALENTS NOT AVAILABLE:

Tablet, Uncoated - Oral - 0.03 mg/4.5 mg/

100's	$8.98	UAA, Embrex Economed	38130-0046-01
100's	$9.05	Urinary Antiseptic, Alphagen Labs	59743-0016-01
100's	$9.42	Urinary Antiseptic, Aligen Independ	00405-4633-01
100's	$9.70	URITIN, Goldline Labs	00182-0850-01
100's	$9.89	URIDON MODIFIED, Rugby	00536-4757-01
100's	$10.45	URINARY ANTISEPTIC NO. 2, Eon Labs Mfg	00185-0230-01
100's	$10.60	Urapine, Major Pharms	00904-3286-60
100's	$11.98	URINARY ANTISEPTIC, Qualitest Pharms	00603-6311-21
100's	$11.99	ATROSEPT, Geneva Pharms	00781-1341-01
100's	$13.89	URI-SEP SC BLUE, HL Moore Drug Exch	00839-7796-06
100's	$17.34	TRAC TABS 2X, Hyrex Pharms	00314-0408-01
100's	$23.00	Urin D.S., Llorens Pharm	54859-0701-10
100's	$24.50	URIMAR-T, Marnel Pharceut	00682-0033-01
100's	$30.94	DOLSED, Amer Urologicals	00539-0708-01
100's	$36.96	PROSED/DS, Star Pharms FL	00076-0108-03
1000's	$60.94	URIDON MODIFIED, Rugby	00536-4757-10
1000's	$71.95	URAPINE, Major Pharms	00904-3286-80
1000's	$79.96	UAA, Embrex Economed	38130-0046-10
1000's	$86.40	Urinary Antiseptic, Alphagen Labs	59743-0016-10
1000's	$89.54	URINARY ANTISEPTIC, Qualitest Pharms	00603-6311-32
1000's	$95.92	ATROSEPT, Geneva Pharms	00781-1341-10
1000's	$143.20	TRAC TABS 2X, Hyrex Pharms	00314-0408-10
1000's	$250.00	DOLSED, Amer Urologicals	00539-0708-10

ATROPINE SULFATE; DIFENOXIN HYDROCHLORIDE *(000338)*

CATEGORIES: Antidiarrhea Agents; Diarrhea; Gastrointestinal Drugs; Pregnancy Category C; DEA Class CIV; FDA Approval Pre 1982

BRAND NAMES: *Lyspafen*; *Lyspafen-E*; *Lyspafena*; **Motofen**
(International brand names outside U.S. in italics)

DESCRIPTION:

Each five-sided dye free Motofen contains: Difenoxin (as the hydrochloride): 1.0 mg

Warning - May be habit forming.

Atropine sulfate: 0.025 mg

Difenoxin hydrochloride, 1-(3-cyano-3,3-diphenylpropyl)-4- phenyl-4-piperidinecarboxylic acid monohydrochloride, is an orally administered antidiarrheal agent which is chemically related to the narcotic meperidine.

Atropine sulfate is present to discourage deliberate overdosage.

Atropine sulfate, an anticholinergic, is endo (±)-α-(hydroxymethyl) benzeneacetic acid 8-methyl-8-azabicyclo[3.2.1] oct-3-yl ester sulfate (2:1) (salt) monohydrate.

Motofen Inactive ingredients: calcium stearate, cellulose, lactose, corn starch.

CLINICAL PHARMACOLOGY:

Animal studies have shown that difenoxin hydrochloride manifests its antidiarrheal effect by slowing intestinal motility. The mechanism of action is by a local effect on the gastrointestinal wall.

Difenoxin is the principal active metabolite of diphenoxylate.

Following oral administration of difenoxin HCl with atropine sulfate is rapidly and extensively absorbed. Mean peak plasma levels of approximately 160 ng/ml occurred within 40 to 60 minutes in most patients following an oral dose of 2 mg. Plasma levels decline to less than 10% of their peak values within 24 hours and to less than 1% of their peak values within 72 hours. This decline parallels the appearance of difenoxin and its metabolites in the urine. Difenoxin is metabolized to an inactive hydroxylated metabolite. Both the drug and its metabolites are excreted, mainly as conjugates, in urine and feces.

INDICATIONS AND USAGE:

Difenoxin HCl with atropine sulfate is indicated as adjunctive therapy in the management of acute nonspecific diarrhea and acute exacerbations of chronic functional diarrhea.

CONTRAINDICATIONS:

Difenoxin HCl with atropine sulfate is contraindicated in patients with diarrhea associated with organisms that penetrate the intestinal mucosa (toxigenic *E. coli, Salmonella* species, *Shigella*) and pseudomembranous colitis associated with broad spectrum antibiotics. Antiperistaltic agents should not be used in these conditions because they may prolong and/or worsen diarrhea.

Difenoxin HCl with atropine sulfate is *contraindicated in children under 2 years of age* because of the decreased margin of safety of drugs in this class in younger age groups.

Difenoxin HCl with atropine sulfate is contraindicated in patients with a known hypersensitivity to difenoxin, atropine, or any of the inactive ingredients, and in patients who are jaundiced.

WARNINGS:

DIFENOXIN HCl WITH ATROPINE SULFATE IS *NOT* AN INNOCUOUS DRUG AND DOSAGE RECOMMENDATIONS SHOULD BE STRICTLY ADHERED TO. DIFENOXIN HCl WITH ATROPINE SULFATE IS NOT RECOMMENDED FOR CHILDREN UNDER 2 YEARS OF AGE. OVERDOSAGE MAY RESULT IN SEVERE RESPIRATORY DEPRESSION AND COMA, POSSIBLY LEADING TO PERMANENT BRAIN DAMAGE OR DEATH (SEE OVERDOSAGE). THEREFORE, KEEP THIS MEDICATION OUT OF THE REACH OF CHILDREN.

FLUID AND ELECTROLYTE BALANCE: THE USE OF DIFENOXIN HCl WITH ATROPINE SULFATE DOES NOT PRECLUDE THE ADMINISTRATION OF APPROPRIATE FLUID AND ELECTROLYTE THERAPY. DEHYDRATION, PARTICULARLY IN CHILDREN, MAY FURTHER INFLUENCE THE VARIABILITY OF RESPONSE TO DIFENOXIN HCl WITH ATROPINE SULFATE AND MAY PREDISPOSE TO DELAYED DIFENOXIN INTOXICATION. DRUG INDUCED INHIBITION OF PERISTALSIS MAY RESULT IN FLUID RETENTION IN THE COLON, AND THIS MAY FURTHER AGGRAVATE DEHYDRATION AND ELECTROLYTE IMBALANCE.

IF SEVERE DEHYDRATION OR ELECTROLYTE IMBALANCE IS MANIFESTED, DIFENOXIN HCl WITH ATROPINE SULFATE SHOULD BE WITHHELD UNTIL APPROPRIATE CORRECTIVE THERAPY HAS BEEN INITIATED.

Ulcerative Colitis: In some patients with acute ulcerative colitis, agents which inhibit intestinal motility or delay intestinal transit time have been reported to induce toxic megacolon. Consequently, patients with acute ulcerative colitis should be carefully observed and difenoxin HCl with atropine sulfate therapy should be discontinued promptly if abdominal distention occurs or if other untoward symptoms develop.

Liver and Kidney Disease: Difenoxin HCl with atropine sulfate should be used with extreme caution in patients with advanced hepatorenal disease and in all patients with abnormal liver function tests since hepatic coma may be precipitated.

Atropine: A subtherapeutic dose of atropine has been added to difenoxin hydrochloride to discourage deliberate overdosage. Usage of difenoxin HCl with atropine sulfate in recommended doses is not likely to cause prominent anticholinergic side effects, but difenoxin HCl with atropine sulfate should be avoided in patients in whom anticholinergic drugs are contraindicated. The warnings and precautions for use of anticholinergic agents should be observed. In children, signs of atropinism may occur even with recommended doses of difenoxin HCl with atropine sulfate, particularly in patients with Down's Syndrome.

PRECAUTIONS:

Information for the Patient: CAUTION PATIENTS TO ADHERE STRICTLY TO RECOMMENDED DOSAGE SCHEDULES. THE MEDICATION SHOULD BE KEPT OUT OF REACH OF CHILDREN SINCE ACCIDENTAL OVERDOSAGE MAY RESULT IN SEVERE, EVEN FATAL, RESPIRATORY DEPRESSION.

Difenoxin HCl with atropine sulfate may produce drowsiness or dizziness. The patient should be cautioned regarding activities requiring mental alertness, such as driving or operating dangerous machinery.

Carcinogenesis, Mutagenesis, and Impairment of Fertility: No evidence of carcinogenesis was found in a long-term study of difenoxin hydrochloride/atropine in the rat. In this 104 week study, rats received dietary doses of 0, 1.25, 2.5, or 5 mg/kg/day difenoxin/atropine (20:1 ratio).

PRECAUTIONS: *(cont'd)*

No experiments have been conducted to determine the mutagenic potential of difenoxin HCl with atropine sulfate. difenoxin HCl with atropine sulfate did not significantly impair fertility in rats.

Pregnancy, Teratogenic Effects, Pregnancy Category C: Reproduction studies in rats and rabbits with doses at 31 and 61 times the human therapeutic dose respectively, on a mg/kg basis, demonstrated no evidence of teratogenesis due to difenoxin HCl with atropine sulfate.

Pregnant rats receiving oral doses of difenoxin hydrochloride/atropine 20 times the maximum human dose had an increase in delivery time as well as a significant increase in the percent of stillbirths.

Neonatal survival in rats was also reduced with most deaths occurring within four days of delivery.

There are no well controlled studies in pregnant women. Difenoxin HCl with atropine sulfate should be used during pregnancy only if the potential benefit justifies the potential risk to the fetus.

Nursing Mothers: Because of the potential for serious adverse reactions in nursing infants from difenoxin HCl with atropine sulfate, a decision should be made whether to discontinue nursing or to discontinue the drug, taking into account the importance of the drug to the mother.

Pediatric Use: SAFETY AND EFFECTIVENESS IN CHILDREN BELOW THE AGE OF 12 HAVE NOT BEEN ESTABLISHED. DIFENOXIN HCl WITH ATROPINE SULFATE IS CONTRAINDICATED IN CHILDREN UNDER 2 YEARS OF AGE. See OVERDOSAGE section for information on hazards from accidental poisoning in children.

DRUG INTERACTIONS:

Since the chemical structure of difenoxin hydrochloride is similar to meperidine hydrochloride, the concurrent use of difenoxin HCl with atropine sulfate with monoamine oxidase inhibitors may, in theory, precipitate a hypertensive crisis.

Difenoxin HCl with atropine sulfate may potentiate the action of barbiturates, tranquilizers, narcotics, and alcohol. When these medications are used concomitantly with difenoxin HCl with atropine sulfate, the patient should be closely monitored.

Diphenoxylate hydrochloride, from which the principal active metabolite difenoxin is derived, was found to inhibit the hepatic microsomal enzyme system at a dose of 2 mg/kg/day in studies conducted with male rats. Therefore, difenoxin has the potential to prolong the biological half-lives of drugs for which the rate of elimination is dependent on the microsomal drug metabolizing enzyme system.

ADVERSE REACTIONS:

In view of the small amount of atropine present (0.025 mg/tablet), effects such as dryness of the skin and mucous membranes, flushing, hyperthermia, tachycardia and urinary retention are very unlikely to occur, except perhaps in children.

Many of the adverse effects reported during clinical investigation of difenoxin HCl with atropine sulfate are difficult to distinguish from symptoms associated with the diarrheal syndrome. However, the following events were reported at the stated frequencies:

Gastrointestinal: Nausea, 1 in 15 patients; vomiting, 1 in 30 patients; dry mouth, 1 in 30 patients; epigastric distress, 1 in 100 patients; and constipation, 1 in 300 patients.

Central Nervous System: Dizziness and light-headedness, 1 in 20 patients, drowsiness, 1 in 25 patients; and headache, 1 in 40 patients; tiredness, nervousness, insomnia and confusion ranged from 1 in 200 to 1 in 600 patients.

Other less frequent reactions: Burning eyes and blurred vision occurred in a few cases.

The following adverse reactions have been reported in patients receiving chemically-related drugs: numbness of extremities, euphoria, depression, sedation, anaphylaxis, angioneurotic edema, urticaria, swelling of the gums, pruritus, toxic megacolon, paralytic ileus, pancreatitis, and anorexia.

THIS MEDICATION SHOULD BE KEPT IN A CHILD-RESISTANT CONTAINER AND OUT OF THE REACH OF CHILDREN SINCE AN OVERDOSAGE MAY RESULT IN SEVERE RESPIRATORY DEPRESSION AND COMA, POSSIBLY LEADING TO PERMANENT BRAIN DAMAGE OR DEATH.

DRUG ABUSE AND DEPENDENCE:

Difenoxin HCl with atropine sulfate tablets are a Schedule IV controlled substance.

Addiction to (dependence on) difenoxin hydrochloride is theoretically possible at high dosage. Therefore, the recommended dosage should not be exceeded. Because of the structural and pharmacological similarities of difenoxin hydrochloride to drugs with a definite addiction potential, difenoxin HCl with atropine sulfate should be administered with considerable caution to patients who are receiving addicting drugs, to individuals known to be addiction prone, or to those in whom histories suggest may increase the dosage on their own initiative.

OVERDOSAGE:

Diagnosis and Treatment: In the event of overdosage (initial signs may include dryness of the skin and mucous membranes, flushing, hyperthermia and tachycardia followed by lethargy or coma, hypotonic reflexes, nystagmus, pinpoint pupils and respiratory depression) gastric lavage, establishment of a patent airway and possibly mechanically assisted respiration are advised.

The narcotic antagonist naloxone may be used in the treatment of respiratory depression caused by narcotic analgesics or pharmacologically related compounds such as difenoxin HCl with atropine sulfate tablets. When naloxone is administered intravenously, the onset of action is generally apparent within two minutes. Naloxone may also be administered subcutaneously or intramuscularly providing a slightly less rapid onset of action but a more prolonged effect.

To counteract respiratory depression caused by difenoxin HCl with atropine sulfate overdosage, the following dosage schedule for naloxone should be followed:

Adult Dosage: The usual initial adult dose of naloxone is 0.4 mg (one ml) administered intravenously. If respiratory function does not adequately improve after the initial dose, the same IV dose may be repeated at two-to-three minute intervals.

Children: The usual adult dose of naloxone for children is 0.01 mg/kg of body weight administered intravenously and repeated at to-to-three minute intervals if necessary.

Since the duration of difenoxin hydrochloride is longer than that of naloxone, improvement of respiration following administration may be followed by recurrent respiratory depression. Consequently, continuous observation is necessary until the effect of difenoxin hydrochloride on respiration (which effect may persist for many hours) has passed. Supplemental intramuscular doses of naloxone may be utilized to produce a longer lasting effect. TREAT ALL POSSIBLE DIFENOXIN HCl WITH ATROPINE SULFATE OVERDOSAGES AS SERIOUS AND MAINTAIN MEDICAL OBSERVATION FOR AT LEAST 48 HOURS, PREFERABLY UNDER CONTINUOUS HOSPITAL CARE.

Although signs of overdosage and respiratory depression may not be evident soon after ingestion of difenoxin hydrochloride, respiratory depression may occur from 12 to 30 hours after later.

DOSAGE AND ADMINISTRATION:

The recommended starting dose of difenoxin HCl with atropine sulfate tablets in adults is 2 tablets (2 mg), then 1 tablet (1 mg) after each loose stool or 1 tablet (1 mg) every 3 to 4 hours as needed, but the total dosage during any 24-hour treatment period should not exceed 8 tablets (8 mg). In the treatment of diarrhea, if clinical improvement is not observed in 48 hours, continued administration of this type medication is not recommended. For acute diarrheas and acute exacerbations of functional diarrhea, treatment beyond 48 hours in usually not necessary.

Studies in children below the age of 12 have been inadequate to evaluate the safety and effectiveness of difenoxin HCl with atropine sulfate in this age group. difenoxin HCl with atropine sulfate is contraindicated in children under 2 years of age.

HOW SUPPLIED:

Motofen is available as a white, dye-free, five-sided, scored tablet with "8674" on the scored side and "C" on the other. Each tablet contains 1.0 mg difenoxin (as the hydrochloride salt) and 0.025 mg atropine sulfate.

Store at controlled room temperature, 15°-30°C (59-86°F).

HOW SUPPLIED - EQUIVALENTS NOT AVAILABLE:

Tablet, Uncoated - Oral - 0.025 mg/1 mg

50's	$23.80	MOTOFEN, Carnrick	00086-0074-05
100's	$42.80	MOTOFEN, Carnrick	00086-0074-10

ATROPINE SULFATE; DIPHENOXYLATE HYDROCHLORIDE *(000339)*

CATEGORIES: Antidiarrhea Agents; Diarrhea; Gastrointestinal Drugs; Pregnancy Category C; DEA Class CV; FDA Approval Pre 1982

BRAND NAMES: *Celidin*; Colonaid; *Dhamotil*; Di-Atro; *Diarase*; *Diarest*; *Diarphen*; *Diarsed* (France); *Diastop*; *Dilomil*; Dimotal; Diphenatol; Diphenoxylate W/Atropine; *Diphensil*; *Ditropine*; *Erlotyl*; *Katevan*; Lo-Rex; Lo-Trol; Lofene; Logen; Lomanate; Lomocot; Lomodix; **Lomotil**; Lomoxate; Lonox; Lotabs; Low-Quel; Nor-Mil; *Protector*; *Reasac*; *Reasec* (Germany); *Retardin*; Romotil; *Sedistal*; *Tropatil* (Mexico); Uni-Lom; Vi-Atro
(International brand names outside U.S. in italics)

FORMULARIES: Aetna; BC-BS; CIGNA; FHP; Humana; Kaiser; Medco; Medi-Cal; PCS; PruCare; United

DESCRIPTION:

Each Lomotil tablet and each 5 ml of Lomotil liquid for oral use contains:

diphenoxylate hydrochloride (abbreviated here as HCl: 2.5 mg)

(Warning—May be habit forming.)

Atropine sulfate: 0.025 mg

Diphenoxylate HCl, an antidiarrheal, is ethyl 1-(3-cyano-3,3- diphenylpropyl)-4-phenylisonipecotate monohydrochloride.

Atropine sulfate, an anticholinergic, is endo-(±)-α-(hydroxymethyl) benzeneacetic acid 8-methyl-8-azabicyclo(3.2.1) oct-3-yl ester sulfate (2:1) (salt) monohydrate.

Inactive ingredients of Lomotil tablets include acacia, corn, starch, magnesium stearate, sorbitol, sucrose, and talc. Inactive ingredients of Lomotil liquid include cherry flavor, citric acid, ethyl alcohol 15%, FD&C Yellow No. 6, glycerin, sodium phosphate, sorbitol, and water.

IMPORTANT INFORMATION

Lomotil is classified as a Schedule V controlled substance by federal law. Diphenoxylate HCl is chemically related to the narcotic meperidine. Therefore, in case of overdosage, treatment is similar to that for meperidine or morphine intoxication, in which prolonged and careful monitoring is essential. Respiratory depression may be evidenced as late as 30 hours after ingestion and may recur in spite of an initial response to narcotic antagonists. A subtherapeutic amount of atropine sulfate is present to discourage deliberate overdosage. LOMOTIL IS *NOT* AN INNOCUOUS DRUG AND DOSAGE RECOMMENDATIONS SHOULD BE STRICTLY ADHERED TO, ESPECIALLY IN CHILDREN, KEEP THIS AND ALL MEDICATIONS OUT OF REACH OF CHILDREN.

CLINICAL PHARMACOLOGY:

Diphenoxylate is rapidly and extensively metabolized in man by ester hydrolysis to diphenoxylic acid (difenoxine), which is biologically active and the major metabolite in the blood. After a 5-mg oral dose of carbon-14 labeled diphenoxylate HCl in ethanolic solution was given to three healthy volunteers, an average of 14% of the drug plus its metabolites was excreted in the urine and 49% in the faces over a four- day period. Urinary excretion of the unmetabolized drug constituted less than 1% of the dose, and diphenoxylic acid plus its glucuronide conjugate constituted about 6% of the dose. In a 16-subject crossover bioavailability study, a liner relationship in the dose range of 2.5 to 10 mg was found between the dose of diphenoxylate HCl (given as atropine sulfate liquid) and the peak plasma concentration, the area under the plasma concentration-time curve, and the amount of diphenoxylic acid excreted in the urine. In the same study the bioavailability of the tablet compared with an equal dose of the liquid was approximately 90%. The average peak plasma concentration of diphenoxylic acid following ingestion of four 2.5-mg tablets was 163 ng/ml at about 2 hours, and the elimination half- life of diphenoxylic acid was approximately 12 to 14 hours.

In dogs, diphenoxylate HCl has a direct effect on circular smooth muscle of the bowel that conceivably results in segmentation and prolongation of gastrointestinal transit time. The clinical antidiarrheal action of diphenoxylate HCl may thus be a consequence of enhanced segmentation that allows increased contact of the intraluminal contents with the intestinal mucosa.

INDICATIONS AND USAGE:

Atropine sulfate is effective as adjunctive therapy in the management of diarrhea.

CONTRAINDICATIONS:

Atropine sulfate is contraindicated in patients with

1. Known hypersensitivity to diphenoxylate or atropine.

2. Obstructive jaundice.

3. Diarrhea associated with pseudomembranous enterocolitis or enterotoxin-producing bacteria.

WARNINGS:

ATROPINE SULFATE IS *NOT* AN INNOCUOUS DRUG AND DOSAGE RECOMMENDATIONS SHOULD BE STRICTLY ADHERED TO, ESPECIALLY IN CHILDREN. ATROPINE SULFATE W/ DIPHENOXYLATE HCl IS NOT RECOMMENDED FOR CHILDREN UNDER 2 YEARS OF AGE. OVERDOSAGE MAY RESULT IN SEVERE RESPIRATORY DEPRESSION AND COMA, POSSIBLY LEADING TO PERMANENT BRAIN DAMAGE OR DEATH (SEE OVERDOSAGE). THEREFORE, KEEP THIS MEDICATION OUT OF THE REACH OF CHILDREN.

THE USE OF ATROPINE SULFATE SHOULD BE ACCOMPANIED BY APPROPRIATE FLUID AND ELECTROLYTE THERAPY, WHEN INDICATED. IF SEVERE DEHYDRATION OR ELECTROLYTE IMBALANCE IS PRESENT, ATROPINE SULFATE SHOULD BE WITHHELD UNTIL APPROPRIATE CORRECTIVE THERAPY HAS BEEN INITIATED. DRUG-INDUCED INHIBITION OF PERISTALSIS MAY RESULT IN FLUID RETENTION IN THE INTESTINE, WHICH MAY FURTHER AGGRAVATE DEHYDRATION AND ELECTROLYTE IMBALANCE.

ATROPINE SULFATE SHOULD BE USED WITH SPECIAL CAUTION IN YOUNG CHILDREN BECAUSE THIS AGE GROUP MAY BE PREDISPOSED TO DELAYED DIPHENOXYLATE TOXICITY AND BECAUSE OF THE GREATER VARIABILITY OF RESPONSE IN THIS AGE GROUP.

Antiperistaltic agents may prolong and/or worsen diarrhea associated with organisms that penetrate the intestinal mucosa (toxigenic *E. coli*, *Salmonella*, *Shigella*), and pseudomembranous enterocolitis associated with broad-spectrum antibiotics. Antiperistaltic agents should not be used in these conditions.

In some patients with acute ulcerative colitis, agents that inhibit intestinal motility or prolong intestinal transit time have been reported to induce toxic megacolon. Consequently, patients with acute ulcerative colitis should be carefully observed and atropine sulfate w/ diphenoxylate HCl therapy should be discontinued promptly if abdominal distention occurs or if other untoward symptoms develop.

Since the chemical structure of diphenoxylate HCl is similar to that of meperidine HCl, the concurrent use of atropine sulfate with monoamine oxidase (MAO) inhibitors may, in theory, precipitate hypertensive crisis.

Atropine sulfate should be used with extreme caution in patients with advanced hepatorenal disease and in all patients with abnormal liver function since hepatic coma may be precipitated.

Diphenoxylate HCl may potentiate the action of barbiturates, tranquilizers, and alcohol. Therefore, the patient should be closely observed when any of these are used concomitantly.

PRECAUTIONS:

General: Since a subtherapeutic dose of atropine has been added to the diphenoxylate HCl, consideration should be given to the precautions relating to the use of atropine. In children, atropine sulfate should be used with caution since signs of atropinism may occur even with recommended doses, particularly in patients with Down's syndrome.

Information for the Patient: INFORM THE PATIENT (PARENT OR GUARDIAN) NOT TO EXCEED THE RECOMMENDED DOSAGE AND TO KEEP ATROPINE SULFATE OUT OF THE REACH OF CHILDREN AND IN A CHILD-RESISTANT CONTAINER. INFORM THE PATIENT OF THE CONSEQUENCES OF OVERDOSAGE, INCLUDING SEVERE RESPIRATORY DEPRESSION AND COMA, POSSIBLY LEADING TO PERMANENT BRAIN DAMAGE OR DEATH. Atropine sulfate may produce drowsiness or dizziness. The patient should be cautioned regarding activities requiring mental alertness, such as driving or operating dangerous machinery. Potentiation of the action of alcohol, barbiturates, and tranquilizers with concomitant use of atropine sulfate should be explained to the patient. The physician should also provide the patient with other information in this labeling, as appropriate.

Carcinogenesis, Mutagenesis, and Impairment of Fertility: No long- term study in animals has been performed to evaluate carcinogenic potential. Diphenoxylate HCl was administered to male and female rats in their diets to provide dose levels of 4 to 20 mg/kg/day throughout a three-litter reproduction study. At 50 times the human dose (20 mg/kg/day), female weight gain was reduced and there was a marked effect on fertility as only 4 of 27 females became pregnant in three test breedings. The relevance of this finding to usage of atropine sulfate in humans is unknown.

Pregnancy Category C: Diphenoxylate HCl has been shown to have an effect on fertility in rats when given in doses 50 times the human dose. Other findings in this study include a decrease in maternal weight gain of 30% at 20 mg/kg/day and of 10% at 4 mg/kg/day. At 10 times the human dose (4 mg/kg/day), average litter size was slightly reduced.

Teratology studies were conducted in rats, rabbits, and mice with diphenoxylate HCl at oral doses of 0.4 to 20 mg/kg/day. Due to experimental design and small numbers of litters, embryotoxic, fetotoxic, or teratogenic effects cannot be adequately assessed. However, examination of the available fetuses did not reveal any indication of teratogenicity.

There are no adequate and well-controlled studies in pregnant women. Atropine sulfate should be used during pregnancy only if the anticipated benefit justifies the potential risk to the fetus.

Nursing Mothers: Caution should be exercised when is administered to a nursing woman, since the physicochemical characteristics of the major metabolite, diphenoxylic acid, are such that it may be excreted in breast milk and since it is known that atropine is excreted in breast milk.

Pediatric Use: Atropine sulfate may be used as an adjunct to the treatment of diarrhea but should be accompanied by appropriate fluid and electrolyte therapy, if needed. Atropine sulfate w/ Diphenoxylate HCl IS NOT RECOMMENDED FOR CHILDREN UNDER 2 YEARS OF AGE. Atropine sulfate should be used with special caution in young children because of the greater variability of response in this age group. See WARNINGS and DOSAGE AND ADMINISTRATION. In case of accidental ingestion by children, see OVERDOSAGE for recommended treatment.

DRUG INTERACTIONS:

Known drug interactions include barbiturates, tranquilizers and alcohol. Atropine sulfate may interact with MAO inhibitors (see WARNINGS.)

In studies with male rats diphenoxylate HCl was found to inhibit the hepatic microsomal enzyme system at a dose of 2 mg/kg/day. Therefore, diphenoxylate has the potential to prolong the biological half-lives of drugs for which the rate of elimination is dependent on the microsomal drug metabolizing enzyme system.

ADVERSE REACTIONS:

At *therapeutic* doses, the following have been reported; they are listed in decreasing order of severity, but not of frequency:

Nervous System: numbness of extremities, euphoria, depression, malaise/lethargy, confusion, sedation/drowsiness, dizziness, restlessness, headache.

Allergic: anaphylaxis, angioneurotic edema, urticaria, swelling of the gums, pruritus.

ADVERSE REACTIONS: *(cont'd)*

Gastrointestinal System: toxic megacolon, paralytic ileus, pancreatitis, vomiting, nausea, anorexia, abdominal discomfort.

The following atropine sulfate effects are listed in decreasing order of severity, but not of frequency: hyperthermia, tachycardia, urinary retention, flushing, dryness of the skin and mucosus membranes. There effects may occur, especially in children.

THIS MEDICATION SHOULD BE KEPT IN A CHILD-RESISTANT CONTAINER AND OUT OF THE REACH OF CHILDREN SINCE AN OVERDOSAGE MAY RESULT IN SEVERE RESPIRATORY DEPRESSION AND COMA, POSSIBLY LEADING TO PERMANENT BRAIN DAMAGE OR DEATH.

DRUG ABUSE AND DEPENDENCE:

Controlled Substance: Atropine sulfate is classified as a Schedule V controlled substance by federal regulation. Diphenoxylate HCl is chemically related to the narcotic analgesic meperidine.

Drug Abuse And Dependence: In doses used for the treatment of diarrhea, whether acute or chronic, diphenoxylate has not produced addiction.

Diphenoxylate HCl is devoid of morphine-like subjective effects at therapeutic doses. At high doses it exhibits codeine-like subjective effects. The dose which produces antidiarrheal action is widely separated from the dose which causes central nervous system effects. The insolubility of diphenoxylate HCl in commonly available aqueous media precludes intravenous self-administration. A dose of 100 to 300 mg/day, which is equivalent to 40 to 120 tablets, administered to humans for 40 to 70 days, produced opiate withdrawal symptoms. Since addition to diphenoxylate HCl is possible at high doses, the recommended dosage should not be exceeded.

OVERDOSAGE:

RECOMMENDED DOSAGE SCHEDULES SHOULD BE STRICTLY FOLLOWED. THIS MEDICATION SHOULD BE KEPT IN A CHILD-RESISTANT CONTAINER AND OUT OF THE REACH OF CHILDREN, SINCE AN OVERDOSAGE MAY RESULT IN SEVERE, EVEN FATAL, RESPIRATORY DEPRESSION.

Diagnosis: Initial signs of overdosage may include dryness of the skin and mucous membranes, mydriasis, restlessness, flushing, hyperthermia, and tachycardia followed by lethargy or coma, hypotonic reflexes, nystagmus, pinpoint pupils, and respiratory depression. Respiratory depression may be evidenced as late as 30 hours after ingestion and may recur despite an initial response to narcotic antagonists. TREAT ALL POSSIBLE ATROPINE SULFATE OVERDOSAGES AS SERIOUS AND MAINTAIN MEDICAL OBSERVATION OF AT LEAST 48 HOURS, PREFERABLY UNDER CONTINUOUS HOSPITAL CARE.

Treatment: In the event of overdose, induction of vomiting, gastric lavage, establishment of a patent airway, and possibly mechanically assisted respiration are advised. *In vitro* and animal studies indicate that activated charcoal may significantly decrease the bioavailability of diphenoxylate. In noncomatose patients, a slurry of 100 g of activated charcoal can be administered immediately after the induction of vomiting or gastric lavage.

A pure narcotic antagonist (*e.g.,* naloxone) should be used in the treatment of respiratory depression caused by atropine sulfate. When a narcotic antagonist is administered intravenously, the onset of action is generally apparent within two minutes. If may also be administered subcutaneously or intramuscularly, providing a slightly less rapid onset of action but a more prolonged effect.

To counteract respiratory depression caused by atropine sulfate overdosage, the following dosage schedule for the narcotic antagonist naloxone HCl should be followed:

Adult dosage: An initial dose of 0.4 mg to 2 mg of naloxone HCl may be administered intravenously. If the desired degree of counteraction and improvement in respiratory functions is not obtained, it may be repeated at 2- to 3-minute intervals. If no response is observed after 10 mg of naloxone HCl has been administered, the diagnosis of narcotic-induced or partial narcotic-induced toxicity should be questioned. Intramuscular or subcutaneous administration may be necessary if the intravenous routs is not available.

Children: The usual initial dose in children is 0.01 mg/kg body weight given IV if this dose does not result in the desired degree of clinical improvement, a subsequent dose of 0.1 mg/kg body weight may be administered. If an IV route of administration if not available, naloxone HCl may be administered IM or SC in divided doses. If necessary, naloxone HCl can be diluted with sterile water for injection.

Following initial improvement of respiratory function, repeated doses of naloxone HCl may be required to counteract recurrent respiratory depression. Supplemental intramuscular doses of naloxone HCl may be utilized to produce a longer-lasting effect.

Since the duration of action of diphenoxylate HCl is longer than that of naloxone HCl, improvement of respiration following administration may be followed by recurrent respiratory depression. Consequently, continuous observation is necessary until the effect of diphenoxylate HCl on respiration has passed. This effect may persist for many hours. The period of observation should extend over at least 48 hours, preferably under continuous hospital care. Although sings of overdosage and respiratory depression may not be evident soon after ingestion of diphenoxylate HCl, respiratory depression may occur from 12 to 30 hours later.

DOSAGE AND ADMINISTRATION:

DO NOT EXCEED RECOMMENDED DOSAGE.

Adults: The recommended initial dosage is two atropine sulfate tablets four times daily or 10 ml (two regular teaspoonfuls) of atropine sulfate liquid four times daily (20 mg per day). Most patients will require this dosage until initial control has been achieved, after which the dosage may be reduced to meet individual requirements. Control may often be maintained with as little as 5 mg (two tablets or 10 ml of liquid) daily.

Clinical improvement of acute diarrhea is usually observed within 48 hours. If clinical improvement of chronic diarrhea after treatment with a maximum daily dose of 20 mg of diphenoxylate HCl is not observed within 10 days, symptoms are unlikely to be controlled by further administration.

Children: atropine sulfate is not recommended in children under 2 years of age and should be used with special caution in young children (see WARNINGS and PRECAUTIONS). The nutritional status and degree of dehydration must be considered. In children under 13 years of age, use atropine sulfate liquid. Do not use atropine sulfate tablets for this age group.

Only the plastic dropper should be used when measuring atropine sulfate liquid for administration to children.

Dosage schedule for children: The recommended initial total daily dosage of atropine sulfate liquid for children is 0.3 to 0.4 mg/kg. administered in four divided doses. TABLE 1 provides an *approximate* initial daily dosage recommendation for children.

These pediatric schedules are the best approximation of an average dose recommendation which may be adjusted downward according to the overall nutritional status and degree of dehydration encountered in the sick child. Reduction of dosage may be made as soon as

DOSAGE AND ADMINISTRATION: *(cont'd)*

TABLE 1

Age (years)	Approximate (kg)	weight (lb)	Dosage in ml (four times daily)
2	11-14	24-31	1.5-3.0
3	12-16	26-35	2.0-3.0
4	14-20	31-44	2.0-4.0
5	16-23	35-51	2.5-4.5
6-8	17-32	38-71	2.5-5.0
9-12	23-55	51-121	3.5-5.0

initial control of symptoms has been achieved. Maintenance dosage may be as low as one-fourth of the initial dosage. If no response occurs within 48 hours, atropine sulfate is unlikely to be effective.

HOW SUPPLIED - RATED THERAPEUTICALLY EQUIVALENT:

Solution - Oral - 0.025 mg/2.5 mg

5 ml x 40	$32.49	Diphenoxylate W/Atropine, Roxane	00054-8191-16
10 ml x 40	$53.54	Diphenoxylate/Atropine, Roxane	00054-8171-16
60 ml	$6.28	Diphenoxylate Hcl & Atropine Sulf, Roxane	00054-3194-46
60 ml	**$12.97**	**LOMOTIL LIQUID 2.5/0.025, Searle**	**00025-0066-02**

Tablet, Uncoated - Oral - 0.025 mg/2.5 mg

100's	$2.42	Diphenoxylate W/Atropine, H.C.F.A. F F P	99999-0339-01
100's	$2.80	LATROPINE, Major Pharms	00904-0032-60
100's	$3.06	Diphenoxylate W/Atropine, Voluntary Hosp	53258-0607-01
100's	$3.15	LOGEN, Goldline Labs	00182-1006-01
100's	$3.80	Diphenoxylate W/Atropine, Qualitest Pharms	00603-3360-21
100's	$4.03	Diphenoxylate/Atropine, Schein Pharm (US)	00364-0449-01
100's	$4.45	Diphenoxylate Hcl & Atropine Sulfate, HL Moore Drug Exch	00839-6120-06
100's	$4.53	Diphenoxylate/Atropine Sulfate Table, Caremark	00339-4037-12
100's	$4.75	Diphenoxylate/Atropine, Halsey Drug	00879-0367-01
100's	$5.91	Diphenoxylate W/Atropine, Voluntary Hosp	53258-0607-13
100's	$6.35	DI-ATRO, MD Pharm	43567-0535-07
100's	$7.50	Diphenoxylate/Atropine, Goldline Labs	00182-8180-89
100's	$8.18	Diphenoxylate/Atropine, Vangard Labs	00615-0429-13
100's	$8.18	Diphenoxylate/Atropine, Vangard Labs	00615-0429-47
100's	$8.39	LONOX, Geneva Pharms	00781-1262-01
100's	$10.92	Diphenoxylate W/Atropine, Roxane	00054-8200-25
100's	$16.25	Diphenoxylate W/Atropine, Roxane	00054-8200-24
100's	**$43.93**	**LOMOTIL 2.5, Searle**	**00025-0061-31**
100's	**$46.52**	**LOMOTIL 2.5, Searle**	**00025-0061-34**
250's	$28.41	Diphenoxylate W/Atropine, Roxane	00054-8196-11
500's	$12.10	Diphenoxylate W/Atropine, H.C.F.A. F F P	99999-0339-02
500's	$12.35	LOGEN, Goldline Labs	00182-1006-05
500's	$17.79	Diphenoxylate Hcl & Atropine Sulfate, Schein Pharm (US)	00364-0449-05
500's	$23.45	DI-ATRO, MD Pharm	43567-0535-11
500's	$40.26	LONOX, Geneva Pharms	00781-1262-05
500's	**$208.51**	**LOMOTIL 2.5, Searle**	**00025-0061-51**
1000's	$16.00	LOMOCOT, C O Truxton	00463-6286-10
1000's	$18.10	Diphenoxylate W/Atropine, Qualitest Pharms	00603-3360-32
1000's	$19.40	LOGEN, Goldline Labs	00182-1006-10
1000's	$19.70	LATROPINE, Major Pharms	00904-0032-80
1000's	$20.86	Diphenoxylate Hcl & Atropine Sulfate, HL Moore Drug Exch	00839-6120-16
1000's	$22.61	Diphenoxylate Hcl 2.5, Aligen Independ	00405-0080-03
1000's	$24.20	Diphenoxylate W/Atropine, H.C.F.A. F F P	99999-0339-03
1000's	$25.00	Diphenoxylate Hcl W/Atropine Sulfate, Halsey Drug	00879-0367-10
1000's	$25.89	Diphenoxylate Hcl & Atropine Sulfate, Schein Pharm (US)	00364-0449-02
1000's	$30.00	DI-ATRO, MD Pharm	43567-0535-12
1000's	$34.28	Diphenoxylate Hcl & Atropine Sulfate, Purepac Pharm	00228-2049-96
1000's	$69.95	Di-Atro, Quality Res Pharms	52765-1131-00
1000's	$72.52	LONOX, Geneva Pharms	00781-1262-10
1000's	$79.95	Diphenoxylate/Atropine Sulfate, Harber Pharm	51432-0262-06
1000's	$85.80	Diphenoxylate Hcl W/ Atropine Sulfate, Mylan	00378-0415-10
1000's	**$388.63**	**LOMOTIL 2.5, Searle**	**00025-0061-52**
2500's	$60.50	Diphenoxylate W/Atropine, H.C.F.A. F F P	99999-0339-04
2500's	**$947.25**	**LOMOTIL 2.5, Searle**	**00025-0061-55**

ATROPINE SULFATE; EDROPHONIUM CHLORIDE *(003101)*

CATEGORIES: Anesthesia; Antagonists and Antidotes; Anti-Muscarinics; Diagnostic Agents; Myasthenia Gravis; Respiratory Depression; Pregnancy Category C; FDA Class 4C ("Little or No Therapeutic Advantage"); FDA Approved 1991 Nov

BRAND NAMES: **Enlon-Plus**

DESCRIPTION:

Enlon-Plus (edrophonium chloride, USP and atropine sulfate, USP) Injection, for intravenous use, is a sterile, nonpyrogenic, nondepolarizing neuromuscular relaxant antagonist. Edrophonium chloride, USP and atropine sulfate, USP is a combination drug containing a rapid acting acetylcholinesterase inhibitor, edrophonium chloride, and an anticholinergic, atropine sulfate. Chemically, edrophonium chloride is ethyl (m-hydroxyphenyl) dimethylammonium chloride.

Molecular Formula: $C_{10}H_{16}ClNO$

Molecular Weight: 201.70

Chemically, atropine sulfate is: endo-(±)-alpha-(hydroxymethyl)-8-methyl-8- azabicyclo (3,2,1) oct-3-yl benzeneacetate sulfate (2:1) monohydrate.

Molecular Formula: $(C_{17}H_{23}NO_3)_2.H_2SO_4.H_2O$

Molecular Weight: 694.84

Edrophonium Chloride, USP and Atropine Sulfate, USP contains in each ml of sterile solution:

5 ml Ampuls: 10 mg edrophonium chloride and 0.14 mg atropine sulfate compounded with 2.0 mg sodium sulfite as a preservative and buffered with sodium citrate and citric acid. The pH is adjusted in the range of 4.4-4.6.

15 ml Multidose Vials: 10 mg edrophonium chloride and 0.14 mg atropine sulfate compounded with 2.0 mg sodium sulfite and 4.5 mg phenol as a preservative and buffered with sodium citrate and citric acid. The pH is adjusted in the range of 4.4-4.6.

CLINICAL PHARMACOLOGY:

PHARMACODYNAMICS

Edrophonium chloride, USP and atropine sulfate, USP Injection is a combination of an anticholinesterase agent, which antagonizes the action of nondepolarizing neuromuscular blocking drugs, and a parasympatholytic (anticholinergic) drug, which prevents the muscarinic effects caused by inhibition of acetylcholine breakdown by the anticholinesterase. Edrophonium chloride antagonizes the effect of nondepolarizing neuromuscular blocking agents primarily by inhibiting or inactivating acetylcholinesterase. By inactivating the acetylcholinesterase enzyme, acetylcholine is not hydrolyzed as rapidly by acetylcholinesterase and is thereby allowed to accumulate. The greater quantity of acetylcholine reaching the sites of nicotinic cholinergic postjunctional receptors improves transmission of impulses across the myoneural junction. The concomitant, unavoidable accumulation of acetylcholine at the sites of muscarinic cholinergic transmission occurring at the parasympathetic, postganglionic receptors of the autonomic nervous system, may cause **bradycardia, bronchoconstriction, increased secretions,** and other parasympathomimetic side effects. The magnitude of these muscarinic side effects can be expected to vary from patient to patient depending upon the amount of vagal nerve activity present. Atropine sulfate counteracts these side effects.

Intravenous edrophonium chloride in doses of 0.5 to 1.0 mg/kg promptly antagonizes the effects of nondepolarizing muscle relaxants reaching the maximum antagonism within 1.2 minutes. A plateau of maximal antagonism is sustained for 70 minutes.[1] Intravenous atropine sulfate has an immediate effect on heart rate which reaches a peak in 2 to 16 minutes and lasts 170 minutes after an average 0.02 mg/kg dose.

PHARMACOKINETICS

Edrophonium Chloride: Edrophonium chloride given intravenously shows first order elimination in a two compartment open pharmacokinetic model.[3] Onset of reversal of muscle relaxant induced depression in twitch tension occurs within three minutes. Edrophonium is primarily renally excreted with 67% of the dose appearing in the urine.[4]Hepatic metabolism and biliary excretion have also been demonstrated in animals[4,8]. While infants and children have been shown to have a reduced plasma half-life and an increased clearance of edrophonium, doses in children are not significantly different from adults on a mg/kg basis although they are more variable in effect. Conversely, elderly subjects (>75 years old) have a prolonged plasma half-life and a reduced clearance. Studies have shown that in spite of these changes the onset and duration of action unchanged in these patients. (TABLE 1)

TABLE 1 Table of Pharmacokinetic Values for Edrophonium Chloride

Population	T 1/2β hr ± S.D.	VD L/kg ± S.D.	Cl ml/kg/min ± S.D.	N	Ref.
Adults	1.8 ± 0.6	1.1 ± 0.2	9.6 ± 2.7	10	3
Anephric Patients*†	3.4 ± 1.0	0.68 ± 0.13	2.7 ± 1.4	6	4
Infants (3 wks-11 mos)	1.2 ± 0.5	1.2 ± 0.2	17.8 ± 1.2	4	5
Children (1-6 yr)	1.6 ± 0.5	1.2 ± 0.7	14.2 ± 7.3	4	5
Adults	‡0.9 ± 0.3	1.1 ± 0.6	13.3 ± 5	5	6
Elderly* (over 75 yr)	‡1.4 ± 0.3	0.6 ± 0.1	5.1 ± 1	5	6

* No adjustments of edrophonium dosage are required because elimination of non-depolarizing muscle relaxants is similarly decreased.
† Values for anephric patients were calculated using a non-compartmental model.
‡ From a study using a different, less sensitive HPLC method and fitting C vs T data to a biexponential curve.
T 1/2β = Elimination half-life
VD = Volume of distribution
Cl = Clearance

Atropine Sulfate: Atropine sulfate given intravenously shows first order elimination in a two compartment open model[7]. Approximately 57% of a dose of atropine appears in the urine as unchanged drug. Tropine is the primary hepatic metabolite of atropine and it accounts for approximately 30% of the dose[2]. Atropine is only 14 ± 9% bound to plasma proteins[7]. Atropine clearance in children under 2 years old and in the elderly is decreased in relation to normal healthy adult males (TABLE 2).

TABLE 2 Table of Pharmacokinetic Values for Atropine Sulfate

Population	T1/2β hr ± S.D.	VD L/kg ± S.D.	Cl ml/kg/min ± S.D.	N	Ref.
Adults	3.0 ± 0.9	1.6 ± 0.4	6.8 ± 2.9	8	7
Children (0.08-10 yrs)	4.8 ± 3.5	2.2 ± 1.5	6.4 ± 3.9	13	7
Elderly (65-75 yrs)*	10.0 ± 7.3	1.8 ± 1.2	2.9 ± 1.9	10	7

* No dose adjustment required because the cardiovascular effect of atropine is diminished in the elderly.
T 1/2β = Elimination half-life
VD = Volume of distribution
Cl = Clearance

INDICATIONS AND USAGE:

Edrophonium chloride, USP and atropine sulfate, USP Injection is recommended as a reversal agent or antagonist of nondepolarizing neuromuscular blocking agents. It is not effective against depolarizing neuromuscular blocking agents. It is also useful if used adjunctively in the treatment of respiratory depression caused by curare overdosage.

The appropriateness of the specific fixed ratio of edrophonium had atropine contained in Edrophonium Chloride, USP and Atropine Sulfate, USP has not been evaluated in myasthenia gravis. Therefore, Edrophonium Chloride, USP and Atropine Sulfate, USP is not recommended for use in the differential diagnosis of this condition.

CONTRAINDICATIONS:

Edrophonium chloride, USP and atropine sulfate, USP Injection is not to be used in patients with known hypersensitivity to either of the components, or in patients with intestinal or urinary obstruction of mechanical type. Atropine sulfate is contraindicated in the presence of acute glaucoma, adhesions (synechiae) between the iris and lens of the eye, and pyloric stenosis.

WARNINGS:

Edrophonium chloride, USP and atropine sulfate, USP Injection should be used with caution in patients with bronchial asthma or cardiac arrhythmias. Cardiac arrest has been reported to occur in digitalized patients as well as in jaundiced subjects receiving cholinesterase inhibitors. In patients with cardiovascular disease, given anesthesia with narcotic and nitrous oxide without a potent inhalational agent, there is increased risk for clinically significant bradycardia. In patients receiving beta-adrenergic blocking agents there is increased risk for

WARNINGS: *(cont'd)*

excessive bradycardia from unopposed parasympathetic vagal tone. Such patients should receives atropine sulfate alone prior to Edrophonium Chloride, USP and Atropine Sulfate, USP. Isolated instances of respiratory arrest have also been reported following the administration of edrophonium chloride. Additional atropine sulfate (1 mg) should be available for immediate use to counteract severe cholinergic reaction which may occur in hypersensitive individuals when Edrophonium Chloride, USP and Atropine Sulfate, USP is used.

Edrophonium Chloride, USP and Atropine Sulfate, USP contains sodium sulfate, a sulfite that may cause allergic- type reactions including anaphylactic symptoms and life-threatening or less severe asthmatic episodes in certain susceptible people. The overall prevalence of sulfite sensitivity in the general population is unknown and probably low. Sulfite sensitivity is seen more frequently in asthmatic than in nonasthmatic people.

There is a potential for tissue irritation by extravascular injection.

PRECAUTIONS:

General: As with any antagonist of nondepolarizing muscle relaxants, adequate recovery of voluntary respiration and neuromuscular transmission must be obtained prior to the discontinuation of respiratory assistance. Should a patient develop "anticholinesterase insensitivity" for brief or prolonged periods, the patient should be carefully monitored and the dosage of anticholinesterase drugs reduced or withheld until the patient again becomes sensitive to them. Use with caution in patients with prostatic hypertrophy and in debilitated patients with chronic lung disease.

When used in therapeutic doses, atropine can cause dryness of the mouth. This effect is additive when the product is administered with other drugs that can cause dryness of the mouth.

Since atropine sulfate slows gastric emptying and gastrointestinal motility, it may interfere with the absorption of other medications. The effect of atropine on dryness of the mouth may be increased if it is given with other drugs that have anticholinergic action (tricyclic antidepressants, antipsychotics, some antihistamines, and antiparkinsonism drugs).

Pregnancy Category C: Animal reproduction studies have not been conducted with Edrophonium Chloride, USP and Atropine Sulfate, USP. It is also not known whether Edrophonium Chloride, USP and Atropine Sulfate, USP can cause fetal harm when administered to a pregnant woman or can affect reproduction capacity. Edrophonium Chloride, USP and Atropine Sulfate, USP should be used during pregnancy only if the potential benefit justifies to potential risk to the fetus.

Labor and Delivery: The effect of Edrophonium Chloride, USP and Atropine Sulfate, USP on the mother and fetus, on the duration of labor or delivery, in the possibility that a forceps delivery or other intervention or resuscitation of the newborn will be necessary, is not known. The effect of the combination drug on the later growth, development and functional maturation of the child is also unknown.

Nursing Mothers: The safety of Edrophonium Chloride, USP and Atropine Sulfate, USP during lactation in humans has not been established.

Pediatric Use: Safety and effectiveness in children have not been established. Pediatric patients may have increased vagal tone. The effect of fixed ratios of edrophonium and atropine on heart rate in such patients has not been evaluated.

DRUG INTERACTIONS:

Edrophonium chloride, USP and atropine sulfate, USP Injection should not be administered prior to the administration of any nondepolarizing muscle relaxants. It should administered with caution to patients with symptoms of myasthenic weakness who are also on anticholinesterase drugs. Anticholinesterase overdosage (cholinergic crisis) symptoms may mimic underdosage (myasthenic weakness), so the use of this drug may worsen the condition of these patients (see OVERDOSAGE for treatment).

Narcotic analgesics, except when combined with potent inhaled anesthetics, appear to potentiate the effect of edrophonium on the sinus node and conduction system, increasing both the frequency and duration of bradycardia. In patients with cardiovascular disease, given anesthesia with narcotic and nitrous oxide without a potent inhalational agent, there is increased risk for clinically significant bradycardia. In patients receiving beta-adrenergic blocking agents there is increased risk for excessive bradycardia from unopposed parasympathetic vagal tone. Such patients should receive atropine sulfate alone prior to Edrophonium Chloride, USP and Atropine Sulfate, USP.

Compared to muscle relaxants with some vagolytic activity, muscle relaxants with no vagolytic effects (*i.e.*, vecuronium) may be associated with a slightly higher incidence of vagotonic effects such as bradycardia and first-degree heart block when reversed with Edrophonium Chloride, USP and Atropine Sulfate, USP.

ADVERSE REACTIONS:

Cardiovascular: Arrhythmias Frequency >10%: junctional rhythm, bradycardia, tachycardia:

Frequency 3-10%: first and second degree A-V block, P Wave changes, atrial premature contractions;

Frequency 1-3%: third degree A-V block, ventricular premature contractions;

Frequency less than 1%: 3 second R-R interval.

Of the patients who experienced any arrhythmias, 85% had the onset within two minutes, 74% on longer had any arrhythmias after 10 minutes. Arrhythmias related to increased vagal tone, bradycardia, second and third degree heart block respond to treatment with 0.2 - 0.4 mg of atropine IV (Bigeminy or ventricular ectopy may be treated with lidocaine 50 mg IV).

Adverse experiences reported for anticholinesterase agents such as edrophonium chloride, but observed in the 235 patients studied with Edrophonium chloride, USP and atropine sulfate, USP Injection:

Cardiovascular: Nonspecific EKG changes, fall in cardiac output leading to hypotension;

Respiratory: Increased tracheobronchial secretions, laryngospasm, bronchiolar constriction and respiratory muscle paralysis;

Neurologic: Convulsions, dysarthria, dysphonia, and dysphagia;

Gastrointestinal: Nausea, vomiting, increased peristalsis, increased gastric and intestinal secretions, diarrhea, abdominal cramps;

Musculoskeletal: Weakness and fasciculations;

Miscellaneous: Increased urinary frequency, diaphoresis, increased lacrimation, pupillary constriction, diplopia, and conjunctival hyperemia.

Untoward reactions to atropine sulfate generally are dose-related. Individual tolerance varies greatly but systemic doses of 0.5 to 10 mg are likely to produce the following effects, which were not observed in the 235 patients treated with Edrophonium Chloride, USP and Atropine Sulfate, USP:

Neurologic: Speech disturbances and restlessness with asthenia;

Dermatologic: Flushed, dry skin, formation of a scarlatiniform rash;

Miscellaneous: Dryness of the nose and mouth, thirst, blurred vision, photophobia, slight mydriasis. Atropine may produce fever through inhibition of heat loss by evaporation.

OVERDOSAGE:

Muscarinic symptoms (nausea, vomiting, diarrhea, sweating, increased bronchial and salivary secretions and bradycardia) may appear with overdosage (cholinergic crisis) of Edrophonium chloride, USP and atropine sulfate, USP Injection, but may be managed by the use of additional atropine sulfate. Obstruction of the airway by bronchial secretions can arise and may be managed with suction (especially if tracheostomy has been performed).

Should edrophonium chloride overdosage occur:

1. Maintain respiratory exchange.

2. Monitor cardiac function.

Appropriate measures should be taken if convulsions occur or shock is present.

Principal manifestations of overdosage (poisoning) with atropine sulfate are delirium, tachycardia and fever. In the treatment of atropine poisoning, respiratory assistance and symptomatic support are indicated. Death is usually due to paralysis of the medullary centers.

In the clinical studies performed with Edrophonium chloride, USP and atropine sulfate, USP Injection, there were no reported overdoses and therefore no clinical information is available regarding overdosing with Edrophonium Chloride, USP and Atropine Sulfate, USP.

DOSAGE AND ADMINISTRATION:

Dosages of Edrophonium chloride, USP and atropine sulfate, USP Injection range from 0.05-0.1 ml/kg given slowly over 45 seconds to 1 minute at a point of at least 5% recovery of twitch response to neuromuscular stimulation (95% block). The dosage delivered is 0.5-1.0 mg/kg of edrophonium chloride and 0.007-0.014 mg/kg of atropine sulfate. A total dosage of 1.0 mg/kg of edrophonium chloride should rarely be exceeded. Response should be monitored carefully and assisted or controlled ventilation secured. Satisfactory reversal permits adequate voluntary respiration and neuromuscular transmission (as tested with a peripheral nerve stimulator). Recurarization had not been reported after satisfactory reversal has been attained.

Parenteral drug products should be inspected visually for particulate matter and discoloration prior to administration.

REFERENCES:

1. Cronnelly R, Morris RB, Miller RD: Edrophonium: Duration of action and atropine requirement in humans during halothane anesthesia. Anesthesiology 1982;57:261-266. **2.** Hinderling PH, Gundert-Remy U, Schmidlin O, Heinzel G: Integrated pharmacokinetics and pharmacodynamics of atropine in healthy humans I: Pharmacokinetics; II: Pharmacodynamics. J Pharmaceutical Sci 1985;74:I-703-710; II-711-717. **3.** Morris RB, Cronnelly R, Miller RD, Stanski DR, Fahey MR: Pharmacokinetics of edrophonium and neostigmine when antagonizing d-tubocurarine neuromuscular blockade in man. Anesthesiology 1981;54:399-402. **4.** Morris RB, Cronnelly R, Miller RD, Stanski DR, Fahey MR: Pharmacokinetics of edrophonium in anephric and renal transplant patients. Br J Anaesth 1981;53:1311-1313. **5.** Fisher DM, Cronnelly R, Sharma M, Miller RD: Clinical pharmacology of edrophonium in infants and children. Anesthesiology 1984;61:428-433. **6.** Silverberg PA, Matteo RS, Ornstein E, Young WL, Diaz J: Pharmacokinetics and pharmacodynamics of edrophonium in the elderly. Anesth Analg 1986;65:S142. **7.** Virtanen R, Kanto J. Iisalo E, Iisalo EU, Salo M, Sjovall S: Pharmacokinetic studies on atropine with special reference to age. Acta Anaesthesiol Scand 1982;26:297-300. **8.** Back DJ, Calvey TN: Excretion of ^{14}C-edrophonium and its metabolites in bile: role of the liver cell and the peribiliary vascular plexus. Br J Pharmacol., 1972; 44:534.

HOW SUPPLIED - EQUIVALENTS NOT AVAILABLE:

Injection, Solution - Intramuscular; - 10 mg/ml

5 ml	**$4.95**	**ENLON-PLUS, Ohmeda Pharm**	**10019-0195-05**
5 ml	**$6.19**	**ENLON-PLUS, Ohmeda Pharm**	**10019-0180-05**
15 ml	**$12.86**	**ENLON-PLUS, Ohmeda Pharm**	**10019-0195-15**

ATROPINE; PHENOBARBITAL *(002006)*

CATEGORIES: Anticholinergic Agents; Antimuscarinics/Antispasmodics; Autonomic Drugs; DESI Drugs; Gastrointestinal Drugs; DEA Class CIV; FDA Pre 1938 Drugs

BRAND NAMES: Antrocol

Prescribing information not available at time of publication.

HOW SUPPLIED - EQUIVALENTS NOT AVAILABLE:

Elixir - Oral - 0.039 mg/3 mg

480 ml	$21.00	ANTROCOL, ECR Pharms	00095-0042-16

ATROPINE; PREDNISOLONE *(000345)*

CATEGORIES: Cycloplegics/Mydriatics; EENT Drugs; Eye, Ear, Nose, & Throat Preparations; Mydriatics; Ocular Infections; Ophthalmics; FDA Pre 1938 Drugs

BRAND NAMES: Mydrapred

Prescribing information not available at time of publication.

HOW SUPPLIED - EQUIVALENTS NOT AVAILABLE:

Suspension - Ophthalmic; Top - 1 %/0.25 %

5 ml	$12.50	MYDRAPRED, Alcon-PR	00998-0619-05

AURANOFIN *(000347)*

CATEGORIES: Antiarthritics; Arthritis; Gold; Nonsteroidal Anti-Inflammatory; Pain; Synovitis; Pregnancy Category C; FDA Approved 1985 May; Patent Expiration 1992 Jan

BRAND NAMES: *Aktil*; *Crisinor*; *Crisofin*; **Ridaura**; *Ridaura Tiltab*; *Ridauran* (France)
(International brand names outside U.S. in italics)

FORMULARIES: Aetna; BC-BS; Medi-Cal; PCS

WARNING:
Auranofin contains gold and, like other gold-containing drugs, can cause gold toxicity, signs of which include fall in hemoglobin, leukopenia below 4,000 WBC/cu mm, granulocytes below 1,500/cu mm, decrease in platelets below 150,000 cu mm, proteinuria, hematuria, pruritus, rash, stomatitis or persistent diarrhea. Therefore, the results of recommended laboratory work (See PRECAUTIONS) should be reviewed before writing each Ridaura prescription. Like other gold preparations, Ridaura is only indicated for use in selected patients with active rheumatoid arthritis. Physicians planning to use Ridaura should be experienced with chrysotherapy and should thoroughly familiarize themselves with the toxicity and benefits of Ridaura.

In addition, the following precautions should be routinely employed:
1. The possibility of adverse reactions should be explained to patients before starting therapy.
2. Patients should be advised to report promptly any symptoms suggesting toxicity. (See PRECAUTIONS, Information for the Patient.)

DESCRIPTION:

Ridaura (auranofin) is available in oral form as capsules containing 3 mg auranofin.

Auranofin is (2,3,4,6-tetra-O-acetyl-1-thio-β-D-glucopyranosato-S-) (triethyl-phosphine) gold.

Auranofin contains 29% gold.

Each Ridaura capsule, with opaque brown cap and opaque tan body, contains auranofin, 3 mg, and is imprinted with the product name RIDAURA and SKF. Inactive ingredients consist of benzyl alcohol, cellulose, cetylpyridinium chloride, D&C Red No. 33, FD&C Blue No. 1, FD&C Red No. 40, FD&C Yellow No. 6, gelatin, lactose, magnesium stearate, povidone, sodium lauryl sulfate, sodium starch glycolate, starch, titanium dioxide and trace amounts of other inactive ingredients.

CLINICAL PHARMACOLOGY:

The mechanism of action of auranofin is not understood. In patients with adult rheumatoid arthritis, auranofin may modify disease activity as manifested by synovitis and associated symptoms, and reflected by laboratory parameters such as ESR. There is no substantial evidence, however, that gold-containing compounds induce remission of rheumatoid arthritis.

Pharmacokinetics: Pharmacokinetic studies were performed in rheumatoid arthritis patients, not in normal volunteers. Auranofin is rapidly metabolized and intact auranofin has never been detected in the blood. Thus, studies of the pharmacokinetics of auranofin have involved measurement of gold concentrations. Approximately 25% of the gold in auranofin is absorbed.

The mean terminal plasma half-life of auranofin gold at steady state was 26 days (range 21 to 31 days, n=5). The mean terminal body half-life was 80 days (range 42 to 128; n=5). Approximately 60% of the absorbed gold (15% of the administered dose) from a single dose of auranofin is excreted in urine; the remainder is excreted in the feces.

In clinical studies, steady state blood-gold concentrations are achieved in about three months. In patients on 6 mg auranofin/day, mean steady state blood-gold concentrations were 0.68 ± 0.45 mcg/ml (n = 63 patients). In blood, approximately 40% of auranofin gold is associated with red cells, and 60% associated with serum proteins. In contrast, 99% of injectable gold is associated with serum proteins.

Mean blood-gold concentrations are proportional to dose; however, no correlation between blood-gold concentrations and safety or efficacy has been established.

INDICATIONS AND USAGE:

Auranofin is indicated in the management of adults with active classical or definite rheumatoid arthritis (ARA criteria) who have had an insufficient therapeutic response to, or are intolerant of, an adequate trial of full doses of one or more nonsteroidal anti-inflammatory drugs. Auranofin should be added to a comprehensive baseline program, including non-drug therapies.

Unlike anti-inflammatory drugs, auranofin does not produce an immediate response. Therapeutic effects may be seen after three to four months of treatment, although improvement has not been seen in some patients before six months.

When cartilage and bone damage has already occurred, gold cannot reverse structural damage to joints caused by previous disease. The greatest potential benefit occurs in patients with active synovitis, particularly in its early stage.

In controlled clinical trials comparing auranofin with injectable gold, auranofin was associated with fewer dropouts due to adverse reactions, while injectable gold was associated with fewer dropouts for inadequate or poor therapeutic effect. Physicians should consider these findings when deciding on the use of auranofin in patients who are candidates for chrysotherapy.

CONTRAINDICATIONS:

Auranofin is contraindicated in patients with a history of any of the following gold-induced disorders: anaphylactic reactions, necrotizing enterocolitis, pulmonary fibrosis, exfoliative dermatitis, bone marrow aplasia or other severe hematologic disorders.

WARNINGS:

Danger signs of possible gold toxicity include fail in hemoglobin, leukopenia below 4,000 WBC/cu mm, granulocytes below 1,500/cu mm, decrease in platelets below 150,000/cu mm, proteinuria, hematuria, pruritus, rash, stomatitis or persistent diarrhea.

Thrombocytopenia has occurred in 1-3% of patients (See ADVERSE REACTIONS) treated with auranofin, some of whom developed bleeding. The thrombocytopenia usually appears to be peripheral in origin and is usually reversible upon withdrawal of auranofin. Its onset bears no relationship to the duration of auranofin therapy and its course may be rapid. While patients' platelet counts should normally be monitored at least monthly (See PRECAUTIONS, Laboratory Tests), the occurrence of a precipitous decline in platelets or a platelet count less than 100,000/cu mm or signs and symptoms (*e.g.,* purpura, ecchymoses or petechiae) suggestive of thrombocytopenia indicates a need to immediately withdraw auranofin and other therapies with the potential to cause thrombocytopenia, and to obtain additional platelet counts. No additional auranofin should be given unless the thrombocytopenia resolves and further studies show it was not due to gold therapy.

Proteinuria has developed in 3-9% of patients (See ADVERSE REACTIONS) treated with auranofin. If clinically significant proteinuria or microscopic hematuria is found (See PRECAUTIONS, Laboratory Tests), auranofin and other therapies with the potential to cause proteinuria or microscopic hematuria should be stopped immediately.

PRECAUTIONS:

GENERAL

The safety of concomitant use of auranofin with injectable gold, hydroxychloroquine, penicillamine, immunosuppressive agents (*e.g.,* cyclophosphamide, azathioprine, or methotrexate) or high doses of corticosteroids has not been established.

Medical problems that might affect the signs or symptoms used to detect auranofin toxicity should be under control before starting auranofin (auranofin).

The potential benefits of using auranofin in patients with progressive renal disease, significant hepatocellular disease, inflammatory bowel disease, skin rash or history of bone marrow depression should be weighed against 1) the potential risks of gold toxicity on organ systems previously compromised or with decreased reserve, and 2) the difficulty in quickly detecting and correctly attributing the toxic effect.

The following adverse reactions have been reported with the use of gold preparations and require modification of auranofin treatment or additional monitoring. See ADVERSE REACTIONS for the approximate incidence of those reactions specifically reported with auranofin.

PRECAUTIONS: *(cont'd)*

Gastrointestinal Reactions: Gastrointestinal reactions reported with gold therapy include diarrhea/loose stools, nausea, vomiting, anorexia and abdominal cramps. The most common reaction to auranofin is diarrhea/loose stools reported in approximately 50% of the patients. This is generally manageable by reducing the dosage (*e.g.*, from 6 mg daily to 3 mg) and in only 6% of the patients is it necessary to discontinue auranofin permanently.

Ulcerative enterocolitis is a rare serious gold reaction. Therefore, patients with gastrointestinal symptoms should be monitored for the appearance of gastrointestinal bleeding.

Cutaneous Reactions: Dermatitis is the most common reaction to injectable gold therapy and the second most common reaction to auranofin.*Any eruption, especially if pruritic, that develops during treatment should be considered a gold reaction until proven otherwise.* Pruritus often exists before dermatitis becomes apparent, and therefore should be considered to be a warning signal of a cutaneous reaction. Gold dermatitis may be aggravated by exposure to sunlight or an actinic rash may develop. The most serious form of cutaneous reaction reported with injectable gold is generalized exfoliative dermatitis.

Mucous Membrane Reactions: Stomatitis, another common gold reaction, may be manifested by shallow ulcers on the buccal membranes, on the borders of the tongue, and on the palate or in the pharynx. Stomatitis may occur as the only adverse reaction or with a dermatitis. Sometimes diffuse glossitis or gingivitis develops. A metallic taste may precede these oral mucous membrane reactions and should be considered a warning signal.

Renal Reactions: Gold can produce a nephrotic syndrome or glomerulitis with proteinuria and hematuria. These renal reactions are usually relatively mild and subside completely if recognized early and treatment is discontinued. They may become severe and chronic if treatment is continued after the onset of the reaction. *Therefore it is important to perform urinalysis regularly* and to discontinue treatment promptly if proteinuria or hematuria develops.

Hematologic Reactions: Blood dyscrasias including leukopenia, granulocytopenia, thrombocytopenia and aplastic anemia have all been reported as reactions to injectable gold and auranofin. These reactions may occur separately or in combination at anytime during treatment. Because they have potentially serious consequences, *blood dyscrasias should be constantly watched for through regular monitoring (at least monthly) of the formed elements of the blood throughout treatment.*

Miscellaneous Reactions: Rare reactions attributed to gold include cholestatic jaundice; gold bronchitis and interstitial pneumonitis and fibrosis; peripheral neuropathy; partial or complete hair loss; fever.

INFORMATION FOR THE PATIENT

Patients should be advised of the possibility of toxicity from auranofin and of the signs and symptoms that they should report promptly. (Patient information sheets are available).

Women of childbearing potential should be warned of the potential risks of auranofin therapy during pregnancy (see PRECAUTIONS, Pregnancy.)

LABORATORY TESTS

CBC with differential, platelet count, urinalysis, and renal and liver function tests should be performed prior to auranofin therapy to establish a baseline and to identify any preexisting conditions.

CBC with differential, platelet count and urinalysis should then be monitored at least monthly; other parameters should be monitored as appropriate.

CARCINOGENESIS, MUTAGENESIS

In a 24-month study in rats, animals treated with auranofin at 0.4, 1.0 or 2.5 mg/kg/day orally (3, 8 or 21 times the human dose) or gold sodium thiomalate at 2 or 6 mg/kg injected twice weekly (4 or 12 times the human dose) were compared to untreated control animals.

There was a significant increase in the frequency of renal tubular cell karyomegaly and cytomegaly and renal adenoma in the animals treated with 1.0 or 2.5 mg/kg/day of auranofin and 2 or 6 mg/kg twice weekly of gold sodium thiomalate. Malignant renal epithelial tumors were seen in the 1.0 mg/kg/day auranofin and in the 2.5 mg/kg/day auranofin and in the 6 mg/kg twice weekly gold sodium thiomalate-treated animals.

In a 12-month study, rats treated with auranofin at 23 mg/kg/day (192 times the human dose) developed tumors of the renal tubular epithelium, whereas those treated with 3.6 mg/kg/day (30 times the human dose) did not.

In an 18-month study in mice given oral auranofin at doses of 1,3, and 9 mg/kg/day (8, 24 and 72 times the human dose), there was no statistically significant increases above controls in the instances of tumors.

In the mouse lymphoma forward mutation assay, auranofin at high concentrations (313 to 700 ng/ml) induced increases in the mutation frequencies in the presence of a rat liver microsomal preparation. Auranofin produced no mutation effects in the AMES test (Salmonella), in the *in vitro* transformation of BALB/T3 cell mouse assay or in the Dominant Lethal Assay.

PREGNANCY, TERATOGENIC EFFECTS, PREGNANCY CATEGORY C

Use of auranofin by pregnant women is not recommended. Furthermore, women of childbearing potential should be warned of the potential risks of auranofin therapy during pregnancy.

Pregnant rabbits given auranofin at doses of 0.5, 3 or 6 mg/kg/day (4.2 to 50 times the human dose) had impaired food intake, decreased maternal and as well as fetal weights, and an increase in controls in the incidence of resorptions, abortions and congenital abnormalities, mainly abdominal defects such as gastroschisis and umbilical hernia.

Pregnant rats given auranofin at a dose of 5 mg/kg/day (42 times the human dose) had an increase above controls in the incidence of resorptions and a decrease in litter size and weight linked to maternal toxicity. No such effects were found in rats given 2.5 mg/kg/day (21 times the human dose).

Pregnant mice given auranofin at a dose of 5 mg/kg/day (42 times the human dose) had no teratogenic effects).

There are no adequate and well-controlled auranofin studies in pregnant women.

NURSING MOTHERS

Nursing during auranofin therapy is not recommended. Following auranofin administration to rats and mice, gold is excreted in milk. Following the administration of injectable gold, gold appears in the milk of nursing women; human data on auranofin are not available.

PEDIATRIC USE

Auranofin is not recommended for use in children because its safety and effectiveness have not been established.

DRUG INTERACTIONS:

In a single patient report, there is the suggestion that concurrent administration of auranofin and phenytoin may have increased phenytoin blood levels.

ADVERSE REACTIONS:

The adverse reactions incidences listed below are based on observations of 1) 4,784 auranofin-treated patients in clinical trials (2,474 U.S. 2,310 foreign), of whom 2,729 were treated more than one year and 573 for more than three years; and 2) postmarketing experience. The highest incidence is during the first six months of treatment; however reactions can occur after many months of therapy. With rare exceptions, all patients were on concomitant nonsteroidal anti-inflammatory therapy; some of them were also taking low dosages of corticosteroids.

Reactions occurring in more than 1% of Auranofin-treated patients

Gastrointestinal: loose stools or diarrhea (47%), abdominal pain (14%), nausea with or without vomiting (10%), constipation, anorexia*, flatulence*, dyspepsia*, dysgeusia

Dermatological: rash (24%), pruritus (17%), hair loss, urticaria

Mucous Membrane: stomatitis (13%), conjunctivitis*, glossitis

Hematological: anemia, leukopenia, thrombocytopenia, eosinophilia

Renal: proteinuria*, hematuria

Hepatic: elevated liver enzymes

*Reactions marked with an asterisk occurred in 3-9% of the patients. The other reactions listed occurred in 1-3%

Reactions occurring in less than 1% of Auranofin-treated patients

Gastrointestinal: dysphagia, gastrointestinal bleeding †, melena †, positive stool for occult blood†, ulcerative enterocolitis

Dermatological: angioedema

Mucous Membrane: gingivitis†

Hematological: aplastic anemia, neutropenia†, agranulocytosis, pure red cell aplasia, pancytopenia

Hepatic: jaundice

Respiratory: interstitial pneumonitis

Neurological: peripheral neuropathy

Ocular: gold deposits in the lens or cornea unassociated clinically with eye disorders or visual impairment

†Reactions marked with a dagger occurred in 0.1-1% of the patients. The other reactions listed occurred in less than 01%

Reactions reported with injectable gold preparations, but not with auranofin (based on clinical trials and on postmarketing experience)

Cutaneous Reactions: generalized exfoliative dermatitis

TABLE 1 Incidence of Adverse Reactions for Specific Categories-18 Comparative Trials:

	Auranofin (Ridaura) (445 patients)	Injectable Gold (445 Patients)
Proteinuria	0.9%	5.4%
Rash	26%	39%
Diarrhea	42.5%	13%
Stomatitis	13%	18%
Anemia	3.1%	2.7%
Leukopenia	1.3%	2.2%
Thrombocytopenia	0.9%	2.2%
Elevated Liver Function Tests	1.9%	1.7%
Pulmonary	0.2%	0.2%

OVERDOSAGE:

The acute oral LD_{50} for auranofin is 310 mg/kg in adult mice and 265 mg/kg in adult rats. The minimum lethal dose in rats is 30 mg/kg.

In case of acute overdosage, immediate induction of emesis or gastric lavage and appropriate supportive therapy is recommended.

Auranofin overdosage experience is limited. A 50-year old female, previously on 6 mg auranofin, took 27 mg (9 capsules) daily for 10 days and developed an encephalopathy and peripheral neuropathy. Auranofin was discontinued and she eventually recovered.

There has been no experience with treating auranofin overdosage with modalities such as chelating agents. However, they have been used with injectable gold and may be considered for auranofin overdosage.

DOSAGE AND ADMINISTRATION:

Usual Adult Dosage: The usual adult dosage of auranofin is 6 mg daily, given either as 3 mg twice daily or 6 mg once daily. Initiation of therapy at dosages exceeding 6 mg daily is not recommended because it is associated with an increased incidence of diarrhea. If response is inadequate after six months, an increase to 9 mg (3 mg three times daily) may be tolerated. If response remains inadequate after a three-month trial of 9 mg daily, auranofin therapy should be discontinued. Safety at dosages exceeding 9 mg daily has not yet been studied.

Transferring from Injectable Gold: In controlled clinical studies, patients on injectable gold have been transferred to auranofin by discontinuing the injectable agent and starting oral therapy with auranofin, 6 mg daily. When patients are transferred to auranofin, they should be informed of its adverse reaction profile, in particular, the gastrointestinal reactions (see PRECAUTIONS, Information for the Patient.) At six months, control of disease activity of patients transferred to auranofin and those maintained on the injectable agent was not different. Data found beyond six months are not available.

HOW SUPPLIED:

Capsules, containing 3 mg auranofin, in bottles of 60.

Storage: Store at controlled room temperature (59°-86°F). Dispense in a tight, light-resistant container.

HOW SUPPLIED - EQUIVALENTS NOT AVAILABLE:

Capsule, Gelatin - Oral - 3 mg

60's $69.00 RIDAURA, SKB Pharms 00007-4879-18

AUROTHIOGLUCOSE *(000348)*

CATEGORIES: Antiarthritics; Arthritis; Gold; Pain; Pregnancy Category C; FDA Pre 1938 Drugs

BRAND NAMES: *Aureotan* (Germany); *Auromyose*; *Gold-50*; *Lomosol*; **Solganal**; *Solganol*

(International brand names outside U.S. in italics)

> **WARNING:**
> Physicians planning to use Solganal Suspension should thoroughly familiarize themselves with its toxicity and its benefits. The possibility of toxic reactions should always be explained to the patient before starting therapy. Patients should be warned to report promptly any symptom suggesting toxicity. Before each injection of Solganal Suspension, the physician should review the results of laboratory work and see the patient to determine the presence or absence of adverse reactions, since some of these can be severe or even fatal.

DESCRIPTION:

Solganal is a sterile suspension, for **intramuscular injection only**. Solganal Suspension is an antiarthritic agent which is absorbed gradually following intramuscular injection, producing a therapeutically desired prolonged effect.

Each ml contains 50 mg of aurothioglucose, USP in sterile sesame oil with 2% aluminum monostearate; 1 mg propylparaben is added as preservative. Aurothioglucose contains approximately 50% gold by weight.

The empirical formula for aurothioglucose is $C_6H_{11}AuO_5S$; the molecular weight is 392.18. Chemically it is (1-Thio-D-glucopyranosato) gold.

Aurothioglucose is a nearly odorless, yellow powder which is stable in air. An aqueous solution is unstable on long standing. Aurothioglucose is freely soluble in water but practically insoluble in acetone, in alcohol, in chloroform, and in ether.

CLINICAL PHARMACOLOGY:

Although the mechanism of action is not well understood, gold compounds have been reported to decrease synovial inflammation and retard cartilage and bone destruction.

Gold is absorbed from injection sites, reaching peak concentration in blood in four to six hours. Following a single intramuscular injection of 50 mg aurothioglucose in each of two patients, peak serum levels were abort 235 mcg/dl in one patient and 450 mcg/dl in other. In plasma, 95% is bound to the albumin fraction. Approximately 70% of the gold is eliminated in the urine and approximately 30% in the feces. When a standard weekly treatment schedule is followed, approximately 40% of the administered dose is excreted each week, and the remainder is excreted over a longer period. The biological half-life of gold salts following a single 50 mg dose has been reported to range from 3 to 27 days. Following successive weekly doses, the half-life increases and may be 14 to 40 days after the third dose and up to 168 days after the eleventh weekly dose.

After the initial injection, the serum level of gold rises sharply and declines over the next week. Peak levels with aqueous preparations are higher and decline faster than those with oily preparations. Weekly administration produces a continuous rise in the basal value for several months, after which the serum level becomes relatively stable. After a standard weekly dose, considerable individual variation in the levels of gold has been found. A steady decline in gold levels occurs when the interval between injections is lengthened, and small amounts may be found in the serum for months after discontinuance of therapy. The incidence of toxic reactions is apparently unrelated to the plasma level of gold, but it may be related to the cumulative body content of gold.

Storage of gold in human tissues is dependent upon organ mass as well as upon the concentration of gold. Therefore, tissues having the highest gold levels (weight/weight) do not necessarily contain the greatest total amounts of gold. The major depots, in decreasing order of total gold content, are the bone marrow, liver, skin, and bone, accounting for approximately 85% of body gold. The highest concentrations of gold are found in the lymph nodes, adrenal glands, liver, kidneys, bone marrow, and spleen. Relatively small concentrations are found in articular structures.

Gold passes the blood-brain barrier in hamsters.

Transfer of gold across the human placenta at the twentieth week of pregnancy has been documented. The placenta showed numerous gold deposits and smaller amounts were detected in the fetal liver and kidneys; other tissues provided no evidence of gold deposition.

Gold is excreted into human milk in significant amounts and trace amounts can be demonstrated in the blood of nursing infants. (See PRECAUTIONS, Nursing Mothers.)

INDICATIONS AND USAGE:

Aurothioglucose is indicated for the adjunctive treatment of early active rheumatoid arthritis (both of the adult and juvenile types) not adequately controlled by other anti-inflammatory agents and conservative measures. In chronic, advanced cases of rheumatoid arthritis, gold therapy is less valuable.

Antirheumatic measures such as salicylates and other antiinflammatory drugs (both steroidal and non-steroidal) may be continued after initiation of gold therapy. After improvement commences, these measures may be discontinued slowly as symptoms permit.

See PRECAUTIONS, Laboratory Tests and DOSAGE AND ADMINISTRATION.

CONTRAINDICATIONS:

A history of known hypersensitivity to any component of aurothioglucose contraindicates its use. Gold therapy is contraindicated in patients with uncontrolled diabetes mellitus, severe debilitation, systemic lupus erythematosus, renal disease, hepatic dysfunction, uncontrolled congestive heart failure, marked hypertension, agranulocytosis, other blood dyscrasias, or hemorrhagic diathesis; or if there is a history of infectious hepatitis. Patients who recently have had radiation, and those who have developed severe toxicity from previous exposure to gold or other heavy metals should not receive aurothioglucose.

Urticaria, eczema, and colitis are also contraindications.

Gold therapy is usually contraindicated in pregnancy. (See PRECAUTIONS, Usage in Pregnancy.)

Gold salts should not be used with penicillamine (see ADVERSE REACTIONS) or antimalarials. The safety of coadministration with immunosuppressive agents other than corticosteroids has not been established.

WARNINGS:

The following signs should be considered danger signals of gold toxicity, and no additional injection should be given unless further studies reveal some other cause for their presence: rapid reduction of hemoglobin, leukopenia (WBC below 400/cu mm), eosinophilia above 5% platelet count below 100,000/cu mm, albuminuria, hematuria, pruritus, dermatitis, stomatitis, jaundice, and petechiae.

Effects that may occur immediately following an injection, or at any time during gold therapy, include: anaphylactic shock, syncope, bradycardia, thickening of the tongue, difficulty in swallowing and breathing, and angioneurotic edema. If such effects are observed, treatment with aurothioglucose should be discontinued.

Tolerance to gold usually decreases with advancing age. Diabetes mellitus or congestive heart failure should be under control before gold therapy is instituted.

WARNINGS: *(cont'd)*

Aurothioglucose should be used with extreme caution in patients with: skin rash, hypersensitivity to other medications, or a history of renal or liver disease.

PRECAUTIONS:

GENERAL

Before **each** injection, the physician should personally check the patient for adverse reactions and inquiry should be made regarding pruritus, rash, sore mouth, indigestion, and metallic taste. The patient should be observed for at least 15 minutes following each injection. (See also Laboratory Tests.)

Patients with HLA-D locus histocompatibility antigens DRw2 and DRw3 have a genetic predisposition to develop certain toxic reactions, such as proteinuria, during treatment with gold or D-penicillamine.

Aurothioglucose should be used with caution in patients with compromised cardiovascular or cerebral circulation.

INFORMATION FOR THE PATIENT

1. Promptly report to the physician any unusual symptoms such as pruritus (itching), rash, sore mouth, indigestion, or metallic taste.

2. Increased joint pain may occur for one or two days after an injection and usually subsides after the first few injections.

3. Exposure to sunlight or artificial ultraviolet light should be minimized.

4. Careful oral hygiene is recommended in conjunction with therapy.

5. Patients should be aware of potential hazards if they become pregnant while receiving gold therapy. (See Usage in Pregnancy.)

LABORATORY TESTS

Before treatment is started, a complete blood count, platelet count, and urinalysis should be done to serve as reference points. Since gold therapy is usually contraindicated in pregnant patients, pregnancy should be ruled out before treatment is started. Throughout the treatment period, urinalysis should be repeated prior to each injection, and complete blood cell and platelet counts should be performed every two weeks. A platelet count is indicated any time that purpura or ecchymosis occurs.

CARCINOGENESIS, MUTAGENESIS, AND IMPAIRMENT OF FERTILITY

Renal adenomas developed in rats receiving an injectable gold product similar to aurothioglucose at doses of 2 mg/kg weekly for 46 weeks, followed by 6 mg/kg daily for 47 weeks. These doses were higher and administered more frequently than the recommended human doses. The adenomas were similar histologically to those produced by chronic administration of other gold compounds and heavy metals, such as lead or nickel.

Renal tubular cell neoplasia consisting of renal adenoma and adenocarcinoma were noted in a dose-response relationship in another study in rats using daily intramuscular doses of 3 mg/kg and 6 mg/kg for up to 2 years. These doses were higher and were administered more frequently than the recommended human doses. In this same study, sarcomas at the injection site occurred in some rats but their numbers were not sufficient to demonstrate a dose-response relationship.

No report of renal adenoma or sarcoma at the injection site in man in association with the use of aurothioglucose has been received.

Gold compounds have not been studied for evaluation of mutagenesis.

Gold sodium thiomalate given subcutaneously did not adversely affect fertility or reproductive performance.

PREGNANCY CATEGORY C

Gold therapy is usually contraindicated in pregnant patients. The patient should be warned about the hazards of becoming pregnant while on gold therapy. Rheumatoid arthritis frequently improves when the patient becomes pregnant, thereby eliminating the need for gold therapy. The potential nephrotoxicity of gold should not be superimposed on the increased renal burden which normally occurs in pregnancy and hence, gold therapy should be discontinued upon recognition of pregnancy unless continued use is required in an individual case. The slow excretion of gold and its persistence in body tissues after discontinuation of treatment should be kept in mind when a woman of child-bearing potential being treated with gold plans to become pregnant.

Gold sodium thiomalate administered subcutaneously, a route not used clinically, has been shown to be teratogenic during the organogenic period in rats and rabbits when given in doses 140 and 175 times, respectively, the usual human dose. Hydrocephalus and microphthalmia were the malformations observed in rats when gold sodium thiomalate was administered at a dose of 25 mg/kg/day from day 6 through day 15 of gestation. In rabbits, limb defects and gastroschisis were the malformations observed when gold sodium thiomalate was administered at doses of 20 to 45 mg/kg/day from day 6 through day 18 of gestation.

Gold compounds administered orally to rabbits from days 6 through 18 of pregnancy resulted in the occurrence of abdominal defects, such as gastroschisis and umbilical hernia; anomalies of the brain, heart, lung and skeleton; and microphthalmia.

The administration of excessive doses of gold-containing compounds during pregnancy in the above studies was toxic to the mothers and their embryos; the embryotoxic effects probably were secondary to maternal toxicity. Therefore, the significance of these findings in relation to human use is unknown.

There are no adequate and well-controlled studies with aurothioglucose in pregnant women. Extensive clinical experience with aurothioglucose has not demonstrated human teratogenicity.

NURSING MOTHERS

Gold has been demonstrated in the milk of lactating mothers. In one patient, a total dose of 135 mg of gold thioglucose was given during the postpartum period. Samples of the maternal milk and urine, and samples of red blood cells and serum of the mother and child were evaluated by atomic absorption spectrophotometry. Trace amounts of gold appeared in the serum and red blood cells of the nursing offspring. It has been postulated that this may be the cause of unexplained rashes, nephritis, hepatitis, and hematologic aberrations in the nursing infants of mothers treated with gold. Because of the potential for serious adverse reactions in nursing infants, a decision should be made whether to discontinue nursing or to discontinue the gold therapy, taking into account the importance of the drug to the mother. The slow excretion of gold and its persistence in the mother after discontinuation of treatment should be kept in mind.

PEDIATRIC USE

Safety and effectiveness in children below the age of six years have not been established.

DRUG INTERACTIONS:

Drug interactions have not been reported (See CONTRAINDICATIONS.)

ADVERSE REACTIONS:

Adverse reactions to gold therapy may occur at any time during treatment or many months after therapy has been discontinued. The incidence of toxic reactions is apparently unrelated to the plasma level of gold. Higher than conventional dosage schedules may increase the occurrence and severity of toxicity. Severe effects are most common after 300 to 500 mg have been administered.

Cutaneous Reactions: Dermatitis is the most common reaction. Pruritus should be considered a warning signal of an impending cutaneous reaction. Erythema and occasionally the more severe reactions such as papular, vesicular, and exfoliative dermatitis leading to alopecia and shedding of the nails may occur. Chrysiasis (gray-to-blue pigmentation) has been reported, especially on photoexposed areas. Gold dermatitis may be aggravated by exposure to sunlight, or an actinic rash may develop.

Mucous Membrane Reactions: Stomatitis is the second most common adverse reaction. Shallow ulcers on the buccal membranes, on the borders of the tongue and on the palate, diffuse glossitis, or gingivitis may be preceded by the sensation of metallic taste. Careful oral hygiene is recommended. Inflammation of the upper respiratory tract, pharyngitis, gastritis, colitis, tracheitis, and vaginitis have also been reported. Conjunctivitis is rare.

Renal Reactions: Nephrotic syndrome or glomerulitis with hematuria, which is usually relatively mild, subsides completely if recognized early and treatment is discontinued. These reactions become severe and chronic if gold therapy is continued after their onset. Therefore, it is important to perform a urinalysis before each injection and to discontinue treatment promptly if proteinuria or hematuria develops.

Hematologic Reactions: Although rare, blood dyscrasias, including granulocytopenia, agranulocytosis, thrombocytopenia with or without purpura, leukopenia, eosinophilia, panmyelopathy, hemorrhagic diathesis, and hypoplastic and aplastic anemia, have been reported. These reactions may occur separately or in combination.

Nitritoid and Allergic Reactions: These reactions, which may rarely occur with aurothioglucose and which resemble anaphylactoid effects, include flushing, fainting, dizziness, sweating, malaise, weakness, nausea, and vomiting.

Miscellaneous Reactions: On rare occasions, gastrointestinal symptoms, i.e., nausea, vomiting, colic, anorexia, abdominal cramps, diarrhea, ulcerative enterocolitis, and headache have been reported.

There have been rare reports of iritis and corneal ulcers. Transient, asymptomatic gold deposits in the cornea or conjunctiva may occur.

Other reported reactions include encephalitis, immunological destruction of the synovia, EEG abnormalities, intrahepatic cholestasis, hepatitis with jaundice, toxic hepatitis, acute yellow atrophy, peripheral neuritis, gold bronchitis, pulmonary injury manifested by interstitial pneumonitis or fibrosis, fever, and partial or complete hair loss.

Less common but more severe effects that may occur shortly after an injection or at any time during gold therapy include: anaphylactic shock, syncope, bradycardia, thickening of the tongue, difficulty in swallowing and breathing, and angioneurotic edema. If they are observed, treatment with aurothioglucose should be discontinued.

Arthralgia may occur for one or two days after an injection and usually subsides after the first few injections. The mechanism of the transient increase in rheumatic symptoms after injection of gold (the so-called nonvasomotor postinjection reaction) is unknown. These reactions are usually mild but occasionally may be so severe that treatment is stopped prematurely.

Management Of Adverse Reactions: In the event of toxic reactions, gold therapy should be discontinued immediately.

In the presence of mild reactions, it may be sufficient to discontinue the administration of aurothioglucose for a short period and then to resume treatment with smaller doses.

Dermatitis and pruritus may respond to soothing lotions, other appropriate antipruritic treatment, or topical glucocorticoids.

If dermatitis or stomatitis becomes severe or spreads, systemic glucocorticoid treatment may be indicated. For renal, hematologic, and most other adverse reactions, glucocorticoids may be required in larger doses and for a longer time than for dermatologic reactions. Often this treatment may be required for many months because of the slow elimination of gold from the body.

If severe adverse reactions do not improve with steroid treatment in patients who receive large doses of gold, a chelating agent, such as dimercaprol (BAL), may be use. In one case, it was reported that penicillamine was beneficial in the treatment of gold-induced thrombocytopenia. Adjunctive use of an anabolic steroid with other drugs (*i.e.,* BAL, penicillamine, and corticosteroids) may contribute to recovery of bone marrow deficiency.

In the presence of severe or idiosyncratic reactions, treatment with aurothioglucose should not be reinstituted.

OVERDOSAGE:

Overdosage resulting from too rapid increase in dosing with aurothioglucose will be manifested by rapid appearance of toxic reactions, particularly those relating to renal damage, such as hematuria, proteinuria, and to hematologic effects, such as thrombocytopenia and granulocytopenia. Other toxic effects, including fever, nausea, vomiting, diarrhea, and various skin disorders such as papulovesicular lesions, urticaria, and exfoliative dermatitis, all attended with severe pruritus, may develop. Treatment consists of prompt discontinuation of the medication, and early administration of dimercaprol. Specific supportive therapy should be given for the renal and hematologic complications. (See also ADVERSE REACTIONS.)

DOSAGE AND ADMINISTRATION:

Adults: The usual dosage schedule for the intramuscular administration of aurothioglucose is as follows: first dose, 10 mg; second and third doses, 25 mg; fourth and subsequent doses, 50 mg. The interval between doses is one week. The 50 mg dose is continued at weekly intervals until 0.8 to 1.0 g aurothioglucose has been given. If the patient has improved and has exhibited no sign of toxicity, the 50 mg dose may be continued many months longer, at three- to four-week intervals. A weekly dose above 50 mg is usually unnecessary and contraindicated; the tendency in gold therapy is toward lower dosage. With this in mind, it may eventually be established that a 25 mg dose is the one of choice. If no improvement has been demonstrated after a total administration of 1.0 g of aurothioglucose, the necessity for gold therapy should be reevaluated.

Children 6 to 12 years: one-fourth of the adult dose, governed chiefly by body weight, not to exceed 25 mg per dose.

Aurothioglucose should be injected **intramuscularly** (preferably intragluteally), **never intravenously**. The patient should be lying down and should remain recumbent for approximately 10 minutes after the injection. The vial should be thoroughly shaken in order to suspend all of the active material. Heating the vial to body temperature (by immersion in warm water) will facilitate drawing the suspension into the syringe. An 18-gauge, 1 1/2-inch needle is recommended for depositing the preparation deep into the muscular tissue. For obese patients, an 18-gauge, 2-inch needle may be used. The site usually selected for injection is the upper outer quadrant of the gluteal region.

DOSAGE AND ADMINISTRATION: *(cont'd)*

NOTE: Shake the vial in horizontal position before the dose is withdrawn. Needle and syringe must be dry. The patient should be observed for at least 15 minutes following each injection.

HOW SUPPLIED:

Solganal Suspension is available in 10 ml multiple-dose vials containing 5% (50 mg/ml) aurothioglucose.

Shake well before using. Store between 0 and 30°C (32 and 86°F). Protect from light. Store in carton until contents are used.

HOW SUPPLIED - EQUIVALENTS NOT AVAILABLE:

Injection, Susp - Intramuscular - 50 mg/ml

10 ml $120.90 SOLGANAL, Schering 00085-0460-03

AZATADINE MALEATE *(000349)*

CATEGORIES: Allergies; Antihistamines; Piperidines; Respiratory & Allergy Medications; Rhinitis; Urticaria; Pregnancy Category B; FDA Approval Pre 1982

BRAND NAMES: *Idulamine* (Mexico); *Idulian*; *Lergocil*; *Nalomet*; **Optimine**; *Verben*; *Zadine* (Australia)

(International brand names outside U.S. in italics)

COST OF THERAPY: $54.72 (Rhinitis; Tablet; 1 mg; 2/day; 30 days)

PRIMARY ICD9: 477.9 (Allergic Rhinitis, Cause Unspecified)

DESCRIPTION:

Optimine Tablets contain azatadine maleate, USP, an antihistamine having the empirical formula, $C_{20}H_{22}N_2 \cdot 2C_4H_4O_4$, the chemical name, 6,11-Dihydro-11-(1-methyl-4-piperidylidene)-5*H*-benzo[5,6] cyclohepta [1,2-b] pyridine maleate (1:2).

The molecular weight of azatadine maleate is 522.55. It is a white to off-white powder and is very soluble in water and soluble in alcohol.

Each Optimine Tablet contains 1 mg azatadine maleate, USP. They also contain: corn starch, lactose, magnesium stearate, and providone.

CLINICAL PHARMACOLOGY:

Azatadine maleate is an antihistamine, related to cyproheptadine, with antiserotonin, anticholinergic (drying), and sedative effects.

Antihistamines competitively antagonize those pharmacological effects of histamine which are mediated through activation of histamine H_1-receptor sites on effector cells. Histamine-related allergic reactions and tissue injury are blocked or diminished in intensity. Antihistamines antagonize the vasodilator effect of endogenously released histamine, especially in small vessels, and mitigate the effect of histamine which results in increased capillary permeability and edema formation. As consequences of these actions, antihistamines antagonize the physiological manifestations of histamine release in the nose following antigen-antibody interactions, such as congestion related to vascular engorgement, mucosal edema, and profuse, watery secretion, and irritation and sneezing resulting from histamine action on afferent nerve terminals.

Pharmacokinetic studies in normal volunteers dosed orally with radio-labeled azatadine maleate show that the drug is readily absorbed with peak plasma levels at about four hours after dosing. Approximately 50% of the drug is excreted in the urine within five days after administration of a single dose, and no evidence of drug accumulation was seen after daily dosing for 30 days. The elimination half-life of azatadine maleate, based on plasma radioactivity, was approximately 9 hours. Approximately 20% of the drug is excreted unchanged and extensive conjugation of the drug and its metabolites occurs. Azatadine maleate is minimally bound to plasma protein.

While the antihistamines have not been studied for passage through the blood-brain and placental barriers, the occurrence of pharmacologic effects in the central nervous system and in the newborn indicate presence of the drug.

INDICATIONS AND USAGE:

Azatadine maleate is indicated for the treatment of perennial and seasonal allergic rhinitis and chronic urticaria.

CONTRAINDICATIONS:

Antihistamines *should NOT* be used to treat lower respiratory tract symptoms, including asthma.

Antihistamines, including azatadine maleate, are also contraindicated in patients hypersensitive to this medication and to other antihistamines of similar chemical structure, and in patients receiving monoamine oxidase inhibitor therapy. (See DRUG INTERACTIONS.)

WARNINGS:

Antihistamines should be used with caution in patients with narrow angle glaucoma, stenosing peptic ulcer; pyloroduodenal obstruction; and urinary bladder obstruction due to symptomatic prostatic hypertrophy and narrowing of the bladder neck.

Use with CNS Depressants: Antihistamines have additive effects with alcohol and other CNS depressants (hypnotics, sedatives, tranquilizers, etc.)

Use in Activities Requiring Mental Alertness: Patients should be warned about engaging in activities requiring mental alertness, such as driving a car or operating certain appliances, machinery, etc., until their response to this medication has been determined.

Use in Patients Approximately 60 Years or Older: Antihistamines are more likely to cause dizziness, sedation, and hypotension in patients over 60 years of age.

PRECAUTIONS:

GENERAL

Azatadine maleate has an atropine-like action and therefore should be used with caution in patients with: a history of bronchial asthma; increased intraocular pressure; hyperthyroidism; cardiovascular disease; hypertension.

INFORMATION FOR THE PATIENT

This information is intended to aid in the safe and effective use of this medication. It is not a disclosure of all possible adverse or intended effects.

1. Antihistamines may cause drowsiness.

2. Patients taking antihistamines should not engage in activities requiring mental alertness, such as driving a car or operating machinery, certain appliances, etc., until their response to this medication has been determined.

3. Alcohol or other sedative drugs may enhance the drowsiness caused by antihistamines.

PRECAUTIONS: *(cont'd)*

4. Patients should not take this medication if they are receiving a monoamine oxidase (MAO) inhibitor, or if they are receiving oral anticoagulants.

5. This medication should not be given to children less than 12 years of age.

DRUG/LABORATORY TEST INTERACTION

Antihistamines should be discontinued about four days prior to skin testing procedures since these drugs may prevent or diminish otherwise positive reactions to dermal reactivity indicators.

CARCINOGENESIS, MUTAGENESIS, AND IMPAIRMENT OF FERTILITY

Long-term oral dosing studies with azatadine maleate in rats and mice showed no evidence or carcinogenesis. No mutagenic effect was seen in a dominant lethal assay study in mice dosed with azatadine maleate orally an intraperitoneally. There was no impairment of fertility in rats fed azatadine maleate at doses greater than 150 times the recommended human daily dose.

PREGNANCY CATEGORY B

Reproduction studies have been performed in rats and rabbits at doses up to 188 times and 38 times, respectively, the human dose and have revealed no evidence of impaired fertility or harm to the fetus due to azatadine maleate. There are, however, no adequate and well-controlled studies in pregnant women. Because animal reproduction studies are not always predictive of human response, this drug should be used during pregnancy only if clearly needed. (See Nonteratogenic Effects.)

Nonteratogenic Effects: Antihistamines should not be used in the third trimester of pregnancy because newborn and premature infants may have severe reactions, such as convulsions, to them.

NURSING MOTHERS

It is not known whether this drug is excreted in human milk. However, certain antihistamines are known to be excreted in human milk in low concentration. Because of the higher risk of antihistamines for infants generally and for newborns and prematures in particular, a decision should be made whether to discontinue nursing or to discontinue the drug, taking into account the importance of the drug to the mother.

PEDIATRIC USE

Safety and effectiveness in children below the age of 12 years have not been established.

DRUG INTERACTIONS:

MAO inhibitors prolong and intensify the anticholinergic and sedative effects of antihistamines. Additive effects may occur from the concomitant use of antihistamines with tricyclic antidepressants. (See also WARNINGS.)

ADVERSE REACTIONS:

Slight to moderate drowsiness may occur with azatadine maleate. Other possible side effects common to antihistamines in general include: (the most frequent are underlined).

General: urticaria, drug rash, anaphylactic shock, photosensitivity, excessive perspiration, chills, dryness of mouth, nose, and throat.

Cardiovascular: hypotension, headache, palpitations, tachycardia, extrasystoles.

Hematologic: hemolytic anemia, hypoplastic anemia, thrombocytopenia, agranulocytosis.

Nervous: sedation, sleepiness, dizziness, vertigo, tinnitus, acute labyrinthitis, disturbed coordination, fatigue, confusion, restlessness, excitation, nervousness, tremor, irritability, insomnia, euphoria, paresthesias, blurred vision, diplopia, hysteria, neuritis, convulsions.

Gastrointestinal: epigastric distress, anorexia, nausea, vomiting, diarrhea, constipation.

Genitourinary: urinary frequency, difficult urination, urinary retention, early menses.

Respiratory: thickening of bronchial secretions, tightness of chest and wheezing, nasal stuffiness.

DRUG ABUSE AND DEPENDENCE:

There is no information to indicate that abuse or dependency occurs with azatadine maleate.

OVERDOSAGE:

In the event of overdosage, emergency treatment should be started immediately.

Manifestations: Antihistamine overdosage effect may vary from central nervous system depression (sedation, apnea, diminished mental alertness, cardiovascular collapse) to stimulation (insomnia, hallucinations, tremors or convulsions) to death. Other signs and symptoms may be dizziness, tinnitus, ataxia, blurred vision, and hypotension. Stimulation is particularly likely in children, as are atropine-like signs and symptoms (dry mouth; fixed dilated pupils; flushing; hyperthermia; and gastrointestinal symptoms).

Treatment: The patient should be induced to vomit, even if emesis has occurred spontaneously. Pharmacologic vomiting by the administration of ipecac syrup is a preferred method. However, vomiting should not be induced in patients with impaired consciousness. The action of ipecac is facilitated by physical activity and by the administration of 8 to 12 fluid ounces of water. If emesis does not occur within fifteen minutes, the dose of ipecac should be repeated. Precautions against aspiration must be taken, especially in infants and children. Following emesis, any drug remaining in the stomach may be adsorbed by activated charcoal administered as a slurry with water. If vomiting is unsuccessful or contraindicated, gastric lavage should be performed. Physiologic saline solution is the lavage solution of choice, particularly in children. In adults, tap water can be used; however, as much as possible of the amount administered should be removed before the next instillation. Saline cathartics, such as milk of magnesia, draw water into the bowel by osmosis and, therefore, may be valuable for their action in rapid dilution of bowel content. Dialysis is of little value in antihistamine poisoning. After emergency treatment, the patient should continue to be medically monitored.

Treatment of the signs and symptoms of overdosage is symptomatic and supportive. Stimulants (analeptic agents) should not be used. Vasopressors may be used to treat hypotension. Short acting barbiturates, diazepam, or paraldehyde may be administered to control seizures. Hyperpyrexia, especially in children, may require treatment with tepid water sponge baths or a hypothermic blanket. Apnea is treated with ventilatory support.

DOSAGE AND ADMINISTRATION:

DOSAGE SHOULD BE INDIVIDUALIZED ACCORDING TO THE NEEDS AND THE RESPONSE OF THE PATIENT.

AZATADINE MALEATE TABLETS ARE NOT RECOMMENDED FOR USE IN CHILDREN UNDER 12 YEARS OF AGE.

The usual adult dosage is 1 or 2 mg, twice a day.

HOW SUPPLIED:

Optimine Tablets, USP, 1 mg, white, compressed, scored tablets impressed with product identification numbers, 282.

Store between 2° and 30°C (36° and 86°F).

HOW SUPPLIED - EQUIVALENTS NOT AVAILABLE:

Tablet, Soluble - Oral - 1 mg

100's	$91.20	OPTIMINE, Schering	00085-0282-03

AZATADINE MALEATE; PSEUDOEPHEDRINE SULFATE *(000350)*

CATEGORIES: Allergies; Antihistamines; Common Cold; Congestion; Decongestants; Nasal Congestion; Respiratory & Allergy Medications; Rhinitis; Influenza*; Pregnancy Category C; FDA Approved 1982 Mar
* Indication not approved by the FDA

BRAND NAMES: *Atiramin*; *Congestan*; *Congesteze* (England); *Idulanex*; **Trinalin**; *Trinalin Repetabs* (Mexico)
(International brand names outside U.S. in italics)

FORMULARIES: Aetna; BC-BS

DESCRIPTION:

Trinalin Long-Acting Antihistamine/Decongestant Repetabs (brand of repeat-action tablets) Tablets contain 1 mg azatadine maleate, USP in the tablet coating and 120 mg pseudoephedrine sulfate, USP, equally distributed between the tablet coating and the barrier-coated core. Following ingestion, the two active components in the coating are quickly liberated; release of the decongestant in the core is delayed for several hours.

Azatadine maleate is an antihistamine having the empirical formula, $C_{20}H_{22}N_2{\cdot}2C_4H_4O_4$, the chemical name, 6,11-Di-hydro-11-(-methyl-4-piperidylidene)-5*H*-benzo (5,6) cyclohepta (1,2-*b*) pyridine maleate (1:2).

The molecular weight of azatadine maleate is 522.54. Azatadine maleate is a white to off-white powder and is very soluble in water and soluble in alcohol.

Pseudoephedrine sulfate, a sympathomimetic amine, is a salt of pseudoephedrine, one of the naturally occurring alkaloids obtained from various species of the plant *Ephedra*. The empirical formula for pseudoephedrine sulfate is $(C_{10}H_{15}NO)_2{\cdot}H_2SO_4$; the chemical name is Benzenemethanol,α-[1-(methylamino)ethyl]-, [S-(R*,R*)]-, sulfate (2:1) (salt).

The molecular weight of pseudoephedrine sulfate is 428.56. It is a white to off-white crystal or powder, very soluble in water, freely soluble in alcohol, and sparingly soluble in chloroform.

The inactive ingredients for Trinalin Repetabs Tablets are: Acacia, Butylparaben, Calcium Sulfate, Carnauba Wax, Corn Starch, D&C Red. No. 30 Al Lake, FD&C Yellow No. 6 Al Lake, Gelatin, Lactose, Magnesium Stearate, Neutral Soap, Oleic Acid, Povidone, Rosin, Sugar, Talc, White Wax, and Zein.

CLINICAL PHARMACOLOGY:

Azatadine maleate is an antihistamine, related to cyproheptadine, with antiserotonin, anticholinergic (drying), and sedative effects. Antihistamines appear to compete with histamine for histamine H_1-receptor sites on effector cells. The antihistamines antagonize those pharmacological effects of histamine which are mediated through activation of H_1-receptor sites and thereby reduce the intensity of allergic reactions and tissue injury response involving histamine release. Antihistamines antagonize the vasodilatory effect of endogenously released histamine, especially in small vessels, and mitigate the effect of histamine which results in increased capillary permeability and edema formation. As consequences of these actions antihistamines antagonize the physiological manifestations of histamine release in the nose following antigen-antibody interaction, such as congestion related to vascular engorgement, mucosal edema, and profuse, watery secretion, and irritation and sneezing resulting from histamine action on afferent nerve terminals.

Pseudoephedrine sulfate (d-isoephedrine sulfate) is an orally effective nasal decongestant which appears to exert its sympathomimetic effect indirectly, predominantly through release of adrenergic mediators from post-ganglionic nerve terminals. In effective recommended oral dosage, pseudoephedrine sulfate produces minimal other sympathomimetic effects, such as pressor activity and CNS stimulation. Use of an orally administered vasoconstrictor for shrinkage of congested nasal mucosa has several advantages: a) it produces a gradual but sustained decongestant effect, causing little, if any "rebound" congestion; b) it facilitates shrinkage of swollen mucosa in upper respiratory areas that are relatively inaccessible to topically applied sprays or drops; c) it relieves nasal obstruction without the additional irritation that may result from local medication.

Pseudoephedrine passes through the blood-brain and placental barriers. While the antihistamines have not been studied systematically for passage through these barriers, the occurrence of pharmacologic effects in the central nervous system and in newborns indicate presence of the drug.

Following administration of the two drugs to normal volunteers in either a single azatadine maleate tablet or similar doses in two conventional pseudoephedrine sulfate tablets and a conventional tablet of azatadine maleate, the blood levels of pseudoephedrine and the urinary excretion of azatadine showed that the azatadine maleate tablets are bioequivalent to the conventional dosage forms. The apparent elimination half-life of pseudoephedrine in azatadine maleate tablets was approximately 6 1/2 hours. The apparent elimination half-life of azatadine maleate (available from the outer layer of the azatadine maleate tablets or from the conventional azatadine maleate tablet) was approximately 12 hours.

INDICATIONS AND USAGE:

Azatadine Maleate Long-Acting Antihistamine/Decongestant Tablets are indicated for the relief of the symptoms of upper respiratory mucosal congestion in perennial and allergic rhinitis, and for the relief of nasal congestion in gestation and eustachian tube congestion. Analgesics, antibiotics, or both may be administered concurrently, when indicated.

CONTRAINDICATIONS:

Antihistamines should not be used to treat lower respiratory tract symptoms, including asthma.

This product is contraindicated in patients with narrow-angle glaucoma or urinary retention, and in patients receiving monoamine oxidase (MAO) inhibitor therapy or within ten days of stopping such treatment. (See DRUG INTERACTIONS) It is also contraindicated in patients with severe hypertension, severe coronary artery disease, hyperthyroidism, and in those who have shown hypersensitivity or idiosyncrasy to its components, to adrenergic agents, or to other drugs of similar chemical structures. Manifestations of patient idiosyncrasy to adrenergic agents include: insomnia, dizziness, weakness, tremor, or arrhythmias.

WARNINGS:

Azatadine maleate tablets should be used with considerable caution in patients with: stenosing peptic ulcer, pyloroduodenal obstruction, urinary bladder obstruction due to symptomatic prostatic hypertrophy, or narrowing of the bladder neck. It should also be administered with

WARNINGS: *(cont'd)*

caution to patients with: cardiovascular disease, including hypertension or ischemic heart disease; increased intraocular pressure (see CONTRAINDICATIONS); diabetes mellitus, or in patients receiving digitalis or oral anticoagulants.

Central nervous system stimulation and convulsions or cardiovascular collapse with accompanying hypotension may be produced by sympathomimetics.

Do not exceed recommended dosage.

Use in Activities Requiring Mental Alertness: Patients should be warned about engaging in activities requiring mental alertness such as driving a car or operating appliances, machinery, etc.

Use in Patients Approximately 60 Years and Older: Antihistamines are more likely to cause dizziness, sedation, and hypotension in patients over 60 years of age. In these patients, sympathomimetics are also more likely to cause adverse reactions, such as confusion, hallucinations, convulsions, CNS depression, and death. For this reason, before, considering the use of a repeat-action formulation, the safe use of a short-acting sympathomimetic in that particular patient should be demonstrated.

PRECAUTIONS:

GENERAL

Because of the atropine-like action of antihistamines, this product should be used with caution in patients with a history of bronchial asthma.

INFORMATION FOR THE PATIENT

1. Products containing antihistamines may cause drowsiness.
2. Patients should not engage in activities requiring mental alertness, such as driving or operating machinery or appliances.
3. Alcohol or other sedative drug may enhance the drowsiness caused by antihistamines.
4. Patients should not take azatadine maleate tablets if they are receiving a monoamine oxidase inhibitor or within 10 days of stopping such treatment, or if they are receiving oral anticoagulants.
5. This medication should not be given to children less than 12 years of age.

DRUG/LABORATORY TEST INTERACTIONS

The *in vitro* addition of pseudoephedrine to sera containing the cardiac isoenzyme MB of serum creatine phosphokinase progressively inhibits the activity of the enzyme. The inhibition becomes complete over six hours.

CARCINOGENESIS, MUTAGENESIS, AND IMPAIRMENT OF FERTILITY

There is no animal or laboratory study of the mixture of azatadine maleate and pseudoephedrine sulfate to evaluate carcinogenesis or mutagenesis. Reproduction studies of this mixture in rats showed no evidence of impaired fertility.

PREGNANCY CATEGORY C

Retarded fetal development and the presence of angulated hyoid wings were seen in the offspring of pregnant rabbits administered azatadine maleate tablets at about 12.5 times the recommended human dosage, respectively; increased resorption was noted at about 25 times the humans dosage. A decreased survival rate at day 21 was seen in rat pups born of mothers given azatadine maleate during pregnancy at a dose about 12.5 times the human dosage. There are no adequate and well-controlled studies in pregnant women. Azatadine maleate tablets should be used during pregnancy only if the potential benefits to the mother justify the potential risks to the infant. (See Nonteratogenic Effects.)

Nonteratogenic Effects: Antihistamines should not be used in the third trimester of pregnancy because newborns and premature infants may have severe reactions to them, such as convulsions.

NURSING MOTHERS

It is not known whether these drug are excreted in human milk. However, certain antihistamines and sympathomimetics are known to be excreted in human milk. Because of the higher risks of antihistamines for infants generally and for newborns and prematures in particular, a decision should be made whether to discontinue nursing or to discontinue the drug, taking into account the importance of the drug to the mother.

There is a report of irritability excessive crying and disturbed sleeping patterns in a nursing infant whose mother had taken a product containing an antihistamine and pseudoephedrine.

PEDIATRIC USE

Safety and effectiveness in children below the age of 12 years have not been established.

DRUG INTERACTIONS:

MAO inhibitors prolong and intensify the effects of antihistamines. Concomitant use of antihistamines with alcohol, tricyclic antidepressants, barbiturates, or other central nervous system depressants may have an additive effect.

When sympathomimetic drugs are given to patients receiving monoamine oxidase inhibitors, hypertensive reactions, including hypertensive crises, may occur. The antihypertensive effects of methyldopa, mecamylamine, reserpine, and veratrum alkaloids may be reduced by sympathomimetics. Beta-adrenergic blocking agents may also interact with sympathomimetics. Increased ectopic pacemaker activity can occur when pseudoephedrine is used concomitantly with digitalis. Antacids increase the rate of absorption of pseudoephedrine, while kaolin decreases it.

ADVERSE REACTIONS:

The following adverse reactions are associated with antihistamine and sympathomimetic drugs. (Those adverse reactions which occur most frequently with the antihistamines are underlined.)

General: Urticaria, drug rash, anaphylactic shock, photosensitivity, excessive perspiration, chills, dryness of mouth, nose, and throat.

Cardiovascular: Hypertension (see CONTRAINDICATIONS and WARNINGS), hypotension, arrhythmias and cardiovascular collapse, headache, palpitations, extrasystoles, tachycardia, angina.

Hematologic: Hemolytic anemia, hypoplastic anemia, thrombocytopenia, agranulocytosis.

Central Nervous System: Sedation, sleepiness, dizziness, vertigo, tinnitus, acute labyrinthitis, disturbed coordination, fatigue, mydriasis, confusion, restlessness, excitation, nervousness, tension, tremor, irritability, insomnia, euphoria, paresthesias, blurred vision, hysteria, neuritis, convulsions, fear, anxiety, hallucinations, CNS depression, weakness, pallor.

Gastrointestinal: Epigastric distress, anorexia, nausea, vomiting, diarrhea, constipation, abdominal cramps.

Genitourinary: Urinary frequency, urinary retention, dysuria, early menses.

Respiratory: Thickening of bronchial secretions, tightness of chest and wheezing, nasal stuffiness, respiratory difficulty.

DRUG ABUSE AND DEPENDENCE:

There is no information to indicate that abuse or dependency occurs with azatadine maleate.

Pseudoephedrine, like the central nervous system stimulants, has been abused. At high doses, subjects commonly experience an elevation of mood, a sense of increased energy and alertness, and decreased appetite. Some individuals become anxious, irritable, and loquacious. In addition to the marked euphoria, the user experiences a sense of markedly enhanced physical strength and mental capacity. With continued use, tolerance develops, the user increases the dose, and toxic signs and symptoms appear. Depression may follow rapid withdrawal.

OVERDOSAGE:

In the event of overdosage, emergency treatment should be started immediately.

Manifestations of Overdose: Manifestations of overdosage may vary from central nervous system depression (sedation, apnea, diminished mental alertness, cyanosis, coma, cardiovascular collapse) to stimulation (insomnia, hallucinations, tremors, or convulsions) to death. Other signs and symptoms may be euphoria, excitement, tachycardia, palpitations, thirst, perspiration, nausea, dizziness, tinnitus, ataxia, blurred vision, and hypertension or hypotension. Stimulation is particularly likely in children, as are atropine-like signs and symptoms (dry mouth; fixed, dilated pupils; flushing; hyperthermia; and gastrointestinal symptoms).

In large doses sympathomimetics may give rise to giddiness, headache, nausea, vomiting, sweating, thirst, tachycardia, precordial pain, palpitations, difficulty in micturition, muscular weakness and tenseness, anxiety, restlessness, and insomnia. Many patients can present a toxic psychosis with delusions and hallucinations. Some may develop cardiac arrhythmias, circulatory collapse, convulsions, coma, and respiratory failure.

The oral LD_{50} of the mixture of the two drugs in mature rats and mice was greater than 1700 mg/kg and 600 mg/kg, respectively.

Treatment: The patient should be induced to vomit, even if emesis has occurred spontaneously. Pharmacologically induced vomiting by the administration of ipecac syrup is a preferred method. However, vomiting should not be induced in patients with impaired consciousness. The action of ipecac is facilitated by physical activity and by the administration of eight to twelve fluid ounces of water. If emesis does not occur within fifteen minutes, the dose of ipecac should be repeated. Precautions against aspiration must be taken, especially in infants and children. Following emesis, any drug remaining in the stomach may be absorbed by activated charcoal administered as a slurry with water. If vomiting is unsuccessful or contraindicated, gastric lavage should be performed. Isotonic and one-half isotonic saline are the lavage solutions of choice. Saline cathartics, such as milk of magnesia, draw water into the bowel by osmosis and therefore may be valuable for their action in rapid dilution of bowel content. Dialysis is of little value in antihistamine poisoning. After emergency treatment the patient should continue to be medically monitored.

Treatment of the signs and symptoms of overdosage is symptomatic and supportive. Stimulants (analeptic agents) should not be used. Vasopressors may be used to treat hypotension. Short-acting barbiturates, diazepam, or paraldehyde, may be administered to control seizures. Hyperpyrexia, especially in children, may require treatment with tepid water sponge baths or a hypothermic blanket. Apnea is treated with ventilatory support.

DOSAGE AND ADMINISTRATION:

AZATADINE MALEATE TABLETS ARE NOT INTENDED FOR USE IN CHILDREN UNDER 12 YEARS OF AGE. The usual adult dosage is one tablet twice a day.

HOW SUPPLIED:

Trinalin Repetabs Tablets contain 1 mg azatadine maleate and 120 mg pseudoephedrine sulfate. Trinalin Repetabs Tablets are coral-colored, sugar coated tablets branded in black with the product name (Trinalin and product identification numbers, 703)

Store between 2 and 30°C (36 and 86°F).

HOW SUPPLIED - EQUIVALENTS NOT AVAILABLE:

Tablet, Coated - Oral - 1 mg/120 mg

100's $95.10 TRINALIN, Schering 00085-0703-04

AZATHIOPRINE *(000351)*

CATEGORIES: Antiarthritics; Antimetabolites; Arthritis; Immunologic; Immunomodulators; Immunosuppressives; Renal Drugs; Renal Transplantation; FDA Approval Pre 1982

BRAND NAMES: *Azamedac* (Germany); *Azamun*; *Azamune* (England); *Azanin* (Japan); *Azapress*; *Azathioprine*; Azathioprine Sodium; *Azatioprina*; *Azatrilem* (Mexico); *Azopi*; *Azoran*; *Immuthera*; *Imuprin*; **Imuran**; *Imurek* (Germany); *Imurel* (France); *Thioprine* (Australia); *Transimune*
(International brand names outside U.S. in italics)

FORMULARIES: Aetna; BC-BS; Medi-Cal; PCS; WHO

> **WARNING:**
> Chronic immunosuppression with this purine antimetabolite increases risk of neoplasia in humans. Physicians using this drug should be very familiar with this risk as well as with the mutagenic potential to both men and women and with possible hematologic toxicities. See WARNINGS.

DESCRIPTION:

Imuran (azathioprine), an immunosuppressive antimetabolite, is available in tablet form for oral administration and 100 mg vials for intravenous injection. Each scored tablet contains 50 mg azathioprine and the inactive ingredients lactose, magnesium stearate, potato starch, povidone, and stearic acid. Each 100 mg vial contains azathioprine, as the sodium salt, equivalent to 100 mg azathioprine sterile lyophilized material and sodium hydroxide to adjust pH.

Azathioprine is chemically 6-[(1-methyl-4-nitroimidazol-5-yl)thio]-1*H*- purine.

It is an imidazolyl derivative of 6-mercaptopurine (Purinethol) and many of its biological effects are similar to those of the parent compound.

Azathioprine is insoluble in water, but may be dissolved with addition of one molar equivalent of alkali. The sodium salt of azathioprine is sufficiently soluble to make a 10 mg/ml water solution which is stable for 24 hours at 59° to 77°F (15° to 25°C). Azathioprine is stable in solution at neutral or acid pH but hydrolysis to mercaptopurine occurs in excess sodium hydroxide (0.1N), especially on warming. Conversion to mercaptopurine also occurs in the presence of sulfhydryl compounds such as cysteine, glutathione and hydrogen sulfide.

CLINICAL PHARMACOLOGY:

Metabolism[1]: Azathioprine is well absorbed following oral administration. Maximum serum radioactivity occurs at one to two hours after oral ^{35}S-azathioprine and decays with a half-life of five hours. This is not an estimate of the half-life of azathioprine itself but is the decay rate for all ^{35}S-containing metabolites of the drug. Because of extensive metabolism, only a fraction of the radioactivity is present as azathioprine. Usual doses produce blood levels of azathioprine, and of mercaptopurine derived from it, which are low (<1 mcg/ml). Blood levels are of little predictive value for therapy since the magnitude and duration of clinical effects correlate with thiopurine nucleotide levels in tissues rather than with plasma drug levels. Azathioprine and mercaptopurine are moderately bound to serum proteins (30%) and are partially dialyzable.

Azathioprine is cleaved *in vivo* to mercaptopurine. Both compounds are rapidly eliminated from blood and are oxidized or methylated in erythrocytes and liver; no azathioprine or mercaptopurine is detectable in urine after eight hours. Conversion to inactive 6-thiouric acid by xanthine oxidase is an important degradative pathway, and the inhibition of this pathway in patients receiving allopurinol (Zyloprim) is the basis for the azathioprine dosage reduction required in these patients (see DRUG INTERACTIONS). Proportions of metabolites are different in individual patients, and this presumably accounts for variable magnitude and duration of drug effects. Renal clearance is probably not important in predicting biological effectiveness or toxicities, although dose reduction is practiced in patients with poor renal function.

Homograft Survival[1,2]: Summary information from transplant centers and registries indicates relatively universal use of azathioprine with or without other immunosuppressive agents.[3,4,5] Although the use of azathioprine for inhibition of renal homograft rejection is well established, the mechanism(s) for this action are somewhat obscure. The drug suppresses hypersensitivities of the cell-mediated type and causes variable alterations in antibody production. Suppression of T-cell effects, including ablation of T-cell suppression, is dependent on the temporal relationship to antigenic stimulus or engraftment. This agent has little effect on established graft rejection or secondary responses.

Alterations in specific immune responses or immunologic functions in transplant recipients are difficult to relate specifically to immunosuppression by azathioprine. These patients have subnormal responses to vaccines, low numbers of T-cells, and abnormal phagocytosis by peripheral blood cells, but their mitogenic responses, serum immunoglobulins and secondary antibody responses are usually normal.

Immunoinflammatory Response: Azathioprine suppresses disease manifestations as well as underlying pathology in animal models of autoimmune disease. For example, the severity of adjuvant arthritis is reduced by azathioprine.

The mechanisms whereby azathioprine affects autoimmune diseases are not known. Azathioprine is immunosuppressive, delayed hypersensitivity and cellular cytotoxicity tests being suppressed to a greater degree than are antibody responses. In the rat model of adjuvant arthritis, azathioprine has been shown to inhibit the lymph node hyperplasia which precedes the onset of the signs of the disease. Both the immunosuppressive and therapeutic effects in animal models are dose-related. Azathioprine is considered a slow-acting drug and effects may persist after the drug has been discontinued.

INDICATIONS AND USAGE:

Azathioprine is indicated as an adjunct for the prevention of rejection in renal homotransplantation. It is also indicated for the management of severe, active rheumatoid arthritis unresponsive to rest, aspirin or other nonsteroidal anti-inflammatory drugs, or to agents in the class of which gold is an example.

Renal Homotransplantation: Azathioprine is indicated as an adjunct for the prevention of rejection in renal homotransplantation. Experience with over 16,000 transplants shows a five-year patient survival of 35% to 55%, but this is dependent on donor, match for HLA antigens, anti-donor or anti B-cell alloantigen antibody and other variables. The effect of azathioprine on these variables has not been tested in controlled trials.

Rheumatoid Arthritis[6,7]: Azathioprine is indicated only in adult patients meeting criteria for classic or definite rheumatoid arthritis as specified by the American Rheumatism Association.[8] Azathioprine should be restricted to patients with severe, active and erosive disease not responsive to conventional management including rest, aspirin or other nonsteroidal drugs or to agents in the class of which gold is an example. Rest, physiotherapy and salicylates should be continued while azathioprine is given, but it may be possible to reduce the dose of corticosteroids in patients on azathioprine. The combined use of azathioprine with gold, antimalarials or penicillamine has not been studied for either added benefit or unexpected adverse effects. The use of azathioprine with these agents cannot be recommended.

CONTRAINDICATIONS:

Azathioprine should not be given to patients who have shown hypersensitivity to the drug.

Azathioprine should not be used for treating rheumatoid arthritis in pregnant women.

Patients with rheumatoid arthritis previously treated with alkylating agents (cyclophosphamide, chlorambucil, melphalan or others) may have a prohibitive risk of neoplasia if treated with azathioprine.[9]

WARNINGS:

Leukopenia and/orThrombocytopenia: Severe leukopenia and/or thrombocytopeniamay occur in patients on azathioprine. Macrocytic anemia and severe bone marrow depression may also occur. Hematologic toxicities are dose related and may be more severe in renal transplant patients whose homograft is undergoing rejection. It is suggested that patients on azathioprine have complete blood counts, including platelet counts, weekly during the first month, twice monthly for the second and third months of treatment, then monthly or more frequently if dosage alterations or other therapy changes are necessary. Delayed hematologic suppression may occur. Prompt reduction in dosage or temporary withdrawal of the drug may be necessary if there is a rapid fall in, or persistently low leukocyte count or other evidence of bone marrow depression. Leukopenia does not correlate with therapeutic effect; therefore the dose should not be increased intentionally to lower the white blood cell count.

Serious Infections: Serious infections are a constant hazard for patients receiving chronic immunosuppression, especially for homograft recipients. Fungal, viral, bacterial and protozoal infections may be fatal and should be treated vigorously. Reduction of azathioprine dosage and/or use of other drugs should be considered.

Risk of Neoplasia: Azathioprine is mutagenic in animals and humans, carcinogenic in animals, and may increase the patient's risk of neoplasia. Renal transplant patients are known to have an increased risk of malignancy, predominantly skin cancer and reticulum cell or lymphomatous tumors.[10] The risk of post-transplant lymphomas may be increased in patients who receive aggressive treatment with immunosuppressive drugs.[11] The degree of immunosuppression is determined not only by the immunosuppressive regimen but also by a number of other patient factors. The number of immunosuppressive agents may not necessarily increase the risk of post-transplant lymphomas. However, transplant patients who receive multiple immunosuppressive agents may be at risk for over-immunosuppression; therefore, immunosuppressive drug therapy should be maintained at the lowest effective levels. Information is available on the spontaneous neoplasia risk in rheumatoid arthritis,[12,13] and on neoplasia

WARNINGS: *(cont'd)*

following immunosuppressive therapy of other autoimmune diseases.[14,15] It has not been possible to define the precise risk of neoplasia due to azathioprine.[16] The data suggest the risk may be elevated in patients with rheumatoid arthritis, though lower than for renal transplant patients.[11,13] However, acute myelogenous leukemia as well as solid tumors have been reported in patients with rheumatoid arthritis who have received azathioprine. Data on neoplasia in patients receiving azathioprine can be found under ADVERSE REACTIONS.

Azathioprine has been reported to cause temporary depression in spermatogenesis and reduction in sperm viability and sperm count in mice at doses 10 times the human therapeutic dose[17]; a reduced percentage of fertile matings occurred when animals received 5 mg/kg.[18]

Use in Pregnancy: Azathioprine can cause fetal harm when administered to a pregnant woman. Azathioprine should not be given during pregnancy without careful weighing of risk versus benefit. Whenever possible, use of azathioprine in pregnant patients should be avoided. This drug should not be used for treating rheumatoid arthritis in pregnant women.[19]

Azathioprine is teratogenic in rabbits and mice when given in doses equivalent to the human dose (5 mg/kg daily). Abnormalities included skeletal malformations and visceral anomalies.[18]

Limited immunologic and other abnormalities have occurred in a few infants born of renal allograft recipients on azathioprine. In a detailed case report,[20] documented lymphopenia, diminished lgG and lgM levels, CMV infection, and a decreased thymic shadow were noted in an infant born to a mother receiving 150 mg azathioprine and 30 mg prednisone daily throughout pregnancy. At ten weeks most features were normalized. DeWitte et al[21]reported pancytopenia and severe immune deficiency in a preterm infant whose mother received 125 mg azathioprine and 12.5 mg prednisone daily. There have been two published reports of abnormal physical findings. Williamson and Karp[22] described an infant born with preaxial polydactyly whose mother received azathioprine 200 mg daily and prednisone 20 mg every other day during pregnancy. Tallent et al[23]described an infant with a large myelomeningocele in the upper lumber region, bilateral dislocated hips, and bilateral talipes equinovarus. The father was on long-term azathioprine therapy.

Benefit versus risk must be weighed carefully before use of azathioprine in patients of reproductive potential. There are no adequate and well-controlled studies in pregnant women. If this drug is used during pregnancy or if the patient becomes pregnant while taking this drug, the patient should be apprised of the potential hazard to the fetus. Women of childbearing age should be advised to avoid becoming pregnant.

PRECAUTIONS:

General: A gastrointestinal hypersensitivity reaction characterized by severe nausea and vomiting has been reported.[24,25,26] These symptoms may also be accompanied by diarrhea, rash, fever, malaise, myalgias, elevations in liver enzymes, and occasionally, hypotension. Symptoms of gastrointestinal toxicity most often develop within the first several weeks of azathioprine therapy and are reversible upon discontinuation of the drug. The reaction can recur within hours after rechallenge with a single dose of azathioprine.

Information for the Patient: Patients being started on azathioprine should be informed of the necessity of periodic blood counts while they are receiving the drug and should be encouraged to report any unusual bleeding or bruising to their physician. They should be informed of the danger of infection while receiving azathioprine and asked to report signs and symptoms of infection to their physician. Careful dosage instructions should be given to the patient, especially when azathioprine is being administered in the presence of impaired renal function or concomitantly with allopurinol (see DOSAGE AND ADMINISTRATIONand DRUG INTERACTIONS). Patients should be advised of the potential risks of the use of azathioprine during pregnancy and during the nursing period. The increased risk of neoplasia following azathioprine therapy should be explained to the patient.

Laboratory Tests: See WARNINGS and ADVERSE REACTIONS.

Carcinogenesis, Mutagenesis, and Impairment of Fertility: See WARNINGSsection.

Pregnancy, Teratogenic Effects, Pregnancy Category D See WARNINGS.

Nursing Mothers: The use of azathioprine in nursing mothers is not recommended. Azathioprine or its metabolites are transferred at low levels, both transplacentally and in breast milk.[29,30,31]Because of the potential for tumorigenicity shown for azathioprine, a decision should be made whether to discontinue nursing or discontinue the drug, taking into account the importance of the drug to the mother.

Pediatric Use: Safety and efficacy of azathioprine in children have not been established.

DRUG INTERACTIONS:

Use with Allopurinol: The principal pathway for detoxification of azathioprine is inhibited by allopurinol. Patients receiving azathioprine and allopurinol concomitantly should have a dose reduction of azathioprine, to approximately 1/3 to 1/4 the usual dose.

Use with Other Agents Effecting Myelopoiesis: Drugs which may affect leukocyte production, including co-trimoxazole, may lead to exaggerated leukopenia, especially in renal transplant recipients.[27]

Use with Angiotensin Converting Enzyme Inhibitors: The use of angiotensin converting enzyme inhibitors to control hypertension in patients on azathioprine has been reported to induce severe leukopenia.[28]

ADVERSE REACTIONS:

The principal and potentially serious toxic effects of azathioprine are hematologic and gastrointestinal. The risks of secondary infection and neoplasia are also significant (see WARNINGS). The frequency and severity of adverse reactions depend on the dose and duration of azathioprine as well as on the patient's underlying disease or concomitant therapies. The incidence of hematologic toxicities and neoplasia encountered in groups of renal homograft recipients is significantly higher than that in studies employing azathioprine for rheumatoid arthritis. The relative incidences in clinical studies are summarized below (TABLE 1):

Hematologic: Leukopenia and/or thrombocytopenia are dose dependent and may occur late in the course of azathioprine therapy. Dose reduction or temporary withdrawal allows reversal of these toxicities. Infection may occur as a secondary manifestation of bone marrow suppression or leukopenia, but the incidence of infection in renal homotransplantation is 30 to 60 times that in rheumatoid arthritis. Macrocytic anemia and/or bleeding have been reported in two patients on azathioprine.

Gastrointestinal: Nausea and vomiting may occur within the first few months of therapy with azathioprine, and occurred in approximately 12% of 676 rheumatoid arthritis patients. The frequency of gastric disturbance often can be reduced by administration of the drug in divided doses and/or after meals. However, in some patients, nausea and vomiting may be severe and may be accompanied by symptoms such as diarrhea, fever, malaise, and myalgias (see PRECAUTIONS). Vomiting with abdominal pain may occur rarely with a hypersensitivity pancreatitis. Hepatotoxicity manifest by elevation of serum alkaline phosphatase, bilirubin and/or serum transaminases is known to occur following azathioprine use, primarily in allograft recipients. Hepatotoxicity has been uncommon (less than 1%) in rheumatoid arthritis patients. Hepatotoxicity following transplantation most often occurs within 6 months of transplantation and is generally reversible after interruption of azathioprine. A rare, but

ADVERSE REACTIONS: *(cont'd)*

TABLE 1

Toxicity	Renal Homograft	Rheumatoid Arthritis
Leukopenia		
Any Degree	$> 50\%$	28
$< 2500/mm^3$	16%	5.3%
Infections	20%	$< 1\%$
Neoplasia		*
Lymphoma	0.5%	
Others	2.8%	

* Data on the rate and risk of neoplasia among persons with rheumatoid arthritis treated with azathioprine are limited. The incidence of lymphoproliferative disease in patients with RA appears to be significantly higher than that in the general population.[12] In one completed study, the rate of lymphoproliferative disease in RA patients receiving higher than recommended doses of azathioprine (5 mg/kg/day) was 1.8 cases per 1000 patient years of follow-up, compared with 0.8 cases per 1000 patient years of follow-up in those not receiving azathioprine.[13] However, the proportion of the increased risk attributable to the azathioprine dosage or to other therapies (*i.e.*, alkylating agents) received by azathioprine-treated patients cannot be determined.

life-threatening hepatic veno-occlusive disease associated with chronic administration of azathioprine has been described in transplant patients and in one patient receiving azathioprine for panuveitis.[32,33,34] Periodic measurement of serum transaminases, alkaline phosphatase and bilirubin is indicated for early detection of hepatotoxicity. If hepatic veno-occlusive disease is clinically suspected, azathioprine should be permanently withdrawn.

Others: Additional side effects of low frequency have been reported. These include skin rashes (approximately 2%), alopecia, fever, arthralgias, diarrhea, steatorrhea and negative nitrogen balance (all less than 1%).

OVERDOSAGE:

The oral LD_{50}s for single doses of azathioprine in mice and rats are 2500 mg/kg and 400 mg/kg, respectively. Very large doses of this antimetabolite may lead to marrow hypoplasia, bleeding, infection, and death. About 30% of azathioprine is bound to serum proteins, but approximately 45% is removed during an 8 hour hemodialysis.[35] A single case has been reported of a renal transplant patient who ingested a single dose of 7500 mg azathioprine. The immediate toxic reactions were nausea, vomiting, and diarrhea, followed by mild abnormalities in liver function. The white blood cell count, SGOT, and bilirubin returned to normal six days after the overdose.

DOSAGE AND ADMINISTRATION:

Renal Homotransplantation: The dose of azathioprine required to prevent rejection and minimize toxicity will vary with individual patients; this necessitates careful management. The initial dose is usually 3 to 5 mg/kg daily, beginning at the time of transplant. Azathioprine is usually given as a single daily dose on the day of, and in a minority of cases one to three days before, transplantation. Azathioprine is often initiated with the intravenous administration of the sodium salt, with subsequent use of tablets (at the same dose level) after the postoperative period. Intravenous administration of the sodium salt is indicated only in patients unable to tolerate oral medications. Dose reduction to maintenance levels of 1 to 3 mg/kg daily is usually possible. The dose of azathioprine should not be increased to toxic levels because of threatened rejection. Discontinuation may be necessary for severe hematologic or other toxicity, even if rejection of the homograft may be a consequence of drug withdrawal.

Rheumatoid Arthritis: Azathioprine is usually given on a daily basis. The initial dose should be approximately 1.0 mg/kg (50 to 100 mg) given as a single dose or on a twice daily schedule. The dose may be increased, beginning at six to eight weeks and thereafter by steps at four-week intervals, if there are no serious toxicities and if initial response is unsatisfactory. Dose increments should be 0.5 mg/kg daily, up to a maximum dose of 2.5 mg/kg/day. Therapeutic response occurs after several weeks of treatment, usually six to eight; an adequate trial should be a minimum of 12 weeks. Patients not improved after twelve weeks can be considered refractory. Azathioprine may be continued long-term in patients with clinical response, but patients should be monitored carefully, and gradual dosage reduction should be attempted to reduce risk of toxicities.

Maintenance therapy should be at the lowest effective dose, and the dose given can be lowered decrementally with changes of 0.5 mg/kg or approximately 25 mg daily every four weeks while other therapy is kept constant. The optimum duration of maintenance azathioprine has not been determined. Azathioprine can be discontinued abruptly, but delayed effects are possible.

Use in Renal Dysfunction: Relatively oliguric patients, especially those with tubular necrosis in the immediate post-cadaveric transplant period, may have delayed clearance of azathioprine or its metabolites, may be particularly sensitive to this drug and are usually given lower doses.

Parenteral Administration: Add 10 ml of Sterile Water for Injection, and swirl until a clear solution results. This solution, equivalent to 100 mg azathioprine, is for intravenous use only; it has a pH of approximately 9.6, and it should be used within twenty-four hours. Further dilution into sterile saline or dextrose is usually made for infusion; the final volume depends on time for the infusion, usually 30 to 60 minutes, but as short as 5 minutes and as long as 8 hours for the daily dose.

Parenteral drug products should be inspected visually for particulate matter and discoloration prior to administration, whenever solution and container permit.

Procedures for proper handling and disposal of this immunosuppressive antimetabolite drug should be considered. Several guidelines on this subject have been published.[36-42] There is no general agreement that all of the procedures recommended in the guidelines are necessary or appropriate.

REFERENCES:

1. Elion GB, Hitchings GH, Azathioprine. In: Sartorelli AC, Johns DG, eds. *Antineoplastic and Immunosuppressive Agents Pt II*. New York, NY: Springer Verlag; 1975:chap 48. **2.** McIntosh J, Hansen P, Ziegler J, et al. Defective immune and phagocytic functions in uraemia and renal transplantation. *Int Arch Allergy Appl Immunol*. 1976;15:544-549. **3.** Renal Transplant Registry Advisory Committee. The 12th report of the Human Renal Transplant Registry. *JAMA*. 1975;233:787-796. **4.** McGeown M. Immunosuppression for kidney transplantation.*Lancet*. 1973;2:310-312. **5.** Simmons RL, Thompson EJ, Yunis EJ, et al. 115 Patients with first cadaver kidney transplants followed two to seven and a half years: a multifactorial analysis. *Am J Med*. 1977;62:234-242. **6.** Fye K, Talal N. Cytotoxic drugs in the treatment of rheumatoid arthritis. *Ration Drug Ther*. 1975;9(4):1-5. **7.** Davis JD, Muss HB, Turner RA. Cytotoxic agents in the treatment of rheumatoid arthritis. *South Med J*. 1978;71:58-64. **8.** McEwen C. The diagnosis and differential diagnosis of rheumatoid arthritis. In: Hollander JL, ed. *Arthritis and Allied Conditions: A Textbook of Rheumatology*. 8th ed. Philadelphia, PA: Lea and Febiger; 1972:403-418. **9.** Hoover R, Fraumeni JF. Drug-induced cancer. *Cancer*. 1981;47(5):1071-1080. **10.** Hoover R, Fraumeni JF Jr. Risk of cancer in renal transplant recipients. *Lancet*. 1973;2:55-57. **11.** Wilkinson AH, Smith JL, Hunsicker LG, et al. Increased frequency of post-transplant lymphomas in patients treated with cyclosporine, azathioprine, and prednisone.*Transplantation*. 1989;47:293-296. **12.** Prior P, Symmons DPM, Hawkins CF, et al. Cancer morbidity in rheumatoid arthritis. *Ann Rheum Dis* 1984;43:128-131. **13.** Silman AJ, Petrie J, Hazelman B, et al. Lymphoproliferative cancer and other malignancy in patients with rheumatoid arthritis treated with azathioprine: a 20 year follow up study. *Ann Rheum Dis.*1988;47:988-992. **14.** Louie S, Schwartz RS. Immunodeficiency and pathogenesis of lymphoma and leukemia. *Semin Hematol*. 1978;15:117-138. **15.** Wang KK, Czaja AJ, Beaver SJ, et al. Extra hepatic malignancy following long-term immunosuppressive therapy of severe hepatitis B surface antigen-negative chronic active hepatitis.*Hepatology*. 1989;10:39-43. **16.** Sieber SM, Adamson RH.

REFERENCES: *(cont'd)*

Toxicity of antineoplastic agents in man: chromosomal aberrations, antifertility effects, congenital malformations, and carcinogenic potential. In: Klein G, Weinhouse S, eds. *Advances in Cancer Research*, v 22. New York, NY: Academic Press; 1975:57-155. **17.** Clark JM. The mutagenicity of azathioprine in mice, *Drosophila Melanogaster* and *Neurospora Crassa*. *Mut Res*. 1975;28(1):87-99. **18.** Data on file, Burroughs Wellcome Co. **19.** Tagatz GE, Simmons RL. Pregnancy after renal transplantation. *Ann Intern Med*. 1975;82:113-144. Editorial Notes. **20.** Cote CJ, Meuwissen HJ, Pickering RJ. Effects on the neonate of prednisone and azathioprine administered to the mother during pregnancy.*J Pediatr*. 1974;85(3):324-328. **21.** DeWitte DB, Buick MK, Stephen EC, et al. Neonatal pancytopenia and severe combined immunodeficiency associated with antenatal administration of azathioprine and prednisone. *J Pediatr*. 1984;105(4):625-628. **22.** Williamson RA, Karp LE. Azathioprine teratogenicity: review of the literature and case report.*Obstet Gynecol*. 1981;58:247-250. **23.** Tallent MB, Simmons RL, Najarian JS. Birth defects in child of male recipient of kidney transplant.*JAMA*. 1970;211(11):1854-1855. **24.** Assini JF, Hamilton R, Strosberg JM. Adverse reactions to azathioprine mimicking gastroenteritis.*J Rheumatol*. 1986;13:1117-1118. **25.** Cochrane D, Adamson AR, Halsey JP. Adverse reactions to azathioprine mimicking gastroenteritis. *J Rheumatol*. 1987;14:1075. **26.** Cox J, Daneshmend JK, Hawkey CJ, et al. Devastating diarrhoea caused by azathioprine: management difficulty in inflammatory bowel disease. *Gut*. 1988;29(5):686-688. **27.** Bradley PP, Warden GD, Maxwell JG, et al. Neutropenia and thrombocytopenia in renal allograft recipients treated with trimethoprim-sulfamethoxazole. *Ann Int Med*. 1980;93:560-562. **28.** Kirchertz EJ, Grone HJ, Rieger J, et al. Successful low dose captopril rechallenge following drug-induced leucopenia. *Lancet*.1981;8234:1362-1363. **29.** Nelson D, Bugge C. Data on file, Burroughs Wellcome Co. **30.** Saarikoski S, Seppala M. Immunosuppression during pregnancy: transmission of azathioprine and its metabolites from the mother to the fetus. *Am J Obstet Gynecol*. 1973;115:1100-1106. **31.** Coulam CB, Moyer TP, Jiang NS, et al. Breast-feeding after renal transplantation. *Transplant Proc*. 1982;14:605-609. **32.** Read AE, Wiesner RH, LaBrecque DR, et al. Hepatic veno-occlusive disease associated with renal transplantation and azathioprine therapy. *Ann Intern Med*. 1986;104:651-655. **33.** Katzka DA, Saul SH, Jorkasky D, et al. Azathioprine and hepatic venocclusive disease in renal transplant patients. *Gastroenterology*. 1986;90:446-454. **34.** Weitz H, Gokel JM, Loeschke K, et al. Veno-occlusive disease of the liver in patients receiving immunosuppressive therapy. *Virchows Arch A*.1982;395:245-256. **35.** Schusziarra V, Ziekursch V, Schlamp R, et al. Pharmacokinetics of azathioprine under haemodialysis. *Int J Clin Pharmacol Biopharm*. 1976;14(4):298-302. **36.** Recommendations for the safe handling of parenteral antineoplastic drugs. Washington, DC: Division of Safety, National Institutes of Health; 1983. US Dept of Health and Human Services, Public Health Service publication NIH 83-2621. **37.** AMA Council on Scientific Affairs. Guidelines for handling parenteral antineoplastics. *JAMA*. 1985;253:1590-1591. **38.** National Study Commission on Cytotoxic Exposure. Recommendations for handling cytotoxic agents. 1984. Available from Louis P. Jeffrey, ScD, Director of Pharmacy Services, Rhode Island Hospital, 593 Eddy Street, Providence, Rhode Island 02902. **39.** Clinical Oncological Society of Australia. Guidelines and recommendations for safe handling of antineoplastic agents. *Med J Australia*. 1983;1:426-428. **40.** Jones RB, Frank R, Mass T. Safe handling of chemotherapeutic agents: a report from the Mount Sinai Medical Center. *CA-A Cancer J for Clin*. 1983;33(Sept/Oct):258-263. **41.** American Society of Hospital Pharmacists. ASHP technical assistance bulletin on handling cytotoxic and hazardous drugs. *Am J Hosp Pharm*.1990;47:1033-1049. **42.** Yodaiken RE, Bennett D. OSHA work-practice guidelines for personnel dealing with cytotoxic (antineoplastic) drugs. *Am J Hosp Pharm*. 1986;43:1193-1204.

HOW SUPPLIED:

50 mg overlapping circle-shaped, yellow to off-white, scored tablets imprinted with "IMURAN" and "50" on each tablet.

Store at 15° to 25°C (59° to 77°F) in a dry place and protect from light.

20 ml vial, each containing the equivalent of 100 mg azathioprine (as the sodium salt).

Store at 15° to 25°C (59° to 77°F) and protect from light. The sterile, lyophilized sodium salt is yellow, and should be dissolved in Sterile Water for Injection (see DOSAGE AND ADMINISTRATION, Parenteral Administration).

HOW SUPPLIED - RATED THERAPEUTICALLY EQUIVALENT:

Injection, Lyphl-Soln - Intravenous - 100 mg/ml

20 ml	$101.18	IMURAN, Glaxo Wellcome	00173-0598-71

Tablet, Uncoated - Oral - 50 mg

100's	$117.89	IMURAN, Glaxo Wellcome	00173-0597-56
100's	$129.72	IMURAN, Glaxo Wellcome	00173-0597-55

HOW SUPPLIED - NOT RATED EQUIVALENT:

Injection, Lyphl-Soln - Intravenous - 100 mg/ml

1's	$81.60	Azathioprine Sodium, Bedford Labs	55390-0600-20

AZELAIC ACID *(003268)*

CATEGORIES: Acne; Anti-Infectives; Antibacterials; Antibiotics; Dermatologicals; Keratolytic Agents; Local Infections; Skin/Mucous Membrane Agents; Topical; FDA Approved 1995 Sep

BRAND NAMES: *Acelain*; *Azalea*; **Azelex**; *Cutacelan* (Mexico); *Skinkoren*; *Skinoderm*; *Skinorem*; *Skinoren* (Australia, Germany, England)
(International brand names outside U.S. in italics)

Prescribing information not available at time of publication.

HOW SUPPLIED - EQUIVALENTS NOT AVAILABLE:

Cream - Topical - 20%

30 g	$22.00	AZELEX, Allergan	00023-8694-30

AZELASTINE *(003278)*

CATEGORIES: Allergies; Antihistamines; FDA Approved 1996 Oct; Pregnancy Category C; Respiratory & Allergy Medications; Rhinitis; Rhinorrhea; Sneezing; Urticaria

BRAND NAMES: *Allergodil* (Germany); **Astelin**; *Azeptin* (Japan)
(International brand names outside U.S. in italics)

DESCRIPTION:

Azelastine hydrochloride nasal spray, 137 micrograms (mcg), is an antihistamine formulated as a metered spray solution for intranasal administration. Azelastine hydrochloride occurs as a white, almost odorless, crystalline powder with a bitter taste. It has a molecular weight of 418.37. It is sparingly soluble in water, methanol, and propylene glycol and slightly soluble in ethanol, octanol, and glycerine. It has a melting point of about 225°C and the pH of a saturated solution is between 5.0 and 5.4. Its chemical name is (±)-1-(2H)-phthalazinone,4-[(4-chlorophenyl)methyl]-2-(hexahydro-1- methyl-1H-azepin-4-yl)-, monohydrochloride. Its molecular formula is $C_{22}H_{24}ClN_3O{\cdot}HCl$.

Astelin Nasal Spray contains 0.1% azelastine hydrochloride in an aqueous solution at pH 6.8 ± 0.3. It also contains benzalkonium chloride (125 mcg/ml), edetate disodium, hydroxypropyl methyl cellulose, citric acid, dibasic sodium phosphate, sodium chloride, and purified water.

After priming, each metered spray delivers a 0.137 ml mean volume containing 137 mcg of azelastine hydrochloride (equivalent to 125 mcg of azelastine base). Each bottle can deliver 100 metered sprays.

CLINICAL PHARMACOLOGY:

Azelastine hydrochloride, a phthalazinone derivative, exhibits histamine H_1 receptor antagonist activity in isolated tissues, animal models, and humans. Azelastine nasal spray is administered as a racemic mixture with no difference in pharmacologic activity noted between the enantiomers in *in vitro* studies. The major metabolite, desmethylazelastine, also possesses H_1-receptor antagonist activity.

CLINICAL PHARMACOLOGY: *(cont'd)*

Pharmacokinetics and Metabolism: After intranasal administration, the systemic bioavailability of azelastine hydrochloride is approximately 40%. Maximum plasma concentrations (C_{max}) are achieved in 2-3 hours. Based on intravenous and oral administration, the elimination half-life, steady-state volume of distribution, and plasma clearance are 22 hours, 14.5 L/kg, and 0.5 L/h/kg, respectively. Approximately 75% of an oral dose of radiolabeled azelastine hydrochloride was excreted in the feces with less than 10% as unchanged azelastine. Azelastine is oxidatively metabolized to the principal active metabolite, desmethylazelastine, by the cytochrome P450 enzyme system. The specific P450 isoforms responsible for the biotransformation of azelastine have not been identified; however, clinical interaction studies with the known CYP3A4 inhibitor erythromycin failed to demonstrate a pharmacokinetic interaction. In a multiple-dose, steady-state drug interaction study in normal volunteers, cimetidine (400 mg twice daily), a non-specific P450 inhibitor, raised orally administered mean azelastine (4 mg twice daily) concentrations by approximately 65%.

The major active metabolite, desmethylazelastine, was not measurable (below assay limits) after single-dose intranasal administration of azelastine hydrochloride. After intranasal dosing of azelastine hydrochloride to steady-state, plasma concentrations of desmethylazelastine range from 20-50% of azelastine concentrations. When azelastine hydrochloride is administered orally, desmethylazelastine has an elimination half-life of 54 hours. Limited data indicate that the metabolite profile is similar when azelastine hydrochloride is administered via the intranasal or oral route.

In vitro studies with human plasma indicate that the plasma protein binding of azelastine and desmethylazelastine are approximately 88% and 97%, respectively.

Azelastine hydrochloride administered intranasally at doses above two sprays per nostril for 29 days resulted in greater than proportional increases in C_{max} and area under the curve (AUC) for azelastine.

Studies in healthy subjects administered oral doses of azelastine hydrochloride demonstrated linear responses in C_{max} and AUC.

Special Populations: Following oral administration, pharmacokinetic parameters were not influenced by age, gender, or hepatic impairment.

Based on oral, single-dose studies, renal insufficiency (creatine clearance <50 ml/min) resulted in a 70-75% higher C_{max} and AUC compared to normal subjects. Time to maximum concentration was unchanged.

Oral azelastine has been safely administered to over 1400 asthmatic subjects, supporting the safety of administering azelastine HCl nasal spray to allergic rhinitis patients with asthma.

Pharmacodynamics: In a placebo-controlled study (95 subjects with allergic rhinitis), there was no evidence of an effect of azelastine nasal spray (2 sprays per nostril twice daily for 56 days) on cardiac repolarization as represented by the corrected QT interval (QTc) of the electrocardiogram. At higher oral exposures (≥4 mg twice daily), a non-clinically significant mean change on the QTc (3-7 millisecond increase) was observed.

Interaction studies investigating the cardiac repolarization effects of concomitanty administered oral azelastine hydrochloride and erythromycin or ketoconazole were conducted. Oral erythromycin had no effect on azelastine pharmacokinetics or QTc based on analysis of serial electrocardiograms. Ketoconazole interfered with the measurement of azelastine plasma levels; however, no effects on QTc were observed (see DRUG INTERACTIONS).

CLINICAL STUDIES:

U.S. placebo-controlled clinical trials of azelastine, included 322 patients with seasonal allergic rhinitis who received two sprays per nostril twice a day for up to 4 weeks. These trials included 55 pediatric patients ages 12 to 16 years. Azelastine significantly improved a complex of symptoms which included rhinorrhea, sneezing, and nasal pruritus.

In dose-ranging trials, azelastine administration resulted in a decrease in symptoms which reached statistical significance from saline placebo within 3 hours after initial dosing and persisted over the 12-hour dosing interval.

There were no findings on nasal examination in an 8-week study that suggested any adverse effect of azelastine on the nasal mucosa.

INDICATIONS AND USAGE:

Azelastine is indicated for the treatment of the symptoms of seasonal allergic rhinitis such as rhinorrhea, sneezing, and nasal pruritus in adults and children 12 years and older.

CONTRAINDICATIONS:

Azelastine is contraindicated n patients with a known hypersensitivity to azelastine hydrochloride or any of its components.

PRECAUTIONS:

Activities Requiring Mental Alertness: In clinical trials, the occurrence of somnolence has been reported in some patients taking azelastine nasal spray: due caution should therefore be exercised when driving a car or operating potentially dangerous machinery. Concurrent use of azelastine nasal spray with alcohol or other CNS depressants should be avoided because additional reductions in alertness and additional impairment of CNS performance may occur.

Information For Patients: Patients should be instructed to use azelastine only as prescribed. For the proper use of the nasal spray and to attain maximum improvement, the patient should read and follow carefully the accompanying patient instructions. Patients should be instructed to prime the delivery system before initial use and after storage for 3 or more days (see PATIENT INSTRUCTIONS FOR USE). Patients should also be instructed to store the bottle upright at room temperature with the pump tightly closed and away from children.

Patients should be advised against the concurrent use of azelastine with other antihistamines without consulting a physician. Patients who are, or may become, pregnant should be told that this product should be used in pregnancy or during lactation only if the potential benefit justifies the potential risks to the fetus or nursing infant. Patients should be advised to assess their individual responses to azelastine before engaging in any activity requiring mental alertness, such as driving a car or operating machinery. Patients should be advised that the concurrent use of azelastine with alcohol or other CNS depressants may lead to additional reductions in alertness and impairment of CNS performance and should be avoided (see DRUG INTERACTIONS).

Geriatric Use: U.S. placebo-controlled clinical trials included 11 patients above the age of 60 years who were treated with azelastine. While this number is very small and no substantial conclusions can be drawn, the adverse events in this group were similar to patients under age 60 years.

Carcinogenesis, Mutagenesis, Impairment of Fertility: Carcinogenicity studies in rats and mice with oral azelastine hydrochloride for 24 months at doses up to 30 mg/kg/day and 25 mg/kg/day, respectively (240 and 100 times the maximum recommended human daily intranasal dose on a mg/m^2 basis), revealed no evidence of carcinogenicity.

Azelastine hydrochloride showed no genotoxic effects in the Ames test, DNA repair test, mouse lymphoma forward mutation assay, mouse micronucleus test, or chromosomal aberration test in rat bone marrow.

PRECAUTIONS: *(cont'd)*

Reproduction and fertility studies in rats showed no effects on male or female fertility at oral doses of up to 30 mg/kg/day (240 times the maximum recommended human daily intranasal dose on a mg/m^2 basis). At 68.6 mg/kg/day (550 times the maximum recommended human daily intranasal dose on a mg/m^2 basis), the duration of estrous cycles was prolonged and copulatory activity and the number of pregnancies were decreased. The numbers of corpora lutea and implantations were decreased; however the implantation ratio was not affected.

Pregnancy Category C: Azelastine hydrochloride has been shown to be embryotoxic fetotoxic, and teratogenic (external and skeletal abnormalities) in mice at an oral dose of 68.6 mg/kg/day (280 times the maximum recommended human daily intranasal dose on a mg/m^2 basis). At an oral dose of 30 mg/kg/day (240 times the maximum recommended human daily intranasal dose on a mg/m^2 basis), delayed ossification (undeveloped metacarpus), and the incidence of 14th rib were increased in rats. At 68.6 mg/kg/day (550 times the maximum recommended human daily intranasal dose on a mg/m^2 basis) azelastine hydrochloride caused abortion and fetotoxic effects in rats.

The relevance to humans of these skeletal findings noted at only high drug exposure levels is unknown. There are no adequate and well-controlled clinical studies in pregnant women. Azelastine should be used during pregnancy only if the potential benefit justifies the potential risk to the fetus.

Nursing Mothers: It is not known whether azelastine hydrochloride is excreted in human milk. Because many drugs are excreted in human milk, caution should be exercised when azelastine is administered to a nursing woman.

Pediatric Use: Safety and efficacy of azelastine in pediatric patients below the age of 12 years have not been established.

DRUG INTERACTIONS:

Concurrent use of azelastine with alcohol or other CNS depressants should be avoided because additional reductions in alertness and additional impairment of CNS performance may occur.

Cimetidine (400 mg twice daily) increased the mean C_{max} and AUC of orally administered azelastine hydrochloride (4 mg twice daily) by approximately 65%. Ranitidine hydrochloride (150 mg twice daily) had no effect on azelastine pharmacokinetics.

Interaction studies investigating the cardiac effects, as measured by the corrected QT interval (QTc), of concomitantly administered azelastine hydrochloride and erythromycin or ketoconazole were conducted. Oral erythromycin (500 mg three times daily for seven days) had no effect on azelastine pharmacokinetics or QTc based on analyses of serial electrocardiograms. Ketoconazole (200 mg twice daily for 7 days) interfered with the measurement of azelastine plasma concentrations; however, no effects on QTc were observed.

No significant pharmacokinetic interaction was observed with the coadministration of an oral 4-mg dose of azelastine hydrochloride twice daily and theophylline 300 mg or 400 mg twice daily.

ADVERSE REACTIONS:

Adverse experience information for azelastine is derived from six well-controlled, 2-day to 8-week clinical studies which included 391 patients who received azelastine at a dose of 2 sprays per nostril twice daily. In placebo-controlled efficacy trials, the incidence of discontinuation due to adverse reactions in patients receiving azelastine was not significantly different from vehicle placebo (2.2% vs 2.8%, respectively).

In these clinical studies, adverse events that occurred statistically significantly more often in patients treated wth azelastine versus vehicle placebo included bitter taste (19.7% vs 0.6%), somnolence (11.5% vs 5.4%), weight increase (2.0% vs 0%), and myalgia (1.5% vs 0%).

The adverse events listed in TABLE 1 were reported with frequencies ≥2% in the azelastine treatment group and more frequently than placebo in short-term (≤2 days) and long-term (2-8 weeks) clinical trials.

TABLE 1

Adverse Event	Azelastine HCl Nasal Spray n=391	Vehicle Placebo n=353
Bitter Taste*	19.7	0.6
Headache	14.8	12.7
Somnolence*	11.5	5.4
Nasal Burning	4.1	1.7
Pharyngitis	3.8	2.8
Dry Mouth	2.8	1.7
Paroxysmal Sneezing	3.1	1.1
Nausea	2.8	1.1
Rhinitis	2.3	1.4
Fatigue	2.3	1.4
Dizziness	2.0	1.4
Epistaxis	2.0	1.4
Weight Increase*	2.0	0.0

* P<0.05, Fisher's Exact Test (two-tailed)

The following events were observed infrequently (<2% and exceeding placebo incidence) in patients who received azelastine (2 sprays/nostril twice daily) in U. S. clinical trials:

Cardiovascular: flushing, hypertension, tachycardia

Dermatological: contact dermatitis, eczema, hair and follicle infecton, furunculosis

Digestive: constipation, gastroenteritis, glossitis, ulcerative stomatitis, vomiting, increased SGPT, aphthous stomatitis

Metabolic and Nutritional: increased appetite

Musculoskeletal: myalgia, temporomandibular dislocation

Neurological: hyperkinesia, hypoesthesia, vertigo

Psychological: anxiety, depersonalization, depression, nervousness, sleep disorder, thinking abnormal

Respiratory: bronchospasm, coughing, throat burning, laryngitis

Special Senses: conjunctivitis, eye abnormality, eye pain, watery eyes, taste loss

Urogenital: albuminuria, amenorrhea, breast pain, hematuria, increased urinary frequency

Whole Body: allergic reaction, back pain, herpes simplex, viral infection, malaise, pain in extremities, abdominal pain

In controlled trials involving nasal and oral azelastine hydrochloride formulations, there were infrequent occurrences of hepatic transaminase elevations. The clinical relevance of these reports has not been established.

OVERDOSAGE:

There have been no reported overdosages with azelastine. Acute overdosage with this dosage form is unlikely to result in clinically significant adverse events, other than increased somnolence, since one bottle of azelastine contains 17 mg of azelastine hydrochloride. Clinical studies with single doses of the oral formulation of azelastine hydrochloride (up to 16

OVERDOSAGE: *(cont'd)*

mg) have not resulted in increased incidence of serious adverse events. General supportive measures should be employed if overdosage occurs. Oral doses greater than 120 mg/kg (480 times the maximum recommended human daily intranasal dose on a mg/m^2 basis) produced a significant mortality in mice. Responses seen prior to mortality were tremor, convulsions, decreased muscle tone, and salivation. Single doses as high as 10 mg/kg (270 times the maximum recommended human daily intranasal dose on a mg/m^2 basis) were well tolerated in dogs, but single doses of 20 mg/kg were lethal.

DOSAGE AND ADMINISTRATION:

The recommended dose of azelastine in adults and children 12 years and older is two sprays per nostril twice daily. Before initial use, the child-resistant screw cap on the bottle should be replaced with the pump unit and the delivery system should be primed with 4 sprays or until a fine mist appears. When 3 or more days have elapsed since the last use, the pump should be reprimed with 2 sprays or until a fine mist appears.

Warning: Avoid spraying in the eyes.

Directions For Use: Illustrated patient instructions for proper use accompany each package of azelastine.

PATIENT INFORMATION:

Azelastine is used for the treatment of symptoms of seasonal allergic rhinitis.

Use with caution in pregnancy and lactation.

May cause drowsiness; use caurion while driving or operating hazardous machinery.

Inform your physician if you are taking any other medications, including over-the-counter products.

Avoid alcohol and other CNS depressants while taking azelastine.

May cause bitter taste, drowsiness, weight gain, and muscle pain.

Patient package insert is available with product.

HOW SUPPLIED:

Astelin Nasal Spray, 137 mcg is supplied as a package containing a total of 200 metered sprays in two high-density polyethylene (HDPE) bottles fitted with child-resistant screw caps. A separate metered-dose spray pump unit and a leaflet of patient instructions are also provided. The spray pump unit is packaged in a polyethylene wrapper and consists of a nasal spray pump fitted with a blue safety clip and a blue plastic dust cover.

Each Astelin Nasal Spray, 137 mcg, bottle contains 17 mg (1 mg/ml) of azelastine hydrochloride to be used with the supplied metered-dose spray pump unit. Each bottle can deliver 100 metered sprays. Each spray delivers a mean of 0.137 ml solution containing 137 mcg of azelastine hydrochloride.

Attention: The imprinted expiration date applies to the product in the bottles with child-resistant screw caps. After the spray pump is inserted into the first bottle of the dispensing package, both bottles of product should be discarded after 6 months, not to exceed the expiration date imprinted on the label.

Storage: Store at controlled room temperature 20°-25°C (68°-77°F). Protect from freezing.

HOW SUPPLIED - EQUIVALENTS NOT AVAILABLE:

Spray - Intranasal - 137 mcg/inh

34 ml $42.60 ASTELIN, Wallace Labs 00037-0241-10

AZITHROMYCIN DIHYDRATE *(003066)*

CATEGORIES: Anti-Infectives; Antibiotics; Azalides; Chlamydia; Erythromycins; Fever; Gram-Negative Antibiotics; Infections; Macrolide; Otitis Media; Pharyngitis; Pneumonia; Pulmonary Disease; Respiratory Tract Infections; Rheumatic Fever; Sexually Transmitted Diseases; Skin Infections; Tonsillitis; Urethritis; FDA Class 1B ("Modest Therapeutic Advantage"); Sales > $100 Million; FDA Approved 1991 Nov; Top 200 Drugs

BRAND NAMES: *Arzomicin*; *Azenil*; *Azithral*; *Azitrocin* (Mexico); *Azitromax*; *Aziwok*; *Aztrin*; *Setron*; *Tobil*; *Tromix*; *Zeto*; *Zifin*; *Zistic*; **Zithromax**; *Zitrim*; *Zitromax*
(International brand names outside U.S. in italics)

FORMULARIES: Aetna; BC-BS; CIGNA; FHP; Humana; Medi-Cal; WellPoint; PCS

COST OF THERAPY: $30.50 (Infections; Capsule; 250 mg; 1/day; 6 days)

PRIMARY ICD9: 136.9 (Unspecified Infections And Parasitic Diseases)

DESCRIPTION:

Azithromycin is an azalide, a subclass of macrolide antibiotics, for oral administration. Azithromycin has the chemical name *(2R,3S,4R,5R,8R,10R,11R,12S,13S,14R)*-13- [(2,6-dideoxy-3-*C*-methyl-3-*O*-methyl-α-*L*-*ribo*-hexopyranosyl)oxy]-2-ethyl-3,4,10-trihydroxy-3,5,6,8,10,12,14-heptamethyl-11-[[3,4,6-trideoxy-3-(dimethylamino)-β-*D*-*xylo*-hexopyranosyl]oxy]-1-oxa-6-azacyclopentadecan-15-one. Azithromycin is derived from erythromycin; however, it differs chemically from erythromycin in that a methyl-substituted nitrogen atom is incorporated into the lactone ring. Its molecular formula is $C_{38}H_{72}N_2O_{12}$, and its molecular weight is 749.00.

Azithromycin, as the dihydrate, is a white crystalline powder with a molecular formula $C_{38}H_{72}N_2O_{12}{\cdot}2H_2O$ and a molecular weight of 785.0.

Zithromax capsules contain azithromycin dihydrate equivalent to 250 mg of azithromycin. The capsules are supplied in red opaque hard-gelatin capsules (containing FD&C Red #40). They also contain the following inactive ingredients: anhydrous lactose, corn starch, magnesium stearate, and sodium lauryl sulfate.

Zithromax tablets contain azithromycin dihydrate equivalent to 600 mg azithromycin. The tablets are supplied as white, modified oval-shaped, film-coated tablets. They also contain the following inactive ingredients: dibasic calcium phosphate anhydrous, pregelatinized starch, sodium croscarmellose, magnesium stearate, sodium lauryl sulfate and an aqueous film coat consisting of hydroxypropyl methyl cellulose, titanium dioxide, lactose and triacetin.

Zithromax for oral suspension is supplied in a single dose packet containing azithromycin dihydrate equivalent to 1 g azithromycin. It also contains the following inactive ingredients: collodial silicon dioxide, sodium phosphate tribasic, anhydrous; spray dried artificial banana flavor, spray dried artificial cherry flavor and sucrose.

CLINICAL PHARMACOLOGY:

PHARMACOKINETICS

Following oral administration, azithromycin is rapidly absorbed and widely distributed throughout the body. Rapid distribution of azithromycin into tissues and high concentration within cells result in significantly higher azithromycin concentrations in tissues than in plasma or serum. The 1 g single dose packet is bioequivalent to four 250 mg capsules.

The pharmacokinetic parameters of azithromycin capsules in plasma after dosing as per labled recommendations in healthy young adults (age 18-40 years old) are portrayed in TABLE 1A and TABLE 1B.

TABLE 1A Mean (CV%) PK Parameter

Dose / Dosage Form	Subject	Day No.	C_{max}(mcg /ml)	T_{max}(hr)	C_{24}(mcg /ml)
500 mg/250 mg capsule	12	Day 1	0.41	2.5	0.05
and 250 mg on Days 2-5	12	Day 5	0.24	3.2	0.05
1200 mg/600 mg tablets	12	Day 1	0.66	2.5	0.074
			(62%)	(79%)	(49%)

TABLE 1B

Dose / Dosage Form	Subject	Day No.	AUC (mcg · hr /ml)	$T_{1/2}$ (hr)	Urinary Excretion (% of dose)
500 mg/250 mg capsule	12	Day 1	2.6[a]	-	4.5
and 250 mg on Days 2-5	12	Day 5	2.1[a]	-	6.5
1200 mg/600 mg tablets	12	Day 1	6.8[b]	40	-
			(64%)	(33%)	

a 0-24 hr
b 0-last

In these studies (500 mg Day 1, 250 mg Days 2-5), there was no significant difference in the disposition of azithromycin between male and female subjects. Plasma concentrations of azithromycin following single 500 mg oral and IV doses declined in a polyphasic pattern resulting in an average terminal half-life of 68 hours. With a regimen of 500 mg on Day 1 and 250 mg/day on Days 2-5, C_{min} and C_{max} remained essentially unchanged from Day 2 through Day 5 of therapy. However, without a loading dose, azithromycin C_{min} levels required 5 to 7 days to reach steady-state.

When azithromycin capsules were administered with food, the rate of absorption (C_{max}) of azithromycin was reduced by 52% and the extent of absorption (AUC) by 43%.

When the oral suspension of azithromycin was administered with food, the C_{max} increased by 46% and the AUC by 14%.

The absolute bioavailability of two 600 mg tablets was 34% (CV=56%). Administration of two 600 mg tablets with food increased $C_{max}$by 31% (CV=43%) while the extent of absorption (AUC) was unchanged (mean ratio of AUCs=1.00; CV=55%).

The AUC of azithromycin in 250 mg capsule was unaffected by coadministration of an antacid containing aluminum and magnesium hydroxide with azithromycin; however, the C_{max} was reduced by 24%. Administration of cimetidine (800 mg) two hours prior to azithromycin had no effect on azithromycin absorption.

When studied in healthy elderly subjects from age 65 to 85 years, the pharmacokinetic parameters of azithromycin (500 mg Day 1, 250 mg Days 2-5) in elderly men were similar to those in young adults; however, in elderly women, although higher peak concentrations (increased by 30 to 50%) were observed, no significant accumulation occurred.

The high values in adults for apparent steady-state volume of distribution (31.1 L/kg) and plasma clearance (630 ml/min) suggest that the prolonged half-life is due to extensive uptake and subsequent release of drug from tissues.

Selected tissue (or fluid) concentration and tissue (or fluid) to plasma/serum concentration ratios are shown in TABLE 2.

TABLE 2 Azithromycin Concentrations Following Two 250 mg (500 mg) Capsules In Adults

Tissue or Fluid	Time After Dose(h)	Tissue or Fluid Concentration (mcg/g or mcg/ml)[1]	Corresponding Plasma or Serum Level (mcg/ml)	Tissue (Fluid) Plasma (Serum) Ration[1]
Skin	72-96	0.4	0.012	35
Lung	72-96	4.0	0.012	>100
Sputum*	2-4	1.0	0.64	2
Sputum**	10-12	2.9	0.1	30
Tonsil***	9-18	4.5	0.03	>100
Tonsil***	180	0.9	0.006	>100
Cervix****	19	2.8	0.04	70

[1]High tissue concentrations should not be interpreted to be quantitatively related to clinical efficacy. The antimicrobial activity of azithromycin is pH related. Azithromycin is concentrated in cell lysosomes which have a low intraorganelle pH, at which the drug's activity is reduced. However, the extensive distribution of drug to tissues may be relevant to clinical activity.
* Sample was obtained 2-4 hours after the first dose.
** Sample was obtained 10-12 hours after the first dose.
*** Dosing regimen of 2 doses of 250 mg each, separated by 12 hours.
**** Sample was obtained 19 hours after a single 500 mg dose.

The extensive tissue distribution was confirmed by examination of additional tissues and fluids (bone, ejaculum, prostate, ovary, uterus, salpinx, stomach, liver, and gallbladder). As there are no data from adequate and well-controlled studies of azithromycin treatment of infections in these additional body sites, the clinical significance of these tissue concentration data is unknown.

Following a regimen of 500 mg on the first day and 250 mg for 4 days, only very low concentrations were noted in cerbrospinal fluid (less than 0.01 mcg/ml) in the presence of non-inflamed meninges.

Following oral administration of a single 1200 mg dose (two 600 mg tablets), the mean maximum concentration in peripheral leukocytes was 140 mcg/ml. Concentrations remained above 32 mcg/ml for approximately 60 hr. The mean half-lives for 6 males and 6 females were 34 hr and 57 hr, respectively. Leukocyte to plasma C_{max} ratios for males and females were 258 (± 77%) and 175 (± 60%), respectively, and the AUC ratios were 804 (± 31%) and 541 (± 28%), respectively. The clinical relevance of these findings is unknown.

CLINICAL PHARMACOLOGY: *(cont'd)*

The serum protein binding of azithromycin is variable in the concentration range approximating human exposure, decreasing from 51% at 0.02 mcg/ml to 7% at 2 mcg/ml. Biliary excretion of azithromycin, predominantly as unchanged drug, is a major route of elimination. Over the course of a week, approximately 6% of the administered dose appears as unchanged drug in urine.

There are no pharmacokinetic data available from studies in hepatically- or renally-impaired individuals.

The effect of azithromycin on the plasma levels or pharmacokinetics of theophylline administered in multiple doses adequate to reach therapeutic steady-state plasma levels is not known. (See PRECAUTIONS.)

MECHANISM OF ACTION

Azithromycin acts by binding to the 50S ribosomal subunit of susceptible microorganisms and, thus, interfering with microbial protein synthesis. Nucleic acid synthesis is not affected.

Azithromycin concentrates in phagocytes and fibroblasts as demonstrated by *in vitro* incubation techniques. Using such methodology, the ratio of intracellular to extracellular concentration was >30 after one hour incubation. *In vivo* studies suggest that concentration in phagocytes may contribute to drug distribution to inflamed tissues.

MICROBIOLOGY

Azithromycin has been shown to be active against most strains of the following microorganisms, both *in vitro* and in clinical infections as described in INDICATIONS AND USAGE.

Aerobic Gram-Positive Microorganisms

Staphylococcus aureus
Streptococcus agalactiae
Streptococcus pneumoniae
Streptococcus pyogenes

NOTE: Azithromycin demonstrates cross-resistance with erythromycin-resistant gram-positive strains. Most strains of *Enterococcus faecalis* and methicillin-resistant staphylococci are resistant to azithromycin.

Aerobic Gram-Negative Microorganisms

Haemophilus influenzae;
Moraxella catarrhalis

"Other" Microorganisms

Chlamydia trachomatis

Beta-lactamase production should have no effect on azithromycin activity.

Azithromycin has been shown to be active *in vitro* and in the prevention of disease caused by the following microorganisms:

Mycobacteria

Mycobacterium avium consisting of:
Mycobacterium avium
Mycobacterium intracellulare.

The following *in vitro* data are available, **but their clinical significance is unknown**.

Azithromycin exhibits *in vitro* minimum inhibitory concentrations (MICs) of 2.0 mcg/ml or less against most (≥90%) strains of the following microorganisms; however, the safety and effectiveness of azithromycin in treating clinical infections due to these microorganisms have not been established in adequate and well-controlled trials.

Aerobic Gram-Positive Microorganisms: Streptococci (Groups C, F, G); Viridans group streptococci

Aerobic Gram-Negative Microorganisms: *Bordetella pertussis; Campylobacter jejuni; Haemophilus ducreyi; Legionella pneumophila*

Anaerobic Microorganisms: *Bacteroides bivius; Clostridium perfringens; Peptostreptococcus* species

"Other" Microorganisms *Borrelia burgdorferi; Mycoplasma pneumoniae; Treponema pallidum; Ureaplasma urealyticum*

SUSCEPTIBILITY TESTING OF BACTERIA EXCLUDING MYCOBACTERIA

The *in vitro* potency of azithromycin is markedly affected by the pH of the microbiological growth medium during incubation. Incubation in a 10% CO_2 atmosphere will result in lowering of media pH (7.2 to 6.6) within 18 hours and in an apparent reduction of the *in vitro* potency of azithromycin. Thus, the initial pH of the growth medium should be 7.2-7.4, and the CO_2content of the incubation atmosphere should be as low as practical.

Azithromycin can be solubilized for *in vitro* susceptibility testing by dissolving in a minimum amount of 95% ethanol and diluting to working concentration with water.

Dilution Techniques: Quantitative methods are used to determine antimicrobial minimal inhibitory concentrations that provide reproducible estimates of the susceptibility of bacteria to antimicrobial compounds. One such standardized procedure uses a standardized dilution method[1] (broth, agar, or microdilution) or equivalent with azithromycin powder. The MIC values should be interpreted according to the criteria enumerated in TABLE 3

TABLE 3

MIC (mcg/ml)	Interpretation
≤ 2	Susceptible (S)
4	Intermediate (I)
≥ 8	Resistant (R)

A report of "Susceptible" indicates that the pathogen is likely to respond to monotherapy with azithromycin. A report of "Intermediate" indicates that the result should be considered equivocal, and, if the microorganism is not fully susceptible to alternative, clinically feasible drugs, the test should be repeated. This category also provides a buffer zone which prevents small uncontrolled technical factors from causing major discrepancies in interpretation. A report of "Resistant" indicates that usually achievable drug concentrations are unlikely to be inhibitory and that other therapy should be selected.

Measurement of MIC or MBC and achieved antimicrobial compound concentrations may be appropriate to guide therapy in some infections. (See CLINICAL PHARMACOLOGYfor further information on drug concentrations achieved in infected body sites and other pharmacokinetic properties of this antimicrobial drug product.)

Standardized susceptibility test procedures require the use of laboratory control microorganisms. Standard azithromycin powder should provide the MIC values found in TABLE 4.

TABLE 4

Microorganism	MIC (mcg/ml)
Escherichia coli ATCC 25922	2.0-8.0
Enterococcus faecalis ATCC 29212	1.0-4.0
Staphylococcus aureus ATCC 29213	0.25-1.0

CLINICAL PHARMACOLOGY: *(cont'd)*

Diffusion Techniques: Quantitative methods that require measurement of zone diameters also provide reproducible estimates of the susceptibility of bacteria to antimicrobial compounds. One such standardized procedure[2] that has been recommended for use with disks to test the susceptibility of microorganisms to azithromycin uses the 15-mcg azithromycin disk. Interpretation involves the correlation of the diameter obtained in the disk test with the minimal inhibitory concentration (MIC) for azithromycin.

Reports from the laboratory providing results of the standard single-disk susceptibility test with a 15-mcg azithromycin disk should be interpreted according to the criteria found in TABLE 5.

TABLE 5

Zone Diameter (mm)	Interpretation
≥ 18	Susceptible (S)
14-17	Intermediate (I)
≤ 13	Resistant (R)

Interpretation should be as stated in TABLE 5 for results using dilution techniques.

As with standardized dilution techniques, diffusion methods require the use of laboratory control microorganisms. The 15-mcg azithromycin disk should provide the diameters found in TABLE 6 in these laboratory test quality control strains.

TABLE 6

Microorganism	Zone Diameter (mm)
Staphylococcus aureus ATCC 25923	21-26

***IN VITRO* ACTIVITY OF AZITHROMYCIN AGAINST MYCOBACTERIA**

Azithromycin has demonstrated *in vitro* activity against *Mycobacterium avium* complex (MAC) organisms. While gene probe techniques may be used to distinguish *M. avium* species from *M. intracellulare*, many studies only report results on *M. avium* complex (MAC) isolates. Azithromycin has also been shown to be active against phagocytized *M. avium* complex (MAC) organisms in mouse and human macrophage cell cultures as well as in the beige mouse infection model.

Various *in vitro* methodologies employing broth or solid media at different pHs, with and without oleic acid-albumin dextrose-catalase (OADC), have been used to determine azithromycin MIC values for *Mycobacterium avium* complex strains. In general, MIC values decreased 4 to 8 fold as the pH of middlebrook 7H11 agar media increased from 6.6 to 7.4, MIC values determined with Mueller-Hinton agar were 4 fold higher than that observed with middlebrook 7H12 media at the same pH. Utilization of oleic acid-albumin-dextrose-catalase (OADC) in these assays has been shown to further alter MIC values. The ability to correlate MIC values and plasma drug levels is difficult as azithromycin concentrates in macrophages and tissues.

A cross resistance relationship between azithromycin and clarithromycin has been observed with some *Mycobacterium avium* complex (MAC) isolates. The various mechanisms of cross resistance between azithromycin and clarithromycin for *M. avium* complex organisms have not been fully characterized. The clinical significance of azithromycin and clarithromycin cross resistance is unknown.

SUSCEPTIBILITY TESTING FOR *MYCOBACTERIUM AVIUM* COMPLEX (MAC)

The disk difusion techniques and dilution methods for susceptibility testing against gram-positive and gram-negative bacteria should not be used for determining azithromycin MIC values against mycobacteria. *In vitro* susceptibility testing methods and diagnostic products currently available for determining minimal inhibitory concentration (MIC) values against *Mycobacterium avium* complex (MAC) organisms have not been established or validated. Azithromycin MIC values will vary depending on the susceptibility testing method employed, composition and pH of media and the utilization of nutritional supplements. Breakpoints to determine whether clinical isolates of *M. intracellulare* are susceptible to azithromycin have not been established.

CLINICAL STUDIES:

TREATMENT OF PATIENTS WITH ADVANCED HIV INFECTION FOR THE PREVENTION OF DISEASE DUE TO DISSEMINATED *MYCOBACTERIUM AVIUM* COMPLEX (MAC) (SEE INDICATIONS AND USAGE)

Two randomized, double blind clinical trials were performed in patients with CD4 counts <100 cells/µl. The first study (155) compared azithromycin (1200 mg once weekly) to placebo and enrolled 182 patients with a mean CD4 count of 35 cells/µl. The second study (174) randomized 723 patients to either azithromycin (1200 mg once weekly), rifabutin (300 mg daily) or the combination of both. The mean CD4 count was 51 cells/µl. The primary endpoint in these studies was disseminated MAC disease. Other endpoints included the incidence of clinically significant MAC disease and discontinuations from therapy for drug-related side effects.

MAC Bacteremia: In trial 155, 85 patients randomized to receive azithromycin and 89 patients randomized to receive placebo met study entrance criteria. Cumulative incidences at 6, 12 and 18 months of the possible outcomes are in TABLE 7.

TABLE 7

Month	MAC Free and Alive	MAC	Adverse Experience	Lost to Follow-up
Cumulative Incidence Rate, %: Placebo (N=89)				
6	69.7	13.5	6.7	10.1
12	47.2	19.1	15.7	18.0
18	37.1	22.5	18.0	22.5
Cumulative Incidence Rate, %; Azithromycin (n=85)				
Month	**MAC Free and Alive**	**MAC**	**Adverse Experience**	**Lost to Follow-up**
6	84.7	3.5	9.4	2.4
12	63.5	8.2	16.5	11.8
18	44.7	11.8	25.9	17.6

The difference in the one year cumulative incidence rates of disseminated MAC disease (placebo—azithromycin) is 10.9%. This difference is statistically significant (p=0.037) with a 95% confidence interval for this difference of (0.8%, 20.9%). The comparable number of patients experiencing adverse events and the fewer number of patients lost to follow-up on azithromycin should be taken into account when interpreting the significance of this difference.

In Study 174, 223 patients randomized to receive rifabutin, 223 patients randomized to receive azithromycin, and 218 patients randomized to receive both rifabutin and azithromycin met study entrance criteria. Cumulative incidences at 6, 12, and 18 months of the possible outcomes are recorded in TABLE 8.

CLINICAL STUDIES: *(cont'd)*

TABLE 8

Month	Cumulative Incidence Rate, %: Rifabutin (n=223) MAC Free and Alive	MAC	Adverse Experience	Lost to Follow-up
6	83.4	7.2	8.1	1.3
12	60.1	15.2	16.1	8.5
18	40.8	21.5	24.2	13.5
Month	**Cumulative Incidence Rate, %; Azithromycin (n=223) MAC Free and Alive**	**MAC**	**Adverse Experience**	**Lost to Follow-up**
6	85.2	3.6	5.8	5.4
12	65.5	7.6	16.1	10.8
18	45.3	12.1	23.8	18.8
Month	**Cumulative Incidence Rate, %; Azithromycin /Rifabutin (n=218) MAC Free and Alive**	**MAC**	**Adverse Experience**	**Lost to Follow-up**
6	89.4	1.8	5.5	3.2
12	71.6	2.8	15.1	10.6
18	49.1	6.4	29.4	15.1

Comparing the cumulative one year incidence rates, azithromycin monotherapy is at least as effective as rifabutin monotherapy. The difference (rifabutin-azithromycin) in the one year rates (7.6%) is statistically significant (p=0.022) with an adjusted 95% confidence interval (0.9%, 14.3%). Additionally azithromycin/rifabutin combination therapy is more effective than rifabutin alone. The difference (rifabutin-azithromycin/rifabutin) in the cumulative one year incidence rates (12.5%) is statisically significant (p<0.001) with an adjusted 95% confidence interval of (6.6%, 18.4%). The comparable number of patients experiencing adverse events and the fewer number of patients lost to follow-up on rifabutin should be taken into account when interpreting the significance of this difference.

In Study 174, sensitivity testing* was performed on all available MAC isolates from subjects randomized to either azithromycin, rifabutin, or the combination. The distribution of MIC values for azithromycin from susceptibility testing of the breakthrough isolates was similar between study arms. As the efficacy of azithromycin in the treatment of disseminated MAC has not been established, the clinical relevance of these *in vitro* MICs as an indicator of susceptibility or resistance is not known. (*Methodology per Inderlied CB, et al. Determination of *In Vitro* Susceptibility of *Mycobacterium avium* Complex Isolates to Antimicrobial Agents by Various Methods. Antimicrob. Agents Chemother 1987; 31: 1697-1702.)

Clinically Significant Disseminated MAC Disease: In association with the decreased incidence of bacteremia, patients in the groups randomized to either azithromycin alone or azithromycin in combination with rifabutin showed reductions in the signs and symptoms of disseminated MAC disease, including fever or night sweats, weight loss and anemia.

Discontinuations From Therapy For Drug-Related Side Effects: In Study 155, discontinuations for drug-related toxicity occurred in 8.2% of subjects treated with azithromycin and 2.3% of those given placebo (p=0.121). In Study 174, more subjects discontinued from the combination of azithromycin and rifabutin (22.7%) than from azithromycin alone (13.5%; p=0.026) or rifabutin alone (15.9%; p=0.209).

Safety: As these patients with advanced HIV disease were taking multiple concomitant medications and experienced a variety of intercurrent illnesses, it was often difficult to attribute adverse events to study medication. Overall, the nature of side effects seen on the weekly dosage regimen of azithromycin over a period of approximately one year in patients with advanced HIV disease was similar to that previously reported for shorter course therapies.

TABLE 9A Incidence of One More Treatment-Related* Adverse Events in HIV Infected Patients Receiving Prophylaxis for Disseminated MAC Over Approximately 1 Year**

	Placebo (N=91)	Study 155 Azithromycin 1200 mg weekly (N=89)
Mean Duration of Therapy (days)	303.8	402.9
Discontinuation of Therapy	2.3	8.2
Autonomic Nervous System		
Mouth Dry	0	0
Central Nervous System		
Dizziness	0	1.1
Headache	0	0
Gastrointestinal		
Diarrhea	15.4	52.8
Loose Stools	6.6	19.1
Abdominal Pain	6.6	27
Dyspepsia	1.1	9
Flatulence	4.4	9
Nausea	11	32.6
Vomiting	1.1	6.7
General		
Fever	1.1	0
Fatigue	0	2.2
Malaise	0	1.1
Musculoskeletal		
Arthralgia	0	0
Psychiatric		
Anorexia	1.1	0
Skin & Appendages		
Pruritis	3.3	0
Rash	3.2	3.4
Skin discoloration	0	0
Special Senses		
Tinnitus	4.4	3.4
Hearing Decreased	2.2	1.1
Uveitis	0	0
Taste Perversion	0	0

* Includes those events considered possibly or probably related to study drug.
** >2% adverse event rates for any group (except uveitis).

Side effects releated to the gastrointestinal tract were seen more frequently in patients receiving azithromycin than in those receiving placebo or rifabutin. In Study 174, 86% of diarrheal episodes were mild to moderate in nature with discontinuation of therapy for this reason occurring in only 9/233 (3.8%) of patients.

Changes in Laboratory Values: In these immunocompromised patients with advanced HIV infection, it was necessary to assess laboratory abnormalities developing on study with additional criteria if baseline values were outside the relevant normal range. See TABLES 10A and 10B.

TABLE 9B

	Azithromycin 1200 mg weekly (N=233)	Study 174 Rifabutine 300 mg daily (N=236)	Azithromycin + Rifabutin (N=224)
Mean Duration of Therapy (days)	315	296.1	344.4
Discontinuation of Therapy	13.5	15.9	22.7
Autonomic Nervous System			
Mouth Dry	0	3.0	2.7
Central Nervous System			
Dizziness	3.9	1.7	0.4
Headache	3.0	5.5	4.5
Gastrointestinal			
Diarrhea	50.2	19.1	50.9
Loose Stools	12.9	3.0	9.4
Abdominal Pain	32.2	12.3	31.7
Dyspepsia	4.7	1.7	1.8
Flatulence	10.7	5.1	5.8
Nausea	27.0	16.5	28.1
Vomiting	9.0	3.8	5.8
General			
Fever	2.1	4.2	4.9
Fatigue	3.9	2.1	3.1
Malaise	0.4	0	2.2
Musculoskeletal			
Arthralgia	3.0	4.2	7.1
Psychiatric			
Anorexia	2.1	2.1	3.1
Skin & Appendages			
Pruritis	3.9	3.4	7.6
Rash	8.1	9.4	11.1
Skin discoloration	0	2.1	2.2
Special Senses			
Tinnitus	0.9	1.3	0.9
Hearing Decreased	0.9	0.4	0
Uveitis	0.4	1.3	1.8
Taste Perversion	1.3	2.5	1.3

* Includes those events considered possibly or probably related to study drug.
** >2% adverse event rates for any group (except uveitis).

TABLE 10A Prophylaxis Against Disseminated MAC Abnormal Laboratory Values*

		Placebo		Azithromycin 1200 mg weekly	
Hemoglobin	<8g/dl	1/51	2%	4/170	2%
Platelet Count	$<50\times10^3/mm^3$	1/71	1%	4/260	2%
WBC Count	$<1\times10^3/mm^3$	0/8	0%	2/70	3%
Neutrophils	$<500/mm^3$	0/26	0%	4/106	4%
SGOT	>5xULN[a]	1/41	2%	8/158	5%
SGPT	>5xULN	0/49	0%	8/166	5%
Alk Phos	>5xULN	1/80	1%	4/247	2%

a Upper Limit of Normal
* excludes subjects outside of the relevant normal range at baseline

TABLE 10B Prophylaxis Against Disseminated MAC Abnormal Laboratory Values*

	Rifabutin 1200 mg weekly		Azithromycin & Rifabutin	
<8g/dl	4/114	4%	8/107	8%
$<50\times10^3/mm^3$	2/182	1%	6/181	3%
$<1\times10^3/mm^3$	2/47	4%	0/43	0%
$<500/mm^3$	3/82	4%	2/78	3%
>5xULN[a]	3/121	3%	6/114	5%
>5xULN	3/130	2%	5/117	4%
>5xULN	2/172	1%	3/164	2%

INDICATIONS AND USAGE:

Azithromycin is indicated for the treatment of patients with mild to moderate infections (pneumonia: see WARNINGS) caused by susceptible strains of the designated microorganisms in the specific conditions listed below.

LOWER RESPIRATORY TRACT

Acute bacterial exacerbations of chronic obstructive pulmonary disease due to *Haemophilus influenzae, Moraxella catarrhalis*, or *Streptococcus pneumoniae.*

Community-acquired pneumonia of mild severity due to *Streptococcus pneumoniae* or *Haemophilus influenzae* in patients appropriate for outpatient oral therapy.

NOTE: Azithromycin should not be used in patients with pneumonia who are judged to be inappropriate for outpatient oral therapy because of moderate to severe illness or risk factors such as any of the following.

patients with nosocomially acquired infections,

patients with known or suspected bacteremia,

patients requiring hospitalization,

eldery or debilitated patients, or

patients with significant underlying health problems that may compromise their ability to respond to their illness (including immunodeficiency or functional asplenia).

UPPER RESPIRATORY TRACT

Streptococcal pharyngitis/tonsilitis: As an alternative to first line therapy of acute pharyngitis/tonsillitis due to *Streptococcus pyogenes* occurring in individuals who cannot use first line therapy.

NOTE: Penicillin is the usual drug of choice in the treatment of *Streptococcus pyogenes* infection and the prophylaxis of rheumatic fever. Azithromycin is often effective in the eradication of susceptible strains of *Streptococcus pyogenes* from the nasopharynx. Data establishing efficacy of azithromycin is subsequent prevention of rheumatic fever are not available.

SKIN AND SKIN STRUCTURE

Uncomplicated skin and skin structure infections due to *Staphylococcus aureus, Streptococcus pyogenes,* or *Streptococcus agalaciae.* Abscesses usually require surgical drainage.

INDICATIONS AND USAGE: *(cont'd)*

SEXUALLY TRANSMITTED DISEASES

Non-gonococcal urethritis and cervicitis due to *Chlamydia trachomatis.*

Azithromycin, at the recommended dose, should not be relied upon to treat gonorrhea or syphilis. Antimicrobial agents used in high doses for short periods of time to treat non-gonococcal urethritis may mask or delay the symptoms of incubating gonorrhea or syphilis. All patients with sexually-transmitted urethritis or cervicitis should have a serologic test for syphilis and appropriate cultures for gonorrhea performed at the time of diagnosis. Appropriate antimicrobial therapy and follow-up tests for these diseases should be initiated if infection is confirmed.

Appropriate culture and susceptibility tests should be performed before treatment to determine the causative organism and its susceptibility to azithromycin. Therapy with azithromycin may be initiated before results of these tests are known; once the results become available, antimicrobial therapy should be adjusted accordingly.

DISSEMINATED *MYCOBACTERIUM AVIUM* COMPLEX (MAC) DISEASE

Azithromycin taken alone or in combination with rifabutin at its approved dose, is indicated for the prevention of disseminated *Mycobacterium avium* complex (MAC) disease is persons with advanced HIV infection. (See CLINICAL STUDIES.)

CONTRAINDICATIONS:

Azithromycin is contraindicated in patients with known hypersensitivity to azithromycin, erythromycin, or any macrolide antibiotic.

WARNINGS:

Rare serious allergic reactions, including angioedema and anaphylaxis, have been reported rarely in patients on azithromycin therapy. (See CONTRAINDICATIONS.) Despite initially successful symptomatic treatment of the allergic symptoms, when symptomatic therapy was discontinued, the allergic symptoms **recurred soon thereafter in some patients without further azithromycin exposure.** These patients required prolonged periods of observation and symptomatic treatment. The relationship of these episodes to the long tissue half-life of azithromycin and subsequent prolonged exposure to antigen is unknown at present.

If an allergic reaction occurs, the drug should be discontinued and appropriate therapy should be instituted. Physicians should be aware that reappearance of the allergic symptoms may occur when symptomatic therapy is discontinued.

In the treatment of pneumonia, azithromycin has only been shown to be safe and effective in the treatment of community-acquired pneumonia of mild severity due to *Streptococcus pneumoniae* or *Haemophilus influenzae* in patients appropriate for outpatient oral therapy. Azithromycin should not be used in patients with pneumonia who are judged to be inappropriate for outpatient oral therapy because of moderate to severe illness or risk factors such as any of the following: patients with nosocomially acquired infections, patients with known or suspected bacteremia, patients requiring hospitalization, elderly or debilitated patients, or patients with significant underlying health problems that may compromise their ability to respond to their illness (including immunodeficiency or functional asplenia). Pseudomembranous colitis has been reported with nearly all antibacterial agents and may range in severity from mild to life-threatening. Therefore, it is important to consider this diagnosis in patients who present with diarrhea subsequent to the administration of antibacterial agents.

Treatment with antibacterial agents alters the normal flora of the colon and may permit overgrowth of clostridia. Studies indicate that a toxin produced by *Clostridium difficile* is a primary cause of "antibiotic-associated colitis."

After the diagnosis of pseudomembranous colitis has been established, therapeutic measures should be initiated. Mild cases of pseudomembranous colitis usually respond to discontinuation of the drug alone. In moderate to severe cases, consideration should be given to management with fluids and electrolytes, protein supplementation, and treatment with an antibacterial drug clinically effective against *Clostridium difficile* colitis.

PRECAUTIONS:

GENERAL

Because azithromycin is principally eliminated via the liver, caution should be exercised when azithromycin is administered to patients with impaired hepatic function. There are no data regarding azithromycin usage in patients with renal impairment; thus, caution should be exercised when prescribing azithromycin in these patients.

The following adverse events have not been reported in clinical trials with azithromycin, an azalide; however, they have been reported with macrolide products; ventricular arrhythmias, including ventricular tachycardia and *torsades de pointes,* in individuals with prolonged QT intervals.

INFORMATION FOR PATIENTS

Patients should be cautioned to take azithromycin capsules at least one hour prior to a meal or at least two hours after a meal. Azithromycin capsules should not be taken with food.

Azithromycin tablets may be taken with or without food. However, increased tolerability has been observed when tablets are taken with food.

Azithromycin for oral suspension in single 1 g packets can be taken with or without food after constitution.

Patients should also be cautioned not to take aluminum- and magnesium-containing antacids and azithromycin simultaneously.

The patient should be directed to discontinue azithromycin immediately and contact a physician if any signs of an allergic reaction occur.

LABORATORY TEST INTERACTIONS

There are no reported laboratory test interactions.

CARCINOGENESIS, MUTAGENESIS, IMPAIRMENT OF FERTILITY

Long-term studies in animals have not been performed to evaluate carcinogenic potential. Azithromycin has shown no mutagenic potential in standard laboratory tests; mouse lymphoma assay, human lymphocyte clastogenic assay, and mouse bone marrow clastogenic assay.

PREGNANCY, TERATOGENIC EFFECTS, PREGNANCY CATEGORY B

Reproduction studies have been performed in rats and mice at doses up to moderately maternally toxic dose levels (*i.e.,* 200 mg/kg/day). These doses, based on a mg/m^2 basis, are estimated to be 4 and 2 times, respectively, the human daily dose of 500 mg.

With regard to the MAC prophylaxis dose of 1200 mg weekly, on a mg/m^2 basis, the doses in rats and mice are approximately 2 and 1 times the human dose, respectively.

No evidence of impaired fertility or harm to the fetus due to azithromycin was found. There are, however, no adequate and well-controlled studies in pregnant women. Because animal reproduction studies are not always predictive of human response, azithromycin should be used during pregnancy only if clearly needed.

NURSING MOTHERS

It is not known whether azithromycin is excreted in human milk. Because many drugs are excreted in human milk, caution should be exercised when azithromycin is administered to a nursing woman.

PRECAUTIONS: *(cont'd)*

PEDIATRIC USE

In controlled clinical studies, azithromycin has been administered to pediatric patients ranging in age from 6 months to 12 years. For information regarding the use of azithromycin for oral suspension in the treatment of pediatric patients, please refer to the INDICATIONS AND USAGEand DOSAGE AND ADMINISTRATION sections.

PREVENTION OF DISSEMINATED *MYCOBACTERIUM AVIUM* COMPLEX (MAC) DISEASE

Safety and efficacy of azithromycin for the prevention of MAC in children have not been established. Limited safety data are available for 24 children 5 months to 14 years of age (mean 4.6 years) who received azithromycin for treatment of opportunistic infections. The mean duration of therapy was 186.7 days (range 13–710 days) at doses <5 to 20 mg/kg/day. Three children were treated for 6 months or more and 4 children were treated for 1 month or more with a dose of >10 mg/kg/day. Adverse events were similar to those observed in the adult population, most of which involved the gastrointestinal tract. While none of these children prematurely discontinued treatment due to a side effect, one child discontinued due to a laboratory abnormality (eosinophilia). The protocols upon which these data are based specified a daily dose of 10-20 mg/kg/day of azithromycin.

GERIATRIC USE

Pharmacokinetic parameters in older volunteers (65-85 years old) were similar to those in younger volunteers (18-40 years old) for the 5-day therapeutic regimen. Dosage adjustment does not appear to be necessary for older patients with normal renal and hepatic function receiving treatment with this dosage regimen. (See CLINICAL PHARMACOLOGY.)

DRUG INTERACTIONS:

Aluminum- and magnesium-containing antacids reduce the peak serum levels (rate) but not the AUC (extent) of azithromycin (500 mg) absorption.

Administration of cimetidine (800 mg) two hours prior to azithromycin had no effect on azithromycin (500 mg) absorption.

Azithromycin (500 mg Day 1, 250 mg Days 2-5) did not affect the plasma levels or pharmacokinetics of theophylline administered as a single intravenous dose. The effect of azithromycin on the plasma levels or pharmacokinetics of theophylline administered in multiple doses resulting in therapeutic steady-state levels of theophylline is not known. However, concurrent use of macrolides and theophylline has been associated with increases in the serum concentrations of theophylline. Therefore, until further data are available, prudent medical practice dictates careful monitoring of plasma theophylline levels in patients receiving azithromycin and theophylline concomitantly.

Azithromycin (500 mg Day 1, 250 mg Days 2-5) did not affect the prothrombin time response to a single dose of warfarin. However, prudent medical practice dictates careful monitoring of prothrombin time in all patients treated with azithromycin and warfarin concomitantly. Concurrent use of macrolides and warfarin in clinical practice has been associated with increased anticoagulant effects.

Dose adjustments are not indicated when azithromycin and zidovudine are coadministered. When zidovudine (100 mg every 3 hours × 5) was coadministered with daily azithromycin (600 mg, n=5 or 1200 mg, n=7), mean C_{max} AUC and Clr increased by 26% (CV 54%), 10% (CV 26%) and 38% (CV 114%), respectively. The mean AUC of phosphorylated zidovudine increased by 75% (CV 95%), while zidovudine glucuronide C_{max} and AUC increased by less than 10%. In another study, addition of 1 gram of azithromycin per week to a regimen of 10 mg/kg daily zidovudine resulted in 25% (CV 70%) and 13% (CV 37%) increases in zidovudine C_{max} and AUC, respectively. Zidovudine glucuronide mean C_{max} and AUC increased by 16% (CV 61%) and 8.0% (CV 32%), respectively.

Doses of 1200 mg/day azithromycin for 14 days in 6 subjects increased C_{max} of concurrently administered didanosine (200 mg every 12 hours) by 44% (CV 54%) and AUC by 14% (CV 23%). However, none of these changes were significantly different from those produced in a parallel placebo control group of subjects.

Preliminary data suggest that coadministration of azithromycin and rifabutin did not markedly affect the mean serum concentrations of either drug. Administration of 250 mg azithromycin daily for 10 days (500 mg on the first day) produced mean concentrations of azithromycin 1 day after the last dose of 53 ng/ml when coadministered with placebo. Mean concentrations 5 days after the last dose were 23 ng/ml and 21 ng/ml in the two groups of subjects. Administration of 300 mg rifabutin for 10 days produced mean concentrations of rifabutin one half day after the last dose of 60 mg/ml when coadministered with daily 250 mg azithromycin and 71 ng/ml when coadministered with placebo. Mean concentrations 5 days after the last dose were 8.1 ng/ml and 9.2 ng/ml in the two groups of subjects.

The following drug interactions have not been reported in clinical trials with azithromycin; however, no specific drug interaction studies have been performed to evaluate potential drug-drug interaction. Nonetheless, they have been observed with macrolide products. Until further data are developed regarding drug interactions when azithromycin and these drugs are used concomitantly, careful monitoring of patients is advised:

Digoxin: elevated digoxin levels.

Ergotamine or dihydroergotamine: acute ergot toxicity characterized by severe peripheral vasospasm and dysesthesia.

Triazolam: decrease the clearance of triazolam and thus may increase the pharmacologic effect of triazolam.

Drugs metabolized by the cytochrome P ^{450} system: elevations of serum carbamazepine, terfenadine, cyclosporine, hexobarbital, and phenytoin levels.

ADVERSE REACTIONS:

In clinical trials, most of the reported side effects were mild to moderate in severity and were reversible upon discontinuation of the drug. Approximately 0.7% of the patients from the multiple-dose clinical trials discontinued azithromycin therapy because of treatment-related side effects. Most of the side effects leading to discontinuation were related to the gastrointestinal tract (*e.g.,* nausea, vomiting, diarrhea, or abdominal pain). Rare but potentially serious side effects were angiodema and cholestatic jaundice.

CLINICAL

Multiple-Dose Regimen: Overall, the most common side effects in adult patients receiving a multiple-dose regimen of azithromycin were related to the gastrointestinal system with diarrhea/loose stools (5%), nausea (3%), and abdominal pain (3%) being the most frequently reported.

No other side effects occurred in patients on the multiple-dose regimen of azithromycin with a frequency greater than 1%. Side effects that occurred with a frequency of 1% or less included the following:

Cardiovascular: Palpitations, chest pain.

Gastrointestinal: Dyspepsia, flatulence, vomiting, melena, and cholestatic jaundice.

Genitourinary: Monilia, vaginitis, and nephritis.

Nervous System: Dizziness, headache, vertigo, and somnolence.

General: Fatigue.

ADVERSE REACTIONS: *(cont'd)*

Allergic: Rash, photosensitivity, and angioedema.

Chronic Therapy with 1200 mg Weekly Regimen: The nature of side effects seen with 1200 mg weekly dosing regiman for the prevention of *Mycobacterium avium* infection in severly immunocompromised HIV-infected patients were similar to those seen with short term dosing regimens. (See CLINICAL STUDIES.)

Single 1-gram Dose Regimen: Overall, the most common side effects in patients receiving a single-dose regimen of 1 gram of azithromycin were related to the gastrointestinal system and were more frequently reported than in patients receiving the multiple-dose regimen.

Side effects that occurred in patients on the single one-gram dosing regimen of azithromycin with a frequency of 1% or greater included diarrhea/loose stools (7%), nausea (5%), abdominal pain (5%), vomiting (2%), dyspepsia (1%), and vaginitis (1%).

LABORATORY ABNORMALITIES

Significant abnormalities (irrespective of drug relationship) occurring during the clinical trials were reported as follows:

With an incidence of 1-2%: elevated serum creatine phosphokinase, potassium, ALT (SGPT), GGT, and AST (SGOT).

With an incidence of less than 1%: leukopenia, neutropenia, decreased platelet count, elevated serum alkaline phosphatase, bilirubin, BUN, creatinine, blood glucose, LDH, and phosphate.

When follow-up was provided, changes in laboratory tests appeared to be reversible.

In multiple-dose clinical trials involving more than 3000 patients, 3 patients discontinued therapy because of treatment-related liver enzyme abnormalities and 1 because of a renal function abnormality.

In a phase I drug interaction study performed in normal volunteers, 1 of 6 subjects given the combination of azithromycin and rifabutin, 1 of 7 given rifabutin alone and 0 of 6 given azithromycin alone developed a clinically significant neutropenia (<500 cells/mm^3).

Laboratory abnormalities seen in clinical trials for the prevention of disseminated *Mycobacterium avium*disease in severely immunocompromised HIV-infected patients are presented in CLINICAL STUDIES.

DOSAGE AND ADMINISTRATION:

(See INDICATIONS AND USAGE.)

Azithromycin capsules should be given at least 1 hour before or 2 hours after a meal. Azithromycin capsules should not be mixed with or taken with food.

Azithromycin for oral suspension (single dose 1 g packet) can be taken with or without food after constitution. Not for pediatric use.

Azithromycin tablets may be taken without regard to food. However, increased tolerability has been observed when tablets are taken with food.

The recommended dose of azithromycin for the treatment of individuals 16 years of age and older with mild to moderate acute bacterial exacerbations of chronic obstructive pulmonary disease, pneumonia, pharyngitis/tonsilitis (as second line therapy), and uncomplicated skin and skin structure infections due to the indicated organisms is: 500 mg as a single dose on the first day followed by 250 mg once daily on Days 2 through 5 for a total dose of 1.5 grams of azithromycin.

The recommended dose of azithromycin for the prevention of disseminated *Mycobacterium avium* complex (MAC) disease is: 1200 mg taken once weekly. This dose of azithromycin may be combined with the approved dosage regimen of rifabutin.

The recommended dose of azithromycin for the treatment of non-gonococcal urethritis and cervicitis due to *C. trachomatis*is: a single 1 gram (1000 mg) dose of azithromycin. This dose can be administered as four 250 mg capsules or as one single dose packet (1 g).

Directions for Administration of Azithromycin for Oral Suspension in The Single Dose Packet (1 g): The entire contents of the packet should be mixed thoroughly with two ounces (approximately 60 ml) of water. Drink the entire contents immediately, add an additional two ounces of water, mix, and drink to assure complete consumption of dosage. **The single dose packet should not be used to administer doses other than 1000 mg of azithromycin. This packet not for pediatric use.**

ANIMAL PHARMACOLOGY:

Toxicity: Phospholipidosis (intracellular phospholipid binding) has been observed in some tissues of mice, rats, and dogs given multiple doses of azithromycin. It has been demonstrated in numerous organ systems (*e.g.*, eye, dorsal root ganglia, liver, gallbladder, kidney, spleen, and pancreas) in dogs administered doses which, based on pharmacokinetics, are as low as 2 times greater than the recommended adult human dose and in rats at doses comparable to the recommended adult human dose. This effect has been reversible after cessation of azithromycin treatment. The significance of these findings for humans is unknown.

REFERENCES:

1. National Committee for Clinical Laboratory Standards, Methods for Dilution Antimicrobial Susceptibility Tests for Bacteria that Grow Aerobically—Third Edition, Approved Standard NCCLS Document M7-A3, Vol. 13, No. 25, NCCLS, Villanova, PA, December, 1993. 2. National Committee for Clinical Laboratory Standards, Performance Standards for Antimicrobial Disk Susceptibility Tests—Fifth Edition. Approved Standard NCCLS Document M2-A5, Vol. 13, No. 24, NCCLS, Villanova, PA, December 1993.

PATIENT INFORMATION:

Azithromycin dihydrate is an antibiotic used to treat infections such as those of the lungs, skin or sexually transmitted diseases. It has been used in combination with other antibiotics for treating and preventing serious infections in some patients. This medication should not be used by patients with true allergies to erythromycin. This does not include upset stomach. This medication should be taken at least one hour before a meal or at least two hours after a meal - it should not be taken with food. Avoid taking antacids within two hours of taking this medication. If you experience signs of allergy, (*e.g.*, itchy watery eyes, skin rash, difficulty breathing), stop taking the medication and call your doctor immediately. You may feel better after a day or so taking this medication; however, to fully cure the infection, you must take all the medication for the entire period of time your doctor has prescribed it.

HOW SUPPLIED:

Capsules: Zithromax capsules (imprinted with "Pfizer 305") are supplied in red opaque hard-gelatin capsules containing azithromycin dihydrate equivalent to 250 mg of azithromycin. These are packaged in bottles and blister cards of 6 capsules (Z-PAKS).

Tablets: Zithromax 600 mg tablets (engraved on front with "PFIZER" and on back with "308" are supplied as white, modified oval-shaped, film-coated tablets containing azithromycin dihydrate equivalent to 600 mg azithromycin. These are packaged in bottles of 30 tablets. *Storage:* Capsules and Tablets should be stored at or below 30°C (86°F).

Oral Suspension: Zithromax for oral suspension is supplied in single dose packs containing azithromycin dihydrate equivalent to 1 gram of azithromycin. *Storage:* Store single dose packs between 5° to 30°C (41° to 86°F).

HOW SUPPLIED - EQUIVALENTS NOT AVAILABLE:

Capsule, Gelatin - Oral - 250 mg

18's	$91.52	ZITHROMAX, Pfizer Labs	00069-3050-34
50's	$254.21	ZITHROMAX, Pfizer Labs	00069-3050-50
50's	$254.21	ZITHROMAX, Pfizer Labs	00069-3050-86

Packet - Oral - 1 gm

3's	$47.37	ZITHROMAX, Pfizer Labs	00069-3051-75
10's	$157.89	ZITHROMAX, Pfizer Labs	00069-3051-07

AZTREONAM *(000354)*

CATEGORIES: Anti-Infectives; Antibacterials; Antibiotics; Antimicrobials; Beta-Lactam Antibiotics; Bronchitis; Burns; Cellulitis; Cystitis; Endometritis; Gynecologic Infections; Infections; Monobactams; Peritonitis; Pneumonia; Pyelonephritis; Respiratory Tract Infections; Septicemia; Skin Infections; Urinary Tract Infections; Pregnancy Category B; Sales > $100 Million; FDA Approved 1986 Dec

BRAND NAMES: **Azactam**; *Primbactam*; *Urobactam*
(International brand names outside U.S. in italics)

FORMULARIES: BC-BS

COST OF THERAPY: $225.37 (Infections; Injection; 500 mg/vial; 3/day; 10 days)

PRIMARY ICD9: 136.9 (Unspecified Infections and Parasitic Diseases)

DESCRIPTION:

Azactam is the first member of a new class of antibiotics developed by the Squibb Institute for Medical Research and classified as monobactams. These agents were originally isolated from *Chromobacterium violaceum.* Azactam is a totally synthetic bactericidal antibiotic with activity against a wide spectrum of gram-negative aerobic pathogens.

The monobactams, having a unique monocyclic beta-lactam nucleus, are structurally different from other beta-lactam antibiotics (*e.g.*, penicillins, cephalosporins, cephamycins). The sulfonic acid substituent in the 1-position of the ring activates the beta-lactam moiety; an aminothiazolyl oxime side chain in the 3-position and a methyl group in the 4-position confer the specific antibacterial spectrum and beta-lactamase stability.

Aztreonam is designated chemically as (Z)-2-[[[(2-amino-4-thiazolyl][[(2S,-3S) -2-methyl-4-oxo-1-sulfo-3-azetidinyl) carbamoyl]methylene]amino]oxy]-2-methylpropionic acid.

Azactam For Injection (Aztreonam for injection) is a sterile, nonpyrogenic, sodium-free, white to yellowish-white lyophilized cake containing approximately 780 mg arginine per gram of aztreonam. Following constitution, the product is for intramuscular or intravenous use. Aqueous solutions of the product have a pH in the range of 4.5 to 7.5.

CLINICAL PHARMACOLOGY:

Single 30-minute intravenous infusions of 500 mg, 1 g and 2 g doses of aztreonam in healthy subjects produced peak serum levels of 54, 90 and 204 mcg/ml, respectively, immediately after administration; at eight hours, serum levels were 1, 3 and 6 mcg/ml, respectively. Single 3-minute intravenous injections of the same doses resulted in serum levels of 58, 125 and 242 mcg/ml at five minutes following completion of injection.

Maximum serum concentrations of aztreonam in healthy subjects following completion of single intramuscular injections of 500 mg and 1 g doses occur at about one hour. After identical single intravenous or intramuscular doses of aztreonam, the serum concentrations of aztreonam are comparable at one hour (1.5 hours from start of intravenous infusion) with similar slopes of serum concentrations thereafter.

The serum levels of aztreonam following single 500 mg or 1 g (intramuscular or intravenous) or 2 g (intravenous) doses of aztreonam exceed the MIC_{90} for *Neisseria* sp., *H. influenzae* and most genera of the *Enterobacteriaceae* for eight hours (for *Enterobacter* sp., the eight hour serum levels exceed the MIC for 80 percent of strains). For *Ps. aeruginosa,* a single 2 g intravenous dose produces serum levels that exceed the MIC_{90} for approximately four to six hours. All of the above doses of aztreonam result in average urine levels of aztreonam that exceed the MIC_{90} for the same pathogens for up to 12 hours.

When aztreonam pharmacokinetics were assessed for adult and pediatric patients, they were found to be comparable (down to 9 months old). The serum half-life of aztreonam averaged 1.7 hours (1.5 to 2.0) in subjects with normal renal function, independent of the dose and route of administration. In healthy subjects, based on a 70 kg person, the serum clearance was 91 ml/min and renal clearance was 56 ml/min; the apparent mean volume of distribution at steady-state averaged 12.6 liters, approximately equivalent to extracellular fluid volume.

In a study of healthy elderly male subjects (65 to 75 years of age), the average elimination half-life of aztreonam was slightly longer than in young healthy males.

In patients with impaired renal function, the serum half-life of aztreonam is prolonged (see DOSAGE AND ADMINISTRATION, Renal Impairment). The serum half-life of aztreonam is only slightly prolonged in patients with hepatic impairment since the liver is a minor pathway of excretion.

Average urine concentrations of aztreonam were approximately 1100, 3500 and 6600 mcg/ml within the first two hours following single 500 mg, 1 g and 2 g intravenous doses of aztreonam (30-minute infusions), respectively. The range of average concentrations for aztreonam in the 8 to 12 hour urine specimens in these studies was 25 to 120 mcg/ml. After intramuscular injection of single 500 mg and 1 g doses of aztreonam, urinary levels were approximately 500 and 1200 mcg/ml, respectively, within the first two hours, declining to 180 and 470 mcg/ml in the six to eight hour specimens. In healthy subjects, aztreonam is excreted in the urine about equally by active tubular secretion and glomerular filtration. Approximately 60 to 70 percent of an intravenous or intramuscular dose was recovered in the urine by eight hours. Urinary excretion of a single parenteral dose was essentially complete by 12 hours after injection. About 12 percent of a single intravenous radiolabeled dose was recovered in the feces. Unchanged aztreonam and the inactive beta-lactam ring hydrolysis product of aztreonam were present in feces and urine.

Intravenous or intramuscular administration of a single 500 mg or 1 g dose of aztreonam every eight hours for seven days to healthy subjects produced no apparent accumulation of aztreonam or modification of its disposition characteristics; serum protein binding averaged 56 percent and was independent of dose. An average of about 6 percent of a 1 g intramuscular dose was excreted as a microbiologically inactive open beta-lactam ring hydrolysis product (serum half-life approximately 26 hours) of aztreonam in the zero to eight hour urine collection on the last day of multiple dosing.

Renal function was monitored in healthy subjects given aztreonam; standard tests (serum creatinine, creatinine clearance, BUN, urinalysis and total urinary protein excretion) as well as special tests (excretion of N-acetyl-β-glucosaminidase, alanine aminopeptidase and β_2-microglobulin) were used. No abnormal results were obtained.

Aztreonam achieves measurable concentrations as seen in TABLE 1.

CLINICAL PHARMACOLOGY: *(cont'd)*

TABLE 1 Extravascular Concentrations Of Aztreonam After A Single Parenteral Dose *

Fluid or Tissue	Dose (g)	Route	Hours Post injection	Number of Patients	Mean Concentration (mcg/ml or µ/g)
Fluids					
bile	1	IV	2	10	39
blister fluid	1	IV	1	6	20
bronchial secretion	2	IV	4	7	5
cerebrospinal fluid (inflamed meninges)	2	IV	0.9-4.3	16	3
pericardial fluid	2	IV	1	6	33
pleural fluid	2	IV	1.1-3.0	3	51
synovial fluid	2	IV	0.8-1.9	11	83
Tissues					
atrial appendage	2	IV	0.9-1.6	12	22
endometrium	2	IV	0.7-1.9	4	9
fallopian tube	2	IV	0.7-1.9	8	12
fat	2	IV	1.3-2.0	10	5
femur	2	IV	1.0-2.1	15	16
gallbladder	2	IV	0.8-1.3	4	23
kidney	2	IV	2.4-5.6	5	67
large intestine	2	IV	0.8-1.9	9	12
liver	2	IV	0.9-2.0	6	47
lung	2	IV	1.2-2.1	6	22
myometrium	2	IV	0.7-1.9	9	11
ovary	2	IV	0.7-1.9	7	13
prostate	1	IM	0.8-3.0	8	8
skeletal muscle	2	IV	0.3-0.7	6	16
skin	2	IV	0.0-1.0	8	25
sternum	2	IV	1	6	6

* Tissue penetration is regarded as essential to therapeutic efficacy, but specific tissue levels have not been correlated with specific therapeutic effects.

The concentration of aztreonam in saliva at 30 minutes after a single 1 g intravenous dose (9 patients) was 0.2 mcg/ml; in breast milk at two hours after a single 1 g intravenous dose (6 patients), 0.2 mcg/ml, and at six hours after a single 1 g intramuscular dose (6 patients), 0.3 mcg/ml; in amniotic fluid at six to eight hours after a single 1 g intravenous dose (5 patients), 2 mcg/ml. The concentration of aztreonam in peritoneal fluid obtained one to six hours after multiple 2 g intravenous doses ranged between 12 and 90 mcg/ml in 7 of 8 patients studied.

Aztreonam given intravenously rapidly reaches therapeutic concentrations in peritoneal dialysis fluid; conversely, aztreonam given intraperitoneally in dialysis fluid rapidly produces therapeutic serum levels.

See DRUG INTERACTIONS.

MICROBIOLOGY

Aztreonam exhibits potent and specific activity *in vitro* against a wide spectrum of gram-negative aerobic pathogens including *Pseudomonas aeruginosa.* The bactericidal action of aztreonam results from the inhibition of bacterial cell wall synthesis due to a high affinity of aztreonam for penicillin binding protein 3 (PBP3). Aztreonam, unlike the majority of beta-lactam antibiotics, does not induce beta-lactamase activity and its molecular structure confers a high degree of resistance to hydrolysis by beta-lactamases (*i.e.,* penicillinases and cephalosporinases) produced by most gram-negative and gram-positive pathogens; it is therefore usually active against gram-negative aerobic organisms that are resistant to antibiotics hydrolyzed by beta-lactamases. Aztreonam maintains its antimicrobial activity over a pH range of 6 to 8 *in vitro,* as well as in the presence of human serum and under anaerobic conditions. Aztreonam is active *in vitro* and is effective in laboratory animal models and clinical infections against most strains of the following organisms, including many that are multiply-resistant to other antibiotics (*i.e.,* certain cephalosporins, penicillins, and aminoglycosides):

Escherichia coli
Enterobacter species
Klebsiella pneumoniae and *K. oxytoca*
Proteus mirabilis
Pseudomonas aeruginosa
Serratia marcescens
Haemophilus influenzae (including ampicillin-resistant and other penicillinase-producing strains)
Citrobacter species

While *in vitro* studies have demonstrated the susceptibility to aztreonam of most strains of the following organisms, clinical efficacy for infections other than those included in INDICATIONS AND USAGEhas not been documented:

Neisseria gonorrhoeae (including penicillinase-producing strains)
Proteus vulgaris
Morganella morganii (formerly *Proteus morganii)*
Providencia species, including *P. stuartii* and *P. rettgeri*(formerly *Proteus rettgeri)*
Pseudomonas species
Shigella species
Pasteurella multocida
Yersinia enterocolitica
Aeromonas hydrophila
Neisseria meningitidis

Aztreonam and aminoglycosides have been shown to be synergistic *in vitro* against most strains of *Ps. aeruginosa,* many strains of *Enterobacteriaceae,* and other gram-negative aerobic bacilli.

Alterations of the anaerobic intestinal flora by broad spectrum antibiotics may decrease colonization resistance, thus permitting overgrowth of potential pathogens (*e.g., Candida* and Clostridia species). Aztreonam has little effect on the anaerobic intestinal microflora in *in vitro* studies. *Clostridium difficile* and its cytotoxin were not found in animal models following administration of aztreonam (see ADVERSE REACTIONS, Gastrointestinal).

SUSCEPTIBILITY TESTING

Diffusion Technique: Quantitative procedures that require measurement of zone diameters give precise estimates of microbial susceptibility to antibiotics. One such method, recommended for use with the aztreonam 30 mcg disk, is the National Committee of Clinical Laboratory Standards (NCCLS) approved procedure. Only a 30 mcg aztreonam disk should be used; there are no suitable surrogate disks.

Results of laboratory tests using 30 mcg aztreonam disks should be interpreted using the criteria found in TABLE 2.

CLINICAL PHARMACOLOGY: *(cont'd)*

TABLE 2

Zone Diameter (mm)	Interpretation
≥ 22	(S) Susceptible
16 - 21	(I) Intermediate (Moderate Susceptibility)
≤ 15	(R) Resistant

Dilution Technique: Broth or agar dilution methods may be used to determine the minimal inhibitory concentration (MIC) of aztreonam.

MIC test results should be interpreted according to the concentrations of aztreonam that can be attained in serum, tissues and body fluids.

TABLE 3

MIC (mcg/ml)	Interpretation
≤8	(S) Susceptible
16	(I) Intermediate (Moderate Susceptibility)
≥32	(R) Resistant

For any susceptibility test, a report of "susceptible" indicates that the pathogen is likely to respond to aztreonam therapy; a report of "resistant" indicates that the pathogen is not likely to respond. A report of "intermediate" (moderate susceptibility) indicates that the pathogen is expected to be susceptible to aztreonam if high dosages are used, or if the infection is confined to tissues and fluids (*e.g.,* urine, bile) in which high aztreonam levels are attained.

The quality control cultures should have the following assigned daily ranges for aztreonam:

TABLE 4

		Disks	Mode MIC (mcg/ml)
E.coli	(ATCC 25922)	28-36 mm	0.06-0.25
Ps. aeruginosa	(ATCC 27853)	23-29 mm	2.0-8.0

CLINICAL STUDIES:

A total of 612 pediatric patients aged 1 month to 12 years were enrolled in uncontrolled clinical trials of aztreonam in the treatment of serious gram-negative infections, including urinary tract, lower respiratory tract, skin and skin-structure, and intra-abdominal infections.

INDICATIONS AND USAGE:

Before initiating treatment with aztreonam, appropriate specimens should be obtained for isolation of the causative organism(s) and for determination of susceptibility to aztreonam. Treatment with aztreonam may be started empirically before results of the susceptibility testing are available; subsequently, appropriate antibiotic therapy should be continued.

Aztreonam For Injection is indicated for the treatment of the following infections caused by susceptible gram-negative microorganisms:

Urinary Tract Infections: (complicated and uncomplicated), including pyelonephritis and cystitis (initial and recurrent) caused by *Escherichia coli, Klebsiella pneumoniae, Proteus mirabilis, Pseudomonas aeruginosa, Enterobacter cloacae, Klebsiella oxytoca**, *Citrobacter* species* and *Serratia marcescens**.

Lower Respiratory Tract Infections: including pneumonia and bronchitis caused by *Escherichia coli, Klebsiella pneumoniae, Pseudomonas aeruginosa, Haemophilus influenzae, Proteus mirabilis, Enterobacter* species and *Serratia marcescens**.

Septicemia: caused by *Escherichia coli, Klebsiella pneumoniae, Pseudomonas aeruginosa, Proteus mirabilis**, *Serratia marcescens** and *Enterobacter* species.

Skin and Skin-Structure Infections: including those associated with postoperative wounds, ulcers and burns caused by *Escherichia coli, Proteus mirabilis, Serratia marcescens, Enterobacter* species, *Pseudomonas aeruginosa, Klebsiella pneumoniae* and *Citrobacter* species*.

Intra-abdominal Infections: including peritonitis caused by *Escherichia coli, Klebsiella* species including *K.pneumoniae, Enterobacter* species including *E. cloacae**, *Pseudomonas aeruginosa, Citrobacter* species* including *C. freundii** and *Serratia*species* including *S. marcescens**.

Gynecologic Infections: including endometritis and pelvic cellulitis caused by *Escherichia coli, Klebsiella pneumoniae**, *Enterobacter* species* including *E. cloacae**and *Proteus mirabilis**.

*Efficacy for this organism in this organ system was studied in fewer than ten infections.

Aztreonam is indicated for adjunctive therapy to surgery in the management of infections caused by susceptible organisms, including abscesses, infections complicating hollow viscus perforations, cutaneous infections and infections of serous surfaces. Aztreonam is effective against most of the commonly encountered gram-negative aerobic pathogens seen in general surgery.

CONCURRENT THERAPY

Concurrent initial therapy with other antimicrobial agents and aztreonam is recommended before the causative organism(s) is known in seriously ill patients who are also at risk of having an infection due to gram-positive aerobic pathogens. If anaerobic organisms are also suspected as etiologic agents, therapy should be initiated using an anti-anaerobic agent concurrently with aztreonam (see DOSAGE AND ADMINISTRATION). Certain antibiotics (*e.g.,* cefoxitin, imipenem) may induce high levels of beta-lactamase *in vitro* in some gram-negative aerobes such as *Enterobacter* and *Pseudomonas* species, resulting in antagonism to many beta-lactam antibiotics including aztreonam. These *in vitro* findings suggest that such beta-lactamase inducing antibiotics not be used concurrently with aztreonam. Following identification and susceptibility testing of the causative organism(s), appropriate antibiotic therapy should be continued.

CONTRAINDICATIONS:

This preparation is contraindicated in patients with known hypersensitivity to aztreonam or any other component in the formulation.

WARNINGS:

Both animial and human data suggest that aztreonam is rarely cross-reactive with other beta-lactam antibiotics and weakly immunogenic. Treatment with aztreonam can result in hypersenisivity reactions with or without prior exposure. (See CONTRAINDICATIONS.)

Careful inquiry should be made to determine whether the patient has any hypersensitivity reactions to any allergens.

While cross-reactivity of aztreonam with other beta-lactma antibiotics is rare, this drug should be administered with caution to any patient with a history of hypersensitivity to beta-lactams (*e.g.,* penicillins, cephalosporins, and/or carbapenems). Treatment with aztreonam can result in hypersensitivity reactions in patients with or without prior exposure to aztreonam. If an allergic reaction to aztreonam occurs, discontinue the drug and institute supportive

WARNINGS: *(cont'd)*

treatment as appropriate (*e.g.,* maintenance of ventilation, pressor amines, antihistamines, corticosteroids). Serious hypersensitivity reactions may require epinephrine and other emergency measures. (See ADVERSE REACTIONS.)

Pseudomembranous colitis has been reported with nearly all antibacterial agents, including aztreonam, and may range in severity from mild to life-threatening. Therefore, it is important to consider this diagnosis in patients who present with diarrhea subsequent to the administration of antibacterial agents.

Treatment with antibacterial agents alters the normal flora of the colon and may permit overgrowth of clostridia. Studies indicate that a toxin produced by *Clostridium difficile* is one primary cause of "antibiotic-associated colitis."

After the diagnosis of pseudomembranous colitis has been established, therapeutic measures should be initiated. Mild cases of pseudomembranous colitis usually respond to drug discontinuation alone. In moderate to severe cases, consideration should be given to management with fluids and electrolytes, protein supplementation, and treatment with an oral antibacterial drug clinically effective against *C. difficile* colitis.

Rare cases of toxic epidermal necrolysis have been reported in association with aztreonam in patients undergoing bone marrow transplant with multiple risk factors including graft versus host disease, sepsis, radiation therapy and other concomitantly administered drugs associated with toxic epidermal necrolysis.

PRECAUTIONS:

GENERAL

In patients with impaired hepatic or renal function, appropriate monitoring is recommended during therapy.

If an aminoglycoside is used concurrently with aztreonam, especially if high dosages of the former are used or if therapy is prolonged, renal function should be monitored because of the potential nephrotoxicity and ototoxicity of aminoglycoside antibiotics.

The use of antibiotics may promote the overgrowth of nonsusceptible organisms, including gram-positive organisms (*Staphylococcus aureus* and *Streptococcus faecalis*) and fungi. Should superinfection occur during therapy, appropriate measures should be taken.

CARCINOGENESIS, MUTAGENESIS, AND IMPAIRMENT OF FERTILITY

Carcinogenicity studies in animals have not been performed.

Genetic toxicology studies performed *in vivo* and *in vitro* with aztreonam in several standard laboratory models revealed no evidence of mutagenic potential at the chromosomal or gene level.

Two-generation reproduction studies in rats at daily doses up to 20 times the maximum recommended human dose, prior to and during gestation and lactation, revealed no evidence of impaired fertility. There was a slightly reduced survival rate during the lactation period in the offspring of rats that received the highest dosage, but not in offspring of rats that received five times the maximum recommended human dose.

PREGNANCY CATEGORY B

Aztreonam crosses the placenta and enters the fetal circulation.

Studies in pregnant rats and rabbits, with daily doses up to 15 and 5 times, respectively, the maximum recommended human dose, revealed no evidence of embryo- or fetotoxicity or teratogenicity. No drug induced changes were seen in any of the maternal, fetal, or neonatal parameters that were monitored in rats receiving 15 times the maximum recommended human dose of aztreonam during late gestation and lactation.

There are no adequate and well-controlled studies in pregnant women. Because animal reproduction studies are not always predictive of human response, aztreonam should be used during pregnancy only if clearly needed.

NURSING MOTHERS

Aztreonam is excreted in breast milk in concentrations that are less than 1 percent of concentrations determined in simultaneously obtained maternal serum; consideration should be given to temporary discontinuation of nursing and use of formula feedings.

PEDIATRIC USE

The satefty and effectiveness of intravenous aztreonam have been established in the age groups 9 months to 16 years. Use of aztreonam in these groups is supported by evidence from adequate and well-controlled studies of aztreonam in adults with additional efficacy, safety, and pharmcokinetic data from non-comparative clinical studies in pediatric patients. Sufficient data are not available for pediatric patients under 9 months of age or for the following treatment indications/ pathogens: septicemia and skin and skin-structure infections (where the skin infection is beleived or known to be due to *H. influenza* type b). In pediatric patients with cyctic fibrosis, higher doses of aztreonam may be warranted. (See CLINICAL PHARMACOLOGY, DOSAGE AND ADMINISTRATION, and CLINICAL STUDIES.)

DRUG INTERACTIONS:

Concomitant administration of probenecid or furosemide and aztreonam causes clinically insignificant increases in the serum levels of aztreonam. Single-dose intravenous pharmacokinetic studies have not shown any significant interaction between aztreonam and concomitantly administered gentamicin, nafcillin sodium, cephradine, clindamycin or metronidazole. No reports of disulfiram-like reactions with alcohol ingestion have been noted; this is not unexpected since aztreonam does not contain a methyl-tetrazole side chain.

ADVERSE REACTIONS:

Local reactions such as phlebitis/thrombophlebitis following IV administration, and discomfort/swelling at the injection site following IM administration occurred at rates of approximately 1.9 percent and 2.4 percent, respectively.

Systemic reactions (considered to be related to therapy or of uncertain etiology) occurring at an incidence of 1 to 1.3 percent include diarrhea, nausea and/or vomiting, and rash. Reactions occurring at an incidence of less than 1 percent are listed within each body system in order of decreasing severity:

Hypersensitivity: anaphylaxis, angioedema, bronchospasm

Hematologic: pancytopenia, neutropenia, thrombocytopenia, anemia, eosinophilia, leukocytosis, thrombocytosis

Gastrointestinal: abdominal cramps; rare cases of *C. difficile:* associated diarrhea, including pseudomembranous colitis, or gastrointestinal bleeding have been reported. Onset of pseudomembranous colitis symptoms may occur during or after antibiotic treatment (see WARNINGS)

Dermatologic: toxic epidermal necrolysis (see WARNINGS) purpura, erythema multiforme, urticaria, exfoliative dermatitis, petechiae, pruritus, diaphoresis

Cardiovascular: hypotension, transient ECG changes (ventricular bigeminy and PVC), flushing

Respiratory: wheezing, dyspnea and chest pain

Hepatobiliary: hepatitis, jaundice

Nervous System: seizure, confusion, vertigo, paresthesia, insomnia, dizziness

Musculoskeletal: muscular aches

ADVERSE REACTIONS: *(cont'd)*

Special Senses: tinnitus, diplopia, mouth ulcer, altered taste, numb tongue, sneezing and nasal congestion, halitosis

Other: vaginal candidiasis, vaginitis, breast tenderness

Body as a Whole: weakness, headache, fever, malaise.

PEDIATRIC ADVERSE REACTIONS

Of the 612 pediatric patients who were treated with aztreonam in clinical trials, less than 1% required discontinuation of therapy due to adverse events. The following systemic adverse events regardless of drug relationship, occurred in at least 1 % of treated patients in domestic clinical trials: rash (4.3%), diarrhea (1.4%), and fever (1.0%). These adverse events were comparable to those observed in adult clinical trials.

In 343 pediatric patients receiving intravenous therapy, the following local reactions were noted: pain (12%), erythema (2.9%), induration (0.9%), and phlebitis (2.1%). In the US population, pain occured in 1.5% of patients while each of the remaining three local reactions had an incidence of 0.5%.

The following laboratory adverse events, regardless of drug relationship, occurred in at least 1% of treated patients: increased eosinophils (6.3%), increased platelets (3.6%), neutropenia (3.2%), increases AST (3.8%), increased ALT (6.5%), and increased serum creatinine (5.8%).

In US pediatric clinical trials, neutropenia (absolute neutrophil count less than $1000/mm^3$) occurred in 11.3% of patients (8/71) younger than 2 years receiving 30 mg/kg every 6 hours. AST and ALT elevations to greater than 3 times the upper limit of normal were noted in 15-20% of patients aged 2 years or above receiving 50 mg/kg every 6 hours. The increased frequency of these reported laboratory adverse events may be due to either increased severity of illness treated or higher doses of aztreonam administered.

ADVERSE LABORATORY CHANGES

Adverse laboratory changes without regard to drug relationship that were reported during clinical trials were:

Hepatic: elevations of AST (SGOT), ALT (SGPT), and alkaline phosphatase; signs or symptoms of hepatobiliary dysfunction occurred in less than 1 percent of recipients.

Hematologic: increases in prothrombin and partial thromboplastin times, positive Coombs test.

Renal: increases in serum creatinine.

OVERDOSAGE:

If necessary, aztreonam may be cleared from the serum by hemodialysis and/or peritoneal dialysis.

DOSAGE AND ADMINISTRATION:

DOSAGE IN ADULT PATIENTS

Aztreonam for injection may be administered intravenously or by intramuscular injection. Dosage and route of administration should be determined by susceptibility of the causative organisms, severity and site of infection, and the condition of the patient.

The intravenous route is recommended for patients requiring single doses greater than 1 g or those with bacterial septicemia, localized parenchymal abscess (*e.g.,* intra-abdominal abscess), peritonitis or other severe systemic or life-threatening infections.

Because of the serious nature of infection due to *Pseudomonas aeruginosa,* dosage of 2 g every 6 to 8 hours is recommended, at least upon initiation of therapy, in systemic infections caused by this organism in adults.

The duration of therapy depends on the severity of infection. Generally, aztreonam should be continued for at least 48 hours after the patient becomes asymptomatic or evidence of bacterial eradication has been obtained. Persistent infections may require treatment for several weeks. Doses smaller than those indicated should not be used.

Renal Impairment in Adult Patients

Prolonged serum levels of aztreonam may occur in patients with transient or persistent renal insufficiency. Therefore, the dosage of aztreonam should be halved in patients with estimated creatinine clearances between 10 and 30 $ml/min/1.73\ m^2$ after an initial loading dose of 1 g or 2 g.

When only the serum creatinine concentration is available, the following formula (based on sex, weight, and age of the patient) may be used to approximate the creatinine clearance (Cl_{cr}). The serum creatinine should represent a steady state of renal function.

TABLE 5

Males: Cl_{cr} = [weight (kg) × (140-age)] ÷ [72 × serum creatinine (mg/dl)]
Females: 0.85 × above value

In patients with severe renal failure (creatinine clearance less than 10 $ml/min/1.73\ m^2$), such as those supported by hemodialysis, the usual dose of 500 mg, 1 g or 2 g should be given initially. The maintenance dose should be one-fourth of the usual initial dose given at the usual fixed interval of 6, 8 or 12 hours. For serious or life-threatening infections, in addition to the maintenance doses, one-eighth of the initial dose should be given after each hemodialysis session.

Dosage In The Elderly

Renal status is a major determinant of dosage in the elderly; these patients in particular may have diminished renal function. Serum creatinine may not be an accurate determinant of renal status. Therefore, as with all antibiotics eliminated by the kidneys, estimates of creatinine clearance should be obtained, and appropriate dosage modifications made if necessary.

DOSAGE IN PEDIATRIC PATIENTS

Aztreonam should be administered intravenously to pediatric patinets with normal renal function. There are insufficient data regarding intramuscular administration to pediatric patients or dosing in pediatric patients with renal impairment. (See PRECAUTIONS, Pediatric Use.)

TABLE 6 Dosage Guidelines

Type of Infection	Dose*	Frequency (hours)
Adults*		
Urinary tract infections	500 mg or 1 g	8 or 12
Moderately severe systemic infections	1 g or 2 g	8 or 12
Severe systemic or life-threatening infections	2 g	6 or 8
Pediatric Patients†		
Mild to moderate infection	30 mg/kg	8
Moderately to severe infections	30 mg/kg	6 or 8

* Maximum recommended adult dose is 8 g per day.
† Maximum recommended pediatric dose is 120 mg/kg/day.

PREPARATION OF PARENTERAL SOLUTIONS

DOSAGE AND ADMINISTRATION: *(cont'd)*

General

Upon the addition of the diluent to the container, contents should be shaken **immediately** and **vigorously**. Constituted solutions are not for multiple-dose use; should the entire volume in the container not be used for a single-dose, the unused solution must be discarded.

Depending upon the concentration of aztreonam and diluent used, constituted aztreonam for injection yields a colorless to light straw yellow solution which may develop a slight pink tint on standing (potency is not affected). Parenteral drug products should be inspected visually for particulate matter and discoloration whenever solution and container permit.

Admixtures With Other Antibiotics

Intravenous infusion solutions of aztreonam for injection not exceeding 2% w/v prepared with Sodium Chloride Injection USP 0.9% or Dextrose Injection USP 5%, to which clindamycin phosphate, gentamicin sulfate, tobramycin sulfate, or cefazolin sodium have been added at concentrations usually used clinically, are stable for up to 48 hours at room temperature or seven days under refrigeration. Ampicillin sodium admixtures with aztreonam in Sodium Chloride Injection USP 0.9% are stable for 24 hours at room temperature and 48 hours under refrigeration; stability in Dextrose Injection USP 5% is two hours at room temperature and eight hours under refrigeration.

Aztreonam-cloxacillin sodium and aztreonam-vancomycin hydrochloride admixtures are stable in Dianeal 137 (Peritoneal Dialysis Solution) with 4.25% Dextrose for up to 24 hours at room temperature.

Aztreonam is incompatible with nafcillin sodium, cephradine, and metronidazole.

Other admixtures are not recommended since compatibility data are not available.

Intravenous (IV) Solutions

For Bolus Injection: The contents of an aztreonam for injection 15 ml or 30 ml capacity vial should be constituted with 6 to 10 ml Sterile Water for Injection USP.

For Infusion: Contents of the 100 ml capacity bottle should be constituted to a final concentration not exceeding 2% w/v (at least 50 ml of any appropriate infusion solution listed below per gram aztreonam). These solutions may be frozen immediately after constitution in the original container. (See Stability.)

If the contents of a 15 ml or 30 ml capacity vial are to be transferred to an appropriate infusion solution, each gram of aztreonam should be initially constituted with at least 3 ml Sterile Water for Injection USP. Further dilution may be obtained with one of the following intravenous infusion solutions:

Sodium Chloride Injection USP, 0.9%

Ringer's Injection USP

Lactated Ringer's Injection USP

Dextrose Injection USP, 5% or 10%

Dextrose and Sodium Chloride Injection USP, 5%:0.9%, 5%:0.45% or 5%:0.2%

Sodium Lactate Injection USP (M/6 Sodium Lactate)

Ionosol B and 5% Dextrose

Isolyte E

Isolyte E with 5% Dextrose

Isolyte M with 5% Dextrose

Normosol-R

Normosol-R and 5% Dextrose

Normosol-M and 5% Dextrose

Mannitol Injection USP, 5% or 10%

Lactated Ringer's and 5% Dextrose Injection

Plasma-Lyte M and 5% Dextrose

10% Travert Injection

10% Travert and Electrolyte No. 1 Injection

10% Travert and Electrolyte No. 2 Injection

10% Travert and Electrolyte No. 3 Injection

Intramuscular (IM) Solutions

The contents of an aztreonam for injection 15 ml or 30 ml capacity vial should be constituted with at least 3 ml of an appropriate diluent per gram aztreonam. The following diluents may be used:

Sterile Water for Injection USP

Bacteriostatic Water for Injection USP (with benzyl alcohol or with methyl- and propylparabens)

Sodium Chloride Injection USP, 0.9%

Bacteriostatic Sodium Chloride Injection USP (with benzyl alcohol)

STABILITY OF IV AND IM SOLUTIONS

Aztreonam solutions for IV infusion at concentrations not exceeding 2% w/v must be used within 48 hours following constitution if kept at controlled room temperature (59°-86°F/15°-30°C) or within seven days if refrigerated (36°-46°F/2°-8°C).

Frozen aztreonam infusion solutions may be stored for up to three months at -4°F/-20°C; frozen solutions may be thawed at controlled room temperature or by overnight refrigeration. Solutions that have been thawed and maintained at controlled room temperature or under refrigeration should be used within 24 or 72 hours after removal from the freezer, respectively. Solutions should not be refrozen.

Aztreonam solutions at concentrations exceeding 2% w/v, except those prepared with Sterile Water for Injection USP or Sodium Chloride Injection USP, should be used promptly after preparation; the two excepted solutions must be used within 48 hours if stored at controlled room temperature or within seven days if refrigerated.

INTRAVENOUS ADMINISTRATION

Bolus Injection: A bolus injection may be used to initiate therapy. The dose should be **slowly** injected directly into a vein, or the tubing of a suitable administration set, over a period of three to five minutes (see Infusion).

Infusion: With any intermittent infusion of aztreonam and another drug with which it is not pharmaceutically compatible, the common delivery tube should be flushed before and after delivery of aztreonam with any appropriate infusion solution compatible with both drug solutions; the drugs should not be delivered simultaneously. Any aztreonam infusion should be completed within a 20 to 60 minute period. With use of a *Y-type administration set,* careful attention should be given to the calculated volume of aztreonam solution required so that the entire dose will be infused. A *volume control administration set* may be used to deliver an initial dilution of aztreonam for injection (see Preparation Of Parenteral Solutions, For Infusion) into a compatible infusion solution during administration; in this case, the final dilution of aztreonam should provide a concentration not exceeding 2% w/v.

DOSAGE AND ADMINISTRATION: *(cont'd)*

INTRAMUSCULAR ADMINISTRATION

The dose should be given by deep injection into a large muscle mass (such as the upper outer quadrant of the gluteus maximus or lateral part of the thigh). Aztreonam is well tolerated and should not be admixed with any local anesthetic agent.

Storage: Store original packages at room temperature; avoid excessive heat.

HOW SUPPLIED - EQUIVALENTS NOT AVAILABLE:

Injection, Lyphl-Soln - Intramuscular; - 1 gm/vial

10's	$149.25	AZACTAM, Bristol Myers Squibb	00003-2560-10
10's	$157.00	AZACTAM, Bristol Myers Squibb	00003-2560-20

Injection, Lyphl-Soln - Intramuscular; - 2 gm/vial

10's	$298.13	AZACTAM, Bristol Myers Squibb	00003-2570-10
10's	$314.25	AZACTAM, Bristol Myers Squibb	00003-2570-20

Injection, Lyphl-Soln - Intramuscular; - 500 mg/vial

10's	$78.13	AZACTAM, Bristol Myers Squibb	00003-2550-10
25's	$187.81	AZACTAM, Bristol Myers Squibb	00003-2550-15

BCG LIVE *(003043)*

CATEGORIES: Antineoplastics; Bladder Carcinoma; Cancer; Chemotherapy; Tumors; Pregnancy Category C; FDA Approved 1991 Dec

BRAND NAMES: **Theracys**

DESCRIPTION:

FOR TREATMENT OF CARCINOMA *IN-SITU* OF THE URINARY BLADDER

BCG Live (Intravesical), TheraCys, is a freeze-dried suspension of an attenuated strain of *Mycobacterium bovis* (Bacillus Calmette and Guerin), which has been grown on Sauton medium (potato and glycerin based medium), used in the non-specific active therapy of carcinoma in-situ of the urinary bladder. CAUTION: BCG live is NOT intended to be used as an immunizing agent for the prevention of tuberculosis. BCG live is NOT a vaccine for the prevention of cancer.

TheraCys is formulated to contain 27 mg (dry weight/vial Bacillus of Calmette and Guerin (BCG) and 5% w/v monosodium glutamate. This product contains no preservative. Each vial of TheraCys is ready for use following reconstitution with the accompanying diluent (1.0 ml), which consists of approximately 0.85% sodium chloride, 0.025% Tween 80, 0.06% w/v sodium dihydrogen phosphate and 0.25% disodium hydrogen phosphate. The diluent contains no preservative. One dose consists of three pooled vials of reconstituted material further diluted in sterile, preservative-free saline. The reconstituted product contains $3.4 \pm 3.0 \times 10^8$ colony forming units (CFU) per vial when resuspended in the diluent provided.

To ensure viability of the product through to its labeled expiration date, it is very important that BCG live and diluent be stored continuously between 2 and 8°C (35 and 46°F) until use (see Storage.) It should be used immediately after reconstitution.

CLINICAL PHARMACOLOGY:

BCG live promotes a local inflammatory reaction with histiocytic and leukocytic infiltration in the urinary bladder.[1,2,3] The local inflammatory effects are associated with an apparent elimination or reduction of superficial cancerous lesions of the urinary bladder. The exact mechanism by which this is accomplished is unknown.

In a randomized, actively controlled multicenter study BCG live was compared to doxorubicin hydrochloride (Adriamycin) in the treatment of carcinoma in-situ of the urinary bladder. The response of 114 eligible patients for evaluation is given in TABLE 1. Among the 54 patients receiving BCG live, 74% had a complete response (negative by cystoscopic examination and by urine cytology). The estimated median time to treatment failure (recurrence, progression or death) was 48.2 months (TABLE 2).[4]

TABLE 1 Response Of Patients With Carcinoma In-Situ To Treatment With BCG Live Or Adriamycin

	BCG (n = 54)	Adriamycin (n = 60)
Complete Response†	74%*	42%*
No Response‡	11%	10%
Progressive Disease††	13%	42%
No Evaluation	2%	7%
Total	100%	100%

* Difference is statistically significant (P <0.01).
† Confirmed by cytology and cystoscopic examination
‡ Less than a CR or stable disease.
†† Increase of stage or grade.

TABLE 2 Time To Recurrence, Progression Or Death: Time To Treatment Failure (TTF)

Treatment	Number Studied	Number Failures	Median TTF
BCG Live	54	27	48.2 months*
Adriamycin	60	46	5.9 months*

* Difference is statistically significant (P <0.01 by stratified logrank test).

The effect of chemotherapy (other than BCG live or Adriamycin) prior to entry into the controlled study was analyzed. Patients in the BCG live treated arm who had receive prior chemotherapy had a complete response rate of 81% (11/26) as compared to 68% (16/28) in the group who had not received prior chemotherapy (TABLE 3). This difference was not statistically significant.

TABLE 3 prior Versus No Prior Treatment

Prior Treatment*	Study Arm	Response Rate	Median TTF (# Events/N)
Yes	BCG Live	81%	Not reached (11/26)
Yes	Adriamycin	53%	7.0 months (22/30)
No	BCG Live	68%	32.8 months (16/28)
No	Adriamycin	30%	3.7 months (24/30)

* Other than BCG Live and Adriamycin.

CLINICAL PHARMACOLOGY: *(cont'd)*

No survival advantage for BCG live therapy[4] over that for Adriamycin[4,5,6] was demonstrated after a 40-72 month follow-up. The median time to death for each group was 23 months and 21 months for BCG live and Adriamycin respectively.

The clinical trials carried out with BCG live included percutaneous administration of 0.5 ml of BCG Live (Intravesical) solution, which was reconstituted in the diluent provided and further diluted in 50 ml sterile preservative-free saline, with each intravesical dose.[4] Some studies have suggested that this may not be necessary[15]and if severe reactions, such as uncertain, occurred the percutaneous treatment was discontinued.

INDICATIONS AND USAGE:

BCG live is indicated for intravesical use in the treatment of primary and relapsed carcinoma in-situ of the urinary bladder to eliminate residual tumor cells and to reduce the frequency of tumor recurrence. It is indicated for the treatment of carcinoma in-situ with or without associated papillary tumors. BCG live is also indicated for the treatment of papillary tumors occurring alone. BCG live is also indicated as a therapy for patients with carcinoma in-situ of the bladder following failure to respond to other treatment regimens. CAUTION: BCG live is NOT a vaccine for the prevention of tuberculosis. BCG live is NOT a vaccine for the prevention of cancer.

CONTRAINDICATIONS:

Patients on immunosuppressive therapy or with compromised immune systems should not be receive BCG live due to the risk of overwhelming systemic mycobacterial sepsis.

BCG live should not be administered to patients with fever unless the caused of the fever is determined and evaluated. If the fever is due to an infection, BCG live should be withheld until the patients is afebrile and off all therapy.

Patients with urinary tract infection should not receive BCG live treatment because administration may result in the risk of disseminated BCG infection or in an increased severity of bladder irritation.

BCG live should NOT be administered as an immunizing agent for the prevention of tuberculosis. BCG live is NOT a vaccine for the prevention of cancer.

WARNINGS:

BCG live should NOT be administered as an immunizing agent for the prevention of tuberculosis. BCG live is NOT vaccine for the prevention of cancer.

Since administration of intravesical BCG live causes in inflammatory response in the bladder and has been associated with hematuria, urinary frequency, dysuria and bacterial urinary tract infection, careful monitoring of urinary status is required. If there is an increase in the patient's existing symptoms, or if their symptoms persist or if any of these symptoms develop, the patient should be evaluated and managed for urinary tract infection or BCG toxicity.

Since death has occurred due to systemic BCG infection, patients should be closely monitored for symptoms of such an infection (see PRECAUTIONS.) BCG therapy should be withheld upon any suspicion of systemic infection (*e.g.*granulomatous hepatitis.

Drug combinations containing bone marrow depressants and/or immunosuppressants and/or radiation may eight impair the response to BCG live or increase the risk of osteomyelitis or disseminated BCG infection (see DRUG INTERACTIONS.)

Patients undergoing antimicrobial therapy for other infections should be evaluated to assess whether the therapy will obviate the effects of BCG live actions.

For patients with small bladder capacity, increased risk of severity of local irritation should be considered in decisions to treat with BCG live.

Intravesical treatment with BCG live may induce a sensitivity to tuberculin which could complicate further interpretations of skin test reactions to tuberculin in the diagnosis of suspected mycobacterial infections. Determination of patient's reactivity to tuberculin prior to administration of BCG live may be desirable in this regard.

In a controlled multi-center clinical trial comparing BCG therapy and doxorubicin hydrochloride (Adriamycin) for the intravesical treatment of superficial transitional cell carcinoma with and without carcinoma in-situ of the bladder, 112 patients received BCG.[4]

In another controlled study using BCG live for the treatment of superficial transitional cell carcinoma, with or without carcinoma in-situ, of the bladder, similar adverse reactions were observed.[13] However, two deaths were noted in this study which may have been associated with traumatic catheterization.

The incidence of adverse reactions associated with intravesical BCG live therapy is given below. Most local adverse reactions occur following the third intravesical instillation. Symptoms usually begin two to four hours after instillation and persist for 24 to 72 hours. Systemic reactions usually last for 1-3 days after each intravesical instillation.[4,13,14]

TABLE 4 Local Reactions (5 Of 112 Patients)

Reaction	Total	Severe*
Dysuria	51.8	3.6
Frequency	40.2	1.8
Hematuria	39.3	17.0
Cystitis	29.5	0.0
Urgency	17.9	0.0
Urinary Tact Infection	17.9	1.0
Urinary Incontinence	6.3	0.0
Cramps/Pain	6.3	0.0
Decreased Bladder Capacity	5.4	0.0
Tissue in Urine	0.9	0.0
Local Infection	0.9	0.0

* Severe is defined as grade 3 (severe) or grade 4 (life threatening).

No fatalities associated with the use of BCG live were reported in this study. Two fatalities have been reported with the use of BCG live in another study after traumatic catheterization or in the presence of urinary infection.[13]

An increased risk of additional primary malignancies has been reported following radiotherapy and chemotherapy for many types of malignancies. No increase in second primary malignancies after treatment with BCG live was reported in these studies.[4]

Irritative bladder symptoms associated with BCG live administration can be managed symptomatically with phenazopyridine hydrochloride (Pyridium), propantheline bromide (Pro-Banthine), and acetaminophen.[4]

PRECAUTIONS:

General: Contains viable attenuated mycobacteria. Handle as infectious. Use aseptic technique.

The possibility of allergic reactions in individuals sensitive to the components of the product should be borne in mind.

PRECAUTIONS: *(cont'd)*

TABLE 5 Systemic Reactions (% Of 112 Patients)

Reaction	Total	Severe*
Malaise	40.2	2.0
Fever (>30°C)	38.4	2.6
Chills	39.9	2.6
Anemia	20.5	0.0
Nausea/Vomiting	16.1	0.0
Anorexia	10.7	0.0
Myalgia/Arthralgia/Arthritis	7.1	1.0
Diarrhea	6.3	0.0
Mild Liver Involvement	2.7	0.0
Mild Abdominal Pain	2.7	0.0
Systemic Infection**	2.7	2.0
Pulmonary Infection**	2.7	0.0
Cardiac	2.7	0.0
Headache	1.8	0.0
Hypersensitivity Skin Rash	1.8	0.0
Constipation	0.9	0.0
Dizziness	0.9	0.0
Fatigue	0.9	0.0
Leukopenia	5.4	0.0
Disseminated Intravascular Coagulation	2.7	0.0
Thrombocytopenia	0.9	0.0
Renal Toxicity	9.8	2.0
Genital Pain	9.8	0.0
Flank Pain	0.9	0.0

* Severe is defined as grade 3 (severe) or grade 4 (life threatening).
** Includes both BCG and other infections.

After usage all equipment and materials (*e.g.*, syringes, catheters and containers that may have come into contact with BCG live) used of instillation of the product into the bladder, should be placed immediately into plastic bags which are labelled "infectious Waste" and disposed of accordingly as biohazardous waste.

Aseptic technique must be used during administration of intravesical BCG live so as not to introduce contaminants into the urinary tract or to traumatize unduly the urinary mucosa.

Urine voided for 6 hours after instillation should be disinfected with an equal volume of 5% hypochlorite solution (undiluted household bleach) and allowed to stand for 15 minutes before flushing.

It is recommended that intravesical BCG live not be administered any sooner than one week following transurethral resection because fatalities due to disseminated BCG infection have been reported with use of BCG live after traumatic catheterization.

If the physician believes that the bladder catheterization has been traumatic (*e.g.*, associated with bleeding or possible false passage), then BCG live should not be administered and there must be a treatment delay of at least one week. Subsequent treatment should be resumed as if no interruption in the schedule had occurred. That is, all doses of BCG live should be administered even after a temporary halt in administration.

If systemic BCG infection is suspected (*i.e.* if patients have fever over 39°C (103°F) or persistent fever above 38°C (101°F) over two days or severe malaise), an infectious disease specialist should be consulted and fast acting antituberculosis therapy should be initiated. It should be noted that BCG systemic infections are rarely evidenced by positive cultures.

Information for the Patient: Patients should be advised to check with their doctor as soon as possible if there is an increase in their existing symptoms, or their symptoms persist even after receiving a number of treatments, or if any of the following symptoms develop (TABLE 6):

TABLE 6

More Common	Rare
Blood in Urine	Cough
Fever and Chills	Skin Rash
Frequent Usage to Urinate	
Increased Frequency of Urination	
Joint Pain	
Nausea and Vomiting	
Painful Urination	

A cough that develops after administration of BCG live could indicate a BCG systemic infection which is life-threatening. If systemic infection occurs it should be treated immediately with antituberculous antibiotics.

All patients should sit while voiding following instillation of solution.

Urine voided for 6 hours after instillation should be disinfected with an equal volume of 5% hypochlorite solution (undiluted household bleach) and allowed to stand for 15 minutes before flushing.

Pregnancy Category C: BCG live. Animal reproduction duties have not been conducted with BCG live. It is also not known whether BCG live can cause fetal harm when administered to a pregnancy woman or can affect reproduction capacity. BCG live should be given to a pregnant woman only if clearly needed. Women should be advised not to become pregnant while on therapy.

Nursing Mothers: It is not known whether BCG live is excreted in human milk. Because many drugs are excreted in human milk, caution should be exercised when BCG live is administered to a nursing mother.

Pediatric Use: Safety and effectiveness for carcinoma in-situ of the urinary bladder in children have not been established.

DRUG INTERACTIONS:

Patients must also be advised that drug combinations containing bone marrow depressants and/or immunosuppressants and/or radiation may impair the response to BCG live or increase the risk of osteomyelitis or disseminated BCG infection.

ADVERSE REACTIONS:

BCG live therapy can affect several organs (or parts) of the body in addition to the cancer cells.

Systemic side effects (such as malaise, fever and chills) may represent hypersensitivity reactions and can be treated with diphenhydramine hydrochloride.[4] Systemic infection as a result of the spread of BCG organisms has occasionally occurred with intravesical BCG live administration. The management of this condition is provided under PRECAUTIONS.

DOSAGE AND ADMINISTRATION:

Intravesical treatment and prophylaxis for carcinoma in-situ of the urinary bladder should begin between 7 to 14 days after biopsy or transurethral resection if this procedure is done. A dose of three (3) trials os BCG live is given intravesically under aseptic conditions once weekly for 6 weeks (induction therapy). Each dose (3 reconstituted vials) is further diluted in an additional 50 ml sterile, preservative-free saline for a total of 53 ml (see DOSAGE AND ADMINISTRATION, Reconstitution of Freeze-Dried Product and Withdrawal from Rubber-Stoppered Vial). A urethral catheter is inserted into the bladder under aseptic conditions, the bladder drained and then the 53 ml suspension of BCG live is instilled slowly by gravity following which the catheter is withdrawn. During the first hour following instillation, the patient should lie for 15 minutes each in the prone and supine positions and also on each side. The patient is then allowed to be up but retains the suspension for another 60 minutes for a total of two hours. All patients may not be able to retain the suspension for the 2 hours and should be instructed to void in less time if necessary. At the end of 2 hours all patients should void in a seated position for safety reasons. Patients should be instructed to maintain adequate hydration.

If the physician believes that the bladder catheterization has been traumatic (*e.g.,* associated with bleeding or possible false passage), then BCG live should not be administered and there must be a treatment delay of at least one week. Subsequent treatment should be resumed as if no interruption in the schedule had occurred. That is, all doses of BCG live should be administered even after a temporary halt in administration.

The indication therapy should be followed by one treatment given 3, 6, 12, 18 and 24 months following the initial treatment.

After use, all equipment, materials and containers that may have come in contact with BCG live should be sterilized or disposed of properly as with any other biohazardous waste (see PRECAUTIONS.)

RECONSTITUTION OF FREEZE-DRIED PRODUCT AND WITHDRAWAL FROM RUBBER-STOPPERED VIAL.

BCG LIVE SHOULD BE USED IMMEDIATELY AFTER RECONSTITUTION. KEEP REFRIGERATED UNTIL USE. DISCARD AFTER 2 HOURS.

DO NOT REMOVE THE RUBBER STOPPER FRO THE VIAL.

Reconstitute and dilute immediately prior to use.

Persons handling product should be masked and gloved.

BCG live should be not be handled by persons with a known immunologic deficiency.

BCG live and dilute using aseptic technique.

BCG live should be reconstituted only with the diluent provided to ensure proper dispersion of the organisms.

Apply a sterile pledget of cotton moistened with a suitable antiseptic to the surface of the rubber stoppers of the vials of diluent and BCG live product. Allow the antiseptic to act for at least 5 minutes. Draw into a sterile syringe a volume of air equal to the volume of the diluent in the vial. Pierce the centre of the rubber stopper in the vial containing diluent with the sterile needle of the syringe, invert the vial, slowly inject into it the air contained in the syringe and, keeping the point of the needle immersed, withdraw into the syringe 1.0 ml of diluent. Then holding the syringe-plunger steady, withdraw the needle from the vial. Injects this volume of diluent into the vial of freeze-dried material. Shake the vial gently until a fine, even suspension results. Withdraw the entire contents of the reconstituted material into the syringe.

The reconstituted material from three vials (1 dose) is further diluted in an additional 50 ml sterile, preservative-free saline to a final volume of 53 ml for intravesical instillation (and percutaneous injection if it is given, see CLINICAL PHARMACOLOGY).

HOW SUPPLIED:

Storage: BCG live and the accompanying diluent should be kept in a refrigerator at a temperature between 2 and 8°C (35 and 46°F). It should not be used after the expiration date marked on the vial, otherwise it may be inactive. The product should be used immediately after reconstitution; however, it must not be used after 2 hours. Any reconstituted product which exhibits flocculation or clumping that cannot be dispersed with gentle shaking should not be used.

At no time should be freeze-fired or reconstituted BCG live be exposed to sunlight, direct or indirect. Exposure to artificial light should be kept to a minimum.[9]

REFERENCES:

1. Old LJ, Clarke DA, Benacerraf B. Effect of bacillus Calmette-Guerin infection on transplanted tumors in the mouse. Nature 1959; 184:291. **2.** Lamm DL, Harris SC, Gittes RF. Bacillus Calmette-Guerin and dinitrochlorobenzene immunotherapy of chemically induced bladder tumors. Investigative Urology 1977; 14: 369. **3.** Morales A, Ottenhof P, Emerson L. Treatment of residual non-infiltrating bladder cancer with bacillus Calmette-Guerin. J Urol 1981; 125: 649. **4.** Unpublished clinical date available from connaught Laboratories Limited. **5.** Horn T, Eidelman A, Walach N, Ilian M. Intravesical chemotherapy in a controlled trial with thiotepa versus doxorubicin hydrochloride. J Urol 1982; 125: 652-654. **6.** Zincke H, Utz DC, Taylor WF, Myers RP, Leary FJ. Influence of thiotepa and doxorubicin instillation at time of transurethral surgical treatment of bladder cancer on tumor recurrence: a prospective, randomized, double-blind, controlled trial. J Urol 1983; 129: 505-509. **7.** Unpublished clinical date available from Connaught Laboratories Limited. **8.** Lamm DL, Et al. Complications of Bacillus Calmette-Guerin immunotherapy: review of 2602 patients and comparison of chemotherapy complications. EORTC GU Group Monograph 1989; 6: 335-355. **9.** Landi S, Barbara C, Przykuta K, Held RH. Effect of light on freeze dried BCG Vaccines. J Biol Stand 1977; 5: 321-6. **10.** Lamm DL, Blumenstein BA, Crawford ED, et al. Sough-West Oncology Group comparison of bacillus Calmette-Guerin and doxorubicin in the treatment and prophylaxis of superficial bladder cancer. J Urol 1987: 178A. **11.** Mori K, Lamm DL, Crawford ED. A trial of Bacillus Calmette-Guerin versus Adriamycin in superficial bladder cancer: a South-West Oncology Group study. Urol Int 1986; 41: 254-259. **12.** Soloway M. Evaluation and management of patients with superficial bladder cancer. Urol Clin North Am 1987; 41: 771. **13.** Lamm DL, BCG in carcinoma in-situ and superficial bladder tumors. EORTC GU Group Monograph 1988; 5: 497. **14.** Lamm DL. Complications of Bacillus Calmette-Guerin immunotherapy in 1,278 patients with bladder cancer. J Urol 1986; 135: 272. **15.** Lamm DL, Sarodosy MS, DeHaven JI. Percutaneous, oral, or intravesical BCG administration: what is the optimal route? EORTC Genitourinary Group Monograph 6: BCG in Superficial Bladder Cancer. 1989; 301-310.

HOW SUPPLIED - EQUIVALENTS NOT AVAILABLE:

Injection, Solution - Irrigation - 27 mg

3's $158.13 THERACYS, Connaught Merieux 11793-8802-01

BCG VACCINE *(000375)*

CATEGORIES: Bladder Carcinoma; Immunologic; Serums, Toxoids and Vaccines; Tuberculosis; Vaccines; Pregnancy Category C; FDA Pre 1938 Drugs

BRAND NAMES: *Immucyst*; *Immun BCG Pasteur* (Germany); Mycobax; *OncoTice*; *Oncotice* (Germany); *OncoTICE*; *Pastimmun*; Theracys; **Tice BCG**
(International brand names outside U.S. in italics)

FORMULARIES: WHO

DESCRIPTION:

FOR INTRAVESICAL OR PERCUTANEOUS USP

Tice BCG, a BCG Vaccine for intravesical or percutaneous use, is attenuated, live culture preparation of the Bacillus of Calmette and Guerin (BCG) strain of *Mycobacterium bovis.*[1] The Tice strain was developed at the University of Illinois from a strain originated at the Pasteur Institute.

The medium in which the BCG organism is grown for preparation of the freeze-dried cake is composed of the following ingredients: glycerin, asparagine, citric acid, potassium phosphate, magnesium sulfate, and iron ammonium citrate. The final preparation prior to freeze-drying also contains lactose. The freeze-dried BCG preparation is delivered in a glass-sealed ampules, each containing 1 to 8 x 10^8 colony forming units (CFU) of Tice BCG which is equivalent to approximately 50 mg net weight.

No preservatives are added.

CLINICAL PHARMACOLOGY:

INTRAVESICAL USE FOR CARCINOMA *IN SITU* OF THE BLADDER

BCG vaccine induces granulomatous reaction at the local site of administration.[2] Intravesical BCG vaccine has been used as a therapy for and prophylaxis against recurrent tumors in patients with carcinoma *in situ* (CIS) of the bladder. The precise mechanism of action is unknown. A variety of different treatment regimens have been used with the Tice[3-6] and other BCG substrains.[7-12]

An evaluation of intravesical administration of BCG vaccine in patients with carcinoma *in situ* of the urinary bladder was recently completed. Bladder cancer patients were identified who had been treated with BCG vaccine under six different Investigational New Drug (IND) applications in which the most important shared aspect was the use of an induction plus maintenance schedule.

Comparison of demographic data between the six INDs revealed uniformity. Among these six studies were 119 evaluable patients who received intravesical treatment of CIS of the bladder. Patients with biopsy-proven CIS received BCG vaccine (50 mg; 1 - 8 x 10^8 CFU) intravesically, once weekly for at least 6 weeks and once monthly thereafter for up to 12 months. A longer maintenance was given in some cases. Follow-up cystoscopies were performed at 3 month intervals, as were urine cytologies for most patients (71 of 119). Urine cytology was obtained at the time of the 1989 follow-up for all patients who responded to BCG vaccine treatment (see CR and CRNC below). The median time post treatment for these follow-up cytologies were 47 months.

The study population consisted of 153 patients; 132 males, 19 females and 2 unidentified as to gender. Thirty patients lacking baseline documentation of CIS and 4 patients lost to follow-up were not evaluable for treatment response. Therefore, 119 patients with biopsy or cystoscopy proven CIS prior to BCG vaccine administration were available for efficacy evaluation. Some of these patients had undergone transurethral resection (TUR) one or more weeks prior to BCG, primarily for the treatment of papillomatous disease. The mean age for CIS population was 68.8 ± 9.7 years s.d. (range: 38-97 years).

Sixty-three evaluable patients had received intravesical chemotherapy treatment for their bladder malignancy prior to BCG vaccine treatment and had been diagnosed as follows: thiotepa (30), mitomycin C (10), doxorubicin (1), mitomycin C (1) and thiotepa, mitomycin C and doxorubicin (2), interferon (1), interferon and thiotepa (1), cyclophosphamide IV (1), and cisplatin and thiotepa (1).

For the 119 patients with biopsy or cytoscopy proven CIS, the BCG vaccine induction dosage consisted of a mean of 6.6 installations (± 1.5 standard error of the mean). These patients also received a mean of 10.0 maintenance installations after completing the induction phase. Twenty patients (16.8%) required BCG vaccine reinduction at some point in the study. Nine patients in one of the six studies received a percutaneous dose along with intravesical instillation. Data from a recent study show that a percutaneous dose with CIS is unnecessary.[13]

Clinical response criteria were defined as follows:

COMPLETE HISTOLOGICAL RESPONSE (CR)

Complete resolution of carcinoma *in situ* documented by biopsy, or, if biopsy was not obtained, then by negative cytoscopy. All patients in this category were required to have urine cytology tests that were negative upon examination.

COMPLETE CLINICAL RESPONSE WITHOUT CYTOLOGY (CRNC)

Patients in this category had an apparent complete disappearance of tumor that was not confirmed by urine cytology tests. Complete resolution of carcinoma *in situ* documented by a biopsy or, if a biopsy was not obtained, then by a negative cystoscopy.

FAILURE/PROGRESSION:

Patients in this category had urine cytology tests that were found to be positive, although biopsy or cystoscopy was negative. This category also included patients who continued to have evidence of malignant legions, or a new progression to a higher stage or grade; the appearance of new lesions; reappearance of old lesions.

A 75.6 percent response rate was reported for 119 evaluable patients (TABLE 1):

TABLE 1 Response Of Patients To BCG Vaccine In CIS Bladder Cancer

	Entered	Evaluable	CR	CRNC	Overall Response
No. of Patients	153	119	54	36	90
% Response		—	45.4%	30.2%	75.6%

The median duration of follow-up for the 1989 update, presented in TABLE 2, is 47 months. Of the 54 patients classified as CR in 1987, 30 remained without evidence of disease (CR) in 1989, whereas 6 patients died of unrelated disease and 18 relapsed. The 15 of 36 patients classified as CRNC in 1987 who remained without evidence of disease in 1989 were all found to meet the criteria of CR status on the basis of negative cytologies. In the interim, 4 CRNC patients died of unrelated diseases, 2 died of unknown causes, and 15 relapsed. Therefore, of the 90 overall responders (75.6%), 36.7 percent of patients relapsed, 13.3 percent died of other diseases, and 50 percent remained in CR. In addition, two patients who relapsed were reinforced in complete response by a second course of BCG vaccine (TABLE 2):

TABLE 2 Therapeutic Efficacy Of BCG Vaccine In CIS Bladder Cancer 1989 Status of 90 Responders (CR or CRNC)

Response	1987/CR n=54	1987/CRNC n=36	1987 Response n=90	Percent
CR	30	15	45	50.0
CRNC	0	0	0	0.0
Unrelated Deaths	6	6	12	13.3
Failure	18	15	33	36.7

CLINICAL PHARMACOLOGY: *(cont'd)*

Among the 119 evaluable patients there was no significant difference in response rates between patients with or without prior intravesical chemotherapy: 45 of 63 (71%) versus 45 of 46 (80%), p >.05. Similarly, for the patient remaining in CR at the time of the 1989 evaluation, there was no significant difference between those with or without prior chemotherapy.

The median duration of response, calculated from the Kaplan-Meier curve as median time to recurrence, is estimated at 4 years or greater. The median duration of follow-up was 47 months. Of the total 90 responders, 45 patients (50%) remained without evidence of disease.

At a median follow-up of 47 months, 85 (71.4%) of the 119 evaluable patients remain alive. Thirteen patients (10.9%) died from causes unrelated to bladder cancer: cardiovascular disease (6 patients), second primary cancer (3 patients), and other (4 patients). Three patients died from unknown causes and bladder cancer cannot be ruled out. The bladder cancer related deaths were 18 (15%) of the 119. Historical data prior to the use of BCG, in a series of CIS patients treated usually with electrofulguration, indicate 82% of the patients developed invasive cancer, and 34% of the patients died of their disease within 5 years.[14]

The incidence of cystectomy for 90 patients who achieved a complete response (CR or CRNC) with BCG vaccine was 11%. For 29 patients who did not achieve CR or CRNC, the incidence of cystectomy was 55% which is consistent with cystectomy rates reported in the literature for CIS patients who were not treated with intravesical therapies.[15]

The median time to cystectomy in patients who achieved a complete response (CR or CRNC) exceeded 74 months, whereas the median time to cystectomy for non-responders was 31 months.

PERCUTANEOUS USE FOR IMMUNIZATION AGAINST TUBERCULOSIS

Immunization with the BCG vaccine lowers the risk of serious complications of primary tuberculosis in children.[16-19] Estimates of efficacy from observational studies in areas where vaccination is performed at birth show that the incidence of tuberculosis meningitis and miliary tuberculosis is 52% - 100% lower and that the incidence of pulmonary tuberculosis is 2% - 80% lower in vaccinated in children less than 15 years of age than in unvaccinated controls.[16-21] However, estimates of vaccine efficacy may be distorted because of the following: vaccination was not allocated randomly in observational studies; there were differences in BCG strains, methods, and routes of administration; and there were differences in the characteristics of the populations and environments in which the vaccines have been studied.[22]

INDICATIONS AND USAGE:

INTRAVESICAL USE FOR CARCINOMA *IN SITU* OF THE BLADDER

Intravesical instillation of BCG vaccine is indicated for the treatment of carcinoma *in situ* of the bladder in the following situations: (1) primary treatment in the absence of an associated invasive cancer without papillary tumors or with papillary tumors after TUR, (2) secondary treatment in the absence of an associated invasive cancer, in patients failing to respond to relapsing after intravesical chemotherapy with other agents, (3) primary or secondary treatment in the absence of invasive cancer for patients with medical contraindications to radical surgery. BCG vaccine is not indicated for the treatment of papillary tumors occurring alone.

Percutaneous Use for Immunization Against Tuberculosis: *Exposed tuberculin skin test-negative infants and children:* BCG vaccination is recommended for infants and children with negative skin test who are (1) at high risk of intimate and prolonged exposure to persistently untreated or ineffectively treated patients who cannot be removed from the source of exposure and cannot be placed on long-term preventative therapy, or (2) continuously exposed to persons with tuberculosis who have bacilli resistant to isoniazid and rifampin.[22]

Groups With An Excessive Rate Of New Infections: BCG vaccination is also recommended for tuberculin-negative infants and children in groups in which the rate of new infections exceeds 1% per year and for whom the usual surveillance and treatment programs have been attempted but are not operationally feasible. These groups include persons without regular access to health care, those for whom usual health care is culturally or socially unacceptable, or groups who have demonstrated an inability to effectively use existing accessible care.

The US Immunization Practices Advisory Committee (IPAC) no longer recommends the use of BCG vaccination of health care workers at risk of repeated exposure to tuberculosis but recommends that these individuals be under tuberculin skin testing surveillance and receive isoniazid prophylaxis in case of tuberculin skin test conversion.[22]

For international travelers, the Center for Disease Control (CDC) recommends that BCG vaccination be considered only for travelers with insignificant reaction to tuberculin skin test who will be in a high-risk environment for prolonged periods of time without access to tuberculin skin test surveillance.[22]

CONTRAINDICATIONS:

INTRAVESICAL USE FOR CARCINOMA *IN SITU* OF THE BLADDER

BCG vaccine should not be used in immunosuppressed patients or persons with congenital or acquired immune deficiencies, whether due to concurrent disease (*e.g.*, AIDS, leukemia, lymphoma) or cancer therapy (*e.g.*, cytotoxic drugs, radiation). BCG vaccine should be avoided in asymptomatic carriers with a positive HIV serology and in patients receiving steroids at immunosuppressive therapies because of the possibility of the vaccine establishing a systemic infection.

Treatment should be postponed until a resolution of a concurrent febrile illness, urinary tract infection, or gross hematuria. Seven to fourteen days should elapse before BCG is administered following biopsy, TUR, or traumatic catheterization.

A positive Mantoux test is a contraindication only if there is evidence of an active tuberculosis infection.

In the absence of safety data, intravesical BCG vaccine should not be given to pregnant or lactating women.

PERCUTANEOUS USE FOR IMMUNIZATION AGAINST TUBERCULOSIS

BCG vaccine for the prevention of tuberculosis should not be given to persons with impaired immune responses, whether they be congenital, disease produced, drug or therapy induced (*i.e.*, cytotoxic drugs and radiation used in cancer therapy). The concurrent use of steroids requires caution because of the possibility of the vaccine establishing a systemic infection. If necessary, the infection can be treated with anti-tuberculous drugs.

WARNINGS:

Intravesical Use for Carcinoma *In Situ* of the Bladder: BCG vaccine is not a vaccine for the prevention of cancer.

There are currently no data on the effectiveness of intravesical instillation of BCG vaccine in the treatment of invasive bladder cancer.

The use of BCG vaccine may cause tuberculin sensitivity. Since this is a valuable aid for the diagnosis of tuberculosis, it may therefore be useful to determine the tuberculin reactivity by PPD skin testing before treatment.

Intravesical instillations should be postponed in the presence of fever, suspected infection, or during treatment with antibiotics, since antimicrobial therapy may interfere with the effectiveness of BCG vaccine.

WARNINGS: *(cont'd)*

Instillation of BCG vaccine onto a bleeding mucosa may promote systemic BCG infection.[23] Death has been reported as a result of systemic BCG infection and sepsis. Patients should be monitored for the presence of symptoms and signs of toxicity after each intravesical treatment. Febrile episodes with flu-like symptoms lasting more than 48 hours, fever ≥ 103°F, systemic manifestations increasing in intensity with repeated instillations, or persistent abnormalities of liver function tests suggest systemic BCG infection and require anti-tuberculous therapy (see ADVERSE REACTIONS).

Small bladder capacity has been associated with increased risk of severe local reactions and should be considered in deciding to use BCG vaccine therapy.

PERCUTANEOUS USE FOR IMMUNIZATION AGAINST TUBERCULOSIS

Administration should be percutaneous with the multiple puncture disc as described below. DO NOT INJECT INTRAVENOUSLY, SUBCUTANEOUSLY, OR INTRADERMALLY. BCG vaccine Vaccine should not be used in infants, children, or adults with severe immune deficiency syndromes. Children with family history of immune deficiency disease should not be vaccinated. If they are, an infectious disease specialist should be consulted and anti-tuberculous therapy[24] administered if clinically indicated.

PRECAUTIONS:

GENERAL

BCG vaccine contains live bacteria and should be used with aseptic technique. All equipment, supplies, and receptacles in contact with BCG vaccine should be handled and disposed of as biohazardous.

The possibility of allergic reactions should be assessed. BCG vaccine administration should not be attempted in individuals with severe deficiency disease. BCG vaccine Vaccine should be administered with caution to persons in groups at high risk for HIV infection.

INTRAVESICAL USE FOR CARCINOMA *IN SITU* OF THE BLADDER

General: Care should be taken not to traumatize the urinary tract or to introduce contaminants into the urinary system. Seven to fourteen days should elapse before BCG is administered following TUR, biopsy, or traumatic catheterization.

Information for the Patient: BCG vaccine is retained in the bladder 2 hours and then voided. Patients should void while seated for safety reasons following installation of suspension. Within 6 hours after treatment, urine voided should be disinfected for 15 minutes with an equal volume of household bleach before flushing. Patients should be instructed to increase fluid intake to "flush" the bladder in the hours following BCG treatment. Patients may experience burning with the first void after treatment. Patients should be attentive to side effects, such as fever, chills, malaise flu-like symptoms, or increased fatigue. If patient experiences severe urinary side effects, such as burning or pain on urination, urgency, frequency of urination, blood in urine, joint pain, cough, or skin rash, the physician should be notified.

Pregnancy Category C: Animal reproduction studies have not been conducted with BCG vaccine. It is not known whether BCG vaccine can cause fetal harm when administered to a pregnant woman or can affect reproduction capacity. BCG vaccine should be given to a pregnant woman only if clearly needed. Women should be advised not to become pregnant while on therapy.

Nursing Mothers: It is not known whether BCG vaccine is excreted in human milk and because of the potential for serious adverse reactions from BCG vaccine in nursing infants, a decision should be made whether to discontinue nursing or to discontinue the drug, taking into account the importance of the drug to the mother.

Pediatric Use: Safety and effectiveness for carcinoma *in situ* of the urinary bladder in children have not been established.

PERCUTANEOUS USE FOR IMMUNIZATION AGAINST TUBERCULOSIS

Normal Reaction: The intensity and duration of the local reaction depends on the depth of penetration of the multi-puncture disc and the individual variations in patient's tissue reactions. The initial skin lesions usually appear within 10-14 days and consist of small red papules at the site. The papules reach maximum diameter (about 3 mm) after 4 to 6 weeks, after which they may scale and then slowly subside.

Six months afterward there is usually no visible sign of the vaccination, but on occasion a faintly discernible pattern of the disc points may be visible. On people whose skin tends to keloid formation, there may be slightly more visible evidence of the vaccination.

Vaccination is recommended only for those who are tuberculin negative to a recent skin test with 5 tuberculin units (5TU). Otherwise, vaccination of persons highly sensitive to mycobacterial antigens can result in hypersensitivity reactions including fever, anorexia, myalgia, and neuralgia, which lasts a few days.

After BCG vaccination, it is usually not possible to clearly distinguish between a tuberculin reaction caused by persistent postvaccination sensitivity and one caused by a virulent suprainfection. Caution is advised in attributing a positive skin test to BCG vaccination. A sharp rise in the tuberculin reaction since the latest test should be further investigated (except in the immediate postvaccination period).

Information for the Patient: Keep the vaccination site clean until the local reaction has disappeared.

Pediatric Use: See DOSAGE AND ADMINISTRATION, Treatment and Schedule. Precautions should be taken with respect to infants vaccinated with BCG and exposed to persons with active tuberculosis.[25]

DRUG INTERACTIONS:

Drug combinations containing immunosuppressants and/or bone marrow depressants and/or radiation interfere with the development of the immune response and should not be used in combination with BCG vaccine. Antimicrobial therapy for other infections may interfere with the effectiveness of BCG vaccine therapy.

Antimicrobial or immunosuppressive agents may interfere with the development of the immune response and should be used only under medical supervision.

ADVERSE REACTIONS:

INTRAVESICAL USE FOR CARCINOMA *IN SITU* OF THE BLADDER

Adverse reactions are often localized to the bladder but may be accompanied by systemic manifestations. Symptoms of bladder irritability related to the inflammatory response induced by intravesical BCG vaccine, are reported in 60 percent of cases. They begin 3-4 hours after instillation and last 24-72 hours. The urinary side effects are usually seen after the third treatment and tend to increase in severity after each administration. There were, however, no long-term urinary complications in this group of patients.

A summary of adverse reactions seen with 674 patients with superficial bladder cancer, including 153 CIS patients treated intravesically with BCG vaccine is shown in TABLE 3-A and TABLE 3-B.[26]

ADVERSE REACTIONS: *(cont'd)*

TABLE 3A Summary of Adverse Effects Seen in 674 Patients With Superficial Bladder Cancer, Including 153 with Carcinoma *In Situ*

Local Adverse Effects	No. of Patients	%	Toxicity Grade (%)* Mild	Moderate	Severe	Not Stated
Dysuria	401	59.5	28.2	18.1	10.7	2.5
Urinary Frequency	272	40.4	17.2	15.7	7.4	—
Hematuria	175	26.0	8.2	9.6	7.4	0.8
Cystitis	40	5.9	1.6	2.4	1.9	—
Urgency	39	5.8	1.2	1.8	1.3	1.5
Nocturia	30	4.5	1.3	1.8	0.6	0.7
Cramps/Pain	27	4.0	0.9	1.3	0.9	0.9
Urinary Incontinence	16	2.4	0.4	0.9	—	1.2
Urinary Debris	15	2.2	0.2	1.0	0.4	0.6
Genital Inflammation/Abscess	12	1.8	0.3	0.4	0.4	0.6
Urinary Tract Infection	10	1.5	0.2	0.3	0.9	0.2
Urethritis	8	1.2	0.3	0.6	—	0.3
Pyuria	5	0.7	0.2	0.1	0.1	0.3
Epididymitis/Prostatitis	2	0.3	—	—	—	0.3
Urinary Obstruction	2	0.3	—	—	—	0.3
Contracted Bladder	1	0.2	—	—	—	0.2
Orchitis	1	0.2	—	—	—	0.2

* Grade was determined using ECOG scale of toxicity criteria, Mild = Grade 1, Moderate = Grade 2, Severe = Grade 3 or 4.

TABLE 3B Summary of Adverse Effects Seen in 674 Patients With Superficial Bladder Cancer, Including 153 with Carcinoma *In Situ*

Local Adverse Effects	No. of Patients	%	Toxicity by Grade (%) Mild	Moderate	Severe	Not Stated
Flu-like Syndrome**	224	33.3	9.3	10.9	9.0	4.0
Fever	134	19.9	6.1	5.3	7.6	0.9
Malaise/ Fatigue	50	7.4	2.7	3.1	—	1.6
Shaking/ Chills	22	3.3	0.2	1.5	1.0	0.6
Nausea/ Vomiting	20	3.0	1.0	1.6	0.3	—
Arthritis/ Myalgia	18	2.7	0.3	1.0	0.4	0.9
Headache/Dizziness	16	2.4	0.3	0.9	—	1.2
Anorexia/Weight Loss	15	2.2	0.4	1.3	0.1	0.5
Allergic	14	2.1	0.6	0.7	0.4	0.3
Cardiac	13	1.9	—	0.3	1.3	0.3
Respiratory (Unclassified)	11	1.6	0.4	0.4	0.2	0.6
Abdominal Pain	10	1.5	—	0.6	0.6	0.3
Anemia	9	1.3	0.2	0.6	0.4	0.1
Diarrhea	8	1.2	0.2	0.6	0.1	0.3
Pneumonitis	8	1.2	0.2	—	0.6	0.4
Gastrointestinal (Unclassified)	7	1.0	0.2	0.1	—	0.7
Neurologic	6	0.9	0.1	—	0.3	0.4
Rash	4	0.6	—	0.4	0.2	—
BCG Sepsis	3	0.4	—	—	0.4	—
Coagulopathy	2	0.3	—	—	0.3	—
Leukopenia	2	0.3	0.2	0.1	—	—
Thrombocytopenia	2	0.3	0.2	0.1	—	—
Hepatic Granuloma	1	0.2	—	—	0.2	—
Hepatitis	1	0.2	—	—	0.2	—

** Flu-like syndrome includes fever, shaking chills, malaise and myalgia.

Irritative bladder adverse effects associated with BCG administration can be managed symptomatically with pyridium, propantheline bromide or oxybutynin chloride, and acetaminophen or ibuprofen.[27] Systemic adverse effects such as malaise, fever, and chills may reflect hypersensitivity reactions and can be treated with antihistamines.[27] The "flu-like" syndrome of 1-2 days' duration that frequently accompanies intravesical BCG administration should be managed by standard symptomatic treatment. Symptoms persisting longer than 2 days suggest continued infection, and consideration should be given to therapy with isoniazid. Localized (*e.g.*, prostatitis epididymitis) as well as systemic infection can occur with intravesical BCG administration. For systemic infection, an infectious diseases specialist should be consulted and the patient promptly treated with anti-tuberculous therapy as advised.[28] At least two deaths have been reported as a result of systemic BCG infection and sepsis.[27] There have been two cases of nephrogenic adenoma, a benign lesion of bladder epithelium, associated with intravesical BCG therapy.[29] In general, the adverse effects of BCG therapy in bladder carcinoma have been of short duration and moderate morbidity.

Percutaneous Use for Immunization Against Tuberculosis: Occasionally, lymphadenopathy of the regional lymph node, which spontaneously resolves itself, is seen in young children. Only rarely does the node create a fistula followed by a short period of drainage. The usually treatment is to maintain cleanliness of the site of drainage and allow the lesion to heal spontaneously without medical intervention.

Other rare events are osteomyelitis, lupoid reactions, disseminated BCG infection, and death. Osteomyelitis has been reported to occur at a rate of about 1 per 1,000,000 vaccinees.[22] Disseminated BCG infection and death are very rare (about 1 per 5,000,000 vaccinees)[30] and occur almost exclusively in children with impaired immune responses.

OVERDOSAGE:

Intravesical Use for Carcinoma in Situ of the Bladder: Overdosage occurs if more than one ampule of BCG vaccine is administered per instillation. The patient should be closely monitored for signs of systemic BCG infection and treated with anti-tuberculous medication (See ADVERSE REACTIONS.)

Percutaneous Use for Immunization Against Tuberculosis: Accidental overdosages if treated immediately with anti-tuberculous drugs have not lead to complications.[31] If the vaccination response is allowed to progress it can still be treated successfully with anti- tuberculous drugs, but complications can include regional adenitis, lupus vulgaris, subcutaneous cold abscesses, ocular lesions, and others.[32]

DOSAGE AND ADMINISTRATION:

Intravesical Use for Carcinoma *In Situ* of the Bladder: The intravesical dose consists of one ampule of BCG vaccine suspended in 50 ml preservative-free saline. *Preparation of Agent:* The preparation of the BCG vaccine suspension should be done using sterile technique. The pharmacist or individual responsible for mixing the agent should wear gloves, mask, and gown to avoid inadvertent exposure of open sores or inhalation of BCG organisms. Draw 1 ml of sterile, preservative-free saline (0.9% Sodium Chloride Injection, USP) at 4-25°C, into a small (*e.g.*, 3 ml) syringe and add to one ampule of BCG vaccine to resuspend. Draw the mixture into the syringe and gently expel back into the ampule three times to ensure thorough mixing. This mixing minimizes the clumping of the mycobacteria. Dispense the cloudy BCG suspension into the top end of a catheter-tip syringe which contains 49 ml saline diluent bringing the total volume to 50 ml. Gently rotate the syringe. The suspended BCG vaccine should be used immediately after preparation. Discard after 2 hours.

Note: DO NOT filter the contents of the BCG vaccine ampule. Precautions should be taken to avoid exposing the BCG vaccine to light. Bacteriostatic solutions must be avoided. In addition, use only sterile preservative-free saline, 0.9% Sodium Chloride Injection, USP, as diluent and perform all mixing operations in sterile glass or thermosetting plastic containers and syringes.

Treatment and Schedule: Allow 7-14 days to elapse after bladder biopsy or TUR before BCG vaccine is administered. Patients should not drink fluids for 4 hours before treatment and should empty their bladder prior to Tice BC administration. The reconstituted BCG vaccine is instilled into the bladder by gravity flow via the catheter. DO NOT depress the plunger and force the flow of the BCG vaccine. The BCG vaccine is retained in the bladder for 2 hours and then voided. Patients unable to retain the suspension for 2 hours should be allowed to void sooner, if necessary. While the BCG vaccine is retained in the bladder, the patient may be repositioned from left side to right side and also may alternately lie upon the back and the abdomen, changing these positions every 15 minutes to maximize bladder surface exposure to the agent.

A standard treatment schedule consists of one intravesical instillation per week for 6 weeks. This schedule may be repeated once if tumor remission has not been achieved and if the clinical circumstances warrant. Thereafter, intravesical BCG vaccine administration should continue at approximately monthly intervals for at least 6-12 months.

Percutaneous Use For Immunization Against Tuberculosis: *Preparation of Agent:* Using sterile methods, 1 ml of sterile water for injection, USP at 4-25°C, is added to one ampule of vaccine. Draw the mixture into a syringe and expel it back into the ampule three times to ensure thorough mixing.

Parenteral drug products should be inspected visually for particulate matter and discoloration prior to administration, whenever solution and container permit. Reconstitution should result in a uniform suspension of the bacilli.

Treatment and Schedule: The vaccine is to be administered after fully explaining the risks and benefits to the vaccinee, parent, or guardian. After the vaccine is prepared, the immunizing dose of 0.2 - 0.3 ml is dropped on the cleansed surface of the skin, and the vaccine is administered percutaneously utilizing a sterile multiple-puncture disc. The multiple-puncture disc is a thin wafer-like stainless steel plate 7/8" x 1 1/8", from which 36 points protrude. The disc is held by a magnet type holder. In this method a drop of vaccine is placed on the arm and spread with the wide edge of disc. The disc is placed gently over the vaccine and the magnet is centered. The arm is grasped firmly from underneath, tensing the skin appreciably. Downward pressure is applied on the magnet so the points of the disc are well buried in skin. With pressure still exerted, the disc is rocked forward and backward and from side to side several times. Pressure underneath the arm is then released and the magnet is slid off the disc. In a successful procedure, the points remain in the skin. If the points are on top of the skin, the procedure must be repeated. Remove the disc after successful puncture and spread vaccine evenly over the puncture area with the wide edge of the disc. Discs should only be used once and discarded after autoclaving. Between individual vaccinations the magnet should be sterilized. Discs may be purchased separately from Organon Teknika Corporation, 115 South Sangamon Street, Chicago, IL 60607; telephone number (800) 662-6842. After vaccination the vaccine should flow into the wounds and dry. No dressing is required; however it is recommended that the site be kept dry for 24 hours. The patient should be advised that the vaccine contains live organisms. Although the vaccine will not survive in a dry state, infection of others is possible.

Reconstituted vaccine should be kept refrigerated, protected from exposure to light, and used within 2 hours. Vaccination should be repeated for those who remain tuberculin negative to 5TU of tuberculin after 2-3 months.

Pediatric Dose: In infants less than 1 month old the dosage of vaccine should be reduced by one-half, by using 2 ml of sterile water when reconstituting. If a vaccinated infant remains tuberculin negative to 5TU on skin testing, and if indications for vaccination persist, the infant should receive a full dose after 1 year of age.

REFERENCES:

1. Guerin C: The history of BCG. In:Rosenthal SR (ed): BCG Vaccine: Tuberculosis-Cancer. Littleton, MA, PSG Publishing C., Inc. 1980, pp. 35-43. **2.** Kelley DR, Haaff E, Becich M, et al.: Prognostic value of purified protein derivative skin test and granuloma fornation in patients treated with intravesical bacillus Calmette-Guerin. J Urol 1986; 135:268-271. **3.** Brosman SA: The use of bacillus Calmette-Guerin in the therapy of bladder carcinoma in situ. J Urol 1985; 134:36-39. **4.** DeKernion JB, Huang M, Linder A, et al.: The Management of superficial bladder tumors and carcinoma in situwith intravesical bacillus Calmette-Guerin. J Urol 1985; 133: 598-601. **5.** Guinan P, Batenhorst R: BCG in the treatment of superficial bladder cancer (Abstract). J Urol 198; 137:180A. **6.** Soloway M, Parry A: Bacillus Calmette-Guerin for treatment of superficial transitional cell carcinoma of the bladder in patients who have failed thiotepa and/or mitomycin C. J Urol 198; 137:871-83. **7.** Morales A: Long-term results and complications of intracavitary bacillus Calmette-Guerin therapy for bladder cancer. J Urol 1984; 132:457-459. **8.** Haaff E, Dresner SM, Ratliff TL, Catalona WJ: Two courses of intravesical bacillus Calmette-Guerin for transitional cell carcinoma of the bladder. J Urol 1986; 136:820-824. **9.** Herr HW, Pinsky CM, Whitmore WF, et al.: Effect of intravesical bacillus Calmette-Guerin (BCG) on carcinoma *in situ*. Cancer 1983; 51:1323-1326. **10.** Kelley DR, Ratliff T, Catalona WJ et al.: Intravesical bacillus Calmette-Guerin therapy for superficial bladder cancer. Effect of bacillus Calmette-Guerin viability on treatment results. J Urol 1985 134:48-53. **11.** Schelhammer PF, Ladaga LE, Fillion MB: Bacillus Calmette-Guerin for therapy of superficial transitional cell carcinoma of the bladder. J Urol 1986; 135:261-264. **12.** Lamm DL: BCG immunotherapy in bladder cancer. In: Urology Annual 198. Vol. 1, Appleton & Lange, Norwalk, CT, 1987; pp. 67-86. **13.** Lamm DL, Sardosy MS, DeHaven JI: Percutaneous, oral, or intravesical BCG administration: What is the optimal route? EORTC Genitourinary Group Monograph 6: BCG in Superficial Bladder Cancer. Alan R. Liss, Inc. New York, NY, 1989; pp 301-310. **14.** Utz DC, Hanash KA, Farrow GM: The plight of the patient with carcinoma *in situ*of the bladder. J Urol 1970; 103:160-164. **15.** Herr HW, Pinsky CM, Whitmore WF Jr., et al.: Long-term effect of intravesical bacillus Calmette-Guerin on flat carcinoma *in situ* of the bladder. J Urol 1986; 135:265-267. **16.** Romanus V: Tuberculosis in bacillus Calmette-Guerin immunized and unimmunized children in Sweden: a ten year evaluation following the cessation of general bacillus Calmette-Guerin immunization of the newborn in 1975. Pediatr Infect Dis 1987; 6:272-280. **17.** Smith PG: Case-control studies of the efficacy of BCG against tuberculosis. In: International Union Against Tuberculosis, Proceedings of the XXVIth IUAT World Conference on Tuberculosis and Respiratory Diseases, Singapore. Professional Postgraduate Services, International, Japan, 1987; 73-79. **18.** Padunchan S, Konjanart S, Kasiratta S, et al.: The effectiveness of BCG vaccination of the newborn against childhood tuberculosis in Bangkok. Bull WHO 1986; 64:247-258. **19.** Tidjani O, Amedone A, ten Dam HG: The protective effect of BCG vaccination of the newborn against childhood tuberculosis in an African community. Tubercule 1986; 67:269-281. **20.** Young TK, Hershfield ES: A case-control study to evaluate the effectiveness of mass neonatal BCG vaccination among Canadian Indians. Am J Public Health 1986; 76:783-786. **21.** Shapiro C, Cook N, Evans D, et al.: A case-control study of BCG and childhood tuberculosis in Cali, Columbia. Int H Epidemiol 1985; 14:441-446. **22.** Morbidity and Mortality Weekly Report 37, No. 43 1988; pp. 663-675. **23.** Rawls WH, Lamm DL, Eyolfson MF: Septic complications in the use of bacillus Calmette-Guerin (BCG) for noninvasive transitional cell carcinoma. Presented at: 1988 Annual Meeting, American Urological Association, Boston, MA. **24.** Lorin MI, Hsu KHK, Jacob SC: Treatment of tuberculosis in children. In: Symposium on anti-infective therapy. Pediatric Clinics of North America, 1983; 30:333-348. **25.** Report if the Committee on the Control of Infectious Diseases. American Academy of Pediatrics 1988; 21st Edition. **26.** Data on file. Organon Teknika Corporation/Biotechnology Research Institute, Rockville. MD. **27.** Lamm DL, Steg A, Boccon-Gibod L, et al.: Complications of bacillus Calmette-Guerin immunotherapy: Review of 2602 patients and comparison of chemotherapy complications. EORTC Genitourinary Group Monograph 6:BCG in Superficial

REFERENCES: *(cont'd)*

Bladder Cancer. Alan R. Liss, Inc., New York, NY, 1989; pp. 335-355. **28.** Standard Therapy for Tuberculosis, 1985. Presented at: National Consensus Conference on Tuberculosis. Chest, 1985; 87 (Suppl):117S- 124S. **29.** Oates R, Siroky M: Nephrogenic adenoma of urinary bladder due to intravesical BCG therapy. J Urol 1986; 135: 186. **20.** Mande R: BCG Vaccination. Dawsons, London, 1968. **31.** Griffith AH: Ten cases of BCG Overdose treated with isoniazid. Tubercle 1963; 44:247-250. **32.** Watkins SM: Unusual complications of BCG Vaccination. Brit Med J 1971; 1:442.

HOW SUPPLIED:

Storage: Storage of the intact ampules of BCG vaccine should be at refrigerated temperatures of 2-8°C (36-46°F). This agent contains live bacteria and should be protect from light. The product should not be used after the expiration date printed on the label.

HOW SUPPLIED - EQUIVALENTS NOT AVAILABLE:

Injection, Solution - Intravenous

1's $147.50 TICE BCG, Organon 00052-0601-01

Injection, Solution - Intravenous - 81 mg

1's $157.31 THERACYS, Connaught Merieux 11793-0880-01

BACAMPICILLIN HYDROCHLORIDE *(000355)*

CATEGORIES: Anti-Infectives; Antibacterials; Antibiotics; Antimicrobials; Bronchitis; Gonorrhea; Infections; Penicillins; Respiratory Tract Infections; Skin Infections; Urinary Tract Infections; Pregnancy Category B; FDA Approval Pre 1982

BRAND NAMES: *Albaxin*; *Ambacamp* (Germany); *Ambacomp*; *Ambaxin* (England); *Ambaxino*; *Amplibac*; *Antibiotic*; *Bacacil* (Japan); *Bacampicilina*; *Bacamcillin*; *Bacampicin*; *Bacampicine* (France); *Campicil*; *Penglobe* (Germany, France, Canada, Mexico, Japan); **Spectrobid**

(International brand names outside U.S. in italics)

DESCRIPTION:

Bacampicillin HCl is a member of the ampicillin class of semi-synthetic penicillins derived from the basic penicillin nucleus: 6-aminopenicillanic acid. Bacampicillin HCl, as well as ampicillin and other ampicillin analogues, is acid resistant and suitable for oral administration.

Bacampicillin HCl is the hydrochloride salt of 1-ethoxycarbonyloxyethyl ester of ampicillin, available either as tablets or as a microencapsulated oral suspension. During the process of absorption from the gastrointestinal tract, bacampicillin HCl is hydrolyzed rapidly to ampicillin, a well characterized and effective antibacterial agent. Each 400 mg tablet of bacampicillin HCl is chemically equivalent to 280 mg of ampicillin.

Chemically, bacampicillin HCl is 1'-ethoxycarbonyloxyethyl-6-(D-α aminophenylacetamide)-penicillinate hydrochloride. It has a molecular weight of 501.96.

Inert ingredients for the tablets are: microcrystalline cellulose, lactose and magnesium stearate. May also include the following: hydroxypropyl methylcellulose; and opaspray white, opadry white and opadry clear (these components may contain other inert ingredients).

CLINICAL PHARMACOLOGY:

Bacampicillin is characterized by its more complete and more rapid absorption from the GI tract than ampicillin. Bacampicillin tablets of 400 mg, 800 mg, and 1600 mg have provided ampicillin peak serum concentrations of 7.9, 12.9, and 20.1 mcg/ml. These peak levels are approximately three times the levels obtained with administration of equivalent amounts of ampicillin. The areas-under-the-serum-concentration curves obtained during the first 6 hours were 24.8 and 12.9 mcg/ml/hr, when bacampicillin HCl 800 mg and ampicillin 500 mg were administered to adults.

In fasting adult volunteers, a 400 mg dose of the tablet gave a peak serum ampicillin concentration of 7.2 mcg/ml. In fasting, pediatric patients a 12.5 mg/kg dose provided a peak of 8.4 mcg/ml.

After oral administration of bacampicillin tablet, ampicillin activity in serum peaks at 0.7-0.9 hours (compared to 1.5-2.0 hours after administration of ampicillin). Serum ampicillin half-life is 1,1 hours after either bacampicillin or ampicillin administration. Peak tissue and body fluid ampicillin concentrations also are higher after administration of bacampicillin. Utilizing a special skin window technique to determine ampicillin levels, therapeutic levels in the interstitial fluid were higher and more prolonged after bacampicillin than after ampicillin administration. Bacampicillin is stable in the presence of gastric acid. Bacampicillin oral suspension absorption is affected by food. Food does not retard absorption of bacampicillin tablets which may be given without regard to meals. Bacampicillin has been shown to be rapidly and well absorbed after oral administration, with about 75% of a given dose being recoverable in the urine as active ampicillin within 8 hours of administration. Urinary excretion can be delayed by concurrent administration of probenecid. The active moiety of bacampicillin (*i.e.,* ampicillin) diffuses readily into most body tissues and fluids. In serum, ampicillin is only 20% protein-bound, compared to 60-90% for other penicillins.

Microbiology: Bacampicillin per se has no *in vitro* antibacterial activity and owes its *in vivo* bactericidal activity to the parent compound, ampicillin. The ampicillin class of penicillins (including bacampicillin) has a broad spectrum of activity against many gram-negative and gram-positive bacteria. Like other penicillins, the ampicillin class of penicillins inhibits the synthesis of cell wall mucopeptide.

Ampicillin class antibiotics are inactivated by β-lactamases produced by certain strains of *Enterobacter, Citrobacter, Haemophilus influenzae*, and *Escherichia coli*, and by most strains of staphylococci and indole-positive *Proteus* spp. Ampicillin class antibiotics are not active against *Pseudomonas, Klebsiella*, or *Serratia* spp.

SUSCEPTIBILITY TESTING

Elution Technique: For the automated method of susceptibility testing (*i.e.,* Autobac TM), gram-negative organisms should be tested with the 4.5 mcg ampicillin elution disk, while gram-positive organisms should be tested with the 0.22 mcg disk.

Diffusion Technique: For the Kirby-Bauer method of susceptibility testing, a 10 mcg ampicillin diffusion disk should be used. With this procedure, a laboratory report of "susceptible" indicates that the infecting organism is likely to respond to bacampicillin therapy, and a report of "resistant" indicates that the infecting organism is not likely to respond to therapy. An "intermediate susceptibility" report suggests that the infecting organism would be susceptible to bacampicillin if a high dosage is used or if the infection is confined to tissues and fluids (*e.g.,* urine) in which high antibiotic levels are attained.

Dilution Techniques: Broth or agar dilution methods may be used to determine the minimal inhibitory concentration (MIC) value for susceptibility of bacterial isolates to bacampicillin. Since bacampicillin per se has no *in vitro* activity, ampicillin powder should be used in a twofold concentration series of the antibiotic prepared in either broth (in tubes) or agar (in petri plates). Tubes should be inoculated to contain 10^4 to 10^5 organisms/ml or plates "spotted" with 10^3 to 10^4 organisms.

INDICATIONS AND USAGE:

Bacampicillin is indicated for the treatment of the following infections when caused by ampicillin-susceptible organisms:

1. Upper and Lower Respiratory Tract Infections (including acute exacerbations of chronic bronchitis) due to streptococci (β-hemolytic streptococci, *Streptococcus pyogenes*), pneumococci (*Streptococcus pneumoniae*), nonpenicillinase-producing staphylococci and *H. influenzae*;
2. Urinary Tract Infections due to *E. coli, Proteus mirabilis*, and *Streptococcus faecalis* (enterococci);
3. Skin and Skin Structure Infections due to streptococci and susceptible staphylococci;
4. Gonorrhea (acute uncomplicated urogenital infections) due to *Neisseria gonorrhoeae*.

Bacteriological studies to determine the causative organisms and their susceptibility to bacampicillin (*i.e.,* ampicillin) should be performed. Therapy may be instituted prior to obtaining results of susceptibility testing. Indicated surgical procedures should be performed.

CONTRAINDICATIONS:

The use of ampicillin class antibiotics is contraindicated in individuals with a history of an allergic reaction to any of the penicillin antibiotics and/or cephalosporins.

WARNINGS:

Serious and occasional fatal hypersensitivity (anaphylactic) reactions have been reported in patients on penicillin therapy. Although anaphylaxis is more frequent following parenteral therapy, it has occurred in patients on oral penicillins. These reactions are more apt to occur in individuals with a history of penicillin hypersensitivity and/or hypersensitivity to multiple allergens.

There have been reports of individuals with a history of penicillin hypersensitivity who have experienced severe reactions when treated with cephalosporins. Before therapy with a penicillin, careful inquiry should be made concerning previous hypersensitivity reactions to penicillins, cephalosporins, and other allergens.

IF AN ALLERGIC REACTION OCCURS, THE DRUG SHOULD BE DISCONTINUED AND THE APPROPRIATE THERAPY INSTITUTED. SERIOUS ANAPHYLACTOID REACTIONS REQUIRE IMMEDIATE EMERGENCY TREATMENT WITH EPINEPHRINE, OXYGEN, INTRAVENOUS STEROIDS, AND AIRWAY MANAGEMENT, INCLUDING INTUBATION, SHOULD ALSO BE ADMINISTERED AS INDICATED.

PRECAUTIONS:

1. General: The possibility of superinfections with mycotic or bacterial pathogens should be kept in mind during therapy. If superinfections occur (usually involving *Aerobacter, Pseudomonas*, or *Candida*), the drug should be discontinued and appropriate therapy instituted.

As with any potent agent, it is advisable to check periodically for organ system dysfunction during prolonged therapy. This includes renal, hepatic, and hematopoietic systems and is particularly important in prematures, neonates, and patients with liver or renal impairments.

A high percentage of patients with mononucleosis who receive ampicillin develop a skin rash. Thus, ampicillin class antibiotics should not be administered to patients with mononucleosis.

2. Drug and Laboratory Test Interactions: When testing for the presence of glucose in urine using Clinitest TM, Benedict's Solution, or Fehling's Solution, high urine concentrations of ampicillin may result in false-positive reactions. Therefore, it is recommended that glucose tests based on enzymatic glucose oxidase reactions (such as Clinistix TM or Testape TM) be used.

Following administration of ampicillin to pregnant women a transient decrease in plasma concentration of total conjugated estriol, estriol-glucuronide, conjugated estrone and estradiol, has been noted.

3. Pregnancy Category B: Reproduction studies have been performed in mice and rats at bacampicillin doses of up to 750 mg/kg (more than 25 times the human dose) and have revealed no evidence of impaired fertility or harm to the fetus due to bacampicillin.

There are, however, no adequate and well controlled studies in pregnant women. Because animal reproduction studies are not always predictive of human response, this drug should be used during pregnancy only if clearly needed.

4. Carcinogenesis, Mutagenesis, Impairment of Fertility: No carcinogenicity or mutagenicity studies were conducted. No impairment of fertility and no significant effect on general reproductive performance was observed in rats administered oral doses of up to 750 mg/kg of bacampicillin HCl per day prior to and during mating and gestation. In addition, bacampicillin HCl caused no drug-related effects on the reproductive organs of rats or dogs receiving daily oral doses of up to 800 and 650 mg/kg respectively for 6 months.

5. Labor and Delivery: Oral ampicillin class antibiotics are generally poorly absorbed during labor. Studies in guinea pigs showed that intravenous administration of ampicillin decreased the uterine tone, frequency of contractions, height of contractions, and duration of contractions. However, it is not known whether use of bacampicillin in humans during labor or delivery has immediate or delayed adverse effects on the fetus, prolongs the duration of labor, or increases the likelihood that forceps delivery or other obstetrical intervention or resuscitation of the newborn will be necessary.

6. Nursing Mothers: Ampicillin class antibiotics are excreted in milk; therefore, caution should be exercised when ampicillin class antibiotics are administered to a nursing woman.

7. Pediatric Use: Bacampicillin tablets are indicated for children weighing 25 kg or more. The bacampicillin oral suspension is indicated for children and infants weighing less than 25 kg or in those children not able to swallow a tablet.

DRUG INTERACTIONS:

The concurrent administration of allopurinol and ampicillin increases substantially the incidence of rashes in patients receiving both drugs as compared to patients receiving ampicillin alone. It is not known whether this potentiation of ampicillin rashes is due to allopurinol or the hyperuricemia present in these patients. There are no data available on the incidence of rash in patients treated concurrently with bacampicillin and allopurinol. Bacampicillin should not be co-administered with Antabuse (disulfiram).

ADVERSE REACTIONS:

As with other penicillins, it may be expected that untoward reactions will be essentially limited to sensitivity phenomena. They are more likely to occur in individuals who have previously demonstrated hypersensitivity to penicillins and in those with a history of allergy, asthma, hay fever, or urticaria.

In well controlled clinical trials conducted in the U.S. the most frequent adverse reactions to bacampicillin were epigastric upset (2%) and diarrhea (2%). Increased dosage may result in an increased incidence of diarrhea. In the same clinical trials the most frequent adverse effects for amoxicillin were diarrhea (4%) and nausea (2%).

The following adverse reactions have been reported for ampicillin.

ADVERSE REACTIONS: *(cont'd)*

Gastrointestinal: diarrhea, gastritis, stomatitis, nausea, vomiting, glossitis, black "hairy" tongue, enterocolitis, and pseudomembranous colitis.

Hypersensitivity Reactions: skin rashes, urticaria, erythema multiforme, and an occasional case of exfoliative dermatitis. These reactions may be controlled with antihistamines and, if necessary, systemic corticosteroids. Whenever such reactions occur, the drug should be discontinued, unless the opinion of the physician dictates otherwise.

Serious and occasional fatal hypersensitivity (anaphylactic) reactions can occur with oral penicillins. (See WARNINGS.)

Liver: A moderate rise in serum glutamic oxaloacetic transaminase (SGOT) has been noted in some ampicillin treated patients, but the significance of this finding is unknown. In well controlled clinical trials no difference was noted between ampicillin and bacampicillin with regard to the incidence of liver function test abnormalities.

Hemic and Lymphatic Systems: Anemia, thrombocytopenia, thrombocytopenic purpura, eosinophilia, leukopenia, and agranulocytosis have been reported during therapy with penicillins. These reactions are usually reversible on discontinuation of therapy and are believed to be hypersensitivity phenomena.

DOSAGE AND ADMINISTRATION:

Bacampicillin tablets may be given without regard to meals. Bacampicillin oral suspension should be administered to fasting patients.

UPPER RESPIRATORY TRACT INFECTIONS (including otitis media) due to streptococci, pneumococci, non-penicillinase-producing staphylococci and *H. influenzae*;

URINARY TRACT INFECTIONS due to *E. coli, Proteus mirabilis,* and *Streptococcus faecalis*;

SKIN AND SKIN STRUCTURES INFECTIONS due to streptococci and susceptible staphylococci:

Usual Dosage: Adults: 1 x 400 mg tablet every 12 hours (for patients weighing 25 kg or more).

Children: 25 mg/kg per day in 2 equally divided doses at 12 hour intervals.

IN SEVERE INFECTIONS OR THOSE CAUSED BY LESS SUSCEPTIBLE ORGANISMS:

Usual Dosage: Adults: 2 x 400 mg tablets every 12 hours (for patients weighing 25 kg or more).

Children: 50 mg/kg per day in 2 equally divided doses at 12 hour intervals.

LOWER RESPIRATORY TRACT INFECTIONS due to streptococci, pneumococci, nonpenicillinase-producing staphylococci, and *H. influenzae*:

Usual Dosage: Adults: 2 × 400 mg tablets every 12 hours (for patients weighing 25 kg or more).

Children: 50 mg/kg per day in 2 equally divided doses at 12 hour intervals.

GONORRHEA - acute uncomplicated urogenital infections due to *N. gonorrhoeae* (males and females):

1.6 grams (4 × 400 mg tablet plus 1 gram probenecid) as a single oral dose.

No pediatric dosage has been established.

Cases of gonorrhea with a suspected lesion of syphilis should have dark field examination before receiving bacampicillin and monthly serological tests for a minimum of four months. Larger doses may be required for stubborn or severe infections.

It should be recognized that in the treatment of chronic urinary tract infections, frequent bacteriological and clinical appraisals are necessary. Smaller doses than those recommended above should not be used. In stubborn infections, therapy may be required for several weeks. It may be necessary to continue clinical and/or bacteriological follow-up for several months after cessation of therapy. Except for gonorrhea, treatment should be continued for a minimum of 48 to 72 hours beyond the time that the patient becomes asymptomatic or evidence of bacterial eradication has been obtained.

IT IS RECOMMENDED THAT THERE BE AT LEAST 10 DAYS' TREATMENT FOR ANY INFECTION CAUSED BY HEMOLYTIC STREPTOCOCCI TO PREVENT THE OCCURRENCE OF ACUTE RHEUMATIC FEVER OR GLOMERULONEPHRITIS.

HOW SUPPLIED:

Spectrobid (bacampicillin HCl) tablets 400 mg: white, film-coated, oblong, unscored are available in bottles of 100.

HOW SUPPLIED - EQUIVALENTS NOT AVAILABLE:

Tablet, Uncoated - Oral - 400 mg

100's $190.12 SPECTROBID, Roerig 00049-0350-66

BACITRACIN *(000356)*

CATEGORIES: Anti-Infectives; Antibiotics; Antimicrobials; EENT Drugs; Eye, Ear, Nose, & Throat Preparations; Ocular Infections; Oncologic Drugs; Ophthalmics; Pharmaceutical Adjuvants; Pneumonia; Skin/Mucous Membrane Agents; FDA Approval Pre 1982

BRAND NAMES: Ak-Tracin; Baci-Rx; Bacticin; *Bacitracine Martinet* (France); Ocu-Tracin; Spectro-Bacitracin

(International brand names outside U.S. in italics)

FORMULARIES: Aetna; BC-BS; DoD; FHP; Medi-Cal; PCS

> WARNING:
> **Nephrotoxicity:** Bacitracin in parenteral (intramuscular) therapy may cause renal failure due to tubular and glomerular necrosis. Its use should be restricted to infants with staphylococcal pneumonia empyema when due to organisms shown to be susceptible to bacitracin. It should be used only where adequate laboratory facilities are available and when constant supervision of the patient is possible.
> Renal function should be carefully determined prior to and daily during therapy. The recommended daily dose should not be exceeded and fluid intake and urinary output maintained at proper levels to avoid kidney toxicity. If renal toxicity occurs the drug should be discontinued. The concurrent use of other nephrotoxic drugs, particularly streptomycin, kanamycin, polymyxin B, polymyxin E colistin, neomycin, and viomycin, should be avoided.

DESCRIPTION:

The chemical structure is $C_{66}H_{103}N_{17}O_{16}S$.

Ophthalmic Ointment: Bacitracin contains anhydrous lanolin, methylparaben, mineral oil, phenethyl alcohol, propylparaben, and white petrolatum.

IM Injection: Bacitracin is a white to pale buff, hygroscopic powder, odorless or having a slight odor. It is freely soluble in water; insoluble in acetone; chloroform, and ether. While soluble in alcohol, methanol, and glacial acetic acid, there is some insoluble residue. It is precipitated from its solutions and inactivated by many heavy metals.

CLINICAL PHARMACOLOGY:

OPHTHALMIC OINTMENT

Bacitracin is an antibiotic that exhibits bactericidal action *in vitro* against certain gram-positive organisms, such as streptococci, some strains of staphylococci, and pneumococci. It is ineffective against most gram-negative organisms.

IM INJECTION

Bacitracin, an antibiotic substance derived from cultures of *Bacillus subtilis* (Tracey), exerts pronounced antibacterial action *in vitro* against a variety of gram-positive and a few gram negative organisms. However, among systemic diseases, only staphylococcal infections qualify for consideration of bacitracin therapy. Bacitracin is assayed against a standard and its activity is expressed in units, 1 mg having a potency of not less than 50 units.

Susceptibility Testing: If the Kirby-Bauer method of disk susceptibility is used, a 10 unit bacitracin disk should give a zone of over 13 mm when tested against a bacitracin-susceptible strain of *Staphylococcus aureus.* Absorption of bacitracin following intramuscular injection is rapid and complete. A dose of 200 or 300 units/kg every 6 hours gives serum levels of 0.2 to 2 mcg/ml in individuals with normal renal function. The drug is excreted slowly by glomerular filtration. It is widely distributed in all body organs and is demonstrable in ascitic and pleural fluids after intramuscular injection.

INDICATIONS AND USAGE:

Ophthalmic Ointment: For the treatment of superficial ocular infections involving the conjunctiva and/or cornea caused by organisms susceptible to bacitracin. *NOTE:* The use of this drug should not replace appropriate surgical management or other concomitant measures. If deep-seated eye infection is suspected or develops, other measures, including systemic antibiotic therapy, should be considered.

IM Injection: In accord with the statements in the BOXED WARNING, the use of intramuscular bacitracin is limited to the treatment of infants with pneumonia and empyema caused by staphylococci shown to be susceptible to the drug.

CONTRAINDICATIONS:

This product should not be used in patients with a history of previous hypersensitivity or toxic reaction to bacitracin.

PRECAUTIONS:

OPHTHALMIC OINTMENT

The use of this product may result in the overgrowth of nonsusceptible organisms. Constant observation of the patient is essential. If new infections due to bacteria or fungi appear during therapy, appropriate measures should be taken.

Information for the Patient: The patient should be advised to discontinue use of this product and consult a physician if symptoms persist or become worse.

If the patient experiences severe eye pain, headache, rapid change in vision (side or straight ahead), sudden appearance of floating spots, acute redness of the eyes, pain on exposure to light, or double vision, a physician should be consulted immediately.

To avoid contamination of this product, the patient should be advised to not let the tip of the container touch any other surface and to replace the cap after use.

IM INJECTION

See BOXED WARNING for precautions in regard to kidney toxicity associated with intramuscular use of bacitracin.

Adequate fluid intake should be maintained orally, or if necessary, by parenteral method.

As with other antibiotics, use of this drug may result in overgrowth of nonsusceptible organisms, including fungi. If superinfection occurs, appropriate therapy should be instituted.

ADVERSE REACTIONS:

OPHTHALMIC OINTMENT

Primary sensitivity to bacitracin is not often seen in patients, and sensitivity does not readily develop with repeated courses of the antibiotic. However, if signs of irritation or sensitivity (for example, itching, burning, or inflammation) occur, the drug should be discontinued.

IM INJECTION

Nephrotoxic Reactions: Albuminuria, cylindruria, azotemia. Rising blood levels without any increase in dosage.

Other Reactions: Nausea and vomiting. Pain at site of injection. Skin rashes.

DOSAGE AND ADMINISTRATION:

OPHTHALMIC OINTMENT

Apply topically 1 or more times daily.

Store at controlled room temperature, 59° to 86° F (15° to 30° C).

IM INJECTION

To Be Aministered Intramuscularly Only

Infant Dose: For infants under 2500 grams - 900 units/kg/24 hours in 2 or 3 divided doses. For infants over 2500 grams =1,000 units/kg/24 hours, in 2 or 3 divided doses. Intramuscular injections of the solution should be given in the upper outer quadrant of the buttocks, alternating right and left and avoiding multiple injections in the same region because of the transient pain following injection.

Preparation of Solutions: Should be dissolved in sodium chloride injection containing 2 percent procaine hydrochloride. The concentration of the antibiotic in the solution should not be less than 5,000 units per ml nor more than 10,000 units per ml.

Diluents containing parabens should not be used to reconstitute bacitracin; cloudy solutions and precipitate formation have occurred.

Reconstitution of the 50,000 unit vial with 9.8 ml of diluent will result in a concentration of 5,000 units per ml.

Storage: Store the unreconstituted product in a refrigerator 2 - 8° C (36 - 46° F). Solutions are stable for one week when stored in a refrigerator 2 - 8° C(36 - 46° F).

HOW SUPPLIED - RATED THERAPEUTICALLY EQUIVALENT:

Injection, Lyphl-Soln - Intramuscular - 50,000 unit/via

1's $9.26 Bacitracin Sterile, Pharmacia & Upjohn 00009-0233-01

HOW SUPPLIED - RATED THERAPEUTICALLY EQUIVALENT: *(cont'd)*

Ointment - Ophthalmic - 500 unit/gm

0.94 gm x 144	$16.00	Bacitracin, Consolidated Midland	00223-0011-09
3.5 gm	$2.20	Bacitracin, Harber Pharm	51432-0704-30
3.5 gm	$2.25	Bacitracin, Raway	00686-0233-35
3.5 gm	$2.59	Bacitracin, Lilly	00002-1861-17
3.5 gm	$3.13	Bacitracin, H.C.F.A. F F P	99999-0356-01
3.5 gm	$3.31	Bacitracin 500U Ophthalmic, HL Moore Drug Exch	00839-5493-43
3.5 gm	$3.40	Bacitracin, Schein Pharm (US)	00364-7174-70
3.5 gm	$3.40	Bacitracin, Major Pharms	00904-2625-38
3.5 gm	$3.50	Bacitracin Opthalmic, Goldline Labs	00182-1698-31
3.5 gm	$3.85	AK-TRACIN, Akorn	17478-0233-35
3.5 gm	$3.90	SPECTRO BACITRACIN, Spectrum Scitfc	53268-0565-55
3.5 gm	$4.95	Bacticin, Ocusoft	54799-0514-35

Powder - 5,000,000 unit

1's	$113.20	Bacitracin, Paddock Labs	00574-0400-05

HOW SUPPLIED - NOT RATED EQUIVALENT:

Injection, Lyphl-Soln - Intramuscular - 50,000 unit/via

1's	$6.81	Bacitracin, Schein Pharm (US)	00364-2419-56

Ointment - Ophthalmic - 500 unit/gm

3.5 gm	$3.64	Bacitracin, Fougera	00168-0026-38

BACITRACIN ZINC; NEOMYCIN SULFATE; POLYMYXIN B SULFATE *(000357)*

CATEGORIES: Anti-Infectives; Antibacterials; Antibiotics; Burns; EENT Drugs; Eye, Ear, Nose, & Throat Preparations; Ocular Infections; Ophthalmics; Skin/Mucous Membrane Agents; Topical; FDA Approval Pre 1982

BRAND NAMES: Ak-Spore Opth; *BNP*; *Baspo*; *Dactrol*; Infa-3; *Multimycin*; *Mycitracin*; Neo-Polycin; *Neobiotic*; Neocidin; **Neosporin**; *Neosporin Dermico* (Mexico); Neotal; Neotricin; Ocu-Spor-B; Ocutricin; *Polixin-Ungena*; *Polixin Ungena*; *Polybamycin*; Spectro-Sporin; *Spersin* (Australia); Tri-Thalmic; Triple Antibiotic
(International brand names outside U.S. in italics)

FORMULARIES: Aetna; BC-BS; Medi-Cal; WHO

DESCRIPTION:

Polymyxin B sulfate-bacitracin zinc-neomycin sulfate (abbreviated here as bacitracin-neo-poly) is a sterile antimicrobial ointment for ophthalmic use. Each gram contains: neomycin sulfate equivalent to 3.5 mg neomycin base, polymyxin B sulfate equivalent to 10,000 polymyxin B units, bacitracin zinc equivalent to 400 bacitracin units, and special white petrolatum, qs.

Neomycin sulfate is the sulfate salt of neomycin B and C, which are produced by the growth of *Streptomyces fradiae* Waksman (Fam. Streptomycetaceae). It has a potency equivalent of not less than 600 mcg of neomycin standard per mg, calculated on an anhydrous basis.

Polymyxin B sulfate is the sulfate salt of polymyxin B_1 and B_2 which are produced by the growth of *Bacillus polymyxa* (Prazmowski) Migula (Fam. Bacillaceae). It has a potency of not less than 6,000 polymyxin B units per mg, calculated on an anhydrous basis.

Bacitracin zinc is the zinc salt of bacitracin, a mixture of related cyclic polypeptides (mainly bacitracin A) produced by the growth of an organism of the *licheniformis* group of *Bacillus subtilis* (var Tracy). It has a potency of not less than 40 bacitracin units per mg.

CLINICAL PHARMACOLOGY:

A wide range of antibacterial action is provided by the overlapping spectra of neomycin, polymyxin B sulfate, and bacitracin.

Neomycin is bactericidal for many gram-positive and gram-negative organisms. It is an aminoglycoside antibiotic which inhibits protein synthesis by binding with ribosomal RNA and causing misreading of the bacterial genetic code.

Polymyxin B is bactericidal for a variety of gram-negative organisms. It increases the permeability of the bacterial cell membrane by interacting with the phospholipid components of the membrane.

Bacitracin is bactericidal for a variety of gram-positive and gram-negative organisms. It interferes with bacterial cell wall synthesis by inhibition of the regeneration of phospholipid receptors involved in peptidoglycan synthesis.

Microbiology: Neomycin Sulfate, Polymyxin B sulfate, and bacitracin zinc together are considered active against the following microorganisms: *Staphylococcus aureus*, streptococci, including*Streptococcus pneumoniae, Escherichia coli, Haemophilus influenzae, Klebsiella-Enterobacter* species, *Neisseria* species and *Pseudomonas aeruginosa*. The product does not provide adequate coverage against *Serratia marcescens*.

INDICATIONS AND USAGE:

Bacitracin-neo-poly is indicated for the topical treatment of superficial infections of the external eye and its adnexa caused by susceptible bacteria. Such infections encompass conjunctivitis, keratitis and keratoconjunctivitis, blepharitis and blepharoconjunctivitis.

CONTRAINDICATIONS:

This product is contraindicated in individuals who have shown hypersensitivity to any of its components.

WARNINGS:

NOT FOR INJECTION INTO THE EYE. Neosporin Ophthalmic Ointment should never be directly introduced into the anterior chamber of the eye. Ophthalmic ointments may retard corneal wound healing.

Topical antibiotics, particularly neomycin sulfate, may cause cutaneous sensitization. A precise incidence of hypersensitivity reactions (primarily skin rash) due to topical antibiotics is not known.

The manifestations of sensitization to topical antibiotics are usually itching, reddening, and edema of the conjunctiva and eyelid. A sensitization reaction of products containing these ingredients may manifest simply as a failure to heal. During long-term use of topical antibiotic products, periodic examination for such signs is advisable, and the patient should be told to discontinue the product if they are observed. Symptoms usually subside quickly on withdrawing the medication. Applications should be avoided for the patient thereafter (see PRECAUTIONS, General).

PRECAUTIONS:

General: As with other antibiotic preparation, prolonged use may result in overgrowth of nonsusceptible organisms including fungi. If superinfection occurs, appropriate measures should be initiated.

Bacterial resistance to this product may also develop. If purulent discharge, inflammation, or pain becomes aggravated, the patient should discontinue use of the medication and consult a physician.

There have been reports of bacterial keratitis associated with the use of topical ophthalmic products in multiple-dose containers which have been inadvertently contaminated by patients, most of whom had a concurrent corneal disease or a disruption of the ocular epithelial surface (see PRECAUTIONS, Information for Patients.)

Allergic cross-reactions may occur which could prevent the use of any or all of the following antibiotics for the treatment of future infections; kanamycin, paromomycin, streptomycin, and possibly gentamicin.

Information for Patients: Patients should be instructed to avoid allowing the tip of the dispensing container to contact the eye, eyelid, fingers, or any other surface. The use of this product by more than one person may spread infection.

Patients should also be instructed that ocular products, if handled improperly, can become contaminated by common bacteria known to cause ocular infections. Serious damage to the eye and subsequent loss of vision may result from using contaminated products (see PRECAUTIONS, General).

If the condition persists or gets worse, or if a rash or allergic reaction develops, the patient should be advised to stop use and consult a physician. Do not use this product if you are allergic to any of the listed ingredients.

Keep tightly closed when not in use. Keep out of reach of children.

Carcinogenesis, Mutagenesis, and Impairment of Fertility: Long-term studies in animals to evaluate carcinogenic or mutagenic potential have not been conducted with polymyxin B sulfate or bacitracin. Treatment of cultured human lymphocytes *in vitro* with neomycin increased the frequency of chromosome aberrations at the highest concentration (80 mcg/ml) tested: however, the effects of neomycin or carcinogenesis and mutagenesis in humans are unknown.

Polymyxin B has been reported to impair the motility of equine sperm, but its effects on male or female fertility are unknown. No adverse effects on male or female fertility, litter size or survival were observed in rabbits given bacitracin zinc 100 gm/ton of diet.

Pregnancy, Teratogenic Effects, Pregnancy Category C: Animal reproduction studies have not been conducted with neomycin sulfate, polymyxin B sulfate, or bacitracin. It is also not known whether this product can cause fetal harm when administered to a pregnant woman or can affect reproduction capacity. This product should be given to a pregnant woman only if clearly needed.

Nursing Mothers: It is not known whether this drug is excreted in human milk. Because many drugs are excreted in human milk, caution should be exercised when this product is administered to a nursing woman.

Pediatric Use: Safety and effectiveness in children have not been established.

ADVERSE REACTIONS:

Adverse reactions have occurred with the anti-infective components of this product. The exact incidence is not known. Reactions occurring most often are allergic sensitization reactions including itching, swelling, and conjunctival erythema (see WARNINGS). More serious hypersensitivity reactions, including anaphylaxis, have been reported rarely.

Local irritation on instillation has also been reported.

DOSAGE AND ADMINISTRATION:

Apply the ointment every 3 or 4 hours for 7 to 10 days, depending on the severity of the infection.

Store at 15° to 25°C (59° to 77°F).

REFERENCES:

1. Leyden JJ, and Kligman AM. Contact Dermatitis to Neomycin Sulfate, *JAMA 242* (12): 1276-1278, 1979. **2.** Prystowsky SD, Allen AM, Smith RW, Nonomura JH, Odom RB, and Akers WA. Allergic Contact Hypersensitivity to Nickle, Neomycin, Ethylenediamine, and Benzocaine.*Arch Dermatol 115:* 959-962, 1979.

HOW SUPPLIED - RATED THERAPEUTICALLY EQUIVALENT:

Ointment - Ophthalmic - 400 unit/3.5 mg

0.94 gm x 144	$16.00	Triple Antibiotic, Consolidated Midland	00223-0012-09
1 gm x 144	$17.40	Triple Antibiotic, Consolidated Midland	00223-4108-01
3.5 gm	$1.94	Bacitracin Neomycin Polymixin, H.C.F.A. F F P	99999-0357-01
3.5 gm	$2.08	Infa-3 Ointment Ophthalmic, Infinity Pharm	58154-0780-55
3.5 gm	$2.50	Ocutricin, Raway	00686-5780-55
3.5 gm	$2.50	Triple Antibiotic, Harber Pharm	51432-0708-30
3.5 gm	$2.75	Triple Antibiotic, Consolidated Midland	00223-4109-03
3.5 gm	$3.22	OCUTRICIN OPHTHALMIC, United Res	00677-0907-18
3.5 gm	$3.63	Triple Antibiotic Opth Oint, HL Moore Drug Exch	00839-6659-43
3.5 gm	$4.32	Bacitracin Neomycin Polymixin, Fougera	00168-0027-38
3.5 gm	$5.10	AK-SPORE OPHTHALMIC, Akorn	17478-0235-35
3.5 gm	$5.95	SPECTRO SPORIN, Spectrum Scitfc	53268-0780-55
3.5 gm	**$17.75**	**NEOSPORIN, Glaxo Wellcome**	**00173-0732-86**
3.5 gm x 12	$29.25	Triple Antibiotic, Rugby	00536-6901-91

HOW SUPPLIED - NOT RATED EQUIVALENT:

Ointment - Ophthalmic - 400 unit/5 mg/5

3.5 gm	$3.25	TRIPLE ANTIBIOTIC, C O Truxton	00463-8049-38

BACITRACIN ZINC; POLYMYXIN B SULFATE *(000358)*

CATEGORIES: Anti-Infectives; Antibacterials; Antibiotics; Burns; Conjunctivitis; EENT Drugs; Eye, Ear, Nose, & Throat Preparations; Ocular Infections; Ophthalmics; Skin/Mucous Membrane Agents; Topical; FDA Approval Pre 1982

BRAND NAMES: Ak-Poly-Bac; Bacitracin Polymyxin; Bacitracin Polymyxin B; Ocumycin; Polycin-B; *Polyfax*; **Polysporin**; Polytracin
(International brand names outside U.S. in italics)

FORMULARIES: FHP; Medi-Cal

DESCRIPTION:

Each gram contains Polymyxin B Sulfate 10,000 units, bacitracin zinc 500 units, special white petrolatum qs.

CLINICAL PHARMACOLOGY:

Polymyxin B attacks gram-negative bacilli, including virtually all strains of *Pseudomonas aeruginosa* and *H influenzae* species.

Bacitracin is active against most gram-positive bacilli and cocci, including hemolytic streptococci.

INDICATIONS AND USAGE:

For the treatment of superficial ocular infections involving the conjunctiva and/or cornea caused by organisms susceptible to polymyxin B sulfate and bacitracin zinc.

CONTRAINDICATIONS:

This product is contraindicated in those individuals who have shown hypersensitivity to any of its components.

WARNINGS:

Ophthalmic ointments may retard corneal healing.

PRECAUTIONS:

As with other antibiotic preparations, prolonged use may result in overgrowth of nonsusceptible organisms, including fungi. Appropriate measures should be taken if this occurs.

DOSAGE AND ADMINISTRATION:

Apply the ointment every 3 or 4 hours, depending on the severity of the infection.

HOW SUPPLIED - RATED THERAPEUTICALLY EQUIVALENT:

Ointment - Ophthalmic - 500 unit/10,000

3.5 gm	$3.90	Bacitracin/Polymyxin, Harber Pharm	51432-0749-30
3.5 gm	$4.15	Bacitracin Zinc/Polymyxin B, Schein Pharm (US)	00364-2552-70
3.5 gm	$4.15	BACITRACIN-POLYMYXIN OPHTHAL, Major Pharms	00904-2968-38
3.5 gm	$4.95	Polycin-B, Ocusoft	54799-0515-35
3.5 gm	$5.95	SPECTRO POLYTRACIN, Spectrum Scitfc	53268-0555-55
3.5 gm	$7.49	OCUMYCIN, Parmed Pharms	00349-8725-38
3.5 gm	$9.73	AK-POLY-BAC, Akorn	17478-0238-35
3.5 gm	$10.79	Bacitracin/Polymyxin B, HL Moore Drug Exch	00839-7983-43
3.5 gm	$10.81	Polytracin, Qualitest Pharms	00603-7262-70
3.5 gm	$10.90	Bacitracin/Polymyxin, Rugby	00536-6204-91
3.5 gm	$10.95	Bacitracin/Polymyxin, Aligen Independ	00405-0640-08
3.5 gm	$11.00	Bacitracin/Polymyxin B, Adv Remedies	57685-0075-61
3.5 gm	**$17.75**	**POLYSPORIN, Glaxo Wellcome**	**00173-0797-86**
30 gm	$3.37	Bacitracin/Polymyxin, Rugby	00536-4121-95

HOW SUPPLIED - NOT RATED EQUIVALENT:

Ointment - Ophthalmic - 500 unit/10,000

15 gm	$2.25	Polytracin, Consolidated Midland	00223-4395-15
30 gm	$3.25	Polytracin, Consolidated Midland	00223-4395-30

BACITRACIN; HYDROCORTISONE ACETATE; NEOMYCIN SULFATE; POLYMYXIN B SULFATE *(000360)*

CATEGORIES: Anti-Infectives; Anti-Inflammatory Agents; Antibacterials; Antibiotics; Burns; Conjunctivitis; Corneal Inflammation; Corneal Injury; Dermatologicals; Dermatoses; EENT Drugs; Edema; Eye, Ear, Nose, & Throat Preparations; Inflammatory Conditions; Ocular Infections; Ophthalmics; Otic Hydrocortisones; Otic Preparations; Otologic; Skin/Mucous Membrane Agents; Steroids; Topical; Uveitis; Pregnancy Category C; FDA Approval Pre 1982

BRAND NAMES: Ak-Spore HC; **Cortisporin**; Infa-3Hc; Neotricin Hc; Ocu-Cort; Ocusporin-Hc; Ocutricin-Hc; Spectro-Sporin; Tri-Thalmic Hc; Triple Antibiotic W/ Hydrocortisone; Vita-Rx

FORMULARIES: Aetna; BC-BS

DESCRIPTION:

In order to avoid confusion, the brand names for these products have been included in the monograph. The monograph contains full information for the topical ointment, and information for the ophthalmic ointment in the sections: DESCRIPTION, INDICATIONS AND USAGE, WARNINGS, and DOSAGE AND ADMINISTRATION.

Topical Ointment: Cortisporin ointment (polymyxin B sulfate-bacitracin zinc-neomycin sulfate-hydrocortisone) is a topical antibacterial ointment. Each gram contains: polymyxin B sulfate 5,000 units, bacitracin zinc 400 units, neomycin sulfate equivalent to 3.5 mg neomycin base, hydrocortisone 10 mg (1%), and special white petrolatum qs.

Ophthalmic Ointment: Cortisporin ophthalmic ointment is a sterile antimicrobial and anti-inflammatory ointment for ophthalmic use. Each gram contains: Polymyxin B sulfate 10,000 units, bacitracin zinc 400 units, neomycin sulfate equivalent to 3.5 mg neomycin base, hydrocortisone 10 mg (1%) and special white petrolatum, q.s.

Polymyxin B sulfate is the sulfate salt of polymyxin B_1 and B_2, which are produced by the growth of *Bacillus polymyxa* (Prazmowski) Migula (Fam. Bacillaceae). It has a potency of not less than 6,000 polymyxin B units per mg, calculated on an anhydrous basis.

Bacitracin zinc is the zinc salt of bacitracin, a mixture of related cyclic polypeptides (mainly bacitracin A) produced by the growth of an organism of the *licheniformis* group of *Bacillus subtilis* (Fam. Bacillaceae). It has a potency of not less than 40 bacitracin units per mg.

Neomycin sulfate is the sulfate salt of neomycin B and C, which are produced by the growth of *Streptomyces fradiae* Waksman (Fam. Streptomycetaceae). It has a potency equivalent of not less than 600 mcg of neomycin standard per mg, calculated on an anhydrous basis.

Hydrocortisone, 11β,17,21-trihydroxypregn-4-ene-3,20-dione, is an anti-inflammatory hormone.

CLINICAL PHARMACOLOGY:

Corticoids suppress the inflammatory response to a variety of agents and they may delay healing. Since corticoids may inhibit the body's defense mechanism against infection, a concomitant antimicrobial drug may be used when this inhibition is considered to be clinically significant in a particular case.

The anti-infective components in the combination are included to provide action against specific organisms susceptible to them. Polymyxin B sulfate, bacitracin zinc and neomycin sulfate together are considered active against the following microorganisms: *Staphylococcus, aureus*, streptococci, including *Streptococcus pneumoniae, Escherichia coli, Haemophilus influenzae, Klebsiella-Enterobacter* species, *Neisseria* species and *Pseudomonas aeruginosa*.

CLINICAL PHARMACOLOGY: *(cont'd)*

The product does not provide adequate coverage against *Serratia marcescens*.

The relative potency of corticosteroids depends on the molecular structure, concentration and release from the vehicle.

INDICATIONS AND USAGE:

TOPICAL OINTMENT

For the treatment of corticosteroid-responsive dermatoses with secondary infection. It has not been demonstrated that this steroid-antibiotic combination provides greater benefit than the steroid component alone after 7 days of treatment (see WARNINGS.)

OPHTHALMIC OINTMENT

For steroid-responsive inflammatory ocular conditions for which a corticosteroid is indicated and where bacterial infection or a risk of bacterial ocular infection exists.

Ocular steroids are indicated in inflammatory conditions of the palpebral and bulbar conjunctiva, cornea and anterior segment of the globe where the inherent risk of steroid use in certain infective conjunctivitides is accepted to obtain a diminution in edema and inflammation. They are also indicated in chronic anterior uveitis and corneal injury from chemical, radiation, or thermal burns, or penetration of foreign bodies.

The use of a combination drug with an anti-infective component is indicated where the risk of infection is high or where there is an expectation that potentially dangerous numbers of bacteria will be present in the eye.

The particular anti-infective drugs in this product are active against the following common bacterial eye pathogens: *Staphylococcus aureus,* streptococci, including *Streptococcus pneumoniae, Escherichia coli, Haemophilus influenzae. Klebsiella-Enterobacter* species, *Neisseria* species, and *Pseudomonas aeruginosa.*

This product does not provide adequate coverage against *Serratia marcescens*.

CONTRAINDICATIONS:

Not for use in the eyes or in the external ear canal if the eardrum is perforated. This product is contraindicated in tuberculous, fungal or viral lesions of the skin (herpes simplex, vaccinia and varicella). This product is contraindicated in those individuals who have shown hypersensitivity to any of its components.

WARNINGS:

TOPICAL OINTMENT

Because of the concern of nephrotoxicity and ototoxicity associated with neomycin, this combination should not be used over a wide area or for extended periods of time.

OPHTHALMIC OINTMENT

Prolonged use may result in glaucoma, with damage to the optic nerve, defects in visual acuity and fields of vision, and posterior subcapsular cataract formation. Prolonged use may suppress the host response and this increase the hazard of secondary ocular infections. In those diseases causing thinning of the cornea or sclera, perforations have been known to occur with the use of topical steroids. In acute purulent conditions of the eye, steroids may mask infection or enhance existing infection. If these products are used for 10 days or longer, intraocular pressure should be routinely monitored even though it may be difficult in children and uncooperative patients.

Employment of steroid medication in the treatment of herpes simplex requires great caution.

Neomycin sulfate may cause cutaneous sensitization. A precise incidence of hypersensitivity reactions (primarily skin rash) due to topical neomycin is not known.

The manifestations of sensitization to neomycin are usually itching, reddening, and edema of the conjunctiva and eyelid. It may be manifest simply as a failure to heal. During long-term use of neomycin-containing products, periodic examination for such signs is advisable, and the patient should be told to discontinue the product is they are observed. These symptoms subside quickly on withdrawing the medication. Neomycin-containing applications should be avoided for the patient thereafter.

PRECAUTIONS:

GENERAL

As with any antibiotic preparation, prolonged use may result in the overgrowth of nonsusceptible organisms, including fungi. Appropriate measures should be taken if this occurs. Use of steroids on infected areas should be supervised with care as anti-inflammatory steroids may encourage spread of infection. If this occurs, steroid therapy should be stopped and appropriate antibacterial drugs used. Generalized dermatological conditions may require systemic corticosteroid therapy.

Signs and symptoms of exogenous hyperadrenocorticism can occur with the use of topical corticosteroids, including adrenal suppression. Systemic absorption of topically applied steroids will be increased if extensive body surface areas are treated or if occlusive dressings are used. Under these circumstances, suitable precautions should be taken when long-term use is anticipated.

INFORMATION FOR THE PATIENT

If redness, irritation, swelling or pain persists or increases, discontinue use and notify physician. Do not use in the eyes.

LABORATORY TESTS

Systemic effects of excessive levels of hydrocortisone may include a reduction in the number of circulating eosinophils and a decrease in urinary excretion of 17-hydroxycorticosteroids.

CARCINOGENESIS, MUTAGENESIS, AND IMPAIRMENT OF FERTILITY

Long-term studies in animals (rats, rabbits, mice) showed no evidence of carcinogenicity attributable to oral administration of corticosteroids.

PREGNANCY, TERATOGENIC EFFECTS

Pregnancy Category C Corticosteroids have been shown to be teratogenic in rabbits when applied topically at concentrations of 0.5% on days 6-18 of gestation and in mice when applied topically at a concentration of 15% on days 10-13 of gestation. There are no adequate and well-controlled studies in pregnant women. Corticosteroids should be used during pregnancy only if the potential benefit justifies the potential risk to the fetus.

NURSING MOTHERS

Hydrocortisone appears in human milk following oral administration of the drug. Since systemic absorption of hydrocortisone may occur when applied topically, caution should be exercised when Cortisporin Ointment is used by a nursing woman.

PEDIATRIC USE

Sufficient percutaneous absorption of hydrocortisone can occur in infants and children during prolonged use to cause cessation of growth, as well as other systemic signs and symptoms of hyperadrenocorticism.

ADVERSE REACTIONS:

Neomycin occasionally causes skin sensitization. Ototoxicity and nephrotoxicity have also been reported (see WARNINGS.) Adverse reactions have occurred with topical use of antibiotic combinations including neomycin, bacitracin and polymyxin B. Exact incidence

ADVERSE REACTIONS: *(cont'd)*

figures are not available since no denominator of treated patients is available. The reaction occurring most often is allergic sensitization. In one clinical study, using a 20% neomycin patch, neomycin-induced allergic skin reactions occurred in two of 2,175 (0.09%) individuals in the general population.[1] In another study, the incidence was found to be approximately 1%.[2]

The following local adverse reactions have been reported with topical corticosteroids, especially under occlusive dressings: burning, itching, irritation, dryness, folliculitis, hypertrichosis, acneiform eruptions, hypopigmentation, perioral dermatitis, allergic contact dermatitis, maceration of the skin, secondary infection, skin atrophy, striae and miliaria.

When steroid preparations are used for long periods of time in intertriginous areas or over extensive body areas, with or without occlusive non-permeable dressings, striae may occur; also there exists the possibility of systemic side effects when steroid preparations are used over larger areas or for a long period of time.

DOSAGE AND ADMINISTRATION:

TOPICAL OINTMENT

A thin film is applied 2 to 4 times daily to the affected area.

Store at 15° to 25°C (59° to 77°F).

OPHTHALMIC OINTMENT

Apply the ointment in the affected eye every 3 or 4 hours, depending in the severity of the condition.

Not more than 8 grams should be prescribed initially and the prescription should not be refilled without evaluation as outlined.

REFERENCES:

1. Leyden JJ, Kligman AM: Contact dermatitis to neomycin sulfate. *JAMA* 1979;242:1276-1278. **2.** Prystowsky SD, Allen AM, Smith RW, et al: Allergic contact hypersensitivity to nickel, neomycin, ethylenediamine, and benzocaine. *Arch Dermatol* 1979;115:959-962.

HOW SUPPLIED - RATED THERAPEUTICALLY EQUIVALENT:

Ointment - Ophthalmic - 400 unit/10 mg/

3.5 gm	$4.20	TRIPLE ANTIBIOTIC/HYDROCORTISONE, C O Truxton	00463-8044-38
3.5 gm	$4.25	Ocusporin-Hc, HL Moore Drug Exch	00839-6658-43
3.5 gm	$4.95	Bacitracin/Neo/Polymyxin/Hc, Fougera	00168-0029-38
3.5 gm	$5.40	AK-SPORE HC, Akorn	17478-0232-35
3.5 gm	**$17.99**	**CORTISPORIN, Glaxo Wellcome**	**00173-0197-86**
3.5 gm x 12	$4.55	TRIPLE ANTIBIOTIC W/HC, Rugby	00536-6401-91
10 ml	$8.10	TRIPLE ANTIBIOTIC OPTHALMIC, Goldline Labs	00182-1549-63

HOW SUPPLIED - NOT RATED EQUIVALENT:

Ointment - Ophthalmic - 400 unit/10 mg/

3.5 gm	$1.65	Ocutricin-Hc, Raway	00686-5785-55
3.5 gm	$3.00	Neomycin/Bacitracin/Poly/Hc, Consolidated Midland	00223-4111-03
3.5 gm	$3.33	Infa-3-Hc Ointment Ophthalmic, Infinity Pharm	58154-0785-55
3.5 gm	$4.25	Bacitracin/Neo/Polymyxin/Hc, Harber Pharm	51432-0864-35
3.5 gm	$5.95	Spectro-Sporin Hc, Spectrum Scitfc	53268-0785-55

Ointment - Topical - 400 unit/10 mg/

15 gm	**$25.60**	**CORTISPORIN, Glaxo Wellcome**	**00173-0196-88**

BACLOFEN *(000361)*

CATEGORIES: Autonomic Drugs; Multiple Sclerosis; Muscle Relaxants; Neuromuscular; Pain; Skeletal Muscle Hyperactivity; Skeletal Muscle Relaxants; Spasticity; Spinal Cord Injury; FDA Approval Pre 1982

BRAND NAMES: *Alpha-Baclofen*; Atrofen; *Baclon*; *Baclosal*; *Baclospas*; *Baklofen*; *Clofen*; *Lebic* (Germany); **Lioresal**; *Mulax*; *Pacifen*; *Spinax*
(International brand names outside U.S. in italics)

FORMULARIES: Aetna; Medi-Cal; PCS

DESCRIPTION:

Baclofen is a muscle relaxant and antispastic. Its chemical name is 4-amino-3-(4-chlorophenyl)-butanoic acid.

Baclofen is a white to off-white, odorless or practically odorless crystalline powder, with a molecular weight of 213.66. It is slightly soluble in water, very slightly soluble in methanol, and insoluble in chloroform.

Baclofen tablets are available as 10-mg and 20-mg tablets for oral administration.

INACTIVE INGREDIENTS

Baclofen tablets: Cellulose compounds, magnesium stearate, povidone, and starch.

Baclofen injection: is a sterile, pyrogen-free, isotonic solution free of antioxidants, preservatives or other potentially neurotoxic additives indicated only for intrathecal administration. The drug is stable in solution at 37° C and compatible with CSF. Each milliliter of baclofen injection contains baclofen U.S.P. 500 mcg or 2000 mcg and sodium chloride 9 mg in Water for Injection; pH range is 5-7. Each ampule is intended for SINGLE USE ONLY. Discard any unused portion. **DO NOT AUTOCLAVE.**

CLINICAL PHARMACOLOGY:

TABLETS

The precise mechanism of action of baclofen is not fully known. Baclofen is capable of inhibiting both monosynaptic and polysynaptic reflexes at the spinal level, possibly by hyperpolarization of afferent terminals, although actions at supraspinal sites may also occur and contribute to its clinical effect. Although baclofen is an analog of the putative inhibitory neurotransmitter gamma-aminobutyric acid (GABA), there is no conclusive evidence that actions on GABA systems are involved in the production of its clinical effects. In studies with animals, baclofen has been shown to have general CNS depressant properties as indicated by the production of sedation with tolerance, somnolence, ataxia, and respiratory and cardiovascular depression. Baclofen is rapidly and extensively absorbed and eliminated. Absorption may be dose-dependent, being reduced with increasing doses. Baclofen is excreted primarily by the kidney in unchanged form and there is relatively large intersubject variation in absorption and/or elimination.

INJECTION

The precise mechanism of action of baclofen as a muscle relaxant and antispasticity agent is not fully understood. Baclofen inhibits both monosynaptic and polysynaptic reflexes at the spinal level, possibly by decreasing excitatory neurotransmitter release from primary afferent terminals, although actions at supraspinal sites may also occur and contribute to its clinical effect. Baclofen is a structural analog of the inhibitory neurotransmitter gamma-aminobutyric acid (GABA) and may exert its effects by stimulation of the $GABA_B$, receptor subtype.

CLINICAL PHARMACOLOGY: *(cont'd)*

Baclofen injection when introduced directly into the intrathecal space permits effective CSF concentrations to be achieved with resultant plasma concentrations 100 times less than those occurring with oral administration.

In people, as well as in animals, baclofen has been shown to have general CNS depressant properties as indicated by the production of sedation with tolerance, somnolence, ataxia, and respiratory and cardiovascular depression.

PHARMACODYNAMICS OF BACLOFEN INJECTION

Adult Patients: The onset of action is generally one-half hour to one hour after an intrathecal bolus. Peak spasmolytic effect is seen at approximately four hours after dosing and effects may last four to eight hours. Onset, peak response, and duration of action may vary with individual patients depending on the dose and severity of symptoms.

Pediatric Patients: The onset, peak, and duration of action is similar to those seen in adult patients.

Continuous Infusion: Baclofen injection's antispastic action is first seen at 6 to 8 hours after initiation of continuous infusion. Maximum activity is observed in 24 to 48 hours.

No additional information is available for pediatric patients.

PHARMACOKINETICS OF BACLOFEN INJECTION

The pharmacokinetics of CSF clearance of baclofen injection calculated from intrathecal bolus or continuous infusion studies approximates CSF turnover, suggesting elimination is by bulk-flow removal of CSF.

Intrathecal Bolus: After a bolus lumbar injection of 50 or 100 mcg baclofen injection in seven patients, the average CSF elimination half-life was 1.51 hours over the first four hours and the average CSF clearance was approximately 30 ml/hour.

Continuous Infusion: The mean CSF clearance for baclofen injection was approximately 30 ml/hour in a study involving ten patients on continuous intrathecal infusion.

Concurrent plasma concentrations of baclofen during intrathecal administration are expected to be low (0-5 ng/ml).

Limited pharmacokinetic data suggest that a lumbar-cisternal concentration gradient of about 4:1 ia established along the neuroaxis during baclofen infusion. This is based upon simultaneous CSF sampling via cisternal and lumbar tap in 5 patients receiving continuous baclofen infusion at the lumbar level at doses associated with therapeutic efficacy; the inter-patient variability was great. The gradient was not altered by position.

Six pediatric patients (age 6-18 years) receiving continuous intrathecal baclofen infusion at doses of 77-400 mcg/day had plasma baclofen levels near or below 10 ng/ml.

INDICATIONS AND USAGE:

TABLETS

Baclofen is useful for the alleviation of signs and symptoms of spasticity resulting from multiple sclerosis, particularly for the relief of flexor spasms and concomitant pain, clonus, and muscular rigidity. Patients should have reversible spasticity so that baclofen treatment will aid in restoring residual function.

Baclofen may also be of some value in patients with spinal cord injuries and other spinal cord diseases.

Baclofen is not indicated in the treatment of skeletal muscle spasm resulting from rheumatic disorders.

The efficacy of baclofen in stroke, cerebral palsy, and Parkinson's disease has not been established and, therefore, it is not recommended for these conditions.

INJECTION

Baclofen injection is indicated for use in the management of severe spasticity. Patients should first respond to a screening dose of intrathecal baclofen prior to consideration for long-term infusion via an implantable pump. For spasticity of spinal cord origin, chronic infusion of baclofen intrathecal via an implantable pump should be reserved for patients unresponsive to oral baclofen therapy, or those who experience intolerable CNS side effects at effective doses. Patients with spasticity due to traumatic brain injury should wait at least one year after the injury before consideration of long-term intrathecal baclofen therapy. Baclofen injection is intended for use by the intrathecal route in single bolus test doses (via spinal catheter or lumbar puncture) and, for chronic use, only in implantable pumps approved by the FDA specifically for the administration of baclofen injection into the intrathecal space.

Spasticity of Spinal Cord Origin: Evidence supporting the efficacy of baclofen injection was obtained in randomized, controlled investigations that compared the effects of either a single intrathecal dose or a three day intrathecal infusion of baclofen injection to placebo. In patients with severe spasticity and spasms due to either spinal cord trauma or multiple sclerosis, baclofen injection was superior to placebo on both principal outcome measures employed: change from baseline in the Ashworth rating of spasticity and the frequency of spasms.

Spasticity of Cerebral Origin: Evidence supporting the efficacy of baclofen injection was obtained in randomized, controlled investigations that compared the effects of a single intrathecal dose of baclofen injection to placebo in patients with severe spasticity associated with cerebral palsy or brain injury. In both cases, an intrathecal dose of baclofen injection was superior to a placebo in reducing spasticity, as measured by the Ashworth scale. In patients with brain injury, baclofen injection was superior to placebo in both principal outcomes of change from baseline in the Ashworth rating of spasticity and the frequency of spasms.

Baclofen injection therapy may be considered an alternative to destructive neurosurgical procedures. Prior to implantation of a device for chronic intrathecal infusion of baclofen intrathecal, patients must show a response to baclofen injection in a screening trial (see DOSAGE AND ADMINISTRATION).

CONTRAINDICATIONS:

TABLETS AND INJECTION

Hypersensitivity to baclofen.

INJECTION

Hypersensitivity to baclofen. Baclofen injection is not recommended for intravenous, intramuscular, or epidural administration

WARNINGS:

TABLETS

a. Abrupt Drug Withdrawal: Hallucinations and seizures have occurred on abrupt withdrawal of baclofen. Therefore, except for serious adverse reactions, the dose should be reduced slowly when the drug is discontinued.

b. Impaired Renal Function: Because baclofen is primarily excreted unchanged through the kidneys, it should be given with caution, and it may be necessary to reduce the dosage.

c. Stroke: Baclofen has not significantly benefited patients with stroke. These patients have also shown poor tolerability to the drug.

WARNINGS: *(cont'd)*

d. Pregnancy: Baclofen has been shown to increase the incidence of omphaloceles (ventral hernias) in fetuses of rats given approximately 13 times the maximum dose recommended for human use, at a dose which caused significant reductions in food intake and weight gain in dams. This abnormality was not seen in mice or rabbits. There was also an increased incidence of incomplete sternebral ossification in fetuses of rats given approximately 13 times the maximum recommended human dose, and an increased incidence of unossified phalangeal nuclei of forelimbs and hindlimbs in fetuses of rabbits given approximately 7 times the maximum recommended human dose. In mice, no teratogenic effects were observed, although reductions in mean fetal weight with consequent delays in skeletal ossification were present when dams were given 17 or 34 times the human daily dose. There are no studies in pregnant women. Baclofen should be used during pregnancy only if the benefit clearly justifies the potential risk to the fetus.

INJECTION

Baclofen injection is for use in single bolus intrathecal injections (via a catheter placed in the lumbar intrathecal space or injection by lumbar puncture) and in implantable pumps approved by the FDA specifically for the intrathecal administration of baclofen. Because of the possibility of potentially life-threatening CNS depression, cardiovascular collapse, and/or respiratory failure, physicians must be adequately trained and educated in chronic intrathecal infusion therapy.

The pump system should not be implanted until the patient's response to bolus baclofen injection is adequately evaluated. Evaluation (consisting of a screening procedure: see DOSAGE AND ADMINISTRATION) requires that baclofen injection be administered into the intrathecal space via a catheter or lumbar puncture. Because of the risks associated with the screening procedure and the adjustment of dosage following pump implantation, these phases must be conducted in a medically supervised and adequately equipped environment following the instructions outlined in the DOSAGE AND ADMINISTRATION.

RESUSCITATIVE EQUIPMENT SHOULD BE AVAILABLE.

Following surgical implantation of the pump, particularly during the initial phases of pump use, the patient should be monitored closely until it is certain that the patient's response to the infusion is acceptable and reasonably stable.

On each occasion that the dosing rate of the pump and/or the concentration of baclofen injection in the reservoir is adjusted, close medical monitoring is required until it is certain that the patient's response to the infusion is acceptable and reasonably stable.

It is mandatory that the patient, all patient care givers, and the physicians responsible for the patient receive adequate information regarding the risks of this mode of treatment. All medical personnel and care givers should be instructed in 1) the signs and symptoms of overdose, 2) procedures to be followed in the event of overdose and 3) proper home care of the pump and insertion site.

Overdose: Signs of overdose may appear suddenly or insidiously. Acute massive overdose may present as coma. Less sudden and/or less severe forms of overdose may present with signs of CNS depression, excessive salivation, dizziness, nausea and/or vomiting, somnolence, and cephalad progression of hypotonia. Should overdose appear likely, the patient should be taken immediately to a hospital for assessment and emptying of the pump reservoir. In the cases reported to date, overdose has generally been related to pump malfunction or dosing error. (See OVERDOSAGE.)

Hallucinations: have occurred after abrupt withdrawal of baclofen injection.

Seizures have been reported during overdose with and withdrawal from baclofen injection as well as in patients maintained on therapeutic doses of baclofen injection.

FATALITIES

Spasticity of Spinal Cord Origin

There were 16 deaths reported among the 576 U.S. patients treated with the baclofen injection, in pre- and post-marketing studies evaluated as of December 1992. Because these patients were treated under uncontrolled clinical settings, it is impossible to determine definitively what role, if any, baclofen injection played in their deaths.

As a group, the patients who died were relatively young [mean age was 47 with a range from 25 to 63], but the majority suffered from severe spasticity of many years duration, were nonambulatory, had various medical complications such as pneumonia, urinary tract infections, and decubiti, and/or had received multiple concomitant medications. A case-by-case review of the clinical course of the 13 patients who died failed to reveal any unique signs, symptoms, or laboratory results that would suggest that treatment with baclofen injection caused their deaths. Two patients, however, did suffer sudden and unexpected death within 2 weeks of pump implantation.

One patient, a 44 year-old male with MS, died in hospital on the second day following pump implantation. An autopsy demonstrated severe fibrosis of the coronary conduction system. A second patient, a 52 year-old woman with MS and a history of an inferior wall myocardial infarction, was found dead in bed 12 days after pump implantation, 2 hours after having had documented normal vital signs. An autopsy revealed pulmonary congestion and bilateral pleural effusions. It is impossible to determine whether baclofen injection contributed to these deaths. The third patient underwent three baclofen screening trials. His medical history included SCI, aspiration pneumonia, septic shock, disseminated intravascular coagulopathy, severe metabolic acidosis, hepatic toxicity, and status epilepticus. Twelve days after screening (he was not implanted), he again experienced status epilepticus with subsequent significant neurological deterioration. Based upon prior instruction, extraordinary resusitative measures were not pursued and the patient died.

Spasticity of Cerebral Origin

There were three deaths occuring among the 211 patients treated with baclofen intrathecal in pre-marketing studies as of March, 1996. These deaths were not attributed to the therapy.

PRECAUTIONS:

TABLETS

Safe use of baclofen in children under 12 has not been established, and it is, therefore, not recommended for use in children. Because of the possibility of sedation, patients should be cautioned regarding the operation of automobiles or other dangerous machinery, and activities made hazardous by decreased alertness. Patients should also be cautioned that the central nervous system effects of baclofen may be additive to those of alcohol and other CNS depressants.

Baclofen should be used with caution where spasticity is utilized to sustain upright posture and balance in locomotion or whenever spasticity is utilized to obtain increased function.

In patients with epilepsy, the clinical state and electroencephalogram should be monitored at regular intervals, since deterioration in seizure control and EEG have been reported occasionally in patients taking baclofen. It is not known whether this drug is excreted in human milk. As a general rule, nursing should not be undertaken while a patient is on a drug since many drugs are excreted in human milk.

A dose-related increase in incidence of ovarian cysts and a less marked increase in enlarged and/or hemorrhagic adrenal glands was observed in female rats treated chronically with baclofen.

PRECAUTIONS: *(cont'd)*

Ovarian cysts have been found by palpation in about 4% of the multiple sclerosis patients that were treated with baclofen for up to one year. In most cases these cysts disappeared spontaneously while patients continued to receive the drug. Ovarian cysts are estimated to occur spontaneously in approximately 1% to 5% of the normal female population.

INJECTION

Children should be sufficient in body mass to accomodate the implantable pump for chronic infusion. Please consult pump manufacturer's manual for specific recommendations.

The safe use of baclofen injection in children under age 4 has not been established.

SCREENING

Patients should be infection-free prior to the screening trial with baclofen injection because the presence of a systemic infection may interfere with an assessment of the patient's response to bolus baclofen injection.

PUMP IMPLANTATION

Patients should be infection-free prior to pump implantation because the presence of infection may increase the risk of surgical complications. Moreover, a systemic infection may complicate dosing.

PUMP DOSE ADJUSTMENT AND TITRATION

In most patients, it will be necessary to increase the dose gradually over time to maintain effectiveness; a sudden requirement for substantial dose escalation typically indicates a catheter complication (*i.e.,* catheter kink or dislodgement).

Reservoir refilling must be performed by fully trained and qualified personnel following the directions provided by the pump manufacturer. Refill intervals should be carefully calculated to prevent depletion of the reservoir, as this would result in the return of severe spasticity and possibly symptoms of withdrawal.

Strict aseptic technique in filling is required to avoid bacterial contamination and serious infection. A period of observation appropriate to the clinical situation should follow each refill or manipulation of the drug reservoir.

Extreme caution must be used when filling an FDA approved implantable pump equipped with an injection port that allows direct access to the intrathecal catheter. Direct injection into the catheter through the access port may cause a life-threatening overdose.

ADDITIONAL CONSIDERATIONS PERTAINING TO DOSAGE ADJUSTMENT

It may be important to titrate the dose to maintain some degree of muscle tone and allow occasional spasms in order to: 1) help support circulatory function, 2) possibly prevent the formation of deep vein thrombosis, and 3) optimize activities of daily living and ease of care.

Except in overdose related emergencies, the dose of baclofen injection should ordinarily be reduced slowly if the drug is discontinued for any reason.

An attempt should be made to discontinue concomitant oral antispasticity medication to avoid possible overdose or adverse drug interactions, preferably prior to initiation of baclofen injection infusion, with careful monitoring by the physician. Abrupt reduction or discontinuation of concomitant antispastics, however, during chronic baclofen injection therapy should be avoided.

Drowsiness: Drowsiness has been reported in patients on baclofen injection. Patients should be cautioned regarding the operation of automobiles or other dangerous machinery, and activities made hazardous by decreased alertness. Patients should also be cautioned that the central nervous system depressant effects of baclofen injection may be additive to those of alcohol and other CNS depressants.

PRECAUTIONS IN SPECIAL PATIENT POPULATIONS

Careful dose titration of baclofen intrathecal is needed when spasticity is necessary to sustain upright posture and balance in locomotion or whenever spasticity is used to obtain optimal function and care.

Patients suffering from psychotic disorders, schizophrenia, or confusional states should be treated cautiously with baclofen injection and kept under careful surveillance, because exacerbations of these conditions have been observed with oral administration.

Baclofen injection should be used with caution in patients with a history of autonomic dysreflexia. The presence of nociceptive stimuli or abrupt withdrawal of baclofen injection may cause an autonomic dysreflexic episode.

Because baclofen injection is primarily excreted unchanged by the kidneys, it should be given with caution in patients with impaired renal function and it may be necessary to reduce the dosage.

LABORATORY TESTS

No specific laboratory tests are deemed essential for the management of patients on baclofen injection.

CARCINOGENESIS, MUTAGENESIS, AND IMPAIRMENT OF FERTILITY

No increase in tumors was seen in rats receiving baclofen USP orally for two years at approximately 30-60 times on a mg/kg basis, or 10-20 times on a mg/m^2 basis, the maximum oral dose recommended for human use. Mutagenicity assays with baclofen have not been performed.

PREGNANCY CATEGORY C

Baclofen USP given orally has been shown to increase the incidence of omphaloceles (ventral hernias) in fetuses of rats given approximately 13 times on a mg/kg basis, or 3 times on a mg/m^2 basis, the maximum oral dose recommended for human use; this dose also caused reductions in food intake and weight gain in the dams.

This abnormality was not seen in mice or rabbits. There are no adequate and well-controlled studies in pregnant women. Baclofen should be used during pregnancy only if the potential benefit justifies the potential risk to the fetus.

NURSING MOTHERS

In mothers treated with oral baclofen USP in therapeutic doses, the active substance passes into the breast milk. It is not known whether detectable levels of drug are present in breast milk of nursing mothers receiving baclofen injection. As a general rule, nursing should be undertaken while a patient is receiving baclofen injection only if the potential benefit justifies the potential risks to the infant.

PEDIATRIC USE

Children should be of sufficient body mass to accomodate the implantable pump for chronic infusion. Please consult pump manufacturer's manual for specific recommendations.

The safe use of baclfen intrathecal in children under age 4 has not been established.

CONSIDERATIONS BASED ON EXPERIENCE WITH ORAL BACLOFEN USP

A dose-related increase in incidence of ovarian cysts was observed in female rats treated chronically with oral baclofen. Ovarian cysts have been found by palpation in about 4% of the multiple sclerosis patients who were treated with oral baclofen for up to one year. In most cases these cysts disappeared spontaneously while patients continued to receive the drug. Ovarian cysts are estimated to occur spontaneously in approximately 1% to 5% of the normal female population.

DRUG INTERACTIONS:

INJECTION

There is inadequate systematic experience with the use of baclofen injection in combination with other medications to predict specific drug-drug interactions. Interactions attributed to the combined use of baclofen injection and epidural morphine include hypotension and dyspnea.

ADVERSE REACTIONS:

TABLETS

The most common is transient drowsiness (10-63%). In one controlled study of 175 patients, transient drowsiness was observed in 63% of those receiving baclofen compared to 36% of those in the placebo group. Other common adverse reactions are dizziness (5-15%), weakness (5-15%) and fatigue (2-4%). Others reported:

Neuropsychiatric: Confusion (1-11%), headache (4-8%), insomnia (2-7%); and, rarely, euphoria, excitement, depression, hallucinations, paresthesia, muscle pain, tinnitus, slurred speech, coordination disorder, tremor, rigidity, dystonia, ataxia, blurred vision, nystagmus, strabismus, miosis, mydriasis, diplopia, dysarthria, epileptic seizure.

Cardiovascular: Hypotension (0.9%). Rare instances of dyspnea, palpitation, chest pain, syncope.

Gastrointestinal: Nausea (4-12%), constipation (2-6%); and, rarely, dry mouth, anorexia, taste disorder, abdominal pain, vomiting, diarrhea, and positive test for occult blood in stool.

Genitourinary: Urinary frequency (2-6%); and, rarely, enuresis, urinary retention, dysuria, impotence, inability to ejaculate, nocturia, hematuria.

Other: Instances of rash, pruritus, ankle edema, excessive perspiration, weight gain, nasal congestion.

Some of the CNS and genitourinary symptoms may be related to the underlying disease rather than to the drug therapy.

The following laboratory tests have been found to be abnormal in a few patients receiving baclofen: increased SGOT, elevated alkaline phosphatase, and elevation of blood sugar.

INJECTION

Commonly Observed in Patients with Spasticity of Spinal Origin: In pre- and post-marketing clinical trials, the most commonly observed adverse events associated with the use of baclofen intrathecal which were not seen at an equivalent incidence among placebo-treated patients were: somnolence, dizziness, nausea, hypotension, headache, convulsions, and hypotonia.

Associated With Discontinuation of Treatment: 8/474 patients with spasticity of spinal cord origin receiving long term infusion of baclofen injection in pre- and post-marketing clinical studies in the U.S. discontinued treatment due to adverse events. These include: pump pocket infections (3), meningitis (2), wound dehiscence (1), gynocological fibroids (1), and pump overpressurization (1) with unknown, if any, sequela. Eleven patients who developed coma secondary to overdose had their reatment temporarily suspended, but all were subsequently re-started and were not, therefore, considered to be true discontinuations.

Fatalities: see WARNINGS.

SPASTICITY OF SPINAL CORD ORIGIN

Incidence in Controlled Trials: Experience with baclofen injection obtained in parallel, placebo-controlled, randomized studies provides only a limited basis for estimating the incidence of adverse events because the studies were of very brief duration (up to three days of infusion) and involved only a total of 63 patients. The following events occurred among the 31 patients receiving baclofen injection in two randomized, placebo-controlled trials: Hypertension (2), dizziness (2), headache (2), dyspnea (1). No adverse events were reported among the 32 patients receiving placebo in these studies.

Events Observed During the Pre- and Post-Marketing Evaluation of Baclofen Injection: Adverse events associated with the use of baclofen injection reflect experience gained with 576 patients followed prospectively in the United States. They received baclofen injection for periods of one day (screening) (N=576) to over eight years (maintenance) (N=10). The usual screening bolus dose administered prior to pump implantation in these studies was typically 50 mcg. The maintenance dose ranged from 12 mcg to 2003 mcg per day.

Because of the open, uncontrolled nature of the experience, a causal linkage between events observed and the administration of baclofen injection cannot be reliably assessed in many cases and many of the adverse events reported are known to occur in association with the underlying conditions being treated. Nonetheless, many of the more commonly reported reactions—drowsiness, dizziness, headache, nausea, hypotension, hypotonia and coma—appear clearly drug-related.

Adverse experiences reported during all domestic studies (both controlled and uncontrolled) are shown in the following table (TABLE 1). None of these adverse experiences led to a discontinuation of treatment.

In addition to the more common (1% or more) adverse events reported in the prospectively followed 576 domestic patients in pre- and post-marketing studies, experience from an additional 194 patients exposed to baclofen injection has been reported. The following adverse events, not described in the table, and arranged in decreasing order of frequency, and classified by body system, were reported:

Central Nervous System: Abnormal gait, thinking abnormal, tremor, amnesia, twitching, vasodilation, cerebrovascular accident, nystagmus, personality disorder, psychotic depression, cerebral ischemia, emotional lability, euphoria, hypertonia, ileus, drug dependance, incoordination, paranoid reaction and ptosis.

Digestive System: Flatulence, dysphagia, dyspepsia and gastroenteritis.

Cardiovascular: Postural Hypotension, bradycardia, palpitations, syncope, arrhythmia ventricular, deep thrombophlebitis, pallor and tachycardia.

Respiratory: Respiratory disorder, aspiration pneumonia, hyperventilation, pulmonary embolus, and rhinitis.

Urogenital: Hematuria and kidney failure.

Skin and Appendages: Alopecia and sweating.

Metabolic and Nutritional Disorders: Weight loss, albuminuria, dehydration, and hyperglycemia.

Special Senses: Abnormal vision, abnormality of accomodation, photophobia, taste loss, and tinnitus.

Body As A Whole: Suicide, lack of drug effect, abdominal pain, hypothermia, neck rigidity, chest pain, chills, face edema, flu syndrome, and overdose.

Hemic and Lymphatic System: Anemia

SPASTICITY OF CEREBRAL ORIGIN

Commonly Observed: In pre-marketing clinical trials, the most commonly observed adverse events associated with the use of baclofen injection which were not seen at an equivalent incidence among placebo-treated patients included: agitation, constipation, somnolence, leukocytosis, chills, fever, urinary retention, and hypotonia.

ADVERSE REACTIONS: *(cont'd)*

TABLE 1 Incidence Of Most Frequent (≥1%) Adverse Events In Patients With Spasticity Of Spinal Origin In Prospectively Monitored Clinical Studies

Adverse Event	Number of Patients Reporting Events N = 576 Screening*	N = 474 Titration†	N = 430 Maintenance‡
Hypotonia	5.4	13.5	25.3
Somnolence	5.7	5.9	20.9
Dizziness	1.7	1.9	7.9
Paresthesia	2.4	2.1	6.7
Nausea/Vomiting	1.6	2.3	5.6
Headache	1.6	2.5	5.1
Constipation	0.2	1.5	5.1
Convulsions	0.5	1.3	4.7
Urinary Retention	0.7	1.7	1.9
Dry Mouth	0.2	0.4	3.3
Accidental Injury	0.0	0.2	3.5
Asthenia	0.7	1.3	1.4
Confusion	0.5	0.6	2.3
Death	0.2	0.4	3.0
Pain	0.0	0.6	3.0
Speech Disorder	0.0	0.2	3.5
Hypotension	1.0	0.2	1.9
Ambylopia	0.5	0.2	2.3
Diarrhea	0.0	0.8	2.3
Hypoventilation	0.2	0.8	2.1
Coma	0.0	1.5	0.9
Impotence	0.2	0.4	1.6
Peripheral Edema	0.0	0.0	2.3
Urinary Incontinence	0.0	0.8	1.4
Insomnia	0.0	0.4	1.6
Anxiety	0.2	0.4	0.9
Depression	0.0	0.0	1.6
Dyspnea	0.3	0.0	1.2
Fever	0.5	0.2	0.7
Pneumonia	0.2	0.2	1.2
Urinary Frequency	0.0	0.6	0.9
Urticaria	0.2	0.2	1.2
Anorexia	0.0	0.4	0.9
Diplopia	0.0	0.4	0.9
Dysaulonomia	0.2	0.2	0.9
Hallucinations	0.3	0.4	0.5
Hypertension	0.2	0.6	0.5

*Following administration of test bolus
†Two month period following implant
‡Beyond two months following implant
(N =Total number of patients entering each period)
% = % of patients evaluated

Associated with Discontinuation of Treatment: Nine of 211 patients receiving baclofen injection in pre-marketing clinical studies in the U.S. discontinued long term infusion due to adverse events associated with intrathecal therapy.

The nine adverseevents leading to discontinuation were: three causes of infection, two cases of CSF leaks, two cases of menigitis, one case of drainage, and one case of unmanageable trunk control.

Fatalities: Three deaths, none of which were attributed to baclofen injection, were reported in patients in clinical trials involving patients with spasticity of cerebral origin. See WARNINGS on other deaths reported in spinal spasticity patients.

Incidence in Controlled Trials: Experience with baclofen injection obtained in parallel, placebo controlled, randomized studies provides only a limited basis for estimating the incidence of adverse events because the studies involved a total of 62 patients exposed to a single 50 mcg intrathecal bolus. The following events occurred among the 62 patients receiving baclofen injection in two randomized, placebo controlled trials involving cerebral palsy and head injury patients, respectively: agitation, constipation, somnolencec, leukocytosis, nausea, vomiting, nystagmus, chills, urinary retention, and hypotonia.

Events observed during the Pre-Marketing Evaluation of Baclofen Injection: Adverse events associated with the use of baclofen injection reflect experience gained with a total of 211 U.S. patients with spasticity of cerebral origin, of whom 112 were pediatric patients (under age 16 at enrollment). They received baclofen injection for periods of one day (screening) (N=211) to 84 months (maintenance) (N=1). The usual screening bolus dose administered prior to pump implantation in these studies was 50–75 mcg. The maintenance dose ranged from 22 mcg to 1400 mcg per day. Doses used in this patient population for long term infusion are generally lower than those required for patients with spasticity of spinal cord origin.

Because of the open, uncontrolled nature of the experience, a causal linkage between events observed and the administration of baclofen injection cannot be reliably assessed in many cases. Nonetheless, many of the more commonly reported reactions - somnolence, dizziness, headache, nausea, hypotension, hypotonia, and coma – appear clealy drug-related.

The most frequent (≥1%) adverse events reported during all clinical trials are shown in the following table. Nine patients discontinued long term treatment due to adverse events.

The more common (1% or more) adverse events reported in the prospectively followed 211 patients exposed to baclofen injection have been reported. In the total cohort, the following adverse events, not described in the table, arranged in decreasing order of frequency, and classified by body system, were reported:

Nervous system: Akathisia, ataxia, confusion, depression, opisthotonos, amnesia, anxiety, halluciantions, hysteria, insomnia, nystagmus, personality disorder, reflexes decreased, and vasodilation.

Digestive System: Dysphagia, fecal incontinence, gastrointestinal hemorrhage, and tongue disorder.

Cardiovascular: Bradycardia.

Respiratory: Apnea, dyspnea, and hyperventilation.

Urogenital: Abnormal ejaculation, kidney calculus, oliguria, and vaginitis.

Skin and Appendages: Rash, sweating, alopecias, contact dermatitis, and skin ulcer.

Special Senses: Abnormality of accomodation.

Body as a Whole: Death, fever, pain, abdominal pain, carcinoma, malaise, and hypothermia.

Hemic and Lymphatic System: Leukocytosis and petechial rash.

OVERDOSAGE:

TABLETS

Signs and Symptoms: Vomiting, muscular hypotonia, drowsiness, accommodation disorders, coma, respiratory depression, and seizures.

OVERDOSAGE: *(cont'd)*

TABLE 2 Incidence Of Most Frequent (≥1%) Adverse Events In Patients With Spasticity Of Spinal Origin In Prospectively Monitored Clinical Studies

Adverse Event	Number of Patients Reporting Events N = 211 Screening*	N = 153 Titration†	N = 150 Maintenance‡
Hypotonia	2.4	14.4	34.7
Somnolence	7.6	10.5	18.7
Headache	6.6	7.8	10.7
Nausea/Vomiting	6.6	10.5	4.0
Vomiting	6.2	8.5	4.0
Urinary Retention	0.9	6.5	8.0
Convulsions	0.2	1.5	5.1
Constipation	0.9	3.3	10.0
Dizziness	2.4	2.6	8.0
Nausea	1.4	3.3	7.3
Hypoventilation	1.4	1.3	4.0
Hypotonia	0.0	0.7	6.0
Paresthesia	1.9	0.7	3.3
Hypotension	1.9	0.7	2.0
Increased Salivation	0.0	2.6	2.7
Back Pain	0.9	0.7	2.0
Constipation	0.5	1.3	2.0
Pain	0.0	0.0	4.0
Pruritus	0.0	0.0	4.0
Diarrhea	0.5	0.7	2.0
Peripheral Edema	0.0	0.0	3.3
Thinking Abnormal	0.5	1.3	0.7
Agitation	0.5	0.0	1.3
Asthenia	0.0	0.0	2.0
Chills	0.5	0.0	1.3
Coma	0.5	0.0	1.3
Dry Mouth	0.5	0.0	1.3
Pneumonia	0.0	0.0	2.0
Speech Disorder	0.5	0.7	0.7
Tremor	0.5	0.0	1.3
Urinary Incontinence	0.0	0.0	2.0
Urticaria	0.2	0.2	1.2
Urination Impaired	0.0	0.0	2.0

*Following administration of test bolus
†Two month period following implant
‡Beyond two months following implant
N = Total number of patients enteringeach period. 211 patients received drug; (1 of 212) received placebo only

Treatment: In the alert patient, empty the stomach promptly by induced emesis followed by lavage. In the obtunded patient, secure the airway with a cuffed endotracheal tube before beginning lavage (do not induce emesis). Maintain adequate respiratory exchange, do not use respiratory stimulants.

INJECTION

Special attention must be given to recognizing the signs and symptoms of overdosage, especially during the initial screening and dose-titration phase of treatment, but also during re-introduction of baclofen injection after a period of interruption in therapy.

SYMPTOMS OF BACLOFEN INJECTION OVERDOSE:

Drowsiness, lightheadedness, dizziness, somnolence, respiratory depression, seizures, rostral progression of hypotonia and loss of consciousness progressing to coma of up to 24 hr duration. In all seven cases reported, coma was reversible without sequelae after infusion was stopped.

Symptoms of baclofen injection overdose were reported in a sensitive adult patient after receiving a 25 mcg intrathecal bolus.

TREATMENT SUGGESTIONS FOR OVERDOSE:

There is no specific antidote for treating overdoses of baclofen injection; however, the following steps should ordinarily be undertaken:

1) Residual baclofen injection solution should be removed from the pump as soon as possible.

2) Patients with respiratory depression should be intubated if necessary, until the drug is eliminated.

Anecdotal reports suggest that intravenous physostigmine may reverse central side effects, notably drowsiness and respiratory depression. Caution in administering physostigmine intravenously is advised, however, because its use has been associated with the induction of seizures, bradycardia, cardiac conduction disturbances.

Physostigmine Doses for Adult Patients: A total dose of 1-2 mg physostigmine may be tried intravenously over 5-10 minutes. Patients should be monitored closely during this time. Repeat doses of 1 mg may be administered at 30-60 minute intervals in an attempt to maintain adequate respiration and alertness if the patient shows a positive response.

Physostigmine Doses for Pediatric Patients: Administer 0.02 mg/kg physostigmine intravenously, do not give more than 0.5 mg per minute. The dosage may be repeated at 5 to 10 minute intervals until a therapeutic effect is obtained or a maximum dose of 2 mg is attained.

Physostigmine may not be effective in reversing large overdoses and patients may need to be maintained with respiratory support.

If lumbar puncture is not contraindicated, consideration should be given to withdrawing 30-40 ml of CSF to reduce CSF baclofen concentration.

DOSAGE AND ADMINISTRATION:

TABLETS

The determination of optimal dosage requires individual titration. Start therapy at a low dosage and increase gradually until optimum effect is achieved (usually between 40-80 mg daily).

The following dosage schedule is suggested:

5 mg t.i.d. for 3 days

10 mg t.i.d. for 3 days

15 mg t.i.d. for 3 days

20 mg t.i.d. for 3 days

Thereafter additional increases may be necessary but the total daily dose should not exceed a maximum of 80 mg daily (20 mg q.i.d.).

The lowest dose compatible with an optimal response is recommended. If benefits are not evident after a reasonable trial period, patients should be slowly withdrawn from the drug (see WARNINGS, Abrupt Drug Withdrawal).

DOSAGE AND ADMINISTRATION: *(cont'd)*

INJECTION

Refer to the manufacturer's manual for the implantable intrathecal infusion pump for specific instructions and precautions for programming the pump and/or refilling the reservoir.

Screening Phase: Prior to pump implantation and initiation of chronic infusion of baclofen injection, patients must demonstrate a positive clinical response to a baclofen injection bolus dose administered intrathecally in a screening trial. The screening trial employs baclofen injection which must be diluted to a concentration of 50 mcg per ml. The screening procedure is as follows. An initial bolus containing 50 micrograms in a volume of 1 milliliter is administered into the intrathecal space by barbotage over a period of not less than one minute. The patient is observed over the ensuing 4 to 8 hours. A positive response consists of a significant decrease in muscle tone and/or frequency and/or severity of spasms. If the initial response is less than desired, a second bolus injection may be administered 24 hours after the first. The second screening bolus dose consists of 75 micrograms in 1.5 milliliters. Again, the patient should be observed for an interval of 4 to 8 hours. If the response is still inadequate, a final bolus screening dose of 100 micrograms in 2 milliliters may be administered 24 hours later.

Pediatric Patients: The starting screening dose for pediatric patients is the same as in adult patients, i.e., 50 mcg. However, for very small patients, a screening dose of 25 mcg may be tried first.

Patients who do not respond to a 100 mcg intrathecal bolus should not be considered candidates for an implanted pump for chronic infusion.

Post-Implant Dose Titration Period: To determine the initial total daily dose of baclofen injection following implant, the screening dose that gave a positive effect should be doubled and administered over a 24-hour period, unless the efficacy of the bolus dose was maintained for more than 12 hours, in which case the starting daily dose should be the screening dose delivered over a 24-hour period. No dose increases should be given in the first 24 hours (*i.e.*, until the steady state is achieved).

Adult Patients with Spasticity of Spinal Cord Origin: After the first 24 hours, the daily dosage should be increased slowly by 10%-30% increments and only once every 24 hours, until the desired clinical effect is achieved.

Adult Patients with Spasticity of Spinal Cord Origin: After the first 224 hours, the daily dose should be increased slowly by 5–15% only once every 24 hours, until the desired clinical effect is achieved.

Pediatric Patients: After the first 24 hours, the daily dose should be increased slowly by 5–15% once every 24 hours, until the desired clinical effect is achieved.

If there is not a substantive clinical response to increases in the daily dose, check for proper pump function and catheter patency.

Patients must be monitored closely in a fully equipped and staffed environment during the screening phase and dose-titration period immediately following implant. Resuscitative equipment should be immediately available for use in case of life-threatening or intolerable side effects.

MAINTENANCE THERAPY

Spasticity of Spinal Cord Origin Patients: The clinical goal is to maintain muscle tone as close to normal as possible, and to minimize the frequency and severity of spasms to the extent possible, without inducing intolerable side effects. Very often the maintenance dose needs to be adjusted during the first few months of therapy while patients adjust to changes in life style due to the alleviation of spasticity. During periodic refills of the pump, the daily dose may be increased by 5–20%, but no more than 20% to maintain adequate symptom control. The daily dose may be reduced by 10–20% if patients experience side effects. Many patients require gradual increases in dose over time to maintain optimal response during chronic therapy. A sudden large requirement for dose escalation suggests a catheter complication (*i.e.*, catheter kink or dislodgement).

Maintenance dosage for long term continuous infusion of baclofen injection has ranged from 12 micrograms/day to 1500 micrograms/day, with most patients adequately maintained on 300 micrograms to 800 micrograms per day. There is limited experience with daily doses greater than 1000 micrograms/day. Determination of the optimal baclofen injection dose requires individual titration. The lowest dose with an optimal response should be used.

Pediatric Patients: Use same dosing recommendations for patients with spasticity of cerebral origin. Pediatric patients under 12 years seemed to require a lower daily dose in clinical trials. Average daily dose for patients under 12 years was 274 mcg/day, with a range of 24 to 1199 mcg/day. Dosage requirement for pediatric patients over 12 years does not seem to be different from that of adult patients. Determination of the optimal baclofen injection dose requires individual titration. The lowest dose with an optimal response should be used.

Potential Need For Dose Adjustments In Chronic Use: During long term treatment approximately 10% of patients become refractory to increasing doses. There is not sufficient experience to make firm recommendations for tolerance treatment; however, this "tolerance" has been treated on occasion, in hospital, by a "drug holiday" consisting of the gradual reduction of baclofen injection over a two week period and switching to alternative methods of spasticity management. After a few days, sensitivity to baclofen may return, and baclofen injection may be restarted at the initial continuous infusion dose.

STABILITY

Parenteral drug products should be inspected for particulate matter and discoloration prior to administration, whenever solution and container permit.

DELIVERY SPECIFICATIONS

The specific concentration that should be used depends on the total daily dose required as well as the delivery rate of the pump. Baclofen injection may require dilution when used with certain implantable pumps. Please consult manufacturer's manual for specific recommendations.

SCREENING

Dilution Instruction: Both strengths of baclofen injection (10 mg/5 ml and 10 mg/20 ml) must be diluted to a 50 mcg/ml concentration for bolus injection into the subarachnoid space.

MAINTENANCE

For patients who require concentrations other than 500 mcg/ml or 2000 mcg/ml, baclofen injection **must be diluted.**

Baclofen injection **must be diluted** with sterile preservative free Sodium Chloride for Injection, U.S.P.

DELIVERY REGIMEN

Baclofen injection is most often administered in a continuous infusion mode immediately following implant. For those patients implanted with programmable pumps who have achieved relatively satisfactory control on continuous infusion, further benefit may be attained using more complex schedules of baclofen injection delivery. For example, patients who have increased spasms at night may require a 20% increase in their hourly infusion rate. Changes in flow rate should be programmed to start two hours before the time of desired clinical effect.

HOW SUPPLIED:

TABLETS AND INJECTION

Tablets: *Dispense in a tight container.*

Injection: Does not require refrigeration. Do not freeze. Do not heat sterilize.

Storage: Do not store above 86°F (30°C).

HOW SUPPLIED - RATED THERAPEUTICALLY EQUIVALENT:

Tablet - Oral - 10 mg

100's	$37.05	Baclofen, Duramed Pharms	51285-0883-02
500's	$175.00	Baclofen, Duramed Pharms	51285-0883-04

Tablet - Oral - 20 mg

100's	$64.10	Baclofen, Duramed Pharms	51285-0884-02
500's	$260.05	Baclofen, Duramed Pharms	51285-0884-04

Tablet, Uncoated - Oral - 10 mg

100's	$10.28	Baclofen, H.C.F.A. F F P	99999-0361-01
100's	$10.88	Baclofen, United Res	00677-1259-01
100's	$15.23	Baclofen, US Trading	56126-0402-11
100's	$25.49	Baclofen, Balan	00304-1959-01
100's	$28.74	Baclofen, Qualitest Pharms	00603-2408-21
100's	$30.98	Baclofen, Squibb-Mark	57783-6980-01
100's	$31.00	Baclofen, Raway	00686-0668-20
100's	$31.75	Baclofen, Major Pharms	00904-3365-60
100's	$32.39	Baclofen, HL Moore Drug Exch	00839-7472-06
100's	$33.50	Atrofen, Athena	59075-0561-10
100's	$34.50	Baclofen, Teva	00332-2234-09
100's	$36.00	Baclofen, Rugby	00536-4959-01
100's	$36.10	Baclofen, Zenith Labs	00172-4096-60
100's	$36.10	Baclofen, Goldline Labs	00182-1295-01
100's	$36.20	Baclofen, Aligen Independ	00405-4110-01
100's	$36.20	Baclofen, Martec Pharms	52555-0513-01
100's	$36.25	Baclofen, Geneva Pharms	00781-1641-01
100's	$36.25	Baclofen, Royce	51875-0255-01
100's	$36.28	Baclofen, Schein Pharm (US)	00364-2312-01
100's	$36.50	Baclofen, Parmed Pharms	00349-8925-01
100's	$38.00	Baclofen, Goldline Labs	00182-1295-89
100's	$39.36	Baclofen, Schein Pharm (US)	00364-2312-90
100's	$41.00	Baclofen, Vangard Labs	00615-3541-13
100's	$41.86	Baclofen, Major Pharms	00904-3365-61
100's	**$48.96**	**LIORESAL, Novartis**	**00028-0023-01**
100's	**$51.83**	**LIORESAL, Novartis**	**00028-0023-61**
250's	$25.70	Baclofen, H.C.F.A. F F P	99999-0361-02
250's	$88.25	Baclofen Tablets 10 Mg, Zenith Labs	00172-4096-65
500's	$51.40	Baclofen, H.C.F.A. F F P	99999-0361-03
500's	$142.85	Baclofen, Major Pharms	00904-3365-40
500's	$142.88	Baclofen, Qualitest Pharms	00603-2408-28
500's	$154.31	Baclofen, HL Moore Drug Exch	00839-7472-12
500's	$162.25	Baclofen, Rugby	00536-4959-05
500's	$172.19	Baclofen, Royce	51875-0255-02
500's	$173.00	Baclofen, Martec Pharms	52555-0513-05
500's	$181.25	Baclofen, Aligen Independ	00405-4110-02
750's	$266.90	Baclofen, Glasgow Pharm	60809-0103-55
750's	$266.90	Baclofen, Glasgow Pharm	60809-0103-72
1000's	$102.80	Baclofen, H.C.F.A. F F P	99999-0361-04
1000's	$289.97	Baclofen, HL Moore Drug Exch	00839-7472-16
1000's	$331.00	Baclofen Tablets 10 Mg, Zenith Labs	00172-4096-80

Tablet, Uncoated - Oral - 20 mg

100's	$20.10	Baclofen, H.C.F.A. F F P	99999-0361-05
100's	$20.93	Baclofen, United Res	00677-1260-01
100's	$24.03	Baclofen, US Trading	56126-0403-11
100's	$43.00	Baclofen, Raway	00686-0669-20
100's	$51.11	Baclofen, Qualitest Pharms	00603-2409-21
100's	$56.69	Baclofen, HL Moore Drug Exch	00839-7473-06
100's	$56.90	Baclofen, Major Pharms	00904-3366-60
100's	$58.50	Atrofen, Athena	59075-0562-10
100's	$60.00	Baclofen, Teva	00332-2236-09
100's	$63.50	Baclofen, Rugby	00536-4960-01
100's	$63.90	Baclofen, Zenith Labs	00172-4097-60
100's	$63.90	Baclofen, Goldline Labs	00182-1296-01
100's	$63.90	Baclofen, Aligen Independ	00405-4111-01
100's	$64.00	Baclofen, Schein Pharm (US)	00364-2313-01
100's	$64.08	Baclofen, Royce	51875-0256-01
100's	$64.30	Baclofen, Martec Pharms	52555-0514-01
100's	$64.67	Baclofen, Geneva Pharms	00781-1642-01
100's	$65.06	Baclofen, Parmed Pharms	00349-8926-01
100's	$69.00	Baclofen, Goldline Labs	00182-1296-89
100's	$70.02	Baclofen, Schein Pharm (US)	00364-2313-90
100's	$73.41	Baclofen, Vangard Labs	00615-3542-13
100's	**$89.68**	**LIORESAL, Novartis**	**00028-0033-01**
100's	**$92.84**	**LIORESAL, Novartis**	**00028-0033-61**
250's	$50.25	Baclofen, H.C.F.A. F F P	99999-0361-06
250's	$157.75	Baclofen Tablets 20 Mg, Zenith Labs	00172-4097-65
500's	$100.50	Baclofen, H.C.F.A. F F P	99999-0361-07
500's	$253.80	Baclofen, Qualitest Pharms	00603-2409-28
500's	$256.05	Baclofen, Major Pharms	00904-3366-40
500's	$268.79	Baclofen, HL Moore Drug Exch	00839-7473-12
500's	$304.38	Baclofen, Royce	51875-0256-02
500's	$320.40	Baclofen, Aligen Independ	00405-4111-02
1000's	$201.00	Baclofen, H.C.F.A. F F P	99999-0361-08
1000's	$499.48	Baclofen, HL Moore Drug Exch	00839-7473-16
1000's	$609.00	Baclofen Tablets 20 Mg, Zenith Labs	00172-4097-80

HOW SUPPLIED - NOT RATED EQUIVALENT:

Kit - Intravenous - 500 mcg/ml

1's	**$198.00**	**LIORESAL INTRATHECAL, Medtronic**	**58281-0560-01**

Kit - Intravenous - 2000 mcg/ml

1's	**$420.00**	**LIORESAL INTRATHECAL, Medtronic**	**58281-0561-02**
1's	**$774.00**	**LIORESAL INTRATHECAL, Medtronic**	**58281-0561-04**

BALANCED SALT SOLUTION *(000363)*

CATEGORIES: EENT Drugs; Electrolyte Solutions; Eye, Ear, Nose, & Throat Preparations; Homeostatic & Nutrient; Ophthalmic Irrigating Solutions; Ophthalmics; FDA Pre 1938 Drugs

BRAND NAMES: Akorn Balanced Salt Solution; *Balanced Salt Solution* (England); Basol-S; **BSS**; I-Sol; Iocare; Spectro-Balanced Salt; Storz B.S.I.S.
(International brand names outside U.S. in italics)

DESCRIPTION:

This monograph contains prescribing information for BSS Sterile Irrigating Solution (250 ml and 500 ml), BSS Sterile Irrigating Solution (15 ml and 30 ml), where noted and BSS Plus Sterile Intraocular Irrigating Solution.

BSS Sterile Irrigating Solution: BSS Sterile Irrigating Solution is a sterile physiological balanced salt solution, each ml, containing Sodium Chloride (NaCl) 0.64%, Potassium Chloride (KCl) 0.075%, Calcium Chloride Dihydrate ($CaCl_2{\cdot}2H_2O$) 0.048%, Magnesium Chloride Hexahydrate ($MgCl_2{\cdot}6H_2O$) 0.03%, Sodium Acetate Trihydrate ($C_2H_3NaO_2{\cdot}3H_2O$) 0.39%, Sodium Citrate Dihydrate ($C_6H_5Na_3O_7{\cdot}2H_2O$) 0.17%, Sodium Hydroxide and/or Hydrochloric Acid (to adjust pH), and Water for Injection.

BSS Sterile Irrigating Solution is isotonic to the tissues of the eyes. It is a lint-free solution containing essential ions for normal cell metabolism.

BSS Plus: BBS Plus is a sterile intraocular irrigating solution for use during all intraocular surgical procedures even those requiring a relatively long intraocular perfusion time (*e.g.,* pars plana vitrectomy, phacoemulsification, extracapsular cataract extraction/lens aspiration, anterior segment reconstruction, etc.). The solution does not contain a preservative and should be prepared just prior to use in surgery.

Part I: Part I is a sterile 480 ml solution in a 500 ml single-dose bottle to which the Part II concentrate is added. Each ml of Part I contains: Sodium Chloride 7.44 mg, Potassium Chloride 0.395 mg, Dibasic Sodium Phosphate 0.433 mg, Sodium Bicarbonate 2.19 mg, Hydrochloric Acid and/or Sodium Hydroxide (to adjust pH), in Water for Injection.

Part II: Part II is a sterile concentrate in a 20 ml single-dose vial addition to Part I. Each ml of Part II contains: Calcium Chloride Dihydrate 3.85 mg, Magnesium Chloride Hexahydrate 5 mg, Dextrose 23 mg, Glutathione Disulfide (Oxidized Glutathione) 4.6 mg, in Water for Injection.

After addition of BSS Plus Part II to the Part I bottle, each ml of the reconstituted product contains: Sodium Chloride 7.14 mg, Potassium Chloride 0.38 mg, Calcium Chloride Dihydrate 0.154 mg, Magnesium Chloride Hexahydrate 0.2 mg, Dibasic Sodium Phosphate 0.42 mg, Sodium Bicarbonate 2.1 mg, Dextrose 0.92 mg, Glutathione Disulfide (Oxidized Glutathione) 0.184 mg, Hydrochloric Acid and/or Sodium Hydroxide (to adjust pH), in Water for Injection.

The reconstituted product has a pH of approximately 7.4. Osmolality is approximately 305 mOsm.

CLINICAL PHARMACOLOGY:

BSS Sterile Irrigating Solution: A physiologic irrigating solution.

BSS Plus: None of the components of BBS Plus are foreign to the eye, and BSS Plus has no pharmacological action. Human perfused cornea studies have shown BBS Plus to be an effective irrigation solution for providing corneal detumescence and maintaining corneal endothelial integrity during intraocular perfusion. An *in vivo* study in rabbits has shown that BSS Plus is more suitable than normal since saline or Balanced Salt Solution for intravitreal irrigation because BBS Plus contains the appropriate bicarbonate pH, and ionic composition necessary for the maintenance of normal retinal electrical activity. Human *in vivo* studies have demonstrated BSS Plus to be safe and effective when used during surgical procedures such as pars plana vitrectomy, phacoemulsification, cataract extraction/lens aspiration, anterior segment reconstruction.

INDICATIONS AND USAGE:

BSS Sterile Irrigating Solution: For irrigation during various surgical procedures of the eyes, ears, nose and/or throat.

BSS Plus: BSS Plus is indicated for use as an intraocular irrigating solution during intraocular surgical procedures involving perfusion of the eye.

CONTRAINDICATIONS:

BSS Plus: There are no specific contraindications to the use of BSS Plus, however, contraindications for the surgical procedure during which BSS Plus is to be used should be strictly adhered to.

WARNINGS:

BSS Sterile Irrigating Solution (250 ml and 500 ml): NOT FOR INJECTION OR INTRAVENOUS INFUSION.

Do not use unless product is clear, seal is intact, vacuum is present and container is undamaged. Do not use if product is discolored or contains a precipitate.

BSS Sterile Irrigating Solution (15 ml and 30 ml): If blister or paper backing is damaged or broken, sterility of the enclosed bottle cannot be assured. Open under aseptic conditions only.

BSS Plus: For irrigation during opthalmic surgery only. Not for injection or intravenous infusion. Do not use unless product is clear, seal is intact, vacuum is present and container is undamaged. Do not use if product is discolored or contains a precipitate.

PRECAUTIONS:

BSS Sterile Irrigating Solution (250 ml and 500 ml): Discard unused contents. **Do not use this container for more than one patient. Do not use additives with this product. Tissue damage could result if other drugs are added to product.**

The solution contains no preservative.

Studies suggest that intraocular irrigating solutions which are isosmotic with normal aqueous fluids should be used with caution in diabetic patients undergoing vitrectomy since intraoperative lens changes have been observed.

There have been reports of corneal clouding or edema following ocular surgery in which BBS sterile irrigating solution was used as an irrigating solution. As in all surgical procedures appropriate measures should be taken to minimize trauma to the cornea and other ocular tissues.

BSS Sterile Irrigating Solution (15 ml and 30 ml): This solution contains no preservative and should not be used for more than one patient. Prior to use, check the following: tip should be firmly in place, irrigating needle should be properly seated; squeeze out several drops before inserting into anterior chamber, The needle shouldbe removed from the anterior chamber prior to releasing pressure to prevent suction.

The addition of any medication to BSS solution may result in damage to intraocular tissue. Studies suggest that intraocular irrigating solutions which are iso-osmotic with normal aqueous fluids should be used with caution in diabetic patients undergoing vitrectomy sonce introperative lens changes have been observed.

There have been reports of corneal clouding or edema following ocular surgery in which BSS solution was used as an irrigating solution. As in all surgical procedures appropriate measures should be taken to minimize trauma to the cornea and other ocular tissues.

BBS Plus: DO NOT USE BSS PLUS UNTIL RECONSTITUTED. Discard unused contents. BBS plus does not contain a preservative, therefore, do not use this container for more than one patient. Do not use additives other than BBS plus concentrate part II (20 ml) with this product. Tissue damage could result if other drugs are added to product. DISCARD ANY UNUSED PORTION SIX HOURS AFTER PREPARATION. Studies suggest that in-

PRECAUTIONS: *(cont'd)*

traocular irrigating solutions which are iso-osmotic with normal aqueous fluids should be used with caution in diabetic patients undergoing vitrectomy since intraoperative lens changes have been observed.

There have been reports of corneal clouding or edema following ocular surgery in which BBS plus was used as an imaging solution. As in all surgical procedures appropriate measures should be taken to minimize trauma to the cornea and other ocular tissues.

Preparation: Reconstitute BBS plus just prior to use in surgery. Follow the same strict aseptic procedures in the reconstitution of BBS plus as is used for intravenous additives. Pull the tab to remove the outer aluminum ring and dust cover from the BSS plus part I (480 ml) bottle. Remove the blue flip-off seal from BSS plus part II (20 ml) vial. Clean and disinfect the rubber stoppers on both containers by using a BSS plus vacuum transfer device (provided). An alternative method of solution transfer may be accomplished by using a 20 ml to the part I container through the target area of the rubber stopper. An excess volume of part II is provided in each vial. Gently agitate the contents to mix the solution. Place a sterile cap on the bottle. Remove the tear-off portion of the label. Record the time and date of reconstitution and the patient's name on the bottle label.

ADVERSE REACTIONS:

BSS Sterile Irrigating Solution: When the corneal endothelium is abnormal, irrigation or any other trauma may result in bullous keratopathy. Post-operative inflammatory reactions as well as incidents of corneal edema and corneal decompensation have been reported. Their relationship to the use of BSS sterile irrigating solution has not been established.

BBS Plus: Postoperative inflammatory reactions as well as incidents of corneal edema and corneal decompensation have been reported. Their relationship to the use of BSS plus has not been established.

OVERDOSAGE:

BSS Plus: The solution has no pharmacological action and thus no potential for overdosage. However, as with any intraocular surgical procedure, the duration of intraocular manipulation should be kept to a minimum.

DOSAGE AND ADMINISTRATION:

BSS Sterile Irrigating Solution (250 ml and 500 ml): This irrigating solution should be used accordingly to standard format for each surgical procedure. **Note:** Use an administration set with an air inlet in the plastic spike since the bottle does not contain a seperate airway tube. Follow directions of the particular administration set to be used. Pull the tab to remove the outer aluminum ring and dust cover. Insert the spike aseptically into the bottle through the target area of the rubber stopper. Allow the fluid to flow and remove air fromt he tubing before irrigation begins.

BSS Sterile Irrigating Solution (15 ml and 30 ml): The adapter plug is designed to accept an irrigating needle. Tissues may irrigated by attaching the needle to the DROP-TAINER bottle as explained below. External irrigation may be done without the irrigating needle.

Method of using Adapter Plug for LUER-LOK* Hub Ophthalmic Irrigating Needle:

1. Aseptically remove DROP-TAINER bottle from blister by peeling paper backing.

2. Snap on surgeon's sterile irrigation needle. Push until firmly in place and twist slightly.

3. Test assembly for proper function before use.

***NOTE:** LUER-LOK is a registered trademark of Becton, Dickinson and Company.

PATIENT PACKAGE INSERT:

BSS Plus: RECONSTITUTION INSTRUCTIONS

Directions: Use Aseptic Technique

1. Pull the tab to remove the outer aluminum ring and dust cover from the BSS plus part I (480 ml) bottle. Remove the blue flip-off seal from the BSS plus part II (20 ml) vial. Prepare the stoppers on both parts by using sterile alcohol wipes.

2. Peel open a BSS plus vacuum transfer device package (supplied) and remove the sterile transfer spike.

NOTE: This device is vented permitting air to enter vial solution transfer, thereby preventing the creation of a vacuum inside the vial. An air-inlet filter is provided to protect the system. Do not remove the air-inlet filter.

3. Remove protector from the white plastic piercing pin.

4. Firmly grasp device from behind the flange and insert the white plastic piercing pin into the upright rubber stopper of the BSS plus part II (20 ml) vial.

5. Remove guard from filter needle. Firmly grasp vial in the palm of one hand and with thumb and index finger, hold plastic flange against top of vial.

6. Invert vial and immediately insert filter needle into the rubber injection site of the BSS plus part I (480 ml) bottle.

7. Fluid will automatically transfer from the vial into the large vacuum bottle unless filter becomes occluded or loss of vacuum occurs. *NOTE:* An excess amount of BSS plus part II is provided in each vial. A non-transferred solution residual of approximately 0.3 ml can be expected to remain in the vial.

8. Immediately remove needle from the BSS plus part I container and discard it after solution transfer has ben completed.

9. Place a sterile safety cap over the rubber stopper of part I if the solution is not going to be used immediately. Mix the solution gently until uniform. Peel off the right-hand side of part I bottle label (fully reconstituted BSS plus solution). Record the patient's name and the date and time of reconstitution. BSS plus solution is now ready for use.

Alternative Transfer Method: If preferred, the contents of the BSS plus part II component may be aspirated with an 18-gauge cannula attached to a 20 ml syringe and then transferred into the Part I bottle.

HOW SUPPLIED:

BSS Sterile Solution (250 ml and 500 ml): In 250 ml and 500 ml bottles.

Storage: Store at 46° to 80°G (8° to 27°C)

BSS Sterile Solution (15 ml and 30 ml): In 15 ml and 30 ml sterile DROP-TAINER bottles.

Storage: Store at 46° to 80°F (8° to 27°C).

BSS Plus: This product is supplied in two packages for reconstitution prior to use: a 500 ml bottle containing 480 ml (Part I) and a 20 ml vial (Part II). See the PRECAUTIONS and Preparation sections for information concerning reconstitution of the solution.

Storage: Store Part I and Part II at 46° - 80°F (8°-27°C). Discard prepared solution after six hours.

HOW SUPPLIED - RATED THERAPEUTICALLY EQUIVALENT:

Solution - Intraocular; Ir

500 ml	**$372.00**	**BSS PLUS, Alcon**	**00065-0800-50**

HOW SUPPLIED - NOT RATED EQUIVALENT:

Solution - Intraocular; Ir

15 ml x 36	**$209.25**	**BSS, Alcon**	**00065-0795-15**
18 ml	$6.56	AKORN BALANCED SALT, Akorn	17478-0920-19
30 ml x 20	**$187.50**	**BSS, Alcon**	**00065-0795-30**
500 ml	$19.31	AKORN BALANCED SALT, Akorn	17478-0920-90
500 ml	$22.00	Balanced Salt, Raway	00686-8100-50
500 ml	$26.34	AMERISAL BALANCED SALT, McGaw	00264-2401-10
500 ml	$28.76	Balanced Salt, Baxter Hlthcare	00338-0058-02
500 ml	$30.20	BALANCED SALT, Abbott	00074-3911-03
500 ml x 6	**$136.50**	**BSS, Alcon**	**00065-0795-50**
1000 ml	$35.47	Balanced Salt, Baxter Hlthcare	00338-0058-03

Solution - Irrigation - 0.9 %

15 ml x 36	$159.59	IOCARE BALANCED SALT, Ciba Vision	00058-0740-15

BALSAM PERU; CASTOR OIL; TRYPSIN *(000366)*

CATEGORIES: Decubitus Ulcer; Dermatologicals; Enzymes; Enzymes & Digestants; Fibrinolytic & Proteolytic; Mucous Membrane Agents; Pain; Skin/Mucous Membrane Agents; Sunburn; Ulcer; Wound Care; FDA Pre 1938 Drugs

BRAND NAMES: Balsa-Derm; Dermuspray; Granulderm; **Granulex**; Granumed; Granusol; Tbc; Topi-Caid

FORMULARIES: Aetna; BC-BS

DESCRIPTION:

To avoid confusion, the brand name for this product is included in the monograph.

Each 0.82 cc contains:

Trypsin: 0.1 mg

Balsam Peru: 72.5 mg

Castor Oil: 650.0 mg

(Water Dispersible Base)

Natural amber in color.

INDICATIONS AND USAGE:

Varicose Ulcers

Decubital Ulcers

Debride Eschar

Dehiscent Wounds

Wound Healing

Sunburn

This combination drug will relieve pain and promote healing; debrides eschar and necrotic tissue physiologically; stimulates vascular bed; improves epithelization by reducing premature epithelial desiccation and cornification; reduces odor from malodorous necrotic wounds.

WARNINGS:

Do not spray on fresh arterial clots. Avoid spraying in eyes. Flammable, do not expose to fire or open flame. Contents under pressure. Do not puncture or incinerate. Do not store at temperatures above 120°F. Keep out of reach of children. Use only as directed. Intentional misuse by deliberately concentrating and inhaling the contents can be harmful or fatal.

DOSAGE AND ADMINISTRATION:

Directions: Shake well before spraying. Hold can upright 12 inches from the area to be treated. Press valve and coat wound quickly. Apply twice daily or as often as necessary. Wound may be left unbandaged or apply a wet dressing. To remove, wash gently with water. When applied to a sensitive area, a temporary stinging may be noted. The nozzle of the canister is designed for large-volume delivery of medication, therefore proper coverage of the wound site is achieved quickly.

HOW SUPPLIED - EQUIVALENTS NOT AVAILABLE:

Aerosol, Spray - Topical - 650 mg/72.5 mg/

2 oz.	**$12.75**	**GRANULEX, Dow Hickam**	**00514-0001-01**
4 oz	$13.45	BALSA-DERM, Major Pharms	00904-3678-22
4 oz	$14.00	GRANULDERM, Copley Pharm	38245-0607-14
4 oz	$15.85	GRANULDERM, Goldline Labs	00182-6056-37
4 oz.	**$17.50**	**GRANULEX, Dow Hickam**	**00514-0001-02**
113.4 ml	$14.68	Granul-Derm, Qualitest Pharms	00603-1270-54
113.4 ml	$15.00	GRANULDERM, Goldline Labs	00182-6119-37
113.4 ml	$15.27	GRANUMED, Rugby	00536-1371-97
113.4 ml	$16.65	Topi-Caid, Topi-Cana	59197-0001-01
113.4 ml	$16.80	TBC, Delta Pharma	53706-1001-01
180 ml	$14.75	GRANUMED, Rugby	00536-1371-58

BARIUM SULFATE *(000371)*

CATEGORIES: Diagnostic Agents; Pharmaceutical Adjuvants; Roentgenography; FDA Pre 1938 Drugs

BRAND NAMES: Bar-Test; Baricon; Baro-Cat; Barobag Enema Kit; Baroflave; Barosperse; Barotrast; Bartest; Bear-E-Bag Pediatric; Bear-E-Yum Gi; E-Z-Cat; Esophotrast; Hd 200 Plus; Imager Ac; Intropaste; Liqui-Coat Hd; Liquid Barosperse; Mede-Scan; Medebar M; Oratrast; Prepcat; Readi-Cat; Tomocat; Tonojug; Tonopaque

FORMULARIES: WHO

Prescribing information not available at time of publication.

HOW SUPPLIED - EQUIVALENTS NOT AVAILABLE:

Cream - Oral - 56 %

454 gm	$29.36	ESOPHOTRAST, Rhone-Poulenc Rorer	00075-0824-01

Kit - Oral

6's	$141.31	IMAGER AC, Lafayette Pharms	59081-0521-65

Kit - Rectal - 95 %

24's	$140.34	BAROBAG ENEMA KIT, Lafayette Pharms	59081-0066-12
24's	$140.34	BAROSPERSE ENEMA KIT, Lafayette Pharms	59081-0621-12
24's	$151.38	BEAR-E-BAG PEDIATRIC, Lafayette Pharms	59081-0522-06
24's	$156.15	BAROBAG ENEMA KIT, Lafayette Pharms	59081-0066-16
24's	$156.15	BAROSPERSE ENEMA KIT, Lafayette Pharms	59081-0621-16

HOW SUPPLIED - EQUIVALENTS NOT AVAILABLE: *(cont'd)*

24's	$217.32	BAROBAG ENEMA KIT, Lafayette Pharms	59081-0067-12
24's	$217.32	BAROSPERSE ENEMA KIT, Lafayette Pharms	59081-0621-32
24's	$233.13	BAROBAG ENEMA KIT, Lafayette Pharms	59081-0067-16
24's	$233.13	BAROSPERSE ENEMA KIT, Lafayette Pharms	59081-0621-36

Paste - Oral - 70 %

454 gm x 2	$59.87	INTROPASTE, Lafayette Pharms	59081-0022-02
454 gm x 12	$316.53	INTROPASTE, Lafayette Pharms	59081-0022-12

Powder, Reconstitution - Oral

6 oz x 36	$90.71	ULTRA-R, E Z Em	10361-0753-01
6 oz x 36	$97.79	POLIBAR, E Z Em	10361-0774-03
6 oz x 36	$102.74	SOL-O-PAKE, E Z Em	10361-0760-02
25 lb	$101.68	E-Z-HD, E Z Em	10361-0764-02
25 lb	$119.94	SOL-O-PAKE, E Z Em	10361-0760-03
340 g x 36	$96.65	E-Z-HD, E Z Em	10361-0764-01
1000 g x 8	$89.95	POLIBAR, E Z Em	10361-0774-01
1000 g x 8	$98.65	SOL-O-PAKE, E Z Em	10361-0760-01
1200 g x 8	$87.95	E-Z-PAQUE (E-Z-JUG), E Z Em	10361-0750-01

Powder, Reconstitution - Rectal - 94 % w/w

340 g x 24	$140.46	POLIBAR, E Z Em	10361-0500-02

Powder, Reconstitution - Rectal - 95 % w/w

340 g x 24	$140.46	E-Z-Paque, E Z Em	10361-0800-01
340 g x 24	$141.47	E-Z-PAQUE, E Z Em	10361-0800-03
340 g x 24	$157.01	E-Z-PAQUE, E Z Em	10361-0800-05
454 g x 24	$156.28	E-Z-PAQUE, E Z Em	10361-0800-02
454 g x 24	$156.28	E-Z-PAQUE, E Z Em	10361-0800-04
454 g x 24	$169.56	E-Z-PAQUE, E Z Em	10361-0800-06

Powder, Reconstitution - Rectal - 97 % w/w

284 g x 24	$132.64	SOLOPAKE, E Z Em	10361-0300-01
340 g x 24	$140.46	SOLOPAKE, E Z Em	10361-0300-02
340 g x 24	$140.46	SOLOPAKE, E Z Em	10361-0300-08
397 g x 24	$149.60	SOLOPAKE, E Z Em	10361-0300-03
454 g x 24	$156.28	SOLOPAKE, E Z Em	10361-0300-04
454 g x 24	$156.28	POLIBAR, E Z Em	10361-0500-04
510 g x 24	$174.08	SOLOPAKE, E Z Em	10361-0300-05
567 x 24	$183.55	SOLOPAKE, E Z Em	10361-0300-06
700 g x 8	$68.53	POLIBAR (LIQUI-JUG), E Z Em	10361-0774-02
11350 gm	$112.93	Barosperse, Lafayette Pharms	59081-0621-25

Suspension - Oral - 1.1 % w/w

225 ml x 24	$77.75	E-Z-CAT, E Z Em	10361-0720-01

Suspension - Oral - 1.2 % w/v

450 ml x 24	$83.81	Readi-Cat, E Z Em	10361-0728-00
450 ml x 24	$83.82	READI-CAT, E Z Em	10361-0728-01
900 ml x 12	$81.00	Readi-Cat, E Z Em	10361-0721-00
900 ml x 12	$81.08	READI-CAT, E Z Em	10361-0728-03
1900 ml x 4	$43.24	Readi-Cat, E Z Em	10361-0724-00
1900 ml x 4	$43.31	READI-CAT, E Z Em	10361-0728-02

Suspension - Oral - 1.5 %

200 ml x 24	$80.30	Bear-E-Yum Ct, Lafayette Pharms	59081-0524-07
300 ml x 24	$81.72	Baro-Cat, Lafayette Pharms	59081-0622-03
450 ml x 24	$83.70	Prepcat, Lafayette Pharms	59081-0126-45
900 ml x 12	$81.00	Baro-Cat, Lafayette Pharms	59081-0622-09
1900 ml x 4	$43.24	Baro-Cat, Lafayette Pharms	59081-0622-19

Suspension - Oral - 2 % w/v

250 ml x 36	$99.00	MEDE-SCAN, Lafayette Pharms	59081-0729-22
450 ml x 24	$83.70	MEDE-SCAN 2.2%, Lafayette Pharms	59081-0729-45
450 ml x 24	$83.81	Readi-Cat 2, E Z Em	10361-0723-00
450 ml x 24	$83.82	READI-CAT 2, E Z Em	10361-0723-01
900 ml x 12	$81.00	Readi-Cat 2, E Z Em	10361-0729-00
900 ml x 12	$81.08	READI-CAT 2, E Z Em	10361-0723-03
1900 ml x 4	$43.21	READI-CAT 2, E Z Em	10361-0723-02
1900 ml x 4	$43.24	Readi-Cat 2, E Z Em	10361-0726-00

Suspension - Oral - 3 % w/v

30 g x 24	$86.23	ESOPHO-CAT, E Z Em	10361-0738-01

Suspension - Oral - 4.6 %

225 ml x 24	$77.71	E-Z-CAT, E Z Em	10361-0720-00

Suspension - Oral - 5 %

145 ml x 24	$78.47	TOMOCAT, Lafayette Pharms	59081-0222-24
225 ml x 24	$77.65	TOMOCAT 1000, Lafayette Pharms	59081-0222-08

Suspension - Oral - 60 % w/v

200 ml x 24	$64.22	BEAR-E-YUM GI, Lafayette Pharms	59081-0525-07
355 ml x 24	$75.74	LIQUID BAROSPERSE, Lafayette Pharms	59081-0325-24
1900 ml x 4	$55.18	LIQUID BAROSPERSE, Lafayette Pharms	59081-0325-19
1900 ml x 4	$55.23	E-Z-PAQUE, E Z Em	10361-0186-01

Suspension - Oral - 72 % w/v

1900 ml x 4	$69.48	SOL-O-PAKE, E Z Em	10361-0172-01

Suspension - Oral - 80 % w/v

1900 ml x 4	$95.22	ENTERO-H, E Z Em	10361-0147-01

Suspension - Oral - 92 %

11350 ml	$212.93	ORATRAST, Rhone-Poulenc Rorer	00075-0812-01

Suspension - Oral - 92.5 %

11350 ml	$212.93	BAROTRAST, Rhone-Poulenc Rorer	00075-0821-01

Suspension - Oral - 95 %

180 ml	$78.28	Tonopaque, Lafayette Pharms	59081-0223-36
225 ml x 36	$104.41	Barosperse, Lafayette Pharms	59081-0621-08
900 ml x 8	$95.69	Barosperse, Lafayette Pharms	59081-0626-09
1200 ml x 8	$87.84	Tonojug, Lafayette Pharms	59081-0223-08
1900 ml x 4	$94.62	IMAGER AC, Lafayette Pharms	59081-0521-19
11350 gm	$88.87	Tonopaque, Lafayette Pharms	59081-0223-01

Suspension - Oral - 98 %

312 ml x 36	$95.14	HD 200 PLUS, Lafayette Pharms	59081-0128-08
340 ml x 36	$96.45	BARICON, Lafayette Pharms	59081-0628-12

Suspension - Oral - 120 % w/v

480 gm x 12	$373.00	E-Z-PASTE, E Z Em	10361-0770-01

Suspension - Oral - 210 %

150 ml x 24	$76.86	LIQUI-COAT HD, Lafayette Pharms	59081-0328-24

Suspension - Oral - 220 % w/v

150 ml x 24	$73.94	LIQUID HD, E Z Em	10361-0155-01

Suspension - Rectal - 1.2 % w/v

400 ml x 10	$73.61	CAT-PAK, E Z Em	10361-0410-01

HOW SUPPLIED - EQUIVALENTS NOT AVAILABLE: *(cont'd)*

Suspension - Rectal - 100 % w/v

1900 ml x 4	$94.74	LIQUID POLIBAR, E Z Em	10361-0164-01
1900 ml x 4	$94.74	E-Z-AC, E Z Em	10361-0178-01

Suspension - Rectal - 105 % w/v

650 ml x 6	$120.80	LIQUID POLIBAR PLUS, E Z Em	10361-0168-01
1900 ml x 4	$94.64	LIQUID POLIBAR PLUS, E Z Em	10361-0168-02

Tablet, Uncoated - Oral - 10 grain

100's	$63.72	BAR-TEST, Glenwood	00516-0130-01
100's	$140.00	E-Z-DISK, E Z Em	10361-0778-01

BECLOMETHASONE DIPROPIONATE *(000376)*

CATEGORIES: Adrenal Corticosteroids; Airway Obstruction; Allergies; Anti-Inflammatory Agents; Antiasthmatics/Bronchodilators; Asthma; Bronchitis; EENT Drugs; Eye, Ear, Nose, & Throat Preparations; Hormones; Nasal Congestion; Nasal Polyps; Respiratory & Allergy Medications; Rhinitis; Steroids; Sales >$500 Million; FDA Approval Pre 1982; Patent Expiration 1994 Dec; Top 200 Drugs

BRAND NAMES: *Aerobec* (Mexico, Germany); *Alanase*; *Aldecin* (Australia); *Aldecina*; *Aldecine* (France); *Andion*; *Atomase*; *Beclate*; *Beclocort Nasel*; *Becloforte*; *Beclomet* (Germany); *Beclomet Nasal*; Beclometasone; *Beclorhinol* (Germany); *Becloturmant* (Germany); **Beclovent**; *Beconase* (Australia, Germany, England, France, Mexico, Canada); Beconase AQ; *Becotide* (Asia, Australia, Europe, Mexico); *Clenil*; *Respocort*; *Rhino Clenil*; *Rhinocort*; Vancenase; Vanceril; *Viarex*; *Viarox*; *Xiten* *(International brand names outside U.S. in italics)*

FORMULARIES: Aetna; BC-BS; CIGNA; DoD; FHP; Humana; Foundation; Kaiser; Medco; Medi-Cal; PCS; PruCare; United; WHO

PRIMARY ICD9: 493.90 (Asthma, Unspecified, Without Mention of Status Asthmaticus)

DESCRIPTION:

Beclomethasone dipropionate, USP, the active component of beclomethasone dipropionate oral and nasal inhalers, is an anti-inflammatory corticosteroid having the chemical name 9-chloro-11β,17,21-trihydroxy-16β-methylpregna-1,4-diene-3,20-doine17,21-dipropionate. Beclomethasone 17, 21-dipropionate is a diester of beclomethasone, a synthetic corticosteroid which is chemically related to dexamethasone. Beclomethasone differs from dexamethasone only in having a chlorine at the 9α carbon in place of fluorine and in having a 16β-methyl group instead of a 16α-methyl group.

INHALATION FORMS

Beclomethasone dipropionate is a white to creamy white, odorless powder with a molecular formula of $C_{28}H_{37}ClO_7$ and a molecular weight of 521.25 (double strength 521.05). It is very slightly soluble in water, very soluble in chloroform, and freely soluble in acetone and in alcohol.

Beclomethasone dipropionate oral and nasal inhalers are pressurized metered-dose aerosol units containing a microcrystalline suspension of beclomethasone dipropionate-trichloromonofluoromethane clathrate in a mixture of propellants (trichloromonofluoromethane and dichlorodifluoromethane) with oleic acid. Each canister contains beclomethasone dipropionate-trichloromonofluoromethane clathrate having a molecular proportion of beclomethasone dipropionate, USP, to trichloromonofluoromethane between 3:1 and 3:2.

Beconase Nasal Inhaler: Each actuation delivers from the compact actuator a quantity of clathrate equivalent to 42 mcg of beclomethasone dipropionate, USP. The contents of one 6.7 g nasal inhaler canister provide at least 80 metered doses and the contents of one 16.8 g nasal inhaler canister provide at least 200 metered doses.

Beclovent Oral Inhaler: Each actuation delivers from the mouthpiece a quantity of clathrate equivalent to 42 mcg of beclomethasone dipropionate, USP. The contents of one 6.7-g oral inhaler canister provide at least 80 oral inhalations, and the contents of one 16.8-g oral inhaler canister provide at least 200 oral inhalations.

Vanceril 84 mcg Oral Inhaler: Each actuation delivers a quantity of clathrate equivalent to 84 mcg of beclomethasone dipropionate, USP, from the mouthpiece and 100 mcg of beclomethasone dipropionate from the valve. The contents of the 5.4 g and 12.2 g canisters provide at 40 and 120 oral inhalations, respectively. (See HOW SUPPLIED.)

NASAL SPRAY

Beclomethasone dipropionate, monohydrate is a white to creamy-white, odorless powder with a molecular weight of 539.06. It is very slightly soluble in water, very soluble in chloroform, and freely soluble in acetone and in alcohol.

This form is a metered-dose, manual pump spray unit containing a microcrystalline suspension of beclomethasone dipropionate, monohydrate equivalent to 0.042% w/ beclomethasone dipropionate calculated on the dried basis in an aqueous medium containing microcrystalline cellulose, carboxymethylcellulose sodium, dextrose, benzalkonium chloride, polysorbate 80, and 0.25% v/w phenylethyl alcohol; hydrochloric acid may be added to adjust pH. The pH is between 4.5 and 7.0.

After initial priming (3 to 4 actuations), each actuation of the pump delivers from the nasal adapter 100 mg of suspension containing beclomethasone dipropionate, monohydrate equivalent to 42 mcg of beclomethasone dipropionate. Each bottle delivers at least 200 metered doses.

CLINICAL PHARMACOLOGY:

NASAL FORMS

The mechanisms responsible for the anti-inflammatory action of beclomethasone dipropionate are unknown. The precise mechanism of the aerosolized drug's action in the nose is also unknown. Biopsies of nasal mucosa obtained during clinical studies showed no histopathologic changes when beclomethasone dipropionate was administered intranasally.

The effect of beclomethasone dipropionate on hypothalamic-pituitary-adrenal (HPA) function have been evaluated in adult volunteers by other routes of administration. Studies with beclomethasone dipropionate by the intranasal route which may demonstrate that there is more or that there is less absorption by this route of administration. There was no suppression of early morning plasma cortisol concentrations when beclomethasone dipropionate was administered in a dose of 1,000 mcg per day for 1 month as an oral aerosol or for 3 days by IM injection. However, partial suppression of plasma cortisol concentration was observed when beclomethasone dipropionate was administered in doses of 2,000 mcg per day either by oral aerosol or intramuscular injection form. Immediate suppression of plasma cortisol concentrations was observed after single doses of 4000 mcg of beclomethasone dipropionate. Suppression of HPA function (reduced early morning plasma cortisol levels) has been reported in adult patients who received 1,600-mcg daily doses of oral beclomethasone dipropionate for 1 month. In clinical studies using beclomethasone dipropionate intranasally, there was no evidence of adrenal insufficiency.

CLINICAL PHARMACOLOGY: *(cont'd)*

The effect of beclomethasone dipropionate nasal spray on HPA function was not evaluated but would not be expected to differ from intranasal beclomethasone dipropionate aerosol.

In one study in asthmatic children, the administration of inhaled beclomethasone at recommended daily doses for at least 1 year was associated with a reduction in nocturnal cortisol secretion. The clinical significance of this finding is not clear. It reinforces other evidence, however, that topical beclomethasone may be absorbed in amounts that can have systemic effects and that physicians should be alert for evidence of sysemic effects, expecially in chronically treated patients (see PRECAUTIONS).

Beclomethasone dipropionate is sparingly soluble. When given by nasal inhalation in the form of an aqueous or aerosolized suspension, the drug is deposited primarily in the nasal passages. A portion of the drug is swallowed. Absorption occurs rapidly from all respiratory and gastrointestinal tissues. There is no evidence of tissue storage of beclomethasone dipropionate or its metabolites. *In vitro* studies have shown that tissue other than the liver (lung slices) can rapidly metabolize beclomethasone dipropionate to beclomethasone 17-monopropionate and more slowly to free becloethasone (which has very weak anti-inflammatory activity). However, irrespective of the route of entry, the principal route of excretion of the drug and its metabolites is the feces. In humans, 12% to 15% of an orally administered dose of beclomethasone dipropionate is excreted in the urine as both conjugated and free metabolites of the drug.

Studies have shown that the degree of binding to plasma proteins is 87%.

42 MCG ORAL INHALATION

Animal studies show that beclomethasone dipropionate has potent anti-inflammatory activity. When administered systemically to mice, the anti-inflammatory activity was accompanied by other typical features of glucocorticoid action, including thymic involution, liver glycogen deposition, and pituitary-adrenal suppression. However, after systemic administration to rats, the anti-inflammatory action was associated with little or no effect on other tests of glucocorticoid activity.

Beclomethasone dipropionate is sparingly soluble and is poorly mobilized from subcutaneous or intramuscular injection sites. However, systemic absorption occurs after all routes of administration. When given to animals in the form of an aerosolized suspension of the trichloromonofluoromethane clathrate, the drug is deposited in the mouth and nasal passages, the trachea and principal bronchi, and in the lung; a considerable portion of the drug is also swallowed. Absorption occurs rapidly from all respiratory and gastrointestinal tissues, as indicated by the rapid clearance of radioactively labeled drug from local tissues and appearance of tracer in the circulation. There is no evidence of tissue storage of beclomethasone dipropionate or its metabolites. Lung slices can metabolize beclomethasone dipropionate rapidly to beclomethasone 17-monopropionate and more slowly to free beclomethasone (which has very weak anti-inflammatory activity). However, irrespective of the route of administration (injection, oral, or aerosol), the principal route of excretion of the drug and its metabolites is the feces. Less than 10% of the drug and its metabolites is excreted in the urine. In humans, 12% to 15% of an orally administered dose of beclomethasone dipropionate was excreted in the urine as both conjugated and free metabolites of the drug.

The mechanisms responsible for the anti-inflammatory action of beclomethasone dipropionate are unknown. The precise mechanism of the aerosolized drug's action in the lung is also unknown.

CLINICAL STUDIES:

ORAL 84 MCG STRENGTH

The efficacy of beclomethasone dipropionate 84 mcg double strength inhalation aerosol was compared with beclomethasone dipropionate inhaler (42 mcg/actuation) in a 28-day randomized parallel group, double-blind, placebo-controlled study in patients with moderate to severe asthma. A total of 336 mcg/day of each beclomethasone dipropionate formulation or placebo was administered based on twice daily dosing. FEV_1 at endpoint (last valid visit for each patient) was regarded as the primary measure of efficacy. Beclomethasone dipropionate 84 mcg double strength inhalation aerosol and beclomethasone dipropionate inhaler were both significantly more effective ($p \leq 0.01$) than placebo in improving FEV_1 at all time points, but were not significantly different from each other at any time point ($p > 0.05$). Thus beclomethasone dipropionate 84 mcg double strength inhalation aerosol administered twice daily to give a total daily dose of 336 mcg was comparable in efficacy to beclomethasone dipropionate inhaler when administered at the same total daily dose.

The effects of beclomethasone dipropionate on hypothalamic-pituitary-adrenal (HPA) function have been evaluated in adult volunteers. There was no suppression of early morning plasma cortisol concentrations when beclomethasone dipropionate was administered at a dose of 840 mcg/day for 1 month as an aerosol or 1000 mcg/day for 3 days by intramuscular injection. However partial suppression of plasma cortisol concentration was observed beclomethasone dipropionate was administered at doses of 2000 mcg/day intramuscularly or 1680 mcg/day by aerosol. Immediate suppression of plasma cortisol concentrations was observed after single doses of 4000 mcg of beclomethasone dipropionate intramuscularly.

The potential for beclomethasone dipropionate 84 mcg double strength inhalation aerosol (84 mcg/actuation) to cause HPA axis suppression was compared with beclomethasone dipropionate inhaler (42 mcg/actuation) in a randomized, parallel, placebo- and positive controlled study. Sixty-four adult patients with moderate asthma received doses of either: 1) 420 mcg twice daily of beclomethasone dipropionate 84 mcg double strength; 2) 420 mcg twice daily of beclomethasone dipropionate inhaler; 3) 10 mg of prednisone orally; or 4) placebo for 35.5 days. The potential for HPA axis suppression was evaluated via a cosyntropin stimulation test administered on the 36th day. In response to a 6-hour cosyntropin 250 mcg infusion, there was no evidence of HPA axis suppression associated with either beclomethasone dipropionate 84 mcg double strength inhalation aerosol or beclomethasone dipropionate inhaler preparations as compared with placebo. However, there were sioniflunt ($p \leq 0.01$) attenuations of the plasma cortisol concentration responses to cosyntropin stimulation in the prednisone-treated group compared with the placebo-treated group.

In another study with beclomethasone dipropionate inhaler, the effects of beclomethasone dipropionate on HPA function were examined in patients with asthma. There was no change in basal early morning plasma cortisol concentrations or in the cortisol responses to tetracosactrin (ACTH 1:24) stimulation after daily aerosol administration of 336, 672, or 1008 mcg of beclomethasone dipropionate for 28 days. After daily aerosol administration of 1344 mcg for 28 days. There was a slight reduction in basal cortisol concentrations and a statistically significant ($p < 0.01$) reduction in plasma cortisol responses to tetracosactrin stimulation. The effects of a more prolonged period of beclomethasone dipropionate administration on HPA function have not been evaluated.

Clinical experience has shown that some patients with asthma who require corticosteroid therapy for control of symptoms can be partially or completely withdrawn from systemic corticosteroid if therapy with beclomethasone dipropionate aerosol is substituted. Beclomethasone dipropionate aerosol is not effective for all patients with asthma or at all stages of the disease in a given patient.

ORAL 42 MCG STRENGTH

The effects of beclomethasone dipropionate on hypothalmic-pituitary-adrenal (HPA) function have been evaluated in adult volunteers. There was no suppression of early morning plasma cortisol concentrations when beclomethasone dipropionate was administered in a dose of

CLINICAL STUDIES: *(cont'd)*

1,000 mcg per day for 1 month as an aerosol or for 3 days by intramuscular injection. However, partial suppression of plasma cortisol concentration was observed when beclomethasone dipropionate was administered in doses of 2,000 mcg per day either intramuscularly or by aerosol. Immediate suppression of plasma cortisol concentrations was observed after single doses of 4,000 mcg of beclomethasone dipropionate.

In one study the effects of beclomethasone dipropionate on HPA function were examined in patients with asthma. There was no change in basal early morning plasma cortisol concentrations or in the cortisol responses to tetracosactin (ACTH 1:24) stimulation after daily administration of 400, 800, or 1,200 mcg of beclomethasone dipropionate for 28 days. After daily administration of 1,600 mcg each day for 28 days, there was a slight reduction in basal cortisol concentrations and a statistically significant ($p < .01$) reduction in plasma cortisol responses to tetracosactrin stimulation. The effects of a more prolonged period of beclomethasone dipropionate administration on HPA function have not been evaluated. However, a number of investigators have noted that when systemic corticosteroid therapy in asthmatic subjects can be replaced with recommended doses of beclomethasone dipropionate, there is gradual recovery of endogenous cortisol concentrations to the normal range. There is still no documented evidence of recovery from other adverse systemic corticosteroid-induced reactions during prolonged therapy of patients with beclomethasone dipropionate.

Clinical experience has shown that some patients with bronchial asthma who require corticosteroid therapy for control of symptoms can be partially or completely withdrawn from systemic corticosteroids if therapy with beclomethasone dipropionate aerosol is substituted. Beclomethasone dipropionate aerosol is not effective for all patients with bronchial asthma or at all stages of the disease in a given patient.

The early clinical experience has revealed several new problems that may be associated with the use of beclomethasone dipropionate by inhalation for treatment of patients with bronchial asthma:

1. There is a risk of adrenal insufficiency when patients are transferred from systemic corticosteroids to aerosol beclomethasone dipropionate. Although the aerosol may provide adequate control of asthma during the transfer period, it does not provide the systemic steroid that is needed during acute stress situations. **Deaths due to adrenal insufficiency have occurred in asthmatic patients during and after transfer from systemic corticosteroids to aerosol beclomethasone dipropionate. (See WARNINGS.)**

2. Transfer of patients from systemic steroid therapy to beclomethasone dipropionate aerosol may unmask allergic conditions that were previously controlled by the systemic steroid therapy (*e.g.*, rhinitis, conjunctivitis, and eczema).

3. Localized infections with *Candida albicans* or *Aspergillus niger* have occurred frequently in the mouth and pharynx and occasionally in the larynx. It has been reported that up to 75% of the patients who receive prolonged treatment with beclomethasone dipropionate have positive oral cultures for *Candida albicans*. The incidence of clinically apparent infection is considerably lower but may require therapy with appropriate antifungal agents or discontinuation of treatment with beclomethasone dipropionate aerosol.

The long-term effects of beclomethasone dipropionate in human subjects are still unknown. In particular, the local effects of the agent on developmental or immunologic processes in the mouth, pharynx, trachea, and lung are unknown. There is also no information about the possible long-term systemic effects of the agent. The possible relevance of the data in animal studies to results in human subjects cannot be evaluated.

INDICATIONS AND USAGE:

84 mcg Oral Inhaler: Double strength inhalation aerosal is indicated in the maintenance treatment of asthma as prophylactic therapy. Double strength inhalation aerosal is also indicated for asthma patients who require systemic corticosteroid administration, where adding beclomethasone dipropionate may reduce or eliminate the need for systemic corticosteroids.

Beclomethasone dipropionate is NOT indicated for the relief of acute bronchospasm.

42 mcg Oral Inhaler: Beclomethasone dipropionate oral inhaler is indicated only for patients who require chronic treatment with corticosteroids for control of the symptoms of bronchial asthma. Such patients would include those already receiving systemic corticosteroids, and selected patients who are inadequately controlled on a nonsteroid regimen and in whom steroid therapy has been withheld because of concern over potential adverse effects.

Beclomethasone dipropionate oral inhaler is NOT indicated:

1. For relief of asthma which can be controlled by bronchodilators and other nonsteroid medications.

2. In patients who require systemic corticosteroid treatment infrequently.

3. In the treatment of nonasthmatic bronchitis.

Nasal Inhaler and Nasal Spray: Beclomethasone dipropionate nasal inhaler and nasal spray is indicated in the relief of the symptoms of seasonal or perennial allergic and nonallergic (vasomotor) rhinitis in those cases poorly responsive to conventional treatment.

Beclomethasone dipropionate nasal inhaler and spray is also indicated for the prevention of recurrence of nasal polyps following surgical removal.

Clinical studies in patients with seasonal or perennial rhinitis have shown that improvement is usually apparent within a few days. However, symptomatic relief may not occur in some patients for as long as 2 weeks. Although systemic effects are minimal at recommended doses, beclomethasone dipropionate nasal inhaler and nasal spray should not be continued beyond 3 weeks in the absence of significant systematic improvement. Beclomethasone dipropionate nasal inhaler and nasal spray should not be used in the presence of untreated localized infection involving the nasal mucosa.

Clinical studies have shown that treatment of the symptoms associated with nasal polyps may be continued for several weeks or more before a therapeutic result can be fully assessed. Recurrence of symptoms due to polyps can occur after stopping treatment, depending on the severity of the disease.

CONTRAINDICATIONS:

Hypersensitivity to any of the ingredients of this preparation contraindicates its use.

Oral Inhalation Forms: Beclomethasone dipropionate inhaler is contraindicated in the primary treatment of status asthmaticus or other acute episodes of asthma where intensive measures are required.

WARNINGS:

Patients who are on drugs which suppress the immune system are more susceptible to infections than healthy individuals. Chickenpox and measles, for example, can have a more serious or even fatal course in non-immune children or adults on corticosteroids. In such children or adults who have not had these diseases, particular care should be taken to avoid exposure of these infectious agents. How the dose, route, and duration of corticosteroid administration affects the risk of developing a disseminated infection is not known. The contribution of the underlying disease and/or prior corticosteroid treatment to the risk of developing a more severe infection is also not known. If exposed to chickenpox, prophylaxis with varicella zoster immune globulin (VZIG) may be indicated. If exposed to measles,

WARNINGS: *(cont'd)*

prophylaxis with pooled intramuscualr immunoglobulin (IG), may be indicated. (See the respective package inserts for complete VZIG and IG prescribing information.) If chickenpox develops, treatment with antiviral agents may be considered.

ORAL INHALERS

Particular care is needed in patients who are transferred from systemically active corticosteroids to beclomethasone dipropionate because *deaths due to adrenal insufficiency have occurred in asthmatic patients during and after transfer from systemic corticosteroids to aerosol beclomethasone dipropionate.* After withdrawal from systemic corticosteroids a number of months are required for recovery of hypothalamic-pituitary-adrenal (HPA) function. During this period of HPA suppression, patients may exhibit signs and symptoms of adrenal insufficiency when exposed to trauma, surgery, or infections, particularly gastroenteritis. Although beclomethasone dipropionate may provide control of asthmatic symptoms during these episodes, it does NOT provide the systemic steroid that is necessary for coping with these emergencies.

During periods of stress or a severe asthmatic attack, patients who have been withdrawn from systemic corticosteroids should be instructed to resume systemic steroids (in large doses) immediately and to contact their physician for further instruction. These patients should also be instructed to carry a warning card indicating that they may need supplementary systemic steroids during periods of stress or a severe asthma attack. To assess the risk of adrenal insufficiency in emergency situations, routine tests of adrenal cortical function, including measurement of early morning resting cortisol levels, should be performed periodically in all patients. An early morning resting cortisol level may be accepted as normal only if it falls at or near the normal mean level.

Localized infections with *Candida albicans* or *Aspergillus niger* have occurred frequently in the mouth and pharynx and occasionally in the larynx. Positive cultures for oral *Candida* may be present in up to 75% of patients. Although the frequency of clinically apparent infection is considerably lower, these infections can develope with any inhaled corticosteroid and may require treatment with appropriate antifungal therapy or discontinuation of treatment with beclomethasone dipropionate inhaler.

Beclomethasone dipropionate inhaler is not to be regarded as a bronchodilator and is not indicated for rapid relief of bronchospasm.

Patients should be instructed to contact their physician immediately when episodes of asthma that are not responsive to bronchodilators occur during the course of treatment with beclomethasone dipropionate. During such episodes, patients may require therapy with systemic corticosteroids.

Transfer of patients from systemic steroid therapy to beclomethasone dipropionate inhaler may unmask allergic conditions previously suppressed by the systemic steroid therapy (*e.g.*, rhinitis, conjunctivitis, and eczema).

Avoid spraying in eyes.

NASAL INHALER AND NASAL SPRAY

The replacement of a systemic corticosteroid with beclomethasone dipropionate nasal inhaler or spray can be accompanied by signs of adrenal insufficiency.

Careful attention must be given when patients previously treated for prolonged periods with systemic corticosteroids are transferred to beclomethasone dipropionate inhaler or spray. This is particularly important in those patients who have associated asthma or other clinical conditions where too rapid a decrease in systemic corticosteroids may cause a severe exacerbation of their symptoms.

Studies have shown that combined administration of alternate-day prednisone systemic treatment and orally inhaled beclomethasone dipropionate increases the likelihood of HPA suppression compared to a therapeutic dose of either one alone. Therefore, these forms of beclomethasone dipropionate should be used with caution in patients already on alternate day prednisone regimens for any disease.

If recommended doses of these forms are exceeded or if individuals are particularly sensitive or predisposed by virtue of recent systemic steroid therapy, symptoms of hypercorticism may occur, including very rare cases of menstrual irregularities, acneform lesions, cataracts, and cushingoid features. If such changes occur, these forms of this drug should be discontinued slowly consistent with accepted procedures for discontinuing oral steroid therapy.

PRECAUTIONS:

GENERAL

Oral Inhalers

During withdrawal from oral steroids, some patients may experience symptoms of systemically active steroid withdrawal (*e.g.*, joint and/or muscular pain, lassitude and depression) despite maintenance or even improvement of respiratory function. (See DOSAGE AND ADMINISTRATIONfor details.)

In responsive patients, beclomethasone dipropionate may permit control of asthmatic symptoms without suppression of HPA function, as discussed below (see CLINICAL PHARMACOLOGY.) Since inhaled beclomethasone dipropionate is absorbed into the circulation and can be systemically active, lack of HPA suppression by beclomethasone dipropionate may be expected only when recommended dosages are not exceeded.

The long-term local and systemic effects of beclomethasone dipropionate in human subjects are still not fully known. In particular, the effects resulting from use of the agent on developmental or immunologic processes in the mouth, pharynx, trachea, and lung are unknown.

This drug should be used with caution, if at all, in patients with active or quiescent tuberculous infection of the respiratory tract; untreated systemic fungal, bacterial, parasitic, or viral infections; or ocular herpes simplex.

Pulmonary infiltrates with eosinophilia may occur in patients receiving orally inhaled beclomethasone dipropionate. Although it is possible that in some patients this state may become manifest because of systemic corticosteroid withdrawal when inhalational corticosteroids are administered, a causative role for beclomethasone dipropionate and/or its vehicle cannot be ruled out.

42 mcg Oral Inhaler: In addition, children should be monitored for a reduction in growth velocity, although the relationship between growth velocity and final adult height is not known.

The potential effects of beclomethasone dipropionate on acute, recurrent, or chronic pulmonary infections, including active or quiescent tuberculosis, are not known. Similarly, the potential effects of long-term administration of the drug on lung or other tissues are unknown.

PRECAUTIONS: *(cont'd)*

Because of the possibility of systemic absorption of orally inhaled corticosteroids, including beclomethasone, patients should be monitored for symptoms of systemic effects such as mental disturbances, increased bruising, weight gain, cushingoid features, and cataracts. Therefore, if such changes occur, this drug should be discontinued slowly, consistent with accepted procedures for discontinuing oral steroids.

Nasal Inhaler and Nasal Spray

During withdrawal from oral steroids, some patients may experience symptoms of withdrawal (*e.g.*, joint and/or muscular pain, lassitude, and depression).

Rare instances of nasal septum perforation have been spontaneously reported.

Rare instances of glaucoma and increased intraocular pressure have been reported following the intranasal application of aerosolized corticosteroids.

In clinical studies with beclomethasone dipropionate administered intranasally, the development of localized infections of the nose and pharynx with *Candida albicans* has occurred only rarely. When such an infection develops, it may require treatment with appropriate local therapy or discontinued use of treatment.

Beclomethasone dipropionate is absorbed into the circulation. Use of excessive doses may suppress HPA function.

This drug should be used with caution, if at all, in patients with active or quiescent tuberculous infections of the respiratory tract; untreated fungal, bacterial, or systemic viral infections; or ocular herpes simplex.

For intranasal forms of beclomethasone dipropionate to be effective in the treatment of nasal polyps, the aerosol or spray must be able to enter the nose. Therefore, treatment of nasal polyps with beclomethasone dipropionate should be considered adjunctive therapy to surgical removal and/or the use of other medications which will permit effective penetration of this drug into the nose. Nasal polyps may recur after any form of treatment.

As with any long-term treatment, patients using intranasal beclomethasone dipropionate over several months or longer should be examined periodically for possible changes in the nasal mucosa.

Because of the inhibitory effect of corticosteroids on wound healing, patients who have experienced recent nasal septal ulcers, nasal surgery, or trauma should not use a nasal corticosteroid until healing has occurred.

Although systemic effects have been minimal with recommended doses, this potential increases with excessive doses. Therefore, larger than recommended doses should be avoided.

Nasal Spray: Rarely, immediate hypersensitivity reactions may occur after the intranasal administration of beclomethasone.

Rare instances of wheezing, glaucoma and increased intraocular pressure have been reported following the intranasal application of aerosolized corticosteroids. Although these have not been observed in clinical trials with these forms, vigilance should be maintained.

If persistent nasopharyngeal irritation occurs, it may be an indication for stopping beclomethasone dipropionate administered intranasally.

PREGNANCY CATEGORY C

84 mcg Oral: Like other corticosteriods, parenteral (subcutaneous) beclomethasone dipropionate was teratogenic and embryocidal in the mouse or rabbit when given at a dose of 0.1 mg/kg/day in mice or at a dose of 0.025 mg/kg/day in rabbits. These doses in rats and rabbits were approximately one-half the maximum recommended human daily inhalation dose on a mg/m_2 basis. No teratogenicity or embryocidal effects were seen in rats when exposed to an inhalation dose of 0.1 mg/kg plus oral doses of up to 10 mg/kg/day for combined daily dose of 10.1 mg/kg (approximately 97 times the maximum recommended human daily inhalation dose on mg/m_2 basis). There are no adequate and well-controlled studies in pregnant women. Beclomethasone dipropionate should be used during pregnancy only if the potential benefit justifies the potential risk to the fetus.

42 mcg Oral: *Teratogenic Effects:* Glucocorticoids are known teratogens in rodent species and beclomethasone dipropionate is no exception.

Teratology studies were done is rats, mice, and rabbits treated with subcutaneous beclomethasone dipropionate. Beclomethasone dipropionate was found to produce fetal resorption, cleft palate, agnathia, microstomia, absence of tongue, delayed ossification and partial agenesis of the thymus. Well-controlled trials relating to fetal risk in humans are not available. Glucocorticoids are secreted in human milk. It is not known whether beclomethasone dipropionate would be secreted in human milk but it is safe to assume that it is likely. The use of beclomethasone dipropionate in pregnant women, nursing mothers, or women of childbearing potential requires that the possible benefits of the drug be weighed against the potential hazards to the mother, embryo, or fetus. Infants born of mothers who have received substantial doses of corticosteroids during pregnancy should be carefully observed for hypoadrenalism.

Nasal: *Teratogenic Effects:* Like other corticoids, parenteral (subcutaneous) beclomethasone dipropionate has shown to be teratogenic and embryocidal in the mouse and rabbit when given in doses approximately 10 times the human dose. In these studies beclomethasone was found to produce fetal resorption, cleft palate, agnathia, microstomia, absence of tongue, delayed ossification, and agenesis of the thymus. No teratogenic or embryocidal effects have been seen in the rat when beclomethasone dipropionate was administered by inhalation at 10 times the human dose or orally at 1,000 times the human dose. There are no adequate and well-controlled studies in pregnant women. Beclomethasone dipropionate should be used during pregnancy only if the potential benefit justifies the potential risk to the fetus. *Nonteratogenic Effects:* Hypoadrenalism may occur in infants born of mothers receiving corticosteroids during pregnancy. Such infants should be carefully observed.

INFORMATION FOR THE PATIENT

Patients being treated with beclomethasone dipropionate should receive the following information and instructions. This information is intended to aid in the safe and effective use of this medication. It is not a disclosure of all possible adverse or intended effects.

Persons who are on immunosuppressant doses of corticosteroids should be warned to avoid exposure to chickenpox or measles and, if exposed, to obtain medical advice without delay.

Nasal and 42 mcg Oral: Patients should use at regular intervals since their effectiveness depends on their regular use. The patient should take the medication as directed. It is not acutely effective, and the prescribed dosage should not be increased. Instead, nasal vasoconstrictors or oral antihistamines may be needed until the effects of this drug are fully manifested. One to 2 weeks may pass before relief is obtained. The patient should contact the doctor if symptoms do not improve, or if the condition worsens, or if sneezing or nasal irritation occurs. For the proper use of this unit and to attain maximum improvement, the patient should read and follow carefully the accompanying patient's instructions.

84 mcg Oral: Patients should use beclomethasone dipropionate double strength inhalation aerosal at regular intervals as directed. Results of clinical trials indicated significant improvement may occur within the first day or two of treatment; however, the full benefit may not be acheived until treatment has been administered for 1 to 2 weeks or longer. The patient should not increase the prescribed dosage but should contact the physician if symptoms do not improve or if condition worsens.

PRECAUTIONS: *(cont'd)*

Patients should also be advised that beclomethasone dipropionate double strength inhalation aerosal is not intended for use in the treatment of acute asthma. Patients should be instructed to contact their physician immediately if there is any deterioration of their asthma.

Patients should be advised to rinse his/her mouth each time after using beclomethasone dipropionate double strength inhalation aerosal.

Beclomethasone dipropionate double strength inhalation aerosal should not be stopped abruptly. If discontinuing use of this product is necessary, the patient's physician should be contacted immediately.

CARCINOGENESIS, MUTAGENESIS, AND IMPAIRMENT OF FERTILITY

The carcinogenicity of beclomethasone dipropionate was evaluated in rats which were exposed for a total of 95 weeks, 13 weeks at inhalation doses up to 0.4 mg/kg/day and the remaining 82 weeks at combined oral and inhalation doses up to 2.4 mg/kg/day. There was no evidence of carcinogenicity in this study at the highest dose which is approximately 23 times the maximum recommended human daily inhalation dose on a mg/m^2 basis. Impairment of fertility, as evidenced by inhibition of the estrous cycle in dogs, was observed following treatment by the oral route at a dose of 0.5 mg/kg/day which is approximately 16 times the maximum recommended human daily inhalation dose on a mg/m^2 basis. No inhibition of the estrous cycle in dogs was seen following 12 months of exposure to beclomethasone dipropionate by the inhaltion route at an estimated daily dose of 0.33 mg/kg (approximately 11 times the maximum recommended human daily inhalation dose on a mg/m^2 basis).

NURSING MOTHERS

Corticosteriods are secreted in human milk. Because of the potential for serious adverse reactions in nursing infants from beclomethasone dipropionate, a decision should be made whether to discontinue nursing or to discontinue the drug, taking into account the importance of the drug to the mother.

PEDIATRIC USE

Safety and effectiveness in children below 6 years of age have not been established.

ADVERSE REACTIONS:

ORAL

In a 4-week, randomized, double-blind, placebo-controlled clinical trial, the incidence of adverse events reported for beclomethasone dipropionate double strength inhalation aerosal was similar to that reported for placebo. Adverse event rates did not appear to differ significantly based on age, sex, or race. Adverse events that were reported by 2% or more of patients receiving this drug (regardless of relationship to treatment) and that occurred more frequently than placebo are displayed in TABLE 1.

In a 4-week, randomized, double-blind clinical study, there were no reports of oral candidasis in patients receiving this drug. (See WARNINGS).

TABLE 1 Adverse Events from 4-Week Placebo-Controlled Clinical Trial in Patients With Asthma

	Percent of Patients Reporting Beclomethasone Dipropionate		
	84 mcg n=103	42 mcg n=104	Placebo n=109
Headache	22	27	18
Pharyngitis	14	11	8
Coughing	9	7	4
Infection (viral)	8	5	6
Nasal congestion	6	5	2
Dysmenorrhea	4	0	3
Sinusitis	4	3	3
Dyspepsia	3	6	2
Fatigue	3	2	2
Influenza-like symptoms	3	<1	0
Sneezing	3	2	0
Eczema	2	0	0
Pruritus	2	0	<1
Respiratory disorder	2	0	0

In addition to those adverse events reported in TABLE 1, the following adverse events have been reported in fewer than 2% of patients receiving double strength beclomethasone dipropionate (regardless of relationship to treatment).

Autonomic Nervous System: Lacrimation.

Body as a Whole: Increased allergy symptoms, chest pain, fever, rigors.

Gastrointestinal: Diarrhea, nausea, rectal hemorrhage.

Hearing and Vestibular: Earache.

Heart Rate and Rhythm: Tachycardia.

Musculoskeletal: Arthralgia, pain.

Psychiatric: Depression, insomnia.

Respiratory: Bronchitis, bronchospasm, chest congestion, dysphonia, upper respiratory infection.

Skin and Appendages: Rash, skin discoloration, urticaria.

Special Senses: Taste perversion.

Urinary: Urinary tract infection.

Vascular (Extracardiac): Migraine.

White Cell and Reticuloendothelial: Lymphadenopathy.

Deaths due to adrenal insufficiency have occurred in asthmatic patients during and after transfer from systemic corticosteroids to aerosol beclomethasone dipropionate. (See WARNINGS.)

Suppression of HPA function (reduction of early morning plasma cortisol levels) has been reported in adult patients who received 1344 mcg daily doses (approximately twice the maximum recommended daily dose) of beclomethasone dipropionate by oral inhalation for one month. Some patients receiving orally inhaled beclomethasone dipropionate have complained of hoarseness or dry mouth.

Rare cases of immediate and delayed hypersensitivity reactions, including urticaria, angioedema, rash, and bronchospasm, have been reported following the oral and intranasal inhalation of beclomethasones.

Rare case of hypercorticism, adrenal insufficiency, growth inhibitory effects, cataracts, glaucoma, and hyperglcemia have been reported with inhaled corticosteriods.

NASAL INHALER

In general, side effects in clinical studies have been primarily associated with the nasal mucous membranes.

ADVERSE REACTIONS: *(cont'd)*

Adverse reactions reported in controlled clinical trials and long-term open studies in patients treated with beclomethasone dipropionate nasal inhaler are described below.

Sensations of irritation and burning in the nose (11 per 100 patients) following the use of beclomethasone dipropionate nasal inhaler have been reported. Also, occasional sneezing attacks (10 per 100 adult patients) have occurred immediately following the use of the intranasal inhaler. This symptom may be more common in children. Rhinorrhea may occur occasionally (1 per 100 patients).

Localized infections of the nose and pharynx with *Candida albicans* have occurred rarely (see PRECAUTIONS).

Transient episodes of epistaxis have been reported in 2 per 100 patients.

Rare cases of ulceration of the nasal mucosa and instances of nasal septum perforation have been spontaneously reported (see PRECAUTIONS). Rare reports of loss of taste and smell have been recieved.

Rare instances of glaucoma and increased intraocular pressure have been reported following the intranasal application of aerosolized corticosteroids (see PRECAUTIONS).

Rare cases of immediate and delayed hypersensitivity reactions, including urticaria, angioedema, rash, and bronchospasm, have been reported following the oral and intranasal inhalation of beclomethasone.

Systemic corticosteroid side effects were not reported during the controlled clinical trials. If recommended doses are exceeded, however, or if individuals are particularly sensitive, symptoms of hypercorticism (*i.e.*, Cushing's syndrome, could occur).

NASAL SPRAY

In general, side effects in clinical studies have been primarily associated with irritation of the nasal mucous membranes. Rarely, immediate hypersensitivity reactions may occur after the intranasal administration of beclomethasone.

Adverse reactions reported in controlled clinical trials and open studies in patients treated with beclomethasone dipropionate nasal spray are described below.

Mild nasopharyngeal irritation following the use of beclomethasone aqueous nasal spray has been reported in up to 24% of patients treated, including occasional sneezing attacks (about 4%) occurring immediately following use of the spray. In patients experiencing these symptoms, none had to discontinue treatment. The incidence of transient irritation and sneezing was approximately the same in the group of patients who received placebo in these studies, implying that these complaints may be related to vehicle components of the formulation.

Fewer than 5 per 100 patients reported headache, nausea, or lightheadedness following the use of beclomethasone dipropionate nasal spray. Fewer than 3 per 100 patients reported nasal stuffiness, nosebleeds, rhinorrhea, or tearing eyes.

Rare cases of ulceration of the nasal mucosa and incidences of nasal septum perforation have been spontaneously reported (see PRECAUTIONS). Rare reports of loss of taste and smell have been received.

Rare instances of wheezing, glaucoma, and increased intraocular pressure have been reported following the intranasal administration of aerosolized corticosteroids (see PRECAUTIONS).

OVERDOSAGE:

84 MCG ORAL

There were no deaths over 15 days following the oral administration of a single dose of 3000 mg/kg in mice, 2000 mg/kg in rats, and 1000 mg/kg in rabiits. The doses in mice, rats, and rabbits were 14,500, 19,300, and 19,300 times, respectively, the maximum recommended human daily inhalation dose on a mg/m^2 basis.

NASAL INHALER AND NASAL SPRAY

When used at excessive doses, systemic corticosteroid effects such as hypercorticism and adrenal suppression may appear. If such changes occur, beclomethasone dipropionate intranasal should be discontinued slowly consistent with accepted procedures for discontinuing oral steroid therapy. The oral LD_{50} of beclomethasone dipropionate is greater that 1 g/kg in rodents. One canister of beclomethasone dipropionate nasal inhaler contains 8.4 mg of beclomethasone dipropionate, and one bottle of beclomethasone dipropionate nasal spray contains beclomethasone dipropionate, monohydrate equivalent to 10.5 mg of beclomethasone dipropionat; therefore, acute overdosage is unlikely.

DOSAGE AND ADMINISTRATION:

84 MCG ORAL INHALER

Double strength oral inhalation aerosal should be test sprayed 2 times into the air before using for the first time and in cases where the product has not been used for more than 7 days.

Adults: The usual recommended dosage is two inhalations (168 mcg) given twice daily. In patients with severe asthma, it is advisable to start with 6 to 8 inhalations a day and adjust the dosage downward according to the response of the patient. *The maximal daily intake should not exceed 10 inhalations, 840 mcg (0.84 mg), in adults.*

Children 6 to 12 Years of Age: The usual recommended dosage is two inhalations (168 mcg) given twice daily. *The maximal daily intake should not exceed 5 inhalations, 420 mcg (0.42 mg), in children 6 to 12 years of age.* Insufficient clinical trial data exist with respect to the administration of beclomethasone dipropionate in children below the age of 6.

Rinsing the mouth after inhalation is advised.

Different considerations must be given to the following groups of patients in order to obtain the full therapeutic benefit of beclomethasone dipropionate inhaler.

Patients Not Receiving Systemic Steroids: Patients who require maintenance therapy of their asthma may benefit from treatment with 84 mcg beclomethasone dipropionate inhalation aerosal at the doses recommended above. In patients who respond to beclomethasone dipropionate, an improvement in pulmonary function is usually apparent within 1 to 4 weeks after the start of beclomethasone dipropionate inhaler. Once the desired effect is acheived, consideration should be given to tapering to the lowest effective dose.

Patients Receiving Systemic Steroids: Clinical studies have shown that beclomethasone dipropionate may be effective in the management of asthmatics dependent or maintained on systemic corticosteriods and may permit replacement or significant reduction in the dosage of systemic corticosteriods.

The patient's asthma should be reasonably stable before treatment with beclomethasone dipropionate inhaler is started. Initially, the aerosol should be used concurrently with the patient's usual maintenance dose of systemic corticosteroid. After approximately 1 week, gradual withdrawal of the systemic corticosteroid is started by reducing the daily or alternate-daily dose. The next reduction is made after an interval of 1 or 2 weeks, depending on the response of the patient. Generally, these decrements should not exceed 2.5 mg of prednisone or its equivalent. A slow rate of withdrawal cannot be overemphasized. During withdrawal some patients may experience symptoms of systemical corticosteroid withdrawal (*e.g.*, joint and/or muscular pain, lassitude, and depression) despite maintenance or even improvement in pulmonary function. Such patients should be encouraged to continue with the inhaler but should be monitored carefully for objective signs of adrenal insufficiency, such as hypoten-

DOSAGE AND ADMINISTRATION: *(cont'd)*

sion and weight loss. If evidence of adrenal insufficiency occurs, the systemic corticosteroid dose should be increased temporarily and thereafter further withdrawal should continue more slowly.

During periods of stress or a severe asthma attack, transfer patients will require supplementary treatment with systemic steroids.

42 MCG ORAL INHALER

Adults and Children 12 Years of Age and Older: The usual recommended dosage is two inhalations (84 mcg) given three or four times a day. Alternatively, four inhalations (168 mcg) given twice daily has been shown to be effective in some patients. In patients with severe asthma, it is advisable to start with 12 to 16 inhalations a day and adjust the dosage downward according to the response of the patient. *The maximal daily intake should not exceed 20 inhalations, 840 mcg (0.84 mg), in adults.*

Children 6 to 12 Years of Age: The usual recommended dosage is one or two inhalations (42 to 84 mcg) given three or four times a day according to the response of the patient. Alternatively, 4 inhalations (168 mcg) given twice daily has been shown to be effective in some patients. *The maximal daily intake should not exceed 10 inhalations, 420 mcg (0.42 mg), in children 6 to 12 years of age.* Insufficient clinical data exist with respect to the administration of beclomethasone dipropionate inhaler in children below the age of 6.

Rinsing the mouth after inhalation is advised.

Patients receiving bronchodilators by inhalation should be advised to use the bronchodilator before beclomethasone dipropionate inhaler in order to enhance penetration of beclomethasone dipropionate into the bronchial tree. After use of an aerosol bronchodilator, several minutes should elapse before use of the beclomethasone dipropionate inhaler to reduce the potential toxicity from the inhaled fluorocarbon propellants in the two aerosols.

Different considerations must be given to the following groups of patients in order to obtain the full therapeutic benefit of beclomethasone dipropionate inhaler.

Patients Not Receiving Systemic Steroids: The use of beclomethasone dipropionate inhaler is straightforward in patients who are inadequately controlled with nonsteroid medications but in whom systemic steroid therapy has been withheld because of concern over potential adverse reactions. In patients who respond to beclomethasone dipropionate, an improvement in pulmonary function is usually apparent within 1 to 4 weeks after the start of beclomethasone dipropionate inhaler.

Patients Receiving Systemic Steroids: In those patients dependent on systemic steroids, transfer to beclomethasone dipropionate and subsequent management may be more difficult because recovery from impaired adrenal function is usually slow. Such suppression has been known to last for up to 12 months. Clinical studies, however, have demonstrated that beclomethasone dipropionate may be effective in the management of these asthmatic patients and may permit replacement or significant reduction in the dosage of systemic corticosteroids.

The patient's asthma should be reasonably stable before treatment with beclomethasone dipropionate inhaler is started. Initially, the aerosol should be used concurrently with the patient's usual maintenance dose of systemic steroid. After approximately 1 week, gradual withdrawal of the systemic steroid is started by reducing the daily or alternate-daily dose. The next reduction is made after an interval of 1 or 2 weeks, depending on the response of the patient. Generally, these decrements should not exceed 2.5 mg of prednisone or its equivalent. A slow rate of withdrawal cannot be overemphasized. During withdrawal some patients may experience symptoms of systemically active steroid withdrawal (*e.g.,* joint and/or muscular pain, lassitude, and depression) despite maintenance or even improvement of respiratory function. Such patients should be encouraged to continue with the inhaler but should be watched carefully for objective signs of adrenal insufficiency, such as hypotension and weight loss. If evidence of adrenal insufficiency occurs, the systemic steroid dose should be boosted temporarily and thereafter further withdrawal should continue more slowly.

During periods of stress or a severe asthma attack, transfer patients will require supplementary treatment with systemic steroids. Exacerbations of asthma that occur during the course of treatment with beclomethasone dipropionate inhaler should be treated with a short course of systemic steroid that is gradually tapered as these symptoms subside. There is no evidence that control of asthma can be achieved by administration of beclomethasone dipropionate in amounts greater than the recommended doses.

NASAL INHALER AND SPRAY

In patients who respond to beclomethasone dipropionate nasal inhaler and nasal spray, an improvement of the symptoms of seasonal or perennial rhinitis usually becomes apparent within a few days after the start of therapy. However, symptomatic relief may not occur in some patients for as long as 2 weeks. Beclomethasone dipropionate nasal inhaler and nasal spray should not be continued beyond 3 weeks in the absence of significant symptomatic improvement.

The therapeutic effect of corticosteroids, unlike those of decongestants, are not immediate. This should be explained to the patient in advance in order to ensure cooperation and continuation of treatment with the prescribed dosage regimen.

In the presence of excessive nasal mucous secretion or edema of the nasal mucosa, the drug may fail to reach the site of intended action. In such cases it is advisable to use a nasal vasoconstrictor during the first 2 to 3 days of beclomethasone dipropionate therapy.

Nasal Inhaler

Adults and Children 12 Years of Age and Over: The usual dosage is one inhalation (42 mcg) in each nostril two to four times a day (total dose, 168 to 336 mcg per day). Patients can often be maintained on a maximum dose of one inhalation in each nostril three times a day (252 mcg per day).

Children 6 to 12 Years of Age: The usual dosage is one inhalation in each nostril three times a day (252 mcg per day). This product is *not* recommended for children under 6 years of age since safety and efficacy studies have not been conducted in this age-group.

Nasal Spray

Adults and Children 6 Years of Age and Over: The usual dosage is one or two inhalations (42 to 84 mcg) in each nostril twice a day (total dose, 168 to 336 mcg per day).

Beclomethasone dipropionate nasal spray is *not* recommended for children below 6 years of age.

ANIMAL PHARMACOLOGY:

42 mcg Oral Inhaler: Studies in a number of animal species, including rats, rabbits, and dogs, have shown no unusual toxicity during acute experiments. However, the effects of beclomethasone dipropionate in producing signs of glucocorticoid excess during chronic administration by various routes were dose related.

PATIENT INFORMATION:

Beclomethasone Dipropionate is a corticosteroid. The oral inhaler is used to prevent the symptoms of asthma. Beclomethasone will not treat an acute asthma attack. The nasal inhaler and nasal spray are used to relieve the symptoms of hayfever and to prevent nasal polyps from growing back after they have been surgically removed. Immediate results do not occur with this medication. To be effective, beclomethasone needs to be used on a regular basis. It is important that beclomethasone oral inhaler, nasal inhaler, and nasal spray are administered using the proper technique. Please obtain detailed administration directions from your pharmacist or physician. Inform your physician if you are pregnant or nursing. Rinse your mouth or drink a glass of water after using the oral inhaler. Blow your nose before using the nasal inhaler or nasal spray. The oral inhaler my cause a sore throat or sore mouth, the nasal inhaler or spray may irritate and dry the nasal mucosa; notify your physician if these occur.

HOW SUPPLIED:

Vanceril 84 mcg Double Strength Inhalation Aerosal: 12.2 g canisters contain 120 metered inhalations. 5.4 g canisters contain 40 metered inhalations for instutional use only. Each canister is supplied with a dark-pink plastic actuator with a maroon cap and Patient's Instructions for Use. Each actuation delivers an amount of beclomethasone dipropionate-trichloromonofluoromethane clathrate equivalent to 84mcg of beclomethasone dipropionate from the mouthpiece and 100 mcg of beclomethasone dipropionate from the valve.

Vanceril 84 mcg Double Strength Inhalation Aerosal should only be used with the Vanceril 84 mcg Double Strength Inhalation Aerosal mouthpiece and this mouthpiece should not be used with any other inhalation drug product.

The correct amount of medication in each inhalation cannot be assured after 120 actuations from the 12.2 g canister or 40 actuations from the 5.4 g canister even thought the canister is not completely empty. The canister should be discarded when the labeled number of actuations have been used.

Store at 15°-30°C (59°-86°F). Protect from moisture and unusual temperature fluctuations. Failure to use the product within this temperature range may result in improper dosing. For optimal results, the canister should be at room temperature before use. Shake well before using. Once canister is removed from the moisture protective package the product must be used within 6 months.

WARNING: Contains trichloromonofluoromethane (CFC-11) and dichlorodifluoromethane (CFC-12), substances which harm public health and environment by destroying ozone in the upper atmosphere.

Oral and Nasal Inhalers: CONTENTS UNDER PRESSURE. Do not puncture. Do not use or store near heat or open flame. Exposure to temperatures above 120°F may cause bursting. Never throw container in fire or incinerator. Keep out of reach of children.

Store between 2° and 30°C (36° and 86°F). As with most inhaled medications in aerosol canisters, the therapeutic effect of this medication may decrease when the canister is cold. Shake well before using.

Nasal Spray: Store between 15° and 30°C (59° and 86°F). Shake well before each use.

HOW SUPPLIED - EQUIVALENTS NOT AVAILABLE:

Aerosol - Inhalation - 42 mcg

6.7 gm	$18.74	BECONASE, Glaxo Wellcome	00173-0468-00
6.7 gm	**$18.90**	**BECLOVENT, Glaxo Wellcome**	**00173-0469-00**
7 gm	$31.36	VANCENASE, Schering	00085-0649-02
16.8 gm	**$28.04**	**BECLOVENT, Glaxo Wellcome**	**00173-0312-98**
16.8 gm	$34.10	BECONASE, Glaxo Wellcome	00173-0336-02
16.8 gm	**$34.39**	**BECLOVENT, Glaxo Wellcome**	**00173-0312-88**

Aerosol - Inhalation - 42 mcg/inh

6.7 gm	$36.16	VANCENASE, Schering	00085-0041-11

Aerosol - Nasal Inhalatio - 42 mcg

16.8 g	$37.36	VANCENASE, Schering	00085-0041-06

Aerosol - Oral Inhalation - 42 mcg

16.8 gm	$31.36	VANCERIL, Schering	00085-0736-04

Aerosol - Oral Inhalation - 84 mcg

12.2 g	$45.46	VANCERIL DOUBLE STRENGTH, Schering	00085-1112-01

Spray - Nasal - 42 mcg

25 g	$36.80	BECONASE AQ, Glaxo Wellcome	00173-0388-79

Spray - Nasal - 42 mcg/spr

25 gm	$33.86	VANCENASE AQ, Schering	00085-0259-02

BELLADONNA *(000382)*

CATEGORIES: Antiarrhythmic Agents; Anticholinergic Agents; Antimuscarinics/Antispasmodics; Autonomic Drugs; Gastrointestinal Drugs; Renal Drugs; FDA Pre 1938 Drugs

BRAND NAMES: *Atrobel*; *Atrobel Forte*; *Belladonna Extract* (England); Painful Menstruation No.31; Simple Throat Irritations; Spacol
(International brand names outside U.S. in italics)

FORMULARIES: Medi-Cal

Prescribing information not available at time of publication.

HOW SUPPLIED - EQUIVALENTS NOT AVAILABLE:

Liquid

120 ml	$6.50	Spacol, Dayton Labs	52041-0043-33

Tablet, Uncoated - Oral

100's	$20.00	SPACOL, Dayton Labs	52041-0044-15

Tincture - Oral - 0.27 mg/ml

500 ml	$18.81	Belladonna, Amend Drug Chem	17317-0044-01

BELLADONNA ALKALOIDS; PHENOBARBITAL *(000383)*

CATEGORIES: Acid/Peptic Disorders; Anticholinergic Agents; Antimuscarinics/Antispasmodics; Antispasmodics & Anticholinergics; Autonomic Drugs; DESI Drugs; Gastrointestinal Drugs; Irritable Bowel Syndrome; Parasympatholytics; Duodenal Ulcer*; Pregnancy Category C; FDA Pre 1938 Drugs
* Indication not approved by the FDA

BRAND NAMES: Antispasmodic; Antispasmodic Compound; Antispasmodil; Barbidonna; *Bardase*; Barophen; Bellabarb; *Belladol*; Belladonna W/Phenobarbital; Bellalphen; Bubarbel; Chardonna-2; Charspast; Colidrops; Dixatal; Donna-Sed; Donnamor; Donnaphen; Donnapine; **Donnatal**; *Espasmoliq*; Haponal; Hyonatal; Hyosophen; Hypersed; Hypnaldyne; Kinesed; Lahey Mixture #3; Malatal; Neoquess; Phenobel; Phenobella; Relaxadon; Sedacord; Sedapar; Sedarex; Seds;

Sparte; Spasmolin; Spasmophen; Spasquid; Spastemms; Spastolate; *Speedtin*; Susano; Tega Donna; *Weyan*
(International brand names outside U.S. in italics)

FORMULARIES: BC-BS; DoD; FHP; Kaiser; Medi-Cal; PruCare

DESCRIPTION:

Each Donnatal tablet, capsule or 5 ml (teaspoonful) of elixir (23% alcohol) contains: *Phenobarbital, USP (1/4 gr):* 16.2 mg (Warning: May be habit forming); *Hyoscyamine Sulfate, USP:* 0.1037 mg; *Atropine Sulfate, USP:* 0.0194 mg; *Scopolamine Hydrobromide, USP:* 0.0065 mg. *Tablets Inactive Ingredients:* Dibasic Calcium Phosphate, Magnesium Stearate, Microcrystalline Cellulose, Silicon Dioxide, Sodium Starch Glycolate, Stearic Acid, Sucrose. May contain Corn Starch, Dextrose or Invert Sugar. *Capsules Inactive Ingredients:* Corn Starch, Edible Ink, D&C Yellow 10 and FD&C Green 3, FD&C Blue 1 and FD&C Yellow 6, FD&C Blue 2 Aluminum Lake, Gelatin, Lactose, Sucrose. May contain FD&C Red 40 and Yellow 6 Aluminum Lakes. *Elixir Inactive Ingredients:* D&C Yellow 10, FD&C Blue 1, FD&C Yellow 6, Flavors, Glucose Saccharin, Sodium, Water.

Each Donnatal Extentabs tablet contains: *Phenobarbital, USP (3/4 gr):* 48.6 mg (Warning: May be habit forming); *Hyoscyamine Sulfate, USP:* 0.3111 mg; *Atropine Sulfate, USP:* 0.0582 mg; *Scopolamine Hydrobromide, USP:* 0.0195 mg.

Each belladonna alkaloids; phenobarbital extentabs tablet contains the equivalent of three belladonna alkaloids; phenobarbital tablets. Extentabs are designed to release the ingredients gradually to provide effects for up to twelve (12) hours. *Inactive Ingredients:* Acacia, Acetylated Monoglycerides, Calcium Sulfate, Carnauba Wax, D&C Yellow 10, Edible Ink, FD&C Blue 1, FD&C Blue 2 Aluminum Lake, FD&C Yellow 6, Gelatin, Guar Gum, Magnesium Stearate, Polysorbates, Shellac, Sodium Phosphate, Sucrose, Titanium Dioxide, Wheat Flour, White Wax and other ingredients, one of which is a corn derivative. May include FD&C Red 40 and Yellow 6 Aluminum Lakes.

CLINICAL PHARMACOLOGY:

This drug combination provides natural belladonna alkaloids in a specific, fixed ratio combined with phenobarbital to provide peripheral anticholinergic/antispasmodic action and mild sedation.

INDICATIONS AND USAGE:

Based on a review of this drug by the National Academy of Sciences —National Research Council and/or other information, FDA has classified the following indications as "possibly" effective:
For use as adjunctive therapy in the treatment of irritable bowel syndrome (irritable colon, spastic colon, mucous colitis) and acute enterocolitis.
May also be useful as adjunctive therapy in the treatment of duodenal ulcer. IT HAS NOT BEEN SHOWN CONCLUSIVELY WHETHER ANTICHOLINERGIC/ANTISPASMODIC DRUGS AID IN THE HEALING OF A DUODENAL ULCER, DECREASE THE RATE OF RECURRENCES OR PREVENT COMPLICATIONS.

CONTRAINDICATIONS:

Glaucoma, obstructive uropathy (for example, bladder neck obstruction due to prostatic hypertrophy); obstructive disease of the gastrointestinal tract (as in achalasia, pyloroduodenal stenosis, etc.); paralytic ileus, intestinal atony of the elderly or debilitated patient; unstable cardiovascular status in acute hemorrhage; severe ulcerative colitis especially if complicated by toxic megacolon; myasthenia gravis; hiatal hernia associated with reflux esophagitis.

Belladonna alkaloids; phenobarbital is contraindicated in patients with known hypersensitivity to any of the ingredients. Phenobarbital is contraindicated in acute intermittent porphyria and in those patients in whom phenobarbital produces restlessness and/or excitement.

WARNINGS:

In the presence of a high environmental temperature, heat prostration can occur with belladonna alkaloids (fever and heatstroke due to decreased sweating).

Diarrhea may be an early symptom of incomplete intestinal obstruction, especially in patients with ileostomy or colostomy. In this instance treatment with this drug would be inappropriate and possibly harmful.

Belladonna alkaloids; phenobarbital may produce drowsiness or blurred vision. The patient should be warned, should these occur, not to engage in activities requiring mental alertness, such as operating a motor vehicle or other machinery, and not to perform hazardous work.

Phenobarbital may decrease the effect of anticoagulants and necessitate larger doses of the anticoagulant for optimal effect. When the phenobarbital is discontinued, the dose of the anticoagulant may have to be decreased.

Phenobarbital may be habit forming and should not be administered to individuals known to be addiction prone or to those with a history of physical and/or psychological dependence upon drugs.

Since barbiturates are metabolized in the liver, they should be used with caution and initial doses should be small in patients with hepatic dysfunction.

PRECAUTIONS:

Use with caution in patients with: autonomic neuropathy, hepatic or renal disease, hyperthyroidism, coronary heart disease, congestive heart failure, cardiac arrhythmias, tachycardia, and hypertension.

Belladonna alkaloids may produce a delay in gastric emptying (antral stasis) which would complicate the management of gastric ulcer.

Theoretically, with overdosage, a curare-like action may occur.

Carcinogenesis, Mutagenesis: Long-term studies in animals have not been performed to evaluate carcinogenic potential.

Pregnancy Category C: Animal reproduction studies have not been conducted with belladonna alkaloids; phenobarbital. It is not known whether Belladonna alkaloids; phenobarbital can cause fetal harm when administered to a pregnant woman or can affect reproduction capacity. Belladonna alkaloids; phenobarbital should be given to a pregnant woman only if clearly needed.

Nursing Mothers: It is not known whether this drug is excreted in human milk. Because many drugs are excreted in human milk, caution should be exercised when belladonna alkaloids; phenobarbital is administered to a nursing mother.

ADVERSE REACTIONS:

Adverse reactions may include xerostomia; urinary hesitancy and retention; blurred vision; tachycardia; palpitation; mydriasis; cycloplegia; increased ocular tension; loss of taste sense; headache; nervousness; drowsiness; weakness; dizziness; insomnia; nausea; vomiting; impotence; suppression of lactation; constipation; bloated feeling; musculoskeletal pain; severe allergic reaction or drug idiosyncracies, including anaphylaxis, urticaria and other dermal manifestations; and decreased sweating. Elderly patients may react with symptoms of excitement, agitation, drowsiness, and other untoward manifestations to even small doses of the drug.

Phenobarbital may produce excitement in some patients, rather than a sedative effect. In patients habituated to barbiturates, abrupt withdrawal may produce delirium or convulsions.

OVERDOSAGE:

The signs and symptoms of overdose are headache, nausea, vomiting, blurred vision, dilated pupils, hot and dry skin, dizziness, dryness of mouth, difficulty in swallowing, CNS stimulation. Treatment should consist of gas-parenteral lavage, emetics, and activated charcoal. If indicated, parenteral cholinergic agents such as physostigmine or bethanechol chloride should be added.

DOSAGE AND ADMINISTRATION:

The dosage of onnatal should be adjusted to the needs of the individual patient to assure symptomatic control with a minimum of adverse effects.

TABLETS AND CAPSULES

Adults: One or two belladonna alkaloids; phenobarbital tablets or capsules three or four times a day according to condition and severity of symptoms.

EXTENDED RELEASE TABLETS

The usual dose is one tablet every twelve (12) hours. If indicated, one tablet every eight (8) hours may be given.

ELIXIR

Adults: One or two teaspoonfuls of elixir three or four times a day according to conditions and severity of symptoms.

Children (Elixir): may be dosed every 4 or 6 hours (TABLE 1):

TABLE 1

Body Weight	Starting Dosage (Kd)	q6h
10 lb (4.5 kg)	0.5 ml	0.75 ml
20 lb (9.1 kg)	1.0 ml	1.5 ml
30 lb (13.6 kg)	1.5 ml	2.0 ml
50 lb (22.7 kg)	1/2 tsp	3/4 tsp
75 lb (34.0 kg)	3/4 tsp	1 tsp
100 lb (45.4 kg)	1 tsp	1 1/2 tsp

HOW SUPPLIED:

Donnatal Tablets: White compressed, scored and embossed "R"; in bottles of 100, 1000 and Dis-co Unit Dose Packs of 100.

Donnatal Extended Release Tablets: Pale green, coated tablets, monogrammed AHR.

Donnatal Capsules: Green and white, monogrammed "AHR" and "4207).

Donnatal Elixir: Green, citrus flavored.

Store at controlled room temperature, between 15°C and 30°C (59°F and 86°F).

Dispense in tight, light resistant container.

HOW SUPPLIED - EQUIVALENTS NOT AVAILABLE:

Capsule, Gelatin - Oral - 0.0194 mg/0.103

100's	**$15.33**	**DONNATAL, AH Robins**	**00031-4207-63**

Elixir - Oral - 16.2 mg/5ml

5 ml x 25	**$101.89**	**DONNATAL, AH Robins**	**00031-4221-13**
120 ml	$2.01	Antispasmodic, HL Moore Drug Exch	00839-5018-65
120 ml	$2.40	Barophen, Consolidated Midland	00223-6419-01
120 ml	$2.50	HYOSCYAMINE COMPOUND, HR Cenci	00556-0053-04
120 ml	$2.55	Donnapine, Major Pharms	00904-0981-20
120 ml	$3.70	Antispasmodic, Morton Grove	60432-0009-04
120 ml	**$6.40**	**DONNATAL, AH Robins**	**00031-4221-12**
240 ml	$7.90	Antispasmodic, Morton Grove	60432-0009-08
473 ml	$6.87	Lahey Clinic Rx 3, Reg Svc	48433-0240-16
480 ml	$4.25	Barophen, Consolidated Midland	00223-6419-02
480 ml	$4.31	DONNAMOR, HL Moore Drug Exch	00839-5018-69
480 ml	$4.50	BELATOL, HR Cenci	00556-0053-16
480 ml	$7.78	Belladonna W/Phenobarbital, Aligen Independ	00405-2350-16
480 ml	$7.95	Donnaphen, Alphagen Labs	59743-0028-16
480 ml	$7.95	Belladonna W/Phenobarbital, Cypress Pharm	60258-0822-16
480 ml	$8.65	DONNAPINE, Major Pharms	00904-0981-16
480 ml	$9.57	HYOSOPHEN, Rugby	00536-0100-85
480 ml	$9.70	ANTISPASMODIC, Goldline Labs	00182-0686-40
480 ml	$9.90	Antispasmodic, HL Moore Drug Exch	00839-7850-69
480 ml	$9.90	SUSANO, Halsey Drug	00879-0059-16
480 ml	$10.50	Antispasmodic, Morton Grove	60432-0009-16
480 ml	$14.75	Belladonna W/Phenobarbital, Qualitest Pharms	00603-1030-58
480 ml	$16.62	Antispasmodic Compound, RID	54807-0125-16
480 ml	$19.95	Hyoscyamine Compound, Harber Pharm	51432-0645-20
480 ml	**$22.68**	**DONNATAL, AH Robins**	**00031-4221-25**
480 ml	$74.05	BARBIDONNA, Wallace Labs	00037-0305-68
3840 ml	$22.45	DONNAPINE, Major Pharms	00904-0981-28
3840 ml	$22.96	BELATOL, HR Cenci	00556-0053-28
3840 ml	$47.46	Barophen, Consolidated Midland	00223-6419-03
3840 ml	$62.63	ANTISPASMODIC, Goldline Labs	00182-0686-41
3840 ml	$64.78	Antispasmodic, HL Moore Drug Exch	00839-7850-70
3840 ml	$67.25	SUSANO, Halsey Drug	00879-0059-28
3840 ml	$68.91	HYOSOPHEN, Rugby	00536-0100-90
3840 ml	$71.77	Antispasmodic, Morton Grove	60432-0009-28
3840 ml	**$160.32**	**DONNATAL, AH Robins**	**00031-4221-29**

Tablet, Uncoated - Oral - 0.0194 mg/0.103

30's	$0.19	Belladonna Alkaloids/Phenobarbital, Talbert Phcy	44514-0134-18
100's	$1.27	Belladonna Alkaloids/Phenobarbital, Talbert Phcy	44514-0134-88
100's	$2.75	BELLALPHEN, Consolidated Midland	00223-0425-01
100's	$5.30	Antispasmodic, HL Moore Drug Exch	00839-5055-06
100's	$10.17	BELLATAL, Richwood Pharm	58521-0162-01
100's	$10.48	Hyosophen, Rugby	00536-3920-01
100's	$11.91	ANTISPASMODIC TABS, RID	54807-0126-01
100's	**$13.75**	**DONNATAL, AH Robins**	**00031-4250-63**
100's	**$15.19**	**DONNATAL, AH Robins**	**00031-4250-64**
100's	$19.06	CHARDONNA-2, Schwarz Pharma (US)	00091-0202-01

HOW SUPPLIED - EQUIVALENTS NOT AVAILABLE: *(cont'd)*

100's	$29.50	Phenobel, Pecos	59879-0110-01
100's	$35.50	Belladonna W/Phenobarbital, Goldline Labs	00182-2611-01
100's	$37.58	Hyosophen, Rugby	00536-5728-01
100's	$42.66	Antispasmodic, HL Moore Drug Exch	00839-7974-06
100's	**$43.81**	**DONNATAL, AH Robins**	**00031-4235-63**
100's	$48.68	BARBIDONNA, Wallace Labs	00037-0301-92
100's	$54.58	BARBIDONNA NO. 2, Wallace Labs	00037-0311-92
500's	**$202.86**	**DONNATAL, AH Robins**	**00031-4235-70**
500's	$207.37	BARBIDONNA, Wallace Labs	00037-0301-96
1000's	$7.47	RELAXADON, Geneva Pharms	00781-1105-10
1000's	$8.25	ANTISPASMODIC, Goldline Labs	00182-0129-10
1000's	$11.50	Phenobarbital & Belladonna, Rexar	00478-5477-10
1000's	$12.50	BUARBEL MODIFIED, C O Truxton	00463-6276-10
1000's	$12.65	SUSANO, Halsey Drug	00879-0058-10
1000's	$23.40	SPASTEMMS, C O Truxton	00463-6181-10
1000's	$24.50	Bellalphen, Consolidated Midland	00223-0425-03
1000's	$29.80	HYPERSED, Embrex Economed	38130-0048-10
1000's	$40.45	Donnapine, Major Pharms	00904-3741-80
1000's	$41.92	HAPONAL, United Res	00677-0074-10
1000's	$53.93	SPASMOLIN, HL Moore Drug Exch	00839-5055-16
1000's	$55.98	Belladonna W/Phenobarbital, Qualitest Pharms	00603-2418-32
1000's	$60.75	Belladonna W/Phenobarbital, Goldline Labs	00182-1048-10
1000's	$63.75	HYOSOPHEN, Rugby	00536-3920-10
1000's	**$77.40**	**DONNATAL NO.2, AH Robins**	**00031-4264-74**
1000's	$81.25	Donnaphen, Alphagen Labs	59743-0027-10
1000's	**$122.86**	**DONNATAL, AH Robins**	**00031-4250-74**
5000's	$52.00	Phenobarbital & Belladonna, Rexar	00478-5477-50
5000's	$255.60	SPASMOLIN, HL Moore Drug Exch	00839-5055-20

BELLADONNA; BUTABARBITAL SODIUM *(000384)*

CATEGORIES: Anticholinergic Agents; Antimuscarinics/Antispasmodics; Autonomic Drugs; DESI Drugs; Gastrointestinal Drugs; FDA Pre 1938 Drugs

BRAND NAMES: **Butibel**

FORMULARIES: Medi-Cal

Prescribing information not available at time of publication.

HOW SUPPLIED - EQUIVALENTS NOT AVAILABLE:

Elixir - Oral - 15 mg/15 mg

480 ml	**$71.87**	**BUTIBEL, Wallace Labs**	**00037-0044-16**

Tablet, Uncoated - Oral - 15 mg/15 mg

100's	**$43.22**	**BUTIBEL, Wallace Labs**	**00037-0046-60**

BELLADONNA; CAFFEINE; ERGOTAMINE; PENTOBARBITAL *(000380)*

CATEGORIES: Antimigraine/Other Headaches; Autonomic Drugs; Ergot Preparations; Pain; Sympatholytic Agents; FDA Pre 1938 Drugs

BRAND NAMES: Belcomp-Pb; Cafergot P-B; Ergo-Caff Pb; Micomp-Pb

FORMULARIES: Aetna

Prescribing information not available at time of publication.

HOW SUPPLIED - EQUIVALENTS NOT AVAILABLE:

Suppository - Rectal

12's	$36.80	Migracet-Pb, Superior	00144-0633-13
12's	$36.89	Ergocaff-Pb, Bio Pharm	59741-0315-15
12's	$37.30	MICOMP-PB, Major Pharms	00904-1751-12
12's	$45.95	E-CAFF P-B, Pecos	59879-0501-12
12's	$49.95	BELCOMP-PB, DSC Labs	52316-0122-12

Tablet, Coated - Oral - 125 mcg/100 mg/

90's	$52.00	MICOMP-PB, Econolab	55053-0525-90
90's	$58.75	EROCOMP-PB, United Res	00677-1382-90
90's	$60.82	ERGOCAFF-PB, Rugby	00536-3801-11

BELLADONNA; CHLORPHENIRAMINE MALEATE; PHENYLPROPANOLAMINE *(000387)*

CATEGORIES: Allergies; Antihistamines; Common Cold; Respiratory & Allergy Medications; FDA Pre 1938 Drugs

BRAND NAMES: Pro-Tuss

Prescribing information not available at time of publication.

HOW SUPPLIED - EQUIVALENTS NOT AVAILABLE:

Tablet, Uncoated, Sustained Action - Oral - 40 mcg/8 mg/190

100's	$20.00	PRO-TUSS, Econolab	55053-0073-01
1000's	$198.00	PRO-TUSS, Econolab	55053-0073-10

BELLADONNA; ENZYME; PHENOBARBITAL *(000389)*

CATEGORIES: Anticholinergic Agents; Antimuscarinics/Antispasmodics; Autonomic Drugs; DESI Drugs; Diarrhea; Digestants; Enzymes & Digestants; Gastrointestinal Drugs; Pregnancy Category C; FDA Pre 1938 Drugs

BRAND NAMES: **Donnazyme**

Prescribing information not available at time of publication.

HOW SUPPLIED - EQUIVALENTS NOT AVAILABLE:

Tablet, Coated - Oral - 0.0097 mg/150 m

100's	**$25.36**	**DONNAZYME, AH Robins**	**00031-4649-63**
500's	**$115.54**	**DONNAZYME, AH Robins**	**00031-4649-70**

BELLADONNA; ERGOTAMINE TARTRATE; PHENOBARBITAL *(000390)*

CATEGORIES: Anticholinergic Agents; Antimigraine/Other Headaches; Antimuscarinics/Antispasmodics; Autonomic Drugs; Cholinergics; DESI Drugs; Diarrhea; Gastrointestinal Drugs; Gastrointestinal Hypermotility; Pain; Parasympatholytics; Sympatholytic Agents; Pregnancy Category X; FDA Pre 1938 Drugs

BRAND NAMES: Bel-Phen-Ergot; Bel-Phen-Ergot S; Bel-Tabs; Bellamine; Bellaphen-S; Bellaspas; **belladonna; ergotamine tartrate; phenobarbital**; *Bellergal Retard; Bellergal Spacetabs* (Canada); Cafatine Pb; Ergobel; Migergot; Phenerbel-S; Phenobarbital Ergotamine Bell; Spastrin; *Trinergot*
(International brand names outside U.S. in italics)

FORMULARIES: Aetna

DESCRIPTION:

Each Tablet Contains: Phenobarbital, USP 40 mg; ergotamine tartrate, USP 0.6 mg; Bellafoline (levorotatory alkaloids of belladonna) 0.2 mg.

belladonna; ergotamine tartrate; phenobarbital Inactive Ingredients: Colloidal silicon dioxide, color additives including FD&C Blue #1, FD&C Red #40, FD&C Yellow #5, FD&C Yellow #6 (Sunset Yellow), gelatin, lactose, magnesium stearate, malic acid, polyvinyl acetate resins, stearic acid, sucrose, and tartaric acid.

CLINICAL PHARMACOLOGY:

Based on the concept that functional disorders frequently involve hyperactivity of both the sympathetic and parasympathetic nervous systems, the ingredients in belladonna; ergotamine tartrate; phenobarbital are combined to provide a balanced preparation designed to correct imbalance of the autonomic nervous system. The integrated action of belladonna; ergotamine tartrate; phenobarbital is effected through the combined administration of ergotamine and the levorotatory alkaloids of belladonna, specific inhibitors of the sympathetic and parasympathetic respectively, reinforced by the synergistic action of phenobarbital in dampening the cortical centers. It should be noted that on a weight basis the levorotatory alkaloids of belladonna have approximately twice the pharmacological effects as do the usual racemic mixtures.

INDICATIONS AND USAGE:

Belladonna; ergotamine tartrate; phenobarbital is employed in the management of disorders characterized by nervous tension and exaggerated autonomic response: **Menopausal disorders** with hot flushes, sweats, restlessness and insomnia; **cardiovascular disorders** with palpitation, tachycardia, chest oppression and vasomotor disturbances; **gastrointestinal disorders** with hypermotility, hypersecretion, "nervous stomach," and alternately diarrhea and constipation; interval treatment of **recurrent, throbbing headache.**

CONTRAINDICATIONS:

Peripheral vascular disease, coronary heart disease, hypertension, impaired hepatic or renal function, sepsis, pregnancy, nursing mothers and glaucoma. The concomitant administration of ergotamine and dopamine should be avoided, due to the increased potential for ischemic vasoconstriction. Phenobarbital is contraindicated in patients with a history of manifest or latent porphyria. Phenobarbital is contraindicated in those patients in whom the drug produces restlessness and/or excitement. belladonna; ergotamine tartrate; phenobarbital is contraindicated in patients with a demonstrated hypersensitivity to any of the components.

WARNINGS:

Total weekly dosage of ergotamine tartrate should not exceed 10 mg. (This dosage corresponds to 16 belladonna; ergotamine tartrate; phenobarbital tablets.) Due to the presence of a barbiturate, may be habit-forming.

PRECAUTIONS:

Even though the ergotamine tartrate content of this product is low and untoward effects have been rare and of minor significance, caution should be exercised if large or prolonged dosage is contemplated, and physicians should be alert to possible peripheral vascular complications in patients sensitive to ergot. Due to the presence of the anticholinergic agent, special caution should be exercised in the use of this drug in patients with bronchial asthma or obstructive uropathy.

Belladonna; ergotamine tartrate; phenobarbital contains FD&C Yellow #5 (tartrazine) which may cause allergic-type reactions (including bronchial asthma) in certain susceptible individuals. Although the overall incidence of FD&C Yellow #5 (tartrazine) sensitivity in the general population is low, it is frequently seen in patients who also have aspirin hypersensitivity.

INFORMATION FOR THE PATIENT

Patients on large or prolonged dosage should be asked to report numbness or tingling of extremities, claudication or other symptoms of peripheral vasoconstriction.

CARCINOGENESIS

No data are available on the long-term potential for carcinogenicity in animals or humans.

PREGNANCY CATEGORY X

Due to the potential uterotonic effects of the ergot alkaloids, the use of belladonna; ergotamine tartrate; phenobarbital during pregnancy is contraindicated (see CONTRAINDICATIONS).

NURSING MOTHERS

A number of ergot alkaloids inhibit the secretion of prolactin. Therefore, belladonna; ergotamine tartrate; phenobarbital is contraindicated in nursing mothers (see CONTRAINDICATIONS.)

PEDIATRIC USE

Safety and effectiveness in children have not been established.

DRUG INTERACTIONS:

Oral Anticoagulants: Phenobarbital may lower the plasma levels of dicumarol (name previously used: bishydroxycoumarin) and may cause a decrease in anticoagulant activity as measured by the prothrombin time. More frequent monitoring of prothrombin time responses is indicated whenever phenobarbital is initiated or discontinued, and the dosage of anticoagulants should be adjusted accordingly.

CNS Depressants: Combined administration of phenobarbital and CNS depressants such as alcohol, tricyclic antidepressants, phenothiazines and narcotic analgesics may result in a potentiation of the depressant action.

Beta Adrenergic Blocking Agents: Although proof is lacking, several reports in the literature suggest a possible interaction between ergot alkaloids and beta adrenergic blocking agents. This interaction may result in excessive vasoconstriction. Although many patients can apparently take propranolol and ergot alkaloids without ill effects, there is enough evidence of an interaction to dictate closer surveillance of patients so treated.

DRUG INTERACTIONS: *(cont'd)*

Hepatic Metabolism: Through the mechanism of enzyme induction caused by phenobarbital, a number of substances have been shown to be metabolized at an increased rate. In these cases, clinical responses should be closely monitored and appropriate dosage adjustments made. Included are such substances as griseofulvin, quinidine, doxycycline and estrogen. Although the meaning of published reports regarding the effects of phenobarbital on estrogen metabolism are unclear at this time, if avoidance of pregnancy is critical, consideration should be given to alternative methods of contraception.

Phenytoin, Sodium Valproate, Valproic Acid: The effect of barbiturates on the metabolism of phenytoin appears to be variable. Some investigators report an accelerating effect, while others report no effect. Because the effect of barbiturates on the metabolism of phenytoin is not predictable, phenytoin and barbiturate blood levels should be monitored more frequently if these drugs are given concurrently. Sodium valproate and valproic acid appear to decrease barbiturate metabolism; therefore, barbiturate blood levels should be monitored and appropriate dosage adjustments made as indicated.

Tricyclic Antidepressants: Due to the presence of levorotatory alkaloids of belladonna, concomitant administration of tricyclic antidepressants may result in additive anticholinergic effects.

ADVERSE REACTIONS:

Tingling and other paresthesias of the extremities, blurred vision, palpitations, dry mouth, decreased sweating, decreased gastrointestinal motility, urinary retention, tachycardia, flushing, and drowsiness occur rarely.

DRUG ABUSE AND DEPENDENCE:

Barbiturates may be habit-forming. Tolerance, psychological dependence, and physical dependence may occur especially following prolonged use of high doses. Daily administration in excess of 400 mg of pentobarbital or secobarbital for approximately 90 days is likely to produce some degree of physical dependence. By way of comparison, the phenobarbital component of belladonna; ergotamine tartrate; phenobarbital at the highest recommended daily dosage amounts to 80 mg.

OVERDOSAGE:

Management of Overdosage: While severe symptoms of overdosage with belladonna; ergotamine tartrate; phenobarbital have not been reported, theoretically they could occur. It is imperative to note that overdosage symptoms with belladonna; ergotamine tartrate; phenobarbital may be attributable to any one or more of the three active ingredients. Which toxic manifestation might predominate in any individual case would be impossible to predict but one should be alert to the various possibilities. When anticholinergic/antispasmodic drugs are taken in sufficient overdose to produce such severe symptoms, prompt treatment should be instituted. Gastric lavage and other measures to limit intestinal absorption should be initiated without delay.

Cholinesterase inhibitors administered parenterally may be necessary for treatment of the serious manifestations of anticholinergic overdosage. Additionally, symptomatic therapy, including oxygen, sedatives and control of hyperthermia may be necessary.

Acute barbiturate overdosage symptoms with belladonna; ergotamine tartrate; phenobarbital, while possible, have not been reported. While the usual procedures for handling barbiturate poisoning should be employed, keep in mind the possibility of anticholinergic overdosing effects.

Acute ergot overdosage symptoms with belladonna; ergotamine tartrate; phenobarbital, while possible, have not been reported. The usual procedures for handling ergot overdosage include the administration of a peripheral vasodilator to counteract the vasospasm.

DOSAGE AND ADMINISTRATION:

One tablet in the morning and one tablet in the evening.

HOW SUPPLIED:

Bellergal-S Tablets: Compressed tablets of tri-colored pattern: dark green, orange and light lemon yellow, scored on one side, embossed "78-31" on other side.

Store and Dispense: Below 77°F (25°C); tight, light-resistant container.

HOW SUPPLIED - EQUIVALENTS NOT AVAILABLE:

Tablet, Uncoated - Oral - 0.2 mg/0.6 mg/4

90's	$63.50	CAFATINE-PB, Major Pharms	00904-1750-89
100's	$37.45	BELLAMINE, Major Pharms	00904-2548-60
100's	$37.95	BELLADONNA/ERGOTAMINE/PHENOB, Harber Pharm	51432-0677-03
100's	$41.56	BELLAMOR, HL Moore Drug Exch	00839-7370-06
100's	$41.75	SPASTRIN, Econolab	55053-0124-01
100's	$43.95	Phenobarbital/Ergotamine/Bell, Aligen Independ	00405-4794-01
100's	$45.40	BEL-TABS, United Res	00677-1171-01
100's	$45.45	BEL-PHEN-ERGOT S, Goldline Labs	00182-1847-01
100's	$45.45	Bel-Phen-Ergot S, Goldline Labs	00182-1990-01
100's	$53.62	PHENERBEL-S, Rugby	00536-4234-01
100's	$53.65	Phenobarbital/Ergotamine/Belladona, Geneva Pharms	00781-1701-01
100's	$56.31	Bellaspas, Qualitest Pharms	00603-2424-21
100's	$59.95	Bellaphen-S, Pecos	59879-0121-01
100's	**$94.86**	**BELLERGAL-S, Novartis**	**00078-0031-05**
500's	$254.69	Phenerbel-S, Rugby	00536-4234-05

BELLADONNA; KAOLIN; PAREGORIC; PECTIN *(000391)*

CATEGORIES: Antidiarrhea Agents; DESI Drugs; Diarrhea; Gastrointestinal Drugs; DEA Class CV; FDA Pre 1938 Drugs

BRAND NAMES: Amogel Pg; Donnachem-Pg; Donnagel-Pg; Donnapectolin-Pg; Kao-Pg; Kapectolin Pg; Quiagel Pg

Prescribing information not available at time of publication.

HOW SUPPLIED - EQUIVALENTS NOT AVAILABLE:

Suspension - Oral

180 ml	$4.25	DONNACHEM-PG, H N Norton Co.	50732-0868-06
180 ml	$5.36	KAOLIN-PECTIN PG, Qualitest Drugs	52446-0825-55
180 ml	$5.69	KAPECTOLIN PG, Balan	00304-0353-77
180 ml	$5.95	KAPECTOLIN PG, Major Pharms	00904-0026-21
480 ml	$10.49	KAPECTOLIN PG, Balan	00304-0353-98
480 ml	$10.50	DONNACHEM-PG, H N Norton Co.	50732-0868-16
480 ml	$12.14	KAOLIN-PECTIN PG, Qualitest Drugs	52446-0825-58
480 ml	$13.44	KAPECTOLIN PG, Major Pharms	00904-0026-16

HOW SUPPLIED - EQUIVALENTS NOT AVAILABLE: *(cont'd)*

3840 ml	$19.97	KAPECTOLIN PG, Century Pharms	00436-0519-28
3840 ml	$75.57	DONNACHEM-PG, H N Norton Co.	50732-0868-28

BELLADONNA; KAOLIN; PECTIN *(000392)*

CATEGORIES: Antidiarrhea Agents; Gastrointestinal Drugs

BRAND NAMES: Kapectolin W/Belladonna

Prescribing information not available at time of publication.

HOW SUPPLIED - EQUIVALENTS NOT AVAILABLE:

Suspension - Oral

480 ml	$6.25	KAPECTOLIN W/BELLADONNA, Harber Pharm	51432-0616-20

BELLADONNA; OPIUM *(000394)*

CATEGORIES: Analgesics; Antidiarrhea Agents; Antispasmodics; Central Nervous System Agents; Gastrointestinal Drugs; Genitourinary Muscle Relaxant; Narcotics, Synthetics & Combinations; Opiate Agonists (Controlled); Opium Preparations; Pain; Sedatives/Hypnotics; Spasm; Hypoglycemia*; Sedation*; Pregnancy Category C; DEA Class CII; FDA Pre 1938 Drugs
* Indication not approved by the FDA

BRAND NAMES: **B & O**; Opium W/Belladonna

FORMULARIES: Aetna; BC-BS

DESCRIPTION:

Each Belladonna and Opium suppositories contains (in the water-soluble Neocera suppository base for rectal administration):

B&O No. 15A: Powdered opium* 30 mg (0.46) (**Warning** - May be habit forming) and Powdered Belladonna Extract 16.2 mg, equivalent to 0.21 mg (0.0032 g) belladonna alkaloids.

B&O No. 16A: Powdered opium* 60 mg (0.92 g) (**Warning** - May be habit forming) and Powdered Belladonna Extract 16.2 mg, equivalent to 0.21 mg (0.0032 g) belladonna alkaloids.

Neocera Base is a blend of Polyethylene Glycols and Polysorbate 60.

*See WARNINGS.

The drug falls into the pharmacological/therapeutic class of narcotic/antispasmodic agents. The pharmacologically active principles present in the belladonna extract component of these rectal suppositories are:

Established Name: Atropine

Chemical Name: dl Tropyl Tropate

Established Name: Scopolamine

Chemical Name: dl Scopolamine

Opium contains more than a score of alkaloids, the principal ones being morphine (10%), narcotine (6%), papaverine (1%) and codeine (0.5%). The major pharmacologically active principle of the powdered opium component of this drug, however, is:

Established Name: Morphine

Morphine Chemical Name: 7,8-Didehydro-4,5-epoxy 17-methyl-morphinan-3,6-diol

CLINICAL PHARMACOLOGY:

Through its parasympatholytic action, atropine relaxes smooth muscle resulting from parasympathetic stimulation. It is the dl isomer of *l*-hyoscyamine and therefore exhibits the same clinical effects. It is, however, approximately one-half as active peripherally as l-hyoscyamine, the latter being the major active plant alkaloid. The dl isomer atropine is formed during the process of isolation of the belladonna extract[1].

Morphine, the major active principle of powdered opium, is responsible for the action of powdered opium although the other alkaloids present also contribute to it. The sedative and analgesic action of morphine, the effect desired by inclusion of belladonna and opium suppositories in powered opium, are thought to be due to its depressant effect on the cerebral cortex, hypothalamus and medullary centers. In large doses, the opiates and their analogs also inhibit synaptic conduction in the spinothalamic tracts, depress the function of the reticular formation, the lemniscus and the thalamic relays, and inhibit spinal reflexes; but these inhibitor actions should not be elicited with therapeutic dose of the drug. Moderate doses of powdered opium should not alter the electroencephalogram.

The action of morphine consists mainly of a descending depression of the central nervous system. It exerts its analgesic action by increasing the pain threshold or the magnitude of stimulus required to evoke pain and by dulling the sensibility or reaction to pain. In addition to its action in abolishing pain, morphine induces a well-being (euphoria) facilitating certain mental processes while retarding others. Upon absorption of morphine, oxidative dealkylation to produce nor-compounds appears to be the first step in the reaction sequence which imparts analgesia. Morphine is conjugated in the liver to form the 3-glucuronide which passes into the bile and is reabsorbed and excreted in the urine. The atropine effect of the belladonna extract serves to eliminate morphine induced smooth muscle spasm without affecting the sedative analgesic action of powdered opium.[2]

INDICATIONS AND USAGE:

Belladonna and opium suppositories are used for relief of moderate to severe pain associated with ureteral spasm not responsive to non-narcotic analgesics and to space intervals between injections of opiates.

CONTRAINDICATIONS:

Do not use belladonna and opium suppositories in patients suffering from glaucoma, severe hepatic or renal disease, bronchial asthma, narcotic idiosyncracies, respiratory depression, convulsion disorders, acute alcoholism, delirium tremens and premature labor.

WARNINGS:

True addiction may result from opium usage. These preparations are not recommended for use in children.

PRECAUTIONS:

Administer with caution to patients with a known idiosyncracy to atropine or atropine-like compounds; to persons known to be sensitive to or addicted to morphine or morphine-like drugs; to persons with cardiac disease, incipient glaucoma or prostatic hypertrophy. Caution should be used in the administration of belladonna and opium rectal suppositories to old and debilitated patients and patients with increased intracranial pressure, toxic psychosis and myxedema.

PRECAUTIONS: *(cont'd)*

PREGNANCY CATEGORY C

Animal studies have not been conducted with belladonna and opium suppositories. It is also not known whether belladonna and opium rectal suppositories can affect reproduction capacity. The active principles in belladonna and opium rectal suppositories, atropine and morphine are known to enter the fetal circulation. Regular use of opium alkaloids during pregnancy has resulted in addiction of the fetus leading to withdrawal symptoms in the neonate. Belladonna and opium suppositories therefore should be used by a pregnant woman with caution and only when clearly indicated.

NURSING MOTHERS

It is not known whether belladonna and opium rectal suppositories are excreted in human milk. Because many drugs are excreted in human milk, caution should be exercised when belladonna and opium suppositories are administered to a nursing woman.

ADVERSE REACTIONS:

Belladonna may cause drowsiness, dry mouth, urinary retention, photophobia, rapid pulse, dizziness, and blurred vision. Opium usage may result in constipation, nausea, or vomiting. Pruritus and urticaria may occur.

DRUG ABUSE AND DEPENDENCE:

Because of their content of opium, belladonna and opium suppositories are considered as schedule II drugs by the drug enforcement administration. No data exists on chronic abuse effects or dependence characteristics of belladonna and opium rectal suppositories.

OVERDOSAGE:

As with morphine and related narcotics, overdosage is characterized by respiratory depression, pinpoint pupils and coma. Respiratory depression may be reversed by intravenous administration of naloxone HCl. In addition, supportive measures such as oxygenation, intravenous fluids and vasopressors should be used as indicated. As with atropine derivatives, hot, dry, flushed skin, dry mouth and hyperpyrexia may occur.

DOSAGE AND ADMINISTRATION:

ADULTS

One belladonna and opium suppository rectally once or twice daily, not to exceed four doses daily or as recommended by the physician. Moisten finger and suppository with water before inserting. Not recommended for use in children 12 and under. Absorption is dependent on body hydration and not on body temperature.

Storage: Store at room temperature. **DO NOT REFRIGERATE.**

REFERENCES:

1.Gilman, A.G., Goodman, L.S. & Gilman A. 6th Edition. *The Pharmacological Basis of Therapeutics*, Macmillan Pub. Co., N.Y. 1980, pp. 121-127. 2. *Ibid*, pp. 494-513

HOW SUPPLIED - EQUIVALENTS NOT AVAILABLE:

Suppository - Rectal - 16.2 mg/30 mg

12's	**$31.88**	**B & O NO. 15A, Alcon-PR**	**00998-5015-75**

Suppository - Rectal - 16.2 mg/60 mg

12's	**$17.35**	**B & O, Paddock Labs**	**00574-7040-12**
12's	$26.35	Opium W/Belladonna, Wyeth Labs	00008-0330-02
12's	**$35.63**	**B & O NO. 16A, Alcon-PR**	**00998-5016-75**
20's	**$28.85**	**B & O, Paddock Labs**	**00574-7040-20**

BELLADONNA; PHENAZO *(000395)*

CATEGORIES: Antimicrobials; Antipruritics/Local Anesthetics; Antiseptics, Urinary Tract; Phenazopyridine; Skin/Mucous Membrane Agents; Urinary Anti-Infectives; FDA Pre 1938 Drugs

BRAND NAMES: Urogesic; Urogesic Blue

Prescribing information not available at time of publication.

HOW SUPPLIED - EQUIVALENTS NOT AVAILABLE:

Tablet, Sugar Coated - Oral - 0.12 mg/81.6 mg

100's	$23.00	Urogesic - Blue Tablets, Edwards Pharms	00485-0051-01

BENACTYZINE HYDROCHLORIDE; MEPROBAMATE *(000399)*

CATEGORIES: Antidepressants; Anxiety; Anxiolytics, Sedatives, Hypnotic; Central Nervous System Agents; DESI Drugs; Depression; Insomnia; Psychotherapeutic Agents; Tranquilizers; DEA Class CIV; FDA Pre 1938 Drugs

BRAND NAMES: **Deprol**; Rexin

Prescribing information not available at time of publication.

HOW SUPPLIED - EQUIVALENTS NOT AVAILABLE:

Tablet, Uncoated - Oral - 1 mg/400 mg

100's	$180.00	Rexin Tablets, Econolab	55053-0175-01
100's	**$312.98**	**DEPROL, Wallace Labs**	**00037-3001-01**
500's	**$1495.98**	**DEPROL, Wallace Labs**	**00037-3001-03**

BENAZEPRIL HYDROCHLORIDE *(003053)*

CATEGORIES: ACE Inhibitors; Angiotensin Converting Enzyme Inhibitors; Antihypertensives; Cardiovascular Drugs; Hypertension; Pregnancy Category D; FDA Class 1C ("Little or No Therapeutic Advantage"); Sales > $100 Million; FDA Approved 1991 Jun

BRAND NAMES: *Cibace*; *Cibacen* (Germany, Japan); *Cibacen CHF*; *Cibacene* (France); **Lotensin**

(International brand names outside U.S. in italics)

FORMULARIES: Aetna; BC-BS; CIGNA; FHP; Humana; Kaiser; Medco; Medi-Cal; PruCare; United

COST OF THERAPY: $232.24 (Hypertension; Tablet; 10 mg; 1/day; 365 days)

PRIMARY ICD9: 401.1 (Essential Hypertension, Benign)

> **WARNING:**
> **Use in Pregnancy:** When used in pregnancy during the second and third trimesters, ACE inhibitors can cause injury and even death to the developing fetus. When pregnancy is detected, benazepril HCl should be discontinued as soon as possible. See WARNINGS, Fetal/Neonatal Morbidity and Mortality.

DESCRIPTION:

Benazepril HCl is a white to off-white crystalline powder, soluble (>100 mg/ml) in water, in ethanol, and in methanol. Benazepril's chemical name is 3-[[1-(ethoxy-carbonyl)-3-phenyl-(1S)-propyl]amino]-2, 3, 4, 5-tetrahydro-2-oxo-1*H*-1-(3S)-benzazepine-1-acetic acid monohydrochloride. Its empirical formula is $C_{24}H_{28}N_2O_5$·HCl, and its molecular weight is 460.96.

Benazeprilat, the active metabolite of benazepril, is a non-sulfhydryl Angiotensin-converting enzyme inhibitor. Benazepril is converted to Benazeprilat by hepatic cleavage of the ester group.

Benazepril HCl is supplied as tablets containing 5 mg, 10 mg, 20 mg, and 40 mg of benazepril for oral administration. The inactive ingredients are cellulose compounds, colloidal silicon dioxide, crospovidone, hydrogenated castor oil (5 mg, 10 mg, and 20 mg tablets), iron oxides, lactose, magnesium stearate (40 mg tablets), polysorbate 80, propylene glycol (5 mg and 40 mg tablets), starch, talc, and titanium dioxide.

CLINICAL PHARMACOLOGY:

MECHANISM OF ACTION

Benazepril and benazeprilat inhibit angiotensin-converting enzyme (ACE) in human subjects and animals. ACE is a peptidyl dipeptidase that catalyzes the conversion of angiotensin I to the vasoconstrictor substance, angiotensin II. Angiotensin II also stimulates aldosterone secretion by the adrenal cortex.

Inhibition of ACE results in decreased plasma angiotensin II, which leads to decreased vasopressor activity and to decreased aldosterone secretion. The latter decrease may result in a small increase of serum potassium. Hypertensive patients treated with benazepril HCl alone for up to 52 weeks had elevations of serum potassium of up to 0.2 mEq/L. Similar patients treated with benazepril HCl and hydrochlorothiazide for up to 24 weeks had no consistent changes in their serum potassium (see PRECAUTIONS).

Removal of angiotensin II negative feedback on renin secretion leads to increased plasma renin activity. In animal studies, benazepril had no inhibitory effect on the vasopressor response to angiotensin II and did not interfere with the hemodynamic effects of the autonomic neurotransmitters acetylcholine, epinephrine, and norepinephrine.

ACE is identical to kininase, an enzyme that degrades bradykinin. Whether increased levels of bradykinin, a potent vasodepressor peptide, play a role in the therapeutic effects of benazepril HCl remains to be elucidated.

While the mechanism through which benazepril lowers blood pressure is believed to be primarily suppression of the renin-angiotensin-aldosterone system, benazepril has an antihypertensive effect even in patients with low-renin hypertension. In particular, benazepril HCl was antihypertensive in all races studied, although it was somewhat less effective in blacks than in nonblacks.

PHARMACOKINETICS AND METABOLISM

Following oral administration of benazepril HCl, peak plasma concentrations of benazepril are reached within 0.5-1.0 hours. The extent of absorption is at least 37% as determined by urinary recovery and is not significantly influenced by the presence of food in the GI tract.

Cleavage of the ester group (primarily in the liver) converts benazepril to its active metabolite, Benazeprilat. Peak plasma concentrations of Benazeprilat are reached 1-2 hours after drug intake in the fasting state and 2-4 hours after drug intake in the nonfasting state. The serum protein binding of benazepril is about 96.7% and that of Benazeprilat about 95.3%, as measured by equilibrium dialysis; on the basis of *in vitro* studies, the degree of protein binding should be unaffected by age, hepatic dysfunction, or concentration (over the concentration range of 0.24-23.6 μmol/L).

Benazepril is almost completely metabolized to benazeprilat, which has much greater ACE inhibitory activity than benazepril, and to the glucuronide conjugates of benazepril and benazeprilat. Only trace amounts of an administered dose of benazepril HCl can be recovered in the urine as unchanged benazepril, while about 20% of the dose is excreted as benazeprilat, 4% as benazepril glucuronide, and 8% as benazeprilat glucuronide.

The kinetics of benazepril are approximately dose-proportional within the dosage range of 10-80 mg.

The effective half-life of accumulation of benazeprilat following multiple dosing of benazepril HCl is 10-11 hours. Thus, steady-state concentrations of benazeprilat should be reached after 2 or 3 doses of benazepril HCl given once daily.

The kinetics did not change, and there was no significant accumulation during chronic administration (28 days) of once-daily doses between 5 mg and 20 mg. Accumulation ratios based on AUC and urinary recovery of benazeprilat were 1.19 and 1.27, respectively.

When dialysis was started two hours after ingestion of 10 mg of benazepril, approximately 6% of benazeprilat was removed in 4 hours of dialysis. The parent compound, benazepril, was not detected in the dialysate.

The disposition of benazepril and benazeprilat in patients with mild-to-moderate renal insufficiency (creatinine clearance >30 ml/min) is similar to that in patients with normal renal function. In patients with creatinine clearance ≤30 ml/min, peak benazeprilat levels and the initial (alpha phase) half-life increase, and time to steady-state may be delayed (see DOSAGE AND ADMINISTRATION).

Benazepril and benazeprilat are cleared predominantly by renal excretion in healthy subjects with normal renal function. Nonrenal (*i.e.*, biliary) excretion accounts for approximately 11-12% of benazeprilat excretion in healthy subjects. In patients with renal failure, biliary clearance may compensate to an extent for deficient renal clearance.

In patients with hepatic dysfunction due to cirrhosis, levels of benazeprilat are essentially unaltered. The pharmacokinetics of benazepril and benazeprilat do not appear to be influenced by age.

In studies in rats given ^{14}C-benazepril, benazepril and its metabolites crossed the blood-brain barrier only to an extremely low extent. Multiple doses of benazepril did not result in accumulation in any tissue except the lung, where, as with other ACE inhibitors in similar studies, there was a slight increase in concentration due to slow elimination in that organ.

Some placental passage occurred when the drug was administered to pregnant rats.

PHARMACODYNAMICS

Single and multiple doses of 10 mg or more of benazepril HCl cause inhibition of plasma ACE activity by at least 80-90% for at least 24 hours after dosing. Pressor responses to exogenous angiotensin I were inhibited by 60-90% (up to 4 hours post-dose) at the 10 mg dose.

CLINICAL PHARMACOLOGY: *(cont'd)*

Administration of benazepril HCl to patients with mild-to-moderate hypertension results in a reduction of both supine and standing blood pressure to about the same extent with no compensatory tachycardia. Symptomatic postural hypotension is infrequent, although it can occur in patients who are salt-and/or volume-depleted (see WARNINGS).

In single-dose studies, benazepril HCl lowered blood pressure within 1 hour, with peak reductions achieved 2-4 hours after dosing. The antihypertensive effect of a single dose persisted for 24 hours. In multiple dose studies, once-daily doses of 20-80 mg decreased seated pressure (systolic/diastolic) 24 hours after dosing by about 6-12/4-7 mmHg. The trough values represent reductions of about 50% of that seen at peak.

Four dose-response studies using once-daily dosing were conducted in 470 mild-to-moderate hypertensive patients not using diuretics. The minimal effective once-daily dose of benazepril HCl was 10 mg; but further falls in blood pressure, especially at morning trough, were seen with higher doses in the studied dosing range (10-80 mg). In studies comparing the same daily dose of benazepril HCl given as a single morning dose or as a twice-daily dose, blood pressure reductions at the time of morning trough blood levels were greater with the divided regimen.

During chronic therapy, the maximum reduction in blood pressure with any dose is generally achieved after 1-2 weeks. The antihypertensive effects of benazepril HCl have continued during therapy for at least two years. Abrupt withdrawal of benazepril HCl has not been associated with a rapid increase in blood pressure.

In patients with mild-to-moderate hypertension, benazepril HCl 10-20 mg was similar in effectiveness to captopril, hydrochlorothiazide, nifedipine SR, and propranolol.

The antihypertensive effects of benazepril HCl were not appreciably different in patients receiving high- or low-sodium diets.

In hemodynamic studies in dogs, blood pressure reduction was accompanied by a reduction in peripheral arterial resistance, with an increase in cardiac output and renal blood flow and little or no change in heart rate. In normal human volunteers, single doses of benazepril caused an increase in renal blood flow but had no effect on glomerular filtration rate.

Use of benazepril HCl in combination with thiazide diuretics gives a blood-pressure-lowering effect greater than that seen with either agent alone. By blocking the renin-angiotensin-aldosterone axis, administration of benazepril HCl tends to reduce the potassium loss associated with the diuretic.

CLINICAL STUDIES:

Creatinine and Blood Urea Nitrogen: Of hypertensive patients with no apparent preexisting renal disease, about 2% have sustained increases in serum creatinine to at least 150% of their baseline values while receiving benazepril HCl, but most of these increases have disappeared despite continuing treatment. A much smaller fraction of these patients (less than 0.1%) developed simultaneous (usually transient) increases in blood urea nitrogen and serum creatinine. None of these increases required discontinuation of treatment. Increases in these laboratory values are more likely to occur in patients with renal insufficiency or those pretreated with a diuretic and, based on experience with other ACE inhibitors, would be expected to be especially likely in patients with renal artery stenosis (see PRECAUTIONS, General).

Potassium: Since benazepril decreases aldosterone secretion, elevation of serum potassium can occur. Potassium supplements and potassium-sparing diuretics should be given with caution, and the patient's serum potassium should be monitored frequently (see PRECAUTIONS).

Hemoglobin: Decreases in hemoglobin (a low value and a decrease of 5 g/dl) were rare, occurring in only 1 of 2014 patients receiving benazepril HCl alone and in 1 of 1357 patients receiving benazepril HCl plus a diuretic. No U.S. patients discontinued treatment because of decreases in hemoglobin.

Other (causal relationships unknown): Clinically important changes in standard laboratory tests were rarely associated with benazepril HCl administration. Elevations of liver enzymes, serum bilirubin, uric acid, and blood glucose have been reported, as have scattered incidents of hyponatremia, electrocardiographic changes, leukopenia, eosinophilia, and proteinuria. In U.S. trials, less than 0.5% of patients discontinued treatment because of laboratory abnormalities.

INDICATIONS AND USAGE:

Benazepril HCl is indicated for the treatment of hypertension. It may be used alone or in combination with thiazide diuretics.

In using benazepril HCl, consideration should be given to the fact that another angiotensin-converting enzyme inhibitor, captopril, has caused agranulocytosis, particularly in patients with renal impairment or collagen-vascular disease. Available data are insufficient to show that benazepril HCl does not have a similar risk (see WARNINGS).

CONTRAINDICATIONS:

Benazepril HCl is contraindicated in patients who are hypersensitive to this product or to any other ACE inhibitor.

WARNINGS:

ANAPHYLACTOID AND POSSIBLY RELATED REACTIONS

Presumably because angiotensin-converting inhibitors affect the metabolism of eicosanoids and polypeptides, including endogenous bradykinin, patients receiving ACE inhibitors (including benazepril HCl) may be subject to a variety of adverse reactions, some of them serious.

Angioedema: Angioedema of the face, extremities, lips, tongue, glottis, and larynx has been reported in patients treated with angiotensin-converting enzyme inhibitors. In U.S. clinical trials, symptoms consistent with angioedema were seen in none of the subjects who received placebo and in about 0.5% of the subjects who received benazepril HCl. Angioedema associated with laryngeal edema can be fatal. If laryngeal stridor or angioedema of the face, tongue, or glottis occurs, treatment with benazepril HCl should be discontinued and appropriate therapy instituted immediately. **Where there is involvement of the tongue, glottis, or larynx, likely to cause airway obstruction, appropriate therapy, *e.g.*, subcutaneous epinephrine injection 1:1000 (0.3 ml to 0.5 ml) should be promptly administered** (see ADVERSE REACTIONS).

Anaphylactoid Reactions During Desensitization: Two patients undergoing desensitizing treatment with hymenoptera venom while receiving ACE inhibitors sustained life-threatening anaphylactoid reactions. In the same patients, these reactions were avoided when ACE inhibitors were temporarily withheld, but they reappeared upon inadvertent rechallenge.

Anaphylactoid Reactions During Membrane Exposure: Anaphylactoid reactions have been reported in patients dialyzed with high-flux membranes and treated concomitantly with an ACE inhibitor. Anaphylactoid reactions have also been reported in patients undergoing low-density lipoprotein apheresis with dextran sulfate absorption (a procedure dependent upon devices not approved in the United States.

WARNINGS: *(cont'd)*

HYPOTENSION

Benazepril HCl can cause symptomatic hypotension. Like other ACE inhibitors, benazepril has been only rarely associated with hypotension in uncomplicated hypertensive patients. Symptomatic hypotension is most likely to occur in patients who have been volume- and/or salt-depleted as a result of prolonged diuretic therapy, dietary salt restriction, dialysis, diarrhea, or vomiting. Volume- and/or salt-depletion should be corrected before initiating therapy with benazepril HCl.

In patients with congestive heart failure, with or without associated renal insufficiency, ACE inhibitor therapy may cause excessive hypotension, which may be associated with oliguria or azotemia and, rarely, with acute renal failure and death. In such patients, benazepril HCl therapy should be started under close medical supervision; they should be followed closely for the first 2 weeks of treatment and whenever the dose of benazepril or diuretic is increased.

If hypotension occurs, the patient should be placed in a supine position, and if necessary, treated with intravenous infusion of physiological saline. benazepril HCl treatment usually can be continued following restoration of blood pressure and volume.

NEUTROPENIA/AGRANULOCYTOSIS

Another angiotensin-converting enzyme inhibitor, captopril, has been shown to cause agranulocytosis and bone marrow depression, rarely in uncomplicated patients, but more frequently in patients with renal impairment, especially if they also have a collagen-vascular disease such as systemic lupus erythematosus or scleroderma. Available data from clinical trials or benazepril are insufficient to show that benazepril does not cause agranulocytosis at similar rates. Monitoring of white blood cell counts should be considered in patients with collagen-vascular disease, especially if the disease is associated with impaired renal function.

FETAL/NEONATAL MORBIDITY AND MORTALITY

ACE inhibitors can cause fetal and neonatal morbidity and death when administered to pregnant women. Several dozen cases have been reported in the world literature. When pregnancy is detected, ACE inhibitors should be discontinued as soon as possible.

The use of ACE inhibitors during the second and third trimesters of pregnancy has been associated with fetal and neonatal injury, including hypotension, neonatal skull hypoplasia, anuria, reversible or irreversible renal failure, and death. Oligohydramnios has also been reported, presumably resulting from decreased fetal renal function; oligohydramnios in this setting has been associated with fetal limb contractures, craniofacial deformation, and hypoplastic lung development. Prematurity, intrauterine growth retardation, and patent ductus arteriosus have also been reported, although it is not clear whether these occurrences were due to the ACE inhibitor exposure.

These adverse effects do not appear to have resulted from intrauterine ACE inhibitor exposure that has been limited to the first trimester. Mothers whose embryos and fetuses are exposed to ACE inhibitors only during the first trimester should be so informed. Nonetheless, when patients become pregnant, physicians should make every effort to discontinue the use of benazepril as soon as possible.

Rarely (probably less often than once in every thousand pregnancies), no alternative to ACE inhibitors will be found. In these rare cases, the mothers should be apprised of the potential hazards to their fetuses, and serial ultrasound examinations should be performed to assess the intraamniotic environment.

If oligohydramnios is observed, benazepril should be discontinued unless it is considered lifesaving for the mother. Contraction stress testing (CST), a nonstress test (NST), or biophysical profiling (BPP) may be appropriate, depending upon the week of pregnancy. Patients and physicians should be aware, however, that oligohydramnios may not appear until after the fetus has sustained irreversible injury.

Infants with histories of *in utero* exposure to ACE inhibitors should be closely observed for hypotension, oliguria, and hyperkalemia. If oliguria occurs, attention should be directed toward support of blood pressure and renal perfusion. Exchange transfusion or dialysis may be required as means of reversing hypotension and/or substituting for disordered renal function. Benazepril, which crosses the placenta, can theoretically be removed from the neonatal circulation by these means; there are occasional reports of benefit from these maneuvers with another ACE inhibitor, but experience is limited.

No teratogenic effects of benazepril were seen in studies of pregnant rats, mice, and rabbits. On a mg/m^2 basis, the doses used in these studies were 60 times (in rats), 9 times (in mice), and more than 0.8 times (in rabbits) the maximum recommended human dose (assuming a 50 kg woman). On a mg/kg basis these multiples are 300 times (in rats), 90 times (in mice) and more than 3 times (in rabbits) the maximum recommended human dose.

HEPATIC FAILURE

Rarely, ACE inhibitors have been associated with a syndrome that starts with cholestatic jaundice and progresses to fulminent hepatic necrosis and (sometimes) death. The mechanism of this syndrome is not understood. Patients receiving ACE inhibitors who develop jaundice or marked elevations of hepatic enzymes should discontinue the ACE inhibitor and receive appropriate medical follow-up.

PRECAUTIONS:

GENERAL

Impaired Renal Function: As a consequence of inhibiting the renin-angiotensin-aldosterone system, changes in renal function may be anticipated in susceptible individuals. In patients with severe congestive heart failure whose renal function may depend on the activity of the renin-angiotensin-aldosterone system, treatment with angiotensin-converting enzyme inhibitors, including benazepril HCl, may be associated with oliguria and/or progressive azotemia and (rarely) with acute renal failure and/or death. In a small study of hypertensive patients with renal artery stenosis in a solitary kidney or bilateral renal artery stenosis, treatment with benazepril HCl was associated with increases in blood urea nitrogen and serum creatinine; these increases were reversible upon discontinuation of benazepril HCl or diuretic therapy, or both. When such patients are treated with ACE inhibitors, renal function should be monitored during the first few weeks of therapy. Some hypertensive patients with no apparent preexisting renal vascular disease have developed increases in blood urea nitrogen and serum creatinine, usually minor and transient, especially when benazepril HCl has been given concomitantly with a diuretic. This is more likely to occur in patients with preexisting renal impairment. Dosage reduction of benazepril HCl and/or discontinuation of the diuretic may be required. **Evaluation of the hypertensive patient should always include assessment of renal function** (see DOSAGE AND ADMINISTRATION).

Hemodialysis: Anaphylactoid reactions have been reported in patients dialyzed with high-flux membranes and treated concomitantly with an ACE inhibitor. In these patients, consideration should be given to using a different type of dialysis membrane or a different class of antihypertensive agent.

Hyperkalemia: In clinical trials, hyperkalemia (serum potassium at least 0.5 mEq/L greater than the upper limit of normal) occurred in approximately 1% of hypertensive patients receiving benazepril HCl. In most cases, these were isolated values which resolved despite continued therapy. Risk factors for the development of hyperkalemia include renal insufficiency, diabetes mellitus, and the concomitant use of potassium-sparing diuretics, potassium supplements, and/or potassium-containing salt substitutes, which should be used cautiously, if at all, with benazepril HCl (see DRUG INTERACTIONS).

PRECAUTIONS: *(cont'd)*

Cough: Cough has been reported with the use of ACE inhibitors. Characteristically, the cough is nonproductive, persistent, and resolves after discontinuation of therapy. ACE inhibitor-induced cough should be considered as part of the differential diagnosis of cough.

Impaired Liver Function: In patients with hepatic dysfunction due to cirrhosis, levels of benazeprilat are essentially unaltered.

Surgery/Anesthesia: In patients undergoing surgery or during anesthesia with agents that produce hypotension, benazepril will block the angiotensin II formation that could otherwise occur secondary to compensatory renin release. Hypotension that occurs as a result of this mechanism can be corrected by volume expansion.

CARCINOGENESIS, MUTAGENESIS, AND IMPAIRMENT OF FERTILITY

No evidence of carcinogenicity was found when benazepril was administered to rats and mice for up to two years at doses of up to 150 mg/kg/day. When compared on the basis of body weights, this dose is 110 times the maximum recommended human dose; When compared on the basis to body surface areas, this dose is 18 and 9 times (rats and mice, respectively) the maximum recommended human dose (calculations assume a patient weight of 60 kg). No mutagenic activity was detected in the Ames test in bacteria (with or without metabolic activation), in an *in vitro* test for forward mutations in cultured mammalian cells, or in a nucleus anomaly test. In doses of 50-500 mg/kg/day (6-60 times the maximum recommended human dose based on mg/m^2 comparison and 37-375 times the maximum recommended human dose based on a mg/kg comparison). Benazepril HCl had no adverse effect on the reproductive performance of male and female rats.

Pregnancy Categories C (first trimester) and D (second and third trimesters) See WARNINGS, Fetal/Neonatal Morbidity and Mortality.

NURSING MOTHERS

Minimal amounts of unchanged benazepril and of benazeprilat are excreted into the breast milk of lactating women treated with benazepril. A newborn child ingesting entirely breast milk would receive less than 0.1% of the mg/kg maternal dose of benazepril and benazeprilat.

GERIATRIC USE

Of the total number of patients who received benazepril in U.S. clinical studies of benazepril HCl, 18% were 65 or older while 2% were 75 or older. No overall differences in effectiveness or safety were observed between these patients and younger patients, and other reported clinical experience has not identified differences in responses between the elderly and younger patients, but greater sensitivity of some older individuals cannot be ruled out.

PEDIATRIC USE

Safety and effectiveness in children have not been established.

DRUG INTERACTIONS:

Diuretics: Patients on diuretics, especially those in whom diuretic therapy was recently instituted, may occasionally experience an excessive reduction of blood pressure after initiation of therapy with benazepril HCl. The possibility of hypotensive effects with benazepril HCl can be minimized by either discontinuing the diuretic or increasing the salt intake prior to initiation of treatment with benazepril HCl. If this is not possible, the starting dose should be reduced (see DOSAGE AND ADMINISTRATION).

POTASSIUM SUPPLEMENTS AND POTASSIUM-SPARING DIURETICS

Benazepril HCl can attenuate potassium loss caused by thiazide diuretics. Potassium-sparing diuretics (spironolactone, amiloride, triamterene, and others) or potassium supplements can increase the risk of hyperkalemia. Therefore, if concomitant use of such agents is indicated, they should be given with caution, and the patient's serum potassium should be monitored frequently.

ORAL ANTICOAGULANTS

Interaction studies with warfarin and acenocoumarol failed to identify any clinically important effects on the serum concentrations or clinical effects of these anticoagulants.

LITHIUM

Increased serum lithium levels and symptoms of lithium toxicity have been reported in patients receiving ACE inhibitors during therapy with lithium. These drugs should be coadministered with caution, and frequent monitoring of serum lithium levels is recommended. If a diuretic is also used, the risk of lithium toxicity may be increased.

OTHER

No clinically important pharmacokinetic interactions occurred when benazepril HCl was administered concomitantly with hydrochlorothiazide, chlorthalidone, furosemide, digoxin, propranolol, atenolol, naproxen, or cimetidine.

Benazepril HCl has been used concomitantly with beta-adrenergic-blocking agents, calcium-channel-blocking agents, diuretics, digoxin, and hydralazine, without evidence of clinically important adverse interactions. Benazepril, like other ACE inhibitors, has had less than additive effects with beta-adrenergic blockers, presumably because both drugs lower blood pressure by inhibiting parts of the renin-angiotensin system.

ADVERSE REACTIONS:

Benazepril HCl has been evaluated for safety in over 6000 patients with hypertension; over 700 of these patients were treated for at least one year. The overall incidence of reported adverse events was comparable in benazepril HCl and placebo patients.

The reported side effects were generally mild and transient, and there was no relation between side effects and age, duration of therapy, or total dosage within the range of 2 to 80 mg.

Discontinuation of therapy because of a side effect was required in approximately 5% of U.S. patients treated with benazepril HCl and in 3% of patients treated with placebo.

The most common reasons for discontinuation were headache (0.6%) and cough (0.5%). See PRECAUTIONS, Cough.

The side effects considered possibly or probably related to study drug that occurred in U.S. placebo-controlled trials in more than 1% of patients treated with benazepril HCl are shown below (TABLE 1).

TABLE 1 Patients In U.S. Placebo-Controlled Studies

	LOTENSIN (N = 964)		PLACEBO (N = 496)	
	%	N	%	N
Headache	60	6.2	21	4.2
Dizziness	35	3.6	12	2.4
Fatigue	23	2.4	11	2.2
Somnolence	15	1.6	2	0.4
Postural Dizziness	14	1.5	1	0.2
Nausea	13	1.3	5	1.0
Cough	12	1.2	5	1.0

Other adverse experiences reported in controlled clinical trials (in less than 1% of benazepril patients), and rarer events seen in postmarketing experience, include the following (in some, a causal relationship to drug use is uncertain):

ADVERSE REACTIONS: *(cont'd)*

Cardiovascular: Symptomatic hypotension was seen in 0.3% of patients, postural hypotension in 0.4%, and syncope in 0.1%; these reactions led to discontinuation of therapy in 4 patients who had received benazepril monotherapy and in 9 patients who had received benazepril with hydrochlorothiazide (see PRECAUTIONS and WARNINGS). Other reports included angina pectoris, palpitations, and peripheral edema.

Renal: Of hypertensive patients with no apparent preexisting renal disease, about 2% have sustained increases in serum creatinine to at least 150% of their baseline values while receiving benazepril HCl, but most of these increases have disappeared despite continuing treatment. A much smaller fraction of these patients (less than 0.1%) developed simultaneous (usually transient) increases in blood urea nitrogen and serum creatinine.

Fetal/Neonatal Morbidity and Mortality: See WARNINGS, Fetal/Neonatal Morbidity and Mortality.

Angioedema: Angioedema has been reported in patients receiving ACE inhibitors. During clinical trials in hypertensive patients with benazepril, 0.5% of patients experienced edema of the lips or face without other manifestations of angioedema. Angioedema associated with laryngeal edema and/or shock may be fatal. If angioedema of the face, extremities, lips, tongue, or glottis and/or larynx occurs, treatment with benazepril HCl should be discontinued and appropriate therapy instituted immediately (see WARNINGS.)

Gastrointestinal: Constipation, gastritis, vomiting, pancreatitis, and melena.

Dermatologic: Apparent hypersensitivity reactions (manifested by dermatitis, pruritus, or rash), photosensitivity, and flushing.

Neurologic and Psychiatric: Anxiety, decreased libido, hypertonia, insomnia, nervousness, and paresthesia.

Hematologic: There have been rare reports of hemolytic anemia in patients receiving ACE inhibitors.

Other: Arthralgia, arthritis, asthenia, asthma, bronchitis, dyspnea, impotence, infection, myalgia, sinusitis, sweating, and urinary tract infection.

OVERDOSAGE:

Single oral doses of 3 g/kg benazepril were associated with significant lethality in mice. Rats however, tolerated single oral doses of up to 6 g/kg. Reduced activity was seen at 1 g/kg in mice and at 5 g/kg in rats. Human overdoses of benazepril have not been reported, but the most common manifestation of human benazepril overdosage is likely to be hypotension.

Laboratory determinations of serum levels of benazepril and its metabolites are not widely available, and such determinations have, in any event, no established role in the management of benazepril overdose.

No data are available to suggest physiological maneuvers (*e.g.*, maneuvers to change the pH of the urine) that might accelerate elimination of benazepril and its metabolites. Benazepril is only slightly dialyzable, but dialysis might be considered in overdosed patients with severely impaired renal function (see WARNINGS.)

Angiotensin II could presumably serve as a specific antagonist-antidote in the setting of benazepril overdose, but angiotensin II is essentially unavailable outside of scattered research facilities. Because the hypotensive effect of benazepril is achieved through vasodilation and effective hypovolemia, it is reasonable to treat benazepril overdose by infusion of normal saline solution.

DOSAGE AND ADMINISTRATION:

The recommended initial dose for patients not receiving a diuretic is 10 mg once-a-day. The usual maintenance dosage range is 20-40 mg per day administered as a single dose or in two equally divided doses. A dose of 80 mg gives an increased response, but experience with this dose is limited. The divided regimen was more effective in controlling trough (pre-dosing) blood pressure than the same dose given as a once-daily regimen. Dosage adjustment should be based on measurement of peak (2-6 hours after dosing) and trough responses. If a once-daily regimen does not give adequate trough response an increase in dosage or divided in dosage or divided administration should be considered. If blood pressure is not controlled with benazepril HCl alone, a diuretic can be added.

Total daily doses above 80 mg have not been evaluated.

Concomitant administration of benazepril HCl with potassium supplements, potassium salt substitutes, or potassium-sparing diuretics can lead to increases of serum potassium (see PRECAUTIONS).

In patients who are currently being treated with a diuretic, symptomatic hypotension occasionally can occur following the initial dose of benazepril HCl. To reduce the likelihood of hypotension, the diuretic should, if possible, be discontinued two to three days prior to beginning therapy with benazepril HCl (see WARNINGS). Then, if blood pressure is not controlled with benazepril HCl alone, diuretic therapy should be resumed.

If the diuretic cannot be discontinued, an initial dose of 5 mg benazepril HCl should be used to avoid excessive hypotension.

DOSAGE ADJUSTMENT IN RENAL IMPAIRMENT

For patients with a creatinine clearance <30 ml/min/1.73 m^2 (serum creatinine >3 mg/dl), the recommended initial dose is 5 mg benazepril HCl once daily. Dosage may be titrated upward until blood pressure is controlled or to a maximum total daily dose of 40 mg (seePRECAUTIONS, Hemodialysis Patients).

PATIENT INFORMATION:

Pregnancy: Female patients of childbearing age should be told about the consequences of second- and third-trimester exposure to ACE inhibitors, and they should also be told that these consequences do not appear to have resulted from intrauterine ACE inhibitor exposure that has been limited to the first trimester. These patients should be asked to report pregnancies to their physicians as soon as possible.

Angioedema: Angioedema, including laryngeal edema, can occur with treatment with ACE inhibitors, especially following the first dose. Patients should be so advised and told to report immediately any signs or symptoms suggesting angioedema (swelling of face, eyes, lips, or tongue, or difficulty in breathing) and to take no more drug until they have consulted with the prescribing physician.

Symptomatic Hypotension: Patients should be cautioned that light-headedness can occur, especially during the first days of therapy, and it should be reported to the prescribing physician. Patients should be told that if syncope occurs, benazepril HCl should be discontinued until the prescribing physician has been consulted.

All patients should be cautioned that inadequate fluid intake or excessive perspiration, diarrhea, or vomiting can lead to an excessive fall in blood pressure, with the same consequences of light-headedness and possible syncope.

Hyperkalemia: Patients should be told not to use potassium supplements or salt substitutes containing potassium without consulting the prescribing physician.

Neutropenia: Patients should be told to promptly report any indication of infection (*e.g.*, sore throat, fever), which could be a sign of neutropenia.

HOW SUPPLIED:

Benazepril HCl is available in tablets of 5 mg, 10 mg, 20 mg, and 40 mg, packaged with a desiccant in bottles of 100 tablets. Benazepril HCl is also supplied in blister packages (1 tablet/blister), in Accu-Pak Unit Dose boxes containing 10 strips of 10 blisters each.

Each tablet is imprinted with "LOTENSIN" on one side and the tablet strength ("5", "10", "20", or "40") on the other. Samples, when available, are identified by the word *SAMPLE* on each tablet.

Storage: Do not store above 86° F (30° C). Protect from moisture. *Dispense in tight container.*

HOW SUPPLIED - EQUIVALENTS NOT AVAILABLE:

Tablet, Uncoated - Oral - 5 mg

100's	$63.63	LOTENSIN, Novartis	00083-0059-30
100's	$63.63	LOTENSIN, Novartis	00083-0059-32

Tablet, Uncoated - Oral - 10 mg

100's	$63.63	LOTENSIN, Novartis	00083-0063-30
100's	$63.63	LOTENSIN, Novartis	00083-0063-32

Tablet, Uncoated - Oral - 20 mg

100's	$63.63	LOTENSIN, Novartis	00083-0079-30
100's	$63.63	LOTENSIN, Novartis	00083-0079-32

Tablet, Uncoated - Oral - 40 mg

100's	$63.63	LOTENSIN, Novartis	00083-0094-30
100's	$63.63	LOTENSIN, Novartis	00083-0094-32

BENAZEPRIL HYDROCHLORIDE; HYDROCHLOROTHIAZIDE *(003124)*

CATEGORIES: ACE Inhibitors; Angiotensin Converting Enzyme Inhibitors; Antihypertensives; Cardiovascular Drugs; Diuretics; Hypertension; Pregnancy Category D; FDA Class 1C ("Little or No Therapeutic Advantage"); FDA Approved 1992 May; Top 200 Drugs; Top 200 Drugs

BRAND NAMES: *Cibacen HCT*; *Cibadrex* (Germany, France); **Lotensin HCT**
(International brand names outside U.S. in italics)

FORMULARIES: Aetna

DESCRIPTION:

This drug is a combination of benazepril and hydrochlorothiazide USP. It is available for oral use in four tablet strengths: Benazepril HCl w/HCTZ 5/6.25, containing 5 mg of benazepril hydrochloride and 6.25 mg of hydrochlorothiazide USP; benazepril HCl w/HCTZ 10/12.5, containing 10 mg of benazepril hydrochloride and 12.5 mg of hydrochlorothiazide USP; and benazepril HCl w/HCTZ 20/12.5, containing 20 mg of benazepril hydrochloride and 12.5 mg of hydrochlorothiazide USP; and benazepril HCl w/HCTZ 20/25, containing 20 mg of benazepril hydrochloride and 25 mg of hydrochlorothiazide USP. The inactive ingredients of the tablets are cellulose compounds, crospovidone, hydrogenated castor oil, iron oxides (10/12.5-mg, 20/12.5-mg, and 20/25-mg tablets), lactose, polyethylene glycol, talc, and titanium dioxide.

INDICATIONS AND USAGE:

Benazepril HCl w/HCTZ is indicated for the treatment of hypertension.

In using benazepril HCl w/HCTZ, consideration should be given to the fact that another angiotensin-converting-enzyme inhibitor, captopril, has caused agranulocytosis, particularly in patients with renal impairment or collagen-vascular disease. Available data are insufficient to show that benazepril does have a similar risk.

FOR COMPLETE PRESCRIBING INFORMATION REFER TO THE INDIVIDUAL DRUG MONOGRAPHS (BENAZEPRIL HCl; HYDROCHLOROTHIAZIDE).

DOSAGE AND ADMINISTRATION:

Benazepril is an effective treatment of hypertension in once-daily doses of 10-80 mg, while hydrochlorothiazide is effective in doses of 25-100 mg. In clinical trials of benazepril/hydrochlorothiazide combination therapy using benazepril doses of 5-20 mg and hydrochlorothiazide doses of 6.25-25 mg, the antihypertensive effects increased with increasing dose of either component.

The side effects of benazepril are generally rare and apparently independent of dose; those of hydrochlorothiazide are a mixture of dose-dependent phenomena (primarily hypokalemia) and dose-independent phenomena (*e.g.*, pancreatitis), the former much more common than the latter. Therapy with any combination of benazepril and hydrochlorothiazide will be associated with both sets of dose-independent side effects, but regimens in which benazepril is combined with low doses of hydrochlorothiazide produce minimal effects on serum potassium. In clinical trials of benazepril HCl w/HCTZ, the average change in serum potassium was near zero in subjects who received 5/6.25 mg or 20/12.5 mg, but the average subject who received 10/12.5 mg or 20/25 mg experienced a mild reduction in serum potassium, similar to that experienced by the average subject receiving the same dose of hydrochlorothiazide monotherapy.

To minimize dose-independent side-effects, it is usually appropriate to begin combination therapy only after a patient has failed to achieve the desired effect with monotherapy.

Therapy Guided by Clinical Effect: A patient whose blood pressure is not adequately controlled with benazepril monotherapy may be switched to benazepril HCl w/HCTZ 10/12.5 or benazepril HCl w/HCTZ 20/12.5. Further increases of either or both components could depend on clinical response. The hydrochlorothiazide dose should generally not be increased until 2-3 weeks have elapsed. Patients whose blood pressures are adequately controlled with 25 mg of daily hydrochlorothiazide, but who experience significant potassium loss with this regimen, may achieve similar blood- pressure control without electrolyte disturbance if they are switched to benazepril HCl w/HCTZ 5/6.25.

Replacement Therapy: The combination may be substituted for the titrated individual components.

Use in Renal Impairment: Regimens of therapy with benazepril HCl w/HCTZ need not take account of renal function as long as the patient's creatinine clearance is >30 ml/min/1.73m^2 (serum creatinine roughly ≤3 mg/dl or 265 µmol/l). In patients with more severe renal impairment, loop diuretics are preferred to thiazides, so benazepril HCl w/HCTZ is not recommended.

Storage: Do not store above 86°F (30°C). Protect from moisture and light. Dispense in tight, light resistance container (USP).

PATIENT INFORMATION:

This product is a combination product containing benazepril (an ACE-inhibitor) and hydrochlorothiazide (a diuretic-water pill). It is used to treat high blood pressure. This medication should not be used during pregnancy and should be discontinued when pregnancy is determined. A nonproductive, persistent cough has been reported with the use of ACE inhibitors. The cough normally disappears when the medication is discontinued. A rare condition called angioedema can occur with ACE inhibitors, especially following the first dose. If you experience swelling of the face, eyes, lips, or tongue, difficulty in breathing) do not take additional medication and contact your physician immediately. Dizziness and lightheaded can result when the mediation is first started. If this persists longer than one week, contact your physician. Signs of infections (sore throat or fever) should be reported to your physician as well to assure these are not drug related.

HOW SUPPLIED - EQUIVALENTS NOT AVAILABLE:

Tablet, Uncoated - Oral - 5 mg/6.25 mg

100's	$63.63	LOTENSIN HCT, Novartis	00083-0057-30

Tablet, Uncoated - Oral - 10 mg/12.5 mg

100's	$63.63	LOTENSIN HCT, Novartis	00083-0072-30

Tablet, Uncoated - Oral - 20 mg/12.5 mg

100's	$63.63	LOTENSIN HCT, Novartis	00083-0074-30

Tablet, Uncoated - Oral - 20 mg/25 mg

100's	$63.63	LOTENSIN HCT, Novartis	00083-0075-30

BENDROFLUMETHIAZIDE *(000401)*

CATEGORIES: Antihypertensives; Cardiovascular Drugs; Cirrhosis; Congestive Heart Failure; Diuretics; Edema; Electrolytic, Caloric-Water Balance; Glomerulonephritis; Heart Failure; Hypertension; Nephrotic Syndrome; Renal Drugs; Renal Failure; Thiazides; Pregnancy Category C; FDA Approval Pre 1982

BRAND NAMES: *Aprinox* (Australia, England); *Bendrofluazide*; *Benzide*; *Berkozide* (England); *Centyl*; *Esberizid*; **Naturetin**; *Naturine* (France); *Neo-Naclex*; *Pluryl*; *Pluryle*; *Salural*; *Sinesalin* (Germany)
(International brand names outside U.S. in italics)

FORMULARIES: Medi-Cal

DESCRIPTION:

Naturetin is a benzothiadiazine derivative containing a benzyl and a trifluoromethyl group. It is a potent oral diuretic and antihypertensive agent. Bendroflumethiazide is designated chemically as 3-benzyl-3,4-dihydro-6-(trifluoromethyl)-2H-1,2,4-benzothiadiazine-7-sulfonamide 1,1-dioxide.

$C_{15}H_{14}F_3N_3O_4S_2$ MW 421.41 CAS-73-48-3

It is available as compressed tablets providing 5 or 10 mg bendroflumethiazide. Inactive ingredients: microcrystalline cellulose, colorants (D&C Yellow No. 10; FD&C Blue No. 1 for 5 mg only, and FD&C Yellow No. 6 for 10 mg only), lactose, magnesium stearate, sodium starch glycolate, and pregelatinized starch.

CLINICAL PHARMACOLOGY:

Thiazides affect the renal tubular mechanism of electrolyte reabsorption. At maximal therapeutic dosage all thiazides are approximately equal in their diuretic potency.

Thiazides increase excretion of sodium and chloride in approximately equivalent amounts. Natriuresis causes a secondary loss of potassium and bicarbonate.

The mechanism of the antihypertensive effect of thiazides is unknown. Thiazides do not affect normal blood pressure.

Onset of action of thiazides occurs in two hours and the peak effect at about four hours. Duration of action persists for approximately six to 12 hours. Thiazides are eliminated rapidly by the kidney.

INDICATIONS AND USAGE:

Naturetin is indicated as adjunctive therapy in edema associated with congestive heart failure, hepatic cirrhosis, and corticosteroid and estrogen therapy.

Naturetin has also been found useful in edema due to various forms of renal dysfunction such as nephrotic syndrome, acute glomerulonephritis, and chronic renal failure.

Naturetin tablets are indicated in the management of hypertension either as the sole therapeutic agent or to enhance the effectiveness of other antihypertensive drugs in the more severe forms of hypertension.

Usage in Pregnancy. The routine use of diuretics in an otherwise healthy woman is inappropriate and exposes mother and fetus to unnecessary hazard. Diuretics do not prevent development of toxemia of pregnancy, and there is no satisfactory evidence that they are useful in the treatment of developed toxemia.

Edema during pregnancy may arise from pathological causes or from the physiologic and mechanical consequences of pregnancy. Thiazides are indicated in pregnancy when edema is due to pathologic causes, just as they are in the absence of pregnancy (however, see PRECAUTIONS, Pregnancy: Nonteratogenic Effects). Dependent edema in pregnancy, resulting from restriction of various return by the expanded uterus, is properly treated through elevation of the lower extremities and use of support hose; use of diuretics to lower intravascular volume in this case is illogical and unnecessary. There is hypervolemia during normal pregnancy which is harmful to neither the fetus nor the mother (in the absence of cardiovascular disease), but which is associated with edema, including generalized edema, in the majority of pregnant women. If this edema produces discomfort, increased recumbency will often provide relief. In rare instances, this edema may cause extreme discomfort which is not relieved by rest. In these cases, a short course of diuretics may provide relief and may be appropriate.

CONTRAINDICATIONS:

Bendroflumethiazide is contraindicated in anuria.

It is also contraindicated in patients who have previously demonstrated hypersensitivity to it or other sulfonamide-derived drugs.

WARNINGS:

Thiazides should be used with caution in severe renal disease. In patients with renal disease,thiazides may precipitate azotemia. Cumulative effects of the drug may develop in patients with impaired renal function.

Thiazides should be used with caution in patients with impaired hepatic function or progressive liver disease, since minor alterations of fluid and electrolyte balance may precipitate hepatic coma.

Sensitivity reactions may occur in patients with or without a history of allergy or bronchial asthma.

The possibility of exacerbation or activation of systemic lupus erythematosus has been reported.

WARNINGS: *(cont'd)*

Lithium generally should not be given with diuretics; diuretic agents reduce the renal clearance of lithium and add a high risk of lithium toxicity. Refer to the package insert for lithium preparations before use of such concomitant therapy.

PRECAUTIONS:

GENERAL

Periodic determination of serum electrolytes to detect possible electrolyte imbalance should be performed at appropriate intervals.

All patients receiving thiazide therapy should be observed for clinical signs of fluid or electrolyte imbalance, namely: hyponatremia, hypochloremic alkalosis, and hypokalemia. Serum and urine electrolyte determinations are particularly important when the patient is vomiting excessively or receiving parenteral fluids. Warning signs or symptoms of fluid and electrolyte imbalance include: dryness of the mouth, thirst, weakness, lethargy, drowsiness, restlessness, muscle pains or cramps, muscular fatigue, hypotension, oligoria, tachycardia, and gastrointestinal disturbances such as nausea and vomiting.

Hypokalemia may develop, especially with brisk diuresis, when severe cirrhosis is present.

Interference with adequate oral electrolyte intake will also contribute to hypokalemia. Hypokalemia can sensitize or exaggerate the response of the heart to the toxic effects of digitalis (*e.g.*, increased ventricular irritability). Concurrent administration of a potassium-sparing diuretic or potassium supplements may be indicated in these patients.

Any chloride deficit is generally mild and usually does not require specific treatment except under extraordinary circumstances (as in liver disease or renal disease). Dilutional hyponatremia may occur in edematous patients in hot weather, appropriate therapy is water restriction, rather than administration of salt, except in rare instances when the hyponatremia is life threatening. In actual salt depiction, appropriate replacement is the therapy of choice.

Hyperuricemia may occur or frank gout may be precipitated in certain patients receiving thiazide therapy.

Latent diabetes mellitus may become manifest during thiazide administration.

The antihypertensive effects of the drug may be enhanced in the postsympathectomy patient.

If progressive renal impairment becomes evident, as indicated by a rising nonprotein nitrogen or blood urea nitrogen (BUN), a careful reappraisal of therapy is necessary with consideration given to withholding or discontinuing diuretic therapy.

Thiazides may decrease serum PBI levels without signs of thyroid disturbance.

Calcium excretion is decreased by thiazides. Pathological changes in the parathyroid gland with hypercalcemia and hypophosphatemia have been observed in a few patients on prolonged thiazide therapy. The common complications of hyperparathyroidism such as renal lithiasis, bone resorption, and peptic ulceration have not been seen. Thiazides should be discontinued before carrying out tests for parathyroid function.

Thiazides have been shown to increase the urinary excretion of magnesium; this may result in hypomagnesemia.

INFORMATION FOR THE PATIENT

The patient should be advised to take the medication at the same time each day as prescribed to minimize the inconvenience of diuresis, warned against interruption or discontinuation of medication even though he may feel well, and advised about a proper course in the event of an inadvertent missed dose.

The patient should be informed of symptoms that would suggest potential adverse effects and told to report them promptly.

LABORATORY TESTS

During therapy, the patient's serum electrolyte levels should be regularly monitored. (See WARNINGS and PRECAUTIONS, General.)

DRUG/LABORATORY TEST INTERACTIONS

Bendroflumethiazide may produce false-negative results with the phentolaine and tyramine tests; may interfere with the phenolsulfonphthalein test due to decreased excretion; and it may cause diagnostic interference of serum electrolyte levels, blood and urine glucose levels, and a decrease in serum PBI levels without signs of thyroid disturbance.

CARCINOGENESIS, MUTAGENESIS, AND IMPAIRMENT OF FERTILITY

Studies have not been performed to evaluate carcinogenic potential, mutagenesis, or whether this drug adversely affects fertility in males or females.

PREGNANCY CATEGORY C:

Teratogenic Effects: Animal reproduction studies have not been conducted with bendroflumethiazide. It is also not known whether bendroflumethiazide can cause fetal harm when administered to a pregnant woman or can affect reproduction capacity. Bendroflumethiazide should be given to a pregnant woman only if clearly needed (see INDICATIONS AND USAGE).

Nonteratogenic Effects: Thiazides cross the placental barrier and appear in cord blood. The use of thiazides in pregnant women requires that the anticipated benefit be weighed against possible hazards to the fetus. These hazards include fetal or neonatal jaundice, thrombocytopenia, and possibly other adverse reactions which have occurred in the adult.

NURSING MOTHERS

Because of the potential for serious adverse reactions in nursing infants from bendroflumethiazide, a decision should be made whether to discontinue nursing or to discontinue the drug, taking into account the importance of the drug to the mother.

PEDIATRIC USE

Safety and effectiveness in children have not been established.

DRUG INTERACTIONS:

When administered concurrently, the following drugs may interact with bendroflumethiazide:

Alcohol, Barbiturates, or Narcotics potentiation of orthostatic hypotension may occur.

Amphotericin B, Corticosteroids, or Corticotropin (ACTH) may intensify electrolyte imbalance, particularly hypokalemia. Monitor potassium levels; use potassium replacements if necessary.

Anticoagulants (Oral) dosage adjustments of anticoagulant medication may be necessary since bendroflumethiazide may decrease their effects.

Antigout Medications dosage adjustments of antigout medication may be necessary since bendroflumethiazide may raise the level of blood uric acid.

Other Antihypertensive Medications (*e.g.*, Ganglionic Or Peripheral Adrenergic Blocking Agents) dosage adjustments may be necessary since bendroflumethiazide may potentiate their effects.

Antidiabetic Drugs (Oral Agents And Insulin) since thiazides may elevate blood glucose levels, dosage adjustments of antidiabetic agents may be necessary.

Calcium Salts increased serum calcium levels due to decreased excretion may occur. If calcium must be prescribed monitor serum calcium levels and adjust calcium dosage accordingly.

Cardiac Glycosides enhanced possibility of digitalis toxicity associated with hypokalemia. Monitor potassium levels; use potassium replacement if necessary.

DRUG INTERACTIONS: *(cont'd)*

Cholestyramine Resin and Colestipol HCL may delay or decrease absorption of bendroflumethiazide. Sulfonamide diuretics should be taken at least one hour before or four to six hours after these medications.

Diazoxide enhanced hyperglycemic, hyperuricemic, and antihypertensive effects. Be cognizant of possible interaction; monitor blood glucose and serum uric acid levels.

Lithium Salts may enhance lithium toxicity due to reduced renal clearance. Avoid concurrent use; if lithium must be prescribed monitor serum lithium levels and adjust lithium dosage accordingly. See WARNINGS.

MAO Inhibitors dosage adjustments of one or both agents may be necessary since hypotensive effects are enhanced.

Nondepolarizing Muscle Relaxants, Preanesthetics and Anesthetics Used in Surgery (*e.g.*, Tubocurarine Chloride and Gallamine Triethiodide) effects of these agents may be potentiated; dosage adjustments may be required. Monitor and correct any fluid and electrolyte imbalances prior to surgery if feasible.

Nonsteroidal Anti-Inflammatory Agents in some patients, the administration of a nonsteroidal anti-inflammatory agent can reduce the diuretic, natriuretic, and anti-hypertensive effect of loop, potassium-sparing or thiazide diuretics. Therefore, when bendroflumethiazide and nonsteroidal anti-inflammatory agents are used concomitantly, the patient should be observed closely to determine if the desired effect of the diuretic is obtained.

Methenamine possible decreased effectiveness due to alkalinization of the urine.

Pressor Amines (*e.g.*, Norepinephrine) decreased arterial responsiveness, but no sufficient to preclude effectiveness of the pressor agent for therapeutic use. Use caution in patients taking both medications who undergo surgery. Administer preanesthetic and anesthetic agents in reduced dosage, and if possible, discontinue bendroflumethiazide one week prior to surgery.

Probenecid or Sulfinpyrazone increased dosage of these agents may be necessary since bendroflumethiazide may have hyperuricemic effects.

ADVERSE REACTIONS:

Gastrointestinal: nausea, vomiting, cramping and anorexia are not uncommon; diarrhea, constipation, gastric irritation, abdominal bloating, jaundice (intrahepatic cholestatic jaundice), hepatitis, and sialadenitis occasionally occur; and pancreatitis has been reported.

Central Nervous System: dizziness, vertigo, paresthesia, headache, and xanthopsia occasionally occur.

Hematologic: leukopenia, agranulocytosis, thrombocytopenia, hemolytic anemia, and aplastic anemia have been reported.

Dermatologic-Hypersensitivity: purpura, exfoliative dermatitis, pruritus, ecchymosis, urticaria, necrotizing angitis (vasculitis, cutaneous vasculitis), respiratory distress including pneumonitis, fever, and anaphylactic reactions occasionally occur; photosensitivity and rash have been reported.

Cardiovascular: orthostatic hypotension may occur and may be potentiated by coadministration with certain other drugs (*e.g.*, alcohol, barbiturates, narcotics, other antihypertensive medications, etc. (See DRUG INTERACTIONS.)

Other: muscle spasm, weakness, or restlessness is not uncommon; hyperglycemia, glycosuria, metabolic acidosis in diabetic patients, hyperuricemia, allergic glomerulonephritis, and transient blurred vision frequently occur.

Whenever adverse reactions are moderate or severe, thiazide dosage should be reduced or therapy withdrawn.

DOSAGE AND ADMINISTRATION:

Therapy should be individualized according to patient response and titrated to obtain maximal therapeutic response as well as the lowest dose possible to maintain that therapeutic response and minimize side effects.

Diuretic: The usual dose is 5 mg once daily, preferably given in the morning. To initiate therapy, doses up to 20 mg may be given once daily or divided into two doses. A single dose of 2.5 mg to 5 mg should suffice for maintenance.

Alternatively, intermittent therapy may be advantageous in many patients. By administering the preparation every other day or on a three to five per week schedule, electrolyte imbalance is less likely to occur; however, the possibility still exists.

In general, the lowest dosage that achieves the therapeutic response should be employed.

Antihypertensive: The suggested initial dosage is 5 to 20 mg daily. Maintenance dosage may range from 2.5 mg to 15 mg per day depending on the individual response of the patient. When the diuretic is used with other antihypertensive agents, lower maintenance doses for each drug are usually sufficient.

HOW SUPPLIED:

Storage: Dispense in tight containers. Store at room temperature; avoid excessive heat.

HOW SUPPLIED - EQUIVALENTS NOT AVAILABLE:

Tablet, Uncoated - Oral - 5 mg

100's	$84.93	NATURETIN, Bristol Myers Squibb	00003-0606-50
1000's	$675.88	NATURETIN, Bristol Myers Squibb	00003-0606-80

Tablet, Uncoated - Oral - 10 mg

100's	$130.70	NATURETIN, Bristol Myers Squibb	00003-0618-50

BENDROFLUMETHIAZIDE; NADOLOL *(000403)*

CATEGORIES: Antihypertensives; Beta Adrenergic Blocking Agents; Beta Blockers; Cardiovascular Drugs; Diuretics; Hypertension; Renal Drugs; Thiazides; Pregnancy Category C; FDA Approved 1983 May

BRAND NAMES: Corgaretic (England, Mexico); *Corgaretic-40*; *Corgaretic-80*; **Corzide**

(International brand names outside U.S. in italics)

COST OF THERAPY: $479.02 (Hypertension; Tablet; 5 mg/40 mg; 1/day; 365 days)

PRIMARY ICD9: 401.1 (Essential Hypertension, Benign)

DESCRIPTION:

Nadolol and bendroflumethiazide tablets for oral administration combine two antihypertensive agents: nadolol, a nonselective beta-adrenergic blocking agent, and bendroflumethiazide, a thiazide diuretic-antihypertensive.

FOR COMPLETE PRESCRIBING INFORMATION REFER TO THE INDIVIDUAL DRUG MONOGRAPHS (BENDROFLUMETHIAZIDE; NADOLOL).

INDICATIONS AND USAGE:

Nadolol and bendroflumethiazide tablets are indicated in the management of hypertension.

This fixed combination drug is not indicated for initial therapy of hypertension. If the fixed combination represents the dose titrated to the individual patient's needs, it may be more convenient than the separate components.

DOSAGE AND ADMINISTRATION:

DOSAGE MUST BE INDIVIDUALIZED (see INDICATIONS AND USAGE), MAY BE ADMINISTERED WITHOUT REGARD TO MEALS.

Bendroflumethiazide is usually given at a dose of 5 mg daily. The usual initial dose of nadolol is 40 mg once daily whether used alone or in combination with a diuretic. Bendroflumethiazide in nadolol and bendroflumethiazide is 30 percent more bioavailable than that of 5 mg bendroflumethiazide tablets. Conversion from nadolol tablets and 5 mg bendroflumethiazide to the combination nadolol and bendroflumethiazide 5 mg tablets represents a 30 percent increase in dose of bendroflumethiazide.

The initial dose of nadolol and bendroflumethiazide tablets may therefore be the 40 mg/5 mg tablet once daily. When the antihypertensive response is not satisfactory the dose may be increased by administering the 80 mg/5mg tablet once daily.

When necessary, another antihypertensive agent may be added gradually beginning with 50 percent of the usual recommended starting dose to avoid an excessive fall in blood pressure.

Dosage Adjustment in Renal Failure: Absorbed nadolol is excreted principally by the kidneys and, although nonrenal elimination does occur, dosage adjustments are necessary in patients with renal impairment. The following dose intervals are recommended (TABLE 1):

TABLE 1

Creatinine Clearance (ml/min (1.73m^2))	Dosage Interval (hours)
>50	24
31-50	24-36
10-30	24-48
<10	40-80

Storage: Keep bottle tightly closed. Store at room temperature; avoid excessive heat.

HOW SUPPLIED - EQUIVALENTS NOT AVAILABLE:

Tablet, Uncoated - Oral - 5 mg/40 mg

100's	**$131.24**	**CORZIDE 40/5, Bristol Myers Squibb**	**00003-0283-50**

Tablet, Uncoated - Oral - 5 mg/80 mg

100's	**$173.15**	**CORZIDE 80/5, Bristol Myers Squibb**	**00003-0284-50**

BENDROFLUMETHIAZIDE; RAUWOLFIA SERPENTINA *(000404)*

CATEGORIES: Antihypertensives; Cardiovascular Drugs; Diuretics; Edema; Hypertension; Rauwolfia Alkaloids; Renal Drugs; Thiazides; Vascular Disorders, Cerebral/ Peripheral; Pregnancy Category C; FDA Pre 1938 Drugs

BRAND NAMES: Flumezide; **Rauzide**

FORMULARIES: Medi-Cal

Prescribing information not available at time of publication.

HOW SUPPLIED - EQUIVALENTS NOT AVAILABLE:

Tablet, Uncoated - Oral - 4 mg/50 mg

100's	$43.28	Rauwolfia w/Bendroflumethiazide, Rugby	00536-4502-01
100's	$44.95	RONDAMETH, Major Pharms	00904-2537-60
100's	$54.89	FLUMEZIDE, Econolab	55053-0069-01
100's	**$113.55**	**RAUZIDE, Bristol Myers Squibb**	**00003-0769-51**
1000's	**$947.13**	**RAUZIDE, Bristol Myers Squibb**	**00003-0769-80**

BENOXINATE HYDROCHLORIDE; FLUORESCEIN SODIUM *(003044)*

CATEGORIES: Anesthesia; Diagnostic Agents

BRAND NAMES: Flurate; **Fluress**; *Thilorbin* (Germany)
(International brand names outside U.S. in italics)

DESCRIPTION:

A sterile ophthalmic solution containing fluorescein sodium 0.25% and benoxinate HCl 0.4% in a boric acid buffer containing povidone, hydrochloric acid to adjust the pH, and purified water. Chlorobutanol 1.0% added as a preservative.

CLINICAL PHARMACOLOGY:

Fluress is a disclosing agent with rapid anesthetic action and short duration. Benoxinate HCl 0.4% produces anesthesia in less than 15 seconds. Using one drop, duration of action averages slightly over 15 minutes. Fluorescein sodium 0.25% produces reproducible results through reliable and uniform fluorescence.

INDICATIONS AND USAGE:

For procedures in which a topical ophthalmic anesthetic agent in conjunction with a disclosing agent are indicated: corneal anesthesia of short duration, *e.g.*, tonometry, gonioscopy, removal of corneal foreign bodies, and for short corneal and conjunctival procedures.

CONTRAINDICATIONS:

Known hypersensitivity to the components of this preparation.

WARNINGS:

Prolonged use of a topical ocular anesthetic is not recommended. It may produce permanent corneal opacification with accompanying visual loss.

ADVERSE REACTIONS:

Occasional temporary stinging, burning, conjunctival redness.

Rare, severe, immediate-type, apparently hyperallergic corneal reaction, with acute, intense, and diffuse epithelial keratitis, a gray, ground-glass appearance, sloughing or large areas of necrotic epithelium, corneal filaments and sometimes, iritis with descemetitis.

DOSAGE AND ADMINISTRATION:

Usual Dosage (removal of foreign bodies and sutures, and for tonometry):

1 to 2 drops (in single installations) in each eye before operating.

Deep ophthalmic anesthesia:

Benoxinate hydrochloride 0.4% solution; 2 drops in each eye at 90 second intervals for 3 instillations.

(NOTE: Because the "blink" reflex is temporarily eliminated, it is suggested that the eye brow be covered with a patch following this procedure.)

HOW SUPPLIED - EQUIVALENTS NOT AVAILABLE:

Solution - Ophthalmic - 0.4 %/0.25 %

5 ml	**$11.44**	**FLURESS, Vision Pharms**	**00077-0628-55**

BENTONITE *(000406)*

CATEGORIES: Pharmaceutical Adjuvants; FDA Pre 1938 Drugs

Prescribing information not available at time of publication.

BENZONATATE *(000446)*

CATEGORIES: Antitussives; Antitussives/Expectorants/Mucolytics; Cough Preparations; Respiratory & Allergy Medications; Pregnancy Category C; FDA Approval Pre 1982

BRAND NAMES: *Beknol* (Mexico); *Benzonal* (Mexico); *Pebegal* (Mexico); *Tesalon* (Mexico); *Tessalon* (Canada); **Tessalon Perles**; *Tusehli* (Mexico)
(International brand names outside U.S. in italics)

FORMULARIES: BC-BS

DESCRIPTION:

Benzonatate, a non-narcotic antitussive agent, is 2, 5, 8, 11, 14, 17, 20, 23, 26-nonaoxaoctacosan-28-yl p-(butylamino) benzoate; with a molecular weight of 603.7.

$C_{30}H_{53}NO_{11}$

Each Perle contains: Benzonatate, USP, 100 mg.

Benzonatate Perles also contain: D&C Yellow 10, gelatin, glycerin, methylparaben and propylparaben.

CLINICAL PHARMACOLOGY:

Benzonatate acts peripherally by anesthetizing the stretch receptors located in the respiratory passages, lungs, and pleura by dampening their activity and thereby reducing the cough reflex at its source. It begins to act within 15 to 20 minutes and its effect lasts for 3 to 8 hours. Benzonatate has no inhibitory effect on the respiratory center in recommended dosage.

INDICATIONS AND USAGE:

Benzonatate is indicated for the symptomatic relief of cough.

CONTRAINDICATIONS:

Hypersensitivity to benzonatate or related compounds.

WARNINGS:

Severe hypersensitivity reactions (including bronchospasm, laryngospasm and cardiovascular collapse) have been reported which are possibly related to local anesthesia from sucking or chewing the perle instead of swallowing it. Severe reactions have required intervention with vasopressor agents and supportive measures.

Isolated instances of bizarre behavior, including mental confusion and visual hallucinations, have also been reported in patients taking Benzonatate in combination with other prescribed drugs.

PRECAUTIONS:

Benzonatate is chemically related to anesthetic agents of the para-amino-benzoic acid class (*e.g.*, procaine; tetracaine) and has been associated with adverse CNS effects possibly related to a prior sensitivity to related agents or interaction with concomitant medication.

INFORMATION FOR THE PATIENT:

Release of benzonatate from the perle in the mouth can produce a temporary local anesthesia of the oral mucosa and choking could occur. Therefore, the perles should be swallowed without chewing.

USAGE IN PREGNANCY:

Pregnancy Category C. Animal reproduction studies have not been conducted with benzonatate. It is also not known whether benzonatate can cause fetal harm when administered to a pregnant woman or can affect reproduction capacity. Benzonatate should be given to a pregnant woman only if clearly needed.

NURSING MOTHERS:

It is not known whether this drug is excreted in human milk. Because many drugs are excreted in human milk caution should be exercised when benzonatate is administered to a nursing woman.

CARCINOGENESIS, MUTAGENESIS, AND IMPAIRMENT OF FERTILITY:

Carcinogenicity, mutagenicity, and reproduction studies have not been conducted with benzonatate.

PEDIATRIC USE:

Safety and effectiveness in children below the age of 10 has not been established.

ADVERSE REACTIONS:

Potential Adverse Reaction to benzonatate may include:

Hypersensitivity reactions including bronchospasm, laryngospasm, cardiovascular collapse possibly related to local anesthesia from chewing or sucking the perle.

CNS: sedation; headache; dizziness; mental confusion; visual hallucinations

GI: constipation; nausea; GI upset

Dermatologic: pruritus; skin eruptions

Other: nasal congestion; sensation of burning in the eyes; vague "chilly" sensation; numbness of the chest; hypersensitivity. Rare instances of deliberate or accidental overdose have resulted in death.

OVERDOSAGE:

Overdose may result in death.

The drug is clinically related to tetracaine and other topical anesthetics and shares various aspects of their pharmacology and toxicology. Drugs of this type are generally well absorbed after ingestion.

SIGNS AND SYMPTOMS

If perles are chewed or dissolved in the mouth, oropharyngeal anesthesia will develop rapidly. CNS stimulation may cause restlessness and tremors which may proceed to clonic convulsions followed by profound CNS depression.

TREATMENT

Evacuate gastric contents and administer copious amounts of activated charcoal slurry. Even in the conscious patient, cough and gag reflexes may be so depressed as to necessitate special attention to protection against aspiration of gastric contents and orally administered materials. Convulsions should be treated with a short-acting barbiturate given intravenously and carefully titrated for the smallest effective dosage. Intensive support of respiration and cardiovascular - renal function is an essential feature of the treatment of severe intoxication from overdosage.

Do not use CNS stimulants.

DOSAGE AND ADMINISTRATION:

Adults and Children over 10: Usual dose is one 100 mg perle t.i.d. as required. If necessary, up to 6 perles daily may be given.

Store at controlled room temperature 15-30°C (59-86°F).

HOW SUPPLIED - RATED THERAPEUTICALLY EQUIVALENT:

Capsule, Elastic - Oral - 100 mg

100's	$48.60	Benzonatate, United Res	00677-1472-01
100's	$48.60	Benzonatate, H.C.F.A. F F P	99999-0446-01
100's	$49.95	Benzonatate, Inwood Labs	00258-3654-01
100's	$54.00	Benzonatate, Goldline Labs	00182-1080-01
100's	$54.12	Benzonatate, Rugby	00536-5566-01
100's	$55.15	Benzonatate, HL Moore Drug Exch	00839-7795-06
100's	$55.15	Benzonatate, HL Moore Drug Exch	00839-7797-06
100's	$55.50	Benzonatate, Aligen Independ	00405-4115-01
100's	$55.50	Benzonatate, Sidmak Labs	50111-0851-01
100's	$55.60	Benzonatate, Qualitest Pharms	00603-2426-21
100's	$56.39	Benzonatate, Schein Pharm (US)	00364-2536-01
100's	$56.90	Benzonatate, Warner Chilcott	00047-0048-24
100's	$56.90	Benzonatate, Teva	00093-0060-01
100's	$57.15	Benzonatate, Major Pharms	00904-7737-60
100's	$57.15	Benzonatate, Martec Pharms	52555-0484-01
100's	$60.15	Benzonatate, Harber Pharm	51432-0803-03
100's	**$92.26**	**TESSALON PERLES, Forest Pharms**	**00456-0688-01**
500's	$243.00	Benzonatate, H.C.F.A. F F P	99999-0446-02
500's	**$459.30**	**TESSALON PERLES, Forest Pharms**	**00456-0688-02**

BENZOYL PEROXIDE *(000447)*

CATEGORIES: Acne; Anti-Infectives; Antibacterials; Antibiotics; Dermatologicals; Keratolytic Agents; Local Infections; Pharmaceutical Adjuvants; Skin/Mucous Membrane Agents; Soaps & Cleansers; Pregnancy Category C; FDA Pre 1938 Drugs

BRAND NAMES: *Acetoxy* (Canada); *Acetoxyl*; *Acnacyl*; Acne-10; *Acnecide*; *Acnefuge*; Acnigel; *Acne Mask*; *Acnie*; *Akneroxid* (Germany); *Aldoacne*; *Altex*; *Antopar*; *Basiron*; Ben-Aqua; *Benoxid*; *Benoxil*; *Benoxyl* (England, Canada); *Benoxyl AQ AL* (Mexico); *Benoxyl 5 Lotion*; Benzac; *Benzac AC*; *Benzac-AC 5*; *Benzac W* (Mexico); *Benzac W5*; *Benzac W10*; Benzagel; Benzashave; *Benzeperox* (Germany); *Benzihex*; *Benzolac*; *Boxazin*; Brevoxyl; Clearplex; *Cutacnyl*; *Dermoxyl* (Canada); Desquam-E; **Desquam-X**; *Eclaran* (France); *Ecuaderm*; *Effacne* (France); *Klinoxid* (Germany); *Mytolac*; *Oxiderma*; *Oxy*; *Oxy-5*; *Oxy 5*; *Oxy 10*; *Oxyderm* (Canada); *Oxy Preps.* (Australia); *Oxy Sensitive Vanishing Gel*; *Oxy Wash*; *PanOxyl*; Panoxyl; *Panoxyl AQ*; *Panoxyl Preps.*; *Panoxyl Wash Lotion* (Mexico); *Panoxylaqua*; *Pansulfox*; *Pernox Gel*; *Peroxiben*; Peroxin; *Persa*; Persa-Gel; *Persol Gel*; *Pimplex*; *Scherogel*; Syoxin; Theroxide; Triaz; *Vixiderm*; Zeroxin

(International brand names outside U.S. in italics)

FORMULARIES: Aetna; BC-BS; FHP; Medi-Cal; WHO

DESCRIPTION:

Each gram of 5 benzoyl peroxide gel and 10 benzoyl peroxide gel contains 50 mg and 100 mg respectively, of benzoyl peroxide in a gel vehicle of purified water, carbomer 940, 14% alcohol, sodium hydroxide, dioctyl sodium sulfosuccinate and fragrance.

Benzoyl peroxide is an antibacterial and keratolytic agent.

CLINICAL PHARMACOLOGY:

Benzoyl peroxide is an antibacterial agent which has been shown to be effective against *Propionibacterium* acnes. This action is believed to be responsible for its usefulness in acne. One study in the rhesus monkey demonstrated a percutaneous absorption of about 1.8 mcg per cm^2 of benzoyl peroxide or 45% of the applied dose in a 24-hour period. The absorbed benzoyl peroxide was completely converted in the skin to benzoic acid.

INDICATIONS AND USAGE:

Benzoyl peroxide may be used alone topically for mild to moderate acne and as an adjunct in acne treatment regimens which might include retinoic acid products, systemic antibiotics, and/or sulfur and salicylic acid containing preparations. The active ingredient, benzoyl peroxide, exerts a desquamative and antibacterial action. It provides mild peeling and keratolytic activity.

CONTRAINDICATIONS:

Benzoyl peroxide gel should not be used by patients having known sensitivity to benzoyl peroxide or any of its components.

WARNINGS:

If itching redness, burning, swelling or undue dryness occurs, discontinue use.

PRECAUTIONS:

For external use only. Not for ophthalmic use. Keep away from eyes and mucosae. Very fair individuals should begin with a single application at bedtime allowing overnight medication. May bleach colored fabrics. Keep this and all medications out of the reach of children.

PRECAUTIONS: *(cont'd)*

CARCINOGENESIS, MUTAGENESIS AND IMPAIRMENT OF FERTILITY:

Long-term studies in animals have not been performed to evaluate carcinogenic potential.

PREGNANCY CATEGORY C:

Animal reproduction studies have not been conducted with benzoyl peroxide. It is also not known whether benzoyl peroxide can cause fetal harm when administered to a pregnant woman or can affect reproduction capacity. Benzoyl peroxide should be given to a pregnant woman only if clearly needed.

NURSING MOTHERS:

It is not known whether this drug is excreted in human milk. Because many drugs are excreted in human milk, caution should be exercised when benzoyl peroxide is administered to a nursing woman.

PEDIATRIC USE:

Safety and effectiveness in children under the age of 12 have not been established.

ADVERSE REACTIONS:

Irritation and contact dermatitis are the most frequent side reactions to benzoyl peroxide.

DOSAGE AND ADMINISTRATION:

Wash and dry affected areas prior to application. Apply sparingly one or more times daily.

HOW SUPPLIED - EQUIVALENTS NOT AVAILABLE:

Bar - Topical - 10 %

4 oz	**$7.68**	**DESQUAM-X, Westwood Squibb**	**00072-2000-04**

Cream - Topical - 5 %

120 gm	$9.50	BENZASHAVE MEDICATED SHAVE, Syosset Labs	47854-0760-09
120 gm	$16.77	Benzashave 5, Medicis	99207-0530-04

Cream - Topical - 10 %

120 gm	$11.50	BENZASHAVE MEDICATED SHAVE, Syosset Labs	47854-0761-09
120 gm	$16.77	Benzashave 10, Medicis	99207-0540-04

Gel - Topical - 2.5 %

1.5 oz	$9.66	DESQUAM-E 2.5, Westwood Squibb	00072-6003-45
45 gm	$7.60	Benzoyl Peroxide, Glades Pharms	59366-2742-02
56.7 gm	$10.35	PANOXYL AQ 2 1/2, Stiefel Labs	00145-2375-06
60 gm	$12.50	BENZAC W 2-1/2, Galderma	00299-3590-60
60 gm	$12.75	BENZAC AC 2 1/2, Galderma	00299-3620-60
90 gm	$15.00	BENZAC W 2-1/2, Galderma	00299-3590-90
90 gm	$15.31	BENZAC AC 2 1/2, Galderma	00299-3620-90
113.4 gm	$13.97	PANOXYL AQ 2 1/2, Stiefel Labs	00145-2375-08

Gel - Topical - 4 %

42.5 gm	$11.80	Brevoxyl Gel 4%, Stiefel Labs	00145-2374-06
90 gm	$16.54	BREVOXYL, Stiefel Labs	00145-2374-08

Gel - Topical - 5 %

1 1/2 oz	$14.90	5-BENZAGEL, Dermik Labs	00066-0430-15
1.5 oz	**$9.58**	**DESQUAM-X, Westwood Squibb**	**00072-6621-01**
1.5 oz	$9.92	DESQUAM-E 5, Westwood Squibb	00072-6103-45
1.5 oz	$10.02	PERSA-GEL, Ortho Pharm	00062-8610-31
1.5 oz	$10.02	PERSA-GEL W, Ortho Pharm	00062-8630-31
2 oz	$11.45	PANOXYL 5 ACNE GEL, Stiefel Labs	00145-2372-06
3 oz	$17.82	PERSA-GEL, Ortho Pharm	00062-8610-03
3 oz	$17.82	PERSA-GEL W, Ortho Pharm	00062-8630-03
3 oz	$20.52	5-BENZAGEL, Dermik Labs	00066-0430-30
3 oz.	**$17.03**	**DESQUAM-X, Westwood Squibb**	**00072-6621-03**
4 oz	$11.62	BENZAC W WASH 5, Galderma	00299-3670-04
4 oz	$15.92	PANOXYL 5 ACNE GEL, Stiefel Labs	00145-2372-08
4 oz	$22.50	FACE UP #2, BPO GEL MEDICATION 5% W/W, Clincl Formula	51822-0002-04
8 oz	$17.37	BENZAC W WASH 5, Galderma	00299-3670-08
42.5 gm	$19.20	TRIAZ, Medicis	99207-0051-01
45 gm	$1.73	Benzoyl Peroxide, Clay Park Labs	45802-0259-42
45 gm	$2.25	Benzoyl Peroxide, Consolidated Midland	00223-4254-45
45 gm	$2.50	Benzoyl Peroxide, Consolidated Midland	00223-4256-45
45 gm	$7.94	Benzoyl Peroxide, Qualitest Pharms	00603-7714-82
45 gm	$7.95	Benzoyl Peroxide, Glades Pharms	59366-2743-02
45 gm	$7.95	Benzoyl Peroxide, Glades Pharms	59366-2745-02
45 gm	$7.96	Benzoyl Peroxide, Qualitest Pharms	00603-7711-82
56.7 gm	$11.45	PANOXYL AQ 5, Stiefel Labs	00145-2376-06
60 gm	$12.87	BENZAC W 5, Galderma	00299-3600-01
60 gm	$13.25	BENZAC AC 5, Galderma	00299-3625-60
60 gm	$13.75	BENZAC 5, Galderma	00299-3655-01
90 gm	$11.55	Benzoyl Peroxide, Glades Pharms	59366-2743-03
90 gm	$11.56	Benzoyl Peroxide, Qualitest Pharms	00603-7714-87
90 gm	$16.88	BENZAC W 5, Galderma	00299-3600-09
90 gm	$17.25	BENZAC AC 5, Galderma	00299-3625-90
113.4 gm	$15.92	PANOXYL AQ 5, Stiefel Labs	00145-2376-08

Gel - Topical - 10 %

1 1/2 oz	$15.34	10-BENZAGEL, Dermik Labs	00066-0431-15
1.5 oz	**$9.77**	**DESQUAM-X, Westwood Squibb**	**00072-6721-01**
1.5 oz	$10.09	DESQUAM-E 10, Westwood Squibb	00072-6203-45
1.5 oz	$10.80	PERSA-GEL W, Ortho Pharm	00062-8620-31
2 oz	$11.91	PANOXYL 10 ACNE GEL, Stiefel Labs	00145-2373-06
3 oz	$18.36	PERSA-GEL, Ortho Pharm	00062-8600-03
3 oz	$18.36	PERSA-GEL W, Ortho Pharm	00062-8620-03
3 oz	$21.17	10-BENZAGEL, Dermik Labs	00066-0431-30
3 oz.	**$17.33**	**DESQUAM-X, Westwood Squibb**	**00072-6721-03**
4 oz	$16.64	PANOXYL 10 ACNE GEL, Stiefel Labs	00145-2373-08
4 oz	$23.50	FACE UP #3, BPO GEL, Clincl Formula	51822-0003-04
8 oz	$19.62	BENZAC W WASH 10, Galderma	00299-3672-08
8 oz	$34.50	FACE UP #3, BPO GEL, Clincl Formula	51822-0003-08
42.5 gm	$19.80	TRIAZ, Medicis	99207-0210-01
45 gm	$2.40	Benzoyl Peroxide, IDE-Interstate	00814-1151-73
45 gm	$8.36	Benzoyl Peroxide, Qualitest Pharms	00603-7712-82
45 gm	$8.36	Benzoyl Peroxide, Glades Pharms	59366-2744-02
45 gm	$8.36	Benzoyl Peroxide, Glades Pharms	59366-2746-02
45 gm	$8.37	Benzoyl Peroxide, Qualitest Pharms	00603-7715-82
56.7 gm	$11.91	PANOXYL AQ 10, Stiefel Labs	00145-2377-06
60 gm	$13.50	BENZAC W 10, Galderma	00299-3610-01
60 gm	$13.62	BENZAC AC 10, Galderma	00299-3630-60
60 gm	$14.25	BENZAC 10, Galderma	00299-3665-01
85.05 gm	$11.00	Acnigel, Ampharco	59015-0100-01
90 gm	$12.08	Benzoyl Peroxide, Qualitest Pharms	00603-7715-87
90 gm	$12.10	Benzoyl Peroxide, Glades Pharms	59366-2744-03
90 gm	$17.69	BENZAC W 10, Galderma	00299-3610-09
90 gm	$18.00	BENZAC AC 10, Galderma	00299-3630-90
113.4 gm	$16.64	PANOXYL AQ 10, Stiefel Labs	00145-2377-08

HOW SUPPLIED - EQUIVALENTS NOT AVAILABLE: *(cont'd)*

Liquid - Topical - 2.5 %

240 ml	$17.94	BENZAC AC WASH, Galderma	00299-3635-08

Liquid - Topical - 5 %

120 ml	$9.19	Benzoyl Peroxide, Glades Pharms	59366-2737-04
150 ml	$7.50	Benzoyl Peroxide, Harber Pharm	51432-0485-17
150 ml	$10.25	Benzoyl Peroxide, Glades Pharms	59366-2739-05
240 ml	$9.50	Benzoyl Peroxide, Harber Pharm	51432-0485-19
240 ml	$13.81	Benzoyl Peroxide, Glades Pharms	59366-2739-08
240 ml	$20.25	BENZAC AC WASH, Galderma	00299-3640-08

Liquid - Topical - 10 %

85.1 gm	$9.90	TRIAZ, Medicis	99207-0106-02
150 ml	$8.50	Benzoyl Peroxide, Harber Pharm	51432-0528-17
150 ml	$10.62	Benzoyl Peroxide, Qualitest Pharms	00603-7717-48
150 ml	$10.95	Benzoyl Peroxide, Glades Pharms	59366-2741-05
240 ml	$11.50	Benzoyl Peroxide, Harber Pharm	51432-0528-19
240 ml	$14.60	Benzoyl Peroxide, Qualitest Pharms	00603-7717-56
240 ml	$15.56	Benzoyl Peroxide, Glades Pharms	59366-2741-08
240 ml	$22.37	BENZAC AC WASH, Galderma	00299-3645-08

Lotion - Topical - 4 %

297 ml x 12	$17.40	BREVOXYL, Stiefel Labs	00145-2310-05

Lotion - Topical - 5 %

30 ml	$2.77	OXY-5, Rugby	00536-0810-95
120 ml	$8.00	BEN AQUA WASH 5%, Syosset Labs	47854-0641-22
240 ml	$10.00	BEN AQUA WASH 5%, Syosset Labs	47854-0641-50

Lotion - Topical - 10 %

30 ml	$1.69	Benzoyl Peroxide, HL Moore Drug Exch	00839-6336-49
30 ml	$3.15	OXY-10, Rugby	00536-0815-95

Soap/Detergent - Topical - 5 %

5 oz	$12.57	**DESQUAM-X WASH 5, Westwood Squibb**	**00072-6905-05**

Soap/Detergent - Topical - 10 %

5 oz	$13.45	**DESQUAM-X WASH 10, Westwood Squibb**	**00072-7000-05**

BENZOYL PEROXIDE; ERYTHROMYCIN

(000448)

CATEGORIES: Acne; Acne Vulgaris; Anti-Infectives; Antibiotics; Dermatologicals; Skin/Mucous Membrane Agents; Topical; Pregnancy Category C; FDA Approved 1984 Oct

BRAND NAMES: **Benzamycin**

FORMULARIES: Aetna; BC-BS

DESCRIPTION:

Reconstitute Before Dispensing.

TAP VIAL UNTIL ALL POWDER FLOWS FREELY.
ADD ETHYL ALCOHOL (70%) TO VIAL (TO THE MARK) AND IMMEDIATELY SHAKE TO DISSOLVE.

Each gram of benzamycin (erythromycin-benzoyl peroxide) topical gel contains, as dispensed, 30 mg (3%) active erythromycin and 50 mg (5%) benzoyl peroxide in a gel vehicle of purified water, carbomer 940, alcohol 16%, sodium hydroxide, docusate sodium and fragrance.

Erythromycin ($C_{37}H_{67}NO_{13}$) is produced by a strain of *Streptomyces erythraeus* and belongs to the macrolide group of antibiotics. Erythromycin has a molecular weight of 733.94.

Benzoyl peroxide ($C_{14}H_{10}O_4$) is an antibacterial and keratolytic agent.

CLINICAL PHARMACOLOGY:

Erythromycin is a bacteriostatic macrolide antibiotic, but may be bactericidal in high concentrations. Although the mechanism by which erythromycin acts in reducing inflammatory lesions of acne vulgaris is unknown, it is presumably due to its antibiotic action. Antagonism has been demonstrated between clindamycin and erythromycin.

Benzoyl peroxide is an antibacterial agent which has been shown to be effective against *Propionibacterium acnes*, an anaerobe found in sebaceous follicles and comedones. The antibacterial action of benzoyl peroxide is believed to be due to the release of active oxygen. Benzoyl peroxide has a keratolytic and desquamative effect which may also contribute to its efficacy.

Benzoyl peroxide has been shown to be absorbed by the skin where it is converted to benzoic acid.

INDICATIONS AND USAGE:

Benzoyl peroxide and erythromycin topical gel is indicated for the topical control of acne vulgaris.

CONTRAINDICATIONS:

Benzoyl peroxide and erythromycin topical gel is contraindicated in those patients with a history of hypersensitivity to erythromycin, benzoyl peroxide or any of the other listed ingredients.

PRECAUTIONS:

General: For external use only. Not for ophthalmic use. Avoid contact with eyes and mucous membranes. Concomitant topical acne therapy should be used with caution because a possible cumulative irritancy effect may occur, especially with peeling, desquamating or abrasive agents. If severe irritation develops, discontinue use and institute appropriate therapy.

The use of antibiotic agents may be associated with the overgrowth of antibiotic-resistant organisms. If this occurs, administration of this drug should be discontinued and appropriate measures taken.

Information for the Patient: Patients using benzoyl peroxide and erythromycin topical gel should receive the following information and instructions:

1. Benzoyl peroxide and erythromycin topical gel is for external use only. Avoid contact with the eyes and mucous membranes.

2. Patient should not use any other topical acne preparation unless otherwise directed by physician.

3. Benzoyl peroxide and erythromycin topical gel may bleach hair or colored fabric.

PRECAUTIONS: *(cont'd)*

4. If excessive irritation or dryness should occur, patient should discontinue medication and consult physician.

5. Discard product after 3 months and obtain fresh material.

Carcinogenesis, Mutagenesis and Impairment of Fertility: Long-term studies in animals have not been performed to evaluate carcinogenic potential or the effect on fertility.

Pregnancy Category C: Animal reproduction studies have not been conducted with benzoyl peroxide and erythromycin topical gel. It is also not known whether benzoyl peroxide and erythromycin topical gel can cause fetal harm when administered to a pregnant woman or can affect reproduction capacity. Benzoyl peroxide and erythromycin topical gel should be given to a pregnant woman only if clearly needed.

Nursing Mothers: It is not known whether this drug is excreted in human milk. Because many drugs are excreted in human milk, caution should be exercised when benzoyl peroxide and erythromycin topical gel is administered to a nursing woman.

Pediatric Use: Safety and effectiveness in children below the age of 12 have not been established.

ADVERSE REACTIONS:

Adverse reactions which may occur include dryness, erythema and pruritus. Of a total of 153 patients treated with benzoyl peroxide and erythromycin topical gel during clinical trials, 4 patients experienced adverse reactions, of whom three experienced dryness and one an urticarial reaction which responded well to symptomatic treatment.

DOSAGE AND ADMINISTRATION:

Benzoyl peroxide and erythromycin topical gel should be applied twice daily, morning and evening, or as directed by physician, to affected areas after the skin is thoroughly washed, rinsed with warm water and gently patted dry.

NOTE: *Prior* to reconstitution, store at room temperature. *After* reconstitution, store under refrigeration. Do not freeze. Keep tightly closed. Keep out of the reach of children.

HOW SUPPLIED - EQUIVALENTS NOT AVAILABLE:

Gel - Topical - 50 mg/30 mg

23.3 gm	**$26.74**	**BENZAMYCIN, Dermik Labs**	**00066-0510-23**
46.6 gm	**$49.17**	**BENZAMYCIN, Dermik Labs**	**00066-0510-46**

BENZOYL PEROXIDE; HYDROCORTISONE

(000449)

CATEGORIES: Acne; Anti-Inflammatory Agents; Dermatologicals; Pruritus; Skin/Mucous Membrane Agents; Steroids; Pregnancy Category C; FDA Pre 1938 Drugs

BRAND NAMES: **Vanoxide-Hc**

Prescribing information not available at time of publication.

HOW SUPPLIED - EQUIVALENTS NOT AVAILABLE:

Lotion - Topical

25 ml	**$23.14**	**VANOXIDE-HC, Dermik Labs**	**00066-0424-25**

BENZOYL PEROXIDE; SULFUR *(000450)*

CATEGORIES: Dermatologicals; Keratolytic Agents; Skin/Mucous Membrane Agents; FDA Pre 1938 Drugs

BRAND NAMES: *Benoxyl Locion* (Mexico); Bpo Sulfur; *Feldixid*; Sulfoxyl
(International brand names outside U.S. in italics)

Prescribing information not available at time of publication.

HOW SUPPLIED - EQUIVALENTS NOT AVAILABLE:

Gel - Topical - 10 %/4 %

4 oz	$23.50	4 FACE UP, Clincl Formula	51822-0004-04
8 oz	$34.50	4 FACE UP, Clincl Formula	51822-0004-08

Gel - Topical - 10 %/8 %

4 oz	$22.50	5 FACE UP, Clincl Formula	51822-0005-04
8 oz	$33.50	5 FACE UP, Clincl Formula	51822-0005-08

Lotion - Topical - 5 %/2 %

60 ml	$12.07	SULFOXYL REGULAR, Stiefel Labs	00145-3518-07

Lotion - Topical - 10 %/5 %

60 ml	$12.89	SULFOXYL STRONG, Stiefel Labs	00145-3519-07

BENZPHETAMINE HYDROCHLORIDE *(000452)*

CATEGORIES: Amphetamines; Anorexients/CNS Stimulants; Appetite Suppressants; Central Nervous System Agents; Obesity; Psychostimulants; Respiratory/Cerebral Stimulant; Sympathomimetic Agents; Pregnancy Category X; DEA Class CIII; FDA Approval Pre 1982

BRAND NAMES: **Didrex**; *Inapetyl*
(International brand names outside U.S. in italics)

DESCRIPTION:

Didrex tablets contain the anorectic agent benzphetamine hydrochloride. Benzphetamine hydrochloride is a white crystalline powder readily soluble in water and 95% ethanol. The chemical name for benzphetamine hydrochloride is*d*-N,α-Dimethyl-N-(phenylmethyl)-benzeneethanamine hydrochloride and its molecular weight is 275.82.

Each Didrex tablet, for oral administration, contains 25 or 50 mg of benzphetamine hydrochloride. Inactive Ingredients:

25 mg: Calcium Stearate, Corn Starch, FD&C Yellow No. 5, Lactose, Povidone, Sorbitol.

50 mg: Calcium Stearate, Corn Starch, Erythrosine Sodium, FD&C Yellow No. 6, Lactose, Povidone, Sorbitol.

CLINICAL PHARMACOLOGY:

Benzphetamine hydrochloride is a sympathomimetic amine with pharmacologic activity similar to the prototype drugs of this class used in obesity, the amphetamines. Actions include central nervous system stimulation and elevation of blood pressure. Tachyphylaxis and tolerance have been demonstrated with all drugs of this class in which these phenomena have been looked for.

Drugs of this class used in obesity are commonly known as "anorectics" or "anorexigenics." It has not been established, however, that the action of such drugs in treating obesity is primarily one of appetite suppression. Other central nervous system actions, or metabolic effects, may be involved.

Adult obese subjects instructed in dietary management and treated with "anorectic" drugs, lose more weight on the average than those treated with placebo and diet, as determined in relatively short-term clinical trials.

The magnitude of increased weight loss of drug-treated patients over placebo-treated patients is only a fraction of a pound a week. The rate of weight loss is the greatest in the first weeks of therapy for both drug and placebo subjects and tends to decrease in succeeding weeks. The possible origins of the increased weight loss due to the various drug effects are not established. The amount of weight loss associated with the use of an "anorectic" drug varies from trial to trial, and the increased weight loss appears to be related in part to variables other than the drug prescribed, such as the physician-investigator, the population treated, and the diet prescribed. Studies do not permit conclusions as to the relative importance of the drug and non-drug factors on weight loss.

The natural history of obesity is measured in years, whereas the studies cited are restricted to a few weeks duration; thus, the total impact of drug-induced weight loss over that of diet alone must be considered to be clinically limited.

Pharmacokinetic data in humans are not available.

INDICATIONS AND USAGE:

Benzphetamine HCl tablets are indicated in the management of exogenous obesity as a short term adjunct (a few weeks) in a regimen of weight reduction based on caloric restriction. The limited usefulness of agents of this class (See CLINICAL PHARMACOLOGY) should be weighed against possible risks inherent in their use such as those described below.

CONTRAINDICATIONS:

Benzphetamine HCl tablets are contraindicated in patients with advanced arteriosclerosis, symptomatic cardiovascular disease, moderate to severe hypertension, hyperthyroidism, known hypersensitivity or idiosyncrasy to sympathomimetic amines, and glaucoma. Benzphetamine should not be given to patients who are in an agitated state or who have a history of drug abuse.

Hypertensive crises have resulted when sympathomimetic amines have been used concomitantly or within 14 days following use of monoamine oxidase inhibitors. Benzphetamine HCl should not be used concomitantly with other CNS stimulants.

Benzphetamine HCl may cause fetal harm when administered to a pregnant woman. Amphetamines have been shown to be teratogenic and embryotoxic in mammals at high multiples of the human dose. Benzphetamine HCl is contraindicated in women who are or may become pregnant. If this drug is used during pregnancy, or if the patient becomes pregnant while taking this drug, the patient should be apprised of the potential hazard to the fetus.

WARNINGS:

When tolerance to the anorectic effect develops, the recommended dose should not be exceeded in an attempt to increase the effect; rather, the drug should be discontinued.

PRECAUTIONS:

General: Insulin requirements in diabetes mellitus may be altered in association with use of anorexigenic drugs and the concomitant dietary restrictions.

Psychological disturbances have been reported in patients who receive an anorectic agent together with a restrictive dietary regime.

Caution is to be exercised in prescribing amphetamines for patients with even mild hypertension. The least amount feasible should be prescribed or dispensed at one time in order to minimize the possibility of overdosage.

Benzphetamine HCl tablets, 25 mg, contain FD&C Yellow No. 5 (tartrazine) which may cause allergic-type reactions (including bronchial asthma) in certain susceptible individuals. Although the overall incidence of FD&C Yellow No. 5 (tartrazine) sensitivity in the general population is low, it is frequently seen in patients who also have aspirin hypersensitivity.

INFORMATION FOR THE PATIENT: Amphetamines may impair the ability of the patient to engage in potentially hazardous activities such as operating machinery or driving a motor vehicle; the patient should therefore be cautioned accordingly.

CARCINOGENESIS, MUTAGENESIS, AND IMPAIRMENT OF FERTILITY: Animal studies to evaluate the potential for carcinogenesis, mutagenesis or impairment of fertility have not been performed.

Pregnancy Category X: (See CONTRAINDICATIONS.)

Nursing Mothers: Amphetamines are excreted in human milk. Mothers taking amphetamines should be advised to refrain from nursing.

Pediatric Use: Use of benzphetamine hydrochloride is not recommended in children under 12 years of age.

DRUG INTERACTIONS:

Hypertensive crises have resulted when sympathomimetic amines have been used concomitantly or within 14 days following use of monoamine oxidase inhibitors. Benzphetamine HCl should not be used concomitantly with other CNS stimulants.

Amphetamines may decrease the hypotensive effect of antihypertensives. Amphetamines may enhance the effects of tricyclic antidepressants.

Urinary alkalinizing agents increase blood levels and decrease excretion of amphetamines. Urinary acidifying agents decrease blood levels and increase excretion of amphetamines.

ADVERSE REACTIONS:

The following have been associated with the use of benzphetamine hydrochloride:

Cardiovascular: Palpitation, tachycardia, elevation of blood pressure. There have been isolated reports of cardiomyopathy associated with chronic amphetamine use.

CNS: Overstimulation, restlessness, dizziness, insomnia, tremor, sweating, headache; rarely, psychotic episodes at recommended doses; depression following withdrawal of the drug.

Gastrointestinal: Dryness of the mouth, unpleasant taste, nausea, diarrhea, other gastrointestinal disturbances.

Allergic: Urticaria and other allergic reactions involving the skin.

Endocrine: Changes in libido

DRUG ABUSE AND DEPENDENCE:

Benzphetamine is a controlled substance under the Controlled Substance Act by the Drug Enforcement Administration and has been assigned to Schedule III.

Benzphetamine hydrochloride is related chemically and pharmacologically to the amphetamines. Amphetamines and related stimulant drugs have been extensively abused, and the possibility of abuse of benzphetamine HCl tablets should be kept in mind when evaluating the desirability of including a drug as part of a weight reduction program. Abuse of amphetamines and related drugs may be associated with intense psychological dependence and severe social dysfunction. There are reports of patients who have increased the dosage to many times that recommended. Abrupt cessation following prolonged high dosage administration results in extreme fatigue and mental depression; changes are also noted on the sleep EEG. Manifestations of chronic intoxication with anorectic drugs include severe dermatoses, marked insomnia, irritability, hyperactivity, and personality changes. The most severe manifestation of chronic intoxication is psychosis, often clinically indistinguishable from schizophrenia.

OVERDOSAGE:

Manifestations of Overdosage: Acute overdosage with amphetamines may result in restlessness, tremor, tachypnea, confusion, assaultiveness and panic states. Fatigue and depression usually follow the central stimulation. Cardiovascular effects include arrhythmias, hypertension or hypotension, and circulatory collapse. Gastrointestinal symptoms include nausea, vomiting, diarrhea, and abdominal cramps. Hyperpyrexia and rhabdomyolysis have been reported and can lead to a number of associated complications. Fatal poisoning is usually preceded by convulsions and coma.

Treatment: See WARNINGS Information concerning the effects of overdosage with benzphetamine HCl tablets is extremely limited. The following is based on experience with other anorexiants.

Management of acute amphetamine intoxication is largely symptomatic and includes sedation with a barbiturate. If hypertension is marked, the use of a nitrite or rapidly acting alpha receptor blocking agent should be considered. Experience with hemodialysis or peritoneal dialysis is inadequate to permit recommendations in this regard.

Acidification of the urine increases amphetamine excretion.

The oral LD_{50} is 174 mg/kg in mice and 104 mg/kg in rats. The intraperitoneal LD_{50} in mice is 153 mg/kg.

DOSAGE AND ADMINISTRATION:

Dosage should be individualized according to the response of the patient. The suggested dosage ranges from 25 to 50 mg one to three times daily. Treatment should begin with 25 to 50 mg once daily with subsequent increase in individual dose or frequency according to response. A single daily dose is preferably given in mid-morning or mid-afternoon, according to the patient's eating habits. In an occasional patient it may be desirable to avoid late afternoon administration. Use of benzphetamine hydrochloride is not recommended in children under 12 years of age.

Store at controlled room temperature 15-30°C (59-86°F).

HOW SUPPLIED - EQUIVALENTS NOT AVAILABLE:

Tablet, Plain Coated - Oral - 50 mg

100's	$48.74	DIDREX, Pharmacia & Upjohn	00009-0024-01
500's	$240.83	DIDREX, Pharmacia & Upjohn	00009-0024-02

BENZTHIAZIDE *(000454)*

CATEGORIES: Antihypertensives; Cardiovascular Drugs; Cirrhosis; Congestive Heart Failure; Diuretics; Edema; Electrolytic, Caloric-Water Balance; Glomerulonephritis; Heart Failure; Hypertension; Nephrotic Syndrome; Renal Drugs; Renal Failure; Thiazides; Pregnancy Category C; FDA Approval Pre 1982

BRAND NAMES: Aquatag; *Diurin*; Exna; *Fovane*; Hydrex; Proaqua; *Regulon*
(International brand names outside U.S. in italics)

FORMULARIES: Medi-Cal

DESCRIPTION:

Benzthiazide is a diuretic for oral administration. Each tablet contains 50 mg benzthiazide.

Benzthiazide Inactive Ingredients: Corn Starch, Dibasic Calcium Phosphate, FD&C Yellow 5, Lactose, Magnesium Stearate, Polyethylene Glycol, Sodium Lauryl Sulfate.

Benzthiazide is a white, crystalline powder with a characteristic odor, freely soluble in alkaline solution. The chemical structure is: 6-chloro-3[((phenylmethyl)thio)methyl]-2H-1,2,4-benzothiadiazine-7-sulfonamide 1,1-dioxide

CLINICAL PHARMACOLOGY:

Benzthiazide is a diuretic and antihypertensive. It affects the renal tubular mechanism of electrolyte reabsorption. At maximal therapeutic dosage, all thiazides are approximately equal in their diuretic potency. The mechanism whereby thiazides function in the control of hypertension is unknown. Benzthiazide increases excretion of sodium and chloride in approximately equivalent amounts. Natriuresis may be accompanied by some loss of potassium and bicarbonate.

In humans, benzthiazide is excreted in the urine almost entirely unchanged. Following a single oral dose of benzthiazide tablets or benzthiazide solution, 1% and 4.3% of the respective doses were recovered in the urine in 24 hr. The relative bioavailability of benzthiazide tablets was determined to be about 25% in reference to benzthiazide solution.

INDICATIONS AND USAGE:

Benzthiazide is indicated as adjunctive therapy in edema associated with congestive heart failure, hepatic cirrhosis and corticosteroid and estrogen therapy.

Benzthiazide has also been found useful in edema due to various forms of renal dysfunction as: nephrotic syndrome; acute glomerulonephritis; and chronic renal failure.

Benzthiazide is indicated in the management of hypertension either as the sole therapeutic agent or to enhance the effectiveness of other antihypertensive drugs in the more severe forms of hypertension.

Use in Pregnancy: The routine use of diuretics in an otherwise healthy woman is inappropriate and exposes mother and fetus to unnecessary hazard. Diuretics do not prevent development of toxemia of pregnancy, and there is no satisfactory evidence that they are useful in the treatment of developed toxemia.

Edema during pregnancy may arise from pathological causes or from the physiologic and mechanical consequences of pregnancy. Thiazides are indicated in pregnancy when edema is due to pathologic causes, just as they are in the absence of pregnancy (however, see WARNINGS). Dependent edema in pregnancy, resulting from restriction of venous return by the expanded uterus, is properly treated through elevation of the lower extremities and use of

INDICATIONS AND USAGE: *(cont'd)*

support hose; use of diuretics to lower intravascular volume in this case is illogical and unnecessary. There is hypervolemia during normal pregnancy which is harmful to neither the fetus nor the mother (in the absence of cardiovascular disease), but which is associated with edema, including generalized edema, in the majority of pregnant women. If this edema produces discomfort, increased recumbency will often provide relief. In rare instances, this edema may cause extreme discomfort which is not relieved by rest. In these cases, a short course of diuretics may provide relief and may be appropriate.

CONTRAINDICATIONS:

Anuria. Hypersensitivity to this or other sulfonamide-derived drugs.

WARNINGS:

Thiazides should be used with caution in severe renal disease. In patients with renal disease, thiazides may precipitate azotemia. Cumulative effects of the drug may develop in patients with impaired renal function.

Thiazides should be used with caution in patients with impaired hepatic function or progressive liver disease, since minor alterations of fluid and electrolyte balance may precipitate hepatic coma.

Thiazides may add to or potentiate the action of other antihypertensive drugs. Potentiation occurs with ganglionic or peripheral adrenergic blocking drugs.

Sensitivity reactions may occur in patients with a history of allergy or bronchial asthma.

The possibility of exacerbation or activation of systemic lupus erythematosus has been reported.

PRECAUTIONS:

General: All patients receiving thiazide therapy should be observed for clinical signs of fluid or electrolyte imbalance; namely, hyponatremia, hypochloremic alkalosis, and hypokalemia. Warning signs are dryness of mouth, thirst, or cramps, muscular fatigue, hypotension, oliguria, tachycardia, and gastrointestinal disturbance such as nausea and vomiting.

Dilutional hyponatremia may occur in edematous patients in hot weather; appropriate therapy is water restriction, rather than administration of salt except in rare instances when hyponatremia is life threatening.

In actual salt depletion, appropriate replacement is the therapy of choice. Any chloride deficit is generally mild and usually does not require specific treatment except under extraordinary circumstances (as in liver disease or renal disease).

Hypokalemia may develop with thiazides as with any other potent diuretic especially with brisk diuresis. Inadequate oral electrolyte intake will also contribute to hypokalemia.

Thiazide diuretics have been shown to increase the urinary excretion of magnesium; this may result in hypomagnesemia.

Calcium excretion is decreased by thiazide diuretics. Pathological changes in the parathyroid gland with hypercalcemia and hypophosphatemia have been observed in a few patients on thiazide therapy. The common complications few patients on thiazide therapy. The common complications of hyperparathyroidism such as renal lithiasis, bone resorption and peptic ulceration have not been seen.

If progressive renal failure becomes evident, a careful reappraisal of therapy is indicated with consideration given to withholding or discontinuing diuretic therapy.

Increases of cholesterol and triglyceride and triglyceride levels may be associated with thiazide diuretic therapy.

Latent diabetes mellitus may become manifest during thiazide administration: hyperuricemia or frank gout may also be precipitated in certain patients. The antihypertensive effect of the drug may be enhanced in the postsympathectomy patient.

This product contains FD&C Yellow No. 5 (tartrazine) which may cause allergic-type reactions (including bronchial asthma) in certain susceptible individuals. Although the overall incidence of FD&C Yellow No. 5 (tartrazine) sensitivity in the general population is low, it is frequently seen in patients who have aspirin hypersensitivity.

Information for the Patient: Warning signs of electrolyte imbalance are: dryness of mouth, thirst, weakness, lethargy, drowsiness, restlessness, muscle pains or cramps, muscular fatigue, hypotension, oliguria, tachycardia, and gastrointestinal disturbances such as nausea and vomiting.

Laboratory Tests: Periodic determination of serum electrolytes to detect possible electrolyte imbalance should be performed at appropriate intervals. When the patient is vomiting excessively or receiving parenteral fluids, serum and urine electrolyte determinations are particularly important.

In patients with renal impairment, nonprotein nitrogen or blood urea nitrogen level should be tested periodically; rising values would indicate progressive renal impairment and careful reappraisal of therapy is necessary with consideration given to withholding or discontinuing diuretic therapy.

Drug/Laboratory Tests Interactions: Thiazides may decrease serum PBI levels without signs of thyroid disturbance.

Thiazides should be discontinued before carrying out tests for parathyroid function (see PRECAUTIONS, General).

Carcinogenesis, Mutagenesis, and Impairment of Fertility: Studies to evaluate the carcinogenic or mutagenic potential of benzthiazide or the potential of the drug to affect fertility adversely have not been performed.

Pregnancy Category C: *Teratogenic Effects:* Benzthiazide has an embryocidal effect in rats when given in doses several hundred times the human dose. There are no adequate and well-controlled studies in pregnant women. Benzthiazide should be used during pregnancy only if clearly needed. *Nonteratogenic Effects:* Thiazides cross the placental barrier and appear in cord blood. There is a risk of fetal or neonatal jaundice, thrombocytopenia and possibly other adverse reactions that have occurred in adults.

Nursing Mothers: It is not known whether this drug is excreted in human milk. Because many drugs are excreted in human milk. Because many drugs are excreted in human milk, caution should be exercised when Exna is administered to a nursing mother.

Pediatric Use: Safety and effectiveness in children have not been established.

DRUG INTERACTIONS:

When given concurrently the following drugs may interact with thiazide diuretics.

Alcohol, Barbiturates, Or Narcotics: potentiation of orthostatic hypotension may occur.

Antidiabetic Drugs: (oral agents and insulin) - dosage adjustment of the antidiabetic drug may be required.

Other Antihypertensive Drugs: additive effect or potentiation occurs with ganglionic or peripheral adrenergic-blocking drugs.

Digitalis: medication such as digitalis may also influence serum electrolytes. Digitalis therapy may exaggerate metabolic effects of hypokalemia especially with reference to myocardial activity (*e.g.,* increased ventricular irritability).

DRUG INTERACTIONS: *(cont'd)*

Pressor Amines (*e.g.,* Norepinephrine): possible decreased response to pressor amines. This diminution is not sufficient to preclude effectiveness of the pressor agent for therapeutic use.

Skeletal Muscle Relaxants, Nondepolarizing (*e.g.,* Tubocurarine): possible increased responsiveness to the muscle relaxant.

Lithium: generally should not be given with diuretics. Diuretic agents reduce the renal clearance of lithium and add a high risk of lithium toxicity. Refer to the package insert for lithium preparations before use of such preparations with Exna.

Nonsteroidal Anti-Inflammatory Drugs: In some patients, the administration of a nonsteroidal anti-inflammatory agent can reduce the diuretic, natriuretic, and antihypertensive effects of loop, potassium-sparing and thiazide diuretics. Therefore, when Exna and nonsteroidal anti-inflammatory agents are used concomitantly, the patient should be observed closely to determine if the desired effect of the diuretic is obtained.

Cholestyramine Resin And Colestipol HCl: may delay decrease absorption of thiazide diuretics.

Amphotericin B, Corticosteroids or Corticotropin: *(ACTH):* may intensify electrolyte imbalance, particularly hypokalemia.

ADVERSE REACTIONS:

The following adverse reactions have been observed, but there is not enough systematic collection of data to support an estimate of their frequency.

Gastrointestinal System: jaundice (intrahepatic cholestatic jaundice); pancreatitis; gastric irritation; vomiting; cramping; nausea; anorexia; diarrhea; constipation.

Central Nervous System: dizziness; restlessness; paresthesia; headache; xanthopsia.

Hematologic: aplastic anemia; thrombocytopenia; agranulocytosis; leukopenia.

Dermatologic-Hypersensitivity: necrotizing angiitis (vasculitis) (cutaneous vasculitis); purpura; urticaria; rash; photosensitivity.

Cardiovascular: Orthostatic hypotension may occur and may be aggravated by alcohol, barbiturates or narcotics.

Other: hyperglycemia; glycosuria; hyperuricemia; weakness; muscle spasm.

Whenever adverse reactions are moderate or severe, thiazide dosage should be reduced or therapy withdrawn.

OVERDOSAGE:

Symptoms of overdosage include electrolyte imbalance and signs of potassium deficiency such as confusion, dizziness, muscular weakness, and gastrointestinal disturbances. General supportive measures including replacement of fluids and electrolytes may be indicated in treatment of overdosage.

DOSAGE AND ADMINISTRATION:

Therapy should be individualized according to patient response. This therapy should be titrated to gain maximal therapeutic response as well as the minimal dose possible to maintain that therapeutic response (TABLE 1):

TABLE 1

	Diuretic	Antihypertensive
Benzthiazide	50 to 200 mg	50 to 200 mg

Edema: *Initiation of diuresis.* 50 to 200 mg daily should be used for several days, or until dry weight is attained. With 100 mg or more daily, it is generally preferable to administer benzthiazide in two doses, following morning and evening meals. *Maintenance of diuresis.* 50 to 150 mg daily depending upon the patient's response. To maintain effectiveness, reduction to minimal effective dosage should be gradual.

Hypertension: *Initiation of antihypertensive therapy.* 50 to 100 mg daily is the average dose. It may be given in two doses of 25 mg or 50 mg each after breakfast and after lunch. This dosage may be continued until a therapeutic drop in blood pressure occurs. *Maintenance of antihypertensive therapy.* Dosage should be adjusted according to the patient response, either upward to as much as 50 mg q.i.d. or downward to the minimal effective dosage level.

Store at controlled room temperature, between 20°C and 25°C (68°F and 77°F).

Dispense in tight container.

For How Supplied Information, Contact AH Robins (NDA# 12489)

BENZTROPINE MESYLATE *(000455)*

CATEGORIES: Analeptics; Antiarthritics; Anticholinergic Agents; Antimuscarinics/ Antispasmodics; Antiparkinson Agents; Autonomic Drugs; Extrapyramidal Movement Disorders; Neuromuscular; Parkinsonism; FDA Approval Pre 1982

BRAND NAMES: *Akitan*; *Apo-Benzthropine* (Canada); *Bensylate*; **Cogentin**; *Cogentine* (France); *Cogentinol* (Germany); Glycopyrrolate; *Phatropine*; *PMS Benztropine* (Canada)
(International brand names outside U.S. in italics)

FORMULARIES: Aetna; BC-BS; FHP; Medi-Cal; PCS

COST OF THERAPY: $9.59 (Parkinsonism; Tablet; 1 mg; 1/day; 365 days)

DESCRIPTION:

Benztropine mesylate is a synthetic compound containing structural features found in atropine and diphenhydramine.

It is designated chemically as 8-azabicyclo(3.2.1) octane, 3-(diphenylmethoxy)-,*endo,* methanesulfonate. Its empirical formula is $C_{21}H_{25}NO{\cdot}CH_4O_3S$.

Benztropine mesylate is a crystalline white powder, very soluble in water, and has a molecular weight of 403.54.

Benztropine mesylate is supplied as tablets in three strengths (0.5 mg, 1 mg, and 2 mg per tablet), and as a sterile injection for intravenous and intramuscular use.

Tablets contain 0.5, 1 or 2 mg of benztropine mesylate. Each tablet contains the following inactive ingredients: calcium phosphate, cellulose, lactose, magnesium stearate and starch.

Each milliliter of the injection contains:

Benztropine Mesylate: 1 mg

Sodium Chloride: 9 mg

Water For Injection Q.S.: 1 ml

CLINICAL PHARMACOLOGY:

Benztropine mesylate possesses both anticholinergic and antihistaminic effects, although only the former have been established as therapeutically significant in the management of parkinsonism.

In the isolated guinea pig ileum, the anticholinergic activity of this drug is about equal to that of atropine; however, when administered orally to unanesthetized cats, it is only about half as active as atropine.

In laboratory animals, its antihistaminic activity and duration of action approach those of pyrilamine maleate.

INDICATIONS AND USAGE:

For use as an adjunct in the therapy of all forms of parkinsonism.

Useful also in the control of extrapyramidal disorders (except tardive dyskinesia — see PRECAUTIONS) due to neuroleptic drugs (*e.g.*, phenothiazines).

CONTRAINDICATIONS:

Hypersensitivity to benztropine mesylate tablets or to any component of benztropine mesylate injection.

Because of its atropine-like side effects, this drug is contraindicated in children under three years of age, and should be used with caution in older children.

WARNINGS:

Safe use in pregnancy has not been established.

Benztropine mesylate may impair mental and/or physical abilities required for performance of hazardous tasks, such as operating machinery or driving a motor vehicle.

When benztropine mesylate is given concomitantly with phenothiazines, haloperidol, or other drugs with anticholinergic or antidopaminergic activity, patients should be advised to report gastrointestinal complaints, fever or heat intolerance promptly. Paralytic ileus, hyperthermia and heat stroke, all of which have sometimes been fatal, have occurred in patients taking anticholinergic-type antiparkinsonism drugs, including benztropine mesylate, in combination with phenothiazines and/or tricyclic antidepressants.

Since benztropine mesylate contains structural features of atropine; it may produce anhidrosis. For this reason, it should be administered with caution during hot weather, especially when given concomitantly with other atropine-like drugs to the chronically ill, the alcoholic, those who have central nervous system disease, and those who do manual labor in a hot environment. Anhidrosis may occur more readily when some disturbance of sweating already exists. If there is evidence of anhidrosis, the possibility of hyperthermia should be considered. Dosage should be decreased at the discretion of the physician so that the ability to maintain body heat equilibrium by perspiration is not impaired. Severe anhidrosis and fatal hyperthermia have occurred.

PRECAUTIONS:

GENERAL

Since benztropine mesylate has cumulative action, continued supervision is advisable. Patients with a tendency to tachycardia and patients with prostatic hypertrophy should be observed closely during treatment.

Dysuria may occur, but rarely becomes a problem. Urinary retention has been reported with benztropine mesylate.

The drug may cause complaints of weakness and inability to move particular muscle groups, especially in large doses. For example, if the neck has been rigid and suddenly relaxes, it may feel weak, causing some concern. In this event, dosage adjustment is required.

Mental confusion and excitement may occur with large doses, or in susceptible patients. Visual hallucinations have been reported occasionally. Furthermore, in the treatment of extrapyramidal disorders due to neuroleptic drugs (*e.g.*, phenothiazines), in patients with mental disorders, occasionally there may be intensification of mental symptoms. In such cases, antiparkinsonian drugs can precipitate a toxic psychosis. Patients with mental disorders should be kept under careful observation, especially at the beginning of treatment or if dosage is increased.

Tardive dyskinesia may appear in some patients on long-term therapy with phenothiazines and related agents, or may occur after therapy with these drugs has been discontinued. Antiparkinsonism agents do not alleviate the symptoms of tardive dyskinesia, and in some instances may aggravate them. Benztropine mesylate is not recommended for use in patients with tardive dyskinesia.

The physician should be aware of the possible occurrence of glaucoma. Although the drug does not appear to have any adverse effect on simple glaucoma, it probably should not be used in angle-closure glaucoma.

DRUG INTERACTIONS:

Antipsychotic drugs such as phenothiazines or haloperidol; tricyclic antidepressants (see WARNINGS.)

ADVERSE REACTIONS:

The adverse reactions below, most of which are anticholinergic in nature, have been reported and within each category are listed in order of decreasing severity.

Cardiovascular: Tachycardia.

Digestive: Paralytic ileus, constipation, vomiting, nausea, dry mouth.

If dry mouth is so severe that there is difficulty in swallowing or speaking, or loss of appetite and weight, reduce dosage, or discontinue the drug temporarily.

Slight reduction in dosage may control nausea and still give sufficient relief of symptoms. Vomiting may be controlled by temporary discontinuation, followed by resumption at a lower dosage.

Nervous System: Toxic psychosis, including confusion, disorientation, memory impairment, visual hallucinations; exacerbation of pre-existing psychotic symptoms; nervousness; depression; listlessness; numbness of fingers.

Special Senses: Blurred vision, dilated pupils.

Urogenital: Urinary retention, dysuria.

Metabolic/Immune or Skin: Occasionally; an allergic reaction, *e.g.*, skin rash develops. If this can not be controlled by dosage reduction, the medication should be discontinued.

Other: Heat stroke, hyperthermia, fever.

OVERDOSAGE:

Manifestations: May be any of those seen in atropine poisoning or antihistamine overdosage: CNS depression, preceded or followed by stimulation; confusion; nervousness; listlessness; intensification of mental symptoms or toxic psychosis in patients with mental illness being treated with neuroleptic drugs (*e.g.*, phenothiazines); hallucinations (especially visual); dizziness; muscle weakness; ataxia; dry mouth; mydriasis; blurred vision; palpitations; tachycardia;

OVERDOSAGE: *(cont'd)*

nausea; vomiting; dysuria; numbness of fingers; dysphagia; allergic reactions, *e.g.*, skin rash; headache; hot, dry, flushed skin; delirium; coma; shock; convulsions; respiratory arrest; anhidrosis; hyperthermia; glaucoma; constipation.

Treatment: Physostigmine salicylate, 1 to 2 mg, SC or IV, reportedly will reverse symptoms of anticholinergic intoxication (Duvoisin, R. C.; Katz, R. J.; Amer. Med. Ass. *206:* 1963-1965, Nov. 25, 1968). A second injection may be given after 2 hours if required. Otherwise treatment is symptomatic and supportive. Induce emesis or perform gastric lavage (contraindicated in precomatose, convulsive, or psychotic states). Maintain respiration. A short-acting barbiturate may be used for CNS excitement, but with caution to avoid subsequent depression; supportive care for depression (avoid convulsant stimulants such as picrotoxin, pentylenetetrazol, or bemegride); artificial respiration for severe respiratory depression; a local miotic for mydriasis and cycloplegia; ice bags or other cold applications and alcohol sponges for hyperpyrexia, a vasopressor and fluids for circulatory collapse. Darken room for photophobia.

DOSAGE AND ADMINISTRATION:

Benztropine mesylate tablets should be used when patients are able to take oral medication.

The injection is especially useful for psychotic patients with acute dystonic reactions or other reaction that make oral medication difficult or impossible. It is recommended also when a more rapid response is desired than can be obtained with the tablets.

Since there is no significant difference in onset of effect after intravenous or intramuscular injection usually there is no need to use the intravenous route. The drug is quickly effective after either route, with improvement sometimes noticeable a few minutes after injection. In emergency situations, when the condition of the patient is alarming, 1 to 2 ml of the injection normally will provide quick relief. If the parkinsonian effect begins to return, the dose can be repeated.

Because of cumulative action, therapy should be initiated with a low dose which is increased gradually at five or six-day intervals to the smallest amount necessary for optimal relief. Increases should be made in increments of 0.5 mg, to a maximum of 6 mg, or until optimal results are obtained without excessive adverse reactions.

POSTENCEPHALITIC AND IDIOPATHIC PARKINSONISM

The usual daily dose is 1 to 2 mg, with a range of 0.5 to 6 mg orally or parenterally.

As with any agent used in parkinsonism, dosage must be individualized according to age and weight, and the type of parkinsonism being treated. Generally, older patients, and thin patients cannot tolerate large doses. Most patients with postencephalitic parkinsonism need fairly large doses and tolerate them well. Patients with a poor mental outlook are usually poor candidates for therapy.

In idiopathic parkinsonism, therapy may be initiated with a single daily dose of 0.5 to 1 mg at bedtime. In some patients, this will be adequate; in others 4 to 6 mg a day may be required.

In postencephalitic parkinsonism, therapy may be initiated in most patients with 2 mg a day in one or more doses. In highly sensitive patients, therapy may be initiated with 0.5 mg at bedtime, and increased as necessary.

Some patients experience greatest relief by taking the entire dose at bedtime; others react more favorably to divided doses, two to four times a day. Frequently, one dose a day is sufficient, and divided doses may be unnecessary or undesirable.

The long duration of action of this drug makes it particularly suitable for bedtime medication when its effects may last throughout the night, enabling patients to turn in bed during the night more easily, and to rise in the morning.

When benztropine mesylate is started, do not terminate therapy with other antiparkinsonian agents abruptly. If the other agents are to be reduced or discontinued, it must be done gradually. Many patients obtain greatest relief with combination therapy.

Benztropine mesylate may be used concomitantly with Carbidopa-Levodopa (Sinemet, MSD), or with levodopa, in which case periodic dosage adjustment may be required in order to maintain optimum response.

DRUG-INDUCED EXTRAPYRAMIDAL DISORDERS

In treating extrapyramidal disorders due to neuroleptic drugs (*e.g.*, phenothiazines), the recommended dosage is 1 to 4 mg once or twice a day orally or parenterally. Dosage must be individualized according to the need of the patient. Some patients require more than recommended; others do not need as much.

In acute dystonic reactions, 1 to 2 ml of the injection usually relieves the condition quickly. After that, the tablets, 1 to 2 mg twice a day, usually prevent recurrence.

When extrapyramidal disorders develop soon after initiation of treatment with neuroleptic drugs (*e.g.*, phenothiazines), they are likely to be transient. One to 2 mg of benztropine mesylate tablets two or three times a day usually provides relief within one or two days. After one or two weeks, the drug should be withdrawn to determine the continued need for it. If such disorders recur, benztropine mesylate can be reinstituted.

Certain drug-induced extrapyramidal disorders that develop slowly may not respond to benztropine mesylate.

HOW SUPPLIED - RATED THERAPEUTICALLY EQUIVALENT:

Tablet, Uncoated - Oral - 0.5 mg

100's	$2.40	Benztropine Mesylate, United Res	00677-0994-01
100's	$2.40	Benztropine, Geneva Pharms	00781-1347-01
100's	$2.40	Benztropine, H.C.F.A. F F P	99999-0455-01
100's	$4.89	Benztropine, US Trading	56126-0164-11
100's	$5.10	Benztropine Mesylate, Qualitest Pharms	00603-2430-21
100's	$5.25	Benztropine, HL Moore Drug Exch	00839-7002-06
100's	$5.70	Benztropine, Invamed	52189-0208-24
100's	$5.80	Benztropine Mesylate, Elkins Sinn	00641-4005-86
100's	$5.95	Benztropine Mesylate, Major Pharms	00904-1055-60
100's	$6.02	Benztropine Mesylate, Vangard Labs	00615-2547-13
100's	$7.00	Benztropine, Schein Pharm (US)	00364-0834-01
100's	$7.05	Benztropine Mesylate, Par Pharm	49884-0164-01
100's	$7.20	Benztropine Mesylate, Martec Pharms	52555-0457-01
100's	$7.36	Benztropine, Parmed Pharms	00349-8941-01
100's	$7.85	Benztropine, Raway	00686-0220-20
100's	$9.21	Benztropine, Duramed Pharms	51285-0827-02
100's	$9.60	Benztropine, Goldline Labs	00182-1299-01
100's	$9.60	Benztropine Mesylate 0.5, Aligen Independ	00405-4116-01
100's	$9.60	Benztropine, Sidmak Labs	50111-0393-01
100's	$9.75	Benztropine, Rugby	00536-3370-01
100's	$12.50	Benztropine, Medirex	57480-0305-01
100's	$14.30	Benztropine, Goldline Labs	00182-1299-89
100's	$15.31	Benztropine, Major Pharms	00904-1055-61
100's	**$17.66**	**COGENTIN, Merck**	**00006-0021-68**
600's	$77.20	Benztropine, Medirex	57480-0305-06
750's	$105.25	Benztropine Mesylate, Glasgow Pharm	60809-0148-55
750's	$105.25	Benztropine Mesylate, Glasgow Pharm	60809-0148-72

HOW SUPPLIED - RATED THERAPEUTICALLY EQUIVALENT: *(cont'd)*

Tablet, Uncoated - Oral - 1 mg

60's	$1.57	Benztropine, H.C.F.A. F F P	99999-0455-02
60's	$3.50	Benztropine Mesylate 1, Major Pharms	00904-1056-52
100's	$2.63	Benztropine, United Res	00677-0993-01
100's	$2.63	Benztropine, Geneva Pharms	00781-1357-01
100's	$2.63	Benztropine, H.C.F.A. F F P	99999-0455-03
100's	$4.88	Benztropine, US Trading	56126-0165-11
100's	$5.40	Benztropine, Qualitest Pharms	00603-2431-21
100's	$6.40	Benztropine, Invamed	52189-0209-24
100's	$7.45	Benztropine Mesylate 1, Major Pharms	00904-1056-60
100's	$7.50	Benztropine, Parmed Pharms	00349-8942-01
100's	$8.10	Benztropine, Mutual Pharm	53489-0183-01
100's	$8.21	Benztropine, Lederle Pharm	00005-3050-23
100's	$8.25	Benztropine Mesylate, Par Pharm	49884-0165-01
100's	$8.40	Benztropine, Schein Pharm (US)	00364-0703-01
100's	$8.40	Benztropine Mesylate, Martec Pharms	52555-0458-01
100's	$9.95	Benztropine, Raway	00686-0221-10
100's	$10.10	Benztropine, Rugby	00536-3371-01
100's	$10.51	Benztropine, Duramed Pharms	51285-0828-02
100's	$10.52	Benztropine, HL Moore Drug Exch	00839-6771-06
100's	$10.90	Benztropine, Goldline Labs	00182-1700-01
100's	$10.90	Benztropine Mesylate 1, Aligen Independ	00405-4117-01
100's	$10.90	Benztropine, Sidmak Labs	50111-0394-01
100's	$13.50	Benztropine, Medirex	57480-0306-01
100's	$19.60	Benztropine, Goldline Labs	00182-1700-89
100's	$20.15	Benztropine Mesylate 1, Major Pharms	00904-1056-61
100's	$20.18	Benztropine Mesylate, Vangard Labs	00615-2548-13
100's	**$20.19**	**COGENTIN, Merck**	**00006-0635-68**
100's	**$24.59**	**COGENTIN, Merck**	**00006-0635-28**
500's	$37.26	Benztropine, Amer Preferred	53445-1700-05
600's	$94.00	Benztropine, Medirex	57480-0306-06
750's	$100.61	Benztropine Mesylate, Glasgow Pharm	60809-0109-55
750's	$100.61	Benztropine Mesylate, Glasgow Pharm	60809-0109-72
1000's	$26.30	Benztropine, United Res	00677-0993-10
1000's	$26.30	Benztropine, Geneva Pharms	00781-1357-10
1000's	$26.30	Benztropine, H.C.F.A. F F P	99999-0455-04
1000's	$37.20	Benztropine Mesylate 1, Major Pharms	00904-1056-80
1000's	$43.15	Benztropine, Qualitest Pharms	00603-2431-32
1000's	$51.00	Benztropine, Goldline Labs	00182-1700-10
1000's	$51.00	Benztropine, Elkins Sinn	00641-4006-89
1000's	$51.00	Benztropine, Invamed	52189-0209-30
1000's	$54.45	Benztropine, Parmed Pharms	00349-8942-10
1000's	$54.50	Benztropine, Mutual Pharm	53489-0183-10
1000's	$65.00	Benztropine, Schein Pharm (US)	00364-0703-02
1000's	$75.50	Benztropine, Rugby	00536-3371-10
1000's	$80.00	Benztropine Mesylate, Par Pharm	49884-0165-10
1000's	$81.60	Benztropine Mesylate, Martec Pharms	52555-0458-10
1000's	$84.21	Benztropine Mesylate, Aligen Independ	00405-4117-03
1000's	$102.97	Benztropine, Duramed Pharms	51285-0828-05
1000's	$102.99	Benztropine Mesylate 1 Mg Tablets, HL Moore Drug Exch	00839-6771-16
1000's	$104.25	Benztropine, Sidmak Labs	50111-0394-03

Tablet, Uncoated - Oral - 2 mg

60's	$1.98	Benztropine, H.C.F.A. F F P	99999-0455-05
60's	$4.10	Benztropine Mesylate, Major Pharms	00904-1057-52
100's	$3.30	Benztropine, United Res	00677-0995-01
100's	$3.30	Benztropine, Geneva Pharms	00781-1367-01
100's	$3.30	Benztropine, H.C.F.A. F F P	99999-0455-06
100's	$5.61	Benztropine, US Trading	56126-0166-11
100's	$6.93	Benztropine, Qualitest Pharms	00603-2432-21
100's	$8.00	Benztropine, Invamed	52189-0210-24
100's	$9.95	Benztropine Mesylate, Major Pharms	00904-1057-60
100's	$10.10	Benztropine Mesylate, Par Pharm	49884-0166-01
100's	$10.30	Benztropine Mesylate, Martec Pharms	52555-0459-01
100's	$10.35	Benztropine, Lederle Pharm	00005-3051-23
100's	$10.55	Benztropine, Raway	00686-0222-20
100's	$10.58	Benztropine, Parmed Pharms	00349-8943-01
100's	$10.75	Benztropine, Mutual Pharm	53489-0184-01
100's	$12.54	Benztropine, HL Moore Drug Exch	00839-6772-06
100's	$12.70	Benztropine, Schein Pharm (US)	00364-0704-01
100's	$13.25	Benztropine, Duramed Pharms	51285-0829-02
100's	$13.75	Benztropine, Goldline Labs	00182-1701-01
100's	$13.75	Benztropine Mesylate 2, Aligen Independ	00405-4118-01
100's	$13.75	Benztropine, Rugby	00536-3372-01
100's	$13.75	Benztropine, Sidmak Labs	50111-0395-01
100's	$16.00	Benztropine, Medirex	57480-0307-01
100's	$20.10	Benztropine, Goldline Labs	00182-1701-89
100's	$20.68	Benztropine Mesylate, Vangard Labs	00615-2549-13
100's	$21.33	Benztropine, Major Pharms	00904-1057-61
100's	**$25.45**	**COGENTIN, Merck**	**00006-0060-68**
100's	**$29.88**	**COGENTIN, Merck**	**00006-0060-28**
500's	$16.50	Benztropine, H.C.F.A. F F P	99999-0455-08
500's	$41.20	Benztropine, Rugby	00536-3372-05
500's	$113.39	Benztropine, HL Moore Drug Exch	00839-6772-16
500's	$130.41	Benztropine, Duramed Pharms	51285-0829-05
500's	$132.00	Benztropine, Goldline Labs	00182-1701-10
600's	$110.80	Benztropine, Medirex	57480-0307-06
750's	$137.66	Benztropine Mesylate, Glasgow Pharm	60809-0110-55
750's	$137.66	Benztropine Mesylate, Glasgow Pharm	60809-0110-72
1000's	$33.00	Benztropine, United Res	00677-0995-10
1000's	$33.00	Benztropine, Geneva Pharms	00781-1367-10
1000's	$33.00	Benztropine, H.C.F.A. F F P	99999-0455-07
1000's	$62.10	Benztropine Mesylate, Major Pharms	00904-1057-80
1000's	$65.11	Benztropine, Qualitest Pharms	00603-2432-32
1000's	$66.00	Benztropine, Invamed	52189-0210-30
1000's	$69.00	Benztropine, Elkins Sinn	00641-4007-89
1000's	$86.41	Benztropine, Lederle Pharm	00005-3051-34
1000's	$89.00	Benztropine, Mutual Pharm	53489-0184-10
1000's	$89.77	Benztropine, Parmed Pharms	00349-8943-10
1000's	$97.97	Benztropine Mesylate, Par Pharm	49884-0166-10
1000's	$99.90	Benztropine Mesylate, Martec Pharms	52555-0459-10
1000's	$132.00	Benztropine, Schein Pharm (US)	00364-0704-02
1000's	$132.00	Benztropine Mesylate 2, Aligen Independ	00405-4118-03
1000's	$132.00	Benztropine, Sidmak Labs	50111-0395-03
1000's	**$212.28**	**COGENTIN, Merck**	**00006-0060-82**

HOW SUPPLIED - NOT RATED EQUIVALENT:

Injection, Solution - Intramuscular; - 1 mg/ml

2 ml x 6	**$40.46**	**COGENTIN, Merck**	**00006-3275-16**

BEPRIDIL HYDROCHLORIDE *(003003)*

CATEGORIES: Angina; Antianginals; Calcium Channel Blockers; Cardiovascular Drugs; Pregnancy Category C; FDA Class 1B ("Modest Therapeutic Advantage"); FDA Approved 1990 Dec

BRAND NAMES: Bepadin; *Bepricol* (Japan); *Cordium* (France); *Cruor*; **Vascor**
(International brand names outside U.S. in italics)

COST OF THERAPY: $984.33 (Angina; Tablet; 200 mg; 1/day; 365 days)

DESCRIPTION:

Bepridil HCl is an anti-anginal agent that inhibits slow calcium as well as fast sodium channels, interferes with calcium binding to calmodulin and blocks both voltage and receptor operated calcium channels. It is not related chemically to other drugs having similar cardioactivity such as diltiazem HCl, nifedipine and verapamil HCl.

Bepridil HCl monohydrate is a white to off-white, crystalline powder with a bitter taste. It is slightly soluble in water, very soluble in ethanol, methanol and chloroform, and freely soluble in acetone. The molecular weight of bepridil HCl monohydrate is 421.02. Its molecular formula is $C_{24}H_{34}N_2O \cdot HCl \cdot H_2O$.

(±)-β[(2-Methylpropoxy)methyl]-*N*-phenyl-*N*-(pheny lmethyl)-1-pyrrolidineethanamine monohydrochloride monohydrate.

Bepridil HCl is available as film-coated tablets for oral use containing 200, 300, or 400 mg of bepridil HCl monohydrate. Inactive ingredients: hydroxypropyl methylcellulose, lactose, magnesium stearate, microcrystalline cellulose, polyethylene glycol, silicon dioxide, pregelatinized corn starch, corn starch, titanium dioxide, FD&C Blue #1.

CLINICAL PHARMACOLOGY:

Bepridil HCl is a calcium channel blocker anti-anginal agent with Type 1 anti-arrhythmic and minimal anti-hypertensive properties. Bepridil HCl has inhibitory effects on both the slow calcium and fast sodium inward currents in myocardial and vascular smooth muscle.

Bepridil HCl inhibits the transmembrane influx of calcium ions into cardiac and vascular smooth muscle. This has been demonstrated in isolated myocardial and vascular smooth muscle preparations in which both the slope of the calcium dose response curve and the maximum calcium-induced inotropic response were significantly reduced by bepridil HCl. In cardiac myocytes *in vitro*, bepridil HCl was shown to be tightly bound to actin. A negative inotropic effect can be seen in the isolated guinea pig atria.

In *in vitro* studies, bepridil HCl has also been demonstrated to inhibit the sodium inward current. Reductions in the maximal upstroke velocity and the amplitude of the action potential, as well as increases in the duration of the normal action potential, have been observed. Additionally, bepridil HCl has been shown to possess local anesthetic activity in isolated myocardial preparations. It effects electrophysiological changes that are observed with several classes of anti-arrhythmic agents.

Mechanism of Action: The precise mechanism of action for bepridil HCl as an anti-anginal agent remains to be fully determined, but is believed to include the following mechanisms:

Bepridil HCl regularly reduces heart rate and arterial pressure at rest and at a given level of exercise by dilating peripheral arterioles and reducing total peripheral resistance (afterload) against which the heart works. In exercise tolerance tests in patients with stable angina the heart rate/blood pressure product was reduced with bepridil HCl for a given work load.

Hemodynamic Effects: Bepridil HCl produces dose dependent slowing of the heart, and reflex tachycardia is not seen. The mean decrease in heart rate in US clinical trials was 3 b.p.m. Orally administered bepridil HCl also produces modest decreases (less than 5 mm Hg) in systolic and diastolic blood pressure in normotensive patients and somewhat larger decreases in hypertensive patients.

Intravenous administration of bepridil HCl is associated with a modest reduction in left ventricular contractility (dP/dt), and increased filling pressure, but radionuclide cineangiography studies in angina patients demonstrated improvement in ejection fraction at rest and during exercise following oral bepridil HCl therapy. Patients with impaired cardiac function (overt heart failure) were not included in these studies.

Electrophysiological Effects: Intravenous administration of bepridil HCl in man prolongs the effective refractory periods of the atria and ventricles, and the functional refractory period of the AV node. There was a tendency for the AV node effective refractory period and A-H interval to be increased as well. Intravenous and oral administration of bepridil HCl slow heart rate, prolong the QT and QT_c intervals, and alter the morphology of the T-wave (indentation). In clinical trials with angina patients, the mean percent prolongation of the QT_c interval was approximately 8%, and QT of about 10%. The prolongation of QT is dose related, varying from about 0.030 sec at doses of 200 mg once a day to 0.055 sec at 400 mg once a day. Upon cessation of therapy, the ECG gradually normalizes. No instances of greater than first-degree heart block have been observed in US controlled or open clinical studies with bepridil HCl, and first-degree heart block occurred in 0.2% of patients in these studies.

Pulmonary Function: In healthy subjects and asthmatic patients, intravenous bepridil HCl did not cause bronchoconstriction. Bepridil HCl has been safely used in asthmatic patients and in patients with chronic obstructive lung disease.

Pharmacokinetics and Metabolism: In studies with healthy volunteers, bepridil HCl is rapidly and completely absorbed after oral administration. The time to peak bepridil plasma concentration is about 2 to 3 hours. Over a ten day period, approximately 70% of a single dose of bepridil HCl is excreted in the urine and 22% in the feces, as metabolites of bepridil. Excretion of unmetabolized drug is negligible. In healthy male volunteers, the relationship between dose and steady-state blood levels of bepridil was linear over the range of 200 to 400 mg/day. Elimination of bepridil is biphasic, with a distribution half-life of about 2 hours. The terminal elimination half-life following the cessation of multiple dosing averaged 42 hours (range 26-64 hours). However, during a given dosing interval, decay from the peak concentration occurs relatively rapidly indicating a dosing interval, decay from the peak concentration occurs relatively rapidly, indicating a dosing interval half-life shorter than 24 hours. Following once-daily dosing with therapeutic doses, steady-state was reached in about 8 days in healthy volunteers. The clearance of bepridil decreases after multiple dosing.

Clearance of bepridil in angina patients was lower than that in healthy volunteers, resulting in higher average plasma bepridil concentrations. At steady state, maximum bepridil concentrations averaged 2332 ng/ml (range 1451 to 3609) and mean minimum concentrations were 1174 ng/ml (range 226 to 2639) in angina patients following 300 mg/day doses of bepridil HCl.

Bepridil HCl is more than 99% bound to plasma proteins. Administration of bepridil HCl after a meal resulted in a clinically insignificant delay in time to peak concentration, but neither peak bepridil plasma levels nor the extent of absorption was changed.

Bepridil HCl passes through the placental barrier. Bepridil HCl may cause uterine hypotonia.

CLINICAL STUDIES:

In controlled studies with 200-400 mg of bepridil HCl, given as a once daily dose, exercise tolerance was improved and angina frequency and daily nitroglycerine use was reduced compared to placebo. Improvement in exercise performance was dose related. In one

CLINICAL STUDIES: *(cont'd)*

controlled clinical study, bepridil HCl as added to propranolol in daily doses of up to 240 mg. The 200-400 mg dose of bepridil HCl was well tolerated (patients entered were not allowed to be in NYHA Class III or IV heart failure) and there was an added effect of bepridil HCl on exercise tolerance.

In another controlled clinical study, bepridil HCl in doses of up to 400 mg/day, significantly improved exercise tolerance compared to diltiazem HCl in patients refractory to diltiazem HCl therapy.

INDICATIONS AND USAGE:

CHRONIC STABLE ANGINA (CLASSIC EFFORT-ASSOCIATED ANGINA)

Bepridil HCl is indicated for the treatment of chronic stable angina (classic effort-associated). Because bepridil HCl has caused serious ventricular arrhythmias, including torsades de pointes type ventricular tachycardia, and the occurrence of cases of agranulocytosis associated with its use (see WARNINGS), it should be reserved for patients who have failed to respond optimally to, or are intolerant of, other anti-anginal medication.

Bepridil HCl may be used alone or in combination with beta blockers and/or nitrates. Controlled clinical studies have shown an added effect when bepridil HCl is administered to patients already receiving propranolol.

CONTRAINDICATIONS:

Bepridil HCl is contraindicated in patients with a known sensitivity to bepridil HCl.

Bepridil HCl is contraindicated in (1) patients with a history of serious ventricular arrhythmias (see WARNINGS, Induction of New Serious Arrhythmias), (2) patients with sick sinus syndrome or patients with second- or third-degree AV block, except in the presence of a functioning ventricular pacemaker, (3) patients with hypotension (less than 90 mm Hg systolic), (4) patients with uncompensated cardiac insufficiency, (5) patients with congenital QT interval prolongation (see WARNINGS), and (6) patients taking other drugs that prolong QT interval (see DRUG INTERACTIONS).

WARNINGS:

Induction Of New Serious Arrhythmias: Bepridil HCl has Class 1 anti-arrhythmic properties and, like other such drugs, can induce new arrhythmias, including VT/VF. In addition, because of its ability to prolong the QT interval, bepridil HCl can cause torsades de pointes type ventricular tachycardia. Because of these properties, bepridil HCl should reserved for patients in whom other anti-anginal agents do not offer a satisfactory effect.

In US clinical trials, the QT and QT_c intervals were commonly prolonged by bepridil HCl in a dose- related fashion. While the mean prolongation of QT_c was 8% and of QT was 10%, QT_c increases of 25% or more were not uncommon, 5%; 8.7% QT. Increased QT and Qt_c may be associated with torsades de pointes type VT, which was seen at least briefly, in about 1.0% of patients in U.S. trials; in many cases, however, patients with marked prolongation of QT_c were taken off bepridil HCl therapy. All of the U.S. patients with torsades de pointes had a prolonged QT interval and relatively low serum potassium. French marketing experience has reported over one hundred verified cases of torsades de pointes. While this number, based on total use, represents a rate of only 0.01%, the true rate is undoubtedly much higher, as spontaneous reporting systems all suffer from substantial under reporting.

Torsades de pointes is a polymorphic ventricular tachycardia often but not always associated with a prolonged QT interval, and often drug induced. The relation between the degree of QT prolongation and the development of torsades de pointes is not linear and the likelihood of torsades appears to be increased by hypokalemia, use of potassium wasting diuretics, and the presence of antecedent bradycardia. While the safe upper limit of QT is not defined, it is suggested that the interval not be permitted to exceed 0.52 seconds during treatment. If dose reduction does not eliminate the excessive prolongation, bepridil should be stopped. Because most domestic and foreign cases of torsades have developed in patients with hypokalemia, usually related to diuretic use or significant liver disease, if concomitant diuretics are needed, low doses and addition or primary use of a potassium sparing diuretic should be considered and the serum potassium should be monitored.

Bepridil HCl has been associated with the usual range of pro-arrhythmic effects characteristic of Class 1 anti-arrhythmics (increased premature ventricular contraction rates, new sustained VT, and VT/VF that is more difficult than previously to convert to sinus rhythm). Use in patients with severe arrhythmias (who are most susceptible to certain pro-arrhythmic effects) has been limited, so that risk in these patients is not defined.

In the National Heart, Lung and Blood Institute's Cardiac Arrhythmia Suppression Trial (CAST), a long-term, multi- centered, randomized, double-blind study in patients with asymptomatic non-life-threatening ventricular arrhythmias who had myocardial infarctions more than six days but less than two years previously, an excess mortality/non-fatal cardiac arrest rate was seen in patients treated with encainide or flecainide (56/730) compared to that seen in patients assigned to matched placebo-treated groups (22/725). The applicability of these results to other populations (*e.g.*, those without recent myocardial infarction) or to other anti-arrhythmic drugs is uncertain, but at present it is prudent to consider any drug documented to provoke new serious arrhythmias or worsening of pre-existing arrhythmias as having a similar risk and to avoid their use in the post-infarction period.

Agranulocytosis: In US clinical trials of over 800 patients treated with bepridil HCl for up to five years, two cases of marked leukopenia and neutropenia were reported. Both patients were diabetic and elderly. One died with overwhelming gram-negative sepsis, itself a possible cause of marked leukopenia. The other patient recovered rapidly when bepridil HCl was stopped.

Congestive Heart Failure: Congestive heart failure has been observed infrequently (about 1%) during US controlled clinical trials, but experience with the use of bepridil HCl in patients with significantly impaired ventricular function is limited. There is little information on the effect of concomitant administration of bepridil HCl and digoxin; therefore, caution should be exercised in treating patients with congestive heart failure.

WARNINGS: *(cont'd)*

Hepatic Enzyme Elevation: In U.S. clinical studies with bepridil HCl in about 1000 patients and subjects, clinically significant (at least 2 times the upper limit of normal) transaminase elevations were observed in approximately 1% of the patients. None of these patients became clinically symptomatic or jaundiced and values returned to normal when the drug was stopped.

Hypokalemia: In clinical trials bepridil HCl has not been reported to reduce serum potassium levels. Because hypokalemia has been associated with ventricular arrhythmias, potassium insufficiency should be corrected before bepridil HCl therapy is initiated and normal potassium concentrations should be maintained during bepridil HCl therapy. Serum potassium should be monitored periodically.

PRECAUTIONS:

General: Caution should be exercised when using bepridil HCl in patients with left bundle branch block or sinus bradycardia (less than 50 b.p.m.). Care should also be exercised in patients with serious hepatic or renal disorders because such patients have not been studied and bepridil is highly metabolized, with metabolites excreted primarily in the urine.

Recent Myocardial Infarction: In U.S. clinical trials with bepridil HCl, patients with myocardial infarctions within three months prior to initiation of drug treatment were excluded. The initiation of bepridil HCl therapy in such patients, therefore, cannot be recommended.

Information for the Patient: Since QT prolongation is not associated with defined symptomatology, patients should be instructed on the importance of maintaining any potassium supplementation or potassium sparing diuretic, and the need for routine electrocardiograms and periodic monitoring of serum potassium.

The following patient information is printed on the carton label of each unit of use bottle of 30 tablets:

As with any medication that you take, you should notify your physician of any changes in your overall condition. Insure that you follow your physician's instructions regarding follow-up visits. Please notify any physician who treats you for a medical condition that you are taking bepridil HCl, as well as any other medications.

Carcinogenesis, Mutagenesis, and Impairment of Fertility: No evidence of carcinogenicity was revealed in one lifetime study in mice at dosages up to 60 times (for a 60 kg subject) the maximum recommended dosage in man. Unilateral follicular adenomas of the thyroid were observed in a study in rats following lifetime administration of high doses of bepridil HCl, (*i.e.*, ≥100 mg/kg/day) (20 times the usual recommended dose in man). No mutagenic or other genotoxic potential of bepridil HCl was found in the following standard laboratory tests: the Micronucleus Test for Chromosomal Effects, the Liver Microsome Activated Bacterial Assay for Mutagenicity, the Chinese Hamster Ovary Cell Assay for Mutagenicity, and the Sister Chromatid Exchange Assay. No intrinsic effect on fertility by bepridil HCl was demonstrated in rats.

In monkeys, at 200 mg/kg/day, there was a decrease in testicular weight and spermatogenesis. There were no systematic studies in man related to this point. In rats, at doses up to 300 mg/kg/day, there was no observed alteration of mating behavior nor of reproductive performance.

Usage in Pregnancy: Pregnancy Category C. Reproductive studies (fertility and peri-postnatal) have been conducted in rats. Reduced litter size at birth and decreased pup survival during lactation were observed at maternal dosages 37 times (on a mg/kg basis) the maximum daily recommended therapeutic dosage.

In teratology studies, no effects were observed in rats or rabbits at these same dosages.

There no well-controlled studies in pregnant women. Use bepridil HCl in pregnant or nursing women only if the potential benefit justifies the potential risk.

Nursing Mothers: Bepridil is excreted in human milk. Bepridil concentration in human milk is estimated to reach about one third the concentration in serum. Because of the potential for serious adverse reactions in nursing infants from bepridil HCl a decision should be made whether to discontinue nursing or to discontinue the drug, taking into account the importance of the drug to the mother.

Pediatric Use: The safety and effectiveness of bepridil HCl in children have not been established.

DRUG INTERACTIONS:

Nitrates: The concomitant use of bepridil HCl with long- and short-acting nitrates has been safely tolerated in patients with stable angina pectoris. Sublingual nitroglycerin may be taken if necessary for the control of acute angina attacks during bepridil HCl therapy.

Beta Blocking Agents: The concomitant use of bepridil HCl and beta-blocking agents has been well tolerated in patients with stable angina. Available data are not sufficient, however, to predict the effects of concomitant medication on patients with impaired ventricular function or cardiac conduction abnormalities (see CLINICAL PHARMACOLOGY and DOSAGE AND ADMINISTRATION).

Dogoxin: In controlled studies in healthy volunteers, bepridil HCl either had no effect (one study) or was associated with modest increases, about 30% (two studies) in steady-state serum digoxin concentrations. Limited clinical data in angina patients receiving concomitant bepridil HCl and digoxin therapy indicate no discernible changes in serum digoxin levels. Available data are neither sufficient to rule out possible increases in serum digoxin with concomitant treatment in some patients, nor other possible interactions, particularly in patients with cardiac conduction abnormalities (also see WARNINGS, Congestive Heart Failure).

Oral Hypoglycemics: Bepridil HCl has been safely used in diabetic patients without significantly lowering their blood glucose levels or altering their need for insulin or oral hypoglycemic agents.

General Interactions: Certain drugs could increase the likelihood of potentially serious adverse effects with bepridil HCl. In general, these are drugs that have one or more pharmacologic activities similar to bepridil HCl, including anti-arrhythmic agents such as quinidine and procainamide, cardiac glycosides and tricyclic anti-depressants. Anti-arrhythmics and tricyclic anti-depressants could exaggerate the prolongation of the QT interval observed with bepridil HCl. Cardiac glycosides could exaggerate the depression of AV nodal conduction observed with bepridil HCl.

ADVERSE REACTIONS:

Adverse reactions were assessed in placebo and active-drug controlled trials of 4-12 weeks duration and longer-term uncontrolled studies. The most common side effects occurring more frequently than in control groups were upper gastrointestinal complaints (nausea, dyspepsia, or GI distress) in about 22%, diarrhea in about 8%, dizziness in about 15%, asthenia in about 10% and nervousness in about 7%. The adverse reactions seen in at least 2% of bepridil patients in controlled trials are shown in the following table: (TABLE 1)

In one twelve week controlled study, daily doses of 200, 300, and 400 mg were compared to placebo. The following table (TABLE 2) shows the rates of more common reactions (at least 5% in at least one bepridil group).

ADVERSE REACTIONS: *(cont'd)*

TABLE 1 Adverse Experiences by Body System and Treatment in Greater Than 2% of Bepridil Patients in Controlled Trials

Adverse Reaction	Bepridil HCL (N=529)	Nifedipine (N=50)	Propanolol (N=88)	Diltiazem (N=41)	Placebo (N=190)
Body As A Whole					
Asthenia	9.83	22.00	22.73	12.20	7.37
Headache	11.34	22.00	13.64	7.32	14.21
Flu Syndrome	2.08	8.00	2.27	*	1.05
Cardiovascular/Respiratory					
Palpitations	2.27	6.00	2.27	0.00	1.58
Dyspnea	3.59	4.00	5.68	4.88	2.11
Respiratory Infection	2.84	4.00	3.41	4.88	3.68
Gastrointestinal					
Dyspepsia	6.81	4.00	5.68	4.88	1.58
GI distress	4.35	10.00	6.82	*	2.11
Nausea	12.29	14.00	11.36	2.44	3.68
Dry Mouth	3.40	0.00	0.00	2.44	2.63
Anorexia	3.02	0.00	2.27	0.00	1.58
Diarrhea	7.75	2.00	9.09	2.44	2.63
Abdominal Pain	3.02	4.00	1.14	*	3.16
Constipation	6.00	1.14	4.88	2.11	2.84
Central Nervous System					
Drowsy	3.78	4.00	4.55	*	3.68
Insomnia	2.65	6.00	3.41	*	1.05
Dizziness	14.74	30.00	10.23	4.88	9.47
Tremor	4.91	4.00	0.00	*	1.05
Tremor of Hand	3.02	4.00	0.00	*	0.53
Paresthesia	2.46	2.00	1.14	4.88	3.16
Psychiatric					
Nervous	7.37	16.00	1.14	2.44	3.68

* No data available

TABLE 2 Adverse Experiences by Body System and Treatment in Greater Than 5% of Bepridil Patients in Controlled Trials

Adverse Reaction	Bepridil HCl 200 mg (N=43)	Bepridil HCl 300 mg (N=46)	Bepridil HCl 400 mg (N=44)	Placebo (N=44)
Body As A Whole				
Asthenia	13.95	6.52	11.36	2.27
Headache	6.88	8.70	13.64	15.91
Cardiovascular/Respiratory				
Palpitations	0.00	6.52	4.55	0.00
Dyspnea	2.33	8.70	0.00	2.27
Gastrointestinal				
GI Distress	6.98	0.00	4.55	4.55
Nausea	6.98	26.09	18.18	2.27
Anorexia	0.00	2.17	6.82	2.27
Diarrhea	0.00	10.87	6.82	0.00
Central Nervous System				
Drowsy	6.98	6.52	0.00	4.55
Dizziness	11.63	15.22	27.27	6.82
Tremor	6.98	0.00	4.55	0.00
Tremor of Hand	9.30	0.00	4.55	0.00
Psychiatric				
Nervous	11.63	8.70	11.36	0.00
Special Senses				
Tinnitus	0.00	6.52	2.27	2.27

Adverse experiences in long-term open studies were generally similar to those seen in controlled trials.

Although adverse experiences were frequent (at least one being reported in 71% of patients participating in controlled clinical trials), most were well-tolerated. About 15% of patients however, left bepridil treatment because of adverse experiences. In controlled clinical trials, these were principally gastrointestinal (1.0%), dizziness (1.0%), ventricular arrhythmias (1.0%), and syncope (0.6%). The major reasons for discontinuation, with comparison to control agents, are shown below. (TABLE 3)

TABLE 3 Most Common Events Resulting in Discontinuation

Adverse Reaction	Bepridil (N=515) n (%)	Placebo (N=288) n (%)	Positive Control (N=119) n (%)
Dizziness	5 (0.97)	0 (0.0)	2 (1.68)
Gastrointestinal Symptoms	5 (0.97)	0 (0.0)	5 (4.20)
Ventricular Arrhythmia	5 (0.97)	0 (0.0)	0 (0.00)
Syncope	3 (0.58)	0 (0.0)	0 (0.00)

Across all controlled and uncontrolled trials, bepridil HCl was evaluated in over 800 patients with chronic angina. In addition to the adverse reactions noted above, the following were observed in 0.5 to 2.0% of the bepridil HCl or are rarer, but potentially important events seen in clinical studies or reported in post marketing experience. In most cases it is not possible to determine whether there is a causal relationship to bepridil treatment.

Body as a Whole: Fever, pain, myalgic asthenia, superinfection, flu syndrome.

Cardiovascular/Respiratory: Sinus tachycardia, sinus bradycardia, hypertension vasodilation, edema, ventricular premature contractions, ventricular tachycardia, prolonged QT interval, rhinitis, cough, pharyngitis.

Gastrointestinal: Flatulence, gastritis, appetite increase, dry mouth, constipation.

Musculoskeletal: Arthritis.

Central Nervous System: Fainting, vertigo, akathisia, drowsiness, insomnia, tremor.

Psychiatric: Depression, anxiousness, adverse behavior effect.

Skin: Rash, sweating, skin irritation.

Special Senses: Blurred vision, tinnitus, taste change.

Urogenital: Loss of libido, impotence.

ADVERSE REACTIONS: *(cont'd)*

Abnormal Lab Values: Abnormal liver function test, SGPT increase.

Certain cardiovascular events, such as acute myocardial infarction (about 3% of patients), worsened heart failure (1.9%), worsened angina (4.5%), severe arrhythmia (about 2.4% VT/VF) and sudden death (1.6%) have occurred in patients receiving bepridil, but have not been included as adverse events because they appear to be, and cannot be distinguished from, manifestations of the patient's underlying cardiac disease. Such events as torsades de pointes arrhythmias, prolonged QT/QT_c, bradycardia, first degree heart block, which are probably related to bepridil, are included in the tables.

OVERDOSAGE:

In the event of overdosage, we recommend close observation in a cardiac care facility for a minimum of 48 hours and use of appropriate supportive measures in addition to gastric lavage. Beta-adrenergic stimulation or parenteral administration of calcium solutions may increase transmembrane calcium ion influx. Clinically significant hypotensive reactions or high-degree AV block should be treated with vasopressor agents or cardiac pacing, respectively. Ventricular tachycardia should be handled by cardioversion and, if persistent, by overdrive pacing.

There has been one experience with overdosage in which a patient inadvertently took a single dose of 1600 mg of bepridil HCl. The patient was observed for 72 hours in intensive care, but no significant adverse experiences were noted.

DOSAGE AND ADMINISTRATION:

Therapy with bepridil HCl should be individualized according to each patient's response and the physician's clinical judgement. The usual starting dose of bepridil HCl is 200 mg once daily. After 10 days, dosage may be adjusted upward depending upon the patient's response (*e.g.*, ability to perform activities of daily living, QT interval, heart rate, and frequency and severity of angina). This long interval for dosage adjustment is needed because steady-state blood levels are not achieved until 8 days of therapy. In clinical trials, most patients were maintained at a dose of bepridil HCl of 300 mg once daily. The maximum daily dose of bepridil HCl is 400 mg and the established minimum effective dose is 200 mg daily.

The starting dose for elderly patients does not differ from that for young patients. After therapeutic response is demonstrated, however, elderly patients may require more frequent monitoring.

Food does not interfere with the absorption of bepridil HCl (see CLINICAL PHARMACOLOGY, Pharmacokinetics and Metabolism). If nausea is experienced with bepridil HCl, the drug may be given at meals or at bedtime.

Bepridil HCl has not been studied adequately in patients with impaired hepatic or renal function. It is therefore possible that dosage adjustments may be necessary in these patients.

Concomitant Use with Other Agents: The concomitant use of bepridil hyrdochloride and beta-blocking agents in patients without heart failure is safely tolerated. Physicians wishing to switch patients from beta-blocker therapy to bepridil HCl therapy may initiate bepridil HCl before terminating the beta-blocker in the usual gradual fashion (see CLINICAL PHARMACOLOGY and PRECAUTIONS).

Store at 15 - 25°C (59 - 77°F). Protect from light.

HOW SUPPLIED - EQUIVALENTS NOT AVAILABLE:

Tablet, Plain Coated - Oral - 200 mg

3 x 30	$220.61	VASCOR 200, McNeil Lab	00045-0682-33
30's	$70.10	VASCOR 200, McNeil Lab	00045-0682-30
100's	$269.68	VASCOR 200, McNeil Lab	00045-0682-10

Tablet, Plain Coated - Oral - 300 mg

3 x 30	$269.15	VASCOR 300, McNeil Lab	00045-0683-33
30's	$85.52	VASCOR 300, McNeil Lab	00045-0683-30
100's	$328.92	VASCOR 300, McNeil Lab	00045-0683-10

Tablet, Plain Coated - Oral - 400 mg

30's	$96.45	VASCOR 400, McNeil Lab	00045-0684-30

BERACTANT *(003045)*

CATEGORIES: Lung Surfactant; Orphan Drugs; Respiratory & Allergy Medications; Respiratory Distress Syndrome, Neonatal; FDA Class 1C ("Little or No Therapeutic Advantage"); FDA Approved 1991 Jul

BRAND NAMES: **Survanta**

COST OF THERAPY: $2,848.96 (RDS; Suspension; 25 mg/ml; 16/day; 2 days)

DESCRIPTION:

Beractant intratracheal suspension is a sterile, non-pyrogenic pulmonary surfactant intended for intratracheal use only. It is a natural bovine lung extract containing phospholipids, neutral lipids, fatty acids, and surfactant-associated proteins to which colfosceril palmitate (dipalmitoylphosphatidylcholine), palmitic acid, and tripalmitin are added to standardize the composition and to mimic surface-tension lowering properties of natural lung surfactant. The resulting composition provides 25 mg/ml phospholipids (including 11.0-15.5 mg/ml desaturated phosphatidylcholine), 0.5-1.75 mg/ml triglycerides, 1.4-3.5 mg/ml free fatty acids, and less than 1.0 mg/ml protein. It is suspended in 0.9% sodium chloride solution, and heat-sterilized. Beractant contains no preservatives. Its protein content consists of two hydrophobic, low molecular weight, surfactant-associated proteins commonly known as SP-B and SP-C. It does not contain the hydrophilic, large molecular weight surfactant-associated protein known as SP-A.

Each ml of beractant contains 25 mg of phospholipids. It is an off-white to light brown liquid supplied in single-use glass vials containing 8 ml (200 mg phospholipids).

CLINICAL PHARMACOLOGY:

Endogenous pulmonary surfactant lowers surface tension on alveolar surfaces during respiration and stabilizes the alveoli against collapse at resting transpulmonary pressures. Deficiency of pulmonary surfactant causes Respiratory Distress Syndrome (RDS) in premature infants. Beractant replenishes surfactant and restores surface activity to the lungs of these infants.

ACTIVITY

*In vitro:*Beractant reproducibly lowers minimum surface tension to less than 8 dynes/cm as measured by the pulsating bubble surfactometer and Wilhelmy Surface Balance. *In situ:* Beractant restores pulmonary compliance to excised rat lungs artificially made surfactant-deficient. *In vivo,* single beractant doses improve lung pressure-volume measurements, lung compliance, and oxygenation in premature rabbits and sheep.

CLINICAL PHARMACOLOGY: *(cont'd)*

ANIMAL METABOLISM

Beractant is administered directly to the target organ, the lungs, where biophysical effects occur at the alveolar surface. In surfactant-deficient premature rabbits and lambs, alveolar clearance of radio-labelled lipid components of beractant is rapid. Most of the dose becomes lung-associated within hours of administration, and the lipids enter endogenous surfactant pathways of reutilization and recycling. In surfactant-sufficient adult animals, beractant clearance is more rapid than in premature and young animals. There is less reutilization and recycling of surfactant in adult animals.

Limited animal experiments have not found effects of beractant on endogenous surfactant metabolism. Precursor incorporation and subsequent secretion of saturated phosphatidylcholine in premature sheep are not changed by beractant treatments.

No information is available about the metabolic fate of the surfactant-associated proteins in beractant. The metabolic disposition in humans has not been studied.

CLINICAL STUDIES:

Clinical effects of beractant were demonstrated in six single-dose and four multiple-dose randomized, multicenter, controlled clinical trials involving approximately 1700 infants. Three open trials, including a treatment IND, involved more than 4800 infants. Each dose of beractant in all studies was 100 mg phospholipids/kg birth weight and was based on published experience with Surfactant TA, a lyophilized powder dosage form of beractant having the same composition.

PREVENTION STUDIES

Infants of 600-1250 g birth weight and 23 to 29 weeks estimated gestational age were enrolled in two multiple-dose studies. A dose of beractant was given within 15 minutes of birth to prevent the development of RDS. Up to three additional doses in the first 48 hours, as often as every 6 hours, were given if RDS subsequently developed and infants required mechanical ventilation with an $FiO_2 \geq 0.30$. Results of the studies at 28 days of age are shown in TABLE 1.

TABLE 1

Study 1	Beractant	Control	*P*-Value
Number infants studied	119	124	
Incidence of RDS (%)	27.6	63.5	<0.001
Death due to RDS (%)	2.5	19.5	<0.001
Death or BPD due to RDS (%)	48.7	52.8	0.536
Death due to any cause (%)	7.6	22.8	0.001
Air Leaks* (%)	5.9	21.7	0.001
Pulmonary interstitial emphysema (%)	20.8	40.0	0.001
Study 2[†]	**Beractant**	**Control**	***P*-Value**
Number infants studied	91	96	
Incidence of RDS (%)	28.6	48.3	0.007
Death due to RDS (%)	1.1	10.5	0.006
Death or BPD due to RDS (%)	27.5	44.2	0.018
Death due to any cause‡(%)	16.5	13.7	0.633
Air Leaks* (%)	14.5	19.6	0.374
Pulmonary interstitial emphysema (%)	26.5	33.2	0.298

‡ No cause of death in the Beractant group was significantly increased; the higher number of deaths in this group was due to the sum of all causes.

RESCUE STUDIES

Infants of 600-1750 g birth weight with RDS requiring mechanical ventilation and an $FiO_2 \geq 0.40$ were enrolled in two multiple-dose rescue studies. The initial dose of Beractant was given after RDS developed and before 8 hours of age. Infants could receive up to three additional doses in the first 48 hours, as often as every 6 hours, if they required mechanical ventilation and an $FiO_2 \geq 0.30$. Results of the studies at 28 days of age are shown in Table 2.

TABLE 2

Study 3*	Beractant	Control	*P*-Value
Number infants studied	198	193	
Death due to RDS (%)	11.6	18.1	0.071
Death or BPD due to RDS (%)	59.1	66.8	0.102
Death due to any cause (%)	21.7	26.4	0.285
Air Leaks† (%)	11.8	29.5	<0.001
Pulmonary interstitial emphysema (%)	16.3	34.0	<0.001
Study 4	**Beractant**	**Control**	***P*-Value**
Number infants studied	204	203	
Death due to RDS (%)	6.4	22.3	0.001
Death or BPD due to RDS (%)	43.6	63.4	<0.001
Death due to any cause (%)	15.2	28.2	0.001
Air Leaks† (%)	11.2	22.2	0.005
Pulmonary interstitial emphysema (%)	20.8	44.4	<0.001

* Study discontinued when treatment IND initiated.
† Pneumothorax or pneumopericardium.

ACUTE CLINICAL EFFECTS

Marked improvements in oxygenation may occur within minutes of administration of beractant.

All controlled clinical studies with beractant provided information regarding the acute effects of beractant on the arterial-alveolar oxygen ratio (a/APO_2), FiO_2, and mean airway pressure (MAP) during the first 48 to 72 hours of life. Significant improvements in these variables were sustained for 48-72 hours in beractant-treated infants in four single-dose and two multiple-dose rescue studies and in two multiple-dose prevention studies. In the single-dose prevention studies, the FiO_2 improved significantly.

INDICATIONS AND USAGE:

Beractant is indicated for prevention and treatment ("rescue") of Respiratory Distress Syndrome (RDS) (hyaline membrane disease) in premature infants. Beractant significantly reduces the incidence of RDS, mortality due to RDS and air leak complications.

PREVENTION

In premature infants less than 1250 g birth weight or with evidence of surfactant deficiency, give beractant as soon as possible, preferably within 15 minutes of birth.

RESCUE

To treat infants with RDS confirmed by x-ray and requiring mechanical ventilation, give beractant as soon as possible, preferably by 8 hours of age.

CONTRAINDICATIONS:

None known.

WARNINGS:

Beractant is intended for intratracheal use only.

BERACTANT CAN RAPIDLY AFFECT OXYGENATION AND LUNG COMPLIANCE. Therefore, its use should be restricted to a highly supervised clinical setting with immediate availability of clinicians experienced with intubation, ventilator management, and general care of premature infants. Infants receiving beractant should be frequently monitored with arterial or transcutaneous measurement of systemic oxygen and carbon dioxide.

DURING THE DOSING PROCEDURE, TRANSIENT EPISODES OF BRADYCARDIA AND DECREASED OXYGEN SATURATION HAVE BEEN REPORTED. If these occur, stop the dosing procedure and initiate appropriate measures to alleviate the condition. After stabilization, resume the dosing procedure.

PRECAUTIONS:

GENERAL

Rales and moist breath sounds can occur transiently after administration. Endotracheal suctioning or other remedial action is not necessary unless clear-cut signs of airway obstruction are present.

Increased probability of post-treatment nosocomial sepsis in BERACTANT-treated infants was observed in the controlled clinical trials in Table 3. The increased risk for sepsis among beractant-treated infants was not associated with increased mortality among these infants. The causative organisms were similar in treated and control infants. There was no significant difference between groups in the rate of post-treatment infections other than sepsis.

Use of beractant in infants less than 600 g birth weight or greater than 1750 g birth weight has not been evaluated in controlled trials. There is no controlled experience with use of beractant in conjunction with experimental therapies for RDS (*e.g.*, high-frequency ventilation or extracorporeal membrane oxygenation).

No information is available on the effects of doses other than 100 mg phospholipids/kg, more than four doses, dosing more frequently than every 6 hours, or administration after 48 hours of age.

CARCINOGENESIS, MUTAGENESIS, AND IMPAIRMENT OF FERTILITY

Reproduction studies in animals have not been completed. Mutagenicity studies were negative. Carcinogenicity studies have not been performed with beractant.

ADVERSE REACTIONS:

The most commonly reported adverse experiences were associated with the dosing procedure. In the multiple-dose controlled clinical trials, transient bradycardia occurred with 11.9% of doses. Oxygen desaturation occurred with 9.8% of doses.

Other reactions during the dosing procedure occurred with fewer than 1% of doses and included endotracheal tube reflux, pallor, vasoconstriction hypotension, endotracheal tube blockage, hypertension, hypocarbia, hypercarbia, and apnea. No deaths occurred during the dosing procedure, and all reactions resolved with symptomatic treatment.

The occurrence of concurrent illnesses common in premature infants was evaluated in the controlled trials. The rates in all controlled studies are in Table 3.

TABLE 3

	All Controlled Studies		
Concurrent Event	Beractant (%)	Control (%)	*P*-Value*
Patent ductus arteriosus	46.9	47.1	0.814
Intracranial hemorrhage	48.1	45.2	0.241
Severe intracranial hemorrhage	24.1	23.3	0.693
Pulmonary air leaks	10.9	24.7	<0.001
Pulmonary interstitial emphysema	20.2	38.4	<0.001
Necrotizing enterocolitis	6.1	5.3	0.427
Apnea	65.4	59.6	0.283
Severe apnea	46.1	42.5	0.114
Post-treatment sepsis	20.7	16.1	0.019
Post-treatment infection	10.2	9.1	0.345
Pulmonary hemorrhage	7.2	5.3	0.166

* *P*-Value comparing groups in controlled studies

When all controlled studies were pooled, there was no difference in intracranial hemorrhage. However, in one of the single-dose rescue studies and one of the multiple-dose prevention studies, the rate of intracranial hemorrhage was significantly higher in beractant patients than control patients (63.3% v 30.8%, P=0.001; and 48.8% v 34.2%, P=0.047, respectively). The rate in a treatment IND involving approximately 4400 infants was lower than in the controlled trials.

In the controlled clinical trials, there was no effect of beractant on results of common laboratory tests: white blood cell count and serum sodium, potassium, bilirubin, creatinine.

More than 3700 pretreatment and post-treatment serum samples were tested by Western Blot immunoassay for antibodies to surfactant-associated proteins SP-B and SP-C. No IgG or IgM antibodies were detected.

Several other complications are known to occur in premature infants. The following conditions were reported in the controlled clinical studies. The rates of the complications were not different in treated and control infants, and none of the complications were attributed to beractant.

Respiratory: lung consolidation, blood from the endotracheal tube, deterioration after weaning, respiratory decompensation, subglottic stenosis, paralyzed diaphragm, respiratory failure.

Cardiovascular: hypotension, hypertension, tachycardia, ventricular tachycardia, aortic thrombosis, cardiac failure, cardio-respiratory arrest, increased apical pulse, persistent fetal circulation, air embolism, total anomalous pulmonary venous return.

Gastrointestinal: abdominal distention, hemorrhage, intestinal perforations, volvulus, bowel infarct, feeding intolerance, hepatic failure, stress ulcer.

Renal: renal failure, hematuria.

Hematologic: coagulopathy, thrombocytopenia, disseminated intravascular coagulation.

Central Nervous System: seizures.

Endocrine/Metabolic: adrenal hemorrhage, inappropriate ADH secretion, hyperphosphatemia.

Musculoskeletal: inguinal hernia.

Systemic: fever, deterioration.

Follow-Up Evaluations: To date, no long-term complications or sequelae of beractant therapy have been found.

ADVERSE REACTIONS: *(cont'd)*

Single Dose Studies: Six-month adjusted-age follow-up evaluations of 232 infants (115 treated) demonstrated no clinically important differences between treatment groups in pulmonary and neurologic sequelae, incidence or severity of retinopathy of prematurity, rehospitalizations, growth, or allergic manifestations.

Multiple-Dose Studies: Six-month adjusted age follow-up evaluations have not been completed. Preliminary, in 605 (333 treated) of 916 surviving infants, there are trends for decreased cerebral palsy and need for supplemental oxygen in beractant infants. Wheezing at the time of examination tended to be more frequent among beractant infants, although there was no difference in bronchodilator therapy.

Twelve-month follow-up data from the multiple-dose studies have been completed in 328 (171 treated) of 909 surviving infants. To date no significant differences between treatments have been found, although there is a trend toward less wheezing in beractant infants in contrast to the six month results.

OVERDOSAGE:

Overdosage with beractant has not been reported. Based on animal data, overdosage might result in acute airway obstruction. Treatment should be symptomatic and supportive.

Rales and moist breath sounds can transiently occur after beractant is given, and do not indicate overdosage. Endotracheal suctioning or other remedial action is not required unless clear-cut signs of airway obstruction are present.

DOSAGE AND ADMINISTRATION:

FOR INTRATRACHEAL ADMINISTRATION ONLY.

BERACTANT SHOULD BE ADMINISTERED BY OR UNDER THE SUPERVISION OF CLINICIANS EXPERIENCED IN INTUBATION, VENTILATOR MANAGEMENT, AND GENERAL CARE OF PREMATURE INFANTS.

MARKED IMPROVEMENTS IN OXYGENATION MAY OCCUR WITHIN MINUTES OF ADMINISTRATION OF BERACTANT. THEREFORE, FREQUENT AND CAREFUL CLINICAL OBSERVATION AND MONITORING OF SYSTEMIC OXYGENATION ARE ESSENTIAL TO AVOID HYPEROXIA.

REVIEW OF AUDIOVISUAL INSTRUCTIONAL MATERIALS DESCRIBING DOSAGE AND ADMINISTRATION PROCEDURES IS RECOMMENDED BEFORE USING BERACTANT. MATERIALS ARE AVAILABLE UPON REQUEST FROM THE MANUFACTURER.

DOSAGE

Each dose of beractant is 100 mg of phospholipids/kg birth weight (4 ml/kg). The beractant dosing chart (Table 4) shows the total dosage for a range of birth weights.

TABLE 4 Beractant Dosing Chart

Weight (grams)	Total Dose (ml)	Weight (grams)	Total Dose (ml)
600- 650	2.6		
1301-1350	5.4		
651- 700	2.8	1351-1400	5.6
701-750	3.0	1401-1450	5.8
751- 800	3.2	1451-1500	6.0
801- 850	3.4	1501-1550	6.2
851- 900	3.6	1551-1600	6.4
901- 950	3.8	1601-1650	6.6
951-1000	4.0	1651-1700	6.8
1001-1050	4.2	1701-1750	7.0
1051-1100	4.4	1751-1800	7.2
1101-1150	4.6	1801-1850	7.4
1151-1200	4.8	1851-1900	7.6
1201-1250	5.0	1901-1950	7.8
1251-1300	5.2	1951-2000	8.0

Four doses of beractant can be administered in the first 48 hours of life. Doses should be given no more frequently than every 6 hours.

DIRECTIONS FOR USE

Beractant should be inspected visually for discoloration prior to administration. The color of beractant is off-white to light brown. If settling occurs during storage, swirl the vial gently (DO NOT SHAKE) to redisperse. Some foaming at the surface may occur during handling and is inherent in the nature of the product.

Beractant is stored refrigerated (2-8° C). Before administration, beractant should be warmed by standing at room temperature for at least 20 minutes or warmed in the hand for at least 8 minutes. ARTIFICIAL WARMING METHODS SHOULD NOT BE USED. If a prevention dose is to be given, preparation of beractant should begin before the infant's birth.

Unopened, unused vials of beractant that have been warmed to room temperature may be returned to the refrigerator within 8 hours of warming, and stored for future use. Drug should not be warmed and returned to the refrigerator more than once. Each single-use vial of beractant should be entered only once. Used vials with residual drug should be discarded.

BERACTANT DOES NOT REQUIRE RECONSTITUTION OR SONICATION BEFORE USE.

DOSING PROCEDURES

General: Beractant is administered intratracheally by instillation through a 5-French end-hole catheter inserted into the infant's endotracheal tube with the tip of the catheter protruding just beyond the end of the endotracheal tube above the infant's carina. Before inserting the catheter through the endotracheal tube, the length of the catheter should be shortened. Beractant should not be instilled into a main-stem bronchus.

It is important to ensure homogenous distribution of beractant throughout the lungs. In the controlled clinical trials, each dose was divided into four quarter doses. Each quarter-dose was administered with the infant in a different position. The sequence of positions was:

Head and body inclined slightly down, head turned to the right

Head and body inclined slightly down, head turned to the left

Head and body inclined slightly up, head turned to the right

Head and body inclined slightly up, head turned to the left

The dosing procedure is facilitated if one person administers the dose while another person positions and monitors the infant.

FIRST DOSE

Determine the total dose of beractant from TABLE 4 based on the infant's birth weight. Slowly withdraw the entire contents of the vial into a plastic syringe through a large-gauge needle (*e.g.,* at least 20 gauge). DO NOT FILTER BERACTANT AND AVOID SHAKING.

Attach the premeasured 5-French end-hole catheter to the syringe. Fill the catheter with beractant. Discard excess beractant through the catheter so that only the total dose to be given remains in the syringe.

DOSAGE AND ADMINISTRATION: *(cont'd)*

BEFORE ADMINISTERING BERACTANT, assure proper placement and patency of the endotracheal tube. At the discretion of the clinician, the endotracheal tube may be suctioned before administering beractant. The infant should be allowed to stabilize before proceeding with dosing.

In the prevention strategy, weigh, intubate and stabilize the infant. Administer the dose as soon as possible after birth, preferably within 15 minutes. Position the infant appropriately and gently inject the first quarter-dose through the catheter over 2-3 seconds.

After administration of the first quarter-dose, remove the catheter from the endotracheal tube. Manually ventilate with a hand-bag with sufficient oxygen to prevent cyanosis, at a rate of 60 breaths/minute, and sufficient positive pressure to provide adequate air exchange and chest wall excursion.

In the rescue strategy, the first dose should be given as soon as possible after the infant is placed on a ventilator for management of RDS. In the clinical trials, immediately before instilling the first quarter-dose, the infant's ventilator settings were changed to rate 60/minute, inspiratory time 0.5 second, and FiO_2 1.0.

Position the infant appropriately and gently inject the first quarter-dose through the catheter over 2-3 seconds. After administration of the first quarter-dose, remove the catheter from the endotracheal tube. Return the infant to the mechanical ventilator.

In both strategies, ventilate the infant for at least 30 seconds or until stable. Reposition the infant for instillation of the next quarter-dose.

Instill the remaining quarter-doses using the same procedures. After instillation of each quarter-dose, remove the catheter and ventilate for at least 30 seconds or until the infant is stabilized. After instillation of the final quarter-dose, remove the catheter without flushing it. Do not suction the infant for 1 hour after dosing unless signs of significant airway obstruction occur.

AFTER COMPLETION OF THE DOSING PROCEDURE, RESUME USUAL VENTILATOR MANAGEMENT AND CLINICAL CARE.

REPEAT DOSES

The dosage of beractant for repeat doses is also 100 mg phospholipids/kg and is based on the infant's birth weight. The infant should not be reweighed for determination of the beractant dosage. Use TABLE 4 to determine the total dosage.

The need for additional doses of beractant is determined by evidence of continuing respiratory distress. Using the following criteria for redosing, significant reductions in mortality due to RDS were observed in the multiple-dose clinical trials with beractant.

Dose no sooner than 6 hours after the preceding dose if the infant remains intubated and requires at least 30% inspired oxygen to maintain a PaO_2 less than or equal to 80 torr. Radiographic confirmation of RDS should be obtained before administering additional doses to those who received a prevention dose.

Prepare beractant and position the infant for administration of each quarter-dose as previously described. After instillation of each quarter-dose, remove the dosing catheter from the endotracheal tube and ventilate the infant for at least 30 seconds or until stable.

In the clinical studies, ventilator settings used to administer repeat doses were different than those used for the first dose. For repeat doses, the FiO_2 was increased by 0.20 or an amount sufficient to prevent cyanosis. The ventilator delivered a rate of 30/minute with an inspiratory time less than 1.0 second. If the infant's pretreatment rate was 30 or greater, it was left unchanged during beractant instillation.

DURING THE DOSING PROCEDURE, VENTILATOR SETTINGS MAY BE ADJUSTED AT THE DISCRETION OF THE CLINICIAN TO MAINTAIN APPROPRIATE OXYGENATION AND VENTILATION.

AFTER COMPLETION OF THE DOSING PROCEDURE, RESUME USUAL VENTILATOR MANAGEMENT AND CLINICAL CARE.

DOSING PRECAUTIONS

If an infant experiences bradycardia or oxygen desaturation during the dosing procedure, stop the dosing procedure and initiate appropriate measures to alleviate the condition. After the infant has stabilized, resume the dosing procedure.

Rales and moist breath sounds can occur transiently after administration of beractant. Endotracheal suctioning or other remedial action is unnecessary unless clear-cut signs of airway obstruction are present.

HOW SUPPLIED - EQUIVALENTS NOT AVAILABLE:

Suspension - Intratracheal - 25 mg/ml

8 ml $712.24 SURVANTA, Abbott 00074-1040-08

BETA-CAROTENE *(000460)*

CATEGORIES: Dermatologicals; Porphyria; Vitamin A; Vitamins; Pregnancy Category C; FDA Approval Pre 1982

BRAND NAMES: *Betavin*; *B-Tene*; *Biocarotine*; *Carotaben* (Germany); *Natural Betacarotene*; **Solatene**; *Solvin*
(International brand names outside U.S. in italics)

DESCRIPTION:

Beta-carotene is available in capsules for oral administration. Each capsule is composed of beadlets containing 30 mg beta-carotene, ascorbyl palmitate, corn starch, dl-α-tocopherol, gelatin, peanut oil and sucrose. Gelatin capsule shells may contain parabens (methyl and propyl), potassium sorbate, FD&C Blue No. 1, D&C Yellow No. 10, FD&C Red No. 3, FD&C Green No. 3 and titanium dioxide.

Beta-carotene, precursor of vitamin A, is a carotenoid pigment occurring naturally in green and yellow vegetables. Chemically, beta-carotene has the empirical formula $C_{40}H_{56}$ and a calculated molecular weight of 536.85. Trans-beta-carotene is a red, crystalline compound which is insoluble in water.

CLINICAL PHARMACOLOGY:

Beta-carotene, a provitamin A, belongs to the class of carotenoid pigments. In terms of its vitamin activity, 6 mcg of dietary beta-carotene is considered equivalent to 1 mcg of vitamin A (retinol). Bio-availability of beta-carotene depends on the presence of fat in the diet to act as a carrier, and bile in the intestinal tract for its absorption. Beta-carotene is metabolized, primarily in the intestine, to vitamin A at a rate of approximately 50% to 60% of normal dietary intake and falls off rapidly as intake goes up. In humans, an appreciable amount of unchanged beta-carotene is absorbed and stored in various tissues, especially the depot fat. Small amounts may be converted to vitamin A in the liver. The vitamin A derived from beta-carotene follows the same metabolic pathway as that from dietary sources. The major route of elimination is fecal excretion. Excessive ingestion of carotenes is not harmful, but it may cause yellow coloration of the skin, which disappears upon reduction or cessation of intake.

INDICATIONS AND USAGE:

Beta-carotene is used to reduce the severity of photosensitivity reactions in patients with erythropoietic protoporphyria (EPP).

CONTRAINDICATIONS:

Beta-carotene is contraindicated in patients with known hypersensitivity to the drug.

WARNINGS:

Beta-carotene has not been shown to be effective as a sunscreen.

PRECAUTIONS:

General Beta-carotene should be used with caution in patients with impaired renal or hepatic function because safe use in the presence of these conditions has not been established.

Information for the Patient Patients receiving beta-carotene should be advised against taking supplementary vitamin A since beta-carotene administration will fulfill normal vitamin A requirements. They should be cautioned to continue sun protection, and forewarned that their skin may appear slightly yellow while receiving beta-carotene.

Carcinogenesis, Mutagenesis, and Impairment of Fertility Long-term studies in animals to determine carcinogenesis have not been completed. *In vitro* and *in vivo* studies to evaluate mutagenic potential were negative. No effects on fertility in male rats were observed at doses as high as 500 mg/kg/day (100 times the recommended human dose).

Pregnancy, Teratogenic Effects, Pregnancy Category C Beta-carotene has been shown to be fetotoxic (*i.e.,* cause an increase in resorption rate), but not teratogenic when given to rats at doses 300 to 400 times the maximum recommended human dose. No such fetotoxicity was observed at 75 times the maximum recommended human dose or less. A three-generation reproduction study in rats receiving beta-carotene at a dietary concentration of 0.1% (1000 ppm) has revealed no evidence of impaired fertility or effect on the fetus. There are no adequate and well-controlled studies in pregnant women. Beta-carotene should be used during pregnancy only if the potential benefit justifies the potential risk to the fetus.

Nursing Mothers It is not known whether this drug is excreted in human milk. Because many drugs are excreted in human milk, caution should be exercised when beta-carotene is administered to a nursing mother.

ADVERSE REACTIONS:

Some patients may have occasional loose stools while taking beta-carotene. This reaction is sporadic and may not require discontinuance of medication. Other reactions which have been reported rarely are ecchymoses and arthralgia.

OVERDOSAGE:

There are no reported cases of overdosage. The oral LD_{50} of beta-carotene (suspended in 5% gum acacia solution) in mice and rats is greater than 20,000 mg/kg. No lethality was observed in mice following administration of 30-mg beadlet capsules (ground and suspended in 5% gum acacia) at a dose of 1200 mg/kg beta-carotene.

DOSAGE AND ADMINISTRATION:

Beta-carotene may be administered either as a single daily dose or in divided doses, preferably with meals.

Usage in Children: The usual dosage for children under 14 is 30 to 150 mg (1 to 5 capsules) per day. Capsules may be opened and the contents mixed in orange or tomato juice to aid administration.

Usage in Adults: The usual adult dosage is 30 to 300 mg (1 to 10 capsules) per day.

Dosage should be adjusted depending on the severity of the symptoms and the response of the patient. Several weeks of therapy are necessary to accumulate enough beta-carotene in the skin to exert its effect. Patients should be instructed not to increase exposure to sunlight until they appear carotenemic (first seen as yellowness of palms and soles). This usually occurs after two to six weeks of therapy. Exposure to the sun may then be increased gradually. The protective effect is not total and each patient should establish his or her own limits of exposure.

HOW SUPPLIED - EQUIVALENTS NOT AVAILABLE:

Capsule, Gelatin - Oral - 30 mg

100's	$59.94	SOLATENE, Roche	00004-0115-01

BETAMETHASONE *(000462)*

CATEGORIES: Adrenal Corticosteroids; Adrenal Hyperplasia; Adrenocortical Insufficiency; Anemia; Ankylosing Spondylitis; Anti-Inflammatory Agents; Antiarthritics; Arthritis; Aspiration Pneumonitis; Asthma; Atopic Dermatitis; Bursitis; Cancer; Carditis; Chemotherapy; Chorioretinitis; Colitis; Conjunctivitis; Dermatitis; Dermatitis Herpetiformis; Dermatologicals; Diuresis; Drug Hypersensitivity; Enteritis; Epicondylitis; Erythema Multiforme; Erythroblastopenia; Gouty Arthritis; Herpes; Herpes Zoster; Hormones; Hypercalcemia; Inflammation; Iridocyclitis; Leukemia; Lupus Erythematosus; Meningitis; Mycosis Fungoides; Nephrotic Syndrome; Oncologic Drugs; Osteoarthritis; Pain; Pemphigus; Pneumonitis; Proteinuria; Psoriasis; Rhinitis; Serum Sickness; Skin/Mucous Membrane Agents; Spondylitis; Synovitis; Tenosynovitis; Thyroiditis; Ulcerative Colitis; Uveitis; FDA Approval Pre 1982

BRAND NAMES: *Benoson*; *Benoson (500 mcg)*; Betaderm; *Betason*; *Betason (500 mcg)*; *Betnelan* (England); *Betnelan (500 mcg)*; *Betnesol*; *Celestamine* (Germany); *Celestan*; *Celestene* (France); *Celeston*; **Celestone**; *Celestone (500 mcg)*; *Rinderon*; *Unicort*; *Walacort*
(International brand names outside U.S. in italics)

FORMULARIES: Aetna; BC-BS; WHO

COST OF THERAPY: $526.07 (Asthma; Tablet; 0.6 mg; 1/day; 365 days)

PRIMARY ICD9: 493.90 (Asthma, Unspecified, Without Mention of Status Asthmaticus)

DESCRIPTION:

Glucocorticoids are adrenocortical steroids, both naturally occurring and synthetic, that are readily absorbed from the gastrointestinal tract. A derivative of prednisolone, Betamethasone has a 16β-methyl group that enhances the anti-inflammatory action of the molecule and reduces the sodium- and water-retaining properties of the fluorine atom bound at carbon 9.

The formula for Betamethasone is $C_{22}H_{29}FO_5$ and has a molecular weight of 329.47. Chemically, it is 9-fluoro-11β,17,21-trihydroxy-16β-methylpregna-1,4-diene-3,20-dione.

DESCRIPTION: *(cont'd)*

Betamethasone is a white to practically white, odorless, crystalline powder. It melts at about 240°C with some decomposition. Betamethasone is sparingly soluble in acetone, alcohol, dioxane, and methanol; very slightly soluble in chloroform and ether; and is insoluble in water.

Each betamethasone tablet contains 0.6 mg betamethasone, NF, betamethasone syrup contains 0.6 mg betamethasone, NF in each 5 ml and less than 1% alcohol.

CLINICAL PHARMACOLOGY:

Naturally occurring glucocorticoids (hydrocortisone or cortisone), which also have salt-retaining properties, are used as replacement therapy in adrenocortical deficiency states. Their synthetic analogs are primarily used for their potent anti-inflammatory effects in disorders of many organ systems. Glucocorticoids, such as betamethasone cause profound and varied metabolic effects. In addition, they modify the body's immune responses to diverse stimuli.

INDICATIONS AND USAGE:

Endocrine Disorders: Primary or secondary adrenocortical insufficiency (hydrocortisone or cortisone is the drug of choice; synthetic analogs may be used in conjunction with mineralocorticoids where applicable; in infancy, mineralocorticoid supplementation is of particular importance).

Congenital adrenal hyperplasia.

Nonsuppurative thyroiditis.

Hypercalcemia associated with cancer.

Rheumatic Disorders: As adjunctive therapy for short-term administration (to tide the patient over an acute episode or exacerbation) in:

Psoriatic arthritis.

Rheumatoid arthritis, including juvenile rheumatoid arthritis (selected cases may require low-dose maintenance therapy).

Ankylosing spondylitis.

Acute and subacute bursitis.

Acute and nonspecific tenosynovitis.

Acute gouty arthritis.

Post-Traumatic osteoarthritis.

Synovitis or osteoarthritis.

Epicondylitis.

Collagen diseases: During an exacerbation or as a maintenance therapy in selected cases of:

Systemic lupus erythematosus.

Acute rheumatic carditis.

Dermatological Diseases

Pemphigus.

Bullous dermatitis herpetiformis.

Severe erythema multiforme (Stevens-Johnson syndrome).

Exfoliative dermatitis.

Mycosis fungoides.

Severe seborrheic dermatitis.

Severe psoriasis.

Systemic lupus erythematosus.

Acute rheumatic carditis.

Allergic States: Control of severe or incapacitating allergic conditions intractable to adequate trials of conventional treatment in:

Bronchial asthma.

Contact dermatitis.

Atopic dermatitis.

Serum sickness.

Seasonal or perennial allergic rhinitis.

Drug hypersensitivity.

Ophthalmic Diseases: Severe, acute and chronic allergic and inflammatory processes involving the eye and its adnexa, such as:

Allergic conjunctivitis.

Herpes zoster ophthalmicus.

Iritis, iridocyclitis.

Chorioretinitis.

Anterior segment inflammation.

Diffuse posterior uveitis and chorditis.

Optic neuritis.

Sympathetic ophthalmia.

Respiratory Diseases

Symptomatic sarcoidosis.

Loftier's syndrome not manageable by any other means.

Berylliosis.

Fulminating or disseminated pulmonary tuberculosis when used concurrently with appropriate antituberculous chemotherapy.

Aspiration pneumonitis.

Hematologic Disorders

Idiopathic thrombocytopenia purpura in adults (IV and IM administration is contraindicated).

Secondary thrombocytopenia in adults.

Acquired (autoimmune) hemolytic amenia.

Erythroblastopenia (RBC anemia).

Congenital (erythroid) hypoplastic anemia.

Neoplastic Diseases: For palliative management of:

Leukemias and lymphomas in adults.

Acute leukemia of childhood.

Edematous States: To induce diuresis or remission of proteinuria in the nephrotic syndrome, without uremia, of the idiopathic type or that due to lupus erythematosus.

Gastrointestinal Diseases: To tide the patient over a critical period of the disease in:

Ulcerative colitis.

INDICATIONS AND USAGE: *(cont'd)*

Regional enteritis.

Miscellaneous

Tuberculous meningitis with subarachnoid block or impending block when used concurrently with appropriate antituberculosis chemotherapy.

Trichinosis with neurologic or myocardial involvement.

CONTRAINDICATIONS:

Betamethasone syrup and tablets contraindicated in systemic fungal infections.

WARNINGS:

In patients on corticosteroid therapy subjected to any unusual stress, increased dosage of rapidly acting corticosteroids before, during, and after the stressful situation is indicated.

Corticosteroids may mask some signs of infection, and new infections may appear during their use.

There may be decreased resistance and inability to localize infection when corticosteroids are used.

Prolonged use of corticosteroids may produce posterior subcapsular cataracts, glaucoma with possible damage to the optic nerves, and may enhance the establishment of secondary ocular infections due to fungi or viruses.

Average and large doses of cortisone or hydrocortisone can cause elevation of blood pressure, salt and water retention, and increased excretion of potassium. These effects are less likely to occur with the synthetic derivatives except when used in large doses. Dietary salt restriction and potassium supplementation may be necessary. All corticosteroids increase calcium excretion.

While on corticosteroid therapy patients should not be vaccinated against smallpox. Other immunization procedures should not be undertaken in patients who are on corticosteroids. Especially in high doses, because of the possible hazards of neurological complications and lack of antibody response.

Children who are on immunosuppressant drugs are more susceptible to infections than healthy children. Chickenpox and measles, for example, can have a more serious or even fatal course in children on immunosuppressant corticosteroids. In such children, or in adults who have not had these diseases, particular care should be taken to avoid exposure. If exposed, therapy with varicella zoster immune globulin (VZIG) or pooled intravenous immunoglobulin (IVIG), as appropriate, may be indicated. If chickenpox develops, treatment with antiviral agents may be considered.

The use of betamethasone syrup and tablets in active tuberculosis should be restricted to those cases of fulminating or disseminated tuberculosis in which the corticosteroid is used for the management of the disease in conjunction with appropriate antituberculosis regimen.

If corticosteroids are indicated in patients with latent tuberculosis or tuberculin reactivity, close observation is necessary as reactivation of the disease may occur. During prolonged corticosteroid therapy, these patients should receive chemoprophylaxis.

Because rare instances of anaphylactoid reactions have occurred in patients receiving parenteral corticosteroid therapy, appropriate precautionary measures should be taken prior to administration, especially when the patient has a history of allergy to any drug.

Usage In Pregnancy: Since adequate human reproduction studies have not been done with corticosteroids, the use of these drugs in pregnancy, nursing mothers, or women of childbearing potential requires that the possible benefits of the drug be weighed against the potential hazards to the mother and embryo or fetus. Infants born to mothers who have received substantial doses of corticosteroids during pregnancy should be carefully observed for signs of hypoadrenalism.

PRECAUTIONS:

Information for the Patient: Patients who are on immunosuppressant doses of corticosteroids should be warned to avoid exposure to chickenpox or measles and, if exposed, to obtain medical advice.

General: Drug-induced secondary adrenocortical insufficiency may be minimized by gradual reduction of dosage. This type of relative insufficiency may persist for months after discontinuation of therapy; therefore, in any situation of stress occurring during that period, hormone therapy should be reinstituted. Since mineralocorticoid secretion may be impaired, salt and/or a mineralocorticoid should be administered concurrently.

There is an enhanced effect of corticosteroids in patients with hypothyroidism and in those with cirrhosis.

Corticosteroids should be used cautiously in patients with ocular herpes simplex for fear of corneal perforation.

The lowest possible dose of corticosteroid should be used to control the condition under treatment, and when reduction in dosage is possible, the reduction in dosage is possible, the reduction must be gradual.

Psychic derangements may appear when corticosteroids are used, ranging from euphoria, insomnia, mood swings, personality changes, and severe depression to frank psychotic manifestations. Also, existing emotional instability or psychotic tendencies may be aggravated by corticosteroids.

Aspirin should be used cautiously in conjunction with corticosteroids in hypothrombinemia.

Steroids should be used with caution in nonspecific ulcerative colitis, if there is a probability of impending perforation, abscess or other pyrogenic infection, also in diverticulitis, fresh Intestinal anastomoses, active or latent peptic ulcer, renal insufficiency, hypertension, osteoporosis, and myasthenia gravis. Growth and development or infants and children on prolonged corticosteroid therapy should be carefully followed.

ADVERSE REACTIONS:

Fluid And Electrolyte Disturbances: Sodium retention; fluid retention; congestive heart failure in susceptible patients; potassium loss; hypokalemic alkalosis; hypertension.

Musculoskeletal: Muscle weakness; steroid myopathy; loss of muscle mass; osteoporosis, vertebral compression fractures; aseptic necrosis of femoral and humeral heads; pathologic fracture of long bones.

Gastrointestinal: Peptic ulcer with possible subsequent perforation and hemorrhage; pancreatitis; abdominal distention; ulcerative esophagitis.

Dermatologic: Impaired wound healing; thin fragile skin; petechiae and ecchymoses; facial erythema; increased sweating; may suppress reactions to skin tests.

Neurological: Convulsions; increased intracranial pressure with papilledema (pseudotumor cerebri) usually after treatment; vertigo; headache.

Endocrine: Menstrual irregularities; development of Cushingoid state; suppression of growth in children; secondary adrenocortical and pituitary unresponsiveness, particularly in times of stress, as in trauma, surgery or illness; decreased carbohydrate tolerance; manifestations of latent diabetes mellitus; increased requirements for insulin or oral hypoglycemic agents in diabetics.

ADVERSE REACTIONS: *(cont'd)*

Ophthalmic: Posterior subcapsular cataracts; increased intraocular pressure; glaucoma; exophthalmos.

Metabolic: Negative nitrogen balance due to protein catabolism.

DOSAGE AND ADMINISTRATION:

The initial dosage of betamethasone may vary from 0.6 mg to 7.2 mg per day depending on the specific disease entity being treated. In situations of less severity lower doses will generally suffice, while in selected patients higher initial doses may be required. The initial dosage should be maintained or adjusted until a satisfactory response is noted. If after a reasonable period of time, there is a lack of satisfactory clinical response, betamethasone should be discontinued and the patient transferred to other therapy. **IT SHOULD BE EMPHASIZED THAT DOSAGE REQUIREMENTS ARE VARIABLE AND MUST BE INDIVIDUALIZED ON THE BASIS OF THE DISEASE UNDER TREATMENT AND RESPONSE OF THE PATIENT.** After a favorable response is noted, the proper maintenance dosage should be determined by decreasing the initial drug dosage in small decrements at appropriate time intervals until the lowest dosage which will maintain an adequate clinical response is reached. It should be kept in mind that constant monitoring is needed in regard to drug dosage. Included in the situations which may make dosage adjustments necessary are changes in clinical status secondary to remissions to exacerbations in the disease process, the patient's individual drug responsiveness, and the effect of patient exposure to stressful situations not directly related to the disease entity under treatment; in this latter situation it may necessary to increase dosage of Bbetamethasone for a period of time consistent with the patient's condition. If after long-term therapy the drug is to be stopped, it is recommended that it be withdrawn gradually rather than abruptly.

Protect **Syrup** from light.

Store tablets between 2 and 30°C (36 and 86°F). Additionally, Protect 21 tablet pack from excessive moisture.

HOW SUPPLIED - EQUIVALENTS NOT AVAILABLE:

Syrup - Oral - 0.6 mg/5ml

120 ml	$36.01	CELESTONE, Schering	00085-0942-05

Tablet, Uncoated - Oral - 0.6 mg

21's	$32.00	CELESTONE, Schering	00085-0011-01
100's	$144.13	CELESTONE, Schering	00085-0011-05

BETAMETHASONE ACETATE; BETAMETHASONE SODIUM PHOSPHATE

(000463)

CATEGORIES: Adrenal Corticosteroids; Adrenal Hyperplasia; Adrenal Insufficiency; Adrenocortical Insufficiency; Airway Obstruction; Allergies; Alopecia; Alopecia Areata; Anemia; Ankylosing Spondylitis; Anti-Inflammatory Agents; Antineoplastics; Arthritis; Asthma; Bursitis; Cancer; Carditis; Chemotherapy; Colitis; Conjunctivitis; Corneal Ulcer; Dermatitis; Diuresis; Drug Hypersensitivity; Edema; Erythema Multiforme; Erythroblastopenia; Glucocorticoids; Granuloma; Granuloma Annulare; Herpes; Herpes Zoster; Hormones; Hypercalcemia; Inflammatory Lesions; Keloids; Keratitis; Laryngeal Edema; Lesions; Leukemia; Lichen Planus; Lichen Simplex Chronicus; Lupus Erythematosus; Lymphoma; Meningitis; Mycosis Fungoides; Necrobiosis Lipoidica; Nephrotic Syndrome; Osteoarthritis; Pneumoconiosis; Proteinuria; Psoriasis; Retinochoroiditis; Rhinitis; Sarcoidosis; Shock; Spondylitis; Steroids; Synovitis; Tenosynovitis; Thrombocytopenia; Thyroiditis; Tumors; Urticaria; Uveitis; FDA Approval Pre 1982

BRAND NAMES: *Celestan Biphase*; *Celestan Depot* (Germany); *Celestene Chronodose* (France); *Celeston*; *Celeston Chronodose*; *Celestone Chronodose* (Australia); *Celestone Cronodose*; *Celestone-Soluspan*; **Celestone Soluspan**
(International brand names outside U.S. in italics)

DESCRIPTION:

Each ml of Celestone Soluspan Suspension contains: 3.0 mg betamethasone as betamethasone sodium phosphate; 3.0 mg betamethasone acetate; 7.1 mg dibasic sodium phosphate; 3.4 mg monobasic sodium phosphate; 0.1 mg edetate disodium; and 0.2 mg benzalkonium chloride. It is a sterile, aqueous suspension with a PH between 6.8 and 7.2.

The formula for betamethasone sodium phosphate is $C_{22}H_{28}FNa_2O_8P$ with a molecular weight of 516.41. Chemically it is 9-Fluoro-11β,17,21-trihydroxy-16β-methylpregna-1,4-diene-3,20-dione 21-acetate.

The formula for betamethasone acetate is $C_{24}H_{31}FO_6$ with a molecular weight of 434.50. chemically it is 9-Fluoro-11β,17,21-trihydroxy-16β-methylpregna-1,4-diene-3,20-dione 21-acetate.

Betamethasone sodium phosphate is a white to practically white, odorless powder, and is hygroscopic. It is freely soluble in water and in methanol, but is practically insoluble in acetone and in chloroform.

Betamethasone acetate is a white to creamy white, odorless powder that sinters and resolidifies at about 165°C, and remelts at about 200°C-220°C with decomposition. It is practically insoluble in water, but freely soluble in acetone, and is soluble in alcohol and in chloroform.

CLINICAL PHARMACOLOGY:

Naturally occurring glucocorticoids (hydrocortisone), which also have salt-retaining properties, are used as replacement therapy in adrenocortical deficiency states. Their synthetic analogs are primarily used for their potent anti-inflammatory effects in disorders of many organ systems.

Betamethasone sodium phosphate, a soluble ester, provides prompt activity, while betamethasone acetate is only slightly soluble and affords sustained activity.

Glucocorticoids cause profound and varied metabolic effects. In addition, they modify the body's immune responses to diverse stimuli.

INDICATIONS AND USAGE:

When oral therapy is not feasible and the strength, dosage form, and route of administration of the drug reasonably lend the preparation to the treatment of the condition, this combination drug for intramuscular use is indicated as follows:

Endocrine Disorders: Primary or secondary adrenocortical insufficiency (hydrocortisone or cortisone is the drug of choice; synthetic analogs may be used in conjunction with mineralocorticoids where applicable; in infancy mineralocorticoid supplementation is of particular importance).

INDICATIONS AND USAGE: *(cont'd)*

Acute adrenocortical insufficiency (hydrocortisone or cortisone is the drug of choice; mineral-ocorticoid supplementation may be necessary, particularly when synthetic analogs are used). Preoperatively and in the event of serious trauma or illness, in patients with known adrenal insufficiency or when adrenocortical reserve is doubtful. Shock unresponsive ot conventional therapy if adrenocortical insufficiency exists or is suspected. Congenital adrenal hyperplasia. Nonsuppurative thyroiditis. Hypercalcemia associated with cancer.

Rheumatic Disorders: As adjunctive therapy for short-term administration (to tide the patient over an acute episode or exacerbation) in: post-traumatic osteoarthritis, synovitis of osteoarthritis; rheumatoid arthritis, including juvenile rheumatoid arthritis (selected cases may require low-dose maintenance therapy); acute and subacute bursitis; epicondylitis; acute nonspecific tenosynovitis; acute gouty arthritis; psoriatic arthritis; ankylosing spondylitis.

Collagen Diseases: During an exacerbation or as maintenance therapy in selected cases of: systemic lupus erythematosus; acute rheumatic carditis.

Dermatologic dDiseases: Pemphigus; severe erythema multiforme (Stevens-Johnson syndrome); exfoliative dermatitis; bullous dermatitis herpetiformis; severe seborrheic dermatitis; severe psoriasis; mycosis fungoides.

Allergic States: Control of severe or incapacitating allergic conditions intractable to adequate trials of conventional treatment in: bronchial asthma; contact dermatitis; atopic dermatitis; serum sickness; seasonal or perennial allergic rhinitis; drug hypersensitivity reactions; urticarial transfusion reactions; acute noninfectious laryngeal edema (epinephrine is the drug of first choice).

Ophthalmic Diseases: Severe, acute and chronic allergic and inflammatory processes involving the eye, such as: herpes zoster ophthalmicus; iritis, iridocyclitis; chorioretinitis; diffuse posterior uveitis and choroiditis; optic neuritis; sympathetic ophthalmia; anterior segment inflammation; allergic conjunctivitis; allergic corneal marginal ulcers; keratitis.

Gastrointestinal Diseases: To tide the patient over a critical period of disease in: ulcerative colitis-(systemic therapy); regional enteritis-(systemic therapy).

Respiratory Diseases: Symptomatic sarcoidosis; berylliosis; fulminating or disseminated pulmonary tuberculosis when used concurrently with appropriate antituberculous chemotherapy; Loeffler's syndrome not manageable by other means; aspiration pneumonitis.

Hematologic Disorders: Acquired (autoimmune) hemolytic anemia. Secondary thrombocytopenia in adults. Erythroblastopenia (RBC anemia). Congenital (erythroid) hypoplastic anemia.

Neoplastic Diseases: For palliative management of: leukemias and lymphomas in adults; acute leukemia of childhood.

Edematous States: To induce diuresis or remission of proteinuria in the nephrotic syndrome, without uremia, of the idiopathic type or that due to lupus erythematosus.

Miscellaneous: Tuberculosis meningitis with subarachnoid block or impending block when used concurrently with appropriate antituberculous chemotherapy. Trichinosis with neurologic or myocardial involvement.

When the strength and dosage form of the drug lend the preparation to the treatment of the condition, the **intra-articular or soft tissue administration** of this combination drug is indicated as adjunctive therapy for short-term administration (to tide the patient over an acute episode or exacerbation) in: synovitis of osteoarthritis; rheumatoid arthritis; acute and subacute bursitis; acute gouty arthritis; epicondylitis; acute nonspecific tenosynovitis; post-traumatic osteoarthritis.

When the strength and dosage form of the drug lend the preparation to the treatment of the condition, the **intralesional administration** of this combination drug is indicated for: keloids, localized hypertrophic, infiltrated, inflammatory lesions of lichen planus, psoriatic plaques, granuloma annulare, and lichen simplex chronicus (neurodermatitis); discoid lupus erythematosus; necrobiosis lipoidica diabeticorum; alopecia areata.

This combination drug may also be useful in cystic tumors of an aponeurosis or tendon (ganglia).

CONTRAINDICATIONS:

This combination drug is contraindicated in systemic fungal infections.

WARNINGS:

This combination drug should not be administered intravenously.

In patients on corticosteroid therapy subjected to any unusual stress, increased dosage of rapidly acting corticosteroids before, during, and after the stressful situation is indicated.

Corticosteroids may mask some signs of infection, and new infections may appear during their use. There may be decreased resistance and inability to localize infection when corticosteroids are used.

Prolonged use of corticosteroids may produce posterior subcapsular cataracts, glaucoma with possible damage to the optic nerves, and may enhance the establishment of secondary ocular infections due to fungi or viruses.

This combination drug contains two betamethasone esters one of which, betamethasone sodium phosphate, disappears rapidly from the injection site. The potential for systemic effect produced by the soluble portion of this combination drug should therefore be taken into account by the physician when using the drug.

Average and large doses of cortisone or hydrocortisone can cause elevation of blood pressure, salt and water retention, and increased excretion of potassium. These effects are less likely to occur with the synthetic derivatives except when used in large doses. Dietary salt restriction and potassium supplementation may be necessary. All corticosteroids increase calcium excretion.

While on Corticosteroid Therapy Patients Should Not Be Vaccinated Against Smallpox. Other Immunization Procedures Should Not Be Undertaken in Patients Who Are on Corticosteroids, Especially in High Doses, Because of Possible Hazards of Neurological Complications and Lack of Antibody Response.

Children who are on immunosuppressant drugs are more susceptible to infections than healthy children. Chickenpox and measles, for example, can have a more serious or even fatal course in children on immunosuppressant corticosteroids. In such children, or in adults who have not had these diseases, particular care should be taken to avoid exposure. If exposed, therapy with varicella zoster immune globulin (VZIG) or pooled intravenous immunoglobulin (IVIG), as appropriate, may be indicated. If chickenpox develops, treatment with antiviral agents may be considered.

The use of this combination drug in active tuberculosis should be restricted ot those cases of fulminating or disseminate tuberculosis in which the corticosteroid is used for the management of the disease in conjunction with appropriate antituberculous regimen.

If corticosteroids are indicated in patients with latent tuberculosis or tuberculin reactivity, close observation is necessary as reactivation of the disease may occur. During prolonged corticosteroid therapy, these patients should receive chemoprophylaxis.

Because rare instances of anaphylactoid reactions have occurred in patients receiving parenteral corticosteroid therapy, appropriate precautionary measures should be taken prior to administration, especially when the patient has a history of allergy to any drug.

WARNINGS: *(cont'd)*

Usage in Pregnancy: Since adequate human reproduction studies have not been done with corticosteroids, the use of these drugs in pregnancy, nursing mothers, or women of childbearing potential requires that the possible benefits of the drug be weighed against the potential hazards to the mother and embryo or fetus. Infants born of mothers who have received substantial doses of corticosteroids during pregnancy should be carefully observed for signs of hypoadrenalism.

PRECAUTIONS:

GENERAL

Drug-induced secondary adrenocortical insufficiency may be minimized by gradual reduction of dosage. This type of relative insufficiency may persist for months after discontinuation of therapy; therefore, in any situation of stress occurring during that period, hormone therapy should be reinstituted. Since mineralocorticoid secretion may be impaired, salt and/or a mineralocorticoid should be administered concurrently.

There is an enhanced effect of corticosteroids in patients with hypothyroidism and in those with cirrhosis.

Corticosteroids should be used cautiously in patients with ocular herpes simplex for fear of corneal perforation.

The lowest possible dose of corticosteroid should be used to control the condition under treatment, and when reduction in dosage is possible, the reduction must be gradual.

Psychic derangements may appear when corticosteroids are used, ranging from euphoria, insomnia, mood swings, personality changes, and severe depression to frank psychotic manifestations. Also, existing emotional instability or psychotic tendencies may be aggravated by corticosteroids.

Aspirin should be used cautiously in conjunction with corticosteroids in hypoprothrombinemia.

Steroids should be used with caution in nonspecific ulcerative colitis, if there is a probability of impending perforation, abscess or other pyogenic infection, also in diverticulitis, fresh intestinal anastomoses, active or latent peptic ulcer, renal insufficiency, hypertension, osteoporosis, and myasthenia gravis.

Growth and development of infants and children on prolonged corticosteroid therapy should be carefully followed.

The following additional precautions also apply for parenteral corticosteroids. **Intra-articular injection of a corticosteroid may produce systemic as well as local effects.**

Appropriate examination of any joint fluid present is necessary to exclude a septic process.

A marked increase in pain accompanied by local swelling, further restriction of joint motion, fever, and malaise are suggestive of septic arthritis. If this complication occurs and the diagnosis of sepsis is confirmed, appropriate antimicrobial therapy should be instituted.

Local injection of a steroid into a previously infected joint is to be avoided.

Corticosteroids should not be injected into unstable joints.

The slower rate of absorption by intramuscular administration should be recognized.

Information for the Patient: who are on immunosuppressant doses of corticosteroids should be warned to avoid exposure to chickenpox or measles and, if exposed, to obtain medical advice.

ADVERSE REACTIONS:

Fluid and Electrolyte Disturbances: sodium retention; fluid retention; congestive heart failure in susceptible patients; potassium loss; hypokalemic alkalosis; hypertension.

Musculoskeletal: muscle weakness; steroid myopathy; loss of muscle mass; osteoporosis; vertebral compression fractures; aseptic necrosis of femoral and humeral heads; pathologic fracture of long bones.

Gastrointestinal: Peptic ulcer with possible subsequent perforation and hemorrhage; pancreatitis; abdominal distention; ulcerative esophagitis.

Dermatologic: impaired wound healing; thin fragile skin; petechiae and ecchymoses; facial erythema; increased sweating may suppress reactions to skin tests.

Neurological: convulsions, increased intracranial pressure with papilledema (pseudotumor cerebri) usually after treatment; vertigo; headache.

Endocrine: menstrual irregularities; development of cushingoid state; suppression of growth in children; secondary adrenocortical and pituitary unresponsiveness, particularly in times of stress, as in trauma, surgery, or illness; decreased carbohydrate tolerance; manifestations of latent diabetes mellitus; increased requirements for insulin or oral hypoglycemic agents in diabetics.

Ophthalmic: posterior subcapsular cataracts; increased intraocular pressure; glaucoma; exophthalmos.

Metabolic: negative nitrogen balance due to protein catabolism.

The following *additional* adverse reactions are related to parenteral corticosteroid therapy: rare instances of blindness associated with intralesional therapy around the face and head; hyperpigmentation or hypopigmentation; subcutaneous and cutaneous atrophy; sterile abscess; post-injection flare (following intra-articular use); charcotlike arthropathy.

DOSAGE AND ADMINISTRATION:

The initial dosage of this combination drug may vary from 0.5 to 9.0 mg per day depending on the specific disease entity being treated. In situations of less severity, lower doses will generally suffice while in selected patients higher initial doses may be required. Usually the parenteral dosage ranges are one-third to one-half the oral dose given every 12 hours. However, in certain overwhelming, acute, life-threatening situations, administration in dosages exceeding the usual dosages may be justified and may be in multiples of the oral dosages.

The initial dosage should be maintained or adjusted until a satisfactory response is noted. If after a reasonable period of time there is a lack of satisfactory clinical response, this combination drug should be discontinued and the patient transferred to other appropriate therapy. *It Should be Emphasized That Dosage Requirements Are Variable and Must Be Individualized on the Basis of the Disease Under Treatment and the Response of the Patient.* After a favorable response is noted, the proper maintenance dosage should be determined by decreasing the initial drug dosage in small decrements at appropriate time intervals until the lowest dosage which will maintain an adequate clinical response is reached. It should be kept in mind that constant monitoring is needed in regard to drug dosage. Included in the situations which may make dosage adjustments necessary are changes in clinical status secondary to remissions or exacerbations in the disease process, the patient's individual drug responsiveness, and the effect of patient exposure to stressful situations not directly related to the disease entity under treatment; in this latter situation it may be necessary to increase the dosage of this combination drug for a period of time consistent with the patient's condition. If after long-term therapy the drug is to be stopped, it is recommended that it be withdrawn gradually rather than abruptly.

DOSAGE AND ADMINISTRATION: *(cont'd)*

If coadministration of a local anesthetic is desired, this combination drug may be mixed with 1% or 2% lidocaine hydrochloride, using the formulations which do not contain parabens. Similar local anesthetics may also be used. Diluents containing methylparaben, propylparaben, phenol, etc. Should be avoided since these compounds may cause flocculation of the steroid. The required dose of this combination drug is first withdrawn from the vial into the syringe. The local anesthetic is then drawn in, and the syringe shaken briefly. **Do not inject local anesthetics into the vial of this combination drug.**

Bursitis, Tenosynovitis, Peritendinitis: In acute subdeltoid, subacromial, olecranon, and prepatellar bursitis, one intrabursal injection of 1.0 ml this combination drug can relieve pain and restore full range of movement. Several intrabursal injections of corticosteroids are usually required in recurrent acute bursitis and in acute exacerbations of chronic bursitis. Partial relief of pain and some increase in mobility can be expected in both conditions after one or two injections. chronic bursitis may be treated with reduced dosage once the acute condition is controlled. In tenosynovitis and tendinitis, three or four local injections at intervals of one to two weeks between injections are given in most cases. Injections should be made into the affected tendon sheaths rather than into the tendons themselves. In ganglions of joint capsules and tendon sheaths, injection of 0.5 ml directly into the ganglion cysts has produced marked reduction in the size of the lesions.

Rheumatoid Arthritis and Osteoarthritis: Following intra-articular administration of 0.5 to 2.0 ml of this combination drug, relief of pain, soreness, and stiffness may be experienced. Duration of relief varies widely in both diseases. Intra-articular Injection of this combination drug is well tolerated in joints and periarticular tissues. There is virtually no pain on injection, and the "secondary flare" that sometimes occurs a few hours after intra-articular injection of corticosteroids has not been reported with this combination drug. Using sterile technique, a 20- to 24-gauge needle on an empty syringe is inserted into the synovial cavity, and a few drops of synovial fluid are withdrawn to confirm that the needle is in the joint. The aspirating syringe is replaced by a syringe containing this combination drug and injection is then made into the joint. (TABLE 1)

TABLE 1 Recommended Doses for Intra-articular Injection

Size of joint	Location	Dose (ml)
Very large	Hip	1.0-2.0
Large	Knee, Ankle, Shoulder	1.0
Medium	Elbow, Wrist	0.5-1.0
Small		
(Metacarpophalangeal, interphalangeal)	Hand	
(Sternoclavicular)	Chest	0.25-0.5

A portion of the administered dose of this combination drug is absorbed systemically following intra-articular injection. In patients being treated concomitantly with oral or parenteral corticosteroids, especially those receiving large doses, the systemic absorption of the drug should be considered in determining intra-articular dosage.

Dermatologic Conditions: In intralesional treatment, 0.2 ml/sq cm of this combination drug is injected intradermally (not subcutaneously) using a tuberculin syringe with a 25-gauge, 1/2-inch needle. Care should be taken to deposit a uniform depot of medication intradermally. A total of no more than 1.0 ml at weekly intervals is recommended.

Disorders of the Foot: A tuberculin syringe with a 25-gauge, 3/4-inch needle is suitable for most injections into the foot. The following doses are recommended at intervals of three days to a week (TABLE 2).

TABLE 2

Diagnosis	Suspension Dose (ml)
Bursitis	
Under heloma durum or heloma molle	0.25-0.5
Under calcaneal spur	0.5
Over hallux rigidus or digiti varus	0.5
Tenosynovitis, periosteitis of cuboid	0.5
Acute gouty arthritis	0.5-1.0

HOW SUPPLIED:

Celestone Soluspan Suspention, 5 ml multiple-dose vial.

Store between 2 and 25°C (36 and 77°F). Protect from light.

HOW SUPPLIED - EQUIVALENTS NOT AVAILABLE:

Injection, Susp - Intra-Articular - 3 mg/ml

5 ml $20.22 CELESTONE SOLUSPAN, Schering 00085-0566-05

BETAMETHASONE DIPROPIONATE *(000465)*

CATEGORIES: Adrenal Corticosteroids; Anti-Inflammatory Agents; Dermatologicals; Glucocorticoids; Pruritus; Skin/Mucous Membrane Agents; Steroids; Pregnancy Category C; Sales > $100 Million; FDA Approval Pre 1982

BRAND NAMES: Alphatrex; *Beprosone*; Betanate; *Cleniderm*; *Dicortin*; *Diprocel*; *Diproderm*; *Diprolen*; Diprolene; Diprolene Af; **Diprosone**; *Diprosone-OV*; *Diprotop*; Maxivate; *Oviskin*; Psorion; *Skizon*; *Tasone*; *Topiderm*; *Valbet*
(International brand names outside U.S. in italics)

FORMULARIES: BC-BS; FHP; PCS

DESCRIPTION:

For Dermatologic Use Only - Not for Ophthalmic Use.

These products contain betamethasone dipropionate, USP, a synthetic adrenocorticosteroid, for dermatologic use. Betamethasone, an analog of prednisolone, has a high degree of corticosteroid activity and a slight degree of mineralocorticoid activity. Betamethasone dipropionate is the 17,21-dipropionate ester of betamethasone.

Chemically, betamethasone dipropionate is 9-fluoro-11β,17,21-trihydroxy-16β-methylpregna-1,4-diene-3,20-dione 17,21-dipropionate, with the empirical formula $C_{28}H_{37}FO_7$, a molecular weight of 504.6.

Betamethasone dipropionate is a white to creamy white, odorless crystalline powder, insoluble in water.

LOTIONS

Each gram of betamethasone diproprionate lotion 0.05% contains: 0.64 mg betamethasone dipropionate, USP (equivalent to 0.5 mg betamethasone), in a lotion base of isopropyl alcohol (46.8%) and purified water slightly thickened with carbomer 934P; the pH is adjusted to approximately 4.7 with sodium hydroxide.

DESCRIPTION: *(cont'd)*

Each gram of Diprolene (augmented betamethasone diproprionate) lotion 0.05% contains: 0.64 mg betamethasone dipropionate, USP (equivalent to 0.5 mg betamethasone), in a lotion base of purified water, isopropyl alcohol (30%), hydroxypropylcellulose, propylene glycol, sodium phosphate, phosphoric acid, and sodium hydroxide used to adjust the pH to 4.5.

CREAM

Each gram of Diprolene AF (augmented betamethasone dipropionate) cream (0.5%) contains: 0.64 mg of betamethasone dipropionate, USP (equivalent to 0.5 mg betamethasone), in an emollient cream base consisting of purified water, chlorocresol, propylene glycol, white petrolatum, white wax, cyclomethicone, sorbitol solution, glyceryl monooleate, ceteareth- 30, carbomer 940 and sodium hydroxide.

OINTMENT

Each gram of Diprolene (augmented betamethasone dipropionate) ointment 0.05% contains: 0.64 mg betamethasone dipropionate, USP (equivalent to 0.5 mg betamethasone), in ACTIBASE, an optimized vehicle of propylene glycol, propylene glycol, propylene glycol stearate, white wax and white petrolatum.

TOPICAL AEROSOL

Betamethasone dipropionate topical aerosol 0.1% contains: 6.4 mg betamethasone dipropionate, USP, equivalent to 5.0 mg betamethasone, in a vehicle of mineral oil and caprylic/capric triglyceride; also containing 10% isopropyl alcohol and sufficient inert hydrocarbon (propane and isobutane) propellant to make 85 grams. The aerosol spray deposits betamethasone dipropionate equivalent to approximately 0.1% betamethasone, in a non-volatile, almost invisible film. A three-second spray delivers betamethasone dipropionate equivalent to approximately 0.06 mg betamethasone.

CLINICAL PHARMACOLOGY:

The corticosteroids are a class of compounds comprising steroid hormones secreted by the adrenal cortex and their synthetic analogs. In pharmacologic doses, corticosteroids are used primarily for their anti-inflammatory, and/or immunosuppressive effects.

Topical corticosteroids, such as betamethasone dipropionate, are effective in the treatment of corticosteroid-responsive dermatoses primarily because of their anti-inflammatory, antipruritic, and vasoconstrictive actions. However, while the physiologic, pharmacologic, and clinical effects of the corticosteroids are well-known, the exact mechanisms of the their actions in each disease are uncertain. Betamethasone dipropionate, a corticosteroid, has been shown to have topical (dermatologic) and systemic pharmacologic and metabolic effects characteristic of this class of drugs.

PHARMACOKINETICS

The extent of percutaneous absorption of topical corticosteroids is determined by many factors including the vehicle, the integrity of the epidermal barrier, and the use of occlusive dressings. (See DOSAGE AND ADMINISTRATION.)

Topical corticosteroids can be absorbed through normal intact skin. Inflammation and/or other disease processes in the skin may increase percutaneous absorption. Occlusive dressings substantially increase the percutaneous absorption of topical corticosteroids. (See DOSAGE AND ADMINISTRATION.)

Once absorbed through the skin, topical corticosteroids enter pharmacokinetic pathways similar to systemically administered corticosteroids. Corticosteroids are bound to plasma proteins in varying degrees. Corticosteroids are metabolized primarily in the liver and excreted by the kidneys. Some of the topical corticosteroids and their metabolites are also excreted into the bile.

AUGMENTED CREAM 0.05%

Augmented betamethasone dipropionate AF cream was applied once daily at 7 grams per day for one week to diseased skin, in patients with psoriasis or atopic dermatitis, to study its effects on the hypothalamic-pituitary-adrenal (HPA) axis. The results suggested that the drug caused a slight lowering of adrenal corticosteroid secretion, although in no case did plasma cortisol levels go below the lower limit of the normal range.

AUGMENTED OINTMENT 0.05%

At 14 g per day, augmented betamethasone dipropionate ointment was shown to depress the plasma levels of adrenal cortical hormones following repeated application to diseased skin in patients with psoriasis. Adrenal depression in these patients was transient, and rapidly returned to normal upon cessation of treatment. At 7 g per day (3.5 g bid). Betamethasone dipropionate ointment was shown to cause minimal inhibition of the hypothalamic-pituitary-adrenal (HPA) axis when applied two times daily for 2 to 3 weeks, in normal patients and in patients with no psoriasis and eczematous disorders.

With 6 or 7 g of betamethasone dipropionate ointment applied once daily for 3 weeks, no significant inhibition of the HPA axis was observed in patients with psoriasis and atopic dermatitis, as measured by plasma cortisol and 24-hour urinary 17-hydroxy-corticosteroid levels.

AUGMENTED LOTION 0.05%

Augmented betamethasone dipropionate lotion was applied once daily at 7 ml per day for 21 days to diseased skin (in patients with scalp psoriasis), to study its effects on the hypothalamic-pituitary-adrenal (HPA) axis. In 2 out of 11 patients, the drug lowered plasma cortisol levels below normal limits. Adrenal depression in these patients was transient, and returned to normal within a week. In one of these patients, plasma cortisol levels returned to normal while treatment continued.

INDICATIONS AND USAGE:

Betamethasone diproprionate products are indicated for relief of the inflammatory and pruritic manifestations of moderate to severe corticosteroid-responsive dermatoses.

ADDITIONAL INFORMATION FOR AUGMENTED LOTION 0.05%

Treatment beyond two weeks is not recommended, and the total dosage should not exceed 50 ml per week because of the potential for the drug to suppress the hypothalamic-pituitary-adrenal axis.

CONTRAINDICATIONS:

Betamethasone diproprionate products is contraindicated in patients who are hypersensitive to betamethasone dipropionate, to other corticosteroids, or to any ingredient in these preparations.

PRECAUTIONS:

GENERAL

Augmented betamethasone dipropionate lotion is a highly potent topical corticosteroid that has been shown to suppress HPA axis at 7 ml per day.

Systemic absorption of topical corticosteroids has produced reversible HPA axis suppression, manifestations of Cushing's syndrome, hyperglycemia, and glucosuria in some patients.

Conditions which augment systemic absorption include the application of the more potent corticosteroids such as betamethasone diproprionate, use over large surface areas, prolonged use, and the addition of occlusive dressings. (See DOSAGE AND ADMINISTRATION.)

PRECAUTIONS: *(cont'd)*

Therefore, patients receiving large doses of potent topical steroid applied to a large surface area should be evaluated periodically for evidence of HPA axis suppression by using the urinary free cortisol and ACTH stimulation tests. If HPA axis suppression is noted, an attempt should be made to withdraw the drug, to reduce the frequency of application, or to substitute with a less potent steroid.

Recovery of HPA axis function is generally prompt and complete upon discontinuation of the drug. Infrequently, signs and symptoms of steroid withdrawal many occur, requiring supplemental systemic corticosteroids.

Children may absorb proportionally large amounts of topical corticosteroids and thus be more susceptible to systemic toxicity. (See PRECAUTIONS, Pediatric Use.)

If irritation develops, topical corticosteroids should be discontinued and appropriate therapy instituted.

In the presence of dermatological infections, the use of an appropriate antifungal or antibacterial agent should be instituted. If a favorable response does not occur promptly, the corticosteroid should be discontinued until the infection has been adequately controlled.

INFORMATION FOR THE PATIENT

Patients using topical corticosteroids should receive the following information and instructions. This information is intended to aid in the safe and effective use of this medication. It is not a disclosure of all possible adverse or intended effects.

1. This medication is to be used as directed by the physician and should not be used longer than the prescribed time period. It is for external use only. Avoid contact with the eyes.

2. Patients should be advised not to use this medication for any disorder other than that for which it was prescribed.

3. The treated skin areas should be not bandaged or otherwise covered or wrapped so as to be occlusive. (See DOSAGE AND ADMINISTRATION.)

4. Patients should report any sign of local adverse reactions.

5. Parents of pediatric patients should be advised not to use tight- fitting diapers or plastic pants on a child being treated in the diaper area, as these garments may constitute occlusive dressing. (See DOSAGE AND ADMINISTRATION.)

LABORATORY TESTS

The following tests may be helpful in evaluating HPA axis suppression:

Urinary free cortisol test

ACTH stimulation test

CARCINOGENESIS, MUTAGENESIS, AND IMPAIRMENT OF FERTILITY

Long-term animal studies have not been performed to evaluate the carcinogenic potential or the effect on fertility of topically applied corticosteroids.

Studies to determine mutagenicity with prednisolone and hydrocortisone have revealed negative results.

PREGNANCY CATEGORY C

Corticosteroids are generally teratogenic in laboratory animal when administered systemically at relatively low dosage levels. The more potent corticosteroids have been shown to be teratogenic after dermal application in laboratory animals. Betamethasone dipropionate has not been tested for teratogenicity by this route; however, it appears to be fairly well-absorbed percutaneously. There are no adequate and well-controlled studies of the teratogenic effects of topically applied corticosteroids in pregnant women. Therefore, topical corticosteroids should be used during pregnancy only if the potential benefit justifies the potential risk to the fetus. Drugs of this class should not be used extensively on pregnant patients, in large amounts, or for prolonged periods of time.

NURSING MOTHERS

It is not known whether topical administration of corticosteroids can result in sufficient systemic absorption to produce detectable quantities in breast milk. Systemically administered corticosteroids are secreted into breast milk in quantities not likely to have deleterious effect on the infant. Nevertheless, a decision should be made whether to discontinue nursing or to discontinue the drug, taking into account the importance of the drug to the mother.

PEDIATRIC USE

The safety and efficacy of betamethasone diproprionate products when used in children 12 years of age have not been established.

Pediatric patients may demonstrate greater susceptibility to topical corticosteroid-induced HPA axis suppression and Cushing's syndrome than mature patients because of a larger skin surface area to body weight ratio.

Hypothalamic-pituitary-adrenal (HPA) axis suppression, Cushing's syndrome, and intracranial hypertension have been reported in children receiving topical corticosteroids. Manifestations of adrenal suppression in children include linear growth retardation, delayed weight gain, low plasma cortisol levels, and absence of response to ACTH stimulation. Manifestations of intracranial hypertension include bulging fontanelles, headaches, and bilateral papilledema.

Administration of topical corticosteroids to children should be limited to the least amount compatible with an effective therapeutic regimen. Chronic corticosteroid therapy may interfere with the growth and development of children.

ADDITIONAL INFORMATION FOR THE TOPICAL AEROSOL

The spray should be kept away from the eyes or other mucous membranes.

Avoid freezing tissues by not spraying for more than three seconds, at a distance of not less than six inches between the nozzle and skin.

Use only as directed; intentional misuse by deliberately concentrating and inhaling the container contents can be harmful or fatal.

The container contents are under pressure; do not puncture the container.

The container mixture is flammable; do not use or store the container near heat or an open flame; exposure to temperature above 120°F may cause bursting; never throw container into a fire or incinerator.

Keep out of reach of children

ADVERSE REACTIONS:

The following local adverse reactions are also reported infrequently when betamethasone dipropionate products are used as recommended in the DOSAGE AND ADMINISTRATION. These reactions are listed in approximate decreasing order of occurrence: burning; itching; irritation; dryness; folliculitis; hypertrichosis; acneiform eruptions; hypopigmentation; perioral dermatitis; allergic contact dermatitis; maceration of the skin; secondary infection; skin atrophy; striae; miliaria.

Systemic absorption of topical corticosteroids has produced reversible hypothalamic-pituitary-adrenal (HPA) axis suppression, manifestations of Cushing's syndrome, hyperglycemia, and glucosuria in some patients.

AUGMENTED CREAM 0.05%

The only local adverse reaction reported to be possibly or probably related to treatment with betamethasone dipropionate cream during controlled clinical studies was stinging. It occurred in 0.4% of the 242 patients or subjects involved in the studies.

ADVERSE REACTIONS: *(cont'd)*

AUGMENTED OINTMENT 0.05%

The local adverse reactions that were reported with betamethasone dipropionate ointment applied either once or twice a day during clinical studies are as follows: erythema, 3 per 767 patients, folliculitis, 2 per 767 patients; pruritus, 2 per 767 patients; vesiculation, 1 per 767 patients.

AUGMENTED LOTION 0.05%

The overall incidence of drug-related adverse reactions in the betamethasone dipropionate lotion clinical studies was 5%. The adverse reactions that were reported to be possibly or probably related to treatment with betamethasone dipropionate lotion during controlled clinical studies involving 327 patients or normal volunteers, were as follows: folliculitis occurred in 2%, burning and acneiform papules each occurred in 1%, and hyperesthesia and irritation each occurred in less than 1% of patients.

OVERDOSAGE:

Topically applied corticosteroids can be absorbed in sufficient amounts to produce systemic effects. (See PRECAUTIONS.)

DOSAGE AND ADMINISTRATION:

CREAM

Apply a thin film of betamethasone dipropionate cream 0.05% to the affected areas once daily. In some cases, a twice daily dosage may be necessary.

AUGMENTED CREAM

Apply a thin film of betamethasone dipropionate cream to the affected skin areas once or twice daily. *Treatment with betamethasone dipropionate cream should be limited to 45 g per week.*

Betamethasone dipropionate cream is not to be used with occlusive dressings.

LOTION

Apply a few drops to the affected areas and massage lightly until it disappears. Apply twice daily, in the morning and at night. For the most effective and economical use, apply nozzle very close to affected area and squeeze bottle gently.

AUGMENTED LOTION

Apply a few drops of betamethasone dipropionate lotion to the affected area once or twice daily and massage lightly until the lotion disappears. Treatment must be limited to 14 days, and amounts greater than 50 ml per week should not be used.

Betamethasone dipropionate lotion is not to be used with occlusive dressings.

OINTMENT

Apply a thin film of betamethasone dipropionate ointment to the affected areas once daily. In some cases, a twice daily dosage may be necessary.

AUGMENTED OINTMENT

Apply a thin film of betamethasone dipropionate ointment to the affected skin areas once or twice daily. Treatment with betamethasone dipropionate ointment should be limited to 45 g per week.

Betamethasone dipropionate ointment is not to be used with occlusive dressings.

TOPICAL AEROSOL

Apply sparingly to the affected skin area three times a day. The container may be held upright or inverted during use. The spray should be directed onto the affected area from a distance of not more than six inches and applied for only three seconds. For the most effective and economical use, a three-second spray is sufficient to cover an area about the size of the hand.

Betamethasone dipropionate products are not to be used with occlusive dressings.

STORAGE

Store all products between 2 and 30°C (36 and 86°F).

HOW SUPPLIED - RATED THERAPEUTICALLY EQUIVALENT:

Cream - Topical - 0.05 %

15 gm	$3.37	Betamethasone Dipropionate, United Res	00677-1569-40
15 gm	$3.37	Betamethasone Dipropionate, H.C.F.A. F F P	99999-0465-01
15 gm	$4.30	Betamethasone Dipropionate, Thames Pharma	49158-0213-20
15 gm	$4.75	Betamethasone Dipropionate, Clay Park Labs	45802-0019-35
15 gm	$5.12	Betamethasone Dipropionate, HL Moore Drug Exch	00839-7049-47
15 gm	$5.31	Betamethasone Dipropionate, Qualitest Pharms	00603-7728-74
15 gm	$5.57	Betamethasone Dipropionate, NMC Labs	23317-0380-15
15 gm	$5.65	Dapronate Betamethasone Dipropionate, Major Pharms	00904-0766-36
15 gm	$5.70	Diprosone, Rugby	00536-5030-20
15 gm	$6.10	Betamethasone Dipropionate, Schein Pharm (US)	00364-7409-72
15 gm	$6.25	Betamethasone Dipropionate, Geneva Pharms	00781-7009-27
15 gm	$6.75	Betamethasone Dipropionate, Fougera	00168-0055-15
15 gm	$6.75	Betamethasone Dipropionate, Taro Pharms (US)	51672-1274-01
15 gm	$6.90	Betamethasone Dipropionate, Goldline Labs	00182-5010-51
15 gm	$15.88	ALPHATREX, Savage Labs	00281-0055-15
15 gm	**$21.26**	**DIPROSONE, Schering**	**00085-0853-02**
45 gm	$6.82	Betamethasone Dipropionate, H.C.F.A. F F P	99999-0465-02
45 gm	$8.60	Betamethasone Dipropionate, Thames Pharma	49158-0213-27
45 gm	$9.07	Betamethasone Dipropionate, Clay Park Labs	45802-0019-42
45 gm	$9.17	Betamethasone Dipropionate, HL Moore Drug Exch	00839-7049-52
45 gm	$10.08	Betamethasone Dipropionate, Qualitest Pharms	00603-7728-83
45 gm	$10.12	Betamethasone Dipropionate, United Res	00677-1569-49
45 gm	$10.43	Betamethasone Dipropionate, NMC Labs	23317-0380-45
45 gm	$10.57	Dapronate Betamethasone Dipropionate, Major Pharms	00904-0766-45
45 gm	$10.71	Betamethasone Dipropionate, Rugby	00536-5030-26
45 gm	$11.50	Betamethasone Dipropionate, Schein Pharm (US)	00364-7409-80
45 gm	$11.50	Betamethasone Dipropionate, Geneva Pharms	00781-7009-19
45 gm	$12.30	Betamethasone Dipropionate, Taro Pharms (US)	51672-1274-06
45 gm	$12.40	Betamethasone Dipropionate, Aligen Independ	00405-0550-64
45 gm	$12.55	Betamethasone Dipropionate, Goldline Labs	00182-5010-60
45 gm	$12.89	Betamethasone Dipropionate, Fougera	00168-0055-46
45 gm	$28.93	ALPHATREX, Savage Labs	00281-0055-46
45 gm	$29.89	MAXIVATE, Westwood Squibb	00072-9410-45
45 gm	**$39.00**	**DIPROSONE, Schering**	**00085-0853-03**

Lotion - Topical - 0.05 %

20 ml	$3.19	Betamethasone Dipropionate, H.C.F.A. F F P	99999-0465-03
20 ml	$4.30	Betamethasone Dipropionate, Thames Pharma	49158-0245-40
20 ml	$4.32	Betamethasone Dipropionate, Clay Park Labs	45802-0021-97
20 ml	$5.00	Betamethasone Dipropionate, Harber Pharm	51432-0701-10
20 ml	$5.64	Betamethasone Dipropionate, NMC Labs	23317-0382-20
20 ml	$6.45	Betamethasone Dipropionate, Teva	00093-0302-60
20 ml	**$26.16**	**DIPROSONE, Schering**	**00085-0028-04**
60 ml	$9.50	Betamethasone Dipropionate, Thames Pharma	49158-0245-32
60 ml	$9.57	Betamethasone Dipropionate, H.C.F.A. F F P	99999-0465-04

HOW SUPPLIED - RATED THERAPEUTICALLY EQUIVALENT:

(cont'd)

60 ml	$9.58	Betamethasone Dipropionate, United Res	00677-1570-31
60 ml	$10.00	Betamethasone Dipropionate, Copley Pharm	38245-0611-12
60 ml	$10.52	Betamethasone Dipropionate, HL Moore Drug Exch	00839-7202-53
60 ml	$10.80	Betamethasone Dipropionate, Clay Park Labs	45802-0021-46
60 ml	$11.55	Dapronate Betamethasone Diprodionate, Major Pharms	00904-0768-03
60 ml	$11.56	Betamethasone Dipropionate, Rugby	00536-5038-61
60 ml	$11.75	Betamethasone Dipropionate, NMC Labs	23317-0382-60
60 ml	$11.88	Betamethasone Dipropionate, Geneva Pharms	00781-7041-61
60 ml	$12.50	Betamethasone Dipropionate, Harber Pharm	51432-0701-17
60 ml	$13.80	Betamethasone Dipropionate, Schein Pharm (US)	00364-2102-58
60 ml	$14.25	Betamethasone Dipropionate, Goldline Labs	00182-1787-68
60 ml	$14.35	Betamethasone Dipropionate, Teva	00093-0302-39
60 ml	$15.14	Betamethasone Dipropionate, Fougera	00168-0057-60
60 ml	$36.77	ALPHATREX, Savage Labs	00281-0057-60
60 ml	$41.11	MAXIVATE, Westwood Squibb	00072-9490-60
60 ml	**$51.50**	**DIPROSONE, Schering**	**00085-0028-06**

Ointment - Topical - 0.05 %

15 gm	$4.75	Betamethasone Dipropionate, Clay Park Labs	45802-0020-35
15 gm	$5.57	Betamethasone Dipropionate, NMC Labs	23317-0381-15
15 gm	$5.62	Betamethasone Dipropionate, H.C.F.A. F F P	99999-0465-05
15 gm	$5.65	Dapronate Betamethasone Dipropionate, Major Pharms	00904-0767-36
15 gm	$5.70	Betamethasone Dipropionate, Rugby	00536-5034-20
15 gm	$5.74	Betamethasone Dipropionate, HL Moore Drug Exch	00839-7110-47
15 gm	$6.60	Betamethasone Dipropionate, Harber Pharm	51432-0707-10
15 gm	$6.70	Betamethasone Dipropionate, Teva	00093-0303-15
15 gm	$7.74	Betamethasone Dipropionate, Fougera	00168-0056-15
15 gm	$13.37	MAXIVATE, Westwood Squibb	00072-9450-15
15 gm	$15.88	ALPHATREX, Savage Labs	00281-0056-15
15 gm	**$21.26**	**DIPROSONE, Schering**	**00085-0510-04**
15 gm	$21.47	Betamethasone Dipropionate, Warrick Pharms	59930-1575-01
45 gm	$9.07	Betamethasone Dipropionate, Clay Park Labs	45802-0020-42
45 gm	$9.44	Betamethasone Dipropionate, HL Moore Drug Exch	00839-7110-52
45 gm	$9.68	Betamethasone Dipropionate, H.C.F.A. F F P	99999-0465-06
45 gm	$10.43	Betamethasone Dipropionate, NMC Labs	23317-0381-45
45 gm	$10.45	Dapronate Betamethasone Dipropionate, Major Pharms	00904-0767-45
45 gm	$12.00	Betamethasone Dipropionate, Harber Pharm	51432-0707-16
45 gm	$12.30	Betamethasone Dipropionate, Teva	00093-0303-95
45 gm	$12.55	Betamethasone Dipropionate, Goldline Labs	00182-5011-60
45 gm	$15.06	Betamethasone Dipropionate, Fougera	00168-0056-46
45 gm	$28.93	ALPHATREX, Savage Labs	00281-0056-46
45 gm	$29.89	MAXIVATE, Westwood Squibb	00072-9450-45
45 gm	**$39.00**	**DIPROSONE, Schering**	**00085-0510-06**
45 gm	$43.20	Betamethasone Dipropionate, Warrick Pharms	59930-1575-02
45 mg	$11.25	Betamethasone Dipropionate, Rugby	00536-5034-26

Ointment, Augmented - Topical - 0.05 %

15 gm	$24.40	DIPROLENE, Schering	00085-0575-02
45 gm	$49.10	DIPROLENE, Schering	00085-0575-03

HOW SUPPLIED - NOT RATED EQUIVALENT:

Aerosol, Spray - Topical - 0.1 %

85 gm	**$21.26**	**DIPROSONE, Schering**	**00085-0475-06**

Cream, Augmented - Topical - 0.05 %

15 gm	$24.40	DIPROLENE AF, Schering	00085-0517-01
45 gm	$49.10	DIPROLENE AF, Schering	00085-0517-02

Gel - Topical - 0.05 %

15 gm	$24.40	DIPROLENE, Schering	00085-0634-01
45 gm	$49.10	DIPROLENE, Schering	00085-0634-02

Lotion, Augmented - Topical - 0.05 %

30 ml	$27.98	DIPROLENE, Schering	00085-0962-01
60 ml	$55.15	DIPROLENE, Schering	00085-0962-02

BETAMETHASONE DIPROPIONATE; CLOTRIMAZOLE *(000466)*

CATEGORIES: Anti-Infectives; Anti-Inflammatory Agents; Antibacterials; Antibiotics; Antifungals; Dermatologicals; Fungal Agents; Glucocorticoids; Hormones; Infections; Pruritus; Skin Infections; Skin/Mucous Membrane Agents; Steroids; Tinea Corporis; Tinea Cruris; Tinea Pedis; Topical; Pregnancy Category C; Sales > $100 Million; FDA Approved 1984 Jul; Top 200 Drugs

BRAND NAMES: *Clotrasone*; *Lotricomb* (Germany); *Lotriderm* (England, Canada); **Lotrisone**; *Sinium*
(International brand names outside U.S. in italics)

FORMULARIES: Aetna; BC-BS

DESCRIPTION:

For Dermatologic Use Only-Not for Ophthalmic Use

Lotrisone Cream contains a combination of clotrimazole, USP, a synthetic antifungal agent, and betamethasone dipropionate, USP, a synthetic corticosteroid, for dermatologic use.

Chemically, clotrimazole is 1-(*o*-Chloro-α,α-diphenyl benzyl) imidazole, with the empirical formula $C_{22}H_{17}ClN_2$, a molecular weight of 344.8.

Clotrimazole is an odorless, white crystalline powder, insoluble in water and soluble in ethanol.

Betamethasone dipropionate has the chemical name 9-Fluoro-11β, 17,21-trihydroxy-16β-methylpregna-1,4-diene-3,20-dione 17,21-dipropionate, with the empirical formula $C_{28}H_{37}FO_7$, a molecular weight of 504.6.

Betamethasone dipropionate is a white to creamy white, odorless crystalline powder, insoluble in water.

Each gram of lotrisone cream contains 10.0 mg clotrimazole, USP and 0.64 mg betamethasone dipropionate, USP (equivalent to 0.5 mg betamethasone), in a hydrophilic emollient cream consisting of purified water, mineral oil, white petrolatum, cetearyl alcohol, ceteareth-30, propylene glycol, sodium phosphate monobasic, and phosphoric acid; benzyl alcohol as preservative.

Lotrisone is a smooth, uniform, white to off-white cream.

CLINICAL PHARMACOLOGY:

CLOTRIMAZOLE

Is a broad-spectrum, antifungal agent that is used for the treatment of dermal infections caused by various species of pathogenic dermatophytes, yeasts, and *Malassezia furfur.* The primary action of clotrimazole is against dividing and growing organisms.

In vitro, clotrimazole exhibits fungistatic and fungicidal activity against isolates of *Trichophyton rubrum, Trichophyton mentagrophytes, Epidermophyton floccosum* and *Microsporum canis.* In general, the *in vitro* activity of clotrimazole corresponds to that of tolnaftate and griseofulvin against the mycelia of dermatophytes *(Trichophyton, Microsporum,* and *Epidermophyton).*

In vivo studies in guinea pigs infected with *Trichophyton mentagrophytes* have shown no measurable loss of clotrimazole activity due to combination with betamethasone dipropionate.

Strains of fungi having a natural resistance to clotrimazole have not been reported.

No single-step or multiple-step resistance to clotrimazole has developed during successive passages of *Trichophyton mentagrophytes.*

In studies of the mechanism of action in fungal cultures, the minimum fungicidal concentration of clotrimazole caused leakage of intracellular phosphorous compounds into the ambient medium with concomitant breakdown of cellular nucleic acids, and accelerated potassium efflux. Both of these events began rapidly and extensively after addition of the drug to the cultures.

Clotrimazole appears to be minimally absorbed following topical application to the skin. Six hours after the application of radioactive clotrimazole 1% cream and 1% solution onto intact and acutely inflamed skin, the concentration of clotrimazole varied from 100 mcg/cm^3 in the stratum corneum, to 0.5 to 1 mcg/cm^3 in the stratum reticulate, and 0.1 mcg/cm^3 in the subcutis. No measurable amount of radioactivity (<0.001 mcg/ml) was found in the serum within 48 hours after application under occlusive dressing of 0.5 ml of the solution or 0.8 g of the cream.

BETAMETHASONE DIPROPIONATE

Betamethasone dipropionate, a corticosteroid, is effective in the treatment of corticosteroid-responsive dermatoses primarily because of its anti-inflammatory, anti-pruritic,and vasoconstrictive actions. However, while the physiologic, pharmacologic, and clinical effects of corticosteroids are well-known, the exact mechanisms of their actions in each disease are uncertain. Betamethasone dipropionate, a corticosteroid, has been shown to have topical (dermatologic) and systemic pharmacologic and metabolic effects characteristic of this class of drugs.

Pharmacokinetics: The extent of percutaneous absorption of topical corticosteroid is determined by many factors including the vehicle, the integrity of the epidermal barrier, and the use of occlusive dressings. (See DOSAGE AND ADMINISTRATION.)

Topical corticosteroids can be absorbed from normal intact skin. Inflammation and/or other disease processes in the skin increase percutaneous absorption. Occlusive dressings substantially increase the percutaneous absorption of topical corticosteroids. (See DOSAGE AND ADMINISTRATION.)

Once absorbed through the skin, topical corticosteroids are handled through pharmacokinetic pathways similar to systemically administered corticosteroids. Corticosteroids are bound to plasma proteins in varying degrees. Corticosteroids are metabolized primarily in the liver and are then excreted by the kidneys. Some of the topical corticosteroids and their metabolites are also excreted into the bile.

Clotrimazole and Betamethasone Dipropionate: In clinical studies of tinea corporis, tinea cruris, and tinea pedis, patients treated with betamethasone dipropionate and clotrimazole cream showed a better clinical response at the first return visit than patients treated with clotrimazole cream. In tinea corporis and tinea cruris, the patient returned 3 days after starting treatment,and in tinea pedis, after 1 week. Mycological cure rates observed in patients treated with betamethasone dipropionate and clotrimazole cream were as good as or better than in those patients treated with clotrimazole cream.

In these same clinical studies, patients treated with betamethasone dipropionate and clotrimazole cream showed statistically significantly better clinical responses and mycological cure rates when compared with patients treated with betamethasone dipropionate cream.

INDICATIONS AND USAGE:

Betamethasone dipropionate and clotrimazole cream is indicated for the topical treatment of the following dermal infections: tinea pedis, tinea cruris, and tinea corporis due to *Trichophyton rubrum, Trichophyton mentagrophytes, Epidermophyton floccosum* and *Microsporum canis.*

CONTRAINDICATIONS:

Betamethasone dipropionate and clotrimazole cream is contraindicated in patients who are sensitive to clotrimazole, betamethasone dipropionate, other corticosteroids or imidazoles, or to any ingredient in this preparation.

PRECAUTIONS:

GENERAL

Systemic absorption of topical corticosteroids has produced reversible hypothalamic-pituitary-adrenal (HPA) axis suppression, manifestations of Cushing's syndrome, hyperglycemia, and glucosuria in some patients.

Conditions which augment systemic absorption include the application of the more potent steroids, use over large surface areas, prolonged use, and the addition of occlusive dressings. (See DOSAGE AND ADMINISTRATION).

Therefore, patients receiving a large dose of a potent topical steroid applied to a large surface area should be evaluated periodically for evidence of HPA axis suppression by using the urinary free cortisol and ACTH simulation tests. If HPA axis suppression is noted, an attempt should be made to withdraw the drug, to reduce the frequency of application, or to substitute a less potent steroid.

Recovery of HPA axis function is generally prompt and complete upon discontinuation of the drug. Infrequently, signs and symptoms of steroid withdrawal may occur, requiring supplemental systemic corticosteroids.

Children may absorb proportionally larger amounts of topical corticosteroids and thus be more susceptible to systemic toxicity. (See PRECAUTIONS, Pediatric Use.)

If irritation or hypersensitivity develops with the use of betamethasone dipropionate and clotrimazole cream, treatment should be discontinued and appropriate therapy instituted.

INFORMATION FOR THE PATIENT

Patients using betamethasone dipropionate and clotrimazole cream should receive the following information and instructions:

1. This medication is to be used as directed by the physician. It is for external use only. Avoid contact with the eyes.

PRECAUTIONS: *(cont'd)*

2. The medication is to be used for the full prescribed treatment time, even though the symptoms may have improved. Notify the physician if there is no improvement after 1 week of treatment for tinea cruris or tinea corporis, or after 2 weeks for tinea pedis.

3. Patients should be advised not to use this medication for any disorder other than for which it was prescribed.

4. The treated skin areas should not be bandaged or otherwise covered or wrapped as to be occluded. (See DOSAGE AND ADMINISTRATION.)

5. When using this medication in the groin area, patients should be advised to use the medication for 2 weeks only, and to apply the cream sparingly. The physician should be notified if the condition persists after 2 weeks. Patients should also be advised to wear loose fitting clothing. (See DOSAGE AND ADMINISTRATION.)

6. Patients should report any signs of local adverse reactions.

7. Patients should avoid sources of infection or reinfection.

LABORATORY TESTS

If there is a lack of response to betamethasone dipropionate and clotrimazole cream, appropriate microbiological studies should be repeated to confirm the diagnosis and rule out other pathogens before instituting another course of anti-mycotic therapy.

The following tests may be helpful in evaluating HPA axis suppression due to the corticosteroid component:

Urinary free cortisol test

ACTH stimulation test

CARCINOGENESIS, MUTAGENESIS, AND IMPAIRMENT OF FERTILITY

There are no animal or laboratory studies with the combination clotrimazole and betamethasone dipropionate to evaluate carcinogenesis, mutagenesis, or impairment of fertility.

An 18-month oral dosing study with clotrimazole in rats has not revealed any carcinogenic effect.

In tests for mutagenesis, chromosomes of the spermatophores of Chinese hamsters which had been exposed to clotrimazole were examined for structural changes during the metaphase. Prior to testing, the hamsters had received five oral clotrimazole doses of 100 mg/kg body weight. The results of this study showed that clotrimazole had no mutagenic effect.

PREGNANCY CATEGORY C

There have been no teratogenic studies performed with the combination Clotrimazole and betamethasone dipropionate.

Studies in pregnant rats with intravaginal doses up to 100 mg/kg have revealed no evidence of harm to the fetus due to clotrimazole.

High oral doses of clotrimazole in rats and mice ranging from 50 to 120 mg/kg resulted in embryotoxicity (possible secondary to maternal toxicity), impairment of mating, decreased litter size and number of viable young and decreased pup survival to weaning. However, clotrimazole was not teratogenic in mice, rabbits, and rats at oral doses up to 200, 180 and 100 mg/kg, respectively. Oral absorption in the rat amounts to approximately 90% of the administered dose.

Corticosteroids are generally teratogenic in laboratory animals when administered systemically at relatively low dosage levels. The more potent corticosteroids have been shown to be teratogenic after dermal application in laboratory animals.

There are no adequate and well-controlled studies in pregnant women on teratogenic effects from a topically applied combination of clotrimazole and betamethasone dipropionate. Therefore, betamethasone dipropionate and clotrimazole cream should be used during pregnancy only if the potential benefit justifies the potential risk to the fetus.

Drugs containing corticosteroids should not be used extensively on pregnant patients, in large amounts, or for prolonged periods of time.

NURSING MOTHERS

It is not known whether this drug is excreted in human milk. Because many drugs are excreted in human milk, caution should be exercised when betamethasone dipropionate and clotrimazole cream is used by a nursing woman.

PEDIATRIC USE

Safety and effectiveness in children below the age of 12 have not been established with betamethasone dipropionate and clotrimazole cream.

Pediatric patients may demonstrate greater susceptibility to topical corticosteroid-induced HPA axis suppression and Cushing's syndrome than mature patients because of a larger skin surface area to body weight ratio.

Hypothalamic-pituitary-adrenal (HPA) axis suppression, Cushing's syndrome,and intracranial hypertension have been reported in children receiving topical corticosteroids. Manifestations of adrenal suppression in children include linear growth retardation, delayed weight gain, low plasma cortisol levels, and absence of response to ACTH stimulation. Manifestations of intracranial hypertension include bulging fontanelles, headaches, and bilateral papilledema.

Administration of topical dermatologics containing a corticosteroid to children should be limited to the least amount compatible with an effective therapeutic regimen. Chronic corticosteroid therapy may interfere with the growth and development of children.

The use of betamethasone dipropionate and clotrimazole cream in diaper dermatitis is not recommended.

ADVERSE REACTIONS:

The following adverse reactions have been reported in connection with the use of betamethasone dipropionate and clotrimazole cream: paresthesia in 5 of 270 patients, maculopapular rash, edema, and secondary infection, each in 1 of 270 patients.

Adverse reactions reported with the use of clotrimazole are as follows: erythema, stinging, blistering, peeling, edema, pruritus, urticaria, and general irritation of the skin.

The following local adverse reactions are reported infrequently when topical corticosteroids are used as recommended. These reactions are listed in an approximate decreasing order of occurrence: burning, itching, irritations, dryness, folliculitis, hypertrichosis, acneiform eruptions, hypopigmentation, perioral dermatitis, allergic contact dermatitis, maceration of the skin, secondary infection, skin atrophy, striae, and miliaria.

OVERDOSAGE:

Acute overdosage with topical application of betamethasone dipropionate and clotrimazole cream is unlikely and would not be expected to lead to a life-threatening situation.

Topically applied corticosteroids can be absorbed in sufficient amounts to produce systemic effects. (See PRECAUTIONS.)

DOSAGE AND ADMINISTRATION:

Gently massage sufficient betamethasone dipropionate and clotrimazole cream into the affected and surrounding skin areas twice a day, in the morning and evening, for 2 weeks in tinea cruris and tinea corporis, and for 4 weeks in tinea pedis. The use of betamethasone dipropionate and clotrimazole cream for longer than 4 weeks is not recommended.

DOSAGE AND ADMINISTRATION: *(cont'd)*

Clinical improvement, with relief of erythema and pruritus, usually occurs within 3 to 5 days of treatment. If a patient with tinea cruris and tinea corporis shows no clinical improvement after one week of treatment with betamethasone dipropionate and clotrimazole cream, the diagnosis should be reviewed. In tinea pedis, the treatment should be applied for 2 weeks prior to making that decision.

Treatment with betamethasone dipropionate and clotrimazole cream should be discontinued if the condition persists after 2 weeks in tinea cruris and tinea corporis, and after 4 weeks in tinea pedis. Alternate therapy may then be instituted with betamethasone dipropionate and clotrimazole cream, a product containing an antifungal only.

Betamethasone dipropionate and clotrimazole cream should not be used with occlusive dressings.

PATIENT INFORMATION:

Betamethasone dipropionate and clotrimazole cream is used for the topical treatment of tinea pedis (Athlete's foot), tinea cruris (jock itch), and tinea corporis (ringworm). This cream is only to be used externally and should not be used in or near the eyes. Gently clean the affected skin before applying the cream. Apply the cream sparingly and rub in gently. Do not apply bandages, dressings, cosmetics or other skin products over the treated area unless directed by your physician. Tight-fitting diapers or plastic pants should not be used on children treated in the diaper area. Avoid applying the cream to the face, genital and rectal areas, armpits, and skin creases for extended lengths of time. Continue to use the cream for the entire treatment time, even though symptoms may have improved. Notify your physician if improvement in jock itch or ringworm has not occurred after two weeks or if improvement in athlete's foot has not occurred after four weeks. Notify your physician if burning, stinging, swelling or redness develop.

HOW SUPPLIED:

Store between 2° and 30° C (36° and 86° F).

HOW SUPPLIED - EQUIVALENTS NOT AVAILABLE:

Cream - Topical - 0.64 mg/10 mg

15 gm	$18.21	LOTRISONE, Schering	00085-0924-01
45 gm	$38.87	LOTRISONE, Schering	00085-0924-02

BETAMETHASONE SODIUM PHOSPHATE

(000467)

CATEGORIES: Adrenal Corticosteroids; Adrenal Hyperplasia; Adrenal Insufficiency; Adrenocortical Insufficiency; Allergies; Alopecia; Alopecia Areata; Anemia; Ankylosing Spondylitis; Arthritis; Asthma; Atopic Dermatitis; Berylliosis; Bursitis; Cancer; Carditis; Chemotherapy; Chorioretinitis; Choroiditis; Colitis; Conjunctivitis; Dermatitis; Dermatitis Herpetiformis; Diuresis; Drug Hypersensitivity; Edema; Enteritis; Epicondylitis; Erythema Multiforme; Gouty Arthritis; Granuloma; Granuloma Annulare; Herpes; Herpes Zoster; Hormones; Hypercalcemia; Inflammation; Inflammatory Lesions; Iridocyclitis; Keloids; Keratitis; Laryngeal Edema; Lesions; Leukemia; Lichen Planus; Lichen Simplex Chronicus; Lupus Erythematosus; Meningitis; Mycosis Fungoides; Necrobiosis Lipoidica; Nephrotic Syndrome; Neuritis; Osteoarthritis; Pemphigus; Proteinuria; Psoriasis; Respiratory & Allergy Medications; Rhinitis; Sarcoidosis; Serum Sickness; Shock; Spondylitis; Synovitis; Synovitis of Osteoarthritis; Tenosynovitis; Thyroiditis; Transfusion Reactions; Tumors; Ulcerative Colitis; Uveitis; FDA Approval Pre 1982

BRAND NAMES: Adbeon; B-S-P; *Betnesol* (England); *Celestone*; **Celestone Phosphate**; *Deltonin*; *Inflacor*; Prelestone; *Rinderon Solution*; Selestoject; Storz-Beta *(International brand names outside U.S. in italics)*

FORMULARIES: BC-BS

DESCRIPTION:

Betamethasone sodium phosphate injection is a sterile, aqueous solution containing in each ml: 4.0 mg betamethasone sodium phosphate, USP, equivalent to 3.0 mg betamethasone alcohol; 10 mg dibasic sodium phosphate; 0.1 mg edetate disodium; 3.2 mg sodium bisulfite; and 5.0 mg phenol as preservative. The pH is adjusted to approximately 8.5 with sodium hydroxide.

The formula for betamethasone sodium phosphate is $C_{22}H_{28}FNA_2O_8P$ and has a molecular weight of 516.41. Chemically, it is 9-fluoro-11β,17,21-trihydroxy-16β-methylpregna-1,4-diene-3,20-dione 21-(disodium phosphate).

Betamethasone sodium phosphate is a white to practically white, odorless powder, and is hygroscopic. Betamethasone sodium phosphate is freely soluble in water and methanol and is practically insoluble in acetone and chloroform.

CLINICAL PHARMACOLOGY:

Naturally occurring glucocorticoids (hydrocortisone), which also have salt-retaining properties, are used as replacement therapy in adrenocortical deficiency states. Their synthetic analogs are primarily used for their potent anti-inflammatory effects in disorders of many organ systems.

Glucocorticoids cause profound and varied metabolic effects. In addition, they modify the body's immune responses to diverse stimuli.

INDICATIONS AND USAGE:

When oral therapy is not feasible and the strength dosage form, and route of administration of the drug reasonably lend the preparation to the treatment of the condition, the **intravenous or intramuscular use** of betamethasone sodium phosphate injection is indicated as follows:

Endocrine Disorders: Primary or secondary adrenocortical insufficiency (hydrocortisone or cortisone is the drug of choice; synthetic analogs may be used in conjunction with mineralocorticoids where applicable; in infancy, mineralocorticoid supplementation is of particular importance), acute adrenocortical insufficiency (hydrocortisone or cortisone is the drug of choice; mineralocorticoid supplementation may be necessary, particularly when synthetic analogs are used), preoperatively and in the event of serious trauma or illness, in patients with known adrenal insufficiency or when adrenocortical insufficiency adrenocortical reserve is doubtful, shock unresponsive to conventional therapy if adrenocortical insufficiency exists or is suspected, congenital adrenal hyperplasia, nonsuppurative thyroiditis, hypercalcemia associated with cancer.

INDICATIONS AND USAGE: *(cont'd)*

Rheumatic Disorders: As adjunctive therapy for short-term administration (to tide the patient over an acute episode or exacerbation) in:

Post-traumatic osteoarthritis, synovitis or osteoarthritis, rheumatoid arthritis, including juvenile rheumatoid arthritis (selected cases may require low-dose maintenance therapy), acute and subacute bursitis, epicondylitis, acute and nonspecific tenosynovitis, acute gouty arthritis, psoriatic arthritis, ankylosing spondylitis.

Collagen Diseases: During an exacerbation or as a maintenance therapy in selected cases of:

Systemic lupus erythematosus and acute rheumatic carditis.

Dermatologic Diseases: Pemphigus, severe erythema multiforme (Stevens-Johnson syndrome), exfoliative dermatitis, bullous dermatitis herpetiformis, severe seborrheic dermatitis, severe psoriasis, severe psoriasis, mycosis fungoides.

Allergic States: Control of severe or incapacitating allergic conditions intractable to adequate trials of conventional treatment in:

Bronchial asthma, contact dermatitis, atopic dermatitis, serum sickness, seasonal or perennial allergic rhinitis, drug hypersensitivity reactions, urticarial transfusion reactions, acute noninfectious laryngeal edema (epinephrine is the drug of first choice).

Ophthalmic Diseases: Severe acute and chronic allergic and inflammatory processes involving the eye such as:

Herpes zoster ophthalmicus, iritis, iridocyclitis, chorioretinitis, diffuse posterior uveitis and choroiditis, optic neuritis, sympathetic ophthalmia, anterior segment inflammation, allergic conjunctivitis, allergic corneal marginal ulcers, keratitis.

Gastrointestinal Diseases: To tide the patient over a critical period of the disease in:

Ulcerative colitis - (Systemic therapy) and regional enteritis - (Systemic therapy).

Respiratory Diseases: Symptomatic sarcoidosis, berylliosis, fulminating or disseminated pulmonary tuberculosis when used concurrently with appropriate antituberculous chemotherapy, Loeffler's syndrome not manageable by other means, aspiration pneumonitis.

Hematologic Disorders: Acquired (autoimmune) hemolytic anemia, idiopathic thrombocytopenia purpura in adults (IV only; IM administration is contraindicated), secondary thrombocytopenia in adults, erythroblastopenia (RBC anemia), congenital (erythroid) hypoplastic anemia.

Neoplastic Diseases: For palliative management of:

Leukemias and lymphomas in adults and acute leukemia of childhood

EDEMATOUS STATES: To induce diuresis or remission of proteinuria in the nephrotic syndrome, without uremia, of the idiopathic type or that due to lupus erythematosus.

Miscellaneous: Tuberculous meningitis with subarachnoid block or impending block when used concurrently with appropriate antituberculosis chemotherapy, trichinosis with neurologic or myocardial involvement.

When the strength and dosage form of the drug lend the preparation to the treatment of the condition, **the intra-articular or soft tissue administration** of betamethasone sodium phosphate injection is indicated as adjunctive therapy for short-term administration (to tide the patient over an acute episode or exacerbation) in:

Synovitis of osteoarthritis, rheumatoid arthritis, acute and subacute bursitis, acute gouty arthritis, epicondylitis, acute nonspecific tenosynovitis, post-traumatic osteoarthritis.

When the strength and dosage form of the drug lend the preparation to the treatment of the condition, the **intralesional administration** of betamethasone sodium phosphate injection is indicated for:

Keloids

Localized hypertrophic, infiltrated, inflammatory lesions of:

lichen planus, psoriatic plaques, granuloma annulare, and lichen simplex chronicus (neurodermatitis), discoid lupus erythematosus, necrobiosis lipoidica diabeticorum, alopecia areata.

BETAMETHASONE SODIUM PHOSPHATE MAY BE USEFUL IN CYSTIC TUMORS OF AN APONEUROSIS OR TENDON (GANGLIA).

CONTRAINDICATIONS:

Betamethasone sodium phosphate injection is contraindicated in systemic fungal infections.

WARNINGS:

In patients on corticosteroid therapy subjected to any unusual stress, increased dosage of rapidly acting corticosteroids before, during, and after the stressful situation is indicated.

Corticosteroids may mask some signs of infection, and new infections may appear during their use. There may be decreased resistance and inability to localize infection when corticosteroids are used.

Prolonged use of corticosteroids may produce posterior subcapsular cataracts, glaucoma with possible damage to the optic nerves, and may enhance the establishment of secondary ocular infections due to fungi or viruses.

Average and large doses of cortisone or hydrocortisone can cause elevation of blood pressure, salt and water retention, and increased excretion of potassium. These effects are less likely to occur with the synthetic derivatives except when used in large doses. Dietary salt restriction and potassium supplementation may be necessary. All corticosteroids increase calcium excretion.

While on Corticosteroid Therapy, Patients Should Not Be Vaccinated Against Smallpox. Other Immunization Procedures Should Not Be Undertaken In Patients Who are on Corticosteroids, Especially In High Doses, Because of Possible Hazards of Neurological Complications and Lack of Antibody Response.

Children who are on immunosuppressant drugs are more susceptible to infections than healthy children. Chickenpox and measles, for example, can have a more serious or even fatal course in children on immunosuppressant corticosteroids. In such children, or in adults who have not had these diseases, particular care should be taken to avoid exposure. If exposed, therapy with varicella zoster immune globulin (VZIG) or pooled intravenous immunoglobulin (IVIG), as appropriate, may be indicated. If chickenpox develops, treatment with antiviral agents may be considered.

The use of betamethasone sodium phosphate injection in active tuberculosis should be restricted to those cases of fulminating or disseminated tuberculosis in which the corticosteroid is used for the management of the disease in conjunction with appropriate antituberculosis regimen.

If corticosteroids are indicated in patients with latent tuberculosis or tuberculin reactivity, close observation is necessary as reactivation of the disease may occur. During prolonged corticosteroid therapy, these patients should chemoprophylaxis.

Because rare instances of anaphylactoid reactions have occurred in patients receiving parenteral corticosteroid therapy, appropriate precautionary measures should be taken prior to administration, especially when the patient has a history of allergy to any drug.

WARNINGS: *(cont'd)*

Usage in Pregnancy: Since adequate human reproduction studies have not been done with corticosteroids, the use of these drugs in pregnancy, nursing mothers, or women of childbearing potential requires that the possible benefits of the drug be weighed against the potential hazards to the mother and embryo or fetus. Infants born to mothers who have received substantial doses of corticosteroids during pregnancy should be carefully observed for signs of hypoadrenalism.

PRECAUTIONS:

INFORMATION FOR THE PATIENT

Patients who are on immunosuppressant doses of corticosteroids should be warned to avoid exposure to chickenpox or measles and, if exposed, to obtain medical advice.

Drug-induced secondary adrenocortical insufficiency may be minimized by gradual reduction of dosage. This type of relative insufficiency may persist for months after discontinuation of therapy; therefore, in any situation of stress occurring during that period, hormone therapy should be reinstituted. Since mineralocorticoid secretion may be impaired, salt and/or a mineralocorticoid should be administered concurrently.

There is an enhanced effect of corticosteroids in patients with hypothyroidism and in those with cirrhosis.

Corticosteroids should be used cautiously in patients with ocular herpes simplex for fear of corneal perforation.

The lowest possible dose of corticosteroid should be used to control the condition under treatment, and when reduction in dosage is possible, the reduction in dosage is possible, the reduction must be gradual.

Psychic derangements may appear when corticosteroids are used, ranging from euphoria, insomnia, mood swings, personality changes, and severe depression to frank psychotic manifestations. Also, existing emotional instability or psychotic tendencies may be aggravated by corticosteroids.

Aspirin should be used cautiously in conjunction with corticosteroids in hypothrombinemia.

Steroids should be used with caution in nonspecific ulcerative colitis, if there is a probability of impending perforation, abscess or other pyrogenic infection, also in diverticulitis, fresh Intestinal anastomoses, active or latent peptic ulcer, renal insufficiency, hypertension, osteoporosis, and myasthenia gravis. Growth and development or infants and children on prolonged corticosteroid therapy should be carefully followed.

THE FOLLOWING ADDITIONAL PRECAUTIONS ALSO APPLY FOR PARENTERAL CORTICOSTEROIDS

Intra-articular Injection of a corticosteroid may produce systemic as well as local effects.

Appropriate examination of any joint fluid present is necessary to exclude a septic process.

A marked increase in pain accompanied by local swelling, further restriction of joint motion, fever, and malaise are suggestive of septic arthritis. If this complication occurs and the diagnosis of sepsis is confirmed, appropriate antimicrobial therapy should be instituted.

Local injection of a steroid into a previously infected joint is to be avoided.

Corticosteroids should not be injected into unstable joints.

The slower rate of absorption by intramuscular administration should be recognized.

ADVERSE REACTIONS:

Fluid And Electrolyte Disturbances: sodium retention; fluid retention; congestive heart failure in susceptible patients; potassium loss; hypokalemic alkalosis; hypertension.

Musculoskeletal: muscle weakness; steroid myopathy; loss of muscle mass; osteoporosis, vertebral compression fractures; aseptic necrosis of femoral and humeral heads; pathologic fracture of long bones.

Gastrointestinal: peptic ulcer with possible subsequent perforation and hemorrhage; pancreatitis; abdominal distention; ulcerative esophagitis.

Dermatologic: impaired wound healing; thin fragile skin; petechiae and ecchymoses; facial erythema; increased sweating; may suppress reactions to skin tests.

Neurological: convulsions; increased intracranial pressure with papilledema (pseudomotor cerebri) usually after treatment; vertigo; headache.

Endocrine: menstrual irregularities; development of cushingoid state; suppression of growth in children; secondary adrenocortical and pituitary unresponsiveness, particularly in times of stress, as in trauma, surgery or illness; decreased carbohydrate tolerance; manifestations of latent diabetes mellitus; increased requirements for insulin or oral hypoglycemic agents in diabetics.

Ophthalmic: posterior subcapsular cataracts; increased intraocular pressure; glaucoma; exophthalmos.

Metabolic: negative nitrogen balance due to protein catabolism.

The following *additional* adverse reactions are also related to parenteral corticosteroid therapy: rare instances of blindness associated with intralesional therapy around the face and head; hyperpigmentation or hypopigmentation; subcutaneous and cutaneous atrophy; sterile abscess; postinjection flare (following intra-articular use); charcot-like arthropathy.

DOSAGE AND ADMINISTRATION:

The initial dosage of parenterally administered betamethasone may vary up to 9.0 mg per day depending on the specific disease entity being treated. In situations of less severity, lower doses will generally suffice while in selected patients higher initial doses may be required. Usually the parenteral dosage are one-third to one-half the 12-hourly oral dose. However, in certain overwhelming acute, life-threatening situations, administration in dosages exceeding the usual dosages may be in multiples of the oral dosages.

The initial dosage should be maintained or adjusted until a satisfactory response is noted. If after a reasonable period of time there is a lack of satisfactory clinical response, betamethasone sodium phosphate injection should be discontinued and the patient transferred to other appropriate therapy. *It Should Be Emphasized that Dosage Requirements are Variable and Must Be Individualized on the Basis of the Disease Under Treatment and Response of the Patient.* After a favorable response is noted, the proper maintenance dosage should be determined by decreasing the initial drug dosage in small decrements at appropriate time intervals until the lowest dosage which will maintain an adequate clinical response is reached. It should be kept in mind that constant monitoring is needed in regard to drug dosage. Included in the situations which may make dosage adjustments necessary are changes in clinical status secondary to remissions to exacerbations in the disease process, the patient's individual drug responsiveness, and the effect of patient exposure to stressful situations not directly related to the disease entity under treatment; in this latter situation it may necessary to increase dosage of betamethasone sodium phosphate injection for a period of time consistent with the patient's condition. If after long-term therapy the drug is to be stopped, it is recommended that it be withdrawn gradually rather than abruptly.

Protect from freezing. Protect from light.

HOW SUPPLIED - RATED THERAPEUTICALLY EQUIVALENT:

Injection, Solution - Intramuscular; - 3 mg/ml

5 ml	$4.25	Betamethasone Sodium Phosphate, Consolidated Midland	00223-7265-05
5 ml	$6.25	Betamethasone Sodium Phsophate, Pasadena	00418-1831-05
5 ml	$6.65	Betamethasone Sodium Phosphate, Insource	58441-0118-05
5 ml	$8.76	Betamethasone Sodium Phosphate, General Inj & Vac	52584-0217-05
5 ml	$8.90	Betamethasone Sodium Phosphate, Hyrex Pharms	00314-6392-75
5 ml	$8.93	ADBEON, UAD Labs	00785-9060-05
5 ml	$9.15	Betamethasone Sodium Phosphate, Steris Labs	00402-0217-05
5 ml	$12.14	Betamethasone Sodium Phosphate, HL Moore Drug Exch	00839-6574-25
5 ml	$13.40	Betamethasone Sodium Phosphate, Goldline Labs	00182-3009-62
5 ml	$13.69	Betamethasone Sodium Phosphate, Schein Pharm (US)	00364-6751-53
5 ml	$14.60	Betamethasone Acet & Na Phos, Major Pharms	00904-0818-05
5 ml	**$15.82**	**CELESTONE PHOSPHATE, Schering**	**00085-0879-05**
5 ml	$20.90	SELESTOJECT, Mayrand Pharms	00259-0349-05

BETAMETHASONE VALERATE *(000468)*

CATEGORIES: Adrenal Corticosteroids; Anti-Inflammatory Agents; Dermatologicals; Dermatoses; Glucocorticoids; Inflammation; Pruritus; Skin/Mucous Membrane Agents; Steroids; Topical; Pregnancy Category C; FDA Approval Pre 1982

BRAND NAMES: *Beavate*; *Bennasone*; *Benoson*; *Besone*; *Bessasone*; *Beta*; Beta-Val; *Beta Scalp*; *Betacort* (Canada); *Betacorten*; Betaderm; *Betagalen* (Germany); *Betamethacot*; *Betasone*; *Betasone DHA*; Betatrex; *Betaval*; *Betnelan*; *Betnelan-V*; *Betnelan V*; *Betnesol-V*; *Betnesol V* (Germany); *Betneval* (France); *Betnevate*; *Betnovat*; *Betnovate* (Australia, England, Canada); *Betopic*; *Betsona*; *Bipro*; *Celestan-V*; *Celestan V* (Germany); *Celestoderm* (France, Canada); *Celestoderm-V*; *Celestoderm V* (Mexico); *Celestone*; *Celestone-M*; *Celestone-V*; *Celeston Valerat*; *Corsaderm*; Dermabet; *Ecoval*; *Ectosone* (Canada); *Inflacor*; *Lenovate*; *Metaderm*; *Muhibeta-V*; *Nolcot*; *Novobetamet* (Canada); Qualisone; *Rinderon-V*; *Setrosone*; **Valisone**; Valnac *(International brand names outside U.S. in italics)*

FORMULARIES: Aetna

DESCRIPTION:

For Dermatologic Use Only-Not for Ophthalmic Use

Betamethasone valerate cream, reduced strength cream, ointment and lotion contains betamethasone valerate, USP, a synthetic adrenocorticoid, for dermatologic use. Betamethasone, an analog of prednisolone, has a slight degree of mineralocorticosteroid activity. Betamethasone valerate is the 17-valerate ester of betamethasone.

Chemically, betamethasone valerate is 9-fluoro-11β,17,21-trihydroxy-16β,methylpregna-1, 4-diene-3,20-dione 17-valerate, with the empirical formula $C_{27}H_{37}FO_6$, and a molecular weight of 476.58. Betamethasone valerate is a white to practically white, oderless crystalline powder, and is practically insoluble in water, freely soluble in acetone and in chloroform, soluble in alcohol and slightly soluble in benzene and either.

Each gram of valisone cream 0.1% contains: 1.2 mg betamethasone valerate, USP (equivalent to 1.0 mg betamethasone), in an aqueous hydrophilic emollient cream consisting of mineral oil, white petrolatum, ceteareth-30, cetearyl alcohol, monobasic sodium phosphate, and phosphoric acid, chlorocresol and propylene glycol as preservatives.

Each gram of valisone ointment 0.1% contains: 1.2 mg betamethasone valerate, USP (equivalent to 1.0 mg betamethasone), in an ointment base of mineral oil, white petrolatum, and hydrogenated lanolin.

Each gram valisone lotion 0.1% contains: 1.2 mg betamethasone valerate, USP (equivalent to 1.0 mg betamethasone), in a lotion base of isopropyl alcohol (47.5%) and water slightly thickened with carbomer 934P, the pH is adjusted to approximately 4.7 with sodium hydroxide.

Each gram of valisone reduced strength cream 0.01% contains: 0.12 mg betamethasone valerate, USP (equivalent to 0.1 mg betamethasone), in an aqueous hydrophilic emollient cream consisting of mineral oil, white petrolatum, cetereth-30, cetearyl alcohol, monobasic sodium phosphate, and phosphoric acid, chlorocresol and propylene glycol as preservatives.

CLINICAL PHARMACOLOGY:

The corticosteroids are a class of compounds comprising steroid hormones secreted by the adrenal cortex and their synthetic analogs. In pharmacologic doses corticosteroids are used primarily for their anti-inflammatory and/or immunosuppressive effects.

Topical corticosteroids, such as betamethasone valerate, are effective in the treatment of corticosteroid-responsive dermatoses primarily because of their anti-inflammatory, anti-pruritic, and vasoconstrictive actions. However, while the physiologic, pharmacologic, and clinical effects of the corticosteroids are well-known, the exact mechanisms of their actions in each disease are uncertain. Betamethasone valerate, a corticosteroid, has been shown to have topical (dermatologic) and systemic pharmacologic and metabolic effects characteristic of this class of drugs.

PHARMACOKINETICS

The extent of percutaneous absorption of topical corticosteroids is determined by many factors including the vehicle, the integrity of the epidermal barrier, and the use of occlusive dressings. Topical corticosteroids can be absorbed from normal intact skin. Inflammation and/or other disease processes in the skin increase percutaneous absorption. Occlusive dressings substantially increase the percutaneous absorption of topical corticosteroids. Thus, occlusive dressings may be a valuable therapeutic adjunct for treatment of resistant dermatoses.

Once absorbed through the skin, topical corticosteroids are handled through pharmacokinetic pathways similar to systemically administered corticosteroids. Corticosteroids are bound to plasma proteins in varying degrees. Corticosteroids are metabolized primarily in the liver and are then excreted by the kidneys. Some of the topical corticosteroids and their metabolites are also excreted into the bile.

INDICATIONS AND USAGE:

Betamethasone valerate cream, reduced strength cream, ointment and lotion indicated for the relief of the inflammatory and pruritic manifestations of corticosteroid-responsive dermatoses.

CONTRAINDICATIONS:

Betamethasone valerate cream, reduced strength cream, ointment and lotion contraindicated in those patients who are hypersensitive to betamethasone valerate, to other corticosteroids, or to any ingredient in this preparation.

PRECAUTIONS:

GENERAL

Systemic absorption of topical corticosteroids has produced reversible hypothalamic-pituitary-adrenal (HPA) axis suppression, manifestations of Cushing's syndrome, hyperglycemia, and glucosuria in some patients.

Conditions which augment systemic absorption include the application of the more potent steroids, use over large surface areas, prolonged use, and the addition of occlusive dressings. Therefore, patients receiving a large dose of a potent topical steroid applied to a large surface area or under an occlusive dressing should be evaluated periodically for evidence of HPA axis suppression by using the urinary free cortisol and ACTH stimulation tests. If HPA axis suppression is noted, an attempt should be made to withdraw the drug, to reduce the frequency of application, or to substitute a less potent steroid.

Recovery of HPA axis function is generally prompt and complete upon discontinuation of the drug. Infrequently, signs and symptoms of steroid withdrawal may occur, requiring supplemental systemic corticosteroids. Children may absorb proportionally larger amounts of topical corticosteroids and thus be more susceptible to systemic toxicity (See PRECAUTIONS, Pediatric Use.)

If irritation develops, topical corticosteroids should be discontinued and appropriate therapy instituted.

In the presence of dermatological infections, the use of an appropriate antifungal or antibacterial agent should be discontinued until the infection has been adequately controlled.

INFORMATION FOR THE PATIENT

Patients using topical corticosteroids should receive the following information and instructions:

1. This medication is to be used as directed by the physician. It is for external use only. Avoid contact with the eyes.

2. Patients should be advised not to use this medication for any disorder other than for which it was prescribed.

3. The treated skin area should not be bandaged or otherwise covered or wrapped as to be occlusive unless directed by the physician.

4. Patients should report any signs of local adverse reactions especially under occlusive dressing.

5. Parents of pediatric patient should be advised not to use tight-fitting diapers or plastic pants on a child being treated in the diaper area, as these garments may constitute occlusive dressings.

LABORATORY TESTS

The following tests may be helpful in evaluating the HPA axis suppression:

Urinary free cortisol test

ACTH stimulation test

CARCINOGENESIS, MUTAGENESIS, AND IMPAIRMENT OF FERTILITY

Long-term animal studies have not been performed to evaluate the carcinogenic potential or the effect on fertility of topical corticosteroids.

Studies to determine mutagenicity with prednisolone and hydrocortisone have revealed negative results.

PREGNANCY CATEGORY C

Corticosteroids are generally teratogenic in laboratory animals when administered systemically at relatively low dosage levels. The more potent corticosteroids have been shown to be teratogenic after dermal application in laboratory animals. There are no adequate and well-controlled studies in pregnant women on teratogenic effects from topically applied corticosteroids. Therefore, topical corticosteroids should be used during pregnancy only if the potential benefit justifies the potential risk to the fetus. Drugs of this class should not be used extensively on pregnant patients, in large amounts, or for prolonged periods of time.

NURSING MOTHERS

It is not know whether topical administration of corticosteroids could result in sufficient systemic absorption to produce detectable quantities in breast milk. Systemically administered corticosteroids are secreted into breast milk in quantities *not*likely to have a deleterious effect on the infant. Nevertheless, caution should be exercised when topical corticosteroids are prescribed to a nursing woman.

PEDIATRIC USE

Pediatric patients may demonstrate greater susceptibility to topical corticosteroid-induced HPA axis suppression and Cushing's syndrome than mature patients because of a larger skin surface area to body weight ratio.

Hypothalamic-pituitary-adrenal (HPA) axis suppression, Cushing's syndrome, and intracranial hypertension have been reported in children receiving topical corticosteroids. Manifestations of adrenal suppression in children include linear growth retardation, delayed weight gain, low plasma cortisol levels, and absence of response to ACTH stimulation. Manifestations of intracranial hypertension include bulging fontanelles, headaches, and bilateral papilledema.

Administration of topical corticosteroids to children should be limited to the least amount compatible with an effective therapeutic regimen. Chronic corticosteroid therapy may interfere with the growth and development of children.

ADVERSE REACTIONS:

The following local adverse reactions are reported infrequently with topical dermatologic corticosteroids, especially under occlusive dressings: burning; itching; irritation; dryness; folliculitis; hypertrichosis; aceneform eruptions; hypopigmentation; periol dermatitis; allergic contact dermatitis; maceration of the skin; secondary infection; skin atrophy; striae; miliaria.

Systemic absorption of topical corticosteroids has produced reversible hypothalamic-pituitary-adrenal (HPA) axis suppression, manifestations of Cushing's syndrome, hyperglycemia, and glucosuria in some patients.

OVERDOSAGE:

Topically applied corticosteroids can be absorbed in sufficient amounts to produce systemic effects (See PRECAUTIONS).

DOSAGE AND ADMINISTRATION:

Betamethasone Valerate Cream and Bethamethasone Valerate Ointment: Apply a thin film to the affected skin areas one to three times a day. Dosage once or twice daily is often effective.

Betamethasone Valerate Lotion: Apply a few drops of betamethasone valerate 0.1% to the affected area and massage lightly until it disappears. Apply twice daily, in the morning and at night. Dosage may be increased in stubborn cases. Following improvement, apply once daily. For the most effective and economical use, apply nozzle very close to affected area and gently squeeze bottle. **Protect from light. Store in carton until contents are used.**

Betamethasone Valerate Reduced Strength Cream: Apply a thin film of betamethasone valerate reduced strength cream to the affected skin areas one to three times daily. Commonly, treatment twice a day is adequate. In some cases, treatment three times a day is necessary; in others, once a day suffices.

DOSAGE AND ADMINISTRATION: *(cont'd)*

Store between 2° and 30°C (36° and 86°F).

HOW SUPPLIED - RATED THERAPEUTICALLY EQUIVALENT:

Cream - Topical - 0.1 %

15 gm	$1.95	Betamethasone Valerate, United Res	00677-0842-40
15 gm	$1.95	Betamethasone Valerate, H.C.F.A. F F P	99999-0468-01
15 gm	$2.48	Betamethasone Valerate, Clay Park Labs	45802-0069-35
15 gm	$2.48	Betamethasone Valerate, Thames Pharma	49158-0184-20
15 gm	$2.55	Betamethasone Valerate, IDE-Interstate	00814-1160-93
15 gm	$2.90	Betamethasone Valerate, NMC Labs	23317-0370-15
15 gm	$3.35	Betamethasone Valerate, Geneva Pharms	00781-7055-27
15 gm	$3.50	Betamethasone Valerate, HL Moore Drug Exch	00839-6371-47
15 gm	$3.95	Betamethasone Valerate, Taro Pharms (US)	51672-1269-01
15 gm	$4.00	Betamethasone Valerate, Consolidated Midland	00223-4259-15
15 gm	$4.20	BETAMETHACOT, C O Truxton	00463-8055-15
15 gm	$4.23	Betamethasone Valerate, Qualitest Pharms	00603-7718-74
15 gm	$4.25	BETA-VAL, Teva	00093-0673-15
15 gm	$4.27	Betamethasone Valerate, Schein Pharm (US)	00364-7269-72
15 gm	$4.30	Betamethasone Valerate, Major Pharms	00904-0776-36
15 gm	$4.47	Betamethasone Valerate, Fougera	00168-0040-15
15 gm	$12.80	BETATREX, Savage Labs	00281-3510-44
15 gm	**$16.26**	**VALISONE, Schering**	**00085-0136-04**
15 mg	$4.25	Betamethasone Valerate, Rugby	00536-4310-20
16 gm	$4.05	Betamethasone Valerate, Goldline Labs	00182-1610-51
45 gm	$3.29	Betamethasone Valerate, H.C.F.A. F F P	99999-0468-02
45 gm	$4.86	Betamethasone Valerate, Thames Pharma	49158-0184-27
45 gm	$5.08	Betamethasone Valerate, Clay Park Labs	45802-0069-42
45 gm	$5.54	Betamethasone Valerate, NMC Labs	23317-0370-45
45 gm	$5.85	Betamethasone Valerate, United Res	00677-0842-49
45 gm	$5.85	Betamethasone Valerate, IDE-Interstate	00814-1160-95
45 gm	$6.25	Betamethasone Valerate, Geneva Pharms	00781-7055-45
45 gm	$6.55	Betamethasone Valerate, HL Moore Drug Exch	00839-6371-52
45 gm	$7.50	Betamethasone Valerate, Goldline Labs	00182-1610-60
45 gm	$7.50	Betamethasone Valerate, Schein Pharm (US)	00364-7269-80
45 gm	$7.51	Betamethasone Valerate, Qualitest Pharms	00603-7718-83
45 gm	$7.65	Betamethasone Valerate, Fougera	00168-0040-46
45 gm	$7.70	Betamethasone Valerate, Major Pharms	00904-0776-45
45 gm	$7.75	BETA-VAL, Teva	00093-0673-95
45 gm	$7.75	Betamethasone Valerate, Consolidated Midland	00223-4259-45
45 gm	$23.25	BETATREX, Savage Labs	00281-3510-50
45 gm	**$29.63**	**VALISONE, Schering**	**00085-0136-06**
45 mg	$7.80	Betamethasone Valerate, Rugby	00536-4310-26
110 gm	$14.30	Betamethasone Valerate, H.C.F.A. F F P	99999-0468-03
110 gm	**$50.87**	**VALISONE, Schering**	**00085-0136-07**
430 gm	$55.90	Betamethasone Valerate, H.C.F.A. F F P	99999-0468-04
430 gm	**$171.06**	**VALISONE, Schering**	**00085-0136-08**
454 gm	$59.02	Betamethasone Valerate, H.C.F.A. F F P	99999-0468-05
454 gm	$62.45	Betamethasone Valerate, Clay Park Labs	45802-0069-05

Lotion - Topical - 0.1 %

20 ml	$2.22	Betamethasone Valerate, H.C.F.A. F F P	99999-0468-06
20 ml	**$20.05**	**VALISONE, Schering**	**00085-0002-03**
60 ml	$6.67	Betamethasone Valerate LotiON, Copley Pharm	38245-0603-12
60 ml	$6.67	Betamethasone Valerate, H.C.F.A. F F P	99999-0468-07
60 ml	$10.10	Betamethasone Valerate, Major Pharms	00904-0778-03
60 ml	$10.20	Betamethasone Valerate, Alpharma	00472-0705-02
60 ml	$10.20	Betamethasone Valerate 0.1 % W/W, NMC Labs	23317-0372-60
60 ml	$10.46	Betamethasone Valerate, Schein Pharm (US)	00364-0778-58
60 ml	$10.50	Betamethasone Valerate, Rugby	00536-4330-61
60 ml	$10.51	Betamethasone Valerate, Qualitest Pharms	00603-7719-49
60 ml	$10.52	Betamethasone Valerate, HL Moore Drug Exch	00839-7022-64
60 ml	$11.25	Betamethasone Valerate, Goldline Labs	00182-1788-68
60 ml	$11.45	BETA-VAL, Teva	00093-0671-39
60 ml	$12.25	Betamethasone Valerate, Fougera	00168-0041-60
60 ml	$12.50	Betamethasone Valerate, Consolidated Midland	00223-6432-60
60 ml	$31.22	BETATREX, Savage Labs	00281-3519-46
60 ml	**$39.62**	**VALISONE, Schering**	**00085-0002-05**

Ointment - Topical - 0.1 %

15 gm	$2.47	Betamethasone Valerate, H.C.F.A. F F P	99999-0468-08
15 gm	$2.59	Betamethasone Valerate, Clay Park Labs	45802-0015-35
15 gm	$2.90	Betamethasone Valerate, NMC Labs	23317-0371-15
15 gm	$3.55	Betamethasone Valerate, Teva	00093-0644-15
15 gm	$4.05	Betamethasone Valerate, Goldline Labs	00182-1735-51
15 gm	$4.24	Betamethasone Valerate 0.1 %, Schein Pharm (US)	00364-2103-72
15 gm	$4.40	Betamethasone Valerate, Harber Pharm	51432-0715-10
15 gm	$4.55	Betamethasone Valerate, Major Pharms	00904-0777-36
15 gm	$4.71	Betamethasone Valerate, HL Moore Drug Exch	00839-6758-47
15 gm	$4.93	Betamethasone Valerate, Fougera	00168-0033-15
15 gm	$12.80	BETATREX, Savage Labs	00281-3516-44
15 gm	**$16.26**	**VALISONE, Schering**	**00085-0898-04**
15 mg	$4.63	Betamethasone Valerate, Rugby	00536-4320-20
45 gm	$5.23	Betamethasone Valerate, H.C.F.A. F F P	99999-0468-09
45 gm	$5.29	Betamethasone Valerate, Clay Park Labs	45802-0015-42
45 gm	$5.54	Betamethasone Valerate, NMC Labs	23317-0371-45
45 gm	$6.60	Betamethasone Valerate, Teva	00093-0644-95
45 gm	$7.29	Betamethasone Valerate, HL Moore Drug Exch	00839-6758-52
45 gm	$7.45	Betamethasone Valerate, United Res	00677-1059-49
45 gm	$7.50	Betamethasone Valerate, Goldline Labs	00182-1735-60
45 gm	$7.50	Betamethasone Valerate 0.1 %, Schein Pharm (US)	00364-2103-80
45 gm	$8.50	Betamethasone Valerate, Harber Pharm	51432-0715-16
45 gm	$8.90	Betamethasone Valerate, Fougera	00168-0033-46
45 gm	$9.10	Betamethasone Valerate, Major Pharms	00904-0777-45
45 gm	$23.25	BETATREX, Savage Labs	00281-3516-50
45 gm	**$29.63**	**VALISONE, Schering**	**00085-0898-06**
45 mg	$8.13	Betamethasone Valerate, Rugby	00536-4320-26
454 gm	$62.45	Betamethasone Valerate, Clay Park Labs	45802-0015-05
454 gm	$74.91	Betamethasone Valerate, H.C.F.A. F F P	99999-0468-10

HOW SUPPLIED - NOT RATED EQUIVALENT:

Cream - Topical - 0.01 %

15 gm	**$9.68**	**VALISONE REDUCED STRENGTH, Schering**	**00085-0929-04**
60 gm	**$22.32**	**VALISONE REDUCED STRENGTH, Schering**	**00085-0929-08**

Powder

5 gm	$98.00	Betamethasone Valerate, Paddock Labs	00574-0480-05

BETAXOLOL HYDROCHLORIDE *(000469)*

CATEGORIES: Antiglaucomatous Agents; Antihypertensives; Beta Adrenergic Blocking Agents; Beta Blockers; Cardiovascular Drugs; EENT Drugs; Eye, Ear, Nose, & Throat Preparations; Glaucoma; Hypertension; Intraocular Pressure; Ocular Hypertension; Ophthalmics; Pregnancy Category C; FDA Approved 1985 Aug

BRAND NAMES: *Alcon Betoptic*; *Abaxon*; *Betasel*; **Betoptic**; *Betoptic S* (Australia); *Betoptima* (Germany); *Kerlon*; Kerlone; *Kerlong* (Japan); *Optipres*; *Optipres 2 x 1*; *Optipress*
(International brand names outside U.S. in italics)

FORMULARIES: Aetna; BC-BS; CIGNA; FHP; Humana; Kaiser; Medco; Medi-Cal; PCS; PruCare; United

COST OF THERAPY: $262.94 (Hypertension; Tablet; 10 mg; 1/day; 365 days)

PRIMARY ICD9: 401.1 (Essential Hypertension, Benign)

DESCRIPTION:

Tablets: Betaxolol HCl is a β_1-selective (cardioselective) adrenergic receptor blocking agent available as 10-mg and 20-mg tablets for oral administration. Kerlone is chemically described as 2-propanol,1-[4-[2-(cyclopropylmethoxy)ethyl]phenoxy]-3-[(1-methylethyl) amino]-, hydrochloride, (±).

Betaxolol HCl is a water-soluble white crystalline powder with a molecular formula of $C_{18}H_{29}NO_3 \cdot HCl$ and a molecular weight of 343.9. It is freely soluble in water, ethanol, chloroform, and methanol, and has a pKa of 9.4.

The inactive ingredients in Kerlone are hydroxypropyl methylcellulose, lactose, magnesium stearate, polyethylene glycol 400, microcrystalline cellulose, colloidal silicon dioxide, sodium starch glycolate, and titanium dioxide.

Ophthalmic Solution: This sterile ophthalmic solution contains betaxolol HCl, a cardioselective beta-adrenergic receptor blocking agent, in a sterile isotonic solution. Betaxolol HCl is a white, crystalline powder, soluble in water, with a molecular weight of 343.89.

Empirical Formula: $C_{18}H_{29}NO_3HCl$

Chemical Name: (±)-1-[p-[2-(Cyclopropylmethoxy)ethyl]phenoxyl]- 3-(isopropylamino)-2-propanol HCl.

Each ml of Betopic ophthalmic solution (0.5%) contains: Active: 5.6 mg betaxolol HCl equivalent to betaxolol base 5 mg. Preservative: Benzalkonium Chloride).01%. Inactive: Edetate Di sodium, Sodium Chloride, Hydrochloric Acid and/or Sodium Hydroxide (to adjust pH), and Purified Water.

CLINICAL PHARMACOLOGY:

TABLETS

Betaxolol HCl is a β_1-selective (cardioselective) adrenergic receptor blocking agent that has weak membrane-stabilizing activity and no intrinsic sympathomimetic (partial agonist) activity. The preferential effect on β_1 receptors is not absolute, however, and some inhibitory effects on β_2 receptors (found chiefly in the bronchial and vascular musculature) can be expected at higher doses.

Pharmacokinetics and Metabolism

In man, absorption of an oral dose is complete. There is a small and consistent first-pass effect resulting in an absolute bioavailability of 89% ± 5% that is unaffected by the concomitant ingestion of food or alcohol. Mean peak blood concentrations of 21.6 ng/ml (range 16.3 to 27.9 ng/ml) are reached between 1.5 and 6 (mean about 3) hours after a single oral dose, in healthy volunteers, of 10 mg of betaxolol HCl. Peak concentrations for 20-mg and 40-mg doses are 2 and 4 times that of a 10-mg dose and have been shown to be linear over the dose range of 5 to 40 mg. The peak to trough ratio of plasma concentrations over 24 hours is 2.7. The mean elimination half-life in various studies in normal volunteers ranged from about 14 to 22 hours after single oral doses and is similar in chronic dosing. Steady state plasma concentrations are attained after 5 to 7 days with once-daily dosing in persons with normal renal function.

Betaxolol HCl is approximately 50% bound to plasma proteins. It is eliminated primarily by liver metabolism and secondarily by renal excretion. Following oral administration, greater than 80% of a dose is recovered in the urine as betaxolol and its metabolites. Approximately 15% of the dose administered is excreted as unchanged drug, the remainder being metabolites whose contribution to the clinical effect is negligible.

Steady state studies in normal volunteers and hypertensive patients found no important differences in kinetics. In patients with hepatic disease, elimination half-life was prolonged by about 33%, but clearance was unchanged, leading to little change in AUC. Dosage reductions have not routinely been necessary in these patients. In patients with chronic renal failure undergoing dialysis, mean elimination half-life was approximately doubled, as was AUC, indicating the need for a lower initial dosage (5 mg) in these patients. The clearance of betaxolol by hemodialysis was 0.015 L/h/kg and by peritoneal dialysis, 0.010 L/h/kg. Patients (n=8) with stable renal failure, not on dialysis, with mean creatinine clearance of 27 ml/min showed slight increases in elimination half-life and AUC, but no change in C_{max}. In a second study of 30 hypertensive patients with mild to severe renal impairment, there was a reduction in clearance of betaxolol with increasing degrees of renal insufficiency. Inulin clearance (ml/min/1.73m^2) ranged from 70 to 107 in 7 patients with mild impairment, 41 to 69 in 14 patients with moderate impairment, and 8 to 37 in 9 patients with severe impairment. Clearance following oral dosing was reduced significantly in patients with moderate and severe renal impairment (26% and 35%, respectively) when compared with those with mildly impaired renal function. In the severely impaired group, the mean C_{max} and the mean elimination half-life tended to increase (28% and 24%, respectively) when compared with the mildly impaired group. A starting dose of 5 mg is recommended in patients with severe renal impairment. (See DOSAGE AND ADMINISTRATION.)

Studies in elderly patients (n=10) gave inconsistent results but suggested some impairment of elimination, with one small study (n=4) finding a mean half-life of 30 hours. A starting dose of 5 mg is suggested in older patients.

Pharmacodynamics

Clinical pharmacology studies have demonstrated the beta-adrenergic receptor blocking activity of betaxolol HCl (1) reduction in resting and exercise heart rate, cardiac output, and cardiac work load, (2) reduction of systolic and diastolic blood pressure at rest and during exercise, (3) inhibition of isoproterenol-induced tachycardia, and (4) reduction of reflex orthostatic tachycardia.

The β_1 selectivity of betaxolol HCl in man was shown in three ways: (1) In normal subjects, 10- and 40-mg oral doses of betaxolol HCl, which reduced resting heart rate at least as much as 40 mg of propranolol, produced less inhibition of isoproterenol-induced increases in forearm blood flow and finger tremor than propranolol. In this study, 10 mg of betaxolol HCl was at least comparable to 50 mg of atenolol. Both doses of betaxolol HCl, and the one dose of atenolol, however, had more effect on the isoproterenol-induced changes than placebo (indicating some β_2 effect at clinical doses) and the higher dose of betaxolol HCl was more inhibitory than the lower. (2) In normal subjects, single intravenous doses of betaxolol and

CLINICAL PHARMACOLOGY: *(cont'd)*

propranolol, which produced equal effects on exercise-induced tachycardia, had differing effects on insulin-induced hypoglycemia, with propranolol, but not betaxolol, prolonging the hypoglycemia compared to placebo. Neither drug affected the maximum extent of the hypoglycemic response (3) In a single-blind crossover study in asthmatics (n=10), intravenous infusion over 30 minutes of low doses of betaxolol (1.5 mg) and propranolol (2 mg) had similar effects on resting heart rate but had differing effects on FEV_1 and forced vital capacity, with propranolol causing statistically significant (10% to 20%) reductions from baseline in mean values for both parameters white betaxolol had no effect on mean values. White blood levels were not measured, the dose of betaxolol used in this study would be expected to produce blood concentrations, at the time of the pulmonary function studies, considerably lower than those achieved during antihypertensive therapy with recommended doses of betaxolol HCl. In a randomized double-blind, placebo-controlled crossover (4 × 4 Latin Square) study in 10 asthmatics, betaxolol (about 5 or 10 mg IV) had little effect on isoproterenol-induced increases in FEV_1; in contrast, propranolol (about 7 mg IV) inhibited the response.

Consistent with its negative chronotropic effect, due to beta-blockade of the SA node, and lack of intrinsic sympathomimetic activity, betaxolol HCl increases sinus cycle length and sinus node recovery time. Conduction in the AV node is also prolonged.

Significant reductions in blood pressure and heart rate were observed 24 hours after dosing in double-blind, placebo-controlled trials with doses of 5 to 40 mg administered once daily. The antihypertensive response to betaxolol was similar at peak blood levels (3 to 4 hours) and at trough (24 hours). In a large randomized, parallel dose-response study of 5, 10, and 20 mg, the antihypertensive effects of the 5-mg dose were roughly half of the effects of the 20-mg dose (after adjustment for placebo effects) and the 10-mg dose gave more than 80% of the antihypertensive response to the 20-mg dose. The effect of increasing the dose from 10 mg to 20 mg was thus small. In this study, while the antihypertensive response to betaxolol showed a dose-response relationship, the heart rate response (reduction in HR) was not dose related. In other trials, there was little evidence of a greater antihypertensive response to 40 mg than to 20 mg. The maximum effect of each dose was achieved within 1 or 2 weeks. In comparative trials against propranolol, atenolol, and chlorthalidone, betaxolol appeared to be at least as effective as the comparative agent.

Betaxolol HCl has been studied in combination with thiazide-type diuretics and the blood pressure effects of the combination appear additive. Betaxolol HCl has also been used concurrently with methyldopa, hydralazine, and prazosin.

The mechanism of the antihypertensive effects of beta-adrenergic receptor blocking agents has not been established. Several possible mechanisms have been proposed, however, including: (1) competitive antagonism of catecholamines at peripheral (especially cardiac) adrenergic-neuronal sites, leading to decreased cardiac output, (2) a central effect leading to reduced sympathetic outflow to the periphery, and (3) suppression of renin activity.

The results from long-term studies have not shown any diminution of the antihypertensive effect of betaxolol HCl with prolonged use.

OPHTHALMIC SOLUTION

Betaxolol HCl, a cardioselective (beta-1-adrenergic) receptor blocking agent, does not have significant membrane-stabilizing (local anesthetic) activity and is devoid of intrinsic sympathomimetic action. Orally administered beta-adrenergic blocking agents reduce cardiac output in healthy subjects and patients with heart disease. In patients with severe impairment of myocardial function beta-adrenergic receptor antagonists may inhibit the sympathetic stimulatory effect necessary to maintain adequate cardiac function.

When instilled in the eye, betaxolol HCl ophthalmic solution has the action of reducing elevated as well as normal intraocular pressure, whether or not accompanied by glaucoma. Ophthalmic betaxolol has minimal effect on pulmonary and cardiovascular parameters.

Ophthalmic betaxolol (one drop in each eye) was compared to timolol and placebo in a three-way crossover study challenging nine patients with reactive airway disease who were selected on the basis of having at least a 15% reduction in the forced expiratory volume in one second (FEV_1) after administration of ophthalmic timolol. Betaxolol HCl had no significant effect on pulmonary function as measured by FEV_1, Forced Vital Capacity (FVC) and FEV_1/VC. Additionally, the action of isoproterenol, a beta stimulant, administered at the end of the study was not inhibited by ophthalmic betaxolol. In contrast, ophthalmic timolol significantly decreased these pulmonary functions (TABLE 1):

TABLE 1 FEV $_1$-Percent Change from Baseline[1]

	Betaxolol 1.0% a	Means Timolol 0.5%	Placebo
Baseline	1.6	1.4	1.4
60 Minutes	2.3	-25.7*	5.8
120 Minutes	1.6	-27.4*	7.5
240 Minutes	- 6.4	-26.9*	6.9
Isoproterenol b	36.1	-12.4*	42.8

1 Schoene, R.B., et al Am. J. Ophthal. 97:86, 1984.
a Twice the clinical concentration.
b Inhaled at 240 minutes; measurement at 270 minutes.
* Timolol statistically different from betaxolol and placebo($p<0.05$).

No evidence of cardiovascular beta-adrenergic blockade during exercise was observed with betaxolol in a double masked, three-way crossover study in 24 normal subjects comparing ophthalmic betaxolol, timolol and placebo for effect on blood pressure and heart rate. Mean arterial blood pressure was not affected by any treatment; however, ophthalmic timolol produced a significant decrease in the mean heart rate (TABLE 2):

TABLE 2 Mean Heart Rates [1]
Treatment, Bruce Stress Exercise Test

Minutes	Betaxolol 1%[a]	Timolol 0.5%	Placebo
0	79.2	79.3	81.2
2	130.2	126.0	130.4
4	133.4	128.0*	134.3
6	136.4	129.0*	137.9
8	139.8	131.8*	139.4
10	140.8	131.8*	141.3

1 Atkins, J.M., *et al* Am. J. Oph. 99:173-175, Feb., 1985.
a Twice the clinical concentration
* Mean pulse rate significantly lower for timolol than betaxolol or placebo ($p<0.05$).

Clinical Studies: Optic nerve head damage and visual field loss are the result of a sustained elevated intraocular pressure and poor ocular perfusion. Betaxolol HCl ophthalmic solution has the action of reducing elevated as well as normal intraocular pressure and the mechanism of ocular hypotensive action appears to be a reduction of aqueous production as demonstrated by tonography and aqueous fluorophotometry. The onset of action with betaxolol HCl ophthalmic solution can generally be noted within 30 minutes and the maximal effect can usually be detected 2 hours after topical administration. A single dose provides a 12-hour reduction in intraocular pressure. Clinical observation of glaucoma patients treated with betaxolol HCl ophthalmic solution for up to three years shows that the intraocular pressure lowering effect is well maintained.

Clinical studies show that topical betaxolol HCl ophthalmic solution reduces mean intraocular pressure 25% from baseline. In trials using 22 mmHg as a generally accepted index of intraocular pressure control, betaxolol HCl ophthalmic solution was effective in more than 94% of the population studied, of which 73% were treated with the beta blocker alone. In controlled, double-masked studies, the magnitude and duration of the ocular hypotensive effect of betaxolol HCl ophthalmic solution and ophthalmic timolol solution were clinically equivalent.

Betaxolol HCl ophthalmic solution has also been used successfully in glaucoma patients who have undergone a laser trabeculoplasty and have needed additional long-term ocular hypotensive therapy.

Betaxolol HCl ophthalmic solution has been well-tolerated in glaucoma patients wearing hard or soft contact lenses and in aphakic patients.

Betaxolol HCl ophthalmic solution does not produce miosis or accommodative spasm which are frequently seen with miotic agents. The blurred vision and night blindness often associated with standard miotic therapy are not associated with betaxolol HCl ophthalmic solution. Thus, patients with central lenticular opacities avoid the visual impairment caused by a constricted pupil.

INDICATIONS AND USAGE:

Tablets: Betaxolol HCl is indicated in the management of hypertension. It may be used alone or concomitantly with other antihypertensive agents, particularly thiazide-type diuretics.

Ophthalmic Solution: Betaxolol HCl ophthalmic solution has been shown to be effective in lowering intraocular pressure and is indicated in the treatment of ocular hypertension and chronic open-angle glaucoma. It may be used alone or in combination with other anti-glaucoma drugs.

In clinical studies Betaxolol HCl safely controlled the intraocular pressure of 47 patients with glaucoma and reactive airway disease followed for a mean period of 15 months. However, caution should be used in treating patients with severe reactive airway disease.

CONTRAINDICATIONS:

Tablets: Betaxolol HCl is contraindicated in patients with known hypersensitivity to the drug. Betaxolol HCl is contraindicated in patients with sinus bradycardia, heart block greater than first degree, cardiogenic shock, and overt cardiac failure (see WARNINGS).

Ophthalmic Solution: Hypersensitivity to any component of this product.

Betaxolol HCl ophthalmic solution is contraindicated in patients with sinus bradycardia, greater than a first degree atrioventricular block, cardiogenic shock, or patients with overt cardiac failure.

WARNINGS:

TABLETS

Cardiac Failure: Sympathetic stimulation may be a vital component supporting circulatory function in congestive heart failure, and beta-adrenergic receptor blockade carries the potential hazard of further depressing myocardial contractility and precipitating more severe heart failure. In hypertensive patients who have congestive heart failure controlled by digitalis and diuretics, beta-blockers should be administered cautiously. Both digitalis and beta-adrenergic receptor blocking agents slow AV conduction.

In Patients Without a History of Cardiac Failure: Continued depression of the myocardium with beta-blocking agents over a period of time can, in some cases, lead to cardiac failure. Therefore, at the first sign or symptom of cardiac failure, discontinuation of betaxolol HCl should be considered. In some cases beta-blocker therapy can be continued while cardiac failure is treated with cardiac glycosides, diuretics, and other agents, as appropriate.

Exacerbation of Angina Pectoris Upon Withdrawal: Abrupt cessation of therapy with certain beta-blocking agents in patients with coronary artery disease has been followed by exacerbations of angina pectoris and, in some cases, myocardial infarction has been reported. Therefore, such patients should be warned against interruption of therapy without the physician's advice. Even in the absence of overt angina pectoris, when discontinuation of betaxolol HCl is planned, the patient should be carefully observed and therapy should be reinstituted, at least temporarily, if withdrawal symptoms occur.

Bronchospastic Diseases: PATIENTS WITH BRONCHOSPASTIC DISEASE SHOULD NOT IN GENERAL RECEIVE BETA-BLOCKERS. Because of its relative β_1 selectively (cardioselectivity), low doses of betaxolol HCl may be used with caution in patients with bronchospastic disease who do not respond to or cannot tolerate alternative treatment. Since β_1 selectivity is not absolute and is inversely related to dose, the lowest possible dose of betaxolol HCl should be used (5 to 10 mg once daily) and a bronchodilator should be made available. If dosage must be increased, divided dosage should be considered to avoid the higher peak blood levels associated with once-daily dosing.

Anesthesia and Major Surgery: The necessary, or desirability, of withdrawal of a beta-blocking therapy prior to major surgery is controversial. Beta-adrenergic receptor blockade impairs the ability of the heart to respond to beta-adrenergically mediated reflex stimuli. While this might be of benefit in preventing arrhythmic response, the risk of excessive myocardial depression during general anesthesia may be increased and difficulty in restarting and maintaining the heart beat has been reported with beta-blockers. If treatment is continued, particular care should be taken when using anesthetic agents which depress the myocardium, such as ether, cyclopropane, and trichloroethylene, and it is prudent to use the lowest possible dose of betaxolol HCl. Betaxolol HCl, like other beta-blockers, is a competitive inhibitor of beta-receptor agonists and its effect on the heart can be reversed by cautious administration of such agents (*e.g.,* dobutamine or isoproterenol—see OVERDOSAGE). Manifestations of excessive vagal tone (*e.g.,* profound bradycardia, hypotension) may be corrected with atropine 1 to 3 mg IV in divided doses.

Diabetes and Hypoglycemia: Beta-blockers should be used with caution in diabetic patients. Beta-blockers may mask tachycardia occurring with hypoglycemia (patients should be warned of this), although other manifestations such as dizziness and sweating may not be significantly affected. Unlike nonselective beta-blockers, betaxolol HCl does not prolong insulin-induced hypoglycemia.

Thyrotoxicosis: Beta-adrenergic blockade may mask certain clinical signs of hyperthyroidism (*e.g.,* tachycardia). Abrupt withdrawal of beta-blockade might precipitate a thyroid storm; therefore, patients known or suspected of being thyrotoxic from whom betaxolol HCl is to be withdrawn should be monitored closely (see DOSAGE AND ADMINISTRATION, Cessation of therapy).

OPHTHALMIC SOLUTION

Although betaxolol HCl ophthalmic solution has had little or no effect on heart rate or blood pressure in clinical studies, caution should be observed in treating patients with a history of cardiac failure. Treatment with betaxolol HCl ophthalmic solution should be discontinued at the first signs of cardiac failure.

PRECAUTIONS:

GENERAL

Tablets

Beta-adrenoceptor blockade can cause reduction of intraocular pressure. Since betaxolol HCl is marketed as an ophthalmic solution for treatment of glaucoma, patients should be told that betaxolol HCl may interfere with the glaucoma-screening test. Withdrawal may lead to a return of increased intraocular pressure. Patients receiving beta-adrenergic blocking agents orally and beta-blocking ophthalmic solutions should be observed for potential additive effects either on the intraocular pressure or on the known systemic effects of beta-blockade.

Impairment Hepatic or Renal Function: Betaxolol HCl is primarily metabolized in the liver to metabolites that are inactive and then excreted by the kidneys; clearance is somewhat reduced in patients with renal failure but little changed in patients with hepatic disease. Dosage reductions have not routinely been necessary when hepatic and/or renal insufficiency is present (see DOSAGE AND ADMINISTRATION) but patients should be observed. Patients with severe renal impairment and those on dialysis require a reduced dose. (See DOSAGE AND ADMINISTRATION.)

Ophthalmic Solution

Patients who are receiving a beta-adrenergic blocking agent orally and betaxolol HCl ophthalmic solution should be observed for a potential additive effect either on the intraocular pressure or on the known systemic effects of beta blockade.

While betaxolol HCl ophthalmic solution has demonstrated a low potential for systemic effect, it should be used with caution in patients with diabetes (especially labile diabetes) because of possible masking of signs and symptoms of acute hypoglycemia. Beta-adrenergic blocking agents may mask certain signs and symptoms of hyperthyroidism and their abrupt withdrawal might precipitate a thyroid storm.

Consideration should be given to the gradual withdrawal of beta-adrenergic blocking agents prior to general anesthesia because of the reduced ability of the heart to respond to beta-adrenergically mediated sympathetic reflex stimuli.

Pulmonary: Betaxolol HCl ophthalmic solution, a cardioselective beta-blocker, has produced only minimal effects in patients with reactive airway disease; however, caution should be exercised in the treatment of patients with excessive restriction of pulmonary function.

Ocular: In patients with angle-closure glaucoma, the immediate treatment objective is to re-open the angle by constriction of the pupil with a miotic agent. Betaxolol has no effect on the pupil; therefore, betaxolol HCl ophthalmic solution should be used with a miotic to reduce elevated intraocular pressure in angle-closure glaucoma.

As with the use of other antiglaucoma drugs, diminished responsiveness to betaxolol HCl ophthalmic solution after prolonged therapy has been reported in some patients. However in one long-term study in which 250 patients have been followed for a mean period of two years, no significant difference in mean intraocular pressure has been observed after initial stabilization.

Animal Studies: No adverse ocular effects were observed following topical ocular administration of betaxolol HCl ophthalmic solution to rabbits for one year.

INFORMATION FOR THE PATIENT

Tablets: Patients, especially those with evidence of coronary artery insufficiency, should be warned against interruption or discontinuation of betaxolol HCl therapy without the physician's advice.

Although cardiac failure rarely occurs in appropriately selected patients, patients being treated with beta-adrenergic blocking agents should be advised to consult a physician at the first sign or symptom of failure.

Patients should know how they react to this medicine before they operate automobiles and machinery or engage in other tasks requiring alertness. Patients should contact their physician if any difficulty in breathing occurs, and before surgery of any type. Patients should inform their physicians or dentists that they are taking betaxolol HCl. Patients with diabetes should be warned that beta-blockers may mask tachycardia occurring with hypoglycemia.

CARCINOGENESIS, MUTAGENESIS, AND IMPAIRMENT OF FERTILITY

Tablets: Lifetime studies with betaxolol HCl in mice at oral dosages of 6, 20, and 60 mg/kg/day (up to 90 × the maximum recommended human dose (MRHD) based on 60-kg body weight) and in rats at 3, 12, or 48 mg/kg/day (up to 72 × MRHD) showed no evidence of a carcinogenic effect. In a variety of *in vitro* and *in vivo* bacterial and mammalian cell assays, betaxolol HCl was nonmutagenic. Betaxolol did not adversely affect fertility or mating performance of male or female rats at doses up to 256 mg/kg/day (380 × MRHD).

Ophthalmic Solution: Lifetime studies with betaxolol HCl have been completed in mice at oral doses of 6, 20 or 60 mg/kg/day and in rats at 3, 12 or 48 mg/kg/day; betaxolol HCl demonstrated no carcinogenic effect. Higher dose levels were not tested. In a variety of *in vitro* and *in vivo* bacterial and mammalian cell assays, betaxolol HCl was nonmutagenic.

PREGNANCY CATEGORY C

Tablets: In a study in which pregnant rats received betaxolol at doses of 4, 40, or 400 mg/kg/day, the highest dose (600 × MRHD) was associated with increased postimplantation loss, reduced litter size and weight, and an increased incidence of skeletal and visceral abnormalities, which may have been a consequence of drug-related maternal toxicity. Other than a possible increased incidence of incomplete descent of testes and sternebral reductions, betaxolol at 4 mg/kg/day and 40 mg/kg/day (6 × MRHD and 60 × MRHD) caused no fetal abnormalities. In a second study with a different strain of rat, 200 mg betaxolol/kg/day (300 × MRHD) was associated with maternal toxicity and an increase in resorptions, but no teratogenicity. In a study in which pregnant rabbits received doses of 1, 4, 12, or 36 mg betaxolol/kg/day (54 × MRHD), a marked increase in postimplantation loss occurred at the highest dose, but no drug-related teratogenicity was observed. The rabbit is more sensitive to betaxolol than other species because of higher bioavailability resulting from saturation on the first-pass effect. In a peri- and postnatal study in rats at doses of 4, 32, and 256 mg betaxolol/kg/day (380 × MRHD), the highest dose was associated with a marked increase in total litter loss within 4 days postpartum. In surviving offspring, growth and development were also affected.

There are no adequate and well-controlled studies in pregnant women. Betaxolol HCl should be used during pregnancy only if the potential benefit justifies the potential risk to the fetus.

Ophthalmic Solution: Reproduction, teratology, and perinatal and postnatal studies have been conducted with orally administered betaxolol HCl in rats and rabbits. There was evidence of drug related post-implantation loss in rabbits and rats at dose levels above 12 mg/kg and 128 mg/kg, respectively. Betaxolol HCl was not shown to be teratogenic, however, and there were no other adverse effects on reproduction at subtoxic dose levels. There are, however, no adequate and well-controlled studies in pregnant women. Because animal reproductive studies are not always predictive of human response, this drug should be used during pregnancy only if clearly indicated.

NURSING MOTHERS

Tablets: Since betaxolol HCl is excreted in human milk in sufficient amounts to have pharmacological effects in the infant, caution should be exercised when betaxolol HCl is administered to a nursing mother.

PRECAUTIONS: *(cont'd)*

Ophthalmic Solution: It is not known whether betaxolol HCl ophthalmic solution is excreted in human milk. Because many drugs are excreted in human milk, caution should be exercised when betaxolol HCl ophthalmic solution is administered to nursing women.

PEDIATRIC USE

Safety and efficacy in children have not been established.

GERIATRIC USE

Tablets: Betaxolol HCl may produce bradycardia more frequently in elderly patients. In general, patients 65 years of age and older had a higher incidence rate of bradycardia (hear rate <50 BPM) than younger patients in U.S. clinical trials. In a double-blind study in Europe, 19 elderly patients (mean age = 82) received betaxolol 20 mg daily. Dosage reduction to 10 mg or discontinuation was required for 6 patients due to bradycardia (See DOSAGE AND ADMINISTRATION).

DRUG INTERACTIONS:

TABLETS

The following drugs have been coadministered with betaxolol HCl and have not altered its pharmacokinetics: cimetidine, nifedipine, chlorthalidone, and hydrochlorothiazide. Concomitant administration of betaxolol HCl with the oral anticoagulant warfarin has been shown not to potentiate the anticoagulant effect of warfarin.

Catecholamine-depleting drugs (*e.g.,* reserpine) may have an additive effect when given with beta-blocking agents. Patients treated with a beta-adrenergic receptor blocking agent plus a catecholamine depletor should therefore be closely observed for evidence of hypotension or marked bradycardia, which may produce vertigo, syncope, or postural hypotension.

Should it be decided to discontinue therapy in patients receiving beta-blockers and clonidine concurrently, the beta-blocker should be discontinued slowly over several days before the gradual withdrawal of clonidine.

Literature reports suggest that oral calcium antagonists may be used in combination with beta-adrenergic blocking agents when heart function is normal, but should be avoided in patients with impaired cardiac function. Hypotension, AV conduction disturbances, and left ventricular failure have been reported in some patients receiving beta-adrenergic blocking agents when an oral calcium antagonist was added to the treatment regimen. Hypotension was more likely to occur if the calcium antagonist were a dihydropyridine derivative, (*e.g.,* nifedipine), while left ventricular failure and AV conduction disturbances, including, complete heart block, were more likely to occur with either verapamil or diltiazem.

Risk of Anaphylactic Reaction: Although it is known that patients on beta-blockers may be refractory to epinephrine in the treatment of anaphylactic shock, beta-blockers can, in addition, interfere with the modulation of allergic reaction and lead to an increased severity and/or frequency of attacks. Severe allergic reactions including anaphylaxis have been reported in patients exposed to a variety of allergens either by repeated challenge, or accidental contact, and with diagnostic or therapeutic agents while receiving beta-blockers. Such patients may be unresponsive to the usual doses of epinephrine used to treat allergic reaction.

OPHTHALMIC SOLUTION

Although betaxolol HCl ophthalmic solution used alone has little or no effect on pupil size, mydriasis resulting from concomitant therapy with betaxolol HCl ophthalmic solution and epinephrine has been reported occasionally. Close observation of the patient is recommended when a beta-blocker is administered to patients receiving catecholamine-depleting drugs such as reserpine, because of possible additive effects and the production of hypotension and/or bradycardia. Caution should be exercised in patients using concomitant adrenergic psychotropic drugs.

ADVERSE REACTIONS:

TABLETS

Most adverse reactions have been mild and transient and are typical of beta-adrenergic blocking agents, (*e.g.,* bradycardia, fatigue, dyspnea, and lethargy). Withdrawal of therapy in U.S. and European controlled clinical trials has been necessary in about 3.5% of patients, principally because of bradycardia, fatigue, dizziness, headache, and impotence. Frequency estimates of adverse events were derived from controlled studies in which adverse reactions were volunteered and elicited in U.S. studies and volunteered and/or elicited in European studies.

In the U.S., the placebo-controlled hypertension studies lasted for 4 weeks, while the active-controlled hypertension studies had a 22- to 24-week double-blind phase. The following doses were studied: betaxolol—5, 10, 20, and 40 mg once daily; atenolol—25, 50, and 100 mg once daily; and propranolol—40, 80, and 160 mg b.i.d.

Betaxolol HCl, like other beta-blockers, has been associated with the development of antinuclear antibodies (ANA). In controlled clinical studies, conversion of ANA from negative to positive occurred in 5.3% of the patients treated with betaxolol, 6.3% of the patients treated with atenolol, 4.9% of the patients treated with propranolol, and 3.2% of the patients treated with placebo.

Betaxolol adverse events reported with a 2% or greater frequency, and selected events with lower frequency, in U.S. controlled studies are in TABLE 3:

Of the above adverse reactions associated with the use of betaxolol, only bradycardia was clearly dose related, but there was a suggestion of dose relatedness for fatigue, lethargy, and dyspepsia.

In Europe, the placebo-controlled study lasted for 4 weeks, while the comparative studies had a 4- to 52-week double-blind phase. The following doses were studied: betaxolol 20 and 40 mg once daily and atenolol 100 mg once daily.

From European controlled clinical trials, the following adverse events reported by 2% or more patients and selected events with lower frequency are presented in TABLE 4:

The only adverse event whose frequency clearly rose with increasing dose was bradycardia. Elderly patients were especially susceptible to bradycardia, which in some cases responded to dose-reduction (see PRECAUTIONS).

The following selected (potentially important) adverse events have been reported at an incidence of less than 2% in U.S. controlled and open, long-term clinical studies, European controlled clinical trials, or in marketing experience. It is not known whether a causal relationship exists between betaxolol and these events; they are listed to alert the physician to a possible relationship:

Autonomic: flushing, salivation, sweating.

Body as a Whole: allergy, fever, malaise, pain, rigors.

Cardiovascular: angina pectoris, arrhythmia, heart failure, hypertension, hypotension, myocardial infarction, thrombosis, syncope.

Central and Peripheral Nervous System: neuropathy, numbness, speech disorder, stupor, tremor, twitching.

Gastrointestinal: anorexia, constipation, dry mouth, increased appetite, mouth ulceration, rectal disorders, vomiting, dysphagia.

Hearing and Vestibular: earache, labyrinth disorders, tinnitus, deafness.

Hematologic: leucocytosis, lymphadenopathy, thrombocytopenia.

ADVERSE REACTIONS: *(cont'd)*

TABLE 3

Body System/Adverse Reaction	Betaxolol (N=509)	Propranolol (N=73)	Atenolol (N=75)	Placebo (N=109)
Dose Range	5-40 mg qd*	40-160 mg bid	25-100 mg qd	
	(%)	(%)	(%)	(%)
Cardiovascular				
Bradycardia (heart rate >50 BPM)	8.1	4.1	12.0	0
Symptomatic Bradycardia	0.8	1.4	0	0
Edema	1.8	0	0	1.8
Central Nervous System				
Headache	6.5	4.1	5.3	15.6
Dizziness	4.5	11.0	2.7	5.5
Fatigue	2.9	9.6	4.0	0
Lethargy	2.8	4.1	2.7	0.9
Psychiatric				
Insomnia	1.2	8.2	2.7	0
Nervousness	0.8	1.4	2.7	0
Bizarre Dreams	1.0	2.7	1.3	0
Depression	0.8	2.7	4.0	0
Autonomic				
Impotence	1.2†	0	0	0
Respiratory				
Dyspnea	2.4	2.7	1.3	0.9
Pharyngitis	2.0	0	4.0	0.9
Rhinitis	1.4	0	4.0	0.9
Upper Respiratory Infection	2.6	0	0	5.5
Gastrointestinal				
Dyspepsia	4.7	6.8	2.7	0.9
Nausea	1.6	1.4	4.0	0
Diarrhea	2.0	6.8	8.0	0.9
Musculoskeletal				
Chest pain	2.4	1.4	2.7	0.9
Arthralgia	3.1	0	4.0	1.8
Skin				
Rash	1.2	0	0	0

* Five patients received 80 mg q.i.d.
† N=336 males; impotence is a known possible adverse effect of this pharmacological class.

TABLE 4

Body System/Adverse Reaction	Betaxolol (N=155)	Atenolol (N=81)	Placebo (N=60)
Dose Range	20-40 mg g.d.	100 mg q.d	
	(%)	(%)	(%)
Cardiovascular			
Bradycardia (heart rate <50 BPM)	5.8	5.0	0
Symptomatic Bradycardia	1.9	2.5	0
Palpitation	1.9	3.7	1.7
Edema	1.3	1.2	0
Cold Extremities	1.9	0	0
Central Nervous System			
Headache	14.8	9.9	23.3
Dizziness	14.8	17.3	15.0
Fatigue	9.7	18.5	0
Asthenia	7.1	0	16.7
Insomnia	5.0	3.7	3.3
Paresthesia	1.9	2.5	0
Gastrointestinal			
Nausea	5.8	1.2	0
Dyspepsia	3.9	7.4	3.3
Diarrhea	1.9	3.7	0
Musculoskeletal			
Chest Pain	7.1	6.2	5.0
Joint Pain	5.2	4.9	1.7
Myalgia	3.2	3.7	3.3

Liver and Biliary: increased AST, increased ALT.

Metabolic and Nutritional: acidosis, diabetes, hypercholesterolemia, hyperglycemia, hyperkalemia, hyperlipemia, hyperuricemia, hypokalemia, weight gain, increased LDH.

Musculoskeletal: arthropathy, neck pain, muscle cramps tendonitis.

Psychiatric: abnormal thinking, amnesia, confusion, emotional lability, hallucinations, decreased libido.

Reproductive Disorders: *Female:*breast pain, breast fibroadenosis, menstrual disorder; *Male:* Peyronie's disease, prostatitis.

Respiratory: bronchitis, bronchospasm, cough, epistaxis, flu, pneumonia, sinusitis.

Skin: alopecia, eczema, erythematous rash, hypertrichosis, pruritus, skin disorders.

Special Senses: abnormal taste, taste loss.

Urinary System: cystitis, dysuria, proteinuria, abnormal renal function, renal pain.

Vascular: cerebrovascular disorder, intermittent claudication, leg cramps, peripheral ischemia, thrombophlebitis.

Vision: abnormal lacrimation, abnormal vision, blepharitis, ocular hemorrhage, conjunctivitis, dry eyes, iritis, cataract, scotoma.

Potential Adverse Effects: Although not reported in clinical studies with betaxolol, a variety of adverse effects have been reported with other beta-adrenergic blocking agents and may be considered potential adverse effects of betaxolol.

Central Nervous System: Reversible mental depression progressing to catatonia, an acute reversible syndrome characterized by disorientation for time and place, short-term memory loss, emotional lability with slightly clouded sensorium, and decreased performance on neuropsychometric tests.

Allergic: Erythematous rash, fever combined with aching and sore throat, laryngospasm, respiratory distress.

Hematologic: Agranulocytosis, thrombocytopenic purpura, and nonthrombocytopenic purpura.

Gastrointestinal: Mesenteric arterial thrombosis, ischemic colitis.

ADVERSE REACTIONS: *(cont'd)*

Miscellaneous: Raynaud's phenomena. There have been reports of skin rashes and/or dry eyes associated with the use of beta-adrenergic blocking drugs. The reported incidence is small, and in most cases, the symptoms have cleared when treatment was withdrawn. Discontinuation of the drug should be considered if any such reaction is not otherwise explicable. Patients should be closely monitored following cessation of therapy.

The oculomucocutaneous syndrome associated with the beta-blocker practolol has not been reported with betaxolol HCl during investigational use and extensive foreign experience. However, dry eyes have been reported.

OPHTHALMIC SOLUTION

The following adverse reactions have been reported in clinical trials with betaxolol HCl ophthalmic solution.

Ocular: Betaxolol HCl ophthalmic solution has been well tolerated. Discomfort of short duration was experienced by one in four patients, but none discontinued therapy; occasional tearing has been reported. Rare instances of decreased corneal sensitivity, erythema, itching sensation, corneal punctate staining, keratitis, anisocoria and photophobia have been reported.

Systemic: Systemic reactions following topical administration of betaxolol HCl ophthalmic solution have been reported rarely (*e.g.*, insomnia and depressive neurosis).

OVERDOSAGE:

TABLETS

No specific information on emergency treatment of overdosage with betaxolol HCl is available. The most common effects expected are bradycardia, congestive heart failure, hypotension, bronchospasm, and hypoglycemia. In one acute overdosage of betaxolol, a 16 year-old female recovered fully after ingesting 460 mg.

Oral LD_{50}s are 350 to 400 mg betaxolol/kg in mice and 860 to 980 mg/kg in rats.

In the case of overdosage, treatment with betaxolol HCl should be stopped and the patient carefully observed. Hemodialysis or peritoneal dialysis does not remove substantial amounts of the drug. In addition to gastric lavage, the following therapeutic measures are suggested if warranted:

Hypotension: Use sympathomimetic pressor drug therapy, such as dopamine, dobutamine, or norepinephrine. If refractory cases of overdosage of other beta-blockers, the use of glucagon HCl has been reported to be useful.

Bradycardia: Atropine should be administered. If there is no response to vagal blockade, isoproterenol should be administered cautiously. If refractory cases the use of a transvenous cardiac pacemaker may be considered.

Acute Cardiac Failure: Conventional therapy including digitalis, diuretics, and oxygen should be instituted immediately.

Bronchospasm: Use a β_2-agonist. Additional therapy with aminophylline may be considered.

Heart Block (2nd- or 3rd-degree): Use isoproterenol or a transvenous cardiac pacemaker.

OPHTHALMIC SOLUTION

No information is available on overdosage of humans. The oral LD_{50} if the drug ranged from 350-920 mg/kg in mice and 860-1050 mg/kg in rats. The symptoms which might be expected with an overdose of a systemically administered beta-1-adrenergic receptor blocker agent are bradycardia, hypotension and acute cardiac failure.

A topical overdose of betaxolol HCl ophthalmic solution may be flushed from the eye(s) with warm tap water.

DOSAGE AND ADMINISTRATION:

TABLETS

The initial dose of betaxolol HCl in hypertension is ordinarily 10 mg once daily either alone or added to diuretic therapy. The full antihypertensive effect is usually seen within 7 to 14 days. If the desired response is not achieved the dose can be doubled after 7 to 14 days. Increasing the dose beyond 20 mg has not been shown to produce a statistically significant additional antihypertensive effect; but the 40-mg dose has been studied and is well tolerated. An increased effect (reduction) on heart rate should be anticipated with increasing dosage. If monotherapy with betaxolol HCl does not produce the desired response, the addition of a diuretic agent or other antihypertensive should be considered (see DRUG INTERACTIONS).

DOSAGE ADJUSTMENT FOR SPECIFIC PATIENTS

Patients With Renal Failure: In patients with renal impairment, clearance of betaxolol declines with decreasing renal function.

In patients with severe renal impairment and those undergoing dialysis, the initial dose of betaxolol HCl is 5 mg once daily. If the desired response in not achieved, dosage may be increased by 5 mg/day increments every 2 weeks to a maximum dose of 20 mg/day.

Patients With Hepatic Disease: Patients with hepatic disease do not have significantly altered clearance. Dosage adjustments are not routinely needed.

Elderly Patients: Consideration should be given to reduction in the starting dose to 5 mg in elderly patients. These patients are especially prone to beta-blocker-induced bradycardia, which appears to be dose related and sometimes responds to reductions in dose.

Cessation of Therapy: If withdrawal of betaxolol HCl therapy is planned, it should be achieved gradually over a period of about 2 weeks. Patients should be carefully observed and advised to limit physical activity to a minimum.

OPHTHALMIC SOLUTION

The usual dose is one drop of betaxolol HCl ophthalmic solution in the affected eye(s) twice daily. In some patients, the intraocular pressure lowering response to betaxolol HCl ophthalmic solution may require a few weeks to stabilize. Clinical follow-up should include a determination of the intraocular pressure during the first month of treatment with betaxolol HCl ophthalmic solution. Thereafter, intraocular pressures should be determined on an individual basis at the judgment of the physician.

When a patient is transferred from a single anti-glaucoma agent, continue the agent already used and add one drop of betaxolol HCl ophthalmic solution in the affected eye(s) twice a day. On the following day, discontinue the previous anti-glaucoma agent completely and continue with betaxolol HCl ophthalmic solution.

Because of diurnal variations of intraocular pressure in individual patients, satisfactory response to twice a day therapy is best determined by measuring intraocular pressure at different times during the day. Intraocular pressures ≤22 mmHg may not be optimal for control of glaucoma in each patient; therefore, therapy should be individualized.

If the intraocular pressure of the patient is not adequately controlled on this regimen, concomitant therapy with pilocarpine, other miotics, epinephrine or systemically administered carbonic anhydrase inhibitors can be instituted.

When a patient is transferred from several concomitantly administered anti-glaucoma agents, individualization is required. Adjustment should involve one agent at a time made at intervals of not less than one week. A recommended approach is to continue the agents being used and add one drop of betaxolol HCl ophthalmic solution in the affected eye(s) twice a day. On the following day, discontinue one of the other anti-glaucoma agents. The remaining

DOSAGE AND ADMINISTRATION: *(cont'd)*

anti-glaucoma agents may be decreased or discontinued according to the patient's response to treatment. The physician may be able to discontinue some or all of the other anti-glaucoma agents.

HOW SUPPLIED:

Kerlone 10-mg tablets are round, white, film coated, with KERLONE 10 debossed on one side and scored on the other.

Kerlone 20–mg tablets are round, white, film coated, with KERLONE 20 debossed on one side and β on the other.

Store at room temperature, below 86°F (30°C).

HOW SUPPLIED - EQUIVALENTS NOT AVAILABLE:

Solution - Ophthalmic - 0.25 %

2.5 ml	$10.00	BETOPTIC S OPHTHALMIC, Alcon	00065-0246-20
5 ml	$19.38	BETOPTIC S, Alcon	00065-0246-05
10 ml	$36.56	BETOPTIC S, Alcon	00065-0246-10
15 ml	$54.06	BETOPTIC S, Alcon	00065-0246-15

Solution - Ophthalmic - 0.5 %

2.5 ml	$10.00	BETOPTIC, Alcon	00065-0245-20
5 ml	$19.38	BETOPTIC, Alcon	00065-0245-05
10 ml	$36.56	BETOPTIC, Alcon	00065-0245-10
15 ml	$54.06	BETOPTIC, Alcon	00065-0245-15

Tablet, Plain Coated - Oral - 10 mg

100's	$72.04	KERLONE 10, Searle	00025-5101-31
100's	$75.64	KERLONE 10, Searle	00025-5101-34

Tablet, Plain Coated - Oral - 20 mg

100's	$108.03	KERLONE 20, Searle	00025-5201-31

BETAXOLOL HYDROCHLORIDE; CHLORTHALIDONE *(003144)*

CATEGORIES: Antihypertensives; Beta Adrenergic Blocking Agents; Beta Blockers; Cardiovascular Drugs; Diuretics; Hypertension; Pregnancy Category C; FDA Approved 1992 Oct

BRAND NAMES: **Kerledex**

Prescribing information not available at time of publication.

BETHANECHOL CHLORIDE *(000470)*

CATEGORIES: Autonomic Drugs; Cholinergics; Parasympathomimetic Agents; Relaxants/Stimulants, Urinary Tract; Renal Drugs; Urinary Retention; Esophagitis*; Pain*; Pregnancy Category C; FDA Approval Pre 1982
* Indication not approved by the FDA

BRAND NAMES: *Besacolin*; Duvoid; *Muscaran*; *Myo Hermes*; *Myocholine*; *Myocholine-Glenwood* (Germany); *Myocholine Glenwood*; Myotonachol; *Myotonine*; *Myotonine Chloride* (England); **Urecholine**; *Urocarb*
(International brand names outside U.S. in italics)

FORMULARIES: Aetna; BC-BS; FHP; Medi-Cal; PCS

DESCRIPTION:

Bethanechol chloride, a cholinergic agent, is a synthetic ester which is structurally and pharmacologically related to acetylcholine.

It is designated chemically as 2-((aminocarbonyl) oxy)-*N,N,N*-trimethyl-1-propanaminium chloride. Its empirical formula is $C_7H_{17}ClN_2O_2$.

It is a white, hygroscopic crystalline compound having a slight amine-like odor, freely soluble in water, and has a molecular weight of 196.68.

Bethanechol chloride is supplied as 5 mg, 10 mg, 25 mg, and 50 mg tablets for oral use. Inactive ingredients in the tablets are calcium phosphate, lactose, magnesium stearate, and starch. Tablets bethanechol chloride 10 mg also contain FD&C Red 3 and FD&C Red 40. Tablets bethanechol chloride 25 mg and 50 mg also contain D&C Yellow 10 and FD&C Yellow 6.

Bethanechol chloride is also supplied as a sterile solution **for subcutaneous use only**. The sterile solution is essentially neutral. Each milliliter contains bethanechol chloride, 5 mg, and Water for Injection, q.s., 1 ml. It may be autoclaved at 120°C for 20 minutes without discoloration or loss of potency.

CLINICAL PHARMACOLOGY:

Bethanechol chloride acts principally by producing the effects of stimulation of the parasympathetic nervous system. It increases the tone of the detrusor urinae muscle, usually producing a contraction sufficiently strong to initiate micturition and empty the bladder. It stimulates gastric motility, increases gastric tone, and often restores impaired rhythmic peristalsis.

Stimulation of the parasympathetic nervous system releases acetylcholine at the nerve endings. When spontaneous stimulation is reduced and therapeutic intervention is required, acetylcholine can be given, but it is rapidly hydrolyzed by cholinesterase, and its effects are transient. Bethanechol chloride is not destroyed by cholinesterase and its effects are more prolonged than those of acetylcholine.

Effects on the GI and urinary tracts sometimes appear within 30 minutes after oral administration of bethanechol chloride, but more often 60-90 minutes are required to reach maximum effectiveness. Following oral administration, the usual duration of action of bethanechol is one hour, although large doses (300-400 mg) have been reported to produce effects for up to six hours. Subcutaneous injection produces a more intense action on bladder muscle than does oral administration of the drug.

Because of the selective action of bethanechol, nicotinic symptoms of cholinergic stimulation are usually absent or minimal when orally or subcutaneously administered in therapeutic doses, while muscarinic effects are prominent. Muscarinic effects usually occur within 5-15 minutes after subcutaneous injection, reach a maximum in 15-30 minutes, and disappear within two hours. Doses that stimulate micturition and defecation and increase peristalsis do not ordinarily stimulate ganglia or voluntary muscles. Therapeutic test doses in normal human subjects have little effect on heart rate, blood pressure, or peripheral circulation.

Bethanechol chloride does not cross the blood-brain barrier because of its charged quaternary amine moiety. The metabolic fate and mode of excretion of the drug have not been elucidated.

CLINICAL PHARMACOLOGY: *(cont'd)*

A clinical study (Diokno, A.C.; Lapides, J., Urol. 10:23-24, July 1977.) was conducted on the relative effectiveness of oral and subcutaneous doses of bethanechol chloride on the stretch response of bladder muscle in patients with urinary retention. Results showed that 5 mg of the drug given subcutaneously stimulated a response that was more rapid in onset and of larger magnitude than an oral dose of 50 mg, 100 mg, or 200 mg. All the oral doses, however, had a longer duration of effect than the subcutaneous dose. Although the 50 mg oral dose caused little change in intravesical pressure in this study, this dose has been found in other studies to be clinically effective in the rehabilitation of patients with decompensated bladders.

INDICATIONS AND USAGE:

For the treatment of acute postoperative and postpartum nonobstructive (functional) urinary retention and for neurogenic atony of the urinary bladder with retention.

CONTRAINDICATIONS:

Hypersensitivity to bethanechol chloride tablets or to any component of bethanechol chloride injection, hyperthyroidism, peptic ulcer, latent or active bronchial asthma, pronounced bradycardia or hypotension, vasomotor instability, coronary artery disease, epilepsy, and parkinsonism.

Bethanechol chloride should not be employed when the strength or integrity of the gastrointestinal or bladder wall is in question, or in the presence of mechanical obstruction; when increased muscular activity of the gastrointestinal tract or urinary bladder might prove harmful, as following recent urinary bladder surgery, gastrointestinal resection and anastomosis, or when there is possible gastrointestinal obstruction; in bladder neck obstruction, spastic gastrointestinal disturbances, acute inflammatory lesions of the gastrointestinal tract, or peritonitis; or in marked vagotonia.

WARNINGS:

The sterile solution is for subcutaneous use only. It should never be given intramuscularly or intravenously. Violent symptoms of cholinergic over-stimulation, such as circulatory collapse, fall in blood pressure, abdominal cramps, bloody diarrhea, shock, or sudden cardiac arrest are likely to occur if the drug is given by either of these routes. Although rare, these same symptoms have occurred after subcutaneous injection, and may occur in cases of hypersensitivity or overdosage.

PRECAUTIONS:

General: In urinary retention, if the sphincter fails to relax as bethanechol chloride contracts the bladder, urine may be forced up the ureter into the kidney pelvis. If there is bacteriuria, this may cause reflux infection.

Information for the Patient: Bethanechol chloride tablets should preferably be taken one hour before or two hours after meals to avoid nausea or vomiting. Dizziness, lightheadedness or fainting may occur, especially when getting up from a lying or sitting position.

Carcinogenesis, Mutagenesis, and Impairment of Fertility: Long-term studies in animals have not been performed to evaluate the effects upon fertility, mutagenic or carcinogenic potential of bethanechol chloride.

Pregnancy Category C: Animal reproduction studies have not been conducted with bethanechol chloride. It is also not known whether bethanechol chloride can cause fetal harm when administered to a pregnant woman or can affect reproduction capacity. Bethanechol chloride should be given to a pregnant woman only if clearly needed.

Nursing Mothers: It is not known whether this drug is secreted in human milk. Because many drugs are secreted in human milk and because of the potential for serious adverse reactions from bethanechol chloride in nursing infants, a decision should be made whether to discontinue nursing or to discontinue the drug, taking into account the importance of the drug to the mother.

Pediatric Use: Safety and effectiveness in children have not been established.

DRUG INTERACTIONS:

Special care is required if this drug is given to patients receiving ganglion blocking compounds because a critical fall in blood pressure may occur. Usually, severe abdominal symptoms appear before there is such a fall in the blood pressure.

ADVERSE REACTIONS:

Adverse reactions are rare following oral administration of bethanechol, but are more common following subcutaneous injection. Adverse reactions are more likely to occur when dosage is increased.

The following adverse reactions have been observed: *Body as a Whole:* malaise; *Digestive:* abdominal cramps or discomfort, colicky pain, nausea and belching, diarrhea, borborygmi, salivation; *Renal:* urinary urgency; *Nervous System:* headache; *Cardiovascular:* a fall in blood pressure with reflex tachycardia, vasomotor response; *Skin:* flushing producing a feeling of warmth, sensation of heat about the face, sweating; *Respiratory:* bronchial constriction, asthmatic attacks; *Special Senses:* lacrimation, miosis.

Causal Relationship Unknown: The following adverse reactions have been reported, and a causal relationship to therapy with bethanechol chloride has not been established: *Body as a Whole:* hypothermia; *Nervous System:* seizures.

OVERDOSAGE:

Early signs of overdosage are abdominal discomfort, salivation, flushing of the skin ("hot feeling"), sweating, nausea and vomiting.

Atropine is a specific antidote. The recommended dose for adults is 0.6 mg (1/100 grain). Repeat doses can be given every two hours, according to clinical response. The recommended dosage in infants and children up to 12 years of age is 0.01 mg/kg (to a maximum single dose of 0.4 mg) repeated every two hours as needed until the desired effect is obtained, or adverse effects of atropine preclude further usage. Subcutaneous injection of atropine is preferred except in emergencies when the intravenous route may be employed.

When bethanechol chloride is administered subcutaneously, a syringe containing a dose of atropine sulfate should always be available to treat symptoms of toxicity.

The oral LD_{50} of bethanechol chloride is 1510 mg/kg in the mouse.

DOSAGE AND ADMINISTRATION:

Dosage and route of administration must be individualized, depending on the type and severity of the condition to be treated.

Preferably give the drug when the stomach is empty. If taken soon after eating, nausea and vomiting may occur.

DOSAGE AND ADMINISTRATION: *(cont'd)*

ORAL

The usual adult dosage is 10 to 50 mg three or four times a day. The minimum effective dose is determined by giving 5 or 10 mg initially and repeating the same amount at hourly intervals until satisfactory response occurs or until a maximum of 50 mg has been given. The effects of the drug sometimes appear within 30 minutes and usually within 60 to 90 minutes. They persist for about an hour.

SUBCUTANEOUS

The usual dose is 1 ml (5 mg), although some patients respond satisfactorily to as little as 0.5 ml (2.5 mg). The minimum effective dose is determined by injecting 0.5 ml (2.5 mg) initially and repeating the same amount at 15 to 30 minute intervals to a maximum of four doses until satisfactory response is obtained, unless disturbing reactions appear. The minimum effective dose may be repeated thereafter three or four times a day as required.

Rarely, single doses up to 2 ml (10 mg) may be required. Such large doses may cause severe reactions and should be used only after adequate trial of single doses of 0.5 to 1 ml (2.5 to 5 mg) has established that smaller doses are not sufficient.

Bethanechol chloride is usually effective in 5 to 15 minutes after subcutaneous injection.

If necessary, the effects of the drug can be abolished promptly by atropine (see OVERDOSAGE.)

Parenteral drug products should be inspected visually for particulate matter and discoloration prior to administration, whenever solution and container permit.

STORAGE

Store bethanechol chloride tablets in a tightly-closed container. Avoid storage at temperatures above 40°C (104°F).

Avoid storage of Injection bethanechol chloride at temperatures below -20°C (-4°F) and above 40°C (104°F).

HOW SUPPLIED - RATED THERAPEUTICALLY EQUIVALENT:

Tablet, Uncoated - Oral - 5 mg

100's	$2.70	Bethanechol, Qualitest Pharms	00603-2455-21
100's	$2.75	Bethanechol Chloride, Consolidated Midland	00223-0430-01
100's	$3.20	Bethanechol Chloride 5, Major Pharms	00904-0590-60
100's	$4.01	Bethanechol, Goldline Labs	00182-0453-01
100's	$4.01	Bethanechol, Sidmak Labs	50111-0323-01
100's	$4.07	Bethanechol, US Trading	56126-0215-11
100's	$4.22	Bethanechol Chloride, Aligen Independ	00405-4123-01
100's	$12.40	Bethanechol Chloride, Goldline Labs	00182-0453-89
100's	$13.02	Bethanechol Chloride, Vangard Labs	00615-2556-13
100's	$13.47	Bethanechol 5, Major Pharms	00904-0590-61
100's	$13.65	Bethanechol, TIE Pharm	55496-1101-09
100's	$14.65	Bethanechol, Medirex	57480-0426-01
100's	**$35.53**	**URECHOLINE, Merck**	**00006-0403-68**
600's	$88.00	Bethanechol, Medirex	57480-0426-06
600's	$94.40	Bethanechol, Medirex	57480-0413-06
1000's	$22.50	Bethanechol Chloride, Consolidated Midland	00223-0430-02
1000's	$37.68	Bethanechol, Sidmak Labs	50111-0323-03

Tablet, Uncoated - Oral - 10 mg

100's	$2.48	Bethanechol Chloride, Geneva Pharms	00781-1254-01
100's	$2.48	Bethanechol, H.C.F.A. F F P	99999-0470-03
100's	$2.95	Bethanechol Chloride, Consolidated Midland	00223-0431-01
100's	$4.15	Bethanechol, United Res	00677-0506-01
100's	$4.44	Bethanechol, US Trading	56126-0216-11
100's	$4.70	Bethanechol, Martec Pharms	52555-0422-01
100's	$4.95	Bethanechol, Rugby	00536-3365-01
100's	$5.01	Bethanechol, Goldline Labs	00182-0454-01
100's	$5.01	Bethanechol, Qualitest Pharms	00603-2456-21
100's	$5.01	Bethanechol, Sidmak Labs	50111-0324-01
100's	$5.27	Bethanechol Chloride 10, Aligen Independ	00405-4124-01
100's	$5.50	Bethanechol, Parmed Pharms	00349-2129-01
100's	$6.01	Bethanechol, HL Moore Drug Exch	00839-6209-06
100's	$8.40	Bethanechol Cl, Schein Pharm (US)	00364-0349-01
100's	$9.50	Bethanecol, Raway	00686-0054-20
100's	$15.75	Bethanechol, Medirex	57480-0413-01
100's	$16.88	Bethanechol, Major Pharms	00904-0591-61
100's	$18.20	Bethanechol, Goldline Labs	00182-0454-89
100's	$18.26	Bethanechol Chloride, Vangard Labs	00615-2557-13
100's	$18.34	Bethanechol, TIE Pharm	55496-1102-09
100's	$19.90	MYOTONACHOL, Glenwood	00516-0021-01
100's	**$66.61**	**URECHOLINE, Merck**	**00006-0412-68**
250's	$6.20	Bethanechol, H.C.F.A. F F P	99999-0470-04
250's	$7.15	Bethanechol Chloride, Major Pharms	00904-0591-70
1000's	$14.54	Bethanechol Chloride 10, Aligen Independ	00405-4124-03
1000's	$17.95	Bethanechol Chloride, Major Pharms	00904-0591-80
1000's	$24.50	Bethanechol Chloride, Consolidated Midland	00223-0431-02
1000's	$24.80	Bethanechol, H.C.F.A. F F P	99999-0470-05
1000's	$25.50	Bethanechol, Rugby	00536-3365-10
1000's	$28.15	Bethanechol, HL Moore Drug Exch	00839-6209-16
1000's	$40.25	Bethanechol, Martec Pharms	52555-0422-10
1000's	$42.99	Bethanechol, Sidmak Labs	50111-0324-03
1000's	$44.55	Bethanechol, Qualitest Pharms	00603-2456-32

Tablet, Uncoated - Oral - 25 mg

100's	$3.45	Bethanechol Chloride, Geneva Pharms	00781-1250-01
100's	$3.45	Bethanechol, H.C.F.A. F F P	99999-0470-06
100's	$3.45	Bethanechol, H.C.F.A. F F P	99999-0470-07
100's	$3.95	Bethanechol Chloride, Consolidated Midland	00223-0432-01
100's	$4.50	Bethanechol Chloride, Major Pharms	00904-0592-60
100's	$5.20	Bethanecol, United Res	00677-0507-01
100's	$5.39	Bethanechol, US Trading	56126-0217-11
100's	$5.90	Bethanechol, Parmed Pharms	00349-2429-01
100's	$6.30	Bethanechol, Martec Pharms	52555-0423-01
100's	$6.40	Bethanechol, Rugby	00536-3369-01
100's	$6.50	Bethanechol, HL Moore Drug Exch	00839-6210-06
100's	$6.73	Bethanechol, Goldline Labs	00182-0455-01
100's	$6.73	Bethanechol, Sidmak Labs	50111-0325-01
100's	$6.74	Bethanechol, Qualitest Pharms	00603-2457-21
100's	$7.08	Bethanechol Chloride 25, Aligen Independ	00405-4125-01
100's	$11.65	Bethanechol Cl, Schein Pharm (US)	00364-0410-01
100's	$12.50	Bethanecol, Raway	00686-0123-20
100's	$13.57	Bethanechol, PRL Enterpr	53633-0217-11
100's	$31.50	Bethanechol, Medirex	57480-0427-01
100's	$32.60	Bethanechol, Goldline Labs	00182-0455-89
100's	$32.73	Bethanechol Chloride, Vangard Labs	00615-2558-13
100's	$34.36	Bethanechol, TIE Pharm	55496-1103-09
100's	$36.82	Bethanechol Chloride, Major Pharms	00904-0592-61
100's	$80.86	DUVOID, Roberts Labs	54092-0101-01
100's	**$100.95**	**URECHOLINE, Merck**	**00006-0457-68**
100's	$125.53	DUVOID, Roberts Labs	54092-0102-01
250's	$8.62	Bethanechol, H.C.F.A. F F P	99999-0470-08

HOW SUPPLIED - RATED THERAPEUTICALLY EQUIVALENT:
(cont'd)

250's	$8.90	Bethanechol Chloride, Major Pharms	00904-0592-70
600's	$189.00	Bethanechol, Medirex	57480-0427-06
1000's	$32.50	Bethanechol Chloride, Consolidated Midland	00223-0432-02
1000's	$34.50	Bethanechol, H.C.F.A. F F P	99999-0470-09
1000's	$34.80	Bethanechol Chloride, Major Pharms	00904-0592-80
1000's	$40.55	Bethanecol, United Res	00677-0507-10
1000's	$44.75	Bethanechol, Rugby	00536-3369-10
1000's	$46.00	Bethanechol, Martec Pharms	52555-0423-10
1000's	$47.52	Bethanechol, HL Moore Drug Exch	00839-6210-16
1000's	$49.10	Bethanechol, Qualitest Pharms	00603-2457-32
1000's	$49.13	Bethanechol, Goldline Labs	00182-0455-10
1000's	$49.13	Bethanechol, Sidmak Labs	50111-0325-03
1000's	$51.72	Bethanechol Chloride 25, Aligen Independ	00405-4125-03

Tablet, Uncoated - Oral - 50 mg

100's	$7.25	Bethanechol Chloride, Consolidated Midland	00223-0433-01
100's	$7.43	Bethanecol Chloride, United Res	00677-0940-01
100's	$7.43	Bethanechol, H.C.F.A. F F P	99999-0470-10
100's	$9.00	Bethanechol Chloride, Major Pharms	00904-0593-60
100's	$10.11	Bethanechol, Qualitest Pharms	00603-2458-21
100's	$10.95	Bethanechol, Rugby	00536-3366-01
100's	$11.46	Bethanechol, Sidmak Labs	50111-0326-01
100's	$12.06	Bethanechol Chloride 50, Aligen Independ	00405-4126-01
100's	$12.41	Bethanechol, HL Moore Drug Exch	00839-6537-06
100's	$13.15	Bethanechol, Parmed Pharms	00349-8009-01
100's	$15.00	Bethanecol, Raway	00686-0056-20
100's	$21.00	Bethanechol Cl, Schein Pharm (US)	00364-0590-01
100's	$38.55	Bethanechol, Medirex	57480-0414-01
100's	$42.00	Bethanechol Chloride, Goldline Labs	00182-1023-89
100's	$44.69	Bethanechol Chloride, Major Pharms	00904-0593-61
100's	$53.93	Bethanechol, TIE Pharm	55496-1104-09
100's	**$142.11**	**URECHOLINE, Merck**	**00006-0460-68**
100's	$194.18	DUVOID, Roberts Labs	54092-0103-01
600's	$213.20	Bethanechol, Medirex	57480-0414-06
1000's	$67.50	Bethanechol Chloride, Consolidated Midland	00223-0433-02
1000's	$74.30	Bethanechol, H.C.F.A. F F P	99999-0470-11
1000's	$107.27	Bethanechol, Sidmak Labs	50111-0326-03
1000's	$117.59	Bethanechol Chloride, HL Moore Drug Exch	00839-6537-16

HOW SUPPLIED - NOT RATED EQUIVALENT:

Injection, Solution - Subcutaneous - 5 mg/ml

1 ml x 6	**$30.84**	**URECHOLINE, Merck**	**00006-7786-29**

BICALUTAMIDE *(003271)*

CATEGORIES: Androgen Inhibitors; Antineoplastics; Cancer; Oncologic Drugs; Oral Androgen Blockers; Prostatic Carcinoma; FDA Class 1P ("Priority Review"); FDA Approved 1995 Oct

BRAND NAMES: **Casodex**

Prescribing information not available at time of publication.

HOW SUPPLIED - EQUIVALENTS NOT AVAILABLE:

Tablet, Uncoated - Oral - 50 mg

30's	**$307.50**	**CASODEX, Zeneca Pharms**	**00310-0705-30**
30's	**$307.50**	**CASODEX, Zeneca Pharms**	**00310-0705-39**
100's	**$1025.00**	**CASODEX, Zeneca Pharms**	**00310-0705-10**

BILE SALTS; PANCREATIN; PEPSIN *(000476)*

CATEGORIES: Digestants; Enzymes & Digestants; Gastrointestinal Drugs; Pancreatic Enzymes; Steatorrhea; Pregnancy Category C; FDA Pre 1938 Drugs

BRAND NAMES: Digestozyme; **Entozyme**

Prescribing information not available at time of publication.

HOW SUPPLIED - EQUIVALENTS NOT AVAILABLE:

Tablet, Enteric Coated - Oral - 150 mg/300 mg/2

100's	$9.75	DIGESTOZYME, Major Pharms	00904-0596-60
100's	**$21.98**	**ENTOZYME, AH Robins**	**00031-5049-63**

BIPERIDEN HYDROCHLORIDE *(000483)*

CATEGORIES: Anticholinergic Agents; Antiparkinson Agents; Autonomic Drugs; Extrapyramidal Movement Disorders; Neuromuscular; Parasympatholytics; Parkinsonism; Pregnancy Category C; FDA Approval Pre 1982

BRAND NAMES: **Akineton**; *Akineton Retard* (France, Germany, Mexico); *Bicamol*; *Biparkin*; *Biperen*; *Biperin*; *Bipiden*; *Dekinet*; *Desiperiden* (Germany); *Dyskinon*; *Tasmolin*
(International brand names outside U.S. in italics)

FORMULARIES: WHO

COST OF THERAPY: $277.14 (Parkinsonism; Tablet; 2 mg; 3/day; 365 days)

DESCRIPTION:

Each Akineton tablet for oral administration contains 2 mg biperiden hydrochloride. Other ingredients may include corn syrup, lactose, magnesium stearate, potato starch and talc. Each 1 ml Akineton ampule for intramuscular or intravenous administration contains 5 mg biperiden lactate in an aqueous 1.4 percent sodium lactate solution. No added preservative.

Biperiden hydrochloride is an anticholinergic agent. Biperiden is α-5- Norbornen-2-yl-α-penyl-1-piperidine-propanol. It is a white, crystalline, odorless powder, slightly soluble in water and alcohol. It is stable in air at normal temperatures.

CLINICAL PHARMACOLOGY:

Biperiden HCl is a weak peripheral anticholinergic agent. It has, therefore, some antisecretory, antispasmodic and mydriatic effects. In addition, biperiden HCl possesses nicotinolytic activity. Parkinsonism is thought to result from an imbalance between the excitatory (cholinergic) and inhibitory (dopaminergic) systems in the corpus striatum. The

CLINICAL PHARMACOLOGY: *(cont'd)*

mechanism of action of centrally active anticholinergic drugs such as biperiden HCl is considered to related to competitive antagonism of acetylcholine at cholinergic receptors in the corpus striatum, which then restores the balance.

The parenteral form of biperiden HCl is an effective and reliable agent for the treatment of acute episodes of extrapyramidal disturbances sometimes seen during treatment with neuroleptic agents. Akathisia, akinesia, dyskinetic tremors, rigor, oculogyric crises, spasmodic torticollis, and profuse sweating are markedly reduced or eliminated. With parenteral biperiden HCl, these drug-induced disturbances are rapidly brought under control. Subsequently, this can usually be maintained with oral doses which may be given with tranquilizer therapy in psychotic and other conditions requiring an uninterrupted therapeutic program.

Pharmacokinetics and Metabolism: Only limited pharmacokinetic studies of biperiden in humans are available. The serum concentration at 1 to 1.5 hours following a single 4 mg oral dose was 4-5 ng/ml. Plasma levels (0.1-0.2 ng/ml) could be determined up to 48 hours after dosing. Six hours after an oral dose of 250 mg/kg in rats, 87% of the drug had been absorbed. The metabolism of biperiden HCl is also incompletely understood, but does involve hydroxylation. In normal volunteers a single 10 mg intravenous dose of biperiden seemed to cause a transient rise in plasma cortisol and prolactin. No change in GH, LH, FSH, or TSH levels were seen. Biperiden lactate (10 mg/ml) was not irritating to the tissue of rabbits when injected intramuscularly (1.0 ml) into the sacrospinalis muscles and intradermally (0.25 ml) and subcutaneously (0.5 ml) into the shaved abdominal skin.

INDICATIONS AND USAGE:

As an adjunct in the therapy of all forms of parkinsonism (idiopathic, post-encephalitic, arteriosclerotic)

Control of extrapyramidal disorders secondary to neuroleptic drug therapy (*e.g.,* phenothiazines).

CONTRAINDICATIONS:

1) Hypersensitivity to biperiden, 2) Narrow angle glaucoma, 3) Bowel obstruction, 4) Megacolon.

WARNINGS:

Isolated instances of mental confusion, euphoria, agitation and disturbed behavior have been reported in susceptible patients. Also, the central anticholinergic syndrome can occur as an adverse reaction to properly prescribed anticholinergic medication, although it is more frequently due to overdosage. It may also result from concomitant administration of an anticholinergic agent and a drug that has secondary anticholinergic actions (See DRUG INTERACTIONS and OVERDOSAGE). Caution should be observed in patients with manifest glaucoma, though no prohibitive rise in intraocular pressure has been noted following either oral or parenteral administration. Patients with prostatism, epilepsy or cardiac arrhythmia should be given this drug with caution.

Occasionally, drowsiness may occur, and patients who drive a car or operate any other potentially dangerous machinery should be warned of this possibility. As with other drugs acting on the central nervous system, the consumption of alcohol should be avoided during biperiden HCl therapy.

PRECAUTIONS:

Pregnancy Category C: Animal reproduction studies have not been conducted with biperiden HCl. It is also not known whether biperiden HCl can cause fetal harm when administered to a pregnant woman or can affect reproduction capacity. Biperiden HCl should be given to a pregnant woman only if clearly needed.

Nursing Mothers: It is not known whether this drug is excreted in human milk. Because many drugs are excreted in human milk, caution should be exercised when biperiden HCl is administered to a nursing woman.

Pediatric Use: Safety and effectiveness in children have not been established.

DRUG INTERACTIONS:

The central anticholinergic syndrome can occur when anticholinergic agents such as Biperiden HCl are administered concomitantly with drugs that have secondary anticholinergic actions, e.g., certain narcotic analgesics such as meperidine, the phenothiazines and other antipsychotics, tricyclic antidepressants, certain antiarrhythmics such as the quinidine salts, and antihistamines. See OVERDOSAGE for signs and symptoms of the central anticholinergic syndrome, and for treatment.

ADVERSE REACTIONS:

Atropine-like side effects such as dry mouth; blurred vision; drowsiness; euphoria or disorientation; urinary retention; postural hypotension; constipation; agitation; disturbed behavior may be seen. There usually are no significant changes in blood pressure or heart rate in patients who have been given the parenteral form of biperiden HCl. Mild transient postural hypotension and bradycardia may occur. These side effects can be minimized or avoided by slow intravenous administration. No local tissue reactions have been reported following intramuscular injection. If gastric irritation occurs following oral administration, it can be avoided by administering the drug during or after meals.

The central anticholinergic syndrome can occur as an adverse reaction to properly prescribed anticholinergic medication. See OVERDOSAGE for signs and symptoms of the central anticholinergic syndrome, and for treatment.

OVERDOSAGE:

Signs and Symptoms: Overdosage with biperiden HCl produces typical central symptoms of atropine intoxication (the central anticholinergic syndrome). Correct diagnosis depends upon recognition of the peripheral signs of parasympathetic blockade including dilated and sluggish pupils; warm, dry skin; facial flushing; decreased secretions of the mouth, pharynx, nose, and bronchi; foul smelling breath; elevated temperature, tachycardia, cardiac arrhythmias, decreased bowel sounds, and urinary retention. Neuropsychiatric signs such as delirium, disorientation, anxiety, hallucinations, illusions, confusion, incoherence, agitation, hyperactivity, ataxia, loss of memory, paranoia, combativeness, and seizures may be present. The condition can progress to stupor, coma, paralysis, and cardiac and respiratory arrest and death.

Treatment: Treatment of acute overdose revolves around symptomatic and supportive therapy. If biperiden HCl was administered orally, gastric lavage or other measures to limit absorption should be instituted. A small dose of diazepam or a short acting barbiturate may be administered if CNS excitation is observed. Phenothiazines are contraindicated because the toxicity may be intensified due to their antimuscarinic action, causing coma. Respiratory support, artificial respiration or vasopressor agents may be necessary. Hyperpyrexia must be reversed, fluid volume replaced and acid-base balance maintained. Urinary catheterization may be necessary.

Routine use of physostigmine for overdose is controversial. Delirium, hallucinations, coma, and supraventricular tachycardia (not ventricular tachycardias or conduction defects) seem to respond. If indicated, 1 mg (half this amount for the children or elderly) may be given intramuscularly or by slow intravenous infusion. If there is no response within 20 minutes, an

OVERDOSAGE: *(cont'd)*

additional 1 mg dose may be given; this may be repeated until a total of 4 mg has been administered, a reversal of the toxic effects occur or excessive cholinergic signs are seen. Frequent monitoring of clinical signs should be done. Since physostigmine is rapidly destroyed, additional injections may be required every one or two hours to maintain control. The relapse intervals tend to lengthens the toxic anticholinergic agent is metabolized, so the patients should be carefully observed for 8 to 12 hours following the last relapse.

DOSAGE AND ADMINISTRATION:

DRUG INDUCED EXTRAPYRAMIDAL SYMPTOMS

Parenteral: The average adult dose is 2 mg intramuscularly or intravenously. May be repeated every half-hour until there is resolution of symptoms, but not more than four consecutive doses should be given in 24-hour period.

Note: Parenteral drug product should be inspected visually for particulate matter and discoloration prior to administration, whenever solution and container permit.

Oral: One tablet one to three times daily.

Parkinson's Disease: Oral the usual beginning dose is one tablet three or four times daily. This dosage should be individualized with the dose titrated upward to a maximum of 8 tablets (16 mg) per 24 hours.

Storage: All dosage forms of Akineton should be stored at 59-86°F(15- 30°C). Dispense in tight, light-resistant container as defined in USP.

(Knoll, 6/87, RE-1/Akin5427B/Rev.(7/21/87))

ANIMAL PHARMACOLOGY:

Toxicity in Animals: The LD_{50} of biperiden in the white mouse is 545 mg/kg orally, 195 mg/kg subcutaneously, and 56 mg/k intravenously. The acute oral toxicity (LD_{50}) in rats is 750 mg/kg. The intraperitoneal toxicity (LD_{50}) of biperiden lactate in rats was 270 mg/kg and the intravenous toxicity (LD_{50}) in dogs was 222 mg/kg. In dogs under general anesthesia, respiratory arrest occurred at 33 mg/kg (intravenous) and circulatory standstill at 45 mg/kg (intravenous). The oral LD_{50} in dogs is 340 mg/kg. Chronic toxicity studies in both rat and dog have been reported.

HOW SUPPLIED - EQUIVALENTS NOT AVAILABLE:

Injection, Solution - Intramuscular; - 5 mg/ml

1 ml x 10	$33.30	AKINETON, Knoll Labs	00044-0110-01

Tablet, Uncoated - Oral - 2 mg

100's	$25.31	AKINETON, Knoll Labs	00044-0120-02
1000's	$187.27	AKINETON, Knoll Labs	00044-0120-04

BISMUTH CITRATE; RANITIDINE *(003314)*

CATEGORIES: Acid/Peptic Disorders; Antacids; Antiulcer Drugs; Duodenal Ulcer; Gastrointestinal Drugs; Histamine H2 Receptor Antagonists; Peptic Ulcer; Pregnancy Category C; FDA Approved 1996 Aug

BRAND NAMES: *Pylorid* (England); *Pylorid 400*; *Pylorisin*; **Tritec**
(International brand names outside U.S. in italics)

PRIMARY ICD9: 533.9 (Ulcer, peptic)

DESCRIPTION:

Tritec tablets contain a complex of ranitidine, trivalent bismuth, and citrate. Chemically, ranitidine bismuth citrate is N-2-[5-Dimethylaminomethyl-2-furanylmethylthio] ethyl-N'-methyl-2- nitoethenediamine 2-hydroxy-1,2,3-propanetricarboxylate, bismuth (III). Analysis shows that ranitidine bismuth citrate is substoichiometric in ranitidine and citrate.

Ranitidine bismuth citrate is a white to off-white amorphous powder. The approximate molecular formula is $[C_{13}H_{22}N_4O_3S]_{0.84}\cdot Bi\cdot [C_6H_5O_7]_{0.94}$ and the approximate molecular weight is 651. It is readily soluble in water. Each Tritec tablet for oral administration contains 400 mg of ranitidine bismuth citrate, equivalent to approximately 162 mg of ranitidine (base), 128 mg of trivalent bismuth, and 110 mg of citrate. Each aqueous film-coated tablet also contains the inactive ingredients FD&C Blue No. 2 Aluminum Lake, magnesium stearate, methyl-hydroxypropylcellulose, microcrystalline cellulose, Povidone K30, sodium carbonate (anhydrous), titanium dioxide, and triacetin.

CLINICAL PHARMACOLOGY:

PHARMACOKINETICS

Following ingestion, ranitidine bismuth citrate dissociates in intragastric fluid, giving rise to ranitidine and soluble and insoluble forms of bismuth.

Absorption: Following a single oral 400 mg dose of ranitidine bismuth citrate to healthy volunteers, mean (±SD) peak ranitidine plasma concentration of 455 (±145.3) ng/ml occurred at 0.5 to 5 hours. The rate and extent of absorption of ranitidine derived from ranitidine bismuth citrate increased proportionally with increasing doses up to 1,600 mg. Ranitidine plasma concentrations showed no evidence of accumulation during a 28-day period.

Oral absorption of bismuth is variable. A mean (±SD) peak bismuth plasma concentration of 3.3 (±2.0) ng/ml occurs at 15 to 60 minutes after a 400 mg dose. The rate and extent of absorption of bismuth from ranitidine bismuth citrate do not increase with increasing doses up to 800 mg, but increase more than proportionally with increasing doses above 800 mg. The rate of absorption of bismuth derived from an 800 mg dose of ranitidine bismuth citrate is decreased by 50%, and the extent of absorption is decreased by 25% when taken 30 minutes after a meal as compared to 30 minutes before a meal. The absorption of bismuth from an 800 mg dose of ranitidine bismuth citrate increased when gastric pH exceeded 6. The increased pH resulted from the administration of an 800 mg dose of ranitidine bismuth citrate given 3 hours previously. Mucosal penetration and absorption of bismuth from ranitidine bismuth citrate is not affected by the degree of gastritis, the presence of *Helicobacter pylori*, or an active ulcer. Small amounts of bismuth accumulate in plasma during twice-daily dosing with ranitidine bismuth citrate. In a 28-day study at 800 mg twice daily (twice the recommended daily dose), peak bismuth concentrations did not exceed 20 ng/ml at any time in any patient, with a median peak concentration of 6.3 ng/ml on day 28. Median peak and trough concentrations on day 28 were 105% and 68% of predicted steady-state peak and trough concentrations. In a study at 400 mg twice daily for 12 weeks (three times the recommended duration), trough bismuth concentrations did not exceed predicted accumulation in any patient, with a median trough concentration of 2.8 ng/ml at week 12.

Distribution: The volume of distribution for ranitidine is 1.7 L/kg. Serum protein binding of ranitidine averages 15%. Bismuth is 98% bound to human plasma proteins, primarily albumin.

Metabolism: Ranitidine is metabolized to the N-oxide, S-oxide, and N-desmethyl metabolites, accounting for approximately 4%, 1%, and 1% of the dose, respectively. It is not known whether bismuth undergoes any biotransformation.

CLINICAL PHARMACOLOGY: *(cont'd)*

Excretion: The elimination half-life of ranitidine derived from ranitidine bismuth citrate is 2.8 to 3.1 hours. The principle route of elimination for ranitidine is renal, accounting for 30% of the dose. Renal clearance averages 530 ml/min, indicating active tubular excretion. Total clearance is 760 ml/min. Elimination of bismuth is polyexponential, with a terminal elimination half-life of 11 to 28 days. Bismuth has an average renal clearance of 30 to 60 ml/min, indicating net tubular secretion. Less than 1% of bismuth derived from ranitidine bismuth citrate is recovered in urine after oral administration. Up to 28% of bismuth was recovered in the feces during a 6-day post-dose period. Bismuth also undergoes minor excretion in the bile.

SPECIAL POPULATIONS

Geriatric: Clinically insignificant increases in plasma concentrations of ranitidine were observed in elderly patients. Bismuth concentrations may be elevated in elderly patients as a result of decreased renal elimination.

Pediatric: No information on the pharmacokinetics of ranitidine or bismuth derived from ranitidine bismuth citrate was obtained in this population.

Gender: There is no evidence of a difference in the pharmacokinetics of ranitidine between males and females when adjusted for body weight. There is no difference in the extent of absorption of bismuth when adjusted for body weight; significant differences are observed for peak plasma concentrations in healthy females.

Race: There is no evidence of any racial differences in the pharmacokinetics of bismuth based on trough concentrations observed in clinical trials.

Renal Insufficiency: The renal clearances of ranitidine and bismuth are correlated with renal function (*i.e.*, creatinine clearance), while nonrenal elimination of ranitidine is unaltered by renal impairment. Thus, ranitidine and bismuth concentrations may be elevated in renally impaired patients as a result of decreased renal elimination.

Hepatic Insufficiency: Elimination of either ranitidine or bismuth by the hepatic route is relatively unimportant. Therefore, the pharmacokinetics of ranitidine or bismuth derived from ranitidine bismuth citrate were not studied in patients with hepatic insufficiency owing to the minimal impact of this condition.

PHARMACODYNAMICS

Antisecretory Activity

1. Effects on Acid Secretion: Ranitidine, derived from ranitidine bismuth citrate, inhibits both daytime and nocturnal basal gastric acid secretions as well as gastric acid secretion stimulated by food, betazole, and pentagastrin.

2. Effects on Other Gastrointestinal Secretions: *Plasma Pepsinogen I and II:* Ranitidine derived from ranitidine bismuth citrate does not alter plasma pepsinogen I and II concentrations or pepsin activity. *Serum Gastrin:* Ranitidine derived from ranitidine bismuth citrate has little or no effect on fasting or postprandial serum gastrin.

There is no information about the gastric mucosal concentrations of ranitidine, bismuth, clarithromycin, or hydroxy-clarithromycin after administration of ranitidine bismuth citrate and clarithromycin.

For information on the clinical pharmacology of clarithromycin, refer to CLINICAL PHARMACOLOGYof the Clarithromycin monograph.

Microbiology: Some *H pylori* isolates obtained from patients treated with clarithromycin plus acid-suppressive regimens demonstrate an increase in clarithromycin MIC's over time, indicating decreasing susceptibility and increasing resistance.

Emerging clarithromycin resistance was not assessed for the ranitidine bismuth citrate plus clarithromycin regimen because there were no patients that had *H pylori* isolates with both pretreatment and post-treatment susceptibility test results. No adequate data were collected during clinical trials or *in vitro* studies to indicate that ranitidine bismuth citrate can either decrease or increase emerging clarithromycin resistance.

It is recommended that all patients, not eradicated of *H pylori* following ranitidine bismuth citrate-plus-clarithromycin treatment be considered to have *H pylori* resistant to clarithromycin.

Patients who fail therapy should not be re-treated with a regimen containing clarithromycin.

CLINICAL STUDIES:

Eradication of *H pylori* Associated with Active Duodenal Ulcer: Ranitidine bismuth citrate alone and in combination with clarithromycin was evaluated in two U.S. double-blind, randomized, multicenter, placebo-controlled trials. 409 patients were enrolled and 265 had *H pylori* infection and active duodenal ulcer prestudy. Ranitidine bismuth citrate 400 mg taken twice daily for 4 weeks plus clarithromycin 500 mg 3 times daily for the first 2 weeks was found to have a significantly higher *H pylori* eradication rate when compared to clarithromycin 500 3 times daily for 2 weeks, ranitidine bismuth citrate 400 mg twice daily for 4 weeks, or placebo. See TABLE 1.

TABLE 1 *H pylori* Eradication Rates
Percent of Patients Cured [95% Confidence Interval] (number of patients)

Study	Ranitidine Bismuth Citrate plus Clarithromycin	Ranitidine Bismuth Citrate	Clarithromycin	Placebo
Study 305	84%† [60%-97%] (n=19)	0% [0%-14%] (n=25)	25% [10%-47%] (n=24)	0% [0%-21%] (n=16)
Study 306	73%† [50%-80%] (n=22)	0% [0%-15%] (n=22)	25% [10%-47%] (n=24)	0% [0%-23%] (n=14)

* *H. pylori*eradication was defined as no positive test (CLOtest™, culture, histology) at 4 weeks following the end of treatment. Patients must have had two tests performed and these must have been negative to be considered eradicated of *H. pylori*. The following patients were excluded: patients not infected with *H. pylori* prestudy, dropouts, patients with major protocol violations, patients with missing *H. pylori* tests, and patients that were not assessed for *H. pylori* eradication 4 weeks after the end of treatment because they were found to have an unhealed ulcer and were *H. pylori*negative at the end of treatment.
† P<0.001 for ranitidine bismuth citrate + clarithromycin versus all other treatment groups.

The relationship between *H pylori* eradication and duodenal ulcer recurrence was assessed in a combined analysis of six U.S. randomized, double-blind, multicenter, placebo-controlled trials using ranitidine bismuth citrate with or without antibiotics. The results from approximately 650 U.S. patients showed that the risk of ulcer recurrence within 6 months of completing treatment was two times less likely in patients whose *H pylori* infection was eradicated compared to patients in whom *H pylori* infection was not eradicated.

Duodenal Ulcer Healing at 4 Weeks (End of Treatment): Ulcer healing rates for the two U.S. double-blind, randomized multicenter, placebo-controlled trials are represented in TABLE 2.

The studies did not evaluate whether bismuth citrate added to the healing effects of ranitidine alone.

TABLE 2 End of Treatment Ulcer Healing Rates*
Percent of Patients Healed [95% Confidence Intervals](Number of Patients)

Study	Ranitidine Bismuth Citrate + Clarithromycin	Ranitidine Bismuth Citrate	Clarithromycin	Placebo
Study 305	75% [53%-90%] (n=24)	73% [54%-88%] (n=30)	70% [50%-86%] (n=27)	56% [30%-80%] (n=16)
Study 306	71%‡ [51%-87%] (n=28)	79% [58%-93%] (n=24)	53% [34%-72%] (n=30)	21% [5%-51%] (n=14)

* This analysis excludes dropouts and patients with major protocol violations
† Ranitidine bismuth citrate alone has not been proven to be superior to ranitidine for duodenal ulcer healing.
‡ P<0.05 for ranitidine bismuth citrate + clarithromycin versus placebo.

INDICATIONS AND USAGE:

Ranitidine bismuth citrate in combination with clarithromycin is indicated for the treatment of patients with an active duodenal ulcer associated with *H pylori* infection. The eradication of *H pylori* has been demonstrated to reduce the risk of duodenal ulcer recurrence. (See DOSAGE AND ADMINISTRATION and CLINICAL STUDIES.)

It is recommended that all patients not eradicated of *H pylori* following ranitidine bismuth citrate plus clarithromycin treatment be considered to have *H pylori* resistant to clarithromycin. (See CLINICAL PHARMACOLOGY, Microbiology.) Patients who fail therapy should not be re-treated with a regimen containing clarithromycin.

Note: Ranitidine bismuth citrate should not be prescribed alone for the treatment of active duodenal ulcer.

CONTRAINDICATIONS:

This product is contraindicated in patients known to have hypersensitivity to ranitidine bismuth citrate or any of its ingredients.

For information on clarithromycin contraindications, see CONTRAINDICATIONS, in the Clarithromycin monograph.

WARNINGS:

The physician should consult the Clarithromycin monograph for information concerning WARNINGSand PRECAUTIONSassociated with this drug.

PRECAUTIONS:

GENERAL

The bismuth derived from ranitidine bismuth citrate may cause a temporary and harmless darkening of the tongue and/or stool. Stool darkening should not be confused with melena (blood in the stool).

Ranitidine bismuth citrate in combination with clarithromycin should not be used in patients with a history of acute porphyria.

This combination therapy is not recommended in patients with creatinine clearance less than 25 ml/min. (See DOSAGE AND ADMINISTRATION.)

LABORATORY TESTS

No specific clinical laboratory tests are recommended for monitoring patients prior to and/or after treatment with ranitidine bismuth citrate plus clarithromycin. False-positive tests for urine protein with Multistix may occur during ranitidine therapy, and, therefore, testing with sulfosalicyclic acid is recommended.

CARCINOGENESIS, MUTAGENESIS, AND IMPAIRMENT OF FERTILITY

In a 24-month oral carcinogenicity study in $B6C3F_1$ mice, ranitidine bismuth citrate at daily doses up to 1000 mg/kg was not carcinogenic. For a 50 kg person of average height (1.46 m^2 body surface area), this dose represents five times the recommended clinical dose of 400 mg twice daily (592 mg/m^2). In a 24-month oral carcinogenicity study in Sprague-Dawley rats, ranitidine bismuth citrate at daily doses up to 500 mg/kg, five times the recommended human dose based on body surface area, was not carcinogenic.

Ranitidine bismuth citrate was not genotoxic in the Ames test, the mouse lymphoma cell (L5178Y/TK+/-) forward mutation test, the *ex vivo* rat gastric mucosal unscheduled DNA synthesis (UDS) test, or the *in vivo* rat micronucleus test. It was positive in *in vitro* human lymphocyte chromosomal aberration assay.

Ranitidine bismuth citrate at oral doses up to 1800 mg/kg per day (18 times the recommended human dose based on an average body surface area of 1.46 m^2) was found to have no effect on impairment of fertility and reproductive performance of male and female rats.

PREGNANCY: PREGNANCY CATEGORY C

Teratogenic Effects: Ranitidine bismuth citrate used in combination with clarithromycin carries a Pregnancy Category C because clarithromycin carries Pregnancy Category C. (See PRECAUTIONS, Pregnancy, Teratogenic Effects, Pregnancy Category C and WARNINGS in the clarithromycin monograph.)

Non-Teratogenic Effects of Ranitidine Bismuth Citrate: Teratology studies have been performed in pregnant rats at oral doses up to 1800 mg/kg per day (18 times the recommended human dose based on body surface area) and pregnant rabbits at oral doses up to 300 mg/kg per day (6 times the recommended human dose, based on body surface area) and have revealed no evidence of harm to the fetus due to ranitidine bismuth citrate.

There are however, no adequate and well-controlled studies in pregnant women. Because animal reproduction studies are not always predictive of human response, this drug should be used during pregnancy only if clearly needed.

Five patients became pregnant while they were receiving ranitidine bismuth citrate alone at varied doses. Three of these patients had normal pregnancies and newborns, one had a voluntary abortion, and one delivered a baby with postaxial polydactyly.

This Caucasian woman had a history of unexplained spontaneous abortions. She had received ranitidine bismuth citrate for 7 days prior to conception and for 20 days after conception. The investigator considered the event unrelated to ranitidine bismuth citrate. Postaxial polydactyly is about 10 times more frequent in blacks than in Caucasians. In American whites, incidence figures vary from 1:3300 to 1:630 live births, and in American blacks figures vary from 1:300 to 1:100 live births. (March of Dimes, 1996.)

NURSING MOTHERS

It is not known whether ranitidine bismuth citrate is excreted in human milk. Because many drugs are excreted in human milk, caution should be exercised when ranitidine bismuth citrate is administered to a nursing woman. It is known that both ranitidine and bismuth are excreted in rat milk.

PEDIATRIC USE

PRECAUTIONS: *(cont'd)*

GERIATRIC USE

Ulcer healing and relapse rates in elderly patients (≥65 years of age) were no different from those in younger age-groups. The incidence rates for adverse events and laboratory abnormalities also were not different from those seen in other age-groups. In a pharmacokinetic study, serum levels of ranitidine were increased in elderly patients, but serum bismuth levels were equivalent to those seen in the overall population.

DRUG INTERACTIONS:

Coadministration or ranitidine bismuth citrate with clarithromycin resulted in increased plasma ranitidine concentrations (57%), increased plasma bismuth trough concentrations (48%), and increased 14-hydroxy-clarithromycin plasma concentrations (31%). Coadministration with aspirin results in a slight decrease in the rate of salicylate absorption that is clinically unimportant. Coadministration with a high dose of antacid (170 mEq) results in a 28% decrease in plasma concentrations of ranitidine and may decrease plasma concentrations of bismuth from ranitidine bismuth citrate. These effects are clinically insignificant.

For information on drug interactions associated with ranitidine, refer to ranitidine, DRUG INTERACTIONS.

ADVERSE REACTIONS:

Placebo-controlled trials in patients with active duodenal ulcer in the United States included 1023 patients given ranitidine bismuth citrate alone or in combination with clarithromycin, 120 patients given clarithromycin alone, and 469 patients given placebo.

Incidence of Drug-Related Adverse Reactions in Placebo-Controlled Clinical Trials: TABLE 3 lists drug-related adverse reactions that occurred at a frequency of ≥1% among patients treated with ranitidine bismuth citrate who participated in U.S. placebo-controlled trials.

TABLE 3 Drug-Related Adverse Reactions During Treatment*

Adverse Reaction	Placebo (n=469)	Ranitidine Bismuth Citrate Tablets 800 mg (n=903)	Clarithromycin 1500 mg (n=120)	Ranitidine Bismuth Citrate Tablets 800 mg + Clarithromycin 1500 mg (n=120)
Gastrointestinal				
Diarrhea	1%	2%	5%	8%
Nausea & vomiting	1%	<1%	2%	3%
Constipation	<1%	1%	0%	0%
Neurological				
Headache	<1%	1%	<1%	5%
Dizziness	<1%	<1%	2%	0%
Miscellaneous				
Disturbance of Taste	<1%	<1%	11%	10%
Sleep disorder	<1%	<1%	<1%	2%
Chest symptoms	<1%	0%	0%	2%
Skin				
Pruritis	0%	<1%	0%	3%
Urogenital				
Gynecological problems	0% (n=159)	<1% (n=267)	6% (n=32)	3% (n=34)

* Total daily doses.

Although seen in US clinical trials at a frequency of <1%, the following adverse events may be associated with the use of ranitidine bismuth citrate:

Gastrointestinal: Abdominal discomfort, gastric pain.

Hepatic: Transient changes in the liver enzymes SGPT (ALT) and SGOT (AST).

Hypersensitivity: There have been rare reports of hypersensitivity reactions, including skin rash and anaphylaxis.

Central Nervous System: Tremors have been reported rarely in patients receiving ranitidine bismuth citrate. The relationship to ranitidine bismuth citrate has been unclear.

For information on ADVERSE REACTIONSassociated with ranitidine, refer to that monograph. For information on ADVERSE REACTIONS associated with clarithromycin, refer to that monograph.

OVERDOSAGE:

There has been limited experience with overdosage. Adverse events related to overdosage with ranitidine are usually reversible, nonspecific, and non-life threatening and result in no adverse sequelae. Although not seen in clinical trials with ranitidine bismuth citrate, bismuth intoxication from prolonged overdosage or deliberate self-poisoning can result in neurotoxicity and nephrotoxicity and possibly other symptoms seen with the use of soluble bismuth compounds. In the event of an overdose or suspected bismuth toxicity, measures should be employed to remove unabsorbed material from the gastrointestinal tract, and symptom monitoring and other supportive therapy should be employed, if indicated.

Single oral doses of ranitidine bismuth citrate at 3000 and 4000 mg/kg in male and female mice, respectively (approximately 15 to 20 times the recommended human dose based on body surface area), and at 2000 and 3000 mg/kg in male and female rats, respectively, (approximately 20 to 30 times the recommended human dose based on body surface area) were lethal. Symptoms of acute toxicity were piloerection, tremors, hunched posture, rapid respiration, and decreased activity.

DOSAGE AND ADMINISTRATION:

Eradication of *H pylori* Infection in Patients With Active Duodenal Ulcer: The recommended dosage of ranitidine bismuth citrate is 400 mg twice daily for 4 weeks (28 days) in conjunction with clarithromycin 500 mg 3 times daily for the first 2 weeks (14 days). Ranitidine bismuth citrate and clarithromycin can be taken with or without food.

Days 1-14	Ranitidine bismuth citrate 2× daily plus clarithromycin 500 mg 3× daily
Days 15-28	Ranitidine bismuth citrate 400 mg 2× daily

Dosage Adjustment in Elderly Patients: No dosage adjustment is necessary in elderly patients. (See PRECAUTIONS, Geriatric Use in the clarithromycin monograph.)

Dosage Adjustment in Renally Impaired Patients: Because the principle route of excretion is renal, care should be exercised when administering this combination therapy to renally impaired patients. This combination therapy is not recommended in patients with creatinine clearance less than 25 ml/min.

PATIENT INFORMATION:

Rinitidine bismuth citrate is used in combination with clarithromycin for the treatment of active duodenal ulcer associated with *H pylori* infection.

Do not use if you have a history of acute porphyria.

Do not take any other prescription or over-the-counter drugs without checking with your physician or pharmacist.

Inform your physician if you are pregnant or nursing or have kidney disease.

May cause diarrhea, nausea/vomiting, dizziness, taste disturbance, or gynecological problems.

May be taken with or without food.

HOW SUPPLIED:

Tritec tablets 400 mg are blue, aqueous film-coated tablets in an elongated octagonal shape engraved with "TRITEC" on one side and a stomach-shaped logo on the other.

Storage: Store between 2° and 30°C (36° and 86°F) in a dry place. Protect from light. Replace cap securely after each opening.

HOW SUPPLIED - EQUIVALENTS NOT AVAILABLE:

Tablet - Oral - 400 mg

100's	$174.00	TRITEC, Glaxo Wellcome	00173-0488-01
100's	$182.70	TRITEC, Glaxo Wellcome	00173-0488-02

BISMUTH; HYDROCORTISONE *(000499)*

CATEGORIES: Anorectal Products; Anti-Inflammatory Agents; Antimicrobials; Antipruritics/Local Anesthetics; Colitis; Cryptitis; DESI Drugs; Mucous Membrane Agents; Skin/Mucous Membrane Agents; Pregnancy Category C; Sales > $100 Million; FDA Pre 1938 Drugs

BRAND NAMES: Anu-Med Hc; Anucort; Anuprep Hc; Anusol-Hc; *Anusol-HC* (England); *Anusol HC*; *Anusol H.C.*; Dixon-Shane; Hemorrhoidal-Hc; **Rectacort**
(International brand names outside U.S. in italics)

FORMULARIES: Aetna

Prescribing information not available at time of publication.

HOW SUPPLIED - EQUIVALENTS NOT AVAILABLE:

Suppository - Rectal - 25 mg

12's	**$5.10**	**RECTACORT, Century Pharms**	**00436-0603-12**
12's	**$5.10**	**RECTACORT, Century Pharms**	**00436-0605-12**
12's	$6.75	Anu-Med Hc, Major Pharms	00904-0160-12
100's	$43.80	Anu-Med Hc, Major Pharms	00904-0160-60

BISMUTH; KAOLIN; PAREGORIC; PECTIN *(000502)*

CATEGORIES: Antidiarrhea Agents; Gastrointestinal Drugs; Otic Preparations; Otologic; Vertigo/Motion Sickness/Vomiting; DEA Class CIII; DEA Class CV; FDA Pre 1938 Drugs

BRAND NAMES: Biskapec; Infantol; Kaodene

Prescribing information not available at time of publication.

HOW SUPPLIED - EQUIVALENTS NOT AVAILABLE:

Tablet, Uncoated - Oral - 65 mg/130 mg/1.

1000's	$50.00	BISKAPEC, C O Truxton	00463-4009-10

BISOPROLOL FUMARATE *(003132)*

CATEGORIES: Antihypertensives; Beta Adrenergic Blocking Agents; Beta Blockers; Cardiovascular Drugs; Hypertension; Renal Drugs; FDA Class 1S ("Standard Review"); FDA Approved 1992 Jul

BRAND NAMES: *Bisobloc*; *Bisomerck* (Germany); *Concor* (Germany); *Concore*; *Cordalin* (Germany); *Detensiel* (France); *Emconcor*; *Emcor* (England); *Euradal*; *Fondril* (Germany); *Isoten*; *Maintate* (Japan); *Monocor* (England); *Pactens*; *Soprol* (France); **Zebeta**
(International brand names outside U.S. in italics)

FORMULARIES: Medi-Cal

DESCRIPTION:

Zebeta (bisoprolol fumarate) is a synthetic, beta$_1$-selective (cardioselective) adrenoreceptor blocking agent. The chemical name for bisoprolol fumarate is (±)-1-(4-((2-(1-Methyl- ethoxy) ethoxy)methyl)phenoxy)-3-((1-methylethyl)amino)-2-propanol(*E*)-2-butenedioate (2:1) (salt). It possesses an asymmetric carbon atom in its structure and is provided as a racemic mixture. The S(-) enantiomer is responsible for most of the beta-blocking activity. Its empirical formula is $(C_{18}H_{31}NO_4)_2 \cdot C_4H_4O_4$.

Bisoprolol fumarate has a molecular weight of 766.97. It is a white crystalline powder which is approximately equally hydrophilic and lipophilic, and is readily soluble in water, methanol, ethanol, and chloroform.

Zebeta is available as 5 and 10 mg tablets for oral administration.

Inactive ingredients include Colloidal Silicon Dioxide, Corn Starch, Crospovidone, Dibasic Calcium Phosphate, Hydroxypropyl Methylcellulose, Magnesium Stearate, Microcrystalline Cellulose, Polyethylene Glycol, Polysorbate 80, and Titanium Dioxide. The 5 mg tablets also contain Red and Yellow Iron Oxide.

CLINICAL PHARMACOLOGY:

Bisoprolol fumarate is a beta$_1$-selective (cardioselective) adrenoreceptor blocking agent without significant membrane stabilizing activity or intrinsic sympathomimetic activity in its therapeutic dosage range. Cardioselectivity is not absolute, however, and at higher doses (≥ 20 mg) bisoprolol fumarate also inhibits beta^2-adrenoreceptors, chiefly located in the bronchial and vascular musculature; to retain selectivity it is therefore important to use the lowest effective dose.

CLINICAL PHARMACOLOGY: *(cont'd)*

PHARMACOKINETICS AND METABOLISM

The absolute bioavailability after a 10 mg oral dose of bisoprolol fumarate is about 80%. Absorption is not affected by the presence of food. The first pass metabolism of bisoprolol fumarate is about 20%.

Binding to serum proteins is approximately 30%. Peak plasma concentrations occur within 2-4 hours of dosing with 5 to 20 mg, and mean peak values range from 16 ng/ml at 5 mg to 70 ng/ml at 20 mg. Once daily dosing with bisoprolol fumarate results in less than twofold intersubject variation in peak plasma levels. The plasma elimination half-life is 9-12 hours and is slightly longer in elderly patients, in part because of decreased renal function in that population. Steady state is attained within 5 days of once daily dosing. In both young and elderly populations, plasma accumulation is low; the accumulation factor ranges from 1.1 to 1.3, and is what would be expected from the first order kinetics and once daily dosing. Plasma concentrations are proportional to the administered dose in the range of 5 to 20 mg. Pharmacokinetic characteristics of the two enantiomers are similar.

Bisoprolol fumarate is eliminated equally by renal and non-renal pathways with about 50% of the dose appearing unchanged in the urine and the remainder appearing in the form of inactive metabolites. In humans, the known metabolites are labile or have no known pharmacologic activity. Less than 2% of the dose is excreted in the feces. Bisoprolol fumarate is not metabolized by cytochrome P450 II D6 (debrisoquin hydroxylase).

In subjects with creatinine clearance less than 40 ml/min, the plasma half-life is increased approximately threefold compared to healthy subjects.

In patients with cirrhosis of the liver, the elimination of bisoprolol fumarate is more variable in rate and significantly slower than that in healthy subjects, with plasma half-life ranging from 8.3 to 21.7 hours.

PHARMACODYNAMICS

The most prominent effect of bisoprolol fumarate is the negative chronotropic effect, resulting in a reduction in resting and exercise heart rate. There is a fall in resting and exercise cardiac output with little observed change in stroke volume, and only a small increase in right atrial pressure, or pulmonary capillary wedge pressure at rest or during exercise.

Findings in short-term clinical hemodynamics studies with bisoprolol fumarate are similar to those observed with other beta-blocking agents.

The mechanism of action of its antihypertensive effects has not been completely established. Factors which may be involved include:

1) Decreased cardiac output,

2) Inhibition of renin release by the kidneys,

3) Diminution of tonic sympathetic outflow from the vasomotor centers in the brain.

In normal volunteers, bisoprolol fumarate therapy resulted in a reduction of exercise- and isoproterenol-induced tachycardia. The maximal effect occurred within 1-4 hours post-dosing. Effects persisted for 24 hours at doses equal to or greater than 5 mg.

Electrophysiology studies in man have demonstrated that bisoprolol fumarate significantly decreases heart rate, increases sinus node recovery time, prolongs AV node refractory periods, and, with rapid atrial stimulation, prolongs AV nodal conduction.

Beta$_1$-selectivity of bisoprolol fumarate has been demonstrated in both animal and human studies. No effects at therapeutic doses on beta$_a$- adrenoreceptor density have been observed. Pulmonary function studies have been conducted in healthy volunteers, asthmatics, and patients with chronic obstructive pulmonary disease (COPD). Doses of bisoprolol fumarate ranged from 5 to 60 mg, atenolol from 50 to 200 mg, metoprolol from 100 to 200 mg, and propranolol from 40 to 80 mg. In some studies, slight, asymptomatic increases in airways resistance (AWR) and decreases in forced expiratory volume (FEV_1) were observed with doses of bisoprolol fumarate 20 mg and higher, similar to the small increases in AWR also noted with the other cardioselective beta-blockers. The changes induced by beta-blockade with all agents were reversed by bronchodilator therapy.

Bisoprolol fumarate has minimal effect on serum lipids during antihypertensive studies. In U.S. placebo-controlled trials, changes in total cholesterol averaged +0.8% for bisoprolol fumarate-treated patients; and +0.7% for placebo. Changes in triglycerides averaged +19% for bisoprolol fumarate- treated patients, and +17% for placebo.

Bisoprolol fumarate has also been given concomitantly with thiazide diuretics. Even very low doses of hydrochlorothiazide (6.25 mg) were found to be additive with bisoprolol fumarate in lowering blood pressure in patients with mild-to-moderate hypertension.

CLINICAL STUDIES:

In two randomized double-blind placebo-controlled trials conducted in the U.S., reductions in systolic and diastolic blood pressure and heart rate 24 hours after dosing in patients with mild-to-moderate hypertension are shown below (TABLE 1). In both studies, mean systolic/diastolic blood pressures at baseline were approximately 150/100 mm Hg, and mean heart rate was 76 bpm. Drug effect is calculated by subtracting the placebo effect from the overall change in blood pressure and heart rate.

TABLE 1 Sitting Systolic/Diastolic Pressure (BP) and Heart Rate (HR) Mean Decrease (Δ) After 3 to 4 Weeks

		Bisoprolol Fumarate		
Study A	**Placebo**	**5 mg**	**10 mg**	**20 mg**
n=	61	61	61	61
Total ΔBP (mm HG)	5.4/3.2	10.4/8.0	11.2/10.9	12.8/11.9
Drug Effect[a]	-	5.0/4.8	5.8/7.7	7.4/8.7
Total ΔHR (bpm)	0.5	7.2	8.7	11.3
Drug Effect[a]	-	6.7	8.2	10.8

[a]Observed total changes from baseline minus placebo.

		Bisoprolol Fumarate	
Study B	**Placebo**	**2.5 mg**	**10 mg**
n=	56	59	62
Total ΔBP (mm Hg)	3.0/3.7	7.6/8.1	13.5/11.2
Drug Effect[a]	-	4.6/4.4	10.5/7.5
Total ΔHR (bpm)	1.6	3.8	10.7
Drug Effect[a]	-	2.2	9.1

[a]Observed total changes from baseline minus placebo.

Blood pressure responses were seen within one week of treatment and changed little thereafter. They were sustained for 12 weeks and for over a year in studies of longer duration. Blood pressure returned to baseline when bisoprolol fumarate was tapered over two weeks in a long-term study.

CLINICAL STUDIES: *(cont'd)*

Overall, significantly greater blood pressure reductions were observed on bisoprolol fumarate than on placebo regardless of race, age, or gender. There were no significant differences in response between black and non- black patients.

INDICATIONS AND USAGE:

Bisoprolol fumarate is indicated in the management of hypertension. It may be used alone or in combination with other antihypertensive agents.

CONTRAINDICATIONS:

Bisoprolol fumarate is containdicated in patients with cardiogenic shock, overt cardiac failure, second or third degree AV block, and marked sinus bradycardia.

WARNINGS:

CARDIAC FAILURE

Sympathetic stimulation is a vital component supporting circulatory function in the setting of congestive heart failure, and beta-blockade may result in further depression of myocardial contractility and precipitate more severe failure. In general, beta-blocking agents should be avoided in patients with overt congestive failure. However, in some patients with compensated cardiac failure it may be necessary to utilize them. In such a situation, they must be used cautiously.

IN PATIENTS WITHOUT A HISTORY OF CARDIAC FAILURE

Continued depression of the myocardium with beta-blockers can, in some patients, precipitate cardiac failure. At the first signs or symptoms of heart failure, discontinuation of bisoprolol fumarate should be considered. In some cases, beta-clocker therapy can be continued while heart failure is treated with other drugs.

ABRUPT CESSATION OF THERAPY

Exacerbation of angina pectoris, and, in some instances, myocardial infarction or ventricular arrhythmia, have been observed in patients with coronary artery disease following abrupt cessation of therapy with beta- blockers. Such patients should, therefore, be cautioned against interruption or discontinuation of therapy without the physician's advice. Even in patients without overt coronary artery disease, it may be advisable to taper therapy with bisoprolol fumarate over approximately one week with the patient under careful observation. If withdrawal symptoms occur, bisoprolol fumarate therapy should be reinstituted, at least temporarily.

PERIPHERAL VASCULAR DISEASE

Beta-blockers can precipitate or aggravate symptoms of arterial insufficiency in patients with peripheral vascular disease. Caution should be exercised in such individuals.

BRONCHOSPASTIC DISEASE

Patients With Bronchospastic Disease Should, In General, Not Receive Beta-Blockers. Because of its relative beta$_1$-selectivity, however, bisoprolol fumarate may be used with caution in patients with bronchospastic disease who do not respond to, or who cannot tolerate other antihypertensive treatment. Since beta$_1$-selectivity is not absolute, the lowest possible dose of bisoprolol fumarate should be used, with therapy starting at 2.5 mg. A beta$_2$ agonist (bronchodilator) should be made available.

ANESTHESIA AND MAJOR SURGERY

If bisoprolol fumarate treatment is to be continued perioperatively, particular care should be taken when anesthetic agents which depress myocardial function, such as ether, cyclopropane, and trichloroethylene, are used. See OVERDOSAGE for information on treatment on bradycardia and hypotension.

DIABETES AND HYPOGLYCEMIA

Beta-blockers may mask some of the manifestations of hypoglycemia, particularly tachycardia.

Nonselective beta-blockers may potentiate insulin-induced hypoglycemia and delay recovery of serum glucose levels. Because of its beta$_1$- selectivity, this is less likely with bisoprolol fumarate. However, patients subject to spontaneous hypoglycemia, or diabetic patients receiving insulin or oral hypoglycemic agents, should be cautioned about these possibilities and bisoprolol fumarate should be used with caution.

THYROTOXICOSIS

Beta-adrenergic blockade may mask clinical signs of hyperthyroidism, such as tachycardia. Abrupt withdrawal of beta-blockade may be followed by an exacerbation of the symptoms of hyperthyroidism or may precipitate thyroid storm.

PRECAUTIONS:

Impaired Renal or Hepatic Function: Use caution in adjusting the dose of bisoprolol fumarate in patients with renal or hepatic impairment (see CLINICAL PHARMACOLOGY and DOSAGE AND ADMINISTRATION).

Information for the Patient: Patients, especially those with coronary artery disease, should be warned about discontinuing use of bisoprolol fumarate without a physician's supervision. Patients should also be advised to consult a physician if any difficulty in breathing occurs, or if they develop signs or symptoms of congestive heart failure or excessive bradycardia.

Patients subject to spontaneous hypoglycemia, or diabetic patients receiving insulin or oral hypoglycemic agents, should be cautioned that beta-blockers may mask some of the manifestations of hypoglycemia, particularly tachycardia, and bisoprolol fumarate should be used with caution.

Patients should know how they react to this medicine before they operate automobiles and machinery or engage in other tasks requiring alertness.

Carcinogenesis, Mutagenesis, and Impairment of Fertility: Long-term studies were conducted with oral bisoprolol fumarate administered in the feed of mice (20 and 24 months) and rats (26 months). No evidence of carcinogenic potential was seen in mice dosed up to 250 mg/kg/day or rats dosed up to 125 mg/kg/day. On a body weight basis, these doses are 625 and 312 times, respectively, the maximum recommended human dose (MRHD) of 20 mg, (or 0.4 mg/kg/day based on a 50 kg individual); on a body-surface-area-basis, these doses are 59 times (mice) and 64 times (rats) the MRHD. The mutagenic potential of bisoprolol fumarate was evaluated in the microbial mutagenicity (Ames) test, the point mutation and chromosome aberration assays in Chinese hamster V79 cells, the uunscheduled DNA synthesis test, the micronucleus test in mice, and the cytogenetics assay in rats. There was no evidence of mutagenic potential in these *in vitro* and *in vitro* assays.

Reproduction studies in rats did not show any impairment of fertility at doses up to 150 mg/kg/day of bisoprolol fumarate, or 375 and 77 times the MRHD on the basis of body-weight and body-surface-area, respectively.

Pregnancy Category C: In rats, bisoprolol fumarate was not teratogenic at doses up to 150 mg/kg/day which is 375 and 77 times the MRHD on the basis of body-weight and body surface area; respectively.

Bisoprolol fumarate was fetotoxic (increased late resorptions) at 50 mg/kg/day and maternotoxic (decreased food intake and body weight gain) at 150 mg/kg/day. The fetotoxicity in rats occurred at 125 times the MRHD on a body-weight-basis and 26 times the MRHD on the basis of body-surface area. The maternotoxicity occurred at 375 times the MRHD on a

PRECAUTIONS: *(cont'd)*

body-weight basis and 77 times the MRHD on the basis of body-surface-area. In rabbits, bisoprolol fumarate was not teratogenic at doses up to 12.5 mg/kg/day, which is 31 and 12 times the MRHD based on body-weight and surface area, respectively, but was embryolethal (increased early resorptions) at 12.5 mg/kg/day.

There are no adequate and well-controlled studies in pregnant women. Bisoprolol fumarate should be used during pregnancy only if the potential benefit justifies the potential risk to the fetus.

Nursing Mothers: Small amounts of bisoprolol fumarate (2% of the dose) have been detected in the milk of lactating rats. It is not known whether this drug is excreted in human milk. Because many drugs are excreted in human milk, caution should be exercised when bisoprolol fumarate is administered to nursing women.

Use in Elderly Patients: Bisoprolol fumarate has been used in elderly patients with hypertension. Response rate and mean decreases in systolic and diastolic blood pressure were similar to the deceases in younger patients in the U.S. clinical studies. Although no dose response study was conducted in elderly patients, there was a tendency for older patients to be maintained on higher doses of bisoprolol fumarate.

Observed reductions in heart rate were slightly greater in the elderly than in the young and tended to increase with starting dose. In general, no disparity in adverse experience reports or dropouts for safety reasons was observed between older and younger patients. Dose adjustment based on age is not necessary.

Pediatric Use: Safety and effectiveness in children have not been established.

DRUG INTERACTIONS:

Bisoprolol fumarate should not be combined with other beta- blocking agents. Patients receiving catecholamine-depleting drugs, such as reserpine or guanethidine, should be closely monitored, because the added beta-adrenergic blocking action of bisoprolol fumarate may produce excessive reduction of sympathetic activity. In patients receiving concurrent therapy with clonidine, if therapy is to be discontinued, it is suggested that bisoprolol fumarate be discontinued for several days before the withdrawal of clonidine.

Bisoprolol fumarate should be used with care when myocardial depressants or inhibitors of AV conduction, such as certain calcium antagonists (particularly of the phenylalkylamine (verapamil) and benzothiazepine (diltiazem) classes), or antiarrhythmic agents, such as disopyramide, are used concurrently.

Concurrent use of rifampin increases the metabolic clearance of bisoprolol fumarate, resulting in a shortened elimination half-life of bisoprolol fumarate. However, initial dose modification is generally not necessary. Pharmacokinetic studies document no clinically relevant interactions with other agents given concomitantly, including thiazide diuretics, digoxin and cimetidine. There was no effect of bisoprolol fumarate on prothrombin time in patients on stable doses of warfarin.

Risk of Anaphylactic Reaction: While taking beta-blockers, patients with a history of severe anaphylactic reaction to a variety of allergens may be more reactive to repeated challenge, either accidental, diagnostic, or therapeutic. Such patients may be unresponsive to the usual doses of epinephrine used to treat allergic reactions.

ADVERSE REACTIONS:

Safety data are available in more than 30,000 patients or volunteers. Frequency estimates and rates of withdrawal of therapy for adverse events were derived from two U.S. placebo-controlled studies.

In study A, doses of 5, 10, and 20 mg bisoprolol fumarate were administered for 4 weeks. In study B, doses of 2.5, 10 and 40 mg of bisoprolol fumarate were administered for 12 weeks. A total of 273 patients were treated with 5-20 mg of bisoprolol, 132 placebo.

Withdrawal of therapy for adverse events was 3.3% for patients receiving bisoprolol fumarate and 6.8% for patients on placebo. Withdrawals were less than 1% for either bradycardia or fatigue/lack of energy.

TABLE 2 presents adverse experiences, whether or not considered drug related, reported in at least 1% of patients in these studies, for all patients studied in placebo controlled clinical trials (2.5-40 mg), as well as for a subgroup that was treated with doses within the recommended dosage range (5-20 mg). Of the adverse events listed in the table, bradycardia, diarrhea, asthenia, fatigue and sinusitis appear to be dose related.

TABLE 2

All Adverse Experiences (%)

Body System/Adverse Experience	Placebo (n=132) %	Bisoprolol Fumarate 5-20 mg (n=273) %	Bisoprolol Fumarate 2.5-40 mg (n=404) %
Skin			
Increased sweating	1.5	0.7	1.0
Musculo-skeletal			
Arthralgia	2.3	2.2	2.7
Central Nervous System			
Dizziness	3.8	2.9	3.5
Headache	11.4	8.8	10.9
Hypoaesthesia	0.8	1.1	1.5
Autonomic Nervous System			
Dry mouth	1.5	0.7	1.3
Heart Rate/Rhythm			
Bradycardia	0	0.4	0.5
Psychiatric			
Vivid dreams	0	0	0
Insomnia	2.3	1.5	2.5
Depression	0.8	0	0.2
Gastrointestinal			
Diarrhea	1.5	2.6	3.5
Nausea	1.5	1.5	2.2
Vomiting	0	1.1	1.5
Respiratory			
Bronchospasm	0	0	0
Cough	4.5	2.6	2.5
Dyspnea	0.8	1.1	1.5
Pharyngitis	2.3	2.2	2.2
Rhinitis	3.0	2.9	4.0
Sinusitis	1.5	2.2	2.2
URI	3.8	4.8	5.0
Body As A Whole			
Asthenia	0	0.4	1.5
Chest pain	0.8	1.1	1.5
Fatigue	1.5	6.6	8.2
Edema (peripheral)	3.8	3.7	3.0

[a] percentage of patients with event

ADVERSE REACTIONS: *(cont'd)*

The following is a comprehensive list of adverse experiences reported with bisoprolol fumarate in worldwide studies, or in post marketing experience (in italics):

Central Nervous System: Dizziness, vertigo, headache, paresthesia, hypoesthesia, somnolence, anxiety/restlessness, decreased, concentration/memory.

Autonomic Nervous System: Dry mouth.

Cardiovascular: Bradycardia; palpitations and other rhythm disturbances, cold extremities, claudication, hypotension, orthostatic hypotension, chest pain, congestive heart failure, dyspnea on exertion.

Psychiatric: Vivid dreams, insomnia, depression.

Gastrointestinal: Gastric/epigastric/abdominal pain, gastritis, dyspepsia, nausea, vomiting, diarrhea, constipation.

Musculoskeletal: Muscle/joint pain, back/neck pain, muscle cramps, twitching/tremor. Skin: rash, acne, eczema, skin irritation, pruritus, flushing, sweating, alopecia, *angioedema, exfoliative dermatitis.*

Special Senses: Visual disturbances, ocular pain/pressure, abnormal lacrimation, tinnitus, earache, taste abnormalities.

Metabolic: Gout.

Respiratory: Asthma/bronchospasm, bronchitis, coughing, dyspnea, pharyngitis, rhinitis, sinusitis, URI.

Genito-urinary: Decreased libido/impotence, *peyronie's disease,* cystitis, renal colic.

Hematologic: Purpura.

General: Fatigue, asthenia, chest pain, malaise, edema, weight gain.

In addition, a variety of adverse effects have been reported with other beta-adrenergic blocking agents and should be considered potential adverse effects of bisoprolol fumarate:

Central Nervous System: Reversible mental depression progressing to catatonia, hallucinations, an acute reversible syndrome characterized by disorientation to time and place, emotional lability, slightly clouded sensorium.

Allergic: Fever, combined with aching and sore throat, laryngospasm, respiratory distress.

Hematologic: Agranulocytosis, thrombocytopenia, thrombocytopenic purpura.

Gastrointestinal: Mesenteric arterial thrombosis, ischemic colitis.

Miscellaneous: The oculomucocutaneous syndrome associated with the beta-blocker practolol has not been reported with bisoprolol fumarate during investigational use or extensive foreign marketing experience.

Laboratory Abnormalities: In clinical trials, the most frequently reported laboratory change was an increase in serum triglycerides, but this was not a consistent finding.

Sporadic liver test abnormalities have been reported. In the U.S. controlled trials experience with bisoprolol fumarate treatment for 4 - 12 weeks, the incidence of concomitant elevations in SGOT and SGPT of between 1-2 times normal was 3.9%, compared to 2.5% for placebo. No patient had concomitant elevations greater than twice normal.

In the long-term, uncontrolled experience with bisoprolol fumarate treatment for 6-18 months, the incidence of one or more concomitant elevations in SGOT and SGPT of between 1-2 times normal was 6.2%. The incidence of multiple occurrences was 1.9%. For concomitant elevations in SGOT and SGPT of greater than twice normal, the incidence was 1.5%. The incidence of multiple occurrences was 0.3%. In many cases these elevations were attributed to underlying disorders, or resolved during continued treatment with bisprolol fumarate.

Other laboratory changes included small increases in uric acid, creatinine, BUN, serum potassium, glucose, and phosphorus and decreases in WBC and platelets. These were generally not of clinical importance and rarely resulted in discontinuation of bisoprolol fumarate.

As with other beta-blockers, ANA conversions have also been reported on bisoprolol fumarate. About 15% of patients in long-term studies converted to a positive titer, although about one-third of these patients subsequently reconverted to a negative toter while on continued therapy.

OVERDOSAGE:

The most common signs expected with overdosage of a beta-blocker are bradycardia, hypotension, congestive heart failure, bronchospasm, and hypoglycemia. To date, a few cases of overdose (maximum: 2000 mg) with bisoprolol fumarate have been reported. Bradycardia and/or hypotension were noted. Sympathomimetic agents were given in some cases, and all patients recovered.

In general, if overdose occurs, bisoprolol fumarate therapy should be stopped and supportive and symptomatic treatment should be provided. Limited data suggest that bisoprolol fumarate is not dialyzable. Based on the expected pharmacologic actions and recommendations for other beta-blockers, the following general measures should be considered when clinically warranted.

Bradycardia: Administer IV atropine. If the response is inadequate, isoproterenol or another gent with positive chronotropic properties may be given cautiously. Under some circumstances, transvenous pacemaker insertion may be necessary.

Hypotension: IV fluids and vasopressors should be administered. Intravenous glucagon may be useful.

Heart Block (second or third degree): Patients should be carefully monitored and treated with isoproterenol infusion or transvenous cardiac pacemaker insertion, as appropriate.

Congestive Heart Failure: Initiate conventional therapy (*i.e.*, digitalis, diuretics, inotropic agents, vasodilating agents).

Bronchospasm: Administer bronchodilator therapy such as isoproterenol and/or aminophylline.

Hypoglycemia: Administer IV glucose.

DOSAGE AND ADMINISTRATION:

The dose of bisoprolol fumarate must be individualized to the needs of the patient. The usual starting dose is 5 mg once daily. In some patients, 2.5 mg may be an appropriate starting dose (see WARNINGS,Bronchospastic Disease). If the antihypertensive effect of 5 mg is inadequate, the dose may be increased to 10 mg and then, if necessary, to 20 mg once daily.

Patients with Renal or Hepatic Impairment: In patients with hepatic impairment (hepatitis or cirrhosis) or renal dysfunction (creatinine clearance less than 40 ml/min), the initial daily dose should be 2.5 mg and caution should be used in dose-titration. Since limited data suggest that bisoprolol fumarate is not dialyzable, drug replacement is not necessary in patients undergoing dialysis.

Elderly Patients: It is not necessary to adjust the dose in the elderly, unless there is also significant renal or hepatic dysfunction (See DOSAGE AND ADMINISTRATION, Patients with Renal or Hepatic Impairment ; PRECAUTIONS, Use in Elderly Patients.

Children: There is no pediatric experience with bisoprolol fumarate.

Storage: Store at Controlled Room Temperature 15-30° (59-86°F). Dispense in tight container as defined in the USP.

HOW SUPPLIED - EQUIVALENTS NOT AVAILABLE:

Tablet, Plain Coated - Oral - 5 mg
30's $26.59 ZEBETA, Lederle Pharm 00005-3816-38

Tablet, Plain Coated - Oral - 10 mg
30's $26.59 ZEBETA, Lederle Pharm 00005-3817-38

BISOPROLOL FUMARATE; HYDROCHLOROTHIAZIDE *(003167)*

CATEGORIES: Antihypertensives; Beta Adrenergic Blocking Agents; Beta Blockers; Cardiovascular Drugs; Hypertension; Renal Drugs; FDA Class 1S ("Standard Review"); FDA Approved 1993 Mar; Top 200 Drugs; Top 200 Drugs

BRAND NAMES: *Concor Plus*; *Concor Plus Forte*; **Ziac**
(International brand names outside U.S. in italics)

DESCRIPTION:

Ziac (bisoprolol fumarate and hydrochlorothiazide) is indicated for the treatment of hypertension. It combines two antihypertensive agents in a once-daily dosage; a synthetic beta$_1$-selective (cardioselective) adrenoceptor blocking agent (bisoprolol fumarate) and a benzothiadiazine diuretic (hydrochlorothiazide).

Bisoprolol fumarate is chemically described as (±)-1-(4-((2-(1-Methylethoxy)ethoxy)methyl) phenoxy)-3-((1-methylethyl)amino)-2-propanol (*E*)-2-butenedioate (2:1) (salt). It possesses an asymmetric carbon atom in its structure and is provided as a racemic mixture. The S(-) enantiomer is responsible for most of the beta-blocking activity. Its empirical formula is $(C_{18}H_{31}NO_4)_2 \cdot C_4H_4O_4$ and it has a molecular weight of 766.97.

Bisoprolol fumarate is a white crystalline powder, approximately equally hydrophilic and lipophilic, and readily soluble in water, methanol, ethanol, and chloroform.

Hydrochlorothiazide (HCTZ) is 6-Chloro-3,4-dihydro-2*H*-1,2,4- benzothiadiazine-7-sulfonamide 1,1-dioxide. It is a white, or practically white, practically odorless crystalline powder. It is slightly soluble in water, sparingly soluble in dilute sodium hydroxide solution, freely soluble in n-butylamine and dimethylformamide, soluble in methanol, and insoluble in ether, chloroform, and dilute mineral acids. Its empirical formula is $C_7H_8ClN_3O_4S_2$ and it has a molecular weight of 297.73.

Each Ziac 2.5 mg/6.25 mg tablet for oral administration contains:Bisoprolol fumarate 2.5 mg,Hydrochlorothiazide 6.25 mg.

Each Ziac 5 mg/6.25 mg tablet for oral administration contains:Bisoprolol fumarate 5 mg,Hydrochlorothiazide 6.25 mg

Each Ziac 10 mg/6.25 mg tablet for oral administration contains:Bisoprolol fumarate 10 mg,Hydrochlorothiazide 6.25 mg

Inactive ingredients include Colloidal Silicon Dioxide, Corn Starch, Dibasic Calcium Phosphate, Hydroxypropyl Methylcellulose, Magnesium Stearate, Microcrystalline Cellulose, Polyethylene Glycol, Polysorbate 80, and Titanium Dioxide. The 5 mg/6.25 mg tablet also contains Red and Yellow Iron Oxide. The 2.5 mg/6.25 mg tablet also contains Crospovidone, Pregelatinized Starch and Yellow Iron Oxide.

CLINICAL PHARMACOLOGY:

Bisoprolol fumarate and HCTZ have been used individually and in combination for the treatment of hypertension. The antihypertensive effects of these agents are additive; HCTZ 6.25 mg significantly increases the antihypertensive effect of bisoprolol fumarate. The incidence of hypokalemia with the bisoprolol fumarate and HCTZ 6.25 mg combination (B/H) is significantly lower than with HCTZ 25 mg. In clinical trials of Ziac, mean changes in serum potassium for patients treated with Ziac 2.5/6.25 mg. 5/6.25 mg or 10/6.25 mg or placebo were less than ± 0.1 mEq/L. Mean changes in serum potassium for patients treated with any dose of bisoprolol in combination with HCTZ 25 mg ranged from -0.1 to -0.3 mEq/L.

Bisoprolol fumarate is a beta$_1$-selective (cardioselective) adrenoceptor blocking agent without significant membrane stabilizing or intrinsic sympathomimetic activities in its therapeutic dose range. At higher doses (≥ 20 mg) bisoprolol fumarate also inhibits beta$_2$-adrenoreceptors located in bronchial and vascular musculature. To retain relative selectivity, it is important to use the lowest effective dose. Hydrochlorothiazide is a benzothiadiazine diuretic. Thiazides affect renal tubular mechanisms of electrolyte reabsorption and increase excretion of sodium and chloride in approximately equivalent amounts. Natriuresis causes a secondary loss of potassium.

PHARMACOKINETICS AND METABOLISM

Ziac: In healthy volunteers, both bisoprolol fumarate and hydrochlorothiazide are well absorbed following oral administration of Ziac. No change is observed in the bioavailability of either agent when given together in a single tablet. Absorption is not affected whether Ziac is taken with or without food. Mean peak bisoprolol fumarate plasma concentrations of about 9.0 ng/ml, 19 ng/ml and 36/ng/ml occur approximately 3 hours after the administration of the 2.5 mg/6.25 mg, 5 mg/6.25 mg and 10 mg/6.25 combination tablets, respectively. Mean peak plasma hydrochlorothiazide concentrations of 30 ng/ml occur approximately 2.5 hours following the administration of the combination. Dose proportional increases in plasma bisoprolol concentrations are observed between the 2.5 and 5, as well as between the 5 and 10 mg doses. The elimination $T_{1/2}$ of bisoprolol ranges from 7 to 15 hours and of hydrochlorothiazide ranges from 4 to 10 hours. The percent of dose excreted unchanged in urine is about 55% for bisoprolol and about 60% for hydrochlorothiazide.

Bisoprolol Fumarate: The absolute bioavailability after a 10 mg oral dose of bisoprolol fumarate is about 80%. The first pass metabolism of bisoprolol fumarate is about 20%.

The pharmacokinetic profile of bisoprolol fumarate has been examined following single doses and at steady state. Binding to serum proteins is approximately 30%. Peak plasma concentrations occur within 2-4 hours of dosing with 2.5 to 20 mg, and mean peak values range from 9.0 ng/ml at 2.5 mg to 70 ng/ml at 20 mg. Once-daily dosing with bisoprolol fumarate results in less than twofold intersubject variation in peak plasma concentrations. Plasma concentrations are proportional to the administered dose in the range of 2.5 to 20 mg. The plasma elimination half-life is 9-12 hours and is slightly longer in elderly patients, in part because of decreased renal function. Steady state is attained within 5 days with once-daily dosing. In both young and elderly populations, plasma accumulation is low; the accumulation factor ranges from 1.1 to 1.3, and is what would be expected from the half-life and once daily-dosing. Bisoprolol is eliminated equally by renal and nonrenal pathways with about 50% of the dose appearing unchanged in the urine and the remainder in the form of inactive metabolites. In humans, the known metabolites are labile or have no known pharmacologic activity. Less than 2% of the dose is excreted in the feces. The pharmacokinetic characteristics of the two enantiomers are similar. Bisoprolol is not metabolized by cytochrome P450 II D6 (debrisoquine hydroxylase).

In subjects with creatinine clearance less than 40 ml/min, the plasma half-life is increased approximately threefold compared to healthy subjects.

CLINICAL PHARMACOLOGY: *(cont'd)*

In patients with liver cirrhosis, the rate of elimination of bisoprolol is more variable and significantly slower than that in healthy subjects, with a plasma half-life ranging from 8 to 22 hours.

In elderly subjects, mean plasma concentrations at steady state are increased, in part attributed to lower creatinine clearance. However, no significant differences in the degree of bisoprolol accumulation is found between young and elderly populations.

Hydrochlorothiazide: Hydrochlorothiazide is well absorbed (65%-75%) following oral administration. Absorption of hydrochlorothiazide is reduced in patients with congestive heart failure.

Peak plasma concentrations are observed within 1-5 hours of dosing, and range from 70-490 ng/ml following oral doses of 12.5-100 mg. Plasma concentrations are linearly related to the administered dose. Concentrations of hydrochlorothiazide are 1.6-1.8 times higher in whole blood than in plasma. Binding to serum proteins has been reported to be approximately 40% to 68%. The plasma elimination half-life has been reported to be 6-15 hours. Hydrochlorothiazide is eliminated primarily by renal pathways. Following oral doses of 12.5-100 mg, 55%-77% of the administered dose appears in urine and greater than 95% of the absorbed dose is excreted in urine as unchanged drug. Plasma concentrations of hydrochlorothiazide are increased and the elimination half-life is prolonged in patients with renal disease.

PHARMACODYNAMICS

Bisoprolol Fumarate: Findings in clinical hemodynamics studies with bisoprolol fumarate are similar to those observed with other beta-blockers. The most prominent effect is the negative chronotropic effect, giving a reduction in resting and exercise heart rate. There is a fall in resting and exercise cardiac output with little observed change in stroke volume, and only a small increase in right atrial pressure, of pulmonary capillary wedge pressure at rest or during exercise.

In normal volunteers, bisoprolol fumarate therapy resulted in a reduction of exercise- and isoproterenol-induced tachycardia.The maximal effect occurred within 1-4 hours post-dosing. Effects generally persisted for 24 hours at doses of 5 ml or greater.

In controlled clinical trials, bisoprolol fumarate given as a single daily dose has been shown to be an effective antihypertensive agent when used alone or concomitantly with thiazide diuretics (see CLINICAL STUDIES).

The mechanism of bisoprolol fumarate's antihypertensive effect has not been completely established. Factors that may be involved include:

1) Decreased cardiac output,

2) Inhibition of renin release by the kidneys,

3) Diminution of tonic sympathetic outflow from vasomotor centers in the brain.

Beta$_1$selectivity of bisoprolol fumarate has been demonstrated in both animal and human studies. No effects at therapeutic doses on beta$_2$-adrenoreceptor density have been observed. Pulmonary function studies have been conducted in healthy volunteers, asthmatics, and patients with chronic obstructive pulmonary disease (COPD). Doses of bisoprolol fumarate ranged from 5 to 60 mg, atenolol from 50 to 200 mg, metoprolol from 100 to 200 mg, and propranolol from 40 to 80 mg. In some studies, slight, asymptomatic increases in airway resistance (AWR) and decreases in forced expiratory volume (FEV_1) were observed with doses of bisoprolol fumarate 20 mg and higher, similar to the small increases in AWR noted with other cardioselective beta-blocking agents. The changes induced by beta-blockade with all agents were reversed by bronchodilator therapy.

Electrophysiology studies in man have demonstrated that bisoprolol fumarate significantly decreases heart rate, increases sinus node recovery time, prolongs AV node refractory periods, and, with rapid atrial stimulation, prolongs AV nodal conduction.

CLINICAL STUDIES:

In controlled clinical trials, bisoprolol fumarate/hydrochlorothiazide 6.25 mg has been shown to reduce systolic and diastolic blood pressure throughout a 24-hour period when administered once daily. The effects on systolic and diastolic blood pressure reduction of the combination of bisoprolol fumarate and hydrochlorothiazide were additive. Further, treatment effects were consistent across age groups (< 60, ≥ 60 years), racial groups (black, nonblack) and gender (male, female).

In two randomized, double-blind, placebo-controlled trials conducted in the U.S., reductions in systolic and diastolic blood pressure and heart rate 24 hours after dosing in patients with mild-to-moderate hypertension are shown below (TABLES 1A and IB). In both studies mean systolic/diastolic blood pressure and heart rate at baseline were approximately 151/101 mm HG and 77 bpm.

TABLE 1A Sitting Systolic/Diastolic Pressure (BP) and Heart Rate (HR)

Mean Decrease (Δ) After 3-4 Weeks	Placebo	Study 1 B5/H6.25 mg
n=	75	150
Total ΔBP (mm Hg)	-2.9/-3.9	-15.8/-12.6
Drug Effect[a]	-/-	-12.9/-8.7
Total ΔHR (bpm)	-0.3	-6.9
Drug Effect[a]	-	-6.6

[a]Observed mean change from baseline minus placebo

TABLE 1B Sitting Systolic/Diastolic Pressure (BP) and Heart Rate (HR)

Mean Decrease (Δ) After 3-4 Weeks	Placebo	H6.25 mg	Study 2 B2.5/H6.25 mg	B10/H6.25 mg
n=	56	23	28	25
Total ΔBP (mm Hg)	-3.0/-3.7	-6.6/-5.8	-14.1/-10.5	-15.3/-14.3
Drug Effect[a]	-/-	-3.6/-2.1	-11.1/-6.8	-12.3/-10.6
Total ΔHR (bpm)	-1.6	-0.8	-3.7	-9.8
Drug Effect[a]	-	+0.8	-2.1	-8.2

[a]Observed mean change from baseline minus placebo.

Blood pressure responses were seen within 1 week of treatment but the maximum effect was apparent after 2 to 3 weeks of treatment. Overall, significantly greater blood pressure reductions were observed on bisoprolol fumarate than on placebo. Further, blood pressure reductions were significantly greater for each of the bisoprolol fumarate plus hydrochlorothiazide combinations than for either of the components used alone regardless of race, age, or gender. There were no significant differences in response between black and nonblack patients.

INDICATIONS AND USAGE:

Bisoprolol fumarate is indicated in the management of hypertension.

CONTRAINDICATIONS:

Bisoprolol fumarate is contraindicated in patients in cardiogenic shock, overt cardiac failure (see WARNINGS), second or third degree AV block, marked sinus bradycardia, anuria, and hypersensitivity to either component of this product or to other sulfonamide-derived drugs.

WARNINGS:

Cardiac Failure: In general, beta-blocking agents should be avoided in patients with overt congestive failure. However, in some patients with compensated cardiac failure, it may be necessary to utilize these agents. In such situations, they must be used cautiously.

Patients Without a History of Cardiac Failure: Continued depression of the myocardium with beta-blockers can, in some patients, precipitate cardiac failure. At the first signs or symptoms of heart failure, discontinuation of bisoprolol fumarate should be considered. In some cases bisoprolol fumarate therapy can be continued while heart failure is treated with other drugs.

Abrupt Cessation of Therapy: Exacerbations of angina pectoris and, in some instances, myocardial infarction or ventricular arrhythmia, have been observed in patients with coronary artery disease following abrupt cessation of therapy with beta-blockers. Such patients should, therefore, be cautioned against interruption or discontinuation of therapy without the physician's advice. Even in patients without overt coronary artery disease, it may be advisable to taper therapy with bisoprolol fumarate over approximately 1 week with the patient under careful observation. If withdrawal symptoms occur, beta-blocking agent therapy should be reinstituted, at least temporarily.

Peripheral Vascular Disease: Beta-blockers can precipitate or aggravate symptoms of arterial insufficiency in patients with peripheral vascular disease. Caution should be exercised in such individuals.

Bronchospastic Disease: PATIENTS WITH BRONCHOSPASTIC PULMONARY DISEASE SHOULD, IN GENERAL, NOT RECEIVE BETA BLOCKERS. Because of the relative beta$_1$-selectivity of bisoprolol fumarate, bisoprolol fumarate may be used with caution in patients with bronchospastic disease who do not respond to, or who cannot tolerate other antihypertensive treatment. Since beta$_1$-selectivity is not absolute, the lowest possible dose of bisoprolol fumarate should be used. A beta$_2$agonist (bronchodilator) should be made available.

Anesthesia and Major Surgery: If bisoprolol fumarate treatment is to be continued perioperatively, particular care should be taken when anesthetic agents that depress myocardial function, such as ether, cyclopropane, and trichloroethylene, are used. See OVERDOSAGE for information on treatment of bradycardia and hypotension.

Diabetes and Hypoglycemia: Beta-blockers may mask some of the manifestations of hypoglycemia, particularly tachycardia. Nonselective beta-blockers may potentiate insulin-induced hypoglycemia and delay recovery of serum glucose levels. Because of its beta$_1$-selectivity, this is less likely with bisoprolol fumarate. However, patients subject to spontaneous hypoglycemia, or diabetic patients receiving insulin or oral hypoglycemic agents, should be cautioned about these possibilities. Also, latent diabetes mellitus may become manifest and diabetic patients given thiazides may require adjustment of their insulin dose. Because of the very low of HCTZ employed, this may be less likely with bisoprolol fumarate.

Thyrotoxicosis: Beta-adrenergic blockade may mask signs of hyperthyroidism, such as tachycardia. Abrupt withdrawal of beta-blockade may be followed by an exacerbation of the symptoms of hyperthyroidism or may precipitate thyroid storm.

Renal Disease: Cumulative effects of the thiazides may develop in patients with impaired renal function.In such patients, thiazides may precipitate azotemia. In subjects with creatinine clearance less than 40 ml/min, the plasma half-life of bisoprolol fumarate is increased up to threefold, as compared to healthy subjects. If progressive renal impairment becomes apparent, bisoprolol fumarate should be discontinued. (See Pharmacokinetics and Metabolism.)

Hepatic Disease: Bisoprolol fumarate should be used with caution in patients with impaired hepatic function or progressive liver disease. Thiazides may alter fluid and electrolyte balance, which may precipitate hepatic coma. Also, elimination of bisoprolol fumarate is significantly slower in patients with cirrhosis than in healthy subjects. (See Pharmacokinetics and Metabolism.)

PRECAUTIONS:

GENERAL

Electrolyte and Fluid Balance Status: Although the probability of developing hypokalemia is reduced with bisoprolol fumarate because of the very low dose of HCTZ employed, periodic determination of serum electrolytes should be performed,and patients should be observed for signs of fluid or electrolyte disturbances, *i.e.*, hyponatremia, hypochloremic alkalosis, and hypokalemia and hypomagnesemia. Thiazides have been shown to increase the urinary excretion of magnesium; this may result in hypomagnesemia.

Warning signs or symptoms of fluid and electrolyte imbalance include dryness of mouth, thirst, weakness, lethargy, drowsiness, restlessness, muscle pains or cramps, muscular fatigue, hypotension, oliguria, tachycardia, and gastrointestinal disturbances such as nausea and vomiting.

Hypokalemia may develop, especially with brisk diuresis when severe cirrhosis is present, during concomitant use of corticosteroids or adrenocorticotropic hormone (ACTH) or after prolonged therapy. Interference with adequate oral electrolyte intake will also contribute to hypokalemia. Hypokalemia and hypomagnesemia can provoke ventricular arrhythmias or sensitize or exaggerate the response of the heart to the toxic effects of digitalis. Hypokalemia may be avoided or treated by potassium supplementation or increased intake of potassium-rich foods.

Dilutional hyponatremia may occur in edematous patients in hot weather; appropriate therapy is water restriction rather than salt administration, except in rare instances when the hyponatremia is life threatening. In actual salt depletion, appropriate replacement is the therapy of choice.

Parathyroid Disease: Calcium excretion is decreased by thiazides, and pathologic changes in the parathyroid glands, with hypercalcemia and hypophosphatemia, have been observed in a few patients on prolonged thiazide therapy.

Hyperuricemia: Hyperuricemia or acute gout may be precipitated in certain patients receiving thiazide diuretics. Bisoprolol fumarate, alone or in combination with HCTZ, has been associated with increases in uric acid. However, in U.S. clinical trials, the incidence of treatment-related increases in uric acid was higher during therapy with HCTZ 25 mg (25%) than with B/H 6.25 mg (10%). Because of the very low dose of HCTZ employed, hyperuricemia may be less likely with bisoprolol fumarate.

Laboratory Test Interactions: Based on reports involving thiazides, bisoprolol fumarate may decrease serum levels of protein-bound iodine without signs of thyroid disturbance.

Because it includes a thiazide, bisoprolol fumarate should be discontinued before carrying out tests for parathyroid function (see PRECAUTIONS, Parathyroid Disease).

INFORMATION FOR THE PATIENT

Patients, especially those with coronary artery disease, should be warned against discontinuing use of bisoprolol fumarate without a physician's supervision. Patients should also be advised to consult a physician if any difficulty in breathing occurs, or if they develop other signs or symptoms of congestive heart failure or excessive bradycardia.

PRECAUTIONS: *(cont'd)*

Patients subject to spontaneous hypoglycemia, or diabetic patients receiving insulin or oral hypoglycemic agents, should be cautioned that beta-blockers may mask some of the manifestations of hypoglycemia, particularly tachycardia, and bisoprolol fumarate should be used with caution.

Patients should know how they react to this medicine before they operate automobiles and machinery or engage in other tasks requiring alertness. Patients should be advised that photosensitivity reactions have been reported with thiazides.

CARCINOGENESIS, MUTAGENESIS, AND IMPAIRMENT OF FERTILITY

Carcinogenesis

Ziac: Long-term studies have not been conducted with the bisoprolol fumarate/hydrochlorothiazide combination.

Bisoprolol Fumarate: Long-term studies were conducted with oral bisoprolol fumarate administered in the feed of mice (20 and 24 months) and rats (26 months). No evidence of carcinogenic potential was seen in mice dosed up to 250 mg/kg/day or rats dosed up to 125 mg/kg/day. On a body-weight basis, these doses are 625 and 312 times, respectively, the maximum recommended human dose (MRHD) of 20 mg, or 0.4 mg/kg/day, based on 50 kg individuals; on a body-surface-area basis, these doses are 59 times (mice) and 64 times (rats) the MRHD.

Hydrochlorothiazide: Two-year feeding studies in mice and rats, conducted under the auspices of the National Toxicology Program (NTP), treated mice and rats with doses of hydrochlorothiazide up to 600 and 100 mg/kg/day, respectively. On a body-weight basis, these doses are 2400 times (in mice) and 400 times (in rats)the MRHD of hydrochlorothiazide (12.5 mg/day) in Ziac. On a body-surface-area basis, these doses are 226 times (in mice) and 82 times (in rats) the MRHD. These studies uncovered no evidence of carcinogenic potential of hydrochlorothiazide in rats or female mice, but there was equivocal evidence of hepatocarcinogenicity in male mice.

Mutagenesis

Ziac: The mutagenic potential of the bisoprolol fumarate/hydrochlorothiazide combination was evaluated in the microbial mutagenicity (Ames) test, the point mutation and chromosomal aberration assays in Chinese hamster V79 cells, and the micronucleus test in mice. There was no evidence of mutagenic potential in these *in vitro* and *in vivo* assays.

Bisoprolol Fumarate: The mutagenic potential of bisoprolol fumarate was evaluated in the microbial mutagenicity (Ames) test, the point mutation and chromosome aberration assays in Chinese hamster V79 cells, the unscheduled DNA synthesis test, the micronucleus test in mice, and the cytogenetics assay in rats. There was no evidence of mutagenic potential in these *in vitro* and *in vivo*assays.

Hydrochlorothiazide: Hydrochlorothiazide was not genotoxic in*in vitro* assays using strains TA 98, TA 100, TA 1535, TA 1537 and TA 1538 of *Salmonella typhimurium* (the Ames test); in the Chinese Hamster Ovary (CHO) test for chromosomal aberrations; or in *in vivo*assays using mouse germinal cell chromosomes, Chinese hamster bone marrow chromosomes, and the *Drosophila* sex-linked recessive lethal trait gene. Positive test results were obtained in the *in vitro* CHO Sister Chromatid Exchange (clastogenicity) test and in the mouse Lymphoma Cell (mutagenicity) assays, using concentrations of hydrochlorothiazide of 43-1300 mcg/ml. Positive test results were also obtained in the *Aspergillus nidulans* nondisjunction assay, using an unspecified concentration of hydrochlorothiazide.

Impairment of Fertility

Ziac: Reproduction studies in rats did not show any impairment of fertility with the bisoprolol fumarate/hydrochlorothiazide combination doses containing up to 30 mg/kg/day of bisoprolol in combination with 75 mg/kg/day of hydrochlorothiazide. On a body-weight basis, these doses are 75 and 300 times, respectively, the MRHD of bisoprolol fumarate and hydrochlorothiazide. On a body-surface-area basis, these study doses are 15 and 62 times, respectively, MRHD.

Bisoprolol Fumarate: Reproduction studies in rats did not show any impairment at dose up to 150 mg/kg/day of bisoprolol fumarate, or 375 and 77 times the MRHD on the basis of body-weight and body-surface-area, respectively.

Hydrochlorothiazide: Hydrochlorothiazide had no adverse effects on the fertility of mice and rats, of either sex in studies wherein these species were exposed, via their diet, to doses of up to 100 and 4 mg/kg/day, respectively, prior to mating and throughout gestation. Corresponding multiples of maximum recommended human doses are 400 (mice) and 16 (rats) on the basis of body-weight and 38 (mice)and 3.3 (rats) on the basis of body-surface-area.

PREGNANCY, TERATOGENIC EFFECTS, PREGNANCY CATEGORY C

Ziac: In rats, the bisoprolol fumarate/hydrochlorothiazide (B/H) combination was not teratogenic at doses up to 51.4 mg/kg/day of bisoprolol fumarate in combination with 128.6 mg/kg/day of hydrochlorothiazide. Bisoprolol fumarate and hydrochlorothiazide doses used in the rat study are, as multiples of the MRHD in the combination, 129 and 514 times greater, respectively, on a body-weight basis, and 26 and 106 times greater, respectively, on the basis of body-surface area. The drug combination was maternotoxic (decreased body weight and food consumption) at B5.7/H14.3 (mg/kg/day) and higher, and fetotoxic (increased late resorptions) at B17.1/H42.9 (mg/kg/day) and higher. Maternotoxicity was present at 14/57 times the MHRD of B/H, respectively, on a body-weight basis, and 3/12 times the MRHD of B/H doses, respectively, on the basis of body-surface area. Fetotoxicity was present at 43/172 times the MHRD of B/H, respectively, on a body-weight basis, and 9/35 times the MRHD of B/H doses, respectively, on the basis of body-surface-area. In rabbits, the B/H combination was not teratogenic at doses of B/10/H25 (mg/kg/day). Bisoprolol fumarate and hydrochlorothiazide used in the rabbit study were not teratogenic at 25/100 times the B/H MRHD, respectively, on a body-weight basis, and 10/40 times the B/H MRHD, respectively, on the basis of body surface area. The drug combination was maternotoxic (decreased body weight) at B1/H2.5 (mg/kg/day) and higher,and fetotoxic (increased resorptions) at B10/H25 (mg/kg/day). The multiples of the MRHD for the B/H combination which were maternotoxic are, respectively, 2.5/10 (on the basis of body-weight) and 1/4 (on the basis of body-surface-area), and for fetotoxicity are, respectively 25/100 (on the basis of body-weight) and 10/40 (on the basis of body surface area).

There are no adequate and well-controlled studies in pregnant women. Ziac should be used during pregnancy only if the potential benefit justifies the risk to the fetus.

Bisoprolol Fumarate: In rats, bisoprolol fumarate was not teratogenic at doses up to 150 mg/kg/day, which are 375 and 77 times the MRHD on the basis of body-weight and body-surface-area, respectively. Bisoprolol fumarate was fetotoxic (increased late resorptions) at 50 mg/kg/day and maternotoxic (decreased food intake and body weight gain) at 150 mg/kg/day. The fetotoxicity in rats occurred at 125 times the MRHD on a body-weight basis and 26 times the MRHD on the basis of body surface area. The maternotoxicity occurred at 375 times the MRHD on a body-weight basis and 77 times the MRHD on the basis of body-surface-area. In rabbits, bisoprolol fumarate was not teratogenic at doses up to 12.5 mg/kg/day, which is 31 and 12 times the MRHD based on body-weight and body-surface-area, respectively, but was embryolethal (increased early resorptions) at 12.5 mg/kg/day.

Hydrochlorothiazide: Hydrochlorothiazide was orally administered to pregnant mice and rats during respective periods of major organogenesis at doses up to 3000 and 1000 mg/kg/day, respectively. At these doses, which are multiples of the MRHD equal to 12,000 for mice and 4000 for rats, based on body-weight, and equal to 1129 for mice and 824 for rats, based on

PRECAUTIONS: *(cont'd)*

body-surface-area, there was no evidence of harm to the fetus. There are, however, no adequate and well-controlled studies in pregnant women. Because animal reproduction studies are not always predictive of human response, this drug should be used during pregnancy only if clearly needed. *Nonteratogenic Effects:* Thiazides cross the placental barrier and appear in the cord blood. The use of thiazides in pregnant women requires that the anticipated benefit be weighed against possible hazards to the fetus. These hazards include fetal or neonatal jaundice, pancreatitis, thrombocytopenia, and possibly other adverse reactions which have occurred in the adult.

NURSING MOTHERS

Bisoprolol fumarate alone or in combination with HCTZ has not been studied in nursing mothers. Thiazides are excreted in human breast milk. Small amounts of bisoprolol fumarate (<2% of the dose) have been detected in the milk of lactating rats. Because of the potential for serious adverse reactions in nursing infants, a decision should be made whether to discontinue nursing or to discontinue the drug, taking into account the importance of the drug to the mother.

GERIATRIC USE

In clinical trials, at least 270 patients treated with bisoprolol fumarate plus HCTZ were 60 years of age or older. HCTZ added significantly to the antihypertensive effect of bisoprolol in elderly hypertensive patients. No overall differences in effectiveness or safety were observed between these patients and younger patients. Other reported clinical experience has not identified differences in responses between the elderly and younger patients, but greater sensitivity of some older individuals cannot be ruled out.

PEDIATRIC USE

Safety and effectiveness of bisoprolol fumarate in children have not been established.

DRUG INTERACTIONS:

Bisoprolol fumarate may potentiate the action of other antihypertensive agents used concomitantly. Bisoprolol fumarate should not be combined with other beta-blocking agents. Patients receiving catecholamine-depleting drugs, such as reserpine or guanethidine, should be closely monitored because the added beta-adrenergic blocking action of bisoprolol fumarate may produce excessive reduction of sympathetic activity. In patients receiving concurrent therapy with clonidine, if therapy is to be discontinued, it is suggested that bisoprolol fumarate be discontinued for several days before the withdrawal of clonidine.

Bisoprolol fumarate should be used with caution when myocardial depressants or inhibitors of AV conduction, such as certain calcium antagonists (particularly of the phenylalkylamine (verapamil) and benzothiazepine (diltiazem) classes), or antiarrhythmic agents, such as disopyramide, are used concurrently.

BISOPROLOL FUMARATE

Concurrent use of rifampin increases the metabolic clearance of bisoprolol fumarate, shortening its elimination half-life. However, initial dose modification is generally not necessary. Pharmacokinetic studies document no clinically relevant interactions with other agents given concomitantly, including thiazide diuretics, digoxin and cimetidine. There was no effect of bisoprolol fumarate on prothrombin times in patients on stable doses of warfarin.

Risk of Anaphylactic Reaction: While taking beta-blockers, patients with a history of severe anaphylactic reaction to a variety of allergens may be more reactive to repeated challenge, either accidental, diagnostic, or therapeutic. Such patients may be unresponsive to the usual doses of epinephrine used to treat allergic reactions.

HYDROCHLOROTHIAZIDE

When given concurrently the following drugs may interact with thiazide diuretics.

Alcohol, barbiturates, or narcotics: potentiation of orthostatic hypotension may occur.

Antidiabetic drugs (oral agents and insulin): dosage adjustment of the antidiabetic drug may be required.

Other antihypertensive drugs: additive effect or potentiation.

Cholestyramine and colestipol resins: Absorption of hydrochlorothiazide is impaired in the presence of anionic exchange resins. Single doses of cholestyramine and colestipol resins bind the hydrochlorothiazide and reduce its absorption in the gastrointestinal tract by up to 85 and 43 percent, respectively.

Corticosteroids, ACTH: Intensified electrolyte depletion, particularly hypokalemia.

Pressor amines (*e.g.,* norepinephrine): possible decreased response to pressor amines but not sufficient to preclude their use.

Skeletal muscle relaxants, nondepolarizing (*e.g.,* tubocurarine): possible increased responsiveness to the muscle relaxant.

Lithium: generally should not be given with diuretics. Diuretic agents reduce the renal clearance of lithium and add a high risk of lithium toxicity. Refer to the package insert for lithium preparation before use of such preparations with bisoprolol fumarate.

Nonsteroidal anti-inflammatory drugs: In some patients, the administration of a nonsteroidal anti-inflammatory agent can reduce the diuretic, natriuretic, and antihypertensive effects of loop, potassium sparing and thiazide diuretics. Therefore, when bisoprolol fumarate and nonsteroidal anti-inflammatory agents are used concomitantly, the patient should be observed closely to determine if the desired effect of the diuretic is obtained.

In patients receiving thiazides, sensitivity reactions may occur with or without a history of allergy or bronchial asthma. Photosensitivity reactions and possible exacerbation or activation of systemic lupus erythematosus have been reported in patients receiving thiazides. The antihypertensive effects of thiazides may be enhanced in the post-sympathectomy patient.

ADVERSE REACTIONS:

ZIAC

Bisoprolol fumarate/H6.25 mg is well tolerated in most patients. Most adverse effects (AEs) have been mild and transient. In more than 65,00 patients treated worldwide with bisoprolol fumarate, occurrences of bronchospasm have been rare. Discontinuation rates for AEs were similar for B/H6.25 mg and placebo-treated patients.

In the United States, 252 patients received bisoprolol fumarate (2.5, 5, 10, or 40 mg)/H6.25 mg and 144 patients received placebo in two controlled trials. In Study 1, bisoprolol fumarate 5/H6.25 mg was administered for 4 weeks. In Study 2, bisoprolol fumarate 2.5, 10 or 40/H6.25 mg was administered for 12 weeks. All adverse experiences, whether drug related or not, and drug related adverse experiences in patients treated with B2.5-10/H6.25 mg, reported during comparable, 4 week treatment periods by at least 2% of bisoprolol fumarate/H6.25 mg-treated patients (plus additional selected adverse experiences) are presented in TABLE 2.

Other adverse experiences that have been reported with the individual components are listed below.

BISOPROLOL FUMARATE

In clinical trials worldwide, a variety of other AEs, in addition to those listed above, have been reported. While in many cases it is not known whether a causal relationship exists between bisoprolol and these AEs, they are listed to alert the physician to a possible relationship.

ADVERSE REACTIONS: *(cont'd)*

TABLE 2 % of Patients with Adverse Experiences*

Body System/Adverse Experience	All Adverse Experiences Placebo† (n=144) %	All Adverse Experiences B2.5-40/H6.25† (n=252) %	Drug Related Adverse Experiences Placebo† (n=144) %	Drug Related Adverse Experiences B2.5-10/H6.25† (n=221) %
Cardiovascular				
Bradycardia	0.7	1.1	0.7	0.9
Arrhythmia	1.4	0.4	0.0	0.0
Peripheral ischemia	0.9	0.7	0.9	0.4
Chest pain	0.7	1.8	0.7	0.9
Respiratory				
Bronchospasm	0.0	0.0	0.0	0.0
Cough	1.0	2.2	0.7	1.5
Rhinitis	2.0	0.7	0.7	0.9
URI	2.3	2.1	0.0	0.0
Body As A Whole				
Asthenia	0.0	0.0	0.0	0.0
Fatigue	2.7	4.6	1.7	3.0
Peripheral edema	0.7	1.1	0.7	0.9
Central Nervous System				
Dizziness	1.8	5.1	1.8	3.2
Headache	4.7	4.5	2.7	0.4
Musculoskeletal				
Muscle cramps	0.7	1.2	0.7	1.1
Myalgia	1.4	2.4	0.0	0.0
Psychiatric				
Insomnia	2.4	1.1	2.0	1.2
Somnolence	0.7	1.1	0.7	0.9
Loss of libido	1.2	0.4	1.2	0.4
Impotence	0.7	1.1	0.7	1.1
Gastrointestinal				
Diarrhea	1.4	4.3	1.2	1.1
Nausea	0.9	1.1	0.9	0.9
Dyspepsia	0.7	1.2	0.7	0.9

* Averages adjusted to combine across studies
† Combined across studies

Central Nervous System: Unsteadiness, vertigo, syncope, paresthesia, hyperesthesia, sleep disturbance/vivid dreams, depression, anxiety/restlessness, decreased concentration/memory.

Cardiovascular: Palpitations and other rhythm disturbances, cold extremities, claudication, hypotension, orthostatic hypotension, chest pain, congestive heart failure.

Gastrointestinal: Gastric/epigastric/abdominal pain, peptic ulcer, gastritis, vomiting, constipation, dry mouth.

Musculoskeletal: Arthralgia, muscle/joint pain, back/neck pain, twitching/tremor.

Skin: Rash, acne, eczema, psoriasis, skin irritation, pruritus, purpura, flushing, sweating, alopecia, dermatitis, exfoliative dermatitis (very rarely).

Special Senses: Visual disturbances, ocular pain/pressure, abnormal lacrimation, tinnitus, decreased hearing, earache, taste abnormalities.

Metabolic: Gout.

Respiratory: Asthma, bronchitis, dyspnea, pharyngitis, sinusitis.

Genito-urinary: Peyronie's disease (very rarely), cystitis, renal colic, polyuria.

General: Malaise, edema, weight gain, angioedema.

In addition, a variety of adverse effects have been reported with other beta-adrenergic blocking agents and should be considered potential adverse effects:

Central Nervous System: Reversible mental depression progressing to catatonia, hallucinations, an acute reversible syndrome characterized by disorientation to time and place, emotional liability, slightly clouded sensorium.

Allergic: Fever, combined with aching and sore throat, laryngospasm, and respiratory distress.

Hematologic: Agranulocytosis, thrombocytopenia.

Gastrointestinal: Mesenteric arterial thrombosis and ischemic colitis.

Miscellaneous: The oculomucocutaneous syndrome associated with the beta-blocker practolol has not been reported with bisoprolol fumarate during investigational use or extensive foreign marketing experience.

HYDROCHLOROTHIAZIDE

The following adverse experiences, in addition to those listed in the above table, have been reported with hydrochlorothiazide (generally with doses of 25 mg or greater).

General: Weakness.

Central Nervous System: Vertigo, paresthesia, restlessness.

Cardiovascular: Orthostatic hypotension (may be potentiated by alcohol, barbiturates, or narcotics).

Gastrointestinal: Anorexia, gastric irritation, cramping, constipation, jaundice (intrahepatic cholestatic jaundice), pancreatitis, cholecystitis, sialadenitis, dry mouth.

Musculoskeletal: Muscle spasm.

Hypersensitive Reactions: Purpura, photosensitivity, rash, urticaria, necrotizing angiitis (vasculitis and cutaneous vasculitis), fever, respiratory pneumonitis and pulmonary edema, anaphylactoid reactions.

Special Senses: Transient blurred vision, xanthopsia.

Metabolic: Gout.

Genito-urinary: Sexual dysfunction, renal failure, renal dysfunction, interstitial nephritis.

LABORATORY ABNORMALITIES

Ziac: Because of the low dose of hydrochlorothiazide in Ziac, adverse metabolic effects with B/H6.25 mg are less frequent and of smaller magnitude than with HCTZ 25 mg. Laboratory data on serum potassium from the U.S. placebo-controlled trials are shown in TABLE 3.

Treatment with both beta blockers and thiazide diuretics is associated with increases in uric acid. However, the magnitude of the change in patients treated with B/H 6.25 mg was smaller than in patients treated with HCTZ 25 mg. Mean increases in serum triglycerides were observed in patients treated with bisoprolol fumarate and hydrochlorothiazide 6.25 mg. Total cholesterol was generally unaffected, but small decreases in HDL cholesterol were noted.

Other laboratory abnormalities that have been reported with the individual components are listed below.

Bisoprolol Fumarate: In clinical trials, the most frequently reported laboratory change was an increase in serum triglycerides, but this was not a consistent finding.

ADVERSE REACTIONS: *(cont'd)*

TABLE 3 Serum Potassium Data from U.S. Placebo Controlled Studies

	Placebo† (n=130*)	B2.5/H6.2 5 mg (n=28*)	B5/H6.25 mg (n=149*)	B10/H6.25 mg (n=28*)	HCTZ25 mg† (n=142*)
Potassium Mean Change[a] (mEq/L)	+0.04	+0.11	-0.08	0.00	-0.30
% Hypokalemia[b]	0.0%	0.0%	0.7%	0.0%	5.5%

* Patients with normal serum potassium at baseline.
[a]Mean change from baseline at Week 4.
[b]Percentage of patients with abnormality at Week 4.
† Combined across studies.

Sporadic liver test abnormalities have been reported. In the U.S. controlled trials experience with bisoprolol fumarate treatment for 4-12 weeks, the incidence of concomitant elevations in SGOT and SGPT of between 1-2 times normal was 3.9%, compared to 2.5% for placebo. No patient had concomitant elevations greater than twice normal.

In the long-term, uncontrolled experience with bisoprolol fumarate treatment for 6-18 months, the incidence of one or more concomitant elevations in SGOT and SGPT of between 1-2 times normal was 6.2%. The incidence of multiple occurrence was 1.9%. For concomitant elevations in SGOT and SGPT of greater than twice normal, the incidence was 1.5%. The incidence of multiple occurrences was 0.35. In many cases these elevations were attributed to underlying disorders, or resolved during continued treatment with bisoprolol fumarate.

Other laboratory changes included small increases in uric acid, creatinine, BUN, serum potassium, glucose, and phosphorus and decreases in WBC and platelets. There have been occasional reports of eosinophilia. These were generally not of clinical importance and rarely resulted in discontinuation of bisoprolol fumarate.

As with other beta-blockers, ANA conversions have also been reported on bisoprolol fumarate. About 15% of patients in long-term studies converted to a positive titer, although about one-third of these patients subsequently reconverted to a negative titer while on continued therapy.

Hydrochlorothiazide: Hyperglycemia, glycosuria, hyperuricemia, hypokalemia and other electrolyte imbalances (see PRECAUTIONS), hyperlipidemia, hypercalcemia, leukopenia, agranulocytosis, thrombocytopenia, aplastic anemia, and hemolytic anemia have been associated with HCTZ therapy.

OVERDOSAGE:

While there have been no reports of overdose with bisoprolol fumarate, several cases of overdose with bisoprolol fumarate have been reported (maximum: 2000 mg). Bradycardia and/or hypotension were noted. Sympathomimetic agents were given in some cases, and all patients recovered.

The most frequently observed signs expected with overdosage of a beta-blocker are bradycardia and hypotension. Lethargy is also common, and with severe overdoses, delirium, coma, convulsions, and respiratory arrest have been reported to occur. Congestive heart failure, bronchospasm, and hypoglycemia may occur, particularly in patients with underlying conditions. With thiazide diuretics, acute intoxication is rare. The most prominent feature of overdose is acute loss of fluid and electrolytes. Signs and symptoms include cardiovascular (tachycardia, hypotension, shock), neuromuscular (weakness, confusion, dizziness, cramps of the calf muscles, paresthesia, fatigue, impairment of consciousness), gastrointestinal (nausea, vomiting, thirst), renal (polyuria, oliguria, or anuria (due to hemoconcentration)), and laboratory findings (hypokalemia, hyponatremia, hypochloremia, alkalosis, increased BUN (especially in patients with renal insufficiency)).

If overdosage of bisoprolol fumarate is suspected, therapy with bisoprolol fumarate should be discontinued and the patient observed closely. Treatment is symptomatic and supportive; there is no specific antidote. Limited data suggest bisoprolol fumarate is not dialyzable. Suggested general measures include induction of emesis and/or gastric lavage, administration of activated charcoal, respiratory support, correction of fluid and electrolyte imbalance, and treatment of convulsions. Based on the expected pharmacologic actions and recommendations for other beta-blockers and hydrochlorothiazide, the following measures should be considered when clinically warranted:

Bradycardia: Administer IV atropine. If the response is inadequate, isoproterenol or another agent with positive chronotropic properties may be given cautiously. Under some circumstances, transvenous pacemaker insertion may be necessary.

Hypotension, Shock: The patient's legs should be elevated. IV fluids should be administered and lost electrolytes (potassium, sodium) replaced. Intravenous glucagon may be useful. Vasopressors should be considered.

Heart Block (second or third degree): Patients should be carefully monitored and treated with isoproterenol infusion or transvenous cardiac pacemaker insertion, as appropriate.

Congestive Heart Failure: Initiate conventional therapy (*i.e.*, digitalis, diuretics, vasodilating agents, inotropic agents).

Bronchospasm: Administer a bronchodilator such as isoproterenol and/or aminophylline.

Hyperglycemia: Administer IV glucose.

Surveillance: Fluid and electrolyte balance (especially serum potassium) and renal function should be monitored until normalized.

DOSAGE AND ADMINISTRATION:

Bisoprolol is an effective treatment of hypertension in once-daily doses of 2.5-40 mg, while hydrochlorothiazide is effective in doses of 15-50 mg. In clinical trials of bisoprolol/hydrochlorothiazide combination therapy using bisoprolol doses of 2.5-20 mg hydrochlorothiazide doses of 6.25-25 mg, the antihypertensive effects increased with increasing doses of either component.

The adverse effects (see WARNINGS) of bisoprolol are a mixture of dose-dependent phenomena (primarily bradycardia, diarrhea, asthenia and fatigue) and dose-independent phenomena (*e.g.*, occasional rash); those of hydrochlorothiazide are a mixture of dose-dependent phenomena (primarily hypokalemia) and dose-independent phenomena (*e.g.*, possibly pancreatitis); the dose-dependent for each being much more common than the dose-independent phenomena. The latter consist of those few that are truly idiosyncratic in nature or those that occur with such low frequency that a dose relationship may be difficult to discern. Therapy with a combination of bisoprolol and hydrochlorothiazide will be associated with both sets of dose-independent adverse effects, and to minimize these, it may be appropriate to begin combination therapy only after a patient has failed to achieve the desired effect with monotherapy. On the other hand, regimens that combine low doses of bisoprolol and hydrochlorothiazide should produce minimal dose dependent adverse effects, e.g., bradycardia, diarrhea, asthenia and fatigue, and minimal dose-dependent adverse metabolic effects, i.e., decreases in serum potassium (see CLINICAL PHARMACOLOGY).

DOSAGE AND ADMINISTRATION: *(cont'd)*

Therapy Guided by Clinical Effect: A patient whose blood pressure is not adequately controlled with 2.5-20 mg bisoprolol daily may instead be given bisoprolol fumarate. Patients whose blood pressures are adequately controlled with 50 mg of hydrochlorothiazide daily, but who experience significant potassium loss with this regimen, may achieve similar blood pressure control with electrolyte disturbance if they are switched to bisoprolol fumarate.

Initial Therapy: Antihypertensive therapy may be initiated with the lowest dose of bisoprolol fumarate, one 2.5/6.25 mg tablet once daily. Subsequent titration (14 day intervals) may be carried out with bisoprolol fumarate tablets up to the maximum recommended dose 20/12.5 mg (two 10/6.25 mg tablets) once daily, as appropriate,

Replacement Therapy: The combination may be substituted for the titrated individual components.

Cessation of Therapy: If withdrawal of bisoprolol fumarate therapy is planned, it should be achieved gradually over a period of about 2 weeks. Patients should be carefully observed.

Patients with Renal or Hepatic Impairment: As noted in the WARNINGS, caution must be used in dosing/titrating patients with hepatic impairment or renal dysfunction. Since there is no indication that hydrochlorothiazide is dialyzable, and limited data suggest that bisoprolol is not dialyzable, drug replacement is not necessary in patients undergoing dialysis.

Elderly Patients: Dosage adjustment on the basis of age is not usually necessary, unless there is also significant renal or hepatic dysfunction. (See DOSAGE AND ADMINISTRATION, WARNINGS.)

Children: There is no pediatric experience with bisoprolol fumarate.

PATIENT INFORMATION:

This tablet is a combination of two drugs, both which lower blood pressure. This combination allows it to be taken once a day. This drug should not be used in patients with very severe heart failure. It may cause an allergic reaction in patients with a sulfa allergy. Any signs of allergy (rash, itching, difficulty breathing) should be reported immediately. This medication should be discontinued abruptly; it may cause the heart to react. Contact your physician immediately if you experience difficulty breathing. This medication may mask signs of low blood sugar in patients with diabetes. This medication can initially cause one to feel drowsy. See how your body reacts before driving or operating machinery. This medication can also cause photosensitivity meaning you may be more sensitive to the sun. Protect your skin accordingly with clothing or sunscreen.

HOW SUPPLIED:

Ziac 2.5 mg/6.25 mg tablets (bisoprolol fumarate 2.5 mg and hydrochlorothiazide 6.25 mg) are yellow, round, convex, film coated tablets, engraved with a script "LL" within an engraved heart shape on one side and "B" above "12" on the other; approximately 1/4" in diameter.

Ziac 5 mg/6.25 mg tablets (bisoprolol fumarate 5 mg and hydrochlorothiazide 6.25 mg) are pink, round, convex, film coated tablets, engraved with a script "LL" within an engraved heart shape on one side and "B" above "13" on the other; approximately 9/32" in diameter.

Ziac 10 mg/6.25 tablets (bisoprolol fumarate 10 mg and hydrochlorothiazide 6.25 mg) are white, round, convex, film coated tablets, engraved with a script "LL" within en engraved heart shape on one side and "B" above "14" on the other; approximately 9/32" in diameter.

Store at Controlled Room Temperature 15-30° (59-86°) in a well-closed container.

HOW SUPPLIED - EQUIVALENTS NOT AVAILABLE:

Tablet, Uncoated - Oral - 6.5 mg/2.5 mg
100's $88.64 ZIAC, Lederle Pharm 00005-3238-23

Tablet, Uncoated - Oral - 6.5 mg/5 mg
100's $88.64 ZIAC, Lederle Pharm 00005-3234-23

Tablet, Uncoated - Oral - 6.5 mg/10 mg
30's $26.59 ZIAC, Lederle Pharm 00005-3235-38

BITOLTEROL MESYLATE *(000505)*

CATEGORIES: Airway Obstruction; Antiasthmatics/Bronchodilators; Asthma; Autonomic Drugs; Beta Adrenergic Stimulators; Bronchial Dilators; Bronchospasm; Sympathomimetic Agents; Sympathomimetics, Beta Agonist; Pregnancy Category C; FDA Approved 1984 Dec

BRAND NAMES: **Tornalate**

COST OF THERAPY: $41.77 (Asthma; Solution; 0.37 mg/0.05ml; 0.3/day; 365 days)

PRIMARY ICD9: 493.90 (Asthma, Unspecified, Without Mention of Status Asthmaticus)

DESCRIPTION:

Bitolterol mesylate is the di-*p*-toluate ester of the β-adrenergic agonist bronchodilator *N*- t-butylarterenol (colterol). It has a molecular weight of 557.7. Bitolterol mesylate is known chemically as 4-[2-[(1,1-dimethylethyl) amino]-1-hydroxyethyl] -1,2 -phenylene 4-methylbenzoate (ester) methanesulfonate (salt).

Tornalate Solution for Inhalation contains 0.2% bitolterol mesylate in an aqueous vehicle containing alcohol 25% (v/v), citric acid, propylene glycol, and sodium hydroxide. Tornalate's pH range is 3.0-3.4.

Each ml of Tornalate Solution for Inhalation, 0.2% contains 0.2% mg of bitolterol mesylate.

Tornalate (bitolterol mesylate) Metered Dose Inhaler is a complete aerosol unit for oral inhalation. It consists of a plastic-coated bottle of ready-to-use aerosol solution and a detachable plastic mouthpiece with built-in-nebulizer. The bottle contains 16.4 g (15 ml) of 0.8% bitolterol mesylate in a vehicle containing 38% alcohol (w/w), inert propellants (dichlorodifluoromethane and dichlorotetrafluoroethane), ascorbic acid, saccharin, and menthol.

Each bottle provides at least 300 actuations. Each actuation delivers a measured dose of 0.37 mg of bitolterol mesylate as a fine, even mist.

CLINICAL PHARMACOLOGY:

Solution for Inhalation: Bitolteral mesylate is administered as a pro-drug which is hydrolyzed by esterases in tissue and blood to the active moiety colterol. Bitolteral mesylate administered by nebulization has a rapid onset of activity (2 to 3 minutes) after administration in most patients based on interpolation between baseline and 5 minutes. The duration of action with bitolteral mesylate administered by nebulization is 6 hours or more in most patients and 8 hours in 40% of patients based on 15% or greater increase in forced expiratory volume in one second (FEV_1), as demonstrated in three-month isoproterenol controlled multicenter trials in non-steroid-dependent patients. Based on mid- maximal expiratory flow (MMEF) measurements, the duration of action is 7.5 to 8 hours in most patients. Median duration of effect in

CLINICAL PHARMACOLOGY: *(cont'd)*

steroid- dependent asthmatic patients ranged from 4.3 to 7.1 hours based on 15% or greater increase in FEV_1. The mean maximum increase in FEV_1 over baseline in patients during the three-month studies was 49% to 55% and occurred by 30 to 60 minutes in most patients.

In vitro studies and *in vivo* pharmacologic studies have demonstrated that bitolteral mesylate has a preferential effect on beta-2 adrenergic receptors compared with isoproterenol. While it is recognized that beta-2 adrenergic receptors are the prominent receptors in bronchial smooth muscle, recent data indicate that there are between 10% to 50% beta-2 receptors in the human heart. The precise mechanism of these, however, is not yet established. Bitolteral mesylate has been shown in most controlled clinical trials to have more effect on the respiratory tract, in the form of bronchial smooth muscle relaxation than isoproterenol at comparable doses, while producing fewer cardiovascular effects. Controlled clinical studies and other clinical experience have shown that inhaled bitolteral mesylate, like other beta-adrenergic agonists, can produce a significant cardiovascular effect in some patients, as measured by pulse rate, blood pressure, symptoms and/or ECG changes.

The incidence of cardiovascular side effects such as tachycardia and palpitation was less in patients treated with bitolterol mesylate as compared with patients treated with isoproterenol hydrochloride. The incidence of tachycardia and palpitation was 3.7% and 3.1%, respectively, in patients treated with bitolterol mesylate as compared with an incidence of 12.3% and 12.6% for tachycardia and palpitation for patients treated with isoproterenol.

Blood levels of colterol formed by gradual release from the pro-drug (bitolterol) in the lungs are too low to be measured by currently available assay methods and the bioavailability, pharmacokinetics and metabolism of bitolterol following administration as a solution for inhalation are not known. Data on disposition are available from oral studies in man. Following oral administration of 5.9 mg titrated bitolterol to man, radioactivity measurements indicated mean maximum colterol concentration in blood of approximately 2.1 mcg/ml one hour after medication. Urinary excretion data indicate that 83% of the radioactivity of this oral dose was excreted within the first 24 hours. By 72 hours, 85.6% of the tritium had been excreted in the urine and 8.1% in the feces. Most of the radioactivity was excreted as conjugated colterol; free colterol accounted for 2.1% to 3.7% of the total radioactivity excreted in the urine. No intact bitolterol was detected in urine.

The pharmacologic effects of β-adrenergic agonist drugs, including bitolterol mesylate, are at least in part attributable to stimulation through beta-adrenergic receptors to intracellular adenyl cyclase, the enzyme which catalyzes the conversion of adenosine to triphosphate (ATP) to cyclic-3', 5'-adenosine monophosphate (c-AMP). Increased c-AMP levels are associated with relaxation of bronchial smooth muscle and inhibition of release of mediators of immediate hypersensitivity from cells, especially from mast cells.

In repetitive dosing studies, continued effectiveness was demonstrated throughout the three-month period of treatment in the majority of patients. In steroid-dependent asthmatics, the median duration of bronchodilator activity as measured by FEV_1 was greater on the first test day as compared with later test days, but patient response remained constant throughout the balance of the three-month period.

Recent studies in laboratory animals (minipigs, rodents, and dogs) recorded the occurrence of cardiac arrhythmias and sudden death (with histologic evidence of myocardial necrosis) when beta-agonists and methylxanthines were administered concurrently. The significance of these findings when applied to humans is currently unknown.

Metered Dose Inhaler: Bitolterol mesylate is administered as a pro-drug which is hydrolyzed by esterases in tissue and blood to the active moiety colterol. Bitolterol mesylate administered as an inhaled aerosol has a rapid (3 to 4 minutes) onset of bronchodilator activity. The duration of action with bitolteral mesylate is at least 5 hours in most patients and 8 or more hours in 25% to 35% of patients, based on 15% or greater increase in forced expiratory volume in one second (FEV_1), as demonstrated in 3-month isoproterenol controlled multicenter trials. Based on mean maximal expiratory flow (MMEF) measurements, the duration of action is 6 to 7 hours. The duration of bronchodilator action with bitolteral mesylate in these trials is longer than that seen with isoproterenol, especially in steroid-dependent patients. Duration of effect was reduced over time in steroid-dependent asthmatic patients where the duration was 3.5 to 5 hours for FEV_1. The mean maximum increase in FEV_1 over baseline in the majority of patients was 39% to 42% and occurred by 30 to 60 minutes, similar to that seen in the isoproterenol group.

Bitolteral mesylate is a beta-adrenergic agonist which has been shown by *in vitro* and *in vivo* pharmacological studies in animals to exert a preferential effect on $beta_2$adrenergic receptors, such as those located in bronchial smooth muscle. However, controlled clinical trials in patients who were administered the drug have not revealed a preferential $beta_2$ adrenergic effect. At doses that produced long duration of bronchodilator activity (up to 8 hours in some patients) with a mean maximum bronchodilating effect of approximately 40% increase in FEV_1 (forced expiratory volume in one second), a less than 10 beat per minute mean maximum increase in heart rate was seen. The effect on the heart rate was transient and similar to the increases seen in the isoproterenol treated patients in these studies.

Although blood levels of colterol formed by gradual release from the pro-drug (bitolterol) in the lungs are too low to be measured by currently available assay methods, data on disposition are available from oral studies in man. Following oral administration of 5.9 mg titrated bitolterol mesylate to man, radioactivity measurements indicated mean maximum colterol concentration in blood of approximately 2.1 mcg/ml one hour after medication. Urinary excretion data indicate that 83 percent of the radioactivity of this oral dose was excreted within the first 24 hours. By 72 hours, 85.6 percent of the tritium had been excreted in the urine and 8.1 percent in the faces. Most of the radioactivity was excreted as conjugated colterol; free colterol accounted for 2.1 to 3.7 percent of the total radioactivity excreted in the urine. No intact bitolterol was detected in urine.

The pharmacologic effects of β-adrenergic drugs including bitolteral mesylate (bitolterol mesylate) are attributable to stimulation of adenyl cyclase, the enzyme which catalyzes the conversion of adenosine triphosphate (ATP) to cyclic-3',5'-adenosine monophosphate (c-AMP). Increased c-AMP levels are associated with relaxation of bronchial smooth muscle and with inhibition of release of mediators of immediate hypersensitivity from cells, especially from mast cells.

In a six-week clinical trial in which 24 asthmatic patients received bitolteral mesylate and theophylline concurrently, improvement in pulmonary function was enhanced over that seen with either drug alone. No potentiation of side effects was observed, and 24-hours ECG recordings (Holter monitoring) indicated no greater degree of cardiac toxicity with bitolteral mesylate alone or in combination with theophylline than that which occurred with theophylline alone.

Bitolteral mesylate did not adversely affect arterial oxygen tension in a blood-gas study in 24 asthmatic patients. However, a decrease in arterial oxygen tension has been reported with other adrenergic bronchodilators and could be anticipated to occur with bitolteral mesylate as well.

In repetitive dosing studies, continued effectiveness was demonstrated throughout the 3-month period of treatment in the majority of patients. However, some overall decrease was observed in steroid-dependent asthmatics.

INDICATIONS AND USAGE:

Solution for Inhalation: Bitolteral mesylate solution for inhalation, 0.2% is indicated for both prophylaxis and treatment of asthma or other conditions characterized by reversible bronchospasm. It may be used with or without concurrent theophylline and/or steroid therapy.

Metered Dose Inhaler: Bitolterol mesylate is indicated for both prophylactic and therapeutic use as a bronchodilator for bronchial asthma and for reversible bronchospasm. It may be used with or without concurrent theophylline and/or steroid therapy.

CONTRAINDICATIONS:

Solution for Inhalation and Metered Dose Inhaler: Bitolteral mesylate is contraindicated in patients who are hypersensitive to bitolterol mesylate or any other ingredients of the formulation.

WARNINGS:

Solution for Inhalation: As with other β-adrenergic agents, bitolterol mesylate should not be used in excess. Fatalities have been reported in association with excessive use of inhaled sympathomimetic drugs. The exact cause of death is unknown. Use of β-adrenergic drugs may have a deleterious cardiac effect. Paradoxical bronchoconstriction (which can be life-threatening) has been reported with administration of β-adrenergic agents. Immediate hypersensitivity reactions can occur after the administration of sympathomimetic agents. In such instances, the drug should be discontinued immediately and alternative therapy instituted.

In controlled clinical studies, clinically significant increases in pulse rate, increases and decreases in systolic and diastolic blood pressure have been demonstrated in individual patients after administration of bitolteral mesylate. Therefore, caution should be exercised when administering bitolterol mesylate to patients with underlying cardiovascular diseases. Even though the changes may be significant in a small number of patients, these changes occur within a short period of time after administration and have not been shown to be persistent.

If an unusual smell or taste is noted with use of this product, the patient should discontinue use in consultation with his/her physician.

Metered Dose Inhaler: As with other β-adrenergic aerosols, bitolterol mesylate should not be used in excess. Fatalities have been reported in association with excessive use of inhaled sympathomimetic drugs. The exact cause of death is unknown. Use of aerosolized β-adrenergic drugs may have a deleterious cardiac effect. Paradoxical bronchoconstriction (which can be life-threatening) has been reported with administration of β-adrenergic agents. Immediate hypersensitivity (allergic) reactions can occur after the administration of bitolteral mesylate. In such instances, the drug should be discontinued immediately and alternative therapy instituted.

The contents of bitolteral mesylate Metered Dose Inhaler are under pressure. Do not puncture. Do not use or store near heat or open flame. Exposure to temperatures above 120° F may cause bursting. Never throw container into fire or incinerator. Keep out of reach of children.

If an unusual smell or taste is noted with use of this product, the patient should discontinue use in consultation with his/her physician.

PRECAUTIONS:

GENERAL

Solution for Inhalation and Metered Dose Inhaler: As with all β-adrenergic stimulating agents, caution should be used when administering bitolterol mesylate to patients with cardiovascular disease such as ischemic heart disease or hypertension. Caution is also advised in patients with hyperthyroidism, diabetes mellitus, cardiac arrhythmias, convulsive disorders or unusual responsiveness to β-adrenergic agonists. Use of any β-adrenergic bronchodilator may produce significant changes in systolic and diastolic blood pressure in some patients. Significant changes in systolic and diastolic blood pressure have been seen in individual patients and could be expected to occur in some patients after use of any β-adrenergic aerosol bronchodilator.

INFORMATION FOR THE PATIENT

Solution for Inhalation: The effects of bitolteral mesylate may last up to eight hours or longer. It should not be used more often than recommended and the patient should not increase the number of treatments or dose without first consulting with the physician. If symptoms of asthma get worse, adverse reactions occur, or the patient does not respond to the usual dose, the patient should be instructed to contact the physician immediately. Drug stability and safety of bitolteral mesylate when mixed with other drugs in a nebulizer have not been established. The patient should be advised as to the proper use of the equipment used for nebulization and to see the Illustrated Patient's Instructions for Use.

Metered Dose Inhaler: The effects of bitolteral mesylate may last up to eight hours or longer. It should not be used more often than recommended and the patient should not increase the number of inhalations or frequency of use without first asking the physician. If symptoms of asthma get worse, adverse reactions occur, or the patient does not respond to the usual dose, the patient should be instructed to contact the physician immediately. The patient should be advised to see the Illustrated Patient's Instructions for Use.

(Note: for all illustrations, please see original package insert).

CARCINOGENESIS, MUTAGENESIS, AND IMPAIRMENT OF FERTILITY

Solution for Inhalation: No tumorigenicity (and specifically no increase in leiomyomas) was observed in a two-year oral study in Sprague-Dawley CD rats at doses of bitolteral mesylate corresponding to 12 or 62 times the maximal total daily human inhalation dose (8.0 mg bitolterol mesylate per day). Bitolteral mesylate was not tumorigenic in an 18-month oral study in Swiss-Webster mice at doses up to 312 times the maximal daily human inhalational dose.

Ames Salmonella and mouse lymphoma mutation assays *in vitro* revealed no mutagenesis due to bitolteral mesylate. Reproductive studies in male and female rats revealed no significant effects on fertility at doses of bitolteral mesylate up to 241 times the maximal daily human inhalational dose.

Metered Dose Inhaler: No tumorigenicity (and specifically no increase in leiomyomas) was observed in a two-year oral study in Sprague-Dawley CD rats at doses of bitolteral mesylate corresponding to 23 or 114 times the maximal daily human inhalation dose. Bitolteral mesylate was not tumorigenic in an 18-month oral study in Swiss-Webster mice at doses up to 568 times the maximal daily human inhalational dose.

Ames Salmonella and mouse lymphoma mutation assays *in vitro* revealed no mutagenesis due to bitolteral mesylate. Reproductive studies in male and female rats revealed no significant effects on fertility at doses of bitolteral mesylate up to 364 times the maximal daily human inhalational dose.

PREGNANCY, TERATOGENIC EFFECTS, PREGNANCY CATEGORY C

Solution for Inhalation: No teratogenic effects were seen in rats and rabbits after oral doses of bitolteral mesylate up to 361 times the maximal daily human inhalational dose and in mice after oral doses up to 188 times the maximal daily human inhalational dose.

PRECAUTIONS: *(cont'd)*

When bitolteral mesylate (as base) was injected subcutaneously into mice in doses of 2 mg/kg, 10 mg/kg, and 20 mg/kg (corresponding to 15, 75, and 151 times the maximal daily human inhalational dose) the incidence of cleft palate was 5.7%, 3.8%, and 3.3%, respectively. Occurrence of cleft palate with isoproterenol (as base) at 10 mg/kg subcutaneously was 10.7%. Since well-controlled studies in pregnant women are not available, bitolteral mesylate should be used during pregnancy only if the potential benefit justifies the potential risk to the fetus.

Metered Dose Inhaler: No teratogenic effects were seen in rats and rabbits after oral doses of bitolteral mesylate up to 557 times the maximal daily human inhalational dose and in mice after oral doses up to 284 times the maximal daily human inhalational dose.

When bitolteral mesylate was injected subcutaneously into mice at doses of 2 mg/kg, 10 mg/kg, and 20 mg/kg (corresponding to 23, 114, and 227 times the maximal daily human inhalational dose) cleft palate incidences of 5.7 percent, 3.8 percent, and 3.3 percent (compared with 0.9 percent in controls) were found. Cleft palate induction with isoproterenol at 10 mg/kg SC as the positive control was 10.7 percent. Since no well-controlled studies in pregnant women are available, bitolteral mesylate should be used during pregnancy only if the potential benefit justifies the potential risk to the fetus.

SOLUTION FOR INHALATION AND METERED DOSE INHALER

Nursing Mothers: It is not known whether bitolteral mesylate is excreted in human milk. Because many drugs are excreted in human milk, caution should be exercised when bitolteral mesylate is administered to a nursing woman.

Pediatric Use: Safety and effectiveness of bitolteral mesylate in children 12 years of age or younger has not been established.

DRUG INTERACTIONS:

Solution for Inhalation: Other sympathomimetic bronchodilators or epinephrine should not be used concomitantly with bitolteral mesylate because they have additive effects.

Bitolteral mesylate should be administered with caution to patients being treated with monoamine oxidase inhibitors or tricyclic antidepressants, since the action of bitolterol on the vascular system may be potentiated.

Metered Dose Inhaler: Other sympathomimetic aerosol bronchodilators should not be used concomitantly with bitolteral mesylate. If additional adrenergic drugs are to be administered by any route, they should be used with caution to avoid deleterious cardiovascular effects.

ADVERSE REACTIONS:

Solution for Inhalation: The adverse reactions observed with bitolteral mesylate are consistent with those seen with other beta-adrenergic agonists. The frequency of most cardiovascular effects was less after bitolterol mesylate than after isoproterenol in 3-month repetitive dose studies.

Like the findings noted after the administration of other beta-adrenergic agonist drugs, infrequent laboratory abnormalities with undetermined clinical significance were noted after administration of bitolteral mesylate. These include decreases in hemoglobin and hematocrit, decreases in WBC, elevation of liver enzymes, increases in blood sugar, decreases in serum potassium and abnormal urinalysis. In addition, one patient in a bitolteral mesylate controlled clinical trial had increased liver function tests and documented hepatomegaly.

The results of all clinical trials with bitolteral mesylate (323 patients) showed the following side effects:

Central/Peripheral Nervous System: Tremors (26.6%), nervousness (11.1%), headache (8.4%), lightheadedness (6.8%), dizziness (4.0%), paresthesia (1.5%), somnolence (1.2%). In three-month studies, the incidence of tremors decreased from 22% during the first month to 9% during the third month.

Cardiovascular: Tachycardia (3.7%), palpitation (3.1%), irregular pulse (1.2%).

Respiratory: Coughing (2.5%), bronchospasm (1.5%), chest discomfort (1.5%), rhinitis (1.5%).

Oro-Pharyngeal: Throat irritation (2.5%), mouth irritation (1.9%).

Gastrointestinal: Nausea (1.9%).

Other: Fatigue (1.5%).

The incidence of the following adverse reactions was less than one percent:

CNS: Vertigo, insomnia, euphoria, incoordination, hyperkinesia, hypoesthesia, anxiety.

Cardiovascular: Transient ECG changes (ventricular premature contractions, atrial arrhythmia, inverted T waves, junctional rhythm), chest discomfort, increase in blood pressure, chills, heart rate decrease, flushing.

Respiratory: Dyspnea, sputum increase.

Gastrointestinal: Vomiting, hepatomegalia.

Others: Pruritus, urticaria, asthenia, arthralgia, eye irritation, facial discomfort, taste loss.

Clinical relevance or relationship to administration of bitolteral mesylate and rarely reported elevations of SGOT, SGPT, LDH are not known.

Metered Dose Inhaler: The results of all clinical trials with bitolteral mesylate (bitolterol mesylate) in 492 patients showed the following side effects.

CNS: Tremors (14%), nervousness (5%), headache (4%), dizziness (3%), lightheadedness (3%), insomnia (<1%), hyperkinesia (<1%).

Gastrointestinal: Nausea (3%).

Oro-Pharyngeal: Throat irritation (5%).

Cardiovascular: The overall incidence of cardiovascular effects was approximately 5% of patients and these effects included palpitations (approximately 3%), and chest discomfort (approximately 1%). Tachycardia was seen in less than 1%. Premature ventricular contractions and flushing were rarely seen.

Respiratory: Coughing (4%), bronchospasm (<1%), dyspnea (<1%), chest tightness (<1%).

Clinical relevance or relationship to bitolteral mesylate administration of rarely reported elevations of SGOT, decrease in patients, decreases in WBC levels or proteinuria are not known.

In comparing the adverse reactions for bitolterol mesylate treated patients to those of isoproterenol treated patients, during three-month clinical trails involving approximately 400 patients, the following moderate to severe reactions, as judged by the investigators, were reported for such steroid and non-steroid dependent patients. The table (TABLE 1) does not include mild reactions or those occurring only with the first dose.

NOTE: In most patients, the total isoproterenol dosage was divided into three equally dosed inhalations, administered at three- minute intervals. This procedure may have reduced the incidence of adverse reactions observed with isoproterenol.

OVERDOSAGE:

Solution for Inhalation and Metered Dose Inhaler: Overdosage with bitolterol mesylate may be expected to result in exaggeration of those drug effects listed in the ADVERSE REACTIONS section. In such cases therapy with bitolteral mesylate and all β-adrenergic stimulating drugs should be stopped, supportive therapy provided, and judicious use of a cardioselective β-adrenergic blocking agent should be considered bearing in mind the possibility that such agents can produce profound bronchospasm. As with all sympathomimetic aerosol medications, cardiac arrest and even death may be associated with abuse.

OVERDOSAGE: *(cont'd)*

TABLE 1 Percent Incidence of Moderate to Severe Adverse Reactions

Reaction	Bitolterol N=197	Isoproterenol N=194
Central Nervous System		
Tremors	9.1%	1.5%
Nervousness	1.5%	1.0%
Headache	3.5%	6.1%
Dizziness	1.0%	1.5%
Insomnia	0.5%	0%
Cardiovascular		
Palpitations	1.5%	0%
PVC—Transient Increase	0.5%	0%
Chest Discomfort	0.5%	0%
Respiratory		
Cough	4.1%	1.0%
Bronchospasm	1.0%	0%
Dyspnea	1.0%	0%
Oro-Pharyngeal		
Throat Irritation	3.0%	3.1%
Gastrointestinal		
Nausea (Dyspepsia)	0.5%	0.5%

With the Solution for Inhalation the oral LD_{50} of bitolteral mesylate in rats was 5,650 mg/kg and in mice it was 6,575 mg/kg.

With the Metered Dose Inhaler the oral LD_{50} of bitolteral mesylate in rats was greater than 5,000 mg/kg and in mice greater than 6,000 mg/kg.

DOSAGE AND ADMINISTRATION:

Solution for Inhalation: Bitolteral mesylate inhalation solution, 0.2% can be administered by nebulization to adults and children over 12 years of age. As with all medications, the physician should begin therapy with the lowest effective dose according to the individual patient's requirements following manufacturer's dosage recommendation. Bitolteral mesylate should be administered during a ten to fifteen minute period. The treatment period can be adjusted by varying the amount of diluent (normal saline solution) placed in the nebulizer with the medication. The total volume (medication plus diluent) is usually adjusted to 2.0 ml to 4.0 ml. Safety of the treatment should be monitored be measuring blood pressure and pulse.

Clinical studies were conducted with two types of nebulizer systems.

Intermittent Aerosol Flow (Patient-Activated Nebulizer): This nebulizer is operated by a patient-activated value to permit the release of aerosol mist during inspiration.

Continuous Aerosol Flow Nebulizer: This nebulizer generates a continuous flow of mist while the patient inhales and exhales through the nebulizer resulting in the loss of some medication through an exhaust port.

When using these types of nebulizer systems the following dosing regimens are recommended (TABLE 2):

TABLE 2 Bitolterol Mesylate for Inhalation, 0.2%

Doses	Continuous Flow Nebulization Volume	Continuous Flow Nebulization Tornalate	Intermittent Flow Nebulization Volume	Intermittent Flow Nebulization Tornalate
Usual Dose	1.25 ml	2.5 mg	0.5 ml	1.0 mg
Decreased Dose	0.75 ml	1.5 mg	0.25 ml	0.5 mg
Increased Dose	1.75 ml	3.5 mg	0.75 ml	1.5 mg

Up to 1.0 ml of bitolteral mesylate Solution for Inhalation, 0.2% (2.0 mg bitolteral mesylate), can be administered with the intermittent flow system to severely- obstructed patients.

The usual frequency of treatments is three times a day. Treatments may be increased up to four times daily, however the interval between treatments should not be less than four hours. For some patients two treatments a day may be adequate. If a previously effective dosage regimen fails to provide the usual relief, the patient should be advised to seek medical advice immediately as this is often a sign of seriously- worsening asthma that would require reassessment of therapy.

The maximum daily dose should not exceed 8.0 mg bitolteral mesylate with an intermittent flow nebulization system or 14.0 mg bitolteral mesylate with a continuous flow nebulization system.

Bitolteral mesylate solution for inhalation, 0.2% should be added to the nebulizer just prior to use and should not be left in the nebulizer.

Bitolteral mesylate solution for inhalation, 0.2% should not be mixed with other drugs such as cromolyn sodium or acetylcysteine at clinically recommended doses due to chemical and/or physical incompatibles.

Metered Dose Inhaler: The usual dose to relieve bronchospasm for adults and children over 12 years of age is two inhalations at an interval of at least one to three minutes followed by a third inhalation if needed. For prevention of bronchospasm, the usual dose is two inhalations every 8 hours. The dose of bitolteral mesylate (bitolterol mesylate) should never exceed 3 inhalations every 6 hours or 2 inhalations every 4 hours. If a previously effective dosage regimen fails to provide the usual relief, the patient should be advised to seek medical advice immediately as this is often a sign of seriously-worsening asthma that would require reassessment of therapy.

PATIENT PACKAGE INSERT:

Solution for Inhalation: Patient's Instructions for Use FOR STANDARD NEBULIZER *Read complete instructions carefully before using.*

1. Withdraw the prescribed dose of bitolteral mesylate Solution for Inhalation into the specially marked dropper that comes with each multi-dose bottle.

2. Squeeze the solution into the nebulizer reservoir through the appropriate opening.

3. Add sterile normal saline solution as directed by your physician. The combined volume (medication plus saline solution) usually equals 2.0 ml to 4.0 ml.

4. Gently swirl the nebulizer to mix the contents and connect it to the mouthpiece or face mask.

5. Connect the nebulizer to the compressor.

6. Sit in a comfortable upright position; place the mouthpiece in your mouth or put on the face mask; and turn on the compressor.

7. Breathe as calmly, deeply and evenly as possible until no more mist is formed in the nebulizer chamber (about 5-15 minutes). At this point, the treatment is finished.

8. Clean the nebulizer.

PATIENT PACKAGE INSERT: *(cont'd)*

Note: Drug stability and safety of bitolteral mesylate solution for inhalation when mixed with other drugs in a nebulizer have not been established. Use only as directed by your physician.

Dosage: Use only as directed by your physician.

Warning: The effects of bitolteral mesylate may last up to eight hours or longer. It should not be used more often than recommended. Do not increase the dose or use more frequently unless directed by your physician. If the recommended dosage does not provide relief of symptoms, if symptoms get worse, or adverse reactions occur, contact your physician immediately.

Store at room temperature between 15°C and 30°C (59°F and 86°F).

Patient's Instructions for Use FOR PARI-JET NEBULIZER *Read complete instructions carefully before using.*

1. Withdraw the prescribed dose of bitolteral mesylate Solution for Inhalation into the specially marked dropper that comes with each multi-dose bottle.

2. Squeeze the solution into the bottom of the nebulizer bowl.

3. Add sterile normal saline solution as directed by your physician. The combined volume (medication plus saline solution) usually equals 2.0 ml to 4.0 ml.

4. Attach top of nebulizer bowl to bottom of nebulizer bowl and gently swirl the nebulizer to mix the contents.

5. Insert nebulizer bowl into handle, close handle, and connect the nebulizer to the compressor using the air hose.

6. Sit in a comfortable upright position; place the mouthpiece in your mouth or put on the face mask; turn on the compressor.

7. Breathe as calmly, deeply and evenly as possible until no more mist is formed in the nebulizer chamber (about 5-15 minutes). At this point, the treatment is finished.

8. Clean the nebulizer.

Note: Drug stability and safety of bitolteral mesylate solution for inhalation when mixed with other drugs in a nebulizer have not been established. Use only as directed by your physician.

Dosage: Use only as directed by your physician.

Warning: The effects of bitolteral mesylate may last up to eight hours or longer. It should not be used more often than recommended. Do not increase the dose or use more frequently unless directed by your physician. If the recommended dosage does not provide relief of symptoms, if symptoms get worse, or adverse reactions occur, contact your physician immediately.

Store at room temperature between 15°C and 30°C (59°F and 86°F).

Metered Dose Inhaler: Patient's Instructions for Use*Read complete instructions carefully before using.*

1. Hold the inhaler upright and pull mouthpiece straight up.

2. Snap mouthpiece into position over the spray opening.

3. Hold inhaler upside down between thumb and forefinger.

4. Breathe out completely. Place the mouthpiece fully into mouth, and close lips loosely around end of mouthpiece.

5. While inhaling, squeeze thumb and forefinger firmly together to actuate. Inhale deeply and slowly for about 10 seconds. Do not activate the aerosol before you begin to inhale or after you have taken as deep a breath as possible.

6. Pause briefly and then exhale slowly. Wait at least one to three full minutes between each additional inhalation as prescribed by your physician.

7. Keep the plastic mouthpiece clean by removing the bottle and rinsing the mouthpiece daily with tap water.

8. As with all aerosol medications, it is recommended to "test spray" into the air before using for the first time and in cases where the product has not been used for a prolonged period of time.

Dosage: Use only as directed by your physician.

WARNING: Contents under pressure. Do not puncture. Do not use or store near heat or open flame. Exposure to temperatures above 120°F may cause bursting. Never throw container into a fire or incinerator. Keep out of reach of children.

Note: The statement below is required by the Federal government's Clean Air Act for all products containing or manufactured with chlorofluorocarbons (CFC's).

This product contains dichlorodifluoromethane and dichlorotetrafluoroethane, substances which harm the environment by destroying ozone in the upper atmosphere.

Your physician has determined that this product is likely to help your personal health. USE THIS PRODUCT AS DIRECTED, UNLESS INSTRUCTED TO DO OTHERWISE BY YOUR PHYSICIAN. If you have any questions about alternatives, consult with your physician.

The effects of bitolteral mesylate may last up to eight hours or longer. It should not be used more often than recommended and the number of inhalations or frequency of use should not be increased without first asking your physician. If the recommended dosage does not provide relief of symptoms, symptoms get worse, or adverse reactions occur, contact your physician immediately. Store between 15°C and 30°C (59°F and 86°F).

Use of this product outside this temperature range may result in improper dosing.

HOW SUPPLIED:

SOLUTION FOR INHALATION

Amber Glass Bottle of 10 ml with.75 cc dropper

Amber Glass Bottle of 30 ml with 1.25 cc dropper

Amber Glass Bottle of 60 ml with 1.25 cc dropper

Included in each carton is an overwrapped graduated medicine dropper for use with bitolteral mesylate solution for inhalation, 0.2%.

Do not use the solution if it is discolored or contains a precipitate.

Store at controlled room temperature between 15°C-30°C (59°F-86°F).

METERED DOSE INHALER

Tornalate (bitolterol mesylate) Metered Dose Inhaler is supplied in 16.4 g (15 ml) self-contained aerosol units. Refill of 16.4 g (15 ml).

Note: The statement below is required by the Federal government's Clean Air Act for all products containing or manufactured with chlorofluorocarbons (CFC's).

WARNING: Contains dichlorodifluoromethane and dichlorotetrafluoroethane, substances which harm public health and environment by destroying ozone in the upper atmosphere.

A notice similar to the above WARNING has been placed in the information for the patient of this product pursuant to EPA regulations.

Store at controlled room temperature between 15°C and 30°C (59°F and 86°F). Use of the product outside this temperature range may result in improper dosing.

(Dura Pharmaceuticals, Inc., 4/94, TS007D1294, TM009E0494)

HOW SUPPLIED - EQUIVALENTS NOT AVAILABLE:

Aerosol - Inhalation - 0.37 mg/0.05ml

15 ml	$34.01	TORNALATE, Dura	51479-0012-01

Solution - Inhalation - 0.37 mg/0.05ml

30 ml	$12.09	TORNALATE, Dura	51479-0011-03
60 ml	$22.89	TORNALATE, Dura	51479-0011-06

BLEOMYCIN SULFATE *(000506)*

CATEGORIES: Antibiotics; Antineoplastics; Cancer; Cervical Carcinoma; Choriocarcinoma; Hodgkin's Disease; Lip Carcinoma; Lymphoma; Lymphosarcoma; Mouth Carcinoma; Oncologic Drugs; Reticulum Cell Sarcoma; Sarcoma; Skin Cancer; Testicular Carcinoma; Throat Cancer; Tongue Cancer; Tonsil Carcinoma; FDA Approval Pre 1982

BRAND NAMES: *Blanoxan* (Mexico); **Blenoxane**; *Bleocin*; *Bleolem* (Mexico); *Bleomicina*; *Bleomycin* (England); *Bleomycine* (France); *Bleomycinum* (Germany) *(International brand names outside U.S. in italics)*

FORMULARIES: BC-BS; Medi-Cal; WHO

> WARNING:
> It is recommended that bleomycin sulfate be administered under the supervision of a qualified physician experienced in the use of cancer chemotherapeutic agents. Appropriate management of therapy and complications is possible only when adequate diagnostic and treatment facilities are readily available.
> Pulmonary fibrosis is the most severe toxicity associated with bleomycin sulfate. The most frequent presentation is pneumonitis occasionally progressing to pulmonary fibrosis. Its occurrence is higher in elderly patients and in those receiving greater than 400 units total dose, but pulmonary toxicity has been observed in young patients and these treated with low doses.
> A severe idiosyncratic reaction consisting of hypotension, mental confusion, fever, chills, and wheezing has been reported in approximately 1% of lymphoma patients treated with bleomycin sulfate.

DESCRIPTION:

Blenoxane (sterile bleomycin sulfate, USP) is a mixture of cytotoxic glycopeptide antibiotics isolated from a strain of *Streptomyces verticillus*. It is freely soluble in water.

Note: A unit of bleomycin is equal to the formerly used milligram activity. The term milligram activity is a misnomer and was changed to units to be more precise.

CLINICAL PHARMACOLOGY:

Although the exact mechanism of action of bleomycin sulfate is unknown, available evidence would seem to indicate that the main mode of action is the inhibition of DNA synthesis with some evidence of lesser inhibition of RNA and protein synthesis.

In mice, high concentrations of bleomycin sulfate are found in the skin, lungs, kidneys, peritoneum and lymphatics. Tumor cells of the skin and lungs have been found to have high concentrations of bleomycin sulfate in contrast to the low concentrations found in hematopoietic tissue. The low concentrations of bleomycin sulfate found in bone marrow may be related to high levels of bleomycin sulfate degradative enzymes found in that tissue.

In patients with normal renal function, 60% to 70% of an administered dose is recovered in the urine as active bleomycin. In patients with a creatinine clearance of > 35 mL per minute, the serum or plasma terminal elimination half-life of bleomycin is approximately 115 minutes. In patients with a creatinine clearance of < 35 mL per minute, the plasma or serum terminal elimination half-life increases exponentially as the creatinine clearance decreases. It was reported that patients with moderately severe renal failure excreted less than 20% of the dose in the urine. This result would suggest that severe renal impairment could lead to accumulation of the drug in blood.

Information on the dose proportionality of bleomycin is not available.

When administered intrapluerally for the treatment of malignant pleural effusion, bleomycin acts as a sclerosing agent.

Following intrapleural administration to a limited number of patients (n=4), the resultant bleomycin plasma concentrations suggest a systemic absorbtion of approximately 45%.

The safety and efficacy of bleomycin and tetracycline (1 gm) as treatment for malignant pleural effusion were evaluated in a multicenter, randomized trial. Patients were required to have cytologically positive pleural effusion, good performance status (0, 1, 2) lung re-expansion following tube thoracostomy with drainage rates of 100 mL/24 hr. or less, no prior intrpleural therapy, prior systemic bleomycin therapy, no chest irradiation and no recent change in systemic therapy. Overall survival did not differ between the bleomycin (n=44) and tetracycline (n=41) groups. Of patients evaluated within 30 days of instillation, the recurrence rate was 36% (10/28) with bleomycin and 67% (18/27) with tetracycline (p=0.023). Toxicity was similar between groups.

INDICATIONS AND USAGE:

Bleomycin sulfate should be considered a palliative treatment. It has been shown to be useful in the management of the following neoplasms either as a single agent or in proven combinations with other approved chemotherapeutic agents:

Squamous Cell Carcinoma: Head and neck (including mouth, tongue, tonsil, nasopharynx, oropharynx, sinus, palate, lip, buccal mucosa, gingiva, epiglottis, skin, larynx), penis, cervix, and vulva. The response to bleomycin sulfate is poorer in patients with head and neck cancer previously irradiated.

Lymphomas: Hodgkin's, reticulum cell sarcoma, lymphosarcoma.

Testicular Carcinoma: Embryonal cell, choriocarcinoma, and teratocarcinoma.

Bleomycin sulfate has also been shown to be useful in the management of:

Malignant Pleural Effusion: Bleomycin sulfate is effective as a sclerosing agent for the treatment of malignant pleural effusion and prevention of recurrent pleural effusions.

CONTRAINDICATIONS:

Bleomycin sulfate is contraindicated in patients who have demonstrated a hypersensitive or an idiosyncratic reaction to it.

WARNINGS:

Patients receiving bleomycin sulfate must be observed carefully and frequently during and after therapy. It should be used with extreme caution in patients with significant impairment of renal function or compromised pulmonary function.

Pulmonary toxicities occur in 10% of treated patients. In approximately 1% the nonspecific pneumonitis induced by bleomycin sulfate progresses to pulmonary fibrosis, and death. Although this is age and dose related, the toxicity is unpredictable. Frequent roentgenograms are recommended.

Idiosyncratic reactions similar to anaphylaxis have been reported in 1% of lymphoma patients treated with bleomycin sulfate. Since these usually occur after the first or second dose, careful monitoring is essential after these doses.

Renal or hepatic toxicity, beginning as a deterioration in renal or liver function tests, have been reported, infrequently. These toxicities may occur, however, at any time after initiation of therapy.

Usage in Pregnancy: Bleomycin can cause fatal harm when administered to a pregnant woman. It has been shown to be teratogenic in rats. Administration of intraperitoneal doses of 1.5 mg/kg/day to rats (about 1.6 times the recommended human dose on a unit/m^2basis) on days 5–15 of gestation caused skeletal malformations, shortened innominate artery and hydroureter. Bleomycin is abortifacient but not teratogenic in rabbits, at i.v. doses of 1.2 mg/kg/day (about 2.4 times the recommended human dose on a unit/m^2 basis) given on gestation days 6–18.

There have been no studies in pregnant women. If bleomycin is used during pregnancy, or if the patient becomes pregnant while receiving this drug, the patient should be apprised of the potential hazard to the fetus. Women of childbearing potential should be advised to avoid becoming pregnant during therapy with bleomycin.

ADVERSE REACTIONS:

Pulmonary: This is potentially the most serious side effect, occurring in approximately 10% of treated patients. The most frequent presentation is pneumonitis occasionally progressing to pulmonary fibrosis. Approximately 1% of patients treated have died of pulmonary fibrosis. Pulmonary toxicity is both dose and age-related, being more common in patients over 70 years of age and in those receiving over 400 units total dose. This toxicity, however, is unpredictable and has been seen occasionally in young patients receiving low doses.

Because of lack of specificity of the clinical syndrome, the identification of patients with pulmonary toxicity due to bleomycin sulfate has been extremely difficult. The earliest symptom associated with bleomycin sulfate pulmonary toxicity is dyspnea. The earliest sign is fine rales.

Radiographically, bleomycin sulfate-induced pneumonitis produces nonspecific patchy opacities, usually of the lower lung fields. The most common changes in pulmonary function tests are a decrease in total lung volume and a decrease in vital capacity. However, these changes are not predictive of the development of pulmonary fibrosis.

The microscopic tissue changes due to bleomycin sulfate toxicity include bronchiolar squamous metaplasia, reactive macrophages, atypical alveolar epithelial cells, fibrinous edema, and interstitial fibrosis. The acute stage may involve capillary changes and subsequent fibrinous exudation into alveoli producing a change similar to hyaline membrane formation and progressing to a diffuse interstitial fibrosis resembling the Hamman-Rich syndrome. These microscopic findings are nonspecific, e.g., similar changes are seen in radiation pneumonitis, pneumocystic pneumonitis.

To monitor the onset of pulmonary toxicity, roentgenograms of the chest should be taken every 1 to 2 weeks. If pulmonary changes are noted, treatment should be discontinued until it can be determined if they are drug related. Recent studies have suggested that sequential measurement of the pulmonary diffusion capacity for carbon monoxide (DL_∞) during treatment with bleomycin sulfate may be an indicator of subclinical pulmonary toxicity. It is recommended that the DL_∞ be monitored monthly if it is to be employed to detect pulmonary toxicities, and thus the drug should be discontinued when the DL_∞ falls below 30% to 35% of the pretreatment value.

Because of bleomycin's sensitization of lung tissue, patients who have received bleomycin are at greater risk of developing pulmonary toxicity when oxygen is administered in surgery. While long exposure to very high oxygen concentrations is a known cause of lung damage, after bleomycin administration, lung damage can occur at lower concentrations that are usually considered safe. Suggested preventive measures are:

1. Maintain Fl O_2at concentrations approximating that of room air (25%) during surgery and the postoperative period.

2. Monitor carefully fluid replacement, focusing more on colloid administration than crystalloid.

Sudden onset of an acute chest pain syndrome suggestive of pleuropericarditis has been rarely reported during bleomycin sulfate infusions. Although each patient must be individually evaluated, further courses of bleomycin sulfate do not appear to be contraindicated.

Idiosyncratic Reactions: In approximately 1% of the lymphoma patients treated with bleomycin sulfate, an idiosyncratic reaction, similar to anaphylaxis clinically, has been reported. The reaction may be immediate or delayed for several hours, and usually occurs after the first or second dose. It consists of hypotension, mental confusion, fever, chills, and wheezing. Treatment is symptomatic including volume expansion, pressor agents, antihistamines and corticosteroids.

Integument and Mucous Membranes: These are the most frequent side effects, being reported in approximately 50% of treated patients. These consist of erythema, rash, striae, vesiculation, hyperpigmentation, and tenderness of the skin. Hyperkeratosis, nail changes, alopecia, pruritus, and stomatitis have also been reported. It was necessary to discontinue bleomycin sulfate therapy in 2% of treated patients because of these toxicities.

Skin toxicity is a relatively late manifestation usually developing in the 2nd and 3rd week of treatment after 150 to 200 units of bleomycin sulfate has been administered and appears to be related to the cumulative dose.

Other: Vascular toxicities coincident with the use of bleomycin sulfate in combination with other antineoplastic agents have been reported rarely. The events are clinically heterogeneous and may include myocardial infarction, cerebrovascular accident, thrombotic microangiopathy (HUS) or cerebral arteritis. Various mechanisms have been proposed for these vascular complications. There are also reports of Raynaud's phenomenon occurring in patients treated with bleomycin sulfate in combination with vinblastine with or without cisplatin or, in a few cases, with bleomycin sulfate as a single agent. It is currently unknown if the case of Raynaud's phenomenon in these cases is the disease, underlying vascular compromise, bleomycin sulfate, vinblastine, hypomagnesemia, or a combination of any of these factors.

Fever, chills, and vomiting were frequently reported side effects. Anorexia and weight loss are common and may persist long after termination of this medication. Pain at tumor site, phlebitis, and other local reactions were reported infrequently.

DOSAGE AND ADMINISTRATION:

DOSAGE

Because of the possibility of an anaphylactoid reaction, lymphoma patients should be treated with 2 units or less for the first 2 doses. If no acute reaction occurs, then the regular dosage schedule may be followed.

The following dose schedule is recommended:

Squamous cell carcinoma, lymphosarcoma, reticulum cell sarcoma, testicular carcinoma: 0.25 to 0.50 units/kg (10 to 20 units/m^2) given intravenously, intramuscularly, or subcutaneously weekly or twice weekly.

Hodgkin's Disease: 0.25 to 0.50 units Kg (10 to 20 units/m^2) given intravenously, intramuscularly, or subcutaneously weekly or twice weekly. After a 50% response, a maintenance dose of 1 units daily or 5 units weekly intravenously or intramuscularly should be given.

Pulmonary toxicity of bleomycin sulfate appears to be dose-related with a striking increase when the total dose is over 400 units. Total doses over 400 units should be given with great caution.**Note: When bleomycin sulfate is used in combination with other antineoplastic agents, pulmonary toxicities may occur at lower doses.**

Improvement of Hodgkin's Disease and testicular tumors is prompt and noted within two weeks. If no improvement is seen by this time, improvement is unlikely. Squamous cell cancers respond more slowly, sometimes requiring as long as three weeks before any improvement is noted.

Malignant Pleural Effusion: 60 units administered as a single dose bolus intrapleural injection.

ADMINISTRATION

Bleomycin sulfate may be given by the intramuscular, intravenous, subcutaneous, intrapleural routes.

Intramuscular or Subcutaneous: The bleomycin 15 units vial should be reconstituted with 1 to 5 mL of Sterile Water for Injection, USP, Sodium Chloride for Injection, 0.9%, USP, or Bacteriostatic Water for Injection, USP. The bleomycin 30 units vial should be reconstituted with 2 to 10 mL of the above diluents.

Intravenous: The contents of the 15 units or 30 units vial should be dissolved in 5 mL or 10 mL, respectively of Sodium Chloride for Injection, 0.9%, USP and administered slowly over a period of 10 minutes.

Intrapleural: 60 units of bleomycin is dissolved in 50–100 mL sodium chloride injection 0.9%, and administered through a thoracostomy tube following drainage of excess pleural fluid and confirmation of complete lung expansion. The literature suggests that successful pleurodesis is, in part, dependent upon complete drainage of the pleural fluid and reestablishment of negative intrapleural pressure prior to instillation of a sclerosing agent. Therefore, the amount of drainage from the chest tube should be as minimal as possible prior to instillaton of bleomycin. Although there is no conclusive evidence to support this contention, it is genrally accepted that chest tube drainage should be less than 100 mL in a 24 hour period prior to sclerosis. However, bleomycin instillation may be appropriate when drainage is between 100–300 mL under clinical conditions that necessitate sclerosis therapy. The thoracostomy tube is clamped after bleomycin instillation. The patient is moved from the supine to the left and right lateral positions several times during the next four hours. The clamp is then removed and suction reestablished. The amount of time the chest tube remains in place following sclerosis is dictated by the clinical situation.

The intrapleural injection of topical anesthetics or systemic narcotic analgesia is generally not required. Parental drug products should be inspected visually for particulate matter and discoloration prior to administration, whenever solution and container permit.

STABILITY

The sterile powder is stable under refrigeration 2°C (36°F) to 8°C (46°F) and should not be used after the expiration date is reached.

Bleomycin should not be reconstituted or diluted with D_5W and analyzed by HPLC, bleomycin demonstrates a loss of A^2 and B^2 potency that does not occur when bleomycin is reconstituted in 0.9% sodium chloride.

Bleomycin sulfate is stable for 24 hours at room temperature in Sodium Chloride.

Procedures for proper handling and disposal of anticancer drugs should be considered. Several guidelines on this subject have been published.[1-7]There is no general agreement that all of the procedures recommended in the guidelines are necessary or appropriate.

REFERENCES:

1. Recommendations for the Safe Handling of Parenteral Antineoplastic Drugs. NIH Publication No. 83-2621. For sale by the Superintendent of Documents, US Government Printing Office, Washington, DC 20402. **2.** AMA Council Report. Guidelines for Handling Parenteral Antineoplastics. JAMA, 1985 March 15. **3.** National Study Commission on Cytotoxic Exposure—Recommendations for Handling Cytotoxic Agents. Available from Louis P. Jeffrey, ScD, Chairman,National Study Commission on Cytotoxic Exposure, Massachusetts College of Pharmacy and Allied Health Sciences, 179 Longwood Avenue, Boston, Massachusetts 02115. **4.** Clinical Oncological Society of Australia: Guidelines and Recommendations for Safe Handling of Antineoplastic Agents. Med J Australia 1983; 1:426-428. **5.** Jones RB, et al: Safe Handling of chemotherapeutic agents: A report from the Mount Sinai Medical Center, CA—A Cancer Journal for Clinicians 1983; (Sept/Oct) 258-263. **6.** American Society for Hospital Pharmacists Technical Assistance Bulletin on Handling Cytotoxic and Hazardous Drugs, Am J Hosp Pharm 1990; 47:1033- 1049. **7.** OSHA Work-Practice Guidelines for Personnel Dealing with Cytotoxic (Antineoplastic) Drugs, Am J Hosp Pharm 1986; 43:1193-1204.

HOW SUPPLIED - EQUIVALENTS NOT AVAILABLE:

Injection, Lyphl-Soln - Intramuscular; - 15 unit/ampul

15 unt $279.87 BLENOXANE, Mead Johnson 00015-3010-20

BOTULINUM TOXIN TYPE A *(000514)*

CATEGORIES: Autonomic Drugs; Blepharospasm; EENT Drugs; Eye, Ear, Nose, & Throat Preparations; Orphan Drugs; Skeletal Muscle Relaxants; Strabismus; Pregnancy Category C; FDA Approved 1989 Dec

BRAND NAMES: Botox; *Botox 100E* (Germany); *Botox (100 U) Injection*; *Botox (Oculinum)*; Oculinum
(International brand names outside U.S. in italics)

DESCRIPTION:

Botulinum toxin type A is a sterile, lyophilized form of botulinum toxin type A, produced from a culture of the Hall strain of*Clostridium botulinum* grown in a medium containing N-Z amine and yeast extract. It is purified from the culture solution by a series of acid precipitations to a crystalline complex consisting of the active high molecular weight toxin protein and an associated hemagglutinin protein. The crystalline complex is re-dissolved in a solution containing saline and albumin and sterile filtered (0.2 microns) prior to lyophilization. Botulinum toxin type A is to be reconstituted with sterile non-preserved saline prior to intramuscular injection.

DESCRIPTION: *(cont'd)*

Each vial of Botox (Botulinum Toxin Type A) contains 100 units (U) of *Clostridium botulinum* toxin type A, 0.5 milligrams of albumin (human), and 0.9 milligrams of sodium chloride in a sterile, lyophilized form without a preservative. One unit (U) corresponds to the calculated median lethal intraperitoneal dose (LD/50) in mice of the reconstituted botulinum toxin type A injected.

CLINICAL PHARMACOLOGY:

Botulinum toxin type A blocks neuromuscular conduction by binding to receptor sites on motor nerve terminals, entering the nerve terminals, and inhibiting the release of acetylcholine. When injected intramuscularly at therapeutic doses, botulinum toxin type A produces localized chemical denervation muscle paralysis. When the muscle is chemically denervated, it atrophies and may develop extrajunctional acetylcholine receptors. There is evidence that the nerve can sprout and reinnervate the muscle, with the weakness thus being reversible.

The paralytic effect on muscles injected with botulinum toxin type A is useful in reducing the excessive, abnormal contractions associated with blepharospasm. When used for the treatment of strabismus, it is postulated that the administration of botulinum toxin type A affects muscle pairs by inducing an atrophic lengthening of the injected muscle and a corresponding shortness of the muscle's antagonist. Following peri-ocular injection of botulinum toxin type A, distant muscles show electrophysiologic changes but no clinical weakness or other clinical changes for a period of several weeks or months, parallel to the duration of local clinical paralysis.[1]

In one study, botulinum toxin was evaluated in 27 patients with essential blepharospasm. Twenty-six of the patients had previously undergone drug treatment using benztropine mesylate, clonazepam and/or baclofen without adequate clinical results. Three of these patients then underwent muscle stripping surgery without an adequate outcome. One patient of the 27 was previously untreated. Upon using botulinum toxin, 25 of the 27 patients reported improvement within 48 hours. One of the other patients was later controlled with higher a dosage. The remaining patient reported only mild improvement but remained functionally impaired.[2]

In another study, twelve patients with blepharospasm were evaluated in a double-blind, placebo-controlled study. All patients receiving botulinum toxin (n = 8) were improved compared with no improvements in the placebo group (n = 4). The mean dystonia score improved by 72%, the self-assessment score rating improved by 61%, and a videotape evaluation rating improved by 39%. The effects of treatment lasted a mean of 12.5 weeks.[3]

One thousand six hundred eighty-four patients with blepharospasm evaluated in an open trial showed clinical improvement lasting an average of 12.5 weeks, prior to the need for retreatment.[4]

Six hundred seventy-seven patients with strabismus treated with one or more injections of botulinum toxin type A were evaluated in an open trial. Fifty-five percent of these patients were improved to an alignment of 10 prism diopters or less when evaluated 6 months or more following injection.[5] These results are consistent with results from additional open label trials which were conducted for this indication.[4]

INDICATIONS AND USAGE:

Botulinum toxin type A is indicated for the treatment of strabismus and blepharospasm associated with dystonia, including benign essential blepharospasm or VII nerve disorders in patients 12 years of age and above.

The efficacy of botulinum toxin type A in deviations over 50 prism diopters, in restrictive strabismus, in Duane's syndrome with lateral rectus weakness, and secondary strabismus caused by prior surgical over-recession of the antagonist is doubtful, or multiple injections overtime may be required. Botulinum toxin type A is ineffective in chronic paralytic strabismus except to reduce antagonist contracture in conjunction with surgical repair.

Presence of antibodies to botulinum toxin type A may reduce the effectiveness of botulinum toxin type A therapy. In clinical studies, reduction in effectiveness due to antibody production has occurred in one patient with blepharospasm receiving 3 doses of botulinum toxin type A over a 6 week period totalling 92 U, and in several patients with torticollis who received multiple doses experimentally, totalling over 300 U in one month period. For this reason, the dose of botulinum toxin type A for strabismus and blepharospasm should be kept as low as possible, in any case below 200 U in a one month period.

CONTRAINDICATIONS:

Botulinum toxin type A is contraindicated in individuals with known hypersensitivity to any ingredient in the formulation.

WARNINGS:

The recommended dosages and frequencies of administration for botulinum toxin type A should not be exceeded. There have not been any reported instances of systemic toxicity resulting from accidental injection or oral ingestion of botulinum toxin type A. Should accidental injection of oral ingestion occur, the person should be medically supervised for several days on an office or outpatient basis for signs and symptoms of systemic weakness or muscle paralysis. The entire contents of a vial is below the estimated dose for systemic toxicity in humans weighing 6 kg or greater.

In the event of overdosage or injection into the wrong muscle, additional information may be obtained by contacting Allergan Pharmaceuticals at (800) 347-5063 from 8:00 a.m. to 4:00 p.m. Pacific Time, or at (714) 724- 5954 for a recorded message at other times.

The effect of botulinum toxin may be potentiated by aminoglycoside antibiotics or any other drugs that interfere with neuromuscular transmission. Caution should be exercised when botulinum toxin type A is used in patients taking any of these drugs.[6]

PRECAUTIONS:

General: The safe and effective use of botulinum toxin type A depends upon proper storage of the product, selection of the correct dose, and proper reconstitution and administration techniques. Physicians administering botulinum toxin type A must understand the relevant neuro-muscular and orbital anatomy and any alterations to the anatomy due to prior surgical procedures, and standard electromyographic techniques.

As with all biologic products, epinephrine and other precautions as necessary should be available should an anaphylactic reaction occur.

During the administration of botulinum toxin type A for the treatment of strabismus, retrobulbar hemorrhages sufficient to compromise retinal circulation have occurred from needle penetrations into the orbit. It is recommended that appropriate instruments to decompress the orbit be accessible. Ocular (globe) penetrations by needles have also occurred. An ophthalmoscope to diagnose this condition should be available.

Reduced blinking from botulinum toxin type A injection of the orbicularis muscle can lead to corneal exposure, persistent epithelial defect and corneal ulceration, especially in patients with VII nerve disorders. One case of corneal perforation in an aphakic eye requiring corneal grafting has occurred because of this effect. Careful testing of corneal sensation in eyes previously operated upon, avoidance of injection into the lower lid area to avoid ectropion, and vigorous treatment of any epithelial defect should be employed. This may require protective drops, ointment, therapeutic soft contact lenses, or closure of the eye by patching or other means.

Information for the Patient: Patients with blepharospasm may have been extremely sedentary for a long time. Sedentary patients should be cautioned to resume activity slowly and carefully following the administration of botulinum toxin type A.

Pregnancy Category C: Animal reproduction studies have not been conducted with botulinum toxin type A. It is also not known whether botulinum toxin type A can cause fetal harm when administered to a pregnant woman or can affect reproduction capacity. Botulinum toxin type A should be administered to a pregnant woman or only if clearly needed.

Carcinogenesis, Mutagenesis, and Impairment of Fertility: Long term studies in animals have not been performed to evaluate carcinogenic potential of botulinum toxin type A.

Nursing Mothers: It is not known whether this drug is excreted in human milk. Because many drugs are excreted in human milk, caution should be exercised when botulinum toxin type A is administered to a nursing woman.

Pediatric Use: Safety and effectiveness in children below the age of 12 have not been established.

DRUG INTERACTIONS:

The effect of botulinum toxin may be potentiated by aminoglycoside antibiotics or other drugs that interfere with neuromuscular transmission. Caution should be exercised when botulinum toxin type A is used in patients taking any of these drugs.[6] (See WARNINGS.)

ADVERSE REACTIONS:

There have been reports of seven cases of diffuse skin rash and two cases of local swelling of the eyelid skin lasting for several days following eyelid injection.

STRABISMUS

Inducing paralysis in one or more extraocular muscles may produce spatial disorientation, double vision, or past-pointing. Converting the affected eye may alleviate these symptoms. Extraocular muscles adjacent to the injection site are often affected, causing ptosis or vertical deviation, especially with higher doses of botulinum toxin type A. The incidence rates of these side effects in 2058 adults who received 3650 injections for injections for horizontal strabismus are listed below:

Ptosis: 15.7%

Vertical deviation: 16.9%

The incidence of ptosis was much less after inferior rectus injection (0.9%) and much greater after superior rectus injection (37.7%).

The incidence rates of these side effects persisting for over 6 months in an enlarged series of 5587 injections of horizontal muscles in 3104 patients are listed below:

Ptosis lasting over 180 days: 0.3%

Vertical deviation greater than 2 prism

Diopters lasting over 180 days: 2.1%

In these patients, the injection procedure itself caused 9 scleral perforations. A vitreous hemorrhage occurred and later cleared in one case. No retinal detachment or visual loss occurred in any case. Sixteen retrobulbar hemorrhages occurred. Decompression of the orbit after 5 minutes was done to restore retinal circulation in one case. No eye lost vision from retrobulbar hemorrhage. Five eyes had pupillary change consistent with ciliary ganglion damage (Adies pupil).

BLEPHAROSPASM

In 1684 patients who received 4258 treatments (involving multiple injections) for blepharospasm, the incidence rates of adverse reactions per treated eye are listed below:

Ptosis: 11.0%

Irritation/Tearing: 10.0%(includes dry eye, lagophthalmos, and photophobia)

Ectropion, keratitis, diplopia and entropion were reported rarely (incidence less than 1%)

Ecchymosis occurs easily in the soft eyelid tissues. This can be prevented by applying pressure at the injection site immediately after the injection.

In two cases of VII nerve disorders (one case of aphakic eye) reduced blinking from botulinum toxin type A injection of the orbicularis muscle led to serious corneal exposure, persistent epithelial defect and corneal ulceration. Perforation requiring corneal grafting occurred in one case, an aphakic eye. Avoidance of injection into the lower lid area to avoid ectropion may reduce this hazard. Vigorous treatment of any corneal epithelial defect should be employed. This may require protective drops, ointment, therapeutic soft contact lenses, or closure of the eye by patching or other means.

Two patients previously incapacitated by blepharospasm experienced cardiac collapse attributed to over-exertion within three weeks following botulinum toxin type A therapy. Sedentary patients should be cautioned to resume activity slowly and carefully following the administration of botulinum toxin type A.

OVERDOSAGE:

In the event of overdosage or injection into the wrong muscle, additional information may be obtained by contacting Allergan Pharmaceuticals at (800) 347-5063 from 8:00 a.m. to 4:00 p.m. Pacific Time, or at (714) 724- 5954 for a recorded message at other times.

DOSAGE AND ADMINISTRATION:

STRABISMUS

Botulinum toxin type A is intended for injection into extraocular muscles utilizing the electrical activity recorded from the tip of the injection needle as a guide to placement within the target muscle. Injection without surgical exposure or electromyographic guidance should not be attempted. Physicians should be familiar with electromyographic technique.

An injection of botulinum toxin type A is prepared by drawing into a sterile 1.0 ml tuberculin syringe an amount of the properly diluted toxin (see TABLE 1) slightly greater than the intended dose. Air bubbles in the syringe barrel are expelled and the syringe is attached to the electromyographic injection needle, preferably a 1.5", 27 gauge needle. Injection volume in excess of the intended dose of the intended dose is expelled through the needle into an appropriate waste container to assure patency of the needle and to confirm that there is no syringe-needle leakage. A new, sterile needle and syringe should be used to enter the vial on each occasion for dilution or removal of botulinum toxin type A.

To prepare the eye for botulinum toxin type A injection, it is recommended that several drops of a local anesthetic and an ocular decongestant be given several minutes prior to injection.

Note: The volume of botulinum toxin type A injected for treatment of strabismus should be between 0.05 ml to 0.15 ml per muscle.

Strabismus Dosage: The initial doses of diluted botulinum toxin type A (see TABLE 1) typically create paralysis of injected muscles beginning one or two days after injection and increasing in intensity during the first week. The paralysis lasts for 2-6 weeks and gradually

DOSAGE AND ADMINISTRATION: *(cont'd)*

resolves over a similar period. Overcorrections lasting over 6 months have been rare. About one half of patients will require subsequent doses because of the lack of binocular motor fusion to stabilize the alignment.

I. Initial doses in units (abbreviate as U). Use the lower listed doses for treatment of small deviations. Use the larger only for large deviations.

A. For vertical muscles, and for horizontal strabismus of less than 20 prism diopters: 1.25 U to 2.5 U in any one muscle.

B. For horizontal strabismus of 20 prism diopters to 50 prism diopters: 2.5 U to 5.0 U in any one muscle.

C. For persistent VI nerve palsy of one month or longer duration: 1.25 U to 2.5 U in the medial rectus muscle.

II. Subsequent doses for residual or recurrent strabismus.

A. It is recommended that patients be re-examined 7-14 days after each injection to assess the effect of that dose.

B. Patients experiencing adequate paralysis of the target muscle that require subsequent injections should receive a dose comparable to the initial dose.

C. Subsequent doses for patients experiencing incomplete paralysis of the target muscle may be increased up to twice the size of the previously administered dose.

D. Subsequent injections should not be administered until the effects of the previous dose have dissipated as evidenced by substantial function in the injected and adjacent muscles.

E. The maximum recommended dose as a single injection for any one muscle is 25 U.

BLEPHAROSPASM

For blepharospasm, diluted botulinum toxin type A (see TABLE 1) is injected using a sterile, 27 - 30 gauge needle without electromyographic guidance. 1.25 U to 2.5 U (0.05 ml to 0.1 ml volume at each site) injected into the medial and lateral pre-tarsal orbicularis oculi of the upper lid and into the lateral pre-tarsal of the lower lid is the recommended dose. In general, the initial effect of the injections is seen within three days and reaches a peak at one to two weeks post-treatment. Each treatment lasts approximately three months, following which the procedure can be repeated indefinitely - usually defined as an effect that does not last longer than two months. However there appears to be little benefit obtainable from injecting more than 5.0 Units per site. Some tolerance may be found when botulinum toxin type A is used in treating blepharospasm if treatments are given any more than every three months, and it is rare to have the effect be permanent.

The cumulative dose of botulinum toxin type A in a 30-day period should not exceed 200 U.

Dilution Technique: To reconstitute lyophilized botulinum toxin type A, use sterile, normal saline **without** a preservative; 0.9% Sodium Chloride Injection is the recommended diluent. Draw up the proper amount of diluent in the appropriate size syringe. Since botulinum toxin type A is denatured by bubbling or similar violent agitation, inject the diluent into the vial gently. Discard the vial if a vacuum does not pull the diluent into the vial. Record the date and time of reconstitution on the space on the label. Botulinum toxin type A should be administered within 4 hours after reconstitution.

During this time period, reconstituted botulinum toxin type A should be stored in a refrigerator (2 to 8°C). Reconstituted botulinum toxin type A should be clear, colorless and free of particulate matter. Parenteral drug products should be inspected visually for particulate matter and discoloration prior to administration and whenever the solution and the container permit. The use of one vial for more than one patient is not recommended because the product and the diluent do not contain a preservative. (TABLE 1):

TABLE 1 Dilution Table

Diluent Added (0.9% Sodium Chloride Injection)	Resulting dose in Units per 0.1 ml
1.0 ml	10.0 U
2.0 ml	5.0 U
4.0 ml	2.5 U
8.0 ml	1.25 U

Note: These dilutions (TABLE 1) are calculated for an injection volume of 0.1 ml. A decrease or increase in the botulinum toxin type A dose is also possible by administering a smaller or larger injection volume - from 0.05 ml (50% decrease in dose) to 0.15 ml (50% increase in dose).

STORAGE

Store the lyophilized product in a freezer at or below -5°C. Administer botulinum toxin type A within 4 hours after the vial is removed from the freezer and reconstituted. During these four hours, reconstituted botulinum toxin type A should be stored in a refrigerator (2 to 8°C). Reconstituted botulinum toxin type A should be clear, colorless, and free of particulate matter.

All vials, including expired vials, or equipment used with the drug should be disposed of carefully as is done with all medical waste.

REFERENCES:

1. Sanders D. Massey W, Buckley E. Botulinum toxin for blepharospasm: single-fiber EMG studies. Neurology 1986; 36: 545-547. **2.** Arthur B, Flanders M, Codere F, Gauthier S, Dresner S, Stone L. Treatment of blepharospasm with medication, surgery and type A botulinum toxin, Can J Ophthalmol 1987; 22:24-28. **3.** Jankovic J, Orman J. Botulinum. A toxin for cranial-cervical dystonia: A double-blind, placebo controlled study. Neurology 1987; 37:616-623. **4.** Data on file, Allergan, Inc. **5.** Scott A.B. Botulinum toxin treatment of strabismus. American Academy of Ophthalmology, Focal Points 1989; Clinical Modules for Ophthalmologists Vol VII Module 12. **6.** Wang Y C, Burr D H, Korthals G J, Sugiyama H. Acute toxicity of aminoglycosides antibiotics as an aid in detecting botulism. Appl Environ Microbiol 1984; 48:951-955.(Allergan, 92/04, 70244 31-1/U)

HOW SUPPLIED - EQUIVALENTS NOT AVAILABLE:

Injection, Lyphl-Soln - Intramuscular; - 100 unit/vial

1's $382.08 BOTOX, Allergan 00023-1145-01

BRETYLIUM TOSYLATE *(000523)*

CATEGORIES: Antiarrhythmic Agents; Arrhythmia; Cardiovascular Drugs; Fibrillation; Tachycardia; Pregnancy Category C; FDA Approval Pre 1982

BRAND NAMES: *Bretylate*; **Bretylol**; *Critifib*
(International brand names outside U.S. in italics)

DESCRIPTION:

Bretylium tosylate is o-bromobenzyl ethyldimethylammonium p-toluene sulfonate. It is an antifibrillatory and antiarrhythmic agent, intended for intravenous or intramuscular use.

Bretylium tosylate is a white, crystalline powder with an extremely bitter taste. It is freely soluble in water and alcohol. Each ml of sterile, non-pyrogenic solution contains bretylium tosylate 50 mg in Water for Injection. pH 5.0 - 7.0; sodium hydroxide and/or hydrochloric acid added, if needed, for pH adjustment. Bretylium tosylate injection contains no preservative.

CLINICAL PHARMACOLOGY:

Bretylium is a bromobenzyl quaternary ammonium compound which selectively accumulates in sympathetic ganglia and their postganglionic adrenergic neurons where it inhibits norepinephrine release by depressing adrenergic nerve terminal excitability.

Bretylium also suppresses ventricular fibrillation and ventricular arrhythmias. The mechanisms of the antifibrillatory and antiarrhythmic actions of bretylium are not established. In efforts to define these mechanisms, the following electrophysiologic actions of bretylium have been demonstrated in animal experiments:

1. Increase in ventricular fibrillation threshold.

2. Increase in action potential duration and effective refractory period without changes in heart rate.

3. Little effect on the rate of rise or amplitude of the cardiac action potential (Phase 0) or in resting membrane potential (Phase 4) in normal myocardium. However, when cell injury slows the rate of rise, decreases amplitude, and lowers resting membrane potential, bretylium transiently restores these parameters toward normal.

4. In canine hearts with infarcted areas, bretylium decreases the disparity in action potential duration between normal and infarcted regions.

5. Increase in impulse formation and spontaneous firing rate of pacemaker tissue as well as increased ventricular conduction velocity.

The restoration of injured myocardial cell electrophysiology toward normal, as well as the increase of the action potential duration and effective refractory period without changing their ratio to each other, may be important factors in suppressing re-entry of aberrant impulses and decreasing induced dispersion of local excitable states.

Bretylium induces a chemical sympathectomy-like state which resembles a surgical sympathectomy. Catecholamine stores are not depleted by bretylium, but catecholamine effects on the myocardium and on peripheral vascular resistance are often seen shortly after administration because bretylium causes an early release of norepinephrine from the adrenergic postganglionic nerve terminals. Subsequently, bretylium blocks the release of norepinephrine in response to neuron stimulation. Peripheral adrenergic blockade regularly causes orthostatic hypotension but has less effect on supine blood pressure. The relationship of adrenergic blockade to the antifibrillatory and antiarrhythmic actions of bretylium is not clear. In a study in patients with frequent ventricular premature beats, peak plasma concentration of bretylium and peak hypotensive effects were seen within one hour of intramuscular administration, presumably reflecting adrenergic neuronal blockade. However, suppression of premature ventricular beats was not maximal until 6 - 9 hours after dosing, when mean plasma concentration had declined to less than one-half of peak level. This suggests a slower mechanism, other than neuronal blockade, was involved in suppression of the arrhythmia. On the other hand, antifibrillatory effects can be seen within minutes of an intravenous injection, suggesting that the effect on the myocardium may occur quite rapidly.

Bretylium has a positive inotropic effect on the myocardium, but it is not yet certain whether this effect is direct or is mediated by catecholamine release.

Bretylium is eliminated intact by the kidneys. No metabolites have been identified following administration of bretylium tosylate injection in man and laboratory animals. In man, approximately 70 to 80% of a ^{14}C-labelled intramuscular dose is excreted in the urine during the first 24 hours, with an additional 10% excreted over the next three days.

The terminal half-life in four normal volunteers averaged 7.8 $\pm$ 0.6 hours (range 6.9 - 8.1). In one patient with a creatinine clearance of 21.0 ml/min x 1.73 m^2, the half-life was 16 hours. In one patient with a creatinine clearance of 1.0 ml/min x 1.73 m^2, the half-life was 31.5 hours. During hemodialysis, this patient's arterial and venous bretylium concentrations declined rapidly, resulting in a half-life of 13 hours. During dialysis there was a two-fold increase in total bretylium clearance.

Effect on Heart Rate: There is sometimes an initial small increase in heart rate when bretylium is administered, but this is an inconsistent and transient occurrence.

Hemodynamic Effects: Following intravenous administration of 5 mg/kg of bretylium tosylate to patients with acute myocardial infarction, there was a mild increase in arterial pressure, followed by a modest decrease, remaining within normal limits throughout. Pulmonary artery pressures, pulmonary capillary wedge pressure, right atrial pressure, cardiac index, stroke volume index and stroke work index were not significantly changed. These hemodynamic effects were not correlated with antiarrhythmic activity.

Onset of Action: Suppression of ventricular fibrillation is rapid, usually occurring within minutes following intravenous administration. Suppression of ventricular tachycardia and other ventricular arrhythmias develops more slowly, usually 20 minutes to 2 hours after parenteral administration.

INDICATIONS AND USAGE:

Bretylium tosylate injection is indicated in the prophylaxis and therapy of ventricular fibrillation.

Bretylium tosylate injection is also indicated in the treatment of life-threatening ventricular arrhythmias, such as ventricular tachycardia, that have failed to respond to adequate doses of a first-line antiarrhythmic agent, such as lidocaine.

Use of bretylium tosylate injection should be limited to intensive care units, coronary care units or other facilities where equipment and personnel for constant monitoring of cardiac arrhythmias and blood pressure are available.

Following injection of bretylium tosylate there may be a delay of 20 minutes to 2 hours in the onset of antiarrhythmic action, although it appears to act within minutes in ventricular fibrillation. The delay in effect appears to be longer after intramuscular than after intravenous injection.

CONTRAINDICATIONS:

There are no contraindications to use in treatment of ventricular fibrillation or life-threatening refractory ventricular arrhythmias.

WARNINGS:

Patients should be kept in the supine position until tolerance to the hypotensive effect of bretylium tosylate injection develops. Tolerance occurs unpredictably but may be present after several days.

1. Hypotension: Administration of bretylium tosylate injection regularly results in postural hypotension, subjectively recognized by dizziness, lightheadedness, vertigo or faintness. Some degree of hypotension is present in about 50% of patients while they are supine. Hypotension may occur at doses lower than those needed to suppress arrhythmias. Hypotension with supine systolic pressure greater than 75 mm hg need not be treated unless there are associated symptoms. If supine systolic pressure falls below 75 mm hg, an infusion of dopamine or norepinephrine may be used to raise blood pressure. When catecholamines are administered, a dilute solution should be employed and blood pressure monitored closely because the pressor effects of the catecholamines are enhanced by bretylium. Volume expansion with blood or plasma and correction of dehydration should be carried out where appropriate.

WARNINGS: *(cont'd)*

2. Transient Hypertension and Increased Frequency of Arrhythmias: Due to the initial release of norepinephrine from adrenergic postganglionic nerve terminals by bretylium, transient hypertension or increased frequency of premature ventricular contractions and other arrhythmias may occur in some patients.

3. Caution During Use with Digitalis Glycosides: The initial release of norepinephrine caused by bretylium may aggravate digitalis toxicity. When a life-threatening cardiac arrhythmia occurs in a digitalized patient, bretylium tosylate injection should be used only if the etiology of the arrhythmia does not appear to be digitalis toxicity and other antiarrhythmic drugs are not effective. Simultaneous initiation of therapy with digitalis glycosides and bretylium tosylate injection should be avoided.

4. Patients with Fixed Cardiac Output: In patients with fixed cardiac output (*i.e.,* severe aortic stenosis or severe pulmonary hypertension) bretylium tosylate injection should be avoided since severe hypotension may result from a fall in peripheral resistance without a compensatory increase in cardiac output. If survival is threatened by the arrhythmia, bretylium tosylate injection may be used but vasoconstrictive catecholamines should be given promptly if severe hypotension occurs.

PRECAUTIONS:

General

1. Dilution for Intravenous Use: One vial/ampul of bretylium tosylate injection should be diluted with a minimum of 50 ml of Dextrose Injection 5%, USP or Sodium Chloride Injection, USP prior to intravenous use. Rapid intravenous administration may cause severe nausea and vomiting. Therefore, the diluted solution should be infused over a period greater than 8 minutes. However, in treating existing ventricular fibrillation, bretylium tosylate injection should be given as rapidly as possible and may be given without dilution.

2. Use Various Sites for Intramuscular Injection: When injected intramuscularly, not more than 5 ml should be given in a site, and injection sites should be varied since repeated intramuscular injection into the same site may cause atrophy and necrosis of muscle tissue, fibrosis, vascular degeneration and inflammatory changes.

3. Reduce Dosage in Impaired Renal Function: Since bretylium is excreted principally via the kidney, the dosage interval should be increased in patients with impaired renal function. See CLINICAL PHARMACOLOGY for information on the effect of reduced renal function on half-life.

CARCINOGENESIS, MUTAGENESIS, AND IMPAIRMENT OF FERTILITY

No data are available on potential for carcinogenicity, mutagenicity or impairment of fertility in animals or humans.

PREGNANCY CATEGORY C

Animal reproduction studies have not been conducted with bretylium tosylate. It is also not known whether bretylium tosylate can cause harm when administered to a pregnant woman or can affect reproduction capacity. Bretylium tosylate should be given to pregnant women only if clearly needed.

PEDIATRIC USE

The safety and efficacy of this drug in children has not been established. Bretylium tosylate has been administered to a limited number of pediatric patients, but such use has been inadequate to define fully proper dosage and limitations for use.

DRUG INTERACTIONS:

1. Digitalis toxicity may be aggravated by the initial release of norepinephrine caused by bretylium.

2. The pressor effects of catecholamines such as dopamine or norepinephrine are enhanced by bretylium. When catecholamines are administered, dilute solutions should be used and blood pressure should be monitored closely. (See WARNINGS.)

3. Although there is little published information on concomitant administration of lidocaine and bretylium, these drugs are often administered concurrently without any evidence of interactions resulting in adverse effects or diminished efficacy.

ADVERSE REACTIONS:

Hypotension and postural hypotension have been the most frequently reported adverse reactions (see WARNINGS.) Nausea and vomiting occurred in about three percent of patients, primarily when bretylium tosylate injection was administered rapidly by the intravenous route (see PRECAUTIONS.) Vertigo, dizziness, light-headedness and syncope, which sometimes accompanied postural hypotension, were reported in about 7 patients in 1000.

Bradycardia, increased frequency of premature ventricular contractions, transitory hypertension, initial increase in arrhythmias (see WARNINGS), precipitation of anginal attacks, and sensation of substernal pressure have also been reported in a small number of patients, i.e. approximately 1 - 2 patients in 1000.

Renal dysfunction, diarrhea, abdominal pain, hiccups, erythematous macular rash, flushing, hyperthermia, confusion, paranoid psychosis, emotional lability, lethargy, generalized tenderness, anxiety, shortness of breath, diaphoresis, nasal stuffiness and mild conjunctivitis, have been reported in about 1 patient in 1000. The relationship of bretylium administration to these reactions has not been clearly established.

OVERDOSAGE:

In the presence of life-threatening arrhythmias, underdosing with bretylium probably presents a greater risk to the patient than potential overdosage. However, one case of accidental overdose has been reported in which a rapidly injected intravenous bolus of 30 mg/kg was given instead of an intended 10 mg/kg dose during an episode of ventricular tachycardia. Marked hypertension resulted, followed by protracted refractory hypotension. The patient expired 18 hours later in asystole, complicated by renal failure and aspiration pneumonitis. Bretylium serum levels were 8,000 ng/ml. The exaggerated hemodynamic response was attributed to the rapid injection of a very large dose while some effective circulation was still present. Neither the total dose nor the serum levels observed in this patient are in themselves associated with toxicity. Total doses of 30 mg/kg are not unusual and do not cause toxicity when given incrementally during cardio-pulmonary resuscitation procedures. Similarly, patients maintained on chronic bretylium therapy have had documented serum levels of 12,000 ng/ml. These levels were achieved after sequential dosage increases over time with no apparent ill effects.

If bretylium tosylate is overdosed and symptoms of toxicity develop, administration of nitroprusside or another short-acting intravenous antihypertensive agent should be considered for the treatment of the hypertensive response. Long-acting drugs that might potentiate the subsequent hypotensive effects of bretylium should not be used. Hypotension should be treated with appropriate fluid therapy and pressor agents such as dopamine or norepinephrine. Dialysis is probably not useful in the treatment of bretylium overdose.

DOSAGE AND ADMINISTRATION:

Bretylium tosylate injection is to be used clinically only for treatment of life-threatening ventricular arrhythmias under constant electrocardiographic monitoring. The clinical use of bretylium tosylate injection is for short-term use only. Patients should either be kept supine during the course of bretylium tosylate therapy or be closely observed for postural hypotension. The optimal dose schedule for parenteral administration of bretylium tosylate injection has not been determined. There is comparatively little experience with dosages greater than 40 mg/kg/day, although such doses have been used without apparent adverse effects. The following schedule is suggested.

FOR IMMEDIATELY LIFE-THREATENING VENTRICULAR ARRHYTHMIAS SUCH AS VENTRICULAR FIBRILLATION OR HEMODYNAMICALLY UNSTABLE VENTRICULAR TACHYCARDIA:

Administer undiluted bretylium tosylate injection at a dosage of 5 mg/kg of body weight by rapid intravenous injection. Other usual cardiopulmonary resuscitative procedures, including electrical cardioversion, should be employed prior to and following the injection in accordance with good medical practice. If ventricular fibrillation persists, the dosage may be increased to 10 mg/kg and repeated as necessary.

For continuous suppression, dilute bretylium tosylate injection with Dextrose Injection, USP or Sodium Chloride Injection, USP using the table below and administer the diluted solution as a constant infusion of 1 to 2 mg bretylium tosylate per minute. When administering bretylium tosylate injection (or any potent medication) by continuous intravenous infusion, it is advisable to use a precision volume control device. An alternative maintenance schedule is to infuse the diluted solution at a dosage of 5 to 10 mg bretylium tosylate per kg body weight, over a period greater than 8 minutes, every 6 hours. More rapid infusion may cause nausea and vomiting.

OTHER VENTRICULAR ARRHYTHMIAS:

Intravenous Use: Bretylium tosylate injection must be diluted as described above before intravenous use. Administer the diluted solution at a dosage of 5 to 10 mg bretylium tosylate per kg of body weight by intravenous infusion over a period greater than 8 minutes. More rapid infusion may cause nausea and vomiting. Subsequent doses may be given at 1 to 2 hour intervals if the arrhythmia persists.

For maintenance therapy, the same dosage may be administered every 6 hours, or a constant infusion of 1 to 2 mg bretylium tosylate per minute may be given. (See TABLE 1.)

TABLE 1 Suggested Bretylium Tosylate Injection Admixture Dilutions and Administration Rates for Continuous Infusion Maintenance Therapy Arranged in Descending Order of Concentration

	Preparation		Final Conc.	Dose	Administration	
Amount of Bretylium Tosylate Injection	Volume of IV Fluid*	Final Volume	mg/ml	mg/min	Micro-drops per min	ml/hr
FOR FLUID RESTRICTED PATIENTS:						
500 mg (10 ml)	50 ml	60 ml	8.3	1	7	7
				1.5	11	11
				2	14	14
2 g (40 ml)	500 ml	540 ml	3.7	1	16	16
1 g (20 ml)	250 ml	270 ml	3.7	1.5	24	24
				2	32	32
1 g (20 ml)	500 ml	520 ml	1.9	1	32	32
500 mg (10 ml)	250 ml	260 ml	1.9	1.5	47	47
				2	63	63

* IV fluid may be either Dextrose Injection, USP or Sodium Chloride Injection, USP. This table does not consider the overfill volume present in the IV fluid.

For Intramuscular Injection: Do not dilute bretylium tosylate injection prior to intramuscular injection. Inject 5 to 10 mg bretylium tosylate per kg of body weight. Subsequent doses may be given at 1 to 2 hour intervals if the arrhythmia persists. Thereafter maintain the same dosage every 6 to 8 hours.

Intramuscular injection should not be made directly into or near a major nerve, and the site of injection should be varied on repeated injections. No more than 5 ml should be injected intramuscularly in one site. (See PRECAUTIONS.)

As soon as possible, and when indicated, patients should be changed to an oral antiarrhythmic agent for maintenance therapy.

Parenteral drug products should be inspected visually for particulate matter and discoloration prior to administration, whenever solution and container permit.

Storage: Store at controlled room temperature 15-30°C (59-86°F).

HOW SUPPLIED - RATED THERAPEUTICALLY EQUIVALENT:

Injection, Solution - Intramuscular; - 50 mg/ml

10 ml	$6.00	Bretylium Tosylate, Voluntary Hosp	53258-0132-03
10 ml	$22.44	Bretylium Tosylate, Am Regent	00517-8810-01
10 ml	$22.56	Bretylium Tosylate, Fujisawa USA	00469-1320-30
10 ml	$24.94	Bretylium Tosylate, Intl Medication	00548-1118-00
10 ml	$33.44	Bretylium Tosylate, Abbott	00074-9263-01
10 ml	$33.44	Bretylium Tosylate, Abbott	00074-9268-01
10 ml	$35.48	Bretylium Tosylate, Abbott	00074-9267-18
10 ml x 1	$23.13	Bretylium Tosylate, Elkins Sinn	00641-2211-41
10 ml x 5	$21.38	Bretylium Tosylate, Astra USA	00186-1131-04
10 ml x 10	$59.38	Bretylium Tosylate, Astra USA	00186-0663-01
10 ml x 10	$186.59	Bretylium Tosylate, Fujisawa USA	00469-9132-87
250 ml	$28.01	Bretylium Tosylate, Baxter Hlthcare	00338-0545-02
250 ml	$34.63	Bretylium Tosylate In 5% Dextrose 2, Abbott	00074-7638-02
250 ml	$38.95	Bretylium Tosylate, Abbott	00074-7638-62
250 ml	$56.58	Bretylium Tosylate In Dextrose, Baxter Hlthcare	00338-0547-02
250 ml	$69.94	Bretylium Tosylate In 5% Dextrose, Abbott	00074-7639-02
250 ml	$78.68	Bretylium Tosylate, Abbott	00074-7639-62
500 ml	$24.00	Bretylium Tosylate, McGaw	00264-6615-10
500 ml	$96.00	BRETYLIUM TOSYLATE, McGaw	00264-6614-10

BRIMONIDINE TARTRATE *(003302)*

CATEGORIES: Alpha Adrenergic Agonists; EENT Drugs; Glaucoma; Miosis; Ocular Hypertension; Ophthalmics; Pregnancy Category B; FDA Approved 1996 Oct

BRAND NAMES: **Alphagan**

DESCRIPTION:

Brimonidine tartrate is a relatively selective alpha-2 adrenergic agonist for ophthalmic use. The chemical name of brimonidine tartrate is 5-bromo-6-(2-imidazolidinylideneamino) quinoxaline L-tartrate. It is an off-white, pale yellow to pale pink powder. In solution,

DESCRIPTION: *(cont'd)*

brimonidine tartrate has a clear, greenish-yellow color. It has a molecular weight of 442.24 as the tartrate salt and is water soluble (34 mg/ml). The molecular formula is $C_{11}H_{10}BrN_5{\cdot}C_4H_6O_6$. Brimonidine tartrate ophthalmic solution 0.2% is a sterile ophthalmic solution.

Each ml of Alphagan Solution contains:*Active:* brimonidine tartrate 2 mg (equivalent to 1.32 mg as brimonidine free base). *Preservative:* benzalkonium chloride (0.05 mg). *Inactives:* polyvinyl alcohol; sodium chloride; sodium citrate; citric acid; and purified water. Hydrochloric acid and/or sodium hydroxide may be added to adjust pH (6.3-6.5).

CLINICAL PHARMACOLOGY:

Mechanism of Action: Brimonidine tartrate is an alpha adrenergic receptor agonist. It has a peak ocular hypotensive effect occurring at two hours post-dosing. Fluorophotometric studies in animals and humans suggest that brimonidine tartrate has a dual mechanism of action by reducing aqueous humor production and increasing uveoscleral outflow.

Pharmacokinetics: After ocular administration of a 0.2% solution, plasma concentrations peaked within 1 to 4 hours and declined with a systemic half-life of approximately 3 hours.

In humans, systemic metabolism of brimonidine tartrate is extensive. It is metabolized primarily by the liver. Urinary excretion is the major route of elimination of the drug and its metabolites. Approximately 87% of an orally-administered radioactive dose was eliminated with 120 hours, with 74% found in the urine.

CLINICAL STUDIES:

Elevated IOP presents a major risk factor in glaucomatous field loss. The higher the level of IOP, the greater the likelihood of optic nerve damage and visual field loss. Brimonidine tartrate has the action of lowering intraocular pressure with minimal effect on cardiovascular and pulmonary parameters.

In comparative clinical studies with timolol 0.5%, lasting up to one year, the IOP lowering effect of brimonidine tartrate 0.2% was approximately 4-6 mm Hg compared with approximately 6 mm Hg for timolol. In these studies, both patient groups were dosed twice daily, however, due to the duration of action of brimonidine tartrate, it is recommended that brimonidine tartrate be dosed three times daily. Eight percent of subjects were discontinued from studies due to inadequately controlled intraocular pressure, which in 30% of these patients occurred during the first month of therapy. Approximately 20% were discontinued due to adverse experiences.

INDICATIONS AND USAGE:

Brimonidine tartrate is indicated for lowering pressure in patients with open-angle glaucoma or ocular hypertension. The IOP lowering efficacy of brimonidine tartrate ophthalmic solution diminishes over time in some patients. This loss of effect appears with a variable time of onset in each patient and should be closely monitored.

CONTRAINDICATIONS:

Brimonidine tartrate is contraindicated in patients with hypersensitivity to brimonidine tartrate or any component of this medication. It is also contraindicated in patients receiving monoamine oxidase (MAO) inhibitor therapy.

PRECAUTIONS:

General: Although brimonidine tartrate had minimal effect on blood pressure of patients in clinical studies, caution should be exercised in treating patients with severe cardiovascular disease.

Brimonidine tartrate has not been studied in patients with hepatic or renal impairment; caution should be used in treating such patients.

Brimonidine tartrate should be used with caution in patients with depression, cerebral or coronary insufficiency, Raynaud's phenomenon, orthostatic hypotension, or thromboangiitis obliterans.

During the studies there was a loss of effect in some patients. The IOP-lowering efficacy with brimonidine tartrate ophthalmic solution during the first month of therapy may not always reflect the long-term level of IOP reduction. Patients prescribed IOP-lowering medication should be routinely monitored for IOP.

Information for the Patient: The preservative in brimonidine tartrate, benzalkonium chloride, may be absorbed by soft contact lenses. Patients wearing soft contact lenses should be instructed to wait at least 15 minutes after instilling brimonidine tartrate to insert soft contact lenses.

As with other drugs in this class, brimonidine tartrate may cause fatigue and/or drowsiness in some patients. Patients who engage in hazardous activities should be cautioned of the potential for a decrease in mental alertness.

Carcinogenesis, Mutagenesis, and Impairment of Fertility: No compound-related carcinogenic effects were observed in 21 month and 2 year studies in mice and rats given oral doses of 2.5 mg/kg/day (as the free base) and 1.0 mg/kg/day, respectively (~77 and 118 times, respectively, the human plasma drug concentration following the recommended ophthalmic dose).

Brimonidine tartrate was not mutagenic or cytogenic in a series of *in vitro* and *in vivo* studies including the Ames test, host-mediated assay, chromosomal aberration assay in Chinese Hamster Ovary (CHO) cells, cytogenic studies in mice and dominant lethal assay.

Pregnancy, Teratogenic Effects, Pregnancy Category B: Reproduction studies performed in rats with oral doses of 0.66 mg base/kg revealed no evidence of impaired fertility or harm to the fetus due to brimonidine tartrate. Dosing at this level produced 100 times the plasma drug concentration level seen in humans following multiple ophthalmic doses. There are no studies of brimonidine tartrate in pregnant women, however in animal studies, brimonidine tartrate crossed the placenta and entered into the fetal circulation to a limited extent. Brimonidine tartrate should be used during pregnancy only if the potential benefit to the mother justifies the potential risk to the fetus.

Nursing Mothers: It is not known whether brimonidine tartrate is excreted in human milk, although in animal studies, brimonidine tartrate has been shown to be excreted in breast milk. A decision should be made whether to discontinue nursing or to discontinue the drug, taking into account the importance of the drug to the mother.

Pediatric Use: Safety and effectiveness in pediatric patients has not been established.

DRUG INTERACTIONS:

Although specific drug interaction studies have not been conducted with brimonidine tartrate, the possibility of an additive or potentiating effect with CNS depressants (alcohol, barbiturates, opiates, sedatives, or anesthetics) should be considered. Brimonidine tartrate did not have significant effects on blood pulse and pressure in clinical studies. However, since alpha-agonists, as a class, may reduce pulse and blood pressure, caution in using concomitant drugs such as beta-blockers (ophthlamic and systemic), antihypertensives, and/or cardiac glycosides is advised.

DRUG INTERACTIONS: *(cont'd)*

Tricyclic antidepressants have been reported to blunt the hypotensive effect of systemic clonidine. It is not known whether the concurrent use of these agents with brimonidine tartrate can lead to an interference in IOP lowering effect. No data on the level of circulating catecholamines after brimonidine tartrate is instilled are available. Caution, however, is advised in patients taking tricyclic antidepressants which can affect the metabolism and uptake of circulating amines.

ADVERSE REACTIONS:

Adverse events occurring in approximately 10-30% of the subjects, in descending order of incidence, included oral dryness, ocular hyperemia, burning and stinging, headache, blurring, foreign body sensation, fatigue/drowsiness, conjunctival follicles, ocular allergic reactions, and ocular pruritus.

Events occurring in approximately 3-9% of the subjects, in descending order included corneal staining/erosion, photophobia, eyelid erythema, ocular ache/pain, ocular dryness, tearing, upper respiratory symptoms, eyelid edema, conjunctival edema, dizziness, blepharitis, ocular irritation, gastrointestinal symptoms, asthenia, conjunctival blanching, abnormal vision and muscular pain.

The following adverse reactions were reported in less than 3% of the patients: lid crusting, conjunctival hemorrhage, abnormal taste, insomnia, conjunctival discharge, depression, hypertension, anxiety, palpitations, nasal dryness, and syncope.

OVERDOSAGE:

No information is available on overdosage in humans. Treatment of an oral overdose includes supportive and symptomatic therapy; a patent airway should be maintained.

DOSAGE AND ADMINISTRATION:

The recommended dose is one drop of brimonidine tartrate in the affected eye(s) three times daily, approximately 8 hours apart.

PATIENT INFORMATION:

Brimonidine tartrate is used for the treatment of open-angle glaucoma and ocular hypertension. Do not take this drug if you are currently taking MAO Inhibitors (*e.g.*, Parnate). Inform your doctor if you are pregnant or nursing.

This product may stain soft contact lenses. Wait at least 15 minutes after instilling brimonidine to insert contact lenses.

May cause drowsiness or tiredness; use caution while driving or operating hazardous machinery. May cause dry mouth, blurring, stinging, or burning of the eyes; headaches, fatigue or drowsiness; allergic or itching of the eyes. Tell your doctor or pharmacist if these effects occur.

HOW SUPPLIED:

Alphagan 0.2% is supplied sterile in white opaque plastic dropper bottles.

Storage: Store at or below 25°C (77°F).

HOW SUPPLIED - EQUIVALENTS NOT AVAILABLE:

Solution - Ophthalmic - 0.2%

5 ml	$21.77	ALPHAGAN, Allergan	00023-8665-05
10 ml	$43.55	ALPHAGAN, Allergan	00023-8665-10

BROMOCRIPTINE MESYLATE *(000527)*

CATEGORIES: Acromegaly; Adenoma; Amenorrhea; Anterior Pituitary/Hypothalmic Function; Anticholinergic Agents; Antiparkinson Agents; Autonomic Drugs; Congestion; Dopamine Receptor Agonists; Extrapyramidal Movement Disorders; Fertility Agents; Galactorrhea Inhibitors; Hypogonadism; Impotence; Infertility; Neuromuscular; Parkinsonism; Tumors; Hyperprolactinemia*; Lactation*; Sales > $100 Million; FDA Approval Pre 1982; Patent Expiration 1990 Aug

* Indication not approved by the FDA

BRAND NAMES: *Alpha-Bromocriptine*; *Apo-Bromocriptine*; *Axialit*; *Barlolin*; *Brameston*; *Bromed*; *Bromergon*; *Bromidine*; *Bromocorn*; *Bromokin*; *Bromopar*; *Cryocriptina* (Mexico); *Demil*; *Deprolac*; *Diken* (Mexico); *Elkrip*; *Kripton*; *Lactismine*; *Lactodel*; *Lactostat*; *Medocriptine*; *Parilac*; **Parlodel**; *Pravidel* (Germany); *Proctinal*; *Serocryptin* (Mexico); *Suplac*; *Syntocriptine*; *Umprel*; *Volbro*
(International brand names outside U.S. in italics)

FORMULARIES: Aetna; BC-BS; Medi-Cal; PCS

COST OF THERAPY: $395.91 (Parkinsonism; Tablet; 2.5 mg; 1/day; 365 days)

DESCRIPTION:

Parlodel (bromocriptine mesylate) is an ergot derivative with potent dopamine receptor agonist activity. Each Parlodel Snap Tabs tablet for oral administration contains 2 1/2 mg and each capsule contains 5 mg bromocriptine (as the mesylate). Bromocriptine mesylate is chemically designated as Ergotaman-3', 6', 18-trione, 2-bromo-12'-hydroxy-2'-(1-methylethyl)-5'-(2-methylpropyl)-, (5'α) monomethanesulfonate (salt).

2 1/2 mg Snap Tabs: *Active Ingredient:* bromocriptine mesylate, USP; *Inactive Ingredients:* colloidal silicon dioxide, lactose, magnesium stearate, povidone, starch, and another ingredient

5 mg Capsules: *Active Ingredient:* bromocriptine mesylate, USP; *Inactive Ingredients:* colloidal silicon dioxide, gelatin, lactose, magnesium stearate, red iron oxide, silicon dioxide, sodium bisulfite, sodium lauryl sulfate, starch, titanium dioxide, yellow iron oxide, and another ingredient.

CLINICAL PHARMACOLOGY:

Parlodel (bromocriptine mesylate) is a dopamine receptor agonist, which activates post-synaptic dopamine receptors. The dopaminergic neurons in the tuberoinfundibular process modulate the secretion of prolactin from the anterior pituitary by secreting a prolactin inhibitory factor (thought to be dopamine); in the corpus striatum the dopaminergic neurons are involved in the control of motor function. Clinically, bromocriptine mesylate significantly reduces plasma levels of prolactin in patients with physiologically elevated prolactin as well as in patients with hyperprolactinemia. The inhibition of physiological lactation as well as galactorrhea in pathological hyperprolactinemic states is obtained at dose levels that do not affect secretion of other tropic hormones from the anterior pituitary. Experiments have demonstrated that bromocriptine induces long lasting stereotyped behavior in rodents and turning behavior in rats having unilateral lesions in the substantia nigra. These actions, characteristic of those produced by dopamine, are inhibited by dopamine antagonists and suggest a direct action of bromocriptine on striatal dopamine receptors.

CLINICAL PHARMACOLOGY: *(cont'd)*

Bromocriptine mesylate is a nonhormonal, nonestrogenic agent that inhibits the secretion of prolactin in humans, with little or no effect on other pituitary hormones, except in patients with acromegaly, where it lowers elevated blood levels of growth hormone in the majority of patients.

In about 75% of cases of amenorrhea and galactorrhea, bromocriptine mesylate therapy suppresses the galactorrhea completely, or almost completely, and reinitiates normal ovulatory menstrual cycles.

Menses are usually reinitiated prior to complete suppression of galactorrhea; the time for this on average is 6-8 weeks. However, some patients respond within a few days, and others may take up to 8 months.

Galactorrhea may take longer to control depending on the degree of stimulation of the mammary tissue prior to therapy. At least a 75% reduction in secretion is usually observed after 8-12 weeks. Some patients may fail to respond even after 12 months of therapy.

In many acromegalic patients, bromocriptine mesylate produces a prompt and sustained reduction in circulating levels of serum growth hormone.

Bromocriptine mesylate produces its therapeutic effect in the treatment of Parkinson's disease, a clinical condition characterized by a progressive deficiency in dopamine synthesis in the substantia nigra, by directly stimulating the dopamine receptors in the corpus striatum. In contrast, levodopa exerts its therapeutic effect only after conversion to dopamine by the neurons of the substantia nigra, which are known to be numerically diminished in this patient population.

Pharmacokinetics: The pharmacokinetics and metabolism of bromocriptine in human subjects were studied with the help of radioactively labeled drug. Twenty-eight percent of an oral dose was absorbed from the gastrointestinal tract. The blood levels following a 2 1/2 mg dose were in the range of 2-3 ng equivalents/ml. Plasma levels were in the range of 4-6 ng equivalents/ml indicating that the red blood cells did not contain appreciable amounts of drug and/or metabolites.*In vitro* experiments showed that the drug was 90%-96% bound to serum albumin.

Bromocriptine was completely metabolized prior to excretion. The major route of excretion of absorbed drug was via the bile. Only 2.5%-5.5% of the dose was excreted in the urine. Almost all (84.6%) of the administered dose was excreted in the feces in 120 hours.

INDICATIONS AND USAGE:

Hyperprolactinemia-Associated Dysfunctions: Bromocriptine mesylate is indicated for the treatment of dysfunctions associated with **hyperprolactinemia** including **amenorrhea**with or without **galactorrhea, infertility or hypogonadism.** Bromocriptine mesylate treatment is indicated in patients with **prolactin-secreting adenomas,**which may be the basic underlying endocrinopathy contributing to the above clinical presentations. **Reduction**in **tumor size** has been demonstrated in both male and female patients with macroadenomas. In cases where adenectomy is elected, a course of bromocriptine mesylate therapy may be used to reduce the tumor mass prior to surgery.

Acromegaly: Bromocriptine mesylate therapy is indicated in the treatment of acromegaly. Bromocriptine mesylate therapy, alone or as adjunctive therapy with pituitary irradiation or surgery, reduces serum growth hormone by 50% or more in approximately 1/2 of patients treated, although not usually to normal levels.

Since the effects of external pituitary radiation may not become maximal for several years, adjunctive therapy with bromocriptine mesylate offers potential benefit before the effects of irradiation are manifested.

Parkinson's Disease: Bromocriptine mesylate tablets or capsules are indicated in the treatment of the signs and symptoms of idiopathic or postencephalitic Parkinson's disease. As adjunctive treatment to levodopa (alone or with a peripheral decarboxylase inhibitor), bromocriptine mesylate therapy may provide additional therapeutic benefits in those patients who are currently maintained on optimal dosages of levodopa, those who are beginning to deteriorate (develop tolerance) to levodopa therapy, and those who are experiencing "end of dose failure" on levodopa therapy. Bromocriptine mesylate therapy may permit a reduction of the maintenance dose of levodopa and, thus may ameliorate the occurrence and/or severity of adverse reactions associated with long-term levodopa therapy such as abnormal involuntary movements (*e.g.,* dyskinesias) and the marked swings in motor function ("on-off" phenomenon). Continued efficacy of bromocriptine mesylate therapy during treatment of more than 2 years has not been established.

Data are insufficient to evaluate potential benefit from treating newly diagnosed Parkinson's disease with bromocriptine mesylate. Studies have shown, however, significantly more adverse reactions (notably nausea, hallucinations, confusion and hypotension) in bromocriptine mesylate treated patients than in levodopa/carbidopa treated patients. Patients unresponsive to levodopa are poor candidates for bromocriptine mesylate therapy.

CONTRAINDICATIONS:

Uncontrolled hypertension and sensitivity to any ergot alkaloids. In patients being treated for hyperprolactinemia bromocriptine mesylate should be withdrawn when pregnancy is diagnosed (see PRECAUTIONS, Hyperprolactinemic States.) In the event that bromocriptine mesylate is reinstituted to control a rapidly expanding macroadenoma (see PRECAUTIONS, Hyperprolactinemic States) and a patient experiences a hypertensive disorder of pregnancy, the benefit of continuing bromocriptine mesylate must be weighted against the possible risk of its use during a hypertensive disorder of pregnancy. When bromocriptine mesylate is being used to treat acromegaly or Parkinson's disease in patients who subsequently become pregnant, a decision should be made as to whether the therapy continues to be medically necessary or can be withdrawn. If it is continued, the drug should be withdrawn in those who may experience hypertensive disorders of pregnancy (including eclampsia, preeclampsia, or pregnancy-induced hypertension) unless withdrawal of bromocriptine mesylate is considered to be medically contraindicated.

WARNINGS:

Since hyperprolactinemia with amenorrhea/galactorrhea and infertility has been found in patients with pituitary tumors, a complete evaluation of the pituitary is indicated before treatment with bromocriptine mesylate.

If pregnancy occurs during bromocriptine mesylate administration, careful observation of these patients is mandatory. Prolactin-secreting adenomas may expand and compression of the optic or other cranial nerves may occur, emergency pituitary surgery becoming necessary. In most cases, the compression resolves following delivery. Reinitiation of bromocriptine mesylate treatment has been reported to produce improvement in the visual fields of patients in whom nerve compression has occurred during pregnancy. The safety of bromocriptine mesylate treatment during pregnancy to the mother and fetus has not been established.

Symptomatic hypotension can occur in patients treated with bromocriptine mesylate for any indication. In postpartum studies with bromocriptine mesylate, decreases in supine systolic and diastolic pressures of greater than 20 mm and 10 mm Hg, respectively, have been observed in almost 30% of patients receiving bromocriptine mesylate. On occasion, the drop in supine systolic pressure was as much as 50-59 mm of Hg. **While hypotension during the start of therapy with bromocriptine mesylate occurs in some patients, in postmarketing experience in the U.S. in postpartum patients 89 cases of hypertension have been reported, sometimes**

WARNINGS: *(cont'd)*

at the initiation of therapy, but often developing in the second week of therapy; seizures have been reported in 72 cases (including 4 cases of status epilepticus), both with and without the prior development of hypertension; 30 cases of stroke have been reported mostly in postpartum patients whose prenatal and obstetric courses had been uncomplicated. Many of these patients experiencing seizures and/or strokes reported developing a constant and often progressively severe headache hours to days prior to the acute event. Some cases of strokes and seizures were also preceded by visual disturbances (blurred vision, and transient cortical blindness). Nine cases of acute myocardial infarction have been reported.

Although a causal relationship between bromocriptine mesylate administration and hypertension, seizures, strokes, and myocardial infarction in postpartum women has not been established, use of the drug for prevention of physiological lactation, or in patients with uncontrolled hypertension is not recommended. In patients being treated for hyperprolactinemia bromocriptine mesylate should be withdrawn when pregnancy is diagnosed (see PRECAUTIONS, Hyperprolactinemic States.) In the event that bromocriptine mesylate is reinstituted to control a rapidly expanding macroadenoma (see PRECAUTIONS, Hyperprolactinemic States)**and a patient experiences a hypertensive disorder of pregnancy, the benefit of continuing bromocriptine mesylate must be weighed against the possible risk of its use during a hypertensive disorder of pregnancy. When bromocriptine mesylate is being used to treat acromegaly or Parkinson's disease in patients who have subsequently become pregnant, a decision should be made as to whether the therapy continues to be medically necessary or can be withdrawn. If it is continued, the drug should be withdrawn in those who may experience hypertensive disorders of pregnancy (including eclampsia, preeclampsia, or pregnancy-induced hypertension) unless withdrawal of bromocriptine mesylate is considered to be medically contraindicated. Because of the possibility of an interaction between bromocriptine mesylate and other ergot alkaloids, the concomitant use of these medications is not recommended. Particular attention should be paid to patients who have recently received other drugs that can alter the blood pressure.** Periodic monitoring of the blood pressure, particularly during the first weeks of therapy is prudent. If hypertension, severe, progressive, or unremitting headache (with or without visual disturbance), or evidence of CNS toxicity develops, drug therapy should be discontinued and the patient should be evaluated promptly.

Long-term treatment (6-36 months) with bromocriptine mesylate in doses ranging from 20-100 mg/day has been associated with pulmonary infiltrates, pleural effusion and thickening of the pleura in a few patients. In those instances in which bromocriptine mesylate treatment was terminated, the changes slowly reverted towards normal.

PRECAUTIONS:

General: Safety and efficacy of bromocriptine mesylate have not been established in patients with renal or hepatic disease. Care should be exercised when administering bromocriptine mesylate therapy concomitantly with other medications known to lower blood pressure.

Hyperprolactinemic States: The relative efficacy of bromocriptine mesylate versus surgery in preserving visual fields is not known. Patients with rapidly progressive visual field loss should be evaluated by a neurosurgeon to help decide on the most appropriate therapy. Since pregnancy is often the therapeutic objective in many hyperprolactinemic patients presenting with amenorrhea/galactorrhea and hypogonadism (infertility), a careful assessment of the pituitary is essential to detect the presence of a prolactin-secreting adenoma. Patients not seeking pregnancy, or those harboring large adenomas, should be advised to use contraceptive measures, other than oral contraceptives, during treatment with bromocriptine mesylate. Since pregnancy may occur prior to reinitiation of menses, a pregnancy test is recommended at least every 4 weeks during the amenorrheic period, and, once menses are reinitiated, every time a patient misses a menstrual period. Treatment with bromocriptine mesylate tablets or capsules should be discontinued as soon as pregnancy has been established. Patients must be monitored closely throughout pregnancy for signs and symptoms that may signal the enlargement of a previously undetected or existing prolactin-secreting tumor. Discontinuation of bromocriptine mesylate treatment in patients with known macroadenomas has been associated with rapid regrowth of tumor and increase in serum prolactin in most cases.

Acromegaly: Cold sensitive digital vasospasm has been observed in some acromegalic patients treated with bromocriptine mesylate. The response, should it occur, can be reversed by reducing the dose of bromocriptine mesylate and may be prevented by keeping the fingers warm. Cases of severe gastrointestinal bleeding from peptic ulcers have been reported, some fatal. Although there is no evidence that bromocriptine mesylate increases the incidence of peptic ulcers in acromegalic patients, symptoms suggestive of peptic ulcer should be investigated thoroughly and treated appropriately.

Possible tumor expansion while receiving bromocriptine mesylate therapy has been reported in a few patients. Since the natural history of growth hormone secreting tumors is unknown, all patients should be carefully monitored and, if evidence of tumor expansion develops, discontinuation of treatment and alternative procedures considered.

Parkinson's Disease: Safety during long-term use for more than 2 years at the doses required for parkinsonism has not been established.

As with any chronic therapy, periodic evaluation of hepatic, hematopoietic, cardiovascular, and renal function is recommended. Symptomatic hypotension can occur and, therefore, caution should be exercised when treating patients receiving antihypertensive drugs.

High doses of bromocriptine mesylate may be associated with confusion and mental disturbances. Since parkinsonian patients may manifest mild degrees of dementia, caution should be used when treating such patients.

Bromocriptine mesylate administered alone or concomitantly with levodopa may cause hallucinations (visual or auditory). Hallucinations usually resolve with dosage reduction; occasionally, discontinuation of bromocriptine mesylate is required. Rarely, after high doses, hallucinations have persisted for several weeks following discontinuation of bromocriptine mesylate.

As with levodopa, caution should be exercised when administering bromocriptine mesylate to patients with a history of myocardial infarction who have a residual atrial, nodal, or ventricular arrhythmia.

Retroperitoneal fibrosis has been reported in a few patients receiving long-term therapy (2-10 years) with bromocriptine mesylate in doses ranging from 30 to 140 mg daily.

Information for the Patient: When initiating therapy, all patients receiving bromocriptine mesylate should be cautioned with regard to engaging in activities requiring rapid and precise responses, such as driving an automobile or operating machinery since dizziness (8%-16%), drowsiness (8%), faintness, fainting (8%), and syncope (less than 1%) have been reported early in the course of therapy. Patients receiving bromocriptine mesylate for hyperprolactinemic states associated with macroadenoma or those who have had previous transsphenoidal surgery, should be told to report any persistent watery nasal discharge to their physician. Patients receiving bromocriptine mesylate for treatment of a macroadenoma should be told that discontinuation of drug may be associated with rapid regrowth of the tumor and recurrence of their original symptoms.

Carcinogenesis, Mutagenesis, and Impairment of Fertility: A 74-week study was conducted in mice using dietary levels of bromocriptine mesylate equivalent to oral doses of 10 and 50 mg/kg/day. A 100-week study in rats was conducted using dietary levels equivalent to oral doses of 1.7, 9.8, and 44 mg/kg/day. The highest doses tested in mice and rats were approximately 2.5 and 4.4 times, respectively, the maximum human dose administered in controlled clinical

PRECAUTIONS: *(cont'd)*

trials (100 mg/day) based on body surface area. Malignant uterine tumors, endometrial and myometrial, were found in rats as follows: 0/50 control females, 2/50 females given 1.7 mg/kg daily, 7/49 females given 9.8 mg/kg daily, and 9/50 females given 44 mg/kg daily. The occurrence of these neoplasms is probably attributable to the high estrogen/progesterone ratio which occurs in rats as a result of the prolactin-inhibiting action of bromocriptine mesylate. The endocrine mechanisms believed to be involved in the rats are not present in humans. There is no known correlation between uterine malignancies occurring in bromocriptine-treated rats and human risk. In contrast to the findings in rats, the uteri from mice killed after 74 weeks treatment did not exhibit evidence of drug-related changes.

Bromocriptine mesylate was evaluated for mutagenic potential in the battery of tests that included Ames bacterial mutation assay, mutagenic activity *in vitro* on V79 Chinese hamster fibroblasts, cytogenetic analysis of Chinese hamster bone marrow cells following*in vivo* treatment, and an *in vivo*micronucleus test for mutagenic potential in mice.

No mutagenic effects were obtained in any of these tests.

Fertility and reproductive performance in female rats were not influenced adversely by treatment with bromocriptine beyond the predicted decrease in the weight of pups due to suppression of lactation. In males treated with 50 mg/kg of this drug, mating and fertility were within the normal range. Increased perinatal loss was produced in the subgroups of dams, sacrificed on day 21 postpartum (p.p.) after mating with males treated with the highest dose (50 mg/kg).

Pregnancy Category B: Administration of 10-30 mg/kg of bromocriptine to 2 strains of rats on days 6-15 post coitum (p.c.) as well as a single dose of 10 mg/kg on day 5 p.c. interfered with nidation. Three mg/kg given on days 6-15 were without effect on nidation, and did not produce any anomalies. In animals treated from day 8-15 p.c., i.e., after implantation, 30 mg/kg produced increased prenatal mortality in the form of increased incidence of embryonic resorption. One anomaly, aplasia of spinal vertebrae and ribs, was found in the group of 262 fetuses derived from the dams treated with 30 mg/kg bromocriptine. No fetotoxic effects were found in offspring of dams treated during the peri- or post-natal period.

Two studies were conducted in rabbits (2 strains) to determine the potential to interfere with nidation. Dose levels of 100 or 300 mg/kg/day from day 1 to day 6 p.c. did not adversely affect nidation. The high dose was approximately 63 times the maximum human dose administered in controlled clinical trials (100 mg/day), based on body surface area. In New Zealand white rabbits some embryo mortality occurred at 300 mg/kg which was a reflection of overt maternal toxicity. Three studies were conducted in 2 strains of rabbits to determine the teratological potential of bromocriptine at dose levels of 3, 10, 30, 100, and 300 mg/kg given from day 6 to day 18 p.c. In 2 studies with the Yellow-silver strain, cleft palate was found in 3 and 2 fetuses at maternally toxic doses of 100 and 300 mg/kg, respectively. One control fetus also exhibited this anomaly. In the third study conducted with New Zealand white rabbits using an identical protocol, no cleft palates were produced.

No teratological or embryo-toxic effects of bromocriptine were produced in any of 6 offspring from 6 monkeys at a dose level of 2 mg/kg.

Information concerning 1276 pregnancies in women taking bromocriptine has been collected. In the majority of cases, bromocriptine was discontinued within 8 weeks into pregnancy (mean 28.7 days), however, 8 patients received the drug continuously throughout pregnancy. The mean daily dose for all patients was 5.8 mg (range 1-40 mg).

Of these 1276 pregnancies, there were 1088 full term deliveries (4 stillborn), 145 spontaneous abortions (11.4%), and 28 induced abortions (2.2%). Moreover, 12 extrauterine gravidities and 3 hydatidiform moles (twice in the same patient) caused early termination of pregnancy. These data compare favorably with the abortion rate (11%-25%) cited for pregnancies induced by clomiphene citrate, menopausal gonadotropin, and chorionic gonadotropin.

Although spontaneous abortions often go unreported, especially prior to 20 weeks of gestation, their frequency has been estimated to be 15%.

The incidence of birth defects in the population at large ranges from 2%-4.5%. The incidence in 1109 live births from patients receiving bromocriptine is 3.3%.

There is no suggestion that bromocriptine contributed to the type or incidence of birth defects in this group of infants.

Nursing Mothers: Bromocriptine mesylate should not be used during lactation in postpartum women.

Pediatric Use: Safety and efficacy of bromocriptine mesylate have not been established in children under the age of 15.

DRUG INTERACTIONS:

Lack or decrease in efficacy may occur in patients receiving bromocriptine mesylate when they are treated concurrently with drugs which have dopamine antagonist activity, e.g., phenothiazines, butyrophenones. This may be a problem particularly for patients treated with bromocriptine mesylate for macroadenomas. Although there is no conclusive evidence demonstrating interactions between bromocriptine mesylate and other ergot derivatives, the concomitant use of these medications is not recommended.

ADVERSE REACTIONS:

Hyperprolactinemic Indications: The incidence of adverse effects is quite high (69%) but these are generally mild to moderate in degree. Therapy was discontinued in approximately 5% of patients because of adverse effects. These in decreasing order of frequency are: nausea (49%), headache (19%), dizziness (17%), fatigue (7%), lightheadedness (5%), vomiting (5%), abdominal cramps (4%), nasal congestion (3%), constipation (3%), diarrhea (3%) and drowsiness (3%).

A slight hypotensive effect may accompany bromocriptine mesylate treatment. The occurrence of adverse reactions may be lessened by temporarily reducing dosage to 1/2 tablet 2 or 3 times daily. A few cases of cerebrospinal fluid rhinorrhea have been reported in patients receiving bromocriptine mesylate for treatment of large prolactinomas. This has occurred rarely, usually only in patients who have received previous transsphenoidal surgery, pituitary radiation, or both, and who were receiving bromocriptine mesylate for tumor recurrence. It may also occur in previously untreated patients whose tumor extends into the sphenoid sinus.

Acromegaly: The most frequent adverse reactions encountered in acromegalic patients treated with bromocriptine mesylate were: nausea (18%), constipation (14%), postural/orthostatic hypotension (6%), anorexia (4%), dry mouth/nasal stuffiness (4%), indigestion/dyspepsia (4%), digital vasospasm (3%), drowsiness/tiredness (3%) and vomiting (2%).

Less frequent adverse reactions (less than 2%) were: gastrointestinal bleeding, dizziness, exacerbation of Raynaud's Syndrome, headache and syncope. Rarely (less than 1%) hair loss, alcohol potentiation, faintness, lightheadedness, arrhythmia, ventricular tachycardia, decreased sleep requirement, visual hallucinations, lassitude, shortness of breath, bradycardia, vertigo, paresthesia, sluggishness, vasovagal attack, delusional psychosis, paranoia, insomnia, heavy headedness, reduced tolerance to cold, tingling of ears, facial pallor and muscle cramps have been reported.

Parkinson's Disease: In clinical trials in which bromocriptine was administered with concomitant reduction in the dose of levodopa/carbidopa, the most common newly appearing adverse reactions were: nausea, abnormal involuntary movements, hallucinations, confusion,

ADVERSE REACTIONS: *(cont'd)*

"on-off" phenomenon, dizziness, drowsiness, faintness/fainting, vomiting, asthenia, abdominal discomfort, visual disturbance, ataxia, insomnia, depression, hypotension, shortness of breath, constipation, and vertigo.

Less common adverse reactions which may be encountered include: anorexia, blepharospasm, dry mouth, dysphagia, edema of the feet and ankles, erythromelalgia, epileptiform seizure, fatigue, headache, lethargy, mottling of skin, nasal stuffiness, nervousness, nightmares, paresthesia, skin rash, urinary frequency, urinary incontinence, urinary retention, and rarely, signs and symptoms of ergotism such as tingling of fingers, cold feet, numbness, muscle cramps of feet and legs or exacerbation of Raynaud's Syndrome.

Abnormalities in laboratory tests may include elevations in blood urea nitrogen, SGOT, SGPT, GGPT, CPK, alkaline phosphatase and uric acid, which are usually transient and not of clinical significance.

ADVERSE EVENTS OBSERVED IN OTHER CONDITIONS

Postpartum Patients: In postpartum studies with bromocriptine mesylate 23 percent of postpartum patients treated had at least 1 side effect, but they were generally mild to moderate in degree. Therapy was discontinued in approximately 3% of patients. The most frequently occurring adverse reactions were: headache (10%), dizziness (8%), nausea (7%), vomiting (3%), fatigue (1.0%), syncope (0.7%), diarrhea (0.4%) and cramps (0.4%). Decreases in blood pressure (≥ 20 mm Hg systolic and ≥ 10 mm Hg diastolic) occurred in 28% of patients at least once during the first 3 postpartum days; these were usually of a transient nature. Reports of fainting in the puerperium may possibly be related to this effect. In postmarketing experience in the U.S. serious adverse reactions reported include 72 cases of seizures (including 4 cases of status epilepticus), 30 cases of stroke, and 9 cases of myocardial infarction among postpartum patients. Seizure cases were not necessarily accompanied by the development of hypertension. An unremitting and often progressively severe headache, sometimes accompanied by visual disturbance, often preceded by hours to days many cases of seizure and or/stroke. Most patients had shown no evidence of any of the hypertensive disorders of pregnancy including eclampsia, preeclampsia or pregnancy induced hypertension. One stroke case was associated with sagittal sinus thrombosis, and another was associated with cerebral and cerebellar vasculitis. One case of myocardial infarction was associated with unexplained disseminated intravascular coagulation and a second occurred in conjunction with use of another ergot alkaloid. The relationship of these adverse reactions to bromocriptine mesylate administration has not been established.

DOSAGE AND ADMINISTRATION:

General: It is recommended that bromocriptine mesylate be taken with food. Patients should be evaluated frequently during dose escalation to determine the lowest dosage that produces a therapeutic response.

Hyperprolactinemic Indications: The initial dosage of bromocriptine mesylate is 1/2 to one 2 1/2 mg tablet daily. An additional 2 1/2 mg tablet may be added to the treatment regimen as tolerated every 3-7 days until an optimal therapeutic response is achieved. The therapeutic dosage usually is 5-7.5 mg and ranges from 2.5-15 mg/day.

In order to reduce the likelihood of prolonged exposure to bromocriptine mesylate should an unsuspected pregnancy occur, a mechanical contraceptive should be used in conjunction with bromocriptine mesylate therapy until normal ovulatory menstrual cycles have been restored. Contraception may then be discontinued in patients desiring pregnancy.

Thereafter, if menstruation does not occur within 3 days of the expected date, bromocriptine mesylate therapy should be discontinued and a pregnancy test performed.

Acromegaly: Virtually all acromegalic patients receiving therapeutic benefit from bromocriptine mesylate also have reductions in circulating levels of growth hormone. Therefore, periodic assessment of circulating levels of growth hormone will, in most cases, serve as a guide in determining the therapeutic potential of bromocriptine mesylate. If, after a brief trial with bromocriptine mesylate therapy, no significant reduction in growth hormone levels has taken place, careful assessment of the clinical features of the disease should be made, and if no change has occurred, dosage adjustment or discontinuation of therapy should be considered.

The initial recommended dosage is 1/2 to one 2 1/2 mg bromocriptine mesylate tablet on retiring (with food) for 3 days. An additional 1/2 to 1 tablet should be added to the treatment regimen as tolerated every 3-7 days until the patient obtains optimal therapeutic benefit. Patients should be reevaluated monthly and the dosage adjusted based on reductions of growth hormone or clinical response. The usual optimal therapeutic dosage range of bromocriptine mesylate varies from 20-30 mg/day in most patients. The maximal dosage should not exceed 100 mg/day.

Patients treated with pituitary irradiation should be withdrawn from bromocriptine mesylate therapy on a yearly basis to assess both the clinical effects of radiation on the disease process as well as the effects of bromocriptine mesylate therapy. Usually a 4-8 week withdrawal period is adequate for this purpose. Recurrence of the signs/symptoms or increases in growth hormone indicate the disease process in still active and further courses of bromocriptine mesylate should be considered.

Parkinson's Disease: The basic principle of bromocriptine mesylate therapy is to initiate treatment at a low dosage and, on an individual basis, increase the daily dosage slowly until a maximum therapeutic response is achieved. The dosage of levodopa during this introductory period should be maintained, if possible. The initial dose of bromocriptine mesylate is 1/2 of a 2 1/2 mg tablet twice daily with meals. Assessments are advised at 2-week intervals during dosage titration to ensure that the lowest dosage producing an optimal therapeutic response is not exceeded. If necessary, the dosage may be increased every 14-28 days by 2 1/2 mg/day with meals. Should it be advisable to reduce the dosage of levodopa because of adverse reactions, the daily dosage of bromocriptine mesylate, if increased, should be accomplished gradually in small (2 1/2 mg) increments.

The safety of bromocriptine mesylate has not been demonstrated in dosages exceeding 100 mg/day.

HOW SUPPLIED:

PARLODEL SNAP TABS

2 1/2 mg Round, white, scored Snap Tabs, each containing 2 1/2 mg bromocriptine (as the mesylate). Engraved "Parlodel 2 1/2" on one side and scored on reverse side.

PARLODEL CAPSULES

5 mg Caramel and white capsules, each containing 5 mg bromocriptine (as the mesylate). Imprinted "Parlodel 5 mg" on one half and "S" on other half.

HOW SUPPLIED - EQUIVALENTS NOT AVAILABLE:

Capsule, Gelatin - Oral - 5 mg

30's	**$76.44**	**PARLODEL, Novartis**	**00078-0102-15**
100's	$166.55	Bromocriptine Mesylate, Athena	59075-0591-10
100's	**$241.50**	**PARLODEL, Novartis**	**00078-0102-05**

HOW SUPPLIED - EQUIVALENTS NOT AVAILABLE: *(cont'd)*

Tablet, Uncoated - Oral - 2.5 mg

30's	**$47.58**	**PARLODEL, Novartis**	**00078-0017-15**
100's	$108.47	Bromocriptine Mesylate, Athena	59075-0590-10
100's	**$158.22**	**PARLODEL, Novartis**	**00078-0017-05**

BROMODIPHENHYDRAMINE HYDROCHLORIDE; CODEINE PHOSPHATE *(000528)*

CATEGORIES: Allergies; Antihistamines; Antitussives; Antitussives/Expectorants/Mucolytics; Common Cold; Cough Preparations; Decongestants; Expectorants; Respiratory & Allergy Medications; Pregnancy Category C; DEA Class CV; FDA Approved 1984 Jan

BRAND NAMES: Ambay; **Ambenyl**; Ambophen; Amgenal; Bromanyl; Bromodiphenhydramine/Codeine; Bromotuss W/Codeine; Mybanil; Myphetane Dc

FORMULARIES: BC-BS

DESCRIPTION:

Each 5 ml of Bromodiphenhydramine HCl w/ codeine phosphate cough syrup contains:

Codeine phosphate (Warning—May be habit-forming) — 10 mg

Bromodiphenhydramine hydrochloride — 12.5 mg

Alcohol — 5%

Chemically codeine phosphate is morphinan-6-ol,7,8-didehydro-4,5-epoxy-3-methoxy-17-methyl-, (5α,6α)-phosphate(1:1)(salt) hemihydrate and bromodiphonhydramine hydrochloride is ethanamine 2-((4-bromophenyl) phenyl-methoxy)-N,N-dimethyl-, hydrochloride.

Bromodiphenhydramine HCl w/ codeine phosphate cough syrup is for oral administration.

CLINICAL PHARMACOLOGY:

Bromodiphenhydramine HCl w/ codeine phosphate is a combination of an antihistaminic agent, along with a well-recognized agent exhibiting antitussive properties.

INDICATIONS AND USAGE:

Bromodiphenhydramine HCl w/ codeine phosphate is indicated for relief of upper respiratory symptoms and coughs associated with allergies or the common cold.

CONTRAINDICATIONS:

Use in Newborn or Premature infants: This drug should *not* be used in newborn or premature infants.

Use in Nursing Mothers: Because of the higher risk of antihistamines for infants generally and for newborns and prematures in particular, antihistamine therapy is contraindicated in nursing mothers.

Use in Lower Respiratory Disease: Antihistamines *should NOT* be used to treat lower respiratory tract symptoms including asthma.

Antihistamines are also contraindicated in the following conditions: Hypersensitivity to bromodiphenhydramine and other antihistamines of similar chemical structure.

Monoamine oxidase inhibitor therapy (see DRUG INTERACTIONS.)

WARNINGS:

Antihistamines should be used with considerable caution in patients with:

Narrow angle glaucoma

Stenosing peptic ulcer

Pyloroduodenal obstruction

Symptomatic prostatic hypertrophy

Bladder neck obstruction

Usage in Children: In infants and children, especially, antihistamines in *overdosage* may cause hallucinations, convulsions, or death. As in adults, antihistamines may diminish mental alertness in children. In the young child, particularly, they may produce excitation.

Use in Pregnancy: Experience with this drug in pregnant women is inadequate to determine whether there exists a potential for harm to the developing fetus.

Use with CNS Depressants: Bromodiphenhydramine HCl w/ codeine phosphate cough syrup has additive effects with alcohol and other CNS depressants (hypnotics, sedatives, tranquilizers, etc.).

Use in Activities Requiring Mental Alertness: Patients should be warned about engaging in activities requiring mental alertness such as driving a car or operating appliances, machinery, etc.

Use in the Elderly (approximately 60 years or older): Antihistamines are more likely to cause dizziness, sedation, and hypotension in elderly patients.

PRECAUTIONS:

Bromodiphenhydramine has an atropine-like action and, therefore, should be used with caution in patients with:

History of bronchial asthma

Increased intraocular pressure

Hyperthyroidism

Cardiovascular disease

Hypertension

DRUG INTERACTIONS:

Codeine may potentiate the effects of other narcotics, general anesthetics, tranquilizers, sedatives and hypnotics, tricyclic antidepressants, MAO inhibitors, alcohol and other CNS depressants.

ADVERSE REACTIONS:

The following side effects may occur in patients taking Bromodiphenhydramine HCl w/ codeine phosphate:

drowsiness
confusion
nervousness
restlessness
nausea
vomiting
diarrhea
dryness of mouth, nose, and throat
tingling, heaviness, weakness of hands
nasal stuffiness
vertigo
palpitation
headache
insomnia

ADVERSE REACTIONS: *(cont'd)*

blurring of vision
diplopia
difficulty in urination
constipation
tightness of the chest and wheezing
thickening of bronchial secretions
urticaria
drug rash
photosensitivity
hemolytic anemia
hypotension
epigastric distress

DRUG ABUSE AND DEPENDENCE:

Codeine can produce drug dependence of the morphine type, and therefore, has the potential for being abused. Psychic dependence, physical dependence and tolerance may develop upon repeated administration of this drug and it should be prescribed and administered with the same degree of caution appropriate to the user of other oral narcose-containing medications. Like other narcotic containing medications, the drug is subject to the Federal Controlled Substances Act.

OVERDOSAGE:

Antihistamine overdosage reactions may vary from central nervous system depression to stimulation. Stimulation is particularly likely in children. Atropine like signs and symptoms—dry mouth; fixed, dilated pupils; flushing; and gastrointestinal symptoms may also occur.

If vomiting has not occurred spontaneously, the patient should be induced to vomit. This is best done by having him drink a glass of water or milk after which he should be made to gag. Precautions against aspiration must be taken, especially in infants and children.

If vomiting is unsuccessful, gastric lavage is indicated within 3 hours after ingestion and even later if large amounts of milk or cream were given beforehand. Isotonic and 1/2 isotonic saline is the lavage solution of choice.

Saline cathartics, as milk of magnesia, by osmosis draw water into the bowel, and therefore, are valuable for their action in rapid dilution of bowel content.

Stimulants should not be used.

Vasopressors may be used to treat hypotension.

DOSAGE AND ADMINISTRATION:

DOSAGE SHOULD BE INDIVIDUALIZED ACCORDING TO THE NEEDS AND THE RESPONSE OF THE PATIENTS.

Adults—one or two teaspoonfuls every four to six hours, not to exceed 12 teaspoonfuls in 24 hours. Children (total intake of codeine phosphate should not exceed 1 mg/kg 24 hours) — Six to under 12 years of age — one-half to one teaspoonful every six hours.

Not recommended for use in children under six years of age.

Store at controlled room temperature (59-86°F).

HOW SUPPLIED - RATED THERAPEUTICALLY EQUIVALENT:

Syrup - Oral - 12.5 mg/10 mg/5

120 ml	$2.23	Bromodiphenhydramine Hcl & Codeine, H.C.F.A. F F P	99999-0528-01
120 ml	$3.09	Bromodiphenhydramine W/Codeine, Aligen Independ	00405-2387-76
120 ml	$3.99	BROMANYL COUGH SYRUP, Alpharma	00472-1634-04
120 ml	**$21.24**	**AMBENYL COUGH SYRUP, Forest Pharms**	**00456-0681-04**
360 ml	**$76.63**	**AMBENYL COUGH SYRUP, Forest Pharms**	**00456-0681-16**
480 ml	$8.93	Bromodiphenhydramine Hcl & Codeine, H.C.F.A. F F P	99999-0528-02
480 ml	$9.93	Bromodiphenhydramine W/Codeine, Aligen Independ	00405-2387-16
480 ml	$11.20	Bromanyl, Harber Pharm	51432-0537-20
480 ml	$11.35	AMBOPHEN, Major Pharms	00904-0067-16
480 ml	$11.75	Bromanyl, Qualitest Pharms	00603-1040-58
480 ml	$11.76	BROMANYL COUGH SYRUP, Alpharma	00472-1634-16
480 ml	$12.50	BROMANYL COUGH SYRUP, Schein Pharm (US)	00364-7405-16
480 ml	$12.50	BROMOTUSS CODEINE, Rugby	00536-0272-85
480 ml	$13.20	Bromodiphenhydramine/Codeine, Morton Grove	60432-0590-16
480 ml	$14.25	AMGENAL COUGH SYRUP, Goldline Labs	00182-1680-40
480 ml	$14.51	BROMANYL, HL Moore Drug Exch	00839-6796-69
3840 ml	$71.42	Bromodiphenhydramine Hcl & Codeine, H.C.F.A. F F P	99999-0528-03
3840 ml	$75.23	AMBOPHEN, Major Pharms	00904-0067-28
3840 ml	$77.38	Bromanyl, Harber Pharm	51432-0537-21
3840 ml	$88.32	BROMANYL COUGH SYRUP, Alpharma	00472-1634-28
3840 ml	**$575.12**	**AMBENYL COUGH SYRUP, Forest Pharms**	**00456-0681-28**

HOW SUPPLIED - NOT RATED EQUIVALENT:

Syrup - Oral - 12.5 mg/10 mg/5

120 ml	$3.50	Bromanyl, Consolidated Midland	00223-6436-04
480 ml	$9.90	Bromanyl, Consolidated Midland	00223-6436-01
3840 ml	$66.97	Bromanyl, Consolidated Midland	00223-6436-02

BROMPHENIRAMINE MALEATE *(000529)*

CATEGORIES: Allergies; Alkylamines; Antihistamines; Cough Preparations; Respiratory & Allergy Medications; FDA Approval Pre 1982

BRAND NAMES: Aller-Brom; Baltane; Bromatane; *Bromine*; *Brommine*; Bromphen; Brotane; Chlor-Phed; Codimal-A; Cophene-B; D-Gestant; *Dimegan* (Germany, France); **Dimetane**; Endafed; Harber-Tane; Hista-Plex; Histafed Im; Histaject; *Ilvin*; K-Histaphed; *Kinmedon*; Med-Hist-Im; Nasahist B; Nd-Stat; *Neo-Meton*; Oraminic II; Pri-Gest R; Prop-A-Tane; U.R.I.; Veltane; Venstat
(International brand names outside U.S. in italics)

FORMULARIES: Medi-Cal

Prescribing information not available at time of publication.

HOW SUPPLIED - RATED THERAPEUTICALLY EQUIVALENT:

Injection, Solution - Intramuscular; - 10 mg/ml

10 ml	$6.40	Brompheniramine Maleate, Pasadena	00418-3001-10

Tablet, Uncoated - Oral - 4 mg

100's	$2.95	Brompheniramine Maleate, Consolidated Midland	00223-0550-01
100's	$4.05	ALLER-BROM, Rugby	00536-3391-01
1000's	$22.42	ALLER-BROM, Rugby	00536-3391-10
1000's	$22.50	Brompheniramine Maleate, Consolidated Midland	00223-0550-02

HOW SUPPLIED - NOT RATED EQUIVALENT:

Injection, Solution - Intramuscular; - 10 mg/ml

10 ml	$7.00	PROP-A-TANE, Bolan Pharm	44437-0602-10
10 ml	$7.05	ENDAFED, UAD Labs	00785-8023-10

HOW SUPPLIED - NOT RATED EQUIVALENT: *(cont'd)*

10 ml	$7.78	N-D STAT, Hyrex Pharms	00314-2236-70
10 ml	$8.78	Brompheniramine Maleate, Steris Labs	00402-0602-10
10 ml	$9.00	Brompheniramine Maleate, Forest Pharms	00456-0623-10
10 ml	$11.00	Brompheniramine Maleate Inj, Schein Pharm (US)	00364-2185-54
10 ml	$20.30	HISTAJECT, Mayrand Pharms	00259-0359-10

BROMPHENIRAMINE MALEATE; CODEINE PHOSPHATE; PHENYLPROPANOLAMINE HYDROCHLORIDE *(000530)*

CATEGORIES: Allergies; Antihistamines; Antitussives; Antitussives/Expectorants/ Mucolytics; Common Cold; Congestion; Cough Preparations; Expectorants; Nasal Congestion; Respiratory & Allergy Medications; Pregnancy Category C; DEA Class CV; FDA Approved 1984 Mar

BRAND NAMES: Baltane Dc; Bromanate-Dc; Bromatane-Dc; Bromphen-Dc; Bromtane D.C.; Delhistine Cs; **Dimetane-Dc**; Liquihistine Cs; M-Tuss; Myphetane-Dc; Normatane Dc; Phenylprop/Cod/Br-Pheniramine; Phenylpropanolamine Dc; Poly-Histine Cs; Polytine Cs; Trihist-Cs; Tusshistine Cs; Uni Multihist Cs

FORMULARIES: Aetna; DoD; Medi-Cal

DESCRIPTION:

Dimetane—DC is a light bluish-pink syrup with a raspberry flavor.

Each 5 ml (1 teaspoonful) contains:

Brompheniramine Maleate, USP 2.0 mg

Phenylpropanolamine Hydrochloride, USP 12.5 mg

Codeine Phosphate, USP 10.0 mg

(Warning: May be habit forming)

Alcohol 0.95 percent

In a palatable aromatic vehicle.

Inactive Ingredients: Citric Acid, FD&C Blue 1, FD&C Red 40 Flavors, Glycerin, Sodium Benzoate, Sorbitol, Water.

Brompheniramine Maleate, USP 2-Pyridinepropanamine, γ-(4-bromophenyl)-N,N-dimethyl-, (Z)-butenedioate (1:1).

Phenylpropanolamine Hydrochloride, USP Benzenemethanol, α-(1-aminoethyl)-, hydrochloride, (R*S*)-,(±)

Codeine Phosphate, USP Morphinan-6-ol, 7,8-didehydro-4,5-epoxy-3-methoxy-17-methyl-, (5α,6α)-, phosphate (1:1) (salt), hemihydrate Antihistamine/Nasal Decongestant/Antitussive syrup for oral administration.

CLINICAL PHARMACOLOGY:

Brompheniramine maleate is a histamine antagonist, specifically an H_1-receptor-blocking agent belonging to the alkylamine class of antihistamines. Antihistamines appear to compete with histamine for receptor sites on effector cells. Brompheniramine also has anticholinergic (drying) and sedative effects. Among the antihistaminic effects, it antagonizes the allergic response (vasodilatation, increased vascular permeability, increased mucus secretion) of nasal tissue. Brompheniramine is well absorbed from the gastrointestinal tract, with peak plasma concentration after a single oral dose of 4 mg reached in 5 hours; urinary excretion is the major route of elimination, mostly as products of biodegradation; the liver is assumed to be the main site of metabolic transformation.

Phenylpropanolamine hydrochloride is a sympathomimetic drug which is readily absorbed from the gastrointestinal tract and produces nasal vasoconstriction (decongestion). Phenylpropanolamine stimulates both α and β-adrenergic receptors, similar to ephedrine. Part of its peripheral action is indirect and is due to the displacement of norepinephrine from storage sites, but it also has direct effect on the adrenergic receptors.

Codeine is an opiate analgesic and antitussive. Codeine calms the cough control center.

INDICATIONS AND USAGE:

For relief of coughs and upper respiratory symptoms, including nasal congestion, associated with allergy or the common cold.

CONTRAINDICATIONS:

Hypersensitivity to any of the ingredients. Do not use in the newborn, in premature infants, in nursing mothers, in patients with severe hypertension or severe coronary artery disease, or in those receiving monoamine oxidase (MAO) inhibitors.

Antihistamines should not be used to treat lower respiratory tract conditions including asthma.

WARNINGS:

Especially in infants and small children, antihistamines in overdosage may cause hallucinations, convulsions, death. Codeine may cause or aggravate constipation.

Antihistamines may diminish mental alertness. In the young child, they may produce excitation.

PRECAUTIONS:

General: Because of its antihistamine component, Brompheniramine/codeine/phenylpropanolamine cough syrup should be used with caution in patients with a history of bronchial asthma, narrow angle glaucoma, gastrointestinal obstruction, or urinary bladder neck obstruction. Because of its sympathomimetic component, brompheniramine/codeine/phenylpropanolamine cough syrup should be used with caution in patients with diabetes, hypertension, heart disease, or thyroid disease.

Information for the Patient: Patients should be warned about engaging in activities requiring mental alertness, such as driving a car or operating dangerous machinery.

Carcinogenesis, Mutagenesis: Long-term studies in animals to evaluate carcinogenic and mutagenic potential have not been performed.

Pregnancy Category C: Animal reproduction studies have not been conducted with brompheniramine/codeine/phenylpropanolamine cough syrup. It is also not known whether brompheniramine/codeine/phenylpropanolamine cough syrup can cause fetal harm when administered to a pregnant woman or can affect reproduction capacity. Brompheniramine/ codeine/phenylpropanolamine cough syrup should be given to a pregnant woman only if clearly needed.

Reproduction studies of brompheniramine maleate (one of the components of the Dimetane formulations) in rats and mice at doses up to 16 times the maximum human dose have revealed no evidence of impaired fertility or harm to the fetus.

PRECAUTIONS: *(cont'd)*

Nursing Mothers: Because of the higher risk of intolerance of antihistamines in small infants generally, and in newborns and prematures in particular, and the fact that codeine appears in human milk, brompheniramine/codeine/phenylpropanolamine cough syrup is contraindicated in nursing mothers.

DRUG INTERACTIONS:

Antihistamines have additive effects with alcohol and other CNS depressants (hypnotics, sedatives, tranquilizers, antianxiety agents, etc.). MAO inhibitors prolong and intensify the anticholinergic (drying) effects of antihistamines. MAO inhibitors may enhance the effect of phenylpropanolamine. Sympathomimetics may reduce the effects of antihypertensive drugs.

ADVERSE REACTIONS:

The most frequent adverse reactions to brompheniramine/codeine/phenylpropanolamine cough syrup are: sedation; dryness of mouth, nose and throat; thickening of bronchial secretions; dizziness. Other adverse reactions may include:

Dermatologic: Urticaria, drug rash, photosensitivity, pruritus.

Cardiovascular System: Hypotension, hypertension, cardiac arrhythmias.

CNS: Disturbed coordination, tremor, irritability, insomnia, visual disturbances, weakness, nervousness, convulsions, headache, euphoria, and dysphoria.

G. U. System: Urinary frequency, difficult urination.

G. I. System: Epigastric discomfort, anorexia, nausea, vomiting, diarrhea, constipation.

Respiratory System: Tightness of chest and wheezing, shortness of breath. At higher doses, codeine has most of the disadvantages of morphine including respiratory depression.

Hematologic System: Hemolytic anemia, thrombocytopenia, agranulocytosis.

DRUG ABUSE AND DEPENDENCE:

Codeine can produce drug dependence of the morphine type, and therefore has the potential for being abused. Psychic dependence, physical dependence and tolerance may develop upon repeated administration of this drug, and it should be prescribed and administered with the same degree of caution appropriate to the use of other oral narcotic medications.

Brompheniramine/codeine/phenylpropanolamine cough syrup is subject to the Federal Controlled Substances Act (Schedule V).

OVERDOSAGE:

Signs and Symptoms: Serious overdose with codeine is characterized by respiratory depression, extreme somnolence progressing to stupor or coma. In severe overdosage, apnea, circulatory collapse, cardiac arrest and death may occur. The central nervous system effects from overdosage of brompheniramine may vary from depression to stimulation. Anticholinergic effects may also occur. Overdosage of phenylpropanolamine may be associated with tachycardia, hypertension and cardiac arrhythmias.

Toxic Doses: Doses of 800 mg or more of codeine have caused partial loss of consciousness, delirium, restlessness, excitement, tremors, convulsions and collapse; or respiratory paralysis with such sequelae as mydriasis, marked vasodilatation, and finally death. A 2-year-old child survived a dose of 300-900 mg of brompheniramine; the lethal dose of phenylpropanolamine is in the range of 50 mg/kg.

Treatment: Respiratory depression should be treated promptly. Oxygen, intravenous fluids, vasopressors and other supportive measures should be employed as indicated. If necessary, reestablishment of adequate respiratory exchange through provision of a patent airway and the institution of assisted or controlled ventilation must be provided. The narcotic antagonist, naloxone, is a specific antidote to codeine-induced respiratory depression, and should be administered by the intravenous route if appropriate (see prescribing information for naloxone). Since the duration of action of codeine may exceed that of the antagonist, the patient should be kept under constant surveillance.

Gastric emptying may be useful in removing unabsorbed drug, either by inducing emesis or lavage; precautions against aspiration must be taken. Stimulants or depressants should be used cautiously and only when specifically indicated. If marked excitement is present, one of the short-acting barbiturates or chloral hydrate may be used.

DOSAGE AND ADMINISTRATION:

Adults and children 12 years of age and over: 2 teaspoonfuls every 4 hours. Children 6 to under 12 years: 1 teaspoonful every 4 hours. Children 2 to under 6 years: 1/2 teaspoonful every 4 hours. Children 6 months to under 2 years: Dosage to be established by physician.

Do not exceed 6 doses during a 24-hour period.

Store at controlled room temperature, between 15 and 30°C (59 and 86°F).

Dispense in tight, light-resistant container.

HOW SUPPLIED - RATED THERAPEUTICALLY EQUIVALENT:

Syrup - Oral - 2 mg/10 mg/12.5

120 ml	$2.75	Bromanate Dc, Harber Pharm	51432-0535-21
120 ml	$2.93	Brompheniramine Dc, H.C.F.A. F F P	99999-0530-01
120 ml	$3.55	Bromanate Dc, Major Pharms	00904-7819-00
120 ml	$3.68	Brompheniramine Dc, Geneva Pharms	00781-6805-04
120 ml	$3.78	Phenylpropanolamine Dc, Aligen Independ	00405-0157-76
120 ml	$3.80	BROMPHEN-DC, Schein Pharm (US)	00364-7387-77
120 ml	$3.85	Brompheniramine Dc, Major Pharms	00904-0716-20
120 ml	$4.00	Myphetane-Dc, Morton Grove	60432-0461-04
120 ml	$4.25	Bromanate Dc, HL Moore Drug Exch	00839-7070-65
120 ml	$7.75	BROMPHEN DC, COUGH SYRUP W/CODEINE, Rugby	00536-0262-97
473 ml	$11.54	Brompheniramine Dc, H.C.F.A. F F P	99999-0530-02
480 ml	$11.71	Brompheniramine Dc, H.C.F.A. F F P	99999-0530-03
480 ml	$13.95	Bromanate Dc, Major Pharms	00904-7819-16
480 ml	$29.85	Bromphen-Dc, Rugby	00536-0262-85
480 ml	$30.40	POLY HISTINE CS, Bock Pharma	00563-1633-16
480 ml	**$35.19**	**DIMETANE-DC, AH Robins**	**00031-1833-25**
3840 ml	$54.99	Bromanate Dc, Harber Pharm	51432-0535-18
3840 ml	$58.94	BROMANATE-DC, HL Moore Drug Exch	00839-7070-70
3840 ml	$71.92	Bromanate Dc, Major Pharms	00904-7819-28
3840 ml	$73.73	Myphetane-Dc, Morton Grove	60432-0461-28
3840 ml	$79.45	Brompheniramine Dc, Major Pharms	00904-0716-28
3840 ml	$93.70	Brompheniramine Dc, H.C.F.A. F F P	99999-0530-04
3840 ml	$113.25	BROMPHEN DC, COUGH SYRUP W/CODEINE, Rugby	00536-0262-90

HOW SUPPLIED - NOT RATED EQUIVALENT:

Syrup - Oral - 2 mg/10 mg/12.5

120 ml	$2.25	Bromanate Dc, Consolidated Midland	00223-6438-01
120 ml	$4.05	BROMANATE-DC, Alpharma	00472-1645-04
473 ml	$26.25	Tusshistine Cs, Econolab	55053-0850-16
473 ml	$26.35	Polytine Cs, Am Generics	58634-0009-01

HOW SUPPLIED - NOT RATED EQUIVALENT: *(cont'd)*

480 ml	$9.95	Bromanate Dc, Consolidated Midland	00223-6438-02
480 ml	$11.71	Uni Multihist Cs, United Res	00677-1526-33
480 ml	$14.05	Bromanate-Dc, Alpharma	00472-1645-16
480 ml	$22.90	Liquihistine Cs, Liquipharm	54198-0176-16
480 ml	$26.95	Trihist-Cs, Cypress Pharm	60258-0748-16
480 ml	$28.37	Phenylprop/Cod/Br-Pheniramine, Aligen Independ	00405-0053-16
3840 ml	$64.97	Bromanate Dc, Consolidated Midland	00223-6438-03
3840 ml	$74.05	BROMANATE-DC, Alpharma	00472-1645-28

BROMPHENIRAMINE MALEATE; DEXTROMETHORPHAN HYDROBROMIDE; PSEUDOEPHEDRINE HYDROCHLORIDE

(000531)

CATEGORIES: Allergies; Antihistamines; Antitussives; Antitussives/Expectorants/Mucolytics; Common Cold; Congestion; Cough Preparations; Nasal Congestion; Respiratory & Allergy Medications; Pregnancy Category C; FDA Approved 1984 Mar

BRAND NAMES: Baltane Dx; Bromanate Dx; Bromarest Dx; Brometane Dx; Bromfed-Dm; Bromophed Dx; Bromphen Dx; Bromtane; Decon-Dm; **Dimetane-Dx**; Gen-Tane Dx; Harber-Tane Dx; Myphetane Dx; Myphetane-Dx; Pseudoephedrine Dx; Tuss-Mine Dm; Veltane

FORMULARIES: Aetna; BC-BS

DESCRIPTION:

Dimetane—Dx is a light- red syrup with a butterscotch flavor.

Each 5 ml (1 teaspoonful) contains:

Brompheniramine Maleate, USP... 2 mg

Pseudoephedrine Hydrochloride, USP... 30 mg

Dextromethorphan Hydrobromide, USP... 10 mg

Alcohol... 0.95 percent

In a palatable, aromatic vehicle.

Dimetane—Dx Inactive Ingredients: Citric Acid, FD&C Red 40, FD&C Yellow 6, Flavors, Glycerin, Saccharin Sodium, Sodium Benzoate, Sorbitol, Water.

Brompheniramine Maleate, USP 2-Pyridinepropanamine, γ-(4-bromophenyl)-N,N-dimethyl-, (Z)-butenedioate (1:1).

Pseudoephedrine Hydrochloride, USP Benzenemethanol, α-(1- (methylamino)ethyl)-,(S-(R*,R*)-, hydrochloride.

Dextromethorphan Hydrobromide, USP Morphinan, 3-methoxy-17-methyl-,(9α, 13α, 14α)-, hydrobromide, monohydrate.

Antihistamine/Nasal Decongestant/Antitussive syrup for oral administration.

CLINICAL PHARMACOLOGY:

Brompheniramine maleate is a histamine antagonist, specifically an H_1-receptor-blocking agent belonging to the alkylamine class of antihistamines. Antihistamines appear to compete with histamine for receptor sites on effector cells. Brompheniramine also has anticholinergic (drying) and sedative effects. Among the antihistaminic effects, it antagonizes the allergic response (vasodilatation, increased vascular permeability, increased mucus secretion) of nasal tissue. Brompheniramine is well absorbed from the gastrointestinal tract, with peak plasma concentration after single, oral dose of 4 mg reached in 5 hours; urinary excretion is the major route of elimination, mostly as products of biodegradation; the liver is assumed to be the main site of metabolic transformation.

Pseudoephedrine acts on sympathetic nerve endings and also on smooth muscle, making it useful as a nasal decongestant. The nasal decongestant effect is mediated by the action of pseudoephedrine on α-sympathetic receptors, producing vasoconstriction of the dilated nasal arterioles. Following oral administration, effects are noted within 30 minutes with peak activity occurring at approximately one hour.

Dextromethorphan acts centrally to elevate the threshold for coughing. It has no analgesic or addictive properties. The onset of antitussive action occurs in 15 to 30 minutes after administration and is of long duration.

INDICATIONS AND USAGE:

For relief of coughs and upper respiratory symptoms, including nasal congestion, associated with allergy or the common cold.

CONTRAINDICATIONS:

Hypersensitivity to any of the ingredients. Do not use in the newborn, in premature infants, in nursing mothers, in patients with severe hypertension or severe coronary artery disease, or in those receiving monoamine oxidase (MAO) inhibitors.

Antihistamines should not be used to treat lower respiratory tract conditions including asthma.

WARNINGS:

Especially in infants and small children, antihistamines in overdosage may cause hallucinations, convulsions, and death.

Antihistamines may diminish mental alertness. In the young child, they may produce excitation.

PRECAUTIONS:

GENERAL

Because of its antihistamine component, brompheniramine/dextromethorphan/psuedoephedrine cough syrup should be used with caution in patients with a history of bronchial asthma, narrow angle glaucoma, gastrointestinal obstruction, or urinary bladder neck obstruction. Because of its sympathomimetic component, brompheniramine/dextromethorphan/psuedoephedrine cough syrup should be used with caution in patients with diabetes, hypertension, heart disease, or thyroid disease.

Information for the Patient: Patients should be warned about engaging in activities requiring mental alertness, such as driving a car or operating dangerous machinery.

Carcinogenesis, Mutagenesis, and Impairment of Fertility: Animal studies of brompheniramine/dextromethorphan/psuedoephedrine cough syrup to assess the carcinogenic and mutagenic potential or the effect on fertility have not been performed.

PRECAUTIONS: *(cont'd)*

Pregnancy, Teratogenic Effects, Pregnancy Category C: Animal reproduction studies have not been conducted with brompheniramine/dextromethorphan/psuedoephedrine cough syrup. It is also not known whether brompheniramine/dextromethorphan/psuedoephedrine cough syrup can cause fetal harm when administered to a pregnant woman or can affect reproduction capacity. Brompheniramine/dextromethorphan/psuedoephedrine cough syrup should be given to a pregnant woman only if clearly needed.

Reproduction studies of brompheniramine maleate (a component of brompheniramine/dextromethorphan/psuedoephedrine cough syrup) in rats and mice at doses up to 16 times the maximum human dose have revealed no evidence of impaired fertility or harm to the fetus.

Nursing Mothers: Because of the higher risk of intolerance of antihistamines in small infants generally, and in newborns and prematures in particular, brompheniramine/dextromethorphan/psuedoephedrine cough syrup is contraindicated in nursing mothers.

DRUG INTERACTIONS:

Antihistamines have additive effects with alcohol and other CNS depressants (hypnotics, sedatives, tranquilizers, antianxiety agents, etc.). MAO inhibitors prolong and intensify the anticholinergic (drying) effects of antihistamines. MAO inhibitors may enhance the effect of pseudoephedrine. Sympathomimetics may reduce the effects of antihypertensive drugs.

ADVERSE REACTIONS:

The most frequent adverse reactions to brompheniramine/dextromethorphan/psuedoephedrine cough syrup are: sedation; dryness of mouth, nose and throat; thickening of bronchial secretions; dizziness. Other adverse reactions may include:

Dermatologic: Urticaria, drug rash, photosensitivity, pruritus.

Cardiovascular System: Hypotension, hypertension, cardiac arrhythmias, palpitation.

CNS: Disturbed coordination, tremor, irritability, insomnia, visual disturbances, weakness, nervousness, convulsions, headache, euphoria, and dysphoria.

Genitourinary System: Urinary frequency, difficult urination.

Gastrointestinal System: Epigastric discomfort, anorexia, nausea, vomiting, diarrhea, constipation.

Respiratory System: Tightness of chest and wheezing, shortness of breath.

Hematologic System: Hemolytic anemia, thrombocytopenia, agranulocytosis.

OVERDOSAGE:

Signs and Symptoms: Central nervous system effects from overdosage of brompheniramine may vary from depression to stimulation, especially in children. Anticholinergic effects may be noted. Toxic doses of pseudoephedrine may result in CNS stimulation, tachycardia, hypertension, and cardiac arrhythmias; signs of CNS depression may occasionally be seen. Dextromethorphan in toxic doses will cause drowsiness, ataxia, nystagmus, opisthotonos, and convulsive seizures.

Toxic Doses: Data suggest that individuals may respond in an unexpected manner to apparently small amounts of a particular drug. A 2 1/2-year-old child survived the ingestion of 21 mg/kg of dextromethorphan exhibiting only ataxia, drowsiness, and fever, but seizures have been reported in 2 children following the ingestion of 13—17 mg/kg. Another 2 1/2 year-old child survived a dose of 300—900 mg of brompheniramine. The toxic dose of pseudoephedrine should be less than that of ephedrine, which is estimated to be 50 mg/kg.

Treatment: Induce emesis if patient is alert and is seen prior to 6 hours following ingestion. Precautions against aspiration must be taken, especially in infants and small children. Gastric lavage may be carried out, although in some instances tracheostomy may be necessary prior to lavage. Naloxone hydrochloride 0.005 mg/kg intravenously may be of value in reversing the CNS depression that may occur from an overdose of dextromethorphan. CNS stimulants may counter CNS depression. Should CNS hyperactivity or convulsive seizures occur, intravenous short-acting barbiturates may be indicated. Hypertensive responses and/or tachycardia should be treated appropriately. Oxygen, intravenous fluids, and other supportive measures should be employed as indicated.

DOSAGE AND ADMINISTRATION:

Adults and children 12 years of age and over: 2 teaspoonfuls every 4 hours.

Children 6 to under 12 years: 1 teaspoonful every 4 hours.

Children 2 to under 6 years: 1/2 teaspoonful every 4 hours.

Children 6 months to under 2 years: Dosage to be established by physician.

Do not exceed 6 doses during a 24-hour period.

Store at controlled room temperature, between 15 and 30°C (59 and 86°F).

HOW SUPPLIED - RATED THERAPEUTICALLY EQUIVALENT:

Syrup - Oral - 2 mg/10 mg/30 m

120 ml	$1.27	Pseudoephedrine Dx, H.C.F.A. F F P	99999-0531-01
120 ml	$4.42	Pseudoephedrine Dx, Aligen Independ	00405-3660-76
120 ml	$5.38	Brompheniramine Cough Syrup Usp, Geneva Pharms	00781-6807-04
120 ml	$8.27	TUSS-MINE DM, Bergmar Pharm	58173-0022-04
473 ml	$27.60	TUSS-MINE DM, Bergmar Pharm	58173-0022-16
480 ml	$4.80	BROMOPHED DX, Qualitest Pharms	00603-1044-58
480 ml	$5.09	Pseudoephedrine Dx, H.C.F.A. F F P	99999-0531-02
480 ml	$5.52	BROMETANE DX CS, HL Moore Drug Exch	00839-7582-69
480 ml	$8.25	BROMANATE DX, Major Pharms	00904-0717-16
480 ml	$8.42	Pseudoephedrine Dx, Aligen Independ	00405-3660-16
480 ml	$12.95	Brompheniramine Cough Syrup Usp, Geneva Pharms	00781-6807-16
480 ml	$13.44	Bromphen Dx Cough Syrup, Rugby	00536-0285-85
480 ml	$15.00	BROMETANE DX, Hi Tech Pharma	50383-0593-16
480 ml	$18.84	Bromphen/Pseudoeph/Dextromethorphan, Schein Pharm (US)	00364-2496-16
480 ml	$30.97	BROMFED DM COUGH SYRUP, Muro Pharm	00451-4101-16
480 ml	**$35.71**	**DIMETANE-DX, AH Robins**	**00031-1836-25**
3840 ml	$40.70	Pseudoephedrine Dx, H.C.F.A. F F P	99999-0531-03
3840 ml	$49.42	BROMANATE DX, Major Pharms	00904-0717-28
3840 ml	$59.98	BROMETANE DX, Hi Tech Pharma	50383-0593-28
3840 ml	**$258.16**	**DIMETANE-DX, AH Robins**	**00031-1836-29**

HOW SUPPLIED - NOT RATED EQUIVALENT:

Syrup - Oral - 2 mg/10 mg/30 m

118 ml	$7.00	DECON-DM, Norega Labs	51724-0017-04
120 ml	$3.31	Myphetane-Dx, HL Moore Drug Exch	00839-7613-65
120 ml	$5.36	Myphetane Dx, Morton Grove	60432-0734-04
480 ml	$9.90	Myphetane Dx, Morton Grove	60432-0734-16
480 ml	$9.95	Harber-Tane Dx, Harber Pharm	51432-0619-20
3840 ml	$73.73	Myphetane Dx, Morton Grove	60432-0734-28
3840 ml	$79.95	Harber-Tane Dx, Harber Pharm	51432-0619-21

BROMPHENIRAMINE MALEATE; PHENYLPROPANOLAMINE HYDROCHLORIDE *(000532)*

CATEGORIES: Allergies; Antihistamines; Common Cold; Cough Preparations; DESI Drugs; Nasal Congestion; Respiratory & Allergy Medications; FDA Approved 1984 Sep

BRAND NAMES: Ami Tapp; Baltapp; Biphetap; Bro-Phen; Brom-Cortann; Bromanate; Bromatapp; Bromophen; Brotep; *Cetafren*; Dimaphen; Dime-Time; *Dimetapp* (Mexico); *Dimetapp New Elixir*; *Dimetapp New Extentabs*; E-Tapp; Ethi-Hist; Harbertapp; *Lunerin*; *Nasapert*; Normatane; Partapp; Phenatapp; Pioten; *Rupton*; *Rupton Chronules* (France); Tamine; Veltap
(International brand names outside U.S. in italics)

Prescribing information not available at time of publication.

HOW SUPPLIED - EQUIVALENTS NOT AVAILABLE:

Elixir - Oral

120 ml	$2.10	Bromanate, Consolidated Midland	00223-6439-01
480 ml	$2.50	BROMOPHEN, Rugby	00536-0290-85
480 ml	$4.50	Bromanate, Consolidated Midland	00223-6439-02
3840 ml	$26.50	Bromanate, Consolidated Midland	00223-6439-03

Tablet, Coated, Sustained Action - Oral

20's	$5.75	DIMAPHEN S.A., Major Pharms	00904-0215-95
100's	$5.39	BROMATAPP TD, HL Moore Drug Exch	00839-1106-06
100's	$6.85	DIMAPHEN S. A., Major Pharms	00904-0215-60
100's	$8.60	BROMOPHEN, Rugby	00536-3397-01
100's	$11.97	Dime-Time, Time-Caps Labs	49483-0039-01
100's	$43.05	E N T, Ion	11808-0031-01
1000's	$40.49	BROMATAPP TD, HL Moore Drug Exch	00839-1106-16
1000's	$44.60	DIMAPHEN S. A., Major Pharms	00904-0215-80
1000's	$52.23	BROMOPHEN, Rugby	00536-3397-10
1000's	$89.85	Dime-Time, Time-Caps Labs	49483-0039-10

BROMPHENIRAMINE MALEATE; PSEUDOEPHEDRINE HYDROCHLORIDE *(000533)*

CATEGORIES: Allergies; Antihistamines; Common Cold; Cough Preparations; Decongestants; Nasal Congestion; Respiratory & Allergy Medications; Rhinitis; FDA Pre 1938 Drugs

BRAND NAMES: Allent; B-Fedrine; B-Fedrine Pd; Brofed; Bromadrine; **Bromfed**; Bromfenex; Bromfenex-Pd; Bromophed; Brompheniramine W/Pseudoephed; Dallergy-Jr; Endafed; Iofed; Iofed-Pd; Lodrane; Lodrane Ld; M-Hist; Nalfed; Nasal Decongestant; Nasal Decongestant Pediatric; Pseubrom; Pseubrom-Pd; Respahist; Shellcap; Touro A & H; Ultrabrom; Ultrabrom Pd

FORMULARIES: Aetna; BC-BS; PCS

Prescribing information not available at time of publication.

HOW SUPPLIED - RATED THERAPEUTICALLY EQUIVALENT:

Capsule, Gelatin, Sustained Action - Oral - 6 mg/60 mg

100's	$46.35	Bromfenex-Pd, Ethex	58177-0020-04

Capsule, Gelatin, Sustained Action - Oral - 12 mg/120 mg

100's	$50.70	Bromfenex, Ethex	58177-0019-04

HOW SUPPLIED - NOT RATED EQUIVALENT:

Capsule, Gelatin, Sustained Action - Oral - 6 mg/60 mg

100's	$28.32	Lodrane LD, ECR Pharms	00095-6006-01
100's	$30.00	Brompheniramine W/Pseudoephed, Goldline Labs	00182-1054-01
100's	$31.44	DALLERGY-JR., Laser	00277-0176-01
100's	$32.22	Bromophed Pd, Qualitest Pharms	00603-2506-21
100's	$35.62	BROMADRINE PD, Rugby	00536-4449-01
100's	$39.95	NALFED-PD, Econolab	55053-0222-01
100's	$39.96	Touro A & H, Dartmouth Pharms	58869-0301-01
100's	$42.05	Brompheniramine W/Pseudoephed, Aligen Independ	00405-4128-01
100's	$44.00	Respahist, Respa Pharms	60575-0825-19
100's	$45.00	ULTRABROM PD, WE Pharm	59196-0004-01
100's	$45.26	Nasal Decongestant Pd, Jerome Stevens	50564-0526-01
100's	$45.95	Pseubrom-Pd, Alphagen Labs	59743-0061-01
100's	$46.30	Nalfed-Pd, Major Pharms	00904-1019-60
100's	$48.25	Nasal Decongestant Pediatric, HL Moore Drug Exch	00839-7973-06
100's	$50.25	B-Fedrine Pd, Pecos	59879-0511-01
100's	**$68.13**	**BROMFED-PD, Muro Pharm**	**00451-4001-50**
500's	**$308.68**	**BROMFED-PD, Muro Pharm**	**00451-4001-60**

Capsule, Gelatin, Sustained Action - Oral - 12 mg/120 mg

100's	$23.86	M-HIST TD, RA McNeil	12830-0200-01
100's	$27.75	Nalfed, Major Pharms	00904-7691-60
100's	$33.90	Bromophed, Qualitest Pharms	00603-2505-21
100's	$34.50	Brompheniramine W/Pseudoephed, Goldline Labs	00182-1053-01
100's	$35.82	ALLENT, Ascher	00225-0480-15
100's	$37.12	BROMADRINE, Rugby	00536-4448-01
100's	$45.65	NALFED, Econolab	55053-0125-01
100's	$47.50	Ultrabrom, WE Pharm	59196-0006-01
100's	$48.36	ENDAFED, UAD Labs	00785-2206-01
100's	$49.51	Nasal Decongestant, Jerome Stevens	50564-0527-01
100's	$49.95	Pseubrom, Alphagen Labs	59743-0060-01
100's	$52.45	Nasal Decongestant, HL Moore Drug Exch	00839-7972-06
100's	$55.00	B-Fedrine, Pecos	59879-0510-01
100's	**$74.53**	**BROMFED, Muro Pharm**	**00451-4000-50**
500's	**$353.41**	**BROMFED, Muro Pharm**	**00451-4000-60**

Elixir - Oral - 4 mg/30 mg

480 ml	$12.40	BROFED, Marnel Pharceut	00682-7777-16

Liquid - Oral - 60 mg/4 mg/5ml

480 ml	$19.80	LODRANE, ECR Pharms	00095-6004-16

Tablet, Uncoated - Oral - 4 mg/60 mg

100's	**$21.90**	**BROMFED, Muro Pharm**	**00451-4060-50**

BROMPHENIRAMINE; DEXTROMETHORPHAN HYDROBROMIDE; PHENYLPROPANOLAMINE *(000534)*

CATEGORIES: Antitussives; Antitussives/Expectorants/Mucolytics; Common Cold; Cough Preparations; Respiratory & Allergy Medications; FDA Pre 1938 Drugs

BRAND NAMES: Bromphen/Ppa Dm; Delhistine Dm; Fenahistine Dm; Hi-Tuss Dm; Highland Dm; Histine Dm; Iohist Dm; Kg-Hist Dm; Liqui-Histine Dm; Poly-Dm; Poly-Histine-Dm; Polytine Dm; Trihist-Dm; Uni Multihist Dm; Uni-Multihist Dm

Prescribing information not available at time of publication.

HOW SUPPLIED - EQUIVALENTS NOT AVAILABLE:

Syrup - Oral - 2 mg/10 mg/12.5

120 ml	$7.33	HISTINEX DM, Ethex	58177-0880-03
473 ml	$24.37	Polytine Dm, Am Generics	58634-0035-01
473 ml	$24.95	Delhistine Dm, Econolab	55053-0820-16
473 ml	$25.50	Liqui-Histine Dm, Liquipharm	54198-0158-16
473 ml	$26.18	Fenahistine Dm, Tmk Pharm	59582-0448-16
480 ml	$22.50	Poly-Dm, Alphagen Labs	59743-0022-16
480 ml	$23.47	HISTINEX DM, Ethex	58177-0880-07
480 ml	$23.94	Highland Dm, Highland Pkging	55782-0103-16
480 ml	$24.12	Delhistine Dm, Rugby	00536-2903-85
480 ml	$24.88	Poly-Dm, Qualitest Pharms	00603-1529-58
480 ml	$24.95	Trihist-Dm, Cypress Pharm	60258-0237-16
480 ml	$24.95	Kg-Hist Dm, King Pharms	60793-0032-16
480 ml	$25.45	Uni Multihist Dm, United Res	00677-1511-33
480 ml	$25.50	Delhistine Dm, HL Moore Drug Exch	00839-7844-69
480 ml	$26.35	Bromphen/Ppa Dm, Major Pharms	00904-5002-16
480 ml	$27.51	Trihist-Dm, Aligen Independ	00405-3879-16
480 ml	$28.52	POLY HISTINE DM SYRUP, Bock Pharma	00563-1686-16

BUDESONIDE *(003201)*

CATEGORIES: Adrenal Corticosteroids; Airway Obstruction; Allergies; Anti-Inflammatory Agents; Antiasthmatics/Bronchodilators; Asthma; Eye, Ear, Nose, & Throat Preparations; Glucocorticoids; Respiratory & Allergy Medications; Rhinitis; FDA Class 1S ("Standard Review"); FDA Approved 1994 Feb

BRAND NAMES: *Budecort*; *Budecort Nasal*; *Budicort Respules*; *Butacort*; *Eltair*; *Nasocort*; Pulmicort; *Pulmicort Nasal Turbohaler*; **Rhinocort**
(International brand names outside U.S. in italics)

FORMULARIES: Medi-Cal; PCS

DESCRIPTION:

Budesonide, the active component of Rhinocort Nasal Inhaler, is an anti-inflammatory glucocorticosteroid. It is designated chemically as 16α, 17α-butylidene-dioxypregna-1, 4-diene-11β, 21-diol-3, 20- dione. Budesonide possesses and asymmetric carbon atom in its structure and is provided as the mixture of the two epimers, 22R and 22S. The empirical formula of budesonide is $C_{25}H_{34}O_6$and its molecular weight is 430.5.

Budesonide is a white to off-white odorless powder that is practically insoluble in water and in heptane, sparingly soluble in ethanol, and freely soluble in chloroform. Its partition coefficient between octanol and water at pH 7.4 is 1.6×10^3.

Rhinocort Nasal Inhaler is a metered-dose pressurized aerosol unit containing a suspension of micronized budesonide in a mixture of propellants, (dichlorodifluoromethane, trichloromonofluoromethane, and dichlorotetrafluoroethane) and sorbitan trioleate.

Each actuation releases 50 mcg budesonide from the valve and delivers approximately 32 mcg budesonide from the nasal adapter (dose to patient). Throughout the package insert 32 mcg per actuation is used to calculate the dose administered. One canister provides at least 200 metered doses.

CLINICAL PHARMACOLOGY:

Budesonide is a glucocorticosteroid having a potent glucocorticoid and weak mineralocorticoid activity. In standard *in vitro* and animal models, budesonide has an approximately 200 fold higher affinity for the glucocorticoid receptor and a 1000 fold higher topical anti-inflammatory potency than cortisol (rat croton oil ear edema assay). As a measure of systemic activity, budesonide is 40 times more potent than cortisol when administered subcutaneously and 25 times more potent when administered orally in the rat thymus involution assay.

The precise mechanism of glucocorticosteroid actions on allergic and nonallergic rhinitis is not known. Glucocorticotrophics have been shown to have a wide range of inhibitory activities against multiple cell types (e.g. mast cells, eosinophils, neutrophils, macrophages and lymphocytes) and mediators (*e.g.*, histamine, eicosanoids, leukotrienes and cytokines) involved in allergic and nonallergic /irritant-mediated inflammation.

Corticoids affect the delayed (6 hour) response to an allergen challenge more than the histamine-associated immediate response (20 minute). The clinical significance of these findings is unknown.

Pharmacokinetics: The pharmacokinetics of budesonide have been studied following nasal, oral and intravenous administration. Pharmacokinetic studies were performed with doses higher than those used clinically because at clinical doses the resulting plasma levels are below the limits of detection. The results are as follows:

TABLE 1

Route of Administration	T_{Max}(hr)	Mean* [range] C_{Max}** (nmol/L)	Systemic Availability ***	V_D (L)	Clearance (L/min)	
Nasal Inhaler	(N=9) [0.3-2]	0.6 [0.24-0.88]	0.52 [16-27]	21	-	-
Oral Capsule	(N=11)	1.0 [0.5-2]	0.33 [0.19-0.50]	12 [8-20]	-	-
I.V.	(N=11)	-	-	100	201 [102-275]	1.2 [0.8-1.5]

* mean of the two epimers
** dose normalized to a 256 mcg dose.
*** % of delivered dose

Only about 20% of an intranasal dose from the budesonide nasal inhaler reaches the systemic circulation.

CLINICAL PHARMACOLOGY: *(cont'd)*

While budesonide is well absorbed from the GI tract, the oral bioavailability of budesonide is low (-10%) primarily due to extensive first pass metabolism in the liver. After reaching the systemic circulation plasma levels decline in a log linear manner with an apparent elimination half-life of approximately 2 hours.

Budesonide has a volume of distribution of approximately 200 L and is 88% protein bound in the plasma. Budesonide is a mixture of two epimers, 22R and 22S. In glucocorticoid receptor affinity studies, the 22R form is two times as active as the 22S epimer. It is also preferentially cleared by the liver with an apparent systemic clearance of 1.4 +/- 0.3 L/min vs. 1.0 +/-0.2 L/min. for the 22S form. *In vitro* studies indicate that the two forms of budesonide do not interconvert.

Budesonide is rapidly and extensively metabolized in man by the liver. *In vitro* studies looking at sites of metabolism showed negligible metabolism in skin, lung, and serum. After intranasal administration of a radiolabeled dose 2/3 of the radioactivity was found in the urine and the remainder in the feces by 96 hours. The primary metabolites of budesonide in the urine following IV administration are 16α-hydroxyprednisolone (24%) and 6β-hydroxybudesonide (5%). An additional 34% of the radioactivity recovered in the urine were conjugates. No unchanged budesonide was found in the urine. These results regarding the metabolic fate of budesonide parallel results obtained in*in vitro* metabolic studies using human liver homogenates.

In vitro studies of the binding of the two primary metabolites to the glucocorticoid receptor indicate that they have less than 1% of the affinity for the receptor as the parent compound budesonide.

Pharmacodynamics: The effect of budesonide nasal inhaler at a dosage of two sprays in each nostril morning and evening (total daily dose of 256 mcg) on hypothalamic-pituitary-adrenal (HPA) axis function has been evaluated in 275 adults and 61 children following short-term use (<2 months) and in 113 adults and 116 children following longer use (6-48 months). Early morning plasma cortisol and the short cosyntropin stimulation test (30-60 minutes) were the most commonly performed assessments of HPA function.

Twenty-four hour urinary cortisol levels were determined in 50 adults (short term) and 96 children (long term). There were no statistically significant changes from baseline measurements in early morning plasma cortisol or 24-hour urinary cortisol excretion or in response to cosyntropin.

In a crossover trial using single doses of 200, 400 and 800 mcg of an aqueous formulation of budesonide administered intranasally at 10 P.M.; a dose-dependent decrease in urinary cortisol excretion was found between 10 P.M. and 8 A.M. the following morning. The same study has not been performed with budesonide nasal inhaler. However, in a study using the budesonide nasal inhaler administered at 10 P.M., doses four (1024 mcg) and eight (2048 mcg) times higher than the recommended daily dose (256 mcg) were followed by a significant decrease in plasma cortisol levels at 8 A.M. the following morning (17% and 22%, respectively).

A 3 week clinical study in seasonal rhinitis, comparing budesonide nasal inhaler and orally ingested budesonide with placebo in 98 patients with allergic rhinitis due to birch pollen, demonstrated that the therapeutic effect of budesonide can be attributed to the topical effects of budesonide. Intranasally, 128 mcg of budesonide applied twice daily (55 mcg) systemically absorbed/day) provided clinically and statistically significant evidence of efficacy, whereas 250 mcg of budesonide ingested twice a day as a capsule (65 mcg systemically absorbed/day) was no different from placebo in reducing nasal symptoms.

CLINICAL STUDIES:

The prophylactic and therapeutic efficacy of budesonide nasal inhaler has been evaluated in 20 controlled clinical trials of seasonal or perennial rhinitis. The number of patients treated with budesonide in these studies was 50 male and 33 female patients ages 6 to 12 years old, 77 males and 62 females ages 13 to 18 years old, 185 males and 246 females ages 19 to 64 and 1 male and 2 females over 64. The patients were predominantly caucasian.

Double-blind clinical trials of two to four weeks duration have shown that, compared with placebo, budesonide nasal inhaler 128 mcg b.i.d. (two sprays in each nostril morning and evening) or 256 mcg q.d. (four sprays in each nostril in the morning) provides statistically significant relief of nasal symptoms such as blockage, rhinorrhea, itching, and sneezing in adults and children with seasonal allergic rhinitis or perennial allergic rhinitis. Similar improvement has also been demonstrated in adults with nonallergic perennial rhinitis.

The therapeutic effect of budesonide nasal inhaler compared with placebo has been demonstrated by rhinoscopic examinations, in children and adults with seasonal or perennial allergic rhinitis and adults with nonallergic perennial rhinitis. Biopsies of the nasal mucosa of 50 adult patients after 12 months of treatment and of 10 patients after 3-5 years of therapy showed no histopathological evidence of adverse effects. The clinical significance of either of these findings is unknown.

Individualization of Dosages: It is recommended that the starting dose for all adults be 256 mcg daily, as either two sprays in each nostril twice per day, morning and evening, or as four sprays in each nostril once a day in the morning. The effect should be assessed 3-7 days after initiating treatment and then periodically until the patient's symptoms are stable. If adequate relief of symptoms is not achieved after 3 weeks of treatment, then budesonide nasal inhaler should be discontinued.

In patients who do achieve a good result it is desirable, once the maximum benefit seems to have been achieved, to titrate and individual patient to the minimum effective dose.

Because of the generally short duration of therapy for seasonal allergic rhinitis, it is usually not necessary to do this.

In patients with perennial allergic rhinitis, once adequate relief has been obtained the dose should be gradually decreased every 2-4 weeks as long as the desired clinical effect is maintained. If symptoms return, the dose may briefly be increased to the patient's starting dose and then returned to the dose the patient was on before symptoms reoccurred.

As with other aerosolized nasal glucocorticotrophics, the vehicle used to deliver the glucocorticosteroid may cause symptoms that are difficult to distinguish from the patient's rhinitis symptoms. The corticoid may suppress symptoms caused by the vehicle at higher doses but as the dose is decreased symptoms from the vehicle may emerge. If a patient needs chronic treatment and the daily dose can not be decreased from the starting dose, it may be advisable to try alternative therapy.

INDICATIONS AND USAGE:

Budesonide nasal inhaler is indicated for the management of symptoms of seasonal or perennial allergic rhinitis in adults and children and nonallergic perennial rhinitis in adults. Budesonide nasal inhaler is not recommended for treatment of nonallergic rhinitis in children because adequate numbers of such children have not been studied.

CONTRAINDICATIONS:

Hypersensitivity to any of the ingredients of this preparation contraindicates its use.

WARNINGS:

The replacement of a systemic glucocorticosteroid with a topical glucocorticosteroid can be accompanied by signs of adrenal insufficiency, and in addition some patients may experience symptoms of withdrawal, e.g. joint and/or muscular pain, lassitude and depression. Patients previously treated for prolonged periods with systemic glucocorticotrophics and transferred to topical glucocorticotrophics should be carefully monitored for acute adrenal insufficiency in response to stress. In those patients who have asthma or other clinical conditions requiring long-term systemic glucocorticosteroid treatment, too rapid a decrease in systemic glucocorticotrophics may cause a severe exacerbation of their symptoms.

The use of budesonide nasal inhaler with alternate-day systemic prednisone could increase the likelihood of hypothalamic-pituitary-adrenal (HPA) suppression compared with a therapeutic dose of either one alone. Therefore, budesonide nasal inhaler should be used with caution in patients already receiving alternate-day prednisone treatment for any disease. In addition, the concomitant use of budesonide nasal inhaler with other inhaled glucocorticotrophics could increase the risk of signs or symptoms of hypercorticism and/or suppression of the HPA-axis.

Patients who are on drugs which suppress the immune system are more susceptible to infections than healthy individuals. Chicken pox and measles, for example, can have a more serious or even fatal course in non-immune children or adults on immunosuppressant doses of corticosteroids. In such children or adults, who have not had these diseases, particular care should be taken to avoid exposure. How the dose, route and duration of corticosteroid administration affects the risk of developing a disseminated infection is not known. The contribution of the underlying disease and/or prior corticosteroid treatment to the risk is also not known. If exposed to chicken pox, prophylaxis with varicella zoster immune globulin (VZIG) may be indicated. If exposed to measles, prophylaxis with pooled intramuscular immunoglobulin (IG) may be indicated. If chicken pox develops, treatment with antiviral agents may be considered.

PRECAUTIONS:

GENERAL

Rarely, immediate hypersensitivity reactions or contact dermatitis may occur after the intranasal administration of budesonide. Rare instances of wheezing, nasal septum perforation and intraocular pressure have been reported following the intranasal application of aerosolized glucocorticotrophics.

Like other glucocorticotrophics, budesonide is absorbed into the circulation. Use of excessive doses of glucocorticotrophics may lead to signs or symptoms of hypercorticism, suppression of HPA function and/or suppression of growth in children or teenagers. In short term studies of the acute effect of inhaled budesonide 256 mcg/day on lower leg growth (knemometry), it like other inhaled and intramuscular corticoids which have been studied showed a decrease in the rate of lower leg growth. The clinical significance of this finding is not known. In two one-year studies in 92 children taking recommended doses of budesonide nasal inhaler, height and skeletal stature were consistent with chronological age. Physicians should closely follow the growth of children taking corticoids, by any route, and weight the benefits of corticoid therapy against the possibility of growth suppression if a child's growth appears slowed.

Although systemic effects have been minimal with recommended doses of budesonide nasal inhaler, this potential risk increases with larger doses. Therefore, larger than recommended doses of budesonide nasal inhaler should be avoided.

When used at larger doses, systemic glucocorticosteroid effects such as hypercorticism and adrenal suppression may appear. if such changes occur, the dosage of budesonide nasal inhaler should be discontinued slowly consistent with accepted procedures for discontinuing oral glucocorticosteroid therapy.

In clinical studies with budesonide administered intranasally, the development of localized infections of the nose and pharynx with *Candida albicans* has occurred only rarely. When such an infection develops, it may require treatment with appropriate local therapy and discontinuation of treatment with budesonide nasal inhaler. Patients using budesonide nasal inhaler over several months or longer should be examined periodically for evidence of *Candida* infection or other signs of adverse effects on the nasal mucosa.

Budesonide nasal inhaler should be used with caution, if at all, in patients with active of quiescent tuberculous infections, untreated fungal, bacterial, or systemic viral infections, or ocular herpes simplex.

Because of the inhibitory effect of glucocorticotrophics on wound healing, patients who have experienced recent nasal septal ulcers, nasal surgery, or nasal trauma should not use a nasal glucocorticosteroid until healing has occurred.

INFORMATION FOR THE PATIENT

Patients being treated with budesonide nasal inhaler should receive the following information and instructions:

Patients should use budesonide nasal inhaler as prescribed. A decrease in symptoms may occur as soon as 24 hours after starting glucocorticosteroid therapy and generally can be expected to occur within a few days of initiating therapy in allergic rhinitis. The patient should contact the physician if symptoms do not improve by three weeks, or if the condition worsens. Nasal irritation and/or burning after use of the spray occur only rarely with this product. The patient should contact the physician if they occur repeatedly.

Patients who are on corticosteroids should be warned to avoid exposure to chicken pox or measles. Patients should also be advised that if they are exposed, they should consult their physician without delay.

For the proper use of this unit and to attain maximum improvement, the patient should read and follow the accompanying patient instructions carefully.

CARCINOGENESIS, MUTAGENESIS, AND IMPAIRMENT OF FERTILITY

Long-term studies were conducted in mice and rats using oral administration to evaluate the carcinogenic potential of budesonide.

There was no evidence of a carcinogenic effect when budesonide was administered orally for 91 weeks to mice at doses up to 200 mcg/kg/day (600 mcg/m^2/day).

In a 104-week carcinogenicity study in Sprague-Dawley rats (41), a statistically significant increase in the incidence of gliomas was observed in male rats receiving 50 mcg/kg/day (300 mcg/m^2/day) orally; no such changes were seen in male rats receiving doses of 10 and 25 mcg/kg/day (60 and 150 mcg/kg/day) or in female rats at any dose. Two additional 104-week carcinogenicity studies have been performed with oral budesonide at doses of 50 mcg/kg/day (300 mcg/m^2/day) in male Sprague-Dawley and Fischer rats. These studies do not demonstrate and increased glioma incidence in budesonide treated animals as compared with concurrent controls or reference glucocorticosteroid treated groups (prednisolone and triamcinolone acetonide).

Compared with concurrent control male Sprague-Dawley rats there was a statistically significant increase in the incidence of hepatocellular tumors. This finding was confirmed in all three steroid groups (budesonide, prednisolone, triamcinolone acetonide) in the second study in male Sprague-Dawley rats.

PRECAUTIONS: *(cont'd)*

The mutagenic potential of budesonide was evaluated in six different test systems: Ames Salmonella/microsome plate test, mouse micronucleus test, mouse lymphoma test, chromosome aberration test in human lymphocytes, sex-linked recessive lethal test in Drosophila melanogaster, and DNA repair analysis in rat hepatocyte culture. No mutagenic or clastogenic properties of budesonide were found in any of the tests.

The effect upon fertility and general reproductive performance was studied in rats given budesonide subcutaneously. At 20 mcg/kg/day (120 mcg/m²/day) and higher dose levels, a decrease in maternal body-weight gain was observed along with a decrease in prenatal viability and viability of the young at birth and during lactation. No such effects were noted at the dose level 5 mcg/kg/day (30 mcg/m²/day).

PREGNANCY CATEGORY C

Teratogenic Effects: As with other glucocorticoids budesonide has been shown to be teratogenic and embryocidal in rabbits and rats when given subcutaneously in doses exceeding 5 and 100 mcg/kg/day (59 and 600 mcg/m²/day), respectively. In these studies budesonide at 25 mcg/kg/day (295 mcg/m²/day) given to rabbits and 500 mcg/kg/day (3000 mcg/m²/day) given to rats was found to produce fetal loss, decreased pup weights and skeletal abnormalities. No teratogenic or embryocidal effects have been seen in rats when budesonide was administered by inhalation at doses of 100-250 mcg/kg/day (600-1500 mcg/m²/day, approximately 27-68 times the human recommended starting dose based on mcg/kg/day or 4-10 times the human dose based on mcg/m²/day).

There are no adequate and well-controlled studies in pregnant women. Budesonide should be used during pregnancy only if the potential benefit justifies the potential risk to the fetus. Experience with oral glucocorticotrophics since their introduction in pharmacologic, as opposed to physiologic, doses suggests that rodents are more prone to teratogenic effects from glucocorticotrophics than humans. In addition, because there is a natural increase in glucocorticosteroid production during pregnancy, most women will require a lower exogenous glucocorticosteroid dose and many will not need glucocorticosteroid treatment during pregnancy.

Nonteratogenic Effects: Hypoadrenalism may occur in infants born of mothers receiving glucocorticotrophics during pregnancy. Such infants should be carefully observed.

NURSING MOTHERS

It is not known whether budesonide is excreted in human milk. Because other glucocorticotrophics are excreted in human milk, caution should be exercised when budesonide nasal inhaler is administered to nursing women.

PEDIATRIC USE

Safety and effectiveness in children below 6 years of age have not been established. Oral glucocorticotrophics have been shown to cause growth suppression in children and teenagers with extended use. If a child or teenager on any glucocorticosteroid appears to have growth suppression, the possibility that they are particularly sensitive to this effect of glucocorticotrophics should be considered (see PRECAUTIONS.)

ADVERSE REACTIONS:

Adverse reaction information is derived from blinded-controlled clinical trials (see CLINICAL PHARMACOLOGY, Clinical Studies), open lab studies and marketing experience. In the description below, rates of rare events are derived principally from marketing experience and publications, and accurate estimates of incidence are not possible.

The incidence of common adverse reactions is based upon controlled clinical trials in 606 patients [101 girls and 145 boys (<19 years of age) and 203 female and 157 male adults] treated with budesonide nasal inhaler 128 mcg twice daily over 2-4 weeks. The most common adverse reactions were symptoms of irritation of the nasal mucous membranes. All common adverse reactions were reported with approximately the same frequency by placebo patients suggesting the possibility that the vehicle of the rhinitis itself was responsible for the symptoms. Sneezing after use of the inhaler occurred in 2% of Rhinocort treated patients and in 11% of patients using the placebo.

Systemic glucocorticosteroid side-effects were not reported during controlled clinical studies with budesonide nasal inhaler. If recommended doses are exceeded, however, or if individuals are particularly sensitive, symptoms of hypercorticism, i.e., Cushing's syndrome, could occur.

Incidence Greater than 1%: (Based on controlled clinical trials)

Respiratory: nasal irritation*, pharyngitis*, cough increased*, epistaxis*

Digestive: dry mouth, dyspepsia

* incidence 3 to 9%; incidence of unmarked reactions 1 to 3%

Incidence Less than 1%: Causal Relationship Probable (Adverse reactions reported only in the literature or from marketing experience, and presumably rarer are *italicized)*

Respiratory: moniliasis, hoarseness, wheezing, nasal pain, *nasal septum mucosal atrophy/necrosis, nasal septum perforation.*

Special Senses: reduced sense of smell, bad taste.

Digestive: nausea.

Skin and Appendages: Facial edema, rash, pruritus, *contact dermatitis,* herpes simplex.

Incidence Less than 1%: Causal Relationship Unknown (Adverse reactions reported only in the literature or from marketing experience, and presumably rarer are *italicized*):

Respiratory: Dyspnea.

Skin and Appendages: *alopecia*

Nervous System: nervousness.

Musculoskeletal: myalgia, arthralgia

OVERDOSAGE:

Acute overdosage with this dosage form is unlikely since once canister of budesonide nasal inhaler only contains approximately 12.7 mg of budesonide. Chronic overdosage may result in signs/symptoms of hypercorticism (see WARNINGS and PRECAUTIONS).

DOSAGE AND ADMINISTRATION:

Adults and children 6 years of age and older: The recommended starting dose is 256 mcg daily, given as either two sprays in each nostril morning and evening or as four sprays in each nostril in the morning.

A decrease in symptoms may occur as soon as 24 hours after onset of treatment with budesonide nasal inhaler but generally it takes 3-7 days to reach maximum benefit.

If no improvement has been obtained by the third week of treatment with budesonide nasal inhaler, treatment should be discontinued.

After the desired clinical effect has been obtained, the maintenance dose should be reduced to the smallest amount necessary for control of symptoms (see Individualization of Dosages).

If glucocorticotrophics are discontinued when they still are needed, symptoms may not recur for several days.

DOSAGE AND ADMINISTRATION: *(cont'd)*

At recommended doses, budesonide's therapeutic effects are localized to the nose, therefore, concomitant treatment may be necessary to counteract allergic eye symptoms. Doses exceeding 256 mcg daily (4 sprays/nostril) are not recommended. Budesonide nasal inhaler is not recommended for children below 6 years of age or for children with nonallergic perennial rhinitis because adequate numbers of these children have not been studied.

Directions for Use: Illustrated Patient's Instructions for Use accompany each package of budesonide nasal inhaler and include the following:

PATIENT'S INSTRUCTIONS FOR USE

Rhinocort Nasal Inhaler: Use a pair of scissors to cut the pouch open. Read the information before using budesonide nasal inhaler. Follow the directions carefully.

1. Blow your nose. Open the nasal adapter by pressing on the arrow on the light gray part. Turn the light gray part into the dark gray transparent part until it is locked.

2. Hold the inhaler and shake it thoroughly.

3. Close one nostril by pressing your finger on the nose. Insert the extreme end of the tube into the other nostril. Hold your breath and actuate a dose by pressing on the canister. Administer the prescribed dose in the other nostril in the same way.

4. Close the nasal adapter by pressing under the tube on the light gray part. Revolve the light gray part until it comes into a locked position.

> **Warning:** Contains trichloromonofluoromethane, dichlorotetrafluoroethane, and dichlorodifluoromethane, substances which harm the environment by destroying ozone in the upper atmosphere. Your physician has determined that this product is likely to help your personal health. USE THIS PRODUCT AS DIRECTED, UNLESS INSTRUCTED TO DO OTHERWISE BY YOUR PHYSICIAN. If you have any questions about alternatives, consult with your physician.

Follow your doctor's directions and do not use budesonide nasal inhaler more often than prescribed. Contact your doctor if you find the effect budesonide nasal inhaler does not give immediate relief. Generally it will take a few days to achieve full effect. It is therefore very important that Rhinocort is used regularly morning and evening.

To be used within 6 months after the aluminum pouch has been opened. After opening the pouch, avoid storage in areas of high humidity.

Cleaning

Remove the aerosol container and wash the plastic parts regularly in warm—not hot—water with addition of mild detergent if necessary. Allow the plastic parts to dry completely and then replace the container.

Contents under pressure

Do not puncture or throw container into incinerator. Using or storing near open flame or heating above 120°F (50°C) may cause container to burst.

HOW SUPPLIED:

Rhinocort Nasal Inhaler is supplied in a 7.0 g canister containing 200 metered doses provided with a metering valve and nasal adapter together with patient's instructions for use. Each actuation delivers approximately 32 mcg of micronized budesonide from the nasal adapter to the patient.

Rhinocort Nasal Inhaler should be stored between 15°C (59°F) and 30°C (86°F) with the valve downwards. Shake well before use.

Each inhaler with actuator is packaged in an aluminum foil pouch to protect the product from moisture. After opening the aluminum pouch, the product should be used within 6 months and storage in an area of high humidity should be avoided.

Contents Under Pressure: Do not puncture. Do not use or store near heat or open flame. Exposure to temperatures above 50°C (120°F) may cause the canister to explode. Never throw the container into fire or an incinerator. Keep out of reach of children.

Note: The statement below is required by the Federal government's Clean Air Act for all products containing or manufactured with chlorofluorocarbons (CFCs).

WARNING: Contains trichloromonofluoromethane, dichlorotetrafluoroethane, and dichlorodifluoromethane, substances which mar public health and environment by destroying ozone in the upper atmosphere.

HOW SUPPLIED - EQUIVALENTS NOT AVAILABLE:

Aerosol - Nasal - 50 mcg

7 gm	$28.34	RHINOCORT, Astra USA	00186-1075-09

BUMETANIDE *(000544)*

CATEGORIES: Congestive Heart Failure; Diuretics; Edema; Electrolytic, Caloric-Water Balance; Heart Failure; Loop Diuretics; Nephrotic Syndrome; Renal Drugs; Pregnancy Category C; FDA Approved 1983 Feb; Patent Expiration 1993 Feb

BRAND NAMES: *Budema*; *Bumedyl* (Mexico); *Bumet*; *Bumetan*; **Bumex**; *Burinax*; *Burinex* (Australia, England, Germany, France); *Busix*; *Butinat*; *Butinon*; *Cambiex*; *Drenural* (Mexico); *Farmadiuril*; *Fluxil*; *Fontego*; *Fordiuran* (Germany); *Lunetoron* (Japan); *Miccil* (Mexico); *Pendock*; *Poliurene*; *Primex*; *Segurex*
(International brand names outside U.S. in italics)

FORMULARIES: Aetna; BC-BS

COST OF THERAPY: $99.20 (Edema; Tablet; 0.5 mg; 1/day; 365 days) vs. Potential Cost of $5,887.41 (Edema)

> **WARNING:**
> Bumetanide is a potent diuretic which, if given in excessive amounts, can lead to a profound diuresis with water and electrolyte depletion. Therefore, careful medical supervision is required, and dose and dosage schedule have to be adjusted to the individual patient's needs. (See DOSAGE AND ADMINISTRATION.)

DESCRIPTION:

Bumex is a loop diuretic, available as scored tablets, 0.5 mg (light green), 1 mg (yellow) and 2 mg (peach) for oral administration; each tablet also contains lactose, magnesium stearate, microcrystalline cellulose, corn starch and talc, with the following dye systems: 0.5 mg—D&C Yellow No. 10 and FD&C Blue No. 1; 1 mg—D&C Yellow No. 10; 2 mg—red iron oxide. Also as 2-ml ampuls, 2-ml vials, 4-ml vials and 10-ml vials (0.25 mg/ml) for intravenous or intramuscular injection as a sterile solution, each 2 ml of which contains 0.5 mg (0.25 mg/ml)

DESCRIPTION: *(cont'd)*

bumetanide compounded with 0.85% sodium chloride and 0.4% ammonium acetate as buffers; 0.01% edetate disodium; 1% benzyl alcohol as preservative, and pH adjusted to approximately 7 with sodium hydroxide.

Chemically, bumetanide is 3-(butylamino)-4-phenoxy-5-sulfamoylbenzoic acid. It is a practically white powder having a calculated molecular weight of 364.41.

CLINICAL PHARMACOLOGY:

Bumetandine is a loop diuretic with a rapid onset and short duration of action. Pharmacological and clinical studies have shown that 1 mg bumetandine has a diuretic potency equivalent to approximately 40 mg furosemide. The major site of bumetandine action is the ascending limb of the loop of Henle.

The mode of action has been determined through various clearance studies in both humans and experimental animals. Bumetandine inhibits sodium reabsorption in the ascending limb of the loop of Henle, as shown by marked reduction of free-water clearance (CH_2O) during hydration and tubular free-water reabsorption (T^cH_2O) during hydropenia. Reabsorption of chloride in the ascending limb is also blocked by bumetandine, and bumetandine is somewhat more chloruretic than natriuretic.

Potassium excretion is also increased by bumetandine, in a dose-related fashion.

Bumetandine may have an additional action in the proximal tubule. Since phosphate reabsorption takes place largely in the proximal tubule, phosphaturia during bumetandine-induced diuresis is indicative of this additional action. This is further supported by the reduction in the renal clearance of bumetandine by probenecid, associated with diminution in the natriuretic response. This proximal tubular activity does not seem to be related to an inhibition of carbonic anhydrase. Bumetandine does not appear to have a noticeable action on the distal tubule.

Bumetandine decreases uric acid excretion and increases serum uric acid. Following oral administration of bumetandine the onset of diuresis occurs in 30 to 60 minutes. Peak activity is reached between 1 and 2 hours. At usual doses (1 to 2 mg) diuresis is largely complete within 4 hours; with higher doses, the diuretic action lasts for 4 to 6 hours. Diuresis starts within minutes following an intravenous injection and reaches maximum levels within 15 to 30 minutes.

Several pharmacokinetic studies have shown that bumetandine, administered orally or parenterally, is eliminated rapidly in humans, with a half-life of between 1 and 1.5 hours. Plasma protein-binding is in the range of 94% to 96%.

Oral administration of carbon-14 labeled bumetandine to human volunteers revealed that 81% of the administered radioactivity was excreted in the urine, 45% of it as unchanged drug. Urinary and biliary metabolites identified in this study were formed by oxidation of the N-butyl side chain. Biliary excretion of bumetandine amounted to only 2% of the administered dose.

INDICATIONS AND USAGE:

Bumetandine is indicated for the treatment of edema associated with congestive heart failure, hepatic and renal disease, including the nephrotic syndrome.

Almost equal diuretic response occurs after oral and parenteral administration of bumetandine. Therefore, if impaired gastrointestinal absorption is suspected or oral administration is not practical, bumetandine should be given by the intramuscular or intravenous route.

Successful treatment with bumetandine following instances of allergic reactions to furosemide suggests a lack of cross-sensitivity.

CONTRAINDICATIONS:

Bumetandine is contraindicated in anuria. Although bumetandine can be used to induce diuresis in renal insufficiency, any marked increase in blood urea nitrogen or creatinine, or the development of oliguria during therapy of patients with progressive renal disease, is an indication for discontinuation of treatment with bumetandine. Bumetandine is also contraindicated in patients in hepatic coma or in states of severe electrolyte depletion until the condition is improved or corrected. Bumetandine is contraindicated in patients hypersensitive to this drug.

WARNINGS:

1. Volume and electrolyte depletion: The dose of bumetandine should be adjusted to the patient's need. Excessive doses or too frequent administration can lead to profound water loss, electrolyte depletion, dehydration, reduction in blood volume and circulatory collapse with the possibility of vascular thrombosis and embolism, particularly in elderly patients.

2. Hypokalemia: Hypokalemia can occur as a consequence of bumetandine administration. Prevention of hypokalemia requires particular attention in the following conditions: patients receiving digitalis and diuretics for congestive heart failure, hepatic cirrhosis and ascites, states of aldosterone excess with normal renal function, potassium-losing nephropathy, certain diarrheal states, or other states where hypokalemia is thought to represent particular added risks to the patient, *i.e.,* history of ventricular arrhythmias. In patients with hepatic cirrhosis and ascites, sudden alterations of electrolyte balance may precipitate hepatic encephalopathy and coma. Treatment in such patients is best initiated in the hospital with small doses and careful monitoring of the patient's clinical status and electrolyte balance. Supplemental potassium and/or spironolactone may prevent hypokalemia and metabolic alkalosis in these patients.

3. Ototoxicity: In cats, dogs and guinea pigs, bumetandine has been shown to produce ototoxicity. In these test animals bumetandine was 5 to 6 times more potent than furosemide and, since the diuretic potency of bumetandine is about 40 to 60 times furosemide, it is anticipated that blood levels necessary to produce ototoxicity will rarely be achieved. The potential exists, however, and must be considered a risk of intravenous therapy, especially at high doses, repeated frequently in the face of renal excretory function impairment. Potentiation of aminoglycoside ototoxicity has not been tested for bumetandine. Like other members of this class of diuretics, bumetandine probably shares this risk.

4. Allergy to sulfonamides: Patients allergic to sulfonamides may show hypersensitivity to bumetandine.

5. Thrombocytopenia: Since there have been rare spontaneous reports of thrombocytopenia from postmarketing experience, patients should be observed regularly for possible occurrence of thrombocytopenia.

PRECAUTIONS:

General: Serum potassium should be measured periodically and potassium supplements or potassium-sparing diuretics added if necessary. Periodic determinations of other electrolytes are advised in patients treated with high doses or for prolonged periods, particularly in those on low salt diets.

Hyperuricemia may occur; it has been asymptomatic in cases reported to date. Reversible elevations of the BUN and creatinine may also occur, especially in association with dehydration and particularly in patients with renal insufficiency. Bumetandine may increase urinary calcium excretion with resultant hypocalcemia.

PRECAUTIONS: *(cont'd)*

Diuretics have been shown to increase the urinary excretion of magnesium; this may result in hypomagnesemia.

Laboratory Tests: Studies in normal subjects receiving bumetandine revealed no adverse effects on glucose tolerance, plasma insulin, glucagon and growth hormone levels, but the possibility of an effect on glucose metabolism exists. Periodic determinations of blood sugar should be done, particularly in patients with diabetes or suspected latent diabetes.

Patients under treatment should be observed regularly for possible occurrence of blood dyscrasias, liver damage or idiosyncratic reactions, which have been reported occasionally in foreign marketing experience. The relationship of these occurrences to bumetandine use is not certain.

Carcinogenesis, Mutagenesis, and Impairment of Fertility: Bumetandine was devoid of mutagenic activity in various strains of *Salmonella typhimurium* when tested in the presence or absence of an *in vitro* metabolic activation system. An 18-month study showed an increase in mammary adenomas of questionable significance in female rats receiving oral doses of 60 mg/kg/day (2000 times a 2-mg human dose). A repeat study at the same doses failed to duplicate this finding.

Reproduction studies were performed to evaluate general reproductive performance and fertility in rats at oral dose levels of 10, 30, 60 or 100 mg/kg/day. The pregnancy rate was slightly decreased in the treated animals; however, the differences were small and not statistically significant.

Pregnancy, Teratogenic Effects, Pregnancy Category C: Bumetandine is neither teratogenic nor embryocidal in mice when given in doses up to 3400 times the maximum human therapeutic dose.

Bumetandine has been shown to be nonteratogenic, but it has a slight embryocidal effect in rats when given in doses of 3400 times the maximum human therapeutic dose and in rabbits at doses of 3.4 times the maximum human therapeutic dose. In one study, moderate growth retardation and increased incidence of delayed ossification of sternebrae were observed in rats at oral doses of 100 mg/kg/day, 3400 times the maximum human therapeutic dose. These effects were associated with maternal weight reductions noted during dosing. No such adverse effects were observed at 30 mg/kg/day (1000 times the maximum human therapeutic dose). No fetotoxicity was observed at 1000 to 2000 times the human therapeutic dose.

In rabbits, a dose-related decrease in litter size and an increase in resorption rate were noted at oral doses of 0.1 and 0.3 mg/kg/day (3.4 and 10 times the maximum human therapeutic dose). A slightly increased incidence of delayed ossification of sternebrae occurred at 0.3 mg/kg/day; however, no such adverse effects were observed at the dose of 0.03 mg/kg/day. The sensitivity of the rabbit to bumetandine parallels the marked pharmacologic and toxicologic effects of the drug in this species.

Bumetandine was not teratogenic in the hamster at an oral dose of 0.5 mg/kg/day (17 times the maximum human therapeutic dose). Bumetandine was not teratogenic when given intravenously to mice and rats at doses up to 140 times the maximum human therapeutic dose.

There are no adequate and well-controlled studies in pregnant women. A small investigational experience in the United States and marketing experience in other countries to date have not indicated any evidence of adverse effects on the fetus, but these data do not rule out the possibility of harmful effects. Bumetandine should be given to a pregnant woman only if the potential benefit justifies the potential risk to the fetus.

Nursing Mothers: It is not known whether this drug is excreted in human milk. As a general rule, nursing should not be undertaken while the patient is on bumetandine since it may be excreted in human milk.

Pediatric Use: Safety and effectiveness in children below the age of 18 have not been established.

DRUG INTERACTIONS:

1. Drugs with ototoxic potential (see WARNINGS): Especially in the presence of impaired renal function, the use of parenterally administered bumetandine in patients to whom aminoglycoside antibiotics are also being given should be avoided, except in life-threatening conditions.

2. Drugs with nephrotoxic potential: There has been no experience on the concurrent use of bumetandine with drugs known to have a nephrotoxic potential. Therefore, the simultaneous administration of these drugs should be avoided.

3. Lithium: Lithium should generally not be given with diuretics (such as bumetandine) because they reduce its renal clearance and add a high risk of lithium toxicity.

4. Probenecid: Pretreatment with probenecid reduces both the natriuresis and hyperreninemia produced by bumetandine. This antagonistic effect of probenecid on bumetandine natriuresis is not due to a direct action on sodium excretion but is probably secondary to its inhibitory effect on renal tubular secretion of bumetanide. Thus, probenecid should not be administered concurrently with bumetandine.

5. Indomethacin: Indomethacin blunts the increases in urine volume and sodium excretion seen during bumetandine treatment and inhibits the bumetanide-induced increase in plasma renin activity. Concurrent therapy with bumetandine is thus not recommended.

6. Antihypertensives: Bumetandine may potentiate the effect of various antihypertensive drugs, necessitating a reduction in the dosage of these drugs.

7. Digoxin: Interaction studies in humans have shown no effect on digoxin blood levels.

8. Anticoagulants: Interaction studies in humans have shown bumetandine to have no effect on warfarin metabolism or on plasma prothrombin activity.

ADVERSE REACTIONS:

The most frequent clinical adverse reactions considered probably or possibly related to bumetandine are muscle cramps (seen in 1.1% of treated patients), dizziness (1.1%), hypotension (0.8%), headache (0.6%), nausea (0.6%), and encephalopathy (in patients with preexisting liver disease) (0.6%). One or more of these adverse reactions have been reported in approximately 4.1% of bumetandine (bumetandine-treated) patients.

Less frequent clinical adverse reactions to bumetandine are impaired hearing (0.5%), pruritus (0.4%), electrocardiogram changes (0.4%), weakness (0.2%), hives (0.2%), abdominal pain (0.2%), arthritic pain (0.2%), musculoskeletal pain (0.2%), rash (0.2%) and vomiting (0.2%). One or more of these adverse reactions have been reported in approximately 2.9% of bumetandine-treated patients.

Other clinical adverse reactions, which have each occurred in approximately 0.1% of patients, are vertigo, chest pain, ear discomfort, fatigue, dehydration, sweating, hyperventilation, dry mouth, upset stomach, renal failure, asterixis, itching, nipple tenderness, diarrhea, premature ejaculation and difficulty maintaining an erection.

Laboratory abnormalities reported have included hyperuricemia (in 18.4% of patients tested), hypochloremia (14.9%), hypokalemia (14.7%), azotemia (10.6%), hyponatremia (9.2%), increased serum creatinine (7.4%), hyperglycemia (6.6%), and variations in phosphorus (4.5%), CO_2 content (4.3%), bicarbonate (3.1%) and calcium (2.4%). Although manifestations of the pharmacologic action of bumetandine, these conditions may become more pronounced by intensive therapy.

ADVERSE REACTIONS: *(cont'd)*

Also reported have been thrombocytopenia (0.2%) and deviations in hemoglobin (0.8%), prothrombin time (0.8%), hematocrit (0.6%), WBC (0.3%) and differential counts (0.1%). There have been rare spontaneous reports of thrombocytopenia from postmarketing experience.

Diuresis induced by bumetandine may also rarely be accompanied by changes in LDH (1.0%), total serum bilirubin (0.8%), serum proteins (0.7%), SGOT (0.6%), SGPT (0.5%), alkaline phosphatase (0.4%), cholesterol (0.4%) and creatinine clearance (0.3%). Increases in urinary glucose (0.7%) and urinary protein (0.3%) have also been seen.

OVERDOSAGE:

Overdosage can lead to acute profound water loss, volume and electrolyte depletion, dehydration, reduction of blood volume and circulatory collapse with a possibility of vascular thrombosis and embolism. Electrolyte depletion may be manifested by weakness, dizziness, mental confusion, anorexia, lethargy, vomiting and cramps. Treatment consists of replacement of fluid and electrolyte losses by careful monitoring of the urine and electrolyte output and serum electrolyte levels.

DOSAGE AND ADMINISTRATION:

Dosage should be individualized with careful monitoring of patient response.

Oral Administration: The usual total daily dosage of bumetandine is 0.5 to 2 mg and in most patients is given as a single dose.

If the diuretic response to an initial dose of bumetandine is not adequate, in view of its rapid onset and short duration of action, a second or third dose may be given at 4- to 5-hour intervals up to a maximum daily dose of 10 mg. An intermittent dose schedule, whereby bumetandine is given on alternate days or for 3 to 4 days with rest periods of 1 to 2 days in between, is recommended as the safest and most effective method for the continued control of edema. In patients with hepatic failure, the dosage should be kept to a minimum, and if necessary, dosage increased very carefully.

Because cross-sensitivity with furosemide has rarely been observed, bumetandine can be substituted at approximately a 1:40 ratio of bumetandine to furosemide in patients allergic to furosemide.

Parenteral Administration: Bumetandine may be administered parenterally (IV or IM) to patients in whom gastrointestinal absorption may be impaired or in whom oral administration is not practical.

Parenteral treatment should be terminated and oral treatment instituted as soon as possible.

The usual initial dose is 0.5 to 1 mg intravenously or intramuscularly. Intravenous administration should be given over a period of 1 to 2 minutes. If the response to an initial dose is deemed insufficient, a second or third dose may be given at intervals of 2 to 3 hours, but should not exceed a daily dosage of 10 mg.

Miscibility and Parenteral Solutions: The compatibility tests of bumetandine injection (0.25 mg/ml, 2-ml ampuls) with 5% dextrose in water, 0.9% sodium chloride, and lactated Ringer's solution in both glass and plasticized PVC (Viaflex) containers have shown no significant absorption effect with either containers, nor a measurable loss of potency due to degradation of the drug. However, solutions should be freshly prepared and used within 24 hours.

Parenteral drug products should be inspected visually for particulate matter and discoloration prior to administration whenever solution and container permit.

HOW SUPPLIED:

Tablets , 0.5 mg (light green), bottles of 100 and 500; Tel-E-Dose packages of 100. 1 mg (yellow), bottles of 100 and 500; Tel-E-Dose packages of 100. 2 mg (peach), bottles of 100; Tel-E-Dose packages of 100.

Imprint on tablets: 0.5 mg-ROCHE BUMEX 0.5; 1 mg-ROCHE BUMEX 1; 2 mg-ROCHE BUMEX 2.

Ampuls (0.25 mg/ml), 2 ml, boxes of 10.

Vials (0.25 mg/ml, 2 ml, boxes of 10; 4 ml, boxes of 10; 10 ml, boxes of 10.

Store all tablets, vials and ampuls at 59° to 86°F.

(Roche, 4/93, 13-06-72913-0493, 13-20-72913-0493)

HOW SUPPLIED - RATED THERAPEUTICALLY EQUIVALENT:

Injection, Solution - Intramuscular; - 0.25 mg/ml

2 ml x 10	$16.20	Bumetanide, Bedford Labs	55390-0500-02
2 ml x 10	**$17.75**	**BUMEX, Roche**	**00004-1944-06**
2 ml x 10	**$17.75**	**BUMEX, Roche**	**00004-1968-01**
4 ml x 10	$27.00	Bumetanide, Bedford Labs	55390-0500-05
4 ml x 10	**$29.80**	**BUMEX, Roche**	**00004-1969-01**
10 ml x 10	$76.80	Bumetanide, Bedford Labs	55390-0500-10
10 ml x 10	**$84.16**	**BUMEX, Roche**	**00004-1970-01**

Tablet, Uncoated - Oral - 0.5 mg

100's	$27.18	Bumetanide, Zenith Labs	00172-4232-60
100's	$27.19	Bumetanide, Rugby	00536-3374-01
100's	$28.02	Bumetanide, Mylan	00378-0245-01
100's	$29.18	Bumetanide, Goldline Labs	00182-2615-89
100's	**$30.22**	**BUMEX, Roche**	**00004-0125-01**
100's	**$32.43**	**BUMEX, Roche**	**00004-0125-49**
500's	$125.58	Bumetanide, Zenith Labs	00172-4232-70
500's	**$139.56**	**BUMEX, Roche**	**00004-0125-14**
1000's	$238.60	Bumetanide, Zenith Labs	00172-4232-80
5000's	**$1253.20**	**BUMEX, Roche**	**00004-0125-11**

Tablet, Uncoated - Oral - 1 mg

100's	$38.15	Bumetanide, Zenith Labs	00172-4233-60
100's	$38.18	Bumetanide, Rugby	00536-3375-01
100's	$39.14	Bumetanide, Mylan	00378-0370-01
100's	$40.15	Bumetanide, Goldline Labs	00182-2616-89
100's	**$42.42**	**BUMEX, Roche**	**00004-0121-01**
100's	**$44.67**	**BUMEX, Roche**	**00004-0121-49**
500's	$176.85	Bumetanide, Zenith Labs	00172-4233-70
500's	**$196.53**	**BUMEX, Roche**	**00004-0121-14**
1000's	$336.00	Bumetanide, Zenith Labs	00172-4233-80
5000's	**$1764.90**	**BUMEX, Roche**	**00004-0121-11**

Tablet, Uncoated - Oral - 2 mg

100's	$64.53	Bumetanide, Zenith Labs	00172-4234-60
100's	$64.56	Bumetanide, Rugby	00536-3376-01
100's	$66.51	Bumetanide, Mylan	00378-0417-01
100's	$66.57	Bumetanide, Goldline Labs	00182-2617-89
100's	**$71.74**	**BUMEX, Roche**	**00004-0162-01**
100's	**$73.97**	**BUMEX, Roche**	**00004-0162-07**
1000's	$610.00	Bumetanide, Zenith Labs	00172-4234-80
5000's	**$3062.40**	**BUMEX, Roche**	**00004-0162-11**

HOW SUPPLIED - NOT RATED EQUIVALENT:

Injection, Solution - Intramuscular; - 0.25 mg/ml

4 ml x 10	$25.20	Bumetanide, Sanofi Winthrop	00024-1012-10

BUPIVACAINE HYDROCHLORIDE *(000545)*

CATEGORIES: Anesthesia; Caudal; Epidural; Injectable Anesthetics; Local Anesthetics; Spinal Anesthetics; Pregnancy Category C; FDA Approval Pre 1982

BRAND NAMES: *Bucain* (Germany); *Bupirop*; Bupivacaine HCl; *Bupivan*; *Buvacaina* (Mexico); *Carbostesin* (Germany); *Macaine*; *Marcain* (Australia, England); **Marcaine**; *Marcaine Plain*; *Markain*; *Picain*; *Pucaine*; Sensorcaine
(International brand names outside U.S. in italics)

FORMULARIES: WHO

DESCRIPTION:

Bupivacaine hydrochloride (abbreviated here as bupivacaine HCl), injections are sterile isotonic solutions that contain a local anesthetic agent with and without epinephrine (as bitartrate) 1:200,000 and are administered parenterally by injection. See INDICATIONS AND USAGE for specific uses. Solutions of bupivacaine HCl may be autoclaved if they do not contain epinephrine.

Bupivacaine HCl injections contain bupivacaine HCl which is chemically designated as 2-piperidinecarboxamide, 1-butyl-N-(2,6-dimethylphenyl)-monohydrochloride, monohydrate.

Epinephrine is (-)-3,4-Dihydroxy-α[(methylamino)methyl] benzyl alcohol.

The pKa of bupivacaine (8.1) is similar to that of lidocaine (7.86). However, bupivacaine possesses a greater degree of lipid solubility and is protein bound to a greater extent than lidocaine.

Bupivacaine is related chemically and pharmacologically to the aminoacyl local anesthetics. It is a homologue of mepivacaine and is chemically related to lidocaine. All three of these anesthetics contain an amide linkage between the aromatic nucleus and the amino or piperidine group. They differ in this respect from the procaine-type local anesthetics, which have an ester linkage. **Dosage forms listed as Bupivacaine HCl-MPF indicates single dose solutions that are Methyl Paraben Free (MPF).**

Bupivacaine HCl-MPF is a sterile isotonic solution containing sodium chloride. Bupivacaine HCl in multiple dose vials, each ml also contains 1 mg methylparaben as antiseptic preservative. The pH of these solutions is adjusted to between 4.0 and 6.5 with sodium hydroxide and/or hydrochloric acid.

Bupivacaine HCl-MPF with Epinephrine 1:200,000 (as bitartrate) is a sterile isotonic solution containing sodium chloride. Each ml contains bupivacaine hydrochloride and 0.005 mg epinephrine, with 0.5 mg sodium metabisulfite as an antioxidant and 0.2 mg citric acid (anhydrous) as stabilizer. Bupivacaine HCl with Epinephrine 1:200,000 (as bitartrate) in multiple dose vials, each ml also contains 1 mg methylparaben as antiseptic preservative. The pH of these solutions is adjusted to between 3.3 to 5.5 with sodium hydroxide and/or hydrochloric acid. Filled under nitrogen.

Note: The user should have an appreciation and awareness of the formulations and their intended uses. (See DOSAGE AND ADMINISTRATION.)

CLINICAL PHARMACOLOGY:

Local anesthetics block the generation and the conduction of nerve impulses, presumably by increasing the threshold for electrical excitation in the nerve, by slowing the propagation of the nerve impulse, and by reducing the rate rise of the action potential. In general, the progression of anesthesia is related to the diameter, myelination and conduction velocity of affected nerve fibers. Clinically, the order of loss of nerve function is as follows: (1) pain, (2) temperature, (3) touch, (4) proprioception, and (5) skeletal muscle tone.

Systemic absorption of local anesthetics produces effects on the cardiovascular and central nervous systems. At blood concentrations achieved with therapeutic doses, changes in cardiac conduction, excitability, refractoriness, contractility, and peripheral vascular resistance are minimal. However, toxic blood concentrations depress cardiac conduction and excitability, which may lead to atrioventricular block, ventricular arrhythmias and to cardiac arrest, sometimes resulting in fatalities. In addition, myocardial contractility is depressed and peripheral vasodilation occurs, leading to decreased cardiac output and arterial blood pressure. Recent clinical reports and animal research suggest that these cardiovascular changes are more likely to occur after unintended intravascular injection of bupivacaine. Therefore, incremental dosing is necessary.

Following systemic absorption, local anesthetics can produce central nervous system stimulation, depression or both. Apparent central stimulation is usually manifested as restlessness, tremors and shivering, progressing to convulsions, followed by depression and coma, progressing ultimately to respiratory arrest. However, the local anesthetics have a primary depressant effect on the medulla and on higher centers. The depressed stage may occur without a prior excited stage.

Pharmacokinetics: The rate of systemic absorption of local anesthetics is dependent upon the total dose and concentration of drug administered, the route of administration, the vascularity of the administration site, and the presence or absence of epinephrine in the anesthetic solution. A dilute concentration of epinephrine (1:200,000 or 5 mcg/ml) usually reduces the rate of absorption and peak plasma concentration of bupivacaine, permitting the use of moderately larger total doses and sometimes prolonging the duration of action.

The onset of action with bupivacaine is rapid and anesthesia is long-lasting. The duration of anesthesia is significantly longer with bupivacaine than with any other commonly used local anesthetic. It has also been noted that there is a period of analgesia that persists after the return of sensation, during which time the need for potent analgesics is reduced.

Local anesthetics are bound to plasma proteins in varying degrees. Generally, the lower the plasma concentration of drug, the higher the percentage of drug bound to plasma proteins.

Local anesthetics appear to cross the placenta by passive diffusion. The rate and degree of diffusion is governed by: (1) the degree of plasma protein binding, (2) the degree of ionization, and (3) the degree of lipid solubility. Fetal/maternal ratios of local anesthetics appear to be inversely related to the degree of plasma protein binding, because only the free, unbound drug is available for placental transfer. Bupivacaine, with a high protein binding capacity (95%), has a low fetal/maternal ratio (0.2-0.4). The extent of placental transfer is also determined by the degree of ionization and lipid solubility of the drug. Lipid soluble, nonionized drugs readily enter the fetal blood from the maternal circulation.

Depending upon the route of administration, local anesthetics are distributed to some extent to all body tissues, with high concentrations found in highly perfused organs such as the liver, lungs, heart, and brain.

Pharmacokinetic studies on the plasma profile of bupivacaine after direct intravenous injection suggest a three-compartment open model. The first compartment is represented by the rapid intravascular distribution of the drug. The second compartment represents the equilibration of the drug throughout the highly perfused organs such as the brain, myocardium, lungs, kidneys, and liver. The third compartment represents an equilibration of the

CLINICAL PHARMACOLOGY: *(cont'd)*

drug with poorly perfused tissues, such as muscle and fat. The elimination of drug from tissue depends largely upon the ability of binding sites in the circulation to carry it to the liver where it is metabolized.

After injection of bupivacaine HCl injection for caudal, epidural or peripheral nerve block in man, peak levels of bupivacaine in the blood are reached in 30 to 45 minutes, followed by a decline to insignificant levels during the next 3 to 6 hours.

Various pharmacokinetic parameters of the local anesthetics can be significantly altered by the presence of hepatic or renal disease, addition of epinephrine, factors affecting urinary pH, renal blood flow, the route of drug administration, and the age of the patient. The half-life of bupivacaine in adults is 3.5 ± 2.0 hours and in neonates 8.1 hours.

Amide-type local anesthetics such as bupivacaine are metabolized primarily in the liver via conjugation with glucuronic acid.

Patients with hepatic disease, especially those with severe hepatic disease, may be more susceptible to the potential toxicities of the amide-type local anesthetics. The major metabolite of bupivacaine is 2,6-pipecoloxylidine.

The kidney is the main excretory organ for most local anesthetics and their metabolites. Urinary excretion is affected by renal perfusion and factors affecting urinary pH. Only 5% of bupivacaine is excreted unchanged in the urine.

When administered in recommended doses and concentrations, bupivacaine HCl injection does not ordinarily produce irritation or tissue damage and does not cause methemoglobinemia.

INDICATIONS AND USAGE:

Bupivacaine HCl injection is indicated for the production of local or regional anesthesia or analgesia for surgery, for oral surgery procedures, for diagnostic and therapeutic procedures, and for obstetrical procedures. Only the 0.25% and 0.5% concentrations are indicated for obstetrical anesthesia. (See WARNINGS.)

Experience with non-obstetrical surgical procedures in pregnant patients is not sufficient to recommend use of the 0.75% concentration in these patients. Bupivacaine HCl injection is not recommended for intravenous regional anesthesia (Bier Block). See WARNINGS.

The routes of administration and indicated bupivacaine HCl concentrations are (TABLE 1):

TABLE 1

local infiltration	0.25%	sympathetic block	0.25%
peripheral nerve block	0.25%, 0.5%	lumber epidural	0.25% 0.5% and 0.75% (non-obstetrical)
retrobulbar block	0.75%	caudal	0.25%, 0.5%
epidural test dose (see PRECAUTIONS)			

See DOSAGE AND ADMINISTRATION for additional information. Standard textbooks should be consulted to determine the accepted procedures and techniques for the administration of bupivacaine HCl.

Use only the single dose ampules and single dose vials for caudal or epidural anesthesia, the multiple dose vials contain a preservative and, therefore, should not be used for these procedures.

CONTRAINDICATIONS:

Bupivacaine HCl injection is contraindicated in obstetrical paracervical block anesthesia. Its use by this technique has resulted in fetal bradycardia and death.

Bupivacaine HCl is contraindicated in patients with a known hypersensitivity to it or to any local anesthetic agent of the amide type or to other components of bupivacaine solutions.

WARNINGS:

THE 0.75% CONCENTRATION OF BUPIVACAINE HYDROCHLORIDE INJECTION IS NOT RECOMMENDED FOR OBSTETRICAL ANESTHESIA. THERE HAVE BEEN REPORTS OF CARDIAC ARREST WITH DIFFICULT RESUSCITATION OR DEATH DURING USE OF BUPIVACAINE FOR EPIDURAL ANESTHESIA IN OBSTETRICAL PATIENTS. IN MOST CASES, THIS HAS FOLLOWED USE OF THE 0.75% CONCENTRATION. RESUSCITATION HAS BEEN DIFFICULT OR IMPOSSIBLE DESPITE APPARENTLY ADEQUATE PREPARATION AND APPROPRIATE MANAGEMENT. CARDIAC ARREST HAS OCCURRED AFTER CONVULSIONS RESULTING FROM SYSTEMIC TOXICITY, PRESUMABLY FOLLOWING UNINTENTIONAL INTRAVASCULAR INJECTION. THE 0.75% CONCENTRATION SHOULD BE RESERVED FOR SURGICAL PROCEDURES WHERE A HIGH DEGREE OF MUSCLE RELAXATION AND PROLONGED EFFECT ARE NECESSARY.

LOCAL ANESTHETICS SHOULD ONLY BE EMPLOYED BY CLINICIANS WHO ARE WELL VERSED IN DIAGNOSIS AND MANAGEMENT OF DOSE-RELATED TOXICITY AND OTHER ACUTE EMERGENCIES WHICH MIGHT ARISE FROM THE BLOCK TO BE EMPLOYED, AND THEN ONLY AFTER INSURING THE *IMMEDIATE* AVAILABILITY OF OXYGEN, OTHER RESUSCITATIVE DRUGS, CARDIOPULMONARY RESUSCITATIVE EQUIPMENT, AND THE PERSONNEL RESOURCES NEEDED FOR PROPER MANAGEMENT OF TOXIC REACTIONS AND RELATED EMERGENCIES. (See also ADVERSE REACTIONS, PRECAUTIONS, and OVERDOSAGE.)DELAY IN PROPER MANAGEMENT OF DOSE-RELATED TOXICITY, UNDERVENTILATION FROM ANY CAUSE AND/OR ALTERED SENSITIVITY MAY LEAD TO THE DEVELOPMENT OF ACIDOSIS, CARDIAC ARREST AND, POSSIBLY, DEATH.

Local anesthetic solutions containing antimicrobial preservatives (*i.e.,* those supplied in multiple dose vials) should not be used for epidural or caudal anesthesia because safety has not been established with regard to intrathecal injection, either intentional or unintentional, of such preservatives.

It is essential that aspiration for blood or cerebrospinal fluid (where applicable) be done prior to injecting any local anesthetic, both the original dose and all subsequent doses, to avoid intravascular or subarachnoid injection. However, a negative aspiration does *not* ensure against an intravascular or subarachnoid injection.

Bupivacaine and epinephrine injection or other vasopressors should not be used concomitantly with ergot-type oxytocic drugs, because a severe persistent hypertension may occur. Likewise, solutions of bupivacaine containing a vasoconstrictor, such as epinephrine, should be used with extreme caution in patients receiving monoamine oxidase (MAO) inhibitors or antidepressants of the triptyline or imipramine types, because severe prolonged hypertension may result.

WARNINGS: *(cont'd)*

Until further experience is gained in children younger than 12 years, administration of bupivacaine in this age group is not recommended.

Reports of cardiac arrest and death have occurred with the use of bupivacaine for intravenous regional anesthesia (Bier Block). Information on safe dosages or techniques of administration of this product are lacking; therefore, bupivacaine is not recommended for use by this technique.

Prior use of chloroprocaine may interfere with subsequent use of bupivacaine. Because of this, and because safety of intercurrent use of bupivacaine and chloroprocaine has not been established, such use is not recommended.

Bupivacaine HCl with epinephrine solutions contain sodium metabisulfite, a sulfite that may cause allergic-type reactions including anaphylactic symptoms and life-threatening or less severe asthmatic episodes in certain susceptible people. The overall prevalence of sulfite sensitivity in the general population is unknown and probably low. Sulfite sensitivity is seen more frequently in asthmatic than in nonasthmatic people.

PRECAUTIONS:

General: The safety and effectiveness of the local anesthetics depend on proper dosage, correct technique, adequate precautions, and readiness for emergencies. Resuscitative equipment, oxygen, and other resuscitative drugs should be available for immediate use. (See WARNINGS, ADVERSE REACTIONS, and OVERDOSAGE.) During major regional nerve blocks, the patient should have IV fluids running via an indwelling catheter to assure a functioning intravenous pathway. The lowest dosage of local anesthetic that results in effective anesthesia should be used to avoid high plasma levels and serious adverse effects. The rapid injection of a large volume of local anesthetic solution should be avoided and fractional (incremental) doses should be used when feasible.

Epidural Anesthesia: During epidural administration of bupivacaine, concentrated solutions (0.5-0.75%) should be administered in incremental doses of 3 to 5 ml with sufficient time between doses to detect toxic manifestations of unintentional intravascular or intrathecal injection. Syringe aspirations should also be performed before and during each supplemental injection in continuous (intermittent) catheter techniques. An intravascular injection is still possible even if aspirations for blood are negative.

During the administration of epidural anesthesia, it is recommended that a test dose be administered initially and the effect monitored before the full dose is given. When using a "continuous" catheter technique, test doses should be given prior to both the original and all reinforcing doses, because plastic tubing in the epidural space can migrate into a blood vessel or through the dura. When clinical conditions permit, the test dose should contain epinephrine (10 to 15 mcg have been suggested) to serve as a warning of unintentional intravascular injection. If injected into a blood vessel, this amount of epinephrine is likely to produce a transient "epinephrine response" within 45 seconds, consisting of an increase in heart rate and systolic blood pressure, circumoral pallor, palpitations and nervousness in the unsedated patient. The sedated patient may exhibit only a pulse rate increase of 20 or more beats per minute for 15 or more seconds. Therefore, following the test dose, the heart rate should be monitored for a heart rate increase. Patients on beta-blockers may not manifest changes in heart rate, but blood pressure monitoring can detect an evanescent rise in systolic blood pressure. The test dose should also contain 10 to 15 mg of bupivacaine HCl injection or an equivalent dose of a short acting amide anesthetic such as 30 to 40 mg of lidocaine, to detect an unintentional intrathecal administration. This will be manifested within a few minutes by signs of spinal block (*e.g.,* decreased sensation of the buttocks, paresis of the legs, or, in the sedated patient, absent knee jerk). An intravascular or subarachnoid injection is still possible even if results of the test dose are negative. The test dose itself may produce a systemic toxic reaction, high spinal or epinephrine-induced cardiovascular effects.

Injection of repeated doses of local anesthetics may cause significant increases in plasma levels with each repeated dose due to slow accumulation of the drug or its metabolites or to slow metabolic degradation. Tolerance to elevated blood levels varies with the physical condition of the patient. Debilitated, elderly patients, acutely ill patients and children should be given reduced doses commensurate with their age and physical condition. Local anesthetics should also be used with caution in patients with hypotension or heart block.

Careful and constant monitoring of cardiovascular and respiratory vital signs (adequacy of ventilation) and the patient's state of consciousness should be performed after each local anesthetic injection. It should be kept in mind at such times that restlessness, anxiety, incoherent speech, light-headedness, numbness and tingling of the mouth and lips, metallic taste, tinnitus, dizziness, blurred vision, tremors, twitching, depression, or drowsiness may be early warning signs of central nervous system toxicity.

Local anesthetic solutions containing a vasoconstrictor should be used cautiously and in carefully restricted quantities in areas of the body supplied by end arteries or having otherwise compromised blood supply such as digits, nose, external ear, penis, etc. Patients with hypertensive vascular disease may exhibit exaggerated vasoconstrictor response. Ischemic injury or necrosis may result.

Because amide-type local anesthetics such as bupivacaine are metabolized by the liver, these drugs, especially repeat doses, should be used cautiously in patients with hepatic disease. Patients with severe hepatic disease, because of their inability to metabolize local anesthetics normally, are at a greater risk of developing toxic plasma concentrations. Local anesthetics should also be used with caution in patients with impaired cardiovascular function because they may be able to compensate for functional changes associated with the prolongation of A-V conduction produced by these drugs.

Serious dose-related cardiac arrhythmias may occur if preparations containing a vasoconstrictor such as epinephrine are employed in patients during or following the administration of potent inhalation anesthetics. In deciding whether to use these products concurrently in the same patient, the combined action of both agents upon the myocardium, the concentration and volume of vasoconstrictor used, and the time since injection, when applicable, should be taken into account.

Many drugs used during the conduct of anesthesia are considered potential triggering agents for familial malignant hyperthermia. Because it is not known whether amide-type local anesthetics may trigger this reaction and because the need for supplemental general anesthesia cannot be predicated in advance, it is suggested that a standard protocol for management should be available. Early unexplained signs of tachycardia, tachypnea, labile blood pressure and metabolic acidosis may precede temperature elevation. Successful outcome is dependent on early diagnosis, prompt discontinuance of the suspect triggering agent(s) and prompt treatment, including oxygen therapy, dantrolene (consult dantrolene sodium intravenous package insert before using) and other supportive measures.

Use in Head and Neck Area: Small doses of local anesthetics injected into the head and neck area, including retrobulbar, dental and stellate ganglion blocks, may produce adverse reactions similar to systemic toxicity seen with unintentional intravascular injections of larger doses. The injection procedures require the utmost care. Confusion, convulsions, respiratory depression, and/or respiratory arrest, and cardiovascular stimulation or depression have been reported. These reactions may be due to intraarterial injection of the local anesthetic with retrograde flow to the cerebral circulation. They may also be due to puncture of the dural sheath of the optic nerve during retrobulbar block with diffusion of any local anesthetic along the subdural space to the midbrain. Patients receiving these blocks should have their

PRECAUTIONS: *(cont'd)*

circulation and respiration monitored and be constantly observed. Resuscitative equipment and personnel for treating adverse reactions should be immediately available. Dosage recommendations should not be exceeded (see DOSAGE AND ADMINISTRATION.)

Use in Ophthalmic Surgery: Clinicians who perform retrobulbar blocks should be aware that there have been reports of respiratory arrest following local anesthetic injection. Prior to retrobulbar block, as with all other regional procedures the immediate availability of equipment, drugs, and personnel to manage respiratory arrest or depression, convulsions, and cardiac stimulation or depression should be assured (see also WARNINGSand Use in Head and Neck Area. As with other anesthetic procedures, patients should be constantly monitored following ophthalmic blocks for signs of these adverse reactions, which may occur following relatively low total doses. A concentration of 0.75% bupivacaine is indicated for retrobulbar block; however, this concentration is not indicated for any other peripheral nerve block, including the facial nerve and not indicated for local infiltration, including the conjunctiva (see INDICATIONS AND USAGEand PRECAUTIONS, General). Mixing bupivacaine HCl with other local anesthetics is not recommended because of insufficient data on the clinical use of such mixtures.

When bupivacaine HCl 0.75% is used for retrobulbar block, complete corneal anesthesia usually precedes onset of clinically acceptable external ocular muscle akinesia. Therefore, presence of akinesia rather than anesthesia alone should determine readiness of the patient for surgery.

Information for the Patient: When appropriate, patients should be informed in advance that they may experience temporary loss of sensation and motor activity, usually in the lower half of the body following proper administration of caudal or lumbar epidural anesthesia. Also, when appropriate, the physician should discuss other information including adverse reactions in the bupivacaine HCl package insert.

Carcinogenesis, Mutagenesis, and Impairment of Fertility: Long-term studies in animals of most local anesthetics, including bupivacaine to evaluate the carcinogenic potential have not been conducted. Mutagenic potential or the effect on fertility have not been determined. There is no evidence from human data that bupivacaine may be carcinogenic or mutagenic or that it impairs fertility.

Pregnancy Category C: Decreased pup survival in rats and embryocidal effect in rabbits have been observed when bupivacaine HCl was administered to these species in doses comparable to nine and five times, respectively, the maximum recommended daily human dose (400 mg). There are no adequate and well-controlled studies in pregnant women of the effect of bupivacaine on the developing fetus. Bupivacaine HCl injection should be used during pregnancy only if the potential benefit justifies the potential risk to the fetus. This does not exclude the use of bupivacaine HCl injection (0.25% and 0.5% concentrations) at term for obstetrical anesthesia or analgesia. See Labor and Delivery.

Labor and Delivery: See WARNINGSregarding obstetrical use in 0.75% concentration.

Bupivacaine HCl injection is contraindicated in obstetrical paracervical block anesthesia.

Local anesthetics rapidly cross the placenta, and when used for epidural, caudal or pudendal block anesthesia, can cause varying degrees of maternal, fetal and neonatal toxicity. See CLINICAL PHARMACOLOGY, Pharmakoinetics. The incidence and degree of toxicity depend upon the procedure performed, the type and amount of drug used, and the technique of drug administration. Adverse reactions in the parturient, fetus and neonate involve alterations of the central nervous system, peripheral vascular tone and cardiac function.

Maternal hypotension has resulted from regional anesthesia. Local anesthetics produce vasodilation by blocking sympathetic nerves. Elevating the patient's legs and positioning her on her left side will help prevent decreases in blood pressure. The fetal heart rate also should be monitored continuously, and electronic fetal monitoring is highly advisable.

Epidural, caudal, or pudendal anesthesia may alter the forces of parturition through changes in uterine contractility of maternal expulsive efforts. Epidural anesthesia has been reported to prolong the second stage of labor by removing the parturient's reflex urge to bear down or by interfering with motor function. The use of obstetrical anesthesia may increase the need for forceps assistance.

The use of some local anesthetic drug products during labor and delivery may be followed by diminished muscle strength and tone for the first day or two of life. This has not been reported with bupivacaine HCl injection.

It is extremely important to avoid aortocaval compression by the gravid uterus during administration of regional block to parturients. To do this, the patient must be maintained in the left lateral decubitus position or a blanket roll or sandbag may be placed beneath the right hip and the gravid uterus displaced to the left.

Nursing Mothers: It is not known whether local anesthetic drugs are excreted in human milk. Because many drugs are excreted in human milk, caution should be exercised when local anesthetics are administered to a nursing mother.

Pediatric Use: Administration of Sensorcaine (bupivacaine HCl) injection is not recommended in children younger than 12 years due to limited experience in controlled clinical trials. Reports in the literature have described an increased risk of toxicity associated with the pediatric use of bupivacaine for regional anesthesia.

DRUG INTERACTIONS:

Clinically Significant Drug Interactions: The administration of local anesthetic solutions containing epinephrine or norepinephrine to patients receiving monoamine oxidase inhibitors or tricyclic antidepressants may produce severe, prolonged hypertension. Concurrent use of these agents should generally be avoided. In situations in which concurrent therapy is necessary, careful patient monitoring is essential.

Concurrent administration of vasopressor drugs and of ergot-type oxytocic drugs may cause severe, persistent hypertension or cerebrovascular accidents. Phenothiazines and butyrophenones may reduce or reverse the pressor effect of epinephrine.

ADVERSE REACTIONS:

Reactions to bupivacaine are characteristic of those associated with other amide-type local anesthetics. A major cause of adverse reactions to this group of drugs may be associated with its excessive plasma levels, which may be due to overdosage, unintentional intravascular injection or slow metabolic degradation.

Systemic: The most commonly encountered acute adverse experiences that demand immediate countermeasures are related to the central nervous system and the cardiovascular system. These adverse experiences are generally dose related and due to high plasma levels which may result from overdosage, rapid absorption from the injection site, diminished tolerance or from unintentional intravascular injection of the local anesthetic solution. In addition to systemic dose-related toxicity, unintentional subarachnoid injection of drug during the intended performance of caudal or lumbar epidural block or nerve blocks near the vertebral column (especially in the head and neck region) may result in underventilation or apnea ("Total or High Spinal"). Also, hypotension due to loss of sympathetic tone and respiratory paralysis or underventilation due to cephalad extension of the motor level of anesthesia may occur. This may lead to secondary cardiac arrest if untreated. Factors

ADVERSE REACTIONS: *(cont'd)*

influencing plasma protein binding, such as acidosis, systemic diseases that alter protein production or competition with other drugs for protein binding sites, may diminish individual tolerance.

Central Nervous System Reactions: These are characterized by excitation and/or depression. Restlessness, anxiety, dizziness, tinnitus, blurred vision or tremors may occur, possibly proceeding to convulsions. However, excitement may be transient or absent, with depression being the first manifestation of an adverse reaction. This may quickly be followed by drowsiness merging into unconsciousness and respiratory arrest. Other central nervous system effects may be nausea, vomiting, chills, and constriction of the pupils.

The incidence of convulsions associated with the use of local anesthetics varies with the procedure used and the total dose administered. In a survey of studies of epidural anesthesia, overt toxicity progressing to convulsions occurred in approximately 0.1 percent of local anesthetic administrations.

Cardiovascular System Reactions: High doses or unintentional intravascular injection may lead to high plasma levels and related depression of the myocardium, decreased cardiac output, heart block, hypotension, bradycardia, ventricular arrhythmias, including ventricular tachycardia and ventricular fibrillation, and cardiac arrest. (See WARNINGS, PRECAUTIONS, and OVERDOSAGE.)

Allergic: Allergic type reactions are rare and may occur as a result of sensitivity to the local anesthetic or to other formulation ingredients, such as the antimicrobial preservative methylparaben contained in multiple dose vials or sulfites in epinephrine-containing solutions (see WARNINGS.) These reactions are characterized by signs such as urticaria, pruritus, erythema, angioneurotic edema (including laryngeal edema), tachycardia, sneezing, nausea, vomiting, dizziness, syncope, excessive sweating, elevated temperature, and possibly, anaphylactoid symptomatology (including severe hypotension). Cross sensitivity among members of the amide-type local anesthetic group has been reported. The usefulness of screening for sensitivity has not been definitely established.

Neurologic: The incidence of adverse neurologic reactions associated with the use of local anesthetics may be related to the total dose of local anesthetic administered and are also dependent upon the particular drug used, and route of administration and the physical status of the patient. Many of these effects may be related to local anesthetic techniques, with or without a contribution from the drug.

In the practice of caudal or lumbar epidural block, occasional unintentional penetration of the subarachnoid space by the catheter or needle may occur. Subsequent adverse effects may depend partially on the amount of drug administered intrathecally and the physiological and physical effects of a dural puncture. A high spinal is characterized by paralysis of the legs, loss of consciousness, respiratory paralysis and bradycardia.

Neurologic effects following unintentional subarachnoid administration during epidural or caudal anesthesia may include spinal block by varying magnitude (including high or total spinal block); hypotension secondary to spinal block; urinary retention; fecal and urinary incontinence; loss of perineal sensation and sexual function; persistent anesthesia, paresthesia, weakness, paralysis of the lower extremities and loss of sphincter control, all of which may have slow, incomplete or no recovery; headache; backache; septic meningitis; meningismus; slowing of labor; increased incidence of forceps delivery; or cranial nerve palsies due to traction on nerves from loss of cerebrospinal fluid.

OVERDOSAGE:

Acute emergencies from local anesthetics are generally related to high plasma levels encountered during therapeutic use of local anesthetics or to unintended subarachnoid injection of local anesthetic solution. (See ADVERSE REACTIONS, WARNINGS, and PRECAUTIONS.)

Management of Local Anesthetic Emergencies: The first consideration is prevention, best accomplished by careful and constant monitoring of cardiovascular and respiratory vital signs and the patient's state of consciousness after each local anesthetic injection. At the first sign of change, oxygen should be administered.

The first step in the management of systemic toxic reactions, as well as under-ventilation or apnea due to unintentional subarachnoid injection of drug solution, consists of ***immediate*** *attention to the establishment and maintenance of a patent airway and effective assisted or controlled ventilation with 100% oxygen with a delivery system capable of permitting immediate positive airway pressure by mask.* This may prevent convulsions if they have not already occurred.

If necessary, use drugs to control the convulsions. A 50 to 100 mg bolus IV injection of succinylcholine will paralyze the patient without depressing the central nervous or cardiovascular systems and facilitate ventilation. A bolus IV dose of 5 to 10 mg of diazepam or 50 to 100 mg of thiopental will permit ventilation and counteract central nervous system stimulation, but these drugs also depress the central nervous system, respiratory and cardiac function, add to postictal depression, and may result in apnea. Intravenous barbiturates, anticonvulsant agents, or muscle relaxants should only be administered by those familiar with their use. Immediately after the institution of these ventilatory measures, the adequacy of the circulation should be evaluated. Supportive treatment of circulatory depression may require administration of intravenous fluids, and, when appropriate, a vasopressor dictated by the clinical situation (such as ephedrine or epinephrine to enhance myocardial contractile force).

If difficulty is encountered in the maintenance of a patent airway or if prolonged ventilatory support (assisted or controlled) is indicated, endotracheal intubation, employing drugs and techniques familiar to the clinician, may be indicated after initial administration of oxygen by mask.

Recent clinical data from patients experiencing local anesthetic induced convulsions demonstrated rapid development of hypoxia, hypercarbia and acidosis with bupivacaine within a minute of the onset of convulsions. These observations suggest that oxygen consumption and carbon dioxide production are greatly increased during local anesthetic convulsions and emphasize the importance of immediate and effective ventilation with oxygen which may avoid cardiac arrest.

If not treated immediately, convulsions with simultaneous hypoxia, hypercarbia and acidosis, plus myocardial depression from the direct effects of the local anesthetic may result in cardiac arrhythmias, bradycardia, asystole, ventricular fibrillation, or cardiac arrest. Respiratory abnormalities, including apnea, may occur. Underventilation or apnea due to unintentional subarachnoid injection of local anesthetic solution may produce these same signs also lead to cardiac arrest if ventilatory support is not instituted. *If cardiac arrest should occur, a successful outcome may require prolonged resuscitative efforts.*

The supine position is dangerous in pregnant women at term because of aortocaval compression by the gravid uterus. Therefore, during treatment of systemic toxicity, maternal hypotension or fetal bradycardia following regional block, the parturient should be maintained in the left lateral decubitus position if possible, or manual displacement of the uterus off the great vessels be accomplished.

The mean seizure dosage of bupivacaine in rhesus monkeys was found to be 4.4 mg/kg with mean arterial plasma concentration of 4.5 mcg/ml. The intravenous subcutaneous LD_{50} in mice is 6 to 8 mg/kg respectively.

DOSAGE AND ADMINISTRATION:

The dose of any local anesthetic administered varies with the anesthetic procedure, the area to be anesthetized, the vascularity of the tissues, the number of neuronal segments to be blocked, the depth of anesthesia and degree of muscle relaxation required, the duration of anesthesia desired, individual tolerance, and the physical condition of the patient. The smallest dose and concentration required to produce the desired result should be administered. Dosages of bupivacaine HCl should be reduced for young, elderly and debilitated patients and patients with cardiac and/or liver disease. The rapid injection of a large volume of local anesthetic solution should be avoided and fractional (incremental) doses should be used when feasible.

The specific techniques and procedures, refer to standard textbooks.

In recommended doses, bupivacaine HCl produces complete sensory block, but the effect on motor function differs among the three concentrations.

0.25%: when used for caudal, epidural, or peripheral nerve block, produces incomplete motor block. Should be used for operations in which muscle relaxation is not important, or when another means of providing muscle relaxation is used concurrently. Onset of action may be slower than with the 0.5% or 0.75% solutions.

0.5%: provides motor blockade for caudal, epidural, or nerve block, but muscle relaxation may be inadequate for operations in which complete muscle relaxation is essential.

0.75%: produces complete motor block. Most useful for epidural block in abdominal operations requiring complete muscle relaxation, and for retrobulbar anesthesia. Not for obstetrical anesthesia.

The duration of anesthesia with bupivacaine HCl is such that for most indications, a single dose is sufficient.

Maximum dosage limit must be individualized in each case after evaluating the size and physical status of the patient, as well as the usual rate of systemic absorption from a particular injection site. Most experience to date is with single doses of bupivacaine HCl up to 225 mg with epinephrine 1:200,000 and 175 mg without epinephrine; more or less drug may be used depending on individualization of each case.

These doses may be repeated up to once every three hours. In clinical studies to date, total daily doses up to 400 mg have been reported. Until further experience is gained, this dose should not be exceeded in 24 hours. The duration of anesthetic effect may be prolonged by the addition of epinephrine.

The dosages in Table 2 have generally proved satisfactory and are recommended as a guide for use in the average adult. These dosages should be reduced for young, elderly or debilitated patients. Until further experience is gained bupivacaine HCl is not recommended for children younger than 12 years. Bupivacaine HCl is contraindicated for obstetrical paracervical blocks, and is not recommended for intravenous regional anesthesia (Bier Block).

Use in Epidural Anesthesia: During epidural administration of bupivacaine HCl, 0.5% and 0.75% solutions should be administered in incremental doses of 3 ml to 5 ml with sufficient time between doses to detect toxic manifestations of unintentional intravascular or intrathecal injection. In obstetrics, only the 0.5% and 0.25% concentrations should be used; incremental doses of 3 ml to 5 ml of the 0.5% solution not exceeding 50 mg to 100 mg at any dosing interval are recommended. Repeat doses should be preceded by a test dose containing epinephrine if not contraindicated. Use only the single dose ampules and single dose vials for caudal or epidural anesthesia; the multiple dose vials contain a preservative and therefore should not be used for these procedures.

Test dose for Caudal and Lumbar Epidural Blocks: See PRECAUTIONS.

Unused portions of solutions in single dose containers should be discarded, since this product form contains no preservatives (TABLE 2):

TABLE 2 Dosage Recommendations - Bupivacaine HCl Injections

Type of Block	Conc.	Each Dose (ml)	(mg)	Motor Block[1]
Local Infiltration	0.25%[4]>	up to max.	up to max.	-
Epidural	0.75%[2,4]	10-20	75-150	complete
	0.5%[4]	10-20	50-100	moderate to complete
	0.25%[4]	10-20	25-50	partial to moderate
Caudal	0.5%[4]	15-30	75-150	moderate to complete
	0.25%[4]	15-30	37.5-75	moderate
Peripheral Nerves	0.5%[4]	5 to max.	25 to max.	moderate to complete
	0.25%[4]	5 to max.	12.5 to max.	moderate to complete
Retrobulbar[3]	0.75%[4]	2-4	15-30	complete
Sympathetic	0.25%	20-50	50-125	-
Epidural[3] Test Dose	0.5% w/epi	2-3	10-15 (SeePRECAUTIONS)	-

[1]With continuous (intermittent) techniques, repeat doses increase the degree of motor block. The first repeat dose of 0.5% may produce complete motor block. Intercostal nerve block with 0.25% may also produce complete motor block for intra-abdominal surgery.
[2]For single dose use, not for intermittent (catheter) epidural techniques. Not for obstetric anesthesia.
[3]See PRECAUTIONS.
[4]Solutions with or without epinephrine.

NOTE: Parenteral drug products should be inspected visually for particulate matter and discoloration prior to administration whenever the solution and container permit. The injection is not to be used if its color is pinkish or darker than slightly yellow or if it contains a precipitate.

Solutions should be stored at controlled room temperature 15-30°C (59-86°F).

Solutions containing epinephrine should be protected from light.

(Astra Pharmaceutical Products, Inc., 94/05)

HOW SUPPLIED - RATED THERAPEUTICALLY EQUIVALENT:

Injection, Solution - Epidural - 0.25 %

10 ml	$4.23	Bupivacaine Hcl, Abbott	00074-1159-01
10 ml x 5	$16.55	SENSORCAINE, Astra USA	00186-1030-12
10 ml x 5	$19.33	SENSORCAINE/EPINEPHRINE, Astra USA	00186-1032-12
10 ml x 10	**$29.84**	**MARCAINE, Sanofi Winthrop**	**00024-1212-10**
20 ml	$9.68	Bupivacaine Hcl, Abbott	00074-4272-01
30 ml	$4.60	SENSORCAINE, Astra USA	00186-1030-01
30 ml	$6.42	Bupivacaine Hcl, Abbott	00074-1159-02
30 ml	$6.59	Bupivacaine Hcl, Abbott	00074-1158-01
30 ml x 5	$24.14	SENSORCAINE, Astra USA	00186-1030-02
30 ml x 5	$32.84	SENSORCAINE, Astra USA	00186-1030-91
30 ml x 5	$34.50	SENSORCAINE, Astra USA	00186-1030-92

HOW SUPPLIED - RATED THERAPEUTICALLY EQUIVALENT: *(cont'd)*

30 ml x 10	**$51.13**	**MARCAINE, Sanofi Winthrop**	**00024-1212-30**
50 ml	**$6.86**	**MARCAINE, Sanofi Winthrop**	**00024-1217-01**
50 ml	$7.66	SENSORCAINE, Astra USA	00186-1031-01
50 ml	$10.02	Bupivacaine Hcl, Abbott	00074-1160-01
50 ml	$10.98	Bupivacaine Hcl, Abbott	00074-1158-02
50 ml	$14.16	Bupivacaine Hcl, Abbott	00074-5749-22
50 ml x 5	**$44.04**	**MARCAINE, Sanofi Winthrop**	**00024-1212-02**

Injection, Solution - Epidural - 0.5 %

10 ml	$4.51	Bupivacaine Hcl 5, Abbott	00074-1162-01
10 ml x 5	$18.06	SENSORCAINE, Astra USA	00186-1033-12
10 ml x 10	**$32.64**	**MARCAINE, Sanofi Winthrop**	**00024-1213-10**
20 ml	$10.40	Bupivacaine Hcl, Abbott	00074-4273-01
30 ml	$4.97	SENSORCAINE, Astra USA	00186-1033-01
30 ml	$6.50	Bupivacaine Hcl 5, Abbott	00074-1162-02
30 ml	$6.74	Bupivacaine Hcl, Abbott	00074-1161-01
30 ml	$13.18	Bupivacaine Hcl, Abbott	00074-5748-01
30 ml x 5	$24.53	SENSORCAINE, Astra USA	00186-1033-02
30 ml x 5	$35.29	SENSORCAINE, Astra USA	00186-1033-91
30 ml x 5	$35.29	SENSORCAINE, Astra USA	00186-1033-92
30 ml x 5	**$37.06**	**MARCAINE, Sanofi Winthrop**	**00024-1213-02**
30 ml x 10	**$55.82**	**MARCAINE, Sanofi Winthrop**	**00024-1213-30**
50 ml	**$7.52**	**MARCAINE, Sanofi Winthrop**	**00024-1218-01**
50 ml	$8.54	SENSORCAINE, Astra USA	00186-1035-01
50 ml	$10.45	Bupivacaine Hcl, Abbott	00074-1163-01

Injection, Solution - Epidural - 0.75 %

10 ml	$5.17	Bupivacaine Hcl, Abbott	00074-1165-01
10 ml	$18.41	BUPIVACAINE HCL, Abbott	00074-4704-01
10 ml x 5	$18.83	SENSORCAINE, Astra USA	00186-1037-12
10 ml x 10	**$35.94**	**MARCAINE, Sanofi Winthrop**	**00024-1214-10**
20 ml	$11.12	Bupivacaine Hcl, Abbott	00074-4274-01
30 ml	$5.20	SENSORCAINE, Astra USA	00186-1037-01
30 ml	$6.92	Bupivacaine Hcl, Abbott	00074-1164-01
30 ml	$7.46	Bupivacaine Hcl, Abbott	00074-1165-02
30 ml x 5	$28.75	SENSORCAINE, Astra USA	00186-1037-02
30 ml x 5	**$37.94**	**MARCAINE, Sanofi Winthrop**	**00024-1214-02**
30 ml x 5	$40.81	SENSORCAINE, Astra USA	00186-1037-92
30 ml x 10	**$57.61**	**MARCAINE, Sanofi Winthrop**	**00024-1214-30**

BUPIVACAINE HYDROCHLORIDE; DEXTROSE *(000547)*

CATEGORIES: Anesthesia; Local Anesthetics; Spinal Anesthetics; Pregnancy Category C; FDA Pre 1938 Drugs

BRAND NAMES: Bupivacaine W/Dextrose; *Buvacaina Pesada* (Mexico); *Marcain Heavy*; *Marcain Heavy Spinal*; *Marcain Spinal 0.5% Heavy*; *Marcain Spinal Tung*; *Marcaine Heavy*; **Marcaine Spinal**; *Marcaine Spinal 0.5% Heavy*; *Marcaine Spinal Heavy*; Sensorcaine W/Dextrose
(International brand names outside U.S. in italics)

DESCRIPTION:

Sterile Hyperbaric Solution for Spinal Anesthesia: Bupivacaine hydrochloride is 1-Butyl-2',6'-pipecoloxylidide monohydrochloride monohydrate, a white crystalline powder that is freely soluble in 95 percent ethanol, soluble in water, and slightly soluble in chloroform or acetone.

Dextrose is D-glucopyranose monohydrate.

Bupivacaine HCl-MPF Spinal (Bupivacaine in Dextrose Injection USP) is available in sterile hyperbaric solution for subarachnoid injection (spinal block). Bupivacaine hydrochloride is related chemically and pharmacologically to the aminoacyl local anesthetics. It is a homologue of mepivacaine and is chemically related to lidocaine. All three of these anesthetics contain an amide linkage between the aromatic nucleus and the amino or piperidine group. They differ in this respect from the procaine-type local anesthetics, which have an ester linkage.

Each 1 ml of Bupivacaine HCl-MPF Spinal contains 7.5 mg bupivacaine hydrochloride and 82.5 mg dextrose. The pH of this solution is adjusted to between 4.0 and 6.5 with sodium hydroxide or hydrochloric acid.

The specific gravity of Bupivacaine HCl-MPF Spinal is between 1.030 at 25°C and 1.03 at 37°C.

Bupivacaine HCl-MPF Spinal does not contain any preservatives.

CLINICAL PHARMACOLOGY:

Local anesthetics block the generation and the conduction of nerve impulses, presumably by increasing the threshold for electrical excitation in the nerve, by slowing the propagation of the nerve impulse, and by reducing the rate of rise of the action potential. In general, the progression of anesthesia is related to the diameter, myelination, and conduction velocity of affected nerve fibers. Clinical, the order of loss of nerve function is as follows: (1) pain, (2) temperature, (3) touch, (4) proprioception, and (5) skeletal muscle tone.

Systemic absorption of local anesthetics produces effects on the cardiovascular and central nervous systems (CNS). At blood concentrations achieved with normal therapeutic doses, changes in cardiac conduction, excitability, refractoriness, contractility, and peripheral vascular resistance are minimal. However, toxic blood concentrations depress cardiac conduction and excitability, which may lead to atrioventricular block, ventricular arrhythmias, and cardiac arrest, sometimes resulting in fatalities. In addition, myocardial contractility is depressed and peripheral vasodilation occurs, leading to decreased cardiac output and arterial blood pressure. Recent clinical reports and animal research suggest that these cardiovascular changes are more likely to occur after unintended direct intravascular injection of bupivacaine. Therefore, when epidural anesthesia with bupivacaine is considered, incremental dosing is necessary.

Following systemic absorption, local anesthetics can produce central nervous system stimulation, depression, or both. Apparent central stimulation is manifested as restlessness, tremors and shivering, progressing to convulsions, followed by depression and coma progressing ultimately to respiratory arrest. However, the local anesthetics have a primary depressant effect on the medulla and on higher centers. The depressed stage may occur without a prior excited stage.

Pharmacokinetics: The rate of systemic absorption of local anesthetics is dependent upon the total dose and concentration of drug administered, the route of administration, the vascularity of the administration site, and the presence or absence of epinephrine in the anesthetic solution. A dilute concentration of epinephrine (1:200,000 or 5 mcg/ml) usually reduces the rate of absorption and peak plasma concentration of bupivacaine HCl injection permitting the use of moderately larger total doses and sometimes prolonging the duration of action.

CLINICAL PHARMACOLOGY: *(cont'd)*

The onset of action with bupivacaine HCl is rapid and anesthesia is long lasting. The duration of anesthesia, is significantly longer with bupivacaine HCl than with any other commonly used local anesthetic. It has also been noted that there is a period of analgesia that persists after the return of sensation, during which time the need for strong analgesics is reduced.

The onset of sensory blockade following spinal block with bupivacaine in dextrose injection is very rapid (within one minute); maximum motor blockade and maximum dermatome level are achieved within 15 minutes in most cases. Duration of sensory blockade (time to return of complete sensation in the operative site or regression of two dermatomes) following a 12 mg dose averages 2 hours with or without 0.2 mg epinephrine. The time to return of complete motor ability with 12 mg bupivacaine HCl and dextrose averages 3 1/2 hours without the addition of epinephrine and 4 1/2 hours if 0.2 mg epinephrine is added. When compared to equal milligram doses of hyperbaric tetracaine, the duration of sensory blockade was the same but the time to complete motor recovery was significantly longer for tetracaine. Addition of 0.2 mg epinephrine significantly prolongs the motor blockade and time to first postoperative narcotic with bupivacaine HCl and dextrose.

Local anesthetics appear to cross the placenta by passive diffusion. The rate and degree of diffusion is governed by (1) the degree of plasma protein binding, (2) the degree of ionization, and (3) the degree of lipid solubility. Fetal/maternal ratios of local anesthetics appear to be inversely related to the degree of plasma protein binding, because only the free, unbound drug is available for placental transfer. Bupivacaine HCl with a high protein binding capacity (95%) has a low fetal/maternal ratio (0.2 to 0.4). The extent of placental transfer is also determined by the degree of ionization and lipid solubility of the drug. Lipid soluble, nonionized drugs readily enter the fetal blood from the maternal circulation.

Depending upon the route of administration, local anesthetics are distributed to some extent to all body tissues, with high concentrations found in highly perfused organs such as the liver, lungs, heart, and brain.

Pharmacokinetic studies on the plasma profiles of bupivacaine HCl after direct intravenous injection suggest a three-compartment open model. The first compartment is represented by the rapid intravascular distribution of the drug. The second compartment represents the equilibration of the drug throughout the highly perfused organs such as the brain, myocardium, lungs, kidneys and liver. The third compartment represents an equilibration of the drug with poorly perfused tissues, such as muscle and fat. The elimination of drug from tissue distribution depends largely upon the ability of binding sites in the circulation to carry to the liver where it is metabolized.

Various pharmacokinetic parameters of the local anesthetics can be significantly altered by the presence of hepatic or renal disease, addition of epinephrine, factors affecting urinary pH, renal blood flow, the route of drug administration, and the age of the patient. The half-life of bupivacaine HCl in adults is 3.5 ± 2.0 hours and in neonates 8.1 hours.

Amide-type local anesthetics such as bupivacaine HCl are metabolized primarily in the liver via conjugation with glucuronic acid. Patients with hepatic disease, especially those with severe hepatic disease, may be more susceptible to the potential toxicities of the amide-type local anesthetics.

Pipecolylxylidine is the major metabolite of bupivacaine HCl.

The kidney is the main excretory organ for most local anesthetics and their metabolites. Urinary excretion is affected by urinary perfusion and factors affecting urinary pH. Only 5% of bupivacaine is excreted unchanged in the urine.

When administered in recommended doses and concentrations, bupivacaine HCl does not ordinarily produce irritation or tissue damage and does not cause methemoglobinemia.

INDICATIONS AND USAGE:

Bupivacaine in dextrose injection USP, is indicated for the production of subarachnoid block (spinal anesthesia). Standard textbooks should be consulted to determine the accepted procedures and techniques for the administration of spinal anesthesia.

CONTRAINDICATIONS:

Bupivacaine in dextrose injection USP is contraindicated in patients with a known hypersensitivity to it or to any local anesthetic agent of the amide type.

The following conditions preclude the use of spinal anesthesia:

1. Severe hemorrhage, severe hypotension or shock and arrhythmias, such as complete heart block, which severely restrict cardiac output.

2. Local infection at the site of proposed lumbar puncture.

3. Septicemia.

WARNINGS:

LOCAL ANESTHETICS SHOULD ONLY BE EMPLOYED BY CLINICIANS WHO ARE WELL VERSED IN DIAGNOSIS AND MANAGEMENT OF DOSE-RELATED TOXICITY AND OTHER ACUTE EMERGENCIES WHICH MIGHT ARISE FROM THE BLOCK TO BE EMPLOYED, AND THEN ONLY AFTER INSURING THE **IMMEDIATE** AVAILABILITY OF OXYGEN, OTHER RESUSCITATIVE DRUGS, CARDIOPULMONARY RESUSCITATIVE EQUIPMENT AND THE PERSONNEL RESOURCES NEEDED FOR PROPER MANAGEMENT OF TOXIC REACTIONS AND RELATED EMERGENCIES (See also ADVERSE REACTIONS and PRECAUTIONS). DELAY IN PROPER MANAGEMENT OF DOSE-RELATED TOXICITY, UNDERVENTILATION FROM ANY CAUSE AND/OR ALTERED SENSITIVITY MAY LEAD TO THE DEVELOPMENT OF ACIDOSIS, CARDIAC ARREST, AND, POSSIBLY, DEATH.

Spinal anesthetics should not be injected during contractions, because spinal fluid current may carry the drug further cephalad than desired.

A free flow of cerebrospinal fluid during the performance of spinal anesthesia is indicative of entry into the subarachnoid space. However, aspiration should be performed before the anesthetic solution is injected to confirm entry into the subarachnoid space and to avoid intravascular injection.

Bupivacaine HCl solutions containing epinephrine or other vasopressors should not be used concomitantly with ergot-type oxytocic drugs, because a severe persistent hypertension may occur. Likewise, solutions of bupivacaine HCl containing a vasoconstrictor, such as epinephrine, should be used with extreme caution in patients receiving monoamine oxidase inhibitors (MAOI) or antidepressants of the triptyline or imipramine types, because severe prolonged hypertension may result.

Until further experience is gained in patients younger 18 years, administration of bupivacaine HCl in this age group is not recommended.

Mixing or the prior or intercurrent use of any other local anesthetic with bupivacaine HCl cannot be recommended because of insufficient data on the clinical use of such mixtures.

PRECAUTIONS:

General: The safety and effectiveness of spinal anesthetics depend on proper dosage, correct technique, adequate precautions, and readiness for emergencies. Resuscitative equipment, oxygen, and other resuscitative drugs should be available for immediate use. (See WARNINGS and ADVERSE REACTIONS.) The patient should have IV fluids running via an indwelling catheter to assure a functioning intravenous pathway. The lowest dosage of local anesthetic that results in effective anesthesia should be used. Aspiration for blood should be performed before injection and injection should be made slowly. Tolerance varies with the status of the patient. Elderly patients and acutely ill patients may require reduced doses. Reduced doses may also be indicated in patients with increased intra-abdominal pressure (including obstetrical patients), if otherwise suitable for spinal anesthesia.

There should be careful and constant monitoring of cardiovascular and respiratory (adequacy of ventilation) vital signs and the patient's state of consciousness after local anesthetic injection. Restlessness, anxiety, incoherent speech, lightheadedness numbness and tingling of the mouth and lips, metallic taste, tinnitus, dizziness, blurred vision, tremors, depression, or drowsiness may be early warning signs of central nervous system toxicity.

Spinal anesthetics should be used with caution in patients with severe disturbances of cardiac rhythm, shock, or heart block.

Sympathetic blockade occurring during spinal anesthesia may result in peripheral vasodilation and hypotension, the extent depending on the number of dermatomes blocked. Blood pressure should, therefore, be carefully monitored especially in the early phases of anesthesia. Hypotension may be controlled by vasoconstrictors in dosages depending on the severity of hypotension and response of treatment. The level of anesthesia should be carefully monitored because it is not always controllable in spinal techniques.

Because amide-type anesthetics such as bupivacaine HCl are metabolized by the liver, these drugs, especially repeat doses, should be used cautiously in patients with hepatic disease. Patients with severe hepatic disease, because of their inability to metabolize local anesthetics normally, are at a greater risk of developing toxic plasma concentrations. Local anesthetics should also be used with caution in patients with impaired cardiovascular function because they may be less able to compensate for functional changes associated with the prolongation of A-V conduction produced by these drugs. However, dosage recommendations for spinal anesthesia are much lower than dosage recommendations for other major blocks and most experience regarding hepatic and cardiovascular disease dose-related toxicity is derived from these other major blocks.

Serious dose-related cardiac arrhythmias may occur if preparations containing a vasoconstrictor such as epinephrine are employed in patients during or following the administration of potent inhalation agents. In deciding whether to use these products concurrently in the same patient, the combined action of both agents upon the myocardium, the concentration of volume of vasoconstrictor used, and the time since injection, when applicable, should be taken into account.

Any drug used during the conduct of anesthesia are considered potential triggering agents for familial malignant hyperthermia. Because it is not known whether amide-type local anesthetics may trigger this reaction and because the need for supplemental general anesthesia cannot be predicted in advance, it is suggested that a standard protocol for management should be available. Early unexplained signs of tachycardia, tachypnea, labile blood pressure, and metabolic acidosis may precede temperature elevation. Successful outcome is dependent on early diagnosis, prompt discontinuance of the suspect triggering agent(s) and institution of treatment, including oxygen therapy, indicated supportive measures, and dantrolene. (Consult dantrolene sodium intravenous package insert before using.)

The following conditions may preclude the use of spinal anesthesia, depending upon the physician's evaluation of the situation and ability to deal with the complications or complaints which may occur.

Preexisting diseases of the central nervous system, such as those attributable to pernicious anemia, poliomyelitis, syphilis, or tumor.

Hematological disorders predisposing to coagulopathies or patients on anticoagulant therapy. Trauma to a blood vessel during the conduct of spinal anesthesia may, in some instances, result in uncontrollable central nervous system hemorrhage or soft tissue hemorrhage.

Chronic backache and preoperative headache.

Hypotension and hypertension.

Technical problems (persistent paresthesias, persistent bloody tap).

Arthritis or spinal deformity.

Extremes of age.

Psychosis or other causes of poor cooperation by the patient.

Information for the Patient: When appropriate, patients should be informed in advance that they may experience temporary loss of sensation and motor activity, usually in the lower half of the body, following proper administration of spinal anesthesia. Also, when appropriate, the physician should discuss other information including adverse reactions in the package insert.

Carcinogenesis, Mutagenesis, and Impairment of Fertility: Long-term studies in animals of most local anesthetics including bupivacaine to evaluate the carcinogenic potential have not been conducted. Mutagenic potential or the effect on fertility have not been determined. There is no evidence from human data that bbupivacaine in dextrose injection USP may be carcinogenic or mutagenic or that it impairs fertility.

Pregnancy Category C: Decreased pup survival in rats and an embryocidal effect in rabbits have been observed when bupivacaine hydrochloride was administered to these species in doses comparable to 230 and 130 times respectively the maximum recommended human spinal dose. There are no adequate and well-controlled studies in pregnant women of the effect of bupivacaine on the developing fetus. Bupivacaine hydrochloride should be used during pregnancy only if the potential benefit justifies the potential risk to the fetus. This does not exclude the use of bupivacaine HCl and dextrose at term for obstetrical anesthesia. See Labor and Delivery.

Labor and Delivery: Spinal anesthesia has a recognized use during labor and delivery. Bupivacaine hydrochloride, when administered properly, via the epidural route in doses 10 to 12 times the amount used in spinal anesthesia has been used for obstetrical analgesia and anesthesia without evidence of adverse effects on the fetus.

Maternal hypotension has resulted from regional anesthesia. Local anesthetics produce vasodilation by blocking sympathetic nerves. Elevating the patients's legs and positioning her on her left side will help prevent decreases in blood pressure. The fetal heart rate also should be monitored continuously and electronic fetal monitoring is highly advisable.

It is extremely important to avoid aortocaval compression by the gravid uterus during administrations of regional block to parturients. To do this, the patient must be maintained in the left lateral decubitus position or a blanket roll or sandbag may be placed beneath the right hip and the gravid uterus displaced to the left.

Spinal anesthesia may alter the forces of parturition through changes in uterine contractility or maternal expulsive efforts. Spinal anesthesia has also been reported to prolong the second stage of labor by removing the parturient's reflex urge to bear down or by interfering with motor function. The use of obstetrical anesthesia may increase the need for forceps assistance.

The use of some local anesthetic drug products during labor and delivery may be followed by diminished muscle strength and tone for the first day or two of life. This has not been reported with bupivacaine.

PRECAUTIONS: *(cont'd)*

There have been reports of cardiac arrest during use of bupivacaine HCl injection 0.75% solution for epidural anesthesia in obstetrical patients. The package insert for bupivacaine HCl injection for epidural, nerve block, etc. has a more complete discussion of preparation for, and management of, this problem.

These cases are compatible with systemic toxicity following unintended intravascular injection of the much larger doses recommended forepidural anesthesia and have not occurred within the dose range of bupivacaine hydrochloride 0.75% recommended for spinal anesthesia in obstetrics. The 0.75% concentration of bupivacaine HCl is therefore not recommended for obstetrical epidural anesthesia. Bupivacaine in dextrose injection USP is recommended for spinal anesthesia in obstetrics.

Nursing Mothers: It is not known whether local anesthetic drugs are excreted in human milk. Because many drugs are excreted in human milk, caution should be exercised when local anesthetics are administered to a nursing woman.

Pediatric Use: Unit further experience is gained in patients younger than 18 years, administration of bupivacaine HCl and dextrose in this age group is not recommended.

DRUG INTERACTIONS:

CLINICALLY SIGNIFICANT DRUG INTERACTIONS

The administration of local anesthetic solutions containing epinephrine or norepinephrine to patients receiving monoamine oxidase inhibitors or tricyclic antidepressants may produce severe, prolonged hypertension. Concurrent use of these agents should generally be avoided. In situations when concurrent therapy is necessary, careful patient monitoring is essential.

Concurrent administration of vasopressor drugs and of ergot-type oxytocic drugs may cause severe persistent hypertension or cerebrovascular accidents.

Phenothiazines and butyrophenones may reduce or reverse the pressor effect of epinephrine.

ADVERSE REACTIONS:

Reactions to bupivacaine are characteristic of those associated with other amide-type local anesthetics.

The most commonly encountered acute adverse experiences which demand immediate countermeasures following the administration of spinal anesthesia are hypotension due to loss of sympathetic tone and respiratory paralysis or underventilation due to cephalad extension of the motor level of anesthesia. These may lead to cardiac arrest if untreated. In addition, dose-related convulsions and cardiovascular collapse may result from diminished tolerance, rapid absorption from the injection site, or from unintentional intravascular injection of local anesthetic solution. Factors influencing plasma protein binding, such as acidosis, systemic diseases which alter protein production, or competition of other drugs for protein binding sites, may diminish individual tolerance.

Respiratory System: Respiratory paralysis or underventilation may be noted as result of upward extension of the level of spinal anesthesia and may lead to secondary hypoxic cardiac arrest if untreated. Preanesthetic medication, intraoperative analgesics and sedatives, as well as surgical manipulation, may contribute to underventilation. This will usually be noted within minutes of the injection of spinal anesthetic solution, but because of differing maximal onset times, differing intercurrent drug usage and differing surgical manipulation, it may occur at any time during surgery or the immediate recovery period.

Cardiovascular System: Hypotension due to loss of sympathetic tone is a commonly encountered extension of the clinical pharmacology of spinal anesthesia. This is more commonly observed in patients with shrunken blood volume, shrunken interstitial fluid volume, cephalad spread of the local anesthetic, and/or mechanical obstruction of venous return. Nausea and vomiting are frequently associated with hypotensive episodes following the administration of spinal anesthesia. High doses, or inadvertent intravascular injection, may lead to high plasma levels and related depression of the myocardium, decreased cardiac output, bradycardia, heart block, ventricular arrhythmias, and possibly, cardiac arrest (See WARNINGS, PRECAUTIONS, and OVERDOSAGE).

Central Nervous System: Respiratory paralysis or underventilation secondary to cephalad spread of the level of spinal anesthesia (see Respiratory System) and hypotension for the same reason (see Cardiovascular System) are the two most commonly encountered central nervous system-related adverse observations which demand immediate countermeasures.

High doses or inadvertent intravascular injection may lead to high plasma levels and related central nervous system toxicity characterized by excitement and/or depression. Restlessness, anxiety, dizziness, tinnitus, blurred vision, or tremors may occur, possibly proceeding to convulsions. However, excitement may be transient or absent, with depression being the first manifestation of an adverse reaction. This may quickly be followed by drowsiness merging into unconsciousness and respiratory arrest.

Neurologic: The incidences of adverse neurologic reactions associated with the use of local anesthetics may be related to the total dose of local anesthetic administered and are also dependent upon the particular drug used, the route of administration, and the physical status of the patient. Many of these effects may be related to local anesthetic techniques, with or without a contribution from the drug.

Neurologic effects following spinal anesthesia may include loss of perineal sensation and sexual function, persistent anesthesia, paresthesia, weakness and paralysis of the lower extremities, and loss of sphincter control all of which may have slow, incomplete, or no recovery; hypotension; high or total spinal block; urinary retention; headache; backache, septic meningitis; meningismus, arachnoiditis; slowing of labor, increased incidence of forceps delivery; shivering; cranial nerve palsies dur to traction on nerves from loss of cerebrospinal fluid; and fecal and urinary incontinence.

Allergic: Allergic-type reactions are rare and may occur as a result of sensitivity to the local anesthetic. These reactions are characterized by signs such as urticaria, pruritus, erythema, angioneurotic edema (including laryngeal edema), tachycardia, sneezing, nausea, vomiting, dizziness, syncope, excessive sweating, elevated temperature, and, possibly, anaphylactoid-like symptomatology (including severe hypotension). Cross sensitivity among members of the amide-type local anesthetic group has been reported. The usefulness of screening for sensitivity has not been definitely established.

Other: Nausea and vomiting may occur during spinal anesthesia.

OVERDOSAGE:

Acute emergencies from local anesthetics are generally related to high plasma levels encountered during therapeutic use or to underventilation (and perhaps apnea) secondary to upward extension of spinal anesthesia. Hypotension is commonly encountered during the conduct of spinal anesthesia due to relaxation of sympathetic tone, and sometimes, contributory mechanical obstruction of venous return.

MANAGEMENT OF LOCAL ANESTHETIC EMERGENCIES

The first consideration is prevention, best accomplished by careful and constant monitoring of cardiovascular rand respiratory vital signs and the patient's state of consciousness after each local anesthetic injection. At the first sign of change, oxygen should be administered.

OVERDOSAGE: *(cont'd)*

The first step in the management of systemic toxic reactions, as well as underventilation or apnea due to a high or total spinal, consists of ***immediate*** *attention to the establishment and maintenance of a patent airway and effective assisted or controlled ventilation with 100% oxygen with a delivery system capable of permitting immediate positive airway pressure by mask.* This may prevent convulsions if they have not already occurred.

If necessary, use drugs to control the convulsion. A 50 mg to 100 mg bolus IV injection of succinylcholine will paralyze the patient without depressing the central nervous or cardiovascular systems and facilitate ventilation. A bolus IV dose of 5 mg to 10 mg of diazepam or 50 mg to 100 mg of thiopental will permit ventilation and counteract central nervous system stimulation, but these drugs also depress central nervous system, respiratory and cardiac function, add to postictal depression and may result in apnea. Intravenous barbiturates, anticonvulsant agents, or muscle relaxants should only be administered by those familiar with their use. Immediately after the institution of these ventilatory measures, the adequacy of the circulation should be evaluated. Supportive treatment of circulatory depression may require administration of intravenous fluids, and, when appropriate, a vasopressor dictated by the clinical situation (such as ephedrine or epinephrine to enhance myocardial contractile force).

Hypotension due to sympathetic relaxation may be managed by giving intravenous fluids (such as Sodium Chloride Injection 0.9% or Lactated Ringer's Injection), in an attempt to relieve mechanical obstruction of venous return, or by using vasopressors (such as ephedrine which increases the force of myocardial contractions) and, if indicated, by giving plasma expanders or whole blood.

Endotracheal intubation, employing drugs and techniques familiar to the clinician, may be indicated after initial administration of oxygen by mask if difficulty is encountered in the maintenance of a patent airway, or if prolonged ventilatory support (assisted or controlled) is indicated.

Recent clinical data from patients experiencing local anesthetic-induced convulsions demonstrated rapid development of hypoxia, hypercarbia, and acidosis with bupivacaine within a minute of the onset of convulsions. These observations suggest that oxygen consumption and carbon dioxide production are greatly increased during local anesthetic convulsions and emphasize the importance of immediate and effective ventilation with oxygen which may avoid cardiac arrest.

If not treated immediately, convulsions with simultaneous hypoxia, hypercarbia, and acidosis plus myocardial depression from the direct effects of the local anesthetic may result in cardiac arrhythmias, bradycardia, asystole, ventricular fibrillation, or cardiac arrest. Respiratory abnormalities, including apnea, may occur. Underventilation or apnea due to a high or total spinal may produce these same signs and also lead to cardiac arrest if ventilatory support is not instituted. If cardiac arrest should occur, standard cardiopulmonary resuscitative measures should be instituted and maintained for a prolonged period if necessary. Recovery has been reported after prolonged resuscitative efforts.

The supine position is dangerous in pregnant women at term because of aortocaval compression by the gravid uterus. Therefore during treatment of systemic toxicity, maternal hypotension, or fetal bradycardia following regional block, the parturient should be maintained in the left lateral decubitus position if possible, or manual displacement of the uterus off the great vessels be accomplished.

The mean seizure dosage of bupivacaine in rhesus monkeys was found to be 4.4 mg/kg with mean arterial plasma concentration of 4.5 mcg/ml. The intravenous and subcutaneous LD_{50} in mice is 6 mg/kg to 8 mg/kg and 38 mg/kg to 50 mg/kg, respectively.

DOSAGE AND ADMINISTRATION:

The dose of any local anesthetic administered varies with the anesthetic procedure, the area to be anesthetized, the vascularity of the tissues, the number of neuronal segments to be blocked, the depth of anesthesia and degree of muscle relaxation required, the duration of anesthesia desired, individual tolerance, and the physical condition of the patient. The smallest dose and concentration required to produce the desired result should be administered. Dosage of bupivacaine HCl and dextrose should be reduced for elderly and debilitated patients and patients with cardiac and/or liver disease.

For specific techniques and procedures, refer to standard textbooks,

The extent and degree of spinal anesthesia depend upon several factors including dosage, specific gravity of the anesthetic solution, volume of solution used, force of injection, level of puncture, and position of the patient during and immediately after injection.

Seven and one-half mg (7.5 mg or 1.0 ml) bupivacaine HCl and dextrose has generally proven satisfactory for spinal anesthesia for lower extremity and perineal procedures including TURP and vaginal hysterectomy. Twelve mg (12 mg or 1.6 ml) has been used for lower abdominal procedures such as abdominal hysterectomy, tubal ligation, and appendectomy. These doses are recommended as a guide for use in the average adult and may be reduced for the elderly or debilitated patients. Because experience with bupivacaine HCl and dextrose is limited in patients below the age of 18 years, dosage recommendation in this age group cannot be made.

OBSTETRICAL USE

Doses as low as 6 mg of bupivacaine hydrochloride have been used for vaginal delivery under spinal anesthesia. The dose range of 7.5 mg to 10.5 mg (1 ml to 1.4 ml) bupivacaine hydrochloride has been used for Cesarean section under spinal anesthesia.

In recommended doses, bupivacaine HCl and dextrose produces complete motor and sensory block.

Unused portions of solutions should be discarded following initial use.

Bupivacaine HCl and dextrose should be inspected visually for discoloration and particulate matter prior to administration; solutions which are discolored or which contain particulate matter should not be administered.

Bupivacaine HCl and dextrose solution may be autoclaved once at 15 pound pressure, 121°C (250°F) for 15 minutes. Do not administer any solution which is discolored or contains particulate matter.

Store at controlled room temperature, between 15°C and 30°C (59°F and 86°F).

(Astra Pharmaceutical Products, Inc., 5/94)

HOW SUPPLIED - RATED THERAPEUTICALLY EQUIVALENT:

Injection, Solution - Caudal Block - 0.75 %

2 ml	$34.33	SENSORCAINE SPINAL, Astra USA	00186-1026-03

Injection, Solution - Intrathecal - 0.75 %

2 ml	$4.76	BUPIVACAINE SPINAL, Abbott	00074-3613-01

Injection, Solution - Intravenous - 0.75 %

2 ml x 10	**$33.13**	**MARCAINE SPINAL, Sanofi Winthrop**	**00024-1229-10**

BUPIVACAINE HYDROCHLORIDE; EPINEPHRINE *(000546)*

CATEGORIES: Anesthesia; Caudal; Epidural; Injectable Anesthetics; Local Anesthetics; FDA Approved 1988 Jun

BRAND NAMES: Anesthesia Tray Various; *Carbostesin mit Adrenalin* (Germany); *Carbostesin mit Epinephrin*; *Macaine with Adrenaline*; *Marcain + Adrenalin*; *Marcain-Adrenalin*; *Marcain Adrenalin*; *Marcain with Adrenaline* (Australia); *Marcaina*; *Marcaina con Adrenalina*; *Marcaine Adrenal* (France); *Marcaine+Adrenaline*; *Marcaine-Adrenaline*; *Marcaine Adrenaline*; *Marcaine met Adrenaline*; *Marcaine with Adrenaline*; **Marcaine W Epinephrine**; *Neocaina*; Sensorcaine W/Epinephrine
(International brand names outside U.S. in italics)

DESCRIPTION:

For Full Prescribing Information See: BUPIVACAINE HYDROCHLORIDE

HOW SUPPLIED - RATED THERAPEUTICALLY EQUIVALENT:

Injection, Solution - Epidural - 0.25 %/5 mcg

10 ml x 10	**$34.34**	**MARCAINE W/EPINEPHRINE, Sanofi Winthrop**	**00024-1222-10**
30 ml	$6.11	SENSORCAINE/EPINEPHRINE, Astra USA	00186-1032-01
30 ml x 10	**$58.80**	**MARCAINE W/EPINEPHRINE, Sanofi Winthrop**	**00024-1222-30**
50 ml	**$7.89**	**MARCAINE W/EPINEPHRINE, Sanofi Winthrop**	**00024-1227-01**
50 ml	$9.40	SENSORCAINE, Astra USA	00186-1027-01
50 ml x 5	**$48.40**	**MARCAINE W/EPINEPHRINE, Sanofi Winthrop**	**00024-1222-02**

Injection, Solution - Epidural - 0.5 %/5 mcg

3 ml x 10	**$22.08**	**MARCAINE W/EPINEPHRINE, Sanofi Winthrop**	**00024-1223-03**
5 ml x 10	$26.41	SENSORCAINE/EPINEPHRINE, Astra USA	00186-1036-03
10 ml x 5	$19.80	SENSORCAINE/EPINEPHRINE, Astra USA	00186-1034-12
10 ml x 10	**$37.48**	**MARCAINE W/EPINEPHRINE, Sanofi Winthrop**	**00024-1223-10**
30 ml	$6.59	SENSORCAINE, Astra USA	00186-1034-01
30 ml x 5	$31.39	SENSORCAINE, Astra USA	00186-1036-02
30 ml x 5	$39.26	SENSORCAINE, Astra USA	00186-1034-91
30 ml x 5	$40.19	SENSORCAINE, Astra USA	00186-1036-92
30 ml x 5	**$42.54**	**MARCAINE W/EPINEPHRINE, Sanofi Winthrop**	**00024-1223-02**
30 ml x 10	**$63.92**	**MARCAINE W/EPINEPHRINE, Sanofi Winthrop**	**00024-1223-30**
50 ml	**$8.60**	**MARCAINE W/EPINEPHRINE, Sanofi Winthrop**	**00024-1228-01**
50 ml	$10.08	SENSORCAINE, Astra USA	00186-1029-01

Injection, Solution - Epidural - 0.75 %/5 mcg

10 ml x 5	$20.30	SENSORCAINE, Astra USA	00186-1038-12
30 ml	$6.77	SENSORCAINE, Astra USA	00186-1038-01
30 ml x 5	$32.67	SENSORCAINE, Astra USA	00186-1038-02
30 ml x 5	$40.26	SENSORCAINE, Astra USA	00186-1038-91
30 ml x 5	$41.42	SENSORCAINE, Astra USA	00186-1038-92
30 ml x 5	**$43.62**	**MARCAINE W/EPINEPHRINE, Sanofi Winthrop**	**00024-1224-02**

HOW SUPPLIED - NOT RATED EQUIVALENT:

Injection, Solution - Dental - 0.5 %

1.8 ml x 10	**$126.00**	**MARCAINE W/EPINEPHRINE, Cook-Waite Labs**	**00961-1230-50**

Injection, Solution - Epidural - 0.25 %/5 mcg

10 ml	$4.98	Bupivacaine Hcl W/Epinephrine, Abbott	00074-9042-01
30 ml	$8.53	BUPIVACAINE HCL & EPINEPHRINE, Abbott	00074-9042-02
50 ml	$11.40	BUPIVACAINE HCL & EPINEPHRINE, Abbott	00074-9043-01
50 ml	$13.97	BUPIVACAINE HCL & EPINEPHRINE, Abbott	00074-9041-01

Injection, Solution - Epidural - 0.5 %/5 mcg

10 ml	$7.03	BUPIVACAINE HCL & EPINEPHRINE, Abbott	00074-9045-01
30 ml	$9.26	BUPIVACAINE HCL & EPINEPHRINE, Abbott	00074-9045-02
30 ml	$13.97	BUPIVACAINE HCL & EPINEPHRINE, Abbott	00074-9044-01
50 ml	$12.42	0.5% BUPIVACAINE HCL & EPINEPHRINE, Abbott	00074-9046-01

Injection, Solution - Epidural - 0.75 %/5 mcg

30 ml	$12.58	0.75% BUPIVACAINE HCL & EPINEPHRINE, Abbott	00074-9047-01

BUPRENORPHINE HYDROCHLORIDE *(000549)*

CATEGORIES: Analgesics; Antipyretics; Central Nervous System Agents; Narcotic Agonist-Antagonist; Narcotics, Synthetics & Combinations; Opiate Agonists (Controlled); Opiate Partial Agonists; Pain; Pregnancy Category C; DEA Class CV; FDA Approval Pre 1982

BRAND NAMES: *Anorfin*; **Buprenex**; *Buprenone*; *Buprex*; *Buprine*; *Finibron*; *Lepetan* (Japan); *Nopan*; *Norphin*; *Pentorel*; *Prefin*; *Temgesic* (Australia, Europe)
(International brand names outside U.S. in italics)

DESCRIPTION:

Buprenex (buprenorphine hydrochloride) is a narcotic under the Controlled Substances Act due to its chemical derivation from thebaine. Chemically, it is 17- (cyclopropylmethyl) -α- (1,1-dimethylethyl) -4,5-epoxy -18, 19-dihydro-3- hydroxy-6-methoxy-α- methyl-6, 14-ethenomorphinan-7- methanol, hydrochloride (5α, 7α(S)). Buprenorphine hydrochloride is a white powder, weakly acidic and with limited solubility in water. Buprenorphine HCl is a clear, sterile, injectable agonist-antagonist analgesic intended for intravenous or intramuscular administration. Each ml of Buprenex contains 0.324 mg buprenorphine hydrochloride (equivalent to 0.3 mg buprenorphine), 500 mg anhydrous dextrose, water for injection and HCl to adjust pH. Buprenorphine hydrochloride has the molecular formula, $C_{29}H_{41}NO_4HCl$.

CLINICAL PHARMACOLOGY:

Buprenorphine HCl is a parenteral opioid analgesic with 0.3 mg buprenorphine HCl being approximately equivalent to 10 mg morphine sulfate in analgesic and respiratory depressant effects in adults. Pharmacological effects occur as soon as 15 minutes after intramuscular injection and persist for 6 hours or longer. Peak pharmacologic effects usually are observed at 1 hour. When used intravenously, the times to onset and peak effect are shortened.

The limits of sensitivity of available analytical methodology precluded demonstration of bioequivalence between intramuscular and intravenous routes of administration. In postoperative adults, pharmacokinetic studies have shown elimination half-lives ranging from 1.2-7.2 hours (mean 2.2 hours) after intravenous administration of 0.3 mg of buprenorphine. A single, ten-patient, pharmacokinetic study of doses of 3mcg/kg in children (age 5-7 years) showed a high inter-patient variability, but suggests that the clearance of the drug may be higher in children than in adults. This is supported by at least one repeat-dose study in postoperative pain that showed an optimal interdose interval of 4-5 hours in pediatric patients as opposed to the recommended 6-8 hours in adults.

CLINICAL PHARMACOLOGY: *(cont'd)*

Buprenorphine, in common with morphine and other phenolic opioid analgesics, is metabolized by the liver and its clearance is related to hepatic blood flow. Studies in patients anesthetized with 0.5% halothane have shown that this anesthetic decreases hepatic blood flow by about 30%.

Mechanism of Analgesic Action: Buprenorphine HCl exerts its analgesic effect via high affinity binding to mc subclass opiate receptors in the central nervous system. Although buprenorphine HCl may be classified as a partial agonist, under the conditions of recommended use it behaves very much like classical mc agonists such as morphine. One unusual property of buprenorphine HCl observed in *in vitro* studies is its very slow rate of dissociation from its receptor. This could account for its longer duration of action than morphine, the unpredictability of its reversal by opioid antagonists, and its low level of manifest physical dependence.

Narcotic Antagonist Activity: Buprenorphine demonstrates narcotic antagonist activity and has been shown to be equipotent with naloxone as an antagonist of morphine in the mouse tail flick test.

Cardiovascular Effects: Buprenorphine HCl may cause a decrease or, rarely, an increase in pulse rate and blood pressure in some patients.

Effects on Respiration: Under usual conditions of use in adults, both buprenorphine HCl and morphine show similar dose-related respiratory depressant effects. At adult therapeutic doses, buprenorphine HCl (0.3 mg buprenorphine) can decrease respiratory rate in an equivalent manner to an equianalgesic dose of morphine (10 mg). (See WARNINGS.)

INDICATIONS AND USAGE:

Buprenorphine HCl is indicated for the relief of moderate to severe pain.

CONTRAINDICATIONS:

Buprenorphine HCl should not be administered to patients who have been shown to be hypertensive to the drug.

WARNINGS:

Impaired Respiration: As with other potent opioids, clinically significant respiratory depression may occur within the recommended dose range in patients receiving therapeutic doses of buprenorphine. Buprenorphine HCl should be used with caution in patients with compromised respiratory function (*e.g.,* chronic obstructive pulmonary disease, corpulmonate, decreased respiratory reserve, hypoxia, hypercapnia, or preexisting respiratory depression). Particular caution is advised if buprenorphine HCl is administered to patients taking or recently receiving drugs with CNS/respiratory depressant effects. In patients with the physical and/or pharmacological risk factors, above, the dose should be reduced by approximately one-half.

NALOXONE MAY NOT BE EFFECTIVE IN REVERSING THE RESPIRATORY DEPRESSION PRODUCED BY BUPRENORPHINE HCl THEREFORE, AS WITH OTHER POTENT OPIOIDS, THE PRIMARY MANAGEMENT OF OVERDOSE SHOULD BE THE REESTABLISHMENT OF ADEQUATE VENTILATION WITH MECHANICAL ASSISTANCE OF RESPIRATION, IF REQUIRED.

Interaction with Other Central Nervous System Depressants: Patients receiving buprenorphine HCl in the presence of other narcotic analgesics, general anesthetics, antihistamines, benzodiazepines, phenothiazines, other tranquilizers, sedative hypnotics or other CNS depressants (including alcohol) may exhibit increased CNS depression. When such combined therapy is contemplated, it is particularly important that the dose of one or both agents be reduced.

Head Injury and Increased Intracranial Pressure: Buprenorphine HCl, like other potent analgesics, may itself elevate cerebrospinal fluid pressure and should be used with caution in head injury, intracranial lesions and other circumstances where cerebrospinal pressure may be increased. Buprenorphine HCl can produce miosis and changes in the level of consciousness which may interfere with patient evaluation.

Use in Ambulatory Patients: Buprenorphine HCl may impair the mental or physical abilities required for the performance of potentially dangerous tasks such as driving a car or operating machinery. Therefore, buprenorphine HCl should be administered with caution to ambulatory patients who should be warned to avoid such hazards.

Use in Narcotic-Dependent Patients: Because of the narcotic antagonist activity of buprenorphine HCl, use in the physically dependent individual may result in withdrawal effects.

PRECAUTIONS:

General: Buprenorphine HCl should be administered with caution in the elderly, debilitated patients, in children and those with severe impairment of hepatic, pulmonary, or renal function, myxedema or hypothyroidism; adrenal cortical insufficiency (*e.g.,* Addison's disease); CNS depression or coma; toxic psychoses; prostatic hypertrophy or urethral stricture; acute alcoholism; delirium tremens; or kyphoscoliosis.

Because buprenorphine HCl is metabolized by the liver, the activity of buprenorphine HCl may be increased and/or extended in those individuals with impaired hepatic function or those receiving other agents known to decrease hepatic clearance.

Buprenorphine HCl has been shown to increase intracholedochal pressure to a similar degree as other opioid analgesics, and thus should be administered with caution to patients with dysfunction of the biliary tract.

Information for the Patient: The effects of buprenorphine HCl, particularly drowsiness, may be potentiated by other centrally acting agents such as alcohol or benzodiazepines. It is particularly important that in these circumstances patients must not drive or operate machinery. Buprenorphine HCl has some pharmacologic effects similar to morphine which in susceptible patients may lead to self administration of the drug when pain no longer exists. Patients must not exceed the dosage of buprenorphine HCl prescribed by their physician. Patients should be urged to consult their physician if other prescription medications are currently being used or are prescribed for future use.

Carcinogenesis, Mutagenesis, and Impairment of Fertility: The effects of buprenorphine HCl on fertility and gestation indices were investigated in rats by the subcutaneous and intramuscular routes at doses 10 to 100 times the proposed human doses. Dystocia was noted in dams treated with 1000 times the human dose. No effects on fertility or gestation were noted in these Segment I studies.

Pregnancy Category C: Reproduction studies have been performed in the rat at doses which ranged from 10 to 1000 times the proposed human dose by the subcutaneous and intramuscular routes and 160 times the proposed human dose by the intravenous route. By the intramuscular route, buprenorphine HCl produced mild but statistically significant ($p < 0.05$) post-implantation losses and early fetal deaths at 10 and 100 but not 1000 times the proposed human dose. No fetal malformations were noted in rats at any dose when buprenorphine HCl was administered by subcutaneous, intramuscular, or intravenous routes. In rabbits, intramuscularly administered buprenorphine HCl produced a dose-related trend for rib formation which attained statistical significance ($p < 0.01$) at 1000 times the proposed human dose. By the intravenous route, doses in rats of 40 and 160 times the proposed

PRECAUTIONS: *(cont'd)*

human dose of buprenorphine HCl caused a slight increase in post-implantation losses that may have been treatment-related. No major fetal malformations were noted in drug treated groups when administered by intramuscular or intravenous routes.

There are no adequate and well-controlled studies in pregnant women. Buprenorphine HCl should be used during pregnancy only if the potential benefit justifies the potential risk to the fetus.

Labor and Delivery: The safety of buprenorphine HCl given during labor and delivery has not been established.

Nursing Mothers: An apparent lack of milk production during general reproduction studies with buprenorphine HCl in rats caused decreased viability and lactation indices. It is unknown at this time whether or not buprenorphine HCl is excreted in human milk. Despite the lack of specific knowledge on this issue, it is reasonable to assume that buprenorphine HCl will enter human milk and caution should be exercised in the sue of buprenorphine HCl when it is administered to nursing mothers.

Pediatric Use: The safety and effectiveness of buprenorphine HCl have been established for children between 2 and 12 years of age. Use of buprenorphine HCl in children is supported by evidence from adequate and well controlled trials of buprenorphine HCl in adults, with additional data from studies of 960 children ranging in age from 9 months to 18 years of age. Data is available from a pharmacokinetic study, several controlled clinical trials, and several large post-marketing studies and case series. The available information provides reasonable evidence that buprenorphine HCl may be used safely in children ranging from 2-12 years of age, and that it is of similar effectiveness in children as in adults.

DRUG INTERACTIONS:

Drug interactions common to other potent opioid analgesics also may occur with buprenorphine HCl. Particular care should be taken when buprenorphine HCl is used in combination with central nervous system depressant drugs (see WARNINGS.) Although specific information is not presently available, caution should be exercised when buprenorphine HCl is used in combination with MAO inhibitors. There have been reports of respiratory and cardiovascular collapse in patients who received therapeutic doses of diazepam and buprenorphine HCl. A suspected interaction between buprenorphine HCl. A suspected interaction between buprenorphine HCl and phenprocoumon resulting in purpura has been reported.

ADVERSE REACTIONS:

The most frequent side effect in clinical studies involving 1133 patients was sedation which occurred in approximately two-thirds of the patients. Although sedated, these patients could be easily aroused to an alert state.

Other less frequent adverse reactions occurring in 5-10% of the patients were:

Nausea

Dizziness/Vertigo

Occurring in 1-5% of the patients:

Sweating	Headache
Hypotension	Nausea/Vomiting
Vomiting	Hypoventilation
Miosis	

The following adverse reactions were reported to have occurred in less than 1% of the patients:

CNS Effect: confusion, blurred vision, euphoria, weakness/fatigue, dry mouth, nervousness, depression, slurred speech, paresthesia.

Cardiovascular: hypertension, tachycardia, bradycardia.

Gastrointestinal: constipation.

Respiratory: dyspnea, cyanosis.

Dermatological: pruritus.

Ophthalmological: diplopia, visual abnormalities.

Miscellaneous: injection site reaction, urinary retention, dreaming, flushing/warmth, chills/cold, tinnitus, conjunctivitis, Wenckebach block, and psychosis.

Other effects observed infrequently include malaise, hallucinations, depersonalization, coma, dyspepsia, flatulence, apnea, rash, amblyopia, tremor and pallor.

The following reactions have been reported to occur rarely: loss of appetite, dysphoria/agitation, diarrhea, urticaria, and convulsions/lack of muscle coordination.

In the United Kingdom, buprenorphine hydrochloride was made available under monitored release regulation during the first year of sale, and yielded data from 1736 physicians on 9123 patients (17,120 administrations). Data on 240 children under the age of 18 years were included in this monitored release program. No important new adverse effects attributable to buprenorphine hydrochloride were observed.

DRUG ABUSE AND DEPENDENCE:

Buprenorphine hydrochloride is a partial agonist of the morphine type; i.e., it has certain opioid properties which may lead to psychic dependence of the morphine type due to an opiate-like euphoric component of the drug. Direct dependence studies have shown little physical dependence upon withdrawal of the drug. However, caution should be used in prescribing to individuals who are known to be drug abusers or ex-narcotic addicts. The drug may not substitute in acutely dependent narcotic addicts due its antagonist component and may induce withdrawal symptoms.

OVERDOSAGE:

Manifestations: Clinical experience with buprenorphine HCl overdosage has been insufficient to define the signs of this condition at this time. Although the antagonist activity of buprenorphine may become manifest at doses somewhat above the recommended therapeutic range, doses in the recommended therapeutic range may produce clinically significant respiratory depression in certain circumstances.

Treatment: The respiratory and cardiac status of the patients should be monitored carefully. Primary attention should be given to the reestablishment of adequate respiratory exchange through provision of a patent airway and institution of assisted or controlled ventilation. Oxygen, intravenous fluids, vasopressors, and other supportive measures should be employed as indicated. Doxapram, a respiratory stimulant, may be used. **NALOXONE MAY NOT BE EFFECTIVE IN REVERSING THE RESPIRATORY DEPRESSION PRODUCED BY BUPRENORPHINE HCl. THEREFORE, AS WITH OTHER POTENT OPIOIDS, THE PRIMARY MANAGEMENT OF OVERDOSE SHOULD BE THE REESTABLISHMENT OF ADEQUATE VENTILATION WITH MECHANICAL ASSISTANCE OF RESPIRATION, IF REQUIRED.**

DOSAGE AND ADMINISTRATION:

Adults: The usual dosage for persons 13 years of age and over is 1 ml of buprenorphine HCl (0.3 mg buprenorphine) given by deep intramuscular or slow (over at least 2 minutes) intravenous injection at up to 6-hour intervals, as needed. Repeat once (up to 0.3 mg) if required, 30 to 60 minutes after initial dosage, giving consideration to previous dose pharmacokinetics, and thereafter only as needed. In high-risk patients (*e.g.,* elderly, debilitated, presence of respiratory disease, etc.) and/or in patients where other CNS depressants are present, such as in the immediate postoperative period, the dose should be reduced by approximately one- half. Extra caution should be exercised with the intravenous route of administration, particularly with the initial dose.

Occasionally, it may be necessary to administer single doses of up to 0.6 mg to adults depending on the severity of the pain and the response of the patient. This dose should only be given I.M. and only to adult patient who are not in a high risk category (see WARNINGS and PRECAUTIONS). At this time, there are insufficient data to recommend single doses greater than 0.6 mg for long-term use.

Children: Buprenorphine HCl has been used in children 2-12 years of age at doses of between 2-6 micrograms/kg of body weight, or the use of a repeat or second dose at 30-60 minutes (such as is used in adults). Since there is some evidence that not all children clear buprenorphine faster than adults, fixed interval or "round-the-clock" dosing should not be undertaken until the proper inter-dose interval has been established by clinical observation of the child. Physicians should recognize that, as with adults, some pediatric patients may not need to be remedicated for 6-8 hours.

Safety And Handling: Buprenorphine HCl is supplied in sealed ampules and poses no known environmental risk to health care providers. Accidental dermal exposure should be treated by removal of any contaminated clothing and rinsing the affected area with water.

Buprenorphine HCl is a potent narcotic, and like all drugs of this class has been associated with abuse and dependence among health care providers. To control the risk of diversion, it is recommended that measures appropriate to the health care setting be taken to provide rigid accounting, control of wastage, and restriction of access.

Parenteral drug products should be inspected visually for particulate matter and discoloration prior to administration, whenever solution and container permit.

HOW SUPPLIED:

Buprenex (buprenorphine hydrochloride) is supplied in clear glass snap-ampuls of 1 ml (0.3 mg buprenorphine).

Avoid excessive heat (over 104°F or 40°C.) Protect from prolonged exposure to light.

HOW SUPPLIED - RATED THERAPEUTICALLY EQUIVALENT:

Injection, Solution - Intramuscular; - 0.3 mg/ml

10's	$24.25	BUPRENEX, Reckitt & Colman	12496-0757-01

BUPROPION HYDROCHLORIDE *(000550)*

CATEGORIES: Aminoketones; Antidepressants; Central Nervous System Agents; Depression; Depressive Disorder; Psychotherapeutic Agents; Seasonal Affective Disorder*; Smoking Cessation; Pregnancy Category B; FDA Approved 1985 Dec

* Indication not approved by the FDA

BRAND NAMES: **Wellbutrin**; Wellbutrin SR; Zyban

FORMULARIES: Aetna; BC-BS; Foundation; Medi-Cal; PCS

COST OF THERAPY: $167.85 (Depression; Tablet; 75 mg; 3/day; 90 days)

PRIMARY ICD9: 311 (Depressive Disorder, Not Elsewhere Classified)

DESCRIPTION:

Bupropion hydrochloride, an antidepressant of the aminoketone class, is chemically unrelated to tricyclic, tetracyclic, selective serotonin re-uptake inhibitor, or other known antidepressant agents. Its structure closely resembles that of diethylpropion; it is related to phenylethylamines. It is (±)-1-(3-chlorophenyl) -2-[(1,1-dimethylethyl)amino]-1-propanone hydrochloride. The molecular weight is 276.2. The empirical formula is $C_{13}H_{18}ClNO{\cdot}HCl$. Bupropion hydrochloride powder is white, crystalline, and highly soluble in water. It has a bitter taste and produces the sensation of local anesthesia on the oral mucosa.

Immediate Release Tablets: Wellbutrin is supplied for oral administration as 75 mg (yellow-gold) and 100 mg (red) film-coated tablets. Each tablet contains the labeled amount of bupropion hydrochloride and the inactive ingredients: *75 mg tablet:* D&C Yellow No. 10 Lake, FD&C Yellow No. 6 Lake, hydroxypropyl cellulose, hydroxypropyl methylcellulose, microcrystalline cellulose, polyethylene glycol, talc, and titanium dioxide; *100 mg tablet:* FD&C Red No. 40 Lake, FD&C Yellow No. 6 Lake, hydroxypropyl cellulose, hydroxypropyl methylcellulose, microcrystalline cellulose, polyethylene glycol, talc, and titanium dioxide.

Sustained Release Tablets: Wellbutrin SR tablets are supplied for oral administration as 100 mg (blue) and 150 mg (purple), film-coated, sustained-release tablets. Each tablet contains the labeled amount of bupropion hydrochloride and the inactive ingredients: carnauba wax, cysteine hydrochloride, hydroxypropyl methylcellulose, magnesium stearate, microcrystalline cellulose, polythylene glycol, and titanium dioxide and is printed with edible black ink. In addition, the 100 mg tablet contains FD&C Blue No.1 Lake and polysorbate 80, and the 150 mg tablet contains FD&C Blue No. 2 Lake, FD&C Red No. 40 Lake, and polysorbate 80.

CLINICAL PHARMACOLOGY:

IMMEDIATE RELEASE AND SUSTAINED RELEASE TABLETS

Pharmacodynamics and Pharmacological Actions

Immediate Release Tablets: The neurochemical mechanism of the antidepressant effect of bupropion is not known. Bupropion does not inhibit monoamine oxidase. Compared to classical tricyclic antidepressants, it is a weak blocker of the neuronal uptake of serotonin and norepinephrine; it also inhibits the neuronal re-uptake of dopamine to some extent. Bupropion produces dose-related CNS stimulant effects in animals, as evidenced by increased locomotor activity, increased rates of responding in various schedule-controlled operant behavior tasks, and, at high doses, induction of mild stereotyped behavior.

Bupropion causes convulsions in rodents and dogs at doses approximately tenfold the dose recommended as the human antidepressant dose.

Sustained Release Tablets: Bupropion is a relatively weak inhibitor of the neuronal uptake or norepinephrine, serotonin, and dopamine, and does not inhibit monoamine oxidase. While the mechanism of action of bupropion, as with other antidepressants, is unknown, it is presumed that this action is mediated by noradrenergic and/or dopaminergic mechanisms.

Pharmacokinetics

Sustained Release Tablets: Following oral administration of bupropion sustained release tablets to healthy volunteers, peak plasma concentrations of bupropion are achieved within 3 hours. Food increased $C_{max}$and AUC of bupropion by 11% and 17%, respectively, indicating that there is no clinically significant food effect.

Oral Bioavailability and Single Dose Pharmacokinetics

In humans, following oral administration of bupropion HCl, peak plasma bupropion concentrations are usually achieved within 2 hours, followed by a biphasic decline. The average half-life of the second (post-distributional) phase is approximately 14 hours, with a range of 8 to 24 hours. Six hours after a single dose, plasma bupropion concentrations are approxi-

CLINICAL PHARMACOLOGY: *(cont'd)*

mately 30% of peak concentrations. Plasma bupropion concentrations are dose-proportional following single doses of 100 to 250 mg; however, it is not known if the proportionality between dose and plasma level is maintained in chronic use.

The absolute bioavailability of bupropion HCl tablets in humans has not been determined because an intravenous formulation for human use is not available.

However, it appears likely that only a small proportion of any orally administered dose reaches the systemic circulation intact. For example, the absolute bioavailability of bupropion in animals (rats and dogs) ranges from 5 to 20%

Metabolism

Following oral administration of 200 mg of ^{14}C-bupropion, 87% and 10% of the radioactive dose were recovered in the urine and feces, respectively. However, the fraction of the oral dose of bupropion HCl excreted unchanged was only 0.5%, a finding documenting the extensive metabolism of bupropion.

Several of the known metabolites of bupropion are pharmacologically active, but their potency and toxicity relative to bupropion have not been fully characterized. However, because of their longer elimination half-lives, the plasma concentrations of at least two of the known metabolites can be expected, especially in chronic use, to be very much higher than the plasma concentration of bupropion. This is of potential clinical importance because factors or conditions altering metabolic capacity (*e.g.,* liver disease, congestive heart failure, age, concomitant medications, etc.) or elimination may be expected to influence the degree and extent of accumulation of these active metabolites.

Furthermore, bupropion has been shown to induce its own metabolism in three animal species (mice, rats, and dogs) following subchronic administration. If induction also occurs in humans, the relative contribution of bupropion and its metabolites to the clinical effects of bupropion HCl may be changed in chronic use.

Plasma and urinary metabolites so far identified include biotransformation products formed via reduction of the carbonyl group and/or hydroxylation of the *tert*-butyl group of bupropion. Four basic metabolites have been identified.

They are the *erythro*-and *threo*-amino alcohols of bupropion, the *erythro*-amino diol of bupropion, and a morpholinol metabolite (formed from hydroxylation of the *tert*-butyl group of bupropion).

The morpholinol metabolite appears in the systemic circulation almost as rapidly as the parent drug following a single oral dose. Its peak level is three times the peak level of the parent drug; it has a half-life on the order of 24 hours; and its AUC 0 to 60 hrs is about 15 times that of bupropion.

The *threo*-amino alcohol metabolite has a plasma concentration-time profile similar to that of the morpholinol metabolite. The *erythro*-amino alcohol and the *erythro*-amino diol metabolites generally cannot be detected in the systemic circulation following a single oral dose of the parent drug. The morpholinol and the*threo*-amino alcohol metabolites have been found to be half as potent as bupropion in animal screening tests for antidepressant drugs.

During a chronic dosing study in 14 depressed patients with left ventricular dysfunction, it was found that there was substantial interpatient variability (two- to fivefold) in the trough steady-state concentrations of bupropion and the morpholinol and *threo*-amino alcohol metabolites. In addition, the steady-state plasma concentrations of these metabolites were 10 to 100 times the steady-state concentrations of the parent drug.

The effect of other disease states and altered organ function on the metabolism and/or elimination of bupropion has not been studied in detail. However, the elimination of the major metabolites of bupropion may be affected by reduced renal or hepatic function because they are moderately polar compounds and are likely to undergo conjugation in the liver prior to urinary excretion. The preliminary results of a comparative single-dose pharmacokinetic study in normal versus cirrhotic patients indicated that half-lives of the metabolites were prolonged by cirrhosis and that the metabolites accumulated to levels two to three times those in normals.

In vitro tests show that bupropion is 80% or more bound to human albumin at plasma concentrations up to 200 mcg/ml. Plasma protein binding of the major metabolites of bupropion has not been studied.

The mean elimination half-life (±SD) of bupropion after chronic dosing is 21 (±9) hours, and steady-state plasma concentrations of bupropion are reached within 8 days.Plasma and urinary metabolites so far identified include biotransformation products formed via reduction of the carbonyl group and/or hydroxylation of the *tert*-butyl group of bupropion. Four basic metabolites have been identified. They are *erythro*- and *threo*-amino alcohols of bupropion, the *erythro*-amino diol of bupropion, and a morpholinol metabolite (formed from hydroxylation of the *tert*- butyl group of bupropion). These metabolites of bupropion are pharmacologically active, but their potency and toxicity relative to bupropion have not been fully characterized. They may be of clinical importance because the plasma concentrations of the metabolites are higher than those of bupropion.

Following a single dose in humans, peak plasma concentrations of the morpholinol metabolite occur approximately 6 hours after administration of bupropion hydrochloride sustained release tablets. Peak plasma concentrations of the morpholinol metabolite are approximately 10 times the peak level of the parent drug at steady state with bupropion HCl sustained release tablets. The elimination half-life of the morpholinol metabolite is approximately 20 (±5) hours, and its AUC at steady state is about 17 times that of bupropion.

The times to peak concentrations for the *erythro* and *threo*-amino alcohol metabolites are similar to that of the morpholinol metabolite. However, their elimination half-lives are longer, 33 (±10) and 37 (±13) hours, respectively, and steady-state AUCs are 1.5 and 7 times that of bupropion.

In a study comparing chronic dosing with bupropion HCl sustained release tablets 150 mg twice a day to the immediate release formulation of bupropion at 100 mg three times a day, peak plasma concentrations of bupropion at steady state for bupropion HCl sustained release tablets were approximately 85% of those achieved with the immediate-release formulation. There was equivalence for both peak plasma concentration and AUCs for all three of the detectable bupropion metabolites. Thus, at steady state, bupropion sustained release tablets and the immediate-release formulation are essentially bioequivalent for both bupropion and the three quantitatively important metabolites.

Bupropion and its metabolites exhibit linear kinetics following chronic administration of 300 to 450 mg/day.

SPECIAL POPULATIONS

Factors or conditions altering metabolic capacity (*e.g.,* liver disease, congestive heart failure, age, concomitant medications, etc.) or elimination may be expected to influence the degree and extent of accumulation of the active metabolites of bupropion. The elimination of the major metabolites of bupropion may be affected by reduced renal or hepatic function because they are moderately polar compounds and are likely to undergo further metabolism or conjugation in the liver prior to urinary excretion.

Hepatic: The effect of hepatic impairment on the pharmacokinetics of bupropion has not been studied. The formation of the major metabolites of bupropion may be affected by reduced hepatic function.

CLINICAL PHARMACOLOGY: *(cont'd)*

Renal: The effect of renal disease on the pharmacokinetics of bupropion has not been studied. The elimination of the major metabolites of bupropion may be affected by reduced renal function.

Left Ventricular Dysfunction: During a chronic dosing study with bupropion in 14 depressed patients with left ventricular dysfunction (history of congestive heart failure or an enlarged heart on x-ray), there was substantial interpatient variability (twofold to fivefold) in the trough steady-state concentrations of bupropion and the morpholinol and *threo*-amino alcohol metabolites. This variability was in the same range of the variability observed in healthy volunteers (threefold to eightfold). In addition, the steady-state plasma concentrations of these metabolites were 10 to 100 times the steady-state concentrations of the parent drug.

Age: The effects of age on the pharmacokinetics of bupropion and its metabolites have not been fully characterized, but an exploration of steady-state bupropion concentrations from several efficacy studies involving patients dosed in a range of 300 to 750 mg/day, on a three-times daily schedule, revealed no relationship between age (18 to 83 years) and plasma concentration of bupropion. These data suggest there is no prominent effect of age on bupropion concentration (see PRECAUTIONS, Geriatric Use).

Gender: A single-dose study involving 12 healthy male and 12 healthy female volunteers revealed no sex-related differences in the pharmacokinetic parameters of bupropion.

CLINICAL STUDIES:

The efficacy of the immediate-release formulation of bupropion as a treatment for depression was established in two 4-week, placebo-controlled trials in adult inpatients with depression and in one 6-week, placebo-controlled trial in adult outpatients with depression. In the first study, patients were titrated in a bupropion dose range of 300 to 600 mg/day on a three times daily schedule; 78% of patients received maximum doses of 450 mg/day or less. This trial demonstrated the effectiveness of the immediate-release formulation of bupropion on the Hamilton Depresssion Rating Scale (HDRS) total score, the depressed mood item (*i.e.,* 1) from that scale, and the Clinical Global Impressions (CGI) severity score. A second study included two fixed doses of the immediate-release formulation of bupropion (300 and 450 mg/day) and placebo. This trial demonstrated the effectiveness of the immediate-release formulation of bupropion, but only at 450-mg/day dose; the results were positive for the HDRS total score and the CGI severity score, but not for HDRS item 1. In the third study, outpatients received 300 mg/day of the immediate-release formulation of bupropion. This study demonstrated the effectiveness of the immediate-release formulation of bupropion on the HDRS total score, HDRS item 1, the Montgomery-Asberg Depression Rating Scale, the CGI severity score, and the CGI improvement score.

Although there are not as yet independent trials demonstrating the antidepressant effectiveness of the sustained-release formulation of bupropion, studies have demonstrated the bioequivalence of the immediate-release and sustained-release forms of bupropion under steasy state conditions, *i.e.,* bupropion sustained-release 150 mg twice daily was shown to be bioequivalent to the 100 mg, three-times daily dose of the immediate-release formulation of bupropion, with regard to both rate and extent of absorption, for parent drug and metabolites.

INDICATIONS AND USAGE:

SUSTAINED RELEASE AND IMMEDIATE RELEASE TABLETS

Bupropion hydrochloride is indicated for the treatment of depression.

A physician considering bupropion SR tablets for the management of a patient's first episode of depression should be aware that the drug may cause generalized seizures in a dose-dependent manner with an approximate incidence of 0.4% (4/1,000) at the upper end of the recommended dose range, *i.e.,* 400 mg/day, and an incidence of 0.1% (1/1,000) at a bupropion dose of 300 mg/day. Bupropion's seizure incidence at the 400-mg/day dose may exceed that of other marketied antidepressants and doses of bupropion sustained release tablets up to 300 mg/day by as much as fourfold. This relative risk is only an approximate estimate because no direct comparative studies have been conducted (see WARNINGS).

The efficacy of bupropion in the treatment of depression was established in two 4-week controlled trials of depressed inpatients and in one 6-week controlled trial of depressed outpatients whose diagnoses corresponded most closely to the Major Depression category of the APA Diagnostic and Statistical Manual (DSM) (see CLINICAL PHARMACOLOGY.)

A major depressive episode (DSM-IV) implies the presence of 1) depressed mood or 2) loss of interest or pleasure; in addition, at least five of the following symptoms have been present during the same 2-week period and represent a change from previous functioning: markedly diminished interest or pleasure in usual activities, significant change in weight and/or appetite, insomnia or hypersomia, psychomotor agitation or retardation, increased fatigue, feeling of guilt or worthlessness, slowed thinking or impaired concentration, a suicide attempt or suicidal ideation.

Effectiveness of bupropion in long-term use (more than 6 weeks) has not been systematically evaluated in controlled trials. Therefore, the physician who elects to use bupropion sustained release tablets for extended periods should periodically reevaluate the long-term usefulness of the drug for the individual patient.

CONTRAINDICATIONS:

IMMEDIATE RELEASE AND SUSTAINED RELEASE TABLETS

Bupropion HCl is contraindicated in patients with a seizure disorder. Bupropion HCl is also contraindicated in patients with a current or prior diagnosis of bulimia or anorexia nervosa because of a higher incidence of seizures noted in such patients treated with bupropion HCl immediate-relase formulation.

The concurrent administration of bupropion HCl and a monoamine oxidase (MAO) inhibitor is contraindicated. At least 14 days should elapse between discontinuation of an MAO inhibitor and initiation of treatment with bupropion HCl.

Bupropion HCl is contraindicated in patients who have shown an allergic response to bupropion or the other ingredients contained in the formulations.

WARNINGS:

SEIZURES

At doses of up to 300 mg/day, the incidence of seizures is approximately 0.1% (1/1,000) but increases to approximately 0.4% (4/1,000) at the recommended dose of 400 mg/day of the sustained-release formulation or 450 mg/day of the immediate-release formulation. The risk of seizure also appears to be strongly associated with the presence of predisposing factors.

Predisposing factors which may increase the risk of seizure with bupropion use include history of head trauma or prior seizures, central nervous system (CNS) tumor, and concomitant medications that lower seizure threshold.

Sustained Release Formulations: Data for bupropion sustained release tablets revealed a seizure incidence of approximately 0.1% (*i.e.,* 3 of 3,100 patients followed propspectively) in patients treated at doses in a range of 100 to 300 mg/day. It is not possible to know if the lower seizure incidence observed in this study involving the sustained-release formulation of bupropion resulted from the different formulation or the lower dose used.

WARNINGS: *(cont'd)*

However, the immediate-release and sustained-release formulations are bioequivalent regarding both rate and extent of absorption during steady-state, the most pertinent condition to estimating seizure incidence since most observed seizures occur under steady-state conditions.

Recommendations for Reducing the Risk of Seizure with the Sustained Release Formulation: Retrospective analysis of clinical experience gained during the development of bupropion suggests that the risk of seizure may be minimized if 1) the total daily dose of bupropion sustained release tablets does not exceed 400 mg, (450 mg for the immediate-release tablet) and 2) the daily dose is administered twice daily, with each single dose *not* to exceed 200 mg (150 mg, immediate-release tablet) to avoid high peak concentrations of bupropion and/or its metabolites, and 3) the rate of incrementation of dose is gradual. Extreme caution should be used when bupropion is 1) administered to patients with a history of seizure, cranial trauma, or other predisposition(s) toward seizure, or 2) prescribed with other agents (*e.g.*, antipsychotics, or other antideperessants, etc.) or treatment regimens (*e.g.*, abrupt discontinuation of a benzodiazepine) that lower seizure threshold.

Immediate Release Formulation: Data for the immediate release bupropion revealed a seizure incidence of approximatley 0.4% (*i.e.*, 13 of 3,200 patients followed propectively) in patients treated at doses in a range of 300 to 450 mg/day. The 450 mg/day upper limit of this dose range is close to the currently recommended maximum dose of 400 mg/day for bupropion sustained release tablets. The seizure incidence (0.4%) may exceed that of other marketed antidepressants and doses of bupropion sustained release tablets up to 300 mg/day by as much as fourfold. This relative risk is only an approximate estimate because no direct comparative studies have been conducted.

Additional data accumulated for the immediate release formulation of bupropion suggested that the estimated seizure incidence increases almost tenfold between 450 and 600 mg/day, which is twice the usual adult target dose and one-half the maximum recommended daily dose (400 mg) of bupropion sustained release tablets. Given the wide variability among individuals and their capacity to metabolize and eliminate drugs, this disproportionate increase in seizure incidence with dose incrementation calls for caution in dosing.

Potential for Hepatotoxicity: In rats receiving large doses of bupropion chronically, there was an increase in incidence of hepatic hyperplastic nodules and hepatocellular hypertrophy. In dogs receiving large doses of bupropion chronically, various histologic changes were seen in the liver, and laboratory tests suggesting mild hepatocellular injury were noted. Although scattered abnormalities in liver function tests were detected in patients participating in clinical trials, there is no clinical evidence that bupropion acts as a hepatotoxin in humans.

PRECAUTIONS:

GENERAL

Agitation and Insomnia: Patients in placebo-controlled trials with bupropion sustained release tablets experienced agitation, anxiety, and insomnia as shown in TABLE 1.

TABLE 1 Incidence of Agitation, Anxiety, and Insomnia in Placebo-Controlled Trials

Adverse Event Term	Bupropion SR 300 mg/day (n=376)	Bupropion SR 400 mg/day (n=114)	Placebo (n=385)
Agitation	3%	9%	2%
Anxiety	5%	6%	3%
Insomnia	11%	16%	6%

In clinical studies of both the immediate and sustained release formulations of bupropion HCl, these symptoms were sometimes of sufficient magnitude to require treatment with sedative/hypnotic drugs.

Symptoms were sufficiently severe to require discontinuation of treatment in 1% and 2.6% of patients treated with 300 and 400 mg/day, respectively, of bupropion sustained release tablets and 0.8% of patients treated with placebo.

Immediate Release Tablets

In approximately 2% of patients, symptoms were sufficiently severe to require discontinuation of treatment with bupropion HCl.

Pyschosis, Confusion, and Other Neuropyschiatric Phenomena: Patients treated with an immediate-release formulation of bupropion or with the sustained release tablets have been reported to show a variety of neuropsychiatric signs and symptoms, including delusions, hallucinations, pyschosis, concentration disturbance, paranoia, and confusion. In some cases, these symptoms abated upon dose reduction and/or withdrawal of treatment.

Activation of Psychosis and/or Mania: Antidepressants can precipitate manic episodes in bipolar disorder patients during the depressed phase of their illness and may activate latent pyschosis in other susceptible patients. Bupropion sustained release formulation is expected to pose similar risks.

Altered Appetite and Weight: In placebo-controlled studies with the sustained release tablets, patients experienced weight gain or weight loss as shown in TABLE 2.

TABLE 2 Incidence of Weight Gain and Weight Loss in Placebo-Controlled Trials

Weight Change	Bupropion Sustained Release 300 mg/day (n=339)	Bupropion Sustained Release 400 mg/day (n=112)	Placebo (n=347)
Gained >5 lbs	3%	2%	4%
Lost >5 lbs	14%	19%	6%

In studies conducted with the immediate-release formulation of bupropion, 35% of patients receiving tricyclic antidepressants gained weight, compared to 9% of patients treated with the immediate-release formulation of bupropion. If weight loss is a major presenting sign of a patient's depressive illness, the anorectic and/or weight-reducing potential of bupropion sustained release tablets should be considered.

A weight loss of greater than 5 pounds occurred in 28% of bupropion HCl patients. This incidence is approximately double that seen in comparable patients treated with tricyclics or placebo.

Suicide: The possibility of a suicide attempt is inherent in depression and may persist until significant remission occurs. Accordingly, prescriptions for bupropion HCl should be written for the smallest number of tablets consistent with good patient management.

Use in Patients With Systemic Illness: There is no clinical experience establishing the safety of bupropion sustained release tablets in patients with a recent history of myocardial infarction or unstable heart disease. Therefore, care should be exercised if it is used in these groups. Bupropion was well tolerated in patients who had previously developed orthostatic hypotension while receiving tricyclic antidepressants, and was also generally well tolerated in a group of 36 depressed inpatients with stable congestive heart failure (CHF). However, bupropion was associated with a rise in supine blood pressure in the study of patients with CHF, resulting is discontinuation of two patients for exacerbation of baseline hypertension.

Because bupropion HCl and its metabolites are almost completely excreted through the kidney and metabolites are likely to undergo conjugation in the liver prior to urinary excretion, treatment of patients with renal or hepatic impairment should be initiated at

PRECAUTIONS: *(cont'd)*

reduced dosage as bupropion and its metabolites may accumulate in such patients to a greater extent than usual. The patient should be closely monitored for possible toxic effects of elevated blood and tissue levels of drug and metabolites.

INFORMATION FOR THE PATIENT

Physicians are advised to discuss the following issues with patients:

As dose is increased during initial titration to doses above 150 mg/day, patients should be instructed to take bupropion sustained release tablets in two divided doses, preferably with at least eight hours between successive doses, to minimize the risk of seizures.

Patients should be told that any CNS-active drug like bupropion sustained release tablets may impair their ability to perform tasks requiring judgement or motor and cognitive skills. Consequently, until they are reasonably certain that bupropion sustained release tablets do not adversely affect their performance, they should refrain from driving an automobile or operating complex, hazardous machinery.

Patients should be told that the use of, and the cessation of use of, alcohol may alter seizure threshold, and, therefore, that the consumption of alcohol should be minimized, and if possible, avoided completely.

Patients should be advised to inform their physicians if they are taking or plan to take any prescription or over-the-counter drugs. Concern is warranted because bupropion sustained release tablets and other drugs may affect each other's metabolism.

Patients should be advised to notify their physicians if they become pregnant or intend to become pregnant during therapy.

Patients should be advised to swallow bupropion sustained release tablets whole so that the release rate is not altered. Do not chew, divide, or crush tablets.

LABORATORY TESTS

There are no specific laboratory tests recommended.

CARCINOGENESIS, MUTAGENESIS, AND IMPAIRMENT OF FERTILITY

Lifetime carcinogenicity studies were performed in rats and mice at doses up to 300 and 150 mg/kg per day, respectively. These doses are approximately seven and two times the maximum recommended dose (MRHD), respectively, on a mg/m^2 basis. In the rat study there was an increase in nodular proliferation lesions of the liver at doses of 100 to 300 mg/kg per day (approximately two to seven times the MRHD on a mg/m^2 basis): lower doses were not tested. The question of whether or not such lesions may be precursors of neoplasms of the liver is currently unresolved. Similar liver lesions were not seen in the mouse study, and no increase in malignant tumors of the liver and other organs was seen in either study.

Bupropion produced a positive response (two to tree times control mutation rate) in two of five strains in the Ames bacterial mutagenicity test and an increase in chromosomal aberrations in one of three *in vivo* rat bone marrow cytogenetic studies.

A fertility study in rats at doses up to 300 mg/kg revealed no evidence of impaired fertility.

PREGNANCY, TERATOGENIC EFFECTS, PREGNANCY CATEGORY B

Teratology studies have been performed at doses up to 450 mg/kg in rats, and at doses up to 150 mg/kg in rabbits (approximately 7 to 11 and 7 times the MRHD, respectively, on a mg/m^2 basis), and have revealed no evidence of harm to the fetus due to bupropion. There are adequate and well-controlled studies in pregnant women. Because animal reproduction studies are not always predictive of human response, this drug should be used during pregnancy only if clearly needed.

LABOR AND DELIVERY

The effect of bupropion sustained release tablets on labor and delivery in humans is unknown.

NURSING MOTHERS

Like many other drugs, bupropion and its metabolites are secreted in human milk. Because of the potential for serious adverse reactions in nursing infants from bupropion, a decision should be made whether to discontinue nursing or to discontinue the drug, taking into account the importance of the drug to the mother.

PEDIATRIC USE

The safety and effectiveness of bupropion sustained release tablets in pediatric patients below 18 years of age have not been established.

GERIATRIC USE

In general, older patients are known to metabolize drugs more slowly and to be more sensitive to the anticholinergic, sedative, and cardiovascular side effects of antidepressant drugs. A single-dose pharmacokinetic study demonstrated that the disposition of bupropion and its metabolites in elderly subjects was similar to that of younger subjects (see CLINICAL PHARMACOLOGY.) Of the approximately 4,100 patients who participated in clinical trials with bupropion sustained release tablets, 204 were 60 to 69 years old and 68 were 70 years of age or older. The experience with patients 60 years of age or older was similar to that in younger patients.

DRUG INTERACTIONS:

Although no systematic data have been collected on the consequences of the concomitant administration of bupropion and other drugs, animal data suggest that bupropion may be an inducer of drug-metabolizing enzymes. This may be of potential clinical importance because the blood levels of coadministered drugs may be altered.

Alternatively, because bupropion is extensively metabolized, the coadministration of other drugs may affect its clinical activity. In particular, certain drugs may induce the metabolism of bupropion (*e.g.*, carbamazepine, phenobarbital, phenytoin), while other drugs may inhibit the metabolism of bupropion (*e.g.*, cimetidine).

In vitro studies indicate that bupropion is primarily metabolized to the morpholinol metabolite by the cytochrome $P_{450}IIB_6$ isoenzyme. Therefore, the potential exists for a drug interaction between bupropion sustained release tablets and drugs that affect the cytochrome $P_{450}IIB_6$ metabolism (*e.g.* orphenadrine and cyclophosphamide). The *threo*-amino alcohol metabolite of bupropion does not appear to be produced by the cytochrome P_{450} system.

Studies in animals demonstrate that the acute toxicity of bupropion is enhanced by the MAO inhibitor phenelzine (see CONTRAINDICATIONS.)

Limited clinical data suggest a higher incidence of adverse experiences in patients receiving concurrent administration of bupropion and levodopa. Administration of bupropion sustained release tablets to patients receiving levodopa concurrently should be undertaken with caution, using small initial doses and gradual dose increases.

Concurrent administration of bupropion sustained release tablets and agents (*e.g.*, antipyschotics, other antidepressants, etc.) or treatment regimens (abrupt discontinuation of benzodiazepines) that lower seizure threshold should be undertaken only with extreme caution (see WARNINGS.) Low initial dosing and gradual dose increases should be employed.

ADVERSE REACTIONS:

(See WARNINGS) and PRECAUTIONS.

ADVERSE REACTIONS: *(cont'd)*

The information included under the Incidence in ADVERSE REACTIONS, Clinical Studies is based on data from controlled clinical trials with bupropion sustained release tablets. Information on additional adverse events associated with bupropion sustained release tablets in the entire development program for that formulation and with the immediate release formulation of bupropion is included in a separate subsection (see Other Events).

INCIDENCE IN CONTROLLED TRIALS WITH BUPROPION SUSTAINED RELEASE TABLETS

Adverse Events Associated With Discontinuation of Treatment Among Patients Treated With Bupropion Sustained Release Tablets: In placebo-controlled clinical trials, 9% and 11% of patients treated with 300 and 400 mg/day, respectively, of bupropion sustained release tablets and 4% of patients treated with placebo discontinued treatment due to adverse events. The specific adverse events in these trials that led to discontinuation in at least 1% of patients treated with either 300 or 400 mg/day of bupropion sustained release tablets and at a rate at least twice the placebo rate are listed in TABLE 3.

TABLE 3 Treatment Discontinuations Due to Adverse Events in Placebo-Controlled Trials

Adverse Event Term	Bupropion Sustained Release 300 mg/day (n=376)	Bupropion Sustained Release 400 mg/day (n=114)	Placebo (n=385)
Rash	2.4%	0.9%	0.0%
Nausea	0.8%	1.8%	0.3%
Agitation	0.3%	1.8%	0.3%
Migraine	0.0%	1.8%	0.3%

Adverse Events Occurring at an Incidence of 1% or More Among Patients Treated With Bupropion Sustained Release Tablets: TABLE 4 enumerates treatment-emergent adverse events that occurred among patients treated with 300 and 400 mg/day of bupropion sustained release tablets and with placebo in placebo-controlled trials. Events that occurred in either the 300- or 400-mg/day group at an incidence of 1% or more and were more frequent than in the placebo are included. Reported adverse events were classified using a COSTART-based Dictionary.

Accurate estimates of the incidence of adverse events associated with the use of any drug are difficult to obtain. Estimates are influenced by drug dose, detection technique, setting, physician judgements, etc. The figures cited cannot be used to predict precisely the incidence of untoward events in the course of usual medical practice where patient characteristics and other factors differ from those that prevailed in the clinical trials. These incidence figures also cannot be compared with those obtained from other clinical studies involving related drug products as each group of drug trials is conducted under a different set of conditions.

Finally, it is important to emphasize that the tabulation does not reflect the relative severity and/or clinical importance of the events. A better perspective on the serious adverse events associated with the use of bupropion sustained release tablets is provided in the WARNINGSand PRECAUTIONS.

Incidence of Commonly Observed Adverse Events in Controlled Clinical Trials: Adverse events from TABLE 4 occurring in at least 5% of patients treated with bupropion sustained release tablets and at a rate at least twice the placebo rate are listed below for the 300- and 400-mg/day dose groups.

Bupropion Sustained Release 300 mg/day: Anorexia, dry mouth, rash, sweating, tinnitus, and tremor.

Bupropion Sustained Release 400 mg/day: Abdominal pain, agitation, anxiety, dizziness, dry mouth, insomnia, myalgia, nausea, palpitation, pharyngitis, sweating, tinnitus, and urinary freqency.

OTHER EVENTS OBSERVED WITH SUSTAINED RELEASE OR WITH IMMEDIATE RELEASE FORMULATION OF BUPROPION

Other Events Observed During the Clinical Development of Bupropion Sustained Release Tablets: In the following enumeration, reported adverse events were classified using a COSTART-based Dictionary.

The frequencies presented represent the proportion of patients who experienced a treatment-emergent adverse event on at least one occasion in placebo-controlled studies (n=987) or patients who experienced an adverse event requiring discontinuation in an open-label surveillance study with bupropion SR tablets (n=3,100). All treatment-emergent adverse events are included except those listed in TABLES 1 through 4, those events listed in other safety-related sections, those events subsumed under COSTART terms that are either overly general or excessively specific so as to be uninformative, those events not reasonably associated with the use of the drug, and those events that were not serious and occurred in only one patient. Events of major clinical importance are described in the WARNINGS and PRECAUTIONS.

Events are further categorized by body system and listed in order of decreasing frequency according to the following definitions of frequency: Frequent adverse events are defined as those occurring in at least 1/100 patients. Infrequent adverse events are those occurring in 1/100 to 1/1,000 patients, while rare events are those occurring in less than 1/1,000 patients.

Body (General): *Infrequent:* Chills, musculskeletal chest pain, and photosensivity. *Rare:* Malaise and facial edema.

Cardiovascular: *Infrequent:* Postural hypotension and tachycardia. *Rare:* Syncope.

Digestive: *Infrequent:* Thirst, bruxism, jaundice, and abnormal liver function. *Rare:* Tongue edema.

Hemic and Lymphatic: *Infrequent:* Ecchymosis.

Metabolic and Nutrional: *Infrequent:* Peripheral edema.

Musculoskeletal: *Infrequent:* Leg cramps.

Nervous system: *Infrequent:* Decreased libido, abnormal coordination, hyperkinesia, hypesthesia, hypertonia, vertigo, and depersonalization. *Rare:* Hypomania, derealization, ataxia, amnesia, and hostility.

Respiratory: *Rare:* Bronchospasm.

Skin: *Rare:* Maculopapular rash.

Special Senses: *Infrequent:* Dry eye.

Urogenital: *Infrequent:* Impotence and polyuria.

EVENTS OBSERVED DURING CLINICAL DEVELOPMENT AND POSTMARKETING EXPERIENCE WITH THE IMMEDIATE RELEASE FORMULATION OF BUPROPION

In addition to the adverse events noted in clinical trials with bupropion sustained release tablets, the following adverse events have been reported in clinical trials and postmarketing clinical experience with the immediate release formulation of bupropion. The extent to which these events may be associated with bupropion sustained release tablets is unkown.

Cardiovascular: Complete AV block, edema, pulmonary embolism, extrasystoles, hypotension, myocardial infarction, and phlebitis.

Digestive: Colitis, esophagitis, gingivitis, gastrointestinal hemorrhage, hepatitis, intestinal perforation, liver damage, increased salivation, and stomach ulcer.

Endocrine: Syndrome of inappropiate antidiuretic hormone.

ADVERSE REACTIONS: *(cont'd)*

TABLE 4 Treatment-Emergent Adverse Events in Placebo-Controlled Trials*

Body System /Adverse Event	Bupropion SR 300 mg/day (n=376)	Bupropion SR 400 mg/day (n=114)	Placebo (n=385)
Body (General)			
Headache	26%	25%	23%
Infection	8%	9%	6%
Abdominal pain	3%	9%	2%
Asthenia	2%	4%	2%
Chest pain	3%	4%	1%
Pain	2%	3%	2%
Fever	1%	2%	-
Cardiovascular			
Palpitation	2%	6%	2%
Flushing	1%	4%	-
Migraine	1%	4%	1%
Hot flashes	1%	3%	1%
Digestive			
Dry mouth	17%	24%	7%
Nausea	13%	18%	8%
Constipation	10%	5%	7%
Diarrhea	5%	7%	6%
Anorexia	5%	3%	2%
Vomiting	4%	2%	2%
Dysphagia	0%	2%	0%
Musculosketal			
Mylagia	2%	6%	3%
Arthralgia	1%	4%	1%
Arthritis	0%	2%	0%
Twitch	1%	2%	-
Nervous system			
Insomnia	11%	16%	6%
Dizziness	7%	11%	5%
Agitation	3%	9%	2%
Anxiety	5%	6%	3%
Tremor	6%	3%	1%
Nervousness	5%	3%	3%
Somnolence	2%	3%	2%
Irritability	3%	2%	2%
Memory decreased	-	3%	1%
Paresthesia	1%	2%	1%
CNS stimulation	2%	1%	1%
Respiratory			
Pharyngitis	3%	11%	2%
Sinsistus	3%	1%	2%
Increased cough	1%	2%	1%
Skin			
Sweating	6%	5%	2%
Rash	5%	4%	1%
Pruritus	2%	4%	2%
Urticaria	2%	1%	0%
Special senses			
Tinnitus	6%	6%	2%
Taste perversion	2%	4%	-
Amblyopia	3%	2%	2%
Urogenital			
Urinary frequency	2%	5%	2%
Urinary urgency	-	2%	0%
Vaginal hemorrhage†	0%	2%	-
Urinary tract infection	1%	0%	-

* Adverse events that occurred in at least 1% of patients treated with either 300 or 400 mg/day of bupropion sustained release tablets, but equally or more frequently in the placebo group, were: abnormal dreams, accidental injury, acne, appetite increased, back pain, bronchitis, dysmenorrhea, flatulence, flu syndrome, hypertension, neck pain, respiratory disorder, rhinitis, and tooth disorder.
† Incidence based on the number of female patients.
- Hyphen denotes adverse events occurring in greater than 0 but less and 0.5% of patients.

Hemic and Lymphatic: Anemia, leukocytosis, leukopenia, lymphadenopathy, and pancytopenia.

Metabolic and Nutritional: Glycosuria.

Musculoskeletal: Arthritis and muscle rigidiy/fever/rhabdomyolysis.

Nervous System: Akinesia, aphasia, coma, delirium, dysarthria, unmasking tardive dyskinesia, dystonia, abnormal electroencephalogram (EEG), labile emotions, euphoria, extrapyramidal syndrome, hypokinesia, increased libido, manic reaction, neuralgia, neuropathy, paranoid reaction, and suicidal ideation.

Respiratory: Bronchitis, dyspnea, and pneumonia.

Skin: Angioedema, exfoliative dermatitis, hirutism, and Stevens-Johnson syndrome.

Special Senses: Deafness, diplopia, and mydriasis.

Urogenital: Cystitis, dyspareunia, dysuria, abnormal ejaculation, gynecomastia, urinary incontinence, menopause, painful erection, salpingitis, urinary retention, and vaginitis.

DRUG ABUSE AND DEPENDENCE:

Controlled Substance Class: Bupropion is not a controlled substance.

HUMANS

Controlled clinical studies of bupropion conducted in normal volunteers, in subjects with a history of multiple drug abuse, and in depressed patients showed some increase in motor activity and agitation/excitement.

In a population of individuals experienced with drugs of abuse, a single dose of 400 mg of bupropion produced mild amphetamine-like activity as compared to placebo on the morphine-Benzedrine subscale of the Addiction Research Center Index (ARCI), and a score intermediate between placebo and amphetimine on the Liking Scale of the ARCI. These scales measure general feelings of euphoria and drug desirability.

Findings in clinical trials, however, are not known to reliably predict the abuse potential of drugs. Nonetheless, evidence from single-dose studies suggest that the recommended daily dosage of bupropion when administered in divided doses is not likely to be especially reinforcing to amphetamine or stimulant abusers. However, higher doses that could not be tested because of the risk of seizure might be modestly attractive to those who abuse stimulant drugs.

ANIMALS

Studies in rodents have shown that bupropion exhibits some pharmacological actions common to psychostimulants, including increases in locomotor activity and the production of a mild, stereotyped behavior and increases in rates of responding in several schedule-controlled

DRUG ABUSE AND DEPENDENCE: *(cont'd)*

behavior paradigms. Drug discrimination studies in rats showed stimulus generalization between bupropion and amphetamine and other psychostimulants. Rhesus monkeys have been shown to self-administer bupropion intravenously.

OVERDOSAGE:

HUMAN OVERDOSAGE EXPERIENCE

Sustained Release Formulation: There has been very limited experience with overdosage of bupropion sustained release tablets; three cases were reported during clinical trials. One patient ingested 3,000 mg of bupropion sustained release tablets and vomited quickly after the overdose; the patient experienced blurred vision and lightheadedness. A second patient ingested a "handful" of bupropion sustained release tablets and experienced confusion, lethargy, nausea, jitteriness, and seizure. A third patient ingested 3,600 mg of bupropion sustained release tablets and a bottle of wine; the patient experienced nausea, visual hallucinations, and "grogginess". None of the patients experienced further sequelae.

Immediate Release Formulation: There has been extensive experience with overdosage of the immediate-release formulation of bupropion. Thirteen overdoses occurred during clinical trials. Twelve patients ingested 850 to 4,200 mg and recovered without significant sequelae. Another patient who ingested 9,000 mg of the immediate-release formulation of bupropion and 300 mg of tranylcypromine experienced a grand mal seizure and recovered without furter sequelae.

Since introduction, overdoses of up to 17,500 mg of the immediate release formulation of bupropion have been reported. Seizure was reported in approximately one third of all cases. Other serious reactions reported with overdoses of the immediate release formulation of bupropion alone included hallucinations, loss of consciousness, and sinus tachycardia. Fever, muscle rigidity, rhabdomyolysis, hypotension, stupor, coma, and respiratory failure have been reported when the immediate release formulation of bupropion was part of multiple drug overdoses.

Although most patients recovered without sequelae, deaths associated with overdoses of the immediate release formulation of bupropion alone have been reported rarely in patients ingesting massive doses of the drug. Multiple uncontrolled seizures, bradycardia, cardiac failure, and cardiac arrest prior to death were reported in these patients.

MANAGEMENT OF OVERDOSAGE

Following suspected overdose, hospitalization is advised. If the patient is conscious, vomiting should be induced by syrup of ipecac. Activated charcoal also may be administered every 6 hours during the first 12 hours after ingestion. Baseline laboratory values should be obtained. Electrocardiogram and EEG monitoring also are recommended for the next 48 hours. Adequate fluid intake should be provided.

If the patient is stuporous, comatose, or convulsing, airway intubation is recommended prior to undertaking gastric lavage. Although there is little clinical experience with lavage following an overdose of the immediate release formulation of bupropion and none with bupropion sustained release tablets, it is likely to be of benefit within the first 12 hours after ingestion since absorption of the drug may not yet be complete.

Although diuresis, dialysis, or hemoperfusion are sometimes used to treat drug overdosage, there is no experience with their use in the management of overdoses of bupropion sustained release tablets. Because diffusion of bupropion and its metabolites from tissue to plasma may be slow, dialysis may be of minimal benefit.

Based on studies in animals, it is recommended that seizures be treated with an intravenous benzodiazepine preparation and other supportive measures, as appropriate.

Further information about the treatment of overdoses may be available from a poison control center.

DOSAGE AND ADMINISTRATION:

General Dosing Considerations: It is particularly important to administer bupropion sustained release tablets in a manner most likely to minimize the risk of seizure (see WARNINGS.) Gradual escalation in dosage is also important if agitation, motor restlessness, and insomnia, often seen during the initial days of treatment, are to be minimized. If necessary, these effects may be managed by temporary reduction of dose or the short-term administration of an intermediate to long-acting sedative hypnotic. A sedative hypnotic usually is not required beyond the first week of treatment. Insomnia may also be minimized by avoiding bedtime doses. If distressing, untoward effects supervene, dose escalation should be stopped.

INITIAL TREATMENT

Sustained Release: The usual adult target dose for bupropion sustained release tablets is 300 mg/day, given as 150 mg, twice daily. Dosing with bupropion sustained release tablets should begin at 150 mg/day given as a sinle daily dose in the morning. If the 150 mg initial dose is adequately tolerated, an increase to the 300 mg/day target dose, given as 150 mg twice daily, may be made as early as day 4 of dosing. There should be an interval of at least 8 hours between successive doses.

Immediate Release: Increases in dose should not exceed 100 mg/day in a 3-day period. No single dose of bupropion HCl should exceed 150 mg. Bupropion HCl should be administered three times daily, preferably with at least 6 hours between successive doses.

The usual adult dose is 300 mg/day, given three times daily. Dosing should begin at 200 mg/day given as 100 mg twice daily. Based on clinical response, this dose may be increased to 300 mg/day, given as 100 mg twice daily, no sooner than 3 days after the beginning of therapy. See TABLE 5

TABLE 5 Dosing Regimen

Treatment Day	Total Daily Dose	Tablet Strength	Number of Tablets		
			Morning	Midday	Evening
1	200 mg	100 mg	1	0	1
4	300 mg	100 mg	1	1	1

Increasing the Dosage Above 300 mg/day: As with other antidepressants, the full antidepressant effect of bupropion sustained release tablets may not be evident until 4 weeks of reatment or longer. An increase in dosage to the maximum of 400 mg/day, given as 200 mg twice daily, (450 mg/day for the immediate release, given as in doses not more than 150 mg each) may be considered for patients in whom no clinical improvement is noted after several weeks if treatment at 300 mg/day. Dosing above 300 mg/day may be accomplished using the 75 or 100 mg tablets (immediate release). The 100 mg tablet must be administered twice daily with at least 4 hours between successive doses, in oder to not exceed the limit og 150 mg in a single dose. Bupropion HCl should be discontinued in patients who do not demonstrate an adequate response after an appropriate period of treatment at 450 mg/day.

Elderly Patients: In general, older patients are known to metabolize drugs more slowly and to be more sensitive to the anticholinergic, sedative, and cardiovascular side effects of antidepressent drugs. Clinical trials enrolled several hundred patients 60 years og age and older. The experience with these patients and younger ones was similar.

DOSAGE AND ADMINISTRATION: *(cont'd)*

Maintenance: The lowest dose that maintains remission is recommended. Although it is not known how long the patient should remain on bupropion HCl, it is generally recognized that acute episodes of depression require several months or longer of antidepressant drug treatment.

HOW SUPPLIED:

Wellbutrin immediate release tablets are supplied as 75 mg (yellow-gold) round, biconvex tablets printed "Wellbutrin" and "75"; and 100 mg (red) round, biconvex tablets printed "Wellbutrin" and "100".

Store at 15° to 25°C (59° to 77°F). Protect from light and moisture.

Wellbutrin SR Sustained Release Tablets, 100 mg of bupropion hydrochloride, are blue, round, biconvex, film-coated tablets printed with "WELLBUTRIN SR 100".

Wellbutrin SR Sustained Release Tablets, 150 mg of bupropion hydrochloride, are purple, round, biconvex, film-coated tablets printed with "WELLBUTRIN SR 150".

Storage: Store at controlled room temperature, 20° to 25°C (68° to 77°F) [see USP]. Dispense in a tight, light-resistant container as defined in the USP.

HOW SUPPLIED - EQUIVALENTS NOT AVAILABLE:

Tablet, Coated - Oral - 75 mg

100's $62.17 WELLBUTRIN, Glaxo Wellcome 00173-0177-55

Tablet, Coated - Oral - 100 mg

100's $82.96 WELLBUTRIN, Glaxo Wellcome 00173-0178-55

BUSPIRONE HYDROCHLORIDE *(000551)*

CATEGORIES: Antianxiety Drugs; Anxiety; Anxiolytics, Sedatives, Hypnotic; Central Nervous System Agents; Tranquilizers; Smoking Cessation*; Pregnancy Category B; Sales >$100 Million; FDA Approved 1986 Sep; Top 200 Drugs
* Indication not approved by the FDA

BRAND NAMES: *Ansial*; *Ansiced*; *Ansitec*; *Anxinil*; *Anxiolan*; *Barpil*; *Bespar* (Germany); *Biron*; *Busirone*; **Buspar**; *Buspirone*; *Kallmiren*; *Narol*; *Nerbet*; *Neurosine* (Mexico); *Normaton*; *Paxon*; *Relac*; *Sburol*; *Tutran*
(International brand names outside U.S. in italics)

FORMULARIES: Aetna; BC-BS; Medi-Cal; PCS

COST OF THERAPY: $214.27 (Anxiety; Tablet; 5 mg; 3/day; 120 days)

DESCRIPTION:

BuSpar (buspirone hydrochloride) is an antianxiety agent that is not chemically or pharmacologically related to the benzodiazepines, barbiturates, or other sedative/anxiolytic drugs.

Buspirone hydrochloride is a white crystalline, water soluble compound with a molecular weight of 422.0. Chemically, buspirone hydrochloride is 8-[4-[4-(2-pyrimidinyl)-1-piperazinyl) butyl)-8-azaspiro [4,5] decane-7,9- dione monohydrochloride. The empirical formula is $C_{21}H_{31}N_5O_2 \cdot HCl$.

BuSpar is supplied for oral administration in 5 mg and 10 mg, white, ovoid-rectangular, scored tablets. BuSpar tablets, 5 mg and 10 mg, contain the following inactive ingredients: colloidal silicon dioxide, lactose, magnesium stearate, microcrystalline cellulose, and sodium starch glycolate.

CLINICAL PHARMACOLOGY:

The mechanism of action of buspirone is unknown. Buspirone differs from typical benzodiazepine anxiolytics in that it does not exert anticonvulsant or muscle relaxant effects. It also lacks the prominent sedative effect that is associated with more typical anxiolytics. *In vitro* preclinical studies have shown that buspirone has a high affinity for serotonin ($5\text{-}HT_{1A}$) receptors. Buspirone has no significant affinity for benzodiazepine receptors and does not affect GABA binding *in vitro* or *in vivo* when tested in preclinical models.

Buspirone has moderate affinity for brain D_2-dopamine receptors. Some studies do suggest that buspirone may have indirect effects on other neurotransmitter systems.

Buspirone HCl is rapidly absorbed in man and undergoes extensive first pass metabolism. In a radiolabeled study, unchanged buspirone in the plasma accounted for only about 1% of the radioactivity in the plasma. Following oral administration, plasma concentrations of unchanged buspirone are very low and variable between subjects. Peak plasma levels of 1 to 6 ng/ml have been observed 40 to 90 minutes after single oral doses of 20 mg. The single-dose bioavailability of unchanged buspirone when taken as a tablet is on the average about 90% of an equivalent dose of solution, but there is large variability.

The effects of food upon the bioavailability of buspirone HCl have been studied in eight subjects. They were given a 20-mg dose with and without food; the area under the plasma concentration-time curve (AUC) and peak plasma concentration (Cmax) of unchanged buspirone increased by 84% and 116% respectively, but the total amount of buspirone immunoreactive material did not change. This suggests that food may decrease the extent of presystemic clearance of buspirone, but the clinical significance of these findings is unknown.

A multiple-dose study conducted in 15 subjects suggests that buspirone has nonlinear pharmacokinetics. Thus, dose increases and repeated dosing may lead to somewhat higher blood levels of unchanged buspirone than would be predicted from results of single-dose studies.

In man, approximately 95% of buspirone is plasma protein bound, but other highly bound drugs, e.g., phenytoin, propranolol, and warfarin are not displaced by buspirone from plasma protein *in vitro*. However,*in vitro* binding studies show that buspirone does displace digoxin.

Buspirone is metabolized primarily by oxidation producing several hydroxylated derivatives and a pharmacologically active metabolite, 1 -pyrimidinylpiperazine (1-PP). In animal models predictive of anxiolytic potential, 1-PP has about one quarter of the activity of buspirone, but is present in up to 20-fold greater amounts. However, this is probably not important in humans: blood samples from humans chronically exposed to buspirone HCl do not exhibit high levels of 1-PP: mean values are approximately 3 ng/ml and the highest human blood level recorded among 108 chronically dosed patients was 17 ng/ml, less than 1/200th of 1-PP levels found in animals given large doses of buspirone without signs of toxicity.

In a single-dose study using 14C-labeled buspirone, 29% to 63% of the dose was excreted in the urine within 24 hours, primarily as metabolites; fecal excretion accounted for 18% to 38% of the dose. The average elimination half-life of unchanged buspirone after single doses of 10 to 40 mg is about 2 to 3 hours.

The pharmacokinetics of buspirone HCl in patients with hepatic or renal dysfunction has not been determined, nor has the effect of age. The effect of buspirone HCl on drug metabolism or concomitant drug disposition has not been investigated.

INDICATIONS AND USAGE:

Buspirone HCl is indicated for the management of anxiety disorders or the short-term relief of the symptoms of anxiety. Anxiety or tension associated with the stress of everyday life usually does not require treatment with an anxiolytic.

The efficacy of buspirone HCl has been demonstrated in controlled clinical trials of outpatients whose diagnosis roughly corresponds to Generalized Anxiety Disorder (GAD). Many of the patients enrolled in these studies also had coexisting depressive symptoms and buspirone HCl relieved anxiety in the presence of these coexisting depressive symptoms. The patients evaluated in these studies had experienced symptoms for periods of 1 month to over 1 year prior to the study, with an average symptom duration of 6 months. Generalized Anxiety Disorder (300.02) is described in the American Psychiatric Association's Diagnostic and Statistical Manual, III[1] as follows:

Generalized, persistent anxiety (of at least one month continual duration), manifested by symptoms from three of the four following categories:

1. Motor tension: shakiness, jitteriness, jumpiness, trembling, tension, muscle aches, fatigability, inability to relax, eyelid twitch, furrowed brow, strained face, fidgeting, restlessness, easy startle.

2. Autonomic hyperactivity: sweating, heart pounding or racing, cold, clammy hands, dry mouth, dizziness, lightheadedness, paresthesias (tingling in hands or feet), upset stomach, hot or cold spells, frequent urination, diarrhea, discomfort in the pit of the stomach, lump in the throat, flushing, pallor, high resting pulse and respiration rate.

3. Apprehensive expectation: anxiety, worry, fear, rumination, and anticipation of misfortune to self or others.

4. Vigilance and scanning: hyperattentiveness resulting in distractibility, difficulty in concentrating, insomnia, feeling "on edge", irritability, impatience.

The above symptoms would not be due to another mental disorder, such as a depressive disorder or schizophrenia. However, mild depressive symptoms are common in GAD.

The effectiveness of buspirone HCl in long-term use, that is, for more than 3 to 4 weeks, has not been demonstrated in controlled trials. There is no body of evidence available that systematically addresses the appropriate duration of treatment for GAD. However, in a study of long-term use, 264 patients were treated with buspirone HCl for 1 year without ill effect. Therefore, the physician who elects to use buspirone HCl for extended periods should periodically reassess the usefulness of the drug for the individual patient.

CONTRAINDICATIONS:

Buspirone HCl is contraindicated in patients hypersensitive to buspirone hydrochloride.

WARNINGS:

The administration of buspirone HCl to a patient taking a monoamine oxidase inhibitor (MAOI) may pose a hazard. There have been reports of the occurrence of elevated blood pressure when buspirone HCl has been added to a regimen including an MAOI. Therefore, it is recommended that buspirone HCl not be used concomitantly with an MAOI.

Because buspirone HCl has no established antipsychotic activity, it should not be employed in lieu of appropriate antipsychotic treatment.

PRECAUTIONS:

GENERAL

Interference with cognitive and motor performance: Studies indicate that buspirone HCl is less sedating than other anxiolytics and that it does not produce significant functional impairment. However, its CNS effects in any individual patient may not be predictable. Therefore, patients should be cautioned about operating an automobile or using complex machinery until they are reasonably certain that buspirone treatment does not affect them adversely.

While formal studies of the interaction of buspirone HCl with alcohol indicate that buspirone does not increase alcohol-induced impairment in motor and mental performance, it is prudent to avoid concomitant use of alcohol and buspirone.

Potential for withdrawal reactions in sedative/hypnotic/anxiolytic drug-dependent patients: Because buspirone HCl does not exhibit cross-tolerance with benzodiazepines and other common sedative/hypnotic drugs, it will not block the withdrawal syndrome often seen with cessation of therapy with these drugs. Therefore, before starting therapy with buspirone HCl, it is advisable to withdraw patients gradually, especially patients who have been using a CNS-depressant drug chronically, from their prior treatment. Rebound or withdrawal symptoms may occur over varying time periods, depending in part on the type of drug, and its effective half-life of elimination.

The syndrome of withdrawal from sedative/hypnotic/anxiolytic drugs can appear as any combination of irritability, anxiety, agitation, insomnia, tremor, abdominal cramps, muscle cramps, vomiting, sweating, flu-like symptoms without fever, and occasionally, even as seizures.

Possible concerns related to buspirone's binding to dopamine receptors: Because buspirone can bind to central dopamine receptors, a question has been raised about its potential to cause acute and chronic changes in dopamine-mediated neurological function (*e.g.,* dystonia, pseudo-parkinsonism, akathisia, and tardive dyskinesia). Clinical experience in controlled trials has failed to identify any significant neuroleptic-like activity; however, a syndrome of restlessness, appearing shortly after initiation of treatment, has been reported in some small fraction of buspirone-treated patients. The syndrome may be explained in several ways. For example, buspirone may increase central noradrenergic activity; alternatively, the effect may be attributable to dopaminergic effects (*i.e.,* represent akathisia). Obviously, the question cannot be totally resolved at this point in time. Generally, long-term sequelae of any drug's use can be identified only after several years of marketing.

INFORMATION FOR THE PATIENT

To assure safe and effective use of buspirone HCl, the following information and instructions should be given to patients:

1. Inform your physician about any medications, prescription or non-prescription, alcohol, or drugs that you are now taking or plan to take during your treatment with buspirone HCl.
2. Inform your physician if you are pregnant, or if you are planning to become pregnant, or if you become pregnant while you are taking buspirone HCl.
3. Inform your physician if you are breast-feeding an infant.
4. Until you experience how this medication affects you, do not drive a car or operate potentially dangerous machinery.

LABORATORY TESTS

There are no specific laboratory tests recommended.

DRUG/LABORATORY TEST INTERACTIONS

Buspirone is not known to interfere with commonly employed clinical laboratory tests.

CARCINOGENESIS, MUTAGENESIS, AND IMPAIRMENT OF FERTILITY

No evidence of carcinogenic potential was observed in rats during a 24-month study at approximately 133 times the maximum recommended human oral dose; or in mice, during an 18-month study at approximately 167 times the maximum recommended human oral dose.

PRECAUTIONS: *(cont'd)*

With or without metabolic activation, buspirone did not induce point mutations in five strains of *Salmonella typhimurium* (Ames Test) or mouse lymphoma L5178YTK$^+$ cell cultures, nor was DNA damage observed with buspirone in Wi-38 human cells. Chromosomal aberrations or abnormalities did not occur in bone marrow cells of mice given one or five daily doses of buspirone.

PREGNANCY, TERATOGENIC EFFECTS, PREGNANCY CATEGORY B:

No fertility impairment or fetal damage was observed in reproduction studies performed in rats and rabbits at buspirone doses of approximately 30 times the maximum recommended human dose. In humans, however, adequate and well-controlled studies during pregnancy have not been performed. Because animal reproduction studies are not always predictive of human response, this drug should be used during pregnancy only if clearly needed.

LABOR AND DELIVERY

The effect of buspirone HCl on labor and delivery in women is unknown. No adverse effects were noted in reproduction studies in rats.

NURSING MOTHERS

The extent of the excretion in human milk of buspirone or its metabolites is not known. In rats, however, buspirone and its metabolites are excreted in milk. Buspirone HCl administration to nursing women should be avoided if clinically possible.

PEDIATRIC USE

The safety and effectiveness of buspirone HCl have not been determined in individuals below 18 years of age.

GERIATRIC USE

Buspirone HCl has not been systematically evaluated in older patients; however, several hundred elderly patients have participated in clinical studies with buspirone HCl and no unusual adverse age-related phenomena have been identified. In 87 elderly patients for whom dosage data were available, the modal total daily dose of buspirone HCl was 15 mg per day, the same as that in the total sample of patients treated with buspirone HCl.

USE IN PATIENTS WITH IMPAIRED HEPATIC OR RENAL FUNCTION

Since buspirone HCl is metabolized by the liver and excreted by the kidneys, its administration to patients with severe hepatic or renal impairment cannot be recommended.

DRUG INTERACTIONS:

It is recommended that buspirone hydrochloride *not* be used concomitantly with MAO inhibitors (See WARNINGS.) Because the effects of concomitant administration of buspirone HCl with most other psychotropic drugs have not been studied, the concomitant use of buspirone HCl with other CNS-active drugs should be approached with caution.

There is one report suggesting that the concomitant use of trazodone hydrochloride (Desyrel) and buspirone HCl may have caused 3-to 6-fold elevations on SGPT (ALT) in a few patients. In a similar study, attempting to replicate this finding, no interactive effect on hepatic transaminases was identified.

In a study in normal volunteers, concomitant administration of buspirone HCl and haloperidol resulted in increased serum haloperidol concentrations. The clinical significance of this finding is not clear.

In vitro, buspirone does not displace tightly bound drugs like phenytoin, propranolol, and warfarin from serum proteins. However, there has been one report of prolonged prothrombin time when buspirone was added to the regimen of a patient treated with warfarin. The patient was also chronically receiving phenytoin, phenobarbital, digoxin, and levothyroxine sodium. *In vitro,* buspirone may displace less firmly bound drugs like digoxin. The clinical significance of this property is unknown.

ADVERSE REACTIONS:

(See also PRECAUTIONS)

COMMONLY OBSERVED

The more commonly observed untoward events associated with the use of buspirone HCl not seen at an equivalent incidence among placebo-treated patients include dizziness, nausea, headache, nervousness, lightheadedness, and excitement.

ASSOCIATED WITH DISCONTINUATION OF TREATMENT

One guide to the relative clinical importance of adverse events associated with buspirone HCl is provided by the frequency with which they caused drug discontinuation during clinical testing. Approximately 10% of the 2200 anxious patients who participated in the buspirone HCl premarketing clinical efficacy trials in anxiety disorders lasting 3 to 4 weeks discontinued treatment due to an adverse event. The more common events causing discontinuation included: central nervous system disturbances (3.4%), primarily dizziness, insomnia, nervousness, drowsiness, and lightheaded feeling; gastrointestinal disturbances (1.2%), primarily nausea; and miscellaneous disturbances (1.1%), primarily headache and fatigue. In addition, 3.4% of patients had multiple complaints, none of which could be characterized as primary.

INCIDENCE IN CONTROLLED CLINICAL TRIALS

The table that follows (TABLE 1) enumerates adverse events that occurred at a frequency of 1% or more among buspirone HCl patients who participated in 4-week, controlled trials comparing buspirone HCl with placebo. The frequencies were obtained from pooled data for 17 trials. The prescriber should be aware that these figures cannot be used to predict the incidence of side effects in the course of usual medical practice where patient characteristics and other factors differ from those which prevailed in the clinical trials. Similarly, the cited frequencies cannot be compared with figures obtained from other clinical investigations involving different treatments, uses, and investigators. Comparison of the cited figures, however, does provide the prescribing physician with some basis for estimating the relative contribution of drug and nondrug factors to the side effect incidence rate in the population studied.

OTHER EVENTS OBSERVED DURING THE ENTIRE PREMARKETING EVALUATION OF BUSPIRONE HCL

During its premarketing assessment, buspirone HCl was evaluated in over 3500 subjects. This section reports event frequencies for adverse events occurring in approximately 3000 subjects from this group who took multiple doses of buspirone HCl in the dose range for which buspirone HCl is being recommended (*i.e.,* the modal daily dose of buspirone HCl fell between 10 and 30 mg for 70% of the patients studied) and for whom safety data were systematically collected. The conditions and duration of exposure to buspirone HCl varied greatly, involving well-controlled studies as well as experience in open and uncontrolled clinical settings. As part of the total experience gained in clinical studies, various adverse events were reported. In the absence of appropriate controls in some of the studies, a causal relationship to buspirone HCl treatment cannot be determined. The list includes all undesirable events reasonably associated with the use of the drug.

The following enumeration by organ system describes events in terms of their relative frequency of reporting in this data base. Events of major clinical importance are also described in the PRECAUTIONS section.

The following definitions of frequency are used: Frequent adverse events are defined as those occurring in at least 1/100 patients. Infrequent adverse events are those occurring in 1/100 to 1/1000 patients, while rare events are those occurring in less than 1/1000 patients.

ADVERSE REACTIONS: *(cont'd)*

TABLE 1 Treatment-Emergent Adverse Experience Incidence In Placebo-Controlled Clinical Studies*
(Percent of Patients Reporting)

Adverse Experience	Buspirone HCl (n = 477)	Placebo (n = 464)
Cardiovascular		
Tachycardia/Palpitations	1	1
CNS		
Dizziness	12	3
Drowsiness	10	9
Nervousness	5	1
Insomnia	3	3
Lightheadedness	3	-
Decreased Concentration	2	2
Excitement	2	-
Anger/Hostility	2	-
Confusion	2	-
Depression	2	2
EENT		
Blurred Vision	2	-
Gastrointestinal		
Nausea	8	5
Dry Mouth	3	4
Abdominal/Gastric Distress	2	2
Diarrhea	2	-
Constipation	1	2
Vomiting	1	2
Musculoskeletal		
Musculoskeletal Aches/Pains	1	-
Neurological		
Numbness	2	-
Paresthesia	1	-
Incoordination	1	-
Tremor	1	-
Skin		
Skin Rash	1	-
Miscellaneous		
Headache	6	3
Fatigue	4	4
Weakness	2	-
Sweating/Clamminess	1	-

* Events reported by at least 1% of BuSpar patients are included. - Incidence less than 1%.

Cardiovascular: Frequent was nonspecific chest pain; infrequent were syncope, hypotension, and hypertension; rare were cerebrovascular accident, congestive heart failure, myocardial infarction, cardiomyopathy, and bradycardia.

Central Nervous System: Frequent were dream disturbances; infrequent were depersonalization, dysphoria, noise intolerance, euphoria, akathisia, fearfulness, loss of interest, dissociative reaction, hallucinations, suicidal ideation, and seizures; rare were feelings of claustrophobia, cold intolerance, stupor, and slurred speech and psychosis.

EENT: Frequent were tinnitus, sore throat, and nasal congestion; infrequent were redness and itching of the eyes, altered taste, altered smell, and conjunctivitis; rare were inner ear abnormality, eye pain, photophobia, and pressure on eyes.

Endocrine: Rare were galactorrhea and thyroid abnormality.

Gastrointestinal: Infrequent were flatulence, anorexia, increased appetite, salivation, irritable colon, and rectal bleeding; rare was burning of the tongue.

Genitourinary: Infrequent were urinary frequency, urinary hesitancy, menstrual irregularity and spotting, and dysuria; rare were amenorrhea, pelvic inflammatory disease, enuresis, and nocturia.

Musculoskeletal: Infrequent were muscle cramps, muscle spasms, rigid/stiff muscles, and arthralgias.

Neurological: Infrequent were involuntary movements and slowed reaction time; rare was muscle weakness.

Respiratory: Infrequent were hyperventilation, shortness of breath, and chest congestion; rare was epistaxis.

Sexual Function: Infrequent were decreased or increased libido; rare were delayed ejaculation and impotence.

Skin: Infrequent were edema, pruritus, flushing, easy bruising, hair loss, dry skin, facial edema, and blisters; rare were acne and thinning of nails.

Clinical Laboratory: Infrequent were increases in hepatic aminotransferases (SGOT, SGPT); rare were eosinophilia, leukopenia, and thrombocytopenia.

Miscellaneous: Infrequent were weight gain, fever, roaring sensation in the head, weight loss, and malaise; rare were alcohol abuse, bleeding disturbance, loss of voice, and hiccoughs.

POST-INTRODUCTION CLINICAL EXPERIENCE

Postmarketing experience has shown an adverse experience profile similar to that given above. Voluntary reports since introduction have included rare occurrences of allergic reactions, cogwheel rigidity, dystonic reactions, ecchymosis, emotional lability, tunnel vision, and urinary retention. Because of the uncontrolled nature of these spontaneous reports, a causal relationship to buspirone HCl treatment has not been determined.

DRUG ABUSE AND DEPENDENCE:

Controlled Substance Class: Buspirone HCl is not a controlled substance.

PHYSICAL AND PSYCHOLOGICAL DEPENDENCE

In human and animal studies, buspirone has shown no potential for abuse or diversion and there is no evidence that it causes tolerance, or either physical or psychological dependence. Human volunteers with a history of recreational drug or alcohol usage were studied in two double-blind clinical investigations. None of the subjects were able to distinguish between buspirone HCl and placebo. By contrast, subjects showed a statistically significant preference for methaqualone and diazepam. Studies in monkeys, mice, and rats have indicated that buspirone lacks potential for abuse.

Following chronic administration in the rat, abrupt withdrawal of buspirone did not result in the loss of body weight commonly observed with substances that cause physical dependency.

Although there is no direct evidence that buspirone HCl causes physical dependence or drug-seeking behavior, it is difficult to predict from experiments the extent to which a CNS-active drug will be misused, diverted, and/or abused once marketed. Consequently, physicians should carefully evaluate patients for a history of drug abuse and follow such patients closely, observing them for signs of buspirone HCl misuse or abuse (eg, development of tolerance, incrementation of dose, drug-seeking behavior).

OVERDOSAGE:

Signs and Symptoms: In clinical pharmacology trials, doses as high as 375 mg/day were administered to healthy male volunteers. As this dose was approached, the following symptoms were observed: nausea, vomiting, dizziness, drowsiness, miosis, and gastric distress. No deaths have been reported in humans either with deliberate or accidental overdosage of buspirone HCl. Toxicology studies of buspirone yielded the following LD_{50} values: mice, 655 mg/kg; rats, 196 mg/kg; dogs, 586 mg/kg; and monkeys, 356 mg/kg. These dosages are 160 to 550 times the recommended human daily dose.

Recommended Overdose Treatment: General symptomatic and supportive measures should be used along with immediate gastric lavage. Respiration, pulse, and blood pressure should be monitored as in all cases of drug overdosage. No specific antidote is known to buspirone, and dialyzability of buspirone has not been determined.

DOSAGE AND ADMINISTRATION:

The recommended initial dose is 15 mg daily (5 mg 3 times a day). To achieve an optimal therapeutic response, at intervals of 2 to 3 days the dosage may be increased 5 mg per day, as needed. The maximum daily dosage should not exceed 60 mg per day. In clinical trials allowing dose titration, divided doses of 20 to 30 mg per day were commonly employed.

PATIENT INFORMATION:

Buspirone is used for the treatment of nervousness and anxiety. Optimum results are usually seen after three to four weeks of treatment. This medication may be taken with or without food. Inform your physican if you are pregnant or nursing. Buspirone may cause dizziness and drowsiness; use caution while driving or operating hazardous machinery. Do not take any other sedating drugs or drink alcohol while taking this medication. Do not take this medication with a monoamine oxidase inhibitor. Notify physician if you develop muscle spasms, uncontrolled twitching in the face and body, or uncontrolled tongue or jaw movements.

HOW SUPPLIED:

BuSpar Tablets, 5 mg and 10 mg (white, ovoid-rectangular with score, MJ logo, strength and the name BuSpar embossed, are available in bottles of 100 and 500, and in cartons containing 100 individually packaged tablets.

U.S. Patent No.4, 182, 763

Store at Room Temperature—Protect from temperatures greater than 86°F (30°C). Dispense in a tight, light-resistant container (USP).

REFERENCES:

1. American Psychiatric Association, Ed.: Diagnostic and Statistical Manual of Mental Disorders—III, American Psychiatric Association, May 1980.

HOW SUPPLIED - EQUIVALENTS NOT AVAILABLE:

Tablet, Uncoated - Oral - 5 mg

100's	$59.52	BUSPAR, Bristol Myers Squibb	00087-0818-41
100's	$65.19	BUSPAR, Bristol Myers Squibb	00087-0818-43
500's	$289.42	BUSPAR, Bristol Myers Squibb	00087-0818-44

Tablet, Uncoated - Oral - 10 mg

100's	$103.83	BUSPAR, Bristol Myers Squibb	00087-0819-41
100's	$113.75	BUSPAR, Bristol Myers Squibb	00087-0819-43
500's	$504.66	BUSPAR, Bristol Myers Squibb	00087-0819-44

BUSULFAN *(000552)*

CATEGORIES: Antineoplastics; Cytotoxic Agents; Leukemia; Oncologic Drugs; Pregnancy Category D; FDA Approval Pre 1982

BRAND NAMES: *Citosulfan*; *Leukosulfan*; *Mablin* (Japan); *Misulban*; **Myleran**
(International brand names outside U.S. in italics)

FORMULARIES: BC-BS; Medi-Cal

WARNING:
Busulfan is a potent drug. It should not be used unless a diagnosis of chronic myelogenous leukemia has been adequately established and the responsible physician is knowledgeable in assessing response to chemotherapy.
Busulfan can induce severe bone marrow hypoplasia. Reduce or discontinue the dosage immediately at the first sign of any unusual depression of bone marrow function as reflected by an abnormal decrease in any of the formed elements of the blood. A bone marrow examination should be performed if the bone marrow status is uncertain.
SEE WARNINGS FOR INFORMATION REGARDING BUSULFAN-INDUCED LEUKEMOGENESIS IN HUMANS.

DESCRIPTION:

Busulfan is a bifunctional alkylating agent. Busulfan is known chemically as 1,4-butanediol dimethanesulfonate and has the following structural formula: $CH_3SO_2O(CH_2)_4OSO_2CH_3$

Busulfan is *not* a structural analog of the nitrogen mustards. Busulfan is available in tablet form for oral administration. Each scored tablet contains 2 mg busulfan and the inactive ingredients magnesium stearate and sodium chloride.

The activity of busulfan in chronic myelogenous leukemia was first reported by D.A.G. Galton in 1953.[1]

CLINICAL PHARMACOLOGY:

No analytical method has been found which permits the quantitation of non-radiolabeled busulfan or its metabolites in biological tissues or plasma. All studies of the pharmacokinetics of busulfan in humans have employed radiolabeled drug using either sulfur-35 (labeling the "carrier" portion of the molecule) or carbon-14 or tritium in the alkane portion of the 4-carbon chain (labels in the "alkylating" portion of the molecule).

Studies with ^{35}S-busulfan.[2]: Following the intravenous administration of a single therapeutic dose of ^{35}S-busulfan, there was rapid disappearance of radioactivity from the blood; 90 to 95% of the ^{35}S-label disappeared within three to five minutes after injection. Thereafter, a constant, low level of radioactivity (1 to 3% of the injected dose) was maintained during the subsequent forty-eight hour period of observation. Following the oral administration of ^{35}S-busulfan, there was a lag period of one-half to two hours prior to the detection of radioactivity in the blood. However, at four hours the (low) level of circulating radioactivity was comparable to that obtained following intravenous administration.

CLINICAL PHARMACOLOGY: *(cont'd)*

After either oral or intravenous administration of ^{35}S-busulfan to humans, 45% to 60% of the radioactivity was recovered in the urine in the forty-eight hours after administration; the majority of the total urinary excretion occurred in the first twenty-four hours. In man, over 95% of the urinary sulfur-35 occurs as ^{35}S-methanesulfonic acid.

The fact that urinary recovery of sulfur-35 was equivalent, irrespective of whether the drug was given intravenously or orally, suggests virtually complete absorption by the oral route.

Studies with ^{14}C-busulfan.[2] Oral and intravenous administration of 1,4-^{14}C-busulfan showed the same rapid initial disappearance of plasma radioactivity with a subsequent low-level plateau as observed following the administration of ^{35}S-labeled drug. Cumulative radioactivity in the urine after forty-eight hours was 25% to 30% of the administered dose (contrasting with 45 to 60% for ^{35}S-busulfan) and suggests a slower excretion of the alkylating portion of the molecule and its metabolites than for the sulfonoxymethyl moieties. Regardless of the route of administration, 1,4-^{14}C-busulfan yielded a complex mixture of at least 12 radiolabeled metabolites in urine; the main metabolite being 3-hydroxytetrahydrothiophene-1, 1-dioxide.

Studies with ^{3}H-busulfan.[3] Human pharmacokinetic studies have been conducted employing busulfan labeled with tritium on the tetramethylene chain. These experiments confirmed a rapid initial clearance of the radioactivity from plasma, irrespective of whether the drug was given orally or intravenously, and showed a gradual accumulation of radioactivity in the plasma after repeated doses. Urinary excretion of less than 50% of the total dose given suggested a slow elimination of the metabolic products from the body.

There is no experience with the use of dialysis in an attempt to modify the clinical toxicity of busulfan. One technical difficulty would derive from the extremely poor water solubility of busulfan. Additionally, all studies of the metabolism of busulfan employing radiolabeled materials indicate rapid chemical reactivity of the parent compound with prolonged retention of some of the metabolites (particularly the metabolites arising from the "alkylating" portion of the molecule). The effectiveness of dialysis at removing significant quantities of unreacted drug would be expected to be minimal in such a situation.

No information is available regarding the penetration of busulfan into brain or cerebrospinal fluid.

Biochemical Pharmacology: In aqueous media, busulfan undergoes a wide range of nucleophilic substitution reactions. While this chemical reactivity is relatively non-specific, alkylation of the DNA is felt to be an important biological mechanism for its cytotoxic effect.[4] Coliphage T7 exposed to busulfan was found to have the DNA crosslinked by intrastrand crosslinkages, but no interstrand linkages were found.

The metabolic fate of busulfan has been studied in rats and humans using ^{14}C- and ^{35}S-labeled materials.[2,5,6] In man,[2] as in the rat,[6] almost all of the radioactivity in ^{35}S-labeled busulfan is excreted in the urine in the form of ^{35}S-methanesulfonic acid. No unchanged drug was found in human urine,[2] although a small amount has been reported in rat urine.[6] Roberts and Warwick demonstrated that the formation of methanesulfonic acid *in vivo* in the rat is not due to a simple hydrolysis of busulfan to 1,4-butanediol, since only about 4% of 2,3-^{14}C-busulfan was excreted as carbon dioxide whereas 2,3-^{14}C-1,4-butanediol was converted almost exclusively to carbon dioxide.[5] The predominant reaction of busulfan in the rat is the alkylation of sulfhydryl groups (particularly cysteine and cysteine-containing compounds) to produce a cyclic sulfonium compound which is the precursor of the major urinary metabolite of the 4-carbon portion of the molecule, 3-hydroxytetrahydrothiophene-1,1-dioxide.[5] This has been termed a "sulfur-stripping" action of busulfan and it may modify the function of certain sulfur-containing amino acids, polypeptides, and proteins; whether this action makes an important contribution to the cytotoxicity of busulfan is unknown.

The biochemical basis for acquired resistance to busulfan is largely a matter of speculation. Although altered transport of busulfan into the cell is one possibility, increased intracellular inactivation of the drug before it reaches the DNA is also possible. Experiments with other alkylating agents have shown that resistance to this class of compounds may reflect an acquired ability of the resistant cell to repair alkylation damage more effectively.[4]

INDICATIONS AND USAGE:

Busulfan is indicated for the palliative treatment of chronic myelogenous (myeloid, myelocytic, granulocytic) leukemia. Although not curative, busulfan reduces the total granulocyte mass, relieves symptoms of the disease, and improves the clinical state of the patient. Approximately 90% of adults with previously untreated chronic myelogenous leukemia will obtain hematologic remission with regression or stabilization of organomegaly following the use of busulfan. It has been shown to be superior to splenic irradiation with respect to survival times and maintenance of hemoglobin levels, and to be equivalent to irradiation at controlling splenomegaly.[7]

It is not clear whether busulfan unequivocally prolongs the survival of responding patients beyond the 31 months experienced by an untreated group of historical controls.[8] Median survival figures of 31-42 months have been reported for several groups of patients treated with busulfan, but concurrent control groups of comparable, untreated patients are not available.[7,9,10,11] The median survival figures reported from different studies will be influenced by the percentage of "poor risk" patients initially entered into the particular study. Patients who are alive two years following the diagnosis of chronic myelogenous leukemia, and who have been treated during that period with busulfan, are estimated to have a mean annual mortality rate during the second to fifth year which is approximately two-thirds that of patients who received either no treatment, conventional x-ray or ^{32}P-irradiation, or chemotherapy with minimally active drugs.[12]

Busulfan is clearly less effective in patients with chronic myelogenous leukemia who lack the Philadelphia (Ph^1) chromosome.[13] Also, the so-called "juvenile" type of chronic myelogenous leukemia, typically occurring in young children and associated with the absence of a Philadelphia chromosome, responds poorly to busulfan.[14] The drug is of no benefit in patients whose chronic myelogenous leukemia has entered a "blastic" phase.

CONTRAINDICATIONS:

Busulfan should not be used unless a diagnosis of chronic myelogenous leukemia has been adequately established and the responsible physician is knowledgeable in assessing response to chemotherapy.

Busulfan should not be used in patients whose chronic myelogenous leukemia has demonstrated prior resistance to this drug.

Busulfan is of no value in chronic lymphocytic leukemia, acute leukemia, or in the "blastic crisis" of chronic myelogenous leukemia.

WARNINGS:

The most frequent, serious side effect of treatment with busulfan is the induction of bone marrow failure (which may or may not be anatomically hypoplastic) resulting in severe pancytopenia. The pancytopenia caused by busulfan may be more prolonged than that induced with other alkylating agents. It is generally felt that the usual cause of busulfan-induced pancytopenia is the failure to stop administration of the drug soon enough; individual idiosyncrasy to the drug does not seem to be an important factor. *Busulfan should be used with extreme caution and exceptional vigilance in patients whose bone marrow reserve may have been compromised by prior irradiation or chemotherapy, or whose marrow function is*

WARNINGS: *(cont'd)*

recovering from previous cytotoxic therapy. Although recovery from busulfan-induced pancytopenia may take from one month to two years, this complication is potentially reversible and the patient should be vigorously supported through any period of severe pancytopenia.[15]

A rare, important complication of busulfan therapy is the development of bronchopulmonary dysplasia with pulmonary fibrosis.[16] Symptoms have been reported to occur within eight months to ten years after initiation of therapy - the average duration of therapy being four years. The histologic findings associated with "busulfan lung" mimic those seen following pulmonary irradiation. Clinically, patients have reported the insidious onset of cough, dyspnea, and low-grade fever. Pulmonary function studies have revealed diminished diffusion capacity and decreased pulmonary compliance. It is important to exclude more common conditions (such as opportunistic infections or leukemic infiltration of the lungs) with appropriate diagnostic techniques. If measures such as sputum cultures, virologic studies, and exfoliative cytology fail to establish an etiology for the pulmonary infiltrates, lung biopsy may be necessary to establish the diagnosis. Treatment of established busulfan-induced pulmonary fibrosis is unsatisfactory; in most cases the patients have died within six months after the diagnosis was established. There is no specific therapy for this complication other than the immediate discontinuation of busulfan. The administration of corticosteroids has been suggested, but the results have not been impressive or uniformly successful.

Busulfan may cause cellular dysplasia in many organs in addition to the lung. Cytologic abnormalities characterized by giant, hyperchromatic nuclei have been reported in lymph nodes, pancreas, thyroid, adrenal glands, liver, and bone marrow. This cytologic dysplasia may be severe enough to cause difficulty in interpretation of exfoliative cytologic examinations from the lung, bladder, breast, and the uterine cervix.

In addition to the widespread epithelial dysplasia that has been observed during busulfan therapy, chromosome aberrations have been reported in cells from patients receiving busulfan.

Busulfan is mutagenic in mice and, possibly, in man.

A number of malignant tumors have been reported in patients on busulfan therapy and this drug may be a human carcinogen. Four cases of acute leukemia occurred among 243 patients treated with busulfan as adjuvant chemotherapy following surgical resection of bronchogenic carcinoma. All four cases were from a subgroup of 19 of these 243 patients who developed pancytopenia while taking busulfan five to eight years before leukemia became clinically apparent. These findings suggest that busulfan is leukemogenic, although its mode of action is uncertain.[17]

Ovarian suppression and amenorrhea with menopausal symptoms commonly occur during busulfan therapy in premenopausal patients. Busulfan interferes with spermatogenesis in experimental animals, and there have been clinical reports of sterility, azoospermia and testicular atrophy in male patients.

A rare but life-threatening hepatic veno-occlusive disease has been reported following the investigational use of very high doses of busulfan in combination with cyclophosphamide or other chemotherapeutic agents prior to bone marrow transplantation.[18-24] A clear cause and effect relationship with busulfan has not been demonstrated. Periodic measurement of serum transaminases, alkaline phosphatase, and bilirubin is indicated for early detection of hepatotoxicity.

Cardiac tamponade has been reported in a small number of patients with thalassemia (2% in one series) who received high doses of busulfan and cyclophosphamide as the preparatory regimen for bone marrow transplantation. In this series, the cardiac tamponade was often fatal. Abdominal pain and vomiting preceded the tamponade in patients.

Pregnancy Category D: Busulfan may cause fetal harm when administered to a pregnant woman. Although there have been a number of cases reported where apparently normal children have been born after busulfan treatment during pregnancy,[25] one case has been cited where a malformed baby was delivered by a mother treated with busulfan. During the pregnancy that resulted in the malformed infant, the mother received x-ray therapy early in the first trimester, mercaptopurine until the third month, then busulfan until delivery.[26] In pregnant rats, busulfan produces sterility in both male and female offspring due to the absence of germinal cells in testes and ovaries.[27] Germinal cell aplasia or sterility in offspring of mothers receiving busulfan during pregnancy has not been reported in humans. There are no adequate and well-controlled studies in pregnant women. If this drug is used during pregnancy, or if the patient becomes pregnant while taking this drug, the patient should be apprised of the potential hazard to the fetus. Women of childbearing potential should be advised to avoid becoming pregnant.

PRECAUTIONS:

GENERAL

The most consistent, dose-related toxicity is bone marrow suppression. This may be manifest by anemia, leukopenia, thrombocytopenia or any combination of these. It is imperative that patients be instructed to report promptly the development of fever, sore throat, signs of local infection, bleeding from any site, or symptoms suggestive of anemia. Any one of these findings may indicate busulfan toxicity; however, they may also indicate transformation of the disease to an acute "blastic" form. Since busulfan may have a delayed effect, it is important to withdraw the medication temporarily at the first sign of an abnormally large or exceptionally rapid fall in any of the formed elements of the blood. *Patients should never be allowed to take the drug without close medical supervision.*

Seizures have been reported in patients receiving very high, investigational doses of busulfan.[18,28-32] As with any potentially epileptogenic drug, caution should be exercised when administering very high doses of busulfan to patients with a history of seizure disorder, head trauma, or receiving other potentially epileptogenic drugs. Some investigators have used prophylactic anticonvulsant therapy in this setting.

INFORMATION FOR THE PATIENT

Patients beginning therapy with busulfan should be informed of the importance of having periodic blood counts and to immediately report any unusual fever or bleeding. Aside from the major toxicity of myelosuppression, patients should be instructed to report any difficulty in breathing, persistent cough or congestion. They should be told that diffuse pulmonary fibrosis is an infrequent but serious and potentially life-threatening complication of long-term busulfan therapy. Patients should be alerted to report any signs of abrupt weakness, unusual fatigue, anorexia, weight loss, nausea and vomiting, and melanoderma that could be associated with a syndrome resembling adrenal insufficiency. Patients should never be allowed to take the drug without medical supervision and they should be informed that other encountered toxicities to busulfan include infertility, amenorrhea, skin hyperpigmentation, drug hypersensitivity, dryness of the mucous membranes and rarely cataract formation. Women of childbearing potential should be advised to avoid becoming pregnant. The increased risk of a second malignancy should be explained to the patient.

LABORATORY TESTS

It is recommended that evaluation of the hemoglobin or hematocrit, total white blood cell count and differential count, and quantitative platelet count be obtained weekly while the patient is on busulfan therapy. In cases where the cause of fluctuation in the formed elements of the peripheral blood is obscure, bone marrow examination may be useful for evaluation of marrow status. A decision to increase, decrease, continue, or discontinue a given dose of busulfan must be based not only on the absolute hematologic values, but also on the rapidity

PRECAUTIONS: *(cont'd)*

with which changes are occurring. The dosage of busulfan may need to be reduced if this agent is combined with other drugs whose primary toxicity is myelosuppression. Occasional patients may be unusually sensitive to busulfan administered at standard dosage and suffer neutropenia or thrombocytopenia after a relatively short exposure to the drug. Busulfan should not be used where facilities for complete blood counts, including quantitative platelet counts, are not available at weekly (or more frequent) intervals.

CARCINOGENESIS, MUTAGENESIS, AND IMPAIRMENT OF FERTILITY

See WARNINGS.

PREGNANCY CATEGORY D

Teratogenic Effects: See WARNINGS section.

Non-Teratogenic Effects: There have been reports in the literature of small infants being born after the mothers received busulfan during pregnancy, in particular, during the third trimester.[34] One case was reported where an infant had mild anemia and neutropenia at birth after busulfan was administered to the mother from the eighth week of pregnancy to term.[25]

NURSING MOTHERS

It is not known whether this drug is excreted in human milk. Because of the potential for tumorigenicity shown for busulfan in animal and human studies, a decision should be made whether to discontinue nursing or to discontinue the drug, taking into account the importance of the drug to the mother.

DRUG INTERACTIONS:

Busulfan may cause additive myelosuppression when used with other myelosuppressive drugs.

In one study, 12 of approximately 330 patients receiving continuous busulfan and thioguanine therapy for treatment of chronic myelogenous leukemia were found to have esophageal varices associated with abnormal liver function tests.[33] Subsequent liver biopsies were performed in four of these patients, all of which showed evidence of nodular regenerative hyperplasia. Duration of combination therapy prior to the appearance of esophageal varices ranged from 6 to 45 months. With the present analysis of the data, no cases of hepatotoxicity have appeared in the busulfan alone arm of the study. Long-term continuous therapy with thioguanine and busulfan should be used with caution.

ADVERSE REACTIONS:

Hematological Effects: The most frequent, serious, toxic effect of busulfan is myelosuppression resulting in leukopenia, thrombocytopenia, and anemia. Myelosuppression is most frequently the result of a failure to discontinue dosage in the face of an undetected decrease in leukocyte or platelet counts.[15]

Pulmonary: Interstitial pulmonary fibrosis has been reported rarely, but it is a clinically significant adverse effect when observed and calls for immediate discontinuation of further administration of the drug. The role of corticosteroids in arresting or reversing the fibrosis has been reported to be beneficial in some cases and without effect in others.[16]

Cardiac: Cardiac tamponade has been reported in a small number of patients with thalassemia who received high doses of busulfan and cyclophamide as the preparatory regimen for bone marrow transplantation (see WARNINGS.)

One case of endocardial fibrosis has been reported in a 79-year-old woman who received a total dose of 7,200 mg of busulfan over a period of nine years for the management of chronic myelogenous leukemia.[35] At autopsy, she was found to have endocardial fibrosis of the left ventricle in addition to interstitial pulmonary fibrosis.

Ocular: Busulfan is capable of inducing cataracts in rats and there have been several reports indicating that this is a rare complication in humans. In the few cases reported in humans, cataracts have occurred only after prolonged administration of busulfan.[36]

Dermatologic: Hyperpigmentation is the most common adverse skin reaction and occurs in 5-10% of patients, particularly those with a dark complexion.

Metabolic: In a few cases, a clinical syndrome closely resembling adrenal insufficiency and characterized by weakness, severe fatigue, anorexia, weight loss, nausea and vomiting, and melanoderma has developed after prolonged busulfan therapy. The symptoms have sometimes been reversible when busulfan was withdrawn. Adrenal responsiveness to exogenously administered ACTH has usually been normal. However, pituitary function testing with metyrapone revealed a blunted urinary 17-hydroxycorticosteroid excretion in two patients.[37] Following the discontinuation of busulfan (which was associated with clinical improvement), rechallenge with metyrapone revealed normal pituitary-adrenal function.

Hyperuricemia and/or hyperuricosuria are not uncommon in patients with chronic myelogenous leukemia. Additional rapid destruction of granulocytes may accompany the initiation of chemotherapy and increase the urate pool. Adverse effects can be minimized by increased hydration, urine alkalinization, and the prophylactic administration of a xanthine oxidase inhibitor such as Zyloprim (allopurinol).

Hepatic Effects: Esophageal varices have been reported in patients receiving continuous busulfan and thioguanine for treatment of chronic myelogenous leukemia (see DRUG INTERACTIONS.) Hepatic veno-occlusive disease has been observed in patients receiving higher than recommended doses of busulfan (see WARNINGS.)

Miscellaneous: Other reported adverse reactions include: urticaria, erythema multiforme, erythema nodosum, alopecia, porphyria cutanea tarda, excessive dryness and fragility of the skin with anhidrosis, dryness of the oral mucous membranes and cheilosis, gynecomastia, cholestatic jaundice and myasthenia gravis. Most of these are single case reports, and in many a clear cause and effect relationship with busulfan has not been demonstrated.

Seizures (see PRECAUTIONS, General) have been observed in patients receiving higher than recommended doses of busulfan.

OVERDOSAGE:

There is no known antidote to busulfan. The principal toxic effect is on the bone marrow. Survival after a single 140 mg dose has been reported in an 18 kg, 4-year-old child,[38] but hematologic toxicity is likely to be more profound with chronic overdosage. The hematologic status should be closely monitored and vigorous supportive measures instituted if necessary. Induction of vomiting or gastric lavage followed by administration of charcoal would be indicated if ingestion were recent. It is not known whether busulfan is dialyzable (see CLINICAL PHARMACOLOGY.)

Oral LD_{50} single doses in mice are 120 mg/kg. Two distinct types of toxic response are seen at median lethal doses given intraperitoneally. Within a matter of hours there are signs of stimulation of the central nervous system with convulsions and death on the first day. Mice are more sensitive to this effect than are rats. With doses at the LD_{50} there is also delayed death due to damage to the bone marrow. At three times the LD_{50}, atrophy of the mucosa of the large intestine is found after a week, whereas that of the small intestine is little affected.[39] After doses in the order of 10 times those used therapeutically were added to the diet of rats, irreversible cataracts were produced after several weeks. Small doses had no such effect.[40]

DOSAGE AND ADMINISTRATION:

Busulfan is administered orally. The usual adult dose range for*remission induction* is four to eight mg, total dose, daily. Dosing on a weight basis is the same for both children and adults, approximately 60 mcg per kg of body weight or 1.8 mg per square meter of body surface, daily. Since the rate of fall of the leukocyte count is dose related, daily doses exceeding four mg per day should be reserved for patients with the most compelling symptoms: the greater the total daily dose, the greater is the possibility of inducing bone marrow aplasia.

A decrease in the leukocyte count is not usually seen during the first ten to fifteen days of treatment; the leukocyte count may actually increase during this period and it should not be interpreted as resistance to the drug, nor should the dose be increased.[41] Since the leukocyte count may continue to fall for more than one month after discontinuing the drug, it is important that busulfan be discontinued *prior* to the total leukocyte count falling into the normal range. When the total leukocyte count has declined to approximately 15,000/μL the drug should be withheld.

With a constant dose of busulfan, the total leukocyte count declines exponentially; a weekly plot of the leukocyte on semi-logarithmic graph paper aids in predicting when therapy should be discontinued.[42]With the recommended dose of busulfan, a normal leukocyte count is usually achieved in twelve to twenty weeks.

During remission, the patient is examined at monthly intervals and treatment resumed with the induction dosage when the total leukocyte count reaches approximately 50,000/μL. When remission is shorter that three months, maintenance therapy of 1 to 3 mg daily may be advisable in order to keep the hematological status under control and prevent rapid relapse.

Procedures for proper handling and disposal of anti-cancer drugs should be considered. Several guidelines on this subject have been published.[43-49]

There is no general agreement that all of the procedures recommended in the guidelines are necessary or appropriate.

Store at 15 to 25°C (59 to 77°F) in a dry place.

REFERENCES:

1. Galton DAG. Myleran in chronic myeloid leukemia: results of treatment. *Lancet.* 1953;1:208-213. **2.** Nadkarni MV, Trams EG, Smith PK. Preliminary studies on the distribution and fate of TEM, TEPA, and Myleran in the human. *Cancer Res.* 1959;19:713-718. **3.** Vodopick H, Hamilton HE, Jackson HL, Peng C-T, Sheets RF. Metabolic fate of tritiated busulfan in man. *J Lab Clin Med.*1969;73:266-276. **4.** Fox BW. Mechanism of action of methane sulfonates. In: Sartorelli AC, Johns DG, eds. *Antineoplastic and Immunosuppressive Agents,* Part II. Berlin: Springer Verlag; 1975:35-36. **5.** Roberts JJ, Warwick GP. The mode of action of alkylating agents, III: the formation of 3-hydroxytetrahydrothiophene-1:1-dioxide from 1:4-dimethane-sulphonyloxybutane (Myleran), S-β-L-alanyltetrahydrothiophenium mesylate, tetrahydrothiophene and tetrahydrothiophene-1:1-dioxide in the rat, rabbit and mouse. *Biochem Pharmacol.* 1961;6:217-227. **6.** Peng C-T. Distribution and metabolic fate of S^{35}-labeled busulfan in normal and tumor-bearing rats.*J Pharmacol Exp Ther.* 1957;120:229-238. **7.** Medical Research Council's Working Party for Therapeutic Trials in Leukemia. Chronic granulocytic leukaemia: comparison of radiotherapy and busulfan therapy. *Br Med J.* 1968;1:201-208. **8.** Minot GR, Buckman TE, Isaacs R. Chronic myelogenous leukemia: age incidence, duration, and benefit derived from irradiation. *JAMA.* 1924;82:1489-1494. **9.** Haut A, Abbott WS, Wintrobe MM, Cartwright GE. Busulfan in the treatment of chronic myelocytic leukemia: the effect of long term intermittent therapy. *Blood.* 1961;17:1-19. **10.** Monfardini S, Gee T, Fried J, Clarkson B. Survival in chronic myelogenous leukemia: influence of treatment and extent of disease at diagnosis. *Cancer.*1973;31;492-501. **11.** Conrad FG. Survival in granulocytic leukemia. *Arch Intern Med.* 1973;131:684-685. **12.** Sokal JE. Evaluation of survival data for chronic myelocytic leukemia. *Am J Hematol.* 1976;1:493-500. **13.** Ezdinli EZ, Sokal JE, Crosswhite L, Sandberg AA. Philadelphia chromosome-positive and -negative chronic myelocytic leukemia. *Ann Intern Med.* 1970;72:175-182. **14.** Smith KL, Johnson W. Classification of chronic myelocytic leukemia in children. *Cancer.* 1974;34:670-679. **15.** Stuart JJ, Crocker DL, Roberts HR. Treatment of busulfan-induced pancytopenia.*Arch Intern Med.* 1977;136:1181-1183. **16.** Sostman HD, Matthay RA, Putman CE. Cytotoxic drug-induced lung disease. *Am J Med.* 1977;62:608-615. **17.** Stott H, Fox W, Griling DJ, Stephens RJ, Gatton DAG. Acute leukaemia after busulfan. *Br Med J.* 1977;2:1513-1517. **18.** Hartmann O, et al. High-dose busulfan and cyclophosphamide with autologous bone marrow transplantation support in advanced malignancies in children: A Phase II study. *J Clin Oncol* 1986;4:1804-10. **19.** Copelan EA, et al. Marrow Transplantation following busulfan and cyclophosphamide for chronic myelogenous leukemia in accelerated or blastic phase. *Br J Haematol*1989;71:487-91. **20.** Kirchner H, et al. Allogeneic and autologous bone marrow transplantation (BMT) after high-dose busulfan and cyclophosphamide treatment. *Blut* 1988;57:198. (abstract) **21.** Thompson J, et al. Allogeneic bone marrow transplantation (BMT) following transplant preparation with cyclophosphamide (CTX) and busulfan (BU). *Proc ASCO* 1989;8:18. (abstract) **22.** Geller RB, et al. Allogeneic bone marrow transplantation after high-dose busulfan cyclophosphamide in patients with acute non-lymphocytic leukemia. *Blood* 1989;73:2209-18. **23.** Lu C, et al. Preliminary results of high-dose busulfan and cyclophosphamide with syngeneic or autologous bone marrow rescue. *Cancer Treat Rep*1984;68:711-7. **24.** Groshow LB, et al. Pharmacokinetics of busulfan: correlation with veno-occlusive disease in patients undergoing bone marrow transplantation. *Cancer Chemother Pharmacol*1989;25:55-61. **25.** Dugdale M, Fort AT. Busulfan treatment of leukemia during pregnancy: case report and review of the literature.*JAMA.*1967;199:131-133. **26.** Diamond I, Anderson MM, McCreadie SR. Transplacental transmission of busulfan (Myleran) in a mother with leukemia: production of fetal malformation and cytomegaly.*Pediatrics.* 1960;25:85-90. **27.** Bollag W. Cytostatica in der Schwangerschaft. *Schweiz Med Wochenschr.* 1954;84:393-395. **28.** Marcus RE, et al. Convulsions due to high-dose busulfan.*Lancet* 1984;2:1463. (letter) **29.** Martell RW, et al. High-dose busulfan and myoclonic epilepsy. *Ann Intern Med*1987;106:173. (letter) **30.** Sureda A, et al. High-dose busulfan and seizures. *Ann Intern Med* 1989;111:543-4. (letter) **31.** Grigg AP, et al. Busulfan and phenytoin. *Ann Intern Med*1989;111:1049-50. (letter) **32.** Beelen DW, et al. Acute toxicity and first clinical results of intensive post-induction therapy using a modified busulfan and cyclophosphamide regimen with autologous bone marrow rescue in first remission of acute myeloid leukemia. *Blood*1989;74:1507-16. **33.** Key NS, Kelly PMA, Emerson PM, Chapman RWG, Allan NC, McGee JO'D. Oesophageal varices associated with busulfan-thioguanine combination therapy for chronic myeloid leukaemia.*Lancet.* 1987;2:1050-1052. **34.** Boros SJ, Reynolds JW. Intrauterine growth retardation following third-trimester exposure to busulfan. *Am J Obstet Gynecol.* 1977;129:111-112. **35.** Weinberger A, Pinkhas J, Sandbank U, Shaklai M, de Vries A. Endocardial fibrosis following busulfan treatment. *JAMA.* 1975;231:495. **36.** Ravindranathan MP, Paul VJ, Kuriakose ET. Cataract after busulfan treatment. *Br. Med J.* 1972;1:218-219. **37.** Vivacqua RJ, Haurani FI, Erslev AJ. "Selective" pituitary insufficiency secondary to busulfan. *Ann Intern Med.* 1967;67:380-387. **38.** DeOliveira HP, Cruz E, Fonseca A de S, Medeiros M. Accidental ingestion of a toxic dose of Myleran by a child. *Acta Haematol* (Basel). 1963;29:249-255. **39.** Sternberg SS, Philips FS, Scholler J. Pharmacological and pathological effects of alkylating agents. *Ann NY Acad Sci.* 1958;68:811-825. **40.** Solomon C, Light AE, deBeer EJ. Cataracts produced in rats by 1,4-dimethanesulfonoxybutane (Myleran). *AMA Arch Ophthal.*1955;54:850-852. **41.** Stryckmans PA: Current concepts in chronic myelogenous leukemia. *Semin Hematol.* 1974;11:101-127. **42.** Galton DAG. Chemotherapy of chronic myelocytic leukemia. *Semin Hematol.* 1969;6:323-343. **43.** Recommendations for the safe handling of parenteral antineoplastic drugs. Washington, DC: Division of Safety, National Institutes of Health; 1983. US Dept of Health and Human Services, Public Health Service publication NIH 83-2621. **44.** AMA Council on Scientific Affairs. Guidelines for handling parenteral antineoplastics. *JAMA.* 1985;253:1590-1591. **45.** National Study Commission on Cytotoxic Exposure. Recommendations for handling cytotoxic agents. 1984. Available from Louis P. Jeffrey, ScD, Director of Pharmacy Services, Rhode Island Hospital, 593 Eddy Street, Providence, Rhode Island 02902. **46.** Clinical Oncological Society of Australia. Guidelines and recommendations for safe handling of antineoplastic agents. *Med J Australia.* 1983;1:426-428. **47.** Jones RB, Frank R, Mass T. Safe handling of chemotherapeutic agents: a report from the Mount Sinai Medical Center. *CA-A Cancer J for Clin.* 1983;33(Sep/Oct);258-263. **48.** American Society of Hospital Pharmacists. ASHP technical assistance bulletin on handling cytotoxic and hazardous drugs. *AM J Hosp Pharm.*1990;47:1033-1049. **49.** Yodaiken RE, Bennett D. OSHA work-practice guidelines for personnel dealing with cytotoxic (antineoplastic) drugs.*Am J Hosp Pharm.* 1986;43:1193-1204.

HOW SUPPLIED:

White, scored tablets containing 2 mg busulfan, imprinted with "Myleran" and "K2A" on each tablet.

HOW SUPPLIED - EQUIVALENTS NOT AVAILABLE:

Tablet, Uncoated - Oral - 2 mg

25's	**$35.70**	**MYLERAN, Glaxo Wellcome**	**00173-0713-25**

BUTABARBITAL SODIUM *(000557)*

CATEGORIES: Anxiolytics, Sedatives, Hypnotic; Barbiturates; Central Nervous System Agents; Insomnia; Sedatives; Sedatives/Hypnotics; Pregnancy Category D; DEA Class CIII; FDA Approval Pre 1982

BRAND NAMES: Barbased; Busodium; Butalan; Butatran; Buticaps; *Butisol* (Canada); **Butisol Sodium**; *Day-Barb* (Canada); Sarisol; Sodium Butabarbital *(International brand names outside U.S. in italics)*

FORMULARIES: BC-BS

COST OF THERAPY: $8.28 (Insomnia; Tablet; 30 mg; 2/day; 7 days)

DESCRIPTION:

Butabarbital sodium is a non-selective central nervous system depressant which is used as a sedative or hypnotic (WARNING: May be habit forming). It is available for oral administration as Tablets containing 15 mg, 30 mg, 50 mg or 100 mg butabarbital sodium, and as Elixir containing 30 mg/5 ml, with alcohol (by volume) 7%. Butabarbital sodium occurs as a white, bitter powder which is freely soluble in water and alcohol, but practically insoluble in benzene and ether.

CLINICAL PHARMACOLOGY:

Butabarbital sodium, like other barbiturates, is capable of producing all levels of CNS mood alteration from excitation to mild sedation, to hypnosis, and deep coma. Overdosage can produce death. Barbiturates depress the sensory cortex, decrease motor activity, alter cerebellar function, and produce drowsiness, sedation, and hypnosis.

Barbiturate-induced sleep differs from physiological sleep. Sleep laboratory studies have demonstrated that barbiturates reduce the amount of time spent in the rapid eye movement (REM) phase of sleep or dreaming stage. Also, Stages III and IV sleep are decreased. Following abrupt cessation of barbiturates used regularly, patients may experience markedly increased dreaming, nightmares, and or insomnia. Therefore, withdrawal of a single therapeutic dose over 5 or 6 days has been recommended to lessen the REM rebound and disturbed sleep which contribute to drug withdrawal syndrome (for example, decrease the dose from 3 to 2 doses a day for 1 week).

In studies, secobarbital sodium and pentobarbital sodium have been found to lose most of their effectiveness for both inducing and maintaining sleep by the end of 2 weeks of continued drug administration even with the use of multiple doses. As with secobarbital sodium and pentobarbital sodium, other barbiturates might be expected to lose their effectiveness for inducing and maintaining sleep after about 2 weeks. The short, intermediate, and, to a lesser degree, long-acting barbiturates have been widely prescribed for treating insomnias. Although the clinical literature abounds with claims that the short-acting barbiturates are superior for producing sleep while the intermediate-acting compounds are more effective in maintaining sleep, controlled studies have failed to demonstrate there differential effects. Therefore, as sleep medications, the barbiturates are of limited value beyond short-term use.

Barbiturates are respiratory depressants. The degree of respiratory depression is dependant upon dose. With hypotonic doses, respiratory depression produced by barbiturates is similar to that which occurs during physiologic sleep with slight decrease in blood pressure and heart rate.

Barbiturates do not impair normal hepatic function, but have been shown to induce liver microsomal enzymes, thus increasing and/or altering the metabolism of barbiturates and other drugs (see DRUG INTERACTIONS.)

Pharmacokinetics: Butabarbital sodium is the sodium salt of a weak acid. Barbiturates are weak acids that are absorbed and rapidly distributed to all tissues and fluids with high concentrations in the brain, liver, and kidneys. Barbiturates are bound to plasma and tissue proteins. The rate of absorption is increased if it is ingested as a dilute solution or taken on an empty stomach.

Barbiturates are metabolized primarily by the hepatic microsomal enzyme system, and most metabolic products are excreted in the urine. The excretion of unchanged butabarbital in the urine is negligible. Butabarbital sodium is classified as an intermediate-acting barbiturate. The average plasma half-life for butabarbital is 100 hours in the adult.

Although variable from patient to patient, butabarbital has an onset of action of about 1/2 to 1 hour, and a duration of action of about 6 to 8 hours.

INDICATIONS AND USAGE:

Butabarbital sodium is indicated for use as a sedative or hypnotic.

Since barbiturates appear to lose their effectiveness for sleep induction and sleep maintenance after 2 weeks, use of Butabarbital Sodium in treating insomnias should be limited to this time (see CLINICAL PHARMACOLOGY.)

CONTRAINDICATIONS:

Barbiturates are contraindicated in patients with known barbiturate sensitivity. Barbiturates are also contraindicated in patients with a history of manifest or latent porphyria.

WARNINGS:

Habit farming: Barbiturates may be habit forming. Tolerance, psychological and physical dependence may occur with continued use (see DRUG ABUSE AND DEPENDENCE.) Patients who have psychological dependance on barbiturates may increase the dosage or decrease the dosage interval without consulting a physician and may subsequently develop a physical dependence on barbiturates. To minimize the possibility of overdosage or the development of dependences, the prescribing and dispensing of sedative-hypnotic barbiturates should be limited to the amount required for the interval until the next appointment. Abrupt cessation after prolonged use in the dependent person may result in withdrawal symptoms, including delirium, convulsions, and possibly death. Barbiturates should be withdrawn gradually from any patient known to be taking excessive dosage over long periods of time. (See DRUG ABUSE AND DEPENDENCE.)

Acute or chronic pain: Caution should be exercised when barbiturates are administered to patients with acute or chronic pain, because paradoxical excitement could be induced, or important symptoms could be masked. However, the use of barbiturates as sedatives in the postoperative surgical period, and as adjuncts to cancer chemotherapy, is well established.

Use in pregnancy: Barbiturates can cause fatal damage when administered to a pregnant woman. Retrospective, case-controlled studies have suggested a connection between the maternal consumption of barbiturates and a higher than expected incidence of fatal abnormalities. Following oral administration, barbiturates readily cross the placental barrier and are distributed throughout fatal tissues with highest concentrations found in the placenta, fatal liver, and brain.

Withdrawal symptoms occur in infants born is mothers who receive barbiturates throughout the last treatment of pregnancy (see DRUG ABUSE AND DEPENDENCE.) If this drug is used during pregnancy, or if the patient becomes pregnant while taking this drug, the patient should be appeared of the potential hazard to the fetus.

PRECAUTIONS:

GENERAL

Barbiturates should be administered with caution, if at all, to patients who are mentally depressed, have suicidal tendencies, or a history of drug abuse.

Elderly or debilitated patients may react to barbiturates with marked excitement, depression, and confusion. In some persons, barbiturates repeatedly produce excitement rather than depression.

PRECAUTIONS: *(cont'd)*

In patients with hepatic damage, barbiturates should be administered with caution and initially in reduced doses. Barbiturates should not be administered to patients showing the premonitory signs of hepatic coma.

butabarbital sodium Tablets, 30 mg and 50 mg, and Elixir contain FD&C Yellow No. 5 (tartrazine) which may cause allergic-type reactions (including bronchial asthma) in certain susceptible individuals. Although the overall incidence of FD&C Yellow No. 5 (tartrazine) sensitivity in the general population is low, it is frequently seen in patients who also have aspirin hypersensitivity.

INFORMATION FOR THE PATIENT

Practitioners should give the following information and instructions to patients receiving barbiturates.

The use of barbiturates carries with it an associated risk of psychological and/or physical dependence. The patient should be warned against increasing the dose of the drug without consulting a physician.

Barbiturates may impair mental and/or physical abilities required for the performance of potentially hazardous tasks, such as driving or operating machinery.

Alcohol should not be consumed while taking barbiturates. Concurrent use of the barbiturates with other CNS depressants, including other sedatives or hypnotics, alcohol, narcotics, tranquilizers, and antihistamines, may result in additional CNS depressant effects.

LABORATORY TESTS

Prolonged therapy with barbiturates should be accompanied by periodic laboratory evaluation of organ systems, including hematopoietic, renal, and hepatic systems (see PRECAUTIONS, General and ADVERSE REACTIONS.

CARCINOGENESIS, MUTAGENESIS, AND IMPAIRMENT OF FERTILITY

No long-term studies in animals have been performed with butabarbital sodium to determine carcinogenic and mutagenic potential, or effects on fertility.

PREGNANCY CATEGORY D

Teratogenic Effects: See WARNINGS, Use in pregnancy.

Nonteratogenic Effects: Infants suffering from long-term barbiturate exposure *in utero* may have an acute withdrawal syndrome of seizures and hyperirritability from birth to a delayed onset of up to 14 days (see DRUG ABUSE AND DEPENDENCE.)

LABOR AND DELIVERY

Hypnotic doses of barbiturates do not appear to significantly impair uterine activity during labor. Administration of sedative-hypnotic barbiturates to the mother during labor may result in respiratory depression in the newborn. Premature infants are particularly susceptible to the depressant effects of barbiturates. If barbiturates are used during labor and delivery, resuscitation equipment should be available.

NURSING MOTHERS

Caution should be exercised when a barbiturate is administered to a nursing woman since small amounts of some barbiturates are excreted in the milk.

DRUG INTERACTIONS:

Most reports of clinically significant drug interactions occurring with the barbiturates have involved phenobarbital. However, the application of these data to other barbiturates appears valid and warrants serial blood level determinations of the relevant drugs when there are multiple therapies.

Anticoagulants: Phenobarbital lowers the plasma levels of dicumarol and causes a decrease in anticoagulant activity as measured by the prothrombin time. Barbiturates can induce hepatic microseme of enzymes resulting in increased metabolism and decreased anticoagulant response of oral anticoagulants (*e.g.,* warfarin, acenocoumarol, dicumarol, and phenprocoumon). Patients stabilized on anticoagulant therapy may require dosage adjustments if barbiturates are added to or withdrawn from their dosage regimen.

Corticosteroids: Barbiturates appear to enhance the metabolism of exogenous corticosteroids probably through the induction of hepatic microsomal enzymes. Patients stabilized on corticosteroid therapy may require dosage adjustments if barbiturates are added to or withdrawn from their dosage regimen.

Griseofulvin: Phenobarbital appears to interfere with the absorption of orally administered griseofulvin, thus decreasing its blood level. The affect of the resultant decreased blood levels of griseofulvin on therapeutic response has not been established. However, it would be preferable to avoid concomitant administration of these drugs.

Doxycycline: Phenobarbital has been shown to shorten the half-life of doxycycline for as long as 2 weeks after barbiturate therapy is discontinued. This mechanism is probably through the induction of hepatic microsomal enzymes that metabolize the antibiotic. If phenobarbital and doxycycline are administered concurrently, the clinical response to doxycycline should be monitored closely.

Phenytoin, Sodium Valproate, Valproic Acid: The effect of barbiturates on the metabolism of phenytoin appears to be variable. Some investigators report an accelerating affect, while others report no effect. Because the effect of barbiturates on the metabolism of phenytoin is not predictable, phenytoin and barbiturate blood levels should be monitored more frequently if those drugs are given concurrently. Sodium valproate and valproic acid appear to decrease barbiturate metabolism; therefore, barbiturate blood levels should be monitored and appropriate adjustments made as indicated.

Central Nervous System: The concomitant use of other central nervous system depressants, including other sedatives or hypnotics, antihistamines, tranquilizers, or alcohol, may produce additive depressant effects.

Monoamine Oxidase Inhibitors (MAOI): MAOI prolong the effects of barbiturates probably because metabolism of the barbiturate is inhibited.

Estradiol, Estrone, Progesterone And Other Steroid Hormones: Pretreatment with or concurrent administration of phenobarbital may decrease the effect of estradiol by increasing its metabolism. There have been reports of patients treated with antiepileptic drugs (e.g. phenobarbital) who become pregnant while taking oral contraceptives. An alternate contraceptive method might be suggested to women taking phenobarbital.

ADVERSE REACTIONS:

The following adverse reactions have been observed with the use of barbiturates in hospitalized patients. Because such patients may be less aware of certain of the milder adverse effects of barbiturates, the incidence of these reactions may be somewhat higher in fully ambulatory patients.

More than 1 in 100 patients: The most common adverse reaction, somnolence, is estimated to occur at a rate of 1 to 3 patients per 100.

Less than 1 in 100 patients: The most common adverse reactions estimated to occur at a rate of less than 1 in 100 patients listed below, grouped by organ system, and by decreasing order of occurrence are:

Central Nervous System/Psychiatric: Agitation, confusion, hyperkinesis, ataxia, CNS depression, nightmares, nervousness, psychiatric disturbance, hallucinations, insomnia, anxiety, dizziness, thinking abnormality.

ADVERSE REACTIONS: *(cont'd)*

Respiratory: Hyperventilation, acnes.

Cardiovascular: Bradycardia, hypotension, syncope.

Gastrointestinal: Nausea, vomiting, constipation.

Other Reported Reactions: Headache, hypersensitivity (angioedema, skin rashes, exfoliative dermatitis), fever, liver damage.

DRUG ABUSE AND DEPENDENCE:

Controlled substance: Schedule III.

Barbiturates may be habit-forming. Tolerance, psychological dependences, and physical dependence may occur especially following prolonged use of high doses of barbiturates. Daily administration in excess of 400 milligrams (mg) of pentobarbital or secobarbital for approximately 96 days is likely to produce some degree of physical dependence. A dosage of from 600 to 800 mg taken for at least 35 days is sufficient to product withdrawal seizures. The average daily dose for the barbiturate addict is usually about 1.5 grams. As tolerance to barbiturates develops, the amount needed to maintain the same level of intoxication increases; tolerance to a fatal dosage, however, does not increase more than two-fold. As this occurs, the margin between an intoxicating dosage and a fatal dosage becomes smaller.

Symptoms of acute intoxication with barbiturates include unsteady gait, slurred speech, and sustained nystagmus. Mental signs of chronic intoxication include confusion, poor judgment, irritability, insomnia, and somatic complaints. Symptoms of barbiturate dependence are similar to those of chronic alcoholism.

If an individual appears to be intoxicated with alcohol to a degree that is radically disproportionate to the amount of alcohol in his or her blood, the use of barbiturates should be suspected. The lethal dose of a barbiturate is far less if alcohol is also ingested.

The symptoms of barbiturate withdrawal can be severe and may cause death. Minor withdrawal symptoms may appear 8 to 12 hours after the last dose of a barbiturate. These symptoms usually appear in the following order: anxiety, muscle twitching, tremor of hands and fingers, progressive weakness, dizziness, distortion in visual perception, nausea, vomiting, insomnia, and orthostatic hypotension. Major withdrawal symptoms convulsions and delirium may occur within 15 hours and last up to 5 days after abrupt cessation of these drugs. Intensity of withdrawal symptoms gradually declines over a period of approximately 15 days.

Drug dependence to barbiturates arises from repeated administration of a barbiturate or agent with barbiturate like effect on a continuous basis, generally in amounts exceeding therapeutic dose levels. The characteristics of drug dependence to barbiturates include; (a) a strong desire or need to continue taking the drug; (b) a tendency to increase the dose; (c) a psychic dependence on the effects of the drug related to subjective and individual appreciation for those effects; and (d) a physical dependence on the effects of the drug requiring its presence for maintenance of homeostasis and resulting in a definite, characteristic, and self-limited abstinence syndrome when the drug is withdrawn.

Treatment of barbiturate dependence consists of cautious and gradual withdrawal of the drug. Barbiturate-dependent patients can be withdrawn by using a number of different withdrawal regimens. In all cases, withdrawal takes an extended period of time. One method involves initiating treatment at the patient's regular dosage level, in 3 to 4 divided doses, and decreasing the daily dose by 10 percent if tolerated by the patient.

Infants physically dependent on barbiturates may be given phenobarbital 3 to 10 mg/kg/day. After withdrawal symptoms (hyperactivity, disturbed sleep, tremors, hyperreflexia) are relieved, the dosage of phenobarbital should be gradually decreased and completely withdrawn after a 1 week period.

OVERDOSAGE:

Signs and Symptoms: The toxic dose of barbiturates varies considerably. In general, an oral dose of 1 gram of more barbiturates produces serious poisoning in an adult. Death commonly occurs after 2 to 10 grams of ingested barbiturates. Symptoms of acute intoxication with barbiturates include unsteady gait, slurred speech, and sustained nystagmus. Mental signs of chronic intoxication include confusion, poor judgment, irritability, insomnia, and somatic complaints. Barbiturate intoxication may be confused with alcoholism, bromide intoxication, and with various neurological disorders.

Acute overdosage with barbiturates is manifested by CNS and respiratory depression which may progress to Cheyne-Stokes respiration, areflexia, constriction of the pupils to a slight degree (though in severe poisoning they may show paralytic dilation), oliguria, tachycardia, hypotension, lowered body temperature, and coma. Typical shock syndrome (apnea, circulatory collapse, respiratory arrest, and death) may occur.

In extreme overdose, all electrical activity in the brain may cease, in which case a 'flat' EEG normally equated with clinical death cannot be accepted. This effect is fully reversible unless hypoxic damage occurs. Consideration should be given to the possibility of barbiturate intoxication even in situations that appear to involve trauma.

Complications: Pneumonia, pulmonary edema, cardiac arrhythmias, congestive heart failure, and renal failure may occur. Uremia may increase CNS sensitivity to barbiturates if renal function is impaired. Differential diagnosis should include hypoglycemia, head trauma, cerebrovascular accidents, convulsive states, and diabetic coma.

Treatment: Treatment of overdosage is mainly supportive and consists of the following:

1. Maintenance of an adequate airway, with assisted respiration and oxygen administration as necessary.

2. Monitoring of vital signs and fluid balance.

3. If the patient is conscious and has not lost the gag reflex, emesis may be induced with ipecac. Care should be taken to prevent pulmonary aspiration of vomitus. After completion of vomiting, 30 grams activated charcoal in a glass of water may be administered.

4. If emesis is contraindicated, gastric lavage may be performed with a cuffed endotracheal tube in place with the patient in the face down position. Activated charcoal may be left in the emptied stomach and a saline cathartic administered.

5. Fluid therapy and other standard treatment for shock, if needed.

6. If renal function is normal, forced diuresis may aid in the elimination of the barbiturate.

7. Although not recommended as a routine procedure, hemodialysis may be used in severe barbiturate intoxications or if the patient is anuric or in shock.

8. Appropriate nursing care, including rolling patients from side-to-side every 30 minutes, to prevent hypostatic pneumonia, decubiti, aspiration, and other complications of patients with altered states of consciousness.

9. Antibiotics should be given if pneumonia is suspected.

DOSAGE AND ADMINISTRATION:

USUAL ADULT DOSAGE

Daytime Sedative: 15 to 30 mg, 3 or 4 times daily.

Bedtime Hypnotic: 50 to 100 mg.

Preoperative Sedative: 50 to 100 mg, 60 to 90 minutes before surgery.

DOSAGE AND ADMINISTRATION: *(cont'd)*

USUAL PEDIATRIC DOSAGE

Preoperative Sedative: 2 to 6 mg/kg maximum 100 mg.

SPECIAL PATIENT POPULATION

Dosage should be reduced in the elderly or debilitated because these patients may be more sensitive to barbiturates. Dosage should be reduced for patients with impaired renal function or hepatic disease (see PRECAUTIONS.)

Storage: Tablets and Elixir - Store at room temperature. Keep bottle tightly closed.

HOW SUPPLIED - RATED THERAPEUTICALLY EQUIVALENT:

Elixir - Oral - 30 mg/5ml

480 ml	$5.93	Butabarbital Sodium, Rugby	00536-0320-85
480 ml	$6.48	Butabarbital Sodium, H.C.F.A. F F P	99999-0557-01
480 ml	$7.30	Butabarbital Sodium, Harber Pharm	51432-0542-20
480 ml	$7.67	Butabarbital Sodium, Alpharma	00472-0933-16
480 ml	$9.90	Butabarbital Sodium, IDE-Interstate	00814-1342-82
480 ml	**$83.39**	**BUTISOL SODIUM, Wallace Labs**	**00037-0110-16**
3840 ml	$27.72	Butabarbital Sodium, Rugby	00536-0320-90
3840 ml	$51.84	Butabarbital Sodium, H.C.F.A. F F P	99999-0557-02
3840 ml	**$567.86**	**BUTISOL SODIUM, Wallace Labs**	**00037-0110-28**

Tablet, Uncoated - Oral - 15 mg

100's	**$44.53**	**BUTISOL SODIUM, Wallace Labs**	**00037-0112-60**
1000's	$11.95	BARBISED, Major Pharms	00904-3883-80
1000's	**$427.86**	**BUTISOL SODIUM, Wallace Labs**	**00037-0112-80**

Tablet, Uncoated - Oral - 30 mg

100's	**$59.15**	**BUTISOL SODIUM, Wallace Labs**	**00037-0113-60**
1000's	**$573.79**	**BUTISOL SODIUM, Wallace Labs**	**00037-0113-80**

Tablet, Uncoated - Oral - 100 mg

100's	**$91.32**	**BUTISOL SODIUM, Wallace Labs**	**00037-0115-60**

HOW SUPPLIED - NOT RATED EQUIVALENT:

Tablet, Uncoated - Oral - 50 mg

100's	**$76.92**	**BUTISOL SODIUM, Wallace Labs**	**00037-0114-60**

BUTABARBITAL; EPHEDRINE; GUAIFENESIN; THEOPHYLLINE *(000553)*

CATEGORIES: DESI Drugs; Respiratory Muscle Relaxant; Smooth Muscle Relaxants; FDA Pre 1938 Drugs

BRAND NAMES: Quibron Plus

Prescribing information not available at time of publication.

HOW SUPPLIED - EQUIVALENTS NOT AVAILABLE:

Capsule, Elastic - Oral - 20 mg/25 mg/100

100's	$32.57	QUIBRON PLUS, Bristol Myers Squibb	00087-0518-01

Elixir - Oral - 20 mg/25 mg/100

480 ml	$31.25	QUIBRON PLUS, Bristol Myers Squibb	00087-0511-01

BUTABARBITAL; GUAIFENESIN; PSEUDOEPHEDRINE; THEOPHYLLINE *(000555)*

CATEGORIES: Antiasthmatics/Bronchodilators; Respiratory & Allergy Medications; Respiratory Muscle Relaxant; Smooth Muscle Relaxants; FDA Pre 1938 Drugs

BRAND NAMES: Broncomar Elixir

Prescribing information not available at time of publication.

HOW SUPPLIED - EQUIVALENTS NOT AVAILABLE:

Elixir - Oral - 15 mg/150 mg/30

480 ml	$20.00	BRONCOMAR, Marlop Pharms	12939-0128-45
3840 ml	$130.00	BRONCOMAR, Marlop Pharms	12939-0128-42

BUTABARBITAL; HYOSCYAMINE HYDROBROMIDE; PHENAZOPYRIDINE HYDROCHLORIDE *(000558)*

CATEGORIES: Antibacterials; Antimicrobials; Antipruritics/Local Anesthetics; Antiseptics, Urinary Tract; Antispasmodics; Dysuria; Pain; Phenazopyridine; Skin/Mucous Membrane Agents; Spasm; Urinary Tract Infections; Pregnancy Category C; FDA Pre 1938 Drugs

BRAND NAMES: **Pyridium Plus**

DESCRIPTION:

Each tablet contains:

150 mg: phenazopyridine hydrochloride

0.3 mg: hyoscyamine hydrobromide

15 mg: butabarbital

Also contains: carnauba wax, NF; corn starch, NF; D&C Red No. 7 Lake; FD&C Blue No. 2 Lake; FD&C Yellow No. 6 Lake; gelatin, NF; lactose, NF; magnesium stearate, NF; sodium starch glycolate, NF; sucrose, NF; titanium dioxide, USP; white wax, NF.

CLINICAL PHARMACOLOGY:

Pyridium Plus relieves lower urinary symptoms of pain, frequency, urgency, burning and dysuria arising from inflammation of the urothelium, the mucosal lining of the lower urinary tract.

Lower urinary tract pain can cause reflex spasm of the detrusor. Pain and spasm are often aggravated by apprehension to promote a pain-spasm-apprehension cycle. Each of the three pharmacologic components acts against a phase of this cycle.

Phenazopyridine hydrochloride, excreted in the urine, is a topical analgesic for the relief of pain and discomfort.

CLINICAL PHARMACOLOGY: *(cont'd)*

Hyoscyamine hydrobromide, a parasympatholytic, acts to relieve detrusor muscle spasm. Butabarbital, a short-to-intermediate acting sedative, helps to allay associated anxiety and apprehension.

INDICATIONS AND USAGE:

This drug is indicated for the symptomatic relief of pain, burning, frequency, urgency and dysuria, particularly when accompanied by detrusor muscle spasm and apprehension.

These symptoms may arise from infection, trauma, surgery, endoscopic procedures, or the passage of sounds or catheters.

Therapy with this drug does not interfere with antibacterial therapy and can help to relieve symptoms of pain and discomfort before definitive treatment is effective. The use of this drug for symptomatic relief should not delay definitive diagnosis and treatment. Treatment of a urinary tract infection with this drug should not exceed 2 days because there is a lack of evidence that the combined administration of phenazopyridine hydrochloride and an antibacterial provides greater benefit than administration of the antibacterial alone after 2 days. (See DOSAGE AND ADMINISTRATION.)

In the absence of infection, this drug may be the only medication required.

CONTRAINDICATIONS:

This drug should not be used in patients who have previously exhibited hypersensitivity to any component. The use of this drug is contraindicated in patients with renal or hepatic insufficiency; glaucoma, bladder neck obstruction, porphyria.

WARNINGS:

BUTABARBITAL MAY BE HABIT-FORMING. Drowsiness or dizziness may occur. Patients should be instructed to use caution in driving or operating machinery.

PRECAUTIONS:

GENERAL

A yellowish tinge of the skin or sclera may indicate accumulation due to impaired renal excretion of phenazopyridine and the need to discontinue therapy.

The decline in renal function associated with advanced age should be kept in mind.

LABORATORY TEST INTERACTIONS

Due to its properties as an azo dye, phenazopyridine hydrochloride may interfere with urinalysis based on spectrometry or color reactions.

INFORMATION FOR THE PATIENT

Phenazopyridine hydrochloride produces an orange to red color in the urine and may stain fabric. Staining of contact lenses has been reported. Butabarbital may cause drowsiness or dizziness; patients should be instructed to use caution in driving or operating machinery.

CARCINOGENESIS, MUTAGENESIS, AND IMPAIRMENT OF FERTILITY

This drug has not undergone adequate studies relating to carcinogenesis, mutagenesis, or impairment of fertility; however, the component phenazopyridine hydrochloride has induced neoplasia in rats (large intestine) and mice (liver). Although no association between phenazopyridine hydrochloride and human neoplasia has been reported, adequate epidemiological studies along these lines have not been conducted.

PREGNANCY CATEGORY C

Animal reproduction studies have not been conducted. It is also not known whether this drug can cause fetal harm when administered to a pregnant woman or can affect reproduction capacity. This drug should be given to a pregnant woman only if clearly needed.

NURSING MOTHERS

No information is available on the appearance of the components in human milk.

ADVERSE REACTIONS:

Methemoglobinemia, hemolytic anemia, renal and hepatic toxicity have been described for phenazopyridine, usually at overdosage levels (see OVERDOSAGE.) Headache, rash, pruritus and occasional gastrointestinal disturbance. An anaphylactoid-like reaction has been described.

Hyoscyamine hydrobromide is an atropinic drug that may produce adverse effects characteristic of this class of drugs. Dry mouth, drowsiness or dizziness is noted in more than one-third of patients (and may occur in half of the patients of older age groups). Other atropine-like effects such as blurred vision may occur. There may be occasional gastrointestinal disturbances.

Butabarbital is a short-to-intermediate acting barbiturate which has the potential for adverse reactions attributable to barbiturates.

OVERDOSAGE:

This drug is a combination of three active drugs, and overdosage can be expected to show the effects related to each ingredient. Management includes the usual measures to empty the stomach by emesis or lavage, administration of a charcoal slurry, and supportive measures as needed.

Toxicity and management suggestions relating to the individual ingredients are as follows:

Phenazopyridine Hydrochloride: Exceeding the recommended dose in patients with good renal function or administering the usual dose to patients with impaired renal function (common in elderly patients), may lead to increased serum levels and toxic reactions. Methemoglobinemia generally follows a massive, acute overdose. Methylene blue, 1 to 2 mg/kg body weight intravenously, should cause prompt reduction of the methemoglobinemia and disappearance of cyanosis which is an aid in diagnosis. Oxidative Heinz body hemolytic anemia may also occur, and "bite cells" (degmacytes) may be present in a chronic overdosage situation. Red blood cell G-6-PD deficiency may predispose to hemolysis. Renal and hepatic impairment and occasional failure, usually due to hypersensitivity, may also occur.

Hyoscyamine Hydrobromide: Overdosage of hyoscyamine, a form of atropine, will cause dilated pupils, blurred vision, rapid pulse, increased intraocular tension, hot, dry, red skin, dry mouth, disorientation, delirium, fever, convulsions, and coma. As an antidote, physostigmine salicylate may be given IV slowly. Dilute 1 mg in 5 ml of saline and use 1 ml of this dilution in children. Repeat every five minutes as needed up to a total of 2 mg in children, or 6 mg in adults every 30 minutes.

Butabarbital: This drug may produce sedation and respiratory depression progressing to coma, depending on the amount ingested. General and supportive measures should be instituted.

DOSAGE AND ADMINISTRATION:

Adult Dosage: One tablet 4 times a day (after meals and at bedtime).

When used concomitantly with an antibacterial agent for the treatment of a urinary tract infection, the administration of this drug should not exceed 2 days.

Store at controlled room temperature 15-30°C (59-86°F).

HOW SUPPLIED - EQUIVALENTS NOT AVAILABLE:

Tablet, Plain Coated - Oral - 15 mg/0.3 mg/15

100's	$56.06	PYRIDIUM PLUS, Parke-Davis	00071-0182-24

BUTOCONAZOLE NITRATE *(000562)*

CATEGORIES: Anti-Infectives; Antibacterials; Antibiotics; Antifungals; Antimicrobials; Candidiasis; Dermatologicals; Fungal Agents; Infections; Skin/Mucous Membrane Agents; Vaginal Preparations; Pregnancy Category C; FDA Approved 1985 Nov

BRAND NAMES: *Femstal* (Mexico); **Femstat**; *Gynomyk* (France)
(International brand names outside U.S. in italics)

FORMULARIES: Aetna; BC-BS; FHP; Foundation; Medi-Cal

DESCRIPTION:

Femstat Vaginal Cream contains butoconazole nitrate 2.0%, an imidazole derivative with antifungal activity. Its chemical name is (±)-1-(4-(*p*-Chlorophenyl)-2-((2,6-dichlorophenyl) thio)buyl)imidazole mononitrate.

Butoconazole nitrate is a white to off-white crystalline powder with a molecular weight of 474.79. It is sparingly soluble in methanol; slightly soluble in chloroform, methylene chloride, acetone, and ethanol; very soluble in ethyl acetate; and practically insoluble in water. It melts at about 159°C with decomposition.

Femstat vaginal cream contains butoconazole nitrate 20 mg/g in a water-washable emollient cream of cetyl alcohol, glyceryl stearate (and) PEG- 100 stearate, methylparaben and propylparaben (preservatives), mineral oil, polysorbate 60, propylene glycol, sorbitan monostearate, stearyl alcohol and water (purified).

CLINICAL PHARMACOLOGY:

Butoconazole nitrate in an imidazole derivative that has fungicidal activity *in vitro* against *Candida, Trichophyton, Microsporum,* and *Epidermophyton.* It is also active against some gram positive bacteria. Clinically, it is highly effective against vaginal infections induced by strains of *Candida albicans, Candida tropicalis,* and other species of this genus.

The primary site of action of imidazoles appears to be the cell membrane. The permeability of the cell membrane is altered, resulting in a reduced osmotic resistance and viability of the fungus. The exact mechanism of antifungal activity of butoconazole nitrate is not known.

Following vaginal administration of butoconazole nitrate, 5.5% of the dose is absorbed on average. After vaginal administration peak plasma levels of the drug and its metabolites are attained at 24 hours and the plasma half-life is approximately 21-24 hours.

INDICATIONS AND USAGE:

Femstat vaginal cream is indicated for the local treatment of vulvovaginal mycotic infections caused by *Candida* species. The diagnosis should be confirmed by KOH smears and/or cultures.

Femstat vaginal cream can be used in association with oral contraceptive and antibiotic therapy. Femstat is effective in both non-pregnant and pregnant women but in pregnant women it should be used only during the second and third trimesters.

CONTRAINDICATIONS:

Femstat vaginal cream 2% is contraindicated in patients with a history of hypersensitivity to any of the components of the cream.

PRECAUTIONS:

General: If clinical symptoms persist, microbiological tests should be repeated to rule out other pathogens and to confirm the diagnosis.

If sensitization or irritation is reported during use, the treatment should be discontinued.

Information for the Patient: The patient should be cautioned against premature discontinuation of the medication during menstruation or in response to relief of symptoms.

Carcinogenesis: Long-term studies in animals have not been performed to evaluate the carcinogenic potential of this drug.

Mutagenesis: Butoconazole nitrate was not mutagenic when tested on microbial indicator organisms.

Impairment of Fertility: No impairment of fertility was seen in rabbits or rats administered butoconazole nitrate in oral doses up to 30 mg/kg/day or 100 mg/kg/day respectively.

Pregnancy Category C: In pregnant rats administered 6 mg/kg/day (3-7 times the human dose) butoconazole nitrate intravaginally during the period of organogenesis, there was an increase in resorption rate and decrease in litter size, but no teratogenicity. Butoconazole nitrate had no apparent adverse effect when administered orally to pregnant rats throughout organogenesis, at dose levels up to 50 mg/kg/day. Daily oral doses of 100, 300, or 750 mg/kg resulted in fetal malformations (abdominal wall defects, cleft palate), but maternal stress was evident at these higher dose levels. There were no adverse effects on litters of rabbits receiving butoconazole nitrate orally, even at maternally stressful dose levels (*e.g.,* 150 mg/kg). There are no adequate and well-controlled studies in pregnant women during the first trimester.

Butoconazole nitrate, like other azole antimycotic agents, causes dystocia in rats when treatment is extended through parturition. However, this effect was not apparent in rabbits treated with as much as 100 mg/kg/day orally.

In clinical studies, over 200 pregnant patients have used butoconazole nitrate cream 2% for 3 or 6 days during the second or third trimester and the drug had no adverse effect in the course of pregnancy. Follow-up reports available on infants born to these women reveal no adverse effects or complication that were attributable to the drug.

Nursing Mothers: It is not known whether this drug is excreted in human milk. Because many drugs are excreted in human milk, caution should be exercised when butoconazole nitrate is administered to a nursing woman.

Pediatric Use: Safety and effectiveness in children have not been established.

ADVERSE REACTIONS:

Of the 561 patients treated with butoconazole nitrate cream 2.0% for 3 or 6 days in controlled clinical trials, 13 (2.3%) reported complaints probably related to therapy. Vulvar/vaginal burning occurred in 2.3%, vulvar itching in 0.9%, and discharge, soreness, swelling, and itching of the fingers each occurred in 0.2%. Nine patients (1.6%) discontinued because of these complaints.

DOSAGE AND ADMINISTRATION:

Non-pregnant patients: The recommended dose is one applicatorful of cream (approximately 5 grams) intravaginally at bedtime for three days. Treatment can be extended for an additional three days if necessary.

DOSAGE AND ADMINISTRATION: *(cont'd)*

Pregnant Patients (2nd and 3rd trimesters only): The recommended dose is one applicatorful of cream (approximately 5 grams) intravaginally at bedtime for six days.

Store at room temperature.

Avoid excessive heat, above 40°C (104°F), and avoid freezing.

(Vaginal Cream: Syntex, 3/90, 02-2280-72-00)

(In Prefilled Applicator: Syntex, 3/88, 02-2280-16-03)

HOW SUPPLIED - EQUIVALENTS NOT AVAILABLE:

Cream - Vaginal - 2 %

3 applicators	$20.36	FEMSTAT PREFILL/, Syntex Labs	00033-2280-16

BUTORPHANOL TARTRATE *(000563)*

CATEGORIES: Analgesics; Anesthesia; Antipyretics; Central Nervous System Agents; Narcotic Agonist-Antagonist; Narcotics, Synthetics & Combinations; Opiate Partial Agonists; Pain; Migraine*; FDA Approval Pre 1982
* Indication not approved by the FDA

BRAND NAMES: *Biforal; Busphen;* **Stadol**; *Stadol NS*
(International brand names outside U.S. in italics)

DESCRIPTION:

Butorphanol tartrate is a synthetically derived opioid agonist-antagonist analgesic of the phenanthrene series. The chemical name is (-)-17-(cy- clobutylmethyl) morphinan-3, 14-diol (S-(R*,R*))-2,3- dihydroxybutanedioate (1:1) (salt). The molecular formula is $C_{21}H_{29}NO_2C_4H_6O_6$ which corresponds to a molecular weight of 477.55.

Butorphanol tartrate is a white crystalline substance. The dose is expressed as the tartrate salt. One milligram of the salt is equivalent to 0.68 mg of the free base. The n-octanol/aqueous buffer partition coefficient of butorphanol is 180:1 at pH 7.5.

Butorphanol tartrate injectable is a sterile, parenteral, aqueous solution of butorphanol tartrate for intravenous or intramuscular administration. In addition to 1 or 2 mg of butorphanol tartrate, each ml of solution contains 3.3 mg of citric acid, 6.4 mg sodium citrate, and 6.4 mg sodium chloride, and 0.1 mg benzethonium chloride (in multiple dose vial only) as a preservative.

Butorphanol tartrate nasal spray is an aqueous solution of butorphanol tartrate for administration as a metered spray to the nasal mucosa. each bottle of butorphanol tartrate nasal spray contains 2.5 ml of a 10 mg/ml solution of butorphanol tartrate with sodium chloride, citric acid, and benzethonium chloride in purified water with sodium hydroxide and/or hydrochloric acid added to adjust the pH to 5.0. The pump reservoir must be fully primed prior to initial use. After initial priming each metered spray delivers an average of 1.0 mg of butorphanol tartrate and the 2.5 ml bottle will deliver an average of 14-15 doses of butorphanol tartrate nasal spray. If not used for 48 hours or longer, the unit must be reprimed (see Patient Information). With intermittent use requiring repriming before each dose, the 2.5 ml bottle will deliver an average of 8-1-doses of butorphanol tartrate nasal spray depending on how much repriming is necessary.

CLINICAL PHARMACOLOGY:

GENERAL PHARMACOLOGY AND MECHANISM OF ACTION

Butorphanol and its major metabolites are agonists at k-opioid receptors and mixed agonist-antagonists at mc-opioid receptors.

Its interactions with these receptors in the central nervous system apparently mediate most of its pharmacologic effects, including analgesia.

In addition to analgesia, CNS effects include depression of spontaneous respiratory activity and cough, stimulation of the emetic center, miosis and sedation. Effects possibly mediated by non-CNS mechanisms include alteration in cardiovascular resistance and capacitance, bronchomotor tone, gastrointestinal secretory and motor activity and bladder spincter activity.

In an animal model, the dose of the butorphanol tartrate required to antagonize morphine analgesia by 50% was similar to that for nalorphine, less than that for pentazocine and more than that for naloxone.

The pharmacological activity of butorphanol metabolites has not been studied in humans; in animal studies, butorphanol metabolites have demonstrated some analgesic activity.

In human studies of butorphanol (see CLINICAL STUDIES), sedation is commonly noted at doses of 0.5 mg or more. Narcosis is produced by 10-12 mg doses of butorphanol administered over 10-15 minutes intravenously.

Butorphanol, like other mixed agonist-antagonists with a high affinity for the kappa receptor, may produce unpleasant psychotomimetic effects in some individuals.

Nausea and/or vomiting may be produced by doses of 1 mg or more administered by any route.

In human studies involving individuals without significant respiratory dysfunction, 2 mg of butorphanol IV and 10 mg of morphine sulfate IV depressed respiration to a comparable degree. At higher doses, the magnitude of respiratory depression with butorphanol is not appreciably increased; however, the duration of respiratory depression is longer. Respiratory depression noted after administration of butorphanol to humans by any route is reversed by treatment with naloxone, a specific opioid antagonist (see Treatment in OVERDOSAGE).

Butorphanol tartrate demonstrates antitussive effects in animals at doses less than those required for analgesia.

Hemodynamic changes noted during cardiac catheterization in patients receiving single 0.025 mg/kg intravenous doses of butorphanol have included increases in pulmonary artery pressure, wedge pressure and vascular resistance, increases in left ventricular end diastolic pressure and in systemic arterial pressure.

PHARMACODYNAMICS

The analgesic effect of butorphanol is influenced by the route of administration. Onset of analgesia is within a few minutes for intravenous administration, within 10-15 minutes for intramuscular injection, and within 15 minutes for the nasal spray doses.

Peak analgesic activity occurs within 30-60 minutes following intravenous and intramuscular administration and within 1-2 hours following the nasal spray administration.

The duration of analgesia varies depending on the pain model as well as the route of administration, but is generally 3-4 hours with IM and IV doses as defined by the time 50% of patients required remedication. In postoperative studies, the duration of analgesia with IV or IM butorphanol was similar to morphine, meperidine and pentazocine when administered in the same fashion at equipotent doses (see CLINICAL STUDIES.) Compared to the injectable form and other drugs in this class, butorphanol tartrate nasal spray has a longer duration of action (4-5 hours) (see CLINICAL STUDIES.)

CLINICAL PHARMACOLOGY: *(cont'd)*

PHARMACOKINETICS

Butorphanol tartrate injectable is rapidly absorbed after IM injection and peak plasma levels are reached in 20-40 minutes.

After nasal administration, mean peak blood levels of 0.9-1.04 ng/ml occur at 30-60 minutes after a 1 mg dose (see TABLE 1.) The absolute bioavailability of butorphanol tartrate nasal spray is 60-70% and is unchanged in patients with allergic rhinitis. In patients using a nasal vasoconstrictor (oxymetazoline) the fraction of the dose absorbed was unchanged, but the rate of absorption was slowed. The peak plasma concentrations were approximately half those achieved in the absence of the vasoconstrictor.

Following its initial absorption/distribution phase, the single dose pharmacokinetics of butorphanol by the intravenous, intramuscular, and nasal routes of administration are similar.

Serum protein binding is independent of concentration over the range achieved in clinical practice (up to 7 ng/ml) with a bound fraction of approximately 80%.

The volume of distribution of butorphanol varies from 305-901 liters and total body clearance from 52-154 liters/hr (see TABLE 1.)

TABLE 1 Mean Pharmacokinetic Parameters of Butorphanol in Young and Elderly Subjects [a]

	Intravenous		Nasal	
Parameters	**Young**	**Elderly**	**Young**	**Elderly**
Tmax[b] (hr)			0.62 (0.32)[e] (0.15-1.50)[g]	1.03 (0.74) (0.25-3.00)
Cmax[c] (ng/ml)			1.04 (0.40) (0.35-1.97)	0.90 (0.57) (0.10-2.68)
AUC (inf)[d] hr. ng/ml)	7.24 (1.57) (4.40-9.77)	8.71 (2.02) (4.76-13.03)	4.93 (1.24) (2.16-7.27)	5.24 (2.27) (0.30-10.34)
Half-life (hr)	4.56 (1.67) (2.06-8.70)	5.61 (1.36) (3.25-8.79)	4.74 (1.57) (2.89-8.79)	6.56 (1.51) (3.75-9.17)
Absolute Bioavailability (%)			69 (16) (44-113)	61 (25) (3-121)
Volume of Distribution[f](L)	487 (155) (305-901)	552 (124) (305-737)		
Total body Clearance(L/hr)	99 (23) (70-154)	82 (21) (52-143)		

[a]Young subjects (n=24) are from 20 to 40 years old and elderly (n=24) are greater than 65 years of age.
[b]Time to peak plasma concentration, median values.
[c]Peak plasma concentration normalized to 1 mg dose.
[d]Area under the plasma concentration-time curve after a 1 mg dose.
[e]Mean (1 S.D.)
[f]Derived from IV data.
[g](range of observed values)

Dose proportionally for butorphanol tartrate nasal spray has been determined at steady state in doses up to 4 mg at 6 hour intervals. Steady state is achieved within 2 days. The mean peak plasma concentration at steady state was 1.8-fold (maximal 3-fold) following a single dose.

The drug is transported across the blood brain and placental barriers and into human milk (see Labor and Delivery and Nursing Mothers).

Butorphanol is extensively metabolized in the liver. Metabolism is qualitatively and quantitatively similar following intravenous, intramuscular, or nasal administration. Oral bioavailability is only 5- 17% because of extensive first pass metabolism of butorphanol.

The major metabolite of butorphanol is hydroxybutorphanol, while norbutorphanol is produced in small amounts. Both have been detected in plasma following administration of butorphanol. Preliminary evidence suggests the elimination half-life of hydroxybutorphanol may be greater than that of its parent.

Elimination occurs by urine and fecal excretion. When ^3H labelled butorphanol is administered to normal subjects, most (70-80%) of the dose is recovered in the urine, while approximately 15% is recovered in the feces.

About 5% of the dose is recovered in the urine as butorphanol. Forty-nine percent is eliminated in the urine as hydroxybutorphanol. Less than 5% is excreted in the urine as norbutorphanol (see CLINICAL PHARMACOLOGY.)

Butorphanol pharmacokinetics in the elderly differ from younger patients(see TABLE 1.) The mean absolute bioavailability of butorphanol tartrate nasal spray in elderly women (48%) was less then that in elderly men (75%), young men (68%) or young women (70%). Elimination half-life is increased in the elderly (6.6 hours as opposed to 4.7 hours in younger subjects).

In renally impaired patients with creatinine clearances <30 ml/min the elimination half-life is approximately doubled and the total body clearance is approximately one-half (10.5 hours (clearance 150 L/h) as compared to 5.8 hours (clearance 260 L/h) in normals). No effect was observed on C_{max} or T_{max} after a single dose.

For further recommendations refer to statements on use in Geriatric Patients, Renal Disease, Hepatic Disease, DRUG INTERACTIONS, and Individualization of Dosage.

USE IN THE MANAGEMENT OF PAIN

Postoperative Analgesia: The analgesic efficacy of butorphanol tartrate injectable in postoperative pain was investigated in several double-blind active-controlled studies involving 958 butorphanol-treated patients. The following doses were found to have approximately equivalent analgesic effect: 2 mg butorphanol, 10 mg morphine 40 mg pentazocine and 80 mg meperidine.

After intravenous administration of butorphanol tartrate injectable, onset and peak analgesic effect occurred by the time of first observation (30 minutes). After intramuscular administration, pain relief onset occurred at 30 minutes or less, and peak effect occurred between 30 minutes and one hour. The duration of action of butorphanol tartrate injectable was 3-4 hours when defined as the time necessary for pain intensity to return to pretreatment level or the time to retreatment.

The analgesic efficacy of butorphanol tartrate nasal spray was evaluated (approximately 35 patients per treatment group in a general and orthopedic surgery trial. Single doses of butorphanol tartrate nasal spray (1 or 2 mg) and IM meperidine (37.5 or 75 mg) were compared. Analgesia provided by 1 and 2 mg doses of butorphanol tartrate nasal spray was similar to 37.5 and 75 mg meperidine, respectively, with onset of analgesia within 15 minutes and peak analgesic effect within 1 hour. the median duration of pain relief was 2.5 hours with 1 mg butorphanol tartrate nasal spray, 3.5 hours with 2 mg butorphanol tartrate nasal spray and 3.3 hours with either dose of meperidine.

In a postcesarean section trial butorphanol tartrate nasal spray administered to 35 patients as two 1 mg doses 60 minutes apart was compared with a single 2 mg dose of butorphanol tartrate nasal spray or a single 2 mg IV dose of butorphanol tartrate injectable (37 patients each). Onset of analgesia was within 15 minutes for all butorphanol tartrate regimens. Peak analgesic effects of 2 mg intravenous butorphanol tartrate injectable and butorphanol tartrate

CLINICAL PHARMACOLOGY: *(cont'd)*

nasal spray were similar in magnitude. The curation of pain relief provided by both 2 mg butorphanol tartrate nasal spray regimens was approximately 4.5 hours and was greater than intravenous butorphanol tartrate injectable (2.6 h).

MIGRAINE HEADACHE PAIN

The analgesic efficacy of two 1 mg doses one hour apart of butorphanol tartrate nasal spray in migraine headache pain was compared with a single dose of 10 mg IM methadone (31 and 32 patients respectively). Significant onset of analgesia occurred within 15 minutes for both butorphanol tartrate nasal spray and IM methadone. Peak analgesic effect occurred at 2 hours for butorphanol tartrate nasal spray and 1.5 hours for methadone. The median duration of pain relief was 6 hours with butorphanol tartrate nasal spray and 4 hours with methadone as judged by the time when approximately half of the patients remedicated.

In two other trials in patients with migraine headache pain, a 2 mg initial dose of Butorphanol tartrate NS followed by an additional 1 mg dose 1 hr later (76 patients) was compared with either 75 mg IM meperidine (24 patients) or placebo (72 patients). Onset, peak activity and duration were similar with both active treatments; however, the incidence of adverse experiences (nausea, vomiting, dizziness) was higher in these two trials with the 2 mg initial dose of Butorphanol Tartrate NS than in the trial with the 1 mg initial dose.

PREANESTHETIC MEDICATION

Butorphanol tartrate injectable (2 mg and 4 mg) and meperidine (80 mg) were studied for use as preanesthetic medication in hospitalized surgical patients. Patients received a single intramuscular dose of either Butorphanol Tartrate injectable or meperidine approximately 90 minutes prior to anesthesia. the anesthesia regimen included barbiturate induction, followed by nitrous oxide and oxygen with halothane or enflurane, with or without a muscle relaxant.

Anesthetic preparation was rated as satisfactory in all 42 Butorphanol Tartrate injectable patients regardless of the type of surgery.

BALANCED ANESTHESIA

Butorphanol Tartrate NS injectable administered intravenously (mean dose 2 mg) was compared to intravenous morphine sulfate (mean dose 10 mg) as premedication shortly before thiopental induction, followed by balanced anesthesia in 50 ASA Class 1 and 2 patients. Anesthesia was then maintained by repeated intravenous doses, averaging 4.6 mg Butorphanol Tartrate NS injectable and 22.8 morphine per patient.

Anesthetic induction and maintenance were generally rated as satisfactory with both Butorphanol Tartrate NS injectable (25 patients) and morphine (25 patients) regardless of the type of surgery performed. Emergence from anesthesia was comparable with both agents.

LABOR AND DELIVERY

(See PRECAUTIONS.) The analgesic efficacy of intravenous Butorphanol Tartrate NS injectable was studied in pain during labor. In a total of 145 patients Butorphanol Tartrate NS injectable (1 mg and 2 mg) was as effective as 40 mg and 80 mg of meperidine (144 patients) in the relief of pain in labor with no effect on the duration or progress of labor. Both drugs readily crossed the placenta and entered fetal circulation. The condition of the infants in these studies, determined by Apgar scores at 1 and 5 minutes (8 or above) and time to sustained respiration, showed that Butorphanol Tartrate NS injectable had the same effects on the infants as meperidine.

In these studies neurobehavioral testing in infants exposed to Butorphanol Tartrate NS injectable at a mean of 18.6 hours after delivery, showed no significant differences between treatment groups.

INDIVIDUALIZATION OF DOSAGE

The usual starting doses of butorphanol are: 1 mg repeated every 3-4 hours IV; 2 mg repeated every 3-4 hours IM; and 1 mg followed by 1 mg in 60-90 minutes nasally repeated every 3-4 hours (see DOSAGE AND ADMINISTRATION.)

Use of butorphanol in geriatric patients, patients with renal impairment, patients with hepatic impairment, and during labor requires extra caution (see PRECAUTIONS.)

BUTORPHANOL INJECTABLE

For pain relief the recommended initial dosage regimen of Butorphanol injectable is 1 mg IV or 2 mg IM with repeated doses every three to four hours, as necessary. This dosage regimen is likely to be effective for the majority of patients. Dosage adjustments of Butorphanol injectable should be based on observations of its beneficial and adverse effects. The initial dose in the elderly and in patients with renal or hepatic impairment should generally be half the recommended adult dose (0.5 mg IV and 1.0 mg IM). Repeat doses in these patients should be determined by the patient's response rather than at fixed intervals but will generally be no less than 6 hours (see PRECAUTIONS.)

The usual preoperative dose is 2 mg IM given 60-90 minutes before surgery or 2 mg IV shortly before induction. This is approximately equivalent in sedative effect to 10 mg morphine or 80 mg of meperidine. This single preoperative dose should be individualized based on age, body weight, physical status, underlying pathological condition, use of other drugs, type of anesthesia to be used and the surgical procedure involved.

During maintenance in balanced anesthesia the usual incremental dose of Butorphanol injectable is 0.5 to 1.0 mg IV. The incremental dose may be higher, up to 0.06 mg/kg (4 mg/70 kg), depending on previous sedative, analgesic, and hypnotic drugs administered. The total dose of Butorphanol injectable will vary; however, patients seldom require less than 4 mg or more than 12.5 mg (approximately 0.06 to 0.18 mg/kg).

As with other opioids of this class, Butorphanol injectable may not provide adequate intraoperative analgesia during balanced anesthesia is commonly reflected by increases in general sympathetic tone. Consequently, if blood pressure or heart rate continue to rise, consideration should be given to adding a potent volatile liquid inhalation anesthetic or another intravenous medication.

In labor, the recommended initial dose of Butorphanol injectable is 1 or 2 mg IM or IV in mothers with fetuses of 37 weeks gestation or beyond and without signs of fetal distress. Dosage adjustments of butorphanol tartrate injectable in labor should be based on initial response with consideration given to concomitant analgesic or sedative drugs and the expected time of delivery. A dose should not be repeated in less than four hours nor administered less than four hours prior to the anticipated delivery (see PRECAUTIONS.)

BUTORPHANOL TARTRATE NASAL SPRAY

Since Butorphanol Tartrate NS does not require an injection, it allows the physician to initiate therapy with a low dose and repeat the dose if needed.

The usual recommended dose for inial nasal administration is 1 mg (1 spray in one nostril). If adequate pain relief is not achieved within 60-90 minutes, an additional 1 mg dose may be given.

The initial dose sequence outlined above may be repeated in 3-4 hours as required.

For the management of severe pain, an initial dose of 2 mg (1 spray in each nostril) may be used in patients who will be able to remain recumbent in the event drowsiness or dizziness occur. In such patients additional doses should not be given for 3-4 hours. The incidence of adverse events is higher with an initial 2 mg dose (see CLINICAL STUDIES.)

The initial dose sequence in elderly patients and patients with renal or hepatic impairment should be limited to 1 mg followed by 1 mg in 90-120 minutes. The repeat dose sequence in these patients should be determined by the patient's response rather than at fixed times but will generally be no less than at 6 hour intervals (see PRECAUTIONS.)

CLINICAL STUDIES:

The effectiveness of opioid analgesics varies in different pain syndromes. Studies with butorphanol tartrate injectable have been performed in postoperative (primarily abdominal and orthopedic) pain and pain during labor and delivery, as preoperative and preanesthetic medication, ans as a supplement to balanced anesthesia.

Studies with butorphanol tartrate NS have been performed in postoperative (general, orthopedic, oral, cesarean section) pain, in postepisiotomy pain, in pain of musculoskeletal origin, and in migraine headache pain.

INDICATIONS AND USAGE:

Butorphanol tartrate injectable and butorphanol tartrate nasal spray are indicated for the management of pain when the use of an opioid analgesic is appropriate.

Butorphanol tartrate injectable is also indicated as a preoperative or preanesthetic medication, as a supplement to balanced anesthesia, and for the relief of pain during labor.

CONTRAINDICATIONS:

Butorphanol tartrate injectable and butorphanol tartrate nasal spray are contraindicated in patients hypersensitive to butorphanol tartrate or the preservative benzethonium chloride in Butorphanol tartrate injectable or butorphanol tartrate nasal spray in the multi-dose vial.

WARNINGS:

PATIENTS DEPENDENT ON NARCOTICS

Because of its opioid antagonist properties, butorphanol is not recommended for use in patients dependent on narcotics. Such patients should have an adequate period of withdrawal from opioid drugs prior to beginning butorphanol therapy. In patients taking opioid analgesics chronically, butorphanol has precipitated withdrawal symptoms such as anxiety, agitation, mood changes, hallucinations, dysphoria, weakness and diarrhea.

Because of the difficulty in assessing opioid tolerance in patients who have recently received repeated doses of narcotic analgesic medication, caution should be used in the administration of butorphanol to such patients.

PRECAUTIONS:

GENERAL

Hypotension associated with syncope during the first hour of dosing with butorphanol tartrate nasal spray has been reported rarely, particularly in patients with past history of similar reactions to opioid analgesics. Therefore, patients should be advised to avoid activities with potential risks.

Head Injury and Increased Intracranial Pressure: As with other opioids, the use of butorphanol in patients with head injury may be associated with carbon dioxide retention and secondary elevation of cerebrospinal fluid pressure, drug-induced miosis, and alterations in mental state that would obscure the interpretation of the clinical course of patients with head injuries. In such patients, butorphanol should be used only if the benefits of use outweigh the potential risks.

Disorders of Respiratory Function or Control: Butorphanol may produce respiratory depression, especially in patients receiving other CNS active agents, or patients suffering from CNS diseases or respiratory impairment.

Hepatic and Renal Disease: In patients with severe hepatic or renal disease the initial dosage interval for butorphanol tartrate injectable and butorphanol tartrate nasal spray should be increased to 6-8 hours until the response has been well characterized. Subsequent doses should be determined by patient response rather than being scheduled at fixed intervals (see Individualization of Dosage.)

Cardiovascular Disease: Because butorphanol may increase the work of the heart, especially the pulmonary circuit (see CLINICAL PHARMACOLOGY), the use of butorphanol in patients with acute myocardial infarction, ventricular dysfunction, or coronary insufficiency should be limited to those situations where the benefits clearly outweigh the risk.

Severe hypertension has been reported rarely during butorphanol therapy. In such cases, butorphanol should be discontinued and the hypertension treated with antihypertensive drugs. In patients who are not opioid dependent, naloxone has also been reported to be effective.

INFORMATION FOR THE PATIENT

1. Drowsiness and dizziness related to the use of butorphanol may impair mental and/or physical abilities required for the performance of potentially hazardous tasks (*e.g.,* driving, operating machinery, etc).

2. Alcohol should not be consumed while using butorphanol. Concurrent use of butorphanol with drugs that affect the central nervous system (*e.g.,* alcohol, barbiturates, tranquilizers, and antihistamines) may result in increased central nervous system depressant effects such as drowsiness, dizziness and impaired mental function.

3. Patients should be instructed on the proper use butorphanol tartrate nasal spray.

USE IN AMBULATORY PATIENTS

Drowsiness and dizziness related to the use of butorphanol may impair mental and/or physical abilities required for the performance of potentially hazardous tasks (*e.g.,* driving, operating machinery, etc.). Patients should be told to use caution in such activities until their individual responses to butorphanol have been well characterized.

Alcohol should not be consumed while using butorphanol. Concurrent use of butorphanol with central nervous system depressants (*e.g.,* alcohol, barbiturates, tranquilizers, and antihistamines) may result in increased central nervous system depressant effects.

Patients should be instructed on the proper use of butorphanol tartrate nasal spray.

CARCINOGENESIS, MUTAGENESIS, AND IMPAIRMENT OF FERTILITY

The carcinogenic potential of butorphanol has not been adequately evaluated.

Butorphanol was not genotoxic in *S. typhimurium* or *E. coli* assays or in unscheduled DNA synthesis and repair assays conducted in cultured human fibroblast cells.

Rats treated orally with 160 mg/kg/day (944 mg/sq. m.) had a reduced pregnancy rate. However, a similar effect was not observed with a 2.5 mg/kg/day (14.75 mg/sq. m.) subcutaneous dose.

PREGNANCY CATEGORY C

Reproduction studies in mice, rats and rabbits during organogenesis did not reveal any teratogenic potential to butorphanol. However, pregnant rats treated subcutaneously with butorphanol at 1 mg/kg (5.9 mg/sq. m.) had a higher frequency of stillbirths than controls. Butorphanol at 30 mg/kg/oral (5.1 mg/sq. m.) and 60 mg/kg/oral (10.2 mg/sq. m.) also showed higher incidences of post-implantation loss in rabbits.

There are no adequate and well-controlled studies of butorphanol tartrate in pregnant women before 37 weeks of gestation. Butorphanol tartrate should be used during pregnancy only if potential benefit justifies the potential risk to the infant.

LABOR AND DELIVERY

Although there have been rare reports of infant respiratory distress/apnea following the administration of butorphanol tartrate injectable during labor, this adverse effect was not attributed to butorphanol tartrate injectable as used during controlled clinical trials. The

PRECAUTIONS: *(cont'd)*

reports of respiratory distress/apnea have been associated with administration of a dose within two hours of delivery, use of multiple doses, use with additional analgesic or sedative drugs, or use in preterm pregnancies.

In a study of 119 patients, the administration of 1 mg of IV butorphanol tartrate injectable during labor was associated with transient (10-90 minutes)sinusoidal fetal heart rate patterns, bur was not associated with adverse neonatal outcomes. In the presence of an abnormal fetal heart rate pattern, butorphanol tartrate injectable should be used with caution.

Butorphanol tartrate nasal spray is not recommended during labor or delivery because there is no clinical experience with its use in this setting.

NURSING MOTHERS

Butorphanol has been detected in milk following administration of butorphanol tartrate injectable to nursing mothers. The amount an infant would receive is probably clinically insignificant (estimated 4 mcg/L of milk in a mother receiving 2 mg IM four times a day).

Although there is no clinical experience with the use of butorphanol tartrate nasal spray in nursing mothers, it should be assumed that butorphanol will appear in the milk in similar amounts following the nasal route of administration.

PEDIATRIC USE

Butorphanol is not recommended for use in patients below 18 years of age because safety and efficacy have not been established in this population.

GERIATRIC USE

The initial dose of butorphanol tartrate injectable recommended for elderly patients is half the usual dose at twice the usual interval. Subsequent doses and intervals should be based on the patient response (see Individualization of Dosage.)

Initially a 1 mg dose of butorphanol tartrate nasal spray should generally be used in geriatric patients and 90-120 minutes should elapse before deciding whether a second 1 mg dose is needed (see Individualization of Dosage.)

Due to changes in clearance, the mean half-life of butorphanol is increased by 25% (to over 6 hours) in patients over the age of 65. Elderly patients may be more sensitive to its side effects. Results from a long-term clinical safety trial suggest that elderly patients may be less tolerant of dizziness due to butorphanol tartrate nasal spray than younger patients.

DRUG INTERACTIONS:

Concurrent use of butorphanol with central nervous system depressants (*e.g.,* alcohol, barbiturates, tranquilizers, and antihistamines) may result in increased central nervous system depressant effects. When used concomitantly with such drugs, the dose of butorphanol should be the smallest effective dose and the frequency of dosing reduced as much as possible when administered concomitantly with drugs that potentiate the action of opioids.

It is not known if the effects of butorphanol are altered by concomitant medications that affect hepatic metabolism of drugs (cimetidine, erythromycin, theophylline, etc.), but physicians should be alert to the possibility that a smaller initial dose and longer intervals between doses may be needed.

The fraction of butorphanol tartrate nasal spray absorbed is unaffected by the concomitant administration of a nasal vasoconstrictor (oxymetazoline), but the rate of absorption is decreased. Therefore, a slower onset can be anticipated if butorphanol tartrate nasal spray is administered concomitantly with, or immediately following, a nasal vasoconstrictor.

No information is available about the use of butorphanol concurrently with MAO inhibitors.

ADVERSE REACTIONS:

A total of 2446 patients were studied in butorphanol clinical trials. Approximately half received butorphanol tartrate injectable with the remainder receiving butorphanol tartrate nasal spray. In nearly all cases the type and incidence of side effects with butorphanol by any route were those commonly observed with opioid analgesics.

The adverse experiences described below are based on data from short- and long-term clinical trials in patients receiving butorphanol by any route and from post-marketing experience with butorphanol tartrate injectable. There has been no attempt to correct for placebo effect or to subtract the frequencies reported by placebo treated patients in controlled trials.

The most frequently reported adverse experiences across all clinical trials with butorphanol tartrate injectable and butorphanol tartrate nasal spray were somnolence (43%), dizziness (19%), nausea and/or vomiting (13%). In long-term trials with butorphanol tartrate nasal spray only, nasal congestion (13%) and insomnia (11%) were frequently reported.

The following adverse experiences were reported at a frequency of 1% or greater, and were considered to be probably related to the use of butorphanol:

Body as a Whole: asthenia/lethargy*, headache*, sensation of heat

Cardiovascular: vasodilation*, palpitations

Digestive: anorexia*, constipation*, dry mouth*, nausea and/or vomiting (13%), stomach pain

Nervous: anxiety, confusion*, dizziness (19%), euphoria, floating feeling, INSOMNIA (11%), nervousness, paresthesia, somnolence (43%), tremor

Respiratory: bronchitis, cough, dyspnea*, epistaxis*, nasal congestion (13%), nasal irritation*, pharyngitis*, rhinitis*, sinus congestion*, sinusitis, upper respiratory infection*

Skin and Appendages: sweating/clammy*, pruritus

Special Senses: blurred vision, ear pain, tinnitus*, unpleasant taste* (also seen in short-term trials with butorphanol tartrate nasal spray.

Reactions occurring with a frequency of 3-9% are marked with an asterisk.* reactions reported predominantly from long-term trials with butorphanol tartrate nasal spray are CAPITALIZED.)

The following adverse experiences were reported with a frequency of less than 1%, in clinical trials or from post-marketing experience, and were considered to be probably related to the use of butorphanol.

Cardiovascular: hypotension, syncope

Nervous: abnormal dreams, agitation, *drug dependence,* dysphoria, hallucination, hostility

Skin and Appendages: rash/hives

Urogenital: Impaired urination

(Reactions reported only from post-marketing experience are *italicized.*)

The following infrequent addition adverse experiences were reported in a frequency of less than 1% of the patients studied in short-term butorphanol tartrate nasal spray trials and from post-marketing experiences under circumstances where the association between these events butorphanol administration is unknown. they are being listed as alerting information for the physician.

Body as a Whole: edema

Cardiovascular: hypertension

Nervous: *convulsion, delusion,* depression

Respiratory: *apnea,* shallow breathing

(Reactions reported only from post-marketing experience are *italicized.*)

DRUG ABUSE AND DEPENDENCE:

Although the mixed agonist-antagonist opioid analgesics, as a class, have lower abuse potential than morphine, all such drugs can be and have been reported to be abused.

Chronic use of butorphanol tartrate injectable has been reported to result in mild withdrawal syndromes, and reports of overuse and self- reported addiction have been received.

Among 161 patients who used butorphanol tartrate nasal spray for 2 months or longer approximately 3% had behavioral symptoms suggestive of possible abuse. Approximately 1% of these patients reported significant overuse. Symptoms such as anxiety, agitation, and diarrhea were observed. Symptoms suggestive of opioid withdrawal occurred in 2 patients who stopped the drug abruptly after using 16 mg a day or more for longer than 3 months.

Special care should be exercised in administering butorphanol to emotionally unstable patients and to those with a history of drug misuse. When long-term therapy is necessary, such patients should be closely supervised.

OVERDOSAGE:

Clinical Manifestations: The clinical manifestations of overdose are those of opioid drugs, the most serious of which are hypoventilation, cardiovascular insufficiency and/or coma.

Overdose can occur due to accidental or intentional misuse of butorphanol, especially in young children who may gain access to the drug in the home.

Treatment: The management of suspected butorphanol overdosage includes maintenance of adequate ventilation, peripheral perfusion, normal body temperature, and protection of the airway. Patients should be under continuous observation with adequate serial measures of mental state, responsiveness, and vital signs. Oxygen and ventilatory assistance should be available with continual monitoring by pulse oximetry if indicated. In the presence of coma, placement of an artificial airway may be required. An adequate intravenous portal should be maintained to facilitate treatment of hypotension associated with vasodilation.

The use of a specific opioid antagonist such as naloxone should be considered. As the duration of butorphanol action usually exceeds the duration of action of naloxone, repeated dosing with naloxone may be required.

DOSAGE AND ADMINISTRATION:

Factors to be considered in determining the dose are age, body weight, physical status, underlying pathological condition, use of other drugs, type of anesthesia to be used, and surgical procedure involved. use in the elderly, patients with hepatic or renal disease or in labor requires extra caution (see PRECAUTIONS and Individualization of Dosage). The following doses are for patients who do not have impaired hepatic or renal function and who are not on CNS active agents.

USE FOR PAIN

Intravenous: The usual recommended single dose for IV administration is 1 mg repeated every three to four hours as necessary. The effective dosage range, depending on the severity of pain, is 0.5 to 2 mg repeated every three to four hours.

Intramuscular: The usual recommended single dose for IV administration is 2 mg in patients who will be able to remain incumbent, in the event drowsiness or dizziness occurs. This may be repeated every three to four hours, as necessary. The effective dosage range depending on the severity of pain is 1 to 4 mg repeated every three to four hours. There are insufficient clinical data to recommend single doses above 4 mg.

Nasal Spray: The usual recommended dose for initial nasal administration is 1 mg (1 spray in one nostril). Adherence to this dose reduces the incidence of drowsiness and dizziness. If adequate pain relief is not achieved within 60-90 minutes, an additional 1 mg dose may be given.

The initial two dose sequence outlined above may be repeated in 3-4 hours as needed.

Depending on the severity of the pain, an initial dose of 2 mg (1 spray in **each** nostril) may be used in patients who will be able to remain incumbent in the event drowsiness or dizziness occur. In such patients single additional 2 mg doses should not be given for 3-4 hours.

USE AS PREOPERATIVE/PREANESTHETIC MEDICATION

The preoperative medication dosage of butorphanol tartrate injectable should be individualized (see Individualization of Dosage.) The usual adult dose is 2 mg IM, administered 60-90 minutes before surgery. This is approximately equivalent in sedative effect to 10 mg morphine or 80 mg meperidine.

USE IN BALANCE ANESTHESIA

The usual dose of butorphanol tartrate injectable is 2 mg IV shortly before induction and/or 0.5 to 1.0 mg IV in increments during anesthesia. The increment may be higher, up to 0.06 mg/kg (4 mg/70 kg), depending on previous sedative, analgesic, and hypnotic drugs administered. The total dose of butorphanol tartrate injectable will vary; however, patients seldom require less than 4 mg or more than 12.5 mg (approximately 0.06 to 0.18 mg/kg).

The use of butorphanol tartrate nasal spray is not recommended, because it has not been studied in induction or maintenance of anesthesia.

LABOR

In patients at full term in early labor a 1-2 mg dose of butorphanol tartrate injectable IV or IM may be administered and repeated after 4 hours. Alternative analgesia should be used for pain associated with delivery or if delivery is expected to occur within 4 hours.

If concomitant use of butorphanol tartrate with drugs that may potentiate its effects is deemed necessary (see DRUG INTERACTIONS) the lowest effective dose should be employed.

The use of butorphanol tartrate nasal spray is not recommended as it has not been studied in labor.

Safety And Handling: Butorphanol tartrate injectable is supplied in sealed delivery systems that have a low risk of accidental exposure to health care workers. ordinary care should be taken to avoid aerosol generation while preparing a syringe for use. Following skin contact, rinsing with cool water is recommended.

Butorphanol tartrate nasal spray is an open delivery system with increased risk of exposure to health care workers.

In the priming process, a certain amount of butorphanol may be aerosolized; therefore, the pump sprayer should be aimed away from the patient or other people or animals.

The unit should be disposed of by unscrewing the cap, rinsing the bottle, and placing the parts in a waste container.

Storage Conditions: Store below 86°F (30°C). Parenteral drug products should be inspected visually for particulate matter and discoloration prior to administration; whenever solution and container permit.

HOW SUPPLIED - EQUIVALENTS NOT AVAILABLE:

Aerosol, Spray - Nasal - 10 mg/ml

2.5 ml $60.52 STADOL NS, Bristol Myers Squibb 00087-5650-41

HOW SUPPLIED - EQUIVALENTS NOT AVAILABLE: *(cont'd)*

Injection, Solution - Intramuscular; - 1 mg/ml

1 ml	$7.31	STADOL, Mead Johnson	00015-5645-20
1 ml	$7.31	STADOL, Mead Johnson	00015-5645-33

Injection, Solution - Intramuscular; - 2 mg/ml

1 ml	$7.62	STADOL, Mead Johnson	00015-5646-20
1 ml	$7.62	STADOL, Mead Johnson	00015-5646-33
2 ml	$12.99	STADOL, Mead Johnson	00015-5644-20
2 ml	$12.99	STADOL, Mead Johnson	00015-5644-33
10 ml	$66.28	STADOL, Mead Johnson	00015-5648-20
10 ml	$66.28	STADOL, Mead Johnson	00015-5648-97

CABERGOLINE *(003323)*

CATEGORIES: Anterior Pituitary/Hypothalmic Function; Dopamine Receptor Agonists; Hyperprolactinemia; Parkinsonism**; FDA Approved 1996 Dec
* Indication not approved by the FDA

BRAND NAMES: **Dostinex**

DESCRIPTION:

Cabergoline is a dopamine receptor agonist. The chemical name for cabergoline is 1-[(6-allylergolin-8β-yl)-carbonyl]-1-[3-(dimethylamino)propyl]-3-ethylurea. Its empirical formula is $C_{26}H_{37}N_5O_2$, and its molecular weight is 451.62.

Cabergoline is a white powder soluble in ethyl alcohol, chloroform, and N,N-dimethylformamide (DMF); slightly soluble in 0.1N hydrochloric acid; very slightly soluble in n-hexane; and insoluble in water.

Dostinex tablets, for oral administration, contain 0.5 mg of cabergoline. Inactive ingredients consist of leucine, USP, and lactose, NF.

Mechanism of Action: The secretion of prolactin by the anterior pituitary is mainly under hypothalmic inhibitory control, likely exerted through release of dopamine by tuberoinfundibular neurons. Cabergoline is a long-acting dopamine receptor agonist with a high affinity for D_2 receptors. Results of *in vitro* studies demonstrate that cabergoline exerts a direct inhibitory effect on the secretion of prolactin by rat pituitary lactotrophs. Cabergoline decreased serum prolactin levels in reserpinized rats. Receptor-binding studies indicate that cabergoline has low affinity for dopamine D_1, α_1- and α_2-adrenergic, and 5-HT_1 and 5-HT_2-serotonin receptors.

PHARMACOKINETICS

Absorption: Following single oral doses of 0.5 mg to 1.5 mg given to 12 healthy adult volunteers, mean peak plasma levels of 30 to 70 picograms (pg)/ml of cabergoline were observed within 2 to 3 hours. Over the 0.5 to 7 mg dose range, cabergoline plasma levels appeared to be dose-proportional in 12 healthy adult volunteers and nine adult parkinsonian patients. A repeat-dose study in 12 healthy volunteers suggests that steady-state levels following a once-weekly dosing schedule are expected to be two-fold to three-fold higher than after a single dose. The absolute bioavailability of cabergoline is unknown. A significant fraction of the administered dose undergoes a first-pass effect. The elimination half-life of cabergoline estimated from urinary data of 12 healthy subjects ranged between 63 to 69 hours. The prolonged prolactin-lowering effect of cabergoline may be related to its slow elimination and long half-life.

Distribution: In animals, based on total radioactivity, cabergoline (and/or its metabolites has shown extensive tissue distribution. Radioactivity in the pituitary exceeded that in plasma by >100-fold and was eliminated with a half-life of approximately 60 hours. This finding is consistent with the long-lasting prolactin-lowering effect of the drug. Whole body autoradiography studies in pregnant rats showed no fetal uptake but high levels in the uterine wall. Significant radioactivity (parent plus metabolites) detected in the milk of lactating rats suggests a potential for exposure to nursing infants. The drug is extensively distributed throughout the body. Cabergoline is moderately bound (40% to 42%) to human plasma proteins in a concentration-independent manner. Concomitant dosing of highly protein-bound drugs is unlikely to affect its disposition.

Metabolism: In both animals and humans, cabergoline is extensively metabolized, predominantly via hydrolysis of the acylurea bond or the urea moiety. Cytochrome P-450 mediated metabolism appears to be minimal. Cabergoline does not cause enzyme induction and/or inhibition in the rat. Hydrolysis of the acylurea or urea moiety abolishes the prolactin-lowering effect of cabgergoline, and major metabolites identified thus far do not contribute to the therapeutic effect.

Excretion: After oral dosing of radioactive cabergoline to five healthy volunteers, approximately 22% and 60% of the dose was excreted within 20 days in the urine and feces, respectively. Less than 4% of the dose was excreted unchanged in the urine. Nonrenal and renal clearances for cabergoline are about 3.2 L/min and 0.08 L/min, respectively. Urinary excretion in hyperprolactinemic patients was similar.

SPECIAL POPULATIONS

Renal Insufficiency: The pharmacokinetics of cabergoline were not altered in 12 patients with moderate-to-severe renal insufficiency as assessed by creatinine clearance.

Hepatic Insufficiency: In 12 patients with mild-to-moderate hepatic dysfunction (Child-Pugh score ≤10), no effect on mean cabergoline C_{max} or area under the plasma concentrations curve (AUC) was observed. However, patients with severe insufficiency (Child-Pugh score >10) show a substantial increase in the mean cabergoline C_{max} and AUC, and thus necessitate caution.

Elderly: Effect on age on the pharmacokinetics of cabergoline has not been studied.

Food-Drug Interaction: In 12 healthy adult volunteers, food did not alter cabergoline kinetics.

PHARMACODYNAMICS

Dose response with inhibition of plasma prolactin, onset of maximal effect, and duration of effect has been documented following single cabergoline doses to healthy volunteers (0.05 to 1.5 mg) and hyperprolactinemic patients (0.3 to 1 mg). In volunteers, prolactin inhibition was evident at doses >0.2 mg, while doses ≥0.5 mg caused maximal suppression in most subjects. Higher doses produce prolactin suppression in a greater proportion of subjects and with an earlier onset and longer duration of action. In 12 healthy volunteers, 0.5, 1, and 1.5 mg doses resulted in complete prolactin inhibition, with a maximum effect within 3 hours in 92% to 100% of subjects after the 1 and 1.5 mg doses compared with 50% of subjects after the 0.5 mg dose.

In hyperprolactinemic patients (N=51), the maximal prolactin decrease after a 0.6 mg single dose of cabergoline was comparable to 2.5 mg bromocriptine; however, the duration of effect was markedly longer (14 days vs 24 hours). The time to maximal effect was shorter for bromocriptine than cabergoline (6 hours vs 48 hours).

In 72 healthy volunteers, single or multiple doses (up to 2 mg) of cabergoline resulted in selective inhibition of prolactin with no apparent effect on other anterior pituitary hormones (GH, FSH, LH, ACTH, and TSH) or cortisol.

CLINICAL STUDIES:

The prolactin-lowering efficacy of cabergoline was demonstrated in hyperprolactinemic women in two randomized, double-blind, comparative studies, one with placebo and the other with bromocriptine. In the placebo-controlled study (placebo n=20; cabergoline n=168), cabergoline produced a dose-related decrease in serum prolactin levels with prolactin normalized after 4 weeks treatment in 29%, 76%, 74%, and 95% of the patients receiving 0.125, 0.5, 0.75, and 1.0 mg twice weekly respectively.

In the 8-week, double-blind period of the comparative trial with bromocriptine (cabergoline n=223; bromocriptine n=236, in the intent-to-treat analysis), prolactin was normalized in 77% of the patients treated with cabergoline at 0.5 mg twice weekly compared with 59% of those treated with bromocriptine at 2.5 mg twice daily. Restoration of menses occurred in 77% of the women treated with cabergoline, compared with 70% of those treated with bromocriptine. Among patients with galactorrhea, this symptom disappeared in 73% of those treated with cabergoline compared with 56% of those treated with bromocriptine.

INDICATIONS AND USAGE:

Cabergoline tablets are indicated for the treatment of hyperprolactinemic disorders, either idiopathic or due to pituitary adenomas.

CONTRAINDICATIONS:

Cabergoline tablets are contraindicated in patients with uncontrolled hypertension or known hypersensitivity to ergot derivatives.

WARNINGS:

Dopamine agonists in general should not be used in patients with pregnancy-induced hypertension, for example, preclampsia and eclampsia, unless the potential benefit is judged to outweigh the possible risk.

PRECAUTIONS:

GENERAL

Initial doses higher than 1.0 mg may produce orthostatic hypotension. Care should be exercised when administering cabergoline with other medications known to lower blood pressure.

Postpartum Lactation Inhibition or Suppression: Cabergoline is not indicated for the inhibition or suppression of physiological lactation. Use of bromocriptine, another dopamine agonist for this purpose, has been associated with cases of hypertension, stroke, and seizures.

Hepatic Impairment: Since cabergoline is extensively metabolized by the liver, caution should be used, and careful monitoring exercised, when administering cabergoline to patients with hepatic impairment.

INFORMATION FOR THE PATIENT

A patient should be instructed to notify her physician if she suspects she is pregnant, becomes pregnant, or intends to become pregnant during therapy. A pregnancy test should be done if there is any suspicion of pregnancy and continuation of treatment should be discussed with her physician.

CARCINOGENESIS, MUTAGENESIS, AND IMPAIRMENT OF FERTILITY

Carcinogenicity studies were conducted in mice and rats with cabergoline given by gavage at doses up to 0.98 mg/kg/day and 0.32 mg/kg/day, respectively. These doses are 7 times and 4 times the maximum recommended human dose calculated on a body surface area basis using total mg/m^2/week in rodents and mg/m^2/week for a 50 kg human.

There was a slight increase in the incidence of cervical and uterine leiomyomas and uterine leiomyosarcomas in mice. In rats, there was a slight increase in malignant tumors of the cervix and uterus and interstitial cell adenomas. The occurrence of tumors in female rodents may be related to the prolonged suppression of prolactin secretion because prolactin is needed in rodents for the maintenance of the corpus luteum. In the absence of prolactin, the estrogen/progesterone ratio is increased, thereby increasing the risk for uterine tumors. In male rodents, the decrease in serum prolactin levels was associated with an increase in serum luteinizing hormone, which is thought to be a compensatory effect to maintain testicular steroid synthesis. Since these hormonal mechanisms are thought to be species-specific, the relevance of these tumors to humans is not known.

The mutagenic potential of cabergoline was evaluated and found to be negative in a battery of *in vitro* tests. These tests included the bacterial mutation (Ames) test with *Salmonella typhimurium*, the gene mutation assay with *Schizosaccharomyces pombe* P_1 and V79 Chinese hamster cells, DNA damage and repair in *Saccharomyces cerevisiae* D_4, and chromosomal aberrations in human lymphocytes. Cabergoline was also negative in the bone marrow micronucleus test in the mouse.

In female rats, a daily dose of 0.003 mg/kg for 2 weeks prior to mating and throughout the mating period inhibited conception. This dose represents approximately 1/28 the maximum recommended human dose calculated on a body surface area basis using total mg/m^2/week in rats and mg/m^2/week for a 50 kg human.

PREGNANCY, TERATOGENIC EFFECTS, PREGNANCY CATEGORY B

Reproduction studies have been performed with cabergoline in mice, rats, and rabbits administered by gavage.

(Multiples of the maximum recommended human dose in this section are calculated on a body surface area basis using total mg/m^2/week for animals and mg/m^2/week for a 50 kg human.

There were maternotoxic effects but no teratogenic effects in mice given cabergoline at doses up to 8 mg/kg/day (approximately 55 times the maximum recommended human dose) during the period of organogenesis.)

A dose of 0.012 mg/kg/day (approximately 1/7 the maximum recommended human dose) during the period of organogenesis in rats caused an increase in post-implantation embryofetal loses. These losses could be due to the prolactin inhibitory properties of cabergoline in rats. At daily doses of 0.5 mg/kg/day (approximately 19 times the maximum recommended human dose) during the period of organogenesis in the rabbit, cabergoline caused maternotoxicity characterized by a loss of body weight and decreased food consumption. Doses of 4 mg/kg/day (approximately 150 times the maximum recommended human dose) during the period of organogenesis in the rabbit caused an increased occurrence of various malformations. However, in another study in rabbits, no treatment-related malformations or embryofetaotoxicity were observed at doses up to 8 mg/kg/day (approximately 300 times the maximum recommended human dose).

In rats, doses higher than 0.003 mg/kg/day (approximately 1/28 the maximum recommended human dose) from 6 days before parturition and throughout the lactation period inhibited growth and caused death of offspring due to decreased milk secretion.

There are, however, no adequate and well-controlled studies in pregnant women. Because animal reproduction studies are not always predictive of human response, this drug should be used during pregnancy only if clearly needed.

PRECAUTIONS: *(cont'd)*

NURSING MOTHERS

It is not known whether this drug is excreted in human milk. Because many drugs are excreted in human milk and because of the potential for serious adverse reactions in nursing infants from cabergoline, a decision should be made whether to discontinue the drug, taking into account the importance of the drug to the mother. Use of cabergoline for the inhibition or suppression of physiologic lactation is not recommended (see PRECAUTIONS).

The prolactin-lowering action of cabergoline suggests that it will interfere with lactation. Due to this interference with lactation, cabergoline should not be given to women postpartum who are breast-feeding or who are planning to breast-feed.

PEDIATRIC USE

Safety and effectiveness of cabergoline in pediatric patients have not been established.

DRUG INTERACTIONS:

Cabergoline should not be administered concurrently with D_2-antagonists, such as phenothiazines, butyrophenones, thioxanthines, or metoclopramide.

ADVERSE REACTIONS:

The safety of cabergoline tablets has been evaluated in more than 900 patients with hyperprolactinemic disorders. Most adverse events were mild or moderate in severity.

In a 4-week, double-blind, placebo controlled study, treatment consisted of placebo or cabergoline at fixed doses of 0.125, 0.5, 0.75, or 1.0 mg twice weekly. Doses were halved during the first week. Since a possible dose-related effect was observed for nausea only, the four cabergoline treatment groups have been combined. The incidence of the most common adverse events during the placebo-controlled study is presented in TABLE 1.

TABLE 1 Incidence of Reported Adverse Events During the 4-Week, Double-Blind, Placebo-Controlled Trial.

Adverse Event*	Cabergoline (n=168) 0.125 to 1 mg two times a week	Placebo (n=20)
	Number (percent)	
Gastrointestinal		
Nausea	45 (27)	4 (20)
Constipation	16 (10)	0
Abdominal pain	9 (5)	1 (5)
Dyspepsia	4 (2)	0
Vomiting	4 (2)	0
Central and Peripheral Nervous System		
Headache	43 (26)	5 (25)
Dizziness	25 (15)	1 (5)
Paresthesia	2 (1)	0
Vertigo	2 (1)	0
Body as a Whole		
Asthenia	15 (9)	2 (10)
Fatigue	12 (7)	0
Hot Flashes	2 (1)	1 (5)
Psychiatric		
Somnolence	9 (5)	1 (5)
Depression	5 (3)	1 (5)
Nervousness	4 (2)	0
Autonomic Nervous System		
Postural hypotension	6 (4)	0
Reproductive - Female		
Breast pain	2 (1)	0
Dysmenorrhea	2 (1)	0
Vision		
Abnormal vision	2 (1)	0

* Reported at ≥1% for cabergoline.

In the 8-week, double-blind period of the comparative trial with bromocriptine, cabergoline (at a dose of 0.5 mg twice weekly) was discontinued because of an adverse event in 4 of 221 patients (2%) while bromocriptine (at a dose of 2.5 mg two times a day) was discontinued in 14 of 231 patients (6%). The most common reasons for discontinuation from cabergoline were headache, nausea and vomiting (3, 2 and 2 patients, respectively); the most common reasons for discontinuation from bromocriptine were nausea, vomiting, headache, and dizziness or vertigo (10, 3, 3, and 3 patients respectively). The incidence of the most common adverse events during the double-blind portion of the comparative trial with bromocriptine is presented in TABLE 2.

Other adverse events that were reported at an incidence of <1.0% in the overall clinical studies follow:

Body as a Whole: facial edema, influenza-like syndrome, malaise

Cardiovascular System: hypotension, syncope, palpitations

Digestive System: dry mouth, flatulence, diarrhea, anorexia

Metabolic and Nutritional System: weight loss, weight gain

Nervous System: somnolence, nervousness, paresthesia, insomnia, anxiety

Respiratory System: nasal stuffiness, epistaxis

Skin and Appendages: acne, pruritus

Special Senses: abnormal vision

Urogenital System: dysmenorrhea, increased libido

The safety of cabergoline has been evaluated in approximately 1200 patients with Parkinson's disease in controlled and uncontrolled studies at dosages of up to 11.5 mg/day which greatly exceeds the maximum recommended dosage of cabergoline for hyperprolactinemic disorders. In addition to the adverse events that occurred in the patients with hyperprolactinemic disorders, the most common adverse events in patients with Parkinson's disease were dyskinesia, hallucinations, confusion, and peripheral edema. Heart failure, pleural effusion, pulmonary fibrosis, and gastric or duodenal ulcer occurred rarely. One case of constrictive pericarditis has been reported.

OVERDOSAGE:

Overdosage might be expected to produce nasal congestion, syncope, or hallucinations. Measures to support blood pressure should be taken if necessary.

DOSAGE AND ADMINISTRATION:

The recommended dosage of cabergoline tablets for initiation of therapy is 0.25 mg twice a week. Dosage may be increased by 0.25 mg twice weekly up to a dosage of 1 mg twice a week according to the patient's serum prolactin level.

DOSAGE AND ADMINISTRATION: *(cont'd)*

TABLE 2 Incidence of Reported Adverse Events During the 8-Week, Double-Blind Period of the Comparative Trial With Bromocriptine

Adverse Event*	Cabergoline (n=221)	Placebo (n=231)
	Number (percent)	
Gastrointestinal		
Nausea	63 (29)	100 (43)
Constipation	15 (7)	21 (9)
Abdominal pain	12 (5)	19 (8)
Dyspepsia	11 (5)	16 (7)
Vomiting	9 (4)	16 (7)
Dry mouth	5 (2)	2 (1)
Diarrhea	4 (2)	7 (3)
Flatulence	4 (2)	3 (1)
Throat irritation	2 (1)	0
Toothache	2 (1)	0
Central and Peripheral Nervous System		
Headache	58 (26)	62 (27)
Dizziness	38 (17)	42 (18)
Vertigo	9 (4)	10 (4)
Paresthesia	5 (2)	6 (3)
Body as a Whole		
Asthenia	13 (6)	15 (6)
Fatigue	10 (5)	18 (8)
Syncope	3 (1)	3 (1)
Influenza-like symptoms	2 (1)	0
Malaise	2 (1)	0
Periorbital edema	2 (1)	2 (1)
Peripheral edema	2 (1)	1
Psychiatric		
Depression	7 (3)	5 (2)
Somnolence	5 (2)	5 (2)
Anorexia	3 (1)	3 (1)
Anxiety	3 (1)	3 (1)
Insomnia	3 (1)	2 (1)
Impaired concentration	2 (1)	1
Nervousness	2 (1)	5 (2)
Cardiovascular		
Hot flashes	6 (3)	3 (1)
Hypotension	3 (1)	4 (2)
Dependent edema	2 (1)	1
Palpitation	2 (1)	5 (2)
Reproductive - Female		
Breast pain	5 (2)	8 (3)
Dysmenorrhea	2 (1)	1
Skin and Appendages		
Acne	3 (1)	0
Pruritits	2 (1)	1
Musculoskeletal		
Pain	4 (2)	6 (3)
Arthralgia	2 (1)	0
Respiratory		
Rhinitis	2 (1)	9 (4)
Vision		
Abnormal vision	2 (1)	2(1)

* Reported at ≥1% for cabergoline.

Dosage increases should not occur more rapidly than every 4 weeks, so that the physician can assess the patient's response to each dosage level. If the patient does not respond adequately, and no additional benefit is observed with higher doses, the lowest dose that achieved maximal response should be used and other therapeutic approaches considered.

After a normal serum prolactin level has been maintained for 6 months, cabergoline may be discontinued, with periodic monitoring of the serum prolactin level to determine whether or when treatment with cabergoline should be reinstituted. The durability of efficacy beyond 24 months of therapy with cabergoline has not been established.

PATIENT INFORMATION:

Cabergoline is used for the treatment of hyperprolactinemia.

Do not use in uncontrolled hypertension or if you have allergies to ergot derivatives.

Inform your physician if you are pregnant, nursing or if you have liver disease.

Inform your physician if you are taking antipsychotic or antidepressant medicine or metoclopramide.

May cause nausea, constipation, headache, dizziness or weakness.

May be taken with or without food.

HOW SUPPLIED:

Dostinex tablets are white, scored, capsule-shaped tablets containing 0.5 mg cabergoline. Each tablet is scored on one side and has the letter P and the letter U on either side of the breakline. The other side of the tablet is engraved with the number 700.

Storage: Store at controlled room temperature 20° to 25°C (68° to 77°F)

CAFFEINE; ERGOTAMINE TARTRATE *(000574)*

CATEGORIES: Antimigraine/Other Headaches; Autonomic Drugs; Cephalalgia; Ergot Preparations; Headache; Migraine; Pain; Sympatholytic Agents; Tension; Pregnancy Category X; FDA Approval Pre 1982

BRAND NAMES: *Avamigran*; Cafatine; **Cafergot**; *Cafergot N* (Germany); Cafermine; Cafetrate; *Degran*; Ercaf; Ercatab; Ergo-Caff; *Ergocaf* (Mexico); *Ergofein*; *Ergoffin* (Germany); *Ergokoffin*; *Ergotamini Tartras Coffeinum*; *Ergoton*; Gotamine; *Gynergene Cafeine* (France); Micomp-Pb; Migergot; *Migranil*; *Polygot*; *Secadol*; *Trinergot* (Mexico); Wigraine

(International brand names outside U.S. in italics)

FORMULARIES: Aetna; BC-BS; DoD; FHP; Medi-Cal; PCS

DESCRIPTION:

Ergotamine tartrate and caffeine tablet:

ergotamine tartrate USP — 1 mg

caffeine USP — 100 mg

DESCRIPTION: *(cont'd)*

Inactive Ingredients: acacia, carnauba wax, lactose, methylparaben, povidone, propylparaben, sodium benzoate, sorbitol, starch, stearic acid, sucrose, synthetic black ferric oxide, synthetic red ferric oxide, synthetic yellow ferric oxide, talc, tartaric acid, and titanium dioxide.

Ergotamine tartrate and caffeine suppository:

ergotamine tartrate USP — 2 mg

caffeine USP — 100 mg

Inactive Ingredients: cocoa butter NF and tartaric acid NF.

Ergotamine tartrate and caffeine suppositories are *sealed* in foil to afford protection from cocoa butter leakage. If an unavoidable period of exposure to heat softens the suppository, it should be chilled in ice-cold water to solidify it before removing the foil.

CLINICAL PHARMACOLOGY:

Ergotamine is an alpha adrenergic blocking agent with a direct stimulating effect on the smooth muscle of peripheral and cranial blood vessels and produces depression of central vasomotor centers. The compound also has the properties of serotonin antagonism. In comparison to hydrogenated ergotamine, the adrenergic blocking actions are less pronounced and vasoconstrictive actions are greater.

Caffeine, also a cranial vasoconstrictor, is added to further enhance the vasoconstrictive effect without the necessity of increasing ergotamine dosage.

Many migraine patients experience excessive nausea and vomiting during attacks, making it impossible for them to retain any oral medication. In such cases, therefore, the only practical means of medication is through the rectal route where medication may reach the cranial vessels directly, evading the splanchnic vasculature and the liver.

INDICATIONS AND USAGE:

Indicated as therapy to abort or prevent vascular headache, e.g., migraine, migraine variants, or so-called "histaminic cephalalgia".

CONTRAINDICATIONS:

Ergotamine tartrate and caffeine may cause fetal harm when administered to pregnant women. Ergotamine tartrate and caffeine is contraindicated in women who are or may become pregnant. If this drug is used during pregnancy or if the patient becomes pregnant while taking this product, the patient should be apprised of the potential hazard to the fetus.

Peripheral vascular disease, coronary heart disease, hypertension, impaired hepatic or renal function and sepsis.

Hypersensitivity to any of the components.

PRECAUTIONS:

GENERAL

Although signs and symptoms of ergotism rarely develop even after long term intermittent use of the orally or rectally administered drugs, care should be exercised to remain within the limits of recommended dosage.

Ergotism is manifested by intense arterial vasoconstriction, producing signs and symptoms of peripheral vascular ischemia. Ergotamine induces vasoconstriction by a direct action on vascular smooth muscle. In chronic intoxication with ergot derivatives, headache, intermittent claudication, muscle pains, numbness, coldness, and pallor of the digits may occur. If the condition is allowed to progress untreated, gangrene can result.

While most cases of ergotism associated with ergotamine treatment result from frank overdosage, some cases have involved apparent hypersensitivity. There are few reports of ergotism among patients taking doses within the recommended limits or for brief periods of time. In rare instances, patients, particularly those who have used the medication indiscriminately over long periods of time, may display withdrawal symptoms consisting of rebound headache upon discontinuation of the drug.

Rare cases of a solitary rectal or anal ulcer have occurred from abuse of ergotamine suppositories usually in higher than recommended doses or with continual use at the recommended dose for many years. Spontaneous healing occurs within usually 4-8 weeks after drug withdrawal.

INFORMATION FOR THE PATIENT

Patients should be advised that two tablets or one suppository of ergotamine tartrate w/caffeine should be taken at the first sign of a migraine headache. No more than 6 tablets or 2 suppositories should be taken for any 7-day period. Ergotamine tartrate w/caffeine should be used only for migraine headaches. It is not effective for other types of headaches and it lacks analgesic properties. Patients should be advised to report to the physician immediately any of the following: numbness or tingling in the fingers and toes, muscle pain in the arms and legs, weakness in the legs, pain in the chest or temporary speeding or slowing of the heart rate, swelling or itching.

PREGNANCY CATEGORY X

Teratogenic Effects: There are no studies on the placental transfer or teratogenicity of the combined products of ergotamine tartrate w/caffeine. Caffeine is known to cross the placenta and has been shown to be teratogenic in animals. Ergotamine crosses the placenta in small amounts, although it does not appear to be embryotoxic in this quantity. However, prolonged vasoconstriction of the uterine vessels and/or increased myometrial tone leading to reduced myometrial and placental blood flow may have contributed to fetal growth retardation observed in animals (see CONTRAINDICATIONS.)

Nonteratogenic Effects: Ergotamine tartrate w/caffeine is contraindicated in pregnancy due to the oxytocic effects of ergotamine (see CONTRAINDICATIONS.)

LABOR AND DELIVERY

Ergotamine tartrate w/caffeine is contraindicated in labor and delivery due to its oxytocic effect which is maximal in the third trimester (see CONTRAINDICATIONS.)

NURSING MOTHERS

Ergot drugs are known to inhibit prolactin but there are no reports of decreased lactation with ergotamine tartrate w/caffeine. Ergotamine is excreted in breast milk and may cause symptoms of vomiting, diarrhea, weak pulse and unstable blood pressure in nursing infants. Because of the potential for serious adverse reactions in nursing infants from ergotamine tartrate w/caffeine, a decision should be made whether to discontinue nursing or discontinue the drug, taking into account the importance of the drug to the mother.

PEDIATRIC USE

Safety and effectiveness in children have not been established.

DRUG INTERACTIONS:

Ergotamine tartrate w/caffeine should not be administered with other vasoconstrictors. Use with sympathomimetics (pressor agents) may cause extreme elevation of blood pressure. The beta-blocker Inderal (propranolol) has been reported to potentiate the vasoconstrictive action of ergotamine tartrate w/caffeine by blocking the vasodilating property of epinephrine. Nicotine may provoke vasoconstriction in some patients, predisposing to a greater ischemic response to ergot therapy.

DRUG INTERACTIONS: *(cont'd)*

The blood levels of ergotamine-containing drugs are reported to be elevated by the concomitant administration of macrolide antibiotics and vasospastic reactions have been reported with therapeutic doses of the ergotamine-containing drugs when coadministered with these antibiotics.

ADVERSE REACTIONS:

Cardiovascular: Vasoconstrictive complications of a serious nature may occur at times. These include ischemia, cyanosis, absence of pulse, cold extremities, gangrene, precordial distress and pain, EKG changes and muscle pains. Although these effects occur most commonly with long-term therapy at relatively high doses, they have also been reported with short-term or normal doses. Other cardiovascular adverse effects include transient tachycardia or bradycardia and hypertension.

Gastrointestinal: Nausea and vomiting, rectal or anal ulcer (from overuse of suppositories).

Allergic: Localized edema and itching.

Fibrotic Complications: There have been a few reports of patients on ergotamine tartrate w/ caffeine therapy developing retroperitoneal and/or pleuropulmonary fibroses. There have also been rare reports of fibrotic thickening of the aortic, mitral, tricuspid, and/or pulmonary valves with long-term, continuous use of ergotamine tartrate w/caffeine.

DRUG ABUSE AND DEPENDENCE:

There have been reports of drug abuse and psychological dependence in patients on ergotamine tartrate w/caffeine therapy. Due to the chronicity of vascular headaches, it is imperative that patients be advised not to exceed recommended dosages with long-term use to avoid ergotism (see PRECAUTIONS.)

OVERDOSAGE:

The toxic effects of an acute overdosage of ergotamine tartrate w/caffeine are due primarily to the ergotamine component. The amount of caffeine is such that its toxic effects will be overshadowed by those of ergotamine. Symptoms include vomiting; numbness, tingling, pain and cyanosis of the extremities associated with diminished or absent peripheral pulses; hypertension or hypotension; drowsiness, stupor, coma, convulsions and shock. A case has been reported of reversible bilateral papillitis with ring scotomata in a patient who received five times the recommended daily adult dose over a period of 14 days.

Treatment consists of removal of the offending drug by induction of emesis, gastric lavage, and catharsis. Maintenance of adequate pulmonary ventilation, correction of hypotension, and control of convulsions are important considerations. Treatment of peripheral vasospasm should consist of warmth, but not heat, and protection of the ischemic limbs. Vasodilators may be beneficial but caution must be exercised to avoid aggravating an already existent hypotension.

DOSAGE AND ADMINISTRATION:

Procedure: For the best results, dosage should start at the first sign of an attack.

MAXIMUM ADULT DOSAGE

Orally: Total dose for any one attack should not exceed 6 tablets.

Rectally: Two suppositories is the maximum dose for an individual attack.

Total weekly dosage should not exceed 10 tablets or 5 suppositories.

In carefully selected patients, with due consideration of maximum dosage recommendations, administration of the drug at bedtime may be an appropriate short-term preventive measure.

HOW SUPPLIED:

Cafergot Tablets: Shell pink colored, sugar coated, imprinted "CAFERGOT" on one side, an "S" contained within a triangle on other side. *Store and Dispense:* Below 77°F (25°C); tight, light-resistant container.

Cafergot Suppositories: Sealed in fuchsia-colored aluminum foil, imprinted "S (contained within a triangle) and SANDOZ underneath the triangle, CAFERGOT SUPPOSITORY 78-33 SANDOZ". *Store and Dispense:* Below 77°F (25°C); tight container (sealed foil).

HOW SUPPLIED - RATED THERAPEUTICALLY EQUIVALENT:

Tablet, Coated - Oral - 100 mg/1 mg

20's	$14.50	WIGRAINE, Organon	00052-0542-20
90's	**$91.08**	**CAFERGOT, Novartis**	**00078-0034-42**
100's	$52.00	ERCAF, Geneva Pharms	00781-1995-01
100's	$60.53	WIGRAINE, Organon	00052-0542-91

HOW SUPPLIED - NOT RATED EQUIVALENT:

Suppository - Rectal - 100 mg/2 mg

12's	$20.94	MIGERGOT, GW Labs	00713-0166-12
12's	$23.32	WIGRAINE, Organon	00052-0548-12
12's	$32.95	CAFATINE, Major Pharms	00904-2595-12
12's	$33.25	CAFETRATE SUPPOSITORIES, Schein Pharm (US)	00364-2177-12
12's	**$49.20**	**CAFERGOT, Novartis**	**00078-0033-02**

CAFFEINE; SODIUM BENZOATE *(000570)*

CATEGORIES: Anorexients/CNS Stimulants; Central Nervous System Agents; Respiratory/Cerebral Stimulant; Stimulants; FDA Pre 1938 Drugs

BRAND NAMES: Caffeine & Sodium Benzoate

Prescribing information not available at time of publication.

HOW SUPPLIED - RATED THERAPEUTICALLY EQUIVALENT:

Injection, Solution - Intramuscular; - 250 mg/ml

2 ml x 10	$137.50	Caffeine & Sodium Benzoate, UDL	51079-0784-11

HOW SUPPLIED - NOT RATED EQUIVALENT:

Injection, Solution - Intramuscular; - 250 mg/ml

2 ml	$24.38	Caffeine & Sodium Benzoate, Yorpharm	61147-8004-01
2 ml x 10	$109.95	Caffeine & Sodium Benzoate, Hope Pharms	60267-0327-02
2 ml x 10	$187.50	CAFFEINE AND SODIUM BENZOATE, Am Regent	00517-2502-10
2 ml x 10	$226.00	CAFFEINE & SODIUM BENZOATE, Pasadena	00418-1531-10
2 ml x 10	$275.00	Caffeine & Sodium Benzoate, Consolidated Midland	00223-7273-10
2 ml x 25	$468.75	CAFFEINE AND SODIUM BENZOATE, Am Regent	00517-2502-25
2 ml x 25	$625.00	Caffeine & Sodium Benzoate, Consolidated Midland	00223-7273-02
25 x 2 ml	$202.50	Caffeine Sodium Benzoate, Pasadena	00418-1531-26

CALCIFEDIOL *(000583)*

CATEGORIES: Calcium Metabolism; Homeostatic & Nutrient; Vitamin D; Vitamins; Pregnancy Category C; FDA Approval Pre 1982

BRAND NAMES: **Calderol**; *Dedrogyl* (France, Germany); *Derdogyl*; *Didrogyl*; *Hidroferol*
(International brand names outside U.S. in italics)

FORMULARIES: Aetna

Prescribing information not available at time of publication.

HOW SUPPLIED - EQUIVALENTS NOT AVAILABLE:

Capsule, Elastic, Sustained Action - Oral - 20 mcg

60's	$50.55	CALDEROL, Organon	00052-0472-60

Capsule, Elastic, Sustained Action - Oral - 50 mcg

60's	$115.28	CALDEROL, Organon	00052-0474-60

CALCIPOTRIENE *(003192)*

CATEGORIES: Dermatologicals; Keratoplastic Agents; Psoriasis; Skin/Mucous Membrane Agents; Topical; Vitamin D; FDA Class 1S ("Standard Review"); FDA Approved 1993 Dec

BRAND NAMES: *Daivonex* (Australia, France, Germany); **Dovonex**; Ditrex; *Psorcutan* (Germany)
(International brand names outside U.S. in italics)

FORMULARIES: Medi-Cal; PCS

DESCRIPTION:

Calcipotriene monohydrate is a synthetic vitamin D_3 derivative for topical dermatological use.

Chemically, calcipotriene is (5Z,7E,22E,24S)-24-cyclopropyl-9,10- secochola-5,7,10(19),22-tetraene-1α, 3β, 24-triol monohydrate, with the empirical formula $C_{27}H_{40}O_3{\cdot}H_2O$, and a molecular weight of 430.6.

Calcipotriene monohydrate is a white or off-white crystalline substance. Dovonex cream contains calcipotriene monohydrate 50 mcg/g anhydrous calcipotrienne in a cream base of cetearyl alcohol, ceteth-20, diazolidinyl urea, dichlorobenzyl alcohol, dibasic sodium phosphate, edetate disodium, glycerin, mineral oil, petrolatum, and water.

CLINICAL PHARMACOLOGY:

In humans, the natural supply of vitamin D depends mainly on exposure to the ultraviolet rays of the sun for conversion of 7-dehydrocholesterol to vitamin D_3 (cholecalciferol) in the skin. Calcipotriene is a synthetic analog of vitamin D_3.

Clinical studies with radiolabeled calcipotriene ointment indicate that approximately 6% (± 3%, SD) of the applied dose of calcipotriene is absorbed systemically when the ointment is applied topically to psoriasis plaques or 5% (± 2.6%,SD) when applied to normal skin, and much of the absorbed active is converted to inactive metabolites within 24 hours of application. Systemic absorption of the cream has not been studied

Vitamin D and its metabolites are transported in the blood, bound to specific plasma proteins. The active form of the vitamin, 1,25-dihydroxy vitamin D_3 (calcitriol), is known to be recycled via the liver and excreted in the bile. Calcipotriene metabolism following systemic uptake is rapid, and occurs via a similar pathway to the natural hormone.

CLINICAL STUDIES:

Adequate and well-controlled trials of patients treated with calcipotriene have demonstrated improvement usually beginning after two weeks of therapy. This improvement continued with approximately 50% of patients showing at least marked improvement in the signs and symptoms of psoriasis after 8 weeks of therapy, but only approximately 4% showed complete clearing.

INDICATIONS AND USAGE:

Calcipotriene ointment, 0.005%, is indicated for the treatment of plaque psoriasis. The safety and effectiveness of topical calcipotriene in dermatoses other than psoriasis have not been established.

CONTRAINDICATIONS:

Calcipotriene cream is contraindicated in those patients with a history of hypersensitivity to any of the components of the preparation. It should not be used by patients with demonstrated hypercalcemia or evidence of vitamin D toxicity. Calcipotriene cream should not be used on the face.

PRECAUTIONS:

General: Use of calcipotriene cream may cause tansient irritation of both lesions and surrounding uninvolved skin. If irritation develops, calcipotriene cream should be discontinued.

Reversible elevation of serum calcium has occurred with use of calcipotriene cream. If elevation in serum calcium outside the normal range should occur, discontinue treatment until normal calcium levels are restored.

Information for the Patient: Patients using calcipotriene cream should receive the following information and instructions:

1. This medication is to be used as directed by the physician. It is for external use only. Avoid contact with the face or eyes. As with any topical medication, patients should wash hands after application.

2. This medication should not be used for any disorder other than that for which it was prescribed.

3. Patients should report to their physician any signs of adverse reactions.

Carcinogenesis, Mutagenesis, and Impairment of Fertility: Animal studies have not been conducted to evaluate the carcinogenic potential of calcipotriene. Studies in rats at doses up to 54 μ/kg/day (318 μ/m²/day) of calcipotriene indicated no impairment of fertility or general reproductive performance.

Calcipotriene did not elicit any mutagenic effects in the Ames mutagenicity assay, the mouse lymphoma TK locus assay, the human lymphocyte chromosome aberration test or the mouse micronucleus test.

Pregnancy, Teratogenic Effects, Pregnancy Category C: Studies of teratogenicity were done by the oral route where bioavailability is expected to be approximately 40-60% of the administered dose. Increased rabbit maternal and fetal toxicity was noted at 12 mcg/kg/day (132 mcg/m²/day). Rabbits administered 36 mcg/kg/day (396 mcg/m²/day) resulted in fetuses with a significant increase in the incidences of pubic bones, forelimb phalanges, and incomplete bone ossification. In a rat study, oral doses of 54 mcg/kg/day (318 mcg/m²/day) resulted in a significantly higher incidence of skeletal abnormalities consisting primarily of enlarged fontanelles and extra ribs. The enlarged fontanelles are most likely due to calcipotriene's effect upon calcium metabolism. The maternal and fetal calculated no-effect exposures in the rat (43.2 mcg/m²/day) and rabbit (17.6 mcg/m²/day) studies are approximately equal to the expected human systemic exposure level (18.5mcg/m²/day) from dermal application. There are no adequate and well-controlled studies in pregnant women. Therefore, calcipotriene cream should be used during pregnancy only if the potential benefit justifies the potential risk to the fetus.

Nursing Mothers: There is evidence that maternal 1,25-dihydroxy vitamin D_3 (calcitriol) may enter the fetal circulation, but it is not known whether it is excreted in human milk. The systemic disposition of calcipotriene is expected to be similar to that of the naturally occurring vitamin. Because many drugs are excreted in human milk, caution should be exercised when calcipotriene cream is administered to a nursing woman.

Pediatric Use: Safety and effectiveness of calcipotriene cream in pediatric patients have not been established. Because of a higher ratio of skin surface area to body mass, children are at greater risk than adults of systemic adverse effects when they are treated with topical medication.

ADVERSE REACTIONS:

In controlled clinical trials, the most frequent adverse experience reported for calcipotriene cream were cases of skin irritation which occurred in approximately 10-15% of patients. Rash, pruritis, dermatitis, and worsening of psoriasis were reported in 1 to 10% of patients.

OVERDOSAGE:

Topically applied calcipotriene cream can be absorbed in sufficient amounts to produce systemic effects. Elevated serum calcium has been observed with excessive use of calcipotriene cream.

If elevation in serum calcium should occur, discontinue treatment until normal calcium levels are restored (See PRECAUTIONS.)

DOSAGE AND ADMINISTRATION:

Apply a thin layer of calcipotriene cream to the affected skin twice daily and rub in gently and completely. The safety and efficacy of calcipotriene cream have been demonstrated in patients treated for eight weeks.

HOW SUPPLIED:

Storage: Store at controlled room temperature 15°- 25°C (59°- 77°F). Do not freeze

HOW SUPPLIED - EQUIVALENTS NOT AVAILABLE:

Ointment - Topical - 0.005 %

30 gm	$36.62	DOVONEX, Westwood Squibb	00072-2540-03
60 gm	$73.25	DOVONEX, Westwood Squibb	00072-2540-06
100 gm	$122.09	DOVONEX, Westwood Squibb	00072-2540-10

CALCITONIN (SALMON) *(000585)*

CATEGORIES: Bone Metabolism Regulators; Calcium Metabolism; Cardiac Output; Homeostatic & Nutrient; Hormones; Hypercalcemia; Hypercalcemic Agents; Hypocalcemic; Lesions; Osteoporosis; Paget's Disease; Pain; Parathyroid; Vitamin D; Pregnancy Category C; Sales > $100 Million; FDA Approval Pre 1982

BRAND NAMES: **Calcimar**; *Calsynar*; *Miacalcic*; Miacalcin; Osteocalcin
(International brand names outside U.S. in italics)

FORMULARIES: Aetna; BC-BS; Medi-Cal

COST OF THERAPY: $411.11 (Osteoporosis; Aerosol; 200 unit/dose; 0.09/day; 365 days)

DESCRIPTION:

Calcitonin is a polypeptide hormone secreted by the parafollicular cells of the thyroid gland in mammals and by the ultimobranchial gland of birds and fish.

Calcitonin-salmon is a synthetic polypeptide of 32 amino acids in the same linear sequence that is found in calcitonin of salmon origin.

Injection: It is provided in sterile solution for subcutaneous or intramuscular injection. Each milliliter contains 200 IU (MRC) of calcitonin-salmon, 5 mg phenol (as preservative), with sodium chloride, sodium acetate, acetic acid, and sodium hydroxide to adjust tonicity and pH.

Nasal Spray: It is provided in 2 ml fill glass bottles as a solution for nasal administration. This is sufficient medication for 14 doses. Each milliliter contains calcitonin-salmon 2200 IU (corresponding to 200 IU per 0.09 ml actuation), sodium chloride 8.5 mg, benzalkonium chloride 0.10 mg, nitrogen, hydrochloric acid (added as necessary to adjust pH) and purified water.

The activity of calcitonin-salmon nasal spray is stated in International Units based on bioassay in comparison with the International Reference Preparation of calcitonin-salmon for Bioassay, distributed by the National Institute of Biologic Standards and Control, Holly Hill, London.

CLINICAL PHARMACOLOGY:

INJECTION

Calcitonin acts primarily on bone, but direct renal effects and actions on the gastrointestinal tract are also recognized. Calcitonin-salmon appears to have actions essentially identical to calcitonins of mammalian origin, but its potency per mg is greater and it has a longer duration of action. The actions of calcitonin on bone and its role in normal human bone physiology are still incompletely understood.

Bone: Single injections of calcitonin cause a marked transient inhibition of the ongoing bone resorptive process. With prolonged use, there is a persistent, smaller decrease in the rate of bone resorption. Histologically, this is associated with a decreased number of osteoclasts and an apparent decrease in their resorptive activity. Decreased osteocytic resorption may also be involved. There is some evidence that initially bone formation may be augmented by calcitonin through increased osteoblastic activity. However, calcitonin will probably not induce a long-term increase in bone formation.

Animal studies indicate that endogenous calcitonin, primarily through its action on bone, participates with parathyroid hormone in the homeostatic regulation of blood calcium. Thus, high blood calcium levels cause increased secretion of calcitonin which, in turn, inhibits bone resorption. This reduces the transfer of calcium from bone to blood and tends to return blood

CLINICAL PHARMACOLOGY: *(cont'd)*

calcium to the normal level. The importance of this process in humans has not been determined. In normal adults, who have a relatively low rate of bone resorption, the administration of exogenous calcitonin results in only a slight decrease in serum calcium. In normal children and in patients with generalized Paget's disease, bone resorption is more rapid and decreases in serum calcium are more pronounced in response to calcitonin.

Paget's Disease of Bone (osteitis deformans): Paget's disease is a disorder of uncertain etiology characterized by abnormal and accelerated bone formation and resorption in one or more bones. In most patients only small areas of bone are involved and the disease is not symptomatic. In a small fraction of patients, however, the abnormal bone may lead to bone pain and bone deformity, cranial and spinal nerve entrapment, or spinal cord compression. The increased vascularity of the abnormal bone may lead to high output congestive heart failure.

Active Paget's disease involving a large mass of bone may increase the urinary hydroxyproline excretion (reflecting breakdown of collagen-containing bone matrix) and serum alkaline phosphatase (reflecting increased bone formation).

Calcitonin-salmon, presumably by an initial blocking effect on bone resorption, causes a decreased rate of bone turnover with a resultant fall in the serum alkaline phosphatase and urinary hydroxyproline excretion in approximately 2/3 of patients treated. These biochemical changes appear to correspond to changes toward more normal bone, as evidenced by a small number of documented examples of: 1) radiologic regression of Pagetic lesions, 2) improvement of impaired auditory nerve and other neurologic function, 3) decreases (measured) in abnormally elevated cardiac output. These improvements occur extremely rarely, if ever, spontaneously (elevated cardiac output may disappear over a period of years when the disease slowly enters a sclerotic phase; in the cases treated with calcitonin, however, the decreases were seen in less than one year.)

Some patients with Paget's disease who have good biochemical and/or symptomatic responses initially, later relapse. Suggested explanations have included the formation of neutralizing antibodies and the development of secondary hyperparathyroidism, but neither suggestion appears to explain adequately the majority of relapses.

Although the parathyroid hormone levels do appear to rise transiently during each hypocalcemic response to calcitonin, most investigators have been unable to demonstrate persistent hypersecretion of parathyroid hormone in patients treated chronically with calcitonin-salmon.

Circulating antibodies to calcitonin after 2-18 months' treatment have been reported in about half of the patients with Paget's disease in whom antibody studies were done, but calcitonin treatment remained effective in many of these cases. Occasionally, patients with high antibody titers are found. These patients usually will have suffered a biochemical relapse of Paget's disease and are unresponsive to the acute hypocalcemic effects of calcitonin.

Hypercalcemia: In clinical trials, calcitonin-salmon has been shown to lower the elevated serum calcium of patients with carcinoma (with or without demonstrated metastases), multiple myeloma or primary hyperparathyroidism (lesser response). Patients with higher values for serum calcium tend to show greater reduction during calcitonin therapy. The decrease in calcium occurs about 2 hours after the first injection and lasts for about 6-8 hours. Calcitonin-salmon given every 12 hours maintained a calcium lowering effect for about 5-8 days, the time period evaluated for most patients during the clinical studies. The average reduction of 8-hour post-injection serum calcium during this period was about 9 percent.

Kidney: Calcitonin increases the excretion of filtered phosphate, calcium, and sodium by decreasing their tubular reabsorption. In some patients, the inhibition of bone resorption by calcitonin is of such magnitude that the consequent reduction of filtered calcium load more than compensates for the decrease in tubular reabsorption of calcium. The result in these patients is a decrease rather than an increase in urinary calcium.

Transient increases in sodium and water excretion may occur after the initial injection of calcitonin. In most patients, these changes return to pretreatment levels with continued therapy.

Gastrointestinal Tract: Increasing evidence indicates that calcitonin has significant actions on the gastrointestinal tract. Short-term administration results in marked transient decreases in the volume and acidity of gastric juice and in the volume and the trypsin and amylase content of pancreatic juice. Whether these effects continue to be elicited after each injection of calcitonin during chronic therapy has not been investigated.

Metabolism: The metabolism of calcitonin-salmon has not yet been studied clinically. Information from animal studies with calcitonin-salmon and from clinical studies with calcitonins of porcine and human origin suggest that calcitonin-salmon is rapidly metabolized by conversion to smaller inactive fragments, primarily in the kidneys, but also in the blood and peripheral tissues. A small amount of unchanged hormone and its inactive metabolites are excreted in the urine.

It appears that calcitonin-salmon cannot cross the placental barrier and its passage to the cerebrospinal fluid or to breast milk has not been determined.

NASAL SPRAY

Calcitonin acts primarily on bone, but direct renal effects and actions on the gastrointestinal tract are also recognized. Calcitonin-salmon appears to have actions essentially identical to calcitonins of mammalian origin, but its potency per mg is greater and it has a longer duration of action.

The information below, describing the clinical pharmacology of calcitonin, has been derived from studies with *injectable* calcitonin. The mean bioavailability of calcitonin-salmon nasal spray is approximately 3% of that of injectable calcitonin in normal subjects and, therefore, the conclusions concerning the CLINICAL PHARMACOLOGY of this preparation may be different.

The actions of calcitonin on bone and its role in normal human bone physiology are still not completely elucidated, although calcitonin receptors have been discovered in osteoclasts and osteoblasts.

Single injections of calcitonin cause a marked transient inhibition of the ongoing bone resorptive process. With prolonged use, there is a persistent, smaller decrease in the rate of bone resorption. Histologically, this is associated with a decreased number of osteoclasts and an apparent decrease in their resorptive activity.*In vitro* studies have shown that calcitonin-salmon causes inhibition of osteoclast function with loss of the ruffled osteoclast border responsible for resorption of bone. This activity resumes following removal of calcitonin-salmon from the test system. There is some evidence from the *in vitro* studies that bone formation may be augmented by calcitonin through increased osteoblastic activity.

Animal studies indicate that endogenous calcitonin, primarily through its action on bone, participates with parathyroid hormone in the homeostatic regulation of blood calcium. Thus, high blood calcium levels cause increased secretion of calcitonin which, in turn, inhibits bone resorption. This reduces the transfer of calcium from bone to blood and tends to return blood calcium towards the normal level. The importance of this process in humans has not been determined. In normal adults, who have a relatively low rate of bone resorption, the administration of exogenous calcitonin results in only a slight decrease in serum calcium in the limits of the normal range. In normal children and in patients with Paget's disease in whom bone resorption is more rapid, decreases in serum calcium are more pronounced in response to calcitonin.

CLINICAL PHARMACOLOGY: *(cont'd)*

Bone biopsy and radial bone mass studies at baseline and after 26 months of daily injectable calcitonin indicate that calcitonin therapy results in formation of normal bone.

Postmenopausal Osteoporosis: Osteoporosis is a disease characterized by low bone mass and architectural deterioration of bone tissue leading to enhanced bone fragility and a consequent increase in fracture risk as patients approach or fall below a bone mineral density associated with increased frequency of fracture. The most common type of osteoporosis occurs in postmenopausal females. Osteoporosis is a result of a disproportionate rate of bone resorption compared to bone formation which disrupts the structural integrity of bone, rendering it more susceptible to fracture. The most common sites of these fractures are the vertebrae, hip, and distal forearm (Colles' fractures). Vertebral fractures occur with the highest frequency and are associated with back pain, spinal deformity and a loss of height.

Calcitonin, given by the intranasal route, has been shown to increase spinal bone mass in postmenopausal women with established osteoporosis but not in early postmenopausal women.

Calcium Homeostasis: In two clinical studies designed to evaluate the pharmacodynamic response to calcitonin-salmon nasal spray, administration of 100-1600 IU to healthy volunteers resulted in rapid and sustained small decreases (but still within the normal range) in both total serum calcium and serum ionized calcium. Single doses greater than 400 IU did not produce any further biological response to the drug. The development of hypocalcemia has not been reported in studies in healthy volunteers or postmenopausal females.

Kidney: Studies with injectable calcitonin show increases in the excretion of filtered phosphate, calcium, and sodium by decreasing their tubular reabsorption. Comparable studies have not been carried out with calcitonin-salmon nasal spray.

Gastrointestinal Tract: Some evidence from studies with injectable preparations suggest that calcitonin may have significant actions on the gastrointestinal tract. Short-term administration of injectable calcitonin results in marked transient decreases in the volume and acidity of gastric juice and in the volume and the trypsin and amylase content of pancreatic juice. Whether these effects continue to be elicited after each injection of calcitonin during chronic therapy has not been investigated. These studies have not been conducted with calcitonin-salmon nasal spray.

Pharmacokinetics and Metabolism: The data on bioavailability of calcitonin-salmon nasal spray obtained by various investigators using different methods show great variability. Calcitonin-salmon nasal spray is absorbed rapidly by the nasal mucosa. Peak plasma concentrations of drug appear 31-39 minutes after nasal administration compared to 16-25 minutes following parenteral dosing. In normal volunteers approximately 3% (range 0.3%-30.6%) of a nasally administered dose is bioavailable compared to the same dose administered by intramuscular injection. The half-life of elimination of calcitonin- salmon is calculated to be 43 minutes. There is no accumulation of the drug on repeated nasal administration at 10 hour intervals for up to 15 days. Absorption of nasally administered calcitonin has not been studied in postmenopausal women.

INDICATIONS AND USAGE:

PAGET'S DISEASE

Calcitonin-salmon injection, synthetic is indicated for the treatment of symptomatic Paget's disease of bone, for the treatment of hypercalcemia, and for the treatment of postmenopausal osteoporosis.

Injection: At the present time, effectiveness has been demonstrated principally in patients with moderate to severe disease characterized by polyostotic involvement with elevated serum alkaline phosphatase and urinary hydroxyproline excretion.

In these patients, the biochemical abnormalities were substantially improved (more than 30% reduction) in about 2/3 of patients studied, and bone pain was improved in a similar fraction. A small number of documented instances of reversal of neurologic deficits has occurred, including improvement in the basilar compression syndrome, and improvement of spinal cord and spinal nerve lesions. At present, there is too little experience to predict the likelihood of improvement of any given neurologic lesion. Hearing loss, the most common neurologic lesion of Paget's disease, is improved infrequently (4 of 29 patients studied audiometrically).

Patients with increased cardiac output due to extensive Paget's disease have had measured decreases in cardiac output while receiving calcitonin. The number of treated patients in this category is still too small to predict how likely such a result will be.

The large majority of patients with localized, especially monostotic disease do not develop symptoms and most patients with mild symptoms can be managed with analgesics. There is no evidence that the prophylactic use of calcitonin is beneficial in asymptomatic patients, although treatment may be considered in exceptional circumstances in which there is extensive involvement of the skull or spinal cord with the possibility of irreversible neurologic damage. In these instances, treatment would be based on the demonstrated effect of calcitonin on Pagetic bone, rather than on clinical studies in the patient population in question.

HYPERCALCEMIA

Injection: Calcitonin-salmon injection, synthetic is indicated for early treatment of hypercalcemic emergencies, along with other appropriate agents, when a rapid decrease in serum calcium is required, until more specific treatment of the underlying disease can be accomplished. It may also be added to existing therapeutic regimens for hypercalcemia such as intravenous fluids and furosemide, oral phosphate or corticosteroids, or other agents.

POSTMENOPAUSAL OSTEOPOROSIS

Injection: Calcitonin-salmon injection, synthetic is indicated for the treatment of postmenopausal osteoporosis in conjunction with adequate calcium and vitamin D intake to prevent the progressive loss of bone mass. No evidence currently exists to indicate whether or not calcitonin-salmon decreases the risk of vertebral crush fractures or spinal deformity. A recent controlled study, which was discontinued prior to completion because of questions regarding its design and implementation, failed to demonstrate any benefit of salmon calcitonin on fracture rate. No adequate controlled trials have examined the effect of salmon calcitonin injection on vertebral bone mineral density beyond 1 year of treatment. Two placebo-controlled studies with salmon calcitonin have shown an increase in total body calcium at 1 year, followed by a trend to decreasing total body calcium (still above baseline) at 2 years. The minimum effective dose of calcitonin-salmon for prevention of vertebral bone mineral density loss has not been established. It has been suggested that those postmenopausal patients having increased rates of bone turnover may be more likely to respond to anti-resorptive agents such as calcitonin-salmon.

Nasal Spray: Calcitonin-salmon nasal spray is indicated for the treatment of postmenopausal osteoporosis in females greater than 5 years postmenopause with low bone mass relative to healthy premenopausal females. Calcitonin-salmon nasal spray should be reserved for patients who refuse or cannot tolerate estrogens or in whom estrogens are contraindicated. Use of calcitonin-salmon nasal spray is recommended in conjunction with an adequate calcium (at least 1000 mg elemental calcium per day) and vitamin D (400 IU per day) intake to retard the progressive loss of bone mass. The evidence of efficacy is based on increases in spinal bone mineral density observed in clinical trials.

INDICATIONS AND USAGE: *(cont'd)*

Two randomized, placebo controlled trials were conducted in 325 postmenopausal females [227 calcitonin-salmon nasal spray treated and 98 placebo treated] with spinal, forearm or femoral bone mineral density (BMD) at least one standard deviation below normal for healthy premenopausal females. These studies conducted over two years demonstrated that 200 IU daily of calcitonin-salmon nasal spray increases lumbar vertebral BMD relative to baseline and relative to placebo in osteoporotic females who were greater than 5 years postmenopause. Calcitonin-salmon nasal spray produced statistically significant increases in lumbar vertebral BMD compared to placebo as early as six months after initiation of therapy with persistance of this level for up to 2 years of observation.

No effects of calcitonin-salmon nasal spray on cortical bone of the forearm or hip were demonstrated. However, in one study, BMD of the hip showed a statistically significant increase compared with placebo in a region composed of predominantly trabecular bone after one year of treatment changing to a trend at 2 years that was no longer statistically significant.

CONTRAINDICATIONS:

Clinical allergy to (synthetic) calcitonin-salmon.

WARNINGS:

ALLERGIC REACTIONS

Injection: Because calcitonin is protein in nature, the possibility of a systemic allergic reaction exists. **Administration of calcitonin-salmon has been reported in a few cases to cause serious allergic-type reactions (*e.g.,* bronchospasm, swelling of the tongue or throat, and anaphylactic shock), and in one case, death attributed to anaphylaxis.** The usual provisions should be made for the emergency treatment of such a reaction should it occur. Allergic reactions should be differentiated from generalized flushing and hypotension.

Skin testing should be considered prior to treatment with calcitonin, particularly for patients with suspected sensitivity to calcitonin. The following procedure is suggested: Prepare a dilution at 10 IU per ml by withdrawing 1/20 ml (0.05 ml) in a tuberculin syringe and filling it to 1.0 ml with Sodium Chloride Injection, USP. Mix well, discard 0.9 ml and inject intracutaneously 0.1 ml (approximately 1 IU) on the inner aspect of the forearm. Observe the injection site 15 minutes after injection. The appearance of more than mild erythema or wheal constitutes a positive response.

The incidence of osteogenic sarcoma is known to be increased in Paget's disease. Pagetic lesions, with or without therapy, may appear by X-ray to progress markedly, possibly with some loss of definition of periosteal margins. Such lesions should be evaluated carefully to differentiate these from osteogenic sarcoma.

Nasal Spray: Because calcitonin is a polypeptide, the possibility of a systemic allergic reaction exists. In clinical trials with calcitonin-salmon nasal spray and foreign marketing experience, no serious allergic-type adverse reactions have been reported. However, with injectable calcitonin-salmon there have been a few reports of serious allergic-type reactions (*e.g.,* bronchospasm, swelling of the tongue or throat, anaphylactic shock, and in one case death attributed to anaphylaxis). The usual provisions should be made for the emergency treatment of such a reaction should it occur. Allergic reactions should be differentiated from generalized flushing and hypotension.

Skin testing should be considered prior to treatment with nasal calcitonin for patients with suspected sensitivity to calcitonin. The following procedure is suggested: Prepare a dilution at 10 IU per ml by withdrawing 1/20 ml (0.05 ml) of injectable calcitonin-salmon in a tuberculin syringe and filling it to 1.0 ml with Sodium Chloride Injection, USP. Mix well, discard 0.9 ml and inject intracutaneously 0.1 ml (approximately 1 IU) on the inner aspect of the forearm. Observe the injection site 15 minutes after injection. The appearance of more than mild erythema or wheal constitutes a positive response.

PRECAUTIONS:

INJECTION

General: The administration of calcitonin possibly could lead to hypocalcemic tetany under special circumstances although no cases have yet been reported. Provisions for parenteral calcium administration should be available during the first several administrations of calcitonin.

Laboratory Tests: Periodic examinations of urine sediment of patients on chronic therapy are recommended.

Coarse granular casts and casts containing renal tubular epithelial cells were reported in young adult volunteers at bed rest who were given calcitonin-salmon to study the effect of immobilization on osteoporosis. There was no other evidence of renal abnormality and the urine sediment became normal after calcitonin was stopped. Urine sediment abnormalities have not been reported by other investigators.

Information for the Patient: Careful instruction in sterile injection technique should be given to the patient, and to other persons who may administer calcitonin-salmon injection, synthetic.

Carcinogenesis, Mutagenesis, and Impairment of Fertility: An increased incidence of pituitary adenomas has been observed in one-year toxicity studies in Sprague-Dawley rats administered calcitonin-salmon at dosages of 20 and 80 IU/kg/day and in Fisher 344 rats given 80 IU/kg/day. The relevance of these findings to humans is unknown. Calcitonin-salmon was not mutagenic in tests using *Salmonella typhimurium, Escherichia coli,* and Chinese Hamster V79 cells.

Pregnancy, Teratogenic Effects, Pregnancy Category C: Calcitonin-salmon has been shown to cause a decrease in fetal birth weights in rabbits when given in doses 14-56 times the dose recommended for human use. Since calcitonin does not cross the placental barrier, this finding may be due to metabolic effects of calcitonin on the pregnant animal. There are no adequate and well-controlled studies in pregnant women. Calcitonin-salmon injection, synthetic should be used during pregnancy only if the potential benefit justifies the potential risk to the fetus.

Nursing Mothers: It is not known whether this drug is excreted in human milk. As a general rule, nursing should not be undertaken while a patient is on this drug since many drugs are excreted in human milk. Calcitonin has been shown to inhibit lactation in animals.

Pediatric Use: Disorders of bone in children referred to as juvenile Paget's disease have been reported rarely. The relationship of these disorders to adult Paget's disease has not been established and experience with the use of calcitonin in these disorders is very limited. There are no adequate data to support the use of calcitonin-salmon injection, synthetic in children.

NASAL SPRAY

Periodic Nasal Examinations: Periodic nasal examinations with visualization of the nasal mucosa, turbinates, septum and mucosal blood vessel status are recommended.

The development of mucosal alterations or transient nasal conditions occurred in up to 9% of patients who received calcitonin-salmon nasal spray and in up to 12% of patients who received placebo nasal spray in studies in postmenopausal females. The majority of patients (approximately 90%) in whom nasal abnormalities were noted also reported nasally related complaints/symptoms as adverse events. Therefore, a nasal examination should be performed prior to start of treatment with nasal calcitonin and at any time nasal complaints occur.

PRECAUTIONS: *(cont'd)*

In all postmenopausal patients treated with calcitonin-salmon nasal spray, the most commonly reported nasal adverse events included rhinitis (12%), epistaxis (3.5%), and sinusitis (2.3%). Smoking was shown not to have any contributory effect on the occurrence of nasal adverse events. One patient (0.3%) treated with calcitonin-salmon nasal spray who was receiving 400 IU daily developed a small nasal wound. In clinical trials in another disorder (Paget's Disease), 2.8% of patients developed nasal ulcerations.

If severe ulceration of the nasal mucosa occurs, as indicated by ulcers greater than 1.5 mm in diameter or penetrating below the mucosa, or those associated with heavy bleeding, calcitonin-salmon nasal spray should be discontinued. Although smaller ulcers often heal without withdrawal of calcitonin-salmon nasal spray, medication should be discontinued temporarily until healing occurs.

Information for the Patient: Careful instructions on pump assembly, priming of the pump and nasal introduction of calcitonin-salmon nasal spray should be given to the patient. Although instructions for patients are supplied with individual bottles, procedures for use should be demonstrated to each patient. Patients should notify their physician if they develop significant nasal irritation.

Carcinogenesis, Mutagenesis, and Impairment of Fertility: An increased incidence of non-functioning pituitary adenomas has been observed in one-year toxicity studies in Sprague-Dawley and Fischer 344 Rats administered (subcutaneously) calcitonin-salmon at dosages of 80 IU per kilogram per day (16-19 times the recommended human parenteral dose and about 130-160 times the human intranasal dose based on body surface area). The findings suggest that calcitonin-salmon reduced the latency period for development of pituitary adenomas that do not produce hormones, probably through the perturbation of physiologic processes involved in the evolution of this commonly occurring endocrine lesion in the rat. Although administration of calcitonin-salmon reduces the latency period of the development of non-functional proliferative lesions in rats, it did not induce the hyperplastic/neoplastic process.

Calcitonin-salmon was tested for mutagenicity using *Salmonella typhimurium* (5 strains) and *Escherichia coli* (2 strains), with and without rat liver metabolic activation, and found to be non- mutagenic. The drug was also not mutagenic in a chromosome aberration test in mammalian V79 cells of the Chinese Hamster *in vitro.*

Laboratory Tests: Urine sediment abnormalities have not been reported in ambulatory volunteers treated with Miacalcin (calcitonin- salmon) Nasal Spray. Coarse granular casts containing renal tubular epithelial cells were reported in young adult volunteers at bed rest who were given injectable calcitonin-salmon to study the effect of immobilization on osteoporosis. There was no evidence of renal abnormality and the urine sediment became normal after calcitonin was stopped. Periodic examinations of urine sediment should be considered.

Pregnancy, Teratogenic Effects, Pregnancy Category C: Calcitonin-salmon has been shown to cause a decrease in fetal birth weights in rabbits when given by injection in doses 8-33 times the parenteral dose and 70-278 times the intranasal dose recommended for human use based on body surface area.

Since calcitonin does not cross the placental barrier, this finding may be due to metabolic effects on the pregnant animal. There are no adequate and well controlled studies in pregnant women with calcitonin-salmon. Calcitonin-salmon nasal spray is *not*indicated for use in pregnancy.

Nursing Mothers: It is not known whether this drug is excreted in human milk. As a general rule, nursing should not be undertaken while a patient is on this drug since many drugs are excreted in human milk. Calcitonin has been shown to inhibit lactation in animals.

Geriatric Use: Clinical trials using Miacalcin (calcitonin- salmon) Nasal Spray have included post-menopausal patients up to 77 years of age. No unusual adverse events or increased incidence of common adverse events have been noted in patients over 65 years of age.

Pediatric Use There are no data to support the use of calcitonin-salmon nasal spray in children. Disorders of bone in children referred to as idiopathic juvenile osteoporosis have been reported rarely. The relationship of these disorders to postmenopausal osteoporosis has not been established and experience with the use of calcitonin in these disorders is very limited.

DRUG INTERACTIONS:

Nasal Spray: Formal studies designed to evaluate drug interactions with calcitonin-salmon have not been done. No drug interaction studies have been performed with calcitonin-salmon nasal spray ingredients.

Currently, no drug interactions with calcitonin-salmon have been observed. The effects of prior use of diphosphonates in postmenopausal osteoporosis patients have not been assessed; however, in patients with Paget's Disease prior diphosphonate use appears to reduce the anti-resorptive response to calcitonin-salmon nasal spray.

ADVERSE REACTIONS:

GASTROINTESTINAL SYSTEM

Injection: Nausea with or without vomiting has been noted in about 10% of patients treated with calcitonin. It is most evident when treatment is first initiated and tends to decrease or disappear with continued administration.

DERMATOLOGIC/HYPERSENSITIVITY

Injection: Local inflammatory reactions at the site of subcutaneous or intramuscular injection have been reported in about 10% of patients. Flushing of face or hands occurred in about 2%-5% of patients. Skin rashes, nocturia, pruritus of the ear lobes, feverish sensation, pain in the eyes, poor appetite, abdominal pain, edema of feet, and salty taste have been reported in patients treated with calcitonin-salmon. Administration of calcitonin-salmon has been reported in a few cases to cause serious allergic-type reactions (*e.g.,* bronchospasm, swelling of the tongue or throat, and anaphylactic shock), and in one case, death attributed to anaphylaxis (see WARNINGS).

Nasal Spray: The incidence of adverse reactions reported in studies involving postmenopausal osteoporotic patients chronically exposed to calcitonin-salmon nasal spray (N=341) and to placebo nasal spray (N=131) and reported in greater than 3% of calcitonin-salmon nasal spray treated patients are presented below in the following table (TABLE 1). Most adverse reactions were mild to moderate in severity. Nasal adverse events were most common with 70% mild, 25% moderate, and 5% severe in nature (placebo rates were 71% mild, 27% moderate, and 2% severe).

† Symptom of nose includes: nasal crusts, dryness, redness or erythema, nasal sores, irritation, itching, thick feeling, soreness, pallor, infection, stenosis, runny/blocked, small wound, bleeding wound, tenderness, uncomfortable feeling and sore across bridge of nose.

In addition, the following adverse events were reported in fewer than 3% of patients during chronic therapy with calcitonin-salmon nasal spray. Adverse events reported in 1%-3% of patients are identified with an asterisk (*). The remainder occurred in less than 1% of patients. Other than flushing, nausea, possible allergic reactions, and possible local irritative effects in the respiratory tract, a relationship to calcitonin-salmon nasal spray has not been established.

Body as a whole (General Disorders): influenza-like symptoms*, fatigue*, periorbital edema, fever

ADVERSE REACTIONS: *(cont'd)*

TABLE 1 Adverse Reactions Occurring in at Least 3% of Postmenopausal Patients Treated Chronically

Miacalcin (calcitonin-salmon)

Adverse Reaction	Nasal Spray N=341 % of Patients	Placebo N=131 % of Patients
Rhinitis	12.0	6.9
Symptom of Nose†	10.6	16.0
Back Pain	5.0	2.3
Arthralgia	3.8	5.3
Epistaxis	3.5	4.6
Headache	3.2	4.6

Integumentary: erythematous rash*, skin ulceration, eczema, alopecia, pruritus, increased sweating

Musculoskeletal/Collagen: arthrosis*, myalgia*, arthritis, polymyalgia rheumatica, stiffness

Respiratory/Special Senses: sinusitis*, upper respiratory tract infection*, bronchospasm*, pharyngitis, bronchitis, pneumonia, coughing, dyspnea, taste perversion, parosmia

Cardiovascular: hypertension*, angina pectoris*, tachycardia, palpitation, bundle branch block, myocardial infarction

Gastrointestinal: dyspepsia*, constipation*, abdominal pain*, nausea*, diarrhea*, vomiting, flatulence, increased appetite, gastritis, dry mouth

Liver/Metabolic: cholelithiasis, hepatitis, thirst, weight increase

Endocrine: goiter, hyperthyroidism

Urinary System: cystitis*, pyelonephritis, hematuria, renal calculus

Central and Peripheral Nervous System: dizziness*, paresthesia*, vertigo, migraine, neuralgia, agitation

Hearing/Vestibular: tinnitus, hearing loss, earache

Vision: abnormal lacrimation*, conjunctivitis*, blurred vision, vitreous floater

Vascular: flushing, cerebrovascular accident, thrombophlebitis

Hematologic/Resistance Mechanisms: lymphadenopathy*, infection*, anemia

Psychiatric: depression*, insomnia, anxiety, anorexia

Common adverse reactions associated with the use of injectable calcitonin-salmon occurred less frequently in patients treated with calcitonin-salmon nasal spray than in those patients treated with injectable calcitonin. Nausea, with or without vomiting, which occurred in 1.8% of patients treated with the nasal spray (and 1.5% of those receiving placebo nasal spray) occurs in about 10% of patients who take injectable calcitonin-salmon. Flushing, which occurred in less than 1% of patients treated with the Nasal Spray, occurs in 2%-5% of patients treated with injectable calcitonin-salmon. Although the administered dosages of injectable and nasal spray calcitonin-salmon are comparable (50-100 units daily of injectable versus 200 units daily of nasal spray), the nasal dosage form has a mean bioavailability of about 3% (range 0.3%- 30.6%) and therefore provides less drug to the systemic circulation, possibly accounting for the decrease in frequency of adverse reactions.

The collective foreign marketing experience with Miacalcin (calcitonin-salmon) Nasal Spray does not show evidence of any notable difference in the incidence profile of reported adverse reactions when compared with that seen in the clinical trials.

OVERDOSAGE:

Injection: A dose of 1000 IU subcutaneously may produce nausea and vomiting as the only adverse effects. Doses of 32 units per kg per day for 1-2 days demonstrate no other adverse effects.

Data on chronic high dose administration are insufficient to judge toxicity.

Nasal Spray: No instances of overdose with calcitonin-salmon nasal spray have been reported and no serious adverse reactions have been associated with high doses. There is no known potential for drug abuse for calcitonin-salmon.

Single doses of calcitonin-salmon nasal spray up to 1600 IU, doses up to 800 IU per day for three days and chronic administration of doses up to 600 IU per day have been studied without serious adverse effects. A dose of 1000 IU of Miacalcin (calcitonin-salmon) injectable solution given subcutaneously may produce nausea and vomiting. A dose of Miacalcin (calcitonin-salmon) injectable solution of 32 IU per kg per day for one or two days demonstrated no additional adverse effects.

There have been no reports of hypocalcemic tetany. However, the pharmacologic actions of calcitonin-salmon nasal spray suggest that this could occur in overdose.

Therefore, provisions for parenteral administration of calcium should be available for the treatment of overdose.

DOSAGE AND ADMINISTRATION:

PAGET'S DISEASE

Injection: The recommended starting dose of calcitonin-salmon in Paget's disease is 100 IU (0.5 ml) per day administered subcutaneously (preferred for outpatient self-administration) or intramuscularly. Drug effect should be monitored by periodic measurement of serum alkaline phosphatase and 24-hour urinary hydroxyproline (if available) and evaluations of symptoms. A decrease toward normal of the biochemical abnormalities is usually seen, if it is going to occur, within the first few months. Bone pain may also decrease during that time. Improvement of neurologic lesions, when it occurs, requires a longer period of treatment, often more than one year.

In many patients, doses of 50 IU (0.25 ml) per day or every other day are sufficient to maintain biochemical and clinical improvement. At the present time, however, there are insufficient data to determine whether this reduced dose will have the same effect as the higher dose on forming more normal bone structure. It appears preferable, therefore, to maintain the higher dose in any patient with serious deformity or neurological involvement.

In any patient with a good response initially who later relapses, either clinically or biochemically, the possibility of antibody formation should be explored. The patient may be tested for antibodies by an appropriate specialized test or evaluated for the possibility of antibody formation by critical clinical evaluation.

Patient compliance should also be assessed in the event of relapse.

In patients who relapse, whether because of antibodies or for unexplained reasons, a dosage increase beyond 100 IU per day does not usually appear to elicit an improved response.

HYPERCALCEMIA

Injection: The recommended starting dose of calcitonin-salmon injection, synthetic in hypercalcemia is 4 IU/kg body weight every 12 hours by subcutaneous or intramuscular injection. If the response to this dose is not satisfactory after one or two days, the dose may be increased to 8 IU/kg every 12 hours. If the response remains unsatisfactory after two more days, the dose may be further increased to a maximum of 8 IU/kg every 6 hours.

DOSAGE AND ADMINISTRATION: *(cont'd)*

POSTMENOPAUSAL OSTEOPOROSIS

Injection: The minimum effective dose of salmon calcitonin for the prevention of vertebral bone mineral density loss has not been established. Data from a single one-year placebo-controlled study with salmon calcitonin injection suggested that 100 IU (subcutaneously or intramuscularly) every other day might be effective in preserving vertebral bone mineral density. Baseline and interval monitoring of biochemical markers of bone resorption/turnover (*e.g.*, fasting AM, second-voided urine hydroxyproline to creatinine ratio) and of bone mineral density may be useful in achieving the minimum effective dose.

The recommended dose of calcitonin is 100 IU per day administered subcutaneously or intramuscularly. Patients should also receive supplemental calcium such as calcium carbonate 1.5 g daily and an adequate vitamin D intake (400 units daily). An adequate diet is also essential.

If the volume of calcitonin-salmon injection, synthetic to be injected exceeds 2 ml, intramuscular injection is preferable and multiple sites of injection should be used.

Parenteral drug products should be inspected visually for particulate matter and discoloration prior to administration whenever solution and container permit.

Nasal Spray: The recommended dose of calcitonin-salmon nasal spray in postmenopausal osteoporotic females is 200 IU per day administered intranasally, alternating nostrils daily.

Drug effect may be monitored by periodic measurements of lumbar vertebral bone mass to document stabilization of bone loss or increases in bone density. Effects of calcitonin-salmon nasal spray on biochemical markers of bone turnover have not been consistently demonstrated in studies in postmenopausal osteoporosis. Therefore, these parameters should not be solely utilized to determine clinical response to calcitonin-salmon nasal spray therapy in these patients.

Activation of Pump: Before the first dose, it is necessary to activate the pump. The bottle should be held upright and the two white side arms depressed toward the bottle six times until a faint spray is emitted. The pump is activated once this first faint spray has been emitted. At this point, the nozzle should be placed firmly into the nostril with the head in the upright position, and the pump depressed toward the bottle. It is not necessary to reactivate the pump before each daily dose.

HOW SUPPLIED:

Nasal Spray: Available as a metered dose solution in 2 ml fill glass bottles. It is available in a dosage strength of 200 IU per activation (0.09 ml/puff). A screw-on pump is provided. This pump, following activation, will deliver 0.09 ml of solution. Miacalcin Nasal Spray contains 2200 IU/ml calcitonin-salmon. Store unopened in refrigerator between 36°-46°F (2°-8°C). Protect from freezing.

Once the pump has been activated, the bottle may be maintained at room temperature until the medication has been finished, which is a period of 2 weeks.

Injection: Store in Refrigerator - Between 2°-8°C (36°-46°F).

(Sandoz Pharmaceuticals Corporation, 95/10, 93/05) (Rhone-Poulenc Rorer Pharmaceuticals Inc., 92/10)

HOW SUPPLIED - RATED THERAPEUTICALLY EQUIVALENT:

Aerosol, Spray - Nasal - 200 unit/dose

2 ml	$25.03	MIACALCIN, Novartis	00078-0149-75

Injection, Solution - Intramuscular; - 200 unit/ml

2 ml	$27.48	MIALCALCIN, Novartis	00078-0149-23
2 ml	$28.50	Calcitonin-Salmon, Astra USA	00186-1608-13
2 ml	$31.35	OSTEOCALCIN, Arcola	00070-4492-01
2 ml	**$42.45**	**CALCIMAR, Rhone-Poulenc Rorer**	**00075-1306-01**

CALCITRIOL *(000586)*

CATEGORIES: Bone Disease; Calcium Metabolism; Homeostatic & Nutrient; Hormones; Hypocalcemia; Hypoparathyroidism; Osteoporosis; Parathyroid; Pseudohypoparathyroidism; Vitamin D; Vitamins; Pregnancy Category C; FDA Approval Pre 1982

BRAND NAMES: *Bonky*; Calcijex; *Calcitriol*; **Rocaltrol**
(International brand names outside U.S. in italics)

FORMULARIES: Aetna; BC-BS; Medi-Cal

COST OF THERAPY: $779.85 (Hypocalcemia; Capsule; 0.25 mcg; 2/day; 365 days)

DESCRIPTION:

Calcitriol is a colorless, crystalline compound which occurs naturally in humans. It is soluble in organic solvents but relatively insoluble in water. Calcitriol is chemically designated (5Z,7E)-9, 10-secocholesta- 5,7,10(19)-triene-1α,3β,25-triol.

Molecular Formula: $C_{27}H_{44}O_3$

The other names frequently used for calcitriol are 1α,25-dihydroxycholecalciferol, 1α,25-dihydroxyvitamin D_3, 1,25-DHCC, 1,25$(OH)_2D_3$ and 1,25-diOHC.

Capsules: Calcitriol is a synthetic vitamin D analog which is active in the regulation of the absorption of calcium from the gastrointestinal tract and its utilization in the body. It is available in capsules containing 0.25 mcg or 0.5 mcg calcitriol. Each capsule also contains butylated hydroxyanisole (BHA), butylated hydroxytoluene (BHT) and fractionated triglyceride of coconut oil. Gelatin capsule shells contain glycerin, parabens (methyl and propyl) and sorbitol, with the following dye systems: 0.25 mcg—FD&C Yellow No. 6 and titanium dioxide; 0.5 mcg- -FD&C Red No. 3, FD&C Yellow No. 6 and titanium dioxide.

Injection: Calcijex (calcitriol injection) is synthetically manufactured calcitriol and is available as a sterile, isotonic, clear, aqueous solution for intravenous injection. Calcijex is available in 1 ml ampuls. Each 1 ml contains calcitriol, 1 or 2 mcg; Polysorbate 20, 4 mg; sodium chloride 1.5 mg; sodium ascorbate 10 mg added; dibasic sodium phosphate, anhydrous 7.6 mg; monobasic sodium phosphate, monohydrate 1.8 mg; edetate disodium, dihydrate 1.1 mg added. pH 7.2 (6.5 to 8.0).

CLINICAL PHARMACOLOGY:

Capsules: Man's natural supply of vitamin D depends mainly on exposure to the ultraviolet rays of the sun for conversion of 7-dehydrocholesterol in the skin to vitamin D_3 (cholecalciferol). Vitamin D_3must be metabolically activated in the liver and the kidney before it is fully active as a regulator of calcium and phosphorus metabolism at target tissues. The initial transformation of vitamin $D_3$is catalyzed by a vitamin D_3-25-hydroxylase enzyme (25-OHase) present in the liver, and the product of this reaction is 25-hydroxyvitamin D_3 [25-$(OH)D_3$]. Hydroxylation of 25-$(OH)D_3$ occurs in the mitochondria of kidney tissue, activated by the renal 25-hydroxyvitamin D_3-1 alpha-hydroxylase (alpha-OHase), to produce 1,25-$(OH)_2D_3$(calcitriol), the active form of vitamin D_3. Several metabolites of calcitriol have been identified which include:

CLINICAL PHARMACOLOGY: *(cont'd)*

1α, 25, $(OH)_2$-24-oxo-D_3; 1α, 23,25$(OH)_3$-24-oxo-D_3; 1α, 24R,25$(OH)_3D_3$; 1α, 25R$(OH)_2$-26-23S-lactone D_3; 1α, 25S,26$(OH)_3D_3$; 1α, 25$(OH)_2$-23-oxo-D_3; 1α, 25R,26$(OH)_3$-23-oxo-D_3; 1α, (OH)24,25,26,27-tetranor-COOH-D_3

The two known sites of action of calcitriol are intestine and bone. A calcitriol receptor-binding protein appears to exist in the mucosa of human intestine. Additional evidence suggests that calcitriol may also act on the kidney and the parathyroid glands. Calcitriol is the most active known form of vitamin D_3 in stimulating intestinal calcium transport. In acutely uremic rats calcitriol has been shown to stimulate intestinal calcium absorption. The kidneys of uremic patients cannot adequately synthesize calcitriol, the active hormone formed from precursor vitamin D. Resultant hypocalcemia and secondary hyperparathyroidism are a major cause of the metabolic bone disease of renal failure. However, other bone-toxic substances which accumulate in uremia (*e.g.,* aluminum) may also contribute.

The beneficial effect of calcitriol in renal osteodystrophy appears to result from correction of hypocalcemia and secondary hyperparathyroidism. It is uncertain whether calcitriol produces other independent beneficial effects.

Calcitriol is rapidly absorbed from the intestine. Peak serum concentrations (above basal values) were reached within 3 to 6 hours following oral administration of single doses of 0.25 to 1.0 mcg of calcitriol. The half-life of calcitriol elimination from serum was found to range from 3 to 6 hours. Following a single oral dose of 0.5 mcg, mean serum concentrations of calcitriol rose from a baseline value of 40.0 ± 4.4 (S.D.) pg/ml to 60.0 ± 4.4 pg/ml at 2 hours, and declined to 53.0 ± 6.9 at 4 hours, 50 ± 7.0 at 8 hours, 44 ± 4.6 at 12 hours and 41.5 ± 5.1 at 24 hours. The duration of pharmacologic activity of a single dose of calcitriol is about 3 to 5 days.

Calcitriol and other vitamin D metabolites are transported in blood, bound to specific plasma proteins. Enterohepatic recycling and biliary excretion of calcitriol occurs. Following intravenous administration of radiolabeled calcitriol in normal subjects, approximately 27% and 7% of the radioactivity appeared in the feces and urine, respectively, within 24 hours. When a 1-mcg oral dose of radiolabeled calcitriol was administered to normals, approximately 10% of the total radioactivity appeared in urine within 24 hours. Cumulative excretion of radioactivity on the sixth day following intravenous administration of radiolabeled calcitriol averaged 16% in urine and 49% in feces.

There is evidence that maternal calcitriol may enter the fetal circulation. Calcitriol may be excreted in human milk.

Injection: Calcitriol is the active form of vitamin D_3 (cholecalciferol). The natural or endogenous supply of vitamin D in man mainly depends on ultraviolet light for conversion of 7-dehydrocholesterol to vitamin D_3in the skin. Vitamin D_3 must be metabolically activated in the liver and the kidney before it is fully active on its target tissues. The initial transformation is catalyzed by a vitamin D_3-25-hydroxylase enzyme present in the liver, and the product of this reaction is 25-$(OH)D_3$ (calcifediol). The latter undergoes hydroxylation in the mitochondria of kidney tissue, and this reaction is activated by the renal 25-hydroxyvitamin D_3-1-α- hydroxylase to produce 1,25-$(OH)_2D_3$ (calcitriol), the active form of vitamin D_3.

The known sites of action of calcitriol are intestine, bone, kidney and parathyroid gland. Calcitriol is the most active known form of vitamin D_3 in stimulating intestinal calcium transport. In acutely uremic rats, calcitriol has been shown to stimulate intestinal calcium absorption. In bone, calcitriol, in conjunction with parathyroid hormone, stimulates resorption of calcium; and in the kidney, calcitriol increases the tubular reabsorption of calcium. *In-vitro* and *in-vivo* studies have shown that calcitriol directly suppresses secretion and synthesis of PTH. A vitamin D-resistant state may exist in uremic patients because of the failure of the kidney to adequately convert precursors to the active compound, calcitriol.

Calcitriol when administered by bolus injection is rapidly available in the blood stream. Vitamin D metabolites are known to be transported in blood, bound to specific plasma proteins. The pharmacologic activity of an administered dose of calcitriol is about 3 to 5 days. Two metabolic pathways for calcitriol have been identified, conversion to 1,24,25-$(OH)_3D_3$ and to calcitroic acid.

INDICATIONS AND USAGE:

Capsules: Calcitriol is indicated in the management of hypocalcemia and the resultant metabolic bone disease in patients undergoing chronic renal dialysis. In these patients, calcitriol administration enhances calcium absorption, reduces serum alkaline phosphatase levels and may reduce elevated parathyroid hormone levels and the histological manifestations of osteitis fibrosa cystica and defective mineralization.

Calcitriol is also indicated in the management of hypocalcemia and its clinical manifestations in patients with postsurgical hypoparathyroidism, idiopathic hypoparathyroidism, and pseudohypoparathyroidism.

Injection: Calcitriol injection is indicated in the management of hypocalcemia in patients undergoing chronic renal dialysis. It has been shown to significantly reduce elevated parathyroid hormone levels. Reduction of PTH has been shown to result in an improvement in renal osteodystrophy.

CONTRAINDICATIONS:

Calcitriol should not be given to patients with hypercalcemia or evidence of vitamin D toxicity.

WARNINGS:

Capsules: Since calcitriol is the most potent metabolite of vitamin D available, pharmacologic doses of vitamin D and its derivatives should be withheld during calcitriol treatment to avoid possible additive effects and hypercalcemia.

Both appropriate oral phosphate-binders and a low phosphate diet should be used to control serum phosphate levels in patients undergoing dialysis.

Magnesium-containing antacids and calcitriol should not be used concomitantly in patients on chronic renal dialysis because such use may lead to the development of hypermagnesemia.

Overdosage of any form of vitamin D is dangerous (see also OVERDOSAGE). Progressive hypercalcemia due to overdosage of vitamin D and its metabolites may be so severe as to require emergency attention. Chronic hypercalcemia can lead to generalized vascular calcification, nephrocalcinosis and other soft-tissue calcification. **The serum calcium times phosphate (Ca × P) product should not be allowed to exceed 70.** Radiographic evaluation of suspect anatomical regions may be useful in the early detection of this condition.

Studies in dogs and rats given calcitriol for up to 26 weeks have shown that small increases of calcitriol above endogenous levels can lead to abnormalities of calcium metabolism with the potential for calcification of many tissues in the body.

Injection: Since calcitriol is the most potent metabolite of vitamin D available, vitamin D and its derivatives should be withheld during treatment.

A non-aluminum phosphate-binding compound should be used to control serum phosphorus levels in patients undergoing dialysis.

Overdosage of any form of vitamin D is dangerous (see also OVERDOSAGE). Progressive hypercalcemia due to overdosage of vitamin D and its metabolites may be so severe as to require emergency attention. Chronic hypercalcemia can lead to generalized vascular calcification, nephrocalcinosis and other soft-tissue calcification. The serum calcium times phosphate (Ca x P) product should not be allowed to exceed 70. Radiographic evaluation of suspect anatomical regions may be useful in the early detection of this condition.

PRECAUTIONS:

GENERAL

Capsules: Excessive dosage of calcitriol induces hypercalcemia and in some instances hypercalciuria; therefore, early in treatment during dosage adjustment, serum calcium should be determined twice weekly. In dialysis patients, a fall in serum alkaline phosphatase levels usually antedates the appearance of hypercalcemia and may be an indication of impending hypercalcemia. Should hypercalcemia develop, the drug should be discontinued immediately. Calcitriol should be given cautiously to patients on digitalis, because hypercalcemia in such patients may precipitate cardiac arrhythmias.

In patients with normal renal function, chronic hypercalcemia may be associated with an increase in serum creatinine. While this is usually reversible, it is important in such patients to pay careful attention to those factors which may lead to hypercalcemia. Calcitriol therapy should always be started at the lowest possible dose and should not be increased without careful monitoring of the serum calcium. An estimate of daily dietary calcium intake should be made and the intake adjusted when indicated.

Patients with normal renal function taking calcitriol should avoid dehydration. Adequate fluid intake should be maintained.

Injection: Excessive dosage of calcitriol injection induces hypercalcemia and in some instances hypercalciuria; therefore, early in treatment during dosage adjustment, serum calcium and phosphorus should be determined at least twice weekly. Should hypercalcemia develop, the drug should be discontinued immediately.

Calcitriol injection should be given cautiously to patients on digitalis, because hypercalcemia in such patients may precipitate cardiac arrhythmias.

INFORMATION FOR THE PATIENT

The patient and his or her parents or spouse should be informed about adherence to instructions about diet and calcium supplementation and avoidance of the use of unapproved nonprescription drugs, including magnesium-containing antacids. Patients should also be carefully informed about the symptoms of hypercalcemia (see ADVERSE REACTIONS.)

LABORATORY TESTS

Capsules: For dialysis patients, serum calcium, phosphorus, magnesium and alkaline phosphatase should be determined periodically. For hypoparathyroid patients, serum calcium, phosphorus and 24-hour urinary calcium should be determined periodically.

Injection: Serum calcium, phosphorus, magnesium and alkaline phosphatase and 24-hour urinary calcium and phosphorus should be determined periodically. During the initial phase of the medication, serum calcium and phosphorus should be determined more frequently (twice weekly).

CARCINOGENESIS, MUTAGENESIS, AND IMPAIRMENT OF FERTILITY

Long-term studies in animals have not been performed to evaluate the carcinogenic potential of calcitriol injection. There was no evidence of mutagenicity as studied by the Ames Method. No significant effects of calcitriol on fertility were reported using oral Calcitriol.

PREGNANCY CATEGORY C

Capsules: *Teratogenic Effects:* Calcitriol has been found to be teratogenic in rabbits when given in doses 4 and 15 times the dose recommended for human use. All 15 fetuses in 3 litters at these doses showed external and skeletal abnormalities. However, none of the other 23 litters (156 fetuses) showed significant abnormalities compared with controls. Teratogenicity studies in rats showed no evidence of teratogenic potential. There are no adequate and well-controlled studies in pregnant women. Calcitriol should be used during pregnancy only if the potential benefit justifies the potential risk to the fetus. *Nonteratogenic Effects:* In the rabbit, dosages of 0.3 mcg/kg/day administered on days 7 to 18 of gestation resulted in 19% maternal mortality, a decrease in mean fetal body weight and a reduced number of newborn surviving to 24 hours. A study of peri- and postnatal development in rats resulted in hypercalcemia in the offspring of dams given calcitriol at doses of 0.08 or 0.3 mcg/kg/day, hypercalcemia and hypophosphatemia in dams at doses of 0.08 or 0.3 mcg/kg/day, and increased serum urea nitrogen in dams given calcitriol at a dose of 0.3 mcg/kg/day. In another study in rats, maternal weight gain was slightly reduced at a dose of 0.3 mcg/kg/day administered on days 7 to 15 of gestation.

The offspring of a woman administered 17 to 36 mcg/day of calcitriol (17 to 144 times the recommended dose) during pregnancy manifested mild hypercalcemia in the first 2 days of life which returned to normal at day 3.

Injection: Calcitriol given orally has been reported to be teratogenic in rabbits when given in doses 4 and 15 times the dose recommended for human use.

All 15 fetuses in 3 litters at these doses showed external and skeletal abnormalities. However, none of the other 23 litters (156 fetuses) showed significant abnormalities compared with controls.

Teratology studies in rats showed no evidence of teratogenic potential. There are no adequate and well-controlled studies in pregnant women. Calcitriol injection should be used during pregnancy only if the potential benefit justifies the potential risk to the fetus.

NURSING MOTHERS

It is not known whether this drug is excreted in human milk. Because many drugs are excreted in human milk and because of the potential for serious adverse reactions in nursing infants from calcitriol, a decision should be made whether to discontinue nursing or to discontinue the drug, taking into account the importance of the drug to the mother.

PEDIATRIC USE

Safety and efficacy of calcitriol in children or children undergoing dialysis have not been established.

DRUG INTERACTIONS:

Capsules: Cholestyramine has been reported to reduce intestinal absorption of fat-soluble vitamins; as such it may impair intestinal absorption of calcitriol. (Also see WARNINGS and PRECAUTIONS [General] sections.)

Injection: Magnesium-containing antacid and calcitriol injection should not be used concomitantly, because such use may lead to the development of hypermagnesemia.

ADVERSE REACTIONS:

Since calcitriol is believed to be the active hormone which exerts vitamin D activity in the body, adverse effects are, in general, similar to those encountered with excessive vitamin D intake. The early and late signs and symptoms of vitamin D intoxication associated with hypercalcemia include:

Early: Weakness, headache, somnolence, nausea, vomiting, dry mouth, constipation, muscle pain, bone pain and metallic taste.

ADVERSE REACTIONS: *(cont'd)*

Late: Polyuria, polydipsia, anorexia, weight loss, nocturia, conjunctivitis (calcific), pancreatitis, photophobia, rhinorrhea, pruritus, hyperthermia, decreased libido, elevated BUN, albuminuria, hypercholesterolemia, elevated SGOT and SGPT, ectopic calcification, nephrocalcinosis, hypertension, cardiac arrhythmias and, rarely, overt psychosis.

In clinical studies on hypoparathyroidism and pseudohypoparathyroidism, hypercalcemia was noted on at least one occasion in about 1 in 3 patients and hypercalciuria in about 1 in 7. Elevated serum creatinine levels were observed in about 1 in 6 patients (approximately one half of whom had normal levels at baseline).

One case of erythema multiforme was confirmed by rechallenge.

OVERDOSAGE:

Administration of calcitriol to patients in excess of their daily requirements can cause hypercalcemia, hypercalciuria and hyperphosphatemia. High intake of calcium and phosphate concomitant with calcitriol may lead to similar abnormalities. High levels of calcium in the dialysate bath may contribute to the hypercalcemia.

Treatment of Hypercalcemia and Overdosage: General treatment of hypercalcemia (greater than 1 mg/dl above the upper limit of the normal range) consists of immediate discontinuation of calcitriol therapy, institution of a low calcium diet and withdrawal of calcium supplements. Serum calcium levels should be determined daily until normocalcemia ensues. Hypercalcemia frequently resolves in 2 to 7 days. When serum calcium levels have returned to within normal limits, calcitriol therapy may be reinstituted at a dose of 0.25 mcg/day less than prior therapy. Serum calcium levels should be obtained at least twice weekly after all dosage changes and subsequent dosage titration. In dialysis patients, persistent or markedly elevated serum calcium levels may be corrected by dialysis against a calcium-free dialysate.

Treatment of Accidental Overdosage of Calcitriol: The treatment of acute accidental overdosage of calcitriol should consist of general supportive measures. If drug ingestion is discovered within a relatively short time, induction of emesis or gastric lavage may be of benefit in preventing further absorption. If the drug has passed through the stomach, the administration of mineral oil may promote its fecal elimination. Serial serum electrolyte determinations (especially calcium), rate of urinary calcium excretion and assessment of electrocardiographic abnormalities due to hypercalcemia should be obtained. Such monitoring is critical in patients receiving digitalis. Discontinuation of supplemental calcium and a low calcium diet are also indicated in accidental overdosage. Due to the relatively short duration of the pharmacological action of calcitriol, further measures are probably unnecessary. Should, however, persistent and markedly elevated serum calcium levels occur, there are a variety of therapeutic alternatives which may be considered, depending on the patient's underlying condition. These include the use of drugs such as phosphates and corticosteroids as well as measures to induce an appropriate forced diuresis. The use of peritoneal dialysis against a calcium-free dialysate has also been reported.

DOSAGE AND ADMINISTRATION:

The optimal daily dose of calcitriol must be carefully determined for each patient.

The effectiveness of calcitriol therapy is predicated on the assumption that each patient is receiving an adequate daily intake of calcium. The U.S. RDA for calcium in adults is 800 to 1200 mg. To ensure that each patient receives an adequate daily intake of calcium, the physician should either prescribe a calcium supplement or instruct the patient in proper dietary measures.

CAPSULES

Dialysis Patients: The recommended initial dose of calcitriol is 0.25 mcg/day. If a satisfactory response in the biochemical parameters and clinical manifestations of the disease state is not observed, dosage may be increased by 0.25 mcg/day at 4- to 8-week intervals. During this titration period, serum calcium levels should be obtained at least twice weekly, and if hypercalcemia is noted, the drug should be immediately discontinued until normocalcemia ensues.

Patients with normal or only slightly reduced serum calcium levels may respond to calcitriol doses of 0.25 mcg every other day. Most patients undergoing hemodialysis respond to doses between 0.5 and 1 mcg/day.

Oral calcitriol may normalize plasma ionized calcium in some uremic patients, yet fail to suppress parathyroid hyperfunction. In these individuals with autonomous parathyroid hyperfunction, oral calcitriol may be useful to maintain normocalcemia, but has not been shown to be adequate treatment for hyperparathyroidism.

Hypoparathyroidism: The recommended initial dose of calcitriol is 0.25 mcg/day given in the morning. If a satisfactory response in the biochemical parameters and clinical manifestations of the disease is not observed, the dose may be increased at 2- to 4-week intervals. During the dosage titration period, serum calcium levels should be obtained at least twice weekly and, if hypercalcemia is noted, calcitriol should be immediately discontinued until normocalcemia ensues. Careful consideration should also be given to lowering the dietary calcium intake.

Most adult patients and pediatric patients age 6 years and older have responded to dosages in the range of 0.5 to 2 mcg daily. Pediatric patients in the 1-5 year age group with hypoparathyroidism have usually been given 0.25 to 0.75 mcg daily. The number of treated patients with pseudohypoparathyroidism less than 6 years of age is too small to make dosage recommendations.

INJECTION

The recommended initial dose of calcitriol injection is 0.5 mcg (0.01 mcg/kg) administered three times weekly, approximately every other day. Calcitriol injection can be administered as a bolus dose intravenously through the catheter at the end of hemodialysis. If a satisfactory response in the biochemical parameters and clinical manifestations of the disease state is not observed, the dose may be increased by 0.25 to 0.50 mcg at two to four week intervals. During this titration period, serum calcium and phosphorus levels should be obtained at least twice weekly, and if hypercalcemia is noted, the drug should be immediately discontinued until normocalcemia ensues. Most patients undergoing hemodialysis respond to doses between 0.5 and 3.0 mcg (0.01 to 0.05 mcg/kg) three times per week.

Parenteral drug products should be inspected visually for particulate matter and discoloration prior to administration, whenever solution and container permit.

Discard unused portion.

HOW SUPPLIED:

CAPSULES

0.25 mcg calcitriol in soft gelatin, light orange, oval capsules, imprinted ROCALTROL 0.25 ROCHE.

0.5 mcg calcitriol in soft gelatin, dark orange, oblong capsules, imprinted ROCALTROL 0.5 ROCHE.

Calcitriol should be protected from heat and light.

INJECTION

Calcijex (calcitriol injection) is supplied in 1 ml ampuls containing 1 mcg (List No. 1200) and 2 mcg (List No. 1210).

HOW SUPPLIED: *(cont'd)*

Protect form light. Store at controlled room temperature 15° to 30°C (59° to 86°F).

(Capsules - Roche Laboratories, 11/93, 13-20-78503-1193)

(Injection - Abbott Laboratories, 10/90, 06-4630-R5)

HOW SUPPLIED - EQUIVALENTS NOT AVAILABLE:

Capsule, Elastic - Oral - 0.25 mcg

30's	**$32.52**	**ROCALTROL, Roche**	**00004-0143-23**
100's	**$106.83**	**ROCALTROL, Roche**	**00004-0143-01**

Capsule, Elastic - Oral - 0.5 mcg

100's	**$170.85**	**ROCALTROL, Roche**	**00004-0144-01**

Injection, Solution - Intravenous - 1 mcg/ml

1 ml	$611.95	CALCIJEX, Abbott	00074-1200-01

Injection, Solution - Intravenous - 2 mcg/ml

1 ml	$1049.80	CALCIJEX, Abbott	00074-1210-01

CALCIUM *(000587)*

CATEGORIES: Calcium Metabolism; Calcium Preparations; Calcium Salts; Electrolytic, Caloric-Water Balance; Homeostatic & Nutrient; Osteoporosis; Replacement Solutions; Vitamins; FDA Pre 1938 Drugs

BRAND NAMES: Alba Lybe; Calcijex; Calcium Levulinate/Glycerol Ph; Calphosan

Prescribing information not available at time of publication.

HOW SUPPLIED - EQUIVALENTS NOT AVAILABLE:

Syrup - Oral

180 ml	$13.75	ALBA-LYBE, Alba Pharma	10023-0101-06

CALCIUM ACETATE *(003004)*

CATEGORIES: Electrolytic, Caloric-Water Balance; Hyperphosphatemia; Orphan Drugs; Renal Failure; Replacement Solutions; Pregnancy Category C; FDA Approved 1990 Dec

BRAND NAMES: Calcate; *Calcetat-GRY* (Germany); *Nephrex*; *Nephrex 600*; **Phoslo**
(International brand names outside U.S. in italics)

DESCRIPTION:

Each tablet contains 667 mg of calcium acetate (anhydrous; $Ca(CH_3COO)_2$; M.W. = 158.17 grams) equal to 169 mg (8.45 mEq) calcium, and 10 mg of the inert binder, polyethylene glycol 8000.

CLINICAL PHARMACOLOGY:

Patients with advanced renal insufficiency (creatinine clearance less than 30 ml/min) exhibit phosphate retention and some degree of hyperphosphatemia. The retention of phosphate plays a pivotal role in causing secondary hyperparathyroidism associated with osteodystrophy, and soft tissue calcification. The mechanism by which phosphate retention leads to hyperparathyroidism is not clearly delineated. Therapeutic efforts directed toward the control of hyperphosphatemia include reduction in the dietary intake of phosphate, inhibition of absorption of phosphate in the intestine with phosphate binders, and removal of phosphate from the body by more efficient methods of dialysis. The rate of removal of phosphate by dietary manipulation or by dialysis is insufficient. Dialysis patients absorb 40% to 80% of dietary phosphorus. Therefore, the fraction of dietary phosphate absorbed form the diet needs to be reduced by using phosphate binders in most renal failure patients on maintenance dialysis. Calcium acetate when taken with meals, combines with dietary phosphate to form insoluble calcium phosphate which is excreted in the feces. Maintenance of serum phosphorus below 6.0 mg/dl is generally considered as a clinically acceptable outcome of treatment with phosphate binders. Calcium acetate is highly soluble at neutral pH, making the calcium readily available for binding to phosphate in the proximal small intestine.

Orally administered calcium acetate from pharmaceutical dosage forms has been demonstrated to be systemically absorbed up to approximately 40% under fasting conditions and up to 30% under nonfasting conditions. This range represents data from both healthy subjects and renal dialysis patients under various conditions.

INDICATIONS AND USAGE:

Calcium acetate is indicated or the control of hyperphosphatemia in end stage renal failure and does not promote aluminum absorption.

CONTRAINDICATIONS:

Patients with hypercalcemia.

WARNINGS:

Patients with end stage renal failure may develop hypercalcemia when given calcium with meals. No other calcium supplements should be given concurrently with calcium acetate.

Progressive hypercalcemia due to overdose of calcium acetate may be severe as to require emergency measures. Chronic hypercalcemia may lead to vascular calcification, and other soft-tissue calcification. The serum calcium level should be monitored twice weekly during the early dose adjustment period. **The serum calcium times phosphate (CaXP) product should not be allowed to exceed 66.** Radiographic evaluation of suspect anatomic region may be helpful in early detection of soft-tissue calcification.

PRECAUTIONS:

General: Excessive dosage of calcium acetate induces hypercalcemia; therefore, early in the treatment during dosage adjustment serum calcium should be determined twice weekly. Should hypercalcemia develop, the dosage should be reduced or the treatment discontinued immediately depending on the severity of hypercalcemia. Calcium acetate should not be given to patients on digitalis, because hypercalcemia may precipitate cardiac arrhythmias. Calcium acetate therapy should always be started at low dose and should not be increased without careful monitoring of serum calcium. An estimate of daily dietary calcium intake should be made initially and the intake adjusted as needed. Serum phosphorus should also be determined periodically.

Information for the Patient: The patient should be informed about compliance with dosage instructions, adherence to instructions about diet and avoidance of the use of nonprescription antacids. Patients should be informed about the symptoms of hypercalcemia (see ADVERSE REACTIONS.)

PRECAUTIONS: *(cont'd)*

Carcinogenesis, Mutagenesis, and Impairment of Fertility: Long term animal studies have not been performed to evaluate the carcinogenic potential or effect on fertility of calcium acetate.

Pregnancy, Teratogenic Effects, Pregnancy Category C: Animal reproduction studies have not been conducted with calcium acetate. It is also not known whether calcium acetate can cause fetal harm when administered to a pregnant woman or can affect reproduction capacity. Calcium acetate should be given to a pregnant woman only if clearly needed.

Pediatric Use: Safety and efficacy of calcium acetate have not been established.

DRUG INTERACTIONS:

Calcium acetate may decrease the bioavailability of tetracyclines.

ADVERSE REACTIONS:

In clinical studies, patients have occasionally experienced nausea during calcium acetate therapy. Hypercalcemia may occur during treatment with calcium acetate. Mild hypercalcemia (Ca L> 10.5 mg/dl) may be asymptomatic or manifest itself as constipation, anorexia, nausea and vomiting. More severe hypercalcemia (Ca > 12 mg/dl) is associated with confusion, delirium, stupor and coma. Mild discontinuing therapy. Severe hypercalcemia can be treated by acute hemodialysis and discontinuing calcium acetate therapy.

Decreasing dialysate calcium concentration could reduce the incidence and severity of calcium acetate induced hypercalcemia. The long-term effect of calcium acetate on the progression of vascular or soft-tissue calcification has not been determined.

OVERDOSAGE:

Administration of calcium acetate in excess of the appropriate daily dosage can cause severe hypercalcemia. (See ADVERSE REACTIONS.)

DOSAGE AND ADMINISTRATION:

The recommended initial dose of calcium acetate for the adult dialysis patient is 2 tablets with each meal. The dosage may be increased gradually to bring the serum phosphate value below 6 mg/dl, as long as hypercalcemia does not develop. Most patients require 3 - 4 tablets with each meal.

Store at controlled room temperature, 15 - 30°C.

HOW SUPPLIED - EQUIVALENTS NOT AVAILABLE:

Injection, Solution - Intravenous - 0.5 meq/ml

10 ml	$1.01	Calcium Acetate, Abbott	00074-2553-01
50 ml	$3.43	Calcium Acetate, Abbott	00074-2553-02
100 ml	$7.71	Calcium Acetate, Abbott	00074-2553-03

Tablet, Uncoated - Oral - 250 mg

120 T/Bottle	$7.00	CALCATE, Nutraceutical Labs	58916-0250-01

Tablet, Uncoated - Oral - 667 mg

200's	$18.50	CALPHRON, Nephro-Tech	59528-0331-02
200's	**$19.60**	**PHOSLO, Braintree**	**52268-0200-01**

CALCIUM CHLORIDE *(000596)*

CATEGORIES: Antimicrobials; Calcium Metabolism; Calcium Salts; Electrolytic, Caloric-Water Balance; Homeostatic & Nutrient; Hyperkalemia; Hypocalcemia; Pharmaceutical Adjuvants; Replacement Solutions; FDA Pre 1938 Drugs

DESCRIPTION:

A HYPERTONIC SOLUTION FOR INTRAVENOUS INJECTION

CAUTION: THIS SOLUTION MUST NOT BE INJECTED INTRAMUSCULARLY OR SUBCUTANEOUSLY.

10% CALCIUM CHLORIDE INJECTION, USP, IS A STERILE, NON-PYROGENIC, HYPERTONIC SOLUTION CONTAINING 100 MG (1.4 MEQ/ML) OF CALCIUM CHLORIDE, DIHYDRATE (1.4 MEQ EACH OF CA^{++} and Cl^-) in water for injection.

THE SOLUTION IS ADMINISTERED ONLY BY INTRAVENOUS OR INTRAVENTRICULAR CAVITY INJECTION AS A CALCIUM REPLENISHER.

THE SOLUTION CONTAINS NO BACTERIOSTAT, ANTIMICROBIAL AGENT OR ADDED BUFFER AND IS INTENDED ONLY FOR USE WITH A SINGLE-DOSE INJECTION. THE PH IS BETWEEN 5.5-7.5 ADJUSTED WITH HYDROCHLORIC ACID. THE OSMOLAR CONCENTRATION IS 2.04 M0SM/ML (CALC.).

CALCIUM CHLORIDE, USP DIHYDRATE IS CHEMICALLY DESIGNATED $CACL_2 \cdot 2H_2O$ (dihydrate) white, odorless fragments or granules freely soluble in water.

CLINICAL PHARMACOLOGY:

Calcium is the fifth most abundant element in the body and the major fraction is in the bony structure. Calcium plays important physiological roles, many of which are poorly understood. It is essential for the functional integrity of the nervous and muscular systems. It is necessary for normal cardiac function and is one of the factors that operates in the mechanisms involved in the coagulation of blood.

Calcium Chloride in water dissociates to provide calcium (Ca^{++}) and chloride (Cl^-) ions. They are normal constituents of the body fluids and are dependent on various physiologic mechanisms for maintenance of balance between intake and output. Approximately 80% of body calcium is excreted in the feces as insoluble salts; urinary excretion accounts for the remaining 20%.

INDICATIONS AND USAGE:

10% Calcium Chloride Injection, USP, is indicated (1) for the treatment of hypocalcemia in those conditions requiring a prompt increase in blood plasma calcium levels, (2) in the treatment of magnesium intoxication due to overdosage of magnesium sulfate and (3) to combat the deleterious effects of hyperkalemia as measured by electrocardiographic (ECG), pending correction of the increased potassium level in the extracellular fluid.

10% Calcium Chloride Injection, USP, also may be used in cardiac resuscitation when weak or inadequate contractions return following defibrillation or when epinephrine injection has failed to strengthen myocardial contractions.

CONTRAINDICATIONS:

Calcium Chloride is contraindicated for cardiac resuscitation in the presence of ventricular fibrillation or in patients with the risk of existing digitalis toxicity.

WARNINGS:

10% Calcium Chloride Injection, USP, is irritating to veins and *must not be injected into tissues,* since severe necrosis and sloughing may occur. Great care should be taken to avoid extravasation or accidental injection into perivascular tissues.

PRECAUTIONS:

Do not administer unless solution is clear. Discard unused portion.

Because of its additive effect, calcium should be administered very cautiously to a patient who is digitalized or who is taking effective doses of digitalis or digitalis-like preparations.

Injections should be made slowly through a small needle into a larger vein to minimize venous irritation and avoid undesirable reactions. It is particularly important to prevent a high concentration of calcium from reaching the heart because of the danger of cardiac syncope. If injected into the ventricular cavity in cardiac resuscitation, it must not be injected into the myocardial tissue.

PREGNANCY CATEGORY C

Animal reproduction studies have not been conducted with calcium chloride. It also is not known whether calcium chloride can cause fetal harm when administered to a pregnant woman or can affect reproduction capacity. Calcium chloride should be given to a pregnant woman only if clearly needed.

ADVERSE REACTIONS:

Rapid injection may cause the patient to complain of tingling sensations, a calcium taste, a sense of oppression or "heat wave".

Injections of calcium chloride are accompanied by peripheral vasodilatation as well as a local "burning" sensation and there may be a moderate fall in blood pressure.

Should perivascular infiltration occur, IV administration at that site should be discontinued at once. Local infiltration of the affected area with 1% procaine hydrochloride, to which hyaluronidase may be added, will often reduce venospasm and dilute the calcium remaining in the tissues locally. Local application of heat may also be helpful.

DRUG ABUSE AND DEPENDENCE:

None known.

OVERDOSAGE:

Too rapid injection may produce lowering of blood pressure and cardiac syncope. Persistent hypercalcemia from overdosage of calcium is unlikely because of rapid excretion. In the event of untoward effects from excessive calcium administration, the drug should be discontinued promptly, the patient reevaluated and appropriate countermeasures instituted, if necessary. See PRECAUTIONS and ADVERSE REACTIONS.

DOSAGE AND ADMINISTRATION:

10% Calcium Chloride Injection, USP, is administered only by *slow* intravenous injection (not to exceed 1 ml/min) and/or in cardiac resuscitation, by injection into the ventricular cavity. It must not be injected into the myocardium.

The usual precautions for intravenous therapy should be observed. If time permits, the solution should be warmed to body temperature. The injection should be halted if the patient complains of any discomfort; it may be resumed when symptoms disappear. Following injection, the patient should remain recumbent for a short time.

The usual adult dosage in hypocalcemic disorders ranges from 500 mg to 1g (5 to 10 ml) at intervals of 1 to 3 days, depending on the response of the patient and/or results of serum calcium determinations. Repeated injections may be required because of rapid excretion of calcium.

In magnesium intoxication, an initial adult dose of 500 mg (5 ml) should be administered promptly and the patient observed for signs or recovery before further doses are given.

In hyperkalemic ECG disturbances of cardiac function, the dosage of calcium chloride injection should be titrated by constant monitoring of ECG changes during administration.

In cardiac resuscitation, the usual adult dosage ranges from 500 mg to 1 g (5 to 10 ml) intravenously.

If there has not been sufficient time to establish an intravenous route, intraventricular injection may be administered by personnel who are well trained in the technique and familiar with possible complications. The intravenous needle supplied with the syringe should be broken off and replaced with a suitable intracardiac needle by affixing it firmly to the Luer taper provided on the syringe. After the injection has been completed, the needle/syringe assembly should be removed from the injection site by grasping the needle at the luer fitting.

The intraventricular dose usually ranges from 200 to 800 mg (2 to 8 ml).

Parenteral drug products should be inspected visually for particulate matter and discoloration prior to administration whenever solution and container permit. See PRECAUTIONS.

The solution should be stored at controlled room temperature 15-30°C (59-86°F).

HOW SUPPLIED - EQUIVALENTS NOT AVAILABLE:

Injection, Solution - Intravenous - 10 %

10 ml	$4.93	Calcium Chloride, Intl Medication	00548-1004-00
10 ml	$5.30	Calcium Chloride, Intl Medication	00548-2004-00
10 ml	$7.09	Calcium Chloride 10%, Intl Medication	00548-1006-00
10 ml	$11.82	CALCIUM CHLORIDE, Abbott	00074-4928-18
10 ml	$12.65	Calcium Chloride, Abbott	00074-4928-23
10 ml	$12.93	Calcium Chloride, Intl Medication	00548-3004-00
10 ml	$13.16	CALCIUM CHLORIDE, Abbott	00074-4928-34
10 ml	$13.31	CALCIUM CHLORIDE, Abbott	00074-4908-18
10 ml x 10	$43.80	Calcium Chloride, Voluntary Hosp	53258-9422-05
10 ml x 10	$62.35	Calcium Chloride, Astra USA	00186-0651-01
10 ml x 10	$70.25	Calcium Chloride, Fujisawa USA	00469-9422-78
10 ml x 10	$79.38	Calcium Chloride, Fujisawa USA	00469-9422-75
10 ml x 25	$17.50	Calcium Chloride, Fujisawa USA	00469-1140-30
10 ml x 25	$19.69	Calcium Chloride, Am Regent	00517-2710-25
10 ml x 25	$20.19	Calcium Chloride, Astra USA	00186-1166-04
10 ml x 25	$37.50	Calcium Chloride, Consolidated Midland	00223-7277-10

CALCIUM GLUCEPTATE *(000599)*

CATEGORIES: Alkalosis; Calcium Metabolism; Calcium Salts; Electrolytic, Caloric-Water Balance; Homeostatic & Nutrient; Hypocalcemia; Parathyroid; Replacement Solutions; Tetany; Vitamin D; Pregnancy Category C; FDA Approval Pre 1982

DESCRIPTION:

FOR INTRAVENOUS OR INTRAMUSCULAR ADMINISTRATION OF CALCIUM

Calcium Gluceptate injection, USP, contains a sterile, aqueous, approximately neutral solution of the calcium salt of d- glucoheptonic acid, stabilized with 0.5% monothioglycerol. Each 5 ml contains 1.1 g of calcium gluceptate representing 90 mg calcium (4.5 mEq) and is equivalent in calcium content to 10 ml of 10% calcium gluconate; the osmolarity is 0.5 mOsm/ml. Sodium hydroxide and/or glucono Delta-lactone may have been added during manufacture to adjust the pH. The empirical formula is $C_{14}H_{26}CaO_{16}$.

CLINICAL PHARMACOLOGY:

Calcium is the fifth most abundant element in the body, and the major fraction is in the bony structure. Calcium plays important physiologic roles, many of which are poorly understood. It is essential for the functional integrity of the nervous and muscular systems, is necessary for normal cardiac function, and is one of the factors involved in the coagulation of blood.

Approximately one third of ingested calcium is absorbed in the upper gastrointestinal tract. It is excreted primarily in the urine and the feces; however, calcium is also lost in milk during lactation and in daily perspiration. After intravenous administration, calcium has a duration of action of 2 to 3 hours; after intramuscular injection, of 1 to 4 hours.

INDICATIONS AND USAGE:

The parenteral administration of calcium is indicated in the treatment of hypocalcemia for those conditions requiring a prompt increase in blood plasma calcium levels, such as neonatal tetany and tetany due to parathyroid deficiency, vitamin D deficiency, and alkalosis. It is also indicated for the prevention of hypocalcemia during exchange transfusions.

CONTRAINDICATIONS:

There are no known contraindications to the use of calcium gluceptate.

WARNINGS:

Because of its additive effect, calcium should be administered with caution to a patient who is digitalized or who is taking effective doses of digitalis or digitalis-like preparations.

Although calcium gluceptate given intramuscularly appears to be well tolerated, this route of administration should be used for very young patients only in emergencies when technical difficulty makes intravenous injection impossible.

PRECAUTIONS:

Calcium gluceptate may be irritating to tissues. Use standard technique for intramuscular injection to avoid injury to subcutaneous tissues and consequent fat necrosis.

Carcinogenesis, Mutagenesis, and Impairment of Fertility: No long-term studies in animals have been performed to evaluate calcium gluceptate.

Usage in Pregnancy: Pregnancy Category C: Animal reproduction studies have not been conducted with calcium gluceptate. It is also not known whether calcium gluceptate can cause fetal harm when administered to a pregnant woman or can affect reproduction capacity. Calcium gluceptate should be given to a pregnant woman only if clearly needed.

Nursing Mothers: Caution should be exercised when calcium gluceptate is administered to a nursing woman.

Pediatric Use: See WARNINGS.

DRUG INTERACTIONS:

See WARNINGS.

ADVERSE REACTIONS:

Following intramuscular administration, mild local reactions may occur; severe inflammatory reactions have not been observed.

Rapid intravenous administration may cause the patient to complain of tingling sensations, a calcium taste, a sense of oppression, or "heat waves".

OVERDOSAGE:

Hypercalcemia is rarely produced by administration of calcium alone but may occur when large doses are given to patients with chronic renal failure. Since hypercalcemia may be more dangerous than hypocalcemia, overtreatment of hypocalcemia should be avoided. Frequent determinations of serum calcium levels should be performed, and serum calcium levels should be maintained at 9 to 10.4 mg/100 ml (4.5 to 5.2 mEq/L). Some clinicians prefer to maintain serum calcium at slightly lower levels. Serum calcium levels usually should not be allowed to exceed 12 mg/100 ml. Administration of calcium in patients who have received transfusions of citrated blood may result in higher than normal total serum calcium levels. In these patients, however, most of the excess calcium is bound to citrate and is inactive; therefore, serious toxicity usually does not result. although determinations of urine calcium have been advised, they are generally unreliable and hypercalciuria can occur in the presence of hypocalcemia. Some clinicians recommend forcing fluids to produce increased urine volume and thus prevent the formation of renal stones in patients with hypercalciuria. When hypercalcemia occurs, discontinuation of the drug is usually sufficient to return serum calcium levels to normal.

DOSAGE AND ADMINISTRATION:

Calcium gluceptate may be given INTRAMUSCULARLY in 2- to 5-ml doses. When 5 ml is administered, the dose should be injected in the gluteal region or, in infants, in the lateral thigh.

The usual INTRAVENOUS dose of calcium gluceptate is 5 to 20 ml. The usual precautions for intravenous therapy should be observed. The solution should be warmed to body temperature and administered slowly (2 ml/min). The injection should be halted if the patient complains of any discomfort; it may be resumed when symptoms disappear. Following injection, the patient should remain recumbent for a short time. Repeated injections may be required because of the rapid excretion of calcium.

During exchange transfusions in newborns, the usual dose is 0.5 ml after every 100 ml of blood exchanged.

HOW SUPPLIED - EQUIVALENTS NOT AVAILABLE:

Injection, Solution - Intramuscular; - 90 mg/5ml

5 ml	$1.89	Calcium Gluceptate 1.1, Abbott	00074-3894-05

CALCIUM GLUCONATE *(000600)*

CATEGORIES: Bites; Black Widow Spider; Calcium Metabolism; Calcium Salts; Colic; Dermatitis; Dermatitis Herpetiformis; Dermatoses; Electrolyte Solutions; Electrolytic, Caloric-Water Balance; Homeostatic & Nutrient; Hypocalcemia; Hypocalcemic; Hypoparathyroidism; Osteomalacia; Pharmaceutical Adjuvants; Pregnancy; Pruritus; Purpura; Replacement Solutions; Rickets; Spider Bites; Tetany; FDA Pre 1938 Drugs

FORMULARIES: WHO

DESCRIPTION:

Calcium gluconate injection, USP 10% is a sterile, nonpyrogenic solution containing 0.465 mEq (9.3 mg) total calcium per each ml equivalent to 0.1 g calcium gluconate as calcium gluconate 94 mg, calcium D-saccharate tetrahydrate 4.5 mg (equivalent to 3.5 mg of calcium

DESCRIPTION: *(cont'd)*

D-saccharate, anhydrous) in water for injection. Calcium D-saccharate provides 6% of the total calcium and stabilizes the supersaturated solution of calcium gluconate. pH adjusted with sodium hydroxide and/or hydrochloric acid to between 6.0-8.2.

CLINICAL PHARMACOLOGY:

Calcium is the fifth most abundant element in the body and is essential for maintenance of the functional integrity of nervous, muscular and skeletal systems and cell membrane and capillary permeability. It is also an important activator in many enzymatic reactions and is essential to a number of physiologic processes including transmission of nerve impulses; contraction of cardiac, smooth and skeletal muscles; renal function; respiration and blood coagulation. Calcium also plays regulatory roles in the release and storage of neurotransmitters and hormones, in the uptake and binding of amino acids, and in cyanocobalamin (vitamin B_{12}) absorption and gastrin secretion.

INDICATIONS AND USAGE:

Calcium gluconate is used to treat conditions arising from calcium deficiencies such as hypocalcemic tetany, hypocalcemia related to hypoparathyroidism and hypocalcemia due to rapid growth or pregnancy. It is also used in the treatment of black widow spider bites to relieve muscle cramping and as an adjunct in the treatment of rickets, osteomalacia, lead colic and magnesium sulfate overdosage. Calcium gluconate has also been employed to decrease capillary permeability in allergic conditions, nonthrombocytopenic purpura and exudative dermatoses such as dermatitis herpetiformis, and for pruritis of eruptions caused by certain drugs. In hyperkalemia, calcium gluconate may aid in antagonizing the cardiac toxicity provided the patient is not receiving digitalis therapy.

CONTRAINDICATIONS:

Calcium salts are contraindicated in patients with ventricular fibrillation or hypercalcemia. Intravenous administration of calcium is contraindicated when serum calcium levels are above normal.

WARNINGS:

For intravenous use only. Subcutaneous or intramuscular injection may cause severe necrosis and sloughing.

PRECAUTIONS:

GENERAL

Supersaturated solutions are prone to precipitation. If precipitation is evident in syringes, do not use syringe. Precipitation if present in vials and ampules may be dissolved by heating to 80°C in a dry heat oven for a minimum of one hour. Shake vigorously. Allow to cool to room temperature before dispensing. The solution should not be used if precipitate remains in vials and ampules after following the above procedure. To avoid undesirable reactions that may follow rapid intravenous administration of calcium gluconate, the drug should be given slowly, e.g. approximately 1.5 ml over a period of 1 minute. When injected intravenously, calcium gluconate should be injected through a small needle into a large vein in order to avoid too rapid increase in serum calcium and extravasation of calcium solution into the surrounding tissue with resulting necrosis.

Rapid injection of calcium gluconate may cause vasodilation, decreased blood pressure, bradycardia, cardiac arrhythmias, syncope and cardiac arrest.

Because of the danger involved in simultaneous use of calcium salts and drugs of the digitalis group, a digitalized patient should not receive an intravenous injection of a calcium compound unless indications are clearly defined.

DRUG/LABORATORY TEST INTERACTIONS

Transient elevations of plasma 11-hydroxycorticosteroid levels (Glenn-Nelson technique) may occur when intravenous calcium is administered, but levels return to control values after 1 hour. In addition, intravenous calcium gluconate can produce false-negative values for serum and urinary magnesium.

PREGNANCY CATEGORY C

Animal reproduction studies have not been conducted with calcium gluconate. It is also not known whether calcium gluconate can cause fetal harm when administered to a pregnant woman or can affect reproduction capacity. Calcium gluconate should be given to a pregnant woman only if clearly needed.

NURSING MOTHERS

It is not known whether this drug is excreted in human milk. Because many drugs are excreted in human milk, caution should be exercised when calcium gluconate is administered to a nursing woman.

DRUG INTERACTIONS:

The inotropic and toxic effects of cardiac glycosides and calcium are synergistic and arrhythmias may occur if these drugs are given together (particularly when calcium is given intravenously). Intravenous administration of calcium should be avoided in patients receiving cardiac glycosides; if necessary, calcium should be given slowly in small amounts.

Calcium complexes tetracycline antibiotics rendering them inactive. The two drugs should not be given at the same time orally nor should they be mixed for parenteral administration.

Calcium gluconate injection has been reported to be incompatible with intravenous solutions containing various drugs. Published data are too varied and/or limited to permit generalizations, and specialized reference should be consulted for specific information.

ADVERSE REACTIONS:

Patients may complain of tingling sensations, a sense of oppression or heat waves and a calcium or chalky taste following the intravenous administration of calcium gluconate.

Rapid intravenous injection of calcium salts may cause vasodilation, decreased blood pressure, bradycardia, cardiac arrhythmias, syncope and cardiac arrest. Use in digitalized patients may precipitate arrhythmias.

Local necrosis and abscess formation may occur with intramuscular injection.

DOSAGE AND ADMINISTRATION:

The dose is dependent on the requirements of the individual patient. Intravenous calcium gluconate injection must be administered slowly.

The usual intravenous dose in adults is 5 ml (500 mg) to 20 ml (2 g).

In children the usual dose is 500 mg/kg/day or 12 g/m²/day well diluted and administered slowly intravenously in divided doses.

Parenteral drug products should be inspected visually for particulate matter and discoloration prior to administration whenever solution and container permit. See PRECAUTIONS.

Store at controlled room temperature 15-30°C (59-86°F).

HOW SUPPLIED - EQUIVALENTS NOT AVAILABLE:

Injection, Solution - Intravenous - 10 %

10 ml	$1.75	Calcium Gluconate, Consolidated Midland	00223-7275-10
10 ml	$1.89	Calcium Gluconate 10%, Abbott	00074-1184-01
10 ml x 25	$12.10	Calcium Gluconate, Americal Pharm	54945-0532-05
10 ml x 25	$15.31	Calcium Gluconate, Elkins Sinn	00641-1390-35
10 ml x 25	$21.00	Calcium Gluconate, Gensia Labs	00703-5344-04
10 ml x 25	$22.19	Calcium Gluconate, Am Regent	00517-3910-25
10 ml x 25	$26.80	Calcium Gluconate, Consolidated Midland	00223-7280-10
10 ml x 25	$32.50	Calcium Gluconate, Pasadena	00418-1691-46
10 ml x 25	$34.06	Calcium Gluconate, Fujisawa USA	00469-0311-10
10 ml x 25	$35.00	Calcium Gluconate, Hyrex Pharms	00314-3910-25
10 ml x 25	$50.00	Calcium Gluconate, C O Truxton	00463-1011-26
10 ml x 100	$55.00	Calcium Gluconate, Elkins Sinn	00641-1390-36
10 ml x 100	$56.87	Calcium Gluconate, Am Regent	00517-0216-70
10 ml x 100	$105.00	Calcium Gluconate, Consolidated Midland	00223-7280-00
25 x 100 ml pha	$93.75	Calcium Gluconate Injection 10 %, Am Regent	00517-3900-25
50 ml x 10	$30.00	Calcium Gluconate, Gensia Labs	00703-5347-03
50 ml x 25	$81.88	Calcium Gluconate, Am Regent	00517-3950-25
50 ml x 25	$100.94	Calcium Gluconate, Fujisawa USA	00469-0311-50
50 ml x 25	$110.50	Calcium Gluconate, Pasadena	00418-1691-50
100 ml	$6.86	Calcium Gluconate, Intl Medication	00548-6524-00
100 ml x 10	$58.80	Calcium Gluconate, Gensia Labs	00703-5348-03
100 ml x 40	$332.00	Calcium Gluconate, Fujisawa USA	00469-0311-61
200 ml	$12.81	Calcium Gluconate, Intl Medication	00548-6538-00
200 ml x 10	$112.80	Calcium Gluconate, Gensia Labs	00703-5340-03
200 ml x 20	$249.48	Calcium Gluconate, Fujisawa USA	00469-0311-63

CALCIUM GLYCEROPHOSPHATE *(000604)*

CATEGORIES: Electrolytic, Caloric-Water Balance; Pharmaceutical Adjuvants; Replacement Solutions; FDA Pre 1938 Drugs

BRAND NAMES: Calphosan; Phos-Cal

DESCRIPTION:

Calcium glycerophosphate is a specially processed solution containing calcium glycerophosphate and calcium lactate. Calcium glycerophosphate is isotonic, with a pH of about 7 or somewhat above. (Other calcium solutions are usually quite acid, with pH values of 4.5 to 5.5). Each 10 ml Calphosan contains calcium glycerophosphate 50 mg. and calcium lactate 50 mg. in a physiological solution of sodium chloride, with 0.25% phenol as a preservative.

CLINICAL PHARMACOLOGY:

Intramuscular injections of calcium glycerophosphate raise blood serum calcium levels, do not raise the calcium levels above normal.

Of conspicuous importance, intramuscular injections of calcium glycerophosphate are without pain, inflammatory reactions or sloughing.

INDICATIONS AND USAGE:

Wherever calcium is indicated or in conditions associated with hypocalcemia.

CONTRAINDICATIONS:

Hypercalcemia: and in view of the fact that hypercalcemia is associated with sarcoidosis and bone metastasis of neoplastic processes. It should not be used in those conditions. As there is a similarity in the actions of calcium and digitals on the contractility and excitability of the heart muscle, calcium glycerophosphate is contraindicated in fully digitalized patients.**Do not use Intramuscularly in infants and young children.**

PRECAUTIONS:

Use in Pregnancy: Safety for use in pregnancy or during lactation has not been established.

DOSAGE AND ADMINISTRATION:

10 ml: one to four times weekly, or as determined by physician.

HOW SUPPLIED - EQUIVALENTS NOT AVAILABLE:

Injection, Solution - Intramuscular;

60 ml	$15.25	CALPHOSAN, Glenwood	00516-0060-60
100 ml	$8.95	PHOS-CAL, Merit Pharms	30727-0344-95

CALCIUM IODIDE; CODEINE PHOSPHATE *(000607)*

CATEGORIES: Antitussives; Antitussives/Expectorants/Mucolytics; Cough Preparations; Iodide Salts; Respiratory & Allergy Medications; Pregnancy Category D; DEA Class CV; FDA Pre 1938 Drugs

BRAND NAMES: **Calcidrine**

DESCRIPTION:

Each 5 ml (teaspoonful) contains:

Codeine, USP — 8.4 mg

Warning- May be habit forming.

Calcium iodide, anhydrous 152 mg

Inactive Ingredients: Alcohol 6%, FD&C Yellow No. 6, glycerin, liquid glucose, sucrose, water, natural and artificial flavors and other ingredients to form a palatable syrup.

Do not accept if band on cap is broken.

Calcium Iodide with Codeine is an oral antitussive, expectorant syrup.

The chemical formula for calcium iodide is CaI_2. Codeine is methylmorphine, a natural alkaloid of opium. The chemical formula for codeine is $C_{18}H_{21}NO_3 \cdot H_2O$

CLINICAL PHARMACOLOGY:

The major effects of codeine in man are on the central nervous system. The antitussive effect is produced by depression of the cough reflex. Codeine is rapidly absorbed from the gastrointestinal tract and is metabolized in the liver.

Iodides are readily absorbed from the gastrointestinal tract and are distributed to extracellular fluid as well as gastric and salivary secretions. Iodides are accumulated by the thyroid gland. Excretion occurs mainly through the kidneys.

INDICATIONS AND USAGE:

In adults and children as an expectorant, and for symptomatic relief of coughs.

CONTRAINDICATIONS:

This preparation should not be used in patients with a history of iodism, or with known hypersensitivity to iodides or codeine. Long-term use of iodide-containing preparations is contraindicated during pregnancy.

WARNINGS:

Physiological dependence may develop with the use of codeine.

Usage During Pregnancy: This syrup can cause fetal harm when administered to a pregnant woman. Maternal ingestion of large amounts of iodides during pregnancy has been associated with development of fetal goiter and resultant acute respiratory distress of the neonate. If this drug is used during pregnancy, or if the patient becomes pregnant while taking this drug, the patient should be apprised of the potential hazard to the fetus.

Severe and occasionally fatal skin eruptions have been reported rarely in patients receiving prolonged administration of iodides.

PRECAUTIONS:

Laboratory Tests: Patients who must receive prolonged iodide therapy should be evaluated periodically for possible depression of thyroid function.

Laboratory Test Interactions: Elevated values may be obtained on thyroid function tests or protein-bound iodine tests when iodide-containing compounds have been ingested. False positive results may be obtained if iodides have been ingested prior to guaiac or benzidine testing.

Carcinogenesis: No data is available on long-term carcinogenicity in animals or humans.

Pregnancy Category D: See WARNINGS.

Nursing Mothers: Iodine is excreted in breast milk. Caution should be exercised when Calcium Iodide with Codeine is administered to a nursing woman.

DRUG INTERACTIONS:

The concurrent administration of calcium iodide and lithium carbonate may enhance the hypothyroid and goitrogenic effects of either drug.

ADVERSE REACTIONS:

In decreasing order of severity: severe and sometimes fatal skin eruptions (ioderma) occur rarely after the prolonged use of iodides. Iodism can occur. Symptoms of iodism include metallic taste, acneform skin lesions, mucous membrane irritation, salivary gland swelling, and gastric distress. These side effects subside quickly upon discontinuance of the iodide-containing drug.

Codeine may produce vomiting, nausea, and constipation.

OVERDOSAGE:

Symptoms of acute codeine poisoning include respiratory and central nervous system depression, pinpoint pupils and coma. Blood pressure and body temperature may fall.

Acute iodide poisoning is associated with gastrointestinal irritation. Angioedema with laryngeal swelling may develop. Shock may also occur.

Treatment for overdose is:

a. Establish a patent airway and ventilate if needed.

b. Gastric evacuation.

c. Treatment for shock.

d. General supportive measures including replacement of fluids and electrolytes may be indicated.

e. The use of naloxone to antagonize the narcotic depression of the central nervous system should be considered.

DOSAGE AND ADMINISTRATION:

Adults and children over ten years of age, usual dose, 1 to 2 teaspoonfuls every 4 hours. Children 6 to 10 years of age, 1/2 to 1 teaspoonful every 4 hours. Children 2 to 6 years of age, 1/2 teaspoonful every 4 hours.

Dispense in a USP tight, light resistant glass container.

HOW SUPPLIED - EQUIVALENTS NOT AVAILABLE:

Syrup - Oral - 152 mg/8.4 mg

480 ml	**$40.88**	**CALCIDRINE, Abbott**	**00074-5763-16**

CALCIUM IODIDE; ISOPROTERENOL HYDROCHLORIDE *(000608)*

CATEGORIES: Antiasthmatics/Bronchodilators; Autonomic Drugs; Expectorants; Iodide Salts; Respiratory & Allergy Medications; Sympathomimetic Agents; FDA Pre 1938 Drugs

BRAND NAMES: Norisodrine W/Calcium Iodide

DESCRIPTION:

Do not accept if band is broken or missing. Norisodrine with Calcium Iodide is a bronchodilator, expectorant in a palatable syrup.

Isoproterenol is a sympathomimetic agent which is chemically related to epinephrine. The chemical formula for isoproterenol sulfate is 1,2- Benzenediol, 4-[1-hydroxy-2[(1-methylethyl) amino] ethyl]-, sulfate (2:1) (salt), dihydrate.

Each 5 ml (teaspoonful) contains:

Isoproterenol Sulfate — 3 mg

Calcium Iodide, Anhydrous — 150 mg

Inactive Ingredients: Alcohol 6%, ascorbic acid, caramel coloring, glycerin, liquid glucose, sucrose, water, artificial flavors and other ingredients forming a palatable aromatic syrup.

CLINICAL PHARMACOLOGY:

Isoproterenol is classified as a catecholamine which acts predominantly on beta receptor sites of peripheral inhibitory and cardiac excitatory sympathetic nerves. It is primary pharmacological actions are to increase both the rate and force of cardiac contractions and to relax the smooth muscle of the bronchi, alimentary tract, and skeletal muscle vasculature. Isoproterenol can prevent or relieve bronchospasm due to drugs, as well as that due to disease. The drug lowers peripheral vascular resistance and reduces the diastolic blood pressure. Systolic pressure is unchanged or slightly increased as a consequence of increased cardiac output.

CLINICAL PHARMACOLOGY: *(cont'd)*

After oral administration, Isoproterenol is extensively converted to its sulfate conjugate in the intestinal walls. This presystemic metabolism explains the higher doses and more variable response to isoproterenol by the oral route compared to parental administration. The primary excretion product found in urine is the sulfate conjugate (50 to 80% of the dose) with only minor fractions of unchanged drug (5 to 15%) and 3-0-methyl isoproterenol (15% or less).

The calorigenic effects of isoproterenol are similar to those of epinephrine. However, it causes less hyperglycemia than epinephrine. Isoproterenol can also cause central excitation.

Calcium iodide is an expectorant.

INDICATIONS AND USAGE:

Indicated in adults and children for the symptomatic control of bronchospasm in asthma and in allied respiratory disorders such as bronchitis and tracheobronchitis.

CONTRAINDICATIONS:

This product should not be used in patients with a history of iodism, or with known hypersensitivity to iodides. It is also contraindicated in rare instances in which a patient has demonstrated hypersensitivity to isoproterenol or other sympathomimetic amines.

Use of Isoproterenol is contraindicated in patients with pre-existing cardiac arrhythmias because the cardiac stimulant effect may aggravate such disorders.

Long-term use of iodide-containing preparations is contraindicated during pregnancy. (see WARNINGS.)

WARNINGS:

Bronchial asthma may mask the presence of cardiac asthma (pulmonary edema). A differential diagnosis should be made before instituting therapy.

Usage in Pregnancy: Norisodrine with Calcium Iodide can cause fetal harm when administered to a pregnant woman, Maternal ingestion of large amount of iodides during pregnancy has been associated with development of fetal goiter and resultant acute respiratory distress of the neonate. If this drug is used during pregnancy, or if the patient becomes pregnant while taking this drug, the patient should be apprised of the potential hazard to the fetus.

PRECAUTIONS:

Isoproterenol should be used cautiously in patients with heart disease, hypertension, hyperthyroidism, diabetes, or unstable vasomotor systems.

Patients who must receive prolonged iodide therapy should be evaluated periodically for possible depression of thyroid function.

Carcinogenesis: No data is available on long-term potential for carcinogenicity in animals or humans.

Pregnancy Category D: (see WARNINGS.)

Nursing Mothers: Iodine is excreted in breast milk, therefore, caution should be exercised when Norisodrine with Calcium Iodide is administered to a nursing woman.

Laboratory Test Interactions: Elevated values may be obtained on thyroid function tests, and then testing for protein-bound iodine, when iodine-containing compounds have been ingested.

The use of iodides may cause false positive results when guaiac testing is performed or when testing for benzidine.

DRUG INTERACTIONS:

The concurrent administration of calcium iodide and lithium carbonate may enhance the hyperthyroid and goitrogenic effects of either drug.

Concomitant use of isoproterenol and MAO inhibitors may induce acute hypertensive crisis.

Propranolol, a beta-adrenergic blocking agent, antagonizes isoproterenol.

Caution should be exercised when Isoproterenol is used concomitantly with a parenteral or inhalation form of *epinephrine* or other*adrenergic agent* since the effects of these drugs are additive.

ADVERSE REACTIONS:

As with other sympathomimetic drugs, isoproterenol may produce undesired side effects. These effects in decreasing order of severity are cardiac arrhythmias, tachycardia, vomiting, dizziness, weakness, nausea, precordial distress and anginal-type pain, headache, palpitation, nervousness, tremor, sweating, and flushing.

Swelling of the parotid glands has been reported with prolonged use of isoproterenol. In such cases the drug should be withdrawn.

Iodism can occur with use of this drug. Symptoms of iodism include metallic taste, acneform skin lesions, mucous membrane irritation, salivary gland swelling, and gastric distress. These side effects subside quickly upon discontinuance of the iodide-containing drug. Severe and sometimes fatal skin eruptions (ioderma) occur rarely after the prolonged use of iodides.

OVERDOSAGE:

Symptoms may include palpitation, tachycardia, restlessness, tremor, sweating, headache, dizziness, weakness, nausea, and vomiting. Blood pressure may at first be elevated slightly. Later, blood pressure may fail and the general picture of "shock" may develop.

Treatment includes general supportive measures. Sedatives may be given for restlessness.

DOSAGE AND ADMINISTRATION:

The following suggestions are offered as a general guide to dosage:

Under 3 years: 1/2 teaspoonful, may be repeated for every four to six hours; 3 to 10 years: 1/2 to 1 teaspoonful, may be repeated every four to six hours; over 10 years and for adults: 1 to 2 teaspoonfuls, may be repeated every four to six hours. Dosage must be adjusted to the response of the patient. Side effects may necessitate dosage reduction.

HOW SUPPLIED:

Store below 77°F (25°C).

Dispense in a USP tight, light-resistant, glass container.

(Abbott Laboratories)

HOW SUPPLIED - EQUIVALENTS NOT AVAILABLE:

Syrup - Oral - 150 mg/3 mg

480 ml $32.18 NORISODRINE WITH CALCIUM IODIDE, Abbott 00074-6953-01

CAPTOPRIL *(000642)*

CATEGORIES: ACE Inhibitors; Angiotensin Converting Enzyme Inhibitors; Antihypertensives; Cardiovascular Drugs; Congestive Heart Failure; Diabetes; Heart Failure; Hypertension; Myocardial Infarction; Nephropathy; Vascular Disease; Pregnancy Category C; Sales > $1 Billion; FDA Approval Pre 1982; Patent Expiration 1996 Feb; Top 200 Drugs

BRAND NAMES: *Acenorm* (Germany); *Acenorm Cor* (Germany); *Acepress*; *Acepril* (England); *Aceten*; *Adocor* (Germany); *Alopresin*; *Angiopril*; *Apuzin*; *Asisten*; *Caftam*; *Capace*; **Capoten**; *Capotena* (Mexico); *Capril*; *Captensin*; *Captoflux* (Germany); *Captolane* (France); *Captolong*; *Captopress* (Germany); *Captopril*; *Captoprilan*; *Captoril* (Japan); *Captral* (Mexico); *Cardipril* (Mexico); *Cesplon*; *Corax*; *Cryopril* (Mexico); *Debax*; *Dexacap*; *Ecapres*; *Ecaten* (Mexico); *Epicordin* (Germany); *Epsitron*; *Farcopril*; *Farmoten*; *Hiperil*; *Hypotensor*; *Inhibace*; *Insucar*; *Isopresol*; *Katopil*; *Lopirin* (Germany); *Lopril* (France); *Medepres*; *Mereprine*; *Minitent*; *Praten*; *Precaptil* (Mexico); *Rilcapton*; *Ropril*; *Smarten*; *Tensicap*; *Tensiomen*; *Tensobon* (Germany); *Tenzib*; *Toprilen*; *Zorkaptil*
(International brand names outside U.S. in italics)

FORMULARIES: Aetna; BC-BS; CIGNA; FHP; Humana; Kaiser; Medco; Medi-Cal; PruCare; United; WHO; PCS

COST OF THERAPY: $48.61 (Hypertension; Tablet; 25 mg; 2/day; 365 days) vs. Potential Cost of $24,027.04 (Coronary Bypass)

PRIMARY ICD9: 401.1 (Essential Hypertension, Benign)

> **WARNING:**
> **USE IN PREGNANCY**
> When used in pregnancy during the second and third trimesters, ACE inhibitors can cause injury and even death to the developing fetus. When pregnancy is detected, captopril should be discontinued as soon as possible. See WARNINGS, Fetal/Neonatal Morbidity and Mortality.

DESCRIPTION:

Captopril is a specific competitive inhibitor of angiotensin I-converting enzyme (ACE), the enzyme responsible for the conversion of angiotensin I to angiotensin II.

Captopril is designated chemically as 1-[(2S)-3-mercapto-2-methylpropionyl]-L-proline [MW 217.29].

Captopril is a white to off-white crystalline powder that may have a slight sulfurous odor; it is soluble in water (approx. 160 mg/ml), methanol, and ethanol and sparingly soluble in chloroform and ethyl acetate.

Captopril is available in potencies of 12.5 mg, 25 mg, 50 mg, and 100 mg as scored tablets for oral administration. Inactive ingredients: microcrystalline cellulose, corn starch, lactose, and stearic acid.

CLINICAL PHARMACOLOGY:

MECHANISM OF ACTION

The mechanism of action of captopril has not yet been fully elucidated. Its beneficial effects in hypertension and heart failure appear to result primarily from suppression of the renin-angiotensin-aldosterone system. However, there is no consistent correlation between renin levels and response to the drug. Renin, an enzyme synthesized by the kidneys, is released into the circulation where it acts on a plasma globulin substrate to produce angiotensin I, a relatively inactive decapeptide. Angiotensin I is then converted by angiotensin converting enzyme (ACE) to angiotensin II, a potent endogenous vasoconstrictor substance. Angiotensin II also stimulates aldosterone secretion from the adrenal cortex, thereby contributing to sodium and fluid retention.

Captopril prevents the conversion of angiotensin I to angiotensin II by inhibition of ACE, a peptidyldipeptide carboxy hydrolase. This inhibition has been demonstrated in both healthy human subjects and in animals by showing that the elevation of blood pressure caused by exogenously administered angiotensin I was attenuated or abolished by captopril. In animal studies, captopril did not alter the pressor responses to a number of other agents, including angiotensin II and norepinephrine, indicating specificity of action.

ACE is identical to "bradykininase", and captopril may also interfere with the degradation of the vasodepressor peptide, bradykinin. Increased concentrations of bradykinin or prostaglandin E_2 may also have a role in the therapeutic effect of captopril.

Inhibition of ACE results in decreased plasma angiotensin II and increased plasma renin activity (PRA), the latter resulting from loss of negative feedback on renin release caused by reduction in angiotensin II. The reduction of angiotensin II leads to decreased aldosterone secretion, and, as a result, small increases in serum potassium may occur along with sodium and fluid loss.

The antihypertensive effects persist for a longer period of time than does demonstrable inhibition of circulating ACE. It is not known whether the ACE present in vascular endothelium is inhibited longer than the ACE in circulating blood.

PHARMACOKINETICS

After oral administration of therapeutic doses of captopril, rapid absorption occurs with peak blood levels at about one hour. The presence of food in the gastrointestinal tract reduces absorption by about 30 to 40 percent; captopril therefore should be given one hour before meals. Based on carbon-14 labeling, average minimal absorption is approximately 75 percent. In a 24-hour period, over 95 percent of the absorbed dose is eliminated in the urine; 40 to 50 percent is unchanged drug; most of the remainder is the disulfide dimer of captopril and captopril-cysteine disulfide.

Approximately 25 to 30 percent of the circulating drug is bound to plasma proteins. The apparent elimination half-life for total radioactivity in blood is probably less than 3 hours. An accurate determination of half-life of unchanged captopril is not, at present, possible, but it is probably less than 2 hours. In patients with renal impairment, however, retention of captopril occurs (see DOSAGE AND ADMINISTRATION.)

PHARMACODYNAMICS

Administration of captopril results in a reduction of peripheral arterial resistance in hypertensive patients with either no change, or an increase, in cardiac output. There is an increase in renal blood flow following administration of captopril and glomerular filtration rate is usually unchanged.

Reductions of blood pressure are usually maximal 60 to 90 minutes after oral administration of an individual dose of captopril. The duration of effect is dose related. The reduction in blood pressure may be progressive, so to achieve maximal therapeutic effects, several weeks of therapy may be required. The blood pressure lowering effects of captopril and thiazide-type diuretics are additive. In contrast, captopril and beta-blockers have a less than additive effect.

CLINICAL PHARMACOLOGY: *(cont'd)*

Blood pressure is lowered to about the same extent in both standing and supine positions. Orthostatic effects and tachycardia are infrequent but may occur in volume-depleted patients. Abrupt withdrawal of captopril has not been associated with a rapid increase in blood pressure.

In patients with heart failure, significantly decreased peripheral (systemic vascular) resistance and blood pressure (afterload), reduced pulmonary capillary wedge pressure (preload) and pulmonary vascular resistance, increased cardiac output, and increased exercise tolerance time (ETT) have been demonstrated. These hemodynamic and clinical effects occur after the first dose and appear to persist for the duration of therapy. Placebo controlled studies of 12 weeks duration in patients who did not respond adequately to diuretics and digitalis show no tolerance to beneficial effects on ETT; open studies, with exposure up to 18 months in some cases, also indicate that ETT benefit is maintained. Clinical improvement has been observed in some patients where acute hemodynamic effects were minimal.

The Survival and Ventricular Enlargement (SAVE) study was a multicenter, randomized, double blind, placebo-controlled trial conducted in 2,231 patients (age 21-79 years) who survived the acute phase of a myocardial infarction and did not have active ischemia. Patients had left ventricular dysfunction (LVD), defined as a resting left ventricular ejection fraction $\leq$ 40%, but at the time of randomization were not sufficiently symptomatic to require ACE inhibitor therapy for heart failure. About half of the patients had had symptoms of heart failure in the past. Patients were given a test dose of 6.25 mg oral captopril and were randomized within 3-16 days post-infarction to receive either captopril or placebo in addition to conventional therapy. Captopril was initiated at 6.25 or 12.5 mg tid and after two weeks titrated to a target maintenance dose of 50 mg tid. About 80% of patients were receiving the target dose at the end of the study. Patients were followed for a minimum of two years and for up to five years, with an average follow-up of 3.5 years.

Baseline blood pressure was 113/70 mm Hg and 112/70 mm Hg for the placebo and captopril groups, respectively. Blood pressure increased slightly in both treatment groups during the study and was somewhat lower in the captopril group (119/74 vs. 125/77 mm Hg at 1 yr).

Therapy with captopril improved long-term survival and clinical outcomes compared to placebo. The risk reduction of all cause mortality was 19% (P = 0.02) and for cardiovascular death was 21% (P = 0.014). Captopril treated subjects had 22% (P = 0.034) fewer first hospitalizations for heart failure. Compared to placebo, 22% fewer patients receiving captopril developed symptoms of overt heart failure. There was no significant difference between groups in total hospitalizations for all cause (2056 placebo; 2036 captopril).

Captopril was well tolerated in the presence of other therapies such as aspirin, beta blockers, nitrates, vasodilators, calcium antagonists and diuretics.

In a multicenter, double-blind, placebo controlled trial, 409 patients, age 18-49 of either gender, with or without hypertension, with type I (juvenile type, onset before age 30) insulin-dependent diabetes mellitus, retinopathy, proteinuria $\geq$ 500 mg per day and serum creatinine $\leq$ 2.5 mg/dl, were randomized to placebo or captopril (25 mg tid) and followed for up to 4.8 years (median 3 years). To achieve blood pressure control, additional hypertensive agents (diuretics, beta blockers, centrally acting agents or vasodilators) were added as needed for patients in both groups.

The captopril group had a 51% reduction in risk of doubling of serum creatinine ($P < 0.01$) and a 51% reduction in risk for the combined endpoint of end-stage renal disease (dialysis or transplantation) or death ($P < 0.01$). Captopril treatment resulted in a 30% reduction in urine protein excretion within the first 3 months ($P < 0.05$), which was maintained throughout the trial. The captopril group had somewhat better blood pressure control than the placebo group, but the effects of captopril on renal function were greater than would be expected from the group differences in blood pressure reduction alone. Captopril was well- tolerated in this patient population.

In two multicenter, double-blind, placebo controlled studies, a total of 235 normotensive patients with insulin-dependent diabetes mellitus, retinopathy and microalbuminuria (20-200 mcg/min) were randomized to placebo or captopril (50 mg bid) and followed for up to 2 years. Captopril delayed the progression to overt nephropathy (proteinuria $\geq$ 500 mg/day) in both studies (risk reduction 67% to 76%; $P < 0.05$). Captopril also reduced the albumin excretion rate. However, the long term clinical benefit of reducing the progression from microalbuminuria to proteinuria has not been established.

Studies in rats and cats indicate that captopril does not cross the blood-brain barrier to any significant extent.

INDICATIONS AND USAGE:

Hypertension: Captopril is indicated for the treatment of hypertension.

In using captopril, consideration should be given to the risk of neutropenia/agranulocytosis (see WARNINGS.)

Captopril may be used as initial therapy for patients with normal renal function, in whom the risk is relatively low. In patients with impaired renal function, particularly those with collagen vascular disease, captopril should be reserved for hypertensives who have either developed unacceptable side effects on other drugs, or have failed to respond satisfactorily to drug combinations.

Captopril is effective alone and in combination with other antihypertensive agents, especially thiazide-type diuretics. The blood pressure lowering effects of captopril and thiazides are approximately additive.

Heart Failure: Captopril is indicated in the treatment of congestive heart failure usually in combination with diuretics and digitalis. The beneficial effect of captopril in heart failure does not require the presence of digitalis, however, most controlled clinical trial experience with captopril has been in patients receiving digitalis, as well as diuretic treatment.

Left Ventricular Dysfunction After Myocardial Infarction: Captopril is indicated to improve survival following myocardial infarction in clinically stable patients with left ventricular dysfunction manifested as an ejection fraction $\leq$ 40% and to reduce the incidence of overt heart failure and subsequent hospitalizations for congestive heart failure in these patients.

Diabetic Nephropathy: Captopril is indicated for the treatment of diabetic nephropathy (proteinuria > 500 mg/day) in patients with type I insulin-dependent diabetes mellitus and retinopathy. Captopril decreases the rate of progression of renal insufficiency and development of serious adverse clinical outcomes (death or need for renal transplantation or dialysis).

CONTRAINDICATIONS:

Captopril is contraindicated in patients who are hypersensitive to this product or any other angiotensin-converting enzyme inhibitor (*e.g.,* a patient who has experienced angioedema during therapy with any other ACE inhibitor).

WARNINGS:

Anaphylactoid and Possibly Related Reactions: Presumably because angiotensin-converting enzyme inhibitors affect metabolism of eicosanoids and polypeptides, including endogenous bradykinin, patients receiving ACE inhibitors (including captopril) may be subject to a variety of adverse reactions, some of them serious.

WARNINGS: *(cont'd)*

Angioedema: Angioedema involving the extremities, face, lips, mucous membranes, tongue, glottis or larynx has been seen in patients treated with ACE inhibitors, including captopril. If angioedema involves the tongue, glottis or larynx, airway obstruction may occur and be fatal. Emergency therapy, including but not necessarily limited to, subcutaneous administration of a 1:1000 solution of epinephrine should be promptly instituted.

Swelling confined to the face, mucous membranes of the mouth, lips and extremities has usually resolved with discontinuation of captopril; some cases required medical therapy. See PRECAUTIONS, Information for Patients and ADVERSE REACTIONS.

Anaphylactoid Reactions During Desensitization: Two patients undergoing desensitizing treatment with hymenoptera while receiving ACE inhibitors sustained life-threatening anaphylactoid reactions. In the same patients, these reactions were avoided when ACE inhibitors were temporarily withheld, but they reappeared upon inadvertent rechallenge.

Anaphylactoid Reactions During Membrane Exposure: Anaphylactoid reactions should have been reported in patients dialyzed with high-flux membranes and treated concomitantly with an ACE inhibitor. Anaphylactoid reactions have also been reported in patients undergoing low-density lipoprotein aphresis with dextran sulfate absorption (a procedure dependent upon devices not approved in the United States).

Neutropenia/Agranulocytosis: Neutropenia (<1000/mm^3) with myeloid hypoplasia has resulted from use of captopril. About half of the neutropenic patients developed systemic or oral cavity infections or other features of the syndrome of agranulocytosis.

The risk of neutropenia is dependent on the clinical status of the patient.

In clinical trials in patients with hypertension who have normal renal function (serum creatinine less than 1.6 mg/dl and no collagen vascular disease), neutropenia has been seen in one patient out of over 8,600 exposed.

In patients with some degree of renal failure (serum creatinine at least 1.6 mg/dl) but no collagen vascular disease, the risk of neutropenia in clinical trials was about 1 per 500, a frequency over 15 times that for uncomplicated hypertension. Daily doses of captopril were relatively high in these patients, particularly in view of their diminished renal function. In foreign marketing experience in patients with renal failure, use of allopurinol concomitantly with captopril has been associated with neutropenia but this association has not appeared in U.S. reports.

In patients with collagen vascular diseases (*e.g.,* systemic lupus erythematosus, scleroderma) and impaired renal function, neutropenia occurred in 3.7 percent of patients in clinical trials.

While none of the over 750 patients in formal clinical trials of heart failure developed neutropenia, it has occurred during the subsequent clinical experience. About half of the reported cases has serum creatinine $\geq$ 1.6 mg/dl and more than 75 percent were in patients also receiving procainamide. In heart failure, it appears that the same risk factors for neutropenia are present.

The neutropenia has usually been detected within three months after captopril was started. Bone marrow examinations in patients with neutropenia consistently showed myeloid hypoplasia, frequently accompanied by erythroid hypoplasia and decreased numbers of megakaryocytes (*e.g.,* hypoplastic bone marrow and pancytopenia); anemia and thrombocytopenia were sometimes seen.

In general, neutrophils returned to normal in about two weeks after captopril was discontinued, and serious infections were limited to clinically complex patients. About 13 percent of the cases of neutropenia have ended fatally, but almost all fatalities were in patients with serious illness, having collagen vascular disease, renal failure, heart failure or immunosuppressant therapy, or a combination of these complicating factors.

Evaluation of the hypertensive or heart failure patient should always include assessment of renal function.

If captopril is used in patients with impaired renal function, white blood cell and differential counts should be evaluated prior to starting treatment and at approximately two-week intervals for about three months, then periodically.

In patients with collagen vascular disease or who are exposed to other drugs known to affect the white cells or immune response, particularly when there is impaired renal function, captopril should be used only after an assessment of benefit and risk, and then with caution.

All patients treated with captopril should be told to report any signs of infection (*e.g.,* sore throat, fever). If infection is suspected, white cell counts should be performed without delay.

Since discontinuation of captopril and other drugs has generally led to prompt return of the white count to normal, upon confirmation of neutropenia (neutrophil count <1000/mm^3) the physician should withdraw captopril and closely follow the patient's course.

PROTEINURIA

Total urinary proteins greater than 1 g per day were seen in about 0.7 percent of patients receiving captopril. About 90 percent of affected patients had evidence of prior renal disease or received relatively high doses of captopril (in excess of 150 mg/day), or both. The nephrotic syndrome occurred in about one-fifth of proteinuric patients. In most cases, proteinuria subsided or cleared within six months whether or not captopril was continued. Parameters of renal function, such as BUN and creatinine, were seldom altered in the patients with proteinuria.

HYPOTENSION

Excessive hypotension was rarely seen in hypertensive patients but is a possible consequence of captopril use in salt/volume depleted persons (such as those treated vigorously with diuretics), patients with heart failure or those patients undergoing renal dialysis. See DRUG INTERACTIONS.

In heart failure, where the blood pressure was either normal or low, transient decreases in mean blood pressure greater than 20 percent were recorded in about half of the patients. This transient hypotension is more likely to occur after any of the first several doses and is usually well tolerated, producing either no symptoms or brief mild lightheadedness, although in rare instances it has been associated with arrhythmia or conduction defects. Hypotension was the reason for discontinuation of drug in 3.6 percent of patients with heart failure.

BECAUSE OF THE POTENTIAL FALL IN BLOOD PRESSURE IN THESE PATIENTS, THERAPY SHOULD BE STARTED UNDER VERY CLOSE MEDICAL SUPERVISION. A starting dose of 6.25 or 12.5 mg tid may minimize the hypotensive effect. Patients should be followed closely for the first two weeks of treatment and whenever the dose of captopril and/or diuretic is increased. In patients with heart failure, reducing the dose of diuretic, if feasible, may minimize the fall in blood pressure.

Hypotension is not *per se* a reason to discontinue captopril. Some decrease of systemic blood pressure is a common and desirable observation upon initiation of captopril treatment in heart failure. The magnitude of the decease is greatest early in the course of treatment; this effect stabilizes within a week or two, and generally returns to pretreatment levels, without a decrease in therapeutic efficacy, within two months.

FETAL/NEONATAL MORBIDITY AND MORTALITY

ACE inhibitors can cause fetal and neonatal morbidity and death when administered to pregnant women. Several dozen cases have been reported in the world literature. When pregnancy is detected, ACE inhibitors should be discontinued as soon as possible.

WARNINGS: *(cont'd)*

The use of ACE inhibitors during the second and third trimesters of pregnancy has been associated with fetal and neonatal injury, including hypotension, neonatal skull hypoplasia, anuria, reversible or irreversible renal failure, and death. Oligohydramnios has also been reported, presumably resulting from decreased fetal renal function; oligohydramnios in this setting has been associated with fetal limb contractures, craniofacial deformation, and hypoplastic lung development. Prematurity, intrauterine growth retardation, and patent ductus arteriosus have also been reported, although it is not clear whether these occurrences where due to the ACE inhibitor exposure.

These adverse effects do not appear to have resulted from intrauterine ACE-inhibitor exposure that has been limited to the first trimester. Mothers whose embryos and fetuses are exposed to ACE inhibitors only during the first trimester should be so informed. Nonetheless, when patients become pregnant, physicians should make every effort to discontinue the use of captopril as soon as possible.

Rarely (probably less often than once in every thousand pregnancies), no alternative to ACE inhibitors will be found. In these rare cases, the mothers should be apprised of the potential hazards to their fetuses, and serial ultrasound examinations should be performed to assess the intraamniotic environment.

If oligohydramnios is observed, captopril should be discontinued unless it is considered life-saving for the mother. Contraction stress testing (CST), a non-stress test (NST), or biophysical profiling (BPP) may be appropriate, depending upon the week of pregnancy. Patients and physicians should be aware, however, that oligohydramnios may not appear until after the fetus has sustained irreversible injury.

Infants with histories of *in utero*exposure to ACE inhibitors should be closely observed for hypotension, oliguria, and hyperkalemia. If oliguria occurs, attention should be directed toward support of blood pressure and renal perfusion. Exchange transfusion or dialysis may be required as a means of reversing hypotension and/or substituting for disordered renal function. While captopril may be removed from the adult circulation by hemodialysis, there is inadequate data concerning the effectiveness of hemodialysis for removing it from the circulation of neonates or children. Peritoneal dialysis is not effective for removing captopril; there is no information concerning exchange transfusion for removing captopril from the general circulation.

When captopril was given to rabbits at doses about 0.8 to 70 times (on a mg/kg basis) the maximum recommended human dose, low incidences of craniofacial malformations were seen. No teratogenic effects of captopril were seen in studies of pregnant rats and hamsters. On a mg/kg basis, the doses used were up to 150 times (in hamsters) and 625 times (in rats) the maximum recommended human dose.

HEPATIC FAILURE

Rarely, ACE inhibitors have been associated with a syndrome that starts with cholestatic jaundice and progresses to fulminant hepatic necrosis and (sometimes) death. The mechanism of this syndrome is not understood. Patients receiving ACE inhibitors who develop jaundice or marked elevations of hepatic enzymes should discontinue the ACE inhibitor and receive appropriate medical follow-up.

PRECAUTIONS:

GENERAL

Impaired Renal Function

Hypertension: Some patients with renal disease, particularly those with severe renal artery stenosis, have developed increases in BUN and serum creatinine after reduction of blood pressure with captopril. Captopril dosage reduction and/or discontinuation of diuretic may be required. For some of these patients, it may not be possible to normalize blood pressure and maintain adequate renal perfusion.

Heart Failure: About 20 percent of patients develop stable elevations of BUN and serum creatinine greater than 20 percent above normal or baseline upon long-term treatment with captopril. Less than 5 percent of patients, generally those with severe preexisting renal disease, required discontinuation of treatment due to progressively increasing creatinine; subsequent improvement probably depends upon the severity of the underlying renal disease.

See CLINICAL PHARMACOLOGY, DOSAGE AND ADMINISTRATIONand ADVERSE REACTIONS: Alerted Laboratory Findings.

Hyperkalemia: Elevations in serum potassium have been observed in some patients treated with ACE inhibitors, including captopril. When treated with ACE inhibitors, patients at risk for the development of hyperkalemia include those with: renal insufficiency; diabetes mellitus; and those using concomitant potassium-sparing diuretics, potassium supplements or potassium-containing salt substitutes; or other drugs associated with increases in serum potassium. In a trial of type I diabetic patients with proteinuria, the incidence of withdrawal of treatment with captopril for hyperkalemia was 2% (4/207). In two trials of normotensive type 1 diabetic patients with microalbuminuria, no captopril group subjects had hyperkalemia (0/116) (See PRECAUTIONS, Information for Patients, DRUG INTERACTIONS and ADVERSE REACTIONS, Altered Laboratory Findings.)

Cough: Cough has been reported with the use of ACE inhibitors. Characteristically, the cough in nonproductive, persistent and resolves after discontinuation of therapy. ACE inhibitor-induced cough should be considered as part of the differential diagnosis of cough.

Valvular Stenosis: There is concern, on theoretical grounds, that patients with aortic stenosis might be at particular risk of decreased coronary perfusion when treated with vasodilators because they do not develop as much afterload reduction as others.

Surgery/Anesthesia: In patients undergoing major surgery or during anesthesia with agents that produce hypotension, captopril will block angiotensin II formation secondary to compensatory renin release. If hypotension occurs and is considered to be due to this mechanism, it can be corrected by volume expansion.

Hemodialysis: Recent clinical observations have shown an association of hypersensitivity-like (anaphylactoid) reactions during hemodialysis with high-flux dialysis membranes (*e.g.,* AN69) in patients receiving ACE inhibitors. In these patients, consideration should be given to using a different type of dialysis membrane or a different class of medication.

INFORMATION FOR PATIENTS

Patients should be advised to immediately report to their physician any signs or symptoms suggesting angioedema (*e.g.,* swelling of face, eyes, lips, tongue, larynx and extremities; difficulty in swallowing or breathing; hoarseness) and to discontinue therapy. (See WARNINGS.)

Patients should be told to report promptly any indication of infection (*e.g.,* sore throat, fever), which may be a sign of neutropenia, or of progressive edema which might be related to proteinuria and nephrotic syndrome.

All patients should be cautioned that excessive perspiration and dehydration may lead to an excessive fall in blood pressure because of reduction in fluid volume. Other causes of volume depletion such as vomiting or diarrhea may also lead to a fall in blood pressure; patients should be advised to consult with the physician.

Patients should be advised not to use potassium-sparing diuretics, potassium supplements or potassium-containing salt substitutes without consulting their physician. See PRECAUTIONS, General; DRUG INTERACTIONS, ADVERSE REACTIONS.

PRECAUTIONS: *(cont'd)*

Patients should be warned against interruption or discontinuation of medication unless instructed by the physician.

Heart failure patients on captopril therapy should be cautioned against rapid increases in physical activity.

Patients should be informed that captopril should be taken one hour before meals (see DOSAGE AND ADMINISTRATION.)

PREGNANCY

Pregnancy Categories C (first trimester) and D (second and third trimesters): See WARNINGS, Fetal/Neonatal Morbidity and Mortality.

Female patients of childbearing age should be told about the consequences of second- and third-trimester exposure to ACE inhibitors, and they should also be told that these consequences do not appear to have resulted from intrauterine ACE-inhibitor exposure that has been limited to the first trimester. These patients should be asked to report pregnancies to their physicians as soon as possible.

DRUG/LABORATORY TEST INTERACTION

Captopril may cause a false-positive urine test for acetone.

CARCINOGENESIS, MUTAGENESIS, AND IMPAIRMENT OF FERTILITY

Two-year studies with doses of 50 to 1350 mg/kg/day in mice and rats failed to show any evidence of carcinogenic potential. The high dose in these studies is 150 times the maximum recommended human dose of 450 mg, assuming a 50-kg subject. On a body-surface-area basis, the high doses for mice and rats are 13 and 26 times the maximum recommended human dose, respectively.

Studies in rats have revealed no impairment of fertility.

NURSING MOTHERS

Concentrations of captopril in human milk are approximately one percent of those in maternal blood. Because of the potential for serious adverse reactions in nursing infants from captopril, a decision should be made whether to discontinue nursing or to discontinue the drug, taking into account the importance of captopril to the mother. (See PRECAUTIONS, Pediatric Use.)

PEDIATRIC USE

Safety and effectiveness in children have not been established. There is limited experience reported in the literature with the use of captopril in the pediatric population; dosage, on a weight basis, was generally reported to be comparable to or less than that used in adults.

Infants, especially newborns, may be more susceptible to the adverse hemodynamic effects of captopril. Excessive, prolonged and unpredictable decreases in blood pressure and associated complications, including oliguria and seizures, have been reported.

Captopril should be used in children only if other measures for controlling blood pressure have not been effective.

DRUG INTERACTIONS:

Hypotension-Patients on Diuretic Therapy: Patients on diuretics and especially those in whom therapy was recently instituted, as well as those on severe dietary salt restriction or dialysis, may occasionally experience a precipitous reduction of blood pressure usually within the first hour after receiving the initial dose of captopril.

The possibility of hypotensive effects with captopril can be minimized by either discontinuing the diuretic or increasing the salt intake approximately one week prior to initiation of treatment with captopril or initiating therapy with small doses (6.25 or 12.5 mg). Alternatively, provide medical supervision for at least one hour after the initial dose. If hypotension occurs, the patient should be placed in a supine position and, if necessary, receive an intravenous infusion of normal saline. This transient hypotensive response is not a contraindication to further doses which can be given without difficulty once the blood pressure has increased after volume expansion.

Agents Having Vasodilator Activity: Data on the effect of concomitant use of other vasodilators in patients receiving captopril for heart failure are not available; therefore, nitroglycerin or other nitrates (as used for management of angina) or other drugs having vasodilator activity should, if possible, be discontinued before starting captopril. If resumed during captopril therapy, such agents should be administered cautiously, and perhaps at lower dosage.

Agents Causing Renin Release: Captopril's effect will be augmented by antihypertensive agents that cause renin release. For example, diuretics (*e.g.,* thiazides) may activate the renin-angiotensin-aldosterone system.

Agents Affecting Sympathetic Activity: The sympathetic nervous system may be especially important in supporting blood pressure in patients receiving captopril alone or with diuretics. Therefore, agents affecting sympathetic activity (*e.g.,* ganglionic blocking agents or adrenergic neuron blocking agents) should be used with caution. Beta-adrenergic blocking drugs add some further antihypertensive effect to captopril, but the overall response is less than additive.

Agents Increasing Serum Potassium: Since captopril decreases aldosterone production, elevation of serum potassium may occur. Potassium-sparing diuretics such as spironolactone, triamterene, or amiloride, or potassium supplements should be given only for documented hypokalemia, and then with caution, since they may lead to a significant increase of serum potassium. Salt substitutes containing potassium should also be used with caution.

Inhibitors Of Endogenous Prostaglandin Synthesis: It has been reported that indomethacin may reduce the antihypertensive effect of captopril, especially in cases of low renin hypertension. Other nonsteroidal anti-inflammatory agents (*e.g.,* aspirin) may also have this effect.

Lithium: Increased serum lithium levels and symptoms of lithium toxicity have been reported in patients receiving concomitant lithium and ACE inhibitor therapy. These drugs should be coadministered with caution and frequent monitoring of serum lithium levels is recommended. If a diuretic is also used, it may increase the risk of lithium toxicity.

ADVERSE REACTIONS:

Reported incidences are based on clinical trials involving approximately 7000 patients.

Renal: About one of 100 patients developed proteinuria (see WARNINGS.)

Each of the following has been reported in approximately 1 to 2 of 1000 patients and are of uncertain relationship to drug use: renal insufficiency, renal failure, nephrotic syndrome, polyuria, oliguria, and urinary frequency.

Hematologic: Neutropenia/agranulocytosis has occurred (see WARNINGS.) Cases of anemia, thrombocytopenia, and pancytopenia have been reported.

Dermatologic: Rash, often with pruritus, and sometimes with fever, arthralgia, and eosinophilia, occurred in about 4 to 7 (depending on renal status and dose) of 100 patients, usually during the first four weeks of therapy. It is usually maculopapular and rarely urticarial. The rash is usually mild and disappears within a few days of dosage reduction, short-term treatment with an antihistaminic agent, and/or discontinuing therapy; remission may occur even if captopril is continued. Pruritus, without rash, occurs in about 2 of 100 patients.

ADVERSE REACTIONS: *(cont'd)*

Between 7 and 10 percent of patients with skin rash have shown an eosinophilia and/or positive ANA titers. A reversible associated pemphigoid-like lesion, and photosensitivity, have also been reported.

Flushing or pallor has been reported in 2 to 5 of 1000 patients.

Cardiovascular: Hypotension may occur; see WARNINGSand DRUG INTERACTIONS for discussion of hypotension with captopril therapy.

Tachycardia, chest pain, and palpitations have each been observed in approximately 1 of 100 patients.

Angina pectoris, myocardial infarction, Raynaud's syndrome, and congestive heart failure have each occurred in 2 to 3 of 1000 patients.

Dysgeusia: Approximately 2 to 4 (depending on renal status and dose) of 100 patients developed a diminution or loss of taste perception. Taste impairment is reversible and usually self-limited (2 to 3 months) even with continued drug administration. Weight loss may be associated with the loss of taste.

Angioedema: Angioedema involving the extremities, face, lips, mucous membranes, tongue, glottis or larynx has been reported in approximately one in 1000 patients. Angioedema involving the upper airways has caused fatal airway obstruction. See WARNINGS and PRECAUTIONS, Information for Patients.

Cough: Cough has been reported in 0.5-2% of patients treated with captopril in clinical trials. See PRECAUTIONS, General, Cough.

The following have been reported in about 0.5 to 2 percent of patients but did not appear at increased frequency compared to placebo or other treatments used in controlled trials: gastric irritation, abdominal pain, nausea, vomiting, diarrhea, anorexia, constipation, aphthous ulcers, peptic ulcer, dizziness, headache, malaise, fatigue, insomnia, dry mouth, dyspnea, alopecia, paresthesias.

Other clinical adverse effects reported since the drug was marketed are listed below by body system. In this setting, an incidence or causal relationship cannot be accurately determined.

Body as a whole: Anaphylactoid reactions (see PRECAUTIONS, Hemodialysis).

General: Asthenia, gynecomastia.

Cardiovascular: Cardiac arrest, cerebrovascular accident/insufficiency, rhythm disturbances, orthostatic hypotension, syncope.

Dermatologic: Bullous pemphigus, erythema multiforme (including Stevens-Johnson syndrome), exfoliative dermatitis.

Gastrointestinal: Pancreatitis, glossitis, dyspepsia.

Hematologic: Anemia, including aplastic and hemolytic.

Hepatobiliary: Jaundic; hepatitis, including rare cases of necrosi; cholestasis.

Metabolic: Symptomatic hyponatremia.

Musculoskeletal: Myalgia, myasthenia.

Nervous/Psychiatric: Ataxia, confusion, depression, nervousness, somnolence.

Respiratory: Bronchospasm, eosinophilic pneumonitis, rhinitis.

Special Senses: Blurred vision.

Urogenital: Impotence.

As with other ACE inhibitors, a syndrome has been reported which may include: fever, myalgia, arthralgia, interstitial nephritis, vasculitis, rash or other dermatologic manifestations, eosinophilia and an elevated ESR.

Fetal/Neonatal Morbidity and Mortality: See WARNINGS, Fetal/Neonatal Morbidity and Mortality

ALTERED LABORATORY FINDINGS

Serum Electrolytes: *Hyperkalemia:* small increases in serum potassium, especially in patients with renal impairment (see PRECAUTIONS.) *Hyponatremia:* particularly in patients receiving a low sodium diet or concomitant diuretics.

BUN/Serum Creatinine: Transient elevations of BUN or serum creatinine especially in volume or salt depleted patients or those with renovascular hypertension may occur. Rapid reduction of longstanding or markedly elevated blood pressure can result in decreases in the glomerular filtration rate and, in turn, lead to increases in BUN or serum creatinine.

Hematologic: A positive ANA has been reported.

Liver Function Tests: Elevations of liver transaminases, alkaline phosphatase, and serum bilirubin have occurred.

OVERDOSAGE:

Correction of hypotension would be of primary concern. Volume expansion with an intravenous infusion of normal saline is the treatment of choice for restoration of blood pressure.

While captopril may be removed from the adult circulation by hemodialysis, there is inadequate data concerning the effectiveness of hemodialysis for removing it from the circulation of neonates or children. Peritoneal dialysis is not effective for removing captopril; there is no information concerning exchange transfusion for removing captopril from the general circulation.

DOSAGE AND ADMINISTRATION:

Captopril should be taken one hour before meals. Dosage must be individualized.

Hypertension: Initiation of therapy requires consideration of recent antihypertensive drug treatment, the extent of blood pressure elevation, salt restriction, and other clinical circumstances. If possible, discontinue the patient's previous antihypertensive drug regimen for one week before starting captopril.

The initial dose of captopril is 25 mg bid or tid. If satisfactory reduction of blood pressure has not been achieved after one or two weeks, the dose may be increased to 50 mg bid or tid. Concomitant sodium restriction may be beneficial when captopril is used alone.

The dose of captopril in hypertension usually does not exceed 50 mg tid. Therefore, if the blood pressure has not been satisfactorily controlled after one to two weeks at this dose, (and the patient is not already receiving a diuretic), a modest dose of a thiazide-type diuretic (*e.g.,* hydrochlorothiazide, 25 mg daily), should be added. The diuretic dose may be increased at one- to two-week intervals until its highest usual antihypertensive dose is reached.

If captopril is being started in a patient already receiving a diuretic, captopril therapy should be initiated under close medical supervision(see WARNINGS and DRUG INTERACTIONS) regarding hypotension, with dosage and titration of captopril as noted above.

If further blood pressure reduction is required, the dose of captopril may be increased to 100 mg bid or tid and then, if necessary, to 150 mg bid or tid (while continuing the diuretic). The usual dose range is 25 to 150 mg bid or tid. A maximum daily dose of 450 mg captopril should not be exceeded.

For patients with severe hypertension (*e.g.,* accelerated or malignant hypertension), when temporary discontinuation of current antihypertensive therapy is not practical or desirable, or when prompt titration to more normotensive blood pressure levels is indicated, diuretic should be continued but other current antihypertensive medication stopped and captopril dosage promptly initiated at 25 mg bid or tid, under close medical supervision.

DOSAGE AND ADMINISTRATION: *(cont'd)*

When necessitated by the patient's clinical condition, the daily dose of captopril may be increased every 24 hours or less under continuous medical supervision until a satisfactory blood pressure response is obtained or the maximum dose of captopril is reached. In this regimen, addition of a more potent diuretic, e.g., furosemide, may also be indicated.

Beta-blockers may also be used in conjunction with captopril therapy (see DRUG INTERACTIONS), but the effects of the two drugs are less than additive.

Heart Failure: Initiation of therapy requires consideration of recent diuretic therapy and the possibility of severe salt/volume depletion. In patients with either normal or low blood pressure, who have been vigorously treated with diuretics and who may be hyponatremic and/or hypovolemic, a starting dose of 6.25 or 12.5 mg tid may minimize the magnitude or duration of the hypotensive effect see WARNINGS, Hypotension ; for these patients, titration to the usual daily dosage can then occur within the next several days.

For most patients the usual initial daily dosage is 25 mg tid. After a dose of 50 mg tid is reached, further increases in dosage should be delayed, where possible, for at least two weeks to determine if a satisfactory response occurs. Most patients studied have had a satisfactory clinical improvement at 50 or 100 mg tid. A maximum daily dose of 450 mg of captopril should not be exceeded.

Captopril should generally be used in conjunction with a diuretic and digitalis. Captopril therapy must be initiated under very close medical supervision.

Left Ventricular Dysfunction After Myocardial Infarction: The recommended dose for long-term use in patients following a myocardial infarction is a target maintenance dose of 50 mg tid.

Therapy may be initiated as early as three days following a myocardial infarction. After a single dose of 6.25 mg. Captopril therapy should be initiated at 12.5 mg tid. Captopril should then be increased to 25 mg tid during the next several days and to a target dose of 50 mg tid over the next several weeks as tolerated (see CLINICAL PHARMACOLOGY.)

Captopril may be used in patients treated with other post-myocardial infarction therapies, e.g., thrombolytics, aspirin, beta blockers.

Diabetic Nephropathy: The recommended dose of captopril for long term use to treat diabetic nephropathy is 25 mg tid.

Other antihypertensives such as diuretics, beta blockers, centrally acting agents or vasodilators may be used in conjunction with captopril if additional therapy is required to further lower blood pressure.

Dosage Adjustment in Renal Impairment: Because captopril is excreted primarily by the kidneys, excretion rates are reduced in patients with impaired renal function. These patients will take longer to reach steady-state captopril levels and will reach higher steady-state levels for a given daily dose than patients with normal renal function. Therefore, these patients may respond to smaller or less frequent doses.

Accordingly, for patients with significant renal impairment, initial daily dosage of captopril should be reduced, and smaller increments utilized for titration, which should be quite slow (one-to two-week intervals). After the desired therapeutic effect has been achieved, the dose should be slowly back-titrated to determine the minimal effective dose. When concomitant diuretic therapy is required, a loop diuretic (*e.g.,* furosemide), rather than a thiazide diuretic, is preferred in patients with severe renal impairment. See also PRECAUTIONS, Hemodialysis.

Do not store above 86° F. Keep bottles tightly closed (protect from moisture).

ANIMAL PHARMACOLOGY:

Animal Toxicology: Chronic oral toxicity studies were conducted in rats (2 years), dogs (47 weeks; 1 year), mice (2 years), and monkeys (1 year). Significant drug-related toxicity included effects on hematopoiesis, renal toxicity, erosion/ulceration of the stomach, and variation of retinal blood vessels.

Reductions in hemoglobin and/or hematocrit values were seen in mice, rats, and monkeys at doses 50 to 150 times the maximum recommended human dose (MRHD) of 450 mg, assuming a 50-mg subject. On a body-surface-area, these doses are 5 to 25 times the maximum recommended human dose (MRHD). Anemia, leukopenia, thrombocytopenia, and bone marrow suppression occurred in dogs at doses 8 to 30 times MRHD on a body-weight basis (4 to 15 times MRHD on a surface-area basis). The reductions in hemoglobin and hematocrit values in rats and mice were only significant at 1 year and returned to normal with continued dosing by the end of the study. Marked anemia was seen at all dose levels (8 to 30 times MRHD) in dogs, whereas moderate to marked leukopenia was noted only at 15 and 30 times the MRHD and thrombocytopenia at 30 times the MRHD. The anemia could be reversed upon discontinuation of dosing. Bone marrow suppression occurred to a varying degree, being associated only with dogs that died or were sacrificed in a moribund condition in the 1 year study. However, in the 47-week study at a dose 30 times MRHD, bone marrow suppression was found to be reversible upon continued drug administration.

Captopril caused hyperplasia of the juxtaglomerular apparatus of the kidneys in mice and rats at doses 7 to 200 times MRHD on a body-weight basis (0.6 to 35 times MRHD on a surface-area basis); in monkeys at 20 to 60 times MRHD on a body-weight basis (7 to 20 times MRHD on a surface- area basis); and in dogs at 30 times MRHD on a body-weight basis (15 times MRHD on a surface-area basis).

Gastric erosions/ulcerations were increased in incidence in male rats at 20 to 200 times MRHD on a body-weight basis (3.5 and 35 times MRHD on a surface-area basis); in dogs at 30 times MRHD on a body-weight basis (15 times on MRHD on a surface-area basis); and in monkeys at 65 times MRHD on a body-weight basis (20 times MRHD on a surface-area basis). Rabbits developed gastric and intestinal ulcers when given oral doses approximately 30 times MRHD on a body-weight basis (10 times MRHD on a surface-area basis) for only 5 to 7 days.

In the two-year rat study, irreversible and progressive variations in the caliber of retinal vessels (focal sacculations and constrictions) occurred at all dose levels (7 to 200 times MRHD) on a body-weight basis; 1 to 35 times MRHD on a surface-area basis in a dose-related fashion. The effect was first observed in the 88th week of dosing, with a progressively increased incidence thereafter, even after cessation of dosing.

PATIENT INFORMATION:

Captopril is an angiotensin-converting enzyme (ACE) inhibitor used for the treatment of high blood pressure or heart failure; following a myocardial infarction (heart attack); or for diabetic nephropathy (kidney disease). Notify your physician if you are pregnant or nursing. The use of captopril during months four through nine of pregnancy may permanently injure or cause the death of the developing fetus. Avoid using potassium containing salt substitutes without notifying your physician. Captopril should be taken on any empty stomach, at least one hour before eating. Dizziness, lightheadedness or fainting may occur after the first dose or during the first week of therapy. Avoid sudden changes in posture. A persistent dry cough or taste alterations may occur while taking captopril. Notify your physician if these become bothersome. Notify your physician if you develop trouble swallowing or breathing; swelling of the face, lips, or tongue; irregular heartbeat; rash, hives or severe itching; unexplained fever; or easy bruising.

HOW SUPPLIED - RATED THERAPEUTICALLY EQUIVALENT:

Tablet - Oral - 12.5 mg

100's	$4.43	Captopril, H.C.F.A. F F P	99999-0642-01
100's	$62.80	Captopril, Mylan	00378-3007-01
100's	$64.51	Captopril, Duramed Pharms	51285-0950-02
1000's	$621.33	Captopril, Mylan	00378-3007-10
1000's	$630.32	Captopril, Duramed Pharms	51285-0950-05

Tablet - Oral - 25 mg

100's	$6.66	Captopril, H.C.F.A. F F P	99999-0642-02
100's	$67.88	Captopril, Mylan	00378-3012-01
100's	$69.74	Captopril, Duramed Pharms	51285-0951-02
1000's	$671.86	Captopril, Mylan	00378-3012-10
1000's	$689.12	Captopril, Duramed Pharms	51285-0951-05

Tablet - Oral - 50 mg

100's	$11.63	Captopril, H.C.F.A. F F P	99999-0642-03
100's	$116.41	Captopril, Mylan	00378-3017-01
100's	$119.50	Captopril, Duramed Pharms	51285-0952-02
1000's	$1151.74	Captopril, Mylan	00378-3017-10
1000's	$1163.23	Captopril, Duramed Pharms	51285-0952-05

Tablet - Oral - 100 mg

100's	$20.82	Captopril, H.C.F.A. F F P	99999-0642-04
100's	$155.02	Captopril, Mylan	00378-3022-01
100's	$159.25	Captopril, Duramed Pharms	51285-0953-02
500's	$796.25	Captopril, Duramed Pharms	51285-0953-04

Tablet, Uncoated - Oral - 12.5 mg

100's	**$66.99**	**CAPOTEN, Bristol Myers Squibb**	**00003-0450-51**
100's	**$67.09**	**CAPOTEN, Bristol Myers Squibb**	**00003-0450-54**
1000's	**$663.86**	**CAPOTEN, Bristol Myers Squibb**	**00003-0450-75**
5000's	**$3485.25**	**Capoten, Bristol Myers Squibb**	**00003-0450-06**

Tablet, Uncoated - Oral - 25 mg

100's	**$72.53**	**CAPOTEN, Bristol Myers Squibb**	**00003-0452-50**
100's	**$73.09**	**CAPOTEN, Bristol Myers Squibb**	**00003-0452-51**
1000's	**$717.83**	**CAPOTEN, Bristol Myers Squibb**	**00003-0452-75**
5000's	**$3768.60**	**CAPOTEN, Bristol Myers Squibb**	**00003-0452-39**

Tablet, Uncoated - Oral - 50 mg

100's	**$124.33**	**CAPOTEN, Bristol Myers Squibb**	**00003-0482-51**
100's	**$124.38**	**CAPOTEN, Bristol Myers Squibb**	**00003-0482-50**
1000's	**$1230.56**	**CAPOTEN, Bristol Myers Squibb**	**00003-0482-75**
5000's	**$6460.40**	**Capoten, Bristol Myers Squibb**	**00003-0482-06**

Tablet, Uncoated - Oral - 100 mg

100's	**$165.63**	**CAPOTEN, Bristol Myers Squibb**	**00003-0485-50**

CAPTOPRIL; HYDROCHLOROTHIAZIDE

(000643)

CATEGORIES: ACE Inhibitors; Angiotensin Converting Enzyme Inhibitors; Antihypertensives; Cardiovascular Drugs; Diuretics; Hypertension; Renal Drugs; Thiazides; Pregnancy Category C; FDA Approved 1984 Oct

BRAND NAMES: *Aceaide*; *Acediur*; *Aceplus*; *Acezide* (England); *Angiopril D.U.*; *Capozid*; **Capozide**; *Capozide Forte*; *Capride*; *Captea* (France); *Captopril-H*; *Captoprilan-D*; *Cesplon Plus*; *Ecapres-D*; *Ecazide* (France); *Lopiretic*
(International brand names outside U.S. in italics)

FORMULARIES: BC-BS; Medi-Cal

COST OF THERAPY: $538.37 (Hypertension; Tablet; 25 mg/15 mg; 2/day; 365 days) vs. Potential Cost of $24,027.04 (Coronary Bypass)

PRIMARY ICD9: 401.1 (Essential Hypertension, Benign)

> WARNING:
> USE IN PREGNANCY: When used in pregnancy during the second and third semesters, ACE inhibitors can cause injury and even death to the developing fetus When pregnancy is detected, captopril hydrochlorothiazide should be discontinued as soon as possible. See WARNINGS, Captopril, Fetal Neonatal Morbidity and Mortality.

DESCRIPTION:

Captopril hydrochlorothiazide for oral administration combines two antihypertensive agents: Capoten (captopril) and hydrochlorothiazide. Captopril, the first of a new class of antihypertensive agents, is a specific competitive inhibitor of angiotensin I-converting enzyme (ACE), the enzyme responsible for the conversion of angiotensin I to angiotensin II. Hydrochlorothiazide is a benzothiadiazide (thiazide) diuretic-antihypertensive. Capozide tablets are available in four combinations of captopril with hydrochlorothiazide: 25 mg with 15 mg, 25 mg with 25 mg, 50 mg with 15 mg, and 50 mg with 25 mg. Inactive ingredients: microcrystalline cellulose, colorant (FD&C Yellow No. 6), lactose, magnesium stearate, pregelatinized starch, and stearic acid.

Captopril is designated chemically a 1-[(2S)-3-mercapto-2-methylpropionyl]-L-proline; hydrochlorothiazide is 6-Chloro-3,4-dihydro-2*H*-1,2,4-benzothiadiazine-7-sulfonamide 1,1-dioxide.

Captopril is a white to off-white crystalline powder that may have a light sulfurous odor; it is soluble in water (approx. 160 mg/ml), methanol, and ethanol and sparingly soluble in chloroform and ethyl acetate.

Hydrochlorothiazide is a white crystalline powder slightly soluble in water but freely soluble in sodium hydroxide solution.

CLINICAL PHARMACOLOGY:

CAPTOPRIL

Mechanism of Action: The mechanism of action of captopril has not yet been fully elucidated. Its beneficial effects in hypertension and heart failure appear to result primarily from suppression of the renin-angiotensin-aldosterone system. However, there is no consistent correlation between renin levels and response to the drug. Renin, an enzyme synthesized by the kidneys, is released into the circulation where it acts on a plasma globulin substrate to produce angiotensin I, a relatively inactive decapeptide. Angiotensin I is then converted by angiotensin converting enzyme (ACE) to angiotensin II, a potent endogenous vasoconstrictor substance. Angiotensin II also stimulates aldosterone secretion from the adrenal cortex, thereby contributing to sodium and fluid retention.

CLINICAL PHARMACOLOGY: *(cont'd)*

Captopril prevents the conversion of angiotensin I to angiotensin II by inhibition of ACE, a peptidyldipeptide carboxy hydrolase. This inhibition has been demonstrated in both healthy human subjects and in animals by showing that the elevation of blood pressure caused by exogenously administered angiotensin I was attenuated or abolished by captopril. In animal studies, captopril did not alter the pressor responses to a number of other agents, including angiotensin II and norepinephrine, indicating specificity of action.

ACE is identical to "bradykininase", and captopril may also interfere with the degradation of the vasodepressor peptide, bradykinin. Increased concentrations of bradykinin or prostaglandin E_2 may also have a role in the therapeutic effect of captopril.

Inhibition of ACE results in decreased plasma angiotensin II and increased plasma renin activity (PRA), the latter resulting from loss of negative feedback on renin release caused by reduction in angiotensin II. The reduction of angiotensin II leads to decreased aldosterone secretion, and, as a result, small increases in serum potassium may occur along with sodium and fluid loss.

The antihypertensive effects persist for a longer period of time than does demonstrable inhibition of circulating ACE. It is not known whether the ACE present in vascular endothelium is inhibited longer than the ACE in circulating blood.

Pharmacokinetics: After oral administration of therapeutic doses of captopril, rapid absorption occurs with peak blood levels at about one hour. The presence of food in the gastrointestinal tract reduces absorption by about 30 to 40 percent; captopril therefore should be given one hour before meals. Based on carbon-14 labeling, average minimal absorption is approximately 75 percent. In a 24-hour period, over 95 percent of the absorbed dose is eliminated in the urine; 40 to 50 percent is unchanged drug; most of the remainder is the disulfide dimer of captopril and captopril-cysteine disulfide.

Approximately 25 to 30 percent of the circulating drug is bound to plasma proteins. The apparent elimination half-life for total radioactivity in blood is probably less than three hours. An accurate determination of half-life of unchanged captopril is not, at present, possible, but it is probably less than two hours. In patients with renal impairment, however, retention of captopril occurs (see DOSAGE AND ADMINISTRATION).

Pharmacodynamics: Administration of captopril results in a reduction of peripheral arterial resistance in hypertensive patients with either no change, or an increase, in cardiac output. There is an increase in renal blood flow following administration of captopril and glomerular filtration rate is usually unchanged. In patients with heart failure, significantly decreased peripheral (systemic vascular) resistance and blood pressure (afterload), reduced pulmonary capillary wedge pressure (preload) and pulmonary vascular resistance, increased cardiac output, and increased exercise tolerance time (ETT) have been demonstrated.

Reductions of blood pressure are usually maximal 60 to 90 minutes after oral administration of an individual dose of captopril. The duration of effect is dose related. The reduction in blood pressure may be progressive, so to achieve maximal therapeutic effects, several weeks of therapy may be required. The blood pressure lowering effects of captopril and thiazide-type diuretics are additive. In contrast, captopril and beta-blockers have a less than additive effect.

Blood pressure is lowered to about the same extent in both standing and supine positions. Orthostatic effects and tachycardia are infrequent but may occur in volume-depleted patients. Abrupt withdrawal of captopril has not been associated with a rapid increase in blood pressure.

Studies in rats and cats indicate that captopril does not cross the blood-brain barrier to any significant extent.

HYDROCHLOROTHIAZIDE

Thiazides affect the renal tubular mechanism of electrolyte reabsorption. At maximal therapeutic dosage all thiazides are approximately equal in their diuretic potency.

Thiazides increase excretion of sodium and chloride in approximately equivalent amounts. Natriuresis causes a secondary loss of potassium and bicarbonate.

The mechanism of the antihypertensive effect of thiazides is unknown. Thiazides do not affect normal blood pressure.

The mean plasma half-life of hydrochlorothiazide in fasted individuals has been reported to be approximately 2.5 hours.

Onset of diuresis occurs in two hours and the peak effect at about four hours. Its action persists for approximately six to twelve hours. Hydrochlorothiazide is eliminated rapidly by the kidney.

INDICATIONS AND USAGE:

Captopril hydrochlorothiazide is indicated for the treatment of hypertension. The blood pressure lowering effects of captopril and thiazides are approximately additive.

This fixed combination drug may be used as initial therapy or substituted for previously titrated doses of the individual components.

When captopril and hydrochlorothiazide are given together it may not be necessary to administer captopril in divided doses to attain blood pressure control at trough (before the next dose). Also, with such a combination, a daily dose of 15 mg of hydrochlorothiazide may be adequate.

Treatment may, therefore, be initiated with captopril hydrochlorothiazide 25 mg/15 mg once daily. Subsequent titration should be with additional doses of the components (captopril, hydrochlorothiazide) as single agents or as captopril hydrochlorothiazide 50 mg/15 mg, 25 mg/25 mg, or 50 mg/25 mg (see DOSAGE AND ADMINISTRATION).

In using captopril hydrochlorothiazide, consideration should be given to the risk of neutropenia/agranulocytosis (see WARNINGS).

Captopril hydrochlorothiazide may be used for patients with normal renal function, in whom the risk is relatively low. In patients with impaired renal function, particularly those with collagen vascular disease, captopril hydrochlorothiazide should be reserved for hypertensives who have either developed unacceptable side effects on other drugs, or have failed to respond satisfactorily to other drug combinations.

CONTRAINDICATIONS:

Captopril: This product is contraindicated in patients who are hypersensitive to captopril or any other angiotensin-converting enzyme inhibitor (*e.g.*, a patient who has experienced angioedema during therapy with any other ACE inhibitor).

Hydrochlorothiazide: Hydrochlorothiazide is contraindicated in anuria. It is also contraindicated in patients who have previously demonstrated hypersensitivity to hydrochlorothiazide or other sulfonamide-derived drugs.

WARNINGS:

CAPTOPRIL

Angioedema: Angioedema involving the extremities, face, lips, mucous membranes, tongue, glottis or larynx has been seen in patients treated with ACE inhibitors, including captopril. If angioedema involves the tongue, glottis or larynx, airway obstruction may occur and be fatal. Emergency therapy, including but not necessarily limited to, subcutaneous administration of a 1:1000 solution of epinephrine should be promptly instituted.

WARNINGS: *(cont'd)*

Swelling confined to the face, mucous membranes of the mouth, lips and extremities has usually resolved with discontinuation of treatment; some cases required medical therapy. (See PRECAUTIONS, Information for Patients and ADVERSE REACTIONS, Captopril).

Neutropenia/Agranulocytosis: Neutropenia(<1000/mm^3) with myeloid hypoplasia has resulted from use of captopril. About half of the neutropenic patients developed systemic or oral cavity infections or other features of the syndrome of agranulocytosis.

The risk of neutropenia is dependent on the clinical status of the patient.

In clinical trials in patients with hypertension who have normal renal function (serum creatinine less than 1.6 mg/dl and no collagen vascular disease), neutropenia has been seen in one patient out of over 8,600 exposed.

In patients with some degree of renal failure (serum creatinine at least 1.6 mg/dl) but no collagen vascular disease, the risk of neutropenia in clinical trials was about 1 per 500, a frequency over 15 times that for uncomplicated hypertension. Daily doses of captopril were relatively high in these patients, particularly in view of their diminished renal function. In foreign marketing experience in patients with renal failure, use of allopurinol concomitantly with captopril has been associated with neutropenia but this association has not appeared in U.S. reports.

In patients with collagen vascular diseases (*e.g.,* systemic lupus erythematosus, scleroderma) and impaired renal function, neutropenia occurred in 3.7 percent of patients in clinical trials.

While none of the over 750 patients in formal clinical trials of heart failure developed neutropenia, it has occurred during the subsequent clinical experience. About half of the reported cases had serum creatinine ≥ 1.6 mg/dl and more than 75 percent were in patients also receiving procainamide. In heart failure, it appears that the same risk factors for neutropenia are present.

The neutropenia has usually been detected within three months after captopril was started. Bone marrow examinations in patients with neutropenia consistently showed myeloid hypoplasia, frequently accompanied by erythroid hypoplasia and decreased numbers of megakaryocytes (*e.g.,* hypoplastic bone marrow and pancytopenia); anemia and thrombocytopenia were sometimes seen.

In general, neutrophils returned to normal in about two weeks after captopril was discontinued, and serious infections were limited to clinically complex patients. About 13 percent of the cases of neutropenia have ended fatally, but almost all fatalities were in patients with serious illness, having collagen vascular disease, renal failure, heart failure or immunosuppressant therapy, or a combination of these complicating factors.

Evaluation of the hypertensive or heart failure patient should always include assessment of renal function. If captopril is used in patients with impaired renal function, white blood cell and differential counts should be evaluated prior to starting treatment and at approximately two-week intervals for about three months, then periodically.

In patients with collagen vascular disease or who are exposed to other drugs known to affect the white cells or immune response, particularly when there is impaired renal function, captopril should be used only after an assessment of benefit and risk, and then with caution.

All patients treated with captopril should be told to report any signs of infection (*e.g.,* sore throat, fever). If infection is suspected, white cell counts should be performed without delay.

Since discontinuation of captopril and other drugs has generally led to prompt return of the white count to normal, upon confirmation of neutropenia (neutrophil count <1000/mm^3) the physician should withdraw captopril and closely follow the patient's course.

Proteinuria: Total urinary proteins greater than 1 g per day were seen in about 0.7 percent of patients receiving captopril. About 90 percent of affected patients had evidence of prior renal disease or received relatively high doses of captopril (in excess of 150 mg/day), or both. The nephrotic syndrome occurred in about one-fifth of proteinuric patients. In most cases, proteinuria subsided or cleared within six months whether or not captopril was continued. Parameters of renal function, such as BUN and creatinine, were seldom altered in the patients with proteinuria.

Since most cases of proteinuria occurred by the eighth month of therapy with captopril, patients with prior renal disease or those receiving captopril at doses greater than 150 mg per day, should have urinary protein estimations (dip-stick on first morning urine) prior to treatment, and periodically thereafter.

Hypotension: Excessive hypotension was rarely seen in hypertensive patients but is a possible consequence of captopril use in salt/volume depleted persons (such as those treated vigorously with diuretics), patients with heart failure or those patients undergoing renal dialysis. See DRUG INTERACTIONS.

Fetal/Neonatal Morbidity and Mortality: ACE inhibitors can cause fetal and neonatal morbidity and mortality when administered to pregnant women. Several dozen cases have been reported in the world literature. When pregnancy is detected, ACE inhibitors should be discontinued as soon as possible.

The use of ACE inhibitors have been used during the second and third trimesters of pregnancy has been associated with fetal and neonatal injury, including hypotension, neonatal skull hypoplasia, anuria, reversible or irreversible renal failure and death. Oligohydramnios has also been reported, presumably representing decreased renal function; oligohydramnios in this setting has been associated with fetal limb contractures, craniofacial deformation, and hypoplastic lung development. Prematurity, intrauterine growth retardation, and patent ductus arteriosus have also been reported, although it is not clear whether these occurrences were due to the ACE inhibitor exposure.

The adverse effects do not appear to have resulted from intrauterine ACE-inhibitor exposure that has been limited to the first trimester. Mothers whose embryos and fetuses are exposed to ACE inhibitors only during the first trimester should be so informed. Nonetheless, when patients become pregnant, physicians should make every effort to discontinue the use of captopril as soon as possible.

Rarely (probably less often than once in every thousand pregnancies), no alternative to ACE inhibitors will be found. In these rare cases, the mothers should be apprised of the potential hazards to their fetuses, and serial ultrasound examinations should be performed to assess the intraamniotic environment.

If oligohydramnios is observed, captopril should be discontinued unless it is considered life-saving to the mother. Contraction stress testing (CST), a non-stress test (NST), or biophysical profiling (BPP) may be appropriate, depending upon the week of pregnancy. Patients and physicians should be aware, however, that oligohydramnios may not appear until after the fetus has sustained irreversible injury.

Infants exposed *in utero* to ACE inhibitors should be closely observed for hypotension, oliguria, and hyperkalemia. If oliguria occurs, attention should be directed toward support of blood pressure and renal perfusion. Exchange transfusion or dialysis may be required as a means of reversing hypotension and/or substituting for disordered renal function. While captopril may be removed from the adult circulation by hemodialysis, there is inadequate data concerning the effectiveness of hemodialysis, there is inadequate data concerning the effectiveness of hemodialysis for removing it from the circulation of neonates or children. Peritoneal dialysis is not effective for removing captopril; there is no information concerning exchange transfusion for removing captopril from the general circulation.

WARNINGS: *(cont'd)*

When captopril was given to rabbits at doses about 0.8 to 70 times (on a mg/kg basis) the maximum recommended human dose, and low incidence of craniofacial malformations were seen. No teratogenic effect of captopril were seen in studies of pregnant rats and hamsters. On a mg/kg basis, the doses used were up to 150 times (in hamsters) and 625 times (in rats) the maximum recommended human dose.

HYDROCHLOROTHIAZIDE

Thiazides should be used with caution in severe renal disease. In patients with renal disease, thiazides may precipitate azotemia. Cumulative effects of the drug may develop in patients with impaired renal function.

Thiazides should be used with caution in patients with impaired hepatic function or progressive liver disease, since minor alterations of fluid and electrolyte balance may precipitate hepatic coma.

Sensitivity reactions may occur in patients with or without a history of allergy or bronchial asthma.

The possibility of exacerbation or activation of systemic lupus erythematosus has been reported.

In general, lithium should not be given with diuretics (see PRECAUTIONS, Hydrochlorothiazide).

PRECAUTIONS:

GENERAL

Captopril

Impaired Renal Function: Some patients with renal disease, particularly those with severe renal artery stenosis, have developed increases in BUN and serum creatinine after reduction of blood pressure with captopril. Captopril dosage reduction and/or discontinuation of diuretic may be required. For some of the patients, it may not be possible to normalize blood pressure and maintain adequate renal perfusion (see CLINICAL PHARMACOLOGY, DOSAGE AND ADMINISTRATION, ADVERSE REACTIONS, Altered Laboratory Findings).

Hyperkalemia: Elevations in serum potassium have been observed in some patients treated with ACE inhibitors, including captopril. When treated it ACE inhibitors, patients at risk for the development of hyperkalemia include those with: renal insufficiency; diabetes mellitus; and those using concomitant potassium-sparing diuretics, potassium supplements or potassium-containing salt substitutes; or other drugs associated with increases in serum potassium. (See PRECAUTIONS, Information for Patient,DRUG INTERACTIONS, Captopril, ADVERSE REACTIONS, Altered Laboratory Findings.)

Cough: Cough has been reported with the use of ACE inhibitors. Characteristically, the cough is non productive, persistent and resolves after discontinuation of therapy. ACE inhibitor-induced cough should be considered as part of the differential diagnosis of cough.

Surgery/Anesthesia: In patients undergoing major surgery or during anesthesia with agents that produce hypotension, captopril will block angiotensin II formation secondary to compensatory renin release. If hypotension occurs and is considered to be due to this mechanism, it can be corrected by volume expansion.

Hydrochlorothiazide

Periodic determination of serum electrolytes to detect possible electrolyte imbalance should be performed at appropriate intervals.

All patients receiving thiazide therapy should be observed for clinical signs of fluid or electrolyte imbalance, namely: hyponatremia, hypochloremic alkalosis, and hypokalemia. Serum and urine electrolyte determinations are particularly important when the patient is vomiting excessively or receiving parenteral fluids. Warning signs or symptoms of fluid and electrolyte imbalance may include: dryness of mouth, thirst, weakness, lethargy, drowsiness, restlessness, muscle pains or cramps, muscular fatigue, hypotension, oliguria, tachycardia, and gastrointestinal disturbances such as nausea and vomiting.

Hypokalemia may develop, especially with brisk diuresis, or when severe cirrhosis is present. Interference with adequate oral electrolyte intake will also contribute to hypokalemia. Hypokalemia can sensitize or exaggerate the response of the heart to the toxic effects of digitalis (e.g., increased ventricular irritability). Because captopril reduces the production of aldosterone, concomitant therapy with captopril reduces the diuretic-induced hypokalemia. Fewer patients may require potassium supplements and/or foods with a high potassium content (see DRUG INTERACTIONS, Agents Increasing Serum Potassium).

Any chloride deficit is generally mild and usually does not require specific treatment except under extraordinary circumstances (as in liver disease or renal disease). Dilutional hyponatremia may occur in edematous patients in hot weather; appropriate therapy is water restriction, rather than administration of salt except in rare instances when the hyponatremia is life-threatening. In actual salt depletion, appropriate replacement is the therapy of choice.

Hyperuricemia may occur or frank gout may be precipitated in certain patients receiving thiazide therapy.

Latent diabetes mellitus may become manifest during thiazide administration.

The antihypertensive effect of thiazide diuretics may be enhanced in the postsympathectomy patient.

If progressive renal impairment becomes evident, as indicated by a rising nonprotein nitrogen or blood urea nitrogen (BUN), a careful reappraisal of therapy is necessary with consideration given to withholding or discontinuing diuretic therapy.

Thiazides may decrease serum PBI levels without signs of thyroid disturbance.

Calcium excretion is decreased by thiazides. Pathological changes in the parathyroid gland with hypercalcemia and hypophosphatemia have been observed in a few patients on prolonged thiazide therapy. The common complications of hyperparathyroidism such as renal lithiasis, bone resorption, and peptic ulceration have not been seen. Thiazides should be discontinued before carrying out tests for parathyroid function.

Thiazides have been shown to increase the urinary excretion of magnesium; this may result in hypomagnesemia.

INFORMATION FOR PATIENTS

Patients should be advised to immediately report to their physician any signs or symptoms suggesting angioedema (*e.g.,* swelling of face, eyes, lips, tongue, larynx and extremities; difficulty in swallowing or breathing; hoarseness) and to discontinue therapy. See WARNINGS, Captopril.

Patients should be told to report promptly any indication of infection (*e.g.,* sore throat, fever), which may be a sign of neutropenia, or of progressive edema which might be related to proteinuria and nephrotic syndrome.

All patients should be cautioned that excessive perspiration and dehydration may lead to an excessive fall in blood pressure because of reduction in fluid volume. Other causes of volume depletion such as vomiting or diarrhea may also lead to a fall in blood pressure; patients should be advised to consult with the physician.

Patients should be advised not to use potassium-sparing diuretics, potassium supplements or potassium-containing salt substitutes without consulting their physician. See PRECAUTIONS, General, DRUG INTERACTIONS, Captopril and ADVERSE REACTIONS, Captopril.

PRECAUTIONS: *(cont'd)*

Patients should be warned against interruption or discontinuation of medication unless instructed by the physician.

Heart failure patients on captopril therapy should be cautioned against rapid increases in physical activity.

Patients should be informed that captopril hydrochlorothiazide should be taken one hour before meals (see DOSAGE AND ADMINISTRATION).

PREGNANCY

Female patients of childbearing age should be told about the consequences of second- and third-trimester exposure to ACE inhibitors, and they should also be told that these consequences do not appear to have resulted from intrauterine ACE-inhibitor exposure that has been limited to the first trimester. These patients should be asked to report pregnancies to their physicians as soon as possible.

LABORATORY TESTS

Serum electrolyte levels should be regularly monitored (see WARNINGS, Captopriland Hydrochlorothiazide, and PRECAUTIONS, General, Hydrochlorothiazide).

DRUG/LABORATORY TEST INTERACTIONS

Captopril: Captopril may cause a false-positive urine test for acetone.

Hydrochlorothiazide: Hydrochlorothiazide may cause diagnostic interference of the bentiromide test.

CARCINOGENESIS, MUTAGENESIS, AND IMPAIRMENT OF FERTILITY

Captopril: Two-year studies with doses of 50 to 1350 mg/kg/day in mice and rats failed to show any evidence of carcinogenic potential.

Studies in rats have revealed no impairment of fertility.

Hydrochlorothiazide: Long-term studies in animals have not been performed to evaluate carcinogenic potential, mutagenesis, or whether this drug affects fertility in males or females.

PREGNANCY

Categories C (first trimester) and D (second and third trimesters): See WARNINGS, Captopril, Fetal/Neonatal Morbidity and Mortality.

Nonteratogenic Effects: *Hydrochlorothiazide:* Thiazides cross the placental barrier and appear in cord blood. The use of thiazides in pregnant women requires that the anticipated benefit be weighed against possible hazards to the fetus. These hazards include fetal or neonatal jaundice, thrombocytopenia, and possibly other adverse reactions which have occurred in the adult.

NURSING MOTHERS

Both captopril and hydrochlorothiazide are excreted in human milk. Because of the potential for serious adverse reactions in nursing infants from both drugs, a decision should be made whether to discontinue nursing or to discontinue therapy taking into account the importance of captopril hydrochlorothiazide to the mother. See PRECAUTIONS, Pediatric Use.

PEDIATRIC USE

Safety and effectiveness in children have not been established. There is limited experience reported in the literature with the use of captopril in the pediatric population; dosage, on a weight basis, was generally reported to be comparable to or less than that used in adults.

Infants, especially newborns, may be more susceptible to the adverse hemodynamic effects of captopril. Excessive, prolonged and unpredictable decreases in blood pressure and associated complications, including oliguria and seizures, have been reported.

Captopril hydrochlorothiazide should be used in children only if other measures for controlling blood pressure have not been effective.

DRUG INTERACTIONS:

CAPTOPRIL

Hypotension—Patients on Diuretic Therapy: Patients on diuretics and especially those in whom diuretic therapy was recently instituted, as well as those on severe dietary salt restriction or dialysis, may occasionally experience a precipitous reduction of blood pressure usually within the first hour after receiving the initial dose of captopril.

The possibility of hypotensive effects with captopril can be minimized by either discontinuing the diuretic or increasing the salt intake approximately one week prior to initiation of treatment with captopril or initiating therapy with small doses (6.25 or 12.5 mg). Alternatively, provide medical supervision for at least one hour after the initial dose. If hypotension occurs, the patient should be placed in a supine position and, if necessary, receive an intravenous infusion of normal saline. This transient hypotensive response is not a contraindication to further doses which can be given without difficulty once the blood pressure has increased after volume expansion.

Agents Having Vasodilator Activity: Data on the effect of concomitant use of other vasodilators in patients receiving captopril for heart failure are not available; therefore, nitroglycerin or other nitrates (as used for management of angina) or other drugs having vasodilator activity should, if possible, be discontinued before starting captopril. If resumed during captopril therapy, such agents should be administered cautiously, and perhaps at lower dosage.

Agents Causing Renin Release: Captopril's effect will be augmented by antihypertensive agents that cause renin release. For example, diuretics (*e.g.,* thiazides) may activate the renin-angiotensin- aldosterone system.

Agents Affecting Sympathetic Activity: The sympathetic nervous system may be especially important in supporting blood pressure in patients receiving captopril alone or with diuretics. Therefore, agents affecting sympathetic activity (*e.g.,* ganglionic blocking agents or adrenergic neuron blocking agents) should be used with caution. Beta-adrenergic blocking drugs add some further antihypertensive effect to captopril, but the overall response is less than additive.

Agents Increasing Serum Potassium: Since captopril decreases aldosterone production, elevation of serum potassium may occur. Potassium-sparing diuretics such as spironolactone, triamterene, or amiloride, or potassium supplements, should be given only for documented hypokalemia, and then with caution, since they may lead to a significant increase of serum potassium. Salt substitutes containing potassium should also be used with caution.

Inhibitors Of Endogenous Prostaglandin Synthesis: It has been reported that indomethacin may reduce the antihypertensive effect of captopril, especially in cases of low renin hypertension. Other nonsteroidal anti-inflammatory agents (*e.g.,* aspirin) may also have this effect.

Lithium: Increased serum lithium levels and symptoms of lithium toxicity have been reported in patients receiving concomitant lithium and ACE inhibitor therapy. These drugs should be coadministered with caution and frequent monitoring of serum lithium levels is recommended. If a diuretic is also used, it may increase the risk of lithium toxicity (see DRUG INTERACTIONS, Hydrochlorothiazide, Lithium).

HYDROCHLOROTHIAZIDE

When administered concurrently the following drugs may interact with thiazide diuretics:

Alcohol, barbiturates, or narcotics: potentiation of orthostatic hypotension may occur.

Amphotericin B, corticosteroids, or corticotropin (ACTH): may intensify electrolyte imbalance, particularly hypokalemia. Monitor potassium levels; use potassium replacements if necessary.

DRUG INTERACTIONS: *(cont'd)*

Anticoagulants (oral): dosage adjustments of anticoagulant medication may be necessary since hydrochlorothiazide may decrease their effects.

Antigout medications: dosage adjustments of antigout medication may be necessary since hydrochlorothiazide may raise the level of blood uric acid.

Other antihypertensive medications (*e.g.,* ganglionic or peripheral adrenergic blocking agents): dosage adjustments may be necessary since hydrochlorothiazide may potentiate their effects.

Antidiabetic drugs (oral agents and insulin): since thiazides may elevate blood glucose levels, dosage adjustments of antidiabetic agents may be necessary.

Calcium salts: increased serum calcium levels due to decreased excretion may occur. If calcium must be prescribed monitor serum calcium levels and adjust calcium dosage accordingly.

Cardiac glycosides: enhanced possibility of digitalis toxicity associated with hypokalemia. Monitor potassium levels (see DRUG INTERACTIONS, Captopril).

Cholestyramine resin and colestipol HCL: may delay or decrease absorption of hydrochlorothiazide. Sulfonamide diuretics should be taken at least one hour before or four to six hours after these medications.

Diazoxide: enhanced hyperglycemic, hyperglycemic, and antihypertensive effects. Be cognizant of possible interaction; monitor blood glucose and serum uric acid levels.

Lithium: diuretic agents reduce the renal clearance of lithium and increase the risk of lithium toxicity. These drugs should be coadministered with caution and frequent monitoring of serum lithium levels is recommended (see DRUG INTERACTIONS, Captopril, Lithium).

MAO inhibitors: dosage adjustments of one or both agents may be necessary since hypotensive effects are enhanced.

Nondepolarizing muscle relaxants, preanesthetics and anesthetics used in surgery (*e.g.,* tubocurarine chloride and gallamine triethiodide): effects of these agents may be potentiated; dosage adjustments may be required. Monitor and correct any fluid and electrolyte imbalances prior to surgery if feasible.

Nonsteroidal anti-inflammatory agents: in some patients, the administration of a nonsteroidal anti-inflammatory agent can reduce the diuretic, natriuretic, and antihypertensive effect of loop, potassium-sparing or thiazide diuretics. Therefore, when hydrochlorothiazide and nonsteroidal anti-inflammatory agents are used concomitantly, the patient should be observed closely to determine if the desired effect of the diuretic is obtained.

Methenamine: possible decreased effectiveness due to alkalinization of the urine.

Pressor amines (*e.g.,* norepinephrine): decreased arterial responsiveness, but not sufficient to preclude effectiveness of the pressor agent for therapeutic use. Use caution in patients taking both medications who undergo surgery. Administer preanesthetic and anesthetic agents in reduced dosage, and if possible, discontinue hydrochlorothiazide therapy one week prior to surgery.

Probenecid or sulfinpyrazone: increased dosage of these agents may be necessary since hydrochlorothiazide may have hyperuricemic effects.

ADVERSE REACTIONS:

CAPTOPRIL

Reported incidences are based on clinical trials involving approximately 7000 patients.

Renal: About one of 100 patients developed proteinuria (see WARNINGS).

Each of the following has been reported in approximately 1 to 2 of 1000 patients and are of uncertain relationship to drug use: renal insufficiency, renal failure, nephrotic syndrome, polyuria, oliguria, and urinary frequency.

Hematologic: Neutropenia/agranulocytosis has occurred (see WARNINGS.) Cases of anemia, thrombocytopenia, and pancytopenia have been reported.

Dermatologic: Rash, often with pruritus, and sometimes with fever, arthralgia, and eosinophilia, occurred in about 4 to 7 (depending on renal status and dose) of 100 patients, usually during the first four weeks of therapy. It is usually maculopapular, and rarely urticarial. The rash is usually mild and disappears within a few days of dosage reduction, short-term treatment with an antihistaminic agent, and/or discontinuing therapy; remission may occur even if captopril is continued. Pruritus. without rash, occurs in about 2 of 100 patients. Between 7 and 10 percent of patients with skin rash have shown eosinophilia and/or positive ANA titers. A reversible associated pemphigoid-like lesion, and photosensitivity, have also been reported.

Flushing or pallor has been reported in 2 to 5 of 1000 patients.

Cardiovascular: Hypotension may occur; see WARNINGS and DRUG INTERACTIONS for discussion of hypotension with captopril therapy.

Tachycardia, chest pain, and palpitations have each been observed in approximately 1 of 100 patients.

Angina pectoris, myocardial infarction, Raynaud's syndrome, and congestive heart failure have each occurred in 2 to 3 of 1000 patients.

Dysgeusia: Approximately 2 to 4 (depending on renal status and dose) of 100 patients developed a diminution or loss of taste perception. Taste impairment is reversible and usually self-limited (2 to 3 months) even with continued drug administration. Weight loss may be associated with the loss of taste.

Angioedema: Angioedema involving the extremities, face, lips, mucous membranes, tongue, glottis or larynx has been reported in approximately one in 1000 patients. Angioedema involving the upper airways has caused fatal airway obstruction. (See WARNINGS, Captopril) and PRECAUTIONS, Information for Patients.

Cough: Cough has been reported in 0.5-2% of patients treated with captopril in clinical trials.

The following have been reported in about 0.5 to 2 percent of patients but did not appear at increased frequency compared to placebo or other treatments used in controlled trials: gastric irritation, abdominal pain, nausea, vomiting, diarrhea, anorexia, constipation, aphthous ulcers, peptic ulcer, dizziness, headache, malaise, fatigue, insomnia, dry mouth, dyspnea, alopecia, paresthesias.

Other clinical adverse effects reported since the drug was marketed are listed below by body system. In this setting, an incidence or causal relationship cannot be accurately determined.

General: asthenia, gynecomastia.

Cardiovascular: cardiac arrest, cerebrovascular accident/insufficiency, rhythm disturbances, orthostatic hypotension, syncope.

Dermatologic: bullous pemphigus, erythema multiforme (including Stevens-Johnson syndrome), exfoliative dermatitis.

Gastrointestinal: pancreatitis, glossitis, dyspepsia.

Hematologic: anemia, including aplastic and hemolytic.

Hepatobiliary: jaundice, hepatitis, including rare cases of necrosis, cholestasis.

Metabolic: symptomatic hyponatremia.

Musculoskeletal: myalgia, myasthenia.

Nervous/Psychiatric: ataxia, confusion, depression, nervousness, somnolence.

Respiratory: bronchospasm, eosinophilic pneumonitis, rhinitis.

ADVERSE REACTIONS: *(cont'd)*

Special Senses: blurred vision.

Urogenital: impotence.

As with other ACE inhibitors, a syndrome has been reported which may include: fever, myalgia, arthralgia, interstitial nephritis, vasculitis, rash or other dermatologic manifestations, eosinophilia and an elevated ESR.

Fetal/Neonatal Morbidity and Mortality: See WARNINGS, Captopril, Fetal/Neonatal Morbidity and Mortality.

HYDROCHLOROTHIAZIDE

Gastrointestinal System: anorexia, gastric irritation, nausea, vomiting, cramping, diarrhea, constipation, jaundice (intrahepatic cholestatic jaundice), pancreatitis, and sialadenitis.

Central Nervous System: dizziness, vertigo, paresthesias, headache, and xanthopsia.

Hematologic: leukopenia, agranulocytosis, thrombocytopenia, aplastic anemia, and hemolytic anemia.

Cardiovascular: orthostatic hypotension.

Hypersensitivity: purpura, photosensitivity, rash, urticaria, necrotizing angiitis (vasculitis; cutaneous vasculitis), fever, respiratory distress including pneumonitis, and anaphylactic reactions.

Other: hyperglycemia, glycosuria, hyperuricemia, muscle spasm, weakness, restlessness, and transient blurred vision.

Whenever adverse reactions are moderate or severe, thiazide dosage should be reduced or therapy withdrawn.

ALTERED LABORATORY FINDINGS

Serum Electrolytes: Hyperkalemia: small increases in serum potassium, especially in patients with renal impairment (see PRECAUTIONS, Captopril).

Hyponatremia: particularly in patients receiving a low sodium diet or concomitant diuretics.

BUN/Serum Creatinine: Transient elevations of BUN or serum creatinine especially in volume or salt depleted patients or those with renovascular hypertension may occur. Rapid reduction of longstanding or markedly elevated blood pressure can result in decreases in the glomerular filtration rate and, in turn, lead to increases in BUN or serum creatinine.

Hematologic: A positive ANA has been reported.

Liver Function Tests: Elevations of liver transaminases, alkaline phosphatase, and serum bilirubin have occurred.

OVERDOSAGE:

Captopril: Correction of hypotension would be of primary concern. Volume expansion with an intravenous infusion of normal saline is the treatment of choice for restoration of blood pressure.

While captopril may be removed from the adult circulation by hemodialysis, there is inadequate data concerning the effectiveness of hemodialysis for removing it from the circulation of neonates or children. Peritoneal dialysis is not effective for removing captopril; there is no information concerning exchange transfusion for removing captopril from the general circulation.

Hydrochlorothiazide: In addition to the expected diuresis, overdosage of thiazides may produce varying degrees of lethargy which may progress to coma within a few hours, with minimal depression of respiration and cardiovascular function and without evidence of serum electrolyte changes or dehydration. The mechanism of thiazide-induced CNS depression is unknown. Gastrointestinal irritation and hypermotility may occur. Transitory increase in BUN has been reported, and serum electrolyte changes may occur, especially in patients with impaired renal function.

In addition to gastric lavage and supportive therapy for stupor or coma, symptomatic treatment of gastrointestinal effects may be needed. The degree to which hydrochlorothiazide is removed by hemodialysis has not been clearly established. Measures as required to maintain hydration, electrolyte balance, respiration, and cardiovascular and renal function should be instituted.

DOSAGE AND ADMINISTRATION:

DOSAGE MUST BE INDIVIDUALIZED ACCORDING TO PATIENT'S RESPONSE.

Captopril hydrochlorothiazide may be substituted for the previously titrated individual components.

Alternatively, therapy may be instituted with a single tablet of captopril hydrochlorothiazide 25 mg/15 mg taken once daily. For patients insufficiently responsive to the initial dose, additional captopril or hydrochlorothiazide may be added as individual components or by using captopril hydrochlorothiazide 50 mg/15 mg, 25 mg/25 mg or 50 mg/25 mg, or divided doses may be used.

Because the full effect of a given dose may not be attained for 6-8 weeks, dosage adjustments should generally be made at 6 week intervals, unless the clinical situation demands more rapid adjustment.

In general, daily doses of captopril should not exceed 150 mg and of hydrochlorothiazide should not exceed 50 mg.

Dosage Adjustment In Renal Impairment: Because captopril and hydrochlorothiazide are excreted primarily by the kidneys, excretion rates are reduced in patients with impaired renal function. These patients will take longer to reach steady-state captopril levels and will reach higher steady-state levels for a given daily dose than patients with normal renal function. Therefore, these patients may respond to smaller or less frequent doses of captopril hydrochlorothiazide.

After the desired therapeutic effect has been achieved, the dose intervals should be increased or the total daily dose reduced until the minimal effective dose is achieved. When concomitant diuretic therapy is required in patients with severe renal impairment, a loop diuretic (*e.g.*, furosemide), rather than a thiazide diuretic is preferred for use with captopril; therefore, for patients with severe renal dysfunction the captopril-hydrochlorothiazide combination tablet is not usually recommended.

ANIMAL PHARMACOLOGY:

Animal Toxicology: Chronic oral toxicity studies were conducted in rats (2 years), dogs (47 weeks; 1 year), mice (2 years), and monkeys (1 year). Significant drug-related toxicity included effects on hematopoiesis, renal toxicity, erosion/ulceration of the stomach, and variation of retinal blood vessels.

Reductions in hemoglobin and/or hematocrit values were seen in mice, rats, and monkeys at doses 50 to 150 times the maximum recommended human dose (MRHD). Anemia, leukopenia, thrombocytopenia, and bone marrow suppression occurred in dogs at doses 8 to 30 times MRHD. The reductions in hemoglobin and hematocrit values in rats and mice were only significant at 1 year and returned to normal with continued dosing by the end of the study. Marked anemia was seen at all dose levels (8 to 30 times MRHD) in dogs, whereas moderate to marked leukopenia was noted only at 15 and 30 times MRHD and thrombocytopenia at 30 times MRHD. The anemia could be reversed upon discontinuation of dosing. Bone marrow suppression occurred to a varying degree, being associated only with dogs that died or were sacrificed in a moribund condition in the 1 year study. However, in the 47-week study at a dose 30 times MRHD, bone marrow suppression was found to be reversible upon continued drug administration.

Captopril caused hyperplasia of the juxtaglomerular apparatus of the kidneys at doses 7 to 200 times the MRHD in rats and mice, at 20 to 60 times MRHD in monkeys, and at 30 times the MRHD in dogs.

Gastric erosions/ulcerations were increased in incidence at 20 and 200 times MRHD in male rats and at 30 and 65 times MRHD in dogs and monkeys, respectively. Rabbits developed gastric and intestinal ulcers when given oral doses approximately 30 times MRHD for only five to seven days.

In the two-year rat study, irreversible and progressive variations in the caliber of retinal vessels (focal sacculations and constrictions) occurred at all dose levels (7 to 200 times MRHD) in a dose-related fashion. The effect was first observed in the 88th week of dosing, with a progressively increased incidence thereafter, even after cessation of dosing.

HOW SUPPLIED:

CAPOZIDE TABLETS

25 mg captopril combined with 15 mg hydrochlorothiazide: Tablets are white and distinct orange mottling; they are biconvex rounded squares with quadrisect bars.

25 mg captopril combined with 25 mg hydrochlorothiazide: Tablets are peach-colored and may show slight mottling; they are biconvex rounded squares with quadrisect bars.

50 mg captopril combined with 15 mg hydrochlorothiazide: Tablets are white with distinct orange mottling; they are biconvex ovals with a bisect bar.

50 mg captopril combined with 25 mg hydrochlorothiazide: Tablets are peach-colored and may show slight mottling; they are biconvex ovals with a bisect bar.

Storage: Keep bottles tightly closed (protect from moisture); do not store above 86°F.

HOW SUPPLIED - EQUIVALENTS NOT AVAILABLE:

Tablet, Uncoated - Oral - 25 mg/15 mg

100's	$73.75	CAPOZIDE 25/15, Bristol Myers Squibb	00003-0338-50

Tablet, Uncoated - Oral - 25 mg/25 mg

100's	$73.75	CAPOZIDE 25/25, Bristol Myers Squibb	00003-0349-50

Tablet, Uncoated - Oral - 50 mg/15 mg

100's	$126.65	CAPOZIDE 50/15, Bristol Myers Squibb	00003-0384-50

Tablet, Uncoated - Oral - 50 mg/25 mg

100's	$126.65	CAPOZIDE 50/25, Bristol Myers Squibb	00003-0390-50

CARAMIPHEN; PHENYLPROPANOLAMINE

(000644)

CATEGORIES: Antitussives; Antitussives/Expectorants/Mucolytics; Common Cold; Cough Preparations; DESI Drugs; Nasal Congestion; Respiratory & Allergy Medications; FDA Pre 1938 Drugs

BRAND NAMES: Anti-Gen; Anti-Tussive; Balnade Dmh; Bionade C; Decongex-D; Detuss; Dixotuss; Oratuss; Ordrine At; Rescaps-D; Tuss Allergine; Tuss Danabe; Tuss Genade; Tuss Vernade T.D.; Tuss-Ade; Tuss-Allergine; Tuss-Genade; **Tuss-Ornade**; Tussadon; Tussogest; Uni-Tuss No. 2

Prescribing information not available at time of publication.

HOW SUPPLIED - EQUIVALENTS NOT AVAILABLE:

Capsule, Gelatin, Sustained Action - Oral - 40 mg/75 mg

50's	$38.95	ORDRINE AT, Eon Labs Mfg	00185-0345-53
100's	$12.50	UNI-TUSS #2, United Res	00677-1100-01
100's	$14.92	TUSS ALLERGINE, Rugby	00536-4741-01
100's	$15.92	DE-TUSS, HL Moore Drug Exch	00839-6372-06
100's	$35.15	RESCAPS-D S.R., Geneva Pharms	00781-2847-01
500's	$67.89	DE-TUSS, HL Moore Drug Exch	00839-6372-12
500's	$324.95	ORDRINE AT, Eon Labs Mfg	00185-0345-05

Liquid - Oral - 6.7 mg/12.5 mg

480 ml	$9.75	Oratuss, Consolidated Midland	00223-6574-01
3840 ml	$58.48	Oratuss, Consolidated Midland	00223-6574-02

CARBACHOL *(000645)*

CATEGORIES: Antiglaucomatous Agents; Cholinesterase Inhibitors; EENT Drugs; Eye, Ear, Nose, & Throat Preparations; Glaucoma; Intraocular Miotic; Intraocular Pressure; Miotics; Ocular Hypertension; Ophthalmics; Parasympathomimetic Agents; Conjunctivitis*; Corneal Ulcer*; FDA Approval Pre 1982

* Indication not approved by the FDA

BRAND NAMES: *Carbachol*; *Carbamann* (Germany); *Carbamil*; Carbastat; *Carbyl*; *Doryl*; *Glaumarin* (Japan); Isopto Carbachol; *Isopto Karbakolin*; *Karbakolin Isopto*; **Miostat**

(International brand names outside U.S. in italics)

FORMULARIES: Aetna; BC-BS; Medi-Cal

COST OF THERAPY: $191.62 (Glaucoma; Solution; 1.5 %; 0.6/day; 365 days) vs. Potential Cost of $1,851.63 (Iredectomy)

PRIMARY ICD9: 365.11 (Primary Open-Angle Glaucoma)

DESCRIPTION:

Please note that the brand names have been used throughout this monograph to avoid confusion.

Isopto (Carbachol) is a cholinergic prepared as a sterile topical ophthalmic solution. The active ingredient is represented by the chemical structure: $(NH_2COOOH_2CH_2N(CH_3)_3)^+Cl^-$

Established name: Carbachol

Chemical Name: 2-[(Aminocarbonyl)oxy]-*N,N,N*- trimethylethanaminium chloride.

Each ml contains: Active: Carbachol 0.75%, 1.5%, 2.25% or 3.0%.**Preservative:**Benzalkonium Chloride 0.005%. **Vehicle:**Hydroxypropyl Methylcellulose 1.0%. **Inactive:** Boric Acid, Sodium Chloride, Sodium Borate, Purified Water.

Miostat (Carbachol 0.01%) is a sterile balanced salt solution of carbachol for intraocular injection.

Established name: Carbachol

DESCRIPTION: *(cont'd)*

Chemical name: Ethanaminium, 2-[(aminocarbonyl)oxy]-N,N,N-trimethyl-chloride.

Each ml contains: Active: Carbachol 0.01%. **Inactives:** Sodium Chloride 0.64%, Potassium Chloride 0.075%, Calcium Chloride Dihydrate 0.048%, Magnesium Chloride Hexahydrate 0.03%, Sodium Acetate Trihydrate 0.39%, Sodium Citrate Dihydrate 0.17%, Sodium Hydroxide and/or Hydrochloric Acid (to adjust pH) and Water for Injection.

CLINICAL PHARMACOLOGY:

A cholinergic (parasympathomimetic) agent. Carbachol has a double action, it not only stimulates the motor endplate of the muscle cell, as do all cholinesters, but it also partially inhibits cholinesterase.

INDICATIONS AND USAGE:

Carbachol Solution: For lowering intraocular pressure in the treatment of glaucoma.

Carbachol Injection: Intraocular use for miosis during surgery.

CONTRAINDICATIONS:

Carbachol Solution: Miotics are contraindicated where constriction is undesirable such as acute iritis. Contraindicated in those persons showing hypersensitivity to any component of this preparation.

Carbachol Injection: This product should not be used in those persons showing hypersensitivity to any of the components of this preparation.

WARNINGS:

Carbachol Solution: For topical use only. Not for injection. Carbachol should be used with caution in the presence of corneal abrasion to avoid excessive penetration which can produce systemic toxicity; and in patients with acute cardiac failure, bronchial asthma, active peptic ulcer, hyperthyroidism, gastrointestinal spasm, urinary tract obstruction, Parkinson's disease, recent myocardial infarct, systemic hypertension or hypotension. As with all miotics, retinal detachment has been reported when used in certain susceptible individuals.

Carbachol Injection: For single-dose intraocular use only. Discard unused portion. Intraocular carbachol 0.01% should be used with caution in patients with acute cardiac failure, bronchial asthma, peptic ulcer, hyperthyroidism, G.I. spasm, urinary tract obstruction and Parkinson's disease.

PRECAUTIONS:

Carbachol Solution: General Avoid overdosage.

Information for the Patient The miosis usually causes difficulty in dark adaptation. Patient should be advised to exercise caution in night driving and other hazardous occupations in poor light. Do not touch dropper tip to any surface, as this may contaminate the solution.

Carcinogenesis, Mutagenesis, and Impairment of Fertility There have been no long-term studies done using carbachol in animals to evaluate carcinogenic potential.

Pregnancy Pregnancy Category C. Animal reproduction studies have not been conducted with carbachol. It is also not known whether carbachol can cause fetal harm when administered to a pregnant woman or can affect reproduction capacity. This drug should be given to a pregnant woman only if clearly needed.

Nursing Mothers It is not known whether this drug is excreted in human milk. Because many drugs are excreted in human milk, caution should be exercised when carbachol is administered to a nursing woman.

ADVERSE REACTIONS:

Carbachol Solution: Transient symptoms of stinging and burning may occur. This preparation is capable of producing systemic symptoms of cholinesterase inhibitor even when the epithelium is intact. Transient ciliary and conjunctival injection, headache, and ciliary spasm with resultant temporary decrease of visual acuity may occur. Salivation, syncope, cardiac arrhythmia, gastrointestinal cramping, vomiting asthma, hypotension, diarrhea, frequent urge to urinate, increased sweating, and irritation of eyes may occur.

Carbachol Injection: Side effects such as flushing, sweating, epigastric distress, abdominal cramps, tightness in urinary bladder, and headache have been reported after systemic or topical use of carbachol. These symptoms were not reported following intraocular use of carbachol 0.01% in pre-marketing studies. Corneal clouding, persistent bullous keratopathy and post-operative iritis following cataract extraction with utilization of intraocular carbachol have been reported in an occasional patient. As with all miotics are used in certain susceptible individuals.

OVERDOSAGE:

Atropine should be administered parenterally (for dosage refer to Goodman & Gilman or other pharmacology reference).

DOSAGE AND ADMINISTRATION:

Carbachol Solution: Instill two drops topically in the eye(s) up to three times daily or as indicated by physician.

Carbachol Injection: Aseptically remove the sterile vial from the blister package by peeling the backing paper and dropping the vial onto a sterile tray. Withdraw the contents into a dry sterile syringe, and replace the needle with an atraumatic cannula prior to intraocular irrigation. **No more than one-half milliliter** should be gently instilled into the anterior chamber for the production of satisfactory miosis. It may be instilled before or after securing sutures. Miosis is usually maximal within two to five minutes after application.

HOW SUPPLIED:

Isopto 15 ml and 30 ml in plastic DROP-TAINER Dispensers.

Storage: Store at 46° - 80°F (8° - 27°C).

Miostat In 1.5 ml sterile glass vials packaged twelve to a carton.

Storage: Store at controlled room temperature 15°-30°C (59° - 86°F).

(Ophthalmic Solution, Alcon, 238325, 9/94)

(Intraocular Solution, Alcon, 342006, 4/95)

HOW SUPPLIED - RATED THERAPEUTICALLY EQUIVALENT:

Solution - Intraocular - 0.01 %

1.5 ml	**$330.00**	**MIOSTAT, Alcon**	**00065-0023-15**

Solution - Intraocular; In - 0.01 %

1.5 ml x 12	$264.24	Carbastat, Ciba Vision	58768-0735-12

HOW SUPPLIED - NOT RATED EQUIVALENT:

Solution - Ophthalmic - 0.75 %

15 ml	$17.50	ISOPTO CARBACHOL, Alcon-PR	00998-0221-15

HOW SUPPLIED - NOT RATED EQUIVALENT: *(cont'd)*

Solution - Ophthalmic - 1.5 %

15 ml	$18.44	ISOPTO CARBACHOL, Alcon-PR	00998-0223-15
30 ml	$26.25	ISOPTO CARBACHOL, Alcon-PR	00998-0223-30

Solution - Ophthalmic - 2.25 %

15 ml	$19.37	ISOPTO CARBACHOL, Alcon-PR	00998-0224-15

Solution - Ophthalmic - 3 %

15 ml	$7.59	Carbachol, Apotex	60505-7507-05
15 ml	$20.31	ISOPTO CARBACHOL, Alcon-PR	00998-0225-15
30 ml	$27.50	ISOPTO CARBACHOL, Alcon-PR	00998-0225-30

CARBAMAZEPINE *(000646)*

CATEGORIES: Analgesics; Anticonvulsants; Antiepileptics; Central Nervous System Agents; Central Pain Syndromes; Convulsions; Epilepsy; Narcotics, Synthetics & Combinations; Neuromuscular; Pain; Seizures; Tonic-Clonic Seizures; Trigeminal Neuralgia; Alcoholism*; Bipolar Disorder*; Depression*; Mania*; Restless Leg Syndrome*; Sedation*; Pregnancy Category C; Sales >$500 Million; FDA Approval Pre 1982; Patent Expiration 1990 Dec; Top 200 Drugs
* Indication not approved by the FDA

BRAND NAMES: *Apo-Carbamazepine* (Canada); Atretol; *Camapine*; *Carbadac*; *Carbatol*; *Carbazene*; *Carbazep* (Mexico); *Carbazina* (Mexico); *Carbazine*; *Carmaz*; *Carmine*; *Carmine CR*; *Carpaz*; *Carzepin*; *Carzepine*; *Convuline*; *Degranol*; *Eleptin*; *Epileptol*; *Epileptol CR*; Epitol; *Foxalepsin* (Germany); *Foxalepsin Retard* (Germany); *Hermolepsin*; *Karbamazepin*; *Kodapan* (Japan); *Lexin* (Japan); *Macrepan*; *Mazepine* (Canada); *Mazetol*; *Neugeron* (Mexico); *Neurotol*; *Neurotop*; *Neurotop Retard*; *Nordotol* (Mexico); *Panitol*; *Prozine*; *Sirtal* (Germany); *Tardotol*; *Taver*; *Tegol*; *Tegretal* (Germany); **Tegretol**; *Tegretol CR* (Australia); *Tegretol-S*; *Telesmin* (Japan); *Temporol*; *Temporal Slow*; *Teril* (Australia); *Timonil* (Germany); *Timonil Retard* (Germany); *Zeptol*
(International brand names outside U.S. in italics)

FORMULARIES: Aetna; BC-BS; CIGNA; FHP; Humana; Kaiser; Medco; Medi-Cal; PCS; PruCare; United; WHO

COST OF THERAPY: $147.16 (Epilepsy; Tablet; 200 mg; 4/day; 365 days)

PRIMARY ICD9: 345.90 (Epilepsy, Unspecified, Without Mention of Intractable)

WARNING:
APLASTIC ANEMIA AND AGRANULOCYTOSIS HAVE BEEN REPORTED IN ASSOCIATION WITH THE USE OF CARBAMAZEPINE. DATA FROM A POPULATION-BASED CASE CONTROL STUDY DEMONSTRATE THAT THE RISK OF DEVELOPING THESE REACTIONS IS 5-8 TIMES GREATER THAN IN THE GENERAL POPULATION. HOWEVER, THE OVERALL RISK OF THESE REACTIONS IN THE UNTREATED GENERAL POPULATION IS LOW, APPROXIMATELY SIX PATIENTS PER ONE MILLION POPULATION PER YEAR FOR AGRANULOCYTOSIS AND TWO PATIENTS PER ONE MILLION POPULATION PER YEAR FOR APLASTIC ANEMIA.
ALTHOUGH REPORTS OF TRANSIENT OR PERSISTENT DECREASED PLATELET OR WHITE BLOOD CELL COUNTS ARE NOT UNCOMMON IN ASSOCIATION WITH THE USE OF CARBAMAZEPINE, DATA ARE NOT AVAILABLE TO ESTIMATE ACCURATELY THEIR INCIDENCE OR OUTCOME. HOWEVER, THE VAST MAJORITY OF THE CASES OF LEUKOPENIA HAVE NOT PROGRESSED TO THE MORE SERIOUS CONDITIONS OF APLASTIC ANEMIA OR AGRANULOCYTOSIS.
BECAUSE OF THE VERY LOW INCIDENCE OF AGRANULOCYTOSIS AND APLASTIC ANEMIA, THE VAST MAJORITY OF MINOR HEMATOLOGIC CHANGES OBSERVED IN MONITORING OF PATIENTS ON CARBAMAZEPINE ARE UNLIKELY TO SIGNAL THE OCCURRENCE OF EITHER ABNORMALITY. NONETHELESS, COMPLETE PRETREATMENT HEMATOLOGICAL TESTING SHOULD BE OBTAINED AS BASELINE. IF A PATIENT IN THE COURSE OF TREATMENT EXHIBITS LOW OR DECREASED WHITE BLOOD CELL OR PLATELET COUNTS, THE PATIENT SHOULD BE MONITORED CLOSELY. DISCONTINUATION OF THE DRUG SHOULD BE CONSIDERED IF ANY EVIDENCE OF SIGNIFICANT BONE MARROW DEPRESSION DEVELOPS.

DESCRIPTION:

Before prescribing carbamazepine, the physician should be thoroughly familiar with the details of this prescribing information, particularly regarding use with other drugs, especially those which accentuate toxicity potential.

Carbamazepine USP is an anticonvulsant and specific analgesic for trigeminal neuralgia, available for oral administration as chewable tablets of 100 mg, tablets of 200 mg, XR tablets of 100, 200, and 400 mg, and as a suspension of 100 mg/5 ml (teaspoon). Its chemical name is 5*H*-dibenz(b,f)azepine-5-carboxamide.

Carbamazepine USP is a white to off-white powder, practically insoluble in water and soluble in alcohol and in acetone. It molecular weight is 236.27.

INACTIVE INGREDIENTS

Tablets: Colloidal silicon dioxide, FD&C Red No. 30 (chewable tablets only), FD&C Red No. 40 (200-mg tablets only), flavoring (chewable tablets only), gelatin, glycerin, magnesium stearate, sodium starch glycolate (chewable tablets only), starch, stearic acid, and sucrose (chewable tablets only).

XR Tablets: cellulose compounds, dextrates, iron oxides, magnesium stearate, mannitol, polyethylene glycol, sodium lauryl sulfate, titanium dioxide (200-mg tablets only).

Suspension: Citric acid, FD&C Yellow No. 6, flavoring, polymer, potassium sorbate, propylene glycol, purified water, sorbitol, sucrose, and xanthan gum.

CLINICAL PHARMACOLOGY:

In controlled clinical trials, carbamazepine has been shown to be effective in the treatment of psychomotor and grand mal seizures, as well as trigeminal neuralgia.

CLINICAL PHARMACOLOGY: *(cont'd)*

MECHANISM OF ACTION

Carbamazepine has demonstrated anticonvulsant properties in rats and mice with electrically and chemically induced seizures. It appears to act by reducing polysynaptic response and blocking the post-tetanic potentiation. Carbamazepine greatly reduces or abolishes pain induced by stimulation of the infraorbital nerve in cats and rats. It depresses thalamic potential and bulbar and polysynaptic reflexes, including the linguomandibular reflex in cats. Carbamazepine is chemically unrelated to other anticonvulsants or other drugs used to control the pain of trigeminal neuralgia. The mechanism of action remains unknown.

The principal metabolite of carbamazepine-10, 11-epoxide, has anticonvulsant activity as demonstrated in several *in vivo* animal models of seizures. Through clinical activity for the epoxide has been postulated, the significance of its activity with respect to the safety and efficacy of carbamazepine has not been established.

PHARMACOKINETICS

In clinical studies suspension, conventional tablets and XR tablets delivered equivalent amounts of drug to the systemic circulation. However, the suspension was absorbed somewhat faster, and the XR tablet slightly slower, than the conventional tablet. The bioavailability of the XR tablet was 89% compared to suspension. Following a twice a day dosage regimen, the suspension provides higher peak levels and lower trough levels than those obtained from the conventional tablet for the same dosage regimen. On the other hand, following a three times a day dosage regimen, carbamazepine suspension affords steady-state plasma levels comparable to carbamazepine tablets given b.i.d. when administered at the same total mg daily dose. Carbamazepine chewable tablets may produce higher peak levels than the same dose given as regular tablets. Carbamazepine in blood is 76% bound to plasma proteins. Plasma levels of carbamazepine are variable and may range from 0.5-25 mcg/ml, with no apparent relationship to the daily intake of the drug. Usual adult therapeutic levels are between 4 and 12 mcg/ml. Following chronic oral administration of suspension, plasma levels peak at approximately 1.5 hours compared to 4 to 5 hours after administration of oral tablets. The CSF/serum ratio is 0.22, similar to the 22% unbound carbamazepine in serum. Because carbamazepine may induce its own metabolism, the half-life is also variable. Initial half-life values range from 25-65 hours, with 12-17 hours on repeated doses. Carbamazepine is metabolized in the liver. After oral administration of ^{14}C-carbamazepine, 72% of the administered radioactivity was found in the urine and 28% in the feces. This urinary radioactivity was composed largely of hydroxylated and conjugated metabolites, with only 3% of unchanged carbamazepine. Transplacental passage of carbamazepine is rapid (30 to 60 minutes), and the drug is accumulated in fetal tissues, with higher levels found in liver and kidney than in brain and lungs.

INDICATIONS AND USAGE:

Epilepsy: Carbamazepine is indicated for use as an anticonvulsant drug. Evidence supporting efficacy of carbamazepine as an anticonvulsant was derived from active drug-controlled studies that enrolled patients with the following seizure types:

1. Partial seizures with complex symptomatology (psychomotor, temporal lobe). Patients with these seizures appear to show greater improvement than those with other types.

2. Generalized tonic-clonic seizures (grand mal).

3. Mixed seizure patterns which include the above, or other partial or generalized seizures. Absence seizures (petit mal) do not appear to be controlled by carbamazepine (see PRECAUTIONS, General).

Trigeminal Neuralgia: Carbamazepine is indicated in the treatment of the pain associated with true trigeminal neuralgia.

Beneficial results have also been reported in glossopharyngeal neuralgia.

This drug is not a simple analgesic and should not be used for the relief of trivial aches or pains.

CONTRAINDICATIONS:

Carbamazepine should not be used in patients with a history of previous bone marrow depression, hypersensitivity to the drug, or known sensitivity to any of the tricyclic compounds such as amitriptyline, desipramine, imipramine, protriptyline, nortriptyline, etc. Likewise, on theoretical grounds its use with monoamine oxidase inhibitors is not recommended. Before administration of carbamazepine, MAO inhibitors should be discontinued for a minimum of fourteen days, or longer if the clinical situation permits.

WARNINGS:

Patients with a history of adverse hematologic reaction to any drug may be particularly at risk.

Severe dermatologic reactions including toxic epidermal necrolysis (Lyell's syndrome) and Stevens-Johnson syndrome, have been reported with carbamazepine. These reactions have been extremely rare. However, a few fatalities have been reported.

Carbamazepine has shown mild anticholinergic activity: therefore, patients with increased intraocular pressure should be closely observed during therapy.

Because of the relationship of the drug to other tricyclic compounds, the possibility of activation of a latent psychosis and, in elderly patients, of confusion or agitation should be borne in mind.

PRECAUTIONS:

GENERAL

Before initiating therapy, a detailed history and physical examination should be made.

Carbamazepine should be used with caution in patients with a mixed seizure disorder that includes atypical absence seizures, since in these patients carbamazepine has been associated with increased frequency of generalized convulsions (see INDICATIONS AND USAGE).

Therapy should be prescribed only after critical benefit-to-risk appraisal in patients with a history of cardiac, hepatic or renal damage, adverse hematologic reaction to other drugs, or interrupted courses of therapy with carbamazepine.

Since a given dose of carbamazepine suspension will produce higher peak levels than the same dose given as the tablet, it is recommended that patients given the suspension be started on lower doses and increased slowly to avoid unwanted side effects (see DOSAGE AND ADMINISTRATION).

INFORMATION FOR THE PATIENT

Patients should be made aware of the early toxic signs and symptoms of a potential hematologic problem, such as fever, sore throat, rash, ulcers in the mouth, easy bruising, petechial or purpuric hemorrhage, and should be advised to report to the physician immediately if any such signs or symptoms appear.

Since dizziness and drowsiness may occur, patients should be cautioned about the hazards of operating machinery or automobiles or engaging in other potentially dangerous tasks.

PRECAUTIONS: *(cont'd)*

LABORATORY TESTS

Complete pretreatment blood counts, including platelets and possibly reticulocytes and serum iron, should be obtained as a baseline. If a patient in the course of treatment exhibits low or decreased white blood cell or platelet counts, the patient should be monitored closely. Discontinuation of the drug should be considered if any evidence of significant bone marrow depression develops.

Baseline and periodic evaluations of liver function, particularly in patients with a history of liver disease, must be performed during treatment with this drug since liver damage may occur. The drug should be discontinued immediately in cases of aggravated liver dysfunction or active liver disease.

Baseline and periodic eye examinations, including slit-lamp, funduscopy and tonometry, are recommended since many phenothiazines and related drugs have been shown to cause eye changes.

Baseline and periodic complete urinalysis and BUN determinations are recommended for patients treated with this agent because of observed renal dysfunction.

Monitoring of blood levels (see CLINICAL PHARMACOLOGY) has increased the efficacy and safety of anticonvulsants. This monitoring may be particularly useful in cases of dramatic increase in seizure frequency and for verification of compliance. In addition, measurement of drug serum levels may aid in determining the cause of toxicity when more than one medication is being used.

Thyroid function tests have been reported to show decreased values with carbamazepine administered alone.

Hyponatremia has been reported in association with carbamazepine use, either alone or in combination with other drugs.

CARCINOGENESIS, MUTAGENESIS, AND IMPAIRMENT OF FERTILITY

Carbamazepine, when administered to Sprague-Dawley rats for two years in the diet at doses of 25, 75, and 250 mg/kg/day, resulted in a dose-related increase in the incidence of hepatocellular tumors in females and of benign interstitial cell adenomas in the testes of males.

Carbamazepine must, therefore, be considered to be carcinogenic in Sprague-Dawley rats. Bacterial and mammalian mutagenicity studies using carbamazepine produced negative results. The significance of these findings relative to the use of carbamazepine in humans is at present, unknown.

PREGNANCY CATEGORY C

Carbamazepine has been shown to have adverse effects in reproduction studies in rats when given orally in dosages 10-25 times the maximum human daily dosage of 1200 mg. In rat teratology studies, 2 of 135 offspring showed kinked ribs at 250 mg/kg and 4 of 119 offspring at 650 mg/kg showed other anomalies (cleft palate, 1;talipes, 1;anophthalmos, 2). In reproduction studies in rats, nursing offspring demonstrated a lack of weight gain and an unkempt appearance at a maternal dosage level of 200 mg/kg.

There are no adequate and well-controlled studies in pregnant women. Epidemiological data suggest that there may be an association between the use of carbamazepine during pregnancy and congenital malformations, including spina bifida. Carbamazepine should be used during pregnancy only if the potential benefit justifies the potential risk to the fetus.

Retrospective case reviews suggest that, compared with monotherapy, there may be a higher prevalence of teratogenic effects associated with the use of anticonvulsants in combination therapy. Therefore, monotherapy is recommended for pregnant women.

It is important to note that anticonvulsant drugs should not be discontinued in patients in whom the drug is administered to prevent major seizures because of the strong possibility of precipitating status epilepticus with attendant hypoxia and threat to life. In individual cases where the severity and frequency of the seizure disorder are such that removal of medication does not pose a serious threat to the patient, discontinuation of the drug may be considered prior to and during pregnancy, although it cannot be said with any confidence that even minor seizures do not pose some hazard to the developing embryo or fetus.

LABOR AND DELIVERY

The effect of carbamazepine on human labor and delivery is unknown.

NURSING MOTHERS

During lactation, concentration of carbamazepine in milk is approximately 60% of the maternal plasma concentration.

Because of the potential of serious adverse reactions in nursing infants from carbamazepine, a decision should be made whether to discontinue nursing or to discontinue the drug, taking into account the importance of the drug to the mother.

PEDIATRIC USE

Safety and effectiveness in children below the age of 6 years have not been established.

DRUG INTERACTIONS:

The simultaneous administration of phenobarbital, phenytoin, or primidone, or a combination of two, produces a marked lowering of serum levels, of carbamazepine. The effect of valproic acid on carbamazepine blood levels is not clearly established, although an increase in the ratio of active 10, 11-epoxide metabolite to parent compound is a consistent finding.

The half-lives of phenytoin, warfarin, doxycycline, and theophylline were significantly shortened when administered concurrently with carbamazepine. Haloperidol and valproic acid serum levels may be reduced when these drugs are administered with carbamazepine. The doses of these drugs may therefore have to be increased when carbamazepine is added to the therapeutic regimen.

Concomitant administration of carbamazepine with erythromycin, cimetidine, propoxyphene, isoniazid, fluoxetine or calcium channel blockers has been reported to result in elevated plasma levels of carbamazepine resulting in toxicity in some cases. Also concomitant administration of carbamazepine and lithium may increase the risk of neurotoxic side effects.

Alterations of thyroid function have been reported in combination therapy with other anticonvulsant medications.

Breakthrough bleeding has been reported among patients receiving concomitant oral contraceptives and their reliability may be adversely affected.

ADVERSE REACTIONS:

If adverse reactions are of such severity that the drug must be discontinued, the physician must be aware that abrupt discontinuation of any anticonvulsant drug in a responsive epileptic patient may lead to seizures or even status epilepticus with its life-threatening hazards.

The most severe adverse reactions have been observed in the hemopoietic system (see BOXED WARNING), the skin and the cardiovascular system.

The most frequently observed adverse reactions, particularly during the initial phases of therapy, are dizziness, drowsiness, unsteadiness, nausea, and vomiting. To minimize the possibility of such reactions, therapy should be initiated at the low dosage recommended.

The following additional adverse reactions have been reported:

ADVERSE REACTIONS: *(cont'd)*

Hemopoietic System: Aplastic anemia, agranulocytosis, pancytopenia, bone marrow depression, thrombocytopenia, leukopenia, leukocytosis, eosinophilia, acute intermittent porphyria.

Skin: Pruritic and erythematous rashes, urticaria, toxic epidermal necrolysis (Lyell's Syndrome) (see WARNINGS), Stevens-Johnson syndrome (see WARNINGS), photosensitivity reactions, alterations in skin pigmentation, exfoliative dermatitis, erythema multiforme and nodosum, purpura, aggravation of disseminated lupus erythematosus, alopecia, and diaphoresis. In certain cases, discontinuation of therapy may be necessary. Isolated cases of hirsutism have been reported, but a causal relationship is not clear.

Cardiovascular System: Congestive heart failure, edema, aggravation of hypertension, hypotension, syncope and collapse, aggravation of coronary artery disease, arrhythmias and AV block, primary thrombophlebitis, recurrence of thrombophlebitis, and adenopathy or lymphadenopathy. Some of these cardiovascular complications have resulted in fatalities. Myocardial infarction has been associated with other tricyclic compounds.

Liver: Abnormalities in liver function tests, cholestatic and hepatocellular jaundice, hepatitis.

Respiratory System: Pulmonary hypersensitivity characterized by fever, dyspnea, pneumonitis or pneumonia.

Genitourinary System: Urinary frequency, acute urinary retention, oliguria with elevated blood pressure, azotemia, renal failure, and impotence. Albuminuria, elevated BUN and microscopic deposits in the urine have also been reported. Testicular atrophy occurred in rats receiving carbamazepine orally from 4 to 52 weeks at dosage levels of 50 to 400 mg/kg/day. Additionally, rats receiving carbamazepine in the diet for two years at dosage levels of 25, 75, and 250 mg/kg/day had a dose related incidence of testicular atrophy and aspermatogenesis. In dogs, it produced a brownish discoloration, presumably a metabolite, in the urinary bladder at dosage levels of 50 mg/kg and higher. Relevance of these findings to humans is unknown.

Nervous System: Dizziness, drowsiness, disturbances of coordination, confusion, headache, fatigue, blurred vision, visual hallucinations, transient diplopia, oculomotor disturbances, nystagmus, speech disturbances, abnormal involuntary movements, peripheral neuritis and paresthesias, depression with agitation, talkativeness, tinnitus, and hyperacusis. There have been reports of associated paralysis and other symptoms of cerebral arterial insufficiency, but the exact relationship of these reactions to the drug has not been established.

Digestive System: Nausea, vomiting, gastric distress and abdominal pain, diarrhea, constipation, anorexia, and dryness of the mouth and pharynx, including glossitis and stomatitis.

Eyes: Scattered punctate cortical lens opacities, as well as conjunctivitis, have been reported. Although a direct causal relationship has not been established, many phenothiazines and related drugs have been shown to cause eye changes.

Musculoskeletal System: Aching joints and muscles, and leg cramps.

Metabolism: Fever and chills. Inappropriate antidiuretic hormone (ADH) secretion syndrome has been reported. Cases of frank water intoxication, with decreased serum sodium (hyponatremia) and confusion, have been reported in association with carbamazepine use (see PRECAUTIONS, Laboratory Tests).

Other: Isolated cases of lupus erythematosus-like syndrome have been reported. There have been occasional reports of elevated levels of cholesterol, HDL cholesterol and triglycerides in patients taking anticonvulsants.

A case of aseptic meningitis, accompanied by myoclonus and peripheral eosinophilia, has been reported in a patient taking carbamazepine in combination with other medications. The patient was successfully dechallenged, and the meningitis reappeared upon rechallenge with carbamazepine.

DRUG ABUSE AND DEPENDENCE:

No evidence of abuse potential has been associated with carbamazepine, nor is there evidence of psychological or physical dependence in humans.

OVERDOSAGE:

ACUTE TOXICITY

Lowest known lethal dose: adults, >60 g (39 year-old man). Highest known doses survived: adults, 30 g (31 year-old woman); children, 10 g (6 year-old boy); small children, 5 g (3 year-old girl).

Oral LD_{50} in animals (mg/kg): mice, 1100-3750; rats, 3850-4025; rabbits, 1500-2680; guinea pigs, 920.

SIGNS AND SYMPTOMS

The first signs and symptoms appear after 1-3 hours. Neuromuscular disturbances are the most prominent. Cardiovascular disorders are generally milder, and severe cardiac complications occur only when very high doses (>60g) have been ingested.

Respiration: Irregular breathing, respiratory depression.

Cardiovascular System: Tachycardia, hypotension or hypertension, shock, conduction disorders.

Nervous System and Muscles: Impairment of consciousness ranging in severity to deep coma. Convulsions, especially in small children. Motor restlessness, muscular twitching, tremor, athetoid movements opisthotonos, ataxia, drowsiness, dizziness, mydriasis, nystagmus, adiadochokinesia, ballism, psychomotor disturbances, dysmetria. Initial hyperreflexia, followed by hyporeflexia.

Gastrointestinal Tract: Nausea, vomiting.

Kidneys and Bladder: Anuria or oliguria, urinary retention.

Laboratory Findings: Isolated instances of overdosage have included leukocytosis, reduced leukocyte count, glycosuria and acetonuria. EEG may show dysrhythmias.

Combined Poisoning: When alcohol, tricyclic antidepressants, barbiturates or hydantoins are taken at the same time, the signs and symptoms of acute poisoning with carbamazepine may be aggravated or modified.

TREATMENT

The prognosis in cases of severe poisoning is critically dependent upon prompt elimination of the drug, which may be achieved by inducing vomiting, irrigating the stomach, and by taking appropriate steps to diminish absorption. If these measures cannot be implemented without risk on the spot, the patient should be transferred at once to a hospital, while ensuring that vital functions are safeguarded. There is no specific antidote.

Elimination of the Drug: Induction of vomiting.

Gastric lavage. Even when more than 4 hours have elapsed following ingestion of the drug, the stomach should be repeatedly irrigated, especially if the patient has also consumed alcohol.

Measures to Reduce Absorption: Activated charcoal, laxatives.

Measures to Accelerate Elimination: Forced diuresis.

Dialysis is indicated only in severe poisoning associated with renal failure. Replacement transfusion is indicated in severe poisoning in small children.

Respiratory Depression: Keep the airways free; resort, if necessary, to endotracheal intubation, artificial respiration, and administration of oxygen.

OVERDOSAGE: *(cont'd)*

Hypotension, Shock: Keep the patient's legs raised and administer a plasma expander. If blood pressure fails to rise despite measures taken to increase plasma volume use of vasoactive substances should be considered.

Convulsions: Diazepam or barbiturates.

Warning: Diazepam or barbiturates may aggravate respiratory depression (especially in children), hypotension, and coma. However, barbiturates should not be used if drugs that inhibit monoamine oxidase have also been taken by the patient either in overdosage or in recent therapy (within on week).

Surveillance: Respiration, cardiac function (ECG monitoring), blood pressure, body temperature, pupillary reflexes, and kidney and bladder function should be monitored for several days.

Treatment of Blood Count Abnormalities: If evidence of significant bone marrow depression develops, the following recommendations are suggested: (1) stop the drug, (2) perform daily CBC, platelet and reticulocyte counts, (3) do a bone marrow aspiration and trephine biopsy immediately and repeat with sufficient frequency to monitor recovery.

Special periodic studies might be helpful as follows: (1) white cell and platelet antibodies, (2) ^{59}Fe - ferrokinetic studies, (3) peripheral blood cell typing, (4) cytogenetic studies on marrow and peripheral blood, (5) bone marrow culture studies for colony - forming units, (6) hemoglobin electrophoresis for A_2 and F hemoglobin, and (7) serum folic acid and B_{12} levels.

A fully developed aplastic anemia will require appropriate, intensive monitoring and therapy, for which specialized consultation should be sought.

DOSAGE AND ADMINISTRATION:

TABLE 1A Dosage Information: Tablets and Suspension

Indication	Initial Dose Tablet	Suspension
Epilepsy		
6-12 years of age	100 mg b.i.d. (200 mg/day)	1/2 teaspoon q.i.d. (200 mg/day)
>12 years of age	200 mg b.i.d. (400 mg/day)	1 teaspoon q.i.d. (400 mg/day)
Trigeminal Neuralgia	100 mg b.i.d. on the first day (200 mg/day)	1/2 teaspoon q.i.d. (200 mg/day)

TABLE 1B Dosage Information: Tablets and Suspension

	Subsequent Dose Tablet	Suspension	Maximum Dose Tablet or Suspension
Epilepsy			
6-12 years of age	Add up to 100 mg per day at weekly intervals, t.i.d. or q.i.d.	Add up to 1 teaspoon (100 mg) per day at weekly intervals, t.i.d. or q.i.d.	1000 mg/24 hours
> 12 years of age	Add up to 200 mg per day at weekly intervals, t.i.d. or q.i.d.	Add up to 2 teaspoons (200 mg) per day at weekly intervals, t.i.d. or q.i.d.	1000 mg/24 hours: 12-15 years
			1200 mg/24 hours: over 15 years 1600 mg/24 hours: adults in rare instances
Trigeminal Neuralgia	Add up to 200 mg per day in increments of 100 mg every 12 hrs.	Add up to 2 teaspoons (mg) per day q.i.d.	1200 mg/24 hours

Monitoring of blood levels has increased the efficacy and safety of anticonvulsants (see PRECAUTIONS, Laboratory Tests). Dosage should be adjusted to the needs of the individual patient. A low initial daily dosage with a gradual increase is advised. As soon as adequate control is achieved, the dosage may be reduced very gradually to the minimum effective level. Medication should be taken with meals.

Since a given dose of carbamazepine suspension will produce higher peak levels than the same dose give as the tablet, it is recommended to start with low doses (children 6-12 years: 1/2 teaspoon four times a day) and to increase slowly to avoid unwanted side effects.

Conversion Of Patients From Oral Carbamazepine Tablets To Carbamazepine Suspension: Patients should be converted by administering the same number of mg per day in smaller, more frequent doses (*i.e.*, twice a day tablets to three times a day suspension).

EPILEPSY

(see INDICATIONS AND USAGE)

Adults And Children Over 12 Years Of Age

Initial: Either 200 mg twice a day for tablets and extended release tablets or 1 teaspoon four times a day for suspension (400 mg per day). Increase at weekly intervals by adding up to 200 mg per day using a twice a day regimen of extened release or three times a day or four times a day regimen until the optimal response is obtained. Dosage generally should not exceed 1000 mg daily in children 12 to 15 years of age, and 1200 mg daily in patients above 15 years of age. Doses up to 1600 mg daily have been used in adults in rare instances.

Maintenance: Adjust dosage to the minimum effective level, usually 800-1200 mg daily.

Children 6 - 12 Years Of Age

Initial: Either 100 mg twice a day for tablets or 1/2 teaspoon four times a day for suspension (200 mg per day). Increase at weekly intervals by adding up to 100 mg per day using a three times a day or four times a day regimen until the optimal response is obtained. Dosage generally should not exceed 1000 mg daily.

Maintenance: Adjust dosage to the minimum effective level, usually 400-800 mg daily.

Combination Therapy: Carbamazepine may be used alone or with other anticonvulsants. When added to existing anticonvulsant therapy, the drug should be added gradually while the other anticonvulsants are maintained or gradually decreased, except phenytoin, which may have to be increased (see PRECAUTIONS and DRUG INTERACTIONS).

TRIGEMINAL NEURALGIA

(see INDICATIONS AND USAGE)

Initial: On the first day, either 100 mg twice a day for tablets or 1/2 teaspoon four times a day for suspension for a total daily dose of 200 mg. This daily dose may be increased by up to 200 mg a day using increments of 100 mg every 12 hours for tablets or 50 mg (1/2 teaspoon) four times a day for suspension, only as needed to achieve freedom from pain. Do not exceed 1200 mg/daily.

DOSAGE AND ADMINISTRATION: *(cont'd)*

Maintenance: Control of pain can be maintained in most patients with 400 mg to 800 mg daily. However, some patients may be maintained on as little as 200 mg daily, while others may require as much as 1200 mg daily. At least once every 3 months throughout the treatment period, attempts should be made to reduce the dose to the minimum effective level or even to discontinue the drug.

STORAGE

Do not store above 86°F (30°C).

Dispense in tight, light-resistant container (USP).

PATIENT INFORMATION:

Carbamazepine is used for the treatment of seizures. It also is used to treat certain types of nerve pain. Inform your physican if you are pregnant or nursing. Inform your physician if you have glaucoma. Do not take this medication with a monoamine oxidase inhibitor. This medication may cause dizziness, drowsiness, or blurred vision; use caution while driving or operating hazardous machinery. Do not stop taking carbamazepine without talking with your physician. Shake the suspension well before each use. This medication should be taken with meals to avoid stomach upset. Notify your physician if you develop unexplained fever, sore throat, unusual bleeding or bruising, or yellow eyes or skin.

HOW SUPPLIED - RATED THERAPEUTICALLY EQUIVALENT:

Tablet, Chewable - Oral - 100 mg

100's	$14.67	Carbamazepine, H.C.F.A. F F P	99999-0646-01
100's	$16.20	Carbamazepine, Goldline Labs	00182-1331-01
100's	$16.30	Carbamazepine, Dupont Pharma	00056-0182-70
100's	$16.86	Carbamazepine, HL Moore Drug Exch	00839-7410-06
100's	$17.25	Carbamazepine Chewable, Schein Pharm (US)	00364-2309-01
100's	$17.30	Carbamazepine, Goldline Labs	00182-1331-89
100's	$17.40	Carbamazepine, Teva	00093-0778-01
100's	$17.55	Carbamazepine, Major Pharms	00904-3854-60
100's	$18.20	Carbamazepine, Aligen Independ	00405-4130-01
100's	$18.75	Carbamazepine, Warner Chilcott	00047-0242-24
100's	$18.75	Carbamazepine, Rugby	00536-3411-01
100's	**$18.90**	**TEGRETOL, Novartis**	**58887-0052-30**
100's	**$21.27**	**TEGRETOL, Novartis**	**58887-0052-32**

Tablet, Uncoated - Oral - 200 mg

100's	$10.08	Carbamazepine, US Trading	56126-0352-11
100's	$14.93	Carbamazepine, United Res	00677-1099-01
100's	$14.93	Carbamazepine, H.C.F.A. F F P	99999-0646-02
100's	$17.27	Carbamazepine, Inwood Labs	00258-3587-01
100's	$23.21	Carbamazepine 200, Purepac Pharm	00228-2143-10
100's	$23.25	Carbamazepine, Major Pharms	00904-3855-60
100's	$23.48	Carbamazepine, Amer Preferred	53445-1233-01
100's	$24.00	Carabamazepine Tabs., 200 Mg, Goldline Labs	00182-1233-01
100's	$24.00	Carbamazepine, Qualitest Pharms	00603-2563-21
100's	$24.91	Carbamazepine, HL Moore Drug Exch	00839-7177-06
100's	$24.98	Carbamazepine, IDE-Interstate	00814-1470-14
100's	$26.80	Atretol, Athena	59075-0554-10
100's	$26.95	Carbamazepine, Sidmak Labs	50111-0410-01
100's	$27.90	Carbamazepine, Aligen Independ	00405-4131-01
100's	$28.68	Carbamazepine, Parmed Pharms	00349-8977-01
100's	$29.50	Carbamazepine, Rugby	00536-3415-01
100's	$29.60	EPITOL, Teva	00093-0090-01
100's	$29.60	Carbamazepine, Teva	00093-0109-01
100's	$29.61	Carbamazepine, Schein Pharm (US)	00364-2106-01
100's	$29.64	Carbamazepine, Dupont Pharma	00056-0183-70
100's	$33.40	Carbamazepine Tabs., 200 Mg, Goldline Labs	00182-1233-89
100's	$33.41	Carbamazepine, Major Pharms	00904-3855-61
100's	$34.96	Carbamazepine 200, Vangard Labs	00615-3505-13
100's	**$36.05**	**TEGRETOL, Novartis**	**58887-0027-30**
100's	**$38.59**	**TEGRETOL, Novartis**	**58887-0027-32**
500's	$74.65	Carbamazepine, H.C.F.A. F F P	99999-0646-03
500's	$116.05	Carbamazepine 200, Purepac Pharm	00228-2143-50
750's	$254.36	Carbamazepine, Glasgow Pharm	60809-0127-55
750's	$254.36	Carbamazepine, Glasgow Pharm	60809-0127-72
1000's	$149.30	Carbamazepine, H.C.F.A. F F P	99999-0646-04
1000's	$161.50	Carbamazepine 200 Mg Tablets, Major Pharms	00904-3855-80
1000's	$213.65	Carbamazepine 200, Purepac Pharm	00228-2143-96
1000's	$220.80	Carbamazepine, Teva	00093-0109-10
1000's	$225.44	CARABAMAZEPINE, HL Moore Drug Exch	00839-7177-16
1000's	**$356.72**	**TEGRETOL, Novartis**	**58887-0027-40**

HOW SUPPLIED - NOT RATED EQUIVALENT:

Suspension - Oral - 100 mg/5ml

5 ml x 10	**$105.24**	**Carbamazepine, Xactdose**	**50962-0227-05**
10 ml x 50	**$93.60**	**TEGRETOL, Xactdose**	**50962-0229-10**
10 ml x 100	**$138.93**	**TEGRETOL, Xactdose**	**50962-0227-10**
450 ml	**$23.21**	**TEGRETOL, Novartis**	**58887-0019-76**

CARBAMIDE PEROXIDE *(000647)*

CATEGORIES: EENT Drugs; Eye, Ear, Nose, & Throat Preparations

BRAND NAMES: Pierre's Ear Wax Remover

FORMULARIES: Aetna

Prescribing information not available at time of publication.

HOW SUPPLIED - EQUIVALENTS NOT AVAILABLE:

Solution - Otic - 6.5 %

15 ml x 12	$24.00	Pierre's Ear Wax Remover, Consolidated Midland	00223-6577-15

CARBENICILLIN INDANYL SODIUM *(000650)*

CATEGORIES: Anti-Infectives; Antibacterials; Antibiotics; Antimicrobials; Broad Spectrum Penicillins; Infections; Penicillins; Prostatitis; Urinary Antibacterial; Urinary Tract Infections; Septicemia*; Pregnancy Category B; FDA Approval Pre 1982
* Indication not approved by the FDA

BRAND NAMES: *Carbachol*; Carbamann (Germany); *Carbamil*; Carbastat; *Carbyl*; *Doryl*; *Glaumarin* (Japan); Isopto Carbachol; *Isopto Karbakolin*; *Karbakolin Isopto* ; **Miostat**
(International brand names outside U.S. in italics)

FORMULARIES: Aetna; FHP; Medi-Cal

DESCRIPTION:

Geocillin, a semisynthetic penicillin, is the sodium salt of the indanyl ester of Geopen (carbenicillin disodium). The chemical name is: 1-(5-Indanyl)-N-(2-carboxy-3,3-dimethyl-7-oxo-4-thia-1-azabicyclo(3.2.0) hept-6-yl)-2-phenylmalonamate monosodium salt.

The empirical formula is: $C_{26}H_{25}N_2NaO_6S$ and mol. wt. is 516.55.

Geocillin tablets are yellow, capsule-shaped and film-coated, made of a white crystalline solid. Carbenicillin is freely soluble in water. Each Geocillin tablet contains 382 mg of carbenicillin, 118 mg of indanyl sodium ester. Each Geocillin tablet contains 23 mg of sodium.

Inert ingredients are: glycine; magnesium stearate and sodium lauryl sulfate. May also include the following: hydroxypropyl cellulose; hydroxypropyl methylcellulose; opaspray (which may include Blue 2 Lake, Yellow 6 Lake, Yellow 10 Lake, and other inert ingredients); opadry light yellow (which may contain D&C Yellow 10 Lake, FD&C Yellow 6 Lake and other inert ingredients); opadry clear (which may contain other inert ingredients).

CLINICAL PHARMACOLOGY:

Free carbenicillin is the predominant pharmacologically active fraction of carbenicillin indanyl sodium. Carbenicillin exerts its antibacterial activity by interference with final cell wall synthesis of susceptible bacteria.

Carbenicillin indanyl sodium is acid stable, and rapidly absorbed from the small intestine following oral administration. It provides relatively low plasma concentrations of antibiotic and is primarily excreted in the urine. After absorption, carbenicillin indanyl sodium is rapidly converted to carbenicillin by hydrolysis of the ester linkage. Following ingestion of a single 500 mg tablet of carbenicillin indanyl sodium, a peak carbenicillin plasma concentration of approximately 6.5 mcg/ml is reached in 1 hour. About 30% of this dose is excreted in the urine unchanged within 12 hours, with another 6% excreted over the next 12 hours.

In a multiple dose study utilizing volunteers with normal renal function, the following mean urine and serum levels of carbenicillin were achieved (TABLE 1):

TABLE 1 Mean Urine Concentration of Carbenicillin mcg/ml Hours After Initial Dose

DRUG	DOSE	0-3	3-6	6-24
Carbenicillin Indanyl Sodium	1 tablet q.6 hr	1130	352	292
Carbenicillin Indanyl Sodium	2 tablets q.6 hr	1428	789	809

Mean serum concentrations of carbenicillin in this study for these dosages are:

TABLE 2 Mean Serum Concentration mcg/ml Hours After Initial Dose

DRUG	DOSE	1/2	1	2	4	6	24	25	26	28
Carbenicillin Indanyl Sodium	1 tablet q.6 hr	5.1	6.5	3.2	1.9	0.0	0.4	8.8	5.4	0.4
Carbenicillin Indanyl Sodium	2 tablets q.6 hr	6.1	9.6	7.9	2.6	0.4	0.8	13.2	12.8	3.8

MICROBIOLOGY

The antibacterial activity of carbenicillin indanyl sodium is due to its rapid conversion to carbenicillin by hydrolysis after absorption. Though carbenicillin indanyl sodium provides substantial *in vitro* activity against a variety of both gram-positive and gram-negative microorganisms, the most important aspect of its profile is in its antipseudomonal and antiproteal activity. Because of the high urine levels obtained following administration, carbenicillin indanyl sodium has demonstrated clinical efficacy in urinary infections due to susceptible strains of:

Escherichia coli
Proteus mirabilis
Proteus vulgaris
Morganella morganii
(formerly *Proteus morganii*)
Pseudomonas species
Providencia rettgeri
(formerly *Proteus rettgeri*)
Enterobacter species
Enterococci (*S. faecalis*)

In addition, *in vitro* data, not substantiated by clinical studies, indicate the following pathogens to be usually susceptible to carbenicillin indanyl sodium:

Staphylococcus species
(nonpenicillinase producing)
Streptococcus species

RESISTANCE

Most *Klebsiella* species are usually resistant to the action of carbenicillin indanyl sodium. Some strains of *Pseudomonas* species have developed resistance to carbenicillin.

SUSCEPTIBILITY TESTING

Geopen (carbenicillin disodium) Susceptibility Powder or 100 mcg Geopen Susceptibility Discs may be used to determine microbial susceptibility to carbenicillin indanyl sodium using one of the following standard methods recommended by the National Committee for Clinical Laboratory Standards:

M2-A3, "Performance Standards for Antimicrobial Disk Susceptibility Tests"

M7-A, "Methods for Dilution Antimicrobial Susceptibility Tests for Bacteria that Grow Aerobically"

M11-A, "Reference Agar Dilution Procedure for Antimicrobial Susceptibility Testing of Anaerobic Bacteria"

M17-P, "Alternative Methods for Antimicrobial Susceptibility Testing of Anaerobic Bacteria"

Tests should be interpreted by the following criteria (TABLE 3):

TABLE 3

Organisms	Disk Diffusion Zone diameter (mm) Susceptible	Intermediate	Resistant
Enterobacter	≥23	18-22	≤17
Pseudomonas sp.	≥17	14-16	≤13
	Dilution MIC (µ/ml)		
Organisms	Susceptible	Moderately Susceptible	Resistant
Enterobacter	≤16	32	≥64
Pseudomonas sp.	≤128	-	≥156

CLINICAL PHARMACOLOGY: *(cont'd)*

Interpretations of susceptible, intermediate, and resistant correlate zone size diameters with MIC values. A laboratory report of "susceptible" indicates that the suspected causative microorganism most likely will respond to therapy with carbenicillin. A laboratory report of "resistant" indicates that the infecting microorganism most likely will not respond to therapy. A laboratory report of "moderately susceptible" indicates that the microorganism is most likely susceptible if a high dosage of carbenicillin is used, or if the infection is such that high levels of carbenicillin may be attained as in urine. A report of "intermediate" using the disk diffusion method may be considered an equivocal result, and dilution tests may be indicated.

INDICATIONS AND USAGE:

Carbenicillin indanyl sodium is indicated in the treatment of acute and chronic infections of the upper and lower urinary tract and in asymptomatic bacteriuria due to susceptible strains of the following organisms:

Escherichia coli
Proteus mirabilis
Morganella morganii (formerly *Proteus morganii*)
Providencia rettgeri (formerly *Proteus rettgeri*)
Proteus vulgaris
Pseudomonas
Enterobacter
Enterococci

Carbenicillin indanyl sodium is also indicated in the treatment of prostatitis due to susceptible strains of the following organisms:

Escherichia coli

Enterococcus (S. faecalis)

Proteus mirabilis

Enterobacter sp.

WHEN HIGH AND RAPID BLOOD AND URINE LEVELS OF ANTIBIOTIC ARE INDICATED, THERAPY WITH GEOPEN (CARBENICILLIN DISODIUM) SHOULD BE INITIATED BY PARENTERAL ADMINISTRATION FOLLOWED, AT THE PHYSICIAN'S DISCRETION, BY ORAL THERAPY.

NOTE: Susceptibility testing should be performed prior to and during the course of therapy to detect the possible emergence of resistant organisms which may develop.

CONTRAINDICATIONS:

Carbenicillin indanyl sodium is ordinarily contraindicated in patients who have a known penicillin allergy.

WARNINGS:

Serious and occasionally fatal hypersensitivity (anaphylactic) reactions have been reported in patients on oral penicillin therapy. Although anaphylaxis is more frequent following parenteral therapy, it has occurred in patients on oral penicillins. These reactions are more apt to occur in individuals with a history of penicillin hypersensitivity and/or a history of sensitivity to multiple allergens.

There have been reports of individuals with a history of penicillin hypersensitivity who have experienced severe hypersensitivity reactions when treated with a cephalosporin, and vice versa. Before initiating therapy with a penicillin, careful inquiry should be made concerning previous hypersensitivity reactions to penicillins, cephalosporins, or other allergens. If an allergic reaction occurs, the drug should be discontinued and the appropriate therapy instituted.

SERIOUS ANAPHYLACTOID REACTIONS REQUIRE IMMEDIATE EMERGENCY TREATMENT WITH EPINEPHRINE. OXYGEN, INTRAVENOUS STEROIDS AND AIRWAY MANAGEMENT, INCLUDING INTUBATION, SHOULD ALSO BE ADMINISTERED AS INDICATED.

PRECAUTIONS:

General: As with any penicillin preparation, an allergic response, including anaphylaxis, may occur particularly in a hypersensitive individual.

Long term use of carbenicillin indanyl sodium may result in the overgrowth of nonsusceptible organisms. If superinfection occurs during therapy, appropriate measures should be taken.

Since carbenicillin is primarily excreted by the kidney, patients with severe renal impairment (creatinine clearance of less than 10 ml/min) will not achieve therapeutic urine levels of carbenicillin.

In patients with creatinine clearance of 10-20 ml/min it may be necessary to adjust dosage to prevent accumulation of drug.

Laboratory Tests: As with other penicillins, periodic assessment of organ system function including renal, hepatic, and hematopoietic systems is recommended during prolonged therapy.

Carcinogenesis, Mutagenesis, and Impairment of Fertility: There are no long-term animal or human studies to evaluate carcinogenic potential. Rats fed 250-1000 mg/kg/day for 18 months developed mild liver pathology (*e.g.,* bile duct hyperplasia) at all dose levels, but there was no evidence of drug-related neoplasia. Carbenicillin indanyl sodium administered at daily doses ranging to 1000 mg/kg had no apparent effect on the fertility or reproductive performance of rats.

Pregnancy Category B: Reproduction studies have been performed at dose levels of 1000 or 500 mg/kg in rats, 200 mg/kg in mice, and at 500 mg/kg in monkeys with no harm to fetus due to carbenicillin indanyl sodium. There are, however, no adequate and well controlled studies in pregnant women. Because animal reproduction studies are not always predictive of human response, this drug should be used during pregnancy only if clearly needed.

Labor and Delivery: It is not known whether the use of carbenicillin indanyl sodium in humans during labor or delivery has immediate or delayed adverse effects on the fetus, prolongs the duration of labor, or increases the likelihood that forceps delivery or other obstetrical intervention or resuscitation of the newborn will be necessary.

Nursing Mothers: Carbenicillin class antibiotics are excreted in milk although the amounts excreted are unknown; therefore, caution should be exercised if administered to a nursing woman.

Pediatric Use: Since only limited clinical data is available to date in children, the safety of carbenicillin indanyl sodium administration in this age group has not yet been established.

DRUG INTERACTIONS:

Carbenicillin indanyl sodium blood levels may be increased and prolonged by concurrent administration of probenecid.

ADVERSE REACTIONS:

The following adverse reactions have been reported as possibly related to carbenicillin indanyl sodium administration in controlled studies which include 344 patients receiving carbenicillin indanyl sodium.

ADVERSE REACTIONS: *(cont'd)*

Gastrointestinal: The most frequent adverse reactions associated with carbenicillin indanyl sodium therapy are related to the gastrointestinal tract. Nausea, bad taste, diarrhea, vomiting, flatulence, and glossitis were reported. Abdominal cramps, dry mouth, furry tongue, rectal bleeding, anorexia, and unspecified epigastric distress were rarely reported.

Dermatologic: Hypersensitivity reactions such as skin rash, urticaria, and less frequently pruritus.

Hematologic: As with other penicillins, anemia, thrombocytopenia, leukopenia, neutropenia, and eosinophilia have infrequently been observed. The clinical significance of these abnormalities is not known.

Miscellaneous: Other reactions rarely reported were hyperthermia, headache, itchy eyes, vaginitis, and loose stools.

Abnormalities of Hepatic Function Tests: Mild SGOT elevations have been observed following carbenicillin indanyl sodium administration.

OVERDOSAGE:

Carbenicillin indanyl sodium is generally nontoxic. Carbenicillin indanyl sodium when taken in excessive amounts may produce mild gastrointestinal irritation. The drug is rapidly excreted in the urine and symptoms are transitory. The usual symptoms of anaphylaxis may occur in hypersensitive individuals.

Carbenicillin blood levels achievable with carbenicillin indanyl sodium are very low, and toxic reactions as a function of overdosage should not occur systematically. The oral LD_{50} in mice is 3,600 mg/kg, in rats 2,000 mg/kg, and in dogs is in excess of 500 mg/kg. The lethal human dose is not known.

Although never reported, the possibility of accumulation of indanyl should be considered when large amounts of carbenicillin indanyl sodium are ingested. Free indole, which is a phenol derivative, may be potentially toxic. In general 8-15 grams of phenol, and presumably a similar amount of indole, are required orally before toxicity (peripheral vascular collapse) may occur. The metabolic by-products of indole are nontoxic. In patients with hepatic failure it may be possible for unmetabolized indole to accumulate.

The metabolic by-products of carbenicillin indanyl sodium, indanyl sulfate and glucuronide, as well as free carbenicillin, are dialyzable.

DOSAGE AND ADMINISTRATION:

Carbenicillin indanyl sodium is available as a coated tablet to be administered orally. (TABLE 4):

TABLE 4 Usual Adult Dose

URINARY TRACT INFECTIONS	
Escherichia coli, Proteus species, and *Enterobacter*	1-2 tablets 4 times daily
Pseudomonas and *Enterococcus*	2 tablets 4 times daily
PROSTATITIS	
Escherichia coli, Proteus mirabilis, Enterobacter and *Enterococcus*	2 tablets 4 times daily

HOW SUPPLIED - EQUIVALENTS NOT AVAILABLE:

Tablet, Uncoated - Oral - 382 mg

100's	**$157.00**	**GEOCILLIN, Roerig**	**00049-1430-66**
100's	**$180.47**	**GEOCILLIN, Roerig**	**00049-1430-41**

CARBETAPENTANE TANNATE; CHLORPHENIRAMINE TANNATE; EPHEDRINE TANNATE; PHENYLEPHRINE HYDROCHLORIDE *(000652)*

CATEGORIES: Allergies; Antihistamines; Antitussives; Antitussives/Expectorants/ Mucolytics; Autonomic Drugs; Bronchial Dilators; Common Cold; Cough Preparations; DESI Drugs; Respiratory & Allergy Medications; Sympathomimetic Agents; Pregnancy Category C; FDA Pre 1938 Drugs

BRAND NAMES: C.C.E.P.; Fen-A-Cough; Fenatuss; Histatuss; Mooretuss; Phenylephrine Compound; Quad-Tuss Tannate; Rentamine; *Rynatus*; **Rynatuss**; Tri-Tannate Plus; Trin Tuss; Tuss-Tan
(International brand names outside U.S. in italics)

Prescribing information not available at time of publication.

HOW SUPPLIED - EQUIVALENTS NOT AVAILABLE:

Suspension - Oral - 30 mg/4 mg/5 mg

240 ml	**$98.38**	**RYNATUSS PEDIATRIC, Wallace Labs**	**00037-0718-67**
473 ml	$41.00	Fen-A-Cough, Tmk Pharm	59582-0449-16
473 ml	$45.52	Phenylephrine Compound, Aligen Independ	00405-3531-16
480 ml	$41.00	Quad-Tuss Tannate, Hi Tech Pharma	50383-0809-16
480 ml	$43.25	Tuss-Tan, Econolab	55053-0112-16
480 ml	$51.00	TRI-TANNATE PLUS, Rugby	00536-2202-85
480 ml	$52.45	Rentamine, Major Pharms	00904-1666-16
480 ml	**$182.29**	**RYNATUSS PEDIATRIC, Wallace Labs**	**00037-0718-68**

Tablet, Uncoated - Oral - 60 mg/5 mg/10 m

100's	$37.60	Tuss-Tan, Econolab	55053-0122-01
100's	$37.90	Fenatuss, Tmk Pharm	59582-0001-02
100's	$43.45	Rentamine, Major Pharms	00904-1665-60
100's	$72.20	TRI-TANNATE PLUS, Rugby	00536-4394-01
100's	**$158.54**	**RYNATUSS, Wallace Labs**	**00037-0717-92**
500's	**$784.02**	**RYNATUSS, Wallace Labs**	**00037-0717-96**
2000's	**$2980.28**	**RYNATUSS, Wallace Labs**	**00037-0717-95**

CARBIDOPA *(003176)*

CATEGORIES: Antiparkinson Agents; Autonomic Drugs; Extrapyramidal Movement Disorders; Neuromuscular; Parkinsonism; FDA Approval Pre 1982

BRAND NAMES: **Lodosyn**

WARNING:
When carbidopa is to be given to patients who are being treated with levodopa, the two drugs should be given at the same time, starting with no more than 20 to 25 percent of the previous daily dosage of levodopa when given without carbidopa. At least eight hours should elapse between the last dose of levodopa and initiation of therapy with carbidopa and levodopa. See WARNINGS and DOSAGE AND ADMINISTRATION before initiating therapy.

DESCRIPTION:

Carbidopa, an inhibitor of aromatic amino acid decarboxylation, is a white, crystalline compound, slightly soluble in water, with a molecular weight of 244.3. It is designated chemically as (-)-L-α-hydrazino- α-methyl-β-(3,4-dihydroxybenzene) propanoic acid monohydrate.

Lodosyn (carbidopa) tablets contain 25 mg of carbidopa. Inactive ingredients are cellulose, FD&C Yellow 6, magnesium stearate and starch.

Tablet content is expressed in terms of anhydrous carbidopa which has a molecular weight of 226.3.

CLINICAL PHARMACOLOGY:

Current evidence indicates that symptoms of Parkinson's disease are related to depletion of dopamine in the corpus striatum. Administration of dopamine is ineffective in the treatment of Parkinson's disease apparently because it does not cross the blood-brain barrier. However, levodopa, the metabolic precursor of dopamine, does cross the blood-brain barrier, and presumably is converted to dopamine in the basal ganglia. This is thought to be the mechanism whereby levodopa relieves symptoms of Parkinson's disease.

When levodopa is administered orally it is rapidly converted to dopamine in extra-cerebral tissues so that only a small portion of a given dose is transported unchanged to the central nervous system. For this reason, large doses of levodopa are required for adequate therapeutic effect and these may often be attended by nausea and other adverse reactions, some of which are attributable to dopamine formed in extracerebral tissues.

Since levodopa competes with certain amino acids, the absorption of levodopa may be impaired in some patients on a high protein diet.

Carbidopa inhibits decarboxylation of peripheral levodopa. It does not cross the blood-brain barrier and does not effect the metabolism of levodopa within the central nervous system. Carbidopa has not been demonstrated to have any overt pharmacodynamic actions in the recommended doses.

Since its decarboxylation inhibiting activity is limited to extracerebral tissues, administration of carbidopa with levodopa makes more levodopa available for transport to the brain. In dogs, reduced formation of dopamine in extracerebral tissues, such as the heart, provides protection against the development of dopamine-induced cardiac arrhythmias. Clinical studies tend to support the hypothesis of a similar protective effort in humans although controlled data are too limited at the present time to draw firm conclusions.

Carbidopa reduces the amount of levodopa required by about 75 percent and, when administered with levodopa, increases both plasma levels and the plasma half-life of levodopa, and decreases plasma and urinary dopamine and homovanillic acid.

In clinical pharmacologic studies, simultaneous administration of carbidopa and levodopa produced greater urinary excretion of levodopa in proportion to the excretion of dopamine than administration of the two drugs at separate times.

Pyridoxine hydrochloride (vitamin B_6) in oral doses of 10 mg to 25 mg, may reverse the effects of levodopa by increasing the rate of aromatic amino acid decarboxylation. Carbidopa inhibits this action of pyridoxine.

Carbidopa is combined with levodopa in carbidopa-levodopa combination tablets. These combination tablets are available in three strengths: 10 mg of carbidopa and 100 mg of levodopa, 25 mg of carbidopa and 250 mg of levodopa (1:10 ratio of carbidopa to levodopa) and 25 mg of carbidopa and 100 mg of levodopa (1:4 ratio of carbidopa to levodopa). Clinical trials show that these ratios of carbidopa and levodopa provide useful therapeutic effects in most patients.

INDICATIONS AND USAGE:

Carbidopa is indicated for use with carbidopa-levodopa combination or with levodopa in the treatment of the symptoms of idiopathic Parkinson's disease (paralysis agitans), postencephalitic parkinsonism, and symptomatic parkinsonism which may follow injury to the nervous system by carbon monoxide intoxications or manganese intoxication.

Carbidopa is for use with carbidopa-levodopa combination in patients who do not have adequate reaction in nausea and vomiting when the dosage of carbidopa-levodopa combination provides less than 70 mg a day of carbidopa.

Carbidopa is for use with levodopa in the occasional patient whose dosage requirement of carbidopa and levodopa necessitates separate titration of each entity.

Carbidopa is used with carbidopa-levodopa combination or with levodopa to permit the administration of lower doses of levodopa with reduced nausea and vomiting, with more rapid dosage titration, and with a somewhat smoother response. However, patients with markedly irregular ("on-off") responses to levodopa have not been shown to benefit from the addition of carbidopa.

The incidence of levodopa-induced nausea and vomiting is less when Lodosyn is used with levodopa than when levodopa is used without Lodosyn. In many patients this reduction in nausea and vomiting will permit more rapid titration.

Since carbidopa prevents the reversal of levodopa effects caused by pyridoxine, supplemental pyridoxine (vitamin B_6), can be given to patients when they are receiving carbidopa and levodopa concomitantly or as carbidopa-levodopa combination.

Although the administration of carbidopa permits control of parkinsonism and Parkinson's disease with much lower doses of levodopa, there is no conclusive evidence at present that this is beneficial other than in reducing nausea and vomiting, permitting more rapid titration, and providing a somewhat smoother response to levodopa.

Carbidopa does not decrease adverse reactions due to central effects of levodopa. By permitting more levodopa to reach the brain, particularly when nausea and vomiting is not a dose-limiting factor, certain adverse CNS effects, e.g., dyskinesias, may occur at lower dosages and sooner during therapy with carbidopa and levodopa than with levodopa alone.

INDICATIONS AND USAGE: *(cont'd)*

Certain patients who responded poorly to levodopa alone have improved when carbidopa and levodopa were given concurrently. This was most likely due to decreased peripheral decarboxylation of the levodopa rather than to a primary effect of carbidopa on the peripheral nervous system. Carbidopa has not been shown to enhance the intrinsic efficacy of levodopa.

In considering whether to give carbidopa with carbidopa-levodopa combination or with levodopa to patients who have nausea and/or vomiting, the physician should be aware that, while many patients may be expected to improve, some may not. Since one cannot predict which patients are likely to improve, this can only be determined by a trial of therapy. It should be further noted that in controlled trials comparing carbidopa and levodopa with levodopa alone, about half the patients with nausea and/or vomiting on levodopa alone improved spontaneously despite being retained on the same dose of levodopa during the controlled portion of the trial.

CONTRAINDICATIONS:

Concomitant therapy with carbidopa and levodopa is contraindicated in patients with known hypersensitivity to either of these drugs.

Monoamine oxidase inhibitors and levodopa, with or without carbidopa, should not be given concomitantly. Monoamine oxidase inhibitors must be discontinued at least two weeks prior to initiating therapy with levodopa.

Levodopa, with or without carbidopa, is contraindicated in narrow angle glaucoma.

Because levodopa may activate a malignant melanoma, it should not be used in patients with suspicious, undiagnosed skin lesions or a history of melanoma.

WARNINGS:

Carbidopa has no antiparkinsonian effect when given alone. It is indicated for use with carbidopa-levodopa combination or levodopa.

When patients are receiving levodopa, it must be discontinued at least eight hours before concomitant therapy with Lodosyn and levodopa is started. When such therapy is given, the dosage of levodopa should be 20 to 25 percent of the previous levodopa dosage (see DOSAGE AND ADMINISTRATION.)

As with levodopa, concomitant administration of carbidopa and levodopa may cause involuntary movements and mental disturbances. These reactions are thought to be due to increased brain dopamine following administration of levodopa. All patients should be observed carefully for the development of depression with concomitant suicidal tendencies. Patients with past or current psychoses should be treated with caution. *Because carbidopa permits more levodopa to reach the brain and, thus, more dopamine to be formed, dyskinesias may occur at lower levodopa dosages and sooner with concomitant use of carbidopa and levodopa than with levodopa.* The occurrence of dyskinesias may require levodopa dosage reduction.

Levodopa, with or without Lodosyn, should be administered cautiously to patients with severe cardiovascular or pulmonary disease, bronchial asthma, renal, hepatic, or endocrine disease.

Care should be exercised in administering levodopa, with or without Lodosyn, to patients with a history of myocardial infarction who have residual atrial, nodal, or ventricular arrhythmias. In such patients, cardiac function should be monitored with particular care during the period of initial dosage adjustment, in a facility with provisions for intensive cardiac care.

As with levodopa alone there is a possibility of upper gastrointestinal hemorrhage in patients with a history of peptic ulcer.

A symptom complex resembling the neuroleptic malignant syndrome including muscular rigidity, elevated body temperature, mental changes, and increased serum creatinine phosphokinase has been reported when antiparkinsonism agents were withdrawn abruptly. Therefore, patients should be observed carefully when the dosage of levodopa is reduced abruptly or discontinued, especially if the patient is receiving neuroleptics.

Use in Pregnancy and Lactation: Although the effects of concomitant use of carbidopa and levodopa on human pregnancy and lactation are unknown, both levodopa and combinations of carbidopa and levodopa have caused visceral and skeletal malformations in rabbits. Use of carbidopa and levodopa in women of childbearing potential requires that the anticipated benefits of the drug be weighed against possible hazards to the mother and child. Levodopa, with or without Lodosyn, should not be given to nursing mothers.

Usage in Children: The safety of concomitant administration of carbidopa and levodopa in patients under 18 years of age has not been established.

PRECAUTIONS:

As with levodopa alone, periodic evaluation of hepatic, hematopoietic, cardiovascular, and renal function are recommended during extended concomitant therapy with carbidopa and levodopa, or with Lodosyn and carbidopa-levodopa combination.

Patients with chronic wide angle glaucoma may be treated cautiously with Lodosyn and levodopa, just as with levodopa alone, provided the intraocular pressure is well controlled and the patient is monitored carefully for changes in intraocular pressure during therapy.

LABORATORY TESTS

Abnormalities in laboratory tests may include elevations of liver function tests such as alkaline phosphatase, SGOT (AST), SGPT (ALT), lactic dehydrogenase, and bilirubin. Abnormalities in protein-bound iodine, blood urea nitrogen, creatinine, and uric acid are lower during concomitant administration of Lodosyn and levodopa than with levodopa alone.

Levodopa may cause a false-positive reaction for urinary ketone bodies when a test tape is used for determination of ketonuria. This reaction will not be altered by boiling the urine specimen. False-negative tests may result with the use of glucose-oxidase methods of testing for glucosuria.

DRUG INTERACTIONS:

Caution should be exercised when the following drugs are administered concomitantly with Carbidopa given with levodopa.

Symptomatic postural hypotension can occur when carbidopa given with levodopa is added to the treatment of a patient receiving antihypertensive drugs. Therefore, when therapy with carbidopa given with levodopa is started, dosage adjustment of the antihypertensive drug may be required. For patients receiving monoamine oxidase inhibitors, (see CONTRAINDICATIONS.)

There have been rare reports of adverse reactions, including hypertension and dyskinesia, resulting from the concomitant use of tricyclic antidepressants and carbidopa-levodopa combination.

Phenothiazines and butyrophenones may reduce the therapeutic effects of levodopa. In addition, the beneficial effects of levodopa in Parkinson's disease have been reported to be reversed by phenytoin and papaverine. Patients taking these drugs with carbidopa and levodopa should be carefully observed for loss of therapeutic response.

ADVERSE REACTIONS:

Carbidopa has not been demonstrated to have any overt pharmacodynamic actions in the recommended doses. The only adverse reactions that have been observed have been with concomitant use of carbidopa and levodopa.

When carbidopa is administered concomitantly with levodopa, the most common serious adverse reactions are choreiform, dystonic, and other involuntary movements. Other serious adverse reactions are mental changes including paranoid ideation and psychotic episodes, depression with or without suicidal tendencies, and dementia. Convulsions also have occurred; however, a causal relationship with concomitant use of Lodosyn and levodopa has not been established.

A common but less serious side effect is nausea.

Less frequent adverse reactions are cardiac irregularities and/or palpitations, orthostatic hypotensive episodes (the "on-off" phenomenon), anorexia, vomiting, and dizziness.

Rarely, gastrointestinal bleeding, development of duodenal ulcer, hypertension, phlebitis, hemolytic and non-hemolytic anemia, thrombocytopenia, leukopenia, and agranulocytosis have occurred.

Laboratory tests which have been reported to be abnormal are alkaline phosphatase, SGOT (AST), SGPT (ALT), lactic dehydrogenase, bilirubin, blood urea nitrogen, protein-bound iodine, and Coombs test.

Other adverse reactions that have been reported with levodopa are:

Nervous System: ataxia, numbness, increased hand tremor, muscle twitching, muscle cramps, blepharospasm (which may be taken as an early sign of excess dosage, consideration of dosage reduction may be made at this time), trismus, activation of latent Horner's syndrome.

Psychiatric: confusion, sleepiness, insomnia, nightmares, hallucinations, delusions, agitation, anxiety, euphoria.

Gastrointestinal: dry mouth, bitter taste, sialorrhea, dysphagia, bruxism, hiccups, abdominal pain and distress, constipation, diarrhea, flatulence, burning sensation of tongue.

Metabolic: weight gain or loss, edema.

Integumentary: malignant melanoma (see also CONTRAINDICATIONS), flushing, increased sweating, dark sweat, skin rash, loss of hair.

Genitourinary: urinary retention, urinary incontinence, dark urine, priapism.

Special Senses: diplopia, blurred vision, dilated pupils, oculogyric crises.

Miscellaneous: weakness, faintness, fatigue, headache, hoarseness, malaise, hot flashes, sense of stimulation, bizarre breathing patterns, neuroleptic malignant syndrome.

OVERDOSAGE:

No reports of overdosage with Lodosyn have been received. For information on overdosage of levodopa or carbidopa-levodopa combination, see the package circulars for levodopa or carbidopa-levodopa combination.

DOSAGE AND ADMINISTRATION:

Whether given with carbidopa-levodopa combination or with levodopa, the optimal daily dosage of Lodosyn must be determined by careful titration. Most patients respond to a 1:10 proportion of carbidopa and levodopa, provided the daily dosage of carbidopa is 70 mg or more a day. The maximum daily dosage of carbidopa should not exceed 200 mg, since clinical experience with larger dosages is limited. If the patient is taking carbidopa-levodopa combination, the amount of carbidopa in carbidopa-levodopa combination should be considered when calculating the total amount of carbidopa to be administered each day.

PATIENTS RECEIVING CARBIDOPA-LEVODOPA COMBINATION WHO REQUIRE ADDITIONAL CARBIDOPA

Some patients taking carbidopa-levodopa combination may not have adequate reduction in nausea and vomiting when the dosage of carbidopa is less than 70 mg a day, and the dosage of levodopa is less than 700 mg a day. When these patients are taking carbidopa(10 mg)-levodopa(100 mg) combination, 25 mg of carbidopa may be given with the first dose of carbidopa-levodopa combination each day. Additional doses of 12.5 mg or 25 mg may be given during the day with each dose of carbidopa-levodopa combination. When patients are taking carbidopa(25 mg)-levodopa (250 mg) combination or carbidopa(25 mg)-levodopa (100 mg) combination, 25 mg of carbidopa may be given with any dose of carbidopa-levodopa combination as required for optimum therapeutic response. The maximum daily dosage of carbidopa, given as carbidopa and as carbidopa-levodopa combination, should not exceed 200 mg.

PATIENTS REQUIRING INDIVIDUAL TITRATION OF CARBIDOPA AND LEVODOPA DOSAGE

Although carbidopa-levodopa combination is the preferred method of carbidopa and levodopa administration, there may be an occasional patient who requires individually titrated doses of these two drugs. **In these patients, carbidopa should be initiated at a dosage of 25 mg three or four times a day. The two drugs should be given at the same time, starting with no more than 20 to 25 percent of the previous or recommended daily dosage of levodopa when given without carbidopa. In patients already receiving levodopa therapy, at least eight hours should elapse between the last dose of levodopa and initiation of therapy with carbidopa and levodopa. A convenient way to initiate therapy in these patients is in the morning following a night when the patient has not taken levodopa.** Physicians who prescribe separate doses of Lodosyn and levodopa should be thoroughly familiar with the direction for use of each drug.

LODOSYN DOSAGE ADJUSTMENT

Dosage of Lodosyn may be adjusted by adding or omitting one-half or one tablet a day. Because both therapeutic and adverse responses occur more rapidly with combined therapy than when only levodopa is given, patients should be monitored closely during the dose adjustment period. Specifically, involuntary movements will occur more rapidly when Lodosyn and levodopa are given concomitantly than when levodopa is given without Lodosyn. The occurrence of involuntary movements may require dosage reduction. Blepharospasm may be a useful early sign of excess dosage in some patients.

Current evidence indicates other standard antiparkinsonian drugs may be continued while carbidopa and levodopa are being administered. However, the dosage of such other standard antiparkinsonian drugs may require adjustment.

If general anesthesia is required, therapy may be continued as long as the patient is permitted to take fluids and medication by mouth. When therapy is interrupted temporarily, the usual daily dosage may be resumed as soon as the patient is able to take medication orally.

For How Supplied Information, Contact Merck (NDA# 017830)

CARBIDOPA; LEVODOPA *(000653)*

CATEGORIES: Anticholinergic Agents; Antiparkinson Agents; Autonomic Drugs; Extrapyramidal Movement Disorders; Neuromuscular; Parkinsonism; Sales > $100 Million; FDA Approval Pre 1982; Patent Expiration 1991 Aug

BRAND NAMES: Atamet; *Dopicar*; *Menesit* (Japan); *Neo Dopaston* (Japan); *Racovel* (Mexico); *Sindopa*; **Sinemet**; *Sinemet CR* (Australia, England, Canada); *Sinemet 25 100*; *Syndopa*; *Tidomet Forte*; *Tidomet L.S.*; *Tidomet Plus*
(International brand names outside U.S. in italics)

FORMULARIES: Aetna; BC-BS; CIGNA; FHP; Humana; Kaiser; Medco; Medi-Cal; PCS; PruCare; United; WHO

COST OF THERAPY: $338.35 (Parkinsonism; Tablet; 25 mg/100 mg; 3/day; 365 days)

> **WARNING:**
> **When carbidopa-levodopa is to be given to patients who are being treated with levodopa, levodopa must be discontinued at least eight hours before therapy with Sinemet is started. In order to reduce adverse reactions, it is necessary to individualize therapy. See WARNINGS and DOSAGE AND ADMINISTRATION before initiating therapy.**

DESCRIPTION:

Carbidopa, an inhibitor of aromatic amino acid decarboxylation, is a white, crystalline compound, slightly soluble in water, with a molecular weight of 244.3. It is designated chemically as (-)-L-α-hydrazino-α-methyl-β-(3,4-dihydroxybenzene) propanoic acid monohydrate.

Tablet content is expressed in terms of anhydrous carbidopa, which has a molecular weight of 226.3.

Levodopa, an aromatic amino acid, is a white, crystalline compound, slightly soluble in water with a molecular weight of 197.2. It is designated chemically as (-)-L-α-amino-β-(3,4-dihydroxybenzene) propanoic acid.

Inactive ingredients are cellulose, magnesium stearate and starch. Tablets Sinemet 10-100 and 25-250 also contain FD&C Blue 2. Tablets Sinemet 25-100 also contain D&C Yellow 10 and FD&C Yellow.

Sinemet CR: Sinemet CR (Carbidopa-Levodopa) is a sustained-release combination of carbidopa and levodopa for the treatment of Parkinson's disease and syndrome.

Inactive ingredients in Sinemet CR 50-200 are: D & C Yellow 10, magnesium stearate, iron oxide, and other ingredients. Inactive ingredients in Sinemet CR 25-100 are: magnesium stearate, red ferric oxide, and other ingredients.

The Sinemet CR tablet is a polymeric-based drug delivery system that controls the release of carbidopa and levodopa as it slowly erodes. Sinemet CR 25-100 is available to facilitate titration and as an alternative to the half- tablet of Sinemet CR 50-200.

CLINICAL PHARMACOLOGY:

Pharmacodynamics: Current evidence indicates that symptoms of Parkinson's disease are related to depletion of dopamine in the corpus striatum. Administration of dopamine is ineffective in the treatment of Parkinson's disease apparently because it does not cross the blood-brain barrier. However, levodopa, the metabolic precursor of dopamine, does cross the blood-brain-barrier, and presumably is converted to dopamine in the basal ganglia or brain. This is thought to be the mechanism whereby levodopa relieves symptoms of Parkinson's disease.

When levodopa is administered orally it is rapidly converted decarboxylated to dopamine in extracerebral tissues so that only a small portion of a given dose is transported unchanged to the central nervous system. For this reason, large doses of levodopa are required for adequate therapeutic effect and these may often be attended by nausea and other adverse reactions, some of which are attributable to dopamine formed in extracerebral tissues.

Since levodopa competes with certain amino acids, the absorption of levodopa may be impaired in some patients on a high protein diet.

Carbidopa inhibits decarboxylation of peripheral levodopa. It does not cross the blood-brain barrier and does not affect the metabolism of levodopa within the central nervous system.

Since its decarboxylase inhibiting activity is limited to extracerebral tissues, administration of carbidopa with levodopa makes more levodopa available for transport to the brain.

Pyridoxine hydrochloride (vitamin B_6), in oral doses of 10 mg to 25 mg, may reverse the effects of levodopa by increasing the rate of aromatic amino acid decarboxylation. Carbidopa inhibits the action of pyridoxine.

TABLETS

In dogs, reduced formation of dopamine in extracerebral tissues, such as the heart, provides protection against the development of dopamine-induced cardiac arrhythmias. Clinical studies tend to support the hypothesis of a similar protective effect in humans although controlled data are too limited at the present time to draw firm conclusions.

Carbidopa reduces the amount of levodopa required by about 75 percent and, when administered with levodopa, increases both plasma levels and the plasma half-life of levodopa, and decreases plasma and urinary dopamine and homovanillic acid.

In clinical pharmacologic studies, simultaneous administration of carbidopa and levodopa produced greater urinary excretion of levodopa in proportion to the excretion of dopamine than administration of the two drugs at separate times.

SUSTAINED RELEASE TABLETS

Patients treated with levodopa therapy for Parkinson's disease may develop motor fluctuations characterized by end-of-dose failure, peak dose dyskinesia, and akinesia. The advanced form of motor fluctuations ('on-off' phenomenon) is characterized by unpredictable swings from mobility to immobility. Although the causes of the motor fluctuations are not completely understood, *in some patients* they may be attenuated by treatment regimens that produce steady plasma levels of levodopa.

Carbidopa-levodopa sustained release tablets contains either 50 mg of carbidopa and 200 mg of levodopa, or 25 mg of carbidopa and 100 mg of levodopa in a sustained-release dosage form designed to release these ingredients over a 4 to 6 hour period. With sustained release tablets there is less variation in plasma levodopa levels than with carbidopa-levodopa, the conventional formulation. *However, carbidopa-levodopa sustained release tablets are less systemically bioavailable than standard carbidopa-levodopa and may require increased daily doses to achieve the same level of symptomatic relief as provided by standard carbidopa-levodopa.*

In clinical trials, patients with moderate to severe motor fluctuations who received carbidopa-levodopa sustained release tablets *did not experience quantitatively significant reductions* in 'off' time when compared to standard carbidopa-levodopa. However, global ratings of improvement as assessed by both patient and physician were better during therapy with carbidopa-levodopa sustained release tablets than with standard carbidopa-levodopa. In patients

CLINICAL PHARMACOLOGY: *(cont'd)*

without motor fluctuations, carbidopa-levodopa sustained release tablets, under controlled conditions, provided the same therapeutic benefit with less frequent dosing when compared to standard carbidopa-levodopa.

PHARMACOKINETICS

Carbidopa reduces the amount of levodopa required to produce a given response by about 75 percent and, when administered with levodopa, increases both plasma levels and the plasma half-life of levodopa, and decreases plasma and urinary dopamine and homovanillic acid.

Sustained Release Tablets

Elimination half-life of levodopa in the presence of carbidopa is about 1.5 hours. Following sustained release tablets, the apparent half-life of levodopa may be prolonged because of continuous absorption.

In healthy elderly subjects (56-67 years old) the mean time to peak concentration of levodopa after a single dose of carbidopa-levodopa sustained release tablets 50 mg/200 mg was about 2 hours as compared to 0.5 hours after standard carbidopa-levodopa. The maximum concentration of levodopa after a single dose of carbidopa-levodopa sustained release was about 35% of the standard carbidopa-levodopa (1151 vs 3256 ng/ml). The extent of availability of levodopa from sustained release tablets was about 70-75% relative to intravenous levodopa or standard carbidopa-levodopa in the elderly. The absolute bioavailability of levodopa from sustained release tablets (relative to IV) in young subjects was shown to be only about 44%. The extent of availability and the peak concentrations of levodopa were comparable in the elderly after a single dose and at steady state after t.i.d. administration of carbidopa-levodopa sustained release tablets 50 mg/200 mg. In elderly subjects, the average trough levels of levodopa at steady state after the CR tablet were about 2 fold higher than after the standard carbidopa-levodopa (163 vs 74 ng/ml).

In these studies, using similar total daily doses of levodopa, plasma levodopa concentrations with sustained release tablets fluctuated in a narrower range than with carbidopa-levodopa. Because the bioavailability of levodopa from sustained release tablets relative to carbidopa-levodopa is approximately 70-75%, the daily dosage of levodopa necessary to produce a given clinical response with the sustained-release formulation will usually be higher.

The extent of availability and peak concentrations of levodopa after a single dose of carbidopa-levodopa sustained release tablets 50 mg/200 mg increased by about 50% and 25%, respectively, when administered with food.

INDICATIONS AND USAGE:

Carbidopa-levodopa is indicated in the treatment of the symptoms of idiopathic Parkinson's disease (paralysis agitans), post-encephalitic parkinsonism, and symptomatic parkinsonism which may follow injury to the nervous system by carbon monoxide intoxication and manganese intoxication.

TABLETS

Carbidopa-levodopa is indicated in these conditions to permit the administration of lower doses of levodopa with reduced nausea and vomiting, with more rapid dosage titration, with a somewhat smoother response, and with supplemental pyridoxine (vitamin B_6).

The incidence of levodopa-induced nausea and vomiting is less with carbidopa-levodopa than with levodopa. In many patients this reduction in nausea and vomiting will permit more rapid dosage titration.

In some patients a somewhat smoother antiparkinsonian effect results from therapy with carbidopa-levodopa than with levodopa. However, patients with markedly irregular ("on-off") responses to levodopa have not been shown to benefit from carbidopa-levodopa.

Since carbidopa prevents the reversal of levodopa effects caused by pyridoxine, carbidopa-levodopa can be given to patients receiving supplemental pyridoxine (vitamin B_6).

Although the administration of carbidopa permits control of parkinsonism and Parkinson's disease with much lower doses of levodopa, there is no conclusive evidence at present that this is beneficial other than in reducing nausea and vomiting, permitting more rapid titration, and providing a somewhat smoother response to levodopa. *Carbidopa does not decrease adverse reactions due to central effects of levodopa. By permitting more levodopa to reach the brain, particularly when nausea and vomiting is not a dose-limiting factor, certain adverse CNS effects, e.g., dyskinesias, may occur at lower dosages and sooner during therapy with carbidopa-levodopa than with levodopa.*

Certain patients who responded poorly to levodopa have improved when carbidopa-levodopa was substituted. This is most likely due to decreased peripheral decarboxylation of levodopa which results from administration of carbidopa rather than to a primary effect of carbidopa on the nervous system. Carbidopa has not been shown to enhance the intrinsic efficacy of levodopa in parkinsonian syndromes.

In considering whether to give carbidopa-levodopa to patients already on levodopa who have nausea and/or vomiting, the practitioner should be aware that, while many patients may be expected to improve, some do not. Since one cannot predict which patients are likely to improve, this can only be determined by a trial of therapy. It should be further noted that in controlled trials comparing carbidopa-levodopa with levodopa, about half of the patients with nausea and/or vomiting on levodopa improved spontaneously despite being retained on the same dose of levodopa during the controlled portion of the trial.

CONTRAINDICATIONS:

Because levodopa may activate a malignant melanoma, it should not be used in patients with suspicious, undiagnosed skin lesions or a history of melanoma.

TABLETS

Monoamine oxidase inhibitors and carbidopa-levodopa should not be given concomitantly.

These inhibitors must be discontinued at least two weeks prior to initiating therapy with carbidopa-levodopa.

SUSTAINED RELEASE TABLETS

Nonselective MAO inhibitors are contraindicated for use with carbidopa-levodopa sustained release tablets. Carbidopa-levodopa sustained release tablets may be administered concomitantly with the manufacture's recommended dose of an MAO inhibitor with selectivity for MAO type B (*e.g.*, selegiline HCl).

Carbidopa-levodopa is contraindicated in patients with known hypersensitivity to any component of this drug and in patients with narrow-angle glaucoma.

WARNINGS:

When patients are receiving levodopa without a decarboxylase inhibitor, levodopa must be discontinued at least eight hours before carbidopa-levodopa is started. In order to reduce adverse reactions, it is necessary to individualize therapy. Carbidopa-levodopa should be substituted at a dosage that will provide approximately 25 percent of the previous levodopa dosage (see DOSAGE AND ADMINISTRATION). Patients who are taking carbidopa-levodopa should be instructed not to take additional levodopa unless it is prescribed by the physician.

WARNINGS: *(cont'd)*

As with levodopa, carbidopa-levodopa may cause involuntary movements and mental disturbances. These reactions are thought to be due to increased brain dopamine following administration of levodopa. All patients should be observed carefully for the development of depression with concomitant suicidal tendencies. Patients with past or current psychoses should be treated with caution. The occurrence of dyskinesias may require dosage reduction.

Carbidopa-levodopa should be administered cautiously to patients with severe cardiovascular or pulmonary disease, bronchial asthma, renal, hepatic or endocrine disease.

As with levodopa, care should be exercised in administering carbidopa-levodopa to patients with a history of myocardial infarction who have residual atrial, nodal, or ventricular arrhythmias. In such patients, cardiac function should be monitored with particular care during the period of initial dosage adjustment, in a facility with provisions for intensive cardiac care.

As with levodopa, treatment with carbidopa-levodopa may increase the possibility of upper gastrointestinal hemorrhage in patients with a history of peptic ulcer.

A symptom complex resembling the neuroleptic malignant syndrome including muscular rigidity, elevated body temperature, mental changes, and increased serum creatine phosphokinase has been reported when anti-parkinsonian agents were withdrawn abruptly. Therefore, patients should be observed carefully when the dosage of carbidopa-levodopa is reduced abruptly or discontinued, especially if the patient is receiving neuroleptics.

SUSTAINED RELEASE TABLETS

Carbidopa does not decrease adverse reactions due to central effects of levodopa. By permitting more levodopa to reach the brain, particularly when nausea and vomiting is not a dose-limiting factor, certain adverse CNS effects, e.g., dyskinesias, will occur at lower dosages and sooner during therapy with carbidopa-levodopa sustained release tablets than with levodopa alone.

Patients receiving carbidopa-levodopa sustained release tablets may develop increased dyskinesia compared to carbidopa-levodopa.

TABLETS

Because carbidopa permits more levodopa to reach the brain and, thus, more dopamine to be formed, dyskinesias may occur at lower dosages and sooner with carbidopa-levodopa than with levodopa. The occurrence of dyskinesias may require dosage reduction.

Usage in Pregnancy and Lactation: Although the effects of carbidopa-levodopa on human pregnancy and lactation are unknown, both levodopa and combinations of carbidopa and levodopa have caused visceral and skeletal malformations in rabbits. Use of carbidopa-levodopa in women of childbearing potential requires that the anticipated benefits of the drug be weighed against possible hazards to mother and child. Carbidopa-levodopa should not be given to nursing mothers.

Usage in Children: The safety of carbidopa-levodopa in patients under 18 years of age has not been established.

PRECAUTIONS:

As with levodopa, periodic evaluations of hepatic, hematopoietic, cardiovascular, and renal function are recommended during extended therapy.

Patients with chronic wide-angle glaucoma may be treated cautiously with carbidopa-levodopa provided the intraocular pressure is well controlled and the patient is monitored carefully for changes in intraocular pressure during therapy.

Laboratory Tests: Abnormalities in laboratory tests may include elevations of liver function tests such a alkaline phosphatase, SGOT (AST), SGPT (ALT), lactic dehydrogenase, and bilirubin. Abnormalities in protein-bound iodine, blood urea nitrogen and positive Coombs test have also been reported. Commonly, levels of blood urea nitrogen, creatinine, and uric acid are lower during administration of carbidopa-levodopa preparations than with levodopa.

Carbidopa-levodopa preparations may cause a false-positive reaction for urinary ketone bodies when a test tape is used for determination of ketonuria. This reaction will not be altered by boiling the urine specimen. False-negative tests may result with the use of glucose-oxidase methods of testing for glucosuria.

SUSTAINED RELEASE TABLETS

Information for the Patient: The patient should be informed that this drug is a sustained-release formulation of carbidopa-levodopa which releases these ingredients over a 4 to 6 hour period. It is important that carbidopa-levodopa sustained release tablets be taken at regular intervals according to the schedule outlined by the physician. The patient should be cautioned not to change the prescribed dosage regimen and not to add any additional anti-parkinson medications, including other carbidopa- levodopa preparations, without first consulting the physician.

If abnormal involuntary movements appear or get worse during treatment with carbidopa-levodopa sustained release tablets, the physician should be notified, as dosage adjustment may be necessary.

Patients should be advised that sometimes the onset of effect of the first morning dose of carbidopa-levodopa sustained release tablets may be delayed for up to 1 hour compared with the response usually obtained from the first morning dose of standard carbidopa-levodopa. The physician should be notified if such delayed responses pose a problem in treatment.

Patients must be advised that the whole or half tablet should be swallowed without chewing or crushing.

NOTE: The suggested advice to patients being treated with carbidopa-levodopa sustained release tablets is intended to aid in the safe and effective use of this medication. It is not a disclosure of all possible adverse or intended effects.

Carcinogenesis, Mutagenesis, and Impairment of Fertility: In a two-year bioassay of carbidopa-levodopa, no evidence of carcinogenicity was found in rats receiving doses of approximately two times the maximum daily human dose of carbidopa and four times the maximum daily human dose of levodopa (equivalent to 8 carbidopa-levodopa sustained release tablets tablets).

In reproduction studies with carbidopa-levodopa, no effects on fertility were found in rats receiving doses of approximately two times the maximum daily human dose of carbidopa and four times the maximum daily human dose of levodopa (equivalent to 8 carbidopa-levodopa sustained release tablets tablets).

Pregnancy Category C: No teratogenic effects were observed in a study in mice receiving up to 20 times the maximum recommended human dose of carbidopa-levodopa. There was a decrease in the number of live pups delivered by rats receiving approximately two times the maximum recommended human dose of carbidopa and approximately five times the maximum recommended human dose of levodopa during organogenesis. Carbidopa-levodopa caused both visceral and skeletal malformations in rabbits at all doses and ratios of carbidopa/levodopa tested, which ranged from 10 times/5 times the maximum recommended human dose of carbidopa/levodopa to 20 times/10 times the maximum recommended human dose of carbidopa/levodopa.

There are no adequate or well-controlled studies in pregnant women. Use of carbidopa-levodopa sustained release tablets in women of childbearing potential requires that the anticipated benefits of the drug be weighted against possible hazards to mother and child.

PRECAUTIONS: *(cont'd)*

Nursing Mothers: It is not known whether this drug is excreted in human milk. Because many drugs are excreted in human milk, caution should be exercised when carbidopa-levodopa sustained release tablets is administered to a nursing mother.

Pediatric Use: Safety and effectiveness in infants and children have not been established, and the use of the drug in patients below the age of 18 is not recommended.

DRUG INTERACTIONS:

Caution should be exercised when the following drugs are administered concomitantly with carbidopa-levodopa.

Symptomatic postural hypotension can occur when carbidopa-levodopa or carbidopa-levodopa sustained release tablets is added to the treatment of a patient receiving antihypertensive drugs. Therefore, when therapy with carbidopa-levodopa is started, dosage adjustment of the antihypertensive drug may be required. For patients receiving monoamine oxidase inhibitors, see CONTRAINDICATIONS.

There have been rare reports of adverse reactions, including hypertension and dyskinesia, resulting from the concomitant use of tricyclic antidepressants and carbidopa-levodopa.

Phenothiazines and butyrophenones may reduce the therapeutic effects of levodopa. In addition, the beneficial effects of levodopa in Parkinson's disease have been reported to be reversed by phenytoin and papaverine. Patients taking these drugs with carbidopa-levodopa should be carefully observed for loss of therapeutic response.

ADVERSE REACTIONS:

TABLETS

The most common serious adverse reactions occurring with carbidopa-levodopa are choreiform, dystonic, and other involuntary movements. Other serious adverse reactions are mental changes including paranoid ideation and psychotic episodes, depression with or without development of suicidal tendencies, and dementia. Convulsions also have occurred; however, a causal relationship with carbidopa-levodopa has not been established.

A common but less serious effect is nausea.

Less frequent adverse reactions are cardiac irregularities and/or palpitation, orthostatic hypotensive episodes, bradykinetic episodes (the "on-off" phenomenon), anorexia, vomiting, and dizziness.

Rarely, gastrointestinal bleeding, development of duodenal ulcer, hypertension, phlebitis, hemolytic and non-hemolytic anemia, thrombocytopenia, leukopenia, and agranulocytosis have occurred.

Laboratory tests which have been reported to be abnormal are alkaline phosphatase, SGOT (AST), SGPT (ALT), lactic dehydrogenase, bilirubin, blood urea nitrogen, protein-bound iodine, and Coombs test.

Other adverse reactions that have been reported with levodopa are:

Nervous System: ataxia, numbness, increased hand tremor, muscle twitching, muscle cramps, blepharospasm (which may be taken as an early sign of excess dosage, consideration of dosage reduction may be made at this time), trismus, activation of latent Horner's syndrome.

Psychiatric: confusion, sleepiness, insomnia, nightmares, hallucinations, delusions, agitation, anxiety, euphoria.

Gastrointestinal: dry mouth, bitter taste, sialorrhea, dysphagia, bruxism, hiccups, abdominal pain and distress, constipation, diarrhea, flatulence, burning sensation of tongue.

Metabolic: weight gain or loss, edema.

Integumentary: malignant melanoma (see also CONTRAINDICATIONS), flushing, increased sweating, dark sweat, skin rash, loss of hair.

Genitourinary: urinary retention, urinary incontinence, dark urine, priapism.

Special Senses: diplopia, blurred vision, dilated pupils, oculogyric crises.

Miscellaneous: weakness, faintness, fatigue, headache, hoarseness, malaise, hot flashes, sense of stimulation, bizarre breathing patterns, neuroleptic malignant syndrome.

SUSTAINED RELEASE TABLETS

In controlled clinical trials, patients predominantly with moderate to severe motor fluctuations while on carbidopa-levodopa were randomized to therapy with either carbidopa-levodopa or carbidopa-levodopa sustained release tablets. The adverse experience frequency profile of carbidopa-levodopa sustained release tablets did not differ substantially from that of carbidopa-levodopa, as shown in TABLE 1.

TABLE 1 Clinical Adverse Experiences Occurring in 1% or Greater of Patients

Adverse Experience	Carbidopa- Levodopa Sustained Release tablets n = 491 %	Carbidopa- Levodopa n = 524 %
Dyskinesia	16.5	12.2
Nausea	5.5	5.7
Hallucinations	3.9	3.2
Confusion	3.7	2.3
Dizziness	2.9	2.3
Depression	2.2	1.3
Urinary tract infection	2.2	2.3
Headache	2.0	1.9
Dream abnormalities	1.8	0.8
Dystonia	1.8	0.8
Vomiting	1.8	1.9
Upper respiratory infection	1.8	1.0
Dyspnea	1.6	0.4
'On-Off' phenomena	1.6	1.1
Back pain	1.6	0.6
Dry Mouth	1.4	1.1
Anorexia	1.2	1.1
Diarrhea	1.2	0.6
Insomnia	1.2	1.0
Orthostatic hypotension	1.0	1.1
Shoulder pain	1.0	0.6
Chest pain	1.0	0.8
Muscle cramps	0.8	1.0
Paresthesia	0.8	1.1
Urinary frequency	0.8	1.1
Dyspepsia	0.6	1.1
Constipation	0.2	1.5

Abnormal laboratory findings occurring at a frequency of 1% or greater in approximately 443 patients who received carbidopa-levodopa sustained release tablets and 475 who received carbidopa-levodopa during controlled clinical trials included: decreased hemoglobin and hematocrit; elevated serum glucose; white blood cells, bacteria and blood in the urine.

ADVERSE REACTIONS: *(cont'd)*

The adverse experiences observed in patients in uncontrolled studies were similar to those seen in controlled clinical studies.

Other adverse experiences reported overall in clinical trials in 748 patients treated with carbidopa-levodopa sustained release tablets, listed by body system in order of decreasing frequency, include:

Nervous System/Psychiatric: Chorea, somnolence, falling, anxiety disorder, disorientation, decreased mental acuity, gait abnormalities, extrapyramidal disorder, agitation, nervousness, sleep disorders, memory impairment.

Body as a Whole: Asthenia, fatigue, abdominal pain, orthostatic effects.

Digestive: Gastrointestinal pain, dysphagia, heartburn.

Cardiovascular: Palpitation, essential hypertension, hypotension, myocardial infarction.

Special Senses: Blurred vision.

Metabolic: Weight loss.

Skin: Rash

Respiratory: Cough, pharyngeal pain, common cold.

Urogenital: Urinary Incontinence.

Musculoskeletal: Leg pain.

Laboratory Tests: Decreased white blood cell count and serum potassium; increased BUN, serum creatinine and serum LDH; protein and glucose in the urine.

Other adverse experiences have been reported with various carbidopa-levodopa formulations and may occur with carbidopa-levodopa sustained release tablets:

Nervous System/Psychiatric: Mental changes including paranoid ideation, psychotic episodes, depression with suicidal tendencies and dementia; convulsions (however, a causal relationship has not been established); bradykinetic episodes.

Gastrointestinal: Gastrointestinal bleeding, development of duodenal ulcer.

Cardiovascular: Cardiac irregularities, phlebitis.

Hematologic: Hemolytic and nonhemolytic anemia, thrombocytopenia, leukopenia, agranulocytosis.

Laboratory Tests: Abnormalities in alkaline phosphatase, SGOT (AST), SGPT (ALT), lactic dehydrogenase, bilirubin, protein-bound iodine, Coombs test.

Other adverse reactions that have been reported with levodopa are:

Nervous System: Numbness, increased hand tremor, muscle twitching, blepharospasm (which may be taken as an early sign of excess dosage, consideration of dosage reduction may be made at this time), trismus, activation of latent Horner's syndrome.

Psychiatric: Delusions, euphoria.

Gastrointestinal: Bitter taste, sialorrhea, bruxism, hiccups, flatulence, burning sensation of tongue.

Metabolic: Weight gain, edema.

Integumentary: Malignant melanoma (see also CONTRAINDICATIONS), flushing, increased sweating, dark sweat, loss of hair.

Genitourinary: Urinary retention, urinary incontinence, dark urine, priapism.

Miscellaneous: Faintness, hoarseness, malaise, hot flashes, sense of stimulation, bizarre breathing patterns, neuroleptic malignant syndrome.

OVERDOSAGE:

Management of acute overdosage with carbidopa-levodopa is basically the same as management of acute overdosage with levodopa; Pyridoxine is not effective in reversing the actions of carbidopa-levodopa.

General supportive measures should be employed, along with immediate gastric lavage. Intravenous fluids should be administered judiciously and an adequate airway maintained. Electrocardiographic monitoring should be instituted and the patient carefully observed for the development of arrhythmias; if required, appropriate antiarrhythmic therapy should be given. The possibility that the patient may have taken other drugs as well as carbidopa-levodopa should be taken into consideration. To date, no experience has been reported with dialysis; hence, its value in overdosage is not known.

Sustained Release Tablets: Based on studies in which high doses of levodopa and/or carbidopa were administered, a significant proportion of rats and mice given single oral doses of levodopa of approximately 1500-2000 mg/kg are expected to die. A significant proportion of infant rats of both sexes are expected to die at a dose of 800 mg/kg. A significant proportion of rats are expected to die after treatment with similar doses of carbidopa. The addition of carbidopa in a 1:10 ratio with levodopa increases the dose at which a significant proportion of mice are expected to die to 3360 mg/kg.

DOSAGE AND ADMINISTRATION:

TABLETS

The optimum daily dosage of carbidopa-levodopa must be determined by careful titration in each patient. Carbidopa-levodopa tablets are available in a 1:4 ratio of carbidopa to levodopa 25 mg/100 mg as well as 1:10 ratio 25 mg/250 mg and 10 mg/100 mg. Tablets of the two ratios may be given separately or combined as needed to provide the optimum dosage.

Studies show that peripheral dopa decarboxylase is saturated by carbidopa at approximately 70 to 100 mg a day. Patients receiving less than this amount of carbidopa are more likely to experience nausea and vomiting.

Usual Initial Dosage: Dosage is best initiated with one tablet of carbidopa-levodopa 25 mg/100 mg three times a day. This dosage schedule provides 75 mg of carbidopa per day. Dosage may be increased by one tablet every day or every other day, as necessary, until a dosage of eight tablets of carbidopa-levodopa 25 mg/100 mg a day is reached.

If carbidopa-levodopa 10 mg/100 mg is used, dosage may be initiated with one tablet three or four times a day. However, this will not provide an adequate amount of carbidopa for many patients. Dosage may be increased by one tablet every day or every other day until a total of eight tablets (2 tablets q.i.d.) is reached.

How to Transfer Patients from Levodopa: Levodopa must be discontinued at least eight hours before starting carbidopa-levodopa combination. A daily dosage of carbidopa-levodopa should be chosen that will provide approximately 25 percent of the previous levodopa dosage. Patients who are taking less than 1500 mg of levodopa a day should be started on one tablet of carbidopa-levodopa 25 mg/100 mg three or four times a day. The suggested starting dosage for most patients taking more than 1500 mg of levodopa is one tablet of carbidopa-levodopa 25 mg/250 mg three or four times a day.

Maintenance: Therapy should be individualized and adjusted according to the desired therapeutic response. At least 70 to 100 mg of carbidopa per day should be provided. When a greater proportion of carbidopa is required, one tablet of carbidopa-levodopa 25 mg/100 mg may be substituted for each tablet of carbidopa-levodopa 10 mg/100 mg. When more levodopa is required, carbidopa-levodopa 25 mg/250 mg should be substituted for carbidopa-levodopa 25 mg/100 mg or carbidopa-levodopa 10 mg/100 mg. If necessary, the dosage of

DOSAGE AND ADMINISTRATION: *(cont'd)*

carbidopa-levodopa 25 mg/250 mg may be increased by one- half or one tablet every day or every other day to a maximum of eight tablets a day. Experience with total daily dosages of carbidopa greater than 200 mg is limited.

Because both therapeutic and adverse responses occur more rapidly with carbidopa-levodopa than with levodopa alone, patients should be monitored closely during the dose adjustment period. Specifically, involuntary movements will occur more rapidly with carbidopa-levodopa than with levodopa. The occurrence of involuntary movements may require dosage reduction. Blepharospasm may be a useful early sign of excess dosage in some patients.

Current evidence indicates that other standard drugs for Parkinson's disease (except levodopa) may be continued while carbidopa-levodopa is being administered, although their dosage may have to be adjusted.

If general anesthesia is required, carbidopa-levodopa may be continued as long as the patient is permitted to take fluids and medication by mouth. If therapy is interrupted temporarily, the usual daily dosage may be administered as soon as the patient is able to take oral medication.

SUSTAINED RELEASE TABLETS

This form contains carbidopa and levodopa in a 1:4 ratio as either the 50 mg/200 mg tablet or the 25 mg/100 mg tablet. The daily dosage of carbidopa-levodopa sustained release tablets must be determined by careful titration. Patients should be monitored closely during the dose adjustment period, particularly with regard to appearance or worsening of involuntary movements, dyskinesias or nausea. Carbidopa-levodopa sustained release tablets 50 mg/200 mg may be administered as whole or as half-tablets which should not be chewed or crushed. Sustained release tablets 25 mg/100 mg may be used in combination with 50 mg/200 mg sustained release tablets to titrate to the optimum dosage, or as an alternative to the 50 mg/200 mg half-tablet.

Standard drugs for Parkinson's disease, other than levodopa without a decarboxylase inhibitor, may be used concomitantly while carbidopa-levodopa sustained release tablets is being administered, although their dosage may have to be adjusted.

Since carbidopa prevents the reversal of levodopa effects caused by pyridoxine, carbidopa-levodopa sustained release tablets can be given to patients receiving supplemental pyridoxine (vitamin B_6).

Initial Dosage: Patients currently treated with conventional carbidopa-levodopa preparations: Dosage with carbidopa-levodopa sustained release tablets should be substituted at an amount that provides approximately 10% more levodopa per day, although this may need to be increased to a dosage that provides up to 30% more levodopa per day depending on clinical response (see DOSAGE AND ADMINISTRATION, Titration). The interval between doses of carbidopa-levodopa sustained release tablets should be 4-8 hours during the waking day. See CLINICAL PHARMACOLOGY, Pharmacodynamics.

A guideline for initiation of carbidopa-levodopa sustained release tablets is shown in TABLE 2.

TABLE 2 Guidelines for Initial Conversion from Carbidopa-Levodopa to Carbidopa-Levodopa Sustained Release Tablets

Carbidopa-Levodopa Total Daily Dose* Levodopa (mg)	Carbidopa-Levodopa Sustained Release Tablets Suggested Dosage Regimen
300-400	200 mg b.i.d.
500-600	300 mg b.i.d. or 200 t.i.d.
700-800	A total of 800 mg in 3 or more divided doses (*e.g.,* 300 mg a.m., 300 mg early p.m., and 200 mg later p.m.)
900-1000	A total of 1000 mg in 3 or more divided doses (*e.g.,* 400 mg a.m., 400 mg early p.m., and 200 mg later p.m.)

* For dosing ranges not shown in the table, see DOSAGE AND ADMINISTRATION, Initial Dosage — Patients currently treated with conventional carbidopa-levodopa preparations.

Patients currently treated with levodopa without a decarboxylase inhibitor: Levodopa must be discontinued at least eight hours before therapy with carbidopa-levodopa sustained release tablets is started. Carbidopa-levodopa sustained release tablets should be substituted at a dosage that will provide approximately 25% of the previous levodopa dosage. In patients with mild to moderate disease, the initial dose is usually 1 tablet of carbidopa-levodopa sustained release tablets 50 mg/200 mg b.i.d.

Patients not receiving levodopa: In patients with mild to moderate disease, the initial recommended dose is 1 tablet of carbidopa-levodopa sustained release tablets 50 mg/200 mg b.i.d. Initial dosage should not be given at intervals of less than 6 hours.

Titration with Sustained Release Tablets: Following initiation of therapy, doses and dosing intervals may be increased or decreased depending upon therapeutic response. Most patients have been adequately treated with doses of carbidopa-levodopa sustained release tablets that provide 400 to 1600 mg of levodopa per day, administered as divided doses at intervals ranging from 4 to 8 hours during the waking day. Higher doses of carbidopa-levodopa sustained release tablets (2400 mg or more of levodopa per day) and shorter intervals (less than 4 hours) have been used, but are not usually recommended.

When doses of carbidopa-levodopa sustained release tablets are given at intervals of less than 4 hours, and/or if the divided doses are not equal, it is recommended that the smaller doses be given at the end of the day.

An interval of at least 3 days between dosage adjustments is recommended.

Maintenance: Because Parkinson's disease is progressive, periodic clinical evaluations are recommended; adjustment of the dosage regimen of carbidopa-levodopa sustained release tablets may be required.

Addition of Other Antiparkinson Medications: Anticholinergic agents, dopamine agonists, and amantadine can be given with carbidopa-levodopa sustained release tablets. Dosage adjustment of carbidopa-levodopa sustained release tablets may be necessary when these agents are added.

A dose of carbidopa-levodopa 25mg/100mg or 10mg/100mg (one half or a whole tablet) can be added to the dosage regimen of carbidopa-levodopa sustained release in selected patients with advanced disease who need additional immediate-release levodopa for a brief time during daytime hours.

Interruption of Therapy: Patients should be observed carefully if abrupt reduction or discontinuation of carbidopa-levodopa sustained release is required, especially if the patient is receiving neuroleptics. (See WARNINGS.)

If general anesthesia is required, carbidopa-levodopa sustained release may be continued as long as the patient is permitted to take oral medication. If therapy is interrupted temporarily, the usual dosage should be administered as soon as the patient is able to take oral medication.

HOW SUPPLIED:

Sinemet: Tablets Sinemet 25-100 are yellow, oval, scored tablets, coded 650.

Tablets Sinemet 10-100 are dark dapple-blue, oval, scored, uncoated tablets, coded 647.

Tablets Sinemet 25-250 are light dapple-blue, oval, scored, uncoated tablets, coded 654.

Sinemet CR: Sinemet CR 50-200 sustained-release tablets containing 50 mg of carbidopa and 200 mg of levodopa, are peach colored, oval, scored, biconvex, compressed tablets, coded 521.

Sinemet CR 25-100 sustained-release tablets containing 25 mg carbidopa and 100 mg of levodopa, are pink colored, oval, biconvex, compressed tablets, coded 601.

Storage: Avoid temperatures above 30°C (86°F). Store in a tightly closed container protected from light.

HOW SUPPLIED - RATED THERAPEUTICALLY EQUIVALENT:

Tablet, Uncoated - Oral - 10 mg/100 mg

30's	$8.48	Carbidopa/Levodopa, H.C.F.A. F F P	99999-0653-01
100's	$28.28	Carbidopa/Levodopa, H.C.F.A. F F P	99999-0653-02
100's	**$50.55**	**SINEMET, Dupont Pharma**	**00056-0647-68**
100's	$51.40	Carbidopa/Levodopa, Harber Pharm	51432-0799-03
100's	$52.10	Carbidopa/Levodopa, West Point Pharma	59591-0247-68
100's	$52.40	Carbidopa/Levodopa, Dupont Pharma	00056-0271-68
100's	$52.40	Carbidopa/Levodpa, Endo Labs	60951-0603-68
100's	$52.60	Carbidopa/Levodopa, Qualitest Pharms	00603-2568-21
100's	$53.15	Carbidopa/Levodopa, Schein Pharm (US)	00364-2538-01
100's	$53.89	Carbidopa/Levodopa, Goldline Labs	00182-1948-01
100's	$53.90	Carbidopa/Levodopa, United Res	00677-1493-01
100's	$53.95	Carbidopa/Levodopa, Major Pharms	00904-7718-60
100's	$54.47	Carbidopa/Levodopa, Purepac Pharm	00228-2538-10
100's	**$55.20**	**SINEMET, Dupont Pharma**	**00056-0647-28**
100's	$55.52	Carbidopa/Levodopa, Geneva Pharms	00781-1626-01
100's	$56.14	Carbidopa/Levodopa, Geneva Pharms	00781-1626-13
100's	$58.04	Carbidopa/Levodopa, HL Moore Drug Exch	00839-7765-06
100's	$58.05	Carbidopa/Levodopa, Teva	00093-0292-01
100's	$58.05	Carbidopa/Levodopa, Rugby	00536-5555-01
100's	$60.65	Carbidopa/Levodopa, Goldline Labs	00182-1948-89
100's	$62.30	Carbidopa/Levodopa, Aligen Independ	00405-4134-01
100's	$65.50	Carbidopa/Levodopa, Vangard Labs	00615-3537-13
500's	$141.40	Carbidopa/Levodopa, H.C.F.A. F F P	99999-0653-03
500's	$262.50	Carbidopa/Levodopa, Goldline Labs	00182-1948-05
500's	$272.35	Carbidopa/Levodopa, Purepac Pharm	00228-2538-50
500's	$272.50	Carbidopa/Levodopa, Teva	00093-0292-05
750's	$462.41	Carbidopa/Levodopa, Glasgow Pharm	60809-0125-55
750's	$462.41	Carbidopa/Levodopa, Glasgow Pharm	60809-0125-72

Tablet, Uncoated - Oral - 25 mg/100 mg

30's	$9.27	Carbidopa/Levodopa, H.C.F.A. F F P	99999-0653-04
100's	$30.90	Carbidopa/Levodopa, H.C.F.A. F F P	99999-0653-05
100's	$31.29	Carbidopa/Levodopa, United Res	00677-1494-01
100's	**$57.05**	**SINEMET, Dupont Pharma**	**00056-0650-68**
100's	$58.15	Carbidopa/Levodopa, Dupont Pharma	00056-0272-68
100's	$58.15	Carbidopa/Levodopa, West Point Pharma	59591-0246-68
100's	$58.15	Carbidopa/Levodpa, Endo Labs	60951-0605-68
100's	$58.50	Carbidopa/Levodopa, HL Moore Drug Exch	00839-7766-06
100's	$58.80	Carbidopa/Levodopa, Qualitest Pharms	00603-2569-21
100's	$59.21	Carbidopa/Levodopa, Schein Pharm (US)	00364-2539-01
100's	$59.40	Carbidopa/Levodopa, Teva	00093-0293-01
100's	$59.40	Carbidopa/Levodopa, Goldline Labs	00182-1949-01
100's	$59.41	Carbidopa/Levodopa, Purepac Pharm	00228-2539-10
100's	$59.95	Carbidopa/Levodopa, Major Pharms	00904-7719-60
100's	**$60.50**	**SINEMET, Dupont Pharma**	**00056-0650-28**
100's	$61.75	Carbidopa/Levodopa, Geneva Pharms	00781-1627-01
100's	$62.44	Carbidopa/Levodopa, Geneva Pharms	00781-1627-13
100's	$62.53	Carbidopa/Levodopa, Aligen Independ	00405-4133-01
100's	$64.17	Carbidopa/Levodopa, Rugby	00536-5556-01
100's	$65.25	Atamet, Athena	59075-0585-10
100's	$65.35	Carbidopa/Levodopa, Goldline Labs	00182-1949-89
100's	$69.51	Carbidopa/Levodopa, Vangard Labs	00615-3561-13
500's	$154.50	Carbidopa/Levodopa, H.C.F.A. F F P	99999-0653-06
500's	$297.00	Carbidopa/Levodopa, Teva	00093-0293-05
500's	$297.05	Carbidopa/Levodopa, Goldline Labs	00182-1949-05
500's	$297.05	Carbidopa/Levodopa, Purepac Pharm	00228-2539-50
750's	$495.19	Carbidopa/Levodopa, Glasgow Pharm	60809-0113-55
750's	$495.19	Carbidopa/Levodopa, Glasgow Pharm	60809-0113-72
1000's	$309.00	Carbidopa/Levodopa, H.C.F.A. F F P	99999-0653-07
1000's	$594.00	Carbidopa/Levodopa, Teva	00093-0293-10
1000's	$594.10	Carbidopa/Levodopa, Goldline Labs	00182-1949-10
1000's	$594.10	Carbidopa/Levodopa, Purepac Pharm	00228-2539-96

Tablet, Uncoated - Oral - 25 mg/250 mg

30's	$11.09	Carbidopa/Levodopa, H.C.F.A. F F P	99999-0653-08
100's	$36.99	Carbidopa/Levodopa, United Res	00677-1495-01
100's	$36.99	Carbidopa/Levodopa, H.C.F.A. F F P	99999-0653-09
100's	$62.50	Carbidopa/Levodopa, Harber Pharm	51432-0764-03
100's	$71.30	Carbidopa/Levodopa, Dupont Pharma	00056-0251-68
100's	$71.30	Carbidopa/Levodopa, West Point Pharma	59591-0250-68
100's	$71.30	Carbidopa/Levodpa, Endo Labs	60951-0607-68
100's	**$72.70**	**SINEMET, Dupont Pharma**	**00056-0654-68**
100's	$73.50	Carbidopa/Levodopa, Schein Pharm (US)	00364-2540-01
100's	$75.14	Carbidopa/Levodopa, Qualitest Pharms	00603-2570-21
100's	$75.25	Carbidopa/Levodopa, Major Pharms	00904-7720-60
100's	$76.10	Carbidopa/Levodopa, Purepac Pharm	00228-2540-10
100's	$76.50	Carbidopa/Levodopa, Goldline Labs	00182-1950-01
100's	**$76.70**	**SINEMET, Dupont Pharma**	**00056-0654-28**
100's	$79.33	Carbidopa/Levodopa, Geneva Pharms	00781-1628-01
100's	$80.22	Carbidopa/Levodopa, Geneva Pharms	00781-1628-13
100's	$80.30	Carbidopa/Levodopa, Teva	00093-0294-01
100's	$80.30	Carbidopa/Levodopa, Rugby	00536-5557-01
100's	$80.31	Carbidopa/Levodopa, HL Moore Drug Exch	00839-7767-06
100's	$83.50	Atamet, Athena	59075-0587-10
100's	$83.70	Carbidopa/Levodopa, Goldline Labs	00182-1950-89
100's	$83.88	Carbidopa/Levodopa, Aligen Independ	00405-4132-01
500's	$184.95	Carbidopa/Levodopa, H.C.F.A. F F P	99999-0653-10
500's	$375.00	Carbidopa/Levodopa, Goldline Labs	00182-1950-05
500's	$380.50	Carbidopa/Levodopa, Purepac Pharm	00228-2540-50
500's	$382.50	Carbidopa/Levodopa, Teva	00093-0294-05
1000's	$369.90	Carbidopa/Levodopa, H.C.F.A. F F P	99999-0653-11
1000's	$750.00	Carbidopa/Levodopa, Goldline Labs	00182-1950-10
1000's	$761.00	Carbidopa/Levodopa, Purepac Pharm	00228-2540-96
1000's	$765.00	Carbidopa/Levodopa, Teva	00093-0294-10

HOW SUPPLIED - NOT RATED EQUIVALENT:

Tablet, Uncoated, Sustained Action - Oral - 25 mg/100 mg

100's	$58.50	SINEMET CR, Dupont Pharma	00056-0601-68
100's	$61.60	SINEMET CR, Dupont Pharma	00056-0601-28

Tablet, Uncoated, Sustained Action - Oral - 50 mg/200 mg

100's	$122.15	SINEMET CR, Dupont Pharma	00056-0521-68
100's	$129.45	SINEMET CR, Dupont Pharma	00056-0521-28

CARBINOXAMINE MALEATE; DEXTROMETHORPHAN HYDROBROMIDE; PSEUDOEPHEDRINE HYDROCHLORIDE

(000655)

CATEGORIES: Antitussives; Antitussives/Expectorants/Mucolytics; Common Cold; Congestion; Cough Preparations; Decongestants; Influenza; Nasal Congestion; Respiratory & Allergy Medications; Pregnancy Category C; FDA Pre 1938 Drugs

BRAND NAMES: Biodec-Dm; Carbinoxamine Compound; Carbodec-Dm; Carbofed-Dm; Cardec Dm; Cardec-Dm; Chemdec Dm; Harberdec-Dm; Maldec-Dm; Mardec Dm; Pseudo-Car Dm; Rondamine-Dm; **Rondec-Dm**; *Rondec-DM*; Sildec-Dm; Tussafed
(International brand names outside U.S. in italics)

FORMULARIES: Aetna; FHP; PCS

PRIMARY ICD9: 477.9 (Allergic Rhinitis, Cause Unspecified)

DESCRIPTION:

NON-ALCOHOLIC

Antihistamine/Decongestant/Antitussive for oral use.

SYRUP

For adults and children: Each 5 ml (teaspoonful) contains carbinoxamine maleate, USP, 4 mg; pseudoephedrine HCl, USP, 60 mg; dextromethorphan hydrobromide, USP, 15 mg.

DROPS

For infants, for oral use: Each 1 ml (dropperful) contains carbinoxamine maleate, USP, 2 mg; pseudoephedrine HCl, USP, 25 mg; dextromethorphan hydrobromide, USP, 4 mg.

Inactive Ingredients: D&C Red #33; FD&C Blue #1; Flavor; Glycerin, USP; Purified Water, Menthol, Sodium Benzoate, and Sorbitol, USP. **It may also contain** Citric Acid, USP and Sodium Citrate, USP.

CLINICAL PHARMACOLOGY:

Antihistaminic, decongestant and antitussive actions.

Carbinoxamine maleate possesses H_1 antihistaminic activity and mild anticholinergic and sedative effects. Serum half-life for carbinoxamine is estimated to be 10 to 20 hours. Virtually, no intact drug is excreted in the urine.

Pseudoephedrine HCl is an oral sympathomimetic amine which acts as a decongestant to respiratory tract mucous membranes. While its vasoconstrictor action is similar to that of ephedrine, pseudoephedrine has less pressor effect in normotensive adults. Serum half-life for pseudoephedrine is 6 to 8 hours. Acidic urine is associated with faster elimination of the drug. About one half of the administered dose is excreted in the urine.

Dextromethorphan hydrobromide is a non-narcotic antitussive with effectiveness equal to codeine. It acts in the medulla oblongata to elevate the cough threshold. Dextromethorphan does not produce analgesia or induce intolerance, and has no potential for addiction. At usual doses, it will not depress respiration or inhibit ciliary activity. Dextromethorphan is rapidly metabolized, with trace amounts of the parent compound and blood urine. About one-half of the administered dose is excreted in the urine as conjugated metabolites.

INDICATIONS AND USAGE:

For relief of cough and upper respiratory symptoms, including nasal congestion, associated with allergy or the common cold.

CONTRAINDICATIONS:

Patients with hypersensitivity or idiosyncrasy to any ingredients, patients taking monoamine oxidase (MAO) inhibitors, patients with narrow-angle glaucoma, urinary retention, peptic ulcer, severe hypertension or coronary artery disease, or patients undergoing an asthmatic attack.

WARNINGS:

Use in Pregnancy: Safety for use during pregnancy has not yet been established.

Nursing Mothers: Use with caution in nursing mothers.

Special Risk Patients: Use with caution in patients with hypertension or ischemic heart disease, and persons over 60 years.

PRECAUTIONS:

Before prescribing medication to suppress or modify cough, identify and provide therapy for the underlying cause of cough.

Use with caution in patients with hypertension, heart disease, asthma, hypothyroidism, increased intraocular pressure, diabetes mellitus, and prostatic hypertrophy.

INFORMATION FOR THE PATIENT

Avoid alcohol and other Central Nervous System (CNS) depressants while taking these products. Patients sensitive to antihistamines may experience moderate to severe drowsiness. Patients sensitive to sympathomimetic amines may note mild CNS stimulation. While taking these products, exercise care in driving or operating appliances, machinery, etc.

PREGNANCY CATEGORY C

Animal reproduction studies have not been conducted with carbinoxamine syrup & drops. It is also not known whether these products can cause fetal harm when administered to a pregnant woman or affect reproduction capacity. Give to pregnant women only if clearly needed.

DRUG INTERACTIONS:

Antihistamines may enhance the effects of tricyclic antidepressants, barbiturates, alcohol, and other CNS depressants. MAO inhibitors prolong and intensify the anticholinergic effects of antihistamines. Sympathomimetic amines may reduce the antihypertensive effects of reserpine, veratrum alkaloids, methyldopa and mecamylamine. Effects of sympathomimetics are increased with MAO inhibitors and beta-adrenergic blockers. The cough suppressant action of dextromethorphan and narcotic antitussives are additive.

ADVERSE REACTIONS:

Antihistamines: Sedation, dizziness, diplopia, vomiting, diarrhea, dry mouth, headache, nervousness, nausea, anorexia, heartburn, weakness, polyuria and dysuria and, rarely, excitability in children.

Sympathomimetic amines: Convulsions, CNS stimulation, cardiac arrhythmias, respiration difficulty, increased heart rate or blood pressure, hallucinations, tremors, nervousness, insomnia, weakness, pallor and dysuria.

Dextromethorphan: Drowsiness and GI disturbance.

OVERDOSAGE:

No information is available as to specific results of an overdose of these products. The signs, symptoms and treatment described below are those of H_1 antihistamine, ephedrine and dextromethorphan overdose.

SYMPTOMS

Should antihistamine effects predominate, central action constitutes the greatest danger. In the small children, predominant symptoms are excitation, hallucination, ataxia, incoordination, tremors, flushed face and fever. Convulsions, fixed and dilated pupils, coma and death may occur in severe cases. In the adult, fever and flushing are uncommon; excitement leading to convulsions and postictal depression is often preceded by drowsiness and coma. Respiration is usually not seriously depressed; blood pressure is usually stable.

Should sympathomimetic symptoms predominate, central effects include restlessness, dizziness, tremor, hyperactive reflexes, talkativeness, irritability and insomnia. Cardiovascular and renal effects include difficulty in micturition, headache, flushing, palpitation, cardiac arrhythmias, hypertension with subsequent hypotension and circulatory collapse. Gastrointestinal effects include dry mouth, metallic taste, anorexia, nausea, vomiting, diarrhea, and abdominal cramps.

Dextromethorphan may cause respiratory depression with a large overdose.

TREATMENT

a. Evacuate stomach as condition warrants. Activated charcoal may be useful.
b. Maintain a non-stimulating environment.
c. Monitor cardiovascular status.
d. Do not give stimulants.
e. Reduce fever with cool sponging.
f. Treat respiratory depression with naloxone if dextromethorphan toxicity is suspected.
g. Use sedatives or anticonvulsants to control CNS excitation and convulsions.
h. Physostigmine may reverse anticholinergic symptoms.
i. Ammonium chloride may acidify the urinary excretion of pseudoephedrine.
j. Further care is symptomatic and supportive.

DOSAGE AND ADMINISTRATION:

TABLE 1

AGE	DOSE*	FREQUENCY*
Syrup		
18 months-6 years adults and children	1/2 teaspoonful (2.5 ml)	q.i.d.
6 years and over	1 teaspoonful (5 ml)	q.i.d.
Drops for oral use only		
1-3 months	1/4 dropperful (1/4 ml)	q.i.d.
3-6 months	1/2 dropperful (1/2 ml)	q.i.d.
6-9 months	3/4 dropperful (3/4 ml)	q.i.d.
9-18 months	1 dropperful (1 ml)	q.i.d.

* In mild cases or in particularly sensitive patients, less frequent or reduced doses may be adequate.

Store at controlled room temperature, 15°-30°C (59°-86°F).

PROTECT FROM FREEZING

AVOID EXCESSIVE HEAT

Dispense in a tight, light-resistant container as defined in the USP.

(91/12)

HOW SUPPLIED - EQUIVALENTS NOT AVAILABLE:

Syrup - Oral - 4 mg/15 mg/60 m

4 fluid ounce	$3.10	MALDEC-DM SYRUP, HR Cenci	00556-0450-04
30 ml	$4.35	RONDAMINE DM, Major Pharms	00904-0702-30
30 ml	$4.40	Carbofed-Dm, Hi Tech Pharma	50383-0754-01
30 ml	$4.44	Cardec-Dm, HL Moore Drug Exch	00839-6404-63
30 ml	$4.66	Cardec-Dm, Vintage Pharms	00254-1113-45
30 ml	$4.66	CARDEC-DM, Qualitest Pharms	00603-1060-45
30 ml	$4.95	CARDEC-DM, Goldline Labs	00182-1342-66
30 ml	$4.95	Cardec-Dm, Goldline Labs	00182-6171-66
30 ml	$4.96	Sildec Dm, Silarx Pharms	54838-0211-30
30 ml	$5.10	Biodec-Dm, Bio Pharm	59741-0134-30
30 ml	$5.15	Carbinoxamine Compound, Morton Grove	60432-0951-30
30 ml	$5.85	CHEMDEC DM DROPS, H N Norton Co.	50732-0866-30
30 ml	$5.90	CARDEC DM, DROPS, Schein Pharm (US)	00364-7277-56
30 ml	$5.93	Carbodec-Dm, Rugby	00536-0454-75
30 ml	$6.95	CARDEC DM DROPS, Alpharma	00472-0733-31
30 ml	$6.95	Harberdec-Dm, Harber Pharm	51432-0795-11
30 ml	$7.00	Carbofed-Dm, Hi Tech Pharma	50383-0750-01
30 ml	$7.52	PSEUDO-CAR DROPS, Geneva Pharms	00781-6541-90
30 ml	$8.97	Cardec-DM Drops, Aligen Independ	00405-2425-53
30 ml	$12.60	TUSSAFED, Everett Labs	00642-0797-30
118 ml	$3.35	CARDEC-DM, Goldline Labs	00182-1204-37
118 ml	$73.90	CARDEC DM SYRUP, Alpharma	00472-0731-28
120 ml	$2.96	Cardec-Dm, HL Moore Drug Exch	00839-6404-65
120 ml	$3.00	Carbofed-Dm, Hi Tech Pharma	50383-0755-04
120 ml	$3.15	RONDAMINE DM, Major Pharms	00904-0703-00
120 ml	$3.15	Rondamine-Dm, Major Pharms	00904-0703-20
120 ml	$3.30	Biodec-Dm, Bio Pharm	59741-0135-04
120 ml	$3.38	CARBODEC, Rugby	00536-0432-97
120 ml	$3.38	Carbodec-Dm, Rugby	00536-0456-97
120 ml	$3.45	CHEMDEC DM, H N Norton Co.	50732-0867-04
120 ml	$3.46	Sildec-Dm, Silarx Pharms	54838-0212-40
120 ml	$3.95	Carbofed-Dm, Hi Tech Pharma	50383-0751-04
120 ml	$7.25	TUSSAFED, Everett Labs	00642-0795-04
480 ml	$8.25	RONDAMINE DM, Major Pharms	00904-0703-16
480 ml	$8.50	Carbofed-Dm, Hi Tech Pharma	50383-0755-16
480 ml	$8.60	MALDEC-DM SYRUP, HR Cenci	00556-0450-16
480 ml	$8.83	Cardec-Dm, Vintage Pharms	00254-1112-58
480 ml	$8.85	Cardec-Dm, United Res	00677-1474-33
480 ml	$8.93	Carbodec-Dm, Rugby	00536-0456-85

HOW SUPPLIED - EQUIVALENTS NOT AVAILABLE: *(cont'd)*

480 ml	$8.97	Cardec-DM Syrup, Aligen Independ	00405-2450-16
480 ml	$9.15	CARDEC-DM, Qualitest Pharms	00603-1061-58
480 ml	$9.20	Biodec-Dm, Bio Pharm	59741-0135-16
480 ml	$9.30	CARDEC DM, Schein Pharm (US)	00364-7318-16
480 ml	$9.50	Sildec-Dm, Silarx Pharms	54838-0212-80
480 ml	$9.90	CARDEC-DM, Goldline Labs	00182-1204-40
480 ml	$10.60	Carbinoxamine Compound, Morton Grove	60432-0202-16
480 ml	$10.94	Cardec Dm, HL Moore Drug Exch	00839-6404-66
480 ml	$10.95	CARDEC DM SYRUP, Alpharma	00472-0731-16
480 ml	$11.00	Carbofed-Dm, Hi Tech Pharma	50383-0751-16
480 ml	$11.88	PSEUDO-CAR DM, Geneva Pharms	00781-6200-16
480 ml	$12.75	CHEMDEC DM SYRUP, H N Norton Co.	50732-0867-16
480 ml	$12.75	Harberdec-Dm, Harber Pharm	51432-0796-20
480 ml	$28.00	TUSSAFED, Everett Labs	00642-0795-16
3785 ml	$67.83	Sildec-Dm, Silarx Pharms	54838-0212-00
3840 ml	$3.96	CARDEC DM SYRUP, Alpharma	00472-0731-04
3840 ml	$55.87	RONDAMINE DM, Major Pharms	00904-0703-28
3840 ml	$58.98	Carbofed-Dm, Hi Tech Pharma	50383-0755-28
3840 ml	$61.48	MALDEC-DM SYRUP, HR Cenci	00556-0450-28
3840 ml	$61.59	CARDEC-DM, Harber Pharm	51432-0544-21
3840 ml	$61.59	Harberdec-Dm, Harber Pharm	51432-0796-21
3840 ml	$62.94	CHEMDEC DM, H N Norton Co.	50732-0867-28
3840 ml	$63.08	Carbodec-Dm, Rugby	00536-0456-90
3840 ml	$63.48	CARDEC-DM, Goldline Labs	00182-1204-41
3840 ml	$63.97	Biodec-Dm, Bio Pharm	59741-0135-20
3840 ml	$74.00	Carbofed-Dm, Hi Tech Pharma	50383-0751-28

CARBINOXAMINE MALEATE; PSEUDOEPHEDRINE HYDROCHLORIDE *(000656)*

CATEGORIES: Allergies; Antihistamines; Antitussives/Expectorants/Mucolytics; Common Cold; Cough Preparations; Respiratory & Allergy Medications; Rhinitis; Sympathomimetic Agents; Pregnancy Category C; FDA Pre 1938 Drugs

BRAND NAMES: Andec-Tr; *Anpirin*; *Became*; Biodec; Biohist-La; Carbiset; Carbiset-Tr; Carbodec; Carbodec Tr; Carbofed; Cardec; Chemdec; *Congestrin*; Cydec; Harberdec; Maldec; Mooredec Tr; Pseudophedrine W/Carbinoxamine; Pseudophedrine Carbinoxamine; Rondamine; **Rondec**; *Rondec-D*; *Rondec-S*; *Rondec-T*; *Rondex*
(International brand names outside U.S. in italics)

FORMULARIES: Aetna; BC-BS; FHP

Prescribing information not available at time of publication.

HOW SUPPLIED - RATED THERAPEUTICALLY EQUIVALENT:

Syrup - Oral - 4 mg/60 mg

480 ml	$10.60	Harberdec, Harber Pharm	51432-0559-20

HOW SUPPLIED - NOT RATED EQUIVALENT:

Syrup - Oral - 4 mg/25 mg

480 ml	$10.60	MALDEC SYRUP, HR Cenci	00556-0451-16

Syrup - Oral - 4 mg/60 mg

30 ml	$6.50	Chemdec, H N Norton Co.	50732-0887-30
30 ml	$12.50	Carbofed, Hi Tech Pharma	50383-0743-01
30 ml	$12.75	Biodec, Bio Pharm	59741-0136-30
30 ml	$14.00	Cydec, Cypress Pharm	60258-0439-30
30 ml	$14.74	Cardec, Aligen Independ	00405-2424-53
30 ml	$14.95	Cardec, Qualitest Pharms	00603-1058-45
30 ml	$14.95	Cp Oral Drops, Pharmacist Choice	54979-0154-03
30 ml	$15.59	Carbodec, Rugby	00536-0439-75
120 ml	$4.76	CHEMDEC, H N Norton Co.	50732-0872-04
120 ml	$6.05	Cydec, Cypress Pharm	60258-0438-04
480 ml	$10.12	CARBODEC SYRUP, Rugby	00536-0440-85
480 ml	$10.30	RONDAMINE SYRUP, Major Pharms	00904-0705-16
480 ml	$10.48	Cardec, Qualitest Pharms	00603-1059-58
480 ml	$10.60	CARDEC S SYRUP, Alpharma	00472-0727-16
480 ml	$10.60	Carbinoxamine W/Pseudoephed, Halsey Drug	00879-0730-16
480 ml	$12.00	Cardec, Goldline Labs	00182-6034-40
480 ml	$19.20	CHEMDEC, H N Norton Co.	50732-0872-16
480 ml	$21.20	Cydec, Cypress Pharm	60258-0438-16

Tablet, Coated, Sustained Action - Oral - 8 mg/120 mg

100's	$18.12	Carbiset-Tr, Palisades Pharms	53159-0512-01
100's	$31.15	RONDAMINE TR, Major Pharms	00904-3250-60
100's	$32.31	CARBODEC TR, Rugby	00536-4453-01
100's	$33.01	MOOREDEC TR, HL Moore Drug Exch	00839-7482-06
100's	$33.50	CARDEC TR, Goldline Labs	00182-1130-01
100's	$36.25	ANDEC-TR, Econolab	55053-0077-01
100's	$38.16	Pseudophedrine/Carbinoxamine, Aligen Independ	00405-4138-01
100's	$46.90	Biohist-La, Wakefield Pharms	59310-0101-10

Tablet, Uncoated - Oral - 4 mg/60 mg

100's	$9.31	Carbiset, Palisades Pharms	53159-0510-01
100's	$16.23	ANDEC, Econolab	55053-0082-01
100's	$17.08	Pseudophedrine W/Carbinoxamine, Aligen Independ	00405-4137-01
100's	$17.35	RONDAMINE, Major Pharms	00904-3248-60
100's	$18.70	Cardec, Goldline Labs	00182-1199-01
100's	$19.07	CARBODEC, Rugby	00536-4452-01
500's	$43.62	Carbiset, Palisades Pharms	53159-0510-50

CARBOL FUCHSIN *(000658)*

CATEGORIES: Anti-Infectives; Antibacterials; Antifungals; Antimicrobials; Dermatologicals; Fungal Agents; Skin/Mucous Membrane Agents; FDA Pre 1938 Drugs

BRAND NAMES: **Castellani Paint**

Prescribing information not available at time of publication.

HOW SUPPLIED - EQUIVALENTS NOT AVAILABLE:

Solution - Topical

30 ml	**$4.75**	**CASTELLANI PAINT, Pedinol Pharma**	**00884-2878-01**
30 ml	**$4.75**	**CASTELLANI PAINT COLORLESS, Pedinol Pharma**	**00884-2978-01**
480 ml	**$45.00**	**CASTELLANI PAINT COLORLESS, Pedinol Pharma**	**00884-2878-16**
480 ml	**$45.00**	**CASTELLANI PAINT, Pedinol Pharma**	**00884-2978-16**

CARBOPLATIN *(000660)*

CATEGORIES: Antineoplastics; Cancer; Cytotoxic Agents; Chemotherapy; Ovarian Carcinoma; Pregnancy Category D; Sales > $100 Million; FDA Approved 1989 Mar

BRAND NAMES: *Blastocarb* (Mexico); *Carboplat* (Germany, Mexico); *Carboplatin* (Australia); *Carboplatin a*; *Carboplatin Abic*; *Carboplatin DBL*; *Carboplatin dbl*; *Carboplatin Lederle*; *Carboplatino*; *Carbosin*; *Carbosin Lundbeck*; *Carplan*; *Delta West Carboplatin*; *Erbakar*; *Ercar*; *Neoplatin*; *Oncocarbin*; **Paraplatin**; *Paraplatin RTU*; *Paraplatine* (France)
(International brand names outside U.S. in italics)

FORMULARIES: BC-BS; Medi-Cal

COST OF THERAPY: $2,803.56 (Ovarian Carcinoma; Injection; 150 mg/vial; 2/day; 6 days)

> WARNING:
> Carboplatin for injection should be administered under the supervision of a qualified physician experienced in the use of cancer chemotherapeutic agents. Appropriate management of therapy and complications is possible only when adequate treatment facilities are readily available.
> Bone marrow suppression is dose related and may be severe, resulting in infection and/or bleeding. Anemia may be cumulative and may require transfusion support. Vomiting is another frequent drug-related side effect. Anaphylactic-like reactions to carboplatin for injection have been reported and may occur within minutes of carboplatin for injection administration. Epinephrine, corticosteroids, and antihistamines have been employed to alleviate symptoms.

DESCRIPTION:

Paraplatin is supplied as a sterile lyophilized powder available in single-dose vials contains 50 mg, 150 mg, and 450 mg of carboplatin for administration by intravenous infusion. Each vial contains equal parts by weight of carboplatin and mannitol.

Carboplatin is a platinum coordination compound that is used as a cancer chemotherapeutic agent. The chemical name for carboplatin is platinum, diammine (1,1-cyclobutane-dicarboxylato(2-)-0,0')-, (*SP*-4-2).

Carboplatin is a white to off-white crystalline powder with the molecular formula of $C_6H_{12}N_2O_4Pt$ and a molecular weight of 371.25. It is soluble in water at a rate of approximately 14 mg/ml, and the pH of a 1% solution is 5-7. It is virtually insoluble in ethanol, acetone, and dimethylacetamide.

CLINICAL PHARMACOLOGY:

Carboplatin, like cisplatin, produces predominantly interstrand DNA cross-links rather than DNA-protein cross-links. This effect is apparently cell-cycle nonspecific. The aquation of carboplatin, which is thought to produce the active species, occurs at a slower rate than in the case of cisplatin. Despite this difference, it appears that both carboplatin and cisplatin induce equal number of drug-DNA cross-links, causing equivalent lesions and biological effects. The differences in potencies for carboplatin and cisplatin appear to be directly related to the difference in aquation rates.

In patients with creatinine clearances of about 60 ml/min or greater, plasma levels of intact carboplatin decay in a biphasic manner after a 30-minute intravenous infusion of 300 to 500 mg/m^2 of carboplatin for injection. The initial plasma half-life (alpha) was found to be 1.1 to 2.0 hours (N=6), and the postdistribution plasma half-life (beta) was found to be 2.6 to 5.9 hours (N=6). The total body clearance, apparent volume of distribution and mean residence time for carboplatin are 4.4 L/hour, 16 L and 3.5 hours, respectively. The Cmax values and areas under the plasma concentration vs time curves from 0 to infinity (AUC inf) increase linearly with dose, although the increase was slightly more than dose proportional. Carboplatin, therefore, exhibits linear pharmacokinetics over the dosing range studied (300-500 mg/m^2).

Carboplatin is not bound to plasma proteins. No significant quantities of protein-free, ultrafiltrable platinum-containing species other than carboplatin are present in plasma. However, platinum from carboplatin becomes irreversibly bound to plasma proteins and is slowly eliminated with a minimum half-life of 5 days.

The major route of elimination of carboplatin is renal excretion. Patients with creatinine clearances of approximately 60 ml/min or greater excrete 65% of the dose in the urine within 12 hours and 71% of the dose within 24 hours. All of the platinum in the 24-hour urine is present as carboplatin. Only 3% to 5% of the administered platinum is excreted in the urine between 24 and 96 hours. There are insufficient data to determine whether biliary excretion occurs.

In patients with creatinine clearances below 60 ml/min the total body and renal clearances of carboplatin decrease as the creatinine clearance decreases. Carboplatin for injection dosages should therefore be reduced in these patients (see DOSAGE AND ADMINISTRATION.)

CLINICAL STUDIES:

Use with cyclophosphamide for initial treatment of ovarian cancer: In two prospectively randomized, controlled studies conducted by the National Cancer Institute of Canada, Clinical Trials Group (NCIC) and the Southwest Oncology Group (SWOG), 789 chemotherapy naive patients with advanced ovarian cancer were treated with carboplatin for injection or cisplatin, both in combination with cyclophosphamide every 28 days for six courses before surgical re-evaluation. The following results were obtained from both studies (TABLE 1):

TABLE 1A Comparative Efficacy Overview of Pivotal Trials

	NCIC	SWOG
Number of patients randomized	447	342
Median age (years)	60	62
Dose of cisplatin	75 mg/M^2	100 mg/M^2
Dose of carboplatin	300 mg/M^2	300 mg/M^2
Dose of cytoxan	600 mg/M^2	600 mg/M^2
Residual tumor < 2 cm (number of patients)	39% (174/447)	4%(49/342)

COMPARATIVE TOXICITY

The pattern of toxicity exerted by the carboplatin for injection-containing regimen was significantly different from that of the cisplatin-containing combinations. Differences between the two studies may be explained by different cisplatin dosages and by different supportive care.

CLINICAL STUDIES: *(cont'd)*

TABLE 1B Clinical Response in Measurable Disease Patients

	NCIC	SWOG
Carboplatin (number of patients)	60% (48/80)	58% (48/83)
Cisplatin (number of patients)	58% (49/85)	43% (33/76)
95% C.I. of difference (Carboplatin - Cisplatin)	(-13.9%, 18.6%)	(-2.3%, 31.1%)

TABLE 1C Pathologic Complete Response*

	NCIC	SWOG
Carboplatin (number of patients)	11% (24/224)	10% (17/171)
Cisplatin (number of patients)	15% (33/223)	10% (17/171)
95% C.I. of difference (Carboplatin - Cisplatin)	(-10.7%, 2.5%)	(-6.9%, 6.9%)

* 114 carboplatin for injection and 109 Cisplatin patients did not undergo second look surgery in NCIC study. 90 carboplatin for injection and 106 Cisplatin patients did not undergo second look surgery in SWOG study.

TABLE 2 Progression-Free Survival (PFS)

	NCIC	SWOG
Median		
Carboplatin	59 weeks	49 weeks
Cisplatin	61 weeks	47 weeks
2-year PFS*		
Carboplatin	31%	21%
Cisplatin	31%	21%
95% C.I. of difference (Carboplatin-Cisplatin)	(-9.3, 8.7)	(-9.0, 9.4)
3-year PFS*		
Carboplatin	19%	8%
Cisplatin	23%	14%
95% C.I. of difference (Carboplatin-Cisplatin)	(-11.5, 4.5)	(-14.1, 0.3)
Hazard Ratio**	1.10	1.02
95% C.I. (Carboplatin-Cisplatin)	(0.89, 1.35)	(0.81, 1.29)

* Kaplan-Meier Estimates Unrelated deaths occurring in the absence of progression were counted as events (progression) in this analysis.
** Analysis adjusted for factors found to be of prognostic significance were consistent with unadjusted analysis.

TABLE 3 Survival

	NCIC	SWOG
Median		
Carboplatin	110 weeks	86 weeks
Cisplatin	99 weeks	79 weeks
2-year Survival*		
Carboplatin	51.9%	40.2%
Cisplatin	48.4%	39.0%
95% C.I. of difference (Carboplatin-Cisplatin)	(-6.2, 13.2)	(-9.8, 12.2)
3-year Survival*		
Carboplatin	34.6%	18.3%
Cisplatin	33.1%	24.9%
95% C.I. of difference (Carboplatin-Cisplatin)	(-7.7, 10.7)	(-15.9, 2.7)
Hazard Ratio**		
95% C.I. (Carboplatin:Cisplatin)	(0.78, 1.23)	(0.78, 1.30)

* Kaplan-Meier Estimates
** Analysis adjusted for factors found to be of prognostic significance were consistent with unadjusted analysis.

The carboplatin for injection-containing regimen induced significantly more thrombocytopenia and, in one study, significantly more leukopenia and more need for transfusional support. The cisplatin-containing regimen produced significantly more anemia in one study. However, no significant differences occurred in incidences of infections and hemorrhagic episodes.

Non-hematologic toxicities (emesis, neurotoxicity, ototoxicity, renal toxicity, hypomagnesemia and alopecia) were significantly more frequent in the cisplatin-containing arms.

Use as a single agent for secondary treatment of advanced ovarian cancer: In two prospective, randomized controlled studies in patients with advanced ovarian cancer previously treated with chemotherapy, carboplatin for injection achieved six clinical complete responses in 47 patients. The duration of these responses ranged from 45 to 71 + weeks.

INDICATIONS AND USAGE:

Initial treatment of advanced ovarian carcinoma: Carboplatin for injection is indicated for the initial treatment of advanced ovarian carcinoma in established combination with other approved chemotherapeutic agents. One established combination regimen consists of carboplatin for injection and cyclophosphamide (Cytoxan). Two randomized controlled studies conducted by the NCIC and SWOG with carboplatin for injection vs. cisplatin, both in combination with cyclophosphamide, have demonstrated equivalent overall survival between the two groups (see CLINICAL STUDIES).

There is limited statistical power to demonstrate equivalence in overall pathologic complete response rates and long-term survival (> 3 years) because of the small number of patients with these outcomes; the small number of patients with residual tumor < 2 cm after initial surgery also limits the statistical power to demonstrate equivalence in this subgroup.

Secondary treatment of advanced ovarian carcinoma: Carboplatin for injection is indicated for the palliative treatment of patients with ovarian carcinoma recurrent after prior chemotherapy, including patients who have been previously treated with cisplatin.

Within the group of patients previously treated with cisplatin, those who have developed progressive disease while receiving cisplatin therapy may have a decreased response rate.

CONTRAINDICATIONS:

Carboplatin for injection is contraindicated in patients with a history of severe allergic reactions to cisplatin or other platinum-containing compounds, or mannitol.

Carboplatin for injection should not be employed in patients with severe bone marrow depression or significant bleeding.

TABLE 4 Adverse Experiences in Patients with Ovarian Cancer

NCIC STUDY

		Carboplatin for Injection Arm Percent*	Cisplatin Arm Percent*	P-Value**
Bone Marrow				
Thrombocytopenia	<100,000/mm^3	70	29	<0.001
	<50,000/mm^3	41	6	<0.001
Neutropenia,	<2,000 cells/mm^3	97	96	n.s.
	<1,000 cells/mm^3	81	79	n.s.
Leukopenia,	<4,000 cells/mm^3	98	97	n.s.
	<2,000 cells/mm^3	68	52	0.001
Anemia,	<11 g/dl	91	91	n.s.
	<8 g/dl	18	12	n.s.
Infections		14	12	n.s.
Bleeding		10	4	n.s.
Transfusions		42	31	0.018
Gastrointestinal				
Nausea and vomiting		93	98	0.010
Vomiting		84	97	<0.001
Other GI side effects		50	62	0.013
Neurological				
Peripheral neuropathies		16	42	<0.001
Ototoxicity		13	33	<0.001
Other sensory side effects		6	10	n.s.
Central neurotoxicity		28	40	0.009
Renal				
Serum creatinine elevations		5	13	0.006
Blood urea elevations		17	31	<0.001
Hepatic				
Bilirubin elevations		5	3	n.s.
SGOT elevations		17	13	n.s.
Alkaline phosphatase elevations		—	—	—
Electrolytes loss				
Sodium		10	20	0.005
Potassium		16	22	n.s.
Calcium		16	19	n.s.
Magnesium		63	88	<0.001
Other Side Effects				
Pain		36	37	n.s.
Asthenia		40	33	n.s.
Cardiovascular		15	19	n.s.
Respiratory		8	9	n.s.
Allergic		12	9	n.s.
Genitourinary		10	10	n.s.
Alopecia +		50	62	0.017
Mucositis		10	9	n.s.

* Values are in percent of evaluable patients
** n.s. = not significant, p>0.05
\+ May have been affected by cyclophosphamide dosage delivered

TABLE 5 Adverse Experiences in Patients with Ovarian Cancer SWOG Study

		Carboplatin for Injection Arm Percent*	Cisplatin Arm Percent*	P-Value**
Bone Marrow				
Thrombocytopenia	<100,000/mm^3	59	35	<0.001
	<50,000/mm^3	22	11	0.006
Neutropenia,	<2,000 cells/mm^3	95	97	n.s.
	<1,000 cells/mm^3	84	78	n.s.
Leukopenia,	<4,000 cells/mm^3	97	97	n.s.
	<2,000 cells/mm^3	7/6	67	n.s.
Anemia,	<11 g/dl	88	87	n.s.
	<8 g/dl	8	24	<0.001
Infections		18	21	n.s.
Bleeding		6	4	n.s.
Transfusions		25	33	n.s.
Gastrointestinal				
Nausea and vomiting		94	96	n.s.
Vomiting		82	91	0.007
Other GI side effects		40	48	n.s.
Neurological				
Peripheral neuropathies		13	28	0.001
Ototoxicity		12	30	<0.001
Other sensory side effects		4	6	n.s.
Central neurotoxicity		23	29	n.s.
Renal				
Serum creatinine elevations		7	38	<0.001
Blood urea elevations		—	—	—
Hepatic				
Bilirubin elevations		5	3	n.s.
SGOT elevations		23	16	n.s.
Alkaline phosphatase elevations		29	20	n.s.
Electrolytes loss				
Sodium		—	—	—
Potassium		—	—	—
Calcium		—	—	—
Magnesium		58	77	<0.001
Other side effects				
Pain		54	52	n.s.
Asthenia		43	46	n.s.
Cardiovascular		23	30	n.s.
Respiratory		12	11	n.s.
Allergic		10	11	n.s.
Genitourinary		11	13	n.s.
Alopecia +		43	57	0.009
Mucositis		6	11	n.s.

* Values are in percent of evaluable patients
** n.s. = not significant, p> 0.05
\+ May have been affected by cyclophosphamide dosage delivered.

WARNINGS:

Bone marrow suppression (leukopenia, neutropenia, and thrombocytopenia) is dose-dependent and is also the dose-limiting toxicity. Peripheral blood counts should be frequently monitored during carboplatin for injection treatment and, when appropriate, until recovery is

WARNINGS: *(cont'd)*

achieved. Median nadir occurs at day 21 in patients receiving single-agent carboplatin for injection. In general, single intermittent courses of carboplatin for injection should not be repeated until leukocyte, neutrophil, and platelet counts have recovered.

Since anemia is cumulative, transfusions may be needed during treatment with carboplatin for injection, particularly in patients receiving prolonged therapy.

Bone marrow suppression is increased in patients who have received prior therapy, especially regimens including cisplatin. Marrow suppression is also increased in patients with impaired kidney function. Initial carboplatin for injection dosages in these patients should be appropriately reduced (see DOSAGE AND ADMINISTRATION) and blood counts should be carefully monitored between courses. The use of carboplatin for injection in combination with other bone marrow suppressing therapies must be carefully managed with respect to dosage and timing in order to minimize additive effects.

Carboplatin for injection has limited nephrotoxic potential, but concomitant treatment with aminoglycosides has resulted in increased renal and/or audiologic toxicity, and caution must be exercised when a patient receives both drugs.

Carboplatin for injection can induce emesis, which can be more severe in patients previously receiving emetogenic therapy. The incidence and intensity of emesis have been reduced by using premedication with antiemetics. Although no conclusive efficacy data exist with the following schedules of carboplatin for injection, lengthening the duration of single intravenous administration to 24 hours or dividing the total dose over five consecutive daily pulse doses has resulted in reduced emesis.

Although peripheral neurotoxicity is infrequent, its incidence is increased in patients older than 65 years and in patients previously treated with cisplatin. Pre-existing cisplatin-induced neurotoxicity does not worsen in about 70% of the patients receiving carboplatin for injection as secondary treatment.

As in the case of other platinum coordination compounds, allergic reactions to carboplatin for injection have been reported. These may occur within minutes of administration and should be managed with appropriate supportive therapy.

High dosages of carboplatin for injection (more than four times the recommended dose) have resulted in severe abnormalities of liver function tests.

Carboplatin for injection may cause fetal harm when administered to a pregnant woman. Carboplatin for injection has been shown to be embryotoxic and teratogenic in rats. There are no adequate and well-controlled studies in pregnant women. If this drug is used during pregnancy, or if the patient becomes pregnant while receiving this drug, the patient should be apprised of the potential hazard to the fetus. Women of childbearing potential should be advised to avoid becoming pregnant.

PRECAUTIONS:

General: Needles or intravenous administration sets containing aluminum parts that may come in contact with carboplatin for injection should not be used for the preparation or administration of the drug. Aluminum can react with carboplatin causing precipitate formation and loss of potency.

Pregnancy: Pregnancy "Category D": (see WARNINGS.)

Nursing Mothers: It is not known whether carboplatin is excreted in human milk. Because there is a possibility of toxicity in nursing infants secondary to carboplatin for injection treatment of the mother, it is recommended that breastfeeding be discontinued if the mother is treated with carboplatin for injection.

Carcinogenesis, Mutagenesis, and Impairment of Fertility: The carcinogenic potential of carboplatin has not been studied, but compounds with similar mechanisms of action and mutagenicity profiles have been reported to be carcinogenic. Carboplatin has been shown to be mutagenic both *in vitro* and *in vivo*. It has also been shown to be embryotoxic and teratogenic in rats receiving the drug during organogenesis.

DRUG INTERACTIONS:

The renal effects of nephrotoxic compounds may be potentiated by carboplatin for injection.

ADVERSE REACTIONS:

For a comparison of toxicities when carboplatin or cisplatin was given in combination with cyclophosphamide, see the COMPARATIVE TOXICITY sub-section of the CLINICAL STUDIES section.

In the narrative section that follows, the incidences of adverse events are based on data from 1,893 patients with various types of tumors who received carboplatin for injection as single-agent therapy.

Hematologic toxicity: Bone marrow suppression is the dose-limiting toxicity of carboplatin for injection. Thrombocytopenia with platelet counts below 50,000/mm^3 occurs in 25% of the patients (35% of pretreated ovarian cancer patients); neutropenia with granulocyte counts below 1,000/mm^3 occurs in 16% of the patients (21% of pretreated ovarian cancer patients); leukopenia with WBC counts below 2,000/mm^3occurs in 15% of the patients (26% of pretreated ovarian cancer patients). The nadir usually occurs about day 21 in patients receiving single-agent therapy. By day 28, 90% of patients have platelet counts above 100,000/mm^3; 74% have neutrophil counts above 2,000/mm^3; 67% have leukocyte counts above 4,000/mm^3.

Marrow suppression is usually more severe in patients with impaired kidney function. Patients with poor performance status have also experienced a higher incidence of severe leukopenia and thrombocytopenia.

The hematologic effects, although usually reversible, have resulted in infectious or hemorrhagic complications in 5% of the patients treated with carboplatin for injection, with drug-related death occurring in less than 1% of the patients.

Anemia with hemoglobin less than 11 g/dl has been observed in 71% of the patients who started therapy with a baseline above that value. The incidence of anemia increases with increasing exposure to carboplatin for injection. Transfusions have been administered to 26% of the patients treated with carboplatin for injection (44% of previously treated ovarian cancer patients).

Bone marrow depression may be more severe when carboplatin for injection is combined with other bone marrow suppressing drugs or with radiotherapy.

Gastrointestinal toxicity: Vomiting occurs in 65% of the patients (81% of previously treated ovarian cancer patients) and in about one-third of these patients it is severe. Carboplatin, as a single agent or in combination, is significantly less emetogenic than cisplatin; however, patients previously treated with emetogenic agents, especially cisplatin, appear to be more prone to vomiting. Nausea alone occurs in an additional 10% to 15% of patients. Both nausea and vomiting usually cease within 24 hours of treatment and are often responsive to antiemetic measures. Although no conclusive efficacy data exist with the following schedules, prolonged administration of carboplatin for injection, either by continuous 24-hour infusion or by daily pulse doses given for 5 consecutive days, was associated with less severe vomiting than the single dose intermittent schedule. Emesis was increased when carboplatin for

ADVERSE REACTIONS: *(cont'd)*

TABLE 6 Adverse Experiences in Patients with Ovarian Cancer

		First Line Combination* Therapy Percent	Second Line Single Agent** Therapy Percent
Bone Marrow			
Thrombocytopenia,	<100,000/mm^3	66	62
	<50,000/mm^3	33	35
Neutropenia,	<2,000 cells/mm^3	96	67
	<1,000 cells/mm^3	82	21
Leukopenia,	<4,000 cells/mm^3	97	85
	<2,000 cells/mm^3	71	26
Anemia,	<11 g/dl	90	90
	<8 g/dl	14	21
Infections		16	5
Bleeding		8	5
Transfusions		35	44
Gastrointestinal			
Nausea and vomiting		93	92
Vomiting		83	81
Other GI side effects		46	21
Neurological			
Peripheral neuropathies		15	6
Ototoxicity		12	1
Other sensory side effects		5	1
Central neurotoxicity		26	5
Renal			
Serum creatinine elevations		6	10
Blood urea elevations		17	22
Hepatic			
Bilirubin elevations		5	5
SGOT elevations		20	19
Alkaline phosphatase elevations		29	37
Electrolytes loss			
Sodium		10	47
Potassium		16	28
Calcium		16	31
Magnesium		61	43
Other side effects			
Pain		44	23
Asthenia		41	11
Cardiovascular		19	6
Respiratory		10	6
Allergic		11	2
Genitourinary		10	2
Alopecia		49	2
Mucositis		8	1

**Use with cyclophosphamide for initial treatment of ovarian cancer:* Data are based on the experience of 393 patients with ovarian cancer (regardless of baseline status) who received initial combination therapy with carboplatin for injection and cyclophosphamide in two randomized controlled studies conducted by SWOG and NCIC (see CLINICAL STUDIESsection). Combination with cyclophosphamide as well as duration of treatment may be responsible for the differences that can be noted in the adverse experience table.

**Single agent use for the secondary treatment of ovarian cancer: Data are based on the experience of 553 patients with previously treated ovarian carcinoma (regardless of baseline status) who received single-agent carboplatin for injection.

injection was used in combination with other emetogenic compounds. Other gastrointestinal effects observed frequently were pain, in 17% of the patients; diarrhea, in 6%; and constipation, also in 6%.

Neurologic toxicity: Peripheral neuropathies have been observed in 4% of the patients receiving carboplatin for injection (6% of pretreated ovarian cancer patients) with mild paresthesias occurring most frequently. Carboplatin therapy produces significantly fewer and less severe neurologic side effects than does therapy with cisplatin. However, patients older than 65 years and/or previously treated with cisplatin appear to have an increased risk (10%) for peripheral neuropathies. In 70% of the patients with pre-existing cisplatin-induced peripheral neurotoxicity, there was no worsening of symptoms during therapy with carboplatin for injection. Clinical ototoxicity and other sensory abnormalities such as visual disturbances and change in taste have been reported in only 1% of the patients. Central nervous system symptoms have been reported in 5% of the patients and appear to be most often related to the use of antiemetics.

Although the overall incidence of peripheral neurologic side effects induced by carboplatin for injection is low, prolonged treatment, particularly in cisplatin pretreated patients, may result in cumulative neurotoxicity.

Nephrotoxicity: Development of abnormal renal function test results is uncommon, despite the fact that carboplatin, unlike cisplatin, has usually been administered without high-volume fluid hydration and/or forced diuresis. The incidences of abnormal renal function tests reported are 6% for serum creatinine and 14% for blood urea nitrogen (10% and 22%, respectively, in pretreated ovarian cancer patients). Most of these reported abnormalities have been mild and about one-half of them were reversible.

Creatinine clearance has proven to be the most sensitive measure of kidney function in patients receiving carboplatin for injection, and it appears to be the most useful test for correlating drug clearance and bone marrow suppression. Twenty-seven percent of the patients who had a baseline value of 60ml/min or more demonstrated a reduction below this value during carboplatin for injection therapy.

Hepatic toxicity: The incidences of abnormal liver function tests in patients with normal baseline values were reported as follows: total bilirubin, 5%; SGOT, 15%; and alkaline phosphatase, 24%; (5%, 19%, and 37%, respectively, in pretreated ovarian cancer patients). These abnormalities have generally been mild and reversible in about one-half of the cases, although the role of metastatic tumor in the liver may complicate the assessment in many patients. In a limited series of patients receiving very high dosages of carboplatin for injection and autologous bone marrow transplantation, severe abnormalities of liver function tests were reported.

Electrolyte changes: The incidences of abnormally decreased serum electrolyte values reported were as follows: sodium, 29%; potassium, 20%; calcium, 22%: and magnesium, 29%; (47%, 28%, 31%, and 43%, respectively, in pretreated ovarian cancer patients). Electrolyte supplementation was not routinely administered concomitantly with carboplatin for injection, and these electrolyte abnormalities were rarely associated with symptoms.

Allergic reactions: Hypersensitivity to carboplatin for injection has been reported in 2% of the patients. These allergic reactions have been similar in nature and severity to those reported with other platinum-containing compounds, i.e., rash, urticaria, erythema, pruritus, and rarely bronchospasm and hypotension. These reactions have been successfully managed with standard epinephrine, corticosteroid, and antihistamine therapy.

ADVERSE REACTIONS: *(cont'd)*

Other events: Pain and asthenia were the most frequently reported miscellaneous adverse effects; their relationship to the tumor and to anemia was likely. Alopecia was reported (3%). Cardiovascular, respiratory, genitourinary, and mucosal side effects have occurred in 6% or less of the patients. Cardiovascular events (cardiac failure, embolism, cerebrovascular accidents) were fatal in less than 1% of the patients and did not appear to be related to chemotherapy. Cancer-associated hemolytic uremic syndrome has been reported rarely.

OVERDOSAGE:

There is no known antidote for carboplatin for injection overdosage. The anticipated complications of overdosage would be secondary to bone marrow suppression and/or hepatic toxicity.

DOSAGE AND ADMINISTRATION:

NOTE: Aluminum reacts with carboplatin causing precipitate formation and loss of potency, therefore, needles or intravenous sets containing aluminum parts that may come in contact with the drug must not be used for the preparation or administration of carboplatin for injection.

Single agent therapy: Carboplatin for injection, as a single agent, has been shown to be effective in patients with recurrent ovarian carcinoma at a dosage of 360 mg/m² IV on day 1 every 4 weeks. In general, however, single intermittent courses of carboplatin for injection should not be repeated until the neutrophil count is at least 2,000 and the platelet count is at least 100.000.

Combination therapy with cyclophosphamide: In the chemotherapy of advanced ovarian cancer, an effective combination for previously untreated patients consists of:

Carboplatin for injection: #300 mg/m² IV on day 1 every 4 weeks for six cycles.

Cyclophosphamide (Cytoxan): 600 mg/m²IV on day 1 every 4 weeks for six cycles. For directions regarding the use and administration of cyclophosphamide (Cytoxan) please refer to its package insert.

(See CLINICAL STUDIES.)

Intermittent courses of carboplatin for injection in combination with cyclophosphamide should not be repeated until the neutrophil count is at least 2,000 and the platelet count is at least 100,000.

Dose Adjustment Recommendations: The suggested dose adjustments for single agent or combination therapy shown in the table below (TABLE 7) are modified from controlled trials in previously treated and untreated patients with ovarian carcinoma. Blood counts were done weekly, and the recommendations are based on the lowest posttreatment platelet or neutrophil value.

TABLE 7

Platelets	Neutrophils	Adjusted Dose* (From Prior Course)
>100,000	>2,000	125%
50-100,000	500-2,000	No adjustment
<50,000	<500	75%

* Percentages apply to carboplatin for injection as a single agent or to both carboplatin for injection and cyclophosphamide in combination. In the controlled studies, dosages were also adjusted at a lower level (50 to 60%) for severe myelosuppression. Escalations above 125% were not recommended for these studies.

Carboplatin for injection is usually administered by an infusion lasting 15 minutes or longer. No pretreatment or posttreatment hydration or forced diuresis is required.

Patients with impaired kidney function: Patients with creatinine clearance values below 60 ml/min are at increased risk of severe bone marrow suppression. In renally-impaired patients who received single agent carboplatin for injection therapy, the incidence of severe leukopenia, neutropenia, or thrombocytopenia has been about 25% when the dosage modifications in the table below (TABLE 8) have been used.

TABLE 8

Baseline Creatinine Clearance	Recommended Dose on Day 1
41-59 ml/min	250 mg/m²
16-40 ml/min	200 mg/m²

The data available for patients with severely impaired kidney function (creatinine clearance below 15 ml/min) are too limited to permit a recommendation for treatment.[1,2]

These dosing recommendations apply to the initial course of treatment. Subsequent dosages should be adjusted according to the patient's tolerance based on the degree of bone marrow suppression.

PREPARATION OF INTRAVENOUS SOLUTION

Immediately before use, the content of each vial must be reconstituted with either Sterile Water for Injection, USP, 5% Dextrose in Water, or 0.9% Sodium Chloride Injection, USP, according to the following schedule:

TABLE 9

Vial Strength	Diluent Volume
50 mg	5 ml
150 mg	15 ml
450 mg	45 ml

These dilutions all produce a carboplatin concentration of 10 mg/ml.

Carboplatin for injection can be further diluted to concentrations as low as 0 5 mg/ml with 5% Dextrose in Water (D_5W) or 0.9% Sodium Chloride Injection, USP.

STABILITY

Unopened vials of carboplatin for injection are stable for the life indicated on the package when stored at controlled room temperature 15°-30°C (59°-86°F), and protected from light.

When prepared as directed, carboplatin for injection solutions are stable for 8 hours at room temperature (25°C). Since no antibacterial preservative is contained in the formulation, it is recommended that carboplatin for injection solutions be discarded 8 hours after dilution.

Parenteral drug products should be inspected visually for particulate matter and discoloration prior to administration.

HOW SUPPLIED:

STORAGE

Store the unopened vials at controlled room temperature 15°-30°C (59°-86°F). Protect from light. Solutions for infusion should be discarded 8 hours after preparation.

HOW SUPPLIED: *(cont'd)*

HANDLING AND DISPOSAL

Procedures for proper handling and disposal of anticancer drugs should be considered. Several guidelines on this subject have been published.[3-9] There is no general agreement that all of the procedures recommended in the guidelines are necessary or appropriate.

REFERENCES:

1. Egorin MJ, et al. Pharmacokinetics and dosage reduction of cis-diammine (1,1-cyclobutanedicarboxylato) platinum in patients with impaired renal function. *Cancer Res.* 1984;44:5432-5438. **2.** Carboplatin, Etoposide, and Bleomycin for Treatment of Stage IIC Seminoma Complicated by Acute Renal Failure. Cancer Treatment Reports. 1987(November); 71(11):1123-1124. **3.** Recommendations for the Safe Handling of Parenteral Antineoplastic Drugs. NIH Publication No. 83-2621. For sale by the Superintendent of Documents. US Government Printing Office, Washington, DC 20402. **4.** AMA Council Report. Guidelines for Handling Parenteral Antineoplastics. *JAMA.* 1985, March 16. **5.** National Study Commission Cytotoxic Exposure—Recommendations for Handling Cytotoxic Agents. Available from Louis P. Jeffrey, Chairman, National Study Commission on Cytotoxic Exposure, Massachusetts College of Pharmacy and Allied Health Sciences. 179 Longwood Avenue, Boston, Massachusetts, 02115. **6.** Clinical Oncological Society of Australia. Guidelines and Recommendations for Safe Handling of Antineoplastic Agents.*Med J Australia.*1983;1:426-428. **7.** Jones RB, et al. Safe Handling of Chemotherapeutic Agents: A report from the Mount Sinai Medical Center, CA — *A Cancer for Clinicians.* 1983; (Sept/Oct) 258-263. **8.** American Society of Hospital Pharmacists Technical Assistance Bulletin on Handling Cytotoxic Drugs in Hospitals.*Am J Hosp Pharm.* 1985;42:131-137. **9.** OSHA Work-Practice Guidelines for Personnel Dealing with Cytotoxic (Antineoplastic) Drugs. *Am J Hosp Pharm.* 1986;43:1193-1204.

HOW SUPPLIED - EQUIVALENTS NOT AVAILABLE:

Injection, Solution - Intravenous - 50 mg/vial

1's $77.89 PARAPLATIN, 10 ML, Mead Johnson 00015-3213-30

Injection, Solution - Intravenous - 150 mg/vial

1's $233.63 PARAPLATIN, 20 ML, Mead Johnson 00015-3214-30

Injection, Solution - Intravenous - 450 mg/vial

1's $700.89 PARAPLATIN, 100 ML, Mead Johnson 00015-3215-30

CARBOPROST TROMETHAMINE *(000661)*

CATEGORIES: Abortion; Bleeding; Hormones; Oxytocics; Pregnancy; Prostaglandins; Relaxants/Stimulants, Uterine; Pregnancy Category C; FDA Approval Pre 1982

BRAND NAMES: Hemabate; *Prostin 15m*; *Prostin 15m*; *Prostinfenem*; *Prostodin* *(International brand names outside U.S. in italics)*

DESCRIPTION:

Carboprost thromethamine sterile solution, an oxytocic, contains the tromethamine salt of the (15S)-15 methyl analogue of naturally occurring prostaglandin F2α in a solution suitable for intramuscular injection.

Carboprost tromethamine is the established name for the active ingredient in Hemabate. Four other chemical names are:

1. (15S)-15-methyl prostaglandin F2α tromethamine salt

2. 7-(3α,5α-dihydroxy-2β-((3S)-3-hydroxy-3-methyl- *trans*-1-octenyl)-1α-cyclopentyl)-*cis*-5-heptenoic acid compound with 2-amino-2-(hydroxymethyl)-1,3-propanediol

3. (15S)-9α, 11α, 15-trihydroxy-15-methylprosta- *cis-5,trans*-13-dienoic acid tromethamine salt

4. (15S)-15-methyl PGF2α-THAM

The molecular formula is $C_{25}H_{47}O_8N$. The molecular weight of carboprost tromethamine is 489.64. It is a white to slightly off-white crystalline powder. It generally melts between 95° and 105°C, depending on the rate of heating.

Carboprost tromethamine dissolves readily in water at room temperature at a concentration greater than 75 mg/ml.

Each ml of carboprost thromethamine sterile solution contains carboprost tromethamine equivalent to 250 mcg of carboprost, 83 mcg tromethamine, 9 mg sodium chloride, and 9.45 mg benzyl alcohol added as preservative. When necessary, pH is adjusted with sodium hydroxide and/or hydrochloric acid. The solution is sterile.

CLINICAL PHARMACOLOGY:

Carboprost tromethamine administered intramuscularly stimulates in the gravid uterus myometrial contractions similar to labor contractions at the end of a full term pregnancy. Whether or not these contractions result from a direct effect of carboprost on the myometrium has not been determined. Nonetheless, they evacuate the products of conception from the uterus in most cases.

Postpartum, the resultant myometrial contractions provide hemostasis at the site of placentation.

Carboprost tromethamine also stimulates the smooth muscle of the human gastrointestinal tract. This activity may produce the vomiting or diarrhea or both that is common when carboprost tromethamine is used to terminate pregnancy and for use postpartum. In laboratory animals and also in humans carboprost tromethamine can elevate body temperature. With the clinical doses of carboprost tromethamine used for the termination of pregnancy, and for use postpartum, some patients do experience transient temperature increases.

In laboratory animals and in humans large doses of carboprost tromethamine can raise blood pressure, probably by contracting the vascular smooth muscle. With the doses of carboprost tromethamine used for terminating pregnancy, this effect has not been clinically significant. In laboratory animals and also in humans carboprost tromethamine can elevate body temperature. With the clinical doses of carboprost tromethamine used for the termination of pregnancy, some patients do experience temperature increases. In some patients, carboprost tromethamine may cause transient bronchoconstriction.

Drug plasma concentrations were determined by radioimmunoassay in peripheral blood samples collected by different investigators from 10 patients undergoing abortion. The patients had been injected intramuscularly with 250 micrograms of carboprost at two hour intervals. Blood levels of drug peaked at an average of 2060 picograms/ml one-half hour after the first injection then declined to an average concentration of 770 picograms/ml two hours after the first injection just before the second injection. The average plasma concentration one-half hour after the second injection was slightly higher (2663 picograms/ml) than that after the first injection and decreased again to an average of 1047 picograms/ml by two hours after the second injection. Plasma samples were collected from 5 of these 10 patients following additional injections of the prostaglandin. The average peak concentrations of drug were slightly higher following each successive injection of the prostaglandin, but always decreased to levels less than the preceding peak values by two hours after each injection.

Five women who had delivery spontaneously at term were treated immediately postpartum with a single injection of 250 micrograms of carboprost tromethamine. Peripheral blood samples were collected at several times during the four hours following treatment and carboprost tromethamine levels were determined by radioimmunoassay. The highest concentration of carboprost tromethamine was observed at 15 minutes in two patients (3009 and 2916) picograms/ml), at 30 minutes in two patients (3097 and 2792 picograms/ml), and at 60 minutes in one patient (2718 picograms/ml).

INDICATIONS AND USAGE:

Carboprost thromethamine sterile solution is indicated for aborting pregnancy between the 13th and 20th weeks of gestation as calculated from the first day of the last normal menstrual period and in the following conditions related to second trimester abortion:

1. Failure of expulsion of the fetus during the course of treatment by another method;

2. Premature rupture of membranes in intrauterine methods with loss of drug and insufficient or absent uterine activity;

3. Requirement of a repeat intrauterine instillation of drug for expulsion of the fetus;

4. Inadvertent or spontaneous rupture of membranes in the presence of a previable fetus and absence of adequate activity for expulsion.

Carboprost thromethamine is indicated for the treatment of postpartum hemorrhage due to uterine atony which has not responded to conventional methods of management. Prior treatment should include the use of intravenously administered oxytocin, manipulative techniques such as uterine massage and, unless contraindicated, intramuscular ergot preparations. Studies have shown that in such cases, the use of carboprost thromethamine has resulted in satisfactory control of hemorrhage, although it is unclear whether or not ongoing or delayed effects of previously administered ecbolic agents have contributed to the outcome. In a high proportion of cases, carboprost thromethamine used in this manner has resulted in the cessation of life threatening bleeding and the avoidance of emergency surgical intervention.

CONTRAINDICATIONS:

1. Hypersensitivity to carboprost thromethamine sterile solution
2. Acute pelvic inflammatory disease
3. Patients with active cardiac, pulmonary, renal or hepatic disease

WARNINGS:

Carboprost thromethamine sterile solution, like other potent oxytocic agents, should be used only with strict adherence to recommended dosages. Carboprost thromethamine should be used by medically trained personnel in a hospital which can provide immediate intensive care and acute surgical facilities.

Carboprost thromethamine does not appear to directly affect the fetoplacental unit. Therefore, the possibility does exist that the previable fetus aborted by carboprost thromethamine could exhibit transient life signs. Carboprost thromethamine is not indicated if the fetus *in utero* has reached the stage of viability. Carboprost thromethamine should not be considered a feticidal agent.

Evidence from animal studies has suggested that certain other prostaglandins have some teratogenic potential. Although these studies do not indicate that carboprost thromethamine is teratogenic, any pregnancy termination with carboprost thromethamine that fails should be completed by some other means.

This product contains benzyl alcohol. Benzyl alcohol has been reported to be associated with a fatal "Gasping Syndrome" in premature infants.

PRECAUTIONS:

GENERAL

Animal studies lasting several weeks at high doses have shown that prostaglandins of the E and F series can induce proliferation of bone. Such effects have also been noted in newborn infants who have received prostaglandin E_1 during prolonged treatment. There is no evidence that short term administration of carboprost thromethamine sterile solution can cause similar bone effects.

As with spontaneous abortion, a process which is sometimes incomplete, carboprost thromethamine induced abortion may be expected to be incomplete in about 20% of cases.

Although the incidence of cervical trauma is extremely small, the cervix should always be carefully examined immediately post-abortion.

Use of carboprost thromethamine is associated with transient pyrexia that may be due to its effect on hypothalamic thermoregulation. Temperature elevations exceeding 2° F (1.1° C) were observed in approximately one-eight of the patients who received the recommended dosage regimen. In all cases, temperature returned to normal when therapy ended. Differentiation of postabortion endometritis from drug-induced temperature elevations is difficult, but with increasing clinical experience, the distinctions become more obvious and are summarized below (TABLE 1):

TABLE 1

Endometritis pyrexia	Carboprost Thromethamine Induced pyrexia
1.**Time of onset:**Typically, on third post-abortional day (38°C or higher).	Within 1 to 16 hours after the injection.
2.**Duration:** Untreated pyrexia and infection continue and may give rise to other pelvic infections.	Temperatures revert to pre-treatment levels after discontinuation of therapy without any other treatment.
3.**Retention:** Products of conception are often retained in the cervical os or uterine cavity.	Temperature elevation occurs whether or not tissue is retained.
4.**Histology:** Endometrium is infiltrated with lymphocytes and some areas are necrotic and hemorrhagic.	Although the endometrial stroma may be edematous and vascular, it is not inflamed.
5.**The uterus:** Often remains boggy and soft with tenderness over the fundus, and pain on moving the cervix on bimanual examination.	Uterine involution normal and uterus is not tender.
6.**Discharge:** Often associated with foul-smelling lochia and leukorrhea.	Lochia normal.
7.**Cervical culture:** The culture of pathological organisms from the cervix or uterine cavity after abortion alone does not warrant the diagnosis of septic abortion in the absence of clinical evidence of sepsis. Pathogens have been cultured soon after abortion in patients with no infections. Persistent positive culture with clear clinical signs of infections are significant in the differential diagnosis.	
8.**Blood count:** Leukocytosis and differential white cell counts do not distinguish between endometritis and carboprost thromethamine hyperthermia since total WBC's may increase during infection and transient leukocytosis may also be drug-induced. Fluids should be forced in patients with drug-induced fever and no clinical or bacteriological evidence of intrauterine infection. Any other simple empirical measures for temperature reduction are unnecessary because all fevers induced by carboprost thromethamine have been transient or self-limiting.	

Increased blood pressure. In the postpartum hemorrhage series, 5/115 (4%) of patients had an increase of blood pressure reported as a side effect. The degree of hypertension was moderate and it is not certain as to whether this was in fact due to a direct effect of carboprost thromethamine or a return to a status of pregnancy associated hypertension manifest by the correction of hypovolemic shock. In any event the cases reported did not require specific therapy for the elevated blood pressure.

Use in patients with chorioamnionitis. During the clinical trials with carboprost thromethamine, chorioamnionitis was identified as a complication contributing to postpartum uterine atony and hemorrhage in 8/115 (7%) of cases, 3 of which failed to respond to carboprost thromethamine. This complication during labor may have an inhibitory effect on the uterine response to carboprost thromethamine similar to what has been reported for other oxytocic agents.[1]

In patients with a history of asthma, hypo- or hypertension, cardiovascular, adrenal, or hepatic disease, anemia, jaundice, diabetes, or epilepsy, carboprost thromethamine should be used cautiously.

As with any oxytocic agent, carboprost thromethamine should be used with caution in patients with compromised (scarred) uteri.

CARCINOGENESIS, MUTAGENESIS, AND IMPAIRMENT OF FERTILITY

Carcinogenic bioassay studies have not been conducted in animals with carboprost thromethamine due to the limited indications for use and short duration of administration. No evidence of mutagenicity was observed in the Micronucleus Test or Ames Assay.

PREGNANCY, TERATOGENIC EFFECTS, PREGNANCY CATEGORY C

Animal studies do not indicate that carboprost thromethamine is teratogenic, however, it has been shown to be embryotoxic in rats and rabbits and any dose which produces increased uterine tone could put the embryo or fetus at risk.

DRUG INTERACTIONS:

Carboprost thromethamine may augment the activity of other oxytocic agents. Concomitant use with other oxytocic agents is not recommended.

ADVERSE REACTIONS:

The adverse effects of carboprost thromethamine sterile solution are generally transient and reversible when therapy ends. The most frequent adverse reactions observed are related to its contractile effect on smooth muscle.

In patients studied, approximately two-thirds experienced vomiting and diarrhea, approximately one-third had nausea, one-eight had a temperature increase greater than 2° F, and one-fourteenth experienced flushing.

The pretreatment or concurrent administration of antiemetic and antidiarrheal drugs decreases considerably the very high incidence of gastrointestinal effects common with all prostaglandins used for abortion. Their use should be considered an integral part of the management of patients undergoing abortion with carboprost thromethamine.

Of those patients experiencing a temperature elevation, approximately one-sixteenth had a clinical diagnosis of endometritis. The remaining temperature elevations returned to normal within several hours after the last injection.

Adverse effects observed during the use of carboprost thromethamine for abortion and for hemorrhage not all of which are clearly drug related, in decreasing order of frequency include

Adverse Effects (In Decreasing Order):

Vomiting
Diarrhea
Nausea
Flushing or hot flashes
Chills or shivering
Coughing
Headaches
Endometritis
Hiccough
Dysmenorrhea-like pain
Paresthesia
Backache
Muscular pain
Breast tenderness
Eye pain
Drowsiness
Dystonia
Asthma
Injection site pain
Tinnitus
Vertigo
Vaso-vagal syndrome
Dryness of mouth
Hyperventilation
Respiratory distress
Hematemesis
Taste alterations
Urinary tract infection
Septic shock
Torticollis
Lethargy
Hypertension
Tachycardia
Pulmonary edema
Endometritis from IUCD
Nervousness
Nosebleed
Sleep disorders
Dyspnea
Tightness in chest
Wheezing
Posterior cervical perforation
Weakness
Diaphoresis
Dizziness
Blurred vision
Epigastric pain
Excessive thirst
Twitching eyelids
Gagging, retching
Dry throat
Sensation of choking
Thyroid storm
Syncope
Palpitations
Rash
Upper respiratory infection
Leg cramps
Perforated uterus
Anxiety
Chest pain
Retained placental fragment
Shortness of breath
Fullness of throat
Uterine sacculation
Faintness, light-headedness
Uterine rupture

The most common complications when carboprost thromethamine was utilized for abortion requiring additional treatment after discharge from the hospital were endometritis, retained placental fragments, and excessive uterine bleeding, occurring in about one in every 50 patients.

DOSAGE AND ADMINISTRATION:

1. Abortion and Indications 1-4: An initial dose of 1 ml of carboprost thromethamine sterile solution (containing the equivalent of 250 micrograms of carboprost) is to be administered deep in the muscle with a tuberculin syringe. Subsequent doses of 250 micrograms should be administered at 1 1/2 to 3 1/2 hour intervals depending on uterine response. An optional test dose of 100 micrograms (0.4 ml) may be administered initially. The dose may be increased to 500 micrograms (2 ml) if uterine contractility is judged to be inadequate after several doses of 250 micrograms (1 ml). The total dose administered of carboprost tromethamine should not exceed 12 milligrams and continuous administration of the drug for more than two days is not recommended.

2. For Refractory Postpartum Uterine Bleeding: An initial dose of 250 micrograms of carboprost thromethamine sterile solution (1 ml of carboprost thromethamine) is to be given deep, intramuscularly. In clinical trials it was found that the majority of successful cases (73%) responded to single injections. In some selected cases, however, multiple dosing at intervals of 15 to 90 minutes was carried out with successful outcome. The need for additional injections and the interval at which these should be given can be determined only by the attending physicians as dictated by the course of clinical events. The total dose of carboprost thromethamine should not exceed 2 milligrams (8 doses).

DOSAGE AND ADMINISTRATION: *(cont'd)*

Parenteral drug products should be inspected visually for particulate matter and discoloration prior to administration, whenever solution and container permit.

Carboprost tromethamine must be refrigerated at 2 to 4° C (36-39° F).

[1] Duff, Sanders, and Gibbs; The course to labor in term patients with chorioamnionitis; *Am.J. Obstet. Gynecol.*; 147, no. 4, October 15, 1983 pp 391-395.

HOW SUPPLIED - EQUIVALENTS NOT AVAILABLE:

Injection, Solution - Intramuscular - 250 mcg/ml

1 ml x 10	$286.23	HEMABATE, Pharmacia & Upjohn	00009-0856-08

CARDIOPLEGIC SOLUTION *(000662)*

CATEGORIES: Cardiovascular Drugs; Electrolytic, Caloric-Water Balance; Replacement Solutions; FDA Pre 1938 Drugs

BRAND NAMES: Plegisol

Prescribing information not available at time of publication.

HOW SUPPLIED - EQUIVALENTS NOT AVAILABLE:

Solution - Intracardiac; I - 17.6 mg/325.3 m

1000 ml	$48.83	PLEGISOL, Abbott	00074-7969-05

CARISOPRODOL *(000664)*

CATEGORIES: Autonomic Drugs; Muscle Relaxants; Neuromuscular; Pain; Skeletal Muscle Hyperactivity; Skeletal Muscle Relaxants; FDA Approval Pre 1982; Top 200 Drugs

BRAND NAMES: *Artifar*; *Caridolin*; *Carisoma* (England); *Chinchen*; *Flexartal*; *Muslax*; *Myolax*; *Neotica*; Rela; *Rotalin*; *Sanoma* (Germany); *Scutamil-C*; Sodol; **Soma**; *Somadril*; Sopridol; Soridol; Vanasom
(International brand names outside U.S. in italics)

FORMULARIES: Aetna; BC-BS; PCS

DESCRIPTION:

Carisoprodol is available as 350 mg tablets. Carisoprodol is 2-methyl-2-propyl-1,3-propanediol carbamate isopropylcarbamate.

Empirical formula: $C_{12}H_{24}N_2O_4$

M.W. = 260.33

Inactive ingredients: Corn starch, lactose, magnesium stearate, povidone, sodium lauryl sulfate, sodium starch glycolate, stearic acid.

CLINICAL PHARMACOLOGY:

Carisoprodol produces muscle relaxation in animals by blocking interneuronal activity in the descending reticular formation and spinal cord. The onset of action is rapid and effects last four to six hours.

INDICATIONS AND USAGE:

Carisoprodol is indicated as an adjunct to rest, physical therapy, and other measures for the relief of discomfort associated with acute, painful, musculoskeletal conditions. The mode of action of this drug has not been clearly identified, but may be related to its sedative properties. Carisoprodol does not directly relax tense skeletal muscles in man.

CONTRAINDICATIONS:

Acute intermittent porphyria as well as allergic or idiosyncratic reactions to carisoprodol or related compounds, such as meprobamate, mebutamate, or tybamate.

WARNINGS:

Idiosyncratic Reactions: On very rare occasions, the first dose of carisoprodol has been followed by idiosyncratic symptoms appearing within minutes or hours. Symptoms reported include: extreme weakness, transient quadriplegia, dizziness, ataxia, temporary loss of vision, diplopia, mydriasis, dysarthria, agitation, euphoria, confusion, and disorientation. Symptoms usually subside over the course of the next several hours. Supportive and symptomatic therapy, including hospitalization, may be necessary.

Usage in Pregnancy and Lactation: Safe usage of this drug in pregnancy or lactation has not been established. Therefore, use of this drug in pregnancy, in nursing mothers, or in women of childbearing potential requires that the potential benefits of the drug be weighed against the potential hazards of the mother and child. Carisoprodol is presenting breast milk of lactating mothers at concentrations two to four times that of maternal plasma. This factor should be taken into account when use of the drug is contemplated in breast-feeding patients.

Usage in Children: Because of limited clinical experience, carisoprodol is not recommended for use in patients under 12 years of age.

Potentially Hazardous Tasks: Patients should be warned that this drug may impair the mental and/or physical abilities required for the performance of potentially hazardous tasks such as driving a motor vehicle or operating machinery.

Additive Effects: Since the effects of carisoprodol and alcohol or carisoprodol and other CNS depressants or psychotropic drugs may be additive, appropriate caution should be exercised with patients who take more than one of these agents simultaneously.

Drug Dependence: In dogs, no withdrawal symptoms occurred after abrupt cessation of carisoprodol from dosages as high as 1 g/kg/day. In a study in man, abrupt cessation of 100 mg/kg/day (about five times the recommended daily adult dosage) was followed in some subjects by mild withdrawal symptoms such as abdominal cramps, insomnia, chilliness, headache, and nausea. Delirium and convulsions did not occur. In clinical use, psychological dependence and abuse have been rare, and there have been no reports of significant abstinence signs. Nevertheless, the drug should be used with caution in addiction-prone individuals.

PRECAUTIONS:

Carisoprodol is metabolized in the liver and excreted by the kidney; to avoid its excess accumulation, caution should be exercised in administration to patients with compromised liver or kidney function.

ADVERSE REACTIONS:

Central Nervous System: Drowsiness and other CNS effects may require dosage reduction. Also observed: dizziness, vertigo, ataxia, tremor, agitation, irritability, headache, depressive reactions, syncope, and insomnia. (See WARNINGS, Idiosyncratic Reactions.)

ADVERSE REACTIONS: *(cont'd)*

Allergic or Idiosyncratic: Allergic or idiosyncratic reactions occasionally develop. They are usually seen within the period of the first to fourth dose in patients having had no previous contact with the drug. Skin rash, erythema multiforme, pruritus, eosinophilia, and fixed drug eruption with cross reaction to meprobamate have been reported with carisoprodol. Severe reactions have been manifested by asthmatic episodes, fever, weakness, dizziness, angioneurotic edema, smarting eyes, hypotension, and anaphylactoid shock. (See WARNINGS, Idiosyncratic Reactions.)

In case of allergic or idiosyncratic reactions to carisoprodol, discontinue the drug and initiate appropriate symptomatic therapy, which may include epinephrine, antihistamines, and in severe cases corticosteroids. In evaluating possible allergic reactions, also consider allergy to excipients (information on excipients is available to physicians on request).

Cardiovascular: Tachycardia, postural hypotension, and facial flushing.

Gastrointestinal: Nausea, vomiting, hiccup, and epigastric distress.

Hematologic: Leukopenia, in which other drugs or viral infection may have been responsible, and pancytopenia, attributed to phenylbutazone, have been reported. No serious blood dyscrasias have been attributed to carisoprodol.

OVERDOSAGE:

Overdosage of carisoprodol has produced stupor, coma. shock, respiratory depression, and, very rarely, death. The effects of an overdosage of carisoprodol and alcohol or other CNS depressants or psychotropic agents can be additive even when one of the drugs has been taken in the usual recommended dosage. Any drug remaining in the stomach should be removed and symptomatic therapy be given. Should respiration or blood pressure become compromised, respiratory assistance, central nervous system stimulants, and pressor agents should be administered cautiously as indicated. Carisoprodol is metabolized in the liver and excreted by the kidney. Although carisoprodol overdosage experience is limited, the following types of treatment have been used successfully with the related drug meprobamate: diuresis, osmotic (mannitol) diuresis, peritoneal dialysis, and hemodialysis (carisoprodol is dialyzable). Careful monitoring of urinary out put is necessary and caution should be taken to avoid overhydration. Observe for possible relapse due to incomplete gastric emptying and delayed absorption. Carisoprodol can be measured in biological fluids by gas chromatography.

DOSAGE AND ADMINISTRATION:

The usual adult dosage of carisoprodol is one 350 mg tablet, three times daily and at bedtime. Usage in patients under age 12 is not recommended.

Store at controlled room temperature 15-30° (59- 86°F).

PATIENT INFORMATION:

Carisoprodol is a muscle relaxant used to relieve the pain and stiffness of muscle spasms and discomfort due to strain and sprain. Inform your physician if you are pregnant or nursing. Do not take this medication with a monoamine oxidase inhibitor. This medication may cause dizziness, drowsiness, or blurred vision; use caution while driving or operating hazardous machinery. Do not take any other sedating drugs or drink alcohol while taking carisoprodol. If dizziness occurs, avoid sudden changes in posture. Take this medication with food to avoid stomach upset. Notify your physician if you develop trouble breathing, unexplained fever, severe weakness, vision changes, swelling, or skin rash. Withdrawal symptoms may occur if therapy is suddenly stopped in a patient on long-term or high-dose therapy.

HOW SUPPLIED - RATED THERAPEUTICALLY EQUIVALENT:

Tablet, Uncoated - Oral - 350 mg

100's	$6.72	Carisoprodol, H.C.F.A. F F P	99999-0664-01
100's	$8.75	Carisoprodol, Consolidated Midland	00223-0657-01
100's	$9.85	Carisoprodol, Aligen Independ	00405-4141-01
100's	$12.20	Carisoprodol, Qualitest Pharms	00603-2582-21
100's	$12.22	Carisoprodol, HL Moore Drug Exch	00839-6246-06
100's	$12.35	Carisoprodol, Rugby	00536-3435-01
100's	$12.35	Carisprodol, Mutual Pharm	53489-0110-01
100's	$12.37	Carisoprodol, Geneva Pharms	00781-1050-01
100's	$12.39	Carisoprodol, United Res	00677-0589-01
100's	$12.40	Carisoprodol, Goldline Labs	00182-1079-01
100's	$12.40	Carisoprodol, Major Pharms	00904-0355-60
100's	$12.87	Carisoprodol, Schein Pharm (US)	00364-0475-01
100's	$35.12	Carisoprodol, Amer Preferred	53445-1079-01
100's	$60.41	Carisoprodol, Bristol Myers Squibb	00003-0386-50
100's	$67.86	RELA, Schering	00085-0160-06
100's	$128.39	VANADOM, GM Pharms	58809-0424-01
100's	**$177.08**	**SOMA, Wallace Labs**	**00037-2001-01**
100's	**$179.11**	**SOMA, Wallace Labs**	**00037-2001-85**
500's	$24.50	Soprodal 350, H & H Labs	46703-0061-05
500's	$33.60	Carisoprodol, H.C.F.A. F F P	99999-0664-02
500's	$40.00	Carisoprodol, Consolidated Midland	00223-0657-05
500's	$59.55	Carisoprodol, Qualitest Pharms	00603-2582-28
500's	$59.90	Carisoprodol, Goldline Labs	00182-1079-05
500's	$59.90	Carisoprodol, Aligen Independ	00405-4141-02
500's	$59.90	Carisprodol, Mutual Pharm	53489-0110-05
500's	$60.19	Carisoprodol, United Res	00677-0589-05
500's	$60.28	Carisoprodol, Rugby	00536-3435-05
500's	$60.30	Carisoprodol, Geneva Pharms	00781-1050-05
500's	$62.42	Carisoprodol, Schein Pharm (US)	00364-0475-05
500's	$66.00	Carisoprodol, Major Pharms	00904-0355-40
500's	**$872.04**	**SOMA, Wallace Labs**	**00037-2001-03**
1000's	$67.20	Carisoprodol, H.C.F.A. F F P	99999-0664-03
1000's	$70.88	Carisoprodol, HL Moore Drug Exch	00839-6246-16
1000's	$77.50	Carisoprodol, Consolidated Midland	00223-0657-02
1000's	$94.60	Carisprodol, Mutual Pharm	53489-0110-10
1000's	$99.90	Carisoprodol, United Res	00677-0589-10
1000's	$99.98	Carisoprodol, Rugby	00536-3435-10
1000's	$112.50	Carisoprodol, Schein Pharm (US)	00364-0475-02
1000's	$113.50	Carisoprodol, Goldline Labs	00182-1079-10

CARMUSTINE *(000665)*

CATEGORIES: Antineoplastics; Astrocytoma; Blastoma; Brain Carcinoma; Chemotherapy; Cytotoxic Agents; Ependymoma; Glioblastoma; Glioma; Hodgkin's Disease; Lymphoma; Medulloblastoma; Multiple Myeloma; Myeloma; Oncologic Drugs; Tumors; Pregnancy Category D; FDA Approval Pre 1982

BRAND NAMES: *Bcnu*; *Becenun*; *BiCNU* (Australia, England, France, Canada, Mexico); **Bicnu**; *Carmubris* (Germany); *Nitrumon* (Germany)
(International brand names outside U.S. in italics)

FORMULARIES: BC-BS; Medi-Cal

WARNING:
Sterile carmustine should be administered under the supervision of a qualified physician experienced in the use of cancer chemotherapeutic agents.
Bone marrow suppression, notably thrombocytopenia and leukopenia, which may contribute to bleeding and overwhelming infections in an already compromised patient, is the most common and severe of the toxic effects of carmustine (see WARNINGS and ADVERSE REACTIONS).
Since the major toxicity is bone marrow suppression, blood counts should be monitored weekly for at least 6 weeks after a dose (see ADVERSE REACTIONS.) At the recommended dosage, courses of carmustine should not be given any more frequently than every 6 weeks.
The bone marrow toxicity of carmustine is cumulative and therefore dosage adjustment must be considered on the basis of nadir blood counts from prior dose (see DOSAGE AND ADMINISTRATION.)
Pulmonary toxicity from carmustine appears to be dose related. Patients receiving greater than 1400 mg/m^2 cumulative dose are at significantly higher risk than those receiving less. Delayed pulmonary toxicity can occur years after treatment, and can result in death, particularly in patients treated in childhood (see ADVERSE REACTIONS.)

DESCRIPTION:

Sterile carmustine [BCNU] is one of the nitrosoureas used in the treatment of neoplastic diseases. It is 1,3-bis (2-chloroethyl)-1-nitrosourea. It is lyophilized pale yellow flakes or congealed mass with a molecular weight of 214.06. It is highly soluble in alcohol and lipids, and poorly soluble in water. Carmustine is administered by intravenous infusion after reconstitution as recommended.

Sterile Bicnu is available in 100 mg single dose vials of lyophilized material.

CLINICAL PHARMACOLOGY:

Although it is generally agreed that carmustine alkylates DNA and RNA, it is not cross resistant with other alkylators. As with other nitrosoureas, it may also inhibit several key enzymatic processes by carbamoylation of amino acids in proteins.

Intravenously administered carmustine is rapidly degraded, with no intact drug detectable after 15 minutes. However, in studies with C^{14}-labeled drug, prolonged levels of the isotope were detected in the plasma and tissue, probably representing radioactive fragments of the parent compound.

It is thought that the antineoplastic and toxic activities of carmustine may be due to metabolites. Approximately 60 to 70% of a total dose is excreted in the urine in 96 hours and about 10% as respiratory CO_2. The fate of the remainder is undetermined.

Because of the high lipid solubility and the relative lack of ionization at physiological pH, carmustine crosses the blood-brain barrier quite effectively. Levels of radioactivity in the CSF are $\geq$ 50% of those measured concurrently in plasma.

INDICATIONS AND USAGE:

Carmustine is indicated as palliative therapy as a single agent or in established combination therapy with other approved chemotherapeutic agents in the following:

1. Brain tumors: glioblastoma, brainstem glioma, medulloblastoma, astrocytoma, ependymoma, and metastatic brain tumors.

2. Multiple myeloma: In combination with prednisone.

3. Hodgkin's Disease: as secondary therapy in combination with other approved drugs in patients who relapse while being treated with primary therapy, or who fail to respond to primary therapy.

4. Non-Hodgkin's lymphomas: as secondary therapy in combination with other approved drugs for patients who relapse while being treated with primary therapy, or who fail to respond to primary therapy.

CONTRAINDICATIONS:

Carmustine should not be given to individuals who have demonstrated a previous hypersensitivity to it.

WARNINGS:

Since the major toxicity is delayed bone marrow suppression, blood counts should be monitored weekly for at least 6 weeks after a dose (see ADVERSE REACTIONS.) At the recommended dosage, courses of carmustine should not be given any more frequently than every 6 weeks.

The bone marrow toxicity of carmustine is cumulative and therefore dosage adjustment must be considered on the basis of nadir blood counts from prior dose (see DOSAGE AND ADMINISTRATION.)

Pulmonary toxicity from carmustine appears to be dose related. Patients receiving greater than 1400 mg/m^2 cumulative dose are at a significantly higher risk than those receiving less. Additionally, delayed onset pulmonary fibrosis occurring up to 15 years after treatment has occurred in patients who received carmustine in childhood and early adolescence (see ADVERSE REACTIONS.)

Long term use of nitrosoureas has been reported to be associated with the development of secondary malignancies.

Liver and renal function tests should be monitored periodically (see ADVERSE REACTIONS.)

Carmustine may cause fetal harm when administered to a pregnant woman. Carmustine has been shown to be embryotoxic in rats and rabbits and teratogenic in rats when given in doses equivalent to the human dose. There are no adequate and well-controlled studies in pregnant women. If this drug is used during pregnancy, or if the patient becomes pregnant while taking (receiving) this drug, the patient should be apprised of the potential hazard to the fetus. Women of childbearing potential should be advised to avoid becoming pregnant.

Carmustine has been administered through an intraarterial intracarotid route; this procedure is investigational and has been associated with ocular toxicity.

PRECAUTIONS:

General: In all instances where the use of carmustine is considered for chemotherapy, the physician must evaluate the need and usefulness of the drug against the risks of toxic effects or adverse reactions. Most such adverse reactions are reversible if detected early. When such effects or reactions do occur, the drug should be reduced in dosage or discontinued and appropriate corrective measures should be taken according to the clinical judgment of the physician. Reinstitution of carmustine therapy should be carried out with caution, and with adequate consideration of the further need for the drug and alertness as to possible recurrence of toxicity.

Laboratory Tests: Due to delayed bone marrow suppression, blood counts should be monitored weekly for at least 6 weeks after a dose.

Baseline pulmonary function studies should be conducted along with frequent pulmonary function tests during treatment. Patients with a baseline below 70% of the predicted Forced Vital Capacity (FVC) or Carbon Monoxide Diffusing Capacity (DL_{co}) are particularly at risk.

Since carmustine may cause liver dysfunction, it is recommended that liver function tests be monitored.

Renal function tests should also be monitored periodically.

Carcinogenesis, Mutagenesis, and Impairment of Fertility: Carmustine is carcinogenic in rats and mice, producing a marked increase in tumor incidence in doses approximating those employed clinically. Nitrosourea therapy does have carcinogenic potential in humans (see ADVERSE REACTIONS.) Carmustine also effects fertility in male rats at doses somewhat higher than the human dose.

Pregnancy: Pregnancy Category D. (see WARNINGS.)

Nursing Mothers: It is not known whether this drug is excreted in human milk. Because many drugs are excreted in human milk and because of the potential for serious adverse reactions in nursing infants from carmustine, a decision should be made whether to discontinue nursing or to discontinue the drug, taking into account the importance of the drug to the mother.

Pediatric Use: Safety and effectiveness in children have not been established.

ADVERSE REACTIONS:

Hematologic Toxicity: The most frequent and most serious toxicity of carmustine is delayed myelosuppression. It usually occurs 4 to 6 weeks after drug administration and is dose related. Thrombocytopenia occurs at about 4 weeks postadministration and persists for 1 to 2 weeks. Leukopenia occurs at 5 to 6 weeks after a dose of carmustine and persists for 1 to 2 weeks. Leukopenia occurs at 5 to 6 weeks after a dose of carmustine and persists for 1 to 2 weeks. Thrombocytopenia is generally more severe than leukopenia. However, both may be dose-limiting toxicities.

Carmustine may produce cumulative myelosuppression, manifested by more depressed indices or longer duration of suppression after repeated doses.

The occurrence of acute leukemia and bone marrow dysplasias have been reported in patients following long term nitrosourea therapy.

Anemia also occurs, but is less frequent and less severe than thrombocytopenia or leukopenia.

Pulmonary Toxicity: Pulmonary toxicity characterized by pulmonary infiltrates and/or fibrosis has been reported to occur from 9 days to 43 months after treatment with carmustine and related nitrosoureas. Most of these patients were receiving prolonged therapy with total doses of carmustine greater than 1400 mg/m^2. However, there have been reports of pulmonary fibrosis in patients receiving lower total doses. Other risk factors include past history of lung disease and duration of treatment. Cases of fatal pulmonary toxicity with carmustine have been reported.

Additionally, delayed onset pulmonary fibrosis occurring up to 15 years after treatment has been reported in a long-term study with 17 patients who received carmustine in childhood and early adolescence in cumulative doses ranging from 770 to 1800 mg/m^2 combined with cranial radiotherapy for intracranial tumors. Chest x-rays have demonstrated pulmonary hypoplasia with upper zone contraction. Gallium scans have been normal in all cases. Thoracic CT scans have demonstrated an unusual pattern of upper zone fibrosis. There appears to be some late reduction of pulmonary function in all long-term survivors. This form of lung fibrosis may be slowly progressive and has resulted in death in some cases. In this long-term study, all those initially treated at less than 5 years of age died of delayed pulmonary fibrosis.

Gastrointestinal Toxicity: Nausea and vomiting after IV administration of carmustine are noted frequently. This toxicity appears within 2 hours of dosing, usually lasting 4 to 6 hours, and is dose related. Prior administration of antiemetics is effective in diminishing and sometimes preventing this side effect.

Hepatotoxicity: A reversible type of hepatic toxicity, manifested by increased transaminase, alkaline phosphatase, and bilirubin levels, has been reported in a small percentage of patients receiving carmustine.

Nephrotoxicity: Renal abnormalities consisting of progressive azotemia, decrease in kidney size, and renal failure have been reported in patients who received large cumulative doses after prolonged therapy with carmustine and related nitrosoureas. Kidney damage has also been reported occasionally in patients receiving lower total doses.

Other Toxicities: Accidental contact of reconstituted carmustine with skin has caused burning and hyperpigmentation of the affected areas.

Rapid IV infusion of carmustine may produce intensive flushing of the skin and suffusion of the conjunctiva within 2 hours, lasting about 4 hours. It is also associated with burning at the site of injection although true thrombosis is rare.

Neuroretinitis has been reported.

OVERDOSAGE:

No proven antidotes have been established for carmustine overdosage.

DOSAGE AND ADMINISTRATION:

The recommended dose of carmustine as a single agent in previously untreated patients is 150 to 200 mg/m^2 intravenously every 6 weeks. This may be given as a single dose or divided into daily injections such as 75 to 100 mg/m^2 on 2 successive days. When carmustine is used in combination with other myelosuppressive drugs or in patients in whom bone marrow reserve is depleted, the doses should be adjusted accordingly.

Doses subsequent to the initial dose should be adjusted according to the hematologic response of the patient to the preceding dose. The following schedule (TABLE 1) is suggested as a guide to dosage adjustment:

TABLE 1

Nadir After Prior Dose Leukocytes/mm^3	Platelets/mm^3	Percentage of Prior Dose to be Given
>4000	>100,000	100%
3000-3999	75,000-99,999	100%
2000-2999	25,000-74,999	70%
<2000	<25,000	50%

DOSAGE AND ADMINISTRATION: *(cont'd)*

A repeat course of carmustine should not be given until circulating blood elements have returned to acceptable levels (platelets above 100,000/mm^3, leukocytes above 4,000/mm^3), and this is usually in 6 weeks. Adequate number of neutrophils should be present on a peripheral blood smear. Blood counts should be monitored weekly and repeat courses should not be given before 6 weeks because the hematologic toxicity is delayed and cumulative.

Administration Precautions: As with other potentially toxic compounds, caution should be exercised in handling carmustine and preparing the solution of carmustine. Accidental contact of reconstituted carmustine with the skin has caused transient hyperpigmentation of the affected areas. The use of gloves is recommended. If carmustine lyophilized material or solution contacts the skin or mucosa, immediately wash the skin or mucosa thoroughly with soap and water.

The reconstituted solution should be used intravenously only and should be administered by IV drip. Injection of carmustine over shorter periods of time than 1 to 2 hours may produce intense pain and burning at the site of injection.

Preparation of Intravenous Solutions: First, dissolve carmustine with 3 ml of the supplied sterile diluent (Dehydrated Alcohol Injection, USP). Second, aseptically add 27 ml Sterile Water for Injection, USP. Each ml of resulting solution contains 3.3 mg of carmustine in 10% ethanol, pH 5.6 to 6.0. Such solutions should be protected from light.

Reconstitution as recommended results in a clear, colorless to yellowish solution which may be further diluted with 5% Dextrose Injection, USP. Parenteral drug products should be inspected visually for particulate matter and discoloration prior to administration, whenever solution and container permit.

Important Note: The lyophilized dosage formulation contains no preservatives and is not intended as a multiple dose vial.

Stability: Unopened vials of the dry drug must be stored in a refrigerator (2°C to 8°C). The recommended storage of unopened vials provides a stable product for 2 years. After reconstitution as recommended, carmustine is stable for 8 hours at room temperature (25°C), protected from light.

Vials reconstituted as directed and further diluted to a concentration of 0.2 mg/ml in 5% Dextrose Injection, USP, should be stored at room temperature, protected from light and utilized within 8 hours.

Glass containers were used for the stability data provided in this section. Only use glass containers for carmustine administration.

Important Note: Carmustine has a low melting point (30.5° to 32.0°C or 86.9° to 89.6°F). Exposure of the drug to this temperature or above will cause the drug to liquefy and appear as an oil film on the vials. This is a sign of decomposition and vials should be discarded. If there is a question of adequate refrigeration upon receipt of this product, immediately inspect the larger vial in each individual carton. Hold the vial to the bright light for inspection. The carmustine will appear as a very small amount of dry flakes or dry congealed mass. If this is evident, the carmustine is suitable for use and should be refrigerated immediately.

Procedures for proper handling and disposal of anticancer drugs should be considered. Several guidelines on this subject have been published.[1-7] There is no general agreement that all of the procedures recommended in the guidelines are necessary or appropriate.

REFERENCES:

1. Recommendations for the Safe Handling of Parenteral Antineoplastic Drugs. NIH Publication No. 83-2621. For sale by the Superintendent of Documents, US Government Printing Office, Washington, DC 20402. **2.** AMA Council Report. Guidelines for Handling Parenteral Antineoplastics. JAMA 1985; 253 (11):1590-1592. **3.** National Study Commission on Cytotoxic Exposure—Recommendations for Handling Cytotoxic Agents. Available from Louis P. Jeffrey, ScD, Chairman, National Study Commission on Cytotoxic Exposure, Massachusetts College of Pharmacy and Allied Health Sciences, 179 Longwood Avenue, Boston, Massachusetts 02115. **4.** Clinical Oncological Society of Australia. Guidelines and Recommendations for Safe Handling of Antineoplastic Agents. Med J Australia 1983; 1:426-428. **5.** Jones RB, et al: Safe Handling of Chemotherapeutic Agents: A Report from the Mount Sinai Medical Center. Ca—A Cancer Journal for Clinicians 1983; (Sept/Oct) 258-263. **6.** American Society of Hospital Pharmacists Technical Assistance Bulletin on Handling Cytotoxic and Hazardous Drugs. Am J Hosp Pharm 1990; 47:1033-1049. **7.** OSHA Work-Practice Guidelines for Personnel Dealing with Cytotoxic (Antineoplastic) Drugs. Am J Hosp Pharm 43:1193-1204.

HOW SUPPLIED:

Bicnu (sterile carmustine [BCNU]). Each package contains a vial containing 100 mg carmustine and a vial containing 3 ml sterile diluent.

Store dry powder in refrigerator (2°C to 8°C).

HOW SUPPLIED - EQUIVALENTS NOT AVAILABLE:

Injection, Dry-Soln - Intravenous - 100 mg/vial

1 vial $794.05 BICNU, Mead Johnson 00015-3012-38

CARTEOLOL HYDROCHLORIDE *(000666)*

CATEGORIES: Antihypertensives; Antiglaucomatous Agents; Beta Adrenergic Blocking Agents; Beta Blockers; Cardiovascular Drugs; EENT Drugs; Eye, Ear, Nose, & Throat Preparations; Glaucoma; Hypertension; Ophthalmics; Pregnancy Category C; FDA Approved 1988 Dec

BRAND NAMES: *Arteolol*; *Arteoptic* (Germany); *Arteoptik*; *Calte*; *Carteol* (France); **Cartrol**; *Endak* (Germany); *Mikelan* (Asia, France); Ocupress; Optipress; *Teoptic* (England)

(International brand names outside U.S. in italics)

FORMULARIES: BC-BS; PCS

COST OF THERAPY: $360.36 (Hypertension; Tablet; 2.5 mg; 1/day; 365 days)

PRIMARY ICD9: 401.1 (Essential Hypertension, Benign)

DESCRIPTION:

TABLETS

Carteolol HCl is a synthetic, nonselective, beta-adrenergic receptor blocking agent with intrinsic sympathomimetic activity. It is chemically described as 5[3-[(1,1-dimethyl-ethyl) amino]- 2-hydroxypropoxy]-3,4-dihydro-2(1H)-quinolinone monohydrochloride.

Carteolol hydrochloride is a stable, white crystalline powder which is soluble in water and slightly soluble in ethanol. The molecular weight is 328.84 and $C_{16}H_{24}N_2O_3 \cdot HCl$ is the empirical formula.

Cartrol (carteolol hydrochloride) is available as tablets containing either 2.5 mg or 5 mg of carteolol hydrochloride for oral administration.

Cartrol Inactive Ingredients: *2.5 mg Tablet:* Cellulosic polymers, corn starch, iron oxide, lactose, magnesium stearate, microcrystalline cellulose, polyethylene glycol, propylene glycol and titanium dioxide. *5 mg Tablet:* Cellulosic polymers, corn starch, lactose, magnesium stearate, microcrystalline cellulose, polyethylene glycol, propylene glycol and titanium dioxide.

DESCRIPTION: *(cont'd)*

OPHTHALMIC SOLUTION

Carteolol HCl ophthalmic solution, 1% is a nonselective beta-adrenoceptor blocking agent for ophthalmic use.

The chemical name for carteolol hydrochloride is (±)-5-(3-((1,1-dimethylethyl)amino)-2-hydroxypropoxy)-3,4-dihydro-2(1H)- quinolinone monohydrochloride.

Each ml contains 10 mg carteolol HCl and the inactive ingredients sodium chloride, monobasic and dibasic sodium phosphate, and Water for injection, USP. Benzalkonium chloride 0.05 mg (0.005%) is added as a preservative. The product has a pH range of 6.2 to 7.2.

CLINICAL PHARMACOLOGY:

Carteolol HCl is a long-acting, nonselective, beta-adrenergic receptor blocking agent with intrinsic sympathomimetic activity (ISA) and without significant membrane stabilizing (local anesthetic) activity.

TABLETS

Pharmacodynamics: Carteolol specifically competes with beta-adrenergic receptor agonists for both beta$_1$-receptors located principally in cardiac muscle and beta$_2$-receptors located in the bronchial and vascular musculature, blocking the chronotropic, inotropic, and vasodilator responses to beta-adrenergic stimulation proportionately. Because of its partial agonist activity, however, carteolol does not reduce resting beta-agonist activity as much as beta-adrenergic blockers lacking this activity. Thus, in clinical trials in man, the decreases in resting pulse rate produced by carteolol (2-5 beats per minute in various studies) were less than those produced by beta-blockers (nadolol and propranolol) without ISA (10-12 beats per minute). There are also equivocal effects on renin secretion, in contrast to beta-blockers without ISA, which inhibit renin secretion.

In controlled clinical trials carteolol, at doses up to 20 mg as monotherapy or in combination with thiazide type diuretics, produced significantly greater reductions in blood pressure than did placebo, with the full effect seen between two and four weeks. The observed differences from placebo ranged from 3.1 to 6.7 mmHg for supine diastolic blood pressure. The antihypertensive effects of carteolol are smaller in black populations but do not seem to be affected by age or sex. Doses of carteolol greater than 10 mg once a day did not produce greater reductions in blood pressure. In fact, doses of 20 mg and above appeared to produce blood pressure reductions less than those produced by 10 mg and below. When carteolol was compared to nadolol and propranolol, although the differences were not statistically significant in relatively small studies, carteolol at doses up to 20 mg produced supine diastolic blood pressure changes consistently 2 mmHg less than that produced by either nadolol or propranolol.

Although the mechanism of the antihypertensive effect of beta-adrenergic blocking agents has not been established, multiple factors are thought to contribute to the lowering of blood pressure, including diminished response to sympathetic nerve outflow from vasomotor centers in the brain, diminished release of renin from the kidneys, and decreased cardiac output. Carteolol does not have a consistent effect on renin and other agents with ISA have been shown to have less effect than other beta-blockers on resting cardiac output (although they cause the usual decrease in exercise cardiac output so that the difference is of uncertain clinical importance), so that the mechanism of its action is particularly uncertain.

Beta-blockade interferes with endogenous adrenergic bronchodilator activity and diminishes the response to exogenous bronchodilators. This is especially important in patients subject to bronchospasm.

Single intravenous doses of carteolol (0.5 mg, 1.0 mg, 2.5 mg and 5.0 mg) produced statistically, but not clinically, significant increases from baseline in AV node conduction time and RR and PR intervals.

Carteolol HCl induced no significant alteration in total serum cholesterol and triglycerides.

Following discontinuation of carteolol treatment in man, pharmacologic activity (evaluated by blockade of the tachycardia induced by isoproterenol or postural changes) is present for 2 to 21 days (median 14 days) after the last dose of carteolol. Following administration of recommended doses of carteolol HCl, both beta-blocking and antihypertensive effects persist for at least 24 hours.

Pharmacokinetics and Metabolism: Following oral administration in man, peak plasma concentrations of carteolol usually occur within one to three hours. Carteolol is well absorbed when administered orally as carteolol HCl tablets. The presence of food in the gastrointestinal tract somewhat slows the rate of absorption, but the extent of absorption is not appreciably affected. Compared to intravenous administration, the absolute bioavailability of carteolol from carteolol HCl tablets is approximately 85%.

The plasma half-life carteolol averages approximately six hours. Steady-state serum levels are achieved within one to two days after initiating therapeutic doses of carteolol in persons with normal renal function. Since approximately 50 to 70% of a carteolol dose is eliminated unchanged by the kidneys, the half-life is increased in patients with impaired renal function. Significant reductions in the rate of carteolol elimination (and prolongations of the half-life) occur in patients as creatinine clearance decreases. Therefore, a reduction in maintenance dose and/or prolongation in dosing interval is appropriate (see DOSAGE AND ADMINISTRATION).

Carteolol is 23-30% bound to plasma proteins in humans. The major metabolites of carteolol are 8-hydroxycarteolol and the glucuronic acid conjugates of both carteolol and 8-hydroxycarteolol. In man, 8-hydroxycarteolol is an active metabolite with a half-life of approximately 8 to 12 hours and represents approximately 5% of the administered dose excreted in the urine.

OPHTHALMIC SOLUTION

Carteolol HCl solution reduces normal and elevated intraocular pressure (IOP) whether or not accompanied by glaucoma. The exact mechanism of the ocular hypotensive effect of beta-blockers has not been definitely demonstrated.

In general, beta-adrenergic blockers reduce cardiac output in patients in good and poor cardiovascular health. In patients with severe impairment of myocardial function, beta-blockers may inhibit the sympathetic stimulation necessary to maintain adequate cardiac function. Beta-adrenergic blockers may also increase airway resistance in the bronchi and bronchioles due to unopposed parasympathetic activity.

Given topically twice daily in controlled clinical trials ranging from 1.5 to 3 months, carteolol HCl solution produced a median percent reduction of IOP 22% to 25%. No significant effects were noted on corneal sensitivity, tear secretion, or pupil size.

INDICATIONS AND USAGE:

Tablets: Carteolol HCl is indicated in the management of hypertension. It may be used alone or in combination with other antihypertensive agents, especially thiazide diuretics. Preliminary data indicate that carteolol does not have a favorable effect on arrhythmias.

Ophthalmic Solution: Carteolol HCl solution, 1%, has been shown to be effective in lowering intraocular pressure and may be used in patients with chronic open-angle glaucoma and intraocular hypertension. It may be used alone or in combination with other intraocular pressure lowering medications.

CONTRAINDICATIONS:

Tablets: Carteolol HCl is contraindicated in patients with: 1) bronchial asthma, 2) severe bradycardia, 3) greater than first degree heart block, 4) cardiogenic shock, and 5) clinically evident congestive heart failure (see WARNINGS).

Ophthalmic Solution: Carteolol HCl solution is contraindicated in those individuals with bronchial asthma or with a history of bronchial asthma, or severe chronic obstructive pulmonary disease (See WARNINGS); sinus bradycardia; second- and third-degree atrioventricular block; overt cardiac failure (see WARNINGS); cardiogenic shock; or hypersensitivity to any component of this product.

WARNINGS:

OPHTHALMIC SOLUTION

Carteolol HCl solution has not been detected in plasma following ocular instillation. However, as with other topically applied ophthalmic preparations, carteolol HCl solution may be absorbed systemically. The same adverse reactions found with systemic administration of beta-adrenergic blocking agents may occur with topical administration. For example, severe respiratory reactions and cardiac reactions, including death due to bronchospasm in patients with asthma, and rarely death in association with cardiac failure, have been reported with topical application of beta-adrenergic blocking agents (see CONTRAINDICATIONS.)

TABLETS AND OPHTHALMIC SOLUTION

Congestive Heart Failure

Sympathetic stimulation may be a vital component supporting circulatory function in patients with congestive heart failure, and impairing that support by beta-blockade may precipitate more severe decompensation.

Although carteolol HCl should be avoided in clinically evident congestive heart failure, it can be used with caution, if necessary, in patients with a history of failure who are well-compensated and are receiving digitalis and diuretics. Beta-adrenergic blocking agents do not abolish the inotropic action of digitalis on heart muscle.

IN PATIENTS WITHOUT A HISTORY OF CONGESTIVE HEART FAILURE, the use of beta-blockers can, in some instances, lead to congestive heart failure. Therefore, at the first sign or symptom of cardiac decompensation, discontinuation of beta-blocker therapy should be considered. The patient should be closely observed and treatment should include a diuretic and/or digitalization as necessary.

Exacerbation of Angina Pectoris Upon Withdrawal

In patients with angina pectoris, exacerbation of angina and, in some cases, myocardial infarction have been reported following abrupt discontinuation of therapy with some beta-blockers. Therefore such patients should be cautioned against interruption of therapy without a physician's advice. The long persistence of beta-adrenergic blockade following abrupt discontinuation of carteolol HCl, however, might be expected to minimize the possibility of this complication. When discontinuation of carteolol HCl is planned, dosage should be tapered gradually as it is with other beta-blockers. If exacerbation of angina occurs when carteolol HCl therapy is interrupted, it is advisable to reinstitute carteolol HCl or other beta-blocker therapy, at least temporarily, and to take other measures appropriate for the management of unstable angina pectoris.

Patients Without Clinically Recognized Angina Pectoris should be carefully monitored after withdrawal of carteolol HCl therapy, since coronary artery disease may be unrecognized.

Nonallergic Bronchospasm (e.g., chronic bronchitis, emphysema)

Patients with bronchospastic disease generally should not receive beta-blocker therapy and carteolol is contraindicated in patients with bronchial asthma. If use of carteolol hydrochloride is essential, it should be administered with caution since it may block bronchodilation produced by endogenous catecholamine stimulation of $beta_2$-receptors or diminish response to therapy with a beta-receptor agonist.

Major Surgery

The necessity, or desirability of withdrawal of beta-blocking therapy prior to major surgery is controversial. Because beta-blockade impairs the ability of the heart to respond to reflex stimuli and may increase risks of general anesthesia and surgical procedures resulting in protracted hypotension or low cardiac output, and difficulty in restarting or maintaining a heartbeat, it has been suggested that beta-blocker therapy should be withdrawn several days prior to surgery. It is also recognized, however, that increased sensitivity to catecholamines of patients recently withdrawn from beta-blocker therapy could increase certain risks. Given the persistence of the beta-blocking activity of carteolol hydrochloride, effective withdrawal would take several weeks and would ordinarily be impractical. When beta-blocker therapy is not discontinued, anesthetic agents that depress the myocardium should be avoided. In one study using intravenous carteolol during surgery, recovery from anesthesia was somewhat delayed in three patients who received carteolol near the end of anesthesia, and respiratory arrest occurred in one of these patients immediately following administration of intravenous carteolol.

In the event that carteolol hydrochloride treatment is not discontinued before surgery, the anesthesiologist should be informed that the patient is receiving carteolol hydrochloride. The effects on the heart of beta-adrenergic blocking agents, such as carteolol HCl, may be reversed by cautious administration of isoproterenol or dobutamine.

Ophthalmic Solution: If necessary during surgery, the effects of beta-adrenergic blocking agents may be reversed by sufficient doses of such agonists as isoproterenol, dopamine, dobutamine or levarterenol (See OVERDOSAGE.)

Diabetes Mellitus and Hypoglycemia

Beta-adrenergic blockade may prevent the appearance of premonitory signs and symptoms (*e.g.,* tachycardia and blood pressure changes) of acute hypoglycemia, and it inhibits glycogenolysis, a normal compensatory mechanism for hypoglycemia. This is especially important for patients with labile diabetes mellitus. Beta-blockade also reduces the release of insulin in response to hyperglycemia; therefore, it may be necessary to adjust the dose of antidiabetic agents used to treat hyperglycemia.

Thyrotoxicosis

Beta-adrenergic blockade may mask certain clinical signs of hyperthyroidism such as tachycardia. Patients suspected of having thyrotoxicosis should be managed carefully to avoid abrupt withdrawal of beta-adrenergic blockade which might precipitate a thyroid storm.

PRECAUTIONS:

GENERAL

Tablets

Impaired Renal Function: Carteolol HCl should be used with caution in patients with impaired renal function. Patients with impaired renal function clear carteolol at a reduced rate, and dosage should be reduced accordingly (see DOSAGE AND ADMINISTRATION).

Beta-adrenoreceptor blockade can cause reduction in intraocular pressure. Therefore, carteolol HCl may interfere with glaucoma testing. Withdrawal may lead to a return of increased intraocular pressure.

Ophthalmic Solution

Carteolol HCl solution should be used with caution in patients with known hypersensitivity to other beta-adrenoceptor blocking agents.

PRECAUTIONS: *(cont'd)*

Use with caution in patients with known diminished pulmonary function.

In patients with angle-closure glaucoma, the immediate objective of treatment is to reopen the angle. This requires constricting the pupil with a miotic. Carteolol HCl solution has little or no effect on the pupil. When carteolol HCl solution is used to reduce elevated intraocular pressure in angle-closure glaucoma, it should be used with a miotic and not alone.

INFORMATION FOR THE PATIENT

Muscle Weakness

Beta-adrenergic blockade has been reported to potentiate muscle weakness consistent with certain myasthenic symptoms (*e.g.,* diplopia, ptosis and generalized weakness).

Risk from Anaphylactic Reaction

While taking beta-blockers, patients with a history of atopy or a history of severe anaphylactic reaction to a variety of allergens may be more reactive to repeated accidental, diagnostic, or therapeutic challenge with such allergens. Such patients may be unresponsive to the usual doses of epinephrine used to treat anaphylactic reactions.

Tablets

Patients, especially those with evidence of coronary artery insufficiency, should be warned against interruption of discontinuation of carteolol HCl therapy without the physician's advice. Although cardiac failure rarely occurs in properly selected patients, patients being treated with beta-adrenergic blocking agents should be advised to consult the physician at the first sign or symptom of impending failure (*i.e.,* fatigue with exertion, difficulty breathing, cough or unusually fast heartbeat).

Ophthalmic Solution

For topical use only. To prevent contaminating the dropper tip and solution, care should be taken not to touch the eyelids or surrounding areas with the dropper tip of the bottle. Keep bottle tightly closed when not in use. Protect from use.

CARCINOGENESIS, MUTAGENESIS, AND IMPAIRMENT OF FERTILITY

Carteolol HCl did not produce carcinogenic effects at doses 280 times the maximum recommended human dose (10 mg/70 kg/day) in two-year oral rat and mouse studies.

Tests of mutagenicity, including the Ames Test, recombinant (rec)-assay,*in vivo* cytogenetics and dominant lethal assay demonstrated no evidence for mutagenic potential.

Fertility of male and female rats and male and female mice was unaffected by administration of carteolol hydrochloride at dosages up to 150 mg/kg/day. This dosage is approximately 1052 times the maximum recommended human dose.

PREGNANCY, TERATOGENIC EFFECTS, PREGNANCY CATEGORY C

Carteolol hydrochloride increased resorptions and decreased fetal weights in rabbits and rats at maternally toxic doses approximately 1052 and 5264 times the maximum recommended human dose (10 mg/70 kg/day), respectively. A dose-related increase in wavy ribs was noted in the developing rat fetus when pregnant females received daily doses of approximately 212 times the maximum recommended human dose. No such effects were noted in pregnant mice subjected to up to 1052 times the maximum recommended human dose. There are no adequate and well-controlled studies in pregnant women. Carteolol hydrochloride should be used during pregnancy only if the potential benefit justifies the potential risk to the fetus.

NURSING MOTHERS

Studies have not been conducted in lactating humans and, therefore, it is not known whether carteolol is excreted in human milk. Studies in lactating rats indicate that carteolol hydrochloride is excreted in milk. Because many drugs are excreted in human milk, caution should be exercised when carteolol hydrochloride is administered to a nursing woman.

PEDIATRIC USE

Safety and effectiveness in children have not been established.

DRUG INTERACTIONS:

TABLETS

Catecholamine-depending drugs (*e.g.,* reserpine) may have an additive effect when given with beta-blocking agents. Therefore, patients treated with carteolol HCl plus a catecholamine-depleting agent must be observed carefully for evidence of hypotension and/or excessive bradycardia, which may produce syncope or postural hypotension.

Concurrent administration of **general anesthetics** and beta-blocking agents may result in exaggeration of the hypotension induced by general anesthetics (see WARNINGS, Major Surgery).

Blunting of the antihypertensive effect of beta-adrenoreceptor blocking agents by **non-steroidal anti-inflammatory drugs** has been reported. When using these agents concomitantly, patients should be observed carefully to confirm that the desired therapeutic effect has been obtained.

Literature reports suggest that **oral calcium antagonists** may be used in combination with beta-adrenergic blocking agents when heart function is normal, but should be avoided in patients with impaired cardiac function. Hypotension, AV conduction disturbances, and left ventricular failure have been reported in some patients receiving beta-adrenergic blocking agents when an oral calcium antagonist was added to the treatment regimen. Hypotension was more likely to occur if the calcium antagonist were a dihydropyridine derivative e.g., nifedipine, while left ventricular failure and AV conduction disturbances were more likely to occur with either verapamil or diltiazem.

Intravenous calcium antagonists should be used with caution in patients receiving beta-adrenergic blocking agents. The concomitant use of beta-adrenergic blocking agents with digitalis and either diltiazem or verapamil may have additive effects in prolonging AV conduction time.

Concomitant use of oral antidiabetic agents or insulin with beta-blocking agents may be associated with hypoglycemia or possibly hyperglycemia. Dosage of the antidiabetic agent should be adjusted accordingly (see WARNINGS, Diabetes Mellitus and Hypoglycemia).

OPHTHALMIC SOLUTION

Carteolol HCl solution should be used with caution in patients who are receiving a beta-adrenergic blocking agent orally, because of the potential for additive effects on systemic beta-blockade.

Close observation of the patient is recommended when a beta-blocker is administered to patients receiving catecholamine-depleting drugs such as reserpine, because of possible additive effects and the production of hypotension and/or marked bradycardia, which may produce vertigo, syncope, or postural hypotension.

ADVERSE REACTIONS:

TABLETS

The prevalence of adverse reactions has been ascertained from clinical studies conducted primarily in the United States. All adverse experiences (events) reported during these studies were recorded as adverse reactions. The prevalence rates presented below are based on combined data from nineteen placebo-controlled studies of patients with hypertension, angina or dysrhythmia, using once-daily carteolol at doses up to 60 mg. Table 1 summarizes those adverse experiences reported for patients in these studies where the prevalence in the carteolol group is 1% or greater and exceeds the prevalence in the placebo group. Asthenia and muscle cramps were the only symptoms that were significantly more common in patients

ADVERSE REACTIONS: *(cont'd)*

receiving carteolol than in patients receiving placebo (TABLE 1). Patients in clinical trials were carefully selected to exclude those, such as patients with asthma or known bronchospasm, or congestive heart failure, who would be at high risk of experiencing beta-adrenergic blocker adverse effect (See WARNINGS and CONTRAINDICATIONS):

TABLE 1 Adverse Reactions During Placebo-Controlled Studies

	Placebo (n=448) %	Carteolol (n=761) %
Body as a Whole		
Asthenia†	4.0	7.1*
Abdominal Pain	0.4	1.3
Back Pain	1.6	2.1
Chest Pain	1.8	2.2
Digestive System		
Diarrhea	2.0	2.1
Nausea	1.8	2.1
Metabolic/Nutritional Disorders		
Abnormal Lab Test	1.1	1.2
Peripheral Edema	1.1	1.7
Musculoskeletal System		
Arthralgia	1.1	1.2
Muscle Cramps	0.2	2.6*
Lower Extremity Pain	0.2	1.2
Nervous System		
Insomnia	0.7	1.7
Paresthesia	1.1	2.0
Respiratory System		
Nasal Congestion	0.9	1.1
Pharyngitis	0.9	1.1
Skin and Appendages		
Rash	1.1	1.3

† Includes weakness, tiredness, lassitude and fatigue.
* Statistically significant at p = 0.05 level.

The adverse experiences were usually mild or moderate in intensity and transient, but sometimes were serious enough to interrupt treatment. The adverse reactions that were most bothersome, as judged by their being reported as reasons for discontinuation of therapy by at least 0.4% of the carteolol group are shown in TABLE 2.

TABLE 2 Discontinuations During Placebo-Controlled Studies

	Placebo (n=448) %	Carteolol (n=761) %
Body as a Whole		
Asthenia	0.2	0.5
Headache	0.7	0.7
Chest Pain	0.2	0.4
Skin and Appendages		
Rash	0.0	0.4
Sweating	0.2	0.4
Digestive System		
Nausea	0.0	0.4
Overall Adverse Reactions	4.2	3.3

Additional adverse reactions have been reported, but these are, in general, not distinguishable from symptoms that might have occurred in the absence of exposure to carteolol. The following additional adverse reactions were reported by at least 1% of 1568 patients who received carteolol in controlled or open, short- or long-term clinical studies, or represent less common, but potentially important, reactions reported in clinical studies or marketing experience (these rare reactions are shown in italics):

Body as a Whole: fever, infection, injury, malaise, pain, neck pain, shoulder pain;

Cardiovascular System: angina pectoris, arrhythmia, *heart failure*, palpitations, *second degree heart block*, vasodilation;

Digestive System: *acute hepatitis with jaundice*, constipation, dyspepsia, flatulence, gastrointestinal disorder;

Metabolic/Nutritional Disorder: gout

Musculoskeletal System: pain in extremity, joint disorder, arthritis;

Nervous System: *abnormal dreams,* anxiety, depression, dizziness, nervousness, somnolence;

Respiratory System: bronchitis, *bronchospasm* cold symptoms, cough, dyspnea, flu symptoms, lung disorder, rhinitis, sinusitis, *wheezing;*

Skin and Appendages: sweating:

Special Senses: blurred vision, conjunctivitis, eye disorder, tinnitus,

Urogenital: impotence, urinary frequency, urinary tract infection.

In studies of patients with hypertension or angina pectoris where carteolol and positive reference beta-adrenergic blocking agents (nadolol (n=82) and propranolol (n=50) have been compared, the differences in prevalence rates between the carteolol group and the reference agent group were statistically significant (p≤0.05) for the adverse reactions listed in TABLE 3.

TABLE 3 Adverse Reactions During Positive-Controlled Studies

	Reference Agents (n=132) %	Carteolol (n=135) %
Body as a Whole		
Chest Pain	5.3	0.7
Cardiovascular System		
Bradycardia	4.5	0.0
Digestive System		
Diarrhea	11.4	4.4
Nervous System		
Somnolence	0.8	7.4
Skin and Appendages		
Sweating	5.3	0.7

POTENTIAL ADVERSE REACTIONS

In addition, other adverse reactions not listed above have been reported with other beta-adrenergic blocking agents and should be considered potential adverse reactions of carteolol HCl.

Body as a Whole: Fever combined with aching and sore throat.

Cardiovascular System: Intensification of AV block. (See CONTRAINDICATIONS).

ADVERSE REACTIONS: *(cont'd)*

Digestive System: Mesenteric arterial thrombosis, ischemia colitis.

Hemic/Lymphatic System: Agranulocytosis, thrombocytopenic and nonthrombocytopenic purpura.

Nervous System: Reversible mental depression progressing to catatonia; an acute reversible syndrome characterized by disorientation to time and place, short-term memory loss, emotional lability, slightly clouded sensorium, and decreased performance on neuropsychometric testing.

Respiratory System: Laryngospasm, respiratory distress.

Skin and Appendages: Erythematous rash, reversible alopecia.

Urogenital System: Peyronie's disease.

The oculomucocutaneous syndrome associated with the beta-adrenergic blocking agent practolol has not been reported with carteolol.

Ophthalmic Solution The following adverse reactions have been reported in clinical trials with carteolol HCl solution:

Ocular: Transient eye irritation, burning, tearing, conjunctival hyperemia and edema occurred in about 1 of 4 patients. Ocular symptoms including blurred and cloudy vision, photophobia, decreased night vision, and ptosis and ocular signs including blepharoconjunctivitis, abnormal corneal staining, and corneal sensitivity occurred occasionally.

Systemic: As a characteristic of nonselective adrenergic blocking agents, carteolol HCl solution may cause bradycardia and decreased blood pressure (see WARNINGS.)

The following systemic events have occasionally been reported with the use of carteolol HCl solution: cardiac arrhythmia, heart palpitation, dyspnea, asthenia, headache, dizziness, insomnia, sinusitis, and taste perversion.

The following additional adverse reactions have been reported with ophthalmic use of $beta_1$ and $beta_2$ (nonselective) adrenergic receptor blocking agents:

Body As a Whole: Headache

Cardiovascular: Arrhythmia, syncope, heart block, cerebral vascular accident, cerebral ischemia, congestive heart failure, palpitation (see WARNINGS.)

Digestive: Nausea

Psychiatric: Depression

Skin: Hypersensitivity, including localized and generalized rash

Respiratory: Bronchospasm (predominantly in patients with pre- existing bronchospastic disease), respiratory failure (see WARNINGS)

Endocrine: Masked symptoms of hypoglycemia in insulin-dependent diabetics (see WARNINGS)

Special Senses: Signs and symptoms of keratitis, blepharoptosis, visual disturbances including refractive changes due to withdrawal of miotic therapy in some cases), diplopia ptosis

Other reactions associated with the oral use of nonselective adrenergic receptor blocking agents should be considered potential effects with ophthalmic use of these agents.

OVERDOSAGE:

TABLETS

No specific information on emergency treatment of overdosage in humans is available. The most common effects expected with overdosage of a beta-adrenergic blocking agent are bradycardia, bronchospasm, congestive heart failure and hypotension.

In case of overdosage, treatment with carteolol HCl should be discontinued and gastric lavage considered. The patient should be closely observed and vital signs carefully monitored. The prolonged effects of carteolol must be considered when determining the duration of corrective therapy. On the basis of the pharmacologic profile, the following additional measures should be considered as appropriate.

OPHTHALMIC SOLUTION

No specific information on emergency treatment of overdosage in humans is available. Should accidental ocular overdosage occur, flush eye(s) with water or normal saline. The most common effects expected with overdosage of a beta-adrenergic blocking agent are bradycardia, bronchospasm, congestive heart failure and hypotension.

In case of ingestion, treatment with carteolol HCl solution should be discontinued and gastric lavage considered. The patient should be closely observed and vital signs carefully monitored. The prolonged effects of carteolol HCl must be considered when determining the duration of corrective therapy. On the basis of the pharmacologic profile, the following additional measures should be considered as appropriate:

TABLETS AND OPHTHALMIC SOLUTION

Symptomatic Bradycardia: Administer atropine. If there is no response to vagal blockade, administer isoproterenol cautiously.

Bronchospasm: Administer a $beta_2$-stimulating agent such as isoproterenol and/or a theophylline derivative.

Congestive Heart Failure: Administer diuretics and digitalis glycosides as necessary.

Hypotension: Administer vasopressors such as intravenous dopamine, epinephrine or norepinephrine bitartrate.

DOSAGE AND ADMINISTRATION:

TABLETS

Dosage must be individualized. The initial dose of carteolol HCl is 2.5 mg given as a single daily oral dose either alone or added to diuretic therapy. If an adequate response is not achieved, the dose can be gradually increased to 5 mg and 10 mg as single daily doses. Increasing the dose above 10 mg per day is unlikely to produce further substantial benefits and, in fact, may decrease the response. The usual maintenance dose of carteolol is 2.5 or 5 mg once daily.

DOSAGE ADJUSTMENT IN RENAL IMPAIRMENT

Carteolol is excreted principally by the kidneys. When administering carteolol HCl to patients with renal impairment, the dosage regimen should be adjusted individually by the physician. Guidelines for dose interval adjustment are shown below (TABLE 4):

TABLE 4

Creatinine Clearance (ml/min)	Dosage Interval (hours)
> 60	24
20 - 60	48
< 20	72

DOSAGE AND ADMINISTRATION: *(cont'd)*

OPHTHALMIC SOLUTION

The usual dose is one drop of carteolol HCl solution, 1%, in the affected eye(s) twice a day. If the patient's IOP is not at a satisfactory level on this regimen, concomitant therapy with pilocarpine and other miotics, and/or epinephrine or dipivefrin, and/or systemically administered carbonic anhydrase inhibitors, such as acetazolamide, can be instituted.

HOW SUPPLIED:

Recommended storage: Avoid exposure to temperatures in excess of 104°F (40°C).
(Tablets: Abbott, 2/89, 07-5664-R1)
Store at 15° to 25°C (59° to 77°F) (room temperature) and protect from light.
(Ophthalmic Solution, Otsuka, 3026/03-92, P/N 570007)

HOW SUPPLIED - EQUIVALENTS NOT AVAILABLE:

Solution - Ophthalmic - 1 %

5 ml	$16.18	OCUPRESS, Otsuka America Pharm	59148-0001-01
10 ml	$30.50	OCUPRESS, Otsuka America Pharm	59148-0001-02

Tablet, Plain Coated - Oral - 2.5 mg

100's	**$98.73**	**CARTROL, Abbott**	**00074-1664-13**

Tablet, Plain Coated - Oral - 5 mg

100's	**$98.73**	**CARTROL, Abbott**	**00074-1665-13**

CARVEDILOL *(003267)*

CATEGORIES: Antihypertensives; Beta Adrenergic Blocking Agents; Beta Blockers; Cardiovascular Drugs; Hypertension; Renal Drugs; Heart Failure*; FDA Class 1S ("Standard Review"); FDA Approved 1995 Sep
* Indication not approved by the FDA

BRAND NAMES: **Coreg**; *Dibloc*; *Dilatrend* (Germany, Mexico); *Dimitone*; *Kredex*; *Querto* (Germany)
(International brand names outside U.S. in italics)

DESCRIPTION:

Carvedilol is a nonselective ϕ-adrenergic blocking agent with α_1 blocking activity. It is (±)-1-(Carbazol-4-yloxy)-3-[(2-(o-methoxyphenoxy)ethyl]amino]-2-propanol. It is a racemic mixture.

Tablets for Oral Administration: Carvedilol is a white, oval, film-coated Tiltab tablet containing 6.25 mg, 12.5 mg or 25 mg of carvedilol. The 6.25 mg tablets are scored. Inactive ingredients consist of colloidal silicon dioxide, crospovidone, hydroxypropyl methylcellulose, lactose, magnesium stearate, polyethylene glycol, polysorbate 80, povidone, sucrose and titanium dioxide.

Carvedilol is a white to off-white powder with a molecular weight of 406.5 and a molecular formula of $C_{24}H_{26}N_2O_4$. It is freely soluble in dimethylsulfoxide; soluble in methylene chloride and methanol; sparingly soluble in 95% ethanol and isopropanol; slightly soluble in ethyl ester; and practically insoluble in water, gastric fluid (simulated, TS, pH 1.1) and intestinal fluid (simulated, TS without pancreatin, pH 7.5).

CLINICAL PHARMACOLOGY:

Carvedilol is a racemic mixture in which nonselective ϕ-adrenoreceptor blocking activity is present in the S(-) enantiomer and α-adrenergic blocking activity is present in both R(+) and S(-) enantiomers at equal potency. Carvedilol has no intrinsic sympathomimetic activity.

PHARMACOKINETICS

Carvedilol is rapidly and extensively absorbed following oral administration, with absolute bioavailability of approximately 25% to 35% due to a significant degree of first-pass metabolism. Following oral administration, the apparent mean terminal elimination half-life of carvedilol generally ranges from 7 to 10 hours. Plasma concentrations achieved are proportional to the oral dose administered. When administered with food, the rate of absorption is slowed, as evidenced by a delay in the time to reach peak plasma levels, with no significant difference in extent of bioavailability. Taking carvedilol with food should minimize the risk of orthostatic hypotension.

Carvedilol is extensively metabolized. Following oral administration of radiolabelled carvedilol to healthy volunteers, carvedilol accounted for only about 7% of the total radioactivity in plasma as measured by area under the curve (AUC). Less than 2% of the dose was excreted unchanged in the urine. Carvedilol is metabolized primarily by aromatic ring oxidation and glucuronidation.

The oxidative metabolites are further metabolized by conjugation via glucuronidation and sulfation. The metabolites of carvedilol are excreted primarily via the bile into the feces. Demethylation and hydroxylation at the phenol ring produce three active metabolites with ϕ-receptor blocking activity. Based on preclinical studies, the 4'-hydroxyphenyl metabolite is approximately 13 times more potent than carvedilol for ϕ-blockade.

Compared to carvedilol, the three active metabolites exhibit weak vasodilating activity. Plasma concentrations of the active metabolites are about one-tenth of those observed for carvedilol and have pharmacokinetics similar to the parent.

Carvedilol undergoes stereoselective first-pass metabolism with plasma levels of R(+)-carvedilol approximately 2 to 3 times higher than S(-)-carvedilol following oral administration in healthy subjects. The mean apparent terminal elimination half-lives for R(+)-carvedilol range from 5 to 9 hours compared with 7 to 11 hours for the S(-)-enantiomer.

Carvedilol is subject to the effects of genetic polymorphism with poor metabolizers of debrisoquin (a marker for cytochrome P450 2D6) exhibiting 2- to 3-fold higher plasma concentrations of R(+) carvedilol compared to extensive metabolizers. In contrast, plasma levels of S(-)-carvedilol are increased only about 20% to 25% in poor metabolizers, indicating this enantiomer is metabolized to a lesser extent by cytochrome P450 2D6 than R(+)-carvedilol. The pharmacokinetics of carvedilol do not appear to be different in poor metabolizers of S-mephenytoin (patients deficient in cytochrome P450 2C19).

Carvedilol is more than 98% bound to plasma proteins, primarily with albumin. The plasma-protein binding is independent of concentration over the therapeutic range. Carvedilol is a basic, lipophilic compound with a steady-state volume of distribution of approximately 115 L, indicating substantial distribution into extravascular tissues. Plasma clearance ranges from 500 to 700 ml/min.

PHARMACOKINETIC DRUG-DRUG INTERACTIONS

Since carvedilol undergoes substantial oxidative metabolism, the metabolism and pharmacokinetics of carvedilol may be affected by induction or inhibition of cytochrome P450 enzymes.

Rifampin: In a pharmacokinetic study conducted in 8 healthy male subjects, rifampin (600 mg daily for 12 days) decreased the AUC and C_{max} of carvedilol by about 70%.

Cimetidine: In a pharmacokinetic study conducted in 10 healthy male subjects, cimetidine (1000 mg/day) increased the steady-state AUC of carvedilol by 30% with no change in C_{max}.

CLINICAL PHARMACOLOGY: *(cont'd)*

Hydrochlorothiazide: A single oral dose of carvedilol 25 mg did not alter the pharmacokinetics of a single oral dose of hydrochlorothiazide 25 mg in 12 patients with hypertension. Likewise, hydrochlorothiazide had no effect on the pharmacokinetics of carvedilol.

Digoxin: Following concomitant administration of carvedilol (25 mg once daily) and digoxin (0.25 mg once daily) for 14 days, steady-state AUC and trough concentrations of digoxin were increased by 14% and 16%, respectively, in 12 hypertensive patients.

Torsemide: In a study of 12 healthy subjects, combined oral administration of carvedilol 25 mg once daily and torsemide 5 mg once daily for 5 days did not result in any significant differences in their pharmacokinetics compared with administration of the drugs alone.

SPECIAL POPULATIONS

Elderly: Plasma levels of carvedilol average about 50% higher in the elderly compared to young subjects.

Hepatic Impairment: Compared to healthy subjects, patients with cirrhotic liver disease exhibit significantly higher concentrations of carvedilol (approximately 4- to 7-fold) following single-dose therapy (see WARNINGS, Hepatic Injury.)

Renal Insufficiency: Although carvedilol is metabolized primarily by the liver, plasma concentrations of carvedilol have been reported to be increased in patients with renal impairment. Based on mean AUC data, approximately 40% to 50% higher plasma concentrations of carvedilol were observed in hypertensive patients with moderate to severe renal impairment compared to a control group of hypertensive patients with normal renal function. However, the ranges of AUC values were similar for both groups. Changes in mean peak plasma levels were less pronounced, approximately 12% to 26% higher in patients with impaired renal function.

Consistent with its high degree of plasma protein-binding, carvedilol does not appear to be cleared significantly by hemodialysis.

PHARMACODYNAMICS

ϕ-adrenoreceptor blocking activity has been demonstrated in animal and human studies showing that carvedilol (1) reduces cardiac output; (2) reduces exercise- and/or isoproterenol-induced tachycardia and (3) reduces reflex orthostatic tachycardia. Significant ϕ-adrenoreceptor blocking effect is usually seen within 1 hour of drug administration. The mechanism by which ϕ-blockade produces an antihypertensive effect has not been established.

α_1-adrenoreceptor blocking activity has been demonstrated in human and animal studies, showing that carvedilol (1) attenuates the pressor effects of phenylephrine; (2) causes vasodilation and (3) reduces peripheral vascular resistance. These effects contribute to the reduction of blood pressure and usually are seen within 30 minutes of drug administration.

Due to the α_1-receptor blocking activity of carvedilol, blood pressure is lowered more in the standing than in the supine position, and symptoms of postural hypotension (1.8%), including rare instances of syncope, can occur. Following oral administration, when postural hypotension has occurred, it has been transient and is uncommon when carvedilol is administered with food at the recommended starting dose and titration increments are closely followed (see DOSAGE AND ADMINISTRATION.)

In hypertensive patients with normal renal function, therapeutic doses of carvedilol decreased renal vascular resistance with no change in glomerular filtration rate or renal plasma flow. Changes in excretion of sodium, potassium, uric acid and phosphorus in hypertensive patients with normal renal function were similar after carvedilol and placebo.

Carvedilol has little effect on plasma catecholamines, plasma aldosterone or electrolyte levels, but it does significantly reduce plasma renin activity when given for at least 4 weeks. It also increases levels of atrial natriuretic peptide.

CLINICAL STUDIES:

Hypertension: Carvedilol was studied in two placebo-controlled trials that utilized twice-daily dosing, at total daily doses of 12.5 to 50 mg. In these and other studies, the starting dose did not exceed 12.5 mg. At 50 mg per day, carvedilol reduced sitting trough (12-hour) blood pressure by about 9/5.5 mm Hg; at 25 mg/day the effect was about 7.5/3.5 mm Hg. Comparisons of trough to peak blood pressure showed a trough to peak ratio for blood pressure response of about 65%. Heart rate fell by about 7.5 beats per minute at 50 mg/day. In general, as is true for other ϕ-blockers, responses were smaller in black than non-black patients. There were no age- or gender-related differences in response.

The peak antihypertensive effect occurred 1 to 2 hours after a dose. The dose-related blood pressure response was accompanied by a dose-related increase in adverse effects (see ADVERSE REACTIONS.)

INDICATIONS AND USAGE:

Carvedilol is indicated for the management of essential hypertension. It can be used alone or in combination with other antihypertensive agents, especially thiazide-type diuretics. (See DRUG INTERACTIONS.)

CONTRAINDICATIONS:

Carvedilol is contraindicated in patients with NYHA Class IV decompensated cardiac failure, bronchial asthma (two cases of death from status asthmaticus have been reported in patients receiving single doses of carvedilol), or related bronchospastic conditions, second- or third-degree AV block, cardiogenic shock, or severe bradycardia.

Use of carvedilol in patients with clinically manifest hepatic impairment is not recommended.

Carvedilol is contraindicated in patients with hypersensitivity to the drug.

WARNINGS:

Cardiac Failure: Sympathetic stimulation is a vital component supporting circulatory function in congestive heart failure, and a ϕ-blockade carries the potential hazard of further depressing myocardial contractility and precipitating more severe failure. Although carvedilol has now been studied in over 1900 patients with heart failure, the dosing and monitoring requirements are different from those for hypertension. In hypertensive patients who have congestive heart failure controlled with digitalis, diuretics and/or an angiotensin-converting enzyme inhibitor, carvedilol should be used with caution. Both digitalis and carvedilol slow AV conduction.

Hepatic Injury: Mild hepatocellular injury, confirmed by rechallenge, has occurred rarely with carvedilol therapy. In controlled studies of hypertensive patients, the incidence of liver function abnormalities reported as adverse experiences was 1.1% (13 of 1,142 patients) in patients receiving carvedilol and 0.9% (4 of 462 patients) in those receiving placebo. One patient receiving carvedilol in a placebo-controlled trial withdrew for abnormal hepatic function. Hepatic injury has been reversible and has occurred after short- and/or long-term therapy with minimal clinical symptomatology. No deaths due to liver function abnormalities have been reported.

At the first symptom/sign of liver dysfunction (*e.g.*, pruritus, dark urine, persistent anorexia, jaundice, right upper quadrant tenderness or unexplained "flu-like" symptoms), laboratory testing should be performed. If the patient has laboratory evidence of liver injury or jaundice, carvedilol should be stopped and not restarted.

WARNINGS: *(cont'd)*

Peripheral Vascular Disease: ϕ-blockers can precipitate or aggravate symptoms of arterial insufficiency in patients with peripheral vascular disease. Caution should be exercised in such individuals.

Anesthesia and Major Surgery: If carvedilol treatment is to be continued perioperatively, particular care should be taken when anesthetic agents which depress myocardial function, such as ether, cyclopropane and trichloroethylene, are used. See OVERDOSAGE for information on treatment of bradycardia and hypertension.

Diabetes and Hypoglycemia: ϕ-blockers may mask some of the manifestations of hypoglycemia, particularly tachycardia. Nonselective ϕ-blockers may potentiate insulin-induced hypoglycemia and delay recovery of serum glucose levels. Patients subject to spontaneous hypoglycemia, or diabetic patients receiving insulin or oral hypoglycemic agents, should be cautioned about these possibilities and carvedilol should be used with caution.

Thyrotoxicosis: ϕ-adrenergic blockade may mask clinical signs of hyperthyroidism, such as tachycardia. Abrupt withdrawal of ϕ-blockade may be followed by an exacerbation of the symptoms of hyperthyroidism or may precipitate thyroid storm.

PRECAUTIONS:

GENERAL

Since carvedilol has ϕ-blocking activity, it should not be discontinued abruptly, particularly in patients with ischemic heart disease. Instead, it should be discontinued over 1 to 2 weeks.

In clinical trials, carvedilol caused bradycardia in about 2% of patients. If pulse rate drops below 55 beats/min., the dosage should be reduced.

Postural hypotension occurred in 1.8% and syncope in 0.1% of patients, especially following the initial dose or at the time of dose increase during repeated dosing. Postural hypotension or syncope was a cause for discontinuation of therapy in 1% of patients.

To decrease the likelihood of syncope or excessive hypotension, treatment should always be initiated with a 6.25 mg dose of carvedilol tablets. Dosage should then be increased slowly, according to recommendations in DOSAGE AND ADMINISTRATION, and the drug should always be taken with food. During initiation of therapy, the patient should be cautioned to avoid situations such as driving or hazardous tasks, where injury could result should syncope occur.

Risk of Anaphylactic Reaction: While taking ϕ-blockers, patients with a history of severe anaphylactic reaction to a variety of allergens may be more reactive to repeated challenge, either accidental, diagnostic or therapeutic. Such patients may be unresponsive to the usual doses of epinephrine used to treat allergic reaction.

Nonallergic Bronchospasm: (*e.g.*, chronic bronchitis and emphysema) Patients with bronchospastic disease should, in general, not receive ϕ-blockers. Carvedilol may be used with caution, however, in patients who do not respond to, or cannot tolerate, other antihypertensive agents. It is prudent, if carvedilol is used, to use the smallest effective dose, so that inhibition of endogenous or exogenous ϕ-agonists is minimized.

INFORMATION FOR THE PATIENT

Patients taking carvedilol should be advised of the following:

they should not interrupt or discontinue using carvedilol without a physician's advice.

they may experience a drop in blood pressure when standing, resulting in dizziness and, rarely, fainting. Patients should sit or lie down when these symptoms of lowered blood pressure occur.

if patients experience dizziness or fatigue, they should avoid driving or hazardous tasks.

they should consult a physician if they experience dizziness or faintness, in case the dosage should be adjusted.

they should take carvedilol with food.

contact lens wearers may experience decreased lacrimation.

CARCINOGENESIS, MUTAGENESIS, AND IMPAIRMENT OF FERTILITY

In 2-year studies conducted in rats given carvedilol at doses up to 75 mg/kg/day (12 times the maximum recommended human dose [MRHD] when compared on a mg/m^2 basis) or in mice given up to 200 mg/kg/day (16 times the MRHD on a mg/m2 basis), carvedilol had no carcinogenic effect.

Carvedilol was negative when tested in a battery of genotoxicity assays, including the Ames and the CHO/HGPRT assays for mutagenicity and the *in vitro* hamster micronucleus and *in vivo* human lymphocyte cell tests for clastogenicity.

At doses ≥200 mg/kg/day (32 times the MRHD as mg/m^2) carvedilol was toxic to adult rats (sedation, reduced weight gain) and was associated with a reduced number of successful matings, prolonged mating time, significantly fewer corpora lutea and implants per dam and complete resorption of 18% of the liters. The no-observed-effect dose level for overt toxicity and impairment of fertility was 60 mg/kg/day (10 times the MRHD as mg/m^2).

PREGNANCY, TERATOGENIC EFFECTS, PREGNANCY CATEGORY C

Studies performed in pregnant rats and rabbits given carvedilol revealed increased post-implantation loss in rats at doses of 300 mg/kg/day (50 times the MRHD as mg/m^2) and in rabbits at doses of 75 mg/kg/day (25 times the MRHD as mg/m^2). In the rats, there was also a decrease in fetal body weight at the maternally toxic dose of 300 mg/kg/day (50 times the MRHD as mg/m^2), which was accompanied by an elevation in the frequency of fetuses with delayed skeletal development (missing or stunted 13th rib). In rats the no-observed-effect level for developmental toxicity was 60 mg/kg/day (10 times the MRHD as mg/m^2); in rabbits it was 15 mg/kg/day (5 times the MRHD as mg/m^2). There are no adequate and well-controlled studies in pregnant women. Carvedilol should be used during pregnancy only if the potential benefit justifies the potential risk to the fetus.

NURSING MOTHERS

It is not known whether this drug is excreted in human milk. Studies in rats have shown that carvedilol and/or its metabolites (as well as other ϕ-blockers) cross the placental barrier and are excreted in breast milk. There was increased mortality at one week post-partum in neonates from rats treated with 60 mg/kg/day (10 times the MRHD as mg/m^2) and above during the last trimester through day 22 of lactation. Because many drugs are excreted in human milk and because of the potential for serious adverse reactions in nursing infants from ϕ-blockers, especially bradycardia, a decision should be made whether to discontinue nursing or to discontinue the drug, taking into account the importance of the drug to the mother. The effects of other α- and ϕ-blocking agents have included perinatal and neonatal distress.

PEDIATRIC USE

Safety and efficacy in patients younger than 18 years of age have not been established.

Geriatric Use: Of the 2065 patients in U.S. clinical trials of efficacy or safety who were treated with carvedilol, 21% (436) were 65 years of age or older. Of 3722 patients receiving carvedilol in hypertension clinical trials conducted worldwide, 24% were 65 years of age or older. There were no notable differences in efficacy or the incidence of adverse events between older and younger patients. With the exception of dizziness (incidence 8.8% in the elderly vs. 6% in younger patients), there were no events for which the incidence in the elderly exceeded that in the younger population by greater than 2.0%.

Similar results were observed in a postmarketing surveillance study of 3328 carvedilol patients, of whom approximately 20% were 65 years of age or older.

DRUG INTERACTIONS:

(Also see CLINICAL PHARMACOLOGY, Pharmacokinetic Drug, Drug Interactions.)

Catecholamine-Depleting Agents: Patients taking both agents with ϕ-blocking properties and a drug that can deplete catecholamines (*e.g.*, reserpine and monoamine oxidase inhibitors) should be observed closely for signs of hypotension and/or severe bradycardia.

Clonidine: Concomitant administration of clonidine with agents with ϕ-blocking properties may potentiate blood-pressure- and heart-rate-lowering effects. When concomitant treatment with agents with ϕ-blocking properties and clonidine is to be terminated, the ϕ-blocking agent should be discontinued first. Clonidine therapy can then be discontinued several days later by gradually decreasing the dosage.

Digoxin: Digoxin concentrations are increased by about 15% when digoxin and carvedilol are administered concomitantly. Therefore, increased monitoring of digoxin is recommended when initiating, adjusting or discontinuing carvedilol.

Inducers and Inhibitors of Hepatic Metabolism: Rifampin reduced plasma concentrations of carvedilol by about 70%. Cimetidine increased AUC by about 30% but caused no change in C_{max}.

Calcium channel blockers: Isolated cases of conduction disturbance (rarely with hemodynamic compromise) have been observed when carvedilol is co-administered with diltiazem. As with other agents with ϕ-blocking properties, if carvedilol is to be administered orally with calcium channel blockers of the verapamil or diltiazem type, it is recommended that ECG and blood pressure be monitored.

Insulin or oral hypoglycemics: Agents with ϕ-blocking properties may enhance the blood-sugar-reducing effect of insulin and oral hypoglycemics. Therefore, in patients taking insulin or oral hypoglycemics, regular monitoring of blood glucose is recommended.

ADVERSE REACTIONS:

Carvedilol has been evaluated for safety in hypertension in more than 2193 patients in U.S. clinical trials and in 2976 patients in international clinical trials. Approximately 36% of the total treated population received carvedilol for at least 6 months. In general, carvedilol was well tolerated at doses up to 50 mg daily. Most adverse events reported during carvedilol therapy were of mild to moderate severity. In U.S. controlled clinical trials directly comparing carvedilol monotherapy in doses up to 50 mg (n=1142) to placebo (n=462), 4.9% of carvedilol patients discontinued for adverse events vs. 5.2% of placebo patients. Although there was no overall difference in discontinuation rates, discontinuations were more common in the carvedilol group for postural hypotension (1% vs. 0). The overall incidence of adverse events in U.S. placebo-controlled trials was found to increase with increasing dose of carvedilol. For individual adverse events this could only be distinguished for dizziness, which increased in frequency from 2% to 5% as total daily dose increased from 6.25 mg to 50 mg.

TABLE 1 shows adverse events in U.S. placebo-controlled clinical trials that occurred with an incidence of greater than 1% regardless of causality, and that were more frequent in drug-treated patients than placebo-treated patients.

TABLE 1 - Carvedilol Adverse Events in U.S. Placebo-Controlled Trials Incidence ≥1% Regardless of Causality; Withdrawal Rates Due to Adverse Events

	Adverse Reactions		Withdrawals	
	Coreg (n=1142) % occurence	Placebo (n=462) % occurence	Coreg (n=1142) % occurence	Placebo (n=462) % occurence
Central Nervous System				
Dizziness	6.2	5.4	0.4	1.3
Insomnia	1.6	0.6	-	0.2
Somnolence	1.8	1.5	-	-
Gastrointestinal				
Abdominal pain	1.4	1.3	0.1	-
Diarrhea	2.2	1.3	0.1	-
Cardiovascular				
Bradycardia	2.1	0.2	0.4	-
Postural Hypotension	1.8	-	1.0	-
Dependent edema	1.7	1.5	0.1	0.4
Peripheral edema	1.4	0.4	0.2	-
Respiratory				
Rhinitis	2.1	1.9	-	-
Pharyngitis	1.5	0.6	-	-
Dyspnea	1.4	0.9	0.4	0.2
Hematologic				
Thrombocytopenia	1.1	0.2	-	-
Metabolic				
Hypertriglyceridemia	1.2	0.2	-	-
Musculoskeletal				
Back pain	2.3	1.5	0.1	-
Urinary / Renal				
Urinary tract infection	1.8	0.6	-	-
Resistance Mechanism				
Viral infection	1.8	1.3	-	-
Body As A Whole				
Fatigue	4.3	3.9	0.3	0.2
Injury	2.9	2.6	0.1	-

In addition to the events in TABLE 1, chest pain, dyspepsia, headache, nausea, pain, sinusitis, and upper respiratory tract infection were also reported, but rates were at least as great in placebo-treated patients.

The following adverse events were reported as possibly or probably related in worldwide open or controlled trials with carvedilol.

Incidence >0.1% to ≤1%

Cardiovascular: AV block (see CONTRAINDICATIONS), extrasystoles, hypertension, hypotension, palpitations, peripheral ischemia, syncope.

Central and Peripheral Nervous System: Ataxia, hypoesthesia, paresthesia, vertigo.

Gastrointestinal: Bilirubinemia, constipation, flatulence, increased hepatic enzymes (0.2% of patients were discontinued from therapy because of increases in hepatic enzymes; see WARNINGS, Hepatic Injury), vomiting.

General: Asthenia, hot flushes, leg cramps, malaise.

Musculoskeletal System: Myalgia.

Psychiatric: Depression, nervousness.

Respiratory System: Asthma (see CONTRAINDICATIONS), cough.

Reproductive: *Male:*decreased libido, impotence.

Skin and Appendages: Pruritus, rash, rash erythematous, rash maculopapular, rash psoriaform.

Special Senses: Abnormal vision, tinnitus.

ADVERSE REACTIONS: *(cont'd)*

Urinary System: Albuminuria, hematuria, micturition frequency.

Autonomic Nervous System: Dry mouth, sweating increased.

Metabolic and Nutritional: Hypercholesterolemia, hyperglycemia, hyperuricemia.

Hematologic: Anemia, leukopenia.

The following events were reported in ≤0.1% of patients and are potentially important: angina, arrhythmia, atrial fibrillation, bundle branch block, cardiac failure, myocardial ischemia, cerebrovascular disorder, migraine, neuralgia, paresis, allergy, alopecia, amnesia, confusion, bronchospasm, decreased hearing, respiratory alkalosis, increased BUN, glycosuria, decreased HDL, hyperkalemia, hypokalemia, increased NPN, increased alkaline phosphatase, increased weight, eosinophilia and atypical lymphocytes.

Other adverse events occurred sporadically in single patients and cannot be distinguished from concurrent disease states or medications.

Carvedilol therapy has not been associated with clinically significant changes in routine laboratory tests. No clinically relevant changes were noted in serum potassium, fasting serum glucose, total triglycerides, total cholesterol, HDL cholesterol, uric acid, blood urea nitrogen or creatinine.

OVERDOSAGE:

The acute oral LD_{50} doses in male and female mice and male and female rats are over 8000 mg/kg.

Overdosage may cause severe hypotension, bradycardia, cardiac insufficiency, cardiogenic shock and cardiac arrest. Respiratory problems, bronchospasms, vomiting, lapses of consciousness and generalized seizures may also occur.

The patient should be placed in a supine position and, where necessary, kept under observation and treated under intensive-care conditions. Gastric lavage or pharmacologically induced emesis may be used shortly after ingestion. The following agents may be administered:

For Excessive Bradycardia: atropine, 2 mg IV.

To Support Cardiovascular Function: glucagon, 5 to 10 mg IV rapidly over 30 seconds, followed by a continuous infusion of 5 mg/hour; sympathomimetics (dobutamine, isoprenaline, adrenaline) at doses according to body weight and effect.

If peripheral vasodilation dominates, it may be necessary to administer adrenaline or noradrenaline with continuous monitoring of circulatory conditions. For therapy-resistant bradycardia, pacemaker therapy should be performed. For bronchospasm ϕ-sympathomimetics (as aerosol or IV) or aminophylline IV should be given. In the event of seizures, slow IV injection of diazepam or clonazepam is recommended.

NOTE: In the event of severe intoxication where there are symptoms of shock, treatment with antidotes must be continued for a sufficiently long period of time consistent with the 7- to 10-hour half-life of carvedilol.

Three cases of overdosage have been reported. A 59-year-old male who ingested 200 mg experienced severe chest pain but recovered completely. A 2-year-old child who ingested an unknown quantity suffered no adverse effects following induced vomiting and observation. A 39-year-old female ingested 400 mg with an unknown amount of benzodiazepine. She was hospitalized in a state of stupor and hypotension, but recovered completely following supportive measures.

DOSAGE AND ADMINISTRATION:

Dosage Must Be Individualized. The recommended starting dose of carvedilol is 6.25 mg twice daily. If this dose is tolerated, using standing systolic pressure measured about 1 hours after dosing as a guide, the dose should be maintained for 7 to 14 days, and then increased to 12.5 mg twice daily if needed, based on trough blood pressure, again using standing systolic pressure one hour after dosing as a guide for tolerance. This dose should also be maintained for 7 to 14 days and can then be adjusted upward to 25 mg twice daily if tolerated and needed. The full antihypertensive effect of carvedilol is seen within 7 to 14 days. Total daily dose should not exceed 50 mg. Carvedilol should be taken with food to slow the rate of absorption and reduce the incidence of orthostatic effects.

Addition of a diuretic to carvedilol, or carvedilol to a diuretic can be expected to produce additive effects and exaggerate the orthostatic component of carvedilol action.

Carvedilol should not be given to patients with severe hepatic impairment (see CONTRAINDICATIONS.)

HOW SUPPLIED:

Tablets: White, oval, film-coated Tiltab tablets: 6.25 mg-scored, imprinted with 4140 and SB; 12.5 mg-imprinted with 4141 and SB; 25 mg-imprinted with 4142 and SB.

Storage: Store between 15° and 30°C (59° and 86°F). Protect from moisture. Dispense in a tight, light-resistant container.

CEFACLOR *(000680)*

CATEGORIES: Anti-Infectives; Antibiotics; Antimicrobials; Cephalosporins; Cystitis; Infections; Otitis Media; Pharyngitis; Pneumonia; Pyelonephritis; Respiratory Tract Infections; Rheumatic Fever; Skin Infections; Streptococcal Infection; Tonsillitis; Urinary Tract Infections; Pregnancy Category B; Sales > $1 Billion; FDA Approval Pre 1982; Patent Expiration 1994 Dec; Top 200 Drugs

BRAND NAMES: *Alfatil* (France); *Capabiotic*; *CEC 500* (Germany); **Ceclor**; *Ceclor AF*; *Ceclor BID*; *Ceclor CD*; *Ceclor MR*; *Ceclor Retard*; *Cefabiocin* (Germany); *Cefallone* (Germany); *Cefaclostad* (Germany); *Cefral*; *Cero*; *Clex*; *Distaclor* (England); *Distaclor MR*; *Especlor*; *Keflor*; *Kefolor*; *Kefral* (Japan); *Kemocin*; *Kerfenmycin*; *Kindoplex*; *Kloclor BD*; *Mediconcef*; *Panacef*; *Panoral* (Germany); *Panoral Forte* (Germany); *Sigacefal* (Germany); *Swiflor*; *Vercef*
(International brand names outside U.S. in italics)

FORMULARIES: Aetna; BC-BS; Medi-Cal; PCS

COST OF THERAPY: $117.48 (Respiratory Infections; Capsule; 500 mg; 3/day; 14 days)

DESCRIPTION:

Cefaclor, USP is a semisynthetic cephalosporin antibiotic for oral administration. It is chemically designated as 3- chloro-7-D-(2-phenylglycinamido)-3-cephem-4-carboxylic acid monohydrate. The chemical formula for cefaclor is $C_{15}H_{14}ClN_3O_4S{\cdot}H_2O$ and the molecular weight is 385.82.

Each Pulvule contains cefaclor monohydrate equivalent to 250 mg (0.68 mmol) or 500 mg (1.36 mmol) anhydrous cefaclor. The Pulvules also contain cornstarch, FD&C Blue No. 1, FD&C Red No. 3, gelatin, magnesium stearate, silicone, titanium dioxide, and other inactive ingredients. The 500-mg Pulvule also contains iron oxide.

DESCRIPTION: *(cont'd)*

After mixing, each 5 ml of Ceclor for Oral Suspension will contain cefaclor monohydrate equivalent to 125 mg (0.34 mmol), 187 mg (0.51 mmol), 250 mg (0.68 mmol), or 375 mg (1.0 mmol) anhydrous cefaclor. The suspensions also contain cellulose, cornstarch, FD &C Red No. 40, flavors, silicone, sodium lauryl sulfate, sucrose, and xanthan gum.

CLINICAL PHARMACOLOGY:

Cefaclor is well absorbed after oral administration to fasting subjects. Total absorption is the same whether the drug is given with or without food; however, when it is taken with food, the peak concentration achieved is 50% to 75% of that observed when the drug is administered to fasting subjects and generally appears from three fourths to 1 hour later. Following administration of 250-mg, 500-mg, and 1-g doses to fasting subjects, average peak serum levels of approximately 7, 13, and 23 mcg/ml respectively were obtained within 30 to 60 minutes. Approximately 60% to 85% of the drug is excreted unchanged in the urine within 8 hours, the greater portion being excreted within the first 2 hours. During this 8-hour period, peak urine concentrations following the 250-mg, 500-mg, and 1-g doses were approximately 600, 900, and 1,900 mcg/ml respectively. The serum half-life in normal subjects is 0.6 to 0.9 hours. In patients with reduced renal function, the serum half-life of cefaclor is slightly prolonged. In those with complete absence of renal function, the biologic half-life of the intact molecule is 2.3 to 2.8 hours. Excretion pathways in patients with markedly impaired renal function have not been determined. Hemodialysis shortens the half-life by 25% to 30%.

Microbiology: In vitro tests demonstrate that the bactericidal action of the cephalosporins results from inhibition of cell-wall synthesis. Cefaclor is active *in vitro* against most strains of clinical isolates of the following organisms:

Staphylococci, including coagulase-positive, coagulase-negative, and penicillinase-producing strains (when tested by *in vitro* methods), exhibit cross-resistance between cefaclor and methicillin; *Streptococcus pyogenes* (group A β-hemolytic streptococci); *Streptococcus pneumoniae*; *Moraxella (Branhamella) catarrhalis; Haemophilus influenzae,* including β-lactamase-producing ampicillin-resistant strains; *Escherichia coli; Proteus mirabilis; Klebsiella* sp; *Citrobacter diversus; Neisseria gonorrhoeae; Propionibacterium acnes* and *Bacteroides* sp (excluding*Bacteroides fragilis*); *Peptococci; Peptostreptococci*

Note: Pseudomonas sp, *Acinetobacter calcoaceticus* (formerly *Mima* sp and *Herellea* sp), and most strains of enterococci (*Enterococcus faecalis* [formerly *Streptococcus faecalis*], group D streptococci), *Enterobacter* sp, indole-positive *Proteus*, and *Serratia* sp are resistant to cefaclor. When tested by *in vitro* methods, staphylococci exhibit cross-resistance between cefaclor and methicillin-type antibiotics.

Disk Susceptibility Tests: Quantitative methods that require measurement of zone diameters give the most precise estimates of antibiotic susceptibility. One such procedure* has been recommended for use with disks for testing susceptibility to cephalothin. The currently accepted zone diameter interpretative criteria for the cephalothin disk are appropriate for determining bacterial susceptibility to cefaclor. With this procedure, a report from the laboratory of "resistant" indicates that the infecting organism is not likely to respond to therapy. A report of "intermediate susceptibility" suggests that the organism would be susceptible if the infection is confined to tissues and fluids (*e.g.,* urine) in which high antibiotic levels can be obtained or if high dosage is used.

* Bauer AW, Kirby WMM, Sherris JC, and Turck M: Antibiotic susceptibility testing by a standardized single disk method. *Am J Clin Pathol*1966;45:493. Standardized disk susceptibility test. *Federal Register* 1974;39:19182-19184.

INDICATIONS AND USAGE:

Cefaclor is indicated in the treatment of the following infections when caused by susceptible strains of the designated microorganisms:

Otitis media caused by *S. pneumoniae, H. influenzae,* staphylococci, and *S. pyogenes* (group A β-hemolytic streptococci)

Lower respiratory infections, including pneumonia, caused by *S. pneumoniae, H. influenzae,* and *S. pyogenes* (group A β-hemolytic streptococci)

Upper respiratory infections, including pharyngitis and tonsillitis, caused by *S. pyogenes* (group A β-hemolytic streptococci)

Note: Penicillin is the usual drug of choice in the treatment and prevention of streptococcal infections, including the prophylaxis of rheumatic fever. Cefaclor is generally effective in the eradication of streptococci from the nasopharynx; however, substantial data establishing the efficacy of cefaclor in the subsequent prevention of rheumatic fever are not available at present.

Urinary tract infections, including pyelonephritis and cystitis, caused by *E. coli, P. mirabilis, Klebsiella* sp, and coagulase-negative staphylococci

Skin and skin structure infections caused by *Staphylococcus aureus* and *S. pyogenes* (group A β-hemolytic streptococci)

Appropriate culture and susceptibility studies should be performed to determine susceptibility of the causative organism to cefaclor.

CONTRAINDICATIONS:

Cefaclor is contraindicated in patients with known allergy to the cephalosporin group of antibiotics.

WARNINGS:

IN PENICILLIN-SENSITIVE PATIENTS, CEPHALOSPORIN ANTIBIOTICS SHOULD BE ADMINISTERED CAUTIOUSLY. THERE IS CLINICAL AND LABORATORY EVIDENCE OF PARTIAL CROSS-ALLERGENICITY OF THE PENICILLINS AND THE CEPHALOSPORINS AND THERE ARE INSTANCES IN WHICH PATIENTS HAVE HAD REACTIONS, INCLUDING ANAPHYLAXIS, TO BOTH DRUG CLASSES.

Antibiotics, including cefaclor, should be administered cautiously to any patient who has demonstrated some form of allergy, particularly to drugs.

Pseudomembranous colitis has been reported with virtually all broad-spectrum antibiotics (including macrolides, semisynthetic penicillins, and cephalosporins); therefore, it is important to consider its diagnosis in patients who develop diarrhea in association with the use of antibiotics. Such colitis may range in severity from mild to life threatening.

Treatment with broad-spectrum antibiotics alters the normal flora of the colon and may permit overgrowth of clostridia. Studies indicate that a toxin produced by *Clostridium difficile* is a primary cause of antibiotic-associated colitis.

Mild cases of pseudomembranous colitis usually respond to drug discontinuance alone. In moderate to severe cases, management should include sigmoidoscopy, appropriate bacteriologic studies, and fluid, electrolyte, and protein supplementation. When the colitis does not improve after the drug has been discontinued, or when it is severe, oral vancomycin is the drug of choice for antibiotic-associated pseudomembranous colitis produced by *C. difficile.* Other causes of colitis should be ruled out.

PRECAUTIONS:

General: If an allergic reaction to cefaclor occurs, the drug should be discontinued, and, if necessary, the patient should be treated with appropriate agents, e.g., pressor amines, antihistamines, or corticosteroids.

Prolonged use of cefaclor may result in the overgrowth of nonsusceptible organisms. Careful observation of the patient is essential. If superinfection occurs during therapy, appropriate measures should be taken.

Positive direct Coombs' tests have been reported during treatment with the cephalosporin antibiotics. In hematologic studies or in transfusion cross-matching procedures when antiglobulin tests are performed on the minor side or in Coombs' testing of newborns whose mothers have received cephalosporin antibiotics before parturition, it should be recognized that a positive Coombs' test may be due to the drug.

Cefaclor should be administered with caution in the presence of markedly impaired renal function. Since the half-life of cefaclor in anuria is 2.3 to 2.8 hours, dosage adjustments for patients with moderate or severe renal impairment are usually not required. Clinical experience with cefaclor under such conditions is limited; therefore, careful clinical observation and laboratory studies should be made.

As with other β-lactam antibiotics, the renal excretion of cefaclor is inhibited by probenecid.

As a result of administration of cefaclor, a false-positive reaction for glucose in the urine may occur. This has been observed with Benedict's and Fehling's solutions and also with Clinitest tablets but not with Tes-Tape (Glucose Enzymatic Test Strip, USP, Lilly).

Broad-spectrum antibiotics should be prescribed with caution in individuals with a history of gastrointestinal disease, particularly colitis.

Pregnancy Category B: Reproduction studies have been performed in mice and rats at doses up to 12 times the human dose and in ferrets given 3 times the maximum human dose and have revealed no evidence of impaired fertility or harm to the fetus due to cefaclor. There are, however, no adequate and well-controlled studies in pregnant women. Because animal reproduction studies are not always predictive of human response, this drug should be used during pregnancy only if clearly needed.

Nursing Mothers: Small amounts of cefaclor have been detected in mother's milk following administration of single 500-mg doses. Average levels were 0.18, 0.20, 0.21, and 0.16 mcg/ml at 2, 3, 4, and 5 hours respectively. Trace amounts were detected at 1 hour. The effect on nursing infants is not known. Caution should be exercised when cefaclor is administered to a nursing woman.

Pediatric Use: Safety and effectiveness of this product for use in infants less than 1 month of age have not been established.

ADVERSE REACTIONS:

Adverse effects considered to be related to therapy with cefaclor are listed below:

Hypersensitivity reactions have been reported in about 1.5% of patients and include morbilliform eruptions (1 in 100). Pruritus, urticaria, and positive Coombs' tests each occur in less than 1 in 200 patients.

Cases of **serum-sickness-like** reactions have been reported with the use of cefaclor. These are characterized by findings of erythema multiforme, rashes, and other skin manifestations accompanied by arthritis/arthralgia, with or without fever, and differ from classic serum sickness in that there is infrequently associated lymphadenopathy and proteinuria, no circulating immune complexes, and no evidence to date of sequelae of the reaction. Occasionally, solitary symptoms may occur, but do not represent a **serum-sickness-like** reaction. While further investigation is ongoing, **serum-sickness-like** reactions appear to be due to hypersensitivity and more often occur during or following a second (or subsequent) course of therapy with cefaclor. Such reactions have been reported more frequently in children than in adults with an overall occurrence ranging from 1 in 200 (0.5%) in one focused trial to 2 in 8,346 (0.024%) in overall clinical trials (with an incidence in children in clinical trials of 0.055%) to 1 in 38,000 (0.003%) in spontaneous event reports. Signs and symptoms usually occur a few days after initiation of therapy and subside within a few days after cessation of therapy; occasionally these reactions have resulted in hospitalization, usually of short duration (median hospitalization = 2 to 3 days, based on postmarketing surveillance studies). In those requiring hospitalization, the symptoms have ranged from mild to severe at the time of admission with more of the severe reactions occurring in children. Antihistamines and glucocorticoids appear to enhance resolution of the signs and symptoms. No serious sequelae have been reported.

More severe hypersensitivity reactions, including Stevens-Johnson syndrome, toxic epidermal necrolysis, and anaphylaxis have been reported rarely. Anaphylactoid events may be manifested by solitary symptoms, including angioedema, asthenia, edema (including face and limbs), dyspnea, paresthesias, syncope, or vasodilation. Anaphylaxis may be more common in patients with a history of penicillin allergy.

Rarely, hypersensitivity symptoms may persist for several months.

Gastrointestinal symptoms occur in about 2.5% of patients and include diarrhea (1 in 70).

Symptoms of pseudomembranous colitis may appear either during or after antibiotic treatment. Nausea and vomiting have been reported rarely. As with some penicillins and some other cephalosporins, transient hepatitis and cholestatic jaundice have been reported rarely.

Other effects considered related to therapy included eosinophilia (1 in 50 patients), genital pruritus or vaginitis (less than 1 in 100 patients), and, rarely, thrombocytopenia or reversible interstitial nephritis.

CASUAL RELATIONSHIP UNCERTAIN

CNS: Rarely, reversible hyperactivity, agitation, nervousness, insomnia, confusion, hypertonia, dizziness, hallucinations, and somnolence have been reported.

Transitory abnormalities in clinical laboratory test results have been reported. Although they were of uncertain etiology, they are listed below to serve as alerting information for the physician.

Hepatic: Slight elevations of AST (SGOT), ALT (SGPT), or alkaline phosphatase values (1 in 40).

Hematopoietic: As has also been reported with other β-lactam antibiotics, transient lymphocytosis, leukopenia, and, rarely, hemolytic anemia and reversible neutropenia of possible clinical significance.

There have been rare reports of increased prothrombin time with or without clinical bleeding in patients receiving cefaclor and warfarin sodium concomitantly.

Renal: Slight elevations in BUN or serum creatinine (less than 1 in 500) or abnormal urinalysis (less than 1 in 200).

OVERDOSAGE:

Signs and Symptoms: The toxic symptoms following an overdose of cefaclor may include nausea, vomiting, epigastric distress, and diarrhea. The severity of the epigastric distress and the diarrhea are dose related. If other symptoms are present, it is probable that they are secondary to an underlying disease state, an allergic reaction, or the effects of other intoxication.

OVERDOSAGE: *(cont'd)*

Treatment: To obtain up-to-date information about the treatment of overdose, a good resource is your certified Regional Poison Control Center. Telephone numbers of certified poison control centers are listed in the *Physicians GenRx*. In managing overdosage, consider the possibility of multiple drug overdoses, interaction among drugs, and unusual drug kinetics in your patient.

Unless 5 times the normal dose of cefaclor has been ingested, gastrointestinal decontamination will not be necessary.

Protect the patient's airway and support ventilation and perfusion. Meticulously monitor and maintain, within acceptable limits, the patient's vital signs, blood gases, serum electrolytes, etc. Absorption of drugs from the gastrointestinal tract may be decreased by giving activated charcoal, which, in many cases, is more effective than emesis or lavage; consider charcoal instead of or in addition to gastric emptying. Repeated doses of charcoal over time may hasten elimination of some drugs that have been absorbed. Safeguard the patient's airway when employing gastric emptying or charcoal.

Forced diuresis, peritoneal dialysis, hemodialysis, or charcoal hemoperfusion have not been established as beneficial for an overdose of cefaclor.

DOSAGE AND ADMINISTRATION:

Cefaclor is administered orally.

Adults: The usual adult dosage is 250 mg every 8 hours. For more severe infections (such as pneumonia) or those caused by less susceptible organisms, doses may be doubled.

Children: The usual recommended daily dosage for children is 20 mg/kg/day in divided doses every 8 hours. In more serious infections, otitis media, and infections caused by less susceptible organisms, 40 mg/kg/day are recommended, with a maximum dosage of 1 g/day (TABLE 1).

TABLE 1 Cefaclor Suspension

Child's Weight	125 mg/5 ml	250 mg/5 ml
20 mg/kg/day		
9 kg	1/2 tsp t.i.d.	
18 kg	1 tsp t.i.d.	1/2 tsp t.i.d.
40 mg/kg/day		
9 kg	1 tsp t.i.d.	1/2 tsp t.i.d.
18 kg		1 tsp t.i.d.

B.I.D. Treatment Option: For the treatment of otitis media and pharyngitis, the total daily dosage may be divided and administered every 12 hours (TABLE 2).

TABLE 2 Cefaclor Suspension

Child's Weight	187 mg/5 ml	375 mg/5 ml
20 mg/kg/day (Pharyngitis)		
9 kg	1/2 tsp b.i.d.	
18 kg	1 tsp b.i.d.	1/2 tsp b.i.d.
40 mg/kg/day (Otitis Media)		
9 kg	1 tsp b.i.d.	1/2 tsp b.i.d.
18 kg		1 tsp b.i.d.

Cefaclor may be administered in the presence of impaired renal function. Under such a condition, the dosage usually is unchanged (see PRECAUTIONS.)

In the treatment of β-hemolytic streptococcal infections, a therapeutic dosage of cefaclor should be administered for at least 10 days.

PATIENT INFORMATION:

Cefaclor is a cephalosporin antibiotic used to treat bacterial infections. Take at regular intervals and complete the entire course of therapy. Do not take this medication if you are allergic to any type of penicillin or cephalosporin. Notify your physician if you are pregnant or nursing. This antibiotic may decrease the effectiveness of birth control pills; use another form of birth control while taking this medication. Shake the suspension well before each use and store it in the refrigerator. May cause nausea, vomiting or diarrhea; notify your physician if these occur. Take with food or milk to avoid stomach upset. Cefaclor may cause a false-positive reaction for nonspecific urine glucose tests in patients with diabetes. This medication does not interfere with enzyme-based urine glucose tests.

HOW SUPPLIED:

CECLOR

Pulvules:

250 mg, purple and white (No. 3061)

500 mg, purple and gray (No. 3062)

For Oral Suspension:

125 mg/5 ml, strawberry flavor (M-5057‡)

187 mg/5 ml, strawberry flavor (M-5130‡)

250 mg/5 ml, strawberry flavor (M-5058‡)

375 mg/5 ml, strawberry flavor (M-5132‡)

‡ After mixing, store in a refrigerator. Shake well before using. Keep tightly closed. The mixture may be kept for 14 days without significant loss of potency. Discard unused portion after 14 days.

Store at controlled room temperature, 59° to 86°F (15° to 30°C).

HOW SUPPLIED - RATED THERAPEUTICALLY EQUIVALENT:

Capsule - Oral - 250 mg

100's	$133.12	Cefaclor, H.C.F.A. F F P	99999-0680-01

Capsule - Oral - 500 mg

100's	$279.73	Cefaclor, H.C.F.A. F F P	99999-0680-02

Capsule, Gelatin - Oral - 250 mg

15's	$30.70	Cefaclor, Zenith Labs	00172-4760-40
15's	$30.70	Cefaclor, Goldline Labs	00182-2606-28
15's	**$34.15**	**CECLOR, Lilly**	**00002-3061-15**
100's	$179.93	Cefaclor, United Res	00677-1540-01
100's	$185.50	Cefaclor, Qualitest Pharms	00603-2586-21
100's	$194.50	Cefaclor, Schein Pharm (US)	00364-2614-01
100's	$194.70	Cefaclor, Zenith Labs	00172-4760-60
100's	$194.70	Cefaclor, Goldline Labs	00182-2606-01
100's	$194.70	Cefaclor, Major Pharms	00904-7932-60
100's	$194.94	Cefaclor, HL Moore Drug Exch	00839-7958-06
100's	$195.83	Cefaclor, Lederle Pharm	00005-3352-23

HOW SUPPLIED - RATED THERAPEUTICALLY EQUIVALENT:
(cont'd)

100's	$198.95	Cefaclor, Mylan	00378-7250-01
100's	$198.95	Cefaclor, Rugby	00536-5706-01
100's	**$216.61**	**CECLOR, Lilly**	**00002-3061-02**
100's	**$220.99**	**CECLOR, Lilly**	**00002-3061-33**
500's	$954.00	Cefaclor, Zenith Labs	00172-4760-70
500's	$954.00	Cefaclor, Goldline Labs	00182-2606-05
1000's	$1850.70	Cefaclor, Zenith Labs	00172-4760-80

Capsule, Gelatin - Oral - 500 mg

15's	$58.30	Cefaclor, Zenith Labs	00172-4761-40
15's	$58.30	Cefaclor, Goldline Labs	00182-2607-28
15's	**$64.81**	**CECLOR, Lilly**	**00002-3062-15**
100's	$364.52	Cefaclor, Qualitest Pharms	00603-2587-21
100's	$382.50	Cefaclor, Schein Pharm (US)	00364-2615-01
100's	$382.65	Cefaclor, Zenith Labs	00172-4761-60
100's	$382.65	Cefaclor, Goldline Labs	00182-2607-01
100's	$382.65	Cefaclor, Major Pharms	00904-7933-60
100's	$383.06	Cefaclor, HL Moore Drug Exch	00839-7961-06
100's	$384.50	Cefaclor, Rugby	00536-5707-01
100's	$384.79	Cefaclor, Lederle Pharm	00005-3353-23
100's	$389.50	Cefaclor, Mylan	00378-7500-01
100's	**$425.65**	**CECLOR, Lilly**	**00002-3062-02**
100's	**$430.03**	**CECLOR, Lilly**	**00002-3062-33**
500's	$1855.85	Cefaclor, Zenith Labs	00172-4761-70
500's	$1855.85	Cefaclor, Goldline Labs	00182-2607-05

Powder, Reconstitution - Oral - 125 mg/5ml

75 ml	$13.39	Cefaclor, Qualitest Pharms	00603-6534-62
75 ml	$13.92	Cefaclor, Schein Pharm (US)	00364-2616-59
75 ml	$14.05	Cefaclor, Zenith Labs	00172-4611-22
75 ml	$14.05	Cefaclor, Goldline Labs	00182-7086-69
75 ml	$14.05	Cefaclor, Major Pharms	00904-7934-71
75 ml	$14.07	Cefaclor, Rugby	00536-5755-62
75 ml	$14.11	Cefaclor, HL Moore Drug Exch	00839-7956-55
75 ml	$14.14	Cefaclor, Lederle Pharm	00005-3354-42
75 ml	$14.15	Cefaclor, Mylan	00378-7602-12
75 ml	$14.92	Cefaclor, United Res	00677-1562-98
75 ml	**$15.64**	**CECLOR, Lilly**	**00002-5057-18**
150 ml	$26.65	Cefaclor, Qualitest Pharms	00603-6534-66
150 ml	$27.95	Cefaclor, Zenith Labs	00172-4611-23
150 ml	$27.95	Cefaclor, Goldline Labs	00182-7086-72
150 ml	$27.95	Cefaclor, Major Pharms	00904-7934-07
150 ml	$27.97	Cefaclor, Schein Pharm (US)	00364-2616-62
150 ml	$28.00	Cefaclor, Rugby	00536-5755-74
150 ml	$28.01	Cefaclor, HL Moore Drug Exch	00839-7956-75
150 ml	$28.28	Cefaclor, Lederle Pharm	00005-3354-49
150 ml	$28.30	Cefaclor, Mylan	00378-7602-06
150 ml	$29.85	Cefaclor, United Res	00677-1562-28
150 ml	**$31.12**	**CECLOR, Lilly**	**00002-5057-68**

Powder, Reconstitution - Oral - 187 mg/5ml

50 ml	$13.39	Cefaclor, Qualitest Pharms	00603-6535-47
50 ml	$14.05	Cefaclor, Zenith Labs	00172-4613-20
50 ml	$14.05	Cefaclor, Goldline Labs	00182-7087-67
50 ml	$14.05	Cefaclor, Schein Pharm (US)	00364-2617-57
50 ml	$14.07	Cefaclor, Rugby	00536-5760-80
50 ml	$14.08	Cefaclor, Major Pharms	00904-7935-50
50 ml	$14.11	Cefaclor, HL Moore Drug Exch	00839-7957-59
50 ml	$14.15	Cefaclor, Mylan	00378-7604-09
50 ml	$14.21	Cefaclor, Lederle Pharm	00005-3355-40
50 ml	**$15.64**	**CECLOR, Lilly**	**00002-5130-87**
100 ml	$26.65	Cefaclor, Qualitest Pharms	00603-6535-64
100 ml	$27.95	Cefaclor, Zenith Labs	00172-4613-21
100 ml	$27.95	Cefaclor, Goldline Labs	00182-7087-70
100 ml	$27.95	Cefaclor, Schein Pharm (US)	00364-2617-61
100 ml	$28.00	Cefaclor, Rugby	00536-5760-82
100 ml	$28.01	Cefaclor, HL Moore Drug Exch	00839-7957-73
100 ml	$28.13	Cefaclor, Lederle Pharm	00005-3355-46
100 ml	$28.30	Cefaclor, Mylan	00378-7604-02
100 ml	**$31.12**	**CECLOR, Lilly**	**00002-5130-48**

Powder, Reconstitution - Oral - 250 mg/5ml

75 ml	$24.85	Cefaclor, Qualitest Pharms	00603-6536-62
75 ml	$26.05	Cefaclor, Zenith Labs	00172-4610-22
75 ml	$26.05	Cefaclor, Goldline Labs	00182-7088-69
75 ml	$26.05	Cefaclor, Major Pharms	00904-7936-71
75 ml	$26.10	Cefaclor, Schein Pharm (US)	00364-2618-59
75 ml	$26.12	Cefaclor, Rugby	00536-5765-62
75 ml	$26.12	Cefaclor, HL Moore Drug Exch	00839-7959-55
75 ml	$26.24	Cefaclor, Lederle Pharm	00005-3356-42
75 ml	$26.40	Cefaclor, Mylan	00378-7610-12
75 ml	$28.42	Cefaclor, United Res	00677-1563-98
75 ml	**$29.03**	**CECLOR, Lilly**	**00002-5058-18**
150 ml	$48.27	Cefaclor, Qualitest Pharms	00603-6536-66
150 ml	$50.65	Cefaclor, Zenith Labs	00172-4610-23
150 ml	$50.65	Cefaclor, Goldline Labs	00182-7088-72
150 ml	$50.65	Cefaclor, Major Pharms	00904-7936-07
150 ml	$50.70	Cefaclor, Schein Pharm (US)	00364-2618-62
150 ml	$50.74	Cefaclor, Rugby	00536-5765-74
150 ml	$50.75	Cefaclor, HL Moore Drug Exch	00839-7959-75
150 ml	$50.99	Cefaclor, Mylan	00378-7610-06
150 ml	$51.21	Cefaclor, Lederle Pharm	00005-3356-49
150 ml	**$56.38**	**CECLOR, Lilly**	**00002-5058-68**
150 ml	$56.85	Cefaclor, United Res	00677-1563-28

Powder, Reconstitution - Oral - 375 mg/5ml

50 ml	$24.85	Cefaclor, Qualitest Pharms	00603-6537-47
50 ml	$25.75	Cefaclor, Schein Pharm (US)	00364-2619-57
50 ml	$26.05	Cefaclor, Zenith Labs	00172-4612-20
50 ml	$26.05	Cefaclor, Goldline Labs	00182-7089-67
50 ml	$26.05	Cefaclor, Major Pharms	00904-7937-50
50 ml	$26.12	Cefaclor, Rugby	00536-5770-80
50 ml	$26.12	Cefaclor, HL Moore Drug Exch	00839-7960-59
50 ml	$26.38	Cefaclor, Lederle Pharm	00005-3357-40
50 ml	$26.40	Cefaclor, Mylan	00378-7612-09
50 ml	**$29.03**	**CECLOR, Lilly**	**00002-5132-87**
100 ml	$48.27	Cefaclor, Qualitest Pharms	00603-6537-64
100 ml	$50.65	Cefaclor, Zenith Labs	00172-4612-21
100 ml	$50.65	Cefaclor, Goldline Labs	00182-7089-70
100 ml	$50.70	Cefaclor, Schein Pharm (US)	00364-2619-61
100 ml	$50.74	Cefaclor, Rugby	00536-5770-82
100 ml	$50.74	Cefaclor, Major Pharms	00904-7937-04
100 ml	$50.75	Cefaclor, HL Moore Drug Exch	00839-7960-73
100 ml	$50.98	Cefaclor, Lederle Pharm	00005-3357-46

HOW SUPPLIED - RATED THERAPEUTICALLY EQUIVALENT:
(cont'd)

100 ml	$50.99	Cefaclor, Mylan	00378-7612-02
100 ml	**$56.38**	**CECLOR, Lilly**	**00002-5132-48**

Powder for reconstitution - Oral - 125 mg/5ml

75 ml	$14.92	Cefaclor, H.C.F.A. F F P	99999-0680-03
150 ml	$29.62	Cefaclor, H.C.F.A. F F P	99999-0680-04

Powder for reconstitution - Oral - 250 mg/5ml

75 ml	$28.42	Cefaclor, H.C.F.A. F F P	99999-0680-05
150 ml	$53.62	Cefaclor, H.C.F.A. F F P	99999-0680-06

Powder for reconstitution - Oral - 375 mg/5ml

50 ml	$28.42	Cefaclor, H.C.F.A. F F P	99999-0680-07
100 ml	$53.63	Cefaclor, H.C.F.A. F F P	99999-0680-08

CEFADROXIL *(000681)*

CATEGORIES: Anti-Infectives; Antibiotics; Antimicrobials; Cephalosporins; Infections; Pharyngitis; Skin Infections; Streptococcal Infection; Tonsillitis; Urinary Tract Infections; Rheumatic Fever*; Pregnancy Category B; Sales > $100 Million; FDA Approval Pre 1982; Patent Expiration 1994 Dec; Top 200 Drugs
* Indication not approved by the FDA

BRAND NAMES: *Baxan* (England); *Bid*; *Bidicef*; *Bidocef* (Germany); *Bidocef Forte* (Germany); *Bidocef S* (Germany); *Biocef*; *Biofaxil*; *Camex*; *Cedrox*; *Cefacar*; *Cefadril*; *Cefadrol*; *Cefadrox*; *Cefadur*; *Cefalom*; *Cefamox* (Mexico); *Cefaroxil*; *Cefat*; *Cefaxil*; *Ceforal*; *Cefra-Om*; *Cefroxil*; *Cefu*; *Cephadrol*; *Cephos*; *Crenodyn*; *Curisafe*; *Cyclomycin-K*; *Droxicef*; *Droxil*; *Droxyl*; *Duracef* (Mexico); **Duricef**; *Egobiotic*; *Eurocef*; *Hafroxil*; *Hanacef*; *Ibidroxyl*; *Kefloxin*; *Kefroxil*; *Kelfex*; *Kleotrat*; *Lesporina*; *Likodin*; *Lydroxil*; *Moxacef*; *Nefalox*; *Odoxil*; *Omnidrox*; *Oracefal* (France); *Oradroxil*; *Sedral* (Japan); *Sumacef* (Japan); *Ucefa*; Ultracef; *Versatic*; *Wincef* *(International brand names outside U.S. in italics)*

COST OF THERAPY: $60.75 (Infections; Tablet; 1 gm; 1/day; 10 days) vs. Potential Cost of $3,912.55 (Urinary Tract Infections)

PRIMARY ICD9: 136.9 (Unspecified Infections and Parasitic Diseases)

DESCRIPTION:

Cefadroxil monohydrate, USP is a semisynthetic cephalosporin antibiotic intended for oral administration. It is a white to yellowish-white crystalline powder. It is soluble in water and it is acid-stable. It is chemically designated as 5-Thia-1-azabicyclo(4.2.0)oct-2-ene-2-carboxylic acid, 7-<[amino(4-hydroxyphenyl)acetyl]amino>-3-methyl-8-oxo-, monohydrate, <6R-[6α, 7β (R*)]>-. It has the formula $C_{16}H_{17}N_3O_5S{\cdot}H_2O$ and the molecular weight of 381.40.

Duricef film-coated tablets, 1 g, contain the following inactive ingredients: microcrystalline cellulose, hydroxypropyl methylcellulose, magnesium stearate, polyethylene glycol, polysorbate 80, simethicone emulsion, and titanium dioxide.

Duricef for Oral Suspension contains the following inactive ingredients: FD&C Yellow #6, flavors (natural and artificial), polysorbate 80, sodium benzoate, sucrose, and xanthan gum.

Duricef capsules contain the following inactive ingredients: FD&C Red #28, FD&C Blue #1, FD&C Red #40, gelatin, magnesium stearate, and titanium dioxide.

CLINICAL PHARMACOLOGY:

Cefadroxil is rapidly absorbed after oral administration. Following single doses of 500 and 1000 mg, average peak serum concentrations were approximately 16 and 28 mcg/ml, respectively. Measurable levels were present 12 hours after administration. Over 90% of the drug is excreted unchanged in the urine within 24 hours. Peak urine concentrations are approximately 1800 mcg/ml during the period following a single 500-mg oral dose. Increases in dosage generally produce a proportionate increase in cefadroxil urinary concentration. The urine antibiotic concentration, following a 1-g dose, was maintained well above the MIC of susceptible urinary pathogens for 20 to 22 hours.

MICROBIOLOGY

In vitro tests demonstrate that the cephalosporins are bactericidal because of their inhibition of cell-wall synthesis. Cefadroxil has been shown to be active against the following organisms both *in vitro* and in clinical infections (see INDICATIONS AND USAGE):

Beta-hemolytic streptococci	*Escherichia coli*
Staphylococci, including penicillinase-producing strains	*Proteus mirabilis*
	Klebsiella spp.
Streptococcus (Diplococcus) pneumoniae	*Moraxella (Branhamella) catarrhalis*

Note: Most strains of *Enterococcus faecalis* spp. (formerly*Streptococcus faecalis*) and *Enterococcus faecium* (formerly *Streptococcus faecium*) are resistant to cefadroxil. It is not active against most strains of *Enterobacter* spp.,*Morganella morganii* (formerly *Proteus morganii*), and *Proteus vulgaris*. It has no activity against *Pseudomonas* spp. and *Acinetobacter calcoaceticus* (formerly *Mima* and *Herellea* spp.).

SUSCEPTIBILITY TESTS

Diffusion Techniques: The use of antibiotic disk susceptibility test methods which measure zone diameter give an accurate estimation of antibiotic susceptibility. One such standard procedure[1] which has been recommended for use with disks to test susceptibility of organisms to cefadroxil uses the cephalosporin class (cephalothin) disk. Interpretation involves the correlation of the diameters obtained in the disk test with the minimum inhibitory concentration (MIC) for cefadroxil.

Reports from the laboratory giving results of the standard single-disk susceptibility test with a 30 mcg cephalothin disk should be interpreted according to specific criteria in Table 1.

TABLE 1

Zone Diameter (mm)	Interpretation
≥ 18	(S) Susceptible
15-17	(I) Intermediate
≤ 14	(R) Resistant

A report of "Susceptible" indicates that the pathogen is likely to be inhibited by generally achievable blood levels. A report of "Intermediate" suggests that the organism would be susceptible if high dosage is used or if the infection is confined to tissue and fluids (*e.g.*, urine) in which high antibiotic levels are attained. A report of "Resistant" indicates that achievable concentrations of the antibiotic are unlikely to be inhibitory and other therapy should be selected.

Standardized procedures require the use of laboratory control organisms. The 30-mcg cephalothin disk should give the zone diameters found in Table 2.

CLINICAL PHARMACOLOGY: *(cont'd)*

TABLE 2

Organism	Zone Diameter (mm)
Staphylococcus aureus ATCC 25923	29-37
Escherichia coli ATCC 25922	17-22

Dilution Techniques: When using the NCCLS agar dilution or broth dilution (including microdilution) method[2] or equivalent, a bacterial isolate may be considered susceptible if the MIC value for cephalothin is 8 mcg/ml or less. Organisms are considered resistant if the MIC is 32 mcg/ml or greater. Organisms with an MIC value of less than 32 mcg/ml but greater than 8 mcg/ml are intermediate.

As with standard diffusion methods, dilution procedures require the use of laboratory control organisms. Standard cephalothin powder should give MIC values in the range of 0.12 mcg/ml to 0.5 mcg/ml for*Staphylococcus aureus* ATCC 29213. For *Escherichia coli* ATCC 25922, the MIC range should be 4.0 mcg/ml to 16.0 mcg/ml. For *Streptococcus faecalis* ATCC 29212, the MIC range should be between 8.0 and 32.0 mcg/ml.

INDICATIONS AND USAGE:

Cefadroxil is indicated for the treatment of patients with infection caused by susceptible strains of the designated organisms in the following diseases:

Urinary tract infections caused by *E. coli, Proteus mirabilis,* and *Klebsiella* spp.

Skin and skin structure infections caused by staphylococci and/or streptococci.

Pharyngitis and tonsillitis caused by Group A beta-hemolytic streptococci. (Penicillin is the usual drug of choice in the treatment and prevention of streptococcal infections, including the prophylaxis of rheumatic fever. Cefadroxil is generally effective in the eradication of streptococci from the nasopharynx; however, substantial data establishing the efficacy of cefadroxil in the subsequent prevention of rheumatic fever are not available at present.)

Note: Culture and susceptibility tests should be initiated prior to and during therapy. Renal function studies should be performed when indicated.

CONTRAINDICATIONS:

Cefadroxil is contraindicated in patients with known allergy to the cephalosporin of antibiotics.

WARNINGS:

BEFORE THERAPY WITH CEFADROXIL IS INSTITUTED, CAREFUL INQUIRY SHOULD BE MADE TO DETERMINE WHETHER THE PATIENT HAS HAD PREVIOUS HYPERSENSITIVITY REACTIONS TO CEFADROXIL, CEPHALOSPORINS, PENICILLINS, OR OTHER DRUGS. IF THIS PRODUCT IS TO BE GIVEN TO PENICILLIN-SENSITIVE PATIENTS, CAUTION SHOULD BE EXERCISED BECAUSE CROSS-SENSITIVITY AMONG BETA-LACTAM ANTIBIOTICS HAS BEEN CLEARLY DOCUMENTED AND MAY OCCUR IN UP TO 10% OF PATIENTS WITH A HISTORY OF PENICILLIN ALLERGY.

IF AN ALLERGIC REACTION TO CEFADROXIL OCCURS, DISCONTINUE THE DRUG. SERIOUS ACUTE HYPERSENSITIVITY REACTIONS MAY REQUIRE TREATMENT WITH EPINEPHRINE AND OTHER EMERGENCY MEASURES, INCLUDING OXYGEN, INTRAVENOUS FLUIDS, INTRAVENOUS ANTIHISTAMINES, CORTICOSTEROIDS, PRESSOR AMINES, AND AIRWAY MANAGEMENT, AS CLINICALLY INDICATED.

Pseudomembranous colitis has been reported with nearly all antibacterial agents, including cefadroxil, and may range from mild to life-threatening. Therefore, it is important to consider this diagnosis in patients who present with diarrhea subsequent to the administration of antibacterial agents.

Treatment with antibacterial agents alters the normal flora of the colon and may permit overgrowth of clostridia. Studies indicate that a toxin produced by *Clostridium difficile* is a primary cause of "antibiotic-associated colitis."

After the diagnosis of pseudomembranous colitis has been established, therapeutic measures should be initiated. Mild cases of pseudomembranous colitis usually respond to discontinuation of the drug alone. In moderate to severe cases, consideration should be given to management with fluids and electrolytes, protein supplementation, and treatment with an antibacterial drug effective against *C. difficile*.

PRECAUTIONS:

General: Cefadroxil should be used with caution in the presence of markedly impaired renal function (creatinine clearance rate of less than 50 ml/min/1.73m^2) (see DOSAGE AND ADMINISTRATION.) In patients with known or suspected renal impairment, careful clinical observation and appropriate laboratory studies should be made prior to and during therapy.

Prolonged use of cefadroxil may result in the overgrowth of nonsusceptible organisms. Careful observation of the patient is essential. If superinfection occurs during therapy, appropriate measures should be taken.

Cefadroxil should be prescribed with caution in individuals with history of gastrointestinal disease, particularly colitis.

Drug/Laboratory Test Interactions: Positive direct Coombs' tests have been reported during treatment with the cephalosporin antibiotics. In hematologic studies or in transfusion cross-matching procedures when antiglobulin tests are performed on the minor side or in Coombs' testing of newborns whose mothers have received cephalosporin antibiotics before parturition, it should be recognized that a positive Coombs' test may be due to the drug.

Carcinogenesis, Mutagenesis, and Impairment of Fertility: No long-term studies have been performed to determine carcinogenic potential. No genetic toxicity tests have been performed.

Pregnancy Category B: Reproduction studies have been performed in mice and rats at doses up to 11 times the human dose and have revealed no evidence of impaired fertility or harm to the fetus due to cefadroxil monohydrate. There are, however, no adequate and well controlled studies in pregnant women. Because animal reproduction studies are not always predictive of human response, this drug should be used during pregnancy only if clearly needed.

Labor and Delivery: Cefadroxil has not been studied for use during labor and delivery. Treatment should only be given if clearly needed.

Nursing Mothers: Caution should be exercised when cefadroxil monohydrate is administered to a nursing mother.

Pediatric Use: (See DOSAGE AND ADMINISTRATION.)

ADVERSE REACTIONS:

Gastrointestinal: Onset of pseudomembranous colitis symptoms may occur during or after antibiotic treatment (See WARNINGS.) Nausea and vomiting have been reported rarely. Diarrhea has also occurred.

ADVERSE REACTIONS: *(cont'd)*

Hypersensitivity: Allergies (in the form of rash, urticaria, and angioedema) have been observed. These reactions usually subsided upon discontinuation of the drug.

Other reactions have included genital pruritus, genital moniliasis, vaginitis, moderate transient neutropenia, and minor elevations in serum transaminase. Stevens-Johnson syndrome has been rarely reported.

In addition to the adverse reactions listed above which have been observed in patients treated with cefadroxil, the following adverse reactions and altered laboratory tests have been reported for cephalosporin-class antibiotics:

Anaphylaxis, erythema multiforme, toxic epidermal necrolysis, fever, abdominal pain, superinfection, renal dysfunction, toxic nephropathy, hepatic dysfunction including cholestasis, aplastic anemia, hemolytic anemia, hemorrhage, prolonged prothrombin time, positive Coombs' test, increased BUN, increased creatinine, elevated alkaline phosphatase, elevated aspartate aminotransferase (AST), elevated alanine aminotransferase (ALT), elevated bilirubin, elevated LDH, eosinophilia, pancytopenia, neutropenia, agranulocytosis, thrombocytopenia.

Several cephalosporins have been implicated in triggering seizures, particularly in patients with renal impairment, when the dosage was not reduced (see DOSAGE AND ADMINISTRATION and OVERDOSAGE). If seizures associated with drug therapy occur, the drug should be discontinued. Anticonvulsant therapy can be given if clinically indicated.

OVERDOSAGE:

A study of children under 6 years of age suggested that ingestion of less than 250 mg/kg of cephalosporins is not associated with significant outcomes. No action is required other than general support and observation. For amounts greater than 250 mg/kg, induce gastric emptying.

In five anuric patients, it was demonstrated that an average of 63% of a 1-g oral dose is extracted from the body during a 6- to 8-hour hemodialysis session.

DOSAGE AND ADMINISTRATION:

Cefadroxil is acid-stable and may be administered orally without regard to meals. Administration with food may be helpful in diminishing potential gastrointestinal complaints occasionally associated with oral cephalosporin therapy.

ADULTS

Urinary Tract Infections: For uncomplicated lower urinary tract infections (*i.e.,* cystitis) the usual dosage is 1 or 2 g per day in single (qd) or divided doses (bid).

For all other urinary tract infections the usual dosage is 2 g per day in divided doses (bid).

Skin and Skin Structure Infections: For skin and skin structure infections the usual dosage is 1 g per day in single (qd) or divided doses (bid).

Pharyngitis and Tonsillitis: Treatment of group A beta-hemolytic streptococcal pharyngitis and tonsillitis—1 g per day in single (qd) or divided doses (bid) for 10 days.

CHILDREN

For urinary tract infections, the recommended daily dosage for children is 30 mg/kg/day in divided doses every 12 hours. For pharyngitis, tonsillitis, and impetigo, the recommended daily dosage for children is 30 mg/kg/day in a single dose or in equally divided doses every 12 hours. For other skin and skin-structure infections, the recommended daily dosage is 30 mg/kg/day in equally divided doses every 12 hours. In the treatment of beta-hemolytic streptococcal infections, a therapeutic dosage of cefadroxil should be administered for at least 10 days.

See TABLE 3 for total daily dosage for children.

TABLE 3 Daily dosage of Cefadroxil Suspension
Child's Weight

lbs	kg	125 mg/5 ml	250 mg/5 ml	500 mg/5 ml
10	4.5	1 tsp	-	
20	9.1	2 tsp	1 tsp	
30	13.6	3 tsp	1.5 tsp	
40	18.2	4 tsp	2 tsp	1 tsp
50	22.7	5 tsp	2.5 tsp	1.25 tsp
60	27.3	6 tsp	3 tsp	1.50 tsp
70 & above	31.8+	-	-	2 tsp

In patients with renal impairment, the dosage of cefadroxil monohydrate should be adjusted according to creatinine clearance rates to prevent drug accumulation. The following schedule is suggested (TABLE 4). In adults, the initial dose is 1000 mg of cefadroxil and the maintenance dose (based on the creatinine clearance rate [ml/min/1.73m^2]) is 500 mg at the time intervals listed below.

TABLE 4

Creatinine Clearances	Dosage Interval
0-10 ml/min	36 hours
10-25 ml/min	24 hours
25-50 ml/min	12 hours

Patients with creatinine clearance rates over 50 ml/min may be treated as if they were patients having normal renal function.

TABLE 5 Reconstitution Directions for Oral Suspension

Bottle Size	Reconstitution Directions
100 ml	Suspend in a total of 66 ml of water. Method: Tap bottle lightly to loosen powder. Add 66 ml of water in two portions. Shake well after each addition.
50 ml	Suspend in a total of 33 ml of water. Method: Tap bottle lightly to loosen powder. Add 33 ml of water in two portions. Shake well after each addition.

STORAGE

After reconstitution, store in refrigerator. Shake well before using. Keep container tightly closed. Discard unused portion after 14 days.

Prior to reconstitution: Store at controlled room temperature (15 to 30° C).

REFERENCES:

1. National Committee for Clinical Laboratory Standards. Approved Standard, *Performance Standards for Antimicrobial Disk Susceptibility Test*, 4th Edition, Vol. 10(7):M2-A4, Villanova, PA, April, 1990. **2.** National Committee for Clinical Laboratory Standards. Approved Standard: *Methods for Dilution Antimicrobial Susceptibility Tests for Bacteria that Grow Aerobically*, 2nd Edition, Vol. 10(8):M7-A2, Villanova, PA, April, 1990.

PATIENT INFORMATION:

Cefadroxil is a cephalosporin antibiotic used to treat bacterial infections.

Take at regular intervals and complete the entire course of therapy. Shake the suspension well before each use and store it in the refrigerator.

Do not take this medication if you are allergic to any type of penicillin or cephalosporin.

Notify your physician if you are pregnant or nursing.

This antibiotic may decrease the effectiveness of birth control pills; use another form of birth control while taking this medication.

May cause nausea, vomiting or diarrhea; notify your physician if these occur.

Take with food or milk to avoid stomach upset.

Cefadroxil may cause a false-positive reaction for nonspecific urine glucose tests in patients with diabetes. This medication does not interfere with enzyme-based urine glucose tests.

HOW SUPPLIED - RATED THERAPEUTICALLY EQUIVALENT:

Capsule - Oral - 500 mg

100's	$276.72	Cefadroxil, H.C.F.A. F F P	99999-0681-01

Capsule, Gelatin - Oral - 500 mg

20's	**$68.81**	**DURICEF, Bristol Myers Squibb**	**00087-0784-07**
50's	**$168.60**	**DURICEF, Bristol Myers Squibb**	**00087-0784-46**
50's	$178.30	ULTRACEF, Mead Johnson	00015-7271-50
100's	**$319.79**	**DURICEF, Bristol Myers Squibb**	**00087-0784-42**
100's	**$325.30**	**DURICEF, Bristol Myers Squibb**	**00087-0784-44**
100's	$338.17	ULTRACEF, Mead Johnson	00015-7271-60
100's	$344.03	ULTRACEF, Mead Johnson	00015-7271-65

Powder, Reconstitution - Oral - 125 mg/5ml

50 ml	**$6.95**	**DURICEF, Bristol Myers Squibb**	**00087-0786-42**
50 ml	$9.46	ULTRACEF, Mead Johnson	00015-7283-25
100 ml	**$12.80**	**DURICEF, Bristol Myers Squibb**	**00087-0786-41**
100 ml	$26.00	ULTRACEF, Mead Johnson	00015-7283-40

Powder, Reconstitution - Oral - 250 mg/5ml

50 ml	**$12.25**	**DURICEF, Bristol Myers Squibb**	**00087-0782-42**
100 ml	**$24.04**	**DURICEF, Bristol Myers Squibb**	**00087-0782-41**
100 ml	$43.40	ULTRACEF, Mead Johnson	00015-7284-40

Powder, Reconstitution - Oral - 500 mg/5ml

50 ml	**$16.63**	**DURICEF, Bristol Myers Squibb**	**00087-0783-42**
75 ml	**$24.93**	**DURICEF, Bristol Myers Squibb**	**00087-0783-05**
100 ml	**$33.28**	**DURICEF, Bristol Myers Squibb**	**00087-0783-41**

Tablet, Uncoated - Oral - 1 gm

24's	$98.73	ULTRACEF, Mead Johnson	00015-7286-30
28's	**$126.27**	**DURICEF, Bristol Myers Squibb**	**00087-0785-46**
40's	**$225.64**	**DURICEF, Bristol Myers Squibb**	**00087-0785-45**
50's	**$317.26**	**DURICEF, Bristol Myers Squibb**	**00087-0785-43**
100's	**$607.57**	**DURICEF, Bristol Myers Squibb**	**00087-0785-42**
100's	**$618.15**	**DURICEF, Bristol Myers Squibb**	**00087-0785-44**

CEFAMANDOLE NAFATE *(000682)*

CATEGORIES: Anti-Infectives; Antibiotics; Antimicrobials; Cephalosporins; Cholecystitis; Infections; Inflammatory Disease; Joint Infections; Pelvic Inflammatory Disease; Perioperative Prophylaxis; Peritonitis; Pneumonia; Renal Function; Respiratory Tract Infections; Septicemia; Skin Infections; Streptococcal Infection; Urinary Tract Infections; Pregnancy Category B; FDA Approval Pre 1982

BRAND NAMES: *Cedol*; *Cefadol*; *Cefiran*; *Dardokef*; *Kefadol* (England); *Kefdole* (Japan); *Kingfamandole*; *Mancef*; *Mandokef*; **Mandol**
(International brand names outside U.S. in italics)

DESCRIPTION:

Cefamandole nafate for injection, USP is a semisynthetic broad-spectrum cephalosporin antibiotic for parenteral administration. It is 5-Thia-azabicyclo(4.2.0)oct-2-ene-2-carboxylic acid, 7 (((formyloxy)phenylacetyl)amino)-3(((1-methyl-1*H*-tetrazol-5- yl)thio)methyl)-8-oxo-, monosodium salt, (6*R*-(6α, 7β(R*))). Cefamandole has the empirical formula $C_{19}H_{17}N_5NaO_6S_2$ representing a molecular weight of 512.49. Mandol also contains 63 mg sodium carbonate per gram of cefamandole activity. The total sodium content is approximately 77 mg (3.3 mEq sodium ion) per gram of cefamandole activity. After addition of diluent, cefamandole nafate rapidly hydrolyzes to cefamandole and both compounds have microbiologic activity *in vivo*. Solutions of Mandol range from light-yellow to amber, depending on concentration and diluent used. The pH of freshly reconstituted solutions usually ranges from 6.0 to 8.5.

CLINICAL PHARMACOLOGY:

After intramuscular administration of a 500 mg dose of cefamandole to normal volunteers, the mean peak serum concentration was 13 mcg/ml. After a 1 gram dose, the mean peak concentration was 25 mcg/ml. These peaks occurred at 30 to 120 minutes. Following intravenous doses of 1, 2 and 3 g, serum concentrations were 139, 240, and 533 mcg/ml respectively at 10 minutes. These concentrations declined to 0.8, 2.2, and 2.9 mcg/ml at 4 hours. Intravenous administration of 4-g doses every 6 hours produced no evidence of accumulation in the serum. The half-life after an intravenous dose is 32 minutes; after intramuscular administration, the half-life is 60 minutes.

Sixty-five percent to 85% of cefamandole is excreted by the kidneys over an 8 hour period, resulting in high urinary concentrations. Following intramuscular doses of 500 mg and 1 g, urinary concentrations averaged 254 and 1,357 mcg/ml respectively. Intravenous doses of 1 and 2 gram produced urinary levels averaging 750 and 1,380 mcg/ml respectively. Probenecid slows tubular excretion and doubles the peak serum level and the duration of measurable serum concentrations.

The antibiotic reaches therapeutic levels in pleural and joint fluids and in bile and bone.

MICROBIOLOGY

The bactericidal action of cefamandole results from inhibition of cell-wall synthesis. Cephalosporins have *in vitro*activity against a wide range of gram-positive and gram-negative organisms. Cefamandole is usually active against the following organisms *in vitro* and in clinical infections:

Gram positive

Staphylococcus aureus, including penicillinase and non-penicillinase-producing strains

Staphylococcus epidermidis

β-hemolytic and other streptococci (Most strains of enterococci, e.g. *Enterococcus faecalis* (formerly *Streptococcus faecalis*), are resistant.)

Streptococcus pneumoniae (formerly *Diplococcus pneumoniae*)

Gram negative

Escherichia coli

CLINICAL PHARMACOLOGY: *(cont'd)*

Klebsiella sp

Enterobacter sp (Initially susceptible organisms occasionally may become resistant during therapy).

Haemophilus influenzae

Proteus mirabilis

Providencia rettgeri (formerly *Proteus rettgeri*)

Morganella morganii (formerly *Proteus morganii*)

Proteus vulgaris (Some strains of *P. vulgaris* have been shown by *in vitro* tests to be resistant to cefamandole and other cephalosporins).

Anaerobic organisms

Gram-positive and gram-negative cocci (including *Peptococcus* and *Peptostreptococcus* sp)

Gram-positive bacilli (including *Clostridium* sp)

Gram-negative bacilli (including *Bacteroides* and *Fusobacterium* sp). Most strains of *Bacteroides fragilis* are resistant.

Pseudomonas, Acinetobacter calcoaceticus (formerly *Mima* and *Herellea* sp), and most *Serratia* strains are resistant to cephalosporins. Cefamandole is resistant to degradation by β-lactamases from certain members of the *Enterobacteriaceae.*

SUSCEPTIBILITY TESTING

Quantitative methods that require measurement of zone diameters give the most precise estimates of antibiotic susceptibility. One such procedure[1] has been recommended for use with disks to test susceptibility to cefamandole. Interpretation involves correlation of the diameters obtained in the disk test with minimum inhibitory concentration (MIC) values for cefamandole.

Reports from the laboratory giving results of the standardized single-disk susceptibility test using a 30 mcg cefamandole disk should be interpreted according to the following criteria:

Susceptible organisms produce zones of 18 mm or greater, indicating that the tested organism is likely to respond to therapy.

Organisms of intermediate susceptibility produce zones of 15 to 17 mm, indicating that the tested organism would be susceptible if high dosage is used or if the infection is confined to tissues and fluids (*e.g.*, urine), in which high antibiotic levels are attained.

Resistant organisms produce zones of 14 mm or less, indicating that other therapy should be selected.

For gram-positive isolates, the test may be performed with either the cephalosporin class disk (30 mcg cephalothin) or the cefamandole disk (30 mcg cefamandole), and a zone of 18 mm indicative of a cefamandole susceptible organism.

Gram-negative organisms should be tested with the cefamandole disk (using the above criteria), since cefamandole has been shown by *in vitro* tests to have activity against certain strains of *Enterobacteriaceae* found resistant when tested with the cephalosporin-class disk. Gram-negative organisms having zones of less than 18 mm around the cephalothin disk are not necessarily of intermediate susceptibility or resistant to cefamandole.

The cefamandole disk should not be used for testing susceptibility to other cephalosporins.

A bacterial isolate may be considered susceptible if the MIC value for cefamandole[2] is not more than 16 mcg/ml. Organisms are considered resistant if the MIC is greater than 32 mcg/ml.

INDICATIONS AND USAGE:

Cefamandole nafate is indicated for the treatment of serious infections caused by susceptible strains of the designated microorganisms in the diseases listed below:

Lower respiratory infections, including pneumonia caused by *S. pneumoniae, H. influenzae, Klebsiella* sp, *S. aureus* (penicillinase and non-penicillinase-producing), β-hemolytic streptococci, and *P mirabilis*

Urinary tract infections caused by *E. coli, Proteus* sp (both indole-negative and indole-positive), *Enterobacter* sp, *Klebsiella* sp, group D *streptococci* (Note: Most enterococci, e.g. *E. faecalis*, are resistant), and *S. epidermidis*

Peritonitis caused by *E. coli* and *Enterobacter* sp

Septicemia caused by *E. coli, S. aureus* (penicillinase and non-penicillinase-producing), *S. pneumoniae, S. pyogenes* (group A β-hemolytic streptococci), *H. influenzae,* and *Klebsiella* sp

Skin and skin-structure infections caused by *S. aureus* (penicillinase and non-penicillinase-producing), *S. pyogenes* (group A β-hemolytic streptococci), *H. influenzae, E. coli, Enterobacter* sp, and *P. mirabilis* Bone and joint infections caused by *S. aureus* (penicillinase and non-penicillinase-producing)

Clinical microbiologic studies in nongonococcal pelvic inflammatory disease in females, lower respiratory infections, and skin infections frequently reveal the growth of susceptible strains of both aerobic and anaerobic organisms. Cefamandole nafate has been used successfully in these infections in which several organisms have been isolated. Most strains of *B. fragilis* are resistant *in vitro*; however, infections caused by susceptible strains have been treated successfully.

Specimens for bacteriologic cultures should be obtained in order to isolate and identify causative organisms and to determine their susceptibilities to cefamandole. Therapy may be instituted before results of susceptibility studies are known; however, once these results become available, the antibiotic treatment should be adjusted accordingly.

In certain cases of confirmed or suspected gram-positive or gram-negative sepsis or in patients with other serious infections in which the causative organism has not been identified, cefamandole nafate may be used concomitantly with an aminoglycoside (see PRECAUTIONS). The recommended doses of both antibiotics may be given, depending on the security of the infection and the patient's condition. The renal function of the patient should be carefully monitored, especially if higher dosages of the antibiotics are to be administered.

Antibiotic therapy of β-hemolytic streptococcal infections should continue for at least 10 days.

Preventive Therapy: The administration of cefamandole nafate preoperatively, intraoperatively, and postoperatively may reduce the incidence of certain postoperative infections in patients undergoing surgical procedures that are classified as contaminated or potentially contaminated (*e.g.,* gastrointestinal surgery, cesarean section, vaginal hysterectomy, or cholecystectomy in high-risk patients such as those with acute cholecystitis, obstructive jaundice, or common-bile-duct stones).

In major surgery in which the risk of postoperative infection is low but serious (cardiovascular surgery, neurosurgery, or prosthetic arthroplasty), cefamandole nafate may be effective in preventing such infections.

The preoperative use of cefamandole nafate should be discontinued after 24 hours; however, in prosthetic arthroplasty, it is recommended that administration be continued for 72 hours. If signs of infection occur, specimens for culture should be obtained for identification of the causative organism so that appropriate antibiotic therapy may be instituted.

CONTRAINDICATIONS:

Cefamandole nafate is contraindicated in patients with known allergy to the cephalosporin group of antibiotics.

WARNINGS:

BEFORE THERAPY WITH CEFAMANDOLE NAFATE IS INSTITUTED, CAREFUL INQUIRY SHOULD BE MADE TO DETERMINE WHETHER THE PATIENT HAS HAD PREVIOUS HYPERSENSITIVITY REACTIONS TO CEPHALOSPORINS, PENICILLINS, OR OTHER DRUGS. THIS PRODUCT SHOULD BE GIVEN CAUTIOUSLY TO PENICILLIN-SENSITIVE PATIENTS. ANTIBIOTICS SHOULD BE ADMINISTERED WITH CAUTION TO ANY PATIENT WHO HAS DEMONSTRATED SOME FORM OF ALLERGY, PARTICULARLY TO DRUGS. SERIOUS ACUTE HYPERSENSITIVITY REACTIONS MAY REQUIRE EPINEPHRINE AND OTHER EMERGENCY MEASURES.

In newborn infants, accumulation of other cephalosporin-class antibiotics (with resulting prolongation of drug half-life) has been reported.

Pseudomembranous colitis has been reported with virtually all broad-spectrum antibiotics (including macrolides, semisynthetic penicillins, and cephalosporins); therefore, it is important to consider its diagnosis in patients who develop diarrhea in association with the use of antibiotics. Such colitis may range in severity from mild to life-threatening.

Treatment with broad-spectrum antibiotics alters the normal flora of the colon and may permit overgrowth of clostridia. Studies indicate that a toxin produced by *Clostridium difficile* is a primary cause of antibiotic-associated colitis.

Mild cases of pseudomembranous colitis usually respond to drug discontinuance alone. In moderate to severe cases, management should include sigmoidoscopy, appropriate bacteriologic studies, and fluid, electrolyte, and protein supplementation. When the colitis does not improve after the drug has been discontinued, or when it is severe, oral vancomycin is the drug of choice for antibiotic-associated pseudomembranous colitis produced by *C difficile*. Other causes of colitis should be ruled out.

PRECAUTIONS:

General: Although cefamandole nafate rarely produces alteration in kidney function, evaluation of renal status is recommended, especially in seriously ill patients receiving maximum doses.

Prolonged use of cefamandole nafate may result in the overgrowth of nonsusceptible organisms. Careful observation of the patient is essential. If superinfection occurs during therapy, appropriate measures should be taken.

Nephrotoxicity has been reported following concomitant administration of aminoglycoside antibiotics and cephalosporins.

A false-positive reaction for glucose in the urine may occur with Benedict's or Fehling's solution or with Clinitest tablets but not with Tes-Tape (Glucose Enzymatic Test Strip, USP). There may be a false-positive test for proteinuria with acid and denaturization-precipitation tests.

As with other broad-spectrum antibiotics, hypoprothrombinemia, with or without bleeding, has been reported rarely, but it has been promptly reversed by administration of vitamin K. Such episodes usually have occurred in elderly, debilitated, or otherwise compromised patients with deficient stores of vitamin K. Treatment of such individuals with antibiotics possessing significant gram-negative and/or anaerobic activity is thought to alter the number and/or type of intestinal bacterial flora, with consequent reduction in synthesis of vitamin K. Prophylactic administration of vitamin K may be indicated in such patients, especially when intestinal sterilization and surgical procedures are performed.

In a few patients receiving Mandol, nausea, vomiting, and vasomotor instability with hypotension and peripheral vasodilatation occurred following the ingestion of ethanol.

Cefamandole inhibits the enzyme acetaldehyde dehydrogenase in laboratory animals. This causes accumulation of acetaldehyde when ethanol is administered concomitantly.

Broad-spectrum antibiotics should be prescribed with caution in individuals with a history of gastrointestinal disease, particularly colitis.

Carcinogenesis, Mutagenesis, and Impairment of Fertility: Certain β-lactam antibiotics containing the N-methylthiotetrazole side chain have been reported to cause delayed maturity of the testicular germinal epithelium when given to neonatal rats during initial spermatogenic development (6 to 36 days of age). In animals that were treated from 6 to 36 days of age with 1,000 mg/kg/day of cefamandole (approximately 5 times the maximum clinical dose), the delayed maturity was pronounced and was associated with decreased testicular weights and a reduced number of germinal cells in the leading waves of spermatogenic development. The effect was slight in rats given 50 or 100 mg/kg/day. Some animals that were given 1,000 mg/kg/day during days 6 to 36 were infertile after becoming sexually mature. No adverse effects have been observed in rats exposed *in utero*, in neonatal rats (4 days of age or younger) treated prior to the initiation of spermatogenesis, or in older rats (more than 36 days of age) after exposure for up to 6 months. The significance to man of these findings in rats is unknown because of differences in the time of initiation of spermatogenesis, rate of spermatogenic development, and duration of puberty.

Pregnancy Category B: Reproduction studies have been performed in rats given doses of 500 or 1,000 mg/kg/day and have revealed no evidence of impaired fertility or harm to the fetus due to Mandol. There are, however, no adequate and well-controlled studies in pregnant women. Because animal reproduction studies are not always predictive of human response, this drug should be used during pregnancy only if clearly needed.

Nursing Mothers: Caution should be exercised when cefamandole nafate is administered to a nursing woman.

Usage in Infancy: Cefamandole nafate has been effectively used in this age group, but all laboratory parameters have not been extensively studied in infants between 1 and 6 months of age; safety of this product has not been established in prematures and infants under 1 month of age. Therefore, if cefamandole nafate is administered to infants, the physician should determine whether the potential benefits outweigh the possible risks involved.

ADVERSE REACTIONS:

Gastrointestinal: Symptoms of pseudomembranous colitis may appear either during or after antibiotic treatment. Nausea and vomiting have been reported rarely. As with some penicillins and some other cephalosporins, transient hepatitis and cholestatic jaundice have been reported rarely.

Hypersensitivity: Anaphylaxis, maculopapular rash, urticaria, eosinophilia, and drug fever have been reported. These reactions are more likely to occur in patients with a history of allergy, particularly to penicillin.

Blood: Thrombocytopenia has been reported rarely. Neutropenia has been reported, especially in long courses of treatment. Some individuals have developed positive direct Coombs' tests during treatment with the cephalosporin antibiotics.

Liver: Transient rise in SGOT, SGPT, and alkaline phosphatase levels has been noted.

ADVERSE REACTIONS: *(cont'd)*

Kidney: Decreased creatinine clearance has been reported in patients with prior renal impairment. As with some other cephalosporins, transitory elevations of BUN have occasionally been observed with Mandol; their frequency increases in patients over 50 years of age. In some of these cases, there was also a mild increase in serum creatinine.

Local Reactions: Pain on intramuscular injection is infrequent. Thrombophlebitis occurs rarely.

OVERDOSAGE:

The administration of inappropriately large doses of parenteral cephalosporins may cause seizures, particularly in patients with renal impairment. Dosage reduction is necessary when renal function is impaired (see DOSAGE AND ADMINISTRATION). If seizures occur, the drug should be promptly discontinued; anticonvulsant therapy may be administered if clinically indicated. Hemodialysis may be considered in cases of overwhelming overdosage.

DOSAGE AND ADMINISTRATION:

Adults: The usual dosage range for cefamandole is 500 mg to 1 gram every 4 to 8 hours.

In infections of skin structures and in uncomplicated pneumonia, a dosage of 500 mg every 6 hours is adequate.

In uncomplicated urinary tract infections, a dosage of 500 mg every 8 hours is sufficient. In more serious urinary tract infections, a dosage of 1 gram every 8 hours may be needed.

In severe infections, 1-g doses may be given at 4 to 6 hour intervals.

In life-threatening infections or infections due to less susceptible organisms, doses up to 2 gram every 4 hours (*i.e.,* 12 g/day) may be needed.

Infants and Children: Administration of 50 to 100 mg/kg/day in equally divided doses every 4 to 8 hours has been effective for most infections susceptible to Mandol. This may be increased to a total daily dose of 150 mg/kg/day (not to exceed the maximum adult dose) for severe infections. (*See* Warnings and Precautions for this age group)

Note: As with antibiotic therapy in general, administration of cefamandole nafate should be continued for a minimum of 48 to 72 hours after the patient becomes asymptomatic or after evidence of bacterial eradication has been obtained; a minimum of 10 days of treatment is recommended in infections caused by group A β-hemolytic streptococci in order to guard against the risk or rheumatic fever or glomerulonephritis; frequent bacteriologic and clinical appraisal is necessary during therapy of chronic urinary tract infection and may be required for several months after therapy has been completed; persistent infections may require treatment for several weeks; and doses smaller than those indicated above should not be used.

For perioperative use of Mandol, the following dosages are recommended:

Adults: 1 or 2 gram intravenously or intramuscularly one-half to 1 hour prior to the surgical incision followed by 1 or 2 gram every 6 hours for 24 to 48 hours.

Children (3 months of age and older): 50 to 100 mg/kg/day in equally divided doses by the routes and schedule designated above.

Note: In patients undergoing prosthetic arthroplasty, administration is recommended for as long as 72 hours.

In patients undergoing cesarean section, the initial dose may be administered just prior surgery or immediately after the cord has been clamped.

Impaired Renal Function: When renal function is impaired, a reduced dosage must be employed and the serum levels closely monitored. After an initial dose of 1 to 2 gram (depending on the severity of infection), a maintenance dosage schedule should be followed (see TABLE 1). Continued dosage should be determined by degree of renal impairment, severity of infection, and susceptibility of the causative organism.

TABLE 1 Maintenance Dosage Guide for Patients with Renal Impairment

Creatinine Clearance (ml/min/1.73 m^2)	Renal Function	Life-Threatening-Maximum Dosage	Less Severe Infections
> 80	Normal	2 g q4h	1-2 g q6h
80-50	Mild Impairment	1.5 g q4h OR 2 g q6h	0.75-1.5 g q6h
50-25	Moderate Impairment	1.5 g q6h OR 2 g q8h	0.75-1.5 g q8h
25-10	Severe Impairment	1 g q6h OR 1.25 g q8h	0.5 -1 g q8h
10-2	Marked Impairment	0.67 g q8h OR 1 g q 12h	0.5-0.75 g q12h
< 2	None	0.5 g q8h OR 0.75 g q 12h	0.25-0.5 g q12h

When only serum creatinine is available, the following formula (based on sex, weight, and age of the patient) may be used to convert this value into creatinine clearance. The serum creatinine should represent a steady state of renal function.

$$\text{Males: [Weight (kg)} \times (140 - \text{age})] \div [72 \times \text{serum creatinine}]$$

$$\text{Females: } 0.9 \times \text{above value}$$

MODES OF ADMINISTRATION

Cefamandole nafate may be given intravenously or by deep intramuscular injection into a large muscle mass (such as the gluteus or lateral part of the thigh) to minimize pain.

INTRAMUSCULAR ADMINISTRATION

Each gram of cefamandole nafate should be diluted with 3 ml of one of the following diluents: Sterile Water for Injection, Bacteriostatic Water for Injection, 0.9% Sodium Chloride Injection, or Bacteriostatic Sodium Chloride Injection. Shake well until dissolved.

INTRAVENOUS ADMINISTRATION

The intravenous route may be preferable for patients with bacterial septicemia, localized parenchymal abscesses (such as intra-abdominal abscess), peritonitis, or other severe or life-threatening infections when they may be poor risks because of lowered resistance. In those with normal renal function, the intravenous dosage for such infections is 3 to 12 gram of cefamandole nafate daily. In conditions such as bacterial septicemia, 6 to 12 g/day may be given initially by the intravenous route for several days, and dosage may then be gradually reduced according to clinical response and laboratory findings.

If combination therapy with cefamandole nafate and an aminoglycoside is indicated, each of these antibiotics should be administered in different sites.*Do not mix an aminoglycoside with cefamandole nafate in the same intravenous fluid container.*

A SOLUTION OF 1 gram OF CEFAMANDOLE NAFATE IN 22 ml OF STERILE WATER FOR INJECTION IS ISOTONIC

The choice of saline, dextrose, or electrolyte solution and the volume to be employed are dictated by fluid and electrolyte management.

DOSAGE AND ADMINISTRATION: *(cont'd)*

For direct intermittent intravenous administration, each gram of cefamandole should be reconstituted with 10 ml of Sterile Water for Injection, 5% Dextrose Injection, or 0.9% Sodium Chloride Injection. Slowly inject the solution into the vein over a period of 3 to 5 minutes, or give it through the tubing of an administration set while the patient is also receiving one of the following intravenous fluids:

0.9% Sodium Chloride Injection; 5% Dextrose Injection; 10% Dextrose Injection; 5% Dextrose and 0.9% Sodium Chloride Injection; 5% Dextrose and 0.45% Sodium Chloride Injection; 5% Dextrose and 0.2% Sodium Chloride Injection; or Sodium Lactate Injection (M/6).

Intermittent intravenous infusion with a Y-type administration set or volume control set can also be accomplished while any of the above-mentioned intravenous fluids are being infused. However, during infusion of the solution containing Mandol, it is desirable to discontinue the other solution. When this technique is employed, careful attention should be paid to the volume of the solution containing cefamandole nafate so that the calculated dose will be infused. When a Y-tube hookup is used, 100 ml of the appropriate diluent should be added to the 1 or 2 gram piggyback (100 ml) vial. If Sterile Water for Injection is used as the diluent, reconstitute with approximately 20 ml/g to avoid a hypotonic solution.

For continuous intravenous infusion , each gram of cefamandole should be diluted with 10 ml of Sterile Water for Injection. An appropriate quantity of the resulting solution may be added to an IV bottle containing one of the following fluids:

0.9% Sodium Chloride Injection; 5% Dextrose Injection; 10% Dextrose Injection; 5% Dextrose and 0.9% Sodium Chloride Injection; 5% Dextrose and 0.45% Sodium Chloride Injection;5% Dextrose and 0.2% Sodium Chloride Injection; or Sodium Lactate Injection (M/6).

STABILITY

Reconstituted cefamandole nafate is stable for 24 hours at room temperature (25°C) and for 96 hours if stored under refrigeration (5°C). *During storage at room temperature, carbon dioxide develops inside the vial after reconstitution. This pressure may be dissipated prior to withdrawal of the vial contents, or it may be used to aid withdrawal if the vial is inverted over the syringe needle and the contents are allowed to flow into the syringe.*

Solutions of cefamandole nafate in Sterile Water for Injection, 5% Dextrose Injection, or 0.9% Sodium Chloride Injection that are frozen immediately after reconstitution in Faspak containers and the conventional vials in which the drugs are supplied are stable for 6 months when stored at -20°C. **If the product is warmed (to a maximum of 37°C), care should be taken to avoid heating it after the thawing is complete. Once thawed, the solution should not be refrozen.**

REFERENCES:

1. Bauer AW, Kirby WMM, Sherris JC, Truck M: Antibiotic susceptibility testing by a standardized single disk method. *AM J Clin Pathol*1966;45:493. Standardized disk susceptibility test. *Federal Register* 1974;39:19182-19184. National Committee for Clinical Laboratory Standards, Approved Standards: M2-A3 Performance Standards for Antimicrobial Disk Susceptibility Tests—Third Edition, December, 1984.

2. Determined by the ICS agar-dilution method (Ericsson HM, Sherris JC:*Acta Pathol Microbiol Scand* (B), Supplement No. 217, 1971) or any other method that has been shown to give equivalent results.

HOW SUPPLIED - EQUIVALENTS NOT AVAILABLE:

Injection, Dry-Soln - Intramuscular; - 1 gm/vial

10 ml x 25	**$226.62**	**MANDOL, Lilly**	**00002-7061-25**
96 x 1	**$1019.65**	**MANDOL, Lilly**	**00002-7208-74**

Injection, Dry-Soln - Intramuscular; - 2 gm/vial

2 gm plastic ba	**$1889.87**	**MANDOL, Lilly**	**00002-7209-74**
20 ml x 10	**$181.30**	**MANDOL, Lilly**	**00002-7064-10**
100 ml x 10	**$187.97**	**MANDOL, Lilly**	**00002-7069-10**

Injection, Dry-Soln - Intramuscular; - 500 mg/vial

10 ml x 25	**$113.32**	**MANDOL, Lilly**	**00002-7060-25**

CEFAZOLIN SODIUM *(000683)*

CATEGORIES: Anti-Infectives; Antibiotics; Antimicrobials; Biliary Tract Infections; Bone Infections; Cephalosporins; Cholecystectomy; Cholecystitis; Endocarditis; Infections; Jaundice; Joint Infections; Perioperative Prophylaxis; Prostatitis; Respiratory Tract Infections; Septicemia; Skin Infections; Streptococcal Infection; Urinary Tract Infections; Rheumatic Fever*; Pregnancy Category B; FDA Approval Pre 1982

* Indication not approved by the FDA

BRAND NAMES: **Ancef**; *Anzolin*; *Basocef* (Germany); *Cefa*; *Cefacidal* (France); *Cefamezin* (Mexico); *Cefarad*; *Cefazin*; Cefazolin; *Cefazol*; *Cefazolina*; *Cefazoline Panpharma* (France); *Elzogram* (Germany); *Fazolin*; *Gramaxin* (Germany); *Izacef*; *Kefarin*; Kefzol; *Kofatol*; *Lupex*; *Lyzolin*; *Megacef*; *Oricef*; *Orizolin*; *Reflin*; *Stancef*; *Stazolin*; *Totacef*; *Surzolin*; *Uzolin*; *Zepilen*; Zolicef; *Zolin*; *Zolkef*
(International brand names outside U.S. in italics)

FORMULARIES: Medi-Cal

DESCRIPTION:

STERILE CEFAZOLIN SODIUM, CEFAZOLIN SODIUM INJECTION, AND STERILE CEFAZOLIN SODIUM (LYOPHILIZED) ADD-VANTAGE VIAL

Sterile cefazolin sodium is a sterile, semi-synthetic cephalosporin for intravenous or intramuscular administration. It is the sodium salt of 3-{[(5-methyl-1,3,4-thiadiazol-2-yl)thio]-methyl}-8-oxo-7-[2-(1H-tetrazo 1-1-yl) acetamido]-5-thia-1-azabicyclo[4.2.O]oct-2-ene-2-carboxylic acid.

STERILE CEFAZOLIN SODIUM AND CEFAZOLIN SODIUM INJECTION

The sodium content is 46 mg per gram of cefazolin.

Cefazolin sodium in lyophilized form is supplied in vials equivalent to 500 mg or 1 gram of cefazolin; in "Piggyback" Vials for intravenous admixture equivalent to 1 gram of cefazolin; and in Pharmacy Bulk Vials equivalent to 5 grams or 10 grams of cefazolin.

Cefazolin sodium is also supplied as a frozen, sterile, nonpyrogenic solution of cefazolin sodium in an iso-osmotic diluent in plastic containers. After thawing, the solution is intended for intravenous use.

The plastic container is fabricated from specially formulated polyvinyl chloride. Solutions in contact with the plastic container can leach out certain of its chemical components in very small amounts within the expiration period, e.g., di 2-ethylhexyl phthalate (DEHP), up to 5 parts per million. However, the suitability of the plastic has been confirmed in tests in animals according to the USP biological tests for plastic containers as well as by tissue culture toxicity studies.

STERILE CEFAZOLIN SODIUM (LYOPHILIZED) ADD-VANTAGE VIAL

Its molecular formula is $C_{14}H_{13}N_8NaO_4S_3$ and the molecular weight is 476.48.

The sodium content is 48 mg per gram of cefazolin.

DESCRIPTION: *(cont'd)*

Sterile cefazolin sodium is supplied as a lyophilized form.

Each ADD-Vantage vial of sterile cefazolin sodium is equivalent to 1 gram cefazolin.

CLINICAL PHARMACOLOGY:

Human Pharmacology: After intramuscular administration of cefazolin to normal volunteers, the mean serum concentrations were 37 mcg/ml at one hour and 3 mcg/ml at eight hours following a 500 mg dose, and 64 mcg/ml at one hour and 7 mcg/ml at eight hours following a 1 gram dose.

Studies have shown that following intravenous administration of cefazolin to normal volunteers, mean serum concentrations peaked at approximately 185 mcg/ml and were approximately 4 mcg/ml at eight hours for a 1 gram dose.

The serum half-life for cefazolin is approximately 1.8 hours following IV administration and approximately 2.0 hours following IM administration.

In a study (using normal volunteers) of constant intravenous infusion with dosages of 3.5 mg/kg for one hour (approximately 250 mg) and 1.5 mg/kg the next two hours (approximately 100 mg), cefazolin produced a steady serum level at the third hour of approximately 28 mcg/ml.

Studies in patients hospitalized with infections indicate that cefazolin produces mean peak serum levels approximately equivalent to those seen in normal volunteers.

Bile levels in patients without obstructive biliary disease can reach or exceed serum levels by up to five times; however, in patients with obstructive biliary disease, bile levels of cefazolin are considerably lower than serum levels (< 1.0 mcg/ml).

In synovial fluid, the cefazolin level becomes comparable to that reached in serum at about four hours after drug administration.

Studies of cord blood show prompt transfer of cefazolin across the placenta. Cefazolin is present in very low concentrations in the milk of nursing mothers.

Cefazolin is excreted unchanged in the urine. In the first six hours approximately 60% of the drug is excreted in the urine and this increases to 70%-80% within 24 hours. Cefazolin achieves peak urine concentrations of approximately 2400 mcg/ml and 4000 mcg/ml respectively following 500 mg and 1 gram intramuscular doses.

In patients undergoing peritoneal dialysis (2 l/hr.), cefazolin produced mean serum levels of approximately 10 and 30 mcg/ml after 24 hours' instillation of a dialyzing solution containing 50 mg/l and 150 mg/l, respectively. Mean peak levels were 29 mcg/ml (range 13-44 mcg/ml) with 50 mg/l (three patients), and 72 mcg/ml (range 26-142 mcg/ml) with 150 mg/l (six patients). Intraperitoneal administration of cefazolin is usually well tolerated.

Controlled studies on adult normal volunteers, receiving 1 gram 4 times a day for 10 days, monitoring CBC, SGOT, SGPT, bilirubin, alkaline phosphatase, BUN, creatinine and urinalysis, indicated no clinically significant changes attributed to cefazolin.

Microbiology: *In vitro* tests demonstrate that the bactericidal action of cephalosporins results from inhibition of cell wall synthesis. Cefazolin is active against the following organisms*in vitro* and in clinical infections:

Staphylococcus aureus (including penicillinase-producing strains); *Staphylococcus epidermidis*

Methicillin-resistant staphylococci are uniformly resistant to cefazolin

Group A beta-hemolytic streptococci and other strains of streptococci (many strains of enterococci are resistant)

Streptococcus pneumoniae; *Escherichia coli*; *Proteus mirabilis*; *Klebsiella* species; *Enterobacter aerogenes*; *Haemophilus influenzae*

Most strains of indole positive Proteus (*Proteus vulgaris*), *Enterobacter cloacae*, *Morganella morganii* and *Providencia rettgeri* are resistant. *Serratia*, *Pseudomonas*, *Mima*, *Herellea* species are almost uniformly resistant to cefazolin.

DISK SUSCEPTIBILITY TESTS

Disk Diffusion Technique: Quantitative methods that require measurement of zone diameters give the most precise estimates of antibiotic susceptibility. One such procedure[1] has been recommended for use with disks to test susceptibility to cefazolin.

Reports from a laboratory using the standardized single-disk susceptibility test[1] with a 30 mcg cefazolin disk should be interpreted according to the following criteria:

Susceptible organisms produce zones of 18 mm or greater, indicating that the tested organism is likely to respond to therapy.

Organisms of intermediate susceptibility produce zones 15 to 17 mm, indicating that the tested organism would be susceptible if high dosage is used or if the infection is confined to tissues and fluids (*e.g.*, urine), in which high antibiotic levels are attained.

Resistant organisms produce zones of 14 mm or less, indicating that other therapy should be selected.

For gram-positive isolates, a zone of 18 mm is indicative of a cefazolin-susceptible organism when tested with either the cephalosporin-class disk (30 mcg cephalothin) or the cefazolin disk (30 mcg cefazolin).

Gram-negative organisms should be tested with the cefazolin disk (using the above criteria), since cefazolin has been shown by *in vitro* tests to have activity against certain strains of *Enterobacteriaceae* found resistant when tested with the cephalothin disk. Gram-negative organisms having zones of less than 18 mm around the cephalothin disk may be susceptible to cefazolin.

Standardized procedures require use of control organisms. The 30 mcg cefazolin disk should give zone diameter between 23 and 29 mm for *E. coli* ATCC 25922 and between 29 and 35 mm for *S. aureus* ATCC 25923.

The cefazolin disk should not be used for testing susceptibility to other cephalosporins.

Dilution Techniques: A bacterial isolate may be considered susceptible if the minimal inhibitory concentration (MIC) for cefazolin is not more than 16 mcg per ml. Organisms are considered resistant if the MIC is equal to or greater than 64 mcg per ml.

The range of MIC's for the control strains are as follows:

S. aureus ATCC 25923, 0.25-1.0 mcg/ml

E. coli ATCC 25922, 1.0-4.0 mcg/ml

INDICATIONS AND USAGE:

Cefazolin is indicated in the treatment of the following serious infections due to susceptible organisms:

Respiratory Tract Infections due to *Streptococcus pneumoniae*, *Klebsiella* species, *Haemophilus influenzae*, *Staphylococcus aureus* (penicillin-sensitive and penicillin-resistant) and group A beta-hemolytic streptococci.

Injectable benzathine penicillin is considered to be the drug of choice in treatment and prevention of streptococcal infections, including the prophylaxis of rheumatic fever.

Cefazolin is effective in the eradication of streptococci from the nasopharynx; however, data establishing the efficacy of cefazolin in the subsequent prevention of rheumatic fever are not available at present.

INDICATIONS AND USAGE: *(cont'd)*

Urinary Tract Infections due to *Escherichia coli, Proteus mirabilis, Klebsiella* species and some strains of enterobacter and enterococci.

Skin and Skin Structure Infections due to *Staphylococcus aureus* (penicillin-sensitive and penicillin-resistant), group A beta-hemolytic streptococci and other strains of streptococci.

Biliary Tract Infections due to *Escherichia coli,* various strains of streptococci, *Proteus mirabilis, Klebsiella* species and *Staphylococcus aureus.*

Bone and Joint Infections due to *Staphylococcus aureus.*

Genital Infections (*i.e.,* prostatitis, epididymitis) due to *Escherichia coli, Proteus mirabilis, Klebsiella* species and some strains of enterococci.

Septicemia due to *Streptococcus pneumoniae, Staphylococcus aureus* (penicillin-sensitive and penicillin-resistant), *Proteus mirabilis, Escherichia coli* and *Klebsiella* species.

Endocarditis due to *Staphylococcus aureus* (penicillin-sensitive and penicillin-resistant) and group A beta-hemolytic streptococci.

Appropriate culture and susceptibility studies should be performed to determine susceptibility of the causative organism to cefazolin.

Perioperative Prophylaxis: The prophylactic administration of cefazolin preoperatively, intraoperatively and postoperatively may reduce the incidence of certain postoperative infections in patients undergoing surgical procedures which are classified as contaminated or potentially contaminated (*e.g.,* vaginal hysterectomy, and cholecystectomy in high-risk patients such as those over 70 years of age, with acute cholecystitis, obstructive jaundice or common duct bile stones).

The perioperative use of cefazolin may also be effective in surgical patients in whom infection at the operative site would present a serious risk (*e.g.,* during open-heart surgery and prosthetic arthroplasty).

The prophylactic administration of cefazolin should usually be discontinued within a 24-hour period after the surgical procedure. In surgery where the occurrence of infection may be particularly devastating (*e.g.,* open-heart surgery and prosthetic arthroplasty), the prophylactic administration of cefazolin may be continued for 3 to 5 days following the completion of surgery.

If there are signs of infection, specimens for cultures should be obtained for the identification of the causative organism so that appropriate therapy may be instituted. (See DOSAGE AND ADMINISTRATION.)

CONTRAINDICATIONS:

CEFAZOLIN IS CONTRAINDICATED IN PATIENTS WITH KNOWN ALLERGY TO THE CEPHALOSPORIN GROUP OF ANTIBIOTICS.

WARNINGS:

STERILE CEFAZOLIN SODIUM AND CEFAZOLIN SODIUM INJECTION

BEFORE CEFAZOLIN THERAPY IS INSTITUTED, CAREFUL INQUIRY SHOULD BE MADE CONCERNING PREVIOUS HYPERSENSITIVITY REACTIONS TO CEPHALOSPORINS AND PENICILLIN. CEPHALOSPORIN C DERIVATIVES SHOULD BE GIVEN CAUTIOUSLY IN PENICILLIN-SENSITIVE PATIENTS.

SERIOUS ACUTE HYPERSENSITIVITY REACTIONS MAY REQUIRE EPINEPHRINE AND OTHER EMERGENCY MEASURES.

There is some clinical and laboratory evidence of partial cross-allergenicity of the penicillins and the cephalosporins. Patients have been reported to have had severe reactions (including anaphylaxis) to both drugs.

Any patient who has demonstrated some form of allergy, particularly to drugs, should receive antibiotics cautiously. No exception should be made with regard to cefazolin sodium.

Pseudomembranous colitis has been reported with nearly all antibacterial agents, including cefazolin, and has ranged in severity from mild to life-threatening. Therefore, it is important to consider this diagnosis in patients who present with diarrhea subsequent to the administration of antibacterial agents.

Treatment with antibacterial agents alters the normal flora of the colon and may permit overgrowth of clostridia. Studies indicate that a toxin produced by *Clostridium difficile* is one primary cause of "antibiotic-associated colitis."

Mild cases of pseudomembranous colitis usually respond to drug discontinuation alone. In moderate to severe cases, consideration should be given to management with fluids and electrolytes, protein supplementation and treatment with an oral antibiotic drug effective against *C. difficile.*

STERILE CEFAZOLIN SODIUM (LYOPHILIZED) ADD-VANTAGE VIAL

SERIOUS AND OCCASIONALLY FATAL HYPERSENSITIVITY (anaphylactic) REACTIONS HAVE BEEN REPORTED IN PATIENTS ON PENICILLIN THERAPY. THESE REACTIONS ARE MORE LIKELY TO OCCUR IN INDIVIDUALS WITH A HISTORY OF PENICILLIN HYPERSENSITIVITY AND/OR A HISTORY OF SENSITIVITY TO MULTIPLE ALLERGENS. THERE HAVE BEEN REPORTS OF INDIVIDUALS WITH A HISTORY OF PENICILLIN HYPERSENSITIVITY WHO HAVE EXPERIENCED SEVERE REACTIONS WHEN TREATED WITH CEPHALOSPORINS. BEFORE INITIATING THERAPY WITH CEFAZOLIN, CAREFUL INQUIRY SHOULD BE MADE CONCERNING PREVIOUS HYPERSENSITIVITY REACTIONS TO PENICILLINS, CEPHALOSPORINS, OR OTHER ALLERGENS. IF AN ALLERGIC REACTION OCCURS, CEFAZOLIN SHOULD BE DISCONTINUED AND APPROPRIATE THERAPY SHOULD BE INSTITUTED. **SERIOUS ANAPHYLACTIC REACTIONS REQUIRE IMMEDIATE EMERGENCY TREATMENT WITH EPINEPHRINE. OXYGEN, INTRAVENOUS STEROIDS, AND AIRWAY MANAGEMENT, INCLUDING INTUBATION, SHOULD ALSO BE ADMINISTERED AS INDICATED.**

Pseudomembranous colitis has been reported with nearly all antibacterial agents, including cefazolin, and may range in severity from mild to life-threatening. Therefore, it is important to consider this diagnosis in patients who present with diarrhea subsequent to the administration of antibacterial agents.

Treatment with antibacterial agents alters the normal flora of the colon and may permit overgrowth of clostridia. Studies indicate that a toxin produced by *Clostridium difficile* is one primary cause of "antibiotic-associated colitis."

After the diagnosis of pseudomembranous colitis has been established, therapeutic measures should be initiated. Mild cases of pseudomembranous colitis usually respond to drug discontinuation alone. In moderate to severe cases, consideration should be given to management with fluids and electrolytes, protein supplementation and treatment with an antibacterial drug clinically effective against *C. difficile* colitis.

PRECAUTIONS:

General: Prolonged use of cefazolin may result in the overgrowth of nonsusceptible organisms. Careful clinical observation of the patient is essential.

When cefazolin is administered to patients with low urinary output because of impaired renal function, lower daily dosage is required. (See DOSAGE AND ADMINISTRATION.)

PRECAUTIONS: *(cont'd)*

As with other beta-lactam antibiotics, seizures may occur if inappropriately high doses are administered to patients with impaired renal function. (See DOSAGE AND ADMINISTRATION.)

Cefazolin, as with all cephalosporins, should be prescribed with caution in individuals with a history of gastrointestinal disease, particularly colitis.

Drug/Laboratory Test Interactions: A false positive reaction for glucose in the urine may occur with Benedict's solution, Fehling's solution or with Clinitest tablets, but not with enzyme-based tests such as Clinistix and Tes-Tape (Glucose Enzymatic Test Strip USP).

Positive direct and indirect antiglobulin (Coombs) tests have occurred; these may also occur in neonates whose mothers received cephalosporins before delivery.

Carcinogenesis/Mutagenesis: Mutagenicity studies and long-term studies in animals to determine the carcinogenic potential of cefazolin have not been performed.

Pregnancy, Teratogenic Effects, Pregnancy Category B: Reproduction studies have been performed in rats, mice and rabbits at doses up to 25 times the human dose and have revealed no evidence of impaired fertility or harm to the fetus due to cefazolin. There are, however, no adequate and well-controlled studies in pregnant women. Because animal reproduction studies are not always predictive of human response, this drug should be used during pregnancy only if clearly needed.

Labor and Delivery: When cefazolin has been administered prior to caesarean section, drug levels in cord blood have been approximately one quarter to one third of maternal drug levels. The drug appears to have no adverse effect on the fetus.

Nursing Mothers: Cefazolin is present in very low concentrations in the milk of nursing mothers. Caution should be exercised when cefazolin is administered to a nursing woman.

Pediatric Use: Safety and effectiveness for use in prematures and infants under one month of age have not been established. See DOSAGE AND ADMINISTRATION for recommended dosage in children over one month.

The potential for the toxic effect in children from chemicals that may leach from the single-dose IV preparation in plastic has not been determined.

DRUG INTERACTIONS:

Probenecid may decrease renal tubular secretion of cephalosporins when used concurrently, resulting in increased and more prolonged cephalosporin blood levels.

ADVERSE REACTIONS:

The following reactions have been reported:

Gastrointestinal: Diarrhea, oral candidiasis (oral thrush), vomiting, nausea, stomach cramps, anorexia and pseudomembranous colitis. Onset of pseudomembranous colitis symptoms may occur during or after antibiotic treatment (see WARNINGS.) Nausea and vomiting have been reported rarely.

Allergic: Anaphylaxis, eosinophilia, itching, drug fever, skin rash, Stevens-Johnson syndrome.

Hematologic: Neutropenia, leukopenia, thrombocytopenia, thrombocythemia.

Hepatic and Renal: Transient rise in SGOT, SGPT, BUN and alkaline phosphatase levels has been observed without clinical evidence of renal or hepatic impairment.

Local Reactions: Rare instances of phlebitis have been reported at site of injection. Pain at the site of injection after intramuscular administration has occurred infrequently. Some induration has occurred.

Other Reactions: Genital and anal pruritus (including vulvar pruritus, genital moniliasis and vaginitis).

DOSAGE AND ADMINISTRATION:

NOTE: Sterile cefazolin sodium in the ADD-Vantage Vial is not intended for direct intravenous or intramuscular injection.

TABLE 1 Usual Adult Dosage

Type of Infection	Dose	Frequency
Moderate to severe infections	500 mg to 1 gram	every 6 to 8 hrs.
Mild infections caused by susceptible gram + cocci	250 mg to 500 mg	every 8 hours
Acute, uncomplicated urinary tract infections	1 gram	every 12 hours
Pneumococcal pneumonia	500 mg	every 12 hours
Severe, life-threatening infections (*e.g.,* endocarditis, septicemia)*	1 gram to 1.5 grams	every 6 hours

* In rare instances, doses of up to 12 grams of cefazolin sodium per day have been used.

Perioperative Prophylactic Use: To prevent postoperative infection in contaminated or potentially contaminated surgery, recommended doses are:

a. 1 gram IV or IM administered 1/2 hour to 1 hour prior to the start of surgery.

b. For lengthy operative procedures (*e.g.,* 2 hours or more), 500 mg to 1 gram IV or IM during surgery (administration modified depending on the duration of the operative procedure).

c. 500 mg to 1 gram IV or IM every 6 to 8 hours for 24 hours postoperatively.

It is important that 1) the preoperative dose be given just (1/2 to 1 hour) prior to the start of surgery so that adequate antibiotic levels are present in the serum and tissues at the time of initial surgical incision; and 2) cefazolin be administered, if necessary, at appropriate intervals during surgery to provide sufficient levels of the antibiotic at the anticipated moments of greatest exposure to infective organisms.

In surgery where the occurrence of infection may be particularly devastating (*e.g.,* open-heart surgery and prosthetic arthroplasty), the prophylactic administration of cefazolin may be continued for 3 to 5 days following the completion of surgery.

Dosage Adjustment for Patients with Reduced Renal Function: Cefazolin may be used in patients with reduced renal function with the following dosage adjustments: Patients with a creatinine clearance of 55 ml/min. or greater or a serum creatinine of 1.5 mg% or less can be given full doses. Patients with creatinine clearance rates of 35 to 54 ml/min. or serum creatinine of 1.6 to 3.0 mg% can also be given full doses but dosage should be restricted to at least 8 hour intervals. Patients with creatinine clearance rates of 11 to 34 ml/min. or serum creatinine of 3.1 to 4.5 mg% should be given 1/2 the usual dose every 12 hours. Patients with creatinine clearance rates of 10 ml/min. or less or serum creatinine of 4.6 mg% or greater should be given 1/2 the usual dose every 18 to 24 hours. All reduced dosage recommendations apply after an initial loading dose appropriate to the severity of the infection. Patients undergoing peritoneal dialysis: See CLINICAL PHARMACOLOGY, Human Pharmacology.

Pediatric Dosage: In children, a total daily dosage of 25 to 50 mg per kg (approximately 10 to 20 mg per pound) of body weight, divided into three or four equal doses, is effective for most mild to moderately severe infections. Total daily dosage may be increased to 100 mg per kg

DOSAGE AND ADMINISTRATION: *(cont'd)*

(45 mg per pound) of body weight for severe infections. Since safety for use in premature infants and in infants under one month has not been established, the use of cefazolin in these patients is not recommended. SeeTABLE 2 and TABLE 3.

TABLE 2 Pediatric Dosage Guide

Weight Lbs	Weight Kg	25 mg/kg/Day Divided into 3 Doses: Approximate Single Dose mg/q8h	Vol. (ml) needed with dilution of 125 mg/ml	25 mg/kg/Day Divided into 4 Doses: Approximate Single Dose mg/q6h	Vol. (ml) needed with dilution of 125 mg/ml
10	4.5	40 mg	0.35 ml	30 mg	0.25 ml
20	9.0	75 mg	0.60 ml	55 mg	0.45 ml
30	13.6	115 mg	0.90 ml	85 mg	0.70 ml
40	18.1	150 mg	1.20 ml	115 mg	0.90 ml
50	22.7	190 mg	1.50 ml	140 mg	1.10 ml

TABLE 3 Pediatric Dosage Guide

Weight Lbs	Weight Kg	50 mg/kg/Day Divided into 3 Doses: Approximate Single Dose mg/q8h	Vol. (ml) needed with dilution of 225 mg/ml	50 mg/kg/Day Divided into 4 Doses: Approximate Single Dose mg/q6h	Vol. (ml) needed with dilution of 225 mg/ml
10	4.5	75 mg	0.35 ml	55 mg	0.25 ml
20	9.0	150 mg	0.70 ml	110 mg	0.50 ml
30	13.6	225 mg	1.00 ml	170 mg	0.75 ml
40	18.1	300 mg	1.35 ml	225 mg	1.00 ml
50	22.7	375 mg	1.70 ml	285 mg	1.25 ml

In children with mild to moderate renal impairment (creatinine clearance of 70 to 40 ml/min.), 60 percent of the normal daily dose given in equally divided doses every 12 hours should be sufficient. In patients with moderate impairment (creatinine clearance of 40 to 20 ml/min.), 25 percent of the normal daily dose given in equally divided doses every 12 hours should be adequate. Children with severe renal impairment (creatinine clearance of 20 to 5 ml/min.), may be given 10 percent of the normal daily dose every 24 hours. All dosage recommendations apply after an initial loading dose.

RECONSTITUTION

Preparation of Parenteral Solution: Parenteral drug products should be SHAKEN WELL when reconstituted, and inspected visually for particulate matter and discoloration prior to administration. If particulate matter is evident in reconstituted fluids, the drug solutions should be discarded.

When reconstituted or diluted according to the instructions below, sterile cefazolin sodium is stable for 24 hours at room temperature or for 96 hours if stored under refrigeration (5°C or 41°F). Reconstituted solutions may range in color from pale yellow to yellow without a change in potency.

STERILE CEFAZOLIN SODIUM AND CEFAZOLIN SODIUM INJECTION

Single-Dose Vials: For IM injection, IV direct (bolus) injection or IV infusion, reconstitute with Sterile Water for Injection according to TABLE 4. SHAKE WELL.

TABLE 4

Vial Size	Amount of Diluent	Approximate Concentration	Approximate Available Volume
500 mg	2.0 ml	225 mg/ml	2.2 ml
1 gram	2.5 ml	330 mg/ml	3.0 ml

Pharmacy Bulk Vials: Add Sterile Water for Injection, Bacteriostatic Water for Injection or Sodium Chloride Injection according to TABLE 5. SHAKE WELL.

TABLE 5

Vial Size	Amount of Diluent	Approximate Concentration	Approximate Available Volume
5 mg	23 ml	1 gram/5 ml	26 ml
	48 ml	1 gram/10 ml	51 ml
10 grams	45 ml	1 gram/5 ml	51 ml
	96 ml	1 gram/10 ml	102 ml

'Piggyback' Vials: Reconstitute with 50 to 100 ml of Sodium Chloride Injection or other IV solution listed under DOSAGE AND ADMINISTRATION. When adding diluent to vial, allow air to escape by using a small vent needle or by pumping the syringe. SHAKE WELL. Administer with primary IV fluids, as a single dose.

ADMINISTRATION

Intramuscular Administration: Reconstitute vials with Sterile Water for Injection according to the dilution table above. Shake well until dissolved. Cefazolin sodium should be injected into a large muscle mass. Pain on injection is infrequent with cefazolin sodium.

Intravenous Administration: Direct (bolus) injection: Following reconstitution according to the above table, further dilute vials with approximately 5 ml Sterile Water for Injection. Inject the solution slowly over 3 to 5 minutes, directly or through tubing for patients receiving parenteral fluids.

Intermittent or continuous infusion: Dilute reconstituted cefazolin sodium in 50 to 100 ml of one of the following solutions:

Sodium Chloride Injection, USP

5% or 10% Dextrose Injection, USP

5% Dextrose in Lactated Ringer's Injection, USP

5% Dextrose and 0.9% Sodium Chloride Injection, USP

5% Dextrose and 0.45% Sodium Chloride Injection, USP

5% Dextrose and 0.2% Sodium Chloride Injection, USP

Lactated Ringer's Injection, USP

Invert Sugar 5% or 10% in Sterile Water for Injection

Ringer's Injection, USP

5% Sodium Bicarbonate Injection, USP

DIRECTIONS FOR USE OF CEFAZOLIN SODIUM INJECTION VIAFLEX PLUS CONTAINER (PL 146 PLASTIC)

Cefazolin sodium in Viaflex Plus Container (PL 146 Plastic) is to be administered either as a continuous or intermittent infusion using sterile equipment.

DOSAGE AND ADMINISTRATION: *(cont'd)*

Storage: Store in a freezer capable of maintaining a temperature of -20°C(-4°F).

Thawing of Plastic Container: Thaw frozen container at room temperature (25°C or 77°F) or under refrigeration (5°C or 41°F). (DO NOT FORCE THAW BY IMMERSION IN WATER BATHS OR BY MICROWAVE IRRADIATION.)

Containers may be thawed individually after separation from the frozen shingle. A shingle consists of stacked frozen containers. Remove frozen shingle from carton and allow to rest at room temperature until the containers can be easily separated (approximately 5 minutes). Then grasp the body of the container (not the ports, corner, or tail flap) to separate individual units. *Promptly* return unneeded frozen containers to freezer.

Check for minute leaks by squeezing container firmly. If leaks are detected, discard solution as sterility may be impaired.

Do not add supplementary medication.

The container should be visually inspected. Components of the solution may precipitate in the frozen state and will dissolve upon reaching room temperature with little or no agitation. Potency is not affected.

Agitate after solution has reached room temperature. If after visual inspection the solution remains cloudy or if an insoluble precipitate is noted or if any seals or outlet ports are not intact, the container should be discarded.

The thawed solution is stable for 10 days under refrigeration (5°C or 41°F) and 48 hours at room temperature (25°C or 77°F). Do not refreeze thawed antibiotics.

Use sterile equipment. It is recommended that the intravenous administration apparatus be replaced at least once every 48 hours.

Caution: Do not use plastic containers in series connections. Such use could result in air embolism due to residual air being drawn from the primary container before administration of the fluid from the secondary container is complete.

Preparation for administration

1. Suspend container from eyelet support.

2. Remove plastic protector from outlet port at bottom of container.

3. Attach administration set. Refer to complete directions accompanying set.

STERILE CEFAZOLIN SODIUM (LYOPHILIZED) ADD-VANTAGE VIAL

ADD-Vantage Vials: ADD-Vantage Vials of sterile cefazolin sodium are to be reconstituted only with 0.9% Sodium Chloride Injection or 5% Dextrose Injection in the 50 ml or 100 ml ADD-Vantage Flexible Diluent Containers or with 0.45% Sodium Chloride Injection in the 50 ml ADD-Vantage Flexible Diluent Container. Sterile cefazolin sodium supplied in single-dose ADD-Vantage Vials should be prepared as directed below.

INSTRUCTIONS FOR USE

To Open Container: Peel overwrap at corner and remove solution container. Some opacity of the plastic due to moisture absorption during the sterilization process may be observed. This is normal and does not affect the solution quality or safety. The opacity will diminish gradually.

TO ASSEMBLE VIAL AND FLEXIBLE DILUENT CONTAINER: (USE ASEPTIC TECHNIQUE)

1. Remove the protective covers from the top of the vial and the vial port on the diluent container as follows:

a. To remove the breakaway vial cap, swing the pull ring over the top of the vial and pull down far enough to start the opening, then pull straight up to remove the cap. *NOTE:*Once the breakaway cap has been removed, do not access vial with syringe.

b. To remove the vial port cover, grasp the tab on the pull ring, pull up to break the three tie strings, then pull back to remove the cover.

2. Screw the vial into the vial port until it will go no further. THE VIAL MUST BE SCREWED IN TIGHTLY TO ASSURE A SEAL. This occurs approximately 1/2 turn (180°) after the first audible click. The clicking sound does not assure a seal; the vial must be turned as far as it will go. *NOTE:*Once vial is seated, do not attempt to remove.

3. Recheck the vial to assure that it is tight by trying to turn it further in the direction of assembly.

4. Label appropriately.

To Reconstitute the Drug

1. Squeeze the bottom of the diluent container gently to inflate the portion of the container surrounding the end of the drug vial.

2. With the other hand, push the drug vial down into the container telescoping the walls of the container. Grasp the inner cap of the vial through the walls of the container.

3. Pull the inner cap from the drug vial. Verify that the rubber stopper has been pulled out, allowing the drug and diluent to mix.

4. Mix container contents thoroughly and use within the specified time.

Preparation for Administration: (Use Aseptic Technique)

1. Confirm the activation and admixture of vial contents.

2. Check for leaks by squeezing container firmly. If leaks are found, discard unit as sterility may be impaired.

3. Close flow control clamp of administration set.

4. Remove cover from outlet port at bottom of container.

5. Insert piercing pin of administration set into port with a twisting motion until the pin is firmly seated. *NOTE:* See full directions on administration set carton.

6. Lift the free end of the hanger loop on the bottom of the vial, breaking the two tie strings. Bend the loop outward to lock it in the upright position, then suspend container from hanger.

7. Squeeze and release drip chamber to establish proper fluid level in chamber.

8. Open flow control clamp and clear air from set. Close clamp.

9. Attach set to venipuncture device. If device is not indwelling, prime and make venipuncture.

10. Regulate rate of administration with flow control clamp.

WARNING: DO NOT USE FLEXIBLE CONTAINER IN SERIES CONNECTIONS.

COMPATIBILITY AND STABILITY: Ordinarily ADD-Vantage Vials should be reconstituted only when it is certain that the patient is ready to receive the drug. However, sterile cefazolin sodium in ADD-Vantage vials is stable for 24 hours at room temperature when reconstituted as directed (see Reconstitution).

STERILE CEFAZOLIN SODIUM, CEFAZOLIN SODIUM INJECTION, AND STERILE CEFAZOLIN SODIUM (LYOPHILIZED) ADD-VANTAGE VIAL

As with other cephalosporins, sterile cefazolin sodium tends to darken depending on storage conditions; within the stated recommendations, however, product potency is not adversely affected.

Before reconstitution protect from light and store at controlled room temperature 15° to 30°C (59° to 86°F).

DOSAGE AND ADMINISTRATION: *(cont'd)*

(Sterile Cefazolin Sodium and Cefazolin Sodium Injection - SmithKline Beecham Pharmaceuticals, 7/92, AF:L48)

(Sterile Cefazolin Sodium (lyophilized) ADD-Vantage Vial - SmithKline Beecham Pharmaceuticals, 8/94, CE:L1AV)

REFERENCES:

1. Bauer, A.W.; Kirby, W.M.M.; Sherris, J.C., and Turck, M.: Antibiotic Testing by a Standardized Single Disc Method, Am. J. Clin. Path. 45:493, 1966. Standardized Disc Susceptibility Test, Federal Register 39:19182-19184, 1974.

HOW SUPPLIED - RATED THERAPEUTICALLY EQUIVALENT:

Injection, Dry-Soln - Intramuscular; - 1 gm/vial

1 gm	$2.48	ZOLICEF 1, Mead Johnson	00015-7339-12
1 gm vial x 1	$3.84	KEFZOL, Lilly	00002-7083-01
1 gm vial x 10	$38.40	KEFZOL, Lilly	00002-7083-10
1 gm x 10	$35.25	Sterile Cefazolin Sodium, Bristol Myers Squibb	00003-2928-30
1 gm x 96	$413.58	KEFZOL, Lilly	00002-7202-74
1's	$2.48	Cefazolin Sodium, Mead Johnson	00015-7339-99
1's	$5.08	Cefazolin, Abbott	00074-4732-03
10 ml	$2.88	KEFZOL, Lilly	00002-1498-01
10 ml x 1	**$3.56**	**ANCEF, SKB Pharms**	**00007-3130-01**
10 ml x 10	$59.00	Cefazolin Sodium, Schein Pharm (US)	00364-2465-33
10 ml x 25	$72.00	KEFZOL, Lilly	00002-1498-25
10 ml x 25	**$75.00**	**ANCEF, SKB Pharms**	**00007-3130-76**
10 ml x 25	**$89.06**	**ANCEF, SKB Pharms**	**00007-3130-16**
10 ml x 100 ml	$52.96	Cefazolin Sodium, Vial, Marsam	00209-0900-22
10's	$22.00	Cefazolin, Raway	00686-0900-22
10's	$30.61	Cefazolin Sodium, Mead Johnson	00015-7339-31
10's	$37.50	Cefazolin Sodium, Solopak Labs	39769-0283-90
10's	$52.96	CEFAZOLIN SODIUM, Marsam	00209-0902-22
10's	$59.89	Cefazolin Sodium, Marsam	00209-1002-42
10's	$66.60	Cefazolin, Teva	00093-0707-03
10's	$70.00	Cefazolin, Goldline Labs	00182-3048-70
10's	$73.25	Cefazolin Sodium, Fujisawa USA	00469-2371-63
25 vials x 1	$84.00	KEFZOL, Lilly	00002-7266-25
25's	$78.13	Cefazolin Sodium, Solopak Labs	39769-0282-10
25's	$147.25	Cefazolin, Teva	00093-0705-07
25's	$162.19	CEFAZOLIN SODIUM, Fujisawa USA	00469-2371-30
100 ml x 10	**$38.85**	**ANCEF, SKB Pharms**	**00007-3137-76**
100 ml x 10	**$46.19**	**ANCEF, SKB Pharms**	**00007-3137-05**
100 ml x 10	$59.89	Cefazolin Sodium, Piggyback, Marsam	00209-1000-42
100 ml x 10	$65.00	Cefazolin Sodium, Schein Pharm (US)	00364-2465-93
500 mg x 10	$18.00	Sterile Cefazolin Sodium, Bristol Myers Squibb	00003-2927-30

Injection, Dry-Soln - Intramuscular; - 5 gm/vial

10's	$176.70	Sterile Cefazolin Sodium, Bristol Myers Squibb	00003-2929-40
100 ml x 10	**$178.13**	**ANCEF, SKB Pharms**	**00007-3136-05**

Injection, Dry-Soln - Intramuscular; - 10 gm/vial

1's	$37.50	Cefazolin, Goldline Labs	00182-3045-70
10's	$189.99	Cefazolin Sodium, Mead Johnson	00015-7346-39
10's	$330.20	Cefazolin, Teva	00093-0709-03
10's	$350.00	Cefazolin Sodium, Solopak Labs	39769-0284-90
20 gm x 10	$720.70	Sterile Cefazolin Sodium 10, Bristol Myers Squibb	00003-2949-30
100 ml x 10	$58.00	Cefazolin Sodium, Schein Pharm (US)	00364-2466-93
100 ml x 10	**$300.00**	**ANCEF, SKB Pharms**	**00007-3135-76**
100 ml x 10	$317.88	Cefazolin Sodium, Bulk, Marsam	00209-1100-52
100 ml x 10	**$356.25**	**ANCEF, SKB Pharms**	**00007-3135-05**

Injection, Dry-Soln - Intramuscular; - 20 gm/vial

100 ml x 6	$345.61	KEFZOL 20, Lilly	00002-7021-16

Injection, Dry-Soln - Intramuscular; - 250 mg/vial

10 ml	$1.36	KEFZOL, Lilly	00002-1496-01
250 mg x 10	$15.10	Sterile Cefazolin Sodium, Bristol Myers Squibb	00003-2926-30

Injection, Dry-Soln - Intramuscular; - 500 mg/vial

1's	$1.31	Cefazolin Sodium, Mead Johnson	00015-7338-99
1's	$2.75	Cefazolin Sodium, Pasadena	00418-2360-30
10 ml	$1.44	KEFZOL, Lilly	00002-1497-01
10 ml x 10	$26.52	Cefazolin Sodium, Vial, Marsam	00209-0800-22
10 ml x 25	$36.00	KEFZOL, Lilly	00002-1497-25
10 ml x 25	**$37.50**	**ANCEF, SKB Pharms**	**00007-3131-76**
10 ml x 25	**$44.53**	**ANCEF, SKB Pharms**	**00007-3131-16**
10's	$13.00	Cefazolin, Raway	00686-0800-20
10's	$22.30	Cefazolin Sodium, Bristol Myers Squibb	00003-2927-35
10's	$25.00	Cefazolin Sodium, Solopak Labs	39769-0281-90
10's	$26.52	Cefazolin Sodium, Marsam	00209-0802-22
10's	$37.10	Cefazolin, Teva	00093-0706-03
10's	$40.88	Cefazolin Sodium, Fujisawa USA	00469-2361-63
10's	$45.00	Cefazolin, Goldline Labs	00182-3047-70
25's	$43.75	Cefazolin Sodium, Solopak Labs	39769-0280-10
25's	$73.75	Cefazolin, Teva	00093-0704-07
25's	$80.94	CEFAZOLIN SODIUM, Fujisawa USA	00469-2361-30
25's	$95.00	Cefazolin Sodium, Pasadena	00418-2360-10
100 ml x 10	$22.92	KEFZOL, Lilly	00002-7018-10
100 ml x 10	$30.14	Cefazolin Sodium, Piggyback, Marsam	00209-0850-42
500 mg plastic	$275.34	KEFZOL, Lilly	00002-7201-74
500 mg x 10	$24.00	KEFZOL 500, Lilly	00002-7082-10
500mg(10 ml)	$1.31	ZOLICEF 500, Mead Johnson	00015-7338-12

HOW SUPPLIED - NOT RATED EQUIVALENT:

Injection, Dry-Soln - Intramuscular; - 1 gm/vial

24's	**$136.80**	**ANCEF IN D5W, SKB Pharms**	**00007-3143-04**

Injection, Dry-Soln - Intramuscular; - 10 gm/vial

10's	$317.88	Cefazolin Sodium, Marsam	00209-1102-52
10's	$367.13	CEFAZOLIN SODIUM, Fujisawa USA	00469-2382-00

Injection, Dry-Soln - Intramuscular; - 500 mg/vial

24's	**$100.80**	**ANCEF IN D5W, SKB Pharms**	**00007-3142-04**

CEFEPIME HYDROCHLORIDE *(003198)*

CATEGORIES: Anti-Infectives; Antibiotics; Antimicrobials; Cephalosporins; Infections; Skin Infections; Urinary Tract Infections; FDA Approved 1996 Apr

BRAND NAMES: *Maxcef*; **Maxipime**
(International brand names outside U.S. in italics)

DESCRIPTION:

Cefepime hydrochloride is a semi-synthetic, broad spectrum, cephalosporin antibiotic for parenteral administration. The chemical name is 1-[[(6R,7R)-7-[2-(2-amino-4-thiazolyl)-glyoxylamido]-2-carboxy-8-oxo-5-thia-1-azabicyclo[4.2.0] oct-2-en-3-yl]methyl]-1-methyl-pyrrolidinium chloride, 7^2-(Z)-(O-methyloxime), monohydrochloride, monohydrate. Cefepime hydrochloride is a white to pale yellow powder with a molecular formula of $C_{19}H_{25}ClN_6O_5S_2 \cdot HCl \cdot H_2O$ and a molecular weight of 571.5. It is highly soluble in water. Cefepime hydrochloride for injection is supplied for intramuscular or intravenous administration in strengths equivalent to 500 mg, 1 g and 2 g of cefepime. (See DOSAGE AND ADMINISTRATION.) Cefepime hydrochloride is a sterile, dry mixture of cefepime hydrochloride and L-arginine. The L-arginine, at an approximate concentration of 725 mg/g of cefepime, is added to control the pH of the constituted solution at 4.0 - 6.0. Freshly constituted solutions of Cefepime hydrochloride will range in color from colorless to amber.

CLINICAL PHARMACOLOGY:

PHARMACOKINETICS

The average plasma concentrations of cefepime observed in healthy adult male volunteers (n=9) at various times following single 30-minute infusions (IV) of cefepime 500 mg, 1 g, and 2 g are summarized in Table 1. Elimination of cefepime is principally via renal excretion with an average (± SD) half-life of 2.0 (± 0.3) hours and total body clearance of 120.0 (± 8.0) mL/min in healthy volunteers. Cefepime pharmacokinetics are linear over the range 250 mg to 2 g. There is no evidence of accumulation in healthy adult male volunteers (n=7) receiving clinically relevant doses for a period of 9 days.

ABSORPTION

The average plasma concentrations of cefepime and its derived pharmacokinetic parameters after intravenous administration are portrayed in Table 1.

TABLE 1 Average Plasma Concentrations in mcg/mL of Cefepime and Derived Pharmacokinetic Parameters (± SD), Intravenous Administration

Parameter	500 mg IV	1 g IV	2 g IV
0.5 hr	38.2	78.7	163.1
1.0 hr	21.6	44.5	85.8
2.0 hr	11.6	24.3	44.8
4.0 hr	5.0	10.5	19.2
8.0 hr	1.4	2.4	3.9
12.0 hr	0.2	0.6	1.1
C_{max}, mcg/mL	39.1 (3.5)	81.7 (5.1)	163.9 (25.3)
AUC, hr·mcg/mL	70.8 (6.7)	148.5 (15.1)	284.8 (30.6)
Number of subjects (male)	9	9	9

Following intramuscular (IM) administration, cefepime is completely absorbed. The average plasma concentrations of cefepime at various times following a single IM injection are summarized in Table 2. The pharmacokinetics of cefepime are linear over the range of 500 mg to 2 g IM and do not vary with respect to treatment duration.

TABLE 2 Average Plasma Concentrations in mcg/mL of Cefepime and Derived Pharmacokinetic Parameters (± SD), Intramuscular Administration

Parameter	500 mg IM	1 g IM	2 g IM
0.5 hr	8.2	14.8	36.1
1.0 hr	12.5	25.9	49.9
2.0 hr	12.0	26.3	51.3
4.0 hr	6.9	16.0	31.5
8.0 hr	1.9	4.5	8.7
12.0 hr	0.7	1.4	2.3
C_{max}, mcg/mL	13.9 (3.4)	29.6 (4.4)	57.5 (9.5)
T_{max}, hr	1.4 (0.9)	1.6 (0.4)	1.5 (0.4)
AUC, hr·mcg/mL	60.0 (8.0)	137.0 (11.0)	262.0 (23.0)
Number of subjects (male)	6	6	12

DISTRIBUTION

The average steady state volume of distribution of cefepime is 18.0 (± 2.0)L. The serum protein binding of cefepime is approximately 20% and is independent of its concentration in serum.

Cefepime is excreted in human milk. A nursing infant consuming approximately 1000 mL of human milk per day would receive approximately 0.5 mg of cefepime per day. (See PRECAUTIONS, Nursing Mothers.)

Concentrations of cefepime achieved in specific tissues and body fluids are listed in Table 3.

TABLE 3 Average Concentrations of Cefepime in Specific Body Fluids (mcg/mL) or Tissues (mcg/g)

Tissue or Fluid	Dose/Route	# of patients	Average Time of Sample Post-Dose (hr)	Average Concentration
Blister Fluid	2 g IV	6	1.5	81.4mcg/mL
Bronchial Mucosa	2 g IV	20	4.8	24.1 mcg/mL
Sputum	2 g IV	5	4.0	7.4 mcg/mL
	500 mg IV	8	0-4	292 mcg/mL
Urine	1 g IV	12	0-4	926 mcg/mL
	2 g IV	12	0-4	3120 mcg/mL

Data suggest that cefepime does cross the inflamed blood-brain barrier. **The clinical relevance of these data are uncertain at this time.**

METABOLISM AND EXCRETION

Cefepime is metabolized to N-methylpyrrolidine (NMP) which is rapidly converted to the N-oxide (NMP-N-oxide). Urinary recovery of unchanged cefepime accounts for approximately 85% of the administered dose. Less than 1% of the administered dose is recovered from urine as NMP, 6.8% as NMP-N-oxide, and 2.5% as an epimer of cefepime. Because renal excretion is a significant pathway of elimination, patients with renal dysfunction and patients undergoing hemodialysis require dosage adjustment. (See DOSAGE AND ADMINISTRATION.)

SPECIAL POPULATIONS

Geriatric patients: Cefepime pharmacokinetics have been investigated in elderly (65 years of age and older) men (n=12) and women (n=12) whose creatinine clearance was 74.0 (±15.0) mL/min. There appeared to be a decrease in cefepime total body clearance as a function of creatinine clearance. Therefore, dosage administration of cefepime in the elderly should be adjusted as appropriate if the patient's creatinine clearance is 60 mL/min or less. (See DOSAGE AND ADMINISTRATION.)

Renal Insufficiency: Cefepime pharmacokinetics have been investigated in patients with various degrees of renal insufficiency (n=30). The average half-life in patients requiring hemodialysis was 13.5 (±2.7) hours and in patients requiring continuous peritoneal dialysis was 19.0 (±2.0) hours. Cefepime total body clearance decreased proportionally with creati-

CLINICAL PHARMACOLOGY: *(cont'd)*

nine clearance in patients with abnormal renal function, which serves as the basis for dosage adjustment recommendations in this group of patients. (See DOSAGE AND ADMINISTRATION.)

Hepatic Insufficiency: The pharmacokinetics of cefepime were unaltered in patients with impaired hepatic function who received a single 1 g dose (n=11).

MICROBIOLOGY

Cefepime is a bactericidal agent that acts by inhibition of bacterial cell wall synthesis. Cefepime has a broad spectrum of *in vitro* activity that encompasses a wide range of gram-positive and gram-negative bacteria. Cefepime has a low affinity for chromosomally-encoded beta-lactamases. Cefepime is highly resistant to hydrolysis by most beta-lactamases and exhibits rapid penetration into gram-negative bacterial cells. Within bacterial cells, the molecular targets of cefepime are the penicillin binding proteins (PBP).

Cefepime has been shown to be active against most strains of the following microorganisms, both*in vitro* and in clinical infections as described in the INDICATIONS AND USAGEsection.

Aerobic Gram-Negative Microorganisms:

Enterobacter spp.
Escherichia coli
Klebsiella pneumoniae
Proteus mirabilis
Pseudomonas aeruginosa

Aerobic Gram-Positive Microorganisms:

Staphylococcus aureus (methicillin-susceptible strains only)
Streptococcus pneumoniae
Streptococcus pyogenes (Lancefield's Group A streptococci)

The following *in vitro* data are available; **but their clinical significance is unknown.**Cefepime has been shown to have*in vitro* activity against most strains of the following microorganisms; however, the safety and effectiveness of cefepime in treating clinical infections due to these microorganisms have not been established in adequate and well-controlled trials.

Aerobic Gram-Positive Microorganisms:

Staphylococcus epidermidis (methicillin-susceptible strains only)
Staphylococcus saprophyticus
Streptococcus agalactiae (Lancefield's Group B streptococci)

NOTE: Most strains of enterococci, *e.g. Enterococcus faecalis,* and methicillin-resistant staphylococci are resistant to cefepime.

Aerobic Gram-Negative Microorganisms:

Acinetobacter calcoaceticus subsp. *lwoffi*
Citrobacter diversus
Citrobacter freundii
Enterobacter agglomerans
Haemophilus influenzae (including beta-lactamase producing strain)
Hafnia alvei
Klebsiella oxytoca
Moraxella (Branhamella) catarrhalis (including beta-lactamase producing strains)
Morganella morganii
Proteus vulgaris
Providencia rettgeri
Providencia stuartii
Serratia marcescens

NOTE: Cefepime is inactive against many strains of *Stenotrophomonas* (formerly *Xanthomonas maltophilia* and *Pseudomonas maltophilia*).

Anaerobic Microorganisms:

NOTE: Cefepime is inactive against most strains of *Clostridium difficile.*

SUSCEPTIBILITY TESTS

Dilution Techniques

Quantitative methods are used to determine antimicrobial minimum inhibitory concentrations (MIC's). These MIC's provide estimates of the susceptibility of bacteria to antimicrobial compounds. The MIC's should be determined using a standardized procedure. Standardized procedures are based on a dilution method[1] (broth or agar) or equivalent with standardized inoculum concentrations and standardized concentrations of cefepime powder. The MIC values should be interpreted according to the following criteria:

TABLE 4

Microorganism	MIC (mcg/ml) Susceptible (S)	Intermediate (I)	Resistant (R)
Microorganisms other than*Haemophilus* spp.* and *S. pneumoniae**	≤8	16	≥32
Haemophilus spp.*	≤2	—*	—*
*Streptococcus pneumoniae**	≤0.5	1	≥2

* NOTE: Isolates from these species should be tested for susceptibility using specialized dilution testing methods.[1] Also, strains of *Haemophilus* spp. with MIC's greater than 2 mcg/mL should be considered equivocal and should be further evaluated.

A report of "Susceptible" indicates that the pathogen is likely to be inhibited if the antimicrobial compound in the blood reaches the concentrations usually achievable. A report of "Intermediate" indicates that the result should be considered equivocal, and, if the microorganism is not fully susceptible to alternative, clinically feasible drugs, the test should be repeated. This category implies possible clinical applicability in body sites where the drug is physiologically concentrated or in situations where high dosage of drug can be used. This category also provides a buffer zone which prevents small uncontrolled technical factors from causing major discrepancies in interpretation. A report of "Resistant" indicates that the pathogen is not likely to be inhibited if the antimicrobial compound in the blood reaches the concentrations usually achievable; other therapy should be selected.

Standardized susceptibility test procedures require the use of laboratory control microorganisms to control the technical aspects of the laboratory procedures. Laboratory control microorganisms are specific strains of microbiological assay organisms with intrinsic biological properties relating to resistance mechanisms and their genetic expression within bacteria; the specific strains are not clinically significant in their current microbiological status. Standard cefepime powder should provide the following MIC values (TABLE 5) when tested against the designated quality control strains:

CLINICAL PHARMACOLOGY: *(cont'd)*

TABLE 5

Microorganism	ATCC	MIC (mcg/ml)
Escherichia coli	25922	0.015-0.06
Staphylococcus aureus	29213	1-4
Pseudomonas aeruginosa	27853	1-4
Haemophilus influenzae	49247	0.5-2
Streptococcus pneumoniae	49619	0.06-0.25

Diffusion techniques

Quantitative methods that require measurement of zone diameters also provide reproducible estimates of the susceptibility of bacteria to antimicrobial compounds. One such standardized procedure[2] requires the use of standardized inoculum concentrations. This procedure uses paper disks impregnated with 30 mcg of cefepime to test the susceptibility of microorganisms to cefepime. Interpretation is identical to that stated above for results using dilution techniques.

Reports from the laboratory providing results of the standard single-disk susceptibility test with a 30-mcg cefepime disk should be interpreted according to the following criteria:

TABLE 6

Microorganism	Zone Diameter (mm) Susceptible (S)	Intermediate (I)	Resistant (R)
Microorganisms other than*Haemophilus* spp.* and *S. pneumoniae**	≥ 18	15-17	≤ 14
Haemophilus spp.*	≥ 26	—*	—*

* NOTE: Isolates from these species should be tested for susceptibility using specialized diffusion testing methods[2]. Isolates of *Haemophilus* spp. with zones smaller than 26 mm should be considered equivocal and should be further evaluated. Isolates of *S. pneumoniae* should be tested against a 1 mcg oxacillin disk; isolates with oxacillin zone sizes larger than or equal to 20 mm may be considered susceptible to cefepime.

As with standardized dilution techniques, diffusion methods require the use of laboratory control microorganisms to control the technical aspects of the laboratory procedures. Laboratory control microorganisms are specific strains of microbiological assay organisms with intrinsic biological properties relating to resistance mechanisms and their genetic expression within bacteria; the specific strains are not clinically significant in their current microbiological status. For the diffusion technique, the 30-mcg cefepime disk should provide the following zone diameters in these laboratory test quality control strains (TABLE 7).

TABLE 7

Microorganism	ATCC	Zone Size Range (mm)
Escherichia coli	25922	29-35
Staphylococcus aureus	25923	23-29
Pseudomonas aeruginosa	27853	24-30
Haemophilus influenzae	49247	25-31

CLINICAL STUDIES:

In clinical trials using multiple doses of cefepime, 4,137 patients were treated with the recommended dosages of cefepime (500 mg to 2 g IV q 12h). There were no deaths or permanent disabilities thought related to drug toxicity. Sixty-four (1.5%) patients discontinued medication due to adverse events thought by the investigators to be possibly, probably, or almost certainly related to drug toxicity. Thirty-three (51%) of these 64 patients who discontinued therapy did so because of rash. The percentage of cefepime-treated patients who discontinued study drug because of drug-related adverse events was very similar at daily doses of 500 mg, 1 g and 2 g q 12h (0.8%, 1.1%, and 2.0%, respectively). However, the incidence of discontinuation due to rash increased with the higher recommended doses.

The following adverse events were thought to be probably related to cefepime during evaluation of the drug in clinical trials conducted in North America (n=3,125 cefepime-treated patients).

TABLE 8 Adverse Clinical Reactions Cefepime Multiple-Dose Dosing Regimens Clinical Studies- North America

Incidence Equal To Or Greater Than 1%	Local reactions (3.0%), including phlebitis (1.3%), pain and/or inflammation (0.6%)*; rash (1.1%)
Incidence Less Than 1% But Greater Than 0.1%	Colitis (including pseudomembranous colitis), diarrhea, fever, headache, nausea, oral moniliasis, pruritus, urticaria, vaginitis, vomiting

* local reactions, irrespective of relationship to cefepime in those patients who received intravenous infusion (n=3.048).

The following adverse laboratory changes, irrespective of relationship to therapy with cefepime, were seen during clinical trials conducted in North America.

TABLE 9 Adverse Laboratory Changes Cefepime Multiple-Dose Dosing Regimens Clinical Studies- North America

Incidence Equal To Or Greater Than 1%	Positive Coombs' test (without hemolysis) (16.2%); decreased phosphorous (2.8%); increased ALT/SGPT (2.8%). AST/SGOT (2.4%), eosinophils (1.7%); abnormal PTT (1.6%), PT
Incidence Less Than 1% But Greater Than 0.1%	Increased alkaline phosphatase, BUN, calcium, creatinine, phosphorous, potassium, total bilirubin; decreased calcium*, hematocrit, neutrophils, platelets, WBC

* Hypocalcemia was more common among elderly patients. Clinical consequences from changes in either calcium or phosphorous were not reported.

IN POSTMARKETING EXPERIENCE

In addition to the events reported during North American clinical trials with cefepime, the following adverse experiences have been reported from foreign sources during worldwide postmarketing experience:

Encephalopathy has been reported in renally impaired patients treated with unadjusted dosing regimens of cefepime. Several cephalosporins have been implicated in triggering seizures, particularly in patients with renal impairment when the dosage was not reduced.

CLINICAL STUDIES: *(cont'd)*

(see DOSAGE AND ADMINISTRATION and OVERDOSAGE.) If seizures associated with drug therapy occur, the drug should be discontinued. Anticonvulsant therapy can be given if clinically indicated.

INDICATIONS AND USAGE:

Cefepime hydrochloride is indicated in the treatment of the following infections when caused by susceptible strains of the designated microorganisms:

Uncomplicated and Complicated Urinary Tract Infections (including pyelonephritis) caused by *Escherichia coli* or *Klebsiella pneumoniae*, when the infection is severe, or caused by *Escherichia coli, Klebsiella pneumoniae,* or *Proteus mirabilis*, when the infection is mild to moderate, including cases associated with concurrent bacteremia with these microorganisms.

Uncomplicated Skin and Skin Structure Infections caused by *Staphylococcus aureus* (methicillin-susceptible strains only) or *Streptococcus pyogenes*.

Pneumonia (moderate to severe) caused by *Streptococcus pneumoniae*, including cases associated with concurrent bacteremia, *Pseudomonas aeruginosa, Klebsiella pneumoniae*, or *Enterobacter species*.

Culture and susceptibility studies should be performed where appropriate to determine the susceptibility of the causative microorganism(s) to cefepime.

Therapy with cefepime hydrochloride may be instituted before results of susceptibility studies are known; however, once these results become available, the antibiotic treatment should be adjusted accordingly.

CONTRAINDICATIONS:

Cefepime hydrochloride is contraindicated in patients who have shown immediate hypersensitivity reactions to cefepime or the cephalosporin class of antibiotics, penicillins or other beta-lactam antibiotics.

WARNINGS:

BEFORE THERAPY WITH CEFEPIME HYDROCHLORIDE FOR INJECTION IS INSTITUTED, CAREFUL INQUIRY SHOULD BE MADE TO DETERMINE WHETHER THE PATIENT HAS HAD PREVIOUS IMMEDIATE HYPERSENSITIVITY REACTIONS TO CEFEPIME, CEPHALOSPORINS, PENICILLINS, OR OTHER DRUGS. IF THIS PRODUCT IS TO BE GIVEN TO PENICILLIN-SENSITIVE PATIENTS, CAUTION SHOULD BE EXERCISED BECAUSE CROSS-HYPERSENSITIVITY AMONG BETA-LACTAM ANTIBIOTICS HAS BEEN CLEARLY DOCUMENTED AND MAY OCCUR IN UP TO 10% OF PATIENTS WITH A HISTORY Of PENICILLIN ALLERGY. IF AN ALLERGIC REACTION TO CEFEPIME HYDROCHLORIDE OCCURS, DISCONTINUE THE DRUG. SERIOUS ACUTE HYPERSENSITIVITY REACTIONS MAY REQUIRE TREATMENT WITH EPINEPHRINE AND OTHER EMERGENCY MEASURES INCLUDING OXYGEN, CORTICOSTEROIDS, INTRAVENOUS FLUIDS, INTRAVENOUS ANTIHISTAMINES, PRESSOR AMINES, AND AIRWAY MANAGEMENT, AS CLINICALLY INDICATED.

Pseudomembranous colitis has been reported with nearly all antibacterial agents, including Cefepime hydrochloride, and may range in severity from mild to life-threatening. Therefore, it is important to consider this diagnosis in patients who present with diarrhea subsequent to the administration of antibacterial agents.

Treatment with antibacterial agents alters the normal flora of the colon and may permit overgrowth clostridia. Studies indicate that a toxin produced by *Clostridium difficile*is a primary cause of "antibiotic-associated colitis".

After the diagnosis of pseudomembranous colitis has been established, therapeutic measures should be initiated. Mild cases of pseudomembranous colitis usually respond to drug discontinuation alone. In moderate-to-severe cases, consideration should be given to management with fluids and electrolytes, protein supplementation, and treatment with an antibacterial drug clinically effective against *Clostridium difficile* colitis.

PRECAUTIONS:

General: As with other antimicrobials, prolonged use of cefepime hydrochloride may result in overgrowth of nonsusceptible microorganisms. Repeated evaluation of the patient's condition is essential. Should superinfection occur during therapy, appropriate measures should be taken.

Many cephalosporins, including cefepime, have been associated with a fall in prothrombin activity. Those at risk include patients with renal or hepatic impairment, or poor nutritional state, as well as patients receiving a protracted course of antimicrobial therapy. Prothrombin time should be monitored in patients at risk, and exogenous vitamin K administered as indicated.

Positive direct Coombs' tests have been reported during treatment with cefepime hydrochloride. In hematologic studies or in transfusion cross-matching procedures when antiglobulin tests are performed on the minor side or in Coombs' testing of newborns whose mothers have received cephalosporin antibiotics before parturition, it should be recognized that a positive Coombs' test may be due to the drug.

Cefepime hydrochloride should be prescribed with caution in individuals with a history of gastrointestinal disease, particularly colitis.

Arginine has been shown to alter glucose metabolism and elevate serum potassium transiently when administered at 50 times the amount provided by the maximum recommended human dose of cefepime hydrochloride. The effect of lower doses is not presently known.

Drug/Laboratory Test Interactions: The administration of cefepime may result in a false-positive reaction for glucose in the urine when using Clinitest tablets. It is recommended that glucose tests based on enzymatic glucose oxidase reactions (such as Clinistix or Tes-Tape) be used.

Carcinogenesis, Mutagenesis, and Impairment of Fertility: No long-term animal carcinogenicity studies have been conducted with cefepime. A battery of *in vivo* and *in vitro* genetic toxicity tests, including the Ames Salmonella reverse mutation assay, CHO/HGPRT mammalian cell forward gene mutation assay, chromosomal aberration and sister chromatid exchange assays in human lymphocytes, CHO fibroblast clastogenesis assay, and cytogenetic and micronucleus assays in mice were conducted. The overall conclusion of these tests indicated no definitive evidence of genotoxic potential. No untoward effects on fertility or reproduction have been observed in rats, mice, and rabbits when cefepime is administered subcutaneously at 1 to 4 times the recommended maximum human dose calculated on a $mg/m^2/day$ basis.

Pregnancy, Teratogenic Effects, Pregnancy Category B: Cefepime was not teratogenic or embryocidal when administered during the period of organogenesis to rats at doses up to 1000 mg/kg/day (4 times the recommended maximum human dose calculated on a $mg/m^2/day$ basis) or to mice at doses up to 1200 mg/kg/day (2 times the recommended maximum human dose calculated on a $mg/m^2/day$ basis) or to rabbits at a dose level of 100 mg/kg/day (approximately equal to the recommended maximum daily human dose calculated on a $mg/m^2/day$ basis).

There are, however, no adequate and well-controlled studies of cefepime use in pregnant women. Because animal reproduction studies are not always predictive of human response, this drug should be used during pregnancy only if clearly needed.

Nursing Mothers: Cefepime is excreted in human breast milk in very low concentrations [0.5 mcg/mL]. Caution should be exercised when cefepime is administered to a nursing woman.

Labor and Deliver: Cefepime has not been studied for use during labor and delivery. Treatment should only be given if clearly indicated.

Pediatric Use : The safety and efficacy of cefepime hydrochloride in pediatric patients below the age of 12 years have not been established. This product is intended for use in patients 12 years of age and older.

Geriatric Use: In clinical studies, when geriatric patients received the usual recommended adult dose, clinical efficacy and safety were comparable to clinical efficacy and safety in non-geriatric adult patients.

In elderly patients, dosage and administration of cefepime should be adjusted in the presence of renal insufficiency. (see DOSAGE AND ADMINISTRATION.)

DRUG INTERACTIONS:

Renal function should be monitored carefully if high doses of aminoglycosides are to be administered with cefepime hydrochloride because of the increased potential of nephrotoxicity and ototoxicity of aminoglycoside antibiotics. Nephrotoxicity has been reported following concomitant administration of other cephalosporins with potent diuretics such as furosemide.

ADVERSE REACTIONS:

CEPHALOSPORIN-CLASS ADVERSE REACTIONS

In addition to the adverse reactions listed above that have been observed in patients treated with cefepime, the following adverse reactions and altered laboratory tests have been reported for cephalosporin-class antibiotics:

Stevens-Johnson syndrome, erythema multiforme, toxic epidermal necrolysis, renal dysfunction, toxic nephropathy, aplastic anemia, hemolytic anemia, hemorrhage and hepatic dysfunction including cholestasis, pancytopenia.

OVERDOSAGE:

In clinical trials, cefepime hydrochloride overdosage occurred in a patient with renal failure (creatinine clearance <11 mL/min) who received 2 g q 24h for seven days. The patient exhibited seizures, encephalopathy, and neuromuscular excitability. Patients who receive an overdose should be carefully observed and given supportive treatment. In the presence of renal insufficiency, hemodialysis, not peritoneal dialysis, is recommended to aid in the removal of cefepime from the body.

DOSAGE AND ADMINISTRATION:

The recommended adult dosages and routes of administration are outlined in the following Table 10. Cefepime hydrochloride should be administered intravenously over approximately 30 minutes.

TABLE 10 Recommended Dosage Schedule for Cefepime HCl

Site and Type of Infection	Dose	Frequency	Duration (days)
Mild to Moderate Uncomplicated or Complicated Urinary Tract Infections, including pyelonephritis, due to *E. coli, K. pneumoniae*, or *P. mirabilis*.*	0.5-1 g IV/IM**	q12 h	7-10
Severe Uncomplicated or Complicated Urinary Tract Infections, including pyelonephritis, due to *E. coli* or *K. pneumoniae*.*	2 g IV	q12 h	10
Moderate to Severe Pneumonia due to *S. pneumoniae**, *Pseudomonas aeruginosa*, Klebsiella pneumoniae, or *Enterobacter* species.	1-2 g IV	q12 h	10
Moderate to Severe Uncomplicated Skin and Skin Structure Infections due to *S. aureus* or *S. pyogenes*.	2 g IV	q12 h	10

* including cases associated with concurrent bacteremia.
** IM route of administration is indicated only for mild to moderate, uncomplicated or complicated UTI's due to E. coli when the IM route is considered to be a more appropriate route of drug administration.

IMPAIRED HEPATIC FUNCTION

No adjustment is necessary for patients with impaired hepatic function.

IMPAIRED RENAL FUNCTION

In patients with impaired renal function (creatinine clearance <60 mL/min), the dose of cefepime hydrochloride should be adjusted to compensate for the slower rate of renal elimination. The recommended initial dose of cefepime hydrochloride should be the same as in patients with normal renal function. The recommended maintenance doses of cefepime hydrochloride in patients with renal insufficiency are presented in Table 11.

TABLE 11 Recommended Maintenance Schedule in Patients with Renal Impairment Relative to Normal Recommended Dosing Schedule

Creatinine Clearance (mL/min)	Recommended Maintenance Schedule		
>60 Normal recommended dosing schedule	500 mg q 12 h	1 g q 12 h	2 g q 12 h
30-60	500 mg q 24 h	1 g q 24 h	2 g q 24 h
11-29	500 mg q 24 h	500 mg q 24 h	1 g q 24 h
≤ 10	250 mg q 24 h	250 mg q 24 h	500 mg q 24 h

When only serum creatinine is available, the following formula (Cockcroft and Gault equation)[3] may be used to estimate creatinine clearance. The serum creatinine should represent a steady state of renal function:

Creatinine Clearance (mL/min)

Males: [Weight (kg) x (140 -age)] ÷ [72 x serum creatinine (mg/dL)]

Females: 0.85 x above value

DOSAGE AND ADMINISTRATION: *(cont'd)*

In patients undergoing hemodialysis, approximately 68% of the total amount of cefepime present in the body at the start of dialysis will be removed during a 3-hour dialysis period. A repeat dose, equivalent to the initial dose, should be given at the completion of each dialysis session.

In patients undergoing continuous ambulatory peritoneal dialysis, cefepime hydrochloride may be administered at normally recommended doses at a dosage interval of every 48 hours.

ADMINISTRATION

For Intravenous Infusion , constitute the 1 g or 2 g piggyback (100 mL) bottle with 50 or 100 mL of a compatible IV fluid listed in the **Compatibility and Stability** subsection. Alternatively, constitute the 500 mg, 1 g, or 2 g vial, and add an appropriate quantity of the resulting solution to an IV container with one of the compatible IV fluids. **THE RESULTING SOLUTION SHOULD BE ADMINISTERED OVER APPROXIMATELY 30 MINUTES.**

Intermittent IV infusion with a Y-type administration set can be accomplished with compatible solutions. However, during infusion of a solution containing cefepime, it is desirable to discontinue the other solution.

ADD-Vantage vials are to be constituted only with 50 or 100 mL of 5% Dextrose Injection or 0.9% Sodium Chloride Injection in Abbott ADD-Vantage flexible diluent containers. (see ADD-Vantage Vial Instructions for Use.)

Intramuscular Administration: For IM administration, cefepime hydrochloride (cefepime hydrochloride) should be constituted with one of the following diluents: Sterile Water for Injection, 0.9% Sodium Chloride, 5% Dextrose Injection, 0.5% or 1.0% Lidocaine Hydrochloride, or Bacteriostatic Water for Injection with Parabens or Benzyl Alcohol (Refer to Table 12).

Preparation of cefepime hydrochloride solutions is summarized in Table 12:

TABLE 12 Preparation Of Solutions Of Cefepime Hydrochloride

Single Dose Vials for Intravenous/Intramuscular Administration	Amount of Diluent to be added (mL)	Approximate Available Volume (mL)	Approximate Cefepime Concentration (mg/mL)
cefepime vial content			
500 mg (iv)	5.0	5.6	100
500 mg (im)	1.3	1.8	280
1 g (iv)	10.0	11.3	100
1 g (im)	2.4	3.6	280
2 g (iv)	10.0	12.5	160
Piggyback (100 mL)			
1 g bottle	50	50	20
1 g bottle	100	100	10
2 g bottle	50	50	40
2 g bottle	100	100	20
ADD-Vantage			
1 g vial	50	50	20
1 g vial	100	100	10

COMPATIBILITY AND STABILITY:

Intravenous Cefepime hydrochloride is compatible at concentrations between 1 and 40 mg/mL with the following IV infusion fluids: 0.9% Sodium Chloride Injection, 5% and 10% Dextrose Injection, M/6 Sodium Lactate Injection, 5% Dextrose and 0.9% Sodium Chloride Injection, Lactated Ringers and 5% Dextrose Injection, Normosol-R, and Normosol-M in 5% Dextrose Injection. These solutions may be stored up to 24 hours at controlled room temperature 20°-25° (68°-77°F) or 7 days in a refrigerator 2°-8°C (36°-46°F). Cefepime hydrochloride in ADD-Vantage vials is stable at concentrations of 10-20 mg/mL in 5% Dextrose Injection or 0.9% Sodium Chloride Injection for 24 hours at controlled room temperature 20°-25°C or 7 days in a refrigerator 2°-8°C.

Cefepime hydrochloride admixture compatibility information is summarized in Table 13.

TABLE 13 Cefepime Admixture Stability

Cefepime Hydrochloride Concentration	Admixture and Concentration	IV Infusion Solutions	Stability Time for RT/L (20°-25° C)	Stability Time for Refrigeration (2°-8° C)
40 mg/mL	Amikacin 6 mg/mL	NS or D5W	24 hours	7 days
40 mg/mL	Ampicillin 1 mg/mL	D5W	8 hours	8 hours
40 mg/mL	Ampicillin 10 mg/mL	D5W	2 hours	8 hours
40 mg/mL	Ampicillin 1 mg/mL	NS	24 hours	48 hours
40 mg/mL	Ampicillin 10 mg/mL	NS	8 hours	48 hours
4 mg/mL	Ampicillin 40 mg/mL	NS	8 hours	8 hours
4-40 mg/mL	Clindamycin Phosphate 0.25-6 mg/mL	NS or D5W	24 hours	7 days
4 mg/mL	Heparin 10-50 units/mL	NS or D5W	24 hours	7 days
4 mg/mL	Potassium Chloride 10-40 mEq/L	NS or D5W	24 hours	7 days
4 mg/mL	Theophylline	D5W	24 hours	7 days
1-4 mg/mL	na	Aminosyn II 4.25% with electrolytes and calcium	8 hours	3 days
0.125-0.25 mg/mL	na	Inpersol with 4.25% dextrose	24 hours	7 days

NS=0.9% Sodium Chloride Injection
D5W=5% Dextrose injection
na=not applicable
RT/L=Ambient room temperature and light

Solutions of cefepime hydrochloride, like those of most beta-lactam antibiotics, should not be added to solutions of ampicillin at a concentration greater than 40 mg/mL, and should not be added to metronidazole, vancomycin, gentamicin, tobramycin, netilmicin sulfate or aminophylline because of potential interaction. However, if concurrent therapy with cefepime hydrochloride is indicated, each of these antibiotics can be administered separately.

DOSAGE AND ADMINISTRATION: *(cont'd)*

Intramuscular: Cefepime hydrochloride constituted as directed is stable for 24 hours at controlled room temperature 20°-25°C (68°-77°F) or for 7 days in a refrigerator 2°-8°C (36°-46°F) with the following diluents: Sterile Water for Injection, 0.9% Sodium Chloride Injection, 5% Dextrose Injection, Bacteriostatic Water for Injection with Parabens or Benzyl Alcohol, or 0.5% or 1% Lidocaine Hydrochloride.

NOTE: PARENTERAL DRUGS SHOULD BE INSPECTED VISUALLY FOR PARTICULATE MATTER BEFORE ADMINISTRATION.

As with other cephalosporins, the color of cefepime hydrochloride powder, as well as its solutions, tend to darken depending on storage conditions; however, when stored as recommended, the product's potency is not adversely affected.

HOW SUPPLIED:

Storage: CEFEPIME HYDROCHLORIDE IN THE DRY STATE SHOULD BE STORED BETWEEN 2°-25°C (36°-77°F) AND PROTECTED FROM LIGHT.

REFERENCES:

1. National Committee for Clinical Laboratory Standards. *Methods for Dilution Antimicrobial Susceptibility Tests for Bacteria that Grow Aerobically* - Third Edition. Approved Standard NCCLS Document M7-A3, Vol. 13, No. 25, NCCLS, Villanova, PA, December, 1993. **2.** National Committee for Clinical Laboratory Standards. *Performance Standards for Antimicrobial Disk Susceptibility Tests* — Fifth Edition. Approved Standard NCCLS Document M2-A5, Vol. 13, No. 24, NCCLS, Villanova, PA, December, 1993. **3.** Cockcroft DW, Gault MH. Prediction of creatinine clearance from serum creatinine. *Nephron.* 1976; 16:31-41.

For How Supplied Information, Contact Bristol Myers Squibb (NDA# 050679)

CEFIXIME *(000684)*

CATEGORIES: Anti-Infectives; Antibiotics; Antimicrobials; Beta-Lactam Antibiotics; Bronchitis; Cephalosporins; Gonorrhea; Infections; Otitis Media; Pharyngitis; Tonsillitis; Urinary Tract Infections; Rheumatic Fever*; Pregnancy Category B; Sales > $100 Million; FDA Approved 1989 Apr; Top 200 Drugs
* Indication not approved by the FDA

BRAND NAMES: *Cefspan*; *Cephoral* (Germany); *Denvar* (Mexico); *Fixime*; *Novacef* (Mexico); *Oroken* (France); *Spancef*; *Supran*; **Suprax**; *Tergecef*; *Topcef*; *Uro-cephoral* (Germany)
(International brand names outside U.S. in italics)

FORMULARIES: Aetna; BC-BS; Foundation; Medi-Cal; PCS

COST OF THERAPY: $63.14 (Infections; Tablet; 400 mg; 1/day; 10 days) vs. Potential Cost of $3,912.55 (Urinary Tract Infections)

PRIMARY ICD9: 136.9 (Unspecified Infections and Parasitic Diseases)

DESCRIPTION:

Cefixime is a semisynthetic, cephalosporin antibiotic for oral administration. Chemically, it is (6*R*,7*R*)-7-[2-(2-Amino-4-thiazolyl) glyoxylamido]-8-oxo-3-vinyl-5-thia-1-azabicyclo[4.2.0]oct-2-ene-2-carboxylic acid, 7^2(*Z*)-[O-(carboxymethyl)oxime]-trihydrate. Molecular weight = 507.50 as the trihydrate.

Suprax is available in scored 200-mg and 400-mg film coated tablets and in a powder for oral suspension which when reconstituted provides 100 mg/5 ml.

Inactive ingredients contained in the 200-mg and 400-mg tablets are: dibasic calcium phosphate, hydroxypropyl methylcellulose 2910, light mineral oil, magnesium stearate, microcrystalline cellulose, pregelatinized starch, sodium lauryl sulfate and titanium dioxide. The powder for oral suspension is strawberry flavored and contains sodium benzoate, sucrose, and xanthan gum.

CLINICAL PHARMACOLOGY:

Cefixime, given orally, is about 40% to 50% absorbed whether administered with or without food; however, time to maximal absorption is increased approximately 0.8 hours when administered with food. A single 200-mg tablet of cefixime produces an average peak serum concentration of approximately 2 mcg/ml (range 1 to 4 mcg/ml); a single 400-mg tablet produces an average peak concentration of approximately 3.7 mcg/ml (range 1.3 to 7.7 mcg/ml). The oral suspension produces average peak concentrations approximately 25% to 50% higher than the tablets. Two hundred and 400-mg doses of oral suspension produce average peak concentrations of 3 mcg/ml (range 1.0 to 4.5 mcg/ml) and 4.6 mcg/ml (range 1.9 to 7.7 mcg/ml), respectively, when tested in normal *adult* volunteers. The area under the time versus concentration curve is greater by approximately 10% to 25% with the oral suspension than with the tablet after doses of 100 to 400 mg, when tested in normal *adult* volunteers. This increased absorption should be taken into consideration if the oral suspension is to be substituted for the tablet. Because of the lack of bioequivalence, tablets should not be substituted for oral suspension in the treatment of otitis media. (See DOSAGE AND ADMINISTRATION.) Crossover studies of tablets versus suspension have not been performed in children.

Peak serum concentrations occur between 2 and 6 hours following oral administration of a single 200-mg tablet, a single 400-mg tablet, or 400 mg of suspension of cefixime. Peak serum concentrations occur between 2 and 5 hours following a single administration of 200 mg of suspension (TABLE 1 and TABLE 2).

TABLE 1 Serum Levels of Cefixime after Administration of Tablets (mcg/ml)

Dose	1 hr	2 hr	4 hr	6 hr	8 hr	12 hr	24 hr
100 mg	0.3	0.8	1.0	0.7	0.4	0.2	0.02
200 mg	0.7	1.4	2.0	1.5	1.0	0.4	0.03
400 mg	1.2	2.5	3.5	2.7	1.7	0.6	0.04

TABLE 2 Serum Levels of Cefixime after Administration of Oral Suspension (mcg/ml)

Dose	1 hr	2 hr	4 hr	6 hr	8 hr	12 hr	24 hr
100 mg	0.7	1.1	1.3	0.9	0.6	0.2	0.02
200 mg	1.2	2.1	2.8	2.0	1.3	0.5	0.07
400 mg	1.8	3.3	4.4	3.3	2.2	0.8	0.07

Approximately 50% of the absorbed dose is excreted unchanged in the urine in 24 hours. In animal studies, it was noted that cefixime is also excreted in the bile in excess of 10% of the administered dose. Serum protein binding is concentration independent with a bound fraction of approximately 65%. In a multiple dose study conducted with a research formulation which is less bioavailable than the tablet or suspension, there was little accumulation of drug in serum or urine after dosing for 14 days.

CLINICAL PHARMACOLOGY: *(cont'd)*

The serum half-life of cefixime in healthy subjects is independent of dosage form and averages 3 to 4 hours but may range up to 9 hours in some normal volunteers. Average AUCs at steady state in elderly patients are approximately 40% higher than average AUCs in other healthy adults.

In subjects with moderate impairment of renal function (20 to 40 ml/min creatinine clearance), the average serum half-life of cefixime is prolonged to 6.4 hours. In severe renal impairment (5 to 20 ml/min creatinine clearance), the half-life increased to an average of 11.5 hours. The drug is not cleared significantly from the blood by hemodialysis or peritoneal dialysis. However, a study indicated that with doses of 400 mg, patients undergoing hemodialysis have similar blood profiles as subjects with creatinine clearances of 21 to 60 ml/min. There is no evidence of metabolism of cefixime *in vivo*.

Adequate date of CSF levels of cefixime are not available.

MICROBIOLOGY

As with other cephalosporins, bactericidal action of cefixime results from inhibition of cell-wall synthesis. Cefixime is highly stable in the presence of beta-lactamase enzymes. As a result, many organisms resistant to penicillins and some cephalosporins, due to the presence of beta- lactamase, may be susceptible to cefixime. Cefixime has been shown to be active against most strains of the following organisms both *in vitro* and in clinical infections (see INDICATIONS AND USAGE).

Gram-Positive Organisms

Streptococcus pneumoniae,
Streptococcus pyogenes.

Gram-Negative Organisms

Haemophilus influenzae (beta-lactamase positive and negative strains),
Moraxella (Branhamella) catarrhalis (most of which are beta-lactamase positive),
Escherichia coli,
Proteus mirabilis.
Neisseria gonorrhoeae (including penicillinase- and non-penicillinase-producing strains)

Cefixime has been shown to be active *in vitro* against most strains of the following organisms; however, clinical efficacy has not been established.

Gram-Positive Organisms

Streptococcus agalactiae.

Gram-Negative Organisms

Haemophilus parainfluenzae (beta-lactamase positive and negative strains),
Proteus vulgaris
Klebsiella pneumoniae,
Klebsiella oxytoca,
Pasteurella multocida,
Providencia spp.,
Salmonella spp.,
Shigella spp.,
Citrobacter amalonaticus,
Citrobacter diversus,
Serratia marcescens.

Note: *Pseudomonas* spp., strains of group D streptococci (including enterococci), *Listeria monocytogenes*, most strains of staphylococci (including methicillin-resistant strains) and most strains of *Enterobacter* are resistant to cefixime. In addition, most strains of *Bacteroides fragilis* and *Clostridium* are resistant to cefixime.

SUSCEPTIBILTY TESTING

Diffusion Techniques: Quantitative methods that require measurement of zone diameters give an estimate of antibiotic susceptibility. One such procedure[1-3] has been recommended for use with disks to test susceptibility to cefixime. Interpretation involves correlation of the diameters obtained in the disk test with minimum inhibitory concentration (MIC) for cefixime.

Reports from the laboratory giving results of the standard single-disk susceptibility test with a 5-mcg cefixime disk should be interpreted according to TABLE 3.

TABLE 3 Recommended Susceptibility Ranges: Agar Disk Diffusion

Organisms	Resistant	Moderately Susceptible	Susceptible
Neisseria gonorrhoeae[a]	—	—	≥ 31 mm
All other organisms	≤ 15 mm	16 - 18 mm	≥ 19 mm

[a]Using GC agar base with a defined 1% supplement without cysteine.

A report of "Susceptible" indicates that the pathogen is likely to be inhibited by generally achievable blood levels. A report of "Moderately Susceptible" indicates that inhibitory concentrations of the antibiotic may well be achieved if high dosage is used or if the infection is confined to tissues and fluids (*e.g.,* urine) in which high antibiotic levels are attained. A report of "Resistant" indicates that achievable concentrations of the antibiotic are unlikely to be inhibitory and other therapy should be selected.

Standardized procedures require the use of laboratory control organisms. The 5-mcg disk should give the following zone diameter (TABLE 4).

TABLE 4

Organism	Zone Diameter (mm)
Escherichia coli ATCC 25922	23-27
Neisseria gonorrhoeae ATCC 49226[a]	37-45

a Using GC agar base with a defined 1% supplement without cysteine.

The class disk for cephalosporin susceptibility testing (the cephalothin disk) is not appropriate because of spectrum differences with cefixime. The 5-mcg cefixime disk should be used for all *in vitro* testing of isolates.

Dilution Techniques: Broth or agar dilution methods can be used to determine the MIC value for susceptibility of bacterial isolates to cefixime. The recommended susceptibility breakpoints are found in TABLE 5.

TABLE 5 MIC Interpretive Standards (mcg/ml)

Organism	Resistant	Moderately Susceptible	Susceptible
Neisseria gonorrhoeae[a]	-	-	≤ 0.25
All other organisms	≥ 4	2	≤ 1

CLINICAL PHARMACOLOGY: *(cont'd)*

As with standard diffusion methods, dilution procedures require the use of laboratory control organisms. Standard cefixime powder should give the following MIC ranges in daily testing of quality control organisms (TABLE 6).

TABLE 6

Organism	MIC Range (mcg/mL)
Escherichia coli ATCC 25922	0.25-1
Staphylococcus aureus ATCC 29213	8-32
Neisseria gonorrhoeae ATCC 49226[a]	0.008-0.03

a Using GC agar base with a defined 1% supplement without cysteine.

CLINICAL STUDIES:

In clinical trials of otitis media in nearly 400 children between the ages of 6 months to 10 years, *Streptococcus pneumoniae* was isolated from 47% of the patients, *Haemophilus influenzae* from 34%, *Moraxella (Branhamella) catarrhalis* from 15% and *Streptococcus pyogenes* from 4%.

The overall response rate of *S. pneumoniae* to cefixime was approximately 10% lower and that of *H. influenzae* or*M. catarrhalis* approximately 7% higher (12% when beta-lactamase positive strains of *H. influenzae* are included) than the response rates of these organisms to the active control drugs.

In these studies, patients were randomized and treated with either cefixime at dose regimens of 4 mg/kg bid or 8 mg/kg qd, or with a standard antibiotic regimen. Sixty-nine to 70% of the patients in each group had resolution of signs and symptoms of otitis media when evaluated 2 to 4 weeks posttreatment, but persistent effusion was found in 15% of the patients. When evaluated at the completion of therapy, 17% of patients receiving cefixime and 14% of patients receiving effective comparative drugs (18% including those patients who had *H. influenzae*resistant to the control drug and who received the control antibiotic) were considered to be treatment failures. By the 2 to 4 week follow-up, a total of 30% to 31% of patients had evidence of either treatment failure or recurrent disease (TABLE 7).

TABLE 7 Bacteriological Outcome of Otitis Media at Two to Four Weeks Posttherapy Based on Repeat Middle Ear Fluid Culture or Extrapolation from Clinical Outcome

Organism	Cefixime[a] 4 mg/kg bid	Cefixim[a] 8 mg/kg qd	Control[a] Drugs
Streptococcus pneumoniae	48/70 (69%)	18/22 (82%)	82/100 (82%)
Haemophilus influenzae beta-lactamase negative	24/34 (71%)	13/17 (76%)	23/34 (68%)
Haemophilus influenzae beta-lactamase positive	17/22 (77%)	9/12 (75%)	1/1[b]
Moraxella (Branhamella) catarrhalis	26/31 (84%)	5/5	18/24 (75%)
Streptococcus pyogenes	5/5	3/3	6/7
All Isolates	120/162 (74%)	48/59 (81%)	130/166 (78%)

a Number eradicated/number isolated.
b An additional 20 beta-lactamase positive strains of *Haemophilus influenzae* were isolated, but were excluded from this analysis because they were resistant to the control antibiotic. In nineteen of these, the clinical course could be assessed and a favorable outcome occurred in 10. When these cases are included in the overall bacteriological evaluation of therapy with the control drugs, 140/185 (76%) of pathogens were considered to be eradicated.

INDICATIONS AND USAGE:

Cefixime is indicated in the treatment of the following infections when caused by susceptible strains of the designated microorganisms:

Uncomplicated Urinary Tract Infections: Caused by *Escherichia coli* and *Proteus mirabilis.*

Otitis Media: Caused by *Haemophilus influenzae* (beta-lactamase positive and negative strains), *Moraxella (Branhamella) catarrhalis* (most of which are beta-lactamase positive) and *Streptococcus pyogenes**.

Note: For information on otitis media caused by *Streptococcus pneumoniae*, see CLINICAL STUDIES.

Pharyngitis and Tonsillitis: Caused by *S. pyogenes.*

Note: Penicillin is the usual drug of choice in the treatment of *S. pyogenes* infections, including the prophylaxis of rheumatic fever. Cefixime is generally effective in the eradication of *S. pyogenes* from the nasopharynx; however, data establishing the efficacy of cefixime in the subsequent prevention of rheumatic fever are not available.

Acute Bronchitis and Acute Exacerbations of Chronic Bronchitis: Caused by *S. pneumoniae* and *H. influenzae* (beta-lactamase positive and negative strains).

Uncomplicated gonorrhea (cervical/urethral): Caused by *Neisseria gonorrhoeae* (penicillinase- and non–penicillinase-producing strains).

Appropriate cultures and susceptibility studies should be performed to determine the causative organism and its susceptibility to cefixime; however, therapy may be started while awaiting the results of these studies. Therapy should be adjusted, if necessary, once these results are known.

*Efficacy for this organism in this organ system was studied in fewer than 10 infections.

CONTRAINDICATIONS:

Cefixime is contraindicated in patients with known allergy to the cephalosporin group of antibiotics.

WARNINGS:

BEFORE THERAPY WITH CEFIXIME IS INSTITUTED, CAREFUL INQUIRY SHOULD BE MADE TO DETERMINE WHETHER THE PATIENT HAS HAD PREVIOUS HYPERSENSITIVITY REACTIONS TO CEPHALOSPORINS, PENICILLINS, OR OTHER DRUGS. IF THIS PRODUCT IS TO BE GIVEN TO PENICILLIN-SENSITIVE PATIENTS, CAUTION SHOULD BE EXERCISED BECAUSE CROSS HYPERSENSITIVITY AMONG BETA-LACTAM ANTIBIOTICS HAS BEEN CLEARLY DOCUMENTED AND MAY OCCUR IN UP TO 10% OF PATIENTS WITH A HISTORY OF PENICILLIN ALLERGY. IF AN ALLERGIC REACTION TO CEFIXIME OCCURS, DISCONTINUE THE DRUG. SERIOUS ACUTE HYPERSENSITIVITY REACTIONS MAY REQUIRE TREATMENT WITH EPINEPHRINE AND OTHER EMERGENCY MEASURES, INCLUDING OXYGEN, INTRAVENOUS FLUIDS, INTRAVENOUS ANTIHISTAMINES, CORTICOSTEROIDS, PRESSOR AMINES, AND AIRWAY MANAGEMENT, AS CLINICALLY INDICATED.

Antibiotics, including cefixime, should be administered cautiously to any patient who has demonstrated some form of allergy, particularly to drugs.

WARNINGS: *(cont'd)*

Treatment with broad, spectrum antibiotics, including cefixime, alters the normal flora of the colon and may permit overgrowth of clostridia. Studies indicate that a toxin produced by *Clostridium difficile* is a primary cause of severe antibiotic-associated diarrhea including pseudomembranous colitis.

Pseudomembranous colitis has been reported with the use of cefixime and other broad-spectrum antibiotics (including macrolides, semisynthetic penicillins, and cephalosporins); therefore, it is important to consider this diagnosis in patients who develop diarrhea in association with the use of antibiotics. Symptoms of pseudomembranous colitis may occur during or after antibiotic treatment and may range in severity from mild to life-threatening. Mild cases of pseudomembranous colitis usually respond to drug discontinuation alone. In moderate to severe cases, management should include fluids, electrolytes, and protein supplementation. If the colitis does not improve after the drug has been discontinued, or if the symptoms are severe, oral vancomycin is the drug of choice for antibiotic-associated pseudomembranous colitis produced by *C. difficile*. Other causes of colitis should be excluded.

PRECAUTIONS:

General: The possibility of the emergence of resistant organisms which might result in overgrowth should be kept in mind, particularly during prolonged treatment. In such use, careful observation of the patient is essential. If superinfection occurs during therapy, appropriate measures should be taken.

The dose of cefixime should be adjusted in patients with renal impairment as well as those undergoing continuous ambulatory peritoneal dialysis (CAPD) and hemodialysis (HD). Patients on dialysis should be monitored carefully. (See DOSAGE AND ADMINISTRATION.)

Cefixime should be prescribed with caution in individuals with a history of gastrointestinal disease, particularly colitis.

Drug/Laboratory Test Interactions: A false-positive reaction for ketones in the urine may occur with tests using nitroprusside but not with those using nitroferricyanide.

The administration of cefixime may result in a false-positive reaction for glucose in the urine using Clinitest, Benedict's solution, or Fehling's solution. It is recommended that glucose tests based on enzymatic glucose oxidase reactions (such as Clinistix or Tes-Tape) be used.

A false-positive direct Coombs' test has been reported during treatment with other cephalosporin antibiotics; therefore, it should be recognized that a positive Coombs' test may be due to the drug.

Carcinogenesis, Mutagenesis, and Impairment of Fertility: Lifetime studies in animals to evaluate carcinogenic potential have not been conducted. Cefixime did not cause point mutations in bacteria or mammalian cells, DNA damage, or chromosome damage *in vitro* and did not exhibit clastogenic potential *in vivo* in the mouse micronucleus test. In rats, fertility and reproductive performance were not affected by cefixime at doses up to 125 times the therapeutic dose.

Pregnancy Category B: Reproduction studies have been performed in mice and rats at doses up to 400 times the human dose and have revealed no evidence of harm to the fetus due to cefixime. There are no adequate and well-controlled studies in pregnant women. Because animal reproduction studies are not always predictive of human response, this drug should be used during pregnancy only if clearly needed.

Labor and Delivery: Cefixime has not been studied for use during labor and delivery. Treatment should only be given if clearly needed.

Nursing Mothers: It is not known whether cefixime is excreted in human milk. Consideration should be given to discontinuing nursing temporarily during treatment with this drug.

Pediatric Use: Safety and effectiveness of cefixime in children aged less than 6 months old have not been established.

The incidence of gastrointestinal adverse reactions, including diarrhea and loose stools, in the pediatric patients receiving the suspension, was comparable to the incidence seen in adult patients receiving tablets.

DRUG INTERACTIONS:

No significant drug interactions have been reported to date.

ADVERSE REACTIONS:

Most of adverse reactions observed in clinical trials were of a mild and transient nature. Five percent of patients in the U.S. trials discontinued therapy because of drug-related adverse reactions. The most commonly seen adverse reactions in U.S. trials of the tablet formulation were gastrointestinal events, which were reported in 30% of adult patients on either the bid or the qd regimen. Clinically mild gastrointestinal side effects occurred in 20% of all patients, moderate events occurred in 9% of all patients, and severe adverse reactions occurred in 2% of all patients. Individual event rates included diarrhea 16%, loose or frequent stools 6%, abdominal pain 3%, nausea 7%, dyspepsia 3%, and flatulence 4%. The incidence of gastrointestinal adverse reactions, including diarrhea and loose stools, in pediatric patients receiving the suspension, was comparable to the incidence seen in adult patients receiving tablets.

These symptoms usually responded to symptomatic therapy or ceased when cefixime was discontinued.

Several patients developed severe diarrhea and/or documented pseudomembranous colitis, and a few required hospitalization.

The following adverse reactions have been reported following the use of cefixime. Incidence rated were less than 1 in 50 (less than 2%), except as noted above for gastrointestinal events.

Gastrointestinal: Diarrhea, loose stools, abdominal pain, dyspepsia, nausea, and vomiting. Several cases of documented pseudomembranous colitis were identified during the studies. The onset of pseudomembranous colitis symptoms may occur during or after therapy.

Hypersensitivity Reactions: Skin rashes, urticaria, drug fever, and pruritus. Erythema multiforme, Stevens-Johnson syndrome, and serum sickness-like reactions have been reported.

Hepatic: Transient elevations is SGPT, SGOT, and alkaline phosphatase.

Renal: Transient elevations in BUN or creatinine.

Central Nervous System: Headaches and/or dizziness.

Hemic and Lymphatic Systems: Transient thrombocytopenia, leukopenia, and eosinophilia. Prolongation in prothrombin time was seen rarely.

Other: Genital pruritus, vaginitis, candidiasis.

In addition to the adverse reactions listed above which have been observed in patients treated with cefixime, the following adverse reactions and altered laboratory tests have been reported for cephalosporin class antibiotics:

Adverse reactions: Allergic reactions including anaphylaxis, toxic epidermal necrolysis, superinfection, renal dysfunction, toxic nephropathy, hepatic dysfunction including cholestasis, aplastic anemia, hemolytic anemia, hemorrhage, and colitis. Several cephalosporins have been implicated in triggering seizures, particularly in patients with renal impairment when the dosage was not reduced (see DOSAGE AND ADMINISTRATION and OVERDOSAGE). If seizures associated with drug therapy occur, the drug should be discontinued. Anticonvulsant therapy can be given if clinically indicated.

ADVERSE REACTIONS: *(cont'd)*

Abnormal Laboratory Tests: Positive direct Coombs' test, elevated bilirubin, elevated LDH, pancytopenia, neutropenia, agranulocytosis.

OVERDOSAGE:

Gastric lavage may be indicated; otherwise, no specific antidote exists. Cefixime is not removed in significant quantities from the circulation by hemodialysis or peritoneal dialysis. Adverse reactions in small numbers of healthy adult volunteers receiving single doses up to 2 g of cefixime did not differ from the profile seen in patients treated at the recommended doses.

DOSAGE AND ADMINISTRATION:

ADULTS

The recommended dose of cefixime is 400 mg daily. This may be given as a 400-mg tablet daily or as 200-mg tablet every 12 hours.

For the treatment of uncomplicated cervical/urethral gonococcal infections, a single oral dose of 400 mg is recommended.

CHILDREN

The recommended dose is 8 mg/kg/day of the suspension. This may be administered as a single daily dose or may be given in two divided doses, as 4 mg/kg every 12 hours (TABLE 8).

TABLE 8 Pediatric Dosage Chart

Patient Weight (kg)	Dose/Day (mg)	Dose/Day (ml)	Dose/Day (tsp of suspension)
6.25	50	2.5	1/2
12.5	100	5.0	1
18.75	150	7.5	1 1/2
25.0	200	10.0	2
31.25	250	12.5	2 1/2
37.5	300	15.0	3

Children weighing more than 50 kg or older than 12 years should be treated with the recommended adult dose.

Otitis media should be treated with the suspension. Clinical studies of otitis media were conducted with the suspension, and the suspension results in higher peak blood levels than the tablet when administered at the same dose. Therefore, the tablet should not be substituted for the suspension in the treatment of otitis media (see CLINICAL PHARMACOLOGY.)

Efficacy and safety in infants aged less than 6 months have not been established.

In the treatment of infections due to *S. pyogenes*, a therapeutic dosage of cefixime should be administered for at least 10 days.

DOSAGE FOR IMPAIRED RENAL FUNCTION

Cefixime may be administered in the presence of impaired renal function. Normal dose and schedule may be employed in patients with creatinine clearances of 60 ml/min or greater. Patients whose clearance is between 21 and 60 ml/min or patients who are on renal hemodialysis may be given 75% of the standard dosage at the standard dosing interval (*i.e.*, 300 mg daily). Patients whose clearance is <20 ml/min, or patients who are on continuous ambulatory peritoneal dialysis may be given half the standard dosage at the standard dosing interval (*i.e.*, 200 mg daily). Neither hemodialysis nor peritoneal dialysis removes significant amounts of drug from the body.

BOTTLE-SIZE RECONSTITUTION DIRECTIONS FOR ORAL SUSPENSION

100 ml: To reconstitute, suspend with **69 ml water**.

Method: Tap the bottle several times to loosen powder contents prior to reconstitution. Add approximately half the total amount of water for reconstitution and shake well. Add the remainder of water and shake well.

75 ml: To reconstitute, suspend with **52 ml water**.

Method: Tap the bottle several times to loosen powder contents prior to reconstitution. Add approximately half the total amount of water for reconstitution and shake well. Add the remainder of water and shake well.

50 ml: To reconstitute, suspend with **36 ml water**.

Method: Tap the bottle several times to loosen powder contents prior to reconstitution. Add approximately half the total amount of water for reconstitution and shake well. Add the remainder of water and shake well.

After reconstitution the suspension may be kept for 14 days either at room temperature, or under refrigeration, without significant loss of potency. Keep tightly closed. Shake well before using. Discard unused portion after 14 days.

REFERENCES:

1. Bauer AW, Kirby WMM, Sherris JC, et al.: Antibiotic susceptibility testing by a standard single disk method. *Am J Clin Pathol* 1966; 45:493. 2. National Committee for Clinical Laboratory Standards, Approved Standard: Performance Standards for Antimicrobial Disk Susceptibility Tests (M2-A3), December 1984. 3. Standardized disk susceptibility test. Federal Register 1974; 39 (May 30): 19182-19184.** Clinitest and Clinistix are registered trademarks of Ames Division, Miles Laboratories, Inc. Tes-Tape is a registered trademark of Eli Lilly and Company.

PATIENT INFORMATION:

Cefixime is a cephalosporin antibiotic used to treat bacterial infections.

Take at regular intervals and complete the entire course of therapy.

Do not take this medication if you are allergic to any type of penicillin or cephalosporin.

Notify your physician if you are pregnant or nursing.

This antibiotic may decrease the effectiveness of birth control pills; use another form of birth control while taking this medication.

Shake the suspension well before each use and store it in the refrigerator.

May cause nausea, vomiting or diarrhea; notify your physician if these occur.

Take with food or milk to avoid stomach upset.

Cefixime may cause a false-positive reaction for nonspecific urine glucose tests in patients with diabetes. This medication does not interfere with enzyme-based urine glucose tests.

HOW SUPPLIED:

Suprax Tablets, 200 mg, are convex, rectangular, white, film-coated tablets with rounded corners and beveled edges and a divided break line on each side, engraved with Suprax across one side and LL to the left and 200 to the right on the other side.

Suprax Tablets, 400 mg, are convex, rectangular, white, film-coated tablets with rounded corners and beveled edges and a divided break line on each side, engraved with Suprax across one side and LL to the left and 400 to the right on the other side.

Store at controlled room temperature 15 to 30° C (59 to 86° F).

HOW SUPPLIED: *(cont'd)*

Suprax for oral suspension is an off-white to cream-colored powder which when reconstituted as directed contains cefixime 100 mg/5 ml.

Prior to reconstitution: Store at controlled room temperature 15 to 30° C (59 to 86° F).

HOW SUPPLIED - EQUIVALENTS NOT AVAILABLE:

Suspension - Oral - 100 mg/5ml

50 ml	$30.96	SUPRAX, Lederle Pharm	00005-3898-40
75 ml	$49.43	SUPRAX, Lederle Pharm	00005-3898-42
100 ml	$62.31	SUPRAX, Lederle Pharm	00005-3898-46

Tablet, Plain Coated - Oral - 200 mg

100's	$322.20	SUPRAX, Lederle Pharm	00005-3899-23

Tablet, Plain Coated - Oral - 400 mg

10's	$67.33	SUPRAX, Lederle Pharm	00005-3897-94
50's	$322.20	SUPRAX, Lederle Pharm	00005-3897-18
100's	$631.45	SUPRAX, Lederle Pharm	00005-3897-23
100's	$663.00	SUPRAX, Lederle Pharm	00005-3897-60

CEFMETAZOLE SODIUM *(000685)*

CATEGORIES: Anti-Infectives; Antibiotics; Bronchitis; Cephalosporins; Gonorrhea; Infections; Intra-Abdominal Infections; Perioperative Prophylaxis; Pneumonia; Respiratory Tract Infections; Sexually Transmitted Diseases; Skin Infections; Urinary Tract Infections; Pregnancy Category B; FDA Class 1C ("Little or No Therapeutic Advantage"); FDA Approved 1989 Dec

BRAND NAMES: *Cefotazol*; *Cefmetazon* (Asia); *Cemetol*; *Cetazone*; *Gomcefa*; *Metalin*; **Zefazone**
(International brand names outside U.S. in italics)

DESCRIPTION:

Cefmetazole sodium is a semisynthetic cephem antibiotic. It was originally derived from cephamycin C, produced by *Streptomyces jumonjinensis*. It is now synthetically produced from 7 -amino-cephalosporanic acid. It is the sodium salt of (6R-cis)-7-((((cyanomethyl)thio) acetyl)amino)-7-methoxy-3-(((1-methyl-1H-tetrazol-5-yl)thio)methyl)-8-oxo-5-thia-1-azabicyclo; (4.2.0)oct-2-ene-2-carboxylic acid. The empirical formula is $C_{15}H_{16}N_7O_5S_3Na$.

The molecular weight of cefmetazole sodium is 493.51.

Zefazone Sterile Powder (sterile cefmetazole sodium) is supplied in vials containing 49 mg (2 milliequivalents) of sodium per gram of cefmetazole activity. Reconstituted solutions of cefmetazole sodium are intended for intravenous and intramuscular administration. the color of the solutions ranges from colorless to light amber. The pH of freshly reconstituted solutions ranges from 4.2 to 6.2

Zefazone IV Solution (cefmetazole sodium injection) in the Galaxy plastic container (PL2040) is a frozen, iso-osmotic, sterile, nonpyrogenic premixed 50 ml solution containing 1 g or 2 g of cefmetazole as cefmetazole sodium. Zefazone IV Solution contains 62 mg (2.7 milliequivalents) of sodium per gram of cefmetazole activity.

Dextrose, USP, has been added to the above dosage to adjust osmolarity (approximately 1.9 g and 1.1 g to the 1 g and 2 g dosages as dextrose hydrous, respectively). Sodium citrate hydrous, USP, has been added as a buffer. Sodium hydroxide is used to adjust pH and to convert cefmetazole free acid to cefmetazole sodium. The pH may have been adjusted with hydrochloric acid if necessary. The pH of thawed solution ranges from 4.2 to 6.2. After thawing to room temperature, cefmetazole sodium injection is intended for intravenous use only.

The Galaxy container is fabricated from a specially designed multilayer plastic (PL2040). Solutions are in contact with the polyethylene layer of this container and can leach out certain chemical components of the plastic in very small amounts within the expiration period. The suitability of the plastic has been confirmed in tests in animals according to USP biologic tests for plastic containers, as well as by tissue culture toxicity studies.

CLINICAL PHARMACOLOGY:

Following an intravenous dose of 2 grams administered over 60 minutes to normal volunteers, the mean maximum serum concentration of cefmetazole was 143 mcg/ml. After intramuscular administration of a 1 g dose to normal volunteers, the mean peak serum concentration was 34 mcg/ml, and the peak occurred at approximately 1.5 hours after administration. (TABLE 1):

TABLE 1 Cefmetazole Serum Levels (mcg/ml)

	Time after beginning of infusion							
Dose	10	20	30 min	1 hr	2 hr	4 hr	6 hr	8 hr
1 gram IV*	-	-	443	73	31	9	3	-
2 gram IV*	-	-	92	143	70	20	6	2
1 gram IM	8	17	25	30	25	13	7	4

* Infused over 60 minutes

Following repeated administration of 2 grams every 6 hours, the mean maximum and trough serum levels of cefmetazole were 138 and 6 mcg/ml, respectively.

After a 5 minute intravenous infusion of 2 grams to normal volunteers, the mean maximum serum concentration of cefmetazole was 290 mcg/ml. (TABLE 2)

TABLE 2 Serum Levels (mcg/ml) After 5 Minute IV Infusions

	Time after beginning of infusion				
Dose	10 min	20 min	1 hr	2 hr	4 hr
1 gram	129	90	43	25	8
2 gram	214	156	91	52	17

The mean plasma or serum elimination half-life after intravenous infusion is approximately 1.2 hours, and the mean plasma clearance is 121 ml/min. Cefmetazole is 65% bound to serum proteins at a concentration of 100 mcg/ml.

Approximately 85% of a dose of cefmetazole is excreted unchanged in the urine over a 12-hour period resulting in high urinary concentrations. Mean urinary concentrations over collection intervals ranged from 9828 to 52 mcg/ml (mean urine volumes - 104 ml and 645 ml, respectively) in a 12 hour period following a 1 hour IV infusion of 2 grams. After a 5 minute IV infusion of 2 grams, analogous mean urinary concentrations ranged from 5138 to 46 mcg/ml (mean urine volumes = 183 ml and 575 ml, respectively).

CLINICAL PHARMACOLOGY: *(cont'd)*

Cefmetazole is excreted by tubular secretion. Probenecid doubles the half-life and increases the duration of measurable plasma concentrations of cefmetazole; however, the maximum plasma concentrations remain unchanged. In patients with reduced renal function, the plasma clearance is decreased and the half-life of cefmetazole is prolonged (see DOSAGE AND ADMINISTRATION.)

After a 1 gram IV dose, mean concentrations in the gallbladder wall and the bile at 2.8 hours were 130 mcg/g and 310 mcg/ml, respectively.

After a 1 gram IV dose, vaginal, uterine and adnexal tissue concentrations were variable and lower than serum concentrations, ranging from 2.7 to 62.5 mcg/g at 0.1 to 2 hours after the dose.

After a 2 gram dose, the mean maximum concentration in interstitial fluid was 4.5 mcg/ml at one hour after administration and was less than 2 mcg/ml by 4 hours after administration.

Data on CSF levels of cefmetazole are not available.

MICROBIOLOGY

The bactericidal action of cefmetazole results from inhibition of cell wall synthesis. Cefmetazole is active *in vitro* against a wide range of aerobic and anaerobic gram-positive and gram-negative organisms. The methoxy group in the 7α position provides cefmetazole sodium with a high degree of stability in the presence of beta lactamases, both penicillinase and cephalosporinase. Cefmetazole is usually active against the following organisms *in vitro* and in clinical infections (see INDICATIONS AND USAGE.)

Gram-positive [a]
Staphylococcus aureus[b] (including penicillinase- and non-penicillinase-producing strains)
Staphylococcus epidermidis[b]
Streptococcus pneumoniae
Streptococcus agalactiae
Streptococcus pyogenes

Gram-negative [c]
Escherichia coli
Klebsiella pneumoniae
Klebsiella oxytoca
Haemophilus influenzae (non-penicillinase-producing strains)
Proteus mirabilis
Proteus vulgaris
Morganella morganii
Providencia stuartii

Anaerobic organisms
Bacteroides fragilis
Bacteroides melaninogenicus
Clostridium perfringens

NOTE:

[a] Most strains of enterococci, e.g. *Enterococcus faecalis* (formerly *Streptococcus faecalis*), are resistant to cefmetazole.

[b] Cefmetazole sodium should not be used for treatment of infections caused by methicillin-resistant staphylococci.

[c] Cefmetazole is inactive *in vitro* against most strains of *Pseudomonas aeruginosa* and many strains of *Enterobacter* species.

Cefmetazole sodium has been shown to be active *in vitro* against most strains of the following organisms; however, clinical efficacy has not been established.

Gram-negative
Citrobacter diversus
Haemophilus influenzae (penicillinase-producing strains)
Moraxella (Branhamella) catarrhalis
Neisseria gonorrhoeae (penicillinase- and non-penicillinase-producing strains)
Providencia rettgeri
Salmonella species
Shigella species

Anaerobic organisms
Bacteroides bivius
Bacteroides disiens
Bacteroides intermedius
Bacteroides ureolyticus
Peptococcus species
Peptostreptococcus species

SUSCEPTIBILITY TESTING

Diffusion Techniques: Quantitative methods that require measurement of zone diameters give an estimate of antibiotic susceptibility. One such procedure has been recommended for use with disks to test susceptibility to cefmetazole used the 30-mcg cefmetazole disk.[1] Interpretation involves correlation of the diameter obtained in the disk test with the minimum inhibitory concentration (MIC) values for cefmetazole.

Reports from the laboratory giving results of the standardized single disk susceptibility test using a 30-mcg cefmetazole disk should be interpreted to the following criteria (TABLE 3):

TABLE 3 Susceptibility Testing

Zone diameter (mm)	Interpretation
≥ 16	(S) Susceptible
13-15	(MS) Moderately Susceptible
≤ 12	(R) Resistant

A report of "Susceptible" indicates that the pathogen is likely to be inhibited by generally achievable blood concentrations.

A report of "Moderately Susceptible" indicates that inhibitory concentrations of the antibiotic may well be achieved if high dosage is used or if the infection is confined to tissues and fluids (*e.g.*, urine) in which high antibiotic levels are attained.

A report of "Resistant" indicates that achievable concentrations of the antibiotic are unlikely to be inhibitory and other therapy should be selected.

Standardized procedures require the use of laboratory control organisms. The 30-mcg disk should give the following zone diameters (TABLE 4):

Cephalosporin class disks should not be used to test for cefmetazole susceptibility.

CLINICAL PHARMACOLOGY: *(cont'd)*

TABLE 4 Susceptibility Testing

Organism	Zone diameter (mm)
E. coli ATCC 25922	26-32
S. aureus ATCC 25923	25-34

Dilution Techniques: Use a with standardized dilution method[2](broth, agar, microdilution) or equivalent with cefmetazole powder. The MIC values obtained should be interpreted according to the following criteria (TABLE 5):

TABLE 5 Dilution Techniques

MIC (mcg/ml)	Interpretation
≤16	(S) Susceptible
32	(MS) Moderately susceptible
≥64	(R) Resistant

As with standard diffusion techniques, dilution methods require the use of laboratory control organisms. Standard cefmetazole powder should provide the following MIC values (TABLE 6).

TABLE 6 Dilution Techniques

Organism	Zone Diameter (mm)
E. coli ATCC	0.25 - 2.0
S. aureus ATCC 29213	0.5 - 2.0

For anaerobic bacteria the MIC of cefmetazole can be determined by agar or broth dilution (including microdilution) techniques.[3]

INDICATIONS AND USAGE:

TREATMENT

Cefmetazole sodium products are indicated for the treatment of serious infections caused by susceptible strains of the designated microorganisms in the following diseases:

Urinary Tract Infections: Complicated or uncomplicated urinary tract infections caused by*Escherichia coli.*

Lower Respiratory Tract Infections: Pneumonia and bronchitis caused by *Streptococcus pneumoniae, Staphylococcus aureus* (penicillinase- and non-penicillinase-producing strains), *Escherichia coli,* and *Haemophilus influenzae* (non-penicillinase producing strains).

Skin and Skin Structure Infections caused by *Staphylococcus aureus* (penicillinase- and non-penicillinase-producing strains),*Staphylococcus epidermidis, Streptococcus pyogenes, Streptococcus agalactiae, Escherichia coli, Proteus mirabilis, Proteus vulgaris**, *Morganella morganii**, *Providencia stuartii**, *Klebsiella pneumoniae, Klebsiella oxytoca**, *Bacteroides fragilis,* and *Bacteroides melaninogenicus**.

Intra-abdominal Infections caused by *Escherichia coli, Klebsiella pneumoniae**, *Klebsiella oxytoca**, *Bacteroides fragilis,* and *Clostridium perfringens**.

Cefmetazole sodium (administered concurrently with oral probenecid) is indicated for the treatment of adults with the following sexually transmitted diseases caused by susceptible strains of the designated organisms.

Sexually Transmitted Diseases: Uncomplicated gonorrhea (urethral/cervical) due to *Neisseria gonorrhoeae* (penicillinase- and non-penicillinase-producing strains).

Uncomplicated rectal infections due to *N. gonorrhoeae* (penicillinase- and non-penicillinase-producing strains) in women. Presently there are no corresponding efficacy data for male patients.

Data do not support the use of cefmetazole sodium in the treatment of pharyngeal infections due to *N. gonorrhoeae* in men or women.

Appropriate specimens for bacteriological examination should be obtained in order to isolate and identify causative organisms and to determine their susceptibility to cefmetazole sodium. Therapy with cefmetazole sodium may be instituted before results of susceptibility studies are known; however, once these results become available, antibiotic treatment should be adjusted accordingly.

PROPHYLAXIS

Preoperative administration of cefmetazole sodium may reduce the incidence of certain postoperative infections in patients who undergo cesarean section, abdominal or vaginal hysterectomy, cholecystectomy (high risk patients), and colorectal surgery. These procedures are classified as clean contaminated or potentially contaminated surgery.

If signs and symptoms of an infection develop after surgery, the causative organism should be identified by culture and appropriate therapeutic measures initiated.

*Efficacy for this organism in this organ system was studied in fewer than 10 infections.

CONTRAINDICATIONS:

Cefmetazole sodium products are contraindicated in patients with known allergy to cefmetazole or to the cephalosporin group of antibiotics.

WARNINGS:

BEFORE THERAPY WITH CEFMETAZOLE SODIUM PRODUCTS IS INSTITUTED, CAREFUL INQUIRY SHOULD BE MADE TO DETERMINE WHETHER THE PATIENT HAS HAD PREVIOUS HYPERSENSITIVITY REACTIONS TO CEFMETAZOLE, CEPHALOSPORINS, PENICILLINS, OR OTHER DRUGS. IF THIS PRODUCT IS TO BE GIVEN TO PENICILLIN-SENSITIVE PATIENTS, CAUTION SHOULD BE EXERCISED BECAUSE CROSS HYPERSENSITIVITY AMONG BETA-LACTAM ANTIBIOTICS HAS BEEN CLEARLY DOCUMENTED AND MAY OCCUR IN UP TO 10% OF PATIENTS WITH A HISTORY OF PENICILLIN ALLERGY. IF AN ALLERGIC REACTION TO CEFMETAZOLE SODIUM OCCURS, DISCONTINUE THE DRUG. SERIOUS ACUTE HYPERSENSITIVITY REACTIONS MAY REQUIRE TREATMENT WITH EPINEPHRINE AND OTHER EMERGENCY MEASURES, INCLUDING OXYGEN, INTRAVENOUS FLUIDS, INTRAVENOUS ANTIHISTAMINES, CORTICOSTEROIDS, PRESSOR AMINES, AND AIRWAY MANAGEMENT, AS CLINICALLY INDICATED.

Pseudomembranous colitis has been reported with nearly all antibacterial agents, including cefmetazole sodium, and may range in severity from mild to life-threatening. Therefore, it is important to consider this diagnosis in patients who present with diarrhea subsequent to the administration of antibacterial agents.

Treatment with antibacterial agents alters the normal flora of the colon and may permit overgrowth of clostridia. Studies indicate that a toxin produced by *Clostridium difficile* is the primary cause of "antibiotic-associated colitis"

WARNINGS: *(cont'd)*

After the diagnosis of pseudomembranous colitis has been established, therapeutic measures should be initiated. Mild cases of pseudomembranous colitis usually respond to drug discontinuation alone. In moderate to severe cases, consideration should be given to management with fluids and electrolytes, protein supplementation and treatment with an oral antibacterial drug effective against *C. difficile.*

PRECAUTIONS:

General: In patients with transient or persistent reduction in urinary output due to renal insufficiency, the total daily dose of cefmetazole sodium products should be reduced (see DOSAGE AND ADMINISTRATION), because high and prolonged serum antibiotic concentrations can occur in such individuals following usual doses.

As with other antibiotics, prolonged use of cefmetazole sodium may result in overgrowth of nonsusceptible organisms. Repeated evaluation of the patient's condition is essential. If superinfection occurs during therapy, appropriate measures should be taken.

As with some other cephalosporins, cefmetazole sodium may be associated with a fall in prothrombin activity. Those at risk include patients with renal or hepatic impairment, or poor nutritional state, as well as patients receiving a protracted course of antimicrobial therapy. Prothrombin time should be monitored for patients at risk and exogenous Vitamin K administered as indicated.

A disulfiram-like reaction has been reported after ingestion of alcohol (see DRUG INTERACTIONS.) Therefore, patients should be advised against the ingestion of alcohol-containing beverages during and for 24 hours after the administration of cefmetazole sodium.

Antibiotics, including cephalosporins, should be prescribed with caution to individuals with a history of gastrointestinal disease, particularly colitis.

Drug/Laboratory Test Interactions: Patients receiving cefmetazole may show a false positive result for glucose in the urine with tests that use Benedict's or Fehling's solution.

Carcinogenesis, Mutagenesis, and Impairment of Fertility: Long-term carcinogenesis studies of cefmetazole sodium have not been performed in animals. Mutagenesis studies of cefmetazole sodium, including the Ames test, the unscheduled DNA synthesis test, the mammalian cell forward gene mutation assay, and the dominant lethal test, were all negative. When administered subcutaneously for 35 days to young (6-41 days of age) rats at dosages of 300 mg/kg/day or 1,000 mg/kg/day, cefmetazole was associated with a reduced number of mature spermatids in the testis and a slight, dose-related reduction of testicular weight. These effects were completely reversible; rats examined 5 and 10 weeks after cessation of the 35 day cefmetazole treatment regimen at the above doses had normal testicular weights and normal spermatogenesis. In an extension of this study, all aspects of reproductive function were normal in male rats allowed to mate at either 4 to 5 weeks or 7 to 8 weeks after cessation of the 300 or 1,000 mg/kg/day cefmetazole sodium treatment regimen. In separate studies, there were no adverse effects on the testicles when cefmetazole sodium was given for 30 days to sexually mature male rats at doses up to 2,500 mg/kg/day. The effects of cefmetazole sodium on the testes of sexually immature rats are probably due to the methylthiotetrazole side chain which is released from the parent compound by nonenzymatic hydrolysis in the intestine. Rats metabolize the parent compound to release the methylthiotetrazole side chain at a greater rate than humans. There are also species differences in age at onset of spermatogenesis and rate of reproductive maturation. The significance for humans of these testicular changes in sexually immature rats treated with high doses of cefmetazole sodium is unknown.

Pregnancy Category B: Cefmetazole sodium was not teratogenic or embryocidal when administered to rats or mice at doses up to 2,000 mg/kg/day (approximately 12.5 times the maximum human dose) during the period of organogenesis. There are, however, no adequate and well-controlled studies of cefmetazole use in pregnant women. Because animal reproduction studies are not always predictive of human response, this drug should be used during pregnancy only if clearly needed.

Nursing Mothers: Trace concentrations of cefmetazole are excreted in human milk: therefore, consideration should be given to temporarily discontinuing nursing during therapy with cefmetazole.

Pediatric Use: Safety and effectiveness in children have not been established. For information concerning testicular changes in prepubertal rats, see the Carcinogenesis, Mutagenesis, Impairment of Fertility subsection.

DRUG INTERACTIONS:

A disulfiram-like reaction, characterized by flushing, sweating, headache, and tachycardia, has been reported when alcohol was ingested after cefmetazole sodium administration. A similar reaction has been reported with other structurally-related cephalosporins.

Although nephrotoxicity has not been noted when cefmetazole sodium was given alone, it is possible that nephrotoxicity may be potentiated if cefmetazole sodium is used concomitantly with an aminoglycoside.

ADVERSE REACTIONS:

Cefmetazole sodium was generally well-tolerated. Adverse reactions that were reported as possibly or probably related to therapy with cefmetazole sodium were:

Gastrointestinal: Diarrhea (3.6%), nausea (1.0%), vomiting, epigastric pain, candidiasis, bleeding. There have been rare reports of pseudomembranous colitis in patients receiving cefmetazole sodium. The onset of pseudomembranous colitis symptoms may occur during or after antibiotic treatment (see WARNINGS.)

Hypersensitivity: Allergic reactions including anaphylaxis and urticaria, periorbital edema.

Dermatologic: Rash (1.1%), pruritus, generalized erythema.

Local: Following intravenous administration: pain and/or swelling at the injection site, phlebitis, thrombophlebitis. Following intramuscular administration: pain (31%), tenderness (26%), induration (3%), bleeding (1.4%), bruising (2%), and/or swelling (1.1%).

Cardiovascular: Shock, hypotension.

Central Nervous System: Headache, hot flashes, dizziness.

Respiratory Tract: Pleural effusion, dyspnea, epistaxis, respiratory distress.

Special Senses: Alteration in color perception, taste alteration.

Musculoskeletal: Joint pain and inflammation.

Other: Fever, superinfection, vaginitis.

ADVERSE LABORATORY CHANGES

Adverse laboratory changes that have been reported, without regard to drug relationship, were:

Hepatic: Transient increases in AST (SGOT), ALT (SGPT), alkaline phosphatase, bilirubin, and LDH.

Hematologic: Eosinophilia, leucocytosis, lymphocytosis, granulocytosis, basophilia, monocytosis, thrombocytosis, decreased hemoglobin, decreased hematocrit, decreased RBC, leucopenia, neutropenia, lymphocytopenia, thrombocytopenia, positive Coombs test, prolonged PT and PTT.

Musculoskeletal: Transient increase in creatinine kinase (CK).

Serum Chemistry: Increased glucose, decreased serum albumin, decreased total serum protein.

ADVERSE REACTIONS: *(cont'd)*

Renal: Increased BUN, increased creatinine.

In addition to the adverse reactions listed above which have been observed in patients treated with cefmetazole sodium, the following adverse reactions and altered laboratory tests have been reported for cephalosporin class antibiotics:

Adverse reactions: Allergic reactions including Stevens-Johnson syndrome, erythema multiforme, toxic epidermal necrolysis, renal dysfunction, toxic nephropathy, hepatic dysfunction including cholestasis, aplastic anemia, hemolytic anemia, hemorrhage.

Several cephalosporins have been implicated in triggering seizures, particularly in patients with renal impairment when the dosage was not reduced (see DOSAGE AND ADMINISTRATION and OVERDOSAGE). If seizures associated with drug therapy occur, the drug should be discontinued. Anticonvulsant therapy can be given if clinically indicated.

Abnormal Laboratory Tests: Agranulocytosis, pancytopenia.

OVERDOSAGE:

Information on overdosage in humans is not available. In the event of serious toxic reactions from overdosage, hemodialysis or peritoneal dialysis may aid in the removal of cefmetazole from the body, particularly if renal function is compromised. In 7 anuric patients, mean hemodialysis clearance for cefmetazole was 104 ml/min.

DOSAGE AND ADMINISTRATION:

Cefmetazole sodium injection should not be used for intramuscular administration.

Efficacy using the intramuscular route of administration has only been established in the treatment of the indicated sexually transmitted diseases. (See INDICATIONS AND USAGE.) For the treatment or prophylaxis of other diseases, the intravenous route of administration should be used.

TREATMENT

The usual adult dosage is 2 grams of cefmetazole sodium powder or cefmetazole sodium injection administered intravenously every 6 to 12 hours for 5 to 14 days. Proper dosage should be determined by the condition of the patient, location and severity of the infection, and susceptibility of the causative organisms (see TABLE 7):

TABLE 7 General Guidelines for Dosage of Cefmetazole Sodium Powder and Cefmetazole Sodium Injection

Type of Infection	Daily Dose	Frequency
Uncomplicated Gonorrhea	1 gram[1]	Single dose IM
Urinary Tract	4 grams	2 grams every 12 hours IV
Other Sites		
Mild to Moderate	6 grams	2 grams every 8 hours IV
Severe to Life-Threatening	8 grams	2 grams every 6 hours IV

[1]with 1 gram of probenecid given by mouth at the same time or up to 1/2 hour before Zefazone Sterile Powder.

PROPHYLAXIS

To reduce the incidence of postoperative infection following vaginal hysterectomy, abdominal hysterectomy, cesarean section, colorectal surgery, or cholecystectomy (high risk) in adults, the recommended doses are (TABLE 8):

TABLE 8

Surgery	Dosing Regimen
Vaginal Hysterectomy	2 grams given as a single dose 30-90 minutes before surgery or
	1 gram doses given 30-90 minutes before surgery and repeated 8 and 16 hours later
Abdominal Hysterectomy	1 gram doses given 30-90 minutes before surgery and repeated 8 and 16 hours later
Cesarean Section	2 grams given as a single dose after clamping the cord or
	1 gram doses given after clamping the cord and repeated 8 and 16 hours later
Colorectal[a] Surgery	2 grams given as a single dose 30-90 minutes before surgery or
	2 gram doses given 30-90 minutes before surgery and repeated 8 and 16 hours later
Cholecystectomy (high risk)	1 g doses given 30-90 minutes before surgery and repeated 8 and 16 hours later

[a]All patients studied received preoperative bowel preparation with mechanical cleansing, oral neomycin or kanamycin and oral erythromycin.

If surgery lasts more than 4 hours, the preoperative dose should be repeated.

IMPAIRED RENAL FUNCTION

For patients with impaired renal function, a reduced dosage schedule should be employed. The following dosage guidelines are derived from clinical pharmacology studies (TABLE 9):

TABLE 9 Dosage Guidelines for Cefmetazole Sodium Powder and Cefmetazole Sodium Injection in Adults With Impaired Renal Function

Renal Function	Creatinine Clearance ($ml/min/1.73M^2$)	Dose (grams)	Frequency
Mild Impairment	90-50	1-2	Q 12 h
Moderate Impairment	49-30	1-2	Q 16 h
Severe Impairment	29-10	1-2	Q 24 h
Essentially No Function	< 10	1-2	Q 48 h*

* administered after hemodialysis

When only the serum creatinine level is available, the following formula (based on sex, weight, and age of the patient) may be used to convert this value into creatinine clearance. The serum creatinine level should represent a steady state of renal function (TABLE 10).

TABLE 10

Males: [Weight (kg) × (140-age)] ÷ [72 × serum creatinine (mg/100 ml)]
Females: 0.85 × above value

GENERAL RECONSTITUTION PROCEDURES FOR STERILE POWDER

For Intravenous Use

Reconstitute with Sterile Water for Injection, Bacteriostatic Water for Injection, or 0.9 Percent Sodium Chloride Injection. Shake to dissolve and let stand until clear (TABLE 11):

DOSAGE AND ADMINISTRATION: *(cont'd)*

TABLE 11 IV Reconstitution

Vial Size	Amount of Diluent to be Added (ml)	Approximate Withdrawable Volume (ml)	Approximate Average Concentration (mg/ml)
1 g	10	10.4	100
1 g	3.7	4.1	250
2 g	15	16	125
2 g	7	8	250

General Reconstitution Procedure for Intramuscular Use

Reconstitute with Sterile Water for Injection, Bacteriostatic Water for Injection, 0.9 Percent Sodium Chloride Injection, or Lidocaine HCl (0.5% or 1.0% without epinephrine). Shake to dissolve and let stand until clear.

TABLE 12 IM Reconstitution

Vial Size	Amount of Diluent to be Added (ml)	Approximate Withdrawable Volume (ml)	Approximate Average Concentration (mg/ml)
1 gram	2.2	2.7	370

INTRAVENOUS ADMINISTRATION

A solution containing 1 g or 2 grams of cefmetazole sodium sterile power in Sterile Water for Injection, Bacteriostatic Water for Injection, or 0.9 Percent Sodium Chloride Injection can be administered by IV infusion over 10 to 60 minutes. For otherwise healthy patients undergoing elective surgical procedure, a solution containing 1 gram or 2 grams of cefmetazole sodium powder in Sterile Water for Injection, Bacteriostatic Water for Injection, or 0.9 Percent Sodium Chloride Injection can also be injected over three to five minutes. During infusion of the solution containing cefmetazole sodium, it is necessary to temporarily discontinue administration of other solutions at the same site.

INTRAMUSCULAR ADMINISTRATION

As with all intramuscular preparations, the solution containing cefmetazole sodium powder should be injected well within the body of a relatively large muscle such as the upper outer quadrant of the buttock (*i.e.,* gluteus maximus). Aspiration is necessary to avoid inadvertent injection into a blood vessel.

IV SOLUTION-DIRECTIONS FOR USE

Zefazone IV Solution in Galaxy plastic container (PL2040) is for intravenous administration only.

Storage: Store in a freezer capable of maintaining a temperature of -20°C (-4°F).

Thawing of Plastic Containers: Thaw frozen container at room temperature (25°C, 77°F) or in a refrigerator (8°, 46°F).

DO NOT FORCE THAW BY IMMERSION IN WATER BATHS OR BY MICROWAVE IRRADIATION. Check for minute leaks by squeezing container firmly. If leaks are detected, discard solution as sterility may be impaired.

The container should be visually inspected. Components of the solution may precipitate in the frozen state and will dissolve upon reaching room temperature with little or no agitation. If after visual inspection the solution remains cloudy or if an insoluble precipitate is noted or if any seals or outlet ports are not intact, the container should be discarded.**DO NOT ADD SUPPLEMENTARY MEDICATION**

The thawed solution in Galaxy container (PL2040 Plastic) is stable for 48 hours at room temperature (25°, 77°F) or for 21 days when stored under refrigeration (8°C, 46°F).**DO NOT REFREEZE.**

PREPARATION FOR INTRAVENOUS ADMINISTRATION (USE ASEPTIC TECHNIQUE)

1. Suspend container(s) from eyelet support.

2. Remove protector from outlet port at bottom of container.

3. Attach administration set. Refer to complete directions accompanying set.

Caution: Do not use plastic containers in series connections. Such use could result in an embolism due to residual air being drawn from the primary container before administration of the fluid from the secondary container is complete.

INTRAVENOUS ADMINISTRATION

Cefmetazole sodium injection can be administered as an intravenous infusion over 10 to 60 minutes.

COMPATIBILITY AND STABILITY

Sterile Powder

When reconstituted as described above (Preparation of Solution), cefmetazole sodium powder maintains satisfactory potency for 24 hours at room temperature (25°C, 77°F), for 7 days under refrigeration (8°C, 46°F), and for 6 weeks in the frozen state (at or below - 20°C, -4°F).

Primary cefmetazole solutions (as described in Preparation of Solution) may be further diluted to concentrations of 1.0 to 20 mg/ml in the following diluents and maintain potency for 24 hours at room temperature (25°C, 77°F), for 7 days under refrigeration (8°C, 46°F), and for 6 weeks in the frozen state (at or below -20°C, -4°F).

0.9 percent Sodium Chloride Injection

5 percent Dextrose Injection

Lactated Ringer's Injection

1% Lidocaine Solution (without epinephrine)

Reconstituted cefmetazole sodium solutions may be stored frozen in glass, Viaflex plastic (PL 146) or McGaw PAB plastic containers, when thawed, remain chemically stable for 24 hours either at room temperature (25°C, 77°F) or under refrigeration (8°C, 46°F).

Use an appropriate storage module in order to avoid unnecessary handling and to prevent surface contact between frozen containers.

Do not refreeze thawed solutions.

Parenteral drug products should be inspected visually for particulate matter and discoloration prior to administration whenever solution and container permit.

Cefmetazole sodium is compatible with clindamycin phosphate and potassium chloride.

Cefmetazole sodium inactivates heparin sodium as determined by USP*in vitro* assay; therefore, the two products should not be admixed.

Solutions of cefmetazole sodium, like those of most beta-lactam antibiotics, should not be added to aminoglycoside solutions. If cefmetazole sodium and aminoglycosides are to be administered to the same patient, they must be administered separately and not admixed.

DOSAGE AND ADMINISTRATION: *(cont'd)*

IV Solution

The thawed solution in Galaxy plastic container (PL 2040) remains chemically stable for 48 hours at room temperature (25°, 77°F) for 21 days when stored under refrigeration (8°C, 46°F).

DO NOT REFREEZE.

REFERENCES:

1. National Committee for Clinical Laboratory Standards: *Performance Standards for Antimicrobial Disk Susceptibility Tests*, 4th Edition, Approved Standard NCCLS Document M2-A4, Vol. 10, No. 7, NCCLS, Villanova, PA, April 1990. **2.** National Committee for Clinical Laboratory Standards, *Methods for Dilution Antimicrobial Susceptibility Tests for Bacteria That Grow Aerobically*, 2nd Edition, Approved Standard NCCLS Document M7-A2, Vol. 10, No. 8, NCCLS, Villanova, PA, April 1990. **3.** National Committee for Clinical Laboratory Standards, *Methods for Antimicrobial Susceptibility Testing of Anaerobic Bacteria*, 2nd Edition, Approved Standard NCCLS Document M11-A2, Vol. 10, No. 15, NCCLS, Villanova, PA, August 1990.

HOW SUPPLIED - EQUIVALENTS NOT AVAILABLE:

Injection, Lyphl-Soln - Intravenous - 1 gm/vial

1 gm x 10	$7.19	ZEFAZONE, Pharmacia & Upjohn	00009-3471-01
50 ml x 24	$240.19	ZEFAZONE, Pharmacia & Upjohn	00009-3512-01

Injection, Lyphl-Soln - Intravenous - 2 gm/vial

2 gm x 10	$14.34	ZEFAZONE, Pharmacia & Upjohn	00009-3477-01
50 ml x 24	$411.62	ZEFAZONE, Pharmacia & Upjohn	00009-3513-01

CEFONICID SODIUM *(000686)*

CATEGORIES: Anti-Infectives; Antibiotics; Antimicrobials; Bone Infections; Cephalosporins; Infections; Joint Infections; Perioperative Prophylaxis; Respiratory Tract Infections; Septicemia; Skin Infections; Urinary Tract Infections; Pregnancy Category B; FDA Approved 1984 May

BRAND NAMES: *Dinacid*; *Monocef*; **Monocid**; *Monocidur* (Mexico)
(International brand names outside U.S. in italics)

FORMULARIES: Medi-Cal

DESCRIPTION:

Monocid (sterile cefonicid sodium), a sterile, lyophilized, semi-synthetic, broad-spectrum cephalosporin antibiotic for intravenous and intramuscular administration, is 5-Thia-1-azabicyclo [4.2.0] oct-2-ene-2-carboxylic acid, 7-[(hydroxyphenyl-acetyl)-amino]-8-oxo-3-[[[1-(sulfomethyl)-1*H*-te trazol-5-yl]thio]methyl]-disodium salt, [6*R*-[6a, 7β,(*R**)]].

Cefonicid sodium contains 85 mg (3.7 mEq) sodium per gram of cefonicid activity.

CLINICAL PHARMACOLOGY:

HUMAN PHARMACOLOGY

The table below (TABLE 1) demonstrates the levels and duration of cefoncid sodium in serum following intravenous and intramuscular administration of 1 gram to normal volunteers.

TABLE 1

Serum Concentrations After 1 Gram Administration (mcg/ml)

Interval	5 min.	15 min.	30 min.	1 hr.	2 hr.	4 hr.
IV	221.3	176.4	147.6	124.2	88.9	61.4
IM	13.5	45.9	73.1	98.6	97.1	77.8
Interval	**6 hr.**	**8 hr.**	**10 hr.**	**12 hr.**	**24 hr.**	
IV	40.0	29.3	20.6	15.2	2.6	
IM	54.9	38.5	28.9	20.6	4.5	

Serum half-life is approximately 4.5 hours with intravenous and intramuscular administration. Cefoncid sodium is highly (greater than 90%) and reversibly protein bound.

Cefoncid sodium is not metabolized; 99% is excreted unchanged in the urine in 24 hours. A 500 mg IM dose provides a high (384 mcg/ml) urinary concentration at 6-8 hours. Probenecid, given concurrently with cefoncid sodium, slows renal excretion, produces higher peak serum levels and significantly increases the serum half-life of the drug (8.2 hours).

Cefoncid sodium reaches therapeutic levels in the following tissues and fluids (TABLE 2):

TABLE 2 Tissue and Body Fluid Levels

Tissue or Body Fluid	Dosage and Route (No. of Patients Sampled)	Time of Sampling After Dose	Average Tissue or Fluid Levels (µ/g or/ml)
Bone	1 g. IM (7)	60-90 min	6.8
	1 g. IV (10)	44-99 min.	14.0
Gallbladder	1 g. IM (10)	60-70 min.	15.5
Bile	1 g. IM (10)	60-70 min.	7.5
Prostate	1 g. IM (10)	50-115 min.	13.0
Uterine Tissue	1 g. IM (6)	60-90 min.	17.5
Wound Fluid	1 g. IM (10)	60-75 min.	37.7
Purulent Wound	1 g. IM (9)	60 min.	11.5
Adipose Tissue	1 g. IM (5)	60 min.	4.0
Atrial	1 g. IM (7)	77-170 min.	7.5
Appendage	2 g. IM (7)	105-170 min.	8.7
	15 mg/kg IV (10)	53-160 min.	15.4

Note: Although cefoncid sodium reaches therapeutic levels in bile, those levels are lower than those seen with other cephalosporins, and amounts of cefoncid sodium released into the gastrointestinal tract are minute. This small amount of cefoncid sodium in the gastrointestinal tract is thought to be the reason for the low incidence of gastrointestinal reactions following therapy with cefoncid sodium.

No disulfiram-like reactions were reported in a crossover study conducted in healthy volunteers receiving cefoncid sodium and alcohol.

MICROBIOLOGY

The bactericidal action of cefoncid sodium results from inhibition of cell-wall synthesis. Cefoncid sodium is highly resistant to beta-lactamases produced by *Staphylococcus aureus, Hemophilus influenzae, Neisseria gonorrhoeae* and Richmond type I beta-lactamases. Cefoncid sodium is resistant to degradation by beta-lactamases from certain members of *Enterobacteriaceae*. Active against a wide range of gram-positive and gram-negative organisms. Cefoncid sodium is usually active against the following organisms *in vitro* and in clinical situations:

Gram-Positive Aerobes: *Staphylococcus aureus* (beta-lactamase producing and non-beta-lactamase producing) and *S. epidermidis* (Note: Methicillin-resistant staphylococci are resistant to cephalosporins, including cefonicid.); *Streptococcus pneumoniae, S. pyogenes* (Group A beta-hemolytic *Streptococcus)*, and *S. agalactiae* (Group B *Streptococcus)*.

CLINICAL PHARMACOLOGY: *(cont'd)*

Gram-Negative Aerobes: *Escherichia coli; Klebsiella pneumoniae; Providencia rettgeri* (formerly *Proteus rettgeri*);*Proteus vulgaris; Morganella morganii* (formerly *Proteus morganii*);*Proteus mirabilis;* and *Hemophilus influenzae* (ampicillin-sensitive and -resistant).

The following *in vitro* data are available but their clinical significance is unknown. Cefoncid sodium is usually active against the following organisms *in vitro:*

Gram-Negative Aerobes: *Moraxella* (formerly *Branhamella*) *catarrhalis*; *Klebsiella oxytoca*; *Enterobacter aerogenes*; *Neisseria gonorrhoeae* (penicillin-sensitive and -resistant): *Citrobacter freundii* and *C. diversus.*

Gram-Positive Anaerobes: *Clostridium perfringens*; *Peptostreptococcus anaerobius*; *Peptococcus magnus*;*P. prevotii*; and *Propionibacterium acnes*.

Gram-Negative Anaerobes: *Fusobacterium nucleatum.*

Cefoncid sodium is usually inactive *in vitro* against most strains of *Pseudomonas*, *Serratia*,*Enterococcus* and *Acinetobacter*. Most strains of *B. fragilis* are resistant.

SUSCEPTIBILITY TESTING

Results from standardized single-disk susceptibility tests using a 30 mcg cefoncid sodium disk should be interpreted according to the following criteria:

Zones of 18 mm or greater indicate that the tested organism is susceptible to cefoncid sodium and is likely to respond to therapy.

Zones from 15 to 17 mm indicate that the tested organism is of intermediate (moderate) susceptibility, and is likely to respond to therapy if a higher dosage is used or if the infection is confined to tissues and fluids in which high antibiotic levels are attained.

Zones of 14 mm or less indicate that the organism is resistant.

Only the cefoncid sodium disk should be used to determine susceptibility, since *in vitro* tests show that cefoncid sodium has activity against certain strains not susceptible to other cephalosporins. The cefoncid sodium disk should not be used for testing susceptibility to other cephalosporins.

A bacterial isolate may be considered susceptible if the MIC value for cefoncid sodium is equal to or less than 8 mcg/ml in accordance with the National Committee for Clinical Laboratory Standards (NCCLS) guidelines. Organisms are considered resistant if the MIC is equal to or greater than 32 mcg/ml For most organisms the MBC value for cefoncid sodium is the same as the MIC value.

The standardized quality control procedure requires use of control organisms. The 30 mcg cefoncid sodium disk should give the zone diameters listed below for the quality control strains.

TABLE 3

Organism	ATCC	Zone Size Range
E. coli	25922	25-29 mm
S. aureus	25923	22-28 mm

INDICATIONS AND USAGE:

Due to the long half-life of cefoncid sodium, a 1 gram dose results in therapeutic serum levels which provide coverage against susceptible organisms (listed below) for 24 hours.

Studies on specimens obtained prior to therapy should be used to determine the susceptibility of the causative organisms to cefoncid sodium. Therapy with cefoncid sodium may be initiated pending results of the studies; however, treatment should be adjusted according to study findings.

TREATMENT

Cefoncid sodium is indicated in the treatment of infections due to susceptible strains of the microorganisms listed below:

Lower Respiratory Tract Infections, due to *Streptococcus pneumoniae*; *Klebsiella pneumoniae**;*Escherichia coli*; and *Hemophilus influenzae* (ampicillin-resistant and ampicillin-sensitive).

Urinary Tract Infections, due to *Escherichia coli*;*Proteus mirabilis* and *Proteus* spp. (which may include the organisms now called *Proteus vulgaris,** *Providencia rettgeri* and *Morganella morganii*); and *Klebsiella pneumoniae.**

Skin and Skin Structure Infections, due to *Staphylococcus aureus* and *S. epidermidis*;*Streptococcus pyogenes* (Group A*Streptococcus*) and *S. agalactiae* (Group B*Streptococcus*).

Septicemia, due to *Streptococcus pneumoniae* (formerly *D. pneumoniae*) and *Escherichia coli.**

Bone and Joint Infections, due to *Staphylococcus aureus.*

SURGICAL PROPHYLAXIS

Administration of a single 1 gram dose of cefoncid sodium before surgery may reduce the incidence of postoperative infections in patients undergoing surgical procedures classified as contaminated or potentially contaminated (*e.g.,* colorectal surgery, vaginal hysterectomy, or cholecystectomy in high-risk patients), or in patients in whom infection at the operative site would present a serious risk (*e.g.,* prosthetic arthroplasty, open heart surgery). Although cefonicid has been shown to be as effective as cefazolin in prevention of infection following coronary artery bypass surgery, no placebo-controlled trials have been conducted to evaluate any cephalosporin antibiotic in the prevention of infection following coronary artery bypass surgery or prosthetic heart valve replacement.

In cesarean section, the use of cefoncid sodium (after the umbilical cord has been clamped) may reduce the incidence of certain postoperative infections.

When administered 1 hour prior to surgical procedures for which it is indicated, a single 1 gram dose of cefoncid sodium provides protection from most infections due to susceptible organisms throughout the course of the procedure. Intraoperative and/or postoperative administrations of cefoncid sodium are not necessary. Daily doses of cefoncid sodium may be administered for two additional days in patients undergoing prosthetic arthroplasty or open heart surgery.

If there are signs of infection, the causative organisms should be identified and appropriate therapy determined through susceptibility testing.

Before using cefoncid sodium concomitantly with other antibiotics, the prescribing information for those agents should be reviewed for contraindications, warnings, precautions and adverse reactions. Renal function should be carefully monitored.

*Efficacy for this organism on this organ system has been demonstrated in fewer than 10 infections.

CONTRAINDICATIONS:

Cefoncid sodium is contraindicated in persons who have shown hypersensitivity to cephalosporin antibiotics.

WARNINGS:

BEFORE THERAPY WITH STERILE CEFONICID SODIUM IS INSTITUTED, CAREFUL INQUIRY SHOULD BE MADE TO DETERMINE WHETHER THE PATIENT HAS HAD PREVIOUS HYPERSENSITIVITY REACTIONS TO CEPHALOSPORINS, PENICILLINS, OR OTHER DRUGS. THIS PRODUCT SHOULD BE GIVEN CAUTIOUSLY TO PENICILLIN-SENSITIVE PATIENTS. ANTIBIOTICS SHOULD BE ADMINISTERED WITH CAUTION TO ANY PATIENT WHO HAS DEMONSTRATED SOME FORM OF ALLERGY, PARTICULARLY TO DRUGS. SERIOUS ACUTE HYPERSENSITIVITY REACTIONS MAY REQUIRE EPINEPHRINE AND OTHER EMERGENCY MEASURES.

Pseudomembranous colitis has been reported with the use of nearly all antibacterial agents, including cefoncid sodium, and has ranged in severity from mild to life-threatening. Therefore, it is important to consider this diagnosis in patients who present with diarrhea subsequent to the administration of antibacterial agents.

Treatment with antibacterial agents alters the normal flora of the colon and may permit overgrowth of clostridia. Studies indicate that a toxin produced by *Clostridium difficile* is one primary cause of "antibiotic-associated colitis."

Mild cases of pseudomembranous colitis usually respond to drug discontinuation alone. In moderate to severe cases, consideration should be given to management with fluids and electrolytes, protein supplementation and treatment with an antibacterial drug clinically effective against *C. difficile* colitis.

PRECAUTIONS:

General: With any antibiotic, prolonged use may result in overgrowth of nonsusceptible organisms. Careful observation is essential, and appropriate measures should be taken if superinfection occurs.

Carcinogenesis, Mutagenesis, and Impairment of Fertility: Beta-lactam antibiotics with methylthio-tetrazole side chains have been shown to cause testicular atrophy in prepubertal rats, which persisted into adulthood and resulted in decreased spermatogenesis and decreased fertility. Cefonicid, which contains a methylsulfonic-thio-tetrazole moiety, has no adverse effect on the male reproductive system of prepubertal, juvenile or adult rats when given under identical conditions.

Carcinogenicity studies of cefonicid have not been conducted, however, results of mutagenicity studies (*i.e.,* Ames/Salmonella/microsome plate assay and the micronucleus test in mice) were negative.

Pregnancy Category B: Reproduction studies have been performed in mice, rabbits and rats at doses up to an equivalent of 40 times the usual adult human dose and have revealed no evidence of impaired fertility or harm to the fetus due to cefoncid sodium. There are, however, no adequate and well-controlled studies in pregnant women. Because animal reproduction studies are not always predictive of human response, this drug should be used in pregnancy only if clearly needed.

Labor and Delivery: In cesarean section, cefoncid sodium should be administered only after the umbilical cord has been clamped.

Nursing Mothers: Cefoncid sodium is excreted in human milk in low concentrations. Caution should be exercised when cefoncid sodium is administered to a nursing woman.

Pediatric Use: Safety and effectiveness in children have not been established.

DRUG INTERACTIONS:

Nephrotoxicity has been reported following concomitant administration of other cephalosporins and aminoglycosides.

ADVERSE REACTIONS:

Cefoncid sodium is generally well tolerated and adverse reactions have occurred infrequently. The most common adverse reaction has been pain on IM injection. On-therapy conditions occurring in greater than 1% of cefoncid sodium-treated patients were:

Injection Site Phenomena Pain and/or discomfort on injection; less often, burning, phlebitis at IV site.

Increased Platelets (1.7%).

Increased Eosinophils (2.9%).

Liver Function Test Alterations (1.6%): Increased alkaline phosphatase, increased SGOT, increased SGPT, increased GGTP, increased LDH. Less frequent on-therapy conditions occurring in less than 1% of cefoncid sodium-treated patients were:

Hypersensitivity Reactions: Fever, rash, pruritus, erythema, myalgia and anaphylactoid-type reactions have been reported.

Hematology: Decreased WBC, neutropenia, thrombocytopenia, positive Coombs' test.

Renal: Increased BUN and creatinine levels have occasionally been seen. Rare reports of acute renal failure associated with interstitial nephritis, observed with other beta-lactam antibiotics, have also occurred with Monocid.

Gastrointestinal: Diarrhea and pseudomembranous colitis. Onset of pseudomembranous colitis symptoms may occur during or after antibiotic treatment (see WARNINGS.)

DOSAGE AND ADMINISTRATION:

GENERAL

The usual adult dosage is 1 gram of cefoncid sodium given once every 24 hours, intravenously or by deep intramuscular injection. Doses in excess of 1 gram daily are rarely necessary; however, in exceptional cases dosage of up to 2 grams given once daily have been well tolerated. When administering 2 gram IM doses once daily, 1/2 the dose should be administered in different large muscle masses.

OUTPATIENT USE

Cefoncid sodium has been used (once daily IM or IV) on an outpatient basis. Individuals responsible for outpatient administration of cefoncid sodium should be instructed thoroughly in appropriate procedures for storage, reconstitution and administration.

SURGICAL PROPHYLAXIS

When administered 1 hour prior to appropriate surgical procedures (see INDICATIONS AND USAGE), a 1 gram dose of cefoncid sodium provides protection from most infections due to susceptible organisms throughout the course of the procedure. Intraoperative and/or postoperative administrations of cefoncid sodium are not necessary. Daily doses of cefoncid sodium may be administered for 2 additional days in patients undergoing prosthetic arthroplasty or open heart surgery.

In cesarean section cefoncid sodium should be administered only after the umbilical cord has been clamped.

IMPAIRED RENAL FUNCTION

Modification of cefoncid sodium dosage is necessary in patients with impaired renal function. Following an initial loading dosage of 7.5 mg/kg IM or IV, the maintenance dosing schedule shown below should be followed. Further dosing should be determined by severity of the infection and susceptibility of the causative organism.

DOSAGE AND ADMINISTRATION: *(cont'd)*

TABLE 4 General Guidelines for Dosage of Cefoncid Sodium, IV or IM

Type of Infection	Daily Dose (grams)	Frequency
Uncomplicated Urinary Tract	0.5	once every 24 hours
Mild to Moderate	1	once every 24 hours
Severe or Life-Threatening	2*	once every 24 hours
Surgical Prophylaxis	1	1 hour preoperatively

* When administering 2 gram IM doses once daily, 1/2 the dose should be administered in different large muscle masses.

TABLE 5 Dosage of Cefoncid Sodium in Adults with Reduced Renal Function

(Monitor renal function and adjust accordingly.)

Creatinine Clearance (ml/min per 1.73 M²)	Dosage Regimen: Mild to Moderate Infections	Severe Infections
79 to 60	10 mg/kg (every 24 hours)	25 mg/kg (every 24 hours)
59 to 40	8 mg/kg (every 24 hours)	20 mg/kg (every 24 hours)
39 to 20	4 mg/kg (every 24 hours)	15 mg/kg (every 24 hours)
19 to 10	4 mg/kg (every 48 hours)	15 mg/kg (every 48 hours)
9 to 5	4 mg/kg (every 3 to 5 days)	15 mg/kg (every 3 to 5 days)
< 5	3 mg/kg (every 3 to 5 days)	4 mg/kg (every 3 to 5 days)

Note: It is not necessary to administer additional dosage following dialysis.

PREPARATION OF PARENTERAL SOLUTION

Parenteral drug products should be SHAKEN WELL when reconstituted, and inspected visually for particulate matter prior to administration. If particulate matter is evident in reconstituted fluids, the drug solutions should be discarded.

RECONSTITUTION

SINGLE-DOSE VIALS

For IM injection, IV direct (bolus) injection, or IV infusion, reconstitute with Sterile Water for Injection according to the following table (TABLE 6). SHAKE WELL.

TABLE 6

Vial Size	Diluent to Be Added	Approx. Avail. Volume	Approx. Avg. Concentration
500 mg	2.0 ml	2.2 ml	225 mg/ml
1 gram	2.5 ml	3.1 ml	325 mg/ml

These solutions of cefoncid sodium are stable 24 hours at room temperature or 72 hours if refrigerated (5°C). Slight yellowing does not affect potency.

For IV infusion, dilute reconstituted solution in 50 to 100 ml of the parenteral fluids listed under ADMINISTRATION.

PHARMACY BULK VIALS (10 GRAMS)

For IM injection, IV direct (bolus) injection or IV infusion, reconstitute with Sterile Water for Injection, Bacteriostatic Water for Injection, or Sodium Chloride Injection according to the following table (TABLE 7):

TABLE 7

Amount of Diluent	Approximate Concentration	Approximate Available Volume
25 ml	1 gram/3 ml	31 ml
45 ml	1 gram/5 ml	51 ml

These solutions of cefoncid sodium are stable 24 hours at room temperature or 72 hours if refrigerated (5°C.) Slight yellowing does not affect potency. For IV infusion add to parenteral fluids listed under ADMINISTRATION.

"PIGGYBACK" VIALS

Reconstitute with 50 to 100 ml of Sodium Chloride Injection or other IV solution listed under ADMINISTRATION. Administer with primary IV fluids, as a single dose. These solutions of cefoncid sodium are stable 24 hours at room temperature or 72 hours if refrigerated (5°C). Slight yellowing does not affect potency.

A solution of 1 gram of cefoncid sodium in 18 ml of Sterile Water for Injection is isotonic.

ADMINISTRATION

IM Injection: Inject well within the body of a relatively large muscle. Aspiration is necessary to avoid inadvertent injection into a blood vessel. When administering 2 gram IM doses once daily, one-half the dose should be given in different large muscle masses.

IV Administration: For direct (bolus) injection, administer reconstituted cefoncid sodium slowly over 3 to 5 minutes, directly or through tubing for patients receiving parenteral fluids. For infusion, dilute reconstituted cefoncid sodium in 50 to 100 ml of one of the following solutions:

0.9% Sodium Chloride Injection, USP

5% Dextrose Injection, USP

5% Dextrose and 0.9% Sodium Chloride Injection, USP

5% Dextrose and 0.45% Sodium Chloride Injection, USP

5% Dextrose and 0.2% Sodium Chloride Injection, USP

10% Dextrose Injection, USP

Ringer's Injection, USP

Lactated Ringer's Injection, USP

5% Dextrose and Lactated Ringer's Injection

10% Invert Sugar in Sterile Water for Injection

5% Dextrose and 0.15% Potassium Chloride Injection

Sodium Lactate Injection, USP

In these fluids cefoncid sodium is stable 24 hours at room temperature or 72 hours if refrigerated (5°C). Slight yellowing does not affect potency.

HOW SUPPLIED:

Monocid (sterile cefonicid sodium) is supplied in vials equivalent to 500 mg and 1 gram of cefonicid, in "Piggyback" Vials for IV admixture equivalent to 1 gram of cefonicid; and in Pharmacy Bulk Vials equivalent to 10 grams of cefonicid.

As with other cephalosporins, cefoncid sodium may darken on storage. However, if stored as recommended, this color change does not affect potency.

Before reconstitution, cefoncid sodium should be protected from light and refrigerated (2° to 8°C).

HOW SUPPLIED - EQUIVALENTS NOT AVAILABLE:

Injection, Lyphl-Soln - Intramuscular; - 0.500 gm

10 ml x 1	$13.10	MONOCID, SKB Pharms	00007-4351-01

Injection, Lyphl-Soln - Intramuscular; - 1 gm

10 ml x 1	$26.10	MONOCID, SKB Pharms	00007-4353-01
10 ml x 1	$26.10	MONOCID, SKB Pharms	00007-4353-76
10's	$271.05	MONOCID, SKB Pharms	00007-4354-76
100 ml x 10	$271.05	MONOCID, SKB Pharms	00007-4354-11

Injection, Lyphl-Soln - Intramuscular; - 10 gm

100 ml x 10	$2607.10	MONOCID, SKB Pharms	00007-4356-11
100 ml x 10	$2607.10	MONOCID, SKB Pharms	00007-4356-76

CEFOPERAZONE SODIUM *(000687)*

CATEGORIES: Anti-Infectives; Antibacterials; Antibiotics; Antimicrobials; Cephalosporins; Endometritis; Infections; Inflammatory Disease; Intra-Abdominal Infections; Pelvic Inflammatory Disease; Peritonitis; Respiratory Tract Infections; Septicemia; Skin Infections; Urinary Tract Infections; Pregnancy Category B; FDA Approved 1982 Nov

BRAND NAMES: *CPZ*; **Cefobid**; *Cefobis* (France, Germany); *Cefogram*; *Cefozone*; *Cezone*; *Dardum*; *Kidazone*; *Magnamycin*; *Mediper*; *Medocef*; *Shinfomycin*; *Tomabef*; *Urazone*; *Zoncef*
(International brand names outside U.S. in italics)

DESCRIPTION:

Cefobid (cefoperazone sodium) is a sterile, semisynthetic, broad-spectrum, parenteral cephalosporin antibiotic for intravenous or intramuscular administration. It is the sodium salt of 7-(D(-)-α- (4-ethyl-2,3-dioxo-1-piperazinecarboxamido)-α - (4-hydroxyphenyl) acetamido)-3-((1-methyl-1H-tetrazol-5-yl)thiomethyl)-3-cephem-4-carboxylic acid. Its chemical formula is $C_{25}H_{26}N_9NaO_8S_2$ with a molecular weight of 667.65.

Cefobid contains 34 mg sodium (1.5 mEq) per gram. Cefobid is a white powder which is freely soluble in water. The pH of a 25% (w/v) freshly reconstituted solution varies between 4.5-6.5 and the solution ranges from colorless to straw yellow depending on the concentration.

Cefobid in crystalline form is supplied in vials equivalent to 1 g or 2 g of cefoperazone and in Piggyback Units for intravenous administration equivalent to 1 g or 2 g cefoperazone. Cefobid is also supplied premixed as a frozen, sterile, nonpyrogenic, iso-osmotic solution equivalent to 1 g or 2 g cefoperazone in plastic containers. After thawing, the solution is intended for intravenous use.

The plastic container is fabricated from specially formulated polyvinyl chloride. Solutions in contact with the plastic container can leach out certain of its chemical components in very small amounts within the expiration period, e.g., di 2-ethylhexyl phthalate (DEHP), up to 5 parts per million. However, the safety of the plastic has been confirmed in tests in animals according to the USP biological tests for plastic containers, as well as by tissue culture toxicity studies.

CLINICAL PHARMACOLOGY:

High serum and bile levels of cefoperazone sodium are attained after a single dose of the drug. Table 1 demonstrates the serum concentrations of cefoperazone sodium in normal volunteers following either a single 15-minute constant rate intravenous infusion of 1,2,3 or 4 grams of the drug, or a single intramuscular injection of 1 or 2 grams of the drug (TABLE 1):

TABLE 1 Cefoperazone Serum Concentrations

Dose/Route	Mean Serum Concentrations (mcg/ml) 0*	0.5 hr	1 hr	2 hr	4 hr	8 hr	12 hr
1 g IV	153	114	73	38	16	4	0.5
2 g IV	252	153	114	70	32	8	2
3 g IV	340	210	142	89	41	9	2
4 g IV	506	325	251	161	71	19	6
1 g IM	32**	52	65	57	33	7	1
2 g IM	40**	69	93	97	58	14	4

* Hours post-administration, with 0 time being the end of the infusion.
** Values obtained 15 minutes post-injection.

The mean serum half-life of cefoperazone sodium is approximately 2.0 hours, independent of the route of administration.

In vitro studies with human serum indicate that the degree of cefoperazone sodium reversible protein binding varies with the serum concentration from 93% at 25 mcg/ml of cefoperazone sodium to 90% at 250 mcg/ml and 82% at 500 mcg/ml.

Cefoperazone sodium achieves therapeutic concentrations in the following body tissues and fluids (TABLE 2):

TABLE 2

Tissue or Fluid	Dose	Concentration
Ascitic Fluid	2 g	64 mcg/ml
Cerebrospinal Fluid (in patients with inflamed meninges)	50 mg/k	1.8 mcg/ml to 8.0 mcg/ml
Urine	2 g	3,286 mcg/ml
Sputum	3 g	6.0 mcg/ml
Endometrium	2 g	74 mcg/g
Myometrium	2 g	54 mcg/g
Palatine Tonsil	1 g	8 mcg/g
Sinus Mucous Membrane	1 g	8 mcg/g
Umbilical Cord Blood	1 g	25 mcg/ml
Amniotic Fluid	1 g	4.8 mcg/ml
Lung	1 g	28 mcg/g
Bone	2 g	40 mcg/g

CLINICAL PHARMACOLOGY: *(cont'd)*

Cefoperazone sodium is excreted mainly in the bile. Maximum bile concentrations are generally obtained between one and three hours following drug administration and exceed concurrent serum concentrations by up to 100 times. Reported biliary concentrations of cefoperazone sodium range from 66 mcg/ml at 30 minutes to as high as 6000 mcg/ml at 3 hours after an intravenous bolus injection of 2 grams.

Following a single intramuscular or intravenous dose, the urinary recovery of cefoperazone sodium over a 12-hour period averages 20-30%. No significant quantity of metabolites has been found in the urine. Urinary concentrations greater than 2200 mcg/ml have been obtained following a 15-minute infusion of a 2 g dose. After an IM injection of 2 g, peak urine concentrations of almost 1000 mcg/ml have been obtained, and therapeutic levels are maintained for 12 hours.

Repeated administration of cefoperazone sodium at 12-hour intervals does not result in accumulation of the drug in normal subjects. Peak serum concentrations, areas under the curve (AUC's), and serum half-lives in patients with severe renal insufficiency are not significantly different from those in normal volunteers. In patients with hepatic dysfunction, the serum half-life is prolonged and urinary excretion is increased. In patients with combined renal and hepatic insufficiencies, cefoperazone sodium may accumulate in the serum.

Cefoperazone sodium has been used in pediatrics, but the safety and effectiveness in children have not been established. The half-life of cefoperazone sodium in serum is 6-10 hours in low birth-weight neonates.

MICROBIOLOGY

Cefoperazone sodium is active *in vitro* against a wide range of aerobic and anaerobic, gram-positive and gram-negative pathogens. The bactericidal action of cefoperazone sodium results from the inhibition of bacterial cell wall synthesis.Cefoperazone sodium has a high degree of stability in the presence of beta-lactamases produced by most gram-negative pathogens. Cefoperazone sodium is usually active against organisms which are resistant to other beta-lactam antibiotics because of beta-lactamase production. Cefoperazone sodium is usually active against the following organisms *in vitro* and in clinical infections:

Gram-Positive Aerobes: *Staphylococcus aureus*, penicillinase and non-penicillinase-producing strains; *Staphylococcus epidermidis*;*Streptococcus pneumoniae* (formerly *Diplococcus pneumoniae*); *Streptococcus pyogenes* (Group A beta-hemolytic streptococci); *Streptococcus agalactiae* (Group B beta-hemolytic streptococci); *Enterococcus* (*Streptococcus faecalis, S. faecium* and *S. durans*)

Gram-Negative Aerobes: *Escherichia coli*;*Klebsiella* species (including *K. pneumoniae*);*Enterobacter* species; *Citrobacter* species;*Haemophilus influenzae*; *Proteus mirabilis*; *Proteus vulgaris*; *Morganella morganii* (formerly *Proteus morganii*); *Providencia stuartii*; *Providencia rettgeri* (formerly *Proteus rettgeri*); *Serratia marcescens*; *Pseudomonas aeruginosa*; *Pseudomonas* species; Some strains of *Acinetobacter calcoaceticus*;*Neisseria gonorrhoeae*

Anaerobic Organisms: Gram-positive cocci (including *Peptococcus* and *Peptostreptococcus*); *Clostridium* species;*Bacteroides fragilis*; other *Bacteroides* species

Cefoperazone sodium is also active *in vitro* against a wide variety of other pathogens although the clinical significance is unknown. These organisms include: *Salmonella* and *Shigella* species, *Serratia liquefaciens, N. meningitidis, Bordetella pertussis, Yersinia enterocolitica, Clostridium difficile, Fusobacterium* species,*Eubacterium* species and beta-lactamase producing strains of*H. influenzae* and *N. gonorrhoeae.*

SUSCEPTIBILITY TESTING

Diffusion Technique: For the disk diffusion method of susceptibility testing, a 75 mcg cefoperazone sodium diffusion disk should be used. Organisms should be tested with the cefoperazone sodium 75 mcg disk since cefoperazone sodium has been shown *in vitro* to be active against organisms which are found to be resistant to other beta-lactam antibiotics.

Tests should be interpreted by the following criteria (TABLE 3):

TABLE 3

Zone Diameter	Interpretation
Greater than or equal to 21 mm	Susceptible
16-20 mm	Moderately Susceptible
Less than or equal to 15 mm	Resistant

Quantitative procedures that require measurement of zone diameters give the most precise estimate of susceptibility. One such method which has been recommended for use with the cefoperazone sodium 75 mcg disk is the NCCLS approved standard. (Performance Standards for Antimicrobic Disk Susceptibility Tests. Second Information Supplement Vol. 2 No. 2 pp. 49-69. Publisher-National Committee for Clinical Laboratory Standards, Villanova, Pennsylvania.)

A report of "susceptible" indicates that the infecting organism is likely to respond to cefoperazone sodium therapy and a report of "resistant" indicates that the infecting organism is not likely to respond to therapy. A "moderately susceptible" report suggests that the infecting organism will be susceptible to cefoperazone sodium if a higher than usual dosage is used or if the infection is confined to tissues and fluids (*e.g.,* urine or bile) in which high antibiotic levels are attained.

Dilution Techniques: Broth or agar dilution methods may be used to determine the minimal inhibitory concentration (MIC) of cefoperazone sodium. Serial twofold dilutions of cefoperazone sodium should be prepared in either broth or agar. Broth should be inoculated to contain 5 X 10^5 organisms/ml and agar "spotted" with 10^4organisms.

MIC test results should be interpreted in light of serum, tissue, and body fluid concentrations of cefoperazone sodium. Organisms inhibited by cefoperazone sodium at 16 mcg/ml or less are considered susceptible, while organisms with MIC's of 17-63 mcg/ml are moderately susceptible. Organisms inhibited at cefoperazone sodium concentrations of greater than or equal to 64 mcg/ml are considered resistant, although clinical cures have been obtained in some patients infected by such organisms.

INDICATIONS AND USAGE:

Cefoperazone sodium is indicated for the treatment of the following infections when caused by susceptible organisms:

Respiratory Tract Infections caused by *S. pneumoniae, H. influenzae, S. aureus* (penicillinase and non-penicillinase producing strains), *S. pyogenes** (Group A beta-hemolytic streptococci),*P. aeruginosa, Klebsiella pneumoniae, E. coli, Proteus mirabilis,* and *Enterobacter* species.

Peritonitis and Other Intra-abdominal Infections caused by*E. coli, P. aeruginosa,** and anaerobic gram-negative bacilli (including *Bacteroides fragilis*).

Bacterial Septicemia caused by *S. pneumoniae, S. agalactiae,** *S. aureus, Pseudomonas aeruginosa,** *E. coli, Klebsiella* spp.,* *Klebsiella pneumoniae,** *Proteus* species* (indole-positive and indole-negative), *Clostridium* spp.* and anaerobic gram-positive cocci.*

Infections of the Skin and Skin Structures caused by *S. aureus* (penicillinase and non-penicillinase producing strains),*S. pyogenes,** and *P. aeruginosa.*

INDICATIONS AND USAGE: *(cont'd)*

Pelvic Inflammatory Disease, Endometritis, and Other Infections of the Female Genital Tract caused by *N. gonorrhoeae, S. epidermidis,** *S. agalactiae, E. coli, Clostridium* spp.,**Bacteroides* species (including *Bacteroides fragilis*), and anaerobic gram-positive cocci.

Urinary Tract Infections caused by *Escherichia coli* and *Pseudomonas aeruginosa*.

Enterococcal Infections: Although cefoperazone has been shown to be clinically effective in the treatment of infections caused by enterococci in cases of **peritonitis and other intra-abdominal infections, infections of the skin and skin structures, pelvic inflammatory disease, endometritis and other infections of the female genital tract, and urinary tract infection,*** the majority of clinical isolates of enterococci tested are not susceptible to cefoperazone but fall just at or in the intermediate zone of susceptibility, and are moderately resistant to cefoperazone. However,*in vitro* susceptibility testing may not correlate directly with*in vivo*results. Despite this, cefoperazone therapy has resulted in clinical cures of enterococcal infections, chiefly in polymicrobial infections. Cefoperazone should be used in enterococcal infections with care and at doses that achieve satisfactory serum levels of cefoperazone.

*Efficacy of this organism in this organ system was studied in fewer than 10 infections.

SUSCEPTIBILITY TESTING

Before instituting treatment with cefoperazone sodium, appropriate specimens should be obtained for isolation of the causative organism and for determination of its susceptibility to the drug. Treatment may be started before results of susceptibility testing are available.

COMBINATION THERAPY

Synergy between cefoperazone sodium and aminoglycosides has been demonstrated with many gram-negative bacilli. However, such enhanced activity of these combinations is not predictable. If such therapy is considered, *in vitro* susceptibility tests should be performed to determine the activity of the drugs in combination, and renal function should be monitored carefully. See PRECAUTIONS, and DOSAGE AND ADMINISTRATION.

CONTRAINDICATIONS:

Cefoperazone sodium is contraindicated in patients with known allergy to the cephalosporin-class of antibiotics.

WARNINGS:

BEFORE THERAPY WITH CEFOPERAZONE SODIUM IS INSTITUTED, CAREFUL INQUIRY SHOULD BE MADE TO DETERMINE WHETHER THE PATIENT HAS HAD PREVIOUS HYPERSENSITIVITY REACTIONS TO CEPHALOSPORINS, PENICILLINS OR OTHER DRUGS. THIS PRODUCT SHOULD BE GIVEN CAUTIOUSLY TO PENICILLIN-SENSITIVE PATIENTS. ANTIBIOTICS SHOULD BE ADMINISTERED WITH CAUTION TO ANY PATIENT WHO HAS DEMONSTRATED SOME FORM OF ALLERGY, PARTICULARLY TO DRUGS. SERIOUS ACUTE HYPERSENSITIVITY REACTIONS MAY REQUIRE THE USE OF SUBCUTANEOUS EPINEPHRINE AND OTHER EMERGENCY MEASURES.

PSEUDOMEMBRANOUS COLITIS HAS BEEN REPORTED WITH THE USE OF CEPHALOSPORINS (AND OTHER BROAD-SPECTRUM ANTIBIOTICS); THEREFORE, IT IS IMPORTANT TO CONSIDER ITS DIAGNOSIS IN PATIENTS WHO DEVELOP DIARRHEA IN ASSOCIATION WITH ANTIBIOTIC USE.

Treatment with broad-spectrum antibiotics alters normal flora of the colon and may permit overgrowth of clostridia. Studies indicate a toxin produced by *Clostridium difficile* is one primary cause of antibiotic-associated colitis. Cholestyramine and colestipol resins have been shown to bind the toxin *in vitro*.

Mild cases of colitis may respond to drug discontinuance alone.

Moderate to severe cases should be managed with fluid, electrolyte, and protein supplementation as indicated.

When the colitis is not relieved by drug discontinuance or when it is severe, oral vancomycin is the treatment of choice for antibiotic-associated pseudomembranous colitis produced by *C. difficile*. Other causes of colitis should also be considered.

PRECAUTIONS:

GENERAL

Although transient elevations of the BUN and serum creatinine have been observed, cefoperazone sodium alone does not appear to cause significant nephrotoxicity. However, concomitant administration of aminoglycosides and other cephalosporins has caused nephrotoxicity.

Cefoperazone sodium is extensively excreted in bile. The serum half-life of cefoperazone sodium is increased 2-4 fold in patients with hepatic disease and/or biliary obstruction. In general, total daily dosage above 4 g should not be necessary in such patients. If higher dosages are used, serum concentrations should be monitored.

Because renal excretion is not the main route of elimination of cefoperazone sodium(see CLINICAL PHARMACOLOGY), patients with renal failure require no adjustment in dosage when usual doses are administered. When high doses of cefoperazone sodium are used, concentrations of drug in the serum should be monitored periodically. If evidence of accumulation exists, dosage should be decreased accordingly.

The half-life of cefoperazone sodium is reduced slightly during hemodialysis. Thus, dosing should be scheduled to follow a dialysis period. In patients with both hepatic dysfunction and significant renal disease, cefoperazone sodium dosage should not exceed 1-2 g daily without close monitoring of serum concentrations.

As with other antibiotics, vitamin K deficiency has occurred rarely in patients treated with cefoperazone sodium. The mechanism is most probably related to the suppression of gut flora which normally synthesize this vitamin. Those at risk include patients with a poor nutritional status, malabsorption states (*e.g.*, cystic fibrosis), alcoholism, and patients on prolonged hyper-alimentation regimens (administered either intravenously or via a naso-gastric tube). Prothrombin time should be monitored in these patients and exogenous vitamin K administered as indicated.

A disulfiram-like reaction characterized by flushing, sweating, headache, and tachycardia has been reported when alcohol (beer, wine) was ingested within 72 hours after cefoperazone sodium administration. Patients should be cautioned about the ingestion of alcoholic beverages following the administration of cefoperazone sodium. A similar reaction has been reported with other cephalosporins.

Prolonged use of cefoperazone sodium may result in the overgrowth of nonsusceptible organisms. Careful observation of the patient is essential. If superinfection occurs during therapy, appropriate measures should be taken.

Cefoperazone sodium should be prescribed with caution in individuals with a history of gastrointestinal disease, particularly colitis.

DRUG LABORATORY TEST INTERACTIONS

A false-positive reaction for glucose in the urine may occur with Benedict's or Fehling's solution.

PRECAUTIONS: *(cont'd)*

CARCINOGENESIS, MUTAGENESIS, IMPAIRMENT OF FERTILITY

Long term studies in animals have not been performed to evaluate carcinogenic potential. The maximum duration of cefoperazone sodium animal toxicity studies is six months. In none of the *in vivo* or *in vitro* genetic toxicology studies did cefoperazone sodium show any mutagenic potential at either the chromosomal or subchromosomal level. Cefoperazone sodium produced no impairment of fertility and had no effects on general reproductive performance or fetal development when administered subcutaneously at daily doses up to 500 to 1000 mg/kg prior to and during mating, and to pregnant female rats during gestation. These doses are 10 to 20 times the estimated usual single clinical dose. Cefoperazone sodium had adverse effects on the testes of prepubertal rats at all doses tested. Subcutaneous administration of 1000 mg/kg per day (approximately 16 times the average adult human dose) resulted in reduced testicular weight, arrested spermatogenesis, reduced germinal cell population and vacuolation of Sertoli cell cytoplasm. The severity of lesions was dose dependent in the 100 to 1000 mg/kg per day range; the low dose caused a minor decrease in spermatocytes. This effect has not been observed in adult rats. Histologically the lesions were reversible at all but the highest dosage levels. However, these studies did not evaluate subsequent development of reproductive function in the rats. The relationship of these findings to humans is unknown.

PREGNANCY

Pregnancy Category B: Reproduction studies have been performed in mice, rats, and monkeys at doses up to 10 times the human dose and have revealed no evidence of impaired fertility or harm to the fetus due to cefoperazone sodium. There are, however, no adequate and well controlled studies in pregnant women. Because animal reproduction studies are not always predictive of human response, this drug should be used during pregnancy only if clearly needed.

NURSING MOTHERS

Only low concentrations of cefoperazone sodium are excreted in human milk. Although cefoperazone sodium passes poorly into breast milk of nursing mothers, caution should be exercised when cefoperazone sodium is administered to a nursing woman.

PEDIATRIC USE

Safety and effectiveness in children have not been established. For information concerning testicular changes in prepubertal rats (see Carcinogenesis, Mutagenesis, Impairment of Fertility.)

ADVERSE REACTIONS:

In clinical studies the following adverse effects were observed and were considered to be related to cefoperazone sodium therapy or of uncertain etiology:

Hypersensitivity: As with all cephalosporins, hypersensitivity manifested by skin reactions (1 patient in 45), drug fever (1 in 260), or a change in Coombs' test (1 in 60) has been reported. These reactions are more likely to occur in patients with a history of allergies, particularly to penicillin.

Hematology: As with other beta-lactam antibiotics, reversible neutropenia may occur with prolonged administration. Slight decreases in neutrophil count (1 patient in 50) have been reported. Decreased hemoglobins (1 in 20) or hematocrits (1 in 20) have been reported, which is consistent with published literature on other cephalosporins. Transient eosinophilia has occurred in 1 patient in 10.

Hepatic: Of 1285 patients treated with cefoperazone in clinical trials, one patient with a history of liver disease developed significantly elevated liver function enzymes during cefoperazone sodium therapy. Clinical signs and symptoms of nonspecific hepatitis accompanied these increases. After cefoperazone sodium therapy was discontinued, the patient's enzymes returned to pre-treatment levels and the symptomatology resolved. As with other antibiotics that achieve high bile levels, mild transient elevations of liver function enzymes have been observed in 5-10% of the patients receiving cefoperazone sodium therapy. The relevance of these findings, which were not accompanied by overt signs or symptoms of hepatic dysfunction, has not been established.

Gastrointestinal: Diarrhea or loose stools have been reported in 1 in 30 patients. Most of these experiences have been mild or moderate in severity and self-limiting in nature. In all cases, these symptoms responded to symptomatic therapy or ceased when cefoperazone therapy was stopped. Nausea and vomiting have been reported rarely.

Symptoms of pseudomembranous colitis can appear during or for several weeks subsequent to antibiotic therapy (see WARNINGS.)

Renal Function Tests: Transient elevations of the BUN (1 in 16) and serum creatinine (1 in 48) have been noted.

Local Reactions: Cefoperazone sodium is well tolerated following intramuscular administration. Occasionally, transient pain (1 in 140) may follow administration by this route. When cefoperazone sodium is administered by intravenous infusion some patients may develop phlebitis (1 in 120) at the infusion site.

DOSAGE AND ADMINISTRATION:

The usual adult daily dose of cefoperazone sodium is 2 to 4 grams per day administered in equally divided doses every 12 hours.

In severe infections or infections caused by less sensitive organisms, the total daily dose and/or frequency may be increased. Patients have been successfully treated with a total daily dosage of 6-12 grams divided into 2, 3 or 4 administrations ranging from 1.5 to 4 grams per dose.

In a pharmacokinetic study, a total daily dose of 16 grams was administered to severely immunocompromised patients by constant infusion without complications. Steady state serum concentrations were approximately 150 mcg/ml in these patients.

When treating infections caused by *Streptococcus pyogenes*, therapy should be continued for at least 10 days.

Solutions of cefoperazone sodium and aminoglycoside should not be directly mixed, since there is a physical incompatibility between them. If combination therapy with cefoperazone sodium and an aminoglycoside is contemplated (see INDICATIONS AND USAGE) this can be accomplished by sequential intermittent intravenous infusion provided that separate secondary intravenous tubing is used, and that the primary intravenous tubing is adequately irrigated with an approved diluent between doses. It is also suggested that cefoperazone sodium be administered prior to the aminoglycoside. *In vitro* testing of the effectiveness of drug combination(s) is recommended.

RECONSTITUTION

The following solutions may be used for the initial reconstitution of cefoperazone sodium sterile powder:

Vehicles for Initial Reconstitution

5% Dextrose Injection (USP)
5% Dextrose and 0.9% Sodium Chloride Injection (USP)
5% Dextrose and 0.2% Sodium Chloride Injection (USP)

DOSAGE AND ADMINISTRATION: *(cont'd)*

10% Dextrose Injection (USP) Bacteriostatic Water for Injection (Benzyl Alcohol or Parabens) (USP)*†
0.9% Sodium Chloride Injection (USP)
Normosol M and 5% Dextrose Injection
Normosol R
Sterile Water for Injection*
* Not to be used as a vehicle for intravenous infusion
† Preparations containing Benzyl Alcohol should not be used in neonates.

GENERAL RECONSTITUTION PROCEDURES

Cefoperazone sodium sterile powder for intravenous or intramuscular use may be initially reconstituted with any compatible solution mentioned above in Table 1. Solutions should be allowed to stand after reconstitution to allow any foaming to dissipate to permit visual inspection for complete solubilization. Vigorous and prolonged agitation may be necessary to solubilize cefoperazone sodium in higher concentrations (above 333 mg cefoperazone/ml). The maximum solubility of cefoperazone sodium sterile powder is approximately 475 mg cefoperazone/ml of compatible diluent.

PREPARATION FOR INTRAVENOUS USE

General: Cefoperazone sodium concentrations between 2 mg/ml and 50 mg/ml are recommended for intravenous administration.

Preparation of Vials: Vials of cefoperazone sodium sterile powder may be initially reconstituted with a minimum of 2.8 ml per gram of cefoperazone of any compatible reconstituting solution appropriate for intravenous administration listed above in TABLE 4. For ease of reconstitution the use of 5 ml of compatible solution per gram of cefoperazone sodium is recommended. The entire quantity of the resulting solution should then be withdrawn for further dilution and administration using any of the following vehicles for intravenous infusion (TABLE 5):

Vehicles for Intravenous Infusion
5% Dextrose Injection (USP)
5% Dextrose and Lactated Ringer's Injection
5% Dextrose and 0.9% Sodium Chloride Injection (USP)
5% Dextrose and 0.2% Sodium Chloride Injection (USP)
10% Dextrose Injection (USP)
Lactated Ringer's Injection (USP)
0.9% Sodium Chloride Injection (USP)
Normosol M and 5% Dextrose Injection
Normosol R

Preparation of Piggy Back Units. Cefoperazone sodium sterile powder in Piggy Back Units for intravenous use may be prepared by adding between 20 ml and 40 ml of any appropriate diluent listed in Table 2 per gram of cefoperazone. If 5% Dextrose and Lactated Ringer's Injection or Lactated Ringer's Injection (USP) is the chosen vehicle for administration the cefoperazone sodium sterile powder should initially be reconstituted using 2.8-5 ml per gram of any compatible reconstituting solution listed in Table 1 prior to the final dilution.

The resulting intravenous solution should be administered in one of the following manners:

Intermittent Infusion: Solutions of cefoperazone sodium should be administered over a 15-30 minute time period.

Continuous Infusion: Cefoperazone sodium can be used for continuous infusion after dilution to a final concentration of between 2 and 25 mg cefoperazone per ml.

PREPARATION FOR INTRAMUSCULAR INJECTION

Any suitable solution listed above may be used to prepare cefoperazone sodium sterile powder for intramuscular injection. When concentrations of 250 mg/ml or more are to be administered, a lidocaine solution should be used. These solutions should be prepared using a combination of Sterile Water for Injection and 2% Lidocaine Hydrochloride Injection (USP) that approximates a 0.5% Lidocaine Hydrochloride Solution. A two-step dilution process as follows is recommended: First, add the required amount of Sterile Water for Injection and agitate until cefoperazone sodium powder is completely dissolved. Second, add the required amount of 2% lidocaine and mix (TABLE 4):

TABLE 4

	Final Cefoperazone Concentration	Step 1 Volume of Sterile Water	Step 2 Volume of 2% Lidocaine	Withdrawable Volume*†
1 g vial	333 mg/ml	2.0 ml	0.6 ml	3 ml
	250 mg/ml	2.8 ml	1.0 ml	4 ml
2 g vial	333 mg/ml	3.8 ml	1.2 ml	6 ml
	250 mg/ml	5.4 ml	1.8 ml	8 ml

* There is sufficient excess present to allow for withdrawal of the stated volume.
† Final lidocaine concentration will approximate that obtained if a 0.5% Lidocaine Hydrochloride Solution is used as diluent.

When a diluent other than Lidocaine HCl Injection (USP) is used reconstitute as follows (TABLE 5):

TABLE 5

	Cefoperazone Concentration	Volume of Diluent to be Added	Withdrawable Volume*
1 g vial	333 mg/ml	2.6 ml	3 ml
	250 mg/ml	3.8 ml	4 ml
2 g vial	333 mg/ml	5.0 ml	6 ml
	250 mg/ml	7.2 ml	8 ml

* There is sufficient excess present to allow for withdrawal of the stated volume.

DIRECTIONS FOR USE OF CEFOPERAZONE SODIUM INJECTION IN PLASTIC CONTAINERS

Cefoperazone sodium supplied premixed as a frozen, sterile, iso-osmotic solution in plastic containers is to be administered either as continuous or intermittent infusion.

Thaw container at room temperature. After thawing, check for minute leaks by squeezing bag firmly. If leaks are found, discard solution as sterility may be impaired. Additives should not be introduced into this solution. Do not use if the solution is cloudy or precipitated or if the seal is not intact.

After thawing, the solution is stable for 10 days if stored under refrigeration (5°C) and for 48 hours at room temperature. DO NOT REFREEZE. Use sterile equipment.

CAUTION: Do not use plastic container in series connections. Such use could result in air embolism due to residual air being drawn from the primary container before administration of the fluid from the secondary container is complete.

DOSAGE AND ADMINISTRATION: *(cont'd)*

PREPARATION FOR ADMINISTRATION

1. Suspend container from eyelet support.
2. Remove plastic protector from outlet port at bottom of container.
3. Attach administration set. Refer to complete directions accompanying set.

STORAGE AND STABILITY

Cefoperazone sodium sterile powder is to be stored at or below 25°C (77°F) and protected from light prior to reconstitution. After reconstitution, protection from light is not necessary.

TABLE 6 Controlled Room Temperature (15-25°C/59-77°F) Approximate

24 Hours	Concentrations
Bacteriostatic Water for Injection (Benzyl Alcohol or Parabens) (USP)	300 mg/ml
5% Dextrose Injection (USP)	2 mg to 50 mg/ml
5% Dextrose and Lactated Ringer's Injection	2 mg to 50 mg/ml
5% Dextrose + 0.9% Sodium Chloride Inj. (USP)	2 mg to 50 mg/ml
5% Dextrose + 0.2% Sodium Chloride Inj. (USP)	2 mg to 50 mg/ml
10% Dextrose Injection (USP)	2 mg to 50 mg/ml
Lactated Ringer's Injection (USP)	2 mg/ml
0.5% Lidocaine Hydrochloride Injection (USP)	300 mg/ml
0.9% Sodium Chloride Injection (USP)	2 mg to 300 mg/ml
Normosol M and 5% Dextrose Injection	2 mg to 50 mg/ml
Normosol	2 mg to 50 mg/ml
Sterile Water for Injection	300 mg/ml

Reconstituted Cefobid solutions may be stored in glass or plastic syringes, or in glass or flexible plastic parenteral solution containers.

TABLE 7 Refrigerator Temperature (2-8°C/36-46°F) Approximate

5 Days	Concentrations
Bacteriostatic Water for Injection (Benzyl Alcohol or Parabens) (USP)	300 mg/ml
5% Dextrose Injection (USP)	2 mg to 50 mg/ml
5% Dextrose + 0.9% Sodium Chloride Inj. (USP)	2 mg to 50 mg/ml
5% Dextrose + 0.2% Sodium Chloride Inj. (USP)	2 mg to 50 mg/ml
Lactated Ringer's Injection (USP)	2 mg/ml
0.5% Lidocaine Hydrochloride Injection (USP)	300 mg/ml
0.9% Sodium Chloride Injection (USP)	2 mg to 300 mg/ml
Normosol M and 5% Dextrose Injection	2 mg to 50 mg/ml
Normosol R	2 mg to 50 mg/ml
Sterile Water for Injection	300 mg/ml

Reconstituted Cefobid solutions may be stored in glass or plastic syringes, or in glass or flexible plastic parenteral solution containers.

TABLE 8 Freezer Temperature (-20 to -10°C/-4 to 14°F) Approximate

3 Weeks	Concentrations
5% Dextrose Injection (USP)	50 mg/ml
5% Dextrose and 0.9% Sodium Chloride Injection (USP)	2 mg/ml
5% Dextrose and 0.2% Sodium Chloride Injection (USP)	2 mg/ml
5 Weeks	
0.9% Sodium Chloride Injection (USP)	300 mg/ml
Sterile Water for Injection	300 mg/ml

Reconstituted Cefobid solutions may be stored in plastic syringes, or in flexible plastic parenteral solution containers.
Frozen samples should be thawed at room temperature before use. After thawing, unused portions should be discarded. Do not refreeze.

The preceding parenteral diluents and approximate concentrations of cefoperazone sodium provide stable solutions under the following conditions for the indicated time periods (TABLE 6, TABLE 7, TABLE 8). (After the indicated time periods, unused portions of solutions should be discarded.)

HOW SUPPLIED - EQUIVALENTS NOT AVAILABLE:

Injection, Solution - Intramuscular; - 1 gm

10's	$164.21	CEFOBID, VIAL, Roerig	00049-1201-83
10's	$175.68	CEFOBID, PIGGYBACK, Roerig	00049-1211-83
50 ml	$16.68	CEFOBID, Roerig	00049-1216-18

Injection, Solution - Intramuscular; - 2 gm

10's	$328.38	CEFOBID, VIAL, Roerig	00049-1202-83
10's	$351.38	CEFOBID, PIGGYBACK, Roerig	00049-1212-83
50 ml	$30.75	CEFOBID, Roerig	00049-1215-18

Injection, Solution - Intramuscular; - 10 gm

1's	$157.28	CEFOBID, BULK, Roerig	00049-1219-28

CEFORANIDE *(000688)*

CATEGORIES: Anti-Infectives; Antibiotics; Antimicrobials; Bone Infections; Cephalosporins; Endocarditis; Infections; Joint Infections; Perioperative Prophylaxis; Respiratory Tract Infections; Septicemia; Skin Infections; Staphyloccocus Aureas; Streptococcal Infection; Urinary Tract Infections; Rheumatic Fever*; Pregnancy Category B; FDA Approved 1984 May
* Indication not approved by the FDA

BRAND NAMES: **Precef**; *Radacef*
(International brand names outside U.S. in italics)

DESCRIPTION:

Ceforanide is a semisynthetic broad spectrum cephalosporin antibiotic for parenteral administration. It is provided as a sterile sodium-free mixture of 7-(o-(aminomethyl) phenylacetamido)-3-(((1-(carboxymethyl)-1H-tetrazol-5-y l)thio)methyl)-3-cephem-4-carboxylic acid and lysine. When reconstituted the lysine salt is formed. Solutions of Precef range in color from light yellow to amber depending on the concentration and diluent used. The pH of the solution ranges from 5.5-8.5.

CLINICAL PHARMACOLOGY:

Mean peak plasma concentrations of 40 and 76 mcg/ml occurred at 1 hr. after intramuscular administration of doses of 0.5 and 1.0 g, respectively, of ceforanideto normal subjects. These concentrations declined to 3.9 and 6.7 mcg/ml at 12 hours. Following 30-minute intravenous infusion of 1.0 and 2.0 g doses of Precef, respectively, the mean plasma concentration were 125 and 240 mcg/ml, declining to 5.9 and 9.0 mcg/ml in 12 hours.

CLINICAL PHARMACOLOGY: *(cont'd)*

The terminal plasma half-life was 2.9 hours after intravenous and intramuscular administration. Plasma protein binding was 80% at plasma concentrations achieved after 0.5-2.0 g doses. There was no evidence of drug accumulation and plasma pharmacokinetics did not change after twice daily administration of 0.5-2.0 g for 9.5 days.

Ceforanidewas not metabolized prior to elimination and was primarily excreted by the kidneys. After intramuscular administration of 0.5 and 1.0 g doses, mean peak urinary concentrations of 1250 and 2900 mcg/ml occurred within 2 hours. Urine levels were 110 and 265 mcg/ml. respectively, at 9-12 hours. Intravenous doses of 1.0 and 2.0 g of ceforanideproduced mean urinary concentrations of 2550 and 5130 mcg/ml, respectively, within 2 hours after administration. Urine levels were 190 and 440 mcg/ml, respectively, at 9-12 hours. Excretion kinetics and clearance rates did not change following twice daily administration of these doses for 9.5 days. Urinary excretion accounted for 78-95% of the 0.5-2.0 g intramuscular and/or intravenous dose in 12 hours.

Probenecid has no effect on serum concentrations of Precef.

Ceforanidereaches therapeutic levels in the gall bladder, myocardium, bone, skeletal muscle, and vaginal tissue. Therapeutic levels are also achieved in pericardial fluid, synovial fluid and bile.

Microbiology: The bactericidal activity of ceforanideresults from inhibition of cell wall synthesis. Ceforanide has a high degree of stability in the presence of some beta-lactamases. Ceforanide is usually active against the following microorganisms *in vitro.*

AEROBES

Gram-negative: *Escherichia coli; Klebsiella* species: *Proteus mirabilis; Providencia* species (including *Providencia rettgeri,* formerly *Proteus rettgeri*); *Citrobacter* species; **Haemophilus influenzae; Haemophilus parainfluenzae; Enterobacter** species; *Salmonella typhi; Neisseria gonorrhoeae.*

Gram-positive: Staphylococci, including penicillinase-producing strains.

Note: Methicillin-resistant staphylococci as well as some strains of *Staphylococcus epidermidis* are resistant.

Streptococcus pneumoniae (Formerly *Diplococcus pneumoniae*) Group A and Group B streptococci, *Streptococcus viridans.*

Note: Most strains of enterococci, e.g., *Streptococcus faecalis,* are resistant.

ANAEROBES

Fusobacterium species, *Clostridium* species.

Note: Most strains of *Clostridium difficile* are resistant.*Peptococcus* species, *Peptostreptococcus* species.

While most strains of *B. fragilis* are resistant, ceforanide demonstrates *in vitro* activity against some bacteroides species.

Note: *Pseudomonas, Acinetobacter calcoaceticus* (formerly*Mima* and *Herellea* species) and most *Serratia* strains are resistant to ceforanide.

Disc susceptibility tests: Quantitative methods that require measurement of zone diameters give the most precise estimate of antibiotic susceptibility. One such procedure† has been recommended for use with discs to test susceptibility to ceforanide.

Reports from the laboratory giving results of the standard single-disc susceptibility test with a 30-mcg cefamandole disc should be interpreted according to the following criteria:

Susceptible organisms produce zones of 18 mm or greater, indicating that the test organism is likely to respond to therapy.

Organisms that produce zones of 15 to 17 mm are expected to be susceptible if high dosage is used or if the infection is confined to tissues and fluids (*e.g.,* urine) in which high antibiotic levels are attained.

Resistant organisms produce zones of 14 mm or less, indicating that other therapy should be selected.

For gram-positive isolates, the test may be performed with either the cephalosporin-class disc (30 mcg cephalothin) or the cefamandole disc (30 mcg cefamandole), and a zone of 18 mm is indicative of a ceforanide-susceptible organism. Gram-negative organisms should be tested with the cefamandole disc (using the above criteria) since ceforanide has been shown by *in vitro* tests to have activity against certain strains of *Enterobacteriaceae* found resistant when tested with the cephalosporin-class disc. Gram-negative organisms having zones of less than 18 mm around the cephalothin disc are not necessarily moderately susceptible or resistant to ceforanide.

In other susceptibility testing procedures, e.g., ICS agar dilution†† or the equivalent, a bacterial isolate may be considered susceptible if the MIC value for ceforanide is not more than 16 mcg/ml. Organisms are considered resistant to ceforanide if the MIC is greater than 32 mcg/ml. Organisms having an MIC value of 32 mcg/ml or less than 32 mcg/ml, but greater than 16 mcg/ml, are expected to be susceptible if high dosage is used or if the infection is confined to tissues and fluids (*e.g.,* urine) in which high antibiotic levels are attained.

† Bauer, et al., Am J Clin Path 1966; 45:493 and Federal Register 1972 Sep 30; 37:20525-20529.

†† Determine by the ICS agar-dilution method (Ericsson H M, and Sherris J C: Acta Pathol Microbiol Scand 1971 (B), Supplement No. 217) or any other method that has been shown to give equivalent results.

INDICATIONS AND USAGE:

Ceforanideis indicated for the treatment of serious infections caused by susceptible strains of the designated microorganisms in the diseases listed below:

1. **Bone and Joint Infections** caused by *Staphylococcus aureus* (penicillinase and non-penicillinase producing strains).
2. **Endocarditis** caused by *Staphylococcus aureus* (penicillinase an non-penicillinase producing strains).
3. **Lower Respiratory Tract Infections** caused by *Staphylococcus aureus* (penicillinase and non-penicillinase producing strains), *Streptococcus pneumoniae* (formerly *D. pneumoniae*), *Klebsiella pneumoniae,* and *Haemophilus influenzae.*
4. **Bacterial Septicemia** caused by *Staphylococcus aureus* (penicillinase and non-penicillinase producing strains), *Streptococcus pneumoniae,* and *Escherichia coli.*
5. **Skin and Skin Structure Infections** caused by *Staphylococcus aureus* (penicillinase and non-penicillinase producing strains), *Staphylococcus epidermidis,* Group A and Group B streptococci, *Escherichia coli, Proteus mirabilis,* and *Klebsiella pneumoniae.*
6. **Urinary Tract Infections** caused by *Escherichia coli, Proteus mirabilis,* and *Klebsiella pneumoniae.*

NOTE: Injectable Penicillin G Benzathine is considered to be the drug of choice in the treatment and prevention of streptococcal infection including prophylaxis of rheumatic fever.

Specimens for bacteriologic cultures should be obtained in order to isolate and identify causative organisms and to determine their susceptibilities to ceforanide. Therapy may be instituted before results of susceptibility studies are known; however, once these results become available, the antibiotic treatment should be adjusted accordingly.

INDICATIONS AND USAGE: *(cont'd)*

Prophylactic Use: Perioperative Phophylaxis: The preoperative prophylactic administration of ceforanide may prevent the growth of susceptible organisms and thereby may reduce the incidence of certain postoperative infections in patients undergoing surgical procedures which are classified as contaminated or potentially contaminated, e.g., vaginal hysterectomy. Effective prophylactic use of an antibiotic in surgery depends upon the time of administration. Ceforanide should usually be administered sixty minutes before the operation to allow sufficient time to achieve an effective antibiotic concentration in the wound tissues during the procedure. Prophylactic administration is usually not required after the surgical procedure ends and should be discontinued within a 24 hour period. In the majority of surgical procedures, continuing prophylactic administration of any antibiotic does not reduce the incidence of subsequent infections but will increase the possibility of adverse reactions and the development of bacterial resistance.

The perioperative use of ceforanide may also be effective in surgical patients in whom infections at the operative site would present a serious risk, e.g., during prosthetic arthroplasty and open-heart surgery. Although ceforanide has been shown to be as effective as cephalothin in the prevention of infections following coronary artery bypass surgery, no placebo controlled trials have been conducted to evaluate any cephalosporin antibiotic in the prevention of infection following either coronary artery bypass surgery or prosthetic heart valve replacement. In these procedures where the occurrence of infection may be particularly devastating, the prophylactic administration of ceforanide may be continued for 2 days, administered every 12 hours following completion of surgery. If there are signs of infection, specimens for culture should be obtained for the identification of the causative organism so that the appropriate therapy may be instituted. (See DOSAGE AND ADMINISTRATION.)

CONTRAINDICATIONS:

Ceforanide is contraindicated in patients with known hypersensitivity to ceforanide and the cephalosporin group of antibiotics.

WARNINGS:

BEFORE THERAPY WITH CEFORANIDE IS INSTITUTED, CAREFUL INQUIRY SHOULD BE MADE TO DETERMINE WHETHER THE PATIENT HAS HAD PREVIOUS HYPERSENSITIVITY REACTIONS TO CEPHALOSPORINS, PENICILLINS, OR OTHER DRUGS. THIS PRODUCT SHOULD BE GIVEN CAUTIOUSLY TO PENICILLIN-SENSITIVE PATIENTS. ANTIBIOTICS SHOULD BE ADMINISTERED WITH CAUTION TO ANY PATIENT WHO HAS DEMONSTRATED SOME FORM OF ALLERGY, PARTICULARLY TO DRUGS. IF AN ALLERGIC REACTION TO CEFORANIDE OCCURS, DISCONTINUE THE DRUG. SERIOUS ACUTE HYPERSENSITIVITY REACTIONS MAY REQUIRE EPINEPHRINE ADMINISTRATION AND OTHER EMERGENCY MEASURES.

Pseudomembranous colitis has been reported with the use of cephalosporins (and other broad spectrum antibiotics); therefore, it is important to consider its diagnosis in patients in whom diarrhea develops in association with cephalosporin use.

Treatment with broad spectrum antibiotics alters the normal flora of the colon and may permit overgrowth of clostridia. Studies indicate a toxin produced by *Clostridium difficile* is one primary cause of antibiotic-associated colitis. Cholestyramine and colestipol HCl resins have been shown to bind the toxin *in vitro.*

Mild cases of colitis may respond to drug discontinuance alone.

Moderate to severe cases should be managed with fluid, electrolyte, and protein supplementation as indicated.

When the colitis is not relieved by drug discontinuance or when it is severe, oral vancomycin is effective in treatment of the antibiotic-associated pseudomembranous colitis produced by *C. difficile.* Other causes of colitis should also be considered.

PRECAUTIONS:

Although ceforanide rarely produces alterations in kidney function, evaluation of renal status during therapy is recommended, especially in seriously ill patients receiving the maximum dosage. The total daily dose of ceforanide should be reduced in patients with transient or persistent renal insufficiency (see DOSAGE AND ADMINISTRATION) because high and prolonged serum antibiotic concentrations can occur in such individuals from usual dosage.

Cephalosporins should be given with caution to patients receiving concurrent treatment with potent diuretics as these regimens are suspected of adversely affecting renal function. Nephrotoxicity has been reported following concomitant administration of cephalosporins and aminoglycoside antibiotics.

Ceforanide should be prescribed with caution in individuals with a history of gastrointestinal disease, particularly colitis.

As with other antibiotics, prolonged use of ceforanide may result in over-growth of non-susceptible organisms. Repeated evaluation of the patient's condition is essential. If superinfection occurs during therapy, appropriate measures should be taken.

Pregnancy Category B: In a study in which rats were treated prior to mating and through pregnancy and lactation at dose levels (1600 mg/kg/day) 50 times the usual ceforanide dose (30 mg/kg/day), there was no evidence of impaired male or female fertility or reproductive performance. Results of teratogenicity tests in mice and rats employing doses as high as 25 times the human dose were also negative. In a peri-postnatal study, female rats treated subcutaneously with ceforanide at 50 times the usual human dose had a higher number of resorption sites than controls and there was a decrease in viability of the offspring. These phenomena may well have been secondary to the effects on the maternal animals of the high volume of solution injected (8 ml/kg/day), rather than representing a direct effect on the conceptus; neither was evident at lower dosage levels (*e.g.,* 25 times human dose). There are, however, no adequate and well controlled studies in pregnant women. Because animal reproduction studies are not always predictive of human response, ceforanide should be used during pregnancy only if clearly needed.

Labor and Delivery: There are no data concerning the administration of ceforanide to women during labor or prior to delivery.

Nursing Mothers: It is not known whether ceforanide is excreted in human milk. Because many drugs are, caution should be exercised when ceforanide is administered to a nursing woman.

Pediatric Use: Safety and effectiveness of ceforanide in children below the age of one year have not been established. Therefore, if ceforanide is administered to infants, the physician should determine if the potential benefits of the product's use outweigh the possible risks of administration. Ceforanide has been effectively used in children between the ages of 1-17 years.

ADVERSE REACTIONS:

Allergic Reactions: Rash (one in 45 patients), pruritus (one in 200 patients) and eosinophilia (in about one in 12 patients) have been reported. Reactions are more likely to occur in patients with a history of hypersensitivity, particularly to penicillins.

ADVERSE REACTIONS: *(cont'd)*

Hematopoietic: As occurs during therapy with other cephalosporin antibiotics, therapy with ceforanide has been associated with transient thrombocytosis (in about one in 5 patients). Some individuals (one in 40 patients) have developed positive direct Coombs Tests during treatment with ceforanide without clinical or laboratory evidence of hemolysis.

Gastrointestinal: Nausea (one in 270 patients), vomiting (one in 2,000 patients) and diarrhea (one in 140 patients) have been reported.

Symptoms of pseudomembranous colitis may appear during or after cephalosporin treatment.

Laboratory Changes: Transient elevation in SGOT (one in 16 patients), SGPT (one in 9 patients), and alkaline phosphatase levels (one in 27 patients) have been reported.

As with other cephalosporins, transient elevations in serum creatinine and BUN levels have been observed (in one in 9 and one in 50 patients, respectively). As may occur with intramuscular injections, and administration of ceforanide by this route has been associated with an elevation of CPK (in about one in 3 patients).

Local Effects: Local effects were reported in less than one percent of patients and included pain (one in 155 patients) and phlebitis (one in 140 patients).

Other reactions which have been reported in less than one percent of patients are local swelling, lethargy, confusion, headache, and, hypotension.

DOSAGE AND ADMINISTRATION:

DOSAGE

Adults: The usual dose range for ceforanide is 0.5 to 1.0 g twice daily depending on the severity of the infection. Ceforanide is administered every 12 hours by either the intramuscular or intravenous route. The route of administration should be dictated by the condition of the patient and anticipated ease of administration.

Children: Administration of 20-40 mg/kg/day in equally divided doses every 12 hours has been effective for most infections susceptible to ceforanide.

Perioperative Prophylactic Use: To prevent postoperative infection in contaminated or potentially contaminated surgery a 0.5 to 1 g IM or IV dose administered 1 hour prior to the start of surgery is recommended.

It is important that the preoperative dose be given 1 hour prior to the start of surgery so that adequate antibiotic levels are present in the serum and tissues at the time of initial surgical incision.

In surgery where the occurrence of infection may be particularly devastating, e.g., prosthetic arthroplasty and open-heart surgery, the prophylactic administration of ceforanide may be continued for 2 days following completion of surgery.

Impaired Renal Function: Dosage should be determined by the degree of renal impairment, the severity of infection, the susceptibility of the causative organism, and therapeutic monitoring. If the creatinine clearance rate (Cl_{cr}) is 60 ml/min/1.73m^{2}or greater, the normal 12-hour dosing interval is maintained. When Cl_{cr} is 20-59 ml/min1.73m^2 a 24-hour dosing interval is recommended, and when Cl_{cr} is 5-19 ml/min/1.73m^2 a 48-hour dosing interval is recommended. If Cl_{cr} is less than 5 ml/min/1.73m^2, a 48-72 hour dosing interval may be used with monitoring of plasma ceforanide concentrations.

If only serum creatinine is available, creatinine clearance may be calculated from the following formula when renal function and serum creatinine levels are at steady state (TABLE 1):

TABLE 1

Males: Cl_{cr} = [(140 - age) × Wt (kg)] ÷ [72 × serum creatinine (mg/100 ml)]
Females: 0.85 of the above value

NOTE: As with antibiotic therapy in general, administration of ceforanide should be continued for minimum of 48 to 72 hours after the patient becomes asymptomatic or after evidence of bacterial eradication has been obtained. A minimum of 10 days of treatment is recommended in infections caused by group A beta-hemolytic streptococci in order to guard against the risk of rheumatic fever or glomerulonephritis.

Administration: Ceforanide may be administered by either the intramuscular or the intravenous routes. Controlled clinical studies performed in normal adult volunteers and patients demonstrated that ceforanide was very well tolerated intramuscularly. In normal volunteers and patients receiving intravenous therapy, a low incidence of venous irritation was attributed to ceforanide.

Intramuscular Injection: The 500 mg, 1 g and 2 g vials should be reconstituted with 1.8 ml, 3.2 ml, and 6.3 ml, respectively, of Bacteriostatic Water for Injection, 0.9% Sodium Chloride Injection, Sterile Water for Injection, or Bacteriostatic Sodium Chloride Injection. Each 1.0 ml contains 250 mg of ceforanide. All injections should be administered deep into the muscle mass.

Intravenous Administration: The intravenous route may be preferable for patients with bacterial septicemia, or other severe or life-threatening infections. These patients may be poor risks because of lowered resistance resulting from such debilitating conditions as malnutrition, trauma, surgery, diabetes, heart failure, or malignancy, particularly if shock is present or impending.

Intravenous Infusion: The contents of the 500 mg, 1 g, and 2 g vials should be diluted in 10 ml or more of the specified diluent and administered slowly by direct IV administration over a 3 to 5 minute period or may be given with intravenous infusions over a 30-minute period.

Intermittent Intravenous Infusion with Y-Tube: Intermittent intravenous infusion with a Y-type administration set can also be accomplished while bulk intravenous solutions are being infused. However, during infusion of the solution containing ceforanide, it is desirable to discontinue the other solution. When this technique is employed, careful attention should be paid to the volume of the solution containing ceforanide so that the calculated dose will be infused. When a Y-tube hookup is used, the contents of the 0.5 g, 1 g, and 2 g vial or StrapKap piggyback ceforanide should be diluted by the addition of the appropriate volume of diluent solution.

STABILITY AND COMPATIBILITY

Intramuscular Solutions: The 500 mg, 1 g, and 2 g vials when reconstituted with 1.8 ml, 3.2 ml, and 6.3 ml, respectively, of (1) Bacteriostatic Water for Injection, (2) 0.9% Sodium Chloride Injection, (3) Sterile Water for Injection, or (4) Bacteriostatic Sodium Chloride Injection, are stable for 48 hours at room temperature (25°C), 14 days at refrigerator temperature (4°C), and 90 days in the frozen state (-15°C). After thawing, the solution is stable for 48 hours at room temperature.

Intravenous Solutions: Ceforanide is stable and compatible for 24 hours at room temperature at concentrations between 0.5 mg/ml and 200 mg/ml in the following infusion solutions:

Sterile Water for Injection; 0.9% Sodium Chloride Injection; 5% Dextrose in Water; 5% Dextrose and 0.45% Sodium Chloride Injection; 5% Dextrose and 0.2% Sodium Chloride Injection; Lactated Ringer's Injection; 5% Dextrose in Lactated Ringer's Injection; 10% Dextrose in Water.

DOSAGE AND ADMINISTRATION: *(cont'd)*

StrapKap Piggyback IV Package: The StrapKap piggyback IV dosage form is available in 500 mg, 1 g and 2 g StrapKap piggyback glass containers. This package is intended for intravenous administration. Reconstitute with 10 ml or more of the appropriate diluent as specified on the container labels. Following reconstitution, the solutions are stable for 24 hours at room temperature.

Hospital Bulk Package: The hospital bulk dosage form is available in 10 and 20 g StrapKap piggyback glass containers. This package is designed for use in the pharmacy in preparing IV additives. The diluents(s) and appropriate reconstitution volumes(s) are specified on the individual container labels. The resulting solution will contain 250 mg of ceforanide activity per ml. Following reconstitution, the solutions are stable for 48 hours at room temperature, 14 days under refrigeration, and 90 days in the frozen state. After thawing, the solutions are stable for 48 hours at room temperature.

Caution: Hospital bulk packages must not be dispensed as a unit.

Upon reconstitution, the initial Precef Injection appears somewhat cloudy but will de-aerate upon brief standing to provide clear solution. Parenteral drug products should be inspected visually for particulate matter and discoloration prior to administration, whenever solution and container permit.

HOW SUPPLIED - EQUIVALENTS NOT AVAILABLE:

Injection, Dry-Soln - Intramuscular; - 1 gm/vial

1 gm	$11.94	PRECEF, Mead Johnson	00015-7352-20
1 gm	$12.54	PRECEF, Mead Johnson	00015-7352-28
10's	$125.42	PRECEF, Mead Johnson	00015-7352-99
10's	$131.66	PRECEF, Mead Johnson	00015-7352-95

Injection, Dry-Soln - Intramuscular; - 10 gm/vial

100's	$113.42	PRECEF, Mead Johnson	00015-7356-94

Injection, Dry-Soln - Intramuscular; - 500 mg/vial

10's	$72.49	PRECEF, Mead Johnson	00015-7351-99
10's	$78.73	PRECEF, Mead Johnson	00015-7351-95
500 mg x 10	$7.50	PRECEF 500, Mead Johnson	00015-7351-28
500 mg x 10	$72.49	PRECEF 500, Mead Johnson	00015-7351-20

CEFOTAXIME SODIUM *(000689)*

CATEGORIES: Anti-Infectives; Antibiotics; Antimicrobials; Cellulitis; Cephalosporins; Endometritis; Genitourinary Tract Infections; Gonorrhea; Infections; Intra-Abdominal Infections; Joint Infections; Meningitis; Pelvic Inflammatory Disease; Perioperative Prophylaxis; Peritonitis; Pneumonia; Respiratory Tract Infections; Septicemia; Skin Infections; Urinary Tract Infections; Ventriculitis; Pregnancy Category B; FDA Approval Pre 1982

BRAND NAMES: *Alfotax* (Mexico); *Benaxima* (Mexico); *Biosint* (Mexico); *Biotax*; *Cefaxim* (Mexico); *Cefirad*; *Cefpiran*; *Cefoclin* (Mexico); *Cefotax* (Japan); *Cefuroxime*; *Cepor*; *Cetax*; *Clacef*; *Claforan*; **Claforan**; *Claraxim*; *Clatax*; *Clavox*; *Fotexina* (Mexico); *Kalfoxim*; *Kidoxim*; *Lyforan*; *Molelant*; *Omnatax*; *Omnicef*; *Oritaxim*; *Primafen*; *Ralopar*; *Spirosine*; *Stoparen*; *Taporin* (Mexico); *Taxcef*; *Viken* (Mexico); *Zariviz*

(International brand names outside U.S. in italics)

FORMULARIES: BC-BS

DESCRIPTION:

Cefotaxime sodium is a semisynthetic, broad spectrum cephalosporin antibiotic for parenteral administration. It is the sodium salt of 7-[2-(2-amino-4-thiazolyl) glyoxylamido]-3-(hydroxymethyl)-8-oxo-5-thia-1-azabicyclo [4.2.0] oct-2-ene-2-carboxylate 7^2(Z)-(o-methyloxime), acetate (ester). Claforan contains approximately 50.5 mg (2.2 mEq) of sodium per gram of cefotaxime activity. Solutions of Claforan range from very pale yellow to light amber depending on the concentration and the diluent used. The pH of the injectable solutions usually ranges from 5.0 to 7.5. The CAS Registry Number is 64485-93-4.

Claforan is supplied as a dry powder in conventional and ADD-Vantage System compatible vials, infusion bottles, pharmacy bulk package bottles, and as a frozen, premixed, iso-osmotic injection in a buffered diluent solution in plastic containers. Claforan, equivalent to 1 gram and 2 grams cefotaxime, is supplied as frozen, premixed, iso-osmotic injections in plastic containers. Solutions range from very pale yellow to light amber. Dextrous Hydrous, USP has been added to adjust osmolality (approximately 1.7 g and 700 mg to the 1 g and 2 g cefotaxime dosages, respectively). The injections are buffered with sodium citrate hydrous, USP. The pH is adjusted with hydrochloric acid and may be adjusted with sodium hydroxide.

The plastic container is fabricated from a specially designed multilayer plastic (PL 2040). Solutions are in contact with the polyethylene layer of this container and can leach out certain chemical components of the plastic in very small amounts within the expiration period. The suitability of the plastic has been confirmed in tests in animals according to the USP biological tests for plastic containers, as well as by tissue culture toxicity studies.

CLINICAL PHARMACOLOGY:

Following IM administration of a single 500 mg or 1 g dose of cefotaxime sodium to normal volunteers, mean peak serum concentrations of 11.7 and 20.5 mcg/ml respectively were attained within 30 minutes and declined with an elimination half-life of approximately 1 hour. There was a dose-dependent increase in serum levels after the IV administration of 500 mg, 1 g, and 2 g of cefotaxime sodium (38.9, 101.7, and 214.4 mcg/ml respectively) without alteration in the elimination half-life. There is no evidence of accumulation following repetitive IV infusion of 1 g doses every 6 hours for 14 days as there are no alterations of serum or renal clearance. About 60% of the administered dose was recovered from urine during the first 6 hours following the start of the infusion.

Approximately 20-36% of an intravenously administered dose of ^{14}C-cefotaxime is excreted by the kidney as unchanged cefotaxime and 15-25% as the desacetyl derivative, the major metabolite. The desacetyl metabolite has been shown to contribute to the bactericidal activity. Two other urinary metabolites (M_2 and M_3) account for about 20-25%. They lack bactericidal activity.

A single 50 mg/kg dose of cefotaxime sodium was administered as an intravenous infusion over a 10- to 15-minute period to 29 newborn infants grouped according to birth weight and age. The mean half-life of cefotaxime in infants with lower birth weights (≤1500 grams), regardless of age, was longer (4.6 hours) than the mean half-life (3.4 hours) in infants whose birth weight was greater than 1500 grams. Mean serum clearance was also smaller in the lower birth weight infants. Although the differences in mean half-life values are statistically significant for weight, they are not clinically important. Therefore, dosage should be based solely on age. (See DOSAGE AND ADMINISTRATION.)

Additionally, no disulfiram-like reactions were reported in a study conducted in 22 healthy volunteers administered cefotaxime sodium and ethanol.

CLINICAL PHARMACOLOGY: *(cont'd)*

MICROBIOLOGY

The bactericidal activity of cefotaxime sodium results from inhibition of cell wall synthesis. Cefotaxime sodium has *in vitro* activity against a wide range of gram-positive and gram-negative organisms. Cefotaxime sodium has a high degree of stability in the presence of beta-lactamases, both penicillinases and cephalosporinases, of gram-negative and gram-positive bacteria. Cefotaxime sodium has been shown to be a potent inhibitor of β-lactamases produced by certain gram-negative bacteria. Cefotaxime sodium is usually active against the following microorganisms both *in vitro* and in clinical infections (see INDICATIONS AND USAGE.)

Aerobes, Gram-positive: *Staphylococcus aureus*, including penicillinase and non-penicillinase producing strains, *Staphylococcus epidermidis, Enterococcus* species, *Streptococcus pyogenes* (group A beta-hemolytic streptococci), *Streptococcus agalactiae* (group B streptococci), *Streptococcus pneumoniae* (formerly *Diplococcus pneumoniae*).

Aerobes, Gram-negative: *Citrobacter* species, *Enterobacter* species, *Escherichia coli, Haemophilus influenzae* (including ampicillin-resistant *H. influenzae*), *Haemophilus parainfluenzae, Klebsiella* species (including *K. pneumoniae*), *Neisseria gonorrhoeae* (including penicillinase and non-penicillinase producing strains), *Neisseria meningitidis, Proteus mirabilis, Proteus vulgaris, Proteus inconstans* group B, *Morganella morganii, Providencia rettgeri, Serratia* species, and *Acinetobacter* species.

NOTE: Many strains of the above organisms that are multiply resistant to other antibiotics (*e.g.,* penicillins, cephalosporins, and aminoglycosides) are susceptible to cefotaxime sodium.

Cefotaxime sodium is active against some strains of *Pseudomonas aeruginosa*.

Anaerobes: *Bacteroides* species, including some strains of *B. fragilis, Clostridium*species (*NOTE:* Most strains of *C. difficile* are resistant.), *Peptococcus* species, *Peptostreptococcus* species, and *Fusobacterium*species (including *F. nucleatum*).

Cefotaxime sodium is highly stable *in vitro* to four of the five major classes of β-lactamases described by Richmond et al., including type IIIa (TEM) which is produced by many gram-negative bacteria. The drug is also stable to β-lactamase (penicillinase) produced by staphylococci. In addition, cefotaxime sodium shows high affinity for penicillin-binding proteins in the cell wall, including PBP: Ib and III.

Cefotaxime sodium also demonstrates *in vitro* activity against the following microorganisms although clinical significance is unknown: *Salmonella* species (including *S. typhi*), *Providencia* species, and *Shigella* species.

Cefotaxime sodium and aminoglycosides have been shown to be synergistic *in vitro* against some strains of *Pseudomonas aeruginosa.*

SUSCEPTIBILITY TESTING

Quantitative methods that require measurement of zone diameters give the most precise estimate of antibiotic susceptibility. One such procedure[1] has been recommended for use with discs to test susceptibility to cefotaxime sodium. Interpretation involves correlation of the diameters obtained in the disc test with minimum inhibitory concentration (MIC) values for cefotaxime sodium.

Reports from the laboratory giving results of the standardized single-disc susceptibility test using a 30 mcg cefotaxime sodium disc should be interpreted according to the following criteria:

Susceptible organisms produce zones of 20 mm or greater, indicating that the tested organism is likely to respond to therapy.

Organisms that produce zones of 15 to 19 mm are expected to be susceptible if high dosage is used or if the infection is confined to tissues and fluids (*e.g.,* urine) in which high antibiotic levels are attained.

Resistant organisms produce zones of 14 mm or less, indicating that other therapy should be selected.

Organisms should be tested with the cefotaxime sodium disc, since cefotaxime sodium has been shown by *in vitro* tests to be active against certain strains found resistant when other beta lactam discs are used. The cefotaxime sodium disc should not be used for testing susceptibility to other cephalosporins. Organisms having zones of less than 18 mm around the cephalothin disc are not necessarily of intermediate susceptibility or resistant to cefotaxime sodium.

A bacterial isolate may be considered susceptible if the MIC value for cefotaxime sodium is not more than 16 mcg/ml. Organisms are considered resistant to cefotaxime sodium if the MIC is equal to or greater than 64 mcg/ml. Organisms having an MIC value of less than 64 mcg/ml but greater than 16 mcg/ml are expected to be susceptible if high dosage is used or if the infection is confined to tissues and fluids (*e.g.,*urine) in which high antibiotic levels are attained.

INDICATIONS AND USAGE:

TREATMENT

Cefotaxime sodium is indicated for the treatment of patients with serious infections caused by susceptible strains of the designated microorganisms in the diseases listed below.

(1) Lower Respiratory Tract Infections: including pneumonia, caused by *Streptococcus pneumoniae* (formerly *Diplococcus pneumoniae*), *Streptococcus pyogenes** (Group A streptococci) and other streptococci (excluding enterococci, *e.g., Streptococcus faecalis*), *Staphylococcus aureus*(penicillinase and non-penicillinase producing), *Escherichia coli, Klebsiella* species, *Haemophilus influenzae*(including ampicillin resistant strains), *Haemophilus parainfluenzae, Proteus mirabilis, Serratia marcescens**, *Enterobacter* species, indole positive *Proteus* and *Pseudomonas* species (including *P. aeruginosa*).

(2) Genitourinary Infections: Urinary tract infections caused by *Enterococcus* species, *Staphylococcus epidermidis, Staphylococcus aureus** (penicillinase and non-penicillinase producing), *Citrobacter* species, *Enterobacter* species, *Escherichia coli, Klebsiella* species, *Proteus mirabilis, Proteus vulgaris**, *Proteus inconstans* group B, *Morganella morganii**, *Providencia rettgeri**, *Serratia marcescens* and *Pseudomonas*species (including *P. aeruginosa*). Also, uncomplicated gonorrhea of single or multiple sites caused by *Neisseria gonorrhoeae*, including penicillinase producing strains.

(3) Gynecologic Infections: including pelvic inflammatory disease, endometritis and pelvic cellulitis caused by *Staphylococcus epidermidis, Streptococcus*species, *Enterococcus* species, *Enterobacter* species*, *Klebsiella* species*, *Escherichia coli, Proteus mirabilis, Bacteroides* species (including *Bacteroides fragilis**), *Clostridium*species, and anaerobic cocci (including *Peptostreptococcus*species and *Peptococcus* species) and *Fusobacterium* species (including *F. nucleatum**).

Cefotaxime sodium, like other cephalosporins, has no activity against *Chlamydia trachomatis.* Therefore, when cephalosporins are used in the treatment of patients with pelvic inflammatory disease and *C. trachomatis* is one of the suspected pathogens, appropriate anti-chlamydial coverage should be added.

(4) Bacteremia/Septicemia: caused by *Escherichia coli, Klebsiella* species, and *Serratia marcescens, Staphylococcus aureus*, and *Streptococcus* species (including *S. pneumoniae*).

(5) Skin and Skin Structure Infections: caused by *Staphylococcus aureus* (penicillinase and non-penicillinase producing), *Staphylococcus epidermidis, Streptococcus pyogenes* (group A streptococci) and other streptococci, *Enterococcus* species, *Acinetobacter* species*, *Escherichia coli, Citrobacter* species (including *C. freundii**), *Enterobacter* species, *Klebsiella* species, *Proteus mirabilis, Proteus vulgaris**, *Morganella morganii, Providencia rettgeri**, *Pseudomonas* species, *Serratia marcescens, Bacteroides* species, and anaerobic cocci (including *Peptostreptococcus** species and *Peptococcus* species).

(6) Intra-Abdominal Infections: including peritonitis caused by *Streptococcus*species*, *Escherichia coli, Klebsiella* species, *Bacteroides* species, and anaerobic cocci (including *Peptostreptococcus** species and *Peptococcus**species), *Proteus mirabilis**, and *Clostridium* species*.

(7) Bone and/or Joint Infections: caused by *Staphylococcus aureus* (penicillinase and non-penicillinase producing strains), *Streptococcus*species (including *S. pyogenes**), *Pseudomonas* species (including *P. aeruginosa**), and *Proteus mirabilis**.

(8) Central Nervous System Infections: (*e.g.,* meningitis and ventriculitis) caused by *Neisseria meningitidis, Haemophilus influenzae, Streptococcus pneumoniae, Klebsiella pneumoniae** and *Escherichia coli**.

(*) Efficacy for this organism, in this organ system, has been studied in fewer than 10 infections.

Although many strains of enterococci (*e.g., S. faecalis*) and *Pseudomonas* species are resistant to cefotaxime sodium *in vitro*, cefotaxime sodium has been used successfully in treating patients with infections caused by susceptible organisms.

Specimens for bacteriologic culture should be obtained prior to therapy in order to isolate and identify causative organisms and to determine their susceptibilities to cefotaxime sodium. Therapy may be instituted before results of susceptibility studies are known; however, once these results become available, the antibiotic treatment should be adjusted accordingly.

In certain cases of confirmed or suspected gram-positive or gram-negative sepsis or in patients with other serious infections in which the causative organism has not been identified, cefotaxime sodium may be used concomitantly with an aminoglycoside. The dosage recommended in the labeling of both antibiotics may be given and depends on the severity of the infection and the patient's condition. Renal function should be carefully monitored, especially if higher dosages of the aminoglycosides are to be administered or if therapy is prolonged, because of the potential nephrotoxicity and ototoxicity of aminoglycoside antibiotics. It is possible that nephrotoxicity may be potentiated if cefotaxime sodium is used concomitantly with an aminoglycoside.

PREVENTION

The administration of cefotaxime sodium preoperatively reduces the incidence of certain infections in patients undergoing surgical procedures (*e.g.,* abdominal or vaginal hysterectomy, gastrointestinal and genitourinary tract surgery) that may be classified as contaminated or potentially contaminated.

In patients undergoing cesarean section, intraoperative (after clamping the umbilical cord) and postoperative use of cefotaxime sodium may also reduce the incidence of certain postoperative infections. (See DOSAGE AND ADMINISTRATION.)

Effective use for elective surgery depends on the time of administration. To achieve effective tissue levels, cefotaxime sodium should be given 1/2 to 1 1/2 hours before surgery. (See DOSAGE AND ADMINISTRATION.)

For patients undergoing gastrointestinal surgery, preoperative bowel preparation by mechanical cleansing as well as with a non-absorbable antibiotic (*e.g.,* neomycin) is recommended.

If there are signs of infection, specimens for culture should be obtained for identification of the causative organism so that appropriate therapy may be instituted.

CONTRAINDICATIONS:

Cefotaxime sodium is contraindicated in patients who have shown hypersensitivity to cefotaxime sodium or the cephalosporin group of antibiotics.

WARNINGS:

BEFORE THERAPY WITH CEFOTAXIME SODIUM IS INSTITUTED, CAREFUL INQUIRY SHOULD BE MADE TO DETERMINE WHETHER THE PATIENT HAS HAD PREVIOUS HYPERSENSITIVITY REACTIONS TO CEFOTAXIME SODIUM, CEPHALOSPORINS, PENICILLINS, OR OTHER DRUGS. THIS PRODUCT SHOULD BE GIVEN WITH CAUTION TO PATIENTS WITH TYPE I HYPERSENSITIVITY REACTIONS TO PENICILLIN. ANTIBIOTICS SHOULD BE ADMINISTERED WITH CAUTION TO ANY PATIENT WHO HAS DEMONSTRATED SOME FORM OF ALLERGY, PARTICULARLY TO DRUGS. IF AN ALLERGIC REACTION TO CEFOTAXIME SODIUM OCCURS, DISCONTINUE TREATMENT WITH THE DRUG. SERIOUS HYPERSENSITIVITY REACTIONS MAY REQUIRE EPINEPHRINE AND OTHER EMERGENCY MEASURES.

During post-marketing surveillance, a potentially life-threatening arrhythmia was reported in each of six patients who received a rapid (less than 60 seconds) bolus injection of cefotaxime through a central venous catheter. Therefore, cefotaxime should only be administered as instructed in DOSAGE AND ADMINISTRATION.

Pseudomembranous colitis has been reported with nearly all antibacterial agents, including cefotaxime, and may range from mild to life-threatening. Therefore, it is important to consider its diagnosis in patients who develop diarrhea subsequent to the administration of antibacterial agents.

Treatment with antibacterial agents alters normal flora of the colon and may permit overgrowth of Clostridia. Studies indicate a toxin produced by *Clostridium difficile* is one primary cause of antibiotic-associated colitis.

After the diagnosis of pseudomembranous colitis has been established, appropriate therapeutic measures should be initiated. Mild cases of colitis may respond to drug discontinuance alone. In moderate to severe cases, consideration should be given to management with fluids and electrolytes, protein supplementation, and treatment with an antibacterial drug clinically effective against *Clostridium difficile* colitis.

When the colitis is not relieved by drug discontinuance or when it is severe, oral vancomycin is the treatment of choice for antibiotic-associated pseudomembranous colitis produced by *C. difficile*. Other causes of colitis should also be considered.

PRECAUTIONS:

Cefotaxime sodium should be prescribed with caution in individuals with a history of gastrointestinal disease, particularly colitis. Because high and prolonged serum antibiotic concentrations can occur from usual doses in patients with transient or persistent reduction of urinary output because of renal insufficiency, the total daily dosage should be reduced when cefotaxime sodium is administered to such patients. Continued dosage should be determined by degree of renal impairment, severity of infection, and susceptibility of the causative organism.

Although there is no clinical evidence supporting the necessity of changing the dosage of cefotaxime sodium in patients with even profound renal dysfunction, it is suggested that, until further data are obtained, the dosage of cefotaxime sodium be halved in patients with estimated creatinine clearances of less than 20 ml/min/1.73 m^2.

PRECAUTIONS: *(cont'd)*

When only serum creatinine is available, the following formula[2] (based on sex, weight, and age of the patient) may be used to convert this value into creatinine clearance. The serum creatinine should represent a steady state of renal function.

TABLE 1
Males: [Weight (kg) × (140 - age)] ÷ [72 × serum creatinine]
Females: 0.85 × above value

As with other antibiotics, prolonged use of cefotaxime sodium may result in overgrowth of nonsusceptible organisms. Repeated evaluation of the patient's condition is essential. If superinfection occurs during therapy, appropriate measures should be taken.

As with other beta-lactam antibiotics, granulocytopenia and, more rarely, agranulocytosis may develop during treatment with cefotaxime sodium, particularly if given over long periods. For courses of treatment lasting longer than 10 days, blood counts should therefore be monitored.

Cefotaxime sodium, like other parenteral anti-infective drugs, may be locally irritating to tissues. In most cases, perivascular extravasation of cefotaxime sodium may result in tissue damage and require surgical treatment. To minimize the potential for tissue inflammation, infusion sites should be monitored regularly and changed when appropriate.

Carcinogenesis, Mutagenesis, and Impairment of Fertility: Long-term studies in animals have not been performed to evaluate carcinogenic potential. Mutagenic tests include a micronucleus and an Ames test. Both tests were negative for mutagenic effects.

Pregnancy: Pregnancy Category B: *Teratogenic Effects:* Reproduction studies have been performed in mice and rats at doses up to 30 times the usual human dose and have revealed no evidence of impaired fertility or harm to the fetus because of cefotaxime sodium. However, there are no well-controlled studies in pregnant women. Because animal reproductive studies are not always predictive of human response, this drug should be used during pregnancy only if clearly needed.

Pregnancy: Pregnancy Category B: *Nonteratogenic Effects:* Use of the drug in women of child-bearing potential requires that the anticipated benefit be weighed against the possible risks.

In perinatal and postnatal studies with rats, the pups in the group given 1200 mg/kg of cefotaxime sodium were significantly lighter in weight at birth and remained smaller than pups in the control group during the 21 days of nursing.

Nursing Mothers: Cefotaxime sodium is excreted in human milk in low concentrations. Caution should be exercised when cefotaxime sodium is administered to a nursing woman.

Pediatric Use: (See PRECAUTIONS regarding perivascular extravasation.) The potential for toxic effects in pediatric patients from chemicals that may leach from the plastic in single dose Galaxy containers (premixed Claforan injection) has not been determined.

DRUG INTERACTIONS:

Increased nephrotoxicity has been reported following concomitant administration of cephalosporins and aminoglycoside antibiotics.

ADVERSE REACTIONS:

Cefotaxime sodium is generally well tolerated. The most common adverse reactions have been local reactions following IM or IV injection. Other adverse reactions have been encountered infrequently.

The most frequent adverse reactions (greater than 1%) are:

Local (4.3%): Injection site inflammation with IV administration. Pain, induration, and tenderness after IM injection.

Hypersensitivity (2.4%): Rash, pruritus, fever, eosinophilia, and less frequently urticaria and anaphylaxis.

Gastrointestinal (1.4%) Colitis, diarrhea, nausea, and vomiting. Symptoms of pseudomembranous colitis can appear during or after antibiotic treatment. Nausea and vomiting have been reported rarely.

Less frequent adverse reactions (less than 1%) are:

Cardiovascular System: Potentially life-threatening arrhymias following rapid (less than 60 seconds) bolus administration via central venous catheter have been observed.

Hematologic System: Neutropenia, transient leukopenia, eosinophilia, thrombocytopenia and agranulocytosis have been reported. Some individuals have developed positive direct Coombs Tests during treatment with cefotaxime sodium and other cephalosporin antibiotics. Rare cases of hemolytic anemia have been reported.

Genitourinary System: Moniliasis, vaginitis.

Central Nervous System: Headache.

Liver: Transient elevations in SGOT, SGPT, serum LDH, and serum alkaline phosphatase levels have been reported.

Kidney: As with some other cephalosporins, interstitial nephritis and transient elevations of BUN and creatinine have been occasionally observed with cefotaxime sodium.

DOSAGE AND ADMINISTRATION:

ADULTS

Dosage and route of administration should be determined by susceptibility of the causative organisms, severity of the infection, and the condition of the patient (see TABLE 2) for dosage guideline. Cefotaxime sodium may be administered IM or IV after reconstitution. Premixed cefotaxime sodium injection is intended for IV administration after thawing. The maximum daily dosage should not exceed 12 grams.

TABLE 2 Guidelines for Dosage of Cefotaxime Sodium

Type of Infection	Daily Dose (grams)	Frequency and Route
Gonorrhea	1	1 gram IM (single dose)
Uncomplicated infections	2	1 gram every 12 hours IM or IV
Moderate to severe infections	3-6	1-2 grams every 8 hours IM or IV
Infections commonly needing antibiotics in higher dosage (*e.g.*, septicemia)	6-8	2 grams every 6-8 hours IV
Life-threatening infections	up to 12	2 grams every 4 hours IV

If *C. trachomatis* is a suspected pathogen, appropriate anti-chlamydial coverage should be added, because cefotaxime sodium has no activity against this oraganism.

To prevent postoperative infection in contaminated or potentially contaminated surgery, the recommended dose is a single 1 gram IM or IV administered 30 to 90 minutes prior to start of surgery.

CESAREAN SECTION PATIENTS

The first dose of 1 gram is administered intravenously as soon as the umbilical cord is clamped. The second and third doses should be given as 1 gram intravenously or intramuscularly at 6 and 12 hours after the first dose.

DOSAGE AND ADMINISTRATION: *(cont'd)*

NEONATES, INFANTS, AND CHILDREN

The dosage schedule in TABLE 3is recommended:

TABLE 3

Neonates (birth to 1 month):	
0-1 week of age	50 mg/kg per dose every 12 hours IV
1-4 weeks of age	50 mg/kg per dose every 8 hours IV

It is not necessary to differentiate between premature and normal-gestational age infants.

Infants and Children (1 month to 12 years): For body weights less than 50 kg, the recommended daily dose is 50 to 180 mg/kg IM or IV of body weight divided into four to six equal doses. The higher dosages should be used for more severe or serious infections, including meningitis. For body weights 50 kg or more, the usual adult dosage should be used; the maximum daily dosage should not exceed 12 grams.

Impaired Renal Function: See PRECAUTIONS.

NOTE: As with antibiotic therapy in general, administration of cefotaxime sodium should be continued for a minimum of 48 to 72 hours after the patient defervesces or after evidence of bacterial eradication has been obtained; a minimum of 10 days of treatment is recommended for infections caused by Group A beta-hemolytic streptococci in order to guard against the risk of rheumatic fever or glomerulonephritis; frequent bacteriologic and clinical appraisal is necessary during therapy of chronic urinary tract infection and may be required for several months after therapy has been completed; persistent infections may require treatment of several weeks and doses smaller than those indicated above should not be used.

TABLE 4 Reconstitution of Sterile Cefotaxime Sodium for IM or IV Administration

Strength	Diluent (ml)	Withdrawable Volume (ml)	Approximate Concentration (mg/ml)
500 mg vial* (IM)	2	2.2	230
1 g vial* (IM)	3	3.4	300
2 g vial* (IM)	5	6.0	330
500 mg vial* (IV)	10	10.2	50
1 g vial* (IV)	10	10.4	95
2 g vial* (IV)	10	11.0	180
1 g infusion	50-100	50-100	20-10
2 g infusion	50-100	50-100	40-20
10 g bottle	47	52.0	200
10 g bottle	97	102.0	100

* in conventional vials

Shake to dissolve; inspect for particulate matter and discoloration prior to use. Solutions of cefotaxime sodium range from very pale yellow to light amber, depending on concentration, diluent used, and length and condition of storage.

For Intramuscular Use: Reconstitute VIALS with Sterile Water for Injection or Bacteriostatic Water for Injection as described in TABLE 4.

For Intravenous Use: Reconstitute VIALS with at least 10 ml of Sterile Water for Injection. Reconstitute INFUSION BOTTLES with 50 or 100 ml of 0.9% Sodium Chloride Injection or 5% Dextrose Injection. For other diluents, see Compatibility and Stability.

Pharmacy Bulk Package: Reconstitute with 47 ml of diluent for an approximate concentration of 200 mg/ml or 97 ml of diluent for an approximate concentration of 100 mg/ml. Stock solutions may be further diluted for IV infusion with diluents as listed in Compatibility and Stability.

NOTE: Solutions of cefotaxime sodium must not be admixed with aminoglycoside solutions. If cefotaxime sodium and aminoglycosides are to be administered to the same patient, they must be administered separately and not as mixed injection.

A SOLUTION OF 1 G CEFOTAXIME SODIUM IN 14 ML OF STERILE WATER FOR INJECTION IS ISOTONIC.

IM Administration: As with all IM preparations, cefotaxime sodium should be injected well within the body of a relatively large muscle such as the upper outer quadrant of the buttock (*i.e.,* gluteus maximus); aspiration is necessary to avoid inadvertent injection into a blood vessel. Individual IM doses of 2 grams may be given if the dose is divided and is administered in different intramuscular sites.

IV Administration: The IV route is preferable for patients with bacteremia, bacterial septicemia, peritonitis, meningitis, or other severe or life-threatening infections, or for patients who may be poor risks because of lowered resistance resulting from such debilitating conditions as malnutrition, trauma, surgery, diabetes, heart failure, or malignancy, particularly if shock is present or impending.

For intermittent IV administration, a solution containing 1 gram or 2 grams in 10 ml of Sterile Water for Injection can be injected over a period of three to five minutes. Cefotaxime should not be administered over a period of less than three minutes. (See WARNINGS.) With an infusion system, it may also be given over a longer period of time through the tubing system by which the patient may be receiving other IV solutions. However, during infusion of the solution containing cefotaxime sodium, it is advisable to discontinue temporarily the administration of other solutions at the same site.

For the administration of higher doses by continuous IV infusion, a solution of cefotaxime sodium may be added to IV bottles containing the solutions discussed below.

DIRECTIONS FOR USE OF CEFOTAXIME SODIUM INJECTION IN GALAXY CONTAINER (PL 2040 PLASTIC)

Claforan Injection in Galaxy containers (PL 2040 plastic) is for continuous or intermittent infusion using sterile equipment.

Storage: Store in a freezer capable of maintaining a temperature of -20°C / -4°F.

Thawing of Plastic Container: Thaw frozen container at room temperature (22°C / 72°F) or under refrigeration (5°C / 41°F). (DO NOT FORCE THAW BY IMMERSION IN WATER BATHS OR BY MICROWAVE IRRADIATION.)

Check for minute leaks by squeezing container firmly. If leaks are detected, discard solution as sterility may be impaired.

DO NOT ADD SUPPLEMENTARY MEDICATION.

The container should be visually inspected. Components of the solution may precipitate in the frozen state and will dissolve upon reaching room temperature with little or no agitation. Potency is not affected. Agitate after solution has reached room temperature. If after visual inspection the solution remains cloudy or if an insoluble precipitate is noted or if any seals or outlet ports are not intact, the container should be discarded.

The thawed solution is stable for 10 days under refrigeration (5°C / 41°F) or 24 hours at room temperature (25°C / 72°F). Do not refreeze thawed antibiotics.

CAUTION: Do not use plastic containers in series connections. Such use could result in air embolism due to residual air being drawn from the primary container before administration of the fluid from the secondary container is complete.

DOSAGE AND ADMINISTRATION: *(cont'd)*

Preparation for Intravenous Administration

1. Suspend container from eyelet support.
2. Remove plastic protector from outlet port at bottom of container.
3. Attach administration set. Refer to complete directions accompanying set.

PREPARATION OF CLAFORAN STERILE IN ADD-VANTAGE SYSTEM**

Claforan Sterile 1 g or 2 g may be reconstituted in 50 ml or 100 ml of 5% Dextrose or 0.9% Sodium Chloride in the ADD-Vantage diluent container.

COMPATIBILITY AND STABILITY

Solutions of cefotaxime sodium sterile reconstituted as described in DOSAGE AND ADMINISTRATION, Preparation of Claforan Sterile in ADD-Vantage System** remain chemically stable (potency remains above 90%) as in TABLE 5 when stored in original containers and disposable plastic syringes.

TABLE 5

Strength	Reconstituted Concentration mg/ml	Stability at or below 22° C	Stability under Refrigeraton (at or below 5° C)	
			Original Containers	Plastic Syringes
500 mg vial IM	200	12 hours	7 days	5 days
1 g vial IM	300	12 hours	7 days	5 days
2 g vial IM	330	12 hours	7 days	5 days
500 mg vial IV	50	24 hours	7 days	5 days
1 g vial IV	95	24 hours	7 days	5 days
2 g vial IV	180	12 hours	7 days	5 days
1 g infusion bottle	10-20	24 hours	10 days	
2 g infusion bottle	20-40	24 hours	10 days	

Reconstituted solutions stored in original containers and plastic syringes remain stable for 13 weeks frozen.

For the 10 g bottle withdraw reconstituted contents immediately. However, if it is not possible, allquoting operations must be completed within four hours of reconstitution. Discard the reconstituted stock solution 4 hours after initial entry.

Reconstituted solutions may be further diluted up to 1000 ml with the following solutions and maintain satisfactory potency for 24 hours at room temperature (at or below 22°C) and at least 5 days under refrigeration (at or below 5°C): 0.9% Sodium Chloride Injection; 5 or 10% Dextrose Injection; 5% Dextrose and 0.9% Sodium Chloride Injection; 5% Dextrose and 0.45% Sodium Chloride Injection; 5% Dextrose and 0.2% Sodium Chloride Injection, Lactated Ringers Solution; Sodium Lactate Injection (M/6); 10% Invert Sugar Injection, 8.5% Travasol (Amino Acid) Injection without Electrolytes.

Solutions of cefotaxime sodium sterile reconstituted in 0.9% Sodium Chloride Injection or 5% Dextrose Injection in Viaflex plastic containers maintain satisfactory potency for 24 hours at room temperature (at or below 22°C), 5 days under refrigeration (at or below 5°C) and 13 weeks frozen. Solutions of cefotaxime sodium sterile reconstituted in 0.9% Sodium Chloride Injection or 5% Dextrose Injection in the ADD-Vantage flexible containers maintain satisfactory potency for 24 hours at room temperature (at or below 22°C). DO NOT FREEZE.

NOTE: Cefotaxime sodium solutions exhibit maximum stability in the pH 5-7 range. Solutions of cefotaxime sodium should not be prepared with diluents having a pH above 7.5, such as Sodium Bicarbonate Injection.

HOW SUPPLIED:

Sterile Claforan is a dry off-white to pale yellow crystalline powder supplied in 500 mg, 1 g, and 2 g vials and 1 g, 2 g, and 10 g bottles.

ADD-Vantage System diluents (5% Dextrose or 0.9% Sodium Chloride) are available from Abbott Laboratories.

NOTE: Claforan in the dry state should be stored below 30°C. The dry material as well as solutions tend to darken depending on storage conditions and should be protected from elevated temperatures and excessive light.

Premixed Claforan Injection is supplied as a frozen, iso-osmotic, sterile, nonpyrogenic solution in 50 ml single dose Galaxy containers (PL 2040 plastic).

NOTE: Store Premixed Claforan Injection at or below -20°C / - 4°F. SeeDOSAGE AND ADMINISTRATION, Directions For Use Of Claforan Injection In Galaxy Containers (Pl 2040 Plastic).

Claforan Injection supplied as a frozen, iso-osmotic, sterile, nonpyrogenic solution in Galaxy containers (PL 2040 plastic) is manufactured for Hoechst-Roussel Pharmaceuticals Inc., by Baxter Healthcare Corporation.

REFERENCES:

1. Bauer, A.W.; Kirby, W.M.M.; Sherris, J.C.; and Turck, M.: Antibiotic Susceptibility Testing by a Standardized Single Disk Method, Am. J. Clin. Pathol., 45:493, 1966; Standardized Disc Susceptibility Test, Federal Register, 39:19182-4, 1974. National Committee for Clinical Laboratory Standards. Approved Standard: ASM-2, Performance Standards for Antimicrobial Disc Susceptibility Tests. July, 1975. 2. Cockcroft, D.W. and Gault, M.H.: Prediction of Creatinine Clearance from Serum Creatinine. Nephron 16:31-41, 1976.

HOW SUPPLIED - EQUIVALENTS NOT AVAILABLE:

Injection, Dry-Soln - Intramuscular; - 1 gm/vial

1 gm x 10	$112.69	CLAFORAN, INFUSION BOTTLE, Hoechst Marion Roussel	00039-0018-11
1 gm x 10	$115.38	CLAFORAN, Hoechst Marion Roussel	00039-0018-10
1 gm x 25	$272.29	CLAFORAN, Hoechst Marion Roussel	00039-0018-25
1 gm x 25	$281.18	CLAFORAN, ADD-VANTAGE, Hoechst Marion Roussel	00039-0023-25
1 gm x 50	$514.08	CLAFORAN, Hoechst Marion Roussel	00039-0018-50
1 gm x 50	$531.88	CLAFORAN, ADD-VANTAGE, Hoechst Marion Roussel	00039-0023-50
50 ml x 24	$306.28	CLAFORAN GALAXY, Hoechst Marion Roussel	00039-0037-05

Injection, Dry-Soln - Intramuscular; - 2 gm/vial

2 gm x 10	$211.63	CLAFORAN, INFUSION BOTTLE, Hoechst Marion Roussel	00039-0019-11
2 gm x 10	$213.46	CLAFORAN, Hoechst Marion Roussel	00039-0019-10
2 gm x 25	$503.75	CLAFORAN, Hoechst Marion Roussel	00039-0019-25
2 gm x 25	$512.65	CLAFORAN, ADD-VANTAGE, Hoechst Marion Roussel	00039-0024-25
2 gm x 50	$951.55	CLAFORAN, Hoechst Marion Roussel	00039-0019-50
2 gm x 50	$969.35	CLAFORAN, ADD-VANTAGE, Hoechst Marion Roussel	00039-0024-50
50 ml x 24	$514.22	CLAFORAN GALAXY, Hoechst Marion Roussel	00039-0038-05

HOW SUPPLIED - EQUIVALENTS NOT AVAILABLE: *(cont'd)*

Injection, Dry-Soln - Intravenous - 10 gm/vial

10 gm x 1	$95.16	CLAFORAN, BOTTLE, Hoechst Marion Roussel	00039-0020-01

Injection, Powder - Intravenous - 500 mg

10's	$69.14	CLAFORAN, Hoechst Marion Roussel	00039-0017-10

CEFOTETAN DISODIUM *(000690)*

CATEGORIES: Anti-Infectives; Antibiotics; Antimicrobials; Bone Infections; Cephalosporins; Gynecologic Infections; Infections; Intra-Abdominal Infections; Joint Infections; Perioperative Prophylaxis; Respiratory Tract Infections; Skin Infections; Urinary Tract Infections; Pregnancy Category B; FDA Approved 1985 Dec

BRAND NAMES: *Apacef* (France); Apatef; **Cefotan**; *Ceftenon*; *Cepan*; *Yamatetan* *(International brand names outside U.S. in italics)*

DESCRIPTION:

Cefotan (sterile cefotetan disodium) and Cefotan (cefotetan disodium injection) in Galaxy™ plastic container (PL 2040) as cefotetan disodium are sterile, semisynthetic, broad-spectrum, beta-lactamase resistant, cephalosporin (cephamycin) antibiotics for parenteral administration. It is the disodium salt of [6*R*-(6α,7α)]-7-[[[4-(2-amino-1-carboxy-2-oxoethylidene)-1,3 -dithietan-2-yl]carbonyl]amino]-7-methoxy-3-[[(1-methyl-1*H*-tetrazol-5-yl)thio]methyl]-8-oxo-5-thia-1-azabicyclo[4.2.0]oct-2-ene-2-carboxylic acid. Its molecular formula is $C_{17}H_{15}N_7Na_2O_8S_4$ with a molecular weight of 619.57.

Cefotan is supplied in vials containing 80 mg (3.5 mEq) of sodium per gram of cefotetan activity. It is a white to pale yellow powder which is very soluble in water. Reconstituted solutions of sterile cefotetan disodium are intended for intravenous and intramuscular administration. The solution varies from colorless to yellow depending on the concentration. The pH of freshly reconstituted solutions is usually between 4.5 to 6.5.

Cefotetan disodium in the ADD-Vantage Vial†: is intended for intravenous use only after dilution with the appropriate volume of ADD-Vantage diluent solution.

Cefotan is available in two vial strengths. Each Cefotan 1 g vial contains cefotetan disodium equivalent to 1 g cefotetan activity. Each Cefotan 2 g vial contains cefotetan disodium equivalent to 2 g cefotetan activity.

Cefotan (cefotetan disodium injection) in the Galaxy plastic container (PL 2040) is a frozen, iso-osmotic, sterile, nonpyrogenic premixed 50 ml solution containing 1 g or 2 g cefotetan as cefotetan disodium. Dextrose, USP has been added to adjust the osmolality to 300 mOsmol/kg (approximately 1.9 g and 1.1 g to the 1 g and 2 g dosages, respectively); sodium bicarbonate has been added to convert cefotetan free acid to the sodium salt. The pH has been adjusted between 4 and 6.5 with sodium bicarbonate and may have been adjusted with hydrochloric acid. Cefotan in the Galaxy plastic container (PL 2040) contains 80 mg (3.5 mEq) of sodium per gram of cefotetan activity. After thawing to room temperature, the solution is intended for intravenous use only.

This Galaxy container is fabricated from a specially designed multilayer plastic (PL 2040). Solutions are in contact with the polyethylene layer of this container and can leach out certain chemical components of the plastic in very small amounts within the expiration dating period. The suitability of the plastic has been confirmed in tests in animals according to the USP biological tests for plastic containers as well as by tissue culture toxicity.

CLINICAL PHARMACOLOGY:

High plasma levels of cefotetan are attained after intravenous and intramuscular administration of single doses to normal volunteers (TABLE 1 and TABLE 2).

TABLE 1 Plasma Concentrations After 1 Gram Iv [A] Or Im Dose Mean Plasma Concentration (mcg/ml)

Route	15 min	30 min	1h	2h	4h	8h	12h
	Time After Injection						
IV	92	158	103	72	42	18	9
IM	34	56	71	68	47	20	9

[a]30-minute infusion

TABLE 2 Plasma Concentrations After 2 Gram Iv [A] Or Im Dose Mean Plasma Concentration (mcg/ml)

Route	5 min	10 min	1h	3h	5h	9h	12h
	Time after Injection						
IV	237	223	135	74	48	22	12[b]
IM	—	20	75	91	69	33	19

[a]Injected over 3 minutes
[b]Concentrations estimated from regression line

The plasma elimination half-life of cefotetan is 3 to 4.6 hours after either intravenous or intramuscular administration.

Repeated administration of cefotetan disodium does not result in accumulation of the drug in normal subjects.

Cefotetan is 88% plasma protein bound.

No active metabolites of cefotetan have been detected; however, small amounts (less than 7%) of cefotetan in plasma and urine may be converted to its tautomer, which has antimicrobial activity similar to the parent drug.

In normal patients, from 51% to 81% of an administered dose of cefotetan disodium is excreted unchanged by the kidneys over a 24 hour period, which results in high and prolonged urinary concentrations. Following intravenous doses of 1 gram and 2 grams, urinary concentrations are highest during the first hour and reach concentrations of approximately 1700 and 3500 mcg/ml respectively.

In volunteers with reduced renal function, the plasma half-life of cefotetan is prolonged. The mean terminal half-life increases with declining renal function, from approximately 4 hours in volunteers with normal renal function to about 10 hours in those with moderate renal impairment. There is a linear correlation between the systemic clearance of cefotetan and creatinine clearance. When renal function is impaired, a reduced dosing schedule based on creatinine clearance must be used (see DOSAGE AND ADMINISTRATION).[1]

Therapeutic levels of cefotetan are achieved in many body tissues and fluids including: skin; muscle; fat; myometrium; endometrium; cervix; ovary; kidney; ureter; bladder; maxillary sinus mucosa; tonsil; bile; peritoneal fluid; umbilical cord serum; amniotic fluid

CLINICAL PHARMACOLOGY: *(cont'd)*

MICROBIOLOGY

The bactericidal action of cefotetan results from inhibition of cell wall synthesis. Cefotetan has *in vitro* activity against a wide range of aerobic and anaerobic gram-positive and gram-negative organisms. The methoxy group in the 7-alpha position provides cefotetan with a high degree of stability in the presence of beta-lactamases including both penicillinases and cephalosporinases of gram-negative bacteria.

Cefotetan has been shown to be active against most strains of the following organisms **both *in vitro* and in clinical infections** (see INDICATIONS AND USAGE).

Gram-Negative Aerobes: *Escherichia coli; Haemophilus influenzae* (including ampicillin-resistant strains); *Klebsiella* species (including *K. pneumoniae*); *Morganella morganii; Neisseria gonorrhoeae* (nonpenicillinase-producing strains); *Proteus mirabilis; Proteus vulgaris; Providencia rettgeri; Serratia marcescens*

NOTE: Approximately one-half of the usually clinically significant strains of *Enterobacter* species (*e.g., E. aerogenes* and *E. cloacae*) are resistant to cefotetan. Most strains of *Pseudomonas aeruginosa* and *Acinetobacter* species are resistant to cefotetan.

Gram-Positive Aerobes: *Staphylococcus aureus* (including penicillinase- and nonpenicillinase-producing strains);*Staphylococcus epidermidis; Streptococcus agalactiae* (group B beta-hemolytic streptococcus); *Streptococcus pneumoniae; Streptococcus pyogenes*

NOTE: Methicillin-resistant staphylococci are resistant to cephalosporins. Some strains of *Staphylococcus epidermidis* and most strains of enterococci, e.g., *Enterococcus faecalis* (formerly *Streptococcus faecalis*), are resistant to cefotetan.

Anaerobes: *Prevotella bivia* (formerly *Bacteroides bivius*); *Prevotella disiens* (formerly *Bacteroides disiens*); *Bacteroides fragilis; Prevotella melaninogenica* (formerly *Bacteroides melaninogenicus*);*Bacteroides vulgatus; Fusobacterium* species; Gram-positive bacilli (including *Clostridium* species; see WARNINGS).

NOTE: Many strains of *C. difficile* are resistant (see WARNINGS).

Peptococcus niger; Peptostreptococcus species

NOTE: Many strains of *B. distasonis, B. ovatus* and *B. thetaiotaomicron* are resistant to cefotetan *in vitro.* However, the therapeutic utility of cefotetan against these organisms cannot be accurately predicted on the basis of *in vitro* susceptibility tests alone.[2]

The following *in vitro* data are available but their clinical significance is unknown. Cefotetan has been shown to be active *in vitro* against most strains of the following organisms:

Gram-Negative Aerobes: *Citrobacter* species (including*C. diversus* and *C. freundii*); *Klebsiella oxytoca; Moraxella (Branhamella) catarrhalis;*

Neisseria gonorrhoeae (penicillinase-producing strains);*Salmonella* species; *Serratia* species; *Shigella* species; *Yersinia enterocolitica*

Anaerobes: *Porphyromonas asaccharolytica* (formerly*Bacteroides asaccharolyticus*); *Prevotella oralis* (formerly *Bacteroides oralis*); *Bacteroides splanchnicus*;*Clostridium difficile*(see WARNINGS); *Propionibacterium* species; *Veillonella* species

SUSCEPTIBILITY TESTING

Diffusion Techniques: Quantitative methods that require measurement of zone diameters provide reproducible estimates of the susceptibility of bacteria to antimicrobial compounds. One such standardized procedure[3] that has been recommended for use with disks to test the susceptibility of microorganisms to cefotetan uses a 30 mcg cefotetan disk. Interpretation involves the correlation of the diameter obtained in the disk test with the minimum inhibitory concentration (MIC) for cefotetan.

Reports from the laboratory providing results of the standard single-disk susceptibility test with a 30 mcg cefotetan disk should be interpreted according to the criteria in TABLE 3.

TABLE 3

Zone Diameter (mm)	Interpretation
≥ 16	Susceptible (S)
13-15	Intermediate (I)
≤ 12	Resistant (R)

A report of "Susceptible" indicates that the pathogen is likely to be inhibited by usually achievable concentrations of the antimicrobial compound in blood. A report of "Intermediate" indicates that the result should be considered equivocal, and, if the microorganism is not fully susceptible to alternative, clinically feasible drugs, the test should be repeated. This category implies possible clinical applicability in body sites where the drug is physiologically concentrated or in situations where high dosage of drug can be used. This category also provides a buffer zone that prevents small uncontrolled technical factors from causing major discrepancies in interpretation. A report of "Resistant" indicates that usually achievable concentrations of the antimicrobial compound in the blood are unlikely to be inhibitory and that other therapy should be selected.

Measurement of MIC or MBC and achieved antimicrobial compound concentrations may be appropriate to guide therapy in some infections. (See CLINICAL PHARMACOLOGYsection for further information on drug concentrations achieved in infected body sites and other pharmacokinetic properties of this antimicrobial drug product.)

Standardized susceptibility test procedures require the use of laboratory control organisms. The 30 mcg cefotetan disk should provide the following zone diameters in these laboratory test quality control strains (TABLE 4).

TABLE 4

Microorganism	Zone Diameter (mm)
E. coli ATCC 25922	28-34
S. aureus ATCC 25923	17-23

Dilution Techniques: Quantitative methods that are used to determine minimum inhibitory concentrations provide reproducible estimates of the susceptibility of bacteria to antimicrobial compounds. One such standardized procedure uses a standardized dilution method[4](broth, agar, or microdilution) or equivalent with cefotetan powder. The MIC values obtained should be interpreted according to the criteria in TABLE 5.

TABLE 5

MIC (mcg/ml)	Interpretation
≤ 16	Susceptible (S)
32	Intermediate (I)
≥ 64	Resistant (R)

Interpretation of S, I, or R should be as stated above for results using diffusion techniques. As with standard diffusion techniques, dilution methods require the use of laboratory control organisms. Standard cefotetan powder should provide the MIC values in TABLE 6.

CLINICAL PHARMACOLOGY: *(cont'd)*

TABLE 6

Microorganism	MIC (mcg/ml)
E. coli ATCC 25922	0.06-0.25
S. aureus ATCC 29213	4-16

Susceptibility Testing Techniques: For anaerobic bacteria, the susceptibility to cefotetan can be determined by the reference agar dilution method or by alternate standardized test methods[5].

The MIC values obtained should be interpreted as in TABLE 7.

TABLE 7

MIC (mcg/ml)	Interpretation
≤ 16	Susceptible (S)
32	Intermediate (I)
≥ 64	Resistant (R)

As with other susceptibility techniques, the use of laboratory control microorganisms is required. Standard cefotetan powder should provide the following MIC values with the reference agar dilution method[5](TABLE 8).

TABLE 8

Microorganism	MIC (mcg/ml)
Bacteroides fragilis ATCC 25285	4-16
Bacteroides thetaiotaomicron ATCC 29741	32-128
Eubacterium lentum ATCC 43055	32-128

INDICATIONS AND USAGE:

Treatment: Cefotetan disodium is indicated for the therapeutic treatment of the following infections when caused by susceptible strains of the designated organisms:

Urinary Tract Infections caused by *E. coli, Klebsiella* spp. (including *K. pneumoniae*), *Proteus mirabilis* and *Proteus* spp. (which may include the organisms now called *Proteus vulgaris, Providencia rettgeri,* and *Morganella morganii*).

Lower Respiratory Tract Infections caused by *Streptococcus pneumoniae, Staphylococcus aureus* (penicillinase- and nonpenicillinase-producing strains), *Haemophilus influenzae* (including ampicillin-resistant strains), *Klebsiella* species (including *K. pneumoniae*), *E. coli, Proteus mirabilis,* and *Serratia marcescens**.

Skin and Skin Structure Infections due to *Staphylococcus aureus* (penicillinase- and nonpenicillinase-producing strains), *Staphylococcus epidermidis, Streptococcus pyogenes, Streptococcus* species (excluding enterococci), *Escherichia coli, Klebsiella pneumoniae, Peptococcus niger**, *Peptostreptococcus* species.

Gynecologic Infections caused by *Staphylococcus aureus* (including penicillinase- and nonpenicillinase-producing strains),*Staphylococcus epidermidis, Streptococcus* species (excluding enterococci), *Streptococcus agalactiae, E. coli, Proteus mirabilis, Neisseria gonorrhoeae, Bacteroides* species (excluding *B. distasonis, B. ovatus, B. thetaiotaomicron*), *Fusobacterium*species*, and gram-positive anaerobic cocci (including*Peptococcus niger* and *Peptostreptococcus* species).

Cefotetan, like other cephalosporins, has no activity against *Chlamydia trachomatis.* Therefore, when cephalosporins are used in the treatment of pelvic inflammatory disease, and *C. trachomatis* is one of the suspected pathogens, appropriate antichlamydial coverage should be added.

Intra-abdominal Infections caused by *E. coli, Klebsiella* species (including *K. pneumoniae*), *Streptococcus* species (excluding enterococci), *Bacteroides* species (excluding *B. distasonis, B. ovatus, B. thetaiotaomicron*) and *Clostridium* species*.

Bone and Joint Infections caused by *Staphylococcus aureus.**

*Efficacy for this organism in this organ system was studied in fewer than ten infections.

Specimens for bacteriological examination should be obtained in order to isolate and identify causative organisms and to determine their susceptibilities to cefotetan. Therapy may be instituted before results of susceptibility studies are known; however, once these results become available, the antibiotic treatment should be adjusted accordingly.

In cases of confirmed or suspected gram-positive or gram-negative sepsis or in patients with other serious infections in which the causative organism has not been identified, it is possible to use cefotetan disodium concomitantly with an aminoglycoside. Cefotetan combinations with aminoglycosides have been shown to be synergistic *in vitro* against many Enterobacteriaceae and also some other gram-negative bacteria. The dosage recommended in the labeling of both antibiotics may be given and depends on the severity of the infection and the patient's condition.

NOTE: Increases in serum creatinine have occurred when cefotetan disodium was given alone. If cefotetan disodium and an aminoglycoside are used concomitantly, renal function should be carefully monitored, because nephrotoxicity may be potentiated.

Prophylaxis: The preoperative administration of cefotetan disodium may reduce the incidence of certain postoperative infections in patients undergoing surgical procedures that are classified as clean contaminated or potentially contaminated (*e.g.,* cesarean section, abdominal or vaginal hysterectomy, transurethral surgery, biliary tract surgery, and gastrointestinal surgery).

If there are signs and symptoms of infection, specimens for culture should be obtained for identification of the causative organism so that appropriate therapeutic measures may be initiated.

CONTRAINDICATIONS:

Cefotetan disodium is contraindicated in patients with known allergy to the cephalosporin group of antibiotics.

WARNINGS:

BEFORE THERAPY WITH CEFOTETAN DISODIUM IS INSTITUTED, CAREFUL INQUIRY SHOULD BE MADE TO DETERMINE WHETHER THE PATIENT HAS HAD PREVIOUS HYPERSENSITIVITY REACTIONS TO CEFOTETAN DISODIUM, CEPHALOSPORINS, PENICILLINS, OR OTHER DRUGS. IF THIS PRODUCT IS TO BE GIVEN TO PENICILLIN-SENSITIVE PATIENTS, CAUTION SHOULD BE EXERCISED BECAUSE CROSS-HYPERSENSITIVITY AMONG BETA-LACTAM ANTIBIOTICS HAS BEEN CLEARLY DOCUMENTED AND MAY OCCUR IN UP TO 10% OF PATIENTS WITH A HISTORY OF PENICILLIN ALLERGY. IF AN ALLERGIC REACTION TO

WARNINGS: *(cont'd)*

CEFOTETAN DISODIUM OCCURS, DISCONTINUE THE DRUG. SERIOUS ACUTE HYPERSENSITIVITY REACTIONS MAY REQUIRE TREATMENT WITH EPINEPHRINE AND OTHER EMERGENCY MEASURES, INCLUDING OXYGEN, INTRAVENOUS FLUIDS, INTRAVENOUS ANTIHISTAMINES, CORTICOSTEROIDS, PRESSOR AMINES, AND AIRWAY MANAGEMENT, AS CLINICALLY INDICATED.

Pseudomembranous colitis has been reported with nearly all antibacterial agents, including cefotetan, and may range from mild to life-threatening. Onset of pseudomembranous colitis symptoms may occur during or after antibiotic treatment or surgical prophylaxis. Therefore, it is important to consider this diagnosis in patients who present with diarrhea subsequent to the administration of antibacterial agents.

Treatment with antibacterial agents alters the normal flora of the colon and may permit overgrowth of clostridia. Studies indicate that a toxin produced by *Clostridium difficile* is a primary cause of "antibiotic-associated colitis".

After the diagnosis of pseudomembranous colitis has been established, therapeutic measures should be initiated. Mild cases of pseudomembranous colitis usually respond to discontinuation of the drug alone. In moderate to severe cases, consideration should be given to management with fluids and electrolytes, protein supplementation, and treatment with an antibacterial drug clinically effective against *Clostridium difficile*. (See ADVERSE REACTIONS.)

In common with many other broad-spectrum antibiotics, cefotetan disodium may be associated with a fall in prothrombin activity and, possibly, subsequent bleeding. Those at increased risk include patients with renal or hepatobiliary impairment or poor nutritional state, the elderly, and patients with cancer. Prothrombin time should be monitored and exogenous vitamin K administered as indicated.

Hemolytic anemia has been reported for cephalosporin-class antibiotics. Severe cases of hemolytic anemia, including fatalities, have been reported in association with the administration of cefotetan disodium. Such reports are uncommon. If a patient develops a hematologic abnormality subsequent to the administration of cefotetan, a diagnosis of drug-induced hemolytic anemia should be considered.

PRECAUTIONS:

General: As with other broad-spectrum antibiotics, prolonged use of cefotetan disodium may result in overgrowth of nonsusceptible organisms. Careful observation of the patient is essential. If superinfection does occur during therapy, appropriate measures should be taken.

Cefotetan disodium should be used with caution in individuals with a history of gastrointestinal disease, particularly colitis.

Information for the Patient: As with some other cephalosporins, a disulfiram-like reaction characterized by flushing, sweating, headache, and tachycardia may occur when alcohol (beer, wine, etc.) is ingested within 72 hours after cefotetan disodium administration. Patients should be cautioned about the ingestion of alcoholic beverages following the administration of cefotetan disodium.

Drug/Laboratory Test Interactions: The administration of cefotetan disodium may result in a false positive reaction for glucose in the urine using Clinitest‡, Benedict's solution, or Fehling's solution. It is recommended that glucose tests based on enzymatic glucose oxidase be used.

As with other cephalosporins, high concentrations of cefotetan may interfere with measurement of serum and urine creatinine levels by Jaffe reaction and produce false increases in the levels of creatinine reported.

Carcinogenesis, Mutagenesis, and Impairment of Fertility: Although long-term studies in animals have not been performed to evaluate carcinogenic potential, no mutagenic potential of cefotetan was found in standard laboratory tests.

Cefotetan has adverse effects on the testes of prepubertal rats. Subcutaneous administration of 500 mg/kg/day (approximately 8-16 times the usual adult human dose) on days 6-35 of life (thought to be developmentally analogous to late childhood and prepuberty in humans) resulted in reduced testicular weight and seminiferous tubule degeneration in 10 of 10 animals. Affected cells included spermatogonia and spermatocytes; Sertoli and Leydig cells were unaffected. Incidence and severity of lesions were dose-dependent; at 120 mg/kg/day (approximately 2-4 times the usual human dose) only 1 of 10 treated animals was affected, and the degree of degeneration was mild.

Similar lesions have been observed in experiments of comparable design with other methylthiotetrazole-containing antibiotics and impaired fertility has been reported, particularly at high dose levels. No testicular effects were observed in 7-week-old rats treated with up to 1000 mg/kg/day SC for 5 weeks, or in infant dogs (3 weeks old) that received up to 300 mg/kg/day IV for 5 weeks. The relevance of these findings to humans is unknown.

Pregnancy, Teratogenic Effects, Pregnancy Category B: Reproduction studies have been performed in rats and monkeys at doses up to 20 times the human dose and have revealed no evidence of impaired fertility or harm to the fetus due to cefotetan. There are, however, no adequate and well-controlled studies in pregnant women. Because animal reproductive studies are not always predictive of human response, this drug should be used during pregnancy only if clearly needed.

Nursing Mothers: Cefotetan is excreted in human milk in very low concentrations. Caution should be exercised when cefotetan is administered to a nursing woman.

Pediatric Use: Safety and effectiveness in children have not been established.

DRUG INTERACTIONS:

Increases in serum creatinine have occurred when cefotetan disodium was given alone. If cefotetan disodium and an aminoglycoside are used concomitantly, renal function should be carefully monitored, because nephrotoxicity may be potentiated.

ADVERSE REACTIONS:

In clinical studies, the following adverse effects were considered related to cefotetan disodium therapy. Those appearing in italics have been reported during postmarketing experience.

Gastrointestinal symptoms occurred in 1.5% of patients, the most frequent were diarrhea (1 in 80) and nausea (1 in 700); *pseudomembranous colitis.* Onset of pseudomembranous colitis symptoms may occur during or after antibiotic treatment or surgical prophylaxis. (See WARNINGS.)

Hematologic laboratory abnormalities occurred in 1.4% of patients and included eosinophilia (1 in 200), positive direct Coombs' test (1 in 250), and thrombocytosis (1 in 300); *agranulocytosis, hemolytic anemia, leukopenia, thrombocytopenia,* and *prolonged prothrombin time with or without bleeding.*

Hepatic enzyme elevations occurred in 1.2% of patients and included a rise in ALT (SGPT) (1 in 150), AST (SGOT) (1 in 300), alkaline phosphatase (1 in 700), and LDH (1 in 700).

Hypersensitivity reactions were reported in 1.2% of patients and included rash (1 in 150) and itching (1 in 700); *anaphylactic reactions and urticaria.*

Local effects were reported in less than 1% of patients and included phlebitis at the site of injection (1 in 300), and discomfort (1 in 500).

Renal: *Elevations in BUN and serum creatinine have been reported.*

ADVERSE REACTIONS: *(cont'd)*

Urogenital: *Nephrotoxicity has rarely been reported.*

Miscellaneous: *Fever*

In addition to the adverse reactions listed above which have been observed in patients treated with cefotetan, the following adverse reactions and altered laboratory tests have been reported for cephalosporin-class antibiotics: pruritus, Stevens-Johnson syndrome, erythema multiforme, toxic epidermal necrolysis, vomiting, abdominal pain, colitis, superinfection, vaginitis including vaginal candidiasis, renal dysfunction, toxic nephropathy, hepatic dysfunction including cholestasis, aplastic anemia, hemorrhage, elevated bilirubin, pancytopenia, and neutropenia.

Several cephalosporins have been implicated in triggering seizures, particularly in patients with renal impairment, when the dosage was not reduced. (See OVERDOSAGE.) If seizures associated with drug therapy occur, the drug should be discontinued. Anticonvulsant therapy can be given if clinically indicated.

OVERDOSAGE:

Information on overdosage with cefotetan disodium in humans is not available. If overdosage should occur, it should be treated symptomatically and hemodialysis considered, particularly if renal function is compromised.

DOSAGE AND ADMINISTRATION:

TREATMENT

Cefotetan disodium injection in Galaxy plastic container should not be used for intramuscular administration.

Cefotetan disodium in the ADD-Vantage Vial is intended for intravenous infusion only, after dilution with the appropriate volume of ADD-Vantage diluent solution.

The usual adult dosage is 1 or 2 grams of cefotetan disodium administered intravenously or intramuscularly or cefotetan disodium injection in the Galaxy plastic container (PL 2040) administered intravenously every 12 hours for 5 to 10 days. Proper dosage and route of administration should be determined by the condition of the patient, severity of the infection, and susceptibility of the causative organism (TABLE 9).

TABLE 9 General Guidelines For Dosage of Cefotetan Disodium

Type of Infection	Daily Dose	Frequency and Route
Urinary Tract	1 - 4 grams	500 mg every 12 hours IV or IM 1 or 2 g every 24 hours IV or IM 1 or 2 g every 12 hours IV or IM
Skin & Skin Structure		
Mild - Moderate[a]	2 grams	2 g every 24 hours IV 1 g every 12 hours IV or IM
Severe	4 grams	2 g every 12 hours IV
Other sites	2 - 4 grams	1 or 2 g every 12 hours IV or IM
Severe	4 grams	2 g every 12 hours IV
Life-Threatening	6 grams[b]	3 g every 12 hours IV

[a] *Klebsiella pneumoniae* skin and skin structure infections should be treated with 1 or 2 grams every 12 hours IV or IM.
[b] Maximum daily dosage should not exceed 6 grams.

If *Chlamydia trachomatis* is a suspected pathogen in gynecologic infections, appropriate antichlamydial coverage should be added, since cefotetan has no activity against this organism.

Prophylaxis: To prevent postoperative infection in clean contaminated or potentially contaminated surgery in adults, the recommended dosage is 1 or 2 g of cefotetan disodium administered once, intravenously, 30 to 60 minutes prior to surgery. In patients undergoing cesarean section, the dose should be administered as soon as the umbilical cord is clamped.

Impaired Renal Function: When renal function is impaired, a reduced dosage schedule must be employed. The dosage guidelines in TABLE 10 may be used.

TABLE 10 Dosage Guidelines For Patients With Impaired Renal Function

Creatinine/ Clearance ml/min	Dose	Frequency
> 30	Usual Recommended Dosage*	Every 12 hours
10 - 30	Usual Recommended Dosage*	Every 24 hours
< 10	Usual Recommended Dosage*	Every 48 hours

* Dose determined by the type and severity of infection, and susceptibility of the causative organism.

Alternatively, the dosing interval may remain constant at 12 hour intervals, but the dose reduced to one-half the usual recommended dose for patients with a creatinine clearance of 10-30 ml/min, and one-quarter the usual recommended dose for patients with a creatinine clearance of less than 10 ml/min.

When only serum creatinine levels are available, creatinine clearance may be calculated from the following formula. The serum creatinine level should represent a steady state of renal function (TABLE 11).

TABLE 11

Males: [Weight (kg) × (140 - age)] ÷ [72 × serum creatinine (mg/100 ml)]
Females: 0.9 × value for males

Cefotetan is dialyzable and it is recommended that for patients undergoing intermittent hemodialysis, one-quarter of the usual recommended dose be given every 24 hours on days between dialysis and one-half the usual recommended dose on the day of dialysis.

PREPARATION OF SOLUTION FROM STERILE CEFOTETAN DISODIUM

For Intravenous Use: Reconstitute with Sterile Water for Injection. Shake to dissolve and let stand until clear (TABLE 12).

TABLE 12

Vial Size	Amount of Diluent Added (ml)	Approximate Withdrawable Vol (ml)	Approximate Average Concentration (mg/ml)
1 gram	10	10.5	95
2 gram	10-20	11-21	182-95

Infusion bottles (100 ml) may be reconstituted with 50 to 100 ml of Dextrose Injection 5% or Sodium Chloride Injection 0.9%.

DOSAGE AND ADMINISTRATION: *(cont'd)*

NOTE: ADD-VANTAGE VIALS ARE NOT TO BE USED IN THIS MANNER

For ADD-Vantage Vials: ADD-Vantage Vials of cefotetan disodium are to be reconstituted only with Sodium Chloride Injection 0.9% or Dextrose Injection 5% in the 50 ml, 100 ml or 250 ml Flexible Diluent Containers. Cefotan supplied in single-use ADD-Vantage Vials should be prepared as directed.

Directions for use of Sterile Cefotetan Disodium in ADD-Vantage Vials

To Open Diluent Container: Peel overwrap from the corner and remove container. Some opacity of the plastic due to moisture absorption during the sterilization process may be observed. This is normal and does not affect the solution quality or safety. The opacity will diminish gradually.

To Assemble ADD-Vantage Vial and Flexible Diluent Container: (Use Aseptic Technique)

1. Remove the protective covers from the top of the vial and the vial port on the diluent container as follows:

a. To remove the breakaway vial cap, swing the pull ring over the top of the vial and pull down far enough to start the opening, then pull straight up to remove the cap. *NOTE:* Once the breakaway cap has been removed, do not access vial with syringe.

b. To remove the vial port cover, grasp the tab on the pull ring, pull up to break the three tie strings, then pull back to remove the cover.

2. Screw the vial into the vial port until it will go no further. THE VIAL MUST BE SCREWED IN TIGHTLY TO ASSURE A SEAL. This occurs approximately 1/2 turn (180°) after the first audible click. The clicking sound does not assure a seal; the vial must be turned as far as it will go. *NOTE:* ONCE VIAL IS SEATED, DO NOT ATTEMPT TO REMOVE.

3. Recheck the vial to assure that it is tight by trying to turn it further in the direction of assembly.

4. Label appropriately.

To Prepare Admixture

1. Squeeze the bottom of the diluent container gently to inflate the portion of the container surrounding the end of the drug vial.

2. With the other hand, push the drug vial down into the container telescoping the walls of the container. Grasp the inner cap of the vial through the walls of the container.

3. Pull the inner cap from the drug vial. Verify that the rubber stopper has been pulled out and invert the system several times, allowing the drug and diluent to mix.

4. Mix contents thoroughly and use within the specified time.

Preparation For Administration: (Use Aseptic Technique)

1. Confirm the activation and admixture of vial contents.

2. Check for leaks by squeezing container firmly. If leaks are found, discard unit as sterility may be impaired.

3. =Close flow control clamp of administration set.

4. Remove cover from outlet port at bottom of container.

5. Insert piercing pin of administration set into port with a twisting motion until the pin is firmly seated. *NOTE:* See full directions on administration set carton.

6. Lift the free end of the hanger loop on the bottom of the vial, breaking the two tie strings. Bend the loop outward to lock it in the upright position, then suspend container from hanger.

7. Squeeze and release drip chamber to establish proper fluid level in chamber.

8. Open flow control clamp and clear air from set. Close clamp.

9. Attach set to venipuncture device. If device is not indwelling, prime and make venipuncture.

10. Regulate rate of administration with flow control clamp.

WARNING: Do not use flexible container in series connections.

For Intramuscular Use: Reconstitute with Sterile Water for Injection; Bacteriostatic Water for Injection; Sodium Chloride Injection 0.9%, USP; 0.5% Lidocaine HCl; or 1% Lidocaine HCl. Shake to dissolve and let stand until clear (TABLE 13).

TABLE 13

Vial Size	Amount of Diluent Added (ml)	Approximate Withdrawable Vol (ml)	Approximate Average Concentration (mg/ml)
1 gram	2	2.5	400
2 gram	3	4	500

Intravenous Administration: The intravenous route is preferable for patients with bacteremia, bacterial septicemia, or other severe or life-threatening infections, or for patients who may be poor risks because of lowered resistance resulting from such debilitating conditions as malnutrition, trauma, surgery, diabetes, heart failure, or malignancy, particularly if shock is present or impending.

For intermittent intravenous administration, a solution containing 1 gram or 2 grams of sterile cefotetan disodium in Sterile Water for Injection can be injected over a period of three to five minutes. Using an infusion system, the solution may also be given over a longer period of time through the tubing system by which the patient may be receiving other intravenous solutions. Butterfly or scalp vein-type needles are preferred for this type of infusion. However, during infusion of the solution containing cefotetan disodium, it is advisable to discontinue temporarily the administration of other solutions at the same site.

NOTE: Solutions of cefotetan disodium must not be admixed with solutions containing aminoglycosides. If cefotetan disodium and aminoglycosides are to be administered to the same patient, they must be administered separately and not as a mixed injection.

Intramuscular Administration: As with all intramuscular preparations, sterile cefotetan disodium should be injected well within the body of a relatively large muscle such as the upper outer quadrant of the buttock (*i.e.,* gluteus maximus); aspiration is necessary to avoid inadvertent injection into a blood vessel.

DIRECTIONS FOR USE OF CEFOTAN INJECTION IN GALAXY PLASTIC CONTAINER (PL 2040)

Cefotan (cefotetan disodium injection) in Galaxy plastic container (PL 2040) is for intravenous administration only.

Storage: Store in a freezer capable of maintaining a temperature of -20°C/-4°F.

Thawing of Plastic Container: Thaw frozen container at room temperature (25°C/77°F) or in a refrigerator (5°C/41°F). **[DO NOT FORCE THAW BY IMMERSION IN WATER BATHS OR BY MICROWAVE IRRADIATION.]**

Check for minute leaks by squeezing container firmly. If leaks are detected, discard solution as sterility may be impaired.

The container should be visually inspected. Components of the solution may precipitate in the frozen state and will dissolve upon reaching room temperature with little or no agitation. Potency is not affected. Agitate after solution has reached room temperature. If after visual inspection the solution remains cloudy or if an insoluble precipitate is noted or if any seals or outlet ports are not intact, the container should be discarded.

DOSAGE AND ADMINISTRATION: *(cont'd)*

Preparation of Intravenous Use (Use aseptic technique)

1. Suspend container from eyelet support.

2. Remove protector from outlet port at bottom of container.

3. Attach administration set. Refer to complete directions accompanying set.

CAUTION: Do not use plastic containers in series connections. Such use could result in air embolism due to residual air being drawn from the primary container before administration of the fluid from the secondary container is complete.

Intravenous Administration: The intravenous route is preferable for patients with bacteremia, bacterial septicemia, or other severe or life threatening infections, or for patients who may be poor risks because of lowered resistance resulting from such debilitating conditions as malnutrition, trauma, surgery, diabetes, heart failure, or malignancy, particularly if shock is present or impending.

Using an infusion system, cefotetan disodium injection in Galaxy plastic container (PL 2040) should be given over 20 to 60 minutes through the tubing system by which the patient may be receiving other intravenous solutions. Butterfly or scalp vein-type needles are preferred for this type of infusion. However, during infusion of the solution containing Cefotan (cefotetan disodium injection) in Galaxy plastic container (PL 2040), it is advisable to discontinue temporarily the administration of other solutions at the same site.

Compatibility and Stability of Products: Frozen samples should be thawed at room temperature before use. After the periods mentioned below, any unused solutions or frozen material should be discarded. **DO NOT REFREEZE.**

NOTE: Solutions of cefotetan disodium must not be admixed-with solutions containing aminoglycosides. If cefotetan disodium and aminoglycosides are to be administered to the same patient, they must be administered separately and not as a mixed injection. **DO NOT ADD SUPPLEMENTARY MEDICATION.**

Sterile Cefotetan Disodium: Sterile cefotetan disodium reconstituted as described above (PREPARATION OF SOLUTION) maintains satisfactory potency for 24 hours at room temperature (25°C/77°F), for 96 hours under refrigeration (5°C/41°F), and for at least 1 week in the frozen state (-20°C/-4°F). After reconstitution and subsequent storage in disposable glass or plastic syringes, sterile cefotetan disodium is stable for 24 hours at room temperature and 96 hours under refrigeration.

ADD-Vantage Vials: Ordinarily, ADD-Vantage Vials should be reconstituted only when it is certain that the patient is ready to receive the drug. However, ADD-Vantage Vials of cefotetan disodium reconstituted as described in Preparation of Solution, for ADD-Vantage Vials, maintains satisfactory potency for 24 hours at room temperature (25°C/77°F).

(DO NOT REFRIGERATE OR FREEZE CEFOTETAN DISODIUM IN ADD-VANTAGE VIALS.)

Cefotetan Disodium Injection: The thawed solution in Galaxy plastic container (PL 2040) remains chemically stable for 48 hours at room temperature (25°C/77°F) or for 21 days under refrigeration (5°C/41°F).

NOTE: Parenteral drug products should be inspected visually for particulate matter and discoloration prior to administration whenever solution and container permit.

REFERENCES:

1 Smith, LeFrock et al. Cefotetan Pharmacokinetics in Volunteers with Various Degrees of Renal Function. Antimicrobial Agents and Chemotherapy. 29(5): 887-893, May 1986. **2** Sheikh and Bobey. Lack of Predictability of Cefotetan *In Vitro* Susceptibility Tests Against Cefotetan-Resistant Anaerobic Bacteria in Determining Clinical and Bacteriological Efficacies. Diagn. Microbiol. Infect. Dis. 15: 595- 600, 1992. **3** National Committee for Clinical Laboratory Standards, Approved Standard: Performance Standards for Antimicrobial Disk Susceptibility Tests, 4th Edition, Vol. 10(7):M2-A4, Villanova, PA, April, 1990. **4** National Committee for Clinical Laboratory Standards, Tentative Standard: Methods for Dilution Antimicrobial Susceptibility Tests for Bacteria That Grow Aerobically, 2nd Edition, Vol. 10(8):M7-A2, Villanova, PA, April, 1990. **5** National Committee for Clinical Laboratory Standards, Approved Standard:Methods for Antimicrobial Susceptibility Testing of Anaerobic Bacteria, 3rd Edition, Vol. 13:M11-A3, Villanova, PA, April 1993. **8** Galaxy is a registered trademark of Baxter Healthcare Corporation. † ADD- Vantage is a registered trademark of Abbott Laboratories Inc. ‡ Clinitest is a registered trademark of Ames Division, Miles Laboratories, Inc.

HOW SUPPLIED:

Cefotan is a dry, white to pale yellow powder supplied in vials containing cefotetan disodium equivalent to 1 g and 2 g cefotetan activity for intravenous and intramuscular administration. The vials should not be stored at temperatures above 22°C (72°F) and should be protected from light.

Cefotan is supplied as a frozen, iso- osmotic, premixed solution in single dose Galaxy plastic containers (PL 2040).

Store containers at or below -20°C/-4°F. **[See DIRECTIONS FOR USE OF CEFOTETAN DISODIUM IN GALAXY PLASTIC CONTAINER (PL 2040)].**

HOW SUPPLIED - EQUIVALENTS NOT AVAILABLE:

Injection, Lyphl-Soln - Intramuscular; - 1 gm/vial

1's	$11.16	CEFOTAN, Zeneca Pharms	00310-0376-10
1's	$11.16	CEFOTAN, Zeneca Pharms	00310-0376-60
1's	$11.58	CEFOTAN, Zeneca Pharms	00310-0376-31
1's	$11.72	CEFOTAN, Zeneca Pharms	00310-0376-11
1's	$11.72	CEFOTAN, Zeneca Pharms	00310-0376-61
50 ml	$13.96	CEFOTAN, Zeneca Pharms	00310-0378-51

Injection, Lyphl-Soln - Intramuscular; - 2 gm/vial

1's	$21.90	CEFOTAN, Zeneca Pharms	00310-0377-20
1's	$21.90	CEFOTAN, Zeneca Pharms	00310-0377-62
1's	$22.32	CEFOTAN, Zeneca Pharms	00310-0377-32
1's	$23.02	CEFOTAN, Zeneca Pharms	00310-0377-21
1's	$23.02	CEFOTAN, Zeneca Pharms	00310-0377-61
50 ml	$24.97	CEFOTAN, Zeneca Pharms	00310-0379-51

Injection, Lyphl-Soln - Intramuscular; - 10 gm

1's	$118.36	CEFOTAN, Zeneca Pharms	00310-0375-10
1's	$118.36	CEFOTAN, Zeneca Pharms	00310-0375-61

CEFOXITIN SODIUM *(000691)*

CATEGORIES: Abdominal Abscess; Anti-Infectives; Antibiotics; Antimicrobials; Beta-Lactam Antibiotics; Bone Infections; Cellulitis; Cephalosporins; Endometritis; Genitourinary Tract Infections; Gonorrhea; Gynecologic Infections; Infections; Joint Infections; Pelvic Inflammatory Disease; Perioperative Prophylaxis; Peritonitis; Pneumonia; Pulmonary Abscess; Respiratory Tract Infections; Septicemia; Skin Infections; Urinary Tract Infections; Pregnancy Category B; Sales > $100 Million; FDA Approval Pre 1982; Patent Expiration 1998 Dec

BRAND NAMES: *Cefmore*; *Cefotin*; *Cefoxin*; *Kinfotin*; *Lephocin*; *Mefoxil*; **Mefoxin**; *Mefoxitin* (Germany)
(International brand names outside U.S. in italics)

FORMULARIES: BC-BS

COST OF THERAPY: $255.75 (Infections; Injection; 1 gm; 3/day; 10 days)

PRIMARY ICD9: 136.9 (Unspecified Infections and Parasitic Diseases)

DESCRIPTION:

Sterile cefoxitin sodium is a semi-synthetic, broad-spectrum cepha antibiotic sealed under nitrogen for parenteral administration. It is derived from cephamycin C, which is produced by*Streptomyces lactamdurans.* It is the sodium salt of 3-(hydroxymethyl)-7α-methoxy-8-oxo-7-(2-(2-thienyl)acetamido)-5-thia-1 -azabicyclo (4.2.0) oct-2-ene-2-carboxylate carbamate (ester). The empirical formula is $C_{16}H_{16}N_3NaO_7S_2$.

Mefoxin contains approximately 53.8 mg (2.3 milliequivalents) of sodium per gram of cefoxitin activity. Solutions of Mefoxin range from colorless to light amber in color. The pH of freshly constituted solutions usually ranges from 4.2 to 7.0.

Premixed Intravenous Solution Only: Premixed Intravenous Solution Mefoxin (Cefoxitin Sodium Injection) is supplied as a sterile, nonpyrogenic, frozen, iso-osmotic solution of cefoxitin sodium. Each 50 ml contains cefoxitin sodium equivalent to either 1 gram or 2 grams cefoxitin. Dextrose hydrous USP has been added to the above dosages to adjust osmolality (approximately 2 grams and 1.1 grams to 1 gram and 2 gram dosages, respectively). The pH is adjusted with sodium bicarbonate and may have been adjusted with hydrochloric acid. The pH is approximately 6.5. After thawing, the solution is intended for intravenous use only. Solutions of cefoxitin sodium range from colorless to light amber.

The plastic container is fabricated from a specially designed multilayer plastic (PL 2040). Solutions are in contact with the polyethylene layer of this container and can leach out certain chemical components of the plastic in very small amounts within the expiration period. The suitability and safety of the plastic have been confirmed in tests in animals according to the USP biological tests for plastic containers, as well as by tissue culture toxicity studies.

CLINICAL PHARMACOLOGY:

After intramuscular administration of a 1 gram dose of cefoxitin sodium to normal volunteers, the mean peak serum concentration was 24 mcg/ml. The peak occurred at 20 to 30 minutes. Following an intravenous dose of 1 gram, serum concentrations were 110 mcg/ml at 5 minutes, declining to less than 1 mcg/ml at 4 hours. The half-life after an intravenous dose is 41 to 59 minutes; after intramuscular administration, the half-life is 64.8 minutes. Approximately 85 percent of cefoxitin is excreted unchanged by the kidneys over a 6-hour period, resulting in high urinary concentrations. Following an intramuscular dose of 1 gram, urinary concentrations greater than 3000 mcg/ml were observed. Probenecid slows tubular excretion and produces higher serum levels and increases the duration of measurable serum concentrations.

Cefoxitin passes into pleural and joint fluids and is detectable in antibacterial concentrations in bile.

Clinical experience has demonstrated that cefoxitin sodium can be administered to patients who are also receiving carbenicillin, kanamycin, gentamicin, tobramycin, or amikacin (see PRECAUTIONS and DOSAGE AND ADMINISTRATION).

MICROBIOLOGY

The bactericidal action of cefoxitin results from inhibition of cell wall synthesis. Cefoxitin has *in vitro* activity against a wide range of gram-positive and gram-negative organisms. The methoxy group in the 7α position provides cefoxitin sodium with a high degree of stability in the presence of beta-lactamases, both penicillinases and cephalosporinases, of gram-negative bacteria. Cefoxitin is usually active against the following organisms *in vitro* and in clinical infections:

Gram-positive

Staphylococcus aureus, including penicillinase and non-penicillinase producing strains

Staphylococcus epidermidis

Beta-hemolytic and other streptococci (most strains of enterococci, e.g., *Streptococcus faecalis* are resistant)

Streptococcus pneumoniae

Gram-negative

Escherichia coli

Klebsiella species (including *K. pneumoniae*)

Hemophilus influenzae

Neisseria gonorrhoeae, including penicillinase and non-penicillinase producing strains

Proteus mirabilis

Morganella morganii

Proteus vulgaris

Providencia species, including *Providencia rettgeri*

Anaerobic organisms

Peptococcus species

Peptostreptococcus species

Clostridium species

Bacteroides species, including the *B. fragilis* group (includes *B. fragilis, B. distasonis, B. ovatus, B. thetaiotaomicron, B. vulgatus*)

Cefoxitin sodium is inactive *in vitro* against most strains of *Pseudomonas aeruginosa* and enterococci and many strains of *Enterobacter cloacae.*

Methicillin-resistant staphylococci are almost uniformly resistant to cefoxitin sodium.

SUSCEPTIBILITY TESTING

For fast-growing aerobic organisms, quantitative methods that require measurements of zone diameters give the most precise estimates of antibiotic susceptibility. One such procedure* has been recommended for use with discs to test susceptibility to cefoxitin. Interpretation involves correlation of the diameters obtained in the disc test with minimal inhibitory concentration (MIC) values for cefoxitin.

Reports from the laboratory giving results of the standardized single disc susceptibility test* using a 30 mcg cefoxitin disc should be interpreted according to the following criteria:

Organisms producing zones of 18 mm or greater are considered susceptible, indicating that the tested organism is likely to respond to therapy.

Organisms of intermediate susceptibility produce zones of 15 to 17 mm, indicating that the tested organism would be susceptible if high dosage is used or if the infection is confined to tissues and fluids (*e.g.,* urine) in which high antibiotic levels are attained.

Resistant organisms produce zones of 14 mm or less, indicating that other therapy should be selected.

The cefoxitin disc should be used for testing cefoxitin susceptibility.

Cefoxitin has been shown by *in vitro* tests to have activity against certain strains of *Enterobacteriaceae* found resistant when tested with the cephalosporin class disc. For this reason, the cefoxitin disc should not be used for testing susceptibility to cephalosporins, and cephalosporin discs should not be used for testing susceptibility to cefoxitin.

CLINICAL PHARMACOLOGY: *(cont'd)*

Dilution methods, preferably the agar plate dilution procedure, are most accurate for susceptibility testing of obligate anaerobes.

A bacterial isolate may be considered susceptible if the MIC value for cefoxitin** is not more than 16 mcg/ml. Organisms are considered resistant if the MIC is greater than 32 mcg/ml

INDICATIONS AND USAGE:

TREATMENT

Cefoxitin sodium is indicated for the treatment of serious infections caused by susceptible strains of the designated microorganisms in the diseases listed below.

(1) Lower respiratory tract infections: Lower respiratory tract infections, including pneumonia and lung abscess, caused by *Streptococcus pneumoniae,* other streptococci (excluding enterococci, e.g., *Streptococcus faecalis*), *Staphylococcus aureus*(penicillinase and non-penicillinase producing), *Escherichia coli, Klebsiella* species, *Hemophilus influenzae,* and *Bacteroides* species.

(2) Genitourinary infections: Urinary tract infections caused by *Escherichia coli, Klebsiella* species, *Proteus mirabilis,* indole-positive Proteus (which include the organisms now called *Morganella morganii* and *Proteus vulgaris*), and *Providencia* species (including *Providencia rettgeri*). Uncomplicated gonorrhea due to *Neisseria gonorrhoeae* (penicillinase and non-penicillinase producing).

(3) Intra-abdominal infections: Intra-abdominal infections, including peritonitis and intra-abdominal abscess, caused by *Escherichia coli, Klebsiella* species, *Bacteroides* species including the *Bacteroides fragilis* group***, and *Clostridium* species.

(4) Gynecological infections: Gynecological infections, including endometritis, pelvic cellulitis, and pelvic inflammatory disease caused by *Escherichia coli, Neisseria gonorrhoeae* (penicillinase and non-penicillinase producing), *Bacteroides* species including the *Bacteroides fragilis* group,*** *Clostridium* species, *Peptococcus* species, *Peptostreptococcus* species, and Group B streptococci.

(5) Septicemia: Septicemia caused by *Streptococcus pneumoniae, Staphylococcus aureus* (penicillinase and non-penicillinase producing), *Escherichia coli, Klebsiella* species, and *Bacteroides* species including the *Bacteroides fragilis* group.***

(6) Bone and joint infections: Bone and joint infections caused by *Staphylococcus aureus* (penicillinase and non-penicillinase producing).

(7) Skin and skin structure infections: Skin and skin structure infections caused by *Staphylococcus aureus* (penicillinase and non-penicillinase producing), *Staphylococcus epidermidis,* streptococci (excluding enterococci *e.g., Streptococcus faecalis*), *Escherichia coli, Proteus mirabilis, Klebsiella* species, *Bacteroides* species including the *Bacteroides fragilis* group,*** *Clostridium* species, *Peptococcus* species, and *Peptostreptococcus* species.

Appropriate culture and susceptibility studies should be performed to determine the susceptibility of the causative organisms to cefoxitin sodium. Therapy may be started while awaiting the results of these studies.

In randomized comparative studies, cefoxitin sodium and cephalothin were comparably safe and effective in the management of infections caused by gram-positive cocci and gram-negative rods susceptible to the cephalosporins. Cefoxitin sodium has a high degree of stability in the presence of bacterial beta-lactamases, both penicillinases and cephalosporinases.

Many infections caused by aerobic and anaerobic gram-negative bacteria resistant to some cephalosporins respond to cefoxitin sodium. Similarly, many infections caused by aerobic and anaerobic bacteria resistant to some penicillin antibiotics (ampicillin, carbenicillin, penicillin G) respond to treatment with cefoxitin sodium. Many infections caused by mixtures of susceptible aerobic and anaerobic bacteria respond to treatment with cefoxitin sodium.

PREVENTION

When compared to placebo in randomized controlled studies in patients undergoing gastrointestinal surgery, vaginal hysterectomy abdominal hysterectomy and cesarean section, the prophylactic use of cefoxitin sodium resulted in a significant reduction in the number of postoperative infections.

The prophylactic administration of cefoxitin sodium may reduce the incidence of certain postoperative infections in patients undergoing surgical procedures (*e.g.,* hysterectomy, gastrointestinal surgery and transurethral prostatectomy) that are classified as contaminated or potentially contaminated.

The perioperative use of cefoxitin sodium may be effective in surgical patients in whom subsequent infection at the operative site would present a serious risk, *e.g.,* prosthetic arthroplasty.

Effective prophylactic use depends on the time of administration. Cefoxitin sodium usually should be given one-half to one hour before the operation which is sufficient time to achieve effective levels in the wound during the procedure. Prophylactic administration should usually be stopped within 24 hours since continuing administration of any antibiotic increases the possibility of adverse reactions but, in the majority of surgical procedures, does not reduce the incidence of subsequent infection. However, in patients undergoing prosthetic arthroplasty, it is recommended that cefoxitin sodium be continued for 72 hours after the surgical procedure.

If there are signs of infection, specimens for culture should be obtained for identification of the causative organism so that appropriate treatment may be instituted.

* Bauer, A. W.; Kirby, W. M. M.; Sherris, J. C.; Turck, M.: Antibiotic susceptibility testing by a standardized single disc method, Amer. J. Clin. Path. *45*: 493-496, Apr. 1966. Standardized disc susceptibility test, Federal Register *37*: 20527-20529, 1972. National Committee for Clinical Laboratory Standards: Approved Standard: ASM-2, Performance Standards for Antimicrobial Disc Susceptibility Tests, July 1975.

** Determined by the ICS agar dilution method (Ericsson and Sherris, Acta Path. Microbiol. Scand. (B) Suppl. No 217, 1971) or any other method that has been shown to give equivalent results.

*** *B. fragilis, B. distasonis, B. ovatus, B. thetaiotaomicron, B. vulgatus.*

CONTRAINDICATIONS:

Cefoxitin sodium is contraindicated in patients who have shown hypersensitivity to cefoxitin and the cephalosporin group of antibiotics.

WARNINGS:

BEFORE THERAPY WITH CEFOXITIN SODIUM IS INSTITUTED, CAREFUL INQUIRY SHOULD BE MADE TO DETERMINE WHETHER THE PATIENT HAS HAD PREVIOUS HYPERSENSITIVITY REACTIONS TO CEFOXITIN, CEPHALOSPORINS, PENICILLINS OR OTHER DRUGS. THIS PRODUCT SHOULD BE GIVEN WITH CAUTION TO PENICILLIN-SENSITIVE PATIENTS. ANTIBIOTICS SHOULD BE ADMINISTERED WITH CAUTION TO ANY PATIENT WHO HAS DEMONSTRATED SOME FORM OF ALLERGY, PARTICULARLY TO DRUGS. IF AN ALLERGIC REACTION TO CEFOXITIN SODIUM OCCURS, DISCONTINUE THE DRUG. SERIOUS HYPERSENSITIVITY REACTIONS MAY REQUIRE EPINEPHRINE AND OTHER EMERGENCY MEASURES.

WARNINGS: *(cont'd)*

Pseudomembranous colitis has been reported with virtually all antibiotics (including cephalosporins); therefore, it is important to consider its diagnosis in patients who develop diarrhea in association with antibiotic use. This colitis may range from mild to life threatening in severity.

Treatment with broad-spectrum antibiotics alters normal flora of the colon and may permit overgrowth of clostridia. Studies indicate a toxin produced by *clostridium difficile* is one primary cause of antibiotic-associated colitis.

Mild cases of pseudomembranous colitis may respond to drug discontinuance alone. In more severe cases, management may include sigmoidoscopy, appropriate bacteriological studies, fluid, electrolyte and protein supplementation, and the use of a drug such as oral vancomycin as indicated. Isolation of the patient may be advisable. Other causes of colitis should also be considered.

PRECAUTIONS:

General: The total daily dose should be reduced when cefoxitin sodium is administered to patients with transient or persistent reduction of urinary output due to renal insufficiency (see DOSAGE AND ADMINISTRATION), because high and prolonged serum antibiotic concentrations can occur in such individuals from usual doses.

Antibiotics (including cephalosporins) should be prescribed with caution in individuals with a history of gastrointestinal disease, particularly colitis.

As with other antibiotics, prolonged use of cefoxitin sodium may result in over-growth of nonsusceptible organisms. Repeated evaluation of the patient's condition is essential. If superinfection occurs during therapy, appropriate measures should be taken.

Drug/Laboratory Test Interactions: As with cephalothin, high concentrations of cefoxitin (>100 micrograms/ml) may interfere with measurement of serum and urine creatinine levels by the Jaffe reaction, and produce false increases of modest degree in the levels of creatinine reported. Serum samples from patients treated with cefoxitin should not be analyzed for creatinine if withdrawn within 2 hours of drug administration.

High concentrations of cefoxitin in the urine may interfere with measurement of urinary 17-hydroxy-corticosteroids by the Porter-Silber reaction, and produce false increases of modest degree in the levels reported.

A false-positive reaction for glucose in the urine may occur. This has been observed with Clinitest reagent tablets.

Carcinogenesis, Mutagenesis, and Impairment of Fertility: Long-term studies in animals have not been performed with cefoxitin to evaluate carcinogenic or mutagenic potential. Studies in rats treated intravenously with 400 mg/kg of cefoxitin (approximately three times the maximum recommended human dose) revealed no effects on fertility or mating ability.

Pregnancy Category B: Reproduction studies performed in rats and mice at parenteral doses of approximately one to seven and one-half times the maximum recommended human dose did not reveal teratogenic or fetal toxic effects, although a slight decrease in fetal weight was observed.

There are, however, no adequate and well-controlled studies in pregnant women. Because animal reproduction studies are not always predictive of human response, this drug should be used during pregnancy only if clearly needed.

In the rabbit, cefoxitin was associated with a high incidence of abortion and maternal death. This was not considered to be a teratogenic effect but an expected consequence of the rabbit's unusual sensitivity to antibiotic-induced changes in the population of the microflora of the intestine.

Nursing Mothers: Cefoxitin sodium is excreted in human milk in low concentrations. Caution should be exercised when cefoxitin sodium is administered to a nursing woman.

Pediatric Use: Safety and efficacy in infants from birth to three months of age have not yet been established. In children three months of age and older, higher doses of cefoxitin sodium have been associated with an increased incidence of eosinophilia and elevated SGOT.

DRUG INTERACTIONS:

Increased nephrotoxicity has been reported following concomitant administration of cephalosporins and aminoglycoside antibiotics.

ADVERSE REACTIONS:

Cefoxitin sodium is generally well tolerated. The most common adverse reactions have been local reactions following intravenous or intramuscular injection. Other adverse reactions have been encountered infrequently.

Local Reactions: Thrombophlebitis has occurred with intravenous administration. Pain, induration and tenderness after intramuscular injections have been reported.

Allergic Reactions: Rash (including exfoliative dermatitis and toxic epidermal necrolysis), pruritus, eosinophilia, fever, dyspnea, and other allergic reactions including anaphylaxis, interstitial nephritis and angioedema have been noted.

Cardiovascular: Hypotension

Gastrointestinal: Diarrhea, including documented pseudomembranous colitis which can appear during or after antibiotic treatment. Nausea and vomiting have been reported rarely.

Neuromuscular: Possible exacerbation of myasthenia gravis

Blood: Eosinophilia, leukopenia including granulocytopenia, neutropenia, anemia, including hemolytic anemia, thrombocytopenia, and bone marrow depression. A positive direct Coombs test may develop in some individuals, especially those with azotemia.

Liver Function: Transient elevations in SGOT, SGPT, serum LDH, and serum alkaline phosphatase; and jaundice have been reported.

Renal Function: Elevations in serum creatinine and/or blood urea nitrogen levels have been observed. As with the cephalosporins, acute renal failure has been reported rarely. The role of cefoxitin sodium in changes in renal function tests is difficult to assess, since factors predisposing to prerenal azotemia or to impaired renal function usually have been present.

OVERDOSAGE:

The acute intravenous LD_{50} in the adult female mouse and rabbit was about 8.0 g/kg and greater than 1.0 g/kg respectively. The acute intraperitoneal LD_{50} in the adult rat was greater than 10.0 g/kg.

DOSAGE AND ADMINISTRATION:

TREATMENT

Adults

The usual adult dosage range is 1 gram to 2 grams every six to eight hours. Dosage and route of administration should be determined by susceptibility of the causative organisms, severity of infection, and the condition of the patient (see TABLE 3) for dosage guidelines.

Cefoxitin sodium may be used in patients with reduced renal function with the following dosage adjustments:

DOSAGE AND ADMINISTRATION: *(cont'd)*

In adults with renal insufficiency, an initial loading dose of 1 gram to 2 grams may be given. After a loading dose, the recommendations for *maintenance dosage* (TABLE 3) may be used as a guide.

When only the serum creatinine level is available, the following formula (based on sex, weight and age of the patient) may be used to convert this value into creatinine clearance. The serum creatinine should represent a steady state of renal function.

TABLE 1

Males: [Weight (kg) × (140 - age)] ÷ [72 × serum creatinine (mg/100 ml)]
Females: 0.85 × above value

In patients undergoing hemodialysis the loading dose of 1 to 2 grams should be given after each hemodialysis, and the maintenance dose should be given as indicated in TABLE 3.

Antibiotic therapy for group A beta-hemolytic streptococcal infections should be maintained for at least 10 days to guard against the risk of rheumatic fever or glomerulonephritis. In staphylococcal and other infections involving a collection of pus, surgical drainage should be carried out where indicated.

The recommended dosage of cefoxitin sodium **for uncomplicated gonorrhea** is 2 grams intramuscularly, with 1 gram of Probenecid given by mouth at the same time or up to 1/2 hour before cefoxitin sodium.

Infants and Children

The recommended dosage in children three months of age and older is 80 to 160 mg/kg of body weight per day divided into four to six equal doses. The higher dosages should be used for more severe or serious infections. The total daily dosage should not exceed 12 grams.

At this time no recommendation is made for children from birth to three months of age (see PRECAUTIONS).

In children with renal insufficiency the dosage and frequency of dosage should be modified consistent with the recommendations for adults (see TABLE 3).

PREVENTION

General

For prophylactic use in surgery, the following doses are recommended:

Adults

(1) 2 grams administered intravenously or intramuscularly just prior to surgery (approximately one-half to one hour before the initial incision).

(2) 2 grams every 6 hours after the first dose for no more than 24 hours (continued for 72 hours after prosthetic arthroplasty).

Children (3 months and older): 30 to 40 mg/kg doses may be given at the times designated above.

Obstetric-Gynecologic

For prophylactic use in vaginal hysterectomy, a single 2.0 gram dose administered intramuscularly one-half to one hour prior to surgery is recommended.

For patients undergoing cesarean section, a single 2.0 gram dose should be administered intravenously as soon as the umbilical cord is clamped. A 3-dose regimen may be more effective than a single dose regimen in preventing postoperative infection (esp. endometritis) following cesarean section. Such a regimen would consist of 2.0 grams given intravenously as soon as the umbilical cord is clamped, followed by 2.0 grams 4 and 8 hours after the initial dose.

Transurethral prostatectomy patients.

One gram administered just prior to surgery; 1 gram every 8 hours for up to five days.

PREPARATION OF SOLUTION

TABLE 4 is provided for convenience in constituting cefoxitin sodium for both intravenous and intramuscular administration.

For intravenous use, 1 gram should be constituted with at least 10 ml of Sterile Water for Injection, and 2 grams, with 10 or 20 ml. The 10 gram, bulk package should be constituted with 43 or 93 ml of Sterile Water for Injection or any of the solutions listed under the *Intravenous* portion of the Compatibility and Stability section. CAUTION: THE 10 GRAM BULK STOCK SOLUTION IS NOT FOR DIRECT INFUSION. One or 2 grams of cefoxitin sodium for infusion may be constituted with 50 or 100 ml of 0.9 percent Sodium Chloride Injection 5 percent or 10 percent Dextrose Injection, or any of the solutions listed under the Intravenous portion of the Compatibility and Stability section.

Benzyl alcohol as a preservative has been associated with toxicity in neonates. While toxicity has not been demonstrated in infants greater than three months of age, in whom use of cefoxitin sodium may be indicated, small infants in this age range may also be at risk for benzyl alcohol toxicity. Therefore, diluents containing benzyl alcohol should not be used when cefoxitin sodium is constituted for administration to infants.

For ADD-Vantage vials, see separate INSTRUCTIONS FOR USE OF CEFOXITIN SODIUM IN ADD-Vantage VIALS. Cefoxitin Sodium in ADD-Vantage vials should be constituted with ADD-Vantage diluent containers containing 50 ml or 100 ml of either 0.9 percent Sodium Chloride Injection or 5 percent Dextrose Injection. Mefoxin in ADD-Vantage vials is for IV use only.

For intramuscular use, each gram of cefoxitin sodium may be constituted with 2 ml of Sterile Water for Injection, *or-*

For intramuscular use ONLY: each gram of cefoxitin sodium may be constituted with 2 ml of 0.5 percent lidocaine hydrochloride solution (without epinephrine) to minimize the discomfort of intramuscular injection.

TABLE 2 Guidelines for Dosage of Cefoxitin Sodium

Type of Infection	Daily Dosage	Frequency and Route
Uncomplicated forms† of infections such as pneumonia, urinary tract infection, cutaneous infection	3-4 grams	1 gram every 6 - 8 hours IV or IM
Moderately severe or severe infections	6-8 grams	1 gram every 4 hours *or* 2 grams every 6-8 hours IV
Infections commonly needing antibiotics in higher dosage (*e.g.,* gas gangrene)	12 grams	2 grams every 4 hours IV *or* 3 grams every 6 hours IV

† Including patients in whom bacteremia is absent or unlikely.

ADMINISTRATION

Cefoxitin Sodium may be administered intravenously or intramuscularly after constitution.

Parenteral drug products should be inspected visually for particulate matter and discoloration prior to administration whenever solution and container permit.

DOSAGE AND ADMINISTRATION: *(cont'd)*

TABLE 3 Maintenance Dosage of Sterile Cefoxitin Sodium in Adults with Reduced Renal Function

Renal Function	Creatinine Clearance (ml/min)	Dose (grams)	Frequency
Mild impairment	50-30	1-2	every 8 - 12 hours
Moderate impairment	29-10	1-2	every 12 - 24 hours
Severe impairment	9-5	0.5-1	every 12 - 24 hours
Essentially no function	< 5	0.5-1	every 24 - 48 hours

TABLE 4 Preparation of Solution

Strength	Amount of Diluent to be Added (ml)‡	Approximate Withdrawable Vol. (ml)	Approximate Average Concentration (mg/ml)
1 gram Vial	2 (Intramuscular)	2.5	400
2 gram Vial	4 (Intramuscular)	5	400
1 gram Vial	10 (IV)	10.5	95
2 gram Vial	10 or 20 (IV)	11.1 or 21.0	180 or 95
1 gram Infusion Bottle	50 or 100 (IV)	50 or 100	20 or 10
2 gram Infusion Bottle	50 or 100 (IV)	50 or 100	40 or 20
10 gram Bulk	43 or 93 (IV)	49 or 98.5	200 or 100

‡ Shake to dissolve and let stand until clear.

INTRAVENOUS ADMINISTRATION

The intravenous route is preferable for patients with bacteremia, bacterial septicemia, or other severe or life-threatening infections, or for patients who may be poor risks because of lowered resistance resulting from such debilitating conditions as malnutrition, trauma, surgery, diabetes, heart failure, or malignancy, particularly if shock is present or impending.

For intermittent intravenous administration, a solution containing 1 gram or 2 grams in 10 ml of Sterile Water for Injection can be injected over a period of three to five minutes. Using an infusion system, it may also be given over a longer period of time through the tubing system by which the patient may be receiving other intravenous solutions. However, during infusion of the solution containing cefoxitin sodium, it is advisable to temporarily discontinue administration of any other solutions at the same site.

For the administration of higher doses by continuous intravenous infusion, a solution of cefoxitin sodium be added to an intravenous bottle containing 5 percent Dextrose Injection, 0.9 percent Sodium Chloride Injection, 5 percent Dextrose and 0.9 percent Sodium Chloride Injection, or 5 percent Dextrose Injection with 0.02 percent sodium bicarbonate solution. Butterfly or scalp vein-type needles are preferred for this type of infusion.

Solutions of cefoxitin sodium, like those of most beta-lactam antibiotics, should not be added to aminoglycoside solutions (*e.g.,* gentamicin sulfate, tobramycin sulfate, amikacin sulfate) because of potential interaction. However, cefoxitin sodium and aminoglycosides may be administered separately to the same patient.

INTRAMUSCULAR ADMINISTRATION

As with all intramuscular preparations, Cefoxitin Sodium should be injected well within the body of a relatively large muscle such as the upper outer quadrant of the buttock (*i.e.,* gluteus maximus); aspiration is necessary to avoid inadvertent injection into a blood vessel.

COMPATIBILITY AND STABILITY

Intravenous

Mefoxin, as supplied in vials or the bulk package and constituted to 1 gram/10 ml with Sterile Water for Injection, Bacteriostatic Water for Injection, (see Preparation of Solution), 0.9 percent Sodium Chloride Injection, or 5 percent Dextrose Injection, maintains satisfactory potency for 24 hours at room temperature, for one week under refrigeration (below 5°C), and for at least 30 weeks in the frozen state.

These primary solutions may be further diluted in 50 to 1000 ml of the following solutions and maintain potency for 24 hours at room temperature and at least 48 hours under refrigeration:

Sterile Water for Injection‡

0.9 percent Sodium Chloride Injection

5 percent or 10 percent Dextrose Injection‡

5 percent Dextrose and 0.9 percent Sodium Chloride Injection

5 percent Dextrose Injection with 0.02 percent Sodium Bicarbonate solution

5 percent Dextrose Injection with 0.2 percent or 0.45 percent saline solution

Ringer's Injection

Lactated Ringer's Injection‡

5 percent Dextrose in Lactated Ringer's Injection‡

5 percent or 10 percent invert sugar in water

10 percent invert sugar in saline solution

5 percent Sodium Bicarbonate Injection

Neut (sodium bicarbonate)‡

M/6 sodium lactate solution

Normosol-M in D5-W‡

Ionosol B w/Dextrose 5 percent‡

Polyonic M 56 in 5 percent Dextrose

Mannitol 5% and 2.5%

Mannitol 10%‡

Isolyt E

Isolyte E with 5% Dextrose

‡In these solutions, cefoxitin sodium has been found to be stable for a period of one week under refrigeration.

Mefoxin, as supplied in infusion bottles and constituted with 50 to 100 ml of 0.9 percent Sodium Chloride Injection, or 5 percent or 10 percent Dextrose Injection, maintains satisfactory potency for 24 hours at room temperature for 1 week under refrigeration (below 5°C).

Mefoxin is supplied in single dose ADD-Vantage vials and should be prepared as directed in the accompanying INSTRUCTIONS FOR USE IN ADD-Vantage VIALS using ADD-Vantage diluent containers containing 50 ml or 100 ml of either 0.9 percent Sodium Chloride Injection or 5 percent Dextrose Injection. When prepared with either of these diluents cefoxitin sodium maintains satisfactory potency for 24 hours at room temperature.

DOSAGE AND ADMINISTRATION: *(cont'd)*

Limited studies with solutions of cefoxitin sodium in 0.9 percent Sodium Chloride Injection, Lactated Ringer's Injection, and 5 percent Dextrose Injection in Viaflex intravenous bags show stability for 24 hours at room temperature, 48 hours under refrigeration or 26 weeks in the frozen state and 24 hours at room temperature thereafter. Also, solutions of cefoxitin sodium in 0.9 percent Sodium Chloride Injection show similar stability in plastic tubing, drip chambers and volume control devices of common intravenous infusion sets.

After constitution with Sterile Water for Injection and subsequent storage in disposable plastic syringes, cefoxitin sodium is stable for 24 hours at room temperature and 48 hours under refrigeration.

After the periods mentioned above, any unused solutions or frozen material should be discarded. Do not refreeze.

Intramuscular

Cefoxitin sodium, as constituted with Sterile Water for Injection, Bacteriostatic Water for Injection, or 0.5 percent or 1 percent lidocaine hydrochloride solution (without epinephrine), maintains satisfactory potency for 24 hours at room temperature, for one week under refrigeration (below 5°C), and for at least 30 weeks in the frozen state.

After the periods mentioned above, any unused solutions or frozen material should be discarded. Do not refreeze.

Cefoxitin sodium has also been found compatible when admixed in intravenous infusions with the following:

Heparin 0.1 units/ml at room temperature—8 hours

Heparin 100 Units/ml at room temperature—24 hours

M.V.I. concentrate at room temperature 24 hours; under refrigeration 48 hours

Berocca C-500 at room temperature 24 hours: under refrigeration 48 hours

Insulin in Normal Saline at room temperature 24 hours; under refrigeration 48 hours

Insulin in 10% invert sugar at room temperature 24 hours; under refrigeration 48 hours

Premixed Intravenous Solution: (See Treatment and Prevention).

ADMINISTRATION

This premixed solution is for intravenous use only. Premixed Intravenous Solution Mefoxin in Galaxy containers (PL 2040 Plastic) is to be administered either as a continuous or intermittent infusion using sterile equipment. Scalp vein-type needles are preferred for this type of infusion. It is recommended that the intravenous administration apparatus is to be replaced at least once every 48 hours.

The intravenous route is preferred for patients with bacteremia, bacterial septicemia, or other severe or life-threatening infections, or for patients who may be poor risks because of lowered resistance resulting from such debilitating conditions as malnutrition, trauma, surgery, diabetes, heart failure, or malignancy, particularly if shock is present or impending.

DIRECTIONS FOR USE OF GALAXY CONTAINERS (PL 2040 PLASTIC)

Thaw frozen container at room temperature, 25°C (77°F), or under refrigeration, 2-8°C (36-46°F. DO NOT FORCE THAW BY IMMERSION IN WATER BATHS OR BY MICROWAVE IRRADIATION.

After thawing, check for minute leaks by squeezing container firmly. If leaks are detected, discard solution as sterility may be impaired.

The container should be visually inspected for particulate matter and discoloration prior to administration. Components of the solution may precipitate in the frozen state and will dissolve upon reaching room temperature with little or no agitation. Agitate after solution has reached room temperature.

Do not use if the solution is cloudy or a precipitate has formed. If any seals or outlet ports are not intact, the container should be discarded. Solutions of cefoxitin sodium tend to darken depending on storage conditions; product potency, however, is not adversely effected. Additives should not be introduced into this solution.

CAUTION: Do not use plastic containers in series connections. Such use would result in air embolism due to residual air being drawn from the primary container before administration of the fluid from the secondary container is complete.

PREPARATION FOR INTRAVENOUS ADMINISTRATION

1. Suspend container from eyelet support.

2. Remove plastic protector from outlet port at bottom of container.

3. Attach administration set. Refer to complete directions accompanying set.

Cefoxitin sodium may be administered through the tubing system by which the patient may be receiving other intravenous solutions. However, during infusion of the solution containing cefoxitin sodium, it is advisable to temporarily discontinue administration of any other solutions at the same site.

Solutions of cefoxitin sodium, like those of most beta-lactam antibiotics, should not be added to aminoglycoside solutions (*e.g.,* gentamicin sulfate, tobramycin sulfate, amikacin sulfate) because of potential interaction. However, cefoxitin sodium and aminoglycosides may be administered separately to the same patient.

STABILITY

Mefoxin, supplied as frozen, premixed, iso-osmotic solution in Galaxy containers (PL 204-Plastic), maintains satisfactory potency after thawing for 24 hours at a room temperature of 25°C (77°F) or 21 days under refrigeration, 2-8°C (36-46°F). After these periods, any unused solutions should be discarded.

DO NOT REFREEZE.

CDC GUIDELINES FOR TREATMENT OF SEXUALLY TRANSMITTED DISEASES

Recommended Treatment Schedules for Gonorrhea and Acute Pelvic Inflammatory Disease (PID):[1,2]

Disseminated gonococcal infection: 1 g cefoxitin IV, 4 times/day for at least 7 days for disseminated infections caused by PPNG.

Gonococcal ophthalmia in adults: For PPNG, use 1 g cefoxitin IV, 4 times/day.

Acute PID: For hospitalized patients, give 100 mg doxycycline, IV, twice/day plus 2 g cefoxitin, IV, 4 times/day. Continue drugs IV for at least 4 days and at least 48 hours after patient improves. Continue 100 mg oral doxycycline, twice/day after discharge to complete 10 to 14 days of therapy. For outpatients, give 2 g cefoxitin IM with 1 g oral probenecid, followed by 100 mg oral doxycycline, twice/day for 10 to 14 days.

[1] *Morbidity and Mortality Weekly Report* 1985 (Oct. 18); 34(Suppl 4S);75S-108S.

[2] *Morbidity and Mortality Weekly Report* 1987 (Sep 11); 36 (Suppl 5S);1S-18S.

HOW SUPPLIED:

Sterile cefoxitin sodium is a dry white to off-white powder supplied in vials and infusion bottles. *Special storage instructions:* Cefoxitin sodium in the dry state should be stored below 30°C. Avoid exposure to temperatures above 50°C. The dry material as well as solutions tend to darken depending on storage conditions; product potency, however, is not adversely affected.

HOW SUPPLIED: *(cont'd)*

Premixed Intravenous Solution: Premixed Intravenous Solution Mefoxin is supplied in single dose Galaxy containers (PL 2040 Plastic). *Special storage instructions:* Store at or below -20°C (-4°F). (See Directions for Use of Galaxy container (PL 2040 Plastic).)

Mefoxin is also available in dry powder form in vials and infusion bottles containing sterile cefoxitin sodium equivalent to either 1 gram or 2 grams of cefoxitin, and in vials for pharmacy bulk use containing sterile cefoxitin sodium equivalent to 10 grams of cefoxitin, for constitution and either intravenous or intramuscular administration.

HOW SUPPLIED - EQUIVALENTS NOT AVAILABLE:

Injection, Dry-Soln - Intramuscular; - 1 gm

10's	$85.25	MEFOXIN, VIALS, Merck	00006-3356-71
10's	$99.53	MEFOXIN, BOTTLES, Merck	00006-3368-71
25's	$228.73	MEFOXIN, VIALS, Merck	00006-3356-45
25's	$238.80	MEFOXIN, ADD-VANTAGE, Merck	00006-3548-45
50 ml x 24	$280.42	MEFOXIN, Merck	00006-3545-24

Injection, Dry-Soln - Intramuscular; - 2 gm

10's	$169.88	MEFOXIN, VIALS, Merck	00006-3357-73
10's	$190.10	MEFOXIN, BOTTLES, Merck	00006-3369-73
25's	$455.81	MEFOXIN, VIALS, Merck	00006-3357-53
25's	$465.86	MEFOXIN, ADD-VANTAGE, Merck	00006-3549-53
50 ml x 24	$498.42	MEFOXIN, Merck	00006-3547-25

Injection, Dry-Soln - Intramuscular; - 10 gm/bottle

100 ml x 6	$546.89	MEFOXIN 10, Merck	00006-3388-67

CEFPODOXIME PROXETIL *(003126)*

CATEGORIES: Anti-Infectives; Antibiotics; Anorectal Products; Bronchitis; Cephalosporins; Cystitis; Gonorrhea; Otitis Media; Pharyngitis; Pneumonia; Respiratory Tract Infections; Sexually Transmitted Diseases; Skin Infections; Tonsillitis; Urinary Tract Infections; Rheumatic Fever*; FDA Class 1S ("Standard Review"); FDA Approved 1992 Aug

* Indication not approved by the FDA

BRAND NAMES: Banan; *Banan Dry Syrup*; *Cefodox* (France); *Celance*; *Orelox* (Australia, Germany, France, England); *Podomexef* (Germany); **Vantin**
(International brand names outside U.S. in italics)

FORMULARIES: PCS

COST OF THERAPY: $40.90 (Pharyngitis; Tablet; 100 mg; 2/day; 10 days)

DESCRIPTION:

Cefpodoxime proxetil is an orally administered, extended spectrum, semi-synthetic antibiotic of the cephalosporin class. The chemical name is (RS)-1-(isopropoxycarbonyloxy)ethyl (+)-(6R,7R)-7-[2-(2-amino-4- thiazolyl)-2-((Z)-methoxyimino)acetamido]-3-methoxymethyl-8-oxo-5-thia-1-azabicyclo[4.2.0]oct-2-ene-2-carboxylate. Its empirical formula is:

$C_{21}H_{27}N_5O_9S_2$.

The molecular weight of cefpodoxime proxetil is 557.61.

Cefpodoxime proxetil is a prodrug; its active metabolite is cefpodoxime. All doses of cefpodoxime proxetil in this insert are expressed in terms of the active cefpodoxime moiety. The drug is supplied both as film-coated tablets and as flavored granules for oral suspension.

Vantin Tablets contain cefpodoxime proxetil equivalent to 100 mg or 200 mg of cefpodoxime activity and the following inactive ingredients: carboxymethylcellulose calcium, carnauba wax, FD&C Yellow No. 6, hydroxypropylcellulose, hydroxypropylmethylcellulose, lactose hydrous, magnesium stearate, propylene glycol, sodium lauryl sulfate and titanium dioxide. In addition, the 100 mg film-coated tablets contain D&C Yellow No. 10 and 200 mg film-coated tablets contain FD&C Red No. 40.

Each 5 ml of Vantin Granules for Oral Suspension contains cefpodoxime proxetil equivalent to 50 mg or 100 mg of cefpodoxime activity after constitution and the following inactive ingredients: artificial flavorings, butylated hydroxy anisole (BHA), carboxymethylcellulose sodium, carrageenan, citric acid, colloidal silicon dioxide, croscarmellose sodium, hydroxypropylcellulose, lactose, lactose hydrous, maltodextrin, microcrystalline cellulose, natural flavorings, propylene glycol alginate, sodium citrate hydrous, sodium benzoate, starch, sucrose, and vegetable oil.

CLINICAL PHARMACOLOGY:

Absorption and Excretion: Cefpodoxime proxetil is a prodrug that is absorbed from the gastrointestinal tract and de-esterified to its active metabolite, cefpodoxime. Following oral administration of 100 mg of cefpodoxime proxetil to fasting subjects, approximately 50% of the administered cefpodoxime dose was absorbed systemically. Over the recommended dosing range (100 to 400 mg), approximately 29 to 33% of the administered cefpodoxime dose was excreted unchanged in the urine in 12 hours. There is minimal metabolism of cefpodoxime *in vivo*.

Effects of food: The extent of absorption (mean AUC) and the mean peak plasma concentration increased when film-coated tablets were administered with food. Following a 200 mg tablet dose taken with food, the AUC was 21 to 33% higher than under fasting conditions, and the peak plasma concentration averaged 3.1 mcg/ml in fed subjects versus 2.6 mcg/ml in fasted subjects. Time to peak concentration was not significantly different between fed and fasted subjects.

When a 200 mg dose of the suspension was taken with food, the extent of absorption (mean AUC) and mean peak plasma concentration in fed subjects were not significantly different from fasted subjects, but the rate of absorption was slower with food (48% increase in T_{max}).

Pharmacokinetics of Cefpodoxime Proxetil Film-coated Tablets: Over the recommended dosing range(100 to 400 mg), the rate and extent of cefpodoxime absorption exhibited dose-dependency; dose-normalized C_{max} and AUC decreased by up to 32% with increasing dose. Over the recommended dosing range, the T_{max} was approximately 2 to 3 hours and the $T_{1/2}$ ranged from 2.09 to 2.84 hours. Mean C_{max} was 1.4 mcg/ml for the 100 mg dose, 2.3 mcg/ml for the 200 mg dose, and 3.9 mcg/ml for the 400 mg dose. In patients with normal renal function, neither accumulation nor significant changes in other pharmacokinetic parameters were noted following multiple oral doses of up to 400 mg Q 12 hours (TABLE 1).

Pharmacokinetics of Cefpodoxime Proxetil Suspension: In adult subjects, a 100 mg dose of oral suspension produced an average peak cefpodoxime concentration of approximately 1.5 mcg/ml (range: 1.1 to 2.1 mcg/ml), which is equivalent to that reported following administration of the 100 mg tablet. Time to peak plasma concentration and area under the plasma concentration-time curve (AUC) for the oral suspension were also equivalent to those produced with film-coated tablets in adults following a 100 mg oral dose.

CLINICAL PHARMACOLOGY: *(cont'd)*

TABLE 1 Cefpodoxime Plasma Levels (mcg/ml) In Fasted Adults After Film-Coated Tablet Administration (Single Dose)

Dose (cefpodoxime equivalents)	Time after oral ingestion 1hr	2hr	3hr	4hr	6hr	8hr	12hr
100 mg	0.98	1.4	1.3	1.0	0.59	0.29	0.08
200 mg	1.5	2.2	2.2	1.8	1.2	0.62	0.18
400 mg	2.2	3.7	3.8	3.3	2.3	1.3	0.38

The pharmacokinetics of cefpodoxime were investigated in 18 patients aged 4 to 17 years. Each patient received a single, oral, 5 mg/kg dose of cefpodoxime oral suspension. Plasma and urine samples were collected for 12 hours after dosing. The plasma levels reported from this study are as follows (TABLE 2):

TABLE 2 Cefpodoxime Plasma Levels (mcg/ml) In Fasted Patients (4 To 17 Years Of Age) After Suspension Administration

Dose (cefpodoxime equivalents)	Time after oral ingestion 1hr	2hr	3hr	4hr	6hr	8hr	12hr
5 mg/kg[1]	1.6	2.4	2.3	1.9	0.96	0.41	0.091

[1] Dose did not exceed 200 mg.

Distribution: Protein binding of cefpodoxime ranges from 22 to 33% in serum and from 21 to 29% in plasma.

Skin Blister: Following multiple-dose administration every 12 hours for 5 days of 200 mg or 400 mg cefpodoxime proxetil, the mean maximum cefpodoxime concentration in skin blister fluid averaged 1.6 and 2.8 mcg/ml, respectively. Skin blister fluid cefpodoxime levels at 12 hours after dosing averaged 0.2 and 0.4 mcg/ml for the 200 mg and 400 mg multiple-dose regimens, respectively.

Tonsil Tissue: Following a single, oral 100 mg cefpodoxime proxetil film-coated tablet, the mean maximum cefpodoxime concentration in tonsil tissue averaged 0.24 mcg/g at 4 hours post-dosing and 0.09 mcg/g at 7 hours post-dosing. Equilibrium was achieved between plasma and tonsil tissue within 4 hours of dosing. No detection of cefpodoxime in tonsillar tissue was reported 12 hours after dosing. These results demonstrated that concentrations of cefpodoxime exceeded the MIC_{90} of *S. pyogenes* for at least 7 hours after dosing of 100 mg of cefpodoxime proxetil.

Lung Tissue: Following a single, oral 200 mg cefpodoxime proxetil film-coated tablet, the mean maximum cefpodoxime concentration in lung tissue averaged 0.63 mcg/g at 3 hours post-dosing, 0.52 mcg/g at 6 hours post-dosing, and 0.19 mcg/g at 12 hours post-dosing. The results of this study indicated that cefpodoxime penetrated into lung tissue and produced sustained drug concentrations for at least 12 hours after dosing at levels at exceeded the MIC_{90} for *S. pneumoniae* and *H. influenzae*.

CSF: Adequate date on CSF levels of cefpodoxime are not available.

Effects of decreased renal function: Elimination of cefpodoxime is reduced in patients with moderate to severe renal impairment (<50 ml/min creatinine clearance). (See PRECAUTIONS and DOSAGE AND ADMINISTRATION.) In subjects with mild impairment for renal function (50 to 80 ml/min creatinine clearance), the average plasma half-life of cefpodoxime was 3.5 hours. In subjects with moderate (30 to 49 ml/min creatinine clearance) or severe renal impairment (5 to 29 ml/min creatinine clearance), the half-life increased to 5.9 and 9.8 hours, respectively. Approximately 23% of the administered dose was cleared from the body during a standard 3-hour hemodialysis procedure.

Effect of hepatic impairment (cirrhosis): Absorption was somewhat diminished and elimination unchanged in patients with cirrhosis. The mean cefpodoxime $T_{1/2}$ and renal clearance in cirrhotic patients were similar to those derived in studies of healthy subjects. Ascites did not appear to affect values in cirrhotic subjects. No dosage adjustment is recommended in this patient population.

Pharmacokinetics in Elderly Subjects: Elderly subjects do not require dosage adjustments unless they have diminished renal function.(See PRECAUTIONS.) In healthy geriatric subjects, cefpodoxime half-life in plasma averaged 4.2 hours (vs 3.3 in younger subjects) and urinary recovery averaged 21% after a 400 mg dose as administered every 12 hours. Other pharmacokinetic parameters (C_{max},AUC, and T_{max}) were unchanged relative to those observed in healthy young subjects.

Microbiology: Cefpodoxime is active *in vitro* against a wide range of gram-positive and gram-negative bacteria. Cefpodoxime is highly stable in the presence of beta-lactamase enzymes. As a result, many organisms resistant to penicillins and some cephalosporins, due to the presence of beta-lactamases, may be susceptible to cefpodoxime.

The bactericidal activity of cefpodoxime results from its inhibition of cell wall synthesis. Cefpodoxime is usually active against the following organisms *in vitro* and in clinical infections. (See INDICATIONS AND USAGE.)

Gram-positive aerobes: *Staphylococcus aureus* (including penicillinase-producing strains)

NOTE: Cefpodoxime is inactive against methicillin-resistant staphylococci.

Staphylococcus saprophyticus; *Streptococcus pneumoniae*;*Streptococcus pyogenes*

Gram-negative aerobes: *Escherichia coli; Haemophilus influenzae (including β-lactamase-producing strains);Klebsiella pneumoniae; Moraxella (Branhamella) catarrhalis; Neisseria gonorrhoeae (including penicillinase-producing strains); Proteus mirabilis*

The following *in vitro* data are available; *however, their clinical significance is unknown.*

Cefpodoxime exhibits *in vitro* minimum inhibitory concentrations of 2.0 mcg/ml or less against most strains of the following organisms. The safety and effectiveness of cefpodoxime proxetil in treating infections due to these organisms have not been established in adequate and well-controlled trials.

Gram-Positive Aerobes: *Streptococcus agalactiae; Streptococcus spp.* (*Groups, C,F,G*)

NOTE: Cefpodoxime is inactive against most strains of*Enterococcus*.

Gram-Negative Aerobes: *Citrobacter diversus; Haemophilus parainfluenzae; Klebsiella oxytoca; Proteus vulgaris; Providencia rettgeri*

NOTE: Cefpodoxime is inactive against most strains of*Pseudomonas* and *Enterobacter*.

Anaerobes: *Peptostreptococcus magnus*

SUSCEPTIBILITY TESTING

Diffusion Techniques: Quantitative methods that require measurement of zone diameters give the most precise estimate of the susceptibility of bacteria to antimicrobial agents. One such standardized procedure[1] recommended for use with the 10 mcg cefpodoxime disk is the National Committee for Clinical Laboratory Standards (NCCLS) approved procedure.

Interpretation involves correlation of the diameters obtained in the disk test with the minimum inhibitory concentration (MIC) for cefpodoxime.

CLINICAL PHARMACOLOGY: *(cont'd)*

Reports from the laboratory giving results of the standardized single disk susceptibility test using a 10 mcg cefpodoxime disk should be interpreted according to the following criteria (TABLE 3):

TABLE 3

Zone diameter (mm)	Interpretation
≥21	(S) Susceptible
18-20	(I) Intermediate
≤17	(R) Resistant

A report of "Susceptible" indicates that the pathogen is likely to be inhibited by generally achievable blood levels. A report of "Intermediate" indicates that the result should be considered equivocal, and, if the organism is not fully susceptible to alternative, clinically feasible drugs, the test should be repeated. This category implies clinical applicability in body sites where the drug is physiologically concentrated or in situations where high dosage of drug can be used. This category provides a buffer zone that prevents small uncontrolled technical factors from causing major discrepancies in interpretation. A report of "Resistant" indicates that achievable concentrations of the antibiotic are unlikely to be inhibitory and other therapy should be selected.

Standardized procedures require the use of laboratory control organisms. The 10 mcg disk should give the following zone diameters (TABLE 4):

TABLE 4

Organism	Zone diameter (mm)
Escherichia coli ATCC 25922	23-28
Staphylococcus aureus ATCC 25923	19-25

Cephalosporin "class disks" should not be used to test for susceptibility to cefpodoxime.

Dilution Technique: Use a standardized dilution method[2] (broth, agar, microdilution) or equivalent with cefpodoxime susceptibility powder. The MIC values should be interpreted according to the following criteria (TABLE 5):

TABLE 5

MIC (mcg/ml)	Interpretation
≤2	(S) Susceptible
4	(I) Intermediate
≥8	(R) Resistant

As with standard diffusion methods, dilution procedures require the use of laboratory control organisms. Standard cefpodoxime susceptibility powder should be give the following MIC values (TABLE 6):

TABLE 6

Organism	MIC range (mcg/ml)
Escherichia coli ATCC 25922	0.25-1
Staphylococcus aureus ATCC 29213	1-8

NOTE: Susceptibility testing by dilution methods requires the use of cefpodoxime susceptibility powder. Cefpodoxime proxetil granules for oral use should **NOT** be used for *in vitro* susceptibility tests.

CLINICAL STUDIES:

Cystitis: In two double-blind, 2:1 randomized, comparative trials performed in adults in the United States, cefpodoxime proxetil was compared to other beta-lactam antibiotics. In these studies, the following bacterial eradication rates were obtained at 5 to 9 days after therapy (TABLE 7):

TABLE 7

Organism	Cefpodoxime	Comparators
E. coli	200/243 (82%)	99/123 (80%)
Other pathogens	34/42 (81%)	23/28 (82%)
K. pneumoniae		
P. mirabilis		
S. saprophyticus		
TOTAL	234/285 (82%)	122/151 (81%)

In these studies, clinical cure rates and bacterial eradication rates for cefpodoxime proxetil were comparable to the comparator agents; however, the clinical cure rates and bacteriologic eradication rates were lower than those observed with some other classes of approved agents for cystitis.

INDICATIONS AND USAGE:

Cefpodoxime proxetil is indicated for the treatment of patients with mild to moderate infections caused by susceptible strains of the designated microorganisms in the conditions listed below. **Recommended dosages, durations of therapy, and applicable patient populations vary among these infections.** Please see DOSAGE AND ADMINISTRATION for specific recommendations.

LOWER RESPIRATORY TRACT

Acute, community-acquired pneumonia caused by *S. pneumoniae* or *H. influenzae* (non-beta-lactamase-producing strains only). Data are insufficient at this time to establish efficacy in patients with pneumonia caused by beta-lactamase-producing strains of*H. influenzae.*

Acute bacterial exacerbation of chronic bronchitis caused by *S. pneumoniae, H. influenzae* (non-beta-lactamase-producing strains only), or *M. catarrhalis.* Data are insufficient at this time to establish efficacy in patients with acute bacterial exacerbations of chronic bronchitis caused by beta-lactamase-producing strains of *H. influenzae.*

SEXUALLY TRANSMITTED DISEASES

Acute, uncomplicated urethral and cervical gonorrhea caused by *Neisseria gonorrhoeae* (including penicillinase-producing strains).

Acute, uncomplicated ano-rectal infections in women due to *Neisseria gonorrhoeae* (including penicillinase-producing strains).

NOTE: The efficacy of cefpodoxime in treating male patients with rectal infections caused by *N. gonorrhoeae* has not been established. Data do not support the use of cefpodoxime proxetil in the treatment of pharyngeal infections due to *N. gonorrhoeae* in men or women.

INDICATIONS AND USAGE: *(cont'd)*

SKIN AND SKIN STRUCTURES

Uncomplicated skin and skin structure infections caused by *Staphylococcus aureus* (including penicillinase-producing strains) or *Streptococcus pyogenes.* Abscesses should be surgically drained as clinically indicated.

NOTE: In clinical trials, successful treatment of uncomplicated skin and skin structure infections was dose-related. The effective therapeutic dose for skin infections was higher than those used in other recommended indications. (See DOSAGE AND ADMINISTRATION.)

UPPER RESPIRATORY TRACT INFECTIONS

Acute otitis media caused by *Streptococcus pneumoniae, Haemophilus influenzae* (Including β-lactamase-producing strains), or *Moraxella (Branhamella) catarrhalis.*

Pharyngitis and/or tonsillitis caused by *Streptococcus pyogenes.*

NOTE: Only penicillin by the intramuscular route of administration has been shown to be effective in the prophylaxis of rheumatic fever. Cefpodoxime proxetil is generally effective in the eradication of streptococci from the oropharynx. However, data establishing the efficacy of cefpodoxime proxetil for the prophylaxis of subsequent rheumatic fever are not available.

URINARY TRACT

Uncomplicated urinary tract infections (cystitis) caused by*Escherichia coli, Klebsiella pneumoniae, Proteus mirabilis,* or *Staphylococcus saprophyticus.*

NOTE: In considering the use of cefpodoxime proxetil in the treatment of cystitis, cefpodoxime proxetil's lower bacterial eradication rates should be weighed against the increased eradication rates and different safety profiles of some other classes of approved agents. (See CLINICAL STUDIES.)

Appropriate specimens for bacteriological examination should be obtained in order to isolate and identify causative organisms and to determine their susceptibility to cefpodoxime. Therapy may be instituted while awaiting the results of these studies. Once these results become available, antimicrobial therapy should be adjusted accordingly.

CONTRAINDICATIONS:

Cefpodoxime proxetil is contraindicated in patients with a known allergy to cefpodoxime or to the cephalosporin group of antibiotics.

WARNINGS:

BEFORE THERAPY WITH CEFPODOXIME PROXETIL IS INSTITUTED, CAREFUL INQUIRY SHOULD BE MADE TO DETERMINE WHETHER THE PATIENT HAS HAD PREVIOUS HYPERSENSITIVITY REACTIONS TO CEFPODOXIME, OTHER CEPHALOSPORINS, PENICILLINS, OR OTHER DRUGS. IF CEFPODOXIME IS TO BE ADMINISTERED TO PENICILLIN-SENSITIVE PATIENTS, CAUTION SHOULD BE EXERCISED BECAUSE CROSS HYPERSENSITIVITY AMONG BETA-LACTAM ANTIBIOTICS HAS BEEN CLEARLY DOCUMENTED AND MAY OCCUR IN UP TO 10% OF PATIENTS WITH A HISTORY OF PENICILLIN ALLERGY. IF AN ALLERGIC REACTION TO CEFPODOXIME PROXETIL OCCURS, DISCONTINUE THE DRUG. SERIOUS ACUTE HYPERSENSITIVITY REACTIONS MAY REQUIRE TREATMENT WITH EPINEPHRINE AND OTHER EMERGENCY MEASURES, INCLUDING OXYGEN, INTRAVENOUS FLUIDS, INTRAVENOUS ANTIHISTAMINE, AND AIRWAY MANAGEMENT, AS CLINICALLY INDICATED. PSEUDOMEMBRANOUS COLITIS HAS BEEN REPORTED WITH NEARLY ALL ANTIBACTERIAL AGENTS, INCLUDING CEFPODOXIME, AND MAY RANGE IN SEVERITY FROM MILD TO LIFE-THREATENING. THEREFORE, IT IS IMPORTANT TO CONSIDER THIS DIAGNOSIS IN PATIENTS WHO PRESENT WITH DIARRHEA SUBSEQUENT TO THE ADMINISTRATION OF ANTIBACTERIAL AGENTS.

Extreme caution should be observed when using this product in patients at increased risk for antibiotic-induced, pseudomembranous colitis because of exposure to institutional settings, such as nursing homes or hospitals with endemic *C. difficile.*

Treatment with broad-spectrum antibiotics, including cefpodoxime proxetil, alters the normal flora of the colon and may permit overgrowth of clostridia. Studies indicate a toxin produced by *Clostridium difficile* is the primary cause of "antibiotic-associated colitis".

After the diagnosis of pseudomembranous colitis has been established, therapeutic measures should be initiated. Mild cases of pseudomembranous colitis usually respond to drug discontinuation alone. In moderate to severe cases, consideration should be given to management with fluids and electrolytes, protein supplementation, and treatment with an oral antibacterial drug effective against *C. difficile.*

A concerted effort to monitor for *C. difficile* in cefpodoxime treated patients with diarrhea was undertaken because of an increased incidence of diarrhea associated with *C. difficile* in early trials in normal subjects. *C. difficile* organisms or toxin was reported in **10%** of the cefpodoxime-treated adult patients with diarrhea; however, no specific diagnosis of pseudomembranous colitis was made in these patients.

In post-marketing experience outside the United States, reports of pseudomembranous colitis associated with the use of cefpodoxime proxetil have been received.

PRECAUTIONS:

General: In patients with transient or persistent reduction in urinary output due to renal insufficiency, the total daily dose of cefpodoxime proxetil should be reduced because high and prolonged serum antibiotic concentrations can occur in such individuals following usual doses. Cefpodoxime, like other cephalosporins, should be administered with caution to patients receiving concurrent treatment with potent diuretics. (See DOSAGE AND ADMINISTRATION.)

As with other antibiotics, prolonged use of cefpodoxime proxetil may result in overgrowth of non-susceptible organisms. Repeated evaluation of the patient's condition is essential. If superinfection occurs during therapy, appropriate measures should be taken.

Drug/Laboratory Test Interactions: Cephalosporins, including cefpodoxime proxetil, are known to occasionally induce a positive direct Coombs' test.

Carcinogenesis, Mutagenesis, and Impairment of Fertility: Long-term animal carcinogenesis studies of cefpodoxime proxetil have not been performed. Mutagenesis studies of cefpodoxime, including the Ames test both with and without metabolic activation, the chromosome aberration test, the unscheduled DNA synthesis assay, mitotic recombination and gene conversion, the forward gene mutation assay and the *in vivo* micronucleus test, were all negative. No untoward effects on fertility or reproduction were noted when 100 mg/kg/day or less (2 times the human dose based on mg/m^2) was administered orally to rats.

Pregnancy, Teratogenic Effects, Pregnancy Category B: Cefpodoxime proxetil was neither teratogenic nor embryocidal when administered to rats during organogenesis at doses up to 100 mg/kg/day (2 times the human dose based on mg/m^2) or to rabbits at doses up to 30 mg/kg/day (1-2 times the human dose based on mg/m^2).

There are, however, no adequate and well-controlled studies of cefpodoxime proxetil use in pregnant women. Because animal reproduction studies are not always predictive of human response, this drug should be used during pregnancy only if clearly needed.

Labor and Delivery: Cefpodoxime proxetil has not been studied for use during labor and delivery. Treatment should only be given if clearly needed.

PRECAUTIONS: *(cont'd)*

Nursing Mothers: Cefpodoxime is excreted in human milk. In a study of 3 lactating women, levels of cefpodoxime in human milk were 0%, 2% and 6% of concomitant serum levels at 4 hours following a 200 mg oral dose of cefpodoxime proxetil. At 6 hours post-dosing, levels were 0%, 9% and 16% of concomitant serum levels. Because of the potential for serious reactions in nursing infants, a decision should be made whether to discontinue nursing or to discontinue the drug, taking into account the importance of the drug to the mother.

Pediatric Use: Safety and efficacy in infants less than 6 months of age have not been established.

Geriatric Use: Of the 3338 patients in multiple-dose clinical studies of cefpodoxime proxetil, film-coated tablets 521 (16%) were 65 and over, while 214 (6%) were 75 and over. No overall differences in effectiveness or safety were observed between the elderly and younger patients. In healthy geriatric subjects with normal renal function, cefpodoxime half-life in plasma averaged 4.2 hours and urinary recovery averaged 21% after a 400 mg dose was given every 12 hours for 15 days. Other pharmacokinetic parameters were unchanged relative to those observed in healthy younger subjects.

Dose adjustment in elderly patients with normal renal function is not necessary.

DRUG INTERACTIONS:

Antacids: Concomitant administration of high doses of antacids (sodium bicarbonate and aluminum hydroxide) or H_2 blockers reduces peak plasma levels by 24% to 42% and the extent of absorption by 27% to 32%, respectively. The rate of absorption is not altered by these concomitant medications. Oral anti-cholinergics (*e.g.*, propantheline) delay peak plasma levels (47% increase in T_{max}), but do not affect the extent of absorption (AUC).

Probenecid: As with other beta-lactam antibiotics, renal excretion of cefpodoxime was inhibited by probenecid and resulted in an approximately 31% increase in AUC and 20% increase in peak cefpodoxime plasma levels.

Nephrotoxic drugs: Although nephrotoxicity has not been noted when cefpodoxime proxetil was given alone, close monitoring of renal function is advised when cefpodoxime proxetil is administered concomitantly with compounds of known nephrotoxic potential.

ADVERSE REACTIONS:

Incidence less than 1%

Cardiovascular: Chest pain, hypotension.

Dermatologic: Fungal skin infection, skin scaling/peeling.

Endocrine: Menstrual irregularity.

Genital: Pruritus.

Gastrointestinal: Flatulence, decreased salivation, candidiasis, pseudomembranous colitis.

Hypersensitivity: Anaphylactic shock.

Metabolic: Decreased appetite.

Miscellaneous: Malaise, fever.

Central Nervous System: Dizziness, fatigue, anxiety, insomnia, flushing, nightmares, weakness.

Respiratory: Cough, epistaxis.

Special Senses: Taste alteration, eye itching, tinnitus.

Film-coated Tablets (Multiple dose): In clinical trials using **multiple doses** of cefpodoxime proxetil film-coated tablets, 3338 patients were treated with the recommended dosages of cefpodoxime (100 to 400 mg Q 12 hours). There were no deaths or permanent disabilities thought related to drug toxicity. Eighty-one (2.4%) patients discontinued medication due to adverse events thought possibly- or probably-related to drug toxicity. Sixty-six (66%) of the 100 patients who discontinued therapy (whether thought related to drug therapy or not) did so because of gastrointestinal disturbances, usually diarrhea. The percentage of cefpodoxime proxetil-treated patients who discontinued study drug because of adverse events was significantly greater at a dose of 800 mg daily than at a dose of 400 mg daily or at a dose of 200 mg daily.

Adverse events thought possibly- or probably-related to cefpodoxime in multiple dose clinical trials (n=3338 cefpodoxime-treated patients) were:

Incidence greater than 1%: Diarrhea: 7.2%

Diarrhea or loose stools were dose related: decreasing from 10.6% of patients receiving 800 mg per day to 5.9% for those receiving 200 mg per day. Of patients with diarrhea, 10% had *C. difficile* organism or toxin in the stool. (See WARNINGS.)

Nausea: 3.8%; Vaginal Fungal Infections: 3.1%; Abdominal Pain: 1.6%; Rash: 1.4%; Headache: 1.1%; Vomiting: 1.1%

Granules for Oral Suspension (Multiple dose): In clinical trials using **multiple doses** of cefpodoxime proxetil granules for oral suspension, pediatric patients (90% of whom were less than 12 years of age) were treated with the recommended dosages of cefpodoxime (10 mg/kg/day divided Q 12 hours to a maximum equivalent adult dose). There were no deaths or permanent disabilities in any of the patients in these studies. Seven patients (<1%) discontinued medication due to adverse events thought possibly- or probably-related to drug toxicity. Primarily, these discontinuations were for gastrointestinal disturbances, usually diarrhea or diaper area rashes.

Adverse events thought possibly- or probably-related to cefpodoxime granules for oral suspension in multiple dose clinical trials (n=758 cefpodoxime-treated patients) were:

Incidence greater than 1%: Diarrhea: 7.0%

The incidence of diarrhea ranged from 17.8% in infants and toddlers to 4.1% in 2 to 12 year olds to 6.0% in adolescents.

Diaper Rash: 3.5%; Other skin rashes: 1.8%; Vomiting: 1.7%

Incidence less than 1%

Central Nervous System: Headache.

Dermatologic: Exacerbation of acne.

Genital: Pruritus or vaginitis.

Gastrointestinal: Nausea, abdominal pain, candidiasis.

Metabolic: Decreased appetite.

Miscellaneous: Fever.

Film-coated tablets (Single dose): In clinical trials using **a single dose** of cefpodoxime proxetil film-coated tablets, 509 patients were treated with the recommended dosage of cefpodoxime (200 mg). There were no deaths or permanent disabilities thought related to drug toxicity in these studies.

Adverse events thought possibly- or probably-related to cefpodoxime in single dose clinical trials conducted in the United States were:

Incidence greater than 1%: Nausea: 1.4%; Diarrhea: 1.2%

Incidence less than 1%

Central Nervous System: Dizziness, headache, syncope.

Dermatologic: Rash.

Genital: Vaginitis.

ADVERSE REACTIONS: *(cont'd)*

Gastrointestinal: Abdominal pain.

Psychiatric: Anxiety.

Laboratory Changes (Adult patients): Significant laboratory changes that have been reported in adult patients in clinical trials of cefpodoxime proxetil, without regard to drug relationship, were:

Hepatic: Transient increases in AST (SGOT), ALT (SGPT), GGT, alkaline phosphatase, bilirubin, and LDH.

Hematologic: Eosinophilia, leukocytosis, lymphocytosis, granulocytosis, basophilia, monocytosis, thrombocytosis, decreased hemoglobin, leukopenia, neutropenia, lymphocytopenia, thrombocytopenia, positive Coombs' test, and prolonged PT and PTT.

Serum Chemistry: Increases in glucose, decreases in glucose, decreases in serum albumin, decreases in serum total protein.

Renal: Increases in BUN and creatinine.

Most of these abnormalities were transient and not clinically significant.

Laboratory Changes (Pediatric patients): Significant laboratory changes that have been reported in pediatric patients in clinical trials of cefpodoxime proxetil, without regard to drug relationship, were:

Hematologic: Eosinophilia, decreased hemoglobin, decreased hematocrit.

Hepatic: Transiently increased ALT (SGPT).

Most of these abnormalities were transient and not clinically significant.

Post-marketing Experience: The following serious adverse experiences have been reported: allergic reactions including Stevens-Johnson syndrome, toxic epidermal necrolysis and erythema multiforme, pseudomembranous colitis, bloody diarrhea with abdominal pain, ulcerative colitis, rectorrhagia with hypotension, anaphylactic shock, acute liver injury, *in utero* exposure with miscarriage, purpuric nephritis, pulmonary infiltrate with eosinophilia, and eyelid dermatitis.

One death was attributed to pseudomembranous colitis and disseminated intravascular coagulation.

Cephalosporin Class Labeling: In addition to the adverse reactions listed above which have been observed in patients treated with cefpodoxime proxetil, the following adverse reactions and altered laboratory tests have been reported for cephalosporin class antibiotics:

Adverse Reactions and Abnormal Laboratory Tests: Renal dysfunction, toxic nephropathy, hepatic dysfunction including cholestasis, aplastic anemia, hemolytic anemia, hemorrhage; agranulocytosis; and pancytopenia.

Several cephalosporins have been implicated in triggering seizures, particularly in patients with renal impairment when the dosage was not reduced. (See DOSAGE AND ADMINISTRATION and OVERDOSAGE.) If seizures associated with drug therapy occur, the drug should be discontinued. Anticonvulsant therapy can be given if clinically indicated.

OVERDOSAGE:

In acute rodent toxicity studies, a single 5 g/kg oral dose produced no adverse effects.

Information on overdosage in humans is not available. In the event of serious toxic reaction from overdosage, hemodialysis or peritoneal dialysis may aid in the removal of cefpodoxime from the body, particularly if renal function is compromised.

The toxic symptoms following an overdose of β-lactam antibiotics may include nausea, vomiting, epigastric distress, and diarrhea.

DOSAGE AND ADMINISTRATION:

(See INDICATIONS AND USAGE for indicated pathogens.)

Film-Coated Tablets: Cefpodoxime proxetil tablets should be administered orally with food to enhance absorption (See CLINICAL PHARMACOLOGY.) The recommended dosages, durations of treatment, and applicable patient population are as described in the following chart (TABLE 8):

TABLE 8 Adults (age 13 years and older)

Type of Infection	Total Daily Dose	Dose Frequency	Duration
Acute community-acquired pneumonia	400 mg	200 mg Q 12 hours	14 days
Acute bacterial exacerbations of chronic bronchitis	400 mg	200 mg Q 12 hours	10 days
Uncomplicated gonorrhea (men and women) and rectal gonococcal infections (women)	200 mg	single dose	
Skin and skin structure	800 mg	400 mg Q 12 hours	7 to 14 days
Pharyngitis and/or tonsillitis	200 mg	100 mg Q 12 hours	10 days
Uncomplicated urinary tract infection	200 mg	100 mg Q 12 hours	7 days

Granules for Oral Suspension: Cefpodoxime proxetil oral suspension may be given without regard to food. The recommended dosages, durations of treatment, and applicable patient populations are as described in the following chart (TABLE 9):

TABLE 9

Type of Infection	Total Daily Dose	Dose Frequency	Duration
Adults (age 13 years and older):			
Acute community-acquired pneumonia	400 mg	200 mg Q 12 hours	14 days
Uncomplicated gonorrhea (men and women) and rectal gonococcal infections (women)	200 mg	single dose	
Skin and skin structure	800 mg	400 mg Q 12 hours	7-14 days
Pharyngitis and/or tonsillitis	200 mg	100 mg Q 12 hours	10 days
Uncomplicated urinary tract infection	200 mg	100 mg Q 12 hours	7 days
Children (age 6 months through 12 years):			
Acute otitis media	10 mg/kg/day divided Q 12 hr Max 400 mg/day	5 mg/kg/dose Max 200 mg/dose	10 days
Pharyngitis and/or tonsillitis	10 mg/kg/day divided Q 12 hr Max 200 mg/day	5 mg/kg/dose Max 100 mg/dose	10 days

DOSAGE AND ADMINISTRATION: *(cont'd)*

Patients with Renal Dysfunction: For patients with severe renal impairment (<30 ml/min creatinine clearance), the dosing intervals should be increased to Q 24 hours. In patients maintained on hemodialysis, the dose frequency should be 3 times/week after hemodialysis.

When only the serum creatinine level is available, the following formula (based on sex, weight, and age of the patient) may be used to estimate creatinine clearance (ml/min). For this estimate to be valid, the serum creatinine level should represent a steady state of renal function (TABLE 9).

TABLE 10

Males: [Weight (kg) × (140 - age)] ÷ [72 × serum creatinine]
Females: 0.85 × above value

Patients with Cirrhosis: Cefpodoxime pharmacokinetics in cirrhotic patients (with or without ascites) are similar to those in healthy subjects. Dose adjustment is not necessary in this population.

Preparation of Suspension (TABLE 10):

TABLE 11 Constitution Directions For Oral Suspension

Bottle Size	Final Concentration	Directions
100 ml	50 mg per 5 ml	Suspend in a total of 58 ml of water. Method: First, tap the bottle to loosen granules. Then add the water in two portions, shaking well after each aliquot of water.
100 ml	100 mg per 5 ml	Suspend in a total of 57 ml of water. Method: First, tap the bottle to loosen granules. Then add the water in two portions, shaking well after each aliquot of water.

After mixing, the suspension should be stored in a refrigerator, 2° to 8°C (36° to 46°F). Shake well before using. Keep container tightly closed. The mixture may be used for 14 days. Discard unused portion after 14 days.

REFERENCES:

1. National Committee for Clinical Laboratory Standards, Approved Standard: Performance Standards for Antimicrobial Disk Susceptibility Tests, 4th Edition, Vol. 10(7):M2-A4, Villanova, PA, April, 1990. 2. National Committee for Clinical Laboratory Standards, Approved Standard: Methods for Dilution Antimicrobial Susceptibility Tests for Bacteria That Grow Aerobically, 2nd Edition, Vol. 10(8):M7-A2, Villanova, PA, April, 1990.

HOW SUPPLIED:

Storage: Store tablets between 15° and 30°C (59° to 86°F). Replace cap securely after each opening. Protect unit dose packs from excessive moisture.

Store unsuspended granules between 15° and 30°C (59° to 86°F).

Directions for mixing are included on the label. After mixing, suspension should be stored in a refrigerator, 2° to 8°C (36° to 46°F). Shake well before using. Keep container tightly closed. The mixture may be used for 14 days. Discard unused portion after 14 days.

HOW SUPPLIED - EQUIVALENTS NOT AVAILABLE:

Suspension - Oral - 50 mg/5ml

100 ml	$30.62	VANTIN, Pharmacia & Upjohn	00009-3531-01

Suspension - Oral - 100 mg/5ml

100 ml	$58.26	VANTIN, Pharmacia & Upjohn	00009-3615-01

Tablet, Uncoated - Oral - 100 mg

20's	$42.97	VANTIN, Pharmacia & Upjohn	00009-3617-01
100's	$204.50	VANTIN, Pharmacia & Upjohn	00009-3617-02
100's	$211.33	VANTIN, Pharmacia & Upjohn	00009-3617-03

Tablet, Uncoated - Oral - 200 mg

20's	$75.16	VANTIN, Pharmacia & Upjohn	00009-3618-01
100's	$357.37	VANTIN, Pharmacia & Upjohn	00009-3618-02
100's	$366.31	VANTIN, Pharmacia & Upjohn	00009-3618-03

CEFPROZIL *(003102)*

CATEGORIES: Anti-Infectives; Antibiotics; Bronchitis; Cephalosporins; Chronic Bronchitis; Otitis Media; Pharyngitis; Respiratory Tract Infections; Skin Infections; Streptococcal Infection; Tonsillitis; Rheumatic Fever*; FDA Class 1C ("Little or No Therapeutic Advantage"); FDA Approved 1991 Dec; Top 200 Drugs
* Indication not approved by the FDA

BRAND NAMES: **Cefzil**; Procef; *Prozef*
(International brand names outside U.S. in italics)

FORMULARIES: PCS

COST OF THERAPY: $155.06 (Respiratory Infections; Tablet; 500 mg; 2/day; 14 days)

DESCRIPTION:

Cefzil (cefprozil) is a semi-synthetic broad-spectrum cephalosporin antibiotic.

Cefprozil is a cis and trans isomeric mixture (≥ 90% cis). The chemical name for the monohydrate is (6R,7R)-7-((R)-2-amino-2-(p-hydroxy-phenyl)acetamido)-8-oxo-3-propenyl-5-thia-1-azabicyclo(4.2.0)oct-2-ene-2-carboxylic acid monohydrate.

Cefprozil is a white to yellowish powder with a molecular formula for the monohydrate of $C_{18}H_{19}N_3O_5S \cdot H_2O$ and a molecular weight of 407.45.

Cefzil tablets and Cefzil for oral suspension are intended for oral administration.

Cefzil tablets contain cefprozil equivalent to 250 mg or 500 mg of anhydrous cefprozil. In addition, each tablet contains the following inactive ingredients: cellulose, hydroxypropyl-methylcellulose, magnesium stearate, methylcellulose, simethicone, sodium starch glycolate, polyethylene glycol, polysorbate 80, sorbic acid and titanium dioxide. The 250 mg tablets also contain FD&C Yellow No. 6.

Cefzil for oral suspension contains cefprozil equivalent to 125 mg or 250 mg anhydrous cefprozil per 5 ml constituted suspension. In addition, the oral suspension contains the following inactive ingredients: aspartame, cellulose, citric acid, colloidal silicone dioxide, FD&C Red No. 3, flavors (natural and artificial), glycine, polysorbate 80, simethicone, sodium benzoate, sodium carboxymethylcellulose, sodium chloride, and sucrose.

CLINICAL PHARMACOLOGY:

Following oral administration of cefprozil to fasting subjects, approximately 95% of the dose was absorbed. Using the investigational capsule formulation, no food effect was observed. The food effect on the tablet and on the suspension formulations has not been studied.

CLINICAL PHARMACOLOGY: *(cont'd)*

The pharmacokinetic data were derived from the capsule dosing; however, bioequivalence has been demonstrated for the oral solution, capsule, tablet and suspension formulations under fasting conditions.

Average peak plasma concentrations after administration of 250 mg, 500 mg, or 1 g doses of cefprozil to fasting subjects were approximately 6.1, 10.5, and 18.3 mcg/ml, respectively, and were obtained within 1.5 hours after dosing. Urinary recovery accounted for approximately 60% of the administered dose. (See TABLE 1):

TABLE 1

Dosage (mg)	Mean Plasma Cefprozil* Concentrations (mcg/ml)			9-hour Urinary Excretion (%)
	Peak appx. 1.5 hr	4hr	8hr	
250 mg	6.1	1.7	0.2	60%
500 mg	10.5	3.2	0.4	62%
1000 mg	18.3	8.4	1.0	54%

* Data represent mean values of 12 healthy volunteers.

During the first four-hour period after drug administration, the average urine concentrations following the 250 mg, 500 mg, and 1 g doses were approximately 700 mcg/ml, 1000 mcg/ml and 2900 mcg/ml.

Plasma protein binding is approximately 36% and is independent of concentration in the range of 2 mcg/ml to 20 mcg/ml.

The average plasma half-life in normal subjects is 1.3 hours.

There was no evidence of accumulation of cefprozil in the plasma in individuals with normal renal function following multiple oral doses of up to 1000 mg every 8 hours for 10 days.

In patients with reduced renal function, the plasma half-life may be prolonged up to 5.2 hours depending on the degree of the renal dysfunction. In patients with complete absence of renal function the plasma half-life of cefprozil has been shown to be as long as 5.9 hours.

The half-life is shortened during hemodialysis. Excretion pathways in patients with markedly impaired renal function have not been determined.(See PRECAUTIONS and DOSAGE AND ADMINISTRATION).

The average AUC observed in elderly subjects (≥65 years of age) is approximately 35-60% higher relative to young adults and the average AUC in females is approximately 15-20% higher than in males. The magnitude of these age and gender related changes in the pharmacokinetics of cefprozil are not sufficient to necessitate dosage adjustments.

In patients with impaired hepatic function, the half-life increases to approximately 2 hours. The magnitude of the changes does not warrant a dosage adjustment for patients with impaired hepatic function.

Adequate data on CSF levels of cefprozil are not available.

MICROBIOLOGY

Cefprozil has *in vitro* activity against a broad range of gram-positive and gram-negative bacteria. The bactericidal action of cefprozil results from inhibition of cell-wall synthesis. Cefprozil has been shown to be active against most strains of the following organisms both *in vitro* and in clinical infections. (See INDICATIONS AND USAGE):

Aerobes, Gram-Positive:

Staphylococcus aureus (including penicillinase-producing strains)

NOTE: Cefprozil is inactive against methicillin-resistant staphylococci.

Streptococcus pneumoniae

Streptococcus pyogenes

Aerobes, Gram-Negative:

Moraxella Branhamella catarrhalis

Haemophilus influenzae (including penicillinase-producing strains)

The following *in vitro* data are available; however, their clinical significance is unknown. Cefprozil exhibits *in vitro* minimum inhibitory concentrations (MIC) of 8 mcg/ml or less against most strains of the following organisms. The safety and efficacy of cefprozil in treating infections due to these organisms have not been established in adequate and well-controlled trials.

Aerobes, Gram-Positive:

Enterococcus durans

Enterococcus faecalis

NOTE: Cefprozil is inactive against *Enterococcus faecium.*

Listeria monocytogenes

Staphylococcus epidermidis

Staphylococcus saprophyticus

Staphylococcus warneri

Aerobes, Gram-Negative:

Streptococci (Groups C, D, F, and G) viridans group streptococci

Citrobacter diversus

Escherichia coli

Klebsiella pneumoniae

Neisseria gonorrhoeae (including penicillinase-producing strains)

Proteus mirabilis

Salmonella spp.

Shigella and

Vibrio spp.

NOTE: Cefprozil is inactive against most strains of *Acinetobacter, Enterobacter, Morganella morganii, Proteus vulgaris, Providencia, Pseudomonas,* and *Serratia.*

Anaerobes:

Bacteroides melaninogenicus

NOTE: Most strains of the *Bacteroides fragilis* group are resistant to cefprozil.

Clostridium perfringens

Clostridium difficile

Fusobacterium spp.

Peptostreptococcus spp.

Propionibacterium acnes

SUSCEPTIBILITY TESTING

Diffusion Techniques: Quantitative methods that require measurement of zone diameters give the most precise estimate of the susceptibility of bacteria to antimicrobial agents. One such standardized procedure recommended for use with the 30-mcg cefprozil disk is the National

CLINICAL PHARMACOLOGY: *(cont'd)*

Committee for Clinical Laboratory Standards (NCCLS) approved procedure[1]. Interpretation involves correlation of the diameter obtained in the disk test with minimum inhibitory concentration (MIC) for cefprozil.

The class disk for cephalosporin susceptibility testing (the cephalothin disk) is not appropriate because of spectrum differences with cefprozil. The 30-mcg cefprozil disk should be used for all *in vitro* testing of isolates.

Reports from the laboratory giving results of the standard single-disk susceptibility test with a 30-mcg cefprozil disk should be interpreted according to the following criteria (TABLE 2):

TABLE 2

Zone diameter (mm)	Interpretation
≥ 18	(S) Susceptible
15-17	(MS) Moderately Susceptible
≤ 14	(R) Resistant

A report of "Susceptible" indicates that the pathogen is likely to be inhibited by generally achievable blood concentrations. A report of "Moderately Susceptible" indicates that the organism would be susceptible if high dosage is used or if the infection is confined to tissues and fluids (*e.g.*, urine) in which high antibiotic levels are attained. A report of "Resistant" indicates that the achievable concentration of the antibiotic is unlikely to be inhibitory and other therapy should be selected.

Standardized procedures require the use of laboratory control organisms. The 30-mcg cefprozil disk should give the following zone diameters (TABLE 3):

TABLE 3

Organism	Zone diameter (mm)
Escherichia coli ATCC 25922	21-27
Staphylococcus aureus ATCC 25923	27-33

Dilution Techniques: Use a standardized dilution method[2] (broth, agar, microdilution) or equivalent with cefprozil powder. The MIC values obtained should be interpreted according to the following criteria (TABLE 4):

TABLE 4

MIC (mcg/ml)	Interpretation
≤8	(S) Susceptible
16	(MS) Moderately Susceptible
≥32	(R) Resistant

As with standard diffusion techniques, dilution techniques require the use of laboratory control organisms. Standard cefprozil powder should give the following MIC values (TABLE 5):

TABLE 5

Organism	MIC (mcg/ml)
Enterococcus faecalis ATCC 29212	4-16
Escherichia coli ATCC 25922	1-4
Pseudomonas aeruginosa ATCC 27853	>32
Staphylococcus aureus ATCC 29213	0.25-1

CLINICAL STUDIES:

STUDY ONE

In a controlled clinical study of **acute otitis media** performed in the United States where significant rates of beta-lactamase producing organisms were found, cefprozil was compared to an oral antimicrobial agent that contained a specific beta-lactamase inhibitor. In this study, using very strict evaluability criteria and microbiologic and clinical response criteria at the 10-16 days post-therapy follow-up, the following presumptive bacterial eradication/clinical cure outcomes (*i.e.*, clinical success) and safety results were obtained (TABLE 6):

TABLE 6 U.S. Acute Otitis Media Study
Cefprozil vs beta-lactamase inhibitor-containing control drug

EFFICACY: Pathogen	% of Cases with Pathogen (n = 155)	Outcome
S. pneumoniae	48.4%	cefprozil success rate 5% better than control
H. influenzae	35.5%	cefprozil success rate 17% less than control
M. catarrhalis	13.5%	cefprozil success rate 12% less than control
S. pyogenes	2.6%	cefprozil equivalent to control
Overall	100.0%	cefprozil success rate 5% less than control

Safety

The incidence of adverse events, primarily diarrhea and rash*, were clinically and statistically significantly higher in the control arm versus the cefprozil arm (TABLE 7):

TABLE 7

Age Group	Cefprozil	Control
6 months - 2 years	21%	41%
3 - 12 years	10%	19%

* The majority of these involved the diaper area in young children.

STUDY TWO

In a controlled clinical study of **acute otitis media** performed in Europe, cefprozil was compared to an oral antimicrobial agent that contained a specific beta-lactamase inhibitor. As expected in a European population, this study population had a lower incidence of beta-lactamase-producing organisms than usually seen in U.S. trials. In this study, using very strict evaluability criteria and microbiologic and clinical response criteria at the 10-16 days post-therapy follow-up, the following presumptive bacterial eradication/clinical cure outcomes (*i.e.*, clinical success) were obtained (TABLE 8):

Safety

The incidence of adverse events in the cefprozil arm was comparable to the incidence of adverse events in the control arm (agent that contained a specific beta-lactamase inhibitor).

INDICATIONS AND USAGE:

Cephprozil is indicated for the treatment of patients with mild to moderate infections caused by susceptible strains of the designated microorganisms in the conditions listed below:

INDICATIONS AND USAGE: *(cont'd)*

TABLE 8 European Acute Otitis Media Study
Cefprozil vs beta-lactamase inhibitor-containing control drug

EFFICACY: Pathogen	% of Cases with Pathogen (n=47)	Outcome
S. pneumoniae	51.0%	cefprozil equivalent to control
H. influenzae	29.8%	cefprozil equivalent to control
M. catarrhalis	6.4%	cefprozil equivalent to control
S. pyogenes	12.8%	cefprozil equivalent to control
Overall	100.0%	cefprozil equivalent to control

Upper Respiratory Tract

Pharyngitis/tonsillitis caused by *Streptococcus pyogenes.*

NOTE: The usual drug of choice in the treatment and prevention of streptococcal infections, including the prophylaxis of rheumatic fever, is penicillin given by the intramuscular route. Cefprozil is generally effective in the eradication of *Streptococcus pyogenes* from the nasopharynx; however, substantial data establishing the efficacy of cefprozil in the subsequent prevention of rheumatic fever are not available at present.

Otitis Media caused by *Streptococcus pneumoniae, Haemophilus influenzae* and *Moraxella (Branhamella) catarrhalis.* (See CLINICAL STUDIES.)

NOTE: In the treatment of otitis media due to beta-lactamase producing organisms, cefprozil had bacteriologic eradication rates somewhat lower than those observed with a product containing a specific beta-lactamase inhibitor. In considering the use of cefprozil, lower overall eradication rates should be balanced against the susceptibility patterns of the common microbes in a given geographic area and the increased potential for toxicity with products containing beta-lactamase inhibitors.

Lower Respiratory Tract

Secondary Bacterial Infection of Acute Bronchitis and Acute Bacterial Exacerbation of Chronic Bronchitis caused by *Streptococcus pneumoniae, Haemophilus influenzae* (beta-lactamase positive and negative strains), and *Moraxella (Branhamella) catarrhalis.*

Skin and Skin Structure

Uncomplicated Skin and Skin-Structure Infections caused by *Staphylococcus aureus* (including penicillinase-producing strains) and *Streptococcus pyogenes.* Abscesses usually require surgical drainage. Culture and susceptibility testing should be performed when appropriate to determine susceptibility of the causative organism to cefprozil.

CONTRAINDICATIONS:

Cephprozil is contraindicated in patients with known allergy to the cephalosporin class of antibiotics.

WARNINGS:

BEFORE THERAPY WITH CEFZIL IS INSTITUTED, CAREFUL INQUIRY SHOULD BE MADE TO DETERMINE WHETHER THE PATIENT HAS HAD PREVIOUS HYPERSENSITIVITY REACTIONS TO CEFZIL, CEPHALOSPORINS, PENICILLINS, OR OTHER DRUGS. IF THIS PRODUCT IS TO BE GIVEN TO PENICILLIN-SENSITIVE PATIENTS, CAUTION SHOULD BE EXERCISED BECAUSE CROSS-SENSITIVITY AMONG BETA-LACTAM ANTIBIOTICS HAS BEEN CLEARLY DOCUMENTED AND MAY OCCUR IN UP TO 10% OF PATIENTS WITH A HISTORY OF PENICILLIN ALLERGY. IF AN ALLERGIC REACTION TO CEFZIL OCCURS, DISCONTINUE THE DRUG. SERIOUS ACUTE HYPERSENSITIVITY REACTIONS MAY REQUIRE TREATMENT WITH EPINEPHRINE AND OTHER EMERGENCY MEASURES, INCLUDING OXYGEN, INTRAVENOUS FLUIDS, INTRAVENOUS ANTIHISTAMINES, CORTICOSTEROIDS, PRESSOR AMINES, AND AIRWAY MANAGEMENT, AS CLINICALLY INDICATED.

Pseudomembranous colitis has been reported with nearly all antibacterial agents, and may range from mild to life-threatening. Therefore, it is important to consider this diagnosis in patients who present with diarrhea subsequent to the administration of antibacterial agents.

Treatment with antibacterial agents alters the normal flora of the colon and may permit overgrowth of clostridia. Studies indicate that a toxin produced by *Clostridium difficile* is a primary cause of "antibiotic-associated colitis".

After the diagnosis of pseudomembranous colitis has been established, therapeutic measures should be initiated. Mild cases of pseudomembranous colitis usually respond to discontinuation of the drug alone. In moderate to severe cases, consideration should be given to management with fluids and electrolytes, protein supplementation and treatment with an antibacterial drug effective against *Clostridium difficile.*

PRECAUTIONS:

GENERAL

Evaluation of renal status before and during therapy is recommended, especially in seriously ill patients. In patients with known or suspected renal impairment (see DOSAGE AND ADMINISTRATION), careful clinical observation and appropriate laboratory studies should be done prior to and during therapy. The total daily dose of cephprozil should be reduced in these patients because high and/or prolonged plasma antibiotic concentrations can occur in such individuals from usual doses. Cephalosporins, including cephprozil, should be given with caution to patients receiving concurrent treatment with potent diuretics since these agents are suspected of adversely affecting renal function.

Prolonged use of cephprozil may result in the overgrowth of nonsusceptible organisms. Careful observation of the patient is essential. If superinfection occurs during therapy, appropriate measures should be taken.

Cefprozil should be prescribed with caution in individuals with a history of gastrointestinal disease particularly colitis.

Positive direct Coombs' tests have been reported during treatment with cephalosporin antibiotics.

INFORMATION FOR THE PATIENT

Phenylketonurics: Cephprozil for oral suspension contains phenylalanine 28 mg per 5 ml (1 teaspoon) constituted suspension for both the 125 mg/5 ml and 250 mg/5 ml dosage forms.

DRUG/LABORATORY TEST INTERACTIONS

Cephalosporin antibiotics may produce a false positive reaction for glucose in the urine with copper reduction tests (Benedict's or Fehling's solution or with Clinitest tablets), but not with enzyme-based tests for glycosuria (*e.g.*, Tes-Tape). A false negative reaction may occur in the ferricyanide test for blood glucose. The presence of cefprozil in the blood does not interfere with the assay of plasma or urine creatinine by the alkaline picrate method.

CARCINOGENESIS, MUTAGENESIS, AND IMPAIRMENT OF FERTILITY

No mutagenic potential of cefprozil was found in appropriate prokaryotic or eukaryotic cells *in vitro* or *in vivo*. No *in vivo* long-term studies have been performed to evaluate carcinogenic potential.

Reproductive studies revealed no impairment of fertility in animals.

PRECAUTIONS: *(cont'd)*

PREGNANCY, TERATOGENIC EFFECTS, PREGNANCY CATEGORY B

Reproduction studies have been performed in mice, rats, and rabbits at doses 14, 7 and 0.7 times the maximum daily human dose (1000 mg) based upon mg/m^2, and have revealed no evidence of harm to the fetus due to cefprozil. There are, however, no adequate and well-controlled studies in pregnant women. Because animal reproduction studies are not always predictive of human response, this drug should be used during pregnancy only if clearly needed.

LABOR AND DELIVERY

Cefprozil has not been studied for use during labor and delivery. Treatment should only be given if clearly needed.

NURSING MOTHERS

It is not known whether cefprozil is excreted in human milk. Because many drugs are excreted in human milk, caution should be exercised when cephprozil is administered to a nursing mother.

PEDIATRIC USE

Safety and effectiveness in children below the age of 6 months have not been established. However, accumulation of other cephalosporin antibiotics in newborn infants (resulting from prolonged drug half-life in this age group) has been reported.

GERIATRIC USE

Healthy geriatric volunteers (≥65 years old) who received a single 1 g dose of cefprozil had 35%-60% higher AUC and 40% lower renal clearance values when compared to healthy adult volunteers 20-40 years of age. In clinical studies, when geriatric patients received the usual recommended adult doses, clinical efficacy and safety were acceptable and comparable to results in non-geriatric adult patients.

DRUG INTERACTIONS:

Nephrotoxicity has been reported following concomitant administration of aminoglycoside antibiotics and cephalosporin antibiotics. Concomitant administration of probenecid doubled the AUC for cefprozil.

ADVERSE REACTIONS:

The adverse reactions to cefprozil are similar to those observed with other orally administered cephalosporins. Cefprozil was usually well tolerated in controlled clinical trials. Approximately 2% of patients discontinued cefprozil therapy due to adverse events.

The most common adverse effects observed in patients treated with cefprozil are:

Gastrointestinal: Diarrhea (2.9%), nausea (3.5%), vomiting (1%) and abdominal pain (1%).

Hepatobiliary: Elevations of AST (SGOT) (2%), ALT (SGPT) (2%), alkaline phosphatase (0.2%), and bilirubin values (<0.1%). As with some penicillins and some other cephalosporin antibiotics, cholestatic jaundice has been reported rarely.

Hypersensitivity: Rash (0.9%), urticaria (0.1%). Such reactions have been reported more frequently in children than in adults. Signs and symptoms usually occur a few days after initiation of therapy and subside within a few days after cessation of therapy.

CNS: Dizziness (1%). Hyperactivity, headache, nervousness, insomnia, confusion, and somnolence have been reported rarely (<1%). All were reversible.

Hematopoietic: Decreased leukocyte count (0.2%), eosinophilia (2.3%).

Renal: Elevated BUN (0.1%), serum creatinine (0.1%).

Other: Diaper rash and superinfection (1.5%), genital pruritus and vaginitis (1.6%).

CEPHALOSPORIN CLASS

In addition to the adverse reactions listed above which have been observed in patients treated with cefprozil, the following adverse reactions and altered laboratory tests have been reported for cephalosporin-class antibiotics:

Anaphylaxis, Stevens-Johnson syndrome, erythema multiforme, toxic epidermal necrolysis, serum-sickness like reaction, fever, renal dysfunction, toxic nephropathy, aplastic anemia, hemolytic anemia, hemorrhage, prolonged prothrombin time, positive Coombs' test, elevated LDH, pancytopenia, neutropenia, agranulocytosis, thrombocytopenia.

Several cephalosporins have been implicated in triggering seizures, particularly in patients with renal impairment, when the dosage was not reduced. (See DOSAGE AND ADMINISTRATION and OVERDOSAGE). If seizures associated with drug therapy occur, the drug should be discontinued. Anticonvulsant therapy can be given if clinically indicated.

OVERDOSAGE:

Cefprozil is eliminated primarily by the kidneys. In case of severe overdosage, especially in patients with compromised renal function, hemodialysis will aid in the removal of cefprozil from the body.

DOSAGE AND ADMINISTRATION:

Cephprozil is administered orally (TABLE 9):

TABLE 9

Population/Infection	Dosage (mg)	Duration (days)
Adults (13 years and older)		
Upper Respiratory Tract		
Pharyngitis/Tonsillitis	500 q 24h	10*
Lower Respiratory Tract		
Secondary Bacterial Infection of Acute Bronchitis and Acute Bacterial Exacerbation of Chronic Bronchitis	500 q 12h	10
Skin And Skin Structure		
Uncomplicated Skin and Skin Structure Infections	250 q 12 h or 500 q 24 h or 500 q 12 h	10
Children (2 Years - 12 Years)		
Upper Respiratory Tract		
Pharyngitis/Tonsillitis	7.5 mg/kg q 12h	10*
Infants & Children (6 months - 12 years)		
Upper Respiratory Tract		
Otitis Media (SeeINDICATIONS AND USAGE and CLINICAL STUDIES)	15 mg/kg q 12h	10

* In the treatment of infections due to *Streptococcus pyogenes*, Cefzil should be administered for at least 10 days.

DOSAGE FOR IMPAIRED RENAL FUNCTION

Cefprozil may be administered to patients with impaired renal function. The following dosage schedule should be used (TABLE 10):

HEPATIC IMPAIRMENT

No dosage adjustment is necessary for patients with impaired hepatic function.

Store at controlled room temperature, 59 to 86°F (15 to 30°C) prior to constitution.

TABLE 10

Creatinine Clearance (ml/min)	Dosage (mg)	Dosing Interval
30 - 120	standard	standard
0 - 30*	50% of standard	standard

* Cefprozil is in part removed by hemodialysis; therefore, cefprozil should be administered after the completion of hemodialysis.

REFERENCES:

1.National Committee for Clinical Laboratory Standards, *Performance Standards for Antimicrobial Disk Susceptibility Tests- Fourth Edition.* Approved Standard NCCLS Document M2-A4, Vol 10, No. 7, NCCLS, Villanova, PA, April, 1990.2.National Committee for Clinical Laboratory Standards, *Methods for Dilution Antimicrobial Susceptibility Tests for Bacteria that Grow Aerobically - Second Edition.* Approved Standard NCCLS Document M7-A2, Vol. 10, No. 8, NCCLS, Villanova, PA, April, 1990.

PATIENT INFORMATION:

Cefprozil is an antibiotic use to treat infections such as tonsillitis, ear infections, bronchitis, pneumonia or skin infections. This drug should not be used by those with allergies to the cephalosporin antibiotics. You should also consult with your pharmacist or physician if you are allergic to penicillin before taking this medication. This medication contains phenylalanine; caution is warranted for phenylketonuric patients. This medication has been known to falsely show glucose (sugar) in the urine. The most common side effects include nausea, vomiting and diarrhea. This medication should be taken for the full period prescribed. Even if you feel better after a day or two of medication, the full prescription should be taken to fully cure the infection.

HOW SUPPLIED - EQUIVALENTS NOT AVAILABLE:

Suspension - Oral - 125 mg/5ml

50 ml	$13.82	CEFZIL, Bristol Myers Squibb	00087-7718-40
75 ml	$20.64	CEFZIL, Bristol Myers Squibb	00087-7718-62
100 ml	$27.47	CEFZIL, Bristol Myers Squibb	00087-7718-64

Suspension - Oral - 250 mg/5ml

50 ml	$25.65	CEFZIL, Bristol Myers Squibb	00087-7719-40
75 ml	$37.71	CEFZIL, Bristol Myers Squibb	00087-7719-62
100 ml	$49.79	CEFZIL, Bristol Myers Squibb	00087-7719-64

Tablet, Uncoated - Oral - 250 mg

100's	$287.53	CEFZIL, Bristol Myers Squibb	00087-7720-60
100's	$317.56	CEFZIL, Bristol Myers Squibb	00087-7720-66

Tablet, Uncoated - Oral - 500 mg

50's	$280.75	CEFZIL, Bristol Myers Squibb	00087-7721-50
100's	$553.82	CEFZIL, Bristol Myers Squibb	00087-7721-60
100's	$612.72	CEFZIL, Bristol Myers Squibb	00087-7721-66

CEFTAZIDIME *(000692)*

CATEGORIES: Anti-Infectives; Antibiotics; Antimicrobials; Bone Infections; Cellulitis; Cephalosporins; Endometritis; Gynecologic Infections; Infections; Intra-Abdominal Infections; Joint Infections; Meningitis; Peritonitis; Pneumonia; Respiratory Tract Infections; Septicemia; Skin Infections; Urinary Tract Infections; Pregnancy Category B; Sales > $500 Million; FDA Approved 1985 Jul; Patent Expiration 1999 Dec

BRAND NAMES: **Fortaz**; Tazicef; Tazidime

FORMULARIES: BC-BS; WHO

PRIMARY ICD9: 136.9 (Unspecified Infections and Parasitic Diseases)

DESCRIPTION:

Ceftazidime is a semisynthetic, broad-spectrum, beta-lactam antibiotic for parenteral administration. It is the pentahydrate of pyridinium, 1-[[7-[[(2-amino-4-thiazolyl)[(1-carboxy-1-methylethoxy)imino]acetyl]amin o]-2-carboxy-8-oxo-5-thia-1-azabicyclo [4.2.0]oct-2-en-3-yl]methyl]-, hydroxide, inner salt, [6R-[6α,7β(Z)]].

The empirical formula is $C_{22}H_{32}N_6O_{12}S_2$, representing a molecular weight of 636.6.

Ceftazidime is a sterile, dry powdered mixture of ceftazidime pentahydrate and sodium carbonate. The sodium carbonate at a concentration of 118 mg/g of ceftazidime activity has been admixed to facilitate dissolution. The total sodium content of the mixture is approximately 54 mg (2.3 mEq)/g of ceftazidime activity.

Ceftazidime in sterile crystalline form is supplied in vials equivalent to 500 mg, 1 g, 2 g, or 6 g of anhydrous ceftazidime and in ADD-Vantage vials equivalent to 1 or 2 g of anhydrous ceftazidime. Solutions of ceftazidime range in color from light yellow to amber, depending on the diluent and volume used. The pH of freshly constituted solutions usually ranges from 5 to 8.

Ceftazidime is available as a frozen, iso-osmotic, sterile, nonpyrogenic solution with 1 or 2 g of ceftazidime as ceftazidime sodium premixed with approximately 2.2 or 1.6 g, respectively, of dextrose hydrous, USP. Dextrose has been added to adjust the osmolality. Sodium hydroxide is used to adjust pH and neutralize ceftazidime pentahydrate free acid to the sodium salt. The pH may have been adjusted with hydrochloric acid. Solutions of premixed ceftazidime range in color from light yellow to amber. The solution is intended for intravenous (IV) use after thawing to room temperature. The osmolality of the solution is approximately 300 mOsmol/kg, and the pH of thawed solutions ranges from 5 to 7.5.

The plastic container for the frozen solution is fabricated from a specially designed multilayer plastic, PL 2040. Solutions are in contact with the polyethylene layer of this container and can leach out certain chemical components of the plastic in very small amounts within the expiration period. The suitability of the plastic has been confirmed in tests in animals according to USP biological tests for plastic containers as well as by tissue culture toxicity studies.

CLINICAL PHARMACOLOGY:

After IV administration of 500-mg and 1-g doses of ceftazidime over 5 minutes to normal adult male volunteers, mean peak serum concentrations of 45 and 90 mcg/ml, respectively, were achieved. After IV infusion of 500-mg, 1-g, and 2-g doses of ceftazidime over 20 to 30 minutes to normal adult male volunteers, mean peak serum concentrations of 42, 69, and 170 mcg/ml, respectively, were achieved. The average serum concentrations following IV infusion of 500-mg, 1-g, and 2-g doses to these volunteers over an 8-hour interval are given in TABLE 1.

The absorption and elimination of ceftazidime were directly proportional to the size of the dose. The half-life following IV administration was approximately 1.9 hours. Less than 10% of ceftazidime was protein bound. The degree of protein binding was independent of

CLINICAL PHARMACOLOGY: *(cont'd)*

TABLE 1

Ceftazidime IV Dose	Serum Concentrations (mcg/ml) 0.5 h	1 h	2 h	4 h	8 h
500 mg	42	25	12	6	2
1 g	60	39	23	11	3
2 g	129	75	42	13	5

concentration. There was no evidence of accumulation of ceftazidime in the serum in individuals with normal renal function following multiple IV doses of 1 and 2 g every 8 hours for 10 days.

Following intramuscular (IM) administration of 500-mg and 1-g doses of ceftazidime to normal adult volunteers, the mean peak serum concentrations were 17 and 39 mcg/ml, respectively, at approximately 1 hour. Serum concentrations remained above 4 mcg/ml for 6 and 8 hours after the IM administration of 500-mg and 1-g doses, respectively. The half-life of ceftazidime in these volunteers was approximately 2 hours.

The presence of hepatic dysfunction had no effect on the pharmacokinetics of ceftazidime in individuals administered 2 g intravenously every 8 hours for 5 days. Therefore, a dosage adjustment from the normal recommended dosage is not required for patients with hepatic dysfunction, provided renal function is not impaired.

Approximately 80% to 90% of an IM or IV dose of ceftazidime is excreted unchanged by the kidneys over a 24-hour period. After the IV administration of single 500-mg or 1-g doses, approximately 50% of the dose appeared in the urine in the first 2 hours. An additional 20% was excreted between 2 and 4 hours after dosing, and approximately another 12% of the dose appeared in the urine between 4 and 8 hours later. The elimination of ceftazidime by the kidneys resulted in high therapeutic concentrations in the urine.

The mean renal clearance of ceftazidime was approximately 100 ml per minute. The calculated plasma clearance of approximately 115 ml per minute indicated nearly complete elimination of ceftazidime by the renal route. Administration of probenecid before dosing had no effect on the elimination kinetics of ceftazidime. This suggested that ceftazidime is eliminated by glomerular filtration and is not actively secreted by renal tubular mechanisms.

Since ceftazidime is eliminated almost solely by the kidneys, its serum half-life is significantly prolonged in patients with impaired renal function. Consequently, dosage adjustments in such patients as described in the DOSAGE AND ADMINISTRATIONsection are suggested.

Therapeutic concentrations of ceftazidime are achieved in the following body tissues and fluids (TABLE 2).

TABLE 2 Ceftazidime Concentrations in Body Tissues and Fluids

Tissue or Fluid	Dose/ Route	No. of Patients	Time of Sample Postdose	Average Tissue or Fluid Level (mcg/ml or mcg/g)
Urine	500 mg IM	6	0-2 h	2,100.0
	2 g IV	6	0-2 h	12,000.0
Bile	2 g IV	3	90 min	36.4
Synovial fluid	2 g IV	13	2 h	25.6
Peritoneal fluid	2 g IV	8	2 h	48.6
Sputum	1 g IV	8	1 h	9.0
Cerebrospinal fluid	2 g q8h IV	5	120 min	9.8
(inflamed meninges)	2 g q8h IV	6	180 min	9.4
Aqueous humor	2 g IV	13	1-3 h	11.0
Blister fluid	1 g IV	7	2-3 h	19.7
Lymphatic fluid	1 g IV	7	2-3 h	23.4
Bone	2 g IV	8	0.67 h	31.1
Heart muscle	2 g IV	35	30-280 min	12.7
Skin	2 g IV	22	30-180 min	6.6
Skeletal muscle	2 g IV	35	30-280 min	9.4
Myometrium	2 g IV	31	1-2 h	18.7

Microbiology: Ceftazidime is bactericidal in action, exerting its effect by inhibition of enzymes responsible for cell-wall synthesis. A wide range of gram-negative organisms is susceptible to ceftazidime*in vitro*, including strains resistant to gentamicin and other aminoglycosides. In addition, ceftazidime has been shown to be active against gram-positive organisms. It is highly stable to most clinically important beta-lactamases, plasmid or chromosomal, which are produced by both gram-negative and gram-positive organisms and, consequently, is active against many strains resistant to ampicillin and other cephalosporins.

Ceftazidime has been shown to be active against the following organisms both *in vitro* and in clinical infections (see INDICATIONS AND USAGE.)

Aerobes, Gram-negative: *Citrobacter* spp., including *Citrobacter freundii* and *Citrobacter diversus; Enterobacter* spp., including *Enterobacter cloacae* and *Enterobacter aerogenes; Escherichia coli; Haemophilus influenzae*, including ampicillin-resistant strains; *Klebsiella* spp. (including *Klebsiella pneumoniae*); *Neisseria meningitidis; Proteus mirabilis; Proteus vulgaris; Pseudomonas* spp. (including *Pseudomonas aeruginosa*); and *Serratia* spp.

Aerobes, Gram-positive: *Staphylococcus aureus*, including penicillinase- and non-penicillinase-producing strains;*Streptococcus agalactiae* (group B streptococci); *Streptococcus pneumoniae;* and *Streptococcus pyogenes* (group A beta-hemolytic streptococci).

Anaerobes: *Bacteroides* spp. (NOTE: many strains of *Bacteroides fragilis* are resistant).

Ceftazidime has been shown to be active *in vitro* against most strains of the following organisms; however, the clinical significance of these data is unknown: *Acinetobacter* spp.; *Clostridium* spp. (not including *Clostridium difficile*); *Haemophilus parainfluenzae; Morganella morganii* (formerly *Proteus morganii); Neisseria gonorrhoeae; Peptococcus* spp.; *Peptostreptococcus* spp.; *Providencia* spp. (including *Providencia rettgeri*, formerly *Proteus rettgeri*); *Salmonella* spp.;*Shigella* spp.; *Staphylococcus epidermis*; and *Yersinia enterocolitica*.

Ceftazidime and the aminoglycosides have been shown to be synergistic*in vitro* against *Pseudomonas aeruginosa* and the Enterobacteriaceae. Ceftazidime and carbenicillin have also been shown to be synergistic *in vitro* against *Pseudomonas aeruginosa*.

Ceftazidime is not active *in vitro* against methicillin-resistant staphylococci; *Streptococcus faecalis* and many other enterococci;*Listeria monocytogenes*; *Campylobacter* spp.; or *Clostridium difficile*.

SUSCEPTIBILITY TESTING

Diffusion Techniques: Quantitative methods that require measurement of zone diameters give an estimate of antibiotic susceptibility. One such procedure[1-3] has been recommended for use with disks to test susceptibility to ceftazidime.

Reports from the laboratory giving results of the standard single-disk susceptibility test with a 30-mcg ceftazidime disk should be interpreted according to the following criteria:

Susceptible organisms produce zones of 18 mm or greater, indicating that the test organism is likely to respond to therapy.

CLINICAL PHARMACOLOGY: *(cont'd)*

Organisms that produce zones of 15 to 17 mm are expected to be susceptible if high dosage is used or if the infection is confined to tissues and fluids (*e.g.,* urine) in which high antibiotic levels are attained.

Resistant organisms produce zones of 14 mm or less, indicating that other therapy should be selected.

Organisms should be tested with the ceftazidime disk since ceftazidime has been shown by *in vitro* tests to be active against certain strains found resistant when other beta-lactam disks are used.

Standardized procedures require the use of laboratory control organisms. The 30-mcg ceftazidime disk should give zone diameters between 25 and 32 mm for *Escherichia coli* ATCC 25922. For *Pseudomonas aeruginosa* ATCC 27853, the zone diameters should be between 22 and 29 mm. For *Staphylococcus aureus* ATCC 25923, the zone diameters should be between 16 and 20 mm.

Dilution Techniques: In other susceptibility testing procedures, e.g., ICS agar dilution or the equivalent, a bacterial isolate may be considered susceptible if the minimum inhibitory concentration (MIC) value for ceftazidime is not more than 16 mcg/ml. Organisms are considered resistant to ceftazidime if the MIC is ≥64 mcg/ml. Organisms having an MIC value of < 64 mcg/ml but > 16 mcg/ml are expected to be susceptible if high dosage is used or if the infection is confined to tissues and fluids (*e.g.,* urine) in which high antibiotic levels are attained.

As with standard diffusion methods, dilution procedures require the use of laboratory control organisms. Standard ceftazidime powder should give MIC values in the range of 4 to 16 mcg/ml for *Staphylococcus aureus* ATCC 25923. For *Escherichia coli* ATCC 25922, the MIC range should be between 0.125 and 0.5 mcg/ml. For *Pseudomonas aeruginosa*ATCC 27853, the MIC range should be between 0.5 and 2 mcg/ml.

INDICATIONS AND USAGE:

Ceftazidime is indicated for the treatment of patients with infections caused by susceptible strains of the designated organisms in the following diseases:

Lower Respiratory Tract Infections, including pneumonia, caused by *Pseudomonas aeruginosa* and other *Pseudomonas* spp.; *Haemophilus influenzae,* including ampicillin-resistant strains; *Klebsiella* spp.; *Enterobacter* spp.; *Proteus mirabilis; Escherichia coli; Serratia* spp.; *Citrobacter* spp.;*Streptococcus pneumoniae*; and *Staphylococcus aureus* (methicillin-susceptible strains).

Skin and Skin-Structure Infections caused by *Pseudomonas aeruginosa; Klebsiella* spp.; *Escherichia coli; Proteus* spp., including *Proteus mirabilis* and indole-positive *Proteus;Enterobacter* spp.; *Serratia* spp.; *Staphylococcus aureus* (methicillin-susceptible strains); and *Streptococcus pyogenes* (group A beta-hemolytic streptococci).

Urinary Tract Infections, both complicated and uncomplicated, caused by *Pseudomonas aeruginosa*; *Enterobacter* spp.;*Proteus* spp., including *Proteus mirabilis* and indole-positive *Proteus; Klebsiella* spp.; and *Escherichia coli.*

Bacterial Septicemia caused by *Pseudomonas aeruginosa; Klebsiella* spp.; *Haemophilus influenzae; Escherichia coli; Serratia* spp.; *Streptococcus pneumoniae*; and *Staphylococcus aureus* (methicillin-susceptible strains).

Bone and Joint Infections caused by *Pseudomonas aeruginosa; Klebsiella* spp.; *Enterobacter* spp.; and *Staphylococcus aureus* (methicillin-susceptible strains).

Gynecologic Infections, including endometritis, pelvic cellulitis, and other infections of the female genital tract caused by*Escherichia coli.*

Intra-abdominal Infections, including peritonitis caused by*Escherichia coli, Klebsiella* spp., and *Staphylococcus aureus* (methicillin-susceptible strains) and polymicrobial infections caused by aerobic and anaerobic organisms and *Bacteroides* spp. (many strains of *Bacteroides fragilis* are resistant).

Central Nervous System Infections, including meningitis, caused by *Haemophilus influenzae* and *Neisseria meningitidis.* Ceftazidime has also been used successfully in a limited number of cases of meningitis due to *Pseudomonas aeruginosa* and *Streptococcus pneumoniae.*

Specimens for bacteria cultures should be obtained before therapy in order to isolate and identify causative organisms and to determine their susceptibility to ceftazidime. Therapy may be instituted before results of susceptibility studies are known; however, once these results become available, the antibiotic treatment should be adjusted accordingly.

As with other extended-spectrum cephalosporins and penicillins, some strains of *Enterobacter* spp. can develop resistance during ceftazidime therapy due to induced type-1 beta-lactamase production. When clinically appropriate during therapy of *Enterobacter* spp. infections, periodic susceptibility testing should be considered.

Ceftazidime may be used alone in cases of confirmed or suspected sepsis. Ceftazidime has been used successfully in clinical trials as empiric therapy in cases where various concomitant therapies with other antibiotics have been used.

Ceftazidime may also be used concomitantly with other antibiotics, such as aminoglycosides, vancomycin, and clindamycin; in severe and life-threatening infections; and in the immunocompromised patient. When such concomitant treatment is appropriate, prescribing information in the labeling for the other antibiotics should be followed. The dose depends on the severity of the infection and the patient's condition.

CONTRAINDICATIONS:

Ceftazidime is contraindicated in patients who have shown hypersensitivity to ceftazidime or the cephalosporin group of antibiotics.

WARNINGS:

BEFORE THERAPY WITH CEFTAZIDIME IS INSTITUTED, CAREFUL INQUIRY SHOULD BE MADE TO DETERMINE WHETHER THE PATIENT HAS HAD PREVIOUS HYPERSENSITIVITY REACTIONS TO CEFTAZIDIME, CEPHALOSPORINS, PENICILLINS, OR OTHER DRUGS. IF THIS PRODUCT IS TO BE GIVEN TO PENICILLIN-SENSITIVE PATIENTS, CAUTION SHOULD BE EXERCISED BECAUSE CROSS-HYPERSENSITIVITY AMONG BETA-LACTAM ANTIBIOTICS HAS BEEN CLEARLY DOCUMENTED AND MAY OCCUR IN UP TO 10% OF PATIENTS WITH A HISTORY OF PENICILLIN ALLERGY. IF AN ALLERGIC REACTION TO CEFTAZIDIME OCCURS, DISCONTINUE THE DRUG. SERIOUS ACUTE HYPERSENSITIVITY REACTIONS MAY REQUIRE TREATMENT WITH EPINEPHRINE AND OTHER EMERGENCY MEASURES, INCLUDING OXYGEN, IV FLUIDS, IV ANTIHISTAMINES, CORTICOSTEROIDS, PRESSOR AMINES, AND AIRWAY MANAGEMENT, AS CLINICALLY INDICATED.

Pseudomembranous colitis has been reported with nearly all antibacterial agents, including ceftazidime, and may range from mild to life threatening. Therefore, it is important to consider this diagnosis in patients who present with diarrhea subsequent to the administration of antibacterial agents.

Treatment with antibacterial agents alters the normal flora of the colon and may permit overgrowth of clostridia. Studies indicate that a toxin produced by *Clostridium difficile* is a primary cause of "antibiotic-associated colitis."

WARNINGS: *(cont'd)*

After the diagnosis of pseudomembranous colitis has been established, therapeutic measures should be initiated. Mild cases of pseudomembranous colitis usually respond to discontinuation of the drug alone. In moderate to severe cases, consideration should be given to management with fluids and electrolytes, protein supplementation, and treatment with an antibacterial drug effective against *Clostridium difficile*.

Elevated levels of ceftazidime in patients with renal insufficiency can lead to seizures, encephalopathy, asterixis, and neuromuscular excitability (see PRECAUTIONS.)

PRECAUTIONS:

General: Ceftazidime has not been shown to be nephrotoxic; however, high and prolonged serum antibiotic concentrations can occur from usual dosages in patients with transient or persistent reduction of urinary output because of renal insufficiency. The total daily dosage should be reduced when ceftazidime is administered to patients with renal insufficiency (see DOSAGE AND ADMINISTRATION.) Elevated levels of ceftazidime in these patients can lead to seizures, encephalopathy, asterixis, and neuromuscular excitability. Continued dosage should be determined by degree of renal impairment, severity of infection, and susceptibility of the causative organisms.

As with other antibiotics, prolonged use of ceftazidime may result in overgrowth of nonsusceptible organisms. Repeated evaluation of the patient's condition is essential. If superinfection occurs during therapy, appropriate measures should be taken.

Cephalosporins may be associated with a fall in prothrombin activity. Those at risk include patients with renal and hepatic impairment, or poor nutritional state, as well as patients receiving a protracted course of antimicrobial therapy. Prothrombin time should be monitored in patients at risk and exogenous vitamin K administered as indicated.

Ceftazidime should be prescribed with caution in individuals with a history of gastrointestinal disease, particularly colitis.

Intra-arterial administration may lead to arteriospasm and necrosis and should therefore be avoided.

Drug/Laboratory Test Interactions: The administration of ceftazidime may result in a false-positive reaction for glucose in the urine when using Clinitest, Benedict's solution, or Fehling's solution. It is recommended that glucose tests based on enzymatic glucose oxidase reactions (such as Clinistix or Tes-Tape) be used.

Carcinogenesis, Mutagenesis, and Impairment of Fertility: Long-term studies in animals have not been performed to evaluate carcinogenic potential. However, a mouse Micronucleus test and an Ames test were both negative for mutagenic effects.

Pregnancy, Teratogenic Effects, Pregnancy Category B: Reproduction studies have been performed in mice and rats at doses up to 40 times the human dose and have revealed no evidence of impaired fertility or harm to the fetus due to ceftazidime. There are, however, no adequate and well-controlled studies in pregnant women. Because animal reproduction studies are not always predictive of human response, this drug should be used during pregnancy only if clearly needed.

Nursing Mothers: Ceftazidime is excreted in human milk in low concentrations. Caution should be exercised when ceftazidime is administered to a nursing woman.

Pediatric Use: (see DOSAGE AND ADMINISTRATION.)

DRUG INTERACTIONS:

Nephrotoxicity has been reported following concomitant administration of cephalosporins with aminoglycoside antibiotics or potent diuretics such as furosemide. Renal function should be carefully monitored, especially if higher dosages of the aminoglycosides are to be administered or if therapy is prolonged, because of the potential nephrotoxicity and ototoxicity of aminoglycosidic antibiotics. Nephrotoxicity and ototoxicity were not noted when ceftazidime was given alone in clinical trials.

Chloramphenicol has been shown to be antagonistic to beta-lactam antibiotics, including ceftazidime, based on *in vitro* studies and time kill curves with enteric gram-negative bacilli. Due to the possibility of antagonism *in vivo*, particularly when bactericidal activity is desired, this drug combination should be avoided.

ADVERSE REACTIONS:

Ceftazidime is generally well tolerated. The incidence of adverse reactions associated with the administration of ceftazidime was low in clinical trials. The most common were local reactions following IV injection and allergic and gastrointestinal reactions. Other adverse reactions were encountered infrequently. No disulfiramlike reactions were reported.

The following adverse effects from clinical trials were considered to be either related to ceftazidime therapy or were of uncertain etiology:

Local Effects: Reported in fewer than 2% of patients, were phlebitis and inflammation at the site of injection (1 in 69 patients).

Hypersensitivity Reactions: Reported in 2% of patients, were pruritus, rash, and fever. Immediate reactions, generally manifested by rash and/or pruritus, occurred in 1 in 285 patients. Toxic epidermal necrolysis, Stevens-Johnson syndrome, and erythema multiforme have also been reported with cephalosporin antibiotics, including ceftazidime. Angioedema and anaphylaxis (bronchospasm and/or hypotension) have been reported very rarely.

Gastrointestinal Symptoms: Reported in fewer than 2% of patients, were diarrhea (1 in 78), nausea (1 in 156), vomiting (1 in 500), and abdominal pain (1 in 416). The onset of pseudomembranous colitis symptoms may occur during or after treatment (see WARNINGS.)

Central Nervous System Reactions: (fewer than 1%) included headache, dizziness, and paresthesia. Seizures have been reported with several cephalosporins, including ceftazidime. In addition, encephalopathy, asterixis, and neuromuscular excitability have been reported in renally impaired patients treated with unadjusted dosing regimens of ceftazidime (see PRECAUTIONS, General.)

Less Frequent Adverse Events: (fewer than 1%) were candidiasis (including oral thrush) and vaginitis. *Hematologic:* Rare cases of hemolytic anemia have been reported.

Laboratory Test Changes: noted during ceftazidime clinical trials were transient and included: eosinophilia (1 in 13), positive Coombs' test without hemolysis (1 in 23), thrombocytosis (1 in 45), and slight elevations in one or more of the hepatic enzymes, aspartate aminotransferase (AST, SGOT) (1 in 16), alanine aminotransferase (ALT, SGPT) (1 in 15), LDH (1 in 18), GGT (1 in 19), and alkaline phosphatase (1 in 23). As with some other cephalosporins, transient elevations of blood urea, blood urea nitrogen, and/or serum creatinine were observed occasionally. Transient leukopenia, neutropenia, agranulocytosis, thrombocytopenia, and lymphocytosis were seen very rarely. Elevations in hepatic enzymes (SGOT, SGPT, LDH, GGT, alkaline phosphatase) have been reported postmarketing.

In addition to the adverse reactions listed above that have been observed in patients treated with ceftazidime, the following adverse reactions and altered laboratory tests have been reported for cephalosporin-class antibiotics:

Adverse Reactions: Urticaria, colitis, renal dysfunction, toxic nephropathy, hepatic dysfunction including cholestasis, aplastic anemia, hemorrhage.

Altered Laboratory Tests: Prolonged prothrombin time, false-positive test for urinary glucose, elevated bilirubin, pancytopenia.

OVERDOSAGE:

Ceftazidime overdosage has occurred in patients with renal failure. Reactions have included seizure activity, encephalopathy, asterixis, and neuromuscular excitability. Patients who receive an acute overdosage should be carefully observed and given supportive treatment. In the presence of renal insufficiency, hemodialysis or peritoneal dialysis may aid in the removal of ceftazidime from the body.

DOSAGE AND ADMINISTRATION:

Dosage: The usual adult dosage is 1 gram administered intravenously or intramuscularly every 8 to 12 hours. The dosage and route should be determined by the susceptibility of the causative organisms, the severity of infection, and the condition and renal function of the patient.

The guidelines for dosage of ceftazidime are listed in TABLE 3. The following dosage schedule is recommended.

TABLE 3 Recommended Dosage Schedule

Adults **Usual recommended dosage**	**Dose** **1 gram IV or IM**	**Frequency** **q8-12h**
Uncomplicated urinary tract infections	250 mg IV or IM	q12h
Bone and joint infections	2 grams IV	q12h
Complicated urinary tract infections	500 mg IV or IM	q8-12h
Uncomplicated pneumonia; mild skin and skin-structure infections	500 mg-1 gram IV or IM	q8h
Serious gynecologic and intra-abdominal infections	2 grams IV	q8h
Meningitis	2 grams IV	q8h
Very severe life-threatening infections, especially in immunocompromised patients	2 grams IV	q8h
Lung infections caused by *Pseudomonas* spp. in patients with cystic fibrosis with normal renal function*	30-50 mg/kg IV to a maximum of 6 grams per day	q8h
Neonates (0-4 weeks)	30 mg/kg IV	q12h
Infants and children (1 month-12 years)	30-50 mg/kg IV to a maximum of 6 grams per day†	q8h

* Although clinical improvement has been shown, bacteriologic cures cannot be expected in patients with chronic respiratory disease and cystic fibrosis.
† The higher dose should be reserved for immunocompromised children or children with cystic fibrosis or meningitis.

Impaired Hepatic Function: No adjustment in dosage is required for patients with hepatic dysfunction.

Impaired Renal Function: Ceftazidime is excreted by the kidneys, almost exclusively by glomerular filtration. Therefore, in patients with impaired renal function (glomerular filtration rate [GFR] <50 ml per minute), it is recommended that the dosage of ceftazidime be reduced to compensate for its slower excretion. In patients with suspected renal insufficiency, an initial loading dose of 1 gram of ceftazidime may be given. An estimate of GFR should be made to determine the appropriate maintenance dose. The recommended dosage is presented in TABLE 4.

TABLE 4 Recommended Maintenance Dosages of Ceftazidime in Renal Insufficiency

Creatinine Clearance (ml/min)	Recommended Unit Dose of Ceftazidime	Frequency of Dosing
50-31	1 gram	q12h
30-16	1 gram	q24h
15-6	500 mg	q24h
<5	500 mg	q48h

NOTE: IF THE DOSE RECOMMENDED IN TABLE 3 ABOVE IS LOWER THAN THAT RECOMMENDED FOR PATIENTS WITH RENAL INSUFFICIENCY AS OUTLINED IN TABLE 4, THE LOWER DOSE SHOULD BE USED.

When only serum creatinine is available, the following formula (Cockcroft's equation)[4] may be used to estimate creatinine clearance. The serum creatinine should represent a steady state of renal function TABLE 5:

TABLE 5

Males: Creatinine clearance (ml/min) = [Weight (kg) × (140 - age)] ÷ [72 × serum creatinine (mg/dl)]
Females: 0.85 × male value

In patients with severe infections who would normally receive 6 grams of ceftazidime daily were it not for renal insufficiency, the unit dose given in the table above may be increased by 50% or the dosing frequency may be increased appropriately. Further dosing should be determined by therapeutic monitoring, severity of the infection, and susceptibility of the causative organism.

In children as for adults, the creatinine clearance should be adjusted for body surface area or lean body mass, and the dosing frequency should be reduced in cases of renal insufficiency.

In patients undergoing hemodialysis, a loading dose of 1 gram is recommended, followed by 1 gram after each hemodialysis period.

Ceftazidime can also be used in patients undergoing intraperitoneal dialysis and continuous ambulatory peritoneal dialysis. In such patients, a loading dose of 1 gram of ceftazidime may be given, followed by 500 mg every 24 hours. In addition to IV use, ceftazidime can be incorporated in the dialysis fluid at a concentration of 250 mg for 2 l of dialysis fluid.

Note: Generally ceftazidime should be continued for 2 days after the signs and symptoms of infection have disappeared, but in complicated infections longer therapy may be required.

Administration: Ceftazidime may be given intravenously or by deep IM injection into a large muscle mass such as the upper outer quadrant of the gluteus maximus or lateral part of the thigh.

Intramuscular Administration: For IM administration, ceftazidime should be constituted with one of the following diluents: sterile water for injection, bacteriostatic water for injection, or 0.5% or 1% lidocaine hydrochloride injection. Refer to TABLE 6.

Intravenous Administration: The IV route is preferable for patients with bacterial septicemia, bacterial meningitis, peritonitis, or other severe or life-threatening infections, or for patients who may be poor risks because of lowered resistance resulting from such debilitating conditions as malnutrition, trauma, surgery, diabetes, heart failure, or malignancy, particularly if shock is present or pending.

For direct intermittent IV administration, constitute ceftazidime as directed in TABLE 6 with sterile water for injection. Slowly inject directly into the vein over a period of 3 to 5 minutes or give through the tubing of an administration set while the patient is also receiving one of the compatible IV fluids (see Compatibility And Stability).

DOSAGE AND ADMINISTRATION: *(cont'd)*

For IV infusion, constitute the 1- or 2-gram infusion pack with 100 ml of sterile water for injection or one of the compatible IV fluids listed under Compatibility And Stability. Alternatively, constitute the 500-mg, 1-gram, or 2-gram vial and add an appropriate quantity of the resulting solution to an IV container with one of the compatible IV fluids.

Intermittent IV infusion with a Y-type administration set can be accomplished with compatible solutions. However, during infusion of a solution containing ceftazidime, it is desirable to discontinue the other solution.

ADD-Vantage vials are to be constituted only with 50 or 100 ml of 5% dextrose injection, 0.9% sodium chloride injection, 0.45% sodium chloride injection in Abbott ADD-Vantage flexible diluent containers (see Instructions for Constitution). ADD-Vantage vials that have been joined to Abbott ADD-Vantage diluent containers and activated to dissolve the drug are stable for 24 hours at room temperature or for 7 days under refrigeration. Joined vials that have not been activated may be used within a 14-day period; this period corresponds to that for use of Abbott ADD-Vantage containers following removal of the outer packaging (overwrap).

Freezing solutions of ceftazidime in the ADD-Vantage system is not recommended.

TABLE 6 Preparation of Ceftazidime Solutions

Size	Amount of Diluent to Be Added (ml)	Approximate Available Volume (ml)	Approximate Ceftazidime Concentration (mg/ml)
Intramuscular			
500-mg vial	1.5	1.8	280
1-gram vial	3.0	3.6	280
Intravenous			
500-mg vial	5.0	5.3	100
1-gram vial	10.0	10.6	100
2-gram vial	10.0	11.5	170
Infusion pack			
1-gram vial	100*	100	10
2-gram vial	100*	100	20
Pharmacy bulk package			
6-gram vial	26	30	200

* **Note:** Addition should be in two stages (see Instructions for Constitution).

All vials of ceftazidime as supplied are under reduced pressure. When ceftazidime is dissolved, carbon dioxide is released and a positive pressure develops. For ease of use please follow the recommended techniques of constitution described on the detachable Instructions for Constitution section of the PATIENT PACKAGE INSERT.

Solutions of ceftazidime, like those of most beta-lactam antibiotics, should not be added to solutions of aminoglycoside antibiotics because of potential interaction.

However, if concurrent therapy with ceftazidime and an aminoglycoside is indicated, each of these antibiotics can be administered separately to the same patient.

Directions for Use of Ceftazidime Frozen in Galaxy Plastic Containers: Ceftazidime supplied as a frozen, sterile, iso-osmotic, nonpyrogenic solution in plastic containers is to be administered after thawing either as a continuous or intermittent IV infusion. The thawed solution is stable for 24 hours at room temperature or for 7 days if stored under refrigeration. **Do not refreeze.**

Thaw container at room temperature (25°C) or under refrigeration (5°C). Do not force thaw by immersion in water baths or by microwave irradiation. Components of the solution may precipitate in the frozen state and will dissolve upon reaching room temperature with little or no agitation. Potency is not affected. Mix after solution has reached room temperature. Check for minute leaks by squeezing bag firmly. Discard bag if leaks are found as sterility may be impaired. Do not add supplementary medication. Do not use unless solution is clear and seal is intact.

Use sterile equipment.

Caution: Do not use plastic containers in series connections. Such use could result in air embolism due to residual air being drawn from the primary container before administration of the fluid from the secondary container is complete.

PREPARATION FOR ADMINISTRATION:

1. Suspend container from eyelet support.

2. Remove protector from outlet port at bottom of container.

3. Attach administration set. Refer to complete directions accompanying set.

COMPATIBILITY AND STABILITY

Intramuscular: Ceftazidime, when constituted as directed with sterile water for injection, bacteriostatic water for injection, or 0.5% or 1% lidocaine hydrochloride injection, maintains satisfactory potency for 24 hours at room temperature or for 7 days under refrigeration. Solutions in sterile water for injection that are frozen immediately after constitution in the original container are stable for 3 months when stored at -20°C. Once thawed, solutions should not be refrozen. Thawed solutions may be stored for up to 8 hours at room temperature or for 4 days in a refrigerator.

Intravenous: Ceftazidime, when constituted as directed with sterile water for injection, maintains satisfactory potency for 24 hours at room temperature or for 7 days under refrigeration. Solutions in sterile water for injection in the infusion vial or in 0.9% sodium chloride injection in Viaflex small-volume containers that are frozen immediately after constitution are stable for 6 months when stored at -20°C. Do not force thaw by immersion in water baths or by microwave irradiation. Once thawed, solutions should not be refrozen. Thawed solutions may be stored for up to 24 hours at room temperature or for 7 days in a refrigerator. More concentrated solutions in sterile water for injection in the original container that are frozen immediately after constitution are stable for 3 months when stored at -20°C. Once thawed, solutions should not be refrozen. Thawed solutions may be stored for up to 8 hours at room temperature or for 4 days in a refrigerator.

Ceftazidime is compatible with the more commonly used IV infusion fluids. Solutions at concentrations between 1 and 40 mg/ml in 0.9% sodium chloride injection; 1/6 M sodium lactate injection; 5% dextrose injection; 5% dextrose and 0.225% sodium chloride injection; 5% dextrose and 0.45% sodium chloride injection; 5% dextrose and 0.9% sodium chloride injection; 10% dextrose injection; Ringer's injection, USP; lactated Ringer's injection, USP; 10% invert sugar in water for injection; and Normosol-M in 5% dextrose injection may be stored for up to 24 hours at room temperature or for 7 days if refrigerated.

The 1- and 2-g ceftazidime ADD-Vantage vials, when diluted in 50 or 100 ml of 5% dextrose injection, 0.9% sodium chloride injection, or 0.45% sodium chloride injection, may be stored for up to 24 hours at room temperature or for 7 days under refrigeration.

Ceftazidime is less stable in sodium bicarbonate injection than in other IV fluids. It is not recommended as a diluent. Solutions of ceftazidime in 5% dextrose injection and 0.9% sodium chloride injection are stable for at least 6 hours at room temperature in plastic tubing, drip chambers, and volume control devices of common IV infusion sets.

DOSAGE AND ADMINISTRATION: *(cont'd)*

Ceftazidime at a concentration of 4 mg/ml has been found compatible for 24 hours at room temperature or for 7 days under refrigeration in 0.9% sodium chloride injection or 5% dextrose injection when admixed with: cefuroxime sodium (Zinacef) 3 mg/ml; heparin 10 or 50 U/ml; or potassium chloride 10 or 40 mEq/l.

Vancomycin solution exhibits a physical incompatibility when mixed with a number of drugs, including ceftazidime. The likelihood of precipitation with ceftazidime is dependent on the concentrations of vancomycin and ceftazidime present. It is therefore recommended, when both drugs are to be administered by intermittent IV infusion, that they be given separately, flushing the IV lines (with one of the compatible IV fluids) between the administration of these two agents.

Note: Parenteral drug products should be inspected visually for particulate matter before administration whenever solution and container permit.

As with other cephalosporins, ceftazidime powder as well as solutions tend to darken, depending on storage conditions; within the stated recommendations, however, product potency is not adversely affected.

Storage: Ceftazidime in the dry state should be stored between 15° and 30°C (59° and 86°F) and protected from light.

Ceftazidime frozen as a premixed solution of ceftazidime sodium should not be stored above -20°C.

REFERENCES:

1. Bauer AW, Kirby WMM, Sherris JC, Turck M. Antibiotic susceptibility testing by a standardized single disk method. *Am J Clin Pathol.* 1966;45:493-496. **2.** National Committee for Clinical Laboratory Standards. *Approved Standard: Performance Standards for Antimicrobial Disc Susceptibility Tests.* (M2-A3). December 1984. **3.** Certification procedure for antibiotic sensitivity discs (21 CFR 460.1). *Federal Register.*May 30, 1974;39:19182-19184. **4.** Cockcroft DW, Gault MH. Prediction of creatinine clearance from serum creatinine. *Nephron.*1976;16:31-41.

PATIENT PACKAGE INSERT:

INSTRUCTIONS FOR CONSTITUTION

Vials: 500 mg IM/IV, 1 g IM/IV, 2 g IV

1. Insert the syringe needle through the vial closure and inject the recommended volume of diluent. The vacuum may assist entry of the diluent. Remove the syringe needle.

2. Shake to dissolve; a clear solution will be obtained in 1 to 2 minutes.

3. Invert the vial. Ensuring that the syringe plunger is fully depressed, insert the needle through the vial closure and withdraw the total volume of solution into the syringe (the pressure in the vial may aid withdrawal).

Ensure that the needle remains within the solution and does not enter the headspace. The withdrawn solution may contain some bubbles of carbon dioxide.

Note: As with the administration of all parenteral products, accumulated gases should be expressed from the syringe immediately before injection of ceftazidime.

Infusion Pack: 1 g, 2 g

1. Insert the syringe needle through the vial closure and inject 10 ml of diluent. The vacuum may assist entry of the diluent. Remove the syringe needle.

2. Shake to dissolve; a clear solution will be obtained in 1 to 2 minutes.

3. Insert a gas-relief needle through the vial closure to relieve the internal pressure. With the gas-relief needle in position, add the remaining 90 ml of diluent. Remove the gas-relief needle and syringe needle; shake the vial and set up the infusion in the normal way.

Note: To preserve product sterility, it is important that a gas-relief needle is *not* inserted through the vial closure before the product has dissolved.

ADD-Vantage Vials: 1 g, 2 g

To Open Diluent Container: Peel the corner of the ADD-Vantage diluent overwrap and remove flexible diluent container. Some opacity of the plastic flexible container due to moisture absorption during the sterilization process may be observed. This is normal and does not affect the solution quality or safety. The opacity will diminish gradually.

To Assemble Vial and Flexible Diluent Container (Use Aseptic Technique):

1. Remove the protective covers from the top of the vial and the vial port on the diluent container as follows:

a. To remove the breakaway vial cap, swing the pull ring over the top of the vial and pull down far enough to start the opening, then pull straight up to remove the cap. *Note:* Once the breakaway cap has been removed, do not access vial with syringe.

b. To remove the vial port cover, grasp the tab on the pull ring, pull up to break the three tie strings, then pull back to remove the cover.

2. Screw the vial into the vial port until it will go no further. THE VIAL MUST BE SCREWED IN TIGHTLY TO ASSURE A SEAL. This occurs approximately one-half turn (180°) after the first audible click. The clicking sound does not assure a seal; the vial must be turned as far as it will go. *Note:* Once vial is seated, do not attempt to remove.

3. Recheck the vial to assure that it is tight by trying to turn it further in the direction of assembly.

4. Label appropriately.

To Prepare Admixture:

1. Squeeze the bottom of the diluent container gently to inflate the portion of the container surrounding the end of the drug vial.

2. With the other hand, push the drug vial down into the container, telescoping the walls of the container. Grasp the inner cap of the vial through the walls of the container.

3. Pull the inner cap from the drug vial. Verify that the rubber stopper has been pulled out, allowing the drug and diluent to mix.

4. Mix container contents thoroughly and use within the specified time.

Preparation for Administration (Use Aseptic Technique):

1. Confirm the activation and admixture of vial contents.

2. Check for leaks by squeezing container firmly. If leaks are found, discard unit as sterility may be impaired.

3. Close flow control clamp of administration set.

4. Remove cover from outlet port at bottom of container.

5. Insert piercing pin of administration set into port with a twisting motion until the pin is firmly seated. *Note:*See full directions on administration set carton.

6. Lift the free end of the hanger loop on the bottom of the vial, breaking the two tie strings. Bend the loop outward to lock it in the upright position, then suspend container from hanger.

7. Squeeze and release drip chamber to establish proper fluid level in chamber.

8. Open flow control clamp and clear air from set. Close clamp.

9. Attach set to venipuncture device. If device is not indwelling, prime and make venipuncture.

10. Regulate rate of administration with flow control clamp.

PATIENT PACKAGE INSERT: *(cont'd)*

WARNING: DO NOT USE FLEXIBLE CONTAINER IN SERIES CONNECTIONS.

Pharmacy Bulk Package: 6 g

1. Insert the syringe needle through the vial closure and inject 26 ml of diluent. The vacuum may assist entry of the diluent. Remove the syringe needle.

2. Shake to dissolve; a clear solution containing approximately 1 g of ceftazidime activity per 5 ml will be obtained in 1 to 2 minutes.

3. Insert a gas-relief needle through the vial closure to relieve the internal pressure. Remove the gas-relief needle before extracting any solution. *Note:*To preserve product sterility, it is important that a gas-relief needle is *not* inserted through the vial closure before the product has dissolved.

HOW SUPPLIED - RATED THERAPEUTICALLY EQUIVALENT:

Injection, Dry-Soln - Intramuscular; - 1 gm

1 gm x 24	$375.72	TAZIDIME, Lilly	00002-7245-24
1 gm x 25	$367.68	TAZIDIME, Lilly	00002-7290-25
10 vials x 1	$145.88	TAZIDIME, Lilly	00002-7238-10

Injection, Dry-Soln - Intramuscular; - 1 gm/vial

10's	**$145.87**	**FORTAZ, Glaxo Wellcome**	**00173-0380-32**
20 ml x 25	$370.50	TAZICEF 1, SKB Pharms	00007-5082-76
20 ml x 25	$439.97	TAZICEF 1, SKB Pharms	00007-5082-16
25 vials	**$355.67**	**FORTAZ, Glaxo Wellcome**	**00173-0378-35**
25 vials x 1	$355.68	TAZIDIME, Lilly	00002-7231-25
25's	**$367.68**	**Fortaz, Glaxo Wellcome**	**00173-0434-00**
25's	$445.31	Tazicef, SKB Pharms	00007-5090-16
50 ml x 24	$402.00	TAZICEF IN DEXTROSE, SKB Pharms	00007-5088-04
50 ml x 24	**$406.24**	**FORTAZ, Glaxo Wellcome**	**00173-0412-00**
100 ml x 10	$152.00	TAZICEF 1, SKB Pharms	00007-5083-76
100 ml x 10	$180.50	TAZICEF 1, SKB Pharms	00007-5083-11

Injection, Dry-Soln - Intramuscular; - 2 gm/vial

trays of 10	**$284.53**	**FORTAZ, Glaxo Wellcome**	**00173-0379-34**
2 gm x 10	$289.34	TAZIDIME, Lilly	00002-7291-10
2 gm x 24	$717.17	TAZIDIME, Lilly	00002-7246-24
10 vials x 1	$284.54	TAZIDIME, Lilly	00002-7234-10
10 vials x 1	$288.14	TAZIDIME, Lilly	00002-7239-10
10's	**$288.13**	**FORTAZ, Glaxo Wellcome**	**00173-0381-32**
10's	**$289.34**	**Fortaz, Glaxo Wellcome**	**00173-0435-00**
10's	$356.25	Tazicef, SKB Pharms	00007-5091-11
50 ml x 24	$739.88	TAZICEF IN DEXTROSE, SKB Pharms	00007-5089-04
50 ml x 24	**$747.67**	**FORTAZ, Glaxo Wellcome**	**00173-0413-00**
60 ml x 10	$296.40	TAZICEF 2, SKB Pharms	00007-5084-76
60 ml x 10	$351.98	TAZICEF 2, SKB Pharms	00007-5084-11
100 ml x 10	$300.15	TAZICEF 2, SKB Pharms	00007-5085-76
100 ml x 10	$356.49	TAZICEF 2, SKB Pharms	00007-5085-11

Injection, Dry-Soln - Intramuscular; - 6 gm/vial

6 vials x 1	$496.82	TAZIDIME, Lilly	00002-7241-16
6's	**$496.80**	**FORTAZ, Glaxo Wellcome**	**00173-0382-37**
100 ml x 10	$862.50	TAZICEF, SKB Pharms	00007-5086-76
100 ml x 10	$1024.22	TAZICEF, SKB Pharms	00007-5086-11

Injection, Dry-Soln - Intramuscular; - 500 mg/vial

25 vials x 1	$177.85	TAZIDIME, Lilly	00002-7230-25
25's	**$177.84**	**FORTAZ, Glaxo Wellcome**	**00173-0377-31**

CEFTAZIDIME (ARGININE) *(003116)*

CATEGORIES: Aminoglycosides; Anti-Infectives; Antibiotics; Antimicrobials; Bone Infections; Cellulitis; Cephalosporins; Endometritis; Gynecologic Infections; Infections; Intra-Abdominal Infections; Joint Infections; Meningitis; Peritonitis; Pneumonia; Respiratory Tract Infections; Sepsis; Septicemia; Skin Infections; Urinary Tract Infections; Pregnancy Category B; FDA Approved 1990 Sep

BRAND NAMES: *Alfacef*; *Cefortam*; *Ceftazim* (Mexico); *Ceftidin*; *Ceftim*; *Ceftum*; **Ceptaz**; *Fortum* (Australia, England, France, Germany, Mexico); *Fortum Pro*; *Ftazidime*; *Kefadim*; *Kefazim*; *Kefzim*; *Glazidim*; *Modacin* (Japan); *Panzid*; *Pentacef*; *Solvetan*; *Spectrum*; *Starcef*; *Tagal* (Mexico); *Taloken* (Mexico); *Tazim*; *Tazime*; *Thidim*; *Waytrax* (Mexico)
(International brand names outside U.S. in italics)

DESCRIPTION:

Ceftazidime is a semisynthetic, broad-spectrum, beta-lactam antibiotic for parenteral administration. It is the pentahydrate of pyridinium, 1-[[7-[[(2-amino-4-thiazolyl)[(1-carboxy-1-methylethoxy)imino]acetyl]amino]-2-carboxy-8-oxo-5-thia-1-azabicyclo[4.2.0]oct-2-en-3-yl]methyl]-, hydroxide, inner salt, [6R-[6α,7β(Z)]].

The empirical formula is $C_{22}H_{32}N_6O_{12}S_2$, representing a molecular weight of 636.6.

Ceptaz is a sterile, dry mixture of ceftazidime pentahydrate and L-arginine. The L-arginine is at a concentration of 349 mg/g of ceftazidime activity. Ceftazidime dissolves without the evolution of gas. The product contains no sodium ion. Solutions of ceftazidime range in color from light yellow to amber, depending on the diluent and volume used. The pH of freshly constituted solutions usually ranges from 5 to 7.5.

CLINICAL PHARMACOLOGY:

After intravenous (IV) administration of 500-mg and 1-g doses of ceftazidime over 5 minutes to normal adult male volunteers, mean peak serum concentrations of 45 and 90 mcg/ml, respectively, were achieved. After IV infusion of 500-mg, 1-g, and 2-g doses of ceftazidime over 20 to 30 minutes to normal adult male volunteers, mean peak serum concentrations of 42, 69, and 170 mcg/ml, respectively, were achieved. The average serum concentrations following IV infusion of 500-mg, 1-g, and 2-g doses to these volunteers over an 8-hour interval are given in TABLE 1.

TABLE 1

Ceftazidime IV Dose	Serum Concentrations (mcg/ml) 0.5 h	1 h	2 h	4 h	8 h
500 mg	42	25	12	6	2
1 g	60	39	23	11	3
2 g	129	75	42	13	5

The absorption and elimination of ceftazidime were directly proportional to the size of the dose. The half-life following IV administration was approximately 1.9 hours. Less than 10% ceftazidime was protein bound. The degree of protein binding was independent of concentration. There was no evidence of accumulation of ceftazidime in the serum in individuals with normal renal function following multiple IV doses of 1 and 2 g every 8 hours for 10 days.

CLINICAL PHARMACOLOGY: *(cont'd)*

Following intramuscular (IM) administration of 500-mg and 1-g doses of ceftazidime to normal adult volunteers, the main peak serum concentrations were 17 and 39 mcg/ml, respectively, at approximately 1 hour. Serum concentrations remained above 4 mcg/ml for 6 and 8 hours after the IM administration of 500-mg and 1-g doses, respectively. The half-life of ceftazidime in these volunteers was approximately 2 hours.

The presence of hepatic dysfunction had no effect on the pharmacokinetics of ceftazidime in individuals administered 2 g intravenously every 8 hours for 5 days. Therefore, a dosage adjustment from the normal recommended dosage is not required for patients with hepatic dysfunction, provided renal function is not impaired.

Approximately 80% to 90% of an IM or IV dose of ceftazidime is excreted unchanged by the kidneys over a 24-hour period. After the IV administration of single 500-mg or 1-g doses, approximately 50% of the dose appeared in the urine in the first 2 hours. An additional 20% was excreted between 2 and 4 hours after dosing, and approximately another 12% of the dose appeared in the urine between 4 and 8 hours later. The elimination of ceftazidime by the kidneys resulted in high therapeutic concentrations in the urine.

The mean renal clearance of ceftazidime was approximately 100 ml per minute. The calculated plasma clearance of approximately 115 ml per minute indicated nearly complete elimination of ceftazidime by the renal route. Administration of probenecid before dosing had no effect on the elimination kinetics of ceftazidime. This suggested that ceftazidime is eliminated by glomerular filtration and is not actively secreted by renal tubular mechanisms.

Since ceftazidime is eliminated almost solely by the kidneys, its serum half-life is significantly prolonged in patients with impaired renal function. Consequently, dosage adjustments in such patients as described in the DOSAGE AND ADMINISTRATIONsection are suggested.

Ceftazidime concentrations achieved in specific body tissues and fluids are depicted in TABLE 2.

TABLE 2 Ceftazidime Concentrations in Body Tissues and Fluids

Tissue or Fluid	Dose/Route	No. of Patients	Time of Sample Postdose	Average Tissue or Fluid Level (mcg/ml or mcg/g)
Urine	500 mg IM	6	0-2 h	2,100.0
	2 g IV	6	0-2 h	12,000.0
Bile	2 g IV	3	90 min	36.4
Synovial fluid	2 g IV	13	2 h	25.6
Peritoneal fluid	2 g IV	8	2 h	48.6
Sputum	1 g IV	8	1 h	9.0
Cerebrospinal fluid	2 g q8h IV	5	120 min	9.8
(inflamed meninges)	2 g q8h IV	6	180 min	9.4
Aqueous humor	2 g IV	13	1-3 h	11.0
Blister fluid	1 g IV	7	2-3 h	19.7
Lymphatic fluid	1 g IV	7	2-3 h	23.4
Bone	2 g IV	8	0.67 h	31.1
Heart muscle	2 g IV	35	30-280 min	12.7
Skin	2 g IV	22	30-180 min	6.6
Skeletal muscle	2 g IV	35	30-280 min	9.4
Myometrium	2 g IV	31	1-2 h	18.7

Microbiology: Ceftazidime is bactericidal in action, exerting its effect by inhibition of enzymes responsible for cell-wall synthesis. A wide range of gram-negative organisms is susceptible to ceftazidime *in vitro,* including strains resistant to gentamicin and other aminoglycosides. In addition, ceftazidime has been shown to be active against gram-positive organisms. It is highly stable to most clinically important beta-lactamases, plasmid or chromosomal, which are produced by both gram-negative and gram-positive organisms and, consequently, is active against many strains resistant to ampicillin and other cephalosporins.

Ceftazidime has been shown to be active against the following organisms both *in vitro* and in clinical infections (see INDICATIONS AND USAGE.)

Aerobes, Gram-negative: *Citrobacter* spp., including *Citrobacter freundii* and *Citrobacter diversus; Enterobacter* spp., including *Enterobacter cloacae* and *Enterobacter aerogenes; Escherichia coli; Haemophilus influenzae,*including ampicillin-resistant strains; *Klebsiella* spp. (including *Klebsiella pneumoniae*); *Neisseria meningitidis; Proteus mirabilis; Proteus vulgaris; Pseudomonas* spp. (including*Pseudomonas aeruginosa*); and *Serratia* spp.

Aerobes, Gram-positive: *Staphylococcus aureus,* including penicillinase-and non-penicillinase-producing strains;*Streptococcus agalactiae* (group B streptococci);*Streptococcus pneumoniae;* and *Streptococcus pyogenes* (group A beta-hemolytic streptococci).

Anaerobes: *Bacteroides* spp. (NOTE: many strains of *Bacteroides fragilis* are resistant).

Ceftazidime has been shown to be active *in vitro* against most strains of the following organisms; however, the clinical significance of this activity is unknown: *Acinetobacter* spp.; *Clostridium* spp. (not including *Clostridium difficile*); *Haemophilus parainfluenzae; Morganella morganii* (formerly *Proteus morganii*); *Neisseria gonorrhoeae; Peptococcus* spp.;*Peptostreptococcus* spp.; *Providencia* spp. (including*Providencia rettgeri,* formerly *Proteus rettgeri*);*Salmonella* spp.; *Shigella* spp.; *Staphylococcus epidermidis;* and *Yersinia enterocolitica.*

Ceftazidime and the aminoglycosides have been shown to be synergistic*in vitro* against *Pseudomonas aeruginosa* and the *Enterobacteriaceae.* Ceftazidime and carbenicillin have also been shown to be synergistic *in vitro* against *Pseudomonas aeruginosa.*

Ceftazidime is not active *in vitro* against methicillin-resistant staphylococci; *Streptococcus faecalis* and many other enterococci;*Listeria monocytogenes; Campylobacter* spp.; or *Clostridium difficile.*

SUSCEPTIBILITY TESTING

Diffusion Techniques: Quantitative methods that require measurement of zone diameters give an estimate of antibiotic susceptibility. One such procedure[1-3] has been recommended for use with disks to test susceptibility to ceftazidime.

Reports from the laboratory giving results of the standard single-disk susceptibility test with a 30-mcg ceftazidime disk should be interpreted according to the following criteria:

Susceptible organisms produce zones of 18 mm or greater, indicating that the test organism is likely to respond to therapy.

Organisms that produce zones of 15 to 17 mm are expected to be susceptible if high dosage is used or if the infection is confined to tissues and fluids (*e.g.,* urine) in which high antibiotic levels are attained.

Resistant organisms produce zones of 14 mm or less, indicating that other therapy should be selected.

Organisms should be tested with the ceftazidime disk since ceftazidime has been shown by *in vitro* tests to be active against certain strains found resistant when other beta-lactam disks are used.

Standardized procedures require the use of laboratory control organisms. The 30-mcg ceftazidime disk should give zone diameters between 25 and 32 mm for *Escherichia coli* ATCC 25922. For *Pseudomonas aeruginosa* ATCC 27853, the zone diameters should be between 22 and 29 mm. For *Staphylococcus aureus* ATCC 25923, the zone diameters should be between 16 and 20 mm.

CLINICAL PHARMACOLOGY: *(cont'd)*

Dilution Techniques: In other susceptibility testing procedures, e.g., ICS agar dilution or the equivalent, a bacterial isolate may be considered susceptible if the minimum inhibitory concentration (MIC) value for ceftazidime is not more than 16 mcg/ml. Organisms are considered resistant to ceftazidime if the MIC is ≥64 mcg/ml. Organisms having an MIC value of <64 mcg/ml but >16 mcg/ml are expected to be susceptible if high dosage is used or if the infection in confined to tissues and fluids (*e.g.,* urine) in which high antibiotic levels are attained.

As with standard diffusion methods, dilution procedures require the use of laboratory control organisms. Standard ceftazidime powder should give MIC values in the range of 4 to 16 mcg/ml for *Staphylococcus aureus* ATCC 25923. For *Escherichia coli* ATCC 25922, the MIC range should be between 0.125 and 0.5 mcg/ml. For *Pseudomonas aeruginosa*ATCC 27853, the MIC range should be between 0.5 and 2 mcg/ml.

INDICATIONS AND USAGE:

Ceftazidime is indicated for the treatment of patients with infections caused by susceptible strains of the designated organisms in the following diseases:

1. Lower Respiratory Tract Infections, including pneumonia, caused by *Pseudomonas aeruginosa* and other *Pseudomonas* spp.; *Haemophilus influenzae,* including ampicillin-resistant strains; *Klebsiella* spp.; *Enterobacter* spp.; *Proteus mirabilis; Escherichia coli; Serratia* spp.; *Citrobacter* spp.; *Streptococcus pneumoniae;* and *Staphylococcus aureus* (methicillin-susceptible strains).

2. Skin and Skin-Structure Infections caused by *Pseudomonas aeruginosa; Klebsiella* spp.; *Escherichia coli; Proteus* spp., including *Proteus mirabilis* and indole-positive *Proteus; Enterobacter* spp.; *Serratia* spp.; *Staphylococcus aureus* (methicillin-susceptible strains); and *Streptococcus pyogenes* (group A beta-hemolytic streptococci).

3. Urinary Tract Infections, both complicated and uncomplicated, caused by *Pseudomonas aeruginosa; Enterobacter* spp.; *Proteus* spp.; including *Proteus mirabilis* and indole-positive *Proteus; Klebsiella* spp.; and *Escherichia coli.*

4. Bacterial Septicemia caused by *Pseudomonas aeruginosa; Klebsiella* spp.; *Haemophilus influenzae; Escherichia coli; Serratia* spp.; *Streptococcus pneumoniae;* and *Staphylococcus aureus* (methicillin-susceptible strains).

5. Bone and Joint Infections caused by *Pseudomonas aeruginosa*; *Klebsiella* spp.; *Enterobacter* spp.; and *Staphylococcus aureus* (methicillin-susceptible strains).

6. Gynecologic Infections, including endometritis, pelvic cellulitis, and other infections of the female genital tract caused by *Escherichia coli.*

7. Intra-abdominal Infections, including peritonitis caused by *Escherichia coli, Klebsiella* spp., and *Staphylococcus aureus* (methicillin-susceptible strains) and polymicrobial infections caused by aerobic and anaerobic organisms and *Bacteroides* spp. (many strains of *Bacteroides fragilis* are resistant).

8. Central Nervous System Infections, including meningitis, caused by *Haemophilus influenzae* and *Neisseria meningitidis.* Ceftazidime has also been used successfully in a limited number of cases of meningitis due to *Pseudomonas aeruginosa* and *Streptococcus pneumoniae.*

Specimens for bacterial cultures should be obtained before therapy in order to isolate and identify causative organisms and to determine their susceptibility to ceftazidime. Therapy may be instituted before results of susceptibility studies are known; however, once these results become available, the antibiotic treatment should be adjusted accordingly.

As with other extended-spectrum cephalosporins and penicillins, some strains of *Enterobacter* spp. can develop resistance during ceftazidime therapy due to induced type-1 beta-lactamase production. When clinically appropriate during therapy of *Enterobacter* spp. infections, periodic susceptibility testing should be considered.

Ceftazidime may be used alone in cases of confirmed or suspected sepsis. Ceftazidime has been used successfully in clinical trials as empiric therapy in cases where various concomitant therapies with other antibiotics have been used.

Ceftazidime may also be used concomitantly with other antibiotics, such as aminoglycosides, vancomycin, and clindamycin; in severe and life-threatening infections; and in the immunocompromised patient (see Compatibility And Stability.) When such concomitant treatment is appropriate, prescribing information in the labeling for the other antibiotics should be followed. The dosage depends on the severity of the infection and the patient's condition.

CONTRAINDICATIONS:

Ceftazidime is contraindicated in patients who have shown hypersensitivity to ceftazidime or the cephalosporin group of antibiotics.

WARNINGS:

BEFORE THERAPY WITH CEPTAZIDIME IS INSTITUTED, CAREFUL INQUIRY SHOULD BE MADE TO DETERMINE WHETHER THE PATIENT HAS HAD PREVIOUS HYPERSENSITIVITY REACTIONS TO CEFTAZIDIME, CEPHALOSPORINS, PENICILLINS, OR OTHER DRUGS. IF THIS PRODUCT IS TO BE GIVEN TO PENICILLIN-SENSITIVE PATIENTS, CAUTION SHOULD BE EXERCISED BECAUSE CROSS-HYPERSENSITIVITY AMONG BETA-LACTAM ANTIBIOTICS HAS BEEN CLEARLY DOCUMENTED AND MAY OCCUR IN UP TO 10% OF PATIENTS WITH A HISTORY OF PENICILLIN ALLERGY. IF AN ALLERGIC REACTION TO CEPTAZIDIME OCCURS, DISCONTINUE THE DRUG. SERIOUS ACUTE HYPERSENSITIVITY REACTIONS MAY REQUIRE TREATMENT WITH EPINEPHRINE AND OTHER EMERGENCY MEASURES, INCLUDING OXYGEN, IV FLUIDS, IV ANTIHISTAMINES, CORTICOSTEROIDS, PRESSOR AMINES, AND AIRWAY MANAGEMENT, AS CLINICALLY INDICATED.

Pseudomembranous colitis has been reported with nearly all antibacterial agents, including ceftazidime, and may range from mild to life threatening. Therefore, it is important to consider this diagnosis in patients who present with diarrhea subsequent to the administration of antibacterial agents.

Treatment with antibacterial agents alters the normal flora of the colon and may permit overgrowth of clostridia. Studies indicate that a toxin produced by *Clostridium difficile* is a primary cause of "antibiotic-associated colitis."

After the diagnosis of pseudomembranous colitis has been established, therapeutic measures should be initiated. Mild cases of pseudomembranous colitis usually respond to discontinuation of the drug alone. In moderate to severe cases, consideration should be given to management with fluids and electrolytes, protein supplementation, and treatment with an antibacterial drug effective against *Clostridium difficile.*

Elevated levels of ceftazidime in patients with renal insufficiency can lead to seizures, encephalopathy, asterixis, and neuromuscular excitability (see PRECAUTIONS.)

PRECAUTIONS:

General: Ceftazidime has not been shown to be nephrotoxic; however, high and prolonged serum antibiotic concentrations can occur from usual dosages in patients with transient or persistent reduction of urinary output because of renal insufficiency. The total daily dosage should be reduced when ceftazidime is administered to patients with renal insufficiency (see

PRECAUTIONS: *(cont'd)*

DOSAGE AND ADMINISTRATION.) Elevated levels of ceftazidime in these patients can lead to seizures, encephalopathy, asterixis, and neuromuscular excitability. Continued dosage should be determined by degree of renal impairment, severity of infection, and susceptibility of the causative organisms.

As with other antibiotics, prolonged use of ceftazidime may result in overgrowth of nonsusceptible organisms. Repeated evaluation of the patient's condition is essential. If superinfection occurs during therapy, appropriate measures should be taken.

Cephalosporins may be associated with a fall in prothrombin activity. Those at risk include patients with renal or hepatic impairment, or poor nutritional state, as well as patients receiving a protracted course of antimicrobial therapy. Prothrombin time should be monitored in patients at risk and exogenous vitamin K administered as indicated.

Ceftazidime should be prescribed with caution in individuals with a history of gastrointestinal disease, particularly colitis.

Arginine has been shown to alter glucose metabolism and elevate serum potassium transiently when administered at 50 times the recommended dose. The effect of lower dosing is not known.

Intra-arterial administration may lead to arteriospasm and necrosis and should therefore be avoided.

Drug/Laboratory Test Interactions: The administration of ceftazidime may result in a false-positive reaction for glucose in the urine when using Clinitest tablets, Benedict's solution, or Fehling's solution. It is recommended that glucose tests based on enzymatic glucose oxidase reactions (such as Clinistix or Tes-Tape) be used.

Carcinogenesis, Mutagenesis, and Impairment of Fertility: Long-term studies in animals have not been performed to evaluate carcinogenic potential. However, a mouse Micronucleus test and an Ames test were both negative for mutagenic effects.

Pregnancy, Teratogenic Effects, Pregnancy Category B: Reproduction studies have been performed in mice and rats at doses up to 40 times the human dose and have revealed no evidence of impaired fertility or harm to the fetus due to ceftazidime. Ceftazidime at 23 times the human dose was not teratogenic or embryotoxic in a rat reproduction study. There are, however, no adequate and well-controlled studies in pregnant women. Because animal reproduction studies are not always predictive of human response, this drug should be used during pregnancy only if clearly needed.

Nursing Mothers: Ceftazidime is excreted in human milk in low concentrations. It is not known whether the arginine component of this product is excreted in human milk. Because many drugs are excreted in human milk and because safety of the arginine component of ceftazidime in nursing infants has not been established, a decision should be made whether to discontinue nursing or to discontinue the drug, taking into account the importance of the drug to the mother.

Pediatric Use: Safety of the arginine component of ceftazidime in children has not been established. This product is for use in patients 12 years and older. If treatment with ceftazidime is indicated for pediatric patients, a sodium carbonate formulation should be used.

DRUG INTERACTIONS:

Nephrotoxicity has been reported following concomitant administration of cephalosporins with aminoglycoside antibiotics or potent diuretics such as furosemide. Renal function should be carefully monitored, especially if higher dosages of the aminoglycosides are to be administered or if therapy is prolonged, because of the potential nephrotoxicity and ototoxicity of aminoglycosidic antibiotics. Nephrotoxicity and ototoxicity were not noted when ceftazidime was given alone in clinical trials.

Chloramphenicol has been shown to be antagonistic to beta-lactam antibiotics, including ceftazidime, based on *in vitro* studies and time kill curves with enteric gram-negative bacilli. Due to the possibility of antagonism*in vivo*, particularly when bactericidal activity is desired, this drug combination should be avoided.

ADVERSE REACTIONS:

The following adverse effects from clinical trials were considered to be either related to ceftazidime therapy or were of uncertain etiology. The most common were local reactions following IV injection and allergic and gastrointestinal reactions. No disulfiramlike reactions were reported.

Local Effects, reported in fewer that 2% of patients, were phlebitis and inflammation at the site of injection (1 in 69 patients).

Hypersensitivity Reactions, reported in 2% of patients, were pruritus, rash, and fever. Immediate reactions, generally manifested by rash and/or pruritus, occurred in 1 in 285 patients. Toxic epidermal necrolysis, Stevens-Johnson syndrome, and erythema multiforme have also been reported with cephalosporin antibiotics, including ceftazidime. Angioedema and anaphylaxis (bronchospasm and/or hypotension) have been reported very rarely.

Gastrointestinal Symptoms, reported in fewer than 2% of patients, were diarrhea (1 in 78), nausea (1 in 156), vomiting (1 in 500), and abdominal pain (1 in 416). The onset of pseudomembranous colitis symptoms may occur during or after treatment (see WARNINGS.)

Central Nervous System Reactions (fewer than 1%) included headache, dizziness, and paresthesia. Seizures have been reported with several cephalosporins, including ceftazidime. In addition, encephalopathy, asterixis, and neuromuscular excitability have been reported in renally impaired patients treated with unadjusted dosing regimens of ceftazidime (see PRECAUTIONS, General.)

Less Frequent Adverse Events (fewer than 1%) were candidiasis (including oral thrush) and vaginitis.

Hematologic: Rare cases of hemolytic anemia have been reported.

Laboratory Test Changes noted during ceftazidime clinical trials were transient and included: eosinophilia (1 in 13), positive Coombs' test without hemolysis (1 in 23), thrombocytosis (1 in 45), and slight elevations in one or more of the hepatic enzymes, aspartate aminotransferase (AST, SGOT) (1 in 16), alanine aminotransferase (ALT, SGPT) (1 in 15), LDH (1 in 18), GGT (1 in 19), and alkaline phosphatase (1 in 23). As with some other cephalosporins, transient elevations of blood urea, blood urea nitrogen, and/or serum creatinine were observed occasionally. Transient leukopenia, neutropenia, agranulocytosis, thrombocytopenia, and lymphocytosis were seen very rarely. Elevations in hepatic enzymes (SGOT, SGPT, LDH, GGT, alkaline phosphatase) have been reported postmarketing.

In addition to the adverse reactions listed above that have been observed in patients treated with ceftazidime, the following adverse reactions and altered laboratory tests have been reported for cephalosporin-class antibiotics.

Adverse Reactions: Urticaria, colitis, renal dysfunction, toxic nephropathy, hepatic dysfunction including cholestasis, aplastic anemia, hemorrhage.

Altered Laboratory Tests: Prolonged prothrombin time, false-positive test for urinary glucose, elevated bilirubin, pancytopenia.

OVERDOSAGE:

Ceftazidime overdosage has occurred in patients with renal failure. Reactions have included seizure activity, encephalopathy, asterixis, and neuromuscular excitability. Patients who receive an acute overdosage should be carefully observed and given supportive treatment. In the presence of renal insufficiency, hemodialysis or peritoneal dialysis may aid in the removal of ceftazidime from the body.

DOSAGE AND ADMINISTRATION:

Dosage: The usual adult dosage is 1 gram administered intravenously or intramuscularly every 8 to 12 hours. The dosage and route should be determined by the susceptibility of the causative organisms, the severity of infection, and the condition and renal function of the patient.

The guidelines for dosage of ceftazidime are listed in TABLE 3. The following dosage schedule is recommended.

TABLE 3 Recommended Dosage Schedule

Adults 12 years and older*	Dose	Frequency
Usual recommended dosage	1 g IV or IM	q8-12h
Uncomplicated urinary tract infections	250 mg IV or IM	q12h
Bone and joint infections	2 grams IV	q12h
Complicated urinary tract infections	500 mg IV or IM	q8-12h
Uncomplicated pneumonia; mild skin and skin-structure infections	500 mg-1 gram IV or IM	q8h
Serious gynecologic and intra-abdominal infections	2 grams IV	q8h
Meningitis	2 grams IV	q8h
Very severe life-threatening infections, especially in immunocompromised patients	2 grams IV	q8h
Lung infections caused by *Pseudomonas* spp. in patients with cystic fibrosis with normal renal function†	30-50 mg/kg IV to a maximum of 6 grams per day	q8h

* This product is for use in patients 12 years and older. If treatment with ceftazidime is indicated for pediatric patients, a sodium carbonate formulation should be used.
† Although clinical improvement has been shown, bacteriologic cures cannot be expected in patients with chronic respiratory disease and cystic fibrosis.

Impaired Hepatic Function: No adjustment in dosage is required for patients with hepatic dysfunction.

Impaired Renal Function: Ceftazidime is excreted by the kidneys, almost exclusively by glomerular filtration. Therefore, in patients with impaired renal function (glomerular filtration rate [GFR] <50 ml per minute), it is recommended that the dosage of ceftazidime be reduced to compensate for its slower excretion. In patients with suspected renal insufficiency, an initial loading dose of 1 gram of ceftazidime may be given. An estimate of GFR should be made to determine the appropriate maintenance dosage. The recommended dosage is presented in TABLE 4.

TABLE 4 Recommended Maintenance Dosages of Ceftazidime in Renal Insufficiency

Creatinine Clearance (ml/min)	Recommended Unit Dose of Ceptaz	Frequency of Dosing
50-31	1 gram	q12h
30-16	1 gram	q24h
15-6	500 mg	q24h
<5	500 mg	q48h

NOTE: IF THE DOSE RECOMMENDED IN TABLE 3 ABOVE IS LOWER THAN THAT RECOMMENDED FOR PATIENTS WITH RENAL INSUFFICIENCY AS OUTLINED IN TABLE 4, THE LOWER DOSE SHOULD BE USED.

When only serum creatinine is available, the following formula (Cockcroft's equation)[4] may be used to estimate creatinine clearance. The serum creatinine should represent a steady state of renal function (TABLE 5):

TABLE 5 Creatinine clearance (ml/min)

Males: [Weight (kg) × (140 - age)] ÷ [72 × serum creatinine (mg/dl)]
Females: 0.85 × male value

In patients with severe infections who would normally receive 6 grams of ceftazidime daily were it not for renal insufficiency, the unit dose given in the table above may be increased by 50% or the dosing frequency may be increased appropriately. Further dosing should be determined by therapeutic monitoring, severity of the infection, and susceptibility of the causative organism.

In patients undergoing hemodialysis, a loading dose of 1 gram is recommended, followed by 1 gram after each hemodialysis period.

Ceftazidime can also be used in patients undergoing intraperitoneal dialysis and continuous ambulatory peritoneal dialysis. In such patients, a loading dose of 1 gram of ceftazidime may be given, followed by 500 mg every 24 hours. It is not known whether or not ceftazidime can be safely incorporated into dialysis fluid.

Note: Generally ceftazidime should be continued for 2 days after the signs and symptoms of infection have disappeared, but in complicated infections longer therapy may be required.

Administration: Ceftazidime may be given intravenously or by deep IM injection into a large muscle mass such as the upper outer quadrant of the gluteus maximus or lateral part of the thigh.

Intramuscular Administration: For IM administration, ceftazidime should be constituted with one of the following diluents: sterile water for injection, bacteriostatic water for injection, or 0.5% or 1% lidocaine hydrochloride injection. Refer to TABLE 6.

Intravenous Administration: The IV route is preferable for patients with bacterial septicemia, bacterial meningitis, peritonitis, or other severe or life-threatening infections, or for patients who may be poor risks because of lowered resistance resulting from such debilitating conditions as malnutrition, trauma, surgery, diabetes, heart failure, or malignancy, particularly if shock is present or pending.

For direct intermittent IV administration, constitute ceftazidime as directed in TABLE 6 with sterile water for injection, 5% dextrose injection, or 0.9% sodium chloride injection. Slowly inject directly into the vein over a period of 3 to 5 minutes or give through the tubing of an administration set while the patient is also receiving one of the compatible IV fluids (see Compatibility And Stability.)

For IV infusion, constitute the 1- or 2-gram infusion pack with 100 ml of sterile water for injection or one of the compatible IV fluids listed under Compatibility And Stability. Alternatively, constitute the 1- or 2-gram vial and add an appropriate quantity of the resulting solution to an IV container with one of the compatible IV fluids.

DOSAGE AND ADMINISTRATION: *(cont'd)*

Intermittent IV infusion with a Y-type administration set can be accomplished with compatible solutions. However, during infusion of a solution containing ceftazidime, it is desirable to discontinue the other solution.

TABLE 6 Preparation of Ceftazidime Solutions

Size	Amount of Diluent to Be Added (ml)	Volume to Be Withdrawn (ml)	Approximate Ceftazidime Concentration (mg/ml)
Intramuscular			
1-gram vial	3.0	Total	250
Intravenous			
1-gram vial	10.0	Total	90
2-gram vial	10.0	Total	170
Infusion pack			
1-gram vial	100	—	10
2-gram vial	100	—	20
Pharmacy bulk package			
10-gram vial	40	Amount needed	200

Solutions of ceftazidime, like those of most beta-lactam antibiotics, should not be added to solutions of aminoglycoside antibiotics because of potential interaction.

However, if concurrent therapy with ceftazidime and an aminoglycoside is indicated, each of these antibiotics can be administered separately to the same patient.

Instructions for Constitution: Vials of ceftazidime as supplied are under a slightly reduced pressure. This may assist entry of the diluent. No gas-relief needle is required when adding the diluent, except for the infusion pack where it is required during the latter stages of addition (in order to preserve product sterility, a gas-relief needle should not be inserted until an overpressure is produced in the vial). No evolution of gas occurs on constitution. When the vial contents are dissolved, vials other than infusion packs may still be under a reduced pressure. This reduced pressure is particularly noticeable for the 10-gram pharmacy bulk package.

COMPATIBILITY AND STABILITY

Intramuscular

Ceftazidime, when constituted as directed with sterile water for injection, bacteriostatic water for injection, or 0.5% or 1% lidocaine hydrochloride injection, maintains satisfactory potency for 18 hours at room temperature or for 7 days under refrigeration. Solutions in sterile water for injection that are frozen immediately after constitution in the original container are stable for 6 months when stored at -20°C. Components of the solution may precipitate in the frozen state and will dissolve on reaching room temperature with little or no agitation. Potency is not affected. Frozen solutions should only be thawed at room temperature. Do not force thaw by immersion in water baths or by microwave irradiation. Once thawed, solutions should not be refrozen. Thawed solutions may be stored for up to 12 hours at room temperature or for 7 days in a refrigerator.

Intravenous

Ceftazidime concentration greater than 100 mg/ml (2-g vial or 10-g pharmacy bulk package): Ceftazidime, when constituted as directed with sterile water for injection, 0.9% sodium chloride injection, or 5% dextrose injection, maintains satisfactory potency for 18 hours at room temperature or for 7 days under refrigeration. Solutions of a similar concentration in sterile water for injection that are frozen immediately after constitution in the original container are stable for 6 months when store at -20°C. Components of the solution may precipitate in the frozen state and will dissolve upon reaching room temperature with little or no agitation. Potency is not affected. Frozen solutions should only be thawed at room temperature. Do not force thaw by immersion in water baths or by microwave irradiation. Once thawed, solutions should not be refrozen. Thawed solutions may be stored for up to 12 hours at room temperature or for 7 days in a refrigerator.

Ceftazidime concentration of 100 mg/ml or less (1-g vial or infusion packs): Ceftazidime, when constituted as directed with sterile water for injection, 0.9% sodium chloride injection, or 5% dextrose injection, maintains satisfactory potency for 24 hours at room temperature or for 7 days under refrigeration. Solutions, prepared by a pharmacist, of the approved arginine formulation of ceftazidime of a similar concentration in sterile water for injection, 0.9% sodium chloride injection, or 5% dextrose injection in the original container or in 0.9% sodium chloride injection in Viaflex (PL 146 Plastic) small-volume containers that are frozen immediately after constitution by the pharmacist are stable for 6 months when stored at -20°C. Solutions in the PL 146 Plastic small-volume containers are in contact with the polyvinyl chloride layer of this container and can leach out certain chemical components of the plastic in very small amounts within the expiration period. The suitability of the plastic has been confirmed in tests in animals according to USP biological tests for plastic containers as well as by tissue culture toxicity studies. Stability of the frozen solution in other containers has not been confirmed. Frozen solutions should only be thawed at room temperature. Do not force thaw by immersion in water baths or by microwave irradiation. For the larger volumes of IV infusion solutions where it may be necessary to warm the frozen product, care should be taken to avoid heating after thawing is complete. Once thawed, solutions should not be refrozen. Thawed solutions may be stored for up to 18 hours at room temperature or for 7 days in a refrigerator.

Components of the solution may precipitate in the frozen state and will dissolve on reaching room temperature with little or no agitation. Potency is not affected. Check for minute leaks in plastic containers by squeezing bag firmly. Discard bag if leaks are found as sterility may be impaired. Do not add supplementary medication to bags. Do not use unless solution is clear and seal is intact.

Use sterile equipment.

Caution: Do not use plastic containers in series connections. Such use could result in air embolism due to residual air being drawn from the primary container before administration of the fluid from the secondary container is complete.

PREPARATION FOR ADMINISTRATION:

1. Suspend container from eyelet support.
2. Remove protector from outlet port at bottom of container.
3. Attach administration set. Refer to complete directions accompanying set.

Ceftazidime is compatible with the more commonly used IV infusion fluids. Solutions at concentrations between 1 and 40 mg/ml in 0.9% sodium chloride injection; 1/6 M sodium lactate injection; 5% dextrose injection; 5% dextrose and 0.225% sodium chloride injection; 5% dextrose and 0.45% sodium chloride injection; 5% dextrose and 0.9% sodium chloride injection; 10% dextrose injection; ringer's injection, USP; lactated ringer's injection, USP; 10% invert sugar in sterile water for injection; and Normosol-M in 5% dextrose injection may be stored for up to 24 hours at room temperature or for 7 days if refrigerated.

Ceftazidime is less stable in sodium bicarbonate injection than in other IV fluids. It is not recommended as a diluent. Solutions of ceftazidime in 5% dextrose injection and 0.9% sodium chloride injection are stable for at least 6 hours at room temperature in plastic tubing, drip chambers, and volume control devices of common IV infusion sets.

DOSAGE AND ADMINISTRATION: *(cont'd)*

Ceftazidime at a concentration of 4 mg/ml has been found compatible for 24 hours at room temperature or for 7 days under refrigeration in 0.9% sodium chloride injection or 5% dextrose injection when admixed with: cefuroxime sodium (Zinacef) 3 mg/ml; heparin sodium in concentrations up to 50 U/ml; or potassium chloride in concentrations up to 40 mEq/l. Ceftazidime may be constituted at a concentration of 20 mg/ml with metronidazole injection 5 mg/ml, and the resultant solution may be stored for 24 hours at room temperature or for 7 days under refrigeration. Ceftazidime at a concentration of 20 mg/ml has been found compatible for 24 hours at room temperature or for 7 days under refrigeration in 0.9% sodium chloride injection or 5% dextrose injection when admixed with 6 mg/ml clindamycin (as clindamycin phosphate).

Vancomycin solution exhibits a physical incompatibility when mixed with a number of drugs, including ceftazidime. The likelihood of precipitation with ceftazidime is dependent on the concentrations of vancomycin and ceftazidime present. It is therefore recommended, when both drugs are to be administered by intermittent IV infusion, that they be given separately, flushing the IV lines (with one of the compatible IV fluids) between the administration of these two agents.

Note: Parenteral drug products should be inspected visually for particulate matter before administration whenever solution and container permit.

As with other cephalosporins, ceftazidime powder as well as solutions tend to darken, depending on storage conditions; within the stated recommendations, however, product potency is not adversely affected.

Directions for Dispensing: *Pharmacy Bulk Package—Not for Direct Infusion.* The pharmacy bulk package is for use in a pharmacy admixture service only under a laminar flow hood. Entry into the vial must be made with a sterile transfer set or other sterile dispensing device, and the contents dispensed in aliquots using aseptic technique. The use of syringe and needle is not recommended as it may cause leakage (see DOSAGE AND ADMINISTRATION). GOOD PHARMACY PRACTICE DICTATES THAT THE CLOSURE BE PENETRATED ONLY ONE TIME AFTER CONSTITUTION. AFTER INITIAL PENETRATION OF THE CLOSURE, USE ENTIRE CONTENTS OF VIAL PROMPTLY. ANY UNUSED PORTION MUST BE DISCARDED WITHIN 18 HOURS OF CONSTITUTION.

REFERENCES:

1. Bauer AW, Kirby WMM, Sherris JC, Turck M. Antibiotic susceptibility testing by a standardized single disk method. *Am J Clin Pathol.* 1966;45:493-496. **2.** National Committee for Clinical Laboratory Standards. *Approved Standard: Performance Standards for Antimicrobial Disc Susceptibility Tests.* (M2-A3). December 1984. **3.** Certification procedure for antibiotic sensitivity discs (21 CFR 460.1). *Federal Register.*May 30, 1974;39:19182-19184. **4.** Cockcroft DW, Gault MH. Prediction of creatinine clearance from serum creatinine. *Nephron.*1976;16: 31-41.

HOW SUPPLIED:

Ceftazidime in the dry state should be stored between 15° and 30°C (59° and 86°F) and protected from light. Ceptaz is a dry, white to off-white powder supplied in vials and infusion packs.

HOW SUPPLIED - RATED THERAPEUTICALLY EQUIVALENT:

Injection, Dry-Soln - Intramuscular; - 1 gm/vial

10's	$157.52	CEPTAZ, Glaxo Wellcome	00173-0416-00
25's	$384.12	CEPTAZ, Glaxo Wellcome	00173-0414-00

Injection, Dry-Soln - Intramuscular; - 2 gm/vial

10's	$311.17	CEPTAZ, Glaxo Wellcome	00173-0417-00
25's	$768.20	CEPTAZ, Glaxo Wellcome	00173-0415-00

Injection, Dry-Soln - Intramuscular; - 10 gm/vial

6's	$894.24	CEPTAZ, Glaxo Wellcome	00173-0418-00

CEFTIBUTEN *(003249)*

CATEGORIES: Anti-Infectives; Antibiotics; Antimicrobials; Cephalosporins; Infections

BRAND NAMES: **Cedax**; *Ceten*; *Cilecef*, *Keimax* (Germany); *Seftem* (Japan) *(International brand names outside U.S. in italics)*

DESCRIPTION:

Ceftibuten capsules and ceftibuten for oral suspension contain the active ingredient ceftibuten as ceftibuten dihydrate. Ceftibuten dihydrate is a semisynthetic cephalosporin antibiotic for oral administration. Chemically, it is (+)-(6R,7R-7– [(Z)–2– (2–Amino–4–thiazolyl)–4 –carboxycrotonamido]– 8– oxo–5–thia–1–azabicyclo [4.2.0]oct– 2–ene–2–carboxylic acid, dihydrate. Its molecular formula is $C_{15}H_{14}N_4O_6S_2{\cdot}2H_2O$. Its molecular weight is 446.43 as a dihydrate.

Cedax contain ceftibuten dihydrate equivalent to 400 mg of ceftibuten. Inactive ingredients contained in the capsule formulation include: magnesium stearate, microcrystalline cellulose, and sodium startch glycolate. The capsule shell and/or band contains gelatin, sodium lauryl sulfate, titanium dioxide, and polysorbate 80. The capsule shell may also contain benzyl alcohol, sodium propionate, edetate calcium disodium, butylparaben, propylparaben, and methylparaben.

Cedax Oral Suspension after reconstitution contains ceftibuten dihydrate equivalent to either 90 mg of ceftibuten per mL or 180 mg of ceftibuten per 5 mL. Cedax Oral Suspension is cherry flavored and contains inactive ingredients: cherry flavoring, polysorbate 80, silicon dioxide, simethicone, sodium benzoate, sucrose (approximately 1 g/5 mL), titanium dioxide, and xanthan gum.

CLINICAL PHARMACOLOGY:

PHARMACOKINETICS

Absorption

Capsules: Ceftibuten is rapidly absorbed after oral administration of capsules. The plasma concentrations and pharmacokinetic parameters of ceftibuten after a single 400–mg dose of ceftibuten capsules to 12 healthy adult male volunteers (20 to 39 years of age) are displayed in the table below. When ceftibuten capsules were administered once daily for 7 days, the average C_{max} was 17.9 mcg/mL on day 7. Therefore, ceftibuten accumulation in plasma is about 20% at steady state.

Oral Suspension: Ceftibuten is rapidly absorbed after oral administration of ceftibuten oral suspension. The plasma concentrations and pharmacokinetic parameters of ceftibuten after a single 9–mg/kg dose of ceftibuten oral suspension to 32 fasting pediatric patients (6 months to 12 years of age) are displayed in TABLE 1.

The absolute bioavailability of ceftibuten oral suspension has not been determined. The plasma concentrations of ceftibuten in pediatric patients are dose proportional following single doses of ceftibuten capsules of 200 mg and 400 mg and of ceftibuten oral suspension between 4.5 mg/kg and 9 mg/kg.

CLINICAL PHARMACOLOGY: *(cont'd)*

TABLE 1

Parameter	Average Plasma Concentration (in mcg/mL of ceftibuten after a single 400-mg dose) and Derived Pharmacokinetic Parameters (± 1 SD) (n=12 healthy males)	Average Plasma Concentration (in mcg/mL of ceftibuten after a single 9-mg/kg dose) and Derived Pharmacokinetic Parameters (± 1 SD) (n=32 pediatric patients)
1.0 h	6.1 (5.1)	9.3 (6.3)
1.5 h	9.9 (5.9)	8.6 (4.4)
2.0 h	11.3 (5.2)	11.2 (4.6)
3.0 h	13.3 (3.0)	9.0 (3.4)
4.0 h	11.2 (2.9)	6.6 (3.1)
6.0 h	5.8 (1.6)	3.8 (2.5)
8.0 h	3.2 (1.0)	1.6 (1.3)
12.0 h	1.1 (0.4)	0.5 (0.4)
C_{MAX},mcg/mL	15.0 (3.3)	13.4 (4.9)
T_{MAX}h	2.6 (0.9)	2.0 (1.0)
AUC, mcg·h/mL	73.7 (16.0)	56.0 (16.9)
$T_{\frac{1}{2}}$, h	2.4 (0.2)	2.0 (0.6)
Total Body Clearance (CI/F) mL/min/kg	1.3 (0.3)	2.9 (0.7)

Distribution

Capsules: The average apparent volume of distribution (V/F) of ceftibuten in 6 adult subjects is 0.21 L/kg (± 1 SD = 0.03 L/kg).

Oral Suspension: The average apparent volume of distribution (V/F) of ceftibuten in 32 fasting pediatric patients is 0.5 L/kg (± 1 SD = 0.2 L/kg).

Protein Binding

Ceftibuten is 65% bound to plasma proteins. The protein binding is independent of plasma ceftibuten concentration.

Tissue Penetration

Bronchial secretions: In a study of 15 adults administered a single 400–mg dose of ceftibuten and scheduled to undergo bronchoscopy, the mean concentrations in epithelial lining fluid and bronchial mucosa were 15% and 37%, respectively, of the plasma concentration.

Sputum: Ceftibuten sputum levels average approximately 7% of the concomitant plasma ceftibuten level. In a study of 24 adults administered ceftibuten 200 mg bid or 400 mg qd, the average C_{max} in sputum (1.5 mcg/mL) occurred at 2 hours postdose and the average C_{max} in plasma (1.5 mcg/mL) occurred at 2 hours postdose.

Middle-ear fluid (MEF): Ceftibuten middle–ear fluid levels average approximately 50% of the concomitant plasma ceftibuten level. In a study of 30 children administered 9 mg/kg of ceftibuten, the average C_{max} in MEF (2.9 ± 0.9 mcg/mL) occurred at 4 hours postdose and the average C_{max} in plasma (6.7 ± 1.9 mcg/mL) occurred at 2 hours postdose.

Tonsillar tissue: Data on ceftibuten penetration into tonsillar tissue are not available.

Cerebrospinal fluid: Data on ceftibuten penetration into cerebrospinal fluid are not available.

Metabolism and Excretion

A study with radiolabeled ceftibuten administered to 6 healthy adult male volunteers demonstrated that *cis*–ceftibuten is the predominant component in both plasma and urine. About 10% of ceftibuten is converted to the *trans*–isomer. The *trans*–isomer is approximately $\frac{1}{8}$ as antimicrobially potent as the*cis*–isomer.

Ceftibuten is excreted in the urine; 95% of the administered radioactivity was recovered either in urine or feces. In 6 healthy adult male volunteers, approximately 56% of the administered dose of ceftibuten was recovered from urine and 39% from the feces within 24 hours. Because renal excretion is a significant pathway of elimination, patients with renal dysfunction and patients undergoing hemodialysis require dosage adjustment (see DOSAGE AND ADMINISTRATION).

Food Effect on Absorption

Food affects the bioavailability of ceftibuten from capsules and oral suspension.

The effect of food on the bioavailablility of ceftibuten capsules was evaluated in 26 healthy adult male volunteers who igested 400 mg of ceftibuten capsules after an overnight fast or immediately after a standardized breakfast. Results showed that food delays the time of C_{max} by 1.75 hours, decreases the C_{max} by 18% and decreases the extent of absorption (AUC) by 8%.

The effect of food on the bioavailability of ceftibuten oral suspension was evaluated in 18 healthy adult male volunteers who ingested 400 mg of ceftibuten oral suspension after an overnight fast or immediately after a standardized breakfast. Results obtained demonstrated a decrease in $C_{max}$of 26% and an AUC of 17% when ceftibuten oral suspension was administered with a high-fat breakfast, and a decrease in C_{max} of 17%and in AUC of 12% when ceftibuten oral suspension was administered with a low-calorie non-fat breakfast (see PRECAUTIONS).

Bioequivalence of Dosage Formulations

A study in 18 healthy adult male volunteers demonstrated that a 400–mg dose of ceftibuten capsules produced equivalent concentrations to a 400–mg dose of ceftibuten oral suspension. Average C_{max} values were 15.6 (3.1) mcg/mL for the capsule and 17.0 (3.2) mcg/mL for the suspension. Average AUC values were 80.1 (14.4) mcg·hr/mL for the capsule and 87.0 (12.2) mcg·hr/mL for the suspension.

Special Populations

Geriatric patients: Ceftibuten pharmacokinetic have been investigated in elderly (65 years of age or older) men (n=8) and women (n=4). Each volunteer received ceftibuten 200–mg capsules twice daily for $3\frac{1}{2}$ days. The average C_{max} was 17.5 (3.7) mcg/mL after $3\frac{1}{2}$ days of dosing compared to 12.9 (2.1) mcg/mL after the first dose; ceftibuten accumulation in plasma was 40% at steady state. Information regarding the renal function of these volunteers was not available; therefore, the significance of this finding for clinical use of ceftibuten capsules in elderly patients is not clear. Ceftibuten dosage adjustment in elderly patients may be necessary (see DOSAGE AND ADMINISTRATION).

Patients with renal insufficiency: Ceftibuten pharmacokinetic have been investigated in adult patients with renal dysfunction. The ceftibuten plasma half-life increased and apparent total clearance (CI/F) decreased proportionally with increasing degree of renal dysfunction. In 6 patients with moderate renal dysfunction (creatinine clearance 30 to 49 mL/min), the plasma half-life of ceftibuten increased to 7.1 hours and CI/F decreased to 30 mL/min. In 6 patients with severe renal dysfunction (creatinine clearance 5 to 29 mL/min), the half-life increased to 13.4 hours and CI/F decreased to 16 mL/min. In 6 functionally anephric patients (creatinine clearance <5 mL/min), the half-life increased to 22.3 hours and CI/F decreased to 11 mL/min (a 7- to 8-fold change compared to healthy volunteers). Hemodialysis removed 65% of the drug from the blood in 2 to 4 hours. These changes serve as the basis for dosage adjustment recommendations in adult patients with mild to severe renal dysfunction (see DOSAGE AND ADMINISTRATION).

CLINICAL PHARMACOLOGY: *(cont'd)*

Microbiology

Ceftibuten exerts its bactericidal action by binding to essential target proteins of the baterial cell wall. This binding leads to inhibition of cell-wall synthesis.

Ceftibuten is stable in the presence of most plasmid-mediated beta-lactamases, but it is not stable in the presence of chromosomally-mediated cephalosporinases, produced in organisms such as *Bacteroides, Citrobacter, Enterobacter, Morganella,* and *Serratia.* Like other beta-lactam agents, ceftibuten should not be used against strains resistant to beta-lactams due to general mechanisms such as permeability or penicillin binding protein changes like penicillin–resistant *S. pneumoniae.*

Ceftibuten has been shown to be active against most strains of the following organisms both *in vitro* and in clinical infections (see INDICATIONS AND USAGE):

Gram-positive aerobes:

Streptococcus pneumoniae (penicillin-suspectible strains only)

Streptococcus pyogenes

Gram-negative aerobes:

Haemophilus influenzae (including β-lactamase-producing strains)

Moraxella catarrhalis (including β–lactamase–producing strains)

There are no known organisms which are potential pathogens in the indications approved for ceftibuten for which ceftibuten exhibits *in vitro* activity but for which the safety and efficacy of ceftibuten in treating clinical infections due to these organisms, have not been established in adequate and well–controlled trials.

NOTE: Ceftibuten is INACTIVE *in vitro* against *Acinetobacter, Bordetella, Campylobacter, Enterobacter, Enterococcus, Flacovacterium, Hafnia, Listeria, Pseudomonas, Staphylococcus,* and *Streptococcus* (except *pneumoniae* and *pyogenes*) species. In addition, it shows little *in vitro* activity against most anaerobes, including most species of *Bacteroides.*

Suspectibility testing

Dilution Techniques: Quantitative methods are used to determine antimicrobial minimal inhibitory concentrations (MICs). These MICs provide estimates of the susceptibility of bacteria to antimicrobial compounds. The MICs should be determined using a standardized procedure. Standardized procedures are based on a dilution method (broth, agar, or microdilution) or equivalent with standardized inoculum concentrations and standardized concentrations of ceftibuten powder. The MIC values should be interpreted according to the following criteria when testing *Haemophilus* species using Haemophilus Test Media (HTM):

TABLE 2

MIC (mcg/mL)	Interpretation
≤2	(S) Susceptible

The current absence of resistant strains precludes defining any categories other than "Susceptible". Strains yielding results suggestive of a "Nonsusceptible" category should be submitted to a reference laboratory for further testing.

A report of a "Susceptible" implies that an infection due to the strain may be appropriately treated with the dosage of antimicrobial agent recommended for that type of infection and infecting species, unless otherwise contraindicated.

Ceftibuten is indicated for penicllin–susceptible only strains of *Streptococcus pneumoniase.* A pneumococcal isolate that is susceptible to penicillin (MIC ≤0.06 mcg/mL) can be considered susceptible to ceftibuten for approved indications. Testing of ceftibuten against penicillin–intermediate or penicillin–resistant isolates is not recommended. Reliable interpretive criteria for ceftibuten are not currently available. Physicians should be informed that clinical response rates with ceftibuten may be lower in strains that are not pencillin–susceptible.

Standardized susceptibility test procedures require the use of laboratory control microorganisms to control the technical aspect of laboratory procedures. Standard ceftibuten powder should provide the following MIC values:

TABLE 3

Organism	MIC range (mcg/mL)
Haemophilus influenzae ATCC 49247	0.25-1.0

Diffusion Techniques: Quantitative methods that require measurement of zone diameters also provide estimates of the susceptibility of bacteria to antimicrobial compounds. One such standardized procedure requires the use of standardized inoculum concentrations. This procedure uses paper disks impregnanted with 30 mcg of ceftibuten to test the susceptibility of microorganisms to ceftibuten.

Reports from the laboratory providing results of the standard single-disk susceptibility test with a 30–mcg ceftibuten disk should be interpreted according to the following criteria when testing *Haemophilus* species using Haemophilus Test Media (HTM):

TABLE 4

Zone diameter (mm)	Interpretation
≥28	(S) Susceptible

The current absence of resistant strains precludes defining any categories other than "Susceptible". Strains yielding results suggestive of a "Nonsusceptible" category should be submitted to a reference laboratory for further testing.

Interpretation should be as stated above for the results using dilution techniques.

Ceftibuten is indicated for penicillin–susceptible only strains of *Streptococcus pnemoniae.* Pneumococcal isolates with oxacillin zone sizes of ≥20 mm are susceptible to penicillin and can be considered susceptible for approved indications. Reliable disk diffusion tests for ceftibuten do not yet exist.

As with standard dilution techniques, diffusion methods require the use of laboratory control microorganisms that are used to control the technical aspects of the laboratory procedures. For the diffusion technique, the 30–mcg ceftibuten disk should provide the following zone diameters in these laboratory quality control strains:

TABLE 5

Organism	Zone diameter (mm)
Haemophilus influenzae ATCC 49247	29–35

Cephalosporin-class disks should not be used to test for susceptibility to ceftibuten.

CLINICAL STUDIES:

ACUTE BACTERIAL EXACERBATIONS OF CHRONIC BRONCHITIS

Three clinical trials (two domestic, the third abroad) have been conducted testing ceftibuten in the treatment of acute exacerbations of chronic bronchitis (AECB). Overall, the clinical outcome among patients who had signs and symptoms of AECB, who had a gram stain showing a predominance of PMNs and a few epithelail cells, and who were evaluated at approximately 1 to 2 weeks after completing therapy is presented in the table below. The bacterial eradication rates of specific pathogens from these three trials are also presented:

TABLE 6 Clinical And Bacteriological Outcome Acute Bacterial Exacerbations Of Chronic Bronchitis

	Ceftibuten 400 mg QD	Control
Clinical Cure Rates	171/271 (63%)	147/216 (68%)
The 95% confidence interval around the difference in the means is (-14%, +4%).		
Bacterial Eradication Rates:		
Haemophilus influenzae	45/62 (73%)	26/36 (72%)
H. parainfluenzae	10/10	4/6
Moraxella catarrhalis	33/46 (72%)	32/34 (94%)
Streptococcus pneumoniae	23/35 (66%)	14/20 (70%)

ACUTE BACTERIAL OTITIS MEDIA

Four clinical trials (three domestic, the fourth abroad) have been conducted testing ceftibuten in the treatment of acute bacterial otitis media. Overall, the clinical outcome among patients who had signs and symptoms of acute bacterial otitis media and who were evaluated approximately 1 to 2 weeks after completing therapy is presented in the table below. Tympanocentesis was performed on patients in three of the above–mentioned studies; the bacterial eradication rates of specific pathogens from these trials are also presented:

TABLE 7 Clinical And Bacteriological Outcome Acute Bacterial Otitis Media

	Ceftibuten 400 mg QD	Control
Clinical Cure Rates	266/365 (73%)	174/226 (7%)
The 95% confidence interval around the difference in the means is (-12%, +4%).		
Bacterial Eradication Rates:		
Haemophilus influenzae	56/67 (81%)	29/38 (76%)
Moraxella catarrhalis	20/26 (77%)	13/17 (77%)
Streptococcus pneumoniae	68/105 (65%)	35/40 (88%)
Streptococcus pyogenes	13/15 (87%)	5/5

INDICATIONS AND USAGE:

Ceftibuten is indicated for the treatment of individuals with mild–to–moderate infections caused by susceptible strains of the designated microorganisms in the specific conditions listed below (see DOSAGE AND ADMINISTRATION and CLINICAL STUDIES).

Acute Bacterial Exacerbations of Chronic Bronchitis due to *Haemophilus influenzae* (including β-lactamase-producing strains), *Moraxella catarrhalis* (including β-lactamase-producing strains), or *Streptococcus pneumoniae* (penicillin-susceptible strains only). **NOTE:**In acute bacterial exacerbations of chronic bronchitis clinical trials where *Moraxella catarrhalis* was isolated from infected sputum at baseline, ceftibuten clinical efficacy was 22% less than control.

Acute Bacterial Otitis Media due to *Haemophilus influenzae* (including β–lactamase–producing strains), *Moraxella catarrhalis* (including β–lactamase–producing strains), or *Streptococcus pyogenes.* **NOTE:**Although ceftibuten used empirically was equivalent to comparators in the treatment of clinically and/or microbiologically documented acute otitis media, the efficacy against *Streptococcus pneumoniae* was 23% less than control. Therefore, ceftibuten should be given empirically only when adequate antimicrobial coverage against *Streptococcus pneumoniae* has been previously administered.

Pharyngitis and Tonsillitis due to *Streptococcus pyogenes.* **NOTE:**Only penicillin by the intramuscular route of administration has been shown to be effective in the prophylaxis of rheumatic fever. Ceftibuten is generally effective in the eradication of *Streptococcus pyogenes* from the oropharynx; however, data establishing the efficacy of ceftibuten for the prophylaxis of subsequent rheumatic fever are not available.

CONTRAINDICATIONS:

Ceftibuten is contraindicated in patients with known allergy to the cephalosporin group of antibiotics.

WARNINGS:

BEFORE THERAPY WITH CEFTIBUTIN IS INSTITUTED, CAREFUL INQUIRY SHOULD BE MADE TO DETERMINE WHETHER THE PATIENT HAS HAD PREVIOUS HYPERSENSITIVITY REACTIONS TO CEFTIBUTIN, OTHER CEPHALOSPORINS, PENICILLINS, OR OTHER DRUGS. IF THIS PRODUCT IS TO BE GIVEN TO PENICILLIN-SENSITIVE PATIENTS, CAUTION SHOULD BE EXERCISED BECAUSE CROSS HYPERSENSITIVITY AMONG BETA-LACTAM ANTIBIOTICS HAS BEEN CLEARLY DOCUMENTED AND MAY OCCUR IN UP TO 10% OF PATIENTS WITH A HISTORY OF PENICILLIN ALLERGY. IF AN ALLERGIC REACTION TO CEFTIBUTIN OCCURS, DISCONTINUE THE DRUG. SERIOUS ACUTE HYPERSENSITIVITY REACTIONS MAY REQUIRE TREATMENT WITH EPINEPHRINE AND OTHER EMERGENCY MEASURES, INCLUDING OXYGEN, INTRAVENOUS FLUIDS, INTRAVENOUS ANTIHISTAMINES, CORTICOSTEROIDS, PRESSOR AMINES, AND AIRWAY MANAGEMENT, AS CLINICALLY INDICATED.

Pseudomembranous colitis has been reported with nearly all antibacterial agents, including ceftibuten, and may range in severity from mild to life threatening. Therefore, it is important to consider this diagnosis in patients who present with diarrhea subsequent to the administration of antibacterial agents.

Treatment with antibacterial agents alters normal flora of the colon and may permit overgrowth of clostridia.. Studies indicate that a toxin produced by *Clostridium difficile* is one primary cause of "antibiotic–associated colitis".

After the diagnosis of pseudomembranous colitis has been established, appropriate therapeutic measures should be initiated. Mild cases of pseudomembranous colitis usually respond to drug discontinuation alone. In moderate to severe cases, consideration should be given to management with fluids and electrolytes, protein supplementation, and treatment with an antibacterial drug clinically effective against *Clostridium difficile.*

PRECAUTIONS:

GENERAL

As with other broad-spectrum antibiotics, prolonged treatment may result in the possible emergence and overgrowth of resistant organisms. Careful observation of the patient is essential. If superinfection occurs during therapy, appropriate measures should be taken.

PRECAUTIONS: *(cont'd)*

The dose of ceftibuten may require adjustment in patients with varying degrees of renal insufficiency, particularly in patients with creatinine clearance less than 50 mL/min or undergoing hemodialysis (see DOSAGE AND ADMINISTRATION).

Ceftibuten is readily dialyzable. Dialysis patients should be monitored carefully, and administration of ceftibuten should occur immediately following dialysis.

Ceftibuten should be prescribed with caution to individuals with a history of gastrointestinal disease, particularly colitis.

INFORMATION TO PATIENTS

Patients should be informed that:

If the patient is diabetic, he/she should be informed that ceftibuten oral suspension contains 1 gram sucrose per teaspoon of suspension.

Ceftibuten oral suspension should be taken at least 2 hours before a meal or at least 1 hour after a meal (see CLINICAL PHARMACOLOGY, Food Effect on Absorption).

CARCINOGENISIS, MUTAGENISIS, IMPAIRMENT OF FERTILITY

Long-term animal studies have not been performed to evaluate the carcinogenic potential of ceftibuten. No mutagenic effects were seen in the following studies:*in vitro* chromosome assay in human lymphocytes, *in vivo* chromosome assay in mouse bone marrow cells, Chinese Hamster Ovary (CHO) cell point mutation assay at the hypoxanthine-guanine phosphoribosyl transferase (HGPRT) locus, and in a bacterial reversion point mutation test (Ames). No impairment of fertility occurred when rats were administered ceftibuten orally up to 2000 mg/kg/day (approximately 43 times the recommended human dose based on mg/m^2/day).

PREGNANCY, TERATOGENIC EFFECTS, PREGNANCY CATEGORY B

Ceftibuten was not teratogenic in the pregnant rat at oral doses up to 400 mg/kg/day (approximately 8.6 times the human dose based on mg/m^2/day). Ceftibuten was not teratogenic in the pregnant rabbit at oral doses up to 40 mg/kg/day (approximately 1.5 times the human dose based on mg/m^2/day) and has revealed no evidence of harm to the fetus. There are no adequate and well-controlled studies in pregnant women. Because animal reproduction studies are not always predictive of human response, this drug should be used during pregnancy only if clearly needed.

LABOR AND DELIVERY

Ceftibuten has not been studied for use during labor and delivery. Its use during such clinical situations should be weighed in terms of potential risk and benefit to both mother and fetus.

NURSING MOTHERS

It is not known whether ceftibuten (at recommended dosages) is excreted in human milk. Because many drugs are excreted in human milk, caution should be exercised when ceftibuten is administered to a nursing woman.

PEDIATRIC USE

The safety and efficacy of ceftibuten in infants less then 6 months of age have not been established.

GERIATRIC USE

The usual adult dosage recommendation may be followed for patients in this age group. However, these patients should be monitored closely, particularly their renal function, as dosage adjustment may be required.

DRUG INTERACTIONS:

Theophylline: Twelve healthy male volunteers were administered one 200–mg ceftibuten capsule twice daily for 6 days. With the morning dose of ceftibuten on day 6, each volunteer received a single intravenous infusion of theophylline (4 mg/kg). The pharmacokinetics of theophylline were not altered. The effect of ceftibuten on the pharmacokinetic of theophylline administered orally has not been investigated,

Antacids or H_2–receptor antagonists: The effect of increases gastric pH on the bioavailability of ceftibuten was evaluated in 18 healthy adult volunteers. Each volunteer was administered one 400–mg ceftibuten capsule. A single dose of liquid antacid did not affect the C_{max} or AUC of ceftibuten; however, 150 mg of ranitidine q12h for 3 days increased the ceftibuten C_{max} by 23% and ceftibuten AUC by 16%. the clinical relevance of these increases is not known.

DRUG/LABORATORY TEST INTERACTIONS

There have been no chemical or laboratory test interactions with ceftibuten noted to date. False-positive direct Coombs' tests have been reported during treatment with other cephalosporins. Therefore, it should be recognized that a positive Coombs' test could be due to the drug. The results of assays using red cells from healthy subjects to determine whether ceftibuten would cause direct Coombs' reactions *in vitro* showed no positive reaction at ceftibuten concentrations as high as 40 mcg/mL.

ADVERSE REACTIONS:

CLINICAL TRIALS

Capsules (adult patients)

In clinical trials, 1728 adult patients (1092 US and 636 international) were treated with the recommended dose of ceftibuten capsules (400 mg per day). There were no deaths or permanent disabilities thought due to drug toxicity in any of the patients in these studies. Thirty-six of the 1728 (2%) patients discontinued medication due to adverse events thought by the investigators to be possibly, probably, or almost certainly related to drug toxicity. The discontinuations were primarily for gastrointestinal disturbances, usually diarrhea, vomiting or nausea. Six of 1728 (0.3%) patients were discontinued due to rash or pruritus thought related to ceftibuten administration.

In the US trials, the following adverse events were thought by the investigators to be possibly, probably, or almost certainly related to ceftibuten capsules in multipe-dose clinical trials (n=1092 ceftibuten-treated patients).

TABLE 8 Adverse Reaction-Ceftibuten Capsules
U.S. Clinical Studies in Adult Patients (n=1092)

Incidence ≥ 1%	Nausea	4%
	Headache	3%
	Diarrhea	3%
	Dyspepsia	2%
	Dizziness	1%
	Abdominal Pain	1%
	Vomiting	1%
0.1% < Incidence < 1%	Anorexia, Constipation, Dry mouth, Dyspnea, Dysuria, Eructation, Fatigue, Flatulence, Loose stools, Moniliasis, Nasal congestion, Paresthesia, Pruritus, Rash, Somnolence, Taste perversion, Urticaria, Vaginitis	

Oral Suspension (pediatric patients)

In clinical trials, 1152 pediatric patients (772 US and 380 international), 97% of whom were younger than 12 years of age, were treated with the recommended dose of ceftibuten (9 mg/kg once daily up to a maximum dose of 400 mg per day) for 10 days. There were no deaths,

ADVERSE REACTIONS: *(cont'd)*

TABLE 9 Laboratory Value Changes*-Ceftibuten Capsules
U.S. Clinical Studies in Adult Patients

Incidence ≥ 1%	↑ BUN	4%
	↑ Eosinophils	3%
	↓ Hemoglobin	2%
	↑ ALT (SGPT)	1%
	↑ Bilirubin	1%
0.1% < Incidence < 1%	↑ Alk phosphatase	
	↑ Creatinine	
	↑ Platelets	
	↓ Platelets	
	↓ Leukocytes	
	↑ AST (SGOT)	

* Changes in laboratory values with possible clinical significance regardless of whether or not the investigator thought that the change was due to drug toxicity.

life-threatening adverse events, or permanent disabilities in any of the patients in these studies. Eight of the 1152 (<1%) patients discontinued medication due to adverse events thought by the investigators to be possibly, probably, or almost certainly related to drug toxicity. These discontinuations were primarily (7 out of 8) for gastrointestinal disturbances, usually diarrhea or vomiting. One patient was discontinued due to a cutaneous rash thought possibly related to ceftibuten administration.

In the US trials, the following adverse events were thought by the investigators to be possibly, probably, or almost certainly related to ceftibuten oral suspension in multiple-dose clinical trials (n=772 ceftibuten–treated patients).

Incidence ≥ 1%

Diarrhea * 4%

Vomiting 2%

Abdominal Pain 2%

Loose stools 2%

0.1% < Incidence < 1%

Agitation, Anorexia, Dehydration, Diaper dermatitis, Dizziness, Dyspepsia, Fever, Headache, Hematuria, Hyperkinesia, Insomnia, Irritability, Nausea, Pruritus, Rash, Rigors, Urticaria

*NOTE: The incidence of diarrhea in children ≤2 years old was 8% (23/301) compared with 2% (9/471) in children >2 years old.

TABLE 10 Laboratory Value Changes-Ceftibutin Oral Suspension
U.S. Clinical Studies in Adult Patients

Incidence ≥ 1%	↑ Eosinophils	3%
	↑ BUN	2%
	↓ Hemoglobin	1%
	↑ Platelets	1%
0.1% < Incidence < 1%	↑ ALT (SGPT)	
	↑ AST (SGOT)	
	↑ Alk phosphatase	
	↑ Bilirubin	
	↑ Creatinine	

* Changes in laboratory values with possible clinical significance regardless of whether or not the investigator thought that the change was due to drug toxicity.

IN POST-MARKETING EXPERIENCE

In addition to the events reported during clinical trials with ceftibuten, the following adverse experiences have been reported during worldwide post–marketing surveillance:

Capsules: Aphasia, jaundice, psychosis, stridor, toxic epidermal necrolysis.

Oral Suspension: Melena.

CEPHALOSPORIN–CLASS ADVERSE REACTIONS

In addition to the adverse reactions listed above that have been observed in patients treated with ceftibutin capsules, the following adverse events and altered laboratory tests have been reported for cephalosporin-class antibiotics: allergic reactions, anaphylaxis, drug fever, Stevens-Johnson syndrome, renal dysfunction, toxic nephropathy, hepatic cholestasis, aplastic anemia, hemolytic anemia, hemorrhage, false-positive test for urinary glucose, neutropenia, pancytopenia, and agranulocytosis. Pseudomembranous colitis; onset of symptoms may occur during or after antibiotic treatment (see WARNINGS).

Several cephalosporins have been implicated in triggering seizures, particularly in patients with renal impairment when the dosage was not reduced (see DOSAGE AND ADMINISTRATION and OVERDOSAGE). If seizures associated with drug therapy occur, the drug should be discontinued. Anticonvulsant therapy can be given if clinically indicated.

OVERDOSAGE:

Overdosage of cephalosporins can cause cerebral irritation leading to convulsions. Ceftibuten is readily dialyzable and significant quantities (65% of plasma concentrations) can be removed from the circulation by a single hemodialysis session. Information does not exist with regard to removal of ceftibuten by peritoneal dialysis.

DOSAGE AND ADMINISTRATION:

The recommended doses of ceftibuten oral suspension are presented in the table below. **Ceftibuten suspension must be administered at least 2 hours before or 1 hour after a meal.**

DOSAGE FOR IMPAIRED RENAL FUNCTION

Ceftibuten capsules and oral suspension may be administered at normal doses in the presence of impaired renal function with creatinine clearance of 50 mL/min or greater. The recommendations for dosing in patients with varying degrees of renal insufficiency are presented in the following table.

HEMODIALYSIS PATIENTS

In patients undergoing hemodialysis two or three times weekly, a single 400–mg dose of ceftibuten capsules or a single dose of 9 mg/kg (maximum of 400 mg of ceftibuten) oral suspension may be administered at the end of each hemodialysis session.

After mixing, the suspension may be kept for 14 days and must be stored in the refrigerator. Keep tightly closed. Shake well before each use. Discard any unused portion after 14 days.

HOW SUPPLIED:

Cedax Capsules, containing 400 mg of ceftibuten (as ceftibuten dihydrate) are white, opaque capsules imprinted with the product name and strength.

Store the capsules between 2° and 25°C (36° and 77°F). Replace cap securely after each opening.

Cedax Oral Suspension is an off-white to cream–colored powder that, when reconstituted as directed, contains either ceftibuten equivalent to 90mg/5 mL or 180 mg/mL.

HOW SUPPLIED: *(cont'd)*

TABLE 11

Type of infection (as qualified in the INDICATIONS AND USAGE section of this labeling)	Daily Maximum Dose	Dose and Frequency	Duration
Adults (12 years of age and older): Acute Bacterial Exaberations of Chronic Bronchitis due to *H. influenza* (including β-lactamase-producing strains), *M. catarrhalis* (including β-lactamas–producing strains), or *Streptococcus pneumoniae* (pencillin–susceptible strains only). (See INDICATIONS AND USAGE, NOTE) Pharyngitis and tonsillitis due to *S. pyogenes*. Acute Bacterial Otitis Media due to by *H. influenza* (including β–lactamase–producing strains), *M. catarrhalis* (including β–lactamase–producing USAGE, NOTE)	400 mg	400 mg QD	10 days
Children: Pharyngitis and tonsillitis due to *S. pyogenes*. Acute Bacterial Otitis Media due to *H. influenza* (including β–lactamase–producing strains), *M. catarrhalis* (including β–lactamase–producing strains), or *S. pyogenes*. (See INDICATIONS AND USAGE, NOTE)	400 mg	9 mg/kg QD	10 days

TABLE 12 Ceftibuten Oral Suspension Pediatric Dosage Chart

Child's Weight		90 mg/5 mL	180 mg/5 mL
10 kg	22 lbs	1 tsp QD	1/2 tsp QD
20 kg	44 lbs	2 tsp QD	1 tsp QD
40 kg	88 lbs	4 tsp QD	2 tsp QD

Children weighing more than 45 kg should receive the maximum daily dose of 400 mg.

TABLE 13

Creatinine Clearance (mL/min)	Recommended Dosing Schedules
>50	9 mg/kg or 400 mg Q24h (normal dosing schedule)
30-49	4.5 mg/kg or 200 mg Q24h
5-29	2.25 mg/kg or 100 mg Q24h

TABLE 14 Directions For Mixing Ceftibuten Oral Suspension

Final Concentration	Bottle Size	Amount of Water
90 mg per 5 mL	30 mL	Suspend in 28 mL of water
	60 mL	Suspend in 53 mL of water
	120 mL	Suspend in 103 mL of water
180 mg per 5 mL	30 mL	Suspend in 28 mL of water
	60 mL	Suspend in 53 mL of water
	120 mL	Suspend in 103 mL of water

Directions: First tap the bottle to loosen powder. Then add water in two portions, shaking well after each aliquot.

Prior to reconsitition, the powder must be stored between 2° and 25°C (36° and 77°F). Once it is reconstituted, the oral suspension is stable for 14 days when stored in a refrigerator between 2° and 8°C (36° and 46°F).

REFERENCES:

1. National Committee for Clinical Laboratory Standards. Methods for Dilution Antimicrobial Susceptibility Tests for Bacteria that Grow Aerobically-Third Edition. Approved Standard NCCLS Document M7–A3, Vol. 13, No. 25, NCCLS, Villanova, PA, December 1993. 2. National Committee for Clinical Laboratory Standards. Performance Standards for Antimicrobial Disk Susceptibility Tests-Fifth Edition. Approved Standard NCCLS Document M2–A5, Vol. 13, No. 24, NCCLS, Villanova, PA. December, 1993.

PATIENT INFORMATION:

Ceftibuten is an antibiotic used for upper respiratory tract and ear infections. Do not use if you are allergic to penicillin or cephalosporin (*e.g.,* Reflux) antibiotics. Inform your doctor if you have gastrointestinal problems, kidney disease or if you are pregnant or nursing. Diabetics should be aware there is 1 gram of sucrose in each teaspoon of oral suspension. Take one time daily as directed by your physician. The oral suspension should be taken at least 2 hours before a meal or at least 1 hour after a meal. May cause diarrhea, nausea, and vomiting. Do not give to children 6 months of age or younger.

HOW SUPPLIED - EQUIVALENTS NOT AVAILABLE:

Capsule - Oral - 400 mg

10 x 4's UD	$251.52	CEDAX, Schering	00085-0691-03
20's	$123.60	CEDAX, Schering	00085-0691-01
100's	$610.00	CEDAX, Schering	00085-0691-02

Oral Suspension - Oral - 18 mg/ml

30 ml	$22.80	CEDAX, Schering	00085-0777-03
60 ml	$29.64	CEDAX, Schering	00085-0777-01

Oral Suspension - Oral - 36 mg/ml

30 ml	$22.80	CEDAX, Schering	00085-0834-03
60 ml	$29.64	CEDAX, Schering	00085-0834-01
120 ml	$59.76	CEDAX, Schering	00085-0834-02

Oral suspension - Oral - 18 mg/ml

120 ml	$59.76	CEDAX, Schering	00085-0777-02

CEFTIZOXIME SODIUM *(000693)*

CATEGORIES: Anti-Infectives; Antibiotics; Antimicrobials; Bone Infections; Cephalosporins; Gonorrhea; Infections; Intra-Abdominal Infections; Joint Infections; Meningitis; Pelvic Inflammatory Disease; Penicillins; Respiratory Tract Infections; Septicemia; Skin Infections; Urinary Tract Infections; Pregnancy Category B; FDA Approved 1983 Sep

BRAND NAMES: *Ceftix* (Germany); **Cefizox**; Cefizox In 5% Dextrose; Cefizox In Dextrose; *Ceftrax*; *Epocelin* (Japan); *Eposerin*; *Lyceft*; *Oframax*; *Rocephin* (Germany); *Tefizox*; *Tergecin*; *Ultracef* (Mexico)
(International brand names outside U.S. in italics)

FORMULARIES: BC-BS

DESCRIPTION:

Cefizox (sterile ceftizoxime sodium) is a sterile, semisynthetic, broad-spectrum, beta-lactamase resistant cephalosporin antibiotic for parenteral (IV, IM) administration. It is the sodium salt of [6R-[6α, 7β(Z)]]-7-[[(2,3-dihydro-2-imino-4-thiazolyl) (methoxyimino) acetyl] amino]-8-oxo-5-thia-1-azabicyclo [4.2.0] oct-2-ene-2-carboxylic acid. Its sodium content is approximately 60 mg (2.6 mEq) per gram of ceftizoxime activity.

Sterile ceftizoxime sodium is a white to pale yellow crystalline powder.

Cefizox is supplied in vials equivalent to 500 mg, 1 gram, 2 grams, or 10 grams of ceftizoxime, and in "Piggyback" Vials for intravenous admixture equivalent to 1 gram or 2 grams of ceftizoxime.

Cefizox, equivalent to 1 gram or 2 grams of ceftizoxime, is also supplied as a frozen, sterile, nonpyrogenic solution of ceftizoxime sodium in an iso-osmotic diluent in plastic containers. After thawing, the solution is intended for intravenous use.

The plastic container is fabricated from specially formulated polyvinyl chloride. Solutions in contact with the plastic container can leach out certain of its chemical components in very small amounts within the expiration period, e.g., di 2-ethylhexyl phthalate (DEHP), up to 5 parts per million. However, the suitability of the plastic has been confirmed in tests in animals according to the USP biological tests for plastic containers as well as by tissue culture toxicity studies.

CLINICAL PHARMACOLOGY:

The table below (TABLE 1) demonstrates the serum levels and duration of ceftizoxime sodium following intramuscular administration of 500 mg and 1 gram doses, respectively, to normal volunteers.

TABLE 1 Serum Concentrations After Intramuscular Administration Serum Concentration (mcg/ml)

Dose	1/2 hr	1 hr	2 hr	4 hr	6 hr	8 hr
500 mg	13.3	13.7	9.2	4.8	1.9	0.7
1 gm	36.0	39.0	31.0	15.0	6.0	3.0

Following intravenous administration of 1, 2, and 3 gram doses of ceftizoxime sodium to normal volunteers, the following serum levels were obtained. (TABLE 2)

TABLE 2 Serum Concentrations After Intravenous Serum Concentration (mcg/ml)

Dose	5 min	10 min	30 min	1 hr	2 hr	4 hr	8 hr
1 g	ND	ND	60.5	38.9	21.5	8.4	1.4
2 g	131.8	110.9	77.5	53.6	33.1	12.1	2.0
3 g	221.1	174.0	112.7	83.9	47.4	26.2	4.8

ND=Not Done

A serum half-life of approximately 1.7 hours was observed after intravenous or intramuscular administration.

Ceftizoxime sodium is 30% protein bound.

Ceftizoxime sodium is not metabolized, and is excreted virtually unchanged by the kidneys in 24 hours. This provides a high urinary concentration. Concentrations greater than 6000 mcg/ml have been achieved in the urine by 2 hours after a 1 gram dose of ceftizoxime sodium intravenously. Probenecid slows tubular secretion and produces even higher serum levels, increasing the duration of measurable serum concentrations.

Ceftizoxime sodium achieves therapeutic levels in various body fluids, e.g., cerebrospinal fluid (in patients with inflamed meninges), bile, surgical wound fluid, pleural fluid, aqueous humor, ascitic fluid, peritoneal fluid, prostatic fluid and saliva, and the following body tissues: heart, gallbladder, bone, biliary, peritoneal, prostatic, and uterine.

In clinical experience to date, no disulfiram-like reactions have been reported with ceftizoxime sodium.

MICROBIOLOGY

The bactericidal action of ceftizoxime sodium results from inhibition of cell-wall synthesis. Ceftizoxime sodium is highly resistant to a broad spectrum of beta-lactamases (penicillinase and cephalosporinase), including Richmond types I, II, III, TEM, and IV, produced by both aerobic and anaerobic gram-positive and gram-negative organisms. Ceftizoxime sodium is active against a wide range of gram-positive and gram-negative organisms, and is usually active against the following organisms *in vitro* and in clinical situations. (See INDICATIONS AND USAGE.)

GRAM-POSITIVE AEROBES

Staphylococcus aureus (including penicillinase- and non-penicillinase- producing strains) Note: Methicillin-resistant staphylococci are resistant to cephalosporins, including ceftizoxime.

Staphylococcus epidermidis (including penicillinase- and non-penicillinase-producing strains) *Streptococcus agalactiae;Streptococcus pneumoniae; Streptococcus pyrogenes* Note: Ceftizoxime is usually inactive against most strains of *Enterococcus faecalis* (formerly *S. faecalis).*

GRAM-NEGATIVE AEROBES

Acinetobacter spp.; *Enterobacter* spp.; *Escherichia coli*; *Haemophilus influenzae* (including ampicillin-resistant strains); *Klebsiella pneumoniae*;*Morganella morganii* (formerly *Proteus morganii*);*Neisseria gonorrhoeae*; *Proteus mirabilis*; *Proteus vulgaris*; *Providencia rettgeri* (formerly *Proteus rettgeri*); *Pseudomonas aeruginosa*; *Serratiamarcescens*

ANAEROBES

Bacteroides spp.; *Peptococcus* spp.;*Peptostreptococcus* spp.

Ceftizoxime is usually active against the following organisms *in vitro*, but the clinical significance of these data is unknown.

GRAM-POSITIVE AEROBES

Corynebacterium diphtheriae

GRAM-NEGATIVE AEROBES

Aeromonas hydrophilia; *Citrobacter* spp.; *Moraxella* spp.; *Neisseria meningitidis*; *Pasteurella multocida*; *Providence stuartii*; *Salmonella* spp.; *Shigella* spp.; *Yersinia enterocolitica*

ANAEROBES

Actinomyces spp.; *Bifidobacterium* spp.; *Clostridium* spp. NOTE: Most strains of *Clostridium difficile* are resistant. *Eubacterium* spp.; Fusobacterium spp.;*Propionibacterium* spp.; *Veillonella* spp.

SUSCEPTIBILITY TESTING

Diffusion Techniques: Quantitative methods that require measurement of zone diameters give the most precise estimate of the susceptibility of bacteria to antimicrobial agents. One such standard procedure[1] has been recommended for use with disks to test susceptibility of organisms to ceftizoxime. Interpretation involves the correlation of the diameters obtained in the disk test with the minimum inhibitory concentration (MIC) for ceftizoxime.

CLINICAL PHARMACOLOGY: *(cont'd)*

Organisms should be tested with the ceftizoxime disk, since ceftizoxime has been shown by *in vitro* tests to be active against certain strains found resistant when other beta-lactam disks are used.

Reports from the laboratory giving results of the standard single-disk susceptibility test with a 30 mcg ceftizoxime disk should be interpreted according to the following criteria (TABLE 3) (with the exception of *Pseudomonas aeruginosa*).

TABLE 3

Zone Diameter (mm)	Interpretation
≥ 20	(S) Susceptible
15-19	(MS) Moderately Susceptible
≤ 14	(R) Resistant

A report of "Susceptible" indicates that the pathogen is likely to be inhibited by generally achievable blood levels. A report of "Moderately Susceptible" suggests that the organism would be susceptible if high dosage is used or if the infection is confined to tissue and fluids (*e.g.*, urine) in which high antibiotic levels are attained. A report of "Resistant" indicates that achievable concentrations of the antibiotic are unlikely to be inhibitory and other therapy should be selected.

Standardized procedures require the use of laboratory control organisms. The 30 mcg ceftizoxime disk should give the following zone diameters. (TABLE 4)

TABLE 4

Organism	ATCC	Zone Diameter (mm)
Escherichia coli	25922	30-36
Pseudomonas aeruginosa	27853	12-17
Staphylococcus aureus	25923	27-35

Pseudomonas in Urinary Tract Infections: Most strains of *Pseudomonas aeruginosa* are moderately susceptible to ceftizoxime. Ceftizoxime achieves high levels in the urine (greater than 6000 mcg/ml at 2 hours with 1 gram IV) and therefore, the following zone sizes should be used when testing ceftizoxime for treatment of urinary tract infections caused by *Pseudomonas aeruginosa*.

Susceptible organisms produce zones of 20 mm or greater, indicating that the test organism is likely to respond to therapy.

Organisms that produce zones of 11 to 19 mm are expected to be susceptible when the infection is confined to the urinary tract (in which high antibiotic levels are attained).

Resistant organisms produce zones of 10 mm or less, indicating that other therapy should be selected.

Dilution Techniques: When using the NCCLS agar dilution or broth dilution (including microdilution) method[2] or equivalent, the following MIC data should be used for interpretation. (TABLE 5)

TABLE 5

MIC (mcg/ml)	Interpretation
≤ 8	(S) Susceptible
16-32	(MS) Moderately Susceptible
≥ 64	(R) Resistant

As with standard disk diffusion methods, dilution procedures require the use of laboratory control organisms. Standard ceftizoxime powder should give MIC values in the following ranges. (TABLE 6)

TABLE 6

Organism	ATCC	MIC (mcg/ml)
Escherichia coli	25922	0.03-0.12
Pseudomonas aeruginosa	27853	16-64
Staphylococcus aureus	29213	2-8

INDICATIONS AND USAGE:

Ceftizoxime sodium is indicated in the treatment of infections due to susceptible strains of the microorganisms listed below:

Lower Respiratory Tract Infections caused by *Klebsiella* spp.;*Proteus mirabilis*; *Escherichia coli*; *Haemophilus influenzae* including ampicillin-resistant strains; *Staphylococcus aureus* (penicillinase- and non-penicillinase producing);*Serratia* spp.; *Enterobacter* spp.; *Bacteroides* spp.; and *Streptococcus* spp. including *S. pneumoniae,* but excluding enterococci.

Urinary Tract Infections caused by *Staphylococcus aureus* (penicillinase- and non-penicillinase-producing); *Escherichia coli*; *Pseudomonas* spp. including *P. aeruginosa; Proteus mirabilis; P. vulgaris; Providencia rettgeri* (formerly *Proteus rettgeri*) and *Morganella morganii* (formerly *Proteus morganii*); *Klebsiella* spp.; *Serratia* spp. including *S. marcescens; and Enterobacter* spp.

Gonorrhea including uncomplicated cervical and urethral gonorrhea caused by *Neisseria gonorrhoeae*.

Pelvic Inflammatory Disease caused by *Neisseria gonorrhoeea,Escherichia coli* or *Streptococcus agalactiae.*NOTE: Ceftizoxime, like other cephalosporins, has no activity against*Chlamydia trachomatis.* Therefore, when cephalosporins are used in the treatment of patients with pelvic inflammatory disease and *C. trachomatis* is one of the suspected pathogens, approximate anti-chlamydial coverage should be added.

Intra-Abdominal Infections caused by *Escherichia coli;Staphylococcus epidermidis*; *Streptococcus* spp. (excluding enterococci); *Enterobacter* spp.; *Klebsiella* spp.; *Bacteroids* spp. including *B. fragilis*; and *anaerobic cocci,* including *Peptococcus* spp. and *Peptostreptococcus* spp.

Septicemia caused by *Streptococcus* spp. including *S. pneumoniae* (but excluding enterococci); *Staphylococcus aureus* (penicillinase- and non-penicillinase-producing); *Escherichia coli*; *Bacteroides* spp. including *B fragilis;Klebsiella* spp.; and *Serratia* spp.

Skin and Skin Structure Infections caused by *Staphylococcus aureus* (penicillinase- and non-penicillinase-producing);*Staphylococcus epidermidis*; *Escherichia coli;Klebsiella* spp.; *Streptococcus* spp. including*Streptococcus pyogenes* (but excluding enterococci); *Proteus mirabilis*; *Serratia* spp.; *Enterobacter* spp.;*Bacteroides* spp. including *B. fragilis*; and anaerobic cocci, including *Peptococcus* spp. and *Peptostreptococcus* spp.

Bone and Joint Infections caused by *Staphylococcus aureus* (penicillinase- and non-penicillinase-producing); *Streptococcus* spp. (excluding enterococci); *Proteus mirabilis,Bacteroids* spp.; and anaerobic cocci, including*Peptococcus* spp. and *Peptostreptococcus* spp.

INDICATIONS AND USAGE: *(cont'd)*

Meningitis caused by *Haemophilus influenzae.* Ceftizoxime sodium has also been used successfully in the treatment of a limited number of pediatric and adult cases of meningitis caused by *Streptococcus pneumoniae.*

Ceftizoxime sodium has been effective in the treatment of seriously ill, compromised patients, including those who were debilitated, immunosuppressed, or neutropenic.

Infections caused by aerobic gram-negative and by mixtures of organisms resistant to other cephalosporins, aminoglycosides, or penicillins have responded to treatment with ceftizoxime sodium.

Because of the serious nature of some urinary tract infections due to*P. aeruginosa* and because many strains of *Pseudomonas* species are only moderately susceptible to ceftizoxime sodium, higher dosage is recommended. Other therapy should be instituted if the response is not prompt.

Susceptibility studies on specimens obtained prior to therapy should be used to determine the response of causative organisms to ceftizoxime sodium. Therapy with ceftizoxime sodium may be initiated pending results of the studies; however, treatment should be adjusted according to study findings. In serious infections, ceftizoxime sodium has been used concomitantly with aminoglycosides (see PRECAUTIONS). Before using ceftizoxime sodium concomitantly with other antibiotics, the prescribing information for those agents should be reviewed for contraindications, warnings, precautions, and adverse reactions. Renal function should be carefully monitored.

CONTRAINDICATIONS:

Ceftizoxime sodium is contraindicated in patients who have known allergy to the drug.

WARNINGS:

BEFORE THERAPY WITH STERILE CEFTIZOXIME SODIUM IS INSTITUTED, CAREFUL INQUIRY SHOULD BE MADE TO DETERMINE WHETHER THE PATIENT HAS HAD PREVIOUS HYPERSENSITIVITY REACTIONS TO CEPHALOSPORINS, PENICILLINS, OR OTHER DRUGS. THIS PRODUCT SHOULD BE GIVEN CAUTIOUSLY TO PENICILLIN-SENSITIVE PATIENTS. CAUTION SHOULD BE EXERCISED BECAUSE CROSS-HYPERSENSITIVITY AMONG BETA-LACTAM ANTIBIOTICS HAS BEEN CLEARLY DOCUMENTED AND MAY OCCUR IN UP TO 10% OF PATIENTS WITH A HISTORY OF PENICILLIN ALLERGY. IF AN ALLERGIC REACTION TO STERILE CEFTIZOXIME SODIUM OCCURS, DISCONTINUE THE DRUG. SERIOUS ACUTE HYPERSENSITIVITY REACTIONS MAY REQUIRE TREATMENT WITH EPINEPHRINE, AND OTHER EMERGENCY MEASURES, INCLUDING OXYGEN, INTRAVENOUS FLUIDS, INTRAVENOUS ANTIHISTAMINES, CORTICOSTEROIDS, PRESSOR AMINES, AND AIRWAY MANAGEMENT, AS CLINICALLY INDICATED.

Pseudomembranous colitis has been reported with the use of cephalosporins (and other broad-spectrum antibiotics); therefore, it is important to consider this diagnosis in patients who develop diarrhea in association with antibiotic use.

Treatment with broad-spectrum antibiotics alters normal flora of the colon and may permit overgrowth of *clostridia.*Studies indicate a toxin produced by *Clostridium difficile* is one primary cause of antibiotic-associated colitis.

Mild cases of colitis may respond to drug discontinuance alone.

Moderate to severe cases should be managed with fluid, electrolyte, and protein supplementation as indicated.

When the colitis is not relieved by drug discontinuance or when it is severe, oral vancomycin is the treatment of choice for antibiotic-associated pseudomembranous colitis produced by *C. difficile.* Other causes of colitis should also be considered.

PRECAUTIONS:

General: As with all broad-spectrum antibiotics, ceftizoxime sodium should be prescribed with caution in individuals with a history of gastrointestinal disease, particularly colitis.

Although ceftizoxime sodium has not been shown to produce an alteration in renal function, renal status should be evaluated, especially in seriously ill patients receiving maximum dose therapy. As with any antibiotic, prolonged use may result in overgrowth of nonsusceptible organisms. Careful observation is essential; appropriate measures should be taken if superinfection occurs.

Carcinogenesis, Mutagenesis, and Impairment of Fertility: Long term studies in animals to evaluate the carcinogenic potential of ceftizoxime have not been conducted. In an *in vitro* bacterial cell assay (*i.e.,* Ames test), there was no evidence of mutagenicity at ceftizoxime concentrations of 0.001-0.5 mcg/plate. Ceftizoxime did not produce increases in micronuclei in the *in vivo* mouse micronucleus test when given to animals at doses up to 7500 mg/kg, approximately six times greater than the maximum daily dose on a mg/m^2 basis.

Ceftizoxime had no effect on fertility when administered subcutaneously to rats at daily doses of up to 1000 mg/kg/day, approximately two times the maximum human daily dose on a mg/m^2 basis. Ceftizoxime produced no histological changes in the sexual organs of male and female dogs when given intravenously for thirteen weeks at a dose of 1000 mg/kg/day, approximately five times greater than the maximum human daily dose on a mg/m^2 basis.

Pregnancy, Teratogenic Effects, Pregnancy Category B: Reproduction studies performed in rats and rabbits have revealed no evidence of impaired fertility or harm to the fetus due to ceftizoxime sodium. There are, however, no adequate and well-controlled studies in pregnant women. Because animal reproduction studies are not always predictive of human effects, this drug should be used during pregnancy only if clearly needed.

Labor and Delivery: Safety of ceftizoxime sodium use during labor and delivery has not been established.

Nursing Mothers: Ceftizoxime sodium is excreted in human milk in low concentrations. Caution should be exercised when ceftizoxime sodium is administered to a nursing woman.

Pediatric Use: Safety and efficacy in infants from birth to six months of age have not been established. In children six months of age and older, treatment with ceftizoxime sodium has been associated with transient elevated levels of eosinophils, AST (SGOT), ALT (SGPT), and CPK (creatine phosphokinase). The CPK elevation may be related to IM administration.

The potential for the toxic effect in children from chemicals that may leach from the single-dose IV preparation in plastic has not been determined.

DRUG INTERACTIONS:

Although the occurrence has not been reported with ceftizoxime sodium, nephrotoxicity has been reported following concomitant administration of other cephalosporins and aminoglycosides.

ADVERSE REACTIONS:

Ceftizoxime sodium is generally well tolerated. The *most* frequent adverse reactions (*greater* than 1% but *less* than 5%) are:

Hypersensitivity: Rash, pruritus, fever.

Hepatic: Transient elevation in AST (SGOT), ALT (SGPT), and alkaline phosphatase.

ADVERSE REACTIONS: *(cont'd)*

Hematologic: Transient eosinophilia, thrombocytosis. Some individuals have developed a positive Coombs test.

Local—Injection site: Burning, cellulitis, phlebitis with IV administration, pain, induration, tenderness, paresthesia.

The *less* frequent adverse reactions (*less* than 1%) are:

Hypersensitivity: Numbness and anaphylaxis have been reported rarely.

Hepatic: Elevation of bilirubin has been reported rarely.

Renal: Transient elevations of BUN and creatinine have been occasionally observed with ceftizoxime sodium.

Hematologic: Anemia, leukopenia, neutropenia, and thrombocytopenia have been reported rarely.

Urogenital: Vaginitis has occurred rarely.

Gastrointestinal: Diarrhea; nausea and vomiting have been reported occasionally.

Symptoms of pseudomembranous colitis can appear during or after antibiotic treatment. (See WARNINGS.)

In addition to the adverse reactions listed above which have been observed in patients treated with ceftizoxime, the following adverse reactions and altered laboratory tests have been reported for cephalosporin-class antibiotics:

Stevens-Johnson syndrome, erythema multiforme, toxic epidermal necrolysis, serum-sickness like reaction, toxic nephropathy, aplastic anemia, hemolytic anemia, hemorrhage, prolonged prothrombin time, elevated LDH, pancytopenia, and agranulocytosis.

Several cephalosporins have been implicated in triggering seizures, particularly in patients with renal impairment, when the dosage was not reduced. (See DOSAGE AND ADMINISTRATION.)If seizures associated with drug therapy occur, the drug should be discontinued. Anticonvulsant therapy can be given if clinically indicated.

DOSAGE AND ADMINISTRATION:

The usual adult dosage is 1 or 2 grams of ceftizoxime sodium every 8 to 12 hours. Proper dosage and route of administration should be determined by the condition of the patient, severity of the infection, and susceptibility of the causative organisms. (TABLE 7)

TABLE 7 General Guidelines for Dosage of Ceftizoxime Sodium

Type of Infection	Daily Dose (Grams)	Frequency and Route
Uncomplicated		
Urinary Tract	1	500 mg q12h IM or IV
Other Sites	2-3	1 gram q8-12h IM or IV
Severe or Refractory	3-6	1 gram q8h IM or IV
		2 grams q8-12h IM[a] or IV
PID[b]	6	2 grams of q8h IV
Life-Threatening[c]	9-12	3-4 grams q8h IV

a When administering 2 gram IM doses, the dose should be divided and given in different large muscle masses.
b If *C. trachomatis* is a suspected pathogen, appropriate anti-chlamydial coverage should be added, because ceftizoxime has no activity against this organism.
c In life-threatening infections, dosages up to 2 grams every 4 hours have been given.

Because of the serious nature of urinary tract infections due to *P. aeruginosa* and because many strains of *Pseudomonas* species are only moderately susceptible to ceftizoxime sodium, higher dosage is recommended. Other therapy should be instituted if the response is not prompt.

A single, 1 gram IM dose is the usual dose for treatment of uncomplicated gonorrhea.

The intravenous route may be preferable for patients with bacterial septicemia, localized parenchymal abscesses (such as intra-abdominal abscess), peritonitis, or other severe or life-threatening infections.

In those with normal renal function, the intravenous dosage for such infections is 2 to 12 grams of ceftizoxime sodium daily. In conditions such as bacterial septicemia, 6 to 12 grams/day may be given initially by the intravenous route for several days, and the dosage may then be gradually reduced according to clinical response and laboratory findings. (TABLE 8)

TABLE 8 Pediatric Dosage Schedule

	Unit Dose	Frequency
Children 6 months and older	50 mg/kg	q6-8h

Dosage may be increased to a total daily dose of 200 mg/kg (not to exceed the maximum adult dose for serious infection).

IMPAIRED RENAL FUNCTION

Modification of ceftizoxime sodium dosage is necessary in patients with impaired renal function. Following an initial loading dose of 500 mg-1 gram IM or IV, the maintenance dosing schedule shown below should be followed. Further dosing should be determined by therapeutic monitoring, severity of the infection, and susceptibility of the causative organisms.

When only the serum creatinine level is available, creatinine clearance may be calculated from the following formula. The serum creatinine level should represent current renal function at the steady state. (TABLE 9)

TABLE 9

Males Clcr = [Weight (kg) × (140 - age)] ÷ [72 × serum creatinine (mg/100 ml)]

Females are 0.85 of the calculated clearance values for males.

In patients undergoing hemodialysis, no additional supplemental dosing is required following hemodialysis; however, dosing should be timed so that the patient receives the dose (according to TABLE 10 below) at the end of the dialysis.

TABLE 10 Dosage in Adults with Reduced Renal Function

Creatinine Clearance ml/min	Renal Function	Less Severe Infections	Life-Threatening Infections
79-50	Mild Impairment	500 mg q8h	0.75-1.5 grams q8h
49-5	Moderate to severe impairment	250-500 mg q12h	0.5-1 gram q12h
4-0	Dialysis patients	500 mg q48h or 250 mg q24h	0.5-1 gram q48h or 0.5 gram q24h

PREPARATION OF PARENTERAL SOLUTION

DOSAGE AND ADMINISTRATION: *(cont'd)*

Reconstitution

IM Administration: Reconstitute with Sterile Water for Injection. SHAKE WELL. (TABLE 11)

TABLE 11

Vial Size	Diluent to Be Added	Approx. Avail. Vol.	Approx. Avg. Concentration
500 mg	1.5 ml	1.8 ml	280 mg/ml
1 gram	3.0 ml	3.7 ml	270 mg/ml
2 grams*	6.0 ml	7.4 ml	270 mg/ml

* When administering 2 gram IM doses, the dose should be divided and given in different large muscle masses.

IV Administration: Reconstitute with Sterile Water for Injection. SHAKE WELL. (TABLE 12)

TABLE 12

Vial Size	Diluent to Be Added	Approx. Avail. Vol.	Approx. Avg. Concentration
500 mg	5 ml	5.3 ml	95 mg/ml
1 gram	10 ml	10.7 ml	95 mg/ml
2 grams	20 ml	21.4 ml	95 mg/ml

These solutions of ceftizoxime sodium are stable 24 hours at room temperature or 96 hours if refrigerated (5°C).

Parenteral drug products should be inspected visually for particulate matter prior to administration. If particulate matter is evident in reconstituted fluids, then the drug solution should be discarded. Reconstituted solutions may range from yellow to amber without changes in potency.

Pharmacy Bulk Vials: For IM or IV direct injection, add Sterile Water for Injection to the 10 gram vial according to table below (TABLE 13). SHAKE WELL. For IV intermittent or continuous infusion, add Sterile Water for Injection according to table below. SHAKE WELL. Add to parenteral fluids listed below under IV Administration.

TABLE 13

Vial Size	Diluent to Be Added	Approx. Avail. Vol.	Approx. Avg. Concentration
10 grams	30 ml	37 ml	1 gram/3.5 ml
	45 ml	51 ml	1 gram/5 ml

These reconstituted solutions of ceftizoxime sodium are stable 24 hours at room temperature or 96 hours if refrigerated (5°C).

"Piggyback" Vials: Reconstitute with 50 to 100 ml of Sodium Chloride Injection or any other IV solution listed below. SHAKE WELL.

Administer with primary IV fluids, as a single dose. These solutions of ceftizoxime sodium are stable 24 hours at room temperature or 96 hours if refrigerated (5°C).

A solution of 1 gram ceftizoxime sodium in 13 ml Sterile Water for Injection is isotonic.

IM INJECTION

Inject well within the body of a relatively large muscle. Aspiration is necessary to avoid inadvertent injection into a blood vessel. When administering 2 gram IM doses, the dose should be divided and given in different large muscle masses.

IV ADMINISTRATION

Direct (bolus) injection, slowly over 3 to 5 minutes, directly or through tubing for patients receiving parenteral fluids (see list below). Intermittent or continuous infusion, dilute reconstituted ceftizoxime sodium in 50 to 100 ml of one of the following solutions:

Sodium Chloride Injection

5% or 10% Dextrose Injection

5% Dextrose and 0.9%, 0.45%, or 0.2% Sodium Chloride Injection

Ringer's Injection

Lactated Ringer's Injection

Invert Sugar 10% in Sterile Water for Injection

5% Sodium Bicarbonate in Sterile Water for Injection

5% Dextrose in Lactated Ringer's Injection (only when reconstituted with 4% Sodium Bicarbonate Injection).

In these fluids, ceftizoxime sodium is stable 24 hours at room temperature or 96 hours if refrigerated (5°C).

REFERENCES:

1. National Committee for Clinical Laboratory Standards, Approved Standard. *Performance Standards for Antimicrobial Disk Susceptibility Test*, 4th Edition, Vol 10 (7): M2-A4. Villanova, PA, April 1990. **2.** National Committee for Clinical Laboratory Standards, Approved Standard. *Methods for Dilution Antimicrobial Susceptibility Tests for Bacteria that Grow Aerobically*, 2nd Edition, Vol 10 (8): M7-A2. Villanova, PA, April 1990.

HOW SUPPLIED:

Unreconstituted ceftizoxime sodium should be protected from excessive light, and stored at controlled room temperature (59°-86°F) in the original package until used.

HOW SUPPLIED - EQUIVALENTS NOT AVAILABLE:

Injection, Solution - Intravenous - 1 gm

1's	$11.86	CEFIZOX, Fujisawa USA	00469-7251-01
10's	$128.13	CEFIZOX, Fujisawa USA	00469-7252-01
10's	$130.00	CEFIZOX, Fujisawa USA	00469-7271-01
50 ml x 24	$349.50	CEFIZOX IN 5% DEXTROSE, Fujisawa USA	00469-7220-01

Injection, Solution - Intravenous - 2 gm

1's	$22.03	CEFIZOX, Fujisawa USA	00469-7253-02
10's	$231.63	CEFIZOX, Fujisawa USA	00469-7272-02
10's	$240.08	CEFIZOX, Fujisawa USA	00469-7254-02
50 ml x 24	$593.40	CEFIZOX IN 5% DEXTROSE, Fujisawa USA	00469-7221-02

Injection, Solution - Intravenous - 10 gm

10's	$1087.96	CEFIZOX, Fujisawa USA	00469-7255-10

Injection, Solution - Intravenous - 500 mg

1's	$6.75	CEFIZOX, Fujisawa USA	00469-7250-01

CEFTRIAXONE SODIUM *(000694)*

CATEGORIES: Anti-Infectives; Antibiotics; Antimicrobials; Bone Infections; Cephalosporins; Gonorrhea; Infections; Intra-Abdominal Infections; Joint Infections; Meningitis; Pelvic Inflammatory Disease; Perioperative Prophylaxis; Respiratory Tract Infections; Septicemia; Sexually Transmitted Diseases; Skin Infections; Urinary Tract Infections; Lyme Disease*; Pregnancy Category B; Sales > $1 Billion; FDA Approved 1984 Dec; Patent Expiration 2000 Dec
* Indication not approved by the FDA

BRAND NAMES: *Benaxona* (Mexico); *Broadced*; *Cefaxona* (Mexico); *Cefaxone*; *Ceftrex*; *Chef*; *Inocef*; *Lendacin*; *Monocef*; *Nakaxone*; *Rocefalin Roche*; *Rocefin*; *Rocephalin*; **Rocephin**; *Rocephin "Biochemie"*; *Rocephin "Roche"*; *Rocephin Roche*; *Rocephine* (France); *Rocephine " Roche"*; *Sintrex*; *Sunflow*; *Tacex* (Mexico); *Triaken* (Mexico); *Tricef*; *Tricephin*; *Zefaxone*; *Zefone 250*
(International brand names outside U.S. in italics)

FORMULARIES: BC-BS; WHO

COST OF THERAPY: $4.00 (Infections; Injection; 1 gm/vial; 1/day; 4 days) vs. Potential Cost of $7,048.46 (DRG 79, Respiratory Infections)

PRIMARY ICD9: 136.9 (Unspecified Infections and Parasitic Diseases)

DESCRIPTION:

Rocephin is a sterile, semisynthetic, broad-spectrum cephalosporin antibiotic for intravenous or intramuscular administration. Ceftriaxone sodium is 5-Thia-1-azabicyclo[4.2.0]oct-2-ene-2-carboxylic acid, 7-[[(2-amino-4-thiazolyl)(methoxyimino)acetyl]-amino]-8-oxo-3-[[(1,2,5,6-tetrahydro-2-methyl-5,6-dioxo-1,2,4-triazin-3-yl)thio]methyl]-, disodium salt, [6R-[6α,7β(Z)]]-.

The chemical formula of ceftriaxone sodium is $C_{18}H_{16}N_8Na_2O_7S_3 3.5H_2O$. It has a calculated molecular weight of 661.59.

Rocephin is a white to yellowish-orange crystalline powder which is readily soluble in water, sparingly soluble in methanol and very slightly soluble in ethanol. The pH of a 1% aqueous solution is approximately 6.7. The color of Rocephin solutions ranges from light yellow to amber, depending on the length of storage, concentration and diluent used.

Rocephin contains approximately 83 mg (3.6 mEq) of sodium per gram of ceftriaxone activity.

CLINICAL PHARMACOLOGY:

Average plasma concentrations of ceftriaxone following a single 30-minute intravenous (IV) infusion of a 0.5, 1 or 2 gm dose and intramuscular (IM) administration of a single 0.5 or 1 gm dose in healthy subjects are presented in TABLE 1.

TABLE 1 Ceftriaxone Plasma Concentrations After Single Dose Administration

Dose/Route	Average Plasma Concentrations (mcg/ml)								
	0.5 hr	1 hr	2 hr	4 hr	6 hr	8 hr	12 hr	16 hr	24 hr
0.5 gm IV*	82	59	48	37	29	23	15	10	5
0.5 gm IM	30	41	43	39	31	25	16	ND†	ND
1 gm IV*	151	111	88	67	53	43	28	18	9
1 gm IM	40	68	76	68	56	44	29	ND	ND
2 gm IV*	257	192	154	117	89	74	46	31	15

* IV doses were infused at a constant rate over 30 minutes.
† ND=Not determined.

Ceftriaxone was completely absorbed following IM administration with mean maximum plasma concentrations occurring between two and three hours postdosing. Multiple IV or IM doses ranging from 0.5 to 2 gm at 12- to 24-hour intervals resulted in 15% to 36% accumulation of ceftriaxone above single dose values.

Ceftriaxone concentrations in urine are high, as shown in TABLE 2.

TABLE 2 Urinary Concentrations of Ceftriaxone After Single Dose Administration

Dose/Route	Average Urinary Concentrations (mcg/ml)					
	0-2 hr	2-4 hr	4-8 hr	8-12 hr	12-24 hr	24-48 hr
0.5 gm IV	526	366	142	87	70	15
0.5 gm IM	115	425	308	127	96	28
1 gm IV	995	855	293	147	132	32
1 gm IM	504	628	418	237	ND*	ND
2 gm IV	2692	1976	757	274	198	40

* ND = Not determined.

Thirty-three percent to 67% of a ceftriaxone dose was excreted in the urine as unchanged drug and the remainder was secreted in the bile and ultimately found in the feces as microbiologically inactive compounds. After a 1 gm IV dose, average concentrations of ceftriaxone, determined from one to three hours after dosing, were 581 mcg/ml in the gallbladder bile, 788 mcg/ml in the common duct bile, 898 mcg/ml in the cystic duct bile, 78.2 mcg/gm in the gallbladder wall and 62.1 mcg/ml in the concurrent plasma.

Over a 0.15 to 3 gm dose range in healthy adult subjects, the values of elimination half-life ranged from 5.8 to 8.7 hours; apparent volume of distribution from 5.78 to 13.5 l; plasma clearance from 0.58 to 1.45 l/hour; and renal clearance from 0.32 to 0.73 l/hour. Ceftriaxone is reversibly bound to human plasma proteins, and the binding decreased from a value of 95% bound at plasma concentrations of <25 mcg/ml to a value of 85% bound at 300 mcg/ml.

The average values of maximum plasma concentration, elimination half-life, plasma clearance and volume of distribution after a 50 mg/kg IV dose and after a 75 mg/kg IV dose in pediatric patients suffering from bacterial meningitis are shown in TABLE 3. Ceftriaxone penetrated the inflamed meninges of infants and children; CSF concentrations after a 50 mg/kg IV dose and after a 75 mg/kg IV dose are also shown in TABLE 3.

TABLE 3 Average Pharmacokinetic Parameters of Ceftriaxone in Pediatric Patients with Meningitis

	50 mg/kg IV	75 mg/kg IV
Maximum Plasma Concentrations (mcg/ml)	216	275
Elimination Half-life (hr)	4.6	4.3
Plasma Clearance (ml/hr/kg)	49	60
Volume of Distribution (ml/kg)	338	373
CSF Concentration—inflamed meninges (mcg/ml)	5.6	6.4
Range (mcg/ml)	1.3-18.5	1.3-44
Time after dose (hr)	3.7-(± 1.6)	3.3(± 1.4)

Compared to that in healthy adult subjects, the pharmacokinetics of ceftriaxone were only minimally altered in elderly subjects and in patients with renal impairment or hepatic dysfunction (TABLE 4); therefore, dosage adjustments are not necessary for these patients

CLINICAL PHARMACOLOGY: *(cont'd)*

with ceftriaxone dosages up to 2 gm per day. Ceftriaxone was not removed to any significant extent from the plasma by hemodialysis. In 6 of 26 dialysis patients, the elimination rate of ceftriaxone was markedly reduced, suggesting that plasma concentrations of ceftriaxone should be monitored in these patients to determine if dosage adjustments are necessary.

TABLE 4 Average Pharmacokinetic Parameters of Ceftriaxone in Humans

Subject Group	Elimination Half-Life (hr)	Plasma Clearance (l/hr)	Volume of Distribution (l)
Healthy Subjects	5.8-8.7	0.58-1.45	5.8-13.5
Elderly Subjects (mean age, 70.5 yr)	8.9	0.83	10.7
Patients with renal impairment			
Hemodialysis patients (0-5 ml/min)*	14.7	0.65	13.7
Severe (5-15 ml/min)	15.7	0.56	12.5
Moderate (16-30 ml/min)	11.4	0.72	11.8
Mild (31-60 ml/min)	12.4	0.70	13.3
Patients with liver disease	8.8	1.1	13.6

* Creatinine clearance.

MICROBIOLOGY

The bactericidal activity of ceftriaxone results from inhibition of cell wall synthesis. Ceftriaxone has a high degree of stability in the presence of beta-lactamases, both penicillinases and cephalosporinases, of gram-negative and gram-positive bacteria. Ceftriaxone is usually active against the following microorganisms *in vitro* and in clinical infections (see INDICATIONS AND USAGE).

Gram-Negative Aerobes: *Acinetobacter calcoaceticus, Enterobacter aerogenes, Enterobacter cloacae, Escherichia coli, Haemophilus influenzae* (including ampicillin-resistant strains), *Haemophilus parainfluenzae, Klebsiella oxytoca, Klebsiella pneumoniae,Morganella morganii, Neisseria gonorrhoeae* (including penicillinase- and nonpenicillinase- producing strains), *Neisseria meningitidis, Proteus mirabilis, Proteus vulgaris, Serratia marcescens.*

Ceftriaxone is also active against many strains of *Pseudomonas aeruginosa.*

Note: Many strains of the above organisms that are multiply resistant to other antibiotics, e.g., penicillins, cephalosporins and aminoglycosides, are susceptible to ceftriaxone.

Gram-Positive Aerobes: *Staphylococcus aureus* (including penicillinase-producing strains), *Staphylococcus epidermidis, Streptococcus pneumoniae, Streptococcus pyogenes,* and *Viridans* group streptococci.

Note: Methicillin-resistant staphylococci are resistant to cephalosporins, including ceftriaxone. Most strains of Group D streptococci and enterococci, e.g., *Enterococcus (Streptococcus) faecalis*, are resistant.

Anaerobes: *Bacteroides fragilis, Clostridium* species, and *Peptostreptococcus* species.

Note: Most strains of *C. difficile* are resistant.

Ceftriaxone also demonstrates *in vitro* activity against most strains of the following microorganisms, although the clinical significance is unknown:

Gram-Negative Aerobes: *Citrobacter diversus, Citrobacter freundii, Providencia* species (including *Providencia rettgeri*), *Salmonella* species (including *S. typhi*), *Shigella* species.

Gram-Positive Aerobes: *Streptococcus agalactiae, Streptococcus agalactiae*

Anaerobes: *Bacteroides bivius, Bacteroides melaninogenicus.*

SUSCEPTIBILITY TESTING

Diffusion Techniques: Quantitative methods that require the measurement of zone diameters give the most precise estimate of the susceptibility of bacteria to antimicrobial agents. One such standard procedure[1] which has been recommended for use with disks to test susceptibility of organisms to ceftriaxone uses a 30-mcg ceftriaxone disk. Interpretation involves the correlation of the diameters obtained in the disk test with the minimum inhibitory concentration (MIC) for ceftriaxone.

Reports from the laboratory giving results of the standardized single disk susceptibility test using a 30-mcg ceftriaxone disk should be interpreted for ceftriaxone according to the criteria listed in TABLE 5.

TABLE 5

Zone Diameter (mm)	Interpretation
≥ 18	(S) Susceptible
14-17	(MS) Moderately Susceptible
≤ 13	(R) Resistant

A report of "Susceptible" indicates that the pathogen is likely to be inhibited by generally achievable levels. A report of "Moderately Susceptible" suggests that the organism would be susceptible if high dosage (not to exceed 4 gm per day) is used or if the infection is confined to tissues and fluids in which high antimicrobial levels are attained. A report of "Resistant" indicates that achievable concentrations are unlikely to be inhibitory, and other therapy should be selected.

Standardized procedures require the use of laboratory control organisms. The 30-mcg ceftriaxone disk should give the zone diameters found in TABLE 6.

TABLE 6

Organism	Zone Diameter
Staphyloccus aureus ATCC 25923	22-28
Escherichia coli ATCC 25922	29-35
Pseudomonas aeruginosa ATCC 27853	17-23

Dilution Techniques: Use a standard dilution method[2] (broth, agar, microdilution) or equivalent with ceftriaxone powder. The MIC values obtained should be interpreted according to the criteria found in TABLE 7.

TABLE 7

MIC (mcg/ml)	Interpretation
≤ 16	Susceptible
>16 - <64	Moderately Susceptible
≥ 64	Resistant

As with standard diffusion techniques, dilution methods require the use of laboratory control organisms. Standard ceftriaxone powder should provide the MIC values as shown in TABLE 8.

TABLE 8 Organism	MIC(mcg/ml)
Staphyloccus aureus ATCC 29213	1-8
Escherichia coli ATCC 25922	0.03-0.12
Pseudomonas aeruginosa ATCC 27853	8-32

INDICATIONS AND USAGE:

Rocephin is indicated for the treatment of the following infections when caused by susceptible organisms:

Lower Respiratory Tract Infections caused by *Streptococcus pneumoniae, Staphylococcus aureus, Haemophilus influenzae, Haemophilus parainfluenzae, Klebsiellapneumoniae, Escherichia coli, Enterobacter aerogenes, Proteus mirabilis*or *Serratia marcescens.*

Skin And Skin Structure Infections caused by *Staphylococcus aureus, Staphylococcus epidermidis, Streptococcus pyogenes, Viridans* group *streptococci, Escherichia coli, Enterobacter cloacae, Klebsiella oxytoca, Klebsiella pneumoniae, Proteus mirabilis, Morganella morganii**, *Pseudomonas aeruginosa, Serratia marcescens, Acinetobacter calcoaceticus, Bacteroides fragilis** or*Peptostreptococcus* species.

Urinary Tract Infections (Complicated And Uncomplicated) caused by *Escherichia coli, Proteus mirabilis, Proteus vulgaris, Morganella morganii* or *Klebsiella pneumoniae.*

Uncomplicated Gonorrhea (Cervical/Urethral And Rectal) caused by*Neisseria gonorrhoeae*, including both penicillinase- and nonpenicillinase-producing strains, and pharyngeal gonorrhea caused by nonpenicillinase-producing strains of *Neisseria gonorrhoeae.*

Pelvic Inflammatory Disease caused by *Neisseria gonorrhoeae.*

Bacterial Septicemia caused by *Staphylococcus aureus, Streptococcus pneumoniae, Escherichia coli, Haemophilus influenzae* or *Klebsiella pneumoniae.*

Bone And Joint Infections caused by *Staphylococcus aureus, Streptococcus pneumoniae, Escherichia coli, Proteus mirabilis, Klebsiella pneumoniae* or *Enterobacter* species.

Intra-Abdominal Infections caused by *Escherichia coli,Klebsiella pneumoniae, Bacteroides fragilis, Clostridium* species

(Note: most strains of *C. difficile* are resistant) or*Peptostreptococcus* species.

Meningitis caused by *Haemophilus influenzae, Neisseria meningitidis* or *Streptococcus pneumoniae.* Rocephin has also been used successfully in a limited number of cases of meningitis and shunt infection caused by *Staphylococcus epidermidis** and *Escherichia coli.**

* Efficacy for this organism in this organ system was studied in fewer than ten infections.

Surgical Prophylaxis: The preoperative administration of a single 1 gm dose of Rocephin may reduce the incidence of postoperative infections in patients undergoing surgical procedures classified as contaminated or potentially contaminated (*e.g.,* vaginal or abdominal hysterectomy or cholecystectomy for chronic calculus cholecystis in high- risk patients, such as those over 70 years of age, with acute cholecystis not requiring therapeutic antimicrobials, obstructive jaundice or common duct bile stones) and in surgical patients for whom infection at the operative site would present serious risk (*e.g.,* during coronary artery bypass surgery). Although Rocephin has been shown to have been as effective as cefazolin in the prevention of infection following coronary artery bypass surgery, no placebo-controlled trials have been conducted to evaluate any cephalosporin antibiotic in the prevention of infection following coronary artery bypass surgery.

When administered prior to surgical procedures for which it is indicated, a single 1 gm dose of Rocephin provides protection from most infections due to susceptible organisms throughout the course of the procedure.

Before instituting treatment with Rocephin, appropriate specimens should be obtained for isolation of the causative organism and for determination of its susceptibility to the drug. Therapy may be instituted prior to obtaining results of susceptibility testing.

CONTRAINDICATIONS:

Rocephin is contraindicated in patients with known allergy to the cephalosporin class of antibiotics.

WARNINGS:

BEFORE THERAPY WITH ROCEPHIN IS INSTITUTED, CAREFUL INQUIRY SHOULD BE MADE TO DETERMINE WHETHER THE PATIENT HAS HAD PREVIOUS HYPERSENSITIVITY REACTIONS TO CEPHALOSPORINS, PENICILLINS OR OTHER DRUGS. THIS PRODUCT SHOULD BE GIVEN CAUTIOUSLY TO PENICILLIN-SENSITIVE PATIENTS. ANTIBIOTICS SHOULD BE ADMINISTERED WITH CAUTION TO ANY PATIENT WHO HAS DEMONSTRATED SOME FORM OF ALLERGY, PARTICULARLY TO DRUGS. SERIOUS ACUTE HYPERSENSITIVITY REACTIONS MAY REQUIRE THE USE OF SUBCUTANEOUS EPINEPHRINE AND OTHER EMERGENCY MEASURES.

Pseudomembranous colitis has been reported with nearly all antibacterial agents, including ceftriaxone, and may range in severity from mild to life-threatening. Therefore, it is important to consider this diagnosis in patients who present with diarrhea subsequent to the administration of antibacterial agents.

Treatment with antibacterial agents alters the normal flora of the colon and may permit overgrowth of clostridia. Studies indicate that a toxin produced by *Clostridium difficile* is one primary cause of "antibiotic-associated colitis."

After the diagnosis of pseudomembranous colitis has been established, therapeutic measures should be initiated. Mild cases of pseudomembranous colitis usually respond to drug discontinuance alone. In moderate to severe cases, consideration should be given to management with fluids and electrolytes, protein supplementation and treatment with an oral antibacterial drug effective against *C. difficile.*

PRECAUTIONS:

GENERAL

Although transient elevations of BUN and serum creatinine have been observed, at the recommended dosages, the nephrotoxic potential of Rocephin is similar to that of other cephalosporins.

Ceftriaxone is excreted via both biliary and renal excretion (see CLINICAL PHARMACOLOGY). Therefore, patients with renal failure normally require no adjustment in dosage when usual doses of Rocephin are administered, but concentrations of drug in the serum should be monitored periodically. If evidence of accumulation exists, dosage should be decreased accordingly.

Dosage adjustments should not be necessary in patients with hepatic dysfunction; however, in patients with both hepatic dysfunction and significant renal disease, Rocephin dosage should not exceed 2 gm daily without close monitoring of serum concentrations.

PRECAUTIONS: *(cont'd)*

Alterations in prothrombin times have occurred rarely in patients treated with Rocephin. Patients with impaired vitamin K synthesis or low vitamin K stores (*e.g.,* chronic hepatic disease and malnutrition) may require monitoring of prothrombin time during Rocephin treatment. Vitamin K administration (10 mg weekly) may be necessary if the prothrombin time is prolonged before or during therapy.

Prolonged use of Rocephin may result in overgrowth of nonsusceptible organisms. Careful observation of the patient is essential. If superinfection occurs during therapy, appropriate measures should be taken.

Rocephin should be prescribed with caution in individuals with a history of gastrointestinal disease, especially colitis.

Rare cases have been reported in which sonographic abnormalities are seen in the gallbladder of patients treated with Rocephin; these patients may also have symptoms of gallbladder disease. These abnormalities are variously described as sludge, precipitations, echoes with shadows, and may be misinterpreted as concretions. The chemical nature of the sonographically-detected material has not been determined. The condition appears to be transient and reversible when Rocephin is discontinued and conservative management employed. Therefore, Rocephin should be discontinued in patients who develop signs and symptoms suggestive of gallbladder disease and/or the sonographic findings described above.

CARCINOGENESIS, MUTAGENESIS, AND IMPAIRMENT OF FERTILITY

Carcinogenesis: Considering the maximum duration of treatment and the class of the compound, carcinogenicity studies with ceftriaxone in animals have not been performed. The maximum duration of animal toxicity studies was six months.

Mutagenesis: Genetic toxicology tests included the Ames test, a micronucleus test and a test for chromosomal aberrations in human lymphocytes cultured *in vitro* with ceftriaxone. Ceftriaxone showed no potential for mutagenic activity in these studies.

Impairment of Fertility: Ceftriaxone produced no impairment of fertility when given intravenously to rats at daily doses up to 586 mg/kg/day, approximately 20 times the recommended clinical dose of 2 gm/day.

PREGNANCY CATEGORY B

Teratogenic Effects: Reproductive studies have been performed in mice and rats at doses up to 20 times the usual human dose and have no evidence of embryotoxicity, fetotoxicity or teratogenicity. In primates, no embryotoxicity or teratogenicity was demonstrated at a dose approximately three times the human dose.

There are, however, no adequate and well-controlled studies in pregnant women. Because animal reproductive studies are not always predictive of human response, this drug should be used during pregnancy only if clearly needed.

Nonteratogenic Effects: In rats, in the Segment I (fertility and general reproduction) and Segment III (perinatal and postnatal) studies with intravenously administered ceftriaxone, no adverse effects were noted on various reproductive parameters during gestation and lactation, including postnatal growth, functional behavior and reproductive ability of the offspring, at doses of 586 mg/kg/day or less.

NURSING MOTHERS

Low concentrations of ceftriaxone are excreted in human milk. Caution should be exercised when Rocephin is administered to a nursing woman.

PEDIATRIC USE

Safety and effectiveness of Rocephin in neonates, infants and children have been established for the dosages described in the DOSAGE AND ADMINISTRATION. *In vitro* studies have shown the ceftriaxone, like some other cephalosporins, can displace bilirubin from serum albumin. Rocephin should not be administered to hyperbilirubinemic neonates, especially prematures.

ADVERSE REACTIONS:

Rocephin is generally well tolerated. In clinical trials, the following adverse reactions, which were considered to be related to Rocephin therapy or of uncertain etiology, were observed:

Local Reactions: pain, induration or tenderness at the site of injection (1%). Less frequently reported (less than 1%) was phlebitis after IV administration.

Hypersensitivity: rash (1.7%). Less frequently reported (less than 1%) were pruritus, fever or chills.

Hematologic: eosinophilia (6%), thrombocytosis (5.1%) and leukopenia (2.1%). Less frequently reported (less than 1%) were anemia, hemolytic anemia, neutropenia, lymphopenia, thrombocytopenia and prolongation of the prothrombin time.

Gastrointestinal: diarrhea (2.7%). Less frequently reported (less than 1%) were nausea or vomiting, and dysgeusia. Onset of pseudomembranous colitis symptoms may occur during or after antibiotic treatment (see WARNINGS).

Hepatic: elevations of SGOT (3.1%) or SGPT (3.3%). Less frequently reported (less than 1%) were elevations of alkaline phosphatase and bilirubin.

Renal: elevations of the BUN (1.2%). Less frequently reported (less than 1%) were elevations of creatinine and the presence of casts in the urine.

Central Nervous System: headache or dizziness were reported occasionally (less than 1%).

Genitourinary: moniliasis or vaginitis were reported occasionally (less than 1%).

Miscellaneous: diaphoresis and flushing were reported occasionally (less than 1%).

Other rarely observed adverse reactions (less than 0.1%) include leukocytosis, lymphocytosis, monocytosis, basophilia, a decrease in the prothrombin time, jaundice, gallbladder sludge, glycosuria, hematuria, anaphylaxis, bronchospasm, serum sickness, abdominal pain, colitis, flatulence, dyspepsia, palpitations and epistaxis.

DOSAGE AND ADMINISTRATION:

Rocephin may be administered intravenously or intramuscularly.

Adults: The usual adult daily dose is 1 to 2 grams given once a day (or in equally divided doses twice a day) depending on the type and severity of infection. The total daily dose should not exceed 4 grams.

For the treatment of uncomplicated gonococcal infections, a single intramuscular dose of 250 mg is recommended.

For preoperative use (surgical prophylaxis), a single dose of 1 gram administered intravenously 1/2 to 2 hours before surgery is recommended.

Children: For the treatment of skin and skin structure infections, the recommended total daily dose is 50 to 75 mg/kg given once a day (or in equally divided doses twice a day). The total daily dose should not exceed 2 grams.

For the treatment of serious miscellaneous infections other than meningitis, the recommended total daily dose is 50 to 75 mg/kg, given in divided doses every 12 hours. The total daily dose should not exceed 2 grams.

In the treatment of meningitis, it is recommended that the initial therapeutic dose be 100 mg/kg (not to exceed 4 grams). Thereafter, a total daily dose of 100 mg/kg/day (not to exceed 4 grams daily) is recommended. The daily dose may be administered once a day (or in equally divided doses every 12 hours). The usual duration of therapy is 7 to 14 days.

DOSAGE AND ADMINISTRATION: *(cont'd)*

Generally, Rocephin therapy should be continued for at least two days after the signs and symptoms of infection have disappeared. The usual duration of therapy is 4 to 14 days; in complicated infections, longer therapy may be required.

When treating infections caused by *Streptococcus pyogenes*, therapy should be continued for at least ten days.

No dosage adjustment is necessary for patients with impairment of renal or hepatic function; however, blood levels should be monitored in patients with severe renal impairment (*e.g.*, dialysis patients) and in patients with both renal and hepatic dysfunctions.

DIRECTIONS FOR USE

Intramuscular Administration: Reconstitute Rocephin powder with the appropriate diluent (see Compatibility and Stability).

TABLE 9

Vial Dosage Size	Amount of Diluent to be Added
250 mg	0.9 ml
500 mg	1.8 ml
1 gm	3.6 ml
2 gm	7.2 ml

After reconstitution, each 1 ml of solution contains approximately 250 mg equivalent of ceftriaxone. If required, more dilute solutions could be utilized. As with all intramuscular preparations, Rocephin should be injected well within the body of a relatively large muscle; aspiration helps to avoid unintentional injection into a blood vessel.

Intravenous Administration: Rocephin should be administered intravenously by infusion over a period of 30 minutes. Concentrations between 10 mg/ml and 40 mg/ml are recommended; however, lower concentrations may be used if desired. Reconstitute vials or "piggyback" bottles with an appropriate IV diluent (see Compatibility and Stability).

TABLE 10

Vial Dosage Size	Amount of Diluent to be Added
250 mg	2.4 ml
500 mg	4.8 ml
1 gm	9.6 ml
2 gm	19.2 ml

After reconstitution, each 1 ml of solution contains approximately 100 mg equivalent of ceftriaxone. Withdraw entire contents and dilute to the desired concentration with the appropriate IV diluent.

TABLE 11

Piggyback Bottle Dosage Size	Amount of Diluent to be Added
1 gm	10 ml
2 gm	20 ml

After reconstitution, further dilute to 50 ml or 100 ml volumes with the appropriate IV diluent.

10 gm Bulk Pharmacy Container: This dosage size is *NOT FOR DIRECT ADMINISTRATION.* Reconstitute powder with 95 ml of an appropriate IV diluent. Before parenteral administration, withdraw the required amount, then further dilute to the desired concentration.

COMPATIBILITY AND STABILITY

Rocephin sterile powder should be stored at room temperature—77°F (25°C)—or below and protected from light. After reconstitution, protection from normal light is not necessary. The color of solutions ranges from light yellow to amber, depending on the length of storage, concentration and diluent used.

TABLE 12 Rocephin *Intramuscular* solutions remain stable (loss of potency less than 10%) for the following time periods:

Diluent	Concentration mg/ml	Storage: Room Temp (25°C)	Storage: Refrigerated (4°C)
Sterile Water for Injection	100	3 days	10 days
	250	24 hours	3 days
0.9% Sodium Chloride Solution	100	3 days	10 days
	250	24 hours	3 days
5% Dextrose Solution	100	3 days	10 days
	250	24 hours	3 days
Bacteriostatic Water + 0.9% Benzyl Alcohol	100	24 hours	10 days
	250	24 hours	3 days
1% Lidocaine Solution (without epinephrine)	100	24 hours	10 days
	250	24 hours	3 days

TABLE 13 Rocephin *Intravenous* solutions, at concentrations of 10, 20 and 40 mg/ml, remain stable (loss of potency less than 10%) for the following time periods stored in glass or PVC containers:

Diluent	Storage: Room Temp (25°C)	Storage: Refrigerated (4°C)
Sterile Water	3 days	10 days
0.9% Sodium Chloride Solution	3 days	10 days
5% Dextrose Solution	3 days	10 days
10% Dextrose Solution	3 days	10 days
5% Dextrose + 0.9% Sodium Chloride Solution*	3 days	Incompatible
5% Dextrose + 0.45% Sodium Chloride Solution	3 days	Incompatible

* Data available for 10-40 mg/ml concentrations in this diluent in PVC containers only.

Similarly, Rocephin *intravenous* solutions, at concentrations of 100 mg/ml, remain stable in the IV piggyback glass containers for the above specified time periods.

The following *intravenous* Rocephin solutions are stable at room temperature (25°C) for 24 hours, at concentrations between 10 mg/ml and 40 mg/ml: Sodium Lactate (PVC container), 10% Invert Sugar (glass container), 5% Sodium Bicarbonate (glass container), Freamine III (glass container), Normosol-M in 5% Dextrose (glass and PVC containers), Ionosol-B in 5% Dextrose (glass container), 5% Mannitol (glass container), 10% Mannitol (glass container).

After the indicated stability time periods, unused portions of solutions should be discarded.

DOSAGE AND ADMINISTRATION: *(cont'd)*

Rocephin reconstituted with 5% Dextrose or 0.9% Sodium Chloride solution at concentrations between 10 mg/ml and 40 mg/ml, and then stored in frozen state (-20°C) in PVC (Viaflex) or polyolefin containers, remains stable for 26 weeks.

Frozen solutions should be thawed at room temperature before use. After thawing, unused portions should be discarded. **DO NOT REFREEZE.**

Rocephin solutions should *not* be physically mixed with or piggybacked into solutions containing other antimicrobial drugs or into diluent solutions other than those listed above, due to possible incompatibility.

CDC GUIDELINES FOR TREATMENT OF SEXUALLY TRANSMITTED DISEASES

Recommended Treatment Schedules for Chancroid, Gonorrhea and Acute Pelvic Inflammatory Disease (PID)†

Chancroid (Haemophilus ducreyi infection): 250 mg IM as a single dose.

Gonococcal Infections: *Uncomplicated:* 125 mg IM once plus doxycycline. *Conjunctivitis:* 1 g IM single dose. *Disseminated:* 1 g IM or IV every 24 hours.

Meningitis/Endocarditis: 1 to 2 g IV every 12 hours for 10 to 14 days (meningitis) or for at least 4 weeks (endocarditis). *Children (<45 kg):* With bacteremia or arthritis, use 50 mg/kg (maximum, 1 g) IM or IV in a single dose for 7 days. For meningitis, increase duration to 10 to 14 days and maximum dose to 2 g. *Infants:* 25 to 50 mg/kg/day IV or IM in a single daily dose, not to exceed 125 mg. For disseminated infection, continue for 7 days, with a duration of 7 to 14 days with documented meningitis.

Acute PID (ambulatory): 250 mg IM plus doxycycline.

† CDC 1993 Sexually Transmitted Diseases Treatment Guidelines. Morbidity and Mortality Weekly Report 1993 Sep. 24; 42 (No. RR-14):1–102.

ANIMAL PHARMACOLOGY:

Concretions consisting of the precipitated calcium salt of ceftriaxone have been found in the gallbladder bile of dogs and baboons treated with ceftriaxone.

These appeared as a gritty sediment in dogs that received 100 mg/kg/day for four weeks. A similar phenomenon has been observed in baboons but only after a protracted dosing period (6 months) at higher dose levels (335 mg/kg/day or more). The likelihood of this occurrence in humans is considered to be low, since ceftriaxone has a greater plasma half-life in humans, the calcium salt of ceftriaxone is more soluble in human gallbladder bile and the calcium content of human gallbladder bile is relatively low.

REFERENCES:

1. National Committee for Clinical Laboratory Standards,*Performance Standards for Antimicrobial Disk Susceptibility Tests.* 4th ed. Villanova, PA: 1990. Approved Standard NCCLS Document M2-A4, Vol. 10, No. 7, NCCLS.
2. National Committee for Clinical Laboratory Standards,*Methods for Dilution Antimicrobial Susceptibility Tests for Bacteria That Grow Aerobically.* 2nd ed. Villanova, PA: 1990. Approved Standard NCCLS Document M7-A2, Vol. 10, No. 8, NCCLS.

HOW SUPPLIED:

Store Rocephin in the frozen state at or below -20°C/- 4°F.

HOW SUPPLIED - EQUIVALENTS NOT AVAILABLE:

Injection, Dry-Soln - Intramuscular; - 1 gm/vial

1 gm	$34.65	ROCEPHIN, Roche	00004-1964-04
1 gm	$40.18	ROCEPHIN, ISO-OSMOTIC DEXTROSE, Roche	00004-2002-78
1 gm x 10	$338.97	ROCEPHIN, Roche	00004-1964-01
1 gm x 10	$349.94	ROCEPHIN, Roche	00004-1964-05
1's	$35.28	ROCEPHIN, Roche	00004-1964-02

Injection, Dry-Soln - Intramuscular; - 2 gm/vial

2 gm x 10	$673.61	ROCEPHIN, Roche	00004-1965-01
2 gm x 10	$691.16	ROCEPHIN, Roche	00004-1965-05
2 gm x 10	$694.04	ROCEPHIN, Roche	00004-1965-03
50 ml	$70.57	ROCEPHIN, ISO-OSMOTIC DEXTROSE, Roche	00004-2003-78

Injection, Dry-Soln - Intramuscular; - 10 gm/vial

10 gm	$330.45	ROCEPHIN, Roche	00004-1971-01

Injection, Dry-Soln - Intramuscular; - 250 mg/vial

250 mg	$11.68	ROCEPHIN, Roche	00004-1962-02
250 mg x 10	$109.24	ROCEPHIN, Roche	00004-1962-01

Injection, Dry-Soln - Intramuscular; - 500 mg/vial

500 mg	$20.57	ROCEPHIN, Roche	00004-1963-02
500 mg x 10	$198.06	ROCEPHIN, Roche	00004-1963-01

CEFUROXIME AXETIL *(000695)*

CATEGORIES: Anti-Infectives; Antibiotics; Antimicrobials; Bronchitis; Cephalosporins; Gonorrhea; Impetigo; Infections; Otitis Media; Pharyngitis; Respiratory Tract Infections; Skin Infections; Streptococcal Infection; Tonsillitis; Urinary Tract Infections; Lyme Disease*; Rheumatic Fever*; Pregnancy Category B; Sales > $500 Million; FDA Approved 1987 Dec; Patent Expiration 2000 Dec; Top 200 Drugs
* Indication not approved by the FDA

BRAND NAMES: *Cefuril*; **Ceftin**; *Cepazine* (France); *Elobact* (Germany); *Furoxime*; *Kalcef*; *Sharox-500*; *Zinacef*; *Zinat*; *Zinnat* (England, France, Germany, Mexico); *Zoref*
(International brand names outside U.S. in italics)

FORMULARIES: Aetna; BC-BS; Foundation; Medi-Cal

COST OF THERAPY: $183.30 (Respiratory Infections; Tablet; 500 mg; 2/day; 14 days)

DESCRIPTION:

Cefuroxime axetil is a semisynthetic, broad-spectrum cephalosporin antibiotic for oral administration.

Chemically, cefuroxime axetil, the 1-(acetyloxy) ethyl ester of cefuroxime, is (*RS*)-1-hydroxyethyl (6*R*,7*R*)-7-[2-(2-furyl)glyoxylamido]-3-hydroxymethyl-8-oxo-5-thia-1-azabicyclo[4.2.0]oct-2-ene-2-carboxylate, 7^2-(*Z*)-(*O*-methyloxime), 1- acetate 3-carbamate. Its molecular formula is $C_{20}H_{22}N_4O_{10}S$, and it has a molecular weight of 510.48.

Cefuroxime axetil is in the amorphous form.

Ceftin Tablets are film-coated and contain the equivalent of 125, 250, or 500 mg of cefuroxime as cefuroxime axetil. Ceftin Tablets contain the inactive ingredients colloidal silicon dioxide, croscarmellose sodium, FD&C Blue No. 1 (250- and 500-mg tablets only), hydrogenated vegetable oil, hydroxypropyl methylcellulose, methylparaben, microcrystalline cellulose, propylene glycol, propylparaben, sodium benzoate (125-mg tablets only), sodium lauryl sulfate, and titanium dioxide.

DESCRIPTION: *(cont'd)*

Ceftin for Oral Suspension, when reconstituted with water, provides the equivalent of 125 mg of cefuroxime (as cefuroxime axetil) per 5 ml of suspension. Ceftin for Oral Suspension contains the inactive ingredients povidone K30, stearic acid, sucrose, and tutti-frutti flavoring.

CLINICAL PHARMACOLOGY:

Absorption and Metabolism: After oral administration, cefuroxime axetil is absorbed from the gastrointestinal tract and rapidly hydrolyzed by nonspecific esterases in the intestinal mucosa and blood to cefuroxime. Cefuroxime is subsequently distributed throughout the extracellular fluids. The axetil moiety is metabolized to acetaldehyde and acetic acid.

Serum Pharmacokinetics: Serum cefuroxime pharmacokinetic parameters for cefuroxime axetil tablets and cefuroxime axetil for oral suspension are shown in the tables (TABLE 1, TABLE 2) below.

TABLE 1 Postprandial Pharmacokinetics of Cefuroxime Administered as Ceftin Tablets to Adults*

Dose† (Cefuroxime Equivalent)	Peak Plasma Concentration (mcg/mL)	Time of Peak Plasma Concentration (h)	Mean Elimination Half-Life (h)	A.U.C. (mcg-h mL)
125 mg	2.1	2.2	1.2	6.7
250 mg	4.1	2.5	1.2	12.9
500 mg	7.0	3.0	1.2	27.4
1,000 mg	13.6	2.5	1.3	50.0

* Mean values of 12 healthy adult volunteers.
† Drug administered immediately after a meal.

TABLE 2 Postprandial Pharmacokinetics of Cefuroxime Administered as Ceftin for Oral Suspension to Pediatric Patients*

Dose† (Cefuroxime Equivalent)	n	Peak Plasma Concentratio n (mcg/ml)	Time of Peak Plasma Concentratio n (h)	Mean Elimination Half-Life (h)	A.U.C. (mcg-h ml)
10 mg/kg	8	3.3	3.6	1.4	12.4
15 mg/kg	12	5.1	2.7	1.9	22.5
20 mg/kg	8	7.0	3.1	1.9	32.8

* Mean age=23 months.
† Drug administered with milk or milk products.

Approximately 50% of serum cefuroxime is bound to protein.

Comparative Pharmacokinetic Properties: Cefuroxime for oral suspension was not bioequivalent to cefuroxime tablets when tested in healthy adults. The tablet and powder for oral suspension formulations are NOT substitutable on a mg/mg basis. The area under the curve for the suspension averaged 91% of that for the tablet, and the peak plasma concentration for the suspension averaged 71% of the peak plasma concentration of the tablets. Therefore, the safety and effectiveness of both the tablet and oral suspension formulations had to be established in separate clinical trials.

Food Effect on Pharmacokinetics: Absorption of the tablet is greater when taken after food (absolute bioavailability of cefuroxime tablets increase from 37% to 52%). Despite this difference in absorption, the clinical and bacteriologic responses of patients were independent of food intake at the time of tablet administration in two studies where this was assessed.

All pharmacokinetic and clinical effectiveness and safety studies in children using the suspension formulation were conducted in the fed state. No data are available on the absorption kinetics of the suspension formulation when administered to fasted pediatric patients.

Renal Excretion: Cefuroxime is excreted unchanged in the urine; in adults, approximately 50% of the administered dose is recovered in the urine within 12 hours. The pharmacokinetics of cefuroxime in the urine of children have not been studied at this time. Until further data are available, the renal pharmacokinetic properties of cefuroxime axetil established in adults should not be extrapolated to children.

Because cefuroxime is renally excreted, the serum half-life is prolonged in patients with reduced renal function. In a study of 20 elderly patients (mean age=83.9 years) having a mean creatinine clearance of 34.9 ml per minute, the mean serum elimination half-life was 3.5 hours. Despite the lower elimination of cefuroxime in geriatric patients, dosage adjustment based on age is not necessary (see PRECAUTIONS, Geriatric Use).

Microbiology: The *in vivo* bactericidal activity of cefuroxime axetil is due to cefuroxime's binding to essential target proteins and the resultant inhibition of cell-wall synthesis.

Cefuroxime has bactericidal activity against a wide range of common pathogens, including many beta-lactamase—producing strains. Cefuroxime is stable to many bacterial beta-lactamases, especially plasmid-mediated enzymes that are commonly found in enterobacteriaceae.

Cefuroxime has been demonstrated to be active against most strains of the following microorganisms both *in vitro* and in clinical infections as described in the INDICATIONS AND USAGE(see INDICATIONS AND USAGE).

Aerobic Gram-positive Microorganisms:

Staphylococcus aureus (including beta-lactamase—producing strains)

Streptococcus pneumoniae

Streptococcus pyogenes

Aerobic Gram-negative Microorganisms:

Escherichia coli; Haemophilus influenzae;(including beta-lactamase— producing strains)

Haemophilus parainfluenzae

Klebsiella pneumoniae

Moraxella catarrhalis (including beta-lactamase— producing strains)

Neisseria gonorrhoeae (beta-lactamase negative strains only)

Cefuroxime has been shown to be active *in vitro* against most strains of the following microorganisms; however, the clinical significance of these findings is unknown.

Cefuroxime exhibits *in vitro* minimum inhibitory concentrations (MICs) of 4.0 mcg/ml or less (systemic susceptible breakpoint) against most (≥90%) strains of the following microorganisms; however, the safety and effectiveness of cefuroxime in treating clinical infections due to these microorganisms have not been established in adequate and well-controlled trials.

Aerobic Gram-positive Microorganisms:

Staphylococcus epidermidis

Staphylococcus saprophyticus

Streptococcus agalactiae

CLINICAL PHARMACOLOGY: *(cont'd)*

NOTE: Certain strains of enterococci, *e.g.,Enterococcus faecalis* (formerly *Streptococcus faecalis*), are resistant to cefuroxime. Methicillin-resistant staphylococci are resistant to cefuroxime.

Aerobic Gram-negative Microorganisms:

Morganella morganii

Neisseria gonorrhoeae (beta-lactamase—producing strains only)

Proteus inconstans

Proteus mirabilis Providencia rettgeri

NOTE:*Pseudomonas* spp., *Campylobacter* spp.,*Acinetobacter calcoaceticus*, and most strains of *Serratia* spp. and *Proteus vulgaris* are resistant to most first- and second-generation cephalosporins. Some strains of *Morganella morganii, Enterobacter cloacae,*and *Citrobacter* spp. have been shown by *in vitro* tests to be resistant to cefuroxime and other cephalosporins.

Anaerobic Microorganisms:

Peptococcus niger

NOTE: Most strains of *Clostridium difficile* and *Bacteroides fragilis* are resistant to cefuroxime.

SUSCEPTIBILITY TESTING

Dilution Techniques: Quantitative methods that are used to determine MICs provide reproducible estimates of the susceptibility of bacteria to antimicrobial compounds. One such standardized procedure uses a standardized dilution method[1] (broth, agar, or microdilution) or equivalent with cefuroxime powder. The MIC values obtained should be interpreted according to the following criteria (TABLE 3):

TABLE 3

MIC (mcg/ml)	Interpretation
≤4	(S) Susceptible
8-16	(I) Intermediate
≥32	(R) Resistant

A report of "Susceptible" indicates that the pathogen, if in the blood, is likely to be inhibited by usually achievable concentrations of the antimicrobial compound in blood. A report of "Intermediate" indicates that inhibitory concentrations of the antibiotic may be achieved if high dosage is used or if the infection is confined to tissues or fluids in which high antibiotic concentrations are attained. This category also provides a buffer zone that prevents small, uncontrolled technical factors from causing major discrepancies in interpretation. A report of "Resistant" indicates that usually achievable concentrations of the antimicrobial compound in the blood are unlikely to be inhibitory and that other therapy should be selected.

Standardized susceptibility test procedures require the use of laboratory control microorganisms. Standard cefuroxime powder should give the following MIC values (TABLE 4):

TABLE 4

Microorganism	MIC (mcg/ml)
Escherichia coli ATCC 25922	2-8
Staphylococcus aureus ATCC 29213	0.5-2

Diffusion Techniques: Quantitative methods that require measurement of zone diameters provide estimates of the susceptibility of bacteria to antimicrobial compounds. One such standardized procedure[2] that has been recommended (for use with disks) to test the susceptibility of microorganisms to cefuroxime uses the 30-mcg cefuroxime disk. Interpretation involves correlation of the diameter obtained in the disk test with the MIC for cefuroxime.

Reports from the laboratory providing results of the standard single-disk susceptibility test with a 30-mcg cefuroxime disk should be interpreted according to the following criteria (TABLE 5):

TABLE 5

Zone diameter (mm)	Interpretation
≥23	(S) Susceptible
15-22	(I) Intermediate
≤14	(R) Resistant

Interpretation should be as stated above for results using dilution techniques.

As with standard dilution techniques, diffusion methods require the use of laboratory control microorganisms. The 30-mcg cefuroxime disk provides the following zone diameters in these laboratory test quality control strains (TABLE 6):

TABLE 6

Microorganism	Zone Diameter (mm)
Escherichia coli ATCC 25922	20-26
Staphylococcus aureus ATCC 25923	27-35

CLINICAL STUDIES:

CEFUROXIME AXETIL TABLETS

Acute Bacterial Maxillary Sinusitis: One adequate and well-controlled study was performed in patients with acute bacterial maxillary sinusitis. In this study each patient had a maxillary sinus aspirate collected by sinus puncture before treatment was initiated for presumptive acute bacterial sinusitis. All patients had to have radiographic and clinical evidence of acute maxillary sinusitis. As shown in the following summary of the study, the general clinical effectiveness of cefuroxime axetil tablets was comparable to an oral antimicrobial agent that contained a specific beta-lactamase inhibitor in treating acute maxillary sinusitis. However, sufficient microbiology data were obtained to demonstrate the effectiveness of cefuroxime axetil tablets in treating acute bacterial maxillary sinusitis due only to *Streptococcus pneumoniae* or non-beta-lactamase-producing *Haemophilus influenzae.* An insufficient number of beta-lactamase-producing *Haemophilus influenzae* and *Moraxella catarrhalis* isolates were obtained in this trial to adequately evaluate the effectiveness of cefuroxime axetil tablets in the treatment of acute bacterial maxillary sinusitis due to these two organisms.

This study enrolled 317 adult patients, 132 patients in the United States and 185 patients in South America. Patients were randomized in a 1:1 ratio to cefuroxime axetil 250 mg b.i.d. or an oral antimicrobial agent that contained a specific beta-lactamase inhibitor. An intent-to-treat analysis of the submitted clinical data yielded the following results:

In this trial and in a supporting maxillary puncture trial, 15 evaluable patients had non-beta-lactamase-producing Haemophilus influenzae as the identified pathogen. Ten (10) of these 15 patients (67%) had their pathogen (non-beta-lactamase-producing *Haemophilus influenzae*)

CLINICAL STUDIES: *(cont'd)*

TABLE 7 Clinical Effectiveness of Cefuroxime Axetil Tablets Compared to Beta-Lactamase Inhibitor-Containing Control Drug in the Treatment of Acute Bacterial Maxillary Sinusitis

	U.S. Patients*		South American Patients†	
	Cefuroxime Axetil (n=43)	Control (n=43)	Cefuroxime Axetil (n=87)	Control (n=89)
Clinical success (cure + improvement	65%	53%	77%	74%
Clinical cure	53%	44%	72%	64%
Clinical improvement	12%	9%	5%	10%

* 95% Confidence interval around the success difference [-0.08, +0.32)]
† 95% Confidence interval around the success difference [-0.10, +0.16].

eradicated. Eighteen (18) evaluable patients had *Streptococcus pneumoniae* as the identified pathogen. Fifteen (15) of these 18 patients (83%) had their pathogen (*Streptococcus pneumoniae*) eradicated.

Safety: The incidence of drug-related gastrointestinal adverse events was statistically significantly higher in the control arm (an oral antimicrobial agent that contained a specific beta-lactamase inhibitor) versus the cefuroxime axetil arm (12% versus 1%, respectively; $p<0.001$), particularly drug-related diarrhea (8% versus 1%, respectively; $p=0.001$).

INDICATIONS AND USAGE:

CEFUROXIME AXETIL IS NOT BIOEQUIVALENT AND IS NOT SUBSTITUTABLE ON A MG/MG BASIS (SEE CLINICAL PHARMACOLOGY).

CEFUROXIME AXETIL TABLETS

Cefuroxime tablets are indicated for the treatment of patients with mild to moderate infections caused by susceptible strains of the designated microorganisms in the conditions listed below:

Pharyngitis/Tonsillitis caused by *Streptococcus pyogenes.*

NOTE: The usual drug of choice in the treatment and prevention of streptococcal infections, including the prophylaxis of rheumatic fever, is penicillin given by the intramuscular route. Cefuroxime tablets are generally effective in the eradication of streptococci from the nasopharynx; however, substantial data establishing the efficacy of cefuroxime in the subsequent prevention of rheumatic fever are not available. Please also note that in all clinical trials, all isolates had to be sensitive to both penicillin and cefuroxime. There are no data from adequate and well-controlled trials to demonstrate the effectiveness of cefuroxime in the treatment of penicillin-resistant strains of*Streptococcus pyogenes.*

Acute Bacterial Otitis Media caused by *Streptococcus pneumoniae, Haemophilus influenzae* (including beta-lactamase— producing strains), *Moraxella catarrhalis* (including beta-lactamase—producing strains), or *Streptococcus pyogenes.*

Acute Bacterial Exacerbations of Chronic Bronchitis and Secondary Bacterial Infections of Acute Bronchitis caused by *Streptococcus pneumoniae, Haemophilus influenzae* (beta-lactamase negative strains), and *Haemophilus parainfluenzae* (beta-lactamase negative strains).

Uncomplicated Skin and Skin-Structure Infections caused by*Staphylococcus aureus* (including beta-lactamase—producing strains) or *Streptococcus pyogenes.*

Uncomplicated Urinary Tract Infections caused by *Escherichia coli* or *Klebsiella pneumoniae.*

Uncomplicated Gonorrhea (urethral and endocervical) caused by non-penicillinase—producing strains of *Neisseria gonorrhoeae.*

CEFUROXIME AXETIL FOR ORAL SUSPENSION

Cefuroxime axetil for oral suspension is indicated for the treatment of children 3 months to 12 years of age with mild to moderate infections caused by susceptible strains of the designated microorganisms in the conditions listed below. The safety and effectiveness of cefuroxime axetil for oral suspension in the treatment of infections other than those specifically listed below have not been established either by adequate and well-controlled trials or by pharmacokinetic data with which to determine an effective and safe dosing regimen.

Pharyngitis/Tonsillitis caused by *Streptococcus pyogenes.*

NOTE: The usual drug of choice in the treatment and prevention of streptococcal infections, including the prophylaxis of rheumatic fever, is penicillin given by the intramuscular route. Cefuroxime for oral suspension is generally effective in the eradication of streptococci from the nasopharynx; however, substantial data establishing the efficacy of cefuroxime in the subsequent prevention of rheumatic fever are not available. Please also note that in all clinical trials, all isolates had to be sensitive to both penicillin and cefuroxime. There are no data from adequate and well-controlled trials to demonstrate the effectiveness of cefuroxime in the treatment of penicillin-resistant strains of*Streptococcus pyogenes.*

Acute Bacterial Otitis Media caused by *Streptococcus pneumoniae, Haemophilus influenzae* (including beta-lactamase-producing strains), *Moraxella catarrhalis* (including beta- lactamase-producing strains), or *Streptococcus pyogenes.*

Impetigo caused by *Staphylococcus aureus*(including beta-lactamase—producing strains) or *Streptococcus pyogenes.*

Culture and susceptibility testing should be performed when appropriate to determine susceptibility of the causative microorganism(s) to cefuroxime. Therapy may be started while awaiting the results of this testing. Antimicrobial therapy should be appropriately adjusted according to the results of such testing.

CONTRAINDICATIONS:

Cefuroxime axetil products are contraindicated in patients with known allergy to the cephalosporin group of antibiotics.

WARNINGS:

CEFUROXIME AXETIL IS NOT BIOEQUIVALENT AND IS THEREFORE NOT SUBSTITUTABLE ON A MG/MG BASIS (SEE CLINICAL PHARMACOLOGY).

BEFORE THERAPY WITH CEFUROXIME AXETIL PRODUCTS IS INSTITUTED, CAREFUL INQUIRY SHOULD BE MADE TO DETERMINE WHETHER THE PATIENT HAS HAD PREVIOUS HYPERSENSITIVITY REACTIONS TO CEFTIN PRODUCTS, OTHER CEPHALOSPORINS, PENICILLINS, OR OTHER DRUGS. IF THIS PRODUCT IS TO BE GIVEN TO PENICILLIN-SENSITIVE PATIENTS, CAUTION SHOULD BE EXERCISED BECAUSE CROSS-HYPERSENSITIVITY AMONG BETA-LACTAM ANTIBIOTICS HAS BEEN CLEARLY DOCUMENTED AND MAY OCCUR IN UP TO 10% OF PATIENTS WITH A HISTORY OF PENICILLIN ALLERGY. IF A CLINICALLY SIGNIFICANT ALLERGIC REACTION TO CEFUROXIME AXETIL PRODUCTS OCCURS, DISCONTINUE THE DRUG AND INSTITUTE APPROPRIATE THERAPY. SERIOUS ACUTE HYPERSENSITIVITY REACTIONS MAY REQUIRE TREATMENT WITH EPINEPHRINE AND OTHER EMERGENCY MEASURES, INCLUDING OXYGEN, INTRAVENOUS FLUIDS, INTRAVENOUS ANTIHISTAMINES, CORTICOSTEROIDS, PRESSOR AMINES, AND AIRWAY MANAGEMENT, AS CLINICALLY INDICATED.

Pseudomembranous colitis has been reported with nearly all antibacterial agents, including cefuroxime, and may range from mild to life threatening. Therefore, it is important to consider this diagnosis in patients who present with diarrhea subsequent to the administration of antibacterial agents.

Treatment with antibacterial agents alters normal flora of the colon and may permit overgrowth of clostridia. Studies indicate that a toxin produced by *Clostridium difficile* is one primary cause of antibiotic-associated colitis.

After the diagnosis of pseudomembranous colitis has been established, appropriate therapeutic measures should be initiated. Mild cases of pseudomembranous colitis usually respond to drug discontinuation alone. In moderate to severe cases, consideration should be given to management with fluids and electrolytes, protein supplementation, and treatment with an antibacterial drug effective against *Clostridium difficile.*

PRECAUTIONS:

General: As with other broad-spectrum antibiotics, prolonged administration of cefuroxime axetil may result in overgrowth of nonsusceptible microorganisms. If superinfection occurs during therapy, appropriate measures should be taken.

Cephalosporins, including cefuroxime axetil, should be given with caution to patients receiving concurrent treatment with potent diuretics because these diuretics are suspected of adversely affecting renal function.

Cefuroxime axetil, as with other broad-spectrum antibiotics, should be prescribed with caution in individuals with a history of colitis. The safety and effectiveness of cefuroxime axetil have not been established in patients with gastrointestinal malabsorption. Patients with gastrointestinal malabsorption were excluded from participating in clinical trials of cefuroxime axetil.

Information for Patients/Caregivers (Pediatric): During clinical trials, the tablet was tolerated by children old enough to swallow the cefuroxime axetil tablet whole. The crushed tablet has a strong, persistent, bitter taste and should not be administered to children in this manner. Children who cannot swallow the tablet whole should receive the oral suspension.

Discontinuation of therapy due to taste and/or problems of administering this drug occurred in 1.4% of children given the oral suspension. Complaints about taste (which may impair compliance) occurred in 5% of children.

Drug/Laboratory Test Interactions: A false-positive reaction for glucose in the urine may occur with copper reduction tests (Benedict's or Fehling's solution or with Clinitest tablets), but not with enzyme-based tests for glycosuria (*e.g.,* Clinistix, Tes-Tape). As a false-negative result may occur in the ferricyanide test, it is recommended that either the glucose oxidase or hexokinase method be used to determine blood/plasma glucose levels in patients receiving cefuroxime axetil. The presence of cefuroxime does not interfere with the assay of serum and urine creatinine by the alkaline picrate method.

Carcinogenesis, Mutagenesis, and Impairment of Fertility: Although lifetime studies in animals have not been performed to evaluate carcinogenic potential, no mutagenic potential was found for cefuroxime axetil in the micronucleus test and a battery of bacterial mutation tests. Reproduction studies in rats at doses up to 1,000 mg/kg per day (nine times the recommended maximum human dose based on mg/mg^2) have revealed no evidence of impaired fertility.

Pregnancy, Teratogenic Effects, Pregnancy Category B: Reproduction studies have been performed in rats and mice at doses up to 3,200 mg/kg per day (23 times the recommended maximum human dose based on mg/m^2) and have revealed no evidence of harm to the fetus due to cefuroxime axetil. There are, however, no adequate and well-controlled studies in pregnant women. Because animal reproduction studies are not always predictive of human response, this drug should be used during pregnancy only if clearly needed.

Labor and Delivery: Cefuroxime axetil has not been studied for use during labor and delivery.

Nursing Mothers: Because cefuroxime is excreted in human milk, consideration should be given to discontinuing nursing temporarily during treatment with cefuroxime axetil.

Pediatric Use: In controlled clinical trials, cefuroxime axetil has been administered to pediatric patients ranging in age from 3 months to 12 years (see INDICATIONS AND USAGE and DOSAGE AND ADMINISTRATION).

Geriatric Use: In clinical trials when 12- to 64-year-old patients and geriatric patients (65 years of age or older) were treated with usual recommended dosages (*i.e.,* 125 to 500 mg b.i.d., depending on type of infections), no overall differences in effectiveness were observed between the two age-groups. The geriatric patients reported somewhat fewer gastrointestinal events and less frequent vaginal candidiasis compared with patients aged 12 to 64 years old; however, no clinically significant differences were reported between the two age- groups. Therefore, no adjustment of the usual adult dose is necessary based on age alone.

DRUG INTERACTIONS:

Concomitant administration of probenecid with cefuroxime axetil tablets increases the area under the serum concentration versus time curve by 50%. The peak serum cefuroxime concentration after a 1.5-g single dose is greater when taken with 1 g of probenecid (mean=14.8 mcg/ml) than without probenecid (mean=12.2 mcg/ml).

Drugs that reduce gastric acidity may result in a lower bioavailability of Ceftin compared with that of fasting state and tend to cancel the effect of postprandial absorption.

ADVERSE REACTIONS:

CEFUROXIME AXETIL TABLETS (MULTIPLE-DOSE DOSING REGIMENS)

In Clinical Trials: In clinical trials using multiple doses of cefuroxime axetil tablets, 912 patients were treated with the recommended dosages of cefuroxime axetil (125 to 500 mg twice a day). There were no deaths or permanent disabilities thought related to drug toxicity. Twenty (2.2%) patients discontinued medication due to adverse events thought by the investigators to be possibly, probably, or almost certainly related to drug toxicity. Seventeen (85%) of the 20 patients who discontinued therapy did so because of gastrointestinal disturbances, including diarrhea, nausea, vomiting, and abdominal pain. The percentage of cefuroxime axetil tablet-treated patients who discontinued study drug because of adverse events was very similar at daily doses of 1,000, 500, and 250 mg (2.3%, 2.1%, and 2.2%, respectively). However, the incidence of gastrointestinal adverse events increased with the higher recommended doses.

The following adverse events (TABLE 8) were thought by the investigators to be possibly, probably, or almost certainly related to cefuroxime axetil tablets in multiple-dose clinical trials (n=912 cefuroxime axetil- treated patients).

In Postmarketing Experience: In addition to the events reported during clinical trials with cefuroxime axetil tablets, the following adverse experiences have been reported from domestic and foreign sources during worldwide postmarketing surveillance: hypersensitivity reactions, including Stevens-Johnson syndrome, erythema multiforme, toxic epidermal necrolysis, serum

ADVERSE REACTIONS: *(cont'd)*

TABLE 8

Incidence ≥1%	Diarrhea/loose stools	3.7%
	Nausea/vomiting	3.0%
	Transient elevation in AST	2.0%
	Transient elevation in ALT	1.6%
	Eosinophilia	1.1%
	Transient elevation in LDH	1.0%
Incidence <1% but >0.1%	Abdominal pain	Dysuria
	Abdominal cramps	Chills
	Flatulence	Chest Pain
	Indigestion	Shortness of breath
	Headache	Mouth ulcers
	Vaginitis	Swollen tongue
	Vulvar itch	Sleepiness
	Rash	Thirst
	Hives	Anorexia
	Itch	Positive Coombs test

sickness—like reactions, anaphylaxis, and angioedema. Jaundice has been reported very rarely. Onset of pseudomembranous colitis symptoms may occur during or after treatment (see WARNINGS).

CEFUROXIME AXETIL TABLETS (SINGLE-DOSE REGIMEN FOR UNCOMPLICATED GONORRHEA):

In Clinical Trials: In clinical trials using a single dose of cefuroxime axetil tablets, 644 patients were treated with the recommended dosage of cefuroxime axetil (1,000 mg) for the treatment of uncomplicated gonorrhea. There were no deaths or permanent disabilities thought related to drug toxicity in these studies.

The following adverse events (TABLE 9) were thought by the investigators to be possibly, probably, or almost certainly related to cefuroxime axetil in 1,000-mg single-dose clinical trials of cefuroxime axetil tablets in the treatment of uncomplicated gonorrhea conducted in the US.

TABLE 9 1-g Single-Dose Regimen for Uncomplicated Gonorrhea-Clinical Trials

Incidence ≥1%	Nausea/vomiting	6.7%
	Diarrhea	4.7%
Incidence <1% but >0.1%	Abdominal pain	Somnolence
	Dyspepsia	Muscle cramps
	Erythema	Muscle stiffness
	Rash	Muscle spasm of neck
	Pruritus	Tightness/pain in chest
	Vaginal candidiasis	Bleeding/pain in urethra
	Vaginal itch	Kidney pain
	Vaginal discharge	Tachycardia
	Headache	Lockjaw-type reaction
	Dizziness	

CEFUROXIME AXETIL FOR ORAL SUSPENSION (MULTIPLE-DOSE DOSING REGIMENS):

In Clinical Trials: In clinical trials using multiple doses of cefuroxime axetil powder for oral suspension, pediatric patients (96.7% of whom were younger than 12 years of age) were treated with the recommended dosages of cefuroxime axetil (20 to 30 mg/kg per day divided twice a day up to a maximum dose of 500 or 1,000 mg per day, respectively). There were no deaths or permanent disabilities in any of the patients in these studies. Eleven US patients (1.2%) discontinued medication due to adverse events thought by the investigators to be possibly, probably, or almost certainly related to drug toxicity. The discontinuations were primarily for gastrointestinal disturbances, usually diarrhea or vomiting. During clinical trials, discontinuation of therapy due to the taste and/or problems with administering this drug occurred in 13 (1.4%) children enrolled at centers in the US.

The following adverse events (TABLE 10) were thought by the investigators to be possibly, probably, or almost certainly related to cefuroxime axetil for oral suspension in multiple-dose clinical trials (n=931 cefuroxime axetil-treated US patients).

TABLE 10 Cefuroxime Axetil for Oral Suspension, Multiple-Dose Dosing Regimens-Clinical Trials

Incidence ≥1%	Diarrhea/loose stools	8.6%
	Dislike of taste	5.0%
	Diaper rash	3.4%
	Nausea/vomiting	2.6%
Incidence <1% but >0.1%	Abdominal pain	Elevated liver enzymes
	Flatulence	Viral illness
	Gastrointestinal infection	Upper respiratory infection
	Candidiasis	
	Vaginal irritation	Sinusitis
	Rash	Cough
	Hyperactivity	Urinary tract infection
	Irritable behavior	Joint swelling
	Eosinophilia	Arthralgia
	Positive direct Coombs' test	Fever Ptyalism

In Postmarketing Experience: In addition to the events reported during clinical trials with cefuroxime axetil for oral suspension, the following adverse experiences have been reported in postmarketing surveillance: hypersensitivity reactions (including rash, pruritus, urticaria, and anaphylaxis).

Cephalosporin-Class Adverse Reactions: In addition to the adverse reactions listed above that have been observed in patients treated with cefuroxime axetil, the following adverse reactions and altered laboratory tests have been reported for cephalosporin-class antibiotics: renal dysfunction, toxic nephropathy, hepatic cholestasis, aplastic anemia, hemolytic anemia, hemorrhage, increased prothrombin time, increased BUN, increased creatinine, false-positive test for urinary glucose, increased alkaline phosphatase, neutropenia, thrombocytopenia, leukopenia, elevated bilirubin, pancytopenia, and agranulocytosis.

Several cephalosporins have been implicated in triggering seizures, particularly in patients with renal impairment when the dosage was not reduced (see DOSAGE AND ADMINISTRATION and OVERDOSAGE). If seizures associated with drug therapy occur, the drug should be discontinued. Anticonvulsant therapy can be given if clinically indicated.

OVERDOSAGE:

Overdosage of cephalosporins can cause cerebral irritation leading to convulsions. Serum levels of cefuroxime can be reduced by hemodialysis and peritoneal dialysis.

DOSAGE AND ADMINISTRATION:

NOTE: CEFUROXIME AXETIL IS NOT BIOEQUIVALENT AND IS NOT SUBSTITUTABLE ON A MG/MG BASIS (See CLINICAL PHARMACOLOGY).

TABLE 11 (May be administered without regard to meals.)

Population/Infection	Dosage	Duration (days)
Adolescents and Adults (13 years and older)		
Pharyngitis/tonsillitis	250 mg b.i.d.	10
Acute bacterial maxillary sinusitis	250 mg b.i.d.	10
Acute bacterial exacerbations of chronic bronchitis and secondary bacterial infections of acute bronchitis	250 or 500 mg b.i.d.	10
Uncomplicated skin and skin-structure infections	250 or 500 mg b.i.d.	10
Uncomplicated urinary tract infections	125 or 250 mg b.i.d.	7-10
Uncomplicated gonorrhea	1,000 mg once	single dose
Children (who can swallow tablets whole)		
Pharyngitis/tonsillitis	125 mg b.i.d.	10
Acute otitis media	250 mg b.i.d.	10

Cefuroxime Axetil for Oral Suspension: Cefuroxime Axetil for oral suspension may be administered to children ranging in age from 3 months to 12 years, according to dosages in the following table (TABLE 12):

TABLE 12 (Must be administered with food. Shake well each time before using.)

Population/Infection	Dosage	Daily Maximum Dose	Duration (days)
Infants and children (3 months to 12 years)			
Pharyngitis/tonsillitis	20 mg/kg/day divided b.i.d.	500 mg	10
Acute otitis media	30 mg/kg/day divided b.i.d.	1,000 mg	10
Impetigo	30 mg/kg/day divided b.i.d.	1,000 mg	10

Patients with Renal Failure: The safety and efficacy of cefuroxime axetil in patients with renal failure have not been established. Since cefuroxime is renally eliminated, its half-life will be prolonged in patients with renal failure.

Directions for Mixing Ceftin for Oral Suspension: Prepare a suspension at the time of dispensing as follows:

1. Shake the bottle to loosen the powder.
2. Remove the cap.
3. Add the total amount of water for reconstitution (see TABLE 13) and replace the cap.
4. Invert the bottle and vigorously rock the bottle from side to side so that water rises through the powder.
5. Once the sound of the powder against the bottle disappears, turn the bottle upright and vigorously shake it in a diagonal direction.

TABLE 13

Bottle Size	Amount of Water Required for Reconstitution
50 ml	20 ml
100 ml	37 ml
200 ml	74 ml

Each teaspoonful (5 ml) will contain the equivalent of 125 mg of cefuroxime as cefuroxime axetil.

NOTE: SHAKE THE ORAL SUSPENSION WELL BEFORE EACH USE. Replace cap securely after each opening. Reconstituted suspension should be stored between 2° and 25°C (36° and 77°F) (either in the refrigerator or at room temperature). DISCARD AFTER 10 DAYS.

REFERENCES:

1. National Committee for Clinical Laboratory Standards. *Methods for Dilution Antimicrobial Susceptibility Tests for Bacteria that Grow Aerobically.* 3rd ed. Approved Standard NCCLS Document M7- A3, Vol. 13, No. 25. Villanova, Pa: NCCLS; 1993. **2.** National Committee for Clinical Laboratory Standards. *Performance Standards for Antimicrobial Disk Susceptibility Tests.* 4th ed. Approved Standard NCCLS Document M2-A4, Vol. 10, No. 7. Villanova, Pa: NCCLS; 1990.

PATIENT INFORMATION:

Cefuroxime axetil is a cephalosporin antibiotic used to treat bacterial infections. Take at regular intervals and complete the entire course of therapy. Do not take this medication if you are allergic to any type of penicillin or cephalosporin. Notify your physician if you are pregnant or nursing. This antibiotic may decrease the effectiveness of birth control pills; use another form of birth control while taking this medication. Shake the suspension well before each use and store it in the refrigerator. Swallow the tablets whole. Do not break, crush, or chew the tablets due to the strongly bitter taste of the medication. May cause nausea, vomiting or diarrhea; notify your physician if these occur. Take with food or milk to avoid stomach upset. Cefuroxime axetil may cause a false-positive reaction for nonspecific urine glucose tests in patients with diabetes. This medication does not interfere with enzyme-based urine glucose tests.

HOW SUPPLIED:

Ceftin Tablets: Ceftin Tablets, 125 mg of cefuroxime (as cefuroxime axetil), are white, capsule-shaped, film-coated tablets engraved with "395" on one side and "Glaxo" on the other side.

Ceftin Tablets, 250 mg of cefuroxime (as cefuroxime axetil), are light blue, capsule-shaped, film-coated tablets engraved with "387" on one side and "Glaxo" on the other side.

Ceftin Tablets, 500 mg of cefuroxime (as cefuroxime axetil), are dark blue, capsule-shaped, film-coated tablets engraved with "394" on one side and "Glaxo" on the other side.

Store the tablets between 15° and 30°C (59° and 86°F). Replace cap securely after each opening. Protect unit dose packs from excessive moisture.

Ceftin for Oral Suspension: Ceftin for Oral Suspension is provided as dry, white to pale yellow, tutti-frutti—flavored powder. When reconstituted as directed, Ceftin for Oral Suspension provides the equivalent of 125 mg of cefuroxime (as cefuroxime axetil) per 5 ml of suspension. It is supplied in amber glass bottles.

Before reconstitution, store dry powder between 2° and 30°C (36° and 86°F).

After reconstitution, store suspension between 2° and 25°C (36° and 77°F), in a refrigerator or at room temperature. DISCARD AFTER 10 DAYS.

HOW SUPPLIED - EQUIVALENTS NOT AVAILABLE:

Powder, Reconstitution - Oral - 125 mg/5ml

50 ml	$15.40	CEFTIN, Glaxo Wellcome	00173-0406-01
100 ml	$30.61	CEFTIN, Glaxo Wellcome	00173-0406-00
200 ml	$53.59	CEFTIN, Glaxo Wellcome	00173-0406-04

Tablet, Coated - Oral - 125 mg

20's	$37.34	CEFTIN, Glaxo Wellcome	00173-0395-00
60's	$106.67	CEFTIN, Glaxo Wellcome	00173-0395-01
100's	$183.25	CEFTIN, Glaxo Wellcome	00173-0395-02

Tablet, Coated - Oral - 250 mg

20's	$70.01	CEFTIN, Glaxo Wellcome	00173-0387-00
60's	$199.82	CEFTIN, Glaxo Wellcome	00173-0387-42
100's	$338.53	CEFTIN, Glaxo Wellcome	00173-0387-01

Tablet, Coated - Oral - 500 mg

20's	$132.84	CEFTIN, Glaxo Wellcome	00173-0394-00
50's	$329.94	CEFTIN, Glaxo Wellcome	00173-0394-01
60's	$392.80	CEFTIN, Glaxo Wellcome	00173-0394-42

CEFUROXIME SODIUM *(000696)*

CATEGORIES: Anti-Infectives; Antibiotics; Antimicrobials; Bone Infections; Cephalosporins; Gonococcal Infections; Gonorrhea; Infections; Joint Infections; Meningitis; Pneumonia; Perioperative Prophylaxis; Respiratory Tract Infections; Septicemia; Sexually Transmitted Diseases; Skin Infections; Urinary Tract Infections; Pregnancy Category B; Sales > $100 Million; FDA Approved 1983 Oct; Patent Expiration 1993 Aug

BRAND NAMES: *Alporin*; *Cefamar*; *Ceflour*; *Cefogen*; *Cefoxin*; *Cekonin*; *Curocef*; *Curoxima*; *Curoxime*; *Froxal* (Mexico); *Furoxime*; Kefurox; *Sencef*; *Seroxin*; *Supacef*; *Ucefaxim*; *Uroxime*; *Vekfazolin*; **Zinacef**; *Zinnat* (France, Mexico)
(International brand names outside U.S. in italics)

FORMULARIES: Aetna; BC-BS

COST OF THERAPY: $90.00 (Infections; Injection; 750 mg/vial; 3/day; 5 days) vs. Potential Cost of $7,048.46 (Respiratory Infections)

PRIMARY ICD9: 136.9 (Unspecified Infections And Parasitic Diseases)

DESCRIPTION:

Cefuroxime is a semisynthetic, broad-spectrum, cephalosporin antibiotic for parenteral administration. It is the sodium salt of (6R,7R)-3-carbamoyloxymethyl-7-[Z-2-methoxyimino-2-(fur-2-yl)acetamido]ce ph-3-em-4-carboxylate.

The empirical formula is $C_{16}H_{15}N_4NaO_8S$, representing a molecular weight of 446.4.

Cefuroxime sodium contains approximately 54.2 mg (2.4 mEq) of sodium per g of cefuroxime activity.

Cefuroxime sodium in sterile crystalline form is supplied in vials equivalent to 750 mg, 1.5 g, or 7.5 g of cefuroxime as cefuroxime sodium and in ADD-Vantage vials equivalent to 750 mg or 1.5 g of cefuroxime as cefuroxime sodium. Solutions of cefuroxime sodium range in color from light yellow to amber, depending on the concentration and diluent used. The pH of freshly constituted solutions usually ranges from 6 to 8.5.

Cefuroxime sodium is available as a frozen, iso-osmotic, sterile, nonpyrogenic solution with 750 mg or 1.5 g of cefuroxime as cefuroxime sodium. Approximately 1.4 g of dextrose hydrous, USP has been added to the 750-mg dose to adjust the osmolality. Sodium citrate hydrous, USP has been added as a buffer (300 mg and 600 mg to the 750-mg and 1.5-g doses, respectively). Cefuroxime sodium contains approximately 111 mg (4.8 mEq) and 222 mg (9.7 mEq) of sodium in the 750-mg and 1.5-g doses, respectively. The pH has been adjusted with hydrochloric acid and may have been adjusted with sodium hydroxide. Solutions of premixed cefuroxime sodium range in color from light yellow to amber. The solution is intended for intravenous (IV) use after thawing to room temperature. The osmolality of the solution is approximately 300 mOsmol/kg, and the pH of thawed solutions ranges from 5 to 7.5.

The plastic container for the frozen solution is fabricated from a specially designed multilayer plastic, PL 2040. Solutions are in contact with the polyethylene layer of this container and can leach out certain chemical components of the plastic in very small amounts within the expiration period. The suitability of the plastic has been confirmed in tests in animals according to USP biologic tests for plastic containers as well as by tissue culture toxicity studies.

CLINICAL PHARMACOLOGY:

After intramuscular (IM) injection of a 750-mg dose of cefuroxime to normal volunteers, the mean peak serum concentration was 27 mcg/ml. The peak occurred at approximately 45 minutes (range, 15 to 60 minutes). Following IV doses of 750 mg and 1.5 g, serum concentrations were approximately 50 and 100 mcg/ml, respectively, at 15 minutes. Therapeutic serum concentrations of approximately 2 mcg/ml or more were maintained for 5.3 hours and 8 hours or more, respectively. There was no evidence of accumulation of cefuroxime in the serum following IV administration of 1.5-g doses every 8 hours to normal volunteers. The serum half-life after either IM or IV injections is approximately 80 minutes.

Approximately 89% of a dose of cefuroxime is excreted by the kidneys over an 8-hour period, resulting in high urinary concentrations.

Following the IM administration of a 750-mg single dose, urinary concentrations averaged 1300 mcg/ml during the first 8 hours. Intravenous doses of 750 mg and 1.5 g produced urinary levels averaging 1150 and 2500 mcg/ml, respectively, during the first 8-hour period.

The concomitant oral administration of probenecid with cefuroxime slows tubular secretion, decreases renal clearance by approximately 40%, increases the peak serum level by approximately 30%, and increases the serum half-life by approximately 30%. Cefuroxime is detectable in therapeutic concentrations in pleural fluid, joint fluid, bile, sputum, bone, cerebrospinal fluid (in patients with meningitis), and aqueous humor.

Cefuroxime is approximately 50% bound to serum protein.

MICROBIOLOGY

Cefuroxime has *in vitro* activity against a wide range of gram-positive and gram-negative organisms, and it is highly stable in the presence of beta-lactamases of certain gram-negative bacteria. The bactericidal action of cefuroxime results from inhibition of cell-wall synthesis.

Cefuroxime is usually active against the following organisms *in vitro*.

Aerobes, Gram-Positive: *Staphylococcus aureus, Staphylococcus epidermidis, Streptococcus pneumoniae*, and *Streptococcus pyogenes* (and other streptococci).

NOTE: Most strains of enterococci (*e.g., Enterococcus faecalis*, formerly *Streptococcus faecalis*) are resistant to cefuroxime. Methicillin-resistant staphylococci and *Listeria monocytogenes* are resistant to cefuroxime.

CLINICAL PHARMACOLOGY: *(cont'd)*

Aerobes, Gram-Negative: *Citrobacter* spp.,*Enterobacter* spp., *Escherichia coli, Haemophilus influenzae* (including ampicillin-resistant strains), *Haemophilus parainfluenzae, Klebsiella* spp. (including *Klebsiella pneumoniae*), *Moraxella (Branhamella) catarrhalis* (including ampicillin- and cephalothin-resistant strains), *Morganella morganii* (formerly *Proteus morganii*), *Neisseria gonorrhoeae* (including penicillinase- and non–penicillinase-producing strains), *Neisseria meningitidis, Proteus mirabilis, Providencia rettgeri* (formerly *Proteus rettgeri*), *Salmonella* spp., and *Shigella* spp.

NOTE: Some strains of *Morganella morganii, Enterobacter cloacae*, and *Citrobacter* spp. have been shown by *in vitro* tests to be resistant to cefuroxime and other cephalosporins. *Pseudomonas* and *Campylobacter* spp., *Acinetobacter calcoaceticus*, and most strains of *Serratia* spp. and *Proteus vulgaris* are resistant to most first- and second-generation cephalosporins.

Anaerobes: Gram-positive and gram-negative cocci (including *Peptococcus* and *Peptostreptococcus* spp.), gram-positive bacilli (including *Clostridium* spp.), and gram-negative bacilli (including *Bacteroides* and *Fusobacterium* spp.).

NOTE: *Clostridium difficile* and most strains of *Bacteroides fragilis* are resistant to cefuroxime.

SUSCEPTIBILITY TESTS

Diffusion Techniques: Quantitative methods that require measurement of zone diameters give an estimate of antibiotic susceptibility. One such standard procedure[1] that has been recommended for use with disks to test susceptibility of organisms to cefuroxime uses the 30-mcg cefuroxime disk. Interpretation involves the correlation of the diameters obtained in the disk test with the minimum inhibitory concentration (MIC) for cefuroxime.

A report of "Susceptible" indicates that the pathogen is likely to be inhibited by generally achievable blood levels. A report of "Moderately Susceptible" suggests that the organism would be susceptible if high dosage is used or if the infection is confined to tissues and fluids in which high antibiotic levels are attained. A report of "Intermediate" suggests an equivocable or indeterminate result. A report of "Resistant" indicates that achievable concentrations of the antibiotic are unlikely to be inhibitory and other therapy should be selected.

Reports from the laboratory giving results of the standard single-disk susceptibility test for organisms other than *Haemophilus* spp. and *Neisseria gonorrhoeae* with a 30-mcg cefuroxime disk should be interpreted according to the criteria found in TABLE 1.

TABLE 1

Zone Diameter (mm)	Interpretation
≥18	(S) Susceptible
15-17	(MS) Moderately Susceptible
≤14	(R) Resistant

Results for *Haemophilus* spp. should be interpreted according to the criteria found in TABLE 2.

TABLE 2

Zone Diameter (mm)	Interpretation
≥24	(S) Susceptible
21-23	(I) Intermediate
≤20	(R) Resistant

Results for *Neisseria gonorrhoeae* should be interpreted according to the criteria found in TABLE 3.

TABLE 3

Zone Diameter (mm)	Interpretation
≥31	(S) Susceptible
26-30	(MS) Moderately Susceptible
≤25	(R) Resistant

Organisms should be tested with the cefuroxime disk since cefuroxime has been shown by *in vitro* tests to be active against certain strains found resistant when other beta-lactam disks are used. The cefuroxime disk should not be used for testing susceptibility to other cephalosporins.

Standardized procedures require the use of laboratory control organisms. The 30-mcg cefuroxime disk should give the zone diameters found in TABLE 4.

TABLE 4

Organism	Zone Diameter (mm)
1. Testing for organisms other than*Haemophilus* spp. and *Neisseria*: *gonorrhoeae:*	
Staphylococcus aureus ATCC 25923	27-35
Escherichia coli ATCC 25922	20-26
2. Testing for*Haemophilus* spp.:	
Haemophilus influenzae ATCC 49766	28-36
3. Testing for*Neisseria gonorrhoeae:*	
Neisseria gonorrhoeae ATCC 49226	33-41
Staphylococcus aureus ATCC 25923	29-33

Dilution Techniques: Use a standardized dilution method[1] (broth, agar, microdilution) or equivalent with cefuroxime powder. The MIC values obtained for bacterial isolates other than *Haemophilus* spp. and *Neisseria gonorrhoeae* should be interpreted according to the criteria found inTABLE 5.

TABLE 5

MIC (mcg/ml)	Interpretation
≤8	(S) Susceptible
16	(MS) Moderately Susceptible
≥32	(R) Resistant

MIC values obtained for *Haemophilus* spp. should be interpreted according to the criteria found in TABLE 6.

MIC values obtained for *Neisseria gonorrhoeae* should be interpreted according to the criteria found in TABLE 7.

As with standard diffusion techniques, dilution methods require the use of laboratory control organisms. Standard cefuroxime powder should provide MIC values found in TABLE 8.

TABLE 6

MIC (mcg/ml)	Interpretation
≤4	(S) Susceptible
8	(I) Intermediate
≥16	(R) Resistant

TABLE 7

MIC (mcg/ml)	Interpretation
≤1	(S) Susceptible
2	(MS) Moderately Susceptible
≥4	(R) Resistant

TABLE 8

Organism	MIC (mcg/ml)
1. For organisms other than *Haemophilus* spp. and *Neisseria gonorrhoeae*:	
Staphylococcus aureus ATCC 29213	0.5-2.0
Escherichia coli ATCC 25922	2.0-8.0
2. For *Haemophilus* spp.:	
Haemophilus influenzae ATCC 49766	0.25-1.0
3. For *Neisseria gonorrhoeae*:	
Neisseria gonorrhoeae ATCC 49226	0.25-1.0
Staphylococcus aureus ATCC 29213	0.25-1.0

INDICATIONS AND USAGE:

Cefuroxime sodium is indicated for the treatment of patients with infections caused by susceptible strains of the designated organisms in the following diseases:

Lower Respiratory Tract Infections Including Pneumonia Caused by *Streptococcus pneumoniae, Haemophilus influenzae* (including ampicillin-resistant strains), *Klebsiella* spp.,*Staphylococcus aureus* (penicillinase- and non–penicillinase-producing strains), *Streptococcus pyogenes*, and *Escherichia coli.*

Urinary Tract Infections Caused by *Escherichia coli* and *Klebsiella* spp.

Skin and Skin Structure Infections Caused by *Staphylococcus aureus* (penicillinase- and non–penicillinase-producing strains), *Streptococcus pyogenes, Escherichia coli, Klebsiella* spp., and *Enterobacter* spp.

Septicemia Caused by *Staphylococcus aureus* (penicillinase- and non–penicillinase-producing strains),*Streptococcus pneumoniae, Escherichia coli, Haemophilus influenzae* (including ampicillin-resistant strains), and *Klebsiella* spp.

Meningitis Caused by *Streptococcus pneumoniae, Haemophilus influenzae* (including ampicillin-resistant strains), *Neisseria meningitidis,* and *Staphylococcus aureus* (penicillinase- and non–penicillinase-producing strains) (see PRECAUTIONS).

Gonorrhea: Uncomplicated and disseminated gonococcal infections due to *Neisseria gonorrhoeae* (penicillinase- and non–penicillinase-producing strains) in both males and females.

Bone and Joint Infections Caused by *Staphylococcus aureus* (penicillinase- and non–penicillinase-producing strains).

Clinical microbiological studies in skin and skin-structure infections frequently reveal the growth of susceptible strains of both aerobic and anaerobic organisms. Cefuroxime sodium has been used successfully in these mixed infections in which several organisms have been isolated. Appropriate cultures and susceptibility studies should be performed to determine the susceptibility of the causative organisms to cefuroxime sodium.

Therapy may be started while awaiting the results of these studies; however, once these results become available, the antibiotic treatment should be adjusted accordingly. In certain cases of confirmed or suspected gram-positive or gram-negative sepsis or in patients with other serious infections in which the causative organism has not been identified, cefuroxime sodium may be used concomitantly with an aminoglycoside (see PRECAUTIONS.) The recommended doses of both antibiotics may be given depending on the severity of the infection and the patient's condition.

Prevention: The preoperative prophylactic administration of cefuroxime sodium may prevent the growth of susceptible disease-causing bacteria and thereby may reduce the incidence of certain postoperative infections in patients undergoing surgical procedures (*e.g.,* vaginal hysterectomy) that are classified as clean-contaminated or potentially contaminated procedures. Effective prophylactic use of antibiotics in surgery depends on the time of administration. Cefuroxime sodium should usually be given one-half to 1 hour before the operation to allow sufficient time to achieve effective antibiotic concentrations in the wound tissues during the procedure. The dose should be repeated intraoperatively if the surgical procedure is lengthy.

Prophylactic administration is usually not required after the surgical procedure ends and should be stopped within 24 hours. In the majority of surgical procedures, continuing prophylactic administration of any antibiotic does not reduce the incidence of subsequent infections but will increase the possibility of adverse reactions and the development of bacterial resistance.

The perioperative use of cefuroxime sodium has also been effective during open heart surgery for surgical patients in whom infections at the operative site would present a serious risk. For these patients it is recommended that cefuroxime sodium therapy be continued for at least 48 hours after the surgical procedure ends. If an infection is present, specimens for culture should be obtained for the identification of the causative organism, and appropriate antimicrobial therapy should be instituted.

CONTRAINDICATIONS:

Cefuroxime sodium is contraindicated in patients with known allergy to the cephalosporin group of antibiotics.

WARNINGS:

BEFORE THERAPY WITH CEFUROXIME SODIUM IS INSTITUTED, CAREFUL INQUIRY SHOULD BE MADE TO DETERMINE WHETHER THE PATIENT HAS HAD PREVIOUS HYPERSENSITIVITY REACTIONS TO CEPHALOSPORINS, PENICILLINS, OR OTHER DRUGS. THIS PRODUCT SHOULD BE GIVEN CAUTIOUSLY TO PENICILLIN-SENSITIVE PATIENTS. ANTIBIOTICS SHOULD BE ADMINISTERED WITH CAUTION TO ANY PATIENT WHO HAS DEMONSTRATED SOME FORM OF ALLERGY, PARTICULARLY TO DRUGS. IF AN ALLERGIC REACTION TO CEFUROXIME SODIUM OCCURS, DISCONTINUE THE DRUG. SERIOUS ACUTE HYPERSENSITIVITY REACTIONS MAY REQUIRE EPINEPHRINE AND OTHER EMERGENCY MEASURES.

WARNINGS: *(cont'd)*

Pseudomembranous colitis has been reported with nearly all antibacterial agents, including cefuroxime, and may range from mild to life threatening. Therefore, it is important to consider this diagnosis in patients who present with diarrhea subsequent to the administration of antibacterial agents.

Treatment with broad-spectrum antibiotics alters the normal flora of the colon and may permit overgrowth of clostridia. Studies indicate that a toxin produced by *Clostridium difficile* is one primary cause of antibiotic-associated colitis. Cholestyramine and colestipol resins have been shown to bind the toxin *in vitro.*

Mild cases of colitis may respond to drug discontinuation alone. Moderate to severe cases should be managed with fluid, electrolyte, and protein supplementation as indicated.

When the colitis is not relieved by drug discontinuation or when it is severe, oral vancomycin is the treatment of choice for antibiotic-associated pseudomembranous colitis produced by*C. difficile*. Other causes of colitis should also be considered.

PRECAUTIONS:

Although cefuroxime sodium rarely produces alterations in kidney function, evaluation of renal status during therapy is recommended, especially in seriously ill patients receiving the maximum doses. Cephalosporins should be given with caution to patients receiving concurrent treatment with potent diuretics as these regimens are suspected of adversely affecting renal function.

The total daily dose of cefuroxime sodium should be reduced in patients with transient or persistent renal insufficiency (see DOSAGE AND ADMINISTRATION), because high and prolonged serum antibiotic concentrations can occur in such individuals from usual doses.

As with other antibiotics, prolonged use of cefuroxime sodium may result in overgrowth of non-susceptible organisms. Careful observation of the patient is essential. If superinfection occurs during therapy, appropriate measures should be taken.

Broad-spectrum antibiotics should be prescribed with caution in individuals with a history of gastrointestinal disease, particularly colitis.

Nephrotoxicity has been reported following concomitant administration of aminoglycoside antibiotics and cephalosporins.

As with other therapeutic regimens used in the treatment of meningitis, mild-to-severe hearing loss has been reported in some pediatric patients treated with cefuroxime sodium. Persistence of positive cerebrospinal fluid (CSF) cultures at 18 to 36 hours, particularly in patients with *Haemophilus influenzae* isolates, has also been noted; however, the precise clinical impact of this is unknown.

Drug/Laboratory Test Interactions: A false-positive reaction for glucose in the urine may occur with copper reduction tests (Benedict's or Fehling's solution or with Clinitest tablets) but not with enzyme-based tests for glycosuria (*e.g.,* Tes-Tape). As a false-negative result may occur in the ferricyanide test, it is recommended that either the glucose oxidase or hexokinase method be used to determine blood plasma glucose levels in patients receiving cefuroxime sodium.

Cefuroxime does not interfere with the assay of serum and urine creatinine by the alkaline picrate method.

Carcinogenesis, Mutagenesis, and Impairment of Fertility: Although no long-term studies in animals have been performed to evaluate carcinogenic potential, no mutagenic potential of cefuroxime was found in standard laboratory tests.

Reproductive studies revealed no impairment of fertility in animals.

Pregnancy, Teratogenic Effects, Pregnancy Category C: Reproduction studies have been performed in mice and rabbits at doses up to 60 times the human dose and have revealed no evidence of impaired fertility or harm to the fetus due to cefuroxime. There are, however, no adequate and well-controlled studies in pregnant women. Because animal reproduction studies are not always predictive of human response, this drug should be used during pregnancy only if clearly needed.

Nursing Mothers: Since cefuroxime is excreted in human milk, caution should be exercised when cefuroxime sodium is administered to a nursing woman.

Pediatric Use: Safety and effectiveness in children below 3 months of age have not been established. Accumulation of other members of the cephalosporin class in newborn infants, with resulting prolongation of drug half-life has been reported.

DRUG INTERACTIONS:

Solutions of cefuroxime sodium, like those of most beta-lactam antibiotics, should not be added to solutions of aminoglycoside antibiotics because of potential interaction.

However, if concurrent therapy with cefuroxime sodium and an aminoglycoside is indicated, each of these antibiotics can be administered separately to the same patient.

ADVERSE REACTIONS:

Cefuroxime sodium is generally well tolerated. The most common adverse effects have been local reactions following IV administration. Other adverse reactions have been encountered only rarely.

Local Reactions: Thrombophlebitis has occurred with IV administration in 1 in 60 patients.

Gastrointestinal: Gastrointestinal symptoms occurred in 1 in 150 patients and included diarrhea (1 in 220 patients) and nausea (1 in 440 patients). Onset of pseudomembranous colitis symptoms may occur during or after treatment (see WARNINGS).

Hypersensitivity Reactions: Hypersensitivity reactions have been reported in fewer than 1% of the patients treated with cefuroxime sodium and include rash (1 in 125). Pruritus, urticaria, and positive Coombs' test each occurred in fewer than 1 in 250 patients, and, as with other cephalosporins, rare cases of anaphylaxis, drug fever, erythema multiforme, interstitial nephritis, toxic epidermal necrolysis, and Stevens-Johnson syndrome have occurred.

Blood: A decrease in hemoglobin and hematocrit has been observed in 1 in 10 patients and transient eosinophilia in 1 in 14 patients. Less common reactions seen were transient neutropenia (fewer than 1 in 100 patients) and leukopenia (1 in 750 patients). A similar pattern and incidence were seen with other cephalosporins used in controlled studies. As with other cephalosporins, there have been rare reports of thrombocytopenia.

Hepatic: Transient rise in SGOT and SGPT (1 in 25 patients), alkaline phosphatase (1 in 50 patients), LDH (1 in 75 patients), and bilirubin (1 in 500 patients) levels has been noted.

Kidney: Elevations in serum creatinine and/or blood urea nitrogen and a decreased creatinine clearance have been observed, but their relationship to cefuroxime is unknown.

In addition to the adverse reactions listed above that have been observed in patients treated with cefuroxime, the following adverse reactions and altered laboratory tests have been reported for cephalosporin-class antibiotics:

Adverse Reactions: Vomiting, abdominal pain, colitis, vaginitis (including vaginal candidiasis), toxic nephropathy, hepatic dysfunction (including cholestasis), aplastic anemia, hemolytic anemia, hemorrhage.

Several cephalosporins have been implicated in triggering seizures, particularly in patients with renal impairment when the dosage was not reduced (see DOSAGE AND ADMINISTRATION). If seizures associated with drug therapy should occur, the drug should be discontinued. Anticonvulsant therapy can be given if clinically indicated.

ADVERSE REACTIONS: *(cont'd)*

Altered Laboratory Tests: Prolonged prothrombin time, pancytopenia, agranulocytosis.

OVERDOSAGE:

Overdosage of cephalosporins can cause cerebral irritation leading to convulsions. Serum levels of cefuroxime can be reduced by hemodialysis and peritoneal dialysis.

DOSAGE AND ADMINISTRATION:

DOSAGE

Adults

The usual adult dosage range for cefuroxime sodium is 750 mg to 1.5 g every 8 hours, usually for 5 to 10 days. In uncomplicated urinary tract infections, skin and skin-structure infections, disseminated gonococcal infections, and uncomplicated pneumonia; a 750-mg dose every 8 hours is recommended. In severe or complicated infections, a 1.5-g dose every 8 hours is recommended.

In bone and joint infections, a 1.5-g dose every 8 hours is recommended. In clinical trials, surgical intervention was performed when indicated as an adjunct to cefuroxime sodium therapy. A course of oral antibiotics was administered when appropriate following the completion of parenteral administration of cefuroxime sodium.

In life-threatening infections or infections due to less susceptible organisms, 1.5 g every 6 hours may be required. In bacterial meningitis, the dosage should not exceed 3 g every 8 hours. The recommended dosage for uncomplicated gonococcal infection is 1.5 g given intramuscularly as a single dose at two different sites together with 1 g of oral probenecid. For preventive use for clean-contaminated or potentially contaminated surgical procedures, a 1.5-g dose administered intravenously just before surgery (approximately one-half to 1 hour before the initial incision) is recommended. Thereafter, give 750 mg intravenously or intramuscularly every 8 hours when the procedure is prolonged.

For preventive use during open heart surgery, a 1.5-g dose administered intravenously at the induction of anesthesia and every 12 hours thereafter for a total of 6 g is recommended.

Impaired Renal Function: A reduced dosage must be employed when renal function is impaired. Dosage should be determined by the degree of renal impairment and the susceptibility of the causative organism (TABLE 9).

TABLE 9 Dosage of Cefuroxime Sodium in Adults With Reduced Renal Function

Creatinine Clearance (ml/min)	Dose	Frequency
>20	750 mg-1.5 g	q8h
10-20	750 mg	q12h
<10	750 mg	q24h*

* Since cefuroxime sodium is dialyzable, patients on hemodialysis should be given a further dose at the end of the dialysis.

When only serum creatinine is available, the following formula[2] (based on sex, weight, and age of the patient) may be used to convert this value into creatinine clearance. The serum creatinine should represent a steady state of renal function (TABLE 10).

TABLE 10

Males: Creatinine clearance (ml/min) = [Weight (kg) × (140 - age)] ÷ [72 × serum creatinine (mg/dl)]
Female: 0.85 × male value

Note: As with antibiotic therapy in general, administration of cefuroxime sodium should be continued for a minimum of 48 to 72 hours after the patient becomes asymptomatic or after evidence of bacterial eradication has been obtained; a minimum of 10 days of treatment is recommended in infections caused by *Streptococcus pyogenes* in order to guard against the risk of rheumatic fever or glomerulonephritis; frequent bacteriologic and clinical appraisal is necessary during therapy of chronic urinary tract infection and may be required for several months after therapy has been completed; persistent infections may require treatment for several weeks; and doses smaller than those indicated above should not be used. In staphylococcal and other infections involving a collection of pus, surgical drainage should be carried out where indicated.

Infants and Children Above 3 Months of Age

Administration of 50 to 100 mg/kg per day in equally divided doses every 6 to 8 hours has been successful for most infections susceptible to cefuroxime. The higher dosage of 100 mg/kg per day (not to exceed the maximum adult dosage) should be used for the more severe or serious infections.

In bone and joint infections, 150 mg/kg per day (not to exceed the maximum adult dosage) is recommended in equally divided doses every 8 hours. In clinical trials, a course of oral antibiotics was administered to children following the completion of parenteral administration of cefuroxime sodium.

In cases of bacterial meningitis, a larger dosage of cefuroxime sodium is recommended: 200 to 240 mg/kg per day intravenously in divided doses every 6 to 8 hours.

In children with renal insufficiency, the frequency of dosing should be modified consistent with the recommendations for adults.

PREPARATION OF SOLUTION AND SUSPENSION

The directions for preparing cefuroxime sodium for both IV and IM use are summarized in TABLE 11.

For Intramuscular Use: Each 750-mg vial of cefuroxime sodium should be constituted with 3.0 ml of sterile water for injection. Shake gently to disperse and withdraw completely the resulting suspension for injection.

For Intravenous Use: Each 750-mg vial should be constituted with 8.0 ml of sterile water for injection. Withdraw completely the resulting solution for injection.

Each 1.5-g vial should be constituted with 16.0 ml of sterile water for injection, and the solution should be completely withdrawn for injection.

The 7.5-g pharmacy bulk vial should be constituted with 77 ml of sterile water for injection; each 8 ml of the resulting solution contains 750 mg of cefuroxime.

Each 750-mg and 1.5-g infusion pack should be constituted with 100 ml of sterile water for injection, 5% dextrose injection, 0.9% sodium chloride injection, or any of the solutions listed under Compatibility And Stability, Intravenous(TABLE 11).

ADMINISTRATION

After constitution, cefuroxime sodium may be given intravenously or by deep IM injection into a large muscle mass (such as the gluteus or lateral part of the thigh). Before injecting intramuscularly, aspiration is necessary to avoid inadvertent injection into a blood vessel.

Intravenous Administration: The IV route may be preferable for patients with bacterial septicemia or other severe or life-threatening infections or for patients who may be poor risks because of lowered resistance, particularly if shock is present or impending.

DOSAGE AND ADMINISTRATION: *(cont'd)*

TABLE 11 Preparation of Solution and Suspension

Strength	Amount of Diluent to Be Added (ml)	Volume to Be Withdrawn	Approximate Cefuroxime Concentration (mg/ml)
750-mg Vial	3.0 (IM)	Total*	220
750-mg Vial	8.0 (IV)	Total	90
1.5-g Vial	16.0 (IV)	Total	90
750-mg Infusion pack	100 (IV)	—	7.5
1.5-g Infusion pack	100 (IV)	—	15
7.5-g Pharmacy bulk package	77 (IV)	Amount Needed†	95

* **Note:** Cefuroxime sodium is a suspension at IM concentrations.
† 8 ml of solution contains 750 mg of cefuroxime; 16 ml of solution contains 1.5 grams of cefuroxime.

For direct intermittent IV administration slowly inject the solution into a vein over a period of 3 to 5 minutes or give it through the tubing system by which the patient is also receiving other IV solutions.

For intermittent IV infusion with a Y-type administration set dosing can be accomplished through the tubing system by which the patient may be receiving other IV solutions. However, during infusion of the solution containing cefuroxime sodium, it is advisable to temporarily discontinue administration of any other solutions at the same site.

ADD-Vantage vials are to be constituted only with 50 or 100 ml of 5% dextrose injection, 0.9% sodium chloride injection, or 0.45% sodium chloride injection in Abbott ADD-Vantage flexible diluent containers (see Patient Package Insert, Instructions for Constitution). ADD-Vantage vials that have been joined to Abbott ADD-Vantage diluent containers and activated to dissolve the drug are stable for 24 hours at room temperature or for 7 days under refrigeration. Joined vials that have not been activated may be used within a 14-day period; this period corresponds to that for use of Abbott ADD-Vantage containers following removal of the outer packaging (overwrap).

Freezing solutions of cefuroxime sodium in the ADD-Vantage system is not recommended.

For continuous IV infusion: a solution of cefuroxime sodium may be added to an IV infusion pack containing one of the following fluids: 0.9% sodium chloride injection; 5% dextrose injection; 10% dextrose injection; 5% dextrose and 0.9% sodium chloride injection; 5% dextrose and 0.45% sodium chloride injection; or 1/6 M sodium lactate injection.

Solutions of cefuroxime sodium, like those of most beta-lactam antibiotics, should not be added to solutions of aminoglycoside antibiotics because of potential interaction.

However, if concurrent therapy with cefuroxime sodium and an aminoglycoside is indicated, each of these antibiotics can be administered separately to the same patient.

Directions for Use of Cefuroxime Sodium Frozen in Galaxy Plastic Containers: Cefuroxime sodium supplied as a frozen, sterile, iso-osmotic, nonpyrogenic solution in plastic containers is to be administered after thawing either as a continuous or intermittent IV infusion. The thawed solution of the premixed product is stable for 28 days if stored under refrigeration (5°C) for 24 hours if stored at room temperature (25°C). **Do not Refreeze.**

Thaw container at room temperature (25°C) or under refrigeration (5°C). Do not force thaw by immersion in water baths or by microwave irradiation. Components of the solution may precipitate in the frozen state and will dissolve upon reaching room temperature with little or no agitation. Potency is not affected. Mix after solution has reached room temperature. Check for minute leaks by squeezing bag firmly. Discard bag if leaks are found as sterility may be impaired. Do not add supplementary medication. Do not use unless solution is clear and seal is intact.

Use sterile equipment.

Caution: Do not use plastic containers in series connections. Such use could result in air embolism due to residual air being drawn from the primary container before administration of the fluid from the secondary container is complete.

Preparation for Administration

1. Suspend container from eyelet support.

2. Remove protector from outlet port at bottom of container

3. Attach administration set. Refer to complete directions accompanying set.

COMPATIBILITY AND STABILITY

Intramuscular: When constituted as directed with sterile water for injection, suspensions of cefuroxime sodium for IM injection maintain satisfactory potency for 24 hours at room temperature and for 48 hours under refrigeration (5°C).

After the periods mentioned above any unused suspensions should be discarded.

Intravenous: When the 750-mg, 1.5-g, and 7.5-g pharmacy bulk vials are constituted as directed with sterile water for injection, the cefuroxime sodium solutions for IV administration maintain satisfactory potency for 24 hours at room temperature and for 48 hours (750-mg and 1.5-g vials) or for 7 days (7.5-g pharmacy bulk vial) under refrigeration (5°C). More dilute solutions, such as 750 mg or 1.5 g plus 100 ml of sterile water for injection, 5% dextrose injection, or 0.9% sodium chloride injection, also maintain satisfactory potency for 24 hours at room temperature and for 7 days under refrigeration.

These solutions may be further diluted to concentrations of between 1 and 30 mg/ml in the following solutions and will lose not more than 10% activity for 24 hours at room temperature or for at least 7 days under refrigeration: 0.9% sodium chloride injection; 1/6 M sodium lactate injection; Ringer's injection, USP; lactated Ringer's injection, USP; 5% dextrose and 0.9% sodium chloride injection; 5% dextrose injection; 5% dextrose and 0.45% sodium chloride injection; 5% dextrose and 0.225% sodium chloride injection; 10% dextrose injection; and 10% invert sugar in water for injection.

Unused solutions should be discarded after the time periods mentioned above.

Cefuroxime sodium has also been found compatible for 24 hours at room temperature when admixed in IV infusion with heparin (10 and 50 U/ml) in 0.9% sodium chloride injection and potassium chloride (10 and 40 mEq/l) in 0.9% sodium chloride injection. Sodium bicarbonate injection, USP is not recommended for the dilution of cefuroxime sodium.

The 750-mg and 1.5-g cefuroxime sodium ADD-Vantage vials, when diluted in 50 or 100 ml of 5% dextrose injection, 0.9% sodium chloride injection, or 0.45% sodium chloride injection, may be stored for up to 24 hours at room temperature or for 7 days under refrigeration.

Frozen Stability: Constitute the 750-mg, 1.5-g, or 7.5-g vial as directed for IV administration in TABLE 11. Immediately withdraw the total contents of the 750-mg or 1.5-g vial or 8 or 16 ml from the 7.5-g bulk vial and add to a Baxter Viaflex Mini-bag containing 50 or 100 ml of 0.9% sodium chloride injection or 5% dextrose injection and freeze. Frozen solutions are stable for 6 months when stored at −20°C. Frozen solutions should be thawed at room temperature and not refrozen. Do not force thaw by immersion in water baths or by microwave irradiation. Thawed solutions may be stored for up to 24 hours at room temperature or for 7 days in a refrigerator.

DOSAGE AND ADMINISTRATION: *(cont'd)*

Note: Parenteral drug products should be inspected visually for particulate matter and discoloration before administration whenever solution and container permit.

As with other cephalosporins, cefuroxime sodium powder as well as solutions and suspensions tend to darken, depending on storage conditions, without adversely affecting product potency.

Directions for Dispensing: Pharmacy Bulk Package—Not for Direct Infusion. The pharmacy bulk package is for use in a pharmacy admixture service only under a laminar flow hood. Entry into the vial must be made with a sterile transfer set or other sterile dispensing device, and the contents dispensed in aliquots using aseptic technique. The use of syringe and needle is not recommended as it may cause leakage (see DOSAGE AND ADMINISTRATION). AFTER INITIAL WITHDRAWAL USE ENTIRE CONTENTS OF VIAL PROMPTLY. ANY UNUSED PORTION MUST BE DISCARDED WITHIN 24 HOURS.

Cefuroxime sodium in the dry state should be stored between 15° – 30° C (59° – 86° F) and protected from light.

Cefuroxime sodium frozen as a premixed solution of cefuroxime sodium should not be stored above –20°C.

REFERENCES:

1. National Committee for Clinical Laboratory Standards.*Performance Standards for Antimicrobial Susceptibility Testing.* Third Informational Supplement. NCCLS Document M100-S3, Vol. 11, No. 17. Villanova, PA: NCCLS; 1991. **2.** Cockcroft DW, Gault MH. Prediction of creatinine clearance from serum creatinine.*Nephron*16:31, 1976.

PATIENT PACKAGE INSERT:

INSTRUCTIONS FOR CONSTITUTION OF ADD-VANTAGE VIALS

To Open Diluent Container: Peel the corner of the ADD-Vantage diluent overwrap and remove flexible diluent container. Some opacity of the plastic flexible container due to moisture absorption during the sterilization process may be observed. This is normal and does not affect the solution quality or safety. The opacity will diminish gradually.

To Assemble Vial and Flexible Diluent Container (Use Aseptic Technique)

1. Remove the protective covers from the top of the vial and the vial port on the diluent container as follows:

a. To remove the breakaway vial cap, swing the pull ring over the top of the vial and pull down far enough to start the opening, then pull straight up to remove the cap.

Note: Once the breakaway cap has been removed, do not access vial with syringe.

b. To remove the vial port cover, grasp the tab on the pull ring, pull up to break the three tie strings, then pull back to remove the cover.

2. Screw the vial into the vial port until it will go no further. THE VIAL MUST BE SCREWED IN TIGHTLY TO ASSURE A SEAL. This occurs approximately one-half turn (180°) after the first audible click. The clicking sound does not assure a seal; the vial must be turned as far as it will go.

Note: Once vial is seated, do not attempt to remove.

3. Recheck the vial to assure that it is tight by trying to turn it further in the direction of assembly.

4. Label appropriately.

To Prepare Admixture

1. Squeeze the bottom of the diluent container gently to inflate the portion of the container surrounding the end of the drug vial.

2. With the other hand, push the drug vial down into the container, telescoping the walls of the container. Grasp the inner cap of the vial through the walls of the container.

3. Pull the inner cap from the drug vial. Verify that the rubber stopper has been pulled out, allowing the drug and diluent to mix.

4. Mix container contents thoroughly and use within the specified time.

Preparation for Administration (Use Aseptic Technique)

1. Confirm the activation and admixture of vial contents.

2. Check for leaks by squeezing container firmly. If leaks are found, discard unit as sterility may be impaired.

3. Close flow control clamp of administration set.

4. Remove cover from outlet port at bottom of container.

5. Insert piercing pin of administration set into port with a twisting motion until the pin is firmly seated.

Note: See full directions on administration set carton.

6. Life the free end of the hanger loop on the bottom of the vial, breaking the two tie strings. Bend the loop outward to lock it in the upright position, then suspend container from hanger.

7. Squeeze and release drip chamber to establish proper fluid level in chamber.

8. Open flow control clamp and clear air from set. Close clamp.

9. Attach set to venipuncture device. If device is not indwelling, prime and make venipuncture.

10. Regulate rate of administration with flow control clamp.

WARNING: Do not use flexible container in series connections.

HOW SUPPLIED - RATED THERAPEUTICALLY EQUIVALENT:

Injection, Dry-Soln - Intramuscular; - 1.5 gm/vial

1.5 gm x 10	$139.39	KEFUROX, Lilly	00002-7279-10
1.5 gm x 24	$357.42	KEFUROX, Lilly	00002-7277-24
10's	$118.00	Cefuroxime Sodium, Raway	00686-1132-22
10's	$121.12	Cefuroxime Sodium, Marsam	00209-1132-22
10's	$124.24	CEFUROXIME SODIUM, Marsam	00209-1133-42
10's	**$139.39**	**ZINACEF, Glaxo Wellcome**	**00173-0437-00**
20 ml x 10	$134.58	KEFUROX 1.5, Lilly	00002-7272-10
25's	**$336.44**	**ZINACEF, Glaxo Wellcome**	**00173-0354-35**
100 ml x 10	$138.04	KEFUROX 1.5, Lilly	00002-7274-10
100 ml x 10	**$138.04**	**ZINACEF, Glaxo Wellcome**	**00173-0356-32**

Injection, Dry-Soln - Intramuscular; - 7.5 gm/vial

6's	**$395.66**	**ZINACEF, Glaxo Wellcome**	**00173-0400-00**
6's	$395.68	KEFUROX, Lilly	00002-7275-16
10's	$593.52	Cefuroxime Sodium, Marsam	00209-1134-52

Injection, Dry-Soln - Intramuscular; - 750 mg/vial

10 ml x 25	$169.10	KEFUROX 750, Lilly	00002-7271-25
10's	$60.00	Cefuroxime Sodium, Raway	00686-1130-22
10's	$60.88	Cefuroxime Sodium, Marsam	00209-1130-22
10's	$63.98	CEFUROXIME SODIUM, Marsam	00209-1131-42
25's	**$169.09**	**ZINACEF, Glaxo Wellcome**	**00173-0352-31**
25's	**$181.10**	**ZINACEF, Glaxo Wellcome**	**00173-0436-00**
100 ml x 10	$71.09	KEFUROX 750, Lilly	00002-7273-10
100 ml x 10	**$71.09**	**ZINACEF, Glaxo Wellcome**	**00173-0353-32**

HOW SUPPLIED - RATED THERAPEUTICALLY EQUIVALENT: *(cont'd)*

750 mg x 24	$196.71	KEFUROX, Lilly	00002-7276-24
750 vials x 25	$181.10	KEFUROX, Lilly	00002-7278-25

HOW SUPPLIED - NOT RATED EQUIVALENT:

Injection, Dry-Soln - Intramuscular; - 1.5 gm/vial

50 ml x 24	**$387.79**	**ZINACEF IV, PREMIXED, Glaxo Wellcome**	**00173-0425-00**

Injection, Dry-Soln - Intramuscular; - 750 mg/vial

50 ml x 24	**$227.12**	**ZINACEF, Glaxo Wellcome**	**00173-0424-00**

CELIPROLOL HYDROCHLORIDE *(003074)*

CATEGORIES: Angina; Antihypertensives; Beta Adrenergic Blocking Agents; Beta Blockers; Cardiovascular Drugs; Hypertension; Renal Drugs; FDA Unapproved

BRAND NAMES: *Cardem*; *Celectol* (England, France); *Corliprol* (Germany); **Selecor**; *Selectol* (Germany, Japan)
(International brand names outside U.S. in italics)

Prescribing information not available at time of publication.

CELLULOSE SODIUM PHOSPHATE *(000697)*

CATEGORIES: Calcium Metabolism; Calcium-Removing Resins; Electrolytic, Caloric-Water Balance; Hypercalciuria; Nephrolithiasis; Parathyroid; Renal Drugs; Renal Stones; Sodium Cellulose Phosphate; Uricosuric Agents; FDA Approved 1982 Dec

BRAND NAMES: *Anacalcit*; **Calcibind**; *Calcisorb* (Australia, Germany)
(International brand names outside U.S. in italics)

DESCRIPTION:

Cellulose Sodium Phosphate (CSP), is a synthetic compound made by phosphorylation of cellulose.

The molecular weight of the CSP monomer is 286.1 and the average molecular weight of the polymer is 858,000.

It has an inorganic bound phosphate of 31-36%, free phosphate of 3.5%, sodium content of approximately 11% and a calcium binding capacity of 1.8 mmol of Ca per gram of the oral powder. It has excellent ion exchange properties, the sodium ion exchanging for calcium. When taken orally, CSP binds calcium, the complex of calcium and cellulose phosphate being excreted in feces. The dosage of Cellulose Sodium Phosphate is powder for oral administration.

CLINICAL PHARMACOLOGY:

CSP alters urinary composition of calcium, magnesium, phosphate and oxalate by affecting their absorption in the intestinal tract. When it is given orally with meals, CSP binds dietary and secreted calcium, and reduces urinary calcium by approximately 50 mg/5 grams of CSP. It also binds dietary magnesium and lowers urinary magnesium. Oral magnesium supplementation given separately from CSP partly overcomes this effect.

CSP administration increases urinary phosphorous (P) and oxalate. The usual rise in urinary P of 15-250 mg/15 grams CSP largely reflects the hydrolysis of 7-30% of CSP in the intestinal tract and absorption of released P. An increase in urinary oxalate occurs. Since CSP binds divalent cations, the cations are not available to complex oxalate and thereby limit its absorption. The rise in urinary oxalate may be largely prevented by moderate dietary oxalate restriction and the use of a modest dose of CSP (10-15 grams/day).

The marked reduction in urinary calcium with only slightly increased urinary phosphorus and oxalate leads to a reduction in urinary saturation and propensity for spontaneous nucleation of calcium oxalate and calcium phosphate (brushite).

CSP does not apparently alter the metabolism of trace metals, since it does not significantly change the serum concentration of copper, zinc, or iron.

INDICATIONS AND USAGE:

CSP is indicated only for absorptive hypercalciuria Type I with recurrent calcium oxalate or calcium in phosphate nephrolithiasis. Appropriate use(see DOSAGE AND ADMINISTRATION) of CSP subtantially reduces the incidence of new stone formation in these patients. Causes of hypercalciuria other than hyperabsorption cannot be expected to respond to CSP. Treatment with CSP is not needed for absorptive hypercalciuria Type II because dietary calcium restriction provides adequate treatment. In patients without hyperabsorption of calcium, CSP would be expected to cause excessive parathyroid hormone secretion and possible hyperparathyroid bone disease.

Absorptive hypercalciuria Type I is characterized by:

a) recurrent passage or formation of calcium oxidate and/or calcium phosphate renal stones,

b) no evidence of bone disease,

c) normal serum calcium and phosphorus,

d) increased intestinal calcium absorption,

e) hypercalciuria,

f) normal urinary calcium during fasting,

g) normal parathyroid function, and

h) lack of renal "leak" or excessive skeletal mobilization of caculi.

MINIMAL DIAGNOSTIC TESTS INCLUDE SERUM CALCIUM AND PHOSPHORUS, PARATHYROID HORMONE (PTH) LEVEL OBTAINED BEFORE BREAKFAST, 24-HOUR URINARY CALCIUM ON A DIET RESTRICTED IN CALCIUM AND SODIUM, AND A FASTING URINARY EXCRETION OF CALCIUM.

The diagnosis of absorptive hypercalciuria Type I can be made if there is:

a) Recurrent calcium nephrolithiasis without clinical evidence of bone disease.

b) Normal serum calcium and phosphorus (borderline values should be repeated).

c) 24-hour urinary calcium greater than 200 mg/day on a diet of 400 mg calcium and 100 mEq sodium/day.

d) Normal serum immunoreactive PTH.

e) Normal fasting urinary calcium.

A definite diagnosis requires, in addition evidence of high intestinal calcium absorption (*e.g.,* urinary calcium > 0.2 mg/mg creatinine after oral load of 1 gram calcium).

CONTRAINDICATIONS:

CSP is contraindicated in:

a) Primary or secondary hyperparathyroidism, including renal hypercalciuria (renal calcium leak).

b) Hypomagnesemic states (serum magnesium < 1.5 mg/dl).

c) Bone disease (osteoporosis, osteomalacia, osteitis).

d) Hypocalcemic states (*e.g.,* hypoparathyroidism, intestinal malabsorption).

e) Normal or low intestinal absorption and renal excretion of calcium.

f) Enteric hyperoxaluria.

It should not be used in patients with high fasting urinary calcium or hypophosphatemia, unless a high skeletal mobilization of calcium can be excluded.

WARNINGS:

In patients with congestive heart failure or ascites, sodium contained in CSP (35-48 mEq exchangeable sodium/15 grams CSP) may represent a hazard.

PRECAUTIONS:

General: By inhibiting intestinal calcium absorption, CSP may stimulate parathyroid function leading to hyperparathyroid hormone levels. CSP treatment has been shown to maintain parathyroid function within normal limits, if it is used only in patients with absorptive hypercalcuria Type I (increased intestinal calcium restricted diet), at a dosage just sufficient to restore normal calcium absorption but not sufficient to cause subnormal absorption.

The following additional complications may potentially develop during long-term use of CSP:

a) Hyperoxaluria and hypomagnesiuria, which would negate the beneficial effect of hypocalciuria on new stone formation.

b) Magnesium depletion.

c) Depletion of trace metals (copper, zinc, iron)

All of these effects may be minimized by restricting the use of CSP to absorptive hypercalciuria Type I only (see INDICATIONS AND USAGE) for diagnostic criteria, and by taking precautionary measures (see DOSAGE AND ADMINISTRATION) and by monitoring serum calcium, magnesium, copper, zinc, iron, parathyroid hormone, and complete blood count every 3 to 6 months. Borderline values for parathyroid hormone and calcium should be repeated promptly. Serum PTH should be obtained at least once between the first 2 weeks to 3 months of treatment and the treatment should be adjusted or stopped if a rise in serum PTH above normal appears. If there is an inadequate hypocalciuric response to CSP treatment (a reduction in urinary calcium of less than 30 mg/5 grams of CSP), while patients are maintained on moderate calcium and sodium restriction, the treatment may be considered ineffective and should be stopped. Cessation of treatment should be considered if urinary oxalate exceeds 55 mg/day on moderate dietary oxalate restriction.

Carcinogenesis, Mutagenesis, and Impairment of Fertility: No long term studies were conducted to determine the carcinogenic potential of CSP.

Pregnancy Category C: Animal reproduction studies have not been conducted with CSP. It is also not known whether CSP can cause fetal harm when administered to a pregnant woman or can affect reproduction capacity. However, because of the increased requirement of dietary calcium in pregnant women, CSP should be given to pregnant women only if clearly needed.

Pediatric Use: Because of the increased requirement for dietary calcium in growing children, the use of CSP in children less than 16 years of age is not recommended.

ADVERSE REACTIONS:

Some patients may have gastrointestinal complaints, manifested by poor taste of the drug, loose bowel movements, diarrhea or dyspepsia.

DOSAGE AND ADMINISTRATION:

THE AMOUNT OF DIETARY CALCIUM BOUND DEPENDS UPON ACTUAL MIXING OF CSP WITH A MEAL. CONSEQUENTLY, CSP SHOULD BE TAKEN WITH A MEAL; THE AMOUNT OF DIETARY CALCIUM BOUND BY CSP IS CONSIDERABLY REDUCED WHEN CSP IS ADMINISTERED MORE THAN 1 HOUR AFTER A MEAL.

Both the initial and maintenance doses of CSP are based on measurements of 24-hour urinary calcium excretion. The recommended initial does of CSP is 15 grams/day (5 grams with each meal) in patients with urinary calcium greater than 300 mg/day (on moderate calcium - restricted diet, i.e., avoidance of dairy products). When urinary calcium declines to less than 150 mg/day, the dosage of CSP should be reduced to 10 grams/day (5 grams with supper, 2.5 grams with each remaining meal). Patients with controlled urinary calcium on moderate calcium - restricted diet of less than 300 mg/day (but greater than 200 mg/day) should begin on CSP 10 grams/day.

The following general measures should be imposed during CSP therapy. A moderate calcium intake is recommended, by avoidance of dairy products. A moderate dietary oxalate restriction should be imposed by discouraging ingestion of spinach (and similar dark greens), rhubarb, chocolate and brewed tea. Vitamin C supplementation should be denied because of its potential metabolism to oxalate. A high sodium intake should be discouraged by advising avoidance of "salty" foods and salt shakers, in an attempt to achieve an intake of less than 150 mEq/day. Fluid intake should be encouraged, to achieve a minimum urine output of 2 liters/day.

The dose of oral magnesium supplements, given as magnesium gluconate, depends upon the dose of CSP. Those receiving 15 grams of CSP/day should take 1.5 grams of magnesium gluconate before breakfast and again at bedtime (separately from CSP). Those taking 10 grams of CSP/day should take 1 gram of magnesium gluconate twice a day. To avoid binding of magnesium by CSP, supplemental magnesium should be given at least 1 hour before or after a dose of CSP.

It is recommended that each dose of CSP (in the powder form) be suspended in a glass of water, soft drink or fruit juice, and ingested within 1/2 hour of the meal. It should not be given with magnesium gluconate.

Store in a dry place at room temperature. 15 - 30 deg. C (59 - 86 deg. F).

TABLE 1A

Criteria	Absorptive Type I	Hypercalciuria Type II	Renal Hypercalciuria
Serum calcium (mg/dl)	normal	normal	normal
Phosphorus (mg/dl)	> 2.5	> 2.5	> 2.5
PTH	normal	normal	normal
Urinary calcium			
Restricted diet (mg/day)	> 200	< 200	> 200
Fasting (mg/100 ml glomerular filtrate)	< 0.11	< 0.11	> 0.11
After calcium load (mg/mg creatinine)	< 0.2	> 0.2	> 0.2

TABLE 1B

Criteria	Primary Hyperparathyroidism	Control Subjects
Serum calcium (mg/dl)	high	normal
Phosphorus (mg/dl)	normal or low	> 2.5
PTH	high	normal
Urinary calcium		
Restricted diet (mg/day)	> 200	< 200
Fasting (mg/100 ml glomerular filtrate)	> 0.11	< 0.11
After calcium load (mg/mg creatinine)	> 0.2	< 0.2

Restricted diet, representing 400 mg calcium and 100 mEq sodium/day, may be imposed in an outpatient setting. The fasting sample is obtained in a 2-hour specimen collected after an overnight fast, and after calcium load sample is obtained in a 4-hour specimen following and oral calcium load (1 gram).

HOW SUPPLIED - EQUIVALENTS NOT AVAILABLE:

Kit - 45 gm

1's $150.00 CALCIBIND, Mission Pharma 00178-0255-45

Powder, Reconstitution - Oral - 2.5 gm/unit

300 gm $82.50 CALCIBIND, Mission Pharma 00178-0255-30

CEPHALEXIN *(000698)*

CATEGORIES: Anti-Infectives; Antibiotics; Antimicrobials; Bone Infections; Cephalosporins; Genitourinary Tract Infections; Ophthalmics; Otitis Media; Prostatitis; Respiratory Tract Infections; Skin Infections; Streptococcal Infection; Sulfonamides; Ocular Infections*; Rheumatic Fever*; Pregnancy Category B; Sales > $100 Million; FDA Approval Pre 1982; Top 200 Drugs

* Indication not approved by the FDA

BRAND NAMES: *Alcephin*; *Alexin*; *Alsporin*; Biocef; C-Lexin; *Carnosporin*; *Cefablan*; *Cefadal*; *Cefadin*; *Cefadina*; *Cefadyl*; *Cefalin*; Cefanex; *Cefaseptin*; *Cefax*; *Ceforal*; *Cefovit*; *Celexin*; *Cepexin*; *Cephaxin*; *Cephin*; *Cepol* (Japan); *Ceporex* (Australia, England, Mexico, Canada); *Ceporex Forte*; *Ceporexin* (Germany); *Ceporexine* (France); *Ceporexin-E*; *Cerexin*; *Check*; *Cophalexin*; *Durantel*; *Durantel DS* (Japan); Ed A-Ceph; *Erocetin*; *Factagard*; *Felexin*; *Fexin*; *Ibilex* (Australia); *Inphalex*; *Ibrexin*; *Kefalex*; *Kefalospes*; *Kefaxin*; *Kefexin* (Germany); Keflet; **Keflex**; *Kefloridina*; *Kefolan*; *Keforal* (France); *Kekrinal*; *Kidolex*; *Lenocef*; *Lexin*; *Lonflex*; *Lopilexin*; *Madlexin*; *Mamlexin*; *Mamalexin* (Japan); *Medoxine*; *Neokef*; *Novolexin* (Canada); *Nufex*; *Oracef* (Germany); *Oriphex*; *Ospexin*; *Palitrex*; *Pectril*; *Pyassan*; *Refosporen*; *Relaxin*; *Roceph*; *Roceph Distab*; *Sanaxin*; *Septilisin*; *Sepexin*; *Servispor*; *Sialexin*; *Sinthecillin*; *Sporicef*; *Sporidex*; *Synecl*; *Syncle* (Japan); *Tepaxin*; *Tokiolexin* (Japan); *Uphalexin*; *Voxxim*; *Winlex*; Zartan; *Zozarine*

(International brand names outside U.S. in italics)

FORMULARIES: Aetna; BC-BS; CIGNA; FHP; Foundation; Humana; Kaiser; Medco; Medi-Cal; PruCare; PCS; United

COST OF THERAPY: $2.83 (Skin Infections; Capsule; 500 mg; 2/day; 7 days)

DESCRIPTION:

Cephalexin, USP is a semisynthetic cephalosporin antibiotic intended for oral administration. It is 7-(D-α-amino-α-phenylacetamido)- 3-methyl-3-cephem-4-carboxylic acid monohydrate. Cephalexin has the molecular formula $C_{16}H_{17}N_3O_4S \cdot H_2O$ and the molecular weight is 365.4.

The nucleus of cephalexin is related to that of other cephalosporin antibiotics. The compound is a zwitterion; i.e., the molecule contains both a basic and an acidic group. The isoelectric point of cephalexin in water is approximately 4.5 to 5.

The crystalline form of cephalexin which is available is a monohydrate. It is a white crystalline solid having a bitter taste. Solubility in water is low at room temperature; 1 or 2 mg/ml may be dissolved readily, but higher concentrations are obtained with increasing difficulty.

The cephalosporins differ from penicillins in the structure of the bicyclic ring system. Cephalexin has a D-phenylglycyl group as substituent at the 7-amino position and an unsubstituted methyl group at the 3-position.

Each Pulvule contains cephalexin monohydrate equivalent to 250 mg (720 μmol) or 500 mg (1,439 μmol) of cephalexin. The Pulvules also contain cellulose, D & C Yellow No. 10, F D & C Blue No. 1, F D & C Yellow No. 6, gelatin, magnesium stearate, silicone, titanium dioxide, and other inactive ingredients.

Each capsule manufactured by Mylan contains cephalexin monohydrate equivalent to 250 mg (720 μmol) or 500 mg (1,439 μmol) of cephalexin. The capsules also contain cellulose, F D & C Blue No. 1, gelatin, magnesium stearate, silicone, titanium dioxide, and other inactive ingredients.

After mixing, each 5 ml of Keflex, for Oral Suspension, will contain cephalexin monohydrate equivalent to 125 mg (360 μmol) or 250 mg (720 μmol) of cephalexin. The suspensions also contain flavors, methylcellulose, silicone, sodium lauryl sulfate, and sucrose. The 125-mg suspension contains F D & C Red No. 40, and the 250-mg suspension contains F D & C Yellow No. 6.

Each capsule manufactured by Biocraft contains cephalexin monohydrate equivalent to 250 mg (720 μmol) or 500 mg (1,439 μmol) of cephalexin. Inactive ingredients: magnesium stearate, silicone dioxide and may contain talc. Capsul shell and print constituents: black iron oxide, D & C Yellow #10 Aluminium Lake, FD & C Blue #1 Aluminium Lake, FD & C Blue #2 Aluminium Lake, FD & C Red #40 Aluminium Lake, gelatin, pharmaceutical glaze modified in SD-45, silcon dioxide or carbomethylcellulose sodium, sodium lauryl sulfate, titanium dioxide and may contian propylene glyceryl. In addition, the 250 mg capsule shell contains yellow iron oxide.

After mixing, each 5 ml of Cephalexin for Oral Suspension by Biocraft, will contain cephalexin monohydrate equivalent to 125 mg (360 μmol) or 250 mg (720 μmol) of cephalexin. The suspensions also contain flavors, methylcellulose, silicone, sodium lauryl sulfate, and sucrose. Inactive ingredients: FD & C Red #40, mixed berry flavor, silcon dioxide, sodium benoate, sugar and xanthan gum.

Each tablet manufactured by Biocraft contains cephalexin monohydrate equivalent to 250 mg (720 μmol) or 500 mg (1,439 μmol) of cephalexin. Inactive ingredients: hydroxypropyl methylcellulose, magnesium stearate, microcrystalline cellulose, polyethylene glycol, polysorbate 90, sodium starch glycolate and titanium dioxide.

CLINICAL PHARMACOLOGY:

HUMAN PHARMACOLOGY

Cephalexin is acid stable and may be given without regard to meals. It is rapidly absorbed after oral administration. Following doses of 250 mg, 500 mg, and 1 g, average peak serum levels of approximately 9, 18, and 32 mcg/ml respectively were obtained at 1 hour. Measurable levels were present 6 hours after administration. Cephalexin is excreted in the urine by glomerular filtration and tubular secretion. Studies showed that over 90% of the drug was excreted unchanged in the urine within 8 hours. During this period, peak urine concentrations following the 250 mg, 500 mg, and 1 g doses were approximately 1,000, 2,200, and 5,000 mcg/ml respectively.

MICROBIOLOGY

In vitro tests demonstrate that the cephalosporins are bactericidal because of their inhibition of cell-wall synthesis. Cephalexin is active against the following organisms both*in vitro* and in clinical infections (see INDICATIONS AND USAGE):

Escherichia coli
Haemophilus influenzae
Klebsiella pneumoniae
Moraxella (Branhamella) catarrhalis
Proteus mirabilis
Staphylococcus aureus (including penicillinase-producing strains)
Staphylococcus epidermidis (penicillin-susceptible strains)
Streptococcus pneumoniae
Streptococcus pyogenes

Note: Methicillin-resistant staphylococci and most strains of enterococci (*Enterococcus faecalis* [formerly *Streptococcus faecalis*]) are resistant to cephalosporins, including cephalexin. It is not active against most strains of *Enterobacter* spp,*Morganella morganii,* and *Proteus vulgaris.* It has no activity against *Pseudomonas* spp or *Acinetobacter calcoaceticus.*

SUSCEPTIBILITY TESTING

Diffusion Techniques: Quantitative methods that require measurement of zone diameters give the most precise estimate of the susceptibility of bacteria to antimicrobial agents. One such standard procedure[1] has been recommended for use with disks to test susceptibility of organisms to cephalexin, using the 30-mcg cephalothin disk. Interpretation involves the correlation of the diameters obtained with the disk test with the minimum inhibitory concentration (MIC) for cephalexin.

Reports from the laboratory giving results of the standard single-disk susceptibility test with a 30-mcg cephalothin disk should be interpreted according to the following criteria (TABLE 1):

TABLE 1

Zone Diameter(mm)	Interpretation
≥18	(S) Susceptible
15-17	(MS) Moderately Susceptible
≤14	(R) Resistant

A report of "Susceptible" indicates that the pathogen is likely to be inhibited by generally achievable blood levels. A report of "Moderately Susceptible" suggests that the organism would be susceptible if high dosage is used or if the infection is confined to tissue and fluids in which high antibiotic levels are obtained. A report of "Resistant" indicates that achievable concentrations of the antibiotic are unlikely to be inhibitory and other therapy should be selected.

Standardized procedures require the use of laboratory control organisms. The 30-mcg cephalothin disk should give the following zone diameters (TABLE 2):

TABLE 2

Organism	Zone Diameter (mm)
E. coli ATCC 25922	17-22
S. aureus ATCC 25923	29-37

Dilution Techniques: Use a standardized dilution method[2](broth, agar, microdilution) or equivalent with cephalothin powder. The MIC values obtained should be interpreted according to the following criteria (TABLE 3):

TABLE 3

MIC (mcg/ml)	Interpretation
≤8	(S) Susceptible
16	(MS) Moderately Susceptible
≥32	(R) Resistant

As with standard diffusion techniques, dilution methods require the use of laboratory control organisms. Standard cephalothin powder should provide the following MIC values (TABLE 4):

TABLE 4

Organism	MIC (mcg/ml)
E. coli ATCC 25922	4.0-16.0
E. faecalis ATCC 29212	8.0-32.0
S. aureus ATCC 29213	0.12-0.5

INDICATIONS AND USAGE:

Cephalexin is indicated for the treatment of the following infections when caused by susceptible strains of the designated microorganisms:

Respiratory tract infections caused by *S. pneumoniae* and *S. pyogenes* (Penicillin is the usual drug of choice in the treatment and prevention of streptococcal infections, including the prophylaxis of rheumatic fever. Cephalexin is generally effective in the eradication of streptococci from the nasopharynx; however, substantial data establishing the efficacy of cephalexin in the subsequent prevention of rheumatic fever are not available at present.)

Otitis media due to *S. pneumoniae, H. influenzae,* staphylococci, streptococci, and *M. catarrhalis*

Skin and skin structure infections caused by staphylococci and/or streptococci

Bone infections caused by staphylococci and/or *P. mirabilis*

Genitourinary tract infections, including acute prostatitis, caused by*E. coli, P. mirabilis,* and *K. pneumoniae*

Note: Culture and susceptibility tests should be initiated prior to and during therapy. Renal function studies should be performed when indicated.

CONTRAINDICATIONS:

Cephalexin is contraindicated in patients with known allergy to the cephalosporin group of antibiotics.

WARNINGS:

BEFORE CEPHALEXIN THERAPY IS INSTITUTED, CAREFUL INQUIRY SHOULD BE MADE CONCERNING PREVIOUS HYPERSENSITIVITY REACTIONS TO CEPHALOSPORINS AND PENICILLIN. CEPHALOSPORIN C DERIVATIVES SHOULD BE GIVEN CAUTIOUSLY TO PENICILLIN-SENSITIVE PATIENTS.

SERIOUS ACUTE HYPERSENSITIVITY REACTIONS MAY REQUIRE EPINEPHRINE AND OTHER EMERGENCY MEASURES.

There is some clinical and laboratory evidence of partial cross-allergenicity of the penicillins and the cephalosporins. Patients have been reported to have had severe reactions (including anaphylaxis) to both drugs.

Any patient who has demonstrated some form of allergy, particularly to drugs, should receive antibiotics cautiously. No exception should be made with regard to cephalexin.

Pseudomembranous colitis has been reported with virtually all broad-spectrum antibiotics (including macrolides, semisynthetic penicillins, and cephalosporins); therefore, it is important to consider its diagnosis in patients who develop diarrhea in association with the use of antibiotics. Such colitis may range in severity from mild to life-threatening.

Treatment with broad-spectrum antibiotics alters the normal flora of the colon and may permit overgrowth of clostridia. Studies indicate that a toxin produced by *Clostridium difficile*is a primary cause of antibiotic-associated colitis.

Mild cases of pseudomembranous colitis usually respond to drug discontinuance alone. In moderate to severe cases, management should include sigmoidoscopy, appropriate bacteriologic studies, and fluid, electrolyte, and protein supplementation. When the colitis does not improve after the drug has been discontinued, or when it is severe, treatment with an oral antibacterial drug effective against *C. difficile* is recommended. Other causes of colitis should be ruled out.

Usage in Pregnancy: Safety of this product for use during pregnancy has not been established.

PRECAUTIONS:

General: Patients should be followed carefully so that any side effects or unusual manifestations of drug idiosyncrasy may be detected. If an allergic reaction to cephalexin occurs, the drug should be discontinued and the patient treated with the usual agents (*e.g.,* epinephrine or other pressor amines, antihistamines, or corticosteroids).

Prolonged use of cephalexin may result in the overgrowth of nonsusceptible organisms. Careful observation of the patient is essential. If superinfection occurs during therapy, appropriate measures should be taken.

Positive direct Coombs' tests have been reported during treatment with the cephalosporin antibiotics. In hematologic studies or in transfusion cross-matching procedures when antiglobulin tests are performed on the minor side or in Coombs' testing of newborns whose mothers have received cephalosporin antibiotics before parturition, it should be recognized that a positive Coombs' test may be due to the drug.

Cephalexin should be administered with caution in the presence of markedly impaired renal function. Under such conditions, careful clinical observation and laboratory studies should be made because safe dosage may be lower than that usually recommended.

Indicated surgical procedures should be performed in conjunction with antibiotic therapy.

As a result of administration of cephalexin, a false-positive reaction for glucose in the urine may occur. This has been observed with Benedict's and Fehling's solutions and also with Clinitest tablets but not with Tes-Tape (Glucose Enzymatic Test Strip, USP, Lilly).

Broad-spectrum antibiotics should be prescribed with caution in individuals with a history of gastrointestinal disease, particularly colitis.

Pregnancy Category B: The daily oral administration of cephalexin to rats in doses of 250 or 500 mg/kg prior to and during pregnancy, or to rats and mice during the period of organogenesis only, had no adverse effect on fertility, fetal viability, fetal weight, or litter size. Note that the safety of cephalexin during pregnancy in humans has not been established.

Cephalexin showed no enhanced toxicity in weanling and newborn rats as compared with adult animals. Nevertheless, because the studies in humans cannot rule out the possibility of harm, cephalexin should be used during pregnancy only if clearly needed.

Nursing Mothers: The excretion of cephalexin in the milk increased up to 4 hours after a 500-mg dose; the drug reached a maximum level of 4 mcg/ml, then decreased gradually, and had disappeared 8 hours after administration. Caution should be exercised when cephalexin is administered to a nursing woman.

ADVERSE REACTIONS:

Gastrointestinal: Symptoms of pseudomembranous colitis may appear either during or after antibiotic treatment. Nausea and vomiting have been reported rarely. The most frequent side effect has been diarrhea. It was very rarely severe enough to warrant cessation of therapy. Dyspepsia, gastritis, and abdominal pain have also occurred. As with some penicillins and some other cephalosporins, transient hepatitis and cholestatic jaundice have been reported rarely.

Hypersensitivity: Allergic reactions in the form of rash, urticaria, angioedema, and, rarely, erythema multiforme, Stevens-Johnson syndrome, or toxic epidermal necrolysis have been observed. These reactions usually subsided upon discontinuation of the drug. In some of these reactions, supportive therapy may be necessary. Anaphylaxis has also been reported.

Other reactions have included genital and anal pruritus, genital moniliasis, vaginitis and vaginal discharge, dizziness, fatigue, headache, agitation, confusion, hallucinations, arthralgia, arthritis, and joint disorder. Reversible interstitial nephritis has been reported rarely. Eosinophilia, neutropenia, thrombocytopenia, and slight elevations in AST (SGOT) and ALT (SGPT) have been reported.

OVERDOSAGE:

Signs and Symptoms: Symptoms of oral overdose may include nausea, vomiting, epigastric distress, diarrhea, and hematuria. If other symptoms are present, it is probably secondary to an underlying disease state, an allergic reaction, or toxicity due to ingestion of a second medication.

Treatment: To obtain up-to-date information about the treatment of overdose, a good resource is your certified Regional Poison Control Center.. In managing overdosage, consider the possibility of multiple drug overdoses, interaction among drugs, and unusual drug kinetics in your patient.

Unless 5 to 10 times the normal dose of cephalexin has been ingested, gastrointestinal decontamination should not be necessary.

Protect the patient's airway and support ventilation and perfusion. Meticulously monitor and maintain, within acceptable limits, the patient's vital signs, blood gases, serum electrolytes, etc. Absorption of drugs from the gastrointestinal tract may be decreased by giving activated charcoal, which, in many cases, is more effective than emesis or lavage; consider charcoal

OVERDOSAGE: *(cont'd)*

instead of or in addition to gastric emptying. Repeated doses of charcoal over time may hasten elimination of some drugs that have been absorbed. Safeguard the patient's airway when employing gastric emptying or charcoal.

Forced diuresis, peritoneal dialysis, hemodialysis, or charcoal hemoperfusion have not been established as beneficial for an overdose of cephalexin; however, it would be extremely unlikely that one of these procedures would be indicated.

The oral median lethal dose of cephalexin in rats is 5,000 mg/kg.

DOSAGE AND ADMINISTRATION:

Cephalexin is administered orally.

Adults: The adult dosage ranges from 1 to 4 g daily in divided doses. The usual adult dose is 250 mg every 6 hours. For the following infections, a dosage of 500 mg may be administered every 12 hours: streptococcal pharyngitis, skin and skin structure infections, and uncomplicated cystitis in patients over 15 years of age. Cystitis therapy should be continued for 7 to 14 days. For more severe infections or those caused by less susceptible organisms, larger doses may be needed. If daily doses of cephalexin greater than 4 g are required, parenteral cephalosporins, in appropriate doses, should be considered.

Children: The usual recommended daily dosage for children is 25 to 50 mg/kg in divided doses. For streptococcal pharyngitis in patients over 1 year of age and for skin and skin structure infections, the total daily dose may be divided and administered every 12 hours (TABLE 5).

TABLE 5 Cephalexin Suspension

Child's Weight	125 mg/5 ml	250 mg/5 ml
10 kg (22 lb)	1/2 to 1 tsp q.i.d.	1/4 to 1/2 tsp q.i.d.
20 kg (44 lb)	1 to 2 tsp q.i.d.	1/2 to 1 tsp q.i.d.
40 kg (88 lb)	2 to 4 tsp q.i.d.	1 to 2 tsp q.i.d.
	OR	
10 kg (22 lb)	1 to 2 tsp b.i.d.	1/2 to 1 tsp b.i.d.
20 kg (44 lb)	2 to 4 tsp b.i.d.	1 to 2 tsp b.i.d.
40 kg (88 lb)	4 to 8 tsp b.i.d.	2 to 4 tsp b.i.d.

In severe infections, the dosage may be doubled.

In the therapy of otitis media, clinical studies have shown that a dosage of 75 to 100 mg/kg/day in 4 divided doses is required.

In the treatment of β-hemolytic streptococcal infections, a therapeutic dosage of cephalexin should be administered for at least 10 days.

Store at controlled room temperature, 15° to 30°C (59° to 86°F).

REFERENCES:

1. National Committee for Clinical Laboratory Standards: Performance standards for antimicrobial disk susceptibility tests—4th ed. Approved Standard NCCLS Document M2-A4, Vol 10, No 7, NCCLS, Villanova, PA, 1990.
2. National Committee for Clinical Laboratory Standards: Methods for dilution antimicrobial susceptibility tests for bacteria that grow aerobically—2nd ed. Approved Standard NCCLS Document M7-A2, Vol 10, No 8, NCCLS, Villanova, PA, 1990.

PATIENT INFORMATION:

Cephalexin is a cephalosporin antibiotic used to treat bacterial infections. Take at regular intervals and complete the entire course of therapy. Do not take this medication if you are allergic to any type of penicillin or cephalosporin. Notify your physician if you are pregnant or nursing. This antibiotic may decrease the effectiveness of birth control pills; use another form of birth control while taking this medication. Shake the suspension well before each use and store it in the refrigerator. May cause nausea, vomiting or diarrhea; notify your physician if these occur. Take with food or milk to avoid stomach upset. Cephalexin may cause a false-positive reaction for nonspecific urine glucose tests in patients with diabetes. This medication does not interfere with enzyme-based urine glucose tests.

HOW SUPPLIED - RATED THERAPEUTICALLY EQUIVALENT:

Capsule, Gelatin - Oral - 250 mg

20's	$2.20	Cephalexin, H.C.F.A. F F P	99999-0698-01
20's	**$2.32**	**KEFLEX, Dista**	**00777-0869-20**
20's	$10.77	Cephalexin, Novopharm (US)	55953-0084-20
40's	$4.41	Cephalexin, H.C.F.A. F F P	99999-0698-02
40's	$17.34	Cephalexin, Talbert Phcy	44514-0490-25
40's	$17.36	Cephalexin, Talbert Phcy	44514-0749-28
100's	$11.03	Cephalexin, H.C.F.A. F F P	99999-0698-03
100's	$11.63	Cephalexin, United Res	00677-1158-01
100's	**$11.63**	**KEFLEX, Dista**	**00777-0869-02**
100's	$14.93	Cephalexin, IDE-Interstate	00814-1605-14
100's	$20.95	Cephalexin, Consolidated Midland	00223-0581-01
100's	$28.00	Cephalexin, Raway	00686-0604-20
100's	$34.95	Cephalexin, Major Pharms	00904-3800-61
100's	$43.75	Cephalexin, Martec Pharms	52555-0970-01
100's	$47.00	Cephalexin, Qualitest Pharms	00603-2595-21
100's	$47.99	CEFANEX, Bristol Myers Squibb	00087-7375-62
100's	$49.40	Cephalexin, Major Pharms	00904-3800-60
100's	$50.07	Cephalexin, HL Moore Drug Exch	00839-7311-06
100's	$51.88	Cephalexin, Schein Pharm (US)	00364-2161-01
100's	$53.85	Cephalexin, Novopharm (US)	55953-0084-40
100's	$56.35	Cephalexin, Novopharm (US)	55953-0084-01
100's	$56.89	Cephalexin, Warner Chilcott	00047-0938-24
100's	$57.70	Cephalexin, Barr	00555-0514-02
100's	$59.38	Cephalexin, Bristol Myers Squibb	00003-0749-50
100's	$62.75	Cephalexin, Amer Preferred	53445-1278-01
100's	$62.97	Cephalexin, Teva	00332-3145-09
100's	$62.97	Cephalexin, Aligen Independ	00405-4152-01
100's	$63.90	Cephalexin, Teva	00093-0541-01
100's	$63.95	Cephalexin, Zenith Labs	00172-4073-60
100's	$63.95	Cephalexin, Goldline Labs	00182-1278-01
100's	$64.00	Cephalexin, Geneva Pharms	00781-2531-01
100's	$64.38	Cephalexin, Lederle Pharm	00005-3413-23
100's	$65.00	Cephalexin, Parmed Pharms	00349-8651-01
100's	$69.26	Cephalexin, Dupont Pharma	00056-0193-70
100's	$69.35	Cephalexin, Mylan	00378-6025-01
100's	$69.45	Cephalexin, Rugby	00536-0120-01
100's	$85.00	Cephalexin, Geneva Pharms	00781-2531-13
100's	$85.44	Cephalexin, Vangard Labs	00615-0353-13
100's	$85.70	Cephalexin, Goldline Labs	00182-1278-89
100's	**$133.16**	**KEFLEX, Dista**	**00777-0869-33**
500's	$55.15	Cephalexin, H.C.F.A. F F P	99999-0698-04
500's	$58.15	Cephalexin, United Res	00677-1158-05
500's	$99.50	Cephalexin, Consolidated Midland	00223-0581-05
500's	$159.70	Cephalexin, Major Pharms	00904-3800-40
500's	$170.47	Cephalexin, Martec Pharms	52555-0970-05
500's	$178.05	Cephalexin, HL Moore Drug Exch	00839-7311-12

HOW SUPPLIED - RATED THERAPEUTICALLY EQUIVALENT: *(cont'd)*

500's	$187.26	Cephalexin, Schein Pharm (US)	00364-2161-05
500's	$195.00	Cephalexin 250 Mg Capsules, Labs Atral	53862-0101-02
500's	$198.96	Cephalexin, Purepac Pharm	00228-2409-50
500's	$204.25	Cephalexin, Bristol Myers Squibb	00003-0749-60
500's	$220.00	Cephalexin, Qualitest Pharms	00603-2595-28
500's	$265.39	Cephalexin, Novopharm (US)	55953-0084-70
500's	$267.62	Cephalexin, Barr	00555-0514-04
500's	$270.00	Cephalexin, Parmed Pharms	00349-8651-05
500's	$282.55	Cephalexin, Warner Chilcott	00047-0938-30
500's	$283.05	Cephalexin, Geneva Pharms	00781-2531-05
500's	$283.25	Cephalexin, Teva	00093-0541-05
500's	$283.37	Cephalexin, Zenith Labs	00172-4073-70
500's	$283.37	Cephalexin, Goldline Labs	00182-1278-05
500's	$283.37	Cephalexin, Teva	00332-3145-13
500's	$283.37	Cephalexin, Aligen Independ	00405-4152-02
500's	$311.70	Cephalexin, Dupont Pharma	00056-0193-85
500's	$311.95	Cephalexin, Mylan	00378-6025-05
500's	$311.95	Cephalexin, Rugby	00536-0120-05
1000's	$110.30	Cephalexin, H.C.F.A. F F P	99999-0698-05
1000's	$300.00	Cephalexin, Parmed Pharms	00349-8651-10
1000's	$504.23	Cephalexin, Novopharm (US)	55953-0084-80

Capsule, Gelatin - Oral - 500 mg

20's	$4.05	Cephalexin, H.C.F.A. F F P	99999-0698-06
20's	**$4.48**	**KEFLEX, Dista**	**00777-0871-20**
20's	$21.54	Cephalexin, Novopharm (US)	55953-0114-20
20's	$23.15	Cephalexin, Rugby	00536-0130-34
40's	$8.10	Cephalexin, H.C.F.A. F F P	99999-0698-07
40's	$35.11	Cephalexin, Talbert Phcy	44514-0491-25
40's	$35.11	Cephalexin, Talbert Phcy	44514-0874-28
100's	$20.25	Cephalexin, H.C.F.A. F F P	99999-0698-08
100's	$22.43	Cephalexin, United Res	00677-1159-01
100's	**$22.43**	**KEFLEX, Dista**	**00777-0871-02**
100's	$30.68	Cephalexin, IDE-Interstate	00814-1606-14
100's	$46.50	Cephalexin, Consolidated Midland	00223-0582-01
100's	$50.00	Cephalexin, Raway	00686-0605-20
100's	$82.32	Cephalexin, Martec Pharms	52555-0971-01
100's	$85.23	Cephalexin, Mova Pharms	55370-0812-07
100's	$90.50	Cephalexin, Qualitest Pharms	00603-2596-21
100's	$93.99	CEFANEX, Bristol Myers Squibb	00087-7376-62
100's	$94.00	ZARTAN, Dartmouth Pharms	58869-0871-01
100's	$96.38	Cephalexin, HL Moore Drug Exch	00839-7312-06
100's	$98.60	Cephalexin, Major Pharms	00904-3801-60
100's	$100.74	Cephalexin, Schein Pharm (US)	00364-2162-01
100's	$103.90	Cephalexin, Zenith Labs	00172-4074-10
100's	$107.69	Cephalexin, Novopharm (US)	55953-0114-40
100's	$110.19	Cephalexin, Novopharm (US)	55953-0114-01
100's	$113.90	Cephalexin, Barr	00555-0515-02
100's	$116.38	Cephalexin, Bristol Myers Squibb	00003-0874-50
100's	$116.38	Cephalexin, Bristol Myers Squibb	00003-0874-51
100's	$123.42	Cephalexin, Amer Preferred	53445-1279-01
100's	$123.76	Cephalexin, Teva	00332-3147-09
100's	$123.76	Cephalexin, Aligen Independ	00405-4153-01
100's	$125.00	Cephalexin, Parmed Pharms	00349-8652-01
100's	$125.12	Cephalexin, Major Pharms	00904-3801-61
100's	$125.95	Cephalexin, Teva	00093-0543-01
100's	$125.95	Cephalexin, Zenith Labs	00172-4074-60
100's	$125.95	Cephalexin, Goldline Labs	00182-1279-01
100's	$125.99	Cephalexin, Geneva Pharms	00781-2532-01
100's	$126.50	Cephalexin, Lederle Pharm	00005-3414-23
100's	$136.13	Cephalexin, Dupont Pharma	00056-0194-70
100's	$137.25	Cephalexin, Warner Chilcott	00047-0939-24
100's	$137.50	Cephalexin, Mylan	00378-6050-01
100's	$137.60	Cephalexin, Rugby	00536-0130-01
100's	$162.00	BIOCEF, Intl Ethical	11584-1034-05
100's	$173.25	Cephalexin, Geneva Pharms	00781-2532-13
100's	$173.88	Cephalexin, Vangard Labs	00615-0354-13
100's	$176.00	Cephalexin, Goldline Labs	00182-1279-89
100's	**$257.49**	**KEFLEX, Dista**	**00777-0871-33**
250's	$50.62	Cephalexin, H.C.F.A. F F P	99999-0698-09
250's	$265.39	Cephalexin, Novopharm (US)	55953-0114-58
500's	$101.25	Cephalexin, H.C.F.A. F F P	99999-0698-10
500's	$112.15	Cephalexin, United Res	00677-1159-05
500's	$225.00	Cephalexin, Consolidated Midland	00223-0582-05
500's	$279.90	Cephalexin, Major Pharms	00904-3801-40
500's	$332.00	Cephalexin, Mova Pharms	55370-0812-08
500's	$351.66	Cephalexin, HL Moore Drug Exch	00839-7312-12
500's	$360.10	Cephalexin, Novopharm (US)	55953-0114-70
500's	$366.74	Cephalexin, Aligen Independ	00405-4153-02
500's	$395.00	Cephalexin 500 Mg Capsules, Labs Atral	53862-0201-03
500's	$399.70	Cephalexin, Martec Pharms	52555-0971-05
500's	$408.50	Cephalexin, Bristol Myers Squibb	00003-0874-60
500's	$435.00	Cephalexin, Qualitest Pharms	00603-2596-28
500's	$445.00	Cephalexin, Parmed Pharms	00349-8652-05
500's	$478.89	Cephalexin, Barr	00555-0515-04
500's	$551.35	Cephalexin, Geneva Pharms	00781-2532-05
500's	$556.93	Cephalexin, Warner Chilcott	00047-0939-30
500's	$556.93	Cephalexin, Teva	00093-0543-05
500's	$556.93	Cephalexin, Zenith Labs	00172-4074-70
500's	$556.93	Cephalexin, Goldline Labs	00182-1279-05
500's	$556.93	Cephalexin, Teva	00332-3147-13
500's	$612.62	Cephalexin, Dupont Pharma	00056-0194-85
500's	$612.95	Cephalexin, Mylan	00378-6050-05
500's	$612.95	Cephalexin, Rugby	00536-0130-05
1000's	$202.50	Cephalexin, H.C.F.A. F F P	99999-0698-11
1000's	$684.23	Cephalexin, Novopharm (US)	55953-0114-80
1000's	$695.00	Cephalexin, Parmed Pharms	00349-8652-10

Powder, Reconstitution - Oral - 125 mg/5ml

60 ml	**$5.40**	**KEFLEX, Dista**	**00777-2321-97**
100 ml	$3.08	Cephalexin, Teva	00332-4175-32
100 ml	$3.08	Cephalexin, United Res	00677-1187-27
100 ml	**$3.08**	**KEFLEX, Dista**	**00777-2321-48**
100 ml	$3.08	Cephalexin, H.C.F.A. F F P	99999-0698-12
100 ml	$6.06	Cephalexin, HL Moore Drug Exch	00839-7313-73
100 ml	$6.20	Cephalexin, Qualitest Pharms	00603-6541-64
100 ml	$6.23	Cephalexin, Bristol Myers Squibb	00003-2201-30
100 ml	$6.36	Cephalexin, Lederle Pharm	00005-3229-46
100 ml	$6.40	Cephalexin, Geneva Pharms	00781-7028-46
100 ml	$6.90	Cephalexin, Major Pharms	00904-3802-04
100 ml	$7.08	Cephalexin, Goldline Labs	00182-7020-70
100 ml	$7.10	Cephalexin, Schein Pharm (US)	00364-2163-61
100 ml	$7.20	Cephalexin, Parmed Pharms	00349-8653-01

HOW SUPPLIED - RATED THERAPEUTICALLY EQUIVALENT:

(cont'd)

100 ml	$7.20	Cephalexin, Rugby	00536-0116-82
100 ml	$7.44	Cephalexin, Warner Chilcott	00047-2375-17
100 ml	$7.65	Cephalexin, Teva	00093-0538-73
100 ml	$7.67	Cephalexin, Barr	00555-0525-22
100 ml	$7.76	Cephalexin, Aligen Independ	00405-2500-60
100 ml	$8.44	Cephalexin, Dupont Pharma	00056-0203-36
100 ml	$10.50	BIOCEF, Intl Ethical	11584-1035-01
150 ml	$4.62	Cephalexin, H.C.F.A. F F P	99999-0698-13
150 ml	$14.25	Ed A-Ceph, Edwards Pharms	00485-0061-15
200 ml	$4.42	Cephalexin, H.C.F.A. F F P	99999-0698-14
200 ml	$6.16	Cephalexin, United Res	00677-1187-29
200 ml	**$6.16**	**KEFLEX, Dista**	**00777-2321-89**
200 ml	$10.50	Cephalexin, Qualitest Pharms	00603-6541-68
200 ml	$11.00	Cephalexin, HL Moore Drug Exch	00839-7313-78
200 ml	$11.58	Cephalexin, Barr	00555-0525-23
200 ml	$11.99	Cephalexin, Geneva Pharms	00781-7028-48
200 ml	$12.35	Cephalexin, Bristol Myers Squibb	00003-2201-40
200 ml	$12.50	Cephalexin, Rugby	00536-0116-84
200 ml	$12.62	Cephalexin, Lederle Pharm	00005-3229-60
200 ml	$12.85	Cephalexin, Major Pharms	00904-3802-08
200 ml	$12.90	Cephalexin, Schein Pharm (US)	00364-2163-63
200 ml	$13.09	Cephalexin, Goldline Labs	00182-7020-73
200 ml	$13.09	Cephalexin, Teva	00332-4175-36
200 ml	$13.45	Cephalexin, Parmed Pharms	00349-8653-02
200 ml	$13.80	Cephalexin, Teva	00093-0538-74
200 ml	$13.83	Cephalexin, Novopharm (US)	55953-0106-53
200 ml	$13.86	Cephalexin, Warner Chilcott	00047-2375-20
200 ml	$15.22	Cephalexin, Dupont Pharma	00056-0203-39
200 ml	$18.13	Cephalexin, Aligen Independ	00405-2500-70

Powder, Reconstitution - Oral - 250 mg/5ml

100 ml	$4.43	Cephalexin, United Res	00677-1188-27
100 ml	**$4.43**	**KEFLEX, Dista**	**00777-2368-48**
100 ml	$4.43	Cephalexin, H.C.F.A. F F P	99999-0698-15
100 ml	$11.19	Cephalexin, HL Moore Drug Exch	00839-7314-73
100 ml	$11.39	Cephalexin, Geneva Pharms	00781-7029-46
100 ml	$11.40	Cephalexin, Martec Pharms	52555-0087-01
100 ml	$11.50	Cephalexin, Qualitest Pharms	00603-6542-64
100 ml	$11.73	Cephalexin, Barr	00555-0526-22
100 ml	$11.81	Cephalexin, Bristol Myers Squibb	00003-2202-30
100 ml	$11.99	Cephalexin, Lederle Pharm	00005-3230-46
100 ml	$12.25	Cephalexin, Major Pharms	00904-3803-04
100 ml	$12.50	Cephalexin, Schein Pharm (US)	00364-2164-61
100 ml	$12.60	Cephalexin, Teva	00093-0540-73
100 ml	$12.62	Cephalexin, Goldline Labs	00182-7021-70
100 ml	$12.62	Cephalexin, Teva	00332-4177-32
100 ml	$12.63	Cephalexin, Warner Chilcott	00047-2376-17
100 ml	$12.75	Cephalexin, Rugby	00536-0118-82
100 ml	$13.44	Cephalexin, Aligen Independ	00405-2525-60
100 ml	$14.00	Cephalexin, Parmed Pharms	00349-8654-01
100 ml	$15.44	Cephalexin, Dupont Pharma	00056-0204-36
100 ml	$20.35	BIOCEF, Intl Ethical	11584-1036-02
100's	**$156.17**	**KEFLEX, Dista**	**00777-2368-33**
150 ml	$27.00	Ed A-Ceph, Edwards Pharms	00485-0063-15
200 ml	$7.72	Cephalexin, H.C.F.A. F F P	99999-0698-17
200 ml	$8.86	Cephalexin, Teva	00332-4177-36
200 ml	$8.86	Cephalexin, United Res	00677-1188-29
200 ml	**$8.86**	**KEFLEX, Dista**	**00777-2368-89**
200 ml	$20.00	Cephalexin, Qualitest Pharms	00603-6542-68
200 ml	$20.47	Cephalexin, Martec Pharms	52555-0087-04
200 ml	$20.56	Cephalexin, Barr	00555-0526-23
200 ml	$20.64	Cephalexin, HL Moore Drug Exch	00839-7314-78
200 ml	$22.57	Cephalexin, Geneva Pharms	00781-7029-48
200 ml	$22.60	Cephalexin, Schein Pharm (US)	00364-2164-63
200 ml	$23.10	Cephalexin, Major Pharms	00904-3803-08
200 ml	$23.30	Cephalexin, Rugby	00536-0118-84
200 ml	$23.56	Cephalexin, Bristol Myers Squibb	00003-2202-40
200 ml	$23.76	Cephalexin, Lederle Pharm	00005-3230-60
200 ml	$24.95	Cephalexin, Parmed Pharms	00349-8654-02
200 ml	$25.00	Cephalexin, Teva	00093-0540-74
200 ml	$25.01	Cephalexin, Goldline Labs	00182-7021-73
200 ml	$25.03	Cephalexin, Warner Chilcott	00047-2376-20
200 ml	$27.02	Cephalexin, Aligen Independ	00405-2525-70
200 ml	$27.61	Cephalexin, Dupont Pharma	00056-0204-39
250 ml	$11.07	Cephalexin, H.C.F.A. F F P	99999-0698-16

Tablet, Plain Coated - Oral - 250 mg

100's	$29.99	Cephalexin, H.C.F.A. F F P	99999-0698-18
100's	$32.33	Cephalexin, HL Moore Drug Exch	00839-7461-06
100's	$35.99	Cephalexin, Balan	00304-1922-01
100's	$36.23	Cephalexin, Barr	00555-0545-02
100's	$37.50	Cephalexin, Consolidated Midland	00223-0583-01
100's	$49.40	Cephalexin, Major Pharms	00904-3795-60
100's	$57.25	Cephalexin, Goldline Labs	00182-1886-01
100's	$57.25	Cephalexin, Teva	00332-2238-09
100's	$62.44	Cephalexin, Lederle Pharm	00005-3331-23
100's	$63.00	Cephalexin, Schein Pharm (US)	00364-2292-01
100's	$95.41	KEFLET, Dista	00777-4202-02
500's	$175.00	Cephalexin, Consolidated Midland	00223-0583-05

Tablet, Plain Coated - Oral - 500 mg

100's	$44.99	Cephalexin, Balan	00304-1923-01
100's	$63.51	Cephalexin, H.C.F.A. F F P	99999-0698-19
100's	$64.73	Cephalexin, HL Moore Drug Exch	00839-7462-06
100's	$72.50	Cephalexin, Consolidated Midland	00223-0584-01
100's	$89.80	Cephalexin, Goldline Labs	00182-1887-01
100's	$112.51	Cephalexin, Teva	00332-2240-09
100's	$122.71	Cephalexin, Lederle Pharm	00005-3332-23
100's	$125.17	Cephalexin, Schein Pharm (US)	00364-2293-01
100's	$187.52	KEFLET, Dista	00777-4203-02
500's	$352.50	Cephalexin, Consolidated Midland	00223-0584-05

HOW SUPPLIED - NOT RATED EQUIVALENT:

Powder, Reconstitution - Oral - 100 mg/ml

10 ml	**$4.94**	**KEFLEX, Dista**	**00777-2322-37**

Powder, Reconstitution - Oral - 125 mg/ 5ml

100 ml	$7.95	Cephalexin, Mylan	00378-6030-02
200 ml	$13.95	Cephalexin, Mylan	00378-6030-04

Powder, Reconstitution - Oral - 250 mg/ 5ml

100 ml	$14.10	Cephalexin, Mylan	00378-6035-02
200 ml	$25.25	Cephalexin, Mylan	00378-6035-04

CEPHALEXIN HYDROCHLORIDE *(000699)*

CATEGORIES: Anti-Infectives; Antibiotics; Antimicrobials; Bone Infections; Cephalosporins; Genitourinary Tract Infections; Infections; Prostatitis; Respiratory Tract Infections; Skin Infections; Streptococcal Infection; Otitis Media*; Rheumatic Fever*; Pregnancy Category B; FDA Approved 1987 Oct
* Indication not approved by the FDA

BRAND NAMES: **Keftab**

FORMULARIES: BC-BS

COST OF THERAPY: $39.34 (Infections; Tablet; 500 mg; 2/day; 10 days)

PRIMARY ICD9: 136.9 (Unspecified Infections And Parasitic Diseases)

DESCRIPTION:

Cephalexin hydrochloride is semisynthetic cephalosporin antibiotic intended for oral administration. Chemically, it is designated 7(D-2-amino-2-phenylacetamido)-3-methyl-3-cephem-4-carboxylic acid hydrochloride monohydrate, and the chemical formula is $C_{16}H_{17}N_3O_4S{\cdot}HCl{\cdot}H_2O$. The molecular weight is 401.86.

The nucleus of cephalexin hydrochloride is related to that of other cephalosporin antibiotics. The compound is the hydrochloride salt of cephalexin. The isoelectric point of cephalexin in water is approximately 4.5 to 5.

Cephalexin hydrochloride is in crystalline form and is a monohydrate. It is a white crystalline solid having a bitter taste. Solubility in water is high at room temperature; greater than 10 mg/ml may be dissolved readily.

The cephalosporins differ from penicillins in the structure of the bicyclic ring system. Cephalexin has *D*-phenylglycyl group as substituent at the 7-amino position and an unsubstituted methyl group at the 3-position.

EachKeftab tablet contains cephalexin hydrochloride equivalent to 500 mg (1,439 μmol) cephalexin. The tablets also contain D & C Yellow No. 10, F D & C Blue No. 1, F D & C Red No. 40, magnesium stearate, silicon dioxide, stearic acid, sucrose, titanium dioxide, and other inactive ingredients.

CLINICAL PHARMACOLOGY:

Human Pharmacology: Cephalexin hydrochloride is acid stable and may be given without regard to meals. It is rapidly absorbed after oral administration. Following doses of 250 mg and 500 mg, average peak serum levels of approximately 9 and 18 mcg/ml respectively were obtained at 1 hour and declined to 1.6 and 3.4 mcg/ml respectively at 3 hours. Measurable levels were present 6 hours after administration. Cephalexin is excreted in the urine by glomerular filtration and tubular secretion. Studies showed that approximately 70% of the drug was excreted unchanged in the urine within 12 hours. During the first 6 hours, average urine concentrations following the 250-mg and 500-mg doses were approximately 200 mcg/ml (range, 54 to 663) and 500 mcg/ml (range, 137 to 1,306) respectively. The average serum half-life is 1.1 hours.

Microbiology: *In vitro* tests demonstrate that the cephalosporins are bactericidal because of their inhibition of cell-wall synthesis. Cephalexin hydrochloride is active against the following organisms *in vitro*:

β-hemolytic streptococci; *Staphylococcus aureus*, including penicillinase-producing strains; *Streptococcus pneumoniae; Escherichia coli; Proteus mirabilis; Klebsiella* sp; *Haemophilus influenzae; Moraxella (Branhamella) catarrhalis*

Note: Most strains of enterococci (*Enterococcus faecalis* [formerly *Streptococcus faecalis*]) and a few strains of staphylococci are resistant to cephalexin hydrochloride. When tested by *in vitro* methods, staphylococci exhibit cross-resistance between cephalexin hydrochloride and methicillin-type antibiotics. Cephalexin hydrochloride is not active against most strains of *Enterobacter* sp, *Morganella morganii* (formerly*Proteus morganii*), *Serratia* sp, and *Proteus vulgaris*. It has no activity against *Pseudomonas*or*Acinetobacter* sp.

Disk Susceptibility Tests: Quantitative methods that require measurement of zone diameters give the most precise estimates of antibiotic susceptibility. One such procedure[1] has been recommended for use with cephalosporin class (cephalothin) disks for testing susceptibility to cephalexin. The currently accepted zone diameter interpretation for the cephalothin disks[1] are appropriate for determining susceptibility to cephalexin. Interpretations correlate zone diameters of the disk test with MIC values for cephalexin. With this procedure, a report from the laboratory of "resistant" indicates a zone diameter of 14 mm or less and suggests that the infecting organism is not likely to respond to therapy. A report of "susceptibility" indicates a zone diameter of 18 mm or greater. A report of "intermediate susceptibility" indicates zone diameters between 15 and 17 mm and suggests that the organism would be susceptible if the infection is confined to the urine, in which high antibiotic levels can be obtained, or if high dosage is used in other types of infection.

Standardized procedures require use of control organisms.[1] The 30-mcg cephalothin disk should give zone diameters between 18 and 23 mm and 25 and 37 mm for the reference strains *E. coli* ATCC 25922 and *S. aureus* ATCC 25923 respectively.

INDICATIONS AND USAGE:

Cephalexin hydrochloride is indicated for the treatment of the following infections when caused by susceptible strains of the designated microorganisms:

Respiratory tract infections caused by *S. pneumoniae* and group A β-hemolytic streptococci (Penicillin is the usual drug of choice in the treatment and prevention of streptococcal infections, including the prophylaxis of rheumatic fever. Cephalexin hydrochloride is generally effective in the eradication of streptococci from the nasopharynx; however, substantial data establishing the efficacy of cephalexin hydrochloride in the subsequent prevention of rheumatic fever are not available at present.)

Skin and skin structure infections caused by *S. aureus* and/or β-hemolytic streptococci.

Bone infections caused by *S. aureus* and/or *P. mirabilis*.

Genitourinary tract infections, including acute prostatitis, caused by *E. coli, P. mirabilis,* and *Klebsiella* sp.

Note: Culture and susceptibility tests should be initiated prior to and during therapy. Renal function studies should be performed when indicated.

CONTRAINDICATIONS:

Cephalexin hydrochloride is contraindicated in patients with known allergy to the cephalosporin group of antibiotics.

WARNINGS:

BEFORE CEPHALEXIN THERAPY IS INSTITUTED, CAREFUL INQUIRY SHOULD BE MADE CONCERNING PREVIOUS HYPERSENSITIVITY REACTIONS TO CEPHALOSPORINS AND PENICILLIN. CEPHALOSPORIN C DERIVATIVES SHOULD BE GIVEN CAUTIOUSLY TO PENICILLIN-SENSITIVE PATIENTS.

WARNINGS: *(cont'd)*

SERIOUS ACUTE HYPERSENSITIVITY REACTIONS MAY REQUIRE EPINEPHRINE AND OTHER EMERGENCY MEASURES.

There is some clinical and laboratory evidence of partial cross-allergenicity of the penicillins and the cephalosporins. Patients have been reported to have had severe reactions (including anaphylaxis) to both drugs.

Any patient who has demonstrated some form of allergy, particularly to drugs, should receive antibiotics cautiously. No exception should be made with regard to cephalexin hydrochloride.

Pseudomembranous colitis has been reported with virtually all broad-spectrum antibiotics (including macrolides, semisynthetic penicillins, and cephalosporins); therefore, it is important to consider its diagnosis in patients who develop diarrhea in association with the use of antibiotics. Such colitis may range in severity from mild to life threatening.

Treatment with broad-spectrum antibiotics alters the normal flora of the colon and may permit overgrowth of clostridia. Studies indicate that a toxin produced by *Clostridium difficile* is a primary cause of antibiotic-associated colitis.

Mild cases of pseudomembranous colitis usually respond to drug discontinuance alone. In moderate to severe cases, management should include sigmoidoscopy, appropriate bacteriologic studies, and fluid, electrolyte, and protein supplementation. When the colitis does not improve after the drug has been discontinued or when it is severe, treatment with an oral antibacterial drug effective against *C. difficile* is recommended. Other causes of colitis should be ruled out.

PRECAUTIONS:

General: Patients should be followed carefully so that any side effects or unusual manifestations of drug idiosyncrasy may be detected. If an allergic reaction to cephalexin hydrochloride occurs, the drug should be discontinued and the patient treated with the usual agents (*e.g.,* epinephrine or other pressor amines, antihistamines, or corticosteroids).

Prolonged use of cephalexin hydrochloride may result in the overgrowth of nonsusceptible organisms. Careful observation of the patient is essential. If superinfection occurs during therapy, appropriate measures should be taken.

Positive direct Coombs' tests have been reported during treatment with the cephalosporin antibiotics. In hematologic studies or in transfusion cross-matching procedures when antiglobulin tests are performed on the minor side or in Coombs' testing of newborns whose mothers have received cephalosporin antibiotics before parturition, it should be recognized that a positive Coombs' test may be due to the drug.

Cephalexin hydrochloride should be administered with caution in the presence of markedly impaired renal function. Under such conditions, careful clinical observation and laboratory studies should be made because safe dosage may be lower than that usually recommended.

As a result of administration of cephalexin hydrochloride, a false-positive reaction for glucose in the urine may occur. This has been observed with Benedict's and Fehling's solutions and also with Clinitest tablets but not with Tes-Tape (Glucose Enzymatic Test Strip, USP).

Broad-spectrum antibiotics should be prescribed with caution in individuals with a history of gastrointestinal disease, particularly colitis.

Pregnancy Category B: Reproduction studies have been performed on rats in doses of 250 or 500 mg/kg/day and have revealed no evidence of impaired fertility or harm to the fetus due to cephalexin. There are, however, no adequate and well-controlled studies in pregnant women. Because animal reproduction studies are not always predictive of human response, this drug should be used during pregnancy only if clearly needed.

Nursing Mothers: The excretion of cephalexin in the milk increased up to 4 hours after a 500-mg dose; the drug reached a maximum level of 4 mcg/ml, then decreased gradually, and had disappeared 8 hours after administration. A decision should be considered to discontinue nursing temporarily during therapy with cephalexin hydrochloride.

Pediatric Use: Safety and effectiveness in children have not been established.

ADVERSE REACTIONS:

Gastrointestinal: Symptoms of pseudomembranous colitis may appear either during or after antibiotic treatment. Nausea and vomiting have been reported rarely. The most frequent side effect has been diarrhea. It was very rarely severe enough to warrant cessation of therapy. Abdominal pain, gastritis, and dyspepsia have also occurred. As with some penicillins and some other cephalosporins, transient hepatitis and cholestatic jaundice have been reported rarely.

Hypersensitivity: Allergic reactions in the form of rash, urticaria, angioedema, and, rarely, erythema multiforme, Stevens-Johnson syndrome, or toxic epidermal necrolysis have been observed. These reactions usually subsided upon discontinuation of the drug. In some of these reactions, supportive therapy may be necessary. Anaphylaxis has also been reported.

Other reactions have included genital and anal pruritus, genital moniliasis, vaginitis and vaginal discharge, dizziness, fatigue, headache agitation, confusion, hallucinations, arthralgia, arthritis, and joint disorder. Reversible interstitial nephritis has been reported rarely. Eosinophilia, neutropenia, thrombocytopenia, slight elevations in aspartate aminotransferase (AST, SGOT) and alanine aminotransferase (ALT, SGPT), and elevated creatinine and BUN have been reported.

In addition to the adverse reactions listed above that have been observed in patients treated with cephalexin hydrochloride, the following adverse reactions and altered laboratory tests have been reported for cephalosporin class antibiotics:

Adverse Reactions: Allergic reactions, including fever, colitis, renal dysfunction, toxic nephropathy, and hepatic dysfunction, including cholestasis.

Several cephalosporins have been implicated in triggering seizures, particularly in patients with renal impairment when the dosage was not reduced (see INDICATIONS AND USAGE and PRECAUTIONS, General. If seizures associated with drug therapy should occur, the drug should be discontinued. Anticonvulsant therapy can be given if clinically indicated.

Altered Laboratory Tests: Increased prothrombin time, increased alkaline phosphatase, and leukopenia.

OVERDOSAGE:

Signs and Symptoms: Symptoms of oral overdose may include nausea, vomiting, epigastric distress, diarrhea, and hematuria. If other symptoms are present, it is probably secondary to an underlying disease state, an allergic reaction, or toxicity due to ingestion of a second medication.

Treatment: To obtain up-to-date information about the treatment of overdose, a good resource is your certified Regional Poison Control Center. Telephone numbers of certified poison control centers are listed in *Physicians GenR$_X$*. In managing overdosage, consider the possibility of multiple drug overdoses, interaction among drugs, and unusual drug kinetics in your patient.

Unless 5 to 10 times the normal dose of cephalexin has been ingested, gastrointestinal decontamination should not be necessary.

Protect the patient's airway and support ventilation and perfusion. Meticulously monitor and maintain, within acceptable limits, the patient's vital signs, blood gases, serum electrolytes, etc. Absorption of drugs from the gastrointestinal tract may be decreased by giving activated

OVERDOSAGE: *(cont'd)*

charcoal, which, in many cases, is more effective than emesis or lavage; consider charcoal instead of or in addition to gastric emptying. Repeated doses of charcoal over time may hasten elimination of some drugs that have been absorbed. Safeguard the patient's airway when employing gastric emptying or charcoal.

Forced diuresis, peritoneal dialysis, hemodialysis, or charcoal hemoperfusion have not been established as beneficial for an overdose of cephalexin; however, it would be extremely unlikely that one of these procedures would be indicated.

The oral median lethal dose of cephalexin in rats is 5,000 mg/kg.

DOSAGE AND ADMINISTRATION:

Cephalexin hydrochloride is administered orally.

The adult dosage ranges from 1 to 4 g daily in divided doses. For the following infections, a dosage of 500 mg may be administered every 12 hours: streptococcal pharyngitis, skin and skin structure infections, and uncomplicated cystitis. Cystitis therapy should be continued for 7 to 14 days. For other infections, the usual dose is 250 mg every 6 hours. For more severe infections or those caused by less susceptible organisms, larger doses may be needed. If daily doses of cephalexin hydrochloride greater than 4 g are required, parenteral cephalosporins, in appropriate doses, should be considered.

REFERENCES:

[1]21 CFR 460.1 *Federal Register* 1987; 838-842.

HOW SUPPLIED:

Tablets (elliptical-shaped): 500 mg* (dark-green) (No. 4143)—(100s)

*Equivalent to cephalexin.

Store at controlled room temperature, 59° to 86°F (15° to 30°C).

HOW SUPPLIED - EQUIVALENTS NOT AVAILABLE:

Tablet, Plain Coated - Oral - 250 mg

100's	$95.34	KEFTAB, Dista	00777-4142-02

Tablet, Plain Coated - Oral - 500 mg

100's	$196.74	KEFTAB, Dista	00777-4143-02

CEPHALOTHIN SODIUM *(000700)*

CATEGORIES: Anti-Infectives; Antibiotics; Antimicrobials; Bone Infections; Cephalosporins; Endocarditis; Genitourinary Tract Infections; Infections; Joint Infections; Meningitis; Perioperative Prophylaxis; Peritonitis; Respiratory Tract Infections; Septicemia; Skin Infections; Pregnancy Category B; FDA Approval Pre 1982

BRAND NAMES: *Cefadin*; *Ceftina* (Mexico); *Ceporacin*; *Cepovenin* (Germany); *Jnflin*; *Kebrothin*; *Keflin-N*; *Keflin -N*; **Keflin**; *Keflin Neutral*; *Keflin Neutro*; *Nafathin*; *Practogen*; Seffin
(International brand names outside U.S. in italics)

DESCRIPTION:

Cephalothin Sodium for Injection, USP, Neutral is a semisynthetic cephalosporin antibiotic for parenteral use. It is 5-thia-1-azabicyclo(4.2.0.(oct-2-ene-2-carboxylic acid, 3-((acetyloxy) methyl)-8- oxo-7-((2-thienylacetyl)amino)-, monosodium salt, (6R-*trans*)-. Cephalothin Sodium, Neutral, contains 30 mg of sodium bicarbonate/g of cephalothin sodium to result in reconstituted solutions having a pH ranging between 6.0 and 8.5. Free cephalothin acid does not form within this range, and the solubility and freezability are thereby enhanced. The total sodium content is approximately 63 mg (2.8 mEq sodium ion) per g of cephalothin sodium.

Cephalothin was synthesized in the Lilly Research Laboratories by the reaction of thiophene-2-acetic-acid with 7-aminocephalosporanic acid. The cephalosporanic acid nucleus is obtained from cephalosporin C, which is produced by the fungus *Cephalosporium,* cephalothin is supplied as the sodium salt of 7-(thiophene-2-acetamido) cephalosporanic acid.

Cephalothin is a cream-colored crystalline solid that is stable in the dry state and moderately soluble in distilled water (250 to 300 mg/ml). Calcium disodium edetate, 0.005%, has been added at the time of manufacture.

The molecular weight of cephalothin sodium is 418.4 and the molecular formula is $C_{16}H_{15}N_2NaO_6S_2$.

CLINICAL PHARMACOLOGY:

Human Pharmacology: Cephalothin is a broad-spectrum antibiotic for parenteral administration. After administration of a 500-mg dose intramuscularly to normal volunteers, the average peak serum antibiotic level at one-half hour was 10 mcg/ml; with a 1 g dose, the average was about 20 mcg/ml. Following a single 1 g intravenous dose of cephalothin, blood levels have been about 30 mcg/ml at 15 minutes, have ranged from 3 to 12 mcg at 1 hour, and have declined to about 1 mcg at 4 hours. With continuous infusion at the rate of 500 mg/hour, levels have been from 14 to 20 mcg/ml of serum. Dosages of 2 g given intravenously over a 30-minute period have produced serum concentrations of 80 to 100 mcg/ml one-half hour after the infusion; levels ranged from 10 to 40 mcg/ml at 1 hour and from 3 to 6 mcg/ml at 2 hours and were not assayable after 5 hours.

Sixty to 70% of an intramuscular dose is excreted by the kidneys in the first 6 hours; this results in high urine levels, e.g., 800 mcg/ml of urine after a 500-mg dose and 2500 mcg/ml following 1 g. Probenecid slows tubular excretion and almost doubles peak blood levels.

Spinal-fluid levels have ranged from 0.4 to 1.4 mcg/ml in a child and from 0.15 to 5 mcg/ml in adults with meningeal inflammatory states. The antibiotic passes readily into other body fluids, e.g., pleural, joint, and ascitic fluids. Studies of amniotic fluid and cord blood show prompt transfer of cephalothin across the placenta.

Following single 1 g intramuscular doses of cephalothin, peak maternal levels were reached between 31 and 45 minutes after injection; the peak levels in the infants occurred about 15 minutes later. All plasma levels in the infants were far below those of the mothers.

Secondary aqueous-humor levels have averaged 0.5 mcg/ml 30 minutes after a single 1 g intravenous dose. The antibiotic has been detected in bile.

Microbiology: The in vitro bactericidal action of cephalothin results from inhibition of cell-wall synthesis.

Cephalothin is usually active against the following organisms *in vitro:*

β-hemolytic and other streptococci (many strains of enterococci, e.g., *Enterococcus* (formerly *Streptococcus) faecalis,* are relatively resistant)

Staphylococci, including coagulase-positive, coagulase-negative, and penicillinase-producing strains

Streptococcus pneumoniae

Haemophilus influenzae

Escherichia coli and other coliform bacteria

CLINICAL PHARMACOLOGY: *(cont'd)*

Klebsiella sp
Proteus mirabilis
Salmonella sp.
Shigella sp.

Pseudomonas organisms are resistant to cephalothin, as are most indole-producing *Proteus* sp and motile *Enterobacter* sp.

Susceptibility Plate Tests: If the Bauer-Kirby-Sherris-Turck method of disc susceptibility testing* is used, a disc containing 30 mcg cephalothin should give a zone of over 17 mm when tested against a cephalothin-susceptible bacterial strain and a zone of over 14 mm with an organism of intermediate susceptibility.

* (Bauer, A.W., Kirby, W.M.M., Sherris, J.C., and Turck, M.: Antibiotic Susceptibility Testing by a Standardized Single Disk Method, Am. J. Clin. Pathol., 45:493, 1966; Standardized Disc Susceptibility Test, Federal Register, 39:19182-19184, 1974).

INDICATIONS AND USAGE:

Cephalothin is indicated for the treatment of serious infections caused by susceptible strains of the designated microorganisms in the diseases listed below. Culture and susceptibility studies should be performed. Therapy may be instituted before results of susceptibility studies are obtained.

Respiratory tract infections caused by *S. pneumoniae*, staphylococci (penicillinase- and non-penicillinase-producing), group A β-hemolytic streptococci, *Klebsiella* sp, and *H. influenzae.*

Skin and soft-tissue infections, including peritonitis, caused by staphylococci (penicillinase- and non-penicillinase-producing), group A β-hemolytic streptococci, *E. coli, P. mirabilis,* and *Klebsiella* sp.

Genitourinary tract infections caused by *E. coli, P. mirabilis,* and *Klebsiella* sp.

Septicemia, including endocarditis, caused by *S. pneumoniae*, staphylococci (penicillinase- and non-penicillinase-producing), group A β-hemolytic streptococci, *S. viridans, E. coli, p. mirabilis,* and *klebsiella* sp.

Gastrointestinal infections caused by *Salmonella* and *Shigella* sp.

Meningitis caused by *S. pneumoniae*, group A β-hemolytic streptococci, and staphylococci (penicillinase- and non-penicillinase-producing)

NOTE: Inasmuch as only low levels of cephalothin are found in the cerebrospinal fluid, the drug is not reliable in the treatment of meningitis and cannot be recommended for that purpose. Cephalothin has, however, proved to be effective in a number of cases of meningitis and may be considered for unusual circumstances in which other, more reliably effective antibiotics cannot be used.

Bone and joint infections caused by staphylococci (penicillinase- and non-penicillinase-producing)

The prophylactic administration of cephalothin preoperatively, intraoperatively, and postoperatively may reduce the incidence of certain postoperative infections in patients undergoing surgical procedures (*e.g.,* vaginal hysterectomy) that are classified as contaminated or potentially contaminated.

The perioperative use of cephalothin also may be effective in surgical patients in whom infection at the operative site would present a serious risk, e.g., during open-heart surgery and prosthetic arthroplasty.

The prophylactic administration of cephalothin should be discontinued within a 24-hour period after the surgical procedure. If there are signs of infection, specimens for culture should be obtained for the identification of the causative organism so that appropriate therapy may be instituted. (See DOSAGE AND ADMINISTRATION.)

NOTE: If the susceptibility tests show that the causative organism is resistant to cephalothin, other appropriate antibiotic therapy should be instituted.

CONTRAINDICATIONS:

Cephalothin is contraindicated in persons who have shown hypersensitivity to cephalosporin antibiotics.

WARNINGS:

BEFORE CEPHALOTHIN THERAPY IS INSTITUTED, CAREFUL INQUIRY SHOULD BE MADE CONCERNING PREVIOUS HYPERSENSITIVITY REACTIONS TO CEPHALOSPORINS AND PENICILLIN. CEPHALOSPORIN C DERIVATIVES SHOULD BE GIVEN CAUTIOUSLY TO PENICILLIN-SENSITIVE PATIENTS.

SERIOUS ACUTE HYPERSENSITIVITY REACTIONS MAY REQUIRE EPINEPHRINE AND OTHER EMERGENCY MEASURES.

There is some clinical and laboratory evidence of partial cross-allergenicity of the penicillins and the cephalosporins. Patients have been reported to have had severe reactions (including anaphylaxis) to both drugs.

Any patient who has demonstrated some form of allergy, particularly to drugs, should receive antibiotics cautiously and then only when absolutely necessary. No exception should be made with regard to cephalothin.

Pseudomembranous colitis has been reported with virtually all broad-spectrum antibiotics (including macrolides, semisynthetic penicillins, and cephalosporins); therefore, it is important to consider its diagnosis in patients who develop diarrhea in association with the use of antibiotics. Such colitis may range in severity from mild to life-threatening.

Treatment with broad-spectrum antibiotics alters the normal flora of the colon and may permit overgrowth of clostridia. Studies indicate that a toxin produced by *Clostridium difficile*is one primary cause of antibiotic-associated colitis.

Mild cases of pseudomembranous colitis usually respond to drug discontinuance alone. In moderate to severe cases, management should include sigmoidoscopy, appropriate bacteriologic studies, and fluid, electrolyte, and protein supplementation. When the colitis does not improve after the drug has been discontinued, or when it is severe, oral vancomycin is the drug of choice of antibiotic-associated pseudomembranous colitis produced by *C. difficile.* Other causes of colitis should be ruled out.

PRECAUTIONS:

General: Patients should be followed carefully so that any side effects or unusual manifestations of drug idiosyncrasy may be detected. If an allergic reaction to cephalothin occurs, the drug should be discontinued and the patient treated with the usual agents (*e.g.,* epinephrine or other pressor amines, antihistamines, or corticosteroids).

Although cephalothin rarely produces alteration in kidney function, evaluation of renal status is recommended, especially in seriously ill patients receiving maximum doses. Patients with impaired renal function should be placed on the dosage schedule recommended under DOSAGE AND ADMINISTRATION. Usual doses in such individuals may result in excessive serum concentrations.

PRECAUTIONS: *(cont'd)*

When intravenous doses of cephalothin larger than 6 g daily are given by infusion for periods longer than 3 days, they may be associated with thrombophlebitis, and the veins may have to be altered. The addition of 10 to 25 mg of hydrocortisone to intravenous solutions containing 4 to 6 g of cephalothin may reduce the incidence of thrombophlebitis. The use of small IV needles in the larger available veins may be preferred.

Prolonged use of cephalothin may result in the overgrowth of nonsusceptible organisms. Constant observation of the patient is essential. If superinfection occurs during therapy, appropriate measures should be taken.

A false-positive reaction for glucose in the urine may occur with Benedict's or Fehling's solution or with Clinitest tablets but not with Glucose Enzymatic Test Strip, USP (Tes-Tape, Lilly).

An increased incidence of nephrotoxicity has been reported following concomitant administration of cephalosporins and aminoglycoside antibiotics.

Broad-spectrum antibiotics should be prescribed with caution in individuals with a history of gastrointestinal disease, particularly colitis.

Pregnancy Category B: Reproduction studies have been performed in rabbits given doses of 200 mg/kg and have revealed no evidence of impaired fertility or harm to the fetus due to cephalothin. There are, however, no adequate and well-controlled studies in pregnant women. Because animal reproduction studies are not always predictive of human response, this drug should be used during pregnancy only if clearly needed.

Nursing Mothers: Caution should be exercised when cephalothin is administered to a nursing woman.

ADVERSE REACTIONS:

Hypersensitivity: Maculopapular rash, urticaria, reactions resembling serum sickness, and anaphylaxis have been reported. Eosinophilia and drug fever have been observed to be associated with other allergic reactions. These reactions are most likely to occur in patients with a history of allergy, particularly to penicillin.

Blood: Neutropenia, thrombocytopenia, and hemolytic anemia have been reported. Some individuals, particularly those with azotemia, have developed positive direct Coombs' tests during cephalothin therapy.

Liver: Transient rise in SGOT and alkaline phosphatase has been noted.

Kidney: Rises in BUN and decreased creatinine clearance have been reported, particularly in patients with prior renal impairment. The role of cephalothin in renal changes is difficult to assess, because other factors predisposing to prerenal azotemia or to acute renal failure usually have been present.

Local Reactions: Pain, induration, tenderness, and elevation of temperature have been reported following repeated intramuscular injections. Thrombophlebitis has occurred and is usually associated with daily doses of more than 6 g given by infusion for longer than 3 days.

Gastrointestinal: Symptoms of pseudomembranous colitis may appear either during or after antibiotic treatment. Nausea and vomiting have been reported rarely.

OVERDOSAGE:

The administration of inappropriately large doses of parenteral cephalosporins may cause seizures, particularly in patients with renal impairment. Dosage reduction is necessary when renal function is impaired (see DOSAGE AND ADMINISTRATION.) If seizures occur, the drug should be promptly discontinued: anticonvulsant therapy may be administered if clinically indicated. Hemodialysis may be considered in cases of overwhelming overdosage.

To obtain up-to-date information about the treatment of overdose, a good resource is your certified Regional Poison Control Center. Telephone number of certified poison control centers are listed in the*Physicians GenR$_x$*). In managing overdosage, consider the possibility of multiple drug overdoses, interaction among drugs, and unusual drug kinetics in your patient.

DOSAGE AND ADMINISTRATION:

IN ADULTS

The usual dosage range is 500 mg to 1 g of cephalothin every 4 to 6 hours. A dosage of 500 mg every 6 hours is adequate in uncomplicated pneumonia, furunculosis with cellulitis, and most urinary tract infections. In severe infections, this may be increased by giving the injections every 4 hours or, when the desired response is not obtained, by raising the dose to 1 g. In life-threatening infections, doses up to 2 g every 4 hours may be required.

For perioperative prophylactic use to prevent postoperative infection in contaminated or potentially contaminated surgery in adults, the following doses are recommended:

a) 1 to 2 g administered IV just prior to surgery (approximately one-half to 1 hour before the initial incision);

b) to 2 g during surgery (administration modified according to the duration of the operative procedure); and

c) 1 to 2 g q. 6 h. postoperatively for 24 hours

In children, 20 to 30 mg/kg may be given at the times designated above.

Since cephalothin has a serum half-life of 30 to 50 minutes, it is important that 1) the preoperative dose be given just prior to the start of surgery so that adequate antibiotic levels are present in the serum and tissues at the time of initial surgical incision; and 2) cephalothin be administered, if necessary, at appropriate intervals during surgery to provide sufficient levels of the antibiotic at the anticipated moments of greatest exposure to infective organisms.

When renal function is reduced, an intravenous loading dose of 1 to 2 g may be given. Continued dosage schedule should be determined by degree of renal impairment, severity of infection, and susceptibility of the causative organism. The maximum doses administered should be based on the following recommendations (TABLE 1):

TABLE 1 Dosage Of Cephalothin Sodium When Renal Function Is Impaired

Status Of Renal Function	Maximum Adult Dosage (Maintenance)
Mild Impairment (Ccr = 80-50 ml/min.)	2 g q.6h
Moderate Impairment (Ccr = 50-25 ml/min.)	1.5 g q.6h
Severe Impairment (Ccr = 25-10 ml/min.)	1 g q.6h
Marked Impairment (Ccr = 10-2 ml/min.)	0.5 g q.6h
Essentially No Function (Ccr = < 2 ml/min.)	0.5 g q.8h

IN INFANTS AND CHILDREN

The dosage should be proportionately less in accordance with age, weight, and severity of infection. Daily administration of 100 mg/kg (80 to 160 mg/kg or 40 to 80 mg/lb) in divided doses has been found effective for most infections susceptible in cephalothin.

Antibiotic therapy in β-hemolytic streptococcal infections should continue for at least 10 days. In staphylococcal infections, surgical procedures, such as incision and drainage, should be carried out in all cases when indicated.

DOSAGE AND ADMINISTRATION: *(cont'd)*

Cephalothin may be given intravenously or by deep intramuscular injection into a large muscle mass, such as the gluteus or lateral aspect of the thigh, to minimize pain and induration.

INTRAMUSCULAR

Each g of cephalothin should be diluted with 4 ml of Sterile Water for Injection. If the vial contents do not completely dissolve, an additional small amount of diluent (*e.g.,* 0.2 to 0.4 ml) may be added and the contents warmed slightly.

INTRAVENOUS

The intravenous route may be preferable for patients with bacteremia, septicemia, or other severe or life-threatening infections who may be poor risks because of lowered resistance resulting from such debilitating conditions as malnutrition, trauma, surgery, diabetes, heart failure, or malignancy, particularly if shock is present or impending. For these infections in patients with normal renal function, the intravenous dosage is 4 to 12 g of cephalothin daily. In conditions such as septicemia, 6 to 8 g/day may be given intravenously for several days at the beginning of therapy; then, depending on the clinical response and laboratory findings, the dosage may gradually be reduced.

For patients who are to receive cephalothin intravenously, it is convenient to use the 1 or 2 g 100-ml-size vial (See PRECAUTIONS.)

For intermittent intravenous administration , a solution containing 1 g cephalothin in 10 ml of diluent may be slowly injected directly into the vein over a period of 3 to 5 minutes or may be given through the tubing when the patient is receiving parenteral solutions.

Intermittent intravenous infusion with a Y-type administration set can also be accomplished while bulk intravenous solutions are being infused. However, during infusion of the solution containing cephalothin, it is desirable to discontinue the other solution. When this technique is employed, careful attention should be paid to the volume of the solution containing cephalothin so that the calculated dose will be infused.

For continuous intravenous infusion , 1 or 2 g of cephalothin, diluted and well mixed with at least 10 ml of Sterile Water for Injection, may be added to an IV bottle containing 1 of the following intravenous solutions: Acetated Ringer's injection, 5% Dextrose injection, 5% Dextrose in Lactated Ringer's injection, Ionosol B in D5-W, Isolyte M with 5% Dextrose, Lactated Ringer's injection, Normosol-M in D5-W, Plasma-Lyte injection, Plasma-Lyte-M injection in 5% Dextrose, Ringer's injection, or 0.9% Sodium chloride injection. The choice of solution and the volume to be employed are dictated by fluid and electrolyte management.

INTRAPERITONEAL

In peritoneal dialysis procedures, cephalothin has been added to dialysis fluid in concentrations up to 6 mg/100 ml and instilled into the peritoneal space throughout an entire dialysis (16 to 30 hours). Careful assay procedures have shown that 44% of the administered drug was absorbed into the bloodstream. Serum levels of 10 mcg/ml were reported, with no evidence of accumulation and no untoward local or systemic reactions.

The intraperitoneal administration of solutions containing 0.1 to 4% cephalothin in saline has been used in treating patients with peritonitis or contaminated peritoneal cavities. (The total daily dosage of cephalothin should take into account the amount given by the intraperitoneal route.)

STABILITY

While stored under *refrigeration*, the solution has a satisfactory potency for 96 hours after reconstitution. Solutions may precipitate; they can be redissolved by being warmed to room temperature with constant agitation. Kept at *room temperature,* solutions for intramuscular injection should be given within 12 hours after being mixed. Intravenous infusions should be started within 12 hours and completed within 24 hours. For prolonged infusions, replace with a freshly prepared solution at least every 24 hours.

The concentrated solution will darken, especially at room temperature. Slight discoloration of the solution is permissible.

Solutions of cephalothin in Sterile Water for injection, 5% Dextrose injection, or 0.9% Sodium chloride injection that are frozen immediately after reconstitution in Faspak containers and the conventional vials in which the drugs are supplied are stable for as long as 12 weeks when stored at -20°C. **If the product is warmed, care should be taken to avoid heating it after the thawing is complete. Once thawed, the solution should not be refrozen.**

HOW SUPPLIED - RATED THERAPEUTICALLY EQUIVALENT:

Injection, Dry-Soln - Intravenous - 1 gm/vial

50 ml	$10.80	Cephalothin Sodium, Baxter Hlthcare	00338-0525-41
100 ml x 6	$172.81	KEFZOL, Lilly	00002-7014-16
100 ml x 10	**$35.32**	**KEFLIN, Lilly**	**00002-7000-10**
100 ml x 10	$37.32	KEFZOL, Lilly	00002-7011-10

Injection, Dry-Soln - Intravenous - 2 gm/vial

10's	**$61.20**	**KEFLIN, Lilly**	**00002-7002-10**
20 ml x 10	**$68.42**	**KEFLIN, Lilly**	**00002-7003-10**
50 ml	$14.30	Cephalothin Sodium, Baxter Hlthcare	00338-0527-41

HOW SUPPLIED - NOT RATED EQUIVALENT:

Injection, Dry-Soln - Intravenous - 20 gm

200 ml x 6	**$376.71**	**KEFLIN, Lilly**	**00002-7020-16**

CEPHAPIRIN SODIUM *(000701)*

CATEGORIES: Anti-Infectives; Antibiotics; Antimicrobials; Cephalosporins; Endocarditis; Infections; Osteomyelitis; Perioperative Prophylaxis; Respiratory Tract Infections; Septicemia; Skin Infections; Urinary Tract Infections; Pregnancy Category B; FDA Approval Pre 1982

BRAND NAMES: *Brisfirina*; **Cefadyl**; *Cefaloject* (France); *Cefatrex*; *Cefatrexyl*; *Lopitrex*; *Unipirin*
(International brand names outside U.S. in italics)

DESCRIPTION:

Cephapirin sodium is a cephalosporin antibiotic intended for intramuscular or intravenous administration only. Each 500 mg contains 1.18 milliequivalents of sodium. Vial headspace contains nitrogen.

Cephapirin is the sodium salt of 7-α-(4-pyridylthio)-acetamido-cephalosporanic acid.

The empirical formula is $C_{17}H_{16}N_3NaO_6S_2$ and the molecular weight is 445.44.

CLINICAL PHARMACOLOGY:

Human Pharmacology

Cephapirin and its metabolites were excreted primarily by the kidneys. Antibiotic activity in the urine was equivalent to 35% of a 500 mg dose 6 hours after IM injection, and to 65% of a 500 mg dose 12 hours after injection. Following an IM dose of 500 mg, peak urine levels averaged 900 mcg/ml within the first 6 hours.

CLINICAL PHARMACOLOGY: *(cont'd)*

TABLE 1 Duration of Blood Levels of Cephapirin in Normal Volunteers (Figures are mcg/ml)

	Time After Injection in Hours		
	1/2	**4**	**6**
Cephapirin 500 mg I.M. (Single dose)	9.0	0.7	0.2
Cephapirin 1 gram I.M. (Single dose)	16.4	1.0	0.3

TABLE 2 Duration of Blood Levels of Cephapirin in Normal Volunteers (Figures are mcg/ml)

	TIME AFTER INJECTION IN MINUTES		
	5	**30**	**180**
Cephapirin 500 mg rapid I.V.	35	6.7	0.27
Cephapirin 1 gram rapid I.V.	67	14.0	0.61
Cephapirin 2 gram rapid I.V.	129	31.7	1.11

Seventy percent of the administered dose was recovered in the urine within 6 hours.

Repetitive intravenous administration of 1 gram doses over 6 hour periods produced serum levels between 4.5 and 5.5 mcg/ml.

At therapeutic drug levels, normal human serum binds cephapirin to the extent of 44 to 50%. The average serum half-life of cephapirin in patients with normal renal function is approximately 36 minutes.

The major metabolite of cephapirin is desacetyl cephapirin which has been shown to contribute to antibacterial activity.

Controlled studies in normal adult volunteers revealed that cephapirin was well tolerated intramuscularly. In controlled studies of volunteers and of patients receiving I.V. cephapirin, the incidence of venous irritation was low.

Microbiology: *In vitro* tests demonstrate that the action of cephalosporins results from inhibition of cell-wall synthesis. Cephapirin is active against the following organisms *in vitro*:

Beta-hemolytic streptococci and other streptococci. (Many strains of enterococci, e.g., *S. faecalis*, are relatively resistant.)

Staphylococcus aureus (penicillinase- and nonpenicillinase-producing); *Staphylococcus epidermis* (methicillin-susceptible strains); *Streptococcus pneumoniae* (formerly *Diplococcus pneumoniae*); *Proteus mirabilis; Haemophilus influenzae; Escherichia coli*; *Klebsiella* species.

Most strains of *Enterobacter* and indole-positive *Proteus* (*P. vulgaris, P. morganii, P. rettgeri*) are resistant to cephapirin. Methicillin-resistant staphylococci, *Serratia, Pseudomonas, Mima, and Herellea* species are almost uniformly resistant to cephapirin.

Disc Susceptibility Tests: Quantitative methods that require measurement of zone diameters give the most precise estimates of antibiotic susceptibility. One such procedure has been recommended or use with discs for testing susceptibility to cephalosporin class antibiotics. Interpretations correlate diameters of the disc test with MIC values for cephapirin. With this procedure, a report from the laboratory of "susceptible" indicates that the infecting organism is not likely to respond to therapy. A report of "intermediate susceptibility" suggests that the organism would be susceptible if high dosage is used, or if the infection is confined to tissues and fluid (*e.g.,* urine), in which high antibiotic levels are attained.

INDICATIONS AND USAGE:

Cephapirin is indicated in the treatment of infections caused by susceptible strains of the designated microorganisms in the diseases listed below. Culture and susceptibility studies should be performed. Therapy may be instituted before results of susceptibility studies are obtained.

Respiratory tract infections caused by *S. pneumoniae* (formerly *D. pneumoniae*). *Staphylococcus aureus* (penicillinase- and nonpenicillinase-producing), *Klebsiella* species,*H. influenzae* and Group A beta-hemolytic streptococci.

Skin and skin structure infections caused by *Staphylococcus aureus* (penicillinase- and nonpenicillinase-producing),*Staphylococcus epidermidis* (methicillin-susceptible strains),*E. coli, P. mirabilis, Klebsiella* species, and Group A beta-hemolytic streptococci.

Urinary tract infections caused by *Staphylococcus aureus* (penicillinase- and nonpenicillinase-producing), *E. coli, P. mirabilis*, and *Klebsiella* species.

Septicemia caused by *Staphylococcus aureus* (penicillinase- and nonpenicillinase-producing), *S. viridans, E. coli, Klebsiella* species and Group A beta-hemolytic streptococci.

Endocarditis caused by *Streptococcus viridans* and *Staphylococcus aureus* (penicillinase- and nonpenicillinase-producing).

Osteomyelitis caused by *Staphylococcus aureus* (penicillinase- and nonpenicillinase-producing), *Klebsiella* species,*P. mirabilis*, and Group A beta-hemolytic streptococci.

Perioperative Prophylaxis: The prophylactic administration of cephapirin preoperatively and postoperatively may reduce the incidence of certain postoperative infections in patients undergoing surgical procedures which are classified as contaminated or potentially contaminated, e.g., vaginal hysterectomy.

The perioperative use of cephapirin may also be effective in surgical patients in whom infection at the operative site would present a serious risk, e.g., during open-heart surgery and prosthetic arthroplasty.

The prophylactic administration of cephapirin should be discontinued within a 24-hour period after the surgical procedure. In surgery where the occurrence of infection may be particularly devastating, e.g., open-heart surgery and prosthetic arthroplasty, the prophylactic administration of cephapirin may be continued for 3 to 5 days following completion of surgery. If there are signs of infection, specimens for culture should be obtained for the identification of the causative organism so that appropriate therapy may be instituted. See DOSAGE AND ADMINISTRATION.

NOTE: If the susceptibility tests show that the causative organism is resistant to cephapirin, other appropriate therapy should be instituted.

CONTRAINDICATIONS:

Cephapirin is contraindicated in persons who have shown hypersensitivity to cephalosporin antibiotics.

WARNINGS:

IN PENICILLIN-ALLERGIC PATIENTS, CEPHALOSPORINS SHOULD BE USED WITH GREAT CAUTION. THERE IS CLINICAL AND LABORATORY EVIDENCE OF PARTIAL CROSS-ALLERGENICITY OF THE PENICILLINS AND THE CEPHALOSPORINS, AND THERE ARE INSTANCES OF PATIENTS WHO HAVE HAD REACTIONS TO BOTH DRUGS (INCLUDING ANAPHYLAXIS AFTER PARENTERAL USE).

Any patient who has demonstrated some form of allergy, particularly to drugs, should receive antibiotics cautiously and then only when absolutely necessary. No exceptions should be made with regard to cephapirin.

WARNINGS: *(cont'd)*

Pseudomembranous colitis has been reported with the use of cephalosporins; therefore, it is important to consider its diagnosis in patients who develop diarrhea in association with antibiotic use.

SERIOUS ANAPHYLACTOID REACTIONS REQUIRE IMMEDIATE EMERGENCY TREATMENT WITH EPINEPHRINE, OXYGEN, INTRAVENOUS STEROIDS, AND AIRWAY MANAGEMENT, INCLUDING INTUBATION, SHOULD ALSO BE ADMINISTERED AS INDICATED.

PRECAUTIONS:

Pregnancy Category B: Reproduction studies have been performed in rats and mice and have revealed no evidence of impaired fertility or harm to the fetus due to cephapirin. There are however no well controlled studies in pregnant women. Because animal studies are not always predictive of human response, this drug should be used during pregnancy only if clearly indicated.

Nursing Mothers: Cephapirin may be present in human milk in small amounts. Caution should be exercised when cephapirin is administered to a nursing woman.

The renal status of the patients should be determined prior to and during cephapirin therapy, since in patients with impaired renal function, a reduced dose may be appropriate (see DOSAGE AND ADMINISTRATION, Adults.) When cephapirin was given to patients with marked reduction in renal function and to renal transplant patients, no adverse effects were reported.

Prolonged use of cephapirin may result in the overgrowth of nonsusceptible organisms. Careful observation of the patient is essential. If superinfection occurs during therapy, appropriate measures should be taken.

With high urine concentrations of cephapirin, false-positive glucose reactions may occur if Clinitest, Benedict's Solution, or Fehling's Solution are used. Therefore, it is recommended that glucose tests based on enzymatic glucose oxidase reactions (such as Clinistix or Tes-Tape) be used.

Increased nephrotoxicity has been reported following concomitant administration of cephalosporins and aminoglycoside antibiotics.

ADVERSE REACTIONS:

Hypersensitivity: Cephalosporins were reported to produce the following reactions: maculopapular rash, urticaria, reactions resembling serum sickness, and anaphylaxis. Eosinophilia and drug fever have been observed to be associated with other allergic reactions. These reactions are most likely to occur in patients with a history of allergy, particularly to penicillin.

Blood: During large scale clinical trials, rare instances of neutropenia, leukopenia, and anemia were reported. Some individuals, particularly those with azotemia, have developed positive direct Coombs' test during therapy with other cephalosporins.

Liver: Elevations in SGPT, or SGOT, alkaline phosphatase, and bilirubin have been reported.

Kidney: Rises in BUN have been observed; their frequency increases in patients over 50 years old.

Gastrointestinal: Symptoms of pseudomembranous colitis can appear during or after antibiotic treatment. See WARNINGS.

DOSAGE AND ADMINISTRATION:

ADULTS

The usual dose is 500 mg to 1 gram every 4 to 6 hours intramuscularly or intravenously. The lower dose of 500 mg is adequate for certain infections, such as skin and skin structure and most urinary tract infections. However, the higher dose is recommended for more serious infections.

Very serious or life-threatening infections may require doses up to 12 grams daily. The intravenous route is preferable when high doses are indicated.

Depending upon the causative organism and the severity of infection, patients with reduced renal function (moderately severe oliguria or serum creatinine above 5.0 mg/100 ml) may be treated adequately with a lower dose, 7.5 to 15 mg/kg of cephapirin every 12 hours. Patients with severely reduced renal function and who are to be dialyzed should receive the same dose just prior to dialysis and every 12 hours thereafter.

PERIOPERATIVE PROPHYLACTIC USE

To prevent postoperative infection in contaminated or potentially contaminated surgery. Recommended doses are:

a. 1 to 2 grams IM or IV administered 1/2 hour to 1 hour prior to the start of surgery.

b. 1 to 2 grams during surgery (administration modified depending on the duration of the operative procedure).

c. 1 to 2 grams IV or IM every 6 hours for 24 hours postoperatively.

It is very important (1) the preoperative dose be given just prior to the start of surgery (1/2 to 1 hour) so that adequate antibiotic levels are present in the serum and tissues at the time of initial surgical incision, and 2) cephapirin be administered, if necessary, at appropriate intervals during surgery to provide sufficient levels of the antibiotic at the anticipated moments of greatest exposure to infective organisms.

In surgery where the occurrence of infection may be particularly devastating, e.g., open-heart surgery and prosthetic arthroplasty, the prophylactic administration of cephapirin may be continued for 3 to 5 days following completion of surgery.

CHILDREN

The dosage is in accordance with age, weight, and severity of infection. The recommended total daily dose is 40 to 80 mg/kg (20 to 40 mg/lb) administered in four equally divided doses.

The drug has not been extensively studied in infants; therefore, in the treatment of children under the age of three months the relative benefit/risk should be considered.

Therapy in beta-hemolytic streptococcal infections should continue for at least 10 days.

Where indicated, surgical procedures should be performed in conjunction with antibiotic therapy.

Cephapirin may be administered by the intramuscular or the intravenous routes.

INTRAMUSCULAR INJECTION

The 500 mg and 1 gram vials should be reconstituted with 1 or 2 ml of sterile water for injection, USP, or Bacteriostatic water for injection, USP, respectively. Each 1.2 ml contains 500 mg of cephapirin. All injections should be deep in the muscle mass.

INTRAVENOUS INJECTION

The intravenous route may be preferable for patients with bacteremia, septicemia, or other severe or life-threatening infections who may be poor risks because of lowered resistance resulting from such debilitating conditions as malnutrition, trauma, surgery, diabetes, heart failure, or malignancy, particularly if shock is present or impending. If patient has impaired renal function, a reduced dose may be indicated See DOSAGE AND ADMINISTRATION,

DOSAGE AND ADMINISTRATION: *(cont'd)*

Adults). In conditions such as septicemia, 6 to 8 grams per day may be given intravenously for several days at the beginning of therapy; then, depending on the clinical response and laboratory findings, the dosage may gradually be reduced.

When the infection has been refractory to previous forms of treatment and multiple sites have been involved, daily doses up to 12 grams have been used.

Intermittent Intravenous Injection: The contents of the 500 mg, 1 gram or 2 gram vial should be diluted with 10 ml or more of the specified diluent and administered slowly over a 3 to 5 minute period or may be given with intravenous infusions.

Intermittent Intravenous Infusion with Y-Tube: Intermittent intravenous infusion with a Y-type administration set can also be accomplished while bulk intravenous solutions are being infused. However, during infusion of the solution containing cephapirin it is desirable to discontinue the other solution. When this technique is employed, careful attention should be paid to the volume of the solution containing cephapirin so that the calculated dose will be infused. When a Y-tube hookup is used, the contents of the 4 gram vial of cephapirin should be diluted by addition of 40 ml of Bacteriostatic water for injection, USP, Dextrose injection, USP, or Sodium chloride injection, USP.

TABLE 3 Stability Utility Time for Cephapirin Sodium In Various Diluents At Concentrations Ranging From 20 to 400 mg/ml

Diluent	Approximate Concentration (mg/ml)	Utility Time 25°C	Utility Time 4°C
Water for injection	50 to 400	12 hrs.	10 days
Bacteriostatic Water for injection with Benzyl Alcohol or Parabens	250 to 400	48 hrs.	10 days
Normal Saline	20 to 100	24 hrs.	10 days
5% Dextrose in water	20 to 100	24 hrs.	10 days

All of the above solutions can be frozen immediately after reconstitution and stored at -15°C. for 60 days before use. After thawing, at room temperature (25°C), all of the solutions are stable for at least 12 hours at room temperature or 10 days under refrigeration (4°C).

The pH of the resultant solution ranges from 6.5 to 8.5. During these storage conditions, no precipitation occurs. A change in solution color during this stage time does not affect the potency.

Compatibility with the Infusion Solution: Cephapirin is stable and compatible for 24 hours at room temperature at concentrations between 2 mg/ml and 30 mg/ml in the following solutions:

Sodium Chloride injection, USP; 5% W/V Dextrose in water, USP; Sodium Lactate injection, USP; 5% Dextrose in normal saline,USP; 10% Invert sugar in normal saline; 10% Invert sugar in water; 5% Dextrose + 0.2% Sodium Chloride injection, USP; Lactated Ringer's injection, USP; Lactated Ringer's with 5% Dextrose; 5% Dextrose + 0.45% Sodium chloride injection, USP; Ringer's injection, USP; 10% Dextrose injection, USP, Sterile water for injection, USP; 20% Dextrose injection, USP; 5% Sodium Chloride in water; 5% Dextrose in Ringer's injection; Normosol R; Normosol R in 5% Dextrose injection; lonosol D-CM; lonosol G in 10% Dextrose injection.

In addition, cephapirin, at a concentration of 4 mg/ml, is stable and compatible for 10 days under refrigeration (4°C) or 14 days in the frozen state (15°C) followed by 24 hours at room temperature (25°C) in all of the intravenous solutions listed above.

'Piggyback' IV Package: This glass vial contains the labeled quantity of cephapirin and is intended for intravenous administration. The diluent and volume are specified on the label.

Parenteral drug products should be inspected visually for particulate matter and discoloration prior to administration, whenever solution and container permit.

STORAGE

Store the dry powder at controlled room temperature, 15°- 30°C (59°-86°F).

HOW SUPPLIED - RATED THERAPEUTICALLY EQUIVALENT:

Injection, Dry-Soln - Intramuscular; - 1 gm/vial

10's	$35.70	Cephapirin Sodium, Fujisawa USA	00469-2663-00
25's	$83.60	Cephapirin Sodium, Fujisawa USA	00469-2630-30

Injection, Dry-Soln - Intramuscular; - 2 gm/vial

2 gm	**$4.84**	**CEFADYL, Mead Johnson**	**00015-7629-28**
10's	$68.78	Cephapirin Sodium, Fujisawa USA	00469-2673-00
25's	$166.30	Cephapirin Sodium, Fujisawa USA	00469-2650-40

Injection, Dry-Soln - Intramuscular; - 4 gm/vial

10's	$133.88	Cephapirin Sodium, Fujisawa USA	00469-2693-00

Injection, Dry-Soln - Intramuscular; - 500 mg/vial

25's	$51.17	Cephapirin Sodium, Fujisawa USA	00469-2590-30

HOW SUPPLIED - NOT RATED EQUIVALENT:

Injection, Dry-Soln - Intramuscular; - 2 gm/vial

1 gm	**$2.35**	**CEFADYL, Mead Johnson**	**00015-7628-28**

Injection, Dry-Soln - Intramuscular; - 20 gm/vial

10's	$641.77	Cephapirin Sodium, Fujisawa USA	00469-2711-00
20 gm	**$45.08**	**CEFADYL, Mead Johnson**	**00015-7613-20**

CEPHRADINE *(000702)*

CATEGORIES: Anti-Infectives; Antibacterials; Antibiotics; Antimicrobials; Cephalosporins; Infections; Otitis Media; Pharyngitis; Pneumonia; Prostatitis; Respiratory Tract Infections; Septicemia; Skin Infections; Streptococcal Infection; Tonsillitis; Urinary Tract Infections; Rheumatic Fever*; Pregnancy Category B; FDA Approval Pre 1982

* Indication not approved by the FDA

BRAND NAMES: Anspor; *Askacef*; *Bactocef*; *Broadcef*; *Cefadin*; *Cefamid*; *Cefra*; *Cefradina*; *Cefradur*; *Cefralin*; *Cefrasol*; *Cefril*; *Cefro* (Japan); *Celex*; *Daicefalin* (Japan); *Doncef* (France); *Drugfradin*; *Duphratex*; *Dynacef*; *Eskacef*; *Eskefrin*; *Fradiceph*; *Lisacef*; *Lovecef*; *Maxisporin*; *Megacef*; *Nakacef-A*; *Noblitina*; *Opebrin*; *Sefril* (Germany); *Sephros*; *Taicefran* (Japan); *U-Save*; *Velocef*; **Velosef**; *Velosef Viol*; *Veracef* (Mexico); *Zolicef*

(International brand names outside U.S. in italics)

FORMULARIES: Aetna; FHP

COST OF THERAPY: $8.76 (Skin Infections; Capsule; 500 mg; 2/day; 7 days)

DESCRIPTION:

Cephradine is a semisynthetic cephalosporin antibiotic; oral dosage forms include capsules containing 250 mg and 500 mg cephradine, and cephradine for oral suspension containing, after constitution, 125 mg and 250 mg per 5 ml dose.

Cephradine is designated chemically as (6R,7R)-7-((R)-2-amino-2-(1,4-cyclohexadien-1-yl) acetamido)-3-methyl-8-oxo-5-thia-1-azabicyclo (4.2.0)oct-2-ene-2-carboxylic acid.

Velosef Inactive Ingredients: Capsules—colorants (D&C Red No. 33 and Yellow No. 10; FD&C Blue No. 1, and, for "250" only, Red No. 3), gelatin, lactose, magnesium stearate, talc, and titanium dioxide. Cephradine for Oral Suspension—citric acid, colorants (FD&C Red No. 40 for "250" only; FD&C Yellow No. 6 for "125" only), flavors, guar gum, methylcellulose, sodium citrate, and sucrose.

CLINICAL PHARMACOLOGY:

Cephradine is acid stable. It is rapidly absorbed after oral administration in the fasting state. Following single doses of 250 mg, 500 mg, and 1 g in normal adult volunteers, average peak serum concentrations within one hour were approximately 9 mcg/ml, 16.5 mcg/ml, and 24.2 mcg/ml, respectively. *In vitro* studies by an ultracentrifugation technique show that at therapeutic serum antibiotic concentrations, cephradine is minimally bound (8 to 17 percent) to normal serum protein. Cephradine does not pass across the blood-brain barrier to any appreciable extent. The presence of food in the gastrointestinal tract delays absorption but does not affect the total amount of cephradine absorbed. Over 90 percent of the drug is excreted unchanged in the urine within six hours. Peak urine concentrations are approximately 1600 mcg/ml, 3200 mcg/ml, and 4000 mcg/ml following single doses of 250 mg, 500 mg, and 1 g, respectively.

MICROBIOLOGY

In vitro tests demonstrate that the cephalosporin are bactericidal because of their inhibition of cell-wall synthesis. Cephradine is active against the following organisms *in vitro:*

Group A beta-hemolytic streptococci

Staphylococci, including coagulase-positive, coagulase-negative, and penicillinase-producing strains

Streptococcus pneumoniae (formerly *Diplococcus pneumoniae*)

Escherichia coli

Proteus mirabilis

Klebsiella species

Haemophilus influenzae

Cephradine is not active against most strains of *Enterobacter* species, *P. morganii,* and *P. vulgaris.* It has no activity against *Pseudomonas* or *Herellea* species. When tested by *in vitro* methods, staphylococci exhibit cross- resistance between cephradine and methicillin-type antibiotics.

Note: Most strains of enterococci (*Streptococcus faecalis*) are resistant to cephradine.

DISC SUSCEPTIBILITY TESTS

Quantitative methods that require measurement of zone diameters give the most precise estimates of antibiotic susceptibility. One recommended procedure (21 CFR 460.1) uses cephalosporin class discs for testing susceptibility; interpretations correlate zone diameters of this disc test with MIC values for cephradine. With this procedure, a report from the laboratory of "resistant" indicates that the infecting organism is not likely to respond to therapy. A report of "intermediate susceptibility" suggests that the organism would be susceptible if the infection is confined to the urinary tract, as high antibiotic levels can be obtained in the urine, or if high dosage is used in other types of infection.

INDICATIONS AND USAGE:

Cephradine capsules and cephradine for oral suspension are indicated in the treatment of the following infections when caused by susceptible strains of the designated microorganisms:

Respiratory Tract Infections: (*e.g.,* tonsillitis, pharyngitis, and lobar pneumonia) caused by group A beta-hemolytic streptococci and *S. pneumoniae* (formerly *D. pneumoniae).*

(Penicillin is the usual drug of choice in the treatment and prevention of streptococcal infections, including the prophylaxis of rheumatic fever. Cephradine is generally effective in the eradication of streptococci from the nasopharynx; substantial data establishing the efficacy of cephradine in the subsequent prevention of rheumatic fever are not available at present.)

Otitis Media: caused by group A beta-hemolytic streptococci, *S. pneumoniae* (formerly *D. pneumoniae), H. influenzae,* and staphylococci.

Skin And Skin Structures Infections: caused by staphylococci (penicillin-susceptible and penicillin-resistant) and beta-hemolytic streptococci.

Urinary Tract Infections: including prostatitis, caused by *E. coli, P. mirabilis, Klebsiella* species, and enterococci (*S. faecalis).* The high concentrations of cephradine achievable in the urinary tract will be effective against many strains of enterococci for which disc susceptibility studies indicate relative resistance. It is to be noted that among beta-lactam antibiotics, ampicillin is the drug of choice for enterococcal urinary tract (*S. faecalis)* infection.

Note: Culture and susceptibility tests should be initiated prior to and during therapy.

Following clinical improvement achieved with parenteral therapy, oral cephradine may be utilized for continuation of treatment of persistent or severe conditions where prolonged therapy is indicated.

CONTRAINDICATIONS:

Cephradine is contraindicated in patients with known hypersensitivity to the cephalosporin group of antibiotics.

WARNINGS:

In penicillin-sensitive patients, cephalosporin derivatives should be used with great caution. There is clinical and laboratory evidence of partial cross-allergenicity of the penicillins and the cephalosporins, and there are instances of patients who have had reactions to both drug classes (including anaphylaxis after parenteral use).

Any patient who has demonstrated some form of allergy, particularly to drugs, should receive antibiotics, including cephradine, cautiously and then only when absolutely necessary.

Pseudomembranous colitis has been reported with the use of cephalosporins (and other broad spectrum antibiotics); therefore, it is important to consider its diagnosis is patients who develop diarrhea in association with antibiotic use. Treatment with broad spectrum antibiotics alters normal flora of the colon and may permit overgrowth of clostridia. Studies indicate a toxin produced by *Clostridium difficile* is one primary cause of antibiotic-associated colitis. Cholestyramine and colestipol resins have been shown to bind the toxin*in vitro.* Mild cases of colitis may respond to drug discontinuance alone. Moderate to severe cases should be managed with fluid, electrolyte and protein supplementation as indicated. When the colitis is not relieved by drug discontinuance or when it is severe, oral vancomycin is the treatment of choice for antibiotic-associated pseudomembranous colitis produced by *C. difficile.* Other causes of colitis should also be considered.

PRECAUTIONS:

General: Patients should be followed carefully so that any side effects or unusual manifestations of drug idiosyncrasy may be detected. If a hypersensitivity reaction occurs, the drug should be discontinued and the patient treated with the usual agents, e.g., pressor amines, antihistamines, or corticosteroids.

Administer cephradine with caution in the presence of markedly impaired function. In patients with known or suspected renal impairment, careful clinical observation and appropriate laboratory studies should be made prior to and during therapy as cephradine accumulates in the serum and tissues. See DOSAGE AND ADMINISTRATION section for information on treatment of patients with impaired renal function.

Cephradine should be prescribed with caution in individuals with a history of gastrointestinal disease, particularly colitis.

Prolonged use of antibiotics may promote the overgrowth of nonsusceptible organisms. Should superinfection occur during therapy, appropriate measures should be taken.

Indicated surgical procedures should be performed in conjunction with antibiotic therapy.

Information for the Patient: Caution diabetic patients that false results may occur with urine glucose tests (see PRECAUTIONS, Drug/Laboratory Test Interactions).

Advise the patient to comply with the full course of therapy even if he begins to feel better and to take a missed dose as soon as possible. Inform the patient that this medication may be taken with food or milk since gastrointestinal upset may be a factor in compliance with the dosage regimen. The patient should report current use of any medicines and should be cautioned not to take other medications unless the physician knows and approves of their use (see DRUG INTERACTIONS.)

Laboratory Tests: In patients with known or suspected renal impairment, it is advisable to monitor renal function (see DOSAGE AND ADMINISTRATION.)

Drug/Laboratory Test Interactions: After treatment with cephradine, a false-positive reaction for glucose in the urine may occur with Benedict's solution, Fehling's solution, or with Clinitest tablets, but not with enzyme-based tests such as Clinistix and Tes-Tape.

False-positive Coombs test results may occur in newborns whose mothers received a cephalosporin prior to delivery.

Cephalosporins have been reported to cause false-positive reactions in tests for urinary proteins which use sulfosalicylic acid, false elevations of urinary 17-ketosteroid values, and prolonged prothrombin times.

Carcinogenesis, Mutagenesis: Long-term studies in animals have not been performed to evaluate carcinogenic potential or mutagenesis.

Pregnancy Category B: Reproduction studies have been performed in mice and rats at doses up to four times the maximum indicated human dose and have revealed no evidence of impaired fertility or harm to fetus due to cephradine. There are, however, no adequate and well-controlled studies in pregnant women. Because animal reproduction studies are not always predictive of human response, this drug should be used during pregnancy only if clearly needed.

Nursing Mothers: Since cephradine is excreted in breast milk during lactation, caution should be exercised when cephradine is administered to a nursing woman.

Pediatric Use: See DOSAGE AND ADMINISTRATION. Adequate information is unavailable on the efficacy of twice daily regimens in children under nine months of age.

DRUG INTERACTIONS:

When administered concurrently, the following drugs may interact with cephalosporins.

Other antibacterial agents Bacteriostats may interfere with the bactericidal action of cephalosporins in acute infection; other agents, *e.g.,* aminoglycosides, colistin, polymyxins, vancomycin, may increase the possibility of nephrotoxicity.

Diuretics (potent "loop diuretics," *e.g.,* furosemide and ethacrynic acid)Enhanced possibility for renal toxicity.

Probenecid Increased and prolonged blood levels of cephalosporins, resulting in increased risk of nephrotoxicity.

ADVERSE REACTIONS:

As with other cephalosporins, untoward reactions are limited essentially to gastrointestinal disturbances and, on occasion, to hypersensitivity phenomena. The latter are more likely to occur in individuals who have previously demonstrated hypersensitivity and those with a history of allergy, asthma, hay fever, or urticaria.

The following adverse reactions have been reported following the use of cephradine:

Gastrointestinal: Symptoms of pseudomembranous colitis can appear during antibiotic treatment. Nausea and vomiting have been reported rarely.

Skin and Hypersensitivity Reactions: Mild urticaria or skin rash, pruritus, and joint pains were reported by very few patients.

Hematologic: Mild, transient eosinophilia, leukopenia, and neutropenia have been reported.

Liver: Transient mild rise of SGOT, SGPT, and total bilirubin have been observed with no evidence of hepatocellular damage.

Renal: Transitory rises in BUN have been observed in some patients treated with cephalosporins; their frequency increases in patients over 50 years old. In adults for whom serum creatinine determinations were performed, the rise in BUN was not accompanied by a rise in serum creatinine.

Other adverse reactions have included dizziness and tightness in the chest and candidal vaginitis.

DOSAGE AND ADMINISTRATION:

Cephradine may be given without regard to meals.

ADULTS

For respiratory tract infections (other than lobar pneumonia) and skin and skin structures infections, the usual dose is 250 mg every 6 hours or 500 mg every 12 hours.

For lobar pneumonia, the usual dose is 500 mg every 6 hours of 1 g every 12 hours.

For uncomplicated urinary tract infections, the usual dose is 500 mg every 12 hours. In more serious urinary tract infections, including prostatitis, 500 mg every 6 hours or 1 g every 12 hours may be administered.

Larger doses (up to 1 g every 6 hours) may be given for severe or chronic infections.

CHILDREN

No adequate information is available on the efficacy of b.i.d. regimens in children under nine months of age. The usual dose in children over nine months of age is 25 to 50 mg/kg/day administered in equally divided doses every 6 or 12 hours. For otitis media due to*H. influenzae,* doses are from 75 to 100 mg/kg/day administered in equally divided doses every 6 or 12 hours, but should not exceed 4 g per day. Dosage for children should not exceed dosage recommended for adults.

All patients, regardless of age and weight: Larger doses (up to 1 q.i.d.) may be given for severe or chronic infections.

DOSAGE AND ADMINISTRATION: *(cont'd)*

As with antibiotic therapy in general, treatment should be continued for a minimum of 48 to 72 hours after the patient becomes asymptomatic or evidence of bacterial eradication has been obtained. In infections caused by group A beta-hemolytic streptococci, a minimum of 10 days of treatment is recommended to guard against the risk of rheumatic fever or glomerulonephritis. In the treatment of chronic urinary tract infection, frequent bacteriologic and clinical appraisal is necessary during therapy and may be necessary for several months afterwards. Persistent infections may require treatment for several weeks. Prolonged intensive therapy is recommended for prostatitis. Doses smaller than those indicated are not recommended.

PATIENTS WITH IMPAIRED RENAL FUNCTION

Not on Dialysis: The following initial dosage schedule (TABLE 1), is suggested as a guideline based on creatinine clearance. Further modification in the dosage schedule may be required because of individual variations in absorption.

TABLE 1

Creatinine Clearance	Dose	Time Interval
>20 ml/min	500 mg	6 hours
5-20 ml/min	250 mg	6 hours
<5 ml/min	250 mg	12 hours

On Chronic, Intermittent Hemodialysis:

250 mg Start

250 mg at 12 hours

250 mg 36-48 hours (after start)

Children may require dosage modification proportional to their weight and severity of infection.

Capsules—Keep tightly closed. Do not store above 86°F.

Oral Suspension—Prior to constitution, store at room temperature; avoid excessive heat. After constitution, when stored at room temperature, discard unused portion after 14 days. Keep tightly closed.

HOW SUPPLIED - RATED THERAPEUTICALLY EQUIVALENT:

Capsule, Gelatin - Oral - 250 mg

24's	$7.87	Cephradine, H.C.F.A. F F P	99999-0702-01
24's	**$21.60**	**VELOSEF, Bristol Myers Squibb**	**00003-0113-24**
40's	$26.00	Cephradine, Teva	00332-3153-06
100's	$32.81	Cephradine, United Res	00677-1135-01
100's	$32.81	Cephradine, H.C.F.A. F F P	99999-0702-02
100's	$35.00	Cephradine, Consolidated Midland	00223-0611-01
100's	$37.00	CEPHADRINE, Raway	00686-0606-20
100's	$42.25	Cephradine, Goldline Labs	00182-1253-89
100's	$46.04	Cephradine, Lederle Pharm	00005-3406-23
100's	$53.00	Cephradine, Qualitest Pharms	00603-2619-21
100's	$53.70	Cephradine, Schein Pharm (US)	00364-2141-01
100's	$54.75	Cephradine, Goldline Labs	00182-1253-01
100's	$55.00	Cephradine, Teva	00332-3153-09
100's	$55.00	Cephradine, Rugby	00536-0180-01
100's	$55.00	Cephradine, Major Pharms	00904-2837-60
100's	$55.05	Cephradine, Geneva Pharms	00781-2533-01
100's	$57.90	Cephradine, HL Moore Drug Exch	00839-7262-06
100's	$59.51	Cephradine, Aligen Independ	00405-4158-01
100's	**$85.99**	**VELOSEF, Bristol Myers Squibb**	**00003-0113-50**
100's	**$85.99**	**VELOSEF, Bristol Myers Squibb**	**00003-0113-52**
500's	$164.05	Cephradine, H.C.F.A. F F P	99999-0702-03

Capsule, Gelatin - Oral - 500 mg

24's	$15.03	Cephradine, H.C.F.A. F F P	99999-0702-04
24's	$30.75	Cephradine, Goldline Labs	00182-1254-16
24's	$31.37	Cephradine, Geneva Pharms	00781-2534-24
24's	**$42.51**	**VELOSEF '500', Bristol Myers Squibb**	**00003-0114-26**
40's	$45.00	Cephradine, Teva	00332-3155-06
100's	$62.63	Cephradine, United Res	00677-1136-01
100's	$62.63	Cephradine, H.C.F.A. F F P	99999-0702-05
100's	$63.00	CEPHADRINE, Raway	00686-0607-20
100's	$65.00	Cephradine, Consolidated Midland	00223-0612-01
100's	$90.84	Cephradine, Rugby	00536-0185-01
100's	$90.90	Cephradine, Lederle Pharm	00005-3407-23
100's	$98.00	Cephradine, Qualitest Pharms	00603-2620-21
100's	$102.00	Cephradine, Teva	00332-3155-09
100's	$102.64	Cephradine, Schein Pharm (US)	00364-2142-01
100's	$104.70	Cephradine, Major Pharms	00904-2838-60
100's	$104.95	Cephradine, Goldline Labs	00182-1254-01
100's	$105.00	Cephradine, Geneva Pharms	00781-2534-01
100's	$105.42	Cephradine, HL Moore Drug Exch	00839-7263-06
100's	$110.90	Cephradine, Goldline Labs	00182-1254-89
100's	$114.45	Cephradine, Aligen Independ	00405-4159-01
100's	**$168.89**	**VELOSEF '500', Bristol Myers Squibb**	**00003-0114-50**
100's	**$168.89**	**VELOSEF '500', Bristol Myers Squibb**	**00003-0114-52**
500's	$313.15	Cephradine, H.C.F.A. F F P	99999-0702-06
500's	$407.25	Cephradine, Rugby	00536-0195-05

Powder, Reconstitution - Oral - 125 mg/5ml

5 ml	**$84.50**	**VELOSEF '125', Bristol Myers Squibb**	**00003-1193-20**
100 ml	$6.69	Cephradine, H.C.F.A. F F P	99999-0702-07
100 ml	$6.74	Cephradine, Balan	00304-1945-63
100 ml	$7.07	Cephradine, Teva	00332-4165-32
100 ml	$7.35	Cephradine, Schein Pharm (US)	00364-2143-61
100 ml	$7.50	Cephradine, Goldline Labs	00182-7014-70
100 ml	**$9.43**	**VELOSEF '125', Bristol Myers Squibb**	**00003-1193-50**
200 ml	$13.38	Cephradine, H.C.F.A. F F P	99999-0702-08
200 ml	**$18.64**	**VELOSEF '125', Bristol Myers Squibb**	**00003-1193-80**

Powder, Reconstitution - Oral - 250 mg/5ml

5 ml	**$127.01**	**VELOSEF 250, Bristol Myers Squibb**	**00003-1194-20**
100 ml	$7.65	Cephradine, Harber Pharm	51432-0541-14
100 ml	$12.50	Cephradine, Goldline Labs	00182-7015-70
100 ml	$12.51	Cephradine, H.C.F.A. F F P	99999-0702-09
100 ml	$12.74	Cephradine, Balan	00304-1946-63
100 ml	$12.75	Cephradine, Schein Pharm (US)	00364-2144-61
100 ml	$12.77	Cephradine, Teva	00332-4167-32
100 ml	**$17.69**	**VELOSEF 250, Bristol Myers Squibb**	**00003-1194-50**
200 ml	$25.02	Cephradine, H.C.F.A. F F P	99999-0702-10
200 ml	**$35.02**	**VELOSEF 250, Bristol Myers Squibb**	**00003-1194-80**

Powder, Reconstitution - Oral - 500 mg/5ml

100 ml	$14.25	Cephradine, Harber Pharm	51432-0545-13

HOW SUPPLIED - NOT RATED EQUIVALENT:

Injection, Dry-Soln - Intramuscular; - 250 mg/vial

250 mg x 10	**$23.36**	**VELOSEF, Bristol Myers Squibb**	**00003-1476-10**

Injection, Dry-Soln - Intravenous - 2 gm/bottle

100 ml	**$15.45**	**VELOSEF, Bristol Myers Squibb**	**00003-1197-20**

Injection, Lyphl-Soln - Intramuscular; - 1 gm/vial

1 gm x 10	**$77.76**	**VELOSEF, Bristol Myers Squibb**	**00003-1199-10**

Injection, Lyphl-Susp - Intramuscular; - 500 mg/vial

500 mg x 10	**$41.34**	**VELOSEF 500, Bristol Myers Squibb**	**00003-1198-10**

CETIRIZINE HYDROCHLORIDE *(003162)*

CATEGORIES: Allergies; Antihistamines; Respiratory & Allergy Medications; Rhinitis; Rhinorrhea; Sneezing; Urticaria; Top 200 Drugs; Top 200 Drugs

BRAND NAMES: *Alercet*; *Alergex*; *Alerid*; *Certex-24*; *Cetrine*; *Cetzine*; *Cezin*; *Riztec*; *Ryzen*; *Triz*; *Virlix* (Mexico); *Xero-sed*; *Zirtin*; **Zyrtec**; *Zyrzine*
(International brand names outside U.S. in italics)

DESCRIPTION:

Cetirizine hydrochloride is an orally active and selective H_1-receptor antagonist. The chemical name is (±)-[2-[4-(p-chloro-α-phenyl-benzyl)-1-piperazinyl)ethoxy] acetic acid, dihydrochloride. Cetirizine hydrochloride is a racemic compound with an empirical formula of $C_{21}H_{25}ClN_2O_3$-2HCl. The molecular weight is 461.82. Cetirizine hydrochloride is a white, crystalline powder and is water soluble. Cetirizine hydrochloride is formulated as a white (dye-free), film-coated, rounded-off rectangular shaped tablet for oral administration and is available in 5 and 10 mg strengths. Inert ingredients are: lactose; magnesium stearate; povidone; titanium dioxide; hydroxypropyl methylcellulose; polyethylene glycol; and corn starch.

CLINICAL PHARMACOLOGY:

MECHANISM OF ACTIONS

Cetirizine, a human metabolite of hydroxyzine, is an antihistamine; its principal effects are mediated via selective inhibition of peripheral H1 receptors. The antihistaminic activity of cetirizine has been clearly documented in a variety of animal and human models. *In vivo* and *ex vivo* animal models have shown negligible anticholinergic and antiserotonergic activity. In clinical studies, however, dry mouth was more common with cetirizine than with placebo. *In vitro* receptor binding studies have shown no measurable affinity for other than H_1 receptors. Autoradiographic studies with radiolabeled cetirizine in the rat have shown negligible penetration into the brain. *Ex vivo* experiments in the mouse have shown that systemically administered cetirizine does not significantly occupy cerebral H_1 receptors. Autoradiographic studies with radiolabeled cetirizine in the rat have shown that systemically administered cetrizine does not significantly occupy cerebral H_1 receptors.

PHARMACOKINETICS

Cetirizine is rapidly absorbed after oral administration of a tablet, which had a bioavailability similar to an oral solution. Food had no effect on the extent of cetirizine absorption, but T_{max} was delayed by 1.7 hours and C_{max} was decreased by 23% in the presence of food. A mass balance study in 6 healthy male volunteers indicated that 70% of the administered radioactive dose was recovered in the urine and 10% in the feces, for a combined total recovery of about 80%. Approximately 50% of the administered radioactive dose was excreted in urine as unchanged drug. Most of the rapid increase in peak plasma radioactivity is associated with parent drug indicating low first pass metabolism. Cetirizine is metabolized to a very limited extent by oxidative O-dealkylation to a metabolite with negligible antihistaminic activity.

Cetirizine exhibits linear kinetics over the dosage range of 5 to 60 mg. In pharmacokinetic studies in 146 healthy volunteers, the mean -n SD terminal half-life was 8.3 ± 1.8 hours, oral clearance was 54 ± 13 mL/min, and the apparent volume of distribution was 0.50 ± 0.08 L/kg. No accumulation was observed for cetirizine following daily doses of 10 mg for 10 days. The steady-state maximum plasma concentration was 311 ± 40 ng/mL and was achieved within 1.0 ± 0.5 hour. Individual histograms of cetirizine C_{max} and AUC showed unimodal distributions with a two- to four-fold variability in healthy subjects. Plasma protein binding of cetirizine is 93 ± 0.3% and is independent of concentration in the range of 0.025 to 1.0 mcg/mL; this concentration range covers the therapeutic plasma levels.

Formal pharmacokinetic interaction studies were conducted with cetirizine and pseudoephedrine, antipyrine, ketoconazole, erythromycin, and azithromycin. No pharmacokinetic interactions were observed. In a multiple dose study of theophylline (400 mg once daily) and cetirizine, there was a small (16%) decrease in clearance of cetirizine.

SPECIAL POPULATIONS

Effect of Age: Following a single 10 mg oral dose, half-life increased by about 50% and clearance decreased by 40% in 16 elderly subjects as compared to the 14 normal subjects. The decrease in cetirizine clearance in these elderly volunteers appeared to be related to their decreased renal function.

Effect of Gender: The effect of gender on cetirizine pharmacokinetics has not been adequately studied.

Effect of Race: No race-related differences were observed in the kinetics of cetirizine between 86 white adult males and 11 black adult males.

Renally Impaired Patients: The kinetics of cetirizine were studied following multiple oral daily doses of 10 mg for 7 days in 7 normal volunteers (creatinine clearance 89-128 mL/min), 8 patients with mild renal function impairment (creatinine clearance 42-77 mL/min) and 7 patients with moderate renal function impairment (creatinine clearance 11-31 mL/min). The pharmacokinetics of the drug were similar in patients with mild impairment and normal volunteers. Moderately renally impaired patients had a 3-fold increase in half-life and 70% decrease in clearance compared to normal volunteers.

Patients (N=5) on hemodialysis (creatinine clearance less than 7 mL/min) given a single oral 10 mg dose of cetirizine had a 3-fold increase in half-life and a 70% decrease in clearance compared to normals. Cetirizine was not completely cleared by hemodialysis as less than 10% of the administered dose was removed during the dialysis session.

Dosing adjustment is necessary in patients with moderate or severe renal impairment and patients on dialysis. (See also DOSAGE AND ADMINISTRATION.)

Hepatically Impaired Patients: Sixteen patients with chronic liver diseases (hepatocellular, cholestatic, and biliary cirrhosis), given 10 or 20 mg of cetirizine as a single oral dose had a 50% increase in half-life along with a 40% decrease in clearance compared to 16 healthy subjects. Dosing adjustment may be necessary in hepatically impaired patients. (See also DOSAGE AND ADMINISTRATION.)

PHARMACODYNAMICS

Studies in normal volunteers show that cetirizine hydrochloride at doses of 5 and 10 mg strongly inhibits the skin wheal and flare caused by the intradermal injection of histamine. The onset of this activity after a single 10 mg dose occurs within 20 minutes in 50% of subjects and within one hour on 95% of subjects; this activity persists for at least 24 hours. In

CLINICAL PHARMACOLOGY: *(cont'd)*

a 35-day study in children ages 5 to 12, no tolerance to the antihistaminic (suppression of wheal and flare response) effects of cetirizine hydrochloride was found. The effects of intradermal injection of various other mediators or histamine releasers are also inhibited by cetirizine, as is response to a cold challenge in patients with a cold-induced urticaria. In mildly asthmatic subjects, cetirizine hydrochloride at 5 to 20 mg blocked bronchoconstriction due to nebulized histamine, with virtually total blockage after a 20 mg dose. In studies conducted for up to 12 hours following cutaneous antigen challenge, the last phase recruitment of eosinophils, neutrophils and basophils, components of the allergic inflammatory response, was inhibited by cetirizine hydrochloride at a dose of 20 mg.

In four clinical studies in healthy adult males, no clinically significant mean increases in QTc were observed in cetirizine hydrochloride treated subjects. In the first study, a placebo-controlled crossover trial, cetirizine hydrochloride was given at doses up to 60 mg per day, 6 times the maximum clinical dose, for 1 week, and no significant mean QTc prolongation occurred. In the second study, a crossover trial, cetirizine hydrochloride 20 mg and erythromycin (500 mg every 8 hours) were given alone and in combination. There was no significant effect on QTc with the combination or with cetirizine hydrochloride alone. In the third trial, also a crossover study, cetirizine hydrochloride 20 mg and ketoconazole (400 mg per day) were given alone and in combination. Cetirizine hydrochloride caused a mean increase in QTc of 9.1 msec from baseline after 10 days of therapy. Ketoconazole also increased QTc by 8.3 msec. The combination caused an increase of 17.4 msec, equal to the sum of the individual effects. Thus, there are no significant drug interaction on QTc with the combination of cetirizine hydrochloride and ketoconazole. In the fourth study, a placebo-controlled parallel trial, cetirizine hydrochloride 20 mg was given alone or in combination with azithromycin (500 mg as a single dose on the first day followed by 250 mg once daily). There was no significant increase in Qtc with cetirizine hydrochloride 20 mg alone or in combination with azithromycin.

In a six-week, placebo-controlled study of 186 patients with allergic rhinitis and mild to moderate asthma, cetirizine hydrochloride 10 mg once daily improved rhinitis symptoms and did not alter pulmonary function. This study supports the safety of administering cetirizine hydrochloride to allergic rhinitis patients with mild to moderate asthma.

CLINICAL STUDIES:

Nine multicenter, randomized, double-blind, clinical trials comparing cetirizine 5 to 20 mg to placebo in patients with seasonal or perennial allergic rhinitis were conducted in the United States. Five of these showed significant reductions in symptoms of allergic rhinitis, 3 in seasonal allergic rhinitis (1 to 4 weeks in duration) and 2 in perennial allergic rhinitis for up to 8 weeks in duration. Two 4-week multicenter, randomized, double-blind, clinical trials comparing cetirizine 5 to 20 mg to placebo in patients with chronic idiopathic urticaria were also conducted and showed significant improvement in symptoms of chronic idiopathic urticaria. In general, the 10 mg dose was more effective than the 5 mg dose and the 20 mg dose gave no added effect. Some of these trials included pediatric patients age 12 to 16 years.

INDICATIONS AND USAGE:

Seasonal Allergic Rhinitis: Cetirizine hydrochloride is indicated for the relief of symptoms associated with seasonal allergic rhinitis due to allergens such as ragweed, grass and tree pollens in adults and children 12 years of age and older. Symptoms treated effectively include sneezing, rhinorrhea, nasal pruritus, ocular pruritus, tearing and redness of the eyes.

Perennial Allergic Rhinitis: Cetirizine hydrochloride is indicated for the relief of symptoms associated with perennial allergic rhinitis due to allergens such as dust mites, animal dander and molds in adults and children 12 years of age and older. Symptoms treated effectively include sneezing, rhinorrhea, post-nasal discharge, nasal pruritus, ocular pruritus and tearing.

Chronic Urticaria: Cetirizine hydrochloride is indicated for the treatment of the uncomplicated skin manifestations of chronic idiopathic urticaria in adults and children 12 years of age and older. It significantly reduces the occurrence, severity and duration of hives and significantly reduces pruritus.

CONTRAINDICATIONS:

Cetirizine hydrochloride is contraindicated in those patients with a known hypersensitivity to it or any of its ingredients or hydroxyzine.

PRECAUTIONS:

Activities Requiring Mental Alertness: In clinical trials, the occurrence of somnolence has been reported in some patients taking cetirizine hydrochloride; due caution should therefore be exercised when driving a car or operating potentially dangerous machinery. Concurrent use of cetirizine hydrochloride with alcohol and other CNS depressants should be avoided because additional reductions in alertness and additional impairment of CNS performance may occur.

Carcinogenesis, Mutagenesis and Impairment of Fertility: No evidence of carcinogenicity was observed in a 2-year carcinogenicity study in rats at dietary doses up to 20 mg/kg/day (15 times the maximum recommended human dose on a mg/m^2/day basis). An increased incidence of benign liver tumors was found in a 2-year carcinogenicity study in male mice at a dietary dose of 16 mg/kg/day (6 times the maximum recommended human dose on a mg/m^2/day basis). The clinical significance of these findings during long-term use of cetirizine hydrochloride is not known. Cetirizine was not mutagenic in the Ames test, and not clastogenic in the human lymphocyte assay, the mouse lymphoma assay, and the *in vivo* micronucleus test in rats. No impairment of fertility was found in a fertility and general reproductive performance study in mice at a dose of 64 mg/kg/day (26 times the maximum recommended human dose on a mg/m^2/day basis).

Pregnancy Category B: Cetirizine was not teratogenic in mice, rats and rabbits at doses up to 96.225 and 135 mg/kg/day (40, 180 and 216 times the maximum recommended human dose on a mg/m^2/day basis), respectively. There are no adequate and well-controlled studies in pregnant women. Because animal studies are not always predictive of human response, cetirizine hydrochloride should be used in pregnancy only if clearly needed.

Nursing Mothers: Retarded pup weight gain was found in mice during lactation when dams were given cetirizine at 96 mg/kg/day (40 times the maximum recommended human dose on a mg/m^2/day basis). Studies in beagle dogs indicate that approximately 3% of the dose is excreted in breast milk. Cetirizine has been reported to be excreted in human breast milk; use of cetirizine hydrochloride in nursing mothers is not recommended.

Geriatric Use In placebo-controlled trials, 186 patients age 65 to 94 years received doses of 5 to 20 mg cetirizine hydrochloride per day. Adverse events were similar in this group to patients under age 65. Subset analysis of efficacy in this group was not done.

Pediatric Use: Safety and effectiveness in children under 12 years of age has not been established.

DRUG INTERACTIONS:

No clinically significant drug interactions have been found with theophylline at a low dose, azithromycin, pseudoephedrine, ketoconazole, or erythromycin. There was a small decrease in the clearance of cetirizine caused by a 400 mg dose of theophylline; it is possible that larger theophylline doses could have a greater effect.

ADVERSE REACTIONS:

Controlled and uncontrolled clinical trials conducted in the United States and Canada included more than 6000 patients, with more than 3900 receiving cetirizine hydrochloride at doses of 5 to 20 mg per day. The duration of treatment ranged from 1 week to 6 months, with a mean exposure of 30 days.

Most adverse reactions reported during therapy with cetirizine hydrochloride were mild or moderate. In placebo-controlled trials, the incidence of discontinuations due to adverse reactions in patients receiving cetirizine hydrochloride 5 mg or 10 mg was not significantly different from placebo (2.9% vs. 2.4%, respectively).

The most common adverse reaction that occurred more frequently on cetirizine than placebo was somnolence. The incidence of somnolence associated with cetirizine hydrochloride was dose related, 6% in placebo, 11% at 5 mg and 14% at 10 mg. Discontinuations due to somnolence for cetirizine hydrochloride were uncommon (1.0% on cetirizine hydrochloride vs. 0.6% on placebo). Fatigue and dry mouth also appeared to be treatment-related adverse reactions. There were no differences by age, race, gender or by body weight with regard to the incidence of adverse reactions.

Table 1 lists adverse experiences which were reported for cetirizine hydrochloride 5 and 10 mg in controlled clinical trials in the United States and that were more common with cetirizine hydrochloride than placebo.

TABLE 1 Adverse Experiences Reported in Placebo-Controlled United States Cetirizine Hydrochloride Trials (Maximum Dose of 10 mg) at Rates of 2% or Greater (Percent Incidence)

Adverse Experience	Cetirizine Hydrochloride	Placebo (N=1612)
Somnolence	13.7	6.3
Fatigue	5.9	2.6
Dry Mouth	5.0	2.3
Pharyngitis	2.0	1.9
Dizziness	2.0	1.2

In addition, headache and nausea occurred in more than 2% of the patients, but were more common in placebo patients.

The following events were observed infrequently (less than 2%). In 3982 patients who received cetirizine hydrochloride in U.S. trials, including an open study of six months duration, a causal relationship with cetirizine hydrochloride administration has not been established.

Autonomic Nervous System: anorexia, urinary retention, flushing, increased salivation

Cardiovascular: palpitation, tachycardia, hypertension, cardiac failure

Central and Peripheral Nervous System: paresthesia, confusion, hyperkinesia, hypertonia, migraine, tremor, vertigo, leg cramps, ataxia, dysphonia, abnormal coordination, hyperesthesia, hypoesthesia, myelitis, paralysis, ptosis, twitching, visual field defect

Gastrointestinal: increased appetite, dyspepsia, abdominal pain, diarrhea, flatulence, constipation, vomiting, ulcerative stomatitis, aggravated tooth caries, stomatitis, tongue discoloration, tongue edema, gastritis, rectal hemorrhage, hemorrhoids, melena, abnormal hepatic function

Genitourinary: polyuria, urinary tract infection, cystitis, dysuria, hematuria

Hearing and Vestibular: earache, tinnitus, deafness, ototoxicity

Metabolic/Nutritional: thirst, dehydration, diabetes mellitus

Musculoskeletal: myalgia, arthralgia, arthrosis, arthritis, muscle weakness

Psychiatric: insomnia, nervousness, depression, emotional lability, impaired concentration, anxiety, depersonalization, paroniria, abnormal thinking, agitation, amnesia, decreased libido, euphoria

Respiratory System: epistaxis, rhinitis, coughing, bronchospasm, dyspnea, upper respiratory tract infection, hyperventilation, sinusitis, increased sputum, bronchitis, pneumonia

Reproductive: dysmenorrhea, female breast pain, intermenstrual bleeding, leukorrhea, menorrhagia, vaginitis

Reticuloendothelial: lymphadenopathy

Skin: pruritus, rash, dry skin, urticaria, acne, dermatitis, erythematous rash, increased sweating, alopecia, angioedema, furunculosis, bullous eruption, eczema, hyperkeratosis, hypertrichosis, photosensitivity reaction, photosensitivity toxic reaction, maculopapular rash, seborrhea, purpura

Special Senses: taste perversion, taste loss, parosmia

Vision: blindness, loss of accommodation, eye pain, conjunctivitis, xerophthalmia, glaucoma, ocular hemorrhage

Body as a Whole: increased weight, back pain, malaise, fever, asthenia, generalized edema, periorbital edema, peripheral edema, rigors, leg edema, face edema, hot flashes, enlarged abdomen, nasal polyp

Occasional instances of transient, reversible hepatic transaminase elevations have occurred during cetirizine therapy. A single case of possible drug-induced hepatitis with significant transaminase elevation (500 to 1000 IU/L) and elevated bilirubin has been reported.

In foreign marketing experience the following additional rare, but potential severe adverse events have been reported: hemolytic anemia, thrombocytopenia, orofacial dyskinesia, severe hypotension, anaphylaxis, hepatitis, glomerulonephritis, stillbirth, and cholestasis.

DRUG ABUSE AND DEPENDENCE:

There is no information to indicate that abuse or dependency occurs with cetirizine hydrochloride.

OVERDOSAGE:

Overdosage has been reported with cetirizine hydrochloride. In one patient who took 150 mg of cetirizine hydrochloride, the patient was somnolent but did not display any other clinical signs or abnormal blood chemistry or hematology results. Should overdose occur, treatment should be symptomatic or supportive, taking into account any concomitantly ingested medications. There is no known specific antidote to cetirizine hydrochloride. Cetirizine hydrochloride is not effectively removed by dialysis, and dialysis will be ineffective unless a dialyzable agent has been concomitantly ingested. The minimal lethal oral dose in rodents is approximately 100 times the maximum recommended clinical dose on a mg/m^2 basis and the liver is the target organ of toxicity.

DOSAGE AND ADMINISTRATION:

The recommended initial dose of cetirizine hydrochloride is 5 or 10 mg per day in adults and children 12 years and older, depending on symptom severity. Most patients in clinical trials started at 10 mg. Cetirizine hydrochloride is given as a single daily dose, with or without food. The time of administration may be varied to suit individual patient needs.

In patients with decreased renal function (creatinine clearance 11-31 ml/min), patients on hemodialysis (creatinine clearance less than 7 ml/min), and in hepatically impaired patients, a dose of 5 mg once daily is recommended.

PATIENT INFORMATION:

Cetirizine is used for allergy and itching due to skin conditions. Take one dose daily, with or without meals, or as directed by your doctor. Inform your doctor if you are pregnant, nursing or have liver or kidney disease. May cause drowsiness; patients should use caution while driving or operating machinery. Inform your doctor if you are taking theophylline. Avoid alcohol and other CNS depressants. May cause sleepiness, tiredness, dry mouth, sore throat, or dizziness. Inform your doctor or pharmacist if these effects occur.

HOW SUPPLIED:

Zyrtec tablets are white (dye-free), film-coated, rounded-off rectangular shaped containing 5 mg or 10 mg cetirizine hydrochloride. 5 mg tablets are engraved with "Pfizer" on one side and with "550" on the other. 10 mg tablets are engraved with "Pfizer" on one side and with "551" on the other.

Storage: Store at room temperature 59° to 86°F (15°-30°C).

HOW SUPPLIED - EQUIVALENTS NOT AVAILABLE:

Tablet, Coated - Oral - 5 mg
100's $144.31 ZYRTEC, Pfizer Labs 00069-5500-66

Tablet, Coated - Oral - 10 mg
100's $144.31 ZYRTEC, Pfizer Labs 00069-5510-66

CETYL ALCOHOL; COLFOSCERIL PALMITATE; TYLOXAPOL *(003005)*

CATEGORIES: Lung Surfactant; Orphan Drugs; Respiratory Distress; Respiratory Distress Syndrome, Neonatal; FDA Class 1A ("Important Therapeutic Advantage"); FDA Approved 1990 Aug

BRAND NAMES: **Exosurf**; *Exosurf Neonatal* (Germany)
(International brand names outside U.S. in italics)

COST OF THERAPY: $20.00 (RDS; Injection; 12 mg/108 mg/47 mg/8 mg; 10/day; 2 days)

DESCRIPTION:

Exosurf Neonatal (colfosceril palmitate, cetyl alcohol, tyloxapol) for Intratracheal Suspension is a protein-free synthetic lung surfactant stored under vacuum as a sterile lyophilized powder. Exosurf Neonatal is reconstituted with preservative-free Sterile Water for Injection prior to administration by intratracheal instillation. Each 10 ml vial contains 108 mg colfosceril palmitate, commonly known as dipalmitoylphosphatidylcholine (DPPC), 12 mg cetyl alcohol, 8 mg tyloxapol, and 47 mg sodium chloride. Sodium hydroxide or hydrochloric acid may have been added to adjust pH. When reconstituted with 8 ml Sterile Water for Injection, the Exosurf Neonatal suspension contains 13.5 mg/ml colfosceril palmitate, 1.5 mg/ml cetyl alcohol, and 1 mg/ml tyloxapol in 0.1 N NaCl. The suspension appears milky white with a pH of 5 to 7 and an osmolality of 185 mOsm/kg.

The chemical names and formulas of the components of Exosurf Neonatal are as follows:

Colfosceril palmitate: (*R*)-4-hydrox y- *N,N,N*- trimethyl- 10-oxo-7- [(1- oxohexadecyl) oxy]-3,5,9-trioxa-4- phosphapentacosan-1-aminium hydroxide inner salt, 4-oxide

Cetyl alcohol: (1-hexadecanol) $CH_3(CH_2)_{14}CH_2OH$

Tyloxapol: (formaldehyde polymer with oxirane and 4-(1,1,3,3-tetramethylbutyl)phenol) [R is $CH_2CH_2O(CH_2CH_2O)_mCH_2CH_2OH$; m is 6 to 8; n is not more than 5]

CLINICAL PHARMACOLOGY:

Surfactant deficiency is an important factor in the development of the neonatal respiratory distress syndrome (RDS). Thus, surfactant replacement therapy early in the course of RDS should ameliorate the disease and improve symptoms. Natural surfactant, a combination of lipids and apoproteins, exhibits not only surface tension reducing properties (conferred by the lipids), but also rapid spreading and adsorption (conferred by the apoproteins). The major fraction of the lipid component of natural surfactant is DPPC, which comprises up to 70% of natural surfactant by weight.

Although DPPC reduces surface tension, DPPC alone is ineffective in RDS because DPPC spreads and adsorbs poorly. In cetyl alcohol; colfosceril palmitate; tyloxapol, which is protein free, cetyl alcohol acts as the spreading agent for the DPPC on the air-fluid interface. Tyloxapol, a polymeric long-chain repeating alcohol, is a nonionic surfactant which acts to disperse both DPPC and cetyl alcohol. Sodium chloride is added to adjust osmolality.

Pharmacokinetics: Cetyl alcohol; colfosceril palmitate; tyloxapol is administered directly into the trachea. Human pharmacokinetic studies of the absorption, biotransformation, and excretion of the components of Cetyl alcohol; colfosceril palmitate; tyloxapol have not been performed. Nonclinical studies, however, have shown that DPPC can be absorbed from the alveolus into lung tissue where it can be catabolized extensively and reutilized for further phospholipid synthesis and secretion. In the developing rabbit, 90% of alveolar phospholipids are recycled. In premature rabbits, the alveolar half-life of intratracheally administered H^3-labeled phosphatidylcholine is approximately 12 hours.

Animal Studies: In animal models of RDS, treatment with cetyl alcohol; colfosceril palmitate; tyloxapol significantly improved lung volume, compliance and gas exchange in premature rabbits and lambs. The amount and distribution of lung water were not affected by cetyl alcohol; colfosceril palmitate; tyloxapol treatment of premature rabbit pups. The extent of lung injury in premature rabbit pups undergoing mechanical ventilation was reduced significantly by cetyl alcohol; colfosceril palmitate; tyloxapol treatment. In premature lambs, neither systemic blood flow nor flow through the ductus arteriosus were affected by cetyl alcohol; colfosceril palmitate; tyloxapol treatment. Survival was significantly better in both premature rabbits and premature lambs treated with cetyl alcohol; colfosceril palmitate; tyloxapol.

CLINICAL STUDIES:

Cetyl alcohol; colfosceril palmitate; tyloxapol has been studied in the U.S. and Canada in controlled clinical trials involving more than 4400 infants. Over 10,000 infants have received cetyl alcohol; colfosceril palmitate; tyloxapol through an open, uncontrolled, North American study designed to provide the drug to premature infants who might benefit and to obtain additional safety information (Exosurf Neonatal Treatment IND).

Prophylactic Treatment: The efficacy of a single dose of cetyl alcohol; colfosceril palmitate; tyloxapol in prophylactic treatment of infants at risk of developing respiratory distress syndrome (RDS) was examined in three double-blind, placebo-controlled studies, one involving 215 infants weighing 500 to 700 grams, one involving 385 infants weighing 700 to 1350 grams, and one involving 446 infants weighing 700 to 1100 grams. The infants were intubated and placed on mechanical ventilation, and received 5 ml/kg cetyl alcohol; colfosceril palmitate; tyloxapol or placebo (air) within 30 minutes of birth.

The efficacy of one versus three doses of cetyl alcohol; colfosceril palmitate; tyloxapol in prophylactic treatment of infants at risk of developing RDS was examined in a double-blind, placebo-controlled study of 823 infants weighing 700 to 1100 grams. The infants were intubated and placed on mechanical ventilation, and received a first 5 ml/kg dose of cetyl alcohol; colfosceril palmitate; tyloxapol within 30 minutes. Repeat 5 ml/kg doses of cetyl alcohol; colfosceril palmitate; tyloxapol or placebo (air) were given to all infants who remained on mechanical ventilation at approximately 12 and 24 hours of age. An initial analysis of 716 infants is available.

The major efficacy parameters from these studies are presented in TABLES 1A and 1B.

TABLE 1A Efficacy Assessments - Prophylactic Treatment

Number of Doses:	Single Dose		Single Dose		Single Dose	
Birth Weight Range:	500 to 700 g		700 to 1350 g		700 to 1100 g	
Treatment Group:	Placebo (Air)	Exosurf	Placebo (Air)	Exosurf	Placebo (Air)	Exosurf
Number of Infants:	N=106	N=109	N=185	N=176	N=222	N=224
	% of Infants		% of Infants		% of Infants	
Death ≤ Day 28[a]	53	50	11	6	21	15
Death through 1 Year[a]	59	60	14	11	30	20*
Death from RDS[b]	25	13*	4	3	10	5***
Intact Cardiopulmonary Survival[a,c]	29	25	69	78*	65	68
Bronchopulmonary Dysplasia (BPD)[a,d]	43	44	23	18	19	21
RDS Incidence[b]	73	81	46	42	55	55

[a] "Intent-to-treat" analyses (as randomized) except for the 700 to 1350 gram,single dose study in which infants with congenital infections and anomalies were excluded
[b] "As-treated" analyses
[c] Defined by survival through 28 days of life without bronchopulmonary dysplasia
[d] Defined by a combination of clinical and radiographic criteria
* $p < 0.05$
*** $p = 0.051$

TABLE 1B Efficacy Assessments - Prophylactic Treatment

One Versus Three Doses 700 to 1100 grams	One Exosurf Dose N=356	Three Exosurf Doses N=360
	% of Infants	
Death ≤ Day 28[a]	16	9*
Death through 1 Year[a]	17	12
Death from RDS[b]	3	2
Intact Cardiopulmonary Survival[a,c]	74	78
Bronchopulmonary Dysplasia (BPP)[a,d]	8	12
RDS Incidence[b]	63	68

[a] "Intent-to-treat" analyses (as randomized) except for the 700 to 1350 gram,single dose study in which infants with congenital infections and anomalies were excluded
[b] "As-treated" analyses
[c] Defined by survival through 28 days of life without bronchopulmonary dysplasia
[d] Defined by a combination of clinical and radiographic criteria
* $p < 0.05$
** $p < 0.01$
*** $p = 0.051$

Rescue Treatment: The efficacy of cetyl alcohol; colfosceril palmitate; tyloxapol in the rescue treatment of infants with RDS was examined in two double-blind, placebo-controlled studies. One study enrolled 419 infants weighing 700 to 1350 grams; the second enrolled 1237 infants weighing 1250 grams and above. In the rescue treatment studies, infants received an initial dose (5 ml/kg) of cetyl alcohol; colfosceril palmitate; tyloxapol or placebo (air) between 2 and 24 hours of life followed by a second dose (5 ml/kg) approximately 12 hours later to infants who remained on mechanical ventilation. The major efficacy parameters from these studies are presented in TABLE 2.

TABLE 2 Efficacy Assessments - Rescue Treatment

Number of Doses:	Two Doses		Two Doses	
Birth Weight Range:	700 to 1350 g		> 1250 g	
Treatment Group:	Placebo (Air)	Exosurf	Placebo (Air)	Exosurf
Number of Infants:	N=213	N=206	N=623	N=614
	% of Infants		% of Infants	
Death ≤ Day 28[a]	23	11†	7	4*
Death through 1 Year[a]	27	15†	9	6†
Death from RDS[b]	10	3**	3	1*
Intact Cardiopulmonary Survival[a,c]	62	75	88	93**
Bronchopulmonary Dysplasia (BPD)[a,d]	18	15	6	3*

[a] "Intent-to-treat" analyses (as randomized)
[b] "As-treated" analyses
[c] Defined by survival through 28 days of life without bronchopulmonary dysplasia
[d] Defined by a combination of clinical and radiographic criteria
* $p < 0.05$
** $p < 0.01$
*** $p < 0.001$
† = 0.067

Clinical Results: In these six controlled clinical studies, infants in the cetyl alcohol; colfosceril palmitate; tyloxapol group showed significant improvements in FiO_2 and ventilator settings which persisted for at least 7 days. Pulmonary air leaks were significantly reduced in each study. Five of these studies also showed a significant reduction in death from RDS. Further, overall mortality was reduced for all infants weighing >700 grams. The one versus three-dose prophylactic treatment study in 700 to 1100 gram infants showed a further reduction in overall mortality with two additional doses.

Safety information is presented in TABLES 3 and 4 (see ADVERSE REACTIONS). Beneficial effects in the cetyl alcohol; colfosceril palmitate; tyloxapol group were observed for some safety assessments. Various forms of pulmonary air leak and use of pancuronium were reduced in infants receiving cetyl alcohol; colfosceril palmitate; tyloxapol in all six studies.

Follow-up data at one year adjusted age are available on 1094 of 2470 surviving infants. Growth and development of infants who received cetyl alcohol; colfosceril palmitate; tyloxapol in this sample were comparable to infants who received placebo.

INDICATIONS AND USAGE:

Cetyl alcohol; colfosceril palmitate; tyloxapol is indicated for:

1. Prophylactic treatment of infants with birth weights of less than 1350 grams who are at risk of developing RDS (see PRECAUTIONS).

INDICATIONS AND USAGE: *(cont'd)*

2. Prophylactic treatment of infants with birth weights greater than 1350 grams who have evidence of pulmonary immaturity, and

3. Rescue treatment of infants who have developed RDS.

For prophylactic treatment, the first dose of cetyl alcohol; colfosceril palmitate; tyloxapol should be administered as soon as possible after birth see DOSAGE AND ADMINISTRATION, General Guidelines for Administration.

Infants considered as candidates for **rescue** treatment with cetyl alcohol; colfosceril palmitate; tyloxapol should be on mechanical ventilation and have a diagnosis of RDS by both of the following criteria:

1. Respiratory distress not attributable to causes other than RDS, based on clinical and laboratory assessments.

2. Chest radiographic findings consistent with the diagnosis of RDS.

During the clinical development of cetyl alcohol; colfosceril palmitate; tyloxapol, all infants who received the drug were intubated and on mechanical ventilation. For three-dose prophylactic treatment with cetyl alcohol; colfosceril palmitate; tyloxapol, the first dose of drug was administered as soon as possible after birth and repeat doses were given at approximately 12 and 24 hours after birth if infants remained on mechanical ventilation at those times. For rescue treatment, two doses were given; one between 2 and 24 hours of life, and a second approximately 12 hours later if infants remained on mechanical ventilation. Infants who received rescue treatment with cetyl alcohol; colfosceril palmitate; tyloxapol had a documented arterial to alveolar oxygen tension ratio (a/A) <0.22.

CONTRAINDICATIONS:

There are no known contraindications to treatment with cetyl alcohol; colfosceril palmitate; tyloxapol.

WARNINGS:

Intratracheal Administration Only: Cetyl alcohol; colfosceril palmitate; tyloxapol should be administered only by instillation into the trachea (see DOSAGE AND ADMINISTRATION).

General: The use of cetyl alcohol; colfosceril palmitate; tyloxapol requires expert clinical care by experienced neonatologists and other clinicians who are accomplished at neonatal intubation and ventilatory management. Adequate personnel, facilities, equipment, and medications are required to optimize perinatal outcome in premature infants.

Instillation of cetyl alcohol; colfosceril palmitate; tyloxapol should be performed **only** by trained medical personnel experienced in airway and clinical management of unstable premature infants. Vigilant clinical attention should be given to all infants prior to, during, and after administration of cetyl alcohol; colfosceril palmitate; tyloxapol.

Acute Effects: Cetyl alcohol; colfosceril palmitate; tyloxapol can rapidly affect oxygenation and lung compliance.

Lung Compliance: If chest expansion improves substantially after dosing, peak ventilator inspiratory pressures should be reduced immediately, without waiting for confirmation of respiratory improvement by blood gas assessment. Failure to reduce inspiratory ventilator pressures rapidly in such instances can result in lung overdistension and fatal pulmonary air leak.

Hyperoxia: If the infant becomes pink and transcutaneous oxygen saturation is in excess of 95%, FiO_2 should be reduced in small but repeated steps (until saturation is 90% to 95%) without waiting for confirmation of elevated arterial pO_2 by blood gas assessment. Failure to reduce FiO_2 in such instances can result in hyperoxia.

Hypocarbia: If arterial or transcutaneous CO_2 measurements are <30 torr, the ventilator rate should be reduced at once. Failure to reduce ventilator rates in such instances can result in marked hypocarbia, which is known to reduce brain blood flow.

Pulmonary Hemorrhage: In the single study conducted in infants weighing <700 grams at birth, the incidence of pulmonary hemorrhage (10% vs 2% in the placebo group) was significantly increased in the cetyl alcohol; colfosceril palmitate; tyloxapol group. None of the five studies involving infants with birth weights >700 grams showed a significant increase in pulmonary hemorrhage in the cetyl alcohol; colfosceril palmitate; tyloxapol group. In a cross-study analysis of these five studies, pulmonary hemorrhage was reported for 1% (14/1420) of infants in the placebo group and 2% (27/1411) of infants in the cetyl alcohol; colfosceril palmitate; tyloxapol group. Fatal pulmonary hemorrhage occurred in three infants; two in the cetyl alcohol; colfosceril palmitate; tyloxapol group and one in the placebo group. Mortality from all causes among infants who developed pulmonary hemorrhage was 43% in the placebo group and 37% in the cetyl alcohol; colfosceril palmitate; tyloxapol group.

Pulmonary hemorrhage in both cetyl alcohol; colfosceril palmitate; tyloxapol and placebo infants was more frequent in infants who were younger, smaller, male, or who had a patent ductus arteriosus. Pulmonary hemorrhage typically occurred in the first 2 days of life in both treatment groups.

In more than 7700 infants in the open, uncontrolled study, pulmonary hemorrhage was reported in 4%, but fatal pulmonary hemorrhage was reported rarely (0.4%).

In the controlled clinical studies, cetyl alcohol; colfosceril palmitate; tyloxapol treated infants who received steroids more than 24 hours prior to delivery or indomethacin postnatally had a lower rate of pulmonary hemorrhage than other cetyl alcohol; colfosceril palmitate; tyloxapol treated infants. Attention should be paid to early and aggressive diagnosis and treatment (unless contraindicated) of patent ductus arteriosus during the first 2 days of life (while the ductus arteriosus is often clinically silent). Other potentially protective measures include attempting to decrease FiO_2 preferentially over ventilator pressures during the first 24 to 48 hours after dosing, and attempting to decrease PEEP minimally for at least 48 hours after dosing.

Mucous Plugs: Infants whose ventilation becomes markedly impaired during or shortly after dosing may have mucous plugging of the endotracheal tube, particularly if pulmonary secretions were prominent prior to drug administration. Suctioning of all infants prior to dosing may lessen the chance of mucous plugs obstructing the endotracheal tube. If endotracheal tube obstruction from such plugs is suspected, and suctioning is unsuccessful in removing the obstruction, the blocked endotracheal tube should be replaced immediately.

PRECAUTIONS:

General: In the controlled clinical studies, infants known prenatally or postnatally to have major congenital anomalies, or who were suspected of having congenital infection, were excluded from entry. However, these disorders cannot be recognized early in life in all cases, and a few infants with these conditions were entered. The benefits of cetyl alcohol; colfosceril palmitate; tyloxapol in the affected infants who received drug appeared to be similar to the benefits observed in infants without anomalies or occult infection.

Prophylactic Treatment—Infants <700 Grams: In infants weighing 500 to 700 grams, a single prophylactic dose of cetyl alcohol; colfosceril palmitate; tyloxapol significantly: improved FiO_2 and ventilator settings, reduced pneumothorax, and reduced death from RDS, but increased pulmonary hemorrhage (see WARNINGS). Overall mortality did not differ significantly between the placebo and cetyl alcohol; colfosceril palmitate; tyloxapol groups (see TABLE 1). Data on multiple doses in infants in this weight class are not yet available. Accordingly, clinicians should carefully evaluate the potential risks and benefits of cetyl alcohol; colfosceril palmitate; tyloxapol administration in these infants.

Rescue Treatment—Number of Doses: A small number of infants with RDS have received more than two doses of cetyl alcohol; colfosceril palmitate; tyloxapol as rescue treatment. Definitive data on the safety and efficacy of these additional doses are not available.

Carcinogenesis, Mutagenesis, Impairment of Fertility: Cetyl alcohol; colfosceril palmitate; tyloxapol at concentrations up to 10,000 mcg/plate was not mutagenic in the Ames *Salmonella* assay.

Long-term studies have not been performed in animals to evaluate the carcinogenic potential of cetyl alcohol; colfosceril palmitate; tyloxapol.

The effects of cetyl alcohol; colfosceril palmitate; tyloxapol on fertility have not been studied.

ADVERSE REACTIONS:

General: Premature birth is associated with a high incidence of morbidity and mortality. Despite significant reductions in overall mortality associated with cetyl alcohol; colfosceril palmitate; tyloxapol, some infants who received cetyl alcohol; colfosceril palmitate; tyloxapol developed severe complications and either survived with permanent handicaps or died.

In controlled clinical studies evaluating the safety and efficacy of cetyl alcohol; colfosceril palmitate; tyloxapol, numerous safety assessments were made. In infants receiving cetyl alcohol; colfosceril palmitate; tyloxapol, pulmonary hemorrhage, apnea and use of methylxanthines were increased. A number of other adverse events were significantly reduced in the cetyl alcohol; colfosceril palmitate; tyloxapol group, particularly various forms of pulmonary air leak and use of pancuronium. (See CLINICAL PHARMACOLOGY, Clinical Results). TABLES 3A, 3B and 4 summarize the results of the major safety evaluations from the controlled clinical studies.

TABLE 3A Safety Assessments [3]-Prophylactic Treatment

Number of Doses:	Single Dose		Single Dose	
Birth Weight Range:	500 to 700 g		700 to 1350 g	
Treatment Group:	Placebo (Air)	EXOSURF	Placebo (Air)	EXOSURF
Number of Infants:	N=108	N=107	N=193	N=192
	% of Infants		% of Infants	
Intraventricular Hemorrhage (IVH)				
Overall	51	57	31	27
Severe IVH	26	25	10	8
Pulmonary Air Leak (PAL)				
Overall	52	48	16	11
Pneumothorax	23	10	5	6
Pneumopericardium	1	4	2	0
Pneumomediastinum	2	1	2	3
Pulmonary Interstitial Emphysema	43	44	1	7*
Death from PAL	4	6	<1	1
Patent Ductus Arteriosus	49	53	66	70
Necrotizing Enterocolitis	2	4	11	13
Pulmonary Hemorrhage	2	10*	2	4
Congenital Pneumonia	4	4	2	4
Nosocomial Pneumonia	10	10		4
Non-Pulmonary Infections	33	35	4	39
Sepsis	30	34	30	34
Death From Sepsis	4	4	3	3
Meningitis	4	6	3	1
Other Infections	7	4	5	3
Major Anomalies	3	1	2	4
Hypotension	70	77	52	47
Hyperbilirubinemia	22	21	63	61
Exchange Transfusion	4	3	1	2
Thrombocytopenia[b]	21	25	n.a.	n.a.
Persistent Fetal Circulation	0	1	1	1
Seizures	11	8	2	2
Apnea	34	33	76	73
Drug Therapy				
Antibiotics	96	99	98	96
Diuretics	55	60	39	37
Anticonvulsants	14	18	23	24
Inotropes	46	40	20	20
Sedatives	62	71	65	64
Pancuronium	19	11	2	14*
Methylxanthines	38	43	7	77

[b]thrombocytopenia requiring platelet transfusion.
* $p<0.05$

Pulmonary Hemorrhage: See WARNINGS.

Abnormal Laboratory Values: Abnormal laboratory values are common in critically ill, mechanically ventilated, premature infants. A higher incidence of abnormal laboratory values in the cetyl alcohol; colfosceril palmitate; tyloxapol group was not reported.

Events During Dosing: Data on events during dosing are available from more than 8800 infants in the open, uncontrolled clinical study (TABLE 5).

REFLUX

Reflux of cetyl alcohol; colfosceril palmitate; tyloxapol into the endotracheal tube during dosing has been observed and may be associated with rapid drug administration. If reflux occurs, drug administration should be halted and, if necessary, peak inspiratory pressure on the ventilator should be increased by 4 to 5 cm H_2O until the endotracheal tube clears.

>20% Drop in Transcutaneous Oxygen Saturation: If transcutaneous oxygen saturation declines during dosing, drug administration should be halted and, if necessary, peak inspiratory pressure on the ventilator should be increased by 4 to 5 cm H_2O for 1 to 2 minutes. In addition, increases of FiO_2 may be required for 1 to 2 minutes.

Mucous Plugs: See WARNINGS.

OVERDOSAGE:

There have been no reports of massive overdosage with cetyl alcohol; colfosceril palmitate; tyloxapol.

TABLE 3B Safety Assessments[3]-Prophylactic Treatment

	Single Dose 700 to 1100 grams		One Versus Three Doses 700 to 1100 grams	
	Placebo (Air) N=222	Exosurf N=224 % of Infants	One Exosurf Dose N=356	Three Exosurf Doses N=360 % of Infants
Intraventricular Hemorrhage (IVH)				
Overall	36	36	38	35
Severe IVH	13	14	9	9
Pulmonary Air Leak (PAL)				
Overall	32	25	29	27
Pneumothorax	19	11*	14	12
Pneumopericardium	<1	1	1	1
Pneumomediastinum	7	1**	3	2
Pulmonary Interstitial Emphysema	26	20	23	22
Death from PAL	2	1	2	1
Patent Ductus Arteriosus	50	55	59	57
Necrotizing Enterocolitis	3	4	6	2
Pulmonary Hemorrhage	1	4	4	6
Congenital Pneumonia	2	2	1	1
Nosocomial Pneumonia	4	7	15	14
Non-Pulmonary Infections	28	29	35	34
Sepsis	23	24	30	27
Death from Sepsis	1	2	3	2
Meningitis	2	3	1	2
Other Infections	6	10	10	11
Major Anomalies	7	4	4	4
Hypotension	59	62	54	50
Hyperbilirubinemia	27	31	20	21
Exchange Transfusion	2	2	3	1
Thrombocytopenia[b]	9	8	12	10
Persistent Fetal Circ.	0	2*	1	<1
Seizures	11	9	6	5
Apnea	55	65*	62	68
Drug Therapy				
Antibiotics	98	99	<99	99
Diuretics	59	63	64	65
Anticonvulsants	20	16	9	8
Inotropes	26	20	28	27
Sedatives	63	57	52	52
Pancuronium	19	13*	15	11
Methylxanthines	61	72	75	82*

[a]All parameters were examined with "as-treated" analyses.
[b]thrombocytopenia requiring platelet transfusion.
* $p<0.05$
** $p<0.01$
*** $p<0.001$

TABLE 4A Safety Assessments[3]-Rescue Treatment

Number of Doses:	Two Doses		Two Doses	
Birth Weight Range:	700 to 1350 grams		1250 grams and above	
Treatment Group:	Placebo (Air)	Exosurf	Placebo (Air)	Exosurf
Number of Infants:	N=213	N=206	N=622	N=615
	% of Infants		% Infants	
Intraventricular Hemorrhage (IVH)				
Overall	48	52	23	18*
Severe IVH	13	9	5	4
Pulmonary Air Leak (PAL)				
Overall	54	34**	30	18***
Pneumothorax	29	20*	20	10***
Pneumoperi	4	1	1	2
Pneumomediastinum	8	4	5	2**
Pulmonary Interstitial Emphysema	48	25	24	13**
Death from PAL	7	3	<1	1
Patent Ductus Arteriosus	66	57	54	45*
Necrotizing Enterocolitis	3	3	1	2
Pulmonary Hemorrhage	3	1	<1	1
Congenital Pneumonia	2	3	2	2
Nosocomial Pneumonia	5	7	2	2
Non-Pulmonary Infections	19	22	13	13
Sepsis	15	17	8	8
Death From Sepsis	<1	<1	1	<1
Meningitis	1	<1	1	<1*
Other Infections	5	8	5	6
Major Anomalies	3	3	4	4
Hypotension	62	57	50	39
Hyperbilirubinemia	17	19	12	10
Exchange Transfusion	3	4	1	2
Thrombocytopenia[b]	10	11	4	<1**
Persistent Fetal Circulation	1	1	6	2**
Seizures	10	10	6	3*
Apnea	48	65**	37	44*
Drug Therapy				
Antibiotics	100	99	98	99
Diuretics	60	65	45	34***
Anticonvulsants	17	17	10	5**
Inotropes	36	31	27	16***
Sedatives	72	68	76	64***
Pancuronium	34	17**	33	15***
Methylxanthines	62	74**	49	53

[a]All parameters were examined with "as-treated" analyses.
[b]Thrombocytopenia requiring platelet transfusion.
* $p < 0.05$
** $p < 0.01$
*** $p < 0.001$

DOSAGE AND ADMINISTRATION:

Preparation of Suspension: Cetyl alcohol; colfosceril palmitate; tyloxapol is best reconstituted immediately before use because it does not contain antibacterial preservatives. However, the reconstituted suspension is chemically and physically stable and remains sterile (when reconstituted using aseptic techniques) when stored at 2° to 30°C (36° to 86°F) for up to 12 hours following reconstitution.

DOSAGE AND ADMINISTRATION: *(cont'd)*

TABLE 5 Events During Dosing in the Open, Uncontrolled Study[2]

Treatment Type: Number of Infants:	Prophylactic Treatment N = 1127 % of Infants	Rescue Treatment N = 7711 % of Infants
Reflux of Exosurf	20	31
Drop in O_2 saturation (≥ 20%)	6	22
Rise in O_2 saturation (≥ 10%)	5	6
Drop in transcutaneous pO_2 (≥ 20 mm Hg)	1	8
Rise in transcutaneous pO_2 (≥ 20 mm Hg)	2	5
Drop in transcutaneous pCO_2 (≥ 20 mm Hg)	<1	1
Rise in transcutaneous pCO_2 (≥ 20 mm Hg)	1	3
Bradycardia (<60 beats/min)	1	3
Tachycardia (>200 beats/min)	<1	<1
Gagging	1	5
Mucous Plugs	<1	<1

[a]Infants may have experienced more than one event. Investigators were prohibited from adjusting FiO_2 and/or ventilator settings during dosing unless significant clinical deterioration occurred.

Solutions containing buffers or preservatives should not be used for reconstitution. **Do Not Use Bacteriostatic Water for Injection, USP.** Each vial of Exosurf Neonatal should be reconstituted only with 8 ml of the accompanying diluent (preservative-free Sterile Water for Injection) as follows:

1. Fill a 10 ml or 12 ml syringe with 8 ml preservative-free Sterile Water for Injection using an 18 or 19 gauge needle;

2. Allow the vacuum in the vial to draw the sterile water into the vial;

3. Aspirate as much as possible of the 8 ml out of the vial into the syringe (while maintaining the vacuum), then SUDDENLY release the syringe plunger.

Step 3 should be repeated three or four times to assure adequate mixing of the vial contents. If vacuum is not present, the vial of cetyl alcohol; colfosceril palmitate; tyloxapol should not be used.

The appropriate dosage volume for the entire dose (5 ml/kg) should then be drawn into the syringe from **below** the froth in the vial (again maintaining the vacuum). If the infant weighs less than 1600 grams, unused cetyl alcohol; colfosceril palmitate; tyloxapol suspension will remain in the vial after the entire dose is drawn into the syringe. If the infant weighs more than 1600 grams, at least two vials will be required for each dose.

Reconstituted cetyl alcohol; colfosceril palmitate; tyloxapol is a milky white suspension with a total volume of 8 ml per vial. Each ml of reconstituted cetyl alcohol; colfosceril palmitate; tyloxapol contains 13.5 mg colfosceril palmitate, 1.5 mg cetyl alcohol, 1 mg tyloxapol, and sodium chloride to provide a 0.1 N concentration. If the suspension appears to separate, gently shake or swirl the vial to resuspend the preparation. The reconstituted product should be inspected visually for homogeneity immediately before administration; if persistent large flakes or particulates are present, the vial should not be used.

Dosage: Accurate determination of weight at birth is the key to accurate dosing.

Prophylactic Treatment: The first dose of cetyl alcohol; colfosceril palmitate; tyloxapol should be administered as a single 5 ml/kg dose as soon as possible after birth. Second and third doses should be administered approximately 12 and 24 hours later to all infants who remain on mechanical ventilation at those times.

Rescue Treatment: Cetyl alcohol; colfosceril palmitate; tyloxapol should be administered in two 5 ml/kg doses. The initial dose should be administered as soon as possible after the diagnosis of RDS is confirmed. The second dose should be administered approximately 12 hours following the first dose, provided the infant remains on mechanical ventilation. A small number of infants with RDS have received more than two doses of cetyl alcohol; colfosceril palmitate; tyloxapol as rescue treatment. Definitive data on the safety and efficacy of these additional doses are not available (see PRECAUTIONS).

Use of Special Endotracheal Tube Adapter: With each vial of cetyl alcohol; colfosceril palmitate; tyloxapol for Intratracheal Suspension, five different sized endotracheal tube adapters each with a special right angle Luer-Lok sideport are supplied. The adapters are clean but not sterile. The adapters should be used as follows:

1. Select an adapter size which corresponds to the inside diameter of the endotracheal tube.

2. Insert the adapter into the endotracheal tube with a firm push-twist motion.

3. Connect the breathing circuit wye to the adapter.

4. Remove the cap from the sideport on the adapter. Attach the syringe containing drug to the sideport.

5. After completion of dosing, remove the syringe and RECAP THE SIDEPORT.

Administration: The infant should be suctioned prior to administration of cetyl alcohol; colfosceril palmitate; tyloxapol.

Cetyl alcohol; colfosceril palmitate; tyloxapol suspension is administered via the sideport on the special endotracheal tube adapter **WITHOUT INTERRUPTING MECHANICAL VENTILATION.**

Each dose of cetyl alcohol; colfosceril palmitate; tyloxapol is administered in two 2.5 ml/kg half-doses. Each half-dose is instilled slowly over 1 to 2 minutes (30 to 50 mechanical breaths) in small bursts timed with inspiration. After the first 2.5 ml/kg half-dose is administered in the midline position, the infant's head and torso are turned 45° to the right for 30 seconds while mechanical ventilation is continued. After the infant is returned to the midline position, the second 2.5 ml/kg half-dose is given in an identical fashion over another 1 to 2 minutes. The infant's head and torso are then turned 45° to the left for 30 seconds while mechanical ventilation is continued, and the infant is then turned back to the midline position. These maneuvers allow gravity to assist in the distribution of cetyl alcohol; colfosceril palmitate; tyloxapol in the lungs.

During dosing, heart rate, color, chest expansion, facial expressions, the oximeter, and the endotracheal tube patency and position should be monitored. If heart rate slows, the infant becomes dusky or agitated, transcutaneous oxygen saturation falls more than 15%, or cetyl alcohol; colfosceril palmitate; tyloxapol backs up in the endotracheal tube, dosing should be slowed or halted and, if necessary, the peak inspiratory pressure, ventilator rate, and/or FiO_2 turned up. On the other hand, rapid improvements in lung function may require immediate reductions in peak inspiratory pressure, ventilator rate, and/or FiO_2. (See WARNINGS and see below for additional information concerning administration.)

Suctioning should not be performed for two hours after cetyl alcohol; colfosceril palmitate; tyloxapol is administered, except when dictated by clinical necessity.

DOSAGE AND ADMINISTRATION: *(cont'd)*

General Guidelines for Administration: Administration of cetyl alcohol; colfosceril palmitate; tyloxapol should not take precedence over clinical assessment and stabilization of critically ill infants.

Intubation: Prior to dosing with cetyl alcohol; colfosceril palmitate; tyloxapol, it is important to ensure that the endotracheal tube tip is in the trachea and not in the esophagus or right or left mainstem bronchus. Brisk and symmetrical chest movement with each mechanical inspiration should be confirmed prior to dosing, as should equal breath sounds in the two axillae. In prophylactic treatment, dosing with cetyl alcohol; colfosceril palmitate; tyloxapol need not be delayed for radiographic confirmation of the endotracheal tube tip position. In rescue treatment, bedside confirmation of endotracheal tube tip position is usually sufficient, if at least one chest radiograph subsequent to the last intubation confirmed proper position of the endotracheal tube tip. Some lung areas will remain undosed if the endotracheal tube tip is too low.

Monitoring: Continuous ECG and transcutaneous oxygen saturation monitoring during dosing are essential. In most infants treated prophylactically, it should be possible to initiate such monitoring prior to administration of the first dose of cetyl alcohol; colfosceril palmitate; tyloxapol. For subsequent prophylactic and all rescue doses, arterial blood pressure monitoring during dosing is also highly desirable. After both prophylactic and rescue dosing, frequent arterial blood gas sampling is required to prevent post-dosing hyperoxia and hypocarbia (see WARNINGS).

Ventilatory Support During Dosing: The 5 ml/kg dosage volume may cause transient impairment of gas exchange by physical blockage of the airway, particularly in infants on low ventilator settings. As a result, infants may exhibit a drop in oxygen saturation during dosing, especially if they are on low ventilator settings prior to dosing. These transient effects are easily overcome by increasing peak inspiratory pressure on the ventilator by 4 to 5 cm H_2O for 1 to 2 minutes during dosing. FiO_2 can also be increased if necessary. In infants who are particularly fragile or reactive to external stimuli, increasing peak inspiratory pressure by 4 to 5 cm H_2O and/or FiO_2 20% just prior to dosing may minimize any transient deterioration in oxygenation. However, in virtually all cases it should be possible to return the infant to pre-dose settings within a very short time of dose completion.

Post-Dosing: At the end of dosing, position of the endotracheal tube should be confirmed by listening for equal breath sounds in the two axillae. Attention should be paid to chest expansion, color, transcutaneous saturation, and arterial blood gases. Some infants who receive cetyl alcohol; colfosceril palmitate; tyloxapol and other surfactants respond with rapid improvements in pulmonary compliance, minute ventilation, and gas exchange (see WARNINGS). Constant bedside attention of an experienced clinician for at least 30 minutes after dosing is essential. Frequent blood gas sampling also is absolutely essential. Rapid changes in lung function require immediate changes in peak inspiratory pressure, ventilator rate, and/or FiO_2.

EDUCATIONAL MATERIAL

A videotape on dosing is available from your Glaxo Wellcome representative. This videotape demonstrates techniques for safe administration of cetyl alcohol; colfosceril palmitate; tyloxapol and should be viewed by health care professionals who will administer the drug.

HOW SUPPLIED:

Cetyl alcohol; colfosceril palmitate; tyloxapol for intratracheal suspension is supplied in a carton containing one 10 ml vial of cetyl alcohol; colfosceril palmitate; tyloxapol for intratracheal suspension, one 10 ml vial of Sterile Water for Injection, and five endotracheal tube adapters (2.5, 3.0, 3.5, 4.0, and 4.5 mm I.D.).

Store cetyl alcohol; colfosceril palmitate; tyloxapol for intratracheal suspension at 15° to 30°C (59° to 86°F) in a dry place.

HOW SUPPLIED - EQUIVALENTS NOT AVAILABLE:

Injection, Lyphl-Susp - Intratracheal - 12 mg/108 mg/47

10 ml vial $719.14 EXOSURF NEONATAL, Glaxo Wellcome 00173-0207-01

CHLORAL HYDRATE *(000715)*

CATEGORIES: Analgesics; Anxiety; Anxiolytics, Sedatives, Hypnotic; Central Nervous System Agents; Sedation; Sedatives/Hypnotics; Pain*; Pregnancy Category C; DEA Class CIV; FDA Pre 1938 Drugs
* Indication not approved by the FDA

BRAND NAMES: *Ansopal*; Aquachloral; *Chloraldurat* (Germany); *Chloralhydrat*; *Chloralhydrat 500*; *Chloralix*; *Dormel*; *Kloral*; *Medianox*; Noctec; *Novochlorhydrate* (Canada); *Pocral*; *Somnox*; *Welldorm* (England)
(International brand names outside U.S. in italics)

FORMULARIES: Aetna; BC-BS; FHP; Medi-Cal; WHO

DESCRIPTION:

> **Chloral Hydrate is genotoxic and may be carcinogenic in mice. Chloral hydrate should not be used when less potentially dangerous agents would be effective.**

Oral Forms: Chloral Hydrate Capsules and Chloral Hydrate Syrup contain chloral hydrate, an effective sedative and hypnotic agent for oral administration.

Chloral Hydrate Capsules provide 250 mg (3 3/4 grains) and 500 mg (7 1/2 grains) chloral hydrate per capsule. Inactive ingredients: colorants (FD&C Red No. 3, Red No. 40, Yellow No. 6), gelatin, glycerin, methylparaben, polyethylene glycol 400, and propylparaben.

Chloral Hydrate Syrup provides 500 mg (7 1/2 grains) chloral hydrate per 5 ml teaspoonful of clear, pink, aromatic, flavored syrup. Inactive ingredients: citric acid, colorants (FD&C Blue No. 2, Red No. 40, Yellow No. 6), flavors, glycerin, purified water, saccharin sodium, sodium citrate, and sucrose.

Chemically, chloral hydrate (MW 165.40; CAS-302-17-0) is 1,1-0Ethanedial,2,2,2-trichloro-; its graphic formula is: $CCl_3CH(OH)_2$. Chloral Hydrate occurs as colorless or white, volatile, hygroscopic crystals very soluble in water and in olive oil and freely soluble in alcohol. It has an aromatic, pungent odor and a slightly bitter, caustic taste.

Suppositories: Chloral Hydrate suppositories are water soluble rectal suppository dosage forms containing Chloral Hydrate, color coded as follows:

Green - Chloral Hydrate 5 g (325 mg)

Blue - Chloral Hydrate 10 g (650 mg)

The Neocera base used to form Chloral Hydrate suppositories is composed of Polyethylene Glycol 400, 1450, 8000, and Polysorbate 60. FD&C Yellow No. 5 (tartrazine) is in the 5 mg suppository.

DESCRIPTION: *(cont'd)*

The active ingredient is represented by: Cl_3CCHOH. The chemical name is 1,1-Ethanedial,2,2,2-trichloro-.

CLINICAL PHARMACOLOGY:

Oral Forms: The mechanism of action by which the central nervous system is affected is not known. Chloral Hydrate is readily absorbed from the gastrointestinal tract following oral administration; however, significant amounts of chloral hydrate have not been detected in the blood after oral administration. It is generally believed that the central depressant effects are due to the principal pharmacologically active metabolite trichloroethanol, which has a plasma half-life of 8 to 10 hours. A portion of the drug is oxidized to trichloroacetic acid (TCA) in the liver and kidneys; TCA is excreted in the urine and bile along with trichloroethanol in free or conjugated form.

Hypnotic dosage produces mild cerebral depression and quiet, deep sleep with little or no "hangover"; blood pressure and respiration are depressed only slightly more than in normal sleep and reflexes are not significantly depressed, so the patient can be awakened and completely aroused. Chloral Hydrate's effect on rapid eye movement (REM) sleep is uncertain.

Chloral Hydrate has been detected in cerebrospinal fluid and human milk, and it crosses the placental barrier.

Suppositories: Chloral Hydrate in the Neocera base is effective when administered rectally as a hypnotic and/or sedative. Irritation has rarely been encountered following correct insertion. Absorption of the drug occurs from the rectum in a short period of time. Somnifacient doses promptly produce drowsiness and/or sedation, followed by quiet sound sleep, generally within an hour. The action of the drug appears to be confined to the cerebral hemispheres. Blood pressures and respiration are depressed only slightly more than in normal REM sleep and reflexes are not greatly depressed so that the patient can be awakened and completely aroused. In contrast to barbiturates and other sedatives, "hangover" and depressant aftereffects are rarely encountered. With the commonly employed therapeutic dosage, the preliminary excitement is rare and tolerance and cumulation are unlikely.

Although the drug is detoxified in the liver and subsequently eliminated by the kidney, moderately impaired function of either organ is not a contraindication for the usual therapeutic doses.

The mechanism of action is not known, but the CNS depressant effects are believed to be due to its active metabolite trichloroethanol.

INDICATIONS AND USAGE:

Chloral Hydrate is indicated for nocturnal sedation in all types of patients and especially for the ill, the young, and the elderly patient. Older patients usually tolerate Chloral Hydrate even when they are intolerant of barbiturates. In candidates for surgery, it is a satisfactory pre-operative sedative that allays anxiety and induces sleep without depressing respiration or cough reflex. In postoperative care and control of pain, it is a valuable adjunct to opiates and analgesics.

CONTRAINDICATIONS:

Chloral Hydrate is contraindicated in patients with marked hepatic or renal impairment and in patients with severe cardiac disease. Oral dosage forms of chloral hydrate are contraindicated in the presence of gastritis. Chloral Hydrate is also contraindicated in patients who have previously exhibited an idiosyncrasy or hypersensitivity to the drug.

WARNINGS:

Chloral Hydrate may be habit forming. Tolerance to the drug is also known to occur. Use with caution in patients who are receiving any of the coumarin or coumarin-related anticoagulants as Chloral Hydrate is known to antagonize the effects of such drugs. When Chloral Hydrate is added to or subtracted from the therapeutic regimen, or when changes in dosage of chloral hydrate are contemplated, the effect of the sedative on prothrombin time deserves special attention.

Tumorigenicity in mice: Chloral Hydrate has shown evidence of carcinogenic activity in studies involving chronic oral administration in mice. Chloral Hydrate has also shown mutagenic and clastogenic activity in a number of *in vitro* assay systems and *in vivo* systems in mammals.

PRECAUTIONS:

ORAL FORMS

General: Chloral Hydrate has been reported to precipitate attacks of acute intermittent porphyria and should be used with caution in susceptible patients.

Continued use of therapeutic doses of chloral hydrate has been shown to be without deleterious effect on the heart. Large doses of chloral hydrate, however, should not be used in patients with *severe* cardiac disease (see CONTRAINDICATIONS).

Information for the Patient: Chloral Hydrate may cause gastrointestinal upset. The capsules should be taken with a full glass of water or fruit juice; capsules should be taken whole, and not chewed. The syrup should be diluted in half a glass of water or fruit juice.

Chloral Hydrate may cause drowsiness; therefore, patients should be instructed to use caution when driving, operating dangerous machinery, or performing any hazardous task.

Patients should avoid alcohol and other CNS depressants. They should also be informed that chloral hydrate may be habit-forming.

Chloral Hydrate and all drugs should be kept out of the reach of children.

Patients should be warned against sudden discontinuation of chloral hydrate except under the advice of the physician; they should also be informed of symptoms that would suggest potential adverse effects.

Drug/Laboratory Test Interactions: Chloral Hydrate may interfere with copper sulfate tests for glycosuria (suspected glycosuria should be confirmed by a glucose oxidase test when the patient is receiving chloral hydrate), fluorometric tests for urine catecholamines (it is recommended that the medication not be administered for 48 hours preceding the test), or urinary 17-hydroxycorticosteroid determinations (when using the Reddy, Jenkins, and Thorn procedure).

Carcinogenesis, Mutagenesis, and Impairment of Fertility: Long-term studies in animals have not been performed.

Pregnancy Category C: Animal reproduction studies have not been conducted with chloral hydrate. Chloral Hydrate crosses the placental barrier and chronic use during pregnancy may cause withdrawal symptoms in the neonate. It is not known whether chloral hydrate can affect reproduction capacity. Chloral Hydrate should be given to a pregnant woman only if clearly needed.

Nursing Mothers: Chloral Hydrate is excreted in human milk; use by nursing mothers may cause sedation in the infant. Caution should be exercised when Chloral Hydrate is administered to a nursing woman

PRECAUTIONS: *(cont'd)*

SUPPOSITORIES

General: The concomitant administration of Chloral Hydrate and alcohol, or other agents which are central nervous system depressants, may significantly potentiate the sedative action of chloral hydrate. Large doses of Chloral Hydrate should not be used in patients with severe cardiac disease. The 5 g suppository contains FD&C Yellow No. 5 (tartrazine) which may cause allergic type reactions (including bronchial asthma) in certain susceptible individuals. Although the overall incidence of FD&C Yellow No. 5 (tartrazine) sensitivity in the general population is low, it is frequently seen in patients who also have a hypersensitivity to aspirin.

Pregnancy Category C: Animal reproduction studies have not been conducted with chloral hydrate. Chloral Hydrate crosses the placental barrier and chronic use during pregnancy may cause withdrawal symptoms in the neonate. It is not known whether chloral hydrate can affect reproduction capacity. Chloral Hydrate should be given to a pregnant woman only if clearly needed.

Nursing Mothers: Chloral Hydrate is excreted in human milk; use by nursing mothers may cause sedation in the infant. Caution should be exercised when Chloral Hydrate is administered to a nursing woman

DRUG INTERACTIONS:

Chloral Hydrate may cause hypoprothrombinemic effects in patients taking oral anticoagulants (see WARNINGS).

Administration of chloral hydrate followed by intravenous furosemide may result in sweating, hot flashes, and variable blood pressure including hypertension due to a hypermetabolic state caused by displacement of thyroid hormone from its bound state.

Caution is recommended in combining chloral hydrate with other CNS depressants such as alcohol, barbiturates, and tranquilizers. Administration of chloral hydrate should be delayed in patients who have ingested significant amounts of alcohol in the preceding 12 to 24 hours. CNS depressants are additive in effect and the dosage should be reduced when such combinations are given concurrently.

ADVERSE REACTIONS:

Central Nervous System: Occasionally a patient becomes somnambulistic and he may be disoriented and incoherent and show paranoid behavior. Rarely, excitement, tolerance, addiction, delirium, drowsiness, staggering gait, ataxia, lightheadedness, vertigo, dizziness, nightmares, malaise, mental confusion, and hallucinations have been reported.

Hematological: Leukopenia and eosinophilia have occasionally occurred.

Dermatological: Allergic skin rashes including hives, erythema, eczematoid dermatitis, urticaria, and scarlatiniform exanthems have occasionally been reported.

Gastrointestinal: Some patients experience gastric irritation and occasionally nausea and vomiting, flatulence, diarrhea, and unpleasant taste occur.

Miscellaneous: Rarely, headache, hangover, idiosyncratic syndrome, and ketonuria have been reported.

DRUG ABUSE AND DEPENDENCE:

Controlled Substance: Drug Enforcement Administration Schedule IV.

Abuse: Chloral Hydrate may be habit-forming. Patients known to be addiction-prone and patients who actively solicit hypnotics in increasing doses are potential addicts. Many patients take higher doses of hypnotics than they admit, and slurring of speech, incoordination, tremulousness, and nystagmus should arouse suspicion. Drowsiness, lethargy, and hangover are frequently observed from excessive drug intake.

Dependence: Prolonged use of larger than usual therapeutic doses may result in psychic and physical dependence. Tolerance and psychologic dependence may develop by the second week of continued administration.

Chloral Hydrate addicts may take huge doses of the drug, i.e., up to 12 g nightly has been reported. This abuse is similar to alcohol addiction and sudden withdrawal may result in central nervous excitation, with tremor, anxiety, hallucination, or even delirium which may be fatal. In patients suffering from chronic chloral hydrate intoxication, gastritis is common and skin eruptions may develop. Parenchymatous renal injury may also occur.

Withdrawal should be undertaken in a hospital and supportive treatment similar to that used during barbiturate withdrawal is recommended.

OVERDOSAGE:

The signs and symptoms of chloral hydrate overdosage resemble those of barbiturate overdosage and especially affect the CNS and cardiovascular system. They may include: hypothermia; pinpoint pupils; blood pressure falls; comatose state; slow, or rapid and shallow breathing. Gastric irritation may result in vomiting and even gastric necrosis. If the patient survives, icterus due to hepatic damage and albuminuria from renal irritation may appear.

The toxic oral dose of chloral hydrate for adults is approximately 10 g; however, death has been reported from a dose of 4 g and some patients have survived after taking as much as 30: : g.

Accidental overdosage should be treated with gastric lavage or by inducing vomiting to empty the stomach. Supportive measures may be used. Hemodialysis is reported to be effective in promoting the clearance of trichloroethanol.

Note: Chloral Hydrate is dialyzable.

DOSAGE AND ADMINISTRATION:

ORAL FORMS

The capsules should be taken with a full glass of liquid. The syrup may be administered in a half glass of water, fruit juice, or ginger ale.

Adults: The usual *hypnotic* dose is 500 mg to 1 g, taken 15 to 30 minutes before bedtime or 1/2 hour before surgery. The usual *sedative*dose is 250 mg three times daily after meals. Generally, single doses or daily dosage should not exceed 2 g.

Children: The usual daily *hypnotic* dosage is 50 mg/kg of body weight, with a maximum of 1 g per single dose. Daily dosage may be given in divided doses, if indicated. The *sedative* dosage is half of the hypnotic dosage.

SUPPOSITORIES

Adults: *Hypnotic Use:* 10 to 20 grains in a single dose on retiring. *Sedative Use:* 5 to 10 grains three times daily. Total daily dose not to exceed 30 grains.

Children: *Hypnotic Use:* 5 grains per 40 lbs. body weight. *Sedative Use:* 1/2 the hypnotic dose. Absorption is dependent on body hydration and not on body temperature. Moisten finger and suppository with water before inserting.

STORAGE

Store Chloral Hydrate **capsules** and syrup at room temperature; avoid excessive heat. Dispense the **syrup** in tight, light-resistant containers.

Store the **suppositories** at room temperature. Do not refrigerate.

(Rectal Suppositories, Polymedica, 3/93)

HOW SUPPLIED - RATED THERAPEUTICALLY EQUIVALENT:

Syrup - Oral - 500 mg/5ml

480 ml	$6.40	Chloral Hydrate, Harber Pharm	51432-0550-20

HOW SUPPLIED - NOT RATED EQUIVALENT:

Capsule, Gelatin - Oral - 250 mg

100's	$7.61	NOCTEC, Bristol Myers Squibb	00003-0623-50

Capsule, Gelatin - Oral - 500 mg

10 cap x 10	$17.10	Chloral Hydrate, Roxane	00054-8140-25
100's	$7.31	Chloral Hydrate, HL Moore Drug Exch	00839-5005-06
100's	$8.25	Chloral Hydrate, Major Pharms	00904-3828-60
100's	$8.50	Chloral Hydrate, United Res	00677-0225-01
100's	$11.48	Chloral Hydrate, IDE-Interstate	00814-1625-14
100's	$12.25	NOCTEC, Bristol Myers Squibb	00003-0626-50
100's	$12.45	Chloral Hydrate, Rugby	00536-3477-01
100's	$13.60	Chloral Hydrate, Goldline Labs	00182-0297-01
100's	$13.60	Chloral Hydrate, Goldline Labs	00182-0324-01
100's	$13.89	Chloral Hydrate S.G., Vangard Labs	00615-0413-13
100's	$15.05	NOCTEC, Bristol Myers Squibb	00003-0626-52
100's	$16.60	Chloral Hydrate, Schein Pharm (US)	00364-0061-01
500's	$33.63	Chloral Hydrate, Caraco Pharm	57664-0204-13

Suppository - Rectal - 500 mg

12's	$27.50	AQUACHLORAL, Alcon-PR	00998-6005-75
12's	$37.50	AQUACHLORAL, Alcon-PR	00998-6010-75
100's	$103.75	Chloral Hydrate, GW Labs	00713-0122-01
100's	$120.00	Chloral Hydrate, Consolidated Midland	00223-5300-00

Syrup - Oral - 250 mg/5ml

10 ml x 40	$23.81	Chloral Hydrate, Roxane	00054-8139-16

Syrup - Oral - 500 mg/5ml

10 ml x 40	$28.10	Chloral Hydrate, Roxane	00054-8138-16
480 ml	$6.50	Chloral Hydrate, H N Norton Co.	50732-0898-16
480 ml	$6.75	NOCTEC, Bristol Myers Squibb	00003-0627-50
480 ml	$8.06	Chloral Hydrate, Qualitest Pharms	00603-1088-58
480 ml	$8.10	Chloral Hydrate, Liquipharm	54198-0140-16
480 ml	$10.45	Chloral Hydrate, United Res	00677-0517-33
480 ml	$10.70	Chloral Hydrate, Morton Grove	60432-0533-16
480 ml	$10.80	Chloral Hydrate, Rugby	00536-0350-85
480 ml	$10.95	Chloral Hydrate, Major Pharms	00904-1300-16
480 ml	$11.26	Chloral Hydrate, Aligen Independ	00405-2550-16
480 ml	$11.49	Chloral Hydrate, Geneva Pharms	00781-6605-16
480 ml	$11.65	Chloral Hydrate, Goldline Labs	00182-0364-40

CHLORAMBUCIL *(000716)*

CATEGORIES: Antineoplastics; Hodgkin's Disease; Leukemia; Lymphoma; Lymphosarcoma; Nitrogen Mustard Derivatives; Oncologic Drugs; Pregnancy Category D; FDA Approval Pre 1982

BRAND NAMES: *Chloraminophene* (France); **Leukeran**; *Linfolysin* *(International brand names outside U.S. in italics)*

FORMULARIES: Aetna; BC-BS; Medi-Cal

WARNING: Chlorambucil can severely suppress bone marrow function. Chlorambucil is a carcinogen in humans. Chlorambucil is probably mutagenic and teratogenic in humans. Chlorambucil produces human infertility. See WARNINGS and PRECAUTIONS.

DESCRIPTION:

Chlorambucil was first synthesized by Everett *et al*[1]. It is a bifunctional alkylating agent of the nitrogen mustard type that has been found active against selected human neoplastic diseases. Chlorambucil is known chemically as 4-[bis(2- chlorethyl)amino]benzenebutanoic acid.

Chlorambucil hydrolyzes in water and has a pKa of 5.8.

Leukeran is available in tablet form for oral administration. Each sugar-coated tablet contains 2 mg chlorambucil and the inactive ingredients corn and wheat starch, gum acacia, lactose, magnesium stearate, polysorbate 60, sucrose, and talc. Printed with edible black ink.

CLINICAL PHARMACOLOGY:

Chlorambucil is rapidly and completely absorbed from the gastrointestinal tract. After single oral doses of 0.6 to 1.2 mg/kg, peak plasma chlorambucil levels are reached within one hour and the terminal half-life of the parent drug is estimated at 1.5 hours. Chlorambucil undergoes rapid metabolism to phenylacetic acid mustard, the major metabolite, and the combined chlorambucil and phenylacetic acid mustard urinary excretion is extremely low - less than 1% in 24 hours. The peak plasma levels of chlorambucil and phenylacetic acid mustard are similar, approximating 1 mcg/ml; however, the metabolite's half-life is 1.6 times greater than the parent drug.[2,3]

Chlorambucil and its metabolites are extensively bound to plasma and tissue proteins. *In vitro,* chlorambucil is 99% bound to plasma proteins, specifically albumin.[4] Cerebrospinal fluid levels of chlorambucil have not been determined. Evidence of human teratogenicity suggests that the drug crosses the placenta.[5,6]

Chlorambucil is extensively metabolized in the liver primarily to phenylacetic acid mustard which has antineoplastic activity.[2,3]Chlorambucil and its major metabolite spontaneously degrade *in vivo* forming monohydroxy and dihydroxy derivatives.[2] After a single dose of radiolabeled chlorambucil (^{14}C) approximately 15% to 60% of the radioactivity appears in the urine after 24 hours. Again, less than 1% of the urinary radioactivity is in the form of chlorambucil or phenylacetic acid mustard.[2] In summary, the pharmacokinetic data suggest that oral chlorambucil undergoes rapid gastrointestinal absorption and plasma clearance and that it is almost completely metabolized, having extremely low urinary excretion.

INDICATIONS AND USAGE:

Chlorambucil is indicated in the treatment of chronic lymphatic (lymphocytic) leukemia, malignant lymphomas including lymphosarcoma, giant follicular lymphoma and Hodgkin's disease. It is not curative in any of these disorders but may produce clinically useful palliation.

CONTRAINDICATIONS:

Chlorambucil should not be used in patients whose disease has demonstrated a prior resistance to the agent. Patients who have demonstrated hypersensitivity to chlorambucil should not be given the drug.[7] There may be cross-hypersensitivity (skin rash) between chlorambucil and other alkylating agents.[8]

WARNINGS:

Because of its carcinogenic properties, chlorambucil should not be given to patients with conditions other than chronic lymphatic leukemia or malignant lymphomas. Convulsions,[9] infertility,[10] leukemia[11,12] and secondary malignancies[13] have been observed when chlorambucil was employed in the therapy of malignant and non-malignant diseases.

There are many reports of acute leukemia arising in patients with both malignant[15] and non-malignant[16] diseases following chlorambucil treatment. In many instances, these patients also received other chemotherapeutic agents or some form of radiation therapy. The quantitation of the risk of chlorambucil-induction of leukemia or carcinoma in humans is not possible. Evaluation of published reports of leukemia developing in patients who have received chlorambucil (and other alkylating agents) suggests that the risk of leukemogenesis increases with both chronicity of treatment and large cumulative doses. However, it has proved impossible to define a cumulative dose below which there is no risk of the induction of secondary malignancy. The potential benefits from chlorambucil therapy must be weighed on an individual basis against the possible risk of the induction of a secondary malignancy.

Chlorambucil has been shown to cause chromatid or chromosome damage in man.[17,18] Both reversible and permanent sterility have been observed in both sexes receiving chlorambucil.

A high incidence of sterility has been documented when chlorambucil is administered to prepubertal and pubertal males.[19] Prolonged or permanent azoospermia has also been observed in adult males.[20] While most reports of gonadal dysfunction secondary to chlorambucil have related to males, the induction of amenorrhea in females with alkylating agents is well documented and chlorambucil is capable of producing amenorrhea. Autopsy studies of the ovaries from women with malignant lymphoma treated with combination chemotherapy including chlorambucil have shown varying degrees of fibrosis, vasculitis, and depletion of primordial follicles.[21,22]

Usage in Pregnancy: Chlorambucil can cause fetal harm when administered to a pregnant woman. Unilateral renal agenesis has been observed in two offspring whose mothers received chlorambucil during the first trimester.[5,6] Urogenital malformations including absence of a kidney were found in fetuses of rats given chlorambucil.[14] There are no adequate and well-controlled studies in pregnant women. If this drug is used during pregnancy, or if the patient becomes pregnant while taking this drug, the patient should be apprised of the potential hazard to the fetus. Women of childbearing potential should be advised to avoid becoming pregnant.

PRECAUTIONS:

General: Many patients develop a slowly progressive lymphopenia during treatment. The lymphocyte count usually rapidly returns to normal levels upon completion of drug therapy. Most patients have some neutropenia after the third week of treatment and this may continue for up to ten days after the last dose. Subsequently, the neutrophil count usually rapidly returns to normal. Severe neutropenia appears to be related to dosage and usually occurs only in patients who have received a total dosage of 6.5 mg/kg or more in one course of therapy with continuous dosing. About one-quarter of all patients receiving the continuous-dose schedule, and one-third of those receiving this dosage in eight weeks or less may be expected to develop severe neutropenia.[23]

While it is not necessary to discontinue chlorambucil at the first evidence of a fall in neutrophil count, it must be remembered that the fall may continue for ten days after the last dose and that as the total dose approaches 6.5 mg/kg there is a risk of causing irreversible bone marrow damage. The dose of chlorambucil should be decreased if leukocyte or platelet counts fall below normal values and should be discontinued for more severe depression.

Chlorambucil should **not** be given at full dosages before four weeks after a full course of radiation therapy or chemotherapy because of the vulnerability of the bone marrow to damage under these conditions. If the pretherapy leukocyte or platelet counts are depressed from bone marrow disease process prior to institution of therapy, the treatment should be instituted at a reduced dosage.

Persistently low neutrophil and platelet counts or peripheral lymphocytosis suggest bone marrow infiltration. If confirmed by bone marrow examination, the daily dosage of chlorambucil should not exceed 0.1 mg/kg. Chlorambucil appears to be relatively free from gastrointestinal side effects or other evidence of toxicity apart from the bone marrow depressant action. In humans, single oral doses of 20 mg or more may produce nausea and vomiting.

Children with nephrotic syndrome[9] and patients receiving high pulse doses of chlorambucil[24] may have an increased risk of seizures. As with any potentially epileptogenic drug, caution should be exercised when administering chlorambucil to patients with a history of seizure disorder, head trauma or receiving other potentially epileptogenic drugs.

Information for the Patient: Patients should be informed that the major toxicities of chlorambucil are related to hypersensitivity, drug fever, myelosuppression, hepatotoxicity, infertility, seizures, gastrointestinal toxicity, and secondary malignancies. Patients should never be allowed to take the drug without medical supervision and should consult their physician if they experience skin rash, bleeding, fever, jaundice, persistent cough, seizures, nausea, vomiting, amenorrhea, or unusual lumps/masses. Women of childbearing potential should be advised to avoid becoming pregnant.

Laboratory Tests: Patients must be followed carefully to avoid life-endangering damage to the bone marrow during treatment. Weekly examination of the blood should be made to determine hemoglobin levels, total and differential leukocyte counts, and quantitative platelet counts. Also, during the first 3 to 6 weeks of therapy, it is recommended that white blood cell counts be made 3 or 4 days after each of the weekly complete blood counts. Galton *et al*[23] have suggested that in following patients it is helpful to plot the blood counts on a chart at the same time that body weight, temperature, spleen size, etc., are recorded. It is considered dangerous to allow a patient to go more than two weeks without hematological and clinical examination during treatment.

Carcinogenesis, Mutagenesis, and Impairment of Fertility: See WARNINGS section for information on carcinogenesis, mutagenesis and impairment of fertility.

Pregnancy, Teratogenic Effects, Pregnancy Category D See WARNINGS.

Nursing Mothers: It is not known whether this drug is excreted in human milk. Because many drugs are excreted in human milk and because of the potential for serious adverse reactions in nursing infants from chlorambucil, a decision should be made whether to discontinue nursing or to discontinue the drug, taking into account the importance of the drug to the mother.

Pediatric Use: The safety and effectiveness in children have not been established.

DRUG INTERACTIONS:

There are no known drug/drug interactions with chlorambucil.

ADVERSE REACTIONS:

Hematologic: The most common side effect is bone marrow suppression.[25] Although bone marrow suppression frequently occurs, it is usually reversible if the chlorambucil is withdrawn early enough. However, irreversible bone marrow failure has been reported.[26,27]

Gastrointestinal: Gastrointestinal disturbances such as nausea and vomiting, diarrhea and oral ulceration occur infrequently.

ADVERSE REACTIONS: *(cont'd)*

CNS: Tremors, muscular twitching, confusion, agitation, ataxia, flaccid paresis and hallucinations have been reported as rare adverse experiences to chlorambucil which resolve upon discontinuation of drug. Rare, focal and/or generalized seizures have been reported to occur in both children[9,28,29] and adults[24,30-33] at both therapeutic daily doses, pulse dosing regimens and in acute overdose (see PRECAUTIONS, General).

Dermatologic: Skin hypersensitivity (including rare reports of skin rash progressing to erythema mutiforme,[9] toxic epidermal necrolysis,[8] and Stevens-Johnson syndrome) has been reported (see**Warnings**).

Miscellaneous: Other reported adverse reactions include: pulmonary fibrosis, hepatotoxicity and jaundice, drug fever, peripheral neuropathy, interstitial pneumonia, sterile cystitis, infertility, leukemia and secondary malignancies (see WARNINGS).

OVERDOSAGE:

Reversible pancytopenia was the main finding of inadvertent overdoses of chlorambucil.[34,35] Neurological toxicity ranging from agitated behavior and ataxia to multiple grand mal seizures has also occurred.[28,34] As there is no known antidote, the blood picture should be closely monitored and general supportive measures should be instituted, together with appropriate blood transfusions if necessary. Chlorambucil is not dialyzable.

Oral LD_{50} single doses in mice are 123 mg/kg. In rats, a single intraperitoneal dose of 12.5 mg/kg of chlorambucil produces typical nitrogen-mustard effects; these include atrophy of the intestinal mucous membrane and lymphoid tissues, severe lymphopenia becoming maximal in four days, anemia and thrombocytopenia. After this dose, the animals begin to recover within three days and appear normal in about a week although the bone marrow may not become completely normal for about three weeks. An intraperitoneal dose of 18.5 mg/kg kills about 50% of the rats with development of convulsions. As much as 50 mg/kg has been given orally to rats as a single dose, with recovery. Such a dose causes bradycardia, excessive salivation, hematuria, convulsions, and respiratory dysfunction.

DOSAGE AND ADMINISTRATION:

The usual oral dosage is 0.1 to 0.2 mg/kg body weight daily for three to six weeks as required. This usually amounts to 4 to 10 mg a day for the average patient. The entire daily dose may be given at one time. These dosages are for initiation of therapy or for short courses of treatment. The dosage must be carefully adjusted according to the response of the patient and must be reduced as soon as there is an abrupt fall in the white blood cell count. Patients with Hodgkin's disease usually require 0.2 mg/kg daily whereas patients with other lymphomas or chronic lymphocytic leukemia usually require only 0.1 mg/kg daily. When lymphocytic infiltration of the bone marrow is present, or when the bone marrow is hypoplastic, the daily dose should not exceed 0.1 mg/kg (about 6 mg for the average patient).

Alternate schedules for the treatment of chronic lymphocytic leukemia employing intermittent, biweekly or once monthly pulse doses of chlorambucil have been reported.[36,37] Intermittent schedules of chlorambucil begin with an initial single dose of 0.4 mg/kg. Doses are generally increased by 0.1 mg/kg until control of lymphocytosis or toxicity is observed. Subsequent doses are modified to produce mild hematologic toxicity. It is felt that the response rate of chronic lymphocytic leukemia to the biweekly or once monthly schedule of chlorambucil administration is similar or better to that previously reported with daily administration and that hematologic toxicity was less than or equal to that encountered in studies using daily chlorambucil.

Radiation and cytotoxic drugs render the bone marrow more vulnerable to damage and chlorambucil should be used with particular caution within four weeks of a full course of radiation therapy or chemotherapy. However, small doses of palliative radiation over isolated foci remote from the bone marrow will not usually depress the neutrophil and platelet count. In these cases chlorambucil may be given in the customary dosage.

It is presently felt that short courses of treatment are safer than continuous maintenance therapy although both methods have been effective. It must be recognized that continuous therapy may give the appearance of "maintenance" in patients who are actually in remission and have no immediate need for further drug. If maintenance dosage is used, it should not exceed 0.1 mg/kg daily and may well be as low as 0.03 mg/kg daily. A typical maintenance dose is 2 mg to 4 mg daily, or less, depending on the status of the blood counts. It may, therefore, be desirable to withdraw the drug after maximal control has been achieved since intermittent therapy reinstituted at time of relapse may be as effective as continuous treatment.

Procedures for proper handling and disposal of anticancer drugs should be considered. Several guidelines on this subject have been published.[38-44]

There is no general agreement that all of the procedures recommended in the guidelines are necessary or appropriate.

HOW SUPPLIED:

White sugar-coated tablet containing 2 mg chlorambucil and printed with "635"; bottle of 50. Store at 15° to 25°C in a dry place.

REFERENCES:

1) Everett JL, Roberts JJ, Ross WCJ: Aryl-2-halogenoalkylamines: Part XII. Some carboxylic derivatives of NN-Di-2-chloroethylaniline.*J Chem Soc* 1953,3:2386-2392.**2**) Alberts DS, Chang SY, Chen H-SG, et al: Pharmacokinetics and metabolism of chlorambucil in man: A preliminary report. *Cancer Treat Rev* 1979;6(suppl):9-17.**3**) Mclean A, Woods RL, Catovsky D, et al: Pharmacokinetics and metabolism of chlorambucil in patients with malignant disease. *Cancer Treat Rev* 1979;6(suppl):33-42. **4**) Ehrsson H, Lonroth U, Wallin I, et al: Degradation of chlorambucil in aqueous solution: Influence of human albumin binding. *J Pharm Pharmacol*1981:33:313-315.**5**) Shotton D, Monie IW: Possible teratogenic effect of chlorambucil on a human fetus. *JAMA* 1963;186:74-75.**6**) Steege JF, Caldwell DS: Renal agenesis after first trimester exposure to chlorambucil. *South Med J* 1980;73:1414-1415.**7**) Knisley RE, Settipane GA, Albala MM: Unusual reaction to chlorambucil in a patient with chronic lymphocytic leukemia. *Arch Dermatol* 1971;104:77-79.**8**) Weiss RB, Bruno S: Hypersensitivity reactions to cancer chemotherapeutic agents. *Ann Intern Med* 1981;94:66-72.**9**) Williams SA, Makker SP, Grupe WE: Seizures: A significant side effect of chlorambucil therapy in children. *J Pediatr* 1978;93:516-518.**10**) Freckman HA, Fry HL, Mendez FL, et al: Chlorambucil-prednisolone therapy for disseminated breast carcinoma. *JAMA* 1964;189:23-26.**11**) Aymard JP, Frustin J, Witz F, et al: Acute leukemia after prolonged chlorambucil treatment for non-malignant disease: A report of a new case and literature survey. *Acta Haematol* 1980;63:283-285.**12**) Berk PD, Goldberg JD, Silverstein MN, et al: Increased incidence of acute leukemia in polycythemia vera associated with chlorambucil therapy. *N Engl J Med* 1981;304:441-447.**13**) Lerner HJ: Acute myelogenous leukemia in patients receiving chlorambucil as long-term adjuvant chemotherapy for stage II breast cancer. *Cancer Treat Rep*1978;62:1135-1138.**14**) Monie IW: Chlorambucil-induced abnormalities of the urogenital system of rat fetuses. *Anat Rec*1961;139:145-153.**15**) Zarrabi MH, Grunwald HW, Rosner F: Chronic lymphocytic leukemia terminating in acute leukemia. *Arch Intern Med* 1977;137:1059-1064. **16**) Cameron S: Chlorambucil and leukemia. *N Eng J Med* 1977;296:1065. **17**) Lawler SD, Lele KP: Chromosomal damage induced by chlorambucil in chronic lymphocytic leukemia. *Scand J Haematol* 1972;9:603-612.**18**) Stevenson AC, Patel C: Effects of chlorambucil on human chromosomes. *Mutat Res* 1973;18:333-351. **19**) Guesry P, Lenoir G, Broyer M: Gonadal effects of chlorambucil given to prepubertal and pubertal boys for nephrotic syndrome. *J Pediatr*1978;92:299-303.**20**) Richter P, Calamera JC, Morgenfeld MC, et al: Effect of chlorambucil on spermatogenesis in the human with malignant lymphoma. *Cancer* 1970;25:1026-1030.**21**) Morgenfeld MC, Goldberg V, Parisier H, et al: Ovarian lesions due to cytostatic agents during the treatment of Hodgkin's disease. *Surg Gynecol Obstet*1972;134:826-828. **22**) Sobrinho LG, Levine RA, DeConti RC: Amenorrhea in patients with Hodgkin's disease treated with antineoplastic agents. *Am J Obstet Gynecol* 1971;109:135-139.**23**) Galton DAG, Israels LG, Nabarro JDN, et al: Clinical trials of p-(Di-2-chloroethylamino)-phenylbutyric acid (CB 1348) in malignant lymphoma.*Br Med J* 1955;2:1172-1176.**24**) Ciobanu N, Runowicz C, Gucalp R, et al: Reversible central nervous system toxicity associated with high-dose chlorambucil in autologous bone marrow transplantation for ovarian cancer. *Cancer Treat Rep*1987;71:1324-1325. **25**) Moore GE, Bross ID, Ausman R, et al: Effects of chlorambucil (NSC-3088) in 374 patients with advanced cancer.*Cancer Chemother Rep* 1968;52 (pt 1):661-666.**26**) Galton DA, Wiltshaw E, Szur L, et al: The use of chlorambucil and steroids in the treatment of chronic lymphocytic leukemia. *Br J Haematol*1961;7:73-98.**27**) Rudd P, Fries JF, Epstein WV: Irreversible bone marrow failure with chlorambucil.*J Rheumatol* 1975;2:421-429.**28**) Wolfson S, Olney MB: Accidental ingestion of a toxic dose of chlorambucil: Report of a case in a

REFERENCES: *(cont'd)*

child. *JAMA*1957;165:239-240.**29**) Byrne TN, Moseley TAE, Finer MA: Myoclonic seizures following chlorambucil overdose. *Ann Neurol*1981;9:191-194. **30**) LaDelfa I, Bayer N, Myers R, Hoffstein V: Chlorambucil-induced myoclonic seizures in an adult. *J Clin Oncol*1985;3:1691-1692. **31**) Naysmith A, Robson RH: Focal fits during chlorambucil therapy. *Postgrad Med J*1979;55:806-807.**32**) Blank DW, Nanji AA, Schreiber DH, et al: Acute renal failure and seizures associated with chlorambucil overdose.*J Toxicol Clin Toxicol* 1983;20:361-365.**33**) Ammenti A, Reitter B, Muller-Wiefel DE: Chlorambucil neurotoxicity: Report of two cases. *Helv Paediatr Acta* 1980;35:281-287.**34**) Green AA, Naiman JL: Chlorambucil poisoning. *Am J Dis Child*1968;116:190-191.**35**) Enck RE, Bennett JM: Inadvertent chlorambucil overdose in adults. *NY State J Med*1977;77:1480-1481.**36**) Knospe WH, Loeb V Jr, Huguley CM: Biweekly chlorambucil treatment of chronic lymphocytic leukemia. *Cancer*1974;33:555-562.**37**) Sawitsky A, Rai KR, Glidewell O, et al: Comparison of daily versus intermittent chlorambucil and prednisone therapy in the treatment of patients with chronic lymphocytic leukemia.*Blood* 1977;50:1049-1059.**38**) Recommendations for the safe handling of parenteral antineoplastic drugs. US Dept of Health and Human Services, publications No. (NIH) 83-2621. Government Printing Office, 1983. **39**) Council on Scientific Affairs: Guidelines for handling parenteral antineoplastic drugs. AMA COUNCIL REPORT. *JAMA* 1985;253:1590-1592. **40**) National Study Commission on Cytotoxic Exposure: Recommendations for Handling Cytotoxic Agents. (Available from L.P. Jeffrey, Director of Pharmacy Services, Rhode Island Hospital, 593 Eddy St, Providence, RI 02902.)**41**) Clinical Oncological Society of Australia: Guidelines and recommendations for safe handling of antineoplastic agents. *Med J Australia* 1983;1:426-428. **42**) Jones RB, Frank R, Mass T: Safe handling of chemotherapeutic agents: A report from the Mount Sinai Medical Center. *CA - A Cancer J for Clin* 1983;33:258-263.**43**) American Society of Hospital Pharmacists technical assistance bulletin on handling cytotoxic drugs in hospitals. *Am J Hosp Pharm* 1985;42:131-137.**44**) Yodaiken RE, Bennett D: OSHA work-practice guidelines for personnel dealing with cytotoxic (antineoplastic) drugs. *Am J Hosp Pharm* 1986;43:1193-1204.

HOW SUPPLIED - EQUIVALENTS NOT AVAILABLE:

Tablet, Plain Coated - Oral - 2 mg

50's	**$61.79**	**LEUKERAN, Glaxo Wellcome**	**00173-0635-35**

CHLORAMPHENICOL *(000717)*

CATEGORIES: Anti-Infectives; Antibiotics; Antimicrobials; Conjunctivitis; Corneal Injury; Dermatologicals; EENT Drugs; Eye, Ear, Nose, & Throat Preparations; Ocular Infections; Ophthalmics; Otic Preparations; Otologic; Skin/Mucous Membrane Agents; Lymphogranuloma*; Meningitis*; Rickettsial Disease*; Septicemia*; Uveitis*; FDA Approval Pre 1982
* Indication not approved by the FDA

BRAND NAMES: *Ak-Chlor* (Canada); *Alchlor*; Amphicol; *Aquamycetin* (Germany); *Archifen*; *Archifen Eye*; *Aromycetin*; *Bekamycetin*; *Biocaf*; *Biomycetin*; *Biophenicol*; *Cadimycetin*; *Cebenicol* (France); *Cetina* (Mexico); *Chemicetina*; *Chloment*; *Chlomin*; *Chlomy* (Japan); *Chlopen*; *Chloracil*; *Chloradrops*; *Chloramex*; *Chloramphenicol* (Germany); *Chloramphenicol "Agepha" Augensalbe*; *Chloramphenicol "Agepha" Ohrentropfen*; *Chloramphenicol Faure, Ophthadoses*; *Chloramphenicol PW Ohrentropfen* (Germany); *Chloramphenicol POS* (Germany); *Chloramphenicol RIT*; *Chloramsaar N* (Germany); *Cloranfenicol McKesson*; *Cloranfenicol N.T.*; *Chlorcol*; *Chlormycin*; *Chlornitromycin*; *Chlorocide*; *Chlorocort*; Chlorofair; **Chloromycetin**; *Chloromycetin Ear Drops* (Australia); *Chloromycetin Eye Drops*; *Chloromycetin Eye Ointment*; *Chloromycetin Eye Preparations*; *Chloromycetine*; *Chloromyxin*; *Chloromyxin Eye Preparation*; *Chloronitrin*; Chloroptic; *Chlorphen*; *Chlorsig*; *Chlorsig Eye Preparations*; *Clorafen* (Mexico); *Cloramfeni*; *Cloramfeni Ofteno* (Mexico); *Cloramfeni Ungena* (Mexico); *Cloramplast*; *Cloromicetin*; *Cloroptic*; *Cogetine*; *Colain*; *Colircusi Cloramfenicol*; *Compacol*; *Comycetin*; *Danmycetin*; *Denicol*; Econochlor; *Enclor*; *Enkacetyn*; *Farmicetina*; *Fen-Alcon*; *Fenicol* (Canada); *Genercin*; *Globenicol*; *Halomycetin Augensalbe*; *Helocetin*; *Heminevrin*; *Hinicol*; I-Chlor; *Ikamicetin*; Infa-Chlor; *Iprobiot*; *Isopto*; *Isopto Fenicol*; *Isotic Salmicol*; *Kemicetin Augensalbe*; *Kemicetine*; *Kemicetine Otologic*; *Kemicetine*; *Keromycin*; *Kimicetina*; *Kloramfenicol*; *Kloramfenikol*; *Kloramphenicol*; *Klorita*; *Leukomycin*; *Levomycetin*; *Metacol*; *Minims Chloramphenicol*; *Minims Eye Drops*; Mychel; *Newlolly*; *Novochlorocap* (Canada); Ocu-Chlor; *Oftan-Akvakol*; *Oleomycetin* (Germany); Ophthochlor; *Opticle*; Optomycin; *Paraxin* (Germany, Mexico); *Pharmacetin Otic*; *Quemicitina* (Mexico); *Reclor*; *Scanicol*; *Silmycetin*; *Sno Phenicol* (England); Spectro-Chlor; *Spersanicol*; *Suismycetin*; *Sunchlormycin*; *Suprachlor*; *Tifomycine* (France); *Troymycetin*; *Vanafen Otologic*; *Vanafen-S*; *Vanafen S*; *Vanmycetin*; *Vernacetin*; *Vitamycetin*; *Xepanicol*; *Ximex Avicol*
(International brand names outside U.S. in italics)

FORMULARIES: Aetna; BC-BS; Medi-Cal; WHO

DESCRIPTION:

Chloramphenicol Ophthalmic Solution, 0.5%, is a sterile, buffered solution containing 0.5% (5 mg/ml) of chloramphenicol. It contains no preservatives.

CLINICAL PHARMACOLOGY:

Chloramphenicol is a broad-spectrum antibiotic originally isolated from *Streptomyces venezuelae*. It is primarily bacteriostatic and acts by inhibition of protein synthesis by interfering with the transfer of activated amino acids from soluble RNA to ribosomes. It has been noted that chloramphenicol is found in measurable amounts in the aqueous humor following local application to the eye. Development of resistance to chloramphenicol can be regarded as minimal for staphylococci and many other species of bacteria.

INDICATIONS AND USAGE:

Chloramphenicol Ophthalmic Solution 0.5% is indicated for the treatment of superficial ocular infections involving the conjunctiva and/or cornea caused by chloramphenicol-susceptible organisms. Bacteriological studies should be performed to determine the causative organisms and their sensitivity to chloramphenicol.

CONTRAINDICATIONS:

This product is contraindicated in persons sensitive to any of its components.

WARNINGS:

Bone marrow hypoplasia including aplastic anemia and death has been reported following the local application of chloramphenicol.

PRECAUTIONS:

The prolonged use of antibiotics may occasionally result in overgrowth of nonsusceptible organisms, including fungi. If new infections appear during medication, the drug should be discontinued and appropriate measures should be taken. In all except very superficial infections the topical use of chloramphenicol should be supplemented by appropriate systemic medication.

ADVERSE REACTIONS:

Blood dyscrasias have been reported in association with the use of chloramphenicol (See WARNINGS).

DOSAGE AND ADMINISTRATION:

Two drops applied to the affected eye every three hours or more frequently if deemed advisable by the prescribing physician. Administration should be continued day and night for the first 48 hours, after which the interval between applications may be increased. Treatment should be continued for at least 48 hours after the eye appears normal.

HOW SUPPLIED - RATED THERAPEUTICALLY EQUIVALENT:

Capsule, Gelatin - Oral - 250 mg

100's	$36.80	Chloramphenicol, Zenith Labs	00172-2960-60
100's	$38.70	Chloramphenicol, H.C.F.A. F F P	99999-0717-01
100's	**$125.42**	**CHLOROMYCETIN, Parke-Davis**	**00071-0379-24**

Ointment - Ophthalmic - 1 %

3.5 gm	$2.44	INFA-CHLOR, Infinity Pharm	58154-0550-55
3.5 gm	$2.50	Chlorofair, Raway	00686-5550-55
3.5 gm	$4.50	AK-CHLOR, Akorn	17478-0280-35
3.5 gm	$5.90	Spectro-Chlor, Spectrum Scitfc	53268-0550-55
3.5 gm	$6.00	Chloramphenicol, Schein Pharm (US)	00364-7373-70
3.5 gm	**$12.50**	**CHLOROMYCETIN, Parke-Davis**	**00071-3070-07**
3.5 gm	$12.69	CHLOROPTIC SOP, Allergan	00023-0301-04

Solution - Ophthalmic - 0.5 %

2.5 ml	$0.95	Chloramphenicol, H.C.F.A. F F P	99999-0717-02
2.5 ml	$2.96	CHLOROPTIC, STERILE OPHTHALMIC, Allergan-Amer	11980-0109-03
7.5 ml	$1.64	I-CHLOR, Americal Pharm	54945-0511-09
7.5 ml	$2.95	Chloramphenicol, Rugby	00536-0405-77
7.5 ml	$3.06	Chloramphenicol, H.C.F.A. F F P	99999-0717-03
7.5 ml	$3.10	Chloramphenicol Ophthalmic, Goldline Labs	00182-1797-83
7.5 ml	$3.29	Chloramphenicol, Aligen Independ	00405-6030-07
7.5 ml	$3.33	Chloramphenicol, Steris Labs	00402-0766-07
7.5 ml	$3.50	Chloramphenicol Ophthalmic, Schein Pharm (US)	00364-7361-75
7.5 ml	$5.63	AK-CHLOR, Akorn	17478-0281-09
7.5 ml	$12.94	CHLOROPTIC, STERILE OPHTHALMIC, Allergan-Amer	11980-0109-08
15 ml	$4.86	Chloramphenicol, H.C.F.A. F F P	99999-0717-04
15 ml	$5.20	Chloramphenicol, Steris Labs	00402-0766-15
15 ml	$5.46	Chloramphenicol Ophthalmic, Schein Pharm (US)	00364-7361-72
15 ml	$5.52	Chloramphenicol, Rugby	00536-0405-72
15 ml	$5.56	AK-CHLOR, Akorn	17478-0281-12
15 ml	$9.96	OPHTHOCHLOR, Parke-Davis	00071-3395-11

HOW SUPPLIED - NOT RATED EQUIVALENT:

Powder - Ophthalmic - 25 mg/vial

kit	**$18.04**	**CHLOROMYCETIN, Parke-Davis**	**00071-3213-35**

Solution - Ophthalmic - 0.5 %

7.5 ml	$2.75	INFA-CHLOR, Infinity Pharm	58154-0690-03
7.5 ml	$5.90	SPECTRO CHLOR, Spectrum Scitfc	53268-0690-03
15 ml	$3.85	Infa-Chlor, Infinity Pharm	58154-0690-06
15 ml	$6.90	SPECTRO CHLOR, Spectrum Scitfc	53268-0690-12

Solution - Otic - 5 mg/ml

15 ml	**$22.09**	**CHLOROMYCETIN, Parke-Davis**	**00071-3313-35**

CHLORAMPHENICOL SODIUM SUCCINATE *(000718)*

CATEGORIES: Anti-Infectives; Antibiotics; Antimicrobials; Bacteremia; Chloramphenicol; Corneal Injury; Cystic Fibrosis; Infections; Lymphogranuloma; Meningitis; Ocular Infections; Rickettsial Disease; Septicemia; Typhoid Fever; Uveitis; FDA Approval Pre 1982

BRAND NAMES: *Acromaxfenicol*; *Berlicetin* (Germany); *Biophenicol*; *Cetina* (Mexico); *Chemicetina*; *Chloracil*; *Chloram-P*; *Chloramphen*; *Chloramphenicol*; *Chlorocide S*; *Chloromycetin* (England, Mexico, Canada); *Chloromycetin Injection*; **Chloromycetin Sodium Succinate**; *Chloromycetin Succinate Injection*; *Chloromycetine*; *Farmicetina*; *Globenicol*; *Helocetin*; *Kemicetin*; *Kemicetine* (England); *Kloramfenicol*; *Lyo-Hinicol*; Mychel-S; *Paraxin* (Germany); *Quemicetina* (Mexico); *Quemicetina Succinato*; *Ranphenicol*; *Solu-Paraxin*; *Synchlolim*; *Synthomycine Succinate*
(International brand names outside U.S. in italics)

> **WARNING:**
> Serious and fatal blood dyscrasias (aplastic anemia, hypoplastic anemia, thrombocytopenia, and granulocytopenia) are known to occur after the administration of chloramphenicol. In addition, there have been reports of aplastic anemia attributed to chloramphenicol which later terminated in leukemia. Blood dyscrasias have occurred after both short term and prolonged therapy with this drug. Chloramphenicol must not be used when less potentially dangerous agents will be effective, as described in the indications section. IT MUST NOT BE USED IN THE TREATMENT OF TRIVIAL INFECTIONS OR WHERE IT IS NOT INDICATED, AS IN COLDS, INFLUENZA, INFECTIONS OF THE THROAT; OR AS A PROPHYLACTIC AGENT TO PREVENT BACTERIAL INFECTIONS.
> **Precautions:** It is essential that adequate blood studies be made during treatment with the drug. While blood studies may detect early peripheral blood changes, such as leukopenia, reticulocytopenia, or granulocytopenia, before they become irreversible, such studies cannot be relied on to detect bone marrow depression prior to development of aplastic anemia. To facilitate appropriate studies and observation during therapy, it is desirable that patients be hospitalized.

DESCRIPTION:

IMPORTANT CONSIDERATIONS IN PRESCRIBING INJECTABLE CHLORAMPHENICOL SODIUM SUCCINATE

CHLORAMPHENICOL SODIUM SUCCINATE IS INTENDED FOR INTRAVENOUS USE ONLY. IT HAS BEEN DEMONSTRATED TO BE INEFFECTIVE WHEN GIVEN INTRAMUSCULARLY.

1. Chloramphenicol sodium succinate must be hydrolyzed to its microbiologically active form and there is a lag in achieving adequate blood levels compared with the base given intravenously.

DESCRIPTION: *(cont'd)*

2. The oral form of chloramphenicol is readily absorbed and adequate blood levels are achieved and maintained on the recommended dosage.

3. Patients started on intravenous chloramphenicol sodium succinate should be changed to the oral form as soon as practicable.

Chloramphenicol is an antibiotic that is clinically useful for, *and should be reserved for,* serious infections caused by organisms susceptible to its antimicrobial effects when less potentially hazardous therapeutic agents are ineffective or contraindicated. Sensitivity testing is essential to determine its indicated use, but may be performed concurrently with therapy initiated on clinical impression that one of the indicated conditions exists (see INDICATIONS AND USAGE).

Each gram (10 ml of a 10% solution) of chloramphenicol sodium succinate contains approximately 52 mg (2.25 mEq) of sodium.

CLINICAL PHARMACOLOGY:

In vitro chloramphenicol exerts mainly a bacteriostatic effect on a wide range of gram-negative and gram-positive bacteria and is active*in vitro* against rickettsias, the lymphogranuloma-psittacosis group and *Vibrio cholerae.* It is particularly active against *Salmonella typhi* and *Haemophilus influenzae.* The mode of action is through interference or inhibition of protein synthesis in intact cells and in cell-free systems.

Chloramphenicol administered orally is absorbed rapidly from the intestinal tract. In controlled studies in adult volunteers using the recommended dosage of 50 mg/kg/day, a dosage of 1 g every 6 hours for 8 doses was given. Using the microbiological assay method, the average peak serum level was 11.2 mcg/ml one hour after the first dose. A cumulative effect gave a peak rise to 18.4 mcg/ml after the fifth dose of 1 g. Mean serum levels ranged from 8 to 14 mcg/ml over the 48-hour period. Total urinary excretion of chloramphenicol in these studies ranged from a low of 68% to a high of 99% over a three-day period. From 8% to 12% of the antibiotic excreted is in the form of free chloramphenicol; the remainder consists of microbiologically inactive metabolites, principally the conjugate with glucuronic acid. Since the glucuronide is excreted rapidly, most chloramphenicol detected in the blood is in the microbiologically active free form. Despite the small proportion of unchanged drug excreted in the urine, the concentration of free chloramphenicol is relatively high, amounting to several hundred mcg/ml in patients receiving divided doses of 50 mg/kg/day. Small amounts of active drug are found in bile and feces. Chloramphenicol diffuses rapidly, but its distribution is not uniform. Highest concentrations are found in liver and kidney, and lowest concentrations are found in brain and cerebrospinal fluid. Chloramphenicol enters cerebrospinal fluid even in the absence of meningeal inflammation, appearing in concentrations about half of those found in the blood. Measurable levels are also detected in pleural and in ascitic fluids, saliva, milk and in the aqueous and vitreous humors. Transport across the placental barrier occurs with somewhat lower concentration in cord blood of newborn infants than in maternal blood.

INDICATIONS AND USAGE:

In accord with the concepts in the BOXED WARNING and INDICATIONS AND USAGE, chloramphenicol must be used only in those serious infections for which less potentially dangerous drugs are ineffective or contraindicated. However, chloramphenicol may be chosen to initiate antibiotic therapy on the clinical impression that one of the conditions below is believed to be present: *in vitro* sensitivity tests should be performed concurrently so that the drug may be discontinued as soon as possible if less potentially dangerous agents are indicated by such tests. The decision to continue use of chloramphenicol rather than another antibiotic when both are suggested by *in vitro* studies to be effective against a specific pathogen should be based upon severity of the infection, susceptibility of the pathogen to the various antimicrobial drugs, efficacy of the various drugs in the infection, and the important additional concepts contained in the BOXED WARNING:

ACUTE INFECTIONS CAUSED BY *SALMONELLA TYPHI**

It is not recommended for the routine treatment of the typhoid carrier state.

*In the treatment of typhoid fever some authorities recommend that chloramphenicol be administered at therapeutic levels for 8 to 10 days after the patient has become afebrile to lessen the possibility of relapse.

Serious infections caused by susceptible strains in accordance with the concepts expressed above:

a) *Salmonella* species

b) *H. influenzae,* specifically meningeal infections

c) *Rickettsia*

d) Lymphogranuloma-psittacosis group

e) Various gram-negative bacteria causing bacteremia, meningitis or other serious gram-negative infections.

f) Other susceptible organisms which have been demonstrated to be resistant to all other appropriate antimicrobial agents.

Cystic fibrosis regimens

CONTRAINDICATIONS:

Chloramphenicol is contraindicated in individuals with a history of previous hypersensitivity and/or toxic reaction to it. *It must not be used in the treatment of trivial infections or where it is not indicated, as in colds, influenza, infections of the throat; or as a prophylactic agent to prevent bacterial infection.*

PRECAUTIONS:

1. Baseline blood studies should be followed by periodic blood studies approximately every two days during therapy. The drug should be discontinued upon appearance of reticulocytopenia, leukopenia, thrombocytopenia, anemia, or any other blood study findings attributable to chloramphenicol. However, it should be noted that such studies do not exclude the possible later appearance of the irreversible type of bone marrow depression.

2. Repeated courses of the drug should be avoided if at all possible. Treatment should not be continued longer than required to produce a cure with little or no risk of relapse of the disease.

3. Concurrent therapy with other drugs that may cause bone marrow depression should be avoided.

4. Excessive blood levels may result from administration of the recommended dose to patients with impaired liver or kidney function, including that due to immature metabolic processes in the infant. The dosage should be adjusted accordingly or, preferably, the blood concentration should be determined at appropriate intervals.

5. There are no studies to establish the safety of this drug in pregnancy.

6. Since chloramphenicol readily crosses the placental barrier, caution in use of the drug is particularly important during pregnancy at term or during labor because of potential toxic effects on the fetus (gray syndrome).

PRECAUTIONS: *(cont'd)*

7. Precaution should be used in therapy of premature and full-term infants to avoid "gray syndrome" toxicity (see ADVERSE REACTIONS). Serum drug levels should be carefully followed during therapy of the newborn infant.

8. Precaution should be used in therapy during lactation because of the possibility of toxic effects on the nursing infant.

9. The use of this antibiotic, as with other antibiotics, may result in an overgrowth of nonsusceptible organisms, including fungi. If infections caused by nonsusceptible organisms appear during therapy, appropriate measures should be taken.

ADVERSE REACTIONS:

Blood Dyscrasias: The most serious adverse effect of chloramphenicol is bone marrow depression. Serious and fatal blood dyscrasias (aplastic anemia, hypoplastic anemia, thrombocytopenia, and granulocytopenia) are known to occur after the administration of chloramphenicol. An irreversible type of marrow depression leading to aplastic anemia with a high rate of mortality is characterized by the appearance weeks or months after therapy of bone marrow aplasia or hypoplasia. Peripherally, pancytopenia is most often observed, but in a small number of cases only one or two of the three major cell types (erythrocytes, leukocytes, platelets) may be depressed.

A reversible type of bone marrow depression, which is dose related, may occur. This type of marrow depression is characterized by vacuolization of the erythroid cells, reduction of reticulocytes and leukopenia, and responds promptly to the withdrawal of chloramphenicol.

An exact determination of the risk of serious and fatal blood dyscrasias is not possible because of lack of accurate information regarding 1) the size of the population at risk, 2) the total number of drug-associated dyscrasias, and 3) the total number of non-drug associated dyscrasias.

In a report to the California State Assembly by the California Medical Association and the State Department of Public Health in January 1967, the risk of fatal aplastic anemia was estimated at 1:24,200 to 1:40,500 based on two dosage levels.

There have been reports of aplastic anemia attributed to chloramphenicol which later terminated in leukemia.

Paroxysmal nocturnal hemoglobinuria has also been reported.

Gastrointestinal Reactions: Nausea, vomiting, glossitis and stomatitis, diarrhea and enterocolitis may occur in low incidence.

Neurotoxic Reactions: Headache, mild depression, mental confusion and delirium have been described in patients receiving chloramphenicol. Optic and peripheral neuritis have been reported, usually following long-term therapy. If this occurs, the drug should be promptly withdrawn.

Hypersensitivity Reactions: Fever, macular and vesicular rashes, angioedema, urticaria and anaphylaxis may occur. Herxheimer reactions have occurred during therapy for typhoid fever.

"Gray Syndrome": Toxic reactions including fatalities have occurred in the premature and newborn; the signs and symptoms associated with these reactions have been referred to as the gray syndrome. One case of gray syndrome has been reported in an infant born to a mother having received chloramphenicol during labor. One case has been reported in a 3-month-old infant. The following summarizes the clinical and laboratory studies that have been made on these patients:

a) In most cases therapy with chloramphenicol had been instituted within the first 48 hours of life.

b) Symptoms first appeared after 3 to 4 days of continued treatment with high doses of chloramphenicol.

c) The symptoms appeared in the following order:

(1) abdominal distention with or without emesis;

(2) progressive pallid cyanosis;

(3) vasomotor collapse, frequently accompanied by irregular respiration;

(4) death within a few hours of onset of these symptoms.

d) The progression of symptoms from onset to exitus was accelerated with higher dose schedules.

e) Preliminary blood serum level studies revealed unusually high concentrations of chloramphenicol (over 90 mcg/ml after repeated doses).

f) Termination of therapy upon early evidence of the associated symptomatology frequently reversed the process with complete recovery.

DOSAGE AND ADMINISTRATION:

ADMINISTRATION

Chloramphenicol, like other potent drugs, should be prescribed at recommended doses known to have therapeutic activity. Administration of 50 mg/kg/day in divided doses will produce blood levels of the magnitude to which the majority of susceptible microorganisms will respond.

As soon as feasible an oral dosage form of chloramphenicol should be substituted for the intravenous form because adequate blood levels are achieved with chloramphenicol by mouth.

The following method of administration is recommended:

Intravenously as a 10% (100 mg/ml) solution to be injected over at least a one-minute interval. This is prepared by the addition of 10 ml of an aqueous diluent such as water for injection or 5% dextrose injection.

DOSAGE

Adults: Adults should receive 50 mg/kg/day in divided doses at 6-hour intervals. In exceptional cases patients with infections due to moderately resistant organisms may require increased dosage up to 100 mg/kg/day to achieve blood levels inhibiting the pathogen, but these high doses should be decreased as soon as possible. Adults with impairment of hepatic or renal function or both may have reduced ability to metabolize and excrete the drug. In instances of impaired metabolic processes, dosages should be adjusted accordingly. (See Newborn Infants.)Precise control of concentration of the drug in the blood should be carefully followed in patients with impaired metabolic processes by the available microtechniques (information available on request).

Children: Dosage of 50 mg/kg/day divided into 4 doses at 6-hour intervals yields blood levels in the range effective against most susceptible organisms. Severe infections (*e.g.,* bacteremia or meningitis), especially when adequate cerebrospinal fluid concentrations are desired, may require dosage up to 100 mg/kg/day; however, it is recommended that dosage be reduced to 50 mg/kg/day as soon as possible. Children with impaired liver or kidney function may retain excessive amounts of the drug.

Newborn Infants: See ADVERSE REACTIONS, Gray Syndrome.

A total of 25 mg/kg/day in 4 equal doses at 6-hour intervals usually produces and maintains concentrations in blood and tissues adequate to control most infections for which the drug is indicated. Increased dosage in these individuals, demanded by severe infections, should be given only to maintain the blood concentration within a therapeutically effective range. After the first two weeks of life, full-term infants ordinarily may receive up to a total of 50 mg/kg/

DOSAGE AND ADMINISTRATION: *(cont'd)*
day equally divided into 4 doses at 6-hour intervals. *These dosage recommendations are extremely important because blood concentration in all premature infants and full-term infants under two weeks of age differs from that of other infants.* This difference is due to variations in the maturity of the metabolic functions of the liver and the kidneys.

When these functions are immature (or seriously impaired in adults), high concentrations of the drug are found which tend to increase with succeeding doses.

Infants and Children with Immature Metabolic Processes: In young infants and other children in whom immature metabolic functions are suspected, a dose of 25 mg/kg/day will usually produce therapeutic concentrations of the drug in the blood. In this group particularly, the concentration of the drug in the blood should be carefully followed by microtechniques. (Information available on request.)

HOW SUPPLIED - RATED THERAPEUTICALLY EQUIVALENT:

Injection, Lyphl-Soln - Intravenous - 10 %

1 gm	**$41.48**	**CHLOROMYCETIN SODIUM SUCCINATE, Parke-Davis**	**00071-4057-03**
15 ml	$52.13	Chloramphenicol Sodium Succinate, Fujisawa USA	00469-1100-90

CHLORAMPHENICOL; DESOXYRIBONUCLEASE; FIBRINOLYSIN

(000719)

CATEGORIES: Anti-Infectives; Antibiotics; Dermatologicals; Enzymes & Digestants; Fibrinolytic & Proteolytic; Mucous Membrane Agents; Skin/Mucous Membrane Agents; FDA Approval Pre 1982

BRAND NAMES: *Clorelase*; **Elase-Chloromycetin**; *Fibrase* (Mexico)
(International brand names outside U.S. in italics)

FORMULARIES: BC-BS

DESCRIPTION:

Elase-Chloromycetin Ointment contains two lytic enzymes, fibrinolysin and desoxyribonuclease, combined with chloramphenicol in an ointment base.

The fibrinolysin component is derived from bovine plasma[1,2] and the desoxyribonuclease is isolated in a purified form from bovine pancreas.

The fibrinolysin used in the combination is activated by chloroform.

Chloramphenicol is a broad-spectrum antibiotic originally isolated from*Streptomyces venezuelae*. It is therapeutically active against a wide variety of susceptible organisms, both gram-positive and gram-negative. Chemically, chloramphenicol may be identified as D(-)-*threo*-1-*p*-nitrophenyl-2-dichloroacetamido-1,3-propanediol.

CLINICAL PHARMACOLOGY:

Combination of the two lytic enzymes is based on the observation that purulent exudates consist largely of fibrinous material and nucleoprotein. Desoxyribonuclease attacks the desoxyribonucleic acid (DNA) and fibrinolysin attacks principally fibrin of blood clots and fibrinous exudates.

The activity of desoxyribonuclease is limited principally to the production of large polynucleotides,[3] which are less likely to be absorbed than the more diffusible protein fractions liberated by certain enzyme preparations obtained from bacteria. The fibrinolytic action of Elase is directed mainly against denatured proteins, such as those found in devitalized tissue, while protein elements of living cells remain relatively unaffected.

Elase-Chloromycetin Ointment contains a combination of active enzymes. This is an important consideration in treating patients suffering from lesions resulting from impaired circulation.

Chloramphenicol is a broad-spectrum antibiotic that is primarily bacteriostatic and acts by inhibition of protein synthesis by interfering with the transfer of activated amino acids from soluble RNA to ribosomes. Development of resistance to chloramphenicol can be regarded as minimal for staphylococci and many other species of bacteria.

The action of Elase-Chloromycetin helps to produce clean surfaces and thus supports healing in a variety of exudative lesions.

INDICATIONS AND USAGE:

Elase-Chloromycetin Ointment is indicated for use in the treatment of infected lesions such as burns, ulcers and wounds where the actions of both a debriding agent and a topical antibiotic are desired. This dual-purpose approach is especially useful in the treatment of infections caused by organisms that utilize a process of fibrin deposition as protective device (*i.e.,* coagulase and the staphylococcus). Appropriate measures should be taken to determine the susceptibility of the pathogen to chloramphenicol.

CONTRAINDICATIONS:

This drug is contraindicated in individuals with a history of hypersensitivity reactions to any of its components.

WARNINGS:

Bone marrow hypoplasia including aplastic anemia and death has been reported following the local application of chloramphenicol.

PRECAUTIONS:

The prolonged use of antibiotics may occasionally result in overgrowth of nonsusceptible organisms, including fungi. If new infections appear during medication, the drug should be discontinued and appropriate measures should be taken.

In all except very superficial infections, the topical use of chloramphenicol should be supplemented by appropriate systemic medication.

The usual precautions against allergic reactions should be observed, particularly in persons with a history of sensitivity to materials of bovine origin.

ADVERSE REACTIONS:

Signs of local irritation, with subjective symptoms of itching or burning, angioneurotic edema, urticaria, vesicular and maculopapular dermatitis have been reported in patients sensitive to chloramphenicol and are causes for discontinuing the medication. Similar sensitivity reactions to other materials in topical preparations may also occur. Blood dyscrasias have been associated with the use of chloramphenicol.

Side effects attributable to the enzymes have not been a problem at the dose and for the indications recommended herein. With higher concentrations, side effects have been minimal, consisting of local hyperemia.

ADVERSE REACTIONS: *(cont'd)*
Chills and fever attributable to antigenic action of profibrinolysin activators of bacterial origin are not a problem with Elase-Chloromycetin.

DOSAGE AND ADMINISTRATION:

Since the conditions for which Elase-Chloromycetin is helpful vary considerably in severity, dosage must be adjusted to the individual case; however, the following general recommendations can be made:

Successful use of enzymatic debridement depends on several factors: (1) dense, dry eschar, if present, should be removed surgically before enzymatic debridement is attempted; (2) the enzyme must be in constant contact with the substrate; (3) accumulated necrotic debris must be periodically removed; (4) the enzyme must be replenished at least once daily; and (5) secondary closure or skin grafting must be employed as soon as possible after optimal debridement has been attained. It is further essential that wound-dressing techniques be performed carefully under aseptic conditions and that appropriate systemically acting antibiotics be administered concomitantly if, in the opinion of the physician, they are indicated. Local application should be repeated at intervals as long as enzymatic action is desired, since the enzymatic activity becomes progressively less after application, and probably is exhausted for practical purposes twenty-four hours after being applied.

Storage: Store at no warmer than 30°C (86°F).

REFERENCES:

1. Seegers WH, Loomis EC: *Science* 104:461, 1946. **2.** Loomis EC, George C Jr, Ryder A: *Arch Biochem* 12:1, 1947. **3.** Smith JD, Markham R: *Biochem et Biophys Acta*8:350, 1952. **4.** Christensen LR: *J Clin Invest* 28:163, 1949.

HOW SUPPLIED:

Elase-Chloromycetin (fibrinolysin-desoxyribonuclease-chloramphenicol) is supplied in 30-g and 10-g ointment tubes. The 10-g tubes have an elongated nozzle to facilitate the application to surface lesions.

Elase-Chloromycetin Ointment, 30-gram.

The 30-g tubes contain 30 units (Loomis) of fibrinolysin (bovine), 20,000 units* of desoxyribonuclease, and 0.3 g** chloramphenicol in a special ointment base of liquid petrolatum and polyethylene.

Elase-Chloromycetin Ointment, 10-gram.

The 10-g tubes contain 10 units (Loomis) of fibrinolysin (bovine), 6,666 units* of desoxyribonuclease, and 0.1 g** chloramphenicol in a special ointment base of liquid petrolatum and polyethylene.

The ointment contains sodium chloride and sucrose used in its manufacture.

*Modified Christensen method.[4]

**10 mg chloramphenicol per gram, or 1%.

HOW SUPPLIED - EQUIVALENTS NOT AVAILABLE:

Ointment - Topical

10 gm	**$17.05**	**ELASE-CHLOROMYCETIN, Fujisawa Pharm (US)**	**57317-0021-12**
30 gm	**$37.45**	**ELASE-CHLOROMYCETIN, Fujisawa Pharm (US)**	**57317-0023-77**

CHLORAMPHENICOL; HYDROCORTISONE ACETATE; POLYMYXIN B SULFATE *(000721)*

CATEGORIES: Anti-Infectives; Antibiotics; Burns; Conjunctivitis; Corneal Injury; EENT Drugs; Eye, Ear, Nose, & Throat Preparations; Inflammation; Inflammatory Conditions; Ocular Infections; Otic Hydrocortisones; Otic Preparations; Otologic; Steroids; Uveitis; FDA Approval Pre 1982

BRAND NAMES: **Ophthocort**

WARNING:
Bone marrow hypoplasia including aplastic anemia and death has been reported following local application of chloramphenicol. Chloramphenicol should not be used when less potentially dangerous agents would be expected to provide effective treatment.

DESCRIPTION:

Ophthocort (Chloramphenicol, Polymyxin B Sulfate, and Hydrocortisone Acetate Ophthalmic Ointment, USP) is a sterile antibiotic/antiinflammatory ointment for ophthalmic administration. Each gram of Ophthocort contains 10 mg chloramphenicol, 10,000 units polymyxin B (as the sulfate), and 5 mg hydrocortisone acetate in a special base of liquid petrolatum and polyethylene. It contains no preservatives.

The chemical names for chloramphenicol are:

(1) Acetamide, 2,2-dichloro-N-(2-hydroxy-1-(hydroxymethyl)-2-(4-nitrophenyl) ethyl)-, and

(2) D- *threo*-(-)-2,2-Dichloro-N-(β-hydroxy-α-(hydroxymethyl)- *p*-nitrophenethyl) acetamide

The chemical names for hydrocortisone acetate are:

(1) Pregn-4-ene-3,20-dione,21-(acetyloxy)-11,17-dihydroxy-,(11β)-, and

(2) 17-Hydroxycorticosterone 21-acetate.

Polymyxin B sulfate is the sulfate salt of an antibiotic substance elaborated by various strains of *Bacillus polymyxa*.

Polymyxin B_1:R = (+)-6-Methyloctanoyl

Polymyxin B_2:R = 6-Methylheptanoyl

DAB = $_{\alpha,\gamma}$Diaminobutyric Acid

CLINICAL PHARMACOLOGY:

Corticoids suppress the inflammatory response to a variety of agents and they probably delay or slow healing. Since corticoids may inhibit the body's defense mechanism against infection, a concomitant antimicrobial drug may be used when this inhibition is considered to be clinically significant in a particular case.

The antiinfective components in this combination are included to provide action against specific organisms susceptible to them. Chloramphenicol is considered active against a wide spectrum of gram-negative and gram-positive organisms such as *Escherichia coli, Haemophilus influenzae, Staphylococcus aureus, Streptococcus hemolyticus,* and *Moraxella lacunata* (Morax-Axenfeld bacillus). Development of resistance to chloramphenicol can be regarded as minimal for staphylococci and many other species of bacteria.

CLINICAL PHARMACOLOGY: *(cont'd)*

Chloramphenicol is primarily bacteriostatic and acts by inhibition of protein synthesis by interfering with the transfer of activated amino acids from soluble RNA to ribosomes. It has been noted that chloramphenicol is found in measurable amounts in the aqueous humor following local application to the eye.

Polymyxin B sulfate has a bactericidal action against almost all gram-negative bacilli except the *Proteus* group. All gram-positive bacteria, fungi, and the gram-negative cocci, *Neisseria gonorrhoeae* and *N. meningitidis*, are resistant.

When a decision to administer both a corticoid and an antimicrobial is made, the administration of such drugs in combination has the advantage of greater patient compliance and convenience, with the added assurance that the appropriate dosage of both drugs is administered, plus assured compatibility of ingredients when both types of drug are in the same formulation and, particularly, that the correct volume of drug is delivered and retained.

The relative potency of corticosteroids depends on the molecular structure, concentration, and release from the vehicle.

INDICATIONS AND USAGE:

Chloramphenicol should be used only in those serious infections for which less potentially dangerous drugs are ineffective or contraindicated. Bacteriological studies should be performed to determine the causative organisms and their sensitivity to chloramphenicol (see BOXED WARNING).

For steroid-responsive inflammatory ocular conditions for which a corticosteroid is indicated and where bacterial infection or a risk of bacterial ocular infection exists.

Ocular steroids are indicated in inflammatory conditions of the palpebral and bulbar conjunctiva, cornea, and anterior segment of the globe where the inherent risk of steroid use in certain infective conjunctivitises is accepted to obtain a diminution in edema and inflammation. They are also indicated in chronic anterior uveitis and corneal injury from chemical radiation, thermal burns, or penetration of foreign bodies.

The use of a combination drug with an antiinfective component is indicated where the risk of infection is high or where there is an expectation that potentially dangerous numbers of bacteria will be present in the eye.

The particular antiinfective drugs in this product are active against the following common bacterial eye pathogens:

Staphylococcus aureus	*Klebsiella/Enterobacterspecies*
Streptococci, includ. *Streptococcus pneumoniae species*	*Neisseria species*
Escherichia coli	*Moraxella lacunata*
Haemophilus influenzae	(*Morax-Axenfeld bacillus*)
	Pseudomonas aeruginosa

The product does not provide adequate coverage against:

Serratia marcescens

CONTRAINDICATIONS:

Epithelial herpes simplex keratitis (dendritic keratitis), vaccinia, varicella, and many other viral diseases of the cornea and conjunctiva. Mycobacterial infection of the eye. Fungal diseases of ocular structures. Hypersensitivity to a component of the medication. (Hypersensitivity to the antibiotic component occurs at a higher rate than for other components.)

The use of these combinations is always contraindicated after uncomplicated removal of a corneal foreign body.

WARNINGS:

See BOXED WARNING.

Prolonged use of steroids may result in glaucoma, with damage to the optic nerve, defects in visual acuity and fields of vision, and posterior subcapsular cataract formation. Prolonged use may suppress the host response and thus increase the hazard of secondary ocular infections. In those diseases causing thinning of the cornea or sclera, perforations have been known to occur with the use of topical steroids. In acute purulent conditions of the eye, steroids may mask infection or enhance existing infection. If these products are used for 10 days or longer, intraocular pressure should be routinely monitored even though it may be difficult in children and uncooperative patients.

Employment of steroid medication in the treatment of herpes simplex requires great caution.

Ophthalmic ointments may retard corneal wound healing.

PRECAUTIONS:

The initial prescription and renewal of the medication order beyond 8 grams should be made by a physician only after examination of the patient with the aid of magnification, such as slit lamp biomicroscopy and, where appropriate, fluorescein staining.

The possibility of persistent fungal infections of the cornea should be considered after prolonged steroid dosing.

The prolonged use of antibiotics may occasionally result in overgrowth of nonsusceptible organisms, including fungi. If new infections appear during medication, the drug should be discontinued and appropriate measures should be taken.

In all serious infections the topical use of chloramphenicol should be supplemented by appropriate systemic medication.

ADVERSE REACTIONS:

There have been reports of punctate staining of the cornea following intensive treatment (every one to two hours during the waking day) of corneal ulcers with Ophthocort. In each reported case, the staining has disappeared after discontinuation of the medication.

Blood dyscrasias have been reported in association with the use of chloramphenicol. (See WARNINGS.)

Adverse reactions have occurred with steroid/antiinfective combination drugs which can be attributed to the steroid component, the antiinfective component, or the combination. Exact incidence figures are not available since no denominator of treated patients is available.

Reactions occurring most often from the presence of the antiinfective ingredient are allergic sensitizations. The reactions due to the steroid component in decreasing order of frequency are: elevation of intraocular pressure (IOP) with possible development of glaucoma, and infrequent optic nerve damage; posterior subcapsular cataract formation; and delayed wound healing.

Secondary Infection: The development of secondary infection has occurred after use of combinations containing steroids and antimicrobials. Fungal infections of the cornea are particularly prone to develop coincidentally with long-term applications of steroid. The possibility of fungal invasion must be considered in any persistent corneal ulceration where steroid treatment has been used.

Secondary bacterial ocular infection following suppression of host responses also occurs.

DOSAGE AND ADMINISTRATION:

Application of a small amount of ointment, placed in the lower conjunctival sac, is made to the affected eye every three hours, or more frequently if deemed advisable by the prescribing physician. Administration should be continued day and night for the first 48 hours, after which the interval between applications may be increased. Treatment should be continued for at least 48 hours after the eye appears normal.

Not more than 8 grams should be prescribed initially and the prescription should not be refilled without further evaluation as outlined in Precautions above.

HOW SUPPLIED - EQUIVALENTS NOT AVAILABLE:

Ointment - Ophthalmic - 10 mg/5 mg

3.5 gm	$15.22	OPHTHOCORT, Parke-Davis	00071-3079-07

CHLORCYCLIZINE HYDROCHLORIDE; HYDROCORTISONE ACETATE *(000725)*

CATEGORIES: Anti-Inflammatory Agents; Antipruritics/Local Anesthetics; Dermatitis; Dermatologicals; Eczema; Insect Bites; Pruritus; Skin/Mucous Membrane Agents; Steroids; Pregnancy Category C; FDA Pre 1938 Drugs

BRAND NAMES: **Mantadil**

DESCRIPTION:

Mantadil Cream contains the antihistamine chlorcyclizine hydrochloride 2% and the corticosteroid hydrocortisone acetate 0.5%, with methylparaben 0.25% (added as a preservative) in a vanishing cream base. The active ingredients are liquid and white petrolatum, emulsifying wax and purified water.

Mantadil Cream is an antipruritic-anti-inflammatory-anesthetic for topical administration.

Chlorcyclizine hydrochloride is known chemically as 1-[(4-chlorophenyl)-phenylmethyl]-4-methylpiperazine monohydrochloride.

Hydrocortisone acetate is the acetate ester of cortisol, known chemically as 21-(acetyloxy)-11β,17-dihydroxypregn-4-ene-3,20 dione.

The pH of this product is approximately 4.5.

CLINICAL PHARMACOLOGY:

Chlorcyclizine hydrochloride is an H_1, histamine-receptor antagonist that will occupy receptor sites in effector cells to the exclusion of histamine. It blocks most of the effects of histamine mediated by H_1 receptors, including contraction of smooth muscle and increased capillary permeability. Absorption of chlorcyclizine hydrochloride into the skin is rapid following topical application, whereas systemic absorption from the skin is minimal. Chlorcyclizine hydrochloride prevents local edema and provides local anesthetic and antipruritic action in the skin.

Hydrocortisone acetate administered topically suppresses most inflammatory and allergic responses in the skin. Following topical application, it is absorbed rapidly into the skin, where it reduces local heat, redness, swelling, and tenderness. A small part of the dose applied to broken skin is absorbed systemically and metabolized by the liver.

INDICATIONS AND USAGE:

Mantadil Cream is indicated for the treatment of pruritic skin eruptions and other dermatoses including: eczema (allergic, nuchal and nummular); dermatitis (atopic, lichenoid and seborrheic); contact dermatitis including poison ivy, poison oak and poison sumac; localized neurodermatitis; insect bites; sunburn; intertrigo; and anogenital pruritus.

CONTRAINDICATIONS:

This preparation is contraindicated in patients who are hypersensitive to any of its components; in tuberculosis of the skin, vaccinia, varicella, and herpes simplex. As with other topical products containing hydrocortisone, the cream should not be used in bacterial infections of the skin unless antibacterial therapy is concomitant.

Not for ophthalmic use.

WARNINGS:

Oral chlorcyclizine is teratogenic in animals. Long-term reproduction studies of topical chlorcyclizine have not been conducted in humans.

PRECAUTIONS:

General: If signs of irritation develop with use of this cream, treatment should be discontinued and appropriate therapy instituted.

Any of the side effects reported following systemic use of corticosteroids, including adrenal suppression, may also occur following their topical use, especially in infants and children. Systemic absorption of topically applied steroids will be increased if extensive body surface areas are treated or if the occlusive technique is used. Under these circumstances, suitable precautions should be taken when long-term use is anticipated, particularly in infants and children.

Carcinogenesis, Mutagenesis, and Impairment of Fertility: Oral chlorcyclizine is teratogenic in animals. Long-term reproduction studies of topical chlorcyclizine have not been conducted. It is poorly absorbed percutaneously.

Pregnancy, Teratogenic Effects, Pregnancy Category C: Animal reproduction studies have not been conducted with Mantadil Cream. It is also not known whether Mantadil Cream can cause fetal harm when administered to a pregnant woman or can affect reproduction capacity. Mantadil Cream should be given to a pregnant woman only if clearly needed.

Nursing Mothers: Hydrocortisone acetate appears in human milk following oral administration of the drug.

Caution should be exercised when hydrocortisone acetate is administered to a nursing woman.

It is not known whether chlorcyclizine hydrochloride is excreted in human milk. Because many drugs are excreted in human milk, caution should be exercised when chlorcyclizine hydrochloride is administered to a nursing woman.

ADVERSE REACTIONS:

Allergic contact dermatitis may occur with topical application of chlorcyclizine hydrochloride. Systemic side effects have been reported after topical application of antihistamines to large areas of skin.

The following local adverse reactions have been reported with topical corticosteroids, especially under occlusive dressings: irritation, folliculitis, hypertrichosis, acneiform eruptions, hypopigmentation, allergic contact dermatitis, secondary infection, skin atrophy, striae and miliaria.

OVERDOSAGE:

With continued application of topical corticosteroid on large areas of damaged skin and under occlusion, there is a remote possibility that sufficient absorption could occur to produce Cushing's syndrome. This is more likely in children.

Systemic toxicity following topical application of chlorcyclizine has never been reported.

The oral LD_{50} of chlorcyclizine hydrochloride in the mouse is 300 mg/kg.

The intraperitoneal LD_{50} of hydrocortisone acetate in the mouse is 2300 mg/kg.

DOSAGE AND ADMINISTRATION:

Apply to the skin two to five times daily. If the condition of the skin will permit, the cream should be well rubbed in.

HOW SUPPLIED:

Mantadil Cream (Chlorcyclizine hydrochloride 2% and hydrocortisone acetate 0.5%) is available in 15 gram tubes.

Store at 15° to 25°C (59° to 77°F).

HOW SUPPLIED - EQUIVALENTS NOT AVAILABLE:

Cream - Topical - 2 %/0.5 %

15 gm $20.22 MANTADIL, Glaxo Wellcome 00173-0650-94

CHLORDIAZEPOXIDE HYDROCHLORIDE

(000726)

CATEGORIES: Alcoholism; Analeptics; Anesthesia; Antianxiety Drugs; Anxiety; Anxiolytics, Sedatives, Hypnotic; Benzodiazepines; Central Nervous System Agents; Tension; Tranquilizers; DEA Class CIV; FDA Approval Pre 1982

BRAND NAMES: *Apo-Chlordiazepoxide* (Canada); *Arsitran*; *Balance* (Japan); *Benpine*; *Benzodiapin*; CDP; *Cetabrium*; Chlordiazachel; *Chlordiazepoxidum*; *Chuichin*; *Contol* (Japan); *Diazebrum*; *Diazepina*; *Dipoxido*; *Disarim*; *Elenium*; *Epoxide*; *Equilibrium*; H-Tran; *Huberplex*; *Kalbrium*; *Karmoplex*; *Klopoxid*; *Lentotran*; *Libnum*; Librelease; Libritabs; **Librium**; *Libulin*; Lipoxide; *Medilium*; Mitran; *Multum* (Germany); *Neo-Gnostorid*; *Neuropax*; *Normide*; *Nova-Pam*; *Novopoxide* (Canada); *O.C.M.*; *Oasil*; *Omnalio*; *Paxium*; Poxi; *Psicofar*; *Radepur* (Germany); *Raysedan*; *Reliberan*; *Reposal*; *Restocalm*; *Retcol* (Japan); *Ripolin*; *Risachief* (Japan); *Risolid*; *Seren*; *Sintesedan*; *Solium* (Canada); Spaz-10; *Taee*; *Tensinyl*; *Tropium* (England); *Vapine*; *Zenecin*

(International brand names outside U.S. in italics)

FORMULARIES: Aetna; BC-BS; FHP; PCS

COST OF THERAPY: $10.65 (Anxiety; Capsule; 5 mg; 3/day; 120 days)

DESCRIPTION:

Tablets: Chlordiazepoxide, the prototype for the benzodiazepine compounds, was synthesized and developed at Hoffmann-La Roche Inc. It is a versatile therapeutic agent of proven value for the relief of anxiety. Chlordiazepoxide is among the safer of the effective psychopharmacologic compounds available, as demonstrated by extensive clinical evidence.

Chlordiazepoxide is available as tablets containing 5 mg, 10 mg or 25 mg. Each tablet also contains corn starch, ethylcellulose, hydroxypropyl methylcellulose, lactose, magnesium stearate, microcrystalline cellulose and triacetin; with FD&C Blue No. 1, D&C Yellow No. 10 and FD&C Yellow No. 6 dyes.

Chlordiazepoxide is 7-chloro-2-(methylamino)-5-phenyl-3H-1,4-benzodiazepine 4-oxide. A yellow crystalline substance, it is insoluble in water. The powder must be protected from light. The molecular weight is 299.76.

Note: Chlordiazepoxide tablets are not in the hydrochloride form.

Capsules: Chlordiazepoxide HCl is available as capsules containing 5 mg, 10 mg, or 25 mg chlordiazepoxide hydrochloride. Each capsule also contains corn starch, lactose and talc. Gelatin capsules may contain methyl and propyl parabens and potassium sorbate, with the following dye systems: 5-mg capsules-FD&C Yellow No. 6 plus D&C Yellow No.10 and either FD&C Blue No.1 or FD&C Green No. 3. 10-mg capsules-FD&C Yellow No.6 plus D&C Yellow No.10 and either FD&C Blue No.1 plus FD&C Red No. 3 plus FD&C Red No.40. 25-mg capsules-D&C Yellow No.10 and either FD&C Green No.3 or FD&C Blue No.1.

Chlordiazepoxide HCl is 7-chloro-2-(methylamino)-5-phenyl-3H-1,4-benzodiazepine 4-oxide hydrochloride. A white to practically white crystalline substance, it is soluble in water. It is unstable in solution and the powder must be protected from light. The molecular weight is 336.22.

Injectable: Chlordiazepoxide HCl injectable is used for the relief of acute anxiety when rapid action is required

CLINICAL PHARMACOLOGY:

Chlordiazepoxide has antianxiety, sedative, appetite-stimulating and weak analgesic actions. The precise mechanism of action is not known. The drug blocks EEG arousal from stimulation of the brain stem reticular formation. It takes several hours for peak blood levels to be reached and the half-life of the drug is between 24 and 48 hours. After the drug is discontinued plasma levels decline slowly over a period of several days. Chlordiazepoxide is excreted in the urine, with 1 to 2% unchanged and 3 to 6% as a conjugate.

INDICATIONS AND USAGE:

Chlordiazepoxide is indicated for the management of anxiety disorders or for the short-term relief of symptoms of anxiety, withdrawal symptoms of acute alcoholism, and preoperative apprehension and anxiety. Anxiety or tension associated with the stress of everyday life usually does not require treatment with an anxiolytic.

The effectiveness of chlordiazepoxide in long-term use, that is, more than 4 months, has not been assessed by systematic clinical studies. The physician should periodically reassess the usefulness of the drug for the individual patient.

CONTRAINDICATIONS:

Chlordiazepoxide is contraindicated in patients with known hypersensitivity to the drug.

WARNINGS:

Chlordiazepoxide and chlordiazepoxide hydrochloride may impair the mental and/or physical abilities required for the performance of potentially hazardous tasks such as driving a vehicle or operating machinery. Similarly, it may impair mental alertness in children. The concomitant use of alcohol or other central nervous system depressants may have an additive effect. PATIENTS SHOULD BE WARNED ACCORDINGLY.

WARNINGS: *(cont'd)*

Usage in Pregnancy: An increased risk of congenital malformations associated with the use of minor tranquilizers (Chlordiazepoxide, diazepam and meprobamate) during the first trimester of pregnancy has been suggested in several studies. Because use of these drugs is rarely a matter of urgency, their use during this period should almost always be avoided. The possibility that a woman of childbearing potential may be pregnant at the time of institution of therapy should be considered. Patients should be advised that if they become pregnant during therapy or intend to become pregnant they should communicate with their physicians about the desirability of discontinuing the drug.

Withdrawal symptoms of the barbiturate type have occurred after the discontinuation of benzodiazepines. (See DRUG ABUSE AND DEPENDENCE.)

PRECAUTIONS:

TABLETS AND CAPSULES

In elderly and debilitated patients, it is recommended that the dosage be limited to the smallest effective amount to preclude the development of ataxia or oversedation (10 mg or less per day initially, to be increased gradually as needed and tolerated). In general, the concomitant administration of chlordiazepoxide and other psychotropic agents is not recommended. If such combination therapy seems indicated, careful consideration should be given to the pharmacology of the agents to be employed - particularly when the known potentiating compounds such as the MAO inhibitors and phenothiazines are to be used. The usual precautions in treating patients with impaired renal or hepatic function should be observed.

Paradoxical reactions, *e.g.,* excitement, stimulation and acute rage, have been reported in psychiatric patients and in hyperactive aggressive children, and should be watched for during chlordiazepoxide therapy. The usual precautions are indicated when chlordiazepoxide is used in the treatment of anxiety states where there is any evidence of impending depression; it should be borne in mind that suicidal tendencies may be present and protective measures may be necessary. Although clinical studies have not established a cause and effect relationship, physicians should be aware that variable effects on blood coagulation have been reported very rarely in patients receiving oral anticoagulants and Chlordiazepoxide. In view of isolated reports associating chlordiazepoxide with exacerbation of porphyria, caution should be exercised in prescribing chlordiazepoxide to patients suffering from this disease.

Information for the Patient: To assure the safe and effective use of benzodiazepines, patients should be informed that, since benzodiazepines may produce psychological and physical dependence it is advisable that they consult with their physician before either increasing the dose or abruptly discontinuing this drug.

INJECTABLE

Injectable chlordiazepoxide (intramuscular or intravenous) is indicated primarily in acute states, and patients receiving this form of therapy should be kept under observation, preferably in bed, for a period of up to three hours. Ambulatory patients should not be permitted to operate a vehicle following an injection. Injectable chlordiazepoxide should not be given to patients in shock or comatose states. Reduced dosage (usually 25 to 50 mg) should be used for elderly or debilitated patients, and for children twelve years or older.

ADVERSE REACTIONS:

TABLETS AND CAPSULES

The necessity of discontinuing therapy because of undesirable effects has been rare. Drowsiness, ataxia and confusion have been reported in some patients - particularly the elderly and debilitated. While these effects can be avoided in almost all instances by proper dosage adjustment, they have occasionally been observed at the lower dosage ranges. In a few instances syncope has been reported.Other adverse reactions reported during therapy include isolated instances of skin eruptions, edema, minor menstrual irregularities, nausea and constipation, extrapyramidal symptoms, as well as increased and decreased libido. Such side effects have been infrequent and are generally controlled with reduction of dosage. Changes in EEG patterns (low-voltage fast activity) have been observed in patients during and after chlordiazepoxide treatment.

Blood dyscrasias (including agranulocytosis), jaundice and hepatic dysfunction have occasionally been reported during therapy. When chlordiazepoxide treatment is protracted, periodic blood counts and liver function tests are advisable.

Similarly, hypotension associated with spinal anesthesia has occurred. Pain following intramuscular injection has been reported. Changes in EEG patterns (low-voltage fast activity) have been reported in patients during and after treatment.

INJECTABLE

Other adverse reactions reported during therapy include isolated instances of syncope, hypotension, tachycardia, skin eruptions, edema, minor menstrual irregularities, nausea and constipation, extrapyramidal symptoms, blurred vision, as well as increased and decreased libido

DRUG ABUSE AND DEPENDENCE:

Chlordiazepoxide and chlordiazepoxide hydrochloride are classified by the Drug Enforcement Administration as a Schedule IV controlled substance.

Withdrawal symptoms, similar in character to those noted with barbiturates and alcohol (convulsions, tremor, abdominal and muscle cramps, vomiting and sweating), have occurred following abrupt discontinuance of Chlordiazepoxide. The more severe withdrawal symptoms have usually been limited to those patients who had received excessive doses over an extended period of time. Generally milder withdrawal symptoms (*e.g.,* dysphoria and insomnia) have been reported following abrupt discontinuance of benzodiazepines taken continuously at therapeutic levels for several months. Consequently, after extended therapy, abrupt discontinuation should generally be avoided and a gradual dosage tapering schedule followed. Addiction-prone individuals (such as drug addicts or alcoholics) should be under careful surveillance when receiving chlordiazepoxide or other psychotropic agents because of the predisposition of such patients to habituation and dependence.

OVERDOSAGE:

Manifestations of chlordiazepoxide overdosage include somnolence, confusion, coma and diminished reflexes. Respiration, pulse and blood pressure should be monitored, as in all cases of drug overdosage, although, in general, these effects have been minimal following chlordiazepoxide overdosage. General supportive measures should be employed, along with immediate gastric lavage. Intravenous fluids should be administered and an adequate airway maintained. Hypotension may be combated by the use of norepinephrine (Levophed) or metaraminol (Aramine). Dialysis is of limited value. There have been occasional reports of excitation in patients following chlordiazepoxide overdosage; if this occurs barbiturates should not be used. As with the management of intentional overdosage with any drug, it should be borne in mind that multiple agents may have been ingested.

DOSAGE AND ADMINISTRATION:

TABLETS AND CAPSULES

Because of the wide range of clinical indications for Chlordiazepoxide, the optimum dosage varies with the diagnosis and response of the individual patient. The dosage, therefore, should be individualized for maximum beneficial effects (See TABLE 1, TABLE 2.

TABLE 1 Adults - Oral Dosage

Adults	Usual Daily Dose
Relief of mild and moderate anxiety disorders and symptoms of anxiety	5 mg or 10 mg, 3 or 4 times daily
Relief of severe anxiety disorders and symptoms of anxiety	20 mg or 25 mg, 3 or 4 times daily
Geriatric patients, or in the presence of debilitating disease	5 mg, 2 to 4 times daily
Preoperative apprehension and anxiety On days preceding surgery, 5 to 10 mg orally, 3 or 4 times daily. If used as preoperative medication, 50 to 100 mg IM*one hour prior to surgery.	
* See TABLE 3	

TABLE 2 Children - Oral Dosage

Children	Usual Daily Dose
Because of the varied response of children to CNS-acting drugs, therapy should be initiated with the lowest dose and increased as required.	5 mg, 2 to 4 times daily (may be increased in some children to 10 mg, 2 or 3 times daily)
Since clinical experience in children under 6 years of age is limited, the use of the drug in this age group is not recommended.	

For the relief of withdrawal symptoms of acute alcoholism, the parenteral form (see TABLE 3)is usually used initially. If the drug is administered orally, the suggested initial dose is 50 to 100 mg, to be followed by repeated doses as needed until agitation is controlled - up to 300 mg per day. Dosage should then be reduced to maintenance levels.

INJECTABLE

Preparation And Administration of Solutions: Solutions of chlordiazepoxide hydrochloride for intramuscular or intravenous use should be prepared aseptically. Sterilization by heating should not be attempted.

Intramuscular: Add 2 ml of *Special Intramuscular Diluent* to contents of 5-ml dry-filled amber ampul of chlordiazepoxide hydrochloride Sterile Powder (100 mg). Avoid excessive pressure in injecting this special diluent into the ampul containing the powder since bubbles will form on the surface of the solution. Agitate gently until completely dissolved. Solution should be prepared immediately before administration. Any unused solution should be discarded. Deep intramuscular injection should be given *slowly* into the upper outer quadrant of the gluteus muscle.

Caution: Chlordiazepoxide hydrochloride solution made with Special Intramuscular Diluent should not be given intravenously because of the air bubbles which form when the intramuscular diluent is added to the chlordiazepoxide hydrochloride powder. Do not use diluent solution if it is opalescent or hazy.

Intravenous: In most cases, intramuscular injection is the preferred route of administration of injectable chlordiazepoxide since beneficial effects are usually seen within 15 to 30 minutes. When, in judgement of the physician, even more rapid action is mandatory, injectable chlordiazepoxide may be administered intravenously. A suitable solution for intravenous administration may be prepared as follows: Add 5 ml or *sterile physiological saline* or *sterile water for injection* to contents of 5-ml dry-filled amber ampul of chlordiazepoxide sterile powder (100 mg). Agitate gently until thoroughly dissolved. Solution should be prepared immediately before administration. Any unused portion should be discarded. *Intravenous solution should be given slowly over a one-minute period.*

Caution: *chlordiazepoxide solution made with physiological saline or sterile water for injection should not be given intramuscularly because of pain on injection.*

Dosage: Dosage should be individualized according to the diagnosis and the response of the patient. While 300 mg may be given during a 6-hour period, this dose should not be exceeded in any 24-hour period (TABLE 3).

TABLE 3 Injectable

Indication	Adult Dosage**
Withdrawal Symptoms of Acute Alcoholism	50 to 100 mg I.M. or I.V. initially; repeat in 2 to 4 hrs, if necessary
Acute or Severe Anxiety Disorders or Symptoms of Anxiety	50 to 100 mg I.M. or I.V. initially; then 25 to 50 mg 3 or 4 times daily, if necessary
Preoperative Apprehension and Anxiety	50 to 100 I.M. one hour prior to surgery
** Lower doses (usually 25 to 50 mg) should be used for elderly or debilitated patients and for older children. Since clinical experience in children under 12 years of age is limited, the use of the drug in this age group is not recommended.	

In most cases, acute symptoms may be rapidly controlled by parenteral administration so that subsequent treatment, if necessary, may be given orally. See Oral Chlordiazepoxide

Caution: Before preparing solution for intramuscular or intravenous administration, please read instructions for PREPARATION AND ADMINISTRATION OF SOLUTIONS.

ANIMAL PHARMACOLOGY:

The drug has been studied extensively in many species of animals and these studies are suggestive of action on the limbic system of the brain, which recent evidence indicates is involved in emotional response.

Hostile monkeys were made tame by oral doses which did not cause sedation. Chlordiazepoxide HCl revealed a "taming" action with the elimination of fear and aggression. The taming effect of chlordiazepoxide hydrochloride was further demonstrated in rats made vicious by lesions in the septal area of the brain. The drug dosage which effectively blocked the vicious reaction was well below the dose which caused sedation in these animals.

The LD_{50} of parenterally administered chlordiazepoxide hydrochloride was determined in mice (72 hours) and rats (5 days), and calculated according to the method of Miller and Tainter, with the following results: mice, IV, 123 ± 12 mg/kg; mice, IM, 366 ± 7 mg/kg; rats, IV, 120 ± 7 mg/kg; rats, IM, >160 mg/kg.

Effects on Reproduction: Reproduction studies in rats fed 10, 20 and 80 mg/kg daily and bred through one or two matings showed no congenital anomalies, nor were there adverse effects on lactation of the dams or growth of the newborn. However, in another study at 100 mg/kg daily there was noted a significant decrease in the fertilization rate and a marked decrease in the viability and body weight of off-spring which may be attributable to sedative activity, thus resulting in lack of interest in mating and lessened maternal nursing and care of the

ANIMAL PHARMACOLOGY: *(cont'd)*

young. One neonate in each of the first and second matings in the rat reproduction study at the 100 mg/kg dose exhibited major skeletal defects. Further studies are in progress to determine the significance of these findings.

HOW SUPPLIED - RATED THERAPEUTICALLY EQUIVALENT:

Capsule, Gelatin - Oral - 5 mg

100's	$2.96	Chlordiazepoxide HCl, H.C.F.A. F F P	99999-0726-01
100's	$3.21	Chlordiazepoxide Hcl, Voluntary Hosp	53258-0601-01
100's	$3.77	Chlordiazepoxide, Parmed Pharms	00349-2032-01
100's	$5.38	Chlordiazepoxide Hcl, Vangard Labs	00615-0435-47
100's	$5.60	Chlordiazepoxide Hcl, HL Moore Drug Exch	00839-1130-06
100's	$5.75	Chlordiazepoxide Hcl, Goldline Labs	00182-0977-01
100's	$5.79	Chlordiazepoxide Hcl, Voluntary Hosp	53258-0601-13
100's	$5.84	Chlordiazepoxide Hcl, Aligen Independ	00405-0040-01
100's	$6.01	Chlordiazepoxide Hcl, Barr	00555-0158-02
100's	$6.15	LIPOXIDE, Major Pharms	00904-0090-60
100's	$6.19	Chlordiazepoxide Hcl, Geneva Pharms	00781-2080-01
100's	$6.20	Chlordiazepoxide Hcl, United Res	00677-0457-01
100's	$6.26	Chlordiazepoxide HCl, Rugby	00536-3487-01
100's	$6.56	Chlordiazepoxide Hcl, Goldline Labs	00182-0977-89
100's	$6.90	Chlordiazepoxide Hcl, Qualitest Pharms	00603-2666-21
100's	**$35.78**	**LIBRIUM, Roche Prod**	**00140-0001-01**
100's	**$37.95**	**LIBRIUM, Roche Prod**	**00140-0001-49**
100's	**$38.48**	**LIBRIUM, Roche Prod**	**00140-0001-50**
500's	$12.20	Chlordiazepoxide Hcl, Halsey Drug	00879-0364-05
500's	$13.84	Chlordiazepoxide, Parmed Pharms	00349-2032-05
500's	$14.80	Chlordiazepoxide HCl, H.C.F.A. F F P	99999-0726-02
500's	$19.65	LIPOXIDE, Major Pharms	00904-0090-40
500's	$23.98	Chlordiazepoxide Hcl, Barr	00555-0158-04
500's	$24.10	Chlordiazepoxide Hcl, Geneva Pharms	00781-2080-05
500's	$25.24	Chlordiazepoxide Hcl, Aligen Independ	00405-0040-02
500's	$25.50	Chlordiazepoxide HCl, Rugby	00536-3487-05
500's	**$177.65**	**LIBRIUM, Roche Prod**	**00140-0001-14**
1000's	$18.75	LIPOXIDE, Major Pharms	00904-0090-80
1000's	$29.60	Chlordiazepoxide HCl, H.C.F.A. F F P	99999-0726-03
1000's	$39.05	Chlordiazepoxide Hcl, Geneva Pharms	00781-2080-10
1000's	$39.14	Chlordiazepoxide Hcl, HL Moore Drug Exch	00839-1130-16
1000's	$48.12	Chlordiazepoxide Hcl, Qualitest Pharms	00603-2666-32

Capsule, Gelatin - Oral - 10 mg

100's	$3.15	Chlordiazepoxide HCl, H.C.F.A. F F P	99999-0726-04
100's	$3.21	Chlordiazepoxide Hcl, Voluntary Hosp	53258-0602-01
100's	$3.40	Chlordiazepoxide Hcl, Halsey Drug	00879-0365-01
100's	$4.18	Chlordiazepoxide Hcl, Barr	00555-0033-02
100's	$5.52	Chlordiazepoxide Hcl 10, Aligen Independ	00405-0041-01
100's	$5.85	LIPOXIDE, Major Pharms	00904-0091-60
100's	$6.00	Chlordiazepoxide Hcl, Goldline Labs	00182-0978-01
100's	$6.00	Chlordiazepoxide Hcl, Voluntary Hosp	53258-0602-13
100's	$6.35	Chlordiazepoxide Hcl, United Res	00677-0458-01
100's	$6.40	Chlordiazepoxide Hcl, Qualitest Pharms	00603-2667-21
100's	$6.49	Chlordiazepoxide HCl, Geneva Pharms	00781-2082-01
100's	$6.68	Chlordiazepoxide Hcl, HL Moore Drug Exch	00839-1131-06
100's	$6.70	Chlordiazepoxide Hcl, Goldline Labs	00182-0978-89
100's	$7.04	Chlordiazepoxide HCl, Rugby	00536-3488-01
100's	$19.92	POXI, Seneca Pharms	47028-0012-01
100's	**$52.08**	**LIBRIUM, Roche Prod**	**00140-0002-01**
100's	**$54.23**	**LIBRIUM, Roche Prod**	**00140-0002-49**
100's	**$54.78**	**LIBRIUM, Roche Prod**	**00140-0002-50**
500's	$13.00	Chlordiazepoxide Hcl, Halsey Drug	00879-0365-05
500's	$15.50	LIPOXIDE, Major Pharms	00904-0091-40
500's	$15.75	Chlordiazepoxide HCl, H.C.F.A. F F P	99999-0726-05
500's	$21.00	Chlordiazepoxide Hcl, Goldline Labs	00182-0978-05
500's	$22.10	Chlordiazepoxide Hcl, United Res	00677-0458-05
500's	$22.97	Chlordiazepoxide HCl, Rugby	00536-3488-05
500's	$25.53	Chlordiazepoxide Hcl, Geneva Pharms	00781-2082-05
500's	**$259.19**	**LIBRIUM, Roche Prod**	**00140-0002-14**
1000's	$13.75	H-Tran 10, H & H Labs	46703-0023-10
1000's	$20.80	Chlordiazepoxide Hcl, Halsey Drug	00879-0365-10
1000's	$21.27	Chlordiazepoxide Hcl, Voluntary Hosp	53258-0602-10
1000's	$22.19	Chlordiazepoxide Hcl, Barr	00555-0033-05
1000's	$29.95	LIPOXIDE, Major Pharms	00904-0091-80
1000's	$31.50	Chlordiazepoxide HCl, H.C.F.A. F F P	99999-0726-06
1000's	$31.75	Chlordiazepoxide Hcl, Goldline Labs	00182-0978-10
1000's	$36.23	Chlordiazepoxide Hcl 10, Aligen Independ	00405-0041-03
1000's	$40.10	Chlordiazepoxide Hcl, United Res	00677-0458-10
1000's	$41.11	Chlordiazepoxide Hcl, Qualitest Pharms	00603-2667-32
1000's	$45.56	Chlordiazepoxide Hcl, HL Moore Drug Exch	00839-1131-16
1000's	$45.60	Chlordiazepoxide Hcl, Geneva Pharms	00781-2082-10
1000's	$46.55	Chlordiazepoxide HCl, Rugby	00536-3488-10
1000's	$99.95	Spaz-10, Quality Res Pharms	52765-2154-00

Capsule, Gelatin - Oral - 25 mg

100's	$3.71	Chlordiazepoxide HCl, H.C.F.A. F F P	99999-0726-07
100's	$4.10	Chlordiazepoxide, Parmed Pharms	00349-2034-01
100's	$4.44	Chlordiazepoxide Hcl, Voluntary Hosp	53258-0603-01
100's	$4.75	Chlordiazepoxide Hcl, Halsey Drug	00879-0366-01
100's	$5.70	LIPOXIDE, Major Pharms	00904-0092-60
100's	$6.24	Chlordiazepoxide Hcl, Aligen Independ	00405-0042-01
100's	$6.70	Chlordiazepoxide Hcl, Goldline Labs	00182-0979-01
100's	$6.95	Chlordiazepoxide Hcl, HL Moore Drug Exch	00839-1132-06
100's	$6.96	Chlordiazepoxide Hcl, Barr	00555-0159-02
100's	$6.96	Chlordiazepoxide Hcl, Voluntary Hosp	53258-0603-13
100's	$7.32	Chlordiazepoxide Hcl, Vangard Labs	00615-0437-47
100's	$7.50	Chlordiazepoxide Hcl, Goldline Labs	00182-0979-89
100's	$7.50	Chlordiazepoxide Hcl, United Res	00677-0459-01
100's	$7.58	Chlordiazepoxide HCl, Rugby	00536-3489-01
100's	$7.60	Chlordiazepoxide HCl, Geneva Pharms	00781-2084-01
100's	$7.80	Chlordiazepoxide Hcl, Qualitest Pharms	00603-2668-21
100's	**$89.28**	**LIBRIUM, Roche Prod**	**00140-0003-01**
500's	$14.10	Chlordiazepoxide Hcl, Halsey Drug	00879-0366-05
500's	$17.07	Chlordiazepoxide, Parmed Pharms	00349-2034-05
500's	$18.21	Chlordiazepoxide Hcl, HL Moore Drug Exch	00839-1132-12
500's	$18.55	Chlordiazepoxide HCl, H.C.F.A. F F P	99999-0726-08
500's	$20.95	LIPOXIDE, Major Pharms	00904-0092-40
500's	$22.71	Chlordiazepoxide Hcl, Aligen Independ	00405-0042-02
500's	$25.25	Chlordiazepoxide Hcl, Barr	00555-0159-04
500's	$27.00	Chlordiazepoxide Hcl, United Res	00677-0459-05
500's	$27.05	Chlordiazepoxide Hcl, Geneva Pharms	00781-2084-05
500's	$27.06	Chlordiazepoxide HCl, Rugby	00536-3489-05
500's	$41.12	Chlordiazepoxide Hcl, Qualitest Pharms	00603-2668-28
500's	**$445.25**	**LIBRIUM, Roche Prod**	**00140-0003-14**
1000's	$24.60	Chlordiazepoxide Hcl, Halsey Drug	00879-0366-10
1000's	$37.10	Chlordiazepoxide HCl, H.C.F.A. F F P	99999-0726-09

HOW SUPPLIED - RATED THERAPEUTICALLY EQUIVALENT: *(cont'd)*

1000's	$41.71	Chlordiazepoxide Hcl, Geneva Pharms	00781-2084-10
1000's	$44.96	Chlordiazepoxide Hcl, HL Moore Drug Exch	00839-1132-16

HOW SUPPLIED - NOT RATED EQUIVALENT:

Injection, Conc, W/Buf - Intramuscular; - 100 mg/ampul

5 ml x 10	**$78.36**	**LIBRIUM, Roche Prod**	**00140-1912-06**

Tablet, Plain Coated - Oral - 5 mg

100's	$33.71	LIBRITABS, Roche Prod	00140-0013-01

Tablet, Plain Coated - Oral - 10 mg

100's	$48.11	LIBRITABS, Roche Prod	00140-0014-01

CHLORDIAZEPOXIDE HYDROCHLORIDE; CLIDINIUM BROMIDE *(000727)*

CATEGORIES: Acid/Peptic Disorders; Antianxiety Drugs; Anticholinergic Agents; Antimuscarinics/Antispasmodics; Antispasmodics & Anticholinergics; Autonomic Drugs; Central Nervous System Agents; Colitis; DESI Drugs; Enterocolitis; Gastrointestinal Drugs; Irritable Bowel Syndrome; Peptic Ulcer; FDA Pre 1938 Drugs

BRAND NAMES: *Bralix*; *Braxidin*; CDP Plus; Chlordinium; Chlorex; Clindex; Clinoxide; *Clioxide*; *Diporax*; *Epirax*; *Equirex*; *Klidibrax*; *Kuanium*; *Lembirax*; Li-Gen; *Liblan*; **Librax**; *Libraxin*; *Librocol*; Lidoxide; *Lonta*; *Nirvaxal*; *Pehaspas*; *Renagas*; *Restolax*; Spazmate; *Spasmoten*; Zebrax
(International brand names outside U.S. in italics)

FORMULARIES: Aetna

DESCRIPTION:

To control emotional and somatic factors in gastrointestinal disorders.

This combination of chlordiazepoxide hydrochloride and clidinium bromide will be abbreviated here as chlordiazepoxide w/ clidinium.

This drug combines in a single capsule formulation the antianxiety action of chlordiazepoxide hydrochloride and the anticholinergic/spasmolytic effects of clidinium bromide, both exclusive developments of Roche research.

FOR COMPLETE PRESCRIBING INFORMATION, REFER TO THE INDIVIDUAL DRUG MONOGRAPHS (CHLORDIAZEPOXIDE HYDROCHLORIDE; CLIDINIUM BROMIDE).

INDICATIONS AND USAGE:

Based on a review of this drug by the National Academy of Sciences - National Research Council and/or other information, FDA has classified the indications as follows:
"Possibly" effective: as adjunctive therapy in the treatment of peptic ulcer and in the treatment of the irritable bowel syndrome (irritable colon, spastic colon, mucous colitis) and acute enterocolitis.
Final classification of the less-than-effective indications requires further investigation.

DOSAGE AND ADMINISTRATION:

Because of the varied individual responses to tranquilizers and anticholinergics, the optimum dosage of Chlordiazepoxide w/ Clidinium varies with the diagnosis and response of the individual patient. The dosage, therefore, should be individualized for maximum beneficial effects. The usual maintenance dose is 1 or 2 capsules, 3 or 4 times a day administered before meals and at bedtime.

HOW SUPPLIED - EQUIVALENTS NOT AVAILABLE:

Capsule, Gelatin - Oral - 5 mg/2.5 mg

100's	$3.25	Chlordiazepoxide Hcl & Clidinium, Eon Labs Mfg	00185-0617-01
100's	$3.25	Chlordiazepoxide Hcl & Clidinium, Eon Labs Mfg	00185-0968-01
100's	$4.35	CLINOXIDE, Halsey Drug	00879-0501-01
100's	$4.55	Chlordiazepoxide/Clidinium Bromide, United Res	00677-1247-01
100's	$4.60	CDP PLUS, Goldline Labs	00182-1856-01
100's	$4.89	CLINOXIDE, Geneva Pharms	00781-2580-01
100's	$4.90	Chlordiazepoxide Hcl & Clidinium Br, Major Pharms	00904-0301-60
100's	$4.94	Clidinium W/Chlordiazepoxide, Vintage Pharms	00254-2732-28
100's	$5.11	Clidinium W/Chlordiazepoxide, Qualitest Pharms	00603-2714-21
100's	$5.25	Chlordiazepoxide/Clidinium Bromide, Major Pharms	00904-2503-60
100's	$5.76	Chlordiazepoxide/Clidinium Bromide, Aligen Independ	00405-0045-01
100's	$5.80	Clordiazinepoxide/Clidinium Bromide, Schein Pharm (US)	00364-0559-01
100's	$5.99	CLINDEX, Rugby	00536-3490-01
100's	$8.87	Clidinium W/Chlordiazepoxide, US Trading	56126-0090-11
100's	$9.95	Chlordiazepoxide/Clidinium, Major Pharms	00904-0301-61
100's	$12.95	Chlordiazepoxide W/Clid Brom, HL Moore Drug Exch	00839-6211-06
100's	$18.75	CLINOXIDE, Geneva Pharms	00781-2580-13
100's	**$68.01**	**LIBRAX, Roche Prod**	**00140-0007-01**
100's	**$70.14**	**LIBRAX, Roche Prod**	**00140-0007-49**
500's	$5.25	Chlordiazepoxide Hcl & Clidinium Br, Major Pharms	00904-0301-40
500's	$14.95	Chlordiazepoxide Hcl & Clidinium, Eon Labs Mfg	00185-0617-05
500's	$14.95	Chlordiazepoxide Hcl & Clidinium, Eon Labs Mfg	00185-0968-05
500's	$17.10	CLINOXIDE, Halsey Drug	00879-0501-05
500's	$17.25	Chlordiazepoxide/Clidinium Bromide, Major Pharms	00904-2503-40
500's	$17.65	CDP PLUS, Goldline Labs	00182-1856-05
500's	$17.65	CLINOXIDE, Geneva Pharms	00781-2580-05
500's	$22.43	CLINDEX, Rugby	00536-3490-05
500's	$22.50	Clordiazinepoxide/Clidinium Bromide, Schein Pharm (US)	00364-0559-05
500's	$42.00	Chlordiazepoxide/Clidinium Bromide, Aligen Independ	00405-0045-02
500's	**$338.88**	**LIBRAX, Roche Prod**	**00140-0007-14**
1000's	$24.95	Chlordiazepoxide Hcl & Clidinium, Eon Labs Mfg	00185-0617-10
1000's	$24.95	Chlordiazepoxide Hcl & Clidinium, Eon Labs Mfg	00185-0968-10
1000's	$28.34	Chlordiazepoxide/Clidinium Bromide, United Res	00677-1247-10
1000's	$29.10	Clidinium W/Chlordiazepoxide, Vintage Pharms	00254-2732-38
1000's	$29.80	Chlordiazepoxide Hcl & Clidinium Br, Major Pharms	00904-0301-80
1000's	$30.85	CDP PLUS, Goldline Labs	00182-1856-10
1000's	$31.20	CLINOXIDE, Halsey Drug	00879-0501-10
1000's	$31.40	Clidinium W/Chlordiazepoxide, Qualitest Pharms	00603-2714-32
1000's	$31.45	Chlordiazepoxide/Clidinium Bromide, Major Pharms	00904-2503-80
1000's	$35.98	Chlordiazepoxide/Clidinium Bromide, Parmed Pharms	00349-8697-10

HOW SUPPLIED - EQUIVALENTS NOT AVAILABLE: *(cont'd)*

1000's	$35.98	Chlordiazepoxide/Clidinium Bromide, Parmed Pharms	00349-8698-10
1000's	$39.95	CLINDEX, Rugby	00536-3490-10
1000's	$115.95	Chlordiazepoxide W/Clid Brom, HL Moore Drug Exch	00839-6211-16

CHLORDIAZEPOXIDE; ESTROGENS, ESTERIFIED *(000728)*

CATEGORIES: Anxiolytics, Sedatives, Hypnotic; Benzodiazepines; Central Nervous System Agents; Hormones; Menopause; Sedatives; Tension; Tranquilizers; Pregnancy Category X; FDA Approval Pre 1982

BRAND NAMES: **Menrium**

DESCRIPTION:

Menrium tablets are available in three strengths: Menrium 5-2, containing 5 mg chlordiazepoxide and 0.2 mg water-soluble esterified estrogens; Menrium 5-4, containing 5 mg chlordiazepoxide and 0.4 mg water-soluble esterified estrogens; and Menrium 10-4, containing 10 mg chlordiazepoxide and 0.4 mg water-soluble esterified estrogens. Each tablet also contains acacia, calcium stearate, calcium sulfate, carnauba wax, corn starch, lactose, pregelatinized starch, sodium bicarbonate, sucrose and flavor, with the following dye systems: Menrium 5-2 and Menrium 5-4 - FD&C Blue No. 1, FD&C Yellow No. 6 and D&C Yellow No. 10; Menrium 10-4 - FD&C Blue No. 1 and FD&C Red No. 3.

Menrium affords in a single formulation the psychotropic action of Librium (chlordiazepoxide) and hormonal replacement in the form of water-soluble esterified estrogens (expressed in terms of sodium estrone sulfate) to provide comprehensive management of the menopausal syndrome or the climacteric.

FOR COMPLETE PRESCRIBING INFORMATION, REFER TO THE INDIVIDUAL DRUG MONOGRAPHS (CHLORDIAZEPOXIDE; ESTROGENS, ESTERIFIED).

INDICATIONS AND USAGE:

Menrium is indicated in the management of the manifestations generally associated with the menopausal syndrome - anxiety and tension, vasomotor complaints and hormonal deficiency states.

DOSAGE AND ADMINISTRATION:

The lowest dose that will control symptoms should be chosen and medication should be discontinued as promptly as possible.

MENRIUM 5-2: For the majority of patients with the menopausal syndrome or the climacteric having anxiety and tension and hormonal deficiency states requiring estrogen replacement - One tablet, t.i.d.

MENRIUM 5-4: For patients with the menopausal syndrome or the climacteric with anxiety and tension and more severe vasomotor manifestations - One tablet, t.i.d.

MENRIUM 10-4: For patients with the menopausal syndrome or the climacteric with pronounced anxiety and tension and marked vasomotor complaints - One tablet, t.i.d.

Therapy should be continued for 21-day courses, followed by one-week rest periods. While these dosage schedules will prove generally satisfactory, individual adjustment of dosage is desirable, since some patients may obtain satisfactory relief with as little as one tablet daily of Menrium 5-2.

Treated patients with an intact uterus should be monitored closely for signs of endometrial cancer and appropriate diagnostic measures should be taken to rule out malignancy in the event of persistent or recurring abnormal vaginal bleeding.

HOW SUPPLIED - EQUIVALENTS NOT AVAILABLE:

Tablet, Uncoated - Oral - 5 mg/0.2 mg

100's	**$53.84**	**MENRIUM, Roche Prod**	**00140-0023-01**

Tablet, Uncoated - Oral - 5 mg/0.4 mg

100's	**$58.72**	**MENRIUM, Roche Prod**	**00140-0024-01**

Tablet, Uncoated - Oral - 10 mg/0.4 mg

100's	**$73.18**	**MENRIUM 10-4, Roche Prod**	**00140-0025-01**

CHLORHEXIDINE GLUCONATE *(000729)*

CATEGORIES: Anti-Infectives; Dental; Gingivitis; Local Infections; Mouthrinse, Antimicrobial; Skin/Mucous Membrane Agents; Pregnancy Category B; FDA Approved 1986 Aug

BRAND NAMES: *Alcloxidine*; *Aubikleen*; *Bactoscrub*; *Bactosept Concentrate*; *Blend-A-Med* (Germany); *Chlorex-a-myl* (France); *Chlorhexamed* (Germany); *Chlorhexidine* (France); *Chlorhexidine Mouthwash*; *Chlorhexidine Obstetric Lotion*; *Chlorhexidinium*; *Chlorohex gel*; *Chlorohex gel Forte*; *Chlorohex Mouth Rinse*; *Corsodyl*; *Hexol*; *Hibiclens Skin Cleanser*; *Hibiclens Solution*; *Hibicol Handrub*; *Hibident* (France); *Hibidil*; *Hibigel*; *Hibiguard*; *Hibiscrub* (France); *Hibisol*; *Hibitan*; *Hibitane* (France); *Hibitane Concentrate*; *Hibitane Cream*; *Hibitane Dental*; *Hibitane Pastillas*; *Hibitane Solution*; *Hidine*; *Improved Phisohex*; *Klorheksidos*; *Klorhexidin*; *Klorhexol*; *Lemocin CX* (Germany); *Novaclens 2*; *Novaclens 4*; **Peridex**; *Perio Chip*; Periogard; *Plakicide*; *Savacol*; *Savlon*; *Septalex*; *Septalone*; *Septol*
(International brand names outside U.S. in italics)

FORMULARIES: BC-BS; WHO

DESCRIPTION:

Peridex is an oral rinse containing 0.12% chlorhexidine gluconate (1, 1'- hexamethylene bis (5-(p-chlorophenyl) biguanide) di-D-gluconate) in a base containing water, 11.6% alcohol, glycerin, PEG-40 sorbitan diisostearate, flavor, sodium saccharin, and FD&C Blue No. 1. Peridex is a near-neutral solution (pH range 5-7). Chlorhexidine gluconate is a salt of chlorhexidine and gluconic acid.

INDICATIONS AND USAGE:

Chlorhexidine gluconate is indicated for use between dental visits as part of a professional program for the treatment of gingivitis as characterized by redness and swelling of the gingivae, including gingival bleeding upon probing. Chlorhexidine gluconate has not been tested among patients with acute necrotizing ulcerative gingivitis (ANUG). For patients having coexisting gingivitis and periodontitis, see PRECAUTIONS.

CONTRAINDICATIONS:

Chlorhexidine gluconate should not be used by persons who are known to be hypersensitive to chlorhexidine gluconate.

WARNINGS:

The effect of chlorhexidine gluconate on periodontitis has not been determined. An increase in supragingival calculus was noted in clinical testing in chlorhexidine gluconate users compared with control users. It is not known if chlorhexidine gluconate use results in an increase in subgingival calculus. Calculus deposits should be removed by a dental prophylaxis at intervals not greater than six months.

Rare hypersensitivity and generalized allergic reactions have also been reported. Chlorhexidine gluconate should not be used by persons who have a sensitivity to it or its components.

PRECAUTIONS:

General: For patients having coexisting gingivitis and periodontitis, the presence of absence or gingival inflammation following treatment with chlorhexidine gluconate should not be used as a major indicator of underlying periodontitis.

Chlorhexidine gluconate can cause staining of oral surfaces, such as tooth surfaces, restorations, and the dorsum of the tongue. Not all patients will experience a visually significant increase in toothstaining. In clinical testing, 56% of chlorhexidine gluconate users exhibited a measurable increase in facial anterior stain, compared to 35% of control users after six months; 15% of chlorhexidine gluconate users developed what was judged to be heavy stain, compared to 1% of control users after six months. Stain will be more pronounced in patients who have heavier accumulations of unremoved plaque.

Stain resulting from use of chlorhexidine gluconate does not adversely affect health of the gingivae of other oral tissues. Stain can be removed from most tooth surfaces by conventional professional prophylactic techniques. Additional time may be required to complete the prophylaxis.

Discretion should be used when prescribing to patients with anterior facial restorations with rough surfaces or margins. If natural stain cannot be removed from these surfaces by a dental prophylaxis, patients should be excluded from chlorhexidine gluconate treatment if permanent discoloration if unacceptable. Stain in these areas may be difficult to remove by dental prophylaxis and on rare occasions may necessitate replacement of these restorations.

Some patients may experience an alteration in taste perception while undergoing treatment with chlorhexidine gluconate. Most patients accommodate to this effect with continued use of chlorhexidine gluconate. No instances of permanent taste alteration due to chlorhexidine gluconate have been reported.

Carcinogenesis, Mutagenesis, and Impairment of Fertility: In a drinking water study in rats, carcinogenesis was not observed. The highest dose of chlorhexidine gluconate used in this study, 38 mg/kg/day, is at least 500 times the amount that would be ingested from the recommended daily dose of chlorhexidine gluconate.

In two mammalian *in vivo* mutagenic studies with chlorhexidine gluconate, mutagenesis was not observed. The highest dose of chlorhexidine gluconate used in a mouse dominant lethal assay was 1000 mg/kg/day and in a hamster cytogenetics test was 250 mg/kg/day, i.e., >3200 times the amount that would be ingested from the recommended daily dose of chlorhexidine gluconate.

Pregnancy Category B Reproduction and fertility studies with chlorhexidine gluconate have been conducted. No evidence of impaired fertility was observed in rats at doses up to 100 mg/kg/day, and no evidence of harm to the fetus was observed in rats and rabbits at doses up to 300 mg/kg/day and 40 mg/kg/day, respectively. These doses are approximately 100, 300, and 40 times that which would result from a person's ingesting 30 ml (2 capfuls) of chlorhexidine gluconate per day. Since controlled studies in pregnant women have not been conducted, the benefits of the drug in pregnant women should be weighed against possible risk to the fetus.

Nursing Mothers: It is not known whether this drug is excreted in human milk. Because many drugs are excreted in human milk, caution should be exercised when chlorhexidine gluconate is administered to a nursing woman.

In parturition and lactation studies with rats, no evidence of impaired parturition or of toxic effects to suckling pups was observed when chlorhexidine gluconate was administered to dams at doses that were over 100 times greater than that which would result from a person's ingesting 30 ml (2 capfuls) of chlorhexidine gluconate per day.

Pediatric Use: Clinical effectiveness and safety of chlorhexidine gluconate have been established in children under the age of 18.

ADVERSE REACTIONS:

The most common side effects associated with chlorhexidine gluconate oral rinses are (1) an increase in staining of teeth and other oral surfaces, (2) an increase in calculus formation, and (3) an alteration in taste perception; see WARNINGS and PRECAUTIONS. No serious systemic adverse reactions associated with use of chlorhexidine gluconate were observed in clinical testing.

Minor irritation and superficial desquamation of the oral mucosa have been noted in patients using chlorhexidine gluconate, particularly among children.

Although there have been no reports of parotitis (inflammation or swelling of salivary glands) among chlorhexidine gluconate users in controlled clinical studies, transient parotitis has been reported in research studies with chlorhexidine-containing mouthrinses.

OVERDOSAGE:

Ingestion of 1 or 2 ounces of chlorhexidine gluconate by a small child (≈10 kg body weight) might result in gastric distress, including nausea, or signs of alcohol intoxication. Medical attention should be sought if more than 4 ounces of chlorhexidine gluconate is ingested by a small child or if signs of alcohol intoxication develop.

DOSAGE AND ADMINISTRATION:

Chlorhexidine gluconate therapy should be initiated directly following a dental prophylaxis. Patients using chlorhexidine gluconate should be reevaluated and given a thorough prophylaxis at intervals no longer than six months.

Recommended use is twice daily oral rinsing for 30 seconds, morning and evening after toothbrushing. Usual dosage is 1/2 fl. oz. (marked in cap) of undiluted chlorhexidine gluconate. Chlorhexidine gluconate is not intended for ingestion and should be expectorated after rinsing.

HOW SUPPLIED - RATED THERAPEUTICALLY EQUIVALENT:

Mouthwash - Oral - 0.12 %

3-16 oz plastic	**$141.81**	**PERIDEX, Procter Gamble Mfg**	**37000-0007-01**
480 ml x 12	$104.83	PERIOGARD, Colgate Oral	00126-0271-16

HOW SUPPLIED - NOT RATED EQUIVALENT:

Mouthwash - Oral - 0.12 %

960 ml	$16.24	Chlorhexidine Gluconate, Harber Pharm	51432-0521-22

CHLOROPROCAINE HYDROCHLORIDE *(000735)*

CATEGORIES: Anesthesia; Dental; Injectable Anesthetics; Local Anesthetics; Pregnancy Category C; FDA Approval Pre 1982

BRAND NAMES: **Nesacaine**; *Nesacaine-CE* (Canada)
(International brand names outside U.S. in italics)

DESCRIPTION:

Chloroprocaine HCl injections are sterile non pyrogenic local anesthetics. The active ingredient in chloroprocaine HCl injections is chloroprocaine HCl (benzoic acid, 4-amino-2-chloro-2-(diethylamino) ethyl ester, monohydrochloride). (TABLE 1):

TABLE 1 Composition of Available Injections
Formula (mg/ml)

Product Identification	Chloroprocaine HCl	Sodium Chloride	Disodium EDTA dihydrate	Methylparaben
Chloroprocaine 1%	10	6.7	0.111	1
Chloroprocaine 2%	20	4.7	0.111	1
Chloroprocaine-M PF 2%	20	4.7	0.111	-
Chloroprocaine-M PF 3%	30	3.3	0.111	-

The solutions are adjusted to pH 2.7-4.0 by means of sodium hydroxide and/or hydrochloric acid. Filled under nitrogen.

Chloroprocaine HCl injections should not be resterilized by autoclaving.

CLINICAL PHARMACOLOGY:

Chloroprocaine, like other local anesthetics, blocks the generation and the conduction of nerve impulses, presumably by increasing the threshold for electrical excitation in the nerve, by slowing the propagation of the nerve impulse and by reducing the rate of rise of the action potential. In general, the progression of anesthesia is related to the diameter, myelination and conduction velocity of affected nerve fibers. Clinically, the order of loss of nerve function is as follows: (1) pain, (2) temperature, (3) touch, (4) proprioception, and (5) skeletal muscle tone.

Systemic absorption of local anesthetics produces effects on the cardiovascular and central nervous systems. At blood concentrations achieved with normal therapeutic doses, changes in cardiac conduction, excitability, refractoriness, contractility, and peripheral vascular resistance are minimal. However, toxic blood concentrations depress cardiac conduction and excitability, which may lead to atrio-ventricular block and ultimately to cardiac arrest. In addition, with toxic blood concentrations myocardial contractility may be depressed and peripheral vasodilation may occur, leading to decreased cardiac output and arterial blood pressure.

Following systemic absorption, toxic blood concentrations of local anesthetics can produce central nervous system stimulation, depression, or both. Apparent central stimulation may be manifested as restlessness, tremors and shivering, which may progress to convulsions. Depression and coma may occur, possibly progressing ultimately to respiratory arrest.

However, the local anesthetics have a primary depressant effect on the medulla and on higher centers. The depressed stage may occur without a prior stage of central nervous system stimulation.

Pharmacokinetics: The rate of systemic absorption of local anesthetic drugs is dependent upon the total dose and concentration of drug administered, the route of administration, the vascularity of the administration site, and the presence or absence of epinephrine in the anesthetic injection. Epinephrine usually reduces the rate of absorption and plasma concentration of local anesthetics and is sometimes added to local anesthetic injections in order to prolong the duration of action.

The onset of action with chloroprocaine is rapid (usually within 6 to 12 minutes), and the duration of anesthesia, depending upon the amount used and the route of administration, may be up to 60 minutes.

Local anesthetics appear to cross the placenta by passive diffusion. However, the rate and degree of diffusion varies considerably among the different drugs as governed by: (1) the degree of plasma protein binding, (2) the degree of ionization, and (3) the degree of lipid solubility. Fetal/maternal ratios of local anesthetics appear to be inversely related to the degree of plasma protein binding, since only the free, unbound drug is available for placental transfer. Thus, drugs with the highest protein binding capacity may have the lowest fetal/maternal ratios. The extent of placental transfer is also determined by the degree of ionization and lipid solubility of the drug. Lipid soluble, nonionized drugs readily enter the fetal blood from the maternal circulation.

Depending upon the route of administration, local anesthetics are distributed to some extent to all body tissues, with high concentrations found in highly perfused organs such as the liver, lungs, heart, and brain.

Various pharmacokinetic parameters of the local anesthetics can be significantly altered by the presence of hepatic or renal disease, addition of epinephrine, factors affecting urinary pH, renal blood flow, the route of administration, and the age of the patient. The *in vitro*plasma half-life of chloroprocaine in adults is 21 ± 2 seconds for males and 25 ± 1 seconds for females. The *in vitro* plasma half-life in neonates is 43 ± 2 seconds.

Chloroprocaine is rapidly metabolized in plasma by hydrolysis of the ester linkage by pseudocholinesterase. The hydrolysis of chloroprocaine results in the production of β-diethylaminoethanol and 2-chloro-4-aminobenzoic acid, which inhibits the action of the sulfonamides (see PRECAUTIONS).

The kidney is the main excretory organ for most local anesthetics and their metabolites. Urinary excretion is affected by urinary perfusion and factors affecting urinary pH.

INDICATIONS AND USAGE:

Chloroprocaine 1% and 2% injections, in multidose vials with methylparaben as preservative, are indicated for the production of local anesthesia by infiltration and peripheral nerve block. They are not to be used for lumbar or caudal epidural anesthesia.

Chloroprocaine-MPF 2% and 3% injections, in single-dose vials without preservative, are indicated for the production of local anesthesia by infiltration, peripheral and central nerve block, including lumbar and caudal epidural blocks.

Chloroprocaine HCl injections are not be used for subarachnoid administration.

CONTRAINDICATIONS:

Chloroprocaine HCl injections are contraindicated in patients hypersensitive (allergic) to drugs of the PABA ester group.

Lumbar and caudal epidural anesthesia should be used with extreme caution in persons with the following conditions: existing neurological disease, spinal deformities, septicemia, and severe hypertension.

WARNINGS:

LOCAL ANESTHETICS SHOULD ONLY BE EMPLOYED BY CLINICIANS WHO ARE WELL VERSED IN DIAGNOSIS AND MANAGEMENT OF DOSE RELATED TOXICITY AND OTHER ACUTE EMERGENCIES WHICH MIGHT ARISE FROM THE BLOCK TO BE EMPLOYED, AND THEN ONLY AFTER ENSURING THE *IMMEDIATE* AVAILABILITY OF OXYGEN, OTHER RESUSCITATIVE DRUGS, CARDIOPULMONARY RESUSCITATIVE EQUIPMENT, AND THE PERSONNEL RESOURCES NEEDED FOR PROPER MANAGEMENT OF TOXIC REACTIONS AND RELATED EMERGENCIES (see also ADVERSE REACTIONS and PRECAUTIONS). DELAY IN PROPER MANAGEMENT OF DOSE RELATED TOXICITY, UNDERVENTILATION FROM ANY CAUSE AND/OR ALTERED SENSITIVITY MAY LEAD TO THE DEVELOPMENT OF ACIDOSIS, CARDIAC ARREST AND, POSSIBLY, DEATH. CHLOROPROCAINE (CHLOROPROCAINE HCl) INJECTION contains methylparaben and should not be used for lumbar or caudal epidural anesthesia because safety of this antimicrobial preservative has not been established with regard to intrathecal injection, either intentional or unintentional. Chloroprocaine-MPF injection contains no preservative; discard unused injection remaining in vial after initial use.

Vasopressors should not be used in the presence of ergot type oxytocic drugs, since a severe persistent hypertension may occur.

To avoid intravascular injection, aspiration should be performed before the anesthetic solution is injected. The needle must be repositioned until no blood return can be elicited. However, the absence of blood in the syringe does not guarantee that intravascular injection has been avoided.

Mixtures of local anesthetics are sometimes employed to compensate for the slower onset of one drug and the shorter duration of action of the second drug. Experiments in primates suggest that toxicity is probably additive when mixtures of local anesthetics are employed, but some experiments in rodents suggest synergism. Caution regarding toxic equivalence should be exercised when mixtures of local anesthetics are employed.

PRECAUTIONS:

GENERAL

The safety and effective use of chloroprocaine depend on proper dosage, correct technique, adequate precautions and readiness for emergencies. Resuscitative equipment, oxygen and other resuscitative drugs should be available for immediate use. (See WARNINGS and ADVERSE REACTIONS). The lowest dosage that results in effective anesthesia should be used to avoid high plasma levels and serious adverse effects. Injections should be made slowly, with frequent aspirations before and during the injection to avoid intravascular injection. Syringe aspirations should also be performed before and during each supplemental injection in continuous (intermittent) catheter techniques. During the administration of epidural anesthesia, it is recommended that a test dose be administered (3 ml of 3% or 5 ml of 2% chloroprocaine-MPF injection) initially and that the patient be monitored for central nervous system toxicity and cardiovascular toxicity, as well as for signs of unintended intrathecal administration, before proceeding. When clinical conditions permit, consideration should be given to employing a chloroprocaine solution that contains epinephrine for the test dose because circulatory changes characteristic of epinephrine may also serve as a warring sign of unintended intravascular injection. An intravascular injection is still possible even if aspirations for blood are negative. With the use of continuous catheter techniques, it is recommended that a fraction of each supplemental dose be administered as a test dose in order to verify proper location of the catheter.

Injection of repeated doses of local anesthetics may cause significant increases in plasma levels with each repeated dose due to slow accumulation of the drug or its metabolites. Tolerance to elevated blood levels varies with the physical condition of the patient. Debilitated, elderly patients, acutely ill patients, and children should be given reduced doses commensurate with their age and physical status. Local anesthetics should also be used with caution in patients with hypotension or heart block.

Careful and constant monitoring of cardiovascular and respiratory (adequacy of ventilation) vital signs and the patient's state of consciousness should be accomplished after each local anesthetic injection. It should be kept in mind at such times that restlessness, anxiety, tinnitus, dizziness, blurred vision, tremors, depression or drowsiness may be early warning signs of central nervous system toxicity.

Local anesthetic injections containing a vasoconstrictor should be used cautiously and in carefully circumscribed quantities in areas of the body supplied by end arteries or having otherwise comprised blood supply. Patients with peripheral vascular disease and those with hypertensive vascular disease may exhibit exaggerated vasoconstrictor response. Ischemic injury or necrosis may result.

Since ester-type local anesthetics are hydrolyzed by plasma cholinesterase produced by the liver, chloroprocaine should be used cautiously in patients with hepatic disease.

Local anesthetics should also be used with caution in patients with impaired cardiovascular function since they may be less able to compensate for functional changes associated with the prolongation of A-V condition produced by these drugs.

Use in Ophthalmic Surgery: When local anesthetic injections are employed for retrobulbar block, lack of corneal sensation should not be relied upon to determine whether or not the patient is ready for surgery. This is because complete lack of corneal sensation usually precedes clinically acceptable external ocular muscle akinesia.

INFORMATION FOR THE PATIENT

When appropriate, patients should be informed in advance that they may experience temporary loss of sensation and motor activity, usually in the lower half of the body, following proper administration of epidural anesthesia.

CARCINOGENESIS, MUTAGENESIS, AND IMPAIRMENT OF FERTILITY

Long-term studies in animals to evaluate carcinogenic potential and reproduction studies to evaluate mutagenesis or impairment of fertility have not been conducted with chloroprocaine.

PREGNANCY CATEGORY C

Animal reproduction studies have not been conducted with chloroprocaine. It is also not known whether chloroprocaine can cause fetal harm when administered to a pregnant woman or can affect reproduction capacity. Chloroprocaine should be given to pregnant woman only if clearly needed. This does not preclude the use of chloroprocaine at term for the production of obstetrical anesthesia.

LABOR AND DELIVERY

Local anesthetics rapidly cross the placenta, and when used for epidural, paracervical, pudendal or caudal block anesthesia, can cause varying degrees of maternal, fetal and neonatal toxicity. See CLINICAL PHARMACOLOGY, Pharmacokinetics.

The incidence and degree of toxicity depend upon the procedure performed, the type amount of drug used, and the technique of drug administration. Adverse reactions in the parturient, fetus and neonate involve alterations of the central nervous system, peripheral vascular tone and cardial function.

Maternal hypotension has resulted from regional anesthesia. Local anesthetics produce vasodilation by blocking sympathetic nerves. Elevating the patient's legs and positioning her on her left side will help prevent decrease in blood pressure. The fetal heart rate also should be monitored continuously, and electronic fetal monitoring is highly advisable.

PRECAUTIONS: *(cont'd)*

Epidural, paracervical, or pudendal anesthesia may alter the forces of parturition through changes in uterine contractility or maternal expulsive efforts. In one study, paracervical block anesthesia was associated with a decrease in the mean duration of first stage labor and facilitation of cervical dilation. However, epidural anesthesia has also been reported to prolong the second stage of labor by removing the parturient's reflex urge to bear down or by interfering with motor function. The use of obstetrical anesthesia may increase the need for forceps assistance.

The use of some local anesthetic drug products during labor and delivery may be followed by diminished muscle strength and tone for the first day or two of life. The long-term significance of these observations in unknown.

Careful adherence to recommended dosage is of the utmost importance in obstetrical paracervical block. Failure to achieve adequate analgesia with recommended doses should arouse suspicion of intravascular or fetal intracranial injection. Cases compatible with unintended fetal intracranial injection of local anesthetic injection have been reported following intended paracervical or pudendal block or both. Babies so affected present with unexplained neonatal depression at birth which correlates with high local anesthetic serum levels and usually manifest seizures within six hours. Prompt use of supportive measures combined with forced urinary excretion of the local anesthetic has been used successfully to manage this complication.

Case reports of maternal convulsions and cardiovascular collapse following use of some local anesthetics for paracervical block in early pregnancy (as anesthesia for elective abortion) suggest that systemic absorption under these circumstances may be rapid. The recommended maximum dose of each drug should not be exceeded. Injection should be made slowly and with frequent aspiration. Allow a 5-minute interval between sides.

There are no data concerning use of chloroprocaine for obstetrical paracervical block when toxemia of pregnancy is present or when fetal distress or prematurity is anticipated in advance of the block; such use is, therefore, not recommended.

The following information should be considered by clinicians who select chloroprocaine for obstetrical paracervical block anesthesia:

1. Fetal bradycardia (generally a heart rate of less than 120 per minute for more than 2 minutes) has been noted by electronic monitoring in about 5 to 10 percent of the cases (various studies) where initial total doses of 120 mg to 400 mg of chloroprocaine were employed. The incidence of bradycardia, within this dose range, might not be dose related.

2. Fetal acidosis has not been demonstrated by blood gas monitoring around the time of bradycardia or afterwards. These data are limited and generally restricted to nontoxemic cases where fetal distress or prematurity was not anticipated in advance of the block.

3. No intact chloroprocaine and only trace quantities of a hydrolysis product, 2-chloro-4-aminobenzoic acid, have been demonstrated in umbilical cord arterial or venous plasma following properly administered paracervical block with chloroprocaine.

4. The role of drug factors and non-drug factors associated with fetal bradycardia following paracervical block is unexplained at this time.

NURSING MOTHERS

It is not known whether this drug is excreted in human milk. Because many drugs are excreted in human milk, caution should be exercised when chloroprocaine is administered to a nursing woman.

PEDIATRIC USE

Guidelines for the administration of chloroprocaine HCl injections to children are presented in DOSAGE AND ADMINISTRATION.

DRUG INTERACTIONS:

The administration of local anesthetic solutions containing epinephrine or norepinephrine to patients receiving monoamine oxidase inhibitors, tricyclic antidepressants or phenothiazines may produce severe, prolonged hypotension or hypertension. Concurrent use of these agents should generally be avoided. In situations when concurrent therapy is necessary, careful patient monitoring is essential.

Concurrent administration of vasopressor drugs (for the treatment of hypotension related to obstetric blocks) and ergot-type oxytocic drugs may cause severe, persistent hypertension or cerebrovascular accidents.

The para-aminobenzoic acid metabolite of chloroprocaine inhibits the action of sulfonamides. Therefore, chloroprocaine should not be used in any condition in which a sulfonamide drug is being employed.

ADVERSE REACTIONS:

Systemic: The most commonly encountered acute adverse experiences that demand immediate countermeasures are related to the central nervous system and the cardiovascular system. These adverse experiences are generally dose related and may result from rapid absorption from the injection site, diminished tolerance, or from unintentional intravascular injection of the local anesthetic solution. In addition to systemic dose-related toxicity, unintentional subarachnoid injection of drug during the intended performance of caudal or lumbar epidural block or nerve blocks near the vertebral column (especially in the head and neck region) may result in underventilation or apnea ("Total Spinal"). Factors influencing plasma protein binding, such as acidosis, systemic diseases that alter protein production, or competition of other drugs for protein binding sites, may diminish individual tolerance. Plasma cholinesterase deficiency may also account for diminished tolerance to ester type local anesthetics.

Central Nervous System Reactions: These are characterized by excitation and/or depression. Restlessness, anxiety, dizziness, tinnitus, blurred vision or tremors may occur, possibly proceeding to convulsions. However, excitement may be transient or absent, with depression being the first manifestation of an adverse reaction. This may quickly be followed by drowsiness merging into unconsciousness and respiratory arrest.

The incidence of convulsions associated with the use of local anesthetics varies with the procedure used and the total dose administered. In a survey of studies of epidural anesthesia, overt toxicity progressing to convulsions occurred in approximately 0.1 percent of local anesthetic administrations.

Cardiovascular System Reactions: High doses, or unintended intravascular injection, may lead to high plasma levels and related depression of the myocardium, hypotension, bradycardia, ventricular arrhythmias, and, possibly, cardiac arrest.

Allergic: Allergic type reactions are rare and may occur as a result of sensitivity to the local anesthetic or to other formulation ingredients, such as the antimicrobial preservative methylparaben, contained in multiple dose vials. These reactions are characterized by signs such as urticaria, pruritus, erythema, angioneurotic edema (including laryngeal edema), tachycardia, sneezing, nausea, vomiting, dizziness, syncope, excessive sweating, elevated temperature, and possibly, anaphylactoid type symptomatology (including severe hypotension). Cross sensitivity among members of the ester-type local anesthetic group has been reported. The usefulness of screening for sensitivity has not been definitely established.

ADVERSE REACTIONS: *(cont'd)*

Neurologic: In the practice of caudal or lumbar epidural block, occasional unintentional penetration of the subarachnoid space by the catheter may occur (see PRECAUTIONS). Subsequent adverse observations may depend partially on the amount of drug administered intrathecally. These observations may include spinal block of varying magnitude (including total spinal block), hypotension secondary to spinal block, loss of bladder and bowel control, and loss of perineal sensation and sexual function. Arachnoiditis, persistent motor, sensory and/or autonomic (sphincter control) deficit of some lower spinal segments with slow recovery (several months) or incomplete recovery have been reported in rare instances. (See DOSAGE AND ADMINISTRATION) discussion of Caudal and Lumbar Epidural Block.Backache and headache have also been noted following lumbar epidural or caudal block.

OVERDOSAGE:

Acute emergencies from local anesthetics are generally related to high plasma levels encountered during therapeutic use of local anesthetics or to unintended subarachnoid injection of local anesthetic solution (see ADVERSE REACTIONS, WARNINGS, and PRECAUTIONS).

In mice, the intravenous LD_{50} of chloroprocaine HCl is 97 mg/kg and the subcutaneous LD_{50} of chloroprocaine HCl is 950 mg/kg.

Management of Local Anesthetic Emergencies: The first consideration is prevention, best accomplished by careful and constant monitoring of cardiovascular and respiratory vital signs and the patient's state of consciousness after each local anesthetic injection. At the first sign of change, oxygen should be administered.

The first step in the management of convulsions, as well as underventilation or apnea due to unintentional subarachnoid injection of drug solution, consists of immediate attention to the maintenance of a patent airway and assisted or controlled ventilation with oxygen and a delivery system capable of permitting immediate positive airway pressure by mask. Immediately after the institution of these ventilatory measures, the adequacy of the circulation should be evaluated, keeping in mind that drugs used to treat convulsions sometimes depress the circulation when administered intravenously. Should convulsions persist despite adequate respiratory support, and if the status of the circulation permits, small increments of an ultra-short acting barbiturate (such as thiopental or thiamylal) or a benzodiazepine (such as diazepam) may be administered intravenously; the clinician should be familiar, prior to the use of anesthetics, with these anticonvulsant drugs. Supportive treatment of circulatory depression may require administration of intravenous fluids and, when appropriate, a vasopressor dictated by the clinical situation (such as ephedrine to enhance myocardial contractile force).

If not treated immediately, both convulsions and cardiovascular depression can result in hypoxia, acidosis, bradycardia, arrhythmias and cardiac arrest. Underventilation or apnea due to unintentional subarachnoid injection of local anesthetic solution may produce these same signs and also lead to cardiac arrest if ventilatory support is not instituted. If cardiac arrest should occur, standard cardiopulmonary resuscitative measures should be instituted. Recovery has been reported after prolonged resuscitative efforts.

Endotracheal intubation, employing drugs and techniques familiar to the clinician, may be indicated, after initial administration of oxygen by mask, if difficulty is encountered in the maintenance of a patent airway of if prolonged ventilatory support (assisted or controlled) is indicated.

DOSAGE AND ADMINISTRATION:

Chloroprocaine may be administered as a single injection or continuously through an indwelling catheter. As with all local anesthetics, the dose administered varies with the anesthetic procedure, the vascularity of the tissues, the depth of anesthesia and degree of muscle relaxation required, the duration of anesthesia desired, and the physical condition of the patient. The smallest dose and concentration required to produce the desired result should be used. Dosage should be reduced for children, elderly and debilitated patients and patients with cardiac and/or liver disease. The maximum single recommended doses of chloroprocaine in adults are: without epinephrine, 11 mg/kg, not to exceed a maximum total dose of 800 mg; with epinephrine (1:200,000), 14 mg/kg, not to exceed a maximum total dose of 1000 mg. For specific techniques and procedures, refer to standard textbooks.

Caudal and Lumbar Epidural Block: In order to guard against adverse experiences sometimes noted following unintended penetration of the subarachnoid space, the following procedure modifications are recommended:

1. Use an adequate test dose (3 ml of chloroprocaine-MPF 3% injection or 5 ml of chloroprocaine-MPF 2% injection) prior to induction of complete block. This test dose should be repeated if the patient is moved in such a fashion as to have displaced the epidural catheter. Allow adequate time for onset of anesthesia following administration of each test dose.

2. Avoid the rapid injection of a large volume of local anesthetic injection through the catheter. Consider fractional doses, when feasible.

3. In the event of the known injection of a large volume of local anesthetic injection into the subarachnoid space, after suitable resuscitation and if the catheter is in place, consider attempting the recovery of drug by draining a moderate amount of cerebrospinal fluid (such as 10 ml) through the epidural catheter.

As a guide for some routine procedures, suggested doses are given below (TABLE 2).

1. Infiltration and Peripheral Nerve Block: chloroprocaine or chloroprocaine-MPF (chloroprocaine HCl) injection

TABLE 2

Anesthetic Procedure	Solution Concentration %	Volume (ml)	Total Dose (mg)
Mandibular	2	2-3	40-60
Infraorbital	2	0.5-1	10-20
Brachial plexus	2	30-40	600-800
Digital (without epinephrine)	1	3-4	30-40
Pudendal	2	10 each side	400
Paracervical (see alsoPRECAUTIONS)	1	3 per each of 4 sites	up to 120

2. Caudal and Lumbar Epidural Block: chloroprocaine-MPF injection. For caudal anesthesia, the initial dose is 15 to 25 ml of a 2% or 3% solution. Repeated doses may be given at 40 to 60 minute intervals.

For lumbar epidural anesthesia, 2 to 2.5 ml per segment of a 2% or 3% solution can be used. The usual total volume of chloroprocaine-MPF injection is from 15 to 25 ml. Repeated doses 2 to 6 ml less than the original dose may be given at 40 to 50 minute intervals.

The above dosages are recommended as a guide for use in the average adult. Maximum dosages of all local anesthetics must be individualized after evaluating the size and physical condition of the patient and the rate of systemic absorption from a particular injection site.

DOSAGE AND ADMINISTRATION: *(cont'd)*

Pediatric Dosage: It is difficult to recommend a maximum dose of any drug for children, since this varies as a function of age and weight. For children over 3 years of age who have a normal lean body mass and normal body development, the maximum dose is determined by the child's age and weight and should not exceed 11 mg/kg (5 mg/lb). For example, in a child of 5 years weighing 50 lbs (23 kg), the dose of chloroprocaine HCl without epinephrine would be 250 mg. Concentrations of 0.5-1.0% are suggested for infiltration and 1.0-1.5% for nerve block. In order to guard against systemic toxicity, the lowest effective concentration and lowest effective dose should be used at all time. Some of other lower concentrations for use in infants and smaller children are not available in pre-packaged containers; it will be necessary to dilute available concentrations with the amount of 0.9% sodium chloride injection necessary to obtain the required final concentration of chloroprocaine injection.

Preparation of Epinephrine Injections: To prepare a 1:200,000 epinephrine-chloroprocaine HCl injection, add 0.15 ml of a 1 to 100 Epinephrine injection USP to 30 ml of chloroprocaine-MPF injection.

Chloroprocaine is incompatible with caustic alkalis and their carbonates, soaps, silver salts, iodine and iodides.

Parenteral drug products should be inspected visually for particulate matter and discoloration prior to administration, whenever injection and container permit. As with other anesthetics having a free aromatic amino group, chloroprocaine HCl injections are slightly photosensitive and may become discolored after prolonged exposure to light. It is recommended that these vials be stored in the original outer containers, protected from direct sunlight. Discolored injection should not be administered. If exposed to low temperatures, chloroprocaine HCl injections may deposit crystals of chloroprocaine HCl which will redissolve with shaking when returned to room temperature. The product should not be used if it contains undissolved (*e.g.,* particulate) material.

Keep from freezing. Protect from light. Store at controlled room temperature 15-30°C (59-86°F).

HOW SUPPLIED - RATED THERAPEUTICALLY EQUIVALENT:

Injection, Solution - Epidural - 2 %

30 ml	$8.21	CHLOROPROCAINE HCL, Abbott	00074-4169-01
30 ml	**$16.04**	**NESACAINE, Astra USA**	**00186-0972-66**
30 ml	**$17.80**	**NESACAINE-MPF, Astra USA**	**00186-0993-66**

Injection, Solution - Epidural - 3 %

30 ml	$9.99	CHLOROPROCAINE HCL, Abbott	00074-4170-01
30 ml	**$18.69**	**NESACAINE MPF 3 %, Astra USA**	**00186-0994-66**

HOW SUPPLIED - NOT RATED EQUIVALENT:

Injection, Solution - Epidural - 1 %

30 ml	**$15.65**	**NESACAINE, Astra USA**	**00186-0971-66**

CHLOROQUINE HYDROCHLORIDE *(000736)*

CATEGORIES: Amebiasis; Aminoquinolines; Anti-Infectives; Antimalarial Agents; Antiprotozoals; Malaria; Parasiticidal; FDA Approval Pre 1982

BRAND NAMES: **Aralen Injection**

FORMULARIES: Aetna; WHO

For Malaria and Extraintestinal Amebiasis

WARNING: PHYSICIANS SHOULD COMPLETELY FAMILIARIZE THEMSELVES WITH THE COMPLETE CONTENTS OF THIS MONOGRAPH BEFORE PRESCRIBING CHLOROQUINE HCl.

Parenteral solution, each ml containing 50 mg of the dihydrochloride salt equivalent to 40 mg of chloroquine base. Chloroquine hydrochloride, a 4-aminoquinoline compound, is chemically 7-(Chloro-[[4-diethylamino)-1-methylbutyl] amino]-quinoline dihydrochloride, a white, crystalline substance, freely soluble in water.

DESCRIPTION:

CLINICAL PHARMACOLOGY:

The compound is a highly active antimalarial and amebicidal agent. Chloroquine hydrochloride has been found to be highly active against the erythrocytic forms of *Plasmodium vivax* and *malariae* and most strains of *Plasmodium falciparum* (but not the gametocytes of *P. falciparum).* The precise mechanism of action of the drug is not known.

Chloroquine hydrochloride does not prevent relapses in patients with vivax or malariae malaria because it is not effective against exoerythrocytic forms of the parasite, nor will it prevent vivax or malariae infection when administered as a prophylactic. It is highly effective as a suppressive agent in patients with vivax or malariae malaria, in terminating acute attacks, and significantly lengthening the interval between treatment and relapse. In patients with falciparum malaria it abolishes the acute attack and effects complete cure of the infection, unless due to a resistant strain of *P. falciparum.*

INDICATIONS AND USAGE:

Chloroquine hydrochloride is indicated for the treatment of extraintestinal amebiasis and for treatment of acute attacks of malaria due to *P. vivax, P. malariae, P. ovale,* and susceptible strains of *P. falciparum* when oral therapy is not feasible.

CONTRAINDICATIONS:

Use of this drug is contraindicated in the presence of retinal or visual field changes, either attributable to 4-aminoquinoline compounds or to any other etiology, and in patients with known hypersensitivity to 4-aminoquinoline compounds, However, in treatment of acute attacks of malaria caused by susceptible strains of plasmodia, the physician may elect to use this drug after carefully weighing the possible benefits and risks to the patient.

WARNINGS:

Children and infants are extremely susceptible to adverse effects from an overdose of parenteral chloroquine HCl and sudden deaths have been recorded after such administration. In no instance should the single dose of parenteral chloroquine HCl administered to infants or children exceed 5 mg base per kg.

In recent years, it has been found that certain strains of *P. falciparum* have become resistant to 4-aminoquinoline compounds (including chloroquine and hydroxychloroquine) as shown by the fact that normally adequate doses have failed to prevent or cure clinical malaria or parasitemia. Treatment with quinine or other specific forms of therapy is therefore advised for patients infected with a resistant strain of parasites.

Use of chloroquine HCl should be avoided in patients with psoriasis, for it may precipitate a severe attack of psoriasis. Some authors consider the use of 4-aminoquinoline compounds contraindicated in patients with porphyria since the condition may be exacerbated.

WARNINGS: *(cont'd)*

Irreversible retinal damage has observed in some patients who had received long-term or high-dosage 4-aminoquinoline therapy. Retinopathy has been reported to be dose related.

If there is any indication (past or present) of abnormality in the visual acuity, visual field, or retinal macular areas (such as pigmentary changes, loss of foveal reflex), or any visual symptoms (such as light flashes and streaks) which are not fully explainable by difficulties of accommodation or corneal opacities, the drug should be discontinued immediately and the patient closely observed for possible progression. Retinal changes (and visual disturbances) may progress even after cessation of therapy.

Usage in Pregnancy: Usage of this drug during pregnancy should be avoided except in the suppression or treatment of malaria when in the judgment of the physician the benefit outweighs the possible hazard. It should be noted that radioactively tagged chloroquine administered intravenously to pregnant pigmented CBA mice passed rapidly across the placenta, accumulated selectively in the melanin structures of the fetal eyes and was retained in the ocular tissues for five months after the drug had been eliminated from the rest of the body.[1]

PRECAUTIONS:

Since the drug is known to concentrate in the liver, it should be used with caution in patients with hepatic disease or alcoholism or in conjunction with known hepatotoxic drugs.

The drug should be administered with caution to patients having G-6-PD (glucose-6-phosphate dehydrogenase) deficiency.

ADVERSE REACTIONS:

Respiratory depression, cardiovascular collapse, shock, convulsions, and death have been reported with overdoses of chloroquine hydrochloride, especially in infants and children.

Any of the adverse reactions associated with short-term oral administration of chloroquine phosphate must be considered a possibility with chloroquine hydrochloride. Cardiovascular effects, such as hypotension and electrocardiographic changes (particularly inversion or depression of the T-wave, widening of the QRS complex), have rarely been noted in patients receiving usual antimalarial doses of the drug. Mild and transient headache, pruritus, psychic stimulation, visual disturbances (blurring vision and difficulty of focusing or accommodation), pleomorphic skin eruptions, and gastrointestinal complaints (anorexia, nausea, vomiting, diarrhea, abdominal cramps) have been observed.

Instances of convulsive seizures associated with oral chloroquine therapy in patients with extraintestinal amebiasis have been reported.

A few cases of a nerve type of deafness have been reported after prolonged therapy, usually high doses. Tinnitus and reduced hearing have been reported, in a patient with preexistent auditory damage, after administration of only 500 mg once a week for a few months. Since neuromyopathy, blood dyscrasias, lichen planus-like eruptions, and skin and mucosal pigmentary changes have been noted during prolonged oral therapy, their occurrence with this dosage form is possible.

Patients with retinal changes may be asymptomatic, especially in early cases, or may complain of nyctalopia and scotomatous vision with field defects of paracentral, pericentral ring types, and typically temporal scotomas, e.g., difficulty in reading with words tending to disappear, seeing only half an object, misty vision, and fog before the eyes. Rarely scotomatous vision may occur without observable retinal changes.

OVERDOSAGE:

Inadvertent toxic doses may produce respiratory depression or shock with hypotension. Respiratory depression is treated by artificial respiration and administration of oxygen. In shock with hypotension, a potent vasopressor, such as Neo-Synephrine hydrochloride, brand of phenylephrine hydrochloride, USP, should be given intramuscularly in doses of 2 mg to 5 mg.

DOSAGE AND ADMINISTRATION:

MALARIA

Adult Dose: An initial dose of 4 ml or 5 ml (160 mg to 200 mg chloroquine base) may be injected intramuscularly and repeated in 6 hours if necessary. The total parenteral dose in the first 24 hours should not exceed 800 mg chloroquine base. Treatment by mouth should be started as soon as practicable and continued until a course of approximately 1.5 g of base in 3 days is complete.

Pediatric Dose: Infants and children are extremely susceptible to overdosage of parenteral chloroquine HCl. Severe reactions and deaths have occurred. In the pediatric age range, parenteral chloroquine HCl dosage should be calculated in proportion to the adult dose based upon body weight. The recommended single dose in infants and children is 5 mg base per kg. This dose may be repeated in 6 hours; however, the total dose in any 24 hour period should not exceed 10 mg base per kg of body weight. Parenteral administration should be terminated and oral therapy instituted as soon as possible.

Extraintenstinal Amebiasis: In adult patients not able to tolerate oral therapy, from 4 ml to 5 ml (160 mg to 200 mg chloroquine base) may be injected daily for 10 to 12 days. Oral administration should be substituted or resumed as soon as possible.

REFERENCES:

1. Ullberg S, Lindquist N G, Sjostrand S E: Accumulation of chorio-retinotoxic drugs in the foetal eye. *Nature* 1970; 227: 1257.

HOW SUPPLIED - EQUIVALENTS NOT AVAILABLE:

Injection, Solution - Intravenous - 50 mg/ml

5 ml x 5 $72.18 ARALEN, Sanofi Winthrop 00024-0074-01

CHLOROQUINE PHOSPHATE *(000738)*

CATEGORIES: Amebiasis; Aminoquinolines; Anti-Infectives; Antimalarial Agents; Antiprotozoals; Malaria; Parasiticidal; FDA Approval Pre 1982

BRAND NAMES: *Anoclor*, **Aralen**; *Avloclor* (England); *Cadiquin*; *Chlorofoz*; *Chlorquin*; *Chloroquini Diphosphas*; *Cidanchin*; *Clo-Kit Junior*; *Clor-Alen*; *Clorkin*; *Delagil*; *Dichinalex*; *Diroquine*; *Emquin*; *Genocin*; *Heliopar*, *Klorokinfosfat*; *Lagaquin*; *Lariago*; *Malarex*; *Malaviron*; *Malarivon*; *Melubrin*; *Mexaquin*; *Nivaquine*; *P Roquine*; *Quinalen*; *Repal*; *Resochin* (Germany); *Resochina*
(International brand names outside U.S. in italics)

FORMULARIES: Medi-Cal; PCS

For Malaria and Extraintestinal Amebiasis

WARNING: PHYSICIANS SHOULD COMPLETELY FAMILIARIZE THEMSELVES WITH THE COMPLETE CONTENTS OF THIS MONOGRAPH BEFORE PRESCRIBING CHLOROQUINE PHOSPHATE.

DESCRIPTION:

Chloroquine phosphate, brand of chloroquine phosphate, USP, is a 4-aminoquinoline compound for oral administration. It is a white, odorless, bitter tasting, crystalline substance, freely soluble in water.

Chloroquine phosphate is an antimalarial and amebicidal drug.

Chemically, it is 7-chloro-4-[[4-(diethylamino)-1-methylbutyl] amino] quinoline phosphate (1: 2). *Aralen Inactive Ingredients:* Carnauba Wax, Colloidal Silicon Dioxide, D&C Red No 27, Dibasic Calcium Phosphate, Hydroxypropyl Methylcellulose, Magnesium Stearate, Microcrystalline Cellulose, Polyethylene Glycol, Polysorbate 80, Pregelatinized Starch, Sodium Starch Glycolate, Stearic Acid, Titanium Dioxide.

CLINICAL PHARMACOLOGY:

Chloroquine phosphate has been found to be active against the erythrocytic forms of *Plasmodium vivax* and *Plasmodium malariae* and most strains of *Plasmodium falciparum* (but not the gametocytes of *P. falciparum).*

The mechanism of plasmodicidal action of chloroquine is not completely certain. While the drug can inhibit certain enzymes, its effect is believed to result, at least in part, from its interaction with DNA.

Chloroquine is rapidly and almost completely absorbed from the gastrointestinal tract, and only a small proportion of the administered dose is found in the stools. Approximately 55% of the drug in the plasma is bound to nondiffusible plasma constituents. Excretion of chloroquine is quite slow, but is increased by acidification of the urine. Chloroquine is deposited in the tissues in considerable amounts. In animals, from 200 to 700 times the plasma concentration may be found in the liver, spleen, kidney, and lung; leukocytes also concentrate the drug. The brain and spinal cord, in contrast, contain only 10 to 30 times the amount present in plasma.

Chloroquine undergoes appreciable degradation in the body. The main metabolite is desethylchloroquine, which accounts for one fourth of the total material appearing in the urine; bisdesethylchloroquine, a carboxylic acid derivative, and other metabolic products as yet uncharacterized are found in small amounts. Slightly more than half of the urinary drug products can be accounted for as unchanged chloroquine.

Microbiology: Chloroquine phosphate has been found to be highly active against the erythrocytic forms of *Plasmodium vivax* and *malariae* and most strains of *Plasmodium falciparum* (but not the gametocytes of *P. falciparum*). The precise mechanism of action of the drug is not known.

In vitro studies with trophozoites of *Entamoeba histolytica* have demonstrated that chloroquine phosphate also possesses amebicidal activity comparable to that of emetine.

INDICATIONS AND USAGE:

Chloroquine phosphate is indicated for the suppressive treatment and for acute attacks of malaria due to *P. vivax, P. malariae, P. ovale,* and susceptible strains of *P. falciparum.* The drug is also indicated for the treatment of extraintestinal amebiasis.

Chloroquine phosphate does not prevent relapses in patients with vivax or malariae malaria because it is not effective against exoerythrocytic forms of the parasite, nor will it prevent vivax or malariae infection when administered as a prophylactic. It is highly effective as a suppressive agent in patients with vivax or malariae malaria, in terminating acute attacks, and significantly lengthening the interval between treatment and relapse. In patients with falciparum malaria it abolishes the acute attack and effects complete cure of the infection, unless due to a resistant strain of *P. falciparum.*

CONTRAINDICATIONS:

Use of this drug is contraindicated in the presence of retinal or visual field changes either attributable to 4-aminoquinoline compounds or to any other etiology, and in patients with known hypersensitivity to 4-aminoquinoline compounds. However, in the treatment of acute attacks of malaria caused by susceptible strains of plasmodia, the physician may elect to use this drug after carefully weighing the possible benefits and risks to the patient.

WARNINGS:

In recent years it has been found that certain strains of *P. falciparum* have become resistant to 4-aminoquinoline compounds (including chloroquine and hydroxy-chloroquine) as shown by the fact that normally adequate doses have failed to prevent or cure clinical malaria or parasitemia. Treatment with quinine or other specific forms of therapy is therefore advised for patients infected with a resistant strain of parasites.

Irreversible retinal damage has been observed in some patients who had received long-term or high-dosage 4-aminoquinoline therapy. Retinopathy has been reported to be dose related.

When prolonged therapy with any antimalarial compound is contemplated, initial (base line) and periodic ophthalmologic examinations (including visual acuity, expert slit-lamp, funduscopic, and visual field tests) should be performed.

If there is any indication (past or present) of abnormality in the visual acuity, visual field, or retinal macular areas (such as pigmentary changes, loss of foveal reflex), or any visual symptoms (such as light flashes and streaks) which are not fully explainable by difficulties of accommodation or corneal opacities, the drug should be discontinued immediately and the patient closely observed for possible progression. Retinal changes (and visual disturbances) may progress even after cessation of therapy.

All patients on long-term therapy with this preparation should be questioned and examined periodically, including testing knee and ankle reflexes, to detect any evidence of muscular weakness. If weakness occurs, discontinue the drug.

A number of fatalities have been reported following the accidental ingestion of chloroquine, sometimes in relatively small doses (0.75 g or 1 g chloroquine phosphate in one 3-year-old child). Patients should be strongly warned to keep this drug out of the reach of children because they are especially sensitive to the 4-aminoquinoline compounds.

Use of chloroquine phosphate in patients with psoriasis may precipitate a severe attack of psoriasis. When used in patients with porphyria the condition may be exacerbated. The drug should not be used in these conditions unless in the judgment of the physician the benefit to the patient outweighs the possible hazard.

PRECAUTIONS:

General: If any severe blood disorder appears which is not attributable to the disease under treatment, discontinuance of the drug should be considered.

Since this drug is known to concentrate in the liver, it should be used with caution in patients with hepatic disease or alcoholism or in conjunction with known hepatotoxic drugs.

The drug should be administered with caution to patients having G-6-PD (glucose-6 phosphate dehydrogenase) deficiency.

Laboratory Tests: Complete blood cell counts should be made periodically if patients are given prolonged therapy.

Nursing Mothers: Because of the potential for serious adverse reactions in nursing infants from chloroquine, a decision should be made whether to discontinue nursing or to discontinue the drug, taking into account the importance of the drug to the mother.

PRECAUTIONS: *(cont'd)*

Pediatric Use: See WARNINGS and DOSAGE AND ADMINISTRATION.

ADVERSE REACTIONS:

Ocular reactions: Irreversible retinal damage in patients receiving long-term or high-dosage 4-aminoquinoline therapy; visual disturbances (blurring of vision and difficulty of focusing or accommodation); nyctalopia; scotomatous vision with field defects of paracentral, pericentral ring types, and typically temporal scotomas, (*e.g.*, difficulty in reading with words tending to disappear, seeing half an object, misty vision, and fog before the eyes).

Neuromuscular reactions: Convulsive seizures.

Auditory reactions: Nerve type deafness; tinnitus, reduced hearing in patients with preexisting auditory damage.

Gastrointestinal reactions: Anorexia, nausea, vomiting, diarrhea, abdominal cramps.

Dermatologic reactions: Pleomorphic skin eruptions, skin and mucosal pigmentary changes; lichen planus-like eruptions, pruritus, and hair loss.

CNS reactions: Mild and transient headache, psychic stimulation.

Cardiovascular reactions: Rarely, hypotension, electrocardiographic change.

OVERDOSAGE:

Symptoms: Chloroquine is very rapidly and completely absorbed after ingestion. Toxic doses of chloroquine can be fatal. As little as 1 g may be fatal in children. Toxic symptoms can occur within minutes. These consist of headache, drowsiness, visual disturbances, nausea and vomiting, cardiovascular collapse, and convulsions followed by sudden and early respiratory and cardiac arrest. The electrocardiogram may reveal atrial standstill, nodal rhythm, prolonged intraventricular conduction time, and progressive bradycardia leading to ventricular fibrillation and/or arrest.

Treatment: Treatment is symptomatic and must be prompt with immediate evacuation of the stomach by emesis (at home, before transportation to the hospital) or gastric lavage until the stomach is completely emptied. If finely powdered, activated charcoal is introduced by stomach tube, after lavage, and within 30 minutes after ingestion of the antimalarial, it may inhibit further intestinal absorption of the drug. To be effective, the dose of activated charcoal should be at least five times the estimated dose of chloroquine ingested.

Convulsions, if present, should be controlled before attempting gastric lavage. If due to cerebral stimulation, cautious administration of an ultra short-acting barbiturate may be tried but, if due to anoxia, it should be corrected by oxygen administration and artificial respiration. In shock with hypotension, a potent vasopressor should be administered. Because of the importance of supporting respiration, tracheal intubation or tracheostomy, followed by gastric lavage, may also be necessary. Peritoneal dialysis and exchange transfusions have also been suggested to reduce the level of the drug in the blood.

A patient who survives the acute phase and is asymptomatic should be closely observed for at least six hours. Fluids may be forced, and sufficient ammonium chloride (8 g daily in divided doses for adults) may be administered for a few days to acidify the urine to help promote urinary excretion in cases of both overdosage or sensitivity.

DOSAGE AND ADMINISTRATION:

The dosage of chloroquine phosphate is often expressed or calculated as the base. Each 500 mg tablet of chloroquine phosphate is equivalent to 300 mg base. In infants and children the dosage is preferably calculated on the body weight.

MALARIA SUPPRESSION

Adult Dose: 500 mg (= 300 mg base) on exactly the same day of each week.

Pediatric Dose: The weekly suppressive dosage is 5 mg calculated as base, per kg of body weight, but should not exceed the adult dose regardless of weight.

If circumstances permit, suppressive therapy should begin two weeks prior to exposure. However, failing this in adults, an initial double (loading) dose of 1 g (= 600 mg base), or in children 10 mg base/kg may be taken in two divided doses, six hours apart. The suppressive therapy should be continued for eight weeks after leaving the endemic area.

FOR TREATMENT OF ACUTE ATTACK

Adults: An initial dose of 1 g (= 600 mg base) followed by an additional 500 mg (= 300 mg base) after six to eight hours and a single dose of 500 mg (= 300 mg base) on each of two consecutive days. This represents a total dose of 2.5 g chloroquine phosphate or 1.5 g base in three days.

The dosage for adults may also be calculated on the basis of body weight; this method is preferred for infants and children. A total dose representing 25 mg of base per kg of body weight is administered in three days, as follows: *First dose:* 10 mg base per kg (but not exceeding a single dose of 600 mg base). *Second dose:* 5 mg base per kg (but not exceeding a single dose of 300 mg base) 6 hours after first dose. *Third dose:* 5 mg base per kg 18 hours after second dose. *Fourth dose:* 5 mg base per kg 24 hours after third dose.

For radical cure of *vivax* and *malariae* malaria concomitant therapy with an 8-aminoquinoline compound is necessary.

Extraintestinal Amebiasis: *Adults:* 1 g (600 mg base) daily for two days, followed by 500 mg (300 mg base) daily for at least two to three weeks. Treatment is usually combined with an effective intestinal amebicide.

HOW SUPPLIED - RATED THERAPEUTICALLY EQUIVALENT:

Tablet, Uncoated - Oral - 250 mg

100's	$7.80	Chloroquine Phosphate, United Res	00677-1011-01
1000's	$49.88	Chloroquine Phosphate, Rugby	00536-3459-10

HOW SUPPLIED - NOT RATED EQUIVALENT:

Tablet, Uncoated - Oral - 250 mg

100's	$17.50	Chloroquine Phosphate, Consolidated Midland	00223-0691-01
1000's	$165.00	Chloroquine Phosphate, Consolidated Midland	00223-0691-02

Tablet, Uncoated - Oral - 500 mg

25's	**$91.60**	**ARALEN PHOSPHATE, Sanofi Winthrop**	**00024-0084-01**

CHLOROTHIAZIDE *(000739)*

CATEGORIES: Antiarrhythmic Agents; Antihypertensives; Cardiovascular Drugs; Cirrhosis; Congestive Heart Failure; Diuretics; Edema; Electrolytic, Caloric-Water Balance; Glomerulonephritis; Heart Failure; Hypertension; Renal Drugs; Renal Failure; Thiazides; Vascular Disorders, Cerebral/Peripheral; Pregnancy Category B; FDA Approval Pre 1982

BRAND NAMES: *Azide*; *Chlothin*; *Chlotride* (Australia, Japan); *Diurazide*; *Diuret*; Diurigen; **Diuril**; *Saluretil*; *Saluric* (England)
(International brand names outside U.S. in italics)

FORMULARIES: Aetna; Medi-Cal

DESCRIPTION:

Chlorothiazide is a diuretic and antihypertensive. It is 6-chloro- 2*H*-1,2,4-benzothiadiazine-7-sulfonamide 1,1-dioxide. Its empirical formula is $C_7H_6ClN_3O_4S_2$.

It is a white, or practically white, crystalline powder with a molecular weight of 295.72, which is very slightly soluble in water, but readily soluble in dilute aqueous sodium hydroxide. It is soluble in urine to the extent of about 150 mg per 100 ml at pH 7.

Chlorothiazide is supplied at 250 mg and 500 mg tablets, for oral use. EachDiuril tablet contains the following inactive ingredients: gelatin, magnesium stearate, starch and talc. The 250 mg tablet also contains lactose.

Oral suspension chlorothiazide contains 250 mg of chlorothiazide per 5 ml, alcohol 0.5 percent, with methylparaben 0.12 percent, propylparaben 0.02 percent, and benzoic acid 0.1 percent added as preservatives. The inactive ingredients are D&C Yellow 10, flavors, glycerin, purified water, sodium saccharin, sucrose and tragacanth.

Intravenous sodium chlorothiazide is a sterile lyophilized white powder and is supplied in a vial containing: Chlorothiazide sodium equivalent to chlorothiazide, 0.5 g; *Inactive ingredients:* Mannitol, 25 g; Sodium hydroxide to adjust pH, with 0.4 mg thimerosal (mercury derivative) added as preservative.

CLINICAL PHARMACOLOGY:

The mechanism of the antihypertensive effect of thiazides is unknown. Chlorothiazide does not usually affect normal blood pressure.

Chlorothiazide affects the distal renal tubular mechanism of electrolyte absorption. At maximal therapeutic dosage all thiazides are approximately equal in their diuretic efficacy.

Chlorothiazide increases excretion of sodium and chloride in approximately equivalent amounts. Natriuresis may be accompanied by some loss of potassium and bicarbonate.

After oral use diuresis begins within 2 hours, peaks in about 4 hours and lasts about 6 to 12 hours. Following intravenous use of sodium chlorothiazide, onset of the diuretic occurs in 15 minutes and the maximal action in 30 minutes.

PHARMACOKINETICS AND METABOLISM

Chlorothiazide is not metabolized but is eliminated rapidly by the kidney. The plasma half-life of chlorothiazide is 45-120 minutes. After oral doses, 10-15 percent of the dose is excreted unchanged in the urine. Chlorothiazide crosses the placental but not the blood-brain barrier and is excreted in breast milk.

INDICATIONS AND USAGE:

Chlorothiazide is indicated as adjunctive therapy in edema associated with congestive heart failure, hepatic cirrhosis, and corticosteroid and estrogen therapy.

Chlorothiazide has also been found useful in edema due to various forms of renal dysfunction such as nephrotic syndrome, acute glomerulonephritis, and chronic renal failure.

Chlorothiazide is indicated in the management of hypertension either as the sole therapeutic agent or to enhance the effectiveness of other antihypertensive drugs in the more severe forms of hypertension.

Use in Pregnancy: Routine use of diuretics during normal pregnancy is inappropriate and exposes mother and fetus to unnecessary hazard. Diuretics do not prevent development of toxemia of pregnancy and there is no satisfactory evidence that they are useful in the treatment of toxemia.

Edema during pregnancy may arise from pathologic causes or from the physiologic and mechanical consequences of pregnancy. Thiazides are indicated in pregnancy when edema is due to pathologic causes, just as they are in the absence of pregnancy (see PRECAUTIONS, Pregnancy). Dependent edema in pregnancy, resulting from the restriction of venous return by the gravid uterus, is properly treated through elevation of the lower extremities and use of support stockings. Use of diuretics to lower intravascular volume in this instance is illogical and unnecessary. During normal pregnancy there is hypervolemia which is not harmful to the fetus or the mother in the absence of cardiovascular disease. However, it may be associated with edema, rarely generalized edema. If such edema causes discomfort, increased recumbency will often provide relief. Rarely this edema may cause extreme discomfort which is not relieved by rest In these instances, a short course of diuretic therapy may provide relief and be appropriate.

CONTRAINDICATIONS:

Anuria: Hypersensitivity to this product or to other sulfonamide-derived drugs.

WARNINGS:

Use with caution in severe renal disease. In patients with renal disease, thiazides may precipitate azotemia. Cumulative effects of the drug may develop in patients with impaired renal function.

Thiazides should be used with caution in patients with impaired hepatic function or progressive liver disease, since minor alterations of fluid and electrolyte balance may precipitate hepatic coma.

Thiazides may add to or potentiate the action of other antihypertensive drugs.

Sensitivity reactions may occur in patients with or without a history of allergy or bronchial asthma.

The possibility of exacerbation or activation of systemic lupus erythematosus has been reported.

Lithium generally should not be given with diuretics (see DRUG INTERACTIONS).

IV ONLY

Intravenous use in infants and children has been limited and is not generally recommended.

PRECAUTIONS:

GENERAL

All patients receiving diuretic therapy should be observed for evidence of fluid or electrolyte imbalance: namely, hyponatremia, hypochloremic alkalosis, and hypokalemia. Serum and urine electrolyte determinations are particularly important when the patient is vomiting excessively or receiving parenteral fluids. Warning signs or symptoms of fluid and electrolyte imbalance, irrespective of cause, include dryness of mouth, thirst, weakness, lethargy, drowsiness, restlessness, confusion, seizures, muscle pains or cramps, muscular fatigue, hypotension, oliguria, tachycardia, and gastrointestinal disturbances such as nausea and vomiting.

Hypokalemia may develop, especially with brisk diuresis, when severe cirrhosis is present or after prolonged therapy.

Interference with adequate oral electrolyte intake will also contribute to hypokalemia. Hypokalemia may cause cardiac arrhythmias and may also sensitize or exaggerate the response of the heart to the toxic effects of digitalis (*e.g.*, increased ventricular irritability). Hypokalemia may be avoided or treated by use of potassium sparing diuretics or potassium supplements such as foods with a high potassium content.

Although any chloride deficit is generally mild and usually does not require specific treatment except under extraordinary circumstances (as in liver disease or renal disease), chloride replacement may be required in the treatment of metabolic alkalosis.

PRECAUTIONS: *(cont'd)*

Dilutional hyponatremia may occur in edematous patients in hot weather; appropriate therapy is water restriction, rather than administration of salt, except in rare instances when the hyponatremia is life-threatening. In actual salt depletion, appropriate replacement is the therapy of choice.

Hyperuricemia may occur or acute gout may be precipitated in certain patients receiving thiazides.

In diabetic patients dosage adjustments of insulin or oral hypoglycemic agents may be required. Hyperglycemia may occur with thiazide diuretics. Thus latent diabetes mellitus may become manifest during thiazide therapy.

The antihypertensive effects of the drug may be enhanced in the post-sympathectomy patient.

If progressive renal impairment becomes evident, consider withholding or discontinuing diuretic therapy.

Thiazides have been shown to increase the urinary excretion of magnesium; this may result in hypo-magnesemia.

Thiazides may decrease urinary calcium excretion. Thiazides may cause intermittent and slight elevation of serum in the absence of known disorders of calcium metabolism. Marked hyperkalemia may be evidence of a hyperparathyroidism. Thiazides should be discontinued before carrying out tests for parathyroid function.

Increases in cholesterol and triglyceride levels may be associated with thiazide diuretic therapy.

LABORATORY TESTS

Periodic determination of serum electrolytes to detect possible electrolyte imbalance should be done at appropriate intervals.

DRUG/LABORATORY TEST INTERACTIONS

Thiazides should be discontinued before carrying out tests for parathyroid function. (See PRECAUTIONS, General.)

CARCINOGENESIS, MUTAGENESIS, AND IMPAIRMENT OF FERTILITY

Carcinogenicity studies have not been done with chlorothiazide.

Chlorothiazide was not mutagenic *in vitro* in the Ames microbial mutagen test (using a maximum concentration of 5 mg/plate and *Salmonella typhimurium* strains TA98 and TA100) and was not mutagenic and did not induce mitotic nondisjunction in diploid strains of *Aspergillus nidulans*.

Chlorothiazide had no adverse effects on fertility in female rats at doses up to 60 mg/kg/day and no adverse effects on fertility in male rats at doses up to 40 mg/kg/day. These doses are 1.5 and 1.0 times* the recommended maximum human dose, respectively, when compared on a body weight basis.

* Calculations based on a human body weight of 50 kg

PREGNANCY

Tablets And Oral Suspension Only

Teratogenic Effects-Pregnancy Category C: Although reproduction studies performed with chlorothiazide doses of 50/mg/kg/day, 60 mg/kg/day in rats and 500 mg/kg/day in mice revealed no external abnormalities of the fetus or impairment of growth and survival of the fetus due to chlorothiazide, such studies did not include complete examinations for visceral and skeletal abnormalities. It is not known whether chlorothiazide can cause fetal harm when administered to a pregnant woman; however, thiazides cross the placental barrier and appear in cord blood. Chlorothiazide should be used during pregnancy only if clearly needed (see INDICATIONS AND USAGE).

IV Only

Teratogenic Effects - Pregnancy Category C: Although reproduction studies performed with chlorothiazide doses of 50mg/kg/day in rabbits, 60mg/kg/day in rats and 500mg/kg/day in mice revealed no external abnormalities of the fetus or impairment of growth and survival of the fetus due to chlorothiazide, such studies did not include complete examinations for visceral and skeletal abnormalities.It is not known whether chlorothiazide can cause fetal harm when administered to a pregnant woman; however, thiazides cross the placental barrier and appear in cord blood. Chlorothiazide should be used during pregnancy only if clearly needed (see INDICATIONS AND USAGE).

All Forms

Nonteratogenic Effects: These may include fetal or neonatal jaundice, thrombocytopenia, and possibly other adverse reactions which have occurred in the adult.

NURSING MOTHERS

Because of the potential for serious adverse reactions in nursing infants from chlorothiazide, a decision should be made whether to discontinue nursing or to discontinue the drug, taking into account the importance of the drug to the mother.

PEDIATRIC USE

Safety and effectiveness of Intravenous Sodium Chlorothiazide in children has not been established.

DRUG INTERACTIONS:

When given concurrently the following drugs may interact with thiazide diuretics.

Alcohol, barbiturates, or narcotics: Potentiation of orthostatic hypotension may occur.

Antidiabetic drugs: (oral agents and insulin) Dosage adjustment of the antidiabetic drug may be required.

Other antihypertensive drugs: Addictive effect or potentiation.

Cholestyramine and colestipol resins: Both cholestyramine and colestipol resins have the potential of binding thiazide diuretics and reducing diuretic absorption from the gastrointestinal tract.

Corticosteroids, ACTH: Intensified electrolyte depletion, particularly hypokalemia.

Pressor amines (*e.g.*, norepinephrine): Possible decreased response to pressor amines but not sufficient to preclude their use.

Skeletal muscle relaxants, nondepolarizing (*e.g.*, tubocurarine) possible increased responsiveness to the muscle relaxant.

Lithium: Generally should not be given with diuretics. Diuretic agents reduce the renal clearance of lithium and add a high risk of lithium toxicity. Refer to the package insert for lithium preparations before use of such preparations with chlorothiazide.

Non-steroidal Anti-inflammatory Drugs: In some patients, the administration of a non-steroidal anti-inflammatory agent can reduce the diuretic, natriuretic, and antihypertensive effects of loop, potassium-sparing and thiazide diuretics. Therefore, when chlorothiazide and non-steroidal anti-inflammatory agents are used concomitantly, the patient should be observed closely to determine if the desired effect of the diuretic is obtained.

ADVERSE REACTIONS:

The following adverse reactions have been reported and, within each category, are listed in order of decreasing severity.

Body as a Whole: Weakness.

ADVERSE REACTIONS: *(cont'd)*

Cardiovascular: Hypotension including orthostatic hypotension (may be aggravated by alcohol, barbiturates, narcotics or antihypertensive drugs).

Digestive: Pancreatitis, jaundice (intrahepatic cholestatic jaundice), diarrhea, vomiting, sialadenitis, cramping, constipation, gastric irritation, nausea, anorexia.

Hematologic: Aplastic anemia, agranulocytosis, leukopenia, hemolytic anemia, thrombocytopenia.

Hypersensitivity: Anaphylactic reactions, necrotizing angiitis (vasculitis and cutaneous vasculitis), respiratory distress including pneumonitis and pulmonary edema, photosensitivity, fever, urticaria, rash, purpura.

Metabolic: Electrolyte imbalance (see PRECAUTIONS), hyperglycemia, glycosuria, hyperuricemia.

Musculoskeletal: Muscle spasm.

Nervous System/Psychiatric: Vertigo, paresthesias, dizziness, headache, restlessness.

Renal: Renal failure, renal dysfunction, interstitial nephritis. (See WARNINGS).

Skin: Erythema multiforme including Stevens-Johnson syndrome, exfoliative dermatitis including toxic epidermal necrolysis, alopecia.

Special Senses: Transient blurred vision, xanthopsia.

Urogenital: Impotence.

Whenever adverse reactions are moderate or severe, thiazide dosage should be reduced or therapy withdrawn.

OVERDOSAGE:

The most common signs and symptoms observed are those caused by electrolyte depletion (hypokalemia, hypochloremia, hyponatremia) and dehydration resulting from excessive diuresis. If digitalis has also been administered, hypokalemia may accentuate cardiac arrhythmias.

In the event of overdosage, symptomatic and supportive measures should be employed. Emesis should be induced or gastric lavage performed. Correct dehydration, electrolyte imbalance, hepatic coma and hypotension by established procedures. If required, give oxygen or artificial respiration for respiratory impairment.

The degree to which chlorothiazide sodium is removed by hemodialysis has not been established.

Tablets And Oral Suspenesion: The oral LD_{50} of chlorothiazide is 8.5 g/kg, greater than 10 g/kg, and greater than 1 g/kg in the mouse, rat, and dog respectively.

IV Only: The intravenous LD_{50} of chlorothiazide in the mouse is 1.1 g/kg.

DOSAGE AND ADMINISTRATION:

TABLETS AND ORAL SUSPENSION

Therapy should be individualized according to patient response. Use the smallest dosage necessary to achieve the required response.

ADULTS

For Edema: The usual adult dosage is 0.5 to 1.0 g once or twice a day. Many patients with edema respond to intermittent therapy, i.e., administration on alternate days or on three to five days each week. With an intermittent schedule, excessive response and the resulting undesirable electrolyte imbalance are less likely to occur.

For Control of Hypertension: The usual adult dosage is 0.5 or 1.0 g a day as a single or divided dose. Dosage is increased or decreased according to blood pressure response. Rarely some patients may require up to 2.0 g a day in divided doses.

INFANTS AND CHILDREN

For Diuresis and For Control of Hypertension: The usual pediatric dosage is 5 to 10 mg per pound (10 to 20 mg/kg) per day in single or two divided doses, not to exceed 375 mg per day (2.5 to 7.5 ml or 1/2 to 1 1/2 teaspoonfuls of the oral suspension daily) in infants up to 2 years of age or 1 g per day in children 2 to 12 years of age. In infants less than 6 months of age, doses up to 15 mg per pound (30 mg/kg per day in two divided) doses may be required.

STORAGE

Tablets: Keep container tightly closed. Protect from moisture, freezing, 20°C (-4°F) and store at room temperature, 15- 30°C (59-86°F).

Oral Suspension: Keep container tightly closed. Protect from freezing, - 20°C (-4°F) and store at room temperature, 15- 30°C (59-86°F).

INTRAVENOUS ROUTE

Intravenous sodium chlorothiazide should be reserved for patients unable to take oral medication or for emergency situations.

Therapy should be individualized according to patient response. Use the smallest dosage necessary to achieve the required response.

Intravenous use in infants and children has been limited and is not generally recommended.

When medication can be taken orally, therapy with chlorothiazide tablets or oral suspension may be substituted for intravenous therapy, using the same dosage schedule as for the parenteral route.

Intravenous Sodium DIURIL may be given slowly by direct intravenous injection or by intravenous infusion.

Add 18 ml of Sterile Water for Injection to the vial to form an isotonic solution for intravenous injection. Never add less than 18 ml. Unused solution may be stored at room temperature for 24 hours, after which it must be discarded. Parenteral drug products should be inspected visually for particulate matter and discoloration prior to use whenever solution and container permit. The solution is compatible with dextrose or sodium chloride solutions for intravenous infusion. Avoid simultaneous administration of solutions of chlorothiazide with whole blood or its derivatives.

EXTRAVASATION MUST BE RIGIDLY AVOIDED. DO NOT GIVE SUBCUTANEOUSLY OR INTRAMUSCULARLY.

The usual adult dosage is 0.5 to 1.0 g once or twice a day. Many patients with edema respond to intermittent therapy, i.e., administration on alternate days or on three or five days each week. With an intermittent schedule, excessive response and the resulting undesirable electrolyte imbalance are less likely to occur.

STORAGE

Store reconstituted solution at room temperature and discard unused portion after 24 hours.

Store lyophilized powder between 2-25°C (36-77°F).

Store reconstituted solution at room temperature, 15-30°C (59- 86°F), and discard unused portion after 24 hours.

(Tablets and Oral Suspension: Merck, 7/93, 7398755)

(IV: Merck, 8/93, 7413532)

HOW SUPPLIED - RATED THERAPEUTICALLY EQUIVALENT:

Tablet, Uncoated - Oral - 250 mg

100's	$4.00	Chlorothiazide, Consolidated Midland	00223-0654-01
100's	$4.98	Chlorothiazide, H.C.F.A. F F P	99999-0739-01
100's	$5.00	Chlorothiazide, Rugby	00536-3460-01
100's	$5.67	Chlorothiazide, West Ward Pharm	00143-1209-01
100's	$5.97	Chlorothiazide, Aligen Independ	00405-4179-01
100's	$6.08	Chlorothiazide, HL Moore Drug Exch	00839-5967-06
100's	$6.20	Chlorothiazide, United Res	00677-0439-01
100's	$6.25	Chlorothiazide, Geneva Pharms	00781-1944-01
100's	$6.31	Chlorothiazide, Qualitest Pharms	00603-2737-21
100's	$7.25	Chlorothiazide, Schein Pharm (US)	00364-0389-01
100's	$7.95	Chlorothiazide, Mylan	00378-0150-01
100's	**$13.48**	**DIURIL, Merck**	**00006-0214-68**
250's	$12.45	Chlorothiazide, H.C.F.A. F F P	99999-0739-02
250's	$13.15	Chlorothiazide, Major Pharms	00904-0183-70
1000's	$23.31	Chlorothiazide, Camall	00147-0144-20
1000's	$35.00	Chlorothiazide, Consolidated Midland	00223-0654-02
1000's	$38.50	Chlorothiazide, West Ward Pharm	00143-1209-10
1000's	$39.31	Chlorothiazide, HL Moore Drug Exch	00839-5967-16
1000's	$39.50	Chlorothiazide, Aligen Independ	00405-4179-03
1000's	$46.90	Chlorothiazide, Major Pharms	00904-0183-80
1000's	$49.80	Chlorothiazide, H.C.F.A. F F P	99999-0739-03
1000's	**$122.71**	**DIURIL, Merck**	**00006-0214-82**

Tablet, Uncoated - Oral - 500 mg

100's	$3.84	Chlorothiazide, Camall	00147-0153-10
100's	$5.76	Chlorothiazide, H.C.F.A. F F P	99999-0739-04
100's	$7.95	Chlorothiazide, Consolidated Midland	00223-0655-01
100's	$8.10	Chlorothiazide, Caremark	00339-5063-12
100's	$8.75	Chlorothiazide, West Ward Pharm	00143-1210-01
100's	$9.71	Chlorothiazide, HL Moore Drug Exch	00839-5930-06
100's	$10.40	Chlorothiazide, Qualitest Pharms	00603-2738-21
100's	$10.48	Chlorothiazide, United Res	00677-0438-01
100's	$10.50	Chlorothiazide, Aligen Independ	00405-4180-01
100's	$10.50	Chlorothiazide, Rugby	00536-3461-01
100's	$10.60	DIURIGEN, Goldline Labs	00182-0790-01
100's	$10.79	Chlorothiazide, HL Moore Drug Exch	00839-7695-06
100's	$10.90	Chlorothiazide, Major Pharms	00904-0184-60
100's	$11.03	Chlorothiazide, Schein Pharm (US)	00364-0390-01
100's	$11.85	Chlorothiazide, Mylan	00378-0162-01
100's	**$21.35**	**DIURIL, Merck**	**00006-0432-68**
500's	$10.09	Chlorothiazide, Geneva Pharms	00781-1940-01
1000's	$36.41	Chlorothiazide, Camall	00147-0153-20
1000's	$57.60	Chlorothiazide, H.C.F.A. F F P	99999-0739-05
1000's	$64.45	Chlorothiazide, United Res	00677-0438-10
1000's	$72.07	Chlorothiazide, West Ward Pharm	00143-1210-10
1000's	$75.00	Chlorothiazide, Consolidated Midland	00223-0655-02
1000's	$80.53	Chlorothiazide, Qualitest Pharms	00603-2738-32
1000's	$99.08	Chlorothiazide, HL Moore Drug Exch	00839-7695-16
1000's	$109.69	Chlorothiazide, HL Moore Drug Exch	00839-5930-16
1000's	$109.90	Chlorothiazide, Mylan	00378-0162-10
1000's	**$191.68**	**DIURIL, Merck**	**00006-0432-82**
5000's	$288.00	Chlorothiazide, H.C.F.A. F F P	99999-0739-06
5000's	**$953.05**	**DIURIL, Merck**	**00006-0432-86**

HOW SUPPLIED - NOT RATED EQUIVALENT:

Injection, Dry-Soln - Intravenous - 500 mg/ml

20 ml	**$8.85**	**DIURIL, Merck**	**00006-3250-32**

Suspension - Oral - 250 mg/5ml

237 ml	**$9.82**	**DIURIL, Merck**	**00006-3239-66**

Tablet, Uncoated - Oral - 250 mg

100's	$6.60	Chlorothiazide, West Point Pharma	59591-0240-68
100's	$6.60	Chlorothiazide, Endo Labs	60951-0765-70

Tablet, Uncoated - Oral - 500 mg

100's	$9.60	Chlorothiazide, West Point Pharma	59591-0245-68
100's	$9.60	Chlorothiazide, Endo Labs	60951-0766-70
1000's	$84.00	Chlorothiazide, West Point Pharma	59591-0245-82
1000's	$84.00	Chlorothiazide, Endo Labs	60951-0766-90

CHLOROTHIAZIDE; METHYLDOPA *(000740)*

CATEGORIES: Antihypertensives; Cardiovascular Drugs; Diuretics; Edema; Hypertension; Renal Drugs; Thiazides; Pregnancy Category B; FDA Approval Pre 1982

BRAND NAMES: Alamethyl; **Aldoclor**; *Supres* (Canada)
(International brand names outside U.S. in italics)

> **WARNING:**
> This fixed combination drug is not indicated for initial therapy of hypertension. Hypertension requires therapy titrated to the individual patient. If the fixed combination represents the dosage so determined, its use may be more convenient in patient management. The treatment of hypertension is not static, but must be re-evaluated as conditions in each patient warrant.

DESCRIPTION:

Methyldopa-chlorothiazide combines two antihypertensives: methyldopa and chlorothiazide.

FOR COMPLETE PRESCRIBING INFORMATION, REFER TO THE INDIVIDUAL DRUG MONOGRAPHS (chlorothiazide; methyldopa).

INDICATIONS AND USAGE:

Hypertension (see BOXED WARNING).

DOSAGE AND ADMINISTRATION:

DOSAGE MUST BE INDIVIDUALIZED, AS DETERMINED BY TITRATION OF THE INDIVIDUAL COMPONENTS (see BOXED WARNING). Once the patient has been successfully titrated, methyldopa-chlorothiazide may be substituted if the previously determined titrated doses are the same as in the combination. The usual starting dosage is one tablet of methyldopa-chlorothiazide 150 or one tablet of methyldopa-chlorothiazide 250 two or three times a day.

When administered individually, the usual daily dosage of chlorothiazide is 0.5 g to 1.0 g in single or divided doses and that of methyldopa is 500 mg to 2 g. To minimize the sedation associated with methyldopa, start dosage increases in the evening.

DOSAGE AND ADMINISTRATION: *(cont'd)*

Occasionally tolerance to methyldopa may occur, usually between the second and third month of therapy. Additional separate doses of methyldopa or replacement of methyldopa-chlorothiazide with single entity agents is necessary until the new effective dose ratio is re-established by titration. The maximum recommended daily dose of methyldopa is 3 g. When methyldopa-chlorothiazide 150 is used to provide 1 g of methyldopa, 0.6 g of chlorothiazide is delivered. When methyldopa-chlorothiazide 250 is used to provide 1 g of methyldopa, 1 g of chlorothiazide is delivered. It is prudent, if greater than 1 g of methyldopa per day is required, to provide the additional methyldopa as methyldopa alone.

If methyldopa-chlorothiazide does not adequately control blood pressure, additional doses of other agents may be given. When methyldopa-chlorothiazide is given with antihypertensives other than thiazides, the initial dosage of methyldopa should be limited to 500 mg daily in divided doses and the dose of these other agents may need to be adjusted to effect a smooth transition.

Since both components of methyldopa-chlorothiazide have a relatively short duration of action, withdrawal is followed by return of hypertension usually within 48 hours. This is not complicated by an overshoot of blood pressure.

Since methyldopa is largely excreted by the kidney, patients with impaired renal function may respond to smaller doses. Syncope in older patients may be related to an increased sensitivity and advanced arteriosclerotic vascular disease. This may be avoided by lower doses.

Storage: Keep container tightly closed. Protect from moisture, light, and freezing, -20°C (-4°F) and store at room temperature, 15-30°C (59-86°F).

HOW SUPPLIED - EQUIVALENTS NOT AVAILABLE:

Tablet, Plain Coated - Oral - 150 mg/250 mg

100's	**$48.28**	**ALDOCLOR 150, Merck**	**00006-0612-68**

Tablet, Plain Coated - Oral - 250 mg/250 mg

100's	**$54.69**	**ALDOCLOR 250, Merck**	**00006-0634-68**

CHLOROTHIAZIDE; RESERPINE *(000741)*

CATEGORIES: Antihypertensives; Cardiovascular Drugs; Diuretics; Edema; Hypertension; Renal Drugs; Thiazides; Vascular Disorders, Cerebral/Peripheral; Pregnancy Category C; FDA Approved 1982 May

BRAND NAMES: Chloroserpine; Chlorothiazide W/Reserpine; Diaserp W/Reserpine; **Diupres**; Diurigen W/Reserpine

FORMULARIES: Medi-Cal

> **WARNING:**
> This fixed combination drug is not indicated for initial therapy for hypertension. Hypertension requires therapy titrated to the individual patient. If the fixed combination represents the dosage so determined, its use may be more convenient in patient management. The treatment of hypertension is not static, but must be re-evaluated as conditions in each patient warrant.

Chlorothiazide w/ reserpine combines two antihypertensives.

FOR COMPLETE PRESCRIBING INFORMATION, REFER TO THE INDIVIDUAL DRUG MONOGRAPHS (CHLOROTHIAZIDE; RESERPINE).

INDICATIONS AND USAGE:

Hypertension (see BOXED WARNING.)

Use in Pregnancy: Routine use of diuretics during normal pregnancy is inappropriate and exposes mother and fetus to unnecessary hazard. Diuretics do not prevent development of toxemia pregnancy and there is no satisfactory evidence that they are useful in the treatment of toxemia.

Edema during pregnancy may arise from pathologic causes or from the physiologic and mechanical consequences of pregnancy. Thiazides are indicated in pregnancy when edema is due to pathologic causes, just as they are in the absence of pregnancy. Dependent edema in pregnancy, resulting from restriction of venous return by the gravid uterus, is properly treated through elevation of the lower extremities and use of support stockings. Use of diuretics to lower intravascular volume in this instance is illogical and unnecessary. During normal pregnancy there is hypervolemia which is not harmful to the fetus or the mother in the absence of cardiovascular disease. However, it may be associated with edema, rarely generalized edema. If such edema causes discomfort, increased recumbency will often provide relief. Rarely this edema may cause extreme discomfort which is not relieved by rest. In these instances, a short course of diuretic therapy may provide relief and be appropriate.

DOSAGE AND ADMINISTRATION:

The initial dosage of chlorothiazide w/ reserpine should conform to the dosages of the individual components established during titration (see BOXED WARNING.)

The usual adult dosage of chlorothiazide w/ reserpine-250 is 1 or 2 tablets once or twice a day; that of chlorothiazide w/ reserpine-500 is 1 tablet once or twice a day. Dosage may require adjustment according to the blood pressure response of the patient.

Storage: Keep container tightly closed. Protect from light.

HOW SUPPLIED - RATED THERAPEUTICALLY EQUIVALENT:

Tablet, Coated - Oral - 325 mg/50 mg

100's	**$29.77**	**DARVOCET-N, Lilly**	**00002-0351-33**

HOW SUPPLIED - NOT RATED EQUIVALENT:

Tablet, Uncoated - Oral - 0.125 mg/500 mg

100's	$21.98	Chlorothiazide W/Reserpine, HL Moore Drug Exch	00839-7942-06

Tablet, Uncoated - Oral - 250 mg/0.125 mg

100's	$5.95	Chlorothiazide W/Reserpine, Consolidated Midland	00223-0656-01
100's	$9.60	Reserpine & Chlorothiazide, Mylan	00378-0175-01
100's	$11.40	DIASERP, Major Pharms	00904-0185-60
100's	$11.48	Chlorothiazide, HL Moore Drug Exch	00839-6031-06
100's	$12.05	Chlorothiazide W/Reserpine, HL Moore Drug Exch	00839-7941-06
100's	**$28.15**	**DIUPRES-250, Merck**	**00006-0230-68**
1000's	$55.50	Chlorothiazide W/Reserpine, Consolidated Midland	00223-0656-02
1000's	**$260.72**	**DIUPRES-250, Merck**	**00006-0230-82**

Tablet, Uncoated - Oral - 500 mg/0.125 mg

100's	$11.35	Chlorothiazide, United Res	00677-0763-01
100's	$14.65	DIASERP, Major Pharms	00904-0186-60
100's	$14.75	Reserpine & Chlorothiazide, Mylan	00378-0176-01

CHLOROTRIANISENE *(000742)*

CATEGORIES: Antineoplastics; Hormones; Hypoestrogenism; Hypogonadism; Kraurosis Vulvae; Menopause; Oncologic Drugs; Ovarian Failure; Prostatic Carcinoma; Vaginitis; Breast Engorgement*; Pregnancy Category X; FDA Approval Pre 1982
* Indication not approved by the FDA

BRAND NAMES: *Estregur* (Mexico); *Merbentul* (Germany); **Tace**
(International brand names outside U.S. in italics)

FORMULARIES: Aetna; Medi-Cal

> WARNING:
>
> 1. ESTROGENS HAVE BEEN REPORTED TO INCREASE THE RISK OF ENDOMETRIAL CARCINOMA IN POSTMENOPAUSAL WOMEN. Close clinical surveillance of all women taking estrogens is important. In all cases of undiagnosed persistent or recurring abnormal vaginal bleeding, adequate diagnostic measures including endometrial sampling when indicated should be undertaken to rule out malignancy. There is currently no evidence that "natural" estrogens are more or less hazardous than "synthetic" estrogens at equiestrogenic doses.
> 2. ESTROGENS SHOULD NOT BE USED DURING PREGNANCY. Estrogen therapy during pregnancy is associated with an increased risk of congenital defects in the reproductive organs of the male and female fetus, an increased risk of vaginal adenosis, squamous cell dysplasia of the uterine cervix, and vaginal cancer in the female later in life. The 1985 Diethylstilbestrol (DES) Task force concluded that women who used DES during their pregnancies may subsequently experience an increased risk of breast cancer. However, a causal relationship is still unproven, and the observed level of risk is similar to that for a number of other breast cancer risk factors. There is no indication for estrogen therapy during pregnancy. Estrogens are ineffective for the prevention or treatment of threatened or habitual abortion.* **If chlorotrianisene is used during pregnancy, or if the patient becomes pregnant while taking this drug, she should be apprised of the potential risks to the fetus, and the advisability of pregnancy continuation.**

DESCRIPTION:

Chlorotrianisene USP is available in capsule form suitable for oral administration. Each green, soft gelatin capsule contains 12 mg of chlorotrianisene. This capsule also contains inactive ingredients: corn oil (solvent), FD&C Blue No. 1, FD&C Yellow No. 5 (tartrazine, see PRECAUTIONS), gelatin, glycerin, methylparaben, propylparaben, titanium dioxide, and water.

Each two-tone green, hard gelatin capsule contains 25 mg of chlorotrianisene. This capsule also contains inactive ingredients: FD&C Blue No. 1 or FD&C Green No. 3, FD&C Blue No. 2, FD&C Red No. 40, FD&C Yellow No. 5 (tartrazine, see PRECAUTIONS), FD&C Yellow No. 6, gelatin, iron oxide, magnesium stearate, titanium dioxide, and tristearin (solvent).

Chlorotrianisene is a long-acting, synthetic estrogen with the chemical name 1,1',1"-(1-chloro-1-ethenyl-2-ylidene)-tris[4-methoxy]-benzene.

Chlorotrianisene occurs as small, white crystals or as a crystalline powder. It is odorless. It is slightly soluble in alcohol and very slightly soluble in water.

INDICATIONS AND USAGE:

Chlorotrianisene is indicated in the treatment of:

1. Advanced androgen-dependent carcinoma of the prostate (for palliation only).

2. Moderate to severe vasomotor symptoms associated with the menopause. There is no adequate evidence that estrogens are effective for nervous symptoms or depression which might occur during menopause and they should not be used to treat these conditions.

3. Atrophic vaginitis.

4. Kraurosis vulvae.

5. Hypoestrogenism due to hypogonadism, castration, or primary ovarian failure.

CONTRAINDICATIONS:

Chlorotrianisene is contraindicated in patients with a known hypersensitivity to chlorotrianisene or other ingredients of the formulation.

Chlorotrianisene should not be used in women or men with any of the following conditions:

1. Known or suspected pregnancy. (See BOXED WARNING.) Estrogen may cause fetal harm when administered to a pregnant woman.

2. Known or suspected cancer of the breast except in appropriately selected patients being treated for metastatic disease.

3. Known or suspected estrogen-dependent neoplasia.

4. Undiagnosed abnormal genital bleeding.

5. Active thrombophlebitis or thromboembolic disorders—Women on estrogen replacement therapy have not been reported to have an increased risk of thrombophlebitis and/or thromboembolic disease. However, there is insufficient information regarding women who have had previous thromboembolic disease.

WARNINGS:

Induction of Malignant Neoplasms: Some studies have suggested a possible increased incidence of breast cancer in those women on estrogen therapy taking higher doses for prolonged periods of time. The majority of studies, however, have not shown an association with the usual doses used for estrogen replacement therapy. Women on this therapy should have regular breast examinations and should be instructed in breast self-examination. The reported endometrial cancer risk among estrogen users was about fourfold or greater than in non-users, and appears dependent on duration of treatment and on estrogen dose. There is no significantly increased risk associated with the use of estrogens for less than one year. The greatest risk appears associated with prolonged use—five years or more. In one study, persistence of risk was demonstrated for 10 years after cessation of estrogen treatment. In another study, a significant decrease in the incidence of endometrial cancer occurred six months after estrogen withdrawal.

Estrogen therapy during pregnancy is associated with an increased risk of fetal congenital reproductive tract disorders. In females, there is an increased risk of vaginal adenosis, squamous cell dysplasia of the cervix, and cancer later in life; in the male, urogenital abnormalities. Although some of these changes are benign, it is not known whether they are precursors of malignancy.

WARNINGS: *(cont'd)*

Gallbladder Disease: The risk of surgically confirmed gallbladder disease has been reported to be 2.5 times higher in women receiving postmenopausal estrogens.

Cardiovascular Disease: Large doses of estrogen (5 mg conjugated estrogens per day), comparable to those used to treat cancer of the prostate and breast, have been shown in a large prospective clinical trial in men to increase the risk of non-fatal myocardial infarction, pulmonary embolism, and thrombophlebitis. It cannot necessarily be extrapolated from men to women. However, to avoid the theoretical cardiovascular risk caused by high estrogen doses, the doses for estrogen replacement therapy should not exceed the recommended dose.

Elevated Blood Pressure: There is no evidence that this may occur with use of estrogens in the menopause. However, blood pressure should be monitored with estrogen use, especially if high doses are used.

Hypercalcemia: Administration of estrogens may lead to severe hypercalcemia in patients with breast cancer and bone metastases. If this occurs, the drug should be stopped and appropriate measures taken to reduce the serum calcium level.

PRECAUTIONS:

GENERAL

Addition of a Progestin: Studies of the addition of a progestin for seven or more days of a cycle of estrogen administration have reported a lowered incidence of endometrial hyperplasia. Morphological and biochemical studies of the endometrium suggest that 10 to 13 days of progestin are needed to provide maximal maturation of the endometrium and to eliminate any hyperplastic changes. Whether this will provide protection from endometrial carcinoma has not been clearly established. There are possible additional risks which may be associated with the inclusion of progestin in estrogen replacement regimens. The potential risks include adverse effects on carbohydrate and lipid metabolism. The choice of progestin and dosage may be important in minimizing these adverse effects.

Physical Examination: A complete medical and family history should be taken prior to the initiation of any estrogen therapy. The pretreatment and periodic physical examinations should include special reference to blood pressure, breasts, abdomen, and pelvic organs, and should include a Papanicolaou smear. As a general rule, estrogen should not be prescribed for longer than 1 year without another physical examination being performed.

Fluid Retention: Because estrogens may cause some degree of fluid retention, conditions which might be influenced by this factor such as asthma, epilepsy, migraine, and cardiac or renal dysfunction, require careful observation.

Uterine Bleeding and Mastodynia: Certain patients may develop undesirable manifestations of estrogenic stimulation, such as abnormal uterine bleeding and mastodynia.

Uterine Fibroids: Pre-existing uterine leiomyomata may increase in size during prolonged high-dose estrogen use.

Impaired Liver Function: Estrogens may be poorly metabolized in patients with impaired liver function and should be administered with caution.

Hypercalcemia and Renal Insufficiency: Prolonged use of estrogens can influence the metabolism of calcium and phosphorus. Estrogens should be used with caution in patients with metabolic bone disease or in patients with renal insufficiency.

INFORMATION FOR THE PATIENT

See PATIENT PACKAGE INSERT which accompanies this drug product.

LABORATORY TESTS

Clinical response at the smallest dose should generally be the guide to estrogen administration for relief of symptoms for those indications in which symptoms are observable. Tests used to measure adequacy of estrogen replacement therapy include serum estrone and estradiol levels and suppression of serum gonadotropin levels.

DRUG/LABORATORY TEST INTERACTIONS

Some of these drug/laboratory test interactions have been observed only with estrogen-progestin combinations (oral contraceptives):

1. Increased prothrombin and factors VII, VIII, IX, and X; decreased antithrombin 3; increased norepinephrine-induced platelet aggregability, decreased fibrinolysis.

2. Increased thyroid-binding globulin (TBG) leading to increased circulating total thyroid hormone, as measured by T_4 levels determined either by column or by radioimmunoassay. Free T_3 resin uptake is decreased, reflecting the elevated TBG; free T_4concentration is unaltered.

3. Impaired glucose tolerance.

4. Reduced response to metyrapone test.

5. Reduced serum folate concentration.

NOTE: *This product contains FD&C Yellow No. 5 (tartrazine), which may cause allergic-type reactions (including bronchial asthma) in certain susceptible individuals. Although the overall incidence of FD&C Yellow No. 5 (tartrazine) sensitivity in the general population is low, it is frequently seen in patients who also have aspirin hypersensitivity.*

MUTAGENESIS AND CARCINOGENESIS

Long-term continuous administration of natural and synthetic estrogens in certain animal species increases the frequency of carcinomas of the breast, cervix, vagina, and liver.

PREGNANCY CATEGORY X

Estrogens should not be used during pregnancy. (See CONTRAINDICATIONSand BOXED WARNING.)

NURSING MOTHERS

As a general principle, the administration of any drug to nursing mothers should be done only when clearly necessary since many drugs are excreted in human milk.

ADVERSE REACTIONS:

See WARNINGS regarding induction of neoplasia, adverse effects on the fetus, increased incidence of gallbladder disease. The following additional adverse reactions have been reported with estrogen therapy:

1. Genitourinary System: Changes in vaginal bleeding pattern and abnormal withdrawal bleeding or flow; breakthrough bleeding, spotting; increase in size of uterine fibromyomata; vaginal candidiasis; change in amount of cervical secretion.

2. Breasts: Tenderness, enlargement.

3. Gastrointestinal: Nausea, vomiting; abdominal cramps, bloating; cholestatic jaundice.

4. Skin: Chloasma or melasma, that may persist when drug is discontinued; erythema multiforme; erythema nodosum; urticaria; hemorrhagic eruption; loss of scalp hair; hirsutism.

5. Eyes: Steepening of corneal curvature; intolerance of contact lenses.

6. CNS: Headache, migraine, dizziness; mental depression; chorea.

7. Miscellaneous: Increase or decrease in weight; reduced carbohydrate tolerance; aggravation of porphyria; edema; changes in libido.

OVERDOSAGE:

ACUTE OVERDOSAGE

Numerous reports of ingestion of large doses of estrogen-containing oral contraceptives by young children indicate that acute serious ill effects do not occur. Overdosage of estrogen may cause nausea and vomiting.

DOSAGE AND ADMINISTRATION:

1. Advanced androgen-dependent carcinoma of the prostate, for palliation only. The usual dosage is 12 to 25 mg daily (one or two 12 mg capsules or one 25 mg capsule).

2. For treatment of moderate to severe vasomotor symptoms, atrophic vaginitis, or kraurosis vulvae associated with the menopause. The lowest dose that will control symptoms should be chosen and medication should be discontinued as promptly as possible. Administration should be cyclic (*e.g.,* 3 weeks on and 1 week off).

Attempts to discontinue or taper medication should be made at 3-month to 6-month intervals.

The usual dosage range for vasomotor symptoms, atrophic vaginitis, or kraurosis vulvae associated with the menopause is 12 to 25 mg daily (one or two 12 mg capsules or one 25 mg capsule) for 30 days; one or more courses may be prescribed.

3. Female hypogonadism; primary ovarian failure.

The usual dosage is 12 to 25 mg daily (one or two 12 mg capsules or one 25 mg capsule) for 21 days. This course may, if desired, be followed immediately by the intramuscular injection of 100 mg of progesterone; alternatively, an oral progesterone such as medroxyprogesterone may be given during the last 5 days of chlorotrianisene therapy. The next course may begin on the 5th day of the induced uterine bleeding.

Treated patients with an intact uterus should be monitored closely for signs of endometrial cancer, and appropriate diagnostic measures should be taken to rule out malignancy in the event of persistent or recurrent abnormal vaginal bleeding.

HOW SUPPLIED - RATED THERAPEUTICALLY EQUIVALENT:

Capsule, Gelatin - Oral - 12 mg

100's $100.38 TACE, Hoechst Marion Roussel 00068-0690-61

CHLOROXINE *(000743)*

CATEGORIES: Anti-Infectives; Dandruff; Dermatitis; Dermatologicals; Local Infections; Seborrhea; Shampoos; Skin/Mucous Membrane Agents; Topical; Pregnancy Category C; FDA Approval Pre 1982

BRAND NAMES: **Capitrol**; *Quixalin*
(International brand names outside U.S. in italics)

DESCRIPTION:

Capitrol is an antibacterial cream shampoo containing 2% chloroxine (each gram contains 20 mg chloroxine) suspended in a base of sodium octoxynol-3 sulfonate, PEG-6 lauramide, dextrin, stearyl alcohol/ceteareth-20, sodium lauryl sulfoacetate, dioctyl sodium sulfosuccinate, magnesium aluminum silicate, PEG-14M, EDTA, citric acid, water, color, fragrance and 1% benzyl alcohol. The pH of the shampoo is 7.0.

Chloroxine is a synthetic antibacterial compound that is effective in the treatment of dandruff and seborrheic dermatitis when incorporated in shampoos.

The chemical name of chloroxine is 5,7-dichloro-8-hydroxyquinoline.

CLINICAL PHARMACOLOGY:

Well controlled studies demonstrate chloroxine effectively reduces the excess scaling in patients with dandruff or seborrheic dermatitis. Though the cause of dandruff is not known it is thought to be the result of accelerated mitotic activity in the epidermis. The presumed mechanism of action to reduce scaling would be to slow down the mitotic activity.

The role of microbes in seborrheic dermatitis is not known; however,*Staphylococcus aureus* and *Pityrosporon* species are often present in increased number during the course of the disease. Chloroxine is antibacterial, inhibiting the growth of Gram-positive as well as some Gram-negative organisms. Antifungal activity against some dermatophytes and yeasts also has been shown.

The absorption, metabolism and pharmacokinetics of chloroxine in humans have not been studied.

INDICATIONS AND USAGE:

Chloroxine is indicated in the treatment of dandruff and mild-to-moderately severe seborrheic dermatitis of the scalp. Clinical studies indicate that improvement may be observed after 14 days of therapy.

CONTRAINDICATIONS:

Chloroxine is contraindicated in those patients with a history of hypersensitivity to any of the listed ingredients.

WARNINGS:

Chloroxine should not be used on acutely inflamed (exudative) lesions of the scalp.

PRECAUTIONS:

Information for the Patient: Exercise care to prevent chloroxine from entering the eyes. If contact occurs, the patient should flush eyes with cool water. Discoloration of light-colored hair (*e.g.,* blond, gray or bleached) may follow use of this preparation.

Irritation and a burning sensation on the scalp and adjacent areas have been reported.

Drug/Laboratory Test Interactions: There is no known interference of chloroxine with laboratory tests.

Carcinogenesis, Mutagenesis: No long term studies in animals have been performed to evaluate the carcinogenic potential of chloroxine.

Results of the *in vitro* Ames Salmonella/Microsome Plate test show that chloroxine does not demonstrate genetic activity and is considered non-mutagenic.

Pregnancy Category C: Animal reproduction studies have not been conducted with chloroxine. It is also not known whether chloroxine can cause fetal harm when administered to a pregnant woman or can affect reproduction capacity. chloroxine should be given to a pregnant woman only if clearly needed.

Nursing Mothers: It is not known whether this drug is excreted in human milk. Because many drugs are excreted in human milk, caution should be exercised when chloroxine is administered to a nursing woman.

Pediatric Use: Specific studies to demonstrate the safety and effectiveness for use of chloroxine in children have not been conducted.

ADVERSE REACTIONS:

One patient out of 225 in clinical studies was reported to have contact dermatitis.

OVERDOSAGE:

The acute oral LD_{50} in mice was found to be 200 mg/kg and in rats 450 mg/kg. On the basis of these animal studies, chloroxine may be considered practically non-toxic.

DOSAGE AND ADMINISTRATION:

Chloroxine should be massaged thoroughly onto the wet scalp, avoiding contact with the eyes. Lather should remain on the scalp for approximately three minutes, then rinsed. The application should be repeated and the scalp rinsed thoroughly. Two treatments per week are usually sufficient.

HOW SUPPLIED - EQUIVALENTS NOT AVAILABLE:

Shampoo - Topical

120 ml $16.60 CAPITROL, Westwood Squibb 00072-6850-04

CHLOROXYLENOL; HYDROCORTISONE; PRAMOXINE HYDROCHLORIDE *(000723)*

CATEGORIES: Anti-Inflammatory Agents; EENT Drugs; Eye, Ear, Nose, & Throat Preparations; Local Anesthetics; Otic Hydrocortisones; Otic Preparations; Otologic; FDA Pre 1938 Drugs

BRAND NAMES: Earsol-HC; Cortane-B; Cortic; Otic-HC; Otomar; Otozone; Tri-Otic; Xotic-Hc; Zoto-HC

DESCRIPTION:

Each 1 ml for otic administration contains:Chloroxylenol 1 mg, Hydrocortisone 10 mg, Pramoxine Hydrochloride 10 mg in a non-aqueous propylene glycol vehicle with 3% propylene glycol diacetate and benzalkonium chloride.

Chloroxylenol: 4-chloro-3.5-dimetyl-phenol is a broad spectrum bactericidal agent which occurs as white crystals with a phenolic odor. It is soluble in alcohol, ether, and alkali hydroxides.

Hydrocortisone: 11, 17,21, trihydroxy, (11B)-Pregn-4-ene-3,20-dione, is an anti-inflammatory and antipruritic agent. It occurs as a white to practically white, odorless, crystalline powder which melts at about 215°C with decomposition. It is very slightly soluble in water and in ether; sparingly soluble in acetone and in alcohol; slightly soluble in chloroform.

Pramoxine hydrochloride: 4 (3 - (4 - butoxyphenoxy) propyl)) - Morphine hydrochloride is a topical anesthetic proven to be safe and effective in hospital tests. It occurs as white to practically white, crystalline powder, having a numbing taste and it may have a slight aromatic odor. The pH of a solution (1 in 100) is about 4.5. It is freely soluble in water and in alcohol; soluble in chloroform; and very slightly soluble in ether.

CLINICAL PHARMACOLOGY:

This product is effective both as an antibacterial and antifungal agent. The special base is a hydrophilic solution having an acid pH and a low surface tension, exerting a drying effect and allowing the medication to spread quickly to all contiguous surfaces, softening and reducing accumulated cerumen.

Chloroxylenol is a halogenated phenol, non-toxic, non-corrosive, non-staining with a high phenol coefficient. It may be applied directly to a wound and shows no chemical reactivity toward blood.

Hydrocortisone is a topical corticosteroid which has anti-inflammatory, antipruritic and vasoconstrictive actions. The mechanism of anti-inflammatory activity of the topical corticosteroids is unclear. Topical corticosteroids can be absorbed from normal intact skin. Inflammation and/or other disease processes in the skin increase percutaneous absorption. Once absorbed through the skin, topical corticosteroids are handled through pharmacokinetic pathways similar to systemically administered corticosteroids. Corticosteroids are bound to plasma proteins in varying degrees. Corticosteroids are metabolized primarily in the liver and are then excreted by the kidneys. Some of the topical corticosteroids and their metabolites are also excreted into the bile.

Pramoxine hydrochloride is a topical anesthetic agent which provides temporary relief from itching and pain. It acts by stabilizing the neuronal membranes of nerve endings with which it comes into contact.

INDICATIONS AND USAGE:

For the treatment of superficial infection of the external auditory canal complicated by inflammation caused by organisms and susceptible to the action of the antimicrobial, or to control itching.

CONTRAINDICATIONS:

Topical steroids are contraindicated in varicella, vaccinia and in patients sensitive to any of the components of this preparation. This or any medication should not be applied in the external auditory canal patients with perforated eardrums.

WARNINGS:

This preparation is not intended for ophthalmic or oral use. If accidental ingestion occurs, seek professional help.

PRECAUTIONS:

GENERAL

If a favorable response does not occur promptly, discontinue the use of this preparation until the infection is controlled by other appropriate measures. Although systemic side effects are not common with topical corticosteroids, the possibility of occurrence must be kept in mind particularly when used for an extended period of time.

Systemic absorption of topical corticosteroids had produced reversible hypothalamic-pituitary-adrenal (HPA) axis suppression, manifestations of Cushing's syndrome, hyperglycemia and glycosuria in some patients. Conditions which augment systemic absorption include the application of more potent steroids. Recovery of HPA axis function is generally prompt and complete upon discontinuation of the drug. Infrequently, signs and symptoms of steroid withdrawal may occur, requiring supplemental corticosteroids. Children may absorb proportionately larger amounts of topical corticosteroids and thus be more susceptible to systemic toxicity (see PRECAUTIONS, Pediatric Use.)

WARNING: If irritation or sensitization occurs, promptly discontinue use of this preparation and institute other measures.

INFORMATION FOR THE PATIENT

Patients using topical corticosteroids should receive the following information and instructions:

PRECAUTIONS: *(cont'd)*

1. This medication is to be used as directed by the physician. It is for external use only. Avoid contact with the eyes.
2. Patients should be advised not to use this medication for any disorder other than that for which it was prescribed.
3. Patients should report any signs of local adverse reactions.

LABORATORY TESTS

The urinary free cortisol test and the ACTH stimulation test may be helpful in evaluating the HPA axis suppression.

CARCINOGENESIS, MUTAGENESIS, AND IMPAIRMENT OF FERTILITY

Long-term animal studies have not been performed to evaluate the carcinogenic potential or the effect of topical corticosteroid on fertility. Studies to determine mutagenicity with prednisolone and hydrocortisone have revealed negative results.

PREGNANCY CATEGORY C

Corticosteroids are generally teratogenic in laboratory animals when administered systemically at low dosage levels. The more potent corticosteroids have been shown to be teratogenic after dermal application in laboratory animals. There are no adequate and well-controlled studies in pregnant women on teratogenic effects from topically applied corticosteroids. Therefore, topical corticosteroids should be used during pregnancy only if the potential benefit justifies the potential risk to the fetus. Drugs of this class should not be used extensively on pregnant patients in large amounts, or for prolonged periods of time.

NURSING MOTHERS

It is not known whether topical administration of corticosteroids could result in sufficient systemic absorption to produce detectable quantities in breast milk. Systemically administered corticosteroids are secreted into breast milk in quantities not likely to have a deleterious effect on the infant. Nevertheless, cautions should be exercised when topical corticosteroids are administered to a nursing woman.

PEDIATRIC USE

Pediatric patients may demonstrate greater susceptibility to topical corticosteroid-induced HPA axis suppression and Cushing's syndrome than mature patients because of a larger skin surface to body weight ratio. Hypothalamic-pituitary-adrenal (HPA) axis suppression, Cushing's syndrome and intracranial hypertension have been reported in children receiving topical corticosteroids. Manifestations of adrenal suppression in children include linear growth retardation, delayed weight gain, low plasma cortisol levels and absence of response to ACTH stimulation. Manifestation of intracranial hypertension include bulging fontanelles, headaches and bilateral papilledema. Administration of topical corticosteroids to children should be limited to the least amount compatible with an effective therapeutic regimen. Chronic corticosteroid therapy may interfere with the growth and development of children.

DRUG INTERACTIONS:

Interaction of other drugs with the hydrocortisone component of this product is possible. Inform your physician of other medication you are currently taking.

ADVERSE REACTIONS:

The following adverse reactions with topical corticosteroids have been observed: itching, burning, irritation, dryness, folliculitis, hypertrichosis, acneform eruptions, hypopigmentations, perioral dermatitis, allergic contact dermatitis, maceration of the skin, secondary infection, skin atrophy, striae and miliaria.

OVERDOSAGE:

Topically applied corticosteroids can be absorbed in sufficient amount to produce systemic effects.

DOSAGE AND ADMINISTRATION:

Carefully remove all cerumen and debris and insert a wick saturated with this product. Instruct the patient to keep the wick moistened for the next 24 hours by occasionally adding a few drops on the wick. Remove the wick after the first 24 hours and continue to instill 5 drops, 3 or 4 times daily thereafter. To prevent infection of the other ear during treatment, this product may be used in the unaffected ear 3 times daily.

Storage: Store at controlled room temperature 15-30° (59-86°F). Protect from light. Dispense in the original container.

HOW SUPPLIED - EQUIVALENTS NOT AVAILABLE:

Solution - Otic

10 ml	$14.95	Oti-Med, Hyrex Pharms	00314-0021-10
10 ml	$15.95	Cortic, Everett Labs	00642-0011-01
10 ml	$17.95	Zoto-Hc, Horizon Pharm	59630-0135-01
10 ml	$19.50	OTOZONE, RA McNeil	12830-0781-10
10 ml	$19.95	Tri-Otic, Pharmics	00813-0393-11

CHLORPHENESIN CARBAMATE *(000747)*

CATEGORIES: Autonomic Drugs; Neuromuscular; Sedatives; Skeletal Muscle Hyperactivity; Skeletal Muscle Relaxants; FDA Approval Pre 1982

BRAND NAMES: **Maolate**; *Rinlaxer*
(International brand names outside U.S. in italics)

DESCRIPTION:

Chlorphenesin carbamate, 3-(p-chlorophenoxy)-2-hydroxypropyl carbamate, is a white to off-white crystalline solid, almost insoluble in cold water, benzene or cyclohexane, fairly readily soluble in dioxane, and readily soluble in ethyl acetate, 95% ethanol and acetone.

CLINICAL PHARMACOLOGY:

The mode of therapeutic action in man has not been identified, but may be related to its sedative properties. It has no direct action on the contractile mechanism of striated muscle, the motor end plate, or the nerve fiber.

ANIMAL TOXICITY

In toxicity studies in rats and dogs, comparison of treated and untreated (control) animals revealed no meaningful changes attributable to chlorphenesin carbamate. Nevertheless, it should be noted that at the high chlorphenesin carbamate dosage levels (100 - 300 mg/kg in rats and 260 - 300 mg/kg in dogs) liver weight : body weight ratios increased.

No hepatocellular changes were noted in the rats, but in dogs, one of three given 300 mg/kg of chlorphenesin carbamate for 28 days and one of four given 260 mg/kg of chlorphenesin carbamate for 174 days showed nonspecific hepatocellular degeneration on microscopic examination. However, attention should be called to the fact that at the high chlorphenesin carbamate dosage levels the dogs involved were markedly obtunded and ate poorly.

INDICATIONS AND USAGE:

Chlorphenesin carbamate is indicated as an adjunct to rest, physical therapy and other measures for the relief of discomfort associated with acute, painful musculoskeletal conditions. The mode of action of this drug has not been completely identified, but may be related to its sedative properties. Chlorphenesin carbamate does not directly relax skeletal muscles in man.

CONTRAINDICATIONS:

Patients who have demonstrated evidence of hypersensitivity to chlorphenesin carbamate, such as skin rash, should not receive further treatment with it.

WARNINGS:

Use In Pregnancy: The safe use of chlorphenesin carbamate in pregnancy has not been established. Therefore, its use during pregnancy, lactation or in women who may become pregnant is not recommended, unless, in the opinion of the physician, potential benefits outweigh possible hazards. Adequate animal reproduction studies have not been done.

Use In Children: The safety and effectiveness of this drug in children have not been established; therefore, chlorphenesin carbamate is not recommended for use in the pediatric age group.

Chlorphenesin carbamate may impair the mental and/or physical abilities required for the performance of potentially hazardous tasks, such as driving a motor vehicle or operating machinery. The patient should be warned accordingly.

PRECAUTIONS:

The safe use of chlorphenesin carbamate for periods exceeding eight weeks has not been established. Chlorphenesin carbamate should be used with caution in patients with pre-existing liver disease or impaired hepatic function.

This product contains FD&C Yellow No. 5 (tartrazine) which may cause allergic-type reactions (including bronchial asthma) in certain susceptible individuals. Although the overall incidence of FD&C Yellow No. 5 (tartrazine) sensitivity in the general population is low, it is frequently seen in patients who also have aspirin hypersensitivity.

ADVERSE REACTIONS:

Hematopoietic: Rare cases of leukopenia, thrombocytopenia, agranulocytosis and pancytopenia have been reported.

Hypersensitivity: Anaphylactoid reactions and drug fever have been observed occasionally. The possibility of other allergic phenomena should be borne in mind. Such reactions are an indication for discontinuing the medication.

Drowsiness, dizziness, confusion, nausea, and epigastric distress have been infrequently reported. While not established as drug related, two cases of gastrointestinal bleeding have been reported.

Occasionally, paradoxical stimulation, insomnia, increased nervousness and headache have been reported. Dose reduction will usually control these symptoms.

OVERDOSAGE:

One patient has been reported who attempted suicide by ingesting 12 grams of chlorphenesin carbamate. He was slightly nauseated and drowsy for about six hours but recovered with only routine supportive therapy.

In treating accidental or intentional overdosage, vomiting may be induced or gastric lavage and/or saline catharsis may be employed. Supportive therapy should suffice in most instances of excessive dosage.

DOSAGE AND ADMINISTRATION:

Initial dosage of 2 tablets three times daily is recommended until the desired effect is obtained. For maintenance, dosage may then be reduced to 1 tablet four times daily, or less as required.

HOW SUPPLIED - EQUIVALENTS NOT AVAILABLE:

Tablet, Uncoated - Oral - 400 mg

50's	$38.04	MAOLATE, Pharmacia & Upjohn	00009-0412-01

CHLORPHENIR; GUAIFENESIN; PHENYLEPHRINE HYDROCHLORIDE *(000748)*

CATEGORIES: Allergies; Antihistamines; Antitussives; Antitussives/Expectorants/Mucolytics; Cough Preparations; Expectorants; Respiratory & Allergy Medications; DEA Class CIV; FDA Pre 1938 Drugs

BRAND NAMES: Amidal; Chemdal; Donatussin; Efasin; Quindal

Prescribing information not available at time of publication.

HOW SUPPLIED - EQUIVALENTS NOT AVAILABLE:

Liquid - Oral - 1 mg/20 mg/2 mg

30 ml	$8.29	DONATUSSIN DROPS, Laser	00277-0106-30

CHLORPHENIRAMINE MALEATE *(000751)*

CATEGORIES: Alkylamines; Allergic Reactions; Allergies; Anaphylactic Reactions; Angioedema; Antihistamines; Conjunctivitis; Cough Preparations; Respiratory & Allergy Medications; Rhinitis; Urticaria; FDA Approval Pre 1982

BRAND NAMES: *Ahiston*; Al-R; *Alergical*; *Aller*; *Allerfin*; *Allergex*; *Allergin* (Japan); *Allergyl*; *Allerhist*; Allerid-Od-12; *Allerkyn*; *Allermin*; *Anaphyl*; Antagonate; *Antamin*; *Cadistan*; Chlo-Amine; *Chlometon* (Japan); *Chlorleate*; Chlorphenamine; *Chlorpheniramine DHA*; *Chlorphenon*; *Chlorpyrimine*; Chlor-100; Chlor-Pro; Chlor-Span-12; Chlor-Trimeton; *Chlor-Tripolon* (Canada); Chloridamine; Chlortab-8; *Chlortrimeton*; *Clometamine*; *Cloro*; *Cloro-Trimeton* (Mexico); *Cloro Trimeton*; *Clorotrimeton*; *Clorten*; *Cohistan*; Com-Time; *Comin*; Cophene-B; *Corometon*; Cpc-Carpenters; *Disoramin 2*; *Evenin*; *Fenaler*; Halortron; *Histacort*; *Histafen*; Histaject; *Histal*; *Histamed*; *Histar* (Japan); *Histatapp*; *Histaton*; Histex; *Istamex*; *Istaminol*; *Kelargine*; Kloromin; *Kobis* (Japan); *Lentostamin*; *Losmanin*; *Methyrit*; *Novopheniram* (Canada); *Pehachlor*; Phenetron; *Piriton*; *Piriton Glaxo*; *Polaramine*; *Polaronil*; *Prof-N-4*; Pyridamal 100; *Reston*; *Reston M* (Japan); Sinunil-R; *Sinvena*; *Trimeton*; *Trimeton Repetabs* (Mexico)
(International brand names outside U.S. in italics)

FORMULARIES: DoD; Medi-Cal; WHO

COST OF THERAPY: $0.76 (Rhinitis; Tablet; 4 mg; 3/day; 30 days)

PRIMARY ICD9: 477.9 (Allergic Rhinitis, Cause Unspecified)

DESCRIPTION:

Chlorpheniramine maleate is an antihistaminic agent. It is a white, odorless, crystalline powder, the solutions of which have a pH between 4 and 5.

CLINICAL PHARMACOLOGY:

Chlorpheniramine maleate is an antihistaminic drug which possesses anticholinergic and sedative effects.

INDICATIONS AND USAGE:

Chlorpheniramine maleate is indicated for the following conditions:

1. Perennial and seasonal allergic rhinitis.
2. Vasomotor rhinitis.
3. Allergic conjunctivitis due to inhalant allergens and foods.
4. Mild, uncomplicated allergic skin manifestations of urticaria and angioedema.
5. Amelioration of allergic reactions to blood or plasma.
6. Dermographism.
7. As therapy for anaphylactic reactions adjunctive to epinephrine and other standard measures after the acute manifestations have been controlled.

CONTRAINDICATIONS:

This drug should not be used in newborn or premature infants.

Antihistamines should NOT be used to treat lower respiratory symptoms.

Do not use this drug in patients with:

Hypersensitivity to preparation
Asthmatic attack
Narrow-angle glaucoma
Prostatic hypertrophy
Stenosing peptic ulcer
Pyloroduodenal obstruction
Bladder neck obstruction
Patients receiving monoamine oxidase inhibitors

WARNINGS:

This drug may impair the mental and/or physical abilities required for the performance of potentially hazardous tasks such as driving a vehicle or operating machinery. This drug may impair mental alertness in children. The concomitant use of alcohol or other central nervous system depressants may have an additive effect. Patients should be warned accordingly.

Usage In Pregnancy: Although there is no evidence that the use of this drug is detrimental to the mother or fetus, the use of any drug in pregnancy should be carefully deliberated. This product may cause an inhibition of lactation.

Usage In Children: In infants and children particularly, antihistamines in overdosage may produce convulsions and/or death.

PRECAUTIONS:

Chlorpheniramine maleate has an atropine-like action and should be used with caution in patients who may have increased intraocular pressure, hyperthyroidism, cardiovascular disease, hypertension or in patients with a history of bronchial asthma.

ADVERSE REACTIONS:

The following adverse reactions have been reported:

Drowsiness	Nasal stuffiness
Confusion	Difficulty in urination
Nervousness	Constipation
Restlessness	Tightness of the chest and wheezing
Nausea	Thickening of bronchial secretions
Vomiting	Dryness of mouth, nose, and throat
Diarrhea	Tingling, heaviness, and weakness of hands
Blurring of vision	Vertigo
Diplopia	Palpitation
Headache	Drug rash
Insomnia	Hemolytic anemia
Urticaria	Hypotension
Epigastric distress	Anaphylaxis

DOSAGE AND ADMINISTRATION:

Adults: The usual adult dose is 4 mg three or four times daily.

Children: For children over 20 pounds the usual dose is 2 mg three or four times daily.

Store at Controlled Room Temperature 15-30 deg. C (59-86 deg. F).

HOW SUPPLIED - RATED THERAPEUTICALLY EQUIVALENT:

Injection, Solution - Intravenous - 10 mg/ml

10 ml	$8.00	COPHENE-B, Dunhall Pharms	00217-0404-08
30 ml	$1.96	PHENETRON, Lannett	00527-0171-58
30 ml	$4.50	Chlorpheniramine Maleate, Consolidated Midland	00223-7310-30
30 ml	$6.68	Chlorpheniramine Maleate, Schein Pharm (US)	00364-6523-56

Tablet, Uncoated - Oral - 4 mg

4's	$.04	Chlorpheniramine Maleate, H.C.F.A. F F P	99999-0751-01
12's	$.12	Chlorpheniramine Maleate, H.C.F.A. F F P	99999-0751-02
24's	$.24	Chlorpheniramine Maleate, H.C.F.A. F F P	99999-0751-03
24's	$2.40	Aller-Chlor, Rugby	00536-3467-35
30's	$.30	Chlorpheniramine Maleate, H.C.F.A. F F P	99999-0751-04
48's	$.49	Chlorpheniramine Maleate, H.C.F.A. F F P	99999-0751-05
100's	$0.85	Chlorpheniramine Maleate, Anabolic	00722-5032-01
100's	$1.03	Chlorpheniramine Maleate, H.C.F.A. F F P	99999-0751-06
100's	$1.50	Chlorpheniramine Maleate, Halsey Drug	00879-0472-01
100's	$1.95	Chlorpheniramine Maleate, Consolidated Midland	00223-0692-01
100's	$5.42	Chlorpheniramine Maleate, Geneva Pharms	00781-1148-01
100's	$5.70	Aller-Chlor, Rugby	00536-3467-01
500's	$5.15	Chlorpheniramine Maleate, H.C.F.A. F F P	99999-0751-07
1000's	$3.20	Chlorpheniramine Maleate, Anabolic	00722-5032-02
1000's	$3.75	Chlorpheniramine Maleate, Halsey Drug	00879-0472-10
1000's	$5.70	CHLOR-PHEN, C O Truxton	00463-6065-10
1000's	$9.75	Chlorpheniramine Maleate, Consolidated Midland	00223-0692-02
1000's	$10.25	Chlorpheniramine, Major Pharms	00904-0012-80
1000's	$10.30	Chlorpheniramine Maleate, H.C.F.A. F F P	99999-0751-08
1000's	$17.17	Aller-Chlor, Rugby	00536-3467-10

HOW SUPPLIED - RATED THERAPEUTICALLY EQUIVALENT: *(cont'd)*

1000's	$65.90	Chlorpheniramine Maleate, Geneva Pharms	00781-1148-10
5000's	$51.50	Chlorpheniramine Maleate, H.C.F.A. F F P	99999-0751-09

HOW SUPPLIED - NOT RATED EQUIVALENT:

Capsule, Gelatin, Sustained Action - Oral - 4 mg

100's	$10.77	COM-TIME, Time-Caps Labs	49483-0036-01

Capsule, Gelatin, Sustained Action - Oral - 8 mg

100's	$6.25	Chlorpheniramine, Major Pharms	00904-2087-60
100's	$9.75	Chlorpheniramine Maleate, Time-Caps Labs	49483-0041-01
100's	$9.95	Chlormate Sa, Alphagen Labs	59743-0052-01
100's	$10.90	Chlorpheniramine Tr, Qualitest Pharms	00603-2784-21
1000's	$38.87	Chlorpheniramine Maleate, HL Moore Drug Exch	00839-1152-16
1000's	$52.50	Chlorpheniramine, Major Pharms	00904-2087-80
1000's	$74.58	Chlorpheniramine Maleate, Time-Caps Labs	49483-0041-10
1000's	$85.00	Chlormate Sa, Alphagen Labs	59743-0052-10
1000's	$90.85	Chlorpheniramine Maleate, Qualitest Pharms	00603-2784-32

Capsule, Gelatin, Sustained Action - Oral - 12 mg

100's	$7.15	Chlorpheniramine Maleate TDC, Major Pharms	00904-2088-60
100's	$7.50	CHLOR-PHEN T.D., C O Truxton	00463-3002-01
100's	$10.74	Chlorpheniramine Maleate, Time-Caps Labs	49483-0043-01
100's	$11.05	Chlormate Sa, Alphagen Labs	59743-0051-01
100's	$11.75	Chlorpheniramine Tr, Qualitest Pharms	00603-2785-21
1000's	$42.65	Chlorpheniramine Maleate, HL Moore Drug Exch	00839-1156-16
1000's	$56.95	Chlorpheniramine Maleate TDC, Major Pharms	00904-2088-80
1000's	$81.36	Chlorpheniramine Maleate, Time-Caps Labs	49483-0043-10
1000's	$98.40	Chlormate Sa, Alphagen Labs	59743-0051-10
1000's	$105.70	Chlorpheniramine Maleate, Qualitest Pharms	00603-2785-32

Injection, Solution - Intravenous - 10 mg/ml

30 ml	$6.64	Chlorpheniramine Maleate, HL Moore Drug Exch	00839-5161-36
30 ml	$6.68	Chlorpheniramine Maleate, Steris Labs	00402-0178-30

Injection, Solution - Intravenous - 100 mg/ml

10 ml	$4.00	Chlorpheniramine Maleate, Consolidated Midland	00223-7310-10

Syrup - Oral - 2 mg/5ml

480 ml	$4.60	Chlorpheniramine Maleate, Consolidated Midland	00223-6244-01
3840 ml	$24.00	Chlorpheniramine Maleate, Consolidated Midland	00223-6244-02

CHLORPHENIRAMINE MALEATE; CODEINE PHOSPHATE; GUAIFENESIN *(000752)*

CATEGORIES: Allergies; Antitussives; Antitussives/Expectorants/Mucolytics; Common Cold; Cough Preparations; DESI Drugs; Decongestants; Nasal Congestion; Respiratory & Allergy Medications; Rhinitis; DEA Class CV; FDA Pre 1938 Drugs

BRAND NAMES: **Tussar**

DESCRIPTION:

Each 5 ml (one teaspoonful) contains:

Codeine Phosphate, U.S.P, 10 mg

WARNING—MAY BE HABIT-FORMING.

Chlorpheniramine Maleate, U.S.P, 2 mg

Guaifenesin, U.S.P, 100 mg

Alcohol, 6%

Tussar Inactive ingredients: artificial flavors, citric acid, D&C Yellow No. 10, FD&C Blue No. 1, glucose, methylparaben, methyl salicylate, propylene glycol, saccharin, sodium citrate, sucrose, water.

INDICATIONS AND USAGE:

Chlorpheniramine maleate with codeine and guaifenesin temporarily relieves cough due to common cold and minor throat and bronchial irritation; provides temporary relief of nasal congestion, runny nose and watery eyes as may occur in allergic rhinitis (such as hay fever). The antitussive, codeine, calms the cough control center and relieves coughing. The expectorant, guaifenesin, increases the flow of natural secretions making a dry cough more productive.

WARNINGS:

A persistent cough may be a sign of a serious condition. If cough persists for more than one week, tends to recur, or is accompanied by fever, rash, or persistent headache, consult a doctor.

May cause or aggravate constipation. Do not take this product if you have a chronic pulmonary disease, shortness of breath, or excessive secretions, unless directed by a doctor. If drowsiness occurs, do not drive a car or operate machinery. Do not exceed recommended dosage. As with any drug, if you are pregnant or nursing a baby, seek the advice of a health professional before using this product.

DOSAGE AND ADMINISTRATION:

Adults and children 12 years of age and over: One teaspoonful (5 ml) every 4 to 6 hours, not to exceed 6 teaspoonfuls in any 24-hour period. Not to be administered to infants or children under 12 unless directed by a doctor.

HOW SUPPLIED - EQUIVALENTS NOT AVAILABLE:

Syrup - Oral - 2 mg/10 mg/100

120 ml	**$91.12**	**TUSSAR SF, Rhone-Poulenc Rorer**	**00075-3665-05**
480 ml	**$50.50**	**TUSSAR SF, Rhone-Poulenc Rorer**	**00075-3665-01**
480 ml	**$50.50**	**TUSSAR-2, Rhone-Poulenc Rorer**	**00075-3666-01**

CHLORPHENIRAMINE MALEATE; CODEINE PHOSPHATE; GUAIFENESIN; PHENYLEPHRINE HYDROCHLORIDE; PHENYLPROPANOLAMINE *(000764)*

CATEGORIES: Antitussives; Cough Preparations; Expectorants; DEA Class CV; FDA Pre 1938 Drugs

BRAND NAMES: Chemdal Expectorant; Quendal

Prescribing information not available at time of publication.

HOW SUPPLIED - EQUIVALENTS NOT AVAILABLE:

Liquid - Oral - 10 mg/100 mg/12

28's	$108.13	CHEMDAL EXPECTORANT, H N Norton Co.	50732-0854-28
480 ml	$15.80	QUENDAL, Qualitest Pharms	00603-1620-58
480 ml	$17.73	CHEMDAL EXPECTORANT, H N Norton Co.	50732-0854-16

CHLORPHENIRAMINE MALEATE; CODEINE PHOSPHATE; PHENYLEPHRINE HYDROCHLORIDE; POTASSIUM IODIDE *(000767)*

CATEGORIES: Allergies; Antitussives; Antitussives/Expectorants/Mucolytics; Bronchitis; Common Cold; Cough Preparations; Croup; Expectorants; Iodide Salts; Pharyngitis; Respiratory & Allergy Medications; Respiratory Tract Infections; Tracheobronchitis; DEA Class CV; FDA Pre 1938 Drugs

BRAND NAMES: Demi-Cof; Pediacof

FORMULARIES: Aetna

DESCRIPTION:

Decongestant and Soothing Cough Syrup for Children: Each teaspoon (5 ml) contains: Codeine phosphate, USP - 5.0 mg (Warning: May be habit forming.) Phenylephrine hydrochloride, USP - 2.5 mg; Chlorpheniramine maleate, USP - 0.75 mg; Potassium iodide, USP - 75.0 mg with sodium benzoate 0.2% as preservative; and alcohol 5%.

Pediacof is a pleasant-tasting, raspberry-flavored cough syrup. It contains four active ingredients in the proper proportion for children. Codeine phosphate is a white crystalline, odorless powder which is freely soluble in water. It is a narcotic analgesic.

Codeine phosphate is 7,8-Didehydro-4,5 α-epoxy-3-methoxy-17 methylmorphinan-6α-ol phosphate.

Phenylephrine hydrochloride is a vasoconstrictor and pressor drug chemically related to epinephrine and ephedrine. It is a synthetic sympathomimetic agent. Chemically, phenylephrine hydrochloride is (-)-*m*-Hydroxy-α-[(methylamino) methyl]-benzyl alcohol hydrochloride.

Chlorpheniramine maleate is an alkylamine H_1-blocking agent (antihistamine) which is chemically 2-Pyridinepropanamine, γ-(4-chlorphenyl)-*N,N*-dimethyl-, *(Z)*-2-butenedioate.

Potassium iodide is an expectorant.

Inactive Ingredients: Alcohol, Citric Acid, FD&C Red #40, Flavor, Glycerin, Liquid Glucose, Purified Water, Saccharin Sodium, Sodium Benzoate.

CLINICAL PHARMACOLOGY:

Codeine phosphate is an antitussive that is well recognized not only because of its efficiency and rapidity of action but also because of its relative safety in clinical use. Thus, irritating, nonproductive cough is suppressed by codeine. The codeine content of this combination drug is reduced to the proportion that is most suitable for children. When codeine is combined with the expectorant potassium iodide, which tends to increase bronchial secretion, coughing, although minimized, is more productive when it does occur. The continuous fatiguing effect of useless coughing is thereby avoided. Codeine is a narcotic analgesic and antitussive which resembles morphine pharmacologically. Codeine is metabolized by the liver and excreted chiefly in the urine, largely in inactive forms. A small fraction (10%) of administered codeine is demethylated to form morphine, and both free and conjugated morphine can be found in the urine after therapeutic doses of codeine. When administered subcutaneously, 120 mg of codeine is approximately equivalent to 10 mg of morphine. The abuse liability of codeine is generally considered to be much lower than that of morphine.

The half-life of codeine in plasma is 2.5 to 3.0 hours.

Codeine has diverse additional actions. It depresses the respiratory center, stimulates the vomiting center, depresses the cough reflex, constricts the pupils, increases the tone of the gastrointestinal and genitourinary tracts, and produces mild vasodilation.

Neo-Synephrine, brand of phenylephrine hydrochloride, produces effective decongestion of the mucous membranes of the respiratory tract via its powerful postsynaptic α-receptor stimulant action. It has little effect on cardiac β-receptors. Most of its effects are due to direct action on receptors and only a small part is due to norepinephrine release. Central stimulant activity is minimal.

Chlorpheniramine maleate helps control allergic coughs and mucosal congestion. The mild anticholinergic action of chlorpheniramine maleate may aid in reducing rhinorrhea, and its mild sedative action may also be beneficial to patients whose excessive coughing has caused them to lose sleep.

Clinical experience with this combination drug has shown it to be a dependable medication for the relief of cough and the reduction of nasal congestion in children.

INDICATIONS AND USAGE:

Coughs due to colds as well as coughs and congestive symptoms associated with upper respiratory tract infections such as tracheobronchitis or laryngobronchitis, croup, pharyngitis, allergic bronchitis, and infectious bronchitis, when accompanied by disturbing and fatiguing cough, have been treated successfully with this combination drug in children.

CONTRAINDICATIONS:

This combination drug is contraindicated in patients who are hypersensitive to any of its ingredients. Due to the component phenylephrine, this combination drug is contraindicated in patients with ventricular tachycardia or severe hypertension.

WARNINGS:

Respiratory Depression: Codeine produces dose-related respiratory depression by acting directly on brain stem respiratory centers. Codeine also affects centers that control respiratory rhythm and may produce irregular and periodic breathing. If significant respiratory depression occurs it may be antagonized by the use of naloxone hydrochloride. (See OVERDOSAGE.)

Head Injury and Increased Intracranial Pressure: The respiratory depressant effects of narcotics and their capacity to elevate cerebrospinal fluid pressure may be markedly exaggerated in the presence of head injury, other intracranial lesions, or a preexisting increase in intracranial pressure. Furthermore, narcotics can produce adverse reactions which may obscure the clinical course of patients with head injuries.

Acute Abdominal Conditions: The administration of narcotics may obscure the diagnosis or clinical course of patients with acute abdominal conditions.

PRECAUTIONS:

Caution should be exercised if this combination drug is administered to patients with cardiac disorders other than ventricular tachycardia, which is contraindicated; mild hypertension and hyperthyroidism.

Special Risk Patients: *Codeine:* should be used with caution in patients with impaired renal or hepatic function, hypothyroidism, Addison's disease, or urethral stricture.In asthma, the indiscriminate use of codeine may, due to its drying action upon the mucosa of the respiratory tract, precipitate severe respiratory insufficiency resulting from increased viscosity of the bronchial secretions and suppression of the cough reflex. As with any narcotic analgesic agent, the usual precautions should be kept in mind. *Phenylephrine hydrochloride:* should be employed only with extreme caution in patients with hyperthyroidism, bradycardia, partial heart block, and myocardial disease.*Chlorpheniramine maleate:* should be used with considerable caution in patients with narrow angle glaucoma, pyloroduodenal obstruction, and bladder neck obstruction. Chlorpheniramine maleate has an atropine-like action and therefore should be used with caution in patients with a history of bronchial asthma, increased intraocular pressure, hyperthyroidism, cardiovascular disease, and hypertension.

Carcinogenesis, Mutagenesis, and Impairment of Fertility: No long-term animal studies have been performed to evaluate the potential of this combination drug in the areas.

Pregnancy: Nonteratogenic Effects: Dependence has been reported in newborns whose mothers received opiates regularly during pregnancy. Withdrawal signs include irritability, excessive crying, tremors, hyperreflexia, fever, vomiting, and diarrhea. Signs usually appear during the fist few days of life.

DRUG INTERACTIONS:

Patients receiving other narcotic analgesics, general anesthetics, phenothiazines, tranquilizers, sedative-hypnotics, MAO inhibitors, tricyclic antidepressants, or other CNS depressants (including alcohol) concomitantly with codeine may exhibit an additive CNS depression. When such combined therapy is contemplated, the dose of one or both agents should be reduced.

ADVERSE REACTIONS:

The only significant untoward effects that have occurred are mild anorexia and an occasional tendency to constipation. However, discontinuance of this combination drug has seldom been required. Mild drowsiness occurs in some patients but, when cough is relieved, the quieting effect of this combination drug is considered beneficial in many instances. Because of its iodide content, this combination drug may cause elevation of the protein bound iodine.

Adverse Reactions To Codeine:

Central Nervous System: Sedation, drowsiness, mental clouding, dizziness, lethargy, impairment of mental and physical performance, anxiety, convulsions, fear, miosis, dysphoria, psychic dependence, mood changes, and respiratory depression.

Gastrointestinal System: Nausea, vomiting, increased pressure in the biliary tract, and constipation.

Cardiovascular System: Orthostatic hypotension, fainting, and tachycardia.

Genitourinary System: Ureteral spasm, spasm of vesical sphincters and urinary retention have been reported.

Other: Flushing, sweating, pruritus, allergic reactions, and suppressed cough reflex. Adverse reactions to phenylephrine hydrochloride include headache, reflex bradycardia, excitability, restlessness, and rarely, arrhythmias.

Adverse Reactions To Chlorpheniramine Maleate:

include slight to moderate drowsiness. Other possible side effects common to antihistamines in general include:

General: Urticaria, drug rash, anaphylactic shock, photosensitivity, excessive perspiration, chills, dryness of mouth, nose, and throat.

Cardiovascular System: Hypotension, headache, palpitations, tachycardia, and extrasystoles.

Hematologic System: Hemolytic anemia, thrombocytopenia, and agranulocytosis.

Nervous System: Sedation, dizziness, disturbed coordination, fatigue, confusion, restlessness, excitation, nervousness, tremor, irritability, insomnia, euphoria, paresthesias, blurred vision, diplopia, vertigo, tinnitus, acute labyrinthitis, hysteria, neuritis, and convulsions.

Gastrointestinal System: Epigastric distress, anorexia, nausea, vomiting, diarrhea, and constipation.

Genitourinary System: Urinary frequency, difficult urination, urinary retention, and early menses.

Respiratory System: Thickening of bronchial secretions, tightness of chest and wheezing, and nasal stuffiness.

OVERDOSAGE:

CODEINE

Signs and Symptoms: Overdosage with codeine is characterized by respiratory depression (a decrease in respiratory rate and/or tidal volume, Cheyne-Stokes respiration, cyanosis), pinpoint pupils, extreme somnolence progressing to stupor or coma, skeletal muscle flaccidity, cold and clammy skin, and sometimes bradycardia and hypotension. In severe overdosage, particularly by the intravenous route, apnea, circulatory collapse, cardiac arrest, and death may occur.

Treatment: Primary attention should be given to the reestablishment of adequate respiratory exchange through provision of a patent airway and institution of assisted or controlled ventilation. Naloxone hydrochloride is a specific and effective antagonist for respiratory depression which may result from overdosage. If the desired degree of counteraction and improvement in respiratory function is not obtained immediately following IV administration, it may be repeated intravenously at 2 or 3 minute intervals. Failure to obtain significant improvement after 2 or 3 doses suggests that the condition may be due partly or completely to other disease processes or nonopioid drugs. The usual initial pediatric dose is 0.01 mg/kg body weight given IV, IM, or SC. If necessary, naloxone can be diluted with Sterile Water for Injection, USP. Oxygen, intravenous fluids, vasopressors, and other supportive measures should be employed as indicated.

Oral LD_{50} in the mouse is 693 mg/kg. Codeine is not dialyzable.

PHENYLEPHRINE HYDROCHLORIDE

Signs and Symptoms: Overdosage may induce ventricular extrasystoles and short paroxysms of ventricular tachycardia, a sensation of fullness in the head, and tingling of the extremities.

Treatment: Should an excessive elevation of blood pressure occur, it may be immediately relieved by an α-adrenergic blocking agent, *e.g.*, phentolamine. The oral LD_{50} in the rat: 350 mg/kg; mouse: 120 mg/kg.

CHLORPHENIRAMINE MALEATE

Signs and Symptoms: Antihistamine overdose may vary from central nervous system depression (sedation, apnea, and cardiovascular collapse) to stimulation (insomnia, hallucinations, tremors or convulsions). Other signs and symptoms may be dizziness, tinnitus, ataxia, blurred vision, and hypotension. Stimulation and atropine-like signs and symptoms (dry mouth; fixed, dilated pupils; flushing; hyperthermia, and gastrointestinal symptoms) are particularly likely in children.

OVERDOSAGE: *(cont'd)*

Treatment: Emergency treatment should be started immediately. Vomiting should be induced, even if it has occurred spontaneously. Vomiting by the administration of ipecac syrup is preferred. Vomiting should **not** be induced in patients with impaired consciousness. The action of ipecac is facilitated by physical activity and by the administration of eight to twelve fluid ounces of water. If emesis does not occur within fifteen minutes, the dose of ipecac should be repeated. Precautions against aspiration must be taken, especially in infants and children. Following emesis, any drug remaining in the stomach may be absorbed by activated charcoal administered as a slurry with water. If vomiting is unsuccessful or contraindicated, gastric lavage should be performed. Isotonic and one-half isotonic saline are the lavage solutions of choice. Saline cathartics, such as milk of magnesia, draw water into the bowel by osmosis and, therefore, may be valuable for their action in rapid dilution of bowel content. After emergency treatment the patient should continue to be medically monitored. Treatment of the signs and symptoms of overdosage is symptomatic and supportive.

Stimulants (analeptic agents) should **not** be used. Vasopressors may be used to treat hypotension. Short-acting barbiturates, diazepam, or paraldehyde may be administered to control seizures. Hyperpyrexia, especially in children, may require treatment with tepid water sponge baths or hypothermic blanket. Apnea is treated with ventilatory support.

DOSAGE AND ADMINISTRATION:

This combination drug should be given in accordance with the needs and age of the patient. Frequency of administration may be adjusted as cough is brought under control. The following doses, to be given at 4 to 6 hour intervals, are suggested for patients under 12 years of age: **from 6 months to 1 year**, 1/4 teaspoon; **from 1 to 3 years**, 1/2 to 1 teaspoon; **from 3 to 6 years**, 1 to 2 teaspoons; and **from 6 to 12 years**, 2 teaspoons.

HOW SUPPLIED - EQUIVALENTS NOT AVAILABLE:

Syrup - Oral

5 ml	$29.95	Demi-Cof Pediatric Cough Syrup, Econolab	55053-0610-16
480 ml	$23.25	PEDITUSS COUGH SYRUP, Major Pharms	00904-1239-16
480 ml	$44.12	PEDIACOF, Sanofi Winthrop	00024-1509-06
3840 ml	$123.99	PEDITUSS COUGH SYRUP, Major Pharms	00904-1239-28

CHLORPHENIRAMINE MALEATE; CODEINE PHOSPHATE; PSEUDOEPHEDRINE HYDROCHLORIDE *(000753)*

CATEGORIES: Allergies; Antihistamines; Antitussives; Antitussives/Expectorants/Mucolytics; Common Cold; Congestion; Cough Preparations; Decongestants; Hay Fever; Influenza; Otitis Media; Pruritus; Respiratory & Allergy Medications; Rhinitis; Sinus Congestion; Sympathomimetic Agents; DEA Class CV; FDA Pre 1938 Drugs

BRAND NAMES: Alamine-C; Co-Histine Dh; Codahist Dh; Codecon-C; Cophene-S; Decohistine Dh; Decongestant-Dh; Dihistine Dh; Histadyl E.C.; Novadyne Dh; Novagest Dh; **Novahistine-Dh**; Novatex-Dh; Phenhist Dh W/Codeine; Phenylhistine Dh; *Rinofed Antitusivo*; Ryna-C
(International brand names outside U.S. in italics)

FORMULARIES: BC-BS; Medi-Cal

Prescribing information not available at time of publication.

HOW SUPPLIED - EQUIVALENTS NOT AVAILABLE:

Liquid - Oral - 2 mg/10 mg/30 m

120 ml	$2.70	NOVAGEST DH, Major Pharms	00904-0922-20
120 ml	$2.80	PHENYLHISTINE DH, HR Cenci	00556-0332-04
120 ml	$2.90	Phenylhistine Dh, Halsey Drug	00879-0728-04
120 ml	$2.90	Co-Histine Dh, Hi Tech Pharma	50383-0084-04
120 ml	$2.94	DIHISTINE DH, Alpharma	00472-1639-04
120 ml	$2.95	Dihistine Dh, Consolidated Midland	00223-6131-01
120 ml	$3.00	Decohistine Dh, Morton Grove	60432-0584-04
120 ml	$3.04	DIHISTINE DH, HL Moore Drug Exch	00839-6694-65
240 ml	$4.96	Dihistine Dh, Alpharma	00472-1639-08
480 ml	$7.75	NOVAGEST DH, Major Pharms	00904-0922-16
480 ml	$7.98	PHENYLHISTINE DH, Qualitest Pharms	00603-1520-58
480 ml	$8.09	DIHISTINE DH, HL Moore Drug Exch	00839-6694-69
480 ml	$8.10	PHENYLHISTINE DH, HR Cenci	00556-0332-16
480 ml	$8.20	Dihistine Dh, Harber Pharm	51432-0520-20
480 ml	$8.48	Decohistine Dh, Morton Grove	60432-0584-16
480 ml	$8.50	Phenylhistine Dh, Halsey Drug	00879-0728-16
480 ml	$8.61	DIHISTINE DH, Alpharma	00472-1639-16
480 ml	$9.00	Co-Histine Dh, Hi Tech Pharma	50383-0084-16
480 ml	$9.50	Dihistine Dh, Consolidated Midland	00223-6131-02
480 ml	$19.06	HISTADYL E.C., Lilly	00002-5126-05
480 ml	$34.50	CODECON-C, Econolab	55053-0550-16
3840 ml	$49.77	Dihistine Dh, HL Moore Drug Exch	00839-6694-70
3840 ml	$51.72	NOVAGEST DH, Major Pharms	00904-0922-28
3840 ml	$54.49	Dihistine Dh, Consolidated Midland	00223-6131-03
3840 ml	$55.49	PHENYLHISTINE DH, HR Cenci	00556-0332-28
3840 ml	$58.50	Phenylhistine Dh, Halsey Drug	00879-0728-28
3840 ml	$58.56	DIHISTINE DH, Alpharma	00472-1639-28

CHLORPHENIRAMINE MALEATE; DEXTROMETHORPHAN HYDROBROMIDE; GUAIFENESIN; PHENPROPANOLAMINE; PSEUDOEPHEDRINE HYDROCHLORIDE *(000773)*

CATEGORIES: Antitussives; Cough Preparations; Expectorants; FDA Pre 1938 Drugs

BRAND NAMES: Lemotussin Dm; Threamine; Threamine Dm

Prescribing information not available at time of publication.

HOW SUPPLIED - EQUIVALENTS NOT AVAILABLE:

Syrup - Oral

120 ml x 12	$27.00	Threamine, Consolidated Midland	00223-6311-01
480 ml	$5.50	Threamine, Consolidated Midland	00223-6311-02
480 ml	$9.50	Threamine Dm, Consolidated Midland	00223-6619-01

HOW SUPPLIED - EQUIVALENTS NOT AVAILABLE: *(cont'd)*

480 ml	$25.52	LEMOTUSSIN DM, Seneca Pharms	47028-0015-16
3840 ml	$31.99	Threamine, Consolidated Midland	00223-6311-03
3840 ml	$55.49	Threamine Dm, Consolidated Midland	00223-6619-02

CHLORPHENIRAMINE MALEATE; DEXTROMETHORPHAN HYDROBROMIDE; GUAIFENESIN; PHENYLEPHRINE HYDROCHLORIDE *(000775)*

CATEGORIES: Antitussives; Antitussives/Expectorants/Mucolytics; Common Cold; Cough Preparations; Expectorants; Respiratory & Allergy Medications; FDA Pre 1938 Drugs

BRAND NAMES: Broncopectol; Chem-Tuss Dme; Donatussin; Neodex

Prescribing information not available at time of publication.

HOW SUPPLIED - EQUIVALENTS NOT AVAILABLE:

Syrup - Oral - 2 mg/7.5 mg/100

480 ml	$19.49	DONATUSSIN, Laser	00277-0139-41
3840 ml	$134.05	DONATUSSIN, Laser	00277-0139-42

CHLORPHENIRAMINE MALEATE; DEXTROMETHORPHAN HYDROBROMIDE; GUAIFENESIN; PHENYLEPHRINE HYDROCHLORIDE; PHENYLPROPANOLAMINE *(000774)*

CATEGORIES: Antitussives; Common Cold; Cough Preparations; Expectorants; Respiratory & Allergy Medications; FDA Pre 1938 Drugs

BRAND NAMES: Anatuss; Anatuss La

Prescribing information not available at time of publication.

CHLORPHENIRAMINE MALEATE; DEXTROMETHORPHAN HYDROBROMIDE; PHENYLEPHRINE HYDROCHLORIDE *(000778)*

CATEGORIES: Antitussives; Antitussives/Expectorants/Mucolytics; Cough Preparations; Respiratory & Allergy Medications; FDA Pre 1938 Drugs

BRAND NAMES: Atuss Dm; Chem-Tuss Dm

Prescribing information not available at time of publication.

HOW SUPPLIED - EQUIVALENTS NOT AVAILABLE:

Elixir - Oral - 4 mg/10 mg/10 m

473 ml	$24.38	Atuss Dm, Atley Pharms	59702-0015-16

CHLORPHENIRAMINE MALEATE; EPHEDRINE; GUAIFENESIN *(000784)*

CATEGORIES: Antitussives/Expectorants/Mucolytics; Expectorants; Respiratory & Allergy Medications; FDA Pre 1938 Drugs

BRAND NAMES: Bronkotuss

Prescribing information not available at time of publication.

HOW SUPPLIED - EQUIVALENTS NOT AVAILABLE:

Liquid - Oral - 4 mg/8.216 mg/1

480 ml	$23.62	BRONKOTUSS, Hyrex Pharms	00314-0001-16
3840 ml	$148.65	BRONKOTUSS, Hyrex Pharms	00314-0001-28

CHLORPHENIRAMINE MALEATE; EPINEPHRINE *(000754)*

CATEGORIES: Airway Obstruction; Allergies; Anaphylactic Shock; Antihistamines; Asthma; Insect Sting Emergency Kits; Pregnancy Category C; FDA Pre 1938 Drugs

BRAND NAMES: Ana-Kit

FORMULARIES: DoD

Prescribing information not available at time of publication.

HOW SUPPLIED - EQUIVALENTS NOT AVAILABLE:

Kit - Misc - 2 mg/1 mg

1 kit	$21.42	ANA-KIT, ANAPHYLAXIS EMERGENCY, Miles Spokane	00118-9988-01
6 kits	$128.50	ANA-KIT, ANAPHYLAXIS EMERGENCY, Miles Spokane	00118-9988-06

CHLORPHENIRAMINE MALEATE; GUAIFENESIN; PHENYLPROPANOLAMINE *(000786)*

CATEGORIES: Allergies; Antihistamines; Common Cold; Expectorants; Respiratory & Allergy Medications; FDA Pre 1938 Drugs

BRAND NAMES: Decongest; Medatussin Plus

Prescribing information not available at time of publication.

HOW SUPPLIED - EQUIVALENTS NOT AVAILABLE:

Tablet, Plain Coated, Sustained Action - Oral - 6 mg/200 mg/75

100's	$20.00	DECONGEST T.D., C O Truxton	00463-3017-01

CHLORPHENIRAMINE MALEATE; GUAIFENESIN; PSEUDOEPHEDRINE *(000788)*

CATEGORIES: Antihistamines; Common Cold; Cough Preparations; Expectorants; Respiratory & Allergy Medications; FDA Pre 1938 Drugs

BRAND NAMES: Lemohist Plus

Prescribing information not available at time of publication.

HOW SUPPLIED - EQUIVALENTS NOT AVAILABLE:

Capsule, Gelatin - Oral - 2 mg/100 mg/32.

100's	$28.68	LEMOHIST PLUS, Seneca Pharms	47028-0019-01
1000's	$195.16	LEMOHIST PLUS, Seneca Pharms	47028-0019-10

CHLORPHENIRAMINE MALEATE; HYDROCODONE BITARTRATE; PSEUDOEPHEDRINE HYDROCHLORIDE *(000790)*

CATEGORIES: Antitussives; Antitussives/Expectorants/Mucolytics; Cough Preparations; Respiratory & Allergy Medications; Pregnancy Category C; DEA Class CIII; FDA Pre 1938 Drugs

BRAND NAMES: Anaplex-Hd; Atuss Hd; Chem-Tuss N; Chemdal Hd; Comtussin Hc; Cytuss Hc; Ed Tuss Hc; Efasin-Hd; Endagen-Hd; Endal-Hd; Guiaphen Hd; Histussin-Hc; Hyphen-Hd; M-End; Maxituss Hc; Med-Hist-Hc; Notuss; Quendal-Hd; Rindal-Hd; S-T Forte Sf; Tussanil oh; Tussend; Uni-Tuss Hc; Vanex-Hd; Ventuss

DESCRIPTION:

Each teaspoonful (5 ml) contains:

Hydocodone Bitratrate*, USP 2.5 mg

*WARNING: May be habit forming

Pseudoephedrine Hydrochloride, USP 30 mg

Chlorpheniramine Maleate, USP 2 mg

Alcohol, USP 5%

Hydrocodone Bitratrate is an opioid analgesic and antitussive and occurs as fine white crystals or as crystalline powder. It is affected by light. The chemical name is 4, 5α-epoxy–3–methoxy–17–methylmorphinanin-6–one–tartrate (1:1) hydrate (2:5). Its molecular formula is $C_{18}H_{21}NO_3{\cdot}C_4H_6O_6{\cdot}2\ 1/2\ H_2O$. Its molecular weight is 494.50.

Pseudoephedrine hydrochloride is an adrenergic (vasoconstrictor) which occurs as fine white to off-white crystals or powder, having a faint characteristic odor. It is very soluble in water, freely soluble in alcohol, and sparingly soluble in chloroform. The chemical name is benzenemethanol,α-[1-(methylamino)ethyl]-[S-(R*,R*)]- hydrochloride. It molecular formula is $C_{10}H_{15}NO\ HCl$. Its molecular weight is 201.70.

Chlorpheniramine maleate is an antihistaminic that occurs as white, odorless crystalline powder. Its solutions have a pH between 4 and 5. It is freely soluble in water, soluble in alcohol and in chloroform, and slightly soluble in ether and benzene. The chemical name is 2-pyridinepropanamine, α-(4–chlorophenyl)–N, N-dimethyl-(Z)-2–butenedioate (1:1). Its molecular formula is $C_{16}H_{19}ClN_2{\cdot}C_4H_4O_4$. It molecular weight is 390.87.

TUSSEND also contains: High Fructose Corn Syrup, Sucrose, Propylene Glycol, Flavor, Methylparaben, Saccharin Sodium, Propylparaben, FD&C Yellow No. 6, and Purified Water, USP.

CLINICAL PHARMACOLOGY:

Hydrocodone is a semisynthetic narcotic antitussive with multiple actions qualitatively similar to those of codeine. Most of these involve the central nervous system and smooth muscle. The precise mechanism of action of hydrocodone and other opiates is not known; however, it is believed to act directly on the cough center. In excessive doses, hydrocodone, like other opium derivatives, will depress respiration. The effects of hydrocodone in therapeutic doses on the cardiovascular system are insignificant. Hydrocodone can produce miosis, euphoria, physical and physiological dependence.

Following a 10 mg oral dose of hydrocodone administered to five adult male subjects, the mean peak concentration was 23.6 +/- 5.2 ng/mL. Maximum serum levels were achieved at 1.3 +/- 0.3 hours and the half-life was determined to be 3.8 +/- 0.3 hours. Hydrocodone exhibits a complex pattern of metabolism including O-demethylation, N-demethylation and 6- keto reduction to the corresponding 6-α- and S-β-hydroxymetabolites.

Pseudoephedrine acts as an indirect sympathomimetic agent by stimulating sympathetic (adrenergic) nerve endings to release norepinephrine. Norepinephrine in turn stimulates alpha and beta receptors throughout the body. The action of pseudoephedrine hydrochloride is apparent in more specific for the blood vessels of the upper respiratory tract and less specific for the blood vessels of the systemic circulation. The vasoconstriction elicited at these sites results in the shrinkage of swollen tissues in the sinuses and nasal passages. Pseudoephedrine is rapidly and almost completely absorbed from the gastrointestinal tract. Considerable variation in half-life has been observed (from about 45 to 10 hours) which is attributed to differences in absorption and excretion. Excretion rates are also altered by urine pH, increasing with acidification and decreasing with alkalinization. As a result, mean half-life falls to about 4 hours at pH 5 and increases to about 12 to 13 hours at pH 8. After administration of a 60 mg tablet, 87 to 97% of the pseudoephedrine is cleared from the body within 24 hours. The drug is distributed to body tissues and fluids, including fetal tissue, breast milk and the central nervous system.

About 55% to 75% of an administered dose is excreted unchanged in the urine: the remainder is apparently metabolized in the liver to inactive compounds by N-demethylation, parahydroxylation, and oxidative deamination.

Chlorpheniramine is an antihistamine that possesses anticholinergic and sedative effects. It is considered one of the most effective and least toxic of the histamine antagonists. Chlorpheniramine is an H_1 receptor antagonist. It antagonizes many of the pharmacologic actions of histamine. It prevents released histamine from dilating capillaries and causing edema of the respiratory mucosa. Chlorpheniramine is well absorbed and has a duration of action of 4 to 6 hours. Its half-life in serum is 12 to 16 hours. Degradation products of chlorpheniramine's metabolic transformation by the liver are almost completely excreted in 24 hours.

INDICATIONS AND USAGE:

This combination drug is indicated for relief of cough and congestion due to colds, acute respiratory infections, laryngeal and pulmonary tuberculosis, acute and chronic bronchitis and hay fever. In addition this combination drug helps relieve the sneezing and itching associated with hay fever.

CONTRAINDICATIONS:

Hypersensitivity To Any Of The Ingredients: Patients known to be hypersensitive to other sympathomimetic amines may exhibit cross sensitivity with pseudoephedrine. Sympathomimetic amines are contraindicated in patients with severe coronary artery disease, and patients on monoamine oxidase (MAO) inhibitor therapy.

Antihistimines are contraindicted in patients with narrow-angle glaucoma, urinary retention, peptic ulcer, during an asthmatic attack and in patients receiving MAO inhibitors.

This combination drug should not be administered to premature or full-term infants.

This combination drug is contraindicated in nursing mothers because of the higher than usual risk for infants from sympathomimetic amines.

WARNINGS:

General: Sympathomimetic amines should be used with caution in patients with hypertension, ischemic heart disease, diabetes mellitus, increased intraocular pressure, hyperthyroidism, or prostatic hypertrophy. Sympathomimetics may produce central nervous system stimulation with convulsions or cardiovascular collapse with accompanying hypotension. DO NOT EXCEED RECOMMENDED DOSAGE.

Hypertensive crises can occur with concurrent use of pseudoephedrine and monoamine oxidase (MAO) inhibitors, indomethacin, or with beta blockers and methyldopa. If a hypertensive crisis occurs, these drugs should be discontinued immediately and therapy to lower blood pressure should be instituted. Fever should be managed by means of external cooling.

Chlorpheniramine has an atropine-like action and should be used with caution in patients with increased intraocular pressure, cardiovascular disease, hypertension or in patients with a history of bronchial asthma.

Head Injury and Increased Intracranial Pressure: The respiratory depressant effects of narcotics and their capacity to elevate cerebrospinal fluid pressure may be markedly exaggerated in the presence of head injury, other intracranial lesions or a pre-existing increase in intracranial pressure. Furthermore, narcotics produce adverse reactions which may obscure clinical course of patients with head injuries.

Acute Abdominal Conditions: The administration of narcotics may obscure the diagnosis or clinical course of patients with acute abdominal conditions.

PRECAUTIONS:

Special Risk Patients: As with any narcotic, this combination drug should be used with caution in elderly or debilitated patients and those with severe impairment of hepatic or renal function, hypothyroidism, Addison's disease, prostatic hypertrophy or urethral stricture. The usual precautions should be observed and the possibility of respiratory depression should be kept in mind.

Information for the Patient: Narcotics and antihistamines may impair the mental and physical abilities required for the performance of potentially hazardous tasks, such as driving a vehicle or operating machinery. Patients should also be warned about the possible additive effects with alcohol and other central nervous system depressants (hypnotics, sedatives, tranquilizers).

Laboratory Test Interactions: Antihistamines may suppress the wheal and flare reactions to antigen skin testing. Considerable interindividual variation in the extent and duration of suppression have been reported, depending on the antigen and test technique, antihistamine and dosage regimen, time since the last dose and individual response to testing. In one study, usual oral dosages of chlorpheniramine suppressed the wheal response for about 2 days after the last dose. Whenever possible antihistamines should be discontinued about 4 days prior to skin testing procedures since they may prevent otherwise positive reactions to dermal reactivity indicators.

Carcinogenesis, Mutagenesis, and Impairment of Fertility: No long term or reproduction studies in animals have been performed with this combination drug to evaluate its carcinogenic, mutagenic and impairment of fertility potential.

Pregnancy, Teratogenic Effects, Pregnancy Category C: Hydrocodone has been shown to be teratogenic in hamsters when given in doses 700 times the human dose. There are no adequate and well-controlled studies in pregnant women. This combination drug should be used during pregnancy only if the potential benefit justifies the potential risk to the fetus.

Nonteratogenic Effects: Babies born to mothers who have been taking opioids regularly prior to delivery will be physically dependent. The withdrawal signs include irritability and excessive crying, tremors, hyperactive reflexes, increased respiratory rate, increased stools, sneezing, yawning, vomiting and fever. The intensity of syndrome does not always correlate with the duration of the maternal opioid use or dose. There is no consensus on the best method of managing withdrawl. Chlorpromazine 0.7–1.0 mg/kg q6h, and paregoric 2–4 drops q4h, have been used to treat withdrawal symptoms in infants. The duration of therapy is 4 to 28 days, with the dosage decreased as tolerated.

Labor and Delivery: As with all narcotics, administration of this combination drug to the mother shortly before delivery may result in some degree of respiratory depression in the newborn, especially if higher doses are used.

Nursing Mothers: This combination drug is contraindicated in nursing mothers because of the higher than usual risk for infants with sympathomimetic amines.

Pediatric Use: Antihistamines may cause excitability, especially in children. Do not exceed recommended dosage because at higher doses nervousness, dizziness or sleeplessness may occur.

In young children, as well as adults, the respiratory center is sensitive to the depressant action of narcotic cough suppressants in a dose-dependent manner. Benefit to risk ratio should be carefully considered especially in children with respiratory embarrassment (*e.g.,* croup).

Geriatric Use: The elderly (60 years and older) are more likely to have adverse reactions to sympathomimetics. Overdose of sympathomimetics in this age group may cause hallucinations, convulsions, CNS depression and death.

DRUG INTERACTIONS:

Patients receiving other narcotics, antipsychotics, antianxiety agents or other CNS depressants (including alcohol) concomitantly with this combination drug may exhibit additive CNS depression. When combined therapy is contemplated, the dose of one or both agents should be reduced.

DRUG INTERACTIONS: *(cont'd)*

The use of MAO inhibitors or tricyclic antidepressants with hydrocodone preparations may increase the effect of either the antidepressant or hydrocodone.

The concurrent use of anticholinergics with hydrocodone may produce paralytic ileus.

Beta-adrenergic blockers and MAO inhibitors may potentiate the pressor effects of pseudoephedrine. Concurrent use of digitalis glycosides may increase the possibility of cardiac arrhythmias. Sympathomimetics may reduce the hypotensive effects of guanethidine, mecamylamine, methyldopa, reserpine, and veratrum alkaloids. Concurrent use of tricyclic antidepressants may antagonize the effects of pseudoephedrine.

ADVERSE REACTIONS:

HYDROCODONE BITARTRATE

The most frequently observed adverse reactions include lightheadedness, dizziness, sedation, nausea and vomiting. These effects seem to be more prominent in ambulatory patients than in nonambulatory patients and some of these adverse reactions may be alleviated if the patient lies down.

Other adverse reactions include:

Central Nervous System: Drowsiness, mental clouding, lethargy, impairment of mental and physical performance, anxiety, fear, dysphoria, psychic dependence, mood changes.

Gastrointestinal System: Prolonged administration may produce constipation.

Genitourinary System: Ureteral spasm, spasm of vesical sphincters and urinary retention have been reported.

PSEUDOEPHEDRINE HYDROCHLORIDE

Psuedoephedrine may cause mild central nervous system stimulation, especially in those patients who are hypersensitive to sympathomimetic drugs. Nervousness, excitability, restlessness, dizziness, weakness and insomnia may also occur. Headache and drowsiness have also been reported. Large doses may cause lightheadedness, nausea and/or vomiting. Sympathimometric drugs have also been associated with certain untoward reactions including fear, anxiety, tenseness, restlessness, tremor, weakness, pallor, respiratory difficulty, dysuria, insomnia, hallucination, convulsion, CNS depression, arrhythmias and cardiovascular collapse with hypotension.

CHLORPHENIRAMINE MALEATE

Slight to moderate drowsiness may occur and is the most frequent side effect.

Other possible side effects of antihistimines in general include:

General: Urticaria, drug rash, anaphylactic shock, photosensitivity, excessive perspiration, chills, dryness of the mouth, nose and throat.

Cardiovascular: Hypotension, headache, palpitation, tachycardia, extrasystoles.

Hematological: Hemolytic anemia, thrombocytopenia, agranulocytosis

CNS: Sedation, dizziness, disturbed coordination, fatigue, convulsion, restlessness, excitation, nervousness, tremor, irritability, insomnia, euphoria, paresthesia, blurred vision, dipilopia, vertigo, tinnitus, hysteria, neuritis, convulsion.

Gastrointestinal: Epigastric distress, anorexia, nausea, vomiting, diarrhea, constipation.

Genitourinary: Urinary frequency, difficult urination, urinary retention, early menses.

Respiratory: Thickening of bronchial secretions, tightness of chest, wheezing and nasal stuffiness.

DRUG ABUSE AND DEPENDENCE:

This combination drug is subject to the Federal Controlled Substances Act (Schedule III).

Psychic dependence and tolerance may develop upon repeated administration of narcotics; therefore, this combination drug should be prescribed and administered with caution. However, psychic dependence is unlikely to develop when this combination drug is used for a short time.

Physical dependence, the condition in which continued administration of the drug is required to prevent the appearance of a withdrawal syndrome, assumes clinically significant proportions only after several weeks of continued narcotic use, although some mild degree of physical dependence may develop after a few days of narcotic therapy. Tolerance, in which increasingly large doses are required to produce the same degree of effectiveness, is manifested initially by a shortened duration of effect, and subsequently by decreases in the intensity of the effect. The rate of development of tolerance varies among patients.

OVERDOSAGE:

SIGNS AND SYMPTOMS

Hydrocodone: Serious overdosage with hydrocodone is characterized by respiratory depression (a decrease in respiratory rate and/or tidal volume, Cheyne- Stokes respiration, cyanosis), extreme somnolence progressing to stupor or coma, skeletal muscle flaccidity, cold and clammy skin, and sometimes bradycardia and hypotension. In severe overdosage, apnea, circulatory collapse, cardiac arrest and death may occur.

Pseudoephedrine: Overdosage with pseudoephedrine can cause excessive central nervous system stimulation resulting in excitement, nervousness, anxiety, tremor, restlessness and insomnia. Other effects include tachycardia, hypertension, pallor, mydriasis, hyperglycemia and urinary retention. Severe overdosage may cause tachypnea or hyperpnea, hallucinations, convulsion, or delirium, but in some individuals there may be central nervous system depression with somnolence, stupor, or respiratory depression. Arrhythmias (including ventricular fibrillation) may lead to hypotension and circulatory collapse. Severe hypokalemia can occur, probably due to compartmental shift rather than depletion of potassium. No organ damage or significant metabolic arrangement is associated with pseudoephedrine overdosage. The toxic and lethal concentration in human biologic fluids are not known. Excretion rates increase with urine acidification and decrease with alkalinization. Few reports of toxicity due to pseudoephedrine have been published, and no case of fatal overdosage is known.

Chlorpheniramine: Manifestations of antihistamine overdosages may vary from central nervous system depression (sedation, apnea, cardiovascular collapse) to stimulation (insomnia, hallucinations, tremors, or convulsions). Other signs and symptoms may be dizziness, tinnitus, ataxia, blurred vision and hypotension. Stimulation is particularly likely in children, as are atropine-like signs and symptoms (dry mouth, dilated pupils, flushing, hyperthermia, and gastrointestinal symptoms).

TREATMENT

Primary attention should be given to the re-establishment of adequate respiratory exchange through provision of a patent airway and institution of assisted or controlled ventilation. The narcotic antagonist naloxone is a specific antidote against respiratory depression which may result from overdosage or unusual sensitivity to narcotics including hydrocodone. Therefore, an appropriate dose of naloxone hydrochloride (see package insert) should be administered, preferably by the intravenous route and simultaneously with efforts at respiratory resuscitation. Since the duration of action of hydrocodone may exceed that of the antagonist, the patient should be kept under continued surveillance and repeated doses of the antagonist should be administered as needed to maintain adequate respiration.

OVERDOSAGE: *(cont'd)*

An antagonist should not be administered in the absence of clinically significant respiratory or cardiovascular depression. Oxygen, intravenous fluids, vasopressors and other supportive measures should be employed as indicated.

Gastric emptying may be useful in removing unabsorbed drug.

The patient should be induced to vomit even if emesis has occurred spontaneously; however, vomiting should not be induced in patients with impaired consciousness. Precautions against aspiration should be taken, especially in infants and children.

Ipecac syrup is the preferred method for inducing vomiting. The action of ipecac is facilitated by physical activity and the administration of eight to twelve fluid ounces of water. If emesis does not occur within fifteen minutes, the dose of ipecac should be repeated. Following emesis, any drug remaining in the stomach may be absorbed by activated charcoal administered as a slurry with water

If vomiting is unsuccessful or contraindicated, gastric lavage should be performed. Isotonic and one-half isotonic saline are the lavage solution of choice. Saline cathartics, such as milk of magnesia, draw water into the bowel by osmosis and, therefore, may be valuable for their action in rapid dilution of bowel content.

Treatment of the signs and symptoms of overdosage is symptomatic and supportive. Vasopressors may be used to treat hypotension. Short-acting barbiturates diazepam or paraldehyde may be administered to control seizures. Hyperpyrexia, especially in children, may require treatment with tepid water sponge baths or a hypothermic blanket. Apnea is treated with ventilatory support. Stimulants (analeptic agents) should not be used.

DOSAGE AND ADMINISTRATION:

Adults: Two teaspoonfuls (10 ml) every 4–6 hours.

Children (6–12 years): One teaspoonful (5 ml) every 4–7 hours.

Do not exceed four doses in a 24 hour period.

HOW SUPPLIED:

TUSSEND syrup is supplied as a clear yellow liquid, banana-flavored, in bottles of one pint (16 fl. oz.)

Storage: Store at a controlled room temperature, 15°–30°C (59°–86°F)

HOW SUPPLIED - EQUIVALENTS NOT AVAILABLE:

Syrup - Oral - 2 mg/2.5 mg/30

pint	$39.79	TUSSEND, Monarch	61570-0004-16

Syrup - Oral - 5 mg/2.5 mg/2 m

473 ml	$27.95	Comtussin Hc, Econolab	55053-0810-16
480 ml	$9.15	ENDAGEN-HD, Abana Pharms	12463-0200-16
480 ml	$14.80	M-End (Sugar/Alcohol Free), RA McNeil	12830-0722-16
480 ml	$15.80	QUENDAL-HD, Qualitest Pharms	00603-1621-58
480 ml	$16.50	CHEMDAL HD, H N Norton Co.	50732-0895-16
480 ml	$16.50	Cytuss Hc, Cypress Pharm	60258-0704-16
480 ml	$16.90	RINDAL-HD, Goldline Labs	00182-0272-40
480 ml	$16.95	Hyphen-Hd, Alphagen Labs	59743-0012-16
480 ml	$17.05	Efasin-HD, Major Pharms	00904-3542-16
480 ml	$17.37	Cytuss Hc, Aligen Independ	00405-0058-16
480 ml	$17.90	Endal-Hd Plus, Alphagen Labs	59743-0008-16
480 ml	$18.89	Comtussin Hc, HL Moore Drug Exch	00839-7845-69
480 ml	$19.50	Ventuss, Venture Pharm	59785-0301-16
480 ml	$20.95	Efasin HD Plus, Major Pharms	00904-7886-16
480 ml	$22.35	Maxituss Hc, Am Pharms	58605-0507-01
480 ml	$22.35	Maxi-Tuss, Am Pharms	58605-0512-01
480 ml	$23.15	GUIAPHEN HD, Rugby	00536-2650-85
480 ml	$24.90	Quendal Hd Plus, Qualitest Pharms	00603-1622-58
480 ml	$25.00	Atuss Hd, Atley Pharms	59702-0025-16
480 ml	$35.27	ENDAL-HD PLUS, UAD Labs	00785-6283-16
480 ml	$38.84	HISTINEX PV, Ethex	58177-0883-07
3840 ml	$105.60	CHEMDAL HD, H N Norton Co.	50732-0895-28

CHLORPHENIRAMINE MALEATE; HYDROCODONE; PHENYLEPHRINE HYDROCHLORIDE *(000749)*

CATEGORIES: Antitussives; Antitussives/Expectorants/Mucolytics; Common Cold; Congestion; Cough Preparations; Respiratory & Allergy Medications; DEA Class CIII; FDA Pre 1938 Drugs

BRAND NAMES: A-G Tussin; Amtussin; Anaplex-Hd; Atuss Ms; Chem-Tuss N; Chlorgest Hd; Chlorphen Hd; Comtussin Hc; Cyndal Hd; Endal-Hd; Exo-Tuss; H-C Tussive; Hi-Tuss Hc; Highland Hc; Hydrocodone/Phenylephrine/Cpm; Hyphed; Iodal Hd; Iotussin Hc; Kg-Dal Hd; Kg-Dal Hd Plus; Kg-Tussin; Med-Hist-Hc; Nasatuss; P-V-Tussin; Para-Hist Hd; Poly-Tussin; Q-V Tussin; Quendal Hd; Tega-Tussin; Tussend; Tussin-V; Uni Tuss Hc; Vanex-Hd

FORMULARIES: Aetna

DESCRIPTION:

Each fluid ounce (30 ml) of this preparation contains:*Hydrocodone Bitartrate:* 10 mg (WARNING. May be habit forming); *Phenylephrine Hydrochloride:* 30 mg; *Chlorpheniramine Maleate:* 12 mg.

CLINICAL PHARMACOLOGY:

This combination drug preparation combines the centrally acting antitussive activity of hydrocodone bitartrate with the nasal decongestant action of phenylephrine hydrochloride with the antihistaminic activity of chlorpheniramine maleate.

INDICATIONS AND USAGE:

To control cough and provide for the temporary symptomatic relief from congestion in the upper respiratory tract due to the common cold.

CONTRAINDICATIONS:

Hypersensitivity to any component of the drug. This product is also contraindicated in patients with bronchial asthma or pulmonary emphysema. It is also contraindicated in pregnant women and nursing mothers.

PRECAUTIONS:

Use this preparation with caution in patients with diabetes, hyperthyroidism, hypertension, cardiovascular disease, who are debilitated, or who have undergone thoracotomies or laparotomies. Patients should be cautioned about participating in activities which require alertness, since drowsiness and dizziness may occur.

Note: Before prescribing medication to suppress or modify cough, it is important to determine the primary cause of the cough and that modification of the cough does not increase the risk of clinical or physiologic complications, and that appropriate concomitant therapy for the primary condition is provided.

ADVERSE REACTIONS:

Occasional drowsiness, cardiac palpitations, dizziness, nervousness, and gastrointestinal upset.

DOSAGE AND ADMINISTRATION:

Adults: 2 teaspoonfuls (10 ml) 3 or 4 times daily.

Children 6 to 12 Years Old: 1 teaspoonful (5 ml) 3 or 4 times daily.

HOW SUPPLIED - EQUIVALENTS NOT AVAILABLE:

Liquid - Oral - 12 mg/10 mg/30

120 ml	$7.08	Anaplex-Hd, ECR Pharms	00095-0130-04
473 ml	$9.75	Nasatuss, Abana Pharms	12463-0230-16
473 ml	$23.75	Atuss Ms, Atley Pharms	59702-0552-16
473 ml	$27.48	Exo-Tuss, Am Generics	58634-0034-01
473 ml	$27.95	H-C Tussive, Qualitest Pharms	00603-1284-58
473 ml	$38.75	Amtussin, Econolab	55053-0940-16
473 ml	$40.58	A-G TUSSIN, Am Generics	58634-0011-01
480 ml	$13.99	Chlorphen Hd, Elge	58298-0430-16
480 ml	$15.09	Hydrocodone/Phenylephrine/Cpm, Aligen Independ	00405-0048-16
480 ml	$15.09	Cyndal Hd, Cypress Pharm	60258-0703-16
480 ml	$16.00	ED-TLC, Edwards Pharms	00485-0052-16
480 ml	$19.50	Anaplex-Hd, ECR Pharms	00095-0130-16
480 ml	$19.80	Kg-Dal Hd, King Pharms	60793-0030-16
480 ml	$22.00	Ed Tuss Hc, Edwards Pharms	00485-0053-16
480 ml	$23.76	VANEX-HD LIQUID, Abana Pharms	12463-0300-16
480 ml	$25.00	Hyphed, Cypress Pharm	60258-0790-16
480 ml	$25.16	HISTINEX HC, Ethex	58177-0877-07
480 ml	$25.20	Kg-Dal Hd Plus, King Pharms	60793-0031-16
480 ml	$25.20	Kg-Tussin, King Pharms	60793-0033-16
480 ml	$25.66	Highland Hc, Highland Pkging	55782-0033-16
480 ml	$26.32	Hyphed, Aligen Independ	00405-0099-16
480 ml	$27.19	Uni Tuss Hc, United Res	00677-1512-33
480 ml	$28.00	Q-V Tussin, Qualitest Pharms	00603-1609-58
480 ml	$28.00	Tussin-V, Alphagen Labs	59743-0001-16
480 ml	$29.43	Comtussin Hc, Rugby	00536-2901-85
480 ml	$29.45	MEDHIST HC WITH HYDROCODONE, Med Tek Pharms	52349-0400-16
480 ml	$29.93	ENDAL-HD, UAD Labs	00785-6200-16
480 ml	$30.10	POLY-TUSSIN, Poly Pharms	50991-0727-16
480 ml	$52.57	P-V-TUSSIN, Solvay Pharms	00032-1083-78
3840 ml	$99.72	Cyndal Hd, Cypress Pharm	60258-0703-28
3840 ml	$397.94	P-V-TUSSIN, Solvay Pharms	00032-1083-79

CHLORPHENIRAMINE MALEATE; HYOSCYAMINE; PHENYLEPHRINE HYDROCHLORIDE; PHENYLPROPANOLAMINE *(000789)*

CATEGORIES: Antitussives; Antitussives/Expectorants/Mucolytics; Cough Preparations; Respiratory & Allergy Medications; DEA Class CIII; DEA Class CV; FDA Pre 1938 Drugs

BRAND NAMES: Chemdal Hd; Cophene-S; Efasin-Hd; Rindal-Hd; Ro-Tussin

FORMULARIES: Aetna

Prescribing information not available at time of publication.

HOW SUPPLIED - EQUIVALENTS NOT AVAILABLE:

Syrup - Oral

480 ml	$15.34	CHEMDAL HD LIQUID, H N Norton Co.	50732-0855-16
480 ml	$18.00	COPHENE-S, Dunhall Pharms	00217-0407-11
3840 ml	$101.68	CHEMDAL HD LIQUID, H N Norton Co.	50732-0855-28

CHLORPHENIRAMINE MALEATE; METHSCOPOLAMINE NITRATE; PHENYLEPHRINE HYDROCHLORIDE *(000755)*

CATEGORIES: Allergies; Antihistamines; Common Cold; Cough Preparations; Decongestants; Nasal Congestion; Respiratory & Allergy Medications; DEA Class CV; FDA Pre 1938 Drugs

BRAND NAMES: Ah-Chew; Alersule; Chem-Tuss; Chlor-Phen Compound; Chlorpheniramine Compound; **Dallergy**; Dihistine; Dura-Vent/Da; Extendryl; Histafed-S.R.; Histaspan-Plus; Histor-D; Nasec; Omnihist L.A.; Phenacon; Phenapp Chlor; Phenchlor S.H.A.; Phenylhistine; Prehist; Rolatuss; Simplet; Sinodec; Sinovan; Tussanil

Prescribing information not available at time of publication.

HOW SUPPLIED - EQUIVALENTS NOT AVAILABLE:

Capsule, Gelatin - Oral - 4 mg/1.25 mg/10

100's	$24.25	EXTENDRYL JR., Fleming	00256-0177-01
1000's	$222.50	EXTENDRYL JR., Fleming	00256-0177-02

Capsule, Gelatin - Oral - 8 mg/2.5 mg/20

100's	$24.20	PREHIST, Marnel Pharceut	00682-0101-01
100's	$26.50	EXTENDRYL, Fleming	00256-0111-01
100's	$28.20	PREHIST D, Marnel Pharceut	00682-0100-01
100's	**$33.41**	**DALLERGY, Laser**	**00277-0101-02**
100's	$55.00	SINOVAN, Drug Industries	00261-0040-01
100's	$100.00	PHENACON, Teral Labs	51234-0135-90
1000's	$244.50	EXTENDRYL, Fleming	00256-0111-02
1000's	**$307.37**	**DALLERGY, Laser**	**00277-0101-03**

HOW SUPPLIED - EQUIVALENTS NOT AVAILABLE: *(cont'd)*

Elixir - Oral - 10 mg/2 mg/0.62

480 ml	**$19.33**	**DALLERGY, Laser**	**00277-0156-01**

Elixir - Oral

480 ml	$4.20	Phenylhistine, HR Cenci	00556-0480-16
480 ml	$4.25	DIHISTINE, Consolidated Midland	00223-6495-01
480 ml	$8.40	ROLATUSS, Major Pharms	00904-1200-16
480 ml	$14.10	EXTENDRYL, Fleming	00256-0127-01
3785 ml	$23.54	Phenylhistine, HR Cenci	00556-0480-28
3840 ml	$102.87	EXTENDRYL, Fleming	00256-0127-02
3840 ml	**$132.90**	**DALLERGY, Laser**	**00277-0156-02**

Tablet, Uncoated - Oral - 4 mg/1.25 mg/10

100's	$20.20	EXTENDRYL, Fleming	00256-0133-01
100's	**$20.37**	**DALLERGY, Laser**	**00277-0160-01**
100's	$37.50	Ah-Chew, WE Pharm	59196-0003-01
100's	**$41.98**	**Dallergy, Laser**	**00277-0180-01**
100's	$43.75	Omnihist L.A., WE Pharm	59196-0002-01
100's	$110.00	PHENACON, Teral Labs	51234-0136-90
1000's	$184.10	EXTENDRYL, Fleming	00256-0133-02

CHLORPHENIRAMINE MALEATE; PHENINDAMINE TARTRATE; PHENYLPROPANOLAMINE HYDROCHLORIDE *(000756)*

CATEGORIES: Allergies; Antihistamines; Common Cold; Cough Preparations; Decongestants; Hay Fever; Nasal Congestion; Respiratory & Allergy Medications; Sinusitis; Sympathomimetic Agents; FDA Pre 1938 Drugs

BRAND NAMES: Amilon Tr; Fenaclor; **Nolamine**; Norphenamine; Prophamine

DESCRIPTION:

Each timed release tablet contains:

Phenindamine tartrate - 24 mg

Chlorpheniramine maleate - 4 mg

Phenylpropanolamine hydrochloride - 50 mg

Formulated to provide 8 to 12 hours continuous relief.

Phenindamine tartrate, a chemically different antihistamine, is effective in suppressing the symptoms of allergic rhinitis.

Chlorpheniramine maleate is an effective antihistamine for runny nose and itchy eyes.

The vasoconstrictive property of phenylpropanolamine hydrochloride, which reduces nasal mucosal edema, has proved itself over the years.

INDICATIONS AND USAGE:

As a nasal decongestant associated with the common cold, sinusitis, hay fever and other allergies.

CONTRAINDICATIONS:

Hypersensitivity to any of the components. Contraindicated in concurrent MAO inhibitor therapy.

PRECAUTIONS:

Antihistamines may cause drowsiness and should be used with caution in patients who operate motor vehicles or dangerous machinery. Use with caution in patients with hypertension, cardiovascular disease, diabetes or hyperthyroidism. This product should be used with caution in patients with prostatic hypertrophy or glaucoma.

ADVERSE REACTIONS:

Nervousness, insomnia, tremors, dizziness and drowsiness may occur occasionally.

DOSAGE AND ADMINISTRATION:

Usual adult dose: Orally, one tablet every 8 hours. In mild cases, one tablet every 10 to 12 hours.

Store at controlled room temperature, 15°-30°C (59-86°F) and keep away from light.

HOW SUPPLIED - EQUIVALENTS NOT AVAILABLE:

Tablet, Coated, Sustained Action - Oral - 4 mg/24 mg/50 m

	$14.40	NORPHENAMINE, Major Pharms	00904-2226-60
100's	$12.69	AMILON TR, HL Moore Drug Exch	00839-7710-06
100's	**$24.65**	**NOLAMINE, Carnrick**	**00086-0204-10**
100's	$39.95	PROPHAMINE, Pecos	59879-0503-01
250's	**$49.15**	**NOLAMINE, Carnrick**	**00086-0204-25**
500's	$64.30	NORPHENAMINE, Major Pharms	00904-2226-40

CHLORPHENIRAMINE MALEATE; PHENYLEPHRINE HYDROCHLORIDE; PHENYLPROPANOLAMINE HYDROCHLORIDE *(000046)*

CATEGORIES: Allergies; Antihistamines; Common Cold; Congestion; Cough Preparations; Decongestants; Influenza; Lacrimation; Nasal Congestion; Otitis Media; Respiratory & Allergy Medications; Rhinitis; Sinus Congestion; DEA Class CV; FDA Pre 1938 Drugs

BRAND NAMES: Atrohist Plus; Chem-Tuss Sr; Cophene; Deca-Stat; Deconhist La; E.N.T.; G-Tuss; Nasahist; Nd-Hist; Novatuss; Pannaz; Phenahist-Tr; Phenchlor S.H.A.; Protid; Q-Tuss; Rolatuss Tablets; Ru-Tab; **Ru-Tuss**; Stahist; Tuss-Delay

DESCRIPTION:

Each yellow, scored Atrohist Plus Tablet provides: 25 mg phenylephrine hydrochloride, 50 mg phenylpropanolamine hydrochloride, 8 mg chlorpheniramine maleate, 0.19 mg hyoscyamine sulfate, 0.04 mg atropine sulfate and 0.01 mg scopolamine hydrobromide in a sustained-release formulation. Atrohist Plus Tablets are intended for oral administration. Atrohist Plus Tablets are an antihistaminic, nasal decongestant and anti-secretory preparation. Inactive ingredients: lactose, stearic acid, sterotex, P.V.P. povidone, magnesium stearate, silicon dioxide, ethyl cellulose, D & C Yellow #10 Lake.

INDICATIONS AND USAGE:

Atrohist Plus Tablets provide relief of the symptoms resulting from irritation of sinus, nasal and upper respiratory tract tissues. Phenylephrine and phenylpropanolamine combine to exert a vasoconstrictive and decongestive action while chlorpheniramine maleate decreases the symptoms of watering eyes, post nasal drip and sneezing which may be associated with an allergic-like response. The belladonna alkaloids, hyoscyamine, atropine and scopolamine further augment the anti-secretory activity of Atrohist Plus Tablets.

CONTRAINDICATIONS:

This product is contraindicated in patients with hypersensitivity to antihistamines or sympathomimetics. Atrohist Plus Tablets are contraindicated in pediatric patients under 12 years of age and in patients with glaucoma, bronchial asthma and women who are pregnant. Concomitant use of monoamine oxidase inhibitors (MAOI) is contraindicated. (See DRUG INTERACTIONS.)

WARNINGS:

Atrohist Plus Tablets may cause drowsiness. Patients should be warned of possible additive effects caused by taking antihistamines with alcohol, hypnotics or tranquilizers.

PRECAUTIONS:

Atrohist Plus Tablets contain belladonna alkaloids, and must be administered with care to those patients with urinary bladder neck obstruction. Caution should be exercised when Atrohist Plus Tablets are given to patients with hypertension, cardiac or peripheral vascular disease or hyperthyroidism. Patients should avoid driving a motor vehicle or operating dangerous machinery. (See WARNINGS.)

DRUG INTERACTIONS:

Do not prescribe this product for use in patients that are now taking a prescription MAO (certain drugs for depression, psychiatric or emotional conditions, or Parkinson's disease), or for 14 days after stopping MAO drug therapy.

ADVERSE REACTIONS:

Hypersensitivity reactions such as rash, urticaria, leukopenia, agranulocytosis, and thrombocytopenia may occur. Large overdoses may cause tachypnea, delirium, fever, stupor, coma and respiratory failure.

Gastrointestinal: nausea, vomiting, diarrhea, constipation, epigastric distress

Genitourinary System: urinary frequency and dysuria

Cardiovascular: tightness of the chest, palpitation, tachycardia, hypotension/hypertension

Central Nervous System: drowsiness, giddiness, faintness, dizziness, headache, incoordination, mydriasis, hyperirritability, nervousness, and insomnia

Metabolic/Endocrine: lassitude, anorexia

Miscellaneous: dryness of mucous membranes, xerostomia

Respiratory: thickening of bronchial secretions

Special Senses: tinnitus, visual disturbances, blurred vision.

OVERDOSAGE:

Since the action of sustained release products may continue for as long as 12 hours, treatment of overdoses directed at reversing the effects of the drug and supporting the patient should be maintained for at least that length of time. In pediatric patients, antihistamine overdosage may produce convulsions and death.

DOSAGE AND ADMINISTRATION:

Adults and children over 12 years of age: One tablet every 12 hours not to exceed 2 tablets in 24 hours. Not recommended for use in children under 12 years of age. Tablets are to be swallowed whole.

HOW SUPPLIED:

Bottles of 100 tablets. Scored, yellow tablets are embossed with "Adams/024". Store at controlled room temperature between 15°C and 30°C (59°F and 86°F). Dispense in tight, light-resistant containers.

(Adams Laboratories, Inc., 4/94, 244/195)

HOW SUPPLIED - EQUIVALENTS NOT AVAILABLE:

Tablet, Coated, Sustained Action - Oral

100's	$11.95	ROLATUSS, Major Pharms	00904-1198-60
100's	$12.35	DECONHIST LA, Goldline Labs	00182-1317-01
100's	$13.00	Pro Tuss, United Res	00677-1418-01
100's	$15.40	Q-TUSS, Qualitest Pharms	00603-5549-21
100's	$20.79	RU-TABS, HL Moore Drug Exch	00839-7440-06
100's	$27.50	STAHIST TABS, Huckaby Pharma	58407-0370-01
100's	$59.88	PROTID, Lunsco	10892-0127-10
100's	$89.34	ATROHIST PLUS, Medeva Pharms	53014-0024-10
500's	$53.95	ROLATUSS, Major Pharms	00904-1198-40
500's	$90.92	PHENCHLOR S.H.A., Rugby	00536-4410-05

CHLORPHENIRAMINE MALEATE; PHENYLEPHRINE HYDROCHLORIDE; PHENYLPROPANOLAMINE; PHENYLTOLOXAMINE *(000792)*

CATEGORIES: Allergies; Antiasthmatics/Bronchodilators; Antihistamines; Common Cold; Congestion; Cough Preparations; DESI Drugs; Decongestants; Hay Fever; Influenza; Nasal Congestion; Otitis Media; Respiratory & Allergy Medications; Rhinitis; Sinusitis; Pregnancy Category C; FDA Pre 1938 Drugs

BRAND NAMES: Allerstat; Amaril D; Ami Decon; Chlortox La; Comhist; Decongestabs; *Decongestant*; Decongestant Compound; Decospan; Hista-Vadrin; Histatest; Nalda-Relief; Naldec; **Naldecon**; Naldelate; Naldelate Pediatric; Naldorin; Nalex-A; Nalgest; Nalphen; Nalspan; Nalspan Pediatric; Nechlorin; New Decongest; Par-Decon; Pedicon; Phena-Chlor; Phenchlor S.H.A.; Phentox Compound; Prop-A-Hist; Quadrahist; Ro-Delate; Sinucon; Sinucon Pediatric; Tri-Phen-Chlor; Tri-Phen-Mine; Tri-Phen-Mine Pediatric; Tuss Delay; Uni Decon; Vi-Tuss Tabs; Vita-Rx; West Decon

(International brand names outside U.S. in italics)

FORMULARIES: FHP

COST OF THERAPY: $5.13 (Rhinitis; Tablet; 5 mg/10 mg/40 mg/15 mg; 3/day; 30 days)

PRIMARY ICD9: 477.9 (Allergic Rhinitis, Cause Unspecified)

DESCRIPTION:

Note: In order to avoid confusion, the brand name of this drug has been included in the monograph.

Each T.D. (sustained action) tablet contains 40 mg phenylpropanolamine hydrochloride, 10 mg phenylephrine hydrochloride, 15 mg of phenyltoloxamine dihydrogen citrate, and 5 mg of chlorpheniramine maleate.

CLINICAL PHARMACOLOGY:

This combination drug is useful for the relief of nasal congestion and eustachian tube congestion associated with the common cold, sinusitis, and acute respiratory infections. It also is useful for symptomatic relief of perennial seasonal allergic rhinitis and vasomotor rhinitis. To relieve eustachian tube congestion associated with eustachian salpingitis, aerotitis and serous otitis media, decongestant-histamine combinations have been used. Orally administered phenylephrine hydrochloride is a vasopressor and relatively non toxic. Phenylpropanolamine hydrochloride acts similarly to phenylephrine though its action is more prolonged. Phenyltoloxamine dihydrogen citrate belongs to the group of antihistaminics exhibiting the amino alkyl ether structure with an H_1blocking action. Chlorpheniramine maleate competitively antagonizes most of the smooth muscle stimulating actions of histamine on the H_1receptors of the G.I. tract, uterus, large blood vessels, and bronchial muscle.

CONTRAINDICATIONS:

Patients with severe hypertension, severe coronary artery disease, or on MAO inhibitor therapy. Patients with urinary retention, narrow angle glaucoma, peptic ulcer, hypersensitivity to sympathomimetic amines or histamines, or during an asthmatic attack.

WARNINGS:

Sympathomimetic amines should be used judiciously and sparingly in patients with hypertension, diabetes mellitus, ischemic heart disease, increased intraocular pressure, hyperthyroidism or prostatic hypertrophy.

Sympathomimetics may produce central nervous system stimulation with convulsions or cardiovascular collapse with accompanying hypotension.

Antihistamines may impair mental and physical abilities required for the performance of potentially hazardous tasks, such as driving a vehicle or operating machinery, and may impair mental alertness in children. Chlorpheniramine and phenyltoloxamine have an atropine-like action and should be used with caution in patients with increased intraocular pressure, cardiovascular disease, hypertension or in patients with a history of bronchial asthma. Do not exceed recommended dosage.

PRECAUTIONS:

The antihistaminics may cause drowsiness and patients who operate machinery or motor vehicles should be cautioned.

Pregnancy Category C: Since animal reproduction studies have not been conducted with this drug, it is not known whether this drug can cause fetal harm when given to pregnant women or whether this drug can affect reproductive capacity. This drug should be given to pregnant women only if clearly needed.

Due to the higher than usual risk of sympathomimetic amines in infants, caution should be exercised when this drug is given to nursing mothers.

DRUG INTERACTIONS:

MAO inhibitors and beta adrenergic blockers increase the effect of sympathomimetics. Sympathomimetics may reduce the antihypertensive effects of methyldopa, mecamylamine, reserpine and veratrum alkaloids. Concomitant use of antihistamines with alcohol, tricyclic antidepressants, barbiturates and other CNS depressants may have an additive effect.

ADVERSE REACTIONS:

Hyperactive individuals may display ephedrine-like reactions such as tachycardia, palpitations, headache, dizziness or nausea. Patients sensitive to antihistamines may experience mild sedation. Sympathomimetics have been associated with certain untoward reactions including restlessness, tremor, weakness, pallor, respiratory difficulty, dysuria, insomnia, hallucinations, convulsions, CNS depression, arrhythmias and cardiovascular collapse with hypotension. Possible side effects of antihistamines are drowsiness, restlessness, dizziness, weakness, dry mouth, anorexia, nausea, vomiting, headache, nervousness, blurring of vision, polyuria, heartburn, dysuria, and very rarely, dermatitis.

DOSAGE AND ADMINISTRATION:

One timed release tablet should be given to children over 12 years and adults on arising, in midafternoon, and at bedtime.

Dispense in a tight, light-resistant container as defined in the USP.

HOW SUPPLIED - EQUIVALENTS NOT AVAILABLE:

Liquid - Oral - 0.5 mg/1.25 mg/

30 ml	$5.39	NALPHEN DX PEDIATRIC DROPS, HL Moore Drug Exch	00839-7753-63
30 ml	$6.50	Pedicon, Pharm Tech	29294-0101-03
30 ml	$7.05	NEW CONGESTANT PEDIATRIC DROPS, Goldline Labs	00182-6091-66
30 ml	$8.73	NALDELATE, HL Moore Drug Exch	00839-7648-63
30 ml	$10.00	Nalphen Pediatric, Hi Tech Pharma	50383-0765-01
30 ml	$10.10	Nalgest Pediatric, Major Pharms	00904-1011-30
30 ml	$10.32	TRI-PHEN-CHLOR PEDIATRIC DROPS, Rugby	00536-2195-75
30 ml	$10.95	Nalspan Pediatric, Morton Grove	60432-0011-30
30 ml	$11.48	NALDELATE PEDIATRIC DROPS, Alpharma	00472-0809-31
30 ml	$12.30	Tri-Phen-Mine, Goldline Labs	00182-6123-66
30 ml	$12.50	Naldelate Pediatric, Vintage Pharms	00254-1551-45
30 ml	$12.70	NALDA-RELIEF DROPS, Liquipharm	54198-0134-30
30 ml	$12.90	NALDELATE, Qualitest Pharms	00603-1465-45
30 ml	$13.75	SINUCON PEDIATRIC, H N Norton Co.	50732-0865-30
30 ml	**$20.42**	**NALDECON, Mead Johnson**	**00015-5615-30**
120 ml	$2.30	Nalphen Pediatric, Hi Tech Pharma	50383-0764-04
120 ml	$2.77	NALDELATE PEDIATRIC SYRUP, Alpharma	00472-1007-04
120 ml	$2.95	Naldelate Pediatric, Consolidated Midland	00223-6567-04
120 ml	$3.63	NALPHEN DX CHILD, HL Moore Drug Exch	00839-7752-65
120 ml	$8.48	SINUCON PEDIATRIC SYRUP, H N Norton Co.	50732-0831-04
480 ml	$5.00	NEW DECONGEST PEDIATRIC SYRUP, Goldline Labs	00182-1495-40
480 ml	$5.00	Tri-Phen-Mine Pediatric, Goldline Labs	00182-6122-40
480 ml	$6.90	Nalgest, Major Pharms	00904-1004-16
480 ml	$6.90	NALGEST PEDIATRIC, Major Pharms	00904-1010-16

HOW SUPPLIED - EQUIVALENTS NOT AVAILABLE: *(cont'd)*

480 ml	$7.00	Nalspan Pediatric, Morton Grove	60432-0012-16
480 ml	$7.02	Naldelate Pediatric, HL Moore Drug Exch	00839-7033-69
480 ml	$7.20	Nalphen, Hi Tech Pharma	50383-0763-16
480 ml	$7.48	NALDELATE PEDIATRIC SYRUP, Alpharma	00472-1007-16
480 ml	$7.50	Naldelate Pediatric, Consolidated Midland	00223-6567-01
480 ml	$7.50	Nalphen Pediatric, Hi Tech Pharma	50383-0764-16
480 ml	$8.00	Naldelate, Harber Pharm	51432-0636-20
480 ml	$8.05	NALDELATE PEDIATRIC SYRUP, United Res	00677-0776-33
480 ml	$8.20	NALDELATE SYRUP, Alpharma	00472-0801-16
480 ml	$8.48	Naldelate Pediatric, Vintage Pharms	00254-9325-58
480 ml	$8.48	Naldelate, Vintage Pharms	00254-9326-58
480 ml	$8.48	NALDELATE, Qualitest Pharms	00603-1464-58
480 ml	$8.75	Naldelate, Consolidated Midland	00223-6565-01
480 ml	$9.30	TRI-PHEN-CHLOR, Rugby	00536-2180-85
480 ml	$9.40	NALDELATE PEDIATRIC, Qualitest Pharms	00603-1466-58
480 ml	$24.52	SINUCON PEDIATRIC SYRUP, H N Norton Co.	50732-0831-16
480 ml	$27.61	SINUCON SYRUP, H N Norton Co.	50732-0832-16
480 ml	**$48.33**	**NALDECON PEDIATRIC, Mead Johnson**	**00015-5616-60**
480 ml	**$51.99**	**NALDECON, Mead Johnson**	**00015-5601-60**
3785 ml	$37.44	NALGEST PEDIATRIC, Major Pharms	00904-1010-28
3840 ml	$38.75	TRI-PHEN-CHLOR, Rugby	00536-2190-90
3840 ml	$39.97	Nalphen, Hi Tech Pharma	50383-0763-28
3840 ml	$39.97	Nalphen Pediatric, Hi Tech Pharma	50383-0764-28
3840 ml	$42.47	Naldelate, Consolidated Midland	00223-6565-02
3840 ml	$42.47	Naldelate Pediatric, Consolidated Midland	00223-6567-02
3840 ml	$46.92	NALDELATE SYRUP, Alpharma	00472-0801-28
3840 ml	$79.30	SINUCON PEDIATRIC SYRUP, H N Norton Co.	50732-0831-28
3840 ml	$91.97	SINUCON SYRUP, H N Norton Co.	50732-0832-28

Tablet, Coated - Oral - 5 mg/10 mg/40 m

100's	$5.70	West Decon, West Ward Pharm	00143-1279-01
100's	$6.30	Decongestant, Qualitest Pharms	00603-3120-21
100's	$6.68	DECONGESTABS, HL Moore Drug Exch	00839-1430-06
100's	$6.85	Tri-Phen-Mine, Goldline Labs	00182-1094-01
100's	$6.85	NALGEST, Major Pharms	00904-1003-60
100's	$6.93	DECONGESTANT S.R., Geneva Pharms	00781-1576-01
100's	$7.75	NALSPAN S.R., Rosemont	00832-1086-00
100's	$9.16	UNI DECON, United Res	00677-0472-01
100's	$9.29	Tri-Phen-Chlor, Rugby	00536-5655-01
100's	$17.28	TUSS-DELAY, H N Norton Co.	50732-0609-01
100's	$23.76	PHENCHLOR S.H.A., Rugby	00536-4410-01
100's	$29.25	Chlortox La, Major Pharms	00904-3545-60
100's	$44.65	Prop-A-Hist, Bolan Pharm	44437-0248-01
100's	**$90.41**	**NALDECON, Mead Johnson**	**00015-5600-60**
500's	$25.60	West Decon, West Ward Pharm	00143-1279-05
500's	$31.80	Tri-Phen-Chlor, Rugby	00536-5655-05
500's	$79.19	TUSS-DELAY, H N Norton Co.	50732-0609-05
500's	$202.95	Prop-A-Hist, Bolan Pharm	44437-0248-05
500's	**$439.95**	**NALDECON, Mead Johnson**	**00015-5600-80**
1000's	$41.34	UNI DECON, United Res	00677-0472-10
1000's	$42.10	Decongestant, Qualitest Pharms	00603-3120-32
1000's	$45.38	Tri-Phen-Chlor, Rugby	00536-5655-10
1000's	$48.99	DECONGESTABS, HL Moore Drug Exch	00839-1430-16
1000's	$53.85	NALGEST, Major Pharms	00904-1003-80
1000's	$53.93	DECONGESTANT S.R., Geneva Pharms	00781-1576-10
1000's	$58.20	Tri-Phen-Mine, Goldline Labs	00182-1094-10
1000's	$77.50	NALSPAN S.R., Rosemont	00832-1086-10
1000's	$150.23	TUSS-DELAY, H N Norton Co.	50732-0609-10
1000's	$391.00	Prop-A-Hist, Bolan Pharm	44437-0248-09
10000's	$33.00	West Decon, West Ward Pharm	00143-1279-10

CHLORPHENIRAMINE MALEATE; PHENYLEPHRINE HYDROCHLORIDE; PHENYLPROPANOLAMINE; PYRILAMINE

(000793)

CATEGORIES: Allergies; Antihistamines; Bronchitis; Bronchospasm; Common Cold; Cough Preparations; Fever; Hay Fever; Nasal Congestion; Respiratory & Allergy Medications; Rhinitis; Sinusitis; FDA Pre 1938 Drugs

BRAND NAMES: Duohist Forte; Histalet Forte; Lantuss Forte; Poly Hist Forte; Prop-A-Hist; Vanex Forte

DESCRIPTION:

Each white with blue dots capsule-shaped scored tablet contains:*Phenylpropanolamine HCl:* 50 mg; *Pyrilamine Maleate:* 25 mg; *Phenylephrine HCl:* 10 mg; *Chlorpheniramine Maleate:* 4 mg.

CLINICAL PHARMACOLOGY:

Phenylpropanolamine Hydrochloride: The drug may directly stimulate adrenergic receptors, but probably indirectly stimulates both alpha (a) and beta (B) adrenergic receptors by releasing norepinephrine from its storage sites. Phenylpropanolamine increases heart rate, force of contraction and cardiac output, and excitability. It acts on alpha receptors in the mucosa of the respiratory tract, producing vasoconstriction which results in shrinkage of swollen mucous membranes, reduction of tissue, hyperemia, edema and nasal congestion, and an increase in nasal airway patency. Phenylpropanolamine causes central nervous system stimulation and reportedly has an anorexigenic effect.

Phenylephrine Hydrochloride: Phenylephrine acts predominately by a direct action on alpha (a) adrenergic receptors. In therapeutic doses, the drug has no significant stimulant effect on the beta (B) adrenergic receptors of the heart. Following oral administration, constriction of the blood vessels in the nasal mucosa may relieve nasal congestion. In therapeutic doses, the drug causes little, if any, central nervous system stimulation.

Chlorpheniramine Maleate: Chlorpheniramine is an antihistamine belonging to the alkylamine class. It possesses anticholinergic and sedative effects. It is considered one of the most effective and least toxic of the histamine antagonists. Chlorpheniramine is an H_1 receptor antagonist. It antagonizes many of the pharmacologic actions of histamine. It prevents released histamine from dilating capillaries and causing edema of the respiratory mucosa. Chlorpheniramine has a duration of action of 4 to 6 hours in clinical studies.

Pyrilamine Maleate: Pyrilamine is an antihistamine belonging to the ethylenediamine class. Pyrilamine is an highly effective H_1 blocker. Pyrilamine is an especially active H_1 blocking drug which possesses local anesthetic activity. Pyrilamine antagonizes most of the smooth muscle stimulating actions of histamine on the H_1 receptors of the gastro-intestinal tract, blood, vessels and bronchial muscle. It also antagonizes the actions of histamine that result in increased capillary permeability and the formation of edema. Pyrilamine has a duration of action of 4 to 6 hours in clinical studies.

INDICATIONS AND USAGE:

This product is indicated for symptomatic relief in allergic rhinitis, allergic bronchitis, bronchospasm, hay fever, common cold, sinusitis and skin allergies.

CONTRAINDICATIONS:

This preparation is contraindicated for individuals sensitive to phenylephrine HCl and antihistamines.

PRECAUTIONS:

General: Administer with caution to patients with hypertension, cardiac, or peripheral vascular disease, hyperthyroidism or diabetes.

Information for the Patient: This medication may cause drowsiness. Patients should be advised not to drive a car or operate dangerous machinery while taking this medication.

Pregnancy Category C: Animal reproduction studies have not been conducted with this product. It is also not known whether this product can cause fetal harm when administered to a pregnant woman or can affect reproductive capacity. This product should be given to a pregnant woman only if clearly needed.

DOSAGE AND ADMINISTRATION:

Adults: One tablet 2 to 3 times daily.

Children 6-12: One-half tablet 2 to 3 times daily.

Children under 6: Only as directed by physician.

DO NOT EXCEED RECOMMENDED DOSAGE. Dispense in a tight, light-resistant container. Store at controlled room temperature 15-30°C (59-86°F)

HOW SUPPLIED - EQUIVALENTS NOT AVAILABLE:

Tablet, Coated, Sustained Action - Oral - 4 mg/10 mg/50 m

100's	$35.75	POLY HIST FORTE, Poly Pharms	50991-0101-01
100's	$54.82	VANEX FORTE, Abana Pharms	12463-0125-01
100's	$79.50	HISTALET FORTE, Solvay Pharms	00032-1039-01
250's	$193.14	HISTALET FORTE, Solvay Pharms	00032-1039-07

CHLORPHENIRAMINE MALEATE; PHENYLEPHRINE HYDROCHLORIDE; PHENYLTOLOXAMINE CITRATE *(000757)*

CATEGORIES: Allergies; Antihistamines; Common Cold; Cough Preparations; Decongestants; Nasal Congestion; Respiratory & Allergy Medications; Rhinitis; Rhinorrhea; Sympathomimetic Agents; Pregnancy Category C; FDA Pre 1938 Drugs

BRAND NAMES: Chlortox; **Comhist LA**; Comtrin La; Ed A-Hist; Linhist-LA; Moorehist La; Q-Hist La

FORMULARIES: Aetna; BC-BS

DESCRIPTION:

Note: the brand name for this drug has not been omitted in order to avoid confusion. All of the following information applies to Comhist LA as well as Comhist (except where stated otherwise).

Each Comhist LA yellow and clear capsule for oral administration contains

chlorpheniramine maleate................4 mg

phenyltoloxamine citrate................50 mg

phenylephrine hydrochloride.............20 mg

in a special base to provide a prolonged therapeutic effect.

Each Comhist yellow, scored tablet for oral administration contains

chlorpheniramine maleate................2 mg

phenyltoloxamine citrate................25 mg

phenylephrine hydrochloride.............10 mg

This product contains ingredients of the following therapeutic classes: antihistamine and decongestant.

Chlorpheniramine maleate is an antihistamine having the chemical name gamma-(4-chlorophenyl)-N,N-dimethyl-2-pyridinepropanamine, (Z)-2-butenedioate (1:1).

Phenyltoloxamine citrate is an antihistamine having the chemical name N,N-dimethyl-2-(α-phenyl-o-tolyloxy) ethylamine dihydrogen citrate.

Phenylephrine hydrochloride is a decongestant having the chemical name 3-hydroxy-α[(methyl-amino)methyl] benzenemethanol hydrochloride.

Inactive Ingredients (Comhist LA): Each capsule contains FD&C Blue #2, edible black ink, gelatin, sugar spheres, D&C Yellow #10, FD&C Yellow #6, and other ingredients.

Inactive Ingredients (Comhist): Each tablet contains compressible sugar, magnesium stearate, macrocrystalline cellulose, and D&C Yellow #10.

CLINICAL PHARMACOLOGY:

Chlorpheniramine maleate is an alkylamine-type antihistamine while phenyltoloxamine citrate belongs to the ethanolamine chemical class. The antihistamines in Comhist/Comhist LA act by competing with histamine for H_1 histamine receptor sites, thereby preventing the action of histamine on the cell. Clinically, chlorpheniramine and phenyltoloxamine suppress the histamine-mediated symptoms of allergic rhinitis, relieving sneezing, rhinorrhea, and itching of the eyes, nose, and throat.

Phenylephrine hydrochloride is an α-adrenergic receptor agonist (sympathomimetic) which produces vasoconstriction by stimulating α-receptors within the mucosa of the respiratory tract. Clinically, phenylephrine shrinks swollen mucous membranes, reduces tissue hyperemia, edema, and nasal congestion, and increases nasal airway patency.

INDICATIONS AND USAGE:

Comhist/Comhist LA is indicated for the relief of rhinorrhea and congestion associated with seasonal and/or perennial allergic rhinitis and vasomotor rhinitis.

CONTRAINDICATIONS:

Comhist/Comhist LA is contraindicated in persons hypersensitive to any of its components. It should not be administered to children under 12 years of age, patients with severe hypertension, narrow angle glaucoma, or asthmatic symptoms, or patients taking monoamine oxidase inhibitors.

WARNINGS:

Chlorpheniramine maleate and phenyltoloxamine citrate should be used with extreme caution in patients with stenosing peptic ulcer, pyloroduodenal obstruction, prostatic hypertrophy, or bladder neck obstruction. These compounds have an atropine-like action and therefore should be used with caution in patients with a history of bronchial asthma, increased intraocular pressure, cardiovascular disease, or hypertension. Sympathomimetic amines should be used with caution in patients with hypertension, diabetes mellitus, heart disease, increased intraocular pressure, hyperthyroidism, or prostatic hypertrophy.

PRECAUTIONS:

Information for the Patient: This product may cause sedation. Patients should be cautioned against engaging in activities requiring mental alertness, such as driving a car or operating machinery.

Pregnancy Category C: Animal reproduction studies have not been conducted with Comhist/Comhist LA. It is also not known whether Comhist/Comhist LA can cause fetal harm when administered to a pregnant woman or can affect reproduction capacity. Comhist/Comhist LA should be given to a pregnant woman only if clearly needed.

Nursing Mothers: It is not known whether the drugs in Comhist/Comhist LA are excreted in human milk. Because many drugs are excreted in human milk and because of the potential for serious adverse reactions in nursing infants, a decision should be made whether to discontinue nursing or to discontinue the product, taking into account the importance of the drug to the mother.

Pediatric Use: Safety and effectiveness of Comhist/Comhist LA in children below the age of 12 have not been established.

DRUG INTERACTIONS:

The sedative effects of chlorpheniramine maleate and phenyltoloxamine citrate are additive to the CNS depressant effects of alcohol, hypnotics, sedatives, and tranquilizers. Comhist/Comhist LA should not be used in patients taking monoamine oxidase inhibitors.

ADVERSE REACTIONS:

General: Urticaria, drug rash, dryness of mouth, nose, and throat.

Cardiovascular System: Hypotension, headache, palpitations.

Hematologic System: Thrombocytopenia, agranulocytosis, leukopenia.

Nervous System: Sedation, dizziness, excitation (especially in children), nervousness, insomnia, blurred vision, convulsions.

Gastrointestinal System: Epigastric distress, anorexia, nausea, vomiting, diarrhea, constipation.

Genitourinary System: Urinary frequency, urinary retention.

Respiratory System: Thickening of bronchial secretions, tightness of chest and wheezing, nasal stuffiness.

OVERDOSAGE:

The treatment of overdosage should provide symptomatic and supportive care. It the amount ingested is considered dangerous or excessive, induce vomiting with ipecac syrup unless the patient is convulsing, comatose, or has lost the gag reflex, in which case perform gastric lavage using a large-bore tube. If indicated, follow with activated charcoal and a saline cathartic. Since the effects of Comhist/Comhist LA may last up to 12 hours, treatment should be continued for at least that length of time.

DOSAGE AND ADMINISTRATION:

COMHIST LA

Adults And Children 12 Years Of Age And Older: 1 capsule every 8 to 12 hours; not recommended for children under 12 years of age.

COMHIST

Adults And Children 12 Years Of Age And Older: 1 to 2 tablets three times daily (every 8 hours)

Children 6 To Under 12 Years Of Age: 1 tablet three times daily (every eight hours); not recommended for children under 6 years of age.

HOW SUPPLIED - EQUIVALENTS NOT AVAILABLE:

Capsule, Gelatin, Sustained Action - Oral - 4/20/50 mg

100's	$89.33	COMHIST LA, Roberts Labs	54092-0065-01

Capsule, Gelatin, Sustained Action - Oral

100's	$24.29	Moorehist La, HL Moore Drug Exch	00839-7506-06
100's	$26.91	Q-HIST LA, Qualitest Pharms	00603-5537-21
100's	$29.95	LINHIST LA, Econolab	55053-0524-01
100's	$30.39	LINHIST LA, Rugby	00536-3975-01
100's	$30.50	C-Hist-Sr, Alphagen Labs	59743-0057-01
100's	$32.00	ED A-HIST, Edwards Pharms	00485-0054-01
100's	$33.00	CPM/PHENYLTOLOX/PE, Goldline Labs	00182-1574-01

Liquid - Oral

480 ml	$19.00	ED A-HIST, Edwards Pharms	00485-0055-16

Tablet, Coated - Oral - 2 mg/10 mg/25 m

100's	$62.98	COMHIST, Roberts Labs	54092-0066-01

CHLORPHENIRAMINE MALEATE; PHENYLPROPANOLAMINE HYDROCHLORIDE *(000758)*

CATEGORIES: Allergies; Antihistamines; Common Cold; Congestion; Cough Preparations; Decongestants; Nasal Congestion; Otitis Media; Respiratory & Allergy Medications; Rhinitis; Sinus Congestion; Sneezing; Influenza*; Lacrimation*; Pregnancy Category C; FDA Approval Pre 1982
* Indication not approved by the FDA

BRAND NAMES: Balnade; C-Nade; Chlornade; Chlorprophen Lanacaps; Condrin-La; Cophene-Pl; Cpa; *Dandum*; *Decidex*; Deconade; Decongen; Decongest; Decongestant; Decongex-3; Dehist; Dixade; *Dristan Ultra*; Drize; Dura-Vent A; *Eazit*; Equi-Nade; Harber-Nade; Hista-Vadrin; Histabid; *Mapesil*; Neatep; Or-Phen-Ade; Orabid; Oragest-Td; Orahist; Oraminic; Ordrine; Ornade; *Ornade-A.F.*; Panadyl Forte; Parhist; Phenade; *Pleoral*; Propade; Propagen; Propanade; Resaid; Rhinolar; *Rinofren A.P.* (Mexico); **Ru-Tuss II**; Sin-U-Span; *Triaminic*; Triphenyl; Truxade; Vernade; Vinade T.D.
(International brand names outside U.S. in italics)

FORMULARIES: Aetna; BC-BS; FHP

COST OF THERAPY: $4.50 (Rhinitis; Capsule; 12 mg/75 mg; 2/day; 30 days)

PRIMARY ICD9: 477.9 (Allergic Rhinitis, Cause Unspecified)

DESCRIPTION:

This drug is a combination of an oral nasal decongestant and an antihistamine.

Each sustained release capsule contains phenylpropanolamine hydrochloride, 75 mg and chlorpheniramine maleate, 12 mg. Inactive ingredients consist of benzyl alcohol, cetylpyridinium chloride, FD&C Blue No. 1, FD&C Red No. 3, FD&C Yellow No. 6, D&C Red No. 27, D&C Red No. 30, gelatin, glyceryl distearate, iron oxide, polyethylene glycol, povidone, silicon dioxide, sodium lauryl sulfate, starch, sucrose, titanium dioxide, wax and trace amounts of other inactive ingredients.

Each sustained release capsule is so prepared that an initial dose is released promptly and the remaining medication is released gradually over a prolonged period.

Chemically, phenylpropanolamine hydrochloride is Benzenemethanol α-(1-amino-ethyl)-, hydrochloride.

Chemically, chlorpheniramine maleate is 2-p-Chloro-α-[2-(dimethylaminoethyl]benzyl]pyridine maleate (1:1).

CLINICAL PHARMACOLOGY:

Phenylpropanolamine Hydrochloride: Phenylpropanolamine hydrochloride is a sympathomimetic agent which is closely related to ephedrine in chemical structure and pharmacologic action, but produces less central nervous system stimulation than ephedrine. It is a vasoconstrictor with decongestant action on nasal and upper respiratory tract mucosal membranes.

Chlorpheniramine Maleate: Chlorpheniramine maleate is an antihistamine with anticholinergic (drying) and sedative side effects. Antihistamines appear to compete with histamine for H_1 cell receptor sites on effector cells.

PHARMACOKINETICS

A single sustained release capsule produces blood levels comparable to those produced by administration of three 25 mg doses of phenylpropanolamine hydrochloride and three 4 mg doses of chlorpheniramine maleate in conventional release form given at four-hour intervals. At steady-state conditions, the following peak levels are reached after the oral administration of an sustained release capsule: 21 ng/ml chlorpheniramine maleate in 7.7 hours; 173 ng/ml phenylpropanolamine hydrochloride in 6.1 hours; under these circumstances, the half-lives are approximately 21 and 7 hours, respectively.

INDICATIONS AND USAGE:

For the treatment of the symptoms of seasonal and perennial allergic rhinitis and vasomotor rhinitis, including nasal obstruction (congestion); also for the treatment of runny nose, sneezing and nasal congestion associated with the common cold.

CONTRAINDICATIONS:

Hypersensitivity to either phenylpropanolamine hydrochloride or chlorpheniramine maleate and other antihistamines of similar chemical structure: severe hypertension; coronary artery disease.

This drug should NOT be used in newborn or premature infants.

Because of the higher risk of antihistamines for infants generally, and for newborns and prematures in particular, antihistamine therapy is contraindicated in nursing mothers.

As with any product containing a sympathomimetic, sustained release capsules should NOT be used in patients taking monoamine oxidase (MAO) inhibitors.

WARNINGS:

Sustained release capsules may potentiate the effects of alcohol and other CNS depressants. Also, this product should not be taken simultaneously with other products containing phenylpropanolamine hydrochloride or amphetamines.

Sustained release capsules should be used with considerable caution in patients with narrow-angle glaucoma, stenosing peptic ulcer, pyloroduodenal obstruction, symptomatic prostatic hypertrophy, or bladder neck obstruction.

Usage in Children: In infants and children, especially, antihistamines in *overdosage* may cause hallucinations, convulsions, or death. As in adults, antihistamines may diminish mental alertness in children. In the young child, particularly, they may produce excitation.

Use in the Elderly (approximately 60 years or older): Antihistamines are more likely to cause dizziness, sedation and hypotension in elderly patients.

PRECAUTIONS:

General: Use with caution in patients with lower respiratory disease including asthma, hypertension, cardiovascular disease, hyperthyroidism, increased intraocular pressure, or diabetes.

Information for the Patient: Caution patients about activities requiring alertness (*e.g.*, operating vehicles or machinery). Also caution patients about the possible additive effects of alcohol and other CNS depressants (hypnotics, sedatives, tranquilizers, etc.), and not to take simultaneously other products containing phenylpropanolamine hydrochloride or amphetamines. Patients should not take sustained release capsules in conjunction with a monoamine oxidase inhibitor or an oral anticoagulant.

Carcinogenesis, Mutagenesis, and Impairment of Fertility: A long-term oncogenic study in rats with the chlorpheniramine maleate component of sustained release capsules did not produce an increase in the incidence of tumors in the drug-treated groups, as compared with the controls. No evidence of mutagenicity was found when chlorpheniramine maleate was evaluated in a battery of mutagenic studies, including the Ames test.

In an early study in rats with chlorpheniramine maleate a reduction in fertility was observed in female rats at doses approximately 67 times the human dose. More recent studies in rabbits and rats, using more appropriate methodology and doses up to approximately 50 and 85 times the human dose, showed no reduction in fertility.

There are no studies available which indicate whether phenylpropanolamine hydrochloride has carcinogenic or mutagenic effects or impairs fertility.

Pregnancy, Teratogenic Effects, Pregnancy Category B: Reproduction studies have been performed with the components of sustained release capsules. Studies with chlorpheniramine maleate in rabbits and rats at doses up to 50 times and 85 times the human dose, respectively, revealed no evidence of harm to the fetus. A study with phenylpropanolamine hydrochloride in rats at doses up to 7 times the human dose revealed no evidence of harm to the fetus. There are, however, no adequate and well-controlled studies in pregnant women. Because animal reproduction studies are not always predictive of human response, sustained release capsules should be used during pregnancy only if clearly needed.

Nonteratogenic Effects: Studies of chlorpheniramine maleate in rats showed a decrease in the postnatal survival rate of offspring of animals dosed with 33 and 67 times the human dose.

PRECAUTIONS: *(cont'd)*

Nursing Mothers: Small amounts of antihistamines are excreted in breast milk. Because of the higher risk with antihistamines in infants generally, and for newborns and prematures in particular. Sustained release capsules should not be administered to a nursing mother (see CONTRAINDICATIONS.)

Pediatric Use: The safety and effectiveness of sustained release capsules in children under 12 years of age have not been established.

In infants and children, especially, antihistamines in *overdosage* may cause hallucinations, convulsions, or death.

As in adults, antihistamines may diminish mental alertness in children. In the young child, particularly, they may produce excitation. (See WARNINGS.)

DRUG INTERACTIONS:

Sustained release capsules may interact with alcohol and other CNS depressants to potentiate their effects.

This product may have additive effects when taken simultaneously with other products containing phenylpropanolamine hydrochloride or amphetamines.

MAO inhibitors prolong and intensify the anticholinergic (drying) effects of antihistamines and potentiate the pressor effects of sympathomimetics such as phenylpropanolamine hydrochloride (see CONTRAINDICATIONS.)

Phenylpropanolamine hydrochloride should not be used with ganglionic blocking drugs - such as mecamylamine - which potentiate reactions of sympathomimetics. It also should not be used with adrenergic blocking drugs, such as guanethidine sulfate or bethanidine, since it antagonizes the hypotensive action of these drugs.

The action of oral anticoagulants may be inhibited by antihistamines.

The CNS depressant and atropine-like effects of anticholinergics may be potentiated by concomitant administration of antihistamines. Concomitant administration of anticholinergics such as trihexyphenidyl, and other drugs with anticholinergic action (such as imipramine), with antihistamines may result in xerostomia.

β-adrenergic blockers may be antagonized by antihistamines.

Concomitant administration of corticosteroids and antihistamines may decrease the effects of the corticosteroids by enzyme induction.

Antihistamines inhibit norepinephrine reuptake by tissues and therefore potentiate the cardiovascular effects of norepinephrine.

Concomitant use of antihistamines with phenothiazines may produce an additive CNS depressant effect; concomitant use also may cause urinary retention or glaucoma.

ADVERSE REACTIONS:

The following adverse reactions have been reported following the use of antihistamines and/or sympathomimetic amines:

General: Anaphylactic shock; chills; drug rash; excessive dryness of mouth, nose and throat; increased intraocular pressure; excessive perspiration; photosensitivity; urticaria; weakness.

Cardiovascular System: Angina pain; extrasystoles; headache; hypertension; hypotension; palpitations; tachycardia.

Hematologic: Agranulocytosis; hemolytic anemia; leukopenia; thrombocytopenia.

Nervous System: Blurred vision; confusion; convulsions; diplopia; disturbed coordination; dizziness; drowsiness; euphoria; excitation; fatigue; hysteria; insomnia; irritability; acute labyrinthitis; nervousness; neuritis; paresthesia; restlessness; sedation; tinnitus; tremor; vertigo.

GI System: Abdominal pain; anorexia; constipation; diarrhea; epigastric distress; nausea; vomiting.

GU System: Dysuria; early menses; urinary frequency; urinary retention.

Respiratory System: Thickening of bronchial secretions; tightness of chest and wheezing; nasal stuffiness.

OVERDOSAGE:

In the event of overdosage, emergency treatment should be started immediately.

Symptoms: Effects of antihistamine overdosage may vary from central nervous system depression (sedation, apnea, diminished mental alertness, cardiovascular collapse) to stimulation (insomnia, hallucinations, tremors, or convulsions) to death.

Other signs and symptoms may be dizziness, tinnitus, ataxia, blurred vision and hypotension. Stimulation is particularly likely in children, as are atropine-like signs and symptoms (dry mouth; fixed, dilated pupils; flushing; hyperthermia; and gastrointestinal symptoms). In large doses, sympathomimetics may cause giddiness, headache, nausea, vomiting, sweating, thirst, tachycardia, precordial pain, palpitations, difficulty in micturition, muscular weakness and tenseness, anxiety, restlessness and insomnia. Many patients can present a toxic psychosis with delusions and hallucinations. Some may develop cardiac arrhythmias, circulatory collapse, convulsions, coma and respiratory failure.

Toxicity: In acute oral toxicity tests in rats, the LD_{50} for the ratio of 75 mg phenylpropanolamine hydrochloride and 12 mg chlorpheniramine maleate was 774.2 mg/kg; in mice, the LD_{50} for the formulation was 757.4 mg/kg.

Treatment: The patient should be induced to vomit even if emesis has occurred spontaneously. Pharmacologically induced vomiting by the administration of ipecac syrup is a preferred method. But vomiting should not be induced in patients with impaired consciousness. The action of ipecac is facilitated by physical activity and by the administration of 8 to 12 fluid ounces of water. If emesis does not occur within 15 minutes, the dose of ipecac should be repeated. Precautions against aspiration must be taken, especially in infants and children.

Following emesis, any drug remaining in the stomach may be adsorbed by activated charcoal administered as a slurry with water. If vomiting is unsuccessful or contraindicated, gastric lavage should be performed. Isotonic and one-half isotonic saline are the lavage solutions of choice. Since much of the capsule medication is coated for gradual release, saline cathartics should be administered to hasten evacuation of pellets that have not already released medication. Saline cathartics, such as milk of magnesia, draw water into the bowel by osmosis and therefore may be valuable for the action in rapid dilution of bowel content. Dialysis has not been reported to be effective in the treatment of phenylpropanolamine hydrochloride and chlorpheniramine maleate overdosage. After emergency treatment, the patient should continue to be medically monitored.

Treatment of the signs and symptoms of overdosage is symptomatic and supportive. *Stimulants* (analeptic agents) should *not* be used. Vasopressors may be used to treat hypotension. Short-acting barbiturates, diazepam, or paraldehyde may be administered to control seizures. Hyperpyrexia, especially in children, may require treatment with tepid water sponge baths or a hypothermic blanket. Apnea is treated with ventilatory support.

DOSAGE AND ADMINISTRATION:

Adults And Children 12 Years Of Age And Over: One capsule every 12 hours.

This drug is not recommended in children under 12.

DOSAGE AND ADMINISTRATION: *(cont'd)*

Capsules should be stored at controlled room temperature (59-86°F).

HOW SUPPLIED - RATED THERAPEUTICALLY EQUIVALENT:

Capsule, Gelatin, Sustained Action - Oral - 12 mg/75 mg

50's	$11.05	Chorphen/Phenylpropanolamine SR, Major Pharms	00904-2132-51
50's	$42.55	ORNADE, SKB Pharms	00007-4421-15
100's	$7.50	HARBER-NADE, Harber Pharm	51432-0194-03
100's	$71.99	RESAID S.R., Geneva Pharms	00781-2427-01
500's	$411.60	ORNADE, SKB Pharms	00007-4421-25
1000's	$703.05	RESAID S.R., Geneva Pharms	00781-2427-10

HOW SUPPLIED - NOT RATED EQUIVALENT:

Capsule, Gelatin, Sustained Action - Oral - 12 mg/75 mg

100's	$6.74	DECONADE, HL Moore Drug Exch	00839-6489-06
100's	$17.85	Ordrine, Pecos	59879-0111-01
100's	$20.65	ORAGEST S.R., Major Pharms	00904-2132-60
100's	$24.50	OR-PHEN-ADE, Qualitest Pharms	00603-4862-21
100's	$44.95	Histade Capsules, Pharmacist Choice	54979-0141-01
1000's	$53.93	DECONADE, HL Moore Drug Exch	00839-6489-16
1000's	$65.95	ORAGEST S.R., Major Pharms	00904-2132-80
1000's	$149.00	Chlornade, Alphagen Labs	59743-0105-10
1000's	$158.40	Or-Phen-Ade, Qualitest Pharms	00603-4862-32
1000's	$364.95	Histade Capsules, Pharmacist Choice	54979-0141-10

Liquid - Oral

480 ml	$4.40	TRIPHENYL, Rugby	00536-2330-85
480 ml	$18.00	COPHENE-PL, Dunhall Pharms	00217-0408-11

Tablet, Coated, Sustained Action - Oral - 12 mg/75 mg

100's	$11.33	HISTA-VADRIN, Scherer	00274-2436-01

CHLORPHENIRAMINE MALEATE; PHENYLPROPANOLAMINE; PSEUDOEPHEDRINE

(000795)

CATEGORIES: Antihistamines; Common Cold; Respiratory & Allergy Medications; FDA Pre 1938 Drugs

BRAND NAMES: Cotofed

Prescribing information not available at time of publication.

HOW SUPPLIED - EQUIVALENTS NOT AVAILABLE:

Syrup - Oral - 2 mg/10 mg/20 m

480 ml	$9.11	COTOFED, C O Truxton	00463-9009-16
3840 ml	$40.00	COTOFED, C O Truxton	00463-9009-28

CHLORPHENIRAMINE MALEATE; PSEUDOEPHEDRINE HYDROCHLORIDE

(000759)

CATEGORIES: Allergies; Angioedema; Antiasthmatics/Bronchodilators; Antibiotics; Antihistamines; Common Cold; Congestion; Conjunctivitis; Cough Preparations; Decongestants; Hay Fever; Nasal Congestion; Otitis Media; Respiratory & Allergy Medications; Rhinitis; Sinusitis; Sympathomimetic Agents; Urticaria; Influenza*; Pregnancy Category C; FDA Pre 1938 Drugs
* Indication not approved by the FDA

BRAND NAMES: Aller-Chlor Decongestant; Allerid-Dc; Anamine; Anaplex; Atrohist; Atrohist Pediatric; Brexin L.A.; Chlor-Ps; Chlorafed; Chlorafed H.S. Timecelles; Chlordrine; Chlorphedrin; Clorfed; *Co-Pyronil 2*; Codimal La; Colfed-A; Cophene No.2 Tr; D-Amine-Sr; D-Congestamine Tr; De-Congestine Tr; Deconamine; Deconamine Sr; Decongestant Sr; Decongestant-Sr; Decongex-8; Deconomed Sr; Desihist; Dura-Tap Pd; Duralex; Dynafed-Er; **Fedahist**; *Fenfedrin*; Histafed-L.A.; Histalet; Histamic; Histaral; Histrin-La; Isophen-Df; Klerist-D; Kronofed-A; Kronofed-A-Jr; Lantuss-La; Med-Hist; Med-Hist-Pl; Mesclor; Nasalspan; *Nastizol*; Nd Clear; Novafed A; *Novahistex* (Canada); Orahist; Orlenta; Probahist; Psenclor-Sa; Pseudo-Chlor; Pseudocot-C; Rescon; Rescon-Gg; Rinade-B.I.D.; Sufedrin Plus; Suphenamine Sr; T-Dry-Jr; Tanafed; Time-Hist
(International brand names outside U.S. in italics)

FORMULARIES: Aetna; BC-BS; FHP; Harvard; Kaiser; PruCare; PCS

DESCRIPTION:

Fedahist Timecaps contain 120 mg pseudoephedrine hydrochloride USP and 8 mg chlorpheniramine maleate USP in an extended-release formulation designed for oral b.i.d. dosage. Pseudoephedrine hydrochloride is a nasal decongestant. The empirical formula is $C_{10}H_{15}NO°HCl$ and the molecular weight is 201.70. Chemically, it is benzenemethanol, α-[1-(methylamino)ethyl]-, [S-(R*, R*)]-, hydrochloride.

Chlorpheniramine maleate is an antihistamine. The empirical formula is $C_{16}H_{19}ClN_2{\cdot}C_4H_4O_4$ and the molecular weight is 390.87. Chemically, it is 2-[*p*-chloro- α-[2-(dimethylamino)ethyl] benzyl] pyridine maleate (1:1).

Each capsule also contains as inactive ingredients: FD&C blue #1, gelatin, pharmaceutical glaze, starch, sucrose, and other ingredients.

CLINICAL PHARMACOLOGY:

Pseudoephedrine is an orally active sympathomimetic amine and exerts a decongestant action on the nasal mucosa. Pseudoephedrine produces peripheral effects similar to those of ephedrine and central effects similar to, but less intense than,amphetamines. It has the potential for excitatory side effects. At the recommended oral dosages it has little or no pressor effect in normotensive adults. The serum half-life of pseudoephedrine is approximately 4 to 6 hours. The serum half-life is decreased with increased excretion of drug at urine pH lower than 6 and may be increased with decreased excretion at urine pH higher than 8.

Chlorpheniramine is an antihistaminic that possesses anticholinergic and sedative effects. It is considered one of the most effective and least toxic of the histamine antagonist. Chlorpheniramine is an H_1 receptor antagonist. It antagonizes many of the pharmacologic actions of histamine. It prevents released histamine from dilating capillaries and causing edema of the respiratory mucosa. Chlorpheniramine has a duration of action of 4 to 6 hours (the

CLINICAL PHARMACOLOGY: *(cont'd)*

formulation provides a continuous therapeutic effect for up to 12 hours). Its half-life in serum is 12-16 hours. Degradation products of chlorpheniramine's metabolic transformation by the liver are almost completely excreted in 24 hours.

This combination drug releases 120 mg pseudoephedrine and 8 mg of chlorpheniramine at a controlled and predictable rate for 12 hours. Peak blood levels occur in 4 hours for pseudoephedrine and 6 hours for chlorpheniramine. The apparent plasma half-life is approximately 6 hours for pseudoephedrine and 16 hours for chlorpheniramine. The relative bioavailability of the extended-release dosage form is approximately 85% and 100% of the immediate-release dosage forms for pseudoephedrine and chlorpheniramine, respectively.

INDICATIONS AND USAGE:

This combination drug is indicated for the relief of nasal congestion and eustachian tube congestion associated with the common cold, sinusitis and acute upper respiratory infections.

This combination drug is also indicated for symptomatic relief of perennial and seasonal allergic rhinitis and vasomotor rhinitis. Decongestants in combination with antihistamines have been used to relieve eustachian tube congestion associated with acute eustachian salpingitis, aerotitis and serous otitis media.

CONTRAINDICATIONS:

Sympathomimetic amines are contraindicated in patients with severe hypertension, severe coronary artery disease and in patients on MAO inhibitor therapy. Antihistamines are contraindicated in patients with narrow-angle glaucoma, urinary retention, peptic ulcer, during an asthmatic attack and in patients receiving MAO inhibitors.

Hypersensitivity: Contraindicated in patients with hypersensitivity or idiosyncrasy to sympathomimetic amines. This combination drug is also contraindicated in patients hypersensitive to chlorpheniramine and other antihistamines of similar chemical structure.

Nursing Mothers: Contraindicated in nursing mothers because of the higher than usual risk for infants from sympathomimetic amines.

Newborn or Premature Infants : This combination drug should not be administered to premature or full-term infants.

WARNINGS:

Sympathomimetic amines should be used judiciously and sparingly in patients with hypertension, diabetes mellitus, ischemic heart disease, increased intraocular pressure, hyperthyroidism, or prostatic hypertrophy(see CONTRAINDICATIONS). Sympathomimetics may produce CNS stimulation and convulsions or cardiovascular collapse with accompanying hypotension.

Chlorpheniramine maleate has an atropine-like action and should be used with caution in patients with increased intraocular pressure, cardiovascular disease, hypertension or in patients with a history of bronchial asthma (see CONTRAINDICATIONS). Antihistamines may cause excitability, especially in children. Do not exceed recommended dosage because of higher doses nervousness, dizziness or sleeplessness may occur.

Use in Elderly: The elderly (60 years and older) are more likely to have adverse reactions to sympathomimetics. Overdosage of sympathomimetics in this age group may cause hallucinations, convulsions, CNS depression and death.

PRECAUTIONS:

General: Should be used with caution in patients with diabetes, hypertension, cardiovascular disease and hyperreactivity to ephedrine. The antihistaminic may cause drowsiness, therefore ambulatory patients who operate machinery or motor vehicles should be cautioned accordingly.

Information for the Patient: Antihistamines may impair mental and physical abilities required for the performance of potentially hazardous tasks, such as driving a vehicle or operating machinery, and mental alertness in children.

Laboratory Test Interactions: Antihistamines may suppress the wheal and flare reactions to antigen skin testing. Considerable interindividual variation in the extent and duration of suppression have been reported, depending on the antigen and test technique, antihistamine and dosage regimen, time since the last dose and individual response to testing. In one study, usual oral dosages of chlorpheniramine suppressed the wheal response for about 2 days after the last dose. Whenever possible, antihistamines should be discontinued about 4 days prior to skin testing procedures since they may prevent otherwise positive reactions to dermal reactivity indicators.

Carcinogenesis, Mutagenesis, and Impairment of Fertility: No long-term or reproduction studies in animals have been performed with this combination drug to evaluate its carcinogenic, mutagenic and impairment of fertility potential.

Pregnancy Category C: Animal reproduction studies have not been conducted with this combination drug. It is not known whether this combination drug can cause fetal harm when administered to a pregnant woman or can affect reproduction capacity. This combination drug may be given to a pregnant woman only if clearly needed.

Nursing Mothers: Pseudoephedrine is contraindicated in nursing mothers because of the higher than usual risk for infants from sympathomimetic amines.

DRUG INTERACTIONS:

MAO inhibitors and beta-adrenergic blockers increase the effect of sympathomimetics. Sympathomimetics may reduce the antihypertensive effects of methyldopa, mecamylamine, reserpine and veratrum alkaloids. Concomitant use of antihistamines with alcohol, tricyclic antidepressants, barbiturates and other CNS depressants may have an additive effect.

ADVERSE REACTIONS:

Hyperreactive individuals may display ephedrine-like reactions such as tachycardia, palpitations, headache, dizziness, or nausea. Patients sensitive to antihistamines may experience mild sedation. Sympathomimetic drugs have been associated with certain untoward reactions including fear, anxiety, tenseness, restlessness, tremor, weakness, pallor, respiratory difficulty, dysuria, insomnia, hallucinations, convulsions, CNS depression, arrhythmias, and cardiovascular collapse with hypotension.

Possible side effects of antihistamines are drowsiness, restlessness, dizziness, weakness, dry mouth, anorexia, nausea, headache, nervousness, blurring of vision, heartburn, dysuria and very rarely dermatitis. Patient idiosyncrasy to adrenergic agents may be manifested by insomnia, dizziness, weakness, tremor or arrhythmias.

OVERDOSAGE:

Symptoms: Manifestations of antihistamine overdosage may vary from central nervous system depression (sedation, apnea, cardiovascular collapse) to stimulation (insomnia, hallucinations, tremors or convulsions). Other signs and symptoms may be dizziness, tinnitus, ataxia, blurred vision and hypotension. Stimulation is particularly likely in children, as are atropine-like signs and symptoms (dry mouth, dilated pupils, flushing, hyperthermia and gastrointestinal symptoms).

OVERDOSAGE: *(cont'd)*

Treatment Recommendations: The patient should be induced to vomit even if emesis has occurred spontaneously; however, vomiting should be taken, especially in infants and children. Ipecac syrup is the preferred method for induced vomiting. The action of ipecac is facilitated by physical activity and by the administration of eight to twelve fluid ounces of water. If emesis does not occur in fifteen minutes, the dose of ipecac should be repeated. Following emesis, any drug remaining in the stomach may be absorbed by activated charcoal administered as a slurry with water.

If vomiting is unsuccessful or contraindicated, gastric lavage should be performed. Isotonic and one-half isotonic saline are the lavage solutions of choice. Saline cathartics, such as milk of magnesia, draw water into the bowel by osmosis and, therefore, may be valuable for their action of rapid dilution of bowel content.

Treatment of the signs and symptoms of overdosage is symptomatic and supportive. Vasopressors may be used to treat hypertension. Short-acting barbiturates, diazepam or paraldehyde may be administered to control seizures. Hyperpyrexia, especially in children, may require treatment with tepid water sponge baths or a hypothermic blanket. Apnea is treated with ventilatory support. Stimulants (analeptic agents) should **not** be used.

The LD_{50} for pseudoephedrine is 202 mg/kg delivered intraperitoneally to rats. When given orally to mice, the LD_{50} for chlorpheniramine is 162 mg/kg.

DOSAGE AND ADMINISTRATION:

Adults and children 12 years of age and older: One capsule every 12 hours not to exceed two capsules in 24 hours. Not recommended for children under 12 years of age.

(Schwarz/Kremers Pharmaceuticals, PC0068D, 6/94)

HOW SUPPLIED - RATED THERAPEUTICALLY EQUIVALENT:

Capsule, Gelatin, Sustained Action - Oral - 8 mg/120 mg

100's	$12.50	Pseudoephedrine W/Chlorphenir, Harber Pharm	51432-0445-03

HOW SUPPLIED - NOT RATED EQUIVALENT:

Capsule, Gelatin, Sustained Action - Oral - 4 mg/60 mg

100's	$23.95	Dynafed-Er, Econolab	55053-0800-01
100's	$27.61	CODIMAL-L.A. HALF, Schwarz Pharma (US)	00131-4501-37
100's	$39.35	KRONOFED- A JR., Ferndale Labs	00496-0434-02
100's	$43.05	RESCON JR, Ion	11808-0082-01
100's	$48.47	Atrohist Pediatric, Medeva Pharms	53014-0400-10
500's	$177.08	KRONOFED- A JR., Ferndale Labs	00496-0434-10

Capsule, Gelatin, Sustained Action - Oral - 8 mg/120 mg

100's	$14.18	Chlorpheniramine/Pseudoephedrine, HL Moore Drug Exch	00839-7178-06
100's	$15.70	Pseudo-Chlor, Major Pharms	00904-7777-60
100's	$16.20	DE-CONGESTINE TR, Qualitest Pharms	00603-3143-21
100's	$16.60	CHLORPHEDRINE SR, Goldline Labs	00182-1151-01
100's	$17.75	Chlorpheniramine/Pseudoephedrine Sr, United Res	00677-1086-01
100's	$18.03	COLFED-A, Parmed Pharms	00349-8782-01
100's	$18.25	D-Amine-Sr, Alphagen Labs	59743-0053-01
100's	$18.25	Psenclor-Sa, Alphagen Labs	59743-0058-01
100's	$19.95	Pseudoephedrine W/Chlorphenir, Aligen Independ	00405-4194-01
100's	$19.95	COLFED-A, Econolab	55053-0740-01
100's	$19.98	RINADE-BID, Embrex Economed	38130-0101-01
100's	$20.00	DURALEX, Amer Urologicals	00539-0903-01
100's	$20.48	Chlorpheniramine Maleate And Pseudoephed, Eon Labs Mfg	00185-1304-01
100's	$22.38	DECONGESTANT SR, Jerome Stevens	50564-0510-01
100's	$22.38	Decongestant-Sr, Pecos	59879-0107-01
100's	$22.50	PSEUDO-CHLOR S R, Geneva Pharms	00781-2915-01
100's	$24.95	Pseudoephedrine W/Chlorphenir, H N Norton Co.	50732-0852-01
100's	$27.50	Med-Hist, Med Tek Pharms	52349-0310-10
100's	$28.28	KRONOFED-A, Ferndale Labs	00496-0382-02
100's	$30.51	CHLORDRINE S.R., Rugby	00536-3420-01
100's	$32.95	TIME-HIST, Am Pharms	58605-0502-01
100's	$33.70	ANAMINE TD, Mayrand Pharms	00259-1234-01
100's	$38.12	CODIMAL LA, Schwarz Pharma (US)	00131-4213-37
100's	$39.09	HISTAFED-LA, Geriatric Pharm	00249-0602-02
100's	$44.60	D-Congestamine Tr, Equipharm	57779-0106-04
100's	$44.94	BREXIN LA, Savage Labs	00281-1934-53
100's	**$47.96**	**FEDAHIST TIMECAPS, Schwarz Pharma (US)**	**00091-0055-01**
100's	$50.40	RESCON-ED, Ion	11808-0089-01
100's	$53.82	NOVAFED A, Hoechst Marion Roussel	00068-0106-61
100's	$68.36	DECONAMINE SR, Bradley Pharms	00482-0181-10
250's	$37.45	Pseudo-Chlor, Major Pharms	00904-0058-70
250's	$37.45	Pseudo-Chlor, Major Pharms	00904-7777-70
250's	$45.00	Psenclor-Sa, Alphagen Labs	59743-0058-25
500's	$92.95	COLFED-A, Econolab	55053-0740-05
500's	$93.05	D-Amine-Sr, Alphagen Labs	59743-0053-05
500's	$122.00	Chlorpheniramine/Pseudoephedrine, H N Norton Co.	50732-0852-05
500's	$126.00	Cophene No.2 Tr, Dunhall Pharms	00217-0409-03
500's	$127.24	KRONOFED-A, Ferndale Labs	00496-0382-10
500's	$215.00	D-Congestamine Tr, Equipharm	57779-0106-06
500's	$329.24	DECONAMINE SR, Bradley Pharms	00482-0181-50
1000's	$99.75	Chlorpheniramine Maleate And Pseudoephed, Eon Labs Mfg	00185-1304-10
1000's	$100.00	DURALEX, Amer Urologicals	00539-0903-10
1000's	$343.28	CODIMAL LA, Schwarz Pharma (US)	00131-4213-43

Capsule, Gelatin, Sustained Action - Oral - 10 mg/65 mg

100's	**$47.96**	**FEDAHIST GYROCAPS, Schwarz Pharma (US)**	**00091-1053-01**

Capsule, Gelatin, Sustained Action - Oral - 12 mg/120 mg

100's	$28.00	Cophene No.2 Tr, Dunhall Pharms	00217-0409-01
100's	$50.40	RESCON, Ion	11808-0087-01

Capsule, Sprinkle - Oral - 4 mg/60 mg

100's	$38.77	ATROHIST, SPRINKLE, Medeva Pharms	53014-0028-10

Syrup - Oral - 2 mg/30 mg

118 ml	$15.25	TANAFED, Horizon Pharm	59630-0120-04
473 ml	$30.32	DECONAMINE, Bradley Pharms	00482-0185-16
473 ml	$52.45	TANAFED, Horizon Pharm	59630-0120-16
480 ml	$23.50	ANAMINE, Mayrand Pharms	00259-2235-16

Syrup - Oral - 3 mg/45 mg

480 ml	$32.27	HISTALET, Solvay Pharms	00032-1035-78

Tablet, Coated, Sustained Action - Oral - 6 mg/120 mg

100's	$8.74	DESIHIST, HL Moore Drug Exch	00839-6471-06
1000's	$71.54	DESIHIST, HL Moore Drug Exch	00839-6471-16

Tablet, Uncoated - Oral - 4 mg/60 mg

24's	$1.87	Klerist-D, Palisades Pharms	53159-0430-24
100's	$4.50	ALLER-CHLOR DECONGESTANT, Rugby	00536-3015-01
100's	$6.68	Klerist-D, Palisades Pharms	53159-0430-01

HOW SUPPLIED - NOT RATED EQUIVALENT: *(cont'd)*

100's	$34.19	DECONAMINE, Bradley Pharms	00482-0184-10
100's	$39.50	MESCLOR, Horizon Pharm	59630-0150-10

CHLORPHENIRAMINE POLISTIREX; HYDROCODONE POLISTIREX *(000760)*

CATEGORIES: Allergies; Antihistamines; Antitussives; Antitussives/Expectorants/Mucolytics; Common Cold; Cough Preparations; Respiratory & Allergy Medications; Influenza*; Pregnancy Category C; DEA Class CIII; FDA Approved 1987 Dec

* Indication not approved by the FDA

BRAND NAMES: *Pennuss*; S-T Forte; **Tussionex**
(International brand names outside U.S. in italics)

FORMULARIES: Aetna; BC-BS

DESCRIPTION:

Each teaspoonful (5 ml) of chlorpheniramine with hydrocodone contains hydrocodone polistirex equivalent to 10 mg of hydrocodone bitartrate (Warning: May be habit forming) and chlorpheniramine polistirex equivalent to 8 mg of chlorpheniramine maleate. Chlorpheniramine with hydrocodone provides up to 12-hour relief per dose. Hydrocodone is a centrally-acting narcotic antitussive. Chlorpheniramine is an antihistamine. Chlorpheniramine with hydrocodone is for oral use only.

Hydrocodone Polistirex: sulfonated styrene-divinylbenzene copolymer complex with 4,5α-epoxy-3-methoxy-17-methylmorphinan-6-one.

Chlorpheniramine Polistirex: sulfonated styrene-divinylbenzene copolymer complex with 2-[*p*-chloro-α-[2-(dimethylamino)ethyl]-benzyl]pyridine.

Inactive Ingredients: Ascorbic acid, D&C Yellow No. 10, ethylcellulose, FD&C Yellow No. 6, flavor, high fructose corn syrup, methylparaben, polyethylene glycol 3350, polysorbate 80, pregelatinized starch, propylene glycol, propylparaben, purified water, sucrose, vegetable oil, xanthan gum.

CLINICAL PHARMACOLOGY:

Hydrocodone is a semisynthetic narcotic antitussive and analgesic with multiple actions qualitatively similar to those of codeine. The precise mechanism of action of hydrocodone and other opiates is not known; however, hydrocodone is believed to act directly on the cough center. In excessive doses, hydrocodone, like other opium derivatives, will depress respiration. The effects of hydrocodone in therapeutic doses on the cardiovascular system are insignificant. Hydrocodone can produce miosis, euphoria, physical and psychological dependence.

Chlorpheniramine is an antihistamine drug (H_1 receptor antagonist) that also possesses anticholinergic and sedative activity. It prevents released histamine from dilating capillaries and causing edema of the respiratory mucosa.

Hydrocodone release from chlorpheniramine with hydrocodone is controlled by the Pennkinetic System, an extended-release drug delivery system which combines an ion-exchange polymer matrix with a diffusion rate-limiting permeable coating. Chlorpheniramine release is prolonged by use of an ion-exchange polymer system.

Following multiple dosing with chlorpheniramine with hydrocodone, hydrocodone mean (S.D.) peak plasma concentrations of 22.8 (5.9) ng/ml occurred at 3.4 hours. Chlorpheniramine mean (S.D.) peak plasma concentrations of 58.4 (14.7) ng/ml occurred at 6.3 hours following multiple dosing. Peak plasma levels obtained with an immediate-release syrup occurred at approximately 1.5 hours for hydrocodone and 2.8 hours for chlorpheniramine. The plasma half-lives of hydrocodone and chlorpheniramine have been reported to be approximately 4 and 16 hours, respectively.

INDICATIONS AND USAGE:

Chlorpheniramine with hydrocodone is indicated for relief of cough and upper respiratory symptoms associated with allergy or a cold.

CONTRAINDICATIONS:

Known allergy or sensitivity to hydrocodone or chlorpheniramine.

WARNINGS:

Respiratory Depression: As with all narcotics, chlorpheniramine with hydrocodone produces dose-related respiratory depression by directly acting on brain stem respiratory centers. Hydrocodone affects the center that controls respiratory rhythm, and may produce irregular and periodic breathing. Caution should be exercised when chlorpheniramine with hydrocodone is used postoperatively and in patients with pulmonary disease or whenever ventilatory function is depressed. If respiratory depression occurs, it may be antagonized by the use of naloxone hydrochloride and other supportive measures when indicated (see OVERDOSAGE.)

Head Injury and Increased Intracranial Pressure: The respiratory depressant effects of narcotics and their capacity to elevate cerebrospinal fluid pressure may be markedly exaggerated in the presence of head injury, other intracranial lesions or a pre-existing increase in intracranial pressure. Furthermore, narcotics produce adverse reactions which may obscure the clinical course of patients with head injuries.

Acute Abdominal Conditions: The administration of narcotics may obscure the diagnosis or clinical course of patients with acute abdominal conditions.

Obstructive Bowel Disease: Chronic use of narcotics may result in obstructive bowel disease especially in patients with underlying intestinal motility disorder.

Pediatric Use: In young children, as well as adults, the respiratory center is sensitive to the depressant action of narcotic cough suppressants in a dose-dependent manner. Benefit to risk ratio should be carefully considered especially in children with respiratory embarrassment (*e.g.,* croup) (see PRECAUTIONS.)

PRECAUTIONS:

GENERAL

Caution is advised when prescribing this drug to patients with narrow-angle glaucoma, asthma or prostatic hypertrophy.

Special Risk Patients: As with any narcotic agent, chlorpheniramine with hydrocodone should be used with caution in elderly or debilitated patients and those with severe impairment of hepatic or renal function, hypothyroidism, Addison's disease, prostatic hypertrophy or urethral stricture. The usual precautions should be observed and the possibility of respiratory depression should be kept in mind.

PRECAUTIONS: *(cont'd)*

INFORMATION FOR THE PATIENT

As with all narcotics, chlorpheniramine with hydrocodone may produce marked drowsiness and impair the mental and/or physical abilities required for the performance of potentially hazardous tasks such as driving a car or operating machinery; patients should be cautioned accordingly. Chlorpheniramine with hydrocodone must not be diluted with fluids or mixed with other drugs as this may alter the resin-binding and change the absorption rate, possibly increasing the toxicity.

Keep out of the reach of children.

Cough Reflex: Hydrocodone suppresses the cough reflex; as with all narcotics, caution should be exercised when chlorpheniramine with hydrocodone is used postoperatively, and in patients with pulmonary disease.

CARCINOGENESIS, MUTAGENESIS, AND IMPAIRMENT OF FERTILITY:

Carcinogenicity, mutagenicity and reproductive studies have not been conducted with chlorpheniramine with hydrocodone.

PREGNANCY, TERATOGENIC EFFECTS, PREGNANCY CATEGORY C

Hydrocodone has been shown to be teratogenic in hamsters when given in doses 700 times the human dose. There are no adequate and well-controlled studies in pregnant women. Chlorpheniramine with hydrocodone should be used during pregnancy only if the potential benefit justifies the potential risk to the fetus.

NONTERATOGENIC EFFECTS

Babies born to mothers who have been taking opioids regularly prior to delivery will be physically dependent. The withdrawal signs include irritability and excessive crying, tremors, hyperactive reflexes, increased respiratory rate, increased stools, sneezing, yawning, vomiting and fever. The intensity of the syndrome does not always correlate with the duration of maternal opioid use or dose.

LABOR AND DELIVERY

As with all narcotics, administration of chlorpheniramine with hydrocodone to the mother shortly before delivery may result in some degree of respiratory depression in the newborn, especially if higher doses are used.

NURSING MOTHERS

It is not known whether this drug is excreted in human milk. Because many drugs are excreted in human milk and because of the potential for serious adverse reactions in nursing infants from chlorpheniramine with hydrocodone, a decision should be made whether to discontinue nursing or to discontinue the drug, taking into account the importance of the drug to the mother.

PEDIATRIC USE

Safety and effectiveness of chlorpheniramine with hydrocodone in children under six have not been established.

DRUG INTERACTIONS:

Patients receiving narcotics, antihistaminics, antipsychotics, antianxiety agents or other CNS depressants (including alcohol) concomitantly with chlorpheniramine with hydrocodone may exhibit an additive CNS depression. When combined therapy is contemplated, the dose of one or both agents should be reduced.

The use of MAO inhibitors or tricyclic antidepressants with hydrocodone preparations may increase the effect of either the antidepressant or hydrocodone.

The concurrent use of other anticholinergics with hydrocodone may produce paralytic ileus.

ADVERSE REACTIONS:

Central Nervous System: Sedation, drowsiness, mental clouding, lethargy, impairment of mental and physical performance, anxiety, fear, dysphoria, euphoria, dizziness, psychic dependence, mood changes.

Dermatologic System: Rash, pruritus.

Gastrointestinal System: Nausea and vomiting may occur; they are more frequent in ambulatory than in recumbent patients. Prolonged administration of chlorpheniramine with hydrocodone may produce constipation.

Genitourinary System: Ureteral spasm, spasm of vesicle sphincters and urinary retention have been reported with opiates.

Respiratory Depression: Chlorpheniramine with hydrocodone may produce dose-related respiratory depression by acting directly on brain stem respiratory centers (see OVERDOSAGE.)

Respiratory System: Dryness of the pharynx, occasional tightness of the chest.

DRUG ABUSE AND DEPENDENCE:

Chlorpheniramine with hydrocodone is a Schedule III narcotic. Psychic dependence, physical dependence and tolerance may develop upon repeated administration of narcotics; therefore, chlorpheniramine with hydrocodone should be prescribed and administered with caution. However, psychic dependence is unlikely to develop when chlorpheniramine with hydrocodone is used for a short time for the treatment of cough. Physical dependence, the condition in which continued administration of the drug is required to prevent the appearance of a withdrawal syndrome, assumes clinically significant proportions only after several weeks of continued oral narcotic use, although some mild degree of physical dependence may develop after a few days of narcotic therapy.

OVERDOSAGE:

Signs and Symptoms: Serious overdosage with hydrocodone is characterized by respiratory depression (a decrease in respiratory rate and/or tidal volume, Cheyne-Stokes respiration, cyanosis), extreme somnolence progressing to stupor or coma, skeletal muscle flaccidity, cold and clammy skin, and sometimes bradycardia and hypotension. Although miosis is characteristic of narcotic overdose, mydriasis may occur in terminal narcosis or severe hypoxia. In severe overdosage apnea, circulatory collapse, cardiac arrest and death may occur. The manifestations of chlorpheniramine overdosage may vary from central nervous system depression to stimulation.

Treatment: Primary attention should be given to the reestablishment of adequate respiratory exchange through provision of a patent airway and the institution of assisted or controlled ventilation. The narcotic antagonist naloxone hydrochloride is a specific antidote for respiratory depression which may result from overdosage or unusual sensitivity to narcotics including hydrocodone. Therefore, an appropriate dose of naloxone hydrochloride should be administered, preferably by the intravenous route, simultaneously with efforts at respiratory resuscitation. Since the duration of action of hydrocodone in this formulation may exceed that of the antagonist, the patient should be kept under continued surveillance and repeated doses of the antagonist should be administered as needed to maintain adequate respiration. For further information, see full prescribing information for naloxone hydrochloride. An antagonist should not be administered in the absence of clinically significant respiratory depression. Oxygen, intravenous fluids, vasopressors and other supportive measures should be employed as indicated. Gastric emptying may be useful in removing unabsorbed drug.

DOSAGE AND ADMINISTRATION:

Shake well before using.

Adults: 1 teaspoonful (5 ml) every 12 hours; do not exceed 2 teaspoonfuls in 24 hours.

Children 6-12: 1/2 teaspoonful every 12 hours; **do not exceed 1 teaspoonful in 24 hours.**

Not recommended for children under 6 years of age (see PRECAUTIONS.)

HOW SUPPLIED:

Tussionex Pennkinetic (hydrocodone polistirex and chlorpheniramine polistirex) Extended-Release Suspension is a gold-colored suspension.

Shake well. Dispense in a well-closed container. Store at 59°-86°F (15°-30°C).

HOW SUPPLIED - EQUIVALENTS NOT AVAILABLE:

Liquid - Oral

120 ml	$7.19	S-T FORTE 2 SF, Scot Tussin	00372-0048-04
240 ml	$12.35	S-T FORTE 2 SF, Scot Tussin	00372-0048-08
473.2 ml	$25.66	S-T FORTE 2 SF, Scot Tussin	00372-0048-16
480 ml	**$82.67**	**TUSSIONEX, Medeva Pharms**	**53014-0548-67**
900 ml	**$141.98**	**TUSSIONEX, Fisons**	**00585-0548-91**
3785 ml	$183.57	S-T FORTE 2 SF, Scot Tussin	00372-0048-28

CHLORPHENIRAMINE TANNATE; PHENYLEPHRINE TANNATE; PYRILAMINE TANNATE *(000761)*

CATEGORIES: Allergies; Antihistamines; Autonomic Drugs; Common Cold; Cough Preparations; Decongestants; Nasal Congestion; Respiratory & Allergy Medications; Rhinitis; Sinusitis; Sympathomimetic Agents; Pregnancy Category C; FDA Pre 1938 Drugs

BRAND NAMES: Atrohist; Equitan; Gelhist; Harber Tannate S; Histatan; Mooretan; Phinatate; R-Tannamine; R-Tannate; Rhinatate; Ricobid; Ryna-Mine; **Rynatan**; Tanamine; Tannate; Tanoral-S; Tri-Tannate; Triotann; Triotann-S; Triple Tannate-S; Tritan; Url-Tannate

FORMULARIES: BC-BS

DESCRIPTION:

This combination drug is an antihistamine/nasal decongestant combination available for oral administration as Tablets and as Pediatric Suspension.

Each Tablet Contains: *Phenylephrine Tannate:* 25 mg; *Chlorpheniramine Tannate:* 8 mg; *Pyrilamine Tannate:* 25 mg; *Other ingredients:* corn starch, dibasic calcium phosphate, magnesium stearate, methylcellulose, polygalacturonic acid, talc.

Each 5 ml (teaspoonful) of the Pediatric Suspension contains: *Phenylephrine Tannate:* 5 mg; *Chlorpheniramine Tannate:* 2 mg; *Pyrilamine Tannate:* 12.5 mg

Other Ingredients: benzoic acid, FD&C Red No. 3, flavors (natural and artificial), glycerin, kaolin, magnesium aluminum silicate, methylparaben, pectin, purified water, saccharin sodium, sucrose.

CLINICAL PHARMACOLOGY:

This combination drug combines the sympathomimetic decongestant effect of phenylephrine with the antihistaminic actions of chlorpheniramine and pyrilamine.

INDICATIONS AND USAGE:

This combination drug is indicated for symptomatic relief of the coryza and nasal congestion associated with the common cold, sinusitis, allergic rhinitis and other upper respiratory tract conditions. Appropriate therapy should be provided for the primary disease.

CONTRAINDICATIONS:

This combination drug is contraindicated for newborns, nursing mothers and patients sensitive to any of the ingredients or related compounds.

WARNINGS:

Use with caution in patients with hypertension, cardiovascular disease, hyperthyroidism, diabetes, narrow angle glaucoma or prostatic hypertrophy. Use with caution or avoid use in patients taking monoamine oxidase (MAO) inhibitors. This product contains antihistamines which may cause drowsiness and may have additive central nervous system (CNS) effects with alcohol or other CNS depressants (*e.g.,* hypnotics, sedatives, tranquilizers).

PRECAUTIONS:

GENERAL

Antihistamines are more likely to cause dizziness, sedation and hypotension in elderly patients. Antihistamines may cause excitation, particularly in children, but their combination with sympathomimetics may cause either mild stimulation or mild sedation.

INFORMATION FOR THE PATIENT

Caution patients against drinking alcoholic beverages or engaging in potentially hazardous activities requiring alertness, such as driving a car or operating machinery, while using this product.

CARCINOGENESIS, MUTAGENESIS, AND IMPAIRMENT OF FERTILITY

No long term animal studies have been performed with this combination drug.

PREGNANCY, TERATOGENIC EFFECTS, PREGNANCY CATEGORY C

Animal reproduction studies have not been conducted with this combination drug. It is also now known whether this combination drug can cause fetal harm when administered to a pregnant woman or can affect reproduction capacity. This combination drug should be given to a pregnant woman only if clearly needed.

NURSING MOTHERS

This combination drug should not be administered to a nursing woman.

DRUG INTERACTIONS:

MAO inhibitors may prolong and intensify the anticholinergic effects of antihistamines and the overall effects of sympathomimetic agents.

ADVERSE REACTIONS:

Adverse effects associated with this combination drug at recommended doses have been minimal. The most common have been drowsiness, sedation, dryness of mucous membranes and gastrointestinal effects. Serious side effects with oral antihistamines or sympathomimetics have been rare.

OVERDOSAGE:

SIGNS AND SYMPTOMS

May vary from CNS depression to stimulation (restlessness to convulsions). Antihistamine overdosage in young children may lead to convulsions and death. Atropine-like signs and symptoms may be prominent.

TREATMENT

Induce vomiting if it has not occurred spontaneously. Precautions must be taken against aspiration especially in infants, children and comatose patients. If gastric lavage is indicated, isotonic or half-isotonic saline solution is preferred. Stimulants should not be used. If hypotension is a problem, vasopressor agents may be considered.

DOSAGE AND ADMINISTRATION:

Administer the recommended dose every 12 hours.

TABLETS

Adults: 1 or 2 tablets.

PEDIATRIC SUSPENSION

Children over six years of age: 5 to 10 ml (1 to 2 teaspoonfuls).

Children two to six years of age: 2.5 to 5 ml (1/2 to 1 teaspoonful).

Children under two years of age: Titrate dose individually.

Storage: Store at controlled room temperature between 15-30°C (59-86°F); protect from freezing.

Dispense in tight container.

(Wallace Labs, 5/92, IN-0713-05)

HOW SUPPLIED - EQUIVALENTS NOT AVAILABLE:

Suspension - Oral - 2 mg/5 mg/12.5

118 ml	$13.95	Gelhist, Econolab	55053-0930-04
118 ml x 4	$52.00	TANORAL-S, Econolab	55053-0190-04
118.3 ml	$22.00	RICOBID-H, Teral Labs	51234-0157-04
118.3 ml	$23.00	RICOBID, Teral Labs	51234-0155-04
120 ml	$7.50	Rhinatate, Major Pharms	00904-7650-20
120 ml	$13.50	R-Tannate, Copley Pharm	38245-0109-14
120 ml	$14.00	R-Tannate, Ethex	58177-0887-03
120 ml	$15.32	Gelhist, HL Moore Drug Exch	00839-7976-65
120 ml	$21.70	ATROHIST, PEDIATRIC, Medeva Pharms	53014-0026-12
120 ml	$63.80	Triotann-S, Duramed Pharms	51285-0717-55
120 ml	**$100.98**	**RYNATAN PEDIATRIC, Wallace Labs**	**00037-0715-67**
120 ml x 4	$21.46	Triotann-S, Aligen Independ	00405-3671-16
120 ml x 4	$26.00	TRIPLE TANNATE-S, Hi Tech Pharma	50383-0808-04
120 ml x 4	$26.45	MOORETAN S, HL Moore Drug Exch	00839-7309-29
120 ml x 4	$29.88	R-TANNAMINE, Qualitest Pharms	00603-1661-54
120 ml x 4	$31.25	Harber Tannate S, Harber Pharm	51432-0613-22
120 ml x 4	$31.50	Triotann-S, Aligen Independ	00405-3671-76
120 ml x 4	$44.25	TRI-TANNATE S, Rugby	00536-2201-97
473 ml	$29.13	Triotann, Duramed Pharms	51285-0717-57
473 ml	$42.00	Ryna-Mine, Bergmar Pharm	58173-0024-16
473 ml	$54.95	Gelhist, Econolab	55053-0930-16
480 ml	$20.62	EQUITAN, Equipharm	57779-0114-09
480 ml	$22.67	MOORETAN PEDIATRIC, HL Moore Drug Exch	00839-7309-69
480 ml	$28.71	R-TANNAMINE, Qualitest Pharms	00603-1661-58
480 ml	$29.40	TRI-TANNATE PED., Rugby	00536-2201-85
480 ml	$30.00	PHENYLEPHRINE/CHLORPHEN/PYRILAMINE, Goldline Labs	00182-6111-40
480 ml	$30.55	RHINATATE PEDIATRIC, Major Pharms	00904-1670-16
480 ml	$30.55	PHINATATE, Major Pharms	00904-7650-16
480 ml	$31.50	R-TANNATE PEDIATRIC, Schein Pharm (US)	00364-2197-16
480 ml	$33.50	R-TANNATE, Copley Pharm	38245-0109-07
480 ml	$34.92	TANORAL PEDIATRIC, Parmed Pharms	00349-8745-16
480 ml	$35.00	URL-TANNATE PED., United Res	00677-1154-33
480 ml	$36.13	TANORAL, Parmed Pharms	00349-8870-16
480 ml	$42.66	R-TANNATE, Warner Chilcott	00047-2885-23
480 ml	$42.66	Phenylephrine/Chlorphen/Pyrilamine, Mikart	46672-0585-16
480 ml	$44.79	R-Tannate, Ethex	58177-0887-07
480 ml	$86.07	ATROHIST, PEDIATRIC, Medeva Pharms	53014-0026-47
480 ml	**$108.25**	**RYNATAN PEDIATRIC, Wallace Labs**	**00037-0715-68**

Tablet, Uncoated - Oral - 8 mg/25 mg/25 m

100's	$13.75	PHENYLEPHRINE/CHLOIRPHEN/PYRILAMINE, Goldline Labs	00182-1912-01
100's	$14.95	TRITAN, Eon Labs Mfg	00185-0700-01
100's	$29.63	MOORETAN, HL Moore Drug Exch	00839-7270-06
100's	$29.80	Tritan, Aligen Independ	00405-4806-01
100's	$34.10	RHINATATE, Major Pharms	00904-1669-60
100's	$34.11	R-TANNAMINE, Qualitest Pharms	00603-5687-21
100's	$34.75	Tanoral, Econolab	55053-0191-01
100's	$35.30	URL-TANNATE, United Res	00677-1153-01
100's	$35.78	TRI-TANNATE, Rugby	00536-4729-01
100's	$40.00	R-TANNATE, Schein Pharm (US)	00364-2196-01
100's	$42.75	R-TANNATE, Copley Pharm	38245-0113-10
100's	$43.00	TRIOTANN, Duramed Pharms	51285-0825-02
100's	$44.36	TANORAL, Parmed Pharms	00349-8681-01
100's	$47.88	HISTATAN, H N Norton Co.	50732-0743-01
100's	$49.76	R-Tannate, Ethex	58177-0234-04
100's	$52.42	R-TANNATE, Warner Chilcott	00047-0940-24
100's	$52.42	Phenylephrine/Chlorphen/Pyrilami, Mikart	46672-0093-10
100's	$115.00	RICOBID, Teral Labs	51234-0154-90
100's	**$128.21**	**RYNATAN, Wallace Labs**	**00037-0713-92**
250's	$72.50	Rhinatate, Major Pharms	00904-1669-70
250's	$86.70	TRI-TANNATE, Rugby	00536-4729-02
500's	$153.75	Tanoral, Econolab	55053-0191-05
500's	$159.45	PHENYLEPHRINE/CHLORPHEN/PYRILAMI, Mikart	46672-0093-50
500's	**$631.63**	**RYNATAN, Wallace Labs**	**00037-0713-96**
1000's	$109.95	TRITAN, Eon Labs Mfg	00185-0700-10
2000's	**$2422.28**	**RYNATAN, Wallace Labs**	**00037-0713-95**

CHLORPROMAZINE HYDROCHLORIDE *(000797)*

CATEGORIES: Analeptics; Anesthesia; Anticonvulsants; Antipsychotics/Antimanics; Anxiety; Central Nervous System Agents; Hiccups; Mania; Nausea and Vomiting; Neuroleptics; Neuromuscular; Phenothiazine Tranquilizers; Porphyria; Psychotherapeutic Agents; Psychotic Disorders; Schizophrenia; Sedatives/Hypnotics; Tetanus; Tranquilizers; Vertigo/Motion Sickness/Vomiting; Depression*; Glaucoma*; Headache*; Migraine*; FDA Approval Pre 1982

* Indication not approved by the FDA

BRAND NAMES: *Ampliactil*; *Artomin*; *Aspersinal*; *Chlomazine* (Japan); *Chloractil* (England); *Chlorazin*; *Chlorpromanyl* (Canada); *Chlorpromed*; *Chlorzine*; *Clonazine*; *Contomin* (Japan); *Esmino* (Japan); *Fenactil*; *Hibernal*; *Klorazin*; *Klorproman*; *Klorpromazin*; *Laractyl*; *Largactil* (Australia, England, France, Canada); *Largactil Forte*; *Matcine*; *Megaphen*; *Meprosetil*; *Neomazine*; *Novochlorpromazine* (Canada); Ormazine; *Plegomazine*; *Proma*; *Promacid*; *Promactil*; *Promazine*; *Promexin* (Japan); *Propaphenin* (Germany); *Protran*; *Prozil*; *Prozin*; *Romazine*; *Sico*; Sonazine; *Taroctyl*; Thor-Prom; **Thorazine**; *Winsumin*; *Wintermin* (Japan)
(International brand names outside U.S. in italics)

FORMULARIES: Aetna; BC-BS; FHP; Medi-Cal; WHO

COST OF THERAPY: $22.10 (Psychotic Disorders; Tablet; 25 mg; 3/day; 120 days)

DESCRIPTION:

Chlorpromazine is 10-(3-dimethylaminopropyl)-2-chlorphenothiazine, a dimethylamine derivative of phenothiazine. It is present in oral and injectable forms as the hydrochloride salt, and in the suppositories as the base.

Thorazine Tablets: Each round, orange, coated tablet contains chlorpromazine hydrochloride as follows: 10 mg imprinted SKF and T73; 25 mg imprinted SKF and T74; 50 mg imprinted SKF and T76; 100 mg imprinted SKF and T77; 200 mg imprinted SKF and T79. Inactive ingredients consist of benzoic acid, croscarmellose sodium, D&C Yellow No. 10, FD&C Blue No. 2, FD&C Yellow No. 6, gelatin, hydroxypropyl methylcellulose, lactose, magnesium stearate, methylparaben, polyethylene glycol, propylparaben, talc, titanium dioxide and trace amounts of other inactive ingredients.

Sustained release capsules: Each chlorpromazine sustained capsule is so prepared that an initial dose is released promptly and the remaining medication is released gradually over a prolonged period.

Each capsule, with opaque orange cap and natural body, contains chlorpromazine hydrochloride as follows: 30 mg imprinted SKF and T63; 75 mg imprinted SKF and T64; 150 mg imprinted SKF and T66. Inactive ingredients consist of benzyl alcohol, calcium sulfate, cetylpyridinium chloride, FD&C Yellow No. 6, gelatin, glyceryl distearate, glyceryl monostearate, iron oxide, povidone, silicon dioxide, sodium lauryl sulfate, starch, sucrose, titanium dioxide, wax and trace amounts of other inactive ingredients.

Thorazine Ampuls: Each ml contains, in aqueous solution, chlorpromazine hydrochloride, 25 mg;ascorbic acid, 2 mg;sodium bisulfite, 1 mg; sodium chloride, 6 mg;sodium sulfite, 1 mg.

Thorazine Multiple-Dose Vials: Each ml contains, in aqueous solution, chlorpromazine hydrochloride, 25 mg; ascorbic acid, 2 mg; sodium bisulfite, 1 mg; sodium chloride, 1 mg; sodium sulfite, 1 mg; benzyl alcohol, 2%, as a preservative.

Thorazine Syrup: Each 5 ml (1 teaspoonful) of clear, orange-custard flavored liquid contains chlorpromazine hydrochloride, 10 mg. Inactive ingredients consist of citric acid, flavors, sodium benzoate, sucrose and water.

Thorazine Suppositories: Each suppository contains chlorpromazine, 25 or 100 mg, glycerin, glyceryl monopalmitate, glyceryl monostearate, hydrogenated coconut oil fatty acids, and hydrogenated palm kernel oil fatty acids.

Thorazine Concentrate: Each ml of clear, custard flavored liquid contains chlorpromazine hydrochloride, 30 or 100 mg. Inactive ingredients consist of calcium disodium edetate, citric acid, flavors, hydroxypropyl methylcellulose, propylene glycol, saccharin sodium, sodium benzoate, water and trace amounts of other inactive ingredients.

CLINICAL PHARMACOLOGY:

The precise mechanism whereby the therapeutic effects of chlorpromazine are produced is not known. The principal pharmacological actions are psychotropic. It also exerts sedative and antiemetic activity. Chlorpromazine has actions at all levels of the central nervous system—primarily at subcortical levels—as well as on multiple organ systems. Chlorpromazine has strong antiadrenergic and weaker, peripheral anticholinergic activity; ganglionic blocking action is relatively slight. It is also possesses slight antihistaminic and antiserotonin activity.

INDICATIONS AND USAGE:

For the management of manifestations of psychotic disorders.

To control nausea and vomiting.

For relief of restlessness and apprehension before surgery.

For acute intermittent porphyria.

As an adjunct in the treatment of tetanus.

To control the manifestations of the manic type of manic-depressive illness.

For relief of intractable hiccups.

For the treatment of severe behavioral problems in children marked by combativeness and/or explosive hyperexcitable behavior (out of proportion to immediate provocations), and in the short-term treatment of hyperactive children who show excessive motor activity with accompanying conduct disorders consisting of some or all of the following symptoms: impulsivity, difficulty sustaining attention, aggressivity, mood lability and poor frustration tolerance.

CONTRAINDICATIONS:

Do not use in patients with known hypersensitivity to phenothiazines.

Do not use in comatose states or in the presence of large amounts of central nervous system depressants (alcohol, barbiturates, narcotics, etc.).

WARNINGS:

The extrapyramidal symptoms which can occur secondary to chlorpromazine may be confused with the central nervous system signs of an undiagnosed primary disease responsible for the vomiting, e.g., Reye's syndrome or other encephalopathy. The use of chlorpromazine and other potential hepatotoxins should be avoided in children and adolescents whose signs and symptoms suggest Reye's syndrome.

Tardive Dyskinesia: Tardive dyskinesia, a syndrome consisting of potentially irreversible, involuntary, dyskinetic movements, may develop in patients treated with neuroleptic (antipsychotic) drugs. Although the prevalence of the syndrome appears to be highest among the elderly, especially elderly women, it is impossible to rely upon prevalence estimates to predict, at the inception of neuroleptic treatment, which patients are likely to develop the syndrome. Whether neuroleptic drug products differ in their potential to cause tardive dyskinesia is unknown.

Both the risk of developing the syndrome and the likelihood that it will become irreversible are believed to increase as the duration of treatment and the total cumulative dose of neuroleptic drugs administered to the patient increase. However, the syndrome can develop, although much less commonly, after relatively brief treatment periods at low doses.

WARNINGS: *(cont'd)*

There is no known treatment for established cases of tardive dyskinesia, although the syndrome may remit, partially or completely, if neuroleptic treatment is withdrawn. Neuroleptic treatment itself, however, may suppress (or partially suppress) the signs and symptoms of the syndrome and thereby may possibly mask the underlying disease process. The effect that symptomatic suppression has upon the long-term course of the syndrome is unknown.

Given these considerations, neuroleptics should be prescribed in a manner that is most likely to minimize the occurrence of tardive dyskinesia. Chronic neuroleptic treatment should generally be reserved for patients who suffer from a chronic illness that, 1) is known to respond to neuroleptic drugs, and, 2) for whom alternative, equally effective, but potentially less harmful treatments are *not* available or appropriate. In patients who do require chronic treatment, the smallest dose and the shortest duration of treatment producing a satisfactory clinical response should be sought. The need for continued treatment should be reassessed periodically.

If signs and symptoms of tardive dyskinesia appear in a patient on neuroleptics, drug discontinuation should be considered. However, some patients may require treatment despite the presence of the syndrome.

For further information about the description of tardive dyskinesia and its clinical detection, please refer to the sections on PRECAUTIONS and ADVERSE REACTIONS.

Neuroleptic Malignant Syndrome (NMS): A potentially fatal symptom complex sometimes referred to as Neuroleptic Malignant Syndrome (NMS) has been reported in association with antipsychotic drugs. Clinical manifestations of NMS are hyperpyrexia, muscle rigidity, altered mental status and evidence of autonomic instability (irregular pulse or blood pressure, tachycardia, diaphoresis, and cardiac dysrhythmias).

The diagnostic evaluation of patients with this syndrome is complicated. In arriving at a diagnosis, it is important to identify cases where the clinical presentation includes both serious medical illness (*e.g.,* pneumonia, systemic infection, etc.) and untreated or inadequately treated extrapyramidal signs and symptoms (EPS). Other important considerations in the differential diagnosis include central anticholinergic toxicity, heat stroke, drug fever and primary central nervous system (CNS) pathology.

The management of NMS should include 1) immediate discontinuation of antipsychotic drugs and other drugs not essential to concurrent therapy, 2) intensive symptomatic treatment and medical monitoring, and 3) treatment of any concomitant serious medical problems for which specific treatments are available. There is no general agreement about specific pharmacological treatment regimens for uncomplicated NMS.

If a patient requires antipsychotic drug treatment after recovery from NMS, the potential reintroduction of drug therapy should be carefully considered. The patient should be carefully monitored, since recurrences of NMS have been reported.

An encephalopathic syndrome (characterized by weakness, lethargy, fever, tremulousness and confusion, extrapyramidal symptoms, leukocytosis, elevated serum enzymes (BUN and FBS) has occurred in a few patients treated with lithium plus a neuroleptic. In some instances, the syndrome was followed by irreversible brain damage. Because of a possible causal relationship between these events and the concomitant administration if lithium and neuroleptics, patients receiving such combined therapy should be monitored closely for early evidnece of neurologic toxicity and treatment discontinued promptly if such signs appear. This encephalopathic syndrome may be similar to or the same as neuroleptic malignant syndrome (NMS).

Chlorpromazine ampuls and multiple-dose vials contain sodium bisulfite and sodium sulfite, sulfites that may cause allergic-type reactions including anaphylactic symptoms and life-threatening or less severe asthmatic episodes in certain susceptible people. The overall prevalence of sulfite sensitivity in the general population is unknown and probably low. Sulfite sensitivity is seen more frequently in asthmatic than in nonasthmatic people.

Patients with bone marrow depression or who have previously demonstrated a hypersensitivity reaction (*e.g.,* blood dyscrasias, jaundice) with a phenothiazine should not receive any phenothiazine, including chlorpromazine, unless in the judgment of the physician the potential benefits of treatment outweigh the possible hazard.

Chlorpromazine may impair mental and/or physical abilities, especially during the first few days of therapy. Therefore, caution patients about activities requiring alertness (*e.g.,* operating vehicles or machinery).

The use of alcohol with this drug should be avoided due to possible additive effects and hypotension.

Chlorpromazine may counteract the antihypertensive effect of guanethidine and related compounds.

Usage in Pregnancy: Safety for the use of chlorpromazine during pregnancy has not been established. Therefore, it is not recommended that the drug be given to pregnant patients except when, in the judgment of the physician, it is essential. The potential benefits should clearly outweigh possible hazards. There are reported instances of prolonged jaundice, extrapyramidal signs, hyperreflexia or hyporeflexia in newborn infants whose mothers received phenothiazines.

Reproductive studies in rodents have demonstrated potential for embryotoxicity, increased neonatal mortality and nursing transfer of the drug. Tests in the offspring of the drug-treated rodents demonstrate decreased performance. The possibility of permanent neurological damage cannot be excluded.

Nursing Mothers: There is evidence that chlorpromazine is excreted in the breast milk of nursing mothers. Because of the potential for serious adverse reactions in nursing infants from chlorpromazine, a decision should be made whether to discontinue nursing or to discontinue the drug, taking into account the importance of the drug to the mother.

PRECAUTIONS:

General: Given the likelihood that some patients exposed chronically to neuroleptics will develop tardive dyskinesia, it is advised that all patients in whom chronic use is contemplated be given, if possible, full information about this risk. The decision to inform patients and/or their guardians must obviously take into account the clinical circumstances and the competency of the patient to understand the information provided.

Chlorpromazine should be administered cautiously to persons with cardiovascular, liver or renal disease. There is evidence that patients with a history of hepatic encephalopathy due to cirrhosis have increased sensitivity to the CNS effects of chlorpromazine (*i.e.,* impaired cerebration and abnormal slowing of the EEG).

Because of its CNS depressant effect, chlorpromazine should be used with caution in patients with chronic respiratory disorders such as severe asthma, emphysema and acute respiratory infections, particularly in children.

Because chlorpromazine can suppress the cough reflex, aspiration of vomitus is possible.

Chlorpromazine prolongs and intensifies the action of CNS depressants such as anesthetics, barbiturates and narcotics. When chlorpromazine is administered concomitantly, about 1/4 to 1/2 the usual dosage of such agents is required. When chlorpromazine is not being administered to reduce requirements of CNS depressants, it is best to stop such depressants before starting chlorpromazine treatment. These agents may subsequently be reinstated at low doses and increased as needed.

PRECAUTIONS: *(cont'd)*

Note: chlorpromazine does *not* intensify the anticonvulsant action of barbiturates. Therefore, dosage of anticonvulsants, including barbiturates, should *not* be reduced if chlorpromazine is started. Instead, start chlorpromazine at low doses and increase as needed.

Use with caution in persons who will be exposed to extreme heat, organophosphorus insecticides, and in persons receiving atropine or related drugs.

Neuroleptic drugs elevate prolactin levels; the elevation persists during chronic administration. Tissue culture experiments indicate that approximately 1/3 of human breast cancers are prolactin-dependent *in vitro,* a factor of potential importance if the prescribing of these drugs is contemplated in a patient with a previously detected breast cancer. Although disturbances such as galactorrhea, amenorrhea, gynecomastia and impotence have been reported, the clinical significance of elevated serum prolactin levels is unknown for most patients. An increase in mammary neoplasms has been found in rodents after chronic administration of neuroleptic drugs. Neither clinical nor epidemiologic studies conducted to date, however, have shown an association between chronic administration of these drugs and mammary tumorigenesis; the available evidence is considered too limited to be conclusive at this time.

Chromosomal aberrations in spermatocytes and abnormal sperm have been demonstrated in rodents treated with certain neuroleptics.

As with all drugs which exert an anticholinergic effect, and/or cause mydriasis, chlorpromazine should be used with caution in patients with glaucoma.

Chlorpromazine diminishes the effect of oral anticoagulants.

Phenothiazines can produce alpha-adrenergic blockade.

Chlorpromazine may lower the convulsive threshold; dosage adjustments of anticonvulsants may be necessary. Potentiation of anticonvulsant effects does not occur. However, it has been reported that chlorpromazine may interfere with the metabolism of phenytoin (Dilantin) and thus precipitate phenytoin toxicity.

Concomitant administration with propranolol results in increased plasma levels of both drugs.

Thiazide diuretics may accentuate the orthostatic hypotension that may occur with phenothiazines.

The presence of phenothiazines may produce false positive phenylketonuria (PKU) test results.

Drugs which lower the seizure threshold, including phenothiazine derivatives, should not be used with metrizamide (Amipaque). As with other phenothiazine derivatives, chlorpromazine should be discontinued at least 48 hours before myelography, should not be resumed for at least 24 hours postprocedure, and should not be used for the control of nausea and vomiting occurring either prior to myelography or postprocedure with metrizamide.

Long-Term Therapy: To lessen the likelihood of adverse reactions related to cumulative drug effect, patients with a history of long-term therapy with chlorpromazine and/or other neuroleptics should be evaluated periodically to decide whether the maintenance dosage could be lowered or drug therapy discontinued.

Antiemetic Effect: The antiemetic action of chlorpromazine may mask the signs and symptoms of overdosage of other drugs and may obscure the diagnosis and treatment of other conditions such as intestinal obstruction, brain tumor and Reye's syndrome. (See WARNINGS.)

When chlorpromazine is used with cancer chemotherapeutic drugs, vomiting as a sign of the toxicity of these agents may be obscured by the antiemetic effect of chlorpromazine.

Abrupt Withdrawal: Like other phenothiazines, chlorpromazine is not known to cause psychic dependence and does not produce tolerance or addiction. There may be, however, following abrupt withdrawal of high-dose therapy, some symptoms resembling those of physical dependence such as gastritis, nausea and vomiting, dizziness and tremulousness. These symptoms can usually be avoided or reduced by gradual reduction of the dosage or by continuing concomitant anti-parkinsonism agents for several weeks after chlorpromazine is withdrawn.

ADVERSE REACTIONS:

Note: Some adverse effects of chlorpromazine may be more likely to occur, or occur with greater intensity, in patients with special medical problems, e.g., patients with mitral insufficiency or pheochromocytoma have experienced severe hypotension following recommended doses.

Drowsiness: Drowsiness, usually mild to moderate, may occur, particularly during the first or second week, after which it generally disappears. If troublesome, dosage may be lowered.

Jaundice: Overall incidence has been low, regardless of indication or dosage. Most investigators conclude it is a sensitivity reaction. Most cases occur between the second and fourth weeks of therapy. The clinical picture resembles infectious hepatitis, with laboratory features of obstructive jaundice, rather than those of parenchymal damage. It is usually promptly reversible on withdrawal of the medication; however, chronic jaundice has been reported.

There is no conclusive evidence that preexisting liver disease makes patients more susceptible to jaundice. Alcoholics with cirrhosis have been successfully treated with chlorpromazine without complications. Nevertheless, the medication should be used cautiously in patients with liver disease. Patients who have experienced jaundice with a phenothiazine should not, if possible, be reexposed to chlorpromazine or other phenothiazines.

If fever with grippe-like symptoms occurs, appropriate liver studies should be conducted. If tests indicate an abnormality, stop treatment.

Liver function tests in jaundice induced by the drug may mimic extrahepatic obstruction; withhold exploratory laparotomy until extrahepatic obstruction is confirmed.

Hematological Disorders: including agranulocytosis, eosinophilia, leukopenia, hemolytic anemia, aplastic anemia, thrombocytopenic purpura and pancytopenia have been reported.

Agranulocytosis: Warn patients to report the sudden appearance of sore throat or other signs of infection. If white blood cell and differential counts indicate cellular depression, stop treatment and start antibiotic and other suitable therapy.

Most cases have occurred between the fourth and tenth weeks of therapy; patients should be watched closely during that period.

Moderate suppression of white blood cells is not an indication for stopping treatment unless accompanied by the symptoms described above.

CARDIOVASCULAR

Hypotensive Effects: Postural hypotension, simple tachycardia, momentary fainting and dizziness may occur after the first injection; occasionally after subsequent injections; rarely, after the first oral dose. Usually recovery is spontaneous and symptoms disappear within 1/2 to 2 hours. Occasionally, these effects may be more severe and prolonged, producing a shock-like condition.

To minimize hypotension after injection, keep patient lying down and observe for at least 1/2 hour. To control hypotension, place patient in head-low position with legs raised. If a vasoconstrictor is required, norepinephrine bitartrate (Levophed) and phenylephrine hydrochloride (Neo-Synephrine) are the most suitable. Other pressor agents, including epinephrine, should not be used as they may cause a paradoxical further lowering of blood pressure.

ADVERSE REACTIONS: *(cont'd)*

EKG Change: particularly nonspecific, usually reversible Q and T wave distortions—have been observed in some patients receiving phenothiazine tranquilizers, including chlorpromazine.

Note: Sudden death, apparently due to cardiac arrest, has been reported.

CNS REACTIONS

Neuromuscular (Extrapyramidal) Reactions: Neuromuscular reactions include dystonias, motor restlessness, pseudo-parkinsonism and tardive dyskinesia, and appear to be dose-related. They are discussed in the following paragraphs:

Dystonias: Symptoms may include spasm of the neck muscles, sometimes progressing to acute, reversible torticollis; extensor rigidity of back muscles, sometimes progressing to opisthotonos; carpopedal spasm, trismus, swallowing difficulty, oculogyric crisis and protrusion of the tongue.

These usually subside within a few hours, and almost always within 24 to 48 hours after the drug has been discontinued.

In mild cases: reassurance or a barbiturate is often sufficient.*In moderate cases:* barbiturates will usually bring rapid relief.*In more severe adult cases:* the administration of an anti-parkinsonism agent, except levodopa (see prescribing information), usually produces rapid reversal of symptoms.*In children:* reassurance and barbiturates will usually control symptoms. (Or, parenteral diphenhydramine HCl (Benadryl) may be useful. See diphenhydramine HCl (Benadryl) prescribing information for appropriate children's dosage.) If appropriate treatment with anti-parkinsonism agents or diphenhydramine HCl (Benadryl) fails to reverse the signs and symptoms, the diagnosis should be reevaluated.

Suitable supportive measures such as maintaining a clear airway and adequate hydration should be employed when needed. If therapy is reinstituted, it should be at a lower dosage. Should these symptoms occur in children or pregnant patients, the drug should not be reinstituted.

Motor Restlessness: Symptoms may include agitation or jitteriness and sometimes insomnia. These symptoms often disappear spontaneously. At times these symptoms may be similar to the original neurotic or psychotic symptoms. Dosage should not be increased until these side effects have subsided.

If these symptoms become too troublesome, they can usually be controlled by a reduction of dosage or change of drug. Treatment with anti-parkinsonian agents, benzodiazepines or propranolol may be helpful.

Pseudo-Parkinsonism: Symptoms may include: mask-like facies, drooling, tremors, pillrolling motion, cogwheel rigidity and shuffling gait. In most cases these symptoms are readily controlled when an anti-parkinsonism agent is administered concomitantly. Anti-parkinsonism agents should be used only when required. Generally, therapy of a few weeks to 2 or 3 months will suffice. After this time patients should be evaluated to determine their need for continued treatment. (Note: Levodopa has not been found effective in neuroleptic-induced pseudo-parkinsonism.) Occasionally it is necessary to lower the dosage of chlorpromazine or to discontinue the drug.

Tardive Dyskinesia: As with all antipsychotic agents, tardive dyskinesia may appear in some patients on long-term therapy or may appear after drug therapy has been discontinued. The syndrome can also develop, although much less frequently, after relatively brief treatment periods at low doses. This syndrome appears in all age groups. Although its prevalence appears to be highest among elderly patients, especially elderly women, it is impossible to rely upon prevalence estimates to predict at the inception of neuroleptic treatment which patients are likely to develop the syndrome. The symptoms are persistent and in some patients appear to be irreversible. The syndrome is characterized by rhythmical involuntary movements of the tongue, face, mouth or jaw (*e.g.,* protrusion of tongue, puffing of cheeks, puckering of mouth, chewing movements). Sometimes these may be accompanied by involuntary movements of extremities. In rare instances, these involuntary movements of the extremities are the only manifestations of tardive dyskinesia. A variant of tardive dyskinesia, tardive dystonia, has also been described.

There is no known effective treatment for tardive dyskinesia; anti-parkinsonism agents do not alleviate the symptoms of this syndrome. If clinically feasible, it is suggested that all antipsychotic agents be discontinued if these symptoms appear. Should it be necessary to reinstitute treatment, or increase the dosage of the agent, or switch to a different antipsychotic agent, the syndrome may be masked.

It has been reported that fine vermicular movements of the tongue may be an early sign of the syndrome and if the medication is stopped at that time the syndrome may not develop.

Adverse Behavioral Effects: Psychotic symptoms and catatonic-like states have been reported rarely.

Other CNS Effects: Neuroleptic Malignant Syndrome (NMS) has been reported in association with antipsychotic drugs. (See WARNINGS.)

Cerebral edema has been reported.

Convulsive seizures (*petit mal* and *grand mal*) have been reported, particularly in patients with EEG abnormalities or history of such disorders.

Abnormality of the cerebrospinal fluid proteins has also been reported.

Allergic Reactions of a mild urticarial type or photosensitivity are seen. Avoid undue exposure to sun. More severe reactions, including exfoliative dermatitis, have been reported occasionally.

Contact dermatitis has been reported in nursing personnel; accordingly, the use of rubber gloves when administering chlorpromazine liquid or injectable is recommended.

In addition, asthma, laryngeal edema, angioneurotic edema and anaphylactoid reactions have been reported.

Endocrine Disorders: Lactation and moderate breast engorgement may occur in females on large doses. If persistent, lower dosage or withdraw drug. False-positive pregnancy tests have been reported, but are less likely to occur when a serum test is used. Amenorrhea and gynecomastia have also been reported. Hyperglycemia, hypoglycemia and glycosuria have been reported.

Autonomic Reactions: Occasional dry mouth; nasal congestion; nausea; obstipation; constipation; adynamic ileus; urinary retention; priapism; miosis and mydriasis, atonic colon, ejaculatory disorders/impotence.

Special Considerations in Long-Term Therapy: Skin pigmentation and ocular changes have occurred in some patients taking substantial doses of chlorpromazine for prolonged periods.

Skin Pigmentation: Rare instances of skin pigmentation have been observed in hospitalized mental patients, primarily females who have received the drug usually for 3 years or more in dosages ranging from 500 mg to 1500 mg daily. The pigmentary changes, restricted to exposed areas of the body, range from an almost imperceptible darkening of the skin to a slate gray color, sometimes with a violet hue. Histological examination reveals a pigment, chiefly in the dermis, which is probably a melanin-like complex. The pigmentation may fade following discontinuance of the drug.

Ocular Changes: Ocular changes have occurred more frequently than skin pigmentation and have been observed both in pigmented and nonpigmented patients receiving chlorpromazine usually for 2 years or more in dosages of 300 mg daily and higher. Eye changes are

ADVERSE REACTIONS: *(cont'd)*

characterized by deposition of fine particulate matter in the lens and cornea. In more advanced cases, star-shaped opacities have also been observed in the anterior portion of the lens. The nature of the eye deposits has not yet been determined. A small number of patients with more severe ocular changes have had some visual impairment. In addition to these corneal and lenticular changes, epithelial keratopathy and pigmentary retinopathy have been reported. Reports suggest that the eye lesions may regress after withdrawal of the drug.

Since the occurrence of eye changes seems to be related to dosage levels and/or duration of therapy, it is suggested that long-term patients on moderate to high dosage levels have periodic ocular examinations.

Etiology: The etiology of both of these reactions is not clear, but exposure to light, along with dosage/duration of therapy, appears to be the most significant factor. If either of these reactions is observed, the physician should weigh the benefits of continued therapy against the possible risks and, on the merits of the individual case, determine whether or not to continue present therapy, lower the dosage, or withdraw the drug.

Other Adverse Reactions: Mild fever may occur after large IM doses. Hyperpyrexia has been reported. Increases in appetite and weight sometimes occur. Peripheral edema and a systemic lupus erythematosus-like syndrome have been reported.

Note: There have been occasional reports of sudden death in patients receiving phenothiazines. In some cases, the cause appeared to be cardiac arrest or asphyxia due to failure of the cough reflex.

OVERDOSAGE:

(See also ADVERSE REACTIONS.)

Symptoms: Primarily symptoms of central nervous system depression to the point of somnolence or coma. Hypotension and extrapyramidal symptoms.

Other possible manifestations include agitation and restlessness, convulsions, fever, autonomic reactions such as dry mouth and ileus, EKG changes and cardiac arrhythmias.

Treatment: It is important to determine other medications taken by the patient since multiple drug therapy is common in overdosage situations. Treatment is essentially symptomatic and supportive. Early gastric lavage is helpful. Keep patient under observation and maintain an open airway, since involvement of the extrapyramidal mechanism may produce dysphagia and respiratory difficulty in severe overdosage. **Do not attempt to induce emesis because a dystonic reaction of the head or neck may develop that could result in aspiration of vomitus.** Extrapyramidal symptoms may be treated with anti-parkinsonism drugs, barbiturates, or diphenhydramine HCl (Benadryl). See prescribing information for these products. Care should be taken to avoid increasing respiratory depression.

If administration of a stimulant is desirable, amphetamine, dextroamphetamine, or caffeine with sodium benzoate is recommended. Stimulants that may cause convulsions (*e.g.*, picrotoxin or pentylenetetrazol) should be avoided.

If hypotension occurs, the standard measures for managing circulatory shock should be initiated. If it is desirable to administer a vasoconstrictor, norepinephrine bitartrate (Levophed) and phenylephrine HCl (Neo-Synephrine) are most suitable. Other pressor agents, including epinephrine, are not recommended because phenothiazine derivatives may reverse the usual elevating action of these agents and cause a further lowering of blood pressure.

Limited experience indicates that phenothiazines are *not*dialyzable.

Special note on sustained release capsules: Since much of the capsule medication is coated for gradual release, therapy directed at reversing the effects of the ingested drug and at supporting the patient should be continued for as long as overdosage symptoms remain. Saline cathartics are useful for hastening evacuation of pellets that have not already released medication.

DOSAGE AND ADMINISTRATION:

ADULTS

Adjust dosage to individual and the severity of his condition, recognizing that the milligram for milligram potency relationship among all dosage forms has not been precisely established clinically. It is important to increase dosage until symptoms are controlled. Dosage should be increased more gradually in debilitated or emaciated patients. In continued therapy, gradually reduce dosage to the lowest effective maintenance level, after symptoms have been controlled for a reasonable period.

In general, dosage recommendations for other oral forms of the drug may be applied to the sustained release capsules on the basis of total daily dosage in milligrams.

The 100 mg and 200 mg tablets are for use in severe neuropsychiatric conditions.

Increase parenteral dosage only if hypotension has not occurred. Before using IM, see IMPORTANT NOTES ON INJECTION.

Elderly Patients: In general, dosages in the lower range are sufficient for most elderly patients. Since they appear to be more susceptible to hypotension and neuromuscular reactions, such patients should be observed closely. Dosage should be tailored to the individual, response carefully monitored, and dosage adjusted accordingly. Dosage should be increased more gradually in elderly patients.

Psychotic Disorders

Increase dosage gradually until symptoms are controlled. Maximum improvement may not be seen for weeks or even months. Continue optimum dosage for 2 weeks; then gradually reduce dosage to the lowest effective maintenance level. Daily dosage of 200 mg is not unusual. Some patients require higher dosages (*e.g.*, 800 mg daily is not uncommon in discharged mental patients).

Hospitalized Patients

Acutely Disturbed or Manic: *IM:* 25 mg (1 ml). If necessary, give additional 25 to 50 mg injection in 1 hour. Increase subsequent IM doses gradually over several days—up to 400 mg q4-6h in exceptionally severe cases—until patient is controlled. Usually patient becomes quiet and cooperative within 24 to 48 hours and oral doses may be substituted and increased until the patient is calm. 500 mg a day is generally sufficient. While gradual increases to 2,000 mg a day or more may be necessary, there is usually little therapeutic gain to be achieved by exceeding 1,000 mg a day for extended periods. In general, dosage levels should be lower in the elderly, the emaciated and the debilitated.

Less Acutely Disturbed: *Oral:* 25 mg t.i.d. Increase gradually until effective dose is reached—usually 400 mg daily.

Outpatients: *Oral:* 10 mg t.i.d. or q.i.d., or 25 mg b.i.d. or t.i.d.

More Severe Cases: *Oral:* 25 mg t.i.d. After 1 or 2 days, daily dosage may be increased by 20 to 50 mg at semiweekly intervals until patient becomes calm and cooperative.

Prompt Control of Severe Symptoms: *IM:* 25 mg (1 ml). If necessary, repeat in 1 hour. Subsequent doses should be oral, 25-50 mg t.i.d.

Nausea and Vomiting

Nausea and Vomiting: *Oral:* 10 to 25 mg q4-6h, p.r.n., increased, if necessary. *IM:* 25 mg (1 ml). If no hypotension occurs, give 25 to 50 mg q3-4h, p.r.n., until vomiting stops. Then switch to oral dosage. *Rectal:* One 100 mg suppository q6-8h, p.r.n. In some patients, half this dose will do.

DOSAGE AND ADMINISTRATION: *(cont'd)*

During Surgery: *IM:* 12.5 mg (0.5 ml). Repeat in 1/2 hour if necessary and if no hypotension occurs. *IV:* 2 mg per fractional injection, at 2-minute intervals. Do not exceed 25 mg. Dilute to 1 mg/ml, *i.e.,* 1 ml (25 mg) mixed with 24 ml of saline.

Presurgical Apprehension

Oral: 25 to 50 mg, 2 to 3 hours before the operation.

IM: 12.5 to 25 mg (0.5-1 ml), 1 to 2 hours before operation.

Intractable Hiccups

Oral: 25 to 50 mg t.i.d. or q.i.d. If symptoms persist for 2-3 days, give 25 to 50 mg (1 to 2 ml) IM. Should symptoms persist, use *slow* IV infusion with patient flat in bed: 25 to 50 mg (1-2 ml) in 500 to 1,000 ml of saline. Follow blood pressure closely.

Acute Intermittent Porphyria

Oral: 25 to 50 mg t.i.d. or q.i.d. Can usually be discontinued after several weeks, but maintenance therapy may be necessary for some patients.

IM: 25 mg (1 ml) t.i.d. or q.i.d. until patient can take oral therapy.

Tetanus

IM: 25 to 50 mg (1-2 ml) given 3 or 4 times daily, usually in conjunction with barbiturates. Total doses and frequency of administration must be determined by the patient's response, starting with low doses and increasing gradually. *IV:* 25 to 50 mg (1 to 2 ml). Dilute to at least 1 mg per ml and administer at a rate of 1 mg per minute.

CHILDREN

Chlorpromazine should generally not be used in children under 6 months of age except where potentially lifesaving. It should not be used in conditions for which specific children's dosages have not been established.

Severe Behavioral Problems

Outpatients: Select route of administration according to severity of patient's condition and increase dosage gradually as required. *Oral:* 1/4 mg/lb body weight q4-6h, p.r.n. (*e.g.,* for 40 lb child—10 mg q4-6h). *Rectal:* 1/2 mg/lb body weight every 6 to 8 hours, p.r.n. (*e.g.,* for 20-30 lb child—half a 25 mg suppositoryevery 6 to 8 hours). *IM:* 1/4 mg/lb body weight every 6 to 8 hours, p.r.n.

Hospitalized Patients: As with outpatients, start with low doses and increase dosage gradually. In severe behavior disorders or psychotic conditions, higher dosages (50 to 100 mg daily, and in older children, 200 mg daily or more) may be necessary. There is little evidence that behavior improvement in severely disturbed mentally retarded patients is further enhanced by doses beyond 500 mg per day. *Maximum IM Dosage:* Children up to 5 years (or 50 lbs), not over 40 mg/day; 5-12 years (or 50-100 lbs), not over 75 mg/day except in unmanageable cases.

Nausea and Vomiting

Dosage and frequency of administration should be adjusted according to the severity of the symptoms and response of the patient. The duration of activity following intramuscular administration may last up to 12 hours. Subsequent doses may be given by the same route if necessary. *Oral:* 1/4 mg/lb body weight (*e.g.,* 40 lb child-10 mg q4-6h). *Rectal:* 1/2 mg/lb body weight q6-8h p.r.n. (*e.g.,* 20 to 30 lb child—half of 25 mg suppository q6-8h). *IM:* 1/4 mg/lb body weight q6-8h, p.r.n.*Maximum IM Dosage:* Children up to 5 yrs. (or 50 lbs), not over 40 mg/day; 5-12 yrs. (or 50-100 lbs), not over 75 mg/day except in severe cases.

During Surgery: *IM:* 1/8 mg/lb body weight. Repeat in 1/2 hour if necessary and if no hypotension occurs.*IV:* 1 mg per fractional injection at 2-minute intervals and not exceeding recommended IM dosage. Always dilute to 1 mg/ml, i.e., 1 ml (25 mg) mixed with 24 ml of saline.

Presurgical Apprehension

1/4 mg/lb body weight, either *orally* 2 to 3 hours before operation, or *IM* 1 to 2 hours before.

Tetanus

IM or IV: 1/4 mg/lb body weight q6-8h. When given IV, dilute to at least 1 mg/ml and administer at rate of 1 mg per 2 minutes. In children up to 50 lbs, do not exceed 40 mg daily; 50 to 100 lbs, do not exceed 75 mg, except in severe cases.

Important Notes On Injection: Inject slowly, deep into upper outer quadrant of buttock.

Because of possible hypotensive effects, reserve parenteral administration for bedfast patients or for acute ambulatory cases, and keep patient lying down for at least 1/2 hour after injection. If irritation is a problem, dilute Injection with saline or 2% procaine; mixing with other agents in the syringe is not recommended. Subcutaneous injection is not advised. Avoid injecting undiluted chlorpromazine into vein. IV route is only for severe hiccups, surgery and tetanus.

Because of the possibility of contact dermatitis, avoid getting solution on hands or clothing. This solution should be protected from light. This is a clear, colorless to pale yellow solution; a slight yellowish discoloration will not alter potency. If markedly discolored, solution should be discarded. For information on sulfite sensitivity, see the WARNINGS section of this labeling.

Note on Concentrate: When the Concentrate is to be used, add the desired dosage of Concentrate to 60 ml (2 fl oz) or more of diluent *just prior to administration.* This will insure palatability and stability. Vehicles suggested for dilution are: tomato or fruit juice, milk, simple syrup, orange syrup, carbonated beverages, coffee, tea, or water. Semisolid foods (soups, puddings, etc.) may also be used. The Concentrate is light sensitive; it should be protected from light and dispensed in amber glass bottles. *Refrigeration is not required.*

HOW SUPPLIED - RATED THERAPEUTICALLY EQUIVALENT:

Concentrate - Oral - 30 mg/ml

120 ml	$5.95	Chlorpromazine Hcl, Roxane	00054-3144-50
120 ml	$8.92	Chlorpromazine Hcl, H.C.F.A. F F P	99999-0797-01
120 ml	**$32.40**	**THORAZINE, SKB Pharms**	**00007-5047-44**

Concentrate - Oral - 100 mg/ml

240 ml	$19.35	Chlorpromazine Hcl, Harber Pharm	51432-0554-19
240 ml	$20.12	Chlorpromazine Hcl, Roxane	00054-3146-58
240 ml	$20.27	Chlorpromazine HCl Concentrate, Alpharma	00472-0742-98
240 ml	$30.16	Chlorpromazine HCl, H.C.F.A. F F P	99999-0797-02
240 ml	**$175.15**	**THORAZINE, SKB Pharms**	**00007-5049-48**

Injection, Solution - Intramuscular; - 25 mg/ml

1 ml x 10	**$72.55**	**THORAZINE, SKB Pharms**	**00007-5060-11**
1 ml x 25	$26.13	Chlorpromazine Hcl, Elkins Sinn	00641-1397-35
2 ml x 10	**$102.50**	**THORAZINE, SKB Pharms**	**00007-5061-11**
2 ml x 25	$28.95	Chlorpromazine Hcl, Elkins Sinn	00641-1398-35
2 ml x 25	$31.25	Chlorpromazine Hcl, Consolidated Midland	00223-7325-02
2 ml x 25	$52.13	Chlorpromazine Hcl, Steris Labs	00402-0350-82
2 ml x 25	$59.10	Chlorpromazine HCl, Schein Pharm (US)	00364-2180-42
2 ml x 100	**$808.20**	**THORAZINE, SKB Pharms**	**00007-5061-20**
10 ml	$6.60	Chlorpromazine Hcl, Steris Labs	00402-0261-10
10 ml	$7.43	Chlorpromazine, Rugby	00536-3850-70
10 ml	$8.67	Chlorpromazine Hcl, Geneva Pharms	00781-3280-70
10 ml	$9.00	Chlorpromazine, IDE-Interstate	00814-1693-40
10 ml	$11.00	Chlorpromazine HCl, Schein Pharm (US)	00364-6664-54

HOW SUPPLIED - RATED THERAPEUTICALLY EQUIVALENT: *(cont'd)*

10 ml	$12.00	Chlorpromazine Hcl, Goldline Labs	00182-0859-63
10 ml	**$47.20**	**THORAZINE, SKB Pharms**	**00007-5062-01**

Syrup - Oral - 10 mg/5ml

120 ml	**$21.90**	**THORAZINE, SKB Pharms**	**00007-5072-44**

HOW SUPPLIED - NOT RATED EQUIVALENT:

Capsule, Gelatin, Sustained Action - Oral - 30 mg

50's	**$49.45**	**THORAZINE, SKB Pharms**	**00007-5063-15**

Capsule, Gelatin, Sustained Action - Oral - 75 mg

50's	**$66.45**	**THORAZINE, SKB Pharms**	**00007-5064-15**

Capsule, Gelatin, Sustained Action - Oral - 150 mg

50's	**$89.55**	**THORAZINE, SKB Pharms**	**00007-5066-15**
500's	**$739.95**	**THORAZINE, SKB Pharms**	**00007-5066-25**

Capsule, Gelatin, Sustained Action - Oral - 200 mg

50's	**$90.50**	**THORAZINE, SKB Pharms**	**00007-5067-15**

Suppository - Rectal - 25 mg

12's	**$35.50**	**THORAZINE, SKB Pharms**	**00007-5070-03**

Suppository - Rectal - 100 mg

12's	**$45.00**	**THORAZINE, SKB Pharms**	**00007-5071-03**

Tablet, Plain Coated - Oral - 10 mg

100's	$4.44	Chlorpromazine, HL Moore Drug Exch	00839-1155-06
100's	$4.54	Chlorpromazine Hcl, Rosemont	00832-0300-00
100's	$4.74	Chlorpromazine Hcl, Aligen Independ	00405-4196-01
100's	$5.45	Chlorpromazine HCl, Rugby	00536-4903-01
100's	$5.60	Chlorpromazine Hcl, Qualitest Pharms	00603-2808-21
100's	$5.73	Chlorpromazine HCl, Schein Pharm (US)	00364-0380-01
100's	$5.90	Chlorpromazine Hcl, United Res	00677-0502-01
100's	$5.95	Chlorpromazine Hcl, Major Pharms	00904-2075-60
100's	$5.95	Chlorpromazine Hcl, Major Pharms	00904-2161-60
100's	$6.70	Chlorpromazine HCl, Geneva Pharms	00781-1715-01
100's	$6.95	Chlorpromazine Hcl, Parmed Pharms	00349-2366-01
100's	$7.76	Chlorpromazine Hcl, Major Pharms	00904-2161-61
100's	$11.48	Chlorpromazine HCl, Geneva Pharms	00781-1715-13
100's	$29.94	Chlorpromazine, RID	54807-0820-01
100's	**$31.70**	**THORAZINE, SKB Pharms**	**00007-5073-21**
100's	**$37.05**	**THORAZINE, SKB Pharms**	**00007-5073-20**
1000's	$19.25	Chlorpromazine Hcl, Major Pharms	00904-2161-80
1000's	$34.88	Chlorpromazine Hcl, Rugby	00536-4903-10
1000's	$36.34	Chlorpromazine Hcl, Rosemont	00832-0300-10
1000's	$38.60	Chlorpromazine Hcl, Qualitest Pharms	00603-2808-32

Tablet, Plain Coated - Oral - 25 mg

100's	$6.14	Chlorpromazine Hcl, HL Moore Drug Exch	00839-1151-06
100's	$7.40	Chlorpromazine Hcl, Qualitest Pharms	00603-2809-21
100's	$7.50	Chlorpromazine Hcl, Goldline Labs	00182-0474-01
100's	$7.50	Chlorpromazine Hcl, Rosemont	00832-0301-00
100's	$7.89	Chlorpromazine Hcl 25, Aligen Independ	00405-4197-01
100's	$8.00	Chlorpromazine HCl, Rugby	00536-4906-01
100's	$8.01	Chlorpromazine Hcl, Major Pharms	00904-2052-61
100's	$8.75	Chlorpromazine Hcl, Major Pharms	00904-2052-60
100's	$8.75	Chlorpromazine Hcl, Major Pharms	00904-2076-60
100's	$8.85	Chlorpromazine Hcl, United Res	00677-0454-01
100's	$8.90	Chlorpromazine HCl, Schein Pharm (US)	00364-0381-01
100's	$9.38	Chlorpromazine HCl, Geneva Pharms	00781-1716-01
100's	$9.45	Chlorpromazine Hcl, Parmed Pharms	00349-2040-01
100's	$10.17	Chlorpromazine HCl, Geneva Pharms	00781-1716-13
100's	$40.50	Chlorpromazine, RID	54807-0821-01
100's	**$47.75**	**THORAZINE, SKB Pharms**	**00007-5074-21**
100's	**$50.15**	**THORAZINE, SKB Pharms**	**00007-5074-20**
100's	$58.80	Chlorpromazine Hcl, Parmed Pharms	00349-2040-10
1000's	$43.00	Chlorpromazine Hcl, Rosemont	00832-0301-10
1000's	$45.00	Chlorpromazine Hcl, Major Pharms	00904-2052-80
1000's	$45.26	Chlorpromazine Hcl, Aligen Independ	00405-4197-03
1000's	$47.36	Chlorpromazine Hcl, Rugby	00536-4906-10
1000's	$51.40	Chlorpromazine Hcl, Qualitest Pharms	00603-2809-32
1000's	$52.45	Chlorpromazine Hcl, United Res	00677-0454-10
1000's	$52.90	Chlorpromazine Hcl, Goldline Labs	00182-0474-10
1000's	$60.68	Chlorpromazine HCl, Geneva Pharms	00781-1716-10
1000's	**$453.80**	**THORAZINE, SKB Pharms**	**00007-5074-30**

Tablet, Plain Coated - Oral - 50 mg

100's	$6.82	Chlorpromazine Hcl, HL Moore Drug Exch	00839-1158-06
100's	$7.98	Chlorpromazine Hcl, Qualitest Pharms	00603-2810-21
100's	$9.39	Chlorpromazine Hcl, Major Pharms	00904-2053-61
100's	$10.85	Chlorpromazine Hcl, Major Pharms	00904-2053-60
100's	$10.85	Chlorpromazine Hcl, Major Pharms	00904-2077-60
100's	$10.95	Chlorpromazine HCl, Rugby	00536-4915-01
100's	$10.95	Chlorpromazine Hcl, United Res	00677-0455-01
100's	$10.97	Chlorpromazine HCl, Schein Pharm (US)	00364-0382-01
100's	$11.85	Chlorpromazine Hcl, Parmed Pharms	00349-2041-01
100's	$13.27	Chlorpromazine Hcl, Goldline Labs	00182-0475-01
100's	$13.27	Chlorpromazine HCl, Geneva Pharms	00781-1717-01
100's	$13.27	Chlorpromazine Hcl, Rosemont	00832-0302-00
100's	$13.30	Chlorpromazine Hcl 50, Aligen Independ	00405-4198-01
100's	$13.59	Chlorpromazine HCl, Geneva Pharms	00781-1717-13
100's	$50.57	Chlorpromazine, RID	54807-0822-01
100's	**$52.00**	**THORAZINE, SKB Pharms**	**00007-5076-21**
100's	**$62.60**	**THORAZINE, SKB Pharms**	**00007-5076-20**
1000's	$29.60	Chlorpromazine Hcl, HL Moore Drug Exch	00839-1158-16
1000's	$49.30	Chlorpromazine Hcl, Major Pharms	00904-2053-80
1000's	$55.86	Chlorpromazine HCl, Rugby	00536-4915-10
1000's	$56.00	Chlorpromazine Hcl, Rosemont	00832-0302-10
1000's	$58.20	Chlorpromazine Hcl, Goldline Labs	00182-0475-10
1000's	$62.20	Chlorpromazine Hcl, United Res	00677-0455-10
1000's	$62.22	Chlorpromazine Hcl, Qualitest Pharms	00603-2810-32
1000's	$69.47	Chlorpromazine Hcl, Aligen Independ	00405-4198-03
1000's	$81.20	Chlorpromazine Hcl, Parmed Pharms	00349-2041-10
1000's	$81.27	Chlorpromazine HCl, Geneva Pharms	00781-1717-10
1000's	**$566.40**	**THORAZINE, SKB Pharms**	**00007-5076-30**

Tablet, Plain Coated - Oral - 100 mg

100's	$10.52	Chlorpromazine Hcl, Major Pharms	00904-2191-61
100's	$10.55	Chlorpromazine Hcl, Goldline Labs	00182-0476-01
100's	$10.55	Chlorpromazine Hcl, Rosemont	00832-0303-00
100's	$11.11	Chlorpromazine Hcl 100, Aligen Independ	00405-4199-01
100's	$12.00	Chlorpromazine HCl, Schein Pharm (US)	00364-0383-01
100's	$12.46	Chlorpromazine Hcl, Qualitest Pharms	00603-2811-21
100's	$12.50	Chlorpromazine Hcl, United Res	00677-0456-01
100's	$12.50	Chlorpromazine Hcl, Major Pharms	00904-2078-60

HOW SUPPLIED - NOT RATED EQUIVALENT: *(cont'd)*

100's	$13.50	Chlorpromazine HCl, Rugby	00536-4916-01
100's	$14.71	Chlorpromazine Hcl, Parmed Pharms	00349-2367-01
100's	$14.71	Chlorpromazine HCl, Geneva Pharms	00781-1718-01
100's	$17.80	Chlorpromazine HCl, Geneva Pharms	00781-1718-13
100's	$31.45	Chlorpromazine Hcl, Major Pharms	00904-2191-60
100's	$65.25	Chlorpromazine, RID	54807-0823-01
100's	**$80.75**	**THORAZINE, SKB Pharms**	**00007-5077-20**
1000's	$69.75	Chlorpromazine Hcl, Major Pharms	00904-2191-80
1000's	$73.85	Chlorpromazine Hcl, Goldline Labs	00182-0476-10
1000's	$73.85	Chlorpromazine Hcl, Rosemont	00832-0303-10
1000's	$77.31	Chlorpromazine Hcl, Rugby	00536-4916-10
1000's	$77.74	Chlorpromazine Hcl, Aligen Independ	00405-4199-03
1000's	$79.51	Chlorpromazine Hcl, Qualitest Pharms	00603-2811-32
1000's	$102.38	Chlorpromazine HCl, Geneva Pharms	00781-1718-10
1000's	**$732.30**	**THORAZINE, SKB Pharms**	**00007-5077-30**

Tablet, Plain Coated - Oral - 200 mg

100's	$9.30	Chlorpromazine, HL Moore Drug Exch	00839-1146-06
100's	$13.00	Chlorpromazine Hcl, Goldline Labs	00182-0477-01
100's	$13.00	Chlorpromazine Hcl, Rosemont	00832-0304-00
100's	$13.68	Chlorpromazine Hcl 200, Aligen Independ	00405-4200-01
100's	$13.95	Chlorpromazine Hcl, Major Pharms	00904-2079-60
100's	$13.95	Chlorpromazine Hcl, Major Pharms	00904-2192-60
100's	$14.23	Chlorpromazine HCl, Schein Pharm (US)	00364-0384-01
100's	$14.95	Chlorpromazine HCl, Rugby	00536-4918-01
100's	$14.96	Chlorpromazine Hcl, Qualitest Pharms	00603-2812-21
100's	$14.98	Chlorpromazine Hcl, United Res	00677-0787-01
100's	$18.95	Chlorpromazine Hcl, Parmed Pharms	00349-2043-01
100's	$18.95	Chlorpromazine HCl, Geneva Pharms	00781-1719-01
100's	$20.57	Chlorpromazine Hcl, Major Pharms	00904-2192-61
100's	$21.99	Chlorpromazine HCl, Geneva Pharms	00781-1719-13
100's	$82.88	Chlorpromazine, RID	54807-0824-01
100's	**$83.85**	**THORAZINE, SKB Pharms**	**00007-5079-21**
100's	**$102.60**	**THORAZINE, SKB Pharms**	**00007-5079-20**
1000's	$94.90	Chlorpromazine Hcl, Major Pharms	00904-2192-80
1000's	$96.20	Chlorpromazine Hcl, Parmed Pharms	00349-2043-10
1000's	$105.00	Chlorpromazine Hcl, Goldline Labs	00182-0477-10
1000's	$105.00	Chlorpromazine Hcl, Rosemont	00832-0304-10
1000's	$106.80	Chlorpromazine Hcl, Rugby	00536-4918-10
1000's	$128.05	Chlorpromazine HCl, Geneva Pharms	00781-1719-10
1000's	**$935.20**	**THORAZINE, SKB Pharms**	**00007-5079-30**

CHLORPROPAMIDE *(000798)*

CATEGORIES: Antidiabetic Agents; Blood Glucose Regulators; Diabetes; Diabetes Mellitus; Hormones; Hyperglycemia; Sulfonylureas; Weight Loss; Pregnancy Category C; FDA Approval Pre 1982

BRAND NAMES: *Abemide* (Japan); *Anti-D*; *Apo-Chlorpropamide* (Canada); *Arodoc*; *Arodoc C* (Japan); Chlorabetic; *Chlordiabet*; *Chlormide* (Japan); *Chlorpropamide Medochemie*; *Chlorprosil*; *Copamide*; *Deavynfar* (Mexico); *Diabeedol*; *Diabemide*; *Diabenil*; *Diabenese* (Canada, England, France, Mexico); *Diabexan*; *Diabiclor* (Mexico); *Diabines*; **Diabinese**; *Diabitex*; *Diamide*; *Diatanpin*; *Dibecon*; *Dibetes*; *Gliconorm*; Glucamide; *Glycemin*; *Glycermin*; *Glymese*; *Hypomide*; *Insilange*; *Insilange C* (Japan); *Insogen* (Mexico); Insulase; *Meldian*; *Mellitos*; *Mellitos C* (Japan); *Melormin*; *Milligon*; *Neo-Toltinon*; *Norgluc*; *Normoglic*; *Novopropamide* (Canada); *Orodiabin*; *Promide*; *Propamide*; *Sucranase*; *Tanpinin*; *Tesmel*
(International brand names outside U.S. in italics)

FORMULARIES: Aetna; BC-BS; CIGNA; FHP; Humana; Kaiser; Medco; Medi-Cal; PruCare; United

DESCRIPTION:

Chlorpropamide, is an oral blood-glucose-lowering drug of the sulfonylurea class. Chlorpropamide is 1-(p-Chlorophenyl) sulfonyl)-3-propylurea, $C_{10}H_{13}ClN_2O_3S$.

Chlorpropamide is a white crystalline powder, that has a slight odor. It is practically insoluble in water at pH 7.3 (solubility at pH 6 is 2.2 mg/ml). It is soluble in alcohol and moderately soluble in chloroform. The molecular weight of chlorpropamide is 276.74. Chlorpropamide is available as 100 mg and 250 mg tablets.

Inert Ingredient: alginic acid; Blue 1 Lake; hydroxypropyl cellulose; magnesium stearate; precipitated calcium carbonate; sodium lauryl sulfate; starch.

CLINICAL PHARMACOLOGY:

Chlorpropamide appears to lower the blood glucose acutely by stimulating the release of insulin from the pancreas, an effect dependent upon functioning beta cells in the pancreatic islets. The mechanism by which Chlorpropamide lowers blood glucose during long-term administration has not been clearly established. Extra-pancreatic effects may play a part in the mechanism of action of oral sulfonylurea hypoglycemic drugs. While chlorpropamide is a sulfonamide derivative, it is devoid of antibacterial activity.

Chlorpropamide may also prove effective in controlling certain patients who have experienced primary or secondary failure to other sulfonylurea agents.

A method developed which permits easy measurement of the drug in blood is available on request.

Chlorpropamide does not interfere with the usual tests to detect albumin in the urine.

Chlorpropamide is absorbed rapidly from the gastrointestinal tract. Within one hour after a single oral dose, it is readily detectable in the blood, and the level reaches a maximum within two to four hours. It undergoes metabolism in humans and it is excreted in the urine as unchanged drug and as hydroxylated or hydrolyzed metabolites. The biological half-life of chlorpropamide averages about 36 hours. Within 96 hours, 80-90% of a single oral dose is excreted in the urine. However, long-term administration of therapeutic doses does not result in undue accumulation in the blood, since absorption and excretion rates become stabilized in about 5 to 7 days after the initiation of therapy.

Chlorpropamide exerts a hypoglycemic effect in normal humans within one hour, becoming maximal at 3 to 6 hours and persisting for at least 24 hours. The potency of Chlorpropamide is approximately six times that of tolbutamide. Some experimental results suggest that its increased duration of action may be the result of slower excretion and absence of significant deactivation.

INDICATIONS AND USAGE:

Chlorpropamide is indicated as an adjunct to diet to lower the blood glucose in patients with non-insulin-dependent diabetes mellitus (type II) whose hyperglycemia cannot be controlled by diet alone.

INDICATIONS AND USAGE: *(cont'd)*

In initiating treatment for non-insulin-dependent diabetes, diet should be emphasized as the primary form of treatment. Caloric restriction and weight loss are essential in the obese diabetic patient. Proper dietary management alone may be effective in controlling the blood glucose and symptoms of hyperglycemia. The importance of regular physical activity should also be stressed, and cardiovascular risk factors should be identified and corrective measures taken where possible.

If this treatment program fails to reduce symptoms and/or blood glucose, the use of an oral sulfonylurea or insulin should be considered. Use of Chlorpropamide must be viewed by both the physician and patient as a treatment in addition to diet, and not as a substitute for diet or as a convenient mechanism for avoiding dietary restraint. Furthermore, loss of blood glucose control on diet alone may be transient, thus requiring only short-term administration of Chlorpropamide.

During maintenance programs, Chlorpropamide should be discontinued if satisfactory lowering of blood glucose is no longer achieved. Judgments should be based on regular clinical and laboratory evaluations.

In considering the use of Chlorpropamide in asymptomatic patients, it should be recognized that controlling the blood glucose in non-insulin-dependent diabetes has not been definitely established to be effective in preventing the long-term cardiovascular or neural complications of diabetes.

CONTRAINDICATIONS:

Chlorpropamide is contraindicated in patients with:

1. Known hypersensitivity to the drug.

2. Diabetic ketoacidosis, with or without coma. This condition should be treated with insulin.

WARNINGS:

SPECIAL WARNING ON INCREASED RISK OF CARDIOVASCULAR MORTALITY

The administration of oral hypoglycemic drugs has been reported to be associated with increased cardiovascular mortality as compared to treatment with diet alone or diet plus insulin. This warning is based on the study conducted by the University Group Diabetes Program (UGDP), a long-term prospective clinical trial designed to evaluate the effectiveness of glucose-lowering drugs in preventing or delaying vascular complications in patients with non-insulin-dependent diabetes. The study involved 823 patients who were randomly assigned to one of four treatment groups (*Diabetes*, 19 (supp. 2): 747-830, 1970.)

UGDP reported that patients treated for 5 to 8 years with diet plus a fixed dose of tolbutamide (1.5 grams per day) had a rate of cardiovascular mortality approximately 2 1/2 times that of patients treated with diet alone. A significant increase in total mortality was not observed, but the use of tolbutamide was discontinued based on the increase in cardiovascular mortality, thus limiting the opportunity for the study to show an increase in overall mortality. Despite controversy regarding the interpretation of these results, the findings of the UGDP study provide an adequate basis for this warning. The patient should be informed of the potential risks and advantages of Chlorpropamide and of alternative modes of therapy.

Although only one drug in the sulfonylurea class (tolbutamide) was included in this study, it is prudent from a safety standpoint to consider that this warning may also apply to other oral hypoglycemic drugs in this class, in view of their close similarities in mode of action and chemical structure.

PRECAUTIONS:

GENERAL

Hypoglycemia: All sulfonylurea drugs are capable of producing severe hypoglycemia. Proper patient selection, dosage, and instructions are important to avoid hypoglycemic episodes. Renal or hepatic insufficiency may cause elevated blood levels of Chlorpropamide and the latter may also diminish gluconeogenic capacity, both of which increase the risk of serious hypoglycemic reactions. Elderly, debilitated or malnourished patients, and those with adrenal or pituitary insufficiency are particularly susceptible to the hypoglycemic action of glucose-lowering drugs. Hypoglycemia may be difficult to recognize in the elderly, and in people who are taking beta-adrenergic blocking drugs. Hypoglycemia is more likely to occur when caloric intake is deficient, after severe or prolonged exercise, when alcohol is ingested, or when more than one glucose-lowering drug is used.

Because of the long half-life of Chlorpropamide, patients who become hypoglycemic during therapy require careful supervision of the dose and frequent feedings for at least 3 to 5 days. Hospitalization and intravenous glucose may be necessary.

Loss Of Control Of Blood Glucose: When a patient stabilized on any diabetic regimen is exposed to stress such as fever, trauma, infection, or surgery, a loss of control may occur. At such times, it may be necessary to discontinue Chlorpropamide and administer insulin.

The effectiveness of any oral hypoglycemic drug, including Chlorpropamide, in lowering blood glucose to a desired level decreases in many patients over a period of time, which may be due to progression of the severity of the diabetes or to diminished responsiveness to the drug. This phenomenon is known as secondary failure, to distinguish it from primary failure in which the drug is ineffective in an individual patient when first given.

INFORMATION FOR THE PATIENT

Patients should be informed of the potential risks and advantages of Chlorpropamide and of alternative modes of therapy. They should also be informed about the importance of adherence to dietary instructions, of a regular exercise program, and of regular testing of urine and/or blood glucose.

The risks of hypoglycemia, its symptoms and treatment, and conditions that predispose to its development should be explained to patients and responsible family members. Primary and secondary failure should also be explained.

Patients should be instructed to contact their physician promptly if they experience symptoms of hypoglycemia or other adverse reactions.

LABORATORY TESTS

Blood and urine glucose should be monitored periodically. Measurement of glycosylated hemoglobin may be useful.

CARCINOGENESIS, MUTAGENESIS, AND IMPAIRMENT OF FERTILITY

Chronic toxicity studies have been carried out in dogs and rats. Dogs treated for 6, 13, or 20 months with doses of Chlorpropamide greater than 20 times the human dose, have not shown any gross histological or pathological abnormalities. After treatment with 100 mg/kg of Chlorpropamide for 20 months, a dog showed no histopathological liver changes.

Rats treated with continuous Chlorpropamide therapy for 6 to 12 months showed varying degrees of suppression of spermatogenesis at higher dosage levels (up to 125 mg/kg). The extent of suppression seemed to follow that of growth retardation associated with chronic administration of high-dose Chlorpropamide in rats.

PREGNANCY, TERATOGENIC EFFECTS, PREGNANCY CATEGORY C

Animal reproductive studies have not been conducted with Chlorpropamide. It is also not known whether Chlorpropamide can cause fetal harm when administered to a pregnant woman or can affect reproduction capacity. Chlorpropamide should be given to a pregnant woman only if clearly needed.

PRECAUTIONS: *(cont'd)*

Because recent information suggests that abnormal blood glucose levels during pregnancy are associated with a higher incidence of congenital abnormalities, many experts recommend that insulin be used during pregnancy to maintain blood glucose levels as close to normal as possible.

NONTERATOGENIC EFFECTS: Prolonged severe hypoglycemia (4 to 10 days) has been reported in neonates born to mothers who were receiving a sulfonylurea drug at the time of delivery. This has been reported more frequently with the use of agents with prolonged half-lives. If Chlorpropamide is used during pregnancy, it should be discontinued at least one month before the expected delivery date.

NURSING MOTHERS

An analysis of a composite of two samples of human breast milk, each taken five hours after ingestion of 500 mg of Chlorpropamide by a patient, revealed a concentration of 5 mcg/ml. For reference, the normal peak blood level of Chlorpropamide after a single 250 mg dose is 30 mcg/ml. Therefore, it is not recommended that a woman breast feed while taking this medication.

PEDIATRIC USE

Safety and effectiveness in children have not been established.

DRUG INTERACTIONS:

The hypoglycemic action of sulfonylurea may be potentiated by certain drugs including nonsteroidal anti-inflammatory agents and other drugs that are highly protein bound, salicylates, sulfonamides, chloramphenicol, probenecid, coumarins, monoamine oxidase inhibitors, and beta adrenergic blocking agents. When such drugs are administered to a patient receiving Chlorpropamide, the patient should be observed closely for hypoglycemia. When such drugs are withdrawn from a patient receiving Chlorpropamide, the patient should be observed closely for loss of control.

Certain drugs tend to produce hyperglycemia and may lead to loss of control. These drugs include the thiazides and other diuretics, corticosteroids, phenothiazines, thyroid products, estrogens, oral contraceptives, phenytoin, nicotinic acid, sympathomimetics, calcium channel blocking drugs, and isoniazid. When such drugs are administered to a patient receiving Chlorpropamide, the patient should be closely observed for loss of control. When such drugs are withdrawn from a patient receiving Chlorpropamide, the patient should be observed closely for hypoglycemia.

Since animal studies suggest that the action of barbiturates may be prolonged by therapy with Chlorpropamide, barbiturates should be employed with caution. In some patients, a disulfiram-like reaction may be produced by the ingestion of alcohol.

A potential interaction between oral miconazole and oral hypoglycemic agents leading to severe hypoglycemia has been reported. Whether this interaction also occurs with the intravenous, topical, or vaginal preparations of miconazole is not known.

ADVERSE REACTIONS:

Hypoglycemia: See PRECAUTIONSand OVERDOSAGE sections.

Gastrointestinal Reactions: Cholestatic jaundice may occur rarely; chlorpropamide should be discontinued if this occurs. Gastrointestinal disturbances are the most common reactions; nausea has been reported in less than 5% of patients, and diarrhea, vomiting, anorexia, and hunger in less than 2%. Other gastrointestinal disturbances have occurred in less than 1% of patients including proctocolitis. They tend to be dose related and may disappear when dosage is reduced.

Dermatologic Reactions: Pruritus has been reported in less than 3% of patients. Other allergic skin reactions, e.g., urticaria and maculopapular eruptions have been reported in approximately 1% or less of patients. These may be transient and may disappear despite continued use of chlorpropamide; if skin reactions persist the drug should be discontinued.

Porphyria cutanea tarda and photosensitivity reactions have been reported with sulfonylureas.

Skin eruptions rarely progressing to erythema multiforme and exfoliative dermatitis have also been reported.

Hematologic Reactions: Leukopenia, agranulocytosis, thrombocytopenia, hemolytic anemia, aplastic anemia, pancytopenia, and eosinophilia have been reported with sulfonylureas.

Metabolic Reactions: Hepatic porphyria and disulfiram-like reactions have been reported with chlorpropamide. See DRUG INTERACTIONS section.

Endocrine Reactions: On rare occasions, chlorpropamide has caused a reaction identical to the syndrome of inappropriate antidiuretic hormone (ADH) secretion. The features of this syndrome result from excessive water retention and include hyponatremia, low serum osmolality, and high urine osmolality. This reaction has also been reported for other sulfonylureas.

OVERDOSAGE:

Overdosage of sulfonylureas including chlorpropamide can produce hypoglycemia. Mild hypoglycemic symptoms without loss of consciousness or neurologic findings should be treated aggressively with oral glucose and adjustments in drug dosage and/or meal patterns. Close monitoring should continue until the physician is assured that the patient is out of danger. Severe hypoglycemic reactions with coma, seizure, or other neurological impairment occur infrequently, but constitute medical emergencies requiring immediate hospitalization. If hypoglycemic coma is diagnosed or suspected, the patient should be given a rapid intravenous injection of concentrated (50%) glucose solution. This should be followed by a continuous infusion of a more dilute (10%) glucose solution at a rate that will maintain the blood glucose at a level above 100 mg/dl. Patients should be closely monitored for a minimum of 24 to 48 hours since hypoglycemia may recur after apparent clinical recovery.

DOSAGE AND ADMINISTRATION:

There is no fixed dosage regimen for the management of diabetes mellitus with chlorpropamide or any other hypoglycemic agent. In addition to the usual monitoring of urinary glucose, the patient's blood glucose must also be monitored periodically to determine the minimum effective dose for the patient; to detect primary failure, i.e., inadequate lowering of blood glucose at the maximum recommended dose of medication; and to detect secondary failure, i.e., loss of an adequate blood glucose lowering response after an initial period of effectiveness. Glycosylated hemoglobin levels may also be of value in monitoring the patient's response to therapy.

Short-term administration of chlorpropamide may be sufficient during periods of transient loss of control in patients usually controlled well on diet.

The total daily dosage is generally taken at a single time each morning with breakfast. Occasionally cases of gastrointestinal intolerance may be relieved by dividing the daily dosage. A LOADING OR PRIMING DOSE IS NOT NECESSARY AND SHOULD NOT BE USED.

INITIAL THERAPY

1. The mild to moderately severe, middle-aged, stable, non-insulin-dependent diabetic patient should be started on 250 mg daily. In elderly patients, debilitated or malnourished patients, and patients with impaired renal or hepatic function, the initial and maintenance dosing

DOSAGE AND ADMINISTRATION: *(cont'd)*

should be conservative to avoid hypoglycemic reactions(see PRECAUTIONS.) Older patients should be started on smaller amounts of chlorpropamide, in the range of 100 to 125 mg daily.

2. No transition period is necessary when transferring patients from other oral hypoglycemic agents to chlorpropamide. The other agent may be discontinued abruptly and chlorpropamide started at once. In prescribing chlorpropamide, due consideration must be given to its greater potency.

Many mild to moderately severe, middle-aged, stable non-insulin-dependent diabetic patients receiving insulin can be placed directly on the oral drug and their insulin abruptly discontinued. For patients requiring more than 40 units of insulin daily, therapy with chlorpropamide may be initiated with a 50 per cent reduction in insulin for the first few days, with subsequent further reductions dependent upon the response.

During the initial period of therapy with chlorpropamide, hypoglycemic reactions may occasionally occur, particularly during the transition from insulin to the oral drug. Hypoglycemia within 24 hours after withdrawal of the intermediate or long-acting types of insulin will usually prove to be the result of insulin carry-over and not primarily due to the effect of chlorpropamide.

During the insulin withdrawal period, the patient should test his urine for sugar and ketone bodies at least three times daily and report the results frequently to his physician. If they are abnormal, the physician should be notified immediately. In some cases, it may be advisable to consider hospitalization during the transition period.

Five to seven days after the initial therapy, the blood level of chlorpropamide reaches a plateau. Dosage may subsequently be adjusted upward or downward by increments of not more than 50 to 125 mg at intervals of three to five days to obtain optimal control. More frequent adjustments are usually undesirable.

Maintenance Therapy: Most moderately severe, middle-aged, stable non-insulin-dependent diabetic patients are controlled by approximately 250 mg daily. Many investigators have found that some milder diabetics do well on daily doses of 100 mg or less. Many of the more severe diabetics may require 500 mg daily for adequate control. PATIENTS WHO DO NOT RESPOND COMPLETELY TO 500 MG DAILY WILL USUALLY NOT RESPOND TO HIGHER DOSES. MAINTENANCE DOSES ABOVE 750 mg DAILY SHOULD BE AVOIDED.

Recommended Storage: Store below 86°F (30°C).

HOW SUPPLIED - RATED THERAPEUTICALLY EQUIVALENT:

Tablet, Uncoated - Oral - 100 mg

100's	$3.06	Chlorpropamide, H.C.F.A. F F P	99999-0798-01
100's	$3.09	Chlorpropamide, United Res	00677-0971-01
100's	$4.20	Chlorpropamide, Major Pharms	00904-0225-60
100's	$6.35	Chlorpropamide, Goldline Labs	00182-1851-01
100's	$6.35	Chlorpropamide, Sidmak Labs	50111-0372-01
100's	$6.36	Chlorpropamide, Parmed Pharms	00349-8929-01
100's	$6.36	Chlorpropamide, Schein Pharm (US)	00364-0699-01
100's	$6.40	Chlorpropamide, Martec Pharms	52555-0077-01
100's	$6.95	Chlorpropamide, Rugby	00536-3462-01
100's	$7.09	Chlorpropamide, Bristol Myers Squibb	00003-0139-50
100's	$7.09	Chlorpropamide 100, Aligen Independ	00405-4205-01
100's	$7.40	Chlorpropamide, Qualitest Pharms	00603-2835-21
100's	$7.97	Chlorpropamide, Geneva Pharms	00781-1613-01
100's	$8.15	Chlorpropamide, Mylan	00378-0197-01
100's	$8.24	Chlorpropamide, HL Moore Drug Exch	00839-7011-06
100's	$8.47	Chlorpropamide, Major Pharms	00904-0225-61
100's	$16.00	Chlorpropamide, Goldline Labs	00182-1851-89
100's	$19.35	Chlorpropamide, TIE Pharm	55496-1501-09
100's	$22.40	Chlorpropamide, Medirex	57480-0316-01
100's	**$35.47**	**DIABINESE, Pfizer Labs**	**00069-3930-66**
500's	$11.20	Chlorpropamide, Major Pharms	00904-0225-40
500's	$15.05	Chlorpropamide, Schein Pharm (US)	00364-0699-05
500's	$15.19	Chlorpropamide, HL Moore Drug Exch	00839-7011-12
500's	$15.30	Chlorpropamide, H.C.F.A. F F P	99999-0798-02
500's	$17.58	Chlorpropamide Tablets 100 Mg, Halsey Drug	00879-0522-05
500's	$19.95	Chlorpropamide, Rugby	00536-3462-05
500's	$22.00	Chlorpropamide, Parmed Pharms	00349-8929-05
500's	$22.10	Chlorpropamide, Geneva Pharms	00781-1613-05
500's	$23.61	Chlorpropamide, Qualitest Pharms	00603-2835-28
500's	$25.00	Chlorpropamide, Sidmak Labs	50111-0372-02
500's	$26.32	Chlorpropamide, Aligen Independ	00405-4205-02
500's	$35.15	Chlorpropamide, Mylan	00378-0197-05
500's	**$174.61**	**DIABINESE, Pfizer Labs**	**00069-3930-73**
600's	$111.00	Chlorpropamide, Medirex	57480-0316-06
1000's	$30.60	Chlorpropamide, H.C.F.A. F F P	99999-0798-03
1000's	$33.16	Chlorpropamide, Halsey Drug	00879-0522-10
1000's	$44.90	Chlorpropamide, Sidmak Labs	50111-0372-03

Tablet, Uncoated - Oral - 250 mg

100's	$4.53	Chlorpropamide, H.C.F.A. F F P	99999-0798-04
100's	$4.83	Chlorpropamide, United Res	00677-0972-01
100's	$4.95	Chlorpropamide, Consolidated Midland	00223-0634-01
100's	$7.00	Chlorpropamide, Raway	00686-0203-20
100's	$7.39	Chlorpropamide, Halsey Drug	00879-0503-01
100's	$7.95	Chlorpropamide, Major Pharms	00904-0226-60
100's	$9.70	Chlorpropamide, Major Pharms	00904-0226-61
100's	$11.50	Chlorpropamide, Rugby	00536-3465-01
100's	$12.30	Chlorpropamide, Schein Pharm (US)	00364-0510-01
100's	$12.50	Chlorpropamide, Goldline Labs	00182-1852-01
100's	$12.50	Chlorpropramide, Sidmak Labs	50111-0373-01
100's	$12.60	Chlorpropamide, Martec Pharms	52555-0078-01
100's	$12.76	Chlorpropamide, Qualitest Pharms	00603-2836-21
100's	$12.95	Chlorpropamide, Parmed Pharms	00349-8928-01
100's	$13.16	Chlorpropamide 250, Aligen Independ	00405-4206-01
100's	$13.40	Chlorpropamide, Geneva Pharms	00781-1623-01
100's	$14.18	Chlorpropamide, HL Moore Drug Exch	00839-7012-06
100's	$14.20	Chlorpropamide, Mylan	00378-0210-01
100's	$14.99	Chlorpropamide, Bristol Myers Squibb	00003-0152-50
100's	$22.39	Chlorpropamide, Vangard Labs	00615-2541-13
100's	$22.40	Chlorpropamide, Medirex	57480-0317-01
100's	$31.29	Chlorpropamide, TIE Pharm	55496-1502-09
100's	$31.70	Chlorpropamide, Goldline Labs	00182-1852-89
100's	**$74.94**	**DIABINESE, Pfizer Labs**	**00069-3940-66**
100's	**$80.17**	**DIABINESE, Pfizer Labs**	**00069-3940-41**
250's	$8.95	Chlorpropamide, Geneva Pharms	00781-1623-25
250's	$11.32	Chlorpropamide, H.C.F.A. F F P	99999-0798-05
250's	$16.00	Chlorpropramide, Sidmak Labs	50111-0373-06
250's	**$181.74**	**DIABINESE, Pfizer Labs**	**00069-3940-71**
500's	$22.65	Chlorpropamide, H.C.F.A. F F P	99999-0798-06
500's	$23.81	Chlorpropamide, Halsey Drug	00879-0503-05
500's	$28.25	Insulase 250, H & H Labs	46703-0075-05
500's	$30.60	Chlorpropamide, Schein Pharm (US)	00364-0510-05

HOW SUPPLIED - RATED THERAPEUTICALLY EQUIVALENT: *(cont'd)*

500's	$42.36	Chlorpropamide, Geneva Pharms	00781-1623-05
500's	$44.25	Chlorpropamide, Rugby	00536-3465-05
500's	$49.40	Chlorpropamide, Qualitest Pharms	00603-2836-28
500's	$55.00	Chlorpropramide, Sidmak Labs	50111-0373-02
600's	$181.60	Chlorpropamide, Medirex	57480-0317-06
1000's	$42.50	Chlorpropamide, Consolidated Midland	00223-0634-02
1000's	$45.30	Chlorpropamide, H.C.F.A. F F P	99999-0798-07
1000's	$48.30	Chlorpropamide, United Res	00677-0972-10
1000's	$51.90	Chlorpropamide, Major Pharms	00904-0226-80
1000's	$53.72	Chlorpropamide, Amer Preferred	53445-1852-00
1000's	$59.62	Chlorpropamide, Halsey Drug	00879-0503-10
1000's	$81.83	Chlorpropamide, Geneva Pharms	00781-1623-10
1000's	$82.00	Chlorpropamide, Rugby	00536-3465-10
1000's	$83.00	Chlorpropamide, Schein Pharm (US)	00364-0510-02
1000's	$96.80	Chlorpropamide, Qualitest Pharms	00603-2836-32
1000's	$99.50	Chlorpropamide, Parmed Pharms	00349-8928-10
1000's	$99.95	Chlorabetic 250, Quality Res Pharms	52765-1076-00
1000's	$102.25	Chlorpropamide, Goldline Labs	00182-1852-10
1000's	$102.25	Chlorpropramide, Sidmak Labs	50111-0373-03
1000's	$103.25	Chlorpropamide, Martec Pharms	52555-0078-10
1000's	$107.39	Chlorpropamide, HL Moore Drug Exch	00839-7012-16
1000's	$109.84	Chlorpropamide 250, Aligen Independ	00405-4206-03
1000's	$126.50	Chlorpropamide, Mylan	00378-0210-10
1000's	**$719.15**	**DIABINESE, Pfizer Labs**	**00069-3940-82**

CHLORTETRACYCLINE HYDROCHLORIDE
(000800)

CATEGORIES: Anti-Infectives; Antibiotics; EENT Drugs; Eye, Ear, Nose, & Throat Preparations; Ocular Infections; Ophthalmics; Tetracyclines; FDA Approval Pre 1982

BRAND NAMES: *Aurecil*; *Aureoftalmina*; *Aureomicina*; **Aureomycin**; *Aureomycine* (France); *Chlortralim*
(International brand names outside U.S. in italics)

FORMULARIES: Medi-Cal

Prescribing information not available at time of publication.

HOW SUPPLIED - EQUIVALENTS NOT AVAILABLE:

Ointment - Ophthalmic - 1 %

3.5 gm	**$14.35**	**AUREOMYCIN, Lederle Pharm**	**00005-3511-51**

CHLORTHALIDONE *(000801)*

CATEGORIES: Antihypertensives; Cardiovascular Drugs; Cirrhosis; Congestive Heart Failure; Diuretics; Edema; Electrolytic, Caloric-Water Balance; Glomerulonephritis; Heart Failure; Hypertension; Nephrotic Syndrome; Pregnancy; Renal Drugs; Renal Failure; Thiazides; FDA Approval Pre 1982

BRAND NAMES: *Apo-Chlorthalidone* (Canada); Biogroton; *Higroton* (Mexico); *Higrotona*; Hydone; *Hydro*; *Hydro-Long* (Germany); **Hygroton**; *Hygroton 50*; *Hypertol*; *Hythalton*; *Igroton*; *Novothalidone* (Canada); *Servidone*; *Thalidone*; *Thalidone-50*; Thalitone; *Urandil*; *Uridon* (Canada); *Urolin*
(International brand names outside U.S. in italics)

FORMULARIES: Aetna; BC-BS; Medi-Cal

COST OF THERAPY: $14.23 (Hypertension; Tablet; 25 mg; 1/day; 365 days)

PRIMARY ICD9: 401.1 (Essential Hypertension, Benign)

DESCRIPTION:

Chlorthalidone is an oral antihypertensive/diuretic. It is a monosulfamyl diuretic that differs chemically from thiazide diuretics in that a double-ring system is incorporated in its structure. It is 2-chloro-5-(1-hydroxy-3-oxo-1-isoindolinyl) benzenesulfonamide.

Chlorthalidone is practically insoluble in water, in ether, and in chloroform: soluble in methanol: slightly soluble in alcohol.

Chlorthalidone tablets also contain colloidal silica, corn starch, gelatin, glycerin, lactose, magnesium stearate, talc, and other ingredients. The 25 mg tablets also contains Yellow 6, methylparaben, and propylparaben. The 50 mg tablets also contain FD&C Blue No. 1, methylparaben, and propylparaben.

CLINICAL PHARMACOLOGY:

Chlorthalidone is an oral diuretic with prolonged action (48-72 hours) and low toxicity. The major portion of the drug is excreted unchanged by the kidneys. The diuretic effect of the drug occurs in approximately 2.6 hours and continues for up to 72 hours. The mean half-life following a 50 to 200 mg dose is 40 hours. In the first order of absorption, the elimination half-life is 53 hours following a 50 mg dose, and 60 hours following a 100 mg dose. Approximately 75 percent of the drug is bound to plasma proteins, 58 percent of the drug being bound to albumin. This is caused by an increased affinity of the drug to erythrocyte carbonic anhydrase. Nonrenal routes of elimination have yet to be clarified. Data are not available regarding percentage of doses as unchanged drug and metabolites, concentration of the drug in body fluids, degree of uptake by a particular organ or in the fetus, or passage across the blood-brain barrier.

The drug produces copious diuresis with greatly increased excretion of sodium and chloride. At maximal therapeutic dosage, chlorthalidone is approximately equal in its diuretic effect to comparable maximal therapeutic doses of benzothiadiazine diuretics. The site of action appears to be the cortical diluting segment of the ascending limb of Henle's loop of the nephron.

INDICATIONS AND USAGE:

Diuretics such as chlorthalidone are indicated in the management of hypertension either as the sole therapeutic agent or to enhance the effect of other antihypertensive drugs in the more severe forms of hypertension.

Chlorthalidone is indicated as adjunctive therapy in edema associated with congestive heart failure, hepatic cirrhosis, and corticosteroid and estrogen therapy.

Chlorthalidone has also been found useful in edema due to various forms of renal dysfunction such as nephrotic syndrome, acute glomerulonephritis, and chronic renal failure.

INDICATIONS AND USAGE: *(cont'd)*

Usage In Pregnancy: The routine use of diuretics in an otherwise healthy woman is inappropriate and exposes mother and fetus to unnecessary hazard. Diuretics do not prevent development of toxemia of pregnancy, and there is no satisfactory evidence that they are useful in the treatment of developed toxemia.

Edema during pregnancy may arise from pathological causes or from the physiologic and mechanical consequences of pregnancy. Chlorthalidone is indicated in pregnancy when edema is due to pathological causes or from the physiologic and mechanical consequences of pregnancy. Chlorthalidone is indicated in pregnancy when edema is due to pathologic causes, just as it is the absence of pregnancy (however, see WARNINGS). Dependent edema in pregnancy, resulting from restriction of venous return by the expanded uterus, is properly treated through elevation of the lower extremities and use of support hose; use of diuretics to lower intravascular volume in this case is illogical and unnecessary. There is hypervolemia during normal pregnancy that is harmful to neither the fetus nor the mother (in the absence of cardiovascular disease), but that is associated with edema, including generalized edema, in the majority of pregnant women. If this edema produces discomfort, increased recumbency will often provide relief. In rare instances, this edema may cause extreme discomfort that is not relieved by rest. In these cases, a short course of diuretics may provide relief and may be appropriate.

CONTRAINDICATIONS:

Anuria.

Hypersensitivity to chlorthalidone or other sulfonamide-derived drugs.

WARNINGS:

Chlorthalidone should be used with caution in severe renal disease. In patients with renal disease, chlorthalidone or related drugs may precipitate azotemia. Cumulative effects of the drug may develop in patients with impaired renal function.

Chlorthalidone should be used with caution in patients with impaired hepatic function or progressive liver disease, because minor alterations of fluid and electrolyte balance may precipitate hepatic coma.

Sensitivity reactions may occur in patients with a history of allergy or bronchial asthma.

The possibility of exacerbation or activation of systemic lupus erythematosus has been reported with thiazide diuretics, which are structurally related to chlorthalidone. However, systemic lupus erythematosus has not been reported following chlorthalidone administration.

PRECAUTIONS:

GENERAL

Hypokalemia may develop with chlorthalidone as with any other potent diuretic, especially with brisk diuresis, when severe cirrhosis is present, or during concomitant use of corticosteroids or ACTH.

Interference with adequate oral electrolyte intake will also contribute to hypokalemia. Digitalis therapy may exaggerate metabolic effects of hypokalemia especially with reference to myocardial activity.

Any chloride deficit is generally mild and usually does not require specific treatment except under extraordinary circumstances (as in liver disease or renal disease). Dilutional hyponatremia may occur in edematous patients in hot weather; appropriate therapy is water restriction, rather than administration of salt except in rare instances when the hyponatremia is life threatening. In actual salt depletion, appropriate replacement is the therapy of choice.

Hyperuricemia may occur or frank gout may be precipitated in certain patients receiving chlorthalidone. Thiazide-like diuretics have been shown to increase the urinary excretion of magnesium; this may result in hypomagnesemia.

The antihypertensive effects of the drug may be enhanced in the postsympathectomy patient.

If progressive renal impairment becomes evident, as indicated by a rising nonprotein nitrogen or blood urea nitrogen, a careful reappraisal of therapy is necessary with consideration given to withholding or discontinuing diuretic therapy.

Calcium excretion is decreased by thiazide-like drugs. Pathological changes in the parathyroid gland with hypercalcemia and hypophosphatemia have been observed in a few patients on thiazide therapy. The common complications of hyperparathyroidism such as renal lithiasis, bone resorption and peptic ulceration have not been seen.

INFORMATION FOR THE PATIENT

Patients should inform their doctor if they have: 1) had an allergic reaction to Hygroton or other diuretics or have asthma 2) kidney disease 3) liver disease 4) gout 5) systemic lupus erythematosus, or 6) been taking other drugs such as cortisone, digitalis, lithium carbonate, or drugs for diabetes.

Patients should be cautioned to contact their physician if they experience any of the following symptoms of potassium loss: excess thirst, tiredness, drowsiness, restlessness, muscle pains or cramps, nausea, vomiting or increased heart rate or pulse.

Patients should also be cautioned that taking alcohol can increase the chance of dizziness occurring.

LABORATORY TESTS

Periodic determination of serum electrolytes to detect possible electrolyte imbalance should be performed at appropriate intervals.

All patients receiving chlorthalidone should be observed for clinical signs of fluid or electrolyte imbalance; namely hyponatremia, hypochloremic alkalosis, and hypokalemia. Serum and urine electrolyte determinations are particularly important when the patient is vomiting excessively or receiving parenteral fluids.

Laboratory Test Interactions: Chlorthalidone and related drugs may decrease serum PBI levels without signs of thyroid disturbance.

CARCINOGENESIS, MUTAGENESIS, AND IMPAIRMENT OF FERTILITY

No information is available.

PREGNANCY, TERATOGENIC EFFECTS, PREGNANCY CATEGORY B:

Reproduction studies have been performed in the rat and rabbit at doses up to 420 times the human dose and have revealed no evidence of impaired fertility or harm to the fetus due to chlorthalidone. There are, however, no adequate and well-controlled studies in pregnant women. Because animal reproduction studies are not always predictive of human response, this drug should be used during pregnancy only if clearly needed.

Nonteratogenic Effects: Thiazides cross the placental barrier and appear in cord blood. The use of chlorthalidone and related drugs in pregnant women requires that the anticipated benefits of the drug be weighed against possible hazards to the fetus. These hazards include fetal or neonatal jaundice, thrombocytopenia, and possibly other adverse reactions that have occurred in the adult.

NURSING MOTHERS

Thiazides are excreted in human milk. Because of the potential for serious adverse reactions in nursing infants from chlorthalidone, a decision should be made whether to discontinue the drug, taking into account the importance of the drug to the mother.

PRECAUTIONS: *(cont'd)*

PEDIATRIC USE

Safety and effectiveness in children have not been established.

DRUG INTERACTIONS:

Chlorthalidone may add to or potentiate the action of other antihypertensive drugs. Potentiation occurs with ganglionic or peripheral adrenergic blocking drugs.

Medication such as digitalis may also influence serum electrolytes. Warning signs, irrespective of cause are: Dryness of mouth, thirst, weakness, lethargy, drowsiness, restlessness, muscle pains or cramps, muscular fatigue, hypotension, oliguria, tachycardia, and gastrointestinal disturbances such as nausea and vomiting.

Insulin requirements in diabetic patients may be increased, decreased, or unchanged. Higher dosage of oral hypoglycemic agents may be required. Latent diabetes mellitus may become manifest during chlorthalidone administration.

Chlorthalidone and related drugs may increase the responsiveness to tubocurarine.

Chlorthalidone and related drugs may decrease arterial responsiveness to norepinephrine. This diminution is not sufficient to preclude effectiveness of the pressor agent for therapeutic use.

ADVERSE REACTIONS:

The following adverse reactions have been observed, but there is not enough systematic collection of data to support an estimate of their frequency.

Gastrointestinal System Reactions: anorexia, gastric irritation, nausea, vomiting, cramping, diarrhea, constipation, jaundice (intrahepatic cholestatic jaundice), pancreatitis

Central Nervous System Reactions: dizziness, vertigo, paresthesias, headache, xanthopsia

Hematologic Reactions: leukopenia, agranulocytosis, thrombocytopenia, aplastic anemia

Dermatologic-Hypersensitivity Reactions: purpura, photosensitivity, rash, urticaria, necrotizing angiitis, (vasculitis), (cutaneous vasculitis), Lyell's syndrome (toxic epidermal necrolysis)

Cardiovascular Reaction: Orthostatic hypotension may occur and may be aggravated by alcohol, barbiturates or narcotics.

Other Adverse Reactions: hyperglycemia, glycosuria, hyperuricemia, muscle spasm, weakness, restlessness, impotence

Whenever adverse reactions are moderate or severe, chlorthalidone dosage should be reduced or therapy withdrawn.

OVERDOSAGE:

Symptoms of acute overdosage include nausea, weakness, dizziness and disturbances of electrolyte balance. The oral LD_{50} of the drug in the mouse and the rat is more than 25,000 mg/kg body weight. The minimum lethal dose (MLD) in humans has not been established. There is no specific antidote, but gastric lavage is recommended, followed by supportive treatment. Where necessary, this may include intravenous dextrose-saline with potassium, administered with caution.

DOSAGE AND ADMINISTRATION:

Therapy should be initiated with the lowest possible dose. This dose should be titrated according to individual patient response to gain maximal therapeutic benefit while maintaining the minimal dosage possible. A single dose given in the morning with food is recommended, divided doses are unnecessary.

HYPERTENSION

Initiation: Therapy, in most patients should be initiated with a single daily dose of 25 mg. If the response is insufficient after a suitable trial, the dosage may be increased to a single daily dose of 50 mg. If additional control is required, the dosage of chlorthalidone may be increased to 100 mg once daily or a second antihypertensive drug (step-2 therapy) may be added. Dosage above 100 mg daily usually does not increase effectiveness. Increases in serum uric acid and decreases in serum potassium are dose-related over the 25-100 mg day range.

Maintenance: Maintenance doses may be lower than initial doses and should be adjusted according to individual patient response. Effectiveness is well sustained during continued use.

EDEMA

Initiation: Adults, initially 50 to 100 mg daily, or 100 mg on alternate days. Some patients may require 150 to 200 mg at these intervals, or up to 200 mg daily. Dosages above this level, however, do not usually produce a greater response.

Maintenance: Maintenance doses may often be lower than initial doses and should be adjusted according to the individual patient. Effectiveness is well sustained during continued use.

Store at controlled room temperature, 15°-30° C (59°-86° F). Avoid excessive heat. Dispense in tight containers as defined in USP.

ANIMAL PHARMACOLOGY:

Biochemical studies in animals have suggested reasons for the prolonged effect of chlorthalidone. Absorption from the gastrointestinal tract is slow, due to its slow solubility. After passage to the liver, some of the drug enters the general circulation, while some is excreted in the bile, to be reabsorbed later. In the general circulation, it is distributed widely to the tissues, but is taken up in highest concentrations by the kidneys, where amounts have been found 72 hours after ingestion, long after it has disappeared from other tissues. The drug is excreted unchanged in the urine.

HOW SUPPLIED - RATED THERAPEUTICALLY EQUIVALENT:

Tablet, Uncoated - Oral - 25 mg

100's	$3.90	Chlorthalidone, H.C.F.A. F F P	99999-0801-01
100's	$5.76	Chlorthalidone, Qualitest Pharms	00603-2860-21
100's	$6.00	Chlorthalidone, Mutual Pharm	53489-0111-01
100's	$6.25	Chlorthalidone, United Res	00677-0682-01
100's	$7.94	Chlorthalidone, Lederle Pharm	00005-3763-23
100's	$7.95	Chlorthalidone, HL Moore Drug Exch	00839-6488-06
100's	$8.27	Chlorthalidone, Major Pharms	00904-1349-61
100's	$8.28	Chlorthalidone, Schein Pharm (US)	00364-0564-01
100's	$8.53	Chlorthalidone, Zenith Labs	00172-2974-60
100's	$8.53	Chlorthalidone, Goldline Labs	00182-1434-01
100's	$8.80	Chlorthalidone, Martec Pharms	52555-0372-01
100's	$8.98	Chlorthalidone 25, Aligen Independ	00405-4211-01
100's	$9.25	Chlorthalidone, Rugby	00536-3485-01
100's	$10.21	Chlorthalidone, Bristol Myers Squibb	00003-0162-50
100's	$11.08	Chlorthalidone, Sidmak Labs	50111-0362-01
100's	$11.97	Chlorthalidone, Geneva Pharms	00781-1726-01
100's	$12.10	Chlorthalidone, Mylan	00378-0222-01
100's	$27.00	Chlorthalidone, Geneva Pharms	00781-1726-13
100's	**$65.81**	**HYGROTON, Rhone-Poulenc Rorer**	**00075-0022-00**
250's	$9.75	Chlorthalidone, H.C.F.A. F F P	99999-0801-02
250's	$11.90	Chlorthalidone 25 Mg Tablets, Major Pharms	00904-1349-70
500's	$10.50	Hydone 25, H & H Labs	46703-0054-05

HOW SUPPLIED - RATED THERAPEUTICALLY EQUIVALENT: *(cont'd)*

500's	$19.50	Chlorthalidone, H.C.F.A. F F P	99999-0801-03
1000's	$39.00	Chlorthalidone, H.C.F.A. F F P	99999-0801-04
1000's	$39.95	Chlorthalidone, Mutual Pharm	53489-0111-10
1000's	$41.05	Chlorthalidone, United Res	00677-0682-10
1000's	$41.55	Chlorthalidone, Major Pharms	00904-1349-80
1000's	$41.55	Chlorthalidone, Major Pharms	00904-7663-80
1000's	$49.75	Chlorthalidone, HL Moore Drug Exch	00839-6488-16
1000's	$54.70	Chlorthalidone, Qualitest Pharms	00603-2860-32
1000's	$59.50	Chlorthalidone, Rugby	00536-3485-10
1000's	$60.89	Chlorthalidone, Zenith Labs	00172-2974-80
1000's	$60.89	Chlorthalidone, Goldline Labs	00182-1434-10
1000's	$62.70	Chlorthalidone, Martec Pharms	52555-0372-10
1000's	$64.09	Chlorthalidone 25, Aligen Independ	00405-4211-03
1000's	$79.16	Chlorthalidone, Sidmak Labs	50111-0362-03
1000's	$98.63	Chlorthalidone, Bristol Myers Squibb	00003-0162-75
1000's	$104.30	Chlorthalidone, Mylan	00378-0222-10

Tablet, Uncoated - Oral - 50 mg

100's	$4.34	Chlorthalidone, H.C.F.A. F F P	99999-0801-05
100's	$6.45	Chlorthalidone, Major Pharms	00904-7665-60
100's	$7.12	Chlorthalidone, Rugby	00536-3468-01
100's	$7.50	Chlorthalidone, Consolidated Midland	00223-0631-01
100's	$7.66	Chlorthalidone, Qualitest Pharms	00603-2861-21
100's	$7.75	Chlorthalidone, Mutual Pharm	53489-0112-01
100's	$8.00	Chlorthalidone, United Res	00677-0683-01
100's	$9.54	Chlorthalidone, Zenith Labs	00172-2999-60
100's	$9.54	Chlorthalidone, Goldline Labs	00182-1435-01
100's	$9.58	Chlorthalidone 50, Aligen Independ	00405-4212-01
100's	$9.85	Chlorthalidone, Martec Pharms	52555-0373-01
100's	$9.95	Chlorthalidone, Rugby	00536-5644-01
100's	$10.11	Chlorthalidone, HL Moore Drug Exch	00839-6369-06
100's	$12.40	Chlorthalidone, Sidmak Labs	50111-0363-01
100's	$12.60	Chlorthalidone, Bristol Myers Squibb	00003-0180-50
100's	$12.97	Chlorthalidone, Geneva Pharms	00781-1728-01
100's	$13.10	Chlorthalidone, Mylan	00378-0213-01
100's	$33.95	Chlorthalidone, Geneva Pharms	00781-1728-13
100's	**$81.15**	**HYGROTON, Rhone-Poulenc Rorer**	**00075-0020-00**
250's	$10.85	Chlorthalidone, H.C.F.A. F F P	99999-0801-06
250's	$15.89	Chlorthalidone 50 Mg Tablets, Major Pharms	00904-1350-70
500's	$29.93	Chlorthalidone, Rugby	00536-3468-05
500's	$121.52	Chlorthalidone, Bristol Myers Squibb	00003-0180-75
1000's	$26.25	Hydone, H & H Labs	46703-0045-10
1000's	$34.80	Chlorthalidone, Mutual Pharm	53489-0112-10
1000's	$43.40	Chlorthalidone, H.C.F.A. F F P	99999-0801-07
1000's	$54.90	Chlorthalidone, Major Pharms	00904-1350-80
1000's	$56.85	Chlorthalidone, Rugby	00536-3468-10
1000's	$59.90	Chlorthalidone, United Res	00677-0683-10
1000's	$67.95	Chlorthalidone 50, Aligen Independ	00405-4212-03
1000's	$68.10	Chlorthalidone, Qualitest Pharms	00603-2861-32
1000's	$70.00	Chlorthalidone, Consolidated Midland	00223-0631-02
1000's	$71.35	Chlorthalidone, Martec Pharms	52555-0373-10
1000's	$71.80	Chlorthalidone, Zenith Labs	00172-2999-80
1000's	$71.82	Chlorthalidone, HL Moore Drug Exch	00839-6369-16
1000's	$90.91	Chlorthalidone, Sidmak Labs	50111-0363-03
1000's	$116.57	Chlorthalidone, Geneva Pharms	00781-1728-10
1000's	$117.25	Chlorthalidone, Mylan	00378-0213-10

HOW SUPPLIED - NOT RATED EQUIVALENT:

Tablet, Uncoated - Oral - 15 mg

100's	$60.03	THALITONE, Horus Therapeutics	59229-0077-01

Tablet, Uncoated - Oral - 25 mg

100's	$6.75	Chlorthalidone, Consolidated Midland	00223-0629-01
100's	$13.20	Chlorthalidone, Raway	00686-2442-13
100's	$36.60	THALITONE, Boehringer Pharms	00597-0076-01
100's	$71.34	THALITONE, Horus Therapeutics	59229-0076-01
1000's	$62.50	Chlorthalidone, Consolidated Midland	00223-0629-02

Tablet, Uncoated - Oral - 100 mg

100's	$8.45	Chlorthalidone, Consolidated Midland	00223-0632-01
100's	$10.35	Chlorthalidone, United Res	00677-1012-01
100's	$10.38	Chlorthalidone, Qualitest Pharms	00603-2862-21
100's	$10.40	HYLIDONE, Major Pharms	00904-1351-60
100's	$10.50	Chlorthalidone, Schein Pharm (US)	00364-0787-01
100's	$10.60	Chlorthalidone, Martec Pharms	52555-0374-01
100's	$10.90	Chlorthalidone, Zenith Labs	00172-2904-60
100's	$10.90	Chlorthalidone, Goldline Labs	00182-1194-01
100's	$11.90	Chlorthalidone, Eon Labs Mfg	00185-0073-01
100's	$12.70	Chlorthalidone, Aligen Independ	00405-4213-01
100's	$13.39	Chlorthalidone, Rugby	00536-3469-01
100's	$13.39	Chlorthalidone, Sidmak Labs	50111-0364-01
100's	$13.76	Chlorthalidone, HL Moore Drug Exch	00839-6370-06
100's	**$135.66**	**HYGROTON, Rhone-Poulenc Rorer**	**00075-0021-00**
1000's	$52.00	HYLIDONE, Major Pharms	00904-1351-80
1000's	$77.50	Chlorthalidone, Consolidated Midland	00223-0632-02
1000's	$92.35	Chlorthalidone, Zenith Labs	00172-2904-80
1000's	$104.00	Chlorthalidone, Sidmak Labs	50111-0364-03
1000's	$110.50	Chlorthalidone, Eon Labs Mfg	00185-0073-10
1000's	$112.05	Chlorthalidone, HL Moore Drug Exch	00839-6370-16

CHLORTHALIDONE; CLONIDINE HYDROCHLORIDE *(000802)*

CATEGORIES: Alpha Adrenoreceptor Agonists; Antihypertensives; Cardiovascular Drugs; Diuretics; Hypertension; Renal Drugs; FDA Approval Pre 1982

BRAND NAMES: *Catapres Diu*; Clonidine Hcl W/Chlorthalidone; Clorodone; *Clothalton*; **Combipres**; *Combipresan* (Germany)
(International brand names outside U.S. in italics)

FORMULARIES: Aetna

DESCRIPTION:

Each tablet contains: 0.1/15 mg, 0.2/15 mg, 0.3/15 mg of clonidine hydrochloride/chlorthalidone, respectively.

FOR COMPLETE PRESCRIBING INFORMATION REFER TO THE INDIVIDUAL DRUG MONOGRAPHS (CHLORTHALIDONE; CLONIDINE HYDROCHLORIDE).

INDICATIONS AND USAGE:

Combipres (clonidine hydrochloride USP/chlorthalidone USP) is indicated in the treatment of hypertension. **This fixed combination drug is not indicated for initial therapy of hypertension. Hypertension requires therapy titrated to the individual patient. If the fixed combination represents the dosage so determined, its use may be more convenient in patient management. The treatment of hypertension is not static, but must be reevaluated as conditions in each patient warrant.**

DOSAGE AND ADMINISTRATION:

The dosage must be determined by individual titration.

Chlorthalidone is usually initiated at a dose of 25 mg once daily and may be increased to 50 mg if the response is insufficient after a suitable trial.

Clonidine hydrochloride is usually initiated at a dose of 0.1 mg twice daily. Elderly patients may benefit from a lower initial dose. Further increments of 0.1 mg/day may be made if necessary until the desired response is achieved. The therapeutic doses most commonly employed have ranged from 0.2 to 0.6 mg per day in divided doses.

One Combipres (clonidine hydrochloride/chlorthalidone) Tablet administered once or twice daily can be used to administer a minimum of 0.1 mg clonidine hydrochloride and 15 mg chlorthalidone to a maximum of 0.6 mg clonidine hydrochloride and 30 mg chlorthalidone.

HOW SUPPLIED - RATED THERAPEUTICALLY EQUIVALENT:

Tablet, Uncoated - Oral - 15 mg/0.1 mg

100's	$20.40	Clonidine Hcl & Chlorthalidone, United Res	00677-1146-01
100's	$20.40	Clonidine HCl & Chlorthalidone, H.C.F.A. F F P	99999-0802-01
100's	$26.10	Clonidine Hcl & Chlorthalidone 0., Goldline Labs	00182-1275-01
100's	$31.43	Clonidine Hcl W/Chlorthalidone, Qualitest Pharms	00603-2978-21
100's	$33.21	Clonidine Hcl & Chlorthalidone, HL Moore Drug Exch	00839-7285-06
100's	$33.82	Clonidine HCl & Chlorthalidone, Schein Pharm (US)	00364-2174-01
100's	$33.83	Clonidine Hcl W/Chlorthalidone, Rugby	00536-3533-01
100's	$33.83	Clonidine Hcl & Chlorthalidone, Rugby	00536-4937-01
100's	$37.50	Clonidine Hcl & Chlorthalidone, Par Pharm	49884-0113-01
100's	$39.47	Clonidine Hcl W/Chlorthalidone, Aligen Independ	00405-4248-01
100's	$39.99	Clonidine & Chlorthalidone, Mylan	00378-0001-01
100's	**$72.73**	**COMBIPRES, Boehringer Pharms**	**00597-0008-01**
500's	$102.00	Clonidine HCl & Chlorthalidone, H.C.F.A. F F P	99999-0802-02
1000's	$204.00	Clonidine HCl & Chlorthalidone, H.C.F.A. F F P	99999-0802-03

Tablet, Uncoated - Oral - 15 mg/0.2 mg

100's	$26.25	Clonidine Hcl & Chlorthalidone, United Res	00677-1147-01
100's	$26.25	Clonidine HCl & Chlorthalidone, H.C.F.A. F F P	99999-0802-04
100's	$37.50	Clonidine Hcl & Chlorthalidone 0., Goldline Labs	00182-1276-01
100's	$39.84	Clonidine Hcl W/Chlorthalidone, Qualitest Pharms	00603-2979-21
100's	$40.45	Clonidine Hcl/Chlorthalidone, Geneva Pharms	00781-1038-01
100's	$43.42	Clonidine Hcl & Chlorthalidone, Rugby	00536-4938-01
100's	$44.00	Clonidine HCl & Chlorthalidone, Schein Pharm (US)	00364-2175-01
100's	$45.75	Clonidine Hcl & Chlorthalidone, HL Moore Drug Exch	00839-7286-06
100's	$46.25	Clonidine Hcl W/Chlorthalidone, Rugby	00536-3535-01
100's	$49.50	Clonidine Hcl & Chlorthalidone, Par Pharm	49884-0115-01
100's	$52.11	Clonidine Hcl W/Chlorthalidone, Aligen Independ	00405-4249-01
100's	$52.20	Clonidine & Chlorthalidone, Mylan	00378-0027-01
100's	**$97.24**	**COMBIPRES, Boehringer Pharms**	**00597-0009-01**
500's	$131.25	Clonidine HCl & Chlorthalidone, H.C.F.A. F F P	99999-0802-05
1000's	$262.50	Clonidine HCl & Chlorthalidone, H.C.F.A. F F P	99999-0802-06

Tablet, Uncoated - Oral - 15 mg/0.3 mg

100's	$32.25	Clonidine HCl & Chlorthalidone, H.C.F.A. F F P	99999-0802-07
100's	$41.00	Clonidine Hcl W/Chlorthalidone, Qualitest Pharms	00603-2980-21
100's	$45.75	Clonidine Hcl & Chlorthalidone 0., Goldline Labs	00182-1277-01
100's	$47.13	Clonidine Hcl & Chlorthalidone, HL Moore Drug Exch	00839-7287-06
100's	$49.49	Clonidine Hcl W/Chlorthalidone, HL Moore Drug Exch	00839-7943-06
100's	$61.50	Clonidine Hcl & Chlorthalidone, Par Pharm	49884-0116-01
100's	$62.99	Clonidine & Chlorthalidone, Mylan	00378-0072-01
100's	**$117.48**	**COMBIPRES, Boehringer Pharms**	**00597-0010-01**

CHLORTHALIDONE; RESERPINE *(000803)*

CATEGORIES: Antihypertensives; Cardiovascular Drugs; Hypertension; Renal Drugs; FDA Approval Pre 1982

BRAND NAMES: Demi-Regroton; *Higroton Reserpina*; *Hygroton*; *Hygroton R* (Japan); *Hygroton-Reserpine* (Mexico); *Hythalton*; **Regroton**
(International brand names outside U.S. in italics)

FORMULARIES: Medi-Cal

> WARNING:
> These fixed combination drugs are not indicated for initial therapy of hypertension. Hypertension requires therapy titrated to the individual patient. If the fixed combination represents the dosage so determined, its use may be more convenient in patient management. The treatment of hypertension is not static, but must be reevaluated as conditions in each patient warrant.

DESCRIPTION:

Chlorthalidone/Reserpine and Demi-Chlorthalidone w/Reserpine are drug combinations of two well-known antihypertensive agents, chlorthalidone and reserpine. Demi-Chlorthalidone w/Reserpine provides one-half the amount of both agents as Chlorthalidone/Reserpine, for flexibility of dosage in patient management.

Chemistry: A monosulfamyl diuretic, chlorthalidone differs from thiazide diuretics in that a double-ring system is incorporated in its structure. Chemically, it is 2-Chloro-5-(1-hydroxy-3-oxo-1-isoindolinyl) benzenesulfonamide.

Chlorthalidone is practically insoluble in water, in ether, and in chloroform; soluble in methanol; slightly soluble in alcohol.

Reserpine is a pure crystalline alkaloid from the root of Rauwolfia serpentina.

Reserpine is insoluble in water; freely soluble in acetic acid and in chloroform; slightly soluble in benzene; very slightly soluble in alcohol and in ether.

Chlorthalidone/Reserpine and Demi-Chlorthalidone w/Reserpine contain the following inactive ingredients: cornstarch, gelatin, glycerin, lactose, magnesium stearate, silica, talc, and other ingredients. Chlorthalidone/Reserpine also contains FD&C Red No. 40 and FD&C Blue No. 1.

CLINICAL PHARMACOLOGY:

The pharmacologic effects are those of the constituent drugs. Chlorthalidone produces a saluretic effect in humans, beginning within two hours after an oral dose and continuing for as long as 72 hours. Copious diuresis is produced, with greatly increased excretion of sodium and chloride.

Reserpine, because it reduces arterial blood pressure and exerts a sedative effect, is particularly useful in the therapy of hypertension with related emotional disturbance.

Reserpine is characterized by slow onset of action and sustained effect. Both its cardiovascular and central nervous system effects may persist following withdrawal of the drug.

(See PRECAUTIONS.)

Both chlorthalidone and reserpine have prolonged action, and the combination is thus able to exert a smooth and concerted effect over a long period.

The two drugs appear to enhance each other, and this gives the combination a high degree of effectiveness. When considered necessary, the combination may be prescribed together with other antihypertensive agents, which may then be given in lower dosage with lessened chance of side reactions.

INDICATIONS AND USAGE:

Treatment of hypertension. (See BOXED WARNING.)

CONTRAINDICATIONS:

Patients with a history of mental depression, demonstrated hypersensitivity, and most cases of severe renal or hepatic diseases are the only contraindications.

WARNINGS:

These drugs should be used with caution in severe renal disease, since products containing chlorthalidone or similar drugs may precipitate azotemia. Cumulative effects of the drug may develop in patients with impaired renal function.

They should be used with caution in patients with impaired hepatic function or progressive liver disease, since minor alterations of fluid and electrolyte balance may precipitate hepatic coma.

Chlorthalidone/Reserpine or Demi-Chlorthalidone w/Reserpine may add to or potentiate the action of other antihypertensive drugs. Potentiation occurs with ganglionic or peripheral adrenergic-blocking drugs.

Sensitivity reactions may occur in patients with a history of allergy or bronchial asthma.

Reserpine may cause mental depression.

Recognition of depression may be difficult because this condition may often be disguised by somatic complaints (Masked Depression). The drug should be discontinued at first signs of depression such as despondency, early morning insomnia, loss of appetite, impotence, or self-deprecation. Drug induced depression may persist for several months after drug withdrawal and may be severe enough to result in suicide. In patients who have had depression, the drug should not be started. Electroshock therapy should not be given to patients taking reserpine, since severe and even fatal reactions have occurred.

The drug should be stopped at least seven days before giving electroshock therapy.

In susceptible patients, peptic ulcer may be precipitated or activated, in which case the drug should be discontinued.

Usage In Pregnancy: Reproduction studies with chlorthalidone in various animal species at multiples of the human dose showed no significant level of teratogenicity; no fetal or congenital abnormalities were observed. Animal data should not be extrapolated for clinical application.

Thiazides cross the placental barrier and appear in cord blood. The use of chlorthalidone and related drugs in pregnant women requires that the anticipated benefits of the drug be weighed against possible hazards to the fetus. These hazards include fetal or neonatal jaundice, thrombocytopenia, and possibly other adverse reactions which have occurred in the adult.

Nursing Mothers: Thiazides and reserpine cross the placental barrier and appear in cord blood and breast milk. Increased respiratory secretions, nasal congestion, cyanosis and anorexia may occur in infants born to reserpine-treated mothers. If use of the drug is deemed essential, the patient should stop nursing.

PRECAUTIONS:

Antihypertensive therapy with chlorthalidone/reserpine combinations should always be initiated cautiously in postsympathectomy patients and in those receiving ganglionic-blocking agents, other potent antihypertensive drugs, or curare. At least a one-half reduction in the usual dosage of such agents may be advisable. Careful and continuous supervision of patients on such multiple-drug regimens is necessary.

Since some patients receiving Rauwolfia preparations have experienced hypotension when undergoing surgery, it may be advisable to discontinue chlorthalidone/reserpine combination drugs about two weeks prior to elective surgical procedures. Emergency surgery may be carried out by using, if necessary, anticholinergic or adrenergic drugs to prevent vagocirculatory responses; other supportive measures may be used as indicated.

Because of the possibility of progression of renal damage, periodic kidney function tests are indicated. In case of a rising BUN, the drug should be stopped.

The drug should be discontinued in cases of aggravated liver dysfunction (hepatic coma may be precipitated).

Periodic determination of serum electrolytes to detect possible electrolyte imbalance should be performed at appropriate intervals.

All patients receiving chlorthalidone should be observed for clinical signs of fluid or electrolyte imbalance; namely, hyponatremia, hypochloremic alkalosis, and hypokalemia. Serum and urine electrolyte determinations are particularly important when the patient is vomiting excessively or receiving parenteral fluids. Medication such as digitalis may also influence serum electrolytes. Warning signs, irrespective of cause, are: Dryness of mouth, thirst, weakness, lethargy, drowsiness, restlessness, muscle pains or cramps, muscular fatigue, hypotension, oliguria, tachycardia, and gastrointestinal disturbances such as nausea and vomiting.

Hypokalemia may develop with chlorthalidone as with any other potent diuretic, especially with brisk diuresis, when severe cirrhosis is present, or during concomitant use of corticosteroids or ACTH.

Interference with adequate oral electrolyte intake will also contribute to hypokalemia.

Digitalis therapy may exaggerate metabolic effects of hypokalemia especially with reference to myocardial activity.

Any chloride deficit is generally mild and usually does not require specific treatment except under extraordinary circumstances (as in liver disease or renal disease). Dilutional hyponatremia may occur in edematous patients in hot weather; appropriate therapy is water restriction, rather than administration of salt except in rare instances when the hyponatremia is life threatening. In actual salt depletion, appropriate replacement is the therapy of choice.

PRECAUTIONS: *(cont'd)*

Hyperuricemia may occur or frank gout may be precipitated in certain patients receiving chlorthalidone.

Insulin requirements in diabetic patients may be increased, decreased, or unchanged. Latent diabetes mellitus may become manifest during chlorthalidone administration.

Chlorthalidone and related drugs may decrease arterial responsiveness to norepinephrine. This diminution is not sufficient to preclude effectiveness of the pressor agent for therapeutic use.

Chlorthalidone and related drugs may decrease serum PBI levels without signs of thyroid disturbance.

Because reserpine increases gastrointestinal motility and secretion, Chlorthalidone/Reserpine or Demi-Chlorthalidone w/Reserpine should be used cautiously in patients with ulcerative colitis or gallstones, where biliary colic may be precipitated. In susceptible patients, bronchial asthma may occur.

Animal Tumorigenicity: Rodent studies have shown that reserpine is an animal tumorigen, causing an increased incidence of mammary fibroadenomas in female mice, malignant tumors of the seminal vesicles in male mice, and malignant adrenal medullary tumors in male rats. These findings arose in two-year studies in which the drug was administered in the feed at concentrations of 5 and 10 ppm- about 100 to 300 times the usual human dose. The breast neoplasms are thought to be related to reserpine's prolactin-elevating effect. Several other prolactin-elevating drugs have also been associated with an increased incidence of mammary neoplasia in rodents.

The extent to which these findings indicate a risk to humans is uncertain. Tissue culture experiments show that about one third of human breast tumors are prolactin-dependent In Vitro, a factor of considerable importance if the use of the drug is contemplated in a patient with previously detected breast cancer. The possibility of an increased risk of breast cancer in reserpine users has been studied extensively; however, no firm conclusion has emerged. Although a few epidemiologic studies have suggested a slightly increased risk (less than twofold in all studies except one) in women who have used reserpine, other studies of generally similar design have not confirmed this. Epidemiologic studies conducted using other drugs (neuroleptic agents) that, like reserpine, increase prolactin levels and, therefore, would be considered rodent mammary carcinogens, have not shown an association between chronic administration of the drug and human mammary tumorigenesis. While long-term clinical observation has not suggested such an association, the available evidence is considered too limited to be conclusive at this time. An association of reserpine intake with pheochromocytoma or tumors of the seminal vesicles has not been explored.

ADVERSE REACTIONS:

Clinical trials indicate that the combination of chlorthalidone with reserpine is generally well tolerated. The adverse reactions most frequently seen include anorexia, gastric irritation, nausea, vomiting, diarrhea, constipation, nasal congestion, muscle cramps, dizziness, weakness, headache, drowsiness, and mental depression. Skin rashes, urticaria, and a case of ecchymosis have been reported. (Other dermatologic manifestations may occur—see below.)

A decreased glucose tolerance evidenced by hyperglycemia and glycosuria may develop inconsistently. This condition, usually reversible on discontinuation of therapy, responds to control with antidiabetic treatment.

Diabetics and those predisposed should be checked regularly.

Hyperuricemia may be observed on occasion and acute attacks of gout have been precipitated. In cases where prolonged and significant elevation of blood uric acid concentration is considered potentially deleterious, concomitant use of a uricosuric agent is effective in reversing hyperuricemia without loss of diuretic and/or antihypertensive activity.

In addition to the reactions listed above, certain adverse reactions attributable to the drugs' components are shown below. Since Chlorthalidone/Reserpine and Demi-Chlorthalidone w/Reserpine combine chlorthalidone and reserpine in relatively small doses, such reactions may be less than when those drugs are used in full dosage.

Chlorthalidone: Idiosyncratic drug reactions such as aplastic anemia, purpura, thrombocytopenia, leukopenia, agranulocytosis, necrotizing angiitis and Lyell's syndrome (toxic epidermal necrolysis) have occurred, but are rare.

The remote possibility of pancreatitis should be considered when epigastric pain or unexplained gastrointestinal symptoms develop after prolonged administration.

Other reported reactions include restlessness, transient myopia, impotence or dysuria, and orthostatic hypotension, which may be potentiated when chlorthalidone is combined with alcohol, barbiturates, or narcotics. Since jaundice, xanthopsia, paresthesia, and photosensitization have been documented in related compounds, the possibility of these reactions should be kept in mind.

Reserpine: The sedative effect of reserpine may lead to drowsiness or lassitude in some patients.

Frequently, this effect disappears with continued administration. Nasal stuffiness sometimes occurs. Gastrointestinal reactions include increased gastric secretions, loose stools, or increased bowel frequency.

Symptoms of mental depression may occur in a small percentage of patients, although the recommended dosage of Chlorthalidone/Reserpine contains substantially less reserpine than that usually implicated in such reactions. The same is true of other rare side effects recorded for reserpine, which include bradycardia and ectopic cardiac rhythms (especially when used with digitalis), pruritus, eruptions and/or flushing of skin, angina pectoris, headache, dizziness, paradoxical anxiety, nightmare, dull sensorium, muscular aches, a reversible paralysis agitans-like syndrome, blurred vision, conjunctival infection, uveitis, optic atrophy and glaucoma, increased susceptibility to colds, dyspnea, weight gain, decreased libido or impotence, dryness of the mouth, deafness, and anorexia.

OVERDOSAGE:

Adverse reactions resulting from accidental acute overdosage may include nausea, weakness, dizziness, syncope, and disturbances of electrolyte balance. There is no specific antidote. However, the following is recommended:

Gastric lavage followed by supportive treatment, including intravenous dextrose-saline with potassium chloride if necessary, to be given with the usual caution. If marked hypotension results from overdosage, it can be treated with vasopressor drugs.

DOSAGE AND ADMINISTRATION:

Selection of drug and dosage should be determined by individual titration. (See BOXED WARNING.)

According to the requirement, the recommended dose of either Chlorthalidone/Reserpine or Demi-Chlorthalidone w/Reserpine is usually One Tablet Once A Day. Some patients may require two tablets once a day. Divided doses are unnecessary, and a single dose given in the morning with food is recommended.

DOSAGE AND ADMINISTRATION: *(cont'd)*

Maintenance: Maintenance dosage must be individually adjusted. Mild cases may be adequately controlled with one Demi-Chlorthalidone w/Reserpine tablet daily. Optimal lowering of elevated blood pressure may require two weeks or more in some cases because of the slow onset of action of reserpine.

Combination With Other Drugs: In more severe cases, if the response to a chlorthalidone/reserpine combination alone is inadequate, potent antihypertensives may be added gradually in dosages at least 50% lower than those usually employed. Such patients should be supervised carefully and continuously. As soon as desired blood pressure levels have been attained, the lowest effective maintenance dosage should be followed.

HOW SUPPLIED - EQUIVALENTS NOT AVAILABLE:

Tablet, Uncoated - Oral - 25 mg/0.125 mg

100 tabs	$133.95	DEMI-REGROTON, Rhone-Poulenc Rorer	00075-0032-00

Tablet, Uncoated - Oral - 50 mg/0.25 mg

100's	**$152.63**	**REGROTON, Rhone-Poulenc Rorer**	**00075-0031-00**

CHLORZOXAZONE *(000804)*

CATEGORIES: Analgesics; Autonomic Drugs; Muscle Relaxants; Neuromuscular; Sedatives; Skeletal Muscle Hyperactivity; Skeletal Muscle Relaxants; FDA Approval Pre 1982

BRAND NAMES: *Biomioran*; *Escoflex*; Eze D.S.; *Klorzoxazon*; *Muscol*; Myoforte; **Paraflex**; *Parafon DSC*; *Parafon Forte*; Parafon Forte Dsc; *Prolax*; Relax-Ds; Relaxazone; Remular; *Solaxin*; Strifon Forte Dsc
(International brand names outside U.S. in italics)

FORMULARIES: BC-BS; FHP

DESCRIPTION:

ThiSmonograph contains information on the 250 mg and 500 mg caplets.

Each caplet (capsule shaped tablet) contains: Chlorzoxazone* - 250 mg

Inactive ingredients: docusate sodium, FD&C Red No. 40, FD&C Yellow No. 6, hydroxypropyl methylcellulose, lactose (hydrous), magnesium stearate, microcrystalline cellulose, polyethylene glycol, polysorbate 80, pregelatinized corn starch, propylene glycol, sodium benzoate, sodium starch glycolate, titanium dioxide.

*5-chlorobenzoxazolinone

Each caplet (capsule shaped tablet) contains: Chlorzoxazone* - 500 mg

Inactive ingredients: FD&C Blue No.1, microcrystalline cellulose, docusate sodium, lactose (hydrous), magnesium stearate, sodium benzoate, sodium starch glycolate, pregelatinized corn starch, D&C Yellow No. 10.

*5-chlorobenzoxazolinone.

CLINICAL PHARMACOLOGY:

Chlorzoxazone is a centrally-acting agent for painful musculoskeletal conditions. Data available from animal experiments as well as human study indicate that chlorzoxazone acts primarily at the level of the spinal cord and subcortical areas of the brain where it inhibits multisynaptic reflex arcs involved in producing and maintaining skeletal muscle spasm of varied etiology. The clinical result is a reduction of the skeletal muscle spasm with relief of pain and increased mobility of the involved muscles. Blood levels of chlorzoxazone can be detected in people during the first 30 minutes and peak levels may be reached, in the majority of the subjects, in about 1 to 2 hours after oral administration of chlorzoxazone. Chlorzoxazone is rapidly metabolized and is excreted in the urine, primarily in a conjugated form as the glucuronide. Less than one percent of a dose of chlorzoxazone is excreted unchanged in the urine in 24 hours.

INDICATIONS AND USAGE:

Chlorzoxazone is indicated as an adjunct to rest, physical therapy, and other measures for the relief of discomfort associated with acute, painful musculoskeletal conditions. The mode of action of this drug has not been clearly identified, but may be related to its sedative properties. Chlorzoxazone does not directly relax tense skeletal muscles in man.

CONTRAINDICATIONS:

Chlorzoxazone is contraindicated in patients with known intolerance to the drug.

WARNINGS:

Serious (including fatal) hepatocellular toxicity has been reported rarely in patients receiving chlorzoxazone. The mechanism is unknown but appears to be idiosyncratic and unpredictable. Factors predisposing patients to this reare event are not known. Patients should be instructed to report early signs and/or symptoms of hepatotoxicity such as fever, rash, anorexia, nausea, vomiting, fatigue, right upper quandrant pain, dark urine, or jaundice. Chlorzoxazone should be discontinued immediately and a physician consulted if any of these signs or symptoms develop. Chlorzoxazone use should also be discontinued if a patient develops abnormal liver enzymes (*e.g.,* AST, ALT, alkaline phosphate and bilirubin).

The concomitant use of alcohol or other central nervous system depressants may have an additive effect.

Usage in Pregnancy: The safe use of chlorzoxazone has not been established with respect to the possible adverse effects upon fetal development. Therefore, it should be used in women of childbearing potential only when, in the judgment of the physician, the potential benefits outweigh the possible risks.

PRECAUTIONS:

Chlorzoxazone should be used with caution in patients with known allergies or with a history of allergic reactions to drugs. If a sensitivity reaction occurs such as urticaria, redness, or itching of the skin, the drug should be stopped.

If any symptoms suggestive of liver dysfunction are observed, the drug should be discontinued.

ADVERSE REACTIONS:

After extensive clinical use of chlorzoxazone-containing products, it is apparent that the drug is well tolerated and seldom produces undesirable side effects. Occasional patients may develop gastrointestinal disturbances. It is possible in rare instances that chlorzoxazone may have been associated with gastrointestinal bleeding. Drowsiness, dizziness, lightheadedness, malaise, or overstimulation may be noted by an occasional patient. Rarely, allergic-type skin rashes, petechiae, or ecchymoses may develop during treatment. Angioneurotic edema or anaphylactic reactions are extremely rare. There is no evidence that the drug will cause renal damage. Rarely, a patient may note discoloration of the urine resulting from a phenolic metabolite of chlorzoxazone. This finding is of no known clinical significance.

OVERDOSAGE:

Symptoms: Initially, gastrointestinal disturbances such as nausea, vomiting, or diarrhea together with drowsiness, dizziness, lightheadedness or headache may occur. Early in the course there may be malaise or sluggishness followed by marked loss of muscle tone, making voluntary movement impossible. The deep tendon reflexes may be decreased or absent. The sensorium remains intact, and there is no peripheral loss of sensation. Respiratory depression may occur with rapid, irregular respiration and intercostal and substernal retraction. The blood pressure is lowered, but shock has not been observed.

Treatment: Gastric lavage or induction of emesis should be carried out, followed by administration of activated charcoal. Thereafter, treatment is entirely supportive. If respirations are depressed, oxygen and artificial respiration should be employed and a patent airway assured by use of an oropharyngeal airway or endotracheal tube. Hypotension may be counteracted by use of dextran, plasma, concentrated albumin or a vasopressor agent such as norepinephrine. Cholinergic drugs or analeptic drugs are of no value and should not be used.

DOSAGE AND ADMINISTRATION:

Usual Adult Dosage: One caplet (250 mg) three or four times daily. Initial dosage for *painful musculoskeletal conditions* should be two caplets (500 mg) three or four times daily. If adequate response is not obtained with this dose, it may be increased to three caplets (750 mg) three or four times daily. As improvement occurs, dosage can usually be reduced.

Store at room controlled room temperature (15°-30°C, 59°-86°F).

HOW SUPPLIED - RATED THERAPEUTICALLY EQUIVALENT:

Tablet - Oral - 500 mg

100's	$46.00	Chlorzoxazone, Duramed Pharms	51285-0886-02
500's	$213.00	Chlorzoxazone, Duramed Pharms	51285-0886-04

Tablet, Uncoated - Oral - 250 mg

100's	$5.25	Chlorzoxazone, Major Pharms	00904-0294-60
100's	$5.28	Chlorzoxazone, Geneva Pharms	00781-1303-01
100's	$5.28	Chlorzoxazone, H.C.F.A. F F P	99999-0804-01
100's	$6.95	Chlorzoxazone, Goldline Labs	00182-1780-01
100's	$9.50	Chlorzoxazone, Par Pharm	49884-0016-01
100's	$30.00	Relax-Ssc 250 Mg Tablets, Deliz	58238-0101-01
100's	$34.90	REMULAR-S, Intl Ethical	11584-1033-01
100's	$35.00	MYOFORTE, Alba Pharma	10023-0220-90
100's	**$57.76**	**PARAFLEX, McNeil Lab**	**00045-0317-60**
1000's	$52.80	Chlorzoxazone, H.C.F.A. F F P	99999-0804-02
1000's	$105.00	Chlorzoxazone, Par Pharm	49884-0016-10

Tablet, Uncoated - Oral - 500 mg

100's	$9.75	Chlorzoxazone, H.C.F.A. F F P	99999-0804-03
100's	$10.43	Chlorzoxazone, United Res	00677-1221-01
100's	$10.43	Chlorzoxazone, Geneva Pharms	00781-1304-01
100's	$20.40	Chlorzoxazone, IDE-Interstate	00814-1714-14
100's	$29.95	EZE D. S., Seneca Pharms	47028-0052-01
100's	$34.00	Relaxazone, Bolan Pharm	44437-0193-01
100's	$42.50	Chlorzoxazone, Sidmak Labs	50111-0861-01
100's	$44.25	Chlorzoxazone, Major Pharms	00904-0302-60
100's	$44.32	Chlorzoxazone, Aligen Independ	00405-4219-01
100's	$44.35	Chlorzoxazone, Qualitest Pharms	00603-2886-21
100's	$44.50	Chlorzoxazone, Mutual Pharm	53489-0193-01
100's	$45.00	Chlorzoxazone, Goldline Labs	00182-1189-01
100's	$45.40	Chlorzoxazone, Royce	51875-0239-01
100's	$45.64	Chlorzoxazone, Schein Pharm (US)	00364-2255-01
100's	$45.68	Chlorzoxazone, Vangard Labs	00615-3511-13
100's	$45.75	Chlorzoxazone, Caraco Pharm	57664-0122-08
100's	$46.30	Chlorzoxazone, Martec Pharms	52555-0263-01
100's	$46.90	Chlorzoxazone, Teva	00093-0542-01
100's	$46.97	Chlorzoxazone, HL Moore Drug Exch	00839-7445-06
100's	$46.97	Chlorzoxazone, HL Moore Drug Exch	00839-7725-06
100's	$47.50	Chlorzoxazone, Harber Pharm	51432-0824-03
100's	$48.00	Chlorzoxazone, Econolab	55053-0787-01
100's	$48.98	Chlorzoxazone, Rugby	00536-3444-01
100's	$48.98	Chlorzoxazone 500, Barr	00555-0585-02
100's	$49.95	Chlorzoxazone, Geneva Pharms	00781-1304-13
100's	$60.00	Relax-Ds, Deliz	58238-0102-01
100's	$99.38	PARAFON FORTE DSC, McNeil Lab	00045-0325-60
100's	$103.93	PARAFON FORTE DSC, McNeil Lab	00045-0325-10
100's	$228.00	Chlorzoxazone, Econolab	55053-0787-05
500's	$48.00	Strifon Forte Dsc, Ferndale Labs	00496-1039-10
500's	$48.75	Chlorzoxazone, H.C.F.A. F F P	99999-0804-04
500's	$52.15	Chlorzoxazone, Geneva Pharms	00781-1304-05
500's	$155.05	Chlorzoxazone, Major Pharms	00904-0302-40
500's	$175.70	Chlorzoxazone, Martec Pharms	52555-0263-05
500's	$195.00	Chlorzoxazone, Goldline Labs	00182-1189-05
500's	$195.00	Chlorzoxazone, Mutual Pharm	53489-0193-05
500's	$195.74	Chlorzoxazone, HL Moore Drug Exch	00839-7445-12
500's	$195.74	Chlorzoxazone, HL Moore Drug Exch	00839-7725-12
500's	$198.70	Chlorzoxazone, Qualitest Pharms	00603-2886-28
500's	$201.50	Chlorzoxazone, Sidmak Labs	50111-0861-02
500's	$211.75	Chlorzoxazone, Royce	51875-0239-02
500's	$211.95	Chlorzoxazone, Caraco Pharm	57664-0122-13
500's	$215.81	Chlorzoxazone 500, Barr	00555-0585-04
500's	$217.74	Chlorzoxazone, Teva	00093-0542-05
500's	$217.74	Chlorzoxazone, Rugby	00536-3444-05
500's	$217.80	Chlorzoxazone, Aligen Independ	00405-4219-02
500's	$475.80	PARAFON FORTE DSC, McNeil Lab	00045-0325-70
1000's	$97.50	Chlorzoxazone, H.C.F.A. F F P	99999-0804-05
1000's	$370.15	Chlorzoxazone, Sidmak Labs	50111-0861-03

CHOLERA VACCINE *(000807)*

CATEGORIES: Cholera; Immunologic; Serums, Toxoids and Vaccines; Vaccines; FDA Pre 1938 Drugs

DESCRIPTION:

CHOLERA VACCINE, USP, is a sterile suspension of equal parts of Ogawa and Inaba serotypes of killed *Vibrio cholerae (V. comma)* in buffered sodium chloride injection. The Inaba and Ogawa strains of *V. cholerae* are grown on trypticase soy agar medium, removed from the medium with buffered sodium chloride injection and killed by the addition of 0.5 percent phenol. Phenol in a concentration of 0.5 percent is also used as the preservative in the finished vaccine. The vaccine contains 8 units of each serotype antigen (Ogawa and Inaba) per milliliter.

Cholera vaccine may be injected intracutaneously (intradermally), subcutaneously or intramuscularly.

CLINICAL PHARMACOLOGY:

Cholera vaccine is used for active immunization against cholera. Field studies carried out in endemic cholera areas have shown cholera vaccines to be approximately 50% effective in reducing incidence of disease and for only 3 to 6 months. Use of cholera vaccine does not prevent transmission of infection.

INDICATIONS AND USAGE:

Active immunization against cholera is indicated only for individuals traveling to or residing in countries where cholera is endemic or epidemic.

CONTRAINDICATIONS:

Use of cholera vaccine should be postponed in the presence of any acute illness.

A history of severe systemic reaction or allergic response following a prior dose of cholera vaccine is a contraindication to further use.

WARNINGS:

DO NOT INJECT INTRAVENOUSLY.

Cholera vaccine should not be administered intramuscularly to persons with thrombocytopenia or any coagulation disorder that would contraindicate intramuscular injection.

PRECAUTIONS:

GENERAL

A separate, sterilized syringe and needle should be used for each patient to prevent transmission of hepatitis B virus and other infectious agents from one person to another.

Before delivering the dose intramuscularly or subcutaneously, aspirate to help avoid inadvertent injection into a blood vessel.

Before the injection of any biological, the physician should take all precautions known for prevention of allergic or other side reactions. This should include: a review of the patient's history regarding possible sensitivity; and a knowledge of the recent literature pertaining to the use of the biological concerned.

Epinephrine (1:1000) should be available for immediate use when this product is injected.

PREGNANCY CATEGORY C

Animal reproduction studies have not been conducted with cholera vaccine. It is also not known whether cholera vaccine can cause fetal harm when administered to a pregnant woman or can affect reproductive capacity. However, as with other inactivated bacterial vaccines, its use is not contraindicated during pregnancy unless the intended recipient has manifested significant systemic or allergic reaction following administration of prior doses. Use of cholera vaccine during pregnancy should be individualized to reflect actual need.[1,3]

DRUG INTERACTIONS:

Some data suggest that administration of cholera and yellow fever vaccines within three weeks of each other may result in decreased levels of antibody response to both vaccines as compared with administration at longer intervals. However, there is no evidence that protection to either disease is diminished following simultaneous administration.[1] It is currently recommended that, when feasible, cholera and yellow fever vaccines should be administered at a minimal interval of three weeks, unless time constraints preclude this. If the vaccines cannot be administered at least three weeks apart, they should be given simultaneously.[2]

ADVERSE REACTIONS:

Local reactions manifested by erythema, induration, pain, and tenderness at the site of injection occur in most recipients, and such local reactions may persist for a few days.

Recipients frequently develop malaise, headache, and mild-to-moderate temperature elevations which may persist for 1 to 2 days.[1,4]

DOSAGE AND ADMINISTRATION:

Shake vial vigorously before withdrawing each dose.

Parenteral drug products should be inspected visually for presence of particulate matter and discoloration prior to use.

The primary immunizing course consists of two doses administered one week to one month or more apart. TABLE 1 summarizes the recommended doses for both primary and booster immunizations by age, volume (ml), and route of administration.[3,5] The intracutaneous (intradermal) route is satisfactory for persons 5 years of age and older, but higher levels of antibody may be achieved in children less than 5 years old by the subcutaneous or intramuscular routes.

TABLE 1 Route & Age

Dose number	Intradermal	Subcutaneous or Intramuscular		
	5 years and over	6 mos-4 years	5-10 years	over 10 years
1 & 2	0.2 ml	0.2 ml	0.3 ml	0.5 ml
Boosters	0.2 ml	0.2 ml	0.3 ml	0.5 ml

In areas where cholera is epidemic or endemic, booster doses should be given every six months.

The primary immunizing series need never be repeated for booster doses to be effective.

Before injection, the rubber diaphragm of the vial and the skin over the site to be injected should be cleansed and prepared with a suitable germicide.

Store between 2° and 8°C (35° and 46°F).

REFERENCES:

1. Recommendation of the Immunization Practices Advisory Committee (ACIP). General recommendations on immunization. MMWR 32(1):1, 1983. **2.** Recommendations of the Immunization Practices Advisory Committee (ACIP). Yellow fever vaccine. MMWR 32(52):679, 1984. **3.** Recommendation of the Public Health Service Advisory Committee on Immunization Practices—Cholera Vaccine. MMWR 27(20):173, 1978. **4.** GANGAROSA, E. and FAICH, G.: Cholera: The risk to American travelers. Ann. Int. Med. *74*:412, 1971. **5.** Report of the Committee on Infectious Diseases, American Academy of Pediatrics, 1982 (Red Book).

HOW SUPPLIED - EQUIVALENTS NOT AVAILABLE:

Injection, Susp - Intramuscular; - 1 unit/ml

1.5 ml	$9.69	Cholera Vaccine, Wyeth Labs	00008-0342-02
20 ml	$34.61	Cholera Vaccine, Wyeth Labs	00008-0342-01

CHOLINE BITARTRATE; DEXPANTHENOL

(000810)

CATEGORIES: Gastrointestinal Drugs; Homeostatic & Nutrient; Vitamins; FDA Pre 1938 Drugs

BRAND NAMES: **Ilopan-Choline**

Prescribing information not available at time of publication.

HOW SUPPLIED - EQUIVALENTS NOT AVAILABLE:

Tablet, Uncoated - Oral - 25 mg/50 mg

100's	$75.73	ILOPAN-CHOLINE, Savage Labs	00281-2311-17

CHOLINE MAGNESIUM TRISALICYLATE

(000811)

CATEGORIES: Analgesics; Anti-Inflammatory Agents; Antiarthritics; Antipyretics; Arthritis; Bursitis; Central Nervous System Agents; Fever; Nonsteroidal Anti-Inflammatory; Osteoarthritis; Pain; Salicylates; Pregnancy Category C; FDA Pre 1938 Drugs

BRAND NAMES: Amilisate; Cmt; Tricosal; **Trilisate**

FORMULARIES: Aetna; BC-BS; FHP; Medi-Cal

DESCRIPTION:

Choline magnesium trisalicylate is nonsteroidal, anti-inflammatory preparations containing choline magnesium trisalicylate which is freely soluble in water. The absolute structure of choline magnesium trisalicylate is not known at this time. Choline magnesium trisalicylate has a molecular formula of $C_{26}H_{29}O_{10}NMg$, a molecular weight of 539.8.

This substance when dissolved in water would appear to form 5 ions (1 choline ion, 1 magnesium ion and 3 salicylate ions).

Trilisate Tablets/Liquid are available in scored, pale pink 500 mg tablets; in scored, white film-coated 750 mg tablets, and in scored, red, film-coated 1000 mg tablets. Trilisate Liquid is a cherry cordial-flavored liquid providing 500 mg salicylate content per teaspoonful (5 ml) for oral administration.

Each Trilisate 500 mg tablet contains 293 mg of choline salicylate combined with 362 mg of magnesium salicylate to provide 500 mg salicylate content. Each 750 mg tablet contains 440 mg of choline salicylate combined with 544 mg of magnesium salicylate to provide 750 mg salicylate content. Each 1000 mg tablet contains 587 mg of choline salicylate combined with 725 mg magnesium salicylate to provide 1000 mg salicylate content.

Trilisate Liquid contains 293 mg of choline salicylate combined with 362 mg of magnesium salicylate to provide 500 mg salicylate per teaspoonful (5 ml) in a clear amber, cherry cordial-flavored vehicle.

Trilisate Inactive Ingredients: *Each 500 mg tablet* contains Carboxymethylcellulose sodium, Corn starch, Edetate disodium, FD&C Yellow No. 6, Stearic acid, and other ingredients. *Each 750 mg tablet contains:* Carboxymethylcellulose sodium, Edetate disodium, Polyethylene glycol, Polysorbate 20, Stearic acid, Talc, Titanium dioxide, and other ingredients. *Each 1000 mg tablet contains:* Carboxymethylcellulose sodium, Edetate disodium, FD&C Red No. 40, FD&C Yellow No. 6, FD&C Blue No. 2, Polyethylene glycol, Polysorbate 20, Stearic acid, Talc, Titanium dioxide, and other ingredients. *Each teaspoonful (5 ml) of Liquid contains:* Caramel, Carboxymethylcellulose sodium, Edetate disodium, FD&C Yellow No. 6, Glycerin, High fructose corn syrup, Potassium sorbate, Water, Artificial flavors.

CLINICAL PHARMACOLOGY:

Choline magnesium trisalicylate contains salicylate with anti-inflammatory, analgesic and antipyretic action. On ingestion of choline magnesium trisalicylate, the salicylate moiety is absorbed rapidly and reaches peak blood levels within an average of one to two hours after single doses of the tablets of liquid. The primary route of excretion is renal: the excretion products are chiefly the glycine and glucuronide conjugates. At higher serum salicylate concentrations, the glycine conjugation pathway becomes rapidly saturated. Thus, the slower glucuronide conjugation pathway becomes the rate limiting step for salicylate excretion. In addition, salicylate excreted in the bile as glucuronide conjugate may be reabsorbed. These factors account for the prolongation of salicylate half-life and the nonlinear increase in plasma salicylate level as the salicylate dose is increased. The serum concentration of salicylate is increased by conditions that decrease glomerular filtration rate or proximal tubular secretion.

The bioequivalence of Trilisate Liquid and Trilisate Tablets 500 mg/750 mg/1000 mg has been established. With the tablets, a steady-state condition is usually reached after 4 to 5 doses, and the half-life of elimination, on repeated administration of tablets, is 9 to 17 hours. This permits a maintenance dosage schedule of once or twice daily. Unlike aspirin and certain other non-steroidal anti-inflammatory agents, such as arylpropionic acid derivatives and arylacetic acid derivatives, choline magnesium trisalicylate, at therapeutic dosage levels, does not affect platelet aggregation, as shown by *in vitro* and *in vivo* studies.

INDICATIONS AND USAGE:

Osteoarthritis, Rheumatoid Arthritis and Acute Painful Shoulder: Salicylates are considered the base therapy of choice in the arthritides; and choline magnesium trisalicylate preparations are indicated for the relief of the signs and symptoms of rheumatoid arthritis, osteoarthritis and other arthritides. Choline magnesium trisalicylate is indicated in the long-term management of these diseases and especially in the acute flare of rheumatoid arthritis. Choline magnesium trisalicylate is also indicated for the treatment of acute painful shoulder.

Choline magnesium trisalicylate preparations are effective and generally well tolerated, and are logical choices whenever salicylate treatment is indicated. They are particularly suitable when a once-a-day or b.i.d. dosage regimen is important to patient compliance; when gastrointestinal intolerance to aspirin is encountered; when gastrointestinal microbleeding or hematologic effects of aspirin are considered a patient hazard; and when interference (or the risk of interference) with normal platelet function by aspirin or by propionic acid derivatives is considered to be clinically undesirable. Use of choline magnesium trisalicylate liquid is appropriate when a liquid dosage form is preferred, as in the elderly patient.

The efficacy of choline magnesium trisalicylate preparations has not been studied in those patients who are designated by the American Rheumatism Association as belonging in Functional Class IV (incapacitated, largely or wholly bedridden or confined to a wheelchair, with little or no self-care). Analgesic and Antipyretic Action: choline magnesium trisalicylate are also indicated for the relief of mild to moderate pain and for antipyresis.

In Children: Choline magnesium trisalicylate preparations are indicated for conditions requiring anti-inflammatory or analgesic action - such as juvenile rheumatoid arthritis and other appropriate conditions.

CONTRAINDICATIONS:

Patients who are hypersensitive to non-acetylated salicylates should not take choline magnesium trisalicylate.

WARNINGS:

Reye Syndrome is a rare but serious disease which may develop in children and teenagers who have chicken pox, influenza, or flu symptoms. While the cause of Reye Syndrome is unknown, some studies suggest a possible association between the development of Reye Syndrome and the use of medicines containing acetylated salicylates or aspirin. Choline magnesium Trisalicylate Tablets and Liquid are a combination of choline salicylate and magnesium salicylate which are nonacetylated salicylates, and there have been no reported cases associating choline magnesium trisalicylate with Reye Syndrome. Nevertheless, choline magnesium trisalicylate, as a salicylate-containing product, is not recommended for use in children and teenagers with chicken pox, influenza or flu symptoms.

PRECAUTIONS:

General: As with other salicylates and non-steroidal anti-inflammatory drugs, choline magnesium trisalicylate preparations should be used with caution in patients with acute or chronic renal insufficiency, with acute or chronic hepatic dysfunction, or with gastritis or peptic ulcer disease.

Although reports exist of cross reactivity, including bronchospasm, with the use of non-acetylated salicylate products in aspirin-sensitive patients, choline magnesium trisalicylate preparations were found to be well tolerated with regard to pulmonary function and respiratory symptoms when these parameters were monitored in a group of documented aspirin-sensitive asthmatics dosed with choline magnesium trisalicylate in both controlled and open label studies.[1]

Concurrent use of other salicylate-containing products and choline magnesium trisalicylate preparations can lead to an increase in plasma salicylate concentration and may result in potentially toxic salicylate levels.

Laboratory Tests: Plasma salicylate levels can be periodically assessed during treatment with choline magnesium trisalicylate preparations to determine whether a therapeutically effective anti-inflammatory concentration of 15 to 30 mg/100 ml (150-300 micrograms/ml) is being maintained. Manifestations of systemic salicylate intoxication are usually not seen until the concentration exceeds 30 mg/100 ml. However, such tests rarely differentiate between the active free and inactive protein bound salicylate components. Since protein binding of salicylate is affected by age, nutritional status, competitive binding of other drugs, and underlying disease (*e.g.,* rheumatoid arthritis), plasma salicylate level determinations may not always accurately reflect efficacious or toxic levels of active free salicylate. Acidification of the urine can significantly diminish the renal clearance of salicylate and increase plasma salicylate concentrations.

Laboratory Test Interactions: Free T4 values may be increased in patients on salicylate drug products due to competitive plasma protein binding; a concurrent decrease in total plasma T4 may be observed. Thyroid function is not affected.

Carcinogenesis, Mutagenesis, and Impairment of Fertility: No long-term animal studies have been performed with choline magnesium trisalicylate to evaluate its carcinogenic potential.

Pregnancy Category C: Animal reproduction studies have not been conducted with choline magnesium trisalicylate preparations. It is also not known whether choline magnesium trisalicylate can cause fetal harm when administered to a pregnant woman or can affect reproduction capacity. choline magnesium trisalicylate should be given to a pregnant woman only if clearly needed. Because of the known effects of other salicylate drug products on the fetal cardiovascular system (closure of ductus arteriosus), use during late pregnancy should be avoided.

Labor and Delivery: The effects of choline magnesium trisalicylate on labor and delivery in pregnant women are unknown. Since prolonged gestation and prolonged labor due to prostaglandin inhibition have been reported with the use of other salicylate products, the use of choline magnesium trisalicylate preparations near term is not recommended. Other salicylate products have also been associated with alterations in maternal and neonatal hemostasis mechanisms and with perinatal mortality.

Nursing Mothers: Salicylate is excreted in human milk. Peak milk salicylate levels are delayed, occurring as long as 9 to 12 hours post dose, and the milk:plasma ratio has been reported to be as high as 0.34. Because of the potential for significant salicylate absorption by the nursing infant, caution should be exercised when choline magnesium trisalicylate is administered to a nursing woman.

Pediatric Use: In a four-week open label pilot study of patients with juvenile rheumatoid arthritis, children from 6 to 16 years of age previously on aspirin received weight adjusted doses (50-60 mg/kg) of choline magnesium trisalicylate 500 mg tablets on a divided b.i.d. schedule with subsequent dose titration to achieve therapeutic serum salicylate levels. Eighty-three percent (83%) of the patients rated the therapeutic effect of choline magnesium trisalicylate as good or excellent. Tinnitus was reported by one patient and elevated SGOT levels at Week 1, which decreased during the trial, were detected in two patients. (See WARNINGS).

DRUG INTERACTIONS:

Foods and drugs that alter urine pH may affect renal clearance of salicylate and plasma salicylate concentrations. Raising urine pH, as with chronic antacid use, can enhance renal salicylate clearance and diminish plasma salicylate concentration; urine acidification can decrease urinary salicylate excretion and increase plasma levels.

When salicylate drug products are concurrently dosed with other plasma protein bound drug products, adverse effects may result. Although choline magnesium trisalicylate preparations are a rational choice for anti-inflammatory and analgesic therapy in patients on oral anticoagulants due to their demonstrated lack of effect *in vivo* and *in vitro* on platelet aggregation, bleeding time, platelet count, prothrombin time, and serum thromboxane B2 generation[1-7]the potential exists for increased levels of unbound warfarin with their concurrent use. Prothrombin time should be closely monitored and warfarin dose appropriately adjusted when therapy with choline magnesium trisalicylate preparations is initiated. The effect of choline magnesium trisalicylate on blood prothrombin levels has not been established.

Salicylates may increase the therapeutic as well as toxic effects of methotrexate, particularly when administered in chemotherapeutic doses, but inhibition of renal methotrexate excretion and by displacement of plasma protein bound methotrexate. Caution should be exercised in administering choline magnesium trisalicylate to rheumatoid arthritis patients on methotrexate. When sulfonylurea oral hypoglycemic agents are co-administered with salicylates, the hypoglycemic effect may be enhanced via increased insulin secretion or by displacement of sulfonylurea agents from binding sites. Insulin-treated diabetics on high doses of salicylates should also be closely monitored for a similar hypoglycemic response. Other drugs with which salicylate competes for protein binding sites, and whose plasma concentration or free fraction may be altered by concurrent salicylate administration, include the following: phenytoin, valproic acid, and carbonic anhydrase inhibitors. The efficacy of uricosuric agents may be decreased when administered with salicylate products. Although low doses of salicylate (1 to 2 grams per day) have been reported to decrease urate excretion and elevate plasma urate concentrations, intermediate doses (2 to 3 grams per day) usually do not alter urate excretion. Larger salicylate doses (over 5 grams per day) can induce uricosuria and lower plasma urate levels.

Corticosteroids can reduce plasma salicylate levels by increasing renal elimination and perhaps by also stimulating hepatic metabolism of salicylates. By monitoring plasma salicylate levels, salicylate dosage may be titrated to accommodate changes in corticosteroid dose or to avoid salicylate toxicity during corticosteroid taper.

ADVERSE REACTIONS:

The most frequent adverse reactions observed with choline magnesium trisalicylate preparations in clinical trials[7-12] are tinnitus and gastrointestinal complaints (including nausea, vomiting, gastric upset, indigestion, heartburn, diarrhea, constipation and epigastric pain). These occur in less than twenty percent (20%) of patients. Should tinnitus develop, reduction of daily dosage is recommended until the tinnitus is resolved. Less frequent adverse reactions, occurring in less than two percent (2%) of patients, are: hearing impairment, headache, lightheadedness, dizziness, drowsiness, and lethargy. Adverse reactions occurring in less than one percent (1%) of patients are: gastric ulceration, positive fecal occult blood, elevation in serum BUN and creatinine, rash, pruritus, anorexia, weight gain, edema, epistaxis and dysgeusia.

Spontaneous reporting has yielded isolated or rare reports of the following adverse experiences: duodenal ulceration, elevated hepatic transaminases, hepatitis, esophagitis, asthma, erythema multiforme, urticaria, ecchymoses, irreversible hearing loss and/or tinnitus, mental confusion, hallucinations.

DRUG ABUSE AND DEPENDENCE:

Drug abuse and dependence have not been reported with choline magnesium trisalicylate preparations.

OVERDOSAGE:

Death in adults has been reported following ingestion of doses of from 10 to 30 grams of salicylate; however, larger doses have been taken without resulting fatality.

Symptoms: Salicylate intoxication, known as salicylism, may occur with large doses or extended therapy. Common symptoms of salicylism include headache, dizziness, tinnitus, hearing impairment, confusion, drowsiness, sweating, vomiting, diarrhea, and hyperventilation. A more severe degree of salicylate intoxication can lead to CNS disturbances, alteration in electrolyte balance, respiratory and metabolic acidosis, hyperthermia, and dehydration.

Treatment: Reduction of further absorption of salicylate from the gastrointestinal tract can be achieved via emesis, gastric lavage, use of activated charcoal, or a combination of the above. Appropriate I.V. fluids should be administered to correct dehydration, electrolyte imbalance, and acidosis and to maintain adequate renal function. To accelerate salicylate excretion, forced diuresis with alkalinizing solution is recommended. In extreme cases, peritoneal dialysis or hemodialysis should be considered for effective salicylate removal.

DOSAGE AND ADMINISTRATION:

Adults: In rheumatoid arthritis, osteoarthritis, the more severe arthritides, and acute painful shoulder, the recommended starting dosage is 1500 mg given b.i.d. Some patients may be treated with 3000 mg given once per day (h.s.) In the elderly patient, a daily dosage of 2250 mg given as 750 mg t.i.d. may be efficacious and well tolerated. Dosage should be adjusted in accordance with the patient's response. For mild to moderate pain or for antipyresis, the usual dosage is 2000 mg to 3000 mg daily in divided doses (b.i.d.). Based on patient response or salicylate blood levels, dosage may be adjusted to achieve optimum therapeutic effect. Salicylate blood levels should be in the range of 15 to 30 mg/100 ml for anti-inflammatory effect and 5 to 15 mg/100 ml for analgesia and antipyresis.

Each 500 mg tablet or teaspoonful is equivalent in salicylate content to 10 gr of aspirin; each 750 mg tablet, to 15 gr of aspirin, and each 1000 mg tablet, to 20 gr of aspirin.

If the physician prefers, the recommended daily dosage may be administered on a t.i.d. schedule.

As with other therapeutic agents, individual dosage adjustment is advisable, and a number of patients may require higher or lower dosages than those recommended. Certain patients require 2 to 3 weeks of therapy for optimal effect.

Children: *Usual daily dose:* for children for anti-inflammatory or analgesic action:

Choline magnesium trisalicylate 500 mg tablets/liquid and choline magnesium trisalicylate 750 mg and 1000 mg tablets, 50 mg/kg/day. (see TABLE 1)

TABLE 1 Usual Daily Dose for Children

Weight (kg):	Total daily dose
12-13:	500 mg
14-17:	750 mg
18-22:	1000 mg
23-27:	1250 mg
28-32:	1500 mg
33-37:	1750 mg

Total daily doses should be administered in divided doses (b.i.d.). Doses of choline magnesium trisalicylate preparations are calculated as the total daily dose of 50 mg/kg/day for children of 37 kg body weight or less and 2250 mg/day for heavier children.

choline magnesium trisalicylate Liquid is available for greater convenience in treating younger patients and those adult patients unable to swallow a solid dosage form.

REFERENCES:

1. Szczeklik, A et al; Choline magnesium trisalicylate in patients with aspirin-induced asthma; *Eur. Respir. J;* 3: 535-539, 1990. **2.** Zucker, MB and Rothwell KB; Differential influences of salicylate compounds in platelet aggregation and serotonin release;*Current Therapeutic Research*; 23(2), Feb 1987. **3.** Stuart, JJ and Pisko, EJ; Choline magnesium trisalicylate does not impair platelet aggregation; *Pharmatherapeutica*; 2(8):547, 1981. **4.** Danesh, BJZ, Saniabadi, AR, Russell, RI et al; Therapeutic potential of choline magnesium trisalicylate as an alternative to aspirin for patients with bleeding tendencies; *Scottish Medical Journal;* 32:167-168, 1987. **5.** Danesh, BJZ, McLaren, M. Russell, Rl et al; Does non-acetylated salicylate inhibit thromboxane biosynthesis in human platelet? *Scottish Medical Journal*; 33:315-316, 1988. **6.** Danesh, BJZ, McLaren, M. Russell, Rl et al; Comparison of the effect of aspirin and choline magnesium trisalicylate on thromboxane biosynthesis in human platelets: role of acetyl moiety;*Haemostasis*; 19:169-173, 1989. **7.** Data on file. Medical Department. The Purdue Frederick Company, 1989. **8.** Blechman, WJ, and Lechner, BL; Clinical comparative evaluation of choline magnesium trisalicylate and acetylsalicylic acid in rheumatoid arthritis;*Rheumatology and Rehabilitation*; 18:119-124, 1979. **9.** McLaughlin, G; Choline magnesium trisalicylate vs. naproxen in rheumatoid arthritis; *Current Therapeutic Research*; 32(4):579- 585, 1982. **10.** Ehrlich, GE; Miller, SB; and Zeiders, RS; Choline magnesium trisalicylate vs. ibuprofen in rheumatoid arthritis;*Rheumatology and Rehabilitation*; 19:30-41, 1980. **11.** Goldenberg, A; Rudnicki, RD, and Koonce, ML; Clinical comparison of efficacy and safety of choline magnesium trisalicylate and indomethacin in treating osteoarthritis; *Current Therapeutic Research*; 24(3):245-260, 1978. **12.** Guerin, BK and Burnstein, SL; Conservative therapy of acute painful shoulder; *Orthopedic Review*; XI(7):29-37, 1982.

HOW SUPPLIED - RATED THERAPEUTICALLY EQUIVALENT:

Capsule - Oral - 750 mg

100's $34.40 Choline Magnesium Trisalicylate, Duramed Pharms 51285-0903-02

HOW SUPPLIED - RATED THERAPEUTICALLY EQUIVALENT: *(cont'd)*

Tablet - Oral - 500 mg

100's	$27.70	Choline Magnesium Trisalicylate, Duramed Pharms	51285-0902-02

Tablet - Oral - 1000 mg

100's	$39.90	Choline Magnesium Trisalicylate, Duramed Pharms	51285-0904-02

HOW SUPPLIED - NOT RATED EQUIVALENT:

Liquid - Oral - 500 mg

240 ml	**$28.67**	**TRILISATE, Purdue Frederick**	**00034-0520-80**

Tablet, Uncoated - Oral - 500 mg

100's	$29.55	Choline Magnesium Trisalicylate, HL Moore Drug Exch	00839-7499-06
100's	$29.84	Choline & Magnesium Salicylate, Major Pharms	00904-3395-61
100's	$29.90	TRICOSAL, United Res	00677-1390-01
100's	$32.00	Choline Mag Trisalicylate, Medirex	57480-0401-01
100's	$33.00	Choline Mag Trisalicylate, Goldline Labs	00182-1899-01
100's	$33.00	Choline Magnesium Trisalicylate, Sidmak Labs	50111-0528-01
100's	$33.43	CHOLINE MAGNESIUM TRISALICYLATE 500, Aligen Independ	00405-4229-01
100's	$34.65	Choline Magnesium Trisalicylate, Martec Pharms	52555-0528-01
100's	$34.90	TRICOSAL, Qualitest Pharms	00603-6215-21
100's	$34.95	Choline Magnesium Trisalicylate 500, Major Pharms	00904-3395-60
100's	$36.41	Choline Mag Trisalicylate, Alpharma	00472-0140-10
100's	$36.45	Choline Magnesium, Geneva Pharms	00781-1637-01
100's	$58.69	Choline Magnesium Trisal, Rugby	00536-3452-01
100's	**$60.31**	**TRILISATE 500, Purdue Frederick**	**00034-0500-80**
100's	**$62.92**	**TRILISATE 500, Purdue Frederick**	**00034-0500-10**
500's	**$301.72**	**TRILISATE 500, Purdue Frederick**	**00034-0500-50**
600's	$192.00	Choline Mag Trisalicylate, Medirex	57480-0401-06

Tablet, Uncoated - Oral - 750 mg

100's	$34.77	Choline & Magnesium Salicylate, Major Pharms	00904-3396-61
100's	$35.09	Choline Magnesium Trisalicylate, HL Moore Drug Exch	00839-7500-06
100's	$39.00	Choline Mag Trisalicylate, Medirex	57480-0402-01
100's	$42.00	Choline Magnesium Trisalicylate, Sidmak Labs	50111-0529-01
100's	$42.80	Choline Magnesium Trisalicylate, Aligen Independ	00405-4230-01
100's	$42.85	TRICOSAL, United Res	00677-1391-01
100's	$42.90	Choline Magnesium Trisalicylate, Goldline Labs	00182-1895-01
100's	$43.50	Choline Magnesium Trisalicylate, Major Pharms	00904-3396-60
100's	$43.51	TRICOSAL, Qualitest Pharms	00603-6216-21
100's	$44.10	Choline Magnesium Trisalicylate, Martec Pharms	52555-0529-01
100's	$45.19	Choline Mag Trisalicylate, Alpharma	00472-0141-10
100's	$45.20	Choline Magnesium, Geneva Pharms	00781-1638-01
100's	$72.87	Choline Magnesium Trisalicylate, Rugby	00536-3453-01
100's	**$74.87**	**TRILISATE 750, Purdue Frederick**	**00034-0505-80**
100's	**$77.61**	**TRILISATE 750, Purdue Frederick**	**00034-0505-10**
500's	**$371.03**	**TRILISATE 750, Purdue Frederick**	**00034-0505-50**
600's	$234.00	Choline Mag Trisalicylate, Medirex	57480-0402-06

Tablet, Uncoated - Oral - 1000 mg

60's	**$49.88**	**TRILISATE 1000, Purdue Frederick**	**00034-0510-60**
100's	$44.80	Choline Mag Trisalicylate, Major Pharms	00904-3397-60
100's	$45.40	TRICOSAL, Qualitest Pharms	00603-6217-21
100's	$47.00	Tricosal, Duramed Pharms	51285-0853-02
100's	$47.00	Choline & Mag Trisalicylate, Invamed	52189-0254-24
100's	$50.06	Choline & Mag Salicylate, Aligen Independ	00405-4231-01
100's	$53.98	Choline Mag Trisalicylate, Alpharma	00472-0142-10
100's	$55.00	Choline Magnesium Trisalicylate, Sidmak Labs	50111-0530-01
100's	$56.01	Choline & Magnesium Salicylate, Major Pharms	00904-3397-61
100's	$57.75	Choline Magnesium Trisalicylate, Martec Pharms	52555-0530-01
100's	**$96.54**	**TRILISATE 1000, Purdue Frederick**	**00034-0510-80**
100's	$98.80	Choline Magnesium Trisal, Rugby	00536-3470-01

CHROMIC CHLORIDE *(000813)*

CATEGORIES: Diagnostic Agents; Electrolytic, Caloric-Water Balance; Homeostatic & Nutrient; Mineral Supplements; Radiopharmaceuticals; Replacement Solutions; Vitamins; Pregnancy Category C; FDA Approved 1986 Jun

BRAND NAMES: Chroma-Pak; **Chromium**

DESCRIPTION:

TRACE ELEMENT ADDITIVE

FOR IV USE ONLY AFTER DILUTION

Chromic Chloride Injection, USP, is a sterile, nonpyrogenic solution of chromic chloride in Water for Injection q.s. It is intended for use as an additive to solutions for total parenteral nutrition (TPN). (See TABLE 1)

TABLE 1 Chromic Chloride, Description

Each ml contains:	10 mg vial (One Withdrawal Only)	30 mg vial (Multiple Dose)
Chromic Chloride Hexahydrate	20.5 mcg	20.5 mcg
(equivalent to Chromium)	(4 mcg)	(4 mcg)
Benzyl Alcohol, NF	-	0.9%
Water for Injection	q.s.	q.s.

Hydrochloric acid and/or sodium hydroxide for pH adjustment (1.5-2.5).

Chromic chloride is chemically designated $CrCl_3$, a greenish compound, soluble in water, Benzyl alcohol is chemically designated $C_6H_5CH_2OH$, a clear liquid with faint aromatic odor and miscible with water.

CLINICAL PHARMACOLOGY:

Trivalent chromic is part of glucose tolerant factor, an essential activator of insulin-mediated reactions. Chromium helps to maintain normal glucose metabolism and peripheral nerve function.

Providing chromium during TPN helps prevent deficiency symptoms including impaired glucose tolerance, ataxia, peripheral neuropathy and a confusional state similar to mild/moderate hepatic encephalopathy.

Serum chromium is bound to transferrin (siderophilin) in the beta-globulin fraction. Typical blood levels for chromium range from 1 to 5 mcg/liter, but blood levels are not considered a meaningful index of tissue stores. Administration of chromium supplements to chromium

CLINICAL PHARMACOLOGY: *(cont'd)*

deficient patients can result in normalization of the glucose tolerance curve from the diabetic-like curve typical of chromium deficiency. This response is viewed as a more meaningful indicator of chromium nutriture than serum chromium levels.

Excretion of chromium is via the kidneys, ranging from 3 to 50 mcg/day. Biliary excretion via the small intestine may be an ancillary route, but it is believed that only small amounts of chromium are excreted in this manner.

INDICATIONS AND USAGE:

Chromic Chloride Injection, USP is indicated for use as a supplement to intravenous solutions given for TPN. Administration of Chromic Chloride Injection helps to maintain chromium serum levels and to prevent depletion of endogenous stores and subsequent deficiency symptoms.

CONTRAINDICATIONS:

Direct intramuscular or intravenous injection of Chromic Chloride Injection is contraindicated, as the acidic pH of the solutio (1.5-2.5) may cause tissue irritation.

WARNINGS:

None known.

PRECAUTIONS:

Do not use unless solution is clear and the seal is intact and undamaged.

The solution is hypotonic and must not be given by direct intramuscular or intravenous route.

Do not use syringes equipped with aluminum needles or hubs, as the solution is acidic.

In assessing the contribution of chromium supplements to maintenance of glucose hemostasis, consideration should be given to the possibility that the patient may be diabetic.

CARCINOGENESIS, MUTAGENESIS, AND IMPAIRMENT OF FERTILITY

Long term animal studies have not been performed to evaluate the carcinogenic potential or the effect of fertility of Chromic Chloride Injection.

PREGNANCY CATEGORY C

Animal reproduction studies have not been conducted with chromic chloride. It is also not known whether chromic chloride can cause fetal harm when administered to a pregnant woman or can affect reproductive capacity. Chromic chloride should be given to a pregnant woman only if clearly indicated.

ADVERSE REACTIONS:

None known.

DRUG ABUSE AND DEPENDENCE:

None known.

OVERDOSAGE:

Trivalent chromium administered intravenously to TPN patients has been shown to be non-toxic when given at dosage levels of up to 250 mcg/day for two consecutive weeks.

Reported toxic reactions to chromium include nausea, vomiting, ulcers of the gastrointestinal tract, renal and hepatic damage, convulsions, and coma. The acute LD_{50} for intravenous trivalent chromium in rats was reported as 10 to 18 mg/kg.

DOSAGE AND ADMINISTRATION:

Chromic Chloride Injection contains 4 mcg chromium/ml. Make only one withdrawal from 10 ml vial. Discard unused portion immediately. It is administered intravenously only after dilution.

ADULT

For the adult receiving TPN, the suggested additive dosage is 10 to 15 mcg (2.5 to 3.75 ml Chromic Chloride Injection) per day. The metabolically stable adult with intestinal fluid losses may require 20 mcg chromium/day, with frequent monitoring of blood levels as a guideline for subsequent administration.

PEDIATRIC

For pediatric patients, the suggested additive dosage is 0.14 to 0.20 mcg (0.035 to 0.05 ml Chromic Chloride Injection)/kg/day. Periodic monitoring of chromic chloride plasma levels is suggested as a guideline for subsequent administration.

Aseptic addition of Chromic Chloride Injection to TPN solutions under a laminar flow hood is recommended. Chromic chloride is physically compatible with the electrolytes and vitamins usually present in the amino acid/dextrose solutions used for TPN.

Parenteral drug products should be inspected visually for particulate matter and discoloration prior to administration, whenever solution and container permit. (See PRECAUTIONS.)

DIRECTIONS FOR DISPENSING IN HOSPITAL PHARMACY

1. Arrange syringes, vials and TPN solutions in the laminar flow hood.

2. Suspend the TPN bags from the hole in the flat plastic extension at the top.

3. Remove the flip-top seal from the vial and swab the exposed rubber stopper with an antiseptic solution.

4. Withdraw the contents of the vial using the sterile syringe and transfer the required volumes through the medication port into the TPN bags. Unused portions in the 10 ml vial should be discarded immediately.

5. Shake the bag gently, to distribute the drug.

6. Check solution for particulate matter.

7. Identify the bag.

Storage: Store at controlled room temperature 15-30°(59-86°F). Do not permit to freeze.

(Lyphomed, 45400B, 9/91)

HOW SUPPLIED - RATED THERAPEUTICALLY EQUIVALENT:

Injection, Conc-Soln - Intravenous - 4 mcg/ml

10 ml	$59.69	CHROMA-PAK, Solopak Labs	39769-0049-10
10 ml x 25	$62.19	Chromic Chloride, Am Regent	00517-6310-25
10 ml x 25	$133.88	Chromic Chloride, Fujisawa USA	00469-9320-30
30 ml	**$14.95**	**CHROMIUM 4 MCG/ML, Abbott**	**00074-4529-03**
30 ml x 5	**$26.56**	**CHROMIUM, Am Regent**	**00517-7330-05**

HOW SUPPLIED - NOT RATED EQUIVALENT:

Injection, Conc-Soln - Intravenous - 4 mcg/ml

10 ml	**$6.06**	**CHROMIUM 4 MCG/ML, Abbott**	**00074-4093-01**

CHYMOPAPAIN *(000814)*

CATEGORIES: Central Pain Syndromes; Chemonucleolysis; Enzymes; Herniated Lumbar Intervertebral Disc; Pain; Sciatica; Pregnancy Category C; FDA Approved 1982 Nov

BRAND NAMES: **Chymodiactin**; *Chymodiactine* (France); *Discase*
(International brand names outside U.S. in italics)

WARNING:
Chymodiactin should only be used in a hospital setting by Physicians experienced and trained in the diagnosis of lumbar disc disease and all standard treatment methods, including surgery. Additionally, these physicians and their support personnel should be competent in the diagnosis and management of all potential complications from the use of Chymopapain.
Anaphylaxis, which can be fatal, is independent of the type of anesthesia used, and occurs in approximately 0.5% of receiving Chymodiactin.
Paraplegia/paraparesis, central nervous system hemorrhage, and other serious neurologic adverse events have been observed within hours or days following chymopapain injection at a rate of less than 1 in 2,000. Onset of paraplegia/paraparesis has also been reported 2 to 3 weeks after chymopapain injection at a much lower rate of less than 1 in 20,000. A cause and effect relationship between these neurological events and chymopapain when properly injected has not been established.
Chymopapain is extremely toxic when injected intravenously intrathecally, as are some radiopaque contrast media used for discography. In many of the reported cases of serious neurologic adverse events, discography was performed as part of the procedure. Great care must be taken to assure that the dura is not penetrated and that chymopapain, or medium if used, does not enter the subarachnoid space. If there is any question regarding needle tip location within the nucleus of the disc or if contrast medium is used and it extravasates into the subarachnoid space, the procedure should not be abandoned and chymopapain should not be injected.
Chemonucleolysis using supplemented local anesthesia whenever possible should be limited to the disc(s) producing the patient's signs and symptoms.

DESCRIPTION:

Chymodiactin is a proteolytic enzyme in the form of a sterile, nonpyrogenic, lyophilized powder. The unit of chymopapain activity is the picoKatal (pKat). One unit (pKat) of enzyme, under the conditions of the assay, forms 1 picomole of p-nitroaniline per second from DL-benzoyl arginine-p-nitroanilide (BAPNA) substrate. In general, 1 mg of chymopapain contains approximately 500 pKat units.

Chymodiactin is available in 2 ml and is accompanied by a vial of Sterile Water for Injection, USP, which is to be used as diluent. The 2 ml vial, which is to be reconstituted with 2 ml of diluent, contains 4,000 pKat units of chymopapain and 1.4 mg of sodium L-cysteinate hydrochloride. The concentration of the solution in a reconstituted vial is 2,000 pKat units of active drug per ml. The vial contains no preservatives.

The proteolytic enzyme chymopapain is derived from the crude latex of*Carica papaya*. Sodium L-cysteinate hydrochloride is added as a reducing agent for this sulphur containing enzyme to maintain the sulphur in the sulphydryl form. The pH of the reconstituted drug is 5.5 to 6.5.

CLINICAL PHARMACOLOGY:

When injected into the herniated nucleus pulposus of the lumbar intervertebral disc, chymopapain causes rapid hydrolysis of the noncollagenous polypeptides or proteins that maintain the tertiary structure of the chondromucoprotein of the nucleus pulposus. By causing degradation of the chondromucoprotein, the intradiscal osmotic activity is lessened, thereby decreasing fluid absorption and reducing intradiscal pressure. The foregoing mechanism of action is based on animal *in vitro* and *in vivo* data. Although the mechanism of action in the human has not been established directly, operative findings in patients who have had surgery following injection have usually revealed the nucleus pulposus to be reduced in size A temporary increase in urinary mucopolysaccharide occurs in humans following intradiscal injection of chymopapain, it appears that the inhibitory activity of the alpha$_2$-macroglobulin prevents expression of any significant proteolytic activity outside the disc.

As chymopapain is injected directly into the herniated lumbar intervertebral disc, absorption, distribution, and metabolism are not necessary for it to achieve its intended purpose. Pharmacological activity has been demonstrated by direct observation both *in vivo* and *in vitro* in animals, *in vitro* in human disc tissue, and pharmacokinetically in the human by observation of increases in urinary excretion of substances known to be in high concentration in the disc.

After injection into the central portion of human lumbar intervertebral discs (*in vivo*), there is an increase in the urinary excretion of glycosaminoglycans of the type known to occur in human intervertebral discs. Chymopapain or its immunologically reactive fragments (CIP) are also detectable by radioimmunoassay in plasma at 30 minutes and are declining at 24 hours. Small amounts of CIP are also detected in the urine. These findings indicate that, after intradiscal injection of Chymopapain, CIP diffuses rapidly into plasma. Due to the inhibitory activity of the plasma alpha$_2$-macroglobulin and the low concentration of CIP, it is unlikely that any proteolytic activity is expressed outside the disc.

In a randomized, double-blind comparison of drug and placebo, approximately 75% of patients responded successfully to Chymodiactin compared to approximately 45% receiving placebo were treated with Chymodiactin, 90% responded with partial or total relief of symptoms. In a multicenter, open-label study involving approximately 1,500 patients, the results were also favorable, with success rates ranging from 80% to 89% depending on the criteria used to determine outcome.

INDICATIONS AND USAGE:

Chymodiactin intradiscal injection is indicated for the treatment of patients with documented herniated lumbar intervertebral discs whose symptoms and signs, particularly sciatica, have not responded to an adequate period or periods of conservative therapy. Chymodiactin has not been studied in the treatment of herniated discs in areas other than the lumber spine.

Chymodiactin should only be used by physicians who are qualified by training and experience to perform laminectomy, discectomy, or other spinal procedures, and who have received specialized training in chemonucleolysis. Appropriate use of Chymodiactin requires experience and training in the use of appropriate diagnostic and treatment methods, including surgical intervention other (laminectomy/discectomy) and all aspects of pre- and post-operative patient management. Proper selection of patients for chemonucleolysis requires extensive

INDICATIONS AND USAGE: *(cont'd)*

training and experience in the diagnosis and management of all spinal disorders and diseases since there are circumstances in which nerve root compression resulting from conditions other than a herniated disc can produce similar signs and symptoms.

Chymodiactin should be used only in hospitals. Support personnel, as well as physicians, must be trained and experienced in the diagnosis and management of all potential complications of the use of Chymodiactin.

CONTRAINDICATIONS:

Chymodiactin is contraindicated in patients with a known sensitivity to chymopapain, papaya or papaya derivatives such as certain papain-containing contact lens cleaners and meat tenderizer preparations. Other contraindications are severe spondylolisthesis; significant spinal stenosis; severe, progressing paralysis as indicated by rapidly progressing neurologic dysfunction; and evidence of spinal cord tumor or other lesions producing spinal motor or sensory dysfunction (*e.g.*, cauda equina lesion).

Chymopapain, a foreign protein, has the potential for generating an immunologic response. Therefore, its is contraindicated in patients who have been previously been injected with any form of chymopapain. It is contraindicated for any patient shown to have circulating chymopapain specific IgE antibodies.

Chymopapain has only been studied in the lumbar spine; therefore, its use is contraindicated in other regions of the spine.

WARNINGS:

(1) Anaphylaxis of a severe to mild nature has been observed after injection of Chymodiactin in about 0.5% of patients and may be life threatening if not treated promptly and correctly. *At least one open intravenous line must always be in place to permit rapid and adequate management.* This reaction can be immediate or delayed up to two hours after injection and can last for minutes to several hours or longer. The patient may present with almost immediate hypotension and/or bronchospasm, (the former being more common), laryngeal edema, cardiac arrhythmia possibly progressing to cardiac arrest, coma, and death. Speed in diagnosis and treatment is essential since the clinical signs, severity, progression, and duration of an anaphylactic reaction are very unpredictable. The patient must also be observed for development of other allergic signs, such as erythema, pilomotor erection, rash, pruritic urticaria, conjunctivitis, vasomotor rhinitis, angioedema, or various gastrointestinal disturbances.

Postmarketing surveillance more than 38,200 patients for whom data are available demonstrate that the incidence of anaphylaxis secondary to Chymodiactin injection varies with gender and race. (TABLE 1).

TABLE 1 Chymopapain, Warnings

	White	Black	Hispanic	Other
Male	0.2%	0.3%	0.3%	0.2%
Female	0.6%	1.7%	0.7%	0.7%

The overall anaphylaxis rate is significantly higher in females (0.7) than in males (0.2%), black females being particularly at risk (1.7%).

Although clinical judgement, choice and speed of therapy enter into the treatment of anaphylaxis, *epinephrine is the definitive therapeutic agent in the immediate treatment of anaphylaxis.*

Substitution of other agents such as steroids should be reserved for cases where epinephrine is not appropriate.

(2) Paraplegia/paraparesis, other serious neurologic adverse events, (*e.g.*, the cauda equina syndrome), subarachnoid/cerebral hemorrhage, and seizures have been observed soon within hours or days following chymopapain injection at a rate of less than 1 in 2,000. Delayed rapid onset of paraplegia/paraparesis has also been reported 2 to 3 weeks after injection of chymopapain at a lower rate of less than 1 in 20,000. Casual relationships to the drug when properly administered have not been established. Needle trauma and/or injection of chymopapain and/or contrast media into the spinal fluid may have been responsible in some of these cases. Other less severe neurologic reactions have included burning sacral or leg pain, hypalgesia, leg weakness, foot drop, cramping in both calves, pain in the opposite leg, paresthesia, tingling in legs, and numbness of legs/toes.

Regarding serious neurologic adverse events, the following should be noted:

(a) In many of the reported cases of serious neurologic adverse events, discography was performed as part of the procedure. Some contrast media approved for use on discography are neurotoxic when introduced intrathecally and such toxicity may be enhanced by intrathecal bleeding. Also, as shown in experimental animals intrathecal chymopapain is highly toxic (see ANIMAL PHARMACOLOGY). Based on this information and to avoid introduction of contrast medium into the spinal fluid, great care should be taken before injection to ensure that the tip of the injection needle is in the center of the nucleus pulposus and that the dura has not been pierced. The transdural or posterior approach for needle placement must be avoided.

(b) Patients receiving injections at two or more disc spaces appear to be at increased risk of serious neurologic adverse events. *Chemonucleolysis should be limited to the disc or discs responsible for the patient's symptoms.*

(c) Nearly all of the patients who experienced a serious neurologic adverse event had the procedure performed under general anesthesia. Local anesthesia provides an awake patient, more likely to experience pain and complain if the needle impinges on nerve tissue. Also, it is unlikely that a patient under local anesthesia will tolerate an excessive number of attempts to place the needle. Although the final choice of anesthetic rests with the patient's physician, *it is recommended that local or supplemented local anesthesia be used for chemonucleolysis whenever possible.*

(d) Patients who have had prior surgery of the lumbar spine appear to be at increased risk of experiencing a serious neurologic adverse event. Therefore, it is recommended that such patients be selected for chemonucleolysis only after careful consideration of the risk/benefit ratio.

(e) A number of patients with a history of hypertension, known or suspected cerebrovascular anomaly, previous cerebrovascular accident, or a strong family history of cerebrovascular accident have experienced extensive, severe, or fatal central nervous system hemorrhage following chemonucleolysis.

(3) Chymopapain is extremely toxic when injected intrathecally in animals. If Chymodiactin is not introduced intrathecally, capillaries can be disrupted potentially resulting in a subarachnoid/cerebral hemorrhage, severe neurological injury and/or death. Great caution must be exercised in assuring that Chymodiactin does not enter the intrathecal space. The transdural or posterior approach for needle placement must be avoided.

(4) Certain radiopaque contrast media used for discography are neurotoxic when injected intrathecally. The toxicity of these materials may be enhanced by intrathecal bleeding. If Chymodiactin is inadvertently administered intrathecally, disruption of the capillaries may occur resulting in intrathecal bleeding.

PRECAUTIONS:

Patient Selection

(1) A careful history should be obtained to determine if the patient has multiple allergies, especially a known allergy to papaya or papaya derivatives or iodine. Absorbable iodine should not be used during myelography (or discography, if performed - See WARNINGS) in patients allergic to iodine.

The use of a preoperative screening test for chymopapain- specific IgE antibody should be considered to identify patients at risk for anaphylaxis.

(2) A number of patients with a history of prior surgery of the lumbar spine, hypertension, known or suspected cerebrovascular anomaly, previous cerebrovascular accident, or strong family history of cerebrovascular accident have experienced a serious neurologic adverse event following chemonucleolysis. (see WARNINGS.)

(3) Females, particularly black females, are more likely to develop anaphylactic reactions secondary to Chymodiactin (chymopapain for injection). (see WARNINGS.)

(4) In case of anaphylaxis, beta-blocker therapy may block the action of epinephrine.

Pretreatment

(1) It is recommended that patients be pretreated prior to the injection of Chymodiactin with histamine receptor (H_1 and H_2) antagonists to lessen the severity of an anaphylactic reaction. (2) Because of the abrupt decrease in intravascular volume during anaphylaxis, patients should be well hydrated by oral or intravenous fluids prior to chemonucleolysis. *At least one open intravenous line must always be in place to permit rapid and adequate management of such an occurrence.*

Procedure

(1) The choice of anesthetic for a specific patient should be made by the attending surgeon and anesthesiologist; however, local or supplemented local anesthetic is recommended whenever possible.

The advantages of local or supplemental local anesthesia include possible early recognition of anaphylaxis, possible recognition of evoked sciatic pain with a specific nerve root, and possible decreased risk of a serious neurologic adverse event secondary to difficult needle placement. (see WARNINGS.)

The advantages of general anesthesia include more precise patient positioning for injection, less patient discomfort and ease of airway management if anaphylaxis should develop. If halothane of any anaphylactic reaction could include cardiac arrhythmia.

(2) Needle placement for the intradiscal administration of Chymodiactin should be made by physicians experienced in needle placement via the lateral approach to avoid puncture of the dura mater. Clinical trials have not been conducted using the posterior approach for needle placement and serious neurologic toxicity has been reported using a posterior transdural approach; therefore, this method of needle placement must be avoided. Prior to injection of Chymodiactin, visualization of the needle tip position in the disc must be confirmed using x-ray image intensifier for both the anteroposterior and lateral views. *If high quality x-ray equipment including an image intensifier is not available, chemonucleolysis should not be performed.*

(3) If discography is deemed essential at the time of the chemonucleolysis procedure (see WARNINGS), at least 15 minutes should elapse after the administration of radiopaque contrast medium to be sure there has been no reaction from the contrast agent.

(4) For 3 minutes prior to Chymodiactin injection, 100% O_2 may be administered to the patient by the anesthesiologist to maximize oxygenation in case of anaphylaxis.

(5) A test dose injection of 0.2 ml of Chymodiactin followed by a 10 to 15 minute wait is recommended prior to the injection of the full therapeutic dose. The purpose of the test dose is to help identify those patients who are most sensitive to chymopapain, and patients who develop signs and/or symptoms of anaphylaxis following the test dose must not receive the therapeutic dose. However, some patients have been reported who failed to react to this test dose, but developed anaphylaxis to the therapeutic dose, suggesting that sensitivity to Chymodiactin may be dose-related.

Patient Instructions

(1) Patients should be instructed that after injection they may experience back pain or involuntary muscle spasm in the lower area of the back for several days. This is not uncommon nor is a residual stiffness or soreness of the low back which may persist for several months.

(2) Patients should be instructed to anticipate the possibility of any of the following delayed allergic reactions which may occur as late as 15 days after injection; rash of any type, urticaria, or itching. If any of these occur, patients should contact their physician.

PREGNANCY CATEGORY C

Animal reproduction studies have not been conducted with Chymodiactin. It is also not known whether Chymodiactin can cause fetal harm when administered to a pregnant woman or can affect reproduction capacity. Chymodiactin should be given to a pregnant woman only if the potential benefits outweigh the possible risks.

PEDIATRIC USE

Safety and effectiveness of Chymodiactin has not been studied in pediatric patients; therefore, the drug should not be used in children.

ADVERSE REACTIONS:

Based on postmarketing surveillance reports, the overall frequency of anaphylaxis is 0.5% or about 1 in 200 patients. The frequency in females is approximately 0.8% and in males approximately 0.3%.

Fatalities have been reported following injection of Chymodiactin. Some, such as those due to anaphylaxis or its complications, to disc space infection, or central nervous system hemorrhage, may be associated with either the drug or the procedure. Others appear to be coincidental. The overall mortality rate after Chymopapain injection has been reported to be approximately 0.025% compared with approximately 0.1% mortality reported following surgery. Paraplegia/paraparesis, other serious neurologic adverse events (*e.g.,* the cauda equina syndrome), subarachnoid/cerebral hemorrhage, and seizures have been observed within hours or days following chymopapain injection at a rate of less than 1 in 2,000. Delayed rapid onset of paraplegia/paraparesis has also been reported 2 to 3 weeks after injection of chymopapain at a lower rate of less than 1 in 20,000. Causal relationships to the drug when properly administered have not been established. Needle trauma and/or injection of chymopapain and/or contrast media into the spinal fluid may have been responsible in some of these cases. Other less severe neurologic reactions have included burning sacral, leg pain, hypalgesia, leg weakness, foot drop, cramping in both calves, pain in the opposite leg, paresthesia, tingling in the legs, and numbness of legs/toes.

Discitis, probably due to bacteria, has been reported.

Less severe, but more frequent adverse reactions include back pain/stiffness/soreness in approximately 50% of treated patients and/or back spasm in approximately 30%. Less frequent adverse reactions, occurring in less than 1% of patients studied include rash, itching, urticaria, nausea, paralytic ileus, urinary retention, headache, and dizziness.

DRUG ABUSE AND DEPENDENCE:

Chymodiactin injection does not lend itself to drug abuse and dependence.

OVERDOSAGE:

Overdosage has not been reported in clinical trials of Chymodiactin or subsequently.

DOSAGE AND ADMINISTRATION:

Each vial of Chymodiactin contains 4,000 pKat units of enzyme and should be reconstituted with 2.0 ml Sterile Water for Injection, USP. The concentration of solution in the reconstituted vial is 2,000 pKat units of chymopapain per ml, with a pH of 5.5 to 6.5. Recommended dosage is 2,000 to 4,000 pKat units per disc, usually 3,000 pKat units per disc, or a volume of injection of 1 to 2 ml, usually 1.5 ml per disc. If more than one disc is to be injected (see WARNINGS), an individual patient should not receive more than 8,000 pKat units.

A 5 ml vial of Sterile Water for Injection, USP is supplied with each vial of Chymodiactin. *This is the only diluent which should be used to reconstitute the drug. Bacteriostatic Water for Injection, USP, must not be used* because it may inactivate the enzyme.

Alcohol should be used to cleanse the vial stopper prior to insertion of needles into the vial. However, since residual alcohol may inactivate the enzyme, it should be allowed to air dry before continuing with the reconstitution process. Parenteral drug products should be inspected visually for particulate matter and discoloration prior to administration. Care should be exercised in the selection of proper size and use of needles inserted into the vials in the reconstitution process to reduce the possibility of coring the stopper. The manufacturing process results in a residual vacuum in the vial; therefore, the use of automatic filling syringes is not recommended.

The drug must be used within two hours of its reconstitution with sterile water for injection, USP. Unused drug must be promptly discarded and not stored for future use.

Appropriate use of Chymodiactin requires precise diagnosis, experience and training and in the use of all appropriate diagnostic and treatment methods, including surgical intervention (laminectomy/discectomy) and a knowledge of all aspects of pre- and post-operative patient management.

The proper selection of patients for chemonucleolysis requires extensive training and experience in the diagnosis and management of all spinal disorders and diseases, since there are circumstances in which nerve root compression resulting from conditions other than the herniated disc can produce similar signs and symptoms.

The use of Chymodiactin, therefore, should be limited to physicians who are trained not only in chemonucleolysis but who are qualified by training and experience to care routinely for such patients in other ways.

Chymodiactin should be used only in a hospital setting with the assistance of trained personnel, and in such a manner as to ensure immediate and proper management of all potential complications.

ANIMAL PHARMACOLOGY:

Injection of Chymodiactin into the lumbar intervertebral disc of mature beagle dogs revealed narrowing of the intervertebral space noted on radiographs obtained at 48 hours and at 14 days. In dogs sacrificed at 14 days following injection, cavitation of the nucleus pulposus was observed, but the endplates were unaffected.

Chymopapain has previously been shown to dissolve the nucleus pulposus of dogs and rabbits at doses as low as 100 pKat units/disc and 50 pKat units/disc, respectively. Doses of 3,000 pKat units/disc cause thinning of only the inner portion of the annulus in rabbits but do not penetrate the entire structure, while doses as high as 24,000 pKat units/disc in dogs resulted in no apparent significant change in the peripheral portion of the annulus. *In vitro* studies demonstrated that chymopapain solubilized the mucopolysaccharide protein complex of human nucleus pulposus, did not attack the collagen of this structure.

When chymopapain is injected into dogs, doses up to 100 times greater than that required to remove the nucleus pulposus were well tolerated when injected intravenously, intradiscally, and epidurally. The drug is extremely toxic when injected intrathecally; the approximate $LD_{50}$is 15 pKat units/kg in rabbits, 150 pKat units/kg in dogs and 200 pKat units/kg in baboons. Therefore, great caution must be exercised in assuring that Chymodiactin is not injected intrathecally.

In baboons the serial injection into the spinal fluid of contrast agents (Renografin, Conray or Amipaque) followed by Chymodiactin 15 minutes later produced serious neurotoxicity, including weakness, paralysis and death. When administered singly at the same doses, Conray, Amipaque, and Chymodiactin were not toxic; Renografin was less toxic singly than in combination with Chymodiactin. This information supports the clinical observation that the documented entry of contrast agent and presumed entry of chymopapain into the spinal fluid can produce serious neurotoxicity including paraplegia and central nervous system hemorrhage.

HOW SUPPLIED:

Chymodiactin is supplied as a sterile. nonpyrogenic, lyophilized powder in single vials containing 4,000 pKat units of enzymatic activity. Each vial of Chymodiactin is accompanied with a 5 ml vial of Sterile Water for Injection, USP, which is to be used as diluent.

4,000 pKat units with Diluent.

Caution: Although a 5 ml vial of Sterile Water for Injection, USP, is supplied, *only 2 ml of diluent is to be used when reconstituting the 4,000 pKat unit vial.*

Chymodiactin can be shipped unrefrigerated; however, it should be stored refrigerated (36° to 46°F or 2° to 8°C) until reconstitution for use.

HOW SUPPLIED - EQUIVALENTS NOT AVAILABLE:

Injection, Solution - Intravenous - 4000 unit

1's $1605.15 CHYMODIACTIN, Knoll Labs 00044-0110-02

CHYMOTRYPSIN *(000815)*

CATEGORIES: EENT Drugs; Eye, Ear, Nose, & Throat Preparations; Ophthalmics; Proteolytic Enzymes, Ophthalmic; Surgical Aid, Ophthalmic; FDA Approval Pre 1982

BRAND NAMES: Alpha Chymar; Catarase; *Chymosin*; *Chymotrypsine Chibret* (France); **Zolyse**
(International brand names outside U.S. in italics)

DESCRIPTION:

Chymotrypsin is a lyophilized form of crystalline chymotrypsin, a proteolytic enzyme obtained from the pancreas of the ox. The diluent is a sterile balanced salt solution to be used for reconstituting crystals. Package includes one vial chymotrypsin, 750 U.S.P. Units; and one 9 mL vial of diluent containing: Sodium Chloride 0.49%, Sodium Acetate 0.39%, Sodium

DESCRIPTION: *(cont'd)*

Citrate 0.17%, Potassium Chloride 0.075%, Calcium Chloride 0.048%, Magnesium Chloride 0.03%,
Hydrochloric Acid and/or Sodium Hydroxide (to adjust pH), Water for Injection.

CLINICAL PHARMACOLOGY:

When instilled into the posterior chamber of the eye, its enzymatic action causes dissolution of zonular fibers attached to the lens.

INDICATIONS AND USAGE:

For enzymatic zonulysis in intracapsular lens extraction.

CONTRAINDICATIONS:

Contraindicated in significant anterior displacement of the lens iris diaphragm with impending vitreous loss or other conditions in which loss of vitreous is a significant problem (*e.g.*, intracapsular extraction of congenital cataracts); and in those persons who have shown hypersensitivity to any component of this preparation.

WARNINGS:

Do not use the reconstituted solution if cloudy or if it contains a precipitate. Do not autoclave the powder or the reconstituted solution-excessive heat, alcohol, and other chemicals used for sterilization inactivate the enzyme. After the operation, discard any unused portion including the diluent. The solution contains no preservative and should not be used for more than one patient.

PRECAUTIONS:

Chymotrypsin may produce an acute rise in intraocular pressure following surgery. This is especially true in patients with poor facility of outflow.

Use of Chymotrypsin is not advised in patients under 20 years of age. Ensure that the synechiae are separated, since this enzyme will not lyse them.

ADVERSE REACTIONS:

Increases in intraocular pressure, moderate uveitis, corneal edema, and striation have been reported.

DOSAGE AND ADMINISTRATION:

Reconstitute immediately prior to the start of surgery. Utilize aseptic technique when inserting a syringe into the rubber stopper of the diluent bottle. It is recommended that the Chymotrypsin be reconstituted with 5mL of the diluent to provide the dilution of 150 units of chymotrypsin per mL which is comparable to a 1:5,000 dilution.

Following cataract section, irrigate the posterior chamber with the reconstituted Chymotrypsin using 0.25 to 0.5 mL (evenly distribute around circumference of the lens). Wait two to four minutes from time of irrigation with Chymotrypsin then irrigate the anterior chamber and the corneal wound edges with at least 2mL of the diluent or balanced salt solution.

NOTE: If zonules are still intact, irrigate with additional Chymotrypsin and wait an additional two minutes before flushing with diluent.

HOW SUPPLIED - EQUIVALENTS NOT AVAILABLE:

Injection, Lyphl-Soln - Intraocular - 300 unit/vial

2 ml	$29.28	CATARASE, OPHTHALMIC CHYMOTRYPSIN, Ciba Vision	00058-2010-45

CICLOPIROX OLAMINE *(000817)*

CATEGORIES: Anti-Infectives; Antifungals; Antimicrobials; Candidiasis; Dermatologicals; Fungal Agents; Infections; Skin Infections; Skin/Mucous Membrane Agents; Tinea Corporis; Tinea Cruris; Tinea Pedis; Tinea Versicolor; Topical; Pregnancy Category B; FDA Approved 1982 Dec; Patent Expiration 1992 May

BRAND NAMES: *Batrafen* (Asia, Germany); *Batrafen Nail Lacquer*; *Brumixol*; *Ciclochem*; *Fungowas*; *Laprox*; **Loprox**; *Miclast*; *Micoxolamina*; *Mycoster* (France); *Nail Batrafen*; *Primax*
(International brand names outside U.S. in italics)

FORMULARIES: Aetna; BC-BS; PCS

COST OF THERAPY: (Tinea Pedis; Cream; 1 %; 2/day; 7 days)

DESCRIPTION:

FOR DERMATOLOGIC USE ONLY. DO NOT USE IN EYES.

Loprox (ciclopirox olamine) Cream 1% and Lotion 1% are for topical use. Each gram of Loprox (ciclopirox olamine) Cream 1% contains 10 mg ciclopirox olamine in a water miscible vanishing cream base consisting of purified water USP, octyldodecanol NF, mineral oil USP, stearyl alcohol NF, cetyl alcohol NF, cocamide DEA, polysorbate 60 NF, myristyl alcohol NF, sorbitan monostearate NF, lactic acid USP, and benzyl alcohol NF (1%) as preservative.

Each gram of Loprox (ciclopirox olamine) Lotion 1% contains 10 mg of ciclopirox olamine in a water miscible lotion base consisting of purified water USP, cocamide DEA, octyldodecanol NF, mineral oil USP, stearyl alcohol NF, cetyl alcohol NF, polysorbate 60 NF, myristyl alcohol NF, sorbitan monostearate NF, lactic acid USP, and benzyl alcohol NF (1%) as preservative. Loprox (ciclopirox olamine) Cream and Lotion contain a synthetic, broad-spectrum, antifungal agent ciclopirox olamine. The chemical name is 6-cyclohexyl-1-hydroxy-4-methyl-2(1*H*)-pyridone, 2-aminoethanol salt.

The CAS Registry Number is 41621-49-2.

Loprox (ciclopirox olamine) Cream 1% and Lotion 1% have a pH of 7.

CLINICAL PHARMACOLOGY:

Ciclopirox olamine is a broad-spectrum, antifungal agent that inhibits the growth of pathogenic dermatophytes, yeasts, and *Malassezia furfur*. Ciclopirox olamine exhibits fungicidal activity *in vitro* against isolates of *Trichophyton rubrum, Trichophyton mentagrophytes, Epidermophyton floccosum, Microsporum canis*, and *Candida albicans*.

Pharmacokinetic studies in men with tagged 1% ciclopirox olamine solution in polyethylene glycol 400 showed an average of 1.3% absorption of the dose when it was applied topically to 750 cm^2 on the back followed by occlusion for 6 hours. The biological half-life was 1.7 hours and excretion occurred via the kidney. Two days after application only 0.01% of the dose applied could be found in the urine. Fecal excretion was negligible.

CLINICAL PHARMACOLOGY: *(cont'd)*

Penetration studies in human cadaverous skin from the back, with Loprox (ciclopirox olamine) Cream 1% with tagged ciclopirox olamine showed the presence of 0.8 to 1.6% of the dose in stratum corneum 1.5 to 6 hours after application. The levels in the dermis were still 10 to 15 times above the minimum inhibitory concentrations.

Autoradiographic studies with human cadaverous skin showed that ciclopirox olamine penetrates into the hair and through the epidermis and hair follicles into the sebaceous glands and dermis, while a portion of the drug remains in the stratum corneum.

Draize Human Sensitization Assay, 21-Day Cumulative Irritancy study, Phototoxicity study, and Photo-Draize study conducted in a total of 142 healthy male subjects showed no contact sensitization of the delayed hypersensitivity type, no irritation, no phototoxicity, and no photo-contact sensitization due to Loprox (ciclopirox olamine) Cream 1%.

In vitro penetration studies in frozen or fresh excised human cadaver and pig skin indicated that the penetration of Loprox (ciclopirox olamine) Lotion 1% is equivalent to that of Loprox (ciclopirox olamine) Cream 1%. Therapeutic equivalence of cream and lotion formulations also was indicated by studies of experimentally induced guinea pig and human trichophytosis.

INDICATIONS AND USAGE:

Loprox (ciclopirox olamine) Cream 1% and Lotion 1% are indicated for the topical treatment of the following dermal infections: tinea pedis, tinea cruris and tinea corporis due to *Trichophyton rubrum, Trichophyton mentagrophytes, Epidermophyton floccosum*, and *Microsporum canis*; cutaneous candidiasis (moniliasis) due to *Candida albicans*; and tinea (pityriasis) versicolor due to *Malassezia furfur*.

CONTRAINDICATIONS:

Loprox (ciclopirox olamine) Cream 1% and Lotion 1% are contraindicated in individuals who have shown hypersensitivity to any of its components.

WARNINGS:

General: Loprox (ciclopirox olamine) Cream 1% and Lotion 1% are not for ophthalmic use.

PRECAUTIONS:

If a reaction suggesting sensitivity or chemical irritation should occur with the use of Loprox (ciclopirox olamine) Cream 1% or Lotion 1%, treatment should be discontinued and appropriate therapy instituted.

Information for the Patient: The patient should be told to:

1. Use the medication for the full treatment time even though symptoms may have improved and notify the physician if there is no improvement after four weeks.

2. Inform the physician if the area of application shows signs of increased irritation (redness, itching, burning, blistering, swelling, oozing) indicative of possible sensitization.

3. Avoid the use of occlusive wrappings or dressings.

Carcinogenesis, Mutagenesis, and Impairment of Fertility: A carcinogenicity study in female mice dosed cutaneously twice per week for 50 weeks followed by a 6-month drug-free observation period prior to necropsy revealed no evidence of tumors at the application site. The following *in vitro* and *in vivo* genotoxicity tests have been conducted with ciclopirox olamine: studies to evaluate gene mutation in the Ames *Salmonella*/Mammalian Microsome Assay (negative) and Yeast Saccharomyces Cerevisiae Assay (negative) and studies to evaluate chromosome aberrations *in vivo* in the Mouse Dominant Lethal Assay and in the Mouse Micronucleus Assay at 500 mg/kg (negative). The following battery of *in vitro* genotoxicity tests were conducted with *ciclopirox*: a chromosome aberration assay in V79 Chinese Hamster Cells, with and without metabolic activation (positive); a gene mutation assay in the HGPRT-test with V79 Chinese Hamster Cells (negative); and a primary DNA damage assay (*i.e.*, unscheduled DNA Synthesis Assay in A549 Human Cells (negative)). An *in vitro* Cell Transformation Assay in BALB/C3T3 Cells was negative for cell transformation. In an *in vivo* Chinese Hamster Bone Marrow Cytogenetic Assay, ciclopirox was negative for chromosome aberrations at 5000 mg/kg.

Pregnancy Category B: Reproduction studies have been performed in the mouse, rat, rabbit, and monkey (via various routes of administration) at doses 10 times or more the topical human dose and have revealed no significant evidence of impaired fertility or harm to the fetus due to ciclopirox olamine. There are, however, no adequate or well-controlled studies in pregnant women. Because animal reproduction studies are not always predictive of human response, this drug should be used during pregnancy only if clearly needed.

Nursing Mothers: It is not known whether this drug is excreted in human milk. Because many drugs are excreted in human milk, caution should be exercised when Loprox (ciclopirox olamine) Cream 1% or Lotion 1% is administered to a nursing woman.

Pediatric Use: Safety and effectiveness in pediatric patients below the age of 10 years have not been established.

ADVERSE REACTIONS:

In all controlled clinical studies with 514 patients using Loprox (ciclopirox olamine) Cream 1% and in 296 patients using the vehicle cream, the incidence of adverse reactions was low. This included pruritus at the site of application in one patient and worsening of the clinical signs and symptoms in another patient using ciclopirox olamine cream 1% and burning in one patient and worsening of the clinical signs and symptoms in another patient using the vehicle cream.

In the controlled clinical trial with 89 patients using Loprox (ciclopirox olamine) Lotion 1% and 89 patients using the vehicle, the incidence of adverse reactions was low. Those considered possibly related to treatment or occurring in more than one patient were pruritus, which occurred in two patients using ciclopirox olamine lotion 1% and one patient using the lotion vehicle, and burning, which occurred in one patient using ciclopirox olamine lotion 1%.

DOSAGE AND ADMINISTRATION:

Gently massage Loprox (ciclopirox olamine) Cream 1% or Lotion 1% into the affected and surrounding skin areas twice daily, in the morning and evening. Clinical improvement with relief of pruritus and other symptoms usually occurs within the first week of treatment. If a patient shows no clinical improvement after four weeks of treatment with Loprox (ciclopirox olamine) Cream 1% or Lotion 1%, the diagnosis should be redetermined. Patients with tinea versicolor usually exhibit clinical and mycological clearing after two weeks of treatment.

REFERENCES:

1. Hanel H, Raether W, Dittmar, W. Evaluation of fungicidal action *in vitro* and in a skin model considering the influence of penetration kinetics of various standard antimycotics. *Ann NY Acad Sci.* 1988;544:329-337. **2.** Lassus A, Nolting KS, Savopoulos C. Comparison of ciclopirox olamine 1% cream with ciclopirox 1%-hydrocortisone acetate 1% cream in the treatment of inflamed superficial mycoses. *Clin Ther.* 1988;10(5):594-599. **3.** Kligman AM, Bogaert H, Cordero C, et al. Evaluation of ciclopirox olamine cream for the treatment of tinea pedis: multicenter, double-blind comparative studies. *Clin Ther.* 1985;7(4):409-417. **4.** Cullen SI, Frost P, Jacobson C, et al. Treatment of tinea versicolor with a new antifungal agent, ciclopirox olamine cream 1%. *Clin Ther.* 1985;7(5):574-583. **5.** Bagatell FK, Bogaert H, Cullen SI, et al. Evaluation of a new antifungal cream, ciclopirox olamine 1% in the treatment of cutaneous candidosis. *Clin Ther.* 1985;8(1):41-48. **6.** Bogaert H, Cordero C, Ollague W, Savin RC, Shalita AR, Zaias N. Multicentre double-blind clinical trials of ciclopirox olamine cream 1% in the treatment of tinea corporis and tinea cruris. *J Int Med Res.* 1986;14(4):210-216.

HOW SUPPLIED:

Loprox (ciclopirox olamine) Cream 1% is supplied in 15 gram (NDC 0039-0009-15); 30 gram (NDC 0039-0009-30); and 90 gram (NDC 0039-0009-90) tubes. Loprox (ciclopirox olamine) Lotion 1% is supplied in 30 ml bottles (NDC 0039-0008-30) and 60 ml bottles (NDC 0039-0008-06).

Bottle space provided to allow for vigorous shaking before each use.

Store Loprox (ciclopirox olamine) Cream 1% at controlled room temperature (59°-86°F).

Store Loprox (ciclopirox olamine) Lotion 1% between 41° and 77°F (5° and 25°C).

HOW SUPPLIED - EQUIVALENTS NOT AVAILABLE:

Cream - Topical - 1 %

15 gm	$10.78	LOPROX, Hoechst Marion Roussel	00039-0009-15
30 gm	$19.27	LOPROX, Hoechst Marion Roussel	00039-0009-30
90 gm	$34.69	LOPROX, Hoechst Marion Roussel	00039-0009-90

Lotion - Topical - 1 %

30 ml	$21.18	LOPROX, Hoechst Marion Roussel	00039-0008-30
60 ml	$40.22	LOPROX, Hoechst Marion Roussel	00039-0008-06

CIDOFOVIR *(003291)*

CATEGORIES: AIDS Related Complex; Anti-Infectives; Antimicrobials; Antivirals; Cytomegalovirus Infections; Herpes Simplex; HIV Infection; Immunodeficiency; Immunodeficiency Syndrome; Infections; Ocular Infections; Retinitis; Viral Agents; Pregnancy Category C; FDA Approved 1996 Jun

BRAND NAMES: **Vistide**

WARNING:
RENAL IMPAIRMENT IS THE MAJOR TOXICITY OF CIDOFOVIR. TO MINIMIZE POSSIBLE NEPHROTOXICITY, INTRAVENOUS PREHYDRATION WITH NORMAL SALINE AND ADMINISTRATION OF PROBENECID MUST BE USED WITH EACH CIDOFOVIR INFUSION. RENAL FUNCTION (SERUM CREATININE AND URINE PROTEIN) SHOULD BE MONITORED PRIOR TO EACH DOSE OF CIDOFOVIR AND THE DOSE OF CIDOFOVIR MODIFIED FOR CHANGES IN RENAL FUNCTION AS APPROPRIATE (SEE DOSAGE AND ADMINISTRATION).
GRANULOCYTOPENIA HAS BEEN OBSERVED IN ASSOCIATION WITH CIDOFOVIR TREATMENT AND NEUTROPHIL COUNTS SHOULD BE MONITORED DURING CIDOFOVIR THERAPY.
CIDOFOVIR IS INDICATED ONLY FOR THE TREATMENT OF CMV RETINITIS IN PATIENTS WITH THE ACQUIRED IMMUNODEFICIENCY SYNDROME.
IN ANIMAL STUDIES CIDOFOVIR WAS CARCINOGENIC, TERATOGENIC, AND CAUSED HYPOSPERMIA (SEE Carcinogenesis, Mutagenesis, and Impairment of Fertility).

DESCRIPTION:

The chemical name of cidofovir is 1-[(*S*)-3-hydroxy-2-(phosphonomethoxy)propyl]cytosine dihydrate (HPMPC), with the molecular formula $C_8H_{14}N_3O_6P\text{-}2H_2O$) and a molecular weight of 315.22 (279.19 for anhydrous).

Cidofovir is a white crystalline powder with an aqueous stability of ≥ 170 mg/mL at pH 6-8 and a log P (octanol/aqueous buffer, pH 7.1) value of −3.3

Cidofovir is a sterile, hypertonic aqueous solution for intravenous infusion only. The solution is clear and colorless. It is supplied in clear glass vials, each containing 375 mg of anhydrous cidofovir in 5 mL aqueous solution at a concentration of 75 mg/mL. The formulation is pH-adjusted to 7.4 with sodium hydroxide and/or hydrochloric acid and contains no preservatives. The appropriate volume of cidofovir must be removed from the single-use vial and diluted prior to administration (see DOSAGE AND ADMINISTRATION).

MICROBIOLOGY

Mechanism of Action: Cidofovir suppresses cytomegalovirus (CMV) replication by selective inhibition of viral DNA synthesis. Biochemical data support selective inhibition of CMV DNA polymerase by cidofovir diphosphate, the active intracellular metabolite of cidofovir. Cidofovir diphosphate inhibits herpesvirus polymerases at concentrations that are 8- to 600-fold lower than those needed to inhibit human cellular DNA polymerases alpha, beta, and gamma[1,2,3].

Incorporation of cidofovir into the growing viral DNA chain results in reductions in the rate of viral DNA synthesis.

In Vitro Susceptibility: Cidofovir is active *in vitro* against a variety of laboratory and clinical isolates of CMV and other herpesviruses (TABLE 1). Controlled clinical studies of efficacy have been limited to patients with AIDS and CMV retinitis.

TABLE 1

Virus	IC_{50}(μM)
Wild-type CMV Isolates	0.5-2.8
HSV-1, HSV-2	12.7-31.7
VZV*	0.79
EBV	0.03
HHV-6	<6.3

* mean result for 4 human VZV strains

Resistance: CMV isolates with reduced susceptibility to cidofovir have been selected *in vitro* in the presence of high concentrations of cidofovir[4]. IC_{50} values for selected resistant isolates ranged from 7-15 μM.

There are insufficient data at this time to assess the frequency or the clinical significance of the development of resistant isolates following cidofovir administration to patients.

Cross Resistance: Cidofovir-resistant isolates selected *in vitro* following exposure to increasing concentrations of cidofovir were assessed for susceptibility to ganciclovir and foscarmet[4]. All were cross resistant to ganciclovir, but remained susceptible to foscarnet. Ganciclovir or ganciclovir/foscarnet —resistant isolates that are cross resistant to cidofovir have been obtained from drug naive patients and from patients following ganciclovir-resistant or ganciclovir/foscarnet therapy. To date, the majority of ganciclovir-resistant isolates are UL97 gene product (phosphokinase) mutants and remain susceptible to cidofovir[5]. Reduced susceptibility to cidofovir, however, has been reported for DNA polymerase mutants of CMV which are resistant to ganciclovir[6-8]. To date, all clinical isolates which exhibit high level resistance to ganciclovir, due to mutations in the DNA polymerase gene, have been shown to be cross

DESCRIPTION: *(cont'd)*

resistant to cidofovir. Cidofovir is active against some, but not all, CMV isolates which are resistant to foscarnet[8-11]. The incidence of foscarnet-resistant isolates that are resistant to cidofovir is not known.

A few triple-drug resistant isolates have been described. Genotypic analysis of two of these triple-resistant isolates revealed several point mutations in the CMV DNA polymerase gene. The clinical significance of the development of these cross-resistant isolates is not known.

CLINICAL PHARMACOLOGY:

PHARMACOKINETICS

Cidofovir must be administered with probenecid. The pharmacokinetics of cidofovir, administered both without and with probenecid, are described below.

The pharmacokinetics of cidofovir without probenecid were evaluated in 27 HIV-infected patients with or without asymptomatic CMV infection. Dose-independent pharmacokinetics were demonstrated after one hr infusions of 1.0 (n=5), 3.0 (n=10), 5.0 (n=2) and 10.0 (n=8) mg/kg (See TABLE 2 for pharmacokinetic parameters). There was no evidence of cidofovir accumulation after 4 weeks of repeated administration of 3 mg/kg/week (n=5) without probenecid. In patients with normal renal function, approximately 80 to 100% of the cidofovir dose was recovered unchanged in urine within 24 hr (n=27). The renal clearance of cidofovir was greater than creatinine clearance, indicating renal tubular secretion contributes to the elimination of cidofovir.

The pharmacokinetics of cidofovir administered with probenecid were evaluated in 12 HIV-infected patients with or without asymptomatic CMV infection and 10 patients with relapsing CMV retinitis. Dose-independent pharmacokinetics were observed for cidofovir, administered with probenecid, after one hr infusions of 3.0 (n=12), 5.0 (n=6), and 7.5 (n=4) mg/kg (See TABLE 2). Approximately 70 to 85% of the cidofovir dose administered with concomitant probenecid was excreted as unchanged drug within 24 hr. When cidofovir was administered with probenecid, the renal clearance of cidofovir was reduced to a level consistent with creatinine clearance, suggesting that probenecid blocks active renal tubular secretion of cidofovir.

TABLE 2 Cidofovir Pharmacokinetic Parameters Following 3.0 and 5.0 mg/kg infusions, Without and With Probenecid*

Parameters	Cidofovir Administered Without Probenecid 3 mg/kg (n=10)	5 mg/kg (n=2)	Cidofovir Administered Without Probenecid 3 mg/kg (n=12)	5 mg/kg (n=6)
AUC (mcg·hr/mL)	20.0 ± 2.3	28.3	25.7 ± 8.5	40.8 ± 9.0
C_{max} (end of infusion) (mcg/mL)	7.3 ± 1.4	11.5	9.8 ± 3.7	19.6 ± 7.2
Vdsm (mL/kg)	537 ± 126 (n=12)		410 ± 102 (n=18)	
Clearance (mL/min/1.73m²)	179 ± 23.1 (n=12)		148 ± 38.8 (n=18)	
Renal Clearance (mL/min/1.73 m²)	150 ± 26.9 (n=12)		98.6 ± 27.9 (n=11)	

* See DOSAGE AND ADMINISTRATION

In vitro, cidofovir was less than 5% bound to plasma or serum proteins over the cidofovir concentration range 0.25 to 25 mcg/mL. CSF concentrations of cidofovir following intravenous infusion of cidofovir 5 mg/kg with concomitant probenecid and intravenous hydration were undetectable (< 0.1 mcg/mL, assay detection threshold) at 15 minutes after the end of a 1 hr infusion in one patient whose corresponding serum concentration was 8.7 mcg/mL.

SPECIAL POPULATIONS

Renal Insufficiency: Cidofovir pharmacokinetics have not been investigated in patients with renal insufficiency. No data are currently available on the pharmacokinetics of cidofovir in patients with creatinine clearance values below 55 mL/min. The effect of dialysis on cidofovir pharmacokinetics is not known.

Geriatric/Gender/Race: The effects of age, gender, and race on cidofovir pharmacokinetics have not been investigated.

CLINICAL STUDIES:

Two phase 2/3 controlled trials of cidofovir have been conducted in HIV-infected patients with CMV retinitis.

Delayed Versus Immediate Therapy (Study 106): In an open-label trial, forty-eight previously untreated patients with peripheral CMV retinitis were randomized to either immediate treatment with cidofovir (5 mg/kg once a week for 2 weeks, then 5 mg/kg every other week), or to have cidofovir delayed until progression of CMV retinitis. Patient baseline characteristics and disposition are shown in Table 3. Of 25 and 23 patients in the immediate and delayed groups respectively, 23 and 21 were evaluable for retinitis progression as determined by retinal photography. Based on masked readings of retinal photographs, the median [95% confidence interval (CI)] times to retinitis progression were 120 days (40, 134) and 22 days (10, 27) for the immediate and delayed therapy groups, respectively. This difference was statistically significant. However, because of the limited number of patients remaining on treatment over time (3 of 25 patients received cidofovir for 120 days or longer), the median time to progression for the immediate therapy group was difficult to precisely estimate. Median (95% CI) times to the alternative endpoint of retinitis progression or study drug discontinuation (including adverse events, withdrawn consent, and systemic CMV disease) were 52 days (37, 85) and 22 days (13, 27) for the immediate and delayed therapy groups, respectively. This difference was statistically significant. Time to progression estimates from this study may not be directly comparable to estimates reported for other therapies.

Dose-response study of cidofovir (Study 107): In an open-label trial, one-hundred patients with relapsing CMV retinitis were randomized to receive 5 mg/kg once a week for 2 weeks and then either 5 mg/kg (n=49) or 3 mg/kg (n=51) every other week. Enrolled patients had been diagnosed with CMV retinitis approximately 1 year prior to randomization and had received a median of 4 prior courses of systemic CMV therapy. Eighty-four of the 100 patients were considered evaluable for progression by serial retinal photographs (43 randomized to 5 mg/kg and 41 randomized to 3 mg/kg). Twenty-three and 20 patients discontinued therapy due to either an adverse event, intercurrent illness, excluded medication, or withdrawn consent in the 5 mg/kg and 3 mg/kg groups, respectively. Based on masked readings of retinal photographs, the median (95% CI) times to retinitis progression for the 5 mg/kg and 3 mg/kg groups were 115 days (70, not reached) and 49 days (35, 52), respectively. This difference was statistically significant. Similar to Study 106, the median time to retinitis progression for the 5 mg/kg group was difficult to precisely estimate due to the limited number of patients remaining on treatment over time (4 of the 49 patients in the 5 mg/kg group were treated for 115 days or longer). Median (95% CI) times to the alternative endpoint of retinitis progression or study drug discontinuation were 49 days (38, 63) and 35 days (27, 39) for the 5 mg/kg and 3 mg/kg groups, respectively. This difference was statistically significant.

TABLE 3 Patient Characteristics and Disposition (Study 106)

	Immediate Therapy (n=25)	Delayed Therapy (n=23)
Baseline Characteristics		
Age (years)	38	38
Sex (M/F)	24/1	22/1
Median CD4 Cell Count	5	9
Endpoints		
CMV Retinitis Progression	10	18
Discontinued Due to Adverse Event	6	0
Withdrew Consent	3[a]	1
Discontinued Due to Intercurrent Illness	2[b]	1[b]
Discontinued Based on Ophthalmological Examination	1[c]	1[c]
No Progression at Study Completion	1	0
Not Evaluable at Baseline	2	2

[a]One patient died 2 weeks after withdrawing consent.
[b]Two patients on immediate therapy were diagnosed with CMV disease and discontinued from study. One patient on delayed therapy was diagnosed with CMV gastrointestinal disease.
[c]CMV retinitis progression not confirmed by retinal photography.

INDICATIONS AND USAGE:

Cidofovir is indicated for the treatment of CMV retinitis in patients with acquired immunodeficiency syndrome (AIDS). THE SAFETY AND EFFICACY OF CIDOFOVIR HAVE NOT BEEN ESTABLISHED FOR TREATMENT OF OTHER CMV INFECTIONS (SUCH AS PNEUMONITIS OR GASTROENTERITIS), CONGENITAL OR NEONATAL CMV DISEASE, OR CMV DISEASE IN NON-HIV-INFECTED INDIVIDUALS).

CONTRAINDICATIONS:

Cidofovir is contraindicated in patients with hypersensitivity to cidofovir.

Cidofovir is contraindicated in patients with a history of clinically severe hypersensitivity to probenecid or other sulfa-containing medications.

Direct intraocular injection of cidofovir is contraindicated; direct injection may be associated with significant decreases in intraocular pressure and impairment of vision.

WARNINGS:

Nephrotoxicity: Dose-dependent nephrotoxicity is the major dose-limiting toxicity related to cidofovir administration. Dose adjustment or discontinuation is required for changes in renal function while on therapy. Proteinuria, as measured by urinalysis in a clinical laboratory, may be an early indicator of cidofovir-related nephrotoxicity. Continued administration of cidofovir may lead to additional proximal tubular cell injury, which may result in glycosuria, and decreases in serum phosphate, uric acid, and bicarbonate, and elevations in serum creatinine. Patients with these adverse events occurring concurrently and meeting a criteria of Fanconi's syndrome have been reported. Renal function that did not return to baseline after drug discontinuation has been observed in clinical studies of cidofovir.

Intravenous normal saline hydration and oral probenecid must accompany each cidofovir infusion. Probenecid is known to interact with the metabolism or renal tubular excretion of many drugs (see PRECAUTIONS). The safety of cidofovir has not been evaluated in patients receiving other known potentially nephrotoxic agents, such as aminoglycosides, amphotericin B, foscarnet, and intravenous pentamidine (see DOSAGE AND ADMINISTRATION).

Preexisting Renal Impairment: Cidofovir has not been studied in patients with baseline serum creatinine concentrations > 1.5 mg/dl or calculated creatinine clearances ≤ 55 ml/min. The most appropriate initial and maintenance doses of cidofovir for patients with moderate to severe renal impairment are not known.

It is recommended that cidofovir not be initiated in patients with baseline serum creatinine > 1.5 mg/dL or creatinine clearances ≤ 55 ml/min. In these patients, cidofovir therapy should only be used when the potential benefits exceed the potential risks.

Hematological Toxicity: Neutropenia may occur during cidofovir therapy. Neutrophil count should be monitored while receiving cidofovir therapy.

Metabolic Acidosis: Fanconi's syndrome and decreases in serum bicarbonate associated with evidence of renal tubular damage have been reported in patients receiving cidofovir (see ADVERSE REACTIONS). Serious metabolic acidosis, in association with liver failure, pancreatitis, mucomycosis, aspergillus, disseminated mycobacterial infection, and progression to death occurred in 1 patient (< 1%) receiving cidofovir.

PRECAUTIONS:

GENERAL

Due to the potential for increased nephrotoxicity, doses greater than the recommended dose should not be administered and the frequency or rate of administration should not be exceeded (see DOSAGE AND ADMINISTRATION).

Cidofovir is formulated for intravenous infusion only and must not be administered by intraocular injection. Administration of cidofovir by infusion must be accompanied by oral probenecid and intravenous saline prehydration (see DOSAGE AND ADMINISTRATION).

INFORMATION FOR THE PATIENT

Patients should be advised that cidofovir is not a cure for CMV retinitis, and that they may continue to experience progression of retinitis during and following treatment. Patients receiving cidofovir should be advised to have regular follow-up ophthalmologic examinations. Patients may also experience other manifestations of CMV disease despite cidofovir therapy.

HIV-infected patients may continue taking antiretroviral therapy, but those taking zidovudine should be advised to temporarily discontinue zidovudine administration or decrease their zidovudine dose by 50%, on days of cidofovir administration only, because probenecid reduces metabolic clearance of zidovudine.

Patients should be informed of the major toxicity of cidofovir, namely renal impairment, and that dose modification, including reduction, interruption, and possibly discontinuation, may be required. Close monitoring of renal function (routine urinalysis and serum creatinine) while on therapy should be emphasized.

The importance of completing a full course of probenecid with each cidofovir dose should be emphasized. Patients should be warned of potential adverse events caused by probenecid (*e.g.,* headache, nausea, vomiting, and hypersensitivity reactions). Hypersensitivity/allergic reactions may include rash, fever, chills and anaphylaxis. Administration of probenecid after a meal or use of antiemetics may decrease the nausea. Prophylactic or therapeutic antihistamines and/or acetaminophen can be used to ameliorate hypersensitivity reactions.

Patients should be advised that cidofovir causes tumors, primarily mammary adenocarcinomas, in rats. Cidofovir should be considered a potential carcinogen in humans (see Carcinogenesis, Mutagenesis, and Impairment of Fertility). Women should be advised of the limited enrollment of women in clinical trials of cidofovir.

PRECAUTIONS: *(cont'd)*

Patients should be advised that cidofovir caused reduced testes weight and hypospermia in animals. Such changes may occur in humans and cause infertility. Women of childbearing potential should be advised that cidofovir is embryotoxic in animals and should not be used during pregnancy. Women of childbearing potential should be advised to use effective contraception during and for 1 month following treatment with cidofovir.

CARCINOGENESIS, MUTAGENESIS, AND IMPAIRMENT OF FERTILITY

Chronic, two-year carcinogenicity studies in rats and mice have not been carried out to evaluate the carcinogenic potential of cidofovir. However, a 26-week toxicology study evaluating once weekly subscapular subcutaneous injections of cidofovir in rats was terminated at 19 weeks because of the induction, in females, of palpable masses, the first of which was detected after six doses. The masses were diagnosed as mammary adenocarcinomas which developed at doses as low as 0.6 mg/kg/week, equivalent to 0.04 times the human systemic exposure at the recommended intravenous cidofovir dose based on AUC comparisons.

In a 26-week intravenous toxicology study in which rats received 0.6, 3, or 15 mg/kg cidofovir once weekly, a significant increase in mammary adenocarcinomas in female rats as well as a significant incidence of Zymbal's gland carcinomas in male and female rats were seen at the high dose but not at the lower two doses. The high dose was equivalent to 1.1 times the human systemic exposure at the recommended dose of cidofovir, based on comparisons of AUC measurements. In light of the results of these studies, cidofovir should be considered to be a carcinogen in rats as well as a potential carcinogen in humans.

Cynomolgus monkeys received intravenous cidofovir, alone and in conjunction with concomitant oral probenecid, intravenously once weekly for 52 weeks at doses resulting in exposures of approximately 0.7 times the human systemic exposure at the recommended dose of cidofovir. No tumors were detected. However, the study was not designed as a carcinogenicity study due to the small number of animals at each dose and the short duration of treatment.

No mutagenic response was observed in microbial mutagenicity assays involving *Salmonella typhimurium* (Ames) and *Escherichia coli* in the presence and absence of metabolic activation. An increase in micronucleated polychromatic erythrocytes *in vivo* was seen in mice receiving ≥ 2000 mg/kg, a dosage approximately 65-fold higher than the maximum recommended clinical intravenous cidofovir dose based on body surface area estimations. Cidofovir induced chromosomal aberrations in human peripheral blood lymphocytes *in vitro* without metabolic activation. At the 4 cidofovir levels tested, the percentage of damaged metaphases and number of aberrations per cell increased in a concentration-dependent manner.

Studies showed that cidofovir caused inhibition of spermatogenesis in rats and monkeys. However, no adverse effects on fertility or reproduction were seen following once weekly intravenous injections of cidofovir in male rats for 13 consecutive weeks at doses up to 15 mg/kg/week (equivalent to 1.1 times the recommended human dose based on AUC comparisons). Female rats dosed intravenously once weekly at 1.2 mg/kg/week (equivalent to 0.09 times the recommended human dose based on AUC) or higher, for up to 6 weeks prior to mating and for 2 weeks post mating had decreased litter sizes and live births per litter and increased early resorptions per litter. Peri- and post-natal development studies in which female rats received subcutaneous injection of cidofovir once daily at dose up to 1.0 mg/kg/day from day 7 of gestation through day 21 postpartum (approximately 5 weeks) resulted in no adverse effects on viability, growth, behavior, sexual maturation or reproductive capacity in the offspring.

PREGNANCY CATEGORY C

Cidofovir was embryotoxic (reduced fetal body weights) in rats at 1.5 mg/kg/day and in rabbits at 1.0 mg/kg/day, doses which were also maternally toxic, following daily intravenous dosing during the period of organogenesis. The no-observable-effect levels for embryotoxicity in rats (0.5 mg/kg/day) and in rabbits (0.25 mg/kg/day) were approximately 0.04 and 0.05 times the clinical dose (5 mg/kg every other week) based on AUC, respectively. An increased incidence of fetal external, soft tissue and skeletal anomalies (meningocele, short snout, and short maxillary bones) occurred in rabbits at the high dose (1.0 mg/kg/day) which was also maternally toxic. There are no adequate and well-controlled studies in pregnant women. Cidofovir should be used during pregnancy only if the potential benefit justifies the potential risk to the fetus.

NURSING MOTHERS

It is not known whether cidofovir is excreted in human milk. Since many drugs are excreted in human milk and because of the potential for adverse reactions as well as the potential for tumorigenicity shown for cidofovir in animal studies, cidofovir should not be administered to nursing mothers. The U.S. Public Health Service Centers for Disease Control and Prevention advises HIV-infected women not to breast-feed to avoid postnatal transmission of HIV to a child who may not yet be infected.

PEDIATRIC USE

Safety and effectiveness in children have not been studied. The use of cidofovir in children with AIDS warrants extreme caution due to the risk of long-term carcinogenicity and reproductive toxicity. Administration of cidofovir to children should be undertaken only after careful evaluation and only if the potential benefits of treatment outweigh the risks.

GERIATRIC USE

No studies of the safety or efficacy of cidofovir in patients over the age of 60 have been conducted. Since elderly individuals frequently have reduced glomerular filtration, particular attention should be paid to assessing renal function before and during cidofovir administration (see DOSAGE AND ADMINISTRATION).

DRUG INTERACTIONS:

Zidovudine: The pharmacokinetics of zidovudine were evaluated in 10 patients receiving zidovudine alone or with intravenous cidofovir (without probenecid). There was no evidence of an effect of cidofovir on the pharmacokinetics of zidovudine.

Probenecid: Probenecid is known to interact with the metabolism or renal tubular excretion of many drugs (*e.g.,* acetaminophen, acyclovir, angiotensin-converting enzyme inhibitors, aminosalicylic acid, barbiturates, benzodiazepines, bumetanide, clofibrate, methotrexate, famoridine, furosemide, nonsteroidal anti-inflammatory agents, theophylline, and zidovudine). Concomitant medications should be carefully assessed.

Nephrotoxic Agents: Concomitant administration of cidofovir and agents with nephrotoxic potential (*e.g.,* amphotericin B, aminoglycosides, foscarnet, and intravenous pentamidine) should be avoided.

ADVERSE REACTIONS:

1. Nephrotoxicity: Renal toxicity, as manifested by >1 + proteinuria, serum creatinine elevations of ≥ 0.4 mg/dL, or decreased creatinine clearance ≤ 55 mL/min, occurred in 47 of 89 (53%) patients receiving cidofovir at a maintenance dose of 5 mg/kg every other week. Maintenance dose reductions from 5 mg/kg to 3 mg/kg due to proteinuria or serum creatinine elevations were made for 12 of 41 (29%) patients who had not received prior therapy for CMV retinitis (Study 106) and 11 of 48 (23%) patients who had received prior therapy for CMV retinitis (Study 107). Prior foscarnet use has been associated with an increased risk of nephrotoxicity, therefore such patients should be monitored closely.

ADVERSE REACTIONS: *(cont'd)*

2. Neutropenia: In clinical trials, at the 5 mg/kg maintenance dose, neutropenia to ≤ 500 cells/mm^3 occurred in 20% of patients. Granulocyte colony stimulating factor (GCSF) was used in 34% of patients.

3. Ocular hypotony: Among the subset of patients monitored for intraocular pressure changes, ocular hypotony (≥ 50% change from baseline) was reported in 5 patients. Hypotony was reported in 1 patient with concomitant diabetes mellitus. Risk of ocular hypotomy may be increased in patients with preexisting diabetes.

4. Metabolic Acidosis: A diagnosis of Fanconi's syndrome, as manifested by multiple abnormalities of proximal tubule function, was reported in 2% of patients. Decreases in serum bicarbonate to ≤ 16 mcg/L associated with evidence of renal tubular damage occurred in approximately 9% of patients. Serious metabolic acidosis, in association with liver failure, pancreatitis, mucormycosis, aspergillus, disseminated mycobacterial infection, and progression to death occurred in 1 patient (< 1%) receiving cidofovir.

In clinical trials, cidofovir was withdrawn due to adverse events in approximately 25% of patients treated with 5 mg/kg every other week as maintenance therapy.

The incidence of adverse reactions reported as serious in two controlled clinical studies in patients with CMV retinitis, regardless of presumed relationship to drug, is listed in TABLE 4.

TABLE 4 Serious Clinical Adverse Events or Laboratory Abnormalities Occurring in > 5% of Patients

	N=89[a]	%
Proteinuria (≥ 100 mg/dL)	42	48
Neutropenia (≤ 500 cells/mm^3)	18	20
Creatinine Elevation	13	15
Fever	13	15
Infection	11	12
Dyspnea	9	10
Pneumonia	8	9
Decreased Serum Bicarbonate (≤ 1 16 mcg/L)	8	9
Creatinine Elevation (to ≥ 2.0 mg/dL)	7	8
Nausea with Vomiting	7	8
Diarrhea	6	7
Asthenia	6	7
Ocular Hypotony[b]	5	12

[a]Patients receiving 5 mg/kg maintenance regimen in Studies 106 and 107.
[b]Incidence based on 42 patients receiving 5 mg/kg maintenance regimen in Studies 106 and 107 with pretreatment baseline intraocular pressure reading and follow-up evaluation ≤ 50% of baseline.

The most frequently reported adverse events regardless of relationship to study drugs (cidofovir or probenecid) or severity are shown in TABLE 5.

TABLE 5 All Clinical Adverse Events, Laboratory Abnormalities or Intercurrent Illnesses Regardless of Severity Occurring in > 15% of Patients

	N=89[a]	%
Any Adverse Event	89	100
Proteinuria	71	80
Nausea +/- Vomiting	58	65
Fever	51	57
Asthenia	41	46
Neutropenia (< 750/mm^3)	28	31
Rash	27	30
Headache	24	27
Diarrhea	24	27
Alopecia	22	25
Infections	22	25
Chills	21	24
Anorexia	20	22
Dyspnea	20	22
Anemia	18	20
Creatinine Elevation (to > 1.5 mg/dL)	16	18
Abdominal Pain	15	17

[a]Patients receiving 5 mg/kg maintenance regimen in Studies 106 and 107.

The following additional list of adverse events/intercurrent illnesses have been observed in clinical studies of cidofovir and are listed below regardless of causal relationship to cidofovir:

Body as a Whole: allergic reaction, face edema, malaise, back pain, chest pain, neck pain, sarcoma, sepsis

Cardiovascular System: hypotension, postural hypotension, pallor, syncope, tachycardia

Digestive System: colitis, constipation, tongue discoloration, dyspepsia, dysphagia, flatulence, gastritis, hepatomegaly, abnormal liver function tests, melena, oral candidiasis, rectal disorder, stomatitis, aphthous stomatitis, mouth ulceration

Hemic & Lymphatic System: thrombocytopenia

Metabolic & Nutritional System: edema, dehydration, hyperglycemia, hyperlipemia, hypocalcemia, hypokalemia, increased alkaline phosphatase, increased SGOT, increased SGPT, weight loss

Musculoskeletal System: arthralgia, myasthenia, myalgia

Nervous System: amnesia, anxiety, confusion, convulsion, depression, dizziness, dry mouth, abnormal gait, hallucinations, insomnia, neuropathy, paresthesia, somnolence, vasodilation

Respiratory System: asthma, bronchitis, coughing, dyspnea, hiccup, increased sputum, lung disorder, pharyngitis, pneumonia, rhinitis, sinusitis

Skin & Appendages: alopecia, acne, skin discoloration, dry skin, herpes simplex, pruritis, rash, sweating, urticaria

Special Senses: amblyopia, conjuctivitis, eye disorder, hypotony, iritis, retinal detachment, taste perversion, uveitis, abnormal vision

Urogenital System: decreased creatinine clearance, glycosuria, hematuria, urinary incontinence, urinary tract infection

REPORTING OF ADVERSE REACTIONS

Malignancies or serious adverse reactions that occur in patients who have received cidofovir should be reported to Gilead in writing to the Director of Clinical Research, Gilead Sciences, Inc., 353 Lakeside Drive, Foster City, CA 94404 or by calling 1-800-GILEAD=5 (445-3235), or to FDA MedWatch 1-800-FDA-1088/fax 1-800-FDA-0178.

OVERDOSAGE:

Overdosage with cidofovir has not been reported; however, hemodialysis and hydration may reduce drug plasma concentrations in patients who receive an overdosage of cidofovir. Probenecid may reduce the potential for nephrotoxicity in patients who receive an overdose of cidofovir through reduction of active tubular secretion.

DOSAGE AND ADMINISTRATION:

CIDOFOVIR MUST NOT BE ADMINISTERED BY INTRAOCULAR INJECTION.

DOSAGE

THE RECOMMENDED DOSAGE, FREQUENCY, OR INFUSION RATE MUST NOT BE EXCEEDED. CIDOFOVIR MUST BE DILUTED IN 100 MILLILITERS 0.9% (NORMAL) SALINE PRIOR TO ADMINISTRATION. TO MINIMIZE POTENTIAL NEPHROTOXICITY, PROBENECID AND INTRAVENOUS SALINE PREHYDRATION MUST BE ADMINISTERED WITH EACH CIDOFOVIR INFUSION.

Induction Treatment: The recommended dose of cidofovir is 5 mg/kg body weight (given as an intravenous infusion at a constant rate over 1 hr) administered once weekly for two consecutive weeks.

Maintenance Treatment: The recommended maintenance dose of cidofovir is 5 mg/kg body weight (given as an intravenous infusion at a constant rate over 1 hr) administered once every two weeks.

Probenecid: Probenecid must be administered orally with each cidofovir dose. Two grams must be administered 3 hr prior to the cidofovir dose and one gram administered at 2 and again at 8 hr after completion of the 1 hr cidofovir infusion (for a total of 4 grams).

Ingestion of food prior to each dose of probenecid may reduce drug-related nausea and vomiting. Administration of an antiemetic may reduce the potential for nausea associated with probenecid ingestion. In patients who develop allergic or hypersensitivity symptoms to probenecid, the use of an appropriate prophylactic or therapeutic antihistamine and/or acetaminophen should be considered (see CONTRAINDICATIONS).

Hydration: Patients should receive a total of one liter of 0.9% (normal) saline solution intravenously with each infusion of cidofovir. The saline solution should be infused over a 1-2 hr period immediately before the cidofovir infusion. Patients who can tolerate the additional fluid load should receive a second liter. If administered, the second liter of saline should be initiated either at the start of the cidofovir infusion or immediately afterwards, and infused over a 1 to 3 hr period.

DOSE ADJUSTMENT

Changes in Renal Function During Cidofovir Therapy: For clinically significant increases in serum creatinine (0.3-0.4 mg/dL), the cidofovir dose should be reduced from 5 mg/kg to 3 mg/kg. Cidofovir therapy should be discontinued for an increase in serum creatinine of ≥ 0.5 mg/dL or development of ≥ 3+ proteinuria.

Preexisting Renal Impairment: Cidofovir has not been studied in patients with preexisting renal impairment. The most appropriate initial and maintenance doses of cidofovir for patients with serum creatinine concentrations > 1.5 mg/dL or creatinine clearances ≤ 55 mL/min are not known. When the potential benefits of therapy exceed the potential risks, dose adjustments should be made based on the following table:

TABLE 6 Cidofovir Dose*

Creatinine Clearance (mL/min)	Induction (once weekly for 2 weeks)	Maintenance (once every 2 weeks)
41-55	2.0 mg/kg	2.0 mg/kg
30-40	1.5 mg/kg	1.5 mg/kg
20-29	1.0 mg/kg	1.0 mg/kg
≤ 19	0.5 mg/kg	0.5 mg/kg

* These recommended dose adjustments are based on pharmacokinetic estimates, not on actual clinical data.

Intravenous normal saline and oral probenecid must accompany each cidofovir infusion. Cidofovir has not been studied in patients receiving dialysis.

Because no clinical efficacy, safety or pharmacokinetic data are available from patients with moderate to severe renal impairment (creatinine clearance ≤ 55 mL/min), careful monitoring of disease progression and patient safety is required.

METHOD OF PREPARATION AND ADMINISTRATION

Inspect vials visually for particulate matter and discoloration prior to administration. If particulate matter or discoloration are observed, the vial should not be used.

With a syringe, extract the appropriate volume of cidofovir from the vial and transfer the dose to an infusion bag containing 100 mL 0.9% (normal) saline solution. Infuse the entire volume intravenously into the patient at a constant rate over a 1 hr period. Use of a standard infusion pump for administration is recommended.

It is recommended that cidofovir infusion admixtures be administered within 24 hr of preparation and that refrigerator or freezer storage not be used to extend this 24 hr limit.

If admixtures are not intended for immediate use, they may be stored under refrigeration (2-8°C) for no more than 24 hr. Refrigerated admixtures should be allowed to equilibrate to room temperature prior to use.

The chemical stability of cidofovir admixtures was demonstrated in polyvinyl chloride composition and ethylene/propylene copolymer composition commercial infusion bags, and in glass bottles. **No data are available to support the addition of other drugs or supplements to the cidofovir admixture for concurrent administration.**

Cidofovir is supplied in single-use vials. Partially used vials should be discarded (see Handling and Disposal).

Compatibility with Ringer's solution, Lactated Ringer's solution or bacteriostatic Infusion fluids has not been evaluated.

HANDLING AND DISPOSAL

Due to the mutagenic properties of cidofovir, adequate precautions including the use of appropriate safety equipment are recommended for the preparation, administration, and disposal of cidofovir. The National Institutes of Health presently recommends that the preparation of such agents be prepared in a Class II laminar flow biological safety cabinet and that personnel preparing drugs of this class wear surgical gloves and a closed front surgical-type gown with knit cuffs. If cidofovir contacts the skin, wash membranes and flush thoroughly with water. Excess cidofovir and all other materials used in the admixture preparation and administration should be placed in a leak-proof, puncture-proof container. The recommended method of disposal is high temperature incineration.

PATIENT MONITORING

Serum creatinine, urine protein, and white blood cell counts with differential should be monitored prior to each dose. In patients with proteinuria, intravenous hydration should be administered and the test repeated. Intraocular pressure, visual acuity and ocular symptoms should be monitored periodically.

REFERENCES:

1. Ho HT, Woods KL, Bronson JJ, De Boeck H, Martin JC and Hitchcock MJM. Intracellular Metabolism of the Antiherpesvirus Agent (S)-1-[3-hydroxy-2-(phosphonylmethoxy)propyl]cytosine. *Mol Pharmacol*, 41;197-202, 1992. **2.** Cherrington JM, Allen SJW, McKee BH, and Chen MS. Kinetic Analysis of the Interaction Between the Diphosphate of (S)-1- (3-hydroxy-2- phosphonylmethoxypropyl)cytosine, zalcitabineTP, zidovudineTP, and FIAUTP with Human DNA Polymerase β and [lgr]. *Biochem Pharmacol*, 48:1986-1988, 1994. **3.** Xiong X, Kim C, Huang E, Smith JL, and Chen MS. Kinetic Analysis of the Interaction of Cidofovir Diphosphate with Human Cytomegalovirus DNA Polymerase. *Biochem Pharmacol*, 1996 (in press). **4.** Cherrington JM, Mulato AS, Fuller MD, Chen MS. *In Vitro* Selection of a Human Cytomegalovirus (HCMV) that is Resistant to Cidofovir. 35th International Conference on Antimicrobial Agents and Chemotherapy (ICAAC), San Francisco, CA, Abstract

REFERENCES: *(cont'd)*

H117, 1995. **5.** Stanat SC, Reardon JE, Brice A, Jordan MC, Drew WL, and Biron KK. Ganciclovir-Resistant Cytomegalovirus Clinical Isolates: Mode of Resistance to Ganciclovir. *Antimicrob Agents Chemother.* 35: 2191–2197, 1991. **6.** Sullivan V, Biron KK, Talarico C, Stanat SC, Davis M, Pozzi M, and Coen DM. A Point Mutation in the Human Cytomegalovirus DNA Polymerase Gene Confers Resistance to Ganciclovir and phosphonylmethoxyalkyl Derivatives. *Antimicrob Agents Chemother.*37:19–25, 1993. **7.** Tatarowicz WA, Lurain NS, and Thompson KD. A Ganciclovir-Resistant Clinical Isolate of Human Cytomegalovirus Exhibiting Cross-Resistance to other DNA Polymerase Inhibitors. *J Infect Dis.* 155:904–907, 1992. **8.** Lurain NS, Thompson KD, Holmes EW, and Read GS. Point Mutations in the DNA Polymerase Gene of Human Cytomegalovirus that Result in Resistance to Antiviral Agents. *J Virol*, 66:7146–7152, 1992. **9.** Sullivan V and Coen DM. Isolation of Foscarnet-Resistant Human Cytomegalovirus Patterns of Resistance and Sensitivity to Other Antiviral Drugs. *J Infect Dis*, 154:781–784, 1991. **10.** Snoeck R, Andrei G, and De Clercq E. Human Cytomegalovirus (HCMV) Strains Selected Under Selective Pressure of Phosphonoformate (PFA) are Resistant for Both PFA and phosphonylmethoxyethyl (PME) Derivatives *In Vitro. Antiviral Res,* 26, Abstract 177, 1995. **11.** Baldanti F, Underwood MR, Stanat SC, Biron KK, Chou S, Sarasini A, Silini E, and Gema G. Single Amino Acid Changes in the DNA Polymerase Confer Foscarnet Resistance and Slow-Growth Phenotype. While Mutations in the UL97–Encoded Phosphotransferase Confer Ganciclovir Resistance in Three Double-Resistant Human Cytomegalovirus Strains Recovered from Patients with AIDS. *J Virol*, 70:1390–1395, 1996.

HOW SUPPLIED:

Vistide 75 mg/mL for intravenous infusion, is supplied as a non-preserved solution in single-use clear glass vials.

Storage: Vistide should be stored at controlled room temperature 20°-25°C (68°-77°F).

Caution: Federal law prohibits dispensing without prescription.

HOW SUPPLIED - EQUIVALENTS NOT AVAILABLE:

Injection - Intravenous - 75 mg/mL

375 mg x 5 mL $706.80 VISTIDE, Gilead Sciences 61958-0101-01

CILASTATIN SODIUM; IMIPENEM *(000819)*

CATEGORIES: Anti-Infectives; Antibiotics; Antimicrobials; Beta-Lactam Antibiotics; Bone Infections; Cystic Fibrosis; Endocarditis; Gynecologic Infections; Infections; Intra-Abdominal Infections; Joint Infections; Pulmonary Disease; Respiratory Tract Infections; Septicemia; Shock; Skin Infections; Urinary Tract Infections; Pregnancy Category C; Sales > $500 Million; FDA Approved 1985 Nov; Patent Expiration 1999 Dec

BRAND NAMES: **Primaxin**; *Tenacid*; *Tienam* (Europe, Asia, Mexico); *Tienam 500*; *Zienam* (Germany)
(International brand names outside U.S. in italics)

FORMULARIES: BC-BS

COST OF THERAPY: $618.00 (Infections; Injection; 500 mg/500 mg; 3/day; 10 days)

PRIMARY ICD9: 136.9 (Unspecified Infections And Parasitic Diseases)

DESCRIPTION:

IV

Primaxin† IV (Imipenem-Cilastatin Sodium for Injection) is a sterile formulation of imipenem, a thienamycin antibiotic, and cilastatin sodium, the inhibitor of the renal dipeptidase, dehydropeptidase I, with sodium bicarbonate added as a buffer. Primaxin IV is a potent broad spectrum antibacterial agent for intravenous administration.

Primaxin IV is buffered to provide solutions in the pH range of 6.5 to 7.5. There is no significant change in pH when solutions are prepared and used as directed. (See DOSAGE AND ADMINISTRATION, Compatibility and Stability.) Primaxin IV 250 contains 18.8 mg of sodium (0.8 mEq) and Primaxin IV 500 contains 37.5 mg of sodium (1.6 mEq). Solutions of Primaxin IV range from colorless to yellow. Variations of color within this range do not affect the potency of the product.

IM

Sterile Primaxin IM (Cilastatin Sodium-Imipenem for Suspension) is a formulation of imipenem (a thienamycin antibiotic) and cilastatin sodium (the inhibitor of the renal dipeptidase, dehydropeptidase l). Primaxin IM is a potent broad spectrum antibacterial agent for intramuscular administration.

Primaxin IM 500 contains 32 mg of sodium (1.4 mEq) and Primaxin 750 contains 48 mg of sodium (2.1 mEq). Prepared Primaxin IM suspensions are white to light tan in color. Variations of color within this range do not effect the potency of the product.

IV AND IM INJECTION

Imipenem (N-formimidoylthienamycin monohydrate) is a crystalline derivative of thienamycin, which is produced by *Streptomyces cattleya.* Its chemical name is (5*R*,6*S*)-3-[[2-(formimidoylamino)ethyl]thio]-6-[(*R*)-1-hydroxyethyl]-7-oxo-1-azabicyclo[3.2.0]hept-2-ene-2-carboxylic acid monohydrate. It is an off-white, nonhygroscopic crystalline compound with a molecular weight of 317.37. It is sparingly soluble in water, and slightly soluble in methanol. Its empirical formula is $C_{12}H_{17}N_3O_4S{\cdot}H_2O$.

Cilastatin sodium is the sodium salt of a derivatized heptenoic acid. Its chemical name is sodium (*Z*)-7-[[(*R*)-2-amino-2- carboxyethyl]thio]-2-[(*S*)-2,2-dimethylcyclopropanecarboxamido]-2- heptenoate. It is an off-white to yellowish-white, hygroscopic, amorphous compound with a molecular weight of 380.43. It is very soluble in water and in methanol. Its empirical formula is $C_{16}H_{25}N_2O_5SNa$.

CLINICAL PHARMACOLOGY:

INTRAVENOUS ADMINISTRATION

Intravenous infusion of Primaxin IV over 20 minutes results in peak plasma levels of imipenem antimicrobial activity that range from 14 to 24 mcg/ml for the 250 mg dose, from 21 to 58 mcg/ml for the 500 mg dose and from 41 to 83 mcg/ml for the 1000 mg dose. At these doses, plasma levels of imipenem antimicrobial activity decline to below 1 mcg/ml or less in 4 to 6 hours. Peak plasma levels of Cilastatin following a 20-minute intravenous infusion of Primaxin IV, range from 15 to 25 mcg/ml for the 250 mg dose, from 31 to 49 mcg/ml for the 500 mg dose and from 56 to 88 mcg/ml for the 1000 mg dose.

GENERAL

The plasma half-life of each component is approximately 1 hour. The binding of imipenem to human serum proteins is approximately 20% and that of cilastatin is approximately 40%. Approximately 70% of the administered imipenem is recovered in the urine within 10 hours after which no further urinary excretion is detectable. Urine concentrations of imipenem in excess of 10 mcg/ml can be maintained for up to 8 hours with Primaxin IV at the 500 mg dose. Approximately 70% of the cilastatin sodium dose is recovered in the urine within 10 hours of administration of Primaxin IV.

No accumulation of Primaxin IV in plasma or urine is observed with regimens administered as frequently as every 6 hours in patients with normal renal function.

CLINICAL PHARMACOLOGY: *(cont'd)*

Imipenem, when administered alone, is metabolized in the kidneys by dehydropeptidase resulting in relatively low levels in urine. Cilastatin sodium, an inhibitor of this enzyme, effectively prevents renal metabolism of imipenem so that when imipenem and cilastatin sodium are given concomitantly fully adequate antibacterial levels of imipenem are achieved in the urine.

After a 1 gram dose of Primaxin IV, the following average levels of imipenem were measured (usually at 1 hour post-dose except where indicated) in the tissues and fluids listed (TABLE 1):

TABLE 1

Tissue or Fluid	n	Imipenem level mcg/ml or mcg/g	Range
Vitreous Humor	3	3.4 (3.5 hours post dose)	2.88-3.6
Aqueous Humor	5	2.99 (2 hours post dose)	2.4-3.9
Lung Tissue	8	5.6 (median)	3.5-15.5
Sputum	1	2.1	—
Pleural	1	22.0	—
Peritoneal	12	23.9 S.D. ± 5.3 (2 hours post dose)	—
Bile	2	5.3 (2.25 hours post dose)	4.6 to 6.0
CSF (uninflamed)	5	1.0 (4 hours post dose)	0.26-2.0
CSF (inflamed)	7	2.6 (2 hours post dose)	0.5-5.5
Fallopian Tubes	1	13.6	—
Endometrium	1	11.1	—
Myometrium	1	5.0	—
Bone	10	2.6	0.4-5.4
Interstitial Fluid	12	16.4	10.0-22.6
Skin	12	4.4	NA
Fascia	12	4.4	NA

Imipenem-cilastatin sodium is hemodialyzable. However, usefulness of this procedure in the overdosage setting is questionable (see OVERDOSAGE.)

IM

Following intramuscular administrations of 500 or 750 mg doses of imipenem-cilastatin sodium in a 1:1 ratio with 1% lidocaine, peak plasma levels of imipenem antimicrobial activity occur within 2 hours and average 10 and 12 mcg/ml, respectively. For cilastatin, peak plasma levels average 24 and 33 mcg/ml respectively, and occur within 1 hour. When compared to intravenous administration of imipenem-cilastatin sodium is approximately 75% bioavailable following intramuscular administration while cilastatin is approximately 95% bioavailable. The absorption of imipenem-cilastatin sodium from the IM injection site continues for 6 to 8 hours while that for cilastatin is essentially complete within 4 hours. This prolonged absorption of imipenem-cilastatin sodium following the administration of the intramuscular formulation of imipenem-cilastatin sodium results in an effective plasma half-life of imipenem of approximately 2 to 3 hours and plasma levels of the antibiotic which remain above 2 mcg/ml for at least 6 to 8 hours, following a 500 mg or 750 mg dose, respectively. This plasma profile for imipenem permits IM administration of the intramuscular formulation of imipenem-cilastatin sodium every 12 hours with no accumulation of cilastatin and only slight accumulation of imipenem.

A comparison of plasma levels of imipenem after a single dose of 500 mg or 750 mg of imipenem-cilastatin sodium (intravenous formulation) administered intravenously or of imipenem-cilastatin sodium (intramuscular formulation) diluted with 1% lidocaine and administered intramuscularly as seen in TABLE 2.

TABLE 2 Plasma Concentrations Of Imipenem (mcg/ml)

	500 mg		750 mg	
TIME	IV	IM	IV	IM
25 min	45.1	6.0	57.0	6.7
1 hr	21.6	9.4	28.1	10.0
2 hr	10.0	9.9	12.0	11.4
4 hr	0.6	2.5	1.1	3.8
12 hr	ND†	0.5	ND†	0.8

† ND: Not Detectable (<0.3 mcg/ml)

Imipenem urine levels remain above 10 mcg/ml for the 12 hour dosing interval following the administration of 500 mg or 750 mg doses of the intramuscular formulation of imipenem-cilastatin sodium. Total urinary excretion of imipenem averages 50% while that for cilastatin averages 75% following either dose of the intramuscular formulation of imipenem- cilastatin sodium.

Imipenem, when administered alone, is metabolized in the kidneys by dehydropeptidase l resulting in relatively low levels in urine. Cilastatin sodium, an inhibitor of this enzyme, effective prevents renal metabolism of imipenem so that when imipenem and cilastatin sodium are given concomitantly increased levels of imipenem are achieved in the urine. The binding of imipenem to human serum proteins is approximately 20% and that of cilastatin is approximately 40%.

In a clinical study in which a 500 mg dose of the intramuscular formulation of imipenem-cilastatin sodium was administered to healthy subjects, the average peak level of imipenem in interstitial fluid (skin blister fluid) was approximately 5.0 mcg/ml within 3.5 hours after administration

Imipenem-cilastatin sodium is hemodialyzable. However, usefulness of this procedure in the overdosage setting is questionable (see OVERDOSAGE.)

MICROBIOLOGY

The bactericidal activity of imipenem results from the inhibition of cell wall synthesis. Its greatest affinity is for penicillin binding proteins (PBPs) 1A, 1B, 2, 4, 5 and 6 of *Escherichia coli,* and 1A, 1B, 2, 4 and 5 of *Pseudomonas aeruginosa.* The lethal effect is related to binding to PBP 2 and PBP 1B.

Imipenem has a high degree of stability in the presence of beta- lactamases, both penicillinases and cephalosporinases produced by gram- negative and gram-positive bacteria. It is a potent inhibitor of beta- lactamases from certain gram-negative bacteria which are inherently resistant to most beta-lactam antibiotics (*e.g., Pseudomonas aeruginosa, Serratia* spp., and *Enterobacter* spp.

Imipenem has *in vitro* activity against a wide range of gram- positive and gram-negative organisms. Imipenem is active against most strains of the following microorganisms *in vitro* and in clinical infections treated with the intramuscular formulation of imipenem- cilastatin sodium (See INDICATIONS AND USAGE.)

Gram-positive aerobes: *Enterococcus faecalis* (formerly *S. faecalis*)
(NOTE: Imipenem is inactive *in vitro* against *Enterococcus faecium* [formerly *S. faecium*].)
Staphylococcus aureus including penicillinase-producing strains
Staphylococcus epidermidis including penicillinase-producing strains
(NOTE: Methicillin-resistant staphylococci should be reported as resistant to imipenem.)

CLINICAL PHARMACOLOGY: *(cont'd)*

Streptococcus agalactiae (Group B streptococcus);*Streptococcus pneumoniae*; *Streptococcus pyogenes*

Gram-negative aerobes

Acinetobacter spp.; *Citrobacter* spp.; *Enterobacter* spp.; *Escherichia coli; Gardnerella vaginalis; Haemophilus influenzae; Haemophilus parainfluenzae; Klebsiella* spp.;*Morganella morganii; Proteus vulgaris; Providencia rettgeri; Pseudomonas aeruginosa*

(NOTE: Imipenem is inactive *in vitro* against *Xanthomonas (Pseudomonas) maltophilia* and some strains of *P. cepacia.*)

Serratia spp., including *S. marcescens*

Gram-positive anaerobes

Bifidobacterium spp.; *Clostridium* spp.; *Eubacterium* spp.; *Peptococcus* spp.; *Peptostreptococcus* spp.;*Propionibacterium* spp.

Gram-negative anaerobes

Bacteroides spp., including *B. fragilis; Fusobacterium* spp.

The following *in vitro* data are available,**but their clinical significance is unknown.**

Imipenem exhibits *in vitro* minimal inhibitory concentrations (MIC's) of 4 mcg/ml or less against most (≥ 90%) strains of the following microorganisms; however, the safety and effectiveness of imipenem in treating clinical infections due to these microorganisms have not been established in adequate and well-controlled clinical trials.

Gram-positive aerobes

Listeria monocytogenes; *Nocardia* spp; Group C streptococcus; Group G streptococcus; Viridans group streptococci

Gram-negative aerobes

Achromobacter spp.; *Aeromonas hydrophila; Alcaligenes* spp.; *Bordetella bronchiseptica; Campylobacter* spp.;*Hafnia alvei; Klebsiella oxytoca; Klebsiella pneumoniae; Moraxella* spp.; *Neisseria gonorrhoeae* including penicillinase-producing strains; *Pasteurella multocida; Plesiomonas shigelloides; Proteus mirabilis; Providencia stuartii; Salmonella* spp.; *Serratia proteamaculans* (formerly *S. liquefaciens*); *Shigella* spp.; *Yersinia* spp., including *Y. enterocolitica* and *Y. pseudotuberculosis*

Gram-positive anaerobes

Actinomyces spp.; *Clostridium perfringens*; *Propionibacterium acnes*

Gram-negative anaerobes:

Bacteroides spp., including *B. bivius, B. disiens, B. distasonis, B. intermedius* (formerly *B. melaninogenicus intermedius*) *B. ovatus, B. thetaiotaomicron, and B. vulgatus Porphyromonas asaccharolytica* (formerly *B.asaccharolyticus*) *Veillonella* spp.

In vitro tests show imipenem to act synergistically with aminoglycoside antibiotics against some isolates of *Pseudomonas aeruginosa.*

SUSCEPTIBILITY TESTS

Measurement of MIC or minimum bactericidal concentration (MBC) and achieved antimicrobial compound concentrations may be appropriate to guide therapy in some infections. (See CLINICAL PHARMACOLOGY section for further information on drug concentrations achieved in infected body sites and other pharmacokinetic properties of this antimicrobial drug product.)

Diffusion techniques: Quantitative methods that require measurement of zone diameters give the most precise estimate of antibiotic susceptibility. One such standard procedure[1], that has been recommended for use with disks to test susceptibility of microorganisms to imipenem, uses the 10-mcg imipenem disk. Interpretation involves the correlation of the diameters obtained in the disk test with the (MIC) for imipenem.

Reports from the laboratory giving results of the standard single-disk susceptibility test with a 10-mcg imipenem disk should be interpreted according to the criteria found in TABLE 3.

TABLE 3

Zone Diameter (mm)	Interpretation
≥16	Susceptible (S)
14-15	Intermediate (I)
≤13	Resistant (R)

A report of "Susceptible" indicates that the pathogen is likely to be inhibited by usually achievable concentrations of the antimicrobial compound in blood. A report of "Intermediate" indicates that the result should be considered equivocal, and, if the microorganism is not fully susceptible to alternative, clinically feasible drugs, the test should be repeated. This category implies possible clinical applicability in body sites where the drug is physiologically concentrated or in situations where high dosage of drug can be used. This category also provides a buffer zone that prevents small uncontrolled technical factors from causing major discrepancies in interpretation. A report of "Resistant" indicates that usually achievable concentrations of the antimicrobial compound in the blood are unlikely to be inhibitory and that other therapy should be selected.

Standardized susceptibility test procedures require the use of laboratory control microorganisms. The 10 mcg imipenem disk should provide diameters (as seen in TABLE 4 in these laboratory test quality control strains.

TABLE 4

Microorganism	Zone Diameter (mm)
E. coli ATCC 25922	26-32
P. aeruginosa ATCC 27853	20-28

Dilution Techniques: Quantitative methods that are used to determine MIC's provide reproducible estimates of the susceptibility of bacteria to antimicrobial compounds. One such procedure uses a standardized dilution method[2] (broth, agar, or microdilution) or equivalent with imipenem powder.

The MIC values obtained should be interpreted according to the criteria found in TABLE 5.

TABLE 5

MIC (mcg/ml)	Interpretation
≤4	Susceptible (S)
8	Intermediate (I)
≥16	Resistant (R)

Interpretation should be as stated above for results using diffusion techniques.

As with standard diffusion techniques, dilution methods require the use of laboratory control organisms. Standard imipenem powder should provide the MIC values as seen in TABLE 6.

Anaerobic Techniques: For anaerobic bacteria, the susceptibility to imipenem can be determined by the reference agar dilution method or by alternate standardized test methods.[3]

CLINICAL PHARMACOLOGY: *(cont'd)*

TABLE 6

Microorganism	MIC (mcg/ml)
E. coli ATCC 25922	0.06 - 0.25
S. aureus ATCC 29213	0.015 - 0.06
E. faecalis ATCC 29212	0.5 - 2.0
P. aeruginosa ATCC 27853	1.0 - 4.0

As with other susceptibility techniques, the use of laboratory control microorganisms is required. Standard imipenem powder should provide the MIC values as seen in TABLE 7 and TABLE 8.

TABLE 7 Reference Agar Dilution Testing

Microorganism	MIC (mcg/ml)
B. fragilis ATCC 25285	0.03-0.12
B. thetaiotaomicron ATCC 29741	0.06-0.25
E. lentum ATCC 43055	0.25-1.0

TABLE 8 Broth Microdilution Testing

Microorganism	MIC (mcg/ml)
B. thetaiotaomicron ATCC 29741	0.06-0.25
E. lentum ATCC 43055	0.12-0.5

INDICATIONS AND USAGE:

IV

Primaxin (Imipenem-Cilastatin Sodium) IV is indicated for the treatment of serious infections caused by susceptible strains of the designated microorganisms in the diseases listed below:

(1) Lower Respiratory Tract Infections: *Staphylococcus aureus* (penicillinase-producing strains), *Acinetobacter* species, *Escherichia coli, Enterobacter* species, *Haemophilus influenzae, Haemophilus parainfluenzae**, *Klebsiella* species, *Serratia marcescens.*

(2) Urinary Tract Infections: (complicated and uncomplicated). *Enterococcus faecalis, Staphylococcus aureus* (penicillinase- producing strains)*, *Enterobacter* species, *Escherichia coli, Klebsiella* species, *Morganella morganii**, *Proteus vulgaris**, *Providencia rettgeri**, *Pseudomonas aeruginosa.*

(3) Intra-Abdominal Infections: *Enterococcus faecalis, Staphylococcus aureus* (penicillinase-producing strains)*, *Staphylococcus epidermidis, Citrobacter* species, *Enterobacter* species, *Escherichia coli, Klebsiella* species, *Morganella morganii**, *Proteus* species (indole positive and indole negative), *Pseudomonas aeruginosa, Bifidobacterium* species, *Clostridium* species, *Eubacterium* species, *Peptococcus* species, *Peptostreptococcus* species, *Propionibacterium* species*, *Bacteroides* species including *B. fragilis, Fusobacterium* species.

(4) Gynecologic Infections: *Enterococcus faecalis, Staphylococcus aureus* (penicillinase-producing strains)*, *Staphylococcus epidermidis, Streptococcus agalactiae* (Group B streptococcus), *Enterobacter* species*, *Escherichia coli, Gardnerella vaginalis, Klebsiella* species*, *Proteus* species (indole positive and indole negative), *Bifidobacterium* species*, *Peptococcus* species*, *Peptostreptococcus* species, *Propionibacterium* species*, *Bacteroides* species including *B.fragilis**.

(5) Bacterial Septicemia: *Enterococcus faecalis, Staphylococcus aureus* (penicillinase-producing strains), *Enterobacter* species, *Escherichia coli, Klebsiella* species, *Pseudomonas aeruginosa, Serratia* species*, *Bacteroides* species including *B. fragilis**.

(6) Bone And Joint Infections: *Enterococcus faecalis, Staphylococcus aureus* (penicillinase-producing strains), *Staphylococcus epidermidis, Enterobacter* species, *Pseudomonas aeruginosa.*

(7) Skin And Skin Structure Infections: *Enterococcus faecalis, Staphylococcus aureus* (penicillinase-producing strains), *Staphylococcus epidermidis, Acinetobacter* species, *Citrobacter* species, *Enterobacter* species, *Escherichia coli, Klebsiella* species, *Morganella morganii, Proteus vulgaris, Providencia rettgeri**, *Pseudomonas aeruginosa, Serratia* species, *Peptococcus* species, *Peptostreptococcus* species, *Bacteroides* species including *B. fragilis, Fusobacterium* species*.

(8) Endocarditis: *Staphylococcus aureus* (penicillinase-producing strains).

(9) Polymicrobic Infections: Primaxin IV is indicated for polymicrobic infections including those in which *S. pneumoniae* (pneumonia, septicemia), Group A beta-hemolytic streptococcus (skin and skin structure), or non penicillinase-producing *S. aureus* is one of the causative organisms. However monobacterial infections due to these organisms are usually treated with narrower spectrum antibiotics, such as penicillin G.

Primaxin IV is not indicated in patients with meningitis because safety and efficacy have not been established.

Because of its broad spectrum of bactericidal activity against gram-positive and gram-negative aerobic and anaerobic bacteria, Primaxin is useful for the treatment of mixed infections and as presumptive therapy prior to the identification of the causative organisms.

Although clinical improvement has been observed in patients with cystic fibrosis, chronic pulmonary disease, and lower respiratory tract infection caused by *Pseudomonas aeruginosa*, bacterial eradication may not necessarily be achieved.

As with other beta-lactam antibiotics, some strains of *Pseudomonas aeruginosa* may develop resistance fairly rapidly on treatment with Primaxin IV. When clinically appropriate during therapy of *Pseudomonas aeruginosa* infections, periodic susceptibility testing should be done.

Infections resistant to other antibiotics, for example, cephalosporins, penicillin, and aminoglycosides, have been shown to respond to treatment with Primaxin IV.

IM

Primaxin IM is indicated for the treatment of serious infections (listed below) of mild to moderate severity for which intramuscular therapy is appropriate. **Primaxin IM is not intended for the therapy of severe or life-threatening infections, including bacterial sepsis or endocarditis, or in instances of major physiological impairments such as shock.**

Primaxin IM is indicated for the treatment of infections caused by susceptible strains of the designated microorganisms in the conditions listed below:

(1) Lower Respiratory Tract Infections: including pneumonia and bronchitis as an exacerbation of COPD, caused by *Streptococcus pneumoniae* and *Haemophilus influenzae.*

(2) Intra-Abdominal Infections: including acute gangrenous or perforated appendicitis and appendicitis with peritonitis, caused by Group D streptococcus including *Enterococcus faecalis**; *Streptococcus viridans* group*; *Escherichia coli*; *Klebsiella pneumoniae**; *Pseudomonas aeruginosa**; *Bacteroides* species including *B fragilis, B. distasonis**, *B. intermedius** and *B. thetaiotaomicron**; *Fusobacterium* species and *Peptostreptococcus** species.

(3) Skin And Skin Structure Infections: including abscesses, cellulitis, infected skin ulcers and wound infections caused by *Staphylococcus aureus* including penicillinase-producing strains; *Streptococcus pyogenes**; Group D streptococcus including *Enterococcus faecalis; Acinetobacter*

INDICATIONS AND USAGE: *(cont'd)*

species* including *A. calcoaceticus**; *Citrobacter* species*; *Escherichia coli; Enterobacter cloacae; Klebsiella pneumoniae**; *Pseudomonas aeruginosa** and *Bacteroides* species* including *B. fragilis**.

(4) Gynecologic Infections: including postpartum endomyometritis, caused by Group D streptococcus including *Enterococcus faecalis**; *Escherichia coli; Klebsiella pneumoniae**; *Bacteroides intermedius**; and *Peptostreptococcus* species*.

As with other beta-lactam antibiotics, some strains of *Pseudomonas aeruginosa* may develop resistance fairly rapidly during treatment with Primaxin IM. During therapy of *Pseudomonas aeruginosa* infections, periodic susceptibility testing should be done when clinically appropriate. Efficacy for this organism in this organ system was studied in fewer than 10 infections.

CONTRAINDICATIONS:

IV AND IM INJECTION

Primaxin IV and IM are contraindicated in patients who have shown hypersensitivity to any component of this product.

IM ONLY

Due to the use of lidocaine HCl diluent, Primaxin IM is contraindicated in patients with a known hypersensitivity to local anesthetics of the amide type and in patients with severe shock or heart block. (Refer to the package circular for lidocaine HCl).

WARNINGS:

SERIOUS AND OCCASIONALLY FATAL HYPERSENSITIVITY (anaphylactic) REACTIONS HAVE BEEN REPORTED IN PATIENTS RECEIVING THERAPY WITH BETA-LACTAMS. THESE REACTIONS ARE MORE APT TO OCCUR IN PERSONS WITH A HISTORY OF SENSITIVITY TO MULTIPLE ALLERGENS.

THERE HAVE BEEN REPORTS OF PATIENTS WITH A HISTORY OF PENICILLIN HYPERSENSITIVITY WHO HAVE EXPERIENCED SEVERE HYPERSENSITIVITY REACTIONS WHEN TREATED WITH ANOTHER BETA-LACTAM. BEFORE INITIATING THERAPY WITH PRIMAXIN IV OR IM, CAREFUL INQUIRY SHOULD BE MADE CONCERNING PREVIOUS HYPERSENSITIVITY REACTIONS TO PENICILLINS, CEPHALOSPORINS, OTHER BETA-LACTAMS, AND OTHER ALLERGENS. IF AN ALLERGIC REACTION OCCURS, PRIMAXIN SHOULD BE DISCONTINUED.

SERIOUS ANAPHYLACTIC REACTIONS REQUIRE IMMEDIATE EMERGENCY TREATMENT WITH EPINEPHRINE. OXYGEN, INTRAVENOUS STEROIDS, AND AIRWAY MANAGEMENT, INCLUDING INTUBATION, MAY ALSO BE ADMINISTERED AS INDICATED.

IV

Seizures and other CNS adverse experiences, such as confusional states and myoclonic activity, have been reported during treatment with Primaxin (See PRECAUTIONS.)

IV AND IM

Pseudomembranous colitis has been reported with nearly all antibacterial agents, including imipenem-cilastatin sodium, and may range in severity from mild to life threatening. Therefore, it is important to consider this diagnosis in patients who present with diarrhea subsequent to the administration of antibacterial agents.

Treatment with antibacterial agents alters the normal flora of the colon and may permit overgrowth of clostridia. Studies indicate that a toxin produced by *Clostridium difficile* is one primary cause of "antibiotic-associated colitis".

After the diagnosis of pseudomembranous colitis has been established, therapeutic measures should be initiated.

Mild cases of pseudomembranous colitis usually respond to drug discontinuation alone. In moderate to severe cases, consideration should be given to management with fluids and electrolytes, protein supplementation and treatment with an antibacterial drug clinically effective against *C. difficile colitis*.

IM

Lidocaine HCl: Refer to the prescribing information for Lidocaine HCl.

PRECAUTIONS:

GENERAL

IV: CNS adverse experiences such as confusional states, myoclonic activity, and seizures have been reported during treatment with Primaxin especially when recommended dosages were exceeded. These experiences occurred most commonly in patients with CNS disorders (*e.g.,* brain lesions or history of seizures) and/or compromised renal function. However, there have been reports of CNS adverse experiences in patients who had no recognized or documented underlying CNS disorder or compromised renal function.

When recommended doses were exceeded, adult patients with creatinine clearances of ≤20 ml/min/1.73 m^2, whether or not underlying hemodialysis, had a higher risk of seizure activity than those without impairment of renal function. Therefore, close adherence to the dosing guidelines for these patients is recommended. (See DOSAGE AND ADMINISTRATION.)

Patients with creatinine clearances of ≤5 ml/min/1.73 m^2 should not receive Primaxin IV unless hemodialysis is instituted within 48 hours.

For patients on hemodialysis, Primaxin IV is recommended only when the benefit outweighs the potential risk of seizures.

Close adherence to the recommended dosage and dosage schedules is urged, especially in patients with known factors that predispose to convulsive activity. Anticonvulsant therapy should be continued in patients with known seizure disorders. If focal tremors, myoclonus, or seizures occur, patients should be evaluated neurologically, placed on anticonvulsant therapy if not already instituted, and the dosage of Primaxin IV re- examined to determine whether it should be decreased or the antibiotic discontinued.

As with other antibiotics, prolonged use of Primaxin IV and IM may result in overgrowth of nonsusceptible organisms. Repeated evaluation of the patient's condition is essential. If superinfection occurs during therapy, appropriate measures should be taken.

IM: CNS adverse experiences such as myoclonic activity, confusional states, or seizures have been reported with Primaxin IV (Imipenem-Cilastatin Sodium for Injection). These experiences have occurred most commonly in patients with CNS disorders (*e.g.,* brain lesions or history of seizures) who also have comprised renal function. However, there were reports in which there was no recognized or documented underlying CNS disorder. These adverse CNS effects have not been seen with Primaxin IM; however, should they occur during treatment, Primaxin IM should be discontinued. Anticonvulsant therapy should be discontinued in patients with a known seizure disorder.

As with other antibiotics, prolonged use of Primaxin IM may result in overgrowth of nonsusceptible organisms. Repeated evaluation of the patient's condition is essential. If superinfection occurs during therapy, approximate measures should be taken.

Caution should be taken to avoid inadvertent injection into a blood vessel(see DOSAGE AND ADMINISTRATION.) For additional precautions, refer to the prescribing information for Lidocaine HCl.

PRECAUTIONS: *(cont'd)*

LABORATORY TESTS

While Primaxin IV possesses the characteristic low toxicity of the beta-lactam group of antibiotics, periodic assessment of organ system functions, including renal, hepatic, and hematopoietic, is advisable during prolonged therapy.

CARCINOGENESIS, MUTAGENESIS, AND IMPAIRMENT OF FERTILITY

Long term studies in animals have not been performed to evaluate carcinogenic potential of imipenem-cilastatin. Genetic toxicity studies were performed in a variety of bacterial and mammalian tests *in vivo* and *in vitro*. The tests used were: V79 mammalian cell mutagenesis assay (imipenem-cilastatin sodium alone and imipenem alone), Ames test (cilastatin sodium alone and imipenem alone), unscheduled DNA synthesis assay (imipenem-cilastatin sodium) and *in vivo* mouse cytogenetics test (imipenem-cilastatin sodium). None of these tests showed any evidence of genetic alterations.

Reproductive tests in male and female rats were performed with imipenem-cilastatin sodium at dosage levels up to 11 times the usual human dose of the intravenous formulation, IM at doses up to 11 times† the maximum daily recommended human dose (on a mg/kg basis). Slight decreases in live fetal body weight were restricted to the highest dosage level. No other adverse effects were observed on fertility, reproductive performance, fetal viability, growth or postnatal development of pups. Similarly, no adverse effects on the fetus or on lactation were observed when imipenem- cilastatin sodium was administered to rats late in gestation.

PREGNANCY, TERATOGENIC EFFECTS, PREGNANCY CATEGORY C

IV: Teratology studies with cilastatin sodium in rabbits and rats at 6 and 20 times† the maximum recommended human dose of the intravenous formulation of imipenem-cilastatin sodium (50 mg/kg/day†), respectively, showed no evidence of adverse effect on the fetus. No evidence of teratogenicity was observed in rabbits and rats given imipenem at doses up to 1 and 18 times† the maximum recommended daily human dose of the intravenous formulation of imipenem-cilastatin sodium, respectively.

Teratology studies with imipenem-cilastatin sodium at doses up to 11 times† the usual recommended dose of the intravenous formulation (30 mg/kg/day†) in pregnant mice and rats during the period of major organogenesis revealed no evidence of teratogenicity.

Imipenem-cilastatin sodium, when administered to pregnant rabbits at dosages equivalent to the usual human dose of the intravenous formulation and higher, caused body weight loss, diarrhea, and maternal deaths. When comparable doses of imipenem-cilastatin sodium were given to non-pregnant rabbits, body weight loss, diarrhea, and deaths were also observed. This intolerance is not unlike that seen with other beta-lactam antibiotics in this species and is probably due to alteration of gut flora.

A teratology study in pregnant cynomolgus monkeys given imipenem-cilastatin sodium at doses of 40 mg/kg/day (bolus intravenous injection) or 160 mg/kg/day (subcutaneous injection) resulted in maternal toxicity including emesis, inappetence, body weight loss, diarrhea, abortion and death in some cases. In contrast, no significant toxicity was observed when non-pregnant cynomolgus monkeys were given doses of imipenem-cilastatin sodium up to 180 mg/kg/day (subcutaneous injection). When doses of imipenem-cilastatin sodium (approximately 100 mg/kg/day or approximately 2 times† the maximum recommended daily human dose of the intravenous formulation) were administered to pregnant cynomolgus monkeys at an intravenous infusion rate which mimics human clinical use, there was minimal maternal intolerance (occasional emesis), no maternal deaths, no evidence of teratogenicity, but an increase in embryonic loss relative to control groups.

There are, however, no adequate and well-controlled studies in pregnant women. Primaxin IV should be used during pregnancy only if the potential benefit justifies the potential risk to the mother and fetus.

IM: Teratology studies with cilastatin sodium in rabbits and rats at 10 and 33 times† the maximum recommended daily human dose of the intramuscular formulation (30 mg/kg/day) of Primaxin, respectively, showed no evidence of adverse effects on the fetus. No evidence of teratogenicity was observed in rabbits and rats given imipenem at doses up to 2 and 30 times† the maximum recommended daily human dose of the intramuscular formulation of Primaxin, respectively.

Teratology studies with imipenem-cilastatin sodium at doses up to 11 times† the maximum recommended human dose in pregnant mice and rats during the period of major organogenesis revealed no evidence of teratogenicity.

Imipenem-cilastatin sodium, when administered to pregnant rabbits at dosages above the usual human dose of the intramuscular formulation (1000-1500 mg/day) caused body weight loss, diarrhea, and maternal deaths. When comparable doses of imipenem-cilastatin sodium were given to non-pregnant rabbits, body weight loss, diarrhea, and deaths were also observed. This intolerance is not unlike that seen with other beta-lactam antibiotics in this species and is probably due to alteration of gut flora.

A teratology study in pregnant cynomolgus monkeys given imipenem- cilastatin sodium at doses of 40 mg/kg/day (bolus intravenous injection) or 160 mg/kg/day (subcutaneous injection) resulted in maternal toxicity including emesis, inappetence, body weight loss, diarrhea, abortion and death in some cases. In contrast, no significant toxicity was observed when non-pregnant cynomolgus monkeys were given doses of imipenem- cilastatin sodium up to 180 mg/kg/day (subcutaneous injection). When doses of imipenem-cilastatin sodium (approximately 100 mg/kg/day or approximately 3 times† the maximum daily recommended human dose of the intramuscular formulation) were administered to pregnant cynomolgus monkeys at an intravenous infusion rate which mimics human clinical use, there was minimal maternal intolerance (occasional emesis), no maternal deaths, no evidence of teratogenicity, but an increase in embryonic loss relative to the control groups.

There are, however, no adequate and well-controlled studies in pregnant women. Primaxin IM should be used during pregnancy only if the potential benefit justifies the potential risk to the mother and fetus.

†Based on patient weight of 50 kg.

NURSING MOTHERS

It is not known whether imipenem-cilastatin sodium is excreted in human milk. Because many drugs are excreted in human milk, caution should be exercised when Primaxin IV or IM is administered to a nursing woman.

PEDIATRIC USE

Safety and effectiveness in infants and children below 12 years of age have not yet been established for Primaxin IV or IM.

DRUG INTERACTIONS:

Since concomitant administration of Primaxin and probenecid results in only minimal increases in plasma levels of imipenem and plasma half-life, it is not recommended that probenecid be given with Primaxin.

Primaxin should not be mixed with or physically added to other antibiotics. However, Primaxin may be administered concomitantly with other antibiotics, such as aminoglycosides.

IV

Generalized seizures have been reported in patients who received ganciclovir and Primaxin. These drugs should not be used concomitantly unless the potential benefits outweigh the risks.

ADVERSE REACTIONS:

Systemic Adverse Reactions: Adverse systemic clinical reactions reported as possibly, probably or definitely drug related occurring in less than 0.2% of the patients or reported since the drug was marketed are listed within each body system in order of decreasing severity: *Gastrointestinal:* pseudomembranous colitis (the onset of pseudomembranous colitis symptoms may occur during or after antibacterial treatment, see WARNINGS), hemorrhagic colitis, hepatitis, jaundice, gastroenteritis, abdominal pain, glossitis, tongue papillar hypertrophy, heartburn, pharyngeal pain, increased salivation;*Hematologic:* thrombocytopenia, neutropenia, leukopenia;*CNS:* encephalopathy, tremor, confusion, myoclonus, paresthesia, vertigo, headache, psychic disturbances; *Special Senses:* transient hearing loss in patients with impaired hearing, tinnitus, taste perversion; *Respiratory:* chest discomfort, dyspnea, hyperventilation, thoracic spine pain;*Cardiovascular:* palpitations, tachycardia; *Skin:* toxic epidermal necrolysis, erythema multiforme, angioneurotic edema, flushing, cyanosis, hyperhidrosis, skin texture changes, candidiasis, pruritus vulvae; *Body as a Whole:* polyarthralgia, asthenia/weakness;*Renal:* acute renal failure, oliguria/anuria, polyuria, urine discoloration. The role of Primaxin (Cilastatin/Imipenem) IV in changes in renal function is difficult to assess, since factors predisposing to pre-renal azotemia or to impaired renal function usually have been present.

IV ONLY

Primaxin IV is generally well tolerated. Many of the 1,723 patients treated in clinical trials were severely ill and had multiple background diseases and physiological impairments, making it difficult to determine causal relationship of adverse experiences to therapy with Primaxin IV.

Local Adverse Reactions: Adverse local clinical reactions that were reported as possibly, probably or definitely related to therapy with Primaxin IV were:

Phlebitis/thrombophlebitis: 3.1%

Pain at the injection site: 0.7%

Erythema at the injection site: 0.4%

Vein induration: 0.2%

Infused vein infection: 0.1%

Systemic Adverse Reactions: The most frequently reported systemic adverse clinical reactions that were reported as possibly, probably, or definitely related to Primaxin IV were nausea (2.0%) (see Granulocytopenic Patients), diarrhea (1.8%), vomiting (1.5%) (see Granulocytopenic Patients), rash (0.9%), fever (0.5%), hypotension (0.4%), seizures (0.4%) (see PRECAUTIONS), dizziness (0.3%), pruritus (0.3%), urticaria (0.2%), somnolence (0.2%).

Granulocytopenic Patients: Drug-related nausea and/or vomiting appear to occur more frequently in granulocytopenic patients than in non-granulocytopenic patients treated with Primaxin IV.

Adverse Laboratory Changes: Adverse laboratory changes without regard to drug relationship that were reported during clinical trials or reported since the drug was marketed were:

Hepatic: Increased ALT (SGPT), AST (SGOT), alkaline phosphatase, bilirubin and LDH.

Hemic: Increased eosinophils, positive Coombs test, increased WBC, increased platelets, decreased hemoglobin and hematocrit, increased monocytes, abnormal prothrombin time, increased lymphocytes, increased basophils.

Electrolytes: Decreased serum sodium, increased potassium, increased chloride.

Renal: Increased BUN, creatinine.

Urinalysis: Presence of urine protein, urine red blood cells, urine white blood cells, urine casts, urine bilirubin, and urine urobilinogen.

IM ONLY

In 686 patients in multiple dose clinical trials of Primaxin IM, the following adverse reactions were reported:

Local Adverse Reactions: The most frequent adverse local clinical reaction that was reported as possibly, probably or definitely related to therapy with Primaxin IM was pain at the injection site (1.2%)

Systemic Adverse Reactions: The most frequently reported systemic adverse clinical reactions that were reported as possibly, probably, or definitely related to therapy with the IM formula were nausea (0.6%), diarrhea (0.6%), vomiting (0.3%) and rash (0.4%).

Adverse Laboratory Changes: Adverse laboratory changes without regard to drug relationship that were reported during clinical trials were:

Hemic: decreased hemoglobin and hematocrit, eosinophil, increased and decreased WBC, increased and decreased platelets, decreased erythrocytes, and increased prothrombin time.

Hepatic: increased AST, ALT, alkaline phosphatase, and bilirubin.

Renal: increased BUN and creatine.

Urinalysis: presence of red blood cells, white blood cells, casts, and bacteria in the urine.

Potential Adverse Effects: In addition, a variety of adverse effects, not observed in clinical trials with Primaxin IM, have been reported with intravenous administration of Primaxin IV (Cilastatin Sodium-Imipenem for Injection). Those listed above are to serve as alerting information to physicians.

Adverse Laboratory Changes: Adverse laboratory changes without regard to drug relationship that were reported during clinical trials or reported since the drug was marketed were: *Hepatic:* increased LDH; *Hemic:* positive Coombs test, decreased neutrophils, agranulocytosis, increased monocytes, abnormal prothrombin time, increased lymphocytes, increased basophils;*Electrolytes:* decreased serum sodium, increased potassium, increased chloride; *Urinalysis:* presence of urine protein, urine bilirubin, and urine urobilinogen.

Lidocaine HCl: Refer to the prescribing information for Lidocaine HCl.

OVERDOSAGE:

The acute intravenous toxicity of imipenem-cilastatin sodium in a ratio of 1:1 was studied in mice at doses of 751 to 1359 mg/mg. Following drug administration, ataxia was rapidly produced and clonic convulsions were noted in about 45 minutes. Deaths occurred within 4-56 minutes at all doses.

The acute intravenous toxicity of imipenem-cilastatin sodium was produced within 5-10 minutes in rats at doses of 771 to 1583 mg/kg. In all dosage groups, females had decreased activity, bradypnea and ptosis with clonic convulsions preceding death; in males, ptosis was seen at all dose levels while tremors and clonic convulsions were seen at all but the lowest dose (771 mg/kg). In another rat study, female rats showed ataxia, bradypnea and decreased activity in all but the lowest dose (550 mg/kg); deaths were preceded by clonic convulsions. Male rats showed tremors at all doses and clonic convulsions and ptosis were seen at the two highest doses (1130 and 1734 mg/kg). Deaths occurred between 6 and 88 minutes within doses of 771 to 1734 mg/kg.

In the case of overdosage, discontinue Primaxin IV, treat symptomatically, and institute supportive measures as required. Imipenem-cilastatin sodium is hemodialyzable. However, usefulness of this procedure in the overdosage setting is questionable.

DOSAGE AND ADMINISTRATION:

IV

The dosage recommendations for Primaxin IV represent the quantity of imipenem to be administered. An equivalent amount of cilastatin is also present in the solution. Each 125 mg, 250 mg or 500 mg dose should be given by intravenous administration over 20 to 30 minutes. Each 750 mg or 1000 mg dose should be infused over 40 to 60 minutes. In patients who develop nausea during the infusion, the rate of infusion may be slowed.

The total daily dosage for Primaxin IV should be based on the type or severity of infection and given in equally divided doses based on consideration of degree of susceptibility of the pathogen(s), renal function and body weight. Patients with impaired renal function, as judged by creatinine clearance ≤ 70 ml/min/1.73 m^2, require adjustment of dosage as described in the succeeding section of these guidelines.

Intravenous Dosage Schedule for Adults with Normal Renal Function and Body Weight ≥ 70 kg: Doses cited in TABLE 9 are based on a patient with normal renal function and a body weight of 70 kg. These doses should be used for a patient with a creatinine clearance of ≥ 71 ml/min/1.73 m^2 and a body weight of ≥ 70 kg. A reduction in dose must be made for a patient with a creatinine clearance ≤ 70 ml/min/1.73 m^2 and/or a body weight less than 70 kg. (See TABLE 11 and TABLE 12).

Dosage regimens in column A in TABLE 9 for Adults with Normal Renal Function are recommended for infections caused by fully susceptible organisms which represent the majority of pathogenic species. Dosage regimens in column B of TABLE 9 are recommended for infections caused by organisms with moderate susceptibility to imipenem, primarily some strains of *P. aeruginosa.*

TABLE 9 Intravenous Dosage Schedule For Adults With Normal Renal Function And Body Weight ≥ 70 kg

A Fully susceptible organisms including gram-positive and gram-negative aerobes and anaerobes	B Moderately susceptible organisms, primarily some strains of *P. aeruginosa*
Mild	
250 mg q6h (TOTAL DAILY DOSE = 1.0g)	500 mg q6h (TOTAL DAILY DOSE = 2.0g)
Moderate	
500 mg q8h (TOTAL DAILY DOSE = 1.5g) or 500 mg q6h (TOTAL DAILY DOSE = 2.0g)	500 mg q6h (TOTAL DAILY DOSE = 2.0g) or 1 g q8h (TOTAL DAILY DOSE = 3.0g)
Severe, life threatening only	
500 mg q6h (TOTAL DAILY DOSE = 2.0g)	1 g q8h (TOTAL DAILY DOSE = 3.0g) or 1 g q6h (TOTAL DAILY DOSE = 4.0g)
Uncomplicated urinary tract infection	
250 mg q6h	250 mg q6h
Complicated urinary tract infection	
(TOTAL DAILY DOSE = 1.0g) 500 mg q6h (TOTAL DAILY DOSE = 2.0g)	(TOTAL DAILY DOSE = 1.0g) 500 mg q6h (TOTAL DAILY DOSE = 2.0g)

Due to the high antimicrobial activity of Primaxin IV, it is recommended that the maximum total daily dosage not exceed 50 mg/kg/day or 4.0 g/day, whichever is lower. There is no evidence that higher doses provide greater efficacy. However, patients over twelve years of age with cystic fibrosis and normal renal function have been treated with Primaxin IV at doses up to 90 mg/kg/day in divided doses, not exceeding 4.0 g/day.

Reduced Intravenous Dosage Schedule for Adults with Impaired Renal Function and/or Body Weight < 70 kg: Patients with creatinine clearance of ≤70 ml/min/1.73 m^2 require adjustment of the dosage of Primaxin IV as indicated in TABLE 10. Creatinine clearance may be calculated from serum creatinine concentration by the equation found in TABLE 10.

TABLE 10

Tcc (Males) = [(wt. in kg) (140 - age)] ÷ [(72) (creatinine in mg/dl)]
Tcc(Females) = 0.85 × above value

To determine the dose for adults with impaired renal function and/or reduced body weight:

1. Choose a total daily dose from TABLE 9 based on infection characteristics.

2. a) If the total daily dose is 1.0 g, 1.5 g or 2.0 g, use the appropriate subsection of TABLE 11 and continue with step 3.

b) If the total daily dose is 3.0 g or 4.0 g, use the appropriate subsection of TABLE 12 and continue with step 3.

3. From TABLE 11 or TABLE 12 :

a) Select the body weight on the far left which is closest to the patient's body weight (kg).

b) Select the patient's creatinine clearance category.

c) Where the row and column intersect is the reduced dosage regimen.

TABLE 11A Reduced Intravenous Dosage Of Primaxin IV In Adult Patients With Impaired Renal Function And/Or Body Weight < 70 kg

If Total Daily Dose from TABLE 9 is: 1.0 g/day and Body Weight (kg) is:	and creatinine clearance (ml/min/1.73m^2) is: ≥ 71	41-70	21-40	6-20
	then the reduced dosage regimen (mg) is:			
≥ 70	250 q6h	250 q8h	250 q12h	250 q12h
60	250 q8h	125 q6h	250 q12h	125 q12h
50	125 q6h	125 q6h	125 q8h	125 q12h
40	125 q6h	125 q8h	125 q12h	125 q12h
30	125 q8h	125 q8h	125 q12h	125 q12h

Patients with creatinine clearances of 6 to 20 ml/min/1.73 m^2 should be treated with Primaxin IV 125 mg or 250 mg every 12 hours for most pathogens. There may be an increased risk of seizures when doses of 500 mg every 12 hours are administered to these patients.

Patients with creatinine clearance ≤ 5 ml/min/1.73 m^2 should not receive Primaxin IV unless hemodialysis is instituted within 48 hours. There is inadequate information to recommended usage of Primaxin IV for patients undergoing peritoneal dialysis.

DOSAGE AND ADMINISTRATION: *(cont'd)*

TABLE 11B Reduced Intravenous Dosage Of Primaxin IV In Adult Patients With Impaired Renal Function And/Or Body Weight < 70 kg

If total daily dose from TABLE 9 is: 1.5 g/day and Body Weight (kg) is: and creatinine clearance (ml/min/1.73m²) is:

	≥ 71	41-70	21-40	6-20
	then the reduced dosage regimen (mg) is:			
≥ 70	500 q8h	250 q6h	250 q8h	250 q12h
60	250 q6h	250 q8h	250 q8h	250 q12h
50	250 q6h	250 q8h	250 q12h	250 q12h
40	250 q8h	125 q6h	125 q8h	125 q12h
30	125 q6h	125 q8h	125 q8h	125 q12h

TABLE 11C Reduced Intravenous Dosage Of Primaxin IV In Adult Patients With Impaired Renal Function And/Or Body Weight < 70 kg

If total daily dose from TABLE 9 is: 2.0 g/day and Body Weight (kg) is: and creatinine clearance (ml/min/1.73m²) is:

	≥ 71	41-70	21-40	6-20
	then the reduced dosage regimen (mg) is:			
≥ 70	500 q6h	500 q8h	250 q6h	250 q12h
60	500 q8h	250 q6h	250 q8h	250 q12h
50	250 q6h	250 q6h	250 q8h	250 q12h
40	250 q6h	250 q8h	250 q12h	250 q12h
30	250 q8h	125 q6h	125 q8h	125 q12h

TABLE 12A Reduced Intravenous Dosage Of Primaxin IV In Adult Patients With Impaired Renal Function And/Or Body Weight < 70 kg

If total daily dose from TABLE 9 is: 3.0 g/day and Body Weight (kg) is: and creatinine clearance (ml/min/1.73m²) is:

	≥ 71	41-70	21-40	6-20
	then the reduced dosage regimen (mg) is:			
≥ 70	1000 q8h	500 q6h	500 q8h	500 q12h
60	750 q8h	500 q8h	500 q8h	500 q12h
50	500 q6h	500 q6h	250 q6h	250 q12h
40	500 q8h	250 q6h	250 q8h	250 q12h
30	250 q6h	250 q8h	250 q8h	250 q12h

TABLE 12B Reduced Intravenous Dosage Of Primaxin IV In Adult Patients With Impaired Renal Function And/Or Body Weight < 70 kg

If total daily dose from TABLE 9 is: 4.0 g/day and Body Weight (kg) is: and creatinine clearance (ml/min/1.73m²) is:

	≥ 71	41 - 70	21 - 40	6 - 20
	then the reduced dosage regimen (mg) is:			
≥ 70	1000 q6h	750 q8h	500 q6h	500 q12h
60	1000 q8h	750 q8h	500 q8h	500 q12h
50	750 q8h	500 q6h	500 q8h	500 q12h
250	40 q6h	500 q8h	500 q6h	250 q12h
30	500 q8h	250 q6h	250 q8h	250 q12h

Hemodialysis: When treating patients with creatinine clearances of ≤ 5 ml/min/1.73 m² who are undergoing hemodialysis,use the dosage recommendations for patients with creatinine clearances of 6 - 20 ml/min/1.73 m². (See TABLE 11.) Both imipenem and cilastatin are cleared form the circulation during hemodialysis. The patient should receive Primaxin IV after hemodialysis and at 12 hour intervals timed from the end of that hemodialysis session. Dialysis patients, especially those with background CNS disease, should be carefully monitored; for patients on hemodialysis, Primaxin IV is recommended only when the benefit outweighs the potential risk of seizures. (See PRECAUTIONS.)

Preparation of Solution

Infusion Bottles: Contents of the infusion bottles of Primaxin IV Powder should be restored with 100 ml of diluent see list of diluents under DOSAGE AND ADMINISTRATION, Compatibility and Stability and shaken until a clear solution is obtained.

Vials: Contents of the vials must be suspended and transferred to 100 ml of an appropriate infusion solution.

A suggested procedure is to add approximately 10 ml from the appropriate infusion solution (see list of diluents under DOSAGE AND ADMINISTRATION, Compatibility and Stability) to the vial. Shake well and transfer the resulting suspension to the infusion solution container.

CAUTION: THE SUSPENSION IS NOT FOR DIRECT INFUSION.

Repeat with an additional 10 ml of infusion solution to ensure complete transfer of vial contents to the infusion solution. **The resulting mixture should be agitated until clear.**

ADD-Vantage Vials: See separate INSTRUCTIONS FOR USE OF PRIMAXIN IV IN ADD-Vantage VIALS, Primaxin IV in ADD-Vantage vials should be reconstituted with ADD-Vantage diluent containers containing 100 ml of either 0.9% Sodium Chloride Injection or 100 ml 5% Dextrose Injection.

DOSAGE AND ADMINISTRATION: *(cont'd)*

Compatibility and Stability:

Before reconstitution: The dry powder should be stored at a temperature below 30°C.

Reconstituted solutions: Solutions of Primaxin IV range from colorless to yellow. Variations of color within this range do not affect the potency of the product.

Primaxin IV, as supplied in infusion bottles and vials and reconstituted as above with the following diluents, maintains satisfactory potency for four hours at room temperature or for 24 hours under refrigeration (5°C) (note exception below). Solutions of Primaxin IV should not be frozen.

0.9% Sodium Chloride Injection††
5% or 10% Dextrose Injection
5% Dextrose Injection with 0.02% sodium bicarbonate solution
5% Dextrose and 0.9% Sodium Chloride Injection
5% Dextrose Injection with 0.225% or 0.45% saline solution
Normosol - M in D5-W**
5% Dextrose Injection with 0.15% potassium chloride solution
Mannitol 2.5%, 5% and 10%

Primaxin IV is supplied in single dose ADD-Vantage vials and should be prepared as directed in the accompanying INSTRUCTIONS FOR USE OF Primaxin IV IN ADD-Vantage VIALS using ADD-Vantage diluent containers containing 100 ml of either 0.9% Sodium Chloride Injection or 5% Dextrose Injection. When prepared with either of these diluents, Primaxin IV maintains satisfactory potency for 8 hours at room temperature.

Primaxin IV should not be mixed with or physically added to other antibiotics. However, Primaxin IV may be administered concomitantly with other antibiotics, such as aminoglycosides.

††Primaxin IV has been found to be stable in 0.9% Sodium Chloride Injections for 10 hours at room temperature or 48 hours under refrigeration.

**Primaxin IV has been found to be stable in Normosol-M in D5-W for 2 hours at room temperature or 9 hours under refrigeration.

IM

Primaxin IM is for intramuscular use only.

The dosage recommendations for Primaxin IM represents the quantity of imipenem to be administered. An equivalent amount of cilastatin is also present.

Patients with lower respiratory tract infections, skin and skin structure infections, and gynecologic infections of mild to moderate severity may be treated with 500 mg or 750 mg administered every 12 hours depending on the severity of the infection.

Intra-abdominal infection may be treated with 750 mg every 12 hours (see TABLE 13.)

TABLE 13 Dosage Guidlines

Type*/Location of Infection	Severity	Dosage Regimen
Lower respiratory tract	Mild/	500 to 750 mg q depending on the severity of infection
Skin and Skin structure Gynecologic	Moderate	
Intra-abdominal	Mild/Moderate	750 mg q12h

* See INDICATIONS AND USAGE

Total daily IM dosages greater than 1500 mg per day are not recommended.

The dosage for any particular patient should be based on the location of and severity of the infection, the susceptibility of the infecting pathogen(s), and renal function.

The duration of therapy depends upon the type and severity of the infection. Generally, Primaxin IM should be continued for at least two days after the signs and symptoms of infection have resolved. Safety and efficacy of treatment beyond fourteen days have not been established.

Primaxin IM should be administered by deep intramuscular injection into a large muscle mass (such as the gluteal muscles or lateral part of the thigh) with a 21 gauge 2" needle. Aspiration is necessary to avoid inadvertent injection into a blood vessel.

Adults With Impaired Renal Function: The safety and efficacy of Primaxin IM has not been studied in patients with creatine clearance of less than 20 ml/min/1.73 m². Serum creatinine alone may not be a sufficiently accurate measure of renal function. Creatinine clearance (T_{cc}) may be estimated from the equation found in TABLE 14.

TABLE 14

$$T_{cc}(\text{Males}) = [(\text{wt. in kg})\ (140\text{-age})] \div [(72)\ (\text{creatinine in mg/dl})]$$
$$T_{cc}(\text{Females}) = 0.85 \times \text{above value}$$

PREPARATION FOR ADMINISTRATION

Primaxin IM should be prepared for use with 1.0% lidocaine HCl solution† (without epinephrine). Primaxin IM 500 should be prepared with 2 ml and Primaxin IM 750 with 3 ml of lidocaine HCl. Agitate to form a suspension then withdraw the entire contents of vial intramuscularly. The suspension of Primaxin IM in lidocaine HCl should be used within one hour of preparation. **Note: The IM formulation is not for IV use.**

COMPATIBILITY AND STABILITY

Before reconstitution: The dry powder should be stored at a temperature below 30°C (86°F).

Suspensions for IM Administration: Suspensions of Primaxin IM are white to light tan in color. Variations of color within this range do not affect the potency of the product.

The suspension of Primaxin IM in lidocaine HCl should be used within one hour after preparation.

Primaxin IM should not be mixed with or physically added to other antibiotics. However, Primaxin IM may be administered concomitantly but at separate sites with other antibiotics, such as aminoglycosides.

†Refer to the monograph for lidocaine HCl for detailed information concerning CONTRAINDICATIONS, WARNINGS, PRECAUTIONS, and ADVERSE REACTIONS.

HOW SUPPLIED:

IV: Primaxin IV is supplied as a sterile powder mixture in vials and infusion bottles containing imipenem (anhydrous equivalent) and cilastatin sodium as follows: No. 3514 — 250 mg imipenem equivalent and 250 mg cilastatin equivalent and 10 mg sodium bicarbonate as a buffer. No. 3516 — 500 mg imipenem equivalent and 500 mg cilastatin equivalent and 20 mg sodium bicarbonate as a buffer. No. 3515 — 250 mg imipenem equivalent and 250 mg cilastatin equivalent and 10 mg sodium bicarbonate as a buffer. No. 3517 — 500 mg imipenem equivalent and 500 mg cilastatin equivalent and 20 mg sodium bicarbonate as a buffer. No. 3551 — 250 mg imipenem equivalent and 250 mg cilastatin equivalent and 10 mg sodium bicarbonate as a buffer. No. 3552 — 500 mg imipenem equivalent and 500 mg cilastatin equivalent and 20 mg sodium bicarbonate as a buffer.

HOW SUPPLIED: *(cont'd)*

IM: Primaxin IM is supplied as a sterile powder mixture in vials for IM administration as follows: No. 3582 — 500 mg imipenem equivalent and 500 mg cilastatin equivalent No. 3583 — 750 mg imipenem equivalent and 750 mg cilastatin equivalent

(IV: Merck, 1/94, 7882120); (IM: Merck, 5/92, 7632904)

HOW SUPPLIED - EQUIVALENTS NOT AVAILABLE:

Injection, Dry-Soln - Intravenous - 250 mg/250 mg

10 ml x 25	$332.39	PRIMAXIN, Merck	00006-3514-58
10's	$111.50	PRIMAXIN, ADD-VANTAGE, Merck	00006-3551-74
25's	$345.13	PRIMAXIN, ADD-VANTAGE, Merck	00006-3551-58
100 ml x 10	$146.20	PRIMAXIN, Merck	00006-3515-74

Injection, Dry-Soln - Intravenous - 500 mg/500 mg

10 ml x 25	$625.58	PRIMAXIN, Merck	00006-3516-59
10's	$206.00	PRIMAXIN, ADD-VANTAGE, Merck	00006-3552-75
25's	$637.89	PRIMAXIN, ADD-VANTAGE, Merck	00006-3552-59
100 ml x 10	$263.53	PRIMAXIN, Merck	00006-3517-75

Injection, Dry-Susp - Intramuscular - 500 mg/500 mg

10's	$250.25	PRIMAXIN IM, Merck	00006-3582-75

Injection, Dry-Susp - Intramuscular - 750 mg/750 mg

10's	$375.39	PRIMAXIN IM, Merck	00006-3583-76

CILAZAPRIL *(003075)*

CATEGORIES: ACE Inhibitors; Angiotensin Converting Enzyme Inhibitors; Antihypertensives; Cardiovascular Drugs; Hypertension; FDA Unapproved

BRAND NAMES: *Dynorm* (Germany); **Inhibace**; *Vascace* (England)
(International brand names outside U.S. in italics)

Prescribing information not available at time of publication.

CIMETIDINE *(000820)*

CATEGORIES: Acid/Peptic Disorders; Adenoma; Antacids; Antiulcer Drugs; Duodenal Ulcer; Endocrine Adenomas; Esophagitis; Gastric Ulcer; Gastroesophagael Reflux Disease; Gastrointestinal Drugs; GERD; Histamine H2 Receptor Antagonists; Hypersecretory Conditions; Mastocytosis; Ulcer; Zollinger-Ellison Syndrome; Warts*; Pregnancy Category B; Sales > $1 Billion; FDA Approval Pre 1982; Patent Expiration 1994 Apr; Top 200 Drugs
* Indication not approved by the FDA

BRAND NAMES: *Acibilin*; *Acidown*; *Aciloc*; *Aci-Med*; *Acinil*; *Altramet*; *Antil*; *Apo-Cimetidine* (Canada); *Asaurex* (Mexico); *Azucimet* (Germany); *Beamat*; *Biomag*; *Brumetidina*; *Campanex*; *Cemedin 200*; *Cemedin 400*; *Cemedin 800*; *Cidine*; *Cigamet*; *Cignatin*; *Cimal*; *Cimebec*; *Cimbene*; *Cimedine*; *Cimehexal* (Germany); *Cimeldine*; *Cimet*; *Cimetag*; *Cimetalgin*; *Cimetase* (Mexico); *Cimetegal*; *Cimetid*; *Cimetidin* (Germany); *Cimetidina*; *Cimetidine*; Cimetidine In Sodium Chloride; *Cimetigal* (Mexico); *Cimetiget*; *Cimetil*; *Cimetin*; *Cimetum*; *Cimewell*; *Cimewet*; *Cimex*; *Cimulcer*; *Cinadine*; *Cinulcus*; *Cismetin*; *Citidine*; *Citius*; *Ciuk* (Germany); *Ciwidine*; *Convenal*; *Corsamet*; *Cymi*; *Cytine*; *Defense*; *Dispamet*; *Duomet*; *Dyspamet* (England); *Edalene*; *Eureceptor*; *Fanimet*; *Fremet*; *Gastidine*; *Gastrobitan*; *Gastrodin*; *Gawei*; *Gerucim*; *H-2*; *Haldin*; *Hexamet*; *Himetin*; *Histodil*; *Inesfay* (Mexico); *Lenamet*; *Lock 2*; *Magicul* (Australia); *Med-Gastramet*; *Montidin*; *Neutronorm*; *Novocimetine* (Canada); *Nulcer*; *Pallia*; *Paoweian*; *Peptol* (Canada); *Piovalen*; *Powegon*; *Procimeti*; *Proctospre*; *Sanmetidin*; *Secapine*; *Shintamet*; *Siamidine*; *Silmet*; *Simalgen*; *Stogamet*; *Stomakon*; *Stomedine* (France); *Stomet*; *Tagagel*; *Tagamed*; **Tagamet**; *Tagamin*; *Tametin*; *Timet*; *Tobymet*; *Tratol*; *Ulcedin*; *Ulcedine*; *Ulcemet*; *Ulcerfen*; *Ulcimet*; *Ulcinfan*; *Ulcodina*; *Ulcomedina*; *Ulcolind H2* (Germany); *Ulcumet*; *Ulpax*; *Ulsikur*; *Valmagen*; *Weisdin*; *Wergen*; *Xepamet*; *Zymerol* (Mexico)
(International brand names outside U.S. in italics)

FORMULARIES: Aetna; BC-BS; CIGNA; FHP; Foundation; Humana; Kaiser; Medco; Medi-Cal; PCS; PruCare; United; WHO

COST OF THERAPY: $16.78 (Duodenal Ulcer; Tablet; 800 mg; 1/day; 28 days)

DESCRIPTION:

Cimetidine is a histamine H_2-receptor antagonist. Chemically it is *N"* cyano-*N*-methyl-*N'*- [2-[((5-methyl-1*H*-imidazol-4-yl)methyl]thio]-ethyl]- guanidine.

The empirical formula for cimetidine is $C_{10}H_{16}N_8S$ and for cimetidine hydrochloride, $C_{10}H_{16}N_6SHCl$; these represent molecular weights of 252.34 and 288.80, respectively.

Cimetidine contains an imidazole ring, and is chemically related to histamine.

(The liquid and injection dosage forms contain cimetidine as the hydrochloride.)

Single-Dose Vials for Intramuscular or Intravenous Administration:

Cimetidine has a bitter taste and characteristic odor.

Solubility Characteristics: Cimetidine is soluble in alcohol, slightly soluble in water, very slightly soluble in chloroform and insoluble in ether. Cimetidine hydrochloride is freely soluble in water, soluble in alcohol, very slightly soluble in chloroform and practically insoluble in ether.

Tablets for Oral Administration: Each light green, film-coated tablet contains cimetidine as follows: 200 mg-round, imprinted with the product name Tagamet, SKF and 200; 300 mg-round, debossed with the product name Tagamet, SB and 300; 400 mg-oval Tiltab tablets, debossed with the product name Tagamet, SB and 400; 800 mg-oval Tiltab tablets, debossed with the product name Tagamet, SB and 800. Inactive ingredients consist of cellulose, D&C Yellow No. 10, FD&C Blue No. 2, FD&C Red No. 40, FD&C Yellow No. 6, hydroxypropyl methylcellulose, iron oxides, magnesium stearate, povidone, propylene glycol, sodium lauryl sulfate, sodium starch glycolate, starch, titanium dioxide and trace amounts of other inactive ingredients.

Liquid for Oral Administration: Each 5 ml (one teaspoonful) of clear, light orange, mint-peach flavored liquid contains cimetidine hydrochloride equivalent to cimetidine, 300 mg; alcohol, 2.8%. Inactive ingredients consist of FD&C Yellow No. 6, flavors, methylparaben, polyoxyethylene polyoxypropylene glycol, propylene glycol, propylparaben, saccharin sodium, sodium chloride, sodium phosphate, sorbitol and water.

INJECTION

Single-Dose Vials for Intramuscular or Intravenous Administration: Each 2 ml contains, in sterile aqueous solution (pH range 3.8 to 6), cimetidine hydrochloride equivalent to cimetidine, 300 mg; phenol, 10 mg.

DESCRIPTION: *(cont'd)*

Multi-Dose Vials for Intramuscular or Intravenous Administration: 8 ml (300 mg/2 ml): Each 2 ml contains, in sterile aqueous solution (pH range 3.8 to 6), cimetidine hydrochloride equivalent to cimetidine, 300 mg; phenol, 10 mg.

Single-Dose Premixed Plastic Containers for Intravenous Administration: Each 50 ml of sterile aqueous solution (pH range 5 to7) contains cimetidine hydrochloride equivalent to 300 mg cimetidine and 0.45 grams sodium chloride.

No preservative has been added.

The plastic container is fabricated from specially formulated polyvinyl chloride. The amount of water that can permeate from inside the container into the overwrap is insufficient to affect the solution significantly. Solutions in contact with the plastic container can leach out certain of its chemical components in very small amounts within the expiration period, e.g., di 2-ethylhexyl phthalate (DEHP), up to 5 parts per million. However, the safety of the plastic has been confirmed in tests in animals according to the USP biological tests for plastic containers as well as by tissue culture toxicity studies.

ADD-Vantage* Vials for Intravenous Administration: Each 2 ml contains, in sterile aqueous solution (pH range 3.8 to 6), cimetidine hydrochloride equivalent to cimetidine, 300 mg; phenol, 10 mg.

All of the above injection formulations are pyrogen free, and sodium hydroxide N.F. is used as an ingredient to adjust the pH.

CLINICAL PHARMACOLOGY:

Cimetidine competitively inhibits the action of histamine at the histamine H_2 receptors of the parietal cells and thus is a histamine H_2-receptor antagonist.

Cimetidine is not an anticholinergic agent. Studies have shown that cimetidine inhibits both daytime and nocturnal basal gastric acid secretion. Cimetidine also inhibits gastric acid secretion stimulated by food, histamine, pentagastrin, caffeine and insulin.

ANTISECRETORY ACTIVITY

1) Acid Secretion: Nocturnal: Cimetidine 800 mg orally at bedtime reduces mean hourly H^+ activity by greater than 85% over an 8-hour period in duodenal ulcer patients, with no effect on daytime acid secretion. Cimetidine 1600 mg orally h.s. produces 100% inhibition of mean hourly H^+ activity over an 8-hour period in duodenal ulcer patients, but also reduces H^+ activity by 35% for an additional 5 hours into the following morning. Cimetidine 400 mg twice daily and 300 mg four times daily decrease nocturnal acid secretion in a dose-related manner, *i.e.,* 47% to 83% over a 6- to 8- hour period and 54% over a 9-hour period, respectively.

Food Stimulated: During the first hour after a standard experimental meal, oral cimetidine 300 mg inhibited gastric acid secretion in duodenal ulcer patients by at least 50%. During the subsequent 2 hours cimetidine inhibited gastric acid secretion by at least 75%.

The effect of a 300 mg breakfast dose of cimetidine continued for at least 4 hours and there was partial suppression of the rise in gastric acid secretion following the luncheon meal in duodenal ulcer patients. This suppression of gastric acid output was enhanced and could be maintained by another 300 mg dose of cimetidine given with lunch.

In another study, cimetidine 300 mg given with the meal increased gastric pH as compared with placebo.

TABLE 1

	Mean Gastric pH	
	Cimetidine	Placebo
1 hour	3.5	2.6
2 hours	3.1	1.6
3 hours	3.8	1.9
4 hours	6.1	2.2

24-Hour Mean H^+ Activity: Cimetidine 800 mg h.s., 400 mg twice dialy and 300 mg four times daily all provide a similar, moderate (less than 60%) level of 24 hour acid suppression. However, the 800 mg h.s. regimen exerts its entire effect on nocturnal acid, and does not affect daytime gastric physiology.

Chemically Stimulated: Oral cimetidine significantly inhibited gastric acid secretion stimulated by betazole (an isomer of histamine), pentagastrin, caffeine and insulin as shown in TABLE 2.

TABLE 2

Stimulant	Stimulant Dose	Tagamet	% Inhibition
Betazole	1.5mg/kg (sc)	300mg (po)	85% at 2.5 hours
Pentagastrin	6mcg/kg/hr (iv)	100mg/hr (iv)	60% at 1 hour
Caffeine	5mg/kg/hr (iv)	300mg (po)	100% at 1 hour
Insulin	0.03 units/kg/hr (iv)	100mg/hr (iv)	82% at 1 hour

When food and betazole were used to stimulate secretion, inhibition of hydrogen ion concentration usually ranged from 45% to 75% and the inhibition of volume ranged from 30% to 65%.

Parenteral administration also significantly inhibits gastric acid secretion. In a crossover study involving patients with active or healed duodenal or gastric ulcers, either continuous IV infusion of cimetidine 37.5 mg/hour (900 mg/day) or intermittent injection of cimetidine 300 mg every 6 hours (1200 mg/day) maintained gastric pH 4.0 for more than 50% of the time under steady-state conditions.

2) Pepsin: Oral cimetidine 300 mg reduced total pepsin output as a result of the decrease in volume of gastric juice.

3) Intrinsic Factor: Intrinsic factor secretion was studied with betazole as a stimulant. Oral cimetidine 300 mg inhibited the rise in intrinsic factor concentration produced by betazole, but some intrinsic factor was secreted at all times.

Other Lower Esophageal Sphincter Pressure and Gastric Emptying: Cimetidine has no effect on lower esophageal sphincter (LES) pressure or the rate of gastric emptying.

Pharmacokinetics: Cimetidine is rapidly absorbed after oral administration and peak levels occur in 45 to 90 minutes. The half-life of cimetidine is approximately 2 hours. Both oral and parenteral (IV or IM) administration provide comparable periods of therapeutically effective blood levels; blood concentrations remain above that required to provide 80% inhibition of basal gastric acid secretion for 4 to 5 hours following a dose of 300 mg.

Steady-state blood concentrations of cimetidine with continuous infusion of cimetidine are determined by the infusion rate and clearance of the drug in the individual patient. In a study of peptic ulcer patients with normal renal function, an infusion rate of 37.5 mg/hour produced average steady-state plasma cimetidine concentrations of about 0.9 mcg/ml. Blood levels with other infusion rates will vary in direct proportion to the infusion rate.

The principal route of excretion of cimetidine is the urine. Following parenteral administration, most of the drug is excreted as the parent compound; following oral administration, the drug is more extensively metabolized, the sulfoxide being the major metabolite. Following a

CLINICAL PHARMACOLOGY: *(cont'd)*

single oral dose, 48% of the drug is recovered from the urine after 24 hours as the parent compound. Following IV or IM administration, approximately 75% of the drug is recovered from the urine after 24 hours as the parent compound.

CLINICAL STUDIES:

ULCERS

Duodenal Ulcer: Cimetidine has been shown to be effective in the treatment of active duodenal ulcer and, at reduced dosage, in maintenance therapy following healing of active ulcers.

Active Duodenal Ulcer: Cimetidine accelerates the rate of duodenal ulcer healing. Healing rates reported in U.S. and foreign controlled trials with cimetidine are summarized below (TABLE 3), beginning with the regimen providing the lowest nocturnal dose.

TABLE 3 Duodenal Ulcer Healing Rates with Various Cimetidine Dosage Regimens*

Regimen	300 mg q.i.d.	400 mg b.i.d	800 mg h.s.	1600 mg h.s.
week 4	68%	73%	80%	86%
week 6	80%	80%	89%	-
week 8	-	92%	94%	-

* Averages from controlled clinical trials.

A U.S., double-blind, placebo-controlled, dose-ranging study demonstrated that all once-daily at bedtime (h.s.) cimetidine regimens were superior to placebo in ulcer healing and that cimetidine 800 mg h.s. healed 75% of patients at 4 weeks. The healing rate with 800 mg h.s. was significantly superior to 400 mg h.s. (66%) and not significantly different from 1600 mg h.s. (81%).

In the U.S. dose-ranging trial, over 80% of patients receiving cimetidine 800 mg h.s. experienced nocturnal pain relief after one day. Relief from daytime pain was reported in approximately 70% of patients after two days. As with ulcer healing, the 800 mg h.s. dose was superior to 400 mg h.s. and not different from 1600 mg h.s.

In foreign, double-blind studies with cimetidine 800 mg h.s., 79 to 85% of patients were healed at 4 weeks.

While short-term treatment with cimetidine can result in complete healing of the duodenal ulcer, acute therapy will not prevent ulcer recurrence after cimetidine has been discontinued. Some follow-up studies have reported that the rate of recurrence once therapy was discontinued was slightly higher for patients healed on cimetidine than for patients healed on other forms of therapy; however, the cimetidine-treated patients generally had more severe disease.

Maintenance Therapy in Duodenal Ulcer: Treatment with a reduced dose of cimetidine has been proven effective as maintenance therapy following healing of active duodenal ulcers.

In numerous placebo-controlled studies conducted worldwide, the percent of patients with observed ulcers at the end of one year's therapy with cimetidine 400 mg h.s. was significantly lower (10%-45%) than in patients receiving placebo (44%-70%). Thus, from 55% to 90% of patients were maintained free of observed ulcers at the end of one year with cimetidine 400 mg h.s.

Factors such as smoking, duration and severity of disease, gender, and genetic traits may contribute to variations in actual percentages.

Trials of other anti-ulcer therapy, whether placebo-controlled, positive-controlled or open, have demonstrated a range of results similar to that seen with cimetidine.

Active Benign Gastric Ulcer: Cimetidine has been shown to be effective in the short-term treatment of active benign gastric ulcer.

In a multicenter, double-blind U.S. study, patients with endoscopically confirmed benign gastric ulcer were treated with cimetidine 300 mg four times a day or with placebo for 6 weeks. Patients were limited to those with ulcers ranging from 0.5 to 2.5 cm in size. Endoscopically confirmed healing at six weeks was seen in significantly* more cimetidine-treated patients than in patients receiving placebo, as shown in TABLE 4.

TABLE 4

	Cimetidine	Placebo
week 2	14/63 (22%)	7/63 (11%)
total at week 6	43/65 (66%)*	30/67 (45%)

* $p<0.05$

In a similar multicenter U.S. study of the 800 mg h.s. oral regimen, the endoscopically confirmed healing rates can be seen in TABLE 5.

TABLE 5

	Cimetidine	Placebo
Total at week 6	63/83 (76%)*	44/80 (55%)

* $p=0.005$

Similarly, in worldwide double-blind clinical studies, endoscopically evaluated benign gastric ulcer healing rates were consistently higher with cimetidine than with placebo.

Gastroesophageal Reflux Disease: In two multicenter, double-blind, placebo-controlled studies in patients with gastroesophageal reflux disease (GERD) and endoscopically proven erosions and/or ulcers, cimetidine was significantly more effective than placebo in healing lesions. The endoscopically confirmed healing rates can be seen in TABLE 6.

TABLE 6

Trial		Tagamet (800 mg b.i.d.)	Tagamet (400 mg q.i.d.)	Placebo	p-Value (800 mg b.i.d. vs. placebo)
1	Week 6	45%	52%	26%	0.02
	Week 12	60%	66%	42%	0.02
2	Week 6	50%		20%	<0.01
	Week 12	67%		36%	<0.01

In these trials cimetidine was superior to placebo by most measures in improving symptoms of day- and night-time heartburn, with many of the differences statistically significant. The q.i.d. regimen was generally somewhat better than the b.i.d. regimen where these were compared.

PREVENTION OF UPPER GASTROINTESTINAL BLEEDING IN CRITICALLY ILL PATIENTS

A double-blind, placebo-controlled randomized study of continuous infusion cimetidine was performed in 131 critically ill patients (mean APACHE II score = 15.99) to compare the incidence of upper gastrointestinal bleeding, manifested as hematemesis or bright red blood which did not clear after adjustment of the nasogastric tube and a 5 to 10 minute lavage, persistent Gastroccult positive coffee grounds for 8 consecutive hours which did not clear

CLINICAL STUDIES: *(cont'd)*

with 100 cc lavage and/or which were accompanied by a drop in hematocrit of 5 percentage points, or melena, with an endoscopically documented upper gastrointestinal source of bleed. 14% (9/65) of patients treated with cimetidine continuous infusion developed bleeding compared to 33% (22/66) of the placebo group. Coffee grounds was the manifestation of bleeding that accounted for the difference between groups. Another randomized, double-blind placebo-controlled study confirmed these results for an end point of upper gastrointestinal bleeding with a confirmed upper gastrointestinal source noted on endoscopy, and by post hoc analyses of bleeding episodes between groups.

Pathological Hypersecretory Conditions: (such as Zollinger-Ellison Syndrome) cimetidine significantly inhibited gastric acid secretion and reduced occurrence of diarrhea, anorexia and pain in patients with pathological hypersecretion associated with Zollinger-Ellison Syndrome, systemic mastocytosis and multiple endocrine adenomas. Use of cimetidine was also followed by healing of intractable ulcers.

INDICATIONS AND USAGE:

Cimetidine is indicated in:

(1) Short-Term Treatment of Active Duodenal Ulcer: Most patients heal within 4 weeks and there is rarely reason to use cimetidine at full dosage for longer than 6 to 8 weeks (see DOSAGE AND ADMINISTRATION, Duodenal Ulcer.) Concomitant antacids should be given as needed for relief of pain. However, simultaneous administration of cimetidine and antacids is not recommended, since antacids have been reported to interfere with the absorption of cimetidine.

(2) Maintenance Therapy for Duodenal Ulcer Patients at Reduced Dosage after Healing of Active Ulcer: Patients have been maintained on continued treatment with cimetidine 400 mg h.s. for periods of up to 5 years.

(3) Short-Term Treatment of Active Benign Gastric Ulcer: There is no information concerning usefulness of treatment periods of longer than 8 weeks.

(4) Erosive Gastroesophageal Reflux Disease (GERD): Erosive esophagitis diagnosed by endoscopy. Treatment is indicated for 12 weeks for healing of lesions and control of symptoms. The use of cimetidine beyond 12 weeks has not been established (see DOSAGE AND ADMINISTRATION, GERD.)

(5) Prevention of Upper Gastrointestinal Bleeding in Critically Ill Patients.

(6) The Treatment of Pathological Hypersecretory Conditions: (*i.e.,* Zollinger-Ellison Syndrome, systemic mastocytosis, multiple endocrine adenomas).

CONTRAINDICATIONS:

cimetidine is contraindicated for patients known to have hypersensitivity to the product.

PRECAUTIONS:

GENERAL

Rare instances of cardiac arrhythmias and hypotension have been reported following the rapid administration of cimetidine hydrochloride injection by intravenous bolus.

Symptomatic response to cimetidine therapy does not preclude the presence of a gastric malignancy. There have been rare reports of transient healing of gastric ulcers despite subsequently documented malignancy.

Reversible confusional states (see ADVERSE REACTIONS) have been observed on occasion, predominantly, but not exclusively, in severely ill patients. Advancing age (50 or more years) and preexisting liver and/or renal disease appear to be contributing factors. In some patients these confusional states have been mild and have not required discontinuation of cimetidine therapy. In cases where discontinuation was judged necessary, the condition usually cleared within 3 to 4 days of drug withdrawal.

CARCINOGENESIS, MUTAGENESIS, AND IMPAIRMENT OF FERTILITY

In a 24- month toxicity study conducted in rats, at dose levels of 150, 378 and 950 mg/kg/day (approximately 8 to 48 times the recommended human dose), there was a small increase in the incidence of benign Leydig cell tumors in each dose group; when the combined drug-treated groups and control groups were compared, this increase reached statistical significance. In a subsequent 24-month study, there were no differences between the rats receiving 150 mg/kg/day and the untreated controls. However, a statistically significant increase in benign Leydig cell tumor incidence was seen in the rats that received 378 and 950 mg/kg/day. These tumors were common in control groups as well as treated groups and the difference became apparent only in aged rats.

Cimetidine has demonstrated a weak antiandrogenic effect. In animal studies this was manifested as reduced prostate and seminal vesicle weights. However, there was no impairment of mating performance or fertility, nor any harm to the fetus in these animals at doses 8 to 48 times the full therapeutic dose of cimetidine, as compared with controls. The cases of gynecomastia seen in patients treated for 1 month or longer may be related to this effect.

In human studies, cimetidine has been shown to have no effect on spermatogenesis, sperm count, motility, morphology or *in vitro* fertilizing capacity.

PREGNANCY, TERATOGENIC EFFECTS, PREGNANCY CATEGORY B

Reproduction studies have been performed in rats, rabbits and mice at doses up to 40 times the normal human dose and have revealed no evidence of impaired fertility or harm to the fetus due to cimetidine. There, are however, no adequate and well-controlled studies in pregnant women. Because animal reproductive studies are not always predictive of human response, this drug should be used during pregnancy only if clearly needed.

NURSING MOTHERS

Cimetidine is secreted in human milk and, as a general rule nursing should not be undertaken while a patient is on a drug.

PEDIATRIC USE

Clinical experience in children is limited. Therefore, cimetidine therapy cannot be recommended for children under 16, unless, in the judgment of the physician, anticipated benefits outweigh the potential risks. In very limited experience, doses of 20 to 40 mg/kg per day have been used.

IMMUNOCOMPROMISED PATIENTS

In immunocompromised patients, decreased gastric acidity, including that produed by acid-suppressing agents such as cimetide, may increase the possibility of a hyperinfection of strongyloidiasis.

DRUG INTERACTIONS:

Cimetidine, apparently through an effect on certain microsomal enzyme systems, has been reported to reduce the hepatic metabolism of warfarin-type anticoagulants, phenytoin, propranolol, nifedipine, chlordiazepoxide, diazepam, certain tricyclic antidepressants, lidocaine, theophylline and metronidazole, thereby delaying elimination and increasing blood levels of these drugs.

DRUG INTERACTIONS: *(cont'd)*

Clinically significant effects have been reported with the warfarin anticoagulants; therefore close monitoring of prothrombin time is recommended, and adjustment of the anticoagulant dose may be necessary when cimetidine is administered concomitantly. Interaction with phenytoin, lidocaine and theophylline has also been reported to produce adverse clinical effects.

However, a crossover study in healthy subjects receiving either cimetidine 300 mg q.i.d. or 800 mg h.s. concomitantly with a 300 mg b.i.d. dosage of theophylline (Theo-Dur, Key Pharmaceuticals, Inc.) demonstrated less alteration in steady-state theophylline peak serum levels with the 800 mg h.s. regimen, particularly in subjects aged 54 years and older. Data beyond 10 days are not available. (Note: All patients receiving theophylline should be monitored appropriately, regardless of concomitant drug therapy.)

Dosage of the drugs mentioned above and other similarly metabolized drugs, particularly those of low therapeutic ratio or in patients with renal and/or hepatic impairment, may require adjustment when starting or stopping concomitantly administered cimetidine to maintain optimum therapeutic blood levels.

Alteration of pH may affect absorption of certain drugs (*e.g.*, ketoconazole). If these products are needed, they should be given at least 2 hours before cimetide administration.

Additional clinical experience may reveal other drugs affected by the concomitant administration of cimetidine.

ADVERSE REACTIONS:

Adverse effects reported in patients taking cimetidine are described below by body system. Incidence figures of 1 in 100 and greater are generally derived from controlled clinical studies.

Gastrointestinal: Diarrhea (usually mild) has been reported in approximately 1 in 100 patients.

CNS: Headaches, ranging from mild to severe, have been reported in 3.5% of 924 patients taking 1600 mg/day, 2.1% of 2,225 patients taking 800 mg/day and 2.3% of 1,897 patients taking placebo. Dizziness and somnolence (usually mild) have been reported in approximately 1 in 100 patients on either 1600 mg/day or 800 mg/day.

Reversible confusional states, e.g., mental confusion, agitation, psychosis, depression, anxiety, hallucinations, disorientation, have been reported predominantly, but not exclusively, in severely ill patients. They have usually developed within 2 to 3 days of initiation of cimetidine therapy and have cleared within 3 to 4 days of discontinuation of the drug.

Endocrine: Gynecomastia has been reported in patients treated for 1 month or longer. In patients being treated for pathological hypersecretory states, this occurred in about 4% of cases while in all others the incidence was 0.3% to 1% in various studies. No evidence of induced endocrine dysfunction was found, and the condition remained unchanged or returned toward normal with continuing cimetidine (cimetidine) treatment.

Reversible impotence has been reported in patients with pathological hypersecretory disorders, e.g., Zollinger Ellison Syndrome, receiving cimetidine, particularly in high doses, for at least 12 months (range 12-79 months, mean 38 months). However, in large scale surveillance studies at regular dosage, the incidence has not exceeded that commonly reported in the general population.

Hematologic: Decreased white blood cell counts in cimetidine-treated patients (approximately 1 per 100,000 patients), including agranulocytosis (approximately 3 per million patients), have been reported, including a few reports of recurrence on rechallenge. Most of these reports were in patients who had serious concomitant illnesses and received drugs and/or treatment known to produce neutropenia. Thrombocytopenia (approximately 3 per million patients) and, very rarely cases of pancytopenia or aplastic anemia have also been reported. As with some other H_2 receptor antagonists, there have been extremely rare reports of immune hemolytic anemia.

Hepatobiliary: Dose-related increases in serum transaminase have been reported. In most cases they did not progress with continued therapy and returned to normal at the end of therapy. There have been rare reports of cholestatic or mixed cholestatic hepatocellular effects. These were usually reversible. Because of the predominance of cholestatic features, severe parenchymal injury is considered highly unlikely. However, as in the occasional liver injury with other H_2-receptor antagonists, in exceedingly rare circumstances fatal outcomes have been reported.

There has been reported a single case of biopsy-proven periportal hepatic fibrosis in a patient receiving cimetidine.

Rare cases of pancreatitis, which cleared on withdrawal of the drug, have been reported.

Hypersensitivity: Rare cases of fever and allergic reactions including anaphylaxis and hypersensitivity vasculitis, which cleared on withdrawal of the drug, have been reported.

Renal: Small, possibly dose-related increases in plasma creatinine, presumably due to competition for renal tubular secretion, are not uncommon and do not signify deteriorating renal function. Rare cases of interstitial nephritis and urinary retention, which cleared on withdrawal of the drug, have been reported.

Cardiovascular: Rare cases of bradycardia, tachycardia and A-V heart block have been reported with H_2-receptor antagonists.

Musculoskeletal: There have been rare reports of reversible arthralgia and myalgia; exacerbation of joint symptoms in patients with preexisting arthritis has also been reported. Such symptoms have usually been alleviated by a reduction in cimetidine dosage. Rare cases of polymyositis have been reported, but no causal relationship has been established.

Integumental: Mild rash and, very rarely, cases of severe generalized skin reactions including Stevens-Johnson syndrome, epidermal necrolysis, erythema multiforme, exfoliative dermatitis and generalized exfoliative erythroderma have been reported with H_2-receptor antagonists. Reversible alopecia has been reported very rarely.

Immune Function: There have been extremely rare reports of strongyloidiasis hyperinfection in immunocompromised patients.

OVERDOSAGE:

Studies in animals indicate that toxic doses are associated with respiratory failure and tachycardia that may be controlled by assisted respiration and the administration of a beta blocker.

Reported acute ingestions orally of up to 20 grams have been associated with transient adverse effects similar to those encountered in normal clinical experience. The usual measures to remove unabsorbed material from the gastrointestinal tract, clinical monitoring, and supportive therapy should be employed.

There have been reports of severe CNS symptoms, including unresponsiveness, following ingestion of between 20 and 40 grams of cimetidine, and extremely rare reports following concomitant use of multiple CNS-active medications and ingestion of cimetidine at doses less than 20 grams. An elderly, terminally ill dehydrated patient with organic brain syndrome receiving concomitant antipsychotic agents and cimetidine 4800 intravenously over a 24-hour period experienced mental deterioration with reversal on cimetidine discontinuation.

There have been two deaths in adults who were reported to have ingested over 40 grams orally on a single occasion.

DOSAGE AND ADMINISTRATION:

Duodenal Ulcer; Active Duodenal Ulcer: Clinical studies have indicated that suppression of nocturnal acid is the most important factor in duodenal ulcer healing (see CLINICAL PHARMACOLOGY, Acid Secretion.) This is supported by recent clinical trials (see CLINICAL STUDIES, Active Duodenal Ulcer.) Therefore, there is no apparent rationale, except for familiarity with use, for treating with anything other than a once-daily at bedtime dosage regimen (h.s.).

In a U.S. dose-ranging study of 400 mg h.s., 800 mg h.s. and 1600 mg h.s., a continuous dose response relationship for ulcer healing was demonstrated.

However, 800 mg h.s. is the dose of choice for most patients, as it provides a high healing rate (the difference between 800 mg h.s. and 1600 mg h.s. being small), maximal pain relief, a decreased potential for drug interactions (see DRUG INTERACTIONS) and maximal patient convenience. Patients unhealed at four weeks, or those with persistent symptoms, have been shown to benefit from 2 to 4 weeks of continued therapy.

It has been shown that patients who both have an endoscopically demonstrated ulcer larger than 1.0 cm and are also heavy smokers (*i.e.*, smoke one pack of cigarettes or more per day) are more difficult to heal. There is some evidence which suggests that more rapid healing can be achieved in this subpopulation with cimetidine 1600 mg at bedtime. While early pain relief with either 800 mg h.s. or 1600 mg h.s. is equivalent in all patients, 1600 mg h.s. provides an appropriate alternative when it is important to ensure healing within four weeks for this subpopulation. Alternatively, approximately 94% of all patients will also heal in eight weeks with cimetidine 800 mg h.s.

Other cimetidine regimens in the U.S. which have been shown to be effective are: 300 mg four times daily, with meals and at bedtime, the original regimen with which U.S. physicians have the most experience and 400 mg twice daily, in the morning and at bedtime (see CLINICAL STUDIES, Active Duodenal Ulcer.)

Concomitant antacids should be given as needed for relief of pain. However, simultaneous administration of cimetidine and antacids is not recommended, since antacids have been reported to interfere with the absorption of cimetidine.

While healing with cimetidine often occurs during the first week or two, treatment should be continued for 4 to 6 weeks unless healing has been demonstrated by endoscopic examination.

Maintenance Therapy for Duodenal Ulcer: In those patients requiring maintenance therapy, the recommended adult oral dose is 400 mg at bedtime.

Active Benign Gastric Ulcer: The recommended adult oral dosage for short-term treatment of active benign gastric ulcer is 800 mg h.s., or 300 mg four times a day with meals and at bedtime. Controlled clinical studies were limited to six weeks of treatment (see CLINICAL STUDIES.) 800 mg h.s. is the preferred regimen for most patients based upon convenience and reduced potential for drug interactions. Symptomatic response to cimetidine does not preclude the presence of a gastric malignancy. It is important to follow gastric ulcer patients to assure rapid progress to complete healing.

Erosive Gastroesophageal Reflux Disease (GERD): The recommended adult oral dosage for the treatment of erosive esophagitis that has been diagnosed by endoscopy is 1600 mg daily in divided doses (800 mg b.i.d. or 400 mg q.i.d.) for 12 weeks. The use of cimetidine beyond 12 weeks has not been established.

Prevention of Upper Gastrointestinal Bleeding: The recommended adult dosing regimen is continuous IV infusion of 50 mg/hour. Patients with creatinine clearance less than 30 cc/min. should receive half the recommended dose. Treatment beyond 7 days has not been studied.

Pathological Hypersecretory Conditions: (such as Zollinger-Ellison Syndrome) Recommended adult oral dosage: 300 mg four times a day with meals and at bedtime. In some patients it may be necessary to administer higher doses more frequently. Doses should be adjusted to individual patient needs, but should not usually exceed 2400 mg per day and should continue as long as clinically indicated.

Parenteral Administration: In hospitalized patients with pathological hypersecretory conditions or intractable ulcers, or in patients who are unable to take oral medication, cimetidine may be administered parenterally.

The doses and regimen for parenteral administration in patients with GERD have not been established.

All parenteral drug products should be inspected visually for particulate matter and discoloration prior to administration.

Recommendations for Parenteral Administration: Intramuscular Injection: 300 mg q 6-8 hours (no dilution necessary).

Transient pain at the site of injection has been reported.

Intravenous Injection: 300 mg q 6-8 hours. In some patients it may be necessary to increase dosage. When this is necessary, the increases should be made by more frequent administration of a 300 mg dose, but should not exceed 2400 mg per day. Dilute cimetidine hydrochloride, Injection, 300 mg, in Sodium Chloride Injection (0.9%) or another compatible IV solution (see Stability of Cimetidine Injection) to a total volume of 20 ml and inject over a period of not less than 5 minutes (see PRECAUTIONS).

INTERMITTENT INTRAVENOUS INFUSION

300 mg q 6-8 hours, infused over 15-20 minutes. In some patients it may be necessary to increase dosage. When this is necessary, the increases should be made by more frequent administration of a 300 mg dose, but should not exceed 2400 mg per day.

Vials: Dilute Cimetidine Injection, 300 mg, in at least 50 ml of 5% Dextrose Injection, or another compatible IV solution (see Stability of Cimetidine Injection).

Plastic Containers: Use premixed Cimetidine Injection, 300 mg, in 0.9% Sodium Chloride in 50 ml plastic containers.

ADD-Vantage Vials: Dilute contents of one vial in an ADD Vantage Diluent Container, available in 50 ml and 100 ml sizes of 0.9% Sodium Chloride Injection, and 5% Dextrose Injection.

CONTINUOUS INTRAVENOUS INFUSION

37.5 mg/hour (900 mg/day). For patients requiring a more rapid elevation of gastric pH, continuous infusion may be preceded by a 150 mg loading dose administered by IV infusion as described above. Dilute 900 mg Cimetidine Injection in a compatible IV fluid (see Stability of Cimetidine Injection for constant rate infusion over a 24 hour period). Note: cimetidine may be diluted in 100-1000 ml; however, a volumetric pump is recommended if the volume for 24 hour infusion is less than 250 ml. In one study in patients with pathological hypersecretory states, the mean infused dose of cimetidine was 160 mg/hour with a range of 40-600 mg/hour.

These doses maintained the intragastric acid secretory rate at 10 mEq/hour or less. The infusion rate should be adjusted to individual patient requirements.

DIRECTIONS FOR USE OF CIMETIDINE HYDROCHLORIDE INJECTION IN PLASTIC CONTAINERS

To Open: Tear overwrap down side at slit and remove solution containers.

Some opacity of the plastic due to moisture absorption during the sterilization process may be observed. This is normal and does not affect solution quality or safety. The opacity will diminish gradually.

Do not add other drugs to premixed Cimetidine Injection in plastic containers.

DOSAGE AND ADMINISTRATION: *(cont'd)*

Caution: Check for minute leaks by squeezing inner bag firmly. If leaks are found, discard solution as sterility may be impaired. Additives should not be introduced into this solution. Do not use if the solution is cloudy or precipitated or if the seal is not intact.

Do not use plastic containers in series connections. Such use could result in air embolism due to residual air being drawn from the primary container before administration of the fluid from the secondary container is complete.

Use sterile equipment.

PREPARATION FOR ADMINISTRATION

1. Suspend container from eyelet support.
2. Remove plastic protector from outlet port at bottom of container.
3. Attach administration set. Refer to complete directions accompanying set.

DIRECTIONS FOR USE OF TAGAMET INJECTION IN ADVANTAGE VIALS are enclosed in ADD Vantage Vial packaging.

Stability of Cimetidine Injection: When added to or diluted with most commonly used intravenous solutions, e.g.,Sodium Chloride Injection (0.9%), Dextrose Injection (5% or 10%), Lactated Ringer's Solution, 5% Sodium Bicarbonate Injection, cimetidine hydrochloride injection should not be used after more than 48 hours of storage at room temperature.

Cimetidine Injection premixed in plastic containers is stable through the labeled expiration date when stored under the recommended conditions.

Dosage Adjustment for Patients with Impaired Renal Function: Patients with severely impaired renal function have been treated with cimetidine. However, such usage has been very limited. On the basis of this experience the recommended dosage is 300 mg q 12 hours orally or by intravenous injection. Should the patient's condition require the frequency of dosing may be increased to q 8 hours or even further with caution. In severe renal failure, accumulation may occur and the lowest frequency of dosing compatible with an adequate patient response should be used. When liver impairment is also present, further reductions in dosage may be necessary. Hemodialysis reduces the level of circulating cimetidine. Ideally, the dosage schedule should be adjusted so that the timing of a scheduled dose coincides with the end of hemodialysis.

Patients with creatinine clearance less than 30 cc/min. who are being treated for prevention of upper gastrointestinal bleeding should receive half the recommended dose.

PATIENT INFORMATION:

Cimetidine is used to treat stomach and duodenal (upper small intestine) ulcers; hypersecretory (increased acid secretion) conditions; heartburn and gastroesophageal reflux disease (stomach contents bubbling into the esophagus causing pain). Notify your physician if you are pregnant or nursing. Cimetidine is involved in several drug interactions; notify your physician and pharmacist of other prescription and over-the-counter medications you are taking. Cimetidine may be taken with or without food. Do not take this medication at the same time you take an antacid; dosing of cimetidine should be staggered at least one hour before or one hour after taking an antacid. Notify your physician if you develop black, tarry stools or coffee-ground vomit.

HOW SUPPLIED:

Tablets: Light green, film-coated as follows: 200 mg-round, imprinted with the product name TAGAMET, SKF and 200—tablets in bottles of 100; 300 mg—round, debossed with the product name TAGAMET, SB and 300—tablets in bottles of 100 and Single Unit Packages of 100 (intended for institutional use only); 400 mg—oval-shaped Tiltab, debossed with the product name. TAGAMET, SB and 400—tablets in bottles of 60 and Single Unit Packages of 100 (intended for institutional use only); 800 mg—oval-shaped Tiltab, debossed with the product name TAGAMET, SB and 800—tablets in bottles of 30 and Single Unit Packages of 100 intended for institutional use only).

Store between 15° to 30°C (59° to 86°F); dispense in a tight light-resistant container.

Liquid: Clear, light orange, mint-peach flavored, as follows: 300 mg/5 ml in 8 fl oz (237 ml) amber glass bottles; 300 mg/5 ml in single-dose units in packages of 10 (intended for institutional use only).

Store between 15° to 30°C (59° to 86°F); dispense in a tight light-resistant container.

Injection: Vials: 300 mg/2 ml in single-dose vials, in packages of 25, and in 8 ml multi-dose vials, in packages of 10 and 25.

Store between 15° to 30°C (59° to 86°F); do not refrigerate.

Single-Dose Premixed Plastic Containers: 300 mg in 50 ml of 0.9% Sodium Chloride in single-dose plastic containers, in packages of 4 units. No preservative has been added.

Exposure of the premixed product to excessive heat should be avoided. It is recommended the product be stored at controlled room temperature 15° to 30°C (59° to 86°F). Brief exposure up to 40°C does not adversely affect the premixed product.

ADD-Vantage Vials: 300 mg/2 ml in a single dose ADD-Vantage Vials, in packages of 25.

Store between 15° to 30°C (59° to 86°F); do not refrigerate.

Cimetidine hydrochloride Injection premixed in single-dose plastic containers is manufactured for SmithKline-Beecham Pharmaceuticals by Baxter Healthcare Corporation, Deerfield, IL 60015

HOW SUPPLIED - RATED THERAPEUTICALLY EQUIVALENT:

Injection, Solution - Intramuscular; - 300 mg/2ml

8 ml vials x 25	**$306.25**	**TAGAMET HCL, SKB Pharms**	**00108-5022-16**
8 ml x 10	**$128.60**	**TAGAMET HCL, SKB Pharms**	**00108-5022-11**

Injection, Solution - Intravenous - 300 mg/2ml

2 ml	$7.05	CIMETIDINE, Abbott	00074-7446-02
2 ml x 10	$18.12	Cimetidine, Endo Labs	60951-0637-53
2 ml x 25	$37.50	Cimetidine, Am Regent	00517-1502-25
2 ml x 25	$44.37	Cimetidine, Endo Labs	60951-0637-57
2 ml x 25	$68.75	Cimetidine, Jordan Pharms	58196-0245-39
2 ml x 25	**$99.05**	**TAGAMET, SKB Pharms**	**00108-5017-16**
2 ml x 25	**$99.05**	**TAGAMET, SKB Pharms**	**00108-5017-77**
2 ml x 25	**$109.70**	**TAGAMET ADD-VANTAGE, SKB Pharms**	**00108-5031-16**
2 ml x 25	**$109.70**	**TAGAMET, SKB Pharms**	**00108-5031-76**
8 ml	$18.17	CIMETIDINE, Abbott	00074-7445-01
8 ml x 10	$54.37	Cimetidine, Endo Labs	60951-0637-69
8 ml x 10	$81.25	Cimetidine, Jordan Pharms	58196-0246-18
8 ml x 10	**$128.60**	**TAGAMET, SKB Pharms**	**00108-5022-76**
8 ml x 25	$112.50	Cimetidine, Am Regent	00517-1508-25
8 ml x 25	$120.62	Cimetidine, Endo Labs	60951-0637-27
8 ml x 25	$218.75	Cimetidine, Jordan Pharms	58196-0246-19
8 ml x 25	**$306.25**	**TAGAMET, SKB Pharms**	**00108-5022-75**

Injection, Solution - Intravenous - 300 mg/50ml

2 ml	$7.48	CIMETIDINE, Abbott	00074-7444-01
48's	**$267.60**	**TAGAMET (IN 0.9% SODIUM), SKB Pharms**	**00108-5029-04**
50 ml	$22.56	CIMETIDINE IN SODIUM CHLORIDE, Abbott	00074-7447-16

HOW SUPPLIED - RATED THERAPEUTICALLY EQUIVALENT: *(cont'd)*

Liquid - Oral - 300 mg/5ml

5 ml x 10	**$25.80**	**TAGAMET HCL, SKB Pharms**	**00108-5014-10**
5 ml x 10	**$25.80**	**TAGAMET, SKB Pharms**	**00108-5014-75**
240 ml	$85.50	Cimetidine, Endo Labs	60951-0635-35
240 ml	$86.20	Cimetidine, Qualitest Pharms	00603-1092-56
240 ml	$86.25	Cimetidine, Goldline Labs	00182-6164-44
240 ml	$86.25	Cimetidine, Alpharma	00472-0514-08
240 ml	$86.52	Cimetidine, Rugby	00536-2975-59
240 ml	$87.00	Cimetidine, Schein Pharm (US)	00364-2602-76
240 ml	$89.75	Cimetidine, Major Pharms	00904-7897-97
240 ml	$89.89	Cimetidine, Geneva Pharms	00781-6527-08
240 ml	$90.79	Cimetidine, Aligen Independ	00405-2531-77
240 ml	**$104.65**	**TAGAMET HCL, SKB Pharms**	**00108-5014-48**
240 ml	**$105.97**	**TAGAMET, SKB Pharms**	**00108-5014-76**
480 ml	$140.95	Cimetidine, Alpharma	00472-0514-16
480 ml	$161.80	Cimetidine, Geneva Pharms	00781-6527-16
480 ml	$170.56	Cimetidine, Rugby	00536-2975-85

Tablet, Coated - Oral - 200 mg

50's	$39.96	Cimetidine, Zenith Labs	00172-7111-48
100's	$19.43	Cimetidine, H.C.F.A. F F P	99999-0820-01
100's	$24.81	Cimetidine, United Res	00677-1527-01
100's	$72.40	Cimetidine, Rosemont	00832-0101-00
100's	$72.48	Cimetidine, Qualitest Pharms	00603-2890-21
100's	$73.40	Cimetidine, Mova Pharms	55370-0536-07
100's	$73.40	Cimetidine, Novopharm (US)	55953-0181-40
100's	$73.49	Cimetidine, West Point Pharma	59591-0259-68
100's	$74.50	Cimetidine, Endo Labs	60951-0630-70
100's	$75.15	Cimetidine, Novopharm (US)	55953-0181-41
100's	$75.42	Cimetidine, Aligen Independ	00405-5370-01
100's	$76.20	Cimetidine, Major Pharms	00904-7866-60
100's	$76.21	Cimetidine, HL Moore Drug Exch	00839-7906-06
100's	$76.30	Cimetidine, Martec Pharms	52555-0515-01
100's	$79.85	Cimetidine, Rugby	00536-5661-01
100's	$79.90	Cimetidine, Teva	00093-0111-01
100's	$79.92	Cimetidine, Zenith Labs	00172-7111-60
100's	$79.92	Cimetidine, Goldline Labs	00182-1983-01
100's	$79.92	Cimetidine, Warrick Pharms	59930-1800-01
100's	$79.95	Cimetidine, Geneva Pharms	00781-1447-01
100's	$81.50	Cimetidine, Goldline Labs	00182-1983-89
100's	$83.15	Cimetidine, Schein Pharm (US)	00364-2591-01
100's	$83.15	Cimetidine, Mylan	00378-0053-01
100's	**$88.85**	**TAGAMET, SKB Pharms**	**00108-5012-20**
500's	$97.15	Cimetidine, H.C.F.A. F F P	99999-0820-02
500's	$348.65	Cimetidine, Novopharm (US)	55953-0181-70
500's	$362.10	Cimetidine, Major Pharms	00904-7866-40
500's	$399.59	Cimetidine, Zenith Labs	00172-7111-70
500's	$399.60	Cimetidine, Warrick Pharms	59930-1800-02
1000's	$194.30	Cimetidine, H.C.F.A. F F P	99999-0820-03
1000's	$562.95	Cimetidine, HL Moore Drug Exch	00839-7906-16
1000's	$662.44	Cimetidine, Novopharm (US)	55953-0181-80
1000's	$686.15	Cimetidine, Major Pharms	00904-7866-80
1000's	$799.20	Cimetidine, Warrick Pharms	59930-1800-03

Tablet, Coated - Oral - 300 mg

30's	$6.27	Cimetidine, H.C.F.A. F F P	99999-0820-04
50's	$43.92	Cimetidine, Zenith Labs	00172-7117-48
60's	$60.00	CIMETIDINE, UDL	51079-0807-98
100's	$20.93	Cimetidine, H.C.F.A. F F P	99999-0820-05
100's	$24.81	Cimetidine, United Res	00677-1528-01
100's	$40.00	Cimetidine, Raway	00686-0813-01
100's	**$44.90**	**TAGAMET, Voluntary Hosp**	**53258-0115-13**
100's	$75.78	Cimetidine, Rosemont	00832-0102-00
100's	$75.85	Cimetidine, Qualitest Pharms	00603-2891-21
100's	$76.80	Cimetidine, Mova Pharms	55370-0537-07
100's	$76.80	Cimetidine, Novopharm (US)	55953-0192-40
100's	$76.87	Cimetidine, West Point Pharma	59591-0260-68
100's	$77.20	Cimetidine, Aligen Independ	00405-5371-01
100's	$77.50	Cimetidine, Lederle Pharm	00005-3416-23
100's	$78.20	Cimetidine, Endo Labs	60951-0631-70
100's	$78.55	Cimetidine, Novopharm (US)	55953-0192-41
100's	$79.75	Cimetidine, Logen Pharm	00820-7867-60
100's	$79.75	Cimetidine, Major Pharms	00904-7867-60
100's	$79.79	Cimetidine, HL Moore Drug Exch	00839-7907-06
100's	$79.80	Cimetidine, Martec Pharms	52555-0516-01
100's	$79.80	Cimetidine, Penn Labs	58437-0001-20
100's	$80.99	Cimetidine, Par Pharm	49884-0405-01
100's	$81.10	Cimetidine, Penn Labs	58437-0001-21
100's	$82.90	Cimetidine, Vangard Labs	00615-2534-13
100's	$83.60	Cimetidine, Teva	00093-0112-01
100's	$83.65	Cimetidine, Zenith Labs	00172-7117-60
100's	$83.65	Cimetidine, Goldline Labs	00182-1984-01
100's	$83.65	Cimetidine, Warrick Pharms	59930-1801-01
100's	$83.70	Cimetidine, Rugby	00536-5662-01
100's	$83.70	Cimetidine, Geneva Pharms	00781-1448-01
100's	$85.00	Cimetidine, Goldline Labs	00182-1984-89
100's	$87.03	Cimetidine, Schein Pharm (US)	00364-2592-01
100's	$87.03	Cimetidine, Mylan	00378-0317-01
100's	**$93.00**	**TAGAMET, SKB Pharms**	**00108-5013-20**
100's	**$93.00**	**TAGAMET, SKB Pharms**	**00108-5013-76**
100's	**$94.50**	**TAGAMET, SKB Pharms**	**00108-5013-21**
100's	**$94.50**	**TAGAMET, SKB Pharms**	**00108-5013-75**
100's	$133.86	Cimetidine, Geneva Pharms	00781-1448-13
500's	$104.65	Cimetidine, H.C.F.A. F F P	99999-0820-06
500's	$359.98	Cimetidine, Rosemont	00832-0102-50
500's	$360.40	Cimetidine, Qualitest Pharms	00603-2891-28
500's	$364.80	Cimetidine, Mova Pharms	55370-0537-08
500's	$364.80	Cimetidine, Novopharm (US)	55953-0192-70
500's	$376.30	Cimetidine, Major Pharms	00904-7867-40
500's	$381.23	Cimetidine, HL Moore Drug Exch	00839-7915-12
500's	$396.32	Cimetidine, Aligen Independ	00405-5371-02
500's	$398.00	Cimetidine, Lederle Pharm	00005-3416-31
500's	$398.95	Cimetidine, Martec Pharms	52555-0516-05
500's	$398.95	Cimetidine, Penn Labs	58437-0001-25
500's	$399.09	Cimetidine, Par Pharm	49884-0405-05
500's	$418.25	Cimetidine, Teva	00093-0112-05
500's	$418.26	Cimetidine, Zenith Labs	00172-7117-70
500's	$418.26	Cimetidine, Goldline Labs	00182-1984-05
500's	$418.26	Cimetidine, Warrick Pharms	59930-1801-02
500's	$418.50	Cimetidine, Endo Labs	60951-0631-85
500's	$435.13	Cimetidine, Schein Pharm (US)	00364-2592-05
500's	$435.13	Cimetidine, Mylan	00378-0317-05
500's	**$465.00**	**TAGAMET, SKB Pharms**	**00108-5013-25**

HOW SUPPLIED - RATED THERAPEUTICALLY EQUIVALENT:

(cont'd)

500's	$681.00	Cimetidine, Geneva Pharms	00781-1448-05
1000's	$209.30	Cimetidine, H.C.F.A. F F P	99999-0820-07
1000's	$693.12	Cimetidine, Mova Pharms	55370-0537-09
1000's	$693.12	Cimetidine, Novopharm (US)	55953-0192-80
1000's	$717.00	Cimetidine, Major Pharms	00904-7867-80
1000's	$718.13	Cimetidine, HL Moore Drug Exch	00839-7907-16
1000's	$797.98	Cimetidine, Teva	00093-0112-10
1000's	$836.52	Cimetidine, Zenith Labs	00172-7117-80
1000's	$836.52	Cimetidine, Goldline Labs	00182-1984-10
1000's	$836.52	Cimetidine, Warrick Pharms	59930-1801-03
1000's	$837.00	Cimetidine, Endo Labs	60951-0631-90
5000's	$1046.50	Cimetidine, H.C.F.A. F F P	99999-0820-08
5000's	$3989.25	Cimetidine, Penn Labs	58437-0001-38
5000's	**$4650.00**	**TAGAMET, SKB Pharms**	**00108-5013-38**

Tablet, Coated - Oral - 400 mg

30's	$10.21	Cimetidine, H.C.F.A. F F P	99999-0820-09
60's	$20.43	Cimetidine, H.C.F.A. F F P	99999-0820-10
60's	$77.25	Cimetidine, Lederle Pharm	00005-3417-32
60's	$79.34	Cimetidine, Geneva Pharms	00781-1449-60
60's	$79.45	Cimetidine, Penn Labs	58437-0002-18
60's	$83.40	Cimetidine, Teva	00093-0113-06
60's	$87.46	Cimetidine, Zenith Labs	00172-7171-49
60's	**$92.60**	**TAGAMET, SKB Pharms**	**00108-5026-18**
60's	**$92.60**	**TAGAMET, SKB Pharms**	**00108-5026-76**
100's	$34.05	Cimetidine, H.C.F.A. F F P	99999-0820-11
100's	$39.54	Cimetidine, United Res	00677-1529-01
100's	$58.00	Cimetidine, Raway	00686-0814-01
100's	$118.70	Cimetidine, Vangard Labs	00615-3566-13
100's	$125.72	Cimetidine, Rosemont	00832-0103-00
100's	$125.85	Cimetidine, Qualitest Pharms	00603-2892-21
100's	$126.86	Cimetidine, West Point Pharma	59591-0261-68
100's	$127.65	Cimetidine, Mova Pharms	55370-0539-07
100's	$127.65	Cimetidine, Novopharm (US)	55953-0204-40
100's	$129.40	Cimetidine, Novopharm (US)	55953-0204-41
100's	$129.50	Cimetidine, Endo Labs	60951-0632-70
100's	$131.05	Cimetidine, Endo Labs	60951-0632-75
100's	$132.37	Cimetidine, HL Moore Drug Exch	00839-7908-06
100's	$133.10	Cimetidine, Aligen Independ	00405-5372-01
100's	$133.23	Cimetidine, HL Moore Drug Exch	00839-7916-06
100's	$133.86	Cimetidine, Geneva Pharms	00781-1449-13
100's	$134.00	Cimetidine, Major Pharms	00904-7868-60
100's	$134.00	Cimetidine, Penn Labs	58437-0002-21
100's	$134.20	Cimetidine, Martec Pharms	52555-0517-01
100's	$135.19	Cimetidine, Par Pharm	49884-0406-01
100's	$138.82	Cimetidine, Zenith Labs	00172-7171-60
100's	$138.82	Cimetidine, Goldline Labs	00182-1985-01
100's	$138.82	Cimetidine, Warrick Pharms	59930-1802-01
100's	$138.90	Cimetidine, Geneva Pharms	00781-1449-01
100's	$138.95	Cimetidine, Teva	00093-0113-01
100's	$139.39	Cimetidine, Rugby	00536-5663-01
100's	$140.55	Cimetidine, Goldline Labs	00182-1985-89
100's	$146.15	Cimetidine, Schein Pharm (US)	00364-2593-01
100's	$146.15	Cimetidine, Mylan	00378-0372-01
100's	**$156.20**	**TAGAMET, SKB Pharms**	**00108-5026-21**
100's	**$156.20**	**TAGAMET, SKB Pharms**	**00108-5026-75**
500's	$170.25	Cimetidine, H.C.F.A. F F P	99999-0820-12
500's	$197.70	Cimetidine, United Res	00677-1529-05
500's	$597.14	Cimetidine, Rosemont	00832-0103-50
500's	$597.80	Cimetidine, Qualitest Pharms	00603-2892-28
500's	$606.34	Cimetidine, Mova Pharms	55370-0539-08
500's	$606.34	Cimetidine, Novopharm (US)	55953-0204-70
500's	$632.33	Cimetidine, HL Moore Drug Exch	00839-7916-12
500's	$640.60	Cimetidine, Major Pharms	00904-7868-40
500's	$661.85	Cimetidine, Penn Labs	58437-0002-25
500's	$665.00	Cimetidine, Lederle Pharm	00005-3417-31
500's	$668.20	Cimetidine, Aligen Independ	00405-5372-02
500's	$671.10	Cimetidine, Martec Pharms	52555-0517-05
500's	$671.29	Cimetidine, Par Pharm	49884-0406-05
500's	$694.10	Cimetidine, Teva	00093-0113-05
500's	$694.10	Cimetidine, Zenith Labs	00172-7171-70
500's	$694.10	Cimetidine, Goldline Labs	00182-1985-05
500's	$694.10	Cimetidine, Warrick Pharms	59930-1802-02
500's	$694.48	Cimetidine, Endo Labs	60951-0632-85
500's	$696.95	Cimetidine, Rugby	00536-5663-05
500's	$722.20	Cimetidine, Schein Pharm (US)	00364-2593-05
500's	$722.20	Cimetidine, Mylan	00378-0372-05
500's	**$771.65**	**TAGAMET, SKB Pharms**	**00108-5026-25**
1000's	$340.50	Cimetidine, H.C.F.A. F F P	99999-0820-13
1000's	$1152.05	Cimetidine, Mova Pharms	55370-0539-09
1000's	$1152.05	Cimetidine, Novopharm (US)	55953-0204-80
1000's	$1191.31	Cimetidine, HL Moore Drug Exch	00839-7908-16
1000's	$1207.90	Cimetidine, Major Pharms	00904-7868-80
1000's	$1342.30	Cimetidine, Teva	00093-0113-10
1000's	$1388.20	Cimetidine, Zenith Labs	00172-7171-80
1000's	$1388.20	Cimetidine, Goldline Labs	00182-1985-10
1000's	$1388.20	Cimetidine, Warrick Pharms	59930-1802-03
1000's	$1388.99	Cimetidine, Endo Labs	60951-0632-90
5000's	$1702.50	Cimetidine, H.C.F.A. F F P	99999-0820-14
5000's	$6618.75	Cimetidine, Penn Labs	58437-0002-38
5000's	**$7716.65**	**TAGAMET, SKB Pharms**	**00108-5026-38**

Tablet, Coated - Oral - 800 mg

30's	$17.97	Cimetidine, H.C.F.A. F F P	99999-0820-15
30's	$67.93	Cimetidine, West Point Pharma	59591-0264-31
30's	$68.80	Cimetidine, Endo Labs	60951-0633-30
30's	$69.50	Cimetidine, Lederle Pharm	00005-3418-38
30's	$70.38	Cimetidine, Geneva Pharms	00781-1444-31
30's	$70.40	Cimetidine, Penn Labs	58437-0003-13
30's	$73.10	Cimetidine, Teva	00093-0122-56
30's	$74.34	Cimetidine, Rugby	00536-5664-07
30's	$77.49	Cimetidine, Zenith Labs	00172-7711-46
30's	**$82.05**	**TAGAMET, SKB Pharms**	**00108-5027-13**
30's	**$82.05**	**TAGAMET, SKB Pharms**	**00108-5027-76**
60's	$131.99	Cimetidine, Par Pharm	49884-0407-02
100's	$59.93	Cimetidine, H.C.F.A. F F P	99999-0820-16
100's	$87.93	Cimetidine, United Res	00677-1530-01
100's	$222.83	Cimetidine, Rosemont	00832-0104-00
100's	$223.08	Cimetidine, Qualitest Pharms	00603-2893-21
100's	$236.26	Cimetidine, Geneva Pharms	00781-1444-13
100's	$236.50	Cimetidine, Major Pharms	00904-7869-60
100's	$236.50	Cimetidine, Penn Labs	58437-0003-21
100's	$245.10	Cimetidine, Novopharm (US)	55953-0235-41

HOW SUPPLIED - RATED THERAPEUTICALLY EQUIVALENT:

(cont'd)

100's	$246.01	Cimetidine, Zenith Labs	00172-7711-60
100's	$246.01	Cimetidine, Goldline Labs	00182-1986-01
100's	$246.01	Cimetidine, Warrick Pharms	59930-1803-01
100's	$248.15	Cimetidine, Goldline Labs	00182-1986-89
100's	$255.21	Cimetidine, Geneva Pharms	00781-1444-01
100's	$256.03	Cimetidine, Schein Pharm (US)	00364-2594-01
100's	$256.03	Cimetidine, Mylan	00378-0541-01
100's	$260.67	Cimetidine, HL Moore Drug Exch	00839-7909-06
100's	$263.75	Cimetidine, Mova Pharms	55370-0540-07
100's	$263.75	Cimetidine, Novopharm (US)	55953-0235-40
100's	$264.20	Cimetidine, Aligen Independ	00405-5373-01
100's	$266.50	Cimetidine, Teva	00093-0122-01
100's	$266.50	Cimetidine, Martec Pharms	52555-0518-01
100's	**$275.75**	**TAGAMET, SKB Pharms**	**00108-5027-21**
100's	**$275.75**	**TAGAMET, SKB Pharms**	**00108-5027-75**
250's	$509.05	Cimetidine, Par Pharm	49884-0407-04
500's	$299.65	Cimetidine, H.C.F.A. F F P	99999-0820-17
500's	$1122.35	Cimetidine, Major Pharms	00904-7869-40
500's	$1173.00	Cimetidine, Penn Labs	58437-0003-25
500's	$1183.75	Cimetidine, Teva	00093-0122-05
500's	$1230.05	Cimetidine, Zenith Labs	00172-7711-70
500's	$1230.05	Cimetidine, Warrick Pharms	59930-1803-02
500's	$1252.89	Cimetidine, Mova Pharms	55370-0540-08
500's	$1252.89	Cimetidine, Novopharm (US)	55953-0235-70
500's	**$1367.50**	**TAGAMET, SKB Pharms**	**00108-5027-25**
1000's	$599.30	Cimetidine, H.C.F.A. F F P	99999-0820-18
1000's	$2126.60	Cimetidine, Major Pharms	00904-7869-80
1000's	$2346.03	Cimetidine, HL Moore Drug Exch	00839-7909-16
1000's	$2380.48	Cimetidine, Mova Pharms	55370-0540-09
1000's	$2380.48	Cimetidine, Novopharm (US)	55953-0235-80
1000's	$2460.10	Cimetidine, Warrick Pharms	59930-1803-03

HOW SUPPLIED - NOT RATED EQUIVALENT:

Injection, Solution - Intravenous - 300 mg/50ml

250 ml	$12.47	CIMETIDINE IN SODIUM CHLORIDE, Abbott	00074-7350-02
250 ml	$14.84	CIMETIDINE IN SODIUM CHLORIDE, Abbott	00074-7351-02
500 ml	$12.47	CIMETIDINE IN SODIUM CHLORIDE, Abbott	00074-7352-03
500 ml	$14.84	CIMETIDINE IN SODIUM CHLORIDE, Abbott	00074-7353-03
1000 ml	$12.46	CIMETIDINE IN SODIUM CHLORIDE, Abbott	00074-7354-09
1000 ml	$14.84	CIMETIDINE IN SODIUM CHLORIDE, Abbott	00074-7355-09

Liquid - Oral - 300 mg/5ml

240 ml	$86.52	Cimetidine, HL Moore Drug Exch	00839-7923-66
480 ml	$173.00	Cimetidine, HL Moore Drug Exch	00839-7923-69

CINOXACIN *(000822)*

CATEGORIES: Anti-Infectives; Antibacterials; Antimicrobials; Antiseptics, Urinary Tract; Quinolones; Urinary Antibacterial; Urinary Tract Infections; Pregnancy Category C; FDA Approval Pre 1982

BRAND NAMES: *Cerexin*; **Cinobac**; *Cinobact* (Japan); *Cinobactin* (Germany); *Gugecin* (Mexico); *Nofrin*; *Nossacin*; *Noxigram*; *Quinoxin*; *Uronorm*
(International brand names outside U.S. in italics)

DESCRIPTION:

Cinoxacin is a synthetic antibacterial agent for oral administration. It is 1-ethyl-1, 4-dihydro-4-oxo-[1,3] dioxolo[4,5-g] cinnoline-3-carboxylic acid and occurs as white or very light-yellow, needle-shaped crystals. Cinoxacin is available as 250- (0.95 mmol) and 500-mg (1.9 mmol) capsules. These capsules also contain D&C Yellow No. 10, FD&C Blue No. 1, FD&C Red No. 3, FD&C Yellow No. 6, gelatin, silicon dioxide, silicon fluid, sodium lauryl sulfate, starch, titanium dioxide, and other inactive ingredients.

The molecular formula is $C_{12}H_{10}N_2O_5$ and the molecular weight is 262.22.

CLINICAL PHARMACOLOGY:

Cinoxacin is rapidly absorbed after oral administration. In fluorometric assay, a 500-mg dose produced a peak serum concentration of 15 mcg/ml, which declined to approximately 1 to 2 mcg/ml 6 hours after administration, as determined by fluorometric assay. A 500 mg dose produced an average urine concentration of approximately 300 mcg/ml during the first 4 hours and approximately 100 mcg/ml during the second 4-hour period. These urine concentrations are many times greater than the minimal inhibitory concentration (MIC) of cinoxacin for most gram-negative organisms commonly found in urinary tract infections.

Ninety-seven percent of a 500-mg oral dose of radiolabeled cinoxacin was recovered in the urine within 24 hours, 60% of which was present as unaltered cinoxacin and the remainder as inactive metabolic products.

The presence of food did not affect the total absorption of cinoxacin. Peak serum concentrations were reduced by 30%, but the 24-hour urinary recovery of antibacterial activity was unaltered. The mean serum half-life is 1.5 hours.

Microbiology: Cinoxacin has *in vitro* activity against many gram-negative aerobic bacteria, particularly strains of *Enterobacteriaceae.* Cinoxacin inhibits bacterial deoxyribonucleic acid (DNA) synthesis, is bactericidal, and is active over the entire urinary pH range. Cross-resistance with nalidixic acid has been demonstrated.

Conventional chromosomal resistance to cinoxacin taken at recommended doses has been reported to emerge in approximately 4% of patients during treatment; however, bactericidal resistance to cinoxacin has not been shown to be transferable via R-factor. Cinoxacin has been shown to be active against most strains of the following organisms both *in vitro* and in clinical infections (see INDICATIONS AND USAGE):

Gram-Negative Aerobes:

Enterobacter species,

Escherichia coli, Klebsiella species,

Proteus mirabilis,

Proteus vulgaris

Note: *Enterococcus* species, *Pseudomonas* species, and *Staphylococcus* species are resistant.

Susceptibility Testing: Diffusion Techniques: Quantitative methods that require measurement of zone diameters give an estimate of bacterial susceptibility. One such procedure is the National Committee for Clinical Laboratory Standards (NCCLS) approved procedure (M2-A4— Performance Standards for Antimicrobial Disk Susceptibility Tests 1990). This method has been recommended for use with the 100-mcg cinoxacin disk to test susceptibility to cinoxacin.

CLINICAL PHARMACOLOGY: *(cont'd)*

Interpretation involves correlation of the diameters, obtained in the disk test with minimum inhibitory concentrations (MIC) for cinoxacin. Reports from the laboratory giving results of the standard single-disk susceptibility test with a 100-mcg cinoxacin disk should be interpreted according to the following criteria **(these criteria apply only to isolates from urinary tract infections):** (TABLE 1)

TABLE 1

Zone diameter (mm)	Interpretation
≥19	(S) Susceptible
15-18	(I) Intermediate
≤14	(R) Resistant

A report of "susceptible" indicates that the pathogen is likely to be inhibited by generally achievable urine levels. A report of "intermediate" indicates that the test results be considered equivocal or indeterminate. A report of "resistant" indicates that achievable concentrations of the antibiotic are unlikely to be inhibitory and other therapy should be selected.

Certain strains of *Enterobacteriaceae* exhibit heterogeneity of resistance to cinoxacin. These strains produce isolated colonies with the inhibition zone. When such strains are encountered, the clear inhibition zone should be measured within the isolated colonies.

Standardized procedures require the use of laboratory control organisms. The 100-mcg cinoxacin disk should give the following zone diameter (TABLE 2):

TABLE 2

Organism	Zone Diameter
E. coli ATCC 25922	26-32

Other quinolone antibacterial disks should not be substituted when performing susceptibility tests for cinoxacin because of spectrum differences between cinoxacin and other quinolones. The 100-mcg cinoxacin disk should be used for all *in vitro* t esting of isolates.

Dilution Techniques: Broth and agar dilution methods, such as those recommended by the NCCLS (M7-A2-Methods for Dilution Antimicrobial Susceptibility Tests for Bacteria that Grow Aerobically 1990), may be used to determine the MIC of cinoxacin. MIC test results should be interpreted according to the following criteria **(these criteria only apply to isolates from urinary tract infections)** (TABLE 3):

TABLE 3

MIC (mcg/ml)	Interpretation
≥16	(S) Susceptible
32	(I) Intermediate
≤64	(R) Resistant

As with standard diffusion methods, dilution require the use of laboratory control organisms. Standard cinoxacin powder should give the following MIC values (TABLE 4):

TABLE 4

Organism	MIC range (mcg/ml)
E. coli ATCC 25922	2.0 - 8.0

INDICATIONS AND USAGE:

Cinoxacin is indicated for the treatment of initial and recurrent urinary tract infections in adults caused by the following susceptible microorganisms:

Escherichia Coli, Proteus Mirabilis, Proteus Vulgaris, Klebsiella species (including *K. Pneumoniae*), and *Enterobacter* species.

Cinoxacin is effective in preventing urinary tract infections for up to 5 months in women with a history of recurrent urinary tract infections.

In vitro susceptibility testing should be performed prior to administration of the drug and, when clinically indicated, during treatment.

CONTRAINDICATIONS:

Cinoxacin is contraindicated in patients with a history of hypersensitivity to cinoxacin or other quinolones.

WARNINGS:

THE SAFETY AND EFFECTIVENESS OF CINOXACIN IN CHILDREN, ADOLESCENT (UNDER THE AGE OF 18 YEARS), PREGNANT WOMEN AND LACTATING WOMEN HAVE NOT BEEN ESTABLISHED. (SEE PEDIATRIC USE, PREGNANCY, AND NURSING MOTHERS SUBSECTIONS IN THE PRECAUTIONS SECTIONS).

The oral administration of a single 250-mg/kg dose of cinoxacin causes lameness in immature dogs. Histopathological examination of the weight-bearing joints of these dogs revealed lesions of the cartilage. Other quinolones also produce erosions of cartilage of weight-bearing joints and other signs of arthropathy in immature animals of various species.

Serious and occasionally fatal hypersensitivity (anaphylactic) reactions, some following the first dose, have been reported in patients receiving quinolone class antimicrobials. Some reactions were accompanied by cardiovascular collapse, loss of consciousness, tingling, pharyngeal or facial edema, dyspnea, urticaria, and itching. Only a few patients had a history of previous hypersensitivity reactions. If an allergic reaction to cinoxacin occurs, discontinue the drug. Serious acute hypersensitivity reactions may require treatment with epinephrine and other resuscitative measures, including oxygen, intravenous fluids, intravenous antihistamines, corticosteroids, pressor amines, and airway management as clinically indicated.

Convulsions and abnormal electroencephalograms have been reported in a few patients receiving quinolone class antimicrobials. No causal relationship has been established. Convulsions, increased intracranial pressure, and toxic psychoses have also been reported in patients receiving other drugs in this class.

Quinolones may also cause central nervous system (CNS) stimulation with tremors, restlessness, light-headedness, confusion, or hallucinations. If these reactions occur in patients receiving cinoxacin, the drug should be discontinued, and appropriate measures instituted. As with all quinolones, cinoxacin should be used with caution in patients with known or suspected CNS disorders, such as severe cerebral arteriosclerosis, epilepsy, and other factors that predispose to seizures (see ADVERSE REACTIONS.)

PRECAUTIONS:

GENERAL

Since Cinoxacin is eliminated primarily by the kidney, the usual dosage should be lower in patients with reduced renal function (See DOSAGE AND ADMINISTRATION.) Administration of cinoxacin is not recommended for anuric patients.

In clinical trials with large doses of quinolones, crystalluria was reported in some volunteers. Although crystalluria is not expected to occur with the usually recommended dosages of cinoxacin, patients should be well hydrated, and alkinalization of urine should be avoided.

Moderate to severe phototoxicity reactions have been observed in patients who were exposed to direction sunlight while receiving some members of this drug class. Excessive sunlight should be avoided. Therapy should be discontinued if phototoxicity occurs.

As with any potent drug, periodic assessment of organ system function, including renal, hepatic, and hematopoietic function, is advisable during prolonged therapy.

INFORMATION FOR THE PATIENT

Patients should be advised that cinoxacin may be taken with or without meals. Patients should drink fluid liberally. Since sucralfate or antacids affect the absorption of certain quinolones, patients should not take sucralfate or antacids within 2 hours of the administration of cinoxacin.

Patients should be advised to avoid excessive sunlight during cinoxacin therapy. If phototoxicity occurs, cinoxacin therapy should be discontinued.

Cinoxacin may be associated with hypersensitivity reactions following even a single dose. The drug should be discontinued at the first signs of skin rash or allergic reaction.

Cinoxacin can cause dizziness and light-headedness; therefore, patients should know how they react to the drug before operating an automobile or machinery or engaging in activity requiring mental alertness or coordination.

Patients should be advised that cinoxacin may increase the effects of theophylline and caffeine. There is a possibility of caffeine accumulation when products containing caffeine are consumed during cinoxacin therapy.

PREGNANCY, TERATOGENIC EFFECTS, PREGNANCY CATEGORY C

Reproduction studies have been performed in rats and rabbits at doses up to 10 times the daily human dose and have revealed no evidence of impaired fertility or harm to the fetus due to cinoxacin. There are, however, no adequate and well-controlled studies in pregnant women. Cinoxacin should be used during pregnancy only if the potential benefit justifies the potential risk to the fetus (see WARNINGS).

NURSING MOTHERS

It is not known whether cinoxacin is excreted in human milk. Because other drugs in this class are excreted in human milk and because of the potential for serious adverse reactions from cinoxacin in nursing infants, a decision should be made whether to discontinue nursing or to discontinue the drug, taking into account the importance of the drug to the mother.

PEDIATRIC USE

Safety and effectiveness in children and adolescents below the age of 18 years have not been established. Cinoxacin causes arthropathy in juvenile animals (see WARNINGS).

DRUG INTERACTIONS:

Elevated plasma levels of theophylline have been reported with concomitant use of some quinolones. There have been reports of theophylline-related side-effects in patients on concomitant theophylline-quinolone therapy. Therefore, monitoring of theophylline plasma levels should be considered and dosage of theophylline adjusted as required.

Quinolones have also been shown to interfere with the metabolism of caffeine. This may lead to reduced clearance of caffeine and a prolongation of its plasma half-life. Although this interaction has not been reported with cinoxacin, caution should be exercised when cinoxacin is given concomitantly with caffeine-containing products.

Antacids or sucralfate substantially interfere with the absorption of some quinolones, resulting in low urine levels. Also, concomitant administration of quinolones with products containing iron or multivitamins containing zinc may result in low urine levels.

Quinolones, including cinoxacin, may enhance the effects of oral anticoagulants, such as warfarin or its derivatives. When these products are administered concomitantly, prothrombin time or other suitable coagulation tests should be closely monitored.

Seizures have been reported in patients taking another quinolone class antimicrobial and the nonsteroidal anti-inflammatory drug fenbufen concurrently. Animal studies also suggest an increased potential for seizures when these 2 drugs are given concomitantly. Fenbufen is not approved in the United States at this time. Physicians are provided this information to increase awareness of the potential for serious interactions when cinoxacin and certain nonsteroidal anti-inflammatory agents are administered concomitantly.

Elevated cyclosporine serum levels have been reported with the concomitant use of quinolone and cyclosporine.

ADVERSE REACTIONS:

In clinical studies involving 1,118 patients, the following adverse effects were considered to be related to cinoxacin therapy:

Gastrointestinal: Nausea was reported most commonly and occurred in less than 3 in 100 patients. Other side effects, occurring less frequently (1 in 100), were anorexia, vomiting, abdominal cramps/pain, perverse taste, and diarrhea.

Central Nervous System: The most frequent side effects were headache and dizziness, reported by 1 in 100 patients. Other adverse reactions possibly related to cinoxacin include insomnia, drowsiness, tingling sensation, perineal burning, photophobia, and tinnitus. These were reported by less than 1 in 100 patients.

Hypersensitivity: Rash, urticaria, pruritus, edema, angioedema, and eosinophilia were reported by less than 3 in 100 patients. Rare cases of anaphylactoid reactions have been reported. Toxic epidermal-necrolysis has been reported very rarely. Erythema multiforme and Stevens-Johnson syndrome have been reported with cinoxacin and other drugs in this class.

Hematologic: Rare reports of thrombocytopenia.

Laboratory values that were reported to be abnormal were, in order of frequency, BUN (1 in 100), AST (SGOT), ALT (SGPT), serum creatinine, alkaline phosphatase, and reduction in hematocrit/hemoglobin (each less than 1 in 100).

Although not observed in the 1,118 patients treated with cinoxacin, the following side effects have been reported for other drugs in the same pharmacologically active and chemically related class: restlessness, nervousness, change in color perception, difficulty in focusing, decrease in visual acuity, double vision, weakness, constipation, erythema and bullae, feelings of disorientation or agitation or acute anxiety, palpitation, soreness of the gums, joint stiffness, swelling of the extremities, and toxic psychosis or convulsions (rare). All adverse reactions observed with drugs in this class were reversible.

The most frequently reported adverse events in postmarketing surveillance of cinoxacin have not been rash and anaphylactic reactions. Other frequently reported reactions have been pruritus, urticaria, allergic reactions, nausea, abdominal pain, and headache.

OVERDOSAGE:

Signs and Symptoms: Symptoms following an overdose of cinoxacin may include anorexia, nausea, vomiting, epigastric distress, and diarrhea. The severity of the epigastric distress and the diarrhea are dose related. Headache, dizziness, insomnia, photophobia, tinnitus, and a tingling sensation have been reported in some patients. If other symptoms are present, they are probably secondary to an underlying disease state, an allergic reaction, or the ingestion of a second medication with toxicity.

Treatment: In all cases of suspected overdosage, call your regional Poison Control Center to obtain the most up-to-date information about the treatment of overdose. This recommendation is made because, in general, information regarding the treatment of overdosage may change more rapidly than do package inserts.

In managing overdosage, consider the possibility of multiple drug overdoses, interaction among drugs, and unusual drug kinetics in your patient.

Patients who have ingested an overdose of cinoxacin should be kept well hydrated to prevent crystalluria.

Protect the patient's airway and support ventilation and perfusion. Meticulously monitor and maintain, within acceptable limits, the patient's vital signs, blood gases, serum electrolytes, etc. Absorption of drugs from the gastrointestinal tract may be decreased by giving activated charcoal, which, in many cases, is more effective than emesis or lavage; consider charcoal instead of, or in addition to, gastric emptying. Repeated doses of charcoal over time may hasten elimination of some drugs that have been absorbed. Safeguard the patient's airway when employing gastric emptying or charcoal.

Forced diuresis, peritoneal dialysis, hemodialysis, or charcoal hemoperfusion have not been established as beneficial for an overdose of cinoxacin.

DOSAGE AND ADMINISTRATION:

The usual adult dosage for the treatment of urinary tract infections is 1 g daily, administered orally in 2 or 4 divided doses (500 mg b.i.d. or 250 mg q.i.d. respectively) for 7 to 14 days. Although susceptible organisms may be eradicated within a few days after therapy has begun, the full treatment course is recommended.

Impaired Renal Function: When renal function is impaired, a reduced dosage must be employed. After an initial dose of 500 mg, a maintenance dosage schedule should be used (See TABLE 5.)

TABLE 5 MAINTENANCE DOSAGE GUIDE FOR PATIENTS WITH RENAL IMPAIRMENT

Creatinine Clearance	Renal Function	Dosage (ml/min/1.73 m^2)
> 80	Normal	500 mg b.i.d.
80-50	Mild Impairment	250 mg t.i.d.
50-20	Moderate Impairment	250 mg b.i.d.
< 20	Marked Impairment	250 mg q.d.

Administration of cinoxacin to anuric patients is not recommended.

When only serum creatinine is available, the following formula (based on sex, weight, and age of the patient) may be used to convert this value into creatinine clearance.

The serum creatinine should represent a steady state of renal function (TABLE 6).

TABLE 6

Males: [Weight (kg) × (140 - age)] ÷ [72 × serum creatinine]
Females: 0.9 × male value

Preventive Therapy: A single dose of 250 mg at bedtime for up to 5 months has been shown to be effective in women with a history of recurrent urinary tract infections.

Store at controlled room temperature, 59° to 86°F (15° to 30°C).

ANIMAL PHARMACOLOGY:

Crystalluria, sometimes associated with secondary urinary tract pathology, occurs in laboratory animals treated orally with cinoxacin. In the rhesus monkey, crystalluria (without urinary tract pathology) has been noted at doses as low as 50 mg/kg/day (lowest dose tested). Cinoxacin-related crystalluria has not been observed in humans receiving twice the recommended daily dosage.

Cinoxacin and other quinolones have been shown to cause arthropathy in immature animals of most species tested (see WARNINGS).

Some drugs of this class have been shown to have occulotoxic potential. Cinoxacin administered to cats at high dosages (200 mg/kg/day) resulted in retinal degeneration and other ocular changes. The dog appeared to be somewhat resistant to these effects to these effects, but high dosages (500 mg/kg/day) resulted in mild retinal atrophy. No cinoxacin-related ocular changes were noted in rabbit, rat, monkey, or human studies. (In one of the studies involving the monkey, cinoxacin was administered for 1 year at 10 times the recommended clinical dose.)

HOW SUPPLIED - RATED THERAPEUTICALLY EQUIVALENT:

Capsule - Oral - 500 mg

50's	**$102.93**	**CINOBAC, Oclassen Pharms**	**55515-0056-04**

Capsule, Gelatin - Oral - 250 mg

40's	$35.70	Cinoxacin, Teva	00332-3179-06
40's	**$45.60**	**CINOBAC, Oclassen Pharms**	**55515-0055-02**

Capsule, Gelatin - Oral - 500 mg

50's	$77.60	Cinoxacin, Teva	00332-3181-07
50's	$85.00	Cinoxacin, Goldline Labs	00182-1957-19
50's	$95.69	Cinoxacin, HL Moore Drug Exch	00839-7757-04

CIPROFLOXACIN HYDROCHLORIDE *(000823)*

CATEGORIES: Anti-Infectives; Antibacterials; Antibiotics; Antimicrobials; Bone Infections; Diarrhea; EENT Drugs; Eye, Ear, Nose, & Throat Preparations; Fluoroquinolones; Gonorrhea; Infections; Joint Infections; Quinolones; Respiratory Tract Infections; Skin Infections; Typhoid Fever; Urinary Antibacterial; Urinary Tract Infections; Cystic Fibrosis*; Tuberculosis*; Pregnancy Category C; Sales > $500 Million; FDA Approved 1987 Oct; Top 200 Drugs

* Indication not approved by the FDA

BRAND NAMES: *Alcon Cilox*; *Bacquinor*; *Baflox*; *Baycip*; *Bernoflox*; *Bi-Cipro*; *Cetraxal*; *Ciflox* (France); *Cifloxin*; *Cifran*; *Cilab*; Ciloxan; *Cimogal* (Mexico); *Ciplox*; *Ciplus*; *Ciprecu*; *Ciprinol*; **Cipro**; *Ciprobay* (Germany); *Ciprobay Uro* (Germany); *Ciprobid*; *Ciprobiotic*; *Ciprocinol*; *Ciprodar*; *Ciproflox* (Mexico); *Ciprogis*; *Ciprok*; *Ciprolin*; *Ciprolon*; *Cipromycin*; *Ciproquinol*; *Ciproxan* (Japan); *Ciproxin* (Australia, England); *Ciproxina* (Mexico); *Ciproxine*; *Ciprowin*; *Ciriax*; *Citopcin*; *Cixan*; *Corsacin*; *Cosflox*; *Cycin*; *Cyprobay*; *Eni* (Mexico); *Fimoflox*; *Italnik* (Mexico); *Ipiflox*; *Kenzoflex* (Mexico); *Loxan*; *Medociprin*; *Mitroken* (Mexico); *Nivoflox* (Mexico); *Probiox*; *Proflaxin*; *Proflox*; *Proksi 250*; *Proksi 500*; *Quinolid*; *Quintor*; *Rancif*; *Roxytal*; *Septicide*; *Sophixin Ofteno* (Mexico); *Spitacin*; *Superocin*; *Unex*; *Uniflox* (France); *Zumaflox*

(International brand names outside U.S. in italics)

FORMULARIES: Aetna; BC-BS; Medi-Cal; PCS; WHO

COST OF THERAPY: $39.20 (Urinary Infections; Tablet; 250 mg; 2/day; 7 days)

DESCRIPTION:

Note: This monograph contains full prescribing information for the tablet form of ciprofloxacin hydrochloride and information for the intravenous form in the DESCRIPTION, CLINICAL PHARMACOLOGY, DOSAGE AND ADMINISTRATION and HOW SUPPLIEDsections.

TABLETS

Ciprofloxacin hydrochloride is a synthetic broad spectrum antibacterial agent for oral administration. Ciprofloxacin, a fluoroquinolone, is available as the monohydrochloride monohydrate salt of 1-cyclopropyl-6-fluoro-1, 4-dihydro -4-oxo-7- (1- piperazinyl) -3-quinolinecarboxylic acid. It is a faintly yellowish to light yellow crystalline substance with a molecular weight of 385.8. Its empirical formula is $C_{17}H_{18}FN_3O_3{\cdot}HCl{\cdot}H_2O$.

Ciprofloxacin is available in 250 mg, 500 mg and 750 mg (ciprofloxacin equivalent) film-coated tablets. The inactive ingredients are starch, microcrystalline cellulose, silicon dioxide, crospovidone, magnesium stearate, hydroxypropyl methylcellulose, titanium dioxide, polyethylene glycol and water. Ciprofloxacin differs from other quinolones in that it has a fluorine atom at the 6-position, a piperazine moiety at the 7-position, and a cyclopropyl ring at the 1-position.

INTRAVENOUS ADMINISTRATION

Ciprofloxacin is a synthetic broad-spectrum antimicrobial agent for IV administration.

Ciprofloxacin is a faint to light yellow crystalline powder with a molecular weight of 331.4. It is soluble in dilute (0.1N) hydrochloric acid and is practically in soluble in water and ethanol. Ciprofloxacin differs from other quinolones in that it has a fluorine atom at the 6- position, a piperazine moiety at the 7-position, and a cyclopropyl ring at the 1-position. Cipro IV solutions are available as 1.0% aqueous concentrates, which are intended for dilution prior to administration, and as a 0.2% ready-for-use infusion solution in 5% Dextrose Injection. All formulas contain lactic acid as a solubilizing agent and hydrochloric acid for pH adjustment. The pH range for the 0.2% ready-for-use infusion solutions is 3.5 to 4.6.

The plastic container is fabricated from a specially formulated polyvinyl chloride. Solutions in contact with the plastic container can leach out of its chemical components in very small amounts within the expiration period, e.g. di(2-ethylhexyl) phthalate (DEHP), up to 5 parts per million. The suitability of the plastic has been confirmed in tests in animals according to USP biological tests for plastic containers as well as by tissue culture toxicity studies.

CLINICAL PHARMACOLOGY:

TABLETS

Cipro tablets are rapidly and well absorbed from the gastrointestinal tract after oral administration. The absolute bioavailability is approximately 70% with no substantial loss by first pass metabolism. Serum concentrations increase proportionately with the dose as shown in TABLE 1.

TABLE 1

Dose (mg)	Maximum Serum Concentration (mcg/ml)	Area Under Curve (AUC) (mcg · hr/ml)
250	1.2	4.8
500	2.4	11.6
750	4.3	20.2
1000	5.4	30.8

Maximum serum concentrations are attained 1 to 2 hours after oral dosing. Mean concentrations 12 hours after dosing with 250, 500, or 750 mg are 0.1, 0.2, and 0.4 mcg/ml, respectively. The serum elimination half-life in subjects with normal renal function is approximately 4 hours.

Approximately 40 to 50% of an orally administered dose is excreted in the urine as unchanged drug. After a 250 mg oral dose, urine concentrations of ciprofloxacin usually exceed 200 mcg/ml during the first two hours and are approximately 30 mcg/ml at 8 to 12 hours after dosing. The urinary excretion of ciprofloxacin is virtually complete within 24 hours after dosing. The renal clearance of ciprofloxacin, which is approximately 300 ml/minute, exceeds the normal glomerular filtration rate of 120 ml/minute. Thus, active tubular secretion would seem to play a significant role in its elimination. Co-administration of probenecid with ciprofloxacin results in about a 50% reduction in the ciprofloxacin renal clearance and a 50% increase in its concentration in the systemic circulation. Although bile concentration of ciprofloxacin are several fold higher than serum concentrations after oral dosing, only a small amount of the dose administrated is recovered from the bile as unchanged drug. An additional 1-2% of the dose is recovered from the bile in the form of metabolites. Approximately 20 to 35% of an oral dose is recovered from the feces within 5 days after dosing. This may arise from either biliary clearance or transintestinal elimination. Four metabolites have been identified in human urine which together account for approximately 15% of an oral dose. The metabolites have antimicrobial activity, but are less active than unchanged ciprofloxacin.

When ciprofloxacin is given concomitantly with food, there is a delay in the absorption of the drug, resulting in peak concentrations that are closer to 2 hours after dosing rather than 1 hour. The overall absorption, however, is not substantially affected. Concurrent administration of antacids containing magnesium hydroxide or aluminum hydroxide may reduce the bioavailability of ciprofloxacin by as much as 90% (see PRECAUTIONS).

Concomitant administration of ciprofloxacin with theophylline decreases the clearance of theophylline resulting in elevated serum theophylline levels, and increased risk of a patient developing CNS or other adverse reactions. Ciprofloxacin also decreases caffeine clearance and inhibits the formation of paraxanthine after caffeine administration. (See PRECAUTIONS.)

In patients with reduced renal function, the half-life of ciprofloxacin is slightly prolonged. Dosage adjustments may be required (See DOSAGE AND ADMINISTRATION.)

In preliminary studies in patients with stable chronic liver cirrhosis, no significant changes in ciprofloxacin pharmacokinetics have been observed. The kinetics for ciprofloxacin in patients with acute hepatic insufficiency, however, have not been fully elucidated.

The binding of ciprofloxacin to serum proteins is 20 to 40% which is not likely to be high enough to cause significant protein binding interactions with other drugs.

CLINICAL PHARMACOLOGY: *(cont'd)*

After oral administration ciprofloxacin is widely distributed throughout the body. Tissue concentrations often exceed serum concentrations in both men and women, particularly in genital tissue including the prostate. Ciprofloxacin is present in active form in the saliva, nasal and bronchial secretions, sputum, skin blister fluid, lymph, peritoneal fluid, bile and prostatic secretions. Ciprofloxacin has also been detected in lung, skin, fat, muscle, cartilage, and bone. The drug diffuses into the cerebrospinal fluid (CSF); however, CSF concentrations are generally less than 10% of peak serum concentrations. Low levels of the drug have been detected in the aqueous and vitreous humors of the eye.

INTRAVENOUS

Following 60-minute intravenous infusions of 200 mg and 400 mg ciprofloxacin to normal volunteers, the mean maximum serum concentrations achieved were 2.1 and 4.6 mcg/ml, respectively; the concentrations at 12 hours were 0.1 and 0.2 mcg/ml respectively. (TABLE 2)

TABLE 2 Steady-state Ciprofloxacin Serum Concentrations (mcg/ml) After 60-minute IV Infusions q 12 h.

	Time after starting the infusion					
Dose	30 min	1 hr	3 hr	6 hr	8 hr	12 hr
200 mg	1.7	2.1	0.6	0.3	0.2	0.1
400 mg	3.7	4.6	1.3	0.7	0.5	0.2

The pharmacokinetics of ciprofloxacin are linear over the dose range of 200 to 400 mg administered intravenously. The serum elimination half-life is approximately 5-6 hours and the total clearance is around 35 l/hr. Comparison of the pharmacokinetic parameters following the 1st and 5th iv dose on a q 12 h regimen indicates no evidence of drug accumulation.

The absolute bioavailability of oral ciprofloxacin is within a range 70- 80% with no substantial loss by first pass metabolism. An intravenous infusion of 400 mg ciprofloxacin given over 60 minutes every 12 hours has been shown to produce an area under the serum concentration time curve (AUC) equivalent to that produced by a 500 mg oral dose given every 12 hours. A 400 mg iv dose administered over 60 minutes every 12 hours results in C_{max} similar to that observed with a 750 mg oral dose. An infusion of 200 mg ciprofloxacin given every 12 hours produces an AUC equivalent to that produced by a 250 mg oral dose given every 12 hours.

After intravenous administration, approximately 50% to 70% of the dose is excreted in the urine as unchanged drug. Following a 200 mg iv dose, concentrations in the urine usually exceed 200 mcg/ml 0-2 hours after dosing and are generally greater than 15 mcg/ml 8-12 hours after dosing. Following a 400 mg IV dose, urine concentrations generally exceed 400 mcg/ml 0-2 hours after dosing and are usually greater than 30 mcg/ml 8-12 hours after dosing. The renal clearance is approximately 22 L/hr. The urinary excretion of ciprofloxacin is virtually complete by 24 hours after dosing.

Co-administration of probenecid with ciprofloxacin results in about a 50% reduction in the ciprofloxacin renal clearance and a 50% increase in its concentration in the systemic circulation. Although bile concentrations of ciprofloxacin are serveralfold higher than serum concentrations after intravenous dosing, only a small amount of the administered dose (<1%) is recovered from the bile as unchanged drug. Approximately 15% of an IV dose is recovered from the feces within 5 days after dosing.

After IV administration, three metabolites of ciprofloxacin have been identified in human urine which together account for approximately 10% of the intravenous dose.

In patients with reduced renal function, the half-life of ciprofloxacin is slightly prolonged and dosage adjustments may be required (See DOSAGE AND ADMINISTRATION.)

In preliminary studies in patients with stable chronic liver cirrhosis, no significant changes in ciprofloxacin pharmacokinetics have been observed. However, the kinetics for ciprofloxacin in patients with acute hepatic insufficiency have not been fully elucidated.

The binding of ciprofloxacin to serum proteins is 20 to 40%.

After intravenous administration, ciprofloxacin is present in saliva, nasal and bronchial secretions, sputum, skin blister fluid, lymph, peritoneal fluid, bile and prostatic secretions. It has also been detected in the lung, skin, fat muscle, cartilage and bone. Although the drug diffuses into cerebrospinal fluid (CSF), CSF concentrations are generally less than 10% of peak serum concentrations. Levels of the drug in the aqueous and vitreous chambers of the eye are lower than in serum.

MICROBIOLOGY

Ciprofloxacin has *in vitro* activity against a wide range of gram-negative and gram-positive organisms. The bactericidal action of ciprofloxacin results from interference with the enzyme DNA gyrase which is needed for the synthesis of bacterial DNA.

Ciprofloxacin has been shown to be active against most strains of the following organisms both *in vitro* and in clinical infections (See INDICATIONS AND USAGE):

Gram-Positive Bacteria:

Enterococcus faecalis, (Many strains are only moderately susceptible)
Staphylococcus aureus
Staphylococcus epidermidis
Streptococcus pneumoniae
Streptococcus pyogenes

Gram-Negative Bacteria:

Campylobacter jejuni
Citrobacter diversus
Citrobacter freundii
Enterobacter cloacae
Escherichia coli
Haemophilus influenzae
Haemophilus parainfluenzae
Klebsiella pneumoniae
Morganella morganii
Neisseria gonorrhoeae
Proteus mirabilis
Proteus vulgaris
Providencia rettgeri
Providencia stuartii
Pseudomonas aeruginosa
Salmonella typhi
Serratia marcescens
Shigella flexneri
Shigella sonnei

Ciprofloxacin has been shown to be active *in vitro* against most strains of the following organisms; however, *the clinical significance of these data is unknown.*

Gram-Positive Bacteria:

Staphylococcus haemolyticus
Staphylococcus hominis
Staphylococcus saprophyticus

Gram-Negative Bacteria:

Acinetobacter calcoaceticus subs. *anitratus*
Acinetobacter calcoaceticus subs. *Iwoffi*
Aeromonas caviae
Aeromonas hydrophila
Brucella melitensis
Campylobacter coli
Edwardsiella tarda
Enterobacter aerogenes
Haemophilus ducreyi
Klebsiella oxytoca
Legionella pneumophila
Moraxella (Branhamella) catarrhalis
Neisseria gonorrhoeae
Neisseria meningitidis
Pasteurella multocida
Salmonella enteritidis
Salmonella typhi
Vibrio cholerae
Vibrio parahaemolyticus
Vibrio vulnificus
Yersinia enterocolitica

Other Organisms:

Chlamydia trachomatis (only moderately susceptible)
Mycobacterium tuberculosis (only moderately susceptible)

CLINICAL PHARMACOLOGY: *(cont'd)*

Most strains of *Pseudomonas cepacia* and some strains of*Pseudomonas maltophilia* are resistant to ciprofloxacin as are most anaerobic bacteria, including *Bacteroides fragilis* and *Clostridium difficile.*

Ciprofloxacin is slightly less active when tested at acidic pH. The inoculum size has little effect when tested *in vitro.* The minimum bactericidal concentration (MBC) generally does not exceed the minimum inhibitory concentration (MIC) by more than a factor of 2. Resistance to ciprofloxacin *in vitro* develops slowly (multiple-step mutation).

Ciprofloxacin does not cross-react with other antimicrobial agents such a beta-lactams or aminoglycosides; therefore, organisms resistant to these drugs may be susceptible to ciprofloxacin.

In vitro studies have shown that additive activity often results when ciprofloxacin is combined with other antimicrobial agents such as beat-lactams, aminoglycosides, clindamycin, or metronidazole. Synergy has been reported particularly with the combination of ciprofloxacin and beta-lactam; antagonism is observed only rarely.

CLINICAL STUDIES:

SUSCEPTIBILITY TESTS

Diffusion Techniques: Quantitative methods that require measurement of zone diameters give the most precise estimates of susceptibility of bacteria to antimicrobial agents. One such standardized procedure[1] which has been recommended for use with disks to test susceptibility of organisms to ciprofloxacin uses the 5-mcg ciprofloxacin disk. Interpretation involves correlation of the diameters obtained in the disk test with the minimum inhibitory concentrations (MICs) for ciprofloxacin.

Reports from the laboratory giving results of the standard single-disk susceptibility test with a 5-mcg ciprofloxacin disk should be interpreted according to the criteria found in TABLE 3.

TABLE 3

Zone Diameter (mm)	Interpretation
≥ 21	(S) Susceptible
16 - 20	(I) Intermediate (Moderately Susceptible)
≤ 15	(R) Resistant

A report of "Susceptible" indicates that the pathogen is likely to be inhibited by generally achievable blood levels. A report of "Intermediate (Moderately Susceptible)" suggests that the organism would be susceptible if high dosage is used or if the infection is confined to tissues and fluids in which high antimicrobial levels are attained. A report of "Resistant" indicates that achievable drug concentrations are unlikely to be inhibitory and other therapy should be selected.

Dilution Techniques: Use a standardized dilution method[2] (broth, agar, microdilution) or equivalent with ciprofloxacin powder. The MIC values obtained should be interpreted according to the criteria in TABLE 4.

TABLE 4

MIC (mcg/ml)	Interpretation
≤ 1	(S) Susceptible
2	(I) Intermediate (Moderately Susceptible)
≥ 4	(R) Resistant

Standardized procedures require the use of laboratory control organisms. This is true for both standardized diffusion techniques and standardized dilution techniques. The 5-mcg ciprofloxacin disk should give the following zone diameters and the standard ciprofloxacin powder should provide the following MIC values: (TABLE 5)

TABLE 5

QC Strains	Disk Zone Diameter (mm)	MIC (mcg/ml)
S. aureus (ATCC 25923)	22 - 30	—
S. aureus (ATCC 29213)	—	0.12 - 0.5
E. coli (ATCC 25922)	30 - 40	0.004 - 0.015
P. aeruginosa (ATCC 27853)	25 - 33	0.25 - 1.0
E. faecalis (ATCC 29212)	—	0.25 - 2.0

For anaerobic bacteria the MIC of ciprofloxacin can be determined by agar or broth dilution (including microdilution) techniques[3].

INDICATIONS AND USAGE:

Ciprofloxacin is indicated for the treatment of infections caused by susceptible strains of the designated microorganisms in the conditions listed below. (Please see DOSAGE AND ADMINISTRATION for specific recommendations.)

Lower Respiratory Infections: *Escherichia coli, Klebsiella pneumoniae, Enterobacter cloacae, Proteus mirabilis, Pseudomonas aeruginosa, Haemophilus influenzae, Haemophilus parainfluenzae,* or *Streptococcus pneumoniae.*

Skin and Skin Structure Infections: *Escherichia coli, Klebsiella pneumoniae, Enterobacter cloacae, Proteus mirabilis, Proteus vulgaris, Providencia stuartii, Morganella morganii, Citrobacter freundii, Pseudomonas aeruginosa, Staphylococcus aureus, Staphylococcus epidermidis,* or *Streptococcus pyogenes*

Bone and Joint Infections: *Enterobacter cloacae, Serratia marcescens,* or *Pseudomonas aeruginosa.*

Urinary Tract Infections: *Escherichia coli, klebsiella pneumoniae, Enterobacter cloacae, Serratia marcescens, proteus mirabilis, Providencia rettgeri, Morganella morganii, Citrobacter diversus, Citrobacter freundii, Pseudomonas aeruginosa, Staphylococcus epidermidis,* or *Enterococcus faecalis*

Typhoid Fever (Enteric Fever): *Salmonella typhi* NOTE: The efficacy of ciprofloxacin in the eradication of the chronic typhoid carrier state has not been demonstrated.

Sexually Transmitted Diseases: (See WARNINGS.) Uncomplicated cervical and urethral gonorrhea due to *Neisseria gonorrhoeae.*

Infectious Diarrhea: *Escherichia coli* (enterotoxigenic strains), *Campylobacter jejuni, Shigella flexneri** or *Shigella sonnei** when antibacterial therapy is indicated.

*Although treatment of infections due to this organism in this organ system demonstrated a clinically significant outcome, efficacy was studied in fewer than 10 patients.

If anaerobic organisms are suspected of contributing to the infection, appropriate therapy should be administered.

Appropriate culture and susceptibility tests should be performed before treatment in order to isolate and identify organisms causing infection and to determine their susceptibility to ciprofloxacin. Therapy with ciprofloxacin may be initiated before results of these tests are known; once results become available appropriate therapy should be continued. As with other

INDICATIONS AND USAGE: *(cont'd)*

drugs, some strains of *Pseudomonas aeruginosa* may develop resistance fairly rapidly during treatment with ciprofloxacin. Culture and susceptibility testing performed periodically during therapy will provide information not only on the therapeutic effect of the antimicrobial agent but also on the possible emergence of bacterial resistance.

CONTRAINDICATIONS:

Ciprofloxacin hydrochloride is contraindicated in persons with a history of hypersensitivity to ciprofloxacin or any member of the quinolone class of antimicrobial agents.

WARNINGS:

THE SAFETY AND EFFECTIVENESS OF CIPROFLOXACIN IN CHILDREN, ADOLESCENTS (LESS THAN 18 YEARS OF AGE), PREGNANT WOMEN, AND LACTATING WOMEN HAVE NOT BEEN ESTABLISHED (SEE,Pediatric Use, Pregnancy, Teratogenic Effects, Pregnancy Category C and Nursing Mothers). The oral administration of ciprofloxacin caused lameness in immature dogs. Histopathological examination of the weight-bearing joints of these dogs revealed permanent lesions of the cartilage. Related drugs such as nalidixic acid, cinoxacin and norfloxacin also produces erosions of cartilage of weight-bearing joints and other signs of arthropathy in immature animals of various species (See ANIMAL PHARMACOLOGY.)

Convulsions have been reported in patients receiving ciprofloxacin. Convulsions, increased intracranial pressure, and toxic psychosis have been reported in patients receiving drugs in this class. Quinolones may also cause central nervous system (CNS) stimulation which may lead to tremors, restlessness, lightheadedness, confusion and hallucinations. If these reactions occur in patients receiving ciprofloxacin, the drug should be discontinued and appropriate measures instituted. As with all quinolones, ciprofloxacin should be used with caution in patients with known or suspected CNS disorders, such as severe cerebral arteriosclerosis, epilepsy, and other factors that predispose to seizures(See ADVERSE REACTIONS.)

SERIOUS AND FATAL REACTIONS HAVE BEEN REPORTED IN PATIENTS RECEIVING CONCURRENT ADMINISTRATION OF CIPROFLOXACIN AND THEOPHYLLINE. These reactions have included cardiac arrest, seizure, status epilepticus and respiratory failure. Although similar serious adverse events have been reported in patients receiving theophylline alone, the possibility that these reactions may be potentiated by ciprofloxacin cannot be eliminated. If concomitant use cannot be avoided, serum levels of theophylline should be monitored and dosage adjustments made as appropriate.

Serious and occasionally fatal hypersensitivity (anaphylactic) reactions, some following the first dose, have been reported in patients receiving quinolone therapy. Some reactions were accompanied by cardiovascular collapse, loss of consciousness, tingling, pharyngeal or facial edema, dyspnea, urticaria, and itching. Only a few patients had a history of hypersensitivity reactions. Serious anaphylactic reactions require immediate emergency treatment with epinephrine. Oxygen, intravenous steroids, and airway management, including intubation, should be administered as indicated.

Ciprofloxacin has not been shown to be effective in the treatment of syphilis. Antimicrobial agents used in high dose for short periods of time to treat gonorrhea may mask or delay the symptoms of incubating syphilis. All patients with gonorrhea should have a serologic test for syphilis at the time of diagnosis. Patients treated with ciprofloxacin should have a follow-up serologic test for syphilis at the time of diagnosis. Patients treated with ciprofloxacin should have a follow-up serologic test for syphilis after three months.

Severe hypersensitivity reactions characterized by rash, fever, eosinophilia, jaundice, and hepatic necrosis with fatal outcome have also been rarely reported in patients receiving ciprofloxacin along with other drugs. The possibility that these reactions were related to ciprofloxacin cannot be excluded. Ciprofloxacin should be discontinued at the first appearance of a skin rash or any other sign of hypersensitivity.

Pseudomembranous colitis has been reported with nearly all antibacterial agents, including ciprofloxacin, and may range in severity from mild to life-threatening. Therefore, it is important to consider this diagnosis in patients who present with diarrhea subsequent to the administration of antibacterial agents.

Treatment with antibacterial agents alters the normal flora of the colon and may permit overgrowth of clostridia. Studies indicate that a toxin produced by *Clostridium difficile* is one primary cause of "antibiotic-associated colitis".

After the diagnosis of pseudomembranous colitis has been established, therapeutic measures should be initiated. Mild cases of pseudomembranous colitis usually respond to drug discontinuation alone. In moderate to severe cases, consideration should be given to management with fluids and electrolytes, protein supplementation and treatment with an antibacterial drug clinically effective against *C. difficile* colitis.

PRECAUTIONS:

GENERAL

Tablets and Intravenous: INTRAVENOUS CIPROFLOXACIN SHOULD BE ADMINISTERED BY SLOW INFUSION OVER A PERIOD OF 60 MINUTES. Local iv site reactions have been reported with intravenous administration of ciprofloxacin. these reactions are more frequent if infusion time is 30 minutes or less or if small veins if the hand are used. (See ADVERSE REACTIONS.)

Crystals of ciprofloxacin have been observed rarely in the urine of human subjects but more frequently in the urine of laboratory animals (See ANIMAL PHARMACOLOGY.) Crystalluria related to ciprofloxacin has been reported only rarely in man because human urine is usually acidic. Alkalinity of the urine should be avoided by patients receiving ciprofloxacin. Patients should be well hydrated to prevent the formation of highly concentrated urine. Alteration of the dosage regimen s necessary for patients with impairment of renal function (See DOSAGE AND ADMINISTRATION.)

Moderate to severe phototoxicity manifested by an exaggerated sunburn reaction has been observed in patients who are exposed to direct sunlight while receiving some members of the quinolone class of drugs. Excessive sunlight should be avoided. Therapy should be discontinued if phototoxicity occurs.

As with any potent drug, periodic assessment of organ system functions, including renal, hepatic, and hematopoietic function, is advisable during prolonged therapy.

INFORMATION FOR THE PATIENT

Patients should be advised that ciprofloxacin may be taken with or without meals. The preferred time of dosing is two hours after a meal. Patients should also be advised to drink fluids liberally and not take antacids containing magnesium, aluminum, or calcium, products containing iron, or multivitamins containing zinc. However, usual dietary intake of calcium has not been shown to alter the absorption of ciprofloxacin.

Patients should be advised that ciprofloxacin may be associated with hypersensitivity reactions, even following a single dose, and to discontinue the drug at the first sign of a skin rash or other allergic reaction.

Ciprofloxacin may cause dizziness and lightheadedness; therefore patients should know how they react to this drug before they operate an automobile or machinery or engage in activities requiring mental alertness or coordination.

PRECAUTIONS: *(cont'd)*

Patients should be advised that ciprofloxacin may increase the effects of theophylline and caffeine. There is a possibility of caffeine accumulation when products containing caffeine are consumed while taking quinolones.

CARCINOGENESIS, MUTAGENESIS, AND IMPAIRMENT OF FERTILITY

Eight*in vitro* mutagenicity tests have been conducted with ciprofloxacin and the test results are listed below:

Salmonella/Microsome Test (Negative)

E. coli DNA Repair Assay (Negative)

Mouse Lymphoma Cell Forward Mutation Assay (Positive)

Chinese Hamster V_{79} Cell HGPRT Test (Negative)

Syrian Hamster Embryo Cell Transformation Assay (Negative)

*Saccharomyces cerevisiae*Point Mutation Assay (Negative)

*Saccharomyces cerevisiae*Mitotic Crossover and Gene Conversion Assay (Negative)

Rat Hepatocyte DNA Repair Assay (Positive)

Thus 2 of the 8 tests were positive but result of the following 3 *in vivo* test systems gave negative results:

Rat Hepatocyte DNA Repair Assay

Micronucleus Test (Mice)

Dominant Lethal Test (Mice)

Long term carcinogenicity studies in mice and rats have been completed. After daily oral dosing for up to 2 years, there is no evidence that ciprofloxacin had any carcinogenic or tumorigenic effects in these species.

PREGNANCY, TERATOGENIC EFFECTS, PREGNANCY CATEGORY C

Reproduction studies have been performed in rats and mice at doses up to 6 times the usual daily human dose and have revealed no evidence of impaired fertility or harm to the fetus due to ciprofloxacin. In rabbits, as with most antimicrobial agents, ciprofloxacin (30 and 100 mg/kg orally) produced gastrointestinal disturbances resulting in maternal weight loss and an increased incidence of abortion. No teratogenicity was observed at either dose. After intravenous administration, at doses up to 20 mg/kg, no maternal toxicity was produced and no embryotoxicity or teratogenicity was observed. There are, however, no adequate and well-controlled studies in pregnant women. Ciprofloxacin should be used during pregnancy only if the potential benefit justifies the potential risk to the fetus (See WARNINGS.)

NURSING MOTHERS

Ciprofloxacin is excreted in human milk. Because of the potential for serious adverse reactions in infants nursing from mothers taking ciprofloxacin, a decision should be made either to discontinue nursing or to discontinue the drug, taking into account the importance of the drug to the mother.

PEDIATRIC USE

Safety and effectiveness in children and adolescents less than 18 years of age have not been established. Ciprofloxacin causes arthropathy in juvenile animals (See WARNINGS.)

DRUG INTERACTIONS:

As with some other quinolones, concurrent administration of ciprofloxacin with theophylline may lead to elevated plasma concentrations of theophylline and prolongation of its elimination half-life. This may result in increased risk of theophylline-related adverse reactions (See WARNINGS.) If concomitant use cannot be avoided, plasma levels of theophylline should be monitored and dosage adjustments made as appropriate.

In rare instances, some quinolones including ciprofloxacin have been reported to interact with phenytoin leading to altered levels of serum phenytoin concentrations.

The concomitant administration of some quinolones, including ciprofloxacin, with the sulfonylurea glyburide has on rare occasions resulted in severe hypoglycemia.

Some quinolones, including ciprofloxacin, have also been shown to interfere with the metabolism of caffeine. This may lead to reduced clearance of caffeine and a prolongation of its serum half-life.

Concurrent administration of ciprofloxacin with antacids containing magnesium, aluminum, or calcium; with sucralfate or divalent and trivalent cautions such as iron may substantially interfere with the absorption of ciprofloxacin resulting in serum and urine levels considerably lower than desired. To a lesser extent this effect is demonstrated with zinc-containing multivitamins. (see DOSAGE AND ADMINISTRATION for concurrent administration of these agents with ciprofloxacin.)

Some quinolones, including ciprofloxacin, have been associated with transient elevations in serum creatinine in patients receiving cyclosporine concomitantly.

Quinolones have been reported to enhance the effects of the oral anticoagulant warfarin or its derivatives. When these products are administered concomitantly, prothrombin time or other suitable coagulation test should be closely monitored.

Probenecid interferes with renal tubular secretion of ciprofloxacin and produces an increase in the level of ciprofloxacin in the serum. This should be considered if patients are receiving both drugs concomitantly.

As with other broad spectrum antimicrobial agents, prolonged use of ciprofloxacin may result in overgrowth of non-susceptible organisms. Repeated evaluation of the patient's condition and microbial susceptibility testing is essential. If superinfection occurs during therapy, appropriate measures should be taken.

ADVERSE REACTIONS:

TABLETS AND INTRAVENOUS

The most frequently reported events, without regard to drug relationship, among patients treated with intravenous ciprofloxacin were nausea, diarrhea, central nervous system disturbance, local i.v. site reactions, abnormalities of liver associated enzymes (hepatic enzymes), and eosinophillia. Headache, restlessness and rash were also noted in greater than 1% of patients treated with the most common doses of ciprofloxacin.

Local iv site reactions have been reported with the intravenous administration of ciprofloxacin. These reactions are more frequent if the infusion time is 30 minutes or less. these may appear as local skin reactions which resolve rapidly upon completion of the infusion. Subsequent intravenous administration is not contraindicated unless the reactions recur or worsen.

During clinical investigation, 2,799 patients received 2,868 courses of the drug. Adverse events that were considered likely to be drug related occurred in 7.3% of patients treated, possibly related in 9.2% (total of 16.5% thought to be possibly or probably related to drug therapy), and remotely related in 3.0%. Ciprofloxacin was discontinued because of an adverse event in 3.5% of patients treated, primarily involving the gastrointestinal system (1.5%), skin (0.6%), and central nervous system (0.4%).

Additional events that occurred in less than 1% of ciprofloxacin courses are listed below:

ADVERSE REACTIONS: *(cont'd)*

Cardiovascular: palpitation, atrial flutter, ventricular ectopy, syncope, hypertension, angina pectoris, myocardial infarction, cardiopulmonary arrest, cerebral thrombosis, cardiovascular collapse, arrhythmia, tachycardia, hypotension

Central Nervous System: dizziness, lightheadedness, insomnia, nightmares, hallucinations, manic reaction, irritability, tremor, ataxia, convulsive seizures, lethargy, drowsiness, weakness, malaise, anorexia, phobia, depersonalization, depression, toxic psychosis, unresponsiveness, paresthesia (See PRECAUTIONS.)

Gastrointestinal: painful oral mucosa, oral candidiasis, dysphagia, intestinal perforation, ileus, gastrointestinal bleeding, *C. difficile* associated diarrhea; pseudomembranous colitis; pancreatitis; hepatic necrosis; intestinal perforation, dyspepsia; epigastric or abdominal pain; vomiting; constipation; oral ulceration; oral candidiasis, mouth dryness; anorexia; flatulence. Cholestatic jaundice has been reported.

Musculoskeletal: joint, arm, jaw or back pain, joint stiffness, achiness, neck or chest pain, flare-up of gout.

Renal/Urogenital: interstitial nephritis, hemorrhagic cystitis, renal calculi, nephritis, renal failure, polyuria, urinary retention, urethral bleeding, vaginitis, acidosis, frequent urination, gynecomastia, candiduria. Crystalluria, cylindruria, hematuria, and albuminuria have also been reported.

Respiratory: dyspnea, epistaxis, laryngeal or pulmonary edema, hiccough, hemoptysis, bronchospasm, pulmonary embolism, respiratory arrest, pulmonary embolism, respiratory distress, pleural effusion.

Skin/Hypersensitivity: pruritus, urticaria, photosensitivity, flushing, fever, chills, angioedema, edema of the face, neck, lips, conjunctivae, hands or lower extremities, cutaneous candidiasis, hyperpigmentation, anaphylactic reactions, erythema multiforme/ Stevens-Johnson syndrome, exfoliative dermatitis, toxic epidermal necrolysis, vasculitis, purpura, vesicles, increased perspiration, hyperpigmentation, angioedema, erythema nodosum,.

Special Senses: blurred vision, disturbed vision (change in color perception, overbrightness of lights), decreased visual acuity, diplopia, eye pain, tinnitus, hearing loss, bad taste.

Allergic reactions ranging from urticaria to anaphylactic reactions have been reported (See WARNINGS.)

IV Infusion Site: thrombophlebitis, burning pain, pruritus, paresthesia, erythema, swelling.

Also reported were agranulocytosis, prolongation of prothrombin time and possible exacerbation of myasthenia gravis.

Most of the adverse events reported were described as only mild or moderate in severity, abated soon after the drug was discontinued, and required no treatment.

In several instances nausea, vomiting, tremor, irritability or palpitation were judged by investigators to be related to elevated serum levels of theophylline possibly as a result of drug interaction with ciprofloxacin.

In domestic clinical trials involving 214 patients receiving a single 250 mg oral dose, approximately 5% of patients reported adverse experiences without reference to drug relationship. The most common adverse experiences were vaginitis (2%0, headache (1%), and vaginal pruritus (1%). Additional reactions, occurring in 0.3%-1% of patients, were abdominal discomfort, lymphadenopathy, foot pain, dizziness, and breast pain. Less than 20% of these patients had laboratory values obtained, and these results were generally consistent with the pattern noted for multi- dose therapy.

Post-Marketing Adverse Events: Additional adverse events regardless of relationship to drug, reported from worldwide marketing experience with quinolones, including ciprofloxacin are anaphylactic reactions, erythema multiforme/Stevens-Johnson syndrome, exfoliative dermatitis, toxic epidermal necrolysis, vasculitis, jaundice, hepatic necrosis, toxic psychosis, postural hypotension, possible exacerbation of myasthenia gravis, anosmia, confusion, dysphasia, nystagmus, pseudomembranous colitis, pancreatitis, dyspepsia, flatulence, and constipation. Also reported were hemolytic anemia; agranulocytosis; elevation of serum triglycerides, serum cholesterol, blood glucose, serum potassium; prolongation of prothrombin time; albuminuria; candiduria, vaginal candidiasis; renal calculi; and change in serum phenytoin (See PRECAUTIONS.)

Adverse Laboratory Changes: Changes in laboratory parameters listed as adverse events without regard to drug relationship were:

Hepatic: Elevations of: ALT (SGPT) (1.9%), AST (SGOT)(1.7%), alkaline Phosphatase (0.8%), LDH (0.4%), serum bilirubin (0.3%).

Hematologic: Eosinophilia (0.6%), leukopenia (0.4%), decreased blood platelets (0.1%), elevated blood platelets (0.1%), pancytopenia (0.1%).

Renal: Elevations of: Serum creatinine (1.1%), BUN (0.9%). CRYSTALLURIA, CYLINDRURIA AND HEMATURIA HAVE BEEN REPORTED.

Other changes occurring in less than 0.1% or courses were: Elevation of serum gammaglutamyl transferase, elevation of serum amylase, reduction in blood glucose, elevated uric acid, decrease in hemoglobin, anemia, bleeding diathesis, increase in blood monocytes, leukocytosis.

OVERDOSAGE:

In the event of acute overdosage, the stomach should be emptied by inducing vomiting or by gastric lavage. The patient should be carefully observed and given supportive treatment. Adequate hydration must be maintained. Only a small amount of ciprofloxacin (<10%) is removed from the body after hemodialysis or peritoneal dialysis.

DOSAGE AND ADMINISTRATION:

TABLETS

The usual adult dosage for patients with urinary tract infections is 250 mg every 12 hours. For patients with complicated infections cause by organisms not highly susceptible, 500 mg may be administered every 12 hours.

Lower respiratory tract infections, skin and skin structure infections, and bone and joint infections may be treated with 500 mg every 12 hours. For more severe of complicated infections, a dosage of 750 mg may be given every 12 hours.

For the treatment of uncomplicated urethral and cervical gonococcal infections, a single 250 mg dose is recommended. (TABLE 6)

The determination of dosage for any particular patient must take into consideration the severity and nature or the infection, the susceptibility of the causative organism, the integrity of the patient's host-defense mechanisms, and the status of renal function and hepatic function.

The duration of treatment depends upon the severity of infection. Generally ciprofloxacin should be continued for at least 2 days after the signs and symptoms of infection have disappeared. The usual duration is 7 to 14 days; however, for severe and complicated infections more prolonged therapy may be required. Bone and joint infections may require treatment for 4 to 6 weeks or longer. Infectious Diarrhea may be treated for 5-7 days. Typhoid fever should be treated for 10 days.

DOSAGE AND ADMINISTRATION: *(cont'd)*

TABLE 6 DOSAGE GUIDELINES

Type of Infection	Type or Severity	Unit Dose	Frequency	Daily Dose
Urinary tract	Mild/Moderate	250 mg	q 12 h	500 mg
	Severe/Complicated	500 mg	q 12 h	1000 mg
Lower respiratory tract;	Mild/Moderate	500 mg	q 12 h	1000 mg
Bone and Joint; Skin or skin Structure	Severe/Complicated	750 mg	q 12 h	1500 mg
Infectious Diarrhea	Mild/moderate/Severe	500 mg	q 12 h	1000 mg
Typhoid Fever	Mild/Moderate	500 mg	q 12 h	1000 mg
Urethral and Cervical Gonococcal Infections	Uncomplicated	250 mg	single dose	—

Concurrent Use With Antacids or Multivalent Cations: Concurrent administration of ciprofloxacin with sucralfate or divalent and trivalent cations such as iron or antacids containing magnesium, aluminum, or calcium may substantially interfere with the absorption of ciprofloxacin, resulting in serum and urine levels considerably lower than desired. Therefore, concurrent administration of these agents with ciprofloxacin should be avoided. However, usual dietary intake of calcium has not been shown to alter the bioavailability of ciprofloxacin. Single dose bioavailability studies have shown that antacids may be administered either 2 hours after or 6 hours before ciprofloxacin dosing without a significant decrease in bioavailability. Histamine H_2-receptor antagonists appear to have no significant effect on the bioavailability of ciprofloxacin.

Impaired Renal Function: Ciprofloxacin is eliminated primarily by renal excretion; however, the drug is also metabolized and partially cleared through the biliary system of the liver the through the intestine. These alternate pathways of drug elimination appear to compensate for the reduced renal excretion in patients with renal impairment. Nonetheless, some modification of dosage is recommended, particularly for patients with severe renal dysfunction. TABLE 7 provides dosage guidelines for use in patients with renal impairment; however, monitoring of serum drug levels provides the most reliable basis for dosage adjustment.

TABLE 7 Recommended Starting And Maintenance Dose For Patients With Impaired Renal Function

Creatinine Clearance (ml/min)	Dose
> 50	See Usual Dosage
30 - 50	250 - 500 mg q 12 h
5 - 29	250 - 500 mg q 18 h
Patients on hemodialysis or Peritoneal dialysis	250 - 500 mg q 24 h (after dialysis)

When only the serum creatinine concentration is known, the following formula may be used to estimate creatinine clearance (TABLE 8).

TABLE 8 Creatine Clearance (ml/min)

Men: [Weight (kg) × (140 - age)] ÷ [72 × serum creatine (mg/dl)]
Women: 0.85 × the value calculated for men.

The serum creatinine should represent a steady state of renal function.

In patients with severe infections and severe renal impairment, a unit dose of 750 mg may be administered at the intervals noted above; however, patients should be carefully monitored and the serum ciprofloxacin concentration should be measured periodically. Peak concentrations (1-2 hours after dosing) should generally range from 2 to 4 mcg/ml.

For patients with changing renal function or for patients with renal impairment and hepatic insufficiency, measurement of serum concentrations of ciprofloxacin will provide additional guidance for adjusting dosage.

INTRAVENOUS

The recommended adult dosage for urinary tract infections of mild to moderate severity is 200 mg every 12 hours. For severe or complicated urinary tract infections the recommended dosage is 400 mg every 12 hours.

The recommended adult dosage for lower respiratory tract infections, skin and skin structure infections and bone and joint infections of mild to moderate severity is 400 mg every 12 hours.

The determination of dosage for any particular patient must take into consideration the severity and nature of the infection, the susceptibility of the causative organism, the integrity of the patient's host-defense mechanisms and the status of renal and hepatic function.

TABLE 9 Dosage Guidelines

Type of Infection	Type or Severity	Intravenous Unit Dose	Frequency	Daily Dose
Urinary tract	Mild/ Moderate	200 mg	q 12 h	400 mg
	Severe/ Complicated	400 mg	q 12 h	800 mg
Lower Respiratory Tract; Bone and Joint; Skin and Skin Structure; Bone and Joint	Mild/ Moderate	400 mg	q 12 h	800 mg

CIPROFLOXACIN IV SHOULD BE ADMINISTERED BY IV INFUSION OVER A PERIOD OF 60 MINUTES.

THE DURATION OF TREATMENT DEPENDS UPON THE SEVERITY OF INFECTION. GENERALLY CIPROFLOXACIN SHOULD BE CONTINUED FOR AT LEAST 2 DAYS AFTER THE SIGNS AND SYMPTOMS OF INFECTION HAVE DISAPPEARED. THE USUAL DURATION IS 7 TO 14 DAYS. BONE AND JOINT INFECTIONS MAY REQUIRE TREATMENT FOR 4 TO 6 WEEKS OR LONGER.

CIPROFLOXACIN HYDROCHLORIDE TABLETS (CIPRO) FOR ORAL ADMINISTRATION ARE AVAILABLE. PARENTERAL THERAPY MAY BE CHANGED TO ORAL CIPROFLOXACIN TABLETS WHEN THE CONDITION WARRANTS, AT THE DISCRETION OF THE PHYSICIAN. FOR COMPLETE DOSAGE AND ADMINISTRATION INFORMATION, SEE CIPROFLOXACIN TABLET PACKAGE INSERT.

IMPAIRED RENAL FUNCTION: TABLE 10 provides dosage guidelines for use in patients with renal impairment; however, monitoring of serum drug levels provides the most reliable basis for dosage adjustment.

DOSAGE AND ADMINISTRATION: *(cont'd)*

TABLE 10 Recommended Starting And Maintenance Doses For Patients With Impaired Renal Function	
Creatinine Clearance (ml/min)	**Dosage**
> 30	See Usual Dosage
5 - 29	200 - 400 mg q 18-24 hr

When only the serum creatinine concentration is known, the following formula may be used to estimate creatinine clearance (TABLE 11).

TABLE 11 Creatinine Clearance (ml/min)

Men: [Weight (kg) × (140 - age)] ÷ [72 × serum creatine (mg/dl)]
Women: 0.85 × the value calculated for men.

The serum creatinine should represent a steady state of renal function.

For patients with changing renal function or for patients with renal impairment and hepatic insufficiency, measurement of serum concentrations of ciprofloxacin will provide additional guidance for adjusting dosage.

Intravenous Administration: Ciprofloxacin IV should be administered by intravenous infusion over a period of 60 minutes. Slow infusion of a dilute solution into a large vein will minimize patient discomfort and reduce the risk of venous irritation.

Vials (Injection Concentrate): .THIS PREPARATION MUST BE DILUTED BEFORE USE. The Intravenous dose should be prepared by aseptically withdrawing the appropriate volume of concentrate from the vials of ciprofloxacin I.V. This should be diluted with a suitable intravenous solution to a final concentration of 1-2 mg/ml (See Compatibility And Stability.) The resulting solution should be infused over a period of 60 minutes by direct infusion or through a Y-type intravenous infusion set which may already be in place.

If this method or the "piggyback" method of administration is used, it is advisable to discontinue temporarily the administration of any other solutions during the infusion of ciprofloxacin IV.

Flexible Containers: Ciprofloxacin IV is also available as a 0.2% premixed solution in 5% dextrose in flexible containers of 100 ml or 200 ml. The solutions in flexible containers may be infused as described above.

Compatibility and Stability: Ciprofloxacin injection 1% (10 mg/ml), when diluted with the following IV solutions to concentrations of 0.5 to 2.0 mg/ml, is stable for up to 14 days at refrigerated or room storage.

0.9% - Sodium Chloride Injection, USP

5% Dextrose Injection, USP

If ciprofloxacin IV is to be given concomitantly with another drug, each drug should be given separately in accordance with the recommended dosage and route of administration for each drug.

ANIMAL PHARMACOLOGY:

Ciprofloxacin and related drugs have been shown to cause arthropathy in immature animal of most species tested (See WARNINGS.) Damage of weight bearing joints was observed in juvenile dogs and rats. In young beagles 100 mg/kg ciprofloxacin given daily for 4 weeks, cause degenerative articular changes of the knee joint. At 30 mg/kg the effect on the joint was minimal. In a subsequent study in beagles removal of weight bearing from the joint reduced the lesions but did not totally prevent them.

Crystalluria, sometimes associated with secondary nephropathy, occurs in laboratory animals dosed with ciprofloxacin. This is primarily related to the reduced solubility of ciprofloxacin under alkaline conditions, which predominate in the urine of test animals; in man, crystalluria is rare since human urine is typically acidic. In rhesus monkeys, crystalluria without nephropathy has been noted after single oral doses as low as 5 mg/kg. After 6 months of intravenous dosing at 10 mg/kg/day, no nephropathological changes were noted; however, nephropathy was observed after dosing at 20 mg/kg/day for the same duration.

In dogs, ciprofloxacin at 3 and 10 mg/kg by rapid IV injection (15 sec.) produces pronounced hypotensive effects. These effects are considered to be related to histamine release since they are partially antagonized by pyrilamine, an antihistamine. In rhesus monkeys, rapid IV injection also produces hypotension but the effect in this species is inconsistent and less pronounced.

In mice, concomitant administration of nonsteroidal anti-inflammatory drugs such as fenbufen, phenylbutazone and indomethacin, with quinolones has been reported to enhance the CNS stimulatory effect or quinolones.

Ocular toxicity seen with some related drugs has not been observed in ciprofloxacin-treated animals.

REFERENCES:

1. National Committee for Clinical Laboratory Standards, Performance Standards for Antimicrobial Disk Susceptibility Tests - Fourth Edition. Approved Standard NCCLS Document M2-A4, Vol. 10, No. 7, NCCLS, Villanova, PA, April, 1990 **2.** National Committee for Clinical Laboratory Standards, Methods for Dilution Antimicrobial Susceptibility Tests for Bacteria that Grow Aerobically - Second Edition. Approved Standard NCCLS Document M7-A2, Vol. 10, No. 8, NCCLS, Villanova, PA, April, 1990. **3.** National Committee for Clinical Laboratory Standards, Methods for Antimicrobial Susceptibility Testing of Anaerobic Bacteria — Second Edition. Approved Standard NCCLS Document M11-A2, Vol.10, No. 15, NCCLS, Villanova, PA, December, 1990.

HOW SUPPLIED:

TABLETS

Ciprofloxacin hydrochloride is available as round, slightly yellowish film-coated tablets containing 250 mg ciprofloxacin. The 250 mg tablet is coded with the word "Cipro" on one side and "250" on the reverse side. Cipro is also available as capsule shaped, slightly yellowish film-coated tablets containing 500 mg or 750 mg ciprofloxacin. The 500 mg tablet is coded with the word "Cipro" on one side and "500" on the reverse side; the 750 mg tablet is coded with the word "Cipro" on one side and "750" on the reverse side. Available in bottles of 50's, 100's and in Unit Dose packages of 100.

TABLE 12

	Strength	Tablet	Identification
Bottles of 50:	750 mg	Cipro	750
Bottles of 100:	250 mg	Cipro	250
	500 mg	Cipro	500
Unit Dose Package of 100:	250 mg	Cipro	250
	500 mg	Cipro	500
	750 mg	Cipro	750

HOW SUPPLIED: *(cont'd)*

INTRAVENOUS

Cipro IV (ciprofloxacin) is available as a clear, colorless to slightly yellowish solution. ciprofloxacin IV is available in 200 mg or 400 mg strengths. The concentrate is supplied in vials while the premixed solution is supplied in flexible containers as seen in TABLE 12

TABLE 12

Container	Size	Strength
Vial:	20 ml	200 mg, 1%
	40 ml	400 mg, 1%
Flexible Container:	100 ml 5% dextrose	200 mg, 0.2%
	200 ml 5% dextrose	400 mg, 0.2%

STORAGE

Tablets: Store below 86°F (30°C).

Vials: Store between 41 - 86°F (5-30°C).

Flexible Containers: Store between 41 - 77°F (5-25°C).

Protect from light, avoid excessive heat, protect from freezing.

PATIENT INFORMATION:

Ciprofloxacin is a fluroquinolone antibiotic used for the treatment of infection. Notify your physician if you are pregnant or nursing. This medication may cause CNS stimulation (tremor, restlessness, confusion); use with caution in patients with seizure disorders. Notify your physician and pharmacist if you are taking theophyllline; ciprofloxacin may alter the clearance of theophylline from your body requiring increased monitoring of theophylline levels. Take at regular intervals and complete the entire course of therapy. Ciprofloxacin may be taken with or without food, however, it is preferable that it be taken two hours after a meal. Drink plenty of fluids while taking this medication. Do not take maganesium or aluminum-containing antacids or iron or zinc-containing products within four hours before or two hours after taking ciprofloxacin. This medication may cause dizziness or lightheadedness; use caution while driving or operating hazardous machinery. Ciprofloxacin may cause increased sensitivity to sunlight. Use sunscreens and wear protective clothing until degree of sensitivity is determined. Notify your physician if you develop a rash while taking ciprofloxacin.

HOW SUPPLIED - EQUIVALENTS NOT AVAILABLE:

Injection, Solution - Intravenous - 10 mg/ml

20 ml x 10	**$144.06**	**CIPRO I.V., Bayer**	**00026-8562-20**
40 ml x 10	**$288.12**	**CIPRO I.V., Bayer**	**00026-8564-64**
120 ml x 6	**$466.38**	**CIPRO I.V., Bayer**	**00026-8566-65**

Injection, Solution - Intravenous - 200 mg/0.1 l

100 ml x 24	**$374.54**	**CIPRO I.V., Bayer**	**00026-8552-36**

Injection, Solution - Intravenous - 400 mg/0.2 l

200 ml x 24	**$720.29**	**CIPRO I.V., Bayer**	**00026-8554-63**

Solution - Ophthalmic; Top - 0.3 %

2.5 ml	$10.94	CILOXAN OPHTHALMIC, Alcon	00065-0656-25
5 ml	$21.88	CILOXAN OPHTHALMIC, Alcon	00065-0656-05

Tablet, Uncoated - Oral - 250 mg

100's	**$280.00**	**CIPRO, Bayer**	**00026-8512-51**
100's	**$290.05**	**CIPRO, Bayer**	**00026-8512-48**

Tablet, Uncoated - Oral - 500 mg

100's	**$324.03**	**CIPRO, Bayer**	**00026-8513-51**
100's	**$334.82**	**CIPRO, Bayer**	**00026-8513-48**

Tablet, Uncoated - Oral - 750 mg

50's	**$281.00**	**CIPRO, Bayer**	**00026-8514-50**
100's	**$571.66**	**CIPRO, Bayer**	**00026-8514-48**

CISAPRIDE MONOHYDRATE *(003164)*

CATEGORIES: Acid/Peptic Disorders; Gastroesophagael Reflux Disease; Gastrointestinal Drugs; GERD; Dyspepsia*; Irritable Bowel Syndrome*; Pregnancy Category C; FDA Class 1S ("Standard Review"); FDA Approved 1993 Jul; Top 200 Drugs
* Indication not approved by the FDA

BRAND NAMES: *Acenalin* (Japan); *Acpulsif*; *Alimix* (England, Germany); *Alimix Forte*; *Calmax*; *Cipride*; *Cisapron*; *Cisawal*; *Dispep*; *Enteropride* (Mexico); *Esorid*; *Gastromet*; *Guptro*; *Kaudalit*; *Kinestase* (Mexico); *Prepulsid* (Australia, Europe, Canada, Mexico); *Presid*; **Propulsid**; *Propulsin* (Germany); *Pulsid*; *Risamol* (Japan); *Sepride*; *Syspride*; *Unamol* (Mexico); *Unipride*; *Vomiprid*
(International brand names outside U.S. in italics)

FORMULARIES: Aetna; BC-BS; CIGNA; Medco; Medi-Cal; PCS; PruCare; United

WARNING:
Serious cardiac arrhythmias including ventricular tachycardia, ventricular fibrillation, torsades de pointes, and QT prolongation have been reported in patients taking cisapride monohydrate with other drugs that inhibit cytochrome P450 3A4, such as ketoconazole, itraconazole, miconazole, troleandomycin, erythromycin, fluconazole, and clarithromycin. Some of these events have been fatal. Cisapride monohydrate is contraindicated in patients taking any of these drugs. (See CONTRAINDICATIONS, WARNINGS, PRECAUTIONS, and DRUG INTERACTIONS.)

DESCRIPTION:

Propulsid (cisapride) Tablets and Suspension contain cisapride as the monohydrate, which is an oral gastrointestinal prokinetic agent chemically designated as (±)-cis-4-amino-5-chloro-N-[1-[3-(4- fluorophenoxy)propyl]-3-methoxy-4-piperidinyl]-2-methoxybenzamide monohydrate. Its empirical formula is $C_{23}H_{29}ClFN_3O_4 \cdot H_2O$. The molecular weight is 483.97.

Cisapride as the monohydrate is a white to slightly beige odorless powder. It is practically insoluble in water, sparingly soluble in methanol, and soluble in acetone. Each 1.04 mg of cisapride as the monohydrate is equivalent to one mg of cisapride.

Propulsid is available for oral use in tablets containing cisapride as the monohydrate equivalent to 10 mg or 20 mg of cisapride and as a suspension containing 1 mg/ml of cisapride. The inactive ingredients in the tablets are colloidal silicon dioxide, lactose monohydrate, magnesium stearate, microcrystalline cellulose, polysorbate 20, povidone, and starch (corn). The 20 mg tablets also contain FD&C Blue No. 2 aluminum lake. The inactive ingredients in the suspension are hydroxypropyl methylcellulose, methylparaben, microcrystal-

DESCRIPTION: *(cont'd)*

line cellulose and carboxymethylcellulose sodium, polysorbate 20, propylparaben, sodium chloride, sorbitol, and water. The 1 mg/ml suspension also contains artificial cherry cream flavor and FD&C Red No. 40.

CLINICAL PHARMACOLOGY:

Pharmacokinetics: Cisapride monohydrate is rapidly absorbed after oral administration; peak plasma concentrations are reached 1 to 1.5 hours after dosing. The absolute bioavailability of cisapride monohydrate is 35-40%. When gastric acidity was reduced by high dose histamine H_2 receptor blocker and sodium bicarbonate in fasting subjects, there was a decrease in the rate, and to a lesser degree the extent, of cisapride monohydrate tablet absorption. (This has not been established for the suspension.) cisapride monohydrate binds to an extent of 97.5-98% to plasma proteins, mainly to albumin. The volume of distribution of cisapride monohydrate is about 180 L, indicating extensive tissue distribution.

The plasma clearance of cisapride monohydrate is about 100 ml/min. The mean terminal half-life reported for cisapride monohydrate ranges from 6 to 12 hours; longer half- lives, up to 20 hours, have been reported following intravenous (IV) administration. Cisapride is metabolized mainly via the cytochrome P450 3A4 enzyme. Cisapride monohydrate is extensively metabolized; unchanged drug accounts for less than 10% of urinary and fecal recovery following oral administration. Norcisapride, formed by N-dealkylation, is the principal metabolite in plasma, feces and urine.

There was no unusual drug accumulation due to time-dependent or non-linear changes in PK. After cessation of the repeated dosing, the elimination half-lives (8 to 10 hr) were in the same order as after single dosing. There is some evidence that the degree of accumulation of cisapride monohydrate and/or its metabolites may be somewhat higher in patients with hepatic or renal impairment and in elderly patients compared to young healthy volunteers, but the differences are not consistent and do not require dosage adjustment.

Pharmacodynamics: The onset of pharmacological action of cisapride is approximately 30 to 60 minutes after oral administration.

The mechanism of action of cisapride is thought to be primarily enhancement of release of acetylcholine at the myenteric plexus. Cisapride does not induce muscarinic or nicotinic receptor stimulation, nor does it inhibit acetylcholinesterase activity. It is less potent than metoclopramide in dopamine receptor-blocking effects in rats. It does not increase or decrease basal or pentagastrin-induced gastric acid secretion.

In vitro studies have shown that cisapride is a serotonin-4 (5- HT_4) receptor agonist. This agonistic action may result in increased gastrointestinal motility and cardiac rate.

Esophagus: Single doses of cisapride (4 to 10 mg IV) increased the lower esophageal sphincter pressure (LESP) and lower esophageal peristalsis compared to placebo and/or metoclopramide. In patients with gastroesophageal reflux disease (GERD) and a LESP of <10 mm Hg, cisapride dose-dependently increased the strength of esophageal peristalsis and more than doubled LESP, raising it to normal values. The increase in LESP was partially reversed by atropine, suggesting that the effect is partly, but not exclusively, cholinergically-mediated. Twenty mg oral cisapride given once to healthy volunteers similarly increased LESP, starting 45 minutes after dosing, with a peak response at 75 minutes. The full duration of the effect was not monitored, and doses smaller than 20 mg were ineffective. Ten mg oral cisapride, administered 3 times daily for several days to patients with GERD, resulted in a significant increase in LESP, and an increased esophageal acid clearance.

Stomach: Cisapride (single 10 mg doses IV or oral or 10 mg given orally 3 times daily up to six weeks) significantly accelerated gastric emptying of both liquids and solids. Acceleration of gastric emptying, measured over a four hour period following a radio-labeled test meal given at lunch time, was greatest when 10 mg cisapride was given both in the morning and again before the test meal, intermediate when 20 mg was given as a single administration in the morning and least when only 10 mg was given on the morning of the test meal. The increases in gastric emptying were proportional to the plasma levels of cisapride measured in these subjects over the same 4 hours that the gastric emptying test was conducted.

CLINICAL STUDIES:

Clinical trials have shown that cisapride can reduce the symptoms of nocturnal heartburn associated with gastroesophageal reflux disease. Two placebo-controlled studies, one using a dose of 10 mg q.i.d., the other both 10 and 20 mg q.i.d., showed effects on nighttime heartburn, although the 10 mg dose in the second study was only marginally effective. There were no consistent effects on daytime heartburn, symptoms of regurgitation, or histopathology of the esophagus. Use of antacids was only infrequently affected and slightly decreased. In a third controlled trial of similar design to the others, neither 10 mg nor 20 mg taken 4 times was superior to placebo.

These clinical trials did not show a significant effect on LESP, perhaps because the majority of these patients had normal LESP's at the beginning and end of the study period. In a clinical trial comparing 10 mg cisapride to placebo, pH probe evaluation, in a relatively small number of patients, did not reveal a significant difference in pH.

INDICATIONS AND USAGE:

Cisapride monohydrate is indicated for the symptomatic treatment of patients with nocturnal heartburn due to gastroesophageal reflux disease.

CONTRAINDICATIONS:

Concomitant administration of ketoconazole tablets, itraconazole capsules, miconazole, fluconazole, erythromycin, clarithromycin, or troleandomycin capsules with cisapride monohydrate is contraindicated. (See WARNINGS and DRUG INTERACTIONS).

Cisapride monohydrate should not be used in patients in whom an increase in gastrointestinal motility could be harmful, e.g., in the presence of gastrointestinal hemorrhage, mechanical obstruction, or perforation. Cisapride monohydrate is contraindicated in patients with known sensitivity or intolerance to the drug.

WARNINGS:

Cisapride monohydrate undergoes metabolism mainly by the hepatic cytochrome P450 3A4 isoenzyme. Drugs which inhibit this enzyme such as ketoconazole, itraconazole, miconazole, clarithromycin, erythromycin, fluconazole, or troleandomycin can lead to elevated cisapride blood levels.

Rare cases of serious cardiac arrhythmias, including ventricular arrhythmias and torsades de pointes associated with QT prolongation, have been reported in patients taking cisapride with ketoconazole, itraconazole, miconazole, erythromycin, clarithromycin, or fluconazole. Some of these patients did not have known cardiac histories; however, most had been receiving multiple other medications and had pre-existing cardiac disease or risk factors for arrhythmias. Some of these cases have been fatal.

PRECAUTIONS:

General: Potential benefits should be weighed against risks prior to administration of cisapride to patients with conditions associated with QT prolongation, such as congenital prolonged QT syndrome, uncorrected electrolyte disturbances or in patients who are taking other medications known to prolong QT interval.

PRECAUTIONS: *(cont'd)*

Information for the Patient: Patients should be warned against concomitant use of oral ketoconazole, itraconazole, miconazole, erythromycin, clarithromycin, fluconazole, or troleandomycin with cisapride monohydrate.

Although cisapride monohydrate does not affect psychomotor function nor does it induce sedation or drowsiness when used alone, patients should be advised that the sedative effects of benzodiazepines and of alcohol may be accelerated by cisapride monohydrate.

Carcinogenesis, Mutagenesis, and Impairment of Fertility: In a twenty-five month oral carcinogenicity study in rats, cisapride at daily doses up to 80 mg/kg was not tumorigenic. For a 50 kg person of average height (1.46 m^2 body surface area), this dose represents 50 times the maximum recommended human dose (1.6 mg/kg/day) on a mg/kg basis and 7 times the maximum recommended human dose (54.4 mg/m^2) on a body surface area basis. In a nineteen month oral carcinogenicity study in mice, cisapride at daily doses up to 80 mg/kg was not tumorigenic. This dose represents 50 times the maximum recommended human dose on a mg/kg basis and about 4 times the maximum recommended human dose on a body surface area basis.

Cisapride was not mutagenic in the *in vitro* Ames test, human lymphocyte chromosomal aberration test, mouse lymphoma cell forward mutation test, and rat hepatocyte UDS test and *in vivo* rat micronucleus test, male and female mouse dominant lethal mutations tests, and sex linked recessive lethal test in male *Drosophila melanogaster.*

Fertility and reproductive performance studies were conducted in male and female rats. Cisapride was found to have no effect on fertility and reproductive performance of male rats at oral doses up to 160 mg/kg/day (100 times the maximum recommended human dose on a mg/kg bases and 14 times the maximum recommended human dose on a mg/m^2 basis). In the female rats, cisapride at oral doses of 40 mg/kg/day and higher prolonged the breeding interval required for impregnation. Similar effects were also observed at maturity in the female offspring (F_1) of the female rats (F_0) treated with oral doses of cisapride at 10 mg/kg/day or higher. Cisapride at an oral dose of 160 mg/kg/day also exerted contragestational/pregnancy disrupting effects in female rats (F_0).

Pregnancy, Teratogenic Effects, Pregnancy Category C: Oral teratology studies have been conducted in rats (doses up to 160 mg/kg/day) and rabbits (doses up to 40 mg/kg/day). There was no evidence of a teratogenic potential of cisapride in rats or rabbits. Cisapride was embryotoxic and fetotoxic in rats at a dose of 160 mg/kg/day (100 times the maximum recommended human dose on a mg/kg basis and 14 times the maximum recommended human dose on a mg/m^2 basis) and in rabbits at a dose of 20 mg/kg/day (approximately 12 times the maximum recommended human dose on a mg/kg basis) or higher. It also produced reduced birth weights of pups in rats at 40 and 160 mg/kg/day and adversely affected the pup survival. There are no adequate and well-controlled studies in pregnant women. Cisapride should be used during pregnancy only if the potential benefit justifies the potential risk to the fetus.

Nursing Mothers: Cisapride is excreted in human milk at concentrations approximately one twentieth of those observed in plasma. Caution should be exercised when cisapride monohydrate is administered to a nursing woman, and particular care must be taken if the nursing infant or the mother is taking a drug that might alter cisapride monohydrate's metabolism. See CONTRAINDICATIONS, WARNINGS, and/or DRUG INTERACTIONS.

Pediatric Use: Safety and effectiveness in children have not been established.

Geriatric Use: Steady-state plasma levels are generally higher in older than in younger patients, due to a moderate prolongation of the elimination half-life. Therapeutic doses, however, are similar to those used in younger adults.

The rate of adverse experiences in patients greater than 65 years of age was similar to that in younger adults.

DRUG INTERACTIONS:

Cisapride is metabolized mainly via the cytochrome P450 3A4 enzyme.

Human pharmacokinetic data indicate that oral ketoconazole potently inhibits the metabolism of cisapride, resulting in a mean eight-fold increase in AUC of cisapride. A study in 14 normal male and female volunteers suggest that coadministration of cisapride monohydrate and ketoconazole can result in prolongation of the QT interval on the ECG.

In vitro data indicate that itraconazole, miconazole, fluconazole, erythromycin, clarithromycin, and troleandomycin also markedly inhibit cytochrome P450 3A4 mainly responsible for the metabolism of cisapride.

In some cases where serious ventricular arrhythmias, QT prolongation, and torsades de pointes have occurred when cisapride was taken in conjunction with one of the cytochrome P450 3A4 inhibitors, elevated blood cisapride levels were noted at the time of the QT prolongation. Normalization of the QT interval after cisapride was discontinued has been observed.

Concurrent administration of anticholinergic compounds would be expected to compromise the beneficial effects of cisapride monohydrate.

The acceleration of gastric emptying by cisapride monohydrate could affect the rate of absorption of other drugs. Patients receiving narrow therapeutic ratio drugs or other drugs that require careful titration should be followed closely; if plasma levels are being monitored, they should be reassessed.

In patients receiving oral anticoagulants, the coagulation times were increased in some cases. It is advisable to check coagulation time within the first few days after the start and discontinuation of cisapride monohydrate therapy, with an appropriate adjustment of the anticoagulant dose, if necessary.

Cimetidine coadministration leads to an increased peak plasma concentration and AUC of cisapride monohydrate; there is no effect on cisapride monohydrate absorption when it is coadministered with ranitidine. The gastrointestinal absorption of cimetidine and ranitidine is accelerated when they are coadministered with cisapride monohydrate.

ADVERSE REACTIONS:

In the U.S. clinical trial population of 1728 patients (comprising 506 with gastroesophageal reflux disorders, and the remainder with other motility disorders) the following adverse experiences were reported in more than 1% of patients treated with cisapride monohydrate and at least as often on cisapride monohydrate as on placebo. The percent of patients who discontinued treatment is displayed in parenthesis in TABLE 1.

The following adverse events also reported in more than 1% of cisapride monohydrate patients were more frequently reported on placebo: dizziness, vomiting, pharyngitis, chest pain, fatigue, back pain, depression, dehydration, and myalgia.

Diarrhea, abdominal pain, constipation, flatulence, and rhinitis all occurred more frequently in patients using 20 mg of cisapride monohydrate than in patients using 10 mg.

Additional adverse experiences reported to occur in 1% or less of patients in the U.S. clinical studies are: dry mouth, somnolence, palpitation, migraine, tremor, and edema.

ADVERSE REACTIONS: *(cont'd)*

TABLE 1

System/Adverse Event	Cisapride Monohydrate N=1042	Placebo N=686
Central & Peripheral Nervous Systems		
Headache	19.3% (1.1%)	17.1% (0.4%)
Gastrointestinal		
Diarrhea	14.2 (0.7)	10.3 (0.1)
Abdominal Pain	10.2 (1.2)	7.7 (0.9)
Nausea	7.6 (1.0)	7.6 (0.3)
Constipation	6.7 (0.1)	3.4 (0.0)
Flatulence	3.5 (0.4)	3.1 (0.4)
Dyspepsia	2.7 (0.1)	1.0 (0.0)
Respiratory System		
Rhinitis	7.3 (0.1)	5.7 (0.1)
Sinusitis	3.6 (0.0)	3.5 (0.0)
Coughing	1.5 (0.2)	1.2 (0.0)
Resistance Mechanism		
Viral infection	3.6 (0.2)	3.2 (0.0)
Upper respiratory tract infection	3.1 (0.1)	2.8 (0.0)
Body as a Whole		
Pain	3.4 (0.0)	2.3 (0.0)
Fever	2.2 (0.1)	1.5 (0.0)
Urinary System		
Urinary tract infection	2.4 (0.0)	1.9 (0.0)
Micturition frequency	1.2 (0.1)	0.6 (0.0)
Psychiatric		
Insomnia	1.9 (0.3)	1.3 (0.4)
Anxiety	1.4 (0.1)	1.0 (0.1)
Nervousness	1.4 (0.2)	0.7 (0.0)
Skin & Appendages		
Rash	1.6 (0.0)	1.6 (0.3)
Pruritus	1.2 (0.1)	1.0 (0.0)
Musculoskeletal System		
Arthralgia	1.4 (0.1)	1.2 (0.0)
Vision		
Abnormal vision	1.4 (0.2)	0.3 (0.0)
Reproductive, Female		
Vaginitis	1.2 (0.0)	0.9 (0.0)

In other U.S. and international trials and in foreign marketing experience, there have been rare reports of seizures and extrapyramidal effects, tachycardia, elevated liver enzymes, hepatitis, thrombocytopenia, leukopenia, aplastic anemia, pancytopenia, and granulocytopenia. The relationship of cisapride monohydrate to the event was not clear in these cases.

There have been rare cases of sinus tachycardia reported. Rechallenge precipitated relapse in some of those patients.

Rare cases of cardiac arrhythmias, including ventricular arrhythmias, torsades de pointes, and QT prolongation, in some cases resulting in death, have been reported. Most of these patients had been receiving multiple other medications and had pre-existing cardiac disease or risk factors for arrhythmias. A casual relationship to cisapride monohydrate has not been established.

OVERDOSAGE:

Reports of overdosage with cisapride monohydrate include an adult who took 540 mg and for 2 hours experienced retching, borborygmi, flatulence, stool frequency and urinary frequency.

A one-month-old male infant received 2 mg/kg of cisapride, 10 times the prescribed dose, four times per day for 5 days. The patient developed third degree heart block and subsequently died of right ventricular perforation caused by pacemaker wire insertion.

Treatment should include gastric lavage and/or activated charcoal, close observation and general supportive measures.

In instances of overdose, patients should be evaluated for possible QT prolongation and for factors that can predispose to the occurrence of ventricular arrhythmias, including torsades de pointes.

Single oral doses of cisapride at 4000 mg/kg, 160 mg/kg, 1280 mg/kg and 640 mg/kg were lethal in adult rats, neonatal rats, mice, and dogs, respectively. Symptoms of acute toxicity were ptosis, tremors, convulsions, dyspnea, loss of righting reflex, catalepsy, catatonia, hypotonia and diarrhea.

DOSAGE AND ADMINISTRATION:

5 ml (1 teaspoon) suspension = 5 mg.

Adults: Initiate therapy with one 10 mg tablet of cisapride monohydrate or 10 ml of the suspension 4 times daily at least 15 minutes before meals and at bedtime. In some patients the dosage will need to be increased to 20 mg, given as above, to obtain a satisfactory result.

In elderly patients, steady-state plasma levels are generally higher due to a moderate prolongation of the elimination half-life. Therapeutic doses, however, are similar to those used in younger adults.

PATIENT INFORMATION:

Cisapride monohydrate is used to treat patients with heartburn and patients with other problems with their gastrointestinal systems. Cisapride helps move food through the gastrointestinal system by increasing movement. Cisapride should not be taken with ketoconazole, itraconazole, miconazole, fluconazole, erythromycin, clarithromycin, or troleandomycin capsules. These drugs inhibit cisapride metabolism and lead to toxicity. Please consult with your pharmacist or physician for specific questions. The most commonly reported side effects include headache, diarrhea, abdominal pain, nausea and constipation. This medication should be taken before meals and at bedtime.

HOW SUPPLIED:

Propulsid Tablets are provided as scored white tablets debossed "Janssen" and P/10 containing the equivalent of 10 mg of cisapride. Propulsid is also provided as blue tablets, debossed "Janssen" and P/20, containing the equivalent of 20 mg cisapride.

Propulsid Suspension is provided as a bright pink homogeneous suspension containing 1 mg/ml of cisapride.

Store at room temperature (59°-86°F)(15°-30°C). Protect the tablets from moisture. The 20 mg tablets should also be protected from light.

HOW SUPPLIED - EQUIVALENTS NOT AVAILABLE:

Suspension - Oral - 1 mg/ml

450 ml	$47.25	PROPULSID, Janssen Phar	50458-0450-45

HOW SUPPLIED - EQUIVALENTS NOT AVAILABLE: *(cont'd)*

Tablet, Uncoated - Oral - 10 mg

100's	$62.94	PROPULSID, Janssen Phar	50458-0430-10
100's	$69.24	PROPULSID, Janssen Phar	50458-0430-01
500's	$314.70	PROPULSID, Janssen Phar	50458-0430-50

Tablet, Uncoated - Oral - 20 mg

100's	$122.10	PROPULSID, Janssen Phar	50458-0440-10

CISATRACURIUM BESYLATE *(003283)*

CATEGORIES: Analeptics; Anesthesia; Autonomic Drugs; Endotracheal Intubation; Muscle Relaxants; Neuromuscular Blocking Agents; Non-Depolarizing Muscle Relaxants; Skeletal Muscle Relaxants; FDA Aproved 1995 Dec; FDA Class 2S ("Standard Review"); Pregnancy Category B

BRAND NAMES: **Nimbex**

DESCRIPTION:

This drug should be administered only by adequately trained individuals familiar with its actions, characteristics, and hazards.

Cisatracurium besylate is a nondepolarizing skeletal muscle relaxant for intravenous administration. Compared to other neuromuscular blocking agents, it is intermediate in its onset and duration of action. Cisatracurium besylate is one of 10 isomers of atracurium besylate and constitutes approximately 15% of that mixture. Cisatracurium besylate is [1*R*-[1 α, 2 α (1 '*R**,2'*R**)]]-2,2'- [1,5-pentanediylbis [oxy (3- oxo- 3,1-propanediyl)]]bis[1-[(3,4-dimethoxyphenyl)methyl] -1,2,3,4- tetrahydro-6,7- dimethoxy-2-methylisoquinolinium] dibenzenesulfonate. The molecular formula of the cisatracurium besylate parent bis-cation is $C_{53}H_{72}N_2O_{12}$ and the molecular weight is 929.2. The molecular formula of cisatracurium as the besylate salt is $C_{65}H_{82}N_2O_{18}S_2$ and the molecular weight is 1243.50. The log of the partition coefficient of cisatracurium besylate is -2.12 in a 1-octanol/distilled water system at 25°C.

Cisatracurium besylate injection is a sterile, non-pyrogenic aqueous solution provided in 5 ml, 10 ml, and 20 ml vials. The pH is adjusted to 3.25 to 3.65 with benzenesulfonic acid. The 5 ml and 10 ml vials each contain cisatracurium besylate, equivalent to 2 mg/ml cisatracurium. The 20 ml vial, **intended for ICU use only**, contains cisatracurium besylate, equivalent to 10 mg/ml cisatracurium. The 10 ml vial, intended for multiple-dose use, contains 0.9% benzyl alcohol as a preservative. The 5 ml and 20 ml vials are single use vials and do not contain benzyl alcohol.

Cisatracurium besylate slowly loses potency with time at a rate of approximately 5% under refrigeration (5°C). Cisatracurium besylate should be refrigerated at 2° to 8°C (36° to 46°F) in the carton to preserve potency. The rate of loss in potency increases to approximately 5% *per month* at 25°C (77°F). Upon removal from refrigeration to room temperature storage conditions (25°C/ 77°F), use cisatracurium besylate within 21 days, even if rerefrigerated.

CLINICAL PHARMACOLOGY:

Cisatracurium besylate binds competitively to cholinergic receptors on the motor endplate to antagonize the action of acetylcholine, resulting in block of neuromuscular transmission. This action is antagonized by acetylcholinesterase inhibitors such as neostigmine.

PHARMACODYNAMICS

The neuromuscular blocking potency of cisatracurium besylate is approximately threefold that of atracurium besylate. The time to maximum block is up to 2 minutes longer for equipotent doses of cisatracurium besylate compared to atracurium besylate. The clinically effective duration of action and rate of spontaneous recovery from equipotent doses of cisatracurium besylate and atracurium besylate are similar.

The average ED_{95} (dose required to produce 95% suppression of the adductor pollicis muscle twitch response to ulnar nerve stimulation) of cisatracurium is 0.05 mg/kg (range: 0.048 to 0.053) in adults receiving opioid/nitrous oxide/oxygen anesthesia. For comparison, the average ED_{95} for atracurium when also expressed as the parent bis-cation is 0.17 mg/kg under similar anesthetic conditions.

The pharmacodynamics of 2 x ED_{95} to 8 x ED_{95} doses of cisatracurium administered over 5 to 10 seconds during opioid/nitrous oxide/oxygen anesthesia are summarized in TABLE 1. When the dose is doubled, the clinically effective duration of block increases by approximately 25 minutes. Once recovery begins, the rate of recovery is independent of dose.

Isoflurane or enflurane administered with nitrous oxide/oxygen to achieve 1.25 MAC [Minimum Alveolar Concentration] may prolong the clinically effective duration of action of initial and maintenance doses, and decrease the average infusion rate requirement of cisatracurium besylate. The magnitude of these effects may depend on the duration of administration of the volatile agents. Fifteen to 30 minutes of exposure to 1.25 MAC isoflurane or enflurane had minimal effects on the duration of action of initial doses of cisatracurium besylate and therefore, no adjustment to the initial dose should be necessary when cisatracurium besylate is administered shortly after initiation of volatile agents. In long surgical procedures during enflurane or isoflurane anesthesia, less frequent maintenance dosing, lower maintenance doses, or reduced infusion rates of cisatracurium besylate may be necessary. The average infusion rate requirement may be decreased by as much as 30% to 40%.

The onset, duration of action, and recovery profiles of cisatracurium besylate during propofol/oxygen or propofol/nitrous oxide/oxygen anesthesia are similar to those during opioid/nitrous oxide/oxygen anesthesia.

When administered during the induction of adequate anesthesia using propofol, nitrous oxide/oxygen, and co-induction agents (*e.g.*, fentanyl and midazolam), good or excellent conditions for tracheal intubation occurred in 67/71 (94%) patients in 1.5 to 2.0 minutes following 0.15 mg/kg cisatracurium and in 69/80 (87%) patients in 1.5 minutes following 0.2 mg/kg cisatracurium.

Repeated administration of maintenance doses or a continuous infusion of cisatracurium besylate for up to 3 hours is not associated with development of tachyphylaxis or cumulative neuromuscular blocking effects. The time needed to recover from successive maintenance doses does not change with the number of doses administered as long as partial recovery is allowed to occur between doses. Maintenance doses can therefore be administered at relatively regular intervals with predictable results. The rate of spontaneous recovery of neuromuscular function after infusion is independent of the duration of infusion and comparable to the rate of recovery following initial doses (TABLE 1).

Long-term infusion (up to 6 days) of cisatracurium besylate during mechanical ventilation in the ICU has been evaluated in two studies. In a randomized, double-blind study using presence of a single twitch during train-of-four (TOF) monitoring to regulate dosage, patients treated with cisatracurium besylate (n=19) recovered neuromuscular function (T_4:T_1 ratio ≥70%) following termination of infusion in approximately 55 minutes (range: 20 to 270) whereas those treated with vecuronium (n=12) recovered in 178 minutes (range: 40 minutes to 33 hours). In another study comparing cisatracurium besylate and atracurium, patients recovered neuromuscular function in approximately 50 minutes for both cisatracurium besylate (range: 20 to 175; n=34) and atracurium (range: 35 to 85; n=15).

CLINICAL PHARMACOLOGY: *(cont'd)*

TABLE 1 Pharmacodynamic Dose Response* of Cisatracurium Besylate During Opioid / Nitrous Oxide / Oxygen Anesthesia

Initial Dose of Nimbex (mg/kg)	Time to 90% Block (min)	Time to Maximum Block (min)	Time To Spontaneous Recovery: 5% Recovery (min)	25% Recovery† (min)	95% Recovery (min)	$T_4:T_1$ ratio‡≥ 70% (min)	25%-75% Recovery Index (min)
Adults							
0.1 (2 x ED_{95}) (n§=98)	3.3 (1.0-8.7)	5.0 (1.2-17.2)	33 (15-51)	42 (22-63)	64 (25-93)	64 (32-91)	13 (5-30)
0.15[11] (3 x ED_{95}) (n=39)	2.6 (1.0-4.4)	3.5 (1.6-6.8)	46 (28-65)	55 (44-74)	76 (60-103	75 (63-98)	13 (2-30)
0.2 (4 x ED_{95}) (n=30)	2.4 (1.5-4.5)	2.9 (1.9-5.2)	59 (31-103)	65 (43-103)	81 (53-114)	85 (55-114)	12 (2-30)
0.25 (5 x ED_{95}) (n=15)	1.6 (0.8-3.3)	2.0 (1.2-3.7)	70 (58-85)	78 (66-86)	91 (76-109)	97 (82-113)	8 (5-12)
0.4 (8 x ED_{95}) (n=15)	1.5 (1.3-1.8)	1.9 (1.4-2.3)	83 (37-103)	91 (59-107)	121 (110-134)	126 (115-137)	14 (10-18)
Children (2-12 yr)							
0.08¶ (2 x ED_{95}) (n=60)	2.2 (1.2-6.8)	3.3 (1.7-9.7)	22 (11-38)	29 (20-46)	52 (37-64)	50 (37-62)	11 (7-15)
0.1 (n=16)	1.7 (1.3-2.7)	2.8 (1.8-6.7)	21 (13-31)	28 (21-38)	46 (37-58)	44 (36-58)	10 (7-12)

* Values shown are medians of means from individual studies. Values in parentheses are ranges of individual patient values.
† Clinically effective duration of block
‡ Train-of-four ratio
§ n = the number of patients with Time to Maximum Block data
11 Propofol anesthesia
¶ Halothane anesthesia

The neuromuscular block produced by cisatracurium besylate is readily antagonized by anticholinesterase agents once recovery has started. As with other nondepolarizing neuromuscular blocking agents, the more profound the neuromuscular block at the time of reversal, the longer the time required for recovery of neuromuscular function.

In children (2 to 12 years) cisatracurium has a lower ED_{95} than in adults (0.04 mg/kg, halothane/nitrous oxide/oxygen anesthesia). At 0.1 mg/kg during opioid anesthesia, cisatracurium had a faster onset and shorter duration of action in children than in adults (TABLE 1). Recovery following reversal is faster in children than in adults.

HEMODYNAMICS PROFILE

Cisatracurium has no dose-related effects on mean arterial blood pressure (MAP) or heart rate (HR) following doses ranging from 2 to 8 x ED_{95} (0.1 to 0.4 mg/kg), administered over 5 to 10 seconds, in healthy adult patients.

In patients with serious cardiovascular disease, cisatracurium besylate has no clinically significant effects on MAP or HR following doses up to and including 6 x ED_{95} (0.3 mg/kg), administered over 5 to 10 seconds. In two comparative studies involving patients undergoing coronary artery bypass grafting (CABG), there were no clinically significant differences in the hemodynamic effects following equipotent doses ranging from 0.1 to 0.3 mg/kg cisatracurium or vecuronium. Doses higher than 6 x ED_{95} have not been studied in patients with serious cardiovascular disease.

Unlike atracurium, cisatracurium, at therapeutic doses of 2 x ED_{95} to 8 x ED_{95} (0.1 to 0.4 mg/kg), administered over 5 to 10 seconds, does not cause dose-related elevations in mean plasma histamine concentration. The cardiovascular profile of cisatracurium besylate allows it to be administered by rapid bolus at higher multiples of the ED_{95} than atracurium.

No clinically significant changes in MAP or HR were observed following administration of doses up to 0.1 mg/kg cisatracurium over 5 to 10 seconds in 2- to 12-year-old children receiving either halothane/nitrous oxide/oxygen or opioid/nitrous oxide/oxygen anesthesia.

PHARMACOKINETICS

General: The neuromuscular blocking activity of cisatracurium besylate is due to parent drug. Cisatracurium plasma concentration-time data following IV bolus administration are best described by a two-compartment open model (with elimination from both compartments) with an elimination half-life ($t_{1/2}$ β) of 22 minutes, a plasma clearance (CL) of 4.57 ml/min/kg, and a volume of distribution at steady state (V_{ss}) of 145 ml/kg. Cisatracurium undergoes organ-independent Hofmann elimination (a chemical process dependent on pH and temperature) to form the monoquaternary acrylate metabolite and laudanosine, neither of which has any neuromuscular blocking activity (see Pharmacokinetics, Metabolism). Following administration of radiolabeled cisatracurium, 95% of the dose was recovered in the urine; less than 10% of the dose was excreted as unchanged parent drug. Laudanosine, a metabolite of cisatracurium (and atracurium) has been noted to cause transient hypotension and, in higher doses, cerebral excitatory effects when administered to several animal species. The relationship between CNS excitation and laudanosine concentrations in humans has not been established (see PRECAUTIONS, Long-term use in the Intensive Care Unit.) Because cisatracurium is three times more potent than atracurium and lower doses are required, the corresponding laudanosine concentrations following cisatracurium are one-third those that would be expected following an equipotent dose of atracurium (see Pharmacokinetics: Special Populations: Intensive Care Unit Patients).

Results from population pharmacokinetic/pharmacodynamic (PK/PD) analyses from 241 healthy surgical patients are summarized in TABLE 2.

The magnitude of interpatient variability in CL was low (16%), as expected based on the importance of Hofmann elimination (see Pharmacokinetics, Elimination). The magnitudes of interpatient variability in CL and volume of distribution were low in comparison to those for k_{eo} and EC_{50}. This suggests that any alterations in the time course of cisatracurium-induced block are more likely to be due to variability in the pharmacodynamic parameters than in the pharmacokinetic parameters. Parameter estimates from the population pharmacokinetic analyses were supported by noncompartmental pharmacokinetic analyses on data from healthy patients and from special patient populations.

CLINICAL PHARMACOLOGY: *(cont'd)*

TABLE 2 Key Population PK/PD Parameter Estimates for Cisatracurium in Healthy Surgical Patients* Following 0.1 (2 x ED 95) to 0.4 mg/kg (8 x ED_{95}) Cisatracurium Besylate

Parameter	Estimate †	Magnitude of Interpatient Variability (CV) ‡
CL (mL/min/kg)	4.57	16%
V_{ss} (mL/kg)§	145	27%
k_{eo} (min^{-1})ll	0.0575	61%
EC_{50} (ng/mL)¶	141	52%

* Healthy male nonobese patients 19-64 years of age with creatinine clearance values greater than 70 mL/min who received cisatracurium during opioid anesthesia and had venous samples collected.
† The percent standard error of the mean (%SEM) ranged from 3 to !12% indicating good precision for the PK/PD estimates
‡ Expressed as a coefficient of variation; the %SEM ranged from 20 to 35% indicating adequate precision for the estimates of interpatient variability.
§ $V_{ss}$is the volume of distribution at steady state estimated using a two-compartment model with elimination from both compartments. V_{ss} is equal to the sum of the volume in the central compartment (V_c) and the volume in the peripheral compartment (V_p); interpatient variability could only be estimated for V
ll Rate constant describing the equilibration between plasma concentrations and neuromuscular block
¶ Concentration required to produce 50% T_1 suppression; an index of patient sensitivity

Conventional pharmacokinetic analyses have shown that the pharmacokinetics of cisatracurium are proportional to dose between 0.1 (2 x ED_{95}) and 0.2 (4 x ED_{95}) mg/kg cisatracurium. In addition, population pharmacokinetic analyses revealed no statistically significant effect of initial dose on CL for doses between 0.1 (2 x ED_{95}) and 0.4 (8 x ED_{95}) mg/kg cisatracurium.

Distribution: The volume of distribution of cisatracurium is limited by its large molecular weight and high polarity. The V_{ss} was equal to 145 ml/kg (TABLE 2) in healthy 19- to 64-year-old surgical patients receiving opioid anesthesia. The $V_{ss}$was 21% larger in similar patients receiving inhalation anesthesia (see Special Populations: Other Patient Factors).

Protein Binding: The binding of cisatracurium to plasma proteins has not been successfully studied due to its rapid degradation at physiologic pH. Inhibition of degradation requires nonphysiological conditions of temperature and pH which are associated with changes in protein binding.

Metabolism: The degradation of cisatracurium is largely independent of liver metabolism. Results from in vitro experiments suggest that cisatracurium undergoes Hofmann elimination (a pH and temperature-dependent chemical process) to form laudanosine (see PRECAUTIONS, Long-Term Use in the Intensive Care Unit) and the monoquaternary acrylate metabolite. The monoquaternary acrylate undergoes hydrolysis by non-specific plasma esterases to form the monoquaternary alcohol (MQA) metabolite. The MQA metabolite can also undergo Hofmann elimination but at a much slower rate than cisatracurium. Laudanosine is further metabolized to desmethyl metabolites which are conjugated with glucuronic acid and excreted in the urine.

Organ-independent Hofmann elimination is the predominant pathway for the elimination of cisatracurium. The liver and kidney play a minor role in the elimination of cisatracurium but are primary pathways for the elimination of metabolites. Therefore, the $t_{1/2}$ β values of metabolites (including laudanosine) are longer in patients with kidney or liver dysfunction and metabolite concentrations may be higher after long-term administration (see PRECAUTIONS, Long-Term Use in the Intensive Care Unit). Most importantly, C_{max} values of laudanosine are significantly lower in healthy surgical patients receiving infusions of cisatracurium than in patients receiving infusions of atracurium (mean ± S.D. C_{max}: 60 ± 52 and 342 ± 93 ng/ml, respectively).

ELIMINATION

Clearance and Half-life: Mean CL values for cisatracurium ranged from 4.5 to 5.7 ml/min/kg in studies of healthy surgical patients. Compartmental pharmacokinetic modeling suggests that approximately 80% of the CL is accounted for by Hofmann elimination and the remaining 20% by renal and hepatic elimination. These findings are consistent with the low magnitude of interpatient variability in CL (16%) estimated as part of the population PK/PD analyses and with the recovery of parent and metabolites in urine. Following ^{14}C-cisatracurium administration to 6 healthy male patients, 95% of the dose was recovered in the urine (mostly as conjugated metabolites) and 4% in the feces; less than 10% of the dose was excreted as unchanged parent drug in the urine. In 12 healthy surgical patients receiving non-radiolabeled cisatracurium who had Foley catheters placed for surgical management, approximately 15% of the dose was excreted unchanged in the urine.

In studies of healthy surgical patients, mean $t_{1/2}$β values of cisatracurium ranged from 22 to 29 minutes and were consistent with the $t_{1/2}$β of cisatracurium in vitro (29 min). The mean ± S.D. $t_{1/2}$β values of laudanosine were 3.1 ± 0.4 and 3.3 ± 2.1 hours in healthy surgical patients receiving cisatracurium besylate (n=10) or atracurium (n=10), respectively. During IV infusions of cisatracurium besylate, peak plasma concentrations (C_{max}) of laudanosine and the MQA metabolite are approximately 6% and 11% of the parent compound, respectively.

SPECIAL POPULATIONS

Elderly Patients (≥65 years): The results of conventional pharmacokinetic analysis from a study of 12 healthy elderly patients and 12 healthy young adult patients receiving a single IV dose of 0.1 mg/kg cisatracurium besylate are summarized in TABLE 3. Plasma clearances of cisatracurium were not affected by age; however, the volumes of distribution were slightly larger in elderly patients than in young patients resulting in slightly longer $t_{1/2}$β values for cisatracurium. The rate of equilibration between plasma cisatracurium concentrations and neuromuscular block was slower in elderly patients than in young patients (mean ± S.D. k_{eo}: 0.071 ± 0.036 and 0.105 ± 0.021 min^{-1}, respectively); there was no difference in the patient sensitivity to cisatracurium-induced block, as indicated by EC_{50} values (mean ± S.D. EC_{50}: 91 ± 22 and 89 ± 23 ng/ml, respectively). These changes were consistent with the one-minute slower times to maximum block in elderly patients receiving 0.1 mg/kg cisatracurium besylate, when compared to young patients receiving the same dose. The minor differences in PK/PD parameters of cisatracurium between elderly patients and young patients were not associated with clinically significant differences in the recovery profile of cisatracurium besylate.

Patients with Hepatic Disease: TABLE 4 summarizes the conventional pharmacokinetic analysis from a study of cisatracurium besylate in 13 patients with end-stage liver disease undergoing liver transplantation and 11 healthy adult patients undergoing elective surgery. The slightly larger volumes of distribution in liver transplant patients were associated with slightly higher plasma clearances of cisatracurium. The parallel changes in these parameters resulted in no difference in $t_{1/2}$β values. There were no differences in k_{eo} or EC_{50} between patient groups. The times to maximum block were approximately one minute faster in liver transplant patients than in healthy adult patients receiving 0.1 mg/kg cisatracurium besylate. These minor differences in pharmacokinetics were not associated with clinically significant differences in the recovery profile of cisatracurium besylate.

CLINICAL PHARMACOLOGY: *(cont'd)*

TABLE 3 Pharmacokinetic Parameters* of Cisatracurium In Healthy Elderly and Young Adult Patients Following 0.1 mg/kg (2xED 95) Cisatracurium Besylate (Isoflurane/Nitrous Oxide/Oxygen Anesthesia)

Parameter	Healthy Elderly Patients	Healthy Young Adult Patients
Elimination Half-Life ($t_{1/2}\beta$, min)	25.8 ± 3.6†	22.1 ± 2.5
Volume of Distribution at Steady State ‡ (mL/kg)	156 ± 17†	133 ± 15
Plasma Clearance (mL/min/kg)	5.7 ± 1.0	5.3 ± 0.9

* Values presented are mean ± S.D.
† P <0.05 for comparisons between healthy elderly and healthy young adult patients
‡ Volume of distribution is underestimated because elimination from the peripheral compartment is ignored.

The $t_{1/2}\beta$ values of metabolites are longer in patients with hepatic disease and concentrations may be higher after long-term administration (see Special Populations: Intensive Care Unit Patients).

TABLE 4 Pharmacokinetic Parameters* of Cisatracurium In Healthy Adult Patients Undergoing Liver Transplantation Following 0.1 mg/kg (2xED 95) Cisatracurium Besylate (Isoflurane/Nitrous Oxide/Oxygen Anesthesia)

Parameter	Liver Transplant Patients	Healthy Adult Patients
Elimination Half-Life ($t_{1/2}\beta$, min)	24.4 ± 2.9	23.5 ± 3.5
Volume of Distribution at Steady State ‡ (mL/kg)	195 ± 38†	161 ± 23
Plasma Clearance (mL/min/kg)	6.6 ± 1.1†	5.7 ± 0.8

* Values presented are mean ± S.D.
† P <0.05 for comparisons between liver transplant patients and healthy adult patients
‡ Volume of distribution is underestimated because elimination from the peripheral compartment is ignored.

Patients with Renal Dysfunction: Results from a conventional pharmacokinetic study of cisatracurium besylate in 13 healthy adult patients and 15 patients with end-stage renal disease (ESRD) undergoing elective surgery are summarized in TABLE 5. The PK/PD parameters of cisatracurium were similar in healthy adult patients and ESRD patients. The times to 90% block were approximately one minute slower in ESRD patients following 0.1 mg/kg cisatracurium besylate. There were no differences in the durations or rates of recovery of cisatracurium besylate between ESRD and healthy adult patients.

The $t_{1/2}\beta$ values of metabolites are longer in patients with renal failure and concentrations may be higher after long-term administration (see Special Populations: Intensive Care Unit Patients).

TABLE 5 Pharmacokinetic Parameters* of Cisatracurium In Healthy Adult Patients and in Patients With End-Stage Renal Disease (ESRD) Following 0.1 mg/kg (2xED 95) Cisatracurium Besylate (Isoflurane/Nitrous Oxide/Oxygen Anesthesia)

Parameter	Healthy Adult Patients	ESRD Patients
Elimination Half-Life ($t_{1/2}\beta$, min)	29.4 ± 4.1	32.3 ± 6.3
Volume of Distribution at Steady State ‡ (mL/kg)	149 ± 35	160 ± 32
Plasma Clearance (mL/min/kg)	4.66 ± 0.86	4.26 ± 0.62

* Values presented are mean ± S.D.
‡ Volume of distribution is underestimated because elimination from the peripheral compartment is ignored.

Population pharmacokinetic analyses revealed that patients with creatinine clearances ≤70 ml/min had a slower rate of equilibration between plasma concentrations and neuromuscular block than patients with normal renal function; this change was associated with a slightly slower (~40 sec) predicted time to 90% T_1 suppression in patients with renal dysfunction following 0.1 mg/kg cisatracurium besylate. There was no clinically significant alteration in the recovery profile of cisatracurium besylate in patients with renal dysfunction. The recovery profile of cisatracurium besylate is unchanged in the presence of renal or hepatic failure, which is consistent with predominantly organ-independent elimination.

Intensive Care Unit (ICU) Patients: The pharmacokinetics of cisatracurium, atracurium, and their metabolites were determined in 6 ICU patients receiving cisatracurium besylate and in 6 ICU patients receiving atracurium and are presented in TABLE 6. The plasma clearances of cisatracurium and atracurium are similar. The volume of distribution was larger and the $t_{\frac{1}{2}}\beta$ was longer for cisatracurium than for atracurium. The relationships between plasma cisatracurium or atracurium concentrations and neuromuscular block have not been evaluated in ICU patients. The minor differences in pharmacokinetics were not associated with any differences in the recovery profiles of cisatracurium besylate and atracurium in ICU patients.

TABLE 6 Parameter Estimates* for Cisatracurium, Atracurium, and Metabolites in ICU Patients After Long-Term (24–48 hr) Administration of Cisatracurium Besylate or Atracurium Besylate

	Parameter	Cisatracurium (n=6)	Atracurium (n=6)
Parent Compound	CL (mL/min/kg)	7.45 ± 1.02	7.49 ± 0.66†
	$t_{1/2}\beta$ (min)	26.8 ± 11.1	16.5 ± 6.0†
	Vβ (mL/kg)‡	280 ± 103	178 ± 71†
Laudanosine	C_{max} (ng/mL)	707 ± 360	2318 ± 1498
$t_{1/2}\beta$ (hrs)	6.6 ± 4.1	8.4 ± 7.3	
MQA metabolite	C_{max} (ng/mL)	152-181§	943 ± 333‖
$t_{1/2}\beta$ (min)	26-31§	21-58§	

* presented as mean ± standard deviation
† n=5
‡ Volume of distribution during the terminal elimination phase, an underestimate because elimination from the peripheral compartment is ignored.
§ n=2, range presented
‖ n=3

Plasma metabolite pharmacokinetics are listed in TABLE 6. Limited pharmacokinetic data are available for patients with liver/kidney dysfunction receiving cisatracurium besylate. Data from studies of atracurium demonstrate that renal/hepatic failure in ICU patients produces little to no effect on its pharmacokinetics, but decreases the biotransformation and elimination of the metabolites. Following atracurium, $t_{1/2}\beta$ values for laudanosine were longer in ICU patients with renal failure than in ICU patients with normal renal function (15 and 6 hrs, respectively). The $t_{1/2}$ β values of laudanosine were 39 ± 14 hrs in ICU patients with liver failure receiving atracurium after an unsuccessful liver transplantation and 5 ± 2 hrs in similar ICU patients after successful liver transplantation. Therefore, relative to ICU patients with normal renal and hepatic function receiving cisatracurium besylate, metabolite concentrations (plasma and tissues) may be higher in ICU patients with renal or hepatic failure (see PRECAUTIONS, Long-term Use in the Intensive Care Unit). Consistent with the decreased infusion rate requirements for cisatracurium besylate, metabolite concentrations were lower in patients receiving cisatracurium besylate than in patients receiving atracurium besylate.

Pediatric Patients: The population PK/PD of cisatracurium were described in 20 healthy pediatric patients during halothane anesthesia, using the same model developed for healthy adult patients. The CL was higher in healthy pediatric patients (5.89 ml/min/kg) than in healthy adult patients (4.57 ml/min/kg) during opioid anesthesia. The rate of equilibration between plasma concentrations and neuromuscular block, as indicated by k_{eo}, was faster in healthy pediatric patients receiving halothane anesthesia (0.1330 min^{-1}) than in healthy adult patients receiving opioid anesthesia (0.0575 min^{-1}). The EC_{50} in healthy pediatric patients (125 ng/ml) was similar to the value in healthy adult patients (141 ng/ml) during opioid anesthesia. The minor differences in the PK/PD parameters of cisatracurium were associated with a faster time to onset and a shorter duration of cisatracurium-induced neuromuscular block in pediatric patients.

Other Patient Factors: Population PK/PD analyses revealed that gender and obesity were associated with statistically significant effects on the pharmacokinetics and/or pharmacodynamics of cisatracurium; these factors were not associated with clinically significant alterations in the predicted onset or recovery profile of cisatracurium besylate. The use of inhalation agents was associated with a 21% larger V_{ss}, a 78% larger k_{eo}, and a 15% lower EC_{50} for cisatracurium. These changes resulted in a slightly faster (~45 sec) predicted time to 90% T_1 suppression in patients receiving 0.1 mg/kg cisatracurium during inhalation anesthesia than in patients receiving the same dose of cisatracurium during opioid anesthesia; however, there were no clinically significant differences in the predicted recovery profile of cisatracurium besylate between patient groups.

Individualization of Dosages: DOSES OF CISATRACURIUM BESYLATE SHOULD BE INDIVIDUALIZED AND A PERIPHERAL NERVE STIMULATOR SHOULD BE USED TO MEASURE NEUROMUSCULAR FUNCTION DURING ADMINISTRATION OF CISATRACURIUM BESYLATE IN ORDER TO MONITOR DRUG EFFECT, TO DETERMINE THE NEED FOR ADDITIONAL DOSES, AND TO CONFIRM RECOVERY FROM NEUROMUSCULAR BLOCK.

Based on the known action of cisatracurium besylate and other neuromuscular blocking agents, the following factors should be considered when administering cisatracurium besylate:

Renal and Hepatic Disease: See PRECAUTIONS.

Long-Term Use in the Intensive Care Unit (ICU): The long-term infusion (up to 6 days) of cisatracurium besylate during mechanical ventilation in the ICU has been evaluated in two studies. Average infusion rates of approximately 3 mcg/kg/min (range: 0.5 to 10.2) were required to achieve adequate neuromuscular block. As with other neuromuscular blocking agents, these data indicate the presence of wide interpatient variability in dosage requirements. In addition, dosage requirements may increase or decrease with time (see PRECAUTIONS). Use of cisatracurium besylate in the ICU for longer than 6 days has not been studied.

Drugs or Conditions Causing Potentiation of or Resistance to Neuromuscular Block: Persons with certain pre-existing conditions or receiving certain drugs may require individualization of dosing (see DRUG INTERACTIONS).

Burns: Patients with burns have been shown to develop resistance to nondepolarizing neuromuscular blocking agents, and may require individualization of dosing (see PRECAUTIONS).

INDICATIONS AND USAGE:

Cisatracurium besylate is an intermediate-onset/intermediate-duration neuromuscular blocking agent indicated for inpatients and outpatients as an adjunct to general anesthesia, to facilitate tracheal intubation, and to provide skeletal muscle relaxation during surgery or mechanical ventilation in the ICU.

CONTRAINDICATIONS:

Cisatracurium besylate is contraindicated in patients known to have an allergic hypersensitivity to cisatracurium besylate or other bis-benzylisoquinolinium agents. Use of cisatracurium besylate from vials containing benzyl alcohol as a preservative is contraindicated in patients with a known hypersensitivity to benzyl alcohol.

WARNINGS:

CISATRACURIUM BESYLATE SHOULD BE ADMINISTERED IN CAREFULLY ADJUSTED DOSAGE BY OR UNDER THE SUPERVISION OF EXPERIENCED CLINICIANS WHO ARE FAMILIAR WITH THE DRUG'S ACTIONS AND THE POSSIBLE COMPLICATIONS OF ITS USE. THE DRUG SHOULD NOT BE ADMINISTERED UNLESS PERSONNEL AND FACILITIES FOR RESUSCITATION AND LIFE SUPPORT (TRACHEAL INTUBATION, ARTIFICIAL VENTILATION, OXYGEN THERAPY), AND AN ANTAGONIST OF CISATRACURIUM BESYLATE ARE IMMEDIATELY AVAILABLE. IT IS RECOMMENDED THAT A PERIPHERAL NERVE STIMULATOR BE USED TO MEASURE NEUROMUSCULAR FUNCTION DURING THE ADMINISTRATION OF CISATRACURIUM BESYLATE IN ORDER TO MONITOR DRUG EFFECT, DETERMINE THE NEED FOR ADDITIONAL DOSES, AND CONFIRM RECOVERY FROM NEUROMUSCULAR BLOCK.

CISATRACURIUM BESYLATE HAS NO KNOWN EFFECT ON CONSCIOUSNESS, PAIN THRESHOLD, OR CEREBRATION. TO AVOID DISTRESS TO THE PATIENT, NEUROMUSCULAR BLOCK SHOULD NOT BE INDUCED BEFORE UNCONSCIOUSNESS.

Cisatracurium besylate injection is acidic (pH 3.25 to 3.65) and may not be compatible with alkaline solutions having a pH greater than 8.5 (*e.g.,* barbiturate solutions).

The 10 ml multiple dose vials of cisatracurium besylate contain benzyl alcohol. In newborn infants, benzyl alcohol has been associated with an increased incidence of neurological and other complications which are sometimes fatal. Single use vials (5 ml and 20 ml) of cisatracurium besylate do not contain benzyl alcohol (see Pediatric Use).

PRECAUTIONS:

Because of its intermediate onset of action, cisatracurium besylate is not recommended for rapid sequence endotracheal intubation.

Recommended doses of cisatracurium besylate have no clinically significant effects on heart rate; therefore, cisatracurium besylate will not counteract the bradycardia produced by many anesthetic agents or by vagal stimulation.

PRECAUTIONS: *(cont'd)*

Neuromuscular blocking agents may have a profound effect in patients with neuromuscular diseases (*e.g.,* myasthenia gravis and the myasthenic syndrome). In these and other conditions in which prolonged neuromuscular block is a possibility (*e.g.,* carcinomatosis), the use of a peripheral nerve stimulator and a dose of not more than 0.02 mg/kg cisatracurium besylate is recommended to assess the level of neuromuscular block and to monitor dosage requirements.

Patients with burns have been shown to develop resistance to nondepolarizing neuromuscular blocking agents, including atracurium. The extent of altered response depends upon the size of the burn and the time elapsed since the burn injury. Cisatracurium besylate has not been studied in patients with burns; however, based on its structural similarity to atracurium, the possibility of increased dosing requirements and shortened duration of action must be considered if cisatracurium besylate is administered to burn patients.

Patients with hemiparesis or paraparesis also may demonstrate resistance to nondepolarizing muscle relaxants in the affected limbs. To avoid inaccurate dosing, neuromuscular monitoring should be performed on a non-paretic limb.

Acid-base and/or serum electrolyte abnormalities may potentiate or antagonize the action of neuromuscular blocking agents.

No data are available to support the use of cisatracurium besylate by intramuscular injection.

Renal and Hepatic Disease: No clinically significant alterations in the recovery profile were observed in patients with renal dysfunction or in patients with end-stage liver disease following a 0.1 mg/kg dose of cisatracurium. The onset time was approximately 1 minute faster in patients with end-stage liver disease and approximately 1 minute slower in patients with renal dysfunction than in healthy adult control patients.

Malignant Hyperthermia (MH): In a study of MH-susceptible pigs, cisatracurium besylate (highest dose 2000 mcg/kg equivalent to 3 x ED_{95} in pigs and 40 x ED_{95}in humans) did not trigger MH. Cisatracurium besylate has not been studied in MH-susceptible patients. Because MH can develop in the absence of established triggering agents, the clinician should be prepared to recognize and treat MH in any patient undergoing general anesthesia.

Long-Term Use in the Intensive Care Unit (ICU): Long term infusion (up to 6 days) of cisatracurium besylate during mechanical ventilation in the ICU has been safely used in two studies. Dosage requirements may increase or decrease with time (see CLINICAL PHARMACOLOGY, Individualization of Doses).

Little information is available on the plasma levels and clinical consequences of cisatracurium metabolites that may accumulate during days to weeks of cisatracurium administration in ICU patients. Laudanosine, a major, biologically active metabolite of atracurium and cisatracurium without neuromuscular blocking activity, produces transient hypotension and, in higher doses, cerebral excitatory effects (generalized muscle twitching and seizures) when administered to several species of animals. There have been rare spontaneous reports of seizures in ICU patients who have received atracurium or other agents. These patients usually had predisposing causes (such as cranial trauma, cerebral edema, hypoxic encephalopathy, viral encephalitis, uremia). There are insufficient data to detemine whether or not laudanosine contributes to seizures in ICU patients. Consistent with the decreased infusion rate requirements for cisatracurium besylate, laudanosine concentrations were lower in patients receiving cisatracurium besylate than in patients receiving atracurium for up to 48 hours (see CLINICAL PHARMACOLOGY).

In a randomized, double-blind study using train-of-four nerve stimulator monitoring to maitain at least one visable twitch, evaluable patients treated with cisatracurium besylate (n=19) recovered neuromuscular function (T_4:T_1 ratio ≥ 70%) following termination of infusion in approximately 55 minutes (range: (range: 20 to 270) whereas evaluable vecuronium-treated patients (n=12) recovered in 178 minutes (range: 40 minutes to 33 hours). In another study comparing cisatracurium besylate and atracurium, patients recovered neuromuscular function in approximately 50 minuts for both cisatracurium besylate (range: 20 to 75; n=34) and atracurium (range: 35 to 85; n=15).

WHENEVER THE USE OF CISATRACURIUM BESYLATE OR ANY OTHER NEUROMUSCULAR BLOCKING AGENT IN THE ICU IS CONTEMPLATED. IT IS RECOMMENDED THAT NEUROMUSCULAR FUNCTION BE MONITORED DURING ADMINISTRATION WITH A NERVE STIMULATOR. ADDITIONAL DOSES OF CISATRACURIUM BESYLATE OR ANY OTHER NEUROMUSCULAR BLOCKING AGENT SHOULD NOT BE GIVEN BEFORE THERE IS A DEFINITE RESPONSE TO NERVE STIMULATION. IF NO RESPONSE IS ELICITED, INFUSION ADMINISTRATION SHOULD BE DISCONTINUED UNTIL A RESPONSE RETURNS.

The effects of hemofiltration, hemodialysis, and hemoperfusion on plasma levels of cisatracurium besylate and its metabolites are unknown.

Drug/Laboratory Test Interactions: None known.

Carcinogenesis, Mutagenesis, and Impairment of Fertility: Carcinogenesis and fertility studies have not been performed. Cisatracurium besylate was evaluated in a battery of four short-term mutagenicity tests. It was non-mutagenic in the Ames Salmonella assay, a rat bone marrow cytogenetic assay, and an *in vitro* human lymphocyte cytogenetics assay. As was the case with atracurium, the mouse lymphoma assay was positive both in the presence and absence of exogenous metabolic activation (rat liver S-9). In the absence of S-9, cisatracurium besylate was positive at *in vitro* cisatracurium concentrations of 40 mcg/ml and higher. The highest non-mutagenic concentration (30 mcg/ml) and incubation time (4 hours) resulted in an AUC approximately 120 times that noted in clinical studies and approximately 8.5 times the mean peak clinical concentration noted. In the presence of S-9, cisatracurium besylate was positive at a cisatracurium concentration of 300 mcg/ml but not at lower or higher concentrations.

Pregnancy, Teratogenic Effects, Pregnancy Category B: Teratology testing in nonventilated pregnant rats treated subcutaneously with maximum subparalyzing doses (4 mg/kg daily; equivalent to 8 x the human ED_{95} following a bolus dose of 0.2 mg/kg IV) and in ventilated rats treated intravenously with paralyzing doses of at 0.5 and 1.0 mg/kg; equivalent to 10 x and 20 x the human ED_{95} dose, respectively, revealed no maternal or fetal toxicity or teratogenic effects. There are no adequate and well-controlled studies of cisatracurium besylate in pregnant women. Because animal studies are not always predictive of human response, cisatracurium besylate should be used during pregnancy only if clearly needed.

Labor and Delivery: The use of cisatracurium besylate during labor, vaginal delivery, or cesarean section has not been studied in humans and it is not known whether cisatracurium besylate administered to the mother has effects on the fetus. Doses of 0.2 or 0.4 mg/kg cisatracurium given to female beagles undergoing cesarean section resulted in negligible levels of cisatracurium in umbilical vessel blood of neonates and no deleterious effects on the puppies. The action of neuromuscular blocking agents may be enhanced by magnesium salts administered for the management of toxemia of pregnancy.

Nursing Mothers: It is not known whether cisatracurium besylate is excreted in human milk. Because many drugs are excreted in human milk, caution should be exercised following administration of cisatracurium besylate to a nursing woman.

Pediatric Use: Cisatracurium besylate has not been studied in pediatric patients below the age of 2 years (see CLINICAL PHARMACOLOGY and DOSAGE AND ADMINISTRATION for clinical experience and recommendations for use in children 2 to 12 years of age).

PRECAUTIONS: *(cont'd)*

Geriatric Use: Cisatracurium besylate was safely administered during clinical trials to 145 elderly (≥65 years) patients, including a subset of patients with significant cardiovascular disease (see Special Populations, elderly and Hemodynamics Profile). Minor differences in the pharmacokinetics of cisatracurium between elderly and young adult patients are not associated with clinically significant differences in the recovery profile of cisatracurium besylate following a single 0.1 mg/kg dose; the time to maximum block is approximately 1 minute slower in elderly patients (see CLINICAL PHARMACOLOGY, Pharmacokinetics).

DRUG INTERACTIONS:

Cisatracurium besylate has been used safely following varying degrees of recovery from succinylcholine-induced neuromuscular block. Administration of 0.1 mg/kg (2 x ED_{95}) cisatracurium besylate at 10% or 95% recovery following an intubating dose of succinylcholine (1 mg/kg) produced ≥95% neuromuscular block. The time to onset of maximum block following cisatracurium besylate is approximately 2 minutes faster with prior administration of succinylcholine. Prior administration of succinylcholine had no effect on the duration of neuromuscular block following initial or maintenance bolus doses of cisatracurium besylate. Infusion requirements of cisatracurium besylate in patients administered succinylcholine prior to infusions of cisatracurium besylate were comparable to or slightly greater than when succinylcholine was not administered.

The use of cisatracurium besylate before succinylcholine to attenuate some of the side effects of succinylcholine has not been studied.

Although not studied systematically in clinical trials, no drug interactions were observed when vecuronium, pancuronium, or atracurium were administered following varying degrees of recovery from single doses or infusions of cisatracurium besylate.

Isoflurane or enflurane administered with nitrous oxide/oxygen to achieve 1.25 MAC [Minimum Alveolar Concentration] may prolong the clinically effective duration of action of initial and maintenance doses of cisatracurium besylate and decrease the required infusion rate of cisatracurium besylate. The magnitude of these effects may depend on the duration of administration of the volatile agents. Fifteen to 30 minutes of exposure to 1.25 MAC isoflurane or enflurane had minimal effects on the duration of action of initial doses of cisatracurium besylate and therefore, no adjustment to the initial dose should be necessary when cisatracurium besylate is administered shortly after initiation of volatile agents. In long surgical procedures during enflurane or isoflurane anesthesia, less frequent maintenance dosing, lower maintenance doses, or reduced infusion rates of cisatracurium besylate may be necessary. The average infusion rate requirement may be decreased by as much as 30% to 40%.

In clinical studies propofol had no effect on the duration of action or dosing requirements for cisatracurium besylate.

Other drugs which may enhance the neuromuscular blocking action of nondepolarizing agents such as cisatracurium besylate include certain antibiotics (*e.g.,* aminoglycosides, tetracyclines, bacitracin, polymyxins, lincomycin, clindamycin, colistin, and sodium colistimethate), magnesium salts, lithium, local anesthetics, procainamide. and quinidine.

Resistance to the neuromuscular blocking action of nondepolarizing neuromuscular blocking agents has been demonstrated in patients chronically administered phenytoin or carbamazepine. While the effects of chronic phenytoin or carbamazepine therapy on the action of cisatracurium besylate are unknown, slightly shorter durations of neuromuscular block may be anticipated and infusion rate requirements may be higher.

ADVERSE REACTIONS:

Observed in Clinical Trials of Surgical Patients: Adverse experiences were uncommon among the 945 surgical patients who received cisatracurium besylate in conjunction with other drugs in U.S. and European clinical studies in the course of a wide variety of procedures in patients receiving opioid, propofol, or inhalation anesthesia. The following adverse experiences were judged by investigators during the clinical trials to have a possible causal relationship to administration of cisatracurium besylate:

Incidence Greater than 1%: None

Incidence Less than 1%:

Cardiovascular: bradycardia (0.4%), hypotension (0.2%), flushing (0.2%)

Respiratory: bronchospasm (0.2%)

Dermatological: rash (0.1%)

Observed in Clinical Trials of Intensive Care Unit Patients: Adverse experiences were uncommon among the 68 ICU patients who received cisatracurium besylate in conjunction with other drugs in U.S. and European clinical studies. One patient experienced bronchospasm. In one of the two ICU studies, a randomized and double-blind study of ICU patients using TOF neuromuscular monitoring, there were 2 reports of prolonged recovery (167 and 270 mins) among 28 patients administered cisatracurium besylate and 13 reports of prolonged recovery (range: 90 mins to 33 hrs) among 30 patients administered vecuronium.

OVERDOSAGE:

Overdosage with neuromuscular blocking agents may result in neuromuscular block beyond the time needed for surgery and anesthesia. The primary treatment is maintenance of a patent airway and controlled ventilation until recovery of normal neuromuscular function is assured. Once recovery from neuromuscular block begins, further recovery may be facilitated by administration of an anticholinesterase agent (*e.g.,* neostigmine, edrophonium) in conjunction with an appropriate anticholinergic agent (see Antagonism of Neuromuscular Block).

Antagonism of Neuromuscular Block: ANTAGONISTS (SUCH AS NEOSTIGMINE AND EDROPHONIUM) SHOULD NOT BE ADMINISTERED WHEN COMPLETE NEUROMUSCULAR BLOCK IS EVIDENT OR SUSPECTED. THE USE OF A PERIPHERAL NERVE STIMULATOR TO EVALUATE RECOVERY AND ANTAGONISM OF NEUROMUSCULAR BLOCK IS RECOMMENDED.

Administration of 0.04 to 0.07 mg/kg neostigmine at approximately 10% recovery from neuromuscular block (range: 0 to 15%) produced 95% recovery of the muscle twitch response and a T_4:T_1 ratio ≥70% in an average of 9 to 10 minutes. The times from 25% recovery of the muscle twitch response to a T_4:T_1 ratio ≥70% following these doses of neostigmine averaged 7 minutes. The mean 25% to 75% recovery index following reversal was 3 to 4 minutes.

Administration of 1.0 mg/kg edrophonium at approximately 25% recovery from neuromuscular block (range: 16% to 30%) produced 95% recovery and a T_4:T_1 ratio ≥70% in an average of 3 to 5 minutes.

Patients administered antagonists should be evaluated for evidence of adequate clinical recovery (*e.g.,* 5-second head lift and grip strength). Ventilation must be supported until no longer required.

The onset of antagonism may be delayed in the presence of debilitation, cachexia, carcinomatosis, and the concomitant use of certain broad spectrum antibiotics, or anesthetic agents and other drugs which enhance neuromuscular block or separately cause respiratory depression (see DRUG INTERACTIONS). Under such circumstances the management is the same as that of prolonged neuromuscular block (see OVERDOSAGE).

DOSAGE AND ADMINISTRATION:

CISATRACURIUM BESYLATE SHOULD ONLY BE ADMINISTERED INTRAVENOUSLY.

The dosage information provided below is intended as a guide only. Doses of cisatracurium besylate should be individualized (see CLINICAL PHARMACOLOGY, Individualization of Dosages). The use of a peripheral nerve stimulator will permit the most advantageous use of cisatracurium besylate, minimize the possibility of overdosage or underdosage, and assist in the evaluation of recovery.

ADULTS

Initial Doses: One of two intubating doses of cisatracurium besylate may be chosen, based on the desired time to intubation and the anticipated length of surgery. Doses of 0.15 (3 x ED_{95}) and 0.20 (4 x ED_{95}) mg/kg cisatracurium besylate, as components of a propofol/nitrous oxide/oxygen induction-intubation technique, may produce generally good or excellent conditions for tracheal intubation in 2.0 and 1.5 minutes, respectively. The clinically effective durations of action for 0.15 and 0.20 mg/kg cisatracurium besylate during propofol anesthesia are 55 minutes (range: 44 to 74 min) and 61 minutes (range: 41 to 81 min), respectively. Lower doses may result in a longer time for the development of satisfactory intubation conditions. In addition to the dose of the neuromuscular blocking agent, the presence of co-induction agents (*e.g.,* fentanyl and midazolam) and the depth of anesthesia are factors that can influence intubation conditions. Doses up to 8 x ED_{95} cisatracurium besylate have been safely administered to healthy adult patients and the larger doses are associated with longer clinically effective durations of action (see CLINICAL PHARMACOLOGY).

Because slower times to onset of complete neuromuscular block were observed in elderly patients and patients with renal dysfunction, extending the interval between administration of cisatracurium besylate and the intubation attempt for these patients may be required to achieve adequate intubation conditions.

A dose of 0.03 mg/kg cisatracurium besylate is recommended for maintenance of neuromuscular block during prolonged surgical procedures. Maintenance doses of 0.03 mg/kg each sustain neuromuscular block for approximately 20 minutes. Maintenance dosing is generally required 40 to 50 minutes following an initial dose of 0.15 mg/kg cisatracurium besylate and 50 to 60 minutes following an initial dose of 0.20 mg/kg cisatracurium besylate, but the need for maintenance doses should be determined by clinical criteria. For shorter or longer durations of action, smaller or larger maintenance doses may be administered.

Isoflurane or enflurane administered with nitrous oxide/oxygen to achieve 1.25 MAC (Minimum Alveolar Concentration) may prolong the clinically effective duration of action of initial and maintenance doses. The magnitude of these effects may depend on the duration of administration of the volatile agents. Fifteen to 30 minutes of exposure to 1.25 MAC isoflurane or enflurane had minimal effects on the duration of action of initial doses of cisatracurium besylate and therefore, no adjustment to the initial dose should be necessary when cisatracurium besylate is administered shortly after initiation of volatile agents. In long surgical procedures during enflurane or isoflurane anesthesia, less frequent maintenance dosing or lower maintenance doses of cisatracurium besylate may be necessary. No adjustments to the initial dose of cisatracurium besylate are required when used in patients receiving propofol anesthesia.

CHILDREN

Initial Doses: The recommended dose of cisatracurium besylate for children 2 to 12 years of age is 0.10 mg/kg administered over 5 to 10 seconds during either halothane or opioid anesthesia. When administered during stable opioid/nitrous oxide/oxygen anesthesia, 0.10 mg/kg cisatracurium besylate produces maximum neuromuscular block in an average of 2.8 minutes (range: 1.8 to 6.7 min) and clinically effective block for 28 minutes (range: 21 to 38 min). Cisatracurium besylate has not been studied in children below the age of 2 years.

USE BY CONTINUOUS INFUSION

Infusion in the Operating Room (OR): After administration of an initial bolus dose of cisatracurium besylate, a diluted solution of cisatracurium besylate can be administered by continuous infusion to adults and children aged 2 or more years for maintenance of neuromuscular block during extended surgical procedures. Infusion of cisatracurium besylate should be individualized for each patient. The rate of administration should be adjusted according to the patient's response as determined by peripheral nerve stimulation. Accurate dosing is best achieved using a precision infusion device.

Infusion of cisatracurium besylate should be initiated only after early evidence of spontaneous recovery from the initial bolus dose. An initial infusion rate of 3 mcg/kg/min may be required to rapidly counteract the spontaneous recovery of neuromuscular function. Thereafter, a rate of 1 to 2 mcg/kg/min should be adequate to maintain continuous neuromuscular block in the range of 89% to 99% in most pediatric and adult patients under opioid/nitrous oxide/oxygen anesthesia.

Reduction of the infusion rate by up to 30% to 40% should be considered when cisatracurium besylate is administered during stable isoflurane or enflurane anesthesia (administered with nitrous oxide/oxygen at the 1.25 MAC level). Greater reductions in the infusion rate of cisatracurium besylate may be required with longer durations of administration of isoflurane or enflurane.

The rate of infusion of atracurium required to maintain adequate surgical relaxation in patients undergoing coronary artery bypass surgery with induced hypothermia (25° to 28°C) is approximately half the rate required during normothermia. Based on the structural similarity between cisatracurium besylate and atracurium, a similar effect on the infusion rate of cisatracurium besylate may be expected.

Spontaneous recovery from neuromuscular block following discontinuation of infusion of cisatracurium besylate may be expected to proceed at a rate comparable to that following administration of a single bolus dose.

INFUSION IN THE INTENSIVE CARE UNIT (ICU)

The principles for infusion of cisatracurium besylate in the OR are also applicable to use in the ICU. An infusion rate of approximately 3 mcg/kg/min (range: 0.5 to 10.2 mcg/kg/min) should provide adequate neuromuscular block in adult patients in the ICU. There may be wide interpatient variability in dosage requirements and these may increase or decrease with time (see PRECAUTIONS, Long-Term Use in the Intensive Care Unit [ICU]). Following recovery from neuromuscular block, readministration of a bolus dose may be necessary to quickly re-establish neuromuscular block prior to reinstitution of the infusion.

INFUSION RATE TABLES

The amount of infusion solution required per minute will depend upon the concentration of cisatracurium besylate in the infusion solution, the desired dose of cisatracurium besylate, and the patient's weight. The contribution of the infusion solution to the fluid requirements of the patient also must be considered. TABLE 7 and TABLE 8 provide guidelines for delivery, in ml/hr (equivalent to microdrops/min when 60 microdrops = 1 ml), of cisatracurium besylate solutions in concentrations of 0.1 mg/ml (10 mg/100 ml) or 0.4 mg/ml (40 mg/100 ml).

CISATRACURIUM BESYLATE INJECTION COMPATIBILITY AND ADMIXTURES

Y-site Administration: Cisatracurium besylate injection is acidic (pH=3.25 to 3.65) and may not be compatible with alkaline solution having a pH greater than 8.5 (*e.g.,* barbiturate solutions). Studies have shown that cisatracurium besylate injection is compatible with:

5% Dextrose Injection USP

DOSAGE AND ADMINISTRATION: *(cont'd)*

TABLE 7 Infusion Rates of Cisatracurium Besylate for Maintainance of Neuromuscular Block During Opioid/Nitrous Oxide/Oxygen Anesthesia for a Concentration of 0.1 mg/ml

Patient Weight (kg)	DRUG DELIVERY RATE (mcg/kg/min) 1.0	1.5	2.0	3.0	5.0
	Infusion Delivery Rate (mL/hr)				
10	6	9	12	18	30
45	27	41	54	81	135
70	42	63	84	126	210
100	60	90	120	180	300

TABLE 8 Infusion Rates of Cisatracurium Besylate for Maintainance of Neuromuscular Block During Opioid/Nitrous Oxide/Oxygen Anesthesia for a Concentration of 0.4 mg/ml

Patient Weight (kg)	DRUG DELIVERY RATE (mcg/kg/min) 1.0	1.5	2.0	3.0	5.0
	Infusion Delivery Rate (mL/hr)				
10	1.5	2.3	3.0	4.5	7.5
45	6.8	10.1	13.5	20.3	33.8
70	10.5	15.8	21.0	31.5	52.5
100	15.0	22.5	30.0	45.0	75.0

0.9% Sodium Chloride Injection USP

5% Dextrose and 0.9% Sodium Chloride Injection USP

Sufenta (sufentanil citrate) Injection, diluted as directed

Alfenta (alfentanil hydrochloride) Injection, diluted as directed

Sublimaze (fentanyl citrate) Injection, diluted as directed

Versed (midazolam hydrochloride) Injection, diluted as directed

Droperidol Injection, diluted as directed

Cisatracurium besylate injection is not compatible with Diprivan (propofol) Injection or Toradol (ketorolac) Injection for Y-site administration. Studies of other parenteral products have not been conducted.

DILUTION STABILITY

Cisatracurium besylate injection diluted in 5% Dextrose Injection USP, 0.9% Sodium Chloride Injection USP, or 5% Dextrose and 0.9% Sodium Chloride Injection USP to 0.1 mg/ml may be stored either under refrigeration or at room temperature for 24 hours without significant loss of potency. Dilutions to 0.1 mg/ml or 0.2 mg/ml in 5% Dextrose and Lactated Ringer's Injection may be stored under refrigeration for 24 hours.

Cisatracurium besylate injection should not be diluted in Lactated Ringer's Injection USP due to chemical instability.

Note: Parenteral drug products should be inspected visually for particulate matter and discoloration prior to administration whenever solution and container permit. Solutions which are not clear, or contain visible particulates, should not be used. Cisatracurium besylate injection is a colorless to slightly yellow or greenish-yellow solution.

HOW SUPPLIED:

Nimbex Injection, 2 mg cisatracurium in each ml.

5 ml Single Use Vials.

10 ml Multiple Dose Vials containing 0.9% w/v benzyl alcohol as a preservative (see WARNINGS concerning newborn infants).

Nimbex Injection, 10 mg cisatracurium in each ml. 20 ml Single Use vials (**intended only for use in the ICU**).

Storage: Nimbex Injection should be refrigerated at 2° to 8°C (36° to 46°F) in the carton to preserve potency.

Protect from light. DO NOT FREEZE. Upon removal from refrigeration to room temperature storage conditions (25°C/77°F), use Nimbex Injection within 21 days even if rerefrigerated.

HOW SUPPLIED - EQUIVALENTS NOT AVAILABLE:

Injection - Intravenous - 5 ml

Vial $99.96 NIMBEX, Glaxo Wellcome 00173-0540-50

Injection - Intravenous - 10 ml

Vial $175.32 NIMBEX, Glaxo Wellcome 00173-0540-47

CISPLATIN *(000824)*

CATEGORIES: Antineoplastics; Bladder Carcinoma; Cancer; Cytotoxic Agents; Oncologic Drugs; Ovarian Carcinoma; Testicular Carcinoma; Tumors; Lung Cancer*; Sales > $100 Million; FDA Approval Pre 1982; Patent Expiration 1996 Dec

* Indication not approved by the FDA

BRAND NAMES: *Abiplatin*; *Asiplatin*; *Blastolem* (Mexico); *Briplatin* (Japan); *Cisplan*; *Cisplatin* (Australia); *Cisplatin-Ebewe*; *Cisplatino*; *Cisplatinum*; *Cisplatyl* (France); *Citoplatino*; *Cytoplatin*; *Kemoplat*; *Lederplatin*; *Medsaplatin* (Mexico); *Neoplatin*; *Niyaplat* (Mexico); *Platamine*; *Platamine RTU*; *Platiblastin* (Germany); *Platidiam*; *Platinex* (Germany); **Platinol**; *Platinol-AQ* (Canada); *Platistil*; *Platistin*; *Platosin* (England); *Tecnoplatin* (Mexico)

(International brand names outside U.S. in italics)

FORMULARIES: BC-BS; Medi-Cal; WHO

COST OF THERAPY: $4,325.75 (Ovarian Carcinoma; Injection; 1 mg/ml; 3.81/day; 365 days)

WARNING:

Cisplatin should be administered under the supervision of a qualified physician experienced in the use of cancer chemotherapeutic agents. Appropriate management of therapy and complications is possible only when adequate diagnostic and treatment facilities are readily available. Cumulative renal toxicity associated with cisplatin is severe. Other major dose-related toxicities are myelosuppression, nausea, and vomiting.

Ototoxicity, which may be more pronounced in children, and is manifested by tinnitus, and/or loss of high frequency hearing and occasionally deafness, is significant.

Anaphylactic-like reactions to cisplatin have been reported. Facial edema, bronchoconstriction, tachycardia, and hypotension may occur within minutes of cisplatin administration. Epinephrine, corticosteroids, and antihistamines have been effectively employed to alleviate symptoms (see WARNINGS and ADVERSE REACTIONS).

DESCRIPTION:

Cisplatin (cis-diamminedichloroplatinum) is a heavy metal complex containing a central atom of platinum surrounded by two chloride atoms and two ammonia molecules in the cis position. It is a white lyophilized powder with the molecular formula $PtCl_2H_6N_2$, and a molecular weight of 300.1. It is soluble in water or saline at 1 mg/ml and in dimethylformamide at 24 mg/ml. It has a melting point of 207°C. Cisplatin-AQ is a sterile aqueous solution, containing 1 mg cisplatin and 9 mg sodium chloride. HCl and/or sodium hydroxide added to adjust pH.

CLINICAL PHARMACOLOGY:

Plasma concentrations of the parent compound, cisplatin, decay monoexponentially with a half-life of about 20 to 30 minutes following bolus administrations of 50 or 100 mg/m^2 doses. Monoexponential decay and plasma half-lives of about 0.5 hour are also seen following two hour or seven hour infusions of 100 mg/m^2. After the latter, the total-body clearances and volumes of distribution at steady-state for cisplatin are about 15 to 16 L/h/m^2.

Due to its unique chemical structure, the chlorine atoms of cisplatin are more subject to chemical displacement reactions by nucleophiles, such as water or sulfhydryl groups, than to enzyme-catalyzed metabolism. At physiological pH in the presence of 0.1M NaCl, the predominant molecular species are cisplatin and monohydroxymonochloro *cis*-dimmamine platinum (II) in nearly equal concentrations. The latter, combined with the possible direct displacement of the chlorine atoms by sulfhydryl groups of amino acids ot proteins, accounts for the instability of cisplatin in biological matrices. The ratios of cisplatin to total free (ultrafiltrable) platinum in the plasma vary considerably between patients and range from 0.5 to 1.1 after a dose of 100 mg/m^2.

Cisplatin does not undergo the instantaneous and reversible binding to plasma proteins that is characteristic of normal drug-binding protein. However, the platinum from cisplatin, but not cisplatin itself, becomes bound to several plasma proteins including albumin, transferrin, and gamma globulin. Three hours after a bolus injection and two hours after the end of a three-hour infusion, 90% of the plasma platinum is protein bound. The complexes between albumin and the platinum from cisplatin do not dissociate to a significant extent and are slowly eliminated with a minimum half-life of five days or more.

Following cisplatin doses of 20 to 120 mg/m^2, the concentrations of platinum are highest in liver, prostate, and kidney, and somewhat lower in bladder, muscle, testicle, pancreas, and spleen and lowest in bowel, adrenal, heart, lung, cerebrum, and cerebellum. Platinum is present in tissues for as long as 180 days after the last administration. With the exception of intracerebral tumors, platinum concentrations in tumors are generally somewhat lower than the concentrations in the organ where the tumor is located. Different metastatic sites in the same patient may have different platinum concentrations. Hepatic metastases have the highest platinum concentrations, but these are similar to the platinum concentrations in normal liver. Maximum red blood cell concentrations of platinum are reached within 90 to 150 minutes after a 100 mg/m^2 dose of cisplatin and decline in a biphasic manner with the terminal half-life of 36 to 47 days.

Over a dose range of 40 to 140 mg cisplatin/m^2 given as a bolus injection or as infusions varying in length from 1 hour to 24 hours, from 10% to about 40% of the administered platinum is excreted within 24 hours, from 10% to about 40% of the administered platinum is excreted in the urine in 24 hours. Over five days following administration of 40 to 100 mg/m^2 doses given as rapid, 2 to 3 hour, or 6 to 8 hour infusions, a mean of 35% to 51% of the dosed platinum is excreted in the urine. Similar mean urinary recoveries of platinum of about 14% to 30% of the dose are found following live daily administrations of 20, 30, or 40 mg/m^2/day. Only a small percentage of the administered platinum is excreted beyond 24 hours post-infusion and most of the platinum excreted in the urine in 24 is excreted within the first few hours. Platinum-containing species excreted in the urine are the same as those found following the incubation of cisplatin with urine from healthy subjects, except that the proportions are different.

The parent compound, cisplatin, is excreted in the urine and accounts for 13% to 17% of the dose excreted within one hour after administration of 50 mg/m^2. The mean renal clearance of cisplatin exceeds creatinine clearance and is 62 and 50 ml/min/m^2 following administration of 100 mg/m^2 as 2 hour or 6 to 7 hour infusions, respectively.

The renal clearance of free (ultrafiltrable) platinum also exceeds the glomerular filtration rate indicating that cisplatin or other platinum-containing molecules are actively secreted by the kidneys. The renal clearance of free platinum is nonlinear and variable and is dependent on dose, urine flow rate, and individual variability in the extent on of active secretion and possible tubular resorption.

There is a potential for accumulation of ultrafiltrable platinum plasma concentration whenever cisplatin is administered on a daily basis but not when dose on an intermittent basis.

No significant relationships exist between the renal clearance of either free platinum and cisplatin and creatinine clearance.

Although small amounts of platinum are present in the bile and large intestine after administration of cisplatin, the fecal excretion of platinum appears to be insignificant.

INDICATIONS AND USAGE:

Cisplatin is indicated as therapy to be employed as follows:

Metastatic Testicular Tumors: In established combination therapy with other approved chemotherapeutic agents in patients with metastatic testicular tumors who have already received appropriate surgical and/or radiotherapeutic procedures.

Metastatic Ovarian Tumors: In established combination therapy with other approved chemotherapeutic agents in patients with metastatic ovarian tumors who have already received appropriate surgical and/or radiotherapeutic procedures. An established combination consists of cisplatin and cyclophosphamide. Cisplatin, as a single agent, is indicated as secondary therapy in patients with metastatic ovarian tumors refractory to standard chemotherapy who have not previously received cisplatin therapy.

Advance Bladder Cancer: Cisplatin is indicated as a single agent for patients with transitional cell bladder cancer which is no longer amenable to local treatments such as surgery and/or radiotherapy.

CONTRAINDICATIONS:

Cisplatin is contraindicated in patients with preexisting renal impairment. Cisplatin should not be employed in myelosuppressed patients, or patients with hearing impairment.

Cisplatin is contraindicated in patients with a history of allergic reactions to cisplatin or other platinum-containing compounds.

WARNINGS:

Cisplatin produces cumulative nephrotoxicity which is potentiated by aminoglycoside antibiotics. The serum creatinine, BUN, creatinine clearance, and magnesium, sodium, potassium, and calcium levels should be measured prior to initiating therapy, and prior to each subsequent course. At the recommended dosage, cisplatin should not be given more frequently than once every 3 to 4 weeks (see ADVERSE REACTIONS).

There are reports of severe neuropathies in patients in whom regimens are employed using higher doses of cisplatin or greater dose frequencies than those recommended. These neuropathies may be irreversible and are seen as paresthesias in a stocking-glove distribution, areflexia, and loss of proprioception and vibratory sensation.

Loss of motor function has also been reported.

Anaphylactic-like reactions to cisplatin have been reported. These reactions have occurred within minutes of administration to patients with prior exposure to cisplatin, and have been alleviated by administration of epinephrine, corticosteroids, and antihistamines.

Since ototoxicity of cisplatin is cumulative, audiometric testing should be performed prior to initiating therapy and prior to each subsequent dose of drug (see ADVERSE REACTIONS).

Cisplatin can cause fetal harm when administered to a pregnant woman. Cisplatin is mutagenic in bacteria and produces chromosome aberrations in animal cells in tissue culture. In mice cisplatin is teratogenic and embryotoxic. If this drug is used during pregnancy or if the patient becomes pregnant while taking this drug, the patient should be apprised of the potential hazard to the fetus. Patients should be advised to avoid becoming pregnant.

The carcinogenic effect of cisplatin was studied in BD IX rats. Cisplatin was administered i.p. to 50 BD IX rats for 3 weeks, 3 x 1 mg/kg body weight per week. Four hundred and fifty-five days after the first application, 33 animals died, 13 of them related to malignancies: 12 leukemias and 1 renal fibrosarcoma.

The development of acute leukemia coincident with the use of cisplatin has rarely been reported in humans. In these reports, cisplatin was generally given in combination with other leukemogenic agents.

PRECAUTIONS:

Peripheral blood counts should be monitored weekly. Liver function should be monitored periodically. Neurologic examination should also be performed regularly (see ADVERSE REACTIONS).

Carcinogenesis, Mutagenesis, and Impairment of Fertility: (See WARNINGS).

Pregnancy: (See WARNINGS).

DRUG INTERACTIONS:

Plasma levels of anticonvulsant agents may become subtherapeutic during cisplatin therapy.

In a randomized trial in advanced ovarian cancer, response duration was adversely affected when pyridoxine was used in combination with altretamine (hexmethylmelamine) and cisplatin.

ADVERSE REACTIONS:

Nephrotoxicity: Dose-related and cumulative renal insufficiency is the major dose-limiting toxicity of cisplatin. Renal toxicity has been noted in 28% to 36% of patients treated with a single dose of 50 mg/m^2. It is first noted during the second week after a dose and is manifested by elevations in BUN and creatinine, serum uric acid and/or a decrease in creatinine clearance. **Renal toxicity becomes more prolonged and severe with repeated courses of the drug. Renal function must return to normal before another dose of cisplatin can be given.**

Impairment of renal function has been associated with renal tubular damage. The administration of cisplatin using a 6- to 8-hour infusion with intravenous hydration, and mannitol has been used to reduce nephrotoxicity. However, renal toxicity still can occur after utilization of these procedures.

Ototoxicity: Ototoxicity has been observed in up to 31% of patients treated with a single dose of cisplatin 50 mg/m^2, and is manifested by tinnitus and/or hearing loss in the high frequency range (4,000 to 8,000 Hz). Decreased ability to hear normal conversational tones may occur occasionally. Deafness after the initial dose of cisplatin has been reported rarely. Ototoxic effects may be more severe in children receiving cisplatin. Hearing loss can be unilateral or bilateral and tends to become more frequent and severe with repeated doses. Ototoxicity may be enhanced with prior or simultaneous cranial irradiation. It is unclear whether cisplatin induced ototoxicity is reversible. Careful monitoring of audiometry should be performed prior to initiation of therapy and prior to subsequent doses of cisplatin.

Vestibular toxicity has also been reported.

Ototoxicity may become more severe in patients being treated with other drugs with nephrotoxic potential.

Hematologic: Myelosuppression occurs in 25% to 30% of patients treated with cisplatin. The nadirs in circulating platelets and leukocytes occur between days 18 to 23 (range 7.5 to 45) with most patients recovering by day 39 (range 13 to 62). Leukopenia and thrombocytopenia are more pronounced at higher doses (>50 mg/m^2). Anemia (decrease of 2 g hemoglobin/100 ml) occurs at approximately the same frequency and with the same timing as leukopenia and thrombocytopenia.

In addition to anemia secondary to myelosuppression, a Coombs' positive hemolytic anemia has been reported. in the presence of cisplatin hemolytic anemia, a further course of treatment may be accompanied by increased hemolysis and this risk should be weighed by the treating physician.

The development of acute leukemia coincident with with the use of cisplatin has rarely been reported in humans. In these report, cisplatin was generally given in combination with other leukemogenic agents.

Gastrointestinal: Marked nausea and vomiting occur in almost all patients treated with cisplatin, and are occasionally so severe that the drug must be discontinued. Nausea and vomiting usually begin within 1 to 4 hours after treatment and last up to 24 hours. Various degrees of nausea and anorexia may persist for up to 1 week after treatment.

Delayed nausea and vomiting (begins or persists 24 hours or more after chemotherapy) has occurred in patients attaining complete emetic control on the day of cisplatin therapy.

Diarrhea has also been reported.

OTHER TOXICITIES

Vascular toxicities coincident with the use of cisplatin in combination with other antineoplastic agents have been reported rarely. The events are clinically heterogeneous and may include myocardial infarction, cerebrovascular accident, thrombotic microangiopathy (HUS), or cerebral arteritis. Various mechanisms have been proposed for these vascular complications. There are also reports of Raynaud's phenomenon occurring in patients treated with the combination of bleomycin, vinblastine with or without cisplatin. It has been suggested that hypomagnesemia developing coincident with the use of cisplatin may be an added, although not essential, factor associated with this event. However, it is currently unknown if the cause of Raynaud's phenomenon in these cases is the disease, underlying vascular compromise, bleomycin, vinblastine, hypomagnesemia, or a combination of any of these factors.

ADVERSE REACTIONS: *(cont'd)*

Serum Electrolyte Disturbances: Hypomagnesemia, hypocalcemia, hyponatremia, hypokalemia, and hypophosphatemia have been reported to occur in patients treated with cisplatin and are probably related to renal tubular damage. Tetany has occasionally been reported in those patients with hypocalcemia and hypomagnesemia. Generally, normal serum electrolyte levels are restored by administering supplemental electrolytes and discontinuing cisplatin.

Inappropriate antidiuretic hormone syndrome has also been reported.

Hyperuricemia: Hyperuricemia has been reported to occur at approximately the same frequency as the increases in BUN and serum creatinine.

It is more pronounced after doses greater than 50 mg/m^2, and peak levels of uric acid generally occur between 3 to 5 days after the dose. Allopurinol therapy for hyperuricemia effectively reduces uric acid levels.

Neurotoxicity: (see WARNINGS) Neurotoxicity, usually characterized by peripheral neuropathies, has been reported. The neuropathies usually occur after prolonged therapy (4 to 7 months); however, neurologic symptoms have been reported to occur after a single dose. Cisplatin therapy should be discontinued when the symptoms are first observed. Preliminary evidence suggests peripheral neuropathy may be irreversible in some patients.

Lhermitte's sign and autonomic neuropathy have also been reported.

Loss of taste and seizures have also been reported.

Muscle cramps, defined as localized, painful, involuntary skeletal muscle contractions of sudden onset and short duration, have been reported and were usually associated in patients receiving a relatively high cumulative dose of cisplatin and with a relatively advanced symptomatic stage of peripheral neuropathy.

Ocular Toxicity: Optic neuritis, papilledema, and cerebral blindness have been reported infrequently in patients receiving standard recommended doses of cisplatin. Improvement and/or total recovery usually occurs after discontinuing cisplatin. Steroids with or without mannitol have been used; however, efficacy has not been established.

Blurred vision and altered color perception have been reported after the use of regimens with higher doses of cisplatin or greater dose frequencies than those recommended in the package insert. The altered color perception manifests as a loss of color discrimination, particularly in the blue-yellow axis. The only finding on funduscopic exam is irregular retinal pigmentation of the macular area.

Anaphylactic-like Reactions: Anaphylactic-like reactions have been occasionally reported in patients previously exposed to cisplatin. The reactions consist of facial edema, wheezing, tachycardia, and hypotension within a few minutes of drug administration. Reactions may be controlled by intravenous epinephrine, corticosteroids, or antihistamines. Patients receiving cisplatin should be observed carefully for possible anaphylactic-like reactions and supportive equipment and medication should be available to treat such a complication.

Other Events: Other toxicities reported to occur infrequently are cardiac abnormalities, anorexia, elevated SGOT, and rash. Alopecia has also been reported.

Local soft tissue toxicity has rarely been reported following extravasation of cisplatin. Severity of the local tissue toxicity appears to be related to the concentration of the cisplatin solution. Infusion of solutions with a cisplatin concentration greater than 0.5 mg/ml may result in tissue cellulitis, fibrosis, and necrosis.

OVERDOSAGE:

Caution should be exercised to prevent inadvertent overdosage with cisplatin. Acute overdosage with this drug may result in kidney failure, liver failure, deafness, ocular toxicity (including detachment of the retina), significant myelosuppression, intractable nausea and vomiting and/or neuritis. In addition, death can occur following overdosage.

No proven antidotes have been established for cisplatin overdosage. Hemodialysis, even when initiated four hours after the overdosage, appears to have little effect on removing platinum from the body because of cisplatin's rapid and high degree of protein binding. Management of overdosage should include general supportive measures to sustain the patient through any period of toxicity that may occur.

DOSAGE AND ADMINISTRATION:

Note: Needles or intravenous sets containing aluminum parts that may come in contact with cisplatin should not be used for preparation or administration. Aluminum reacts with cisplatin, causing precipitate formation and a loss of potency.

Metastatic Testicular Tumors: The usual cisplatin dose for the treatment of testicular cancer in combination with other approved chemotherapeutic agents is 20 mg/m^2 IV daily for 5 days.

Metastatic Ovarian Tumors: The usual cisplatin dose for the treatment of metastatic ovarian tumors in combination with Cytoxan is 75- 100 mg/m^2 IV once every 4 weeks (DAY 1).[2,3]

The dose of Cytoxan when used in combination with cisplatin is 600 mg/m^2 IV once every 4 weeks (DAY 1).[2,3]

For directions for the administration of Cytoxan, refer to the Cytoxan monograph.

In combination therapy, cisplatin and Cytoxan are administered sequentially.

As a single agent, cisplatin should be administered at a dose of 100 mg/m^2 IV once every 4 weeks.

Advanced Bladder Cancer: Cisplatin should be administered as a single agent at a dose of 50-70 mg/m^2 IV once every 3 to 4 weeks depending on the extent of prior exposure to radiation therapy and/or prior chemotherapy. For heavily pretreated patients an initial dose of 50 mg/m^2 repeated every 4 weeks is recommended.

Pretreatment hydration with 1 to 2 liters of fluid infused for 8 to 12 hours prior to a cisplatin dose is recommended. The drug is then diluted in 2 liters of 5% Dextrose in 1/2 or 1/3 normal saline containing 37.5 g of mannitol, and infused over a 6- to 8-hour period. If diluted solution is not to be used within 6 hours, protect solution from light. Adequate hydration and urinary output must be maintained during the following 24 hours.

A repeat course of cisplatin should not be given until the serum creatinine is below 1.5 mg/100 ml, and/or the BUN is below 25 mg/100 ml. A repeat course should not be given until circulating blood elements are at an acceptable level (platelets $\geq$100,000/mm^3, WBC $\geq$4,000/mm^3). Subsequent doses of cisplatin should not be given until an audiometric analysis indicates that auditory acuity is within normal limits.

As with other potentially toxic compounds, caution should be exercised in handling the powder and preparing the solution of cisplatin. Skin reactions associated with accidental exposure to cisplatin may occur. The use of gloves is recommended. If cisplatin powder or solution contact the skin or mucosae, immediately wash the skin or mucosae thoroughly with soap and water.

The aqueous solution should be used intravenously only and be administered by IV infusion over 6- to 8-hour period.

STABILITY

Cisplatin is a sterile, multidose vial without preservatives.

Store at 15°-25°C. Do not refrigerate. Protect unopened container from light.

DOSAGE AND ADMINISTRATION: *(cont'd)*

The cisplatin remaining in the amber vial following initial entry is stable for 28 days protected from light or for 7 days under fluorescent room light.

Procedures For Proper Handling And Disposal: Anticancer drugs should be considered. Several guidelines on this subject have been published.[4-10] There is no general agreement that all of the procedures recommended in the guidelines are necessary or appropriate.

REFERENCES:

1. Wiernik PH: Hexamethylmelamine and Low or Moderate Dose Cisplatin With or Without Pyridoxine for Treatment of Advanced Ovarian Carcinoma: A Study of the Eastern Oncology Group. Cancer Invest. 1992: 10: 1-9. 2. Alberts DS, et al: Improved Therapeutic Index of Carboplatin Plus Cyclophosphamide versus Cisplatin Plus Cyclophosphamide: Final Report by the Southwest Oncology Group of a Phase III Randomized Trial in Stages III and IV Ovarian Cancer. J Clin Oncol 1992: 10 706-717. 3. Swenerton K, et al: Cisplatin-Cyclophosphamide versus Carboplatin-Cycvlophosphamide in Advanced Ovarian Cancer: A Randomized Phase II Study of the National Cancer Institute of Canada Clinical Trials Group. J Clin Oncol 1992: 10: 718-726. 4. Recommendations for the Safe Handling of Parenteral Antineoplastic Drugs, NIH Publication No. 83-2621. For sale by the Superintendent of Documents, US Government Printing Office, Washington, DC 20402. 5. AMA Council Report. Guidelines for Handling Parenteral Antineoplastic Drugs. NIH Publication No. 83-2621. For sale by the Superintendent of Documents. US Government Printing Office. Washington, DC 20402. 6. National Study Commission on Cytotoxic Exposure-Recommendations for Handling Cytotoxic Agents. Available from Louis P. Jeffrey, Sc.D., Chairman, National Study Commission on Cytotoxic Exposure. Massachusetts College of Pharmacy and Allied Health Sciences, 179 Longwood Avenue, Boston, Massachusetts 02115. 7. Clinical Oncological Society of Australia, Guidelines and Recommendations for Safe Handling of Antineoplastic Agents. Med J Australia 1983; 1:426-428. 8. Jones RB, et al: Safe Handling of Chemotherapeutic Agents: A report from the Mount Sinai Medical Center. CA - A Cancer Journal for Clinicians 1983; (Sept/Oct) 258-263. 9. American Society of Hospital Pharmacists Technical Assistance Bulletin on Handling Cytotoxic and Hazardous Drugs. Am J Hosp Pharm 1990; 47:1033-1049. 10. OSHA Work-Practice Guidelines for Personnel Dealing with Cytotoxic (Antineoplastic) Drugs. Am J Hosp Pharm 1986; 43:1193-1204.

HOW SUPPLIED - EQUIVALENTS NOT AVAILABLE:

Injection, Dry-Soln - Intravenous - 1 mg/ml

50 ml	**$155.53**	**PLATINOL, Mead Johnson**	**00015-3072-20**
50 ml	$162.52	PLATIMOL-AQ, Mead Johnson	00015-3220-22
100 ml	**$325.01**	**PLATINOL-AQ, Mead Johnson**	**00015-3221-22**

Injection, Lyphl-Soln - Intravenous - 10 mg/vial

20 ml	**$33.28**	**PLATINOL, Mead Johnson**	**00015-3070-20**

CITRATE PHOSPHATE DEXTROSE *(000825)*

CATEGORIES: Alkalinizing Agents; Anticoagulants; Anticoagulants/Thrombolytics; Blood Formation/Coagulation; Coagulants and Anticoagulants; Electrolytic, Caloric-Water Balance; FDA Pre 1938 Drugs

BRAND NAMES: Anticoagulant Citrate Phosphate Dex; Citra Ph

Prescribing information not available at time of publication.

HOW SUPPLIED - EQUIVALENTS NOT AVAILABLE:

Solution - Misc - 300 mg/2.55 gm/

500 ml	$24.93	CITRATE PHOSPHATE DEXTROSE, Abbott	00074-1967-04

CITRIC ACID; GLUCONOLACTONE; MAGNESIUM CARBONATE *(000826)*

CATEGORIES: Electrolytic, Caloric-Water Balance; Irrigating Solutions; Kidney Stones; Urinary Tract Infections; FDA Approved 1990 Oct

BRAND NAMES: D-Gluconic Acid; **Renacidin**

DESCRIPTION:

Renacidin (Citric Acid, Glucono-delta-lactone, and Magnesium Carbonate) Irrigation is a sterile, non-pyrogenic irrigation for use within the urinary tract in the prevention of calculi.

Each 100 Ml Of Renacidin Irrigation Contains:

Citric Acid (anhydrous), USP, 6.602 grams, $C_6H_8O_7$

Glucono-delta-lactone, 0.198 grams, $C_6H_{10}O_6$.

Magnesium Carbonate, U.S.P., 3.177 grams, $(MgCO_3)_4 \cdot Mg(OH)_2 \cdot 3H_2O$

Inert Ingredients: Benzoic Acid, U.S.P., 0.023 grams

Solution pH: 3.85 (3.50-4.20)

CLINICAL PHARMACOLOGY:

This combination irrigation's action on susceptible apatite calculi results from an exchange of magnesium from the irrigating solution for calcium contained in the stone matrix. The magnesium salts thereby formed are soluble in the gluconocitrate irrigating solution resulting in the dissolution of the calculus. Struvite calculi are composed mainly of magnesium ammonium phosphates which are solubilized by this combination irrigation due to its acidic pH.

This combination irrigation is not effective for dissolution of calcium oxalate, uric acid or cysteine stones.

INDICATIONS AND USAGE:

This combination irrigation is indicated for use by local irrigation in the dissolution of renal calculi composed of apatite (a calcium carbonate - phosphate compound) or struvite (magnesium aluminum phosphates) in patients who are not candidates for surgical removal of the calculi.

It may also be used as adjunctive therapy to dissolve residual apatite or struvite calculi and fragments after surgery or to achieve a partial dissolution of renal calculi to facilitate surgical removal.

This combination irrigation is also indicated for dissolution of bladder calculi of the struvite or apatite variety by local intermittent irrigation through a urethral catheter or cystostomy catheter as an alternative or adjunct to surgical procedures.

This combination irrigation is also for use as an intermittent irrigating solution to prevent or minimize encrustation of indwelling urinary tract catheters.

Since many complications are experienced by patients receiving infusions of this combination irrigation into the renal pelvis, considerable caution must be employed. Additionally, hospitalization is prolonged for days to weeks when chemolytic therapy is used in lieu of, or following surgery. For these reasons, use of this therapy should be reserved for selected patients.

This combination irrigation is not indicated for dissolution of calcium oxalate, uric acid or cysteine calculi.

CONTRAINDICATIONS:

The use of this combination irrigation in the treatment of renal calculi is contraindicated in patients with urinary tract infections.Urea-splitting bacteria reside within struvite and apatite stones which therefore serve as a source of infection. Dissolution therapy with this combination irrigation in the presence of an infected urinary tract may lead to sepsis and death. Urine specimens should be obtained for culture prior to initiating chemolytic therapy of the renal pelvis. Appropriate antibiotic therapy should be instituted to treat any infection detected. A sterile urine must be present prior to initiating therapy. An infected stone can serve as a continual source for infection and, therefore, antibiotic therapy should be continued throughout the course of dissolution therapy.

This combination irrigation is contraindicated in the presence of demonstrable urinary tract extravasation.

WARNINGS:

This combination irrigation use should be stopped immediately if the patient develops fever, urinary tract infection, signs and symptoms consistent with urinary tract infection, or persistent flank pain. Irrigation should be stopped if hypermagnesemia or elevated serum creatinine develops.

Severe hypermagnesemia has been reported with this combination irrigation. Caution should be employed when irrigating the renal pelvis of patients with impaired renal function. Patients should be observed for early signs and symptoms of hypermagnesemia including nausea, lethargy, confusion and hypotension. Severe hypermagnesemia may result in hyporeflexia, dyspnea, apnea, coma, cardiac arrest and subsequent death. Serum magnesium levels should be monitored and deep tendon reflexes should be evaluated. Treatment of hypermagnesemia should include discontinuation of this combination irrigation followed by medical therapy with intravenous calcium gluconate, fluids and diuresis in severe cases.

PRECAUTIONS:

Care must be taken during chemolysis of renal calculi with this combination irrigation to maintain the patency of the irrigating catheter. Calculus fragments and debris may obstruct the outflow catheter. Continued irrigation under those circumstances leads to increased intrapelvic pressure with a danger of tissue damage or absorption of the irrigating solution. Catheter outflow blockage may be prevented by flushing the catheter with saline and repositioning of the catheter. Frequent monitoring of the system should be performed by a nurse, an aide or any person with sufficient skills to be able to detect any problems with the patency of the catheter. At the first sign of obstruction, irrigation should be discontinued and the system disconnected.

Intrapelvic pressures must be maintained at or below 25 cm of water. The preferred method of pressure control is the insertion of an open Y connection pop-off valve into the infusion line allowing immediate decompression if pressure exceeds 25 cm of water. An alternative method has been proposed to direct or stop the flow of the irrigating solution to prevent increased intrapelvic pressure: placement of a pinch clamp on the inflow line which can be used by the patient or nurse to stop the irrigation at the first sign of flank pain. However, extreme caution must be taken when relying on cooperation of the patient. Patients may not be sufficiently alert to detect signs and symptoms of out-flow obstruction. This is especially true in elderly patients or patients who have been sedated or who have severe neurological dysfunction with varying degrees of sensory loss and/or motor paralysis.

Patients with indwelling urethral or cystostomy catheters frequently have vesicoureteral reflux. Cystogram prior to initiation of this combination irrigation is essential for such patients. If reflux is demonstrated, all precautions recommended for renal pelvis irrigation must be taken.

Throughout the course of therapy, patients should be monitored to assure safety. Serum creatinine, phosphate and magnesium should be obtained every several days. Urine specimens should be collected for culture and antibacterial sensitivity every three days or less and at the first sign of fever. The irrigation should be stopped if any culture exhibits growth and appropriate antibacterial therapy should be initiated. The irrigation may be started again after a course of antibacterial therapy upon demonstration of a sterile urine. Struvite calculi frequently contain bacteria within the stone and antibacterial therapy should therefore be continued throughout the course of dissolution therapy. Hypermagnesemia or an elevated serum creatinine level are indications to halt the irrigation until they return to pre-irrigation levels. Evidence of severe urothelial edema on x-ray is also an indication for temporarily halting the irrigation until the complication resolves.

Concurrent use of magnesium containing medications may contribute to production of hypermagnesemia and is not recommended.

Carcinogenesis, Mutagenesis, and Impairment of Fertility: Long term studies to evaluate carcinogenic potential of this combination irrigation in animals have not been conducted. Mutagenicity studies have not been conducted.

Pregnancy Category C: Animal reproduction studies have not been conducted with Renacidin Injection. It is also not known whether this combination irrigation can cause fetal harm when administered to a pregnant woman or can effect reproduction capacity. This combination irrigation should be given to a pregnant woman only if clearly needed.

Nursing Mothers: Magnesium is known to be excreted into human milk. it is not known whether this combination irrigation is excreted in human milk. Because many drugs are excreted in human milk, caution should be exercised when this combination irrigation is administered to a nursing woman.

ADVERSE REACTIONS:

The most common adverse reaction in selected case series is transient flank pain which occurs in most patients. Additional common reactions include urothelial ulceration and/or edema (13%) or fever (20% but up to 40% in some case series). Other adverse reactions which occur in 1-10% of cases include: urinary tract infection, back pain, dysuria, transient hematuria, nausea, hypermagnesemia, hyperphosphatemia, elevated serum creatinine, candidiasis, and bladder irritability. Adverse reactions which occur in less than 1% of patients include: septicemia, ileus, vomiting and thrombophlebitis. Death from sepsis has been reported.

OVERDOSAGE:

See WARNINGS.

DOSAGE AND ADMINISTRATION:

This combination irrigation (sterile, non-pyogenic) in water for local irrigation within the urinary tract.

The action of this combination irrigation in the prevention and dissolution of calculi results from an ion exchange mechanism or solvent action. (See CLINICAL PHARMACOLOGY)

Parenteral drug products should be inspected visually for particulate matter and discoloration prior to administration whenever solution and container permit.

Renal Calculi: See PRECAUTIONS. It is essential that patients be free from urinary tract infections prior to initiating chemolytic therapy. Urine specimens should be collected for culture and appropriate antibiotic therapy should be initiated for any bacteria identified. A nephrostomy tube is placed at surgery or percutaneously to permit lavage of the calculi. A

DOSAGE AND ADMINISTRATION: *(cont'd)*

single catheter may be sufficient if the calculus is not obstructing the ureter or uteropelvic junction. In patients with an obstructed ureter, a retrograde catheter can be placed through the ureter to he renal pelvis via a cystoscope. The second catheter is used to irrigate the calculus while the percutaneous nephrostomy tube is used for drainage.

Plain radiographs and nephrotomograms are performed to assure proper placement of the catheter(s). Pressure measurements are made under fluoroscopy to assure that 2-3 ml/min can be infused without causing pain, pyelovenous or pyelotubular backflow or manometric evidence of elevated pressure within the collecting system.

For postoperative patients irrigation should not be started before the fourth or fifth postoperative day. Irrigation of the renal pelvis is begun with sterile saline only after a sterile urine has been demonstrated. The saline is infused at a rate of 60 ml/hr initially and the rate is increased until pain or an elevated pressure (25 cm H_2O) appears, or until a maximum flowrate of 120 ml/hr is achieved. Th site of insertion should be inspected for leakage. if leakage occurs, the irrigation is discontinued temporarily to allow for complete healing around the nephrostomy tube.

If no leakage or flank pain occur, irrigation is then started with this combination irrigation with a flow rate equal to the maximum rate achieved with the saline solution. A clamp should be placed on the inflow tube and patients (see PRECAUTIONS) and nursing personnel should be instructed to stop the irrigating solution whenever pain develops. Nursing personnel who are responsible for performing the irrigation must be instructed concerning the location of the nephrostomy tube(s) and the direction of lw of the irrigating solution to insure against misconnection of the inflowing and egress tubes. Nephrotomograms should be performed periodically to assure proper placement of the catheter tip and to assess efficacy. If stones fail to change size after several days of adequate irrigation the procedure should be discontinued.

Upon demonstration of complete dissolution of the calculus the inflow tube is clamped and left in place for a few days to ensure that no obstruction exists, after which time the nephrostomy tube is removed.

Bladder Calculi: Chemolysis of bladder calculi is used as an alternative to cystoscopic or surgical removal or in whom these procedures constitute an unwarranted risk. Following appropriate studies to evaluate possible vesicoureteral reflux, thirty ml of this combination irrigation is instilled through a urinary catheter into the bladder and the catheter is clamped for 30-60 minutes. The clamp is then released and the bladder is drained. This is repeated 4-6 times a day. A continuous drip through a 3-way Foley catheter is an alternative means of dissolving bladder stones. In the presence of bladder spasm and associated high pressure reflux, all precautions required for irrigation of the renal pelvis must be observed.

Indwelling Urinary Tract Catheter Encrustation: Periodic instillation of this combination irrigation is indicated to minimize or prevent encrustation of indwelling catheters which frequently results in plugging of the catheter and discomfort to the patient. This is accomplished by instilling 30 ml of the solution through the catheter and than clamping the catheter for 10 minutes, after which the clamp is removed to allow drainage of the bladder. This process is repeated 3 times a day.

HOW SUPPLIED:

Renacidin irrigation is available as a sterile, non-pyrogenic solution in 500 ml containers, packaged in cartons of six. Exposure of renacidin irrigation to heat or cold should be minimized. Renacidin irrigation should be stored at controlled room temperature, 59° F to 86° F (15° C to 30° C). Avoid excessive heat or cold (keep from freezing). Brief exposure to temperatures of up to 40° C or temperatures down to 5° C does not adversely affect the product.

HOW SUPPLIED - EQUIVALENTS NOT AVAILABLE:

Powder, Reconstitution - Irrigation

300 gm $32.10 RENACIDIN, Guardian Labs 00327-0007-03

Solution - Irrigation

500 ml $23.60 RENACIDIN, Guardian Labs 00327-0011-05

CITRIC ACID; MAGNESIUM OXIDE; SODIUM CARBONATE *(000827)*

CATEGORIES: Electrolytic, Caloric-Water Balance; Irrigating Solutions; Urinary Bladder Calculi; Pregnancy Category C; FDA Approved 1982 Jun

BRAND NAMES: Irrigating Solution G; **Urologic G**

DESCRIPTION:

Urologic G irrigation is a sterile, nonpyrogenic, solution of the ingredients listed below, in water for irrigation.

The solution is administered only by transurethral irrigation for dissolving phosphatic calculi in the urinary bladder. It must not be used for transurethral surgical procedures involving electrical instrumentation.

Each 100 ml of urologic G irrigation contains:

Citric Acid, hydrous 3.24 g

Sodium Carbonate, anhydrous 0.43 g

Magnesium Oxide, anhydrous 0.38 g

The pH is 4 (approx.).

It contains no bacteriostat, antimicrobial agent or added buffer.

Citric acid, USP, hydrous (monohydrate) is chemically designated $C_6H_8O_7$-H_2O, colorless, translucent crystals or white crystalline powder very soluble in water.

Sodium Carbonate, NF, anhydrous is chemically designated Na_2CO_3, odorless hygroscopic powder freely soluble in water.

Magnesium Oxide, USP, anhydrous is chemically designated MgO, white powder soluble in dilute acids.

Water for injection, USP is chemically designated H_2O.

The semi-rigid container is fabricated from a specially formulated polyolefin. It is a copolymer of ethylene and propylene. The safety of the plastic has been confirmed by tests in animals according to USP biological standards for plastic containers. The container requires no vapor barrier to maintain the proper drug concentration.

CLINICAL PHARMACOLOGY:

The dissolution of urinary calculi by this irrigating solution derives primarily from the ability of the citrate ion to complex with calcium in the calculi, forming soluble calcium citrates. This effect provided by citric acid in the formula, is limited to urinary bladder stones composed of calcium phosphate, with or without magnesium ammonium phosphate and/or calcium carbonate.

Sodium carbonate in the formula serves as a mild alkali to control acidity of the solution.

CLINICAL PHARMACOLOGY: *(cont'd)*

Magnesium oxide in the formula serves to diminish irritation of the bladder mucosa caused by the citric acid.

INDICATIONS AND USAGE:

This irrigating solution is indicated for use as an irrigating solution to help dissolve calculi of phosphatic origin in the urinary bladder in patients for whom other methods of treatment are impractical or contraindicated.

CONTRAINDICATIONS:

Not for injection into body tissue.

Contraindicated for irrigation during transurethral surgical procedures. This solution is conductive and should not be used in the presence of electrical instrumentation.

WARNINGS:

FOR IRRIGATION ONLY. NOT FOR INJECTION.

This irrigating solution is not recommended for dissolving phosphatic calculi in the renal pelvis because of the risk of creating back pressure that may reactivate an existing pyelonephritis.

This solution should not be used to replace other indicated measures, including correction of underlying metabolic disorders, surgical intervention and treatment of infection.

The contents of an opened container should be used promptly to minimize the possibility of bacterial growth or pyrogen formation.

Do not heat over 66 ° C (150 ° F).

PRECAUTIONS:

Do not open container until ready to use. Dilute aqueous solutions of citric acid not kept in tightly closed containers are susceptible to fermentation, fungus growth and/or bacterial contamination on standing.

Do not use unless solution is clear and seal is intact. Discard unused portion.

Pregnancy Category C: Animal reproduction studies have not been conducted with this irrigating solution. It is also not known whether this irrigation solution can cause fetal harm when given to a pregnant woman or can affect reproduction capacity. This irrigation solution should be given to a pregnant woman only if clearly needed.

ADVERSE REACTIONS:

Patients may complain of some discomfort or pain due to bladder irritation during irrigation, or irrigation may initiate bleeding from the bladder in the presence of undetected mucosal lesions. In such cases the physician should re-evaluate the basis for irrigation therapy versus other indicated methods of treatment.

DOSAGE AND ADMINISTRATION:

This irrigating solution may be administered by intermittent irrigation or by tidal instillation and drainage to allow continuous irrigation of the bladder for periods of several hours. The usual dose is one to three liters daily.

Intermittent irrigation of the bladder (after the manner of intermittent peritoneal dialysis) may be preferred to promote more prolonged contact of the irrigation with bladder stones; tidal (continuous in and out flow) irrigation may be less efficient and require larger amounts of irrigation fluid.

The LD_{50} intraperitoneal dose of citric acid in rats is 975 mg/kg.

Parenteral drug products should be inspected visually for particulate matter and discoloration prior to administration, whenever container and solution permit. See PRECAUTIONS.

Storage: Protect from freezing and extreme heat. Do not store above 40 ° C (104 ° F).

HOW SUPPLIED - RATED THERAPEUTICALLY EQUIVALENT:

Solution - Irrigation - 3.24 gm/0.38 gm

1000 ml $29.68 UROLOGIC G, Abbott 00074-7168-09

CITRIC ACID; POTASSIUM CITRATE *(000828)*

CATEGORIES: Acidosis; Alkalinizing Agents; Alkalosis; Antagonists and Antidotes; Antidotes; Electrolyte Solutions; Electrolytic, Caloric-Water Balance; Gout; Homeostatic & Nutrient; Replacement Solutions; Urinary Tract Infections; FDA Pre 1938 Drugs

BRAND NAMES: **Polycitra K**; Urocit-K

FORMULARIES: Aetna

DESCRIPTION:

Polycitra-K Crystals is a pleasant tasting oral systemic alkalizer, containing potassium citrate and citric acid, sugar-free, for reconstitution, and supplied as single dose packets. The contents of each packet, when reconstituted, will provide the same amount of active ingredient as is contained in 15 ml (one tablespoonful) Polycitra-K (Potassium Citrate and Citric Oral Solution U.S.P.).

Composition: Each single dose packet contains:

Potassium citrate-monohydrate 3300 mg

Citric Acid-monohydrate 1002 mg

Each packet provides 30 mEq Potassium equivalent to 30 meq bicarbonate (HCO_3)

CLINICAL PHARMACOLOGY:

Potassium citrate is absorbed and metabolized to potassium bicarbonate, thus acting as a systemic alkalizer. The effects are essentially those of chlorides before absorption and those of bicarbonates subsequently.

INDICATIONS AND USAGE:

Citric acid/potassium citrate is an effective alkalinizing agent useful in those conditions where long term maintenance of an alkaline urine is desirable, such as in patients with uric acid and cystine calculi of the urinary tract, especially when the administration of sodium salts is undesirable or contraindicated.

In addition, it is a valuable adjuvant when administered with uricosuric agents in gout therapy, since urates tend to crystalize out of an acid urine. It is also effective in correcting the acidosis of certain renal tubular disorders where the administration of potassium citrate may be preferable. Citric acid/potassium citrate, when administered after meals and before bedtime, allows one to maintain an alkaline urinary pH around the clock, usually without the necessity of a 2 a.m. dose. Citric acid/potassium citrate alkalinizes the urine without producing systemic alkalosis in the recommended dosage. It is highly palatable, pleasant tasting and tolerable, even when administered for long periods.

CONTRAINDICATIONS:

Severe renal impairment with oliguria or azotemia, untreated Addison's disease, adynamia episodica hereditaria, acute dehydration, heat cramps, anuria, severe myocardial damage, and hyperkalemia from any cause.

WARNINGS:

Large doses may cause hypercalcemia and alkalosis, especially in the presence of renal disease. Concurrent administration of potassium-containing medication, potassium sparring diuretics, or cardiac-glycosides may lead to toxicity.

PRECAUTIONS:

Should be used with caution by patients with low urinary output unless under the constant supervision of a physician. As with all products containing a high concentration of potassium, patients should be directed to dilute adequately with water to minimize the possibility of gastrointestinal injury associated by the oral ingestion of concentrated potassium salt preparations; and preferably, to take each dose after meals and avoid saline laxative effect.

Pregnancy: Citric acid/potassium citrate is not expected to cause fetal harm when administered in dosages which will not result in hyperkalemia.

Nursing Mothers: Caution should be exercised when administered to a nursing women.

Pediatric Use: Citric acid/potassium citrate solution is recommended for pediatric administration since dosage can be more easily regulated.

ADVERSE REACTIONS:

Citric acid/potassium citrate is generally well tolerated without any unpleasant side effects when given in recommended doses to patients with normal renal function and urinary output. However, as with any alkalinizing agent, caution must be used in certain patients with abnormal renal mechanisms to avoid development of hyperkalemia or alkalosis. Potassium intoxication causes listlessness, weakness, mental confusion, tingling of extremities, and other symptoms associated with a high concentration of potassium in the serum. Periodic determination of serum electrolytes should be carried out in those patients with renal disease in order to avoid these complications. Hyperkalemia may exhibit the following electrocardiographic abnormalities: Disappearance of the P wave, widening and slurring of QRS complex, changes of the S-T segment, tall peaked T waves, etc.

OVERDOSAGE:

The administration of oral potassium salts to persons with normal excretory mechanisms for potassium rarely causes serious hyperkalemia. However, if excretory mechanisms are impaired hypercalcemia can result (see CONTRAINDICATIONS and WARNINGS). Hyperkalemia, when detected, must be treated immediately because lethal levels can be reached in a few hours.

TREATMENT OF HYPERKALEMIA

Should hyperkalemia occur, treatment measures include the following: (1) elimination of foods or medications containing potassium. (2) The IV administration of 300 to 500 ml/hr of dextrose solution (10 to 25%) containing 10 units of insulin/20 gm dextrose. (3) The use of exchange resins, hemodialysis, or peritoneal dialysis. (4) Correction of acidosis, if present, with IV sodium bicarbonate. In treating hypercalcemia, it should be recalled that in patients who have been stabilized on digitalis, too rapid a lowering of the plasma potassium concentration can produce digitalis toxicity.

DOSAGE AND ADMINISTRATION:

Citric acid/potassium citrate should be taken mixed in cool water or fruit juice according to directions, followed by additional water, if desired.

Usual Adult Dose: Contents of 1 packet mixed with at least 6 ounces of cool water or fruit juice, after meals and at bedtime, or as directed by physician.

Usual Dosage Range: Contents of 1 packet mixed with 6 ounces of cool water or juice taken three times a day will usually maintain a urinary pH of 6.5-7.4. This provides the same amount of active ingredients as is contained in equivalent doses of citric acid/potassium citrate solution.

HOW SUPPLIED - EQUIVALENTS NOT AVAILABLE:

Powder

500 gm $12.11 Potassium Citrate, Mallinckrodt 00406-0714-03

CITRIC ACID; SODIUM CITRATE *(000830)*

CATEGORIES: Acidosis; Alkalinizing Agents; Anticoagulants/Thrombolytics; Blood Formation/Coagulation; Electrolytic, Caloric-Water Balance; FDA Pre 1938 Drugs

BRAND NAMES: **Bicitra**; Citra pH; Oracit; Shohl's Modified

FORMULARIES: BC-BS

DESCRIPTION:

Bicitra is a stable and pleasant-tasting oral systemic alkalizer solution containing sodium citrate and citric acid in a sugar-free base. It is a nonparticulate neutralizing buffer.

Bicitra contains in each teaspoonful (5 ml):

Sodium citrate dihydrate 500 mg (0.34 Molar)

Citric acid monohydrate 334 mg (0.32 Molar)

Each ml contains 1 mEq sodium ion and is equivalent to 1 mEq sodium ion and is equivalent to 1 mEq bicarbonate (HCO_3). Bicitra also contains butylparaben, flavoring, maltitol, and sodium saccharin.

CLINICAL PHARMACOLOGY:

Sodium citrate is absorbed and metabolized to sodium bicarbonate, thus acting as a systemic alkalizer. The effects are essentially those of chlorides before absorption and those of bicarbonates subsequently. Oxidation is virtually complete so that less than 5% of sodium citrate is excreted in the urine unchanged.

INDICATIONS AND USAGE:

Sodium citrate; citric acid is an effective alkalizing agent. It is useful in those conditions where long-term maintenance of an alkaline urine is desirable, and is of value in the alleviation of chronic metabolic acidosis, such as results from chronic renal insufficiency or

INDICATIONS AND USAGE: *(cont'd)*

the syndrome of renal tubular acidosis, especially when the administration of potassium salts is undesirable or contraindicated. Sodium citrate; citric acid is also useful for buffering and neutralizing gastric hydrochloric acid quickly and effectively.

Sodium citrate; citric acid is concentrated, and when administered after meals and before bedtime, allows one to maintain an alkaline urinary pH around the clock, usually without the necessity of a 2 a.m. dose. Sodium citrate; citric acid alkalinizes the urine without producing a systemic alkalosis in the recommended dosage. Sodium citrate; citric acid is highly palatable, pleasant tasting, and tolerable, even when administered for long periods. Sodium citrate; citric acid is sugar-free.

CONTRAINDICATIONS:

Patients on sodium-restricted diets or with severe renal impairment. In certain situations, potassium citrate, as contained in polycitra-K, may be preferable.

PRECAUTIONS:

Should be used with caution by patients with low urinary output unless under the supervision of a physician. Sodium citrate; citric acid should not be administered concurrently with aluminum-based antacids. Patients should be directed to dilate adequately with water and, preferably, to take each dose after meals to avoid saline laxative effect. Sodium salts should be used cautiously in patients with cardiac failure, hypertension, impaired renal function, peripheral and pulmonary edema, and toxemia of pregnancy. Periodic examinations and determinations of serum electrolytes, particularly serum bicarbonate level, should be carried out in those patients with renal disease in order to avoid these complications.

ADVERSE REACTIONS:

Sodium citrate; citric acid is generally well tolerated, without any unpleasant side effects, when given in recommended doses to patients with normal renal function and urinary output. However, as with any alkalinizing agent, caution must be used in certain patients with abnormal renal mechanisms to avoid development of alkalosis, especially in the presence of hypocalcemia.

OVERDOSAGE:

Overdosage with sodium salts may cause diarrhea, nausea and vomiting, hypernoia, and convulsions.

DOSAGE AND ADMINISTRATION:

Sodium citrate; citric acid should be taken diluted in water, followed by additional water, if desired. Palatability is enhanced if chilled before taking.

FOR SYSTEMIC ALKALIZATION

Usual Adult Dose: 2 to 6 teaspoonfuls (10 to 30 ml), diluted in 1 to 3 ounces of water, after meals and at bedtime, or as directed by a physician.

Usual Pediatric Dose: 1 to 3 teaspoonfuls (5 to 15 ml), diluted in 1 to 3 ounces of water, after meals and at bedtime, or as directed by a physician. For children under two years of age, use is based on a consultation with a physician.

As A Neutralizing Buffer: 3 teaspoonfuls (15 ml), diluted with 15 ml water, taken as a single dose, or as directed by a physician.

Keep tightly closed and protect from excessive heat or freezing.

HOW SUPPLIED - EQUIVALENTS NOT AVAILABLE:

Solution - Oral

15 ml x 100	**$59.00**	**BICITRA, Baker Norton Pharms**	**00575-0225-15**
15 ml x 100	$75.00	ORACIT, Carolina Med	46287-0014-15
30 ml x 100	$49.00	CITRA PH, 450 MG/5ML (0.3 MOLAR), SODIUM, Valmed	54627-0502-30
30 ml x 100	**$79.00**	**BICITRA, Baker Norton Pharms**	**00575-0225-30**
30 ml x 100	$93.00	ORACIT, Carolina Med	46287-0014-30
480 ml	$7.20	ORACIT, Carolina Med	46287-0014-01
3840 ml	$18.74	ORACIT, Carolina Med	46287-0014-99

CLADRIBINE *(003137)*

CATEGORIES: Anemia; Antineoplastics; Hairy Cell Leukemia; Leukemia; Orphan Drugs; Thrombocytopenia; Pregnancy Category D; FDA Class 1P ("Priority Review"); FDA Approved 1993 Feb

BRAND NAMES: CdA; Chlorodeoxyadenosine; **Leustatin**

FORMULARIES: Medi-Cal

> WARNING:
> For Intravenous Infusion Only
> Cladribine injection should be administered under the supervision of a qualified physician experienced in the use of antineoplastic therapy. Suppression of bone marrow function should be anticipated. This is usually reversible and appears to be dose dependent. High doses (4 to 9 times the recommended dose for Hairy Cell Leukemia), in conjunction with cyclophosphamide and total body irradiation as preparation for bone marrow transplantation, have been associated with severe, irreversible, neurologic toxicity (paraparesis/quadriparesis) and/or acute renal insufficiency in 45% of patients treated for 7-14 days.

DESCRIPTION:

Cladribine injection (also commonly known as 2-chloro-2'-deoxy-β-D-adenosine) is a synthetic antineoplastic agent for continuous intravenous infusion. It is a clear, colorless, sterile, preservative-free, isotonic solution. Leustatin injection is available in single-use vials containing 10 mg (1 mg/ml) of cladribine, a chlorinated purine nucleoside analog. Each milliliter of leustatin injection contains 1 mg of the active ingredient and 9 mg (0.15 mEq) of sodium chloride as an inactive ingredient. The solution has a pH range of 5.5 to 8.0. Phosphoric acid and/or dibasic sodium phosphate may have been added to adjust the pH to 6.3 ± 0.6.

The chemical name for cladribine is 2-chloro-6-amino-9-(2-deoxy-β-D-erythropento-furanosyl) purine. Molecular Weight: 285.7.

CLINICAL PHARMACOLOGY:

CELLULAR RESISTANCE AND SENSITIVITY

The selective toxicity of 2-chloro-2'-deoxy-β-D-adenosine towards certain normal and malignant lymphocyte and monocyte populations is based on the relative activities of deoxycytidine kinase, deoxynucleotidase and adenosine deaminase. In cells with a high ratio of deoxycytidine kinase to deoxynucleotidase, 2-chloro-2'-deoxy-β-D-adenosine, a purine nucleoside analog, passively crosses the cell membrane. It is phosphorylated by deoxycytidine kinase to 2-chloro-2'-deoxy-β-D-adenosine monophosphate (2-CdAMP). Since 2-chloro-2'-deoxy-β-D-adenosine is resistant to deamination by adenosine deaminase and there is little deoxynucleotide deaminase in lymphocytes and monocytes, 2-CdAMP accumulates intracellularly and is subsequently converted into the active triphosphate deoxynucleotide, 2-chloro-2'-deoxy-β-D-adenosine triphosphate (2-CdATP). It is postulated that cells with high deoxycytidine kinase and low deoxynucleotidase activities will be selectively killed by 2-chloro-2'-deoxy-β-D-adenosine as toxic deoxynucleotides accumulate intracellularly.

Cells containing high concentrations of deoxynucleotides are unable to properly repair single-strand DNA breaks. The broken ends of DNA activate the enzyme poly (ADP-ribose) polymerase resulting in NAD and ATP depletion and disruption of cellular metabolism. There is evidence, also, that 2-CdATP is incorporated into the DNA of dividing cells, resulting in impairment of DNA synthesis. Thus, 2-chloro-2'-deoxy-β-D- adenosine can be distinguished from other chemotherapeutic agents affecting purine metabolism in that it is cytotoxic to both actively dividing and quiescent lymphocytes and monocytes, inhibiting both DNA synthesis and repair.

HUMAN PHARMACOLOGY

In a clinical investigation, 17 patients with Hairy Cell Leukemia and normal renal function were treated for 7 days with the recommended treatment regimen of cladribine injection (0.09 mg/kg/day) by continuous intravenous infusion. The mean steady-state serum concentration was estimated to be 5.7 ng/ml with an estimated systemic clearance of 663.5 ml/h/kg when cladribine was given by continuous infusion over 7 days. Accumulation of cladribine over the seven day treatment period was not noted. In Hairy Cell leukemia patients, there does not appear to be a relationship between serum concentrations and ultimate clinical outcome.

In another study, 8 patients with hematologic malignancies received a two (2) hour infusion of cladribine injection (0.12 mg/kg). The mean end-of-infusion plasma cladribine concentration was 48 ± 19 ng/ml. For 5 of these patients, the disappearance of cladribine could be described by either a biphasic or triphasic decline. For these patients with normal renal function, the mean terminal half-life was 5.4 hours. Mean values for clearance and steady-state volume of distribution were 978 ± 422 ml/h/kg and 4.5 ± 2.8 l/kg, respectively.

Cladribine is bound approximately 20% to plasma proteins.

Except for some understanding of the mechanism of cellular toxicity, no other information is available on the metabolism or route of excretion of cladribine in humans. In a pilot study in rats treated with radiolabeled cladribine, approximately 41% to 44% of the administered label was recovered in the urine in the first 6 hours from 1 mg/kg bolus or infusion. Only small amounts of radioactivity were recovered after 6 hours. Less than 1% of the administered radioactivity was excreted in the feces following a bolus dose to rats. The effect of renal and hepatic impairment on the elimination of cladribine has not been investigated in humans.

Two single-center open label studies of cladribine have been conducted in patients with Hairy Cell Leukemia with evidence of active disease requiring therapy. In the study conducted at the Scripps Clinic and Research Foundation (Study A), 89 patients were treated with a single course of cladribine injection given by continuous intravenous infusion for 7 days at a dose of 0.09 mg/kg/day. In the study conducted at the M.D. Anderson Cancer Center (Study B), 35 patients were treated with a 7-day continuous intravenous infusion of cladribine injection at a comparable dose of 3.6 mg/m²/day. A complete response (CR) required clearing of the peripheral blood and bone marrow of hairy cells and recovery of the hemoglobin to 12 g/dl, platelet count to 100×10^9/L, and absolute neutrophil count to 1500×10^6/L. A good partial response (GPR) required the same hematologic parameters as a complete response, and that fewer than 5% hairy cells remain in the bone marrow. A partial response (PR) required that hairy cells in the bone marrow be decreased by at least 50% from baseline and the same response for hematologic parameters as for complete response. A pathologic relapse was defined as an increase in bone marrow hairy cells to 25% of pretreatment levels. A clinical relapse was defined as the recurrence of cytopenias, specifically, decreases in hemoglobin ≥2 g/dl, ANC ≥25% or platelet counts ≥50,000. Patients who met the criteria for a complete response but subsequently were found to have evidence of bone marrow hairy cells (<25% of pretreatment levels) were reclassified as partial responses and were not considered to be complete responses with relapse.

Among patients evaluable for efficacy (N=106), using the hematologic and bone marrow response criteria described above, the complete response rates in patients treated with cladribine injection were 65% and 68% for Study A and Study B, respectively, yielding a combined complete response rate of 66%. Overall response rates (*i.e.,* Complete plus Good Partial plus Partial Responses) were 89% and 86% in Study A and Study B, respectively, for a combined overall response rate of 88% in evaluable patients treated with cladribine injection.

Using an intent-to-treat analysis (N=123) and further requiring no evidence of splenomegaly as a criterion for CR (*i.e.,* no palpable spleen on physical examination and ≤13 cm on CT scan), the complete response rates for Study A and Study B were 54% and 53%, respectively, giving a combined CR rate of 54%. The overall response rates (CR + GPR + PR) were 90% and 85%, for Studies A and B respectively, yielding a combined overall response rate of 89% (TABLE 1).

TABLE 1 RESPONSE RATES TO CLADRIBINE TREATMENT IN PATIENTS WITH HAIRY CELL LEUKEMIA

	CR	Overall
Evaluable Patients N = 106	66%	88%
Intent-to-treat Population N = 123	54%	89%

In these studies, 60% of the patients had not received prior chemotherapy for HCl or had undergone splenectomy as the only prior treatment and were receiving cladribine as a first-line treatment. The remaining 40% of the patients received cladribine as a second-line treatment, having been treated previously with other agents, including α-interferon and/or deoxycoformycin. The overall response rate for patients without prior chemotherapy was 92%, compared with 84% for previously treated patients. Cladribine is active in previously treated patients, however, retrospective analysis suggests that the overall response rate is decreased in patients previously treated with splenectomy or deoxycoformycin and in patients refractory to α-interferon (TABLE 2).

After a reversible decline, normalization of peripheral blood counts (Hemoglobin >12.0 g/dl, Platelets $>100 \times 10^9$/L, Absolute Neutrophil Count (ANC) $>1500 \times 10^6$/L) was achieved by 92% of evaluable patients. The median time to normalization of peripheral counts was 9 weeks from the start of treatment (Range: 2 to 72). The median time to normalization of platelet count was 2 weeks, the median time to normalization of ANC was 5 weeks and the median time to normalization of hemoglobin was 8 weeks. With normalization of platelet count and hemoglobin, requirements for platelet and RBC transfusions were abolished after months 1 and 2, respectively, in those patients with complete response. Platelet recovery may be delayed in a minority of patients with severe baseline thrombocytopenia. Corresponding to

CLINICAL PHARMACOLOGY: *(cont'd)*

TABLE 2 Overall Response Rates (CR + GPR + PR) to Cladribine Treatment in Patients With Hairy Cell Leukemia

	Overall Response (N=123)	NR + Relapse
No Prior Chemotherapy	68/74 92%	6 + 4 14%
Any Prior Chemotherapy	41/49 84%	8 + 3 22%
Previous Splenectomy	32/41* 78%	9 + 1 24%
Previous Interferon	40/48 83%	8 + 3 23%
Interferon Refractory	6/11* 55%	5 + 2 64%
Previous Deoxycoformycin	3/6* 50%	3 + 1 66%

* P<0.05
NR=No Response

normalization of ANC, a trend toward a reduced incidence of infection was seen after the third month, when compared to the months immediately preceding cladribine therapy. (See also WARNINGS, PRECAUTIONS, and ADVERSE REACTIONS). (TABLE 3).

TABLE 3 CLADRIBINE TREATMENT IN PATIENTS WITH HAIRY CELL LEUKEMIA TIME TO NORMALIZATION OF PERIPHERAL BLOOD COUNTS

Parameter	Median Time to Normalization of Count*
Platelet Count	2 weeks
Absolute Neutrophil Count	5 weeks
Hemoglobin	8 weeks
ANC, Hemoglobin and Platelet Count	9 weeks

* Day 1=First day of infusion

For patients achieving a complete response, the median time to response (*i.e.,* absence of hairy cells in bone marrow and peripheral blood together with normalization of peripheral blood parameters), measured from treatment start, was approximately 4 months. Since bone marrow aspiration and biopsy were frequently not performed at the time of peripheral blood normalization, the median time to complete response may actually be shorter than that which was recorded. At the time of data cut-off, the median duration of complete response was greater than 8 months and ranged to 25+ months. Among 93 responding patients, seven had shown evidence of disease progression at the time of data cut-off. In four of these patients, disease was limited to the bone marrow, without peripheral blood abnormalities (pathologic progression), while in three patients there were also peripheral blood abnormalities (clinical progression). Seven patients who did not respond to a first course of cladribine received a second course of therapy. In the five patients who has adequate follow-up, additional courses did not appear to improve their overall response.

INDICATIONS AND USAGE:

Cladribine is indicated for the treatment of active Hairy Cell Leukemia as defined by clinically significant anemia, neutropenia, thrombocytopenia or disease-related symptoms.

CONTRAINDICATIONS:

Cladribine injection is contraindicated in those patients who are hypersensitive to this drug or any of its components.

WARNINGS:

Severe bone marrow suppression, including neutropenia, anemia, and thrombocytopenia, has been commonly observed in patients treated with cladribine, especially at high doses. At initiation of treatment, most patients in the clinical studies had hematologic impairment as a manifestation of active Hairy Cell Leukemia. Following treatment with cladribine, further hematologic impairment occurred before recovery of peripheral blood counts began. During the first two weeks after treatment initiation, mean platelet count, ANC, and Hemoglobin concentration declined and subsequently increased with normalization of mean counts by Day 12, Week 5 and Week 8, respectively. The myelosuppressive effects of cladribine were most notable during the first month following treatment. Forty-four percent (44%) of patients received transfusions with RBCs and 14% received transfusions with platelets during Month 1. Careful hematologic monitoring, especially during the first 4 to 8 weeks after treatment with cladribine injection, is recommended. (See PRECAUTIONS.)

Fever (T≥100° F) was associated with the use of cladribine in approximately two-thirds of patients (131/196) in the first month of therapy. Virtually all of these patients were treated empirically with parenteral antibiotics. Overall, 47% (93/196) of all patients had fever in the setting of neutropenia (ANC≤1000), including 62 patients (32%) with severe neutropenia (*i.e.,* ANC≤500).

In a Phase I investigational study using cladribine in high doses (4 to 9 times the recommended dose for Hairy Cell Leukemia) as part of a bone marrow transplant conditioning regimen, which also included high dose cyclophosphamide and total body irradiation, acute nephrotoxicity and delayed onset neurotoxicity were observed. Thirty-one (31) poor-risk patients with drug-resistant acute leukemia in relapse (29 cases) or non-Hodgkins Lymphoma (2 cases) received cladribine for 7 to 14 days prior to bone marrow transplantation. During infusion, 8 patients experienced gastrointestinal symptoms. While the bone marrow was initially cleared of all hematopoietic elements, including tumor cells, leukemia eventually recurred in all treated patients. Within 7 to 13 days after starting treatment with cladribine, 6 patients (19%) developed manifestations of renal dysfunction (*e.g.,* acidosis, anuria, elevated serum creatinine, etc.) and 5 required dialysis. Several of these patients were also being treated with other medications having known nephrotoxic potential. Renal dysfunction was reversible in 2 of these patients. In the 4 patients whose renal function had not recovered at the time of death, autopsies were performed; in 2 of these, evidence of tubular damage was noted. Eleven (11) patients (35%) experienced delayed onset neurologic toxicity. In the majority, this was characterized by progressive irreversible motor weakness (paraparesis/quadriparesis), of the upper and/or lower extremities, first noted 35 to 84 days after starting high dose therapy with cladribine. Non-invasive testing (electromyography and nerve conduction studies) was consistent with demyelinating disease. Severe neurologic toxicity has also been noted with high doses of another drug in this class.

In patients with Hairy Cell Leukemia treated with the recommended treatment regimen (0.09 mg/kg/day for 7 consecutive days), there have been no reports of similar nephro- or neurologic toxicities. Mild neurologic toxicities, specifically paresthesias and dizziness, have been reported rarely.

WARNINGS: *(cont'd)*

Of the 196 Hairy Cell Leukemia patients entered in the two trials, there were 8 deaths following treatment. Of these, 6 were of infectious etiology, including 3 pneumonias, and 2 occurred in the first month following cladribine therapy. Of the 8 deaths, 6 occurred in previously treated patients who were refractory to α-interferon.

Benzyl alcohol is a constituent of the recommended diluent for the 7-day infusion solution. Benzyl alcohol has been reported to be associated with a fatal "Gasping Syndrome" in premature infants. (See DOSAGE AND ADMINISTRATION.)

PREGNANCY CATEGORY D

Cladribine is teratogenic in mice and rabbits and consequently has the potential to cause fetal harm when administered to a pregnant woman. A significant increase in fetal variations was observed in mice receiving 1.5 mg/kg/day (4.5 mg/m^2) and increased resorptions, reduced litter size and increased fetal malformations were observed when mice received 3.0 mg/kg/day (9 mg/m^2). Fetal death and malformations were observed in rabbits that received 3.0 mg/kg/day (33.0 mg/m^2). No fetal effects were seen in mice at 0.5 mg/kg/day (1.5 mg/m^2) or in rabbits at 1.0 mg/kg/day (11.0 mg/m^2).

Although there is no evidence of teratogenicity in humans due to cladribine, other drugs which inhibit DNA synthesis (*e.g.,* methotrexate and aminopterin) have been reported to be teratogenic in humans. Cladribine has been shown to be embryotoxic in mice when given at doses equivalent to the recommended dose. If cladribine is used during pregnancy, or if the patient becomes pregnant while taking this drug, the patient should be apprised of the potential hazard to the fetus. Women of childbearing age should be advised to avoid becoming pregnant. Cladribine should be used during pregnancy only if the potential benefit justifies the potential risk to the fetus.

PRECAUTIONS:

GENERAL

Cladribine injection is a potent antineoplastic agent with potentially significant toxic side effects. It should be administered only under the supervision of a physician experienced with the use of cancer chemotherapeutic agents. Patients undergoing therapy should be closely observed for signs of hematologic and non-hematologic toxicity. Periodic assessment of peripheral blood counts, particularly during the first 4 to 8 weeks post-treatment, is recommended to detect the development of anemia, neutropenia and thrombocytopenia and for early detection of any potential sequelae (*e.g.,* infection or bleeding). As with other potent chemotherapeutic agents, monitoring of renal and hepatic function is also recommended, especially in patients with underlying kidney or liver dysfunction. (see WARNINGS and ADVERSE REACTIONS).

Fever was a frequently observed side effect during the first month on study. Since the majority of fevers occurred in neutropenic patients, patients should be closely monitored during the first month of treatment and empiric antibiotics should be initiated as clinically indicated. Although 69% of patients developed fevers, less than 1/3 of febrile events were associated with documented infection. Given the known myelosuppressive effects of cladribine, practitioners should carefully evaluate the risks and benefits of administering this drug to patients with active infections. (See WARNINGS and ADVERSE REACTIONS).

The kidney has not been established as the organ of excretion for cladribine. There are inadequate data on dosing of patients with renal or hepatic insufficiency. Development of acute renal insufficiency in some patients receiving high doses of cladribine has been described. Until more information is available, caution is advised when administering the drug to patients with known or suspected renal or hepatic insufficiency. (See WARNINGS.)

While hyperuricemia and tumor lysis syndrome is always possible in patients with large tumor burdens, patients in these studies were treated empirically with allopurinol and no episodes of tumor lysis were reported.

Cladribine injection must be diluted in designated intravenous solutions prior to administration. (See DOSAGE AND ADMINISTRATION.)

LABORATORY TESTS

During and following treatment, the patient's hematologic profile should be monitored regularly to determine the degree of hematopoietic suppression. In the clinical studies, following reversible declines in all cell counts, the mean platelet count reached 100×10^9/L by Day 12, the mean absolute neutrophil count reached 1500×10^6/L by Week 5 and the mean hemoglobin reached 12 g/dl by Week 8. After peripheral counts have normalized, bone marrow aspiration and biopsy should be performed to confirm response to treatment with cladribine. Febrile events should be investigated with appropriate laboratory and radiologic studies. Periodic assessment of renal function and hepatic function should be performed as clinically indicated.

CARCINOGENESIS, MUTAGENESIS, AND IMPAIRMENT OF FERTILITY

No animal carcinogenicity studies have been conducted with cladribine.

As expected for compounds in this class, the actions of cladribine have been shown to yield DNA damage. In mammalian cells in culture, cladribine has been shown to cause an imbalance of intracellular deoxyribonucleotide triphosphate pools. This imbalance results in the inhibition of DNA synthesis and DNA repair, yielding DNA strand breaks and subsequently cell death. Inhibition of thymidine incorporation into human lymphoblastic cells was 90% at concentrations of 0.3 μM. Cladribine was also incorporated into DNA of these cells. Cladribine was not mutagenic to bacteria and did not induce unscheduled DNA synthesis in primary rat hepatocyte cultures.

When administered intravenously to Cynomolgus monkeys, cladribine has been shown to cause suppression of rapidly generating cells, including testicular cells. The effect on human fertility is unknown.

PREGNANCY CATEGORY C:

(see WARNINGS.)

NURSING MOTHERS

It is not known whether this drug is excreted in human milk. Because many drugs are excreted in human milk and because of the potential for serious adverse reactions in nursing infants from cladribine, a decision should be made whether to discontinue nursing or discontinue the drug, taking into account the importance of the drug for the mother.

PEDIATRIC USE

Safety and effectiveness in children has not been established. In a Phase I study involving patients 1-21 years old with relapsed acute leukemia, cladribine was given by continuous intravenous infusion in doses ranging from 3 to 10.7 mg/m^2/day for 5 days (one-half to twice the dose recommended in Hairy Cell Leukemia). In this study, the dose-limiting toxicity was severe myelosuppression with profound neutropenia and thrombocytopenia. At the highest dose (10.7 mg/m^2/day), 3 of 7 patients developed irreversible myelosuppression and fatal systemic bacterial or fungal infection. No unique toxicities were noted in this study.[1] (See WARNINGS and ADVERSE REACTIONS.)

DRUG INTERACTIONS:

There are no known drug interactions with cladribine injection. Caution should be exercised if cladribine injection is administered following or in conjunction with other drugs known to cause myelosuppression.

ADVERSE REACTIONS:

Safety Data Are Based On 196 Patients With HCl: The original cohort of 124 patients plus an additional 72 patients enrolled at the same 2 centers after the original enrollment cutoff. In Month 1 of the Hairy Cell Leukemia clinical trials, severe neutropenia was noted in 70% of patients, fever in 69% and infection was documented in 28%. Other adverse experiences reported frequently during the first 14 days after initiating treatment included: fatigue (45%), nausea (28%), rash (27%), headache (22%) and injection site reactions (19%). Most non-hematologic adverse experiences were mild to moderate in severity.

Myelosuppression was frequently observed during the first month after starting treatment. Neutropenia (ANC <500 × 10⁶/L) was noted in 70% of patients, compared with 26% in whom it was present initially. Severe anemia (Hemoglobin <8.5 g/dl) developed in 37% of patients, compared with 10% initially and thrombocytopenia (Platelets <20 × 10⁹/L) developed in 12% of patients,compared to 4% in whom it was noted initially.

During the first month, 54 of 196 patients (28%) exhibited documented evidence of infection. Serious infections (*e.g.*, septicemia, pneumonia) were reported in 6% of all patients; the remainder were mild or moderate. Several deaths were attributable to infection and/or complications related to the underlying disease. During the second month, the overall rate of documented infection was 6%; these infections were mild to moderate and no severe systemic infections were seen. After the third month, the monthly incidence of infection was either less than or equal to that of the months immediately preceding cladribine therapy.

During the first month, 11% of patients experienced severe fever (*i.e.*, ≥104°F). Documented infections were noted in fewer than one-third of febrile episodes. Of the 196 patients studied, 19 were noted to have a documented infection in the month prior to treatment. In the month following treatment, there were 54 episodes of documented infection: 23 (42%) were bacterial, 11 (20%) were viral and 11 (20%) were fungal. Seven (7) of 8 documented episodes of herpes zoster occurred during the month following treatment. Fourteen (14) of 16 episodes of documented fungal infection occurred in the first two months following treatment. Virtually all of these patients were treated empirically with antibiotics. (See WARNINGS and PRECAUTIONS)

Analysis of lymphocyte subsets indicates that treatment with cladribine is associated with prolonged depression of the CD4 counts. Prior to treatment, the mean CD4 count was 766/µl. The mean CD4 count nadir, which occurred 4 to 6 months following treatment, was 272/µl. Fifteen (15) months after treatment, mean CD4 counts remained below 500/µl. CD8 counts behaved similarly, though increasing counts were observed after 9 months. There were no associated opportunistic infections reported during this time.

Another event of unknown clinical significance includes the observation of prolonged bone marrow hypocellularity. Bone marrow cellularity of <35% was noted after 4 months in 42 of 124 patients (34%) treated in the two pivotal trials. This hypocellularity was noted as late as day 1010. It is not known whether the hypocellularity is the result of disease related marrow fibrosis or if it is the result of cladribine toxicity. There was no apparent clinical effect on the peripheral blood counts.

The vast majority of rashes were mild and occurred in patients who were receiving or had recently been treated with other medications (*e.g.*, allopurinol or antibiotics) known to cause rash.

Most episodes of nausea were mild, not accompanied by vomiting, and did not require treatment with antiemetics. In patients requiring antiemetics, nausea was easily controlled, most frequently with chlorpromazine.

Adverse reactions reported during the first 2 weeks following treatment initiation (regardless of relationship to drug) by >5% of patients included.

Body as a Whole: fever (69%), fatigue (45%), chills (9%), asthenia (9%), diaphoresis (9%), malaise (7%), trunk pain (6%)

Gastrointestinal: nausea (28%), decreased appetite (17%), vomiting (13%), diarrhea (10%), constipation (9%), abdominal pain (6%)

Hemic/Lymphatic: purpura (10%), petechiae (8%), epistaxis (5%)

Nervous System: headache (22%), dizziness (9%), insomnia (7%)

Cardiovascular System: edema (6%), tachycardia (6%)

Respiratory System: abnormal breath sounds (11%), cough (10%), abnormal chest sounds (9%), shortness of breath (7%)

Skin/Subcutaneous Tissue: rash (27%), injection site reactions (19%), pruritus (6%), pain (6%), erythema (6%)

Musculoskeletal System: myalgia (7%), arthralgia (5%)

Adverse experiences related to intravenous administration included: injection site reactions (9%) (*i.e.*, redness, swelling, pain), thrombosis (2%), phlebitis (2%), and a broken catheter (1%). These appear to be related to the infusion procedure and/or indwelling catheter, rather than the medication or the vehicle.

From Day 15 to the last follow-up visit, the only events reported by > 5% cf patients were: fatigue (11%), rash (10%), headache (7%), cough (7%), and malaise (5%).

For a description of adverse reactions associated with use of high doses in non-Hairy Cell Leukemia patients, see WARNINGS.

OVERDOSAGE:

High doses of cladribine have been associated with: irreversible neurologic toxicity (paraparesis/quadriparesis), acute nephrotoxicity, and severe bone marrow suppression resulting in neutropenia, anemia and thrombocytopenia. (See WARNINGS.) There is no known specific antidote to overdosage. Treatment of overdosage consists of discontinuation of cladribine, careful observation and appropriate supportive measures. It is not known whether the drug can be removed from the circulation by dialysis or hemofiltration.

DOSAGE AND ADMINISTRATION:

Usual Dose: The recommended dose and schedule of cladribine injection for active Hairy Cell Leukemia is as a single course given by continuous infusion for 7 consecutive days at a dose of 0.09 mg/kg/day. Deviations from this dosage regimen are not advised. Physicians should consider delaying or discontinuing the drug if neurotoxicity or renal toxicity occurs. (See WARNINGS.)

Specific risk factors predisposing to increased toxicity from cladribine have not been defined. In view of the known toxicities of agents of this class, it would be prudent to proceed carefully in patients with known or suspected renal insufficiency or severe bone marrow impairment of any etiology. Patients should be monitored closely for hematologic and non-hematologic toxicity. (See WARNINGS and PRECAUTIONS.)

Preparation and Administration of Intravenous Solutions: Cladribine injection must be diluted with the designated diluent prior to administration. Since the drug product does not contain any anti-microbial preservative or bacteriostatic agent, **aseptic technique and proper environmental precautions must be observed in preparation of cladribine injection solutions.**

To Prepare A Single Daily Dose: Add the calculated dose (0.09 mg/kg or 0.09 ml/kg) of cladribine injection to an infusion bag containing 500 ml of 0.9% Sodium Chloride Injection, USP. Infuse continuously over 24 hours. Repeat daily for a total of 7 consecutive days. **The use of 5% dextrose as a diluent is not recommended because of increased degradation of cladribine.** Admixtures of cladribine injection are chemically and physically stable for at least

DOSAGE AND ADMINISTRATION: *(cont'd)*

24 hours at room temperature under normal room fluorescent light in Baxter Viaflex† PVC infusion containers. **Since limited compatibility data are available, adherence to the recommended diluents and infusion systems is advised.** (TABLE 4).

TABLE 4

	Dose of Leustatin Injection	Recommended Diluent	Quantity of Diluent
24-hour infusion method	1 (day) × 0.09 mg/kg	0.9% Sodium Chloride Injection, USP	500 ml

To Prepare A 7-Day Infusion: The 7-day infusion solution should only be prepared with Bacteriostatic 0.9% Sodium Chloride Injection, USP (0.9% benzyl alcohol preserved). In order to minimize the risk of microbial contamination, both cladribine injection and the diluent should be passed through a sterile 0.22 µ disposable hydrophilic syringe filter as each solution is being introduced into the infusion reservoir. First add the calculated dose of cladribine Injection (days × 0.09 mg/kg or ml/kg) to the infusion reservoir through the sterile filter. Then add a calculated amount of Bacteriostatic 0.9% Sodium Chloride Injection, USP (0.9% benzyl alcohol preserved) also through the filter to bring the total volume of the solution to 100 ml. After completing solution preparation, clamp off the line, disconnect and discard the filter. Aseptically aspirate air bubbles from the reservoir as necessary using the syringe and a dry second sterile filter or a sterile vent filter assembly. Reclamp the line and discard the syringe and filter assembly. Infuse continuously over 7 days. Solutions prepared with Bacteriostatic Sodium Chloride Injection for individuals weighing more than 85 kg may have reduced preservative effectiveness due to greater dilution of the benzyl alcohol preservative. Admixtures for the 7 day infusion have demonstrated acceptable chemical and physical stability for at least 7 days in Pharmacia Deltec MEDICATION CASSETTES‡. (TABLE 5)

TABLE 5

	Dose of Leustatin Injection	Recommended Diluent	Quantity of Diluent
7-day infusion method (use sterile 0.22 µ filter when preparing infusion solution)	7 (days) × 0.09 mg/kg	Bacteriostatic 0.9% Sodium Chloride Injection, USP (0.9% benzyl alcohol)	q.s. to 100 ml

Since limited compatibility data are available, adherence to the recommended diluents and infusion systems is advised. Solutions containing cladribine injection should not be mixed with other intravenous drugs or additives or infused simultaneously via a common intravenous line, since compatibility testing has not been performed. Preparations containing benzyl alcohol should not be used in neonates (See WARNINGS.)

Care must be taken to assure the sterility of prepared solutions. Once diluted, solutions of cladribine Injection should be administered promptly or stored in the refrigerator (2° to 8° C) for no more than 8 hours prior to start of administration. Vials of cladribine injection are for single-use only. Any unused portion should be discarded in an appropriate manner. (See Handling and Disposal.)

Parenteral drug products should be inspected visually for particulate matter and discoloration prior to administration, whenever solution and container permit. A precipitate may occur during the exposure of cladribine injection to low temperatures; it may be resolubilized by allowing the solution to warm naturally to room temperature and by shaking vigorously. **DO NOT HEAT OR MICROWAVE.**

Chemical Stability of Vials: When stored in refrigerated conditions between 2° to 8° C (36° to 46° F) protected from light, unopened vials of cladribine injection are stable until the expiration date indicated on the package. Freezing does not adversely affect the solution. If freezing occurs, thaw naturally to room temperature. DO NOT heat or microwave. Once thawed, the vial of cladribine injection is stable until expiry if refrigerated. DO NOT refreeze. Once diluted, solutions containing cladribine injection should be administered promptly or stored in the refrigerator (2° to 8° C) for no more than 8 hours prior to administration.

Handling and Disposal: The potential hazards associated with cytotoxic agents are well established and proper precautions should be taken when handling, preparing, and administering cladribine injection. The use of disposable gloves and protective garments is recommended. If cladribine injection contacts the skin or mucous membranes, wash the involved surface immediately with copious amounts of water. Several guidelines on this subject have been published.[2-8] There is no general agreement that all of the procedures recommended in the guidelines are necessary or appropriate. Refer to your institution's guidelines and all applicable state/local regulations for disposal of cytotoxic waste.

Store refrigerated 2° to 8° C (36° to 46° F). Protect from light during storage.

† Viaflex containers, manufactured by Baxter Healthcare Corporation - Code No. 2B8013 (tested in 1991)

‡ MEDICATION CASSETTE Reservoir, manufactured by Pharmacia Deltec, Inc. - Model No. 602100A (tested in 1991)

REFERENCES:

1. Santana VM. Mirro J, Harwood FC, *et al:* A phase I clinical trial of 2-Chloro-deoxyadenosine in pediatric patients with acute leukemia. J. Clin. Onc., 9:416 (1991). **2.** Recommendations for the Safe Handling of Parenteral Antineoplastic Drugs. NIH Publication No. 83-2621. For sale by the Superintendent of Documents, U.S. Government Printing Office, Washington, D.C. 20402. **3.** AMA Council Report, Guidelines for Handling Parenteral Antineoplastics,JAMA, March 15 (1985). **4.** National Study Commission on Cytotoxic Exposure - Recommendations for Handling Cytotoxic Agents. Available from Louis P. Jeffery, Sc.D., Chairman, National Study Commission on Cytotoxic Exposure, Massachusetts College of Pharmacy and Allied Health Sciences, 179 Longwood Avenue, Boston, MA 02115. **5.** Clinical Oncological Society of Australia: Guidelines and Recommendations for Safe Handling f Antineoplastic Agents, Med. J. Australia1:425 (1983). **6.** Jones RB, *et al.* Safe Handling of Chemotherapeutic Agents: A Report from the Mount Sinai Medical Center.Ca- A Cancer Journal for Clinicians, Sept/Oct. 258-263 (1983). **7.** American Society of Hospital Pharmacists Technical Assistance Bulletin on Handling Cytotoxic Drugs in Hospitals, Am J. Hosp. Pharm, **42:** 131 (1985). **8.** OSHA Work-Practice Guidelines for Personnel Dealing with Cytotoxic (antineoplastic) DrugsAm J Hosp Pharm, **43:** 1193 (1986).

HOW SUPPLIED - EQUIVALENTS NOT AVAILABLE:

Injection, Solution - Intravenous - 1 mg/ml

10 ml $480.00 LEUSTATIN, Ortho Biotech 59676-0201-01

CLARITHROMYCIN *(003068)*

CATEGORIES: AIDS Related Complex; Anti-Infectives; Antibiotics; Bronchitis; Chronic Bronchitis; Erythromycins; Macrolide; Mycobacterium Avium Complex; Otitis Media; Pharyngitis; Pneumonia; Respiratory Tract Infections; Sinusitis; Skin Infections; Tonsillitis; Ulcer*; Pregnancy Category C; FDA Class 1B ("Modest Therapeutic Advantage"); Sales > $1 Billion; FDA Approved 1991 Oct; Top 200 Drugs

* Indication not approved by the FDA

BRAND NAMES: *Abbotic*; **Biaxin**; *Biaxin HP* (Germany); *Bicrolid*; *Clacine*; *Clambiotic*; *Claribid*; *Clarith* (Japan); *Klacid* (Australia, Germany); *Klaricid* (England, Mexico, Japan); *Klaricid H.P.* (Mexico); *Klaricid Pediatric*; *Macladin*; *Veclam* *(International brand names outside U.S. in italics)*

FORMULARIES: BC-BS; Medi-Cal; PCS

COST OF THERAPY: $43.47 (Infections; Tablet; 250 mg; 2/day; 7 days)

PRIMARY ICD9: 136.9 (Unspecified Infections And Parasitic Diseases)

DESCRIPTION:

Clarithromycin is a semi-synthetic macrolide antibiotic. Chemically, it is 6-*0*-methylerythromycin. The molecular formula is $C_{38}H_{69}NO_{13}$, and the molecular weight is 747.96.

Clarithromycin is a white to off-white crystalline powder. It is soluble in acetone, slightly soluble in methanol, ethanol, and acetonitrile, and practically insoluble in water.

Biaxin is available as tablets and granules for oral suspension.

Each yellow oval film-coated Biaxin tablet contains 250 mg or 500 mg of clarithromycin and the following inactive ingredients: cellulosic polymers, croscarmellose sodium, D&C Yellow No.10, FD&C Blue No. 1, magnesium stearate, povidone, propylene glycol, silicon dioxide, sorbic acid, sorbitan monooleate, stearic acid, talc, titanium dioxide, and vanillin. The 250 mg tablet also contains pregelatinized starch.

After constitution, each 5 ml of Biaxin suspension contains 125 mg or 250 mg of clarithromycin. Each bottle of Biaxin granules contains 1250 mg (50 ml size), 2500 mg (50 and 100 ml sizes) or 5000 mg (100 ml size) of clarithromycin and the following inactive ingredients: carbomer, castor oil, citric acid, hydroxypropyl methylcellulose phthalate, maltodextrin, potassium sorbate, povidone, silicon dioxide, sucrose, xanthan gum, titanium dioxide and fruit punch flavor.

CLINICAL PHARMACOLOGY:

Pharmacokinetics: Clarithromycin is rapidly absorbed from the gastrointestinal tract after oral administration. The absolute bioavailability of 250 mg clarithromycin tablets was approximately 50%. Food slightly delays both the onset of clarithromycin absorption and the formation of the antimicrobially active metabolite, 14-OH clarithromycin, but does not affect the extent of bioavailability. Therefore, clarithromycin tablets may be given without regard to food.

In fasting healthy human subjects, peak serum concentrations were attained within 2 hours after oral dosing. Steady-state peak serum clarithromycin concentrations were attained in 2 to 3 days and were approximately 1 mcg/ml with a 250 mg dose administered every 12 hours, 2 to 3 mcg/ml with a 500 mg dose administered every 12 hours, and 3 to 4 mcg/ml with a 500 mg dose administered every 8 hours. The elimination half-life of clarithromycin was about 3 to 4 hours with 250 mg administered every 12 hours but increased to 5 to 7 hours with 500 mg administered every 8-12 hours. The nonlinearity of clarithromycin pharmacokinetics is slight at the recommended doses of 250 mg and 500 mg administered every 8-12 hours. With a 250 mg every 12 hours dosing, the principal metabolite, 14-OH clarithromycin, attains a peak steady-state concentration of about 0.6 mcg/ml and has an elimination half-life of 5 to 6 hours. With a 500 mg every 8-12 hours dosing, the peak steady-state concentration of 14-OH clarithromycin is slightly higher (up to 1 mcg/ml), and its elimination half-life is about 7-9 hours. With any of these dosing regimens, the steady-state concentration of this metabolite is generally attained within 2 to 3 days.

After a 250 mg tablet every 12 hours, approximately 20% of the dose is excreted in the urine as clarithromycin, while after a 500 mg tablet every 12 hours, the urinary excretion of clarithromycin is somewhat greater, approximately 30%. In comparison, after an oral dose of 250 mg (125 mg/5 ml) suspension every 12 hours, approximately 40% is excreted in urine as clarithromycin. The renal clearance of clarithromycin is, however, relatively independent of the dose size and approximates the normal glomerular filtration rate. The major metabolite found in urine is 14-OH clarithromycin, which accounts for an additional 10% to 15% of the dose with either a 250 mg or a 500 mg tablet administered every 12 hours.

Steady-state concentrations of clarithromycin and 14-OH clarithromycin observed following administration of 500 mg doses of clarithromycin every 12 hours to adult patients with HIV infection were similar to those observed in healthy volunteers. In adult HIV-infected patients taking 500 or 1000 mg doses of clarithromycin every 12 hours, steady-state clarithromycin C_{max} values ranged from 2-4 mcg/ml and 5-10 mcg/ml, respectively.

The steady-state concentrations of clarithromycin in subjects with impaired hepatic function did not differ from those in normal subjects; however, the 14-OH clarithromycin concentrations were lower in the hepatically impaired subjects. The decreased formation of 14-OH clarithromycin was at least partially offset by an increase in renal clearance of clarithromycin in the subjects with impaired hepatic function when compared to healthy subjects.

The pharmacokinetics of clarithromycin was also altered in subjects with impaired renal function. (See PRECAUTIONSand DOSAGE AND ADMINISTRATION.)

Clarithromycin and the 14-OH clarithromycin metabolite distribute readily into body tissues and fluids. There are no data available on cerebrospinal fluid penetration. Because of high intracellular concentrations, tissue concentrations are higher than serum concentrations. Examples of tissue and serum concentrations are presented in TABLE 1.

TABLE 1 Concentration (after 250 mg every 12 hours)

Tissue Type	Tissue (mcg/g)	Serum (mcg/ml)
Tonsil	1.6	0.8
Lung	8.8	1.7

When 250 mg doses of clarithromycin as Biaxin suspension were administered to fasting healthy adult subjects, peak plasma concentrations were attained around 3 hours after dosing. Steady-state peak plasma concentrations were attained in 2 to 3 days and were approximately 2 mcg/ml for clarithromycin and 0.7 mcg/ml for 14-OH clarithromycin when 250 mg doses of the clarithromycin suspension were administered every 12 hours. Elimination half-life of clarithromycin (3 to 4 hours) and that of 14-OH clarithromycin (5 to 7 hours) were similar to those observed at steady state following administration of equivalent doses of clarithromycin tablets.

For adult patients, the bioavailability of 10 ml of the 125 mg/5 ml suspension or 10 ml of the 250 mg/5 ml suspension is similar to a 250 mg or 500 mg tablet, respectively.

In children requiring antibiotic therapy, administration of 7.5 mg/kg every 12 hours, doses of clarithromycin as the suspension generally resulted in steady-state peak plasma concentrations of 3-7 mcg/ml for clarithromycin and 1 to 2 mcg/ml for 14-OH clarithromycin.

In HIV-infected children taking 15 mg/kg every 12 hours, steady-state clarithromycin peak concentrations generally ranged from 6-15 mcg/ml.

Clarithromycin penetrates into the middle ear fluid of children with secretory otitis media (TABLE 2).

CLINICAL PHARMACOLOGY: *(cont'd)*

TABLE 2 Concentration (after 7.5 mg/kg every 12 hours for 5 doses)

Analyte	Middle Ear Fluid (mcg/ml)	Serum (mcg/ml)
Clarithromycin	2.5	1.7
14-OH Clarithromycin	1.3	0.8

In adults given 250 mg clarithromycin as suspension (n=22), food appeared to decrease mean peak plasma clarithromycin concentrations from 1.2 (±0.4) mcg/ml to 1.0 (±0.4) mcg/ml and the extent of absorption from 7.2 (±2.5) hr·mcg/ml to 6.5 (±3.7) hr·mcg/ml. When children (n=10) were administered a single oral dose of 7.5 mg/kg suspension, food increased mean peak plasma clarithromycin concentration from 3.6 (±1.5) mcg/ml to 4.6 (±2.8) mcg/ml and the extent of absorption from 10.0 (±5.5) hr·mcg/ml to 14.2 (±9.4) hr·mcg/ml.

Clarithromycin 500 mg every 8 hours was given in combination with omeprazole 40 mg daily to healthy adult males. The plasma levels of clarithromycin and 14-hydroxy-clarithromycin were increased by the concomitant administration of omeprazole. For clarithromycin, the mean C_{max} was 10% greater, the mean C_{min} was 27% greater, and the mean $AUC_{0\text{-}8}$ was 15% greater when clarithromycin was administered with omeprazole than when clarithromycin was administered alone. Similiar results were seen for 14-hydroxy-clarithromycin, the mean C_{max} was 45% greater. Clarithromycin concentrations in the gastric tissue and mucus were also increased by concomitant administration of omeprazole.

TABLE 3 Clarithromycin Tissue Concentrations 2 hours after Dose (mcg/ml)(mcg/g)

Treatment	N	antrum	fundus	N	mucus
Clarithromycin	5	10.48±2.01	20.81±7.64	4	4.15±7.74
Clarithromycin + Omeprazole	5	19.96±4.71	24.25±6.37	4	39.29±32.79

For information on omeprazole refer to its prescribing information.

MICROBIOLOGY

Clarithromycin exerts its antibacterial action by binding to the 50S ribosomal subunit of susceptible microorganisms resulting in inhibition of protein synthesis.

Clarithromycin is active *in vitro* against a variety of aerobic and anaerobic gram-positive and gram-negative microorganisms as well as most *Mycobacterium avium* complex (MAC) microorganisms.

Additionally, the 14-OH clarithromycin metabolite also has clinically significant antimicrobial activity. Against *Haemophilus influenzae* microorganisms, 14-OH clarithromycin is twice as active as the parent compound. However, for *Mycobacterium avium* complex (MAC) isolates the 14-OH metabolite is 4 to 7 times less active than clarithromycin. The clinical significance of this activity against *Mycobacterium avium* complex is unknown.

Clarithromycin has been shown to be active against most strains of the following microorganisms both *in vitro* and in clinical infections as described in INDICATIONS AND USAGE.

Aerobic Gram-Positive Microorganisms: *Staphylococcus aureus; Streptococcus pneumoniae; Streptococcus pyrogenes*

Aerobic Gram-Negative Microorganisms: *Haemophilus influenzae; Moraxella catarrhalis*

Other Microorganisms: *Mycoplasma pneumoniae; Chlamydia pneumoniae (TWAR)*

Mycobacteria: *Mycobacterium avium* complex (MAC) consisting of: *Mycobacterium avium; Mycobacterium intracellulare*

Beta-lactamase production should have no effect on clarithromycin activity.

NOTE: Most strains of methicillin-resistant and oxacillin-resistant staphylococci are resistant to clarithromycin.

Clarithromycin has been shown to be active against most strains of *Helicobacter pylori in vitro* and in clinical infections when combined with omeprazole as described in INDICATIONS AND USAGE.

HELICOBACTER

Helicobacter pylori: Some *Helicobacter pylori* isolates obtained from patinets treated with clarithromycin plus omeprazole demonstrated an increase in clarithromycin MIC's over time, indicating decreasing susceptibility and increasing resistance. In the two U.S. clarithromycin plus omeprazole clinical trials, 104 patients had *H. pylori* isolated and clarithromycin MIC's determined pre-treatment. Of these, 4 patients had resistant strains, 2 patients had strains with intermediate susceptibility, and 98 patients had susceptible strains. Of the patients with susceptible *H. pylori* pre-treatment, 72 patients were eradicated of the *H. pylori* and 26 patients had *H. pylori* present post-treatment. Isolates from 25 of these 26 patients became resistant to clarithromycin. The six patients with resistant or intermediate *H. pylori* strains pre-treatment had resistant strains isolated post-treatment.

The following *in vitro* data are available, **but their clinical significance is unknown.**Clarithromycin exhibits *in vitro* against most strains of the following microorganisms; however, the safety and effectiveness of clarithromycin in treating clinical infections due to these microorganisms have not been established in adequate and well-controlled clinical trials.

Aerobic Gram-Positive Microorganisms: *Listeria monocytogenes; Streptococcus agalactiae; Streptococci (Groups C, F, G);* Viridans group streptococci

Aerobic Gram-Negative Microorganisms: *Bordetella pertussis; Campylobacter jejuni; Legionella pneumophila; Neisseria gonorrhoeae; Pasteurella multocida*

Other Microorganisms: *Chlamydia trachomatis*

Anaerobic Gram-Positive Microorganisms: *Clostridium perfringens; Peptococcus niger; Propionibacterium acnes*

Anaerobic Gram-Negative Microorganisms: *Prevotella melaninogenica* (formerly **Bacteriodes melaninogenicus)**

SUSCEPTIBILITY TESTING EXCLUDING MYCOBACTERIA AND HELICOBACTER

Dilution Techniques: Quantitative methods are used to determine minimum inhibitory concentrations (MIC's). These MIC's provide estimates of the susceptibility of bacteria to antimicrobial compounds. The MIC's should be determined using a standardized procedure. Standardized procedures are based on a dilution method[1] (broth or agar) or equivalent with standardized inoculum concentrations and standardized concentrations of clarithromycin powder. The MIC values should be interpreted according to the criteria in TABLE 4.

TABLE 4

MIC (mcg/ml)	Interpretation
≤2.0	Susceptible (S)
4.0	Intermediate (I)
≥8.0	Resistant (R)

A report of "Susceptible" indicates that the pathogen is likely to be inhibited if the antimicrobial compound in the blood reached the concentrations usually achievable.

CLINICAL PHARMACOLOGY: *(cont'd)*

A report of "Intermediate" indicates that the result should be considered equivocal, and, if the microorganism is not fully susceptible to alternative, clinically feasible drugs, the test should be repeated. This category implies possible clinical applicability in body sites where the drug is physiologically concentrated or in situations where high dosage of drug can be used. This category also provides a buffer zone which prevents small uncontrolled technical factors from causing major discrepancies in interpretation.

A report of "Resistant" indicates the pathogen is not likely to be inhibited if the antimicrobial compound in the blood reaches the concentrations usually achievable; other therapy should be selected.

Standardized susceptibility test procedures require the use of laboratory control microorganisms to contrl the technical aspects of the laboratory procedures. Standard clarithromycin powder should provide the MIC values found in TABLE 5.

TABLE 5

Microorganism		MIC(mcg/ml)
S. aureus	ATCC 29213	0.12-0.5

Diffusion Techniques: Quantitative methods that require measurement of zone diameters also provide reproducible estimates of the susceptibility of bacteria to antimicrobial compounds. One such standardized procedure[2] requires the use of standardized inoculum concentrations. This procedure uses paper disks impregnated with 15-mcg clarithromycin to test the susceptibility of microorganisms to clarithromycin.

Reports from the laboratory providing results of the standard single-disk susceptibility test with a 15-mcg clarithromycin disk should be interpreted according to the criteria found in TABLE 6.

TABLE 6

Zone Diameter (mm)	Interpretation
≥18	Susceptible (S)
14-17	Intermediate (I)
≤13	Resistant (R)

Interpretation should be as stated above for results using dilution techniques. Interpretation involves correlation of the diameter obtained in the disk test with the MIC for clarithromycin. However, standardized diffusion methods for routine *in vitro* susceptibility testing, using the 15-mcg clarithromycin disk, do not measure the additive antimicrobial activity of the 14-OH metabolite and, thus, may underestimate the drug's potential activity against *Haemophilus influenzae. Haemophilus influenzae* isolates falling into the "Intermediate" category often respond to treatment.

As with standardized dilution techniques, diffusion methods require the use of laboratory control microorganisms that are used to control the technical aspects of the laboratory procedures. For the diffusion technique, the 15-mcg clarithromycin disk should provide the zone diameters in the laboratory test quality control strain found in TABLE 7.

TABLE 7

Organism		Zone Diameter (mm)
S. aureus	ATCC 25923	26-32

IN VITRO ACTIVITY OF CLARITHROMYCIN AGAINST MYCOBACTERIA

Clarithromycin has demonstrated *in vitro* activity against *Mycobacterium avium* complex (MAC) microorganisms isolated from both AIDS and non-AIDS patients. While gene probe techniques may be used to distinguish *M. avium* species from *M. intracellulare*, many studies only reported results on *M. avium* complex (MAC) isolates.

Various *in vitro* methodologies employing broth or solid media at different pH's, with and without oleic acid-albumin-dextrose-catalase (OADC), have been used to determine clarithromycin MIC values for mycobacterial species. In general, MIC values decrease more than 16-fold as the pH of Middlebrook 7H12 broth media increases from 5.0 to 7.4. At pH 7.4, MIC values determined with Mueller-Hinton agar were 4- to 8-fold higher than those observed with Middlebrook 7H12 media. Utilization of oleic acid-albumin-dextrose-catalase (OADC) in these assays has been shown to further alter MIC values.

Clarithromycin activity against 80 MAC isolates from AIDS patients and 211 MAC isolates from non-AIDS patients was evaluated using a microdilution method with Middlebrook 7H9 broth. Results showed an MIC value of ≤4.0 mcg/ml in 81% and 89% of the AIDS and non-AIDS MAC isolates, respectively. Twelve percent of the non-AIDS isolates had an MIC value ≤0.5 mcg/ml. Clarithromycin was also shown to be active against phagocytized *M. avium* complex (MAC) in mouse and human macrophage cell cultures as well as in the beige mouse infection model.

Clarithromycin activity was evaluated against *Mycobacterium tuberculosis* microorganisms. In one study utilizing the agar dilution method with Middlebrook 7H10 media, 3 of 30 clinical isolates had an MIC of 2.5 mcg/ml. Clarithromycin inhibited all isolates at >10.0 mcg/ml.

SUSCEPTIBILITY TESTING FOR *MYCOBACTERIUM AVIUM* COMPLEX (MAC)

The disk diffusion and dilution techniques for susceptibility testing against gram-positive and gram-negative bacteria should not be used for determining clarithromycin MIC values against mycobacteria. *In vitro* susceptibility testing methods and diagnostic products currently available for determining minimum inhibitory concentration (MIC) values against *Mycobacterium avium* complex (MAC) organisms have not been standardized or validated. Clarithromycin MIC values will vary depending on the susceptibility testing method employed, composition and pH of the media, and the utilization of nutritional supplements. Breakpoints to determine whether clinical isolates of *M. avium* or *M. intracellulare* are susceptible or resistant to clarithromycin have not been established.

IN VITRO ACTIVITY OF CLARITHROMYCIN AGAINST *HELICOBACTER PYLORI*

Clarithromycin has demonstrated *in vitro* activity against *Helicobacter pylori* isolated from patients with duodenal ulcers. *In vitro* susceptibility testing methods (broth microdilution, agar dilution, E-test, and disk diffusion) and diagnostic products currently available for determining minimum inhibitory concentrations (MIC's) and zone sizes have not been standardized, validated, or approved for testing *H. pylori*. The clarithromycin MIC values and zone sizes will vary depending on the susceptibility testing methodology employed, media, growth additives, pH, inoculum concentration tested, growth phase, incubation atmosphere, and time.

SUSCEPTIBILITY TEST FOR *HELICOBACTER PYLORI*

In vitro susceptibility testing methods and diagnostic products currently available for determining minimum inhibitory concentrations (MIC's) and zone sizes have not been standardized, validated, or approved for testing *H. pylori* microorganisms. MIC values for *H. pylori* isolates collected during the two U.S. clinical trials evaluating clarithromycin plus omeprazole, were determined by broth microdilution MIC methodology[3]. Results obtained during the clarithromycin plus omeprazole clinical trials fell into a distinct bimodal distribution of susceptible and resistant clarithromycin MIC's.

If the broth microdilution MIC methodology published in Hachem, et al.[3] is used and the following tentative breakpoints are employed, there should be reasonable correlation between MIC results and clinical and microbiological outcomes for patients treated with clarithromycin plus omeprazole.

TABLE 8

MIC (mcg/mL)	Interpretation
≤0.06	Susceptible (S)
0.12-2.0	Intermediate (I)
≥4	Resistant (R)

These breakpoints should not be used to interpret results obtained using alternative methods.

CLINICAL STUDIES:

MYCOBACTERIAL INFECTIONS

Prophylaxis: A randomized, double-blind study (561) compared clarithromycin 500 mg twice a day to placebo in patients with CDC-defined AIDS and CD_4 counts <100 cells/µl. This study accrued 682 patients from November 1992 to January 1994, with a median CD_4 cell count at study entry of 30 cells/µl. Median duration of clarithromycin was 10.6 months vs. 8.2 months for placebo. More patients in the placebo arm than the clarithromycin arm discontinued prematurely from the study (75.6% and 67.4%, respectively). However, if premature discontinuations due to MAC or death are excluded, approximately equal percentages of patients on each arm (54.8% on clarithromycin and 52.5% on placebo) discontinued study drug early for other reasons. The study was designed to evaluate the following endpoints:

1. MAC bacteremia, defined as at least one positive culture for **M. avium** complex bacteria from blood or another normally sterile site.

2. Survival.

3. Clinically significant disseminated MAC disease, defined as MAC bacteremia accompanied by signs or symptoms of serious MAC infection, including fever, night sweats, weight loss, anemia, or elevations in liver function tests.

MAC Bacteremia: In patients randomized to claithromycin, the risk of MAC bacteremia was reduced by 69% compared to placebo. The difference between groups was statistically significant (p<0.001). On an intent-to-treat basis, the one-year cumulative incidence of MAC bacteremia was 5.0% for patients randomized to clarithromycin and 19.4% for patients randomized to placebo. While only 19 of the 341 patients randomized to clarithromycin developed MAC, 11 of these cases were resistant to clarithromycin. The patients with resistant MAC bacteremia had a median baseline CD_4 count of 10 cells/mm^3 (range 2-25 cells/mm^3). Information regarding the clinical course and response to treatment of the patients with resistant MAC bacteremia is limited. The 8 patients who received clarithromycin and developed susceptible MAC bacteremia had a median baseline CD_4 count of 25 cells/mm^3 (range 10-80 cells/mm^3). Comparatively, 53 of the 341 placebo patients developed MAC; none of these isolates were resistant to clarithromycin. The median baseline CD_4 count was 15 cells/mm^3 (range 2-130 cells/mm^3) for placebo patients that developed MAC.

Survival: A statistically significant survival benefit was observed.

TABLE 9

	Mortality		Reduction in Mortality on Clarithromycin
	Placebo	Clarithromycin	
6 month	9.4%	6.5%	31%
12 month	29.7%	20.5%	31%
18 month	46.4%	37.5%	20%

Since the analysis at 18 months includes patients no longer receiving prophylaxis the survival benefit of clarithromycin may be underestimated.

Clinically significant disseminated MAC disease: In association with the decreased incidence of bacteremia, patients in the group randomized to clarithromycin showed reductions in the signs and symptoms of disseminated MAC disease, inlcuding fever, night sweats, weight loss, and anemia.

Safety: In AIDS patients treated with clarithromycin over long periods of time for prophylaxis against *M. avium*, it was often difficult to distinguish adverse events possibly associated with clarithromycin administration from underlying HIV disease or intercurrent illness. Median duration of treatment was 10.6 months for the clarithromycin group and 8.2 months for the clarithromycin group and 8.2 months for the placebo group.

TABLE 10 Treatment-related* Adverse Event Incidence Rates (%) in Immunocompromised Adult Patients Receiving Prophylaxis Against *M. Avium* Complex

BODY SYSTEM‡; Adverse Event	Clarithromycin (n=339) %	Placebo (n=339) %
Body As A Whole		
Abdominal pain	5.0%	3.5%
Headache	2.7%	0.9%
Digestive		
Diarrhea	7.7%	4.1%
Dyspepsia	3.8%	2.7%
Flatulence	2.4%	0.9%
Nausea	11.2%	7.1%
Vomiting	5.9%	3.2%
Skin & Appendages		
Rash	3.2%	3.5%
Special Senses		
Taste Perversion	8.0%	0.3%

* Includes those events possibly or probably related to study drug and excludes concurrent conditions.
‡ ≥2% Adverse Event Incidence Rates for either treatment group.

Among these events, taste perversion was the only event that had significantly higher incidence in the clarithromycin-treated group compared to the placebo-treated group.

Discontinuation due to adverse events was required in 18% of patients receiving clarithromycin compared to 17% of patients receiving placebo in this trial. Primary reasons for discontinuation in clarithromycin-treated patients include headache, nausea, vomiting, depression and taste perversion.

CLINICAL STUDIES: *(cont'd)*

Changes in Laboratory Values of Potential Clinical Importance: In immunocompromised patients receiving prophylaxis against *M. avium*, evaluations of laboratory values were made by analyzing those values outside the seriously abnormal value (*i.e.*, the extreme high or low limit) for the specified test.

TABLE 11 Percentage of Patients [a]Exceeding Extreme Laboratory Value in Patients Receiving Prophylaxis Against *M. avium* Complex

		Clarithromycin 500 mg twice a day		Placebo	
Hemoglobin	<8g/dl	4/118	3%	5/103	5%
Platelet Count	$<50x10^9/L$	11/249	4%	12/250	5%
WBC Count	$<1x10^9/L$	2/103	4%	0/95	0%
SGOT	>5xULN[b]	7/196	4%	5/208	2%
SGPT	>5xULN[b]	6/217	3%	4/232	2%
Alk. Phos.	>5xULN[b]	5/220	2%	5/218	2%

(a) Includes only patients with baseline values within the normal range or borderline high (hematology variables) and within the normal range or boderline low (chemistry variables).
(b) ULN=Upper Limit of Normal

Treatment: Three randomized studies (500, 577, and 521) compared different dosages of clarithromycin in patients with CDC-defined AIDS and CD_4 counts <100 cells/μl. These studies accrued patients from May 1991 to March 1992. Study 500 was randomized, double-blind; Study 577 was open-label compassionate use. Both studies used 500 and 1000 mg twice a day doses; Study 500 also had a 2000 mg twice a day group. Study 521 was a pediatric study at 3.75, 7.5, and 15 mg/kg twice a day. Study 500 enrolled 154 adult patients, Study 577 enrolled 469 adult patients, and Study 521 enrolled 25 patients between the ages of 1 to 20. The majority of patients had CD_4 cell counts <50/μl at study entry. The studies were designed to evaluate the following end points:

1. Change in MAC bacteremia or blood cultures negative for *M. avium*.

2. Change in clinical signs and symptoms of MAC infection including one or more of the following: fever, night sweats, weight loss, diarrhea, splenomegaly, and hepatomegaly.

The results for the 500 study are described below. The 577 study results were similar to the results of the 500 study. Results with the 7.5 mg/kg twice a day dose in the pediatric study were comparable to those for the 500 mg twice a day regimen in the adult studies.

MAC Bacteremia: Decreases in MAC bacteremia or negative blood cultures were seen in the majority of patients in all dose groups. Mean reductions in colony forming units (CFU) are shown in TABLE 12. Included in the table are results from a separate study with a four drug regimen[5] (ciprofloxacin, ethambutol, rifampicin, and clofazimine). Since patient populations and study procedures may vary between these two studies, comparisons between the clarithromycin results and the combination therapy results should be interpreted cautiously.

TABLE 12 Mean Reductions in Log CFU from Baseline (After 4 Weeks of Therapy)

500 mg twice a day (N=35)	1000 mg twice a day (N=32)	2000 mg twice a day (N=26)	Four Drug Regimen (N=24)
1.5	2.3	2.3	1.4

Although the 1000 mg and 2000 mg twice a day doses showed significantly better control of bacteremia during the first four weeks of therapy, no significant differences were seen beyond that point. The percent of patients whose blood was sterilized as shown by one or more negative cultures at any time during acute therapy was 61% (30/49) for the 500 mg twice a day group and 59% (29/49) and 52% (25/48) for the 1000 and 2000 mg twice a day groups, respectively. The percent of patients who had 2 or more negative cultures during acute therapy that were sustained through study Day 84 was 25% (12/49) in both the 500 and 1000 mg twice a day groups and 8% (4/48) for the 2000 mg twice a day group. By Day 84, 23% (11/49), 37% (18/49), and 56% (27/48) of patients had died or discontinued from the study, and 14% (7/49), 12% (6/49), and 13% (6/48) of patients had relapsed in the 500, 1000, and 2000 mg twice a day dose groups, respectively. All of the isolates had an MIC <8 mcg/ml at pretreatment. Relapse was almost always accompanied by an increase in MIC. The median time to first negative culture was 54, 41, and 29 days for the 500, 1000, and 2000 mg twice a day groups, respectively. The time to first decrease of at least 1 log in CFU count was significantly shorter with the 1000 and 2000 mg twice a day doses (median equal to 16 and 15 days, respectively) in comparison to the 500 mg twice a day group (median equal to 29 days). The median time to first positive culture or study discontinuation following the first negative culture was 43, 59 and 43 days for the 500, 1000, and 2000 mg twice a day groups, respectively.

Clinically Significant Disseminated MAC Disease: Among patients experiencing night sweats prior to therapy, 84% showed resolution or improvement at some point during the 12 weeks of clarithromycin at 500-2000 mg twice a day doses. Similarly, 77% of patients reported resolution or improvement in fevers at some point. Response rates for clinical signs of MAC are given in TABLE 13A and TABLE 13B.

TABLE 13A

Resolution of Fever			Resolution of Night Sweats		
twice a day dosing (mg)	% ever afebrile	% afebrile ≥6 weeks	twice a day dosing (mg)	% ever resolving	% resolving ≥6 weeks
500	67%	23%	500	85%	42%
1000	67%	12%	1000	70%	33%
2000	62%	22%	2000	72%	36%

TABLE 13B

Weight Gain >3%			Hemoglobin Increase >1 gm		
twice a day dosing (mg)	% ever gaining	% gaining ≥6 weeks	twice a day dosing (mg)	% ever increasing	% increasing ≥6 weeks
500	33%	14%	500	58%	26%
1000	26%	17%	1000	37%	6%
2000	26%	12%	2000	62%	18%

The median duration of response, defined as improvement or resolution of clinical signs and symptoms, was 2-6 weeks.

Since the study was not designed to determine the benefit of monotherapy beyond 12 weeks, the duration of response may be underestimated for the 25-33% of patients who continued to show clinical response after 12 weeks.

Survival: Median survival time from study entry (Study 500) was 249 days at the 500 mg twice a day dose compared to 215 days with the 1000 mg twice a day dose. However, during the first 12 weeks of therapy, there were 2 deaths in 53 patients in the 500 mg twice a day group versus 13 deaths in 51 patients in the 1000 mg twice a day group. The reason for this apparent mortality difference is not known. Survival in the two groups was similar beyond 12 weeks. The median survival times for these dosages were similar to recent historical controls with MAC when treated with combination therapies.[5]

Median survival time from study entry in Study 577 was 199 days for the 500 mg twice a day dose and 179 days for the 1000 mg twice a day dose. During the first four weeks of therapy, while patients were maintained on their originally assigned dose, there were 11 deaths in 255 patients taking 500 mg twice a day and 18 deaths in 214 patients taking 1000 mg twice a day.

Safety: The adverse event profiles showed that both the 500 and 1000 mg twice a day doses were well tolerated. The 2000 mg twice a day dose was poorly tolerated and resulted in a higher proportion of premature discontinuations.

In AIDS patients and other immunocompromised patients treated with the higher doses of clarithromycin over long periods of time for mycobacterial infections, it was often difficult to distinguish adverse events possibly associated with clarithromycin administration from underlying signs of HIV disease or intercurrent illness.

The following analyses summarize experience during the first 12 weeks of therapy with clarithromycin. Data are reported separately for Study 500 (randomized, double-blind) and Study 577 (open-label, compassionate use) and also combined. Adverse events were reported less frequently in Study 577, which may be due in part to differences in monitoring between the two studies. In adult patients receiving clarithromycin 500 mg twice a day, the most frequently reported adverse events, considered possibly or probably related to study drug, with an incidence of 5% or greater, are listed below. Most of these events were mild to moderate in severity, although 5% (Study 500: 8%; Study 577: 4%) of patients receiving 500 mg twice a day and 5% (Study 500: 4%; Study 577: 6%) of patients receiving 1000 mg twice a day reported severe adverse events. Excluding those patients who discontinued therapy or died due to complications of their underlying non-mycobacterial disease, approximately 8% (Study 500: 15%; Study 577: 7%) of the patients who received 500 mg twice a day and 12% (Study 500: 14%; Study 577: 12%) of the patients who received 1000 mg twice a day discontinued therapy due to drug-related events during the first 12 weeks of therapy. Overall, the 500 and 1000 mg twice a day doses had similar adverse event profiles (TABLE 14).

TABLE 14 Treatment-related* Adverse Event Incidence Rates (%) In Immunocompromised Adult Patients During the First 12 Weeks of Therapy with 500 mg Twice a Day Clarithromycin Dose

Adverse Event	Study 500 (n=53)	Study 577 (n=255)	Combined (n=308)
Abdominal Pain	7.5	2.4	3.2
Diarrhea	9.4	1.6	2.9
Flatulence	7.5	0.0	1.3
Headache	7.5	0.4	1.6
Nausea	28.3	9.0	12.3
Rash	9.4	2.0	3.2
Taste Perversion	18.9	0.4	3.6
Vomiting	24.5	3.9	7.5

* Includes those events possibly or probably related to study drug and excludes concurrent conditions.

A limited number of pediatric AIDS patients have been treated with clarithromycin suspension for mycobacterial infections. The most frequently reported adverse events, excluding those due to the patient's concurrent condition, were consistent with those observed in adult patients.

Changes in Laboratory Values: In immunocompromised patients treated with clarithromycin for mycobacterial infections, evaluations of laboratory values were made by analyzing those values outside the seriously abnormal level (*i.e.*, the extreme high or low limit) for the specified test (TABLE 15).

TABLE 15 Percentage of Patients [(a)]Exceeding Extreme Laboratory Value Limits During First 12 Weeks of Treatment 500 mg Twice a Day Dose[(b)]

		Study 500	Study 577	Combined
BUN	>50 mg/dl	0%	<1%	<1%
Platelet Count	$<50 \times 10^9/L$	0%	<1%	<1%
SGOT	>5 x ULN[c]	0%	3%	2%
SGPT	>5 ULN[c]	0%	2%	1%
WBC	<1 xx $10^9/L$	0%	1%	1%

a Includes only patients with baseline values within the normal range or borderline high (hematology variables) and within normal range or borderline low (chemistry variables)
b Includes all values within first 12 weeks for patients who start on 500 mg twice a day.
c ULN=Upper Limit of Normal

OTITIS MEDIA

In a controlled clinical study of acute otitis media performed in the United States, where significant rates of beta-lactamase producing organisms were found, clarithromycin was compared to an oral cephalosporin. In this study, very strict evaluability criteria were used to determine clinical response. For the 223 patients who were evaluated for clinical efficacy, the clinical success rate (*i.e.*, cure plus improvement) at the post-therapy visit was 88% for clarithromycin and 91% for the cephalosporin.

In a smaller number of patients, microbiologic determinations were made at the pre-treatment visit. The presumptive bacterial eradication/clinical cure outcomes (*i.e.*, clinical success) were obtained and are found in TABLE 16.

TABLE 16 U.S. Acute Otitis Media Study Clarithromycin vs. Oral Cephalosporin: EFFICACY RESULTS

PATHOGEN	OUTCOME
S. pneumoniae	clarithromycin success rate, 13/15 (87%), control 4/5
*H. influenzae**	clarithromycin success rate, 10/14 (71%), control 3/4
M. catarrhalis	clarithromycin success rate, 4/5, control 1/1
S. pyrogenes	clarithromycin success rate, 3/3, control 0/1
Overall	clarithromycin success rate, 30/37 (81%), control 8/11 (73%)

* None of the *H. influenzae* isolated pre-treatment was resistant to clarithromycin; 6% were resistant to the control agent.

Safety: The incidence of adverse events in all patients treated, primarily diarrhea and vomiting, did not differ clinically or statistically for the two agents.

CLINICAL STUDIES: *(cont'd)*

In two other controlled clinical trials of acute otitis media performed in the United States, where significant rates of beta-lactamase producing organisms were found, clarithromycin was compared to an oral antimicrobial agent that contained a specific beta-lactamase inhibitor. In these studies, very strict evaluability criteria were used to determine the clinical responses. In the 233 patients who were evaluated for clinical efficacy, the combined clinical success rate (*i.e.*, cure and improvement) at the post-therapy visit was 91% for both clarithromycin and the control.

For the patients who had microbiologic determinations at the pre-treatment visit, the following presumptive bacterial eradication/clinical cure outcomes (*i.e.*, clinical success) were obtained and can be found in TABLE 17.

TABLE 17 Two U.S. Acute Otitis Media Studies Clarithromycin vs. Antimicrobial/Beta-lactamase Inhibitor: EFFICACY RESULTS

PATHOGEN	OUTCOME
S. pneumoniae	clarithromycin success rate, 43/51 (84%), control 55/56 (98%)
*H. influenzae**	clarithromycin success rate, 36/45 (80%), control 31/33 (94%)
M. catarrhalis	clarithromycin success rate, 9/10 (90%), control 6/6
S. pyrogenes	clarithromycin success rate, 3/3, control 5/5
Overall	clarithromycin success rate, 91/109 (83%), control 97/100 (97%)

* Of the *H. influenzae*isolated pre-treatment, 3% were resistant to clarithromycin and 10% were resistant to the control agent.

Safety: The incidence of adverse events in all patients treated, primarily diarrhea (15% vs. 38%) and diaper rash (3% vs. 11%) in young children, was clinically and statistically lower in the clarithromycin arm versus the control arm.

Duodenal Ulcer Associated with *H. Pylori* Infection: Four randomized, double-blind, multi-center studies (067, 100, 812b, and 058) evaluated clarithromycin 500 mg twice a day plus omeprazole 40 mg every day for 14 days, follwed by omeprazole 20 mg every day (067, 100, and 058) or by omeprazole 40 mg every day (812b) for an additional 14 days in patients with active duodenal ulcer associated with *H. pylori*. Studies 067 and 100 were conducted in the U.S. and Canada and enrolled 242 and 256 patients, respectively. *H. pylori* infection and duodenal ulcer were confirmed in 219 patients in Study 067 and 228 patients in Study 100. These studies compared the combination regimen to omeprazole and clarithromycin mon-therapies. Studies 812b and 058 were conducted in Europe and enrolled 154 and 215 patients, respectively. *H. pylori* infection and duodenal ulcer were confirmed in 148 patients in Study 812b and 208 patients in Study 058. These studies compared the combination regimen to omeprazole monotherapy. The results for the efficacy analyses for these studies are described below.

Duodenal Ulcer Healing: The combination of clarithromycin and omeprazole was as effective as omeprazole alone for healing duodenal ulcer.

TABLE 18 End-of-Treatment Ulcer Healing Rates

Study	Clarithromycin + Omeprazole	Omeprazole	Clarithromycin
U.S. Studies			
Study 100	94% (58/62)†	88% (60/68)	71% (49/69)
Study 067	88% (56/64)	85% (55/65)	64% (44/69)
Non-U.S. Studies			
Study 058	99% (81/85)	95% (82/86)	N/A
Study 812b[1]	100% (64/64)	99% (71/72)	N/A

† p<0.05 for clarithromycin + omeprazole versus clarithromycin monotherapy.
[1]In Study 812b patients received omeprazole 40 mg daily for days 15 to 28.

Eradication of *H. Pylori* Associated with Duodenal Ulcer: The combination of clarithromycin and omeprazle was effective in eradicating *H. pylori*.

TABLE 19 *H. pylori*Eradication Rates (Per-Protocol Analysis) at 4 to 6 Weeks

Study	Clarithromycin + Omeprazole	Omeprazole	Clarithromycin
U.S. Studies			
Study 100	64% (39/61)†‡	0% (0/59)	39% (17/44)
Study 067	74% (39/53)†‡	0% (0/54)	31% (13/42)
Non-U.S. Studies			
Study 058	74% (64/86)‡	1%	N/A
Study 812b	83% (50/60)‡	1%	N/A

† Statistically significantly higher than clarithromycin monotherapy (p<0.05).
‡ Statistically significantly higher than omeprazole monotherapy (p<0.5).

H. pylori eradication was defined as no positive test (culture or histology) at 4 weeks following the end of treatment, and two negative tests were required to be considered eradicated. In the per-protocol analysis, the following patients were excluded: dropouts, patients with major protocol violations, patients with missing *H. pylori* tests post-treatment, and patients that were not assessed for *H. pylori* eradication at 4 weeks after the end of treatment because they were found to have an unhealed ulcer at the end of treatment.

Ulcer recurrence at 6–months following the end of treatment was assessed for patients in whom ulcers were healed post-treatment.

Thus, in patients with duodenal ulcer associated with *H. pylori* infection, eradication of *H. pylori* reduced ulcer recurrence.

Safety: The adverse event profiles for the four studies showed that the combination of clarithromycin 500 mg three times a day and omeprazole 40 mg every day for 14 days, followed by omeprazole 20 mg every day (067, 100, and 058) or 40 mg every day (812b) for an additional 14 days was well tolerated. Of the 346 patients who received the combination. 12 (3.5%) patients discontinued study drug due to adverse events.

Changes in Laboratory Values: Changes in laboratory values with possible clinical significance in patients taking clarithromycin and omeprazole were as follows:

Hepatic: Elevated direct bilirubin <1%; GGT <1%; SGOT (AST) <1%; SGPT (ALT) <1%.

Renal: Elevated serum creatinine <1%.

For information on omeprazole refer to its prescribing information.

INDICATIONS AND USAGE:

Clarithromycin is indicated for the treatment of mild to moderate infections caused by susceptible strains of the designated microorganisms in the conditions listed below:

INDICATIONS AND USAGE: *(cont'd)*

TABLE 20 Ulcer Recurrence at 6 months by *H. Pylori* Status at 4 to 6 Weeks

	H. pylori Negative	*H. pylori* Positive
U.S. Studies		
Study 100		
Clarithromycin + Omeprazole	6% (2/34)	56% (9/16)
Omeprazole	- (0/0)	71% (35/49)
Clarithromycin	12% (2/17)	32% (7/22)
Study 067		
Clarithromycin + Omeprazole	38% (11/29)	50% (6/12)
Omeprazole	- (0/0)	67% (31/46)
Clarithromycin	18% (2/11)	52% (14/27)
Non-U.S. Studies		
Study 058		
Clarithromycin + Omeprazole	6% (3/53)	24% (4/17)
Omeprazole	0% (0/3)	55% (39/71)
Study 812b*		
Clarithromycin + Omeprazole	5% (2/42)	0% (0/7)
Omeprazole	0% (0/1)	54% (32/59)
* 12-month recurrence rates:		
Clarithromycin + Omeprazole	3% (1/40)	0% (0/6)
Omeprazole	0% (0/1)	67% (29/43)

TABLE 21 Adverse Events with an Incidence of 3% or Greater

Adverse Event	Clarithromycin + Omeprazole (N=346) % of Patients	Omeprazole (N=355) % of Patients	Clarithromycin (N=166) % of Patients*
Taste Perversion	15%	1%	16%
Nausea	5%	1%	3%
Headache	5%	6%	9%
Diarrhea	4%	3%	7%
Vomiting	4%	<1%	1%
Abdominal Pain	3%	2%	1%
Infection	3%	4%	2%

* Studies 067 and 100, only

Most of these events were mild to moderate in severity.

Adults: Pharyngitis/Tonsillitis due to *Streptococcus pyogenes* (The usual drug of choice in the treatment and prevention of streptococcal infections and the prophylaxis of rheumatic fever is penicillin administered by either the intramuscular or the oral route. Clarithromycin is generally effective in the eradication of *S. pyrogenes* from the nasopharynx; however, data establishing the efficacy of clarithromycin in the subsequent prevention of rheumatic fever are not available at present.)

Acute maxillary sinusitis due to *Haemophilus influenzae, Moraxella catarrhalis*, or *Streptococcus pneumoniae*.

Acute bacterial exacerbation of chronic bronchitis due to *Haemophilus influenzae, Moraxella catarrhalis*, or *Streptococcus pneumoniae*

Pneumonia due to *Mycoplasma pneumoniae, Streptococcus pneumoniae*, or *Chlamydia pneumoniae* (TWAR).

Uncomplicated skin and skin structure infections due to *Staphylococcus aureus*, or *Streptococcus pyogenes*. (Abscesses usually require surgical drainage.)

Disseminated mycobacterial infections due to *Mycobacterium avium*, or *Mycobacterium intracellulare*.

Clarithromycin in combination with omeprazole is indicated for the treatment of patients with an active duodenal ulcer associated with *H. pylori* infection. The eradication of *H. pylori* has been demonstrated to reduce the risk of duodenal ulcer recurrence.

In patients who fail therapy, susceptibility testing should be done if possible. If resistence is demonstrated, alternative therapy is recommended. (For information on development of resistance (see Microbiology.)

Children: Pharyngitis/Tonsillitis due to *Streptococcus pyogenes*Pneumonia due to *Mycoplasma pneumoniae, Streptococcus pneumoniae*, or *Chlamydia pneumoniae* (TWAR).

Acute maxillary sinusitis due to *Haemophilus influenzae, Moraxella catarrhalis*, or *Streptococcus pneumoniae*.

Acute otitis media due to *Haemophilus influenzae, Moraxella catarrhalis*, or *Streptococcus pneumoniae*

NOTE: For information on otitis media, see CLINICAL STUDIES, Otitis Media.

Uncomplicated skin and skin structure infections due to *Staphylococcus aureus*, or *Streptococcus pyogenes* (Abscesses usually require surgical drainage.)

Disseminated mycobacterial infections due to *Mycobacterium avium*, or *Mycobacterium intracellulare*.

Prophylaxis: Clarithromycin tablets and granules for oral suspension are indicated for the prevention of disseminated *Mycobacterium avium* complex (MAC) disease in patients with advanced HIV infection.

CONTRAINDICATIONS:

Clarithromycin is contraindicated in patients with a known hypersensitivity to clarithromycin, erythromycin, or any of the macrolide antibiotics.

Clarithromycin is contraindicated in patients receiving terfenadine therapy who have pre-existing cardiac abnormalities (arrhythmia, bradycardia, QT interval prolongation, ischemic heart disease, congestive heart failure, etc.) or electrolyte disturbances. (See DRUG INTERACTIONS.)

For information on omeprazole refer to its prescribing information.

WARNINGS:

CLARITHROMYCIN SHOULD NOT BE USED IN PREGNANT WOMEN EXCEPT IN CLINICAL CIRCUMSTANCES WHERE NO ALTERNATIVE THERAPY IS APPROPRIATE. IF PREGNANCY OCCURS WHILE TAKING THIS DRUG, THE PATIENT SHOULD BE APPRISED OF THE POTENTIAL HAZARD TO THE FETUS. CLARITHROMYCIN HAS DEMONSTRATED ADVERSE EFFECTS OF PREGNANCY OUTCOME AND/OR EMBRYO-FETAL DEVELOPMENT IN MONKEYS, RATS, MICE, AND RABBITS AT DOSES THAT PRODUCED PLASMA LEVELS 2 TO 17 TIMES THE SERUM LEVELS ACHIEVED IN HUMANS TREATED AT THE MAXIMUM RECOMMENDED HUMAN DOSES. (See PRECAUTIONS, Pregnancy.)

WARNINGS: *(cont'd)*

Pseudomembranous colitis has been reported with nearly all antibacterial agents, including clarithromycin, and may range in severity from mild to life threatening. Therefore, it is important to consider this diagnosis in patients who present with diarrhea subsequent to the administration of antibacterial agents.

Treatment with antibacterial agents alters the normal flora of the colon and may permit overgrowth of clostridia. Studies indicate that a toxin produced by *Clostridium difficile* is a primary cause of "antibiotic-associated colitis".

After the diagnosis of pseudomembranous colitis has been established, therapeutic measures should be initiated. Mild cases of pseudomembranous colitis usually respond to discontinuation of the drug alone. In moderate to severe cases, consideration should be given to management with fluids and electrolytes, protein supplementation, and treatment with an antibacterial drug clinically effective against *Clostridium difficile* colitis.

For information on Omeprazole, please refer to its prescribing information.

PRECAUTIONS:

GENERAL

Clarithromycin is principally excreted via the liver and kidney. Clarithromycin may be administered without dosage adjustment to patients with hepatic impairment and normal renal function. However, in the presence of severe renal impairment with or without coexisting hepatic impairment, decreased dosage or prolonged dosing intervals may be appropriate.

For information on omeprazole, please refer to its prescribing information.

INFORMATION FOR PATIENTS

Clarithromycin tablets and oral suspension can be taken with or without food and can be taken with milk. Do **NOT** refrigerate the suspension.

CARCINOGENESIS, MUTAGENESIS, IMPAIRMENT OF FERTILITY

The following *in vitro* mutagenicity tests have been conducted with clarithromycin:

Salmonella/Mammalian Microsomes Test;

Bacterial Induced Mutation Frequency Test;

In Vitro Chromosome Aberration Test;

Rat Hepatocyte DNA Synthesis Assay;

Mouse Lymphoma Assay;

Mouse Dominant Lethal Study;

Mouse Micronucleus Test

All tests had negative results except the *In Vitro* Chromosome Aberration Test which was weakly positive in one test and negative in another.

In addition, a Bacterial Reverse-Mutation Test (Ames Test) has been performed on clarithromycin metabolites with negative results.

Fertility and reproduction studies have shown that daily doses of up to 160 mg/kg/day (1.3 times the recommended maximum human dose based on mg/m^2) to male and female rats caused no adverse effects on the estrous cycle, fertility, parturition, or number and viability of offspring. Plasma levels in rats after 150 mg/kg/day were 2 times the human serum levels.

In the 150 mg/kg/day monkey studies, plasma levels were 3 times the human serum levels. When given orally at 150 mg/kg/day (2.4 times the recommended maximum human dose based on mg/m^2), clarithromycin was shown to produce embryonic loss in monkeys. This effect has been attributed to marked maternal toxicity of the drug at this high dose.

In rabbits, *in utero* fetal loss occurred at an intravenous dose of 33 mg/m^2, which is 17 times less than the maximum proposed human oral daily dose of 618 mg/m^2.

Long-term studies in animals have not been performed to evaluate the carcinogenic potential of clarithromycin.

PREGNANCY

Teratogenic Effects: Pregnancy Category C: Four teratogenicity studies in rats (three with oral doses and one with intravenous doses up to 160 mg/kg/day administered during the period of major organogenesis) and two in rabbits at oral doses up to 125 mg/kg/day (approximately 2 times the recommended maximum human dose based on mg/m^2), or intravenous doses of 30 mg/kg/day administered during gestation days 6 to 18 failed to demonstrate any teratogenicity from clarithromycin. Two additional oral studies in a different rat strain at similar doses and similar conditions demonstrated a low incidence of cardiovascular anomalies at doses of 150 mg/kg/day administered during gestation days 6 to 15. Plasma levels after 150 mg/kg/day were 2 times the human serum levels. Four studies in mice revealed a variable incidence of cleft palate following oral doses of 1000 mg/kg/day (2 and 4 times the recommended maximum human dose based on mg/m^2, respectively) during gestation days 6 to 15. Cleft palate was also seen at 500 mg/kg/day. The 1000 mg/kg/day exposure resulted in plasma levels 17 times the human serum levels. In monkeys, an oral dose of 70 mg/kg/day (an approximate equidose of the recommended maximum human dose based on mg/m^2) produced fetal growth retardation at plasma levels that were 2 times the human serum levels.

There are no adequate and well-controlled studies in pregnant women. Clarithromycin should be used during pregnancy only if the potential benefit justifies the potential risk to the fetus. (See WARNINGS.)

NURSING MOTHERS

It is not known whether clarithromycin is excreted in human milk. Because many drugs are excreted in human milk, caution should be exercised when clarithromycin is administered to a nursing woman. It is known that clarithromycin is excreted in the milk of lactating animals and that other drugs of this class are excreted in human milk. Preweaned rats, exposed indirectly via consumption of milk from dams treated with 150 mg/kg/day for 3 weeks, were not adversely affected, despite data indicating higher drug levels in milk than in plasma.

PEDIATRIC USE

Safety and effectiveness of clarithromycin in children under 6 months of age have not been established. The safety of clarithromycin has not been studied in MAC patients under the age of 20 months. Neonatal and juvenile animals tolerated clarithromycin in a manner similar to adult animals. Young animals were slightly more intolerant to acute overdosage and to subtle reductions in erythrocytes, platelets and leukocytes but were less sensitive to toxicity in the liver, kidney, thymus, and genitalia.

GERIATRIC USE

In a steady-state study in which healthy elderly subjects (age 65 to 81 years old) were given 500 mg every 12 hours, the maximum serum concentrations and area under the curves of clarithromycin and 14-OH clarithromycin were increased compared to those achieved in healthy young adults. These changes in pharmacokinetics parallel known age-related decreases in renal function. In clinical trials, elderly patients did not have an increased incidence of adverse events when compared to younger patients. Dosage adjustment should be considered in elderly patients with severe renal impairment.

DRUG INTERACTIONS:

Clarithromycin use in patients who are receiving theophylline may be associated with an increase of serum theophylline concentrations. Monitoring of serum theophylline concentrations should be considered for patients receiving high doses of theophylline or with baseline concentrations in the upper therapeutic range. In two studies in which theophylline was administered with clarithromycin (a theophylline sustained-release formulation was dosed at either 6.5 mg/kg or 12 mg/kg together with 250 or 500 mg clarithromycin every 12 hours), the steady-state levels of C_{max}, C_{min}, and the area under the serum concentration time curve (AUC) of theophylline increased about 20%.

Concomitant administration of single doses of clarithromycin and carbamazepine has been shown to result in increased plasma concentrations of carbamazepine. Blood level monitoring of carbamazepine may be considered.

When clarithromycin and terfenadine were coadministered, plasma concentrations of the active acid metabolite of terfenadine were threefold higher, on average, than the values observed when terfenadine was administered alone. The pharmacokinetics of clarithromycin and the 14-hydroxy-clarithromycin were not significantly affected by coadministration of terfenadine once clarithromycin reached steady-state conditions. The increase in the QT interval seen in association with the elevated terfenadine acid metabolite level is unlikely to be of clinical significance in healthy individuals. Clarithromycin should not be given to patients receiving terfenadine therapy who have preexisting cardiac abnormalities (arrhythmia, bradycardia, QT interval prolongation, ischemic heart disease, congestive heart failure, etc.) or electrolyte disturbances. (See CONTRAINDICATIONS.)

Clarithromycin 500 mg every 8 hours was given in combination with omeprazole 40 mg daily to healthy adult subjects. The steady-state plasma concentrations of omeprazole were increased (C_{max}, AUC_{0-24}, and $T_{1/2}$ increases of 30%, 89%, and 34%, respectively), by the concomitant administration of clarithromycin. The mean 24–hour gastric pH value was 5.2 when omeprazole was administered alone and 5.7 when co-administered with clarithromycin.

Simultaneous oral administration of clarithromycin and zidovudine to HIV-infected adult patients resulted in decreased steady-state zidovudine concentrations. When 500 mg of clarithromycin were administered twice daily, steady-state zidovudine AUC was reduced by a mean of 12% (n=4). Individual values ranged from a decrease of 34% to an increase of 14%. Based on limited data in 24 patients, when clarithromycin was administered two to four hours prior to oral zidovudine, the steady-state zidovudine C_{max} was increased by approximately 2–fold, whereas the AUC was unaffected.

Simultaneous administration of clarithromycin and didanosine to 12 HIV-infected adult patients resulted in no statistically significant change in didanosine pharmacokinetics.

Concomitant administration of fluconazole 200 mg daily and clarithromycin 500 mg twice daily to 21 healthy volunteers led to increases in the mean steady-state clarithromycin C_{min} and AUC of 33% and 18%, respectively. Steady-state concentrations of 14–OH clarithromycin were not significantly affected by concomitant administration of fluconazole.

Spontaneous reports in the post-marketing period suggest that concomitant administration of clarithromycin and oral anticoagulants may potentiate the effects of the oral anticoagulants. Prothrombin times should be carefully monitored while patients are receiving clarithromycin and oral anticoagulants simultaneously.

Elevated digoxin serum concentrations in patients receiving clarithromycin and digoxin concomitantly have also been reported in post-marketing surveillance. Some patients have shown clinical signs consistent with digoxin toxicity, including arrhythmias. Serum digoxin levels should be carefully monitored while patients are receiving digoxin and clarithromycin simultaneously.

The following drug interactions, other than increased serum concentrations of carbamazepine and active acid metabolite of terfenadine, have not been reported in clinical trials with clarithromycin; however, they have been observed with erythromycin products and/or with clarithromycin in post-marketing experience.

Concurrent use of erythromycin or clarithromycin and ergotamine or dihydroergotamine has been associated in some patients with acute ergot toxicity characterized by severe peripheral vasospasm and dysesthesia.

Erythromycin has been reported to decrease the clearance of triazolam and, thus, may increase the pharmacologic effect of triazolam. There have been post-marketing reports of drug interactions and CNS effects (*e.g.*, somnolence and confusion) with the concomitant use of clarithromycin and triazolam.

The use of erythromycin and clarithromycin in patients concurrently taking drugs metabolized by the cytochrome P450 system may be associated with elevations in serum levels of these other drugs. There have been reports of interactions of erythromycin and/or clarithromycin with carbamazepine, cyclosporine, hexobarbital, phenytoin, alfentanil, disopyramide, lovastatin, bromocriptine, valproate, terfenadine, cisapride, pimozide, and astemizole. Serum concentrations of drugs metabolized by the cytochrome P450 system should be monitored closely in patients concurrently receiving these drugs.

ADVERSE REACTIONS:

The majority of side effects observed in clinical trials were of a mild and transient nature. Fewer than 3% of adult patients without mycobacterial infections and fewer than 2% of pediatric patients without mycobacterial infections discontinued therapy because of drug-related side effects.

The most frequently reported events in adults were diarrhea (3%), nausea (3%), abnormal taste (3%), dyspepsia (2%), abdominal pain/discomfort (2%), and headache (2%). In pediatric patients, the most frequently reported events were diarrhea (6%), vomiting (6%), abdominal pain (3%), rash (3%), and headache (2%). Most of these events were described as mild or moderate in severity. Of the reported adverse events, only 1% were described as severe.

In pneumonia studies conducted in adults comparing clarithromycin to erythromycin base or erythromycin stearate, there were fewer adverse events involving the digestive system in clarithromycin-treated patients compared to erythromycin-treated patients (13% vs. 32%; $p<0.01$). Twenty percent of erythromycin-treated patients discontinued therapy due to adverse events compared to 4% of clarithromycin-treated patients.

In two U.S. studies of acute otitis media comparing clarithromycin to amoxicillin/potassium clavulanate in pediatric patients, there were fewer adverse events involving the digestive system in clarithromycin-treated patients compared to amoxicillin/potassium clavulanate-treated patients (21% vs. 40%, $p<0.001$). One-third as many clarithromycin-treated patients reported diarrhea as did amoxicillin/potassium clavulanate-treated patients.

POST-MARKETING EXPERIENCE

Allergic reactions ranging from urticaria and mild skin eruptions to rare cases of anaphylaxis and Stevens-Johnson syndrome have occurred. Other spontaneously reported adverse events include glossitis, stomatitis, oral moniliasis, vomiting and dizziness. There have been isolated reports of hearing loss, which is usually reversible, occurring chiefly in elderly women. Reports of alterations of the sense of smell, usually in conjunction with taste perversion have also been reported.

Transient CNS events including behavioral changes, confusional states, depersonalization, disorientation, hallucinations, insomnia, nightmares, tinnitus, and vertigo have been reported during post-marketing surveillance. Events usually resolve quickly with discontinuation of the drug.

ADVERSE REACTIONS: *(cont'd)*

Hepatic dysfunction, including increased liver enzymes, and hepatocellular and/or cholestatic hepatitis, with or without jaundice, has been infrequently reported with clarithromycin. This hepatic dysfunction may be severe and is usually reversible. In very rare instances, hepatic failure with fatal outcome has been reported and generally has been associated with serious underlying diseases and/or concomitant medications.

Rarely, erythromycin and clarithromycin have been associated with ventricular arrhythmias, including ventricular tachycardia and torsades de pointes, in individuals with prolonged QT_c intervals.

CHANGES IN LABORATORY VALUES

Changes in laboratory values with possible clinical significance were as follows:

Hepatic: elevated SGPT (ALT) <1%; SGOT (AST) <1%; GGT <1%; alkaline phosphatase <1%; LDH <1%; total bilirubin <1%

Hematologic: decreased WBC <1%; elevated prothrombin time 1%

Renal: elevated BUN 4%; elevated serum creatinine <1%

GGT, alkaline phosphatase, and prothrombin time data are from adult studies only.

DOSAGE AND ADMINISTRATION:

Clarithromycin may be given with or without food (TABLE 22).

TABLE 22 Adult Dosage Guidelines

Infection	Dosage (every 12 hours)	Normal Duration (days)
Pharyngitis/Tonsillitis	250 mg	10
Acute maxillary sinusitis	500 mg	14
Acute exacerbation of chronic bronchitis due to:		
S. pneumoniae	250 mg	7-14
M. catarrhalis	250 mg	7-14
H. influenzae	500 mg	7-14
Pneumonia due to:		
S. pneumoniae	250 mg	7-14
M. pneumoniae	250 mg	7-14
Uncomplicated skin and skin structure	250 mg	7-14

TABLE 23 Active Duodenal Ulcer Associated with *H. pylori* Infection (28 day therapy)

Days 1 to 14	Days 15 to 28
Clarithromycin 500 mg tablet three times a day plus Omeprazole 2 × 20 mg capsules every morning	Omeprazole 20 mg capsule every morning

For information on omeprazole refer to its prescribing information.

Children: The usual recommended daily dosage is 15 mg/kg/day divided every 12 hours for 10 days (TABLE 24).

TABLE 24 Pediatric Dosage Guidelines: Based on Body Weight

Weight		Dosing Calculated on 7.5 mg/kg every 12 hours		
Kg	lbs	Dose (every 12 hours)	125 mg/ 5 ml	250 mg/ 5 ml
9	20	62.5 mg	2.5 ml every 12 hours	1.25 ml every 12 hours
17	37	125 mg	5 ml every 12 hours	2.5 ml every 12 hours
25	55	187.5 mg	7.5 ml every 12 hours	3.75 ml every 12 hours
33	73	250 mg	10 ml every 12 hours	5 ml everu 12 hours

Clarithromycin may be administered without dosage adjustment in the presence of hepatic impairment if there is normal renal function. However, in the presence of severe renal impairment (CR_{CL} <30 ml/min), with or without coexisting hepatic impairment, the dose should be halved or the dosing interval doubled.

MYCOBACTERIAL INFECTIONS

Prophylaxis: The recommended dose of clarithromycin for the prevention of dissemindated *Mycobacterium avium* disease is 500 mg twice a day. In children, the recommended dose is 7.5 mg/kg twice a day up to 500 mg twice a day. No studies of clarithromycin for MAC prophylaxis have been performed in pediatric populations and the doses recommended for prophylaxis are derived from MAC treatment studies in children. Dosing recommendations for children are in TABLE 24.

Treatment: Clarithromycin is recommended as the primary agent for the treatment of disseminated infection due to *Mycobacterium avium* complex. Clarithromycin should be used in combination with other antimycobacterial drugs that have shown *in vitro* activity against MAC, including ethambutol, clofazimine, and rifampin. Although no controlled clinical trial information is available for combination therapy with clarithromycin, the U.S. Public Health Service Task Force has provided recommendations for the treatment of MAC.[3] The recommended dose for mycobacterial infections in adults is 500 mg twice a day. In children, the recommended dose is 7.5 mg/kg twice a day up to 500 mg twice a day. Dosing recommendations for children are in TABLE 24.

Clarithromycin therapy should continue for life if clinical and mycobacterial improvements are observed.

CONSTITUTING INSTRUCTIONS

TABLE 25 indicates the volume of water to be added when constituting.

TABLE 25

Total volume after constitution	Clarithromycin concentration after constitution	Amount of water to be added*
50 ml	125 mg/5 ml	27 ml
100 ml	125 mg/5 ml	55 ml
50 ml	250 mg/5 ml	27 ml
100 ml	250 mg/5 ml	55 ml

* See instructions below.

Add half the volume of water to the bottle and shake vigorously. Add the remainder of water to the bottle and shake.

Shake well before each use. Oversize bottle provides shake space. Keep tightly closed.

Do not refrigerate. After mixing, store at 15° to 30° C (59° to 86° F) and use within 14 days.

ANIMAL PHARMACOLOGY:

Clarithromycin is rapidly and well-absorbed with dose-linear kinetics, low protein binding, and a high volume of distribution. Plasma half-life ranged from 1-6 hours and was species dependent. High tissue concentrations were achieved, but negligible accumulation was observed. Fecal clearance predominated. Hepatotoxicity occurred in all species tested (*i.e.*, in rats and monkeys at doses 2 times greater than and in dogs at doses comparable to the maximum human daily dose, based on mg/m^2). Renal tubular degeneration (calculated on a mg/m^2 basis) occurred in rats at doses 2 times, in monkeys at doses 8 times, and in dogs at doses 12 times greater than the maximum human daily dose. Testicular atrophy (on a mg/m^2 basis) occurred in rats at doses 7 times, in dogs at doses 3 times, and in monkeys at doses 8 times greater than the maximum human daily dose. Corneal opacity (on a mg/m^2 basis) occurred in dogs at doses 12 times and in monkeys at doses 8 times greater than the maximum human daily dose. Lymphoid depletion (on a mg/m^2 basis) occurred in dogs at doses 3 times greater than and in monkeys at doses 2 times greater than the maximum human daily dose. These adverse events were absent during clinical trials.

REFERENCES:

1. National Committee for Clinical Laboratory Standards, Methods for Dilution Antimicrobial Susceptibility Tests for Bacteria that Grow Aerobically -Third Edition. Approved Standard NCCLS Document M7-A3, Vol. 13, No. 25, NCCLS, Villanova, PA, December 1993. **2.** National Committee for Clinical Laboratory Standards, Performance Standards for Antimicrobial Disk Susceptibility Tests -Fifth Edition. Approved Standard NCCLS Document M2-A5, Vol. 13, No. 24, NCCLS, Villanova, PA, December, 1993. **3.** Hachem, C. Y., J. E. Claridge, R. Reckly, R. Flamm, D. G. Evans, S. K. Tanaka, and D. Y. Graham. Antimicrobial susceptibility testing of *Helicobacter pylori*: comparison of E-test, broth microdilution, and disk diffusion for ampicillin, clarithromycin, and metronidazole. *Diagnost. Microbial Infect. Dis.* 1996: 24:37–41. **4.** Public Health Service Task Force on Prophylaxis and Therapy for Disseminated *Mycobacterium avium* complex. Recommendations on Prophylaxis and Therapy for *Mycobacterium avium* Complex Disease in Patients Infected With The Human Immunodeficiency Virus. *NEJM.* 1993; 329:898-904. **5.** Kemper CA, et al. Treatment of*Mycobacterium avium* Complex Bacteremia in AIDS with a Four-Drug Oral Regimen.*Ann Intern Med.* 1992;116:466-472.

PATIENT INFORMATION:

Clarithromycin is an antibiotic used to treat infections such as sinus infections, throat infections, tonsil infections and other lung related infections. It can be used by some patients to prevent infections. It is important that you take this medication for the full period of time your doctor has prescribed it, even if you feel better after a day or two. This medication should not be taken by those with an allergy to erythromycin. There are several significant drug interactions with clarithromycin. Make sure to have your doctor or pharmacist fully evaluate all medications you might be taking and ask them about drug interactions. The most common side effects reported include taste disturbances, diarrhea and nausea, occurring in approximately 3% of patients. Clarithromycin can be taken with or without food. Unlike other suspensions (liquid forms), this suspension should not be refrigerated.

HOW SUPPLIED:

Biaxin Filmtab (clarithromycin tablets) are supplied as yellow oval film-coated tablets imprinted (on one side) in blue with the Abbott logo and a two-letter Abbo-Code designation, KT for the 250 mg tablet and KL for the 500 mg tablet.

Storage: Store tablets and granules for oral suspension at controlled room temperature 15° to 30° C (59° to 86° F) in a well-closed container. Protect from light. Do not refrigerate Biaxin suspension.

HOW SUPPLIED - EQUIVALENTS NOT AVAILABLE:

Powder, Reconstitution - Oral - 125 mg/5ml

100 ml $25.90 BIAXIN, Abbott 00074-3163-13

Powder, Reconstitution - Oral - 250 mg/5ml

100 ml $49.33 BIAXIN, Abbott 00074-3188-13

Tablet, Coated - Oral - 250 mg

60's $185.26 BIAXIN, Abbott 00074-3368-60

Tablet, Coated - Oral - 500 mg

60's $185.26 BIAXIN, Abbott 00074-2586-60

Tablet, Uncoated - Oral - 250 mg

100's $310.56 BIAXIN, Abbott 00074-3368-11

Tablet, Uncoated - Oral - 500 mg

100's $310.56 BIAXIN, Abbott 00074-2586-11

CLAVULANATE POTASSIUM; TICARCILLIN DISODIUM *(000833)*

CATEGORIES: Anti-Infectives; Antibiotics; Antimicrobials; Bacteremia; Bone Infections; Broad Spectrum Penicillins; Endometritis; Gynecologic Infections; Infections; Intra-Abdominal Infections; Joint Infections; Penicillins; Peritonitis; Respiratory Tract Infections; Septicemia; Skin Infections; Urinary Tract Infections; Pregnancy Category B; Sales > $100 Million; FDA Approved 1985 Apr

BRAND NAMES: **Timentin**

FORMULARIES: BC-BS

DESCRIPTION:

Intravenous Administration, Intravenous Administration - ADD-Vantage Antibiotic Vial, Intravenous Administration - Pharmacy Bulk Package-Not For Direct Infusion, Injection - Galaxy (PL 2040) Plastic Container (Product Package)

Timentin is an injectable antibacterial combination consisting of the semisynthetic antibiotic, ticarcillin disodium, and the β-lactamase inhibitor, clavulanate potassium (the potassium salt of clavulanic acid), for intravenous administration. Ticarcillin is derived from the basic penicillin nucleus, 6-amino-penicillanic acid.

Chemically, it is 4-Thia-1-azabicyclo[3.2 0]heptane-2-carboxylic acid, 6-[(carboxy-3-thienylacetyl)amino]-3,3-dimethyl-7-oxo-, disodium salt, [2*S*-[2α,5α,6β(*S**)]].

Clavulanic acid is produced by the fermentation of *Streptomyces clavuligerus.* It is a β-lactam structurally related to the penicillins and possesses the ability to inactivate a wide variety of β-lactamases by blocking the active sites of these enzymes. Clavulanic acid is particularly active against the clinically important plasmid-mediated β-lactamases frequently responsible for transferred drug resistance to penicillins and cephalosporins.

Chemically, clavulanate potassium is potassium 4-Oxa-1-azabicyclo[3.2.0]heptane-2-carboxylic acid, 3-(2-hydroxyethylidene)-7-oxo-, monopotassium salt [2*R*-(2α,3*Z*,5α)].

Timentin is supplied as a white to pale yellow powder for reconstitution. Clavulanate potassium/ticarcillin disodium is very soluble in water, its solubility being greater than 600 mg/ml. The reconstituted solution is clear, colorless or pale yellow, having a pH of 5.5 to 7.5.

For the Timentin 3.1 gram and 3.2 gram dosages, the theoretical sodium content is 4.75 mEq (109 mg) per gram of clavulanate potassium; ticarcillin disodium. The theoretical potassium content is 0.15 mEq (6 mg) and 0.3 mEq (11.9 mg) per gram of clavulanate potassium; ticarcillin disodium for the 3.1 gram and 3.2 gram dosages, respectively.

DESCRIPTION: *(cont'd)*

PHARMACY BULK PACKAGE (NOT FOR DIRECT INFUSION)

RECONSTITUTED STOCK SOLUTION MUST BE TRANSFERRED AND FURTHER DILUTED FOR IV INFUSION.

Timentin is available in a 31 gram pharmacy bulk package. This sterile dosage form contains multiple-single doses for use in a pharmacy admixture program for the preparation of parenteral fluids.

GALAXY (PL 2040) PLASTIC CONTAINER (PRODUCT PACKAGE)

Timentin is an iso-osmotic, sterile, nonpyrogenic, frozen solution consisting of 3.0 grams ticarcillin as ticarcillin disodium and 0.1 gram clavulanic acid as clavulanate potassium. Approximately 0.3 grams sodium citrate hydrous, USP, is added as a buffer. Sodium hydroxide is used to adjust pH and convert ticarcillin monosodium to ticarcillin disodium. The pH may have been adjusted with hydrochloric acid. The solution is intended for intravenous use after thawing to room temperature. The pH of thawed solution ranges from 5.5 to 7.5.

For the clavulanate potassium; ticarcillin disodium 3.1 gram in the Galaxy (PL 2040) plastic container, the theoretical total sodium content of the 100 ml solution is 18.7 mEq (429 mg), of which 15.6 mEq (359 mg) is contributed by the ticarcillin disodium component of clavulanate potassium; ticarcillin disodium. The total theoretical potassium content of the 100 ml solution is 0.50 mEq (19.63 mg).

The plastic container is fabricated from a specially designed multilayer plastic (PL 2040). Solutions are in contact with the polyethylene layer of this container and can leach out certain chemical components of the plastic in very small amounts within the expiration period. The suitability of the plastic has been confirmed in tests in animals according to USP biological tests for plastic containers, as well as by tissue culture toxicity studies.

CLINICAL PHARMACOLOGY:

After an intravenous infusion (30 min) of 3.1 grams or 3.2 grams clavulanate potassium/ticarcillin disodium, peak serum concentrations of both ticarcillin and clavulanic acid are attained immediately after completion of infusion. Ticarcillin serum levels are similar to those produced by the administration of equivalent amounts of ticarcillin alone with a mean peak serum level of 330 mcg/ml for the 3.1 gram and 3.2 gram formulations. The corresponding mean peak serum levels for clavulanic acid were 8 mcg/ml and 16 mcg/ml for the 3.1 gram and 3.2 gram formulations, respectively. (See TABLE 1.)

TABLE 1 Serum Levels in Adults After A 30-Minute IV Infusion of Clavulanate Potassium; Ticarcillin Disodium

Ticarcillin Serum Levels (mcg/ml)				
Dose	**0**	**15 min.**	**30 min.**	**1 hr.**
3.1 g	324 (293 to 388)	223 (184 to 293)	176 (135 to 235)	131 (102 to 195)
Dose	**1.5 hr.**	**3.5 hr.**	**5.5 hr.**	
	90 (85 to 119)	27 (19 to 37)	6 (5 to 7)	
3.2 g	336 (301 to 386)	214 (180 to 258)	186 (160 to 218)	122 (108 to 136)
	78 (33 to 113)	29 (19 to 44)	10 (5 to 15)	
Clavulanic Acid Serum Levels (mcg/ml)				
Dose	**0**	**15 min.**	**30 min.**	**1 hr.**
3.1 g	8.0 (5.3 to 10.3)	4.6 (3.0 to 7.6)	2.6 (1.8 to 3.4)	1.8 (1.6 to 2.2)
Dose	**1.5 hr.**	**3.5 hr.**	**5.5 hr.**	
	1.2 (0.8 to 1.6)	0.3 (0.2 to 0.3)	0	
3.2 g	15.8 (11.7 to 21.0)	8.3 (6.4 to 10.0)	5.2 (3.5 to 6.3)	3.4 (1.9 to 4.0)
	2.5 (1.3 to 3.4)	0.5 (0.2 to 0.8)	0	

The mean area under the serum concentration curves for ticarcillin was 485 mcg/ml.hr. for the clavulanate potassium/ticarcillin disodium 3.1 gram and 3.2 gram formulations. The corresponding areas under the serum concentration curves for clavulanic acid were 8.2 mcg/ml.hr. and 15.6 mcg/ml.hr. for the clavulanate potassium/ticarcillin disodium 3.1 gram and 3.2 gram formulations, respectively.

The mean serum half-lives of ticarcillin and clavulanic acid in healthy volunteers are 68 minutes and 64 minutes, respectively, following administration of 3.1 grams or 3.2 grams of clavulanate potassium/ticarcillin disodium.

Approximately 60% to 70% of ticarcillin and approximately 35% to 45% of clavulanic acid are excreted unchanged in urine during the first 6 hours after administration of a single dose of clavulanate potassium/ticarcillin disodium to normal volunteers with normal renal function. Two hours after an intravenous injection of 3.1 grams or 3.2 grams clavulanate potassium/ticarcillin disodium, concentrations of ticarcillin in urine generally exceed 1500 mcg/ml. The corresponding concentrations of clavulanic acid in urine generally exceed 40 mcg/ml and 70 mcg/ml following administration of the 3.1 gram and 3.2 gram doses, respectively. By 4 to 6 hours after injection, the urine concentrations of ticarcillin and clavulanic acid usually decline to approximately 190 mcg/ml and 2 mcg/ml, respectively, for both doses. Neither component of clavulanate potassium/ticarcillin disodium is highly protein bound; ticarcillin has been found to be approximately 45% bound to human serum protein and clavulanic acid approximately 9% bound.

Somewhat higher and more prolonged serum levels of ticarcillin can be achieved with the concurrent administration of probenecid; however, probenecid does not enhance the serum levels of clavulanic acid.

Ticarcillin can be detected in tissues and interstitial fluid following parenteral administration.

Penetration of ticarcillin into the bile, pleural fluid and cerebrospinal fluid with inflamed meninges has been demonstrated. The results of experiments involving the administration of clavulanic acid to animals suggest that this compound, like ticarcillin, is well distributed in body tissues.

An inverse relationship exists between the serum half-life of ticarcillin and creatinine clearance. The dosage of clavulanate potassium/ticarcillin disodium need only be adjusted in cases of severe renal impairment (see DOSAGE AND ADMINISTRATION.)

Ticarcillin may be removed from patients undergoing dialysis; the actual amount removed depends on the duration and type of dialysis.

MICROBIOLOGY

Ticarcillin is a semisynthetic antibiotic with a broad spectrum of bactericidal activity against many gram-positive and gram-negative aerobic and anaerobic bacteria.

Ticarcillin is, however, susceptible to degradation by β-lactamases and therefore the spectrum of activity does not normally include organisms which produce these enzymes.

CLINICAL PHARMACOLOGY: *(cont'd)*

Clavulanic acid is a β-lactam, structurally related to the penicillins, which possesses the ability to inactivate a wide range of β-lactamase enzymes commonly found in microorganisms resistant to penicillins and cephalosporins. In particular, it has good activity against the clinically important plasmid-mediated β-lactamases frequently responsible for transferred drug resistance.

The formulation of ticarcillin with clavulanic acid in clavulanate potassium/ticarcillin disodium protects ticarcillin from degradation by β-lactamase enzymes and effectively extends the antibiotic spectrum of ticarcillin to include many bacteria normally resistant to ticarcillin and other β-lactam antibiotics. Thus clavulanate potassium/ticarcillin disodium possesses the distinctive properties of a broad-spectrum antibiotic and a β-lactamase inhibitor.

While *in vitro* studies have demonstrated the susceptibility of most strains of the following organisms, clinical efficacy for infections other than those included in the INDICATIONS AND USAGE section has not been documented:

Gram-Negative Bacteria: *Pseudomonas aeruginosa* (β-lactamase and non-β-lactamase producing), *Pseudomonas* species including *P. maltophilia* (β-lactamase and non-β-lactamase producing), *Escherichia coli* (β-lactamase and non-β-lactamase producing), *Proteus mirabilis* (β-lactamase and non-β-lactamase producing), *Proteus vulgaris* (β-lactamase and non-β-lactamase producing), *Providencia rettgeri* (formerly *Proteus rettgeri*) (β-lactamase and non-β-lactamase producing), *Providencia stuartii* (β-lactamase and non-β-lactamase producing), *Morganella morganii* (formerly *Proteus morganii*) (β-lactamase and non-β-lactamase producing), *Enterobacter* species (Although most strains of *Enterobacter* species are resistant *in vitro*, clinical efficacy has been demonstrated with clavulanate potassium/ticarcillin disodium in urinary tract infections caused by these organisms.), *Acinetobacter* species (β-lactamase and non-β-lactamase producing), *Hemophilus influenzae* (β-lactamase and non-β-lactamase producing), *Branhamella catarrhalis* (β-lactamase and non-β-lactamase producing), *Serratia* species including *S. marcescens* (β-lactamase and non-β-lactamase producing), *Neisseria gonorrhoeae* (β-lactamase and non-β-lactamase producing), *Neisseria meningitidis**, *Salmonella* species (β-lactamase and non-β-lactamase producing), *Klebsiella* species including *K. pneumoniae* (β-lactamase and non-β-lactamase producing), *Citrobacter* species including *C. freundii, C. diversus* and *C. amalonaticus* (β-lactamase and non-β-lactamase producing).

Gram-Positive Bacteria: *Staphylococcus aureus* (β-lactamase and non-β-lactamase producing), *Staphylococcus saprophyticus, Staphylococcus epidermidis* (coagulase-negative staphylococci) (β-lactamase and non-β-lactamase producing), *Streptococcus pneumoniae* (D. pneumoniae), Streptococcus bovis**, *Streptococcus agalactiae** (Group B), *Streptococcus faecalis** (*Enterococcus*), *Streptococcus pyogenes** (Group A, β-hemolytic), Viridans group streptococci*.

Anaerobic Bacteria: *Bacteroides* species, including *B. fragilis* group (*B. fragilis, B. vulgatus*) (β-lactamase and non-β-lactamase producing), non-*B. fragilis* (*β-melaninogenicus*) (β-lactamase and non-β-lactamase producing), *B. thetaiotaomicron, B. ovatus, B. distasonis* (β-lactamase and non-β-lactamase producing), *Clostridium* species including *C. perfringens, C. difficile, C. sporogenes, C. ramosum* and *C. bifermentans**, *Eubacterium* species, *Fusobacterium* species including *F. nucleatum* and *F. necrophorum**, *Peptococcus* species*, *Peptostreptococcus* species*, *Veillonella* species.

* These are non-β-lactamase-producing strains and therefore are susceptible to ticarcillin alone. Some of the β-lactamase-producing strains are also susceptible to ticarcillin alone.

In vitro synergism between clavulanate potassium/ticarcillin disodium and gentamicin, tobramycin or amikacin against multiresistant strains of *Pseudomonas aeruginosa* has been demonstrated.

SUSCEPTIBILITY TESTING

Diffusion Technique: An 85 mcg clavulanate potassium/ticarcillin disodium (75 mcg ticarcillin plus 10 mcg clavulanic acid) diffusion disk is available for use with the Kirby-Bauer method. Based on the zone sizes given below, a report of "Susceptible" indicates that the infecting organism is likely to respond to clavulanate potassium/ticarcillin disodium therapy, while a report of "Resistant" indicates that the organism is not likely to respond to therapy with this antibiotic. A report of "Intermediate" susceptibility indicates that the organism would be susceptible to clavulanate potassium/ticarcillin disodium at a higher dosage or if the infection is confined to tissues or fluids (*e.g.*, urine) in which high antibiotic levels are attained.

Dilution Technique: Broth or agar dilution methods may be used to determine the minimal inhibitory concentration (MIC) values for bacterial isolates to clavulanate potassium/ticarcillin disodium. Tubes should be inoculated with the test culture containing 10^4 to 10^5 CFU/ml or plates spotted with a test solution containing 10^3 to 10^4CFU/ml.

The recommended dilution pattern utilizes a constant level of clavulanic acid, 2 mcg/ml, in all tubes together with varying amounts of ticarcillin. MICs are expressed in terms of the ticarcillin concentration in the presence of 2 mcg/ml clavulanic acid (TABLE 2).

TABLE 2 Recommended Ranges For Susceptibility Testing *, †, ‡

Diffusion Method Disk Zone Size, mm			Dilution Method MIC Correlates§, mcg/ml	
Res.	**Inter.**	**Susc.**	**Res.**	**Susc.**
≤11	12 to 14	≥15	≥128	≤64

*The non-β-lactamase-producing organisms which are normally susceptible to ticarcillin will have similar zone sizes as for ticarcillin.
†Staphylococci which are susceptible to Timentin but resistant to methicillin, oxacillin or nafcillin must be considered as resistant.
‡The quality control cultures should have the following assigned daily ranges for Timentin:
§Expressed as concentration of ticarcillin in the presence of a constant 2.0 mcg/ml concentration of clavulanic acid.

TABLE 3

		Disks	MIC Range (mcg/ml)
E. coli	(ATCC 25922)	24 to 30 mm	2/2 to 8/2
S. aureus	(ATCC 25923)	32 to 40 mm	—
Ps. aeruginosa	(ATCC 27853)	20 to 28 mm	8/2 to 32/2
E. coli	(ATCC 35218)	21 to 25 mm	4/2 to 16/2
S. aureus	(ATCC 29213)	—	0.5/2 to 2/2

INDICATIONS AND USAGE:

Clavulanate potassium/ticarcillin disodium is indicated in the treatment of infections caused by susceptible strains of the designated organisms in the conditions listed below:

Septicemia: including bacteremia, caused by β-lactamase-producing strains of *Klebsiella spp.**, *E. coli**, *Staphylococcus aureus** or *Pseudomonas aeruginosa** (or other *Pseudomonas* species*).

Lower Respiratory Infections: caused by β-lactamase-producing strains of *Staphylococcus aureus, Hemophilus influenzae** or *Klebsiella* spp.*

Bone and Joint Infections: caused by β-lactamase-producing strains of *Staphylococcus aureus.*

INDICATIONS AND USAGE: *(cont'd)*

Skin and Skin Structure Infections: caused by β-lactamase-producing strains of *Staphylococcus aureus, Klebsiella spp.** or *E. coli**.

Urinary Tract Infections: (complicated and uncomplicated) caused by β-lactamase-producing strains of *E. coli, Klebsiella* spp, *Pseudomonas aeruginosa** (or other *Pseudomonas* spp.*), *Citrobacter* spp.*, *Enterobacter cloacae**, *Serratia marcescens** and *Staphylococcus aureus**.

Gynecologic Infections: Endometritis caused by β-lactamase-producing strains of *B. melaninogenicus**, *Enterobacter* spp. (including *E. cloacae**), *Escherichia coli, Klebsiella pneumoniae*, Staphylococcus aureus* and *Staphylococcus epidermidis.*

Intra-abdominal Infections: Peritonitis caused by β-lactamase-producing strains of *Escherichia coli, Klebsiella pneumoniae* or *Bacteroides fragilis** group.

* Efficacy for this organism in this organ system was studied in fewer than 10 infections.

While clavulanate potassium/ticarcillin disodium is indicated only for the conditions listed above, infections caused by ticarcillin-susceptible organisms are also amenable to clavulanate potassium/ticarcillin disodium treatment due to its ticarcillin content. Therefore, mixed infections caused by ticarcillin-susceptible organisms and β-lactamase-producing organisms susceptible to clavulanate potassium/ticarcillin disodium should not require the addition of another antibiotic.

Appropriate culture and susceptibility tests should be performed before treatment in order to isolate and identify organisms causing infection and to determine their susceptibility to clavulanate potassium/ticarcillin disodium. Because of its broad spectrum of bactericidal activity against gram-positive and gram-negative bacteria, clavulanate potassium/ticarcillin disodium is particularly useful for the treatment of mixed infections and for presumptive therapy prior to the identification of the causative organisms. Clavulanate potassium/ticarcillin disodium has been shown to be effective as single drug therapy in the treatment of some serious infections where normally combination antibiotic therapy might be employed. Therapy with clavulanate potassium/ticarcillin disodium may be initiated before results of such tests are known when there is reason to believe the infection may involve any of the β-lactamase-producing organisms listed above; however, once these results become available, appropriate therapy should be continued.

Based on the *in vitro* synergism between clavulanate potassium/ticarcillin disodium and aminoglycosides against certain strains of *Pseudomonas aeruginosa*, combined therapy has been successful, especially in patients with impaired host defenses. Both drugs should be used in full therapeutic doses. As soon as results of culture and susceptibility tests become available, antimicrobial therapy should be adjusted as indicated.

CONTRAINDICATIONS:

Cavulanate potassium/ticarcillin disodium is contraindicated in patients with a history of hypersensitivity reactions to any of the penicillins.

WARNINGS:

SERIOUS AND OCCASIONALLY FATAL HYPERSENSITIVITY (ANAPHYLACTOID) REACTIONS HAVE BEEN REPORTED IN PATIENTS ON PENICILLIN THERAPY. THESE REACTIONS ARE MORE LIKELY TO OCCUR IN INDIVIDUALS WITH A HISTORY OF PENICILLIN HYPERSENSITIVITY AND/OR A HISTORY OF SENSITIVITY TO MULTIPLE ALLERGENS. THERE HAVE BEEN REPORTS OF INDIVIDUALS WITH A HISTORY OF PENICILLIN HYPERSENSITIVITY WHO HAVE EXPERIENCED SEVERE REACTIONS WHEN TREATED WITH CEPHALOSPORINS. BEFORE INITIATING THERAPY WITH CLAVULANTE POTASSIUM AND TICARCILLIN DISODIUM CAREFUL INQUIRY SHOULD BE MADE CONCERNING PREVIOUS HYPERSENSITIVITY REACTIONS TO PENICILLINS, CEPHALOSPORINS OR OTHER ALLERGENS. IF AN ALLERGIC REACTION OCCURS, CLAVULANTE POTASSIUM AND TICARCILLIN DISODIUM SHOULD BE DISCONTINUED AND THE APPROPRIATE THERAPY INSTITUTED. **SERIOUS ANAPHYLACTOID REACTIONS REQUIRE IMMEDIATE EMERGENCY TREATMENT WITH EPINEPHRINE. OXYGEN, INTRAVENOUS STEROIDS AND AIRWAY MANAGEMENT, INCLUDING INTUBATION, SHOULD ALSO BE PROVIDED AS INDICATED.**

Pseudomembranous colitis has been reported with nearly all antibacterial agents, including clavulanate potassium/ticarcillin disodium, and may range in severity from mild to life-threatening. Therefore, it is important to consider this diagnosis in patients who present with diarrhea subsequent to the administration of antibacterial agents.

Treatment with antibacterial agents alters the normal flora of the colon and may permit overgrowth of clostridia. Studies indicate that a toxin produced by *Clostridium difficile* is one primary cause of "antibiotic-associated colitis."

After the diagnosis of pseudomembranous colitis has been established, therapeutic measures should be initiated. Mild cases of pseudomembranous colitis usually respond to drug discontinuation alone. In moderate to severe cases, consideration should be given to management with fluids and electrolytes, protein supplementation and treatment with an antibacterial drug clinically effective against *C. difficile* colitis.

PRECAUTIONS:

General: While clavulanate potassium/ticarcillin disodium possesses the characteristic low toxicity of the penicillin group of antibiotics, periodic assessment of organ system functions, including renal, hepatic and hematopoietic function, is advisable during prolonged therapy.

Bleeding manifestations have occurred in some patients receiving β-lactam antibiotics. These reactions have been associated with abnormalities of coagulation tests such as clotting time, platelet aggregation and prothrombin time and are more likely to occur in patients with renal impairment.

If bleeding manifestations appear, clavulanate potassium/ticarcillin disodium treatment should be discontinued and appropriate therapy instituted.

Clavulanate potassium/ticarcillin disodium has only rarely been reported to cause hypokalemia; however, the possibility of this occurring should be kept in mind particularly when treating patients with fluid and electrolyte imbalance. Periodic monitoring of serum potassium may be advisable in patients receiving prolonged therapy.

The theoretical sodium content is 4.75 mEq (109 mg) per gram of clavulanate potassium/ticarcillin disodium. This should be considered when treating patients requiring restricted salt intake.

As with any penicillin, an allergic reaction, including anaphylaxis, may occur during clavulanate potassium/ticarcillin disodium administration, particularly in a hypersensitive individual.

The possibility of superinfections with mycotic or bacterial pathogens should be kept in mind, particularly during prolonged treatment. If superinfections occur, appropriate measures should be taken.

DRUG/LABORATORY TEST INTERACTIONS

As with other penicillins, the mixing of clavulanate potassium/ticarcillin disodium with an aminoglycoside in solutions for parenteral administration can result in substantial inactivation of the aminoglycoside.

PRECAUTIONS: *(cont'd)*

Probenecid interferes with the renal tubular secretion of ticarcillin, thereby increasing serum concentrations and prolonging serum half-life of the antibiotic.

High urine concentrations of ticarcillin may produce false-positive protein reactions (pseudoproteinuria) with the following methods: sulfosalicylic acid and boiling test, acetic acid test, biuret reaction and nitric acid test. The bromphenol blue (Multi-stix) reagent strip test has been reported to be reliable.

The presence of clavulanic acid in clavulanate potassium/ticarcillin disodium may cause a nonspecific binding of IgG and albumin by red cell membranes leading to a false-positive Coombs test.

CARCINOGENESIS, MUTAGENESIS, IMPAIRMENT OF FERTILITY

Long-term studies in animals have not been performed to evaluate carcinogenic potential. Results of studies performed with clavulanate potassium/ticarcillin disodium *in vitro* and *in vivo* did not indicate a potential for mutagenicity.

PREGNANCY CATEGORY B

Reproduction studies have been performed in rats given doses up to 1050 mg/kg/day and have revealed no evidence of impaired fertility or harm to the fetus due to clavulanate potassium/ticarcillin disodium. There are, however, no adequate and well-controlled studies in pregnant women. Because animal reproduction studies are not always predictive of human response, this drug should be used during pregnancy only if clearly needed.

NURSING MOTHERS

Caution should be exercised when clavulanate potassium/ticarcillin disodium is administered to a nursing woman.

PEDIATRIC USE

The efficacy and safety of clavulanate potassium/ticarcillin disodium have not been established in infants and children under the age of 12.

ADVERSE REACTIONS:

As with other penicillins, the following adverse reactions may occur:

Hypersensitivity Reactions: Skin rash, pruritus, urticaria, arthralgia, myalgia, drug fever, chills, chest discomfort and anaphylactic reactions.

Central Nervous System: Headache, giddiness, neuromuscular hyperirritability or convulsive seizures.

Gastrointestinal Disturbances: Disturbances of taste and smell, stomatitis, flatulence, nausea, vomiting and diarrhea, epigastric pain and pseudomembranous colitis. Onset of pseudomembranous colitis symptoms may occur during or after antibiotic treatment (see WARNINGS.)

Hemic and Lymphatic Systems: Thrombocytopenia, leukopenia, neutropenia, eosinophilia and reduction of hemoglobin or hematocrit. Prolongation of prothrombin time and bleeding time.

Abnormalities Of Hepatic And Renal Function Tests: Elevation of serum aspartate aminotransferase (SGOT), serum alanine aminotransferase (SGPT), serum alkaline phosphatase, serum LDH, serum bilirubin. Rarely, transient hepatitis and cholestatic jaundice—as with some other penicillins and some cephalosporins. Elevation of serum creatinine and/or BUN, hypernatremia. Reduction in serum potassium and uric acid.

Local Reactions: pain, burning, swelling and induration at the injection site and thrombophlebitis with intravenous administration.

DRUG ABUSE AND DEPENDENCE:

Neither clavulanate potassium/ticarcillin disodium abuse nor clavulanate potassium/ticarcillin disodium dependence has been reported.

OVERDOSAGE:

As with other penicillins, clavulanate potassium/ticarcillin disodium in overdosage has the potential to cause neuromuscular hyperirritability or convulsive seizures. Ticarcillin may be removed from circulation by hemodialysis. The molecular weight, degree of protein binding and pharmacokinetic profile of clavulanic acid together with information from a single patient with renal insufficiency all suggest that this compound may also be removed by hemodialysis.

DOSAGE AND ADMINISTRATION:

Intravenous Administration, Intravenous Administration - ADD-Vantage Antibiotic Vial, Intravenous Administration - Pharmacy Bulk Package-Not For Direct Infusion, Injection - Galaxy (PL 2040) Plastic Container (Product Package)

Clavulanate potassium/ticarcillin disodium should be administered by intravenous infusion (30 min.).

Adults: The usual recommended dosage for systemic and urinary tract infections for average (60 kg) adults is 3.1 grams clavulanate potassium; ticarcillin disodium (3.1 gram vial containing 3 grams ticarcillin and 100 mg clavulanic acid) given every 4 to 6 hours. For gynecologic infections, clavulanate potassium/ticarcillin disodium should be administered as follows: Moderate infections 200 mg/kg/day in divided doses every 6 hours and for severe infections 300 mg/kg/day in divided doses every 4 hours. For patients weighing less than 60 kg, the recommended dosage is 200 to 300 mg/kg/day, based on ticarcillin content, given in divided doses every 4 to 6 hours.

In urinary tract infections, a dosage of 3.2 grams clavulanate potassium; ticarcillin disodium (3.2 gram vial containing 3 grams ticarcillin and 200 mg clavulanic acid) given every 8 hours is adequate.

For infections complicated by renal insufficiency[1], an initial loading dose of 3.1 grams should be followed by doses based on creatinine clearance and type of dialysis as indicated below (TABLE 4):

TABLE 4

Creatinine clearance ml/min.	Dosage
over 60	3.1 grams every 4 hrs.
30 to 60	2 grams every 4 hrs.
10 to 30	2 grams every 8 hrs.
less than 10	2 grams every 12 hrs.
less than 10 with hepatic dysfunction	2 grams every 24 hrs.
patients on peritoneal dialysis	3.1 grams every 12 hrs.
patients on hemodialysis	2 grams every 12 hrs. supplemented with 3.1 grams after each dialysis

To calculate creatinine clearance* from a serum creatinine value use the following formula.
$C_{cr} = [(140\text{-Age})\ (\text{wt. in kg})] \div [72 \times S_{cr}\ (\text{mg/100 ml})]$
This is the calculated creatinine clearance for adult males; for females it is 15% less.
* Cockcroft, D.W., et al: Prediction of Creatinine Clearance from Serum Creatinine, Nephron 16:31-41, 1976.

[1] The half-life of ticarcillin in patients with renal failure is approximately 13 hours.

DOSAGE AND ADMINISTRATION: *(cont'd)*

Dosage for any individual patient must take into consideration the site and severity of infection, the susceptibility of the organisms causing infection and the status of the patient's host defense mechanisms.

The duration of therapy depends upon the severity of infection. Generally, clavulanate potassium/ticarcillin disodium should be continued for at least 2 days after the signs and symptoms of infection have disappeared. The usual duration is 10 to 14 days; however, in difficult and complicated infections, more prolonged therapy may be required.

Frequent bacteriologic and clinical appraisal is necessary during therapy of chronic urinary tract infection and may be required for several months after therapy has been completed; persistent infections may require treatment for several weeks and doses smaller than those indicated above should not be used.

In certain infections, involving abscess formation, appropriate surgical drainage should be performed in conjunction with antimicrobial therapy.

INTRAVENOUS ADMINISTRATION-DIRECTIONS FOR USE

3.1 gram and 3.2 gram Vials and Piggyback Bottles: The 3.1 gram or 3.2 gram vial should be reconstituted by adding approximately 13 ml of Sterile Water for Injection, USP, or sodium chloride injection, USP, and shaking well. When dissolved, the concentration of ticarcillin will be approximately 200 mg/ml with corresponding concentrations of 6.7 mg/ml and 13.4 mg/ml clavulanic acid for the 3.1 gram and 3.2 gram respective doses. Conversely, each 5.0 ml of the 3.1 gram dose reconstituted with approximately 13 ml of diluent will contain approximately 1 gram of ticarcillin and 33 mg of clavulanic acid. For the 3.2 gram dose reconstituted with 13 ml of diluent, each 5.0 ml will contain 1 gram of ticarcillin and 66 mg of clavulanic acid.

Intravenous Infusion: The dissolved drug should be further diluted to desired volume using the recommended solution listed in the COMPATIBILITY AND STABILITY SECTION (STABILITY PERIOD) to a concentration between 10 mg/ml to 100 mg/ml. The solution of reconstituted drug may then be administered over a period of 30 minutes by direct infusion or through a Y-type intravenous infusion set. If this method or the "piggyback" method of administration is used, it is advisable to discontinue temporarily the administration of any other solutions during the infusion of clavulanate potassium/ticarcillin disodium.

Stability: For IV solutions, see STABILITY PERIOD.

When clavulanate potassium/ticarcillin disodium is given in combination with another antimicrobial, such as an aminoglycoside, each drug should be given separately in accordance with the recommended dosage and routes of administration for each drug.

After reconstitution and prior to administration, clavulanate potassium/ticarcillin disodium, as with other parenteral drugs, should be inspected visually for particulate matter. If this condition is evident, the solution should be discarded.

The color of reconstituted solutions of clavulanate potassium/ticarcillin disodium normally ranges from light to dark yellow depending on concentration, duration and temperature of storage while maintaining label claim characteristics.

COMPATIBILTY AND STABILITY

3.1 gram and 3.2 gram Vials and Piggyback Bottles

(Dilutions derived from a stock solution of 200 mg/ml)

The concentrated stock solution at 200 mg/ml is stable for up to 6 hours at room temperature 21° to 24°C (70° to 75°F) or up to 72 hours under refrigeration 4°C (40°F).

If the concentrated stock solution (200 mg/ml) is held for up to 6 hours at room temperature 21° to 24°C (70° to 75°F) or up to 72 hours under refrigeration 4°C (40°F) and further diluted to a concentration between 10 mg/ml and 100 mg/ml with any of the diluents listed below, then the following stability periods apply.

TABLE 5 Stability Period

(3.1 gram and 3.2 gram Vials and Piggyback Bottles)

Intravenous Solution (ticarcillin concentrations	Room Temperature 21° to 24°C	Refrigerated 4°C
of 10 mg/ml to 100 mg/ml)	(70° to 75°F)	(40°F)
Dextrose Injection 5%, USP	24 hours	3 days
Sodium Chloride, Injection, USP	24 hours	7 days
Lactated Ringer's Injection, USP	24 hours	7 days

If the concentrated stock solution (200 mg/ml) is stored for up to 6 hours at room temperature and then further diluted to a concentration between 10 mg/ml and 100 mg/ml, solutions of sodium chloride injection, USP, and Lactated Ringer's Injection, USP, may be stored frozen -18°C (0°F) for up to 30 days. Solutions prepared with Dextrose Injection 5%, USP, may be stored frozen -18°C (0°F) for up to 7 days. All thawed solutions should be used within 8 hours or discarded. Once thawed, solutions should not be refrozen.

NOTE: Clavulanate potassium/ticarcillin disodium is incompatible with sodium bicarbonate.

Unused solutions must be discarded after the time periods listed above.

ADD-Vantage Antibiotic Vial

NOTE: Clavulanate potassium/ticarcillin disodium in the ADD-Vantage system should only be administered for 3.1 gram dosing.

INSTRUCTIONS FOR USE

To Open Diluent Container: Peel overwrap at corner and remove solution container. Some opacity of the plastic due to moisture absorption during the sterilization process may be observed. This is normal and does not affect the solution quality or safety. The opacity will diminish gradually.

TO ASSEMBLE VIAL AND FLEXIBLE DILUENT CONTAINER (USE ASEPTIC TECHNIQUE)

1. Remove the protective covers from the top of the vial and the vial port on the diluent container as follows:

a. To remove the breakaway vial cap, swing the pull ring over the top of the vial and pull down far enough to start the opening, then pull straight up to remove the cap.

NOTE: Do not access vial with syringe.

b. To remove the vial port cover, grasp the tab on the pull ring, pull up to break the three tie strings, then pull back to remove the cover.

2. Screw the vial into the vial port until it will go no further. THE VIAL MUST BE SCREWED IN TIGHTLY TO ASSURE A SEAL. This occurs approximately 1/2 turn (180°) after the first audible click. The clicking sound does not assure a seal; the vial must be turned as far as it will go.

3. Recheck the vial to assure that it is tight by trying to turn it further in the direction of assembly.

4. Label appropriately.

TO RECONSTITUTE THE DRUG

1. Squeeze the bottom of the diluent container gently to inflate the portion of the container surrounding the end of the drug vial.

DOSAGE AND ADMINISTRATION: *(cont'd)*

2. With the other hand, push the drug vial down into the container telescoping the walls of the container. Grasp the inner cap of the vial through the walls of the container.

3. Pull the inner cap from the drug vial. Verify that the rubber stopper has been pulled out, allowing the drug and diluent to mix.

4. Mix container contents thoroughly and use within the specified time.

PREPARATION FOR ADMINISTRATION (USE ASEPTIC TECHNIQUE)

1. Confirm the activation and admixture of vial contents.

2. Check for leaks by squeezing container firmly. If leaks are found discard unit as sterility may be impaired.

3. Close flow control clamp of administration set.

4. Remove cover from outlet port at bottom of container.

5. Insert piercing pin of administration set into port with a twisting motion until the pin is firmly seated. **NOTE:** See full directions on administration set carton.

6. Lift the free end of the hanger loop on the bottom of the vial, breaking the two tie strings. Bend the loop outward to lock it in the upright position, then suspend container from hanger.

7. Squeeze and release drip chamber to establish proper fluid level in chamber.

8. Open flow control clamp and clear air from set. Close clamp.

9. Attach set to venipuncture device. If device is not indwelling, prime and make venipuncture.

10. Regulate rate of administration with flow control clamp.

WARNING: Do not use flexible container in series connections.

RECONSTITUTION DIRECTIONS

Intravenous Infusion: Use a 50 ml or 100 ml Add-Vantage DILUENT CONTAINER containing either Sodium Chloride Injection, USP, or 5% Dextrose in Water (refer to INSTRUCTIONS FOR USE section). The resulting concentration of the 3.1 gram dose reconstituted in 50 ml of diluent is approximately 60 mg/ml of ticarcillin and approximately 2 mg/ml of clavulanic acid. The resulting concentration of the 3.1 gram dose reconstituted in 100 ml of diluent is approximately 30 mg/ml of ticarcillin and approximately 1 mg/ml of clavulanic acid.

The solution of reconstituted drug may then be administered over a period of 30 minutes by direct infusion or through a Y-type intravenous infusion set which may already be in place. If this method or the "piggyback" method of administration is used, it is advisable to discontinue temporarily the administration of any other solutions during the infusion of clavulanate potassium/ticarcillin disodium. When clavulanate potassium/ticarcillin disodium is given in combination with another antimicrobial, such as an aminoglycoside, each drug should be given separately in accordance with the recommended dosage and routes of administration for each drug. After reconstitution and prior to administration, clavulanate potassium/ticarcillin disodium, as with other parenteral drugs, should be inspected visually for particulate matter. If this condition is evident, the solution should be discarded.

The color of reconstituted solution of clavulanate potassium/ticarcillin disodium normally ranges from light to dark yellow depending on concentration, duration and temperature of storage while maintaining label claim characteristics.

NOTE:

Intravenous Solution	Room Temperature
(ticarcillin concentration of ≈30 mg/ml or ≈60 mg/ml)	21° to 24°C (70 to 75°F)
Sodium Chloride Injection, USP	24 hours
5% Dextrose in Water	12 hours

NOTE: Clavulanate potassium/ticarillin disodium is incompatible with Sodium Bicarbonate. Unused portions of solutions should be discarded after the time periods listed above.

Avoid excessive heat.

Protect from freezing.

INTRAVENOUS ADMINISTRATION

DIRECTIONS FOR PROPER USE OF PHARMACY BULK PACKAGE

RECONSTITUTED STOCK SOLUTION MUST BE TRANSFERRED AND FURTHER DILUTED FOR IV INFUSION.

The container closure may be penetrated only one time utilizing a suitable sterile transfer device or dispensing set that allows measured distribution of the contents. A sterile substance that must be reconstituted prior to use may require a separate closure entry.

Restrict use of Pharmacy Bulk Packages to an aseptic area such as a laminar flow hood.

Reconstituted contents of the vial should be withdrawn immediately. However, if this is not possible, aliquoting operations must be completed within 4 hours of reconstitution. **Discard the reconstituted stock solution 4 hours after initial entry.**

Add 76 ml of Sterile Water for Injection, USP, or sodium chloride Injection, USP, to the 31 gram Pharmacy Bulk Package and shake well. For ease of reconstitution, the diluent may be added in two portions. Each 1.0 ml of the resulting concentrated stock solution contains approximately 300 mg of ticarcillin and 10 mg of clavulanic acid.

Intravenous Infusion: The desired dosage should be withdrawn from the stock solution and further diluted to desired volume using the recommended solution listed in the COMPATIBILITY AND STABILITY SECTION (STABILITY PERIOD) to a concentration between 10 mg/ml to 100 mg/ml. The solution of reconstituted drug may then be administered over a period of 30 minutes by direct infusion, or through a Y-type intravenous infusion set. If this method, or the "piggyback" method of administration is used, it is advisable to discontinue temporarily the administration of any other solution during the infusion of clavulanate potassium/ticarcillin disodium.

Stability: For I.V. solutions, see STABILITY PERIOD.

When clavulanate potassium/ticarcillin disodium is given in combination with another antimicrobial, such as an aminoglycoside, each drug should be given separately in accordance with the recommended dosage and routes of administration for each drug.

After reconstitution and prior to administration, clavulanate potassium/ticarcillin disodium, as with other parenteral drugs, should be inspected visually for particulate matter. If this condition is evident, the solution should be discarded.

The color of reconstituted solutions of clavulanate potassium/ticarcillin disodium normally ranges from light to dark yellow depending on concentration, duration and temperature of storage while maintaining label claim characteristics.

COMPATIBILTY AND STABILITY

31 gram Pharmacy Bulk Package

(Dilutions derived from a stock solution of 300 mg/ml)

Aliquots of the reconstituted stock solution at 300 mg/ml are stable for up to 6 hours between 21° and 24°C (70° and 75°F) or up to 72 hours under refrigeration 4°C (40°F). The reconstituted stock solution should be held under refrigeration 4°C (40°F).

DOSAGE AND ADMINISTRATION: *(cont'd)*

If the aliquots of the reconstituted stock solution (300 mg/ml) are held up to 6 hours between 21° and 24°C (70° and 75°F) or up to 72 hours under refrigeration 4°C (40°F) and further diluted to a concentration between 10 mg/ml and 100 mg/ml with any of the diluents listed below, then the following stability periods apply.

TABLE 7 Stability

(31 gram Pharmacy Bulk Package) Intravenous Solution (ticarcillin concentrations of 10 mg/ml to 100 mg/ml)	Room Temperature 21° to 24°C (70° to 75°F)	Refrigerated 4°C (40°F)
Dextrose Injection 5%, USP	24 hours	3 days
Sodium Chloride Injection 0.9%, USP	24 hours	4 days
Lactated Ringer's Injection, USP	24 hours	4 days
Sterile Water for Injection, USP	24 hours	4 days

If an aliquot of concentrated stock solution (300 mg/ml) is stored for up to 6 hours between 21° and 24°C (70° and 75°F) and then further diluted to a concentration between 10 mg/ml and 100 mg/ml, solutions of sodium chloride injection, USP, lactated ringer's injection, USP, and Sterile Water for Injection, USP, may be stored frozen -18°C (0°F) for up to 30 days. Solutions prepared with dextrose injection 5%, USP, may be stored frozen (0°F) for up to 7 days. All thawed solutions should be used within 8 hours or discarded. Once thawed, solutions should not be refrozen.

NOTE: Clavulanate potassium/ticarcillin disodium is incompatible with Sodium Bicarbonate.

Unused solutions must be discarded after the time periods listed above.

GALAXY (PL 2040) PLASTIC CONTAINER

Timentin supplied as an iso-osmotic, sterile, nonpyrogenic, frozen solution in Galaxy (PL 2040) Plastic Containers is for intravenous administration only.

Storage: Avoid unnecessary handling of bags. Store in a freezer capable of maintaining a temperature -20°C (-4°F).

Thawing of Plastic Containers: Thaw frozen bag at room temperature 22°C (72°F) or in a refrigerator 4°C (39°F). [DO NOT FORCE THAW BY IMMERSION IN WATER BATHS OR BY MICROWAVE IRRADIATION.] Check for minute leaks by squeezing bag firmly. If leaks are detected discard solution as sterility may be impaired. Do not add supplementary medication.

The bag should be visually inspected. Thawed solutions should not be used unless clear; solutions will be light to dark yellow in color. Components of the solution may precipitate in the frozen state and will dissolve upon reaching room temperature with little or no agitation. If, after visual inspection, the solution remains cloudy or if an insoluble precipitate is noted or if any seals or outlet ports are not intact, the bag should be discarded.

Use Sterile Equipment: The thawed solution is stable for 24 hours at room temperature 22°C (72°F) or for seven days under refrigeration 4°C (39°F).

DO NOT REFREEZE*Caution:* Do not use plastic containers in series connections. Such use could result in an embolism due to residual air being drawn from the primary container before administration of the fluid from the secondary container is complete.

Preparation for Administration:

1. Suspend container from eyelet support.
2. Remove protector from outlet port at bottom of container.
3. Attach administration set. Refer to complete directions accompanying set.

REFERENCES:

1. National Committee for Clinical Laboratory Standards, Approved Standard: Performance Standards for Antimicrobial Disk Susceptibility Tests. 3rd Edition. Vol. 4(16): M2-A3. Villanova, PA. December 1984. 2. National Committee for Clinical Laboratory Standards, Approved Standard: Methods for Dilution Antimicrobial Susceptibility Tests for Bacteria That Grow Aerobically. Vol. 5(22): M7-A. Villanova, PA. December 1985.

HOW SUPPLIED:

Timentin (sterile ticarcillin disodium and clavulanate potassium).

Each 3.1 gram vial contains sterile ticarcillin disodium equivalent to 3 grams ticarcillin and sterile clavulanate potassium equivalent to 0.1 gram clavulanic acid.

Each 31 gram pharmacy bulk package contains sterile ticarcillin disodium equivalent to 30 grams ticarcillin and sterile clavulanate potassium equivalent to 1 gram clavulanic acid.

Vials should be stored at or below 24°C (75°F).

* ADD-Vantage is a trademark of Abbott Laboratories.

† Galaxy is a trademark of Baxter International Inc.

HOW SUPPLIED - EQUIVALENTS NOT AVAILABLE:

Injection, Dry-Soln - Intravenous - 0.1 gm/3 gm

21 ml x 10	$13.65	TIMENTIN 3.1 ADD-VANTAGE, Beecham	00029-6571-40
50 ml x 10	$13.35	TIMENTIN 3.1, Beecham	00029-6571-26
100 ml x 10	$14.20	TIMENTIN 3.1, Beecham	00029-6571-21
100 ml x 10	$133.50	TIMENTIN, Beecham	00029-6579-21
100 ml x 12	$188.70	TIMENTIN ISO OSMOTIC, Beecham	00029-6571-31

CLEMASTINE FUMARATE *(000835)*

CATEGORIES: Allergies; Angioedema; Antihistamines; Ethanolamines; Hay Fever; Lacrimation; Pruritus; Respiratory & Allergy Medications; Rhinitis; Sneezing; Urticaria; Pregnancy Category B; FDA Approval Pre 1982

BRAND NAMES: *Aller-Eze* (England); *Clema*; *Darvine*; *Histaverin*; *Martine*; *Tavegil* (Germany); *Tavegyl* (France); **Tavist**
(International brand names outside U.S. in italics)

FORMULARIES: Aetna; BC-BS

COST OF THERAPY: $43.50 (Rhinitis; Tablet; 2.68 mg; 2/day; 30 days)

PRIMARY ICD9: 477.9 (Allergic Rhinitis, Cause Unspecified)

DESCRIPTION:

TABLETS

Clemastine fumarate belongs to the benzhydryl ether group of antihistaminic compounds. The chemical name is (+)-2-[2]-[(p-chloro-α-methyl-α-phenylbenzyl)oxy]ethyl]-1-methylpyrrolidine* hydrogen fumarate. 1.34 mg and 2.68 tablets. Active Ingredient: clemastine fumarate, USP. Inactive Ingredients: lactose, povidone, starch, stearic acid and talc.

DESCRIPTION: *(cont'd)*

SYRUP

Each teaspoonful (5 ml) of clemastine fumarate syrup for oral administration contains clemastine 0.5 mg (present as clemastine fumarate 0.67 mg). Other ingredients: alcohol 5.5%, flavors, methylparaben, propylene glycol, propylparaben, purified water, saccharin sodium, sorbitol in a buffered solution. Clemastine fumarate belongs to the benzhydryl ether group of antihistamine compounds. the chemical name is (+)-(2R)-2-[2-[[(R)-p-Chloro-α-methyl-α-phenylbenzyl]-oxy]-ethyl]-1-methylpyrrolidine fumarate*.

Clemastine fumarate occurs as a colorless to faintly yellow, practically odorless, crystalline powder. Clemastine fumarate syrup has an approximate pH of 6.2

CLINICAL PHARMACOLOGY:

TABLETS

Clemastine fumarate is an antihistamine with anticholinergic (drying) and sedative side effects. Antihistamines appear to compete with histamine for cell receptor sites on effector cells. The inherently long duration of antihistaminic effects of clemastine fumarate has been demonstrated in wheal and flare studies. In normal human subjects who received histamine injections over a 24-hour period, the antihistaminic activity of clemastine fumarate reached a peak at 5-7 hours, persisted for 10-12 hours, and, in some cases, for as long as 24 hours. Pharmacokinetic studies in man utilizing ^{3}H and ^{14}C labeled compound demonstrates that: clemastine fumarate is rapidly absorbed from the gastrointestinal tract, peak plasma concentrations are attained in 2-4 hours, and urinary excretion is the major mode of elimination.

SYRUP

Clemastine fumarate is an antihistamine with anticholinergic (drying) and sedative side effects. Antihistamines competitively antagonize various physiological effects of histamine including increased capillary permeability and dilation, the formation of edema, the "flare" and "itch" response, and gastrointestinal and respiratory smooth muscle constriction. Within the vascular tree, H_1-receptor antagonists inhibit both the vasoconstrictor and vasodilator effects of histamine. Depending on the dose, H_1 receptor antagonists can produce CNS stimulation or depression. Most antihistamines exhibit central and/or peripheral anticholinergic activity. Antihistamines act by competitively blocking H_1-receptor sites. Antihistamines do not pharmacologically antagonize or chemically inactivate histamine, nor do they prevent the release of histamine.

Pharmacokinetics: Antihistamines are well-absorbed following oral administration. Chlorpheniramine maleate, clemastine fumarate, and diphenhydramine hydrochloride active peak blood levels within 2-5 hours following oral administration. The absorption of antihistamines is often partially delayed by the use of controlled release dosage forms. In these instances, plasma concentrations from identical doses of the immediate and controlled release dosage forms will not be similar. Tissue distribution of the antihistamines in humans has not been established.

Antihistamines appear to be metabolized in the liver chiefly via mono- and didemethylation and glucuronide conjugation. Antihistamine metabolites and small amounts of unchanged drug excreted in the urine. Small amounts of the drugs may also be excreted in breast milk.

In normal human subjects who received histamine injections over a 24-hour period, the antihistaminic activity of clemastine fumarate reach peak at 5-7 hours, persisted for 10-12 hours and, in some cases, for as long as 24 hours. Pharmacokinetic studies in man utilizing ^{3}H and ^{14}C labeled compound demonstrate that: clemastine fumarate is rapidly absorbed from the gastrointestinal tract, peak plasma concentrations are attained in 2-4 hours, and urinary excretion is the major mode of elimination.

INDICATIONS AND USAGE:

TABLETS

Clemastine fumarate tablets, 1.34 mg are indicated for the relief symptoms associated with allergic rhinitis such as sneezing, rhinorrhea, pruritus, and lacrimation.

Clemastine fumarate tablets 2.68 mg are indicated for the relief symptoms associated with allergic rhinitis such as sneezing, rhinorrhea, pruritus, and lacrimation. Clemastine fumarate tablets 2.68 mg are also indicated for the relief of mild, uncomplicated allergic skin manifestations of urticaria and angioedema.

It should be noted that clemastine fumarate USP is indicated for the dermatologic indications at the 2.68 mg dosage level only.

SYRUP

Clemastine fumarate syrup is indicated for the relief of symptoms associated with allergic rhinitis such as sneezing, rhinorrhea, pruritus and lacrimation. Clemastine fumarate syrup is indicated for use in pediatric populations (age 6 years through 12) and adults (see DOSAGE AND ADMINISTRATION.)

It should be noted that clemastine fumarate is indicated for the relief of mild uncomplicated allergic skin manifestations of urticaria and angioedema at the 2 mg dosage level only.

CONTRAINDICATIONS:

TABLETS

Use in Nursing Mothers: Because of the higher risk of antihistamines for infants generally and for newborns and prematures in particular antihistamine therapy is contraindicated in nursing mothers.

Use in Lower Respiratory Disease: Antihistamines **should not** be used to treat lower respiratory tract symptoms including asthma.

Antihistamines are also contraindicated in the following conditions:

Hypersensitivity to clemastine fumarate USP or other antihistamines of similar chemical structure.

Monamine oxidase inhibitor therapy (see DRUG INTERACTIONS.)

SYRUP

Antihistamines are contraindicated in patients hypersensitive to the drug or to other antihistamines of similar chemical structure (see DRUG INTERACTIONS.)

Antihistamines **should not** be used **in newborn or premature infants.** Because of the higher risk of antihistamines for infants generally and for newborns and prematures in particular, antihistamine therapy is contraindicated **in nursing mothers** (see CONTRAINDICATIONS, Nursing Mothers.)

WARNINGS:

TABLETS AND SYRUP

Antihistamines should be used with considerable caution in patients with narrow angle glaucoma, stenosing peptic ulcer, pyloroduodenal obstruction, symptomatic prostatic hypertrophy, and bladder neck obstruction.

SYRUP

Usage in Children: Safety and efficacy of clemastine fumarate have not been established in children under the age of 12.

Use in Pregnancy: Experience with this drug in pregnant women is inadequate to determine whether there exists a potential for harm to the developing fetus.

Clemastine Fumarate

WARNINGS: *(cont'd)*

Use with CNS Depressants: Clemastine fumarate has addictive effects with alcohol and other CNS depressants (hypnotics, sedatives, tranquilizers, etc.).

Use in Activities Requiring Mental Alertness: Patients should be warned about engaging in activities requiring mental alertness such as driving a car or operating appliances, machinery, etc.

Use in the Elderly (approximately 60 years or older): Antihistamines are more likely to cause dizziness, sedation, and hypotension in elderly patients.

PRECAUTIONS:

TABLETS AND SYRUP

General: Clemastine fumarate should be used with caution in patients with: history of bronchial asthma, increased intraocular pressure, hyperthyroidism, cardiovascular disease, and hypertension.

Information for the Patient: Patients taking antihistamines should receive the following information and instructions:

1. Antihistamines are prescribed to reduce allergic symptoms.

2. Patients should be questioned regarding a history of glaucoma, peptic ulcer, urinary retention or pregnancy before starting antihistamine therapy.

3. Patients should be told not to take alcohol, sleeping pills, sedatives, tranquilizers while taking antihistamines.

4. Antihistamines may cause drowsiness, dizziness, dry mouth, blurred vision, weakness, nausea, headache, or nervousness in some patients.

5. Patients should avoid driving a car or working with hazardous machinery until they assess the effects of this medicine.

6. Patients should be told to store this medicine in a tightly closed container in a dry, cool place away from heat or direct sunlight and out of the reach for children.

DRUG INTERACTIONS:

TABLETS

MAO inhibitors prolong and intensify the anticholinergic (drying) effects of antihistamines.

SYRUP

Additive CNS depressions may occur when antihistamines are administered concomitantly with other CNS depressants including barbiturates, tranquilizers, and alcohol. Patients receiving antihistamines should be advised against the concurrent use of other CNS depressant drugs.

Monoamine oxidase (MAO) inhibitors prolong and intensify the anticholinergic effects of antihistamines.

ADVERSE REACTIONS:

TABLETS AND SYRUP

Transient drowsiness, the most common adverse reaction associated with clemastine fumarate, USP, occurs relatively frequently and may require discontinuation of therapy in some instances.

Antihistaminic Compounds: It should be noted that the following reactions have occurred with one or more antihistamines and, therefore, should be kept in mind when prescribing drugs belonging to this class, including clemastine fumarate. The most frequent adverse reactions are underlined.

1. General : Urticaria, drug rash, anaphylactic shock, photosensitivity, excessive perspiration, chills, dryness of mouth, nose, and throat.

2. Cardiovascular System: Hypotension, headache, palpitations, tachycardia, extrasystoles.

3. Hematologic System : Hemolytic anemia, thrombocytopenia, agranulocytosis.

4. Nervous System: Sedation, sleepiness, dizziness, disturbedcoordination, fatigue, confusion, restlessness, excitation, nervousness, tremor, irritability, insomnia, euphoria, paresthesia, blurred vision, diplopia, vertigo, tinnitus, acute labyrinthitis, hysteria, neuritis, convulsions.

5. GI System: Epigastric distress, anorexia, nausea, vomiting, diarrhea, constipation.

6. GU System: Urinary frequency, difficult urination, urinary retention, early menses.

7. Respiratory System: Thickening of bronchial secretions, tightness of chest and wheezing, nasal stuffiness.

OVERDOSAGE:

TABLETS

Antihistamine overdosage reactions may vary from central nervous system depression to stimulation. Stimulation is particularly likely in children. Atropine-like signs and symptoms; dry mouth, fixed, dilated pupils: flushing: and gastrointestinal symptoms may also occur.

If Vomiting Has Not Occurred Spontaneously: The conscious patient should be induced to vomit. This is best done by having him drink a glass of water or milk after which he should be made to gag. Precautions against aspiration must be taken, especially infants and children.

If vomiting is unsuccessful gastric lavage is indicated within 3 hours after ingestion and even later if large amounts of milk or cream were given beforehand. Isotonic and $\frac{1}{2}$ isotonic saline is the lavage solution of choice.

Saline Cathartics: such as milk of magnesia, by osmosis draw water into the bowel and therefore, are valuable for their action in rapid dilution of bowel content.

Stimulants: should **not** be used.

Vasopressors may be used to treat hypotension.

SYRUP

Antihistamine overdosage reactions may vary from central nervous system depression to stimulation. In children, stimulation predominates initially in a syndrome which may include excitement hallucinations, ataxia, incoordination, muscle twitching, athetosis, hyperthermia, cyanosis convulsions, tremors, and hyperreflexia followed by postictal depression and cardiorespiratory arrest. Convulsions in children may be preceded by mild depression. Dry mouth, fixed dilated pupils, flushing of the face, and fever are common. In adults, CNS depression, ranging from drowsiness to coma, is more common. The convulsant dose of antihistamines lies near the lethal dose. Convulsions indicate a poor prognosis.

In both children and adults, coma and cardiovascular collapse may occur. Deaths are reported especially in infants and children.

There is no specific therapy for acute overdosage with antihistamines. the latent period from ingestion to appearance of toxic effects is characteristically short ($\frac{1}{2}$-2 hours). General symptomatic and supportive measures should be instituted promptly and maintained for as long as necessary.

Since overdoses of other classes of drugs (*i.e.,* tricyclic antidepressants) may also present anticholinergic symptomatology, appropriate toxicological analysis should be performed as soon as possible to identify the causative agent.

OVERDOSAGE: *(cont'd)*

In the conscious patient, vomiting should be induced even though it may have occurred spontaneously. If vomiting cannot be induced, gastric lavage is indicated. Adequate precautions must be taken to protect against aspiration, especially in infants and children. Charcoal slurry or other suitable agents should be instilled into the stomach after vomiting or lavage. Saline cathartics or milk of magnesia may be of additional benefit.

In the unconscious patient, the airway should be secured with a cuffed endotracheal tube before attempting to evacuate the gastric contents. Intensive supportive and nursing care is indicated, as for any comatose patient.

If breathing is significantly impaired, maintenance of an adequate airway and mechanical support of respiration is the most effective means of providing adequate oxygenation.

Hypotension is an early sign of impending cardiovascular collapse and should be treated vigorously. Although general supportive measures are important, specific treatment with intravenous infusion of a vasopressor titrated with intravenous infusion of a vasopressor titrated to maintain adequate blood pressure may be necessary.

Do not use with CNS stimulants.

Convulsions should be controlled by careful administration of diazepam or a short-acting barbiturate, repeated as necessary. Physostigmine may also be considered for use in controlling centrally mediated convulsions.

Ice packs and cooling sponge baths, not alcohol, can aid in reducing fever commonly seen in children. A more detailed review of antihistamine toxicology and overdose management is available in Gosselin, R.E., et al., "Clinical Toxicology of Commercial Products."

DOSAGE AND ADMINISTRATION:

DOSAGE SHOULD BE INDIVIDUALIZED ACCORDING TO THE NEEDS AND RESPONSE OF THE PATIENT.

TABLETS

Clemastine Fumarate Tablets 1.34 mg: The recommended starting dose is one tablet twice daily. Dosage may be increased as required, but not to exceed six tablets daily.

Clemastine Fumarate Tablets 2.68 mg: The maximum recommended dosage is one tablet three times daily. Many patients respond favorably to a single dose which may be repeated as required, but not to exceed three tablets daily.

SYRUP

Pediatric: *Children aged 6 to 12 years:*

For Symptoms Of Allergic Rhinitis: The starting dose is 1 teaspoonful (0.5 mg clemastine) twice daily. Since single doses of up to 2.25 mg clemastine were well tolerated by this age group, dosage may be increased as required, but not to exceed 6 teaspoonfuls daily (3 mg clemastine).

For Urticaria and Angioedema: The starting dose is 2 teaspoonfuls (1 mg clemastine) twice daily, not to exceed 6 teaspoonfuls daily (3 mg clemastine).

ADULTS AND CHILDREN 12 YEARS AND OVER

For Symptoms of Allergic Rhinitis: The starting dose is 2 teaspoonful (1.0 mg clemastine) twice daily. Dosage may be increased as required, but not to exceed 12 teaspoonful daily (6 mg clemastine).

For Urticaria and Angioedema: The starting dose is 4 teaspoonful (2 mg clemastine) twice daily, not to exceed 12 teaspoonful (2 mg clemastine) twice daily, not to exceed 12 teaspoonful daily (6 mg clemastine).

HOW SUPPLIED - RATED THERAPEUTICALLY EQUIVALENT:

Syrup - Oral - 0.67 mg/5ml

120 ml	$16.50	Clemastine Fumarate, Qualitest Pharms	00603-1096-54
120 ml	$16.58	Clemastine Fumarate, Geneva Pharms	00781-6128-04
120 ml	$18.37	Clemastine Fumarate, United Res	00677-1441-41
120 ml	$18.50	Clemastine Fumarate, Goldline Labs	00182-6036-37
120 ml	$18.52	Clemastine Fumarate, Schein Pharm (US)	00364-2445-77
120 ml	$19.00	Clemastine Fumarate, Rugby	00536-0735-97
120 ml	$19.25	Clemastine Fumarate, Copley Pharm	38245-0268-14
120 ml	$19.50	Clemastine Fumarate, Teva	00093-0309-12
120 ml	$20.10	Clemastine Fumarate, Aligen Independ	00405-2529-76
120 ml	$20.41	Clemastine Fumarate, HL Moore Drug Exch	00839-7625-65
120 ml	$22.45	Clemastine Fumarate, Major Pharms	00904-1524-00
120 ml	$22.45	Clemastine Fumarate, Major Pharms	00904-1524-20
120 ml	**$25.08**	**TAVIST, Novartis**	**00078-0222-31**

Tablet, Uncoated - Oral - 1.34 mg

100's	$31.25	Clemastine Fumarate, Major Pharms	00904-7678-60
100's	$36.20	Clemastine Fumarate, Aligen Independ	00405-5355-01
100's	$37.17	Clemastine Fumarate, HL Moore Drug Exch	00839-7739-06
100's	$54.25	Clemastine Fumarate, Harber Pharm	51432-0426-03
100's	**$63.84**	**TAVIST-1, Novartis**	**00078-0075-05**

Tablet, Uncoated - Oral - 2.68 mg

100's	$72.50	Clemastine Fumarate, Aligen Independ	00405-5356-01
100's	$72.50	Clemastine Fumarate, Harber Pharm	51432-0427-03
100's	$74.20	Clemastine Fumarate, Qualitest Pharms	00603-2900-21
100's	$76.50	Clemastine Fumarate, Goldline Labs	00182-1936-01
100's	$76.95	Clemastine Fumarate, Schein Pharm (US)	00364-2521-01
100's	$77.05	Clemastine Fumarate, Teva	00093-0308-01
100's	$82.10	Clemastine Fumarate, Major Pharms	00904-7679-60
100's	$82.13	Clemastine Fumarate, United Res	00677-1443-01
100's	$82.13	Clemastine Fumarate, H.C.F.A. F F P	99999-0835-01
100's	$82.50	Clemastine Fumarate, Rugby	00536-3506-01
100's	$86.05	Clemastine Fumarate, Geneva Pharms	00781-1359-01
100's	$86.08	Clemastine Fumarate, HL Moore Drug Exch	00839-7740-06
100's	**$109.14**	**TAVIST, Novartis**	**00078-0072-05**
100's	$111.99	CLEMASTINE FUMARATE, Vangard Labs	00615-4502-13

HOW SUPPLIED - NOT RATED EQUIVALENT:

Syrup - Oral - 0.67 mg/5ml

120 ml	$16.50	Clemastine Syrup, Harber Pharm	51432-0524-18
120 ml	$19.00	Clemastine Fumarate, Alpharma	00472-0857-04
120 ml	$19.95	Clemastine Fumarate, Geneva Pharms	50752-0284-31
480 ml	$75.81	Clemastine Fumarate, Geneva Pharms	50752-0284-33

Tablet, Uncoated - Oral - 1.34 mg

100's	$33.00	Clemastine Fumarate, Geneva Pharms	00781-1358-01
100's	$51.34	CLEMASTINE FUMARATE, Vangard Labs	00615-4501-13

CLEMASTINE FUMARATE; PHENYLPROPANOLAMINE HYDROCHLORIDE *(000836)*

CATEGORIES: Allergies; Antihistamines; Common Cold; Cough Preparations; Decongestants; Hay Fever; Lacrimation; Nasal Congestion; Pruritus; Respiratory & Allergy Medications; Rhinitis; Sinusitis; Sneezing; Pregnancy Category B; Sales > $100 Million; FDA Approved 1982 Dec

BRAND NAMES: *Rhinalgan*; *Rhinergal*; *Tavegyl-D*; **Tavist-D**
(International brand names outside U.S. in italics)

FORMULARIES: Aetna; BC-BS

DESCRIPTION:

Active Ingredients: Each clemastine fumarate w/ phenylpropanolamine tablet contains clemastine fumarate, USP, 1.34 mg (equivalent to 1 mg clemastine) immediate release and 75 mg phenylpropanolamine hydrochloride, USP, extended release.

Inactive Ingredients: Colloidal silicon dioxide, dibasic calcium phosphate, lactose, magnesium stearate, methylcellulose, polyethylene glycol, povidone, starch, synthetic polymers, titanium dioxide and Yellow 10.

INDICATIONS AND USAGE:

For the temporary relief of nasal congestion associated with upper respiratory allergies or sinusitis when accompanied by other symptoms of hay fever or allergies, including runny nose, sneezing, itchy nose or throat or itchy, watery eyes.

WARNINGS:

May cause drowsiness; alcohol, sedatives, and tranquilizers may increase the drowsiness effect. Avoid alcoholic beverages while taking this product. Do not take this product if you are taking sedatives or tranquilizers without first consulting your doctor. Use caution when driving a motor vehicle or operating machinery. May cause excitability especially in children.

Do not exceed recommended dosage because at higher doses nervousness, dizziness, or sleeplessness may occur. Do not take this product for more than 7 days. If symptoms do not improve or are accompanied by fever, consult a doctor. Do not take this product if you have asthma, diabetes, glaucoma, heart disease, high blood pressure, thyroid disease, emphysema, chronic pulmonary disease, shortness of breath, difficulty in breathing or difficulty in urination due to enlargement of the prostate gland unless directed by a doctor. As with any drug, if you are pregnant or nursing a baby, seek the advice of a health professional before using this product. Keep this and all drugs out of the reach of children. In case of accidental overdose, seek professional assistance or contact a Poison Control Center immediately.

DRUG INTERACTIONS:

Do not take this product if you are presently taking a decongestant or prescription drug for high blood pressure or depression, without first consulting your doctor.

DOSAGE AND ADMINISTRATION:

Directions: Adults and children 12 years of age and over: Take one tablet swallowed whole every 12 hours, not to exceed 2 tablets in 24 hours, or as directed by a doctor. Children under 12 years: Consult a doctor.

Store in a dry place at controlled room temperature, 15-30°C (59-86°F).

HOW SUPPLIED - EQUIVALENTS NOT AVAILABLE:

Tablet, Plain Coated - Oral - 1.34 mg/75 mg

100's	$79.50	TAVIST-D, Novartis	00078-0221-05

CLIDINIUM BROMIDE *(000837)*

CATEGORIES: Anticholinergic Agents; Antimuscarinics/Antispasmodics; Antispasmodics & Anticholinergics; Autonomic Drugs; Gastrointestinal Drugs; Peptic Ulcer; FDA Approval Pre 1982

BRAND NAMES: **Quarzan**

DESCRIPTION:

Clidinium bromide is 3-hydroxy-1-methyl-quinuclidinium bromide benzilate. A white or nearly white crystalline compound, it is soluble in water and has a calculated molecular weight of 432.36.

Clidinium bromide is a quaternary ammonium compound with anticholinergic and antispasmodic activity. Quarzan is available as green and red opaque capsules each containing 2.5 mg clidinium bromide, and green and grey opaque capsules each containing 5 mg clidinium bromide. Each capsule also contains corn starch, lactose and talc. Gelatin capsule shells contain methyl and propyl parabens and potassium sorbate, with the following dye systems: 2.5-mg capsules—FD&C Blue No. 1, FD&C Green No. 3, FD&C Red No. 3, D&C Red No. 33 and D&C Yellow No. 10. 5-mg capsules-FD&C Green No. 3, D&C Red No. 33, FD&C Yellow No. 6 and D&C Yellow No. 10.

CLINICAL PHARMACOLOGY:

Clidinium bromide inhibits gastrointestinal motility and diminishes gastric acid secretion. Its anticholinergic activity approximates that of atropine sulfate and propantheline bromide.

INDICATIONS AND USAGE:

Clidinium bromide is effective as adjunctive therapy in peptic ulcer disease. **Clidinium bromide has not been shown to be effective in contributing to the healing of peptic ulcer, decreasing the rate of recurrence or preventing complications.**

CONTRAINDICATIONS:

Known hypersensitivity to clidinium bromide or to other anticholinergic drugs, glaucoma, obstructive uropathy (for example, bladder neck obstruction due to prostatic hypertrophy), obstructive disease of the gastrointestinal tract (for example, pyloroduodenal stenosis), paralytic ileus, intestinal atony of the elderly or debilitated patient, unstable cardiovascular status in acute hemorrhage, severe ulcerative colitis, toxic megacolon complicating ulcerative colitis, myasthenia gravis.

WARNINGS:

Clidinium bromide may produce drowsiness or blurred vision. The patient should be cautioned regarding activities requiring mental alertness such as operating a motor vehicle or other machinery or performing hazardous work while taking this drug. In the presence of high environmental temperature, heat prostration (fever and heat stroke) may occur with the

WARNINGS: *(cont'd)*

use of anticholinergics due to decreased sweating. Diarrhea may be an early symptom of incomplete intestinal obstruction, especially in patients with ileostomy or colostomy. Use of anticholinergics in patients with suspected intestinal obstruction would be inappropriate and possibly harmful. With overdosage, a curare-like action may occur, *i.e.,*neuromuscular blockade leading to muscular weakness and possible paralysis.

Usage in Pregnancy: No controlled studies in humans have been performed to establish the safety of the drug in pregnancy. Uncontrolled data derived from clinical usage have failed to show abnormalities attributable to its use. Reproduction studies in rats have failed to show any impaired fertility or abnormality in the fetuses that might be associated with the use of clidinium bromide. Use of any drug in pregnancy or in women of childbearing potential requires that the potential benefit of the drug be weighed against the possible hazards to mother and fetus.

Nursing Mothers: As with all anticholinergic drugs, clidinium bromide may be secreted in human milk and may inhibit lactation. As a general rule, nursing should not be undertaken while a patient is on clidinium bromide, or the drug should not be used by nursing mothers.

Pediatric Use: Since there is no adequate experience in children who have received this drug, safety and efficacy in children have not been established.

PRECAUTIONS:

Use clidinium bromide with caution in the elderly and in all patients with autonomic neuropathy, hepatic or renal disease, ulcerative colitis - large doses may suppress intestinal motility to the point of producing a paralytic ileus and for this reason precipitate or aggravate "toxic megacolon," a serious complication of the disease; hyperthyroidism; coronary heart disease; congestive heart failure; cardiac tachy-arrhythmias; tachycardia; hypertension; prostatic hypertrophy; hiatal hernia associated with reflux esophagitis, since anticholinergic drugs may aggravate this condition.

DRUG INTERACTIONS:

No specific drug interactions are known.

ADVERSE REACTIONS:

As with other anticholinergic drugs, the most frequently reported adverse effects are dryness of mouth, blurring of vision, urinary hesitancy and constipation. Other adverse effects reported with the use of anticholinergic drugs include decreased sweating, urinary retention, tachycardia, palpitations, dilatation of the pupils, cycloplegia, increased ocular tension, loss of taste, headaches, nervousness, mental confusion, drowsiness, weakness, dizziness, insomnia, nausea, vomiting, bloated feeling, impotence, suppression of lactation and severe allergic reactions or drug idiosyncrasies including anaphylaxis, urticaria and other dermal manifestations.

OVERDOSAGE:

The symptoms of overdosage with clidinium bromide progress from an intensification of the usual side effects to CNS disturbances (from restlessness and excitement to psychotic behavior), circulatory changes (flushing, tachycardia, fall in blood pressure, circulatory failure), respiratory failure, paralysis and coma.

Treatment should consist of:

General Measures: (1) gastric lavage, (2) maintenance of adequate airway, using artificial respiration if needed, (3) administration of IV fluids, and (4) for fever: alcohol sponging or ice packs.

Specific Measures: *Antidotes:* physostigmine (Antilirium) 0.5 to 2 mg, IV, repeated as needed up to a total of 5 mg; or pilocarpine, 5 mg, s.c. at intervals until mouth is moist; neostigmine may also be useful. *Against Excitement:* sodium pentothal 2% may be given IV or chloral hydrate chloral hydrate (100 to 200 ml, 2% solution) *rectally. Against Hypotension And Circulatory Collapse:* levarterenol (Levophed) or metaraminol (Aramine) infusions. *Against CNS Depression:* caffeine and sodium benzoate.

The usefulness of dialysis in not known.

DOSAGE AND ADMINISTRATION:

For maximum efficacy, dosage should be individualized according to severity of symptoms and occurrence of side effects. The usual dosage is 2.5 to 5 mg three or four times daily before meals and at bedtime. Dosage in excess of 20 mg daily is usually not required to obtain maximum effectiveness. For the aged or debilitated, one 2.5-mg capsule three times daily before meals is recommended. The desired pharmacological effect of the drug is unlikely to be attained without occasional side effects.

HOW SUPPLIED:

Quarzan opaque capsules, 2.5 mg, green and red; 5 mg, green and grey.

HOW SUPPLIED - EQUIVALENTS NOT AVAILABLE:

Capsule, Gelatin - Oral - 2.5 mg

100's	$19.62	QUARZAN, Roche Prod	00140-0119-01

Capsule, Gelatin - Oral - 5 mg

100's	$26.74	QUARZAN, Roche Prod	00140-0120-01

CLINDAMYCIN HYDROCHLORIDE *(000838)*

CATEGORIES: Abdominal Abscess; Anti-Infectives; Antibiotics; Antimicrobials; Cellulitis; Colitis; Dermatologicals; Empyema; Endometritis; Gynecologic Infections; Infections; Intra-Abdominal Infections; Lincosamides/Macrolides; Peritonitis; Pneumonitis; Pulmonary Abscess; Respiratory Tract Infections; Septicemia; Skin Infections; Skin/Mucous Membrane Agents; Acne*; Sales > $100 Million; FDA Approval Pre 1982
* Indication not approved by the FDA

BRAND NAMES: *Aclinda* (Germany); *Albiotin*; *BB*; **Cleocin**; *Climadon*; *Clincin*; Clinda-Derm; *Clindacin*; Clindamycin Phosphate; *Dalacin* (Japan); *Dalacin C* (Australia, England, Canada, Mexico); *Dalacine* (France); *Dalcap*; *Klimicin*; *Lacin*; *Librodan*; *Lindan*; *Sobelin* (Germany); *Tidact*; *Turimycin*
(International brand names outside U.S. in italics)

FORMULARIES: Aetna; BC-BS; Medi-Cal; PCS; WHO

COST OF THERAPY: $28.17 (Infections; Capsule; 150 mg; 4/day; 10 days)

PRIMARY ICD9: 136.9 (Unspecified Infections And Parasitic Diseases)

WARNING:
Clindamycin therapy has been associated with severe colitis which may end fatally. Therefore, it should be reserved for serious infections where less toxic antimicrobial agents are inappropriate, as described in the INDICATIONS AND USAGEsection. It should not be used in patients with nonbacterial infections, such as most upper respiratory tract infections. Studies indicate a toxin(s) produced by Clostridia is one primary cause of antibiotic-associated colitis. Cholestyramine and colestipol resins have been shown to bind the toxin in vitro. See WARNINGS. The colitis is usually characterized by severe, persistent diarrhea and severe abdominal cramps and may be associated with the passage of blood and mucus. Endoscopic examination may reveal pseudomembranous colitis. Stool culture for Clostridium difficile and stool assay for C. difficile toxin may be helpful diagnostically.
When significant diarrhea occurs, the drug should be discontinued or, if necessary, continued only with close observation of the patient. Large bowel endoscopy has been recommended.
Antiperistaltic agents such as opiates and diphenoxylate with atropine may prolong and/or worsen the condition. Vancomycin has been found to be effective in the treatment of antibiotic associated pseudomembranous colitis produced by Clostridium difficile. The usual adult dose is 500 milligrams to 2 grams of vancomycin orally per day in three to four divided doses administered for 7 to 10 days. Cholestyramine or colestipol resins bind vancomycin in vitro. If both a resin and vancomycin are to be administered concurrently, it may be advisable to separate the time of administration of each drug.
Diarrhea, colitis, and pseudomembranous colitis have been observed to begin up to several weeks following cessation of therapy with clindamycin.

DESCRIPTION:

CAPSULES

Clindamycin hydrochloride is the hydrated hydrochloride salt of clindamycin. Clindamycin is a semisynthetic antibiotic produced by a 7(S)-chloro-substitution of the 7(R)-hydroxyl group of the parent compound lincomycin.

Clindamycin HCl capsules contain clindamycin hydrochloride equivalent to 75 mg, 150 mg or 300 mg of clindamycin.

Inactive ingredients: 75 mg—corn starch, erythrosine sodium, FD&C blue no. 1, FD&C yellow no. 5, gelatin, lactose, magnesium stearate and talc; 150 mg—corn starch, erythrosine sodium, FD&C blue no. 1, FD&C yellow no. 5, gelatin, lactose, magnesium stearate, talc and titanium dioxide; 300 mg—corn starch, erythrosine sodium, FD&C blue no. 1, gelatin, lactose, magnesium stearate, talc and titanium dioxide.

The chemical name for clindamycin hydrochloride is Methyl 7-chloro-6,7,8-trideoxy-6-(1-methyl-*trans*-4-propyl-L-2-pyrrolidin ecarbox-amido)-1-thio-L-*threo*-α-D-*galacto*-octopyranoside monohydrochloride.

GRANULES

Clindamycin palmitate hydrochloride is a water soluble hydrochloride salt of the ester of clindamycin and palmitic acid. Clindamycin is a semisynthetic antibiotic produced by a 7(S)-chloro-substitution of the 7(R)-hydroxyl group of the parent compound lincomycin.

The chemical name for clindamycin palmitate hydrochloride is Methyl 7-chloro-6,7,8-trideoxy-6-(1-methyl-*trans*-4-propyl-L-2-pyrrolidin ecarbox-amido)-1-thio-L-*threo*-α-D-*galacto*-octopyranoside 2-palmitate monohydrochloride.

Clindamycin palmitate HCl pediatric flavored granules contain clindamycin palmitate hydrochloride for reconstitution. Each 5 ml contains the equivalent of 75 mg clindamycin. *Inactive ingredients:* artificial cherry flavor, dextrin, ethylparaben, pluronic F68, polymethylsiloxane, sucrose.

CLINICAL PHARMACOLOGY:

CAPSULES

Microbiology: Clindamycin has been shown to have *in vitro* activity against isolates of the following organisms:

Aerobic Gram-Positive Cocci, Including: *Staphylococcus aureus*; *Staphylococcus epidermidis (penicillinase and nonpenicillinase producing strains)*. When tested by *in vitro* methods some staphylococcal strains originally resistant to erythromycin rapidly develop resistance to clindamycin.

Streptococci (except *Streptococcus faecalis*); Pneumococci

Anaerobic Gram-Negative Bacilli, Including: Bacteroides species (including *Bacteroides fragilis* group and *Bacteroides melaninogenicus* group); Fusobacterium species

Anaerobic Gram-Positive Nonsporeforming Bacilli, Including: *Propionibacterium; Eubacterium; Actinomyces* species

Anaerobic And Microaerophilic Gram-Positive Cocci, Including: *Peptococcus* species; *Peptostreptococcus* species; *Microaerophilic streptococci*

Clostridia: Clostridia are more resistant than most anaerobes to clindamycin. Most *Clostridium perfringens* are susceptible, but other species, (*e.g., Clostridium sporogenes* and *Clostridium tertium*) are frequently resistant to clindamycin. Susceptibility testing should be done.

Cross resistance has been demonstrated between clindamycin and lincomycin.

Antagonism has been demonstrated between clindamycin and erythromycin.

Human Pharmacology

Serum level studies with a 150 mg oral dose of clindamycin hydrochloride in 24 normal adult volunteers showed that clindamycin was rapidly absorbed after oral administration. An average peak serum level of 2.50 mcg/ml was reached in 45 minutes; serum levels averaged 1.51 mcg/ml at 3 hours and 0.70 mcg/ml at 6 hours. Absorption of an oral dose is virtually complete (90%), and the concomitant administration of food does not appreciably modify the serum concentrations; serum levels have been uniform and predictable from person to person and dose to dose. Serum level studies following multiple doses of clindamycin HCl for up to 14 days show no evidence of accumulation or altered metabolism of drug.

Serum half-life of clindamycin is increased slightly in patients with markedly reduced renal function. Hemodialysis and peritoneal dialysis are not effective in removing clindamycin from the serum.

Concentrations of clindamycin in the serum increased linearly with increased dose. Serum levels exceed the MIC (minimum inhibitory concentration) for most indicated organisms for at least six hours following administration of the usually recommended doses. Clindamycin is widely distributed in body fluids and tissues (including bones). The average biological half-life is 2.4 hours. Approximately 10% of the bioactivity is excreted in the urine and 3.6% in the feces; the remainder is excreted as bioinactive metabolites.

Doses of up to 2 grams of clindamycin per day for 14 days have been well tolerated by healthy volunteers, except that the incidence of gastrointestinal side effects is greater with the higher doses.

No significant levels of clindamycin are attained in the cerebrospinal fluid, even in the presence of inflamed meninges.

GRANULES

Microbiology: Although clindamycin palmitate HCl is inactive *in vitro*, rapid *in vivo* hydrolysis converts this compound to the antibacterially active clindamycin.

Clindamycin has been shown to have *in vitro* activity against isolates of the following organisms:

Aerobic Gram Positive Cocci, Including: *Staphylococcus aureus; Staphylococcus epidermis* (penicillinase and non-penicillinase producing strains). When tested by *in vitro* methods some staphylococcal strains originally resistant to erythromycin rapidly develop resistance to clindamycin.

Streptococci (except *Streptococcus faecalis*); *Pneumococci.*

Anaerobic Gram Negative Bacilli, Including: Bacteroides species (including *Bacteroides fragilis* group and *Bacteroides melaninogenicus* group); *Fusobacterium* species.

Anaerobic Gram Positive Nonsporeforming Bacilli, Including: *Propionibacterium; Eubacterium; Actinomyces* species.

Anaerobic And Microaerophilic Gram Positive Cocci, Including: *Peptococcus* species; *Peptostreptococcus* species; *Microaerophilic streptococci.*

Clostridia: Clostridia are more resistant than most anaerobes to clindamycin. Most *Clostridium perfringens* are susceptible, but other species, (*e.g., Clostridium sporogenes* and *Clostridium tertium*) are frequently resistant to clindamycin. Susceptibility testing should be done.

Cross resistance has been demonstrated between clindamycin and lincomycin.

Antagonism has been demonstrated between clindamycin and erythromycin.

Human Pharmacology

Blood level studies comparing clindamycin palmitate HCl with clindamycin hydrochloride show that both drugs reach their peak active serum levels at the same time, indicating a rapid hydrolysis of the palmitate to the clindamycin.

Clindamycin is widely distributed in body fluids and tissues (including bones). Approximately 10% of the biological activity is excreted in the urine. The average biological half-life after doses of clindamycin Palmitate HCl Pediatric is approximately two hours in children.

Serum half-life of clindamycin is increased slightly in patients with markedly reduced renal function. Hemodialysis and peritoneal dialysis do not appreciably affect the half-life of clindamycin in the serum.

Serum level studies with clindamycin palmitate HCl in normal children weighing 50-100 lbs given 2, 3 or 4 mg/kg every 6 hours (8, 12 or 16 mg/kg/day) demonstrated mean peak clindamycin serum levels of 1.24, 2.25 and 2.44 mcg/ml respectively, one hour after the first dose. By the fifth dose, the 6-hour serum concentration had reached equilibrium. Peak serum concentrations after this time would be about 2.46, 2.98 and 3.79 mcg/ml with doses of 8, 12 and 16 mg/kg/day, respectively. Serum levels have been uniform and predictable from person to person and dose to dose. Multiple-dose studies in newborns and infants up to 6 months of age show that the drug does not accumulate in the serum and is excreted rapidly. Serum levels exceed the MIC's for most indicated organisms for at least six hours following administration of the usually recommended doses of clindamycin palmitate HCl pediatric in adults and children.

No significant levels of clindamycin are attained in the cerebrospinal fluid, even in the presence of inflamed meninges.

INDICATIONS AND USAGE:

Clindamycin is indicated in the treatment of serious infections caused by susceptible anaerobic bacteria.

Clindamycin is also indicated in the treatment of serious infections due to susceptible strains of streptococci, pneumococci, and staphylococci. Its use should be reserved for penicillin-allergic patients or other patients for whom, in the judgment of the physician, a penicillin is inappropriate. Because of the risk of colitis, as described in the BOXED WARNING, before selecting clindamycin the physician should consider the nature of the infection and the suitability of less toxic alternatives (*e.g.,* erythromycin).

Anaerobes: Serious respiratory tract infections such as empyema, anaerobic pneumonitis and lung abscess; serious skin and soft tissue infections; septicemia; intra-abdominal infections such as peritonitis and intra-abdominal abscess (typically resulting from anaerobic organisms resident in the normal gastrointestinal tract); infections of the female pelvis and genital tract such as endometritis, nongonococcal tubo-ovarian abscess, pelvic cellulitis and postsurgical vaginal cuff infection.

Streptococci: Serious respiratory tract infections; serious skin and soft tissue infections.

Staphylococci: Serious respiratory tract infections; serious skin and soft tissue infections.

Pneumococci: Serious respiratory tract infections.

Bacteriologic studies should be performed to determine the causative organisms and their susceptibility to clindamycin.

IN VITRO

Susceptibility Testing: A standardized disk testing procedure* is recommended for determining susceptibility of aerobic bacteria to clindamycin. Using this method, the laboratory can designate isolates as resistant, intermediate, or susceptible. Tube or agar dilution methods may be used for both anaerobic and aerobic bacteria. An MIC of 1.6 mcg/ml may be considered susceptible; MICs of 1.6 to 4.8 mcg/ml may be considered intermediate and MICs greater than 4.8 mcg/ml may be considered resistant.

*Bauer AW, Kirby WMM, Sherris JC, et al: Antibiotic susceptibility testing by a standardized single disc method. *Am J Clin Pathol*45:493-496, 1966. Standardized disc susceptibility test.*Federal Register* 37:20527-29, 1972.

For anaerobic bacteria the minimal inhibitory concentration (MIC) of clindamycin can be determined by agar dilution and broth dilution (including microdilution) techniques. If MICs are not determined routinely, the disk broth method is recommended for routine use. THE KIRBY-BAUER DISK DIFFUSION METHOD AND ITS INTERPRETIVE STANDARDS ARE NOT RECOMMENDED FOR ANAEROBES.

CONTRAINDICATIONS:

Clindamycin is contraindicated in individuals with a history of hypersensitivity to preparations containing clindamycin or lincomycin.

WARNINGS:

See BOXED WARNING. Studies indicate a toxin(s) produced by*Clostridia* is one primary cause of antibiotic associated colitis.[1-5] Cholestyramine and colestipol resins have been shown to bind the toxin *in vitro*. Mild cases of colitis may respond to drug discontinuance alone. Moderate to severe cases should be managed promptly with fluid, electrolyte and protein supplementation as indicated. Vancomycin has been found to be effective in the treatment of antibiotic associated pseudomembranous colitis produced by *Clostridium difficile*. The usual adult dose is 500 milligrams to 2 grams of vancomycin orally per day in three to four divided doses administered for 7 to 10 days. Cholestyramine or colestipol resins bind vancomycin *in vitro*. If both a resin and vancomycin are to be administered concurrently, it may be advisable to separate the time of administration of each drug. Systemic corticoids and corticoid retention enemas may help relieve the colitis. Other causes of colitis should also be considered.

A careful inquiry should be made concerning previous sensitivities to drugs and other allergens.

Usage in Pregnancy: Safety for use in pregnancy has not been established.

Usage in Newborns and Infants: When clindamycin is administered to newborns and infants, appropriate monitoring of organ system functions is desirable.

Nursing Mothers: Clindamycin has been reported to appear in breast milk in ranges of 0.7 to 3.8 mcg/ml.

Usage in Meningitis: Since clindamycin does not diffuse adequately into the cerebrospinal fluid, the drug should not be used in the treatment of meningitis.

Antagonism has been demonstrated between clindamycin and erythromycin *in vitro*. Because of possible clinical significance, these two drugs should not be administered concurrently.

PRECAUTIONS:

Review of experience to date suggests that a subgroup of older patients with associated severe illness may tolerate diarrhea less well. When clindamycin is indicated in these patients, they should be carefully monitored for change in bowel frequency.

Clindamycin should be prescribed with caution in individuals with a history of gastrointestinal disease, particularly colitis.

Clindamycin should be prescribed with caution in atopic individuals.

During prolonged therapy, periodic liver and kidney function tests and blood counts should be performed.

Indicated surgical procedures should be performed in conjunction with antibiotic therapy.

The use of clindamycin occasionally results in overgrowth of nonsusceptible organisms—particularly yeasts. Should superinfections occur, appropriate measures should be taken as indicated by the clinical situation.

Patients with very severe renal disease and/or very severe hepatic disease accompanied by severe metabolic aberrations should be dosed with caution, and serum clindamycin levels monitored during high-dose therapy.

Clindamycin has been shown to have neuromuscular blocking properties that may enhance the action of other neuromuscular blocking agents. Therefore, it should be used with caution in patients receiving such agents.

CAPSULES

The 75 mg and 150 mg capsules contain FD&C yellow no. 5 (tartrazine) which may cause allergic-type reactions (including bronchial asthma) in certain susceptible individuals. Although the overall incidence of FD&C yellow no. 5 (tartrazine) sensitivity in the general population is low, it is frequently seen in patients who also have aspirin hypersensitivity.

ADVERSE REACTIONS:

The following reactions have been reported with the use of clindamycin.

Gastrointestinal: Abdominal pain, esophagitis, nausea, vomiting and diarrhea (see BOXED WARNING.)

Hypersensitivity Reactions: Maculopapular rash and urticaria have been observed during drug therapy. Generalized mild to moderate morbilliform-like skin rashes are the most frequently reported of all adverse reactions. Rare instances of erythema multiforme, some resembling Stevens-Johnson syndrome, have been associated with clindamycin. A few cases of anaphylactoid reactions have been reported. If a hypersensitivity reaction occurs, the drug should be discontinued. The usual agents (epinephrine, corticosteroids, antihistamines) should be available for emergency treatment of serious reactions.

Liver: Jaundice and abnormalities in liver function tests have been observed during clindamycin therapy.

Renal: Although no direct relationship of clindamycin to renal damage has been established, renal dysfunction as evidenced by azotemia, oliguria, and/or proteinuria has been observed in rare instances.

Hematopoietic: Transient neutropenia (leukopenia) and eosinophilia have been reported. Reports of agranulocytosis and thrombocytopenia have been made. No direct etiologic relationship to concurrent clindamycin therapy could be made in any of the foregoing.

Musculoskeletal: Rare instances of polyarthritis have been reported.

DOSAGE AND ADMINISTRATION:

CAPSULES

If significant diarrhea occurs during therapy, this antibiotic should be discontinued (see BOXED WARNING.)

Adults: *Serious infections:* 150 to 300 mg every 6 hours. *More severe infections:* 300 to 450 mg every 6 hours.

Children: *Serious infections:* 8 to 16 mg/kg/day (4 to 8 mg/lb/day) divided into three or four equal doses. *More severe infections:* 16 to 20 mg/kg/day (8 to 10 mg/lb/day) divided into three or four equal doses.

To avoid the possibility of esophageal irritation, clindamycin HCl capsules should be taken with a full glass of water.

Serious infections due to anaerobic bacteria are usually treated with clindamycin phosphate sterile solution. However, in clinically appropriate circumstances, the physician may elect to initiate treatment or continue treatment with clindamycin HCl capsules.

In cases of β-hemolytic streptococcal infections, treatment should continue for at least 10 days.

Store at controlled room temperature 15°-30° C (59°-86° F).

Toxicology: Animal toxicity studies showed the following:

LD_{50}I.P. Administration: Mouse 361 mg/kg

LD_{50}I.V. Administration: Mouse 245 mg/kg

LD_{50}Oral Administration: Rat 2,618 mg/kg

One year oral toxicity studies in Spartan Sprague-Dawley rats and Beagle dogs at levels of 30, 100, and 300 mg/kg/day (3 grams/day per dog) have shown clindamycin HCl to be well tolerated. No appreciable difference in pathological findings has been obtained in groups of

DOSAGE AND ADMINISTRATION: *(cont'd)*

animals treated with clindamycin HCl from comparable control groups. Rats receiving clindamycin hydrochloride at 600 mg/kg/day for six months tolerated the drug well; however, dogs dosed at this level vomited, would not eat and lost weight.

GRANULES

If significant diarrhea occurs during therapy, this antibiotic should be discontinued (see BOXED WARNING.)

Concomitant administration of food does not adversely affect the absorption of clindamycin palmitate HCl contained in clindamycin palmitate HCl pediatric flavored granules.

Serious Infections: 8-12 mg/kg/day (4-6 mg/lb/day) divided into 3 or 4 equal doses.

Severe Infections: 13-16 mg/kg/day (6.5-8 mg/lb/day) divided into 3 or 4 equal doses.

More Severe Infections: 17-25 mg/kg/day (8.5-12.5 mg/lb/day) divided into 3 or 4 equal doses.

In children weighing 10 kg or less, ½ teaspoon (37.5 mg) three times a day should be considered the minimum recommended dose.

Serious infections due to anaerobic bacteria are usually treated with clindamycin palmitate HCl phosphate sterile solution. However, in clinically appropriate circumstances, the physician may elect to initiate treatment or continue treatment with clindamycin palmitate HCl pediatric.

NOTE: In cases of β-hemolytic streptococcal infections, treatment should be continued for at least 10 days.

Reconstitution Instructions: When reconstituted with water as follows, each 5 ml (teaspoon) of solution contains clindamycin palmitate HCl equivalent to 75 mg clindamycin.

Reconstitute bottles of 100 ml with **75 ml** of water. Add a large portion of the water and shake vigorously; add the remainder of the water and shake until the solution is uniform.

Storage Conditions: Store at controlled room temperature 15°-30° C (59°-86° F).

Do **NOT** refrigerate the reconstituted solution; when chilled, the solution may thicken and be difficult to pour. The solution is stable for 2 weeks at room temperature.

REFERENCES:

1. Bartlett JG, et al: Antibiotic associated pseudomembranous colitis due to toxin-producing *Clostridia. N Engl J Med*298(10):531-534, 1978. **2.** George RH, et al: Identification of *Clostridium difficile* as a cause of pseudomembranous colitis. *Br Med J* 6114:669-671, 1978. **3.** Larson HE, Price AB: Pseudomembranous colitis presence of clostridial toxin. *Lancet* 8052/3:1312-1314, 1977. **4.** Rifkin GD, Fekety FR, Silva J: Antibiotic-induced colitis implication of a toxin neutralized by *Clostridium sordellii* antitoxin. *Lancet* 8048:1103-1106, 1977. **5.** Bailey WR, Scott EG: Diagnostic Microbiology, The CV Mosby Company, St. Louis, 1978.

HOW SUPPLIED - RATED THERAPEUTICALLY EQUIVALENT:

Capsule, Gelatin - Oral - 75 mg

100's	$44.50	Clindamycin Hcl, Harber Pharm	51432-0910-03
100's	$48.80	Clindamycin Hydrochloride, United Res	00677-1332-01
100's	**$62.89**	**CLEOCIN HCL, Pharmacia & Upjohn**	**00009-0331-02**

Capsule, Gelatin - Oral - 150 mg

16's	$11.26	Clindamycin HCl, H.C.F.A. F F P	99999-0838-01
16's	**$19.75**	**CLEOCIN HCL, Pharmacia & Upjohn**	**00009-0225-01**
100's	$70.43	Clindamycin Hcl, United Res	00677-1333-01
100's	$70.43	Clindamycin HCl, H.C.F.A. F F P	99999-0838-02
100's	$83.76	Clindamycin Hcl, US Trading	56126-0418-11
100's	$85.00	Clindamycin HCl, Teva	00332-3171-09
100's	$96.20	Clindamycin Hcl, Goldline Labs	00182-1202-01
100's	$96.20	Clindamycin Hcl, Aligen Independ	00405-4233-01
100's	$96.29	Clindamycin HCl, Greenstone	59762-3328-01
100's	$96.43	Clindamycin Hcl, Qualitest Pharms	00603-2909-21
100's	$97.64	Clindamycin HCl, Schein Pharm (US)	00364-2337-01
100's	$97.90	Clindamycin Hcl, Major Pharms	00904-3838-60
100's	$99.10	Clindamycin Hcl, Geneva Pharms	00781-2937-01
100's	$103.73	Clindamycin HCl, Rugby	00536-0155-01
100's	$104.96	Clindamycin HCl, HL Moore Drug Exch	00839-7534-06
100's	$112.39	Clindamycin Hcl, Vangard Labs	00615-1310-13
100's	**$116.11**	**CLEOCIN HCL, Pharmacia & Upjohn**	**00009-0225-02**
100's	**$119.75**	**CLEOCIN HCL, Pharmacia & Upjohn**	**00009-0225-03**

HOW SUPPLIED - NOT RATED EQUIVALENT:

Capsule, Gelatin - Oral - 300 mg

16's	**$39.38**	**CLEOCIN HCL, Pharmacia & Upjohn**	**00009-0395-13**
100's	**$231.41**	**CLEOCIN HCL, Pharmacia & Upjohn**	**00009-0395-14**
100's	**$236.14**	**CLEOCIN HCL, Pharmacia & Upjohn**	**00009-0395-02**

Granule, Reconstitution - Oral - 75 mg/5ml

100 ml	**$12.90**	**CLEOCIN PEDIATRIC, Pharmacia & Upjohn**	**00009-0760-04**

CLINDAMYCIN PHOSPHATE *(003129)*

CATEGORIES: Abdominal Abscess; Acne; Acne Vulgaris; Anti-Infectives; Antibiotics; Antimicrobials; Bacterial Vaginosis; Bone Infections; Cellulitis; Dermatologicals; Endometritis; Gynecologic Infections; Infections; Intra-Abdominal Infections; Joint Infections; Lincosamides/Macrolides; Lung Abscess; Osteomyelitis; Peritonitis; Pneumonia; Pulmonary Abscess; Respiratory Tract Infections; Septicemia; Skin Infections; Skin/Mucous Membrane Agents; Topical; Trichomonas; Vaginitis; Vaginosis; Chlamydia*; Herpes*; Herpes Simplex*; FDA Approved 1987 Jan

* Indication not approved by the FDA

BRAND NAMES: *Basocin Akne Gel* (Germany); *Basocin Akne Losung* (Germany); *Cleocin*; Cleocin T; **Cleocin Phosphate**; *Cleocin Vaginal*; *Cindala*; *Clicinin*; *Clinac*; *Dalacin* (England); *Dalacin 2% Vaginal Cream*; *Dalacin T* (Canada, Mexico, England); *Dalacin T Lotion*; *Dalacin T Topical Solution*; *Dalacin V* (Mexico); *Dalacin VC 2%*; *Dalacine T* (France); *Dalagis T*; *Euroclin*; *Sobelin Vaginal Creme* (Germany)

(International brand names outside U.S. in italics)

FORMULARIES: Aetna; BC-BS; CIGNA; FHP; Humana; Kaiser; Medco; Medi-Cal; PruCare; United

WARNING:

Sterile Solution and IV Solution

Clindamycin therapy has been associated with severe colitis which may end fatally. Therefore, it should be reserved for serious infections where less toxic antimicrobial agents are inappropriate, as described in INDICATIONS AND USAGE. It should not be used in patients with nonbacterial infections, such as most upper respiratory tract infections. Studies indicate a toxin(s) produced by Clostridia is one primary cause of antibiotic-associated colitis. Cholestyramine and colestipol resins have been shown to bind the toxin in vitro. See WARNINGS section. The

colitis is usually characterized by severe, persistent diarrhea and severe abdominal cramps and may be associated with the passage of blood and mucus. Endoscopic examination may reveal pseudomembranous colitis. Stool culture for Clostridium difficile and stool assay for C. difficile toxin may be helpful diagnostically.
When significant diarrhea occurs, the drug should be discontinued or, if necessary, continued only with close observation of the patient. Large bowel endoscopy has been recommended.
Antiperistaltic agents such as opiates and diphenoxylate with atropine may prolong and/or worsen the condition. Vancomycin has been found to be effective in the treatment of antibiotic-associated pseudomembranous colitis produced by Clostridium difficile. The usual adult dose is 500 milligrams to 2 grams of vancomycin orally per day in three to four divided doses administered for 7 to 10 days. Cholestyramine or colestipol resins bind vancomycin *in vitro*. If both a resin and vancomycin are to be administered concurrently, it may be advisable to separate the time of administration of each drug.
Diarrhea, colitis, and pseudomembranous colitis have been observed to begin up to several weeks following cessation of therapy with clindamycin.

DESCRIPTION:

Clindamycin phosphate sterile solution in vials contains clindamycin phosphate, a water soluble ester of clindamycin and phosphoric acid. Each ml contains the equivalent of 150 mg clindamycin, 0.5 mg disodium edetate and 9.45 mg benzyl alcohol added as preservative in each ml. Clindamycin is a semisynthetic antibiotic produced by a 7(S)-chloro-substitution of the 7(R)-hydroxyl group of the parent compound lincomycin.

The chemical name of clindamycin phosphate is L-*threo*-α-D-*galacto*-Octopyranoside, methyl 7-chloro-6,7,8-trideoxy-6-[[(1-methyl-4-propyl-2-pyrrolidinyl) carbonyl] amino]-1-thio-, 2-(dihydrogen phosphate), (2S-trans)-.

The molecular formula is $C_{18}H_{34}ClN_2O_8PS$ and the molecular weight is 504.96.

STERILE SOLUTION AND IV SOLUTION

Clindamycin phosphate in the ADD-Vantage Vial is intended for intravenous use only after further dilution with appropriate volume of ADD-Vantage diluent base solution.

Clindamycin phosphate IV solution in the Galaxy plastic container for intravenous use is composed of clindamycin phosphate equivalent to 300, 600 and 900 mg of clindamycin premixed with 5% dextrose as a sterile solution. Disodium edetate has been added at a concentration of 0.04 mg/ml. The pH has been adjusted with sodium hydroxide and/or hydrochloric acid.

The plastic container is fabricated from a specially designed multilayer plastic, PL 2501. Solutions in contact with the plastic container can leach out certain of its chemical components in very small amounts within the expiration period. The suitability of the plastic has been confirmed in tests in animals according to the USP biological tests for plastic containers, as well as by tissue culture toxicity studies.

VAGINAL CREAM

FOR INTRAVAGINAL USE ONLY

NOT FOR OPHTHALMIC, DERMAL, OR ORAL USE

Clindamycin phosphate is a water soluble ester of the semi-synthetic antibiotic produced by a 7(S)-chloro-substitution of the 7(R)-hydroxyl group of the parent antibiotic lincomycin.

Clindamycin phosphate vaginal cream, is a semi-solid, white cream, which contains 2% clindamycin phosphate, USP, at a concentration equivalent to 20 mg clindamycin per gram. The pH of the cream is between 3.0 and 6.0. The cream also contains benzyl alcohol, cetostearyl alcohol, cetyl palmitate, mineral oil, polysorbate 60, propylene glycol, purified water, sorbitan monostearate, and stearic acid.

Each applicator of 5 grams of vaginal cream contains approximately 100 mg of clindamycin phosphate.

TOPICAL SOLUTION, GEL AND LOTION

Clindamycin phosphate topical solution, gel and lotion contain clindamycin phosphate, USP, at a concentration equivalent to 10 mg clindamycin per milliliter. Each Clindamycin Topical Solution pledget applicator contains approximately 1 ml of topical solution.

Clindamycin phosphate is a water soluble ester of the semi-synthetic antibiotic produced by a 7(S)-chloro-substitution of the 7(R)-hydroxyl group of the parent antibiotic lincomycin.

The solution contains isopropyl alcohol 50% v/v, propylene glycol, and water.

The gel contains allantoin, carbomer 934P, methylparaben, polyethylene glycol 400, propylene glycol, sodium hydroxide, and purified water.

The lotion contains cetostearyl alcohol (2.5%); glycerin; glyceryl stearate SE (with potassium monostearate); isostearyl alcohol (2.5%); methylparaben (0.3%); sodium lauroyl sarcosinate; stearic acid; and purified water.

VAGINAL CREAM, TOPICAL SOLUTION, GEL AND LOTION

The chemical name for clindamycin phosphate is Methyl 7-chloro-6,7,8-trideoxy-6-(1-methyl-*trans*-4-propyl-L- 2-pyrrolidinecarboxamido)-1-thio-L-*threo*-α-D-*galacto*-octopyranoside 2-(dihydrogen phosphate).

CLINICAL PHARMACOLOGY:

STERILE SOLUTION AND IV SOLUTION

Biologically inactive clindamycin phosphate is rapidly converted to active clindamycin.

By the end of short-term intravenous infusion, peak serum levels of active clindamycin are reached. Biologically inactive clindamycin phosphate disappears rapidly from the serum; the average disappearance half-life is 6 minutes; however, the serum disappearance half-life of active clindamycin is about 3 hours in adults and 2 ½ hours in children.

After intramuscular injection of clindamycin phosphate, peak levels of active clindamycin are reached within 3 hours in adults and 1 hour in children. Serum level curves may be constructed from IV peak serum levels as given in TABLE 1 by application of disappearance half-lives listed above.

Serum levels of clindamycin can be maintained above the *in vitro* minimum inhibitory concentrations for most indicated organisms by administration of clindamycin phosphate every 8 to 12 hours in adults and every 6 to 8 hours in children, or by continuous intravenous infusion. An equilibrium state is reached by the third dose.

The disappearance half-life of clindamycin is increased slightly in patients with markedly reduced renal or hepatic function. Hemodialysis and peritoneal dialysis are not effective in removing clindamycin from the serum. Dosage schedules need not be modified in the presence of mild or moderate renal or hepatic disease.

No significant levels of clindamycin are attained in the cerebrospinal fluid even in the presence of inflamed meninges.

Serum assays for active clindamycin require an inhibitor to prevent *in vitro* hydrolysis of clindamycin phosphate (TABLE 1).

CLINICAL PHARMACOLOGY: *(cont'd)*

TABLE 1 Average Peak Serum Concentrations After Dosing With Clindamycin Phosphate

Dosage Regimen	Clindamycin mcg/ml	Clindamycin Phosphate mcg/ml
Healthy Adult Males (Post equilibrium)		
300 mg IV in 10 min q8h	7	15
600 mg IV in 20 min q8h**	10	23
900 mg IV in 30 min q12h**	11	29
1200 mg IV in 45 min q12h	14	49
300 mg IM q8h	6	3
600 mg IM q12h*	9	3
Children (first dose)*		
5-7 mg/kg IV in 1 hr	10	
3-5 mg/kg IM	4	
5-7 mg/kg IM	8	

* Data in this group from patients being treated for infection.
** Clindamycin Phosphate in the ADD-Vantage Vial is For Intravenous Use Only

Microbiology: Although clindamycin phosphate is inactive *in vitro*, rapid *in vivo* hydrolysis converts this compound to the antibacterially active clindamycin.

Clindamycin has been shown to have *in vitro* activity against isolates of the following organisms:

Aerobic gram positive cocci, including: *Staphylococcus aureus; Staphylococcus epidermidis* (penicillinase and non-penicillinase producing strains). When tested by *in vitro* methods, some staphylococcal strains originally resistant to erythromycin rapidly develop resistance to clindamycin.

Streptococci (except *Enterococcus faecalis*); Pneumococci

Anaerobic Gram Negative Bacilli, Including: *Bacteroides* species (including *Bacteroides fragilis* group and *Bacteroides melaninogenicus* group); *Fusobacterium* species

Anaerobic Gram Positive Nonsporeforming Bacilli, Including: *Propionibacterium; Eubacterium; Actinomyces* species

Anaerobic and Microaerophilic Gram Positive Cocci, Including: *Peptococcus* species; *Peptostreptococcus* species; Microaerophilic streptococci

Clostridia: Clostridia are more resistant than most anaerobes to clindamycin. Most *Clostridium perfringens* are susceptible, but other species, (*e.g., Clostridium sporogenes* and *Clostridium tertium*) are frequently resistant to clindamycin. Susceptibility testing should be done.

Cross resistance has been demonstrated between clindamycin and lincomycin.

Antagonism has been demonstrated between clindamycin and erythromycin.

***IN VITRO* SUSCEPTIBILITY TESTING**

Disk Diffusion Technique: Quantitative methods that require measurement of zone diameters give the most precise estimates of antibiotic susceptibility. One such procedure[1] has been recommended for use with disks to test susceptibility to clindamycin.

Reports from a laboratory using the standardized single-disk susceptibility test[1] with a 2 mcg clindamycin disk should be interpreted according to the following criteria:

Susceptible organisms produce zones of 17 mm or greater, indicating that the tested organism is likely to respond to therapy.

Organisms of intermediate susceptibility produce zones of 15-16 mm, indicating that the tested organism would be susceptible if a high dosage is used or if the infection is confined to tissues and fluids (*e.g.,* urine), in which high antibiotic levels are attained.

Resistant organisms produce zones of 14 mm or less, indicating that other therapy should be selected.

Standardized procedures require the use of control organisms. The 2 mcg clindamycin disk should give a zone diameter between 24 and 30 mm for*S. aureus* ATCC 25923.

Dilution Techniques: A bacterial isolate may be considered susceptible if the minimum inhibitory concentration (MIC) for clindamycin is not more than 1.6 mcg/ml. Organisms are considered moderately susceptible if the MIC is greater than 1.6 mcg/ml and less than or equal to 4.8 mcg/ml. Organisms are considered resistant if the MIC is greater than 4.8 mcg per ml.

The range of MIC's for the control strains are as follows:

S. aureus ATCC 29213, 0.06—0.25 mcg/ml.

E. faecalis ATCC 29212, 4.0—16 mcg/ml.

For anaerobic bacteria the minimum inhibitory concentration (MIC) of clindamycin can be determined by agar dilution and broth dilution (including microdilution) techniques.[2] If MICs are not determined routinely, the disk broth method is recommended for routine use. THE KIRBY-BAUER DISK DIFFUSION METHOD AND ITS INTERPRETIVE STANDARDS ARE NOT RECOMMENDED FOR ANAEROBES.

VAGINAL CREAM

Following a once a day intravaginal dose of 100 mg of clindamycin phosphate vaginal cream 2%, administered to 6 healthy female volunteers for 7 days, approximately 5% (range 0.6% to 11%) of the administered dose was absorbed systemically. The peak serum clindamycin concentration observed on the first day averaged 18 ng/ml (range 4 to 47 ng/ml) and averaged 25 ng/ml (range 6 to 61 ng/ml) on day 7. These peak concentrations were attained in approximately 10 hours post-dosing (range 4-24 hours).

Following a once a day intravaginal dose of 100 mg of clindamycin phosphate vaginal cream 2%, administered for 7 consecutive days to 5 women with bacterial vaginosis, absorption was slower and less variable than that observed in healthy females. Approximately 5% (range 2% to 8%) of the dose was absorbed systemically. The peak serum clindamycin concentration observed on the first day averaged 13 ng/ml (range 3 to 34 ng/ml) and averaged 16 ng/ml (range 7 to 26 ng/ml) on day 7. These peak concentrations were attained in approximately 16 hours post-dosing (range 8-24 hours).

There was little or no systemic accumulation of clindamycin after repeated vaginal dosing of clindamycin phosphate vaginal cream 2%. The systemic $t_{1/2}$ was 1.5 to 2.6 hours.

Microbiology: Clindamycin inhibits bacterial protein synthesis by its action at the bacterial ribosome. The antibiotic binds preferentially to the 50S ribosomal subunit and affects the process of peptide chain initiation. Although clindamycin phosphate is inactive *in vitro*, rapid *in vivo* hydrolysis converts this compound to the antibacterially active clindamycin.

Culture and sensitivity testing of bacteria are not routinely performed to establish the diagnosis of bacterial vaginosis. (See INDICATIONS AND USAGE.) Standard methodology for the susceptibility testing of the potential bacterial vaginosis pathogens, *Gardnerella vaginalis, Mobiluncus* spp., or *Mycoplasma hominis*, has not been defined.

Nonetheless, clindamycin is an antimicrobial agent active *in vitro* against most strains of the following organisms that have been reported to be associated with bacterial vaginosis: *Bacteroides* spp.;*Gardnerella vaginalis; Mobiluncus* spp.; *Mycoplasma hominis; Peptostreptococcus* spp.

CLINICAL PHARMACOLOGY: *(cont'd)*

TOPICAL SOLUTION, GEL AND LOTION

Although clindamycin phosphate is inactive *in vitro,* rapid *in vivo* hydrolysis converts this compound to the antibacterially active clindamycin.

Cross resistance has been demonstrated between clindamycin and lincomycin.

Antagonism has been demonstrated between clindamycin and erythromycin.

Following multiple topical applications of clindamycin phosphate at a concentration equivalent to 10 mg clindamycin per ml in an isopropyl alcohol and water solution, very low levels of clindamycin are present in the serum (0.3 ng/ml) and less than 0.2% of the dose is recovered in urine as clindamycin.

Clindamycin activity has been demonstrated in comedones from acne patients. The mean concentration of antibiotic activity in extracted comedones after application of clindamycin Phosphate Topical Solution for 4 weeks was 597 mcg/g of comedonal material (range 0-1490). Clindamycin *in vitro* inhibits all *Propionibacterium acnes* cultures tested (MICs 0.4 mcg/ml). Free fatty acids on the skin surface have been decreased from approximately 14% to 2% following application of clindamycin.

CLINICAL STUDIES:

VAGINAL CREAM

In clinical trials, approximately 4% of non-pregnant patients treated with clindamycin phosphate vaginal cream, discontinued therapy due to drug-related adverse events. Medical events judged to be related, probably related, or possibly related to vaginally administered clindamycin phosphate vaginal cream 2%, were reported for 249/1020 (24%) non-pregnant patients. Unless percentage are otherwise stipulated, the incidence of individual adverse reactions listed below was less than 1%:

Genital Tract: Cervicitis/vaginitis, symptomatic (16%): *Candida albicans* (11%); *Trichomonas vaginalis* (1%); Vulvar irritation (6%)

Central Nervous System: Dizziness, headache, vertigo

Dermatologic: Rash

Gastrointestinal: Heartburn, nausea, vomiting, diarrhea, constipation, abdominal pain

Hypersensitivity: Urticaria

Other Clindamycin Formulations: Other effects that have been reported in association with the use of topical (dermal) formulations of clindamycin include severe colitis (including pseudomembranous colitis), contact dermatitis, skin irritation (*e.g.,* erythema, peeling and burning) oily skin, gram-negative folliculitis, abdominal pain, and gastrointestinal disturbances.

Clindamycin vaginal cream affords minimal peak serum levels and systemic exposure (A.U.C.'s) of clindamycin compared to 100 mg oral clindamycin dosing. Although these lower levels of exposure are less likely to produce the common reactions seen with oral clindamycin, the possibility of these and other reactions cannot be excluded presently. Data from well-controlled trials directly comparing clindamycin administered orally to clindamycin administered vaginally are not available.

The following adverse reactions and altered laboratory tests have been reported with the oral or parenteral use of clindamycin:

Gastrointestinal: Abdominal pain, esophagitis, nausea, vomiting, and diarrhea. (See WARNINGS.)

Hematopoietic: Transient neutropenia (leukopenia), eosinophilia, agranulocytosis, and thrombocytopenia have been reported. No direct etiologic relationship to concurrent clindamycin therapy could be made in any of these reports.

Hypersensitivity Reactions: Maculopapular rash and urticaria have been observed during drug therapy. Generalized mild to moderate morbilliform-like skin rashes are the most frequently reported of all adverse reactions. Rare instances of erythema multiforme, some resembling Stevens-Johnson syndrome, have been associated with clindamycin. A few cases of anaphylactoid reactions have been reported. If a hypersensitivity reaction occurs, the drug should be discontinued.

Liver: Jaundice and abnormalities in liver function tests have been observed during clindamycin therapy.

Musculoskeletal: Rare instances of polyarthritis have been reported.

Renal: Although no direct relationship of clindamycin to renal damage has been established, renal dysfunction as evidenced by azotemia, oliguria, and/or proteinuria has been observed in rare instances.

TOPICAL SOLUTION, GEL AND LOTION

In 18 clinical studies of various formulations of clindamycin phosphate using placebo vehicle and/or active comparator drugs as controls, patients experienced a number of treatment emergent adverse dermatologic events (see TABLE 2).

TABLE 2 Number of Patients Reporting Events

Treatment Emergent Adverse Event	Solution n=553 (%)	Gel n=148 (%)	Lotion n=160 (%)
Burning	62 (11)	15 (10)	17 (11)
Itching	36 (7)	15 (10)	17 (11)
Burning/Itching	60 (11)	* (-)	* (-)
Dryness	105 (19)	34 (23)	29 (18)
Erythema	86 (16)	10 (7)	22 (14)
Oiliness/Oily Skin	8 (1)	26 (18)	12†(10)
Peeling	61 (11)	*(-)	11 (7)

* not recorded
† of 126 subjects

Orally and parenterally administered clindamycin has been associated with severe colitis which may end fatally. Cases of diarrhea, bloody diarrhea and colitis (including pseudomembranous colitis) have been reported as adverse reactions in patients treated with oral and parenteral formulations of clindamycin and rarely with topical clindamycin (see WARNINGS.)

Abdominal pain and gastrointestinal disturbances as well as gram-negative folliculitis have also been reported in association with the use of topical formulations of clindamycin.

INDICATIONS AND USAGE:

STERILE SOLUTION AND IV SOLUTION

Clindamycin phosphate products are indicated in the treatment of serious infections caused by susceptible anaerobic bacteria.

Clindamycin phosphate products are also indicated in the treatment of serious infections due to susceptible strains of streptococci, pneumococci, and staphylococci. Its use should be reserved for penicillin-allergic patients or other patients for whom, in the judgment of the physician, a penicillin is inappropriate. Because of the risk of antibiotic-associated

INDICATIONS AND USAGE: *(cont'd)*

pseudomembranous colitis, as described in the BOXED WARNING, before selecting clindamycin the physician should consider the nature of the infection and the suitability of less toxic alternatives (*e.g.,* erythromycin).

Bacteriologic studies should be performed to determine the causative organisms and their susceptibility to clindamycin.

Indicated surgical procedures should be performed in conjunction with antibiotic therapy.

Clindamycin phosphate is indicated in the treatment of serious infections caused by susceptible strains of the designated organisms in the conditions listed below:

Lower respiratory tract infections including pneumonia, empyema, and lung abscess caused by anaerobes, *Streptococcus pneumoniae,* other streptococci (except *E. faecalis*), and *Staphylococcus aureus.*

Skin and skin structure infections caused by *Streptococcus pyogenes, Staphylococcus aureus,* and anaerobes.

Gynecological infections including endometritis, nongonococcal tubo-ovarian abscess, pelvic cellulitis, and postsurgical vaginal cuff infection caused by susceptible anaerobes.

Intra-abdominal infections including peritonitis and intra-abdominal abscess caused by susceptible anaerobic organisms.

Septicemia caused by *Staphylococcus aureus,* streptococci (except *Enterococcus faecalis*), and susceptible anaerobes.

Bone and joint infections including acute hematogenous osteomyelitis caused by *Staphylococcus aureus* and as adjunctive therapy in the surgical treatment of chronic bone and joint infections due to susceptible organisms.

VAGINAL CREAM

Clindamycin phosphate vaginal cream, is indicated in the treatment of bacterial vaginosis (formerly referred to as *Haemophilus* vaginitis, *Gardnerella* vaginitis, nonspecific vaginitis, *Corynebacterium* vaginitis, or anaerobic vaginosis).

NOTE: For purposes of this indication, a clinical diagnosis of bacterial vaginosis is defined by the presence of a homogeneous vaginal discharge that (a) has a pH of greater than 4.5, (b) emits a "fishy" amine odor when mixed with a 10% KOH solution, and (c) contains clue cells on microscopic examination. Gram's stain results consistent with a diagnosis of bacterial vaginosis include (a) markedly reduced or absent *Lactobacillus* morphology, (b) predominance of *Gardnerella* morphotype, and (c) absent or few white blood cells.

Other pathogens commonly associated with vulvovaginitis, (*e.g., Trichomonas vaginalis, Chlamydia trachomatis, N. gonorrhoeae, Candida albicans,* and *Herpes simplex* virus) should be ruled out.

TOPICAL SOLUTION, GEL AND LOTION

Clindamycin phosphate topical solution, gel and lotion are indicated in the treatment of acne vulgaris. In view of the potential for diarrhea, bloody diarrhea and pseudomembranous colitis, the physician should consider whether other agents are more appropriate. (See CONTRAINDICATIONS, WARNINGS, and ADVERSE REACTIONS.)

CONTRAINDICATIONS:

STERILE SOLUTION AND IV SOLUTION

This drug is contraindicated in individuals with a history of hypersensitivity to preparations containing clindamycin or lincomycin.

VAGINAL CREAM

Clindamycin phosphate vaginal cream, is contraindicated in individuals with a history of hypersensitivity to clindamycin, lincomycin, or any of the components of this vaginal cream. Clindamycin phosphate vaginal cream, is also contraindicated in individuals with a history of regional enteritis, ulcerative colitis, or a history of "antibiotic-associated" colitis.

TOPICAL SOLUTION, GEL AND LOTION

Clindamycin phosphate topical solution, gel and lotion are contraindicated in individuals with a history of hypersensitivity to preparations containing clindamycin or lincomycin, a history of regional enteritis or ulcerative colitis, or a history of antibiotic-associated colitis.

WARNINGS:

STERILE SOLUTION AND IV SOLUTION

See BOXED WARNING. Studies indicate a toxin(s) produced by Clostridia is one primary cause of antibiotic-associated colitis.[3-7] Cholestyramine and colestipol resins have been shown to bind the toxin *in vitro.* Mild cases of colitis may respond to drug discontinuance alone. Moderate to severe cases should be managed promptly with fluid, electrolyte and protein supplementation as indicated. Vancomycin has been found to be effective in the treatment of antibiotic-associated pseudomembranous colitis produced by *Clostridium difficile.* The usual adult dose is 500 milligrams to 2 grams of vancomycin orally per day in three to four divided doses administered for 7 to 10 days. Cholestyramine or colestipol resins bind vancomycin *in vitro.* If both a resin and vancomycin are to be administered concurrently, it may be advisable to separate the time of administration of each drug. Systemic corticoids and corticoid retention enemas may help relieve the colitis. Other causes of colitis should also be considered.

A careful inquiry should be made concerning previous sensitivities to drugs and other allergens.

This product contains benzyl alcohol as a preservative. Benzyl alcohol has been associated with a fatal "Gasping Syndrome" in premature infants. (See PRECAUTIONS, Pediatric Use.)

Usage in Meningitis: Since clindamycin does not diffuse adequately into the cerebrospinal fluid, the drug should not be used in the treatment of meningitis.

SERIOUS ANAPHYLACTOID REACTIONS REQUIRE IMMEDIATE EMERGENCY TREATMENT WITH EPINEPHRINE. OXYGEN AND INTRAVENOUS CORTICOSTEROIDS SHOULD ALSO BE ADMINISTERED AS INDICATED.

VAGINAL CREAM

Pseudomembranous colitis has been reported with nearly all antibacterial agents, including clindamycin, and may range in severity from mild to life-threatening. Orally and parenterally administered clindamycin has been associated with severe colitis which may end fatally. Diarrhea, bloody diarrhea, and colitis (including pseudomembranous colitis) have been reported with the use of orally and parenterally administered clindamycin, as well as with topical (dermal) formulations of clindamycin. Therefore, it is important to consider this diagnosis in patients who present with diarrhea subsequent to the administration of clindamycin, even when administered by the vaginal route, because approximately 5% of the clindamycin dose is systemically absorbed from the vagina.

Treatment with antibacterial agents alters the normal flora of the colon and may permit overgrowth of clostridia. Studies indicate that a toxin produced by *Clostridium difficile* is a primary cause of "antibiotic-associated colitis".

After the diagnosis of pseudomembranous colitis has been established, therapeutic measures should be initiated. Mild cases of pseudomembranous colitis usually respond to discontinuation of the drug alone. In moderate to severe cases, consideration should be given to management with fluids and electrolytes, protein supplementation, and treatment with an antibacterial drug clinically effective against *Clostridium difficile* colitis.

WARNINGS: *(cont'd)*

Onset of pseudomembranous colitis symptoms may occur during or after antimicrobial treatment.

This cream contains mineral oil. Mineral oil may weaken latex or rubber products such as condoms or vaginal contraceptive diaphragms; therefore, use of such products within 72 hours following treatment with clindamycin phosphate vaginal cream, is not recommended.

TOPICAL SOLUTION, GEL AND LOTION

Orally and parenterally administered clindamycin has been associated with severe colitis which may result in patient death. Use of the topical formulation of clindamycin results in absorption of the antibiotic from the skin surface. Diarrhea, bloody diarrhea, and colitis (including pseudomembranous colitis) have been reported with the use of topical and systemic clindamycin.

Studies indicate a toxin(s) produced by clostridia is one primary cause of antibiotic-associated colitis. The colitis is usually characterized by severe persistent diarrhea and severe abdominal cramps and may be associated with the passage of blood and mucus. Endoscopic examination may reveal pseudomembranous colitis. Stool culture for *Clostridium difficile* and stool assay for *C. difficile* toxin may be helpful diagnostically.

When significant diarrhea occurs, the drug should be discontinued. Large bowel endoscopy should be considered to establish a definitive diagnosis in cases of severe diarrhea.

Antiperistaltic agents such as opiates and diphenoxylate with atropine may prolong and/or worsen the condition. Vancomycin has been found to be effective in the treatment of antibiotic-associated pseudomembranous colitis produced by *Clostridium difficile*. The usual adult dosage is 500 milligrams to 2 grams of vancomycin orally per day in three to four divided doses administered for 7 to 10 days. Cholestyramine or colestipol resins bind vancomycin *in vitro*. If both a resin and vancomycin are to be administered concurrently, it may be advisable to separate the time of administration of each drug.

Diarrhea, colitis, and pseudomembranous colitis have been observed to begin up to several weeks following cessation of oral and parenteral therapy with clindamycin.

PRECAUTIONS:

GENERAL

Sterile Solution and IV Solution

Review of experience to date suggests that a subgroup of older patients with associated severe illness may tolerate diarrhea less well. When clindamycin is indicated in these patients, they should be carefully monitored for change in bowel frequency.

Clindamycin phosphate products should be prescribed with caution in individuals with a history of gastrointestinal disease, particularly colitis.

Clindamycin phosphate should be prescribed with caution in atopic individuals.

Certain infections may require incision and drainage or other indicated surgical procedures in addition to antibiotic therapy.

The use of clindamycin phosphate may result in overgrowth of nonsusceptible organisms—particularly yeasts. Should superinfections occur, appropriate measures should be taken as indicated by the clinical situation.

Clindamycin phosphate should not be injected intravenously undiluted as a bolus, but should be infused over a least 10-60 minutes as directed in the DOSAGE AND ADMINISTRATION section.

Patients with very severe renal disease and/or very severe hepatic disease accompanied by severe metabolic aberrations should be dosed with caution, and serum clindamycin levels monitored during high-dose therapy (see OVERDOSAGE).

Vaginal Cream

Clindamycin phosphate vaginal cream, contains ingredients that will cause burning and irritation of the eye. In the event of accidental contact with the eye, rinse the eye with copious amounts of cool tap water.

The use of clindamycin phosphate vaginal cream may result in the overgrowth of nonsusceptible organisms—particularly yeasts—in the vagina. Approximately 16% of patients treated with clindamycin phosphate vaginal cream developed symptomatic cervicitis/vaginitis with 11% of patients developing cervicitis/vaginitis secondary to *C. albicans*.

Topical Solution, Gel and Lotion

Clindamycin phosphate topical solution contains an alcohol base which will cause burning and irritation of the eye. In the event of accidental contact with sensitive surfaces (eye, abraded skin, mucous membranes), bathe with copious amounts of cool tap water. The solution has an unpleasant taste and caution should be exercised when applying medication around the mouth.

Clindamycin phosphate should be prescribed with caution in atopic individuals.

VAGINAL CREAM

Information for the Patient: The patient should be instructed not to engage in vaginal intercourse during treatment with this product.

Carcinogenesis, Mutagenesis, and Impairment of Fertility: Long term studies in animals have not been performed with clindamycin to evaluate carcinogenic potential. Genotoxicity tests performed included a rat micronucleus test and an Ames test. Both tests were negative. Fertility studies in rats treated orally with up to 300 mg/kg/day (31 times the human exposure based on mg/m^2) revealed no effects on fertility or mating ability.

Pregnancy, Teratogenic Effects, Pregnancy Category B: Reproduction studies have been performed in rats and mice using oral and parenteral doses of clindamycin up to 600 mg/kg/day (62 and 25 times, respectively, the maximum human exposure based on mg/m^2) and have revealed no evidence of harm to the fetus due to clindamycin. In one mouse strain, cleft palates were observed in treated fetuses; this outcome was not produced in other mouse strains or in other species and is, therefore, considered to be a strain specific effect.

There are, however, no adequate and well-controlled studies in pregnant women. Because animal reproduction studies are not always predictive of human response, this drug should be used during pregnancy only if clearly needed.

Nursing Mothers: It is not known if clindamycin is excreted in human milk following the use of vaginally administered clindamycin phosphate. However, after oral or parenteral administration, clindamycin has been detected in human milk.

Because of the potential for serious adverse reactions in nursing infants from clindamycin phosphate, a decision should be made whether to discontinue nursing or to discontinue the drug, taking into account the importance of the drug to the mother.

Pediatric Use: Safety and effectiveness in children have not been established.

STERILE SOLUTION AND IV SOLUTION

Laboratory Tests: During prolonged therapy periodic liver and kidney function tests and blood counts should be performed.

Usage in Pregnancy: Safety for use in pregnancy has not been established.

Nursing Mothers: Clindamycin has been reported to appear in breast milk in the range of 0.7 to 3.8 mcg/ml at dosages of 150 mg orally to 600 mg intravenously. Because of the potential for adverse reactions due to clindamycin in neonates (see Pediatric Use), the decision to discontinue the drug should be made, taking into account the importance of the drug to the mother.

PRECAUTIONS: *(cont'd)*

Pediatric Use: When clindamycin phosphate sterile solution is administered to newborns, infants, and children, appropriate monitoring of organ system functions is desirable.

This product contains benzyl alcohol as a preservative. Benzyl alcohol has been associated with a fatal "Gasping Syndrome" in premature infants.

The potential for the toxic effect in children from chemicals that may leach from the single dose premixed IV preparation in plastic has not been evaluated.

TOPICAL SOLUTION, GEL AND LOTION

Pregnancy, Teratogenic Effects, Pregnancy Category B: Reproduction studies have been performed in rats and mice using subcutaneous and oral doses of clindamycin ranging from 100 to 600 mg/kg/day and have revealed no evidence of impaired fertility or harm to the fetus due to clindamycin. There are, however, no adequate and well-controlled studies in pregnant women. Because animal reproduction studies are not always predictive of human response, this drug should be used during pregnancy only if clearly needed.

Nursing Mothers: It is not known whether clindamycin is excreted in human milk following use of clindamycin phosphate. However, orally and parenterally administered clindamycin has been reported to appear in breast milk. Because of the potential for serious adverse reactions in nursing infants, a decision should be made whether to discontinue nursing or to discontinue the drug, taking into account the importance of the drug to the mother.

Pediatric Use: Safety and effectiveness in children under the age of 12 has not been established.

DRUG INTERACTIONS:

Clindamycin has been shown to have neuromuscular blocking properties that may enhance the action of other neuromuscular blocking agents. Therefore, it should be used with caution in patients receiving such agents.

Antagonism has been demonstrated between clindamycin and erythromycin *in vitro*. Because of possible clinical significance, the two drugs should not be administered concurrently.

ADVERSE REACTIONS:

STERILE SOLUTION AND IV SOLUTION

The following reactions have been reported with the use of clindamycin.

Gastrointestinal: Antibiotic-associated colitis (see WARNINGS), abdominal pain, nausea, and vomiting. An unpleasant or metallic taste occasionally has been reported after intravenous administration of the higher doses of clindamycin phosphate.

Hypersensitivity Reactions: Maculopapular rash and urticaria have been observed during drug therapy. Generalized mild to moderate morbilliform-like skin rashes are the most frequently reported of all adverse reactions. Rare instances of erythema multiforme, some resembling Stevens-Johnson syndrome, have been associated with clindamycin. A few cases of anaphylactoid reactions have been reported. If a hypersensitivity reaction occurs, the drug should be discontinued. The usual agents (epinephrine, corticosteroids, antihistamines) should be available for emergency treatment of serious reactions.

Liver: Jaundice and abnormalities in liver function tests have been observed during clindamycin therapy.

Renal: Although no direct relationship of clindamycin to renal damage has been established, renal dysfunction as evidenced by azotemia, oliguria, and/or proteinuria has been observed in rare instances.

Hematopoietic: Transient neutropenia (leukopenia) and eosinophilia have been reported. Reports of agranulocytosis and thrombocytopenia have been made. No direct etiologic relationship to concurrent clindamycin therapy could be made in any of the foregoing.

Local Reactions: Pain, induration and sterile abscess have been reported after intramuscular injection and thrombophlebitis after intravenous infusion. Reactions can be minimized or avoided by giving deep intramuscular injections and avoiding prolonged use of indwelling intravenous catheters.

Musculoskeletal: Rare instances of polyarthritis have been reported.

Cardiovascular: Rare instances of cardiopulmonary arrest and hypotension have been reported following too rapid intravenous administration. (See DOSAGE AND ADMINISTRATION).

OVERDOSAGE:

STERILE SOLUTION AND IV SOLUTION

Hemodialysis and peritoneal dialysis are not effective in removing clindamycin from the serum.

VAGINAL CREAM

Vaginally applied clindamycin phosphate vaginal cream 2%, could be absorbed in sufficient amounts to produce systemic effects. (See WARNINGS.)

TOPICAL SOLUTION, GEL AND LOTION

Topically applied clindamycin phosphate can be absorbed in sufficient amounts to produce systemic effects. (See WARNINGS.)

DOSAGE AND ADMINISTRATION:

STERILE SOLUTION AND IV SOLUTION

If diarrhea occurs during therapy, this antibiotic should be discontinued (see BOXED WARNING).

Adults: *Parenteral (IM or IV Administration):* Serious infections due to aerobic gram-positive cocci and the more susceptible anaerobes (NOT generally including *Bacteroides fragilis, Peptococcus* species and *Clostridium* species other than *Clostridium perfringens*): 600-1200 mg/day in 2, 3 or 4 equal doses.

More severe infections, particularly those due to proven or suspected *Bacteroides fragilis, Peptococcus* species, or *Clostridium* species other than *Clostridium perfringens:* 1200-2700 mg/day in 2, 3 or 4 equal doses.

For more serious infections, these doses may have to be increased. In life-threatening situations due to either aerobes or anaerobes these doses may be increased. Doses of as much as 4800 mg daily have been given intravenously to adults. See Dilution and Infusion Rates section.

Single intramuscular injections of greater than 600 mg are not recommended.

Alternatively, drug may be administered in the form of a single rapid infusion of the first dose followed by continuous IV infusion as follows (TABLE 3):

TABLE 3

To maintain serum clindamycin levels	Rapid infusion rate	Maintenance infusion rate
Above 4 mcg/ml	10 mg/min for 30 min	0.75 mg/min
Above 5 mcg/ml	15 mg/min for 30 min	1.00 mg/min
Above 6 mcg/ml	20 mg/min for 30 min	1.25 mg/min

DOSAGE AND ADMINISTRATION: *(cont'd)*

Neonates (less than 1 month): 15 to 20 mg/kg/day in 3 to 4 equal doses. The lower dosage may be adequate for small prematures.

Children (over 1 month of age): Parenteral (IM or IV) administration: 20 to 40 mg/kg/day in 3 or 4 equal doses. The higher doses would be used for more severe infections. As an alternative to dosing on a body weight basis, children may be dosed on the basis of square meters body surface: 350 mg/m^2/day for serious infections and 450 mg/m^2/day for more severe infections.

Parenteral therapy may be changed to oral clindamycin palmitate hydrochloride or clindamycin hydrochloride when the condition warrants and at the discretion of the physician.

In cases of β-hemolytic streptococcal infections, treatment should be continued for at least 10 days.

Dilution and Infusion Rates: Clindamycin phosphate must be diluted prior to IV administration. The concentration of clindamycin in diluent for infusion should not exceed 18 mg per ml. Infusion rates should not exceed 30 mg per minute. The usual infusion dilutions and rates are as follows (TABLE 4):

TABLE 4

Dose	Diluent	Time
300 mg	50 ml	10 min
600 mg	50 ml	20 min
900 mg	50-100 ml	30 min
1200 mg	100 ml	40 min

Administration of more than 1200 mg in a single 1-hour infusion is not recommended.

Parenteral drug products should be inspected visually for particulate matter and discoloration prior to administration, whenever solution and container permit.

Dilution and Compatibility: Physical and biological compatibility studies monitored for 24 hours at room temperature have demonstrated no inactivation or incompatibility with the use of clindamycin phosphate sterile solution in IV solutions containing sodium chloride, glucose, calcium or potassium, and solutions containing vitamin B complex in concentrations usually used clinically. No incompatibility has been demonstrated with the antibiotics cephalothin, kanamycin, gentamicin, penicillin or carbenicillin.

The following drugs are physically incompatible with clindamycin phosphate: ampicillin sodium, phenytoin sodium, barbiturates, aminophylline, calcium gluconate, and magnesium sulfate.

The compatibility and duration of stability of drug admixtures will vary depending on concentration and other conditions. For current information regarding compatibilities of clindamycin phosphate under specific conditions, please contact the Medical Correspondence Unit, The Upjohn Company.

PHYSICO-CHEMICAL STABILITY OF DILUTED SOLUTIONS OF CLINDAMYCIN PHOSPHATE

Room Temperature: 6, 9 and 12 mg/ml (equivalent to clindamycin base) in dextrose 5% in water, sodium chloride 0.9%, or lactated ringers in glass bottles or minibags, demonstrated physical and chemical stability for at least 16 days at 25°C. Also, 18 mg/ml (equivalent to clindamycin base) in dextrose 5% in water, in minibags, demonstrated physical and chemical stability for at least 16 days at 25°C.

Refrigeration: 6, 9 and 12 mg/ml (equivalent to clindamycin base) in dextrose 5% in water, sodium chloride 0.9%, or Lactated Ringers in glass bottles or minibags, demonstrated physical and chemical stability for at least 32 days at 4° C.

Frozen: 6, 9 and 12 mg/ml (equivalent to clindamycin base) in dextrose 5% in water, sodium chloride 0.9%, or Lactated Ringers in minibags demonstrated physical and chemical stability for at least eight weeks at -10° C.

Frozen solutions should be thawed at room temperature and not refrozen.

DIRECTIONS FOR DISPENSING

Pharmacy Bulk Package: Not for direct infusion

The pharmacy bulk package is for use in a pharmacy admixture service only under a laminar flow hood. Entry into the vial should be made with a small diameter sterile transfer set or other small diameter sterile dispensing device, and contents dispensed in aliquots using aseptic technique. Multiple entries with a needle and syringe are not recommended. AFTER ENTRY USE ENTIRE CONTENTS OF VIAL PROMPTLY. ANY UNUSED PORTION MUST BE DISCARDED WITHIN 24 HOURS AFTER INITIAL ENTRY.

DIRECTIONS FOR USE

Clindamycin Phosphate IV Solution in Galaxy Plastic Container

Premixed clindamycin phosphate IV Solution is for intravenous administration using sterile equipment. Check for minute leaks prior to use by squeezing bag firmly. If leaks are found, discard solution as sterility may be impaired. Do not add supplementary medication. Parenteral drug products should be inspected visually for particulate matter and discoloration prior to administration whenever solution and container permit. Do not use unless solution is clear and seal is intact.

Caution: Do not use plastic containers in series connections. Such use could result in air embolism due to residual air being drawn from the primary container before administration of the fluid from the secondary container is complete.

Preparation for Administration:

1. Suspend container from eyelet support.

2. Remove protector from outlet port at bottom of container.

3. Attach administration set. Refer to complete directions accompanying set.

Preparation of clindamycin phosphate in ADD-Vantage‡ System-For IV Use Only. Clindamycin phosphate 600 mg and 900 mg may be reconstituted in 50 ml or 100 ml, respectively, of 5% Dextrose or 0.9% Sodium Chloride in the ADD-diluent container. Refer to separate instructions for ADD-Vantage System.

Store at controlled room temperature 15°-30° C (59°-86° F).

Exposure of pharmaceutical products to heat should be minimized. It is recommended that Galaxy plastic containers be stored at room temperature (25°C). Avoid temperatures above 30°C.

Vaginal Cream

The recommended dose is one applicatorful of clindamycin phosphate vaginal cream 2%, (5 grams containing approximately 100 mg of clindamycin phosphate) intravaginally, preferably at bedtime, for seven consecutive days.

Store at controlled room temperature 15° to 30° C (59° to 86° F). Protect from freezing.

Topical Solution, Gel and Lotion

Apply a thin film of clindamycin phosphate topical solution, lotion, gel, or use a clindamycin phosphate topical solution pledget for the application of clindamycin phosphate twice daily to affected area. More than one pledget may be used. Each pledget should be used only once and then be discarded.

Lotion: Shake well immediately before using.

DOSAGE AND ADMINISTRATION: *(cont'd)*

Pledget: Remove pledget from foil just before use. Do not use if seal is broken. Discard after single use. Keep all liquid dosage forms in containers tightly closed.

Store at controlled room temperature 15° to 30° C (59° to 86° F).

Protect from freezing.

REFERENCES:

1. Bauer AW, Kirby WMM, Sherris JC, Turck M; Antibiotic susceptibility testing by a standardized single disk method. *Am. J. Clin. Path.,* **45**:493-496; 1966. Standardized Disk Susceptibility Test, *Federal Register*, **37**:20527-29, 1972. **2.** National Committee for Clinical Lab. Standards. Methods for Antimicrobial Susceptibility Testing of Anaerobic Bacteria—Second Edition; Tentative Standard. NCCLS publication M11-T2. Villanova, PA; NCCLS; 1988. **3.** Bartlett JG, et al: Antibiotic associated pseudomembranous colitis due to toxin-producing *Clostridia. N Eng J Med* **298** (10): 531-534, 1978. **4.** George RH, et al: Identification of *Clostridium difficile* as a cause of pseudomembranous colitis. *Br Med J* **6114**:669-671, 1978. **5.** Larson HE, Price AB: Pseudomembranous colitis presence of clostridial toxin. *Lancet* **8052/3**:1312-1314, 1977. **6.** Rifkin GD, Fekety FR, Silva J: Antibiotic-induced colitis-implication of a toxin neutralized by *Clostridium sordellii* antitoxin. *Lancet* **8048**:1103-1106, 1977. **7.** Bailey WR, Scott EG: Diagnostic Microbiology. The CV Mosby Company, St. Louis, 1978.

HOW SUPPLIED - RATED THERAPEUTICALLY EQUIVALENT:

Injection, Solution - Intramuscular; - 150 mg/ml

2 ml	$10.69	Clindamycin Phosphate 300, Abbott	00074-4050-01
2 ml	$10.78	Clindamycin Phosphate 300, Abbott	00074-4053-03
2 ml	$140.63	Clindamycin Phosphate, Solopak Labs	39769-0226-02
2 ml x 25	$130.53	Clindamycin Phosphate, Vial, Marsam	00209-2052-24
2 ml x 25	$130.63	Clindamycin Phosphate, Bristol Myers Squibb	00003-2942-11
2 ml x 25	$140.63	Clindamycin Phosphate, Astra USA	00186-1450-04
2 ml x 25	$150.60	Clindamycin Phosphate, Gensia Labs	00703-9102-04
2 ml x 25	**$189.53**	**CLEOCIN PHOSPHATE, Pharmacia & Upjohn**	**00009-0870-26**
4 ml	**$14.71**	**CLEOCIN PHOSPHATE, Pharmacia & Upjohn**	**00009-3124-01**
4 ml	$19.59	Clindamycin Phosphate 600, Abbott	00074-4051-01
4 ml	$19.81	Clindamycin Phosphate 600, Abbott	00074-4054-03
4 ml	$260.94	Clindamycin Phosphate, Solopak Labs	39769-0226-04
4 ml x 25	$196.88	Clindamycin Phosphate, Du Pont Merck	00590-5110-65
4 ml x 25	$242.40	Clindamycin Phosphate, Vial, Marsam	00209-2102-24
4 ml x 25	$242.50	Clindamycin Phosphate, Bristol Myers Squibb	00003-2942-21
4 ml x 25	$250.00	Clindamycin Phosphate, Astra USA	00186-1451-04
4 ml x 25	$268.80	Clindamycin Phosphate, Gensia Labs	00703-9110-04
4 ml x 25	**$346.84**	**CLEOCIN PHOSPHATE, Pharmacia & Upjohn**	**00009-0775-26**
6 ml	$26.23	Clindamycin Phosphate 900, Abbott	00074-4052-01
6 ml	$26.48	CLINDAMYLIN PHOSPHATE 900, Abbott	00074-4055-03
6 ml	$346.88	Clindamycin Phosphate, Solopak Labs	39769-0226-06
6 ml x 25	$262.50	Clindamycin Phosphate, Du Pont Merck	00590-5110-73
6 ml x 25	$315.78	Clindamycin Phosphate, Vial, Marsam	00209-2106-24
6 ml x 25	$315.87	Clindamycin Phosphate, Bristol Myers Squibb	00003-2942-22
6 ml x 25	$328.13	Clindamycin Phosphate, Astra USA	00186-1452-04
6 ml x 25	$351.60	Clindamycin Phosphate, Gensia Labs	00703-9120-04
6 ml x 25	**$462.56**	**CLEOCIN PHOSPHATE, Pharmacia & Upjohn**	**00009-0902-18**
6 ml x 25	**$485.70**	**CLEOCIN PHOSPHATE, Pharmacia & Upjohn**	**00009-3447-03**
25 x 2 ml	$180.31	Clindamycin Phosphate, Lederle Parenterals	00205-2801-83
25 x 4 ml	$328.13	Clindamycin Phosphate, Lederle Parenterals	00205-2801-93
25 x 6 ml	$501.87	Clindamycin Phosphate, Lederle Parenterals	00205-2801-47
50 ml	**$6.07**	**CLEOCIN PHOSPHATE IN D5W, Pharmacia & Upjohn**	**00009-3382-01**
50 ml x 24	**$4.12**	**CLEOCIN PHOSPHATE IV, Pharmacia & Upjohn**	**00009-3381-01**
50 ml x 24	**$5.80**	**CLEOCIN PHOSPHATE IV, Pharmacia & Upjohn**	**00009-3375-01**
60 ml	$107.40	Clindamycin Phosphate, Gensia Labs	00703-9138-01
60 ml	**$181.32**	**CLEOCIN PHOSPHATE, Pharmacia & Upjohn**	**00009-0728-05**
60 ml	$215.09	Clindamycin Phosphate, Abbott	00074-4197-01
60 ml x 5	$343.75	Clindamycin Phosphate, Astra USA	00186-1453-01
60 ml x 10	$1743.75	Clindamycin Phosphate, Lederle Parenterals	00205-2801-24
100 ml	$178.92	Clindamycin Phosphate, Gensia Labs	00703-9148-01

Solution - Topical - 1 %

30 ml	$9.17	Clindamycin Phosphate, Qualitest Pharms	00603-1098-45
30 ml	$9.20	Clindamycin Phosphate, Copley Pharm	38245-0628-11
30 ml	$9.74	Clindamycin Phosphate, Alpharma	00472-0987-91
30 ml	$10.07	Clindamycin Phosphate, Greenstone	59762-3728-01
30 ml	$10.31	Clindamycin Phosphate, Rugby	00536-0336-75
30 ml	$10.31	Clindamycin Phosphate, Rugby	00536-0366-75
30 ml	$10.80	Clindamycin Phosphate, Goldline Labs	00182-6028-66
30 ml	$10.95	Clindamycin Phosphate, Major Pharms	00904-7733-30
30 ml	$10.97	Clindamycin Phosphate, Geneva Pharms	00781-6800-90
30 ml	$11.82	CLEOCIN T, Pharmacia & Upjohn	00009-3116-01
60 ml	$17.90	Clindamycin Phosphate, Copley Pharm	38245-0628-12
60 ml	$17.94	Clindamycin Phosphate, Qualitest Pharms	00603-1098-49
60 ml	$18.00	Clindamycin Phosphate, Goldline Labs	00182-6028-68
60 ml	$19.04	Clindamycin Phosphate, Alpharma	00472-0987-92
60 ml	$19.44	Clinda-Derm, Paddock Labs	00574-0016-02
60 ml	$19.70	Clindamycin Phosphate, Greenstone	59762-3728-02
60 ml	$19.85	Clindamycin Phosphate, HL Moore Drug Exch	00839-7815-64
60 ml	$20.16	Clindamycin Phosphate, Rugby	00536-0366-96
60 ml	$20.18	Clindamycin Phosphate, Teva	00093-0413-39
60 ml	$21.45	Clindamycin Phosphate, Geneva Pharms	00781-6800-61
60 ml	$21.55	Clindamycin Phosphate, Major Pharms	00904-7733-03
60 ml	$23.12	CLEOCIN T, Pharmacia & Upjohn	00009-3116-02

Swab, Medicated - Topical - 1 %

60's	$28.71	CLEOCIN T, Pharmacia & Upjohn	00009-3116-14

HOW SUPPLIED - NOT RATED EQUIVALENT:

Cream - Vaginal - 2 %

40 gm	$30.54	CLEOCIN, Pharmacia & Upjohn	00009-3448-01

Gel - Topical - 1 %

30 gm	$20.00	CLEOCIN T, Pharmacia & Upjohn	00009-3331-02
60 gm	$36.03	CLEOCIN T, Pharmacia & Upjohn	00009-3331-01

Lotion - Topical - 1 %

60 ml	$27.81	CLEOCIN T, Pharmacia & Upjohn	00009-3329-01

Powder

5 gm	$50.62	Clindamycin Phosphate, Paddock Labs	00574-0415-05
10 gm	$75.00	Clindamycin Phosphate, Paddock Labs	00574-0415-10

CLIOQUINOL *(001563)*

CATEGORIES: Anti-Infectives; Local Infections; Pharmaceutical Adjuvants; Skin/Mucous Membrane Agents; FDA Pre 1938 Drugs

BRAND NAMES: Iodochlorhydroxyquin; *Vioform*; Yodoxin
(International brand names outside U.S. in italics)

Prescribing information not available at time of publication.

HOW SUPPLIED - EQUIVALENTS NOT AVAILABLE:

Powder - Oral

30 gm	$18.20	Iodochlorhydroxyquin, Millgood	53118-0303-01
100 gm	$33.60	Clioquinol, Paddock Labs	00574-0598-01
120 gm	$49.00	Iodochlorhydroxyquin, Millgood	53118-0303-04

CLIOQUINOL; HYDROCORTISONE *(001487)*

CATEGORIES: Acne; Anti-Infectives; Anti-Inflammatory Agents; Antibacterials; Antifungals; Antimicrobials; DESI Drugs; Dermatitis; Dermatologicals; Dermatoses; Eczema; Intertrigo; Otic Hydrocortisones; Pruritus; Skin Infections; Skin/Mucous Membrane Agents; Steroids; Tinea Capitis; Tinea Cruris; Tinea Corporis; Tinea Pedis; FDA Pre 1938 Drugs

BRAND NAMES: Ala-Quin; Albaform Hc; *Barquinol*; Caquin; Corque; Cortin; Dek-Quin; Epiform-Hc; Hysone; Iodo-Hc; Iodochlor W/Hc; *Kalviocort*; Lanvisone; Pedi-Cort V; Pricort; Steroform; Topiquin; Uad Cream; Vio-Tex Hc; *Viocortiderm*; **Vioform-Hc**; Viosone
(International brand names outside U.S. in italics)

FORMULARIES: Aetna; BC-BS; FHP

DESCRIPTION:

Vioform-Hydrocortisone, a topical compound for dermatologic use, combines the antifungal and antibacterial actions of clioquinol USP and the anti-inflammatory and antipruritic effects of hydrocortisone USP to provide broad control of acute and chronic dermatoses. It is available as cream, or ointment, containing 3% clioquinol USP and 1% hydrocortisone USP and as mild cream containing 3% clioquinol USP and 0.5% hydrocortisone USP.

Vioform is 5-chloro-7-iodo-8-quinolinol. Hydrocortisone is 11β, 17, 21-trihydroxypregn-4-ene-3,20-dione.

CLINICAL PHARMACOLOGY:

In vitro studies have demonstrated than clioquinol and hydrocorisone effectively inhibits the growth of various mycotic organisms such as *Microsporons, Trichophytons, and Candida albicans* and gram positive cocci such as *staphylococci and enterococci.*

The role of steroids in alleviating the inflammation and pruritus associated with many dermatoses has been well established.

INDICATIONS AND USAGE:

Based on a review of this drug by the National Academy of Sciences-National Research Council and/or other information, FDA has classified the indications as follows:
"Possibly" Effective: Contact or atopic dermatitis; impetiginized eczema; nummular eczema; infantile eczema; endogenous chronic infectious dermatitis; stasis dermatitis; pyoderma; nuchal eczema and chronic eczematoid otitis externa; acne urticata; localized or disseminated neurodermatitis; lichen simplex chronicus; anogenital pruritus (vulvae, scroti, ani); folliculitis; bacterial dermatoses; mycotic dermatoses such as tinea (capitis, cruris, corporis, pedis); moniliasis; intertrigo.
Final classification of the less-than-effective indications requires further investigation.

CONTRAINDICATIONS:

Hypersensitivity to clioquinol and hydrocorisone, or any of its ingredients or related compounds; lesions of the eye; tuberculosis of the skin; most viral skin lesions (including herpes simplex, vaccinia, and varicella).

Clioquinol and hydrocorisone should not be used in children under 2 years of age. Clioquinol and hydrocorisone should not be used for diaper rash.

WARNINGS:

This product is not for ophthalmic use.

In the presence of systemic infections, appropriate systemic antibiotics should be used.

USAGE IN PREGNANCY

Although topical steroids have not been reported to have an adverse effect on pregnancy, the safety of their use in pregnant women has not been absolutely established. In laboratory animals, increases in incidence of fetal abnormalities have been associated with exposure of gestating females to topical corticosteroids, in some cases at rather low dosage levels. Therefore, drugs of this class should not be used extensively on pregnant patients in large amounts or for prolonged periods of time.

PRECAUTIONS:

May prove irritating to sensitized skin in rare cases. If irritation occurs, discontinue therapy. Staining of skin and fabrics may occur. Additionally, there are rare reports of discoloration of hair and nails.

Signs and symptoms of systemic toxicity, electrolyte imbalance, or adrenal suppression have not been reported with clioquinol and hydrocorisone. Nevertheless, the possibility of suppression of the pituitary-adrenal axis during therapy should be kept in mind, especially when the drug is used under occlusive dressings, for a prolonged period, or for treating extensive cutaneous areas since significant absorption of corticosteroid may occur under these conditions, particularly in children and infants.

Clioquinol and hydrocorisone may be absorbed through the skin and interfere with thyroid function tests. If such tests are contemplated, wait at least one month between discontinuation of therapy and performance of these tests. The ferric chloride test for phenylketonuria (PKU) can yield a false-positive result if clioquinol and hydrocorisone is present in the diaper or urine.

Prolonged use may result in overgrowth of nonsusceptible organism requiring appropriate therapy.

ADVERSE REACTIONS:

There have been a few reports of rash and hypersensitivity.

ADVERSE REACTIONS: *(cont'd)*

The following local adverse reactions have been reported with topical corticosteroids, especially under occlusive dressings: burning; itching; irritation; dryness; folliculitis; hypertrichosis; acneiform eruptions; hypopigmentation; perioral dermatitis; allergic contact dermatitis; maceration of the skin; secondary infection; skin atrophy; striae; miliaria. Discontinue therapy if any untoward reaction occurs.

DOSAGE AND ADMINISTRATION:

Apply a thin layer to the affected part 3 or 4 times daily.

The cream, because of its slight drying effect, is primarily useful for moist, weeping lesions; the ointment is best used for lesions accompanied by thickening and scaling of the skin.

The mild cream should be used when treating lesions involving extensive body areas or less severe dermatoses.

Do not store above 86° F.

HOW SUPPLIED - RATED THERAPEUTICALLY EQUIVALENT:

Cream - Topical - 3 %/1 %

20 gm	$2.79	CORQUE, Geneva Pharms	00781-7007-22

HOW SUPPLIED - NOT RATED EQUIVALENT:

Cream - Topical - 1 %/0.5 %

30 gm	$2.13	Hydrocortisone/Iodochlorhydroxyquin, Rugby	00536-0991-95
30 gm	$2.70	Hydrocortisone/Iodochlorhydroxyquin, Clay Park Labs	45802-0007-03

Cream - Topical - 1 mg/1 mg

30 gm	$7.00	1 + 1-F, Dunhall Pharms	00217-8409-80

Cream - Topical - 3 %/0.5 %

15 gm	$2.75	Iodochlorhydroxyquin W/Hc, Consolidated Midland	00223-4127-15
15 gm	$3.00	DEK QUIN, C O Truxton	00463-8003-15
28.4 gm	$1.99	Hydrocortisone/Iodochlorhydroxyquin, HL Moore Drug Exch	00839-5513-49
30 gm	$1.94	Hydrocortisone/Iodochlorhydroxyquin, Rugby	00536-0990-95
30 gm	$2.27	Hydrocortisone/Iodochlorhydroxyquin, Clay Park Labs	45802-0005-03
30 gm	$2.65	Iodochlorhydroxyquin W/Hc, Major Pharms	00904-2679-31
30 gm	$3.00	Iodochlorhydroxyquin W/Hc, Consolidated Midland	00223-4127-30
30 gm	$5.68	ALA QUIN WITH HYDROCORTISONE 0.5%, Del Ray Lab	00316-0123-01
454 gm	$21.60	Hydrocortisone/Iodochlorhydroxyquin, Clay Park Labs	45802-0005-05

Cream - Topical - 3 %/1 %

20 g	$3.10	Hydrocortisone/Iodochlorhyroxyquin, Goldline Labs	00182-0875-48
20 g	$4.28	Hydrocortisone/Iodochlorhydroxyquin, Rugby	00536-1001-99
20 gm	$2.01	Hydrocortisone w/Iodochlorhyroxyquin, HL Moore Drug Exch	00839-5508-45
20 gm	$2.10	Clioquinol 3% W/ Hydrocortisone 1%, Thames Pharma	49158-0104-07
20 gm	$2.16	Hydrocortisone/Iodochlorhydroxyquin, Clay Park Labs	45802-0006-02
20 gm	$2.43	Iodochlorhydroxyquin W/Hc, Qualitest Pharms	00603-7801-76
20 gm	$2.75	Hydrocortisone/Iodochlorhydroxyquin, United Res	00677-0726-38
20 gm	$2.82	Iodochlorhydroxyquin/Hydrocortisone, NMC Labs	23317-0341-20
20 gm	$2.85	IODOCHLORHYDROXYQUIN W/HC, Major Pharms	00904-0753-29
20 gm	$3.25	Hydrocortisone W/Iodochlor, Consolidated Midland	00223-4128-20
30 gm	$2.80	Clioquinol 3% W/ Hydrocortisone 1%, Thames Pharma	49158-0104-08
30 gm	$3.24	Hydrocortisone/Iodochlorhydroxyquin, Clay Park Labs	45802-0006-03
30 gm	$3.25	Hydrocortisone W/Iodochlor, Consolidated Midland	00223-4128-30
300 gm	$4.25	Hydrocortisone/Iodochlorhyroxyquin, Goldline Labs	00182-0875-34
454 gm	$30.69	Hydrocortisone/Iodochlorhydroxyquin, Rugby	00536-2480-98
454 gm	$32.94	Hydrocortisone/Iodochlorhydroxyquin, Clay Park Labs	45802-0006-05

Ointment - Topical - 3 %/1 %

20 gm	$2.01	Hydrocortisone/Iodochlorhydroxyquin, HL Moore Drug Exch	00839-5509-45
20 gm	$2.16	Hydrocortisone/Iodochlorhydroxyquin, Clay Park Labs	45802-0016-02
20 gm	$15.25	ALBAFORM HC, Alba Pharma	10023-0125-20
30 gm	$3.24	Hydrocortisone/Iodochlorhydroxyquin, Clay Park Labs	45802-0016-03
454 gm	$32.94	Hydrocortisone/Iodochlorhydroxyquin, Clay Park Labs	45802-0016-05

CLOBETASOL PROPIONATE *(000839)*

CATEGORIES: Anti-Inflammatory Agents; Dermatologicals; Dermatoses; Pruritus; Skin/Mucous Membrane Agents; Steroids; Topical; Psoriasis*; Pregnancy Category C; FDA Approved 1985 Dec; Patent Expiration 1992 Mar
* Indication not approved by the FDA

BRAND NAMES: *Betasol*; *Betavate*; *Butavate*; *Clobasone*; *Clobesol*; *Clobeson*; *Clobet*; *Clobezan*; *Cloderm*; *Clovate*; *Decloban*; *Dermatovate* (Mexico); *Dermocure*; *Dermol*; *Dermotyl*; *Dermoval* (France); *Dermovat*; *Dermovate* (Asia, England, Canada); *Dermoxin* (Germany); *Dermoxinale* (Germany); *Domo-Horn*; *Karison Creme* (Germany); *Karison Salbe* (Germany); *Kloderma*; *Lamodex*; *Lobate*; *Lobesol*; *Medodermone*; *Rubocort*; *S.Z.*; **Temovate**; *Tenovate*; *Topifort*; *Univate*; *Yihfu*; *Yugofin*
(International brand names outside U.S. in italics)

FORMULARIES: Aetna; BC-BS

DESCRIPTION:

Cream, Ointment and Scalp Application: FOR DERMATOLOGIC USE ONLY-NOT FOR OPHTHALMIC USE.

Emollient Cream and Gel: FOR TOPICAL DERMATOLOGIC USE ONLY - NOT FOR OPHTHALMIC, ORAL, OR INTRAVAGINAL USE

All Forms: All forms of clobetasol propionate contain the active compound clobetasol propionate, a synthetic corticosteroid, for topical dermatologic use. Clobetasol, an analog of prednisolone, has a high degree of glucocorticoid activity and a slight degree of mineralocorticoid activity.

Clobetasol propionate has the empirical formula $C_{25}H_{32}ClFO_5$ and a molecular weight of 467. It is a white to cream-colored crystalline powder insoluble in water.

Clobetasol propionate cream contains clobetasol propionate 0.5 mg/g in a cream base of propylene glycol, glyceryl monostearate, cetostearyl alcohol, glyceryl stearate, PEG 100 stearate, white wax, chlorocresol, sodium citrate, citric acid monohydrate, and purified water.

Clobetasol propionate ointment contains clobetasol propionate 0.5 mg/g in a base of propylene glycol, sorbitan sesquioleate, and white petrolatum.

Clobetasol propionate scalp application contains clobetasol propionate 0.5 mg/g in a base compound of purified water, isopropyl alcohol (39.3%), carbomer 934P, and sodium hydroxide.

DESCRIPTION: *(cont'd)*

Clobetasol propionate emollient cream contains clobetasol propionate 0.5 mg/g in an emollient base of cetostearyl alcohol, isopropyl myristate, propylene glycol, cetomacrogol 1000, dimethicone 360, citric acid, sodium citrate, purified water, and imidurea as a preservative.

Clobetasol propionate gel contains clobetasol propionate 0.5 mg/g in a base of propylene glycol, carbomer 934P, sodium hydroxide, and purified water.

Scalp Application Emollient Cream and Gel: Chemically, clobetasol propionate is (11β,16β)-21-chloro-9-fluoro-11-hydroxy-16-methyl-17-(1-oxo-propoxy)pregna-1,4-diene-3,20-dione.

Cream and Ointment: Chemically, clobetasol propionate is (11β,16β)-21-chloro-9-fluoro-11-dihydroxy-16-methyl-17-(1-oxo-propoxy)pregna-1,4-diene-3,20-dione.

CLINICAL PHARMACOLOGY:

Cream, Ointment and Scalp Application: The corticosteroids are a class of compounds comprising steroid hormones secreted by the adrenal cortex and their synthetic analogs. In pharmacologic doses, corticosteroids are used primarily for their anti-inflammatory and/or immunosuppressive effects. Topical corticosteroids such as clobetasol propionate are effective in the treatment of corticosteroid-responsive dermatoses primarily because of their anti-inflammatory, antipruritic, and vasoconstrictive actions. However, while the physiologic, pharmacologic, and clinical effects of the corticosteroids are well known, the exact mechanisms of their actions in each disease are uncertain.

Clobetasol propionate, a corticosteroid, has been shown to have topical (dermatologic) and systemic pharmacologic and metabolic effects characteristic of this class of drugs.

Emollient Cream and Gel: Like other topical corticosteroids, clobetasol propionate has anti-inflammatory, antipruritic, and vasoconstrictive properties. The mechanism of the anti- inflammatory activity of the topical steroids, in general, is unclear. However, corticosteroids are thought to act by the induction of phospholipase A_2 inhibitory proteins, collectively called lipocortins. It is postulated that these proteins control the biosynthesis of potent mediators of inflammation such as prostaglandins and leukotrienes by inhibiting the release of their common precursor, arachidonic acid. Arachidonic acid is released from membrane phospholipids by phospholipase A_2.

PHARMACOKINETICS

Cream, Ointment and Scalp Application: The extent of percutaneous absorption of topical corticosteroids, including clobetasol propionate, is determined by many factors, including the vehicle, the integrity of the epidermal barrier, and the use of occlusive dressings (see DOSAGE AND ADMINISTRATION.)

As with all topical corticosteroids, clobetasol propionate can be absorbed from normal intact skin. Inflammation and/or other disease processes in the skin may increase percutaneous absorption. Occlusive dressings substantially increase the percutaneous absorption of topical corticosteroids (see DOSAGE AND ADMINISTRATION.)

Once absorbed through the skin, topical corticosteroids enter pharmacokinetic pathways similarly to systemically administered corticosteroids. Corticosteroids are bound to plasma proteins in varying degrees. Corticosteroids are metabolized primarily in the liver and are then excreted by the kidneys. Some of the topical corticosteroids, including clobetasol propionate and its metabolites, are also excreted into the bile.

Cream and Ointment: Clobetasol propionate has been shown to depress the plasma levels of adrenal cortical hormones following repeated nonocclusive application to diseased skin in patients with psoriasis and eczematous dermatitis. These effects have been shown to be transient and reversible upon completion of a two-week course of treatment.

Scalp Application: Following repeated nonocclusive application in the treatment of scalp psoriasis, there is some evidence that clobetasol propionate scalp application has the potential to depress plasma cortisol levels in some patients. However, hypothalamic-pituitary-adrenal (HPA) axis effects produced by systemically absorbed clobetasol propionate have been shown to be transient and reversible upon completion of a two-week course treatment.

Emollient Cream and Gel: The extent of percutaneous absorption of topical steroids is determined by many factors, including the vehicle and the integrity of the epidermal barrier. Occlusive dressing with hydrocortisone for up to 24 hours has not been demonstrated to increase penetration; however, occlusion of hydrocortisone for 96 hours markedly enhances penetration. Topical corticosteroids can be absorbed from normal intact skin, while inflammation and/or other disease processes in the skin may increase percutaneous absorption.

Studies performed with clobetasol propionate emollient cream and gel indicate that it is in the super-high range of potency as compared with other topical steroids.

Gel: Greater absorption was observed for the clobetasol propionate gel formulation as compared to the cream formulation in *in vitro* human skin penetration studies.

INDICATIONS AND USAGE:

Cream and Ointment: Clobetasol propionate cream and ointment are indicated for short-term treatment of inflammatory and pruritic manifestations of moderate to severe corticosteroid-responsive dermatoses.

Emollient Cream and Gel: Clobetasol propionate emollient cream and gel are a super- high potency corticosteroid formulation indicated for the relief and pruritic manifestations of corticosteroid-responsive dermatoses.

Scalp Application: Clobetasol propionate scalp application is indicated for short-term topical treatment of inflammatory and pruritic manifestations of moderate to severe corticosteroid-responsive dermatoses of the scalp. Treatment beyond 2 consecutive weeks is not recommended, and the total dosage should not exceed 50 ml per week because of the potential for the drug to suppress the HPA axis.

Cream, Ointment, Emollient Cream and Gel: Treatment beyond 2 consecutive weeks is not recommended, and the total dosage should not exceed 50 g per week because of the potential for the drug to suppress the hypothalamic-pituitary-adrenal (HPA) axis.

All Forms: These products are not recommended for use in children under 12 years of age.

CONTRAINDICATIONS:

Cream and Ointment: Clobetasol propionate cream and ointment are contraindicated in patients who are hypersensitive to clobetasol propionate, to other corticosteroids, or to any ingredient in these preparations.

Scalp Application: Clobetasol propionate scalp application is contraindicated in patients with primary infections of the scalp, or in patients who are hypersensitive to clobetasol propionate, other corticosteroids or any ingredient in this preparation.

Emollient Cream and Gel: Clobetasol propionate emollient cream and gel is contraindicated in those patients with a history of hypersensitivity to any of the components of the preparation.

PRECAUTIONS:

GENERAL

Cream, Ointment, and Scalp Application: Clobetasol propionate is a highly potent topical corticosteroid that has been shown to suppress the HPA axis at doses as low as 2 g (of ointment) per day.

PRECAUTIONS: *(cont'd)*

Systemic absorption of topical corticosteroids has resulted in reversible HPA axis suppression, manifestations of Cushing's syndrome, hyperglycemia, and glucosuria in some patients.

Conditions that augment systemic absorption include the application of the more potent corticosteroids, use over large surface areas, prolonged use, and the addition of occlusive dressings. Therefore, patients receiving a large dose of a potent topical steroid applied to a large surface area should be evaluated periodically for evidence of HPA axis suppression by using the urinary free cortisol and ACTH stimulation tests. If HPA axis suppression is noted, an attempt should be made to withdraw the drug, to reduce the frequency of application, or to substitute a less potent steroid.

Recovery of HPA axis function is generally prompt and complete upon discontinuation of the drug. Infrequently, signs and symptoms of steroid withdrawal may occur, requiring supplemental systemic corticosteroids.

Children may absorb proportionally larger amounts of topical corticosteroids and thus be more susceptible to systemic toxicity (see PRECAUTIONS, Pediatric Use.)

If irritation develops, topical corticosteroids should be discontinued and appropriate therapy instituted.

As with other potent topical corticosteroids, clobetasol propionate cream, ointment or scalp application should not be used in the treatment of rosacea and perioral dermatitis. Topical corticosteroids in general should not be used in the treatment of acne or as sole therapy in widespread plaque psoriasis.

Additional Information for Cream and Ointment: In the presence of dermatologic infections, the use of an appropriate antifungal or antibacterial agent should be instituted. If a favorable response does not occur promptly, the corticosteroid should be discontinued until the infection has been adequately controlled.

Certain areas of the body, such as the face, groin, and axillae, are more prone to atrophic changes than other areas of the body following treatment with corticosteroids. Frequent observation of the patient is important if these areas are to be treated.

Additional Information for Scalp Application: Irritation is possible if clobetasol propionate scalp application contacts the eye. If that should occur, immediate flushing of the eye with large volume of water is recommended.

If the inflammatory lesion becomes infected, the use of an appropriate antifungal or antibacterial agent should be instituted. If a favorable response does not occur promptly, the corticosteroid should be discontinued until the infection has been adequately controlled.

Although clobetasol propionate scalp application is intended for the treatment of inflammatory conditions of the scalp, it should be noted that certain areas of the body, such as the face, groin, and axillae, are more prone to atrophic changes than other areas of the body following treatment with corticosteroids. Frequent observation of the patient is important if these areas are to be treated.

Emollient Cream and Gel: Clobetasol propionate is a highly potent topical corticosteroid that has been shown to suppress the HPA axis as low as 2 g per day.

Systemic absorption of topical corticosteroids can produce reversible HPA axis suppression with the potential for glucocorticosteroid insufficiency after withdrawal from treatment. Manifestations of Cushing's syndrome, hyperglycemia, and glucosuria can also be produced in some patients by systemic absorption of topical corticosteroids while on therapy.

Patients receiving a large dose applied to a large surface area should be evaluated periodically for evidence of HPA axis suppression. This may be done by using the ACTH stimulation, a.m. plasma cortisol, and urinary free cortisol tests. Patients receiving super-potent corticosteroids should not be treated for more than 2 weeks at a time, and only small areas should be treated at any one time due to the increased risk of HPA suppression.

If HPA axis suppression is noted, an attempt should be made to withdraw the drug, to reduce the frequency of application, or to substitute a less potent corticosteroid. Recovery of HPA axis function is generally prompt and complete upon discontinuation of topical corticosteroids. Infrequently, signs and symptoms of glucocorticosteroid insufficiency, may occur that require supplemental systemic corticosteroids. For information on systemic supplementation, see prescribing information for those products.

Children may be more susceptible to systemic toxicity from equivalent doses due to their larger skin surface to body mass ratios (see PRECAUTIONS, Pediatric Use.)

If irritation develops, clobetasol propionate emollient cream and gel should be discontinued and appropriate therapy instituted. Allergic contact dermatitis with corticosteroids is usually diagnosed by observing *failure to heal* rather than noting a clinical exacerbations as with most topical products not containing corticosteroids. Such an observation should be corroborated with appropriate diagnostic patch testing.

If concomitant skin infections are present or develop, an appropriate antifungal or antibacterial agent should be used. If a favorable response does not occur promptly, use of clobetasol propionate emollient cream and gel should be discontinued until the infection has been adequately controlled.

Clobetasol propionate emollient cream and gel should not be used in the treatment of rosacea or perioral dermatititis, and should not be used on the face, groin or axillae.

Information for the Patient: Patients using clobetasol propionate should receive the following information and instructions:

1. This medication is to be used as directed by the physician and should not be used longer than the prescribed time period. It is for external use only. Avoid contact with the eyes.

2. This medication should not be used for any disorder other than that for which it was prescribed.

3. The treated skin area should not be bandaged or otherwise covered or wrapped so as to be occlusive unless directed by a physician.

4. Patients should report any signs of local adverse reactions to the physician.

5. Patients should inform their physicians that they are using clobetasol propionate if surgery is contemplated. (emollient cream and gel only)

Laboratory Tests: The following tests may be helpful in evaluating HPA axis suppression:

Urinary free cortisol test

ACTH stimulation test

A.M. plasma cortisol test (emollient cream and gel only)

CARCINOGENESIS, MUTAGENESIS, AND IMPAIRMENT OF FERTILITY

Cream, Ointment and Scalp Application: Long-term animal studies have not been performed to evaluate the carcinogenic potential or the effect on fertility of topical corticosteroids.

Studies to determine mutagenicity with prednisolone have revealed negative results.

Emollient Cream and Gel: Long-term animal studies have not been performed to evaluate the carcinogenic potential of clobetasol propionate.

Studies in the rat following oral administration at dosage levels up to 50 mg/kg per day revealed no significant effect on the males. The females exhibited an increase in the number of resorbed embryos and a decrease in the number of living fetuses at the highest dose.

Clobetasol propionate was nonmutagenic in three different test systems: the Ames test, the *Saccharomyces cerevisiae*gene conversion assay, and the *E. coli* B WP2 fluctuation test.

PRECAUTIONS: *(cont'd)*

PREGNANCY, TERATOGENIC EFFECTS, PREGNANCY CATEGORY C

Cream, Ointment and Scalp Application: The more potent corticosteroids have been shown to be teratogenic in animals after dermal application. Clobetasol propionate has not been tested for teratogenicity by this route; however, it is absorbed percutaneously, and when administered subcutaneously it was a significant teratogen in both the rabbit and the mouse. Clobetasol propionate has greater teratogenic potential than steroids that are less potent.

There are no adequate and well-controlled studies of the teratogenic effects of topically applied corticosteroids, including clobetasol, in pregnant women. Therefore, clobetasol and other topical corticosteroids should be used during pregnancy only if the potential benefit justifies the potential risk to the fetus, and they should not be used extensively on pregnant patients, in large amounts, or for prolonged periods of time.

Emollient Cream and Gel: Corticosteroids have been shown to be teratogenic in laboratory animals when administered systematically at relatively low dosage levels. Some corticosteroids have been shown to be teratogenic after dermal application to laboratory animals.

Clobetasol propionate has not been tested for teratogenicity by this route; however, it is absorbed percutaneously, and when administered subcutaneously it was a significant teratogen in both the rabbit and mouse.

Clobetasol propionate has greater teratogenic potential than steroids that are less potent.

Teratogenicity studies in mice using the subcutaneous route resulted in fetotoxicity at the highest dose tested (1 mg/kg) and teratogenicity at all dose levels tested down to 0.03 mg/kg. These doses are approximately 0.33 and 0.01 times, respectively, the human topical dose of clobetasol propionate emollient cream or gel. Abnormalities seen included cleft palate, cranioschisis, and other skeletal abnormalities.

In rabbits, clobestasol propionate given by the same route was teratogenic at doses of 3 and 10 mcg/kg.

These doses are approximately 0.001 and 0.003 times, respectively, the human topical dose of clobetasol propionate emollient cream and gel. Abnormalities included cleft palate, cranioschisis, and other skeletal abnormalities.

There are no adequate and well-controlled studies of the teratogenic potential of clobetasol propionate in pregnant women. Clobetasol propionate emollient cream and gel should be used during pregnancy only if the potential benefit justifies the potential risk of the fetus.

NURSING MOTHERS

Cream, Ointment and Scalp Application: It is not known whether topical administration of corticosteroids could result in sufficient systemic absorption to produce detectable quantities in breast milk. Systemically administered corticosteroids are secreted into breast milk in quantities not likely to have a deleterious effect on the infant. Nevertheless, caution should be exercised when topical corticosteroids are prescribed for a nursing woman.

Emollient Cream and Gel: Systemically administered corticosteroids appear in human milk and could suppress growth, interfere with endogenous corticosteroid production, or cause other untoward effects. It is not known whether topical administration of corticosteroids could result in sufficient systemic absorption to produce detectable quantities in human milk. Because many drugs are excreted in human milk, caution should be exercised when clobetasol propionate emollient cream and gel is administered to a nursing woman.

PEDIATRIC USE

Cream, Ointment and Scalp Application: Use of clobetasol propionate in children under 12 years of age is not recommended.

Pediatric patients may demonstrate greater susceptibility to topical corticosteroid-induced HPA axis suppression and Cushing's syndrome than mature patients because of a large skin surface area to body weight ratio.

Emollient Cream and Gel: Safety and effectiveness of clobetasol propionate emollient cream and gel in children and infants have not been established; therefore, use in children under 12 years of ae is not recommended. Because of a higher ratio of skin area to body mass, children are at a greater risk than adults of HPA axis suppression when they are treated with topical corticosteroids.

They are therefore also at greater risk of glucocorticosteroid insufficiency after withdrawal of treatment and of Cushing's syndrome while on treatment.

Adverse effects including striae have been reported with inappropriate use of topical corticosteroids in infants and children (see PRECAUTIONS.)

All Forms: HPA axis suppression, Cushing's syndrome, and intracranial hypertension have been reported in children receiving topical corticosteroids. Manifestations of adrenal suppression in children include linear growth retardation, delayed weight gain, low plasma cortisol levels, and absence of response to ACTH stimulation. Manifestations of intracranial hypertension include bulging fontanelles, headaches, and bilateral papilledema.

ADVERSE REACTIONS:

Cream, Ointment, and Scalp Application: Clobetasol propionate cream, ointment, and scalp application are generally well tolerated when used for 2-week treatment periods.

The following local adverse reactions are reported infrequently when topical corticosteroids are used as recommended. These reactions are listed in an approximately decreasing order of occurrence: burning, itching, irritation, dryness, folliculitis, hypertrichosis, acneiform eruptions, hypopigmentation, perioral dermatitis, allergic contact dermatitis, maceration of the skin, secondary infection, skin atrophy, striae, and miliaria. Systemic absorption of topical corticosteroids has produced reversible HPA axis suppression, manifestations of Cushing's syndrome, hyperglycemia, and glucosuria in some patients. In rare instances, treatment (or withdrawal of treatment) of psoriasis with corticosteroids is thought to have exacerbated the disease or provoked the pustular form of the disease, so careful patient supervision is recommended.

Cream and Ointment: The most frequent adverse reactions reported for clobetasol propionate cream have been local and have included burning sensation in 4 of 421 patients and stinging sensation in 3 of 421 patients. Less frequent adverse reactions were itching, skin atrophy, and cracking and fissuring of the skin, which occurred in 1 of 421 patients.

Ointment: The most frequent adverse events reported for clobetasol propionate ointment have been local and have included burning sensation, irritation, and itching. These occurred in 2 of 366 patients. Less frequent adverse reactions were stinging, cracking, erythema, folliculitis, numbness of fingers, skin atrophy, and telangiectasia, which occurred in 1 of 366 patients.

Scalp Application: The most frequent adverse events reported for clobetasol propionate scalp application have been local and have included burning and/or stinging sensation, which occurred in 29 of 294 patients; scalp pustules, which occurred in 3 of 294 patients; and tingling and folliculitis each of which occurred in 2 of 294 patients. Less frequent adverse events were itching and tightness of the scalp, dermatitis, tenderness, headache, hair loss, and eye irritation, each of which occurred in 1 of 294 patients.

Emollient Cream: In a 2-week controlled trial with clobetasol propionate emollient cream, the only reported adverse reaction that was considered to be drug related was a report of burning sensation (1.9% of treated patients).

ADVERSE REACTIONS: *(cont'd)*

In two 4-week controlled trials with clobetasol propionate emollient cream, the only reported adverse reactions considered to be drug related were burning/stinging (5% of treated patients), pruritus (2%), and tenderness in the elbow (1%).

The following additional local adverse reactions are reported infrequently with topical corticosteroids, but may occur more frequently with super-high potency corticosteroids such as clobetasol propionate emollient cream. These reactions are listed in approximate decreasing order of occurrence: dryness, hypertrichosis, acneiform eruptions, hypopigmentation, perioral dermatitis, allergic contact, dermatitis, secondary infection, irritation, striae, and miliaria.

Gel: In a controlled trial with clobetasol propionate gel, the only reported adverse reaction that was considered to be drug related was a report of burning sensation (1.8% of treated patients).

Emollient Cream and Gel: In larger controlled clinical trials with other clobetasol propionate formulations, the most frequently reported adverse reactions have included burning, stinging, irritation, pruritus, erythema, folliculitis, cracking and fissuring of the skin, numbness of fingers, skin atrophy, and telangiectasia (all less than 2%).

Cushing's syndrome has been reported in infants and adults as a result of prolonged use of topical clobetasol propionate formulations.

OVERDOSAGE:

Topically applied clobetasol propionate can be absorbed in sufficient amounts to produce systemic effects (see PRECAUTIONS.)

DOSAGE AND ADMINISTRATION:

Cream and Ointment: A thin layer of clobetasol propionate cream or ointment should be applied with gentle rubbing to the affected skin areas twice daily, once in the morning and once at night.

Clobetasol propionate cream and ointment are potent; therefore, **treatment must be limited to 2 consecutive weeks, and amounts greater than 50 g per week should not be used.**

Scalp Application: Clobetasol propionate scalp application should be applied to the affected scalp areas twice daily, once in the morning and once at night.

Clobetasol propionate scalp application is potent; therefore, **treatment must be limited to 2 consecutive weeks, and amounts greater than 50 ml per week should not be used.**

Emollient Cream: Apply a thin layer of clobetasol propionate emollient cream to the affected skin areas twice daily and rub in gently and completely. (see INDICATIONS AND USAGE)

Clobetasol propionate emollient cream is a super-high potency topical corticosteroid; therefore, **treatment should be limited to 2 consecutive weeks, and amounts greater than 50 g per week should not be used.**

As with other highly active corticosteroids, therapy should be discontinued when control has been achieved. If no improvement is seen within 2 weeks, reassessment of diagnosis may be necessary.

Gel: Apply a thin layer of clobetasol propionate gel to the affected areas twice daily and rub in gently and completely (see INDICATIONS AND USAGE)

Clobetasol propionate gel is a super-high potency topical corticosteroid; therefore, **treatment should be limited to 2 consecutive weeks, and amounts greater than 50 g per week should not be used.**

Emollient Cream and Gel: As with other highly active corticosteroids, therapy should be discontinued when control has been achieved. If no improvement is seen within 2 weeks, reassessment of diagnosis may be necessary.

ALL FORMS OF CLOBETASOL PROPIONATE ARE NOT TO BE USED WITH OCCLUSIVE DRESSINGS.

HOW SUPPLIED:

Store between 15° and 30°C (59° and 86° F). Clobetasol propionate cream, ointment emollient cream and gel should not be refrigerated.

Scalp Application: Store between 4° and 25° C (39° and 77° F). Do not use near an open flame.

HOW SUPPLIED - RATED THERAPEUTICALLY EQUIVALENT:

Cream - Topical - 0.05 %

15 gm	$18.35	Clobetasol Propionate, Copley Pharm	38245-0650-70
15 gm	$18.40	Clobetasol Propionate, Goldline Labs	00182-5113-51
15 gm	$18.40	Clobetasol Propionate, NMC Labs	23317-0400-15
15 gm	$19.31	CLOBETASOL PROPIONATE, HL Moore Drug Exch	00839-7944-47
15 gm	$21.45	Clobetasol Propionate, H.C.F.A. F F P	99999-0839-01
15 gm	**$22.33**	**TEMOVATE, Glaxo Wellcome**	**00173-0375-73**
30 gm	$25.40	Clobetasol Propionate, Copley Pharm	38245-0650-71
30 gm	$25.45	Clobetasol Propionate, Goldline Labs	00182-5113-56
30 gm	$25.45	Clobetasol Propionate, NMC Labs	23317-0400-30
30 gm	$26.72	CLOBETASOL PROPIONATE, HL Moore Drug Exch	00839-7944-49
30 gm	$29.68	Clobetasol Propionate, H.C.F.A. F F P	99999-0839-02
30 gm	**$30.89**	**TEMOVATE, Glaxo Wellcome**	**00173-0375-72**
45 gm	$37.00	Clobetasol Propionate, Copley Pharm	38245-0650-72
45 gm	$37.05	Clobetasol Propionate, NMC Labs	23317-0400-45
45 gm	$38.88	CLOBETASOL PROPIONATE, HL Moore Drug Exch	00839-7944-52
45 gm	$43.20	Clobetasol Propionate, H.C.F.A. F F P	99999-0839-03
45 gm	**$44.95**	**TEMOVATE, Glaxo Wellcome**	**00173-0375-01**
60 gm	**$56.11**	**TEMOVATE, Glaxo Wellcome**	**00173-0375-02**

Liquid - Topical - 0.05 %

25 ml	**$25.57**	**TEMOVATE, SCALP APPLICATION, Glaxo Wellcome**	**00173-0432-00**
50 ml	**$49.19**	**TEMOVATE, SCALP APPLICATION, Glaxo Wellcome**	**00173-0432-01**

Ointment - Topical - 0.05 %

15 gm	$18.35	Clobetasol Propionate, Copley Pharm	38245-0128-70
15 gm	$18.40	Clobetasol Propionate, Goldline Labs	00182-5114-51
15 gm	$18.40	Clobetasol Propionate, NMC Labs	23317-0401-15
15 gm	$19.31	CLOBETASOL PROPIONATE, HL Moore Drug Exch	00839-7945-47
15 gm	$21.45	Clobetasol Propionate, H.C.F.A. F F P	99999-0839-04
30 gm	$25.40	Clobetasol Propionate, Copley Pharm	38245-0128-71
30 gm	$25.45	Clobetasol Propionate, Goldline Labs	00182-5114-56
30 gm	$25.45	Clobetasol Propionate, NMC Labs	23317-0401-30
30 gm	$26.72	CLOBETASOL PROPIONATE, HL Moore Drug Exch	00839-7945-49
30 gm	$29.68	Clobetasol Propionate, H.C.F.A. F F P	99999-0839-05
45 gm	$37.00	Clobetasol Propionate, Copley Pharm	38245-0128-72
45 gm	$37.05	Clobetasol Propionate, NMC Labs	23317-0401-45
45 gm	$38.88	CLOBETASOL PROPIONATE, HL Moore Drug Exch	00839-7945-52
45 gm	$43.20	Clobetasol Propionate, H.C.F.A. F F P	99999-0839-06
45 gm	**$44.95**	**TEMOVATE, Glaxo Wellcome**	**00173-0376-01**
60 gm	**$56.11**	**TEMOVATE, Glaxo Wellcome**	**00173-0376-02**

HOW SUPPLIED - NOT RATED EQUIVALENT:

Cream - Topical - 0.05 %

15 gm	$22.33	TEMOVATE EMOLLIENT, Glaxo Wellcome	00173-0454-01
30 gm	$30.89	TEMOVATE EMOLLIENT, Glaxo Wellcome	00173-0454-02
60 gm	$56.11	TEMOVATE EMOLLIENT, Glaxo Wellcome	00173-0454-03

Gel - Topical - 0.05 %

15 gm	$22.33	TEMOVATE, Glaxo Wellcome	00173-0455-01
30 gm	$30.89	TEMOVATE, Glaxo Wellcome	00173-0455-02

CLOCORTOLONE PIVALATE *(000840)*

CATEGORIES: Anti-Inflammatory Agents; Dermatologicals; Dermatoses; Skin/Mucous Membrane Agents; Steroids; Topical; FDA Approval Pre 1982

BRAND NAMES: **Cloderm**; *Kaban* (Germany); *Lenen*
(International brand names outside U.S. in italics)

DESCRIPTION:

Cloderm Cream 0.1% contains the medium potency topical corticosteroid, clocortolone pivalate, in a specially formulated water-washable emollient cream base consisting of purified water, white petrolatum, mineral oil, stearyl alcohol, polyoxyl 40 stearate, carbomer 934P, edetate disodium, sodium hydroxide, with methylparaben and propylparaben as preservatives.

The chemical name is 9-chloro-6α-fluoro-11β,21-dihydroxy-16α-methylpregna-1, 4-diene-3,20-dione 21-pivalate.

CLINICAL PHARMACOLOGY:

Topical corticosteroids share anti-inflammatory, anti-pruritic and vasoconstrictive actions.

The mechanism of anti-inflammatory activity of the topical corticosteroids is unclear. Various laboratory methods, including vasoconstrictor assays, are used to compare and predict potencies and/or clinical efficacies of the topical corticosteroids. There is some evidence to suggest that a recognizable correlation exists between vasoconstrictor potency and therapeutic efficacy in man.

Pharmacokinetics: The extent of percutaneous absorption of topical corticosteroids is determined by many factors including the vehicle, the integrity of the epidermal barrier, and the use of occlusive dressings.

Topical corticosteroids can be absorbed from normal intact skin. Inflammation and/or other disease processes in the skin increase percutaneous absorption. Occlusive dressings substantially increase the percutaneous absorption of topical corticosteroids. Thus, occlusive dressings may be a valuable therapeutic adjunct for treatment of resistant dermatoses. (See DOSAGE AND ADMINISTRATION.)

Once absorbed through the skin, topical corticosteroids are handled through pharmacokinetic pathways similar to systemically administered corticosteroids. Corticosteroids are bound to plasma proteins in varying degrees. Corticosteroids are metabolized primarily in the liver and are then excreted by the kidneys. Some of the topical corticosteroids and their metabolites are also excreted in the bile.

INDICATIONS AND USAGE:

Topical corticosteroids are indicated for the relief of the inflammatory and pruritic manifestations of corticosteroid-responsive dermatoses.

CONTRAINDICATIONS:

Topical corticosteroids are contraindicated in those patients with a history of hypersensitivity to any of the components of the preparation.

PRECAUTIONS:

General: Systemic absorption of topical corticosteroids has produced reversible hypothalamic-pituitary-adrenal (HPA) axis suppression, manifestations of Cushing's syndrome, hyperglycemia, and glucosuria in some patients.

Conditions which augment systemic absorption include the application of the more potent steroids, use over large surface areas, prolonged use, and the addition of occlusive dressings.

Therefore, patients receiving a large dose of a potent topical steroid applied to a large surface area or under an occlusive dressing should be evaluated periodically for evidence of HPA axis suppression by using the urinary free cortisol and ACTH stimulation tests. If HPA axis suppression is noted, an attempt should be made to withdraw the drug, to reduce the frequency of application, or to substitute a less potent steroid.

Recovery of HPA axis function is generally prompt and complete upon discontinuation of the drug. Infrequently, signs and symptoms of steroid withdrawal may occur, requiring supplemental systemic corticosteroids.

Children may absorb proportionally larger amounts of topical corticosteroids and thus be more susceptible to systemic toxicity (See PRECAUTIONS, Pediatric Use.)

If irritation develops, topical corticosteroids should be discontinued and appropriate therapy instituted.

In the presence of dermatological infections, the use of an appropriate antifungal or antibacterial agent should be instituted. If a favorable response does not occur promptly, the corticosteroid should be discontinued until the infection has been adequately controlled.

Information for the Patient: Patients using topical corticosteroids should receive the following information and instructions:

1. This medication is to be used as directed by the physician. It is for external use only. Avoid contact with the eyes.

2. Patients should be advised not to use this medication for any disorder other than for which it was prescribed.

3. The treated skin area should not be bandaged or otherwise covered or wrapped as to be occlusive unless directed by the physician.

4. Patients should report any signs of local adverse reactions especially under occlusive dressing.

5. Parents of pediatric patients should be advised not to use tight- fitting diapers or plastic pants on a child being treated in the diaper area, as these garments may constitute occlusive dressings.

Laboratory Tests: The following tests may be helpful in evaluating the HPA axis suppression:

Urinary free cortisol test

ACTH stimulation test

Carcinogenesis, Mutagenesis, and Impairment of Fertility: Long-term animal studies have not been performed to evaluate the carcinogenic potential or the effect on fertility of topical corticosteroids.

Studies to determine mutagenicity with prednisolone and hydrocortisone have revealed negative results.

PRECAUTIONS: *(cont'd)*

Pregnancy Category C: Corticosteroids are generally teratogenic in laboratory animals when administered systematically at relatively low dosage levels. The more potent corticosteroids have been shown to be teratogenic after dermal application in laboratory animals. There are no adequate and well-controlled studies in pregnant women on teratogenic effects from topically applied corticosteroids. Therefore, topical corticosteroids should be used during pregnancy only if the potential benefit justifies the potential risk to the fetus. Drugs of this class should not be used extensively on pregnant patients, in large amounts, or for prolonged periods of time.

Nursing Mothers: It is not known whether topical administration of corticosteroids could result in sufficient systemic absorption to produce detectable quantities in breast milk. Systematically administered corticosteroids are secreted into breast milk in quantities *not* likely to have a deleterious effect on the infant. Nevertheless, caution should be exercised when topical corticosteroids are administered to a nursing woman.

Pediatric Use: *Pediatric patients may demonstrate greater susceptibility to topical corticosteroid-induced HPA axis suppression and Cushing's syndrome than mature patients because of a larger skin surface area to body weight ratio.*

Hypothalamic-pituitary-adrenal (HPA) axis suppression, Cushing's syndrome, and intracranial hypertension have been reported in children receiving topical corticosteroids. Manifestations of adrenal suppression in children include linear growth retardation, delayed weight gain, low plasma cortisol levels, and absence of response to ACTH stimulation. Manifestations of intracranial hypertension include bulging fontanelles, headaches, and bilateral papilledema.

Administration of topical corticosteroids to children should be limited to the least amount compatible with an effective therapeutic regimen. Chronic corticosteroid therapy may interfere with the growth and development of children.

ADVERSE REACTIONS:

The following local adverse reactions are reported infrequently with topical corticosteroids, but may occur more frequently with the use of occlusive dressings. These reaction are listed in an appropriate decreasing order of occurrence: burning, itching, irritation, dryness, folliculitis, hypertrichosis, acneform eruptions, hypopigmentation, perioral dermatitis, allergic contact dermatitis, maceration of the skin, secondary infection, skin atrophy, striae, and miliaria.

OVERDOSAGE:

Topically applied corticosteroids can be absorbed in sufficient amounts to produce systemic effects (see PRECAUTIONS.)

DOSAGE AND ADMINISTRATION:

Apply clocortolone pivalate cream sparingly to the affected areas three times a day and rub in gently.

Occlusive dressings may be used for the management of psoriasis or recalcitrant conditions.

If an infection develops, the use of occlusive dressings should be discontinued and appropriate antimicrobial therapy instituted.

HOW SUPPLIED:

Cloderm Cream 0.1% is supplied in tubes containing 15 grams and 45 grams.

Store clocortolone pivalate cream between 59° and 86° F. Avoid freezing.

HOW SUPPLIED - EQUIVALENTS NOT AVAILABLE:

Cream - Topical - 0.1 %

15 g	$13.75	CLODERM, Ctr Labs Hermal	48017-1375-02
45 g	$24.50	CLODERM, Ctr Labs Hermal	48017-1375-06

CLOFAZIMINE *(000841)*

CATEGORIES: Anti-Infectives; Antimicrobials; Antimycobacterials; Laprostatics; Leprosy; Orphan Drugs; Tuberculosis*; Pregnancy Category C; FDA Approved 1986 Dec

* Indication not approved by the FDA

BRAND NAMES: *Clofozine*; *Hansepran*; *Lampren*; **Lamprene**; *Lapren*
(International brand names outside U.S. in italics)

FORMULARIES: Medi-Cal; WHO

DESCRIPTION:

Lamprene, clofazimine, is an antileprosy agent available as capsules for oral administration. Each capsule contains 50 mg or 100 mg of micronized clofazimine suspended in an oil-wax base. Clofazimine is a substituted iminophenazine bright-red dye. Its chemical name is 3-(*p*-chloroanilino)-10-(*p*-chlorophenyl)-2,10-dihydro-2-isopropyliminophenazine.

Clofazimine is a reddish-brown powder. It is readily soluble in benzene; soluble in chloroform; poorly soluble in acetone and in ethyl acetate; sparingly soluble in methanol and in ethanol; and virtually insoluble in water. Its molecular weight is 473.4.

Inactive Ingredients: Beeswax, butylated hydroxytoluene, citric acid, ethyl vanillin, gelatin, glycerin, iron oxide, lecithin, p-methoxy acetophenone, parabens, plant oils, propylene glycol.

CLINICAL PHARMACOLOGY:

Clofazimine exerts a slow bactericidal effect on *Mycobacterium leprae* (Hansen's Bacillus). Clofazimine inhibits mycobacterial growth and binds preferentially to mycobacterial DNA. Clofazimine also exerts anti-inflammatory properties in controlling erythema nodosum leprosum reactions. However, its precise mechanisms of action are unknown.

PHARMACOKINETICS

Clofazimine has a variable absorption rate in leprosy patients, ranging from 45-62% after oral administration. The average serum concentrations in leprosy patients treated with 100 mg and 300 mg daily were 0.7 mcg/ml and 1.0 mcg/ml, respectively. After ingestion of a single dose of 300 mg, elimination of unchanged clofazimine and its metabolites in a 24-hour urine collection was negligible. Clofazimine is retained in the human body for a long time. The half-life of clofazimine following repeated oral doses is estimated to be at least 70 days. Part of the ingested drug recovered from the feces may represent excretion via the bile. A small amount is also eliminated in the sputum, sebum and sweat.

Clofazimine is highly lipophilic and tends to be deposited predominantly in fatty tissue and in cells of the reticuloendothelial system. It is taken up by macrophages throughout the body. In autopsies performed on leprosy patients, clofazimine crystals were found predominantly in the mesenteric lymph nodes, adrenals, subcutaneous fat, liver, bile, gall bladder, spleen, small intestine, muscles, bones, and skin.

CLINICAL PHARMACOLOGY: *(cont'd)*

MICROBIOLOGY

Measurement of the minimum inhibitory concentration (MIC) of clofazimine against leprosy bacilli *in vitro* is not yet feasible. In the mouse footpad system, the multiplication of *M. leprae* is inhibited by introducing 0.0001-0.001% clofazimine in the diet. Although bacterial killing may begin shortly after starting the drug, it cannot be measured in biopsy tissues taken from patients for mouse footpad studies until approximately 50 days after the start of therapy.

Clofazimine does not show cross-resistance with dapsone or rifampin.

The following *in vitro* data are available, but their clinical significance is unknown. Clofazimine has been shown *in vitro* to inhibit *M. avium* and *M. bovis* at concentrations of approximately 0.1-1.0 mcg/ml. The MIC for *M. avium-intracellulare* isolated from patients with acquired immuno-deficiency syndrome (AIDS) ranged from 1.0 to 5.0 mcg/ml. With a few exceptions, microorganisms other than mycobacteria are not uninhibited by clofazimine.

INDICATIONS AND USAGE:

Clofazimine is indicated in the treatment of lepromatous leprosy, including dapsone-resistant lepromatous leprosy and lepromatous leprosy complicated by erythema nodosum leprosum. Clofazimine has not been demonstrated to be effective in the treatment of other leprosy-associated inflammatory reactions.

Combination drug therapy has been recommended for initial treatment of multibacillary leprosy to prevent the development of drug resistance.

CONTRAINDICATIONS:

There are no known contraindications.

WARNINGS:

Severe abdominal symptoms have necessitated exploratory laparotomies in some patients receiving clofazimine. Rare reports have included splenic infarction, bowel obstruction, and gastrointestinal bleeding. There have also been reports of death following severe abdominal symptoms. Autopsies have revealed crystalline deposits of clofazimine in various tissues including the intestinal mucosa, liver, spleen, and mesenteric lymph nodes.

Clofazimine should be used with caution in patients who have gastrointestinal problems such as abdominal pain and diarrhea. Dosages of clofazimine of more than 100 mg daily should be given for as short a period as possible and only under close medical supervision. If a patient complains of colicky or burning pain in the abdomen, nausea, vomiting, or diarrhea, the dose should be reduced, and if necessary, the interval between doses should be increased, or the drug should be discontinued.

PRECAUTIONS:

GENERAL

Physicians should be aware that skin discoloration due to clofazimine may result in depression. Two suicides have been reported in patients receiving clofazimine.

For skin dryness and ichthyosis, oil can be applied to the skin.

INFORMATION FOR THE PATIENT

Patients should be warned that clofazimine may cause a discoloration of the skin from red to brownish black, as well as discoloration of the conjunctivae, lacrimal fluid, sweat, sputum, urine, and feces. Patients should be advised that skin discoloration, although reversible, may take several months or years to disappear after the conclusion of therapy with clofazimine.

Patients should be told to take clofazimine with meals.

CARCINOGENESIS, MUTAGENESIS, AND IMPAIRMENT OF FERTILITY

Long-term carcinogenicity studies in animals have not been conducted with clofazimine. Results of mutagenicity studies (Ames test) were negative. There was some evidence of impaired fertility in one study in rats treated at a dose 25 times time usual human dose; the number of offspring was reduced and there was a lower proportion of implantations.

PREGNANCY CATEGORY C

Clofazimine was not teratogenic in laboratory animals at dose levels equivalent to 8 times (rabbit) and 25 times (rat) the usual human daily dose. However, there was evidence of fetotoxicity in the mouse at 12-25 times the human dose, (*i.e.,* retardation of fetal skull ossification, increased incidence of abortions and stillbirths, and impaired neonatal survival). The skin and fatty tissue of offspring became discolored approximately 3 days after birth, which was attributed to the presence of clofazimine in the maternal milk.

It has been found that clofazimine crosses the human placenta. The skin of infants born to women who had received the drug during pregnancy was found to be deeply pigmented at birth. No evidence of teratogenicity was found in these infants. There are no adequate and well-controlled studies in pregnant women. Clofazimine should be used during pregnancy only if the potential benefit justifies the risk to the fetus.

NURSING MOTHERS

Clofazimine is excreted in the milk of nursing mothers. Clofazimine should not be administered to a nursing woman unless clearly indicated.

PEDIATRIC USE

Safety and effectiveness in children have not been established. Several cases of children treated with clofazimine have been reported in the literature.

DRUG INTERACTIONS:

Preliminary data which suggest that dapsone may inhibit the anti-inflammatory activity of clofazimine have not been confirmed. If leprosy-associated inflammatory reactions develop in patients being treated with dapsone and clofazimine, it is still advisable to continue treatment with both drugs.

ADVERSE REACTIONS:

In general, clofazimine is well tolerated when administered in dosages no greater than 100 mg daily. The most consistent adverse reactions are usually dose related and are usually reversible when clofazimine is discontinued.

ADVERSE REACTIONS OCCURRING IN MORE THAN 1% OF PATIENTS

Skin: Pigmentation from pink to brownish-black in 75-100% of the patients within a few weeks of treatment; ichthyosis and dryness (8-28%); rash and pruritus (1-5%).

Gastrointestinal: Abdominal and epigastric pain, diarrhea, nausea, vomiting, gastrointestinal intolerance (40-50%).

Ocular: Conjunctival and corneal pigmentation due to clofazimine crystal deposits; dryness; burning; itching; irritation.

Other: Discoloration of urine, feces, sputum, sweat; elevated blood sugar; elevated ESR.

ADVERSE REACTIONS: *(cont'd)*

ADVERSE REACTIONS OCCURRING IN LESS THAN 1% OF PATIENTS

Skin: Phototoxicity, erythroderma, acneiform eruptions, monilial cheilosis.

Gastrointestinal: Bowel obstruction (see WARNINGS), Gastrointestinal Bleeding (see WARNINGS), anorexia, constipation, weight loss, hepatitis, jaundice, eosinophilic enteritis, enlarged liver.

Ocular: Diminished vision.

Nervous: Dizziness, drowsiness, fatigue, headache, giddiness, neuralgia, taste disorder.

Psychiatric: Depression secondary to skin discoloration; two suicides have been reported.

Laboratory: Elevated levels of albumin, serum bilirubin, and AST (SGOT); eosinophilia; hypokalemia.

Other: Splenic infarction (see WARNINGS), thromboembolism, anemia, cystitis, bone pain, edema, fever, lymphadenopathy, vascular pain.

OVERDOSAGE:

No specific data are available on the treatment of overdosage with clofazimine. However, in case of overdose, the stomach should be emptied by inducing vomiting or by gastric lavage, and supportive symptomatic treatment should be employed.

DOSAGE AND ADMINISTRATION:

Clofazimine should be taken with meals.

Clofazimine should be used preferably in combination with one or more other antileprosy agents to prevent the emergence of drug resistance.

For the treatment of proven dapsone-resistant leprosy, clofazimine should be given at a dosage of 100 mg daily in combination with one or more other antileprosy drugs for 3 years, followed by monotherapy with 100 mg of clofazimine daily. Clinical improvement usually can be detected between the first and third months of treatment and is usually clearly evident by the sixth month.

For dapsone-sensitive multibacillary leprosy, a combination therapy with two other antileprosy drugs is recommended. The triple-drug regimen should be given for at least 2 years and continued, if possible, until negative skin smears are obtained. At this time, monotherapy with an appropriate antileprosy drug can be instituted.

The treatment of erythema nodosum leprosum reactions depends on the severity of symptoms. In general, the basic antileprosy treatment should be continued, and if nerve injury or skin ulceration is threatened, corticosteroids should be given. Where prolonged corticosteroid therapy becomes necessary, clofazimine administered at dosages of 100 mg to 200 mg daily for up to 3 months may be useful in eliminating or reducing corticosteroid requirements. Dosages above 200 mg daily are not recommended, and the dosage should be tapered to 100 mg daily as quickly as possible after the reactive episode is controlled. The patient must remain under medical surveillance.

For advice about combination drug regimens, contact the USPHS Gillis W.Long Hansen's Disease Center, Carville, LA (504-642-7771).

Do not store above 86°F. Protect from moisture.

Dispense in tight container (USP).

HOW SUPPLIED - EQUIVALENTS NOT AVAILABLE:

Capsule, Elastic - Oral - 50 mg

100's $13.02 LAMPRENE, Novartis 00028-0108-01

CLOFIBRATE *(000842)*

CATEGORIES: Antilipemic Agents; Cardiovascular Drugs; Cholesterol; Fibrates; Hyperlipidemia; Hyperlipoproteinemia; Hypertriglyceridemia; Hypolipidemics; Pregnancy Category C; FDA Approval Pre 1982

BRAND NAMES: *Amadol* (Japan); *Apoterin*; *Apoterin A* (Japan); *Arterioflexin*; *Arterol*; *Artes*; **Atromid-S**; *Atromid-S 500*; *Atromidin*; *Cartagyl*; *Cholenal*; *Claripex* (Canada); *Clobrate*; *Clofi ICN*; *Clofibral*; *Clofibrato*; *Clofibrato Procaps*; *Clofipront*; *Col*; *Colebron*; *Coles*; *Kalipion*; *Lipavlon* (France); *Lipilim*; *Lipomid*; *Miscleron*; *Neo Atromid*; *Novofibrate* (Canada); *Regelan*; *Regelan N* (Germany); *Skleromexe* (Germany); *Triglicer*; *Yuclo* (Japan)

(International brand names outside U.S. in italics)

COST OF THERAPY: $191.69 (Hyperlipidemia; Capsule; 500 mg; 4/day; 365 days)

DESCRIPTION:

Clofibrate capsules, ethyl 2-(p-chlorophenoxy)-2-methyl-propionate, an antilipidemic agent.

Its molecular formula is $C_{12}H_{15}O_3Cl$, molecular weight 242.7, and boiling point 148-150° C at 25 mm Hg. It is a stable, colorless to pale-yellow liquid with a faint odor and characteristic taste, soluble in common solvents but not in water. Each clofibrate capsule contains 500 mg clofibrate for oral administration.

Atromid-S Capsules contain the following inactive ingredients: D&C Red No. 28, D&C Red No. 30, D&C Yellow No. 10, FD&C Blue No. 1, FD&C Red No. 3, FD&C Yellow No. 6, gelatin.

CLINICAL PHARMACOLOGY:

Clofibrate is an antilipidemic agent. It acts to lower elevated serum lipids by reducing the very low-density lipoprotein fraction (S_f20-400) rich in triglycerides. Serum cholesterol may be decreased, particularly in those patients whose cholesterol elevation is due to the presence of IDL as a result of Type III hyperlipoproteinemia.

The mechanism of action has not been established definitively. Clofibrate may inhibit the hepatic release of lipoproteins (particularly VLDL), potentiate the action of lipoprotein lipase, and increase the fecal excretion of neutral sterols.

Between 95% and 99% of an oral dose of clofibrate is excreted in the urine as free and conjugated clofibric acid; thus, the absorption of clofibrate is virtually complete. The half-life of clofibric acid in normal volunteers averages 18 to 22 hours (range 14 to 35 hours) but can vary by up to 7 hours in the same subject at different times. Clofibric acid is highly protein-bound (95% to 97%). In subjects undergoing continuous clofibrate treatment, 1 g q12h, plasma concentrations of clofibric acid range from 120 to 125 mcg/ml to an approximate peak of 200 mcg/ml.

Several investigators have observed in their studies that clofibrate may produce a decrease in cholesterol linoleate but an increase in palmitoleate and oleate, the latter being considered atherogenic in experimental animals. The significance of this finding is unknown at this time.

Reduction of triglycerides in some patients treated with clofibrate or certain of its chemically and clinically similar analogs may be associated with an increase in LDL cholesterol. Increase in LDL cholesterol has been observed in patients whose cholesterol is initially normal.

CLINICAL PHARMACOLOGY: *(cont'd)*

Animal studies suggest that clofibrate interrupts cholesterol biosynthesis prior to mevalonate formation.

INDICATIONS AND USAGE:

The initial treatment of choice for hyperlipidemia is dietary therapy specific for the type of hyperlipidemia.[1]

Excess body weight and alcoholic intake may be important factors in hypertriglyceridemia and should be addressed prior to any drug therapy. Physical exercise can be an important ancillary measure. Estrogen therapy, some beta-blockers, and thiazide diuretics may also be associated with increases in plasma triglycerides. Discontinuation of such products may obviate the need for specific antilipidemic therapy. Contributory diseases such as hypothyroidism or diabetes mellitus should be looked for and adequately treated. The use of drugs should be considered only when reasonable attempts have been made to obtain satisfactory results with non-drug methods. If the decision ultimately is to use drugs, the patient should be instructed that this does not reduce the importance of adhering to diet.

Because clofibrate is associated with certain serious adverse findings reported in two large clinical trials (see WARNINGS), agents other than clofibrate may be more suitable for a particular patient.

Clofibrate is indicated for Primary Dysbetalipoproteinemia (Type III hyperlipidemia) that does not respond adequately to diet.

Clofibrate may be considered for the treatment of adult patients with very high serum-triglyceride levels (Type IV and V hyperlipidemia) who present a risk of abdominal pain and pancreatitis and who do not respond adequately to a determined dietary effort to control them. Patients who present such risk typically have serum triglycerides over 2000 mg/dl and have elevations of VLDL-cholesterol as well as fasting chylomicrons (Type V hyperlipidemia). Subjects who consistently have total serum or plasma triglycerides below 1000 mg/dl are unlikely to present a risk of pancreatitis. Clofibrate therapy may be considered for those subjects with triglyceride elevations between 1000 and 2000 mg/dl who have a history of pancreatitis or of recurrent abdominal pain typical of pancreatitis. It is recognized that some Type IV patients with triglycerides under 1000 mg/dl may, through dietary or alcoholic indiscretion, convert to a Type V pattern with massive triglyceride elevations accompanying fasting chylomicronemia, but the influence of clofibrate therapy on the risk of pancreatitis in such situations has not been adequately studied.

Clofibrate is not useful for the hypertriglyceridemia of Type I hyperlipidemia, where elevations of chylomicrons and plasma triglycerides are accompanied by normal levels of very low-density lipoprotein (VLDL). Inspection of plasma refrigerated for 12 to 14 hours is helpful in distinguishing Types I, IV, and V hyperlipoproteinemia.[2]

Clofibrate has not been shown to be effective for prevention of coronary heart disease.

The biochemical response to clofibrate is variable, and it is not always possible to predict from the lipoprotein type or other factors which patients will obtain favorable results. LDL cholesterol, as well as triglycerides, should be rechecked during the first several months of therapy in order to detect rises in LDL cholesterol that often accompany fibric-acid-type drug-induced reductions in elevated triglycerides. It is essential that lipid levels be reassessed periodically and that the drug be discontinued in any patient in whom lipids do not show significant improvement.

CONTRAINDICATIONS:

Clofibrate is contraindicated in pregnant women. While teratogenic studies have not demonstrated any effect attributable to clofibrate, it is known that serum of the rabbit fetus accumulates a higher concentration of clofibrate than that found in maternal serum, and it is possible that the fetus may not have developed the enzyme system required for the excretion of clofibrate.

It is contraindicated in patients with clinically significant hepatic or renal dysfunction. Rhabdomyolysis and severe hyperkalemia have been reported in association with preexisting renal insufficiency.

It is contraindicated in patients with primary biliary cirrhosis, since it may raise the already elevated cholesterol in these cases.

It is contraindicated in patients with a known hypersensitivity to clofibrate.

It is contraindicated in nursing women (see PRECAUTIONS.)

WARNINGS:

In a large prospective study involving 5,000 patients in a clofibrate-treated group and 5,000 in a placebo-treated group followed for an average of five years on drug or placebo and one year beyond (the WHO study), there was a statistically significant 36% higher mortality due to noncardiovascular causes in the clofibrate-treated group than in a comparable placebo group. Half of this difference was due to malignancy; other causes of death included postcholecystectomy complications and pancreatitis.[3] In another prospective study involving 1,000 clofibrate- and 3,000 placebo-treated patients followed for an average of six years on drug or placebo (the Coronary Drug Project study), the noncardiovascular mortality rate, including that of malignancy, was not significantly different in the clofibrate- and placebo-treated groups.[4] This should not be interpreted to mean that clofibrate is not associated with an increased risk of noncardiovascular death, because the patients in the Coronary Drug Project were much older than those in the WHO study and they all had had a previous myocardial infarction, so that the deaths in the Coronary Drug Project were overwhelmingly due to cardiovascular causes, and it would have been very difficult to discern a clofibrate-associated risk of death due to noncardiovascular causes if it existed. Both studies demonstrated that clofibrate users have twice the risk of developing cholelithiasis and cholecystitis requiring surgery as do non-users.

A potential benefit of clofibrate was, however, reported in the WHO study which involved patients with hypercholesterolemia and no history of myocardial infarction or angina pectoris. In this study, there was a statistically significant 25% decrease in subsequent nonfatal myocardial infarctions in the clofibrate-treated group when compared with the placebo group. There was no difference in incidence of fatal myocardial infarction in the two groups. In the Coronary Drug Project study, which involved patients with or without hypercholesterolemia and/or hypertriglyceridemia and with a history of previous myocardial infarction, there was no significant difference in incidence of either nonfatal or fatal myocardial infarction between the clofibrate- and placebo-treated groups.[3] As a result of these and other studies, the following can be stated:

1. Clofibrate, in general, causes a relatively modest reduction of serum cholesterol and somewhat greater reduction of serum triglycerides. In Type III hyperlipidemia, however, substantial reductions of both cholesterol and triglycerides can occur with clofibrate use.

2. No study to date has shown a convincing reduction in incidence of FATAL myocardial infarction.

3. A significantly increased incidence of cholelithiasis has been demonstrated consistently in clofibrate-treated groups, and an increase in morbidity from this complication and mortality from cholecystectomy must be anticipated during clofibrate treatment.

4. Several types of other undesirable events have been associated in a statistically significant way with clofibrate administration in the WHO and the Coronary Drug Project studies. There was an increase in incidence of noncardiovascular deaths reported in the WHO study. There was an increase in cardiac arrhythmias, intermittent claudication, and definite or suspected thromboembolic events, and angina reported in the Coronary Drug Project, which was not, however, reported in the WHO study.

5. Administration of clofibrate to mice and rats in long-term studies at eight times the human dose, and to rats at five times the human dose, resulted in a higher incidence of benign and malignant liver tumors than in controls. Lower doses were not included in these studies. An increase in benign Leydig-cell tumors in male rats treated at 400 mg/kg (10 times the estimated human dose) was observed in a single study with clofibrate; similar increases were not observed in other studies conducted with clofibrate although they have been observed with other fibric-acid derivatives.

6. Administration of clofibrate to male monkeys at dosages of 2 to 6 times the human dose resulted in increases in mortality of 2- to 5-fold. As in the case of men in the WHO study, no single cause of death was identified.

BECAUSE OF THE TUMORIGENICITY OF CLOFIBRATE IN RODENTS AND THE POSSIBLE INCREASED RISK OF MALIGNANCY ASSOCIATED WITH CLOFIBRATE IN THE HUMAN, AS WELL AS THE INCREASED RISK OF CHOLELITHIASIS, AND BECAUSE THERE IS NOT, TO DATE, SUBSTANTIAL EVIDENCE OF A BENEFICIAL EFFECT ON CARDIOVASCULAR MORTALITY FROM CLOFIBRATE, THIS DRUG SHOULD BE UTILIZED ONLY FOR THOSE PATIENTS DESCRIBED IN THE "INDICATIONS AND USAGE" SECTION, AND SHOULD BE DISCONTINUED IF SIGNIFICANT LIPID RESPONSE IS NOT OBTAINED.

CONCOMITANT ANTICOAGULANTS

CAUTION SHOULD BE EXERCISED WHEN ANTICOAGULANTS ARE GIVEN IN CONJUNCTION WITH CLOFIBRATE. THE DOSAGE OF THE ANTICOAGULANT SHOULD BE REDUCED USUALLY BY ONE-HALF (DEPENDING ON THE INDIVIDUAL CASE) TO MAINTAIN THE PROTHROMBIN TIME AT THE DESIRED LEVEL TO PREVENT BLEEDING COMPLICATIONS. FREQUENT PROTHROMBIN DETERMINATIONS ARE ADVISABLE UNTIL IT HAS BEEN DEFINITELY DETERMINED THAT THE PROTHROMBIN LEVEL HAS BEEN STABILIZED.

SKELETAL MUSCLE

Myalgia, myositis, myopathy, and rhabdomyolysis with or without elevation of CPK have been associated with clofibrate therapy. Consideration should be given to withholding or discontinuing drug therapy in any patient with a risk factor predisposing to the development of renal failure secondary to rhabdomyolysis, including: severe acute infection; hypotension; major surgery; trauma; severe metabolic, endocrine, or electrolyte disorders; and uncontrolled seizures.

Clofibrate therapy should be discontinued if markedly elevated CPK levels occur or myositis is diagnosed.

AVOIDANCE OF PREGNANCY

Strict birth-control procedures must be exercised by women of child-bearing potential. In patients who plan to become pregnant, clofibrate should be withdrawn several months before conception. Because of the possibility of pregnancy occurring despite birth-control precautions in patients taking clofibrate, the possible benefits of the drug to the patient must be weighed against possible hazards to the fetus. (See Pregnancy.)

PRECAUTIONS:

GENERAL

Before instituting therapy with clofibrate, attempts should be made to control serum lipids with appropriate dietary regimens, weight loss in obese patients, control of diabetes mellitus, etc.

Because of the long-term administration of a drug of this nature, adequate baseline studies should be performed to determine that the patient has significantly elevated serum-lipid levels. Frequent determinations of serum lipids should be obtained during the first few months of clofibrate administration, and periodic determinations made thereafter. The drug should be withdrawn after three months if response is inadequate. However, in the case of xanthoma tuberosum, the drug should be employed for longer periods (even up to one year) provided that there is a reduction in the size and/or number of the xanthomata.

Since cholelithiasis is a possible side effect of clofibrate therapy, appropriate diagnostic procedures should be performed if signs and symptoms related to disease of the biliary system should occur.

Clofibrate may produce "flu-like" symptoms (muscular aching, soreness, cramping) associated with increased creatine kinase levels indicative of drug-induced myopathy. The physician should differentiate this from actual viral and/or bacterial disease.

Use with caution in patients with peptic ulcer, since reactivation has been reported. Whether this is drug related is unknown.

Various cardiac arrhythmias have been reported with the use of clofibrate.

LABORATORY TESTS

Subsequent serum lipid determinations should be done to detect a paradoxical rise in serum cholesterol or triglyceride levels. Clofibrate will not alter the seasonal variations of serum cholesterol: peak elevations in midwinter and late summer and decreases in fall and spring. If the drug is discontinued, the patient should be continued on an appropriate hypolipidemic diet, and serum lipids should be monitored until stabilized, as a rise in these values to or above the original baseline may occur.

During clofibrate therapy, frequent serum-transaminase determinations and other liver-function tests should be performed, since the drug may produce abnormalities in these parameters. These effects are usually reversible when the drug is discontinued. Hepatic biopsies are

PRECAUTIONS: *(cont'd)*

usually within normal limits. If the hepatic-function tests steadily rise or show excessive abnormalities, the drug should be withdrawn. Therefore, use with caution in those patients with a past history of jaundice or hepatic disease.

Complete blood counts should be done periodically since anemia, and more frequently, leukopenia have been reported in patients who have been taking clofibrate.

CARCINOGENESIS, MUTAGENESIS, AND IMPAIRMENT OF FERTILITY

See WARNINGS section for information on carcinogenesis and mutagenesis.

Arrest of spermatogenesis has been seen in both dogs and monkeys at doses approximately 4 to 6 times the human therapeutic dose.

PREGNANCY, TERATOGENIC EFFECTS, PREGNANCY CATEGORY C

Animal reproduction studies have not been conducted with clofibrate. It is also not known whether clofibrate can cause fetal harm when administered to a pregnant woman or can affect reproductive capacity. However, animal reproduction studies with clofibrate plus androsterone showed increases in neonatal deaths and pup mortality during lactation.

NURSING MOTHERS

Clofibrate is contraindicated in lactating women, since an active metabolite (CPIB) has been measured in breast milk.

PEDIATRIC USE

Safety and efficacy in children have not been established.

DRUG INTERACTIONS:

Caution should be exercised when anticoagulants are given in conjunction with clofibrate. Usually, the dosage of the anticoagulant should be reduced by one-half (depending on the individual case) to maintain the prothrombin time at the desired level to prevent bleeding complications. Frequent prothrombin determinations are advisable until it has been determined definitely that the prothrombin level has been stabilized.

Clofibrate may displace acidic drugs such as phenytoin or tolbutamide from their binding sites. Caution should be exercised when treating patients with either of these drugs or other highly protein-bound drugs and clofibrate. The hypoglycemic effect of tolbutamide has been reported to increase when clofibrate is given concurrently.

Fulminant rhabdomyolysis has been seen as early as three weeks after initiation of combined therapy with another fibrate and lovastatin but may be seen after several months. For these reasons, it is felt that, in most subjects who have had an unsatisfactory lipid response to either drug alone, the possible benefits of combined therapy with lovastatin and a fibrate do not outweigh the risks of severe myopathy, rhabdomyolysis, and acute renal failure. While it is not known whether this interaction occurs with fibrates other than gemfibrozil, myopathy and rhabdomyolysis have occasionally been associated with the use of fibrates alone, including clofibrate. Therefore, the combined use of lovastatin with fibrates should generally be avoided.

ADVERSE REACTIONS:

The most common is nausea. Less frequently encountered gastrointestinal reactions are vomiting, loose stools, dyspepsia, flatulence, and abdominal distress. Reactions reported less often than gastrointestinal ones are headache, dizziness, and fatigue; muscle cramping, aching, and weakness; skin rash, urticaria, and pruritus; dry, brittle hair, and alopecia.

The following reported adverse reactions are listed alphabetically by systems:

Cardiovascular: Increased or decreased angina, cardiac arrhythmias, both swelling and phlebitis at site of xanthomas.

Dermatologic: Allergic reaction including urticaria, skin rash, pruritus, dry skin and dry, brittle hair, alopecia, toxic epidermal necrolysis.

Gastrointestinal: Gallstones, nausea, vomiting, diarrhea, gastrointestinal upset (bloating, flatulence, abdominal distress), hepatomegaly (not associated with hepatotoxicity), stomatitis and gastritis.

Genitourinary: Findings consistent with renal dysfunction as evidenced by dysuria, hematuria, proteinuria, decreased urine output. One patient's renal biopsy suggested "allergic reaction," impotence and decreased libido.

Hematologic: Leukopenia, potentiation of anticoagulant effect, anemia, eosinophilia, agranulocytosis.

Musculoskeletal: Myalgia (muscle cramping, aching, weakness), "flu-like" symptoms, myositis, myopathy, rhabdomyolysis in the setting of preexisting renal insufficiency, aarthralgia.

Neurologic: Fatigue, weakness, drowsiness; dizziness; headache.

Miscellaneous: Weight gain, polyphagia.

Laboratory Findings: Abnormal liver-function tests as evidenced by increased transaminase (SGOT and SGPT), BSP retention, and increased thymol turbidity; Proteinuria; Increased creatine phosphokinase; Hyperkalemia in association with renal insufficiency and continuous ambulatory peritoneal dialysis treatment.

Reported adverse reactions whose direct relationship with the drug has not been established: peptic ulcer, gastrointestinal hemorrhage, rheumatoid arthritis, tremors, increased perspiration, systemic lupus erythematosus, blurred vision, gynecomastia, thrombocytopenic purpura.

OVERDOSAGE:

While there has been no reported case of overdosage, should it occur, symptomatic supportive measures should be taken.

DOSAGE AND ADMINISTRATION:

Initial: The recommended dosage for adults is 2 g daily in divided doses. Some patients may respond to a lower dosage.

Maintenance: Same as for initial dosage.

Store at room temperature (approximately 25° C).

Avoid freezing and excessive heat.

REFERENCES:

1. Coronary Risk Handbook (1973). American Heart Association. **2.** Nikkila, E.A.: Familial lipoprotein lipase deficiency and related disorders of chylomicron metabolism. In Stanbury J.B. et al (eds): The Metabolic Basis of Inherited Disease, 5th ed., McGraw-Hill, 1983, Chap. 30 p.622-642. **3.** Report from the Committee of Principal Investigators: A cooperative trial in the primary prevention of ischaemia heart disease using clofibrate. Br Heart J *40*:1069, 1978. **4.** The Coronary Drug Project Research Group: Clofibrate and niacin in coronary heart disease. JAMA *231*:360, 1975.

HOW SUPPLIED - RATED THERAPEUTICALLY EQUIVALENT:

Capsule, Elastic - Oral - 500 mg

100's	$13.13	Clofibrate, United Res	00677-1111-01
100's	$13.13	Clofibrate, H.C.F.A. F F P	99999-0842-01
100's	$23.31	Clofibrate, Qualitest Pharms	00603-2932-21
100's	$24.50	Clofibrate, Aligen Independ	00405-4236-01
100's	$25.23	Clofibrate, HL Moore Drug Exch	00839-7228-06
100's	$25.48	Clofibrate, Novopharm (US)	55953-0382-40

HOW SUPPLIED - RATED THERAPEUTICALLY EQUIVALENT: *(cont'd)*

100's	$25.75	Clofibrate, Schein Pharm (US)	00364-2136-01
100's	$25.81	Clofibrate, Caremark	00339-5651-12
100's	$26.00	Clofibrate, Goldline Labs	00182-1269-01
100's	$26.08	Clofibrate Capsules 500 Mg, Geneva Pharms	00781-2600-01
100's	$26.24	Clofibrate, Rugby	00536-3466-01
100's	$26.40	Clofibrate, Major Pharms	00904-2916-60
100's	$26.70	Clofibrate, Parmed Pharms	00349-8604-01
100's	$28.43	Clofibrate, Martec Pharms	52555-0111-01
100's	**$88.75**	**ATROMID-S, Ayerst**	**00046-0243-81**

CLOMIPHENE CITRATE *(000843)*

CATEGORIES: Anterior Pituitary/Hypothalmic Function; Fertility Agents; Infertility; Ovarian Failure; Ovulation Stimulants; Pregnancy; FDA Approval Pre 1982

BRAND NAMES: *Arcafen*; *Clom 50* (Germany); Clomid; *Clomifen*; *Clomifen-Ratiopharm* (Germany); Clomifene; *Clomin*; *Clomiphene Serono*; *Clomivid*; *Clomoval*; *Clonin*; *Clostil*; *Clostilbegyt*; *Dufine*; *Duinum*; *Dyneric* (Germany); *Fertilan*; *Fertomid*; *Fertotab*; *Ikaclomin*; *Indovar*; *Mestrolin*; Milophene; *Nefimol* (Mexico); *Omicite*; *Omifin* (Mexico); *Ova-Mit*; *Ovamit*; *Pergotime* (France); *Phemilon* (Japan); *Phenate*; *Profertil*; *Serofene* (Mexico); **Serophene**; *Serpafar*
(International brand names outside U.S. in italics)

FORMULARIES: Aetna; BC-BS; WHO

DESCRIPTION:

Clomiphene citrate tablets USP is an orally administered, non steroidal, ovulatory stimulant designated chemically as 2-[p-(2-chloro-l,2-diphenylvinyl) phenoxy] triethylamine dihydrogen citrate (1:1). It has the molecular formula of $C_{26}H_{28}ClNO{\cdot}C_6H_8O_7$ and a molecular weight of 598.09.

Clomiphene citrate is a white to pale yellow, essentially odorless, crystalline powder. It is freely soluble in methanol; soluble in ethanol; slightly soluble in acetone, water, and chloroform; and insoluble in ether.

Each white scored tablet contains 50 mg clomiphene citrate USP. The tablet also contains the following inactive ingredients: corn starch, lactose, magnesium stearate, pregelatinized corn starch, and sucrose.

CLINICAL PHARMACOLOGY:

Action: Clomiphene citrate is a drug of considerable pharmacologic potency. With careful selection and proper management of the patient, clomiphene citrate has been demonstrated to be a useful therapy for the anovulatory patient desiring pregnancy.

Clomiphene citrate is capable of interacting with estrogen-receptor-containing tissues, including the hypothalamus, pituitary, ovary, endometrium, vagina, and cervix. It may compete with estrogen-receptor-binding sites and may delay replenishment of intracellular estrogen receptors. Clomiphene citrate initiates a series if endocrine events culminating in a preovulatory gonadotropin surge and subsequent follicular rupture. The first endocrine event in response to a course of clomiphene therapy is an increase in the release of pituitary gonadotropins. This initiates steroidogenesis and folliculogenesis, resulting in growth of the ovarian follicle and an increase in the circulating level of estradiol. Following ovulation, plasma progesterone and estradiol rise and fall as they would in a normal ovulatory cycle.

Available data suggest that both the estrogenic and antiestrogenic properties of clomiphene may participate in the initiation of ovulation. The two clomiphene isomers have been found to have mixed estrogenic and antiestrogenic effects, which may vary from one species to another. Some data suggest that zuclomiphene has greater estrogenic activity than enclomiphene.

Clomiphene citrate has no apparent progestational, androgenic, or antiandrogenic effects and does not appear to interfere with pituitary-adrenal or pituitary-thyroid function.

Although there is no evidence of a "carryover effect" of clomiphene citrate, spontaneous ovulatory menses have been noted in some patients after clomiphene citrate therapy.

Pharmacokinetics: Based on early studies with ^{14}C-labeled clomiphene citrate, the drug was shown to be readily absorbed orally in humans and excreted principally in the feces. Cumulative urinary and fecal excretion if the ^{14}C averaged about 50% of the oral dose and 37% of an intravenous dose after 5 days. Mean urinary excretion was approximately 8% with fecal excretion of about 42%.

Some ^{14}C label was still present in the feces 6 weeks after administration. Subsequent single-dose studies in normal volunteers showed that zuclomiphene (cis) has a longer half-life than enclomiphene (trans). Detectable levels of zuclomiphene persisted for longer than a month in these subjects. This may be suggestive of stereo-specific enterohepatic recycling or sequestering of the zuclomiphene. Thus, it is possible that some active drug may remain in the body during early pregnancy in women who conceive in the menstrual cycle during clomiphene citrate therapy.

CLINICAL STUDIES:

During clinical investigations, 7578 patients received clomiphene citrate, some of whom had impediments to ovulation other than ovulatory dysfunction (see INDICATIONS AND USAGE.) In those clinical trials, successful therapy characterized by pregnancy occurred in approximately 30% of these patients.

There were a total of 2635 pregnancies reported during the clinical trial period. Of those pregnancies, information on outcome was only available for 2369 of the cases. TABLE 1 summarizes the outcome of these cases.

Of the reported pregnancies, the incidence of multiple pregnancies was 7.98%: 6.9% twin, 0.5% triplet, 0.3% quadruplet, and 0.1% quintuplet. Of the 165 twin pregnancies for which sufficient information was available, the ratio of monozygotic to dizygotic twins was about 1: 5. TABLE 1 reports the survival rate of the live multiple births.

A sextuplet birth was reported after completion of original clinical studies; none of the sextuplets survived (each weighed less than 400 g), although each appeared grossly normal.

TABLE 1 Outcome of Reported Pregnancies in Clinical Trials (n=2369)

Outcome	Total Number of Pregnancies	Survival Rate
Pregnancy Wastage		
Spontaneous Abortions	483*	
Stillbirths	24	
Live Births		
Single Births	1697	98.16%†
Multiple Births	165	26%†

* Includes 28 ectopic pregnancies, 4 hydatiform moles, and 1 fetus papyraceous
†Indicates percentage of surviving infants from these pregnancies.

CLINICAL STUDIES: *(cont'd)*

The overall survival of infants from multiple pregnancies including spontaneous abortions, stillbirths, and neonatal deaths is 73%.

INDICATIONS AND USAGE:

Clomiphene citrate is indicated for the treatment of ovulatory dysfunction in women desiring pregnancy. Impediments to achieving this goal of therapy must be excluded or adequately treated before beginning clomiphene citrate therapy. Those patients most likely to achieve success with clomiphene therapy include patients with polycystic ovary syndrome (see WARNINGS, Ovarian Hyperstimulation Syndrome), amenorrhea-galactorrhea syndrome, psychogenic amenorrhea, post-oral-contraceptive amenorrhea, and certain cases of secondary amenorrhea of undetermined etiology.

Properly timed coitus in relationship to ovulation is important. A basal body temperature graph or other appropriate tests may help the patient and her physician determine if ovulation occurred. Once ovulation has been established, each course of clomiphene citrate should be started on or about the 5th day of the cycle. If pregnancy has not been achieved after three ovulatory responses to clomiphene citrate, further treatment is not recommended.

Clomiphene citrate is indicated only in patients with demonstrated ovulatory dysfunction who meet the conditions described below (see CONTRAINDICATIONS):

1. Patients who are not pregnant.

2. Patients without ovarian cysts. Clomiphene citrate should not be used in patients with ovarian enlargement except those with polycystic ovary syndrome. Pelvic examination is necessary prior to the first and each subsequent course of clomiphene citrate.

3. Patients without abnormal vaginal bleeding. If abnormal vaginal bleeding is present, the patient should be carefully evaluated to ensure that neoplastic lesions are not present.

4. Patients with normal liver function.

In addition, patients selected for clomiphene citrate therapy should be evaluated in regard to the following:

1. Estrogen Levels: Patients should have adequate levels of endogenous estrogen (as estimated from vaginal smears, endometrial biopsy, assay of urinary estrogen, or from bleeding in response to progesterone). Reduced estrogen levels, while less favorable, do not preclude successful therapy.

2. Primary Pituitary or Ovarian Failure: Clomiphene citrate therapy cannot be expected to substitute for specific treatment of other causes of ovulatory failure.

3. Endometriosis and Endometrial Carcinoma: The incidence of endometriosis and endometrial carcinoma increases with age as does the incidence of ovulatory disorders. Endometrial biopsy should always be performed prior to clomiphene citrate therapy in this population.

4. Other Impediments to Pregnancy: Impediments to pregnancy can include thyroid disorders, adrenal disorders, hyperprolactinemia, and male factor infertility.

5. Uterine Fibroids: Caution should be exercised when using clomiphene citrate in patients with uterine fibroids due to the potential for further enlargement of the fibroids.

There are no adequate or well-controlled studies that demonstrate the effectiveness of clomiphene citrate in the treatment of male infertility. In addition, testicular tumors and gynecomastia have been reported in males using clomiphene. The cause and effect relationship between reports of testicular tumors and the administration of clomiphene is not known.

Although the medical literature suggests various methods, there is no universally accepted standard regimen for combined therapy (*i.e.,* clomiphene citrate in conjunction with other ovulation-inducing drugs). Similarly, there is no standard clomiphene citrate regimen for ovulation induction in *in vitro* fertilization programs to produce ova for fertilization and reintroduction. Therefore, clomiphene is not recommended for these users.

CONTRAINDICATIONS:

Hypersensitivity: Clomiphene citrate is contraindicated in patients with a known hypersensitivity or allergy to clomiphene citrate or to any of its ingredients.

Pregnancy: Clomiphene should not be administered during pregnancy. Clomiphene citrate may cause fetal harm in animals (see Animal Fetotoxicity.) Although no causative evidence of a deleterious effect of clomiphene therapy on the human fetus has been established, there have been reports of birth anomalies which, during clinicals studies, occurred at an incidence within the range reported for the general population (see Fetal/Neonatal Anomalies and Mortality; ADVERSE REACTIONS.)

To avoid inadvertent clomiphene administration during early pregnancy, appropriate tests should be utilized during each treatment cycle to determine whether ovulation occurs. The patient should be evaluated carefully to exclude pregnancy, ovarian enlargement, or ovarian cyst formation between each treatment cycle. The next course of clomiphene citrate therapy should be delayed until these conditions have been excluded.

Fetal/Neonatal Anomalies and Mortality: The following fetal abnormalities have been reported subsequent to pregnancies following ovulation induction therapy with clomiphene citrate during clinical trials. Each of the following fetal abnormalities were reported at a rate <1% (experiences are listed in order of decreasing frequency): Congenital heart lesions, Down syndrome, club foot, congenital gut lesions, hypospadias, microcephaly, harelip and cleft palate, congenital hip, hemangioma, undescended testicles, polydactyly, conjoined twins and teratomatous malformation, patient ductus arteriosus, amaurosis, arteriovenous fistula, inguinal hernia, umbilical hernia, syndactyly, pectus excavatum, myopathy, dermoid cyst of scalp, omphalocele, spina bifida occulta, ichthyosis, and persistent lingual frenulum. Neonatal death and fetal death/stillbirth infants with birth in infants with birth defects have also been reported at a rate of <1%. The overall incidence of reported birth anomalies from pregnancies associated with maternal clomiphene citrate ingestion during clinical studies was within the range of that reported for the general population.

In addition, reports of birth anomalies have been received during postmarketing surveillance of clomiphene citrate (see ADVERSE REACTIONS).

Animal Fetotoxicity: Oral administration of clomiphene citrate to pregnant rats during organogenesis at doses of 1 to 2 mg/kg/day resulted in hydramnion and weak, edematous fetuses with wavy ribs and other temporary bone changes. Doses of 8 mg/kg/day or more also caused increased resorptions and dead fetuses, dystocia, and delayed parturition, and 40 mg/kg/day resulted in increased maternal mortality. Single doses of 50 mg/kg/day caused fetal cataracts, while 200 mg/kg caused cleft palate.

Following injection of clomiphene citrate 2 mg/kg to mice and rats during pregnancy, the offspring exhibited metaplastic changes of the reproductive tract. Newborn mice and rats injected during the first few days of life also developed metaplastic changes in uterine and vaginal mucosa, as well as premature vaginal opening and anovulatory ovaries. these findings are similar to the abnormal reproductive behavior and sterility described with other estrogens and antiestrogens.

In rabbits, some temporary bone alterations were seen in fetuses from dams given oral doses or 20 or 40 mg/kg/day during pregnancy, but not following 8 mg/kg/day. No permanent malformations were observed in those studies. Also, rhesus monkeys given oral doses of 1.5 to 4.5 mg/kg/day for various periods during pregnancy did not have any abnormal offspring.

CONTRAINDICATIONS: *(cont'd)*

Liver Disease: Clomiphene citrate therapy is contraindicated in patients with liver disease or a history of liver dysfunction. (see also INDICATIONS AND USAGE and ADVERSE REACTIONS)

Abnormal Uterine Bleeding: Clomiphene citrate is contraindicated in patients with abnormal uterine bleeding of undetermined origin (see INDICATIONS AND USAGE).

Ovarian Cysts: Clomiphene citrate is contraindicated in patients with ovarian cysts or enlargement not due to polycystic ovarian syndrome (see INDICATIONS AND USAGE and WARNINGS).

Other: Clomiphene citrate is contraindicated in patients with uncontrolled thyroid or adrenal dysfunction or in the presence of an organic intracranial lesion such as pituitary tumor (see INDICATIONS AND USAGE).

WARNINGS:

Visual Symptoms: Patients should be advised that blurring and/or other visual symptoms such as spots or flashes (scintillating scotomata) may occasionally occur during therapy with clomiphene citrate. These visual symptoms increase in incidence with increasing total dose or therapy duration and generally disappear within a few days or weeks after clomiphene citrate is discontinued. Patients should be warned that these visual symptoms may render such activities as driving a car or operating machinery more hazardous than usual, particularly under conditions of variable lighting.

These visual symptoms appear to be due to intensification and prolongation of afterimages. Symptoms often first appear or are accentuated with exposure to a brightly lit environment. While measured visually acuity usually has not been affected, a study patient taking 200 mg clomiphene citrate daily developed visual blurring on the 7th day of treatment, which progressed to severe diminution of visual acuity by the 10th day. No other abnormality was found, and the visual activity returned to normal on the 3rd day after treatment was stopped.

Ophthalmologically definable scotomata and retinal cell function (electroretinographic) changes have also been reported. A patient treated during clinical studies developed phosphenes and scotomata during prolonged clomiphene citrate administration, which disappeared by the 32nd day after stopping therapy.

Postmarketing surveillance of adverse events has also revealed other visual signs and symptoms during clomiphene citrate therapy, (see ADVERSE REACTIONS).

While the etiology of these visual symptoms is not yet understood, patients with any visual symptoms should discontinue treatment and have a complete ophthalmological evaluation carried out promptly.

Ovarian Hyperstimulation Syndrome: The ovarian hyperstimulation syndrome (OHSS) has been reported to occur in patients receiving clomiphene citrate therapy for ovulation induction. In some cases, OHSS occurred following cyclic use of clomiphene citrate therapy or when clomiphene citrate was used in combination with gonadotropins. Transient liver function test abnormalities suggestive of hepatic dysfunction, which may be accompanied by morphologic changes on liver biopsy, have been reported in association with ovarian hyperstimulation syndrome (OHSS).

OHSS is a medical event distinct from uncomplicated ovarian enlargement. The clinical signs of this syndrome in severe cases can include gross ovarian enlargement, gastrointestinal symptoms, ascites, dyspnea, oliguria, and pleural effusion. In addition, the following symptoms have been reported in association with this syndrome: pericardial effusion, anasarca, hydrothorax, acute abdomen, hypotension, renal failure, pulmonary edema, intraperitoneal and ovarian hemorrhage, deep venous thrombosis, torsion of the ovary, and acute respiratory distress. The early warning signs of OHSS are abdominal pain and distention, nausea, vomiting, diarrhea, and weight gain. Elevated urinary steroid levels, varying degrees of electrolyte imbalance, hypovolemia, hemoconcentration, and hypoproteinemia may occur. Death due to hypovolemic shock, hemoconcentration, or thromboembolism has occurred. Due to fragility of enlarged ovaries in severe cases, abdominal and pelvic examination should be performed very cautiously. If conception results, rapid progression to the severe form of the syndrome may occur.

To minimize the hazard associated with occasional abnormal ovarian enlargement associated with clomiphene citrate therapy, the lowest dose consistent with expected clinical results should be used. Maximal enlargement of the ovary, whether physiologic or abnormal, may not occur until several days after discontinuation of the recommended dose of clomiphene citrate. Some patients with polycystic ovary syndrome who are unusually sensitive to gonadotropin may have an exaggerated response to usual doses of clomiphene citrate. Therefore, patients with polycystic ovary syndrome should be started on the lowest recommended dose and shortest treatment duration for the first course of therapy (see DOSAGE AND ADMINISTRATION).

If enlargement of the ovary occurs, additional clomiphene citrate therapy should not be given until the ovaries have returned to pretreatment size, and the dosage or duration of the next course should be reduced. Ovarian enlargement and cyst formation associated with clomiphene citrate therapy usually regress spontaneously within a few days or weeks after discontinuing treatment. The potential benefit of subsequent clomiphene citrate therapy in these cases should exceed the risk. Unless surgical indication for laparotomy exists, such cystic enlargement should always be managed conservatively.

A casual relationship between ovarian hyperstimulation and ovarian cancer has not been determined. However, because correlation between ovarian cancer and nulliparity, infertility, and age has been suggested, if ovarian cysts do not regret spontaneously, a thorough elevation should be performed to rule out the presence of ovarian neoplasia.

PRECAUTIONS:

General: Careful attention should be given to the selection of candidates for clomiphene citrate therapy. Pelvic examination is necessary prior to clomiphene citrate treatment and before each subsequent course. (see CONTRAINDICATIONS and WARNINGS).

Information for the Patient: The purpose and risks of clomiphene citrate therapy should be presented to the patient before starting treatment. It should be emphasized that the goal of clomiphene citrate therapy is ovulation for subsequent pregnancy. The physician should counsel the patient with special regard to the following potential risks:

Visual Symptoms: Advise that blurring or other visual symptoms occasionally may occur during or shortly after clomiphene citrate therapy. Warn that visual symptoms may render such activities as driving a car or operating machinery more hazardous than usual, particularly under conditions of variable lighting (see WARNINGS).

The patient should be instructed to inform the physician whenever any unusual visual symptoms occur. If the patient has any visual symptoms, treatment should be discontinued and complete ophthalmologic evaluation performed.

Abdominal/Pelvic Pain or Distention: Ovarian enlargement may occur during or shortly after therapy with clomiphene citrate. To minimize the risk associated with ovarian enlargement, the patient should be instructed to inform the physician of any abdominal or pelvic pain, weight gain, discomfort, or distention after taking clomiphene citrate (see WARNINGS).

PRECAUTIONS: *(cont'd)*

Multiple Pregnancy: Inform the patient that there is an increased chance of multiple pregnancy, including bilateral tubal pregnancy and coexisting tubal and intrauterine pregnancy, when conception occurs in relation to clomiphene citrate therapy. The potential complications and hazards of multiple pregnancy should be explained.

Pregnancy Wastage and Birth Anomalies: The physician should explain the assumed risk of any pregnancy, whether ovulation is induced with the aid of clomiphene citrate or occurs naturally. The patient should be informed of the greater risks associated with certain characteristics or conditions of any pregnant woman, (*e.g.*, age of female and male partner, history of spontaneous abortions. Rh genotype, abnormal menstrual history, infertility history, organic heart disease, diabetes, exposure to infectious agents such as rubella, familial history of birth anomaly), that may be pertinent to the patient for whom clomiphene citrate is being considered. Based upon the evaluation of the patient, genetic counseling may be indicated.

The overall incidence of reported birth anomalies from pregnancies associated with maternal clomiphene citrate ingestion during the investigational studies was within the range of that reported in published references for the general population. (see CONTRAINDICATIONS, Pregnancy)

During clinical investigation, the experience from patients with known pregnancy outcome TABLE 1 shows a spontaneous abortion rate of 20.4% and stillbirth rate of 1.0%. (See CLINICAL PHARMACOLOGY.)

Carcinogenesis, Mutagenesis, and Impairment of Fertility: Long-term toxicity studies in animals have not been performed to evaluate the carcinogenic or mutagenic potential of clomiphene citrate.

Oral administration of clomiphene citrate to male rats at doses of 0.3 or 1 mg/kg/day caused decreased fertility, while higher doses caused temporary infertility. Oral doses of 0.1 mg/kg/day in female rats temporarily interrupted the normal cyclic vaginal smear pattern and prevented conception. Doses of 0.3 mg/kg/day slightly reduced the number of ovulated ova and corpora lutea, while 3 mg/kg/day inhibited ovulation.

Pregnancy Category X: (See CONTRAINDICATIONS.)

Nursing Mothers: It is not known whether clomiphene citrate is excreted in human milk. Because many drugs are excreted in human milk, caution should be excercised if clomiphene citrate is administered to a nursing woman. In some patients, clomiphene citrate may reduce lactation.

Ovarian Cancer: Prolonged use of clomiphene citrate tablets USP may increase the risk of a borderline or invasive ovarian tumor (see ADVERSE REACTIONS).

DRUG INTERACTIONS:

Drug Interactions with clomiphene citrate have not been documented.

ADVERSE REACTIONS:

Clinical Trial Adverse Events: Clomiphene citrate, at recommended dosages, is generally well tolerated. Adverse reactions usually have been mild and transient and most have disappeared promptly after treatment has been discontinued. Adverse experiences reported in patients treated with clomiphene citrate during clinical studies are shown in TABLE 2.

TABLE 2 Incidence of Adverse Events in Clinical Studies (Events Greater than 1%) (n = 8029*)

Adverse Event	%
Ovarian Enlargement	13.6
Vasomotor Flushes	10.4
Abdominal-Pelvic Discomfort/Distention/Bloating	5.5
Nausea and Vomiting	2.2
Breast Discomfort	2.1
Visual Symptoms	1.5
Blurred vision, lights, floaters, waves unspecified visual complaints, photophobia, diplopia, scotomata, phosphenes	
Headache	1.3
Abnormal Uterine Bleeding Intermenstrual spotting, menorrhagia	1.3

* Includes 498 patients whose reports may have been duplicated in the event totals and could not be distinguished as such. Also, excludes 47 patients who did not report symptom data.

The following adverse events have been reported in fewer than 1% of patients in clinical trials: Acute abdomen, appetite increase, constipation, dermatitis or rash, depression, diarrhea, dizziness, fatigue, hair loss/dry hair, increased urinary frequency/volume, insomnia, lightheadedness, nervous tension, vaginal mucosa dry, vertigo, weight gain/loss.

Patients on prolonged clomiphene citrate therapy may show elevated serum levels of desmosterol. This is most likely due to a direct interference with cholesterol synthesis. However, the serum sterols in patients receiving the recommended dose of clomiphene citrate are not significantly altered. Ovarian cancer has been infrequently reported with fertility drugs. However, because infertility is a primary risk factor for ovarian cancer, it cannot be determined if the use of fertility drugs increases the risk beyond that associated with infertility.

Postmarketing Adverse Events: The following adverse experiences were reported spontaneously with clomiphene citrate. The cause and effect relationship of the listed events to the administration of clomiphene citrate is not known.

Dermatologic: Acne, allergic reaction, erythema, erythema multiforme, erythema nodosum, hypertrichosis, pruritus.

Central Nervous System: Migraine headache, paresthesia, seizure, stroke, syncope.

Psychiatry: Anxiety, irritability, mood changes, psychosis.

Visual Disorders: Abnormal, accommodation, cataract, eye pain, macular edema, optic neuritis, photopsia, posterior vitreous detachment, retinal hemorrhage, retinal thrombosis, retinal vascular spasm, temporary loss of vision.

Cardiovascular: Arrhythmia, chest pain, edema, hypertension, palpitation, phlebitis, pulmonary embolism, shortness of breath, tachycardia, thrombophlebitis.

Musculoskeletal: Arthralgia, back pain, myalgia.

Hepatic: Transaminases increased, hepatitis.

Neoplasms: Liver (hepatic hemangiosarcoma, liver cell adenoma, hepatocellular carcinoma); breast (fibrocystic disease, breast carcinoma); endometrium (endometrial carcinoma); nervous system (astrocytoma, pituitary tumor, prolactinoma, neurofibromatosis, glioblastoma multiforme, brain abcess); ovary (luteoma of pregnancy, dermoid cyst of the ovary, ovarian carcinoma); trophoblastic (hydatiform mole, choriocarcinoma); miscellaneous (melanoma, myeloma, perianal cysts, renal cell carcinoma, Hodgkin's lymphoma, tongue carcinoma, bladder carcinoma); and neoplasms of offspring (neuroectodermal tumor, thyroid tumor, hepatoblastoma, lymphocytic leukemia).

Genitourinary: Endometriosis, ovarian cyst (ovarian enlargement or cysts could, as such be complicated by adnexal torsion), ovarian hemorrhage, tubal pregnancy, uterine hemorrhage.

Body as a Whole: Fever, tinnitus, weakness.

ADVERSE REACTIONS: *(cont'd)*

Other: Leukocytosis, thyroid disorder.

Fetal/Neonatal Anomalies: The following fetal abnormalities have also been reported during postmarketing surveillance: delayed development; abnormal bone development including skeletal malformations of the skull, face, nasal passages, jaw, hand, limb (ectromelia including amelia, hemimelia, and phocomelia), foot, and joints: tissue malformations including imperforate anus, tracheoesophageal fistula, diaphragmatic hernia, renal agenesis and dysgenesis, and malformations of the eye and lens (cataract), ear, lung, heart (ventricular septal defect and tetrology of Fallot), and genitalia; as well as dwarfism, deafness, mental retardation, chromosomal disorders, and neural tube defects (including anencephaly).

DRUG ABUSE AND DEPENDENCE:

Tolerance, abuse, or dependence with clomiphene citrate has not been reported.

OVERDOSAGE:

Signs and Symptoms: Toxic effects accompanying acute overdosage of clomiphene citrate have not been reported. Signs and symptoms of overdosage as a result of the use of more than the recommended dose during the clomiphene therapy include nausea, vomiting, vasomotor flushes, visual blurring, spots or flashes, scotomata, ovarian enlargement with pelvic or abdominal pain. (See CONTRAINDICATIONS, Ovarian Cyst.)

Oral LD_{50}: The acute oral LD_{50} of clomiphene citrate is 1700 mg/kg in mice and 5750 mg/kg in rats. The toxic dose in humans is not known.

Dialysis: It is not known if clomiphene citrate is dialyzable.

Treatment: In the event of overdose, appropriate supportive measures should be employed in addition to gastrointestinal decontamination.

DOSAGE AND ADMINISTRATION:

General Considerations: The workup and treatment of candidates for clomiphene citrate therapy should be supervised by physicians experienced in management of gynecologic or endocrine disorders. Patients should be chosen for therapy with clomiphene citrate only after careful diagnostic evaluation (see INDICATIONS AND USAGE). The plan of therapy should be outlined in advance. Impediments to achieving the goal of therapy must be excluded or adequately treated before beginning clomiphene citrate. The therapeutic objective should be balanced with potential risks and discussed with the patient and other involved in the achievement of a pregnancy.

Ovulation most often occurs from 5 to 10 days after a course of clomiphene citrate. Coitus should be timed to coincide with the expected time of ovulation. Appropriate tests to determine ovulation may be useful during this time.

Recommended Dosage: Treatment of the selected patient should begin with a low dose, 50 mg daily (1 tablet) for 5 days. The dose should be increased only in those patients who do not ovulate in response to cyclic 50 mg clomiphene citrate. A low dosage or duration of treatment course is particularly recommended if unusual sensitivity to pituitary gonadotropin is suspected, such as in patients with polycystic ovary syndrome (see WARNINGS, Ovarian Hyperstimulation Syndrome).

The patient should evaluated carefully to exclude pregnancy, ovarian enlargement, or ovarian cyst formation between each treatment cycle.

If progestin-induced bleeding is planned, or if spontaneous uterine bleeding occurs prior to therapy, the regimen of 50 mg daily for 5 days should be started on or about the 5th day of the cycle. Therapy may be started at any time in the patient who has had no recent uterine bleeding. When ovulation occurs at this dosage, there is no advantage to increasing the dose in subsequent cycles of treatment.

If ovulation does not appear to occur the first course of therapy, a second course of 100 mg daily (two 50 mg tablets given as a single daily dose) for 5 days should be given. This course may be started as early as 30 days after the previous one after precautions are taken to exclude the presence of pregnancy. Increasing the dosage or duration of therapy beyond 100 mg/day for 5 days is not recommended.

The majority of patients who are going to respond will respond to the first course of therapy. If pregnancy has not achieved after three ovulatory responses to clomiphene citrate, further treatment is not recommended. Long-term clomiphene citrate therapy is not advised. If ovulatory menses do not occur, the patient should be reevaluated. Further clomiphene citrate treatment beyond this is not recommended in the patient who does not exhibit evidence of ovulation.

Store tablets at controlled room temperature 59-86° F (15-30° C). Protect from heat, light, and excessive humidity, and store in closed containers.

HOW SUPPLIED - RATED THERAPEUTICALLY EQUIVALENT:

Tablet, Uncoated - Oral - 50 mg

10's	$57.32	Clomiphene, Teva	00093-0041-03
10's	**$63.32**	**SEROPHENE, Serono Labs**	**44087-8090-06**
30's	$164.27	Clomiphene, Teva	00093-0041-56
30's	**$181.44**	**SEROPHENE, Serono Labs**	**44087-8090-01**
30's	$185.00	Clomiphene Citrate, Harber Pharm	51432-0825-02
30's	$207.60	Clomiphene Citrate, Rugby	00536-3109-07
30's	$222.24	CLOMID, Hoechst Marion Roussel	00068-0226-30

CLOMIPRAMINE HYDROCHLORIDE *(000844)*

CATEGORIES: Antidepressants; Central Nervous System Agents; Obsessive-Compulsive Disorder; Psychotherapeutic Agents; Tricyclics; Tricyclic Antidepressants; Pregnancy Category C; FDA Class 1A ("Important Therapeutic Advantage"); Sales > $100 Million; FDA Approved 1989 Dec

BRAND NAMES: **Anafranil**; *Anafranil 25*; *Anafranil Retard*; *Anafranil SR*; *Clofranil*; *Clomifril*; *Clopress*; *Gromin*; *Placil*
(International brand names outside U.S. in italics)

FORMULARIES: Aetna; BC-BS; Medi-Cal; WHO

COST OF THERAPY: $54.80 (Obsessive-Compulsive Disorder; Capsule; 25 mg; 1/day; 70 days)

PRIMARY ICD9: 300.3 (Obsessive-Compulsive Disorders)

DESCRIPTION:

Clomipramine hydrochloride is an antiobsessional drug that belongs to the class (dibenzazepine) of pharmacologic agents known as tricyclic antidepressants. Anafranil is available as capsules of 25, 50, and 75 mg for oral administration.

Clomipramine hydrochloride is 3-chloro-5-(3-(dimethylamino)propyl)-10,11-dihydro-5H-dibenz(b,f)azepine monohydrochloride.

DESCRIPTION: *(cont'd)*

Clomipramine hydrochloride is a white to off-white crystalline powder. It is freely soluble in water, in methanol, and in methylene chloride, and insoluble in ethyl ether and in hexane. Its molecular weight is 351.3.

Anafranil inactive ingredients: D&C Red No.33 (25-mg capsules only), D&C Yellow No. 10, FD&C Blue No.1 (50-mg capsules only), FD&C Yellow No. 6, gelatin, magnesium stearate, methylparaben, propylparaben, silicon dioxide, sodium lauryl sulfate, starch, and titanium dioxide.

CLINICAL PHARMACOLOGY:

PHARMACODYNAMICS

Clomipramine (CMI) is presumed to influence obsessive and compulsive behaviors through its effects on serotonergic neuronal transmission. The actual neurochemical mechanism is unknown, but CMI's capacity to inhibit the reuptake of serotonin (5-HT) is thought to be important.

PHARMACOKINETICS

Absorption/Bioavailability: CMI from clomipramine HCl capsules is as bioavailable as CMI from a solution. The bioavailability of CMI from capsules is not significantly affected by food.

In a dose proportionality study involving multiple CMI doses, steady-state plasma concentrations (C_{ss}) and area-under-plasma-concentration-time curves (AUC) of CMI and CMI's major active metabolite, desmethylclomipramine (DMI), were not proportional to dose over the ranges evaluated, (*i.e.,* between 25-100 mg/day and between 25-150 mg/day), although C_{ss} and AUC are approximately linearly related to dose between 100-150 mg/day. The relationship between dose and CMI/DMI concentrations at higher daily doses has not been systematically assessed, but if there is significant dose dependency at doses above 150 mg/day, there is the potential for dramatically higher C_{ss} and AUC even for patients dosed within the recommended range. This may pose a potential risk to some patients (see WARNINGS and DRUG INTERACTIONS).

After a single 50-mg oral dose, maximum plasma concentrations of CMI occur within 2-6 hours (mean, 4.7 hr) and range from 56 ng/ml to 154 ng/ml (mean, 92 ng/ml). After multiple daily doses of 150 mg of clomipramine HCl, steady-state maximum plasma concentrations range from 94 ng/ml to 339 ng/ml (mean, 218 ng/ml) for CMI and from 134 ng/ml to 532 ng/ml (mean, 274 ng/ml) for DMI. No pharmacokinetic information is available for doses ranging from 150 mg/day to 250 mg/day, the maximum recommended daily dose.

Distribution: CMI distributes into cerebrospinal fluid (CSF) and brain and into breast milk. DMI also distributes into CSF, with a mean CSF/plasma ratio of 2.6. The protein binding of CMI is approximately 97%, principally to albumin, and is independent of CMI concentration. The interaction between CMI and other highly protein-bound drugs has not been fully evaluated, but may be important (see DRUG INTERACTIONS).

Metabolism: CMI is extensively biotransformed to DMI and other metabolites and their glucuronide conjugates. DMI is pharmacologically active, but its effects on OCD behaviors are unknown. These metabolites are excreted in urine and feces, following biliary elimination. After a 25-mg radiolabeled dose of CMI in two subjects, 60% and 51%, respectively, of the dose were recovered in the urine and 32% and 24%, respectively, in feces. In the same study, the combined urinary recoveries of CMI and DMI were only about 0.8-1.3% of the dose administered. CMI does not induce drug-metabolizing enzymes, as measured by antipyrine half-life.

Elimination: Evidence that the C_{ss} and AUC for CMI and DMI may increase disproportionately with increasing oral doses suggests that the metabolism of CMI and DMI may be capacity limited. This fact must be considered in assessing the estimates of the pharmacokinetic parameters presented below, as these were obtained in individuals exposed to doses of 150 mg. If the pharmacokinetics of CMI and DMI are nonlinear at doses above 150 mg, their elimination half-lives may be considerably lengthened at doses near the upper end of the recommended dosing range (*i.e.,* 200 mg/day to 250 mg/day). Consequently, CMI and DMI may accumulate, and this accumulation may increase the incidence of any dose- or plasma-concentration-dependent adverse reactions, in particular seizures (see WARNINGS).

After a 150-mg dose, the half-life of CMI ranges from 19 hours to 37 hours (mean, 32 hr) and that of DMI ranges from 54 hours to 77 hours (mean, 69 hr). Steady-state levels after multiple dosing are typically reached within 7-14 days for CMI. Plasma concentrations of the metabolite exceed the parent drug on multiple dosing. After multiple dosing with 150 mg/day, the accumulation factor for CMI is approximately 2.5 and for DMI is 4.6. Importantly, it may take two weeks or longer to achieve this extent of accumulation at constant dosing because of the relatively long elimination half-lives of CMI and DMI (see DOSAGE AND ADMINISTRATION). The effects of hepatic and renal impairment on the disposition of clomipramine HCl have not been determined.

Interactions: Coadministration of haloperidol with CMI increases plasma concentrations of CMI. Coadministration of CMI with phenobarbital increases plasma concentrations of phenobarbital (see DRUG INTERACTIONS). Younger subjects (18-40 years of age) tolerated CMI better and had significantly lower steady-state plasma concentrations, compared with subjects over 65 years of age. Children under 15 years of age had significantly lower plasma concentration/dose ratios, compared with adults. Plasma concentrations of CMI were significantly lower in smokers than in nonsmokers.

INDICATIONS AND USAGE:

Clomipramine HCl is indicated for the treatment of obsessions and compulsions in patients with Obsessive-Compulsive Disorder (OCD). The obsessions or compulsions must cause marked distress, be time-consuming, or significantly interfere with social or occupational functioning, in order to meet the DSM-III-R (circa 1989) diagnosis of OCD.

Obsessions are recurrent, persistent ideas, thoughts, images, or impulses that are ego-dystonic. Compulsions are repetitive, purposeful, and intentional behaviors performed in response to an obsession or in a stereotyped fashion, and are recognized by the person as excessive or unreasonable.

The effectiveness of clomipramine HCl for the treatment of OCD was demonstrated in multicenter, placebo-controlled, parallel-group studies, including two 10-week studies in adults and one 8-week study in children and adolescents 10-17 years of age. Patients in all studies had moderate-to-severe OCD (DSM-III), with mean baseline ratings on the Yale-Brown Obsessive Compulsive Scale (YBOCS) ranging from 26 to 28 and a mean baseline rating of 10 on the NIMH Clinical Global Obsessive Compulsive Scale (NIMH-OC). Patients taking CMI experienced a mean reduction of approximately 10 on the YBOCS, representing an average improvement on this scale of 35% to 42% among adults and 37% among children and adolescents. CMI treated patients experienced a 3.5 unit decrement on the NIMH-OC. Patients on placebo showed no important clinical response on either scale. The maximum dose was 250 mg/day for most adults and 3 mg/kg/day (up to 200 mg) for all children and adolescents.

The effectiveness of clomipramine HCl for long-term use (*i.e.,* for more than 10 weeks) has not been systematically evaluated in placebo-controlled trials. The physician who elects to use clomipramine HCl for extended periods should periodically reevaluate the long-term usefulness of the drug for the individual patient (see DOSAGE AND ADMINISTRATION).

CONTRAINDICATIONS:

Clomipramine HCl is contraindicated in patients with a history of hypersensitivity to clomipramine HCl or other tricyclic antidepressants.

Clomipramine HCl should not be given in combination, or within 14 days before or after treatment, with a monoamine oxidase (MAO) inhibitor. Hyperpyretic crisis, seizures, coma, and death have been reported in patients receiving such combinations.

Clomipramine HCl is contraindicated during the acute recovery period after a myocardial infarction.

WARNINGS:

SEIZURES

During premarket evaluation, seizure was identified as the most significant risk of clomipramine HCl use.

The observed cumulative incidence of seizures among patients exposed to clomipramine HCl at doses up to 300 mg/day was 0.64% at 90 days, 1.12% at 180 days, and 1.45% at 365 days. The cumulative rates correct the crude rate of 0.7%, (25 of 3519 patients) for the variable duration of exposure in clinical trials.

Although dose appears to be a predictor of seizure, there is a confounding of dose and duration of exposure, making it difficult to assess independently the effect of either factor alone. The ability to predict the occurrence of seizures in subjects exposed to doses of CMI greater than 250 mg is limited, given that the plasma concentration of CMI may be dose-dependent and may vary among subjects given the same dose. Nevertheless, prescribers are advised to limit the daily dose to a maximum of 250 mg in adults and 3 mg/kg (or 200 mg) in children and adolescents (see DOSAGE AND ADMINISTRATION.)

Caution should be used in administering clomipramine HCl to patients with a history of seizures or other predisposing factors. (*e.g.,* brain damage of varying etiology), alcoholism, and concomitant use with other drugs that lower the seizure threshold.

Rare reports of fatalities in association with seizures have been reported by foreign post-marketing surveillance, but not in U.S. clinical trials. In some of these cases, clomipramine HCl had been administered with other epileptogenic agents: in others, the patients involved had possibly predisposing medical conditions. Thus a causal association between clomipramine HCl treatment and these fatalities has not been established.

Physicians should discuss with patients the risk of taking clomipramine HCl while engaging in activities in which sudden loss of consciousness could result in serious injury to the patient or others, (*e.g.,* the operation of complex machinery, driving, swimming, climbing).

PRECAUTIONS:

GENERAL

Suicide: Since depression is a commonly associated feature of OCD, the risk of suicide must be considered. Prescriptions for clomipramine HCl should be written for the smallest quantity of capsules consistent with good patient management, in order to reduce the risk of overdose.

Cardiovascular Effects: Modest orthostatic decreases in blood pressure and modest tachycardia were each seen in approximately 20% of patients taking clomipramine HCl in clinical trials; but patients were frequently asymptomatic. Among approximately 1400 patients treated with CMI in the premarketing experience who had ECGs, 1.5% developed abnormalities during treatment, compared with 3.1% of patients receiving active control drugs and 0.7% of patients receiving placebo. The most common ECG changes were PVCs, ST-T wave changes, and intraventricular conduction abnormalities. These changes were rarely associated with significant clinical symptoms. Nevertheless, caution is necessary in treating patients with known cardiovascular disease, and gradual dose titration is recommended.

Psychosis, Confusion, And Other Neuropsychiatric Phenomena: Patients treated with clomipramine HCl have been reported to show a variety of neuropsychiatric signs and symptoms including delusions, hallucinations, psychotic episodes, confusion, and paranoia. Because of the uncontrolled nature of many of the studies, its is impossible to provide a precise estimate of the extent of risk imposed by treatment with clomipramine HCl. As with tricyclic antidepressants to which it is closely related, clomipramine HCl may precipitate an acute psychotic episode in patients with unrecognized schizophrenia.

Mania/Hypomania: During premarketing testing of clomipramine HCl in patients with affective disorder, hypomania or mania was precipitated in several patients. Activation of mania or hypomania has also been reported in a small proportion of patients with affective disorder treated with marketed tricyclic antidepressants, which are closely related to clomipramine HCl.

Hepatic Changes: During premarketing testing, clomipramine HCl was occasionally associated with elevations in SGOT and SGPT (pooled incidence of approximately 1% and 3% respectively) of potential clinical importance (*i.e.,* values greater than 3 times the upper limit of normal). In the vast majority of instances these enzyme increases were not associated with other clinical findings suggestive of hepatic injury; none were jaundiced. Rare reports of more severe liver injury, some fatal, have been recorded in foreign post-marketing experience. Caution is indicated in treating patients with known liver disease, and periodic monitoring of hepatic enzyme levels is recommended in such patients.

Hematologic Changes: Although no instances of severe hematologic toxicity were seen in the premarketing experience with clomipramine HCl, there have been post-marketing reports of leukopenia, agranulocytosis, thrombocytopenia, anemia, and pancytopenia in association with clomipramine HCl use. As is the case with tricyclic antidepressants to which clomipramine HCl is closely related, leukocyte and differential blood counts should be obtained in patients who develop fever and sore throat during treatment with clomipramine HCl.

Central Nervous System: More than 30 cases of hyperthermia have been recorded by nondomestic post-marketing surveillance systems. Most cases occurred when clomipramine HCl was used in combination with other drugs. When clomipramine HCl and a neuroleptic were used concomitantly, the cases were sometimes considered to be examples of a neuroleptic malignant syndrome.

Sexual Dysfunction: The rate of sexual dysfunction in male patients with OCD who were treated with clomipramine HCl in the premarketing experience was markedly increased compared with placebo controls (*i.e.,* 42% experienced ejaculatory failure and 20% experienced impotence, compared with 2.0% and 2.6% respectively, in the placebo group). Approximately 85% of males with sexual dysfunction chose to continue treatment.

Weight Changes: In controlled studies of OCD, weight gain was reported in 18% of patients receiving clomipramine HCl, compared with 1% of patients receiving placebo. In these studies, 28% of patients receiving clomipramine HCl had a weight gain of at least 7% of their initial body weight, compared with 4% of patients receiving placebo. Several patients had weight gains in excess of 25% of their initial body weight. Conversely, 5% of patients receiving placebo had weight losses of at least 7% of their initial body weight.

Electroconvulsive Therapy: As with closely related tricyclic antidepressants, concurrent administration of clomipramine HCl with electroconvulsive therapy may increase the risks; such treatment should be limited to those patients for whom it is essential, since there is limited clinical experience.

PRECAUTIONS: *(cont'd)*

Surgery: Prior to elective surgery with general anesthetics, therapy with clomipramine HCl should be discontinued for as long as is clinically feasible, and the anesthetist should be advised.

Use in Concomitant Illness: As with closely related tricyclic antidepressants, clomipramine HCl should be used with caution in the following:

(1) Hyperthyroid patients or patients receiving thyroid medication, because of the possibility of cardiac toxicity:

(2) Patients with increased intraocular pressure, a history of narrow-angle glaucoma, or urinary retention, because of the anticholinergic properties of the drug;

(3) Patients with tumors of the adrenal medulla (*e.g.,* pheochromocytoma, neuroblastoma) in whom the drug may provoke hypertensive crises;

(4) Patients with significantly impaired renal function.

Withdrawal Symptoms: A variety of withdrawal symptoms have been reported in association with abrupt discontinuation of clomipramine HCl, including dizziness, nausea, vomiting, headache, malaise, sleep disturbance, hyperthermia, and irritability. In addition, such patients may experience a worsening of psychiatric status. While the withdrawal effects of clomipramine HCl have not been systematically evaluated in controlled trials, they are well known with closely related tricyclic antidepressants, and it is recommended that the dosage be tapered gradually and the patient monitored carefully during discontinuation (see DRUG ABUSE AND DEPENDENCE).

INFORMATION FOR PATIENTS

Physicians are advised to discuss the following issues with patients for whom they prescribe clomipramine HCl:

(1) The risk of seizure (see WARNINGS);

(2) The relatively high incidence of sexual dysfunction among males (see Sexual Dysfunction) ;

(3) Since clomipramine HCl may impair the mental and/or physical abilities required for the performance of complex and hazardous tasks and since clomipramine HCl is associated with a risk of seizures, patients should be cautioned about the performance of complex and hazardous tasks (see WARNINGS);

(4) Patients should be cautioned about using alcohol, barbiturates, or other CNS depressants concurrently, since clomipramine HCl may exaggerate their response to these drugs;

(5) Patients should notify their physician if they become pregnant or intend to become pregnant during therapy;

(6) Patients should notify their physician if they are breast-feeding.

CARCINOGENESIS, MUTAGENESIS, IMPAIRMENT OF FERTILITY

In a 2-year bioassay, no clear evidence of carcinogenicity was found in rats given doses 20 times the maximum daily human dose. Three out of 235 treated rats had a rare tumor (hemangioendothelioma); it is unknown if these neoplasms are compound related.

In reproduction studies, no effects on fertility were found in rats given doses approximately 5 times the maximum daily human dose.

PREGNANCY CATEGORY C

No teratogenic effects were observed in studies performed in rats and mice at doses up to 20 times the maximum daily human dose. Slight nonspecific fetotoxic effects were seen in the offspring of pregnant mice given doses 10 times the maximum daily human dose. Slight nonspecific embryotoxicity was observed in rats given doses 5-10 times the maximum daily human dose.

There are no adequate or well-controlled studies in pregnant women. Withdrawal symptoms, including jitteriness, tremor, and seizures, have been reported in neonates whose mothers had taken clomipramine HCl until delivery. Clomipramine HCl should be used during pregnancy only if the potential benefit justifies the potential risk to the fetus.

NURSING MOTHERS

Clomipramine HCl has been found in human milk. Because of the potential for adverse reactions, a decision should be made whether to discontinue nursing or to discontinue the drug, taking into account the importance of the drug to the mother.

PEDIATRIC USE

In a controlled clinical trial in children and adolescents (10-17 years of age), 46 outpatients received clomipramine HCl for up to 8 weeks. In addition, 150 adolescent patients have received clomipramine HCl in open-label protocols for periods of several months to several years. Of the 196 adolescents studies, 50 were 13 years of age or less and 146 were 14-17 years of age. While the adverse reaction profile in this age group (see ADVERSE REACTIONS) is similar to that in adults, it is unknown what, if any, effects long-term treatment with clomipramine HCl may have on the growth and development of children.

The safety and effectiveness in children below the age of 10 have not been established. Therefore, specific recommendations cannot be made for the use of clomipramine HCl in children under the age of 10.

USE IN ELDERLY

Clomipramine HCl has not been systematically studied in older patients; but 152 patients at least 60 years of age participating in U.S. clinical trials received clomipramine HCl for periods of several months to several years. No unusual age-related adverse events have been identified in this elderly population, but these data are insufficient to rule out possible age-related differences, particularly in elderly patients who have concomitant systemic illnesses or who are receiving other drugs concomitantly.

DRUG INTERACTIONS:

The risks of using clomipramine HCl in combination with other drugs have not been systematically evaluated. Given the primary CNS effects of clomipramine HCl, caution is advised in using it concomitantly with other CNS-active drugs (see Information for Patients). Clomipramine HCl should not be used with MAO inhibitors (see CONTRAINDICATIONS.)

Close supervision and careful adjustment of dosage are required when clomipramine HCl is administered with anticholinergic or sympathomimetic drugs.

Several tricyclic antidepressants have been reported to block the pharmacologic effects of guanethidine, clonidine, or similar agents, and such an effect may be anticipated with CMI because of its structural similarity to other tricyclic antidepressants.

The plasma concentration of CMI has been reported to be increased by the concomitant administration of haloperidol; plasma levels of several closely related tricyclic antidepressants have been reported to be increased by the concomitant administration of methylphenidate or hepatic enzyme inhibitors (*e.g.,* cimetidine, fluoxetine) and decreased by the concomitant administration of hepatic enzyme inducers (*e.g.,* barbiturates, phenytoin), and such an effect may be anticipated with CMI as well. Administration of CMI has been reported to increase the plasma levels of phenobarbital, if given concomitantly (see CLINICAL PHARMACOLOGY, Interactions).

Because clomipramine HCl is highly bound to serum protein, the administration of clomipramine HCl to patients taking other drugs that are highly bound to protein (*e.g.,* warfarin, digoxin) may cause an increase in plasma concentrations of these drugs, potentially resulting

DRUG INTERACTIONS: *(cont'd)*

in adverse effects. Conversely, adverse effects may result from displacement of protein-bound clomipramine HCl by other highly bound drugs (see CLINICAL PHARMACOLOGY, Distribution).

ADVERSE REACTIONS:

COMMONLY OBSERVED

The most commonly observed adverse events associated with the use of clomipramine HCl and not seen at an equivalent incidence among placebo-treated patients were gastrointestinal complaints, including dry mouth, constipation, nausea, dyspepsia, and anorexia; nervous system complaints, including somnolence, tremor, dizziness, nervousness, and myoclonus; genitourinary complaints, including changed libido, ejaculatory failure, impotence, and micturition disorder; and other miscellaneous complaints, including fatigue, sweating, increased appetite, weight gain, and visual changes.

LEADING TO DISCONTINUATION OF TREATMENT

Approximately 20% of 3616 patients who received clomipramine HCl in U.S. premarketing clinical trials discontinued treatment because of an adverse event. Approximately one-half of the patients who discontinued (9% of the total) had multiple complaints, none of which could be classified as primary. Where a primary reason for discontinuation could be identified, most patients discontinued because of nervous system complaints (5.4%), primarily somnolence. The secondmost-frequent reason for discontinuation was digestive system complaints (1.3%), primarily vomiting and nausea.

INCIDENCE IN CONTROLLED CLINICAL TRIALS

The following tables (TABLE 1A, TABLE 1B) enumerates adverse events that occurred at an incidence of 1% or greater among patients with OCD who received clomipramine HCl in adult or pediatric placebo-controlled clinical trials. The frequencies were obtained from pooled data of clinical trials involving either adults receiving clomipramine HCl (N=322) or placebo (N=319) or children treated with clomipramine HCl (N=46) or placebo (N=44). The prescriber should be aware that these figures cannot be used to predict the incidence of side effects in the course of usual medical practice, in which patient characteristics and other factors differ from those which prevailed in the clinical trials. Similarly, the cited frequencies cannot be compared with figures obtained from other clinical investigations involving different treatment, uses, and investigators. The cited figures, however, provide the physician with a basis for estimating the relative contribution of drug and nondrug factors to the incidence of side effects in the populations studied.

OTHER EVENTS OBSERVED DURING THE PREMARKETING EVALUATION OF CLOMIPRAMINE HCL

During clinical testing in the U.S., multiple doses of clomipramine HCl were administered to approximately 3600 subjects. Untoward events associated with this exposure were recorded by clinical investigators using terminology of their own choosing. Consequently, it is not possible to provide a meaningful estimate of the proportion of individuals experiencing adverse events without first grouping similar types of untoward events into a smaller number of standardized event categories.

In the tabulations that follow, a modified World Health Organization dictionary of terminology has been used to classify reported adverse events. The frequencies presented, therefore, represent the proportion of the 3525 individuals exposed to clomipramine HCl who experienced an event of the type cited on at least one occasion while receiving clomipramine HCl. All events are included except those already listed in the previous table, those reported in terms so general as to be uninformative, and those in which an association with the drug was remote. It is important to emphasize that although the events reported occurred during treatment with clomipramine HCl, they were not necessarily caused by it.

Events are further categorized by body system and listed in order of decreasing frequency according to the following definitions: frequent adverse events are those occurring on one or more occasions in at least 1/100 patients; infrequent adverse events are those occurring in 1/100 to 1/1000 patients; rare events are those occurring in less than 1/1000 patients.

Body as a Whole: *Infrequent:*general edema, increased susceptibility to infection, malaise. *Rare:*dependent edema, withdrawal syndrome.

Cardiovascular System: *Infrequent:*abnormal ECG, arrhythmia, bradycardia, cardiac arrest, extrasystoles, pallor. *Rare:*aneurysm, atrial flutter, bundle branch block, cardiac failure, cerebral hemorrhage, heart block, myocardial infarction, myocardial ischemia, peripheral ischemia, thrombophlebitis, vasospasm, ventricular tachycardia.

Digestive System: *Infrequent:*abnormal hepatic function, blood in stool, colitis, duodenitis, gastric ulcer, gastritis, gastroesophageal reflux, gingivitis, glossitis, hemorrhoids, hepatitis, increased saliva, irritable bowel syndrome, peptic ulcer, rectal hemorrhage, tongue ulceration, tooth caries. *Rare:*cheilitis, chronic enteritis, discolored feces, gastric dilatation, gingival bleeding, hiccup, intestinal obstruction, oral/pharyngeal edema, paralytic ileus, salivary gland enlargement.

Endocrine System: *Infrequent:*hypothyroidism. *Rare:*goiter, gynecomastia, hyperthyroidism.

Hemic and Lymphatic System: *Infrequent:*lymphadenopathy. *Rare:*leukemoid reaction, lymphoma-like disorder, marrow depression.

Metabolic and Nutritional Disorder: *Infrequent:*dehydration, diabetes mellitus, gout, hypercholesterolemia, hyperglycemia, hyperuricemia, hypokalemia. *Rare:*fat intolerance, glycosuria.

Musculoskeletal System: *Infrequent:*arthrosis. *Rare:*dystonia, exostosis, lupus erythematosus rash, bruising, myopathy, myositis, polyarteritis nodosa, torticollis.

Nervous System: *Frequent:*abnormal thinking, vertigo. *Infrequent:*abnormal coordination, abnormal EEG, abnormal gait, apathy, ataxia, coma, convulsions, delirium, delusion, dysphonia, encephalopathy, euphoria, extrapyramidal disorder, hallucination, hostility, hyperkinesia, hypnagogic hallucinations, hypokinesia, leg cramps, manic reaction, neuralgia, paranoia, phobic disorder, psychosis, sensory disturbance, somnambulism, stimulation, suicidal ideation, suicide attempt, teeth-grinding. *Rare:*anticholinergic syndrome, aphasia, apraxia, catalepsy, cholinergic syndrome, choreoathetosis, generalized spasm, hemiparesis, hyperesthesia, hyperreflexia, hypoesthesia, illusion, impaired impulse control, indecisiveness, mutism, neuropathy, nystagmus, oculogyric crisis, oculomotor nerve paralysis, schizophrenic reaction, stupor, suicide.

Respiratory System: *Infrequent:*bronchitis, hyperventilation, increased sputum, pneumonia. *Rare:*cyanosis, hemoptysis, hypoventilation, laryngismus.

Skin and Appendages: *Infrequent:*alopecia, cellulitis, cyst, eczema, erythematous rash, genital pruritus, maculopapular rash, photosensitivity reaction, psoriasis, pustular rash, skin discoloration. *Rare:*chloasma, folliculitis, hypertrichosis, piloerection, seborrhea, skin hypertrophy, skin ulceration.

Special Senses: *Infrequent:*abnormal accommodation, deafness, diplopia, earache eye pain, foreign body sensation, hyperacusis, parosmia, photophobia, scleritis, taste loss. *Rare:* blepharitis, chromatopsia, conjunctival hemorrhage, exophthalmos, glaucoma, keratitis, labyrinth disorder, night blindness, retinal disorder, strabismus, visual field defect.

Urogenital System: *Infrequent:*endometriosis, epididymitis, hematuria, nocturia, oliguria, ovarian cyst, perineal pain, polyuria, prostatic disorder, renal calculus, renal pain, urethral disorder, urinary incontinence, uterine hemorrhage, vaginal hemorrhage. *Rare:*albuminuria,

ADVERSE REACTIONS: *(cont'd)*

TABLE 1A Incidence of Treatment-Emergent Adverse (Percentage of Patients Reporting Event)

Body System/ Adverse Event*	Adults: Clomipramine HCl (N=322)	Adults: Placebo (N=319)	Children and Adolescents: Clomipramine HCl (N=46)	Children and Adolescents: Placebo (N=44)
Nervous System				
Somnolence	54	16	46	11
Tremor	54	2	33	2
Dizziness	54	14	41	14
Headache	52	41	28	34
Insomnia	25	15	11	7
Libido change	21	3	-	-
Nervousness	18	2	4	2
Myoclonus	13	-	2	-
Increased appetite	11	2	-	2
Paresthesia	9	3	2	2
Memory impairment	9	1	7	2
Anxiety	9	4	2	-
Twitching	7	1	4	5
Impaired concentration	5	2	-	-
Depression	5	1	-	-
Hypertonia	4	1	2	-
Sleep disorder	4	-	9	5
Psychosomatic disorder	3	-	-	-
Yawning	3	-	-	-
Confusion	3	-	2	-
Speech disorder	3	-	-	-
Abnormal dreaming	3	-	-	2
Agitation	3	-	-	-
Migraine	3	-	-	-
Depersonalization	2	-	2	-
Irritability	2	2	2	-
Emotional lability	2	-	-	2
Panic reaction	1	-	2	-
Aggressive reaction	-	-	2	-
Paresis	-	-	2	-
Skin and Appendages				
Increased sweating	29	3	9	-
Rash	8	1	4	2
Pruritus	6	-	2	2
Dermatitis	2	-	-	2
Acne	2	2	-	5
Dry skin	2	-	-	5
Urticaria	1	-	-	-
Abnormal skin odor	-	-	2	-
Digestive System				
Dry mouth	84	17	63	16
Constipation	47	11	22	9
Nausea	33	14	9	11
Dyspepsia	22	10	13	2
Diarrhea	13	9	7	5
Anorexia	12	-	22	2
Abdominal pain	11	9	13	16
Vomiting	7	2	7	-
Flatulence	6	3	-	2
Tooth disorder	5	-	-	-
Gastrointestinal disorder	2	-	-	2
Dysphagia	2	-	-	-
Esophagitis	1	-	-	-
Eructation	-	-	2	2
Ulcertative stomatitis	-	-	2	-
Body as a Whole				
Fatigue	39	18	35	9
Weight increase	18	1	2	-
Flushing	8	-	7	-
Hot flushes	5	-	2	-
Chest pain	4	4	7	-
Fever	4	-	2	7
Allergy	3	3	7	5
Pain	3	2	4	2
Local edema	2	4	-	-
Chills	2	1	-	-
Weight decrease	-	-	7	-
Otitis media	-	-	4	5
Asthenia	-	-	2	-
Halitosis	-	-	2	-

* Events reported by at least 1% of clomipramine HCl patients are included

anorgasmy, breast engorgement, breast fibroadenosis, cervical dysplasia, endometrial hyperplasia, premature ejaculation, pyelonephritis, pyuria, renal cyst, uterine inflammation, vulvar disorder.

DRUG ABUSE AND DEPENDENCE:

Clomipramine HCl has not been systematically studied in animals or humans for its potential for abuse, tolerance, or physical dependence. While a variety of withdrawal symptoms have been described in association with clomipramine HCl discontinuation (see PRECAUTIONS, Withdrawal Symptoms), there is no evidence for drug-seeking behavior, except for a single report of potential clomipramine HCl abuse by a patient with a history of dependence on codeine, benzodiazepines, and multiple psychoactive drugs. The patient received clomipramine HCl for depression and panic attacks and appeared to become dependent after hospital discharge.

Despite the lack of evidence suggesting an abuse liability for clomipramine HCl in foreign marketing, it is not possible to predict the extent to which clomipramine HCl might be misused or abused once marketed in the U.S. Consequently, physicians should carefully evaluate patients for a history of drug abuse and follow such patients closely.

OVERDOSAGE:

HUMAN EXPERIENCE

In U.S. clinical trials, 2 deaths occurred in 12 reported cases of acute overdosage with clomipramine HCl either alone or in combination with other drugs. One death involved a patient suspected of ingesting a dose of 7000 m The second death involved a patient suspected of ingesting a dose of 5750 mg. The 10 nonfatal cases involved doses of up to 5000 mg, accompanied by plasma levels of up to 1010 ng/ml. All 10 patients completely recovered. Among reports from other countries of clomipramine HCl overdose, the lowest dose associated with a fatality was 750 mg. Based upon post-marketing reports in the United Kingdom, CMI's lethality in overdose is considered to be similar to that reported for closely related tricyclic compounds marketed as antidepressants.

OVERDOSAGE: *(cont'd)*

TABLE 1B

Body System/ Adverse Event*	Adults: Clomipramine HCl (N=322)	Adults: Placebo (N=319)	Children and Adolescents: Clomipramine HCl (N=46)	Children and Adolescents: Placebo (N=44)
Cardiovascular System				
Postural hypotension	6	-	4	-
Palpitation	4	2	4	-
Tachycardia	4	-	2	-
Syncope	-	-	2	-
Respiratory System				
Pharyngitis	14	9	-	5
Rhinitis	12	10	7	9
Sinusitis	6	4	2	5
Coughing	6	6	4	5
Bronchospasm	2	-	7	2
Epistaxis	2	-	-	2
Dyspnea	-	-	2	-
Laryngitis	-	1	2	-
Urogenital System				
Male and Female Patients Combined				
Micturition disorder	14	2	4	2
Urinary tract infection	6	1	-	-
Micturition frequency	5	3	-	-
Urinary retention	2	-	7	-
Dysuria	2	2	-	-
Cystitis	2	-	-	-
Female Patients Only	(N=182)	(N=167)	(N=10)	(N=21)
Dysmenorrhea	12	14	10	10
Lactation (nonpuerperal)	4	-	-	-
Menstrual disorder	4	2	-	-
Vaginitis	2	-	-	-
Leukorrhea	2	-	-	-
Breast enlargement	2	-	-	-
Breast pain	1	-	-	-
Amenorrhea	1	-	-	-
Male Patients Only	(N=140)	(N=152)	(N=36)	(N=23)
Ejaculation failure	42	2	6	-
Impotence	20	3	-	-
Special Senses				
Abnormal vision	18	4	7	2
Taste perversion	8	-	4	-
Tinnitus	6	-	4	-
Abnormal lacrimation	3	2	-	-
Mydriasis	2	-	-	-
Conjunctivitis	1	-	-	-
Anisocoria	-	-	2	-
Blepharospasm	-	-	2	-
Ocular allergy	-	-	2	-
Vestibular disorder	-	-	2	2
Musculoskeletal				
Myalgia	13	9	-	-
Back pain	6	6	-	-
Arthralgia	3	5	-	-
Muscle weakness	1	-	2	-
Hemic and Lymphatic				
Purpura	3	-	-	-
Anemia	-	-	2	2
Metabolic and Nutritional				
Thirst	2	2	-	2

* Events reported by at least 1% of clomipramine HCl patients are included

SIGNS AND SYMPTOMS

Signs and symptoms vary in severity depending upon factors such as the amount of drug absorbed, the age of the patient, and the time elapsed since drug ingestion. Blood and urine levels of clomipramine HCl may not reflect the severity of poisoning: they have chiefly a qualitative rather than quantitative value, and they are unreliable indicators in the clinical management of the patient. The first signs and symptoms of poisoning with tricyclic antidepressants are generally severe anticholinergic reactions. CNS abnormalities may include drowsiness, stupor, coma, ataxia, restlessness, agitation, delirium, severe perspiration, hyperactive reflexes, muscle rigidity, athetoid and choreiform movement, and convulsions. Cardiac abnormalities may include arrhythmia, tachycardia, ECG evidence of impaired conduction, and signs of congestive heart failure, and in very rare cases, cardiac arrest. Respiratory depression, cyanosis, hypotension, shock, vomiting, hyperpyrexia, mydriasis, oliguria or anuria, and diaphoresis may also be present.

TREATMENT

The recommended treatment for tricyclic overdose may change periodically. Therefore, it is recommended that the physician contact a poison control center for current information on treatment.

Because CNS involvement, respiratory depression, and cardiac arrhythmia can occur suddenly, hospitalization and close observation may be necessary, even when the amount ingested is thought to be small or the initial degree of intoxication appears slight or moderate. All patients with ECG abnormalities should have continuous cardiac monitoring and be closely observed until well after the cardiac status has returned to normal; relapses may occur after apparent recovery.

In the alert patient, the stomach should be emptied promptly by lavage. In the obtunded patient, the airway should be secured with a cuffed endotracheal tube before beginning lavage (do not induce emesis). Instillation of activated charcoal slurry may help reduce absorption of CMI.

External stimulation should be minimized to reduce the tendency for convulsions. If anticonvulsants are necessary, diazepam and phenytoin may be useful. Adequate respiratory exchange should be maintained, including intubation and artificial respiration, if necessary. Respiratory stimulants should not be used.

In severe hypotension or shock, the patient should be placed in an appropriate position and given a plasma expander, and, if necessary, a vasopressor agent by intravenous drip. The use of corticosteroids in shock is controversial and may be contraindicated in case of overdosage with tricyclic antidepressants. Digitalis may increase conduction abnormalities and further irritate an already sensitized myocardium. If congestive heart failure necessitates rapid digitalization, particular care must be exercised. Hyperpyrexia should be controlled by whatever external means are available, including ice packs and cooling sponge baths, if

OVERDOSAGE: *(cont'd)*

necessary. Hemodialysis, peritoneal dialysis, exchange transfusions, and forced diuresis have generally been reported as ineffective because of the rapid fixation of clomipramine HCl in tissues.

The slow intravenous administration of physostigmine salicylate has been used as a last resort to reverse severe CNS anticholinergic manifestations of overdosage with tricyclic antidepressants; however, it should not be used routinely, since it may induce seizures and cholinergic crises.

DOSAGE AND ADMINISTRATION:

The treatment regimens described below are based on those used in controlled clinical trials of clomipramine HCl in 520 adults, and 91 children and adolescents with OCD. During initial titration, clomipramine HCl should be given in divided doses with meals to reduce gastrointestinal side effects. The goal of this initial titration phase is to minimize side effects by permitting tolerance to side effects to develop or allowing the patient time to adapt if tolerance does not develop.

Because both CMI and its active metabolite, DMI, have long elimination half-lives, the prescriber should take into consideration the fact that steady-state plasma levels may not be achieved until 2-3 weeks after dosage change (see CLINICAL PHARMACOLOGY). Therefore, after initial titration, it may be appropriate to wait 2-3 weeks between further dosage adjustments.

INITIAL TREATMENT/DOSE ADJUSTMENT (ADULTS)

Treatment with clomipramine HCl should be initiated at a dosage of 25 mg daily and gradually increased, as tolerated, to approximately 100 mg during the first 2 weeks. During initial titration, clomipramine HCl should be given in divided doses with meals to reduce gastrointestinal side effects. Thereafter, the dosage may be increased gradually over the next several weeks, up to a maximum of 250 mg daily. After titration, the total daily dose may be given once daily at bedtime to minimize daytime sedation.

INITIAL TREATMENT/DOSE ADJUSTMENT (CHILDREN AND ADOLESCENTS)

As with adults, the starting dose is 25 mg daily and should be gradually increased (also given in divided doses with meals to reduce gastrointestinal side effects) during the first 2 weeks, as tolerated, up to a daily maximum of 3 mg/kg or 100 mg, whichever is smaller. Thereafter, the dosage may be increased gradually over the next several weeks up to a daily maximum of 3 mg/kg or 200 mg, whichever is smaller (see PRECAUTIONS, Pediatric Use). As with adults, after titration, the total daily dose may be given once daily at bedtime to minimize daytime sedation.

MAINTENANCE/CONTINUATION TREATMENT (ADULTS, CHILDREN, AND ADOLESCENTS)

While there are no systematic studies that answer the question of how long to continue clomipramine HCl, OCD is a chronic condition and it is reasonable to consider continuation for a responding patient. Although the efficacy of clomipramine HCl after 10 weeks has not been documented in controlled trials, patients have been continued in therapy under double-blind conditions for up to 1 year without loss of benefit. However, dosage adjustments should be made to maintain the patient on the lowest effective dosage, and patients should be periodically reassessed to determine the need for treatment. During maintenance, the total daily dose may be given once daily at bedtime.

ANIMAL PHARMACOLOGY:

ANIMAL TOXICOLOGY

Testicular and lung changes commonly associated with tricyclic compounds have been observed with clomipramine HCl. In 1- and 2-year studies in rats, changes in the testes (atrophy, aspermatogenesis, and calcification) and drug-induced phospholipidosis in the lungs were observed at doses 4 times the maximum daily human dose. Testicular atrophy was also observed in a 1-year oral toxicity study in dogs at 10 times the maximum daily human dose.

Do not store above 86° F (30° C). Protect from moisture.

Dispense in tight container (USP).

HOW SUPPLIED - RATED THERAPEUTICALLY EQUIVALENT:

Capsule, Gelatin - Oral - 25 mg

100's	$78.29	ANAFRANIL, Novartis	58887-0115-30
100's	$81.62	ANAFRANIL, Novartis	58887-0115-32

Capsule, Gelatin - Oral - 50 mg

100's	$105.57	ANAFRANIL, Novartis	58887-0116-30
100's	$109.46	ANAFRANIL, Novartis	58887-0116-32

Capsule, Gelatin - Oral - 75 mg

100's	$138.97	ANAFRANIL, Novartis	58887-0117-30
100's	$145.29	ANAFRANIL, Novartis	58887-0117-32

CLONAZEPAM *(000845)*

CATEGORIES: Anticonvulsants; Benzodiazepine Anticonvulsants; Central Nervous System Agents; Convulsions; Lennox-Gastaut Syndrome; Neuromuscular; Seizures; Anxiety*; Mania*; Panic Disorder*; Schizophrenia*; DEA Class CIV; FDA Approval Pre 1982; Top 200 Drugs
* Indication not approved by the FDA

BRAND NAMES: *Clonex*; *Iktorivil*; **Klonopin**; *Landsen* (Japan); *Lonazep*; *Rivotril* (Australia, Asia, England, France, Germany)
(International brand names outside U.S. in italics)

FORMULARIES: Aetna; BC-BS; Medi-Cal; PCS; WHO

DESCRIPTION:

Klonopin is available as scored tablets containing 0.5 mg, 1 mg or 2 mg clonazepam. Each tablet also contains lactose, magnesium stearate, microcrystalline cellulose and corn starch, with the following dye systems: 0.5 mg—FD&C Yellow No. 6; 1 mg—FD&C Blue No. 1 and FD&C Blue No. 2.

Chemically, clonazepam is 5-(2-chlorophenyl)-1,3-dihydro-7-nitro-2H-1,4-benzodiazepin-2-one. It is a light yellow crystalline powder. It has a molecular weight of 315.7.

CLINICAL PHARMACOLOGY:

In laboratory animals, clonazepam exhibits several pharmacologic properties which are characteristic of the benzodiazepine class of drugs. Convulsions produced in rodents by pentylenetetrazol or electrical stimulation are antagonized, as are convulsions produced by photic stimulation in susceptible baboons. A taming effect in aggressive primates, muscle weakness and hypnosis are likewise produced by clonazepam. In humans it is capable of suppressing the spike and wave discharge in absence seizures (petit mal) and decreasing the frequency, amplitude, duration and spread of discharge in minor motor seizures.

CLINICAL PHARMACOLOGY: *(cont'd)*

Single oral dose administration of clonazepam to humans gave maximum blood levels of drug, in most cases, within one to two hours. The half-life of the parent compound varied from approximately 18 to 50 hours, and the major route of excretion was in the urine. In humans, five metabolites have been identified. In general, the biotransformation of clonazepam followed two pathways: oxidative hydroxylation at the C-3 position and reduction of the 7-nitro function to form 7-amino and/or 7-acetyl-amino derivatives.

INDICATIONS AND USAGE:

Clonazepam is useful alone or as an adjunct in the treatment of the Lennox-Gastaut syndrome (petit mal variant), akinetic and myoclonic seizures. In patients with absence seizures (petit mal) who have failed to respond to succinimides, clonazepam may be useful.

In some studies, up to 30% of patients have shown a loss of anticonvulsant activity, often within three months of administration. In some cases, dosage adjustment may reestablish efficacy.

CONTRAINDICATIONS:

Clonazepam should not be used in patients with a history of sensitivity to benzodiazepines, nor in patients with clinical or biochemical evidence of significant liver disease. It may be used in patients with open angle glaucoma who are receiving appropriate therapy, but is contraindicated in acute narrow angle glaucoma.

WARNINGS:

Since clonazepam produces CNS depression, patients receiving this drug should be cautioned against engaging in hazardous occupations requiring mental alertness, such as operating machinery or driving a motor vehicle. They should also be warned about the concomitant use of alcohol or other CNS-depressant drugs during clonazepam therapy (see DRUG INTERACTIONS).

USAGE IN PREGNANCY

The effects of clonazepam in human pregnancy and nursing infants are unknown.

Recent reports suggest an association between the use of anticonvulsant drugs by women with epilepsy and an elevated incidence of birth defects in children born to these women. Data are more extensive with respect to diphenylhydantoin and phenobarbital, but these are also the most commonly prescribed anticonvulsants; less systematic or anecdotal reports suggest a possible similar association with the use of all known anticonvulsant drugs.

The reports suggesting an elevated incidence of birth defects in children of drug-treated epileptic women cannot be regarded as adequate to prove a definite cause and effect relationship. There are intrinsic methodologic problems in obtaining adequate data on drug teratogenicity in humans; the possibility also exists that other factors, *e.g.*, genetic factors or the epileptic condition itself, may be more important than drug therapy in leading to birth defects. The great majority of mothers on anticonvulsant medication deliver normal infants. It is important to note that anticonvulsant drugs should not be discontinued in patients in whom the drug is administered to prevent seizures because of the strong possibility of precipitating status epilepticus with attendant hypoxia and threat to life. In individual cases where the severity and frequency of the seizure disorder are such that the removal of medication does not pose a serious threat to the patient, discontinuation of the drug may be considered prior to and during pregnancy, although it cannot be said with any confidence that even mild seizures do not pose some hazards to the developing embryo or fetus.

These considerations should be weighed in treating or counseling epileptic women of childbearing potential.

Use of clonazepam in women of childbearing potential should be considered only when the clinical situation warrants the risk. Mothers receiving clonazepam should not breast feed their infants.

In a two-generation reproduction study with clonazepam given orally to rats at 10 or 100 mg/kg/day, there was a decrease in the number of pregnancies and a decrease in the number of offspring surviving until weaning. When clonazepam was administered orally to pregnant rabbits at 0.2, 1.0, 5.0 or 10.0 mg/kg/day, a nondose-related incidence of cleft palates, open eyelids, fused sternebrae and limb defects was observed at the 0.2 and 5.0 mg/kg/day levels. Nearly all of the malformations were seen from one dam in each of the affected dosages.

USAGE IN CHILDREN

Because of the possibility that adverse effects on physical or mental development could become apparent only after many years, a benefit-risk consideration of the long-term use of clonazepam is important in pediatric patients.

Withdrawal symptoms of the barbiturate type have occurred after the discontinuation of benzodiazepines. (See DRUG ABUSE AND DEPENDENCE.)

PRECAUTIONS:

When used in patients in whom several different types of seizure disorders coexist, clonazepam may increase the incidence or precipitate the onset of generalized tonic-clonic seizures (grand mal). This may require the addition of appropriate anticonvulsants or an increase in their dosages. The concomitant use of valproic acid and clonazepam may produce absence status.

Periodic blood counts and liver function tests are advisable during long term therapy with clonazepam.

The abrupt withdrawal of clonazepam, particularly in those patients on long-term, high-dose therapy, may precipitate status epilepticus. Therefore, when discontinuing clonazepam, gradual withdrawal is essential. While clonazepam is being gradually withdrawn, the simultaneous substitution of another anticonvulsant may be indicated. Metabolites of clonazepam are excreted by the kidneys; to avoid their excess accumulation, caution should be exercised in the administration of the drug to patients with impaired renal function.

Clonazepam may produce an increase in salivation. This should be considered before giving the drug to patients who have difficulty handling secretions. Because of this and the possibility of respiratory depression, clonazepam should be used with caution in patients with chronic respiratory diseases.

INFORMATION FOR THE PATIENT

To assure the safe and effective use of benzodiazepines, patients should be informed that, since benzodiazepines may produce psychological and physical dependence, it is advisable that they consult with their physician before either increasing the dose or abruptly discontinuing this drug.

DRUG INTERACTIONS:

The CNS-depressant action of the benzodiazepine class of drugs may be potentiated by alcohol, narcotics, barbiturates, nonbarbiturate hypnotics, antianxiety agents, the phenothiazines, thioxanthene and butyrophenone classes of antipsychotic agents, monoamine oxidase inhibitors and the tricyclic antidepressants, and by other anticonvulsant drugs.

ADVERSE REACTIONS:

The most frequently occurring side effects of clonazepam are referable to CNS depression. Experience to date has shown that drowsiness has occurred in approximately 50% of patients and ataxia in approximately 30%. In some cases, these may diminish with time; behavior problems have been noted in approximately 25% of patients. Others, listed by system are:

Neurologic: Abnormal eye movements, aphonia, choreiform movements, coma, diplopia, dysarthria, dysdiadochokinesis, "glassy-eyed" appearance, headache, hemiparesis, hypotonia, nystagmus, respiratory depression, slurred speech, tremor, vertigo.

Psychiatric: Confusion, depression, amnesia, hallucinations, hysteria, increased libido, insomnia, psychosis, suicidal attempt (the behavior effects are more likely to occur in patients with a history of psychiatric disturbances).

Respiratory: Chest congestion, rhinorrhea, shortness of breath, hypersecretion in upper respiratory passages.

Cardiovascular: Palpitations.

Dermatologic: Hair loss, hirsutism, skin rash, ankle and facial edema.

Gastrointestinal: Anorexia, coated tongue, constipation, diarrhea, dry mouth, encopresis, gastritis, hepatomegaly, increased appetite, nausea, sore gums.

Genitourinary: Dysuria, enuresis, nocturia, urinary retention.

Musculoskeletal: Muscle weakness, pains.

Miscellaneous: Dehydration, general deterioration, fever, lymphadenopathy, weight loss or gain.

Hematopoietic: Anemia, leukopenia, thrombocytopenia, eosinophilia.

Hepatic: Transient elevations of serum transaminases and alkaline phosphatase.

DRUG ABUSE AND DEPENDENCE:

Withdrawal symptoms, similar in character to those noted with barbiturates and alcohol (*e.g.,* convulsions, psychosis, hallucinations, behavioral disorder, tremor, abdominal and muscle cramps) have occurred following abrupt discontinuance of clonazepam. The more severe withdrawal symptoms have usually been limited to those patients who received excessive doses over an extended period of time. Generally milder withdrawal symptoms (*e.g.,* dysphoria and insomnia) have been reported following abrupt discontinuance of benzodiazepines taken continuously at therapeutic levels for several months. Consequently, after extended therapy, abrupt discontinuation should generally be avoided and a gradual dosage tapering schedule followed. Addiction-prone individuals (such as drug addicts or alcoholics) should be under careful surveillance when receiving clonazepam or other psychotropic agents because of the predisposition of such patients to habituation and dependence.

OVERDOSAGE:

Symptoms of clonazepam overdosage, like those produced by other CNS depressants, include somnolence, confusion, coma and diminished reflexes. Treatment includes monitoring of respiration, pulse and blood pressure, general supportive measures and immediate gastric lavage. Intravenous fluids should be administered and an adequate airway maintained. Hypotension may be combated by the use of levarterenol or metaraminol. Methylphenidate or caffeine and sodium benzoate may be given to combat CNS depression. Dialysis is of no known value.

DOSAGE AND ADMINISTRATION:

INFANTS AND CHILDREN

Clonazepam is administered orally. In order to minimize drowsiness, the initial dose for infants and children (up to 10 years of age or 30 kg of body weight) should be between 0.01 and 0.03 mg/kg/day but not to exceed 0.05 mg/kg/day given in two or three divided doses. Dosage should be increased by no more than 0.25 to 0.5 mg every third day until a daily maintenance dose of 0.1 to 0.2 mg/kg of body weight has been reached unless seizures are controlled or side effects preclude further increase. Whenever possible, the daily dose should be divided into three equal doses. If doses are not equally divided, the largest dose should be given before retiring.

ADULTS

The initial dose for adults should not exceed 1.5 mg/day divided into three doses. Dosage may be increased in increments of 0.5 to 1 mg every three days until seizures are adequately controlled or until side effects preclude any further increase. Maintenance dosage must be individualized for each patient depending upon response. Maximum recommended daily dose is 20 mg.

The use of multiple anticonvulsants may result in an increase of depressant adverse effects. This should be considered before adding clonazepam to an existing anticonvulsant regimen.

PATIENT INFORMATION:

Clonazepam is used for the treatment of seizures. Notify your physician if you are pregnant or nursing. This medication may cause dizziness, drowsiness, or blurred vision; use caution while driving or operating hazardous machinery. Do not take any other sedating drugs or drink alcohol while taking clonazepam. Do not change the dose or stop taking clonazepam without talking with your physician. This medication may be habit forming. Seizures or withdrawal symptoms may occur after you stop taking it. This medication should be taken with meals to avoid stomach upset.

HOW SUPPLIED - RATED THERAPEUTICALLY EQUIVALENT:

Tablet, Uncoated - Oral - 0.5 mg

100 (4x25)	$78.36	KLONOPIN, Roche	00004-0068-50
100's	$74.82	KLONOPIN, Roche	00004-0068-01

Tablet, Uncoated - Oral - 1 mg

100 (4x25)	$88.92	KLONOPIN, Roche	00004-0058-50
100's	$85.35	KLONOPIN, Roche	00004-0058-01

Tablet, Uncoated - Oral - 2 mg

100 (4x25)	$121.83	KLONOPIN, Roche	00004-0098-50
100's	$118.28	KLONOPIN, Roche	00004-0098-01

CLONIDINE *(003243)*

CATEGORIES: Alpha Adrenoreceptor Agonists; Antihypertensives; Cardiovascular Drugs; Hypertension; Pregnancy Category C; FDA Approved 1984 Oct; Patent Expiration 1997 May

BRAND NAMES: *Arkamin*; *Barclyd* (France); *Capril*; *Caprysin*; *Catapres* (Australia, Asia, England, Canada); **Catapres-TTS**; *Catapres TTS*; *Catapresan* (Germany); *Catapresan 100* (Mexico); *Catapresan Depot* (Germany); *Catapresan TTS*; *Catapresan* (France); *Clonidine*; *Daipres* (Japan); *Dixarit*; *Haemiton* (Germany); *Normopresan*; *Paracefan*; *Sulmidine* (Japan); *Taitecin* (Japan)
(International brand names outside U.S. in italics)

DESCRIPTION:

TRANSDERMAL THERAPEUTIC SYSTEM

Programmed delivery *in vivo* of 0.1, 0.2, or 0.3 mg clonidine per day, for one week.

Catapres-TTS (clonidine) is a transdermal system providing continuous systemic delivery of clonidine for 7 days at an approximately constant rate. Clonidine is a centrally acting alpha agonist and is an antihypertensive agent. It is an imidazoline derivative whose chemical name is 2,6-dichloro-N-2-imidazolidinylidenebenzenamine.

System Structure and Components: Catapres-TTS is a multilayered film, 0.2 mm thick, containing clonidine as the active agent. System area is 3.5, 7.0, or 10.5 cm^2 and the amount of drug released is directly proportional to area. (See DESCRIPTION, Release Rate Concept). The composition per unit area of all three dosages is identical.

Proceeding from the visible surface towards the surface attached to the skin, are four layers 1) a backing layer of pigmented polyester film; 2) a drug reservoir of clonidine, mineral oil, polyisobutylene, and colloidal silicon dioxide; 3) a microporous polypropylene membrane that controls the rate of delivery of clonidine from the system to the skin surface; 4) an adhesive formulation of clonidine, mineral oil, polyisobutylene, and colloidal silicon dioxide. Prior to use, a protective peel strip of polyester that covers layer 4 is removed.

Cross Section of the System - Backing; Drug Reservoir; Control Membrane; Adhesive; Protective Peel Strip

Release Rate Concept: Clonidine film is programmed to release clonidine at an approximately constant rate for 7 days. The energy source for drug release derives from the concentration gradient existing between a saturated solution of drug in the system and the much lower concentration prevailing in the skin. Clonidine flows in the direction of the lower concentration at a constant rate, limited by the rate- controlling membrane, so long as a saturated solution is maintained in the drug reservoir.

Following system application to intact skin, clonidine in the adhesive layer saturates the skin sites below the system. Clonidine from the drug reservoir then begins to flow through the rate-controlling membrane and the adhesive layer of the system into the systemic circulation via the capillaries beneath the skin. Therapeutic plasma clonidine levels are achieved 2 to 3 days after initial application of clonidine film.

The 3.5, 7.0, and 10.5 cm^2 systems respectively deliver 0.1, 0.2, and 0.3 mg clonidine per day. To ensure constant release of drug over 7 days, the total drug content of the system is greater than the total amount of drug delivered. Application of a new system to a fresh skin site at weekly intervals continuously maintains therapeutic plasma concentrations of clonidine. If the clonidine film is removed and not replaced with a new system, therapeutic plasma clonidine levels will persist for about 8 hours and than decline slowly over several days. Over this time period, blood plasma returns gradually to pretreatment levels. If the patient experiences localized skin irritation before completing 7 days of use, the system may be removed and replaced with a new one applied on a fresh skin site.

CLINICAL PHARMACOLOGY:

The plasma half-life of clonidine is 12.7 $\pm$7 hours. Following oral administration about 40-60% of the absorbed dose is recovered in the urine as unchanged drug in 24 hours. About 50% of the absorbed dose is metabolized in the liver.

Clonidine stimulates alpha-adrenoreceptors in the brain stem, resulting in reduced sympathetic outflow from the central nervous system and a decrease in peripheral resistance, renal vascular resistance, heart rate, and blood pressure. Renal blood flow and glomerular filtration rate remain essentially unchanged. Normal postural reflexes are intact, and therefore orthostatic symptoms are mild and infrequent.

Acute studies with clonidine hydrochloride in human have demonstrated a moderate reduction (15% to 20%) of cardiac output in the supine position with no change in the peripheral resistance; at a 45° tilt there is a smaller reduction in cardiac output and a decrease of peripheral resistance. During long-term therapy, cardiac output tends to return to control values, while peripheral resistance remains decreased. Slowing of the pulse rate has been observed in most patients given clonidine, but the drug does not alter normal hemodynamic response to exercise.

Other studies in patients have provided evidence of a reduction in plasma renin activity and in the excretion of aldosterone and catecholamines, but the exact relationship of these pharmacologic actions to the antihypertensive effect has not been fully elucidated.

Clonidine acutely stimulates growth hormone release in both children and adults, but does not produce a chronic elevation of growth hormone with long-term use.

Tolerance may develop in some patients, necessitating a reevaluation of therapy.

INDICATIONS AND USAGE:

Clonidine film is indicated in the treatment of hypertension. It may be employed alone or concomitantly with other antihypertensive agents.

CONTRAINDICATIONS:

Clonidine film should not be used in patients with known hypersensitivity to clonidine or to any other component of the adhesive layer of the therapeutic system.

PRECAUTIONS:

General: In patients who have developed localized contact sensitization to clonidine film, substitution of oral clonidine hydrochloride therapy may be associated with development of a generalized skin rash.

In patients who develop an allergic reaction to clonidine film that extends beyond the local patch site (such as generalized skin rash, urticaria, or angioedema) oral clonidine hydrochloride substitution may elicit a similar reaction.

As with all antihypertensive therapy, clonidine film should be used with caution in patients with severe coronary insufficiency, recent myocardial infarction, cerebrovascular disease, or chronic renal failure.

Transdermal clonidine systems should be removed before attempting defibrillation or cardioversion because of the potential for altered electrical conductivity which may enhance the possibility of arcing, a phenomenon associated with the use of defibrillators.

Withdrawal: Patients should be instructed not to discontinue therapy without consulting their physician. Sudden cessation of clonidine treatment has resulted in subjective symptoms such as nervousness, agitation and headache, accompanied or followed by a rapid rise in blood pressure and elevated catecholamine concentrations in the plasma, but such occurrences have usually been associated with previous administration of high oral doses (exceeding 1.2 mg/day) and/or with continuation of concomitant beta-blocker therapy. Rare instances of hypertensive encephalopathy and death have been reported.

An excessive rise in blood pressure following clonidine film discontinuance can be reversed by administration of oral clonidine or by intravenous phentolamine. If therapy is to be discontinued in patients receiving beta-blockers and clonidine concurrently, beta-blockers should be discontinued several days before cessation of clonidine film administration.

Perioperative Use: As with oral clonidine therapy, clonidine film therapy should not be interrupted during the surgical period. Blood pressure should be carefully monitored during surgery and additional measures to control blood pressure should be available if required.

PRECAUTIONS: *(cont'd)*

Physicians considering starting clonidine film therapy during the perioperative period must be aware that therapeutic plasma clonidine levels are not achieved until 2 to 3 days after initial application of clonidine film (see DOSAGE AND ADMINISTRATION.)

Information for the Patient: Patients who engage in potentially hazardous activities, such as operating machinery or driving, should be advised of a potential sedative effect of clonidine. Patients should be cautioned against interruption of clonidine film therapy without a physician's advice. Patients should be advised that if the system begins to loosen from the skin after application, the adhesive overlay should be applied directly over the system to ensure good adhesion over its 7-day lifetime. Instructions for using the system are provided. Patients who develop moderate or severe erythema and/or localized vesicle formation at the site of application, or a generalized skin rash, should consult their physician promptly about the possible need to remove the patch.

Carcinogenesis, Mutagenesis, and Impairment of Fertility: In a 132-week (fixed concentration) dietary administration study in rats, clonidine HCl administered at 32 to 46 times the oral maximum recommended daily human dose (MRDHD) was unassociated with evidence of carcinogenic potential. Results from the Ames test with clonidine hydrochloride reveled no evidence of mutagenesis. Fertility of male or female rats was unaffected by clonidine doses as high as 150 mcg/kg or about 3 times the oral MRDHD. Fertility of female rats did, however, appear to be affected (in another experiment) at the dose levels of 500 to 2000 mcg/kg or 10 to 40 times the oral MRDHD.

Pregnancy, Teratogenic Effects, Pregnancy Category C: Reproduction studies performed in rabbits at doses up to approximately 3 times the oral maximum recommended daily human dose (MRDHD) of Catapres (clonidine HCl) have revealed no evidence of teratogenic or embryotoxic potential in rabbits. In rats, however, doses as low as 1/3 the MRDHD of clonidine were associated with increased resorptions in a study in which dams were treated continuously from 2 months prior to mating. Increased resorptions were not associated with treatment at the same or at higher dose levels (up to 3 times the oral MRDHD) when dams were treated days 6-15 of gestation. Increased resorptions were observed at much higher levels (40 times the MRDHD) in rats and mice treated days 1-14 of gestation (lowest dose employed in the study was 500 mcg/kg). There are, however, no adequate and well-controlled studies in pregnant women. Because animal reproduction studies are not always predictive of human response, this drug should be used during pregnancy only if clearly needed.

Nursing Mothers: As clonidine is excreted in human milk, caution should be exercised when clonidine film is administered to a nursing woman.

Pediatric Use: Safety and effectiveness in children below the age of twelve have not been established.

DRUG INTERACTIONS:

If a patient receiving clonidine is also taking tricyclic antidepressants, the effect of clonidine may be reduced, thus necessitating an increase in dosage. Clonidine may enhance the CNS-depressive effects of alcohol, barbiturates or other sedatives. Amitriptyline in combination with clonidine enhances the manifestation of corneal lesions in rats (see DOSAGE AND ADMINISTRATION, TOXICOLOGY).

ADVERSE REACTIONS:

Most systemic adverse effects during therapy with clonidine film have been mild and have tended to diminish with continued therapy. In a 3-month, multiclinic trial of clonidine film in 101 hypertensive patients, the most frequent systemic reactions were dry mouth (25 patients) and drowsiness (12 patients).

Transient localized skin reactions, primarily localized pruritus, occurred in 51 patients. Twenty-six patients experienced localized erythema. This erythema and pruritus were more common in patients utilizing an adhesive overlay for the entire 7-day treatment period. Allergic contact sensitization to clonidine film was observed in 5 patients.

In additional clinical experience contact dermatitis resulting in treatment discontinuation was observed in 128 of 673 patients (about 19 in 100) after a mean duration of treatment of 37 weeks. The incidence in white females was about 34 in 100; in white males about 18 in 100; in black females about 14 in 100; and in black males about 8 in 100.

The following less frequent adverse experiences were also reported in patients involved in the multiclinic trial with clonidine film.

Gastrointestinal: Constipation (1 patient); nausea (1); and change in taste (1).

Central Nervous System: Fatigue (6 patients); headache (5); lethargy (3); sedation (3); insomnia (2); dizziness (2); and nervousness (1).

Genitourinary: Impotence/sexual dysfunction (2 patients).

Dermatological: Localized vesiculation (7 patients); hyperpigmentation (5); edema (3); excoriation (3); burning (3); papules (1); throbbing (1); blanching (1); and generalized macular rash (1). In additional clinical experience involving 3539 patients, less common dermatological reactions have occurred, where a causal relationship to clonidine film was not established: maculopapular skin rash (10 cases); urticaria (2 cases); angioedema involving the face (2 cases), one of which also involved the tongue.

Oro-otolaryngeal: Dry throat (2 patients). In long experience with oral Catapres, the most common adverse reactions have been dry mouth (about 40%), drowsiness (about 35%) and sedation (about 8%). In addition, the following adverse reactions have been reported less frequently:

Gastrointestinal: Nausea and vomiting, about 5 in 100 patients; anorexia and malaise, each about 1 in 100; mild transient abnormalities in liver function tests, about 1 in 100; rare reports of hepatitis; parotitis, rarely.

Metabolic: Weight gain, about 1 in 100 patients; gynecomastia, about 1 in 1000; transient elevation of blood glucose or serum creatine phosphokinase, rarely.

Central Nervous System: Nervousness and agitation, about 3 in 100 patients; mental depression, about 1 in 100 and insomnia, about 5 in 1000. Vivid dreams or nightmares, other behavioral changes, restlessness, anxiety, visual and auditory hallucinations and delirium have been reported.

Cardiovascular: Orthostatic symptoms, about 3 in 100 patients; palpitations and tachycardia, and bradycardia, each about 5 in 1000. Raynaud's phenomenon, congestive heart failure, and electrocardiographic abnormalities (*i.e.,* conduction disturbances and arrhythmias) have been reported rarely. Rare cases of sinus bradycardia and atrioventricular block have been reported, both with and without the use of concomitant digitalis.

Dermatological: Rash, about 1 in 100 patients; pruritus, about 7 in 1000; hives; angioneurotic edema and urticaria, about 5 in 100; alopecia, about 2 in 1000.

Genitourinary: Decreased sexual activity, impotence and loss of libido, about 3 in 100 patients; nocturia, about 1 in 100; difficulty in micturition, about 2 in 1000; urinary retention, about 1 in 1000.

ADVERSE REACTIONS: *(cont'd)*

Other: Weakness, about 10 in 100 patients; fatigue, about 4 in 100; headache, and discontinuation syndrome, each about 1 in 100; muscle or joint pain, about 6 in 1000 and cramps of the lower limbs, about 3 in 1000. Dryness, burning of the eyes, blurred vision, dryness of the nasal mucosa, pallor, weakly positive Coombs' test, increased sensitivity to alcohol and fever have been reported.

OVERDOSAGE:

If symptoms of overdosage occur, remove all clonidine film systems. The signs and symptoms of clonidine overdosage include hypotension, bradycardia, lethargy, irritability, weakness, somnolence, diminished or absent reflexes, miosis, vomiting and hypoventilation. With large overdoses, reversible cardiac conduction defects or arrhythmias, apnea, seizures and transient hypertension have been reported. The oral LD_{50} of clonidine in rats was 465 mg/kg, and in mice 206 mg/kg.

The general treatment of clonidine film overdosage may include intravenous fluids as indicated. Bradycardia can be treated with intravenous atropine sulfate and hypotension with dopamine infusion in addition to intravenous fluids. Hypertension associated with overdosage has been treated with intravenous furosemide or diazoxide or alpha-blocking agents such as phentolamine. Tolazoline, an alpha-blocker, in intravenous doses of 10 mg at 30-minute intervals, may reverse clonidine's effects if other efforts fail. Routine hemodialysis is of limited benefit, since a maximum of 5% of circulating clonidine is removed.

In a patient who ingested 100 mg clonidine hydrochloride, plasma clonidine levels were 60 ng/ml (1 hour), 190 ng/ml (1.5 hours), 370 ng/ml (2 hours) and 120 ng/ml (5.5 and 6.5 hours). This patient developed hypertension followed by hypotension, bradycardia, apnea, hallucinations, semicoma, and premature ventricular contractions. The patient fully recovered after intensive treatment.

DOSAGE AND ADMINISTRATION:

Apply clonidine film to a hairless area of intact skin on the upper arm or torso, once every 7 days. Each new application of clonidine film should be on a different skin site from the previous location. If the system loosens during 7-day wearing, the adhesive overlay should be applied directly over the system to ensure good adhesion.

To initiate therapy, clonidine film dosage should be titrated according to individual therapeutic requirements, starting with clonidine film 0.1 mg. If after one or two weeks the desired reduction in blood pressure is not achieved, increase the dosage by adding an additional clonidine film 0.1 mg or changing to a larger system. An increase in dosage above the two clonidine film 0.3 mg is usually not associated with additional efficacy.

When substituting clonidine film in patients on prior antihypertensive therapy, physicians should be aware that the antihypertensive effect of clonidine film may not commence until 2 to 3 days after initial application. Therefore, gradual reduction of prior drug dosage is advised. Some or all previous antihypertensive treatment may have to be continued, particularly in patients with more severe forms of hypertension.

Toxicology: In several studies, oral clonidine hydrochloride produced a dose-dependent increase in the incidence and severity of spontaneously occurring retinal degeneration in albino rats treated for six months or longer. Tissue distribution studies in dogs and monkeys revealed that clonidine hydrochloride was concentrated in the choroid of the eye. In view of the retinal degeneration observed in rats, eye examinations were performed in 908 patients prior to the start of clonidine hydrochloride therapy, who were then examined periodically thereafter. In 353 of these 908 patients, examinations were performed for periods of 24 months or longer. Except for some dryness of the eyes, no drug-related abnormal ophthalmologic findings were recorded and clonidine hydrochloride did not alter retinal function as shown by specialized tests such as the electroretinogram and macular dazzle.

In rats, clonidine hydrochloride in combination with amitriptyline produced corneal lesions within 5 days.

TABLE 1

Programmed Delivery	Clonidine *in vivo* /day over 1 week	Clonidine Content	Size	Code
Catapres-TTS-1	0.1 mg	2.5 mg	3.5 cm^2	BI-31
Catapres-TTS-2	0.2 mg	5.0 mg	7.0 cm^2	BI-32
Catapres-TTS-3	0.3 mg	7.5 mg	10.5 cm^2	BI-33

PATIENT PACKAGE INSERT:

(Read the following instructions carefully before using this medication. If you have any questions, please consult your doctor.)

GENERAL INFORMATION

Catapres-TTS is a square, tan adhesive patch containing an active blood pressure lowering medication. It is designed to deliver the drug into the body through the skin smoothly and consistently for one full week. Normal exposure to water, as in showering, bathing, and swimming, should not affect the patch. However, should the patch begin to separate from the skin, the white, round, adhesive overlay should be applied directly over it to ensure adhesion for seven full days. The Catapres-TTS patch must be replaced with a new one on a fresh skin site if the one in use significantly loosens or falls off.

HOW TO APPLY THE CATAPRES-TTS PATCH

1) Apply the square, tan Catapres-TTS patch once a week, preferably at a convenient time on the same day of the week (*i.e.,* prior to bedtime on Tuesday of week one; prior to bedtime on Tuesday of week two, etc.).

2) Select a hairless area such as on the upper, outer arm or upper chest. The area chosen should be free of cuts, abrasions, irritation, scars or calluses and should not be shaved before applying the Catapres-TTS patch. Do not place the Catapres-TTS patch on skin folds or under tight undergarments, since premature loosening may occur.

3) Wash hands with soap and water and thoroughly dry them.

4) Clean the area chosen with soap and water. Rinse and wipe dry with a clean, dry tissue.

5) Select the pouch labeled Catapres-TTS (clonidine) and open it. Remove the square, tan patch from the pouch.

6) Remove the clear plastic protective backing from the patch by gently peeling off one half of the backing at a time. Avoid touching the sticky side of the Catapres-TTS patch.

7) Place the Catapres-TTS patch on the prepared skin site (sticky side down) by applying firm pressure over the patch to ensure good contact with the skin, especially around the edges. Discard the clear plastic protective backing and wash your hands with soap and water to remove any drug from your hands.

8) Next week, remove the old patch and discard it (refer to **Instructions for Disposal**). After choosing a different skin site, repeat instructions 2 through 7 for the application of your next Catapres-TTS patch.

PATIENT PACKAGE INSERT: *(cont'd)*

HOW TO APPLY THE OVERLAY

Note: The white, round, adhesive overlay does not contain any drug and should not be used alone. The overlay should be applied directly over the Catapres-TTS patch only if the patch begins to separate from the skin, thereby ensuring adhesion for seven full days.

1) Wash hands with soap and water and thoroughly dry them.

2) Using a clean, dry tissue, make sure that the area around the square, tan Catapres-TTS patch is clean and dry. Press gently on the Catapres-TTS patch to ensure that the edges are in good contact with the skin.

3) Take the white, round, adhesive overlay from its pouch and remove the paper liner backing from the overlay.

4) Carefully center the adhesive overlay over the square, tan Catapres-TTS patch and apply firm pressure, especially around the edges in contact with the skin.

INSTRUCTIONS FOR DISPOSAL

KEEP OUT OF REACH OF CHILDREN

During or even after use, a patch contains active medication which may be harmful to infants and children if accidentally applied or ingested. After use, fold in half with the sticky sides together. Dispose of carefully out of reach of children.

HOW SUPPLIED:

Catapres-TTS-1 (clonidine) and Catapres-TTS-2 are supplied as 4 pouched systems and 4 adhesive overlays per carton, 3 cartons per shipper. Catapres-TTS-3 is supplied as 4 pouched systems and 4 adhesive overlays per carton.

See chart above.

Storage and Handling: Store below 86°F (30°C).

HOW SUPPLIED - EQUIVALENTS NOT AVAILABLE:

Film, Continuous Release - Percutaneous - 2.5 mg/unit

3 x 4 $90.11 CATAPRES-TTS-1, Boehringer Pharms 00597-0031-12

Film, Continuous Release - Percutaneous - 5 mg/unit

3 x 4 $152.15 CATAPRES-TTS-2, Boehringer Pharms 00597-0032-12

Film, Continuous Release - Percutaneous - 7.5 mg/unit

4's $70.14 CATAPRES-TTS-3, Boehringer Pharms 00597-0033-34

CLONIDINE HYDROCHLORIDE *(000846)*

CATEGORIES: Alpha Adrenoreceptor Agonists; Analgesics; Alcohol Withdrawal*; Attention Deficit Disorders*; Antihypertensives; Cardiovascular Drugs; Hypertension; Herpes Zoster*; Menopause*; Pheochromocytoma Test*; Smoking Cessation*; Tourette Syndrome*; Ulcerative Colitis*; FDA Approved 1996 Sep; Pregnancy Category C; Sales > $100 Million; FDA Approval Pre 1982; Top 200 Drugs
* Indication not approved by the FDA

BRAND NAMES: *Aclon*; *Arkamin*; *Cares*; **Catapres**; *Clinolou*; *Clonnirit*; *Daipres*; *Dixarit*; *Drylon*; **Duraclon**; *Hyposyn*; *Ipotensium*; *Isoglaucon*; *Josechazu*; *Normopresan*; *Sulmidine*; *Taltecin*; *Tinya*; *Winpress*
(International brand names outside U.S. in italics)

FORMULARIES: Aetna; BC-BS; CIGNA; DoD; FHP; Humana; Kaiser; Medco; Medi-Cal; PCS; PruCare; United

COST OF THERAPY: $17.52 (Hypertension; Tablet; 0.1 mg; 2/day; 365 days)

PRIMARY ICD9: 401.1 (Essential Hypertension, Benign)

WARNING:
Note: Epidural clonidine is not recommended for obsetrical, post-partum, or peri-operative pain management. The risk of hemodynamic instability, especially hypotension and bradycardia, from epidural clonidine may be unacceptable in these patients. However, in a rare obstetrical, post-partum or peri-operative patient, potential benefits may outweigh the possible risks.

DESCRIPTION:

TABLET

Clonidine hydrochloride USP is a centrally acting antihypertensive agent available as tablets for oral administration in three dosage strengths: 0.1 mg, 0.2 mg and 0.3 mg. The 0.1 mg tablet is equivalent to 0.087 mg of the free base.

The inactive ingredients in Catapres are colloidal silicon dioxide, corn starch, dibasic calcium phosphate, FD&C Yellow No. 6, gelatin, glycerin, lactose, magnesium stearate, methylparaben, propylparaben. The Catapres 0.1 mg tablet also contains FD&C Blue No. 1 and FD&C Red No. 3.

Clonidine hydrochloride is an imidazoline derivative and exists as a mesomeric compound. The chemical name is 2-(2,6-dichlorophenylamino)-2- imidazoline hydrochloride. It has the following molecular formula: $C_9H_9Cl_2N_3 \cdot HCl$, with molecular weight of 266.56.

Clonidine hydrochloride is an odorless, bitter, white, crystalline substance soluble in water and alcohol.

EPIDURAL INJECTION

Clonidine hydrochloride injection is a centrally-acting analgesic solution for use in continuous epidural infusion devices.

Clonidine hydrochloride is an imidazoline derivative and exists as a mesomeric compound. The chemical names are Benzenamine, 2,6-dichloro-N-2-imidazolidinylidene-monohydrochloride and 2-[(2,6-dichlorophenyl) imino]imidazolidine monohydrochloride. Its molecular formula is $C_9H_9Cl_2N_3 \cdot HCl$, with molecular weight of 266.56.

Clonidine hydrochloride injection is supplied as a clear, colorless, preservative-free, pyrogen-free, aqueous sterile solution (pH 5 to 7) in a single-dose, 10 ml vial. Each ml of solution contains 100 mcg of clonidine hydrochloride, USP and 9 mg sodium chloride, USP in water for injection, USP. Hydrochloric acid and/or sodium hydroxide may have been added for pH adjustment. Each 10 ml vial contains 1 mg (1000 mcg) of clonidine hydrochloride.

CLINICAL PHARMACOLOGY:

TABLET

Clonidine hydrochloride acts relatively rapidly. The patient's blood pressure declines within 30 to 60 minutes after an oral dose, the maximum decrease occurring within 2 to 4 hours. The plasma level of clonidine hydrochloride peaks in approximately 3 to 5 hours and the plasma half-life ranges from 12 to 16 hours. The half-life increases up to 41 hours in patients with severe impairment of renal function. Following oral administration about 40-60% of the absorbed dose is recovered in the urine as unchanged drug in 24 hours. About 50% of the absorbed dose is metabolized in the liver.

Clonidine stimulates alpha-adrenoreceptors in the brain stem, resulting in reduced sympathetic outflow from the central nervous system and a decrease in peripheral resistance: at a 45° tilt there is a smaller reduction in cardiac output and a decrease of peripheral resistance. During long-term therapy, cardiac output tends to return to control values, while peripheral resistance remains decreased. Slowing of the pulse rate has been observed in most patients given clonidine, but the drug does not alter normal hemodynamic response to exercise.

Other studies in patients have provided evidence of a reduction in plasma renin activity and in the excretion of aldosterone and catecholamines, but the exact relationship of these pharmacologic actions to the antihypertensive effect has not been fully elucidated.

Clonidine acutely stimulates growth hormone release in both children and adults, but does not produce a chronic elevation of growth hormone with long-term use.

Tolerance may develop in some patients, necessitating a reevaluation of therapy.

EPIDURAL INJECTION

Mechanism of Action: Epidurally administered clonidine produces dose-dependent analgesia not antagonized by opiate antagonists. The analgesia is limited to the body regions innervated by the spinal segments where analgesic concentrations of clonidine are present. Clonidine is thought to produce analgesia at presynaptic and postjunctional alpha-2-adrenoceptors in the spinal cord by preventing pain signal transmission to the brain.

Pharmacokinetics: Following a 10 minute intravenous infusion of 300 mcg clonidine HCl to five male volunteers, plasma clonidine levels showed an initial rapid distribution phase (mean $\pm$ SD $t_{\frac{1}{2}} = 11 \pm 9$ minutes) followed by a slower elimination phase ($t_{\frac{1}{2}} = 9 \pm 2$ hours) over 24 hours. Clonidine's total body clearance (CL) was 219 ± 92 ml/min.

Following a 700 mcg clonidine HCl epidural dose given over five minutes to four male and five female volunteers, peak clonidine plasma levels (4.4 ± 1.4 ng/ml) were obtained in 19 ± 27 minutes. The plasma elimination half-life was determined to be 22 ± 15 hours following sample collection for 24 hours. CL was 190 ± 70 ml/min. In cerebral spinal fluid (CSF), peak clonidine levels (418 ± 255 ng/ml) were achieved in 26 ± 11 minutes. The clonidine CSF elimination half-life was 1.3 ± 0.5 hours when samples were collected for 6 hours. Compared to men, women had a lower mean plasma clearance, longer mean plasma half-life, and higher mean peak level of clonidine in both plasma and CSF.

In cancer patients who received 14 days of clonidine HCl epidural infusion (rate=30 mcg/hr) plus morphine by patient-controlled analgesia (PCA), steady state clonidine plasma concentrations of 2.2 ± 1.1 and 2.4 ± 1.4 ng/ml were obtained on dosing days 7 and 14 respectively. CL was 279 ± 184 and 272 ± 163 ml/min on these days. CSF concentrations were not determined in these patients.

Distribution: Clonidine is highly lipid soluble and readily distributes into extravascular sites including the central nervous system. Clonidine's volume of distribution is 2.1 ± 0.4 L/kg. The binding of clonidine to plasma protein is primarily to albumin and varies between 20 and 40% *in vitro*. Epidurally administered clonidine readily partitions into plasma via the epidural veins and attains systemic concentrations (0.5–2.0 ng/ml) that are associated with a hypotensive effect mediated by the central nervous system.

Excretion: Following an intravenous dose of ^{14}C-clonidine, 72% of the administered dose was excreted in urine in 96 hours of which 40–50% was unchanged clonidine. Renal clearance for clonidine was determined to be 133 ± 66 ml/min. In a study where ^{14}C-clonidine was given to subjects with varying degrees of kidney function, elimination half-lives varied (17.5 to 41 hours) as a function of creatinine clearance. In subjects undergoing hemodialysis only 5% of body clonidine stores was removed.

Metabolism: In humans, clonidine metabolism follows minor pathways with the major metabolite, p-hydroxyclonidine, being present at less than 10% of the concentration of unchanged drug in urine.

Special Populations: The pharmacokinetics of epidurally administered clonidine has not been studied in the pediatric population or in patients with renal or hepatic disease.

CLINICAL STUDIES:

EPIDURAL INJECTION

In a double-blind, randomized study of cancer patients with severe intractable pain below the C4 dermatome not controlled by morphine, 38 patients were randomized to an epidural infusion of clonidine HCl plus epidural morphine, whereas 47 subjects received epidural placebo plus epidural morphine. Both groups were allowed rescue doses of epidural morphine. Successful analgesia, defined as a decrease in either morphine use or Visual Analog Score (VAS) pain, was significantly more common with epidural clonidine than placebo (45% vs 21%, p=0.016). Only the subgroup of 36 patients with "neuropathic" pain, characterized by the investigator as well-localized, burning, shooting, or electric-like pain in a dermatomal or peripheral nerve distribution had significant analgesic effects relative to placebo in this study.

The most frequent adverse events with clonidine were hypotension (45% vs 11% for placebo, p<0.001), postural hypotension (32% vs 0%, p<0.001), dizziness (13% vs 4%, p=0.234), anxiety (11% vs 2%, p=0.168) and dry mouth (13% vs 9%, p=0.505). Both mean blood pressure and heart rate were reduced in the clonidine group. At the conclusion of the two week study period in the clinical trial, all patients were abruptly withdrawn from study drug or placebo. Four patients of the clonidine group suffered rebound hypertension upon withdrawl of clonidine; one of these patients suffered a cerebrovascular accident. Asymptomatic bradycardia was noted in one clonidine patient.

INDICATIONS AND USAGE:

TABLET

Clonidine hydrochloride is indicated in the treatment of hypertension. Clonidine hydrochloride may be employed alone or concomitantly with other antihypertensive agents.

EPIDURAL INJECTION

Epidural clonidine HCl is indicated in combination with opiates for the treatment of severe pain in cancer patients that is not adequately relieved by opioid analgesics alone. Epidural clonidine is more likely to be effective in patients with neuropathic pain than somatic or visceral pain (see CLINICAL STUDIES).

The safety of this drug product has only been established in a highly selected group of cancer patients, and only after an adequate trial of opioid analgesia. Other use is of unproven safety and is not recommended. In a rare patient, the potential benefits may outweigh the known risks (see WARNINGS).

CONTRAINDICATIONS:

TABLET

None known.

CONTRAINDICATIONS: *(cont'd)*

EPIDURAL INJECTION

Clonidine HCl is contraindicated in patients with a history of sensitization or allergic reactions to clonidine. Epidural administration is contraindicated in the presence of an injection site infection, in patients on anticoagulant therapy, and in those with a bleeding diathesis. Administration of epidural clonidine HCl above the C4 dermatome is contraindicated since there are no adequate data to support such use (see WARNINGS).

WARNINGS:

EPIDURAL INJECTION

Use in Postoperative or Obstetrical Analgesia: Epidural clonidine is not recommended for obstetrical, post-partum, or peri-operative pain management. The risk of hemodynamic instability, especially hypotension and bradycardia, from epidural clonidine may be unacceptable in these patients.

Hypotension: Because severe hypotension may follow the administration of clonidine, it should be used with caution in all patients. It is not recommended in most patients with severe cardiovascular disease or in those who are otherwise hemodynamically unstable. The benefit of its administration in these patients should be carefully balanced against the potential risks resulting from hypotension.

Vital signs should be monitored frequently, especially during the first few days of epidural clonidine therapy. When clonidine is infused into the upper thoracic spinal segments, more pronounced decreases in the blood pressure may be seen.

Clonidine decreases sympathetic outflow from the central nervous system resulting in decreases in peripheral resistance, renal vascular resistance, heart rate, and blood pressure. However, in the absence of profound hypotension, renal blood flow and glomerular filtration rate remain essentially unchanged.

In the pivotal double-blind, randomized study of cancer patients, where 38 subjects were administered epidural clonidine HCl at 30 mcg/hr in addition to epidural morphine, hypertension occurred in 45% of subjects. Most episodes of hypotension occurred within the first fours days after beginning epidural clonidine. However, hypotensive episodes occurred throughout the duration of the trial. There was a tendency for these episodes to occur more commonly in women, and in those with higher serum clonidine levels. Patients experiencing hypotension also tended to weigh less than those who did not experience hypotension. The hypotension usually responded to intravenous fluids and, if necessary, parenteral ephedrine.

Published reports on the use of epidural clonidine for intraoperative or postoperative analgesia also show a consistent and marked hypotensive response to clonidine. Severe hypotension may occur if intravenous fluid pretreatment is given.

Withdrawl: Sudden cessation of clonidine treatment, regardless of the route of administration, has, in some cases, resulted in symptoms such as nervousness, agitation, headache, and tremor, accompanied or followed by a rapid rise in blood pressure. The likelihood of such reactions appears to be greater after administration of higher doses or with concomitant beta-blocker treatment. Special caution is therefore advised in these situations. Rare instances of hypertensive encephalopathy, cerebrovascular accidents and death have been reported after abrupt clonidine withdrawl. Patients with a history of hypertension and/or other underlying cardiovascular conditions may be at risk of the consequences of abrupt discontinuation of clonidine. In the pivotal double-blind, randomized cancer pain study, four of 38 subjects receiving 720 mcg of clonidine per day experienced rebound hypertension following abrupt withdrawl. One of these patients with rebound hypertension subsequently experienced a cerebrovascular accident.

Careful monitoring of infusion pump function and inspection of catheter tubing for obstruction or dislodgement can help reduce the risk of inadvertent abrupt withdrawl of epidural clonidine. Patients should notify their physician immediately if clonidine administration is inadvertently interrupted for any reason. Patients should also be instructed not to discontinue therapy without consulting their physician.

When discontinuing therapy with epidural clonidine, the physician should reduce the dose gradually over 2 to 4 days to avoid withdrawl symptoms.

An excessive rise in blood pressure following discontinuation of epidural clonidine can be treated by administration of clonidine or by intravenous phentolamine. If therapy is to be discontinued in patients receiving a beta-blocker and clonidine concurrently, the beta-blocker should be withdrawn several days before the gradual discontinuation of epidural clonidine.

Infections: Infections related to implantable epidural catheters pose a serious risk. Evaluation of fever in a patient receiving epidural clonidine should include the possibility of catheter-related infection such as meningitis or epidural abscess.

PRECAUTIONS:

TABLET

General: In patients who have developed localized contact sensitization to clonidine film, substitution of oral clonidine hydrochloride therapy may be associated with the development of a generalized skin rash.

In patients who develop an allergic reaction from clonidine film that extends beyond the local patch site (such as generalized skin rash, urticaria, or angioedema), oral clonidine hydrochloride substitution may elicit a similar reaction.

As with all antihypertensive therapy, clonidine hydrochloride should be used with caution in patients with severe coronary insufficiency, recent myocardial infarction, cerebrovascular disease or chronic renal failure.

Withdrawal: Patients should be instructed not to discontinue therapy without consulting their physician. Sudden cessation of clonidine treatment has resulted in subjective symptoms such as nervousness, agitation and headache, accompanied or followed by a rapid rise in blood pressure and elevated catecholamine concentrations in the plasma, but such occurrences have usually been associated with previous administration of high oral doses (exceeding 1.2 mg/day) and/or with continuation of concomitant beta-blocker therapy. Rare instances of hypertensive encephalopathy and death have been reported. When discontinuing therapy with clonidine hydrochloride, the physician should reduce the dose gradually over 2 to 4 days withdrawal symptomatology.

An excessive rise in blood pressure following clonidine hydrochloride discontinuance can be reversed by administration of oral clonidine or by intravenous phentolamine. If therapy is to be discontinued in patients receiving beta-blockers and clonidine concurrently, beta-blockers should be discontinued several days before the gradual withdrawal of clonidine hydrochloride.

Perioperative Use: Administration of clonidine hydrochloride should be continued to within four hours of surgery and resumed as soon as possible thereafter. The blood pressure should be carefully monitored and appropriate measures instituted to control it as necessary.

Information for Patients: Patients who engage in potentially hazardous activities, such as operating machinery or driving, should be advised of a potential sedative effect of clonidine. Patients should be cautioned against interruption of clonidine hydrochloride therapy without a physician's advice.

PRECAUTIONS: *(cont'd)*

Carcinogenesis, Mutagenesis, Impairment of Fertility: In a 132-week (fixed concentration) dietary administration study in rats, clonidine hydrochloride administered at 32 to 46 times the maximum recommended daily human dose was unassociated with evidence of carcinogenic potential.

Fertility of male or female rats was unaffected by clonidine hydrochloride doses as high as 150 mcg/kg or about 3 times the maximum recommended daily human dose (MRDHD). Fertility of female rats did, however, appear to be affected (in another experiment) at dose levels of 500 to 2000 mcg/kg or 10 to 40 times the MRDHD.

Usage in Pregnancy: Teratogenic Effects: Pregnancy Category C: Reproduction studies performed in rabbits at doses up to approximately 3 times the maximum recommended daily human dose (MRDHD) of clonidine hydrochloride have revealed no evidence of teratogenic or embryotoxic potential in rabbits. In rats, however, doses as low as 1/3 the MRDHD were associated with increased resorptions in a study in which dams were treated continuously from 2 months prior to mating. Increased resorptions were not associated with treatment at the same or at higher dose levels (up to 3 times the MRDHD) when dams were treated days 6-15 of gestation. Increased resorptions were observed at much higher levels (40 times the MRDHD) in rats and mice treated days 1-14 of gestation (lowest dose employed in that study was 500 mcg/kg). There are, however, no adequate and well-controlled studies in pregnant women. Because animal reproduction studies are not always predictive of human response, this drug should be used during pregnancy only if clearly needed.

Nursing Mothers: As clonidine hydrochloride is excreted in human milk, caution should be exercised when clonidine hydrochloride is administered to a nursing woman.

Pediatric Use: Safety and effectiveness in children have not been established.

EPIDURAL INJECTION

General

Cardiac Effects: Epidural clonidine frequently causes decreases in heart rate. Symptomatic bradycardia can be treated with atropine. Rarely, atrioventricular block greater than first degree has been reported. Clonidine does not alter the hemodynamic response to exercise, but may mask the increase in heart rate associated with hypovolemia.

Respiratory Depression and Sedation: Clonidine administration may result in sedation through the activation of alpha-adrenoceptors in the brainstem. High doses of clonidine cause sedation and ventilatory abnormalities that are usually mild. Tolerance to these effects can develop with chronic administration. These effects have been reported with bolus doses that are significantly larger than the infusion rate recommended for treating cancer pain.

Depression: Depression has been seen in a small percentage of patients treated with oral or transdermal clonidine. Depression commonly occurs in cancer patients and may be exacerbated by treatment with clonidine. Patients, especially those with a known history of affective disorders, should be monitored for the signs and symptoms of depression.

Pain of Visceral or Somatic Origin: In the clinical investigations, at doses tested, epidural clonidine HCl was most effective in well-localized, "neuropathic" pain that was characterized as electrical, burning, or shooting in nature, and which was localized to a dermatomal or peripheral nerve distribution. Epidural clonidine HCl may be less effective, or possibly ineffective in the treatment of pain that is diffuse, poorly localized, or visceral in origin.

Information for the Patient

Patients should be instructed about the risks of rebound hypertension and warned not to discontinue clonidine except under the supervision of a physician. Patients should notify their physician immediately if clonidine administration is inadvertently interrupted for any reason. Patients who engage in potentially hazardous activities, such as operating machinery or driving, should be advised of the potential sedative and hypotensive effects of epidural clonidine. They should also be informed that sedative effects may be increased by CNS-depressing drugs such as alcohol and barbiturates, and that hypotensive effects may be increased by opiates.

Carcinogenesis, Mutagenesis, and Impairment of Fertility

In a 132-week study in rats, clonidine HCl administered as a dietary admixture at 5–8 times (based on body surface area) the 50 mcg/kg maximum recommended daily human dose (MRDHD) for hypertension did not show any carcinogenic potential. Clonidine was inactive in the Ames test of mutagenicity. Fertility of male and female rats was unaffected by oral clonidine HCl doses as high as 150 mcg/kg, or about 0.5 times the MRDHD. Fertility of female rats did, however, appear to be affected in another experiment at oral dose levels of 500–2000 mcg/kg, or 2–7 times the MRDHD.

Usage in Pregnancy: Teratogenic Effects: Pregnancy Category C

Reproduction studies in rabbits at clonidine HCl doses up to approximately the MRDHD revealed no evidence of teratogenic or embryotoxic potential. In rats, however, doses as low as one-third the MRDHD were associated with increased resorptions in a study in which dams were treated continuously from 2 months prior to mating. Increased resorptions were not associated with treatment with the same or higher doses up to 0.5 times the MRDHD when dams were treated on days 6–15 of gestation. Increased resorptions were observed at higher levels (7–times the MRDHD) in rats and mice treated on days 1–14 of gestation.

Clonidine readily crosses the placenta and its concentrations are equal in maternal and umbilical cord plasma; amniotic fluid concentrations can be 4–times those found in serum. There are no adequate and well-controlled studies in pregnant women during early gestation when organ formation takes place. Studies using epidural clonidine during labor have demonstrated no apparent adverse effects on the infant at the time of delivery. However, these studies did not monitor the infants for hemodynamic effects in the days following delivery. Clonidine HCl injection should be used during pregnancy only if the potential benefits justify the potential risk to the fetus.

Labor and Delivery

There are no adequate controlled clinical trials evaluating the safety, efficacy, and dosing of epidural clonidine HCl in obstetrical settings. Because maternal perfusion of the placenta is critically dependent on blood pressure, use of epidural clonidine HCl as an analgesic during labor and delivery is not indicated (see WARNINGS.)

Nursing Mothers

Concentrations of clonidine in human breast milk are approximately twice those found in maternal plasma. Caution should be exercised when clonidine is administered to a nursing woman. Because of the potential for severe adverse reactions in nursing infants, a decision should be made to either discontinue nursing or to discontinue clonidine.

Pediatric Use

The safety and effectiveness of epidural clonidine HCl in this limited indication and clinical population have been established in patients old enough to tolerate placement and management of an epidural catheter, based on evidence from adequate and well controlled studies in adults and experience with the use of clonidine in the pediatric age group for other indications. The use of epidural clonidine HCl should be restricted to pediatric patients with severe intractable pain from malignancy that is unresponsive to epidural or spinal opiates or other more conventional analgesic techniques. The starting dose of epidural clonidine HCl should be selected on per kilogram basis (0.5 mcg per kg per hour) and cautiously adjusted based on the clinical response.

DRUG INTERACTIONS:

TABLET

If a patient receiving clonidine hydrochloride is also taking tricyclic antidepressants, the effect of clonidine may be reduced, thus necessitating an increase in dosage. Clonidine hydrochloride may enhance the CNS-depressive effects of alcohol, barbiturates or other sedatives. Amitriptyline in combination with clonidine enhances the manifestation of corneal lesions in rats (See DOSAGE AND ADMINISTRATION, Toxicology).

EPIDURAL INJECTION

Clonidine may potentiate the CNS-depressive effect of alcohol, barbiturates or other sedating drugs. Narcotic analgesics may potentiate the hypotensive effects of clonidine. Tricyclic antidepressants may antagonize the hypotensive effects of clonidine. The effects of tricyclic antidepressants on clonidine's analgesic actions are not known.

Beta blockers may exacerbate the hypertensive response seen with clonidine withdrawl. Also, due to the potential for additive effects such as bradycardia and AV block, caution is warranted in patients receiving clonidine with agents known to affect sinus node function or AV nodal conduction (*e.g.,* digitalis, calcium channel blockers, and beta-blockers).

There is one reported case of a patient with acute delirium associated with the simultaneous use of fluphenazine and oral clonidine. Symptoms resolved when clonidine was withdrawn and recurred when the patient was rechallenged with clonidine.

Epidural clonidine may prolong the duration of pharmacologic effects of epidural local anesthetics, including both sensory and motor blockade.

ADVERSE REACTIONS:

TABLET

Most adverse effects are mild and tend to diminish with continued therapy. The most frequent (which appear to be dose-related) are dry mouth, occurring in about 40 to 100 patients; drowsiness, about 33 in 100; dizziness, about 16 in 100; constipation and sedation, each about 10 in 100.

The following less frequent adverse experiences have also been reported in patients receiving clonidine hydrochloride, but in many cases patients were receiving concomitant medication and a causal relationship has not been established.

Gastrointestinal: Nausea and vomiting, about 5 in 100 patients; anorexia and malaise, each about 1 in 100; mild transient abnormalities in liver function tests, about 1 in 100; rare reports of hepatitis; parotitis, rarely.

Metabolic: Weight gain, about 1 in 100 patients; gynecomastia, about 1 in 1000; transient elevation of blood glucose or serum creatine phosphokinase, rarely.

Central Nervous System: Nervousness and agitation, about 3 in 100 patients; mental depression, about 1 in 100; headache, about 1 in 100; insomnia, about 5 in 1000. Vivid dreams or nightmares, other behavioral changes, restlessness, anxiety, visual and auditory hallucinations and delirium have been reported.

Cardiovascular: Orthostatic symptoms, about 3 in 100 patients; palpitations and tachycardia, and bradycardia, each about 5 in 1000. Raynaud's phenomenon, congestive heart failure, and electrocardiographic abnormalities (*i.e.,* conduction disturbances and arrhythmias) have been reported rarely. Rare cases of sinus bradycardia and atrioventricular block have been reported, both with and without the use of concomitant digitalis.

Dermatological: Rash, about 1 in 100 patients; pruritus, about 7 in 1000; hives, angioneurotic edema and urticaria, about 5 in 1000; alopecia, about 2 in 1000.

Genitourinary: Decreased sexual activity, impotence and loss of libido, about 3 in 100 patients; nocturia, about 1 in 100; difficulty in micturition, about 2 in 1000; urinary retention, about 1 in 1000.

Other: Weakness, about 10 in 100 patients; fatigue, about 4 in 100; discontinuation syndrome, about 1 in 100; muscle or joint pain, about 6 in 1000 and cramps of the lower limbs, about 3 in 1000. Dryness, burning of the eyes, blurred vision, dryness of the nasal mucosa, pallor, weakly positive Coombs' test, increased sensitivity to alcohol and fever have been reported.

EPIDURAL INJECTION

Adverse reactions seen during continuous epidural clonidine infusion are dose dependent and typical for a compound of this pharmacologic class. The adverse events most frequently reported in the pivotal controlled clinical trial of continuous epidural clonidine administration consisted of hypotension, postural hypotension, decreased heart rate, rebound hypertension, dry mouth, nausea, confusion, dizziness, somnolence, and fever. Hypotension is the adverse event that most frequently requires treatment. The hypotension is usually responsive to intravenous fluids and, if necessary, parenterally-administered ephedrine. Hypotension was observed more frequently in women and in lower weight patients, but no dose-related response was established.

Implantable epidural catheters are associated with a risk of catheter-related infections, including meningitis and/or epidural abscess. The risk depends on the clinical situation and the type of catheter used, but catheter related infections occur in 5%-20% of patients, depending on the kind of catheter used, catheter placement technique, quality of catheter care, and length of catheter placement.

The inadvertent intrathecal administration of clonidine has not been associated with a significantly increased risk of adverse events, but there are inadequate safety and efficacy data to support the use of intrathecal clonidine.

Epidural clonidine was compared to placebo in a two-week double-blind study of 85 terminal cancer patients with intractable pain receiving epidural morphine. The adverse events in TABLE 1 were reported in two or more patients and may be related to administration of either epidural clonidine HCl or morphine.

An open label long-term extension of the trial was performed. Thirty-two subjects received epidural clonidine and morphine for up to 94 weeks with a median dosing period of 10 weeks. The following adverse events (and percent incidence) were reported: hypotension/postural hypotension (47%); nausea (13%); anxiety/confusion (38%); somnolence (25%); urinary tract infection (22%); constipation, dyspnea, fever, infection (6% each); asthenia, hyperaesthesia, pain, skin ulcer, and vomiting (5% each). Eighteen percent of subjects discontinued this study as a result of catheter-related problems (infections, accidental dislodging, etc.), and one subject developed meningitis, possibly as a result of a catheter-related infection. In this study, rebound hypertension was not assessed, and ECG and laboratory data were not systemically sought.

The following adverse reactions have also been reported with the use of any dosage form of clonidine. In many cases patients were receiving concomitant medication and a causal relationship has not been established:

Body as a Whole: Weakness, 10%; fatigue, 4%; headache and withdrawl syndrome, each 1%. Also reported were pallor, a weakly positive Coomb's test, and increased sensitivity to alcohol.

Cardiovascular: Palpitations and tachycardia, and bradycardia, each 0.5%. Syncope, Raynaud's phenomenon, congestive heart failure, and electrocardiographic abnormalities (*i.e.,* sinus node arrest, functional bradycardia, high degree AV block) have been reported rarely. Rare case of sinus bradycardia and atrioventricular block have been reported, both with and without the use of concomitant digitalis.

ADVERSE REACTIONS: *(cont'd)*

TABLE 1 Incidence of Adverse Events in the Two-Week Trial

Adverse Events	Clonidine N=38 n (%)	Placebo N=47 n (%)
Total number of patients who experienced at least one adverse event.	37 (97.4)	38 (80.5)
Hypotension	17 (44.8)	5 (10.6)
Postural Hypotension	12 (31.6)	0 (0)
Dry Mouth	5 (13.2)	4 (8.5)
Nausea	5 (13.2)	10 (21.3)
Somnolence	5 (13.2)	10 (21.3)
Dizziness	5 (13.2)	2 (4.3)
Confusion	5 (13.2)	5 (10.6)
Vomiting	4 (10.5)	7 (14.9)
Nausea/ Vomiting	3 (7.9)	1 (2.1)
Sweating	2 (5.3)	0 (0)
Chest Pain	2 (5.3)	0 (0)
Hallucination	2 (5.3)	1 (2.1)
Tinnitus	2 (5.3)	0 (0)
Constipation	1 (2.6)	2 (4.3)
Tachycardia	1 (2.6)	2 (4.3)
Hypoventilation	1 (2.6)	2 (4.3)

Central Nervous System: Nervousness and agitation, 3%; mental depression, 1%; insomnia, 0.5%. Cerebrovascular accidents, other behavioral changes, vivid dreams or nightmares, restlessness, and delirium have been reported rarely.

Dermatological: Rash, 1%; pruritus, 0.7%; hives, angioneurotic edema and urticaria, 0.5%; alopecia, 0.2%.

Gastrointestinal: Anorexia and malaise, each 1%; mild transient abnormalities in liver function tests, 1%; hepatitis, parotitis, ileus and pseudoobstruction, and abdominal pain, rarely.

Genitourinary: Decreased sexual activity, impotence, and libido, 3%; nocturia, about 1%; difficulty in maicturition, about 0.2%; urinary retention, about 0.1%.

Hematologic: Theombocytopenia, rarely.

Metabolic: Weight gain, 0.1%; gynecomastia, 1%; transient elevation of glucose or serum phosphatase, rarely.

Musculoskeletal: Muscle or joint pain, about 0.6%; leg cramps, 0.3%.

Oro-otolaryngeal: Dryness of the nasal mucosa was rarely reported.

Ophthalmological: Dryness of the eyes, burning of the eyes and blurred vision were rarely reported.

OVERDOSAGE:

TABLET

The signs and symptoms of clonidine hydrochloride overdosage include hypotension, bradycardia, lethargy, irritability, weakness, somnolence, diminished or absent reflexes, miosis, vomiting and hypoventilation. With large overdoses, reversible cardiac conduction defects or arrhythmias, apnea, seizures and transient hypertension have been reported. The oral LD_{50} of clonidine in rats was 465 mg/kg, and in mice 206 mg/kg.

The general treatment of clonidine hydrochloride overdosage may include intravenous fluids as indicated. Bradycardia can be treated with intravenous fluids as indicated. Bradycardia can be treated with intravenous atropine sulfate and hypotension with dopamine infusion in addition to intravenous fluids. Hypertension, associated with overdosage, has been treated with intravenous furosemide or diazoxide or alpha-blocking agents such as phentolamine. Tolazoline, an alpha-blocker, in intravenous doses of 10 mg at 30-minute intervals, may reverse clonidine's effects if other efforts fail. Routine hemodialysis is of limited benefit, since a maximum of 5% of circulating clonidine is removed.

In a patient who ingested 100 mg clonidine hydrochloride, plasma clonidine levels were 60 ng/ml (one hour), 190 ng/ml (1.5 hours), 370 ng/ml (two hours) and 120 ng/ml (5.5 and 6.5 hours). This patient developed hypertension followed by hypotension, bradycardia, apnea, hallucinations, semicoma, and premature ventricular contractions. The patient fully recovered after intensive treatment.

EPIDURAL INJECTION

Hypertension may develop early and may be followed by hypotension, bradycardia, respiratory depression, hypothermia, drowsiness, decreased or absent reflexes, irritability, and miosis. With large oral overdoses, reversible cardiac conduction defects or arrhythmias, apnea, coma, and seizures have been reported. As little as 100 mcg of oral clonidine has produced signs of toxicity in pediatric patients.

There is no specific antidote for clonidine overdosage. Supportive care may include atropine sulfate for bradycardia, intravenous fluids and/or vasopressor agents for hypotension. Hypertension associated with overdosage has been treated with intravenous furosemide, diazoxide or alpha-blocking agents such as phentolamine. Naloxone may be useful adjunct in the treatment of clonidine-induced respiratory depression, hypotension, and/or coma; blood pressure should be monitored since administration of naloxone has occasionally resulted in paradoxical hypertension. Tolazoline administration has yielded inconsistent results and is not recommended as first-line therapy. Dialysis is not likely to significantly enhance the elimination of clonidine.

The largest overdose reported to date involved a 28–year old white male who ingested 100 mg of clonidine HCl powder. This patient developed hypertension followed by hypotension, bradycardia, apnea, hallucinations, semicoma, and premature ventricular contractions. The patient fully recovered after intensive treatment. Plasma clonidine levels were 60 ng/ml after 1 hour, 190 ng/ml after 1.5 hours, 370 ng/ml after 2 hours, and 120 ng/ml after 5.5 and 6.5 hours. In mice and rats, the oral LD_{50} of clonidine is 206 and 465 mg/kg, respectively.

DOSAGE AND ADMINISTRATION:

TABLET

Adults: The dose of clonidine hydrochloride must be adjusted according to the patient's individual blood pressure response. The following is a general guide to its administration.

Initial Dose: 0.1 mg tablet twice daily (morning and bedtime). Elderly patients may benefit from a lower initial dose.

Maintenance Dose: Further increments of 0.1 mg per day may be made if necessary until the desired response is achieved. Taking the larger portion of the oral daily dose at bedtime may minimize transient adjustment effects of dry mouth and drowsiness. The therapeutic doses most commonly employed have ranged from 0.2 mg to 0.6 mg per day given in divided doses. Studies have indicated that 2.4 mg is the maximum effective daily dose, but doses as high as this have rarely been employed.

Renal Impairment: Dosage must be adjusted according to the degree of impairment, and patients should be carefully monitored. Since only a minimal amount of clonidine is removed during routine hemodialysis, there is no need to give supplemental clonidine following dialysis.

DOSAGE AND ADMINISTRATION: *(cont'd)*

Toxicology: In several studies, oral clonidine hydrochloride produced a dose-dependent increase in the incidence and severity of spontaneously occurring retinal degeneration in albino rats treated for six months or longer. Tissue distribution studies in dogs and monkeys revealed that clonidine hydrochloride was concentrated in the choroid of the eye. In view of the retinal degeneration observed in rats, eye examinations were performed in 908 patients prior to the start of clonidine hydrochloride therapy, who were then examined periodically thereafter. In 353 of these 908 patients, examinations were performed for periods of 24 months or longer. Except for some dryness of the eyes, no drug-related abnormal ophthalmologic findings were recorded and clonidine hydrochloride did not alter retinal function as shown by specialized tests such as the electroretinogram and macular dazzle. In rats, clonidine hydrochloride in combination with amitriptyline produced corneal lesions within 5 days.

EPIDURAL INJECTION

The recommended starting dose of epidural clonidine HCl for continuous epidural infusion is 30 mcg/hr. Although dosage may be titrated up or down depending on pain relief and occurrence of adverse events, experience with dosage rates above 40 mcg/hr is limited.

Familiarization with the continuous epidural infusion device is essential. Patients receiving epidural clonidine from a continuous infusion device should be closely monitored for the first few days to assess their response.

Dosage for Impaired Renal Function: Dosage should be adjusted according to the degree of renal impairment, and patients should be carefully monitored. Since only a minimal amount of clonidine is removed during routine hemodialysis, there is no need to give supplemental clonidine following dialysis.

Epidural clonidine HCl must *not* be used with a preservative.

PATIENT INFORMATION:

Clonidine is used for the treatment of high blood pressure. This medication should be taken even if you feel fine because high blood pressure may not produce physical symptoms. Do not discontinue this medication suddenly without consulting your physician. Inform your physician if you are pregnant or nursing. This medication may cause dizziness or drowsiness, especially during the first days of therapy; use caution while driving or operating hazardous machinery. Avoid sudden changes in posture. Clonidine may be taken with food or milk to prevent stomach upset. Apply the clonidine trandermal patch to a hairless area of skin on your upper arm or torso. Do not cut or trim the patch. When changing patches, use a different place on your skin. Leave the patch in place even when showering, bathing, or swimming. If the patch becomes loose apply the adhesive overlay directly over the patch.

HOW SUPPLIED:

TABLET

Store below 86°F (30°).

Dispense in tight, light-resistant container.

EPIDURAL INJECTION

Store at controlled room temperature 15°-30°C (59°-86°F). **Preservative Free**. Discard unused portion.

HOW SUPPLIED - RATED THERAPEUTICALLY EQUIVALENT:

Tablet, Uncoated - Oral - 0.1 mg

60's	$2.10	Clonidine Hcl, Goldline Labs	00182-1133-26
100's	$2.40	Clonidine HCl, H.C.F.A. F F P	99999-0846-01
100's	$3.25	Clonidine Hcl, Consolidated Midland	00223-0660-01
100's	$3.41	Clonidine Hydrochloride, US Trading	56126-0110-11
100's	$5.00	Clonidine Hcl, Voluntary Hosp	53258-0191-01
100's	$5.76	Clonidine Hcl, Martec Pharms	52555-0328-01
100's	$6.10	Clonidine Hcl, United Res	00677-1077-01
100's	$6.45	Clonidine, Major Pharms	00904-1025-60
100's	$7.00	Clonidine Hcl, Voluntary Hosp	53258-0191-13
100's	$10.38	Clonidine Hcl, Qualitest Pharms	00603-2954-21
100's	$10.40	Clonidine Hcl, HL Moore Drug Exch	00839-7182-06
100's	$10.43	Clonidine Hcl, Goldline Labs	00182-1250-01
100's	$10.43	Clonidine Hcl, Purepac Pharm	00228-2127-10
100's	$10.45	Clonidine HCl, Schein Pharm (US)	00364-0820-01
100's	$10.45	Clonidine HCl, Rugby	00536-5621-01
100's	$11.19	Clonidine, Major Pharms	00904-1025-61
100's	$11.52	Clonidine Hcl, Aligen Independ	00405-4241-01
100's	$13.09	Clonidine Hcl, Geneva Pharms	00781-1471-01
100's	$15.19	Clonidine Hcl, TIE Pharm	55496-1401-09
100's	$15.89	Clonidine HCl, Bristol Myers Squibb	00003-0289-50
100's	$16.59	Clonidine Hcl, Lederle Pharm	00005-3180-23
100's	$18.00	Clonidine Hcl, Parmed Pharms	00349-8921-01
100's	$18.10	Clonidine Hcl, Mylan	00378-0152-01
100's	$19.05	Clonidine Hcl, Vangard Labs	00615-2572-13
100's	$19.35	Clonidine Hcl, Medirex	57480-0309-01
100's	$24.00	Clonidine Hcl, Geneva Pharms	00781-1471-13
100's	$26.00	Clonidine Hcl, Goldline Labs	00182-1250-89
100's	**$56.16**	**CATAPRES, Boehringer Pharms**	**00597-0006-01**
100's	**$60.46**	**CATAPRES, Boehringer Pharms**	**00597-0006-61**
500's	$12.00	Clonidine HCl, H.C.F.A. F F P	99999-0846-02
500's	$46.88	Clonidine Hcl, Qualitest Pharms	00603-2954-28
500's	$48.50	Clonidine Hcl, Goldline Labs	00182-1250-05
500's	$49.54	Clonidine Hcl, Aligen Independ	00405-4241-02
500's	$52.15	Clonidine Hcl, Purepac Pharm	00228-2127-50
500's	$69.55	Clonidine Hcl, Parmed Pharms	00349-8921-05
500's	$80.97	Clonidine HCl, Rugby	00536-5621-05
600's	$139.20	Clonidine Hcl, Medirex	57480-0309-06
750's	$168.29	Clonidine Hcl, Glasgow Pharm	60809-0114-55
750's	$168.29	Clonidine Hcl, Glasgow Pharm	60809-0114-72
1000's	$16.98	Clonidine Hcl, Balan	00304-1685-00
1000's	$24.00	Clonidine HCl, H.C.F.A. F F P	99999-0846-03
1000's	$24.50	Clonidine Hcl, Consolidated Midland	00223-0660-02
1000's	$41.95	Clonidine Hcl, Aligen Independ	00405-4241-03
1000's	$48.45	Clonidine Hcl, Martec Pharms	52555-0328-10
1000's	$49.05	Clonidine Hcl, Rugby	00536-3523-10
1000's	$51.00	Clonidine Hcl, United Res	00677-1077-10
1000's	$51.50	Clonidine, Major Pharms	00904-1025-80
1000's	$73.97	Clonidine Hcl, HL Moore Drug Exch	00839-7182-16
1000's	$92.46	Clonidine HCl, Geneva Pharms	00781-1471-10
1000's	$94.25	Clonidine HCl, Schein Pharm (US)	00364-0820-02
1000's	$144.28	Clonidine Hcl, Amer Preferred	53445-1767-00
1000's	$156.75	Clonidine Hcl, Lederle Pharm	00005-3180-34
1000's	$161.95	Clonidine Hcl, Mylan	00378-0152-10
1000's	**$543.52**	**CATAPRES, Boehringer Pharms**	**00597-0006-10**

Tablet, Uncoated - Oral - 0.2 mg

100's	$2.70	Clonidine HCl, H.C.F.A. F F P	99999-0846-04
100's	$3.57	Clonidine Hydrochloride, US Trading	56126-0111-11
100's	$4.25	Clonidine Hcl, Consolidated Midland	00223-0661-01

HOW SUPPLIED - RATED THERAPEUTICALLY EQUIVALENT: *(cont'd)*

100's	$7.00	Clonidine Hcl, Voluntary Hosp	53258-0221-01
100's	$7.65	Clonidine Hcl, Martec Pharms	52555-0329-01
100's	$9.30	Clonidine Hcl, Voluntary Hosp	53258-0221-13
100's	$9.80	Clonidine Hcl, United Res	00677-1078-01
100's	$9.95	Clonidine, Major Pharms	00904-1026-60
100's	$10.92	Clonidine Hcl, HL Moore Drug Exch	00839-7183-06
100's	$11.48	Clonidine Hcl, Qualitest Pharms	00603-2955-21
100's	$12.85	Clonidine, Major Pharms	00904-1026-61
100's	$13.50	Clonidine HCl, Schein Pharm (US)	00364-0821-01
100's	$14.25	Clonidine HCl, Rugby	00536-5622-01
100's	$14.33	Clonidine Hcl, Goldline Labs	00182-1251-01
100's	$14.33	Clonidine Hcl, Purepac Pharm	00228-2128-10
100's	$15.86	Clonidine Hcl, Aligen Independ	00405-4242-01
100's	$17.96	Clonidine HCl, Geneva Pharms	00781-1472-01
100's	$19.01	Clonidine Hcl, TIE Pharm	55496-1402-09
100's	$20.00	Clonidine Hcl, Parmed Pharms	00349-8922-01
100's	$23.01	Clonidine Hcl, Vangard Labs	00615-2573-13
100's	$23.30	Clonindine Hcl, Medirex	57480-0310-01
100's	$24.28	Clonidine HCl, Bristol Myers Squibb	00003-0520-50
100's	$26.06	Clonidine Hcl, Lederle Pharm	00005-3181-23
100's	$26.95	Clonidine Hcl, Mylan	00378-0186-01
100's	$34.20	Clonidine Hcl, Goldline Labs	00182-1251-89
100's	$35.00	Clonidine Hcl, Geneva Pharms	00781-1472-13
100's	**$85.76**	**CATAPRES, Boehringer Pharms**	**00597-0007-01**
100's	**$90.29**	**CATAPRES, Boehringer Pharms**	**00597-0007-61**
500's	$13.50	Clonidine HCl, H.C.F.A. F F P	99999-0846-05
500's	$51.66	Clonidine Hcl, Qualitest Pharms	00603-2955-28
500's	$66.80	Clonidine Hcl, Goldline Labs	00182-1251-05
500's	$70.40	Clonidine Hcl, Aligen Independ	00405-4242-02
500's	$71.65	Clonidine Hcl, Purepac Pharm	00228-2128-50
500's	$80.25	Clonidine Hcl, Parmed Pharms	00349-8922-05
500's	$128.97	Clonidine HCl, Rugby	00536-5622-05
600's	$198.40	Clonidine Hcl, Medirex	57480-0310-06
1000's	$27.00	Clonidine HCl, H.C.F.A. F F P	99999-0846-06
1000's	$29.50	Clonidine Hcl, Consolidated Midland	00223-0661-02
1000's	$50.95	Clonidine Hcl, Aligen Independ	00405-4242-03
1000's	$60.47	Clonidine Hcl, Rugby	00536-3524-10
1000's	$62.48	Clonidine Hcl, United Res	00677-1078-10
1000's	$62.90	Clonidine, Major Pharms	00904-1026-80
1000's	$66.40	Clonidine Hcl, Martec Pharms	52555-0329-10
1000's	$86.79	Clonidine Hcl, HL Moore Drug Exch	00839-7183-16
1000's	$109.09	Clonidine HCl, Geneva Pharms	00781-1472-10
1000's	$126.00	Clonidine HCl, Schein Pharm (US)	00364-0821-02
1000's	$239.87	Clonidine Hcl, Amer Preferred	53445-1768-00
1000's	$250.06	Clonidine Hcl, Lederle Pharm	00005-3181-34
1000's	$257.95	Clonidine Hcl, Mylan	00378-0186-10
1000's	**$831.16**	**CATAPRES, Boehringer Pharms**	**00597-0007-10**

Tablet, Uncoated - Oral - 0.3 mg

100's	$3.38	Clonidine HCl, H.C.F.A. F F P	99999-0846-07
100's	$3.98	Clonidine Hcl, Balan	00304-1687-01
100's	$4.75	Clonidine Hcl, Consolidated Midland	00223-0662-01
100's	$6.00	Clonidine Hydrochloride, US Trading	56126-0112-11
100's	$10.00	Clonidine Hcl, Voluntary Hosp	53258-0193-01
100's	$11.68	Clonidine Hcl, Qualitest Pharms	00603-2956-21
100's	$11.73	Clonidine Hcl, HL Moore Drug Exch	00839-7184-06
100's	$12.40	Clonidine, Major Pharms	00904-1027-60
100's	$17.00	Clonidine Hcl, Voluntary Hosp	53258-0193-13
100's	$18.04	Clonidine Hcl, Goldline Labs	00182-1252-01
100's	$18.04	Clonidine Hcl, Purepac Pharm	00228-2129-10
100's	$18.49	Clonidine Hcl, Major Pharms	00904-1027-61
100's	$20.01	Clonidine Hcl, Aligen Independ	00405-4243-01
100's	$22.50	Clonidine Hcl, Goldline Labs	00182-1769-89
100's	$22.84	Clonidine HCl, Geneva Pharms	00781-1473-01
100's	$24.55	Clonidine Hcl, Vangard Labs	00615-2574-13
100's	$26.49	Clonidine HCl, Schein Pharm (US)	00364-0824-01
100's	$28.50	Clonidine Hcl, Medirex	57480-0311-01
100's	$30.50	Clonidine HCl, Bristol Myers Squibb	00003-0534-50
100's	$32.56	Clonidine Hcl, Lederle Pharm	00005-3182-23
100's	$33.96	Clonidine Hcl, Amer Preferred	53445-1769-01
100's	$38.30	Clonidine Hcl, Goldline Labs	00182-1252-89
100's	$39.64	Clonidine Hcl, Parmed Pharms	00349-8923-01
100's	$39.75	Clonidine Hcl, Mylan	00378-0199-01
100's	$39.75	Clonidine HCl, Rugby	00536-5623-01
100's	**$107.76**	**CATAPRES, Boehringer Pharms**	**00597-0011-01**
500's	$16.90	Clonidine HCl, H.C.F.A. F F P	99999-0846-08
500's	$29.20	Clonidine Hcl, Major Pharms	00904-1027-40
600's	$202.00	Clonidine Hcl, Medirex	57480-0311-06
1000's	$32.50	Clonidine Hcl, Consolidated Midland	00223-0662-02
1000's	$33.96	Clonidine Hcl, Amer Preferred	53445-1769-00

HOW SUPPLIED - NOT RATED EQUIVALENT:

Injection - Epidural - 100 mcg

10 ml	$51.00	DURACLON, Fujisawa USA	00469-4001-10

CLORAZEPATE DIPOTASSIUM *(000847)*

CATEGORIES: Alcohol Withdrawal; Alcoholism; Antianxiety Drugs; Antipsychotics/Antimanics; Anxiety; Anxiolytics, Sedatives, Hypnotic; Benzodiazepines; Central Nervous System Agents; Convulsions; Seizures; Tranquilizers; DEA Class CIV; FDA Approval Pre 1982

BRAND NAMES: *Ansiopaz*; *Anxidin*; *Audilex*; *Covengar*; *Clozene*; *Dipot*; *Enadine*; *Flulium*; Gen-Xene; *Justum*; *Mendon*; *Moderane*; *Nansius*; *Nevracten*; *Novoclopate* (Canada); *Sanor*; *Serene*; *Tencilan*; *Trancon*; *Transene*; *Tranxal*; *Tranxen*; **Tranxene**; *Tranxilen*; *Tranxilium* (Germany); *Travex*; *Zetran-5*
(International brand names outside U.S. in italics)

FORMULARIES: Aetna

COST OF THERAPY: $5.76 (Anxiety; Tablet; 15 mg; 1/day; 120 days)

DESCRIPTION:

Clorazepate dipotassium is a benzodiazepine. The molecular formula is $C_{16}H_{11}ClK_2N_2O_4$; the molecular weight is 408.92.

It is a fine, light yellow, practically odorless compound insoluble in the common organic solvents, but very soluble in water. Aqueous solutions are unstable, clear, light yellow, and alkaline.

DESCRIPTION: *(cont'd)*

It is available for oral administration as 3.75 mg, 7.5 mg, 11.25 mg, 15 mg and 22.5 mg tablets.

The inactive ingredients include lactose anhydrous, magnesium stearate, microcrystalline cellulose, polacrilin potassium, silicon dioxide colloidal and talc. In addition, the following coloring agents are used: 3.75 mg tablets - FD&C Blue No. 2, 7.5 mg tablets - FD&C Yellow No. 6, 15 mg tablets - FD&C Red No. 3.

CLINICAL PHARMACOLOGY:

Pharmacologically, clorazepate dipotassium has the characteristics of benzodiazepines. It has depressant effects on the central nervous system. The primary metabolite, nordiazepam, quickly appears in the blood stream. The serum half-life is about 2 days. The drug is metabolized in the liver and excreted primarily in the urine.

(See also ANIMAL PHARMACOLOGY.)

Studies in healthy men have shown that clorazepate has depressant effects on the central nervous system. Prolonged administration of single daily doses as high as 120 mg was without toxic effects. Abrupt cessation of high doses was followed in some patients by nervousness, insomnia, irritability, diarrhea, muscle aches, or memory impairment.

Absorption—Excretion: After oral administration of clorazepate dipotassium, there is essentially no circulating parent drug. Nordiazepam, its primary metabolite, quickly appears in the blood stream. In 2 volunteers given 15 mg of (50 microcuries) of ^{14}C-clorazepate dipotassium, about 80% was recovered in the urine and feces within 10 days. Excretion was primarily in the urine with about 1% excreted per day on day 10.

INDICATIONS AND USAGE:

Clorazepate dipotassium is indicated for the management of anxiety disorders or for the short-term relief of the symptoms of anxiety. Anxiety or tension associated with the stress of everyday life usually does not require treatment with an anxiolytic.

Clorazepate dipotassium is indicated as adjunctive therapy in the management of partial seizures.

The effectiveness of clorazepate in the long-term management of anxiety, that is, for more than 4 months, has not been assessed by systematic clinical studies. Long-term studies in epileptic patients, however, have shown continued therapeutic activity. The physician should reassess periodically the usefulness of the drug for the individual patient.

Clorazepate dipotassium is indicated for the symptomatic relief of acute alcohol withdrawal.

CONTRAINDICATIONS:

Clorazepate dipotassium is contraindicated in patients with a known hypersensitivity to the drug, and in those with acute narrow angle glaucoma.

WARNINGS:

Clorazepate is not recommended for use in depressive neuroses or in psychotic reactions.

Patients on clorazepate dipotassium should be cautioned against engaging in hazardous occupations requiring mental alertness, such as operating dangerous machinery, including motor vehicles.

Since clorazepate has a central nervous system depressant effect, patients should be advised against the simultaneous use of other CNS-depressant drugs, and cautioned that the effects of alcohol may be increased.

Because of the lack of sufficient clinical experience, clorazepate dipotassium is not recommended for use in patients less than 9 years of age.

USAGE IN PREGNANCY

An increased risk of congenital malformations associated with the use of minor tranquilizers (chlordiazepoxide, diazepam, and meprobamate) during the first trimester of pregnancy has been suggested in several studies. Clorazepate, a benzodiazepine derivative, has not been studied adequately to determine whether it, too, may be associated with an increased risk of fetal abnormality. Because use of these drugs is rarely a matter of urgency, their use during this period should almost always be avoided. The possibility that a woman of childbearing potential may be pregnant at the time of institution of therapy should be considered. Patients should be advised that if they become pregnant during therapy or intend to become pregnant they should communicate with their physician about the desirability of discontinuing the drug.

USAGE DURING LACTATION

Clorazepate dipotassium should not be given to nursing mothers since it has been reported that nordiazepam is excreted in human breast milk.

PRECAUTIONS:

In those patients in which a degree of depression accompanies the anxiety, suicidal tendencies may be present and protective measures may be required. The least amount of drug that is feasible should be available to the patients.

Patients on clorazepate for prolonged periods should have blood counts and liver function tests periodically. The usual precautions in treating patients with impaired renal or hepatic function should also be observed.

In elderly or debilitated patients, initial dose should be small, and increments should be made gradually, in accordance with the response of the patient, to preclude ataxia or excessive sedation.

DRUG INTERACTIONS:

If clorazepate dipotassium is to be combined with other drugs acting on the central nervous system, careful consideration should be given to the pharmacology of the agents to be employed. Animal experience indicates that clorazepate prolongs the sleeping time after hexobarbital or after ethyl alcohol, increases the inhibitory effects of chlorpromazine, but does not exhibit monoamine oxidase inhibition. Clinical studies have shown increased sedation with concurrent hypnotic medications. The actions of the benzodiazepines may be potentiated by barbiturates, narcotics, phenothiazines, monoamine oxidase inhibitors or other antidepressants.

If clorazepate dipotassium is used to treat anxiety associated with somatic disease states, careful attention must be paid to possible drug interaction with concomitant medication.

In bioavailability studies with normal subjects, the concurrent administration of antacids at therapeutic levels did not significantly influence the bioavailability of clorazepate.

ADVERSE REACTIONS:

The side effect most frequently reported was drowsiness. Less commonly reported (in descending order of occurrence) were: dizziness, various gastrointestinal complaints, nervousness, blurred vision, dry mouth, headache, and mental confusion. Other side effects included insomnia, transient skin rashes, fatigue, ataxia, genitourinary complaints, irritability, diplopia, depression and slurred speech.

There have been reports of abnormal liver and kidney function tests and decrease in hematocrit.

ADVERSE REACTIONS: *(cont'd)*

Decrease in systolic blood pressure has been observed.

DRUG ABUSE AND DEPENDENCE:

Clorazepate dipotassium tablets are a Schedule IV controlled substance.

Withdrawal symptoms (similar in character to those noted with barbiturates and alcohol) have occurred following abrupt discontinuance of clorazepate. Symptoms of nervousness, insomnia, irritability, diarrhea, muscle aches and memory impairment have followed abrupt withdrawal after long-term use of high dosage. Withdrawal symptoms have also been reported following abrupt discontinuance of benzodiazepines taken continuously at therapeutic levels for several months.

Caution should be observed in patients who are considered to have a psychological potential for drug dependence.

Evidence of drug dependence has been observed in dogs and rabbits which was characterized by convulsive seizures when the drug has abruptly withdrawn or the dose was reduced; the syndrome in dogs could be abolished by administration of clorazepate.

OVERDOSAGE:

MANAGEMENT OF OVERDOSAGE

Overdosage is usually manifested by varying degrees of CNS depression ranging from slight sedation to coma. As in the management of overdosage with any drug, it should be borne in mind that multiple agents may have been taken.

There are no specific antidotes for the benzodiazepines. The treatment of overdosage should consist of the general measures employed in the management of overdosage of any CNS depressant. Gastric evacuation either by the induction of emesis, lavage, or both, should be performed immediately. General supportive care, including frequent monitoring of the vital signs and close observation of the patients, is indicated. Hypotension, though rarely reported, may occur with large overdoses. In such cases the use of agents such as norepinephrine bitartrate injection or metaraminol bitartrate injection should be considered.

While reports indicate that individuals have survived overdoses of clorazepate dipotassium as high as 450 to 675 mg, these doses are not necessarily an accurate indication of the amount of drug absorbed since the time interval between ingestion and the institution of treatment was not always known. Sedation in varying degrees was the most common physiological manifestation of clorazepate overdosage. Deep coma, when it occurred, was usually associated with the ingestion of other drugs in addition to clorazepate.

DOSAGE AND ADMINISTRATION:

For The Symptomatic Relief Of Anxiety: Clorazepate dipotassium T-TABS tablets are administered orally in divided doses. The usual daily dose is 30 mg. The dose should be adjusted gradually within the range of 15 to 60 mg daily in accordance with the response of the patient. In elderly or debilitated patients, it is advisable to initiate treatment at a daily dose of 7.5 to 15 mg.

Clorazepate dipotassium tablets may also be administered in a single dose daily at bedtime; the recommended initial dose is 15 mg. After the initial dose, the response of the patient may require adjustment of subsequent dosage. Lower doses may be indicated in the elderly patient. Drowsiness may occur at the initiation of treatment and with dosage increment.

Clorazepate dipotassium-SD (22.5 mg tablet) may be administered as a single dose every 24 hours. The tablet is intended as an alternative form for the convenience of patients stabilized on a dose of 7.5 mg tablets three times a day. Clorazepate dipotassium-SD should not be used to initiate therapy.

Clorazepate dipotassium-SD half strength (11.25 mg tablet) may be administered as a single dose every 24 hours. This tablet is intended as an alternate dosage form for the convenience of patients stabilized on a dose of 3.75 mg tablets three times a day. Clorazepate dipotassium-SD half strength should not be used to initiate therapy.

For the symptomatic relief of acute alcohol withdrawal: The following dosage schedule is recommended (TABLE 1):

TABLE 1

1st 24 hours (Day 1)	30 mg clorazepate dipotassium initially; followed by 30 to 60 mg in divided doses
2nd 24 hours (Day 2)	45 to 90 mg in divided doses
3rd 24 hours (Day 3)	22.5 to 45 mg in divided doses
Day 4	15 to 30 mg in divided doses

Thereafter, gradually reduce the daily dose to 7.5 to 15 mg. Discontinue drug therapy as soon as patient's condition is stable.

The maximum recommended total daily dose is 90 mg. Avoid excessive reductions in the total amount of drug administered on successive days.

AS AN ADJUNCT TO ANTIEPILEPTIC DRUGS

In order to minimize drowsiness, the recommended initial dosages and dosage increments should not be exceeded.

Adults: The maximum recommended initial dose in patients over 12 years old is 7.5 mg three times a day. Dosage should be increased by no more than 7.5 mg every week and should not exceed 90 mg/day.

Children (9-12 years): The maximum recommended initial dose is 7.5 mg two times a day. Dosage should be increased by no more than 7.5 mg every week and should not exceed 60 mg/day.

Recommended Storage: Store below 77°F (25°C)

ANIMAL PHARMACOLOGY:

Studies in rats and monkeys have shown a substantial difference between doses producing tranquilizing, sedative and toxic effects. In rats, conditioned avoidance response was inhibited at an oral dose of 10 mg/kg; sedation was induced at 32 mg/kg; the LD_{50} was 1320 mg/kg. In monkeys, aggressive behavior was reduced at an oral dose of 0.25 mg/kg; sedation (ataxia) was induced at 7.5 mg/kg; the LD_{50} could not be determined because of the emetic effect of large doses, but the LD_{50} exceeds 1600 mg/kg.

Twenty-four dogs were given clorazepate dipotassium orally in a 22-month toxicity study; doses up to 75 mg/kg were given. Drug-related changes occurred in the liver; weight was increased and cholestasis with minimal hepatocellular damage was found, but lobular architecture remained well preserved.

Eighteen rhesus monkeys were given oral doses of clorazepate dipotassium from 3 to 36 mg/kg daily for 52 weeks. All treated animals remained similar to control animals. Although total leucocyte count remained within normal limits it tended to fall in the female animals on the highest doses.

Examination of all organs revealed no alterations attributable to clorazepate. There was no damage to liver function or structure.

ANIMAL PHARMACOLOGY: *(cont'd)*

REPRODUCTION STUDIES

Standard fertility, reproduction, and teratology studies were conducted in rats and rabbits. Oral doses in rats up to 150 mg/kg and in rabbits up to 15 mg/kg produced no abnormalities in the fetuses. Clorazepate dipotassium did not alter the fertility indices or reproductive capacity of adult animals. As expected, the sedative effect of high doses interfered with care of the young by their mothers (see Usage in Pregnancy).

HOW SUPPLIED - RATED THERAPEUTICALLY EQUIVALENT:

Tablet, Uncoated - Oral - 3.75 mg

30's	$1.12	Clorazepate, H.C.F.A. F F P	99999-0847-01
100's	$3.75	Clorazepate, United Res	00677-1175-01
100's	$3.75	Clorazepate, H.C.F.A. F F P	99999-0847-02
100's	$22.50	Clorazepate Dipotassium, Elkins Sinn	00641-4025-86
100's	$24.19	Clorazepate, Bristol Myers Squibb	00003-0133-50
100's	$24.56	Clorazepate, Rugby	00536-4940-01
100's	$24.60	TAZEPATE, Major Pharms	00904-3970-60
100's	$24.95	Clorazepate, Watson Labs	52544-0363-01
100's	$25.18	Clorazepate, HL Moore Drug Exch	00839-7335-06
100's	$25.70	Clorazepate, Qualitest Pharms	00603-3004-21
100's	$26.95	Clorazepate, Goldline Labs	00182-0009-01
100's	$26.97	Clorazepate, Geneva Pharms	00781-1865-01
100's	$27.50	Clorazepate, Warner Chilcott	00047-0451-24
100's	$28.28	Clorazepate Dipotassium, Harber Pharm	51432-0547-03
100's	$31.46	Clorazepate Dipotassium, Parmed Pharms	00349-8984-01
100's	$31.95	Clorazepate, Martec Pharms	52555-0986-01
100's	$58.85	Clorazepate Dipotassium, Alpharma	00472-0047-10
100's	$58.95	Clorazepate Dipotassium, Mylan	00378-0030-01
100's	$78.47	Clorazepate Dipotassium, Aligen Independ	00405-0050-01
100's	**$116.13**	**TRANXENE, Abbott**	**00074-4389-13**
100's	**$118.50**	**TRANXENE T-TAB, Abbott**	**00074-4389-11**
500's	$18.75	Clorazepate, H.C.F.A. F F P	99999-0847-03
500's	$69.45	TAZEPATE, Major Pharms	00904-3970-40
500's	$96.55	Clorazepate, Elkins Sinn	00641-4025-88
500's	$118.13	Clorazepate, Bristol Myers Squibb	00003-0133-60
500's	$118.73	Clorazepate, HL Moore Drug Exch	00839-7335-12
500's	$119.95	Clorazepate, Watson Labs	52544-0363-05
500's	$122.01	Clorazepate, Qualitest Pharms	00603-3004-28
500's	$125.75	Clorazepate, Goldline Labs	00182-0009-05
500's	$125.77	Clorazepate, Geneva Pharms	00781-1865-05
500's	$126.50	Clorazepate, Warner Chilcott	00047-0451-30
500's	$159.95	Clorazepate, Rugby	00536-4940-05
500's	$159.95	Clorazepate, Martec Pharms	52555-0986-05
500's	$288.38	Clorazepate Dipotassium, Alpharma	00472-0047-50
500's	$288.50	Clorazepate Dipotassium, Mylan	00378-0030-05
500's	$384.51	Clorazepate Dipotassium, Aligen Independ	00405-0050-02
500's	**$569.01**	**TRANXENE T-TAB, Abbott**	**00074-4389-53**

Tablet, Uncoated - Oral - 7.5 mg

30's	$1.23	Clorazepate, H.C.F.A. F F P	99999-0847-04
100's	$4.13	Clorazepate, United Res	00677-1176-01
100's	$4.13	Clorazepate, H.C.F.A. F F P	99999-0847-05
100's	$28.10	Clorazepate Dipotassium, Elkins Sinn	00641-4026-86
100's	$30.05	Clorazepate, Bristol Myers Squibb	00003-0157-50
100's	$31.45	Clorazepate Dipotassium, Major Pharms	00904-3971-60
100's	$31.95	Clorazepate, Qualitest Pharms	00603-3005-21
100's	$31.95	Clorazepate, Watson Labs	52544-0364-01
100's	$31.98	Clorazepate Civ, HL Moore Drug Exch	00839-7336-06
100's	$32.80	Clorazepate, Schein Pharm (US)	00364-2202-01
100's	$33.50	Clorazepate, Rugby	00536-4941-01
100's	$34.25	Clorazepate, Goldline Labs	00182-0010-01
100's	$34.27	Clorazepate, Geneva Pharms	00781-1866-01
100's	$34.95	Clorazepate, Warner Chilcott	00047-0452-24
100's	$35.18	Clorazepate Dipotassium, Harber Pharm	51432-0549-03
100's	$39.27	Clorazepate Dipotassium, Parmed Pharms	00349-8985-01
100's	$39.95	Clorazepate, Martec Pharms	52555-0987-01
100's	$73.20	Clorazepate Dipotassium, Alpharma	00472-0049-10
100's	$73.50	Clorazepate Dipotassium, Mylan	00378-0040-01
100's	$97.61	Clorazepate Dipotassium, Aligen Independ	00405-0051-01
100's	**$144.45**	**TRANXENE T-TAB, Abbott**	**00074-4390-13**
100's	**$146.82**	**TRANXENE T-TAB, Abbott**	**00074-4390-11**
500's	$20.65	Clorazepate, H.C.F.A. F F P	99999-0847-06
500's	$69.10	Clorazepate Dipotassium, Major Pharms	00904-3971-40
500's	$120.60	Clorazepate, Elkins Sinn	00641-4026-88
500's	$145.06	Clorazepate Civ, HL Moore Drug Exch	00839-7336-12
500's	$148.31	Clorazepate, Bristol Myers Squibb	00003-0157-60
500's	$151.11	Clorazepate, Qualitest Pharms	00603-3005-28
500's	$151.95	Clorazepate, Watson Labs	52544-0364-05
500's	$158.95	Clorazepate, Goldline Labs	00182-0010-05
500's	$158.97	Clorazepate, Geneva Pharms	00781-1866-05
500's	$159.95	Clorazepate, Warner Chilcott	00047-0452-30
500's	$159.95	Clorazepate, Schein Pharm (US)	00364-2202-05
500's	$189.95	Clorazepate, Rugby	00536-4941-05
500's	$189.95	Clorazepate, Martec Pharms	52555-0987-05
500's	$358.69	Clorazepate Dipotassium, Alpharma	00472-0049-50
500's	$359.95	Clorazepate Dipotassium, Mylan	00378-0040-05
500's	$478.26	Clorazepate Dipotassium, Aligen Independ	00405-0051-02
500's	**$707.80**	**TRANXENE T-TAB, Abbott**	**00074-4390-53**

Tablet, Uncoated - Oral - 15 mg

30's	$1.44	Clorazepate, H.C.F.A. F F P	99999-0847-07
100's	$4.80	Clorazepate, United Res	00677-1177-01
100's	$4.80	Clorazepate, H.C.F.A. F F P	99999-0847-08
100's	$44.11	Clorazepate, Qualitest Pharms	00603-3006-21
100's	$44.58	Clorazepate, Bristol Myers Squibb	00003-0163-50
100's	$45.06	CLORAZEPATE DIPOTASSIUM, Rugby	00536-5595-01
100's	$45.35	Clorazepate, HL Moore Drug Exch	00839-7337-06
100's	$45.75	Clorazepate Dipotassium, Major Pharms	00904-3973-60
100's	$46.95	Clorazepate, Watson Labs	52544-0365-01
100's	$49.85	Clorazepate, Warner Chilcott	00047-0453-24
100's	$49.85	Clorazepate, Goldline Labs	00182-0014-01
100's	$49.87	Clorazepate Dipotasium, Geneva Pharms	00781-1867-01
100's	$55.47	Clorazepate, Lederle Pharm	00005-3436-23
100's	$59.55	Clorazepate, Martec Pharms	52555-0988-01
100's	$64.39	Clorazepate Dipotassium, Parmed Pharms	00349-8986-01
100's	$69.90	Chlorazepate, Major Pharms	00904-3973-61
100's	$99.33	Clorazepate Dipotassium, Alpharma	00472-0051-10
100's	$101.95	Clorazepate Dipotassium, Mylan	00378-0070-01
100's	$132.44	Clorazepate Dipotassium, Aligen Independ	00405-0052-01
100's	**$196.00**	**TRANXENE T-TAB, Abbott**	**00074-4391-13**
100's	**$198.37**	**TRANXENE T-TAB, Abbott**	**00074-4391-11**
500's	$24.00	Clorazepate, H.C.F.A. F F P	99999-0847-09
500's	$222.95	Clorazepate, Watson Labs	52544-0365-05
500's	**$960.39**	**TRANXENE T-TAB, Abbott**	**00074-4391-53**

HOW SUPPLIED - NOT RATED EQUIVALENT:

Tablet, Uncoated, Sustained Action - Oral - 11.25 mg

100's	**$307.27**	**TRANXENE SD, HALF STRENGTH, Abbott**	**00074-2699-13**

Tablet, Uncoated, Sustained Action - Oral - 22.5 mg

100's	**$393.51**	**TRANXENE SD, Abbott**	**00074-2997-13**

CLOTRIMAZOLE *(000848)*

CATEGORIES: Anti-Infectives; Antibacterials; Antibiotics; Antifungals; Antimicrobials; Candidiasis; Dermatologicals; Fungal Agents; Infections; Oropharyngeal Candidiasis; Skin/Mucous Membrane Agents; Tinea Corporis; Tinea Cruris; Tinea Pedis; Tinea Versicolor; Topical; Vaginal Preparations; Pregnancy Category B; FDA Approval Pre 1982

BRAND NAMES: *Agisten*; *Apocanda* (Germany); *Baby Agisten*; *Calcrem*; *Canastene*; *Canazol*; *Candespor*; *Candid*; *Candimon* (Mexico); *Candinox*; *Candizole*; *Canesten* (Australia, Europe, Asia, Asia); *Canestene*; *Canifug* (Germany); *Canifunga*; *Cinabel* (Mexico); *Clocreme*; *Clomaderm*; *Clomaz*; *Clomine*; *Clomizol*; *Clonea*; *Clostrin* (Japan); *Clotrizol*; *Cloxy*; *Clozole*; *Comyer*; *Cotren*; *Covospor*; *Dermatin*; *Durafungol* (Germany); *Dynaspor*; *Elcid* (Japan); *Empecid* (Japan); *Factodin*; *Fungicide*; *Fungiderm*; *Fungistin*; *Fungizid*; *Gino-Lotrimin*; *Gyne-Lotremin*; *Gyne Lotremin*; Gyne-Lotrimin; *Gyne Lotrimin*; *Gyno Canesten*; *Gyno-Canestene*; *Holfungin* (Germany); *Jenamazol* (Germany); *Kanezin*; *Lotramina*; *Lotremin*; **Lotrimin**; *Micoter*; Mycelex; Mycelex-G; *Myclo* (Canada); *Myco-Hermal*; *Mycoban*; *Mycocid*; *Mycoril*; *Nalbix*; *Once*; *Pan-Fungex*; *Sinium*; *Panmicol*; *Taon* (Japan); *Timazol*; *Tinaderm Extra*; *Trimadan*; *Trimysten* (France); *Vanesten*; *Xeraspor V*
(International brand names outside U.S. in italics)

FORMULARIES: Aetna; BC-BS; CIGNA; FHP; Foundation; Humana; Kaiser; Medco; Medi-Cal; PCS; PruCare; United

COST OF THERAPY: $5.14 (Tinea Pedis; Cream; 1 %; 2/day; 7 days)

DESCRIPTION:

FOR DERMATOLOGIC USE ONLY NOT FOR OPHTHALMIC USE

THESE PREPARATIONS ARE ALSO AVAILABLE WITHOUT A PRESCRIPTION

CLOTRIMAZOLE PRODUCTS CONTAIN CLOTRIMAZOLE, USP, A SYNTHETIC ANTIFUNGAL AGENT HAVING THE CHEMICAL NAME [1-(*O*-CHLORO-æ,æDIPHENYLBENZYL)IMIDAZOLE]; THE EMPIRICAL FORMULA, $C_{22}H_{17}ClN_2$; a molecular weight of 344.84.

CLOTRIMAZOLE IS AN ODORLESS, WHITE CRYSTALLINE SUBSTANCE. IT IS PRACTICALLY INSOLUBLE IN WATER, SPARINGLY SOLUBLE IN ETHER, AND VERY SOLUBLE IN POLYETHYLENE GLYCOL 400, ETHANOL, AND CHLOROFORM.

EACH GRAM OF CLOTRIMAZOLE CREAM CONTAINS 10 MG CLOTRIMAZOLE, USP IN VANISHING CREAM BASE OF BENZYL ALCOHOL, CETEARYL ALCOHOL, CETYL ESTERS WAX, OCTYLDODECANOL, POLYSORBATE, SORBITAN MONOSTEARATE, AND WATER.

EACH GRAM OF CLOTRIMAZOLE LOTION CONTAINS 10 MG CLOTRIMAZOLE, USP DISPERSED IN AN EMULSION VEHICLE COMPOSED OF BENZYL ALCOHOL, CETEARYL ALCOHOL, CETYL ESTERS WAX, OCTYLDODECANOL, POLYSORBATE, SODIUM PHOSPHATE, SORBITAN MONOSTEARATE, AND WATER.

EACH ML OF CLOTRIMAZOLE TOPICAL SOLUTION CONTAINS 10 MG CLOTRIMAZOLE, USP IN A NONAQUEOUS VEHICLE OF PEG.

CLINICAL PHARMACOLOGY:

Clotrimazole is a broad-spectrum antifungal agent that is used for the treatment of dermal infections caused by various species of pathogenic dermatophytes, yeasts, and *Malassezia furfur*. The primary action of clotrimazole is against dividing and growing organisms.

In vitro, clotrimazole exhibits fungistatic and fungicidal activity against isolates of *Trichophyton rubrum, Trichophyton mentagrophytes, Epidermophyton floccosum, Microsporum canis,* and *Candida* species, including *Candida albicans*. In general, the *in vitro* activity of clotrimazole corresponds to that of tolnaftate and griseofulvin against the mycelia of dermatophytes (*Trichophyton, Microsporum,* and *Epidermophyton*), and to that of the polyenes (amphotericin B and nystatin) against budding fungi (*Candida*). Using an *in vitro* (mouse) and an *in vitro* (mouse kidney homogenate) testing system, clotrimazole and miconazole were equally effective in preventing the growth of the pseudomycelia and mycelia of *Candida albicans*.

Strains of fungi having a natural resistance to clotrimazole are rare. Only a single isolate of *Candida guilliermondi* has been reported to have primary resistance to clotrimazole.

No single-step or multiple-step resistance to clotrimazole has developed during successive passages of *Candida albicans* and *Trichophyton mentagrophytes*. No appreciable change in sensitivity was detected after successive passages of isolates of *C. albicans, C. krusei,* or *C. pseudotropicalis* in liquid or solid media containing clotrimazole. Also, resistance could not be developed in chemically induced mutant strains of polyene-resistant isolates of *C. albicans*. Slight, reversible resistance was noted in three isolates of *C. albicans* tested by one investigator. There is a single report that records the clinical emergence of a *C. albicans* strain with considerable resistance of flucytosine and miconazole, and with cross-resistance to clotrimazole; the strain remained sensitive to nystatin and amphotericin B.

In studies of the mechanism of action, the minimum fungicidal concentration of clotrimazole caused leakage of intracellular phosphorus compounds into the ambient medium with concomitant breakdown of cellular nucleic acids and accelerated potassium efflux. Both these events began rapidly and extensively after addition of the drug.

Clotrimazole appears to be well absorbed in humans following oral administration and is eliminated mainly as inactive metabolites. Following topical and vaginal administration, however, clotrimazole appears to be minimally absorbed.

Six hours after the application of radioactive clotrimazole 1% cream and 1% solution onto intact and acutely inflamed skin, the concentration of clotrimazole varied from 100 mcg/cm^3 in the stratum corneum to 0.5 to 1 mcg/cm^3 in the stratum reticulare and 0.1 mcg/cm^3 in the subcutis. No measurable amount of radioactivity (≤0.001 mcg/ml) was found in the serum within 48 hours after application under occlusive dressing of 0.5 ml of the solution or 0.8 g of the cream. Only 0.5% or less of the applied radioactivity was excreted in the urine.

Following intravaginal administration of 100 mg ^{14}C-clotrimazole vaginal tablets to nine adult females, an average peak serum level, corresponding to only 0.03 mcg equivalents/ml of clotrimazole, was reached 1 to 2 days after application. After intravaginal administration of 5 g of 1% ^{14}C-clotrimazole vaginal cream containing 50 mg active drug to five subjects (one with candidal colpitis), serum levels corresponding to approximately 0.01 mcg equivalents/ml were reached between 8 and 24 hours after application.

INDICATIONS AND USAGE:

Prescription clotrimazole cream, lotion and solution 1% products are indicated for the topical treatment of candidiasis due to *Candida albicans* and tinea versicolor due to *Malassezia furfur.*

These formulations are also available as the clotrimazole (cream, lotion, and solution 1%) line of nonprescription products which are indicated for the topical treatment of the following dermal infections: tinea pedis, tinea cruris, and tinea corporis due to *Trichophyton rubrum, Trichophyton mentagrophytes, Epidermophyton floccosum,* and *Microsporum canis.*

CONTRAINDICATIONS:

Clotrimazole products are contraindicated in individuals who have shown hypersensitivity to any of their components.

WARNINGS:

Clotrimazole products are not for ophthalmic use.

PRECAUTIONS:

General: If irritation of sensitivity develops with the use of clotrimazole, treatment should be discontinued and appropriate therapy instituted.

Information for the Patient: This information is intended to aid in the safe and effective use of this medication. It is not a disclosure of all possible adverse or intended effects.

The patient should be advised to:

1. Use the medication for the full treatment time even though the symptoms may have improved. Notify the physician if there is no improvement after 4 weeks of treatment.

2. Inform the physician if the area of application shows signs of increased irritation (redness, itching, burning, blistering, oozing) indicative of possible sensitization.

3. Avoid sources of infection or reinfection.

Laboratory Tests: If there is lack of response to clotrimazole, appropriate microbiological studies should be repeated to confirm the diagnosis and rule out other pathogens before instituting another course of antimycotic therapy.

Carcinogenesis, Mutagenesis, and Impairment of Fertility: An 18-month oral dosing study with clotrimazole in rats has not revealed any carcinogenic effect.

In tests for mutagenesis, chromosomes of the spermatophores of Chinese hamsters which had been exposed to clotrimazole were examined for structural changes during the metaphase. Prior to testing, the hamsters had received five oral clotrimazole doses of 100 mg/kg body weight. The results of this study showed that clotrimazole had no mutagenic effect.

Usage in Pregnancy: Pregnancy Category B: The disposition of ^{14}C-clotrimazole has been studied in humans and animals. Clotrimazole is very poorly absorbed following dermal application or intravaginal administration to humans. (See CLINICAL PHARMACOLOGY.)

In clinical trials, use of vaginally applied clotrimazole in pregnant women in their second and third trimesters has not been associated with ill effects. There are, however, no adequate and well-controlled studies in pregnant women during the first trimester of pregnancy.

Studies in pregnant rats with **intravaginal** doses up to 100 mg/kg have revealed no evidence of harm to the fetus due to clotrimazole.

High **oral** doses of clotrimazole in rats and mice ranging from 50 to 120 mg/kg resulted in embryotoxicity (possible secondary to maternal toxicity) impairment of mating, decreased litter size and number of viable young and decreased pup survival to weaning. However, clotrimazole was **not** teratogenic in mice, rabbits and rats at oral doses up to 200, 180 and 100 mg/kg, respectively. Oral absorption in the rat amounts to approximately 90% of the administered dose.

Because animal reproduction studies are not always predictive of human response, this drug should be used only if clearly indicated during the first trimester of pregnancy.

Nursing Mothers: It is not known whether this drug is excreted in human milk. Because many drugs are excreted in human milk, caution should be exercised when clotrimazole is used by a nursing women.

Pediatric Use: Safety and effectiveness in children have been established for clotrimazole when used as indicated and in the recommended dosage.

DRUG INTERACTIONS:

Synergism or antagonism between clotrimazole and nystatin, or amphotericin B, or flucytosine against strains of *C. albicans* has not been reported.

ADVERSE REACTIONS:

The following adverse reactions have been reported in connection with the use of clotrimazole: erythema, stinging, blistering, peeling, edema, pruritus, urticaria, burning, and general irritation of the skin.

OVERDOSAGE:

Acute overdosage with topical application of clotrimazole is unlikely and would not be expected to lead to a life-threatening situation.

DOSAGE AND ADMINISTRATION:

Gently massage sufficient clotrimazole into the affected and surrounding skin areas twice a day, in the morning and evening.

Clinical improvement, with relief of pruritus, usually occurs within the first week of treatment with clotrimazole. If the patient shows no clinical improvement after 4 weeks of treatment with clotrimazole, the diagnosis should be reviewed.

Cream and Topical Solution: Store between 2° and 30°C (36° and 86°F).

Lotion: Store between 2° and 25°C (36° and 77°F).

Shake well before using.

HOW SUPPLIED - RATED THERAPEUTICALLY EQUIVALENT:

Cream - Topical - 1 %

15 gm	$7.85	Clotrimazole, Qualitest Pharms	00603-7730-74
15 gm	$8.85	Clotrimazole, Major Pharms	00904-7794-36
15 gm	$9.35	Clotrimazole, Goldline Labs	00182-5094-51
15 gm	**$11.74**	**LOTRIMIN, Schering**	**00085-0613-02**
30 gm	$13.40	Clotrimazole, Qualitest Pharms	00603-7730-78
30 gm	$15.05	Clotrimazole, Major Pharms	00904-7794-31
30 gm	$15.90	Clotrimazole, Goldline Labs	00182-5094-56
30 gm	**$19.92**	**LOTRIMIN, Schering**	**00085-0613-05**
45 gm	$16.75	Clotrimazole, Qualitest Pharms	00603-7730-83
45 gm	$18.25	Clotrimazole, Major Pharms	00904-7794-45
45 gm	$19.00	Clotrimazole, Goldline Labs	00182-5094-60
45 gm	**$24.16**	**LOTRIMIN, Schering**	**00085-0613-04**
90 gm	**$33.10**	**LOTRIMIN, Schering**	**00085-0613-03**

HOW SUPPLIED - RATED THERAPEUTICALLY EQUIVALENT: *(cont'd)*

Cream - Vaginal - 50 mg/tube

45 gm	$14.00	MYCELEX-G, Bayer	00026-3094-45
90 gm	$24.44	MYCELEX-G, Bayer	00026-3094-46

Solution - Topical - 1 %

10 ml	$8.21	MYCELEX, Bayer	00026-3092-10
10 ml	**$10.33**	**LOTRIMIN, Schering**	**00085-0182-02**
30 ml	$17.24	MYCELEX, Bayer	00026-3092-30
30 ml	**$21.50**	**LOTRIMIN, Schering**	**00085-0182-04**

HOW SUPPLIED - NOT RATED EQUIVALENT:

Cream - Topical - 1 %

15 gm	$7.85	Clotrimazole, Warrick Pharms	59930-1570-01
15 gm	$9.30	MYCELEX, Bayer	00026-3091-61
15 gm	$9.37	Clotrimazole, Rugby	00536-2990-20
15 gm	$9.44	Clotrimazole, HL Moore Drug Exch	00839-7836-47
30 gm	$13.40	Clotrimazole, Warrick Pharms	59930-1570-02
30 gm	$15.89	MYCELEX, Bayer	00026-3091-59
30 gm	$15.91	Clotrimazole, Rugby	00536-2990-28
30 gm	$16.05	Clotrimazole, HL Moore Drug Exch	00839-7836-49
45 gm	$16.25	Clotrimazole, Warrick Pharms	59930-1570-03
45 gm	$19.29	Clotrimazole, Rugby	00536-2990-26
45 gm	$19.43	Clotrimazole, HL Moore Drug Exch	00839-7836-52
45 gm x 2	$26.57	MYCELEX, Bayer	00026-3091-67
90 gm	$22.25	Clotrimazole, Warrick Pharms	59930-1570-09

Lotion - Topical - 1 %

30 ml	**$22.50**	**LOTRIMIN, Schering**	**00085-0707-02**

Tablet, Uncoated, Sustained Action - Vaginal - 11 mg

7's	$14.71	MYCELEX-G, Bayer	00026-3093-17
500 mg tablet x	$15.17	MYCELEX TWIN PACK, Bayer	00026-3098-22

Tablet, Uncoated, Sustained Action - Vaginal - 500 mg

1's	$13.35	MYCELEX-G, Bayer	00026-3097-01

Troche - Buccal - 10 mg

70's	$55.22	MYCELEX, Bayer	00026-3095-55
70's	$58.99	MYCELEX, Bayer	00026-3095-38
140's	$100.30	MYCELEX, Bayer	00026-3095-56

CLOXACILLIN SODIUM *(000850)*

CATEGORIES: Anti-Infectives; Antiarthritics; Antibiotics; Antimicrobials; Infections; Penicillins; FDA Approval Pre 1982

BRAND NAMES: *Alclox*; *Ampiclox*; *Amplium*; *Anaclosil*; *Apo-Cloxi* (Canada); *Austrastaph*; *Bactopen*; *Bioclox*; *Chuckin*; *Clocillin*; *Cloxacap*; *Cloxadar*; Cloxapen; *Cloxgen*; *Cloxillin*; *Cloxin*; *Cloxypen*; *Diclocil*; *Ekvacillin*; *Isoxacillin*; *Klox*; *Loxavit*; *Meikam*; *Methocillin*; *Methocillin S* (Japan); *Monoclox*; *Novocloxin* (Canada); *Orbenil*; *Orbenin* (Asia, England, Canada); *Orbenine* (France); *Orbrex*; *Penstapho N*; *Prostafilina*; *Prostafilina A*; *Prostafilina-A*; *Prostaphlin*; *Prostaphlin-A*; *Serviclox*; *Staflocil*; **Tegopen**; *Vaclox*

(International brand names outside U.S. in italics)

FORMULARIES: Aetna; Medi-Cal; WHO

DESCRIPTION:

Cloxacillin sodium is an antibacterial agent of the isoxazolyl penicillin series. It is a penicillinase-resistant, acid resistant semisynthetic penicillin suitable for oral administration. Cloxacillin sodium is available as an oral solution and capsules.

Inactive ingredient in Tegopen Capsules is: magnesium stearate.

Inactive ingredients in Tegopen Oral Solution are: FD&C Red No. 3, natural & artificial flavorings, sodium benzoate, sodium chloride, sodium citrate, sodium saccharin and sucrose.

$C_{19}H_{17}ClN_3NaO_5S.H_20$ 475.88(CAS 7081449)

4-Thia-1-azabicyclo(3.2.0)heptane-2-carboxylic acid,6[[[3(2-chlorophenyl)-5-methyl-4-isoxazolyl]carbonyl]amino]3,3-dimethyl-7-oxo-,monosodium salt, monohydrate,2*S*(2α5α,6β)-.

CLINICAL PHARMACOLOGY:

MICROBIOLOGY

Penicillinase-resistant penicillins exert a bactericidal action against penicillin-susceptible microorganisms during the state of active multiplication. All penicillins inhibit the biosynthesis of the bactericidal cell wall.

The drugs in this class are highly resistant to inactivation by staphylococcal penicillinase and are active against penicillinase producing and non-penicillinase producing strains of **Staphylococcus aureus.** The penicillinase-resistant penicillins are active *in vitro* against a variety of other bacteria.

SUSCEPTIBILITY TESTING

Quantitative methods of susceptibility testing that require measurement of zone diameters or minimal inhibitory concentration (MIC's) give the most precise estimates of antibiotic susceptibility. One such procedure has been recommended for use with discs to test susceptibility to this class of drugs.

Interpretations correlate diameters on the disc test with MIC values. A penicillinase-resistant class disc may be used to determine microbial susceptibility to cloxacillin, dicloxacillin, methicillin, nafcillin, and oxacillin. With this procedure, employing a 5 microgram methicillin sodium disc, a report from the laboratory of "susceptible" (zone of at least 14 mm) indicates that the infecting organism is likely to respond early to therapy. A report of "resistant" (zone of less than 10 mm) indicates that the infecting organism is not likely to respond to therapy. A report of "intermediate susceptibility" (zone of 10 to 13 mm) suggests that the organism might be susceptible if high doses of the antibiotic are used, or if the infection is confined to tissues and fluids (*e.g.,* urine), in which high antibiotic levels are attained.

In general, all staphylococci should be tested against the penicillin G disc and against the methicillin disc. Routine methods of antibiotic susceptibility testing may fail to detect strains of organisms resistant to the penicillinase-resistant penicillins. For this reason, the use of large inocula and 48-hour incubation periods may be necessary to obtain accurate susceptibility studies with these antibiotics. Bacterial strains which are resistant to one of the penicillinase-resistant penicillins should be considered resistant to all of the drugs in the class.

PHARMACOKINETICS

Cloxacillin sodium is resistant to destruction by acid. Absorption of cloxacillin sodium after oral administration is rapid but incomplete. Studies with an oral dose of 1 gram gave average serum levels at 60 minutes of 14.4 mcg/ml. At four hours, average levels were 2 mcg/ml. In one study, single oral doses of cloxacillin sodium 500 mg produced peak serum concentrations of 7.5 to 14.4 mcg/ml at 1 to 1.5 hours.

CLINICAL PHARMACOLOGY: *(cont'd)*

Once absorbed, cloxacillin sodium binds to serum protein, mainly albumin. The degree of protein binding reported varies with the method of study and the investigator, but generally has been found to be 95.2 ± 0.5%. Oral absorption of cloxacillin is delayed when the drug is administered after meals.

Cloxacillin sodium, with normal doses, has insignificant concentrations in the cerebrospinal and ascitic fluids. It is found in therapeutic concentrations in the pleural, bile, and amniotic fluids. Cloxacillin sodium is rapidly excreted as unchanged drug in the urine by glomerular filtration and active tubular secretion.

INDICATIONS AND USAGE:

The penicillinase-resistant penicillins are indicated in the treatment of infections caused by penicillinase-producing staphylococci which have demonstrated susceptibility to the drugs. Cultures and susceptibility tests should be performed initially to determine the causative organism and their sensitivity to the drug (see CLINICAL PHARMACOLOGY, Susceptibility Testing).

The penicillinase-resistant penicillins may be used to initiate therapy in suspected cases of resistant staphylococcal infections prior to the availability of laboratory test results. The penicillinase-resistant penicillins should not be used in infections caused by organisms susceptible to penicillin G. If the susceptibility tests indicate that the infection is due to an organism other than a resistant staphylococcus, therapy should not be continued with a penicillinase-resistant penicillin.

CONTRAINDICATIONS:

A history of hypersensitivity (anaphylactic) reaction to any penicillin is a contraindication.

WARNINGS:

Serious and occasionally fatal hypersensitivity (anaphylactic shock with collapse) reactions have occurred in patients receiving penicillin. The incidence of anaphylactic shock in all penicillin-treated patients is between 0.015 and 0.04 percent. Anaphylactic shock resulting in death has occurred in approximately 0.002 percent of the patients treated. Although anaphylaxis is more frequent following a parenteral administration, it has occurred in patients receiving oral penicillins.

When penicillin therapy is indicated, it should be initiated only after a comprehensive patient drug and allergy history has been obtained. If an allergic reaction occurs, the drug should be discontinued and the patient should receive supportive treatment, e.g., artificial maintenance of ventilation, pressor amines, antihistamines, and corticosteroids. Individuals with a history of penicillin hypersensitivity may also experience allergic reactions when treated with a cephalosporin.

PRECAUTIONS:

General: Penicillinase-resistant penicillins should generally not be administered to patients with a history of sensitivity to any penicillin.

Penicillin should be used with caution in individuals with histories of significant allergies and/or asthma. Whenever allergic reactions occur, penicillin should be withdrawn unless, in the opinion of the physician, the condition being treated is life-threatening and amenable only to penicillin therapy.

The oral route of administration should not be relied upon in patients with severe illness, or with nausea, vomiting, gastric dilation, cardiospasm, or intestinal hypermotility. Occasionally patients will not absorb therapeutic amounts of orally administered penicillin.

The use of antibiotics may result in overgrowth of nonsusceptible organisms. If new infections due to bacteria of fungi occur, the drug should be discontinued and appropriate measures taken.

Information for the Patient: Patients receiving penicillins should be given the following information and instructions by the physician:

1. Patients should be told that penicillin is an antibacterial agent which will work with the body's natural defenses to control certain types of infections. They should be told that the drug should not be taken if they have had an allergic reaction to any form of penicillin previously, and to inform the physician of any allergies or previous allergic reactions to any drugs they may have had (see WARNINGS.)

2. Patients who have previously experienced an anaphylactic reaction to penicillin should be instructed to wear a medical identification tag or bracelet.

3. Because most antibacterial drugs taken by mouth are best absorbed on an empty stomach, patients should be directed, unless circumstances warrant otherwise, to take penicillin one hour before meals or two hours after eating (see CLINICAL PHARMACOLOGY, Pharmacokinetics).

4. Patients should be told to take the entire course of therapy prescribed, even if fever and other symptoms have been stopped (see PRECAUTIONS, General).

5. If any of the following reactions occur, stop taking your prescription and notify the physician: shortness of breath, wheezing, skin rash, mouth irritation, black tongue, sore throat, nausea, vomiting, diarrhea, fever, swollen joints, or any unusual bleeding or bruising (see ADVERSE REACTIONS).

6. Do not take any additional medications without physician approval, including non-prescription drugs such as antacids, laxatives or vitamins.

7. Discard any liquid forms of penicillin after 7 days if stored at room temperature or after 14 days if refrigerated.

Laboratory Tests: Bacteriologic studies to determine the causative organisms and their susceptibility to the penicillinase-resistant penicillins should be performed (see CLINICAL PHARMACOLOGY, Microbiology). In the treatment of suspected staphylococcal infections, therapy should be changed to another active agent if culture tests fail to demonstrate the presence of staphylococci.

Periodic assessment of organ system function including renal, hepatic, and hematopoietic should be made during prolonged therapy with the penicillinase-resistant penicillins.

Blood cultures, white blood cell, and differential cell counts should be obtained prior to initiation of therapy and at least weekly during therapy with penicillinase-resistant penicillins.

Periodic urinalysis, blood urea nitrogen, and creatinine determinations should be performed during therapy with the penicillinase-resistant penicillins and dosage alterations should be considered if these values become elevated. If any impairment of renal function is suspected or known to exist, a reduction in the total dosage should be considered and blood levels monitored to avoid possible neurotoxic reactions (See DOSAGE AND ADMINISTRATION).

SGOT and SGPT values should be obtained periodically during therapy to monitor for possible liver function abnormalities.

Carcinogenesis, Mutagenesis, and Impairment of Fertility: No long-term animal studies have been conducted with these drugs.

Studies on reproduction (Nafcillin) in rats and rabbits reveal no fetal or maternal abnormalities before conception and continuously through weaning (one generation).

PRECAUTIONS: *(cont'd)*

Pregnancy Category B: Reproduction studies performed in the mouse, rat, and rabbit have revealed no evidence of impaired fertility or harm to the fetus due to the penicillinase-resistant penicillins. Human experience with the penicillins during pregnancy has not shown any positive evidence of adverse effects on the fetus. There are, however, no adequate or well-controlled studies in pregnant women showing conclusively that harmful effects of these drugs on the fetus can be excluded. Because animal reproduction studies are not always predictive of human response, this drug should be used during pregnancy only if clearly needed.

Nursing Mothers: Penicillins are excreted in breast milk. Caution should be exercised when penicillins are administered to a nursing woman.

Pediatric Use: Because of incompletely developed renal function in newborns, penicillinase-resistant penicillins (especially methicillin) may not be completely excreted, with abnormally high blood resulting. Frequent blood levels are advisable in this group with dosage adjustments when necessary. All newborns treated with penicillins should be monitored closely for clinical and laboratory evidence of toxic or adverse effects (see DOSAGE AND ADMINISTRATION).

DRUG INTERACTIONS:

Tetracycline, a bacteriostatic antibiotic, may antagonize the bactericidal effect of penicillin and concurrent use of these drugs should be avoided.

ADVERSE REACTIONS:

Body as a Whole: The reported incidence of allergic reactions to penicillin ranges from 0.7 to 10 percent (see WARNINGS). Sensitization is usually the result of treatment but some individuals have had immediate reactions to penicillin when first treated. In such cases, it is thought that the patients may have had prior exposure to the drug via trace amounts present in milk and vaccines.

Two types of allergic reactions to penicillin are noted clinically, immediate and delayed.

Immediately reactions usually occur within 20 minutes of administration and range in severity from urticaria and pruritus to angioneurotic edema, laryngospasm, bronchospasm, hypotension, vascular collapse, and death. Such immediate anaphylactic reactions are very rare (see WARNINGS) and usually occur after parenteral therapy but have occurred in patients receiving oral therapy. Another type of immediate reaction, an accelerated reaction, may occur between 20 minutes and 48 hours after administration and may include urticaria, pruritus, and fever. Although laryngeal edema, laryngospasm, and hypotension occasionally occur, fatality is uncommon.

Delayed allergic reactions to penicillin therapy usually occur after 48 hours and sometimes as late as 2 to 4 weeks after initiation of therapy. Manifestations of this type of reaction include serum sickness-like symptoms (*i.e.,* fever, malaise, urticaria, myalgia, arthralgia, abdominal pain) and various skin rashes. Nausea, vomiting, diarrhea, stomatitis, black or hairy tongue, and other symptoms of gastrointestinal irritation may occur, especially during oral penicillin therapy.

Nervous System Reactions: Neurotoxic reactions similar to those observed with penicillin G may occur with large intravenous doses of the penicillinase-resistant penicillins especially in patients with renal insufficiency.

Urogenital Reactions: Renal tubular damage and interstitial nephritis have been associated with the administration of nafcillin and oxacillin. Manifestations of this reaction may include rash, fever, eosinophilia, hematuria, proteinuria, and renal insufficiency. Methicillin-induced nephropathy does not appear to be dose-related and is generally reversible upon prompt discontinuation of therapy.

Metabolic Reactions: Agranulocytosis, neutropenia, and bone marrow depression have been associated with the use of methicillin sodium, nafcillin, oxacillin, and cloxacillin. Hepatotoxicity, characterized by fever, nausea, and vomiting associated with abnormal liver function tests, mainly elevated SGOT levels, has been associated with the use of oxacillin and cloxacillin.

DOSAGE AND ADMINISTRATION:

The penicillinase-resistant penicillins are available for oral administration and for intramuscular and intravenous injection. The sodium salts of methicillin, oxacillin, and nafcillin may be administered parenterally and the sodium salts of cloxacillin, dicloxacillin, oxacillin, and nafcillin are available for oral use.

Bacteriologic studies to determine the causative organisms and their sensitivity to the penicillinase-resistant penicillins should always be performed. Duration of therapy varies with the type and severity of infection as well as the overall condition of the patient, therefore it should be determined by the clinical and bacteriological response of the patient. In severe staphylococcal infections, therapy with penicillinase-resistant penicillins should be continued for at least 14 days. Therapy should be continued for at least 48 hours after the patient has become afebrile, asymptomatic, and cultures are negative. The treatment of endocarditis and osteomyelitis may require a longer term of therapy.

Concurrent administration of the penicillinase-resistant penicillins and probenecid increases and prolongs serum penicillin levels. Probenecid decreases the apparent volume of distribution and slows the rate of excretion by competitively inhibiting renal tubular secretion of penicillin. Penicillin-probenecid therapy is generally limited to those infections where very high serum levels of penicillin are necessary.

Oral preparations of the penicillinase-resistant penicillins should not be used as initial therapy in serious, life-threatening infections (see PRECAUTIONS, General). Oral therapy with the penicillinase-resistant penicillins may be used to follow-up the previous use of a parenteral agent as soon as the clinical condition warrants. For intramuscular gluteal injections, care should be taken to avoid sciatic nerve injury. With intravenous administration, particularly in elderly patients, care should be taken because of the possibility of thrombophlebitis.

TABLE 1 RECOMMENDED DOSAGES FOR CLOXACILLIN SODIUM IN MILD TO MODERATE AND SEVERE INFECTIONS

DRUG	ADULTS Mild to moderate	Severe	CHILDREN Mild to moderate	Severe
Cloxacillin	250 mg every 6 hours	500 mg or higher every 6 hours	50 mg/kg/day[a] in equally divided doses	100mg/kg/day[a] or higher in equally divided doses every 6 hours

[a]Patients weighing less than 20 kg (44 lbs)

DIRECTIONS FOR DISPENSING ORAL SOLUTION

Prepare solution at the time of dispensing. For ease in preparation, add the water in two portions, shaking well after each addition. Add the total amount of water as directed on the labeling of the package being dispensed. Refrigerated, the solution is stable for 14 days.

HOW SUPPLIED - RATED THERAPEUTICALLY EQUIVALENT:

Capsule, Gelatin - Oral - 250 mg

100's	$20.95	Cloxacillin Sodium, Raway	00686-0311-09
100's	$21.75	Cloxacillin Sodium, H.C.F.A. F F P	99999-0850-01
100's	$34.70	Cloxacillin Sodium, Lederle Pharm	00005-3779-23
100's	$35.43	Cloxacillin Sodium, Squibb-Mark	57783-6028-01
100's	$35.49	Cloxacillin Sodium, HL Moore Drug Exch	00839-6436-06
100's	$35.52	Cloxacillin Sodium, Aligen Independ	00405-4255-01
100's	$36.60	CLOXAPEN, Beecham	00029-6250-30
100's	$36.83	Cloxacillin Sodium, Rugby	00536-1130-01
100's	$37.96	Cloxacillin Sodium, Goldline Labs	00182-1358-01
100's	$37.96	Cloxacillin, Teva	00332-3119-09
100's	$37.96	Cloxacillin Sodium, Qualitest Pharms	00603-3029-21

Capsule, Gelatin - Oral - 500 mg

100's	$38.90	Cloxacillin Sodium, Raway	00686-3121-09
100's	$38.93	Cloxacillin Sodium, United Res	00677-0929-01
100's	$38.93	Cloxacillin Sodium, H.C.F.A. F F P	99999-0850-02
100's	$61.40	Cloxacillin Sodium, Qualitest Pharms	00603-3030-21
100's	$63.71	Cloxacillin Sodium, HL Moore Drug Exch	00839-6437-06
100's	$71.90	Cloxacillin Sodium, Squibb-Mark	57783-6038-01
100's	$72.65	CLOXAPEN, Beecham	00029-6255-30
100's	$75.65	Cloxacillin, Goldline Labs	00182-1359-01
100's	$75.65	Cloxacillin, Teva	00332-3121-09
100's	$79.63	Cloxacillin Sodium, Aligen Independ	00405-4256-01
100's	**$150.69**	**TEGOPEN, Mead Johnson**	**00015-7496-60**

Powder, Reconstitution - Oral - 125 mg/5ml

100 ml	$3.25	Cloxacillin Sodium, Raway	00686-4159-32
100 ml	$4.62	Cloxacillin Sodium, H.C.F.A. F F P	99999-0850-03
100 ml	$4.90	Cloxacillin Sodium, Major Pharms	00904-1619-04
100 ml	$5.35	Cloxacillin Sodium, Goldline Labs	00182-1720-70
100 ml	$5.43	Cloxacillin, Teva	00332-4159-32
100 ml	$5.65	Cloxacillin Sodium, Harber Pharm	51432-0655-14
100 ml	$5.72	Cloxacillin Sodium, Aligen Independ	00405-2530-60
100 ml	$6.38	Cloxacillin Sodium, Rugby	00536-1110-82
100 ml	**$10.80**	**TEGOPEN, Mead Johnson**	**00015-7941-40**
200 ml	$5.95	Cloxacillin Sodium, Raway	00686-4159-36
200 ml	$8.75	Cloxacillin Sodium, Major Pharms	00904-1619-08
200 ml	$9.24	Cloxacillin Sodium, H.C.F.A. F F P	99999-0850-04
200 ml	$9.82	Cloxacilln, Rugby	00536-1120-84
200 ml	$9.95	Cloxacillin Sodium, Harber Pharm	51432-0655-16
200 ml	$10.49	Cloxacillin Sodium, Goldline Labs	00182-1720-73
200 ml	$10.49	Cloxacillin, Teva	00332-4159-36
200 ml	$11.04	Cloxacillin Sodium, Aligen Independ	00405-2530-70
200 ml	**$20.89**	**TEGOPEN, Mead Johnson**	**00015-7941-64**

CLOZAPINE *(000851)*

CATEGORIES: Antipsychotics/Antimanics; Central Nervous System Agents; Psychotherapeutic Agents; Schizophrenia; Pregnancy Category B; FDA Class 1A ("Important Therapeutic Advantage"); Sales > $100 Million; FDA Approved 1989 Sep; Patent Expiration 1994 Dec

BRAND NAMES: **Clozaril**; *Entumin*; *Etumine*; *Leponex* (Germany, France, Mexico); *Lozapin*; *Sizopin*
(International brand names outside U.S. in italics)

FORMULARIES: Aetna; PCS

COST OF THERAPY: $3,744.90 (Schizophrenia; Tablet; 100 mg; 3/day; 365 days)

DESCRIPTION:

Clozapine, an atypical antipsychotic drug, is a tricyclic dibenzodiazepine derivative, 8-chloro-11-(4-methyl-1-piperazinyl)-*5H*-dibenzo[*b,e*][1,4]diazepine.

Clazaril 25 mg and 100 mg Tablets: *Active Ingredient:* clozapine is a yellow, crystalline powder, very slightly soluble in water. *Inactive Ingredients:* colloidal silicon dioxide, lactose, magnesium stearate, mineral oil, povidone, starch and talc.

CLINICAL PHARMACOLOGY:

Pharmacodynamics: Clozapine is classified as an 'atypical' antipsychotic drug because its profile of binding to dopamine receptors and its effects on various dopamine mediated behaviors differ from those exhibited by more typical antipsychotic drug products. In particular, although clozapine does interfere with the binding of dopamine at both D-1 and D-2 receptors, it does not induce catalepsy nor inhibit apomorphine-induced stereotypy. This evidence, consistent with the view that clozapine is preferentially more active at limbic than at striatal dopamine receptors, may explain the relative freedom of clozapine from extrapyramidal side effects.

Clozapine also acts as an antagonist at adrenergic, cholinergic, histaminergic and serotonergic receptors.

Absorption, Distribution, Metabolism and Excretion: In man, clozapine tablets (25 mg and 100 mg) are equally bioavailable relative to a clozapine solution. Following a dosage of 100 mg b.i.d., the average steady state peak plasma concentration was 319 ng/ml (range: 102-771 ng/ml), occurring at the average of 2.5 hours (range: 1-6 hours) after dosing. The average minimum concentration at steady state was 122 ng/ml (range: 41-343 ng/ml), after 100 mg b.i.d. dosing. Food does not appear to affect the systemic bioavailability of clozapine. Thus, clozapine may be administered with or without food.

Clozapine is approximately 95% bound to serum proteins. The interaction between clozapine and other highly protein-bound drugs has not been fully evaluated but may be important. (See PRECAUTIONS)

Clozapine is almost completely metabolized prior to excretion and only trace amounts of unchanged drug are detected in the urine and feces. Approximately 50% of the administered dose is excreted in the urine and 30% in the feces. The demethylated, hydroxylated and N-oxide derivatives are components in both urine and feces. Pharmacological testing has shown the desmethyl metabolite to have only limited activity, while the hydroxylated and N-oxide derivatives were inactive.

The mean elimination half-life of clozapine after a single 75 mg dose was 8 hours (range: 4-12 hours), compared to a mean elimination half-life, after achieving steady state with 100 mg b.i.d. dosing, of 12 hours (range: 4-66 hours). A comparison of single-dose and multiple-dose administration of clozapine showed that the elimination half-life increased significantly after multiple dosing relative to that after single-dose administration, suggesting the possibility of concentration dependent pharmacokinetics. However, at steady state, linearly dose-proportional changes with respect to AUC (area under the curve), peak and minimum clozapine plasma concentrations were observed after administration of 37.5 mg, 75 mg, and 150 mg b.i.d.

CLINICAL PHARMACOLOGY: *(cont'd)*

Human Pharmacology: In contrast to more typical antipsychotic drugs, clozapine therapy produces little or no prolactin elevation.

As is true of more typical antipsychotic drugs, clinical EEG studies have shown that clozapine increases delta and theta activity and slows dominant alpha frequencies. Enhanced synchronization occurs, and sharp wave activity and spike and wave complexes may also develop. Patients on rare occasions may report an intensification of dream activity during clozapine therapy. REM sleep was found to be increased to 85% of the total sleep time. In these patients, the onset of REM sleep occurred almost immediately after falling asleep.

INDICATIONS AND USAGE:

Clozapine is indicated for the management of severely ill schizophrenic patients who fail to respond adequately to standard antipsychotic drug treatment. Because of the significant risk of agranulocytosis and seizure associated with its use, clozapine should be used only in patients who have failed to respond adequately to treatment with appropriate courses of standard antipsychotic drugs, either because of insufficient effectiveness or the inability to achieve an effective dose due to intolerable adverse effects from those drugs. (See WARNINGS)

The effectiveness of clozapine in a treatment resistant schizophrenic population was demonstrated in a 6-week study comparing clozapine and chlorpromazine. Patients meeting DSM-III criteria for schizophrenia and having a mean BPRS total score of 61 were demonstrated to be treatment resistant by history and by open, prospective treatment with haloperidol before entering into the double-blind phase of the study. The superiority of clozapine to chlorpromazine was documented in statistical analyses employing both categorical and continuous measures of treatment effect.

Because of the significant risk of agranulocytosis and seizure, events which both present a continuing risk over time, the extended treatment of patients failing to show an acceptable level of clinical response should ordinarily be avoided. In addition, the need for continuing treatment in patients exhibiting beneficial clinical responses should be periodically re-evaluated.

CONTRAINDICATIONS:

Clozapine is contraindicated in patients with myeloproliferative disorders, uncontrolled epilepsy, or a history of clozapine-induced agranulocytosis or severe granulocytopenia. Clozapine should not be used simultaneously with other agents reported to cause agranulocytosis or otherwise suppress bone marrow function. As with more typical antipsychotic drugs, clozapine is contraindicated in severe central nervous system depression or comatose states from any cause.

WARNINGS:

GENERAL

BECAUSE OF THE SIGNIFICANT RISK OF AGRANULOCYTOSIS, A POTENTIALLY LIFE-THREATENING ADVERSE EVENT (SEE FOLLOWING), CLOZAPINE SHOULD BE RESERVED FOR USE IN THE TREATMENT OF SEVERELY ILL SCHIZOPHRENIC PATIENTS WHO FAIL TO SHOW AN ACCEPTABLE RESPONSE TO ADEQUATE COURSES OF STANDARD ANTIPSYCHOTIC DRUG TREATMENT, EITHER BECAUSE OF INSUFFICIENT EFFECTIVENESS OR THE INABILITY TO ACHIEVE AN EFFECTIVE DOSE DUE TO INTOLERABLE ADVERSE EFFECTS FROM THOSE DRUGS. CONSEQUENTLY, BEFORE INITIATING TREATMENT WITH CLOZAPINE, IT IS STRONGLY RECOMMENDED THAT A PATIENT BE GIVEN AT LEAST 2 TRIALS, EACH WITH A DIFFERENT STANDARD ANTIPSYCHOTIC DRUG PRODUCT, AT AN ADEQUATE DOSE, AND FOR AN ADEQUATE DURATION.

PATIENTS WHO ARE BEING TREATED WITH CLOZAPINE MUST HAVE A BASELINE WHITE BLOOD CELL (WBC) AND DIFFERENTIAL COUNT BEFORE INITIATION OF TREATMENT, AND A WBC COUNT EVERY WEEK THROUGHOUT TREATMENT, AND FOR 4 WEEKS AFTER THE DISCONTINUATION OF CLOZAPINE.

CLOZAPINE IS AVAILABLE ONLY THROUGH A DISTRIBUTION SYSTEM THAT ENSURES WEEKLY WBC TESTING PRIOR TO DELIVERY OF THE NEXT WEEK'S SUPPLY OF MEDICATION.

Agranulocytosis

Agranulocytosis, defined as an absolute neutrophil count (ANC) of less than 500/mm^3, has been estimated to occur in association with clozapine use at a cumulative incidence at 1 year of approximately 1.3%, based on the occurrence of 15 US cases out of 1743 patients exposed to clozapine during its clinical testing prior to domestic marketing. All of these cases occurred at a time when the need for close monitoring of WBC counts was already recognized. This reaction could prove fatal if not detected early and therapy interrupted. Of the 149 cases of agranulocytosis reported worldwide in association with Clozaril (clozapine) use as of December 31, 1989, 32% were fatal. However, few of these deaths occurred since 1977, at which time the knowledge of clozapine-induced agranulocytosis became more widespread, and close monitoring of WBC counts more widely practiced. Nevertheless, it is unknown at present what the case fatality rate will be for clozapine-induced agranulocytosis, despite strict adherence to the recommendation for weekly monitoring of WBC counts. In the US, under a weekly WBC monitoring system with clozapine, there have been 317 cases of agranulocytosis as of January 1, 1994; 11 were fatal. During this period, over 68,000 patients received Clozaril (clozapine).

Because of the substantial risk of agranulocytosis in association with clozapine use, which may persist over an extended period of time, patients must have a blood sample drawn for a WBC count before initiation of treatment with clozapine, and must have subsequent WBC counts done at least weekly for the duration of therapy, as well as for 4 weeks thereafter. The distribution of clozapine is contingent upon performance of the required blood tests.

Treatment should not be initiated if the WBC count is less than 3500/mm^3, or if the patient has a history of a myeloproliferative disorder, or previous clozapine-induced agranulocytosis or granulocytopenia. Patients should be advised to report immediately the appearance of lethargy, weakness, fever, sore throat or any other signs of infection. If, after the initiation of treatment, the total WBC count has dropped below 3500/mm^3 or it has dropped by a substantial amount from baseline, even if the count is above 3500/mm^3, or if immature forms are present, a repeat WBC count and a differential count should be done. A substantial drop is defined as a single drop of 3,000 or more in the WBC count or a cumulative drop of 3,000 or more within 3 weeks. If subsequent WBC counts and the differential count

WARNINGS: *(cont'd)*

reveal a total WBC count between 3000 and 3500/mm³ and an ANC above 1500/mm³, twice weekly WBC counts and differential counts should be performed.

If the total WBC count falls below 3000/mm³ or the ANC below 1500/mm³, clozapine therapy should be interrupted, WBC count and differential should be performed daily, and patients should be carefully monitored for flu-like symptoms or other symptoms suggestive of infection. Clozapine therapy may be resumed if no symptoms of infection develop, and if the total WBC count returns to levels above 3000/mm³ and the ANC returns to levels above 1500/mm³. However, in this event, twice-weekly WBC counts and differential counts should continue until total WBC counts return to levels above 3500/mm³.

If the total WBC count falls below 2000/mm³ or the ANC falls below 1000/mm³, bone narrow aspiration should be considered to ascertain granulopoietic status. Protective isolation with close observation may be indicated if granulopoiesis is determined to be deficient. Should evidence of infection develop, the patient should have appropriate cultures performed and an appropriate antibiotic regimen instituted.

Patients whose total WBC counts fall below 2000/mm³, or ANCs below 1000/mm³ during clozapine therapy should have daily WBC count and differential. These patients should not be re-challanged with clozapine. Patients discontinued from Clozaril (clozapine) therapy due to significant WBC suppression have been found to develop agranulocytosis upon re-challenge, often with a shorter latency on re-exposure. To reduce the chances of re-challenge occurring in patients who have experienced significant bone marrow suppression during clozapine therapy, a single, national master file will be maintained confidentially.

Except for evidence of significant bone marrow suppression during initial clozapine therapy, there are no established risk factors, based on world-wide experience, for the development of agranulocytosis in association with clozapine use. However, a disproportionate number of the U.S. cases of agranulocytosis occurred in patients of Jewish background compared to the overall proportion of such patients exposed during domestic development of clozapine. Most of the U.S. cases occurred within 4-10 weeks of exposure, but neither dose nor duration is a reliable predictor of this problem. No patient characteristics have been clearly linked to the development of agranulocytosis in association with clozapine use, but agranulocytosis associated with other antipsychotic drugs has been reported to occur with a greater frequency in women, the elderly and in patients who are cachectic or have serious underlying medical illness; such patients may also be at particular risk with clozapine.

To reduce the risk of agranulocytosis developing undetected, clozapine is available only through a distribution system that ensures weekly WBC testing prior to delivery of the next week's supply of medication.

Eosinophilia: In clinical trials, 1% of patients developed eosinophilia, which, in rare cases, can be substantial. If a differential count reveals a total eosinophil count above 4,000/mm³, clozapine therapy should be interrupted until the eosinophil count falls below 3,000/mm³.

Seizures

Seizure has been estimated to occur in association with clozapine use at a cumulative incidence at one year of approximately 5%, based on the occurrence of one or more seizures in 61 of 1743 patients exposed to clozapine during its clinical testing prior to domestic marketing (*i.e.,* a crude rate of 3.5%). Dose appears to be an important predictor of seizure, with a greater likelihood of seizure at the higher clozapine doses used.

Caution should be used in administering clozapine to patients having a history of seizures or other predisposing factors. Because of the substantial risk of seizure associated with clozapine use, patients should be advised not to engage in any activity where sudden loss of consciousness could cause serious risk to themselves or others, (*e.g.,* the operation of complex machinery, driving an automobile, swimming, climbing, etc.).

Adverse Cardiovascular and Respiratory Effects

Orthostatic hypotension with or without syncope can occur with clozapine treatment and may represent a continuing risk in some patients. Rarely (approximately 1 case per 3,000 patients), collapse can be profound and be accompanied by respiratory and/or cardiac arrest. Orthostatic hypotension is more likely to occur during initial titration in association with rapid dose escalation and may even occur on first dose. In one report, initial doses as low as 12.5 mg were associated with collapse and respiratory arrest. When restarting patients who have had even a brief interval off clozapine, (*i.e.,* 2 days or more since the last dose), it is recommended that treatment be reinitiated with one-half of a 25 mg tablet (12.5 mg) once or twice daily (see DOSAGE AND ADMINISTRATION).

Some of the cases of collapse/respiratory arrest/cardiac arrest during initial treatment occurred in patients who were being administered benzodiazepines; similar events have been reported in patients taking other psychotropic drugs or even clozapine by itself. Although it has not been established that there is an interaction between clozapine and benzodiazepines or other psychotropics, caution is advised when clozapine is initiated in patients taking a benzodiazepine or any other psychotropic drug.

Tachycardia, which may be sustained, has also been observed in approximately 25% of patients taking clozapine, with patients having an average increase in pulse rate of 10-15 bpm. The sustained tachycardia is not simply a reflex response to hypotension, and is present in all positions monitored. Either tachycardia or hypotension may pose a serious risk for an individual with compromised cardiovascular function.

A minority of clozapine treated patients experience ECG repolarization changes similar to those seen with other antipsychotic drugs, including S-T segment depression and flattening or inversion of T waves, which all normalize after discontinuation of clozapine. The clinical significance of these changes is unclear. However, in clinical trials with clozapine, several patients experienced significant cardiac events, including ischemic changes, myocardial infarction, arrhythmias and sudden death. In addition there have been postmarketing reports of congestive heart failure, myocarditis, and pericarditis/pericardial effusions in association with clozapine use. Causality assessment was difficult in many of these cases because of serious

WARNINGS: *(cont'd)*

preexisting cardiac disease and plausible alternative causes. Rare instances of sudden death have been reported in psychiatric patients, with or without associated antipsychotic drug treatment, and the relationship of these events to antipsychotic drug use is unknown.

Clozapine should be used with caution in patients with known cardiovascular and/or pulmonary disease, and the recommendation for gradual titration of dose should be carefully observed.

Neuroleptic Malignant Syndrome (NMS): A potentially fatal symptom complex sometimes referred to as Neuroleptic Malignant Syndrome (NMS) has been reported in association with antipsychotic drugs. Clinical manifestations of NMS are hyperpyrexia, muscle rigidity, altered mental status and evidence of autonomic instability (irregular pulse or blood pressure, tachycardia, diaphoresis, and cardiac dysrhythmias).

The diagnostic evaluation of patients with this syndrome is complicated. In arriving at a diagnosis, it is important to identify cases where the clinical presentation includes both serious medical illness (*e.g.,* pneumonia, systemic infection, etc.) and untreated or inadequately treated extrapyramidal signs and symptoms (EPS). Other important considerations in the differential diagnosis include central anticholinergic toxicity, heat stroke, drug fever and primary central nervous system (CNS) pathology.

The management of NMS should include 1) immediate discontinuation of antipsychotic drugs and other drugs not essential to concurrent therapy, 2) intensive symptomatic treatment and medical monitoring, and 3) treatment of any concomitant serious medical problems for which specific treatments are available. There is no general agreement about specific pharmacological treatment regimens for uncomplicated NMS.

If a patient requires antipsychotic drug treatment after recovery from NMS, the potential reintroduction of drug therapy should be carefully considered. The patient should be carefully monitored, since recurrences of NMS have been reported.

There have been several reported cases of NMS in patients receiving clozapine alone or in combination with lithium or other CNS-active agents.

Tardive Dyskinesia: A syndrome consisting of potentially irreversible, involuntary, dyskinetic movements may develop in patients treated with antipsychotic drugs. Although the prevalence of the syndrome appears to be highest among the elderly, especially elderly women, it is impossible to rely upon prevalence estimates to predict, at the inception of treatment, which patients are likely to develop the syndrome.

There are several reasons for predicting that clozapine may be different from other antipsychotic drugs in its potential for inducing tardive dyskinesia, including the preclinical finding that it has a relatively weak dopamine blocking effect and the clinical finding of a virtual absence of certain acute extrapyramidal symptoms, (*e.g.,* dystonia). A few cases of tardive dyskinesia have been reported in patients on clozapine who had been previously treated with other antipsychotic agents, so that a causal relationship cannot be established. There have been no reports of tardive dyskinesia directly attributable to clozapine alone. Nevertheless, it cannot be concluded, without more extended experience, that clozapine is incapable of inducing this syndrome.

Both the risk of developing the syndrome and the likelihood that it will become irreversible are believed to increase as the duration of treatment and the total cumulative dose of antipsychotic drugs administered to the patient increase. However, the syndrome can develop, although much less commonly, after relatively brief treatment periods at low doses. There is no known treatment for established cases of tardive dyskinesia, although the syndrome may remit, partially or completely, if antipsychotic drug treatment is withdrawn. Antipsychotic drug treatment, itself, however, may suppress (or partially suppress) the signs and symptoms of the syndrome and thereby may possibly mask the underlying process. The effect that symptom suppression has upon the long-term course of the syndrome is unknown.

Given these considerations, clozapine should be prescribed in a manner that is most likely to minimize the occurrence of tardive dyskinesia. As with any antipsychotic drug, chronic clozapine use should be reserved for patients who appear to be obtaining substantial benefit from the drug. In such patients, the smallest dose and the shortest duration of treatment should be sought. The need for continued treatment should be reassessed periodically.

If signs and symptoms of tardive dyskinesia appear in a patient on clozapine, drug discontinuation should be considered. However, some patients may require treatment with clozapine despite the presence of the syndrome.

PRECAUTIONS:

General: Because of the significant risk of agranulocytosis and seizure, both of which present a continuing risk over time, the extended treatment of patients failing to show an acceptable level of clinical response should ordinarily be avoided. In addition, the need for continuing treatment in patients exhibiting beneficial clinical responses should be periodically re-evaluated.

The mechanism of clozapine-induced agranulocytosis is unknown; nonetheless, the possibility that causative factors may interact synergistically to increase the risk and/or severity of bone marrow suppression warrants consideration. Therefore, clozapine should not be used with other agents reported to cause agranulocytosis or otherwise suppress bone marrow function.

Fever: During clozapine therapy, patients may experience transient temperature elevations above 100.4°F (38°C), with the peak incidence within the first 3 weeks of treatment. While this fever is generally benign and self limiting, it may necessitate discontinuing patients from treatment. On occasion, there may be an associated increase or decrease in WBC count. Patients with fever should be carefully evaluated to rule out the possibility of an underlying infectious process or the development of agranulocytosis. In the presence of high fever, the possibility of Neuroleptic Malignant Syndrome (NMS) must be considered. There have been several reports of NMS in patients receiving clozapine, usually in combination with lithium or other CNS-active drugs. [See Neuroleptic Malignant Syndrome (NMS), under WARNINGS].

Anticholinergic Toxicity: Clozapine has very potent anticholinergic effects and great care should be exercised in using this drug in the presence of prostatic enlargement or narrow angle glaucoma.

Interference with Cognitive and Motor Performance: Because of initial sedation, clozapine may impair mental and/or physical abilities, especially during the first few days of therapy. The recommendations for gradual dose escalation should be carefully adhered to, and patients cautioned about activities requiring alertness.

Use in Patients with Concomitant Illness: Clinical experience with clozapine in patients with concomitant systemic diseases is limited. Nevertheless, caution is advisable in using clozapine in patients with hepatic, renal or cardiac disease.

Use in Patients Undergoing General Anesthesia: Caution is advised in patients being administered general anesthesia because of the CNS effects of clozapine. Check with the anesthesiologist regarding continuation of clozapine therapy in a patient scheduled for surgery.

Information for the Patient: Physicians are advised to discuss the following issues with patients for whom they prescribe clozapine:

Patients who are to receive clozapine should be warned about the significant risk of developing agranulocytosis. They should be informed that weekly blood tests are required to monitor for the occurrence of agranulocytosis, and that clozapine tablets will be made available only through a special program designed to ensure the required blood monitoring.

PRECAUTIONS: *(cont'd)*

Patients should be advised to report immediately the appearance of lethargy, weakness, fever, sore throat, malaise, mucous membrane ulceration or other possible signs of infection. Particular attention should be paid to any flu-like complaints or other symptoms that might suggest infection.

Patients should be informed of the significant risk of seizure during clozapine treatment, and they should be advised to avoid driving and any other potentially hazardous activity while taking clozapine.

Patients should be advised of the risk of orthostatic hypotension, especially during the period of initial dose titration.

Patients should be informed that if they stop taking clozapine for more than 2 days, they should not restart their medication at the same dosage, but should contact their physician for dosing instructions.

Patients should notify their physician if they are taking, or plan to take, any prescription or over-the-counter drugs or alcohol.

Patients should notify their physician if they become pregnant or intend to become pregnant during therapy.

Patients should not breast feed an infant if they are taking clozapine.

Carcinogenesis, Mutagenesis, and Impairment of Fertility: No carcinogenic potential was demonstrated in long-term studies in mice and rats at doses approximately 7 times the typical human dose on a mg/kg basis. Fertility in male and female rats was not adversely affected by clozapine. Clozapine did not produce genotoxic or mutagenic effects when assayed in appropriate bacterial and mammalian tests.

Pregnancy Category B: Reproduction studies have been performed in rats and rabbits at doses of approximately 2-4 times the human dose and have revealed no evidence of impaired fertility or harm to the fetus due to clozapine. There are, however, no adequate and well-controlled studies in pregnant women. Because animal reproduction studies are not always predictive of human response, and in view of the desirability of keeping the administration of all drugs to a minimum during pregnancy, this drug should be used only if clearly needed.

Nursing Mothers: Animal studies suggest that clozapine may be excreted in breast milk and have an effect on the nursing infant. Therefore, women receiving clozapine should not breast feed.

Pediatric Use: Safety and effectiveness in children below age 16 have not been established.

DRUG INTERACTIONS:

The risks of using clozapine in combination with other drugs have not been systematically evaluated.

The mechanism of clozapine-induced agranulocytosis is unknown; nonetheless, the possibility that causative factors may interact synergistically to increase the risk and/or severity of bone marrow suppression warrants consideration. Therefore, clozapine should not be used with other agents having a well-known potential to suppress bone marrow function.

Given the primary CNS effects of clozapine, caution is advised in using it concomitantly with other CNS-active drugs.

Orthostatic hypotension in patients taking clozapine can, in rare cases (approximately 1 case per 3,000 patients), be accompanied by profound collapse and respiratory and/or cardiac arrest. Some of the cases of collapse/respiratory arrest/cardiac arrest during initial treatment occurred in patients who were being administered benzodiazepines; similar events have been reported in patients taking other psychotropic drugs or even clozapine by itself. Although it has not been established that there is an interaction between clozapine and benzodiazepines or other psychotropics, caution is advised when clozapine is initiated in patients taking a benzodiazepine or any other psychotropic drug.

Because clozapine is highly bound to serum protein, the administration of clozapine to a patient taking another drug which is highly bound to protein (*e.g.*, warfarin, digitoxin) may cause an increase in plasma concentrations of these drugs, potentially resulting in adverse effects. Conversely, adverse effects may result from displacement of protein-bound clozapine by other highly bound drugs.

Cimetidine may increase plasma levels of clozapine, potentially resulting in adverse effects. Phenytoin may decrease clozapine plasma levels, resulting in a decrease in effectiveness of a previously effective clozapine dose.

A subset (3%-10%) of the population has reduced activity of certain drug metabolizing enzymes such as the cytochrome P450 isozyme P450 2D6. Such individuals are referred to as "poor metabolizers" of drugs such as debrisoquin, dextromethorphan, the tricyclic antidepressants, and clozapine. These individuals may develop higher than expected plasma concentrations of clozapine when given usual doses. In addition, certain drugs that are metabolized by this isozyme, including many antidepressants (clozapine, selective serotonin reuptake inhibitors, and others), may inhibit the activity of this isozyme, and thus may make normal metabolizers resemble poor metabolizers with regard to concomitant therapy with other drugs metabolized by this enzyme system, leading to drug interaction.

Concomitant use of clozapine with other drugs metabolized by cytochrome P450 2D6 may require lower doses than usually prescribed for either clozapine or the other drug. Therefore, co-administration of clozapine with other drugs that are metabolized by this isozyme, including antidepressants, phenothiazines, and carbamazepine, and Type 1C antiarrhythmics (*e.g.*, propafenone, flecainide and encainide), or that inhibit this enzyme (*e.g.*, quinidine), should be approached with caution.

Clozapine may also potentiate the hypotensive effects of antihypertensive drugs and the anticholinergic effects of atropine-type drugs. The administration of epinephrine should be avoided in the treatment of drug-induced hypotension because of a possible reverse epinephrine effect.

Use in Patients Undergoing General Anesthesia: Caution is advised in patients being administered general anesthesia because of the CNS effects of clozapine. Check with the anesthesiologist regarding continuation of clozapine therapy in a patient scheduled for surgery.

ADVERSE REACTIONS:

Associated with Discontinuation of Treatment: Sixteen percent of 1080 patients who received clozapine in premarketing clinical trials discontinued treatment due to an adverse event, including both those that could be reasonably attributed to clozapine treatment and those that might more appropriately be considered intercurrent illness. The more common events considered to be causes of discontinuation included: CNS, primarily drowsiness/sedation, seizures, dizziness/syncope; cardiovascular, primarily tachycardia, hypotension and ECG changes; gastrointestinal, primarily nausea/vomiting; hematologic, primarily leukopenia/granulocytopenia/agranulocytosis; and fever. None of the events enumerated accounts for more than 1.7% of all discontinuations attributed to adverse clinical events.

Commonly Observed: Adverse events observed in association with the use of clozapine in clinical trials at an incidence of greater than 5% were: central nervous system complaints, including drowsiness/sedation, dizziness/vertigo, headache and tremor; autonomic nervous system complaints, including salivation, sweating, dry mouth and visual disturbances; cardiovascular findings, including tachycardia, hypotension and syncope; and gastrointestinal complaints, including constipation and nausea; and fever. Complaints of drowsiness/sedation tend to subside with continued therapy or dose reduction. Salivation may be profuse, especially during sleep, but may be diminished with dose reduction.

Incidence in Clinical Trials: The following table (TABLE 1) enumerates adverse events that occurred at a frequency of 1% or greater among clozapine patients who participated in clinical trials. These rates are not adjusted for duration of exposure.

TABLE 1 Treatment-Emergent Adverse Experience Incidence Among Patients Taking Clozapine in Clinical Trials (N=842) Percentage of Patients Reporting

Body System Adverse Event[a]	Percent
Central Nervous System	
Drowsiness/Sedation	39
Dizziness/Vertigo	19
Headache	7
Tremor	6
Syncope	6
Disturbed sleep/Nightmares	4
Restlessness	4
Hypokinesia/Akinesia	4
Agitation	4
Seizures (convulsions)	3[b]
Rigidity	3
Akathisia	3
Confusion	3
Fatigue	2
Insomnia	2
Hyperkinesia	1
Weakness	1
Lethargy	1
Ataxia	1
Slurred speech	1
Depression	1
Epileptiform movements/Myoclonic jerks	1
Anxiety	1
Cardiovascular	
Tachycardia	25[b]
Hypotension	9
Hypertension	4
Chest pain/Angina	1
ECG change/Cardiac abnormality	1
Gastrointestinal	
Constipation	14
Nausea	5
Abdominal discomfort/Heartburn	4
Nausea/Vomiting	3
Vomiting	3
Diarrhea	2
Liver test abnormality	1
Anorexia	1
Urogenital	
Urinary abnormalities	2
Incontinence	1
Abnormal ejaculation	1
Urinary urgency/frequency	1
Urinary retention	1
Autonomic Nervous System	
Salivation	31
Sweating	6
Dry mouth	6
Visual disturbances	5
Integumentary (Skin)	
Rash	2
Musculoskeletal	
Muscle weakness	1
Pain (back, neck, legs)	1
Muscle spasm	1
Muscle pain, ache	1
Respiratory	
Throat discomfort	1
Dyspnea, shortness of breath	1
Nasal congestion	1
Hemic/Lymphatic	
Leukopenia/Decreased WBC/Neutropenia	3
Agranulocytosis	1[b]
Eosinophilia	1
Miscellaneous	
Fever	5
Weight gain	4
Tongue numb/sore	1

[a] Events reported by at least 1% of clozapine patients are included.
[b] Rate based on population of approximately 1700 exposed during premarket clinical evaluation of clozapine.

Other Events Observed During the Premarketing Evaluation of Clozapine: This section reports additional, less frequent adverse events which occurred among the patients taking clozapine in clinical trials. Various adverse events were reported as part of the total experience in these clinical studies; a causal relationship to clozapine treatment cannot be determined in the absence of appropriate controls in some of the studies. The table (TABLE 1) above enumerates adverse events that occurred at a frequency of at least 1% of patients treated with clozapine. The list below includes all additional adverse experiences reported as being temporally associated with the use of the drug which occurred at a frequency less than 1% enumerated by organ system.

Central Nervous System: loss of speech, amentia, tics, poor coordination, delusions/hallucinations, involuntary movement, stuttering, dysarthria, amnesia/memory loss, histrionic movements, libido increase or decrease, paranoia, shakiness, Parkinsonism, and irritability.

Cardiovascular System: edema, palpitations, phlebitis/thrombophlebitis, cyanosis, premature ventricular contraction, bradycardia, and nose bleed.

Gastrointestinal System: abdominal distention, gastroenteritis, rectal bleeding, nervous stomach, abnormal stools, hematemesis, gastric ulcer, bitter taste, and eructation.

Urogenital System: dysmenorrhea, impotence, breast pain/discomfort, and vaginal itch/infection.

Autonomic Nervous System: numbness, polydipsia, hot flashes, dry throat, and mydriasis.

Integumentary (Skin): pruritus, pallor, eczema, erythema, bruise, dermatitis, petechiae, and urticaria.

Musculoskeletal System: twitching and joint pain.

ADVERSE REACTIONS: *(cont'd)*

Respiratory System: coughing, pneumonia/ pneumonia-like symptoms, rhinorrhea, hyperventilation, wheezing, bronchitis, laryngitis, and sneezing.

Hemic and Lymphatic System: anemia and leukocytosis.

Miscellaneous: chills/chills with fever, malaise, appetite increase, ear disorder, hypothermia, eyelid disorder, bloodshot eyes, and nystagmus.

Postmarketing Clinical Experience: Postmarketing experience has shown an adverse experience profile similar to that presented above. Voluntary reports of adverse events temporally associated with clozapine not mentioned above that have been received since market introduction and that may have no causal relationship with the drug include the following:

Central Nervous System: delirium; EEG abnormal; exacerbation of psychosis; myoclonus; overdose; paresthesia; and status epilepticus.

Cardiovascular System: atrial or ventricular fibrillation and periorbital edema.

Gastrointestinal System: acute pancreatitis; dysphagia; fecal impaction; hepatitis; intestinal obstruction/paralytic ileus; jaundice; and salivary gland swelling.

Urogenital System: priapism.

Integumentary (Skin): hypersensitivity reactions: photosensitivity, vasculitis, erythema multiforme, and Stevens-Johnson Syndrome.

Respiratory System: aspiration and pleural effusion.

Hemic and Lymphatic System: deep vein thrombosis; elevated hemoglobin/hematocrit; ESR increased; pulmonary embolism; sepsis; thrombocytosis; and thrombocytopenia.

Miscellaneous: CPK elevation; hyperglycemia; hyperuricemia; hyponatremia; and weight loss.

DRUG ABUSE AND DEPENDENCE:

Physical and psychological dependence have not been reported or observed in patients taking clozapine.

OVERDOSAGE:

Human Experience: The most commonly reported signs and symptoms associated with clozapine overdose are: altered states of consciousness, including drowsiness, delirium and coma; tachycardia; hypotension; respiratory depression or failure; hypersalivation. Aspiration pneumonia and cardiac arrhythmias have also been reported. Seizures have occurred in a minority of reported cases. Fatal overdoses have been reported with clozapine, generally at doses above 2500 mgs. There have also been reports of patients recovering from overdoses well in excess of 4 gms.

Management of Overdose: Establish and maintain an airway; ensure adequate oxygenation and ventilation. Activated charcoal, which may be used with sorbitol, may be as or more effective than emesis or lavage, and should be considered in treating overdosage. Cardiac and vital signs monitoring is recommended along with general symptomatic and supportive measures. Additional surveillance should be continued for several days because of the risk of delayed effects. Avoid epinephrine and derivatives when treating hypotension, and quinidine and procainamide when treating cardiac arrhythmia.

There are no specific antidotes for clozapine. Forced diuresis, dialysis, hemoperfusion and exchange transfusion are unlikely to be of benefit.

In managing overdosage, the physician should consider the possibility of multiple drug involvement.

Up-to-date information about the treatment of overdose can often be obtained from a certified Regional Poison Control Center. Telephone numbers of certified Poison Control Centers are listed in the Physicians GenRx.

DOSAGE AND ADMINISTRATION:

In order to minimize the risk of agranulocytosis, clozapine is available only through a distribution system that ensures weekly WBC testing prior to delivery of the next week's supply of medication. Upon initiation of clozapine therapy, up to a 1 week supply of additional clozapine tablets may be provided to the patient to be held for emergencies (*e.g.*, weather, holidays).

Initial Treatment: It is recommended that treatment with clozapine begin with one-half of a 25 mg (12.5 mg) once or twice daily and then be continued with daily dosage increments of 25-50 mg/day, if well-tolerated, to achieve a target dose of 300-450 mg/day by the end of 2 weeks. Subsequent dosage increments should be made no more than once or twice-weekly, in increments not to exceed 100 mg. Cautious titration and a divided dosage schedule are necessary to minimize the risks of hypotension, seizure, and sedation.

In the multicenter study that provides primary support for the effectiveness of clozapine in patients resistant to standard antipsychotic drug treatment, patients were titrated during the first 2 weeks up to a maximum dose of 500 mg/day, on a t.i.d. basis, and were then dosed in a total daily dose range of 100-900 mg/day, on a t.i.d. basis thereafter, with clinical response and adverse effects as guides to correct dosing.

Therapeutic Dose Adjustment: Daily dosing should continue on a divided basis as an effective and tolerable dose level is sought. While many patients may respond adequately at doses between 300-600 mg/day, it may be necessary to raise the dose to the 600-900 mg/day range to obtain an acceptable response. [*Note:* In the multicenter study providing the primary support for the superiority of clozapine in treatment resistant patients, the mean and median clozapine doses were both approximately 600 mg/day.]

Because of the possibility of increased adverse reactions at higher doses, particularly seizures, patients should ordinarily be given adequate time to respond to a given dose level before escalation to a higher dose is contemplated.

Dosing should not exceed 900 mg/day.

Because of the significant risk of agranulocytosis and seizure, events which both present a continuing risk over time, the extended treatment of patients failing to show an acceptable level of clinical response should ordinarily be avoided.

Maintenance Treatment: While the maintenance effectiveness of clozapine in schizophrenia is still under study, the effectiveness of maintenance treatment is well established for many other antipsychotic drugs. It is recommended that responding patients be continued on clozapine, but at the lowest level needed to maintain remission. Because of the significant risk associated with the use of clozapine, patients should be periodically reassessed to determine the need for maintenance treatment.

Discontinuation of Treatment: In the event of planned termination of clozapine therapy, gradual reduction in dose is recommended over a 1-2 week period. However, should a patient's medical condition require abrupt discontinuation (*e.g.*, leukopenia), the patient should be carefully observed for the recurrence of psychotic symptoms.

Re-initiation of Treatment in Patients Previously Discontinued: When restarting patients who have had even a brief interval off clozapine, (*i.e.*, 2 days or more since the last dose), it is recommended that treatment be reinitiated with one-half of a 25 mg tablet (12.5 mg) once or twice daily (see WARNINGS.) If that dose is well tolerated, it may be feasible to titrate patients back to a therapeutic dose more quickly than is recommended for initial treatment.

DOSAGE AND ADMINISTRATION: *(cont'd)*

However, any patient who has previously experienced respiratory or cardiac arrest with initial dosing, but was then able to be successfully titrated to a therapeutic dose, should be re-titrated with extreme caution after even 24 hours of discontinuation.

Certain additional precautions seem prudent when re-initiating treatment. The mechanisms underlying clozapine-induced adverse reactions are unknown. It is conceivable, however, that re-exposure of a patient might enhance the risk of an untoward event's occurrence and increase its severity. Such phenomena, for example, occur when immune mediated mechanisms are responsible. Consequently, during the re-initiation of treatment, additional caution is advised. Patients discontinued for WBC counts below 2000/mm^3 or an ANC below 1000/mm^3 must *not* be restarted on clozapine. (See WARNINGS)

Store and Dispense: Storage temperature should not exceed 86°F (30°C). Drug dispensing should not ordinarily exceed a weekly supply. Dispensing should be contingent upon the results of a WBC count.

HOW SUPPLIED:

Clozaril is available only through a distribution system that ensures weekly WBC testing prior to delivery of the next week's supply of medication.

25 mg: Round, pale yellow, scored, uncoated tablets, engraved with "CLOZARIL" (on the periphery) on one side, and "25" on the scored side.

100 mg: Round, pale yellow, compressed tablets, engraved with "CLOZARIL" (on the periphery) on one side, and "100" on the other side.

HOW SUPPLIED - RATED THERAPEUTICALLY EQUIVALENT:

Tablet, Uncoated - Oral - 25 mg

100's	$132.00	CLOZARIL, Novartis	00078-0126-05
100's	$132.00	CLOZARIL, Novartis	00078-0126-06

Tablet, Uncoated - Oral - 100 mg

100's	$342.00	CLOZARIL, Novartis	00078-0127-05
100's	$342.00	CLOZARIL, Novartis	00078-0127-06

COAL TAR *(000852)*

CATEGORIES: Atopic Dermatitis; Dermatitis; Dermatoses; Eczema; Keratoplastic Agents; Psoriasis; Skin/Mucous Membrane Agents; Pregnancy Category C; FDA Pre 1938 Drugs

BRAND NAMES: *Alphosyl* (Canada); *Balnetar* (Canada); *Basotar*; *Berniter* (Germany); *Carbo-Dome*; *Doak Tar*; *Estar* (Canada); *Linotar*; *Linotar Gel 1*; *Linotar Gel 2*; *Linotar Gel 3*; *Meditar*; *Pentrax*; *Polytar*; *Psorigel* (Canada); *Psoriasdin*; *Psoriderm*; *T-Gel* (Canada); *T Gel Shampoo*; *Tar Doak* (Canada); *Tarpaste* (Canada); **Zetar**

(International brand names outside U.S. in italics)

FORMULARIES: WHO

DESCRIPTION:

Coal tar emulsion is a liquid for topical application, following dilution in aqueous media. Each ml contains 300 mg whole coal tar in polysorbates. It is a topical anti-eczematic. The complete chemical composition of coal tar has not been ascertained; components are grouped into six categories: aromatic hydrocarbons, acidic phenolic compounds, cyclic nitrogen compounds, organic sulfur compounds, non-acidic phenolics and nonbasic nitrogen compounds.

CLINICAL PHARMACOLOGY:

There is no confirmed scientific evidence as to the clinical pharmacologic effects of coal tar. Its actions in humans have been reported in the literature as antiseptic, antipruritic, antiparasitic, antifungal, antibacterial, keratoplastic and antiacanthotic. Vasoconstrictive activity of coal tar has also been reported.

INDICATIONS AND USAGE:

Coal tar emulsion is indicated for the relief of symptoms associated with generalized, persistent dermatoses, such as psoriasis, eczema, atopic dermatitis and seborrheic dermatitis.

CONTRAINDICATIONS:

Not to be used on open or infected lesions.

WARNINGS:

Application of coal tar may elicit a pustular eruption or a cyst (epidermal) like reaction.

Patients who have previously exhibited sensitivity to tars must be under careful and continuous supervision by the physician.

PRECAUTIONS:

For external (topical) use only. Keep away from eyes. When used in the bath, add lukewarm water (not hot water). For 72 hours following treatment with coal tar, patients should avoid exposure to either direct sunlight or sunlamps (ultra-violet A and/or B) unless directed by physician, as this drug may photoactivate the skin. Prior to exposure to sunlight, completely remove all tar from skin. Sensitization or dermatitis may occur after prolonged use. If irritation develops or increases, discontinue use and consult physician. Keep out of the reach of children.

Carcinogenesis: Coal tar applied to the skin of mice resulted in an increase in epidermal carcinomas. Painting rabbit ears with coal tar appears to increase self-limiting keratoacanthomas. To date, existing reports do not suggest an increased incidence of skin cancer in psoriatics treated with coal tar.

Pregnancy Category C: Animal reproduction studies have not been conducted with Coal tar emulsion. It is also not known whether coal tar emulsion can cause fetal harm when administered to a pregnant woman or can affect reproduction capacity. Coal tar emulsion should be given to a pregnant woman only if clearly needed.

Nursing Mothers: It is not known whether this drug is excreted in human milk. Because of the tumorigenicity shown for coal tar in animal studies, a decision should be made whether to discontinue nursing or to discontinue the drug, taking into account the importance of the drug to the mother.

DRUG INTERACTIONS:

While no known drug interactions have been reported pertaining to the clinical use of this drug in patients, the concomitant use of drugs with phototoxic and/or photoactivating potential is not recommended (*i.e.*, tetracyclines, psoralens, topical retinoic acid).

ADVERSE REACTIONS:

Application of coal tar may result in superficial folliculitis. Patients hypersensitive to coal tar may exhibit a pustular or keratocystic response.

DOSAGE AND ADMINISTRATION:

Add 3 to 5 teaspoonfuls of coal tar emulsion to a bath of lukewarm water. This is mixed throughout the bath. The patient immerses in the bath for 15 to 20 minutes. The interval recommended between dosing is from once-a-day to once every third day, and usual duration of treatment is 30 to 45 days.

If the physician decides to administer supplemental ultraviolet irradiation (Goeckerman treatment) to the patient (ultraviolet B; A or A/B), this may be accomplished between 2 and 72 hours. A determination of minimal erythemal dosage (MED) should be made for each patient; initial irradiation should be suberythemal, not to exceed MED.

Compounding: Coal tar emulsion may be utilized in compounding prescriptions in aqueous based vehicles requiring coal tar. Each ml of coal tar Emulsion contains 300 mg whole coal tar.

HOW SUPPLIED - EQUIVALENTS NOT AVAILABLE:

Emulsion - Topical - 300 mg/ml

6 oz	$25.45	ZETAR, Dermik Labs	00066-0062-06

COAL TAR; SALICYLIC ACID *(000860)*

CATEGORIES: Dermatologicals; Keratolytic Agents; Skin/Mucous Membrane Agents; FDA Pre 1938 Drugs

BRAND NAMES: Coalgel (France); *Inoxa T*; *Ionax T* (France); Salatar; *Tarisdin*
(International brand names outside U.S. in italics)

Prescribing information not available at time of publication.

HOW SUPPLIED - EQUIVALENTS NOT AVAILABLE:

Cream - Topical - 5 %/3 %

120 gm	$4.00	SALATAR, Lannett	00527-0419-04
454 gm	$11.00	SALATAR, Lannett	00527-0419-16

COCAINE HYDROCHLORIDE *(000861)*

CATEGORIES: Anesthesia; Antipruritics/Local Anesthetics; EENT Drugs; Eye, Ear, Nose, & Throat Preparations; Local Anesthetics; Skin/Mucous Membrane Agents; Topical; Pregnancy Category C; DEA Class CII; FDA Pre 1938 Drugs

DESCRIPTION:

An aqueous solution.

Each ml Contains: Cocaine hydrochloride 40 mg or 100 mg

WARNING: MAY BE HABIT FORMING

NOT FOR INJECTION OR OPHTHALMIC USE.

NOTE: External surface of unopened bottle may be sterilized by ethylene oxide only. Do not steam autoclave.

Cocaine hydrochloride USP is a crystalline, granular, or powder substance, having a saline, slightly bitter taste that numbs tongue and lips. Cocaine hydrochloride is a local anesthetic.

CLINICAL PHARMACOLOGY:

Cocaine blocks the initiation or conduction of the nerve impulse following local application, thereby effecting local anesthetic action.

Cocaine is absorbed from all sites of application, including mucous membranes and gastrointestinal mucosa. Cocaine is degraded by plasma esterases, with the half-life in the plasma being, approximately one hour.

INDICATIONS AND USAGE:

Cocaine hydrochloride topical solution is indicated for the introduction of local (topical) anesthesia of accessible mucous membranes of the oral, laryngeal and nasal cavities.

CONTRAINDICATIONS:

Cocaine hydrochloride is contraindicated in patients with a known history of hypersensitivity to the drug or to the components of the solution.

WARNINGS:

RESUSCITATIVE EQUIPMENT AND DRUGS SHOULD BE IMMEDIATELY AVAILABLE WHEN ANY LOCAL ANESTHETIC IS USED.

Carcinogenesis, Mutagenesis: Long-term studies to determine the carcinogenic and mutagenic potential of cocaine are not available.

Pregnancy, Teratogenic Effects, Pregnancy Category C: Animal reproduction studies have not been conducted with cocaine. It is also not known whether the cocaine can cause fetal harm when administered to a pregnant woman or can affect reproduction capacity. Cocaine should be given to a pregnant woman only if needed.

PRECAUTIONS:

The safety and effectiveness of cocaine hydrochloride topical solution depends on proper dosage, correct technique, adequate precautions, and readiness for emergencies. Standard textbooks should be consulted for specific techniques and precautions for various anesthetic procedures.

The lowest dosage that results in effective anesthesia should be used to avoid high plasma levels and serious adverse effects. Debilitated, elderly patients, acutely ill patients, and children should be given reduced doses commensurate with their age and physical status.

Cocaine hydrochloride topical solution should be used with caution in patients with severely traumatized mucosa and sepsis in the region of the proposed application. Use with caution in persons with known drug sensitivities.

ADVERSE REACTIONS:

Adverse reactions may be due to high plasma levels as a result of excessive and rapid absorption of the drug. Reactions are systemic in nature and involve the central nervous system and/or the cardiovascular system. A small number of reactions may result from hypersensitivity, idiosyncrasy or diminished tolerance on the part of the patient.

ADVERSE REACTIONS: *(cont'd)*

CNS reactions are excitatory and/or depressant, and may be characterized by nervousness, restlessness and excitement. Tremors and eventually clonicotonic convulsions may result. Emesis may occur. Central stimulation is followed by depression, with death resulting from respiratory failure.

Small doses of cocaine slow the heart rate, but after moderate doses, the rate is increased due to central sympathetic stimulation.

Cocaine is pyrogenic, augmenting heat production in stimulating muscular activity and causing vasoconstriction which decreases heat loss. Cocaine is known to interfere with the uptake of norepinephrine by adrenergic nerve terminals, producing sensitization to catecholamines, causing vasoconstriction and mydriasis.

Cocaine causes sloughing of the corneal epithelium, causing clouding, pitting, and occasionally ulceration of the cornea. The drug is not meant for ophthalmic use.

OVERDOSAGE:

The fatal dose of cocaine has been approximated 1.2 g, although severe toxic effects have been reported from doses as low as 20 mg.

Symptoms: The symptoms of cocaine poisoning are referable to the CNS, namely the patient becomes excited, restless, garrulous, anxious and confused. Enhanced reflexes, headache, rapid pulse, irregular respiration, chills, rise in body temperature, mydriasis, exophthalmos, nausea, vomiting, and abdominal pain are noticed in severe overdoses, delirium, Cheyne-Stokes respiration, convulsions, unconsciousness and death from respiratory arrest result. Acute poisoning by cocaine is rapid in developing.

Treatment: The specific treatment of acute cocaine poisoning is the intravenous administration of a short-acting barbiturate or diazepam. Artificial respiration may be necessary. It is important to limit absorption of the drug. If entrance of the drug into circulation can be checked, and respiratory exchange maintained, the progress is favorable since cocaine is eliminated fairly rapidly.

DOSAGE AND ADMINISTRATION:

The dosage varies and depends upon the area to be anesthetized, vascularity of the tissues, individual tolerance, and the technique of anesthesia. The lowest dosage needed to provide effective anesthesia should be administered. Dosages should be reduced for children and for elderly and debilitated patients. Cocaine hydrochloride topical solution can be administered by means of cotton applicators or packs, instilled into a cavity, or a spray.

Store at controlled room temperature 15° - 30° C (59° - 89° F).

HOW SUPPLIED - EQUIVALENTS NOT AVAILABLE:

Crystals

5 gm	$293.50	Cocaine Hcl, Mallinckrodt	00406-1520-53
25 gm	$1467.50	Cocaine Hcl, Mallinckrodt	00406-1520-55

Solution - Topical - 4 %

4 ml x 5	$87.89	Cocaine Hcl, Roxane	00054-8211-03
4 ml x 5	$98.88	COCAINE HCL VISCOUS, Roxane	00054-8110-03
4 ml x 5	$98.88	Cocaine Hcl, Roxane	00054-8163-03
4 ml x 5	$113.55	Cocaine Hcl, Schein Pharm (US)	00364-3023-26
4 ml x 5	$124.38	COCAINE HCL VISCOUS, Astra USA	00186-1794-35
10 ml	$48.88	Cocaine Hcl, Roxane	00054-3091-40
10 ml	$48.88	COCAINE HCL VISCOUS, Roxane	00054-3110-40
10 ml	$48.88	Cocaine Hcl, Roxane	00054-3154-40
10 ml	$55.35	Cocaine Hcl, Schein Pharm (US)	00364-3023-54
10 ml	$291.31	Cocaine Hcl Topical, Astra USA	00186-1791-13
10 ml x 5	$308.63	COCAINE HCL VISCOUS, Astra USA	00186-1794-45

Solution - Topical - 10 %

4 ml	$201.31	Cocaine Hcl Topical, Astra USA	00186-1792-78
4 ml x 5	$168.92	COCAINE HCL VISCOUS, Roxane	00054-8111-03
4 ml x 5	$168.92	Cocaine Hcl, Roxane	00054-8164-03
4 ml x 5	$168.92	Cocaine Hcl, Roxane	00054-8212-03
4 ml x 5	$195.30	Cocaine Hcl, Schein Pharm (US)	00364-3024-26
4 ml x 5	$212.81	COCAINE HCL VISCOUS, Astra USA	00186-1795-35
10 ml	$83.85	Cocaine Hcl, Roxane	00054-3092-40
10 ml	$83.85	COCAINE HCL VISCOUS, Roxane	00054-3111-40
10 ml	$83.85	Cocaine Hcl, Roxane	00054-3155-40
10 ml	$98.10	Cocaine Hcl, Schein Pharm (US)	00364-3024-54
10 ml	$499.69	Cocaine Hcl Topical, Astra USA	00186-1793-13
10 ml x 5	$529.06	COCAINE HCL VISCOUS, Astra USA	00186-1795-45

Tablet, Soluble - Misc - 135 mg

100's	$1144.80	Cocaine Hcl, Lilly	00002-2514-02

COD LIVER OIL *(000871)*

CATEGORIES: Vitamin D; Vitamins

BRAND NAMES: *Cod Liver Oil* ; *Cod Liver Oil Capsules*; *Gelosellan* (Germany); *Merluzzina*; *Torskelevertran*
(International brand names outside U.S. in italics)

Prescribing information not available at time of publication.

HOW SUPPLIED - EQUIVALENTS NOT AVAILABLE:

Oil - Oral

480 ml x 12	$54.89	Cod Liver Oil, Purepac Pharm	00228-1249-16

CODEINE PHOSPHATE *(000870)*

CATEGORIES: Analgesics; Antipyretics; Central Nervous System Agents; Narcotic Analgesics; Opiate Agonists (Controlled); Pain; DEA Class CII; FDA Pre 1938 Drugs

BRAND NAMES: *Actacode*; *Codate*; *Codein Knoll*; *Codein Kwizda*; *Codein Phosphate*; *Codein Slovakofarma*; *Codeine Linctus*; *Codeine Phosphate* (Australia); **Codeine Phosphate Injection**; Codeine Sulfate; *Codeinum Phosphorcum*; *Codeisan*; *Codephos*; *Codicept* (Germany); *Codicompren Retard* (Germany); *Codiforton* (Germany); *Colinctus 10*; *Melrosum*; *Paveral* (Canada); *Solcodein*; *Tricodein* (Germany); *Tricodein Solco*
(International brand names outside U.S. in italics)

FORMULARIES: Aetna; Medi-Cal; WHO

DESCRIPTION:

WARNING - MAY BE HABIT FORMING

Codeine is an alkaloid obtained from opium or prepared from morphine by methylation and occurs as white crystals. Codeine effloresces slowly in dry air and is effected by light.

The chemical name of codeine phosphate is 7,8-Didehydro-4,5α-epoxy-3-methoxy-17-methylmorphinan-6α-ol phosphate (1:1)(salt) hemihydrate and has the empirical formula of $C_{18}H_{21}NO_3 \cdot H_3PO_4 \cdot 1/2H_20$. Its molecular weight is 406.4.

Each soluble tablet contains 30 mg (0.074 mmol) or 60 mg (0.15 mmol) of codeine phosphate. These tablets also contain lactose and sucrose.

Soluble tablets of codeine phosphate are freely soluble in water. They are intended for the preparation of solutions for parenteral administration. These tablets are not sterile. Codeine phosphate is an analgesic.

CLINICAL PHARMACOLOGY:

Codeine phosphate is a centrally active analgesic. When administered parenterally, 120 mg of codeine phosphate produces an analgesic response equivalent to that from 10 mg of morphine. Other actions include respiratory depression; depression of the cough center; release of antidiuretic hormone; activation of the vomiting center; pupillary constriction; a decrease in gastric, pancreatic, and biliary secretion; a reduction in intestinal motility; an increase in biliary tract pressure; and an increased amplitude of ureteral contractions.

Onset of analgesia following intramuscular or subcutaneous administration occurs within 10 to 30 minutes. The effect persists for 4 to 6 hours.

Most of a dose of codeine is excreted within 24 hours, 5% to 15% as unchanged codeine and the remainder as a product of glucuronide conjugates of codeine and its metabolites.

INDICATIONS AND USAGE:

Codeine phosphate is an analgesic indicated for the relief of mild to moderate pain.

CONTRAINDICATIONS:

Hypersensitivity to codeine.

PRECAUTIONS:

GENERAL

Head Injury and Increased Intracranial Pressure: The respiratory depressant effects of narcotics and their capacity to elevate cerebrospinal-fluid pressure may be markedly exaggerated in the presence of head injury, other intracranial lesions, or a preexisting increase in intracranial pressure. Furthermore, narcotics produce adverse reactions that may obscure the clinical course in patients with head injuries.

Acute Abdominal Conditions: The administration of codeine or other narcotics may obscure the diagnosis or clinical course in patients with acute abdominal conditions.

Special-Risk Patients: Codeine should be given with caution to certain patients, such as the elderly or debilitated and those with severe impairment of hepatic or renal function, hypothyroidism, Addison's disease, and prostatic hypertrophy or urethral stricture.

Kidney or Liver Dysfunction: Codeine phosphate may have a prolonged cumulative effect in patients with kidney or liver dysfunction.

INFORMATION FOR THE PATIENT

Codeine may impair the mental and/or physical abilities required for the performance of potentially hazardous tasks, such as driving a car or operating machinery. Codeine in combination with other narcotic analgesics, phenothiazines, sedative hypnotics, and alcohol has additive depressant effects.

PREGNANCY CATEGORY C

Animal reproduction studies have not been conducted with codeine phosphate. It is also not known whether codeine phosphate can cause fetal harm when administered to a pregnant woman or can affect reproduction capacity. On the basis of the historical use of codeine phosphate during all stages of pregnancy, there is no known risk of fetal abnormality. Codeine phosphate should be given to a pregnant woman only if clearly needed.

LABOR AND DELIVERY

The use of codeine phosphate in obstetrics may prolong labor. It passes the placental barrier and may produce depression of respiration in the newborn. Resuscitation and, in severe depression, the administration of naloxone may be required.

NURSING MOTHERS

Codeine appears in the milk of nursing mothers. Caution should be exercised when it is administered to a nursing woman.

DRUG INTERACTIONS:

Codeine in combination with other narcotic analgesics, general anesthetics, phenothiazines, tranquilizers, sedative-hypnotics, or other CNS depressants (including alcohol) has additive depressant effects. When such combination therapy is contemplated, the dosage of one or both agents should be reduced.

ADVERSE REACTIONS:

The most frequent adverse reactions include lightheadedness, dizziness, sedation, nausea, and vomiting. These effects seem to be more prominent in ambulatory than in non ambulatory patients, and some of these adverse reactions may be alleviated if the patient lies down.

Other adverse reactions include euphoria, dysphoria, constipation, and pruritus.

DRUG ABUSE AND DEPENDENCE:

Controlled Substance: Codeine phosphate is a Schedule II narcotic.

DEPENDENCE

Although much less potent in this regard than morphine, codeine can produce drug dependence and, therefore, has the potential for being abused. Patients given 60 mg codeine every 6 hours for 2 months usually show some tolerance and mild withdrawal symptoms. Development of the dependent state is recognized by an increased tolerance to the analgesic effect and the appearance of purposive phenomena (complaints, pleas, demands, or manipulative actions) shortly before the time of the next scheduled dose. A patient in withdrawal should be treated in a hospital environment. Usually, it is necessary only to provide supportive care with administration of a tranquilizer to suppress anxiety. Severe symptoms of withdrawal may require administration of a replacement narcotic.

OVERDOSAGE:

SIGNS AND SYMPTOMS

Codeine is metabolized to morphine and its effects are similar to those of morphine and other opiate analgesics. Respiratory depression, sedation and miosis and common symptoms of overdose. Other symptoms include nausea, vomiting, skeletal muscle flaccidity, bradycardia, hypotension, and cool, clammy skin. Apnea and death may ensue; children have had apnea after doses as small as 5 mg/kg. Noncardiac pulmonary edema may develop opioid overdose, and monitoring of heart filling pressure may be helpful.

OVERDOSAGE: *(cont'd)*

TREATMENT

To obtain up-to-date information about the treatment of overdose, a good resource is your Certified Regional Control Center. Telephone numbers of certified poison control centers are listed in the beginning of *Physicians GenRx.* In managing overdosage, consider the possibility of multiple drug overdoses, interaction among drugs, and unusual drug kinetics in your patient.

Naloxone antagonizes most effects of codeine. Protect the airway as Naloxone may induce vomiting. Naloxone has a shorter duration of action than codeine; repeated doses may be needed. In patients who abuse opioids chronically, a withdrawal syndrome may be manifest on administration of naloxone. This may include yawning, tearing, restlessness, sweating, dilated pupils, piloerection, vomiting, diarrhea, and abdominal cramps. This syndrome usually abates quickly as the effect of naloxone dissipates.

Protect the patient's airway and support ventilation and perfusion. Meticulously monitor and maintain, within acceptable limits, the patient's vital signs, blood gases, serum electrolytes, etc. Absorption of drugs from the gastrointestinal tract may be decreased by giving activated charcoal, which in many cases, is more effective than emesis or lavage; consider charcoal instead of or in addition to gastric emptying. Repeated doses of charcoal over time may hasten elimination of some drugs that have been absorbed. Safeguard the patient's airway when employing gastric emptying or charcoal.

Forced diuresis, peritoneal dialysis, hemodialysis, or charcoal hemoperfusion have not been established as beneficial for an overdose of codeine phosphate.

DOSAGE AND ADMINISTRATION:

For Analgesia: Dosage should be adjusted according to the severity of the pain and the response of the patient.

Adults: 15 to 60 mg every 4 to 6 hours (usual adult dose, 30 mg).

Children: 1 Year of Age and Older - 0.5 mg/kg of body weight or 15 mg/m^2 of body surface every 4 to 6 hours.

Soluble tablets codeine phosphate are administered subcutaneously or intramuscularly.

Solutions for injection should be prepared with sterile water and filtered through a 0.22 μ membrane filter.

Note: Do not use the solution if it is more than slightly discolored or contains a precipitate.

HOW SUPPLIED - EQUIVALENTS NOT AVAILABLE:

Injection, Solution - Intramuscular; - 15 mg/ml

2 ml x 10	$8.21	Codeine Carpuject 2Ml, Sanofi Winthrop	00024-0272-02
2 ml x 10	$12.80	Codeine Phosphate, Sanofi Winthrop	00024-0272-03

Injection, Solution - Intramuscular; - 30 mg/ml

1 ml x 10	$8.24	Codeine Phosphate, Wyeth Labs	00008-0728-01
1 ml x 10	$11.99	Codeine Phosphate, Wyeth Labs	00008-0728-50
1 ml x 25	$15.00	Codeine Phosphate, Elkins Sinn	00641-0100-25
2 ml x 10	$9.04	Codeine Carpuject 2Ml, Sanofi Winthrop	00024-0274-02
2 ml x 10	$13.53	Codeine Phosphate, Sanofi Winthrop	00024-0274-04
10 1 ml x 10	$60.00	Codeine Phosphate, Elkins Sinn	00641-0100-26

Injection, Solution - Intramuscular; - 60 mg/ml

1 ml x 10	$9.14	Codeine Phosphate, Wyeth Labs	00008-0729-01
1 ml x 10	$12.89	Codeine Phosphate, Wyeth Labs	00008-0729-50
1 ml x 25	$17.50	Codeine Phosphate, Elkins Sinn	00641-0110-25
10 1 ml x 10	$70.00	Codeine Phosphate, Elkins Sinn	00641-0110-26

Powder

10 gm	$68.88	Codeine Phosphate, Mallinckrodt	00406-1548-32
25 gm	$172.06	Codeine Phosphate, Mallinckrodt	00406-1548-35

Solution - Oral - 15 mg/5ml

5 ml x 40	$52.14	CODEINE PHOSPHATE, Roxane	00054-8160-16
500 ml	$31.58	CODEINE PHOSPHATE, Roxane	00054-3161-63

Tablet, Hypodermic - Intramuscular - 30 mg

100's	$50.34	Codeine Phosphate, Lilly	00002-2557-02

Tablet, Hypodermic - Intramuscular - 60 mg

100's	$96.20	Codeine Phosphate, Lilly	00002-2558-02

Tablet, Uncoated - Oral - 15 mg

25 reverse numb	$33.02	Codeine Sulfate, Roxane	00054-8155-24
100's	$21.35	Codeine Sulfate, Lilly	00002-1009-02

Tablet, Uncoated - Oral - 30 mg

100's	$35.54	Codeine Sulfate, Roxane	00054-4156-25
100's	$35.68	Codeine Sulfate, Lilly	00002-2546-02
100's	$39.36	Codeine Sulfate, Roxane	00054-8156-24
100's	$42.39	Codeine Sulfate, Lilly	00002-1010-02
100's	$46.04	Codeine Sulfate, Knoll Labs	00044-0623-02
1000's	$205.50	Codeine Sulfate, Halsey Drug	00879-0002-10

Tablet, Uncoated - Oral - 60 mg

100's	$65.11	Codeine Sulfate, Roxane	00054-4157-25
100's	$71.47	Codeine Sulfate, Roxane	00054-8157-24
100's	$80.97	Codeine Sulfate, Lilly	00002-1011-02
100's	$87.78	Codeine Sulfate, Knoll Labs	00044-0626-02
250's	$58.50	Codeine Sulfate, Roxane	00054-8157-11

CODEINE PHOSPHATE; GUAIFENESIN *(000881)*

CATEGORIES: Allergies; Antipsychotics/Antimanics; Antitussives; Antitussives/Expectorants/Mucolytics; Central Nervous System Agents; Common Cold; Congestion; Cough Preparations; Expectorants; Respiratory & Allergy Medications; Vertigo/Motion Sickness/Vomiting; DEA Class CIII; DEA Class CV; FDA Pre 1938 Drugs

BRAND NAMES: Baytussin A.C.; Biotussin Ac; Bitex; Bron-Tuss; Brontex; Cheracol; Cheratussin Ac; Cherospect; Cherralex W/Codeine; Codefen; *Codesia;* Gani-Tuss Nr; Glyatuss Ac; Glydeine; Guaifen-C; Guaifenesin Ac; Guaifenesin W/Codeine; Guaituss Ac; Guiatuss Ac; Guiatussin Ac; Guiatussin W/Codeine; Halotussin-Dac; Iofen-C Nf; Marcof; Medi-Tuss W/Codeine; Mytussin Ac; Nortussin; Robafen Ac; Robichem Ac; **Robitussin-Ac**; Robolene Ac; Tolu-Sed; Tussi-Organidin Nr; Tussi-Organidin-S Nr; Tussidin Nr; Tussin Ac

(International brand names outside U.S. in italics)

FORMULARIES: Aetna; BC-BS; FHP; Medi-Cal; PCS

DESCRIPTION:

GUAIFENESIN AND CODEINE

Each 5 ml (1 teaspoonful) Contains: Guaifenesin, USP 100 mg and codeine Phosphate, USP 10 mg and alcohol 3.5 percent. In a palatable, aromatic syrup.

(Warning: May be habit forming)

Inactive Ingredients: Caramel, Citric Acid, FD&C Red 40, Flavors, Glycerin, Saccharin Sodium, Sodium Benzoate, Sorbitol, Water.

CLINICAL PHARMACOLOGY:

This syrup preparation combines the expectorant, guaifenesin, with the cough suppressant, codeine. Guaifenesin enhances the output of lower respiratory tract fluid. The enhanced flow of less viscid secretions promotes and facilitates the removal of mucus. Codeine is a centrally acting agent which elevates the threshold for cough. As a result, dry, unproductive coughs become more productive and less frequent.

Under Federal law, this preparation is available without a prescription. Certain state laws may differ. The container label contains the following indications, warnings and drug interaction precaution statements and directions:

INDICATIONS AND USAGE:

Temporarily controls cough due to minor throat and bronchial irritation as may occur with the common cold or inhaled irritants. Helps loosen phlegm (mucus) and thin bronchial secretions to make coughs more productive.

WARNINGS:

A persistent cough may be a sign of a serious condition. If cough persists for more than 1 week, tends to recur, or is accompanied by fever, rash, or persistent headache, consult a doctor. Do not take this product for persistent or chronic cough such as occurs with smoking, asthma, chronic bronchitis, emphysema, or if cough is accompanied by excessive phlegm (mucus) unless directed by a doctor. Adults and children who have a chronic pulmonary disease or shortness of breath, or children who are taking other drugs, should not take this product unless directed by a doctor. May cause or aggravate constipation. As with any drug, if you are pregnant or nursing a baby, seek the advice of a health professional before using this product.

Professional Note: Guaifenesin has been shown to produce a color interference with certain clinical laboratory determinations of 5-hydroxyindoleacetic acid (5-HIAA) and vanillylmandelic acid (VMA).

DRUG INTERACTIONS:

Caution should be used when taking this product with sedatives, tranquilizers and drugs used for depression, especially monoamine oxidase inhibitors (MAOIs). These combinations may cause greater sedation (drowsiness) than is caused by the products used alone.

Directions: Take orally as stated below or use as directed by a doctor. *Adults and Children 12 Years of Age and Over:* 2 teaspoonfuls every 4 hours, not to exceed 12 teaspoonfuls in a 24-hour period; *Children 6 to Under 12 Years:* 1 teaspoonful every 4 hours, not to exceed 6 teaspoonfuls in a 24-hour period; *Children Under 6 Years:* consult a doctor. A special measuring device should be used to give an accurate dose of this product to children under 6 years of age. Giving a higher dose than recommended by a doctor could result in serious side effects for a child. Use of codeine-containing preparations is not recommended for children under 2 years of age. Do not exceed recommended dosage.

HOW SUPPLIED - EQUIVALENTS NOT AVAILABLE:

Syrup - Oral - 10 mg/100 mg/5m

118 ml	$3.20	Guaifenesin W/Codeine, Schein Pharm (US)	00364-2621-77
120 ml	$2.50	HALOTUSSIN-DAC, Halsey Drug	00879-0682-04
120 ml	$2.55	Guaituss Ac, HL Moore Drug Exch	00839-7953-79
120 ml	$2.70	Robafen Ac, Major Pharms	00904-0054-20
120 ml	$2.78	Cheratussin Ac, Qualitest Pharms	00603-1075-54
120 ml	$2.82	Halotussin AC Sugar Free, HL Moore Drug Exch	00839-7784-65
120 ml	$2.84	Guiatuss Ac, Alpharma	00472-0012-04
120 ml	$2.85	GUIATUSS AC, Consolidated Midland	00223-6515-01
120 ml	$2.90	HALOTUSSIN-AC, Halsey Drug	00879-0660-04
120 ml	$2.90	Biotussin Ac, Bio Pharm	59741-0113-04
120 ml	$2.90	Mytussin Ac, Morton Grove	60432-0045-04
120 ml	$2.95	Guaifenesin Ac, HR Cenci	00556-0477-04
120 ml	$3.00	Guiatussin Ac, Hi Tech Pharma	50383-0087-04
120 ml	$3.00	ROBICHEM AC, H N Norton Co.	50732-0883-04
120 ml	$3.04	Guaituss Ac, HL Moore Drug Exch	00839-7953-65
120 ml	$3.38	Guaifenesin W/Codeine, IDE-Interstate	00814-3580-76
120 ml	$3.55	Guaifenesin W/Codeine, Aligen Independ	00405-0090-76
120 ml	$3.72	Guiatussin W/Codeine, Rugby	00536-0981-97
120 ml	$6.60	MEDI-TUSS W/CODEINE, Medi-Plex Pharm	59010-0150-04
120 ml x 4	$57.01	TUSSI-ORGANIDIN-S NR, Wallace Labs	00037-4814-01
240 ml	$3.20	Guaifenesin Ac, HR Cenci	00556-0477-08
240 ml	$4.60	HALOTUSSIN-AC, Halsey Drug	00879-0660-08
240 ml	$4.85	Guiatuss Ac, Alpharma	00472-0012-08
240 ml	$5.20	HALOTUSSIN-DAC, Halsey Drug	00879-0682-08
473 ml	$7.50	Guaifenesin Ac, United Res	00677-1492-33
473 ml	$21.25	Guaifen-C, Qualitest Pharms	00603-1276-58
473 ml	$23.16	BRON-TUSS, Am Generics	58634-0012-01
473 ml	$24.95	BITEX, Econolab	55053-0600-16
473 ml	$28.37	BRONTEX, Procter Gamble Pharm	00149-0441-16
480 ml	$7.30	Cheratussin Ac, Qualitest Pharms	00603-1075-58
480 ml	$7.60	TUSSCIDIN A-C EXPECTORANT, HR Cenci	00556-0196-16
480 ml	$7.65	Guaifenesin Ac, HR Cenci	00556-0477-16
480 ml	$7.90	Halotussin AC Sugar Free, HL Moore Drug Exch	00839-7784-69
480 ml	$7.90	Guiatuss Ac, Harber Pharm	51432-0602-20
480 ml	$8.05	ROBAFEN AC, Major Pharms	00904-0054-16
480 ml	$8.19	Guiatuss Ac, Alpharma	00472-0012-16
480 ml	$8.27	GLYDEINE COUGH SYRUP, Geneva Pharms	00781-6899-16
480 ml	$8.34	Guaifenesin W/Codeine, Schein Pharm (US)	00364-2621-16
480 ml	$8.50	GUIATUSS AC, Consolidated Midland	00223-6515-02
480 ml	$8.50	HALOTUSSIN-AC, Halsey Drug	00879-0660-16
480 ml	$8.50	ROBICHEM AC, H N Norton Co.	50732-0883-16
480 ml	$8.50	Biotussin Ac, Bio Pharm	59741-0113-16
480 ml	$8.73	Guiatussin W/Codeine, Rugby	00536-0981-85
480 ml	$8.90	Mytussin Ac, Morton Grove	60432-0045-16
480 ml	$9.17	Guaituss Ac, HL Moore Drug Exch	00839-7953-69
480 ml	$9.20	Guiatussin Ac, Hi Tech Pharma	50383-0087-16
480 ml	$9.38	GUAICOLATE W/CODEINE, IDE-Interstate	00814-3580-82
480 ml	$10.12	Guaifenesin W/Codeine, Aligen Independ	00405-0090-16
480 ml	$22.30	MARCOF EXPECTORANT, Marnel Pharceut	00682-0445-16
480 ml	$24.90	Codefen, Alphagen Labs	59743-0023-16
480 ml	$39.95	Gani-Tuss Nr, Cypress Pharm	60258-0261-16
480 ml	$47.86	Iofen-C Nf, Superior	00144-0637-16
480 ml	$59.83	TUSSI-ORGANIDIN NR, Wallace Labs	00037-4814-10
3785 ml	$52.50	Guaifenesin Ac, HR Cenci	00556-0477-28

HOW SUPPLIED - EQUIVALENTS NOT AVAILABLE: *(cont'd)*

3840 ml	$41.43	Guiatussin W/Codeine, Rugby	00536-0981-90
3840 ml	$49.00	GUIATUSS AC, Consolidated Midland	00223-6515-03
3840 ml	$50.38	ROBAFEN AC, Major Pharms	00904-0054-28
3840 ml	$51.00	Guiatuss Ac, Harber Pharm	51432-0602-21
3840 ml	$51.19	TUSSCIDIN A-C EXPECTORANT, HR Cenci	00556-0196-28
3840 ml	$51.23	Halotussin AC Sugar Free, HL Moore Drug Exch	00839-7784-70
3840 ml	$51.99	ROBICHEM AC, H N Norton Co.	50732-0883-28
3840 ml	$51.99	Mytussin Ac, Morton Grove	60432-0045-28
3840 ml	$53.41	Guiatuss Ac, HL Moore Drug Exch	00839-7953-70
3840 ml	$53.57	Cheratussin Ac, Qualitest Pharms	00603-1075-60
3840 ml	$55.72	HALOTUSSIN-AC, Halsey Drug	00879-0660-28
3840 ml	$55.80	Guiatuss Ac, Alpharma	00472-0012-28

Tablet, Uncoated - Oral - 300 mg/10 mg

100's	$49.95	Guaifenesin/Codeine Phosphate, Pecos	59879-0512-01
100's	$53.99	Guaifenesin/Codeine Phosphate, Rugby	00536-5676-01
100's	$53.99	Guaifenesin/Codeine Phosphate, Ethex	58177-0223-04
100's	$59.99	BRONTEX, Procter Gamble Pharm	00149-0440-01

CODEINE PHOSPHATE; GUAIFENESIN; PHENYLPROPANOLAMINE *(000883)*

CATEGORIES: Antitussives; Antitussives/Expectorants/Mucolytics; Cough Preparations; Expectorants; Respiratory & Allergy Medications; DEA Class CV; FDA Pre 1938 Drugs

BRAND NAMES: Alphen; C-Tussin; Chemdal; Codegest; Codeine/Phenylprop/Guaifenesin; Codemine; Conex W/Codeine; Cyndal; Dihistine; Efasin; **Endal**; Naldecon-Cx; Novagest; Statuss; Triaminic W/Codeine

Prescribing information not available at time of publication.

HOW SUPPLIED - RATED THERAPEUTICALLY EQUIVALENT:

Liquid - Oral - 10 mg/100 mg/12

480 ml	$18.25	Alphen, Alphagen Labs	59743-0112-16

HOW SUPPLIED - NOT RATED EQUIVALENT:

Liquid - Oral - 10 mg/100 mg/12

120 ml	$2.90	Dihistine, HL Moore Drug Exch	00839-6695-65
120 ml	$3.00	Novagest, Major Pharms	00904-0923-20
120 ml	$3.50	Dihistine, Consolidated Midland	00223-6132-01
473 ml	$28.74	Statuss, Huckaby Pharma	58407-0376-16
480 ml	$10.95	Dihistine, Consolidated Midland	00223-6132-02
480 ml	$15.99	Codemine, Elge	58298-0435-16
480 ml	$17.95	Efasin, Major Pharms	00904-3541-16
480 ml	$19.80	Cyndal, Cypress Pharm	60258-0695-16
480 ml	$20.95	Codeine/Phenylprop/Guaifenesin, Aligen Independ	00405-0059-16
480 ml	$22.90	Codeine/Phenylprop/Guaifenesin, Goldline Labs	00182-0153-40
480 ml	$23.39	NALDECON-CX ADULT, Mead Johnson	00015-5661-60
480 ml	**$38.44**	**ENDAL EXPECTORANT LIQUID, UAD Labs**	**00785-6226-16**
3840 ml	$59.48	Dihistine, Consolidated Midland	00223-6132-03

CODEINE PHOSPHATE; GUAIFENESIN; PSEUDOEPHEDRINE HYDROCHLORIDE *(000873)*

CATEGORIES: Allergies; Antihistamines; Antitussives; Antitussives/Expectorants/Mucolytics; Bronchitis; Common Cold; Congestion; Cough Preparations; Decongestants; Expectorants; Hay Fever; Infections; Influenza; Nasal Congestion; Otitis Media; Pruritus; Respiratory & Allergy Medications; Rhinitis; Sinus Congestion; Sinusitis; Sympathomimetic Agents; Pregnancy Category C; DEA Class CIII; DEA Class CIV; DEA Class CV; FDA Pre 1938 Drugs

BRAND NAMES: Alamine Expectorant; Biotussin Dac; Cheratussin Dac; Co-Histine; Codafed; Cophene Xp; Cycofed; Decohistine; Decongestant; Deconsal C; Deproist W/Codeine; Dihistine; Glyatuss Dac; Guaifenesin Dac; Guaifenesin/P-Ephedrine/Cod; Guaituss Dac; Guiatuss Dac; Guiatuss-Dac; Guiatussin Dac; Isoclor; Isoclor Expectorant; Kg-Fed; Kg-Fed Pediatric; Medi-Tuss Dac; Mytussin Dac; Novadyne; Novagest; Novahistine; Nucochem; Nucodine Exp; Nucodine Ped; **Nucofed**; Nucotuss; Phenhist; Phenylhistine; Robafen-Dac; Robichem Dac; Robitussin-Dac; Ryna-Cx; Tussar-2; Tussar-Sf; Tussin Dac

FORMULARIES: FHP; PCS

DESCRIPTION:

Codeine Phosphate, Pseudoephedrine Hydrochloride and Guaifenesin may be represented by the following chemical names:

7,8-didehydro-4,5α-epoxy-3-methoxy-17-methylmorphinan-6α-ol Phosphate (1:1) salt hemihydrate; *(S-(R*,R*))*-α-[1-(methylamino)ethyl]benzene methanol hydrochloride; 3-(O-methoxyphenoxy)-1,2-propanediol.

FOR COMPLETE PRESCRIBING INFORMATION, REFER TO INDIVIDUAL DRUG MONOGRAPHS (CODEINE PHOSPHATE; GUAIFENESIN; PSEUDOEPHEDRINE HYDROCHLORIDE).

INDICATIONS AND USAGE:

This drug is indicated for symptomatic relief when both coughing and congestion are associated with upper respiratory infections and related conditions such as common cold, bronchitis, influenza, and sinusitis.

DOSAGE AND ADMINISTRATION:

EXPECTORANT-RECOMMENDED DOSAGE

Adults: 1 teaspoonful every 6 hours, not to exceed 4 teaspoonfuls in 24 hours.

Children: *6 to Under 12 Years:* 1/2 teaspoonful every 6 hours, not to exceed 2 teaspoonfuls in 24 hours. *2 to Under 6 Years:* 1/4 teaspoonful every 6 hours, not to exceed 1 teaspoonful in 24 hours.

Do not give this product to children under **2 years,** except under the advice and supervision of physician.

PEDIATRIC EXPECTORANT

6 to Under 12 Years: 1 teaspoonful every 6 hours, not to exceed 4 teaspoonfuls in 24 hours.

2 to Under 6 Years: ½ teaspoonful every 6 hours, not to exceed 2 teaspoonful in 24 hours.

DOSAGE AND ADMINISTRATION: *(cont'd)*

Do not give this product to children under **2 years,** except under the advice and supervision of physician.

HOW SUPPLIED - EQUIVALENTS NOT AVAILABLE:

Syrup - Oral - 10 mg/100 mg/30

120 ml	$2.62	DEPROIST W/CODEINE, Geneva Pharms	00781-6606-04
120 ml	$2.90	PHENYLHISTINE EXPECTORANT, HR Cenci	00556-0333-04
120 ml	$2.90	Decohistine, Morton Grove	60432-0585-04
120 ml	$3.09	Halotussin DAC Sugar Free, HL Moore Drug Exch	00839-7785-65
120 ml	$3.10	Phenylhistine, Halsey Drug	00879-0729-04
120 ml	$3.15	DIHISTINE, Alpharma	00472-1640-04
120 ml	$3.15	Co-Histine, Hi Tech Pharma	50383-0086-04
120 ml	$4.00	ROBICHEM DAC, H N Norton Co.	50732-0885-04
120 ml	$4.20	Biotussin Dac, Bio Pharm	59741-0115-04
120 ml	$4.79	PHENHIST, Rugby	00536-1910-97
120 ml	$5.00	Mytussin Dac, Morton Grove	60432-0541-04
120 ml x 6	$118.43	TUSSAR-SF, Rhone-Poulenc Rorer	00075-1700-05
473 ml	$13.00	Guiatussin Dac, Hi Tech Pharma	50383-0088-16
473 ml	$20.00	Cophene Xp, Dunhall Pharms	00217-2834-11
473 ml	$21.58	Nucodine Ped, Am Generics	58634-0007-01
473 ml	**$34.50**	**NUCOFED, Roberts Labs**	**54092-0405-16**
480 ml	$8.77	DEPROIST W/CODEINE, Geneva Pharms	00781-6606-16
480 ml	$8.90	Phenylhistine, Qualitest Pharms	00603-1521-58
480 ml	$9.50	PHENYLHISTINE EXPECTORANT, HR Cenci	00556-0333-16
480 ml	$10.30	Decohistine, Morton Grove	60432-0585-16
480 ml	$10.38	GUIATUSSIN DAC, Rugby	00536-0790-85
480 ml	$10.38	Guiatussin Dac, Rugby	00536-0945-85
480 ml	$10.40	Phenylhistine, Halsey Drug	00879-0729-16
480 ml	$10.46	DIHISTINE, Alpharma	00472-1640-16
480 ml	$10.50	Co-Histine, Hi Tech Pharma	50383-0086-16
480 ml	$11.39	PHENHIST, Rugby	00536-1910-85
480 ml	$12.70	ROBAFEN-DAC, Major Pharms	00904-0042-16
480 ml	$12.75	Biotussin Dac, Bio Pharm	59741-0115-16
480 ml	$12.80	Guaifenesin Dac, HR Cenci	00556-0432-16
480 ml	$12.90	Guiatuss Dac, Harber Pharm	51432-0603-20
480 ml	$13.00	Guiatuss Dac, United Res	00677-1438-33
480 ml	$13.29	GUIATUSS DAC, TX Drug Reps	47202-1255-01
480 ml	$13.40	Mytussin Dac, Morton Grove	60432-0541-16
480 ml	$13.50	ROBICHEM DAC, H N Norton Co.	50732-0885-16
480 ml	$13.55	Guiatuss Dac, Alpharma	00472-0011-16
480 ml	$14.87	Pseudoephedrine G W/Codeine, Rugby	00536-1519-85
480 ml	$15.73	Halotussin DAC Sugar Free, HL Moore Drug Exch	00839-7785-69
480 ml	$16.27	Guaituss Dac, HL Moore Drug Exch	00839-7954-69
480 ml	$16.81	Guaifenesin/P-Ephed/Codeine, Aligen Independ	00405-0093-16
480 ml	$18.46	NUCOCHEM PEDIATRIC EXPECTORANT SYRUP, H N Norton Co.	50732-0858-16
480 ml	$18.50	NUCOTUSS PEDIATRIC EXPECTORANT SYRUP, Alpharma	00472-1240-16
480 ml	$18.50	Antitussive/Decongestant, Major Pharms	00904-7756-16
480 ml	$18.50	Cycofed, Cypress Pharm	60258-0603-16
480 ml	$19.47	Guaifenesin/P-Ephedrine/Cod, Aligen Independ	00405-0057-16
480 ml	$19.94	Kg-Fed Pediatric, King Pharms	60793-0029-16
480 ml	$20.85	Guaifenesin/P-Ephedrine/Cod, Goldline Labs	00182-0155-40
480 ml	$30.13	Deconsal, Medeva Pharms	53014-0046-47
480 ml	$65.63	TUSSAR-SF, Rhone-Poulenc Rorer	00075-1700-01
480 ml	$65.63	TUSSAR-2, Rhone-Poulenc Rorer	00075-1702-01
3840 ml	$41.97	C-TUSSIN, Century Pharms	00436-0920-28
3840 ml	$49.84	PHENHIST, Rugby	00536-1910-90
3840 ml	$55.45	Novagest, Major Pharms	00904-0923-28
3840 ml	$58.60	PHENYLHISTINE EXPECTORANT, HR Cenci	00556-0333-28
3840 ml	$58.60	Phenylhistine, Halsey Drug	00879-0729-28
3840 ml	$73.00	ROBICHEM DAC, H N Norton Co.	50732-0885-28

Syrup - Oral - 20 mg/200 mg/60

473 ml	$31.44	Nucodine Exp, Am Generics	58634-0006-01
473 ml	**$50.26**	**NUCOFED, Roberts Labs**	**54092-0404-16**
480 ml	$22.00	Pseudoephedrine G W/Codeine, Rugby	00536-1518-85
480 ml	$26.95	NUCOTUSS EXPECTORANT SYRUP, Alpharma	00472-1245-16
480 ml	$26.98	NUCOCHEM EXPECTORANT SYRUP, H N Norton Co.	50732-0857-16
480 ml	$27.00	Antitussive/Decongestant, Major Pharms	00904-7757-16
480 ml	$27.10	Cycofed, Cypress Pharm	60258-0602-16
480 ml	$28.50	Kg-Fed, King Pharms	60793-0028-16
480 ml	$28.52	Guaifenesin/P-Ephedrine/Cod, Aligen Independ	00405-0056-16
480 ml	$30.40	Guaifenesin/P-Ephedrine/Cod, Goldline Labs	00182-0154-40
480 ml	$43.87	Deconsal C, Medeva Pharms	53014-0040-47

CODEINE PHOSPHATE; IODINATED GLYCEROL *(000874)*

CATEGORIES: Antitussives; Antitussives/Expectorants/Mucolytics; Asthma; Bronchitis; Chronic Bronchitis; Cough Preparations; Croup; Decongestants; Emphysema; Iodide Salts; Mucolytic Agents; Pertussis; Pharyngitis; Respiratory & Allergy Medications; Tracheobronchitis; Pregnancy Category X; DEA Class CV; FDA Pre 1938 Drugs

BRAND NAMES: Bio-Tuss C; Io Tuss; Iocen-C; Iodur W/Codeine; Iophen-C; Iotuss; Myodine C; Oridol C; Roganidin; **Tussi-Organidin**; Tussi-R-Gen

COST OF THERAPY: $154.83 (Asthma; Solution; 10 mg/30 mg; 30/day; 365 days) vs. Potential Cost of $3,576.99 (DRG 96, Bronchitis & Asthma)

PRIMARY ICD9: 493.90 (Asthma, Unspecified, Without Mention of Status Asthmaticus)

DESCRIPTION:

Active Ingredients: Each 5 ml (one teaspoonful) contains:

Iodinated Glycerol 30 mg

(Containing 15 mg organically bound iodine)

Codeine Phosphate 10 mg

Warning: May Be Habit Forming.

Inactive Ingredients: Citric Acid, FD & C Red # 40, Flavor (artificial), Glycerin, Propylene Glycol, Purified Water, Sodium Benzoate, Sodium Citrate, Sodium Saccharin, Sorbitol Solution.

DESCRIPTION: *(cont'd)*

Iodinated glycerol, a mucolytic-expectorant, is an isomeric mixture formed by the interaction of iodine and glycerol, whose structural and chemical formulas have not been precisely established. Iodinated glycerol is a viscous, amber liquid stable in acid media, including gastric juice, which contains virtually no inorganic iodide and no free iodine. Contains codeine phosphate an antitussive.

CLINICAL PHARMACOLOGY:

Codeine phosphate w/iodinated glycerol liquid combines the antitussive action of codeine with the mucolytic-expectorant action of iodinated glycerol.

INDICATIONS AND USAGE:

Codeine phosphate w/iodinated glycerol liquid is indicated for the symptomatic relief of irritating, nonproductive cough associated with respiratory tract conditions such as chronic bronchitis, bronchial asthma, tracheobronchitis and the common cold; also for the symptomatic relief of cough accompanying other respiratory tract conditions such as laryngitis, pharyngitis, croup, pertussis and emphysema. Appropriate therapy should be provided for the primary disease.

CONTRAINDICATIONS:

History of marked sensitivity to inorganic iodides; hypersensitivity to any of the ingredients or related compounds; pregnancy; newborns; and nursing mothers.

The human fetal thyroid begins to concentrate iodine in the 12th to 14th week of gestation and the use of inorganic iodides in pregnant women during this period and thereafter has rarely been reported to induce fetal goiter (with or without hypothyroidism) with the potential for airway obstruction. If the patient becomes pregnant while taking codeine phosphate w/iodinated glycerol liquid, the drug should be discontinued and the patient should be apprised of the potential risk to the fetus.

WARNINGS:

Discontinue use if rash or other evidence of hypersensitivity appears. Use with caution or avoid use in patients with history or evidence of thyroid disease.

PRECAUTIONS:

General: Iodides have been reported to cause a flare-up of adolescent acne. Children with cystic fibrosis appear to have an exaggerated susceptibility to the goitrogenic effect of iodides. Dermatitis and other reversible manifestation of iodism have been reported with chronic use of inorganic iodides. Although these have not been reported to be a problem clinically with iodinated glycerol formulations, they should be kept in mind in patients receiving these preparations for prolonged periods.

Carcinogenesis, Mutagenesis, and Impairment of Fertility: No long-term animal studies have been performed with Codeine phosphate w/iodinated glycerol liquid.

Pregnancy, Teratogenic Effects, Pregnancy Category X: (see CONTRAINDICATIONS)

Nursing Mothers: Codeine phosphate w/iodinated glycerol liquid should not be administered to a nursing mother.

DRUG INTERACTIONS:

Iodides may potentiate the hypothyroid effect of lithium and other antithyroid drugs.

ADVERSE REACTIONS:

Side effects have been rare, including those which may occur with the individual active ingredients and which may be modified as a result of their combination. *Iodinated Glycerol:* Rare side effects include gastrointestinal irritation, rash, hypersensitivity, thyroid gland enlargement, and acute parotitis, *Codeine:* Nausea, vomiting, constipation, drowsiness, and miosis have been reported.

DRUG ABUSE AND DEPENDENCE:

Controlled Substance-Schedule V Dependence: Codeine may be habit forming.

OVERDOSAGE:

Acute overdose experience with iodinated glycerol has been rare and there have been no reports of any serious problems.

DOSAGE AND ADMINISTRATION:

Adults: 1 to 2 teaspoonfuls every 4 hours.

Children: $\frac{1}{2}$ to 1 teaspoonful every 4 hours.

Dispense in a tight container. Store at controlled room temperature 15 - 30°C (59-86°F); avoid excessive heat. Keep bottle tightly closed.

HOW SUPPLIED - EQUIVALENTS NOT AVAILABLE:

Solution - Oral - 10 mg/30 mg

5 ml x 40	$17.58	Iodinated Glycerol/Codeine, Roxane	00054-8398-16
120 ml	$2.70	IOCEN-DM LIQUID, HR Cenci	00556-0457-04
120 ml	$3.10	IOCEN-C LIQUID, HR Cenci	00556-0456-04
120 ml	**$8.18**	**TUSSI-ORGANIDIN, Wallace Labs**	**00037-4812-01**
480 ml	$8.30	IOCEN-DM LIQUID, HR Cenci	00556-0457-16
480 ml	$9.60	IOCEN-C, HR Cenci	00556-0456-16
480 ml	$10.45	TORGANIC-C, Major Pharms	00904-1546-16
480 ml	$12.20	Iodur W/Codeine, Aligen Independ	00405-0103-16
480 ml	$12.25	Iodinated Glycerol W/Codeine, Geneva Pharms	00781-6300-16
500 ml	$7.07	Iodinated Glycerol/Codeine Phosphate, Roxane	00054-3398-63
3840 ml	$55.87	IOCEN-DM LIQUID, HR Cenci	00556-0457-28
3840 ml	$64.97	IOCEN-C, HR Cenci	00556-0456-28

Solution - Oral - 20 mg/60 mg

10 ml x 40	$23.90	Iodinated Glycerol/Codeine, Roxane	00054-8399-16

CODEINE PHOSPHATE; PHENYLEPHRINE HYDROCHLORIDE; PHENIRAMINE; POTASSIUM CITRATE *(000868)*

CATEGORIES: Antitussives; Antitussives/Expectorants/Mucolytics; Cough Preparations; Expectorants; Respiratory & Allergy Medications; DEA Class CV; FDA Pre 1938 Drugs

BRAND NAMES: Tussirex

Prescribing information not available at time of publication.

HOW SUPPLIED - EQUIVALENTS NOT AVAILABLE:

Liquid - Oral

120 ml	$7.19	TUSSIREX WITH CODEINE, Scot Tussin	00372-0017-04
120 ml	$7.19	TUSSIREX, SUGAR-FREE, Scot Tussin	00372-0018-04
240 ml	$12.35	TUSSIREX WITH CODEINE, Scot Tussin	00372-0017-08
240 ml	$12.35	TUSSIREX, SUGAR-FREE, Scot Tussin	00372-0018-08
480 ml	$25.66	TUSSIREX WITH CODEINE, Scot Tussin	00372-0017-16
480 ml	$28.31	TUSSIREX, Scot Tussin	00372-0018-16
840 ml	$183.57	TUSSIREX WITH CODEINE, Scot Tussin	00372-0017-28
3785 ml	$183.57	TUSSIREX, Scot Tussin	00372-0018-28

CODEINE PHOSPHATE; PHENYLEPHRINE HYDROCHLORIDE; PROMETHAZINE HYDROCHLORIDE *(000875)*

CATEGORIES: Allergies; Anaphylactic Shock; Anesthesia; Angioedema; Antihistamines; Antitussives; Antitussives/Expectorants/Mucolytics; Anxiety; Common Cold; Congestion; Conjunctivitis; Cough Preparations; Decongestants; Expectorants; Influenza; Nasal Congestion; Nausea; Respiratory & Allergy Medications; Rhinitis; Urticaria; Pregnancy Category C; DEA Class CV; FDA Approved 1984 Apr

BRAND NAMES: M-Phen; Mallergan Vc; Para-Hist; **Phenergan Vc W/Codeine**; Pherazine Vc W/Codeine; Promethazine Vc W/Codeine

FORMULARIES: Aetna; BC-BS

DESCRIPTION:

FOR COMPLETE PRESCRIBING INFORMATION, REFER TO THE INDIVIDUAL DRUG MONOGRAPHS (CODEINE PHOSPHATE; PHENYLEPHRINE HYDROCHLORIDE; PROMETHAZINE HYDROCHLORIDE).

INDICATIONS AND USAGE:

Promethazine/phenylephrine with codeine is indicated for the temporary relief of coughs and upper respiratory symptoms, including nasal congestion, associated with allergy or the common cold.

DOSAGE AND ADMINISTRATION:

The average effective dose is given in TABLE 1:

TABLE 1

Adults	1 teaspoon (5 ml) every 4 to 6 hours, not to exceed 30.0 ml in 24 hours.
Children 6 years to under 12 years	1/2 to 1 teaspoon (2.5 to 5 ml) every 4 to 6 hours, not to exceed 30.0 ml in 24 hours.
Children under 6 years (weight: 18 kg or 40 lbs)	1/4 to 1/2 teaspoon (1.25 to 2.5 ml) every 4 to 6 hours, not to exceed 9.0 ml in 24 hours.
Children under 6 years (weight: 16 kg or 35 lbs)	1/4 to 1/2 teaspoon (1.25 to 2.5 ml) every 4 to 6 hours, not to exceed 8.0 ml in 24 hours.
Children under 6 years (weight: 14 kg or 30 lbs)	1/4 to 1/2 teaspoon (1.25 to 2.5 ml) every 4 to 6 hours, not to exceed 7.0 ml in 24 hours.
Children under 6 years (weight: 12 kg or 25 lbs)	1/4 to 1/2 teaspoon (1.25 to 2.5 ml) every 4 to 6 hours, not to exceed 6.0 ml in 24 hours.

Promethazine/phenylephrine with codeine is not recommended for children under 2 years of age.

Store at Room Temperature, between 15 and 25° C (59 and 77° F).

HOW SUPPLIED - RATED THERAPEUTICALLY EQUIVALENT:

Syrup - Oral - 10 mg/5 mg/6.25

4 oz	$4.70	Prometh Vc With Codeine Cough Syrup, Alpharma	00472-1629-04
16 oz	$12.34	Prometh Vc With Codeine Cough Syrup, Alpharma	00472-1629-16
120 ml	$1.50	Promethazine Vc With Codeine, H.C.F.A. F F P	99999-0875-01
120 ml	$2.60	Promethazine Vc/Codeine Cough Syrup, HR Cenci	00556-0345-04
120 ml	$3.50	Promethazine Vc With Codeine, HL Moore Drug Exch	00839-7061-65
120 ml	$3.95	Promethazine Vc With Codeine, Rugby	00536-1872-97
120 ml	$4.00	Promethazine Vc W/Codeine, Morton Grove	60432-0607-04
120 ml	$4.10	PHENAMETH VC W/CODEINE COUGH SYRUP, Major Pharms	00904-1514-00
120 ml	$4.10	Promethazine Vc W/Codeine, Major Pharms	00904-1514-20
120 ml	$4.38	Promethazine Vc W/Codeine, Qualitest Pharms	00603-1581-54
120 ml	$4.65	PHERAZINE VC WITH CODEINE SYRUP, Halsey Drug	00879-0515-04
120 ml x 24	**$229.25**	**PHENERGAN VC WITH CODEINE, Wyeth Labs**	**00008-0552-02**
473 ml	$8.74	Promethazine Vc W/Codeine, Aligen Independ	00405-0170-16
480 ml	$6.00	Promethazine Vc With Codeine, H.C.F.A. F F P	99999-0875-02
480 ml	$6.24	Promethazine Vc With Codeine, United Res	00677-0965-33
480 ml	$8.30	Promethazine Vc/Codeine Cough Syrup, HR Cenci	00556-0345-16
480 ml	$8.49	Promethazine Vc With Codeine, HL Moore Drug Exch	00839-7061-69
480 ml	$9.95	Prometh VC With Codeine Syrup, Schein Pharm (US)	00364-7389-16
480 ml	$10.50	Prometh Vc With Codeine Cough Syrup, Goldline Labs	00182-1713-40
480 ml	$10.88	PHENAMETH VC W/CODEINE, Major Pharms	00904-1514-16
480 ml	$11.32	Promethazine Vc W/Codeine, Morton Grove	60432-0607-16
480 ml	$11.80	Promethazine Vc W/Codeine, Qualitest Pharms	00603-1581-58
480 ml	$11.90	M-PHEN, RA McNeil	12830-0656-02
480 ml	$11.95	Promethazine Vc With Codeine, Rugby	00536-1872-85
480 ml	$12.25	PHERAZINE VC WITH CODEINE SYRUP, Halsey Drug	00879-0515-16
480 ml	$17.70	Promethazine Vc With Codeine, Geneva Pharms	00781-6950-16
480 ml	**$34.48**	**PHENERGAN VC WITH CODEINE, Wyeth Labs**	**00008-0552-03**
3785 ml	$70.35	PHENAMETH VC W/CODEINE, Major Pharms	00904-1514-28
3840 ml	$48.00	Promethazine Vc With Codeine, H.C.F.A. F F P	99999-0875-03
3840 ml	$54.29	Promethazine Vc With Codeine, Rugby	00536-1872-90
3840 ml	$58.98	Promethazine Vc/Codeine Cough Syrup, HR Cenci	00556-0345-28
3840 ml	$61.48	Prometh Vc With Codeine Cough Syrup, Goldline Labs	00182-1713-41
3840 ml	$63.20	Prometh Vc With Codeine Cough Syrup, Alpharma	00472-1629-28
3840 ml	$63.48	PHERAZINE VC WITH CODEINE SYRUP, Halsey Drug	00879-0515-28
3840 ml	$65.78	Promethazine Vc With Codeine, HL Moore Drug Exch	00839-7061-70
4000 ml	$50.00	Promethazine Vc With Codeine, H.C.F.A. F F P	99999-0875-04

HOW SUPPLIED - NOT RATED EQUIVALENT:

Syrup - Oral - 10 mg/5 mg/6.25

120 ml	$2.65	Promethazine Vc W/Codeine, Harber Pharm	51432-0665-18
480 ml	$7.97	Promethazine Vc W/Codeine, Harber Pharm	51432-0665-20

HOW SUPPLIED - NOT RATED EQUIVALENT: *(cont'd)*

480 ml	$9.50	Promethazine Vc W/Codeine, ESI Lederle	59911-5821-03
3840 ml	$56.03	Promethazine Vc W/Codeine, Harber Pharm	51432-0665-21

CODEINE PHOSPHATE; PHENYLEPHRINE HYDROCHLORIDE; PYRILAMINE MALEATE *(000885)*

CATEGORIES: Allergies; Antihistamines; Antitussives; Antitussives/Expectorants/Mucolytics; Cough Preparations; Decongestants; Hay Fever; Respiratory & Allergy Medications; Rhinitis; Pregnancy Category C; DEA Class CV; FDA Pre 1938 Drugs

BRAND NAMES: Codatuss-Ph; **Codimal Ph**

Prescribing information not available at time of publication.

HOW SUPPLIED - EQUIVALENTS NOT AVAILABLE:

Syrup - Oral

118 ml	$5.50	Dicomal-Ph, Econolab	55053-0920-04
120 ml x 12	**$97.81**	**CODIMAL PH, Schwarz Pharma (US)**	**00131-5038-64**
473 ml	$19.95	Dicomal-Ph, Econolab	55053-0920-16
480 ml	**$26.44**	**CODIMAL PH, Schwarz Pharma (US)**	**00131-5038-70**
3840 ml	**$180.47**	**CODIMAL PH, Schwarz Pharma (US)**	**00131-5038-72**

CODEINE PHOSPHATE; PROMETHAZINE HYDROCHLORIDE *(000876)*

CATEGORIES: Allergies; Antihistamines; Antitussives; Antitussives/Expectorants/Mucolytics; Common Cold; Cough Preparations; Expectorants; Influenza; Respiratory & Allergy Medications; Rhinitis; Anaphylactic Shock*; Anesthesia*; Angioedema*; Anxiety*; Conjunctivitis*; Nausea*; Urticaria*; DEA Class CV; FDA Approved 1984 Apr; Top 200 Drugs

* Indication not approved by the FDA

BRAND NAMES: Dectuss; **Phenergan W Codeine**; *Phensedyl*; Pherazine W/Codeine; Promethazine W/Codeine; Prothazine

(International brand names outside U.S. in italics)

FORMULARIES: Aetna; BC-BS; CIGNA; FHP; Humana; Kaiser; Medco; Medi-Cal; PCS; PruCare; United

COST OF THERAPY: $6.64 (Rhinitis; Syrup; 10 mg/6.25 mg/5ml; 20/day; 30 days)

PRIMARY ICD9: 477.9 (Allergic Rhinitis, Cause Unspecified)

DESCRIPTION:

FOR COMPLETE PRESCRIBING INFORMATION, REFER TO THE INDIVIDUAL DRUG MONOGRAPHS (CODEINE PHOSPHATE; PROMETHAZINE HYDROCHLORIDE).

INDICATIONS AND USAGE:

Codeine phosphate with promethazine HCl is indicated for the temporary relief of coughs and upper respiratory symptoms associated with allergy or the common cold.

DOSAGE AND ADMINISTRATION:

The average effective dose is given in TABLE 1:

TABLE 1

Adults	1 teaspoon (5 ml) every 4 to 6 hours, not to exceed 30.0 ml in 24 hours.
Children 6 years to under 12 years	1/2 to 1 teaspoon (2.5 to 5 ml) every 4 to 6 hours, not to exceed 30.0 ml in 24 hours.
Children under 6 years (weight: 18 kg or 40 lbs)	1/4 to 1/2 teaspoon (1.25 to 2.5 ml) every 4 to 6 hours, not to exceed 9.0 ml in 24 hours.
Children under 6 years (weight: 16 kg or 35 lbs)	1/4 to 1/2 teaspoon (1.25 to 2.5 ml) every 4 to 6 hours, not to exceed 8.0 ml in 24 hours.
Children under 6 years (weight: 14 kg or 30 lbs)	1/4 to 1/2 teaspoon (1.25 to 2.5 ml) every 4 to 6 hours, not to exceed 7.0 ml in 24 hours.
Children under 6 years (weight: 12 kg or 25 lbs)	1/4 to 1/2 teaspoon (1.25 to 2.5 ml) every 4 to 6 hours, not to exceed 6.0 ml in 24 hours.

Codeine phosphate with promethazine HCl is not recommended for children under 2 years of age.

Keep bottles tightly closed—Store at Room Temperature, between 15 and 25°C (59 and 77°F). Protect from light.

Dispense in light-resistant, glass, tight containers.

PATIENT INFORMATION:

Codeine phosphate with promethazine is used for the temporary relief of coughs and upper respiratory symptoms associated with an allergy or the common cold. Notify your physician if you are pregnant or nursing. Do not take this medication with monoamine oxidase inhibitors. This medication may cause dizziness, drowsiness, or blurred vision; use caution while driving or operating hazardous machinery. Do not take any other sedating drugs or drink alcohol while taking codeine with promethazine. This medication may be habit forming. Withdrawal symptoms may occur after you stop taking it. May cause nausea, vomiting or constipation; notify your physician if these occur. Notify physician if you develop muscle spasms, uncontrolled twitching in the face and body, or uncontrolled tongue or jaw movements. This medication may cause increased sensitivity to sunlight. Use sunscreens and wear protective clothing until degree of sensitivity is determined. This medication may be taken with food to avoid stomach upset.

HOW SUPPLIED - RATED THERAPEUTICALLY EQUIVALENT:

Syrup - Oral - 10 mg/6.25 mg/5

5 ml x 100	$59.13	Promethazine W/Codeine, Xactdose	50962-0550-05
118 ml	$2.80	Prometh With Codeine Cough Syrup, Goldline Labs	00182-1712-37
118 ml	$3.44	Promethazine With Codeine, HL Moore Drug Exch	00839-7059-65
118 ml	$3.83	PHENAMETH W/CODEINE COUGH SYRUP, Major Pharms	00904-1510-00
120 ml	$1.33	Promethazine With Codeine, H.C.F.A. F F P	99999-0876-01
120 ml	$2.50	Promethazine/Codeine Cough Syrup, HR Cenci	00556-0343-04
120 ml	$2.60	Promethazine W/Codeine, Major Pharms	00904-1510-20

HOW SUPPLIED - RATED THERAPEUTICALLY EQUIVALENT:
(cont'd)

120 ml	$2.95	Promethazine W/Codeine, Qualitest Pharms	00603-1578-54
120 ml	$3.90	Promethazine With Codeine, Rugby	00536-1805-97
120 ml	$3.98	Promethazine W/Codeine, Morton Grove	60432-0606-04
120 ml	$4.30	Promethazine W/Codeine, Goldline Labs	00182-0346-37
120 ml	$4.30	Prometh With Codeine Cough Syrup, Alpharma	00472-1627-04
120 ml	$4.45	PHERAZINE WITH CODEINE SYRUP, Halsey Drug	00879-0513-04
120 ml	$6.03	Promethazine With Codeine, Geneva Pharms	00781-6930-04
120 ml x 24	**$212.54**	**PHENERGAN WITH CODEINE, Wyeth Labs**	**00008-0550-02**
480 ml	$5.32	Promethazine With Codeine, United Res	00677-0963-33
480 ml	$5.33	Promethazine With Codeine, H.C.F.A. F F P	99999-0876-02
480 ml	$7.10	Promethazine/Codeine Cough Syrup, HR Cenci	00556-0343-16
480 ml	$7.30	Promethazine W/Codeine, Aligen Independ	00405-0166-16
480 ml	$7.80	Prometh With Codeine Cough Syrup, Goldline Labs	00182-1712-40
480 ml	$8.45	Prometh With Codeine Syrup, Schein Pharm (US)	00364-7390-16
480 ml	$9.38	Promethazine With Codeine, HL Moore Drug Exch	00839-7059-69
480 ml	$9.75	PHENAMETH W/CODEINE, Major Pharms	00904-1510-16
480 ml	$9.96	Promethazine W/Codeine, Morton Grove	60432-0606-16
480 ml	$10.50	Promethazine W/Codeine, Qualitest Pharms	00603-1578-58
480 ml	$10.64	Prometh With Codeine Cough Syrup, Alpharma	00472-1627-16
480 ml	$10.95	PHERAZINE WITH CODEINE SYRUP, Halsey Drug	00879-0513-16
480 ml	$14.83	Promethazine With Codeine, Rugby	00536-1805-85
480 ml	$14.83	Promethazine With Codeine, Geneva Pharms	00781-6930-16
480 ml	**$31.95**	**PHENERGAN WITH CODEINE, Wyeth Labs**	**00008-0550-03**
3785 ml	$52.49	Prometh With Codeine Cough Syrup, Goldline Labs	00182-1712-41
3840 ml	$42.62	Promethazine With Codeine, H.C.F.A. F F P	99999-0876-03
3840 ml	$49.50	Promethazine/Codeine Cough Syrup, HR Cenci	00556-0343-28
3840 ml	$50.48	Promethazine With Codeine, Rugby	00536-1805-90
3840 ml	$52.20	Prometh With Codeine Cough Syrup, Alpharma	00472-1627-28
3840 ml	$53.22	PHERAZINE WITH CODEINE SYRUP, Halsey Drug	00879-0513-28
3840 ml	$53.41	Promethazine With Codeine, HL Moore Drug Exch	00839-7059-70
3840 ml	$55.45	Promethazine With Codeine, Geneva Pharms	00781-6930-28
3840 ml	$58.18	PHENAMETH W/CODEINE, Major Pharms	00904-1510-28
4000 ml	$44.40	Promethazine With Codeine, H.C.F.A. F F P	99999-0876-04

HOW SUPPLIED - NOT RATED EQUIVALENT:
Syrup - Oral - 10 mg/6.25 mg/5

480 ml	$7.40	Promethazine W/Codeine, ESI Lederle	59911-5819-03

CODEINE PHOSPHATE; PSEUDOEPHEDRINE HYDROCHLORIDE *(000877)*

CATEGORIES: Antitussives; Antitussives/Expectorants/Mucolytics; Bronchitis; Common Cold; Congestion; Cough Preparations; Decongestants; Infections; Influenza; Respiratory & Allergy Medications; Sinusitis; Pregnancy Category C; DEA Class CIII; FDA Pre 1938 Drugs

BRAND NAMES: Cycofed; Kg-Fed; Nucochem; Nucodine Syr; **Nucofed**; Pseudoephedrine W/Codeine

DESCRIPTION:
FOR COMPLETE PRESCRIBING INFORMATION, REFER TO THE INDIVIDUAL DRUG MONOGRAPHS (CODEINE PHOSPHATE, PSEUDOEPHEDRINE HYDROCHLORIDE).

INDICATIONS AND USAGE:
Codeine phosphate with pseudoephedrine HCl is indicated for symptomatic relief when both coughing and congestion are associated with upper respiratory infections and related conditions such as common cold, bronchitis, influenza, and sinusitis.

DOSAGE AND ADMINISTRATION:
ADULTS
Capsule: 1 capsule every 6 hours, not to exceed 4 capsules in 24 hours.

Syrup: 1 teaspoonful every 6 hours, not to exceed 4 teaspoonfuls in 24 hours.

CHILDREN
6 to under 12 years: 1/2 teaspoonful every 6 hours, not to exceed 2 teaspoonfuls in 24 hours.

2 to under 6 years: 1/4 teaspoonful every 6 hours, not to exceed 1 teaspoonful in 24 hours.

Do not give this product to children under 2 years, except under the advice and supervision of a physician.

HOW SUPPLIED - EQUIVALENTS NOT AVAILABLE:
Capsule, Gelatin - Oral - 20 mg/60 mg

60's	**$35.84**	**NUCOFED, Roberts Labs**	**54092-0005-60**
100's	$27.53	NUCOCHEM, H N Norton Co.	50732-0860-01

Liquid - Oral - 20 mg/60 mg

473 ml	$30.19	Nucodine Syr, Am Generics	58634-0008-01
473 ml	**$48.27**	**NUCOFED, Roberts Labs**	**54092-0403-16**
480 ml	$26.02	NUCOCHEM SYRUP, H N Norton Co.	50732-0859-16
480 ml	$26.25	Kg-Fed, King Pharms	60793-0027-16
480 ml	$26.50	Cycofed, Cypress Pharm	60258-0601-16
480 ml	$27.90	Pseudoephedrine W/Codeine, Aligen Independ	00405-0054-16

CODEINE PHOSPHATE; PSEUDOEPHEDRINE HYDROCHLORIDE; TRIPROLIDINE HYDROCHLORIDE *(000878)*

CATEGORIES: Allergies; Antihistamines; Antitussives; Antitussives/Expectorants/Mucolytics; Common Cold; Cough Preparations; Decongestants; Expectorants; Hay Fever; Influenza; Nasal Congestion; Respiratory & Allergy Medications; Rhinitis; Sinus Congestion; Sympathomimetic Agents; Pregnancy Category C; DEA Class CV; FDA Approved 1984 Apr

BRAND NAMES: Actagen-C; *Actifed Antitusivo*; *Actifed Compound*; *Actifed Compound Linctus*; **Actifed W/ Codeine**; Allerfrin W/Codeine; *Fedac Compound*; Histafed C; Triafed With Codeine; Triafed-C; Triaphed-C; Triprolidine P-Ephed Codeine; *Unitified*
(International brand names outside U.S. in italics)

FORMULARIES: Aetna; Medi-Cal

DESCRIPTION:
Each 5 ml (1 teaspoonful) contains: codeine phosphate 10 mg (Warning—may be habit forming). Triprolidine HCl 1.25 mg, pseudoephedrine HCl 30 mg and alcohol 4.3%. Sodium benzoate 0.1% and methylparaben 0.1% are added as preservatives. This medication is intended for oral administration. Codeine phosphate w/ pseudoephedrine HCl and triprolidine HCl cough syrup has antitussive, antihistaminic and nasal decongestant effects. The components of codeine phosphate w/ pseudoephedrine HCl and triprolidine HCl cough syrup have the following chemical names and structural formulae:

Codeine Phosphate, USP: 7.8-didehydro-4,5α-epoxy-3-methoxy-17-methylmorphinan-6α-ol phosphate (1:1) (salt) hemihydrate

Triprolidine HCl Monohydrate: (*E*)-2-[3-(1-pyrrolidinyl)-1-(*p-tolyl*)propenyl]pyridine monohydrochloride monohydrate

Pseudoephedrine HCl: (S-(R*,R*))-α-(1-(methylamino)ethyl)benzenemethanol HCl

CLINICAL PHARMACOLOGY:
CODEINE
Codeine probably exerts its antitussive activity by depressing the medullary (brain) cough center, thereby raising its threshold for incoming cough impulses.

Codeine is readily absorbed from the gastrointestinal tract, with a therapeutic dose reaching peak antitussive in about 2 hours and persisting for 4 to 6 hours. Codeine is rapidly distributed from blood to body tissues and taken up preferentially by parenchymatous organs such as liver, spleen and kidney. It passes the blood brain barrier and is found in fetal tissue and breast milk.

The drug is not bound by plasma proteins nor is it accumulated in body tissues. Codeine is metabolized in the liver to morphine and norcodeine, each representing about 10 percent of the administered codeine dose. About 90 percent of the dose is excreted within 24 hours, primarily through the kidneys. Urinary excretion products are free and glucuronide-conjugated codeine (about 70%), free and conjugated norcodeine (about 10%) free and conjugated morphine (about 10%), normorphine (under 4%) and hydrocodone (<1%). The remainder of the dose appears in the faces.

TRIPROLIDINE
Antihistamines such as triprolidine HCl act as antagonists of the H_1 histamine receptor. Consequently, they prevent histamine from eliciting typical immediate hypersensitivity responses in the nose, eyes, lungs and skin.

Animal distribution studies have shown localization of triprolidine in lung. Spleen and kidney tissue. Liver microsome studies have revealed the presence of several metabolites with an oxidized product of the toluene methyl group predominating.

PSEUDOEPHEDRINE
Pseudoephedrine acts as an indirect sympathomimetic agent by stimulating sympathetic (adrenergic) nerve endings to release norepinephrine. Norepinephrine in turn stimulates alpha and beta receptors throughout the body. The action of pseudoephedrine HCl is apparently more specific for the blood vessels of the upper respiratory tract and less specific for the blood vessels of the systemic circulation. The vasoconstriction elicited at these sites results in the shrinkage of swollen tissues in the sinuses and nasal passages. Pseudoephedrine is rapidly and almost completely absorbed from the gastrointestinal tract. Considerable variation in half-life has been observed (from about 4 1/2 to 10 hours), which is attributed to individual differences in absorption and excretion. Excretion rates are also altered by urine pH, increasing with acidification and decreasing with alkalinization. As a result, mean half-life falls to about 4 hours at pH 5 and increases to 12 to 13 hours at pH 8. After administration of a 60 mg tablet, 87 to 96% of the pseudoephedrine is cleared from the body within 24 hours. The drug is distributed to body tissues and fluids, including fetal tissue, breast milk and the central nervous system (CNS). About 55 to 75% of an administered dose is excreted unchanged in the urine; the remainder is apparently metabolized in the liver to inactive compounds by N-demethylation, parahydroxylation and oxidative deamination.

The pharmacokinetic properties of codeine, triprolidine and pseudoephedrine from 10 ml of codeine phosphate w/pseudoephedrine HCl and triprolidine HCl cough syrup were investigated compared to a reference preparation of equal component doses in 18 healthy adults. The results of this study showed that codeine phosphate w/ pseudoephedrine HCl and triprolidine HCl cough syrup and the reference preparation were bioequivalent. Pharmacokinetic parameters for codeine phosphate w/ pseudoephedrine HCl and triprolidine HCl cough syrup are as follows (TABLE 1):

TABLE 1

Parameter	Codeine*	Triprolidine†	Pseudoephedrine‡
Elimination Half-life (hr)	2.7 ± 0.4**	4.0 ± 2.2	5.5 ± 0.9
Time to Maximum Concentration (hr)	1.2 ± 0.5	1.8 ± 0.7	2.6 ± 1.0
Maximum Plasma Concentration (mg/ml)	44.8 ± 11.7	4.9 ± 1.8	189 ± 44
Area Under Plasma Curve from 1=0 to 1=infinity (mg/ml.hr)	226 ± 41	42.5 ± 34.0	1938 ± 440

* 20 mg Codeine Phosphate hemihydrate (equivalent to 14.7 mg free base)
† 2.5 mg Triprolidine HCl monohydrate (equivalent to 2.1 mg free base)
‡ 60 mg Pseudoephedrine HCl (equivalent to 49.1 mg free base)
** Means ± S.D.

INDICATIONS AND USAGE:
Codeine phosphate w/ pseudoephedrine HCl and triprolidine HCl cough syrup is indicated for temporary relief of coughs and upper respiratory symptoms, including nasal congestion, associated with allergy or the common cold.

CONTRAINDICATIONS:
Codeine phosphate w/ pseudoephedrine HCl and triprolidine HCl cough syrup is contraindicated under the following conditions:

Use in Newborn or Premature Infants: This drug should *not* be used in newborn or premature infants.

Use in Lower Respiratory Disease: Antihistamines should *not* be used to treat lower respiratory tract symptoms, including asthma.

Hypersensitivity To:

(1) codeine phosphate or other narcotics;

(2) triprolidine HCl or other antihistamines of similar chemical structure;

(3) sympathomimetic amines, including pseudoephedrine. Sympathomimetic amines are contraindicated in patients with severe hypertension, severe coronary artery disease and in patients on monoamine oxidase (MAO) inhibitor therapy (see DRUG INTERACTIONS).

WARNINGS:

Codeine phosphate w/ pseudoephedrine HCl and triprolidine HCl cough syrup should be used with considerable caution in patients with increased intraocular pressure (narrow angle glaucoma), stenosing peptic ulcer, pyloroduodenal obstruction, symptomatic prostatic hypertrophy, bladder neck obstruction, hypertension, diabetes mellitus, ischemic heart disease, and hyperthyroidism.

In the presence of head injury or other intracranial lesions, the respiratory depressant effects of codeine and other narcotics may be markedly enhanced, as well as their capacity for elevating cerebrospinal fluid pressure.

Narcotics also produce other CNS depressant effects. Such as drowsiness, that may further obscure the clinical course of patients with head injuries.

Codeine or other narcotics may obscure signs on which to judge the diagnosis or clinical course of patients with acute abdominal conditions.

PRECAUTIONS:

GENERAL

Codeine phosphate w/ pseudoephedrine HCl and triprolidine HCl cough syrup should be prescribed with caution for certain special-risk patients, such as the elderly or debilitated, and for those with severe impairment of renal or hepatic function, gallbladder disease or gallstones, respiratory impairment, cardiac arrhythmias, history of bronchial asthma, prostatic hypertrophy or urethral stricture and in patients known to be taking other antitussive, antihistamine or decongestant medications. Patients' self-medication habits should be investigated to determine their use of such medications. Codeine phosphate w/ pseudoephedrine HCl and triprolidine HCl cough syrup is intended for short-term use only.

INFORMATION FOR THE PATIENT

1. Patients should be warned about engaging in activities requiring mental alertness such as driving a car, operating dangerous machinery or hazardous appliances.

2. Patients with a history of glaucoma, peptic ulcer, urinary retention or pregnancy should be cautioned before starting codeine phosphate w/ pseudoephedrine HCl and triprolidine HCl.

3. Patients should be told not to take alcohol, sleeping pills, sedatives or tranquilizers while taking codeine phosphate w/ pseudoephedrine HCl and triprolidine HCl.

4. Antihistamines as in codeine phosphate w/ pseudoephedrine HCl and triprolidine HCl, may cause dizziness, drowsiness, dry mouth, blurred vision, weakness, nausea, headache or nervousness in some patients.

5. Patients should be told to store this medicine in a tightly closed container in a dry, cool place away from heat or direct sunlight and out of the reach of children.

6. Nursing mothers refer to PRECAUTIONS.

Codeine phosphate w/ pseudoephedrine HCl and triprolidine HCl cough syrup should not be used by persons intolerant to sympathomimetics used for the relief of nasal or sinus congestion. Such drugs include ephedrine, epinephrine, phenylpropanolamine, and phenylephrine. Symptoms of intolerance include drowsiness, dizziness, weakness, difficulty in breathing, tenseness, muscle tremors or palpitations.

Codeine may be habit-forming when used over long periods or in high doses. Patients should take the drug only for as long, in the amounts, and as frequently as prescribed.

DRUG/LABORATORY TEST INTERACTIONS

Codeine: Narcotic administration may increase serum amylase levels.

CARCINOGENESIS, MUTAGENESIS, AND IMPAIRMENT OF FERTILITY

No adequate studies have been conducted in animals to determine whether the components of codeine phosphate w/ pseudoephedrine HCl and triprolidine HCl cough syrup have a potential for carcinogenesis, mutagenesis or impairment of fertility.

PREGNANCY, TERATOGENIC EFFECTS, PREGNANCY CATEGORY C

Animal reproduction studies have not been conducted with codeine phosphate w/ pseudoephedrine HCl and triprolidine HCl cough syrup. It is also not known whether codeine phosphate w/ pseudoephedrine HCl and triprolidine HCl cough syrup can cause fetal harm when administered to a pregnant woman or can affect reproduction capacity. Codeine phosphate w/ pseudoephedrine HCl and triprolidine HCl cough syrup should be given a pregnant woman only if clearly needed.

Teratology studies have been conducted with the three ingredients of codeine phosphate w/ pseudoephedrine HCl and triprolidine HCl cough syrup. Pseudoephedrine studies were conducted in rats at doses up to 150 times the human dose; triprolidine was studied in rats and rabbits at doses up to 125 times the human dose, and codeine studies were conducted in rats and rabbits at doses up to 150 times the human dose. No evidence of teratogenic harm to the fetus was revealed in any of these studies. However, overt signs of toxicity were observed in the dams which received pseudoephedrine. This was reflected in reduced average weight and length and rate of skeletal ossification in their fetuses.

NURSING MOTHERS

The components of codeine phosphate w/ pseudoephedrine HCl and triprolidine HCl cough syrup are excreted in breast milk in small amounts, but the significance of their effects on nursing infants is not known. Because of the potential for serious adverse reactions in nursing infants from maternal ingestion of codeine phosphate w/ pseudoephedrine HCl and triprolidine HCl cough syrup, a decision should be made whether to discontinue nursing or to discontinue the drug, taking into account the importance of the drug to the mother.

PEDIATRIC USE

As in adults, the combination of an antihistamine, sympathomimetic amine and codeine can elicit either mild stimulation or mild sedation in children. In infants and children particularly, the ingredients in this drug product in overdosage may produce hallucinations, convulsions and death. Symptoms of toxicity in children may include fixed dilated pupils, flushed face, dry mouth, fever, excitation, hallucinations, ataxia, incoordination, athetosis, tonic clonic convulsions and postictal depression, (see CONTRAINDICATIONS and OVERDOSAGE).

Geriatric Use

Use in Elderly (approximately 60 years or older): The ingredients in codeine phosphate w/ pseudoephedrine HCl and triprolidine HCl cough syrup are more likely to cause adverse reactions in elderly patients.

DRUG INTERACTIONS:

CODEINE PHOSPHATE W/ PSEUDOEPHEDRINE HCL AND TRIPROLIDINE HCL COUGH SYRUP MAY ENHANCE THE EFFECTS OF:

1. Monoamine oxidase (MAO) inhibitors.

2. Other narcotic analgesics, alcohol, general anesthetics, tranquilizers, sedative-hypnotics, surgical skeletal muscle relaxants, or other CNS depressants, by causing increased CNS depression.

CODEINE PHOSPHATE W/ PSEUDOEPHEDRINE HCL AND TRIPROLIDINE HCL COUGH SYRUP MAY DIMINISH: THE ANTIHYPERTENSIVE EFFECTS OF GUANETHIDINE, BETHANIDINE, METHYLDOPA, AND RESERPINE.

ADVERSE REACTIONS:

(The most frequent adverse reactions are underlined.)

General: Dryness of mouth, dryness of nose, dryness of throat, urticaria, drug rash, anaphylactic shock, photosensitivity, excessive perspiration and chills.

Cardiovascular System: Hypotension, headache, palpitations, tachycardia, extrasystoles.

Hematologic System: Hemolytic anemia, thrombocytopenia, agranulocytosis.

Nervous System: Sedation, sleepiness, dizziness, disturbed coordination, fatigue, confusion, restlessness, excitation, anxiety, nervousness, tremor, irritability, insomnia, euphoria, paresthesias, blurred vision, diplopia, vertigo, tinnitus, acute labyrinthitis, hysteria, neuritis, convulsions, CNS depression, hallucination.

G.I. System: Epigastric distress, anorexia, nausea, vomiting, diarrhea, constipation.

G.U.System: Urinary frequency, difficult urination, urinary retention, early menses.

Respiratory system: Thickening of bronchial secretions, tightness of chest and wheezing, nasal stuffiness, respiratory depression.

DRUG ABUSE AND DEPENDENCE:

Like other medications containing a narcotic, codeine phosphate w/ pseudoephedrine HCl and triprolidine HCl cough syrup is controlled by the Drug Enforcement Administration. It is classified under Schedule V.

Codeine phosphate w/ pseudoephedrine HCl and triprolidine HCl cough syrup can produce drug dependence of the morphine type, and therefore it has a potential for being abused. Psychic dependence, physical dependence and tolerance may develop on repeated administration.

The dependence liability of codeine has been found to be too small to permit a full definition of its characteristics. Studies indicate that addiction to codeine is extremely uncommon and requires very high parenteral doses.

When dependence on codeine occurs at therapeutic doses, it appears to require from one to two months to develop, and withdrawal symptoms are mild. Most patients on long-term oral codeine therapy show no signs of physical dependence upon abrupt withdrawal.

OVERDOSAGE:

Since codeine phosphate w/ pseudoephedrine HCl and triprolidine HCl cough syrup is comprised of three pharmacologically different compounds, it is difficult to predict the exact manifestation of symptoms in a given individual. Reaction to an overdosage of codeine phosphate w/ pseudoephedrine HCl and triprolidine HCl cough syrup may vary from CNS depression to stimulation. A detailed description of symptoms which are likely to appear after ingestion of an excess of individual components follows.

Overdosage with codeine can cause transient euphoria, drowsiness, dizziness, weariness, diminution of sensibility, loss of sensation, vomiting, transient excitement in children and occasionally in adult women, miosis progressing to nonreactive pinpoint pupils. Itching sometimes with skin rashes and urticaria, and clammy skin with mottled cyanosis. In more severe cases, muscular relaxation with depressed or absent superficial and deep reflexes and a positive Babinski sign may appear. Marked slowing of the respiratory rate with inadequate pulmonary ventilation and consequent cyanosis may occur. Terminal signs include shock, pulmonary edema, hypostatic or aspiration pneumonia and respiratory arrest, with death occurring within 6-12 hours following ingestion.

Overdoses of antihistamines may cause hallucinations, convulsions, or possible death, especially in infants and children. Antihistamines are more likely to cause dizziness, sedation, and hypotension in elderly patients.

Overdosage with triprolidine may produce reactions varying from depression to stimulation of the Central Nervous System(CNS); the latter is particularly likely in children. Atropine-like signs and symptoms (dry mouth, fixed dilated pupils, flushing, tachycardia, hallucinations, convulsions, urinary retention, cardiac arrhythmias and coma) may occur.

Overdosage with pseudoephedrine can cause excessive CNS stimulation resulting in excitement, nervousness, anxiety, tremor, restlessness and insomnia. Other effects include tachycardia, hypertension, pallor, mydriasis, hyperglycemia and urinary retention. Severe overdosage may cause tachypnea or hyperpnea, hallucinations, convulsions, or delirium, but in some individuals there may be CNS depression with somnolence, stupor or respiratory depression. Arrhythmias (including ventricular fibrillation) may lead to hypotension and circulatory collapse. Severe hypokalemia can occur, probably due to compartmental shift rather than depletion of potassium. No organ damage or significant metabolic derangement is associated with pseudoephedrine overdosage.

The toxic plasma concentration of codeine is not known with certainty. Experimental production of mild to moderate CNS depression in healthy, non-tolerant subjects occurs at plasma concentrations of 0.5-1.9 mcg/ml when codeine is given by intravenous infusion. The single lethal dose of codeine in adults is estimated to be from 0.5 to 1.0 gram. It is also estimated that 5 mg/kg could be fatal in children.

The LD_{50} (single, oral dose) of triprolidine is 163 to 308 mg/kg in the mouse (depending upon strain) and 840 mg/kg in the rat.

Insufficient data are available to estimate the toxic and lethal doses of triprolidine in humans. No reports of acute poisoning with triprolidine have appeared.

The LD_{50} (single, oral dose) of pseudoephedrine is 726 mg/kg in the mouse. 2206 mg/kg in the rat and 1177 mg/kg in the rabbit. The toxic and lethal concentrations in human biologic fluids ar not known. Excretion rates increase with urine acidification and decrease with alkalinization. Few reports of toxicity due to pseudoephedrine have been published and no case of fatal overdosage is known.

Therapy, if instituted within 4 hours of overdosage, is aimed at reducing further absorption of the drug. In the conscious patient, vomiting should be induced even though it may have occurred spontaneously. If vomiting cannot be induced, gastric lavage is indicated. Adequate precautions must be taken to protect against aspiration, especially in infants and children. Charcoal slurry or other suitable agents should be instilled into the stomach after vomiting or lavage. Saline cathartics or milk of magnesia may be of additional benefit.

In the unconscious patient, the airway should be secured with a cuffed endotracheal tube before attempting to evaluate the gastric contents. Intensive supportive and nursing care is indicated, as for any comatose patient.

If breathing is significantly impaired, maintenance of an adequate airway and mechanical support of respiration is the most effective means of providing adequate oxygenation.

Hypotension is an early sign of impending cardiovascular collapse and should be treated vigorously. Do not use CNS stimulants. Convulsions should be controlled by careful administration of diazepam or short-acting barbiturate repeated as necessary. Physostigmine may be also considered for use in controlling centrally mediated convulsions.

Ice packs and cooling sponge baths, not alcohol, can aid in reducing the fever commonly seen in children. For codeine, continuous stimulation that arouses, but does not exhaust, the patient is useful in preventing coma. Continuous or intermittent oxygen therapy is usually indicated, while Naloxone is useful as a codeine antidote. Close nursing care is essential. Saline cathartics, such as Milk of Magnesia, help to dilute the concentration of the drugs in the bowel by drawing water into the gut, thereby hastening drug elimination.

OVERDOSAGE: *(cont'd)*

Adrenergic receptor blocking agents are antidotes to pseudoephedrine. In practice, the most useful is the beta-blocker propranolol, which is indicated when there are signs of cardiac toxicity.

There are no specific antidotes to triprolidine. Histamine should not be given.

Pseudoephedrine and codeine are theoretically dialyzable, but the procedures have not been clinically established.

In severe cases of overdosage, it is essential to monitor both the heart (by electrocardiograph) and plasma electrolytes and to give intravenous potassium as indicated by these continuous controls. Vasopressors may be used to treat hypotension, and excessive CNS stimulation may be counteracted with parenteral diazepam. Stimulants should not be used.

DOSAGE AND ADMINISTRATION:

Dosage should be individualized according to the needs and response of the patient (TABLE 2):

TABLE 2 Usual Dose

Adults and Children	Teaspoonfuls (5 ml)	
12 years and older	2	(every 4-6 hours not to exceed 4 doses in a 24-hours period)
Children 6 to under 12 years	1	
Children 2 to under 6 years	½	

Store at 15-30°C (59-86°F) and protect from light.

HOW SUPPLIED - RATED THERAPEUTICALLY EQUIVALENT:

Syrup - Oral - 10 mg/30 mg/1.2

120 ml	$1.24	Triprolidine/P-Ephed/Codeine, H.C.F.A. F F P	99999-0878-01
120 ml	$2.30	Triprolidine/Pseudoephed/Codeine, HR Cenci	00556-0471-04
120 ml	$3.40	Triprolidine/P-Ephed/Codeine, Morton Grove	60432-0462-04
120 ml	$3.57	TRIACIN-C COUGH SYRUP, Alpharma	00472-1633-04
240 ml	$2.47	Triprolidine/P-Ephed/Codeine, H.C.F.A. F F P	99999-0878-02
240 ml	$3.40	Triprolidine/P-Ephed/Codeine, HR Cenci	00556-0471-08
480 ml	$4.94	Triprolidine/P-Ephed/Codeine, H.C.F.A. F F P	99999-0878-03
480 ml	$6.60	Triprolidine/Pseudoephed/Codeine, HR Cenci	00556-0471-16
480 ml	$9.15	APRODINE WITH CODEINE COUGH SYRUP, Major Pharms	00904-1579-16
480 ml	$9.20	TRIACIN-C COUGH SYRUP, Alpharma	00472-1633-16
480 ml	$9.31	Triprolidine/P-Ephed/Codeine, Aligen Independ	00405-0191-16
480 ml	$9.70	TRIACIN-C-COUGH SYRUP, HL Moore Drug Exch	00839-7079-69
480 ml	$9.70	Triprolidine/P-Ephed/Codeine, Morton Grove	60432-0462-16
480 ml	$10.18	Triprolidine-C, Qualitest Pharms	00603-1771-58
480 ml	$10.50	ACTAGEN-C COUGH SYRUP, Goldline Labs	00182-1710-40
480 ml	$12.75	ACTIFED C, Rugby	00536-0065-85
480 ml	$13.00	TRIAFED WITH CODEINE, Schein Pharm (US)	00364-7385-16
480 ml	$23.09	TRIFED-C COUGH SYRUP, Geneva Pharms	00781-6550-16
480 ml	$50.27	ACTIFED WITH CODEINE, Glaxo Wellcome	00173-0025-96
3785 ml	$38.99	Triprolidine/P-Ephed/Codeine, H.C.F.A. F F P	99999-0878-05
3840 ml	$39.55	Triprolidine/P-Ephed/Codeine, H.C.F.A. F F P	99999-0878-04
3840 ml	$44.17	Triprolidine/Pseudoephed/Codeine, HR Cenci	00556-0471-28
3840 ml	$65.59	TRIACIN C, HL Moore Drug Exch	00839-7079-70
3840 ml	$67.43	Triprolidine/P-Ephed/Codeine, Major Pharms	00904-1579-28
3840 ml	$68.20	Triprolidine/P-Ephed/Codeine, Morton Grove	60432-0462-28
3840 ml	$68.60	TRIACIN-C COUGH SYRUP, Alpharma	00472-1633-28
3840 ml	$75.72	ACTAGEN-C COUGH SYRUP, Goldline Labs	00182-1710-41

HOW SUPPLIED - NOT RATED EQUIVALENT:

Syrup - Oral - 10 mg/30 mg/1.2

120 ml	$2.95	Triacin C, Consolidated Midland	00223-6198-01
120 ml	$3.10	Triacin C, Harber Pharm	51432-0685-18
120 ml	$3.55	Triprolidine/P-Ephed/Codeine, Halsey Drug	00879-0750-04
480 ml	$8.95	Triacin C, Consolidated Midland	00223-6198-02
480 ml	$9.10	Triprolidine/P-Ephed/Codeine, Halsey Drug	00879-0750-16
480 ml	$9.20	Triacin C, Harber Pharm	51432-0685-20
3840 ml	$63.90	Triacin C, Harber Pharm	51432-0685-21
3840 ml	$64.97	Triacin C, Consolidated Midland	00223-6198-03
3840 ml	$68.43	Triprolidine/P-Ephed/Codeine, Halsey Drug	00879-0750-28

CODEINE PHOSPHATE; TERPIN HYDRATE

(000888)

CATEGORIES: Antitussives; Antitussives/Expectorants/Mucolytics; Cough Preparations; Respiratory & Allergy Medications; DEA Class CV; FDA Pre 1938 Drugs

BRAND NAMES: Prunicodeine; *Terpin*
(International brand names outside U.S. in italics)

FORMULARIES: Aetna; Medi-Cal

Prescribing information not available at time of publication.

HOW SUPPLIED - EQUIVALENTS NOT AVAILABLE:

Elixir - Oral - 10 mg/85 mg

480 ml	$4.96	Terpin Hydrate W/Codeine, Lannett	00527-0774-27
3840 ml	$34.79	Terpin Hydrate W/Codeine, Lannett	00527-0774-28

COLCHICINE *(000890)*

CATEGORIES: Antigout; Arthritis; Back Pain; Electrolytic, Caloric-Water Balance; Gout; Gouty Arthritis; Pain; Uricosuric Agents; Pregnancy Category D; FDA Pre 1938 Drugs

BRAND NAMES: *Artrichine; Colchicine; Colchicinecapsules; Colchicine Evans; Colchicine Houde; Colchicine MR; Colchicum-Dispert; Colchimedio; Colchineos* (France); *Colchiquim* (Mexico); *Colgout;* Colsalide Improved; *Coluric; Conicine; Goutnil; Kolkicin; Tolchicine*
(International brand names outside U.S. in italics)

FORMULARIES: Aetna; BC-BS; FHP; Medi-Cal; WHO; PCS

DESCRIPTION:

THIS PRODUCT IS TO BE USED BY OR UNDER THE DIRECTION OF A PHYSICIAN.

A PHENANTHRENE DERIVATIVE, COLCHICINE IS THE ACTIVE ALKALOIDAL PRINCIPLE DERIVED FROM VARIOUS SPECIES OF *COLCHICUM;* IT APPEARS AS PALE-YELLOW AMORPHOUS SCALES OR POWDER THAT DARKENS ON EXPOSURE TO LIGHT. ONE G DISSOLVES IN 25 ML OF WATER AND IN 220 ML OF ETHER. COLCHICINE IS FREELY SOLUBLE IN ALCOHOL AND CHLOROFORM.

CHEMICALLY IT IS ACETAMIDE, *N*-(5,6,7,9-TETRAHYDRO-1,2,3,10-TETRAMETHOXY-9-OXOBENZO(æ)HEPTALEN-7-YL)-,(*S*)-. THE MOLECULAR WEIGHT IS 399.44, THE EMPIRICAL FORMULA IS $C_{22}H_{25}NO_6$.

COLCHICINE, AN ACETYLTRIMETHYLCOLCHICINIC ACID, IS HYDROLYZED IN THE PRESENCE OF DILUTE ACIDS OR ALKALIES, WITH CLEAVAGE OF A METHYL GROUP AS METHANOL AND FORMATION OF *COLCHICEINE,* WHICH HAS VERY LITTLE THERAPEUTIC ACTIVITY. ON HYDROLYSIS WITH STRONG ACIDS, COLCHICINE IS CONVERTED TO TRIMETHYLCOLCHICINIC ACID.

AMPOULES COLCHICINE INJECTION, USP, PROVIDE A STERILE AQUEOUS SOLUTION OF COLCHICINE FOR INTRAVENOUS USE. EACH AMPOULE CONTAINS 1 MG (2.5 ßMOL) OF COLCHICINE IN 2 ML OF SOLUTION. SODIUM HYDROXIDE MAY HAVE BEEN ADDED DURING MANUFACTURE TO ADJUST THE PH.

CLINICAL PHARMACOLOGY:

The mechanism of the relief afforded by colchicine in acute attacks of gouty arthritis is not completely known, but studies on the processes involved in precipitation of an acute attack have helped elucidate how this drug may exert its effects. The drug is not an analgesic, does not relieve other types of pain or inflammation, and is of no value in other types of arthritis. It is not a diuretic and does not influence the renal excretion of uric acid or its level in the blood or the magnitude of the "miscible pool" of uric acid. It also does not alter the solubility of urate in the plasma.

Colchicine is not a uricosuric agent. An acute attack of gout apparently occurs as a result of an inflammatory reaction to crystals of monosodium urate that are deposited in the joint tissue from hyperuric body fluids; the reaction is aggravated as more urate crystals accumulate. The initial inflammatory response involves local infiltration of granulocytes that phagocytize the urate crystals. Interference with these processes will prevent the development of an acute attack. Colchicine apparently exerts its effect by reducing the inflammatory response to the deposited crystals and also by diminishing phagocytosis. The deposition of uric acid is favored by an acid pH. In synovial tissues and in leukocytes associated with inflammatory processes, lactic acid production is high; this favors a local decrease in pH that enhances uric acid deposition. Colchicine diminishes lactic acid production by leukocytes both directly and by diminishing phagocytosis, thereby interrupting the cycle of urate crystal deposition and inflammatory response that sustains the acute attack. The oxidation of glucose in phagocytizing as well as in nonphagocytizing leukocytes *in vitro* is suppressed by colchicine; this suppression may explain the diminished lactic acid production. The precise biochemical step that is affected by colchicine is not yet known. The antimitotic activity of colchicine is unrelated to its effectiveness in the treatment of acute gout, as indicated by the fact that trimethylcolchicinic acid, an analog of colchicine, has no antimitotic activity except in extremely high doses.

INDICATIONS AND USAGE:

Colchicine is indicated for the treatment of gout. It is effective in relieving the pain of acute attacks, especially if therapy is begun early in the attack and in adequate dosage. Many therapists use colchicine as interval therapy to prevent acute attacks of gout. It has no effect on nongouty arthritis or on uric acid metabolism.

The intravenous use of colchicine is advantageous when a rapid response is desired or when gastrointestinal side effects interfere with oral administration of the medication. Occasionally, intravenous colchicine is effective when the oral preparation is not. After the acute attack has subsided, the patient can usually be given colchicine tablets by mouth.

CONTRAINDICATIONS:

Colchicine is contraindicated in patients with gout who also have serious gastrointestinal, renal, hepatic, or cardiac disorders. Colchicine should not be given in the presence of combined renal and hepatic disease.

WARNINGS:

Colchicine can cause fetal harm when administered to a pregnant woman. If this drug is used during pregnancy, or if the patient becomes pregnant while taking it, the woman should be apprised of the potential hazard to the fetus.

Mortality Related to Overdosage: Cumulative intravenous doses of colchicine above 4 mg hav resulted in irreversible multiple organ failure and death (see OVERDOSAGE and DOSAGE AND ADMINISTRATION).

PRECAUTIONS:

General: Reduction in dosage is indicated if weakness, anorexia, nausea, vomiting or diarrhea occurs. Rarely, thrombophlebitis occurs at the site of injection. Colchicine should be with great caution to aged and debilitated patients, especially those with renal, hepatic, gastrointestinal, or heart disease.

Pregnancy Category C: See WARNINGS.

Nursing Mothers: It is not known whether this drug is excreted in human milk. Because many drugs are excreted in human milk, caution should be exercised when colchicine is administered to a nursing woman.

Usage in Children: Safety and effectiveness in children have not been established.

DRUG INTERACTIONS:

Colchicine has been shown to induce reversible malabsorption of vitamin B_{12}, apparently by altering the function of ileal mucosa. The possibility that colchicine may increase response to central nervous system depressants and to sympathomimetic agents is suggested by the results of experiments on animals.

ADVERSE REACTIONS:

These are usually gastrointestinal in nature and consist of abdominal pain, nausea, vomiting, and diarrhea. The diarrhea may be severe. The gastrointestinal symptoms may occur even though the drug is given intravenously; however, such symptoms are unusual unless the recommended dose is exceeded.

Prolonged administration may cause bone marrow depression, with agranulocytosis, thrombocytopenia, and aplastic anemia. Peripheral neuritis and epilation have also been reported.

Myopathy may occur in patients on usual maintenance doses, especially in the presence of renal impairment.

OVERDOSAGE:

SIGNS AND SYMPTOMS

Symptoms, the onset of which may be delayed, include nausea, vomiting, diarrhea, abdominal pain, hemorrhagic gastroenteritis, and burning pain in the throat, stomach, and skin. Fluid extravasation may lead to shock. Myocardial injury may be accompanied by ST-segment elevation, decreased contractility, and profound shock. Muscle weakness or paralysis may occur and progress to respiratory failure. Hepatocellular damage, renal failure, and lung parenchymal infiltrates may occur and, by the fifth day after overdose, leukopenia, thrombocytopenia, and coagulopathy may also occur. if the patient survives, alopecia and stomatitis may be experienced. There is no clear separation of nontoxic, toxic, and lethal doses of colchicine. The lethal dose of colchicine has been estimated to be 65 mg; however, **death has resulted from intravenous doses as small as 7 mg acutely (see WARNINGS and DOSAGE AND ADMINISTRATION).** Serum concentrations that may be toxic or lethal are not defined. The intravenous median lethal dose in rats is 1.7 mg/kg.

TREATMENT

To obtain up-to-date information about the treatment of overdose, a good resource is your certified Regional Poison Control Center. Telephone numbers certified poison control centers are listed in the *Physicians GenRx*. In managing overdosage, consider the possibility of multiple drug overdoses, interaction among drugs, and unusual drug kinetics in your patient.

Protect the patient's airway and support ventilation and perfusion. Meticulously monitor and maintain, within acceptable limits, the patient's vital signs, blood gases, serum electrolytes, etc. If colchicine was recently ingested and vomiting has not occurred, perform gastric lavage once the patient is stabilized. Absorption of drugs from the gastrointestinal tract may be decreased by giving activated charcoal, which, in many cases, is more effective than emesis or lavage; consider charcoal instead of or in addition to gastric emptying. repeated doses of charcoal over time may hasten elimination of some drugs that have been absorbed. Safeguard the patient's airway when employing gastric emptying or charcoal.

Forced diuresis, peritoneal dialysis, hemodialysis, or charcoal hemoperfusion have not been established as beneficial for an overdose of colchicine.

DOSAGE AND ADMINISTRATION:

Colchicine injection is for intravenous use only. Severe local irritation occurs if it is administered subcutaneously or intramuscularly.

It is extremely important that the needle be properly positioned in the vein before colchicine is injected. If leakage into surrounding tissue or outside the vein along its course should occur during intravenous administration, considerable irritation and possible tissue damage may follow. There is no specific antidote for the prevention of this irritation. Local application of heat or cold, as well as the administration of analgesics, may afford relief.

The injection should take 2 to 5 minutes for completion. To minimize the risk of extravasation, it is recommended that the injection be made into an established intravenous line into a large vein using normal saline as the intravenous fluid. Colchicine injection should not be diluted with 5% Dextrose in Water. If a decrease in concentration of colchicine in solution is required, 0.9% Sodium Chloride Injection, which does not contain a bacteriostatic agent, should be used. Solutions that become turbid should not be used.

In the treatment of acute gouty arthritis, rhe average initial dose of colchicine injection is 2 mg (4 ml). This may be followed by 0.5 (1 ml) every 6 hours until a satisfactory response is achieved. In general, a total dosage for the first 24-hour period should is achieved. In general, the total dosage for the first 24-hour period should not exceed 4 mg (8 ml). Cumulative doses of colchicine above 4 mg have resulted in irreversible multiple organ failure and death. The total dosage for a single course of treatment should not exceed 4 mg. Some clinicians recommend a single intravenous dose of 3 mg, whereas others recommend an initial dose of not more than 1 mg of colchicine intravenously, followed by 0.5 mg once or twice daily if needed.

If pain recurs, it may be necessary to administer a daily dose of 1 to 2 mg (2 to 4 ml) for several days; however, **no more colchicine should be given by any route** for at least 7 days after a full course of IV therapy (4 mg).[1,2] Many patients can be transferred to oral colchicine at a dosage similar to that being given intravenously.

In the prophylactic or maintenance therapy of recurrent or chronic gouty arthritis, a dosage of 0.,5 to 1 mg (1 to 2 ml) once or twice daily may be used. However, in these cases, oral administration of colchicine is preferable, usually taken in conjunction with a uricosuric agent. If an acute attack of gout occurs while the patient is taking colchicine as maintenance therapy, an alternative drug should be instituted in preference to increasing the dose of colchicine.

Parenteral drug products should be inspected visually for particulate matter and discoloration prior to administration, whenever solution and container permit.

Storage: Store at controlled room temperature, 59 to 86°F (15 to 30°C).

REFERENCES:

1. Wallace SL, Singer JZ: Review: systemic toxicity associated with the intravenous administration of colchicine - guidelines for use. *J Rheumatol 1988;* 15:495-499. **2.** Simons RJ, Kingma DW: Fatal colchicine toxicity. *Am J Med*1989; 86:356-357.

HOW SUPPLIED - EQUIVALENTS NOT AVAILABLE:

Injection, Solution - Intravenous - 1 mg/2ml

2 ml x 6	$19.55	Colchicine, Lilly	00002-1443-16
2 ml x 10	$45.60	COLCHICINE, Bedford Labs	55390-0605-02

Tablet, Uncoated - Oral - 0.5 mg

100's	$26.03	Colchicine, Abbott	00074-0074-02

Tablet, Uncoated - Oral - 0.6 mg

100's	$3.80	Colchicine, West Ward Pharm	00143-1201-01
100's	$4.30	Colchicine, Major Pharms	00904-2047-60
100's	$4.60	Colchicine, United Res	00677-0040-01
100's	$4.70	Colchicine, Qualitest Pharms	00603-3052-21
100's	$4.76	Colchicine, Schein Pharm (US)	00364-0074-01
100's	$5.00	Colchicine, Trinity Technologies	61355-0001-10
100's	$5.78	Colchicine, US Trading	56126-0472-11
100's	$19.95	Colchicine, Abbott	00074-3781-01
1000's	$16.80	Colchicine, West Ward Pharm	00143-1201-10
1000's	$17.47	Colchicine, Aligen Independ	00405-4266-03
1000's	$18.90	Colchicine, Rugby	00536-3494-10
1000's	$19.90	Colchicine, Qualitest Pharms	00603-3052-32
1000's	$20.30	Colchicine, United Res	00677-0040-10
1000's	$21.40	Colchicine, Major Pharms	00904-2047-80
1000's	$23.58	Colchicine, Schein Pharm (US)	00364-0074-02
1000's	$23.60	Colchicine, Goldline Labs	00182-0174-10
1000's	$23.60	Colchicine, Trinity Technologies	61355-0001-11
1000's	$24.50	Colchicine, HL Moore Drug Exch	00839-5152-16
1000's	$88.12	Colchicine, Lilly	00002-1013-04

Tablet, Uncoated - Oral - 1 mg

100's	$3.95	Colchicine, Consolidated Midland	00223-0703-01
1000's	$19.75	Colchicine, Consolidated Midland	00223-0703-02

COLCHICINE; PROBENECID *(000891)*

CATEGORIES: Antiarthritics; Antigout; Arthritis; Electrolytic, Caloric-Water Balance; Gout; Gouty Arthritis; Pain; Renal Drugs; Uricosuric Agents; FDA Approval Pre 1982

BRAND NAMES: Col-Probenecid; **Colbenemid**; Proben-C

FORMULARIES: BC-BS; Medi-Cal

DESCRIPTION:

Probenecid-colchicine contains probenecid, which is a uricosuric agent, and colchicine, which has antigout activity, the mechanism of which is unknown.

FOR COMPLETE PRESCRIBING INFORMATION REFER TO THE INDIVIDUAL DRUG MONOGRAPHS (COLCHICINE; PROBENECID).

INDICATIONS AND USAGE:

For the treatment of chronic gouty arthritis when complicated by frequent, recurrent acute attacks of gout.

DOSAGE AND ADMINISTRATION:

Therapy with probenecid-colchicine should not be *started* until an acute gouty attack has subsided. However, if an acute attack is precipitated *during* therapy, probenecid-colchicine may be continued without changing the dosage, and additional colchicine or other appropriate therapy should be given to control the acute attack.

The recommended adult dosage is 1 tablet of probenecid-colchicine daily for one week, followed by 1 tablet twice a day thereafter.

Some degree of renal impairment may be present in patients with gout. A daily dosage of 2 tablets may be adequate. However, if necessary, the daily dosage may be increased by 1 tablet every four weeks within tolerance (and usually not above 4 tablets per day) if symptoms of gouty arthritis are not controlled or the 24 hour uric acid excretion is not above 700 mg. As noted, probenecid may not be effective in chronic renal insufficiency particularly when the glomerular filtration rate is 30 ml/minute or less.

Gastric intolerance may be indicative of overdosage, and may be corrected by decreasing the dosage.

As uric acid tends to crystallize out of an acid urine, a liberal fluid intake is recommended, as well as sufficient sodium bicarbonate (3 to 7.5 g daily) or potassium citrate (7.5 g daily) to maintain an alkaline urine (see PRECAUTIONS in Colchicine and Probenecid).

Alkalization of the urine is recommended until the serum urate level returns to normal limits and tophaceous deposits disappear, i.e., during the period when urinary excretion of uric acid is at a high level. Thereafter, alkalization of the urine and the usual restriction of purine-producing foods may be somewhat relaxed.

Probenecid-colchicine (or probenecid) should be continued at the dosage that will maintain normal serum urate levels. When acute attacks have been absent for six months or more and serum urate levels remain within normal limits, the daily dosage of probenecid-colchicine may be decreased by 1 tablet every six months. The maintenance dosage should not be reduced to the point where serum urate levels tend to rise.

Storage: Protect from light.

HOW SUPPLIED - EQUIVALENTS NOT AVAILABLE:

Tablet, Uncoated - Oral - 0.5 mg/500 mg

100 tablet	$18.50	Probenecid & Colchicine, Parmed Pharms	00349-8875-01
100's	$13.05	Probenecid With Colchicine, Harber Pharm	51432-0368-03
100's	$14.65	Colchicine & Probenicid, HL Moore Drug Exch	00839-1172-06
100's	$16.60	Col Probenecid, United Res	00677-0339-01
100's	$16.65	PROBEN-C, Rugby	00536-4365-01
100's	$16.70	Probenecid W/ Colchicine, Major Pharms	00904-2193-60
100's	$17.10	Probenecid W/Colchicine, Qualitest Pharms	00603-5382-21
100's	$17.45	Probenecid & Colchicine, Zenith Labs	00172-2193-60
100's	$17.45	COL-PROBENECID, Goldline Labs	00182-0478-01
100's	$17.50	Probenecid And Colchicine Tablets, Aligen Independ	00405-4846-01
100's	$18.50	Probenecid With Colchicine, Schein Pharm (US)	00364-0315-01
100's	$18.50	Probenecid & Colchicine, Geneva Pharms	00781-1023-01
100's	$18.75	Probenecid W/Colchicine, Consolidated Midland	00223-1473-01
100's	**$35.63**	**COLBENEMID, Merck**	**00006-0614-68**
1000's	$158.30	Probenicid W/Colchicine, Parmed Pharms	00349-8875-10
1000's	$160.70	Probenecid & Colchicine, Zenith Labs	00172-2193-80
1000's	$167.50	Probenecid W/Colchicine, Consolidated Midland	00223-1473-02

COLESTIPOL HYDROCHLORIDE *(000892)*

CATEGORIES: Antilipemic Agents; Bile Acid Sequestrants; Cardiovascular Drugs; Cholesterol; Coronary Artery Disease; Heart Disease; Hypercholesterolemia; Hyperlipidemia; Hyperlipoproteinemia; Hypolipidemics; Resins, Ion Exchange; FDA Approval Pre 1982

BRAND NAMES: *Cholestabyl* (Germany); **Colestid**; *Lestid*
(International brand names outside U.S. in italics)

FORMULARIES: Aetna; BC-BS; FHP; Medi-Cal; PCS

COST OF THERAPY: $760.95 (Hypercholesterolemia; Granule; 5 gm; 20/day; 365 days) vs. Potential Cost of $24,027.04 (DRG 106, Coronary Bypass)

DESCRIPTION:

Colestid Granules consist of colestipol HCl, which is a lipid lowering agent for oral use. Colestipol HCl is an insoluble, high molecular weight basic anion-exchange copolymer of diethylenetriamine and 1-chloro-2,3-epoxypropane, with approximately 1 out of 5 amine nitrogens protonated (chloride form). It is a light yellow water-insoluble resin which is hygroscopic and swells when suspended in water or aqueous fluids. Colestid is tasteless and odorless. Inactive ingredient: Silicon dioxide.

CLINICAL PHARMACOLOGY:

Cholesterol is the major, and probably the sole precursor of bile acids. During normal digestion, bile acids are secreted via the bile from the liver and gall bladder into the intestines. Bile acids emulsify the fat and lipid materials present in food, thus facilitating absorption. A major portion of the bile acids secreted is reabsorbed from the intestines and returned via the portal circulation to the liver, thus completing the enterohepatic cycle. Only very small amounts of bile acids are found in normal serum.

CLINICAL PHARMACOLOGY: *(cont'd)*

Colestipol HCl binds bile acids in the intestine forming a complex that is excreted in the feces. This nonsystemic action results in a partial removal of the bile acids from the enterohepatic circulation, preventing their reabsorption. Since colestipol HCl is an anion exchange resin, the chloride anions of the resin can be replaced by other anions, usually those with a greater affinity for the resin than chloride ion.

Colestipol HCl is hydrophilic, but it is virtually water insoluble (99.75%) and it is not hydrolyzed by digestive enzymes. The high molecular weight polymer in colestipol HCl apparently is not absorbed. Less than 0.05% of ^{14}C-labeled colestipol HCl is excreted in the urine.

The increased fecal loss of bile acids due to colestipol HCl administration leads to an increased oxidation of cholesterol to bile acids. This results in an increase in the number of LDL receptors, increased hepatic uptake of LDL and a decrease in beta lipoprotein or low density lipoprotein serum levels, and a decrease in serum cholesterol levels. Although colestipol HCl produces an increase in the hepatic synthesis of cholesterol in man, serum cholesterol levels fall.

There is evidence to show that this fall in cholesterol is secondary to an increased rate of clearance of cholesterol rich lipoproteins (beta or low density lipoproteins) from the plasma. Serum triglyceride levels may increase or remain unchanged in colestipol treated patients.

The decline in serum cholesterol levels with colestipol HCl treatment is usually evident by one month. When colestipol HCl is discontinued, serum cholesterol levels usually return to baseline levels within one month. Periodic determinations of serum cholesterol levels as outlined in the National Cholesterol Education Program (NCEP) guidelines should be done to confirm a favorable initial and long-term response.[1]

In patients with heterozygous familial hypercholesterolemia who have not obtained an optimal response to colestipol HCl alone in maximal doses, the combination of colestipol HCl and nicotinic acid has been shown to provide effective further lowering of serum cholesterol, triglyceride, and LDL cholesterol values. Simultaneously, HDL cholesterol values increased significantly. In many such patients it is possible to normalize serum lipid values.[2-4] Preliminary evidence suggests that the cholesterol-lowering effects of lovastatin and the bile acid sequestrant, colestipol, are additive.

The effect of intensive lipid-lowering therapy on coronary atherosclerosis has been assessed by arteriography in hyperlipidemic patients. In these randomized, controlled clinical trials, patients were treated for two to four years by either conventional measures (diet, placebo, or in some cases low-dose resin), or with intensive combination therapy using diet plus colestipol HCl granules plus either nicotinic acid or lovastatin. When compared to conventional measures, intensive lipid-lowering combination therapy significantly reduced the frequency of progression and increased the frequency of regression of coronary atherosclerotic lesions in patients with or at risk for coronary artery disease.[5-8]

INDICATIONS AND USAGE:

Since no drug is innocuous, strict attention should be paid to the indications and contraindications, particularly when selecting drugs for chronic long-term use.

Colestipol HCl is indicated as adjunctive therapy to diet for the reduction of elevated serum total and low-density lipoprotein (LDL) cholesterol in patients with primary hypercholesterolemia (elevated low density lipoproteins (LDL) cholesterol) who do not respond adequately to diet. Generally, colestipol HCl has no clinically significant effect on serum triglycerides, but with its use triglyceride levels may be raised in some patients.

In a large, placebo-controlled, multiclinic study, the LRC-CPPT[9], hypercholesterolemic subjects treated with cholestyramine, a bile acid sequestrant with a mechanism of action and an effect on serum cholesterol similar to that of colestipol HCl, had reductions in total and low-density lipoprotein cholesterol (LDL-C). Over the seven-year study period the cholestyramine group experienced a 19% reduction in the combined rate of coronary heart disease death plus non-fatal myocardial infarction (cumulative incidences of 7% cholestyramine and 8.6% placebo). The subjects included in the study were middle-aged men (age 35-59) with serum cholesterol levels above 265 mg/dl, LDL-C above 175 mg/dl on a moderate cholesterol lowering diet, and no history of heart disease. It is not clear to what extent these findings can be extrapolated to other segments of the hypercholesterolemic population not studied.

Treatment for elevated serum cholesterol (>200 mg/dl) should begin with dietary therapy and carried out in two steps (*i.e.,* Step-One and Step-Two Diets). A minimum of six months of intensive dietary therapy and counseling should be carried out prior to initiation of drug therapy. Shorter periods can be considered in patients with severe elevations of LDL-cholesterol (>225 mg/dl) or with definite CHD.

CONTRAINDICATIONS:

Colestipol HCl is contraindicated in those individuals who have shown hypersensitivity to any of its components.

WARNINGS:

TO AVOID ACCIDENTAL INHALATION OR ESOPHAGEAL DISTRESS, COLESTIPOL HCl SHOULD NOT BE TAKEN IN ITS DRY FORM. ALWAYS MIX COLESTIPOL HCl WITH WATER OR OTHER FLUIDS BEFORE INGESTING.

PRECAUTIONS:

Before instituting therapy with colestipol HCl, diseases contributing to increased blood cholesterol such as hypothyroidism, diabetes mellitus, nephrotic syndrome, dysproteinemias and obstructive liver disease should be looked for and specifically treated. The patient's current medications should be reviewed for their potential to increase serum LDL-cholesterol or total cholesterol. It should be verified that an elevated LDL-C level is responsible for high total cholesterol, especially in those patients with marked elevations of high density lipoprotein (HDL) cholesterol and those with triglycerides over 400 mg/dl whose total cholesterol elevation may be due to very low density lipoprotein (VLDL) cholesterol rather than LDL-C. In most patients, LDL-C may be estimated according to the following equation:

$$\text{LDL - C} = \text{total cholesterol} - (0.16 \times (\text{triglycerides}) + \text{HDL - C})$$

When the total triglycerides are greater than 400, this equation is less accurate.

Because it sequesters bile acids, colestipol HCl may interfere with normal fat absorption and thus may prevent absorption of fat soluble vitamins such as A, D, and K.

Chronic use of colestipol HCl may be associated with an increased bleeding tendency due to hypoprothrombinemia from vitamin K deficiency. This will usually respond promptly to parenteral vitamin K_1 and recurrences can be prevented by oral administration of vitamin K_1.

Serum cholesterol and triglyceride levels should be determined periodically based on NCEP guidelines to confirm a favorable initial and adequate long-term response.

Colestipol HCl may produce or severely worsen pre-existing constipation. The dosage should be increased gradually in patients to minimize the risk of developing fecal impaction. In patients with preexisting constipation, the starting dose should be 5 grams (1 packet or 1 scoop) once daily for 5-7 days, increasing to 5 grams twice daily with monitoring of constipation and of serum lipoproteins, at least twice, 4-6 weeks apart. Increased fluid and fiber intake should be encouraged to alleviate constipation and a stool softener may occasionally be indicated. If the initial dose is well tolerated, the dose may be increased as needed by a further 5 grams/day (at monthly intervals) with periodic monitoring of serum lipoproteins. If constipation worsens or the desired therapeutic response is not achieved at 5-30 grams/day, combination therapy or alternate therapy should be considered. Particular effort should be made to avoid constipation in patients with symptomatic coronary artery disease. Constipation associated with colestipol HCl may aggravate hemorrhoids.

While there have been no reports of hypothyroidism induced in individuals with normal thyroid function, the theoretical possibility exists, particularly in patients with limited thyroid reserve.

Since colestipol HCl is a chloride form of an anion exchange resin, there is a possibility that prolonged use may lead to the development of hyperchloremic acidosis.

CARCINOGENESIS, MUTAGENESIS AND IMPAIRMENT OF FERTILITY

In studies conducted in rats in which cholestyramine resin (a bile acid sequestering agent similar to colestipol HCl) was used as a tool to investigate the role of various intestinal factors, such as fat, bile salts and microbial flora, in the development of intestinal tumors induced by potent carcinogens, the incidence of such tumors was observed to be greater in cholestyramine resin treated rats than in control rats.

The relevance of this laboratory observation from studies in rats with cholestyramine resin to the clinical use of colestipol HCl is not known. In the LRC-CPPT study referred to above, the total incidence of fatal and non-fatal neoplasms was similar in both treatment groups. When the many different categories of tumors are examined, various alimentary system cancers were somewhat more prevalent in the cholestyramine group. The small numbers and the multiple categories prevent conclusions from being drawn. Further follow-up of the LRC-CPPT participants by the sponsors of that study is planned for cause-specific mortality and cancer morbidity.

When colestipol HCl was administered in the diet to rats for 18 months, there was no evidence of any drug related intestinal tumor formation. In the Ames assay, colestipol HCl was not mutagenic.

USE IN PREGNANCY

The use of colestipol HCl in pregnancy or lactation or by women of childbearing age requires that the potential benefits of drug therapy be weighed against the possible hazards to the mother and child. The safe use of colestipol HCl resin by pregnant women has not been established.

USE IN CHILDREN

Safety and effectiveness in children have not been established.

DRUG INTERACTIONS:

Since colestipol HCl is an anion exchange resin, it may have a strong affinity for anions other than the bile acids. Therefore colestipol HCl resin may delay or reduce the absorption of concomitant oral medication. The interval between the administration of colestipol HCl and any other medication should be as long as possible. Patients should take other drugs at least one hour before or four hours after colestipol HCl to avoid impeding their absorption.

Human studies have demonstrated that colestipol HCl may decrease propranolol absorption. Effects on the absorption of other beta-blockers have not been determined. Therefore, patients on propranolol should be observed when colestipol HCl is either added or deleted from a therapeutic regimen.

In vitro studies have indicated that colestipol HCl binds a number of drugs. Studies in humans show that the absorption of chlorothiazide as reflected in urinary excretion is markedly decreased even when administered one hour before colestipol HCl. The absorption of tetracycline, furosemide, penicillin G and gemfibrozil was significantly decreased when given simultaneously with colestipol HCl brand of colestipol HCl granules colestipol HCl; these drugs were not tested to determine the effect of administration one hour before colestipol HCl.

No depressant effect on blood levels in humans was noted when colestipol HCl was administered with any of the following drugs: aspirin, clindamycin, clofibrate, methyldopa, tolbutamide, phenytoin or warfarin. Particular caution should be observed with digitalis preparations since there are conflicting results for the effect of colestipol HCl on the availability of digoxin and digitoxin. The potential for binding of these drugs if given concomitantly is present. Discontinuing colestipol HCl could pose a hazard to health if a potentially toxic drug that is significantly bound to the resin has been titrated to a maintenance level while the patient was taking colestipol HCl.

ADVERSE REACTIONS:

Gastrointestinal: The most common adverse reactions are confined to the gastrointestinal tract. To achieve minimal GI disturbance with an optimal LDL-cholesterol lowering effect, a gradual increase of dosage starting with 5 grams once daily is recommended. Constipation, reported by about one patient in 10, is the major single complaint and at times is severe and occasionally accompanied by impaction. Most instances of constipation are mild, transient, and controlled with standard treatment. Increased fluid intake and inclusion of additional dietary fiber should be the first step; a stool softener may be added if needed. Some patients require decreased dosage or discontinuation of therapy. Hemorrhoids may be aggravated.

Less frequent gastrointestinal complaints occurring in about one in 30 to one in 100 patients, are abdominal discomfort (abdominal pain and distention), belching, flatulence, nausea, vomiting, and diarrhea. Peptic ulceration, gastrointestinal irritation and bleeding, cholecystitis, and cholelithiasis have been reported by fewer than one in 500 patients and are not necessarily drug related.

Hypersensitivity: Urticaria and dermatitis were noted in fewer than one in 1,000 patients. Asthma and wheezing were not reported in the colestipol HCl studies but have been noted during treatment with other cholesterol-lowering agents.

Musculoskeletal: Muscle and joint pains, and arthritis have had a reported incidence of less than one in 1,000 patients.

Neurologic: Headache and dizziness were noted in about one in 300 patients: anxiety, vertigo, and drowsiness were reported in fewer than one in 1,000.

Miscellaneous: Anorexia, fatigue, weakness, and shortness of breath have been seen in 1-3 patients in 1,000. Transient and modest elevations of serum glutamic oxaloacetic transaminase and of alkaline phosphatase were observed on one or more occasions in various patients treated with colestipol HCl. Some patients have shown an increase in serum phosphorus and chloride with a decrease in sodium and potassium.

OVERDOSAGE:

Overdosage of colestipol HCl has not been reported. Should overdosage occur, however, the chief potential harm would be obstruction of the gastrointestinal tract. The location of such potential obstruction, the degree of obstruction and the presence or absence of normal gut motility would determine treatment.

DOSAGE AND ADMINISTRATION:

For adults, colestipol HCl is recommended in doses of 5-30 grams/day given once or in divided doses. The starting dose should be 5 grams once or twice daily with a daily increment of 5 grams at one- or two-month intervals. Appropriate use of lipid profiles as per NCEP guidelines including LDL-cholesterol and triglycerides is advised so that optimal, but not excessive doses are used to obtain the desired therapeutic effect on LDL-cholesterol level. If the desired therapeutic effect is not obtained at a dose of 5-30 grams/day with good compliance and acceptable side effects, combined therapy or alternate treatment should be considered.

To avoid accidental inhalation or esophageal distress colestipol HCl should not be taken in its dry form. Colestipol HCl should always be mixed with water or other fluids before ingesting. Patients should take other drugs at least one hour before or four hours after colestipol HCl to minimize possible interference with their absorption. (See DRUG INTERACTIONS).

BEFORE COLESTIPOL HCL ADMINISTRATION

1. Define the type of hyperlipoproteinemia, as described in NCEP guidelines.
2. Institute a trial of diet and weight reduction.
3. Establish baseline serum total and LDL-cholesterol and triglyceride levels.

DURING COLESTIPOL HCL ADMINISTRATION

1. The patient should be carefully monitored clinically, including serum cholesterol and triglyceride levels. Periodic determinations of serum cholesterol levels as outlined in the NCEP guidelines should be done to confirm a favorable initial and long-term response.

2. Failure of total or LDL-cholesterol to fall within the desired range should lead one to first examine dietary and drug compliance. If these are deemed acceptable, combined therapy or alternate treatment should be considered.

3. Significant rise in triglyceride level should be considered as indication for dose reduction, drug discontinuation, or combined or alternate therapy.

MIXING AND ADMINISTRATION GUIDE

Colestipol HCl should always be taken mixed in a liquid such as orange or tomato juice, milk, carbonated beverage, or water. It may also be taken in soups or with cereals or pulpy fruits. Colestipol HCl *should never be taken in its dry form.*

WITH BEVERAGES

1. Add the prescribed amount of colestipol HCl to a glassful (three ounces or more) of water, milk, flavored drink, or a favorite juice (orange, tomato, pineapple, or other fruit juice). A heavy or pulpy juice may minimize complaints relative to consistency. An unsweetened juice may improve palatability.

2. Stir the mixture until the medication is completely mixed. (colestipol HCl will not dissolve in the liquid.) Colestipol HCl may also be mixed with carbonated beverages, slowly stirred in large glass; however, this mixture may be associated with GI complaints.

Rinse the glass with a small amount of additional beverage to make sure all the medication is taken.

WITH CEREALS, SOUPS, AND FRUITS

Colestipol HCl may be taken mixed with milk in hot or regular breakfast cereals, or even mixed in soups that have a high fluid content (tomato or chicken noodle soup). It may also be added to fruits that are pulpy such as crushed pineapple, pears, peaches, or fruit cocktail.

Store at controlled room temperature 15°-30°C (59°-86°F).

REFERENCES:

1. National Cholesterol Education Program (NCEP), The Expert Panel. Report of the National Cholesterol Education Program Expert Panel on Detection, Evaluation, and Treatment of High Blood Cholesterol in Adults.*Arch Intern Med* 148:36-69, 1988. **2.** Kane JP, Malloy MJ, Tun P et al: Normalization of low-density-lipoprotein levels in heterozygous familial hypercholesterolemia with a combined drug regimen. *N Engl. J. Med*304:251-258, 1981. **3.** Illingworth DR, Phillipson BE. JH Rapp et al: Colestipol plus nicotinic acid in treatment of heterozygous familial hypercholesterolemia. *Lancet* 1:296-298, 1981. **4.** Kuo PT, Kostis JB, Moreyra AE et al: Familial type II hyperlipoproteinemia with coronary heart disease: Effect of diet-colestipol-nicotinic acid treatment. *Chest* 79:286-291, 1981. **5.** Blankenhorn DH, et al. Beneficial Effects of Combined Colestipol-Niacin Therapy on Coronary Atherosclerosis and Coronary Venous Bypass Grafts. *JAMA* 257(23):3233-3240, 1987. **6.** Cashin-Hemphill L, et al. Beneficial Effects of Colestipol-Niacin on Coronary Atherosclerosis: A 4-Year Follow-up. *JAMA* 264:3013-3017, 1990. **7.** Brown G, et al. Regression of Coronary Artery Disease as a Result of Intensive Lipid-Lowering Therapy in Men with High Levels of Apolipoprotein B. *N Engl. J. Med* 323:1289-1298, 1990. **8.** Kane JP, Malloy MJ, et al. Regression of Coronary Atherosclerosis During Treatment of Familial Hypercholesterolemia with Combined Drug Regimens. *JAMA* 264:3007-3012, 1990. **9.** Lipid Metabolism-Atherogenesis Branch, National Heart, Lung, and Blood Institute, Bethesda, MD: The Lipid Research Clinics Coronary Primary Prevention Trial Results. I. Reduction in Incidence of Coronary Heart Disease. *JAMA* 251: 351-364, 1984.

HOW SUPPLIED - EQUIVALENTS NOT AVAILABLE:

Granule - Oral - 5 gm

30's	$37.50	COLESTID, PACKETS, Pharmacia & Upjohn	00009-0260-01
90's	$110.25	COLESTID, PACKETS, Pharmacia & Upjohn	00009-0260-04
300 gm	$46.91	COLESTID, Pharmacia & Upjohn	00009-0260-17
450 gm	$46.91	COLESTID, Pharmacia & Upjohn	00009-0370-05
500 gm	$78.19	COLESTID, Pharmacia & Upjohn	00009-0260-02

Packet - Oral - 7.5 gm

60's	$73.50	COLESTID, Pharmacia & Upjohn	00009-0370-03

Tablet, Uncoated - Oral - 1 gm

120's	$34.40	COLESTID, Pharmacia & Upjohn	00009-0450-03

COLISTIMETHATE SODIUM *(000893)*

CATEGORIES: Anti-Infectives; Antibiotics; Antimicrobials; Diarrhea; Infections; Polymyxins; FDA Approval Pre 1982

BRAND NAMES: *Coliracin*; **Coly-Mycin M**
(International brand names outside U.S. in italics)

DESCRIPTION:

Coly-Mycin M Parenteral (Sterile Colistimethate Sodium, USP) is a sterile parenteral antibiotic product which, when reconstituted (see Reconstitution), is suitable for intramuscular or intravenous administration. Each vial contains 150 mg colistin base equivalent. Colistimethate sodium is a polypeptide antibiotic with an approximate molecular weight of 1750; The empirical formula is $C_{58}H_{105}N_{16}Na_5O_{28}S_5$.

CLINICAL PHARMACOLOGY:

Microbiology: Colistimethate sodium has bactericidal activity against the following gram-negative bacilli: *Enterobacter aerogenes, Escherichia coli, Klebsiella pneumoniae,* and *Pseudomonas aeruginosa.*

HUMAN PHARMACOLOGY

Higher serum levels were obtained at 10 minutes following IV administration. Serum concentration declined with a half-life of 2-3 hours following either intravenous or intramuscular administration in adults and children including premature infants.

CLINICAL PHARMACOLOGY: *(cont'd)*

Colistimethate sodium is transferred across the placental barrier, and blood levels of about 1 mcg/ml are obtained in the fetus following intravenous administration to the mother.

Average urine levels ranged from about 270 mcg/ml at 2 hours to about 15 mcg/ml at 8 hours after intravenous administration and from 200 to about 25 mcg/ml during a similar period following intramuscular administration.

CLINICAL STUDIES:

Clinically, colistimethate sodium has been of particular therapeutic value in acute and chronic urinary tract infections caused by sensitive strains of *Pseudomonas aeruginosa.* Colistimethate sodium is clinically effective in the treatment of infections due to other sensitive gram-negative pathogenic bacilli which have become resistant to broad spectrum antibiotics.

Colistimethate sodium has been used to treat bacteriuria and overt urinary infections in pregnant women during the third trimester. However, in view of the evidence of possible embryotoxic and teratogenic effects of colistimethate sodium in pregnant rabbits, caution should be exercised in use of this drug in women of childbearing potential.

INDICATIONS AND USAGE:

Colistimethate sodium is indicated for the treatment of acute or chronic infections due to sensitive strains of certain gram-negative bacilli. It is particularly indicated when the infection is caused by sensitive strains of *Pseudomonas aeruginosa.* This antibiotic is not indicated for infections due to *Proteus or Neisseria.* Colistimethate sodium has proven clinically effective in treatment of infections due to the following gram-negative organisms: *Enterobacter aerogenes, Escherichia coli, Klebsiella pneumoniae,* and *Pseudomonas aeruginosa.*

Pending results of appropriate bacteriologic cultures and sensitivity tests, colistimethate sodium may be used to initiate therapy in serious infections that are suspected to be due to gram-negative organisms.

CONTRAINDICATIONS:

The use of colistimethate sodium is contraindicated for patients with a history of sensitivity to the drug.

WARNINGS:

Maximum daily dose should not exceed 5 mg/kg/day (2.3 mg/lb) with normal renal function.

Transient neurological disturbances may occur. These include circumoral paresthesias or numbness, tingling or formication of the extremities, generalized pruritus, vertigo, dizziness, and slurring of speech. For these reasons, patients should be warned not to drive vehicles or use hazardous machinery while on therapy. Reduction of dosage may alleviate symptoms. Therapy need not be discontinued, but such patients should be observed with particular care. Overdosage can result in renal insufficiency, muscle weakness and apnea. See PRECAUTIONS for use concomitantly with curariform drugs, and DOSAGE AND ADMINISTRATIONSection for use in renal impairment.

PRECAUTIONS:

Since colistimethate sodium is eliminated mainly by renal excretion, it should be used with caution when the possibility of impaired renal function exists. The decline in renal function with advanced age should be considered.

When actual renal impairment is present, colistimethate sodium may be used, but the greatest caution should be exercised and the dosage should be reduced in proportion to the extent of the impairment. Administration of amounts of colistimethate sodium in excess of renal excretory capacity will lead to high serum levels and can result in further impairment of renal function, initiating a cycle which, if not recognized, can lead to acute renal insufficiency, renal shutdown and further concentration of the antibiotic to toxic levels in the body. At this point, interference of nerve transmission at neuromuscular junctions may occur and result in muscle weakness and apnea.

Easily recognized signs indicating the development of impaired renal function are diminishing urine output, rising BUN and serum creatinine. If present, therapy with colistimethate sodium should be discontinued immediately.

If a life-threatening situation exists, therapy may be reinstated at a lower dosage after blood levels have fallen.

Certain other antibiotics (kanamycin, streptomycin, dihydrostreptomycin, polymyxin, neomycin) have also been reported to interfere with the nerve transmission at the neuromuscular junction. Based on this reported activity, they should not be given concomitantly with colistimethate sodium except with the greatest caution. The antibiotics with a gram-positive antimicrobial spectrum, e.g. penicillin, tetracycline, sodium cephalothin, have not been reported to interfere with nerve transmission and, accordingly, would not be expected to potentiate this activity of colistimethate sodium.

Other drugs, including curariform muscle relaxants (ether, tubocurarine, succinylcholine, gallamine, decamethonium and sodium citrate) potentiate the neuromuscular blocking effect and should be used with extreme caution in patients being treated with colistimethate sodium.

If apnea occurs, it may be treated with assisted respiration, oxygen, and calcium chloride injections.

Use in Pregnancy: The safety of colistimethate sodium during human pregnancy has not been established.

ADVERSE REACTIONS:

Respiratory arrest has been reported following intramuscular administration of colistimethate sodium. Impaired renal function increases the possibility of apnea and neuromuscular blockade following administration of colistimethate sodium. This has been generally due to failure to follow recommended guidelines, usually overdosage, failure to reduce dose commensurate with degree of renal impairment, and/or concomitant use of other antibiotics or drugs with neuromuscular blocking potential.

A decrease in urine output or increase in blood urea nitrogen or serum creatinine can be interpreted as signs of nephrotoxicity, which is probably a dose-dependent effect of colistimethate sodium. These manifestations of nephrotoxicity are reversible following discontinuation of the antibiotic.

Increases of blood urea nitrogen have been reported for patients receiving colistimethate sodium at dose levels of 1.6-5 mg/kg per day. The BUN values returned to normal following cessation of colistimethate sodium administration.

Paresthesia, tingling of the extremities or tingling of the tongue and generalized itching or urticaria have been reported by patients who received colistimethate sodium by intravenous or intramuscular injection. In addition, the following adverse reactions have been reported for colistimethate sodium: drug fever and gastrointestinal upset, vertigo, and slurring of speech. The subjective symptoms reported by the adult may not be manifest in infants or young children, thus requiring close attention to renal function.

DOSAGE AND ADMINISTRATION:

Important: Colistimethate sodium is supplied in vials containing colistimethate sodium equivalent to 150 mg colistin base activity per vial.

Reconstitution: The **150-mg** vial should be reconstituted with **2.0 ml** Sterile Water for Injection, USP. The reconstituted solution provides colistimethate sodium at a concentration of 75 mg/ml.

During reconstitution swirl **gently** to avoid frothing.

DOSAGE ADULTS AND CHILDREN

Intravenous or Intramuscular Administration: Colistimethate sodium should be given in 2 to 4 divided doses at dose levels of 2.5 to 5 mg/kg per day for patients with normal renal function, depending on the severity of the infection.

In obese individuals, dosage should be based on ideal body weight.

The daily dose should be reduced in the presence of any renal impairment, which can often be anticipated from the history.

Modifications of dosage in the presence of renal impairment are presented in TABLE 1.

TABLE 1 Suggested Modification of Dosage Schedules of Colistimethate Sodium for Adults with Impaired Renal Function

Renal Function	Degree of Impairment: Normal	Mild	Moderate	Considerable
Plasma creatinine, mg/100 ml	0.7-1.2	1.3-1.5	1.6-2.5	2.6-4.0
Urea clearance, % of normal	80-100	40-70	25-40	10-25
Dosage Unit dose of Coly-Mycin M, mg	100-150	75-115	66-150	100-150
Frequency, times/day	4 to 2	2	2 or 1	every 36 hr
Total daily dose, mg	300	150-230	133-150	100
Approximate daily dose, mg/kg/day	5.0	2.5-3.8	2.5	1.5

Note: The suggested unit dose is 2.5-5 mg/kg; however, the time INTERVAL between injections should be increased in the presence of impaired renal function.

Intravenous Administration

1. Direct Intermittent Administration: slowly inject one-half of the total daily dose over a period of 3 to 5 minutes every 12 hours.

2. Continuous Infusion:

- 0.9% NaCl
- 5% dextrose in 0.9% NaCl
- 5% dextrose in water
- 5% dextrose in 0.45% NaCl
- 5% dextrose in 0.225% NaCl
- Lactated Ringer's solution
- 10% invert sugar solution.

There are not sufficient data to recommend usage of colistimethate sodium with other drugs or other than the above listed infusion solutions.

Administer the second half of the total daily dose by slow intravenous infusion, starting 1 to 2 hours after the initial dose, over the next 22 to 23 hours. In the presence of impaired renal function, reduce the infusion rate depending on the degree of renal impairment.

The choice of intravenous solution and the volume to be employed are dictated by the requirements of fluid and electrolyte management.

ANY INFUSION SOLUTION CONTAINING COLISTIMETHATE SODIUM SHOULD BE FRESHLY PREPARED AND USED FOR NO LONGER THAN 24 HOURS.

Store at controlled room temperature 15°-30°C (59°-86°F).

Store reconstituted solution in refrigerator 2°-8°C (36°-46°F) or at controlled room temperature 15°-30°C (59°-86°F) and use within 7 days.

ANIMAL PHARMACOLOGY:

TOXICOLOGY

Acute Toxicity: The intravenous LD_{50} was 41.5 mg/kg in the dog and 739 mg/kg in the mouse; intramuscular toxicity was 42 mg/kg in the dog and 267 mg/kg in the mouse.

Subacute Toxicity: In albino rabbits and beagle dogs, IV doses of 5, 10 and 20 mg/kg/day for 28 days resulted in elevated blood urea nitrogen in the dog (10 mg/kg/day dose group) and in both 20 mg/kg dose groups.

HOW SUPPLIED - EQUIVALENTS NOT AVAILABLE:

Injection, Lyphl-Soln - Intramuscular; - 150 mg/vial

5 ml	$32.56	COLY-MYCIN M, Parke-Davis	00071-4145-01
5 ml x 10	$1232.32	COLY-MYCIN M, Parke-Davis	00071-4145-47

COLISTIN SULFATE; HYDROCORTISONE ACETATE; NEOMYCIN SULFATE; THONZONIUM BROMIDE *(000894)*

CATEGORIES: Anti-Infectives; Antibiotics; EENT Drugs; Eye, Ear, Nose, & Throat Preparations; Infections; Otic Hydrocortisones; Otic Preparations; Otologic; FDA Pre 1938 Drugs

BRAND NAMES: *Colimycin F; Coly-Mycin Otic* (Canada); **Coly-Mycin S**; *Coly-Mycin S Otic*
(International brand names outside U.S. in italics)

FORMULARIES: Aetna

DESCRIPTION:

Coly-Mycin S Otic with neomycin and hydrocortisone (colistin sulfate-neomycin sulfate-thonzonium bromide-hydrocortisone acetate otic suspension) is a sterile aqueous suspension containing in each ml: colistin base activity, 3 mg (as the sulfate); neomycin base activity, 3.3 mg (as the sulfate); hydrocortisone acetate, 10 mg (1%); thonzonium bromide, 0.5 mg (0.05%); polysorbate 80, acetic acid, and sodium acetate in a buffered aqueous vehicle.

DESCRIPTION: *(cont'd)*

Thimerosal (mercury derivative) 0.002%, added as a preservative. It is a nonviscous liquid, buffered at pH 5, for instillation into the canal of the external ear or direct application to the affected aural skin.

CLINICAL PHARMACOLOGY:

1. Colistin Sulfate: an antibiotic with bactericidal action against most gram-negative organisms, notably *Pseudomonas aeruginosa, E coli* and *Klebsiella-Aerobacter.*

2. Neomycin Sulfate: a broad-spectrum antibiotic bactericidal to many pathogens, notably *Staph aureus* and *Proteus* sp.

3. Hydrocortisone Acetate: a corticosteroid that controls inflammation, edema, pruritus and other dermal reactions.

4. Thonzonium Bromide: a surface-active agent that promotes tissue contact by dispersion and penetration of the cellular debris and exudate.

INDICATIONS AND USAGE:

For the treatment of superficial bacterial infections of the external auditory canal, caused by organisms susceptible to the action of the antibiotics; and for the treatment of infections of mastoidectomy and fenestration cavities, caused by organisms susceptible to the antibiotics.

CONTRAINDICATIONS:

This product is contraindicated in those individuals who have shown hypersensitivity to any of its components, and in herpes simplex, vaccinia and varicella.

WARNINGS:

As with other antibiotic preparations, prolonged treatment may result in overgrowth of nonsusceptible organisms and fungi.

If the infection is not improved after one week, cultures and susceptibility tests should be repeated to verify the identity of the organism and to determine whether therapy should be changed.

Patients who prefer to warm the medication before using should be cautioned against heating the suspension above body temperature, in order to avoid loss of potency.

PRECAUTIONS:

GENERAL

If sensitization or irritation occurs, medication should be discontinued promptly.

This drug should be used with care in cases of perforated eardrum and in long-standing cases of chronic otitis media because of the possibility of ototoxicity caused by neomycin.

Treatment should not be continued for longer than ten days.

Allergic cross-reactions may occur which could prevent the use of any or all of the following antibiotics for the treatment of future infections: kanamycin, paromomycin, streptomycin, and possibly gentamicin.

ADVERSE REACTIONS:

Neomycin is a not uncommon cutaneous sensitizer. There are articles in the current literature that indicate an increase in the prevalence of persons sensitive to neomycin.

DOSAGE AND ADMINISTRATION:

The external auditory canal should be thoroughly cleansed and dried with a sterile cotton applicator.

When using the calibrated dropper:

For adults, 5 drops of the suspension should be instilled into the affected ear 3 or 4 times daily. For infants and children, 4 drops are suggested because of the smaller capacity of the ear canal.

This dosage correlates to the 4 drops (for adults) and 3 drops (for children) recommended when using the dropper-bottle container for this product.

The patient should lie with the affected ear upward and then the drops should be instilled. This position should be maintained for 5 minutes to facilitate penetration of the drops into the ear canal. Repeat, if necessary, for the opposite ear.

If preferred, a cotton wick may be inserted into the canal and then the cotton may be saturated with the suspension. This wick should be kept moist by adding further solution every 4 hours. The wick should be replaced at least once every 24 hours.

Shake well before using.

Store at controlled room temperature 15°-30°C (59°-86°F). Stable for 18 months at room temperature; prolonged exposure to higher temperatures should be avoided.

HOW SUPPLIED - EQUIVALENTS NOT AVAILABLE:

Suspension - Otic - /10 mg

5 ml	$13.97	COLY-MYCIN S, Parke-Davis	00071-3141-35
10 ml	$22.39	COLY-MYCIN S, Parke-Davis	00071-3141-36

COLLAGEN HEMOSTAT *(000895)*

CATEGORIES: Bleeding; Blood Formation/Coagulation; Coagulants and Anticoagulants; EENT Drugs; Eye, Ear, Nose, & Throat Preparations; Hemostatics; Mucous Membrane Agents; Skin/Mucous Membrane Agents; FDA Pre 1938 Drugs

BRAND NAMES: Avitene; Endo-Avitene; Ent Avitene; **Hemopad**; Hemotene; Instat; Neuro Avitene

DESCRIPTION:

Hemopad Absorbable Collagen Hemostat is a purified bovine collagen. The material, prepared as a textured pad, is sterile nonpyrogenic, and absorbable. Hemostatic activity, which is an inherent property of collagen, is largely dependent on the basic helical structure of this protein. The helical structure of native collagen is preserved during the manufacture of Hemopad Hemostat. When collagen comes into contact with blood, platelets aggregate on the collagen and release coagulation factors which, together with plasma factors result in the formation of fibrin, and finally in the formation of a clot.

CLINICAL STUDIES:

The safety effectiveness and handling characteristics of collagen hemostat pad were evaluated in a variety of surgical procedures. The average time to hemostasis for collagen hemostat pad was 4.4 minutes. Passive Hemagglutination Assay (PHA) and Enzyme-Linked Immunoabsorbent Assay (ELISA) methods have been used to evaluate the immunological potential for collagen hemostat pad to produce antibodies in animals. These assays revealed little if any elevation of antibody titers in collagen hemostat pad treated animals while in animals treated

CLINICAL STUDIES: *(cont'd)*

with a collagen control hemostat, mild elevation of antibodies occurred. The handling properties of collagen hemostat pad were judged superior to those of the collagen control hemostat.

INDICATIONS AND USAGE:

Collagen hemostat pad is indicated in surgical procedures (other than in neurological, urological and ophthalmological surgery) for use as an adjunct to hemostasis when control of bleeding by ligature or other conventional methods is ineffective or impractical.

CONTRAINDICATIONS:

Collagen hemostat pad is contraindicated in the closure of skin incisions as it may interfere with the healing of skin edges. This interference is due to simple mechanical interposition of dry collagen and not due to any intrinsic interference with wound healing.

Collagen hemostat pad is contraindicated on bone surfaces to which prosthetic materials are to be attached with methylmethacrylate adhesives. It has been reported with another absorbable collagen hemostat pad, that by filling porosities of cancellous bone, collagen may reduce the bonding strength of methylmethacrylate.

WARNINGS:

Collagen hemostat pad is inactivated by autoclaving. It should not be resterilized. As with any foreign substance, use in contaminated wounds may enhance infection.

Collagen hemostat pad should not be used in instances of pumping arterial hemorrhage.

Collagen hemostat pad should not be used where blood or other fluids have pooled or in cases where the point of hemorrhage is submerged. Collagen hemostat pad will not act as a tampon or plug in a bleeding site nor will it close off an area of blood collecting behind a tampon.

Only the amount of collagen hemostat necessary to provide hemostasis should be used. The long-term effects of leaving collagen hemostat *in situ* are unknown. Opened, unused collagen hemostat pad should be discarded because it cannot be resterilized.

PRECAUTIONS:

As with other hemostatic agents, it is not recommended that collagen hemostat pad be left in an infected or contaminated space, nor is it recommended for use in persons known to be sensitive to material of bovine origin. When placed into cavities or closed spaces, care should be exercised to avoid overpacking collagen hemostat pad as it may absorb fluid and expand and press against neighboring structures.

Safety of this products has not been established in children and pregnant women: therefore, collagen hemostat pad should only be used when benefit to risk clearly warrants its use.

Collagen hemostat pad is not intended to be used to treat systemic coagulation disorders.

ADVERSE REACTIONS:

Collagen hemostat pad is a collagen product. Although several types of postoperative complications were observed in collagen hemostat pad treated patients, none were attributed to collagen hemostat pad by the investigator. Adverse reactions reported for other collagen hemostats include hematoma, potentiation of infection, would dehiscence, inflammation and edema. Other reported adverse reactions that may be related to the use of collagen hemostats include adhesion formation, allergic reaction, foreign body reaction and subgaleal seroma (in a single case). The use of microfibrillar collagen in dental extraction sockets has been reported to increase the incidence of alveolalgia. The possibility that all of the above reaction may occur with collagen hemostat pad cannot be excluded.

DOSAGE AND ADMINISTRATION:

Collagen hemostat pad is applied directly to the bleeding surface with pressure. Collagen hemostat pad can be cut to size. The amount needed and the period of time necessary to apply pressure will vary with the type and amount of bleeding to be controlled. Hemostasis time depends upon the type of surgery and degree of pretreatment bleeding. It usually occurred between 2 to 6 minutes with collagen hemostat pad.

Collagen hemostat pad maintains its integrity in the presence of blood and is not dispersed when wet. It is easily removed from the site following hemostasis. It is most effective when used dry.

Collagen hemostat pad may be left *in situ* whenever necessary. However, the surgeon, at his discretion, should remove any excess of collagen hemostat pad prior to wound closure. Animal implant studies have demonstrated that absorption and tissue reaction to collagen hemostat pad are similar to those observed with another absorbable collagen hemostatic agent.

HOW SUPPLIED - EQUIVALENTS NOT AVAILABLE:

Topical - 1 gm

5's	$466.13	HEMOTENE, Astra USA	00186-2005-02

Pad, Medicated - Topical

10's	**$503.25**	**HEMOPAD, Astra USA**	**00186-2001-00**
10's	**$1097.25**	**HEMOPAD, Astra USA**	**00186-2002-00**
10's	**$1974.50**	**HEMOPAD, Astra USA**	**00186-2003-00**

COLLAGENASE *(000896)*

CATEGORIES: Dermatologicals; Mucous Membrane Agents; Pressure Ulcers; Skin/Mucous Membrane Agents; FDA Pre 1938 Drugs

BRAND NAMES: Biozyme-C; *Iruxol Mono*; *Iruxol Simplex*; Santyl
(International brand names outside U.S. in italics)

DESCRIPTION:

Collagenase ointment is a sterile enzymatic debriding ointment which contains 250 collagenase units per gram of white petrolatum USP. The enzyme collagenase is derived from the fermentation by *Clostridium histolyticum.* It possesses the unique ability to digest native and denatured collagen in necrotic tissue.

CLINICAL PHARMACOLOGY:

Since collagen accounts for 75% of the dry weight of skin tissue, the ability of collagenase to digest collagen in the physiological pH range and temperature makes it particularly effective in the removal of detritus.[1] Collagenase thus contributes towards the formation of granulation tissue and subsequent epithelization of dermal ulcers and severely burned areas.[2-6] Collagen in healthy tissue or in newly formed granulation tissue is not attacked.[2-8]

INDICATIONS AND USAGE:

Collagenase ointment is indicated for debriding chronic dermal ulcers[2-6,8-18] and severely burned areas.[3-5,7,16,19,20,21]

CONTRAINDICATIONS:

Collagenase ointment is contraindicated in patients who have shown local or systemic hypersensitivity to collagenase.

PRECAUTIONS:

The optimal pH range of collagenase is 6 to 8. Higher or lower pH conditions will decrease the enzyme's activity and appropriate precautions should be taken. The enzymatic activity is also adversely affected by detergents, hexachlorophene and heavy metal ions such as mercury and silver which are used in some antiseptics. When it is suspected such materials have been used, the site should be carefully cleansed by repeated washings with normal saline before collagenase ointment is applied. Soaks containing metal ions or acidic solutions such as Burow's solution should be avoided because of the metal ion and low pH. Cleansing materials such as hydrogen peroxide, Dakin's solution, and sterile saline are compatible with collagenase ointment.

Debilitated patients should be closely monitored for systemic bacterial infections because of the theoretical possibility that debriding enzymes may increase the risk of bacteremia.

A slight transient erythema has been noted occasionally in the surrounding tissue, particularly when collagenase ointment was not confined to the lesion. Therefore, the ointment should be applied carefully within the area of the lesion.

ADVERSE REACTIONS:

No allergic sensitivity or toxic reactions have been noted in the recorded clinical investigations. However, one case of systemic manifestations of hypersensitivity to collagenase in a patient treated for more than one year with a combination of collagenase and cortisone has been reported to us.

OVERDOSAGE:

Action of the enzyme may be stopped, should this be desired, by the application of Burow's solution USP (pH 3.6-4.4) to the lesion.

DOSAGE AND ADMINISTRATION:

Collagenase ointment should be applied once daily (or more frequently if the dressing becomes soiled, as from incontinence) in the following manner:

(1) Prior to application the lesion should be cleansed of debris and digested material by gently rubbing with a gauze pad saturated with hydrogen peroxide or Dakin's solution followed by sterile normal saline.

(2) Whenever infection is present it is desirable to use an appropriate topical antibiotic powder. The antibiotic should be applied to the lesion prior to the application of collagenase ointment. Should the infection not respond, therapy with collagenase ointment should be discontinued until remission of the infection.

(3) Collagenase ointment should be applied directly to deep lesions with a wooden tongue depressor or spatula. For shallow lesions, collagenase ointment may be applied to a sterile gauze pad which is then applied to the wound and properly secured.

(4) Crosshatching thick eschar with a #10 blade allows collagenase more surface contact with necrotic debris. It is also desirable to remove, with forceps and scissors, as much loosened detritus as can be done readily.

(5) All excess ointment should be removed each time dressing is changed.

(6) Use of collagenase ointment should be terminated when debridement of necrotic tissue is complete and granulation tissue is well established.

HOW SUPPLIED:

Collagenase ointment contains 250 units of collagenase enzyme per gram of white petrolatum USP. The potency assay of collagenase is based on the digestion of undenatured collagen (from bovine Achilles tendon) at pH 7.2 and 37°C for 24 hours. The number of peptide bonds cleaved are measured by reaction with ninhydrin. Amino groups released by a trypsin digestion control are subtracted. One net collagenase unit will solubilize ninhydrin reactive material equivalent to 4 micromoles of leucine.

REFERENCES:

1. Mandl, I., Adv. Enzymol. 23:163, 1961. **2.** Boxer, A.M., Gottesman, N., Bernstein, H., & Mandl, I., Geriatrics 24:75, 1969. **3.** Mazurek, I., Med. Welt 22:150, 1971. **4.** Zimmerman, W.E., in "Collagenase," I., Mandl, ed., Gordon & Breach, Science Publishers, New York, 1971, p. 131, p.185. **5.** Vetra, H., Whittaker, D., Geriatrics 30: 53, 1975. **6.** Rao, D.B., Sane, P.G., & Georgiev, E.L., J. Am. Geriatrics Soc. 23:22, 1975. **7.** Vrabec, R., Moserova, J., Konickova, Z., Behounkova, E., & Blaha, J., J. Hyg. Epidemiol. Microbiol. Immunol. 18:496, 1974. **8.** Lippmann, H.I., Arch. Phys. Med. Rehabil. 54:588, 1973. **9.** German, F.M., in "Collagenase," I. Mandl, ed., Gordon & Breach, Science Publishers, New York, 1971, p. 165. **10.** Haimovici, H. & Strauch, B., in "Collagenase," I. Mandl, ed., Gordon & Breach, Science Publishers, New York, 1971, p. 177. **11.** Lee, L.K., & Ambrus, J.L., Geriatrics 30:91, 1975. **12.** Locke, R.K., & Heiflitz, N.M., J. Am. Pod. Assoc. 65:242, 1975. **13.** Varma, A.O., Bugatch, E., & German, F.M., Surg. Gynecol. Obstet. 136:281, 1973. **14.** Barrett D., Jr., & Klibanski, A., Am. J. Nurs. 733:849, 1973. **15.** Bardfeld, L.A., J. Pod. Ed. 1:41, 1970. **16.** Blum, G., Schweiz, Rundschau Med. Praxis 62:820, 1973, Abstr. in Dermatology Digest, Feb. 1974, p. 36. **17.** Zaruba, F., Lettl, A., Brozkova, L., Skrdlantova, H., & Krs, V., J. Hyg. Epidemiol. Microbiol. Immunol. 18:499, 1974. **18.** Altman, M.I., Goldstein, L., Horowitz, S., J. Am. Pod. Assoc. 68:11, 1978. **19.** Rehn, V.J., Med. Klin. 58:799, 1963. **20.** Krauss, H., Koslowski, L., & Zimmerman W.E., Langenbecks Arch. Klin. Chir. 303:23, 1963. **21.** Gruenagel, H.H., Med. Klin. 58:442, 1963.

HOW SUPPLIED - EQUIVALENTS NOT AVAILABLE:

Ointment - Topical - 250 unit/gm

15 gm	$27.89	SANTYL, Knoll Labs	00044-5270-02
30 gm	$53.03	SANTYL, Knoll Labs	00044-5270-03

COLLODION *(000897)*

CATEGORIES: Skin/Mucous Membrane Agents; FDA Pre 1938 Drugs

BRAND NAMES: *Collodion B.P.* (England); Flexible Collodion
(International brand names outside U.S. in italics)

Prescribing information not available at time of publication.

HOW SUPPLIED - EQUIVALENTS NOT AVAILABLE:

Liquid

480 ml	$13.55	Flexible Collodion, Millgood	53118-0319-01

COPPER *(000903)*

CATEGORIES: Electrolytic, Caloric-Water Balance; Replacement Solutions; FDA Approved 1988 Apr

BRAND NAMES: *Anticon 300*; *Copper T 380A*; *Copper-T*; *Copper T 200B*; *Copper T 200 Schering*; *Cuprocept CCL*; *Dalcept Cu 260*; *Gene T 380 Slimline*; *Gravigard* (England, Germany); *Gyne-T* (France, Germany); *Gyne-T 380 Slimline*; *Gyne T 200*; *Gyne T*; *Gyne T 380*; Intrauterine Copper Contraceptive; *Mini-Gravigard* (England);

Multiload (Mexico); *Multiload (Cu 250)*; *Multiload Cu 250* (Germany); *Multiload Cu 250 Short*; *Multiload Cu 375*; *Multiload Cu 375 SL*; *Multiload Cu 375-X* (Germany); *Multiload CU 250*; *Multiload CU 375*; *Nova-T*; *Nova T* (Mexico); *Nova T Cu 200 Ag*; *Nova T Schering Intrauterine Device*; *Ortho Gyne-T 380 Slimline*; *Protec T* (Mexico); *Sof-T*; *Tricept*
(International brand names outside U.S. in italics)

Prescribing information not available at time of publication.

HOW SUPPLIED - EQUIVALENTS NOT AVAILABLE:

Iud - Intrauterine - 176 mg

1's	$176.00	PARAGARD, Gynopharma	54765-0380-01
5's	$835.00	PARAGARD, Gynopharma	54765-0380-05

CORTICOTROPIN *(000904)*

CATEGORIES: ACTH; Adrenal Function; Adrenal Insufficiency; Adrenocortical Insufficiency; Allergic Reactions; Allergies; Anemia; Anterior Pituitary/Hypothalmic Function; Anti-Inflammatory Agents; Arthritis; Aspiration Pneumonitis; Asthma; Cancer; Carditis; Dermatitis; Dermatomyositis; Diagnostic Agents; Diuresis; Edema; Endocrine Disorders; Enteritis; Epicondylitis; Erythema Multiforme; Erythroblastopenia; Herpes; Herpes Zoster; Hormones; Hypercalcemia; Leukemia; Lupus Erythematosus; Lymphoma; Meningitis; Multiple Sclerosis; Mycosis Fungoides; Nephrotic Syndrome; Pituitary; Pneumonitis; Proteinuria; Psoriasis; Serum Sickness; Synovitis; Thrombocytopenia; Trichinosis; Uveitis; FDA Approval Pre 1982

BRAND NAMES: ACTH; *ACTH Lannacher*; *ACTH Vitoria*; **Acthar**; **H P Acthar Gel**; *Acthar Gel*; *Acthelea*; *Acton Prolongatum*
(International brand names outside U.S. in italics)

FORMULARIES: BC-BS; Medi-Cal

DESCRIPTION:

Repository corticotropin injection is a highly purified sterile preparation of the adrenocorticotropic hormone in 16% gelatin to provide a prolonged release after intramuscular or subcutaneous injection. Also contains 0.5% phenol, not more than 0.1% cysteine (added), sodium hydroxide and/or acetic acid to adjust pH, and water for injection, q.s.

Corticotropin for injection is a sterile lyophilized ACTH which in dry form is stable at room temperature. Each vial contains 25 or 40 Units of Corticotropin U.S.P. and approximately 9 and 14 milligrams of hydrolyzed gelatin respectively. After reconstitution, this product is administered in the intravenous, intramuscular, or subcutaneous route.

ACTH is a 39 amino acid peptide with the following chemical formula:

H-	Ser- 1	Tyr- 2	Ser- 3	Met- 4	Glu- 5	His- 6	Phe- 7	Arg- 8	Trp- 9
Gly- 10	Lys- 11	Pro- 12	Val- 13	Gly- 14	Lys- 15	Lys- 16	Arg- 17	Arg- 18	Pro 19
Val- 20	Lys- 21	Val- 22	Try- 23	Pro- 24	Asp- 25	Gly- 26	Ala- 27	Glu- 28	Asp- 29
Gin- 30	Leu- 31	Ala- 32	Glu- 33	Ala- 34	Phe- 35	Pro- 36	Leu- 37	Glu- 38	
Phe- 39	OH								

CLINICAL PHARMACOLOGY:

ACTH stimulates the adrenal cortex to secrete cortisol, corticosterone, aldosterone, and a number of weakly androgenic substances. Although ACTH does stimulate secretion of aldosterone, the rate is relatively independent. Prolonged administration of large doses of ACTH induces hyperplasia and hypertrophy of the adrenal cortex and continuous high output of cortisol, corticosterone, and weak androgens. The release of ACTH is under the influence of the nervous system via the corticotropin regulatory hormone released from the hypothalamus and by a negative corticosteroid feedback mechanism. Elevated plasma cortisol suppresses ACTH release.

The trophic effects of ACTH on the adrenal cortex are not understood beyond the fact that they appear to be mediated by cyclic AMP.

ACTH rapidly disappears from the circulation following its intravenous administration; in man the plasma half-life is about 15 minutes.

The maximal effects of a trophic hormone on a target organ are achieved when optimal amounts of hormone are acting continuously. Thus, a fixed dose of ACTH will demonstrate a linear increase in adrenocortical secretion with increasing duration of the infusion.

INDICATIONS AND USAGE:

Corticotropin for injection and repository corticotropin injection are indicated for diagnostic testing of adrenocortical function.

Corticotropin for injection and repository corticotropin injection have limited therapeutic value in those conditions responsive to corticosteroid therapy; in such cases, corticosteroid therapy is considered to be the treatment of choice.

Corticotropin for injection and repository corticotropin injection may be employed in the following disorders:

Endocrine Disorders: Nonsuppurative thyroiditis; Hypercalcemia associated with cancer.

Nervous System Diseases: Acute exacerbations of multiple sclerosis.

Rheumatic Disorders: As adjunctive therapy for short-term administration (to tide the patient over an acute episode or exacerbation) in: psoriatic arthritis; rheumatoid arthritis, including juvenile rheumatoid arthritis (selected cases may require low-dose maintenance therapy); ankylosing spondylitis; acute and subacute bursitis; acute nonspecific tenosynovitis; acute gouty arthritis; post-traumatic arthritis; synovitis of osteoarthritis; epicondylitis.

Collagen Diseases: During an exacerbation or as maintenance therapy in selected cases of: systemic lupus erythematosus; systemic dermatomyositis (polymyositis); Acute rheumatic carditis.

Dermatologic Diseases: Pemphigus; bullous dermatitis herpetiformis; severe erythema multiforme (Stevens-Johnson syndrome); exfoliative dermatitis; severe psoriasis; severe seborrheic dermatitis; mycosis fungoides.

Allergic States: Control of severe or incapacitating allergic conditions intractable to adequate trials of conventional treatment: seasonal or perennial allergic rhinitis; bronchial asthma; contact dermatitis; atopic dermatitis; serum sickness.

Opthalmic Diseases: Severe acute and chronic allergic and inflammatory processes involving the eye and its adnexa such as: allergic conjunctivitis; keratitis; herpes zoster ophthalmicus; iritis and iridocyclitis; diffuse posterior uveitis and choroiditis; optic neuritis; sympathetic ophthalmia; chorioretinitis; anterior segment inflammation; allergic corneal marginal ulcers.

INDICATIONS AND USAGE: *(cont'd)*

Respiratory Diseases: Symptomatic sarcoidosis; loeffler's syndrome not manageable by other means; berylliosis; fulminating or disseminated pulmonary tuberculosis when used concurrently with antituberculous chemotherapy; aspiration pneumonitis.

Hematologic Disorders: Acquired (autoimmune) hemolytic anemia; secondary thrombocytopenia in adults; erythroblastopenia (rbc anemia); congenital (erythroid) hypoplastic anemia.

Neoplastic Diseases: For palliative management of: leukemias and lymphomas in adults; acute leukemia of childhood.

Edematous State: To induce a diuresis or a remission of proteinuria in the nephrotic syndrome without uremia of the idiopathic type or that due to lupus erythematosus.

Gastrointestinal Diseases: *To Tide the Patient Over a Critical Period of the Disease In:* ulcerative colitis; regional enteritis.

Miscellaneous: Tuberculous meningitis with subarachnoid block or impending block when used concurrently with appropriate anti-tuberculous chemotherapy; trichinosis with neurologic or myocardial involvement.

CONTRAINDICATIONS:

Corticotropin is contraindicated in patients with scleroderma, osteoporosis, systemic fungal infections, ocular herpes simplex, recent surgery, history of or the presence of a peptic ulcer, congestive heart failure, hypertension, or sensitivity to proteins of porcine origin.

Treatment of conditions listed within the INDICATIONS AND USAGE is contraindicated when they are accompanied by primary adrenocortical insufficiency or adrenocortical hyperfunction.

Intravenous administration of corticotropin is contraindicated for treatment of conditions listed within INDICATIONS AND USAGE, but Corticotropin is used intravenously for diagnostic purposes (see DOSAGE AND ADMINISTRATION).

WARNINGS:

Chronic administration of corticotropin may lead to adverse effects which are not reversible. Corticotropin may only suppress symptoms and signs of chronic diseases without altering the natural course of the disease. Neither repository corticotropin injection nor corticotropin for injection should be administered for treatment until adrenal responsiveness has been verified with the route of administration which will be utilized during treatment, intramuscularly or subcutaneously. A rise in urinary and plasma corticosteroid values provides direct evidence of a stimulatory effect. Prolonged administration of corticotropin increases the risk of hypersensitivity reactions. Although the action of corticotropin is similar to that of exogenous adrenocortical steroids the quantity of adrenocorticoid may be variable. In patients who receive prolonged corticotropin therapy the additional use of rapidly acting corticosteroids before, during, and after an unusual stressful situation is indicated.

Prolonged use of corticotropin may produce posterior subcapsular cataracts and glaucoma with possible damage to the optic nerves.

Corticotropin may mask some signs of infection, and new infections including those of the eye due to fungi or viruses may appear during its use. There may be decreased resistance and inability to localize infection when corticotropin is used.

Corticotropin can cause elevation of blood pressure, salt and water retention, and increased excretion of potassium. Dietary salt restriction and potassium supplementation may be necessary. Corticotropin increases calcium excretion.

While on corticotropin therapy, patients should not be vaccinated against smallpox. Other immunization procedures should be undertaken with caution in patients who are receiving corticotropin, especially when high doses are administered because of the possible hazards of neurological complications and lack of antibody response.

PRECAUTIONS:

General: Corticotropin injection should be used in the lowest dose for the shortest period of time to accomplish the therapeutic goal. Corticotropin should be used for treatment only when the disease is intractable to non-steroid treatment.

There is an enhanced effect in patients with hypothyroidism and in those with cirrhosis of the liver. Sensitivity to porcine protein should be considered before starting therapy and during the course of treatment should symptoms arise.

Then an infection is present, appropriate antibiotic therapy should be given. Patients with latent tuberculosis should be observed closely and if therapy is prolonged, chemoprophylaxis should be instituted.

Psychic symptoms may appear with use of corticotropin or pre-existing symptoms may be enhanced. These may range from mood alteration to a psychotic state.

Patients with a secondary disease may have that disease worsened. Caution should be used when prescribing corticotropin in patients with diabetes, renal insufficiency, diverticulitis, and myasthenia gravis.

Corticotropin often acts by suppressing symptoms without altering the course of the underlying disease. Since complications with corticotropin use are dependent on the dose and duration of treatment, a risk/benefit decision must be made in each case.

Suppression of the pituitary adrenal axis occurs following prolonged therapy which may be slow in returning to normal. Patients should be protected from the stress of trauma or surgery by the use of corticosteroids during the period of stress.

Since maximal corticotropin stimulation of the adrenals may be limited during the first few days of treatment, other drugs should be administered when an immediate therapeutic effect is desirable.

Although controlled clinical trials have shown ACTH to be effective in speeding the resolution of acute exacerbations of multiple sclerosis they do not show that it affects the ultimate outcome or natural history of the disease. The studies do show that relatively high doses of ACTH are necessary to demonstrate a significant effect. (See DOSAGE AND ADMINISTRATION.)

Treatment of acute gouty arthritis should be limited to a few days. Since rebound attacks may occur when corticotropin is discontinued, conventional concomitant therapy should be administered during corticotropin treatment and for several days after it is stopped.

Aspirin should be used cautiously in conjunction with corticotropin in hypoprothrombinemia.

Carcinogenesis, Mutagenesis, and Impairment of Fertility: Adequate and well-controlled studies have not been done in animals. Human use has not been associated with an increase in malignant disease. See Pregnancy warning below.

Pregnancy Category C: Corticotropin has been shown to have an embryocidal effect. There are no adequate and well-controlled studies in pregnant women. Corticotropin should be used during pregnancy only if the potential benefit justifies the potential risk to the fetus.

Nursing Mothers: It is not known whether this drug is excreted in human milk. Because many drugs are excreted in human milk and because of the potential for serious adverse reactions in nursing infants from corticotropin, a decision should be made whether to discontinue nursing or to discontinue the drug, taking into account the importance of the drug to the mother.

PRECAUTIONS: *(cont'd)*

Pediatric Use: Prolonged use of corticotropin in children will inhibit skeletal growth. If use is necessary, it should be given intermittently and the child carefully observed.

DRUG INTERACTIONS:

Corticotropin may accentuate the electrolyte loss associated with diuretic therapy.

ADVERSE REACTIONS:

Fluid and Electrolyte Disturbances: Sodium retention; fluid retention; potassium loss; hypokalemic alkalosis; calcium loss.

Musculoskeletal: Muscle weakness; steroid myopathy; loss of muscle mass; osteoporosis; vertebral compression fractures; aseptic necrosis of femoral and humeral heads; pathologic fracture of long bones.

Gastrointestinal: Peptic ulcer with possible perforation and hemorrhage; pancreatitis; abdominal distention; ulcerative esophagitis.

Dermatologic: Impaired wound healing; thin fragile skin; petechiae and ecchymoses; facial erythema; increased sweating; suppression of skin test reactions; acne; hyperpigmentation.

Cardiovascular: Hypertension, necrotizing angitis; congestive heart failure.

Neurological: Convulsions; increased intracranial pressure with papilledema, (pseudo-tumor cerebri) usually after treatment; headache, vertigo.

Endocrine: Menstrual irregularities; development of Cushingoid state; suppression of growth in children; secondary adrenocortical and pituitary unresponsiveness, particularly in times of stress, as in trauma, surgery or illness; decreased carbohydrate tolerance; manifestations of latent diabetes mellitus; increased requirements for insulin or oral hypoglycemic agents in diabetics; hirsutism.

Ophthalmic: Posterior subcapsular cataracts; increased intraocular pressure; glaucoma with possible damage to optic nerve; exophthalmos.

Metabolic: Negative nitrogen balance due to protein catabolism.

Allergic reactions: Especially in patients with allergic responses to proteins manifesting as dizziness, nausea and vomiting, shock, skin reactions.

Miscellaneous: Abscess: prolonged use of ACTH may result in antibodies to it and resulting loss of stimulatory effect.

DRUG ABUSE AND DEPENDENCE:

Although drug dependence does not occur, sudden withdrawal of corticotropin after prolonged use may lead to recurrent symptoms which make it difficult to stop. It may be necessary to taper the dose and increase the injection interval to gradually discontinue the medication.

OVERDOSAGE:

An acute overdose would present no different adverse reactions.

DOSAGE AND ADMINISTRATION:

Standard tests for verification of adrenal responsiveness to corticotropin may utilize as much as 80 units as a single injection or one or more injections of a lesser dosage. Verification tests should be performed prior to treatment with corticotropins. The test should utilize the route (s) of administration proposed for treatment. Following verification, dosage should be individualized according to the disease under treatment and the general medical condition of each patient. Frequency and dose of the drug should be determined by considering severity of the disease, plasma and urine corticosteroid levels and the initial response of the patient. Only gradual change in dosage schedules should be attempted, after full drug effects have become apparent.

The chronic administration of more than 40 units daily may be associated with uncontrollable adverse effects.

When reduction in dosage is indicated this should be done gradually by either reducing the amount of each injection, administering injections at longer intervals, or by a combination of both of the above. During reduction of dosage careful consideration should be given to the disease being treated, the general medical conditions of the patient and the duration over which corticotropin was administered.

Acthar must be reconstituted at the time of use by dissolving in a convenient volume of Sterile Water for Injection or Sodium Chloride Injection in such a manner that the individual dose will be contained in 1-2 ml of solution. The reconstituted solution should be refrigerated and used within 24 hours.

Repository corticotropin injection and corticotropin for injection may be administered intramuscularly or subcutaneously.

Repository corticotropin injection is given intramuscularly or subcutaneously every 24-72 hours in doses of 40-80 units.

The usual intramuscular or subcutaneous dose for corticotropin for injection is 20 units four times a day.

In the treatment of acute exacerbations of multiple sclerosis daily intramuscular doses of 80-120 units for 2-3 weeks may be administered.

For diagnostic purposes, corticotropin for injection may be given intravenously in doses of 10-25 units dissolved in 500 ml of 5% glucose infused over an 8-hour period.

Repository corticotropin injection is stable for the period indicated on the label when stored under refrigeration between 2°- 8°C (36°-46°F).

Corticotropin for injection is stable for the period indicated on the label when stored at controlled room temperature, 15°-30°C (59°-86°F).

HOW SUPPLIED - RATED THERAPEUTICALLY EQUIVALENT:

Injection, Lyphl-Soln - Intramuscular; - 25 unit/vial

1's	**$21.64**	**ACTHAR, Rhone-Poulenc Rorer**	**00075-1025-01**

Injection, Lyphl-Soln - Intramuscular; - 40 unit/vial

1's	**$31.84**	**ACTHAR, Rhone-Poulenc Rorer**	**00075-1040-01**
40 unt	$17.38	ACTH, Parke-Davis	00071-4198-01

HOW SUPPLIED - NOT RATED EQUIVALENT:

Injection, Repository - Intramuscular; - 40 unit/ml

1 ml x 10	**$154.90**	**H P ACTHAR GEL, Rhone-Poulenc Rorer**	**00075-1330-02**
5 ml	**$21.96**	**H P ACTHAR GEL, Rhone-Poulenc Rorer**	**00075-1330-01**

Injection, Solution - Intravenous - 40 unit/ml

5 ml	$34.95	ACTH, Hyrex Pharms	00314-7101-05

Injection, Solution - Intravenous - 80 unit/ml

1 ml x 10	**$266.25**	**H P ACTHAR GEL, Rhone-Poulenc Rorer**	**00075-1350-02**
5 ml	**$43.59**	**H P ACTHAR GEL, Rhone-Poulenc Rorer**	**00075-1350-01**
5 ml	$55.35	ACTH, Hyrex Pharms	00314-7102-05

CORTISONE ACETATE *(000907)*

CATEGORIES: Adrenal Corticosteroids; Adrenal Hyperplasia; Adrenal Insufficiency; Adrenocortical Insufficiency; Airway Obstruction; Allergies; Anemia; Ankylosing Spondylitis; Anti-Inflammatory Agents; Antiarthritics; Arthritis; Aspiration Pneumonitis; Asthma; Atopic Dermatitis; Berylliosis; Bursitis; Cancer; Carditis; Chemotherapy; Choroiditis; Colitis; Conjunctivitis; Corneal Ulcer; Dermatitis; Dermatitis Herpetiformis; Dermatomyositis; Diuresis; Drug Hypersensitivity; Enteritis; Epicondylitis; Erythema Multiforme; Erythroblastopenia; Glucocorticoids; Gouty Arthritis; Herpes; Herpes Zoster; Hormones; Hypercalcemia; Inflammation; Iridocyclitis; Keratitis; Laryngeal Edema; Leukemia; Lupus Erythematosus; Lymphoma; Meningitis; Mycosis Fungoides; Nephrotic Syndrome; Neuritis; Osteoarthritis; Pain; Pemphigus; Pneumoconiosis; Pneumonitis; Proteinuria; Psoriasis; Purpura; Retinochoroiditis; Rhinitis; Sarcoidosis; Serum Sickness; Shock; Spondylitis; Steroids; Synovitis; Synovitis of Osteoarthritis; Tenosynovitis; Thrombocytopenia; Thrombocytopenic Purpura; Thyroiditis; Trichinosis; Tuberculosis; Ulcerative Colitis; Urticaria; Uveitis; FDA Approval Pre 1982

BRAND NAMES: *Adreson*; *Altesona*; *Cortate*; *Cortelan* (England); *Cortison Ciba* (Germany); *Cortison Nycomed*; *Cortisone* (France); *Cortisone Acetate*; *Cortisoni Acetas*; *Cortistab* (England); *Cortisyl*; *Cortogen*; **Cortone**; *Cortone Acetato*; *Cortone-Azetat*; *Scheroson* (Japan)
(International brand names outside U.S. in italics)

FORMULARIES: BC-BS; Medi-Cal

COST OF THERAPY: $155.12 (Asthma; Tablet; 25 mg; 1/day; 365 days)

PRIMARY ICD9: 493.90 (Asthma, Unspecified, Without Mention of Status Asthmaticus)

DESCRIPTION:

Cortisone acetate is a white to practically white, odorless, crystalline powder. It is stable in air. It is insoluble in water. The molecular weight is 402.49. It is designated chemically as 21-(acetyloxy)-17-hydroxy-pregn-4-ene-3,11,20-trione. The empirical formula is $C_{23}H_{30}O_6$.

Tablets: Glucocorticoids are adrenocortical steroids, both naturally occurring and synthetic, which are readily absorbed from the gastrointestinal tract.

Cortone (Cortisone Acetate) tablets contain 25 mg of cortisone acetate in each tablet. Inactive ingredients are lactose, magnesium stearate, and starch.

IM Injection: Cortone sterile suspension is a sterile suspension containing 50 mg per milliliter of cortisone acetate in an aqueous medium (pH 5.0 to 7.0). Inactive ingredients per ml: sodium chloride, 9 mg; polysorbate 80, 4 mg; sodium carboxymethylcellulose, 5 mg; Water for Injection q.s. 1 ml. Benzyl alcohol, 9 mg, added as preservative.

No attempt should be made to alter Cortone Acetate sterile suspension. Diluting it or mixing it with other substances may affect the state of suspension or change the rate of absorption and reduce its effectiveness.

CLINICAL PHARMACOLOGY:

Naturally occurring glucocorticoids (hydrocortisone & cortisone), which also have salt-retaining properties, are used as replacement therapy in adrenocortical deficiency states. They are also used for their potent anti-inflammatory effects in disorders of many organ systems.

Glucocorticoids cause profound and varied metabolic effects. In addition, they modify the body's immune responses to diverse stimuli.

IM Injection: Cortisone acetate sterile suspension has a slow onset but long duration of action when compared with more soluble preparations. When daily corticosteroid therapy is required and oral therapy is not feasible, the required daily dosage may be given in a single intramuscular injection of this preparation.

INDICATIONS AND USAGE:

Endocrine Disorders: Primary or secondary adrenocortical insufficiency (hydrocortisone or cortisone is the first choice; synthetic analogs may be used in conjunction with mineralocorticoids where applicable; in infancy mineralocorticoid supplementation is of particular importance)

Congenital adrenal hyperplasia, nonsuppurative thyroiditis, hypercalcemia associated with cancer.

Rheumatic Disorders: As adjunctive therapy for short-term administration (to tide the patient over an acute episode or exacerbation) in:

Psoriatic arthritis, rheumatoid arthritis, including juvenile rheumatoid arthritis (selected cases may require low-dose maintenance therapy), ankylosing spondylitis, acute and subacute bursitis, acute nonspecific tenosynovitis, acute gouty arthritis, post-traumatic osteoarthritis, synovitis of osteoarthritis, epicondylitis

Collagen Diseases: During an exacerbation or as maintenance therapy in selected cases of:

Systemic lupus erythematosus, acute rheumatic carditis, systemic dermatomyositis (polymyositis).

Dermatologic Diseases:

Pemphigus, bullous dermatitis herpetiformis, severe erythema multiforme (Stevens-Johnson syndrome), exfoliative dermatitis, mycosis fungoides, severe psoriasis, severe seborrheic dermatitis.

Allergic States: Control of severe or incapacitating allergic conditions intractable to adequate trials of conventional treatment:

Seasonal or perennial allergic rhinitis, bronchial asthma, contact dermatitis, atopic dermatitis, serum sickness, drug hypersensitivity reactions.

Ophthalmic Diseases: Severe acute and chronic allergic and inflammatory processes involving the eye and its adnexa such as:

Allergic conjunctivitis, keratitis, allergic corneal marginal ulcers, herpes zoster ophthalmicus, iritis and iridocyclitis, chorioretinitis, anterior segment inflammation, diffuse posterior uveitis and choroiditis, optic neuritis, sympathetic ophthalmia.

Respiratory Diseases:

Symptomatic sarcoidosis, loeffler's syndrome not manageable by other means, berylliosis, fulminating or disseminated pulmonary tuberculosis when used concurrently with appropriate antituberculous chemotherapy, aspiration pneumonitis

Hematologic Disorders:

Acquired (autoimmune) hemolytic anemia, erythroblastopenia (RBC anemia), congenital (erythroid) hypoplastic anemia

Neoplastic Diseases: For palliative management of:

Leukemias and lymphomas in adults, acute leukemia of childhood

Edematous States: To induce a diuresis or remission of protein-uria in the nephrotic syndrome, without uremia, of the idiopathic type or that due to lupus erythematosus

INDICATIONS AND USAGE: *(cont'd)*

Gastrointestinal Diseases: To tide the patient over a critical period of the disease in:

Ulcerative colitis, regional enteritis

Miscellaneous: Tuberculous meningitis with subarachnoid block or impending block when used concurrently with appropriate antituberculous chemotherapy, trichinosis with neurologic or myocardial involvement

TABLETS ONLY

Hematologic Disorders: Idiopathic thrombocytopenic purpura in adults, secondary thrombocytopenia in adults

IM INJECTION ONLY

Endocrine Disorders: Acute adrenocortical insufficiency (hydrocortisone or cortisone is the drug of choice; mineralocorticoid supplementation may be necessary, particularly when synthetic analogs are used)

Preoperatively, and in the event of serious trauma or illness, in patients with known adrenal insufficiency or when adrenocortical reserve is doubtful.

Shock unresponsive to conventional therapy if adrenocortical insufficiency exists or is suspected.

Allergic States: Urticarial transfusion reactions

Acute noninfectious laryngeal edema (epinephrine is the drug of first choice)

CONTRAINDICATIONS:

Systemic fungal infections

Hypersensitivity to this product

WARNINGS:

In patients on corticosteroid therapy subjected to unusual stress, increased dosage of rapidly acting corticosteroids before, during, and after the stressful situation is indicated.

Drug-induced secondary adrenocortical insufficiency may result from too rapid withdrawal of corticosteroids and may be minimized by gradual reduction of dosage. This type of relative insufficiency may persist for months after discontinuation of therapy; therefore, in any situation of stress occurring during that period, hormone therapy should be reinstituted. If the patient is receiving steroids already, dosage may have to be increased. Since mineralocorticoid secretion may be impaired, salt and/or a mineralocorticoid should be administered concurrently.

Corticosteroids may mask some signs of infection, and new infections may appear during their use. There may be decreased resistance and inability to localize infection when corticosteroids are used. Moreover, corticosteroids may affect the nitrobluetetrazolium test for bacterial infection and produce false negative results.

In cerebral malaria, a double-blind trial has shown that the use of corticosteroids is associated with prolongation of coma and a higher incidence of pneumonia and gastrointestinal bleeding.

Corticosteroids may activate latent amebiasis. Therefore, it is recommended that latent or active amebiasis be ruled out before initiating corticosteroid therapy in any patient who has spent time in the tropics or any patient with unexplained diarrhea.

Prolonged use of corticosteroids may produce posterior subcapsular cataracts, glaucoma with possible damage to the optic nerves, and may enhance the establishment of secondary ocular infections due to fungi or viruses.

Usage in Pregnancy: Since adequate human reproduction studies have not been done with corticosteroids, use of these drugs in pregnancy or in women of childbearing potential requires that the anticipated benefits be weighed against the potential hazards to the mother and embryo or fetus. Infants born of mothers who have received substantial doses of corticosteroids during pregnancy should be carefully observed for signs of hypoadrenalism.

Corticosteroids appear in breast milk and could suppress growth, interfere with endogenous corticosteroid production, or cause other unwanted effects. Mothers taking pharmacologic doses of corticosteroids should be advised not to nurse.

Average and large doses of hydrocortisone or cortisone can cause elevation of blood pressure, salt and water retention, and increased excretion of potassium. These effects are less likely to occur with the synthetic derivatives except when used in large doses. Dietary salt restriction and potassium supplementation may be necessary. All corticosteroids increase calcium excretion.

Administration of live virus vaccines, including smallpox, is contraindicated in individuals receiving immunosuppressive doses of corticosteroids. If inactivated viral or bacterial vaccines are administered to individuals receiving immunosuppressive doses of corticosteroids, the expected serum antibody response may not be obtained. However, immunization procedures may be undertaken in patients who are receiving corticosteroids as replacement therapy, e.g., for Addison's disease.

The use of cortisone acetate tablets or sterile suspension in active tuberculosis should be restricted to those cases of fulminating or disseminated tuberculosis in which the corticosteroid is used for the management of the disease in conjunction with an appropriate antituberculosis regimen.

If corticosteroids are indicated in patients with latent tuberculosis or tuberculin reactivity, close observation is necessary as reactivation of the disease may occur. During prolonged corticosteroid therapy, these patients should receive chemoprophylaxis.

Literature reports suggest an apparent association between use of corticosteroids and left ventricular free wall rupture after a recent myocardial infarction; therefore, therapy with corticosteroids should be used with great caution in these patients.

IM INJECTION ONLY

Because rare instances of anaphylactoid reactions have occurred in patients receiving parenteral corticosteroid therapy, appropriate precautionary measures should be taken prior to administration, especially when the patient has a history of allergy to any drug. Anaphylactoid and hypersensitivity reactions have been reported for sterile suspension cortisone acetate (see ADVERSE REACTIONS).

PRECAUTIONS:

Following prolonged therapy, withdrawal of corticosteroids may result in symptoms of the corticosteroid withdrawal syndrome including fever, myalgia, arthralgia, and malaise. This may occur in patients even without evidence of adrenal insufficiency.

There is an enhanced effect of corticosteroids on patients with hypothyroidism and in those with cirrhosis.

Corticosteroids should be used cautiously in patients with ocular herpes simplex because of possible corneal perforation.

The lowest possible dose of corticosteroid should be used to control the condition under treatment, and when reduction in dosage is possible, the reduction should be gradual.

PRECAUTIONS: *(cont'd)*

Psychic derangements may appear when corticosteroids are used, ranging from euphoria, insomnia, mood swings, personality changes, and severe depression, to frank psychotic manifestations. Also, existing emotional instability or psychotic tendencies may be aggravated by corticosteroids.

Aspirin should be used cautiously in conjunction with corticosteroids in hypoprothrombinemia.

Steroids should be used with caution in nonspecific ulcerative colitis, if there is a probability of impending perforation, abscess or other pyogenic infection, diverticulitis, fresh intestinal anastomoses, active or latent peptic ulcer, renal insufficiency, hypertension, osteoporosis, and myasthenia gravis. Signs of peritoneal irritation following gastrointestinal perforation in patients receiving large doses of corticosteroids may be minimal or absent. Fat embolism has been reported as a possible complication of hypercortisonism.

When large doses are given, some authorities advise that corticosteroids be taken with meals and antacids be taken between meals to help to prevent peptic ulcer.

Growth and development of infants and children on prolonged corticosteroid therapy should be carefully observed.

Steroids may increase or decrease motility and number of spermatozoa in some patients.

Phenytoin, phenobarbital, ephedrine, and rifampin may enhance the metabolic clearance of corticosteroids, resulting in decreased blood levels and lessened physiologic activity, thus requiring adjustment in corticosteroid dosage.

The prothrombin time should be checked frequently in patients who are receiving corticosteroids and coumarin anticoagulants at the same time because of reports that corticosteroids have altered the response to these anticoagulants. Studies have shown that the usual effect produced by adding corticosteroids is inhibition of response to coumarins, although there have been some conflicting reports of potentiation not substantiated by studies.

When corticosteroids are administered concomitantly with potassium-depleting diuretics, patients should be observed closely for the development of hypokalemia.

IM INJECTION ONLY

Cortisone acetate sterile suspension, like many other steroid formulations, is sensitive to heat. Therefore, it should not be autoclaved when it is desirable to sterilize the exterior of the vial.

ADVERSE REACTIONS:

Fluid and Electrolyte Disturbances

Sodium retention, fluid retention, congestive heart failure in susceptible patients, potassium loss, hypokalemic alkalosis, hypertension

Musculoskeletal

Muscle weakness, steroid myopathy, loss of muscle mass, osteoporosis, vertebral compression fractures, aseptic necrosis of femoral and humeral heads, pathologic fracture of long bones, tendon rupture

Gastrointestinal

Peptic ulcer with possible perforation and hemorrhage, perforation of the small and large bowel, particularly in patients with inflammatory bowel disease, pancreatitis, abdominal distention, ulcerative esophagitis

Dermatologic

Impaired wound healing, Thin fragile skin, Thin fragile skin, Petechiae and ecchymoses, Erythema, Increased sweating, May suppress reactions to skin tests, Other cutaneous reactions, such as allergic dermatitis, urticaria, angioneurotic edema

Neurological

Convulsions, increased intracranial pressure with papilledema (pseudotumor cerebri) usually after treatment, vertigo, headache, psychic disturbances

Endocrine

Menstrual irregularities, development of cushingoid state, suppression of growth in children, secondary adrenocortical and pituitary unresponsiveness, particularly in times of stress, as in trauma, surgery or illness, decreased carbohydrate tolerance, manifestations of latent diabetes mellitus, increased requirements for insulin or oral hypoglycemic agents in diabetics, hirsutism

Ophthalmic: Posterior subcapsular cataracts, increased intraocular pressure, glaucoma, exophthalmos

Metabolic: Negative nitrogen balance due to protein catabolism.

Cardiovascular: Myocardial rupture following recent myocardial infarction (see WARNINGS).

Other: Hypersensitivity, thromboembolism, weight gain, increased appetite, nausea

OVERDOSAGE:

Reports of acute toxicity and/or death following overdosage of glucocorticoids are rare. In the event of overdosage, no specific antidote is available; treatment is supportive and symptomatic.

The intraperitoneal LD_{50} of cortisone acetate in female mice was 1405 mg/kg.

DOSAGE AND ADMINISTRATION:

Tablets: For oral administration

IM Injection: For intramuscular injection only.NOT FOR INTRAVENOUS USE.

The initial dosage of cortisone acetate may vary from 25 to 300 mg per day depending on the disease being treated. In less severe diseases doses lower than 25 mg may suffice, while in severe diseases doses higher than 300 mg may be required. The initial dosage should be maintained or adjusted until the patient's response is satisfactory. If satisfactory clinical response does not occur after a reasonable period of time, discontinue cortisone acetate tablets or sterile suspension and transfer the patient to other therapy.

After a favorable initial response, the proper maintenance dosage should be determined by decreasing the initial drug dosage in small amounts to the lowest dosage that maintains an adequate clinical response.

Patients should be observed closely for signs that might require dosage adjustment, including changes in clinical status resulting from remissions or exacerbations of the disease, individual drug responsiveness, and the effect of stress (*e.g.*, surgery, infection, trauma). During stress it may be necessary to increase dosage temporarily

If the drug is to be stopped after more than a few days of treatment, it usually should be withdrawn gradually.

HOW SUPPLIED - EQUIVALENTS NOT AVAILABLE:

Injection, Solution - Intramuscular - 50 mg/ml

10 ml	$9.50	Cortisone Acetate, Hyrex Pharms	00314-0620-70
10 ml	**$26.20**	**CORTONE ACETATE, Merck**	**00006-7069-10**

Tablet, Uncoated - Oral - 5 mg

50's	$6.51	Cortisone Acetate, Pharmacia & Upjohn	00009-0015-01

HOW SUPPLIED - EQUIVALENTS NOT AVAILABLE: *(cont'd)*

Tablet, Uncoated - Oral - 10 mg

100's	$24.01	Cortisone Acetate, Pharmacia & Upjohn	00009-0023-01

Tablet, Uncoated - Oral - 25 mg

100's	$42.50	Cortisone Acetate, West Ward Pharm	00143-1202-01
100's	$42.50	Cortisone Acetate, Qualitest Pharms	00603-3062-21
100's	$43.50	Cortisone Acetate, Major Pharms	00904-2043-60
100's	$45.48	Cortisone Acetate, HL Moore Drug Exch	00839-5084-06
100's	$47.95	Cortisone Acetate, United Res	00677-0046-01
100's	$48.00	Cortisone Acetate, Goldline Labs	00182-1648-01
100's	$50.48	Cortisone Acetate, Rugby	00536-3530-01
100's	$58.03	Cortisone Acetate, Pharmacia & Upjohn	00009-0034-01
100's	**$62.40**	**CORTONE ACETATE, Merck**	**00006-0219-68**

COSYNTROPIN *(000908)*

CATEGORIES: ACTH; Adrenal Function; Adrenal Insufficiency; Adrenocortical Insufficiency; Anterior Pituitary/Hypothalmic Function; Diagnostic Agents; Hormones; Tumors; Tuberculosis*; FDA Approval Pre 1982
* Indication not approved by the FDA

BRAND NAMES: *Cortrosinta Depot*; **Cortrosyn**; *Cortrosyn Depot* (France); *Nuvacthen Depot*; *Synacthen* (Australia, England, Germany); *Synacthen Deposito*; *Synacthen Depot* (Australia, England, Germany, Canada); *Synacthene* (France)
(International brand names outside U.S. in italics)

FORMULARIES: BC-BS

DESCRIPTION:

Cosyntropin for injection is a sterile lyophilized powder in vials containing 0.25 mg of cosyntropin and 10 mg of mannitol to be reconstituted with 1 ml sodium chloride for injection, USP as a solvent. Administration is by intravenous or intramuscular injection. Cosyntropin is alpha 1-24 corticotropin, a synthetic subunit of ACTH. It is an open chain polypeptide containing, from the N terminus, the first 24 of the 39 amino acids of natural ACTH.

The sequence of amino acids in the 1-24 compound is found in TABLE 1

TABLE 1

Ser- 1	Tyr- 2	Ser- 3	Met- 4	Glu- 5	acid-	His- 6	Phe- 7	Arg- 8	Trp- 9	Gly 10
Lys- 11	Pro- 12	Val- 13	Gly- 14	Lys- 15	Lys- 16	Arg- 17	Arg- 18	Pro- 19	Val- 20	Lys 21
Val- 22	Try- 23	Pro- 24								

CLINICAL PHARMACOLOGY:

Cosyntropin exhibits the full corticosteroidogenic activity of natural ACTH. Various studies have shown that the biologic activity of ACTH resides in the N-terminal portion of the molecule and that the 1-20 amino acid residue is the minimal sequence retaining full activity. Partial or complete loss of activity is noted with progressive shortening of the chain beyond 20 amino acid residue. For example, the decrement from 20 to 19 results in a 70% loss of potency.

The pharmacologic profile of cosyntropin is similar to that of purified natural ACTH. It has been established that 0.25 mg of cosyntropin will stimulate the adrenal cortex maximally and to the same extent as 25 units of natural ACTH. This dose of cosyntropin will produce maximal secretion of 17-OH corticosteroids, 17- ketosteroids and/or 17-ketogenic steroids.

The extra-adrenal effects which natural ACTH and cosyntropin have in common include increased melanotropic activity, increased growth hormone secretion and an adipokinetic effect. These are considered to be without physiological or clinical significance.

Animal, human and synthetic ACTH (1-39) which all contain 39 amino acids exhibit similar immunologic activity. This activity resides in the C-terminal portion of the molecule and the 22-39 amino acid residues exhibit the greatest degree of antigenicity. In contrast, synthetic polypeptide containing 1-19 or fewer amino acids have no detectable immunologic activity. Those containing 1-26, 1-24, or 1-23 amino acids have very little immunologic although full biologic activity. This property of cosyntropin assumes added importance in view of the known antigenicity of natural ACTH.

INDICATIONS AND USAGE:

Cosyntropin is intended for use as a diagnostic agent in the screening of patients presumed to have adrenocortical insufficiency. Because of its rapid effect on the adrenal cortex it may be utilized to perform a 30-minute test of adrenal function (plasma cortisol response) as an office or outpatient procedure, using only 2 venipunctures. (See DOSAGE AND ADMINISTRATIONfor details.)

Severe hypofunction of the pituitary-adrenal axis is usually associated with subnormal plasma cortisol values but a low basal level is not per se evidence of adrenal insufficiency and does not suffice to make the diagnosis. Many patients with proven insufficiency will have normal basal levels and will develop signs of insufficiency only when stressed. For this reason the only criterion which should be used in establishing the diagnosis is the failure to respond to adequate corticotropin stimulation as provided by 0.25 mg of cosyntropin for injection. When presumptive adrenal insufficiency is diagnosed by a subnormal cosyntropin test, further studies are indicated to determine if it is primary or secondary.

Primary adrenal insufficiency (Addison's Disease) is the result of an intrinsic disease process, such as tuberculosis within the gland. The production of adrenocortical hormones is deficient despite high ACTH levels (feedback mechanism). Secondary or relative insufficiency arises as the result of defective production of ACTH leading in turn to disuse atrophy of the adrenal cortex. It is commonly seen, for example, as a result of corticosteroid therapy, Sheehan's syndrome and pituitary tumors or ablation.

The differentiation of both types is based on the premise that a primarily defective gland cannot be stimulated by ACTH whereas a secondarily defective gland is potentially functional and will respond to adequate stimulation with ACTH. Patients selected for further study as the result of a subnormal cosyntropin test should be given a 3 or 4 day course of treatment with Repository Corticotropin Injection USP and then retested. Suggested doses are 40 USP units twice daily for 4 days or 60 USP units twice daily for 3 days. Under these conditions little or no increase in plasma cortisol levels will be seen in Addison's disease whereas higher or even normal levels will be seen in cases with secondary adrenal insufficiency.

CONTRAINDICATIONS:

The only contraindication to cosyntropin is a history of a previous adverse reaction to it.

PRECAUTIONS:

General: Cosyntropin exhibits slight immunologic activity, does not contain foreign animal protein and is therefore less risky to use than natural ACTH. Patients known to be sensitized to natural ACTH with markedly positive skin tests will, with few exceptions, react negatively when tested intradermally with cosyntropin. Further, most patients with a history of a previous hypersensitivity reaction to natural ACTH or a preexisting allergic disease will tolerate cosyntropin without incident. Despite this however, cosyntropin is not completely devoid of immunologic activity and hypersensitivity reactions are possible, at least in susceptible patients.

Therefore, the physician should be prepared, prior to injection, to treat any possible acute hypersensitivity reaction.

Carcinogenesis, Mutagenesis, and Impairment of Fertility: Long term studies in animals have not been performed to evaluate carcinogenic or mutagenic potential or impairment of fertility. A study in rats noted inhibition of reproductive function like natural ACTH.

Pregnancy Category C: Animal reproduction studies have not been conducted with cosyntropin. It is also not known whether cosyntropin can cause fetal harm when administered to a pregnant woman or can affect reproduction capacity. Cosyntropin should be given to a pregnant woman only if clearly needed.

Nursing Mothers: It is not known whether this drug is excreted in human milk. Because many drugs are excreted in human milk, caution should be exercised when cosyntropin is administered to a nursing woman.

Pediatric Usage: (See DOSAGE AND ADMINISTRATION for details).

DRUG INTERACTIONS:

Corticotropin may accentuate the electrolyte loss associated with diuretic therapy.

ADVERSE REACTIONS:

Since cosyntropin for injection is intended for diagnostic and not therapeutic use, adverse reactions other than a rare hypersensitivity reaction are not anticipated. To date only 3 such reactions have been reported in the literature and in each instance the patient had a preexisting allergic disease and/or a previous reaction to natural ACTH. One investigator reported a single instance of slight whealing with splotchy erythema at the injection site. A similar but more marked reaction was also noted in the same patient following an injection of natural ACTH.

DOSAGE AND ADMINISTRATION:

Cosyntropin may be administered intramuscularly or as a direct intravenous injection when used as a rapid screening test of adrenal function. It may also be given as an intravenous infusion over a 4 to 8 hour period to provide a greater stimulus to the adrenal glands. Doses of cosyntropin 0.25 to 0.75 mg have been used in clinical studies and a maximal response noted with the smallest dose.

A suggested method for a rapid screening test of adrenal function has been described by Wood and associates. A control blood sample of 6 to 7 ml is collected in a heparinized tube. Reconstitute 0.25 mg of cosyntropin in solvent (ampul of 1 ml sodium chloride injection USP 0.9%) and inject intramuscularly. In children aged 2 years or less, a dose of 0.125 mg will often suffice. A second blood sample is collected exactly 30 minutes later. Both blood samples should be refrigerated until sent to the laboratory for determination of the plasma cortisol response by some appropriate method. If it is not possible to send them to the laboratory or to perform the fluorometric procedure within 12 hours, then the plasma should be separated and refrigerated or frozen according to need.

The usual normal response in most cases is an approximate doubling of the basal level, provided that the basal level does not exceed the normal range. Patients taking inadvertent doses of cortisone or hydrocortisone on the test day and patients taking spironolactone or women taking drugs which contain estrogen may exhibit abnormally high basal plasma cortisol levels. A paradoxical response may be noted in the former group as seen in a decrease in plasma cortisol values following a stimulating dose of cosyntropin. In the latter group only a normal incremental response is to be expected. Many patients with normal adrenal function, however, do not respond to the expected degree so that the following criteria have been established to denote a normal response:

1. The control plasma cortisol level should exceed 5 micrograms/100 ml.

2. The 30-minute level should show an increment of at least 7 micrograms/100 ml above the basal level.

3. The 30-minute level should exceed 18 micrograms/100 ml. Comparable figures have been reported by Grieg and co-workers. These criteria also apply when the drug is injected intravenously in 2 to 5 ml of saline over a 2-minute period.

Plasma cortisol levels usually peak about 45 to 60 minutes after an injection of cosyntropin for injection and some prefer the 60-minute interval for testing for this reason. While it is true that the 60-minute values are usually higher than the 30-minute values, the difference may not be significant enough in most cases to outweigh the disadvantage of a longer testing period. If the 60-minute test period is used, the criterion for a normal response is an approximate doubling of the basal plasma cortisol value.

When given as an intravenous infusion: cosyntropin, 0.25 mg may be added to glucose or saline solutions and given at the rate of approximately 40 micrograms per hour over a 6-hour period. It should not be added to blood or plasma as it is apt to be inactivated by enzymes. Adrenal response may be measured in the usual manner by determining urinary steroid excretion before and after treatment or by measuring plasma cortisol levels before and at the end of the infusion. The latter is preferable because the urinary steroid excretion does not always accurately reflect the adrenal or plasma cortisol response to ACTH. Patients receiving cortisone, hydrocortisone or spironolactone should omit their pre- test doses on the day selected for testing. In patients with a raised plasma bilirubin or in patients where the plasma contains free hemoglobin, falsely high fluorescence measurements will result. The test may be performed at any time during the day but because of the physiological diurnal variation of plasma cortisol the criteria listed by Wood cannot apply. It has been shown that basal plasma cortisol levels and the post cosyntropin increment exhibit diurnal changes. However, the 30-minute plasma cortisol level remains unchanged throughout the day so that only this single criterion should be used.

Parenteral drug products should be inspected visually for particulate matter and discoloration whenever solution and container permit. Reconstituted cosyntropin should not be retained.

HOW SUPPLIED - EQUIVALENTS NOT AVAILABLE:

Injection, Dry-Soln - Intramuscular; - 0.25 mg/10 mg

1 ml x 10	**$126.29**	**CORTROSYN, Organon**	**00052-0731-10**

CROMOLYN SODIUM *(000916)*

CATEGORIES: Airway Obstruction; Allergies; Antiasthmatics/Bronchodilators; Asthma; Bronchospasm; Conjunctivitis; Diarrhea; EENT Drugs; Eye, Ear, Nose, & Throat Preparations; Headache; Keratitis; Keratoconjunctivitis; Lacrimation; Mastocytosis; Nausea; Ophthalmics; Orphan Drugs; Pain; Respiratory & Allergy Medications; Rhinitis; Urticaria; Vomiting; Pregnancy Category B; Sales > $100 Million; FDA Approval Pre 1982; Patent Expiration 1993 May

BRAND NAMES: *Alecrom*; *Clesin*; *Colimune* (Germany); *Cromal-5 Inhaler*; *Cromo-Asma*; Cromoglicic Acid; *Cromogloz*; *Cromolyn*; *Cromoptic* (France); *Cromunal*; *Fintal*; *Fivent* (Canada); *Frenal*; Gastrocrom; *Ifiral*; *Inostral*; **Intal**; *Intal Forte*; *Lomudal* (France); *Lomudal Gastrointestinum*; *Lomudal Nasal*; *Lomudal Nesespray*; *Lomupren* (Germany); *Lomupren-Nasenspray*; *Lomusol* (France); *Lomusol Forte*; *Lomusol Nasenspray*; *Maxicrom*; *Nalcrom* (England, Canada); Nasalcrom; *Nazotral*; Opticrom; *Opticron* (France); *Rynacrom* (Australia, Canada, Mexico); *Rynacrom M*; *Sificrom*; *Vicrom*; *Vistacrom* (Canada); *Vividrin*
(International brand names outside U.S. in italics)

FORMULARIES: Aetna; BC-BS; CIGNA; FHP; Humana; Kaiser; Medco; Medi-Cal; PCS; PruCare; United; WHO

PRIMARY ICD9: 493.90 (Asthma, Unspecified, Without Mention of Status Asthmaticus)

DESCRIPTION:

Chemically, cromolyn sodium is the disodium salt of 1,3-bis(2-carboxychromon-5-yloxy)-2-hydroxypropane. The empirical formula is $C_{23}H_{14}Na_2O_{11}$; the molecular weight is 512.34.

GELATIN CAPSULES

Each gelatin capsule of Gastrocrom (cromolyn sodium, USP) contains 100 mg cromolyn sodium. Cromolyn sodium is a hygroscopic, white powder having little odor. It may leave a slightly bitter aftertaste. It is soluble in water (1 part in 20) and the resulting solution is neutral. It is intended for oral use.

Pharmacologic Category: Mast cell stabilizer

Therapeutic Category: Antiallergic

CAPSULES FOR INHALATION, INHALATION AEROSOL, AND INHALATION SOLUTION

The active ingredient is cromolyn sodium, USP. It is an inhaled anti-inflammatory agent for the preventive management of asthma. Cromolyn sodium is a water-soluble, odorless, white, hydrated crystalline powder. It is tasteless at first, but leaves a slightly bitter aftertaste.

Capsules for Inhalation: Each cromolyn sodium for inhalation capsule contains 20 mg cromolyn sodium and 20 mg lactose. The contents of the capsule are intended for inhalation use only, with the Spinhaler turbo-inhaler.

Inhalation Aerosol: Cromolyn sodium Inhaler is a metered dose aerosol unit for oral inhalation containing micronized cromolyn sodium, sorbitan trioleate with dichlorotetrafluoroethane and dichlorodifluoromethane as propellants. Each metered inhalation delivers approximately 800 mcg cromolyn sodium through the mouthpiece to the patient. Each 8.1 g canister delivers at least 112 metered inhalations (56 doses); each 14.2 g canister delivers at least 200 metered inhalations (100 doses).

Inhalation Solution: Cromolyn sodium inhalation solution is clear, colorless, sterile, and has a target pH of 5.5.

Each 2 ml ampule of Intal Nebulizer Solution contains 20 mg cromolyn sodium, USP, in purified water.

NASAL SOLUTION

Each milliliter of Nasalcrom Nasal Solution contains 40 mg cromolyn sodium in purified water with 0.01% benzalkonium chloride to preserve and 0.01% EDTA (edetate disodium) to stabilize the solution. Cromolyn sodium nasal solution possesses a natural pH of 4.5-6.5 and negligible titratable acidity.

Pharmacologic Category: Mast cell stabilizer/antiallergic.

Therapeutic Category: Antiallergic.

After priming the delivery system for Nasalcrom, each actuation of the unit delivers a metered spray containing 5.2 mg of cromolyn sodium. The contents of one bottle delivers at least 100 sprays (13 ml bottle) or 200 sprays (26 ml bottle).

CLINICAL PHARMACOLOGY:

Gelatin Capsules: *In vitro* and *in vivo* animal studies have shown that cromolyn sodium inhibits the release of mediators from sensitized mast cells. Cromolyn sodium acts by inhibiting the release of histamine and leukotrienes (SRS-A) from the mast cell.

Cromolyn sodium has no intrinsic vasoconstrictor, antihistaminic or anti-inflammatory activity.

Cromolyn sodium is poorly absorbed from the gastrointestinal tract. No more than 1% of an administered dose is absorbed by humans after oral administration, the remainder being excreted in the feces. Very little absorption of cromolyn sodium was seen after oral administration of 500 mg by mouth to each of 12 volunteers. From 0.28 to 0.50% of the administered dose was recovered in the first 24 hours of urinary excretion in 3 subjects. The mean urinary excretion of an administered dose over 24 hours in the remaining 9 subjects was 0.45%.

Capsules for Inhalation, Inhalation Aerosol, and Inhalation Solution: *In vitro* and *in vivo* animal studies have shown that cromolyn sodium inhibits sensitized mast cell degranulation which occurs after exposure to specific antigens. Cromolyn sodium acts by inhibiting the release of mediators from mast cells. Studies show that cromolyn sodium indirectly blocks calcium ions from entering the mast cell, thereby preventing mediator release.

Cromolyn sodium inhibits both the immediate and non-immediate bronchoconstrictive reactions to inhaled antigen. Cromolyn sodium also attenuates bronchospasm caused by exercise, toluene diisocyanate, aspirin, cold air, sulfur dioxide, and environmental pollutants, at least in some patients - (Inhalation Aerosol).

Cromolyn sodium has no intrinsic bronchodilator or antihistaminic activity.

After administration by inhalation, approximately 8% of the total cromolyn sodium dose administered is absorbed and rapidly excreted unchanged, approximately equally divided between urine and bile. The remainder of the dose is either exhaled or deposited in the oropharynx, swallowed, and excreted via the alimentary tract.

Nasal Solution: *In vitro* and *in vivo* animal studies have shown that cromolyn sodium inhibits the degranulation of sensitized mast cells which occurs after exposure to specific antigens. Cromolyn sodium inhibits the release of histamine and SRS-A (the slow-acting substance of anaphylaxis). Rhinitis induced by the inhalation of specific antigens can be inhibited to varying degrees by pretreatment with cromolyn sodium nasal solution.

CLINICAL PHARMACOLOGY: *(cont'd)*

Another activity demonstrated *in vitro* is the capacity of cromolyn sodium to inhibit the degranulation of non-sensitized rat mast cells by phospholipase A and the subsequent release of chemical mediators. An additional *in vitro* study showed that cromolyn sodium did not inhibit the enzymatic activity of released phospholipase A on its specific substrate.

Cromolyn sodium has no intrinsic bronchodilator, antihistaminic or anti-inflammatory activity.

Cromolyn sodium is poorly absorbed from the gastrointestinal tract. After instillation of cromolyn sodium nasal solution, less than 7% of the total dose administered is absorbed and is rapidly excreted unchanged in the bile and urine. The remainder of the dose is expelled from the nose, or swallowed and excreted via the alimentary tract.

INDICATIONS AND USAGE:

Gelatin Capsules: Gelatin capsules are indicated in the management of patients with mastocytosis. Use of this product has been associated with improvement in diarrhea, flushing, headaches, vomiting, urticaria, abdominal pain, nausea, and itching in some patients.

Capsules for Inhalation, Inhalation Aerosol, and Inhalation Solution: Cromolyn sodium is a prophylactic agent indicated in the management of patients with bronchial asthma.

In patients whose symptoms are sufficiently frequent to require a continuous program of medication, cromolyn sodium is given by inhalation on a regular daily basis (see DOSAGE AND ADMINISTRATION). The effect of cromolyn sodium is usually evident after several weeks of treatment, although some patients show an almost immediate response.

Capsules for Inhalation and Inhalation Solution: In patients who develop acute bronchoconstriction in response to exposure to exercise, toluene diisocyanate, environmental pollutants, etc., cromolyn sodium should be given shortly before exposure to the precipitating factor (see DOSAGE AND ADMINISTRATION).

Inhalation Aerosol: If improvement occurs, it will ordinarily occur within the first 4 weeks of administration as manifested by a decrease in the severity of clinical symptoms of asthma, or in the need for concomitant therapy, or both.

In patients who develop acute bronchoconstriction in response to exposure to exercise, toluene diisocyanate, environmental pollutants, known antigens, etc., cromolyn sodium inhaler should be used shortly before exposure to the precipitating factor, (*i.e.,* within 10-15 minutes but not more than 60 minutes) (see DOSAGE AND ADMINISTRATION) Cromolyn sodium inhaler may be effective in relieving bronchospasm in some, but not all, patients with exercise induced bronchospasm.

Nasal Solution: Cromolyn sodium nasal solution is indicated for the prevention and treatment of the symptoms of allergic rhinitis.

CONTRAINDICATIONS:

Gelatin Capsules and Inhalation Solution: Capsules and Inhalation Solution are contraindicated in those patients who have shown hypersensitivity to cromolyn sodium.

Capsules for Inhalation: Cromolyn sodium is contraindicated in those patients who have shown hypersensitivity to cromolyn sodium or to lactose.

Inhalation Aerosol: Cromolyn sodium inhaler is contraindicated in those patients who have shown hypersensitivity to cromolyn sodium or other ingredients in this preparation.

Nasal Solution: Cromolyn sodium nasal solution is contraindicated in those patients who have shown hypersensitivity to any of the ingredients.

WARNINGS:

Gelatin Capsules: The recommended dosage should be decreased in patients with decreased renal or hepatic function. Severe anaphylactic reactions may occur rarely in association with cromolyn sodium administration.

Capsules for Inhalation and Inhalation Solution: Cromolyn sodium has no role in the treatment of status asthmaticus.

Inhalation Aerosol: Cromolyn sodium inhaler has no role in the treatment of an acute attack of asthma, especially status asthmaticus. Severe anaphylactic reactions can occur after cromolyn sodium administration. The recommended dosage should be decreased in patients with decreased renal or hepatic function. Cromolyn sodium inhaler should be discontinued if the patient develops eosinophilic pneumonia (or pulmonary infiltrates with eosinophilia). Because of the propellants in this preparation, it should be used with caution in patients with coronary artery disease or a history of cardiac arrhythmias.

PRECAUTIONS:

GENERAL

Gelatin Capsules: In view of the biliary and renal routes of excretion of cromolyn sodium, consideration should be given to decreasing the dosage of the drug in patients with impaired renal or hepatic function.

Inhalation Aerosol and Nasal Solution: In view of the biliary and renal routes of excretion for cromolyn sodium, consideration should be given to decreasing the dosage or discontinuing the administration of the drug in patients with impaired renal or hepatic function.

Capsules for Inhalation, Inhalation Aerosol, and Inhalation Solution: Occasionally, patients may experience cough and/or bronchospasm following cromolyn sodium inhalation. At times, patients who develop bronchospasm may not be able to continue cromolyn sodium administration despite prior bronchodilator administration. Rarely, very severe bronchospasm has been encountered.

Capsules for Inhalation and Inhalation Solution: Symptoms of asthma may recur if cromolyn sodium is reduced below the recommended dosage or discontinued.

Nasal Solution: Some patients may experience transient nasal stinging and/or sneezing immediately following instillation of cromolyn sodium nasal solution. Except in rare occurrences, these experiences have not caused discontinuation of therapy.

INFORMATION FOR THE PATIENT

Capsules for Inhalation and Inhalation Solution: Cromolyn sodium is to be taken as directed by the physician. Because it is preventive medication, it may take up to four weeks before the patient experiences maximum benefit.

Capsules for Inhalation: Patients may experience irritation of the throat or coughing after inhalation of the powder. In some cases, rinsing the mouth or taking a drink of water immediately before and/or after using the Spinhaler will eliminate the throat irritation or cough.

If the patient experiences difficulty in emptying the capsule, which may require several deep inhalations, check to make certain the patient is following the directions carefully. A light dusting of powder remaining in the capsule is normal, and is not an indication that the Spinhaler or capsule is faulty or that the proper dose was not delivered. The Spinhaler should be washed in clean, warm water at least once a week, and dried thoroughly before use.

Inhalation Solution: Cromolyn sodium inhalation solution should be used in a power-driven nebulizer with an adequate airflow rate equipped with a suitable face mask or mouthpiece.

For additional information, see the accompanying leaflet entitled "Living a Full Life with Asthma."

PRECAUTIONS: *(cont'd)*

CARCINOGENESIS, MUTAGENESIS, AND IMPAIRMENT OF FERTILITY

Long term studies in mice (12 months intraperitoneal treatment followed by 6 months observation), hamsters (12 months intraperitoneal treatment followed by 12 months observation), and rats (18 months subcutaneous treatment) showed no neoplastic effect of cromolyn sodium.

No evidence of chromosomal damage or cytotoxicity was obtained in various mutagenesis studies.

No evidence of impaired fertility was shown in laboratory animal reproduction studies.

PREGNANCY CATEGORY B

Reproduction studies with cromolyn sodium administered parenterally to pregnant mice, rats, and rabbits in doses up to 338 times the human clinical dose produced no evidence of fetal malformations. Adverse fetal effects (increased resorptions and decreased fetal weight) were noted only at the very high parenteral doses that produced maternal toxicity. There are, however, no adequate and well controlled studies in pregnant women. Because animal reproduction studies are not always predictive of human response, this drug should be used during pregnancy only if clearly needed.

NURSING MOTHERS

Gelatin Capsules, Capsules for Inhalation, Inhalation Solution, and Nasal Solution: It is not known whether this drug is excreted in human milk. Because many drugs are excreted in human milk, caution should be exercised when cromolyn sodium is administered to a nursing woman.

Inhalation Aerosol: It is not known whether this drug is excreted in human milk, therefore, caution should be exercised when cromolyn sodium inhaler is administered to a nursing woman and the attending physician must make a benefit/risk assessment in regard to its use in this situation.

PEDIATRIC USE

Gelatin Capsules: Animal studies suggest increased risk of toxicity in premature animals when given doses much higher than clinically recommended. In term infants up to six months of age, available clinical data suggest that the dose should not exceed 20 mg/kg/day. The use of this product in children less than two years should be reserved for patients with severe disease in which the potential benefits clearly outweigh the risks.

Capsules for Inhalation: Safety and effectiveness in children below the age of 2 years have not been established. For young children unable to utilize the Spinhaler, cromolyn sodium inhalation solution is recommended.

Inhalation Aerosol: Safety and effectiveness in children below the age of 5 years have not been established. For young children unable to utilize the inhaler, cromolyn sodium inhalation solution is recommended. Because of the possibility that adverse effects of this drug could become apparent only after many years, a benefit/risk consideration of the long-term use of cromolyn sodium inhaler is particularly important in pediatric patients.

Inhalation Solution: Safety and effectiveness in children below the age of 2 years have not been established.

Nasal Solution: Safety and effectiveness in children below the age of 6 years have not been established.

DRUG INTERACTIONS:

DRUG INTERACTION DURING PREGNANCY

Cromolyn sodium and isoproterenol were studied following subcutaneous injections in pregnant mice. Cromolyn sodium alone in doses of 60 to 540 mg/kg (38 to 338 times the human dose) did not cause significant increases in resorptions or major malformations. Isoproterenol alone at a dose of 2.7 mg/kg (90 times the human dose) increased both resorptions and malformations. The addition of cromolyn sodium (338 times the human dose) to isoproterenol (90 times the human dose) appears to have increased the incidence of both resorptions and malformations.

ADVERSE REACTIONS:

GELATIN CAPSULES

Most of the adverse events reported in mastocytosis patients have been transient and could represent symptoms of the disease. The most frequently reported adverse events in mastocytosis patients who have received oral cromolyn sodium capsules during clinical studies were headache and diarrhea. Each occurred in 4 of the 87 patients. Pruritus, nausea, and myalgia were each reported in 3 patients and abdominal pain, rash, and irritability in 2 patients each. One report of malaise was also recorded.

A generally similar profile of adverse events has been reported during studies in other clinical conditions. Additional reports which have been received during the course of these studies and spontaneous reports during foreign marketing include: flushing, urticaria/angioedema, arthralgia, dizziness, fatigue, paresthesia, taste perversion, migraine, psychosis, anxiety, depression, insomnia, behavior change, esophagospasm, flatulence, dysphagia, hepatic function test abnormal, edema, dyspnea, polycythemia, neutropenia, dysuria, hallucinations, skin erythema and burning, burning mouth and throat, stiffness and weakness of the legs, and postprandial lightheadedness and lethargy. These events are infrequent, the majority representing only a single report, and in many cases the causal relationship to oral cromolyn sodium capsules is uncertain.

CAPSULES FOR INHALATION

Clinical experience with the use of cromolyn sodium suggests that adverse reactions are rare events. The most common side effects are associated with inhalation of the powder and include transient cough (1 in 5 patients) and mild wheezing (1 in 25 patients). These effects rarely require treatment or discontinuation of the drug.

INHALATION SOLUTION

Clinical experience with the use of cromolyn sodium suggests that adverse reactions are rare events. The following adverse reactions have been associated with cromolyn sodium inhalation solution: cough, nasal congestion, nausea, sneezing, and wheezing.

Other reactions have been reported in clinical trials; however, a causal relationship could not be established: drowsiness, nasal itching, nose bleed, nose burning, serum sickness, and stomachache.

In addition, adverse reactions have been reported with cromolyn sodium capsules for inhalation. The most common side effects are associated with inhalation of the powder and include transient cough (1 in 5 patients) and mild wheezing (1 in 25 patients). These effects rarely require treatment or discontinuation of the drug.

CAPSULES FOR INHALATION AND INHALATION SOLUTION

Information on the incidence of adverse reactions to cromolyn sodium has been derived from U.S. postmarketing surveillance experience. The following adverse reactions attributed to cromolyn sodium, based upon recurrence following readministration, have been reported in less than 1 in 10,000 patients: laryngeal edema, swollen parotid gland, angioedema, bronchospasm, joint swelling and pain, dizziness, dysuria and urinary frequency, nausea, cough, wheezing, headache, nasal congestion, rash, urticaria and lacrimation.

ADVERSE REACTIONS: *(cont'd)*

Other adverse reactions have been reported in less than 1 in 100,000 patients, and it is unclear whether these are attributable to the drug: anaphylaxis, nephrosis, periarteritic vasculitis, pericarditis, peripheral neuritis, pulmonary infiltrates with eosinophilia, polymyositis, exfoliative dermatitis, hemoptysis, anemia, myalgia, hoarseness, photodermatitis and vertigo.

CAPSULES FOR INHALATION

The following adverse effects have been reported in less than 1 in 10,000 patients, and are a consequence of the Spinhaler delivery system: inhalation of (capsule) gelatin particles and inhalation of mouthpiece or propeller.

INHALATION AEROSOL

In controlled clinical studies of cromolyn sodium inhaler, the most frequently reported adverse reactions attributed to cromolyn sodium treatment were: Throat irritation or dryness, Bad taste, Cough, Wheeze, Nausea.

The most frequently reported adverse reactions attributed to other forms of cromolyn sodium (on the basis of recurrence following readministration) involve the respiratory tract and are: bronchospasm [sometimes severe, associated with a precipitous fall in pulmonary function (FEV_1)], cough, laryngeal edema (rare), nasal congestion (sometimes severe), pharyngeal irritation, and wheezing.

Adverse reactions which occur infrequently and are associated with administration of the drug are: anaphylaxis, angioedema, dizziness, dysuria and urinary frequency, joint swelling and pain, lacrimation, nausea and headache, rash, swollen parotid gland, urticaria, pulmonary infiltrates with eosinophilia, substernal burning, and myopathy.

The following adverse reactions have been reported as rare events and it is unclear whether they are attributable to the drug: anemia, exfoliative dermatitis, hemoptysis, hoarseness, myalgia, nephrosis, periarteritic vasculitis, pericarditis, peripheral neuritis, photodermatitis, sneezing, drowsiness, nasal itching, nasal bleeding, nasal burning, serum sickness, stomach ache, polymyositis, vertigo, and liver disease.

NASAL SOLUTION

The most frequent adverse reactions occurring in the 430 patients included in the clinical trials with cromolyn sodium nasal solution were sneezing (1 in 10 patients), nasal stinging (1 in 20), nasal burning (1 in 25), and nasal irritation (1 in 40). Headaches and bad taste were reported in about 1 in 50 patients. Epistaxis, postnasal drip, and rash were reported in less than one percent of the patients. One patient in the clinical trials developed anaphylaxis.

Adverse reactions which have occurred in the use of other cromolyn sodium formulations for inhalation include angioedema, joint pain and swelling, urticaria, cough, and wheezing. Other reactions reported rarely are serum sickness, periarteritic vasculitis, polymyositis, pericarditis, photodermatitis, exfoliative dermatitis, peripheral neuritis, and nephrosis.

OVERDOSAGE:

There is no clinical syndrome associated with an overdosage of cromolyn sodium. Acute toxicity testing in a wide variety of species has demonstrated an extremely low order of toxicity for cromolyn sodium, regardless of whether administration was parenteral, oral or by inhalation. Parenteral administration in mice, rats, guinea pigs, hamsters and rabbits demonstrated an LD_{50} in the region of 4000 mg/kg. Intravenous administration in monkeys also indicated a similar order of toxicity. The highest dose administered by the oral route in rats and mice was 8000 mg/kg and at this dose level no deaths occurred. By inhalation, even in long term studies, it proved impossible to achieve toxic dose levels of cromolyn sodium in a range of mammalian species.

DOSAGE AND ADMINISTRATION:

GELATIN CAPSULES

NOT FOR INHALATION. SEE DIRECTIONS FOR USE.

The usual starting dose is as follows:

Adults: Two capsules four times daily one-half hour before meals and at bedtime.

Premature to Term Infants: Not recommended.

Term to 2 years: 20 mg/kg/day in four divided doses. Use of this product in children less than 2 years is not recommended and should be attempted only in those patients with severe incapacitating diseases where the benefits clearly outweigh the risks.

Children 2-12 years: One capsule four times daily one-half hour before meals and bedtime.

If satisfactory control of symptoms is not achieved within two to three weeks the dosage may be increased but should not exceed 40 mg/kg/day (30 mg/kg/day for children six months to two years).

Patients should be advised that the effect of oral cromolyn sodium capsule therapy is dependent upon its administration at regular intervals, as directed.

Maintenance Dose: Once a therapeutic response has been achieved the dose may be reduced to the minimum required to maintain the patient with a lower degree of symptomatology. To prevent relapses, the dosage should be maintained.

Administration: Oral cromolyn sodium capsules should be administered as a solution in water at least $\frac{1}{2}$ hour before meals after preparation according to the following directions:

1. Open capsule(s) and pour powder contents of capsule(s) into $\frac{1}{2}$ glass of hot water.
2. Stir until completely dissolved (clear solution).
3. Add equal quantity of cold water while stirring.
4. DO NOT MIX WITH FRUIT JUICE, MILK OR FOODS.
5. Drink all of the liquid.

CAPSULES FOR INHALATION

For management of bronchial asthma in adults and children (two years of age and over) who are able to use the Spinhaler turbo-inhaler, the usual starting dosage is the contents of one cromolyn sodium Capsule inhaled four times daily at regular intervals.

INHALATION AEROSOL

For management of bronchial asthma in adults and young children (5 years of age and over) who are able to use the inhaler, the usual starting dosage is two metered inhalations four times daily at regular intervals. This dose should not be exceeded. Not all patients will respond to the recommended dose and there is evidence to suggest, at least in younger patients, that a lower dose may provide efficacy.

INHALATION SOLUTION

For management of bronchial asthma in adults and children (two years of age and over), the usual starting dosage is the contents of one ampule administered by nebulization four times a day at regular intervals.

CAPSULES FOR INHALATION, INHALATION AEROSOL, AND INHALATION SOLUTION

Patients with chronic asthma should be advised that the effect of cromolyn sodium therapy is dependent upon its administration at regular intervals, as directed. Cromolyn episode should be introduced into the patient's therapeutic regimen when the acute episode has been controlled, the airway has been cleared, and the patient is able to inhale adequately.

DOSAGE AND ADMINISTRATION: *(cont'd)*

CAPSULES FOR INHALATION

For the prevention of acute bronchospasm which follows exercise or exposure to cold dry air, environmental agents (*e.g.,* animal danders, toluene diisocyanate, pollutants), etc., the usual dose is the contents of one cromolyn sodium Capsule inhaled shortly before exposure to the precipitating factor.

It should be emphasized to the patient that the drug is poorly absorbed when swallowed and is not effective by this route of administration.

INHALATION AEROSOL

For the prevention of acute bronchospasm which follows exercise, exposure to cold dry air or environmental agents, the usual dose is two metered inhalations shortly,(*i.e.,* 10-15 minutes but not more than 60 minutes), before exposure to the precipitating factor.

INHALATION SOLUTION

For the prevention of acute bronchospasm which follows exercise or exposure to cold dry air, environmental agents (*e.g.,* animal danders, toluene diisocyanate, pollutants), etc., the usual dose is the contents of one ampule administered by nebulization shortly before exposure to the precipitating factor.

It should be emphasized to the patient that the drug is poorly absorbed when swallowed and is not effective by this route of administration.

CAPSULES FOR INHALATION, INHALATION AEROSOL, AND INHALATION SOLUTION

Cromolyn Sodium Therapy in Relation to Other Treatments for Asthma: *Non-Steroidal Agents:* Cromolyn sodium should be *added* to the patient's existing treatment regimen (*e.g.,* bronchodilators). When a clinical response to cromolyn sodium is evident, usually within two to four weeks, and if the asthma is under good control, an attempt may be made to decrease concomitant medication usage gradually.

CAPSULES FOR INHALATION

If concomitant medications are eliminated or required on no more than a p.r.n. basis, the frequency of administration of cromolyn sodium may be titrated downward to the lowest level consistent with the desired effect. The usual decrease is from four capsules to three to two capsules per day. It is important that the dosage be reduced gradually to avoid exacerbation of asthma. It is emphasized that in patients whose dosage has been titrated to fewer than four capsules per day, an increase in the dosage of cromolyn sodium and the introduction of, or increase in, symptomatic medications may be needed if the patient's clinical condition deteriorates.

INHALATION AEROSOL

If concomitant medications are eliminated or required on no more than a prn basis, the frequency of administration of cromolyn sodium inhaler may be titrated downward to the lowest level consistent with the desired effect. The usual decrease is from two metered inhalations four times daily to three times daily to twice daily. It is important that the dosage be reduced gradually to avoid exacerbation of asthma. It is emphasized that in patients whose dosage has been titrated to fewer than four inhalations per day, an increase in the dosage of cromolyn sodium inhaler and the introduction of, or increase in, symptomatic medications may be needed if the patient's clinical condition deteriorates.

INHALATION SOLUTION

If concomitant medications are eliminated or required on no more than a prn basis, the frequency of administration of cromolyn sodium may be titrated downward to the lowest level consistent with the desired effect. The usual decrease is from four to three ampules per day. It is important that the dosage be reduced gradually to avoid exacerbation of asthma. It is emphasized that in patients whose dosage has been titrated to fewer than four ampules per day, an increase in the dose of cromolyn sodium and the introduction of, or increase in, symptomatic medications may be needed if the patient's clinical condition deteriorates.

CAPSULES FOR INHALATION, INHALATION AEROSOL, AND INHALATION SOLUTION

Corticosteroids: In patients chronically receiving corticosteroids for the management of bronchial asthma, the dosage should be maintained following the introduction of cromolyn sodium. If the patient improves, an attempt to decrease corticosteroids should be made. Even if the corticosteroid-dependent patient fails to show symptomatic improvement following cromolyn sodium administration, the potential to reduce corticosteroids may nonetheless be present. Thus, gradual tapering of corticosteroid dosage may be attempted. It is important that the dose be reduced slowly, maintaining close supervision of the patient to avoid an exacerbation of asthma.

It should be borne in mind that prolonged corticosteroid therapy frequently causes an impairment in the activity of the hypothalamic- pituitary-adrenal axis and a reduction in the size of the adrenal cortex. A potentially critical degree of impairment or insufficiency may persist asymptomatically for some time even after gradual discontinuation of adrenocortical steroids. Therefore, if a patient is subjected to significant stress, such as a severe asthmatic attack, surgery, trauma or severe illness while being treated or within one year (occasionally up to two years) after corticosteroid treatment has been terminated, consideration should be given to reinstituting corticosteroid therapy. When respiratory function is impaired, as may occur in severe exacerbation of asthma, a temporary increase in the amount of corticosteroids may be required to regain control of the patient's asthma.

It is particularly important that great care be exercised if, for any reason, cromolyn sodium is withdrawn in cases where its use has permitted a reduction in the maintenance dose of corticosteroids. In such cases, continued close supervision of the patient is essential since there may be sudden reappearance of severe manifestations of asthma which will require immediate therapy and possible reintroduction of corticosteroids.

NASAL SOLUTION

The dose for adults and children 6 years and older is **one spray in each nostril** 3-4 times daily at regular intervals. If needed, this dose may be increased to one spray to each nostril 6 times daily. The patient should be instructed to clear the nasal passages before administering the spray and should inhale through the nose during administration.

In the management of seasonal (pollenotic) rhinitis, and for prevention of rhinitis caused by exposure to other types of specific inhalant allergens, treatment with cromolyn sodium nasal solution will be more effective if started prior to expected contact with the offending allergen. Treatment should be continued throughout the period of exposure i.e., until the pollen season is over or until exposure to the offending allergen is terminated.

In the management of perennial allergic rhinitis, the effects of treatment with cromolyn sodium nasal solution may become apparent only after two to four weeks of treatment. The concomitant use of antihistamines and/or nasal decongestants may be necessary during the initial phase of treatment, but the need for this type of medication should diminish and may be eliminated when the full benefit of cromolyn sodium nasal solution is achieved.

PATIENT PACKAGE INSERT:

GELATIN CAPSULES

How to Use Cromolyn Sodium Capsules: As with all prescription drugs, follow the directions for dosage that your physician recommends.

PATIENT PACKAGE INSERT: *(cont'd)*

The effect of oral cromolyn sodium capsule therapy is dependent upon its administration at REGULAR intervals, for as long as recommended by your physician.

USUAL STARTING DOSE

Adults: Two capsules four times daily one-half hour before meals and at bedtime.

Children 2-12 years: One capsule four times daily one-half hour before meals and at bedtime.

Note: Your physician may decide to increase OR decrease your dosage to achieve optimum results with oral cromolyn sodium capsules. However, do not change your dose or stop taking oral cromolyn sodium capsules without first consulting your physician.

DIRECTIONS FOR USE

1. Open capsule(s) and pour powder contents into $\frac{1}{2}$ glass of hot water.
2. Stir until completely dissolved (clear solution).
3. Add $\frac{1}{2}$ glass of cold water while stirring.
4. Drink all of the liquid.

Note: Mix the powder only with water. **Do not mix with fruit juice, milk or foods.**

Gelatin capsules are most effective when taken in a liquid form. It is not recommended that the capsules be swallowed whole.

Each capsule contains a precisely measured dose. The capsules are intentionally oversized to prevent the powder from spilling when the capsule is opened.

NOT FOR INHALATION

INHALATION AEROSOL

Patient Instructions for Use of Intal Inhaler (cromolyn sodium inhalation aerosol) Metered Dose Inhaler

1. Make sure the canister is properly inserted into the Inhaler unit. Take the cover off the mouthpiece. **Shake the inhaler gently.**
2. Hold Inhaler and breathe out slowly. *Do Not Breathe Into the Inhaler:* it could clog the Inhaler valve.
3. Place the mouthpiece into your mouth, close your lips around it, and tilt your head back. Keep your tongue below the opening of the Inhaler.
4. Press the top of the metal canister down firmly and breathe in through your mouth **at the same time.**
5. Remove the Inhaler from your mouth. Hold your breath for several seconds, then breathe out slowly. This step is very important. It allows the cromolyn sodium to spread throughout your lungs.

Repeat steps 2-5, then replace the mouthpiece cover.

HINTS

1. Keep the cap on the Inhaler while not in use so that dirt can't get into it. You can clean the Inhaler by removing the metal canister and rinsing the plastic mouthpiece in warm water.
2. Before using the Inhaler for the first time, or if it has not been used for a while, it's a good idea to test it. Just give the canister one press.
3. It is essential that the canister be pressed at exactly the same time as you breathe in, so it's worth some time practicing this.
4. The dose delivered from the Inhaler can be seen as a fine white mist. If any of this can be seen escaping from your mouth or nose, then you are not using the Inhaler correctly.
5. To keep your Inhaler in good working order, do not exhale into the mouthpiece.

Important: *Remember:* A little time spent taking cromolyn sodium correctly and regularly can save you from countless attacks of asthma and the upheaval they cause.

It must be used everyday as directed by your doctor. Do not stop the treatment or even reduce the dose without consulting your doctor.

Dosage: For management of bronchial asthma in adults and children, the usual starting dosage is two metered inhalations four times a day at regular intervals. When asthma symptoms are well controlled, your doctor may reduce the dose to three times a day, and sometimes two times a day.

For the prevention of acute bronchospasm which follows exercise, exposure to cold dry air, or environmental agents, the usual dosage is two metered inhalations shortly **before exposure** to the offending factor.

Use as directed by your physician.

Cleaning: Twice a week, remove the metal canister from the plastic mouthpiece. Wash the mouthpiece in warm water and **dry thoroughly** before replacing the metal canister. **Never immerse the metal canister in water.**

Storage: Store between 15°-30°C (59°-86°F). Contents under pressure. Do not puncture, incinerate, or place near sources of heat. Keep out of the reach of children.

Note: The indented statement below is required by the Federal government's Clean Air Act for all products containing or manufactured with chlorofluorocarbons (CFC's).

This product contains CFC-12 and CFC-114, substances which harm the environment by destroying ozone in the upper atmosphere.

Your physician has determined that this product is likely to help your personal health. USE THIS PRODUCT AS DIRECTED, UNLESS INSTRUCTED TO DO OTHERWISE BY YOUR PHYSICIAN. If you have any questions about alternatives, consult with your physician.

NASAL SOLUTION: 40 mg/ml

How to Use Your Nasalmatic Unit

1. Remove the clear plastic Dust Cap from the Tip.
2. Remove the yellow Safety Clip beneath the Finger Rests.
3. Holding the Unit, place your index and second finger on either side of the Finger Rests and your thumb underneath the Unit.
4. Press the Finger Rests down firmly and allow to return *until* a single spray is delivered. It is only necessary to do this the first time you use the Unit.
5. Place the Tip into one nostril and inhale deeply as you press the Finger Rests down firmly. This will release one dose of medication. *NOTE:*Dose only as directed by your physician.
6. Repeat the process in your other nostril.
7. Replace Dust Cap and Safety Clip before storing.

SPECIAL TIPS

1. Clear nasal passages before using your Nasalmatic Unit. Your doctor will instruct you if any other medication is required.
2. Keep out of the reach of children.

HOW SUPPLIED:

GELATIN CAPSULES

Each capsules contains 100 mg of cromolyn sodium and is supplied in aluminum cans containing 100 capsules.

HOW SUPPLIED: *(cont'd)*

Each capsule contains a precisely measured dose. The capsules are intentionally oversized to prevent the powder from spilling when the capsule is opened.

Keep tightly closed and out of the reach of children.

Store between 15°-30°C (59°-86°F).

CAPSULES FOR INHALATION

Capsules for inhalation, each containing 20 mg of cromolyn sodium, are available in foil strip packs of 120 capsules. Each yellow and clear capsule is imprinted with the product identification code: Fisons 670

Store capsules between 15°-30°C (59°-86°F). Keep out of the reach of children. Spinhaler turbo-inhalers are supplied separately in individual containers. The Spinhaler should be replaced after 6 months of use.

INHALATION AEROSOL

Intal Inhaler, 8.1 g or 14.2 g canister, box of one. Supplied with mouthpiece and patient instructions.

Store between 15°-30°C (59°-86°F). Contents under pressure. Do not puncture, incinerate, or place near sources of heat. Keep out of the reach of children.

Note: The indented statement below is required by the Federal government's Clean Air Act for all products containing or manufactured with chlorofluorocarbons (CFC's).

Warning: Contains CFC-12 and CFC-114, substances which harm public health and environment by destroying ozone in the upper atmosphere.

A notice similar to the above WARNING has been placed in the "Patient Instructions for Use" portion of this package circular pursuant to EPA regulations.

INHALATION SOLUTION

Intal inhalation solution is a colorless solution supplied in a low density polyethylene plastic unit dose ampule with 12 ampules per foil pouch. Each 2 ml ampule contains 20 mg cromolyn sodium, USP, in purified water.

Intal inhalation solution should be stored between 15°-30°C (59°-86°F) and protected from light. Do not use if it contains a precipitate or becomes discolored. Keep out of the reach of children. Store ampules in foil pouch until ready for use.

NASAL SOLUTION

Nasalcrom is available in bottles of 13 ml and 26 ml. Each fully assembled unit consists of a pump unit and actuator with cover in position on the bottle of nasal solution. The amount of cromolyn sodium in each bottle is: 13 ml - 520 mg (40 mg/ml); 26 ml - 1040 mg (40 mg/ml). Nasalcrom should be stored between 15°-30°C (59°-86°F). Protect from light.

HOW SUPPLIED - RATED THERAPEUTICALLY EQUIVALENT:

Solution - Inhalation - 10 mg/ml

2 ml x 60	$42.00	Cromolyn Sodium, Dey Labs	49502-0689-02
2 ml x 60	**$48.25**	**INTAL NEBULIZER, Fisons**	**00585-0673-02**
2 ml x 120	$84.00	Cromolyn Sodium, Dey Labs	49502-0689-12
2 ml x 120	**$90.13**	**INTAL NEBULIZER, Fisons**	**00585-0673-03**

HOW SUPPLIED - NOT RATED EQUIVALENT:

Aerosol, Spray - Inhalation - 800 mcg/spr

112 spr's	**$39.50**	**INTAL, 8.1 GM CANISTER, Fisons**	**00585-0675-02**
200 spr's	**$62.86**	**INTAL, 14.2 GM CANISTER, Fisons**	**00585-0675-01**

Capsule, Gelatin - Inhalation - 20 mg

60's	**$35.44**	**INTAL, Fisons**	**00585-0670-60**

Capsule, Gelatin - Oral - 100 mg

100's	$94.10	GASTROCROM, Fisons	00585-0677-01

Powder

100 gm	$230.00	Cromolyn Sodium, Elge	58298-0520-01

Solution - Nasal - 40 mg

13 ml	$22.28	NASALCROM, Fisons	00585-0671-03
26 ml	$40.82	NASALCROM, Fisons	00585-0671-04

CROTAMITON *(000917)*

CATEGORIES: Anti-Infectives; Antiparasitics; Arthropods; Dermatologicals; Parasiticidal; Pruritus; Scabicides/Pediculicides; Skin/Mucous Membrane Agents; Topical; Pregnancy Category C; FDA Approval Pre 1982

BRAND NAMES: *Bestloid* (Japan); *Coltrum*; *Congen*; *Crotaderm*; *Crotamitex* (Germany); Crotan; *Crotorax*; **Eurax**; *Eurax-Lotio*; *Euraxil* (Germany); *Scabicin*; *Topicrom*; *Ulex Sinphar*, *Uracin*
(International brand names outside U.S. in italics)

FORMULARIES: FHP; Medi-Cal

DESCRIPTION:

Crotamiton USP, is a scabicidal and antipruritic agent available as a cream or lotion for topical use only. Crotamiton provides 10% (w/w) of the synthetic, crotamiton USP, in a vanishing-cream or emollient-lotion base containing: water, petrolatum, propylene glycol, steareth-2, cetyl alcohol, dimethicone, laureth-23, fragrance, magnesium aluminum silicate, carbomer-934, sodium hydroxide, diazolidinyl urea, methylchloroisothiazolinone, methylisothiazolinone and magnesium nitrate. In addition, the cream contains glyceryl stearate. Crotamiton is N-ethyl-N-(*o*-methylphenyl)-2-butenamide.

Crotamiton USP is a colorless to slightly yellowish oil, having a faint amine-like odor. It is miscible with alcohol and with methanol. Crotamiton is a mixture of the *cis* and *trans* isomers. Its molecular weight is 203.28.

CLINICAL PHARMACOLOGY:

Crotamiton has scabicidal and antipruritic actions. The mechanisms of these actions are not known.

INDICATIONS AND USAGE:

For eradication of scabies (*Sarcoptes scabiei*) and for symptomatic treatment of pruritic skin.

CONTRAINDICATIONS:

Crotamiton should not be applied topically to patients who develop a sensitivity or are allergic to it or who manifest a primary irritation response to topical medications.

WARNINGS:

If severe irritation or sensitization develops, treatment with this product should be discontinued and appropriate therapy instituted.

PRECAUTIONS:

General: Crotamiton should not be applied in the eyes or mouth because it may cause irritation. It should not be applied to acutely inflamed skin or raw or weeping surfaces until the acute inflammation has subsided.

Information for the Patient: See "Directions for patients with scabies".

Carcinogenesis, Mutagenesis, and Impairment of Fertility: Long-term carcinogenicity studies in animals have not been conducted.

Pregnancy Category C: Animal reproduction studies have not been conducted with Crotamiton. It is also not known whether Crotamiton can cause fetal harm when applied topically to a pregnant woman or can affect reproduction capacity. Crotamiton should be given to a pregnant woman only if clearly needed.

Pediatric Use: Safety and effectiveness in children have not been established.

DRUG INTERACTIONS:

None known.

ADVERSE REACTIONS:

Allergic sensitivity or primary irritation reactions may occur in some patients.

OVERDOSAGE:

There is no specific information on the effect of overtreatment with repeated topical applications in humans. *Acute toxicity (after accidental oral administration in children):* Highest known doses ingested: *Cream:* Children 2 g (age 1 ½ years); *Lotion:* 1 ounce (age 2 years.) A death was reported but cause was not confirmed.

Oral LD_{50} in animals (mg/kg): rats, 2212; mice, 2011

Signs and Symptoms (of oral ingestion): Burning sensation in the mouth, irritation of the buccal, esophageal and gastric mucosa, nausea, vomiting, abdominal pain.

Treatment: There is no specific antidote if taken orally. General measures to eliminate the drug and reduce its absorption, combined with symptomatic treatment, are recommended.

DOSAGE AND ADMINISTRATION:

LOTION

Shake well before using.

In Scabies: Thoroughly massage into the skin of the whole body from the chin down, paying particular attention to all folds and creases. A second application is advisable 24 hours later. Clothing and bed linen should be changed the next morning. A cleansing bath should be taken 48 hours after the last application.

In Pruritus: Massage gently into affected areas until medication is completely absorbed. Repeat as needed.

Directions for Patients with Scabies

1. Take a routine bath or shower. Thoroughly massage Crotamiton cream or lotion into the skin from the chin to the toes including folds and creases.

2. A second application is advisable 24 hours later.

3. The 60 gram tube or bottle is sufficient for two applications.

4. Clothing and bed linen should be changed the next day. Contaminated clothing and bed linen may be dry-cleaned, or washed in the hot cycle of the washing machine.

5. A cleansing bath should be taken 48 hours after the last application.

STORE AT ROOM TEMPERATURE.

HOW SUPPLIED - RATED THERAPEUTICALLY EQUIVALENT:

Lotion - Topical - 10 %

60 g	**$11.05**	**EURAX, Westwood Squibb**	**00072-2203-60**
480 ml	**$71.95**	**EURAX, Westwood Squibb**	**00072-2203-16**

HOW SUPPLIED - NOT RATED EQUIVALENT:

Cream - Topical - 10 %

60 gm	**$10.36**	**EURAX, Westwood Squibb**	**00072-2103-60**

CUPRIC CHLORIDE *(000919)*

CATEGORIES: Electrolytic, Caloric-Water Balance; Homeostatic & Nutrient; Mineral Supplements; Pharmaceutical Adjuvants; Replacement Solutions; Vitamins; Pregnancy Category C; FDA Approved 1986 Jun

BRAND NAMES: **Copper Chloride**

DESCRIPTION:

Cupric chloride 0.4 mg/ml is a sterile, nonpyrogenic solution intended for use as an additive to intravenous solutions for total parenteral nutrition (TPN). Each ml of solution contains 1.07 mg cupric chloride, dihydrate and 9 mg sodium chloride.

The solution contains no bacteriostat, antimicrobial agent or added buffer. The pH is 2 (approx.); may contain hydrochloric acid and sodium hydroxide for pH adjustment. The osmolarity is 0.327 mOsm/ml (calc.).

Cupric chloride, USP is chemically designated cupric chloride, dihydrate ($CuCl_2{\cdot}2H_20$), a crystalline compound freely soluble in water.

Sodium Chloride, USP is chemically designated NaCl, a white crystalline compound freely soluble in water.

The semi-rigid vial is fabricated from a specially formulated polyolefin.

It is a copolymer of ethylene and propylene. The safety of the plastic has been confirmed by tests in animals according to USP biological standards for plastic containers. The small amount of water vapor that can pass through the plastic container wall will not significantly alter the drug concentration.

CLINICAL PHARMACOLOGY:

Cupric chloride is an essential nutrient which serves as a cofactor for serum ceruloplasmin, an oxidase necessary for proper formation of the iron carrier protein, transferrin. Cupric chloride also helps maintain normal rates of red and white blood cell formation.

Providing copper during TPN helps prevent development of the following deficiency symptoms: Leukopenia, neutropenia, anemia, depressed ceruloplasmin levels, impaired transferrin formation and secondary iron deficiency.

Normal serum copper values range from 80 to 163 mcg/dl (mean, approximately 110 mcg/dl). The serum copper level at which deficiency symptoms appear is not precisely defined. A serum value of 9 mcg copper/dl was reported for one TPN patient who received no copper. The daily turnover of copper through ceruloplasmin is approximately 0.5 mg. Excretion of copper is through the bile (80%), directly through the intestinal wall (16%) and in urine (4%).

INDICATIONS AND USAGE:

Cupric chloride 0.4 mg/ml is indicated for use as a supplement to intravenous solutions given for total parenteral nutrition (TPN). Administration helps to maintain copper serum levels and to prevent depletion of endogenous stores and subsequent deficiency symptoms.

CONTRAINDICATIONS:

None known.

WARNINGS:

Direct intramuscular or intravenous injection of cupric chloride 0.4 mg/ml is contraindicated, as the acidic pH of the solution (2) may cause considerable tissue irritation. Liver and/or biliary tract dysfunction may require omission or reduction of copper and manganese doses because these elements are primarily eliminated in the bile.

PRECAUTIONS:

GENERAL

Do not use unless the solution is clear and the seal is intact. Administration of zinc in the absence of copper may cause a decrease in serum copper levels. Cupric chloride 0.4 mg/ml should only be used in conjunction with a pharmacy directed admixture program using aseptic technique in a laminar flow environment; it should be used promptly and in a single operation without any repeated penetrations. Solution contains no preservatives; discard unused portion immediately after admixture procedure is completed. It is not recommended to administer copper to a patient with Wilson's Disease, a genetic disease of copper metabolism.

LABORATORY TESTS

Twice monthly serum assays for copper and/or ceruloplasmin are suggested for monitoring copper concentrations in long-term TPN patients. As ceruloplasmin is a cuproenzyme, ceruloplasmin assays may be depressed secondary to copper deficiency.

CARCINOGENESIS, MUTAGENESIS, AND IMPAIRMENT OF FERTILITY

Long-term animal studies to evaluate the carcinogenic potential of cupric chloride 0.4 mg/ml have not been performed, nor have studies been done to assess mutagenesis or impairment of fertility.

NURSING MOTHERS

It is not known whether this drug is excreted in human milk. Because many drugs are excreted in human milk, caution should be exercised when cupric chloride 0.4 mg/ml is administered to a nursing woman.

PEDIATRIC USE

See DOSAGE AND ADMINISTRATION section. Safety and effectiveness in children have not been established.

PREGNANCY CATEGORY C

Animal reproduction studies have not been conducted with cupric chloride. It is also not known whether cupric chloride can cause fetal harm when administered to a pregnant woman or can affect reproductive capacity. Cupric chloride should be given to a pregnant woman only if clearly indicated.

DRUG INTERACTIONS:

Cupric ion may degrade ascorbic acid in total parenteral nutrition (TPN) solutions. In order to avoid this loss of ascorbate, multivitamin additives should be added to TPN solutions immediately prior to infusion. Alternatively, the multivitamin additive may be added to one container of TPN solution, followed by copper in a subsequent container.

ADVERSE REACTIONS:

None known.

DRUG ABUSE AND DEPENDENCE:

None known.

OVERDOSAGE:

Cupric chloride toxicity can produce prostration, behavior change, diarrhea, progressive marasmus, hypotonia, photophobia and peripheral edema. Such symptoms have been reported with a serum copper level of 286 mcg/dl. D-penicillamine has been reported effective as an antidote.

DOSAGE AND ADMINISTRATION:

Cupric chloride 0.4 mg/ml contains 0.4 mg copper/ml and is administered intravenously only after dilution. The additive should be diluted in a volume of fluid not less than 100 ml. For the adult receiving TPN, the suggested additive dosage is 0.5 to 1.5 mg copper/day. (1.25 to 3.75 ml/day). For pediatric patients, the suggested additive dosage is 20 mcg copper/kg/day (0.05 ml/kg/day). Parenteral drug products should be inspected visually for particulate matter and discoloration prior to administration, whenever solution and container permit. See PRECAUTIONS.

Exposure of pharmaceutical products to heat should be minimized. Avoid excessive heat. Protect from freezing. It is recommended that the product be stored at room temperature (25°C); however, brief exposure up to 40°C does not adversely affect the product.

HOW SUPPLIED - EQUIVALENTS NOT AVAILABLE:

Injection, Conc-Soln - Intravenous - 0.4 mg/ml

10 ml	**$1.65**	**COPPER CHLORIDE, Consolidated Midland**	**00223-7346-10**
30 ml	$15.71	COPPER 0.4, Abbott	00074-4528-03

Injection, Conc-Soln - Intravenous - 0.85 mg/ml

10 ml	$6.37	COPPER 0.4, Abbott	00074-4092-01
30 ml	$13.45	COPPER 0.4, Abbott	00074-4092-03

CUPRIC SULFATE *(000920)*

CATEGORIES: Copper Deficiency; Electrolyte Solutions; Electrolytic, Caloric-Water Balance; Homeostatic & Nutrient; Mineral Supplements; Replacement Solutions; Vitamins; Pregnancy Category C; FDA Approved 1987 May

BRAND NAMES: Copper Sulfate; Cupri-Pak

DESCRIPTION:

Trace Element Additive

FOR IV USE ONLY AFTER DILUTION

Cupric sulfate injection is a sterile, nonpyrogenic solution of cupric sulfate in water for injection. It is intended for use as an additive to solutions for total parenteral nutrition (TPN). See TABLE 1 for ingredients. **Each ml Contains**

DESCRIPTION: *(cont'd)*

TABLE 1

Each ml contains:	10 ml VIAL (One Withdrawal Only)	30 ml VIAL (Multiple Dose)
Cupric Sulfate Pentahydrate, USP	1.57 mg	1.57 mg
Benzyl Alcohol, NF	—	0.9%
Water for Injection, USP	q.s.	q.s.

Sulfuric acid and/or sodium hydroxide for pH adjustment (2.0 - 3.5).

Cupric sulfate is chemically designated as $CuSO_4$. Its pentahydrate form ($CuSO_4$-$5H_2O$) is a blue or ultramarine crystals or blue granules, or light blue powder which slowly effloresces in air. It is very soluble in water, soluble in methanol, glycerol, and slightly soluble in ethanol. Benzyl alcohol is chemically designated $C_6H_5CH_2OH$, a clear liquid with faint aromatic odor and miscible with water.

CLINICAL PHARMACOLOGY:

Copper is an essential nutrient which serves as a cofactor for several metalloenzymes including ceruloplasmin, cytochrome *c* oxidase, superoxide dismutase and lysyl oxidase. The stomach and duodenum absorb 40 to 60% of dietary copper which rapidly accumulates in the liver, where it is incorporated into ceruloplasmin and released into the circulation. In normal adults, 90 to 95% of plasma copper is in ceruloplasmin, 1 to 2% complexed with amino acids or free, and the remainder reversibly bound to albumin. Copper is secreted in saliva, gastric and pancreatic juice, and bile. A copper-metallothionein complex present in intestinal mucosal cells is shed into the intestinal lumen. Although much of this copper is reabsorbed, about 1 mg/day of body copper is lost through fecal excretion and a slightly greater amount of dietary copper is absorbed each day. Urinary copper excretion is usually less than 0.05 mg/day. Loss due to sweat and epidermal shedding averages 0.2 mg/day although loss in very hot environments may exceed 1 mg/day. Biliary excretion is the major route for elimination of excess copper.

Copper deficiency may develop in premature infants due to dietary copper deficiency and in children and adults with malabsorption due to chronic gastrointestinal disease. Anemia and neutropenia refractory to iron and other nutrients occur when plasma copper and ceruloplasmin are reduced to 10 to 30% of normal levels. Defective bone mineralization and growth develop in small children with chronic copper deficiency. These sequelae begin to resolve within one week after therapy with copper is begun.

INDICATIONS AND USAGE:

Cupric sulfate injection is indicated for use as a supplement to intravenous solutions given for TPN, to prevent and treat copper deficiency.

CONTRAINDICATIONS:

The multiple dose preparation should not be used in patients with known sensitivity to benzyl alcohol.

WARNINGS:

LIVER AND/OR BILIARY TRACT DYSFUNCTION

Copper is eliminated in bile; therefore, patients with severe liver and/or biliary tract disease may require a decrease or elimination of TPN copper supplements.

WILSON'S DISEASE

Copper supplements should be avoided in patients with this genetic disorder of copper metabolism.

Direct intramuscular or intravenous injection of cupric sulfate injection is contraindicated, as the acidic pH of the solution (2.0-3.5) may cause considerable tissue irritation.

PRECAUTIONS:

1. Do not use unless the solution is clear and the seal is intact.

2. The solution is hypotonic and must not be given by direct intramuscular or intravenous route.

3. Do not use syringes equipped with aluminum needles or hubs, as the solution is acidic.

LABORATORY TESTS

Serum or plasma copper and ceruloplasmin should be monitored periodically during intravenous cupric sulfate therapy. Normal ranges of tests for these substances should be adjusted for the age and sex of the patient, and the assay method used. Normal infants have slightly lower circulating copper levels than children greater than one year old, and both copper and ceruloplasmin levels are slightly higher in women than in men. In patients with chronic hepatobiliary disease, serum copper is frequently low due to impaired ceruloplasmin synthesis in spite of greatly increased liver copper levels. Serum ceruloplasmin is increased by hyperthyroidism, estrogen therapy and during the third trimester of pregnancy. Ceruloplasmin level also increases in diseases associated with chronic inflammation including rheumatoid arthritis, chronic infection and some neoplasms.

CARCINOGENESIS, MUTAGENESIS, AND IMPAIRMENT OF FERTILITY

Long-term animal studies have not been performed to evaluate the carcinogenic potential or the effect on fertility of cupric sulfate injection.

PREGNANCY CATEGORY C

Animal reproduction studies have not been conducted with cupric sulfate. It is also not known whether cupric sulfate can cause fetal harm when administered to a pregnant woman or can affect reproductive capacity. Cupric sulfate should be given to a pregnant woman only if clearly indicated.

DRUG INTERACTIONS:

Cupric ion will degrade ascorbic acid in TPN solutions. To avoid loss of ascorbate and other sensitive vitamins, cupric sulfate and other trace nutrient metal ions should be added to TPN solutions immediately prior to infusion.

ADVERSE REACTIONS:

None known.

OVERDOSAGE:

No toxicity data are available for this intravenous cupric sulfate product.

Acute ingestion of 1000 mg or more cupric sulfate is associated with epigastric distress, vomiting and diarrhea. Hemolysis, renal failure and shock may follow. Chronic toxicity can include prostration, behavioral change, diarrhea, progressive marasmus, hypotonia, photophobia, hepatic damage and peripheral edema. The parenteral copper dose producing chronic toxicity has not been established but may be as low as 10 times that needed to prevent deficiency.

DOSAGE AND ADMINISTRATION:

THE DAILY REQUIREMENT FOR COPPER TO PREVENT OR TREAT COPPER DEFICIENCY HAS NOT BEEN PRECISELY DETERMINED FOR PATIENTS RECEIVING PARENTERAL NUTRIENTS AS THEIR SOLE OR PRIMARY NUTRIENT SOURCE. THE FOLLOWING DOSAGES ARE PROVIDED AS GUIDELINES. THE ADEQUACY FOR THERAPY SHOULD BE MONITORED BY PERIODIC MEASUREMENTS OF CIRCULATING COPPER AND CERULOPLASMIN LEVELS.

ADULT

For the metabolically stable adult receiving TPN, 0.5 to 1.5 mg copper/day should be added to the TPN solution.

PEDIATRIC

For full-term infants and children, 20 mcg/kg/day should be added to the TPN solution. Limited data are available for premature infants who may require larger doses.

Copper deficient patients with documented high rates of gastrointestinal loss may require higher doses adjusted to compensate for the loss.

Cupric sulfate injection provides 0.4 mg copper/ml, in both single use and multiple dose preparations. The solution is hypotonic and must not be given by direct intramuscular or intravenous route. It is administered intravenously only after dilution. Do not use syringes equipped with aluminum needles or hubs as the solution is acidic.

Aseptic addition of cupric sulfate injection to TPN solutions under a laminar flow hood is recommended. Cupric sulfate is physically compatible with the electrolytes and most vitamins usually present in the amino acid/dextrose solutions used for TPN; however chemical degradation of ascorbic acid and possibly other nutrients may occur. Cupric sulfate and other trace nutrient metal ions should be added to TPN solutions immediately prior to infusion.

Parenteral drug products should be inspected visually for particulate matter and discoloration prior to administration, whenever solution and container permit.

DIRECTIONS FOR DISPENSING IN HOSPITAL PHARMACY

1. Arrange syringes, vials and TPN solutions in the laminar flow hood.

2. Suspend the TPN bags from the hole in the flat plastic extension at the top.

3. Remove the flip-top seal from the vial and swab the exposed rubber stopper with an antiseptic solution.

4. Withdraw the contents of the vial using the sterile syringe and transfer the required volumes through the medication port into the TPN bags. Unused portions in the 10 ml vial should be discarded immediately.

5. Shake the bag gently to distribute the drug.

6. Check solution for particulate matter.

7. Identify the bag.

Make only one withdrawal from the 10 ml vial.

Store at controlled room temperature 15 - 30°C (59 - 86°F). Do not permit to freeze.

REFERENCES:

1. Expert Panel for Nutrition Advisory Group, AMA Department of Foods and Nutrition. Guidelines for Essential trace element preparations for parenteral use: a statement by an expert panel. *JAMA* 241:2051- 2054, 1979.

HOW SUPPLIED - EQUIVALENTS NOT AVAILABLE:

Injection, Solution - Intravenous - 0.4 mg/ml

10 ml x 25	$62.19	Cupric Sulfate, Am Regent	00517-6210-25
30 ml x 5	$26.56	Cupric Sulfate, Am Regent	00517-7230-05

Injection, Solution - Intravenous - 2 mg/ml

5 ml	$3.90	COPPER SULFATE, Fujisawa USA	00469-7320-20
10 ml x 25	$133.88	COPPER SULFATE, Fujisawa USA	00469-7320-30

CYANIDE ANTIDOTE *(000921)*

CATEGORIES: Antagonists and Antidotes; Antidotes; Heavy Metal Antagonists; FDA Pre 1938 Drugs

BRAND NAMES: Cyanide Antidote Package

Prescribing information not available at time of publication.

HOW SUPPLIED - EQUIVALENTS NOT AVAILABLE:

Kit - Inhalation; Int - 5 drop/300 mg/1

1's	$99.00	Cyanide Antidote Package, Pasadena	00418-4030-01
1's	$182.88	CYANIDE ANTIDOTE PACKAGE, Yorpharm	61147-8601-00

CYANOCOBALAMIN *(000922)*

CATEGORIES: Anemia; Antibiotics; Blood Formation/Coagulation; Deficiency Anemias; Fish Tapeworm; Folic Acid Deficiency; Homeostatic & Nutrient; Lesions; Thyrotoxicosis; Vitamin B Complex; Vitamin B12; Vitamins; Chronic Fatigue Syndrome*; Hemorrhage*; Pregnancy Category C; FDA Approval Pre 1982
* Indication not approved by the FDA

BRAND NAMES: *Anacobin* (Canada); *Antipernicin*; *Arcored*; B-12-1000; *Bedoc*; *Bedodeka*; *Behepan*; Berubigen; Betalin 12; *Betlovex*; *Betolvex*; Blu-12; Cobal; *Cobalin*; *Cobalmed*; *Cobalparen*; Cobavite; Cobex; Cobolin-M; *Compensal*; *Compensal 25,000* (Mexico); Corubeen; *Corubin*; Cpc-Carpenters; Crystamine; Crysti-12; Cyano-Plex; Cyanocob; Cyanoject; Cyomin; *Cytacon*; *Cytaman*; *Cytamen* (England); *Depinar*; Depo-Cobolin; *Dobetin*; *Docemine*; Dodecamin; *Hematolamin* (Japan); *Iloban*; La-12; *Lagavit B12*; *Lifaton*; *Lifaton B12*; Nascobal; Neurin-12; *Neurodex*; Neuroforte-R; *Norivite*; *Norivite-12*; *Ottovit*; Pan B-12; Primabalt; *Redisol* (Japan); *Rojamin*; Rubesol-1000; *Rubisol*; Rubivite; *Rubramin* (Canada); Rubramin Pc; *Rubranova* (Mexico); Ruvite; Shovite; Sytobex; Vibal; Vibisone; *Vicapan N* (Germany); Vita Liver; Vita-Plus B-12; Vitabee 12; **Vitamin B-12**; *Vitarubin*; *Yobramin*
(International brand names outside U.S. in italics)

FORMULARIES: Aetna; BC-BS; Medi-Cal

DESCRIPTION:

Cyanocobalamin Injection, USP is a sterile solution of cyanocobalamin. Each ml contains 100 or 1000 mcg cyanocobalamin. The vials also contain sodium chloride, 0.25%. Benzyl alcohol, 2% is present as a preservative. Sodium hydroxide and/or hydrochloric acid may have been added during manufacture to adjust the pH.

DESCRIPTION: *(cont'd)*

Cyanocobalamin appears as dark-red crystals or as an amorphous or crystalline red powder. It is very hygroscopic in the anhydrous form and sparingly soluble in water (1:80). It is stable to autoclaving for short periods at 121°C. The vitamin B_{12} coenzymes are very unstable in light.

The chemical name is 5, 6-dimethyl-benzimidazolyl cyanocobalamine; the empirical formula is $C_{63}H_{88}CoN_{14}O_{14}P$. The cobalt content is 4.34%. The molecular weight is 1355.38

GEL FOR INTRANASAL ADMINISTRATION

Cyanocobalamin, USP gel for Intranasal Administration is a solution of cyanocobalamin, USP (vitamin B_{12}) for administration as a metered gel to the nasal mucosa. Each bottle of Nascobal contains 5ml of a 500 mcg/ 0. 1 ml gel solution of cyanocobalamin with methylcellulose, sodium citrate, citric acid, glycerin, benzalkonium chloride in purified water. The gel solution has a pH between 4.5 and 5.5. The gel pump unit must be fully primed (see HOW SUPPLIED) prior to initial use. After initial priming, each metered gel delivers an average of 500mcg of cyanocobalamin and the 5ml bottle will deliver 8 doses of Nascobal. If not used for 48 hours or longer, the unit must be reprimed (see HOW SUPPLIED).

CLINICAL PHARMACOLOGY:

Vitamin B_{12} is essential to growth, cell reproduction, hematopoiesis, and nucleoprotein and myelin synthesis. Cyanocobalamin is quantitatively and rapidly absorbed from intramuscular and subcutaneous sites of injection; the plasma level of the compound reaches its peak within 1 hour after intramuscular injection. Absorbed vitamin B_{12} is transported via specific B_{12}-binding proteins, transcobalamin I and II, to the various tissues. The liver is the main organ for vitamin B_{12} storage.

Within 48 hours after injection of 100 or 1000 mcg of vitamin B_{12}, 50 to 98% of the injected dose may appear in the urine. The major portion is excreted within the first 8 hours. Intravenous administration results in even more rapid excretion with little opportunity for liver storage. Gastrointestinal absorption of vitamin B_{12} depends on the presence of sufficient intrinsic factor and calcium ions. Intrinsic factor deficiency causes pernicious anemia, which may be associated with subacute combined degeneration of the spinal cord. Prompt parenteral administration of vitamin B_{12} prevents progression of neurologic damage.

The average diet supplies about 5 to 15 mcg/day of vitamin B_{12} in a protein-bound form that is available for absorption after normal digestion. Vitamin B_{12} is not present in foods of plant origin but is abundant in foods of animal origin. In people with normal absorption, deficiencies have been reported only in strict vegetarians who consume no products of animal origin (including no milk products or eggs).

Vitamin B_{12} is bound to intrinsic factor during transit through the stomach; separation occurs in the terminal ileum in the presence of calcium, and vitamin B_{12} enters the mucosal cell for absorption. It is then transported by the transcobalamin-binding proteins. A small amount (approximately 1% of the total amount ingested) is absorbed by simple diffusion, but this mechanism is adequate only with very large doses. Oral absorption is considered too undependable to rely on in patients with pernicious anemia or other conditions resulting in malabsorption of vitamin B_{12}.

Cyanocobalamin is the most widely used form of vitamin B_{12} and has hematopoietic activity apparently identical to that of the antianemia factor in purified liver extract. Hydroxycobalamin is equally as effective as cyanocobalamin, and they share the cobalamin molecular structure.

Colchicine, para-aminosalicylic acid, and heavy alcohol intake for longer than 2 weeks may produce malabsorption of vitamin B_{12}.

GEL FOR INTRANASAL ADMINISTRATION

Cells characterized by rapid division (*e.g.,* epithelial cells, bone marrow, myeloid cells) appear to have the greatest requirement for vitamin B_{12}. Vitamin B_{12} can be converted to coenzyrne B_{12} in tissues, and as such is essential for conversion of methylmalonate to succinate and synthesis of methionine from homocysteine, a reaction which also requires folate. In the absence of coenzyme B_{12}, tetrahydrofolate cannot be regenerated from its inactive storage form, 5-methyl tetrahydrofolate, and a functional folate deficiency occurs. Vitamin B_{12} also may be involved in maintaining sulfhydryl (SH) groups in the reduced form required by many SH-activated enzyme systems. Through these reactions, vitamin B_{12} is associated with fat and carbohydrate metabolism and protein synthesis. Vitamin B_{12} deficiency results in megaloblastic anemia, GI lesions, and neurologic damage that begins with an inability to produce myelin and is followed by gradual degeneration of the axon and nerve head.

Cyanocobalamin is the most stable and widely used form of vitamin B_{12}, and has hematopoietic activity apparently identical to that of the antianemia factor in purified liver extract. The information below, describing the clinical pharmacology of cyanocobalamin, has been derived from studies with injectable vitamin B_{12}.

Vitamin B_{12} is quantitatively and rapidly absorbed from intramuscular and subcutaneous sites of injection. It is bound to plasma proteins and stored in the liver. Vitamin B_{12} is excreted in the bile and undergoes some enterohepatic recycling. Absorbed vitamin B_{12} is transported via specific B_{12} binding proteins, transcobalamin I and II, to the various tissues. The liver is the main organ for vitamin B_{12} storage.

Parenteral (intramuscular) administration of vitamin B_{12} completely reverses the megaloblastic anemia and GI symptoms of vitamin B_{12} deficiency; the degree of improvement in neurologic symptoms depends on the duration and severity of the lesions, although progression of the lesions is immediately arrested.

Gastrointestinal absorption of vitamin B_{12} depends on the presence of sufficient intrinsic factor and calcium ions. Intrinsic factor deficiency causes pernicious anemia, which may be associated with subacute combined degeneration of the spinal cord. Prompt parenteral administration of vitamin B 12 prevents progression of neurologic damage.

The average diet supplies about 4 to 15 mcg/day of vitamin B_{12} in a protein-bound form that is available for absorption after normal digestion. Vitamin B_{12} is not present in foods of plant origin, but is abundant in foods of animal origin. In people with normal absorption, deficiencies have been reported only in strict vegetarians who consume no products of animal origin (including no milk products or eggs).

Vitamin B12 is bound to intrinsic factor during transit through the stomach; separation occurs in the terminal ileum in the presence of calcium, and vitamin B_{12} enters the mucosal cell for absorption. It is then transported by the transcobalamin binding proteins. A small amount (approximately 1% of the total amount ingested) is absorbed by simple diffusion, but this mechanism is adequate only with very large doses. Oral absorption is considered too undependable to rely on in patients with pernicious anemia or other conditions resulting in malabsorption of vitamin B_{12}.

Colchicine, para-aminosalicylic acid, and heavy alcohol intake for longer than weeks may produce malabsorption of vitamin B_{12}.

Pharmacokinetics

Absorption: In a bioavailability study in 23 pernicious anernia patients comparing B 12 nasal gel to intramuscular B_{12}, peak concentrations of B_{12} after intranasal administration were reached in 1-2 hours. The average peak concentration of B12 after intranasal adrninistration was 1387 ±971 kg/ml. The bioavailability of the nasal gel relative to an intramuscular injection was found to be 8.9% (90% confidence intervals 7.1 1 1.2%).

CLINICAL PHARMACOLOGY: *(cont'd)*

In pernicious anemia patients, once weekly intranasal dosing with 500 mcg B_{12} resulted in a consistent increase in pre-dose serum B_{12} levels during one month of treatment ($p<0.003$) above that seen one month after 100 mcg intramuscular dose.

Distribution: In the blood, B_{12} is bound to transcobalamin II, a specific B-globulin carrier protein, and is distributed and stored primarily in the liver and bone marrow.

Elimination: About 3-8 mcg of B_{12} is secreted into the GI tract daily via the bile; in normal subjects with sufficient intrinsic factor, all but about 1 mcg is re-absorbed. When B_{12} is administered in doses which saturate the binding capacity of plasma proteins and the liver, the unbound B_{12} is rapidly eliminated in the urine. Retention of B_{12} in the body is dose-dependent. About 80-90% of an intramuscular dose up to 50 mcg is retained in the body; this percentage drops to 55% for a 100 mcg dose, and decreases to 15% when a 1000 mcg dose is given.

INDICATIONS AND USAGE:

Cyanocobalamin is indicated for vitamin B_{12} deficiencies due to malabsorption which may be associated with the following conditions: Addisonian (pernicious) anemia Gastrointestinal pathology, dysfunction, or surgery, including gluten enteropathy or sprue, small-bowel bacterial overgrowth, total or partial gastrectomy fish tapeworm infestation.

Malignancy of pancreas or bowel folic acid deficiency.

It may be possible to treat the underlying disease by surgical correction of anatomic lesions leading to small-bowel bacterial overgrowth, expulsion of fish tapeworm, discontinuation of drugs leading to vitamin malabsorption (See CLINICAL PHARMACOLOGY and Drug/Laboratory Test Interactions), use of a gluten-free diet in nontropical sprue, or administration of antibiotics in tropical sprue. Such measures remove the need for long-term administration of cyanocobalamin.

Requirements of vitamin B_{12} in excess of normal (due to pregnancy, thyrotoxicosis, hemolytic anemia, hemorrhage, malignancy, hepatic and renal disease) can usually be met with oral supplementation.

Cyanocobalamin injection is also suitable for the vitamin B_{12} absorption test (Schilling test).

GEL FOR INTRANASAL ADMINISTRATION

Cyanocobalamin, USP gel for Intranasal Administration is indicated for the maintenance of the hematologic status of patients who are in remission following intramuscular vitamin B_{12} therapy for the following conditions:

1. Pernicious anemia. Indicated only in patients who are in hematologic remission with no nervous system involvement.

2. Dietary deficiency of vitamin B_{12} occurring in strict vegetarians. (Isolated vitamin B_{12} deficiency is very rare).

3. Malabsorption of vitamin B_{12} resulting from structural or functional damage to the stomach, where intrinsic factor is secreted or to the ileum, where intrinsic factor facilitates vitamin B_{12} absorption. These conditions include tropical sprue, and nontropical sprue (Idiopathic steatorrhea, gluten-induced enteropathy). Folate deficiency in these patients is usually more severe than vitamin B_{12} deficiency.

4. Inadequate secretion of intrinsic factor, resulting from lesions that destroy the gastric mucosa (ingestion of corrosives, extensive neoplasia), and a number of conditions associated with a variable degree of gastric atrophy (such as multiple sclerosis, certain endocrine disorders, iron deficiency, and subtotal gastrectomy). Total gastrectomy always produces vitamin B_{12} deficiency. Structural lesions leading to vitamin B_{12} deficiency include regional ileitis, ileal resections, malignancies, etc.

5. Competition for vitamin B_{12} by intestinal parasites or bacteria. The fish tapeworm (I) iphyllobothrium latum) absorbs huge quantities of vitamin B_{12} and infested patients often have associated gastric atrophy. The blind-loop syndrome may produce deficiency of vitamin B_{12} or folate.

6. Inadequate utilization of vitamin B_{12}. This may occur if antimetabolites for the vitamin are employed in the treatment of neoplasia. It may be possible to treat the underlying disease by surgical correction of anatomic lesions leading to small bowel bacterial overgrowth, expulsion of fish tapeworm, discontinuation of drugs leading to vitamin malabsorption (see Drug/Laboratory Test Interactions), use of a gluten-free diet in nontropical sprue, or administration of antibiotics in tropical sprue. Such measures remove the need for long-term administration of vitamin B_{12}. Requirements of vitamin B_{12} in excess of normal (due to pregnancy, thyrotoxicosis, hemolytic anemia, hemorrhage, malignancy, hepatic and renal disease) can usually be met with intranasal or oral supplementation.

Cyanocobalamin, USP gel for Intranasal Administration has only been tested in patients with vitamin B_{12} malabsorption who have received prior intramuscular cyanocobalamin treatment and are in hematologic remission. Cyanocobalamin, USP gel for Intranasal Administration is not suitable for the vitamin B_{12} absorption test (Schilling Test).

CONTRAINDICATIONS:

Sensitivity to cobalt and/or vitamin B_{12}, or any component of the mediaction is a contraindication.

WARNINGS:

Patients with early Leber's disease (hereditary optic nerve atrophy) who were treated with cyanocobalamin suffered severe and swift optic atrophy.

Hypokalemia and sudden death may occur in severe megaloblastic anemia which is treated intensively with vitamin B_{12}. Folic acid is not a substitute for vitamin B_{12} although it may improve vitamin B_{12} deficient megaloblastic anemia. Exclusive use of folic acid in treating vitamin B_{12}-deficient megaloblastic anemia could result in progressive and irreversible neurologic damage.

Anaphylactic shock and death have been reported after parenteral vitamin B_{12} administration. No such reactions have been reported in clinical trials with cyanocobalamin, USP gel for Intranasal Administration.

Blunted or impeded therapeutic response to vitamin B_{12} may be due to such conditions as infection, uremia, drugs having bone marrow suppressant properties such as chloramphenicol, and concurrent iron or folic acid deficiency.

This product contains benzyl alcohol. Benzyl alcohol has been reported to be associated with a fatal "gasping syndrome" in premature infants.

PRECAUTIONS:

General: Vitamin B_{12} deficiency that is allowed to progress for longer than 3 months may produce permanent degenerative lesions of the spinal cord. Doses of folic acid greater than 0.1 mg/day may result in hematologic remission in patients with vitamin B_{12} deficiency. Neurologic manifestations will not be prevented with folic acid, and if they are not treated with vitamin B_{12}, irreversible damage will result. Doses of cyanocobalamin exceeding 10 mcg daily may produce hematologic response in patients with folate deficiency. Indiscriminate administration may mask the true diagnosis.

PRECAUTIONS: *(cont'd)*

GEL FOR INTRANASAL ADMINISTRATION

An intradermal test dose of parenteral vitamin B_{12} is recommended before cyanocobalamin, USP gel for Intranasal Administration is administered to patients suspected of cyanocobalamin sensitivity. Vitamin B_{12} deficiency that is allowed to progress for longer than three months may produce permanent degenerative lesions of the spinal cord. Doses of folic acid greater than 0. 1 mg per day may result in hematologic remission in patients with vitamin B_{12} deficiency. Neurologic manifestations will not be prevented with folic acid, and if not treated with vitamin B_{12}, irreversible damage will result.

Doses of vitamin B_{12} exceeding 10 mcg daily may produce hematologic response in patients with folate deficiency. Indiscriminate administration may mask the true diagnosis.

The validity of diagnostic vitamin B_{12} or folic acid blood assays could be compromised by medications, and this should be considered before relying on such tests for therapy.

Vitamin B_{12} is not a substitute for folic acid and since it might improve folic acid deficient megaloblastic anemia, indiscriminate use of vitamin B_{12} could mask the true diagnosis.

Hypokalemia and thrombocytosis could occur upon conversion of severe megaloblastic to normal erythropoiesis with vitamin B_{12} therapy. Therefore, serum potassium levels and the platelet count should be monitored carefully during therapy.

Vitamin B_{12} deficiency may suppress the signs of polycythemia vera. Treatment with vitamin B_{12} may unmask this condition.

If a patient is not properly maintained with cyanocobalamin, USP gel for Intranasal Administration, intramuscular vitamin B_{12} is necessary for adequate treatment of the patient. No single regimen fits all cases, and the status of the patient observed in follow-up is the final criterion for adequacy of therapy.

The effectiveness of cyanocobalamin, USP gel for Intranasal Administration in patients with nasal congestion, allergic rhinitis and upper respiratory infections has not been determined. Therefore, treatment with cyanocobalamin, USP gel for Intranasal Administration should be deferred until symptoms have subsided.

Information for the Patient: Patients with pernicious anemia should be informed that they will require monthly injections of vitamin B_{12} for the remainder of their lives. Failure to do so will result in return of the anemia and in development of incapacitating and irreversible damage to the nerves of the spinal chord. Also, patients should be warned about the danger of taking folic acid in place of vitamin B_{12}, because the former may prevent anemia but allow progression of subacute combined degeneration.

A vegetarian diet which contains no animal products (including milk products or eggs) does not supply any vitamin B_{12}. Patients following such a diet should be advised to take oral vitamin B_{12} regularly. The need for vitamin B_{12} is increased by pregnancy and lactation. Deficiency has been recognized in infants of vegetarian mothers who were breast fed, even though the mothers had no symptoms of deficiency at the time.

GEL FOR INTRANASAL ADMINISTRATION

Patients with pernicious anemia should be instructed that they will require weekly intranasal administration of cyanocobalamin, USP gel for Intranasal Administration for the remainder of their lives. Failure to do so will result in return of the anemia and in development of incapacitating and irreversible damage to the nerves of the spinal cord. Also, patients should be warned about the danger of taking folic acid in place of vitamin B_{12}, because the former may prevent anemia but allow progression of subacute combined degeneration of the spinal cord. (Hot foods may cause nasal secretions and a resulting loss of medication; therefore, patients should be told to administer cyanocobalamin, USP gel for Intranasal Administration at least one hour before or one hour after ingestion of hot foods or liquids).

A vegetarian diet which contains no animal products (including milk products or eggs) does not supply any vitamin B_{12}. Therefore, patients following such a diet should be advised to take cyanocobalamin, USP gel for Intranasal Administration weekly. The need for vitamin B_{12} is increased by pregnancy and lactation. Deficiency has been recognized in infants of vegetarian mothers who were breast fed, even though the mothers had no symptoms of deficiency at the time.

The patient should also understand the importance of returning for follow-up blood tests every 3 to 6 months to confirm adequacy of the therapy. Careful instructions on the actuator assembly, priming of the actuator and nasal administration of cyanocobalamin, USP gel for Intranasal Administration should be given to the patient. Although instructions for patients are supplied with individual bottles, procedures for use should be demonstrated to each patient.

Laboratory Tests: During the initial treatment of patients with pernicious anemia, serum potassium must be observed closely during the first 48 hours and potassium should be replaced, if necessary.

Hematocrit, reticulocyte count, and vitamin B_{12}, folate, and iron levels should be obtained prior to treatment. Hematocrit and reticulocyte counts should be repeated daily from the fifth to seventh days of therapy and then frequently until the hematocrit is normal. If folate levels are low, folic acid should also be administered. If reticulocytes have not increased after treatment or if reticulocyte counts do not continue at least twice the normal level (as long as the hematocrit is less than 35%), diagnosis or treatment should be reevaluated. Repeat determinations of iron and folic acid may reveal a complicating illness that might inhibit the response of the marrow. Since patients with pernicious anemia have about 3 times the incidence of carcinoma of the stomach as the general population, appropriate tests for this condition should be carried out when indicated.

Hematocrit, reticulocyte count, vitamin B_{12}, folate and iron levels should be obtained prior to treatment. If folate levels are low, folic acid should also be administered. All hematologic parameters should be normal when beginning treatment with cyanocobalamin, USP gel for Intranasal Administration.

Vitamin B_{12} blood levels and peripheral blood counts must be monitored initially at one month after the start of treatment with cyanocobalamin, USP gel for Intranasal Administration, and then at intervals of 3 to 6 months.

A decline in the serum levels of B_{12} after one month after treatment with B_{12} nasal gel may indicate that the dose may need to be adjusted upward. Patients should be seen one month after each dose adjustment, continued low levels of serum B_{12} may indicate that the patient is not a candidate for this mode of administration.

Patients with pernicious anemia have about 3 times the incidence of carcinoma of the stomach as in the general population, so appropriate tests for this condition should be carried out when indicated.

Drug/Laboratory Test Interactions: Persons taking most antibiotics, methotrexate, and pyrimethamine invalidate folic acid and vitamin B_{12} diagnostic blood assays.

GEL FOR INTRANASAL ADMINISTRATION

Colchicine, para-aminosalicylic acid and heavy alcohol intake for longer than 2 weeks may produce malabsorption of vitamin B_{12}.

Carcinogenesis, Mutagenesis, and Impairment of Fertility: Long-term studies in animals to evaluate carcinogenic potential have not been done. There is no evidence from long-term use in patients with pernicious anemia that cyanocobalamin is carcinogenic. Pernicious anemia is associated with an increased incidence of carcinoma of the stomach, but this is believed to be related to the underlying pathology and not to treatment with cyanocobalamin.

PRECAUTIONS: *(cont'd)*

Usage in Pregnancy: Pregnancy Category C: Adequate and well-controlled studies have not been done in pregnant women. However, vitamin B_{12} is an essential vitamin, and requirements are increased during pregnancy. Amounts of vitamin B_{12} that are recommended by the Food and Nutrition Board, National Academy of Science-National Research Council, for pregnant women (4 mcg daily) should be consumed during pregnancy.

GEL FOR INTRANASAL ADMINISTRATION

Pregnancy Category C: Animal reproduction studies have not been conducted with vitamin B_{12}. It is also not known whether vitamin B_{12} can cause fetal harm when adrministered to a pregnant woman or can affect reproduction capacity. However, vitamin B_{12} is an essential vitamin, and requirements are increased during pregnancy. Amounts of vitamin B_{12} that are recommended by the Food and Nutrition Board, National Academy of Science-National Research Council, for pregnant women (4 mcg daily) should be consumed during pregnancy.

Nursing Mothers: Vitamin B_{12} appears in the milk of nursing mothers in concentrations which approximate the mother's level of vitamin B_{12} in the blood. Amounts of vitamin B_{12} that are recommended by the Food and Nutrition Board, National Academy of Science-National Research Council, for lactating women (4 mcg daily) should be consumed during lactation.

Pediatric Use: Intake for children should be the amount (0.5 to 3 mcg daily) recommended by the Food and Nutrition Board, National Academy of Science-National Research Council.

ADVERSE REACTIONS:

GEL FOR INTRANASAL ADMINISTRATION

The incidence of adverse experiences described in TABLE 1 are based on data from a short-term clinical trial in vitamin B_{12} deficient patients in hematologic remission receiving cyanocobalamin, USP gel for Intranasal Administration (N=24) and intramuscular vitamin B_{12} (N=25).

TABLE 1 Adverse Experiences by Body System, Number of Patients and Number of Occurrences by Treatment Following Intramuscular and Intranasal Administration of Cyanocobalamin

Body System (Adverse Experience)	Number of Patients (Occurrences)	
	Vitamin B12 Nasal Gel, 500 mcg (N=24)	Intramuscular Vitamin B12 100 mcg (N=25)
Body as a Whole		
Asthenia	1 (1)	4 (4)
Back Pain	0 (0)	1 (1)
Generalized Pain	0 (0)	2 (3)
Headache	1 (2)*	5 (11)
Infection†	3 (4)	3 (3)
Cardiovascular System		
Peripheral vascular disorder	0 (0)	1 (1)
Digestive System		
Dyspepsia	0 (0)	1 (2)
Glossitis	1 (1)	0 (0)
Nausea	1 (1)*	1 (1)
Nausea & vomiting	0 (0)	1 (1)
Vomiting	0 (0)	1 (1)
Musculoskeletal System		
Arthritis	0 (0)	2 (2)
Myalgia	0 (0)	1 (1)
Nervous System		
Abnormal gait	0 (0)	1 (1)
Anxiety	0 (0)	1 (1)*
Dizziness	0 (0)	3 (3)
Hypesthesia	0 (0)	1 (1)
Incoordination	0 (0)	1 (2)*
Nervousness	0 (0)	1 (3)*
Paresthesia	1 (1)	1 (1)
Respiratory System		
Dyspnea	0 (0)	1 (1)
Rhinitis	1 (1)	2 (2)

* There may be a possible relationship between these adverse experiences and the study drugs. These adverse experiences could also have been produced by the patient's clinical state or other concomitant therapy.
† Sore throat, common cold.

The intensity of the reported adverse experiences following the adrninistration of cyanocobalamin, USP gel for Intranasal Adrninistration and intramuscular vitamin B_{12} were generally rnild. One patient reported severe headache following intramuscular dosing. Similarly, a few adverse experiences of moderate intensity were reported following intramuscular dosing (two headaches and rhinitis; one dyspepsia, arthritis, and dizziness), and dosing with cyanocobalamin, USP gel for Intranasal Administration (one headache, infection, and paresthesia).

The majority of the reported adverse experiences following dosing with cyanocobalamin, USP gel for Intranasal Administration and intramuscular vitamin B_{12} were judged to be intercurrent events. For the other reported adverse experiences, the relationship to study drug was judged as "possible" or "remote". Of the adverse experiences judged to be of "possible" relationship to the study drug, anxiety, incoordination, and nervousness were reported following intramuscular vitamin B12 and headache, nausea, and rhinitis were reported following dosing with cyanocobalamin, USP gel for Intranasal Administration.

The following adverse reactions have been reported with *parenteral* vitamin B_{12}:

Generalized: Anaphylactic shock and death have been reported with administration of parenteral vitamin B_{12} (See WARNINGS.)

Cardiovascular: Pulmonary edema and congestive heart failure early in treatment; peripheral vascular thrombosis

Hematologic: Polycythemia vera

Gastrointestinal: Mild transient diarrhea

Dermatologic: Itching; transitory exanthema

Miscellaneous: Feeling of swelling of entire body

OVERDOSAGE:

No overdosage has been reported with this drug.

DOSAGE AND ADMINISTRATION:

Avoid using the intravenous route. Use of this product intravenously will result in almost all of the vitamin being lost in the urine. Pernicious Anemia: Parenteral vitamin B_{12} is the recommended treatment and will be required for the remainder of the patient's life. The oral form is not dependable. A dose of 100 mcg daily for 6 or 7 days should be administered by intramuscular or deep subcutaneous injection.

DOSAGE AND ADMINISTRATION: *(cont'd)*

If there is clinical improvement and if a reticulocyte response is observed, the same amount may be given on alternate days for 7 doses, then every 3 to 4 days for another 2 to 3 weeks. By this time, hematologic values should have become normal. This regimen should be followed by 100 mcg monthly for life. Folic acid should be administered concomitantly, if needed.

Patients With Normal Intestinal Absorption: When the oral route is not deemed adequate, initial treatment similar to that for patients with pernicious anemia may be indicated, depending on the severity of the deficiency. Chronic treatment should be with an oral B_{12}preparation.

If other vitamin deficiencies are present, they should be treated.

Other Indications In Patients With Inadequate Intestinal Absorption: Doses similar to those for pernicious anemia are generally appropriate.

The individual patient and specific condition must be assessed to help guide needs and dosage.

Schilling Test: The flushing dose is 1000 mcg.

GEL FOR INTRANASAL ADMINISTRATION

The recommended initial dose of cyanocobalamin, USP gel for Intranasal Administration in patients with vitamin B_{12} malabsorption who are in remission following injectable vitamin B_{12} therapy is 500 mcg administered intranasally once weekly. Patients should be in hematologic remission before treatment with cyanocobalamin, USP gel for Intranasal Adrninistration. See Laboratory Tests for monitoring B_{12} levels and adjustment of dosage.

HOW SUPPLIED:

Parenteral drug products should be inspected visually for particulate matter and discoloration prior to administration, whenever solution and container permit.

Cyanocobalamin Injection should be protected from light. Vials should be stored at controlled room temperature, 59° to 86°F (15° to 30°C).

GEL FOR INTRANASAL ADMINISTRATION

Nascobal (cyanocobalamin, USP) gel for Intranasal Administration is available as a metered dose gel in 5ml glass bottles. It is available in a dosage strength of 500 mcg per actuation (0.1 ml/ actuation). A screw-on actuator is provided. This actuator, following priming, will deliver 0.1ml of the gel. Nascobal (cyanocobalamin, USP) gel for Intranasal Administration is provided in a sealed prescription vial containing a metered dose nasal gel actuator with dust cover, a bottle of nasal gel solution, and a patient instruction leaflet. One bottle will deliver 8 doses.

Pharmacist Assembly Instructions for Nasocobal (Cyanocobalamin, USP) Gel for Intranasal Administration

The pharmacist should assemble Nascobal (cyanocobalamin, USP) gel for Intranasal Administration prior to dispensing to the patient, according to the following instructions:

1. Break the protective seal, open the prescription vial, and remove the gel actuator and gel solution bottle.

2. Assemble Nascobal by first unscrewing the white cap from the gel solution bottle and screwing the actuator unit tightly onto the bottle. Make sure the clear dust cover is on the pump unit.

3. Return the Nascobal bottle to the prescription vial for dispensing to the patient.

Storage: Protect from light. Keep covered in prescription vial until ready to use. Store at room temperature 15°C to 30°C (59°F to 86°F). Protect from freezing.

HOW SUPPLIED - RATED THERAPEUTICALLY EQUIVALENT:

Injection, Solution - Intramuscular; - 0.1 mg/ml

1 ml	$3.33	RUBRAMIN PC, Bristol Myers Squibb	00003-0516-16
10 ml	$3.80	RUBRAMIN PC, Bristol Myers Squibb	00003-0516-40
30 ml	$1.95	Cyanocobalamin, Steris Labs	00402-0090-30
30 ml	$2.00	CRYSTAL B 12, C O Truxton	00463-1021-30
30 ml	$2.40	Cyanocobalamin, Consolidated Midland	00223-8868-30
30 ml	$2.69	VITAMIN B 12, HL Moore Drug Exch	00839-5660-36
30 ml	$3.85	Cyanocobalamin, Goldline Labs	00182-0693-66
30 ml	$3.85	Cyanocobalamin Crystalline, United Res	00677-0322-23
30 ml	**$7.20**	**Vitamin B-12, Rugby**	**00536-2080-75**

Injection, Solution - Intramuscular; - 1 mg/ml

1 ml	$2.55	RUBRAMIN PC, Bristol Myers Squibb	00003-0519-10
1 ml	$3.43	RUBRAMIN PC, Bristol Myers Squibb	00003-0519-16
1 ml x 25	$17.04	Cyanocobalamin, Elkins Sinn	00641-0370-25
1 ml x 25	$31.25	Cyanocobalamin, Consolidated Midland	00223-8861-01
1 ml x 25	$35.63	Cyanocobalamin, Fujisawa USA	00469-1044-25
10 ml	$1.10	B 12 Vitamin Crystalline, Lannett	00527-0160-55
10 ml	$1.49	VITAMIN B12, AF Hauser	52637-0282-10
10 ml	$1.89	VITAMIN B 12, HL Moore Drug Exch	00839-5661-30
10 ml	$2.05	Cyanocobalamin, Geneva Pharms	00781-3020-70
10 ml	$2.10	Cyanocobalamin (B-12), Pasadena	00418-0151-41
10 ml	**$2.30**	**Vitamin B-12, UAD Labs**	**00785-8010-10**
10 ml	$2.30	Cyanocobalamin, Major Pharms	00904-0889-10
10 ml	$2.40	Cyanocobalamin, Hyrex Pharms	00314-0622-70
10 ml	$2.44	Cyanocobalamin, Elkins Sinn	00641-2260-41
10 ml	$2.63	VIT. B12, IDE-Interstate	00814-8449-40
10 ml	$2.80	Cyanocobalamin, Goldline Labs	00182-0202-63
10 ml	**$3.00**	**Vitamin B-12, Schein Pharm (US)**	**00364-6651-54**
10 ml	$3.00	Cyanocobalamin, Steris Labs	00402-0091-10
10 ml	$3.15	Cyanocobalamin, United Res	00677-0323-21
10 ml	**$3.17**	**VITAMIN B-12, Purepac Pharm**	**00228-2862-60**
10 ml	$3.90	Cyanocobalamin, Consolidated Midland	00223-8859-10
10 ml	$4.70	CYANOJECT, Mayrand Pharms	00259-0295-10
10 ml	$4.94	Cyanocobalamin Vitamin B-12, Rugby	00536-2041-70
10 ml	$5.00	Neurin-12, Sorter	53879-0301-10
10 ml	$10.00	NEUROFORTE-R, Intl Ethical	11584-1025-01
10 ml x 25	$35.94	Cyanocobalamin, Am Regent	00517-0032-25
30 ml	$1.56	Cyanocobalamin, Am Regent	00517-0130-01
30 ml	$1.69	Cyanocobalamin, McGuff	49072-0145-30
30 ml	$1.88	B 12 Vitamin Crystalline, Lannett	00527-0160-58
30 ml	$1.98	VITAMIN B12, AF Hauser	52637-0312-30
30 ml	$2.00	Cyanocobalamin, Calvin Scott	17224-0709-10
30 ml	**$2.00**	**VITAMIN B-12, Americal Pharm**	**54945-0559-43**
30 ml	$2.25	CRYSTAL B 12, C O Truxton	00463-1015-30
30 ml	$2.25	Cyanocobalamin, Geneva Pharms	00781-3021-90
30 ml	$2.28	VITAMIN B 12, HL Moore Drug Exch	00839-5661-36
30 ml	$2.40	Cobal-1000 Im Injection 1000 Mg/Ml, Merit Pharms	30727-0314-80
30 ml	$2.55	Cyanocobalamin (B-12), Pasadena	00418-0151-61
30 ml	**$2.77**	**Vitamin B-12, UAD Labs**	**00785-8010-30**
30 ml	$3.15	VIT. B12, IDE-Interstate	00814-8449-46
30 ml	$3.25	Cyanocobalamin, Major Pharms	00904-0889-30
30 ml	**$3.35**	**Vitamin B-12, Schein Pharm (US)**	**00364-6651-56**
30 ml	$3.35	Cyanocobalamin, Steris Labs	00402-0091-30
30 ml	$3.99	Cyanocobalamin, United Res	00677-0323-23

HOW SUPPLIED - RATED THERAPEUTICALLY EQUIVALENT: *(cont'd)*

30 ml	$4.05	Cyanocobalamin, Goldline Labs	00182-0202-66
30 ml	$4.50	Cyanocobalamin, Hyrex Pharms	00314-0622-30
30 ml	$4.50	CYOMIN, Forest Pharms	00456-1015-30
30 ml	$6.25	Cyanocobalamin, Elkins Sinn	00641-2270-41
30 ml	$7.35	Cyanocobalamin Vitamin B-12, Rugby	00536-2041-75
30 ml	$8.00	CYANOJECT, Mayrand Pharms	00259-0295-30

HOW SUPPLIED - NOT RATED EQUIVALENT:

Injection, Solution - Intramuscular - 75 mg

10 ml	$0.74	B 12 Vitamin Crystalline, Lannett	00527-0154-55
30 ml	$1.10	B 12 Vitamin Crystalline, Lannett	00527-0154-58

CYANOCOBALAMIN; FERROUS FUMARATE; VITAMIN C *(001269)*

CATEGORIES: Anemia; Antianemia Drugs; Blood Formation/Coagulation; Deficiency Anemias; Hematinics; Homeostatic & Nutrient; Iron Preparations; Pregnancy; Vitamins; FDA Pre 1938 Drugs

BRAND NAMES: Fetrin; **Chromagen**; Tolfrinic; Vitamin B-12

FORMULARIES: Aetna

DESCRIPTION:

Contents: Each Chromagen maroon soft gelatin capsule contains: ferrous fumarate USP 200 mg, ascorbic acid USP 250 mg, cyanocobalamin USP 10 mcg, desiccated stomach substance 100 mg.

Discussion: The amount of elemental iron and the absorption of the iron components of commercial iron preparations vary widely. It is further established that certain "accessory components" may be included to enhance absorption and utilization of iron. These capsules are formulated to provide the essential factors for a complete, versatile hematinic.

CLINICAL PHARMACOLOGY:

High Elemental Iron Content: Ferrous fumarate, used in these capsules, is an organic iron complex which has a higher elemental iron content than any other hematinic salt—33%. This compares with 20% for ferrous sulfate and 12% for ferrous gluconate.

More Complete Absorption: It has been repeatedly shown that ascorbic acid, when given in sufficient amounts, can increase the absorption of ferrous iron from the gastrointestinal tract.

The absorption-promoting effect is mainly due to the reducing action of ascorbic acid within the gastrointestinal lumen, which helps to prevent or delay the formation of insoluble or less dissociated ferric compounds.

Iron absorption has been shown to increase sharply with increasing amounts of ascorbic acid, showing a gain in absorption of approximately 40% at 250 mg. Above 250 mg, the gain becomes insignificant, with an additional gain of only approximately 8% at 500 mg. Each Chromagen Capsule contains 250 mg of ascorbic acid, believed to be the optimal amount.

Promotes Movement of Plasma Iron: Ascorbic acid also plays an important role in the movement of plasma iron to storage depots in the tissues.

The action, which leads to the transport of plasma iron to ferritin, presumably involves its reducing effect, converting transferrin iron from the ferric to the ferrous state. There is also evidence that ascorbic acid improves iron utilization, presumably as a further result of its reducing action, and some evidence that it may have a direct effect upon erythropoiesis.

Ascorbic acid is further alleged to enhance the conversion of folic acid to a more physiologically active form, folinic acid, which would make it even more important in the treatment of anemia since it would aid in the utilization of dietary folic acid.

Excellent Oral Toleration: Ferrous fumarate is used in These capsules because it is less likely to cause the gastric disturbances so often associated with oral iron therapy. Ferrous fumarate has a low ionization constant and high solubility in the entire pH range of the gastrointestinal tract. It does not precipitate proteins or have the astringency of more ionizable forms of iron, and does not interfere with proteolytic or diastatic activities of the digestive system. Because of excellent oral toleration, These capsules can usually be administered between meals when iron absorption is maximal.

Facilitates Absorption of Vitamin B_{12}: It is now known that "Intrinsic Factor" is essential for the adequate alimentary absorption of vitamin B_{12} The chemical structure of intrinsic factor is still undetermined and it has not yet been isolated in pure form; however,the inclusion of desiccated stomach substance with oral vitamin B_{12} will furnish sufficient intrinsic factor to assure absorption of the vitamin.

Toxicity: Ferrous fumarate was found to be the least toxic of three popular oral iron salts, with an oral LD_{50} of 630 mg/kg. In the same report, the LD_{50} of ferrous gluconate was reported to be 320 mg/kg and ferrous sulfate 230 mg/kg.

INDICATIONS AND USAGE:

For the treatment of all anemias responsive to oral iron therapy, such as hypochromic anemia associated with pregnancy, chronic or acute blood loss, dietary restriction, metabolic disease and post-surgical convalescence.

CONTRAINDICATIONS:

Hemochromatosis and hemosiderosis are contraindications to iron therapy.

ADVERSE REACTIONS:

Average capsule doses in sensitive individuals or excessive dosage may cause nausea, skin rash, vomiting, diarrhea, precordial pain, or flushing of the face and extremities.

DOSAGE AND ADMINISTRATION:

Usual adult dose is 1 soft gelatin capsule daily.

HOW SUPPLIED - EQUIVALENTS NOT AVAILABLE:

Capsule, Gelatin - Oral - 250 mg/10 mcg/2

100's	**$26.99**	**CHROMAGEN, Savage Labs**	**00281-4285-53**
500's	**$120.53**	**CHROMAGEN, Savage Labs**	**00281-4285-56**

Capsule, Gelatin, Sustained Action - Oral - 60 mg/5 mcg/200

100's	$35.88	FETRIN, Lunsco	10892-0114-10

Tablet, Coated - Oral - 100 mg/25 mcg/6

100's	$31.56	TOLFRINIC, Ascher	00225-0105-15

CYANOCOBALAMIN; FERROUS GLUCONATE; FOLIC ACID *(001270)*

CATEGORIES: Antianemia Drugs; Blood Formation/Coagulation; Deficiency Anemias; Homeostatic & Nutrient; Iron Preparations; Vitamins; FDA Pre 1938 Drugs

BRAND NAMES: Hytinic; Vitamin B-12

Prescribing information not available at time of publication.

HOW SUPPLIED - EQUIVALENTS NOT AVAILABLE:

Injection, Solution - Intramuscular - 1.25 mg/8.2 mg/

30 ml	$9.95	HYTINIC, Hyrex Pharms	00314-0674-30

CYANOCOBALAMIN; FOLIC ACID *(001336)*

CATEGORIES: Homeostatic & Nutrient; Vitamins; FDA Pre 1938 Drugs

BRAND NAMES: Vicam; Vitamin B-12

Prescribing information not available at time of publication.

HOW SUPPLIED - EQUIVALENTS NOT AVAILABLE:

Injection, Lyphl-Soln - Intramuscular; - 50 mg/1000 mcg/

10 ml	$8.00	VICAM, Keene Pharms	00588-5255-70

CYANOCOBALAMIN; FOLIC ACID; IRON POLYSACCHARIDE COMPLEX *(001332)*

CATEGORIES: Antianemia Drugs; Blood Formation/Coagulation; Deficiency Anemias; Iron Preparations; Polysaccharide-Iron Complex; Vitamin B Complex; Vitamins; FDA Pre 1938 Drugs

BRAND NAMES: Fercon; Niferex Forte; Nu-Iron Plus

Prescribing information not available at time of publication.

HOW SUPPLIED - EQUIVALENTS NOT AVAILABLE:

Capsule, Gelatin - Oral - 25 mcg/150 mg/1

100's	$11.45	Fercon, Aligen Independ	00405-4432-01
100's	$23.55	NIFEREX-150 FORTE, Schwarz Pharma (US)	00131-4330-37
1000's	$218.41	NIFEREX-150 FORTE, Schwarz Pharma (US)	00131-4330-43

Elixir - Oral

240 ml	$15.50	NU-IRON PLUS, Mayrand Pharms	00259-0342-08

CYANOCOBALAMIN; FOLIC ACID; LIVER EXTRACT *(001333)*

CATEGORIES: Antianemia Drugs; Blood Formation/Coagulation; Deficiency Anemias; Homeostatic & Nutrient; Liver/Stomach Preparations; Vitamin B Complex; Vitamins; FDA Pre 1938 Drugs

BRAND NAMES: Folabee; Hepfomin-R; Hyliver-Plus; Lifoject; Lifolbex; Lifolex-Plus; Liverfol-B12; Livifol; Livroben; Pernivit-R; Primafort; Sanguis-R

Prescribing information not available at time of publication.

HOW SUPPLIED - EQUIVALENTS NOT AVAILABLE:

Injection, Solution - Intramuscular

10 ml	$2.50	LIVER, FOLIC ACID & B-12, Lannett	00527-0100-55
10 ml	$4.25	LIVER, FOLIC ACID & B-12, Harber Pharm	51432-0621-10
10 ml	$7.50	Liver,Folic Acid & B-12, Consolidated Midland	00223-7956-10
10 ml	$9.80	LIFOLEX, Pasadena	00418-0411-10
10 ml	$9.90	HYLIVER PLUS R, Hyrex Pharms	00314-0666-70

CYANOCOBALAMIN; FOLIC ACID; PEPTO-FERROUS SULFATE *(001335)*

CATEGORIES: Antianemia Drugs; Blood Formation/Coagulation; Deficiency Anemias; Homeostatic & Nutrient; Hyperlipidemia; Iron Preparations; FDA Pre 1938 Drugs

BRAND NAMES: Hemocyte-V; Vitamin B-12

Prescribing information not available at time of publication.

HOW SUPPLIED - EQUIVALENTS NOT AVAILABLE:

Injection, Solution - Intramuscular - 1 mg/15 mcg/31.

10 ml	$30.00	HEMOCYTE-V, US Pharm	52747-0190-10

CYANOCOBALAMIN; PEPTO-FERROUS SULFATE *(001984)*

CATEGORIES: Antianemia Drugs; Blood Formation/Coagulation; Deficiency Anemias; Homeostatic & Nutrient; Iron Preparations; Vitamins; FDA Pre 1938 Drugs

BRAND NAMES: Livaid-Plus; Rogenic

Prescribing information not available at time of publication.

HOW SUPPLIED - EQUIVALENTS NOT AVAILABLE:

Injection, Solution - Intramuscular - 1.25 mg/15 mcg/

30 ml	$13.50	Livaid-Plus, Teregen Labs	52384-0035-30

CYANOCOBALAMIN; THIAMINE HYDROCHLORIDE *(002334)*

CATEGORIES: Vitamin B Complex; Vitamins; FDA Pre 1938 Drugs

BRAND NAMES: Bexibee; Nervidox; Neuro B12; Neurobion; Tia Doce

Prescribing information not available at time of publication.

HOW SUPPLIED - EQUIVALENTS NOT AVAILABLE:

Injection, Solution - Intravenous

10 ml	$22.50	TIA DOCE, Alba Pharma	10023-0185-10
10 ml	$22.50	Neurobion, AJ Bart	49326-0111-10
10 ml	$22.50	NEURO B12, AJ Bart	49326-0114-10
10 ml	$22.50	NERVIDOX, Teral Labs	51234-0100-10

CYCLANDELATE *(000924)*

CATEGORIES: Cardiovascular Drugs; Claudication; DESI Drugs; Ischemia; Leg Cramps; Peripheral Vasodilators; Renal Drugs; Vascular Disorders, Cerebral/Peripheral; Vasodilating Agents; FDA Pre 1938 Drugs

BRAND NAMES: *Anticen* (Japan); *Beriup* (Japan); *Capilan* (Japan); *Cepidan* (Japan); *Ciclol*; *Ciclospasmol*; *Cyclan* (Japan); *Cyclasyn*; *Cyclat*; *Cycleate*; *Cyclergine* (France); *Cyclidon*; *Cyclobral*; *Cyclolyt*; *Cyclomandol* (Mexico); **Cyclospasmol**; *Kabirone*; *Martispasmol*; *Mitalon* (Japan); *Natil* (Germany); *Novodil* (France); *Spasmocyclon* (Germany); *Takabran* (Japan); *Vasonal*; *Venala* (Japan)
(International brand names outside U.S. in italics)

FORMULARIES: Aetna

DESCRIPTION:

Each capsule contains 200 mg or 400 mg of cyclandelate. The inactive ingredients present are FD&C Blue 1, gelatin, magnesium stearate, methylcellulose, titanium dioxide, and other ingredients. The 200 mg strength also contains D&C Red 28. The 400 mg strength also contains FD&C Red 40 and FD&C Yellow 6.

Cyclandelate is a white amorphous powder having a faint menthol-like odor. It is slightly soluble in water and highly soluble in ethyl alcohol and organic solvents.

CLINICAL PHARMACOLOGY:

Cyclandelate is an orally acting vasodilator. The activity of this drug, as measured by pharmacological tests against various types of smooth muscle spasm produced by acetylcholine, histamine, and barium chloride, exceeds that of papaverine, particularly in regard to the neurotropic component produced by the acetylcholine. Cyclandelate is musculotropic, acting directly on vascular smooth muscle, and has no significant adrenergic stimulating or blocking actions.

The drug is not intended to substitute for other appropriate medical or surgical programs in the treatment of peripheral- or cerebral-vascular disease.

INDICATIONS AND USAGE:

Based on a review of this drug by the Nation Academy of Sciences - National Research Council and/or other information, FDA has classified the indications as follows:
"Possibly" effective: Cyclandelate is indicated for adjunctive therapy in intermittent claudication; arteriosclerosis obliterans; thrombophlebitis (to control associated vasospasm and muscular ischemia); nocturnal leg cramps; Raynaud's phenomenon; and for selected cases of ischemic cerebral-vascular disease.
Final classification of the less-than-effective indication requires further investigation.

CONTRAINDICATIONS:

Cyclandelate is contraindicated in cases of known hypersensitivity to the drug.

WARNINGS:

1. Cyclandelate should be used with extreme caution in patients with severe obliterative coronary-artery or cerebral-vascular disease, since there is a possibility that these diseased areas may be compromised by vasodilatory effects of the drug elsewhere.

2. Use in Pregnancy :The safety of cyclandelate for use during pregnancy or lactation has not been established; therefore, it should not be used in pregnant women or in women of childbearing age unless, in the judgement of the physician, its use is deemed absolutely essential to the welfare of the patient.

3. Although no prolongation of bleeding time has been demonstrated in humans in therapeutic dosages, it has been demonstrated in animals at very large doses. Therefore, the hazard of a prolonged bleeding time should be carefully considered when administering cyclandelate to a patient with active bleeding or a bleeding tendency.

PRECAUTIONS:

Since cyclandelate is a vasodilator, it should be used with caution in patients having glaucoma.

ADVERSE REACTIONS:

Gastrointestinal distress (pyrosis, pain, and eructation) may occur with cyclandelate. These symptoms occur infrequently and are usually mild. Relief can often be obtained by taking the medication with meals or by the concomitant use of antacids.

Mild flush, headache, feeling of weakness, or tachycardia may occur, especially during the first weeks of administration.

DOSAGE AND ADMINISTRATION:

It is often advantageous to initiate therapy at higher dosage; e.g.: 1200 to 1600 mg per day, given in divided doses before meals and at bedtime. When a clinical response is noted, the dosage can be decreased in 200 mg decrements until the maintenance dosage is reached. The usual maintenance dosage of cyclandelate is between 400 mg and 800 mg per day given in two to four divided doses.

DOSAGE AND ADMINISTRATION: *(cont'd)*

Although objective signs of therapeutic benefit may be rapid and dramatic, more often, this improvement occurs gradually over weeks of therapy. It is strongly recommended that the patient be educated to the fact that prolonged use may be necessary. Short-term use of cyclandelate is rarely beneficial, nor is it likely to be of any permanent value.

Storage: Keep Tightly closed. Protect From light. Dispense in light- resistant, tight container.

HOW SUPPLIED - RATED THERAPEUTICALLY EQUIVALENT:

Capsule, Gelatin - Oral - 200 mg

1000's	$36.95	Cyclandelate, Harber Pharm	51432-0116-06

Capsule, Gelatin - Oral - 400 mg

1000's	$55.95	Cyclandelate, Harber Pharm	51432-0118-06

HOW SUPPLIED - NOT RATED EQUIVALENT:

Capsule, Gelatin - Oral - 200 mg

100's	$5.66	Cyclandelate, HL Moore Drug Exch	00839-1217-06
100's	$5.90	CYCLAN, Major Pharms	00904-0238-60
100's	$13.50	Cyclandelate, Qualitest Pharms	00603-3075-21
100's	$14.21	Cyclandelate, Aligen Independ	00405-4284-01
100's	$14.30	Cyclandelate, Goldline Labs	00182-1540-01
100's	$14.30	Cyclandelate, Rugby	00536-3531-01
100's	$14.35	Cyclandelate, Major Pharms	00904-5008-60
100's	**$54.95**	**CYCLOSPASMOL, Wyeth Labs**	**00008-4124-01**
1000's	$30.25	Cyclandelate, Rugby	00536-3531-10
1000's	$36.79	Cyclandelate, HL Moore Drug Exch	00839-1217-16
1000's	$39.80	CYCLAN, Major Pharms	00904-0238-80

Capsule, Gelatin - Oral - 400 mg

100's	$7.00	CYCLAN, Major Pharms	00904-0239-60
100's	$7.75	Cyclandelate, Consolidated Midland	00223-0707-01
100's	$8.22	Cyclandelate, HL Moore Drug Exch	00839-6027-06
100's	$17.65	Cyclandelate, Goldline Labs	00182-1541-01
100's	$17.75	Cyclandelate, Qualitest Pharms	00603-3076-21
100's	$17.80	Cyclandelate, Aligen Independ	00405-4285-01
100's	$17.87	Cyclandelate, Rugby	00536-3529-01
100's	$18.95	Cyclandelate, Major Pharms	00904-5009-60
100's	**$99.36**	**CYCLOSPASMOL, Wyeth Labs**	**00008-4148-04**
500's	$24.88	Cyclandelate, Rugby	00536-3529-05
1000's	$48.50	Cyclandelate, Rugby	00536-3529-10
1000's	$50.95	CYCLAN, Major Pharms	00904-0239-80
1000's	$57.98	Cyclandelate, HL Moore Drug Exch	00839-6027-16
1000's	$67.50	Cyclandelate, Consolidated Midland	00223-0707-02

CYCLOBENZAPRINE HYDROCHLORIDE *(000926)*

CATEGORIES: Autonomic Drugs; Muscle Relaxants; Neuromuscular; Pain; Skeletal Muscle Hyperactivity; Skeletal Muscle Relaxants; Spasm; Cerebral Palsy*; Pregnancy Category B; Sales > $100 Million; FDA Approval Pre 1982; Patent Expiration 1992 Dec; Top 200 Drugs
* Indication not approved by the FDA

BRAND NAMES: *Benzamin*; *Cloben*; *Cyben*; Cycoflex; **Flexeril**; *Flexiban*; *Yurelax*
(International brand names outside U.S. in italics)

FORMULARIES: Aetna; BC-BS; PCS

DESCRIPTION:

Cyclobenzaprine hydrochloride is a white, crystalline tricyclic amine salt with the empirical formula $C_{20}H_{21}N{\cdot}HCl$ and a molecular weight of 311.9. It has a melting point of 217°C, and a pK_a of 8.47 at 25° C. It is freely soluble in water and alcohol, sparingly soluble in isopropanol, and insoluble in hydrocarbon solvents. If aqueous solutions are made alkaline, the free base separates. Cyclobenzaprine HCl is designated chemically as 3-(5*H*-dibenzo(*a,d*) cyclohepten-5-ylidene)-*N*, *N*-dimethyl-1-propanamine hydrochloride.

Cyclobenzaprine HCl is supplied as 10 mg tablets for oral administration.

Cyclobenzaprine HCl tablets contain the following inactive ingredients: hydroxypropyl cellulose, hydroxypropyl methylcellulose, iron oxide, lactose, magnesium stearate, starch, and titanium dioxide.

CLINICAL PHARMACOLOGY:

Cyclobenzaprine HCl relieves skeletal muscle spasm of local origin without interfering with muscle function. It is ineffective in muscle spasm due to central nervous system disease.

Cyclobenzaprine reduced or abolished skeletal muscle hyperactivity in several animal models. Animal studies indicate that cyclobenzaprine does not act at the neuromuscular junction or directly on skeletal muscle. Such studies show that cyclobenzaprine acts primarily within the central nervous system at brain stem as opposed to spinal cord levels, although its action on the latter may contribute to its overall skeletal muscle relaxant activity. Evidence suggests that the net effect of cyclobenzaprine is a reduction of tonic somatic motor activity, influencing both gamma (γ) and alpha (α) motor systems.

Pharmacological studies in animals showed a similarity between the effects of cyclobenzaprine and the structurally related tricyclic antidepressants, including reserpine antagonism, norepinephrine potentiation, potent peripheral and central anticholinergic effects, and sedation. Cyclobenzaprine caused slight to moderate increase in heart rate in animals.

Cyclobenzaprine is well absorbed after oral administration, but there is a large intersubject variation in plasma levels. Cyclobenzaprine is eliminated quite slowly with a half-life as long as one to three days. It is highly bound to plasma proteins, is extensively metabolized primarily to glucuronide-like conjugates, and is excreted primarily via the kidneys.

No significant effect on plasma levels or bioavailability of cyclobenzaprine HCl or aspirin was noted when single or multiple doses of the two drugs were administered concomitantly. Concomitant administration of cyclobenzaprine HCl and aspirin is usually well tolerated and no unexpected or serious clinical or laboratory adverse effects have been observed. No studies have been performed to indicate whether cyclobenzaprine HCl enhances the clinical effect of aspirin or other analgesics, or whether analgesics enhance the clinical effect of cyclobenzaprine HCl in acute musculoskeletal conditions.

CLINICAL STUDIES:

Controlled clinical studies show that cyclobenzaprine HCl significantly improves the signs and symptoms of skeletal muscle spasm as compared with placebo. The clinical responses include improvement in muscle spasm as determined by palpation, reduction in local pain and tenderness, increased range of motion, and less restriction in activities of daily living. When daily observations were made, clinical improvement was observed as early as the first day of therapy.

CLINICAL STUDIES: *(cont'd)*

Eight double-blind controlled clinical studies were performed in 642 patients comparing cyclobenzaprine HCl, diazepam, and placebo. Muscle spasm, local pain and tenderness, limitation of motion, and restriction in activities of daily living were evaluated. In three of these studies there was a significantly greater improvement with cyclobenzaprine HCl than with diazepam, while in the other studies the improvement following both treatments was comparable.

Although the frequency and severity of adverse reactions observed in patients treated with cyclobenzaprine HCl were comparable to those observed in patients treated with diazepam, dry mouth was observed more frequently in patients treated with cyclobenzaprine HCl and dizziness more frequently in those treated with diazepam. The incidence of drowsiness, the most frequent adverse reaction, was similar with both drugs.

Analysis of the data from controlled studies shows that cyclobenzaprine HCl produces clinical improvement whether or not sedation occurs.

SURVEILLANCE PROGRAM

A post-marketing surveillance program was carried out in 7607 patients with acute musculoskeletal disorders, and included 297 patients treated for 30 days or longer. The overall effectiveness of cyclobenzaprine HCl was similar to that observed in the double-blind controlled studies; the overall incidence of adverse effects was less (see ADVERSE REACTIONS).

INDICATIONS AND USAGE:

Cyclobenzaprine HCl is indicated as an adjunct to rest and physical therapy for relief of muscle spasm associated with acute, painful musculoskeletal conditions.

Improvement is manifested by relief of muscle spasm and its associated signs and symptoms, namely, pain, tenderness, limitation of motion, and restriction in activities of daily living.

Cyclobenzaprine HCl should Be used only for short periods (up to two or three weeks) because adequate evidence of effectiveness for more prolonged use is not available and because muscle spasm associated with acute, painful musculoskeletal conditions is generally of short duration and specific therapy for longer periods is seldom warranted.

Cyclobenzaprine HCl has not been found effective in the treatment of spasticity associated with cerebral or spinal cord disease, or in children with cerebral palsy.

CONTRAINDICATIONS:

Hypersensitivity to the drug.

Concomitant use of monoamine oxidase inhibitors or within 14 days after their discontinuation.

Acute recovery phase of myocardial infarction, and patients with arrhythmias, heart block or conduction disturbances, or congestive heart failure.

Hyperthyroidism.

WARNINGS:

Cyclobenzaprine is closely related to the tricyclic antidepressants, *e.g.,* amitriptyline and imipramine. In short term studies for indications other than muscle spasm associated with acute musculoskeletal conditions, and usually at doses somewhat greater than those recommended for skeletal muscle spasm, some of the more serious central nervous system reactions noted with the tricyclic antidepressants have occurred (see WARNINGS, and ADVERSE REACTIONS).

Cyclobenzaprine HCl may interact with monoamine oxidase (MAO) inhibitors. Hyperpyretic crisis, severe convulsions, and deaths have occurred in patients receiving tricyclic antidepressants and MAO inhibitor drugs.

Tricyclic antidepressants have been reported to produce arrhythmias, sinus tachycardia, prolongation of the conduction time leading to myocardial infarction and stroke.

Cyclobenzaprine may enhance the effects of alcohol, barbiturates, and other CNS depressants.

PRECAUTIONS:

GENERAL

Because of its atropine-like action, cyclobenzaprine HCl should be used with caution in patients with a history of urinary retention, angle-closure glaucoma, increased intraocular pressure, and in patients taking anticholinergic medication.

INFORMATION FOR THE PATIENT

Cyclobenzaprine HCl may impair mental and/or physical abilities required for performance of hazardous tasks, such as operating machinery or driving a motor vehicle.

CARCINOGENESIS, MUTAGENESIS, AND IMPAIRMENT OF FERTILITY

In rats treated with cyclobenzaprine for up to 67 weeks at doses of approximately 5 to 40 times the maximum recommended human dose, pale, sometimes enlarged, livers were noted and there was a dose-related hepatocyte vacuolation with lipidosis. In the higher dose groups this microscopic change was seen after 26 weeks and even earlier in rats which died prior to 26 weeks; at lower doses, the change was not seen until after 26 weeks.

Cyclobenzaprine did not affect the onset, incidence or distribution of neoplasia in an 81-week study in the mouse or in a 105-week study in the rat.

At oral doses of up to 10 times the human dose, cyclobenzaprine did not adversely affect the reproductive performance or fertility of male or female rats. Cyclobenzaprine did not demonstrate mutagenic activity in the male mouse at dose levels of up to 20 times the human dose.

PREGNANCY

Pregnancy Category B: Reproduction studies have been performed in rats, mice and rabbits at doses up to 20 times the human dose, and have revealed no evidence of impaired fertility or harm to the fetus due to cyclobenzaprine HCl. There are, however, no adequate and well-controlled studies in pregnant women. Because animal reproduction studies are not always predictive of human response, this drug should be used during pregnancy only if clearly needed.

NURSING MOTHERS

It is not known whether this drug is excreted in human milk. Because cyclobenzaprine is closely related to the tricyclic antidepressants, some of which are known to be excreted in human milk, caution should be exercised when cyclobenzaprine HCl is administered to a nursing woman.

PEDIATRIC USE

Safety and effectiveness of cyclobenzaprine HCl in children below the age of 15 have not been established.

DRUG INTERACTIONS:

Cyclobenzaprine HCl may enhance the effects of alcohol, barbiturates, and other CNS depressants.

Tricyclic antidepressants may block the antihypertensive action of guanethidine and similarly acting compounds.

ADVERSE REACTIONS:

The following list of adverse reactions is based on the experience in 473 patients treated with cyclobenzaprine HCl in controlled clinical studies, 7607 patients in the post-marketing surveillance program, and reports received since the drug was marketed. The overall incidence of adverse reactions among patients in the surveillance program was less than the incidence in the controlled clinical studies.

The adverse reactions reported most frequently with cyclobenzaprine HCl were drowsiness, dry mouth and dizziness. The incidence of these common adverse reactions was lower in the surveillance program than in the controlled clinical studies (see TABLE 1.)

TABLE 1

	Clinical Studies	Surveillance Program
drowsiness	39%	16%
dry mouth	27%	7%
dizziness	11%	3%

Among the less frequent adverse reactions, there was no appreciable difference in incidence in controlled clinical studies or in the surveillance program. Adverse reactions which were reported in 1% to 3% of the patients were fatigue/tiredness, asthenia, nausea, constipation, dyspepsia, unpleasant taste, blurred vision, headache, nervousness, and confusion.

INCIDENCE LESS THAN 1 IN 100

The following adverse reactions have been reported at an incidence of less than 1 in 100:

Body As A Whole: Syncope; malaise, facial edema.

Cardiovascular: Tachycardia; arrhythmia; vasodilation; palpitation; hypotension.

Digestive: Vomiting; anorexia; diarrhea; gastrointestinal pain; gastritis; thirst; flatulence; edema of the tongue; abnormal liver function and rare reports of hepatitis, jaundice and cholestasis.

Hypersensitivity: Anaphylaxis; angioedema; pruritus; facial edema; urticaria; rash.

Musculoskeletal: Local weakness.

Nervous System And Psychiatric: Ataxia; vertigo; dysarthria; tremors; hypertonia; convulsions; muscle twitching; disorientation; insomnia; depressed mood; abnormal sensations; anxiety; agitation; abnormal thinking and dreaming; hallucinations; excitement; paresthesia; diplopia.

Skin: Sweating.

Special Senses: Ageusia; tinnitus.

Urogenital: Urinary frequency and/or retention.

CAUSAL RELATIONSHIP UNKNOWN

Other reactions, reported rarely for cyclobenzaprine HCl under circumstances where a causal relationship could not be established or reported for other tricyclic drugs, are listed to serve as alerting information to physicians:

Body As A Whole: Chest pain; edema.

Cardiovascular: Hypertension; myocardial infarction; heart block; stroke.

Digestive: Paralytic ileus; tongue discoloration; stomatitis; parotid swelling.

Endocrine: Inappropriate ADH syndrome.

Hematic And Lymphatic: Purpura; bone marrow depression; leukopenia; eosinophilia; thrombocytopenia.

Metabolic, Nutritional And Immune: Elevation and lowering of blood sugar levels; weight gain or loss.

Musculoskeletal: Myalgia.

Nervous System And Psychiatric: Decreased or increased libido; delusions; abnormal gait; peripheral neuropathy; Bell's palsy; alteration in EEG patterns; extrapyramidal symptoms.

Respiratory: Dyspnea.

Skin: Photosensitization; alopecia, pruritus.

Urogenital: Impaired urination; dilatation of urinary tract; impotence; testicular swelling; gynecomastia; breast enlargement; galactorrhea.

DRUG ABUSE AND DEPENDENCE:

Pharmacologic similarities among the tricyclic drugs require that certain withdrawal symptoms be considered when cyclobenzaprine HCl is administered, even though they have not been reported to occur with this drug. Abrupt cessation of treatment after prolonged administration may produce nausea, headache, and malaise. These are not indicative of addiction.

OVERDOSAGE:

MANIFESTATIONS

High doses may cause temporary confusion, disturbed concentration, transient visual hallucinations, agitation, hyperactive reflexes, muscle rigidity, vomiting, or hyperpyrexia, in addition to anything listed under **ADVERSE REACTIONS**. Based on the known pharmacologic actions of the drug, overdosage may cause drowsiness, hypothermia, tachycardia and other cardiac rhythm abnormalities such as bundle branch block, ECG evidence of impaired conduction, and congestive heart failure. Other manifestations may be dilated pupils, convulsions, severe hypotension, stupor, and coma.

The acute oral LD_{50} of cyclobenzaprine HCl is approximately 338 and 425 mg/kg in mice and rats, respectively.

TREATMENT

Treatment is symptomatic and supportive. Empty the stomach as quickly as possible by emesis, followed by gastric lavage. After gastric lavage, activated charcoal may be administered. Twenty to 30 g of activated charcoal may be given every four to six hours during the first 24 to 48 hours after ingestion. An ECG should be taken and close monitoring of cardiac function must be instituted if there is any evidence of dysrhythmia. Maintenance of an open airway, adequate fluid intake, and regulation of body temperature are necessary.

The intravenous administration of 1-3 mg of physostigmine salicylate is reported to reverse symptoms of poisoning by atropine and other drugs with anticholinergic activity. Physostigmine may be helpful in the treatment of cyclobenzaprine overdose. Because physostigmine is rapidly metabolized, the dosage of physostigmine should be repeated as required, particularly if life-threatening signs such as arrhythmias, convulsions, and deep coma recur or persist after the initial dosage of physostigmine. Because physostigmine itself may be toxic, it is not recommended for routine use.

Standard medical measures should be used to manage circulatory shock and metabolic acidosis. Cardiac arrhythmias may be treated with neostigmine, pyridostigmine, or propranolol. When signs of cardiac failure occur, the use of a short-acting digitalis preparation should be considered. Close monitoring of cardiac function for not less than five days is advisable.

Anticonvulsants may be given to control seizures.

Dialysis is probably of no value because of low plasma concentrations of the drug.

OVERDOSAGE: *(cont'd)*

Since overdosage is often deliberate, patients may attempt suicide by other means during the recovery phase. Deaths by deliberate or accidental overdosage have occurred with this class of drugs.

DOSAGE AND ADMINISTRATION:

The usual dosage of cyclobenzaprine HCl is 10 mg three times a day, with a range of 20 to 40 mg a day in divided doses. Dosage should not exceed 60 mg a day. Use of cyclobenzaprine for periods longer than two or three weeks is not recommended. (See INDICATIONS AND USAGE.)

PATIENT INFORMATION:

Cyclobenzaprine is a muscle relaxant used to relieve the pain and stiffness of muscle spasms and discomfort due to strain and sprain. It should not be taken longer than two to three weeks. Inform your physician if you are pregnant or nursing. Inform your physician if you have glaucoma or difficulty urinating. Do not take this medication with a monoamine oxidase inhibitor. This medication may cause dizziness, drowsiness, or blurred vision; use caution while driving or operating hazardous machinery. Do not take any other sedating drugs or drink alcohol while taking cyclobenzaprine. If dizziness occurs, avoid sudden changes in posture. Take this medication with food to avoid stomach upset.

HOW SUPPLIED - RATED THERAPEUTICALLY EQUIVALENT:

Tablet - Oral - 10 mg

100's	$73.00	Cyclobenzaprine Hcl, Duramed Pharms	51285-0913-02
1000's	$727.00	Cyclobenzaprine Hcl, Duramed Pharms	51285-0913-05

Tablet, Coated - Oral - 10 mg

30's	$3.98	Cyclobenzaprine HCl, H.C.F.A. F F P	99999-0926-01
30's	$24.95	Cyclobenzaprine Hcl, Schein Pharm (US)	00364-2348-30
30's	**$27.66**	**FLEXERIL, Merck**	**00006-0931-30**
100's	$13.28	Cyclobenzaprine Hcl, United Res	00677-1429-01
100's	$13.28	Cyclobenzaprine HCl, H.C.F.A. F F P	99999-0926-02
100's	$70.66	Cyclobenzaprine Hcl, Qualitest Pharms	00603-3077-21
100's	$72.75	Cyclobenzaprine Hcl, Harber Pharm	51432-0367-03
100's	$73.99	Cyclobenzaprine Hcl, Watson Labs	52544-0418-01
100's	$74.87	Cyclobenzaprine Hcl, Martec Pharms	52555-0441-10
100's	$75.90	Cyclobenzaprine Hcl, West Point Pharma	59591-0156-68
100's	$75.90	Cyclobenzaprine Hcl, Endo Labs	60951-0767-70
100's	$77.61	Cyclobenzaprine Hcl, HL Moore Drug Exch	00839-7566-06
100's	$78.20	Cyclobenzaprine Hcl, Aligen Independ	00405-4290-01
100's	$78.55	Cyclobenzaprine Hcl, Martec Pharms	52555-0441-01
100's	$79.25	Cyclobenzaprine Hcl, Major Pharms	00904-7586-60
100's	$79.25	Cyclobenzaprine Hcl, Major Pharms	00904-7809-60
100's	$79.95	Cyclobenzaprine Hcl, HL Moore Drug Exch	00839-7711-06
100's	$81.68	Cyclobenzaprine Hcl, Royce	51875-0257-01
100's	$83.10	Cyclobenzaprine Hydrochoride, Goldline Labs	00182-1919-01
100's	$84.50	Cyclobenzaprine HCl, Geneva Pharms	50752-0285-05
100's	$85.00	Cyclobenzaprine Hcl, Vangard Labs	00615-3520-13
100's	$86.10	Cyclobenzaprine HCl, Schein Pharm (US)	00364-2348-01
100's	$86.30	Cyclobenzaprine HCl, Warner Chilcott	00047-0057-24
100's	$86.30	Cyclobenzaprine HCl, Rugby	00536-4840-01
100's	$86.30	Cyclobenzaprine HCl, Geneva Pharms	00781-1324-01
100's	$86.95	Cyclobenzaprine Hcl, Mylan	00378-0751-01
100's	**$87.10**	**FLEXERIL, Merck**	**00006-0931-54**
100's	$87.10	Cyclobenzaprine Hcl, Invamed	52189-0252-24
100's	$88.42	Cyclobenzaprine Hcl, Major Pharms	00904-7586-61
100's	$90.41	Cyclobenzaprine HCl, Geneva Pharms	00781-1324-13
100's	$92.00	Cyclobenzaprine HCl, Schein Pharm (US)	00364-2348-90
100's	$92.07	Cyclobenzaprine Hcl, Major Pharms	00904-2221-61
100's	**$95.89**	**FLEXERIL, Merck**	**00006-0931-68**
100's	$96.00	Cyclobenzaprine Hcl, Goldline Labs	00182-1919-89
100's	**$100.46**	**FLEXERIL, Merck**	**00006-0931-28**
500's	$66.40	Cyclobenzaprine Hcl, United Res	00677-1429-05
500's	$66.40	Cyclobenzaprine HCl, H.C.F.A. F F P	99999-0926-03
500's	$325.25	Cyclobenzaprine Hcl, Major Pharms	00904-7586-40
500's	$350.00	Cyclobenzaprine Hcl, Goldline Labs	00182-1919-05
500's	$352.25	Cyclobenzaprine Hcl, Major Pharms	00904-7809-40
500's	$356.80	Cyclobenzaprine Hcl, Martec Pharms	52555-0441-05
500's	$365.08	Cyclobenzaprine Hcl, Qualitest Pharms	00603-3077-28
500's	$365.08	Cyclobenzaprine Hcl, Watson Labs	52544-0418-05
500's	$367.56	Cyclobenzaprine Hcl, Royce	51875-0257-02
500's	$369.75	Cyclobenzaprine HCl, Schein Pharm (US)	00364-2348-05
500's	$393.75	Cyclobenzaprine HCl, Warner Chilcott	00047-0057-30
500's	$395.95	Cyclobenzaprine HCl, Geneva Pharms	00781-1324-05
500's	$414.05	Cyclobenzaprine HCl, Geneva Pharms	50752-0285-08
500's	$422.87	Cyclobenzaprine HCl, Rugby	00536-4840-05
1000's	$11.55	Cyclobenzaprine HCl, Rugby	00536-4540-10
1000's	$132.80	Cyclobenzaprine HCl, H.C.F.A. F F P	99999-0926-04
1000's	$528.40	Cyclobenzaprine Hcl, Major Pharms	00904-7586-80
1000's	$528.40	Cyclobenzaprine Hcl, Major Pharms	00904-7809-80
1000's	$602.00	Cyclobenzaprine Hcl, Aligen Independ	00405-4290-03
1000's	$670.43	Cyclobenzaprine Hcl, Qualitest Pharms	00603-3077-32
1000's	$674.99	Cyclobenzaprine Hcl, HL Moore Drug Exch	00839-7566-16
1000's	$683.00	Cyclobenzaprine Hcl, West Point Pharma	59591-0156-82
1000's	$683.00	Cyclobenzaprine Hcl, Endo Labs	60951-0767-90
1000's	$725.00	Cyclobenzaprine Hcl, Watson Labs	52544-0418-10
1000's	$727.00	Cyclobenzaprine Hcl, Invamed	52189-0252-30
1000's	$727.77	Cyclobenzaprine Hcl, Royce	51875-0257-04
1000's	$745.00	Cyclobenzaprine HCl, Schein Pharm (US)	00364-2348-02
1000's	$764.99	Cyclobenzaprine Hcl, HL Moore Drug Exch	00839-7711-16
1000's	$811.00	Cyclobenzaprine HCl, Rugby	00536-4840-10
1000's	$811.00	Cyclobenzaprine HCl, Geneva Pharms	50752-0285-09
1000's	$812.00	Cyclobenzaprine Hcl, Mylan	00378-0751-10

CYCLOPENTOLATE HYDROCHLORIDE *(000928)*

CATEGORIES: Cycloplegics/Mydriatics; Dermatologicals; EENT Drugs; Eye, Ear, Nose, & Throat Preparations; Mydriasis; Mydriatics; Mydriatics & Cycloplegics; Ophthalmics; Pregnancy Category C; FDA Approval Pre 1982

BRAND NAMES: Ak-Pentolate; *Alnide*; *Ciclolux*; *Ciclopleg*; *Cicloplegic*; Cyclate; **Cyclogyl**; *Cyclomidri*; *Cyclomydri*; *Cyclopentol*; *Cyclopentolat*; *Cyclopentolat Thilo* (Germany); *Cyclopentolate*; *Cyclopentolate Eye Drops*; Cylate; *Cyplegin* (Japan); I-Pentolate; *Midriodavi*; *Minims Cyclopentolate Hydrocloride* (Australia); *Mydrilate* (England, Japan); Ocu-Pentolate; *Oftan-Syklo*; Pentolair; *Refractyl*; *Refractyl Ofeno* (Mexico); *Skiacol* (France); Spectro-Pentolate; *Zyklolat*; *Zyklolat-Edo* (Germany) *(International brand names outside U.S. in italics)*

FORMULARIES: Aetna; BC-BS; Medi-Cal

DESCRIPTION:

Cyclopentolate hydrochloride ophthalmic solution is an anticholinergic prepared as a sterile, borate buffered, solution for topical ocular use. It is supplied in three strengths.

The chemical formula is $C_{17}H_{25}NO_3 \cdot HCl$ and the molecular weight is 327.85.

Established name: Cyclopentolate Hydrochloride

Chemical name: 2-(Dimethylamino)ethyl 1-hydroxy-α- phenylcyclopentaneacetate hydrochloride

Each ml contains: **Active:** Cyclopentolate Hydrochloride 0.5%, 1% or 2%. **Preservative:** Benzalkonium Chloride 0.01%.**Inactive:** Boric Acid, Edetate Disodium, Potassium Chloride (except 2% strength). Sodium Carbonate and/or Hydrochloric Acid (to adjust pH). Purified Water The pH range is between 3.0 and 5.5.

CLINICAL PHARMACOLOGY:

This anticholinergic preparation blocks the responses of the sphincter muscle of the iris and the accommodative muscle of the ciliary body to cholinergic stimulation, producing pupillary dilation (mydriasis) and paralysis of accommodation (cycloplegia). It acts rapidly, but has a shorter duration than atropine. Maximal cycloplegia occurs within 25 to 75 minutes after instillation. Complete recovery of accommodation usually takes 6 to 24 hours. Complete recovery from mydriasis in some individuals may require several days.

INDICATIONS AND USAGE:

Cyclopentolate hydrochloride is used to produce mydriasis and cycloplegia.

CONTRAINDICATIONS:

Should not be used when narrow-angle glaucoma or anatomical narrow angles are present, or where there is hypersensitivity to any component of this preparation.

WARNINGS:

For topical use only — not for injection. This preparation may cause CNS disturbances. This is especially true in younger age groups but may occur at any age, especially with the stronger solutions. Premature and small infants are especially prone to CNS and cardiopulmonary side effects from systemic absorption of cyclopentolate. To minimize absorption, use only one drop of 0.5% cyclopentolate hydrochloride solution per eye followed by pressure applied over the nasolacrimal sac for two to three minutes. Observe infants closely for at least 30 minutes following instillation.

PRECAUTIONS:

General: To avoid inducing angle closure glaucoma an estimation of the depth of the angle of the anterior chamber should be made. The lacrimal sac should be compressed by digital pressure for two to three minutes after instillation to avoid excessive systemic absorption. Caution should be observed when considering use of this medication in the presence of Down's syndrome or mongolism, and in those predisposed to angle-closure glaucoma.

Patient Information: Do not touch dropper tip to any surface, as this may contaminate the solution. A transient burning sensation may occur upon instillation. Patients should be advised not to drive or engage in other hazardous activities while pupils are dilated. Patients may experience sensitivity to light and should protect eyes in bright illumination during dilation. Patients should be warned not to get this preparation in their child's mouth and to wash their own hands and the child's hands following administration.

Carcinogenesis, Mutagenesis, and Impairment of Fertility: Studies in animals or humans have not been conducted to evaluate the potential of these effects.

Pregnancy Category C: Animal reproduction studies have not been conducted with cyclopentolate. It is also not known whether cyclopentolate can cause fetal harm when administered to a pregnant woman or can affect reproduction capacity. Cyclopentolate should be administered to a pregnant woman only if clearly needed.

Nursing Mothers: It is not known whether this drug is excreted in human milk. Because many drugs are excreted in human milk, caution should be exercised when cyclopentolate hydrochloride is administered to a nursing woman.

Pediatrics: Increased susceptibility to cyclopentolate has been reported in infants, young children, and in children with spastic paralysis or brain damage. Therefore, cyclopentolate should be used with great caution in these patients. Feeding intolerance may follow ophthalmic use of this product in neonates. It is recommended that feeding be withheld for four (4) hours after examination. Do not use in concentrations higher than 0.5% in small infants (see WARNINGS.)

Geriatrics: In the elderly and others where increased intraocular pressure may be encountered, mydriatics and cycloplegics should be used cautiously.

DRUG INTERACTIONS:

Cyclopentolate may interfere with the anti-glaucoma action of carbachol or pilocarpine, also, concurrent use of these medications may antagonize the anti-glaucoma and miotic actions of ophthalmic cholinesterase inhibitors.

ADVERSE REACTIONS:

Ocular: Increased intraocular pressure, burning, photophobia, blurred vision, irritation, hyperemia, conjunctivitis, blepharoconjunctivitis, punctate keratitis, synechiae.

Systemic: Use of cyclopentolate has been associated with psychotic reactions and behavioral disturbances, usually in children especially with 2% concentration. These disturbances include ataxia, incoherent speech, restlessness, hallucinations, hyperactivity, seizures, disorientation as to time and place, and failure to recognize people. This drug produces reactions similar to those of other anticholinergic drugs, but the central nervous system manifestations as noted above are more common. Other toxic manifestations of anticholinergic drugs are skin rash, abdominal discretion in infants, unusual drowsiness, tachycardia, hyperpyrexia, vasodilation, urinary retention, diminished gastrointestinal motility and decreased secretion in salivary and sweat glands, pharynx, bronchii and nasal passages. Severe manifestations of toxicity include coma, medullary paralysis and death.

OVERDOSAGE:

Excessive dosage may produce exaggerated symptoms as noted in ADVERSE REACTIONS. When administration of the drug product is discontinued the patient usually recovers spontaneously. In case of severe manifestations of toxicity the antidote of choice is physostigmine salicylate.

Pediatric Dose: As an antidote, slowly inject intravenously 0.5 mg physostigmine salicylate if toxic symptoms persist and no cholinergic symptoms are produced repeat at five minute intervals to a maximum cumulative dose of 2 mg.

Adolescent and Adult: As an antidote, slowly inject 2 mg physostigmine salicylate intravenously. A second dose of 1 to 2 mg may be given after 20 minutes if no reversal of toxic manifestations has occurred.[1,2,3]

DOSAGE AND ADMINISTRATION:

Adults: One or two drops of 0.5%, 1% or 2% solution in the eye which may be repeated in five to ten minutes if necessary. Complete recovery usually occurs in 24 hours.

Children: One or two drops of 0.5%, 1% or 2% solution in the eye which may be repeated five to ten minutes later by a second application or 0.5% or 1% solution if necessary.

Small Infants: A single instillation of one drop of 0.5% cyclopentolate hydrochloride in the eye. To minimize absorption apply pressure over the nasolacrimal sac for two to three minutes. Observe infant closely for at least 30 minutes following instillation. Individuals with heavily pigmented indies may require higher strengths.

Storage: Store at 8° - 27°C (46° - 80°F).

REFERENCES:

1. Rumack B H: Anticholinergic Poisoning: Treatment with Physostigmine **Pediatrics** 52(6): 449-51, 1973. **2.** Duvoisin, R.C. and Katz, R.: Reversal of Central Anticholinergic Syndromes in Man by Physostigmine. J. Am. Med. Assn. 206(9); 1963-65, 1968. **3.** Grant, W.M. **Toxicology of the Eye.** Second Edition. Volume 1. Springfield, Illinois, Charles C. Thomas: 1974.(Alcon Laboratories, 342086, 4/95)

HOW SUPPLIED - RATED THERAPEUTICALLY EQUIVALENT:

Solution - Ophthalmic - 0.5 %

2 ml	**$5.94**	**CYCLOGYL, Alcon**	**00065-0395-02**
5 ml	**$11.25**	**CYCLOGYL, Alcon**	**00065-0395-05**
15 ml	**$21.56**	**CYCLOGYL, Alcon**	**00065-0395-15**

Solution - Ophthalmic - 1 %

2 ml	$1.25	I-PENTOLATE, Americal Pharm	54945-0501-20
2 ml	$1.30	Cyclopentolate Hcl, H.C.F.A. F F P	99999-0928-01
2 ml	$2.75	Cyclopentolate Hcl, Rugby	00536-0602-67
2 ml	$4.65	Cyclate, Ocusoft	54799-0501-02
2 ml	$4.69	AK-PENTOLATE, Akorn	17478-0100-20
2 ml	**$7.19**	**CYCLOGYL, Alcon**	**00065-0396-02**
5 ml	$3.25	Cyclopentolate Hcl, H.C.F.A. F F P	99999-0928-02
5 ml	$5.25	Cyclopentolate Hcl, Rugby	00536-0602-72
5 ml	**$13.13**	**CYCLOGYL, Alcon**	**00065-0396-05**
15 ml	$3.49	I-PENTOLATE, Americal Pharm	54945-0501-12
15 ml	$3.81	Cyclopentolate Hcl, Rugby	00536-0602-65
15 ml	$7.45	CYLATE 1% OPHTHALMIC, Ocusoft	54799-0501-12
15 ml	$7.95	Cyclopentolate HCl, Aligen Independ	00405-6040-15
15 ml	$7.95	SPECTRO PENTOLATE, Spectrum Scitfc	53268-0332-12
15 ml	$8.50	Cyclopentolate Hcl, Steris Labs	00402-0777-15
15 ml	$9.25	Cyclopentolate Hcl, HL Moore Drug Exch	00839-6679-31
15 ml	$9.75	Cyclopentolate HCl, H.C.F.A. F F P	99999-0928-03
15 ml	$12.19	AK-PENTOLATE, Akorn	17478-0100-12
15 ml	**$22.81**	**CYCLOGYL, Alcon**	**00065-0396-15**

HOW SUPPLIED - NOT RATED EQUIVALENT:

Solution - Ophthalmic - 1 %

2 ml	$1.50	Pentolair, Raway	00686-0735-01
2 ml	$2.75	In-Pentolate, Infinity Pharm	58154-0735-01
2 ml	$4.75	Spectro-Pentolate, Spectrum Scitfc	53268-0332-59
15 ml	$2.95	Pentolair, Raway	00686-0735-06
15 ml	$5.85	IN-PENTOLATE, Infinity Pharm	58154-0735-06

Solution - Ophthalmic - 2 %

2 ml	**$9.69**	**CYCLOGYL, Alcon**	**00065-0397-02**
5 ml	**$15.94**	**CYCLOGYL, Alcon**	**00065-0397-05**
15 ml	**$26.87**	**CYCLOGYL, Alcon**	**00065-0397-15**

CYCLOPENTOLATE HYDROCHLORIDE; PHENYLEPHRINE HYDROCHLORIDE *(000929)*

CATEGORIES: Cycloplegics/Mydriatics; EENT Drugs; Eye, Ear, Nose, & Throat Preparations; Mydriasis; Mydriatics; Mydriatics & Cycloplegics; Ophthalmics; FDA Approval Pre 1982

BRAND NAMES: *Cyclomidril*; **Cyclomydril**; Murocoll-2 Solution
(International brand names outside U.S. in italics)

FORMULARIES: Aetna

DESCRIPTION:

Cyclomydril (Cyclopentolate Hydrochloride, Phenylephrine Hydrochloride) is a mydriatic prepared as a sterile topical ophthalmic solution.

Established name: Cyclopentolate Hydrochloride

Chemical name: Benzeneacetic acid, α-(1-hydroxy-cyclopentyl)-, 2-(dimethylamino)ethyl ester, hydrochloride.

Established name: Phenylephrine Hydrochloride

Chemical name: 3-hydroxy-α-[(methylamino)-methyl]-,Benzenemethanol, hydrochloride (*S*)-.

Each ml contains: Active: Cyclopentolate Hydrochloride 0.2%, Phenylephrine Hydrochloride 1%. Preservative: Benzalkonium Chloride 0.01%. Inactive: Edetate Disodium, Boric Acid, Hydrochloric Acid and/or Sodium Carbonate (to adjust pH), Purified Water.

CLINICAL PHARMACOLOGY:

Cyclopentolate HCl is an anticholinergic drug and phenylephrine hydrochloride is an adrenergic drug. This combination induces mydriasis that is considerably greater than that of either drug alone. The concentrations of cyclopentolate hydrochloride and of phenylephrine hydrochloride have been selected to induce safe and rapid mydriasis with little or no accompanying cycloplegia.

INDICATIONS AND USAGE:

For the production of mydriasis.

CONTRAINDICATIONS:

Do not use in patients with narrow-angle glaucoma or with anatomically narrow angles or where there is hypersensitivity to any component of this preparation.

WARNINGS:

For topical use only — not for injection. The use of this combination may have an adverse effect on individuals suffering from cardiovascular disease, hypertension, and hyperthyroidism; and it may cause CNS disturbances. Small infants are especially prone to CNS and cardiopulmonary side effects from systemic absorption of cyclopentolate.

PRECAUTIONS:

To avoid inducing angle closure glaucoma, an estimation of the depth of the angle of the anterior chamber should be made. The lacrimal sac should be compressed by digital pressure for two to three minutes after instillation to avoid excessive system absorption. The effect of long-term use of this preparation has not been established, therefore it should be restricted to short-term use.

Patient Warning: Patient should be advised not to drive or engage in other hazardous activities while pupils are dilated. Patient may experience sensitivity to light and should protect eyes in bright illumination during dilation. Parents should be warned not to get this preparation in their child's mouth and to wash their own hands and the child's hands following administration.

ADVERSE REACTIONS:

Increased intraocular pressure. Use of cyclopentolate has been associated with psychotic reactions and behavioral disturbances in children, especially with 2% concentration. These disturbances include ataxia, incoherent speech, restlessness, hallucinations, hyperactivity, seizures, disorientation as to time and place, and failure to recognize people. This drug produces reactions similar to those of other anticholinergic drugs. However, the central nervous system manifestations as noted above are more common. Other toxic manifestations of anticholinergic drugs are tachycardia, hyperpyrexia, vasodilation, urinary retention, diminished gastrointestinal motility and decreased secretion in salivary and sweat glands, pharynx, bronchii and nasal passages. Severe manifestations of toxicity include coma, medullary paralysis and death.

OVERDOSAGE:

In case of severe manifestations of toxicity, the antidote of choice is physostigmine salicylate.

Pediatric Dose: Slowly inject intravenously 0.5 mg. If toxic symptoms persist and no cholinergic symptoms are produces repeat at five minute intervals to a maximum dose of 2.0 mg.

Adolescent and Adult Dose: Slowly inject 2.0 mg intravenously. A second dose of 1-2 mg may be given after 20 minutes if no reversal of toxic manifestations has occurred. Physostigmine salicylate can be administered subcutaneously.[1,2]

DOSAGE AND ADMINISTRATION:

For fundus-copy, instill one drop in each eye every five to ten minutes, not to exceed three times, to produce rapid mydriasis, permitting ready visual access to the fundus. Heavily pigmented irides may require larger doses. To minimize absorption in premature and small infants, apply pressure over the nasolacrimal sac for two to three minutes following instillation. Observe infants closely for at least 30 minutes.

REFERENCES:

1. Rumack, B. H.: Anticholinergic Poisoning: Treatment with Physostigmine. Pediatrics 52(6):449-51, 1973. **2.** Duvoisin, R. C. and Katz, R.: Reversal of Central Anticholinergic Syndromes in Man by Physostigmine. J. Am. Med. Assn. 206(9):1963-65, 1968.

HOW SUPPLIED - EQUIVALENTS NOT AVAILABLE:

Solution - Ophthalmic - 0.2 %/1 %

2 ml	**$7.19**	**CYCLOMYDRIL, Alcon**	**00065-0359-02**
5 ml	**$12.81**	**CYCLOMYDRIL, Alcon**	**00065-0359-05**

CYCLOPHOSPHAMIDE *(000930)*

CATEGORIES: Antineoplastics; Breast Carcinoma; Burkitt's Lymphoma; Cytotoxic Agents; Hodgkin's Disease; Immunologic; Immunomodulators; Leukemia; Lymphoma; Mycosis Fungoides; Myeloma; Nephrotic Syndrome; Neuroblastoma; Oncologic Drugs; Ovarian Carcinoma; Pregnancy Category D; FDA Approval Pre 1982

BRAND NAMES: *Alkyloxan*; *Carloxan*; *Ciclofosfamida*; *Ciclolen* (Mexico); *Cicloxal*; *Cycloblastin* (Australia); *Cycloblastine*; *Cyclomide*; *Cyclophar*; *Cyclostin* (Germany); *Cyclostin N* (Germany); *Cycloxan*; *Cytokan*; *Cytophosphan*; **Cytoxan**; *Endoxan* (Germany, Japan); *Endoxan Asta*; *Endoxan-Asta* (France); *Endoxana* (England); *Endoxon*; *Endoxon-Asta*; *Enduxan*; *Genoxal* (Mexico); *Ledoxina* (Mexico); *Lyophilisate*; Neosar; Neosar For Injection; *Procytox* (Canada); *Sendoxan*; *Syklofosfamid*
(International brand names outside U.S. in italics)

FORMULARIES: Aetna; BC-BS; Medi-Cal; WHO

COST OF THERAPY: $1,020.28 (Ovarian Carcinoma; Tablet; 50 mg; 1/day; 365 days)

DESCRIPTION:

Cyclophosphamide for injection is a sterile white powder blend consisting of 45 mg sodium chloride per 100 mg cyclophosphamide (anhydrous). Lyophilized cyclophosphamide for injection is a sterile white lyophilized cake, or partially broken cake, containing 75 mg mannitol per 100 mg cyclophosphamide (anhydrous). Cyclophosphamide tablets are for oral use and contain 25 mg or 50 mg cyclophosphamide (anhydrous). Inactive ingredients in cyclophosphamide tablets are: acacia, FD&C Blue No. 1, D&C Yellow No. 10 Aluminum Lake, lactose, magnesium stearate, starch, stearic acid and talc. Cyclophosphamide is a synthetic antineoplastic drug chemically related to the nitrogen mustards. Cyclophosphamide is a white crystalline powder with the molecular formula $C_7H_{15}Cl_2N_2O_2P{\cdot}H_2O$ and a molecular weight of 279.1. The chemical name for cyclophosphamide is 2-[bis(2-chloroethyl)amino] tetrahydro-2H-1,3,2-oxazaphosphorine 2-oxide monohydrate. Cyclophosphamide is soluble in water, saline, or ethanol.

CLINICAL PHARMACOLOGY:

Cyclophosphamide is biotransformed principally in the liver to active alkylating metabolites by a mixed function microsomal oxidase system. These metabolites interfere with the growth of susceptible rapidly proliferating malignant cells. The mechanism of action is thought to involve cross-linking of tumor cell DNA.

Cyclophosphamide is well absorbed after oral administration with a bioavailability greater than 75%. The unchanged drug has an elimination half-life of 3 to 12 hours. It is eliminated primarily in the form of metabolites, but from 5 to 25% of the dose is excreted in urine as unchanged drug. Several cytotoxic and noncytotoxic metabolites have been identified in urine and in plasma. Concentrations of metabolites reach a maximum in plasma 2 to 3 hours after an intravenous dose. Plasma protein binding of unchanged drug is low but some metabolites are bound to an extent greater than 60%. It has not been demonstrated that any single metabolite is responsible for either the therapeutic or toxic effects of cyclophosphamide. Although elevated levels of metabolites of cyclophosphamide have been observed in patients with renal failure, increased clinical toxicity in such patients has not been demonstrated.

INDICATIONS AND USAGE:

MALIGNANT DISEASES

Cyclophosphamide, although effective alone in susceptible malignancies, is more frequently used concurrently or sequentially with other antineoplastic drugs. The following malignancies are often susceptible to cyclophosphamide treatment:

1. Malignant lymphomas (Stages III and IV of the Ann Arbor staging system), Hodgkin's disease, lymphocytic lymphoma, Burkitt's lymphoma.

2. Multiple myeloma.

3. Leukemias: Chronic lymphocytic leukemia, chronic granulocytic leukemia (it is usually ineffective in acute blastic crisis), acute myelogenous and monocytic leukemia, acute lymphoblastic (stemcell) leukemia in children cyclophosphamide given during remission is effective in prolonging its duration).

4. Mycosis fungoides (advanced disease).

5. Neuroblastoma (disseminated disease).

6. Adenocarcinoma of the ovary.

7. Retinoblastoma.

8. Carcinoma of the breast.

NONMALIGNANT DISEASE

Biopsy Proven "Minimal Change" Nephrotic Syndrome in Children: Cyclophosphamide is useful in carefully selected cases of biopsy proven "minimal change" nephrotic syndrome in children but should not be used as primary therapy. In children whose disease fails to respond adequately to appropriate adrenocorticosteroid therapy or in whom the adrenocorticosteroid therapy produces or threatens to produce intolerable side effects, cyclophosphamide may induce a remission. Cyclophosphamide is not indicated for the nephrotic syndrome in adults or for any other renal disease.

CONTRAINDICATIONS:

Continued use of cyclophosphamide is contraindicated in patients with severely depressed bone marrow function. Cyclophosphamide is contraindicated in patients who have demonstrated a previous hypersensitivity to it (see WARNINGS and PRECAUTIONS).

WARNINGS:

CARCINOGENESIS, MUTAGENESIS, IMPAIRMENT OF FERTILITY

Second malignancies have developed in some patients treated with cyclophosphamide used alone or in association with other antineoplastic drugs and/or modalities. Most frequently, they have been urinary bladder, myeloproliferative, or lymphoproliferative malignancies. Second malignancies most frequently were detected in patients treated for primary myeloproliferative or lymphoproliferative malignancies or non-malignant disease in which immune processes are believed to be involved pathologically. In some cases, the second malignancy developed several years after cyclophosphamide treatment had been discontinued. Urinary bladder malignancies generally have occurred in patients who previously had hemorrhagic cystitis. One case of carcinoma of the renal pelvis was reported in a patient receiving long-term cyclophosphamide therapy for cerebral vasculitis. The possibility of cyclophosphamide-induced malignancy should be considered in an benefit-to-risk assessment for use of the drug.

Cyclophosphamide can cause fetal harm when administered to a pregnant woman and such abnormalities have been reported following cyclophosphamide therapy in pregnant women. Abnormalities were found in two infants and a six-month old fetus born to women treated with cyclophosphamide. Ectrodactylia was found in two of the three cases. Normal infants have also been born to women treated with cyclophosphamide during pregnancy, including the first trimester. If this drug is used during pregnancy, or if the patient becomes pregnant while taking (receiving) this drug, the patient should be apprised of the potential hazard to the fetus. Women of childbearing potential should be advised to avoid becoming pregnant.

Cyclophosphamide interferes with oogenesis and spermatogenesis. It may cause sterility in both sexes. Development of sterility appears to depend on the dose of cyclophosphamide, duration of therapy, and the state of gonadal function at the time of treatment. Cyclophosphamide induced sterility may be irreversible in some patients.

Amenorrhea associated with decreased estrogen and increased gonadotropin secretion develops in a significant proportion of women treated with cyclophosphamide. Affected patients generally resume regular menses within a few months after cessation of therapy. Girls treated with cyclophosphamide during prepubescence generally develop secondary sexual characteristics normally, and have regular menses. Ovarian fibrosis with apparently complete loss of germ cells after prolonged cyclophosphamide treatment in late prepubescence has been reported. Girls treated with cyclophosphamide during prepubescence subsequently have conceived.

Men treated with cyclophosphamide may develop oligospermia or azoospermia associated with increased gonadotropin but normal testosterone secretion. Sexual potency and libido are unimpaired in these patients. Boys treated with cyclophosphamide during prepubescence develop secondary sexual characteristics normally, but may have oligospermia or azoospermia and increased gonadotropin secretion. Some degree of testicular atrophy may occur. Cyclophosphamide induced azoospermia is reversible in some patients, though the reversibility may not occur for several years after cessation of therapy. Men temporarily rendered sterile by cyclophosphamide have subsequently fathered normal children.

URINARY SYSTEM

Hemorrhagic cystitis may develop in patients treated with cyclophosphamide. Rarely, this condition can be severe and even fatal. Fibrosis of the urinary bladder, sometimes extensive, also may develop with or without accompanying cystitis. Atypical urinary bladder epithelial cells may appear in the urine. These adverse effects appear to depend on the dose of cyclophosphamide and the duration of therapy. Such bladder injury is thought to be due to cyclophosphamide metabolites excreted in the urine. Forced fluid intake helps to assure an ample output of urine, necessitates frequent voiding, and reduces the time the drug remains in the bladder. This helps to prevent cystitis. Hematuria usually resolves in a few days after cyclophosphamide treatment is stopped, but it may persist. Medical and/or surgical supportive treatment may be required, rarely, to treat protracted cases of severe hemorrhagic cystitis. It is usually necessary to discontinue cyclophosphamide therapy in instances of severe hemorrhagic cystitis.

CARDIAC TOXICITY

Although a few instances of cardiac dysfunction have been reported following use of recommended doses of cyclophosphamide, no causal relationship has been established. Cardiotoxicity has been observed in some patients receiving high doses of cyclophosphamide ranging from 120 to 270 mg/kg administered over a period of a few days, usually as a portion of an intensive antineoplastic multi-drug regimen or in conjunction with transplantation procedures. In a few instances with high doses of cyclophosphamide, severe, and sometimes fatal, congestive heart failure has occurred within a few days after the first cyclophosphamide dose. Histopathologic examination has primarily shown hemorrhagic myocarditis. Hemopericardium has occurred secondary to hemorrhagic myocarditis and myocardial necrosis. Pericarditis has been reported independent of any hemopericardium.

WARNINGS: *(cont'd)*

No residual cardiac abnormalities, as evidenced by electrocardiogram or echocardiogram appear to be present in patients surviving episodes of apparent cardiac toxicity associated with high doses of cyclophosphamide.

Cyclophosphamide has been reported to potentiate doxorubicin induced cardiotoxicity.

INFECTIONS

Treatment with cyclophosphamide may cause significant suppression of immune responses. Serious, sometimes fatal, infections may develop in severely immunosuppressed patients. Cyclophosphamide treatment may not be indicated or should be interrupted or the dose reduced in patients who have or who develop viral, bacterial, fungal, protozoan, or helminthic infections.

OTHER

Rare instances of anaphylactic reaction including one death have been reported. One instance of possible cross-sensitivity with other alkylating agents has been reported.

PRECAUTIONS:

GENERAL

Special attention to the possible development of toxicity should be exercised in patients being treated with cyclophosphamide if any of the following conditions are present.

1. Leukopenia

2. Thrombocytopenia

3. Tumor cell infiltration of bone marrow

4. Previous X-ray therapy

5. Previous therapy with other cytotoxic agents

6. Impaired hepatic function

7. Impaired renal function

Laboratory Tests: During treatment, the patient's hematologic profile (particularly neutrophils and platelets) should be monitored regularly to determine the degree of hematopoietic suppression. Urine should also be examined regularly for red cells which may precede hemorrhagic cystitis.

Adrenalectomy: Since cyclophosphamide has been reported to be more toxic in adrenalectomized dogs, adjustment of the doses of both replacement steroids and cyclophosphamide may be necessary for the adrenalectomized patient.

Wound Healing: Cyclophosphamide may interfere with normal wound healing.

Carcinogenesis, Mutagenesis, and Impairment of Fertility: See WARNINGS section for information on carcinogenesis, mutagenesis, and impairment of fertility.

Pregnancy Category C: See WARNINGS.

Nursing Mothers: Cyclophosphamide is excreted in breast milk. Because of the potential for serious adverse reactions and the potential for tumorigenicity shown for cyclophosphamide in humans, a decision should be made whether to discontinue nursing or to discontinue the drug, taking into account the importance of the drug to the mother.

DRUG INTERACTIONS:

The rate of metabolism and the leukopenic activity of cyclophosphamide reportedly are increased by chronic administration of high doses of phenobarbital.

The physician should be alert for possible combined drug actions, desirable or undesirable, involving cyclophosphamide even though cyclophosphamide has been used successfully concurrently with other drugs, including other cytotoxic drugs.

Cyclophosphamide treatment, which causes a marked and persistent inhibition of cholinesterase activity, potentiates the effect of succinylcholine chloride.

If a patient has been treated with cyclophosphamide within 10 days of general anesthesia, the anesthesiologist should be alerted.

ADVERSE REACTIONS:

Information on adverse reactions associated with the use of cyclophosphamide is arranged according to body system affected or type of reaction. The adverse reactions are listed in order of decreasing incidence. The most serious adverse reactions are described in the WARNINGS section.

Reproductive System: See WARNINGS section for information on impairment of fertility.

Digestive System: Nausea and vomiting commonly occur with cyclophosphamide therapy. Anorexia and, less frequently, abdominal discomfort or pain and diarrhea may occur. There are isolated reports of hemorrhagic colitis, oral mucosal ulceration and jaundice occurring during therapy. These adverse drug effects generally remit when cyclophosphamide treatment is stopped.

Skin and Its Structures: Alopecia occurs commonly in patients treated with cyclophosphamide. The hair can be expected to grow back after treatment with the drug or even during continued drug treatment, though it may be different in texture or color. Skin rash occurs occasionally in patients receiving the drug. Pigmentation of the skin and changes in nails can occur.

Hematopoietic System: Leukopenia occurs in patients treated with cyclophosphamide, is related to the dose of drug, and can be used as a dosage guide. Leukopenia of less than 2000 cells/mm^3 develops commonly in patients treated with an initial loading dose of the drug, and less frequently in patients maintained on smaller doses. The degree of neutropenia is particularly important because it correlates with a reduction in resistance to infections.

Thrombocytopenia or anemia develop occasionally in patients treated with cyclophosphamide. These hematologic effects usually can be reversed by reducing the drug dose or by interrupting treatment. Recovery from leukopenia usually begins in 7 to 10 days after cessation of therapy.

Urinary System: See WARNINGS section for information on cystitis and urinary bladder fibrosis.

Hemorrhagic ureteritis and renal tubular necrosis have been reported to occur in patients treated with cyclophosphamide. Such lesions usually resolve following cessation of therapy.

Infections: See WARNINGS section for information on reduced host resistance to infections.

Carcinogenesis: See WARNINGS section for information on carcinogenesis.

Respiratory System: Interstitial pulmonary fibrosis has been reported in patients receiving high doses of cyclophosphamide over a prolonged period.

Other: Rare instances of anaphylactic reaction including one death have been reported. One instance of possible cross-sensitivity with other alkylating agents has been reported.

OVERDOSAGE:

No specific antidote for cyclophosphamide is known. Overdosage should be managed with supportive measures, including appropriate treatment for any concurrent infection, myelosuppression, or cardiac toxicity should it occur.

DOSAGE AND ADMINISTRATION:

TREATMENT OF MALIGNANT DISEASES

Adults and Children: When used as the only oncolytic drug therapy, the initial course of cyclophosphamide for patients with no hematologic deficiency usually consists of 40 to 50 mg/kg given intravenously in divided doses over a period of 2 to 5 days. Other intravenous regimens include 10 to 15 mg/kg given every 7 to 10 days or 3 to 5 mg/kg twice weekly.

Oral cyclophosphamide dosing is usually in the range of 1 to 5 mg/kg/day for both initial and maintenance dosing.

Many other regimens of intravenous and oral cyclophosphamide have been reported. Dosages must be adjusted in accord with evidence of antitumor activity and/or leukopenia. The total leukocyte count is a good, objective guide for regulating dosage. Transient decreases in the total white blood cell count to 2000 cells/mm^3 (following short courses) or more persistent reduction to 3000 cells/mm^3 (with continuing therapy) are tolerated without serious risk of infection if there is no marked granulocytopenia.

When cyclophosphamide is included in combined cytotoxic regimens, it may be necessary to reduce the dose of cyclophosphamide as well as that of the other drugs.

Cyclophosphamide and its metabolites are dialyzable although there are probably quantitative differences depending upon the dialysis system being used. Patients with compromised renal function may show some measurable changes in pharmacokinetic parameters of cyclophosphamide metabolism, but there is no consistent evidence indicating a need for cyclophosphamide dosage modification in patients with renal function impairment.

TREATMENT OF NONMALIGNANT DISEASES

Biopsy Proven "Minimal Change" Nephrotic Syndrome in Children

An oral dose of 2.5 to 3 mg/kg daily for a period of 60 to 90 days is recommended. In males, the incidence of oligospermia and azoospermia increases if the duration of cyclophosphamide treatment exceeds 60 days. Treatment beyond 90 days increases the probability of sterility. Adrenocorticosteroid therapy may be tapered and discontinued during the course of cyclophosphamide therapy. See PRECAUTIONS section concerning hematologic monitoring.

PREPARATION AND HANDLING OF SOLUTIONS

Parenteral drug products should be inspected visually for particulate matter and discoloration prior to administration, whenever solution and container permit.

Cyclophosphamide for injection and lyophilized cyclophosphamide for injection should be prepared for parenteral use by adding Sterile Water for Injection, USP, to the vial and shaking to dissolve. Use the quantity of diluent shown below to reconstitute the product (TABLE 1):

TABLE 1

Dosage Strength	Cyclophosphamide for Injection Quantity of Diluent	Lyophilized Cyclophosphamide for Injection Quantity of Diluent
100 mg	5 ml	5 ml
200 mg	10 ml	10 ml
500 mg	25 ml	20-25 ml
1 g	50 ml	50 ml
2 g	100 ml	80-100 ml

Solutions of cyclophosphamide for injection and lyophilized cyclophosphamide for injection may be injected intravenously, intramuscularly, intraperitoneally, or intrapleurally or they may be infused intravenously in the following:

Dextrose Injection, USP (5% dextrose)

Dextrose and Sodium Chloride Injection, USP (5% dextrose and 0.9% sodium chloride)

5% Dextrose and Ringer's Injection

Lactated Ringer's Injection, USP

Sodium Chloride Injection, USP (0.45% sodium chloride)

Sodium Lactate Injection, USP (1/6 molar sodium lactate)

Reconstituted cyclophosphamide for injection and lyophilized cyclophosphamide for injection are chemically and physically stable for 24 hours at room temperature or for six days in the refrigerator; it does not contain any antimicrobial preservative and thus care must be taken to assure the sterility of prepared solutions.

The osmolarities of solutions of cyclophosphamide for injection, lyophilized cyclophosphamide for injection, and normal saline are compared in the following table (TABLE 2):

TABLE 2

	mOsm/L
Lyophilized Cyclophosphamide for Injection	431
Cyclophosphamide for Injection	352
4 mL diluent per 100 mg cyclophosphamide	219
5 mL diluent per 100 mg cyclophosphamide	172
Normal saline	287

Lyophilized cyclophosphamide for injection is slightly hypotonic while cyclophosphamide for injection is slightly hypertonic with respect to normal saline.

Extemporaneous liquid preparations of cyclophosphamide for oral administration may be prepared by dissolving cyclophosphamide for injection or lyophilized cyclophosphamide for injection in Aromatic Elixir, N.F. Such preparations should be stored under refrigeration in glass containers and used within 14 days.

HOW SUPPLIED:

CYTOXAN for Injection contains 45 mg of sodium chloride per 100 mg of cyclophosphamide (anhydrous) and is supplied in vials for single dose use.

Lyophilized CYTOXAN for Injection contains 75 mg of mannitol per 100 mg of cyclophosphamide (anhydrous) and is supplied in vials for single-dose use.

CYTOXAN Tablets, 25 mg and CYTOXAN Tablets, 50 mg, are white tablets with blue flecks containing 25 mg and 50 mg cyclophosphamide (anhydrous), respectively.

Storage at or below 77°F (25°C) is recommended; this product will withstand brief exposure to temperatures up to 86°F (30°C) but should be protected from temperatures above 86°F (30°C).

Procedures For Proper Handling And Disposal of anticancer drugs should be considered. Several guidelines on this subject have been published.[1-7] There is no general agreement that all of the procedures recommended in the guidelines are necessary or appropriate.

REFERENCES:

1. Recommendations for the Safe Handling of Parenteral Antineoplastic Drugs. NIH Publication No.83-2621. For sale by the Superintendent of Documents, US Government Printing Office, Washington, DC 20402. **2.** AMA Council Report, Guidelines for Handling Parenteral Antineoplastics, JAMA 1985 March 15. **3.** National Study Commission on Cytotoxic Exposure-Recommendations for Handling Cytotoxic Agents. Available from Louis P. Jeffrey, Sc.D., Chairman, National Study Commission on Cytotoxic Exposure, Massachusetts College of Pharmacy and Allied Health Sciences, 179 Longwood Avenue, Boston, Massachusetts 02115. **4.** Clinical Oncological

REFERENCES: *(cont'd)*

Society of Australia. Guidelines and Recommendations for Safe Handling of Antineoplastic Agents. Med J Australia 1983; 1:426-428. **5.** Jones RB, et al: Safe handling of chemotherapeutic agents: A report from the Mount Sinai Medical Center. CA-A Cancer Journal for Clinicians 1983; (Sept/Oct)258-263. **6.** American Society of Hospital Pharmacists Technical Assistance Bulletin on Handling Cytotoxic and Hazardous Drugs. Am J Hosp Pharm 1990; 47:1033-1049. **7.** OSHA Work-Practice Guidelines for Personnel Dealing with Cytotoxic (Antineoplastic) Drugs. Am J Hosp Pharm 1986; 43:1193-1204.

HOW SUPPLIED - RATED THERAPEUTICALLY EQUIVALENT:

Injection, Lyphl-Soln - Intravenous - 1 gm/vial

1 g x 6	$43.01	NEOSAR, Pharmacia & Upjohn	00013-5636-70
1 gm x 6	**$244.77**	**CYTOXAN, Mead Johnson**	**00015-0505-41**

Injection, Lyphl-Soln - Intravenous - 2 gm/vial

1's	$86.00	NEOSAR, Pharmacia & Upjohn	00013-5676-70
2 gm x 6	**$489.68**	**CYTOXAN, Mead Johnson**	**00015-0506-41**
6 x 2 gm	$86.00	Neosar For Injection 2 Gm/Vial, Pharmacia & Upjohn	00013-5646-70
100 ml x 6	**$592.73**	**CYTOXAN, Mead Johnson**	**00015-0549-41**

Injection, Lyphl-Soln - Intravenous - 100 mg/vial

12's	**$74.32**	**CYTOXAN, Mead Johnson**	**00015-0539-41**
100 mg x 12	$5.39	NEOSAR, Pharmacia & Upjohn	00013-5606-93
100 mg x 12	**$61.21**	**CYTOXAN, Mead Johnson**	**00015-0500-41**

Injection, Lyphl-Soln - Intravenous - 200 mg/vial

200 mg x 12	$10.24	NEOSAR, Pharmacia & Upjohn	00013-5616-93
200 mg x 12	**$116.52**	**CYTOXAN, Mead Johnson**	**00015-0501-41**
200 mg x 12	**$141.14**	**CYTOXAN, Mead Johnson**	**00015-0546-41**

Injection, Lyphl-Soln - Intravenous - 500 mg/vial

12's	**$244.70**	**CYTOXAN 500, Mead Johnson**	**00015-0502-41**
30 ml x 12	**$296.26**	**CYTOXAN, Mead Johnson**	**00015-0547-41**
500 mg x 12	$21.50	NEOSAR, Pharmacia & Upjohn	00013-5626-93

Injection, Lyphl-Soln - Intravenous - 750 mg/vial

1 g x 6	**$296.26**	**CYTOXAN, Mead Johnson**	**00015-0548-41**

HOW SUPPLIED - NOT RATED EQUIVALENT:

Tablet, Uncoated - Oral - 25 mg

100's	**$152.31**	**CYTOXAN, Mead Johnson**	**00015-0504-01**

Tablet, Uncoated - Oral - 50 mg

100's	**$279.53**	**CYTOXAN, Mead Johnson**	**00015-0503-01**
1000's	**$2662.27**	**CYTOXAN, Mead Johnson**	**00015-0503-02**

CYCLOSPORINE *(000932)*

CATEGORIES: Adrenal Corticosteroids; Immunologic; Immunomodulators; Immunosuppressives; Psoriasis; Renal Transplantation; Transplantation; Pregnancy Category C; Sales > $1 Billion; FDA Approved 1983 Nov; Patent Expiration 1995 Sep

BRAND NAMES: Ciclosporin; *Consupren* (Mexico); *Implanta*; Neoral; *Sandimmun* (Australia, Europe, Asia, Mexico, Canada); *Sandimmun Neoral* (Mexico); **Sandimmune**

(International brand names outside U.S. in italics)

FORMULARIES: BC-BS; WHO

COST OF THERAPY: $3,863.16 (Transplantation; Capsule; 100 mg; 2/day; 365 days)

WARNING:

Only physicians experienced in immunosuppressive therapy and management of organ transplant patients should prescribe cyclosporine. Patients receiving the drug should be managed in facilities equipped and staffed with adequate laboratory and supportive medical resources. The physician responsible for maintenance therapy should have complete information requisite for the follow-up of the patient.

CYCLOSPORINE

Cyclosporine should be administered with adrenal corticosteroids but not with other immunosuppressive agents. Increased susceptibility to infection and the possible development of lymphoma may result from immunosuppression.

The absorption of cyclosporine during chronic administration of cyclosporine soft gelatin capsules and oral solution was found to be erratic. It is recommended that patients taking the soft gelatin capsules or oral solution over a period of time be monitored at repeated intervals for cyclosporine blood levels and subsequent dose adjustments be made in order to avoid toxicity due to high levels and possible organ rejection due to low absorption of cyclosporine. This is of special importance in liver transplants. Numerous assays are being developed to measure blood levels of cyclosporine. Comparison of levels in published literature to patient levels using current assays must be done with detailed knowledge of the assay methods employed. See DOSAGE AND ADMINISTRATION, Blood Level Monitoring.

NEORAL

Neoral may be administered with other immunosuppressive agents. Increased susceptibility to infection and the possible development of lymphoma and other neoplasms may result from the degree of immunosuppression.

Neoral Soft Gelatin Capsules (cyclosporine capsules for microemulsion) and Neoral Oral Solution (cyclosporine oral solution for microemulsion) have increased bioavailability in comparison to Sandimmune Soft Gelatin Capsules (cyclosporine capsules, USP) and Sandimmune Oral Solution (cyclosporine oral solution, USP). Neoral and Sandimmune are not bioequivalent and cannot be used interchangeably without physician supervision. It is recommended that cyclosporine blood concentrations be monitored in patients taking Neoral and that dose adjustments be made in order to avoid toxicity due to high concentrations and possible organ rejection due to low concentrations. For a given trough concentration, cyclosporine exposure will be greater with Neoral than with Sandimmune. If a patient who is receiving exceptionally high doses of Sandimmune is converted to Neoral, particular caution should be exercised. Comparison of blood concentrations in the published literature with blood concentrations obtained using current assays must be done with detailed knowledge of the assay methods employed. See DOSAGE AND ADMINISTRATION, Blood Concentration Monitoring.

DESCRIPTION:

Cyclosporine is a cyclic polypeptide immunosuppressant agent consisting of 11 amino acids. It is produced as a metabolite by the fungus species Tolypocladium inflatum Gams.

Chemically, cyclosporine is designated as *[R-[R*,R*-(E)]]*-cyclic(L-alanyl-D-alanyl-*N*-methyl-L-leucyl-*N*-methyl-L-leucyl-*N*-methyl-L-va lyl-3-hydroxy-*N*,4-dimethyl-L-2-amino-6-octenoyl-L-α-amino-buty ryl-*N*-methylglycyl-*N*-methyl-L-leucyl-L-valyl-*N*-methyl-L-leucyl).

Sandimmune Soft Gelatin Capsules: (cyclosporine capsules, USP) are available in 25 mg, 50 mg, and 100 mg strengths.

Each 25 mg capsule contains:

Cyclosporine, USP... 25 mg

Alcohol, USP dehydrate... max 12.7% by volume

Each 50 mg capsule contains:

Cyclosporine, USP... 50 mg

Alcohol, USP dehydrate... max 12.7% by volume

Each 100 mg capsule contains:

Cyclosporine, USP... 100 mg

Alcohol, USP dehydrate... max 12.7% by volume

Sandimmune Inactive Ingredients: corn oil, gelatin, glycerol, Labrafil M 2125 CS (polyoxyethylated glycolysed glycerides), red iron oxide (25 mg and 100 mg capsule only), sorbitol, titanium dioxide, yellow iron oxide (50 mg capsule only), and other ingredients.

Sandimmune Oral Solution: (cyclosporine oral solution, USP) is available in 50 ml bottles.

Each ml contains:

Cyclosporine, USP... 100 mg

Alcohol, USP dehydrate... max 12.5% by volume

It is dissolved in an olive oil, Ph. Helv./Labrafil M 1944 CS (polyoxyethylated oleic glycerides) vehicle which must be further diluted with milk, chocolate milk, or orange juice before oral administration.

Sandimmune Injection: (cyclosporine concentrate for injection, USP) is available in a 5 ml sterile ampul for IV administration.

Each ml contains:

Cyclosporine, USP... 50 mg

Polyoxyethylated castor oil... 650 mg

Alcohol, Ph. Helv... 32.9% by volume

Nitrogen... qs

It must be diluted further with 0.9% Sodium Chloride Injection or 5% Dextrose Injection before use.

NEORAL

Neoral is an oral formulation of cyclosporine that immediately forms a microemulsion in an aqueous environment.

Cyclosporine, the active principle in Neoral, is a cyclic polypeptide immunosuppressant agent consisting of 11 amino acids. It is produced as a metabolite by the fungus species *Beauveria nivea.*

Chemically, cyclosporine is designated as *[R-[R*,R*-(E)]]*-cyclic(L-alanyl-D-alanyl-*N*-methyl-L-leucyl-*N*-methyl-L-leucyl-*N*-methyl-L-va lyl-3-hydroxy-*N*,4-dimethyl-L-2-amino-6-octenoyl-L-α-amino-buty ryl-*N*-methylglycyl-*N*-methyl-L-leucyl-L-valyl-*N*-me thyl-L-leucyl).

Neoral Soft Gelatin Capsules: (cyclosporine capsules for microemulsion) are available in 25 mg and 100 mg strengths.

Each 25 mg capsule contains:

Cyclosporine... 25 mg

Alcohol, USP dehydrated... 9.5% wt/vol.

Each 100 mg capsule contains:

Cyclosporine... 100 mg

Alcohol, USP dehydrated... 9.5% wt/vol.

Neoral Inactive Ingredients: Corn oil-mono-di-triglycerides, polyoxyl 40 hydrogenated castor oil NF, DL-α-tocopherol USP, gelatin NF, glycerol, iron oxide black, propylene glycol USP, titanium dioxide USP, carmine, and other ingredients.

Neoral Oral Solution: (cyclosporine oral solution for microemulsion) is available in 50 ml bottles.

Each ml contains:

Cyclosporine... 100 mg/ml

Alcohol, USP dehydrated... 9.5% wt/vol.

Neoral Inactive Ingredients: Corn oil-mono-di-triglycerides, polyoxyl 40 hydrogenated castor oil NF, DL-α-tocopherol USP, propylene glycol USP.

CLINICAL PHARMACOLOGY:

SANDIMMUNE

Sandimmune is a potent immunosuppressive agent which in animals prolongs survival of allogeneic transplants involving skin, heart, kidney, pancreas, bone marrow, small intestine, and lung. Sandimmune has been demonstrated to suppress some humoral immunity and to a greater extent, cell-mediated reactions such as allograft rejection, delayed hypersensitivity, experimental allergic encephalomyelitis, Freund's adjuvant arthritis, and graft vs. host disease in many animal species for a variety of organs.

Successful kidney, liver, and heart allogeneic transplants have been performed in man using Sandimmune.

The exact mechanism of action of Sandimmune is not known. Experimental evidence suggests that the effectiveness of cyclosporine is due to specific and reversible inhibition of immunocompetent lymphocytes in the G_0- or G_1- phase of the cell cycle. T-lymphocytes are preferentially inhibited. The T-helper cell is the main target, although the T-suppressor cell may also be suppressed. Sandimmune also inhibits lymphokine production and release including interleukin-2 or T-cell growth factor (TCGF).

No functional effects on phagocytic (changes in enzyme secretions not altered, chemotactic migration of granulocytes, macrophage migration, carbon clearance *in vivo*) or tumor cells (growth rate, metastasis) can be detected in animals. Sandimmune does not cause bone marrow suppression in animal models or man.

The absorption of cyclosporine from the gastrointestinal tract is incomplete and variable. Peak concentrations (C_{max}) in blood and plasma are achieved at about 3.5 hours. C_{max} and area under the plasma or blood concentration/time curve (AUC) increase with the administered dose; for blood the relationship is curvilinear (parabolic) between 0 and 1400 mg. As determined by a specific assay, C_{max} is approximately 1.0 ng/ml/mg of dose for plasma and 2.7-1.4 ng/ml/mg of dose for blood (for low to high doses). Compared to an intravenous infusion, the absolute bioavailability of the oral solution is approximately 30% based upon the results in 2 patients. The bioavailability of Sandimmune soft gelatin capsules (cyclosporine capsules, USP) is equivalent to Sandimmune oral solution, (cyclosporine oral solution, USP).

CLINICAL PHARMACOLOGY: *(cont'd)*

Cyclosporine is distributed largely outside the blood volume. In blood the distribution is concentration dependent. Approximately 33%-47% is in plasma, 4%-9% in lymphocytes, 5%-12% in granulocytes, and 41%-58% in erythrocytes. At high concentrations, the uptake by leukocytes and erythrocytes becomes saturated. In plasma, approximately 90% is bound to proteins, primarily lipoproteins.

The disposition of cyclosporine from blood is biphasic with a terminal half-life of approximately 19 hours (range: 10-27 hours). Elimination is primarily biliary with only 6% of the dose excreted in the urine.

Cyclosporine is extensively metabolized but there is no major metabolic pathway. Only 0.1% of the dose is excreted in the urine as unchanged drug. Of 15 metabolites characterized in human urine, 9 have been assigned structures. The major pathways consist of hydroxylation of the Cγ-carbon of 2 of the leucine residues, C eta-carbon hydroxylation, and cyclic ether formation (with oxidation of the double bond) in the side chain of the amino acid 3-hydroxyl-*N*,4-dimethyl-L-2-amino-6-octenoic acid and *N*-demethylation of *N*-methyl leucine residues. Hydrolysis of the cyclic peptide chain or conjugation of the aforementioned metabolites do not appear to be important biotransformation pathways.

NEORAL

Cyclosporine is a potent immunosuppressive agent that in animals prolongs survival of allogeneic transplants involving skin, kidney, liver, heart, pancreas, bone marrow, small intestine, and lung. Cyclosporine has been demonstrated to suppress some humoral immunity and to a greater extent, cell-mediated immune reactions such as allograft rejection, delayed hypersensitivity, experimental allergic encephalomyelitis, Freund's adjuvant arthritis, and graft vs. host disease in many animal species for a variety of organs.

The effectiveness of cyclosporine results from specific and reversible inhibition of immunocompetent lymphocytes in the G_0- or G_1-phase of the cell cycle. T-lymphocytes are preferentially inhibited. The T-helper cell is the main target, although the T-suppressor cell may also be suppressed. Cyclosporine also inhibits lymphokine production and release including interleukin-2.

No effects on phagocytic function (changes in enzyme secretions, chemotactic migration of granulocytes, macrophage migration, carbon clearance *in vivo*) or tumor cells (growth rate, metastasis) have been detected in animals. Cyclosporine does not cause bone marrow suppression in animal models or man.

Pharmacokinetics: The immunosuppressive activity of cyclosporine is primarily due to parent drug. Following oral administration, absorption of cyclosporine is incomplete. The extent of absorption of cyclosporine is dependent on the individual patient, the patient population, and the formulation. Elimination of cyclosporine is primarily biliary with only 6% of the dose (parent drug and metabolites) excreted in urine. The disposition of cyclosporine from blood is generally biphasic, with a terminal half-life of approximately 8.4 hours (range 5 to 18 hours). Following intravenous administration, the blood clearance of cyclosporine (assay: HPLC) is approximately 5 to 7 ml/min/kg in adult recipients of renal or liver allografts. Blood cyclosporine clearance appears to be slightly slower in cardiac transplant patients.

The Neoral Soft Gelatin Capsules (cyclosporine capsules for microemulsion) and Neoral Oral Solution (cyclosporine oral solution for microemulsion) are bioequivalent.

The relationship between administered dose and exposure (area under the concentration versus time curve, AUC) is linear within the therapeutic dose range. The intersubject variability (total, %CV) of cyclosporine exposure (AUC) when Neoral or Sandimmune is administered ranges from approximately 20% to 50% in renal transplant patients. This intersubject variability contributes to the need for individualization of the dosing regimen for optimal therapy (see DOSAGE AND ADMINISTRATION.) Intrasubject variability of AUC in renal transplant recipients (%CV) was 9-21% for Neoral and 19-26% for Sandimmune. In the same studies, intrasubject variability of trough concentrations (%CV) was 17-30% for Neoral and 16- 38% for Sandimmune.

Absorption: Neoral has increased bioavailability compared to Sandimmune. The absolute bioavailability of cyclosporine administered as Sandimmune is dependent on the patient population, estimated to be less than 10% in liver transplant patients and as great as 89% in renal patients. The increased bioavailability of Neoral relative to Sandimmune varies across patient populations; however, the absolute bioavailability of cyclosporine administered as Neoral has not been determined in adults. In crossover studies where stable renal transplant patients received both Neoral and Sandimmune, the mean relative AUC of Neoral to Sandimmune ranged from 1.24 ± 0.34 to 1.51 ± 0.59. The dose normalized AUC in *de novo* renal transplant patients dosed with Neoral was 23% greater than in those patients dosed with Sandimmune. The dose normalized AUC in *de novo* liver transplant patients administered Neoral 28 days after transplantation was 50% greater than in those patients administered Sandimmune. The increase in AUC is accompanied by an increase in peak blood cyclosporine concentration (C_{max}) in the range of 40% to 106% in renal transplant patients and approximately 90% in liver transplant patients. AUC and C_{max} are also increased (Neoral relative to Sandimmune) in heart transplant patients, but data are very limited. Although the AUC and C_{max} values are higher on Neoral relative to Sandimmune, the pre-dose trough concentrations (dose-normalized) are similar for the two formulations.

Following oral administration of Neoral, the time to peak blood cyclosporine concentrations (T_{max}) ranged from 1.5 to 2.0 hours in renal transplant patients. The administration of food with Neoral decreases the AUC and C_{max} of cyclosporine. A high fat meal (669 kcal, 45 grams fat) consumed within one-half hour before Neoral administration decreased the AUC by 13% and C_{max} by 33%. The effects of a low fat meal (667 kcal, 15 grams fat) were similar.

The effects of T-tube diversion of bile on the absorption of cyclosporine from Neoral was investigated in eleven *de novo* liver transplant patients. When the patients were administered Neoral with and without T- tube diversion of bile, very little difference in absorption was observed, as measured by the change in maximal cyclosporine blood concentrations from pre-dose values with the T-tube closed relative to when it was open: $6.9 \pm 41\%$ (range -55% to 68%).

Distribution: Cyclosporine is distributed largely outside the blood volume. The steady state volume of distribution during intravenous dosing has been reported as 3-5 L/kg in solid organ transplant recipients. In blood, the distribution is concentration dependent. Approximately 33-47% is in plasma, 4-9% in lymphocytes, 5-12% in granulocytes, and 41-58% in erythrocytes. At high concentrations, the binding capacity of leukocytes and erythrocytes becomes saturated. In plasma, approximately 90% is bound to proteins, primarily lipoproteins. Cyclosporine is excreted in human milk. (See PRECAUTIONS.)

Metabolism: Cyclosporine is extensively metabolized by the cytochrome P-450 III-A enzyme system in the liver, and to a lesser degree in the gastrointestinal tract, and the kidney. At least 25 metabolites have been identified from human bile, feces, blood, and urine. The biological activity of the metabolites and their contributions to toxicity are considerably less than those of the parent compound. The major metabolites (M1, M9, and M4N) result from oxidation

CLINICAL PHARMACOLOGY: *(cont'd)*

TABLE 1 Pharmacokinetic Parameters in Adult Patients (mean ± SD)

Patient Population	Dose/day (mg/d)	Dose/weight (mg/kg/d)	AUC[1] (ng·hr/ml)	C_{max} (ng/ml)
[3]*De novo* renal transplant Week 4 (N=37)	597 ± 174	7.95 ± 2.81	8772 ± 2089	1802 ± 428
[3]Stable renal transplant (N=55)	344 ± 122	4.10 ± 1.58	6035 ± 2194	1333 ± 469
[4]*De novo* renal transplant Week 4 (N=18)	458 ± 190	6.89 ± 3.68	7187 ± 2816	1555 ± 740

Patient Population	Trough[2] (ng/ml)	Cl/F (ml/min)	Cl/F (ml/min/kg)
[3]*De novo* renal transplant Week 4 (N=37)	361 ± 129	593 ± 204	7.8 ± 2.9
[3]Stable (N=55)	251 ± 116	492 ± 140	5.9 ± 2.1
[4]*De novo* liver transplant Week 4 (N=18)	268 ± 101	577 ± 309	8.6 ± 5.7

[1]AUC was measured over one dosing interval
[2]Trough concentration was measured just prior to the morning Neoral dose, approximately 12 hours after the previous dose
[3]Assay: TDx specific monoclonal fluorescence polarization immunoassay
[4]Assay: Cyclo-trac specific monoclonal radioimmunoassay

at the 1-beta, 9-gamma, and 4-N-desmethylated positions, respectively. At steady state following the oral administration of Sandimmune, the mean AUCs for blood concentrations of M1, M9 and M4N are about 70%, 21%, and 7.5% of the AUC for blood cyclosporine concentrations, respectively. Based on blood concentration data from stable renal transplant patients (13 patients administered Neoral and Sandimmune in a crossover study), and bile concentration data from *de novo* liver transplant patients (4 administered Neoral, 3 administered Sandimmune), the percentage of dose present as M1, M9, and M4N metabolites is similar when either Neoral or Sandimmune is administered.

Excretion: Only 0.1% of a cyclosporine dose is excreted unchanged in the urine. Elimination is primarily biliary with only 6% of the dose (parent drug and metabolites) excreted in the urine. Neither dialysis nor renal failure alter cyclosporine clearance significantly.

Patient Population: Pharmacokinetic data from pediatric patients administered Neoral or Sandimmune are very limited. In 15 renal transplant patients aged 3-16 years, cyclosporine whole blood clearance after IV administration of Sandimmune was 10.6 ± 3.7 ml/min/kg (assay: Cyclo-trac specific RIA). In a study of 7 renal transplant patients aged 2-16, the cyclosporine clearance ranged from 9.8 to 15.5 ml/min/kg. In 9 liver transplant patients aged 0.6 to 5.6 years, clearance was 9.3 ± 5.4 ml/min/kg (assay: HPLC).

In the pediatric population, Neoral also demonstrates an increased bioavailability as compared to Sandimmune. In 7 liver *de novo* transplant patients aged 1.4 to 10 years, the absolute bioavailability of Neoral was 43% (range 30% to 68%) and for Sandimmune in the same individuals absolute bioavailability was 28% (range 17% to 42%).

TABLE 2 Pediatric Pharmacokinetic Parameters (mean ± SD)

Patient Population	Dose/day (mg/d)	Dose/Weight (mg/kg/d)	AUC[1] (ng·hr/ml)	C_{max} (ng/ml)
[2]Stable liver transplant				
Age 2-8, Dosed TID (N=9)	101 ± 25	5.95 ± 1.32	2163 ± 801	629 ± 219
Age 8-15, Dosed BID (N=8)	188 ± 55	4.96 ± 2.09	4272 ± 1462	975 ± 281
[3]Stable liver transplant				
Age 3, Dosed BID (N=1)	120	8.33	5832	1050
Age 8-15, Dosed BID (N=5)	158 ± 55	5.51 ± 1.91	4452 ± 2475	1013 ± 635
[3]Stable renal transplant Age 7-15, Dosed BID (N=5)	328 ± 83	7.37 ± 4.11	6922 ± 1988	1827 ± 487

Patient Population	Cl/F (ml/min)	Cl/F (ml/min/kg)
[2]Stable liver transplant		
Age 2-8, Dosed TID (N=9)	285 ± 94	16.6 ± 4.3
Age 8-15, Dosed BID (N=8)	378 ± 80	10.2 ± 4.0
[3]Stable liver transplant		
Age 3, Dosed BID (N=1)	171	11.9
Age 8-15, Dosed BID (N=5)	328 ± 121	11.0 ± 1.9
[3]Stable renal transplant Age 7-15, Dosed BID (N=5)	418 ± 143	8.7 ± 2.9

[1]AUC was measured over one dosing interval
[2]Assay: Cyclo-trac specific monoclonal radioimmunoassay
[3]Assay: TDx specific monoclonal fluorescence polarization immunoassay

INDICATIONS AND USAGE:

Sandimmune: Sandimmune is indicated for the prophylaxis of organ rejection in kidney, liver, and heart allogeneic transplants. It is always to be used with adrenal corticosteroids. The drug may also be used in the treatment of chronic rejection in patients previously treated with other immunosuppressive agents.

INDICATIONS AND USAGE: *(cont'd)*

Because of the risk of anaphylaxis, Sandimmune injection (cyclosporine concentrate for injection, USP) should be reserved for patients who are unable to take the soft gelatin capsules or oral solution.

Neoral: Neoral is indicated for the prophylaxis of organ rejection in kidney, liver, and heart allogeneic transplants. Neoral has been used in combination with azathioprine and corticosteroids.

CONTRAINDICATIONS:

Sandimmune: Sandimmune injection (cyclosporine concentrate for injection, USP) is contraindicated in patients with a hypersensitivity to Sandimmune and/or Cremophor EL (polyoxyethylated castor oil).

Neoral: Neoral is contraindicated in patients with a hypersensitivity to cyclosporine or to any of the ingredients of the formulation.

WARNINGS:

(See BOXED WARNING.) Sandimmune, when used in high doses, can cause hepatotoxicity and nephrotoxicity.

Cyclosporine, the active ingredient of Neoral, can cause nephrotoxicity and hepatotoxicity when used in high doses.

It is not unusual for serum creatinine and BUN levels to be elevated during cyclosporine therapy. These elevations in renal transplant patients do not necessarily indicate rejection, and each patient must be fully evaluated before dosage adjustment is initiated.

Based on the historical Sandimmune experience with oral solution, nephrotoxicity associated with cyclosporine had been noted in 25% of cases of renal transplantation, 38% of cases of cardiac transplantation, and 37% of cases of liver transplantation. Mild nephrotoxicity was generally noted 2-3 months after renal transplant and consisted of an arrest in the fall of the pre-operative elevations of BUN and creatinine at a range of 35-45 mg/dl and 2.0-2.5 mg/dl respectively. These elevations were often responsive to cyclosporine dosage reduction.

More overt nephrotoxicity was seen early after transplantation and was characterized by a rapidly rising BUN and creatinine. Since these events are similar to renal rejection episodes, care must be taken to differentiate between them. This form of nephrotoxicity is usually responsive to cyclosporine dosage reduction.

Although specific diagnostic criteria which reliably differentiate renal graft rejection from drug toxicity have not been found, a number of parameters have been significantly associated with one or the other. It should be noted however, that up to 20% of patients may have simultaneous nephrotoxicity and rejection.

TABLE 3

Nephrotoxicity vs Rejection Parameter/Nephrotoxicity	Rejection
History	
Donor >50 years old or hypotensive	Antidonor immune response
Prolonged kidney preservation	Retransplant patient
Prolonged anastomosis time	
Concomitant nephrotoxic drugs	
Clinical	
Often >6 weeks postop[b]	Often <4 weeks postop[b]
Prolonged initial nonfunction (acute tubular necrosis)	Fever >37.5°C
	Weight gain >0.5 kg
	Graft swelling and tenderness
	Decrease in daily urine volume >500 ml (or 50%)
Laboratory	
CyA serum trough level >200 ng/ml	CyA serum trough level <150 ng/ml
Gradual rise in Cr (<0.15 mg/dl/day)[a]	Rapid rise in Cr (>0.3 mg/dl/day)[a]
Cr plateau <25% above baseline	Cr >25% above baseline
BUN/Cr ≥20	BUN/Cr <20
Biopsy	
Arteriolopathy (medial hypertrophy[a], hyalinosis, nodular deposits, intimal thickening, endothelial vacuolization, progressive scarring)	Endovasculitis[c] (proliferation[a], intimal arteritis[b], necrosis, sclerosis)
Tubular atrophy, isometric vacuolization, isolated calcifications	Tubulitis with RBC[b] and WBC[b] casts, some irregular vacuolization
Minimal edema	Interstitial edema[c] and hemorrhage[b]
Mild focal infiltrates[c]	Diffuse moderate to severe mononuclear infiltrates[d]
Diffuse interstitial fibrosis, often striped form	Glomerulitis (mononuclear cells)[c]
Aspiration Cytology	
CyA deposits in tubular and endothelial cells	Inflammatory infiltrate with mononuclear phagocytes, macrophages, lymphoblastoid cells, and activated T-cells
Fine isometric vacuolization of tubular cells	These strongly express HLA-DR antigens
Urine Cytology	
Tubular cells with vacuolization and granularization	Degenerative tubular cells, plasma cells, and lymphocyturia >20% of sediment
Manometry	
Intracapsular pressure <40 mm Hg[b]	Intracapsular pressure >40 mm Hg[b]
Ultrasonography	
Unchanged graft cross sectional area	Increase in graft cross sectional area AP diameter ≥Transverse diameter
Magnetic Resonance Imagery	
Normal appearance	Loss of distinct cortionmedullary junction, swelling imge intensity of parachyma approaching that of psoas, loss of hilar fat
Radionuclide	
Normal or generally decreased perfusion	Patchy arterial flow
Scan	
Decrease in tubular function	Decrease in perfusion >decrease in tubular function
(^{131}I-hippuran)> decrease in perfusion (^{99m}Tc DTPA)	Increased uptake of Indium 111 labeled platelets or Tc-99m in colloid
Therapy	
Responds to decreased Sandimmune (cyclosporine)	Responds to increased steroids or antilymphocyte globulin

a p <0.05
b p <0.01
c p <0.001
d p <0.0001

WARNINGS: *(cont'd)*

SANDIMMUNE

A form of chronic progressive cyclosporine-associated nephrotoxicity is characterized by serial deterioration in renal function and morphologic changes in the kidneys. From 5%-15% of transplant recipients will fail to show a reduction in a rising serum creatinine despite a decrease or discontinuation of cyclosporine therapy. Renal biopsies from these patients will demonstrate an interstitial fibrosis with tubular atrophy. In addition, toxic tubulopathy, peritubular capillary congestion, arteriolopathy, and a striped form of interstitial fibrosis with tubular atrophy may be present. Though none of these morphologic changes is entirely specific, a histologic diagnosis of chronic progressive cyclosporine-associated nephrotoxicity requires evidence of these.

When considering the development of chronic nephrotoxicity it is noteworthy that several authors have reported an association between the appearance of interstitial fibrosis and higher cumulative doses or persistently high circulating trough levels of cyclosporine. This is particularly true during the first 6 post-transplant months when the dosage tends to be highest and when, in kidney recipients, the organ appears to be most vulnerable to the toxic effects of cyclosporine. Among other contributing factors to the development of interstitial fibrosis in these patients must be included, prolonged perfusion time, warm ischemia time, as well as episodes of acute toxicity, and acute and chronic rejection. The reversibility of interstitial fibrosis and its correlation to renal function have not yet been determined.

Impaired renal function at any time requires close monitoring, and frequent dosage adjustment may be indicated. In patients with persistent high elevations of BUN and creatinine who are unresponsive to dosage adjustments, consideration should be given to switching to other immunosuppressive therapy. In the event of severe and unremitting rejection, it is preferable to allow the kidney transplant to be rejected and removed rather than increase the Sandimmune dosage to a very high level in an attempt to reverse the rejection.

Occasionally patients have developed a syndrome of thrombocytopenia and microangiopathic hemolytic anemia which may result in graft failure. The vasculopathy can occur in the absence of rejection and is accompanied by avid platelet consumption within the graft as demonstrated by Indium 111 labeled platelet studies. Neither the pathogenesis nor the management of this syndrome is clear. Though resolution has occurred after reduction or discontinuation of Sandimmune and 1) administration of streptokinase and heparin or 2) plasmapheresis, this appears to depend upon early detection with Indium 111 labeled platelet scans. (See ADVERSE REACTIONS.)

Significant hyperkalemia (sometimes associated with hyperchloremic metabolic acidosis) and hyperuricemia have been seen occasionally in individual patients.

Hepatotoxicity has been noted in 4% of cases of renal transplantation, 7% of cases of cardiac transplantation, and 4% of cases of liver transplantation. This was usually noted during the first month of therapy when high doses of Sandimmune were used and consisted of elevations of hepatic enzymes and bilirubin. The chemistry elevations usually decreased with a reduction in dosage.

As in patients receiving other immunosuppressants, those patients receiving Sandimmune are at increased risk for development of lymphomas and other malignancies, particularly those of the skin. The increased risk appears related to the intensity and duration of immunosuppression rather than to the use of specific agents. Because of the danger of oversuppression of the immune system, which can also increase susceptibility to infection, Sandimmune should not be administered with other immunosuppressive agents except adrenal corticosteroids. The efficacy and safety of cyclosporine in combination with other immunosuppressive agents have not been determined.

There have been reports of convulsions in adult and pediatric patients receiving cyclosporine, particularly in combination with high dose methylprednisolone.

Rarely (approximately 1 in 1000), patients receiving Sandimmune injection (cyclosporine concentrate for injection, USP) have experienced anaphylactic reactions. Although the exact cause of these reactions is unknown, it is believed to be due to the Cremophor EL (polyoxyethylated castor oil) used as the vehicle for the IV formulation. These reactions have consisted of flushing of the face and upper thorax, acute respiratory distress with dyspnea and wheezing, blood pressure changes, and tachycardia. One patient died after respiratory arrest and aspiration pneumonia. In some cases, the reaction subsided after the infusion was stopped.

Patients receiving Sandimmune injection (cyclosporine concentrate for Injection, USP) should be under continuous observation for at least the first 30 minutes following the start of the infusion and at frequent intervals thereafter. If anaphylaxis occurs, the infusion should be stopped. An aqueous solution of epinephrine 1:1000 should be available at the bedside as well as a source of oxygen.

Anaphylactic reactions have not been reported with the soft gelatin capsules or oral solution which lack Cremophor EL (polyoxyethylated castor oil). In fact, patients experiencing anaphylactic reactions have been treated subsequently with the soft gelatin capsules or oral solution without incident.

Care should be taken in using Sandimmune with nephrotoxic drugs. (See PRECAUTIONS.)

NEORAL

A form of a cyclosporine-associated nephropathy is characterized by serial deterioration in renal function and morphologic changes in the kidneys. From 5% to 15% of transplant recipients who have received cyclosporine will fail to show a reduction in rising serum creatinine despite a decrease or discontinuation of cyclosporine therapy. Renal biopsies from these patients will demonstrate one or several of the following alterations: tubular vacuolization, tubular microcalcifications, peritubular capillary congestion, arteriolopathy, and a striped form of interstitial fibrosis with tubular atrophy. Though none of these morphologic changes is entirely specific, a diagnosis of cyclosporine-associated structural nephrotoxicity requires evidence of these findings.

When considering the development of cyclosporine-associated nephropathy, it is noteworthy that several authors have reported an association between the appearance of interstitial fibrosis and higher cumulative doses or persistently high circulating trough levels of cyclosporine. This is particularly true during the first 6 posttransplant months when the dosage tends to be highest and when, in kidney recipients, the organ appears to be most vulnerable to the toxic effects of cyclosporine. Among other contributing factors to the development of interstitial fibrosis in these patients are prolonged perfusion time, warm ischemia time, as well as episodes of acute toxicity, and acute and chronic rejection. The reversibility of interstitial fibrosis and its correlation to renal function have not yet been determined. Reversibility of arteriolopathy has been reported after stopping cyclosporine or lowering the dosage.

Impaired renal function at any time requires close monitoring, and frequent dosage adjustment may be indicated.

In the event of severe and unremitting rejection, when rescue therapy with pulse steroids and monoclonal antibodies fail to reverse the rejection episode, it may be preferable to switch to alternative immunosuppressive therapy rather than increase the Neoral dose to excessive levels.

Occasionally patients have developed a syndrome of thrombocytopenia and microangiopathic hemolytic anemia which may result in graft failure. The vasculopathy can occur in the absence of rejection and is accompanied by avid platelet consumption within the graft as

WARNINGS: *(cont'd)*

demonstrated by Indium 111 labeled platelet studies. Neither the pathogenesis nor the management of this syndrome is clear. Though resolution has occurred after reduction or discontinuation of cyclosporine and 1) administration of streptokinase and heparin or 2) plasmapheresis, this appears to depend upon early detection with Indium 111 labeled platelet scans. (See ADVERSE REACTIONS.)

Significant hyperkalemia (sometimes associated with hyperchloremic metabolic acidosis) and hyperuricemia have been seen occasionally in individual patients.

Hepatotoxicity associated with cyclosporine use had been noted in 4% of cases of renal transplantation, 7% of cases of cardiac transplantation, and 4% of cases of liver transplantation. This was usually noted during the first month of therapy when high doses of cyclosporine were used and consisted of elevations of hepatic enzymes and bilirubin. The chemistry elevations usually decreased with a reduction in dosage.

As in patients receiving other immunosuppressants, those patients receiving cyclosporine are at increased risk for development of lymphomas and other malignancies, particularly those of the skin. The increased risk appears related to the intensity and duration of immunosuppression rather than to the use of specific agents. Because of the danger of oversuppression of the immune system resulting in increased risk of infection or malignancy, a treatment regimen containing multiple immunosuppressants should be used with caution.

There have been reports of convulsions in adult and pediatric patients receiving cyclosporine, particularly in combination with high dose methylprednisolone.

Care should be taken in using cyclosporine with nephrotoxic drugs. (See PRECAUTIONS.)

Because Neoral is not bioequivalent to Sandimmune, conversion from Neoral to Sandimmune using a 1:1 ratio (mg/kg/day) may result in lower cyclosporine blood concentrations. Conversion from Neoral to Sandimmune should be made with increased monitoring to avoid the potential of underdosing.

PRECAUTIONS:

SANDIMMUNE

General: Patients with malabsorption may have difficulty in achieving therapeutic levels with Sandimmune soft gelatin capsules or oral solution.

Hypertension is a common side effect of Sandimmune therapy. (See ADVERSE REACTIONS.) Mild or moderate hypertension is more frequently encountered than severe hypertension and the incidence decreases over time. Antihypertensive therapy may be required. Control of blood pressure can be accomplished with any of the common antihypertensive agents. However, since cyclosporine may cause hyperkalemia, potassium-sparing diuretics should not be used. While calcium antagonists can be effective agents in treating cyclosporine-associated hypertension, care should be taken since interference with cyclosporine metabolism may require a dosage adjustment. (See DRUG INTERACTIONS.)

During treatment with Sandimmune, vaccination may be less effective; and the use of live attenuated vaccines should be avoided.

Information for Patients: Patients should be informed of the necessity of repeated laboratory tests while they are receiving the drug. They should be given careful dosage instructions, advised of the potential risks during pregnancy, and informed of the increased risk of neoplasia.

Laboratory Tests: Renal and liver functions should be assessed repeatedly by measurement of BUN, serum creatinine, serum bilirubin, and liver enzymes.

Carcinogenesis, Mutagenesis, and Impairment of Fertility: Cyclosporine gave no evidence of mutagenic or teratogenic effects in appropriate test systems. Only at dose levels toxic to dams, were adverse effects seen in reproduction studies in rats. (See Pregnancy.)

Carcinogenicity studies were carried out in male and female rats and mice. In the 78-week mouse study, at doses of 1, 4, and 16 mg/kg/day, evidence of a statistically significant trend was found for lymphocytic lymphomas in females, and the incidence of hepatocellular carcinomas in mid-dose males significantly exceeded the control value. In the 24-month rat study, conducted at 0.5, 2, and 8 mg/kg/day, pancreatic islet cell adenomas significantly exceeded the control rate in the low dose level. The hepatocellular carcinomas and pancreatic islet cell adenomas were not dose related.

No impairment in fertility was demonstrated in studies in male and female rats.

Cyclosporine has not been found mutagenic/genotoxic in the Ames Test, the V79-HGPRT Test, the micronucleus test in mice and Chinese hamsters, the chromosome-aberration tests in Chinese hamster bone-marrow, the mouse dominant lethal assay, and the DNA-repair test in sperm from treated mice. A recent study analyzing sister chromatid exchange (SCE) induction by cyclosporine using human lymphocytes *in vitro* gave indication of a positive effect (*i.e.,* induction of SCE), at high concentrations in this system.

An increased incidence of malignancy is a recognized complication of immunosuppression in recipients of organ transplants. The most common forms of neoplasms are non-Hodgkin's lymphoma and carcinomas of the skin. The risk of malignancies in cyclosporine recipients is higher than in the normal, healthy population but similar to that in patients receiving other immunosuppressive therapies. It has been reported that reduction or discontinuance of immunosuppression may cause the lesions to regress.

Pregnancy Category C: Sandimmune oral solution (cyclosporine oral solution, USP) has been shown to be embryo- and fetotoxic in rats and rabbits when given in doses 2-5 times the human dose. At toxic doses (rats at 30 mg/kg/day and rabbits at 100 mg/kg/day), Sandimmune oral solution (cyclosporine oral solution, USP) was embryo- and fetotoxic as indicated by increased pre- and postnatal mortality and reduced fetal weight together with related skeletal retardations. In the well-tolerated dose range (rats at up to 17 mg/kg/day and rabbits at up to 30 mg/kg/day), Sandimmune oral solution (cyclosporine oral solution, USP) proved to be without any embryolethal or teratogenic effects.

There are no adequate and well-controlled studies in pregnant women. Sandimmune should be used during pregnancy only if the potential benefit justifies the potential risk to the fetus.

The following data represent the reported outcomes of 116 pregnancies in women receiving Sandimmune during pregnancy, 90% of whom were transplant patients, and most of whom received Sandimmune throughout the entire gestational period. Since most of the patients were not prospectively identified, the results are likely to be biased toward negative outcomes. The only consistent patterns of abnormality were premature birth (gestational period of 28 to 36 weeks) and low birth weight for gestational age. It is not possible to separate the effects of Sandimmune on these pregnancies from the effects of the other immunosuppressants, the underlying maternal disorders, or other aspects of the transplantation milieu. Sixteen fetal losses occurred. Most of the pregnancies (85 of 100) were complicated by disorders; including, pre-eclampsia, eclampsia, premature labor, abruptio placentae, oligohydramnios, Rh incompatibility and fetoplacental dysfunction. Preterm delivery occurred in 47%. Seven malformations were reported in 5 viable infants and in 2 cases of fetal loss. Twenty-eight percent of the infants were small for gestational age. Neonatal complications occurred in 27%. In a report of 23 children followed up to 4 years, postnatal development was said to be normal. More information on cyclosporine use in pregnancy is available from Sandoz Pharmaceuticals Corporation.

Nursing Mothers: Since Sandimmune is excreted in human milk, nursing should be avoided.

PRECAUTIONS: *(cont'd)*

Pediatric Use: Although no adequate and well controlled studies have been conducted in children, patients as young as 6 months of age have received the drug with no unusual adverse effects.

NEORAL

General: Cyclosporine is the active ingredient of Neoral. Hypertension is a common side effect of cyclosporine therapy. (See ADVERSE REACTIONS.) Mild or moderate hypertension is encountered more frequently than severe hypertension and the incidence decreases over time. Antihypertensive therapy may be required. Control of blood pressure can be accomplished with any of the common antihypertensive agents. However, since cyclosporine may cause hyperkalemia, potassium-sparing diuretics should not be used. Calcium antagonists can be effective agents in treating cyclosporine-associated hypertension. However, care should be taken since interference with cyclosporine metabolism may require a dosage adjustment. (See DRUG INTERACTIONS.)

During treatment with cyclosporine, vaccination may be less effective; and the use of live attenuated vaccines should be avoided.

Information for the Patient: Patients should be advised that any change of cyclosporine formulation should be made cautiously and only under physician supervision because it may result in the need for a change in dosage.

Patients should be informed of the necessity of repeated laboratory tests while they are receiving the drug. Patients should be advised of the potential risks during pregnancy and informed of the increased risk of neoplasia.

Patients should be given careful dosage instructions. Neoral Oral Solution (cyclosporine oral solution for microemulsion) should be diluted, preferably with orange or apple juice that is at room temperature. Grapefruit and grapefruit juice affect metabolism of cyclosporine and should be avoided. The combination of Neoral Oral Solution (cyclosporine oral solution for microemulsion) with milk can be unpalatable.

Patients should be advised to take Neoral on a consistent schedule with regard to time of day and relation to meals.

Laboratory Tests: Renal and liver functions should be assessed repeatedly by measurement of BUN, serum creatinine, serum bilirubin, and liver enzymes.

Carcinogenesis, Mutagenesis, and Impairment of Fertility: Cyclosporine gave no evidence of mutagenic or teratogenic effects in appropriate test systems. Only at dose levels toxic to dams, were adverse effects seen in reproduction studies in rats. (See Pregnancy.)

Carcinogenicity studies were carried out in male and female rats and mice. In the 78-week mouse study, evidence of a statistically significant trend was found for lymphocytic lymphomas in females, and the incidence of hepatocellular carcinomas in mid-dose males significantly exceeded the control value. In the 24-month rat study, pancreatic islet cell adenomas significantly exceeded the control rate in the low dose level. Doses used in the mouse and rat studies were 0.01 to 0.16 times the clinical maintenance dose. The hepatocellular carcinomas and pancreatic islet cell adenomas were not dose related.

No impairment in fertility was demonstrated in studies in male and female rats.

Cyclosporine has not been found to be mutagenic/genotoxic in the Ames Test, the V79-HGPRT Test, the micronucleus test in mice and Chinese hamsters, the chromosome-aberration tests in Chinese hamster bone-marrow, the mouse dominant lethal assay, and the DNA-repair test in sperm from treated mice. A recent study analyzing sister chromatid exchange (SCE) induction by cyclosporine using human lymphocytes *in vitro* gave indication of a positive effect (*i.e.,* induction of SCE), at high concentrations in this system.

An increased incidence of malignancy is a recognized complication of immunosuppression in recipients of organ transplants. The most common forms of neoplasms are non-Hodgkin's lymphoma and carcinomas of the skin. The risk of malignancies in cyclosporine recipients is higher than in the normal, healthy population but similar to that in patients receiving other immunosuppressive therapies. Reduction or discontinuance of immunosuppression may cause the lesions to regress.

Pregnancy Category C: Cyclosporine has been shown to be embryo- and fetotoxic in rats and rabbits following oral administration at maternally toxic doses. Fetal toxicity was noted in rats at 0.8 and rabbits at 5.4 times the human maintenance dose of 6.0 mg/kg, where dose corrections are based on body surface area. Cyclosporine was embryo- and fetotoxic as indicated by increased pre- and postnatal mortality and reduced fetal weight together with related skeletal retardations.

There are no adequate and well-controlled studies in pregnant women. Neoral should be used during pregnancy only if the potential benefit justifies the potential risk to the fetus.

The following data represent the reported outcomes of 116 pregnancies in women receiving cyclosporine during pregnancy, 90% of whom were transplant patients, and most of whom received cyclosporine throughout the entire gestational period. The only consistent patterns of abnormality were premature birth (gestational period of 28 to 36 weeks) and low birth weight for gestational age. Sixteen fetal losses occurred. Most of the pregnancies (85 of 100) were complicated by disorders, including pre-eclampsia, eclampsia, premature labor, abruptio placentae, oligohydramnios, Rh incompatibility and fetoplacental dysfunction. Preterm delivery occurred in 47%. Seven malformations were reported in 5 viable infants and in 2 cases of fetal loss. Twenty-eight percent of the infants were small for gestational age. Neonatal complications occurred in 27%. Therefore, the risks and benefits of using Neoral during pregnancy should be carefully weighed.

Nursing Mothers: Since cyclosporine is excreted in human milk, nursing should be avoided.

Pediatric Use: Although no adequate and well controlled studies have been completed in children, patients as young as one year of age have received Neoral with no unusual adverse effects.

DRUG INTERACTIONS:

SANDIMMUNE

All of the individual drugs cited below (TABLE 4) are well substantiated to interact with Sandimmune.

Drugs That Exhibit Nephrotoxic Synergy

gentamicin	cimetidine
tobramycin	ranitidine
vancomycin	diclofenac
amphotericin B	trimethoprim with sulfamethoxazole
ketoconazole	azapropazon
melphalan	

Careful monitoring of renal function should be practiced when Sandimmune is used with nephrotoxic drugs.

Drugs That Alter Cyclosporine Levels: Cyclosporine is extensively metabolized by the liver. Therefore, circulating cyclosporine levels may be influenced by drugs that affect hepatic microsomal enzymes, particularly the cytochrome P-450 system. Substances known to inhibit these enzymes will decrease hepatic metabolism and increase cyclosporine levels. Substances that are inducers of cytochrome P-450 activity will increase hepatic metabolism and decrease cyclosporine levels. Monitoring of circulating cyclosporine levels and appropriate Sandimmune dosage adjustment are essential when these drugs are used concomitantly (see Blood Level Monitoring.)

DRUG INTERACTIONS: *(cont'd)*

Drugs That Increase Cyclosporine Levels

diltiazem	danazol
nicardipine	bromocriptine
verapamil	metoclopramide
ketoconazole	erythromycin
fluconazole	methylprednisolone
itraconazole	

Other Drug Interactions: Reduced clearance of prednisolone, digoxin, and lovastatin have been observed when these drugs are administered with Sandimmune. In addition, a decrease in the apparent volume of distribution of digoxin has been reported after Sandimmune administration. Severe digitalis toxicity has been seen within days of starting cyclosporine in several patients taking digoxin. Sandimmune should not be used with potassium-sparing diuretics because hyperkalemia can occur. During treatment with Sandimmune, vaccination may be less effective; and the use of live vaccines should be avoided. Myositis has occurred with concomitant lovastatin, frequent gingival hyperplasia with nifedipine, and convulsions with high dose methylprednisolone. Further information on drugs that have been reported to interact with Sandimmune is available from Sandoz Pharmaceuticals Corporation.

NEORAL

All of the individual drugs cited below (TABLE 6) are well substantiated to interact with cyclosporine.

Drugs That May Potentiate Renal Dysfunction

Antibiotics: gentamicin, tobramycin, vancomycin, trimethoprim with sulfamethoxazole.

Antineoplastics: melphalan.

Antifungals: amphotericin B, ketoconazole.

Anti-inflammatory Drugs: azapropazon, diclofenac.

Gastrointestinal Agents: cimetidine, ranitidine.

Immunosuppressives: tracolimus.

Careful monitoring of renal function should be practiced when Neoral is used with nephrotoxic drugs.

Drugs That Alter Cyclosporine Levels: Cyclosporine is extensively metabolized. Cyclosporine concentrations may be influenced by drugs that affect microsomal enzymes, particularly cytochrome P-450 III-A. Substances that inhibit this enzyme could decrease metabolism and increase cyclosporine concentrations. Substances that are inducers of cytochrome P-450 activity could increase metabolism and decrease cyclosporine concentrations. Monitoring of circulating cyclosporine concentrations and appropriate Neoral dosage adjustment are essential when these drugs are used concomitantly. (See Blood Concentration Monitoring.)

Drugs That Increase Cyclosporine Concentrations

Calcium Channel Blockers: diltiazem, nicardipine, verapamil

Antifungals: fluconazole, itraconazole, ketoconazole

Antibiotics: clarithromycin, erythromycin

Glucocorticoids: methylprednisolone

Other Drugs: allopurinol, bromocriptine, danazol, metoclopramide

Drugs That Decrease Cyclosporine Concentrations

Antibiotics: nafcillin, rifampin

Anticonvulsants: carbamazepine, phenobarbital, phenytoin

Other Drugs: octreotide, ticlopidine

Rifabutin is known to increase the metabolism of other drugs metabolized by the cytochrome P-450 system. The interaction between rifabutin and cyclosporine has not been studied. Care should be exercised when these two drugs are administered concomitantly.

Other Drug Interactions: Reduced clearance of prednisolone, digoxin, and lovastatin have been observed when these drugs are administered with cyclosporine. In addition, a decrease in the apparent volume of distribution of digoxin has been reported after cyclosporine administration. Severe digitalis toxicity has been seen within days of starting cyclosporine in several patients taking digoxin. Cyclosporine should not be used with potassium-sparing diuretics because hyperkalemia can occur. During treatment with cyclosporine, vaccination may be less effective. The use of live vaccines should be avoided. Myositis has occurred with concomitant lovastatin, frequent gingival hyperplasia with nifedipine, and convulsions with high dose methylprednisolone. Further information on drugs that have been reported to interact with cyclosporine is available from Sandoz Pharmaceuticals Corporation.

ADVERSE REACTIONS:

The principal adverse reactions of cyclosporine therapy are renal dysfunction, tremor, hirsutism, hypertension, and gum hyperplasia.

Hypertension, which is usually mild to moderate, may occur in approximately 50% of patients following renal transplantation and in most cardiac transplant patients.

Glomerular capillary thrombosis has been found in patients treated with cyclosporine and may progress to graft failure. The pathologic changes resemble those seen in the hemolytic-uremic syndrome and include thrombosis of the renal microvasculature, with platelet-fibrin thrombi occluding glomerular capillaries and afferent arterioles, microangiopathic hemolytic anemia, thrombocytopenia, and decreased renal function. Similar findings have been observed when other immunosuppressives have been employed posttransplantation.

Hypomagnesemia has been reported in some, but not all, patients exhibiting convulsions while on cyclosporine therapy. Although magnesium-depletion studies in normal subjects suggest that hypomagnesemia is associated with neurologic disorders, multiple factors, including hypertension, high dose methylprednisolone, hypocholesterolemia, and nephrotoxicity associated with high plasma concentrations of cyclosporine appear to be related to the neurological manifestations of cyclosporine toxicity.

NEORAL

In controlled studies, the nature, severity and incidence of the adverse events that were observed in 493 transplanted patients treated with Neoral were comparable with those observed in 208 transplanted patients who received Sandimmune in these same studies when the dosage of the two drugs was adjusted to achieve the same cyclosporine blood trough concentrations.

SANDIMMUNE AND NEORAL

Based on the historical experience with Sandimmune, the following reactions occurred in 3% or greater of 892 patients involved in clinical trials of kidney, heart, and liver transplants.

The following reactions occurred in 2% or less of Sandimmune-treated patients: allergic reactions, anemia, anorexia, confusion, conjunctivitis, edema, fever, brittle fingernails, gastritis, hearing loss, hiccups, hyperglycemia, muscle pain, peptic ulcer, thrombocytopenia, tinnitus.

The following reactions occurred rarely: anxiety, chest pain, constipation, depression, hair breaking, hematuria, joint pain, lethargy, mouth sores, myocardial infarction, night sweats, pancreatitis, pruritus, swallowing difficulty, tingling, upper GI bleeding, visual disturbance, weakness, weight loss.

ADVERSE REACTIONS: *(cont'd)*

TABLE 4

Body System/ Adverse Reactions	Randomized Kidney Patients: Sandimmune N=227 %	Randomized Kidney Patients: Azathioprine N=228 %	Cyclosporine Patients: Kidney N=705 %	Cyclosporine Patients: Heart N=112 %	Cyclosporine Patients: Liver N=75 %
Genitourinary					
Renal Dysfunction	32	6	25	38	37
Cardiovascular					
Hypertension	26	18	13	53	27
Cramps	4	<1	2	<1	0
Skin					
Hirsutism	21	<1	21	28	45
Acne	6	8	2	2	1
Central Nervous System					
Tremor	12	0	21	31	55
Convulsions	3	1	1	4	5
Headache	2	<1	2	15	4
Gastrointestinal					
Gum Hyperplasia	4	0	9	5	16
Diarrhea	3	<1	3	4	8
Nausea/Vomiting	2	<1	4	10	4
Hepatotoxicity	<1	<1	4	7	4
Abdominal Discomfort	<1	0	<1	7	0
Autonomic Nervous System					
Paresthesia	3	0	1	2	1
Flushing	<1	0	4	0	4
Hematopoietic					
Leukopenia	2	19	<1	6	0
Lymphoma	<1	0	1	6	1
Respiratory					
Sinusitis	<1	0	4	3	7
Miscellaneous					
Gynecomastia	<1	0	<1	4	3

Among 705 kidney transplant patients treated with cyclosporine oral solution (Sandimmune in clinical trials, the reason for treatment discontinuation was renal toxicity in 5.4%, infection in 0.9%, lack of efficacy in 1.4%, acute tubular necrosis in 1.0%, lymphoproliferative disorders in 0.3%, hypertension in 0.3%, and other reasons in 0.7%.

TABLE 5 Renal Transplant Patients in Whom Therapy Was Discontinued

Reason for Discontinuation	Randomized Patients Sandimmune (N=227) %	Azathioprine (N=228) %	All Sandimmune Patients (N=705) %
Renal Toxicity	5.7	0	5.4
Infection	0	0.4	0.9
Lack of Efficacy	2.6	0.9	1.4
Acute Tubular Necrosis	2.6	0	1.0
Lymphoma/ Lymphoproliferative Disease	0.4	0	0.3
Hypertension	0	0	0.3
Hematological Abnormalities	0	0.4	0
Other	0	0	0.7

Sandimmune was discontinued on a temporary basis and then restarted in 18 additional patients.

TABLE 6 Infectious Complications in Historical Randomized Studies in Renal Transplant Patients Using Sandimmune

Cyclosporine Treatment / Complication	Azathioprine with Steroids* (N=227) % of Complications	(N=228) % of Complications
Septicemia	5.3	4.8
Abscesses	4.4	5.3
Systemic Fungal Infection	2.2	3.9
Local Fungal Infection	7.5	9.6
Cytomegalovirus	4.8	12.3
Other Viral Infections	15.9	18.4
Urinary Tract Infections	21.1	20.2
Wound and Skin Infections	7.0	10.1
Pneumonia	6.2	9.2

* Some patients also received ALG.

SANDIMMUNE

Cremophor EL (polyoxyethylated castor oil) is known to cause hyperlipemia and electrophoretic abnormalities of lipoproteins. These effects are reversible upon discontinuation of treatment but are usually not a reason to stop treatment.

OVERDOSAGE:

SANDIMMUNE

There is a minimal experience with overdosage. Because of the slow absorption of Sandimmune soft gelatin capsules or oral solution, forced emesis would be of value up to 2 hours after administration. Transient hepatotoxicity and nephrotoxicity may occur which should resolve following drug withdrawal. General supportive measures and symptomatic treatment should be followed in all cases of overdosage. Sandimmune is not dialyzable to any great extent, nor is it cleared well by charcoal hemoperfusion. The oral LD_{50} is 2329 mg/kg in mice, 1480 mg/kg in rats, and >1000 mg/kg in rabbits. The IV LD_{50} is 148 mg/kg in mice, 104 mg/kg in rats, and 46 mg/kg in rabbits.

NEORAL

There is a minimal experience with cyclosporine overdosage. Forced emesis can be of value up to 2 hours after administration of Neoral. Transient hepatotoxicity and nephrotoxicity may occur which should resolve following drug withdrawal. General supportive measures and symptomatic treatment should be followed in all cases of overdosage. Cyclosporine is not dialyzable to any great extent, nor is it cleared well by charcoal hemoperfusion. The oral dosage at which half of experimental animals are estimated to die is 31 times, 39 times and >54 times the human maintenance dose (6 mg/kg; corrections based on body surface area) in mice, rats, and rabbits.

DOSAGE AND ADMINISTRATION:

SANDIMMUNE

Sandimmune Soft Gelatin Capsules (cyclosporine capsules, USP) and Sandimmune Oral Solution (cyclosporine oral solution, USP)

The initial oral dose of Sandimmune should be given 4-12 hours prior to transplantation as a single dose of 15 mg/kg. Although a daily single dose of 14-18 mg/kg was used in most clinical trials, few centers continue to use the highest dose, most favoring the lower end of the scale. There is a trend towards use of even lower initial doses for renal transplantation in the ranges of 10-14 mg/kg/day. The initial single daily dose is continued postoperatively for 1-2 weeks and then tapered by 5% per week to a maintenance dose of 5-10 mg/kg/day. Some centers have successfully tapered the maintenance dose to as low as 3 mg/kg/day in selected *renal* transplant patients without an apparent rise in rejection rate. (See Blood Level Monitoring.)

In pediatric usage, the same dose and dosing regimen may be used as in adults although in several studies children have required and tolerated higher doses than those used in adults.

Adjunct therapy with adrenal corticosteroids is recommended. Different tapering dosage schedules of prednisone appear to achieve similar results. A dosage schedule based on the patient's weight started with 2.0 mg/kg/day for the first 4 days tapered to 1.0 mg/kg/day by 1 week, 0.6 mg/kg/day by 2 weeks, 0.3 mg/kg/day by 1 month, and 0.15 mg/kg/day by 2 months and thereafter as a maintenance dose. Another center started with an initial dose of 200 mg tapered by 40 mg/day until reaching 20 mg/day. After 2 months at this dose, a further reduction to 10 mg/day was made. Adjustments in dosage of prednisone must be made according to the clinical situation.

To make Sandimmune oral solution (cyclosporine oral solution, USP) more palatable, the oral solution may be diluted with milk, chocolate milk, or orange juice preferably at room temperature. Patients should avoid switching diluents frequently. Sandimmune soft gelatin capsules and oral solution should be administered on a consistent schedule with regard to time of day and relation to meals.

Take the prescribed amount of Sandimmune from the container using the dosage syringe supplied. Transfer the solution to a glass of milk, chocolate milk, or orange juice. Stir well and drink at once. Do not allow to stand before drinking. It is best to use a glass container and rinse it with more diluent to ensure that the total dose is taken. After use, replace the dosage syringe in the protective cover. To avoid cloudiness, do not rinse the dosage syringe with water or other cleaning agents. If the dosage syringe requires cleaning, it must be completely dry before resuming use.

SANDIMMUNE INJECTION FOR INFUSION ONLY

Note: Anaphylactic reactions have occurred with Sandimmune injection (cyclosporine concentrate for injection, USP). (See WARNINGS.)

Patients unable to take Sandimmune soft gelatin capsules or oral solution pre- or postoperatively may be treated with the IV concentrate.**Sandimmune injection (cyclosporine concentrate for injection, USP) is administered at 1/3 the oral dose.** The initial dose of Sandimmune injection (cyclosporine concentrate for injection, USP) should be given 4-12 hours prior to transplantation as a single IV dose of 5-6 mg/kg/day. This daily single dose is continued postoperatively until the patient can tolerate the soft gelatin capsules or oral solution. Patients should be switched to Sandimmune soft gelatin capsules or oral solution as soon as possible after surgery. In pediatric usage, the same dose and dosing regimen may be used, although higher doses may be required.

Adjunct steroid therapy is to be used.

Immediately before use, the IV concentrate should be diluted 1 ml Sandimmune injection (cyclosporine concentrate for injection, USP) in 20 ml-100 ml 0.9% Sodium Chloride Injection or 5% Dextrose Injection and given in a slow intravenous infusion over approximately 2-6 hours.

Diluted infusion solutions should be discarded after 24 hours.

The Cremophor EL (polyoxyethylated castor oil) contained in the concentrate for intravenous infusion can cause phthalate stripping from PVC.

Parenteral drug products should be inspected visually for particulate matter and discoloration prior to administration, whenever solution and container permit.

Blood Level Monitoring: Several study centers have found blood level monitoring of cyclosporine useful in patient management. While no fixed relationships have yet been established, in one series of 375 consecutive cadaveric renal transplant recipients, dosage was adjusted to achieve specific whole blood 24-hour trough levels of 100-200 ng/ml as determined by high-pressure liquid chromatography (HPLC).

Of major importance to blood level analysis is the type of assay used. The above levels are specific to the parent cyclosporine molecule and correlate directly to the new monoclonal specific radioimmunoassays (mRIA-sp). Nonspecific assays are also available which detect the parent compound molecule and various of its metabolites. Older studies often cited levels using a nonspecific assay which were roughly twice those of specific assays. Assay results are not interchangeable and their use should be guided by their approved labeling. If plasma specimens are employed, levels will vary with the temperature at the time of separation from whole blood. Plasma levels may range from 1/2-1/5 of whole blood levels. Refer to individual assay labeling for complete instructions. In addition, *Transplantation Proceedings* (June 1990) contains position papers and a broad consensus generated at the Cyclosporine-Therapeutic Drug Monitoring conference that year. Blood level monitoring is not a replacement for renal function monitoring or tissue biopsies.

NEORAL

Neoral has increased bioavailability in comparison to Sandimmune. Neoral and Sandimmune are not bioequivalent and cannot be used interchangeably without physician supervision.

The daily dose of Neoral should always be given in two divided doses (BID). It is recommended that Neoral be administered on a consistent schedule with regard to time of day and relation to meals.

Newly Transplanted Patients: The initial oral dose of Neoral can be given 4-12 hours prior to transplantation or be given postoperatively. The initial dose of Neoral varies depending on the transplanted organ and the other immunosuppressive agents included in the immunosuppressive protocol. In newly transplanted patients, the initial oral dose of Neoral is the same as the initial oral dose of Sandimmune.

Suggested initial doses are available from the results of a 1994 survey of the use of Sandimmune in US transplant centers. The mean ±SD initial doses were 9±3 mg/kg/day for renal transplant patients (75 centers), 8±4 mg/kg/day for liver transplant patients (30 centers), and 7±3 mg/kg/day for heart transplant patients (24 centers). Total daily doses were divided into two equal daily doses. The Neoral dose is subsequently adjusted to achieve a pre-defined cyclosporine blood concentration. (See Blood Concentration Monitoring.) If cyclosporine trough blood concentrations are used, the target range is the same for Neoral as for Sandimmune. Using the same trough concentration target range for Neoral as for Sandimmune results in greater cyclosporine exposure when Neoral is administered. See CLINICAL PHARMACOLOGY, Pharmacokinetics, Absorption. Dosing should be titrated based on clinical assessment of rejection and tolerability. Lower Neoral doses may be sufficient as maintenance therapy.

DOSAGE AND ADMINISTRATION: *(cont'd)*

Adjunct therapy with adrenal corticosteroids is recommended initially. Different tapering dosage schedules of prednisone appear to achieve similar results. A representative dosage schedule based on the patient's weight started with 2.0 mg/kg/day for the first 4 days tapered to 1.0 mg/kg/day by 1 week, 0.6 mg/kg/day by 2 weeks, 0.3 mg/kg/day by 1 month, and 0.15 mg/kg/day by 2 months and thereafter as a maintenance dose. Steroid doses may be further tapered on an individualized basis depending on status of patient and function of graft. Adjustments in dosage of prednisone must be made according to the clinical situation.

Conversion from Sandimmune to Neoral: In transplanted patients who are considered for conversion to Neoral from Sandimmune, Neoral should be started with the same daily dose as was previously used with Sandimmune (1:1 dose conversion). The Neoral dose should subsequently be adjusted to attain the pre-conversion cyclosporine blood trough concentration. Using the same trough concentration target range for Neoral as for Sandimmune results in greater cyclosporine exposure when Neoral is administered. See CLINICAL PHARMACOLOGY, Pharmacokinetics, Absorption. Patients with suspected poor absorption of Sandimmune require different dosing strategies. See Patients with Poor Absorption of Sandimmune In some patients, the increase in blood trough concentration is more pronounced and may be of clinical significance.

Until the blood trough concentration attains the pre-conversion value, it is strongly recommended that the cyclosporine blood trough concentration be monitored every 4 to 7 days after conversion to Neoral. In addition, clinical safety parameters such as serum creatinine and blood pressure should be monitored every two weeks during the first two months after conversion. If the blood trough concentrations are outside the desired range and/or if the clinical safety parameters worsen, the dosage of Neoral must be adjusted accordingly.

Patients with Poor Absorption of Sandimmune: Patients with lower than expected cyclosporine blood trough concentrations in relation to the oral dose of Sandimmune may have poor or inconsistent absorption of cyclosporine from Sandimmune. After conversion to Neoral, patients tend to have higher cyclosporine concentrations. **Due to the increase in bioavailability of cyclosporine following conversion to Neoral, the cyclosporine blood trough concentration may exceed the target range. Particular caution should be exercised when converting patients to Neoral at doses greater than 10 mg/kg/day.** The dose of Neoral should be titrated individually based on cyclosporine trough concentrations, tolerability, and clinical response. In this population the cyclosporine blood trough concentration should be measured more frequently, at least twice a week (daily, if initial dose exceeds 10 mg/kg/day) until the concentration stabilizes within the desired range.

Neoral Oral Solution (cyclosporine oral solution for microemulsion) -Recommendations for Administration: To make Neoral Oral Solution (cyclosporine oral solution for microemulsion) more palatable, it should be diluted preferably with orange or apple juice that is at room temperature. Grapefruit juice affects metabolism of cyclosporine and should be avoided. The combination of Neoral Oral Solution (cyclosporine oral solution for microemulsion) with milk can be unpalatable.

Take the prescribed amount of Neoral Oral Solution (cyclosporine oral solution for microemulsion) from the container using the dosing syringe supplied, after removal of the protective cover, and transfer the solution to a glass of orange or apple juice. Stir well and drink at once. Do not allow diluted oral solution to stand before drinking. Use a glass container (not plastic). Rinse the glass with more diluent to ensure that the total dose is consumed. After use, dry the outside of the dosing syringe with a clean towel and replace the protective cover. Do not rinse the dosing syringe with water or other cleaning agents. If the syringe requires cleaning, it must be completely dry before resuming use.

Blood Concentration Monitoring: Transplant centers have found blood concentration monitoring of cyclosporine to be an essential component of patient management. Of importance to blood concentration analysis are the type of assay used, the transplanted organ, and other immunosuppressant agents being administered. While no fixed relationship has been established, blood concentration monitoring may assist in the clinical evaluation of rejection and toxicity, dose adjustments, and the assessment of compliance.

Various assays have been used to measure blood concentrations of cyclosporine. Older studies using a non-specific assay often cited concentrations that were roughly twice those of specific assays, thus comparison of the concentrations in published literature to patient concentrations using current assays must be made with detailed knowledge of the assay methods employed. Current assay results are also not interchangeable and their use should be guided by their approved labeling. A discussion of the different assay methods is contained in *Annals of Clinical Biochemistry* 1994;31:420-446. While several assays and assay matrices are available, there is a consensus that parent-compound-specific assays correlate best with clinical events. Of these, HPLC is the standard reference, but the monoclonal antibody RIAs and the monoclonal antibody FPIA offer sensitivity, reproducibility, and convenience. Most clinicians base their monitoring on trough cyclosporine concentrations. *Applied Pharmacokinetics, Principles of Therapeutic Drug Monitoring* (1992) contains a broad discussion of cyclosporine pharmacokinetics and drug monitoring techniques. Blood concentration monitoring is not a replacement for renal function monitoring or tissue biopsies.

HOW SUPPLIED:

SANDIMMUNE SOFT GELATIN CAPSULES

25 mg: Oblong, pink, branded "78/240".

50 mg: Oblong, corn-yellow, branded "78/242".

100 mg: Oblong, dusty rose, branded "78/241".

Store and Dispense: In the original unit-dose container at temperatures below 86°F (30°C).

SANDIMMUNE ORAL SOLUTION

Supplied in 50 ml bottles containing 100 mg of cyclosporine per ml. A dosage syringe is provided for dispensing.

Store and Dispense: In the original container at temperatures below 86°F (30°C). Do not store in the refrigerator. Once opened, the contents must be used within 2 months.

SANDIMMUNE INJECTION

FOR INTRAVENOUS INFUSION

Supplied as a 5 ml sterile ampul containing 50 mg of cyclosporine per ml.

Store and Dispense: At temperatures below 86°F (30°C) and protected from light. Protect from freezing.

NEORAL SOFT GELATIN CAPSULES

25 mg: Oval, blue-gray imprinted in red, "Neoral" over "25 mg."

100 mg: Oblong, blue-gray imprinted in red, "Neoral" over "100 mg."

Store and Dispense: In the original unit-dose container at controlled room temperature 77°F (25°C).

NEORAL ORAL SOLUTION

A clear, yellow liquid supplied in 50 ml bottles containing 100 mg/ml.

Store and Dispense: In the original container at controlled room temperature 77°F (25°C). Do not store in the refrigerator. Once opened, the contents must be used within two months. At temperatures below 68°F (20°C) the solution may gel; light flocculation or the formation of a

HOW SUPPLIED: *(cont'd)*

light sediment may also occur. There is no impact on product performance or dosing using the syringe provided. Allow to warm to room temperature 77°F (25°C) to reverse these changes.

HOW SUPPLIED - EQUIVALENTS NOT AVAILABLE:

Capsule, Elastic - Oral - 25 mg

30's	$39.72	NEORAL, Novartis	00078-0246-15
30's	**$42.12**	**SANDIMMUNE SOFT GELATIN, Novartis**	**00078-0240-15**

Capsule, Elastic - Oral - 50 mg

30's	**$84.18**	**SANDIMMUNE, Novartis**	**00078-0242-15**

Capsule, Elastic - Oral - 100 mg

30's	$158.76	NEORAL, Novartis	00078-0248-15
30's	**$168.30**	**SANDIMMUNE SOFT GELATIN, Novartis**	**00078-0241-15**

Injection, Solution - Intravenous - 250 mg/5ml

10's	**$250.08**	**SANDIMMUNE, Novartis**	**00078-0109-01**

Solution - Oral - 100 mg/5ml

50 ml	$264.42	NEORAL, Novartis	00078-0274-22
50 ml	**$280.32**	**SANDIMMUNE, Novartis**	**00078-0110-22**

CYCLOTHIAZIDE *(000933)*

CATEGORIES: Antihypertensives; Cirrhosis; Congestive Heart Failure; Diuretics; Edema; Electrolytic, Caloric-Water Balance; Glomerulonephritis; Heart Failure; Hypertension; Nephrotic Syndrome; Pregnancy; Renal Drugs; Renal Failure; Thiazides; Pregnancy Category C; FDA Approval Pre 1982

BRAND NAMES: **Anhydron**; *Doburil*; *Valmiran* (Japan)
(International brand names outside U.S. in italics)

FORMULARIES: Medi-Cal

DESCRIPTION:

Anhydron (Cyclothiazide, USP, Lilly) is 6-chloro-3,4-dihydro-3-(5-norbornen-2-yl)-2*H*-1,2,4-benzothiadiazine-7-sulfonamide 1,1-dioxide.

Cyclothiazide is a white crystalline solid with a melting point of approximately 220°C. It is moderately soluble in hot ethyl alcohol and hot dilute alcohol, very soluble in cold ethyl acetate (an ethyl acetate solvate is formed), and relatively insoluble in ether, benzene, or chloroform.

Anhydron is an orally effective diuretic-antihypertensive agent. It is available in 2 mg (5 μmol) tablets. These tablets also contain D & C Yellow No. 10, FD&C Red No. 40, FD&C Yellow No. 6, lactose, magnesium stearate, and starch.

CLINICAL PHARMACOLOGY:

The diuretic effect of cyclothiazide results from inhibition of renal tubular reabsorption of sodium and chloride in the distal portion of the nephron. Cyclothiazide increases the urinary excretion of sodium and chloride in approximately equal proportion. The excretion of potassium is generally increased to a lesser extent than that of sodium. The excretion of bicarbonate is slightly increased by cyclothiazide, although not enough to change urinary pH. At maximum therapeutic dosage, all thiazides have approximately equal diuretic efficacy.

Like other benzothiazides, cyclothiazide also has antihypertensive properties. The mechanism of the antihypertensive effect of benzothiazides is not known.

During chronic administration of cyclothiazide, as with other benzothiazides, some patients develop hypokalemia, hyperuricemia, and hyperglycemia. Hyponatremia and hypochloremia also occur, particularly in edematous patients, and appear to be related to positive water balance.

Thiazides are rapidly absorbed from the gastrointestinal tract. All thiazides probably undergo active secretion in the proximal tubule. The renal clearance of thiazides is high. Most compounds are rapidly excreted within 3 to 6 hours.

The diuretic effect of cyclothiazide starts within 2 to 4 hours, peaks between 7 and 12 hours, and has a total duration of 18 to 24 hours following the administration of a single dose.

INDICATIONS AND USAGE:

Cyclothiazide is indicated as adjunctive therapy in edema associated with congestive heart failure, hepatic cirrhosis, and corticosteroid and estrogen therapy.

Cyclothiazide has also been found useful in edema due to various forms of renal dysfunction, such as nephrotic syndrome, acute glomerulonephritis, and chronic renal failure.

Cyclothiazide is indicated in the management of hypertension either as the sole therapeutic agent or to enhance the effectiveness of other antihypertensive drugs in the more severe forms of hypertension.

Usage in Pregnancy: The routine use of diuretics in an otherwise healthy woman is inappropriate and exposes mother and fetus to unnecessary hazard. Diuretics do not prevent development of toxemia of pregnancy, and there is no satisfactory evidence that they are useful in the treatment of developed toxemia.

Edema during pregnancy may arise from pathologic causes or from the physiologic and mechanical consequences of pregnancy. Thiazides are indicated in pregnancy, as in the absence of pregnancy, when edema is due to pathologic causes (however, see PRECAUTIONS, Pregnancy). Dependent edema in pregnancy, resulting from restriction of venous return caused by the expanded uterus, is properly treated through elevation of the lower extremities and use of support hose; in such cases, use of diuretics to lower intravascular volume is illogical and unnecessary. In the majority of pregnant women, hypervolemia occurs during normal pregnancy and is not harmful to either the fetus or the mother (in the absence of cardiovascular disease) but is associated with edema, including generalized edema. If this edema produces discomfort, increased recumbency will often provide relief. In rare instances, such edema may cause extreme discomfort that is not relieved by rest. In these cases, a short course of diuretics may provide relief and may be appropriate.

CONTRAINDICATIONS:

Cyclothiazide is contraindicated in anuria and in patients who are hypersensitive to cyclothiazide or other sulfonamide-derived drugs.

WARNINGS:

Thiazides should be used with caution in severe renal disease. In patients with renal disease, thiazides may precipitate azotemia. Cumulative effects of the drug may develop in patients with impaired renal function.

Thiazides should be used with caution in patients with impaired hepatic function or progressive liver disease, since minor alterations of fluid and electrolyte balance may precipitate hepatic coma.

PRECAUTIONS:

General: All patients receiving thiazides should be observed for clinical signs of fluid or electrolyte imbalance, e.g., hyponatremia, hypochloremic alkalosis, and hypokalemia. Serum and urine electrolyte determinations are particularly important when the patient is vomiting excessively or receiving parenteral fluids. Medication such as digitalis may also influence serum electrolytes. Warning signs, irrespective of cause, are dryness of mouth, thirst, weakness, lethargy, drowsiness, restlessness, muscle pains or cramps, muscular fatigue, hypotension oliguria, tachycardia, and gastrointestinal disturbances, such as nausea and vomiting.

Hypokalemia may develop with use of thiazides as with any other potent diuretic, especially with brisk diuresis, in the presence of severe cirrhosis, or during concomitant use of corticosteroids or ACTH. Interference with adequate oral electrolyte intake will also contribute to hypokalemia.

Any chloride deficit is generally mild and does not require specific treatment except under extraordinary circumstances (as in liver or renal disease). Dilutional hyponatremia may occur in edematous patients in hot weather. The appropriate therapy is water restriction instead of administration of salt (except in rare instances when the hyponatremia is life threatening). In actual salt depletion, appropriate replacement is the therapy of choice.

In certain patients receiving thiazide therapy, hyperuricemia or hypercalcemia may occur or frank gout may be precipitated.

Hypomagnesemia may also occur in some patients, especially the elderly, during thiazide therapy.

The antihypertensive effects of the drug may be enhanced in postsympathectomy patients.

Thiazides may decrease arterial responsiveness to norepinephrine. This diminution is not sufficient to preclude effectiveness of the pressor agent for therapeutic use.

If progressive renal impairment becomes evident, as indicated by a rising nonprotein nitrogen or blood urea nitrogen, therapy should be carefully reappraised, because it may be necessary to withhold or discontinue diuretic therapy.

Sensitivity reactions may occur in patients with a history of allergy or bronchial asthma.

The possibility of exacerbation or activation of systemic lupus erythematosus has been reported.

Information for the Patient: Patients should be informed about the possible additive effects of treatment with corticosteroids, excessive gastrointestinal fluid losses (vomiting, diarrhea), and the effect of treatment with thiazides on potassium depletion. Patients should also be informed about the potential risk of drug-related potassium depletion and hypokalemia with regard to the enhancement of digitalis toxicity. When the weather is hot, diuretic-receiving patients, especially the elderly, should be warned of the increased risk of heatstroke.

Laboratory Tests: Determination of serum electrolytes to detect possible imbalance should be performed at appropriate intervals.

Drug/Laboratory Test Interactions: Thiazides may decrease serum PBI levels without signs of thyroid disturbance.

Carcinogenesis, Mutagenesis, and Impairment of Fertility: No studies have been performed in animals to evaluate the carcinogenic or mutagenic potential of cyclothiazide. No animal studies have been conducted to determine whether cyclothiazide has the potential to impair fertility.

Pregnancy, Teratogenic Effects, Pregnancy Category C: Animal reproduction studies have not been conducted with cyclothiazide. It is also not known whether this drug can cause fetal harm when administered to a pregnant woman or can affect reproduction capacity. Cyclothiazide should be given to a pregnant woman only if clearly needed (see INDICATIONS AND USAGE).

Nonteratogenic Effects: Thiazides cross the placental barrier and appear in cord blood. The use of thiazides in pregnant women requires that the anticipated benefit be weighed against possible hazards to the fetus. These hazards include fetal or neonatal jaundice, thrombocytopenia, and possibly other adverse reactions that have occurred in the adult.

Nursing Mothers: Thiazides appear in breast milk. If use of the drug is deemed essential, the patient should stop nursing.

Pediatric Use: Safety and effectiveness in children have not been established.

DRUG INTERACTIONS:

Thiazides may add to or potentiate the action of other antihypertensive drugs. Potentiation occurs with ganglionic or peripheral adrenergic blocking drugs.

The concurrent use of ACTH or corticosteroids and thiazide diuretics may enhance urinary potassium loss.

Potassium depletion and hypokalemia secondary to the use of thiazide diuretics may potentiate the effects of digitalis on the heart, thus enhancing the possibility of digitalis toxicity.

Insulin requirements in diabetic patients may be increased, decreased or unchanged. Latent diabetes mellitus may become manifest during thiazide administration.

Thiazide drugs may increase the responsiveness of tubocurarine.

The renal clearance of lithium may be reduced during administration of thiazide derivatives, thus enhancing lithium toxicity.

Concurrent administration of some nonsteroidal anti-inflammatory agents may reduce the diuretic, natriuretic, and antihypertensive effects of thiazide diuretics.

ADVERSE REACTIONS:

The following adverse reactions have been observed but there is not enough systematic collection of data to support an estimate of their frequency.

Gastrointestinal: Anorexia, gastric irritation, nausea, vomiting, cramping, diarrhea, constipation, jaundice (intrahepatic cholestatic jaundice), pancreatitis

Central Nervous System: Dizziness, vertigo, paresthesias, headache, xanthopsia

Hematologic: Leukopenia, agranulocytosis, thrombocytopenia, aplastic anemia

Dermatologic and Hypersensitivity: Purpura, photosensitivity, rash, urticaria, necrotizing angitis (vasculitis or cutaneous vasculitis)

Cardiovascular: Orthostatic hypotension may occur and may be aggravated by alcohol, barbiturates, or narcotics

Other: Hyperglycemia, glycosuria, hyperuricemia, muscle spasm, weakness, restlessness

Whenever adverse reactions are moderate or severe, thiazide dosage should be reduced or therapy withdrawn.

OVERDOSAGE:

Signs and Symptoms: Symptoms of overdose from cyclothiazide are often related to hypovolemia, hypokalemia, and other types of electrolyte imbalance. Symptoms may also include orthostatic hypotension, weakness, confusion, dizziness, hyporeflexia, impaired urinary concentrating ability and cardiac arrhythmias. Cyclothiazide may also cause hyperglycemia, hypercalcemia, and hyperuricemia.

OVERDOSAGE: *(cont'd)*

Treatment: To obtain up-to-date information about the treatment of overdose, a good resource is your certified Regional Poison Control Center Telephone numbers of certified poison control centers are listed in the *Physicians GenR$_x$ (PGX)*. In managing overdosage, consider the possibility of multiple drug overdoses, interaction among drugs, and unusual drug kinetics in your patient.

For small overdoses, correct fluid and electrolyte balance and monitor electrolytes frequently.

Protect the patient's airway and support ventilation and perfusion. Meticulously monitor and maintain, within acceptable limits, the patient's vital signs, blood gases, serum electrolytes, etc. Absorption of drugs from the gut may be decreased by giving activated charcoal, which in many cases, is more effective than emesis or lavage; consider charcoal instead of or in addition to gastric emptying. Repeated doses of charcoal over time may hasten elimination of some drugs that have been absorbed. Safeguard the patient's airway when employing gastric emptying or charcoal.

Absorption of drugs from the gut may be decreased by giving activated charcoal, which in many cases, is more effective than emesis or lavage; consider charcoal instead of or in addition to gastric emptying. Repeated doses of charcoal over time may hasten elimination of some drugs that have been absorbed. Safeguard the patient's airway when employing gastric emptying or charcoal.

DOSAGE AND ADMINISTRATION:

Therapy should be individualized according to patient response. This therapy should be titrated to gain maximum therapeutic response with the minimum dose possible to maintain that response.

For Diuretic Effect: The usual adult dosage of cyclothiazide is 1/2 or 1 tablet (1 or 2 mg) once a day, preferably given early in the morning in order to obtain diuresis predominantly during the day and avoid disturbing the patient's rest at night. After the edema is eliminated, the dosage should be reduced according to the patient's need; body weight is usually a very helpful guide. For maintenance therapy, 1/2 to 1 tablet given on alternate days or 2 or 3 times a week may be sufficient. Such an intermittent dosage schedule reduces the possibility of excessive depletion of body sodium and chloride or of potassium deficiency.

For Antihypertensive Effect: The dosage of cyclothiazide, like that of other thiazides, if often greater than that required for diuresis. The usual dosage of cyclothiazide is 1 tablet (2 mg) once a day; in some cases, it may be necessary to give 1 tablet 2 or 3 times a day.

Since cyclothiazide augments the action of other antihypertensive drugs, dosage of the latter should be reduced-perhaps to 50% of the usually recommended dosage-at the start of treatment and carefully readjusted upward or downward according to the patient's response and need.

Store at controlled room temperature, 59 to 86°F (15 to 30°C).

HOW SUPPLIED - EQUIVALENTS NOT AVAILABLE:

Tablet, Plain Coated - Oral - 2 mg

100's $29.28 ANHYDRON, Lilly 00002-2109-02

CYPROHEPTADINE HYDROCHLORIDE *(000934)*

CATEGORIES: Allergic Reactions; Allergies; Anaphylactic Reactions; Anaphylactic Shock; Angioedema; Antihistamines; Caloric Agents; Cold Urticaria; Conjunctivitis; Dermatographism; Electrolytic, Caloric-Water Balance; Piperidines; Respiratory & Allergy Medications; Rhinitis; Urticaria; Migraine*; Pregnancy Category B; FDA Approval Pre 1982

* Indication not approved by the FDA

BRAND NAMES: *Actinal*; *Adekin*; *Alphahist*; *Anapeptol*; *Anapromine*; *Aperitol*; *Aptide*; *Arsigran*; *Ciplactin*; *Ciproral* (Germany); *Cyheptin*; *Cyheptine*; *Cyproatin* (Japan); *Cyprodin*; *Cyprogin*; Cypromar; *Cypromin* (Japan); *Cyprosian*; *Cytadine*; *Ennamax*; *Heptasan*; *Huavine*; *Ifrasal* (Japan); *Ioukmin*; *Istam-Far*; *Klarivitina*; *Kulinet*; *Nekomin*; *Nelactin*; *Nuran* (Germany); *Oractine*; **Periactin**; *Periactine* (France); *Periactinol* (Germany); Periavit; *Peritol* (Germany); *Petina*; *Pilian*; *Pronicy*; Pyrohep; *Setomin*; *Sigloton*

(International brand names outside U.S. in italics)

FORMULARIES: BC-BS; FHP; PCS

COST OF THERAPY: $1.56 (Rhinitis; Tablet; 4 mg; 3/day; 30 days)

PRIMARY ICD9: 477.9 (Allergic Rhinitis, Cause Unspecified)

DESCRIPTION:

Cyproheptadine Hydrochloride (Cyproheptadine HCl) is an antihistaminic and antiserotonergic agent.

Cyproheptadine hydrochloride is a white to slightly yellowish, crystalline solid, with a molecular weight of 350.89, which is soluble in water, freely soluble in methanol, sparingly soluble in ethanol, soluble in chloroform, and practically insoluble in ether. It is the sesquihydrate of 4-(5*H*-dibenzo *(a,d)* cyclohepten-5-ylidene)-1-methylpiperidine hydrochloride. The empirical formula of the anhydrous salt is $C_{21}H_{21}N{\cdot}HCl$.

Cyproheptadine HCl is available in tablets, containing 4 mg of cyproheptadine hydrochloride, and as a syrup in which 5 ml contains 2 mg of cyproheptadine hydrochloride, with a pH range of 3.5 to 4.5.

The tablets also contain the following inactive ingredients: calcium phosphate, lactose, magnesium stearate, and starch. The syrup contains the following inactive ingredients: D & C Yellow 10, artificial flavors, glycerin, purified water, sodium saccharin, and sucrose, with sorbic acid 0.1% added as preservative.

CLINICAL PHARMACOLOGY:

Cyproheptadine HCl is a serotonin and histamine antagonist with anticholinergic and sedative effects. Antiserotonin and antihistamine drugs appear to compete with serotonin and histamine, respectively, for receptor sites.

PHARMACOKINETICS AND METABOLISM

After a single 4 mg oral dose of ^{14}C-labelled cyproheptadine HCI in normal subjects, given as tablets or syrup, 2-20% of the radioactivity was excreted in the stools. Only about 34% of the stool radioactivity was unchanged drug, corresponding to less than 5.7% of the dose. At least 40% of the administered radioactivity was excreted in the urine. No significant difference in the mean urinary excretion exists between the tablet and syrup formulations. No detectable amounts of unchanged drug were present in the urine of patients on chronic 12-20 mg daily doses of cyproheptadine HCl Syrup. The principle metabolite found in human urine has been identified as a quaternary ammonium glucuronide conjugate of cyproheptadine. Elimination is diminished in renal insufficiency.

INDICATIONS AND USAGE:

Perennial and seasonal allergic rhinitis
Vasomotor rhinitis
Allergic conjunctivitis due to inhalant allergens and foods
Mild, uncomplicated allergic skin manifestations of urticaria and angioedema
Amelioration of allergic reactions to blood or plasma
Cold urticaria
Dermatographism
As therapy for anaphylactic reactions *adjunctive* to epinephrine and other standard measures after the acute manifestations have been controlled.

CONTRAINDICATIONS:

NEWBORN OR PREMATURE INFANTS

This drug should not be used in newborn or premature infants.

NURSING MOTHERS

Because of the higher risk of antihistamines for infants generally and for newborns and prematures in particular, antihistamine therapy is contraindicated in nursing mothers.

Other Conditions

Hypersensitivity to cyproheptadine and other drugs of similar chemical structure: Monoamine oxidase inhibitor therapy (see DRUG INTERACTIONS)
Angle-closure glaucoma
Stenosing peptic ulcer
Symptomatic prostatic hypertrophy
Bladder neck obstruction
Pyloroduodenal obstruction
Elderly, debilitated patients

WARNINGS:

CHILDREN

Overdosage: Of antihistamines, particularly in infants and children, may produce hallucinations, central nervous system depression, convulsions, and death.

Antihistamines may diminish mental alertness; conversely, particularly, in the young child, they may occasionally produce excitation.

CNS DEPRESSANTS

Antihistamines may have additive effects with alcohol and other CNS depressants, e.g., hypnotics, sedatives, tranquilizers, antianxiety agents.

ACTIVITIES REQUIRING MENTAL ALERTNESS

Patients should be warned about engaging in activities requiring mental alertness and motor coordination, such as driving a car or operating machinery.

Antihistamines are more likely to cause dizziness, sedation, and hypotension in elderly patients.

PRECAUTIONS:

GENERAL

Cyproheptadine has an atropine-like action and, therefore, should be used with caution in patients with:
History of bronchial asthma
Increased intraocular pressure
Hyperthyroidism
Cardiovascular disease
Hypertension

INFORMATION FOR THE PATIENT

Antihistamines may diminish mental alertness; conversely, particularly, in the young child, they may occasionally produce excitation.

Patients should be warned about engaging in activities requiring mental alertness and motor coordination, such as driving a car or operating machinery.

CARCINOGENESIS, MUTAGENESIS, AND IMPAIRMENT OF FERTILITY

Long-term carcinogenic studies have not been done with cyproheptadine.

Cyproheptadine had no effect on fertility in a two-litter study in rats or a two generation study in mice at about 10 times the human dose.

Cyproheptadine did not produce chromosome damage in human lymphocytes or fibroblasts *in vitro*; high doses (10^{-4}M) were cytotoxic. Cyproheptadine did not have any mutagenic effect in the Ames microbial mutagen test; concentrations of above 500 mcg/plate inhibited bacterial growth.

PREGNANCY CATEGORY B

Reproduction studies have been performed in rabbits, mice, and rats at oral or subcutaneous doses up to 32 times the maximum recommended human oral dose and have revealed no evidence of impaired fertility or harm to the fetus due to cyproheptadine. Cyproheptadine has been shown to be fetotoxic in rats when given by intraperitoneal injection in doses four times the maximum recommended human oral dose. Two studies in pregnant women, however, have not shown that cyproheptadine increases the risk of abnormalities when administered during the first, second and third trimesters of pregnancy. No teratogenic effects were observed in any of the newborns. Nevertheless, because the studies in humans cannot rule out the possibility of harm, cyproheptadine should be used during pregnancy only if clearly needed.

NURSING MOTHERS

It is not known whether this drug is excreted in human milk. Because many drugs are excreted in human milk, and because of the potential for serious adverse reactions in nursing infants from cyproheptadine HCl, a decision should be made whether to discontinue nursing or to discontinue the drug, taking into account the importance of the drug to the mother (see CONTRAINDICATIONS).

PEDIATRIC USE

Safety and effectiveness in children below the age of two have not been established. See CONTRAINDICATIONS, Newborn Premature Infants, and WARNINGS, Children.

DRUG INTERACTIONS:

MAO inhibitors prolong and intensify the anticholinergic effects of antihistamines.

Antihistamines may have additive effect with alcohol and other CNS depressants, e.g. hypnotics, sedatives, tranquilizers, antianxiety agents.

ADVERSE REACTIONS:

Adverse reactions which have been reported with the use of antihistamines are as follows:

Central Nervous System: Sedation and sleepiness (often transient), dizziness, disturbed coordination, confusion, restlessness, excitation, nervousness, tremor, irritability, insomnia, paresthesias, neuritis, convulsions, euphoria, hallucinations, hysteria, faintness.

Integumentary: Allergic manifestation of rash and edema, excessive perspiration, urticaria, photosensitivity.

Special Senses: Acute labyrinthitis, blurred vision, diplopia, vertigo, tinnitus.

Cardiovascular: Hypotension, palpitation, tachycardia, extrasystoles, anaphylactic shock.

Hematologic: Hemolytic anemia, leukopenia, agranulocytosis, thrombocytopenia.

Digestive System: Dryness of mouth, epigastric distress, anorexia, nausea, vomiting, diarrhea, constipation, jaundice.

Genitourinary: Urinary frequency, difficult urination, urinary retention, early menses.

Respiratory: Dryness of nose and throat, thickening of bronchial secretions, tightness of chest and wheezing, nasal stuffiness.

Miscellaneous: Fatigue, chills, headache.

OVERDOSAGE:

Antihistamine overdosage reactions may vary from central nervous system depression to stimulation especially in children. Also, atropine-like signs and symptoms (dry mouth; fixed, dilated pupils; flushing, etc.) as well as gastrointestinal symptoms may occur.

If Vomiting Has Not Occurred Spontaneously: The patient should be induced to vomit with syrup of ipecac.

If The Patient Is Unable To Vomit: Perform gastric lavage followed by activated charcoal. Isotonic or 1/2 isotonic saline is the lavage of choice. Precautions against aspiration must be taken especially in infants and children.

When life threatening CNS signs and symptoms are present, intravenous physostigmine salicylate may be considered. Dosage and frequency of administration are dependent on age, clinical response, and recurrence after response.

Saline Cathartics: Milk of magnesia, by osmosis draw water into the bowel and, therefore, are valuable for their action in rapid dilution of bowel content.

Stimulants: Should *not* be used.

Vasopressors may be used to treat hypotension.

The oral LD_{50} of cyproheptadine is 123 mg/kg, and 295 mg/kg in the mouse and rat, respectively.

DOSAGE AND ADMINISTRATION:

DOSAGE SHOULD BE INDIVIDUALIZED ACCORDING TO THE NEEDS AND THE RESPONSE OF THE PATIENT.

Each cyproheptadine HCl tablet contains 4 mg of cyproheptadine hydrochloride. Each 5 ml of cyproheptadine HCl syrup contains 2 mg of cyproheptadine hydrochloride.

Although intended primarily for administration to children, the syrup is also useful for administration to adults who cannot swallow tablets.

CHILDREN

The total daily dosage for children may be calculated on the basis of body weight or body area using approximately 0.25 mg/kg/day (0.11 mg/lb/day) or 8 mg per square meter of body surface (8 mg/M²). In small children for whom the calculation of dosage based upon body size is most important, it may be necessary to use cyproheptadine HCl syrup to permit accurate dosage.

AGE 2 TO 6 YEARS

The usual dose is 2 mg ($\frac{1}{2}$ tablet or 1 teaspoon) two or three times a day, adjusted as necessary to the size and response of the patient. The dose is not to exceed 12 mg a day.

AGE 7 TO 14 YEARS

The usual dose is 4 mg (1 tablet or 2 teaspoons) two or three times a day, adjusted as necessary to the size and response of the patient. The dose is not to exceed 16 mg a day.

ADULTS

The total daily dose for adults should not exceed 0.5 mg/kg/day (0.23 mg/lb/day).

The therapeutic range is 4 to 20 mg a day, with the majority of patients requiring 12 to 16 mg a day. An occasional patient may require as much as 32 mg a day for adequate relief. It is suggested that dosage be initiated with 4 mg (1 tablet or 2 teaspoons) three times a day and adjusted according to the size and response of the patient.

STORAGE

Store tablets cyproheptadine HCl in a well-closed container. Avoid storage at temperatures above 40°C (104°F).

Store syrup cyproheptadine HCl in a container which is kept tightly closed. Avoid storage at temperatures below -20°C (-4°F) and above 40°C (104°F).

HOW SUPPLIED - RATED THERAPEUTICALLY EQUIVALENT:

Syrup - Oral - 2 mg/5ml

5 ml	$0.07	Cyproheptadine Hcl, H.C.F.A. F F P	99999-0934-01
480 ml	$4.55	Cyproheptadine Hcl, Raway	00686-0755-16
480 ml	$6.38	Cyproheptadine HCl, H.C.F.A. F F P	99999-0934-02
480 ml	$6.74	Cyproheptadine Hcl, HL Moore Drug Exch	00839-6493-69
480 ml	$8.50	Cyproheptadine Hcl, Consolidated Midland	00223-6489-01
480 ml	$8.90	PYROHEP, Major Pharms	00904-1146-16
480 ml	$9.45	Cyproheptadine HCl, Schein Pharm (US)	00364-7272-16
480 ml	$9.50	Cyproheptadine Hcl Syrup, Harber Pharm	51432-0556-20
480 ml	$10.49	Cyproheptadine Hcl, Qualitest Pharms	00603-1117-58
480 ml	$10.50	Cyproheptadine Hcl, Goldline Labs	00182-1355-40
480 ml	$10.71	Cyproheptadine HCl, Alpharma	00472-0755-16
480 ml	$10.75	Cyproheptadine HCl, Rugby	00536-1930-85
480 ml	$10.75	Cyproheptadine Hcl Syrup 2, Halsey Drug	00879-0473-16
480 ml	$12.65	Cyproheptadine Hcl, Aligen Independ	00405-2600-16
480 ml	**$31.12**	**PERIACTIN, Merck**	**00006-3289-74**
3840 ml	$51.07	Cyproheptadine Hcl, H.C.F.A. F F P	99999-0934-03
3840 ml	$57.48	Cyproheptadine Hcl, Consolidated Midland	00223-6489-02
3840 ml	$62.25	Cyproheptadine Hcl Syrup 2, Halsey Drug	00879-0473-28
3840 ml	$69.35	Cyproheptadine Hcl, Rugby	00536-1930-90

Tablet, Uncoated - Oral - 4 mg

100's	$1.74	Cyproheptadine HCl, H.C.F.A. F F P	99999-0934-04
100's	$3.59	Cyproheptadine Hcl, US Trading	56126-0043-11
100's	$3.95	Cyproheptadine Hcl, Squibb-Mark	57783-6780-01
100's	$4.20	Cyproheptadine Hcl, United Res	00677-0623-01
100's	$4.25	Cyproheptadine Hcl, Major Pharms	00904-1145-60
100's	$4.27	Cyproheptadine HCl, Camall	00147-0236-10
100's	$4.30	Cyproheptadine Hcl, Halsey Drug	00879-0524-01
100's	$4.31	Cyproheptadine Hcl, Qualitest Pharms	00603-3098-21
100's	$4.71	Cyproheptadine Hcl, HL Moore Drug Exch	00839-6300-06

HOW SUPPLIED - RATED THERAPEUTICALLY EQUIVALENT:
(cont'd)

100's	$4.71	Cyproheptadine Hcl, HL Moore Drug Exch	00839-7866-06
100's	$5.05	Cyproheptadine Hcl, Par Pharm	49884-0043-01
100's	$5.25	Cyproheptadine Hydrochloride, MD Pharm	43567-0547-07
100's	$5.30	Cyproheptadine HCl, Schein Pharm (US)	00364-0499-01
100's	$5.75	Cyproheptadine Hcl, Consolidated Midland	00223-0709-01
100's	$6.25	Cyproheptadine Hcl, Rugby	00536-3515-01
100's	$6.55	Cyproheptadine, Zenith Labs	00172-2929-60
100's	$6.55	Cyproheptadine Hcl, Goldline Labs	00182-1132-01
100's	$6.55	Cyproheptadine Hcl, Aligen Independ	00405-4295-01
100's	$6.55	Cyproheptadine Hcl, Sidmak Labs	50111-0314-01
100's	$6.55	Cyproheptadine Hcl, Martec Pharms	52555-0043-01
100's	$8.25	Cyproheptadine, Raway	00686-0159-20
100's	$16.50	Cyproheptadine Hcl, Medirex	57480-0428-01
100's	$18.70	Cyproheptadine Hcl, Goldline Labs	00182-1132-89
100's	$19.12	Cyproheptadine Hcl, Major Pharms	00904-1145-61
100's	$19.45	Cyproheptadine Hcl, Vangard Labs	00615-1536-13
100's	**$40.68**	**PERIACTIN, Merck**	**00006-0062-68**
500's	$6.63	Cyproheptadine Hydrochloride, MD Pharm	43567-0547-11
500's	$8.70	Cyproheptadine HCl, H.C.F.A. F F P	99999-0934-05
500's	$11.80	Cyproheptadine HCl, Camall	00147-0236-05
500's	$19.54	Cyproheptadine HCl, Schein Pharm (US)	00364-0499-05
500's	$22.75	Cyproheptadine Hcl, Rugby	00536-3515-05
600's	$68.80	Cyproheptadine Hcl, Medirex	57480-0428-06
1000's	$17.40	Cyproheptadine HCl, H.C.F.A. F F P	99999-0934-06
1000's	$18.53	Cyproheptadine HCl, Camall	00147-0236-20
1000's	$29.40	Cyproheptadine Hcl, United Res	00677-0623-10
1000's	$29.75	Cyproheptadine Hcl, Squibb-Mark	57783-6780-03
1000's	$29.75	Cyproheptadine Hcl, Squibb-Mark	57783-6783-03
1000's	$30.10	Cyproheptadine Hcl, Major Pharms	00904-1145-80
1000's	$30.50	Cyproheptadine Hcl, HL Moore Drug Exch	00839-6300-16
1000's	$30.50	Cyproheptadine Hcl, HL Moore Drug Exch	00839-7866-16
1000's	$31.90	Cyproheptadine Hcl, Halsey Drug	00879-0524-10
1000's	$32.50	Cyproheptadine Hcl, Consolidated Midland	00223-0708-02
1000's	$43.50	Cyproheptadine Hcl, Rugby	00536-3515-10
1000's	$43.91	Cyproheptadine Hcl, Qualitest Pharms	00603-3098-32
1000's	$44.28	Cyproheptadine, Zenith Labs	00172-2929-80
1000's	$44.28	Cyproheptadine Hcl, Goldline Labs	00182-1132-10
1000's	$44.28	Cyproheptadine Hcl, Aligen Independ	00405-4295-03
1000's	$44.28	Cyproheptadine Hcl, Sidmak Labs	50111-0314-03
1000's	$46.25	Cyproheptadine Hydrochloride, MD Pharm	43567-0547-12
1000's	$49.50	Cyproheptadine Hcl, Martec Pharms	52555-0043-10
1000's	$53.03	Cyproheptadine Hcl, Par Pharm	49884-0043-10

HOW SUPPLIED - NOT RATED EQUIVALENT:
Kit - Oral

1's	$10.00	PERIAVIT, Dayton Labs	52041-0033-36

CYSTEAMINE BITARTRATE *(003216)*

CATEGORIES: Nephropathic Cystinosis; Orphan Drugs; FDA Class 1P ("Priority Review"); FDA Approved 1994 Aug

BRAND NAMES: **Cystagon**

COST OF THERAPY: $2,942.65 (Cystinosis; Capsule; 150 mg; 8/day; 365 days)

PRIMARY ICD9: 270.0 (Disturbances of Amino-Acid Transport)

DESCRIPTION:

Cystagon (cysteamine bitartrate) capsules for oral administration, contain cysteamine bitartrate, a cystine depleting agent which lowers the cystine content of cells in patients with cystinosis, an inherited defect of lysosomal transport. Cystagon is the bitartrate salt of cysteamine, an aminothiol, beta-mercaptoethylamine. Cysteamine bitartrate is a highly water soluble white powder with a molecular weight of 227 and the molecular formula C_2H_7NS $C_4H_6O_6$.

Each Cystagon capsule contains 50 mg or 150 mg of cysteamine free base as cysteamine bitartrate. Cystagon capsules contain the following inactive ingredients: colloidal silicon dioxide, croscarmellose sodium, D&C yellow #10 aluminum lake, FD&C blue #1 aluminum lake, FD&C blue #2 aluminum lake, FD&C red #40 aluminum lake, gelatin, magnesium stearate, microcrystalline cellulose, pharmaceutical glaze, pregelatinized starch, sodium lauryl sulfate, synthetic black iron oxide and titanium dioxide.

CLINICAL PHARMACOLOGY:

Mechanism of Action: Cystinosis is an autosomal recessive inborn error of metabolism in which the transport of cystine out of lysosomes is abnormal; in the nephropathic form, accumulation of cystine and formation of crystals damage various organs, especially the kidney, leading to renal tubular Fanconi Syndrome and progressive glomerular failure, with end stage renal failure by the end of the first decade of life. In four studies of cystinosis patients before cysteamine was available, renal death (need for transplant or dialysis) occurred at median age of less than 10 years. Patients with cystinosis also experience growth failure, rickets, and photophobia due to cystine deposits in the cornea. With time most organs are damaged, including the retina, muscles and central nervous system.

Cysteamine is an aminothiol that participates within lysosomes in a thiol-disulfide interchange reaction converting cystine into cysteine and cysteine-cysteamine mixed disulfide, both of which can exit the lysosome in patients with cystinosis.

Pharmacodynamics: Normal individuals and persons heterozygous for cystinosis have white cell cystine levels of < 0.2 and usually below 1 nmol/1/2 cystine/mg protein, respectively. Individuals with nephropathic cystinosis have elevations of white cell cystine above 2 nmol/1/2 cystine/mg protein. White cell cystine is monitored in these patients to determine adequacy of dosing, levels being measured 5 to 6 hours after dosing. In the Long-Term Study entry white cell cystine levels were 3.73 nmol/1/2 cystine/mg protein (range 0.13 to 19.80 nmol/1/2 cystine/mg protein) and were maintained close to 1 nmol/1/2 cystine/mg protein with a cysteamine dose range of 1.3 to 1.95 g/m^2/day. After administration of cysteamine HCI, leukocyte cystine levels fall, with minimum levels at approximately 1 hour.

Because cysteamine HCI has an unpleasant taste and odor, other formulations have been developed, including phosphocysteamine, the phosphorothioester of cysteamine that is rapidly converted to cysteamine in the gut, and cysteamine bitartrate. Cysteamine bitartrate has been shown in a transfer study in 8 patients to maintain white cell cystine levels below 1 nmol/1/2 cystine/mg protein when substituted for cysteamine HCl or phosphocysteamine. Total cysteamine levels 2 and 6 hours post-dosing were higher after cysteamine bitartrate than for the solutions. Most clinical data have been developed using cysteamine HCI or phosphocysteamine solutions. In all discussions that follow, administered amounts of various cysteamine salts will be expressed as amounts of cysteamine free base.

CLINICAL STUDIES:

There are approximately 200 pre-transplant cystinosis patients in the United States with nephropathic cystinosis and clinical studies have included almost all of them, in addition to about 40 studies in the United Kingdom. For all patients, mean age at entry into studies was just under 4 years. Patients were approximately equally divided between genders and about 85% were white, 9% were black, and 3% were hispanic.

The National Collaborative Cysteamine Study (NCCS) treated 94 children (mainly from the United States) with nephropathic cystinosis with increasing doses of cysteamine HCI (mean dose 54 mg/kg/day) to attain white cell cystine levels of less than 2 nmol/1/2 cystine/mg protein 5 to 6 hours post-dose, and compared their outcome with an historical control group of 17 children who had been in the placebo group of a randomized placebo-controlled trial of ascorbic acid. Cysteamine treated patients had been diagnosed at a mean age of 22 months and were a mean age of 46 months old at study entry; placebo patients had been diagnosed at about 29 months and were a mean age of about 52 months old at study entry. The principal measures of effectiveness were serum creatinine and calculated creatinine clearance and growth (height).

The average median white cell cystine level attained during treatment in the NCCS was 1.7 ± 0.2 nmol/1/2 cystine/mg protein. There were 70 cysteamine patients with baseline serum creatinine less than 2 mg/dl who were followed for at least a year and 17 placebo patients. Twelve of the 94 cysteamine treated patients required early dialysis or renal transplant. Median follow-up of cysteamine patients was over 32 months and 20% were followed more than 5 years. For the placebo group median follow-up was 20 months and only one was followed more than 24 months. Among cysteamine patients glomerular function was maintained over time despite the longer period of treatment and follow-up. Placebo treated patients, in contrast, experienced a gradual rise is serum creatinine. Height, corrected for age, was compared for treated patients with the height, at the various ages patients appeared, of the 143 patients initially screened for inclusion in the NCCS. Patients on treatment maintained growth (did not show increasing growth failure compared to normals) although growth velocity did not increase enough to allow patients to catch up to age norms. Renal tubular function was not affected by treatment.

Calculated creatinine clearances were evaluated for two groups of children, one with poor white cell cystine depletion and one with good white cell cystine depletion as shown in Table 3. The final mean creatinine clearance of the good depletion group was 20.8 ml/min/1.73 m^2 greater than the mean for the poor depletion group, despite the older mean age of the good depletion group.

TABLE 3 CREATININE CLEARANCE CHANGES BY WHITE CELL CYSTINE DEPLETION

	Age (years) Initial	Final	Creatinine Clearance (ml/min/1.73m^2) Initial	Final
Poor Depletion[1] (n=18)	4.2 ± 1.8	6.5 ± 0.5	33.6 ± 17.0	29.7 ± 5.4
Good Depletion[2] (n=19)	3.3 ± 2.2	7.2 ± 0.7	44.3 ± 15.0	50.5 ± 5.1

[1] Median leukocyte cystine levels were over 3 nmol/1/2 cystine/mg protein or were not measured at least 2 times per year. Patients did receive cysteamine for at least 1 year.
[2] Median leukocyte cystine levels were less than 1 nmol/1/2 cystine/mg protein and received cysteamine for at least 1 year.

The Long Term Study, initiated in 1988, utilized both cysteamine HCI and phosphocysteamine (patient's choice) in 46 patients who had completed the NCCS (averaging 6.5 years of treatment) and 93 new patients. Patients had cystinosis diagnosed by elevated white cell cystine (mean 3.63 nmol/1/2 cystine/mg). New patients and 46 continuing patients were required to have serum creatinine less than 3.0 mg/dl and 4.0 mg/dl, respectively. Patients were randomized to doses of 1.3 or 1.95 g/m^2/day and stratified according to whether the serum creatinine was above 1.2 mg/dl or not. Doses could be raised if white cell cystine levels were approximately 2 nmol/1/2 cystine/mg protein and lowered due to intolerance.

Mean doses were 1.27 g/m^2/day and 1.87 g/m^2/day in the two groups and white cell cystine levels averaged 1.72 ± 1.65 nmol/1/2 cystine/mg protein and 1.86 ± 0.92 nmol/1/2 cystine/mg protein in the 1.3 and 1.95 g/m^2/day groups, respectively. In new patients, a group similar in age to the NCCS group, serum creatinine was essentially unchanged over the period of follow-up (about half of the patients were followed for 24 months) and phosphocysteamine and cysteamine HCI had similar effects. The long-term follow-up group, about nine years old on average at entry, stayed in the study (almost 80% were followed at least 2 years) and had essentially no change in renal function. In four studies of untreated cystinosis, renal death (need for transplant or dialysis) occurred at median age of less than 10 years. Both groups maintained height (although they did not catch up from baseline). There was no apparent difference between the two doses.

INDICATIONS AND USAGE:

Cysteamine bitartrate is indicated for the management of nephropathic cystinosis in children and adults.

CONTRAINDICATIONS:

Cysteamine bitartrate is contraindicated in patients who have developed hypersensitivity to it or to cysteamine or penicillamine.

WARNINGS:

If a skin rash develops, cysteamine bitartrate should be withheld until the rash clears. Cysteamine bitartrate may be restarted at a lower dose under close supervision, then slowly titrated to the therapeutic dose. If a severe skin rash develops such as erythema multiforme bullosa or toxic epidermal necrolysis, cysteamine bitartrate should not be readministered.

CNS symptoms such as seizures, lethargy, somnolence, depression, and encephalopathy have been associated with cysteamine. If CNS symptoms develop, the patient should be carefully evaluated and the dose adjusted as necessary. Neurological complications have been described in some cystinotic patients not on cysteamine treatment. This may be a manifestation of the primary disorder. Patients should not engage in hazardous activities until the effects of cysteamine bitartrate on mental performance are known.

PRECAUTIONS:

General: Gastrointestinal tract symptoms including nausea, vomiting, anorexia and abdominal pain have been associated with cysteamine, sometimes severe. If these develop, therapy may have to be interrupted and the dose adjusted. A cysteamine dose of 1.95 grams/m^2/day (approximately 80 to 90 mg/kg/day) was associated with an increased number of withdrawals from treatment due to intolerance and an increased incidence of adverse events.

Cysteamine has occasionally been associated with reversible leukopenia and abnormal liver function studies. Therefore, blood counts and liver function studies should be monitored.

PRECAUTIONS: *(cont'd)*

Information for Patients and Parents and/or Guardians: See attached information for patients and parents and/or guardians.

Laboratory Tests: Leukocyte cystine measurements are useful to determine adequate dosage and compliance. When measured 5 to 6 hours after cysteamine bitartrate administration, the goal should be a level <1 nmol/1/2 cystine/mg protein. In some patients with poorer tolerability for cysteamine bitartrate, patients may still receive benefit with a white cell cystine level of less than 2 nmol/1/2 cystine/mg protein. Measurements should be done every three months, more frequently when patients are transferred from cysteamine hydrochloride or phosphocysteamine solutions to cysteamine bitartrate.

Carcinogenesis, Mutagenesis, and Impairment of Fertility: Cysteamine has not been tested for its carcinogenic potential in long-term animal studies.

Cysteamine was not mutagenic in the Ames test. It produced a negative response in an *in-vitro* sister chromatid exchange assay in human lymphocytes, but a positive response in a similar assay in hamster ovarian cells.

Repeat breeding reproduction studies were conducted in male and female rats. Cysteamine was found to have no effect on fertility and reproductive performance at an oral dose of 75 mg/kg/day (450 mg/m^2/day, 0.4 times the recommended human dose based on body surface area). At an oral dose of 375 mg/kg/day (2,250 mg/m^2/day 1.7 times the recommended human dose based on body surface area), it reduced the fertility of the adult rats and the survival of their offspring.

Pregnancy, Teratogenic Effects, Pregnancy Category C: It is not known whether cysteamine can cause fetal harm when administered to a pregnant woman or can affect reproduction capacity.

Nursing Mothers: It is not known whether cysteamine is excreted in human milk. Because many drugs are excreted in human milk and because of the manifested potential of cysteamine for developmental toxicity in suckling rat pups when it was administered to their lactating mothers at an oral dose of 375 mg/kg/day (2,250 mg/m^2/day, 1.7 times the recommended human dose based on body surface area), a decision should be made whether to discontinue nursing or to discontinue the drug, taking into account the importance of the drug to the mother.

Pediatric Use: The safety and effectiveness of cysteamine bitartrate for cystinotic children have been established. Cysteamine therapy should be initiated as soon as the diagnosis of nephropathic cystinosis has been confirmed.

DRUG INTERACTIONS:

None have been described. Cysteamine bitartrate can be administered with electrolyte and mineral replacements necessary for management of the Fanconi Syndrome as well as vitamin D and thyroid hormone.

ADVERSE REACTIONS:

In three clinical trials, cysteamine or phosphocysteamine have been administered to 246 children with cystinosis. Causality of side effects is sometimes difficult to determine because adverse effects may result from the underlying disease.

The most frequent adverse reactions seen involve the gastrointestinal and central nervous systems. These are especially prominent at the initiation of cysteamine therapy. Temporarily suspending treatment, then gradual re-introduction may be effective in improving tolerance.

Adverse reactions were not collected systematically in the NCCS, but were often listed by investigators. The following rates may therefore be underestimated. The most common events (>5%) were vomiting 35%, anorexia 31%, fever 22%, diarrhea 16%, lethargy 11%, and rash 7%.

Less common adverse events are:

Body as a whole: Dehydration.

Cardiovascular: Hypertension.

Digestive: Nausea, bad breath, abdominal pain, dyspepsia, constipation, gastroenteritis, duodenitis, duodenal ulceration.

Central Nervous System: Somnolence, encephalopathy, headache, seizures, ataxia, confusion, tremor, hyperkinesia, decreasing hearing, dizziness, jitteriness.

Psychiatric: Nervousness, abnormal thinking, depression, emotional lability, hallucinations, nightmares.

Integumentary: Urticaria.

Clinical Laboratory: Abnormal liver function, anemia, leukopenia.

Adverse reactions or intolerance leading to cessation of treatment occurred in 8% of patients in the U.S. Studies.

Withdrawals due to intolerance, vomiting associated with medication, anorexia, lethargy, and fever appeared dose related, occurring more frequently in those patients receiving 1.95 grams/m^2/day as compared to 1.30 grams/m^2/day.

TABLE 1 Dose in grams/m ^{2}/day

	1.30 (n=42) %	1.95 (n=51) %
Vomiting Considered Related to Medicine	31	67
Anorexia	33	51
Lethargy	17	27
Diarrhea	31	31
Fever	28	45

Sudden deaths have been reported in this disease state.

DRUG ABUSE AND DEPENDENCE:

Cysteamine bitartrate has not been associated with abuse potential, psychological or physical dependence in humans.

OVERDOSAGE:

A single oral dose of cysteamine at 660 mg/kg was lethal to rats. Symptoms of acute toxicity were reduction of motor activity and generalized hemorrhage in gastrointestinal tract and kidneys.

One case of massive human overdosage has been reported. The patient immediately vomited the drug and did not develop any symptoms. Should overdose occur, the respiratory and cardiovascular systems should be supported appropriately. No specific antidote is known. Hemodialysis may be considered since cysteamine is poorly bound to plasma proteins.

DOSAGE AND ADMINISTRATION:

For the management of nephropathic cystinosis, cysteamine therapy should be initiated promptly once the diagnosis is confirmed (*i.e.,* increased white cell cystine).

New patients should be started on 1/4 to 1/6 of the maintenance dose of cysteamine bitartrate. The dose should then be raised gradually over four to six weeks to avoid intolerance.

The recommended cysteamine bitartrate maintenance dose for children up to age 12 years is 1.30 grams/m^2/day of the free base, given in four divided doses. Intact cysteamine bitartrate capsules should not be administered to children under the age of approximately six years due to the risk of aspiration. Cysteamine bitartrate capsules may be administered to children under the age of approximately six years by sprinkling the capsule contents over food. Patients over age 12 and over 110 pounds weight should receive 2.0 grams/day, divided four times daily.

When cysteamine bitartrate is well tolerated, the goal of therapy is to keep leukocyte cystine levels below 1 nmol/1/2 cystine/mg protein five to six hours following administration of cysteamine bitartrate. Patients with poorer tolerability still receive significant benefit if white cell cystine levels are below 2 nmol/1/2 cystine/mg protein. The cysteamine bitartrate dose can be increased to a maximum of 1.95 grams/m^2/day to achieve this level. The dose of 1.95 grams/m^2/day has been associated with an increased rate of withdrawal from treatment due to intolerance and an increased incidence of adverse events.

Cystinotic patients taking cysteamine hydrochloride or phosphocysteamine solutions may be transferred to equimolar doses of cysteamine bitartrate capsules.

The recommended maintenance dose of 1.30 grams/m^2/day can be approximated by administering cysteamine bitartrate according to the following table, which takes surface area as well as weight into consideration.

TABLE 2

Weight in Pounds	mg of Cysteamine Free Base Every 6 Hours
0-10	100
11-20	150
21-30	200
31-40	250
41-50	300
51-70	350
71-90	400
91-110	450
>110	500

Patients over age 12 and over 110 pounds should receive 2.0 grams/day given in four divided doses as a starting maintenance dose. This dose should be reached after 4 to 6 weeks of incremental dosage increases as stated above. The dose should be raised if the leukocyte cystine level remains >2 nmol/1/2 cystine/mg/protein.

Leukocyte cystine measurements, taken 5 to 6 hours after dose administration, are recommended for new patients after the maintenance dose is achieved. Patients being transferred from cysteamine hydrochloride or phosphocysteamine solutions to capsules should have their white cell cystine levels measured in 2 weeks, and thereafter every 3 months to assess optimal dosage as described above.

If cysteamine bitartrate is poorly tolerated initially due to gastrointestinal tract symptoms or transient skin rashes, therapy should be temporarily stopped, then re-instituted at a lower dose and gradually increased to the proper dose.

PATIENT PACKAGE INSERT:

WHAT IS THE MOST IMPORTANT INFORMATION I SHOULD KNOW ABOUT CYSTEAMINE BITARTRATE?

Cysteamine bitartrate is prescribed to manage nephropathic cystinosis. Cysteamine bitartrate can only be obtained with a prescription from your or your child's doctor.

It is important to take or give cysteamine bitartrate and other cystinosis medications exactly as your or your child's doctor prescribes. Do not increase or decrease these medications without your doctor's approval. There have been reports of unexpected deaths in children with cystinosis. Some of these children were receiving cysteamine/phosphocysteamine treatment for their cystinosis while others were not.

WHAT IS NEPHROPATHIC CYSTINOSIS?

Nephropathic cystinosis is a rare inherited disorder characterized by the build up of cystine in organs, such as kidneys. Cystine build up causes kidney damage and excretion of excess amounts of glucose, proteins and electrolytes. Cystinosis can be detected by measuring the amount of cystine in white blood cells and other body cells. The results of cystinosis are slow body growth, weak bones, and progressive kidney failure. Replacement of electrolytes (like potassium) are still required during therapy with cysteamine bitartrate.

WHAT IS CYSTEAMINE BITARTRATE?

Cysteamine bitartrate is a medication that reacts with cystine so that the cystine level in cells is decreased.

WHO SHOULD NOT TAKE CYSTEAMINE BITARTRATE?

This medication has been prescribed for a specific patient with cystinosis. Do not give this drug to others who may have similar symptoms. Do not use it for any other reason.

Keep the medicine in a safe place where children cannot reach it.

HOW SHOULD I OR MY CHILD TAKE CYSTEAMINE BITARTRATE?

The dose of cysteamine bitartrate prescribed for you or your child will be based on you or your child's weight. In order for cysteamine bitartrate to work correctly, you must do the following:

Follow your doctor's directions exactly. Do not increase or decrease the amount of medicine without your doctor's approval.

If a dose of medicine is missed, it should be taken as soon as possible. However, if it is within two hours of the next dose, skip the missed dose and go back to the regular dosing schedule. Do not double dose.

Capsules should not be given to children under approximately six years of age because they may not be able to swallow them and they may choke. For children under approximately six years of age, the capsule may be opened and the contents sprinkled on food or mixed in formula.

Consult the doctor for complete directions.

You or your child's medical treatment will include, in addition to cysteamine bitartrate, one or more supplements to replace important electrolytes lost through the kidneys. It is important to take or give these supplements exactly as instructed. If a dose of one of these supplements is missed, do not take or give extra doses to make up for the missed dose. If several doses of the supplements are missed or weakness or drowsiness develops, call the doctor for instructions.

PATIENT PACKAGE INSERT: *(cont'd)*

Regular blood tests to measure the amount of cystine inside white blood cells are necessary to help determine the correct dose of cysteamine bitartrate. Your or your child's doctor will arrange for the blood tests to be done. Regular blood and urine tests to measure the levels of the body's important electrolytes are also necessary to help your or your child's doctor correctly adjust the doses of these supplements.

WHAT SHOULD MY CHILD OR I AVOID WHILE TAKING CYSTEAMINE BITARTRATE?

Cysteamine bitartrate may cause some people to become drowsy or less alert than they are normally. Make sure you know how you or your child (the patient) reacts to this medicine before doing anything that could be dangerous if not alert.

Cysteamine bitartrate should be taken or given exactly as your or your child's doctor directs. Do not increase or decrease the amount of medicine without your doctor's approval.

If a dose of cysteamine bitartrate is missed, do not take or give twice as much the next time.

WHAT ARE THE POSSIBLE SIDE EFFECTS OF CYSTEAMINE BITARTRATE?

The most common side effects of cysteamine bitartrate include:

Nausea
Vomiting
Loss of appetite
Diarrhea
Drowsiness
Rash
Unpleasant breath odor

You should contact your or your child's doctor or the hospital emergency department immediately if more medicine has been taken than has been prescribed, lethargy develops or persistent vomiting occurs.

HOW SHOULD I STORE CYSTEAMINE BITARTRATE?

Store the medicine in a dry place away from light.

This leaflet provides a summary of the information available on cysteamine bitartrate. This leaflet should be kept until the medicine is finished; you may read it again. This leaflet does not contain all of the information on cysteamine bitartrate capsules and is not meant to take the place of your doctor's instructions. If you have any questions about this medicine, be sure to ask your or your child's doctor.

HOW SUPPLIED:

Cystagon (cysteamine bitartrate) is supplied in hard gelatin capsules which provide 50 mg or 150 mg of cysteamine free base as cysteamine bitartrate:

Cystagon 50 mg capsules (cysteamine bitartrate) are white, opaque capsules printed with CYSTA 50 on the body and MYLAN on the cap.

Cystagon 150 mg capsules (cysteamine bitartrate) are white, opaque capsules printed with Cystagon 150 on the body and MYLAN on the cap.

STORE AT CONTROLLED ROOM TEMPERATURE 15°-30°C (59°-86°F).

PROTECT FROM LIGHT AND MOISTURE.

HOW SUPPLIED - EQUIVALENTS NOT AVAILABLE:

Capsule - Oral - 50 mg

500's $172.90 CYSTAGON, Mylan 00378-9040-05

Capsule - Oral - 150 mg

500's $503.88 CYSTAGON, Mylan 00378-9045-05

CYTARABINE *(000935)*

CATEGORIES: Antineoplastics; Cytotoxic Agents; Leukemia; Oncologic Drugs; Lymphoma*; Pregnancy Category D; FDA Approval Pre 1982
* Indication not approved by the FDA

BRAND NAMES: *Alexan* (England, Germany, Mexico); *Arabitin* (Japan); *Arace*; *Aracytin*; *Aracytine* (France); *Cytarabin*; *Cytarabine*; *Cytarabine Injection* (Australia); *Cytarbel* (France); *Cytosar* (England, Canada); *Cytosar U*; **Cytosar-U**; *Erbabin*; *Iretin* (Japan); *Mack Cytarabine*; Tarabine Pfs; *Udicil* (Germany)
(International brand names outside U.S. in italics)

FORMULARIES: BC-BS; Medi-Cal; WHO

WARNING:

Only physicians experienced in cancer chemotherapy should use Cytosar-U Sterile Powder.

For induction therapy patients should be treated in a facility with laboratory and supportive resources sufficient to monitor drug tolerance and protect and maintain a patient compromised by drug toxicity. The main toxic effect of Cytosar-U is bone marrow suppression with leukopenia, thrombocytopenia and anemia. Less serious toxicity includes nausea, vomiting, diarrhea and abdominal pain, oral ulceration, and hepatic dysfunction.

The physician must judge possible benefit to the patient against known toxic effects of this drug in considering the advisability of therapy with cytarabine. Before making this judgment or beginning treatment, the physician should be familiar with the following text.

DESCRIPTION:

Cytarabine, commonly known as ara-C, an antineoplastic, is a sterile lyophilized material for reconstitution and intravenous, intrathecal or subcutaneous administration. It is available in multi-dose vials containing 100 mg, 500 mg, 1 g or 2 g sterile cytarabine. The pH of cytarabine was adjusted, when necessary, with hydrochloric acid and/or sodium hydroxide.

Cytarabine is chemically 4-amino-1-β-D-arabinofuranosyl-2 (IH)-pyrimidinone.

Cytarabine is an odorless, white to off-white, crystalline powder which is freely soluble in water and slightly soluble in alcohol and in chloroform.

CLINICAL PHARMACOLOGY:

CELL CULTURE STUDIES

Cytarabine is cytotoxic to a wide variety of proliferating mammalian cells in culture. It exhibits cell phase specificity, primarily killing cells undergoing DNA synthesis (S-phase) and under certain conditions blocking the progression of cells from the G_1 phase to the S-phase. Although the mechanism of action is not completely understood, it appears that cytarabine acts through the inhibition of DNA polymerase. A limited, but significant, incorporation of cytarabine into both DNA and RNA has also been reported. Extensive chromosomal damage, including chromatoid breaks, have been produced by cytarabine and malignant transformation of rodent cells in culture has been reported. Deoxycytidine prevents or delays (but does not reverse) the cytotoxic activity.

Cell culture studies have shown an antiviral effect.[1] However, efficacy against herpes zoster or smallpox could not be demonstrated in controlled clinical trials.[2-4]

CELLULAR RESISTANCE AND SENSITIVITY

Cytarabine is metabolized by deoxycytidine kinase and other nucleotide kinases to the nucleotide triphosphate, an effective inhibitor of DNA polymerase; it is inactivated by a pyrimidine nucleoside deaminase which converts it to the nontoxic uracil derivative. It appears that the balance of kinase and deaminase levels may be an important factor in determining sensitivity or resistance of the cell to cytarabine.

ANIMAL STUDIES

In experimental studies with mouse tumors, cytarabine was most effective in those tumors with a high growth fraction. The effect was dependent on the treatment schedule; optimal effects were achieved when the schedule (multiple closely spaced doses or constant infusion) ensured contact of the drug with the tumor cells when the maximum number of cells were in the susceptible S-phase. The best results were obtained when courses of therapy were separated by intervals sufficient to permit adequate host recovery.

HUMAN PHARMACOLOGY

Cytarabine is rapidly metabolized and is not effective orally; less than 20 percent of the orally administered dose is absorbed from the gastrointestinal tract.

Following rapid intravenous injection of cytarabine labeled with tritium, the disappearance from plasma is biphasic. There is an initial distributive phase with a half-life of about 10 minutes, followed by a second elimination phase with a half-life of about 1 to 3 hours. After the distributive phase, more than 80 percent of plasma radioactivity can be accounted for by the inactive metabolite 1-β-D-arabinofuranosyluracil (ara-U). Within 24 hours about 80 percent of the administered radioactivity can be recovered in the urine, approximately 90 percent of which is excreted as ara-U.

Relatively constant plasma levels can be achieved by continuous intravenous infusion.

After subcutaneous or intramuscular administration of cytarabine labeled with tritium, peak-plasma levels of radioactivity are achieved about 20 to 60 minutes after injection and are considerably lower than those after intravenous administration.

Cerebrospinal fluid levels of cytarabine are low in comparison to plasma levels after single intravenous injection. However, in one patient in whom cerebrospinal levels were examined after 2 hours of constant intravenous infusion, levels approached 40 percent of the steady state plasma level. With intrathecal administration, levels of cytarabine in the cerebrospinal fluid declined with a first order half-life of about 2 hours. Because cerebrospinal fluid levels of deaminase are low, little conversion to ara-U was observed.

IMMUNOSUPPRESSIVE ACTION

Cytarabine is capable of obliterating immune responses in man during administration with little or no accompanying toxicity.[5,6] Suppression of antibody responses to E-coli-VI antigen and tetanus toxoid have been demonstrated. This suppression was obtained during both primary and secondary antibody responses.

Cytarabine also suppressed the development of cell-mediated immune responses such as delayed hypersensitivity skin reaction to dinitrochlorobenzene. However, it had no effect on already established delayed hypersensitivity reactions.

Following 5-day courses of intensive therapy with cytarabine the immune response was suppressed, as indicated by the following parameters: macrophage ingress into skin windows; circulating antibody response following primary antigenic stimulation; lymphocyte blastogenesis with phytohemagglutinin. A few days after termination of therapy there was a rapid return to normal.[7]

INDICATIONS AND USAGE:

Cytarabine in combination with other approved anticancer drugs is indicated for remission induction in acute non-lymphocytic leukemia of adults and children. It has also been found useful in the treatment of acute lymphocytic leukemia and the blast phase of chronic myelocytic leukemia. Intrathecal administration of cytarabine is indicated in the prophylaxis and treatment of meningeal leukemia.

CONTRAINDICATIONS:

Cytarabine is contraindicated in those patients who are hypersensitive to the drug.

WARNINGS:

(See BOXED WARNING)

Cytarabine is a potent bone marrow suppressant. Therapy should be started cautiously in patients with pre-existing drug-induced bone marrow suppression. Patients receiving this drug must be under close medical supervision and, during induction therapy, should have leukocyte and platelet counts performed daily. Bone marrow examinations should be performed frequently after blasts have disappeared from the peripheral blood. Facilities should be available for management of complications, possibly fatal, of bone marrow suppression (infection resulting from granulocytopenia and other impaired body defenses, and hemorrhage secondary to thrombocytopenia). One case of anaphylaxis that resulted in acute cardiopulmonary arrest and required resuscitation has been reported. This occurred immediately after the intravenous administration of cytarabine.

Severe and at times fatal CNS, GI and pulmonary toxicity (different from that seen with conventional therapy regimens of cytarabine) has been reported following some experimental dose schedules for cytarabine.[8-11] These reactions include reversible corneal toxicity, and hemorrhagic conjunctivitis, which may be prevented or diminished by prophylaxis with a local corticosteroid eye drop; cerebral and cerebellar dysfunction, including personality changes, somnolence and coma, usually reversible; severe gastrointestinal ulceration, including pneumatosis cystoides intestinalis leading to peritonitis; sepsis and liver abscess; pulmonary edema, liver damage with increased hyperbilirubinemia; bowel necrosis; and necrotizing colitis. Rarely, severe skin rash, leading to desquamation has been reported. Complete alopecia is more commonly seen with experimental high dose therapy than with standard treatment programs using cytarabine. If experimental high dose therapy is used, do not use a diluent containing benzyl alcohol.

An increase in cardiomyopathy with subsequent death has been reported following experimental high dose therapy with cytarabine in combination with cyclophosphamide when used for bone marrow transplant preparation.[12]

A syndrome of sudden respiratory distress, rapidly progressing to pulmonary edema and radio-graphically pronounced cardiomegaly has been reported following experimental high dose therapy with cytarabine used for the treatment of relapsed leukemia from one institution in 16/72 patients. The outcome of this syndrome can be fatal.[13]

Benzyl alcohol is contained in the diluent for this product. Benzyl alcohol has been reported to be associated with a fatal "Gasping Syndrome" in premature infants.

WARNINGS: *(cont'd)*

Two patients with childhood acute myelogenous leukemia who received intrathecal and intravenous cytarabine at conventional doses (in addition to a number of other concomitantly administered drugs) developed delayed progressive ascending paralysis resulting in death in one of the two patients.[14]

USE IN PREGNANCY

Cytarabine can cause fetal harm when administered to a pregnant woman. (See ANIMAL PHARMACOLOGY.) There are no adequate and well-controlled studies in pregnant women. If cytarabine is used during pregnancy, or if the patient becomes pregnant while taking cytarabine, the patient should be apprised of the potential hazard to the fetus. Women of childbearing potential should be advised to avoid becoming pregnant.

PRECAUTIONS:

General: Patients receiving cytarabine must be monitored closely. Frequent platelet and leukocyte counts and bone marrow examinations are mandatory. Consider suspending or modifying therapy when drug-induced marrow depression has resulted in a platelet count under 50,000 or a polymorphonuclear granulocyte count under 1000/mm^3. Counts of formed elements in the peripheral blood may continue to fall after the drug is stopped and reach lowest values after drug-free intervals of 12 to 24 days. When indicated, restart therapy when definite signs of marrow recovery appear (on successive bone marrow studies). Patients whose drug is withheld until "normal" peripheral blood values are attained may escape from control.

When large intravenous doses are given quickly, patients are frequently nauseated and may vomit for several hours postinjection. This problem tends to be less severe when the drug is infused.

The human liver apparently detoxifies a substantial fraction of an administered dose. Use the drug with caution and at reduced dose in patients whose liver function is poor.

Periodic checks of bone marrow, liver and kidney functions should be performed in patients receiving cytarabine.

Like other cytotoxic drugs, cytarabine may induce hyperuricemia secondary to rapid lysis of neoplastic cells. The clinician should monitor the patients's blood uric acid level and be prepared to use such supportive and pharmacologic measures as might be necessary to control this problem.

Acute pancreatitis has been reported to occur in patients being treated with cytarabine who have had prior treatment with L-asparaginase.[15]

Information for the Patient: Not applicable

Laboratory Tests: See General

Carcinogenesis, Mutagenesis, and Impairment of Fertility: Extensive chromosomal damage, including chromatoid breaks have been produced by cytarabine and malignant transformation of rodent cells in culture has been reported.

Pregnancy Category D See WARNINGS. A review of the literature has shown 32 reported cases where cytarabine was given during pregnancy, either alone or in combination with other cytotoxic agents:

Eighteen normal infants were delivered. Four of these had first trimester exposure. Five infants were premature or of low birth weight. Twelve of the 18 normal infants were followed up at ages ranging from six weeks to seven years, and showed no abnormalities. One apparently normal infant died at 90 days of gastroenteritis.

Two cases of congenital abnormalities have been reported, one with upper and lower distal limb defects,[16] and the other with extremity and ear deformities.[17] Both of these cases had first trimester exposure.

There were seven infants with various problems in the neonatal period, including pancytopenia; transient depression of WBC, hematocrit or platelets; electrolyte abnormalities; transient eosinophilia; and one case of increased IgM levels and hyperpyrexia possible due to sepsis. Six of the seven infants were also premature. The child with pancytopenia died at 21 days of sepsis.

Therapeutic abortions were done in five cases. Four fetuses were grossly normal, but one had an enlarged spleen and another showed Trisomy C chromosome abnormality in the chorionic tissue.

Because of the potential for abnormalities with cytotoxic therapy, particularly during the first trimester, a patient who is or who may become pregnant while on cytarabine should be apprised of the potential risk to the fetus and the advisability of pregnancy continuation. There is a definite, but considerably reduced risk if therapy is initiated during the second or third trimester. Although normal infants have been delivered to patients treated in all three trimesters of pregnancy, follow-up of such infants would be advisable.

Labor and Delivery: Not applicable

Nursing Mothers: It is not known whether this drug is excreted in human milk. Because many drugs are excreted in human milk and because of the potential for serious adverse reactions in nursing infants from cytarabine, a decision should be made whether to discontinue nursing or to discontinue the drug, taking into account the importance of the drug to the mother.

Pediatric Use: See INDICATIONS AND USAGE.

DRUG INTERACTIONS:

Reversible decreases in steady-state plasma digoxin concentrations and renal glycoside excretion were observed in patients receiving beta-acetyldigoxin and chemotherapy regimens containing cyclophosphamide, vincristine and prednisone with or without cytarabine or procarbazine.[39] Steady-state plasma digitoxin concentrations did not appear to change. Therefore, monitoring of plasma digoxin levels may be indicated in patients receiving similar combination chemotherapy regimens. The utilization of digitoxin for such patients may be considered as an alternative.

An *in vitro* interaction study between gentamicin and cytarabine showed a cytarabine related antagonism for the susceptibility of *K. pneumoniae* strains. This study suggests that in patients on cytarabine being treated with gentamicin for a *K. pneumoniae* infection, the lack of a prompt therapeutic response may indicate the need for reevaluation of antibacterial therapy.[40]

Clinical evidence in one patient showed possible inhibition of fluorocytosine efficacy during therapy with cytarabine.[41] This may be due to potential competitive inhibition of its uptake.[42]

ADVERSE REACTIONS:

EXPECTED REACTIONS

Because cytarabine is a bone marrow suppressant, anemia, leukopenia, thrombocytopenia, megaloblastosis and reduced reticulocytes can be expected as a result of administration with cytarabine. The severity of these reactions are dose and schedule dependent.[18] Cellular changes in the morphology of bone marrow and peripheral smears can be expected.[19]

Following 5-day constant infusions or acute injections of 50 mg/m^2 to 600 mg/m^2, white cell depression follows a biphasic course. Regardless of initial count, dosage level, or schedule, there is an initial fall starting the first 24 hours with a nadir at days 7-9. This is followed by a brief rise which peaks around the twelfth day. A second and deeper fall reaches nadir at days 15-24. Then there is rapid rise to above baseline in the next 10 days. Platelet depression is noticeable at 5 days with a peak depression occurring between days 12-15. Thereupon, a rapid rise to above baseline occurs in the next 10 days.[20]

INFECTIOUS COMPLICATIONS

Infection: Viral, bacterial, fungal, parasitic, or saprophytic infections, in any location in the body may be associated with the use of cytarabine alone or in combination with other immunosuppressive agents following immunosuppressant doses that affect cellular or humoral immunity. These infections may be mild, but can be severe and at times fatal.

The Cytarabine (Ara-C) Syndrome: A cytarabine syndrome has been described by Castleberry.[21] It is characterized by fever, myalgia, bone pain, occasionally chest pain, maculopapular rash, conjunctivitis and malaise. It usually occurs 6-12 hours following drug administration. Corticosteroids have been shown to be beneficial in treating or preventing this syndrome. If the symptoms of the syndrome are deemed treatable, corticosteroids should be contemplated as well as continuation of therapy with cytarabine.

Most Frequent Adverse Reactions: Anorexia, nausea, vomiting, diarrhea, oral and anal inflammation, or ulceration, hepatic dysfunction, fever, rash, thrombophlebitis, bleeding (all sites).

Nausea and vomiting are most frequent following rapid intravenous injection.

Less Frequent Adverse Reactions: Sepsis, pneumonia, cellulitis at injection site, skin ulceration, urinary retention, renal dysfunction, neuritis, neural toxicity, sore throat, esophageal ulceration, esophagitis, chest pain, bowel necrosis, abdominal pain, freckling, jaundice, conjunctivitis (may occur with rash), dizziness, alopecia, anaphylaxis (See WARNINGS), allergic edema, pruritus, shortness of breath, urticaria, headache

EXPERIMENTAL DOSES

Severe and at times fatal CNS, GI and pulmonary toxicity (different from that seen with conventional therapy regimens of cytarabine) has been reported following some experimental dose schedules of cytarabine.[8-11] These reactions include reversible corneal toxicity and hemorrhagic conjunctivitis, which may be prevented or diminished by prophylaxis with a local corticosteroid eye drop; cerebral and cerebellar dysfunction, including personality changes, somnolence and coma, usually reversible; severe gastrointestinal ulceration, including pneumatosis cystoides intestinalis leading to peritonitis; sepsis and liver abscess; pulmonary edema, liver damage with increased hyperbilirubinemia; bowel necrosis; and necrotizing colitis. Rarely, severe skin rash, leading to desquamation has been reported. Complete alopecia is more commonly seen with experimental high dose therapy than with standard treatment programs using cytarabine. If experimental high dose therapy is used, do not use a diluent containing benzyl alcohol.

An increase in cardiomyopathy with subsequent death has been reported following experimental high dose therapy with cytarabine in combination with cyclophosphamide when used for bone marrow transplant preparation.[12] **This cardiac toxicity may be schedule dependent.[45]**

A syndrome of sudden respiratory distress, rapidly progressing to pulmonary edema and radiographically pronounced cardiomegaly has been reported following experimental high dose therapy with cytarabine used for the treatment of relapsed leukemia from one institution in 16/72 patients. The outcome of this syndrome can be fatal.[13]

Two patients with adult acute non-lymphocytic leukemia developed peripheral motor and sensory neuropathies after consolidation with high-dose cytarabine, daunorubicin, and asparaginase. Patients treated with high-dose cytarabine should be observed for neuropathy since dose schedule alterations may be needed to avoid irreversible neurologic disorders.[22]

Ten patients treated with experimental intermediate doses of cytarabine (1 g/m^2) with and without other chemotherapeutic agents (meta-AMSA, daunorubicin, etoposide) at various dose regimes developed a diffuse interstitial pneumonitis without clear cause that may have been related to the cytarabine.[43]

Two cases of pancreatitis have been reported following experimental doses of cytarabine and numerous other drugs. Cytarabine could have been the causative agent.[44]

OVERDOSAGE:

There is no antidote for overdosage of cytarabine. Doses of 4.5 g/m^2 by intravenous infusion over 1 hour every 12 hours for 12 doses has caused an unacceptable increase in irreversible CNS toxicity and death.[9]

Single doses as high as 3 g/m^2 have been administered by rapid intravenous infusion without apparent toxicity.[23]

DOSAGE AND ADMINISTRATION:

Cytarabine is not active orally. The schedule and method of administration varies with the program of therapy to be used. Cytarabine may be given by intravenous infusion or injection, subcutaneously, or intrathecally. Thrombophlebitis has occurred at the site of drug injection or infusion in some patients, and rarely patients have noted pain and inflammation at subcutaneous injection sites. In most instances, however, the drug has been well tolerated.

Patients can tolerate higher total doses when they receive the drug by rapid intravenous injection as compared with slow infusion. This phenomenon is related to the drug's rapid inactivation and brief exposure of susceptible normal and neoplastic cells to significant levels after rapid injection. Normal and neoplastic cells seem to respond in somewhat parallel fashion to these different modes of administration and no clear-cut clinical advantage has been demonstrated for either.

In the induction therapy of acute non-lymphocytic leukemia, the usual cytarabine dose in combination with other anti-cancer drugs is 100 mg/m^2/day by continuous IV infusion (Days 1-7) or 100 mg/m^2 IV every 12 hours (Days 1-7).

The literature should be consulted for the current recommendations for use in acute lymphocytic leukemia.

INTRATHECAL USE IN MENINGEAL LEUKEMIA

Cytarabine has been used intrathecally in acute leukemia in doses ranging from 5 mg/m^2 to 75 mg/m^2 of body surface area. The frequency of administration varied from once a day for 4 days to once every 4 days. The most frequently used dose was 30 mg/m^2 every 4 days until cerebrospinal fluid findings were normal, followed by one additional treatment.[24-28] The dosage schedule is usually governed by the type and severity of central nervous system manifestations and the response to previous therapy.

If used intrathecally, do not use a diluent containing benzyl alcohol. Many clinicians reconstitute with autologous spinal fluid or preservative-free 0.9% Sodium chloride, USP, for Injection and use immediately.

Cytarabine given intrathecally may cause systemic toxicity and careful monitoring of the hemopoietic system is indicated. Modification of other anti-leukemia therapy may be necessary. Major toxicity is rare. The most frequently reported reactions after intrathecal administration were nausea, vomiting and fever; these reactions are mild and self-limiting. Paraplegia has been reported.[29] Necrotizing leukoencephalopathy occurred in 5 children; these patients had also been treated with intrathecal methotrexate and hydrocortisone, as well as by central nervous system radiation.[30] Isolated neurotoxicity has been reported.[31] Blindness occurred in two patients in remission whose treatment had consisted of combination systemic chemotherapy, prophylactic central nervous system radiation and intrathecal cytarabine.[32]

DOSAGE AND ADMINISTRATION: *(cont'd)*

Focal leukemic involvement of the central nervous system may not respond to intrathecal cytarabine and may better be treated with radiotherapy.

The 100 mg vial may be reconstituted with 5 ml of Bacteriostatic Water for Injection with Benzyl Alcohol 0.945% w/v added as preservative. The resulting solution contains 20 mg of cytarabine per ml. (Do not use Bacteriostatic Water for Injection with Benzyl Alcohol 0.945% w/v as a diluent for intrathecal use. See WARNINGS).

The 500 mg vial may be reconstituted with 10 ml Bacteriostatic Water for Injection with Benzyl Alcohol 0.945% w/v added as preservative. The resulting solution contains 50 mg of cytarabine per ml. (Do not use Bacteriostatic Water for Injection with Benzyl Alcohol 0.945% w/v as a diluent for intrathecal use. See WARNINGS).

The 1 gram vial may be reconstituted with 10 ml of Bacteriostatic Water for Injection with Benzyl Alcohol 0.945% w/v added as preservative. The resulting solution contains 100 mg of cytarabine per ml. (Do not use Bacteriostatic Water for Injection with Benzyl Alcohol 0.945% w/v as a diluent for intrathecal use. See WARNINGS).

The 2 gram vial may be reconstituted with 20 ml of Bacteriostatic Water for Injection with Benzyl Alcohol 0.945% w/v added as preservative. The resulting solution contains 100 mg of cytarabine per ml. (Do not use Bacteriostatic Water for Injection with Benzyl Alcohol 0.945% w/v as a diluent for intrathecal use. See WARNINGS).

If used intrathecally many clinicians reconstitute with preservative-free 0.9% Sodium Chloride for Injection and use immediately.

The pH of the reconstituted solutions is about 5. Solutions reconstituted with Bacteriostatic Water for Injection with Benzyl Alcohol 0.945% w/v may be stored at controlled room temperature, 15-30°C (59-86°F) for 48 hours. Discard any solutions in which a slight haze develops.

Solutions reconstituted without a preservative should be used immediately.

CHEMICAL STABILITY OF INFUSION SOLUTIONS

Chemical stability studies were performed by ultraviolet assay on cytarabine in infusion solutions. These studies showed that when reconstituted cytarabine was added to Water for Injection, 5% Dextrose in Water or Sodium Chloride Injection, 94 to 96 percent of the cytarabine was present after 192 hours storage at room temperature.

Parenteral drugs should be inspected visually for particulate matter and discoloration, prior to administration, whenever solution and container permit.

Procedures for proper handling and disposal of anticancer drugs should be considered. Several guidelines on this subject have been published.[33-38] There is no general agreement that all of the procedures recommended in the guidelines are necessary or appropriate.

Store the product at controlled room temperature 15-30°C (59-86°F).

REFERENCES:

1. Zaky DA, Betts RF, Douglas RG, et al: Varicella-Zoster Virus and Subcutaneous Cytarabine: Correlation of In Vitro Sensitivities to Blood Levels. *Antimicrob Agents Chemother*1975; *7*:229-232. **2.** Davis CM, VanDersarl JV, Coltman CA Jr: Failure of Cytarabine in Varicella-Zoster Infections. *JAMA*1973; *224*: 122-123. **3.** Betts RF, Zaky DA, Douglas RG, et al: Ineffectiveness of Subcutaneous Cytosine Arabinoside in Localized Herpes Zoster. *Ann Intern Med* 1975: *82*:778-783. **4.** Dennis DT, Doberstyn EB, Awoke S, et al: Failure of Cytosine Arabinoside in Treatment Smallpox; A Double-blind Study, *Lancet* 1974; *2*:377-379. **5.** Gray GD: ARA-C and Derivatives as Examples of Immunosuppressive Nucleoside Analogs. *Ann NY Acad Sci*1975; *255*:372-379. **6.** Mitchell MS, Wade ME, DeConti RC, et al: Immunosuppressive Effects of Cytosine Arabinoside and Methotrexate in Man. *Ann Intern Med* 1969; *70*:535-547. **7.** Frei E, Ho DHW, Bodey GP, et al: Pharmacologic and Cytokinetic Studies of Arabinosyl Cytosine, *In Unifying Concepts of Leukemia. Bibl. Hematol.* No. 39. Karger, Basel 1973, pp 1085-1097. **8.** Hopen G, Mondino BJ, Johnson BL, et al: Corneal Toxicity with Systemic Cytarabine. *Am J Ophthalmol*1981; *91*:500-504. **9.** Lazarus HM, Herzig RH, Herzig GP, et al: Central Nervous System Toxicity of High-Dose Systemic Cytosine Arabinoside. *Cancer* 1981; *48*:2577-2582. **10.** Slavin RE, Dias MA, Soral R: Cytosine Arabinoside Induced Gastrointestinal Toxic Alterations in Sequential Chemotherapeutic Protocols-A Clinical Pathologic Study of 33 Patients. *Cancer*1978; *42*:1747-1759. **11.** Haupt HM, Hutchins GM, Moore GW: Ara-C Lung: Noncardiogenic Pulmonary Edema Complicating Cytosine Arabinoside Therapy of Leukemia. *Am J Med* 1981; *70*:256-261. **12.** Takvorian T, Anderson K, Ritz J: A Fatal Cardiomyopathy Associated with High Dosage Ara-C (HIDAC) and Cyclophosphamide (CTX) in Bone Marrow Transplantation (BMTx). (Abstract submitted for 1985 AACR Meetings in Houston, Texas.) **13.** Andersson BS, Cogan B, Keating MJ, Estey EH, et al: Subacute Pulmonary Failure Complicating Therapy with High-Dose Ara-C in Acute Leukemia. *Cancer* 1985; *56*:2181-2184. **14.** Dunton SF, Ruprecht N, Spruce W, et al: Progressive Ascending Paralysis Following Administration of Intrathecal and Intravenous Cytosine Arabinoside. *Cancer* 1986; *57*:1083-1088. **15.** Altman AJ, Dinndorf P, Quinn JJ: Acute Pancreatitis in Association with Cytosine Arabinoside Therapy. *Cancer*1982; *49*:1384-1386. **16.** Shafer Al: Teratogenic Effects of Antileukemic Chemotherapy. *Arch Intern Med* 1981; *141*:514-515. **17.** Wagner VM, et al: Congenital Abnormalities in Baby Born to Cytarabine Treated Mother. *Lancet* 1980; *2*:98-99. **18.** Frei E III, Bickers JN, Hewlett JS, et al: Dose Schedule and Antitumor Studies of Arabinosyl Cytosine (NSC 63878). *Cancer Res* 1969; *29*:1325-1332. **19.** Bell WR, Wang JJ, Carbone PP, et al: Cytogenetic and Morphologic Abnormalities in Human Bone Marrow Cells during Cytosine Arabinoside Therapy. *J Hematol* 1966; *27*:771-781. **20.** Burke PJ, Serpick AA, Carbone PP, et al: A Clinical Evaluation of Dose and Schedule of Administration of Cytosine Arabinoside (NSC 63878). *Cancer Res* 1968; *28*:274-279. **21.** Castleberry RP, Crist WM, Holbrook T, et al: The Cytosine Arabinoside (Ara-C) Syndrome. *Med Pediatr Oncol*1981; *9*:257-264. **22.** Powell BL, Capizzi RL, Lyerly EW, et al: Peripheral Neuropathy After High-Dose Cytosine Arabinoside, Daunorubicin, and Asparaginase Consolidation for Acute Nonlymphocytic Leukemia. *J Clin Oncol* 1986; *4* (1): 95-97. **23.** Rudnick SA, et al: High Dose Cytosine Arabinoside (HDARAC) In Refractory Acute Leukemia. *Cancer* 1979; *44*:1189-1193. **24.** Proceedings of the Chemotherapy Conference on ARA-C: Development and Application (Cytosine Arabinoside Hydrochloride-NSC 63878), Oct. 10, 1969 **25.** Lay HN, Colebatch JH, Ekert H: Experiences with Cytosine Arabinoside in Childhood Leukemia and Lymphoma. *Med J Aust*1971; *2*:187-192. **26.** Halikowski B, Cyklis R, Armata J, et al: Cytosine Arabinoside Administered Intrathecally in Cerebromeningeal Leukemia, *Acta Paediat Scand* 1970; *59*:164-168. **27.** Wang JJ, Pratt CB: Intrathecal Arabinosyl Cytosine in Meningeal Leukemia. *Cancer* 1970; *25*:531-534. **28.** Band PR, Holland JF, Bernard J, et al: Treatment of Central Nervous System Leukemia with Intrathecal Cytosine Arabinoside. *Cancer* 1973; *32*:744-748. **29.** Saiki JH, Thompson S, Smith F, et al: Paraplegia Following Intrathecal Chemotherapy. *Cancer* 1972; *29*:370-374. **30.** Rubinstein LJ, Herman MM, Long TF, et al: Disseminated Necrotizing Leukoencephalopathy: A Complication of Treated Central System Leukemia and Lymphoma. *Cancer* 1975; *35*:291-305. **31.** Marmont AM, Damasio EE: Neurotoxicity of Intrathecal Chemotherapy for Leukemia. *Brit Med J* 1973; *4*:47. **32.** Margileth DA, Poplack DG, Pizzo PA, et al: Blindness During Remission in Two Patients with Acute Lymphoblastic Leukemia. *Cancer* 1977; *39*:58-61. **33.** Recommendations for the Safe Handling of Parenteral Antineoplastic Drugs. NIH Publication No. 83-2621. For sale by the Superintendent of Documents, US Government Printing Office, Washington, DC 20402. **34.** AMA Council Report. Guidelines for Handling Parenteral Antineoplastics. JAMA, March 15, 1985. **35.** National Study Commission on Cytotoxic Exposure-Recommendations for Handling Cytotoxic Agents. Available from Louis P. Jeffrey, ScD, Director of Pharmacy Services, Rhode Island Hospital, 593 Eddy Street, Providence, Rhode Island 02902. **36.** Clinical Oncological Society of Australia: Guidelines and recommendations for safe handling of antineoplastic agents. *Med J Australia* 1983; *1*:426-428. **37.** Jones, RB, et al: Safe handling of chemotherapeutic agents: A report from the Mount Sinai Medical Center CA-A *Cancer Journal for Clinicians* Sept/Oct., pp. 258-263. **38.** American Society of Hospital Pharmacists Technical assistance bulletin on handling cytotoxic drugs in hospitals. *Am J Hosp Pharm* 1985; *42*:131-137. **39.** Kuhlman J: Inhibition of Digoxin Absorption but not of Digitoxin During Cytostatic Drug Therapy. *Arzneim Forsch*1982; *32*:698-704. **40.** Moody MR, Morris JJ, Yang VM, et al: Effect of Two Cancer Chemotherapeutic Agents on the Antibacterial Activity of Three Antimicrobial Agents. *Antimicrob Agents Chemother* 1978; *14*:737-742. **41.** Holt RJ: Clinical Problems with 5-Fluorocytosine. *Mykosen* 1978; *21* (11):363-369. **42.** Polak A, Grenson M: Interference Between the Uptake of Pyrimidines and Purines in Yeasts. *Path Microbiol*1973; *39*:37-38. **43.** Peters WG. Willemze R, Colly LP: Results of Induction and Consolidation Treatment with Intermediate and High-Dose Ara-C and m-AMSA Containing Regimens in Patients with Primarily Failed or Relapsed Acute Leukemia and Non-Hodgkin's Lymphoma. *Scan J Hemat* 1986; *36* (Suppl 44):7-16. **44.** Siemers RF, Friedenberg WR, Norfleet RG: High-Dose Cytosine Arabinoside-Associated Pancreatitis. *Cancer*1985; *56*:1940-1942. **45.** Paul S, et al: "High Dose Ara-C Does Not Increase the Cardiotoxicity of cyclophosphamide-Total Body Irradiation Conditioning Regimes for Bone Marrow Transplantation". *Proceeding of ASCO* 1989; 8:16, abstract 60.

ANIMAL PHARMACOLOGY:

Toxicity of cytarabine in experimental animals, as well as activity, is markedly influenced by the schedule of administration. For example, in mice, the LD_{10} for single intraperitoneal administration is greater than 6000 mg/m^2. However, when administered as 8 doses, each separated by 3 hours, the LD_{10} is less than 750 mg/m^2 total dose. Similarly, although a total dose of 1920 mg/m^2 administered as 12 injections at 6-hour intervals was lethal to beagle dogs (severe bone marrow hypoplasia with evidence of liver and kidney damage), dogs receiving the same total dose administered in 8 injections (again at 6-hour intervals) over a 48-hour period survived with minimal signs of toxicity. The most consistent observation in

ANIMAL PHARMACOLOGY: *(cont'd)*

surviving dogs was elevated transaminase levels. In all experimental species the primary limiting toxic effect is marrow suppression with leukopenia. In addition, cytarabine causes abnormal cerebellar development in the neonatal hamster and is teratogenic to the rat fetus.

HOW SUPPLIED - RATED THERAPEUTICALLY EQUIVALENT:

Injection, Lyphl-Soln - Intrathecal; In - 1 gm/vial

1 gm	**$50.83**	**CYTOSAR-U, Pharmacia & Upjohn**	**00009-3295-01**

Injection, Lyphl-Soln - Intrathecal; In - 2 gm/vial

2 gm	**$99.50**	**CYTOSAR-U, Pharmacia & Upjohn**	**00009-3296-01**

Injection, Lyphl-Soln - Intrathecal; In - 100 mg/vial

1's	$6.07	Cytarabine, Fujisawa USA	00469-2410-20
5 ml	$6.00	Cytarabine, Schein Pharm (US)	00364-2467-53
100 mg	**$6.73**	**CYTOSAR-U, Pharmacia & Upjohn**	**00009-0373-01**

Injection, Lyphl-Soln - Intrathecal; In - 500 mg/vial

1's	$24.16	Cytarabine, Fujisawa USA	00469-2420-30
10 ml	$23.06	Cytarabine, Schein Pharm (US)	00364-2468-54
500 mg	**$26.75**	**CYTOSAR-U, Pharmacia & Upjohn**	**00009-0473-01**

HOW SUPPLIED - NOT RATED EQUIVALENT:

Injection, Solution - Intrathecal; In - 20 mg/ml

5 ml x 10	$6.73	TARABINE PFS, Pharmacia & Upjohn	00013-7106-78
50 ml	$50.79	TARABINE PFS, Pharmacia & Upjohn	00013-7091-73

CYTOMEGALOVIRUS IMMUNE GLOBULIN

(003055)

CATEGORIES: CMV Disease; Cytomegalovirus Disease; Immune Globulin; Orphan Drugs; Renal Transplantation; Serums, Toxoids and Vaccines; Transplantation; Pregnancy Category C; FDA Approved 1991 Jul

BRAND NAMES: **Cytogam**

DESCRIPTION:

CytoGam, Cytomegalovirus Immune Globulin Intravenous (Human) (CMV-IGIV), is an immunoglobulin G (IgG) containing a standardized amount of antibody to Cytomegalovirus (CMV). CMV-IGIV is formulated in final vial as a sterile liquid. The globulin is stabilized with 5% sucrose and 1% Albumin (Human). CMV-IGIV contains no preservative. The purified immunoglobulin is derived from pooled adult human plasma selected for high titers of antibody for Cytomegalovirus (CMV).[1] Source material for fractionation may be obtained from another U.S. licensed manufacturer. Pooled plasma was fractioned by ethanol precipitation of the proteins according to Cohn Methods 6 and 9, modified to yield a product suitable for intravenous administration. A widely utilized solvent- detergent viral inactivation process is also used.[2] Each milliliter contains 50 ± 10 mg of immunoglobulin, primarily IgG, and trace amounts of IgA and IgM; 50 mg sucrose; 10 mg of Albumin (Human). The sodium content is 20-30 mEq per liter, i.e., 1.0-1.5 mEq per 50 ml. The solution should appear colorless and translucent.

CLINICAL PHARMACOLOGY:

CMV-IGIV contains IgG antibodies representative of the large number of normal persons who contributed to the plasma pools from which the product was derived. The globulin contains a relatively high concentration of antibodies directed against Cytomegalovirus (CMV). In the case of persons who may be exposed to CMV, CMV-IGIV can raise the relevant antibodies to levels sufficient to attenuate or reduce the incidence of serious CMV disease.

In two separate clinical trials, CMV-IGIV was shown to provide effective prophylaxis in renal-transplant recipients at risk for primary CMV disease. In the first randomized trial, the incidence of virologically confirmed CMV-associated syndromes was reduced from 60% in controls (n=35) to 21% in recipients of CMV immune globulin (n=24) (P <0.01); marked leukopenia was reduced from 37% in controls to 4% in globulin recipients (P <0.01); and fungal or parasitic superinfections were not seen in globulin recipients but occurred in 20% of controls (P=0.05). Serious CMV disease was reduced from 46% to 13%. There was a concomitant but not statistically significant reduction in the incidence of CMV pneumonia (17% of controls as compared with 4% of globulin recipients). There was no effect on rates of viral isolation or seroconversion although the rate of viremia was less in CMV-IGIV recipients. In a subsequent non-randomized trial in renal transplant recipients (n=36), the incidence of virologically confirmed CMV-associated syndrome was reduced to 36% in the globulin recipients. The rates of CMV-associated pneumonia. CMV- associated hepatitis, and concomitant fungal and parasitic superinfection were similar to those in the first trial.

INDICATIONS AND USAGE:

Cytomegalovirus Immune Globulin Intravenous (Human) is indicated for the attenuation of primary (1st deg.) Cytomegalovirus disease associated with kidney transplantation. Specifically, the product is indicated for kidney transplant recipients who are seronegative for CMV and who receive a kidney from a CMV seropositive donor. In a population of seronegative recipients of seropositive kidneys approximately 75% of the untreated recipients would be expected to develop CMV disease. Clinical studies have shown a 50% reduction in 1st deg. CMV disease in renal transplant patients given Cytomegalovirus Immune Globulin Intravenous (Human).

CONTRAINDICATIONS:

CMV-IGIV should not be used in individuals with a history of a prior severe reaction associated with the administration of this or other human immunoglobulin preparations. Persons with selective immunoglobulin A deficiency have the potential for developing antibodies to immunoglobulin A and could have anaphylactic reactions to subsequent administration of blood products that contain immunoglobulin A.

WARNINGS:

During administration, the patient's vital signs should be monitored continuously and careful observation made for any symptoms throughout the infusion. Epinephrine should be available for the treatment of an acute anaphylactic reaction (See PRECAUTIONS.)

PRECAUTIONS:

Although systemic allergic reactions are rare (See ADVERSE REACTIONS), epinephrine and diphenhydramine should be available for treatment of acute allergic symptoms. If hypotension or anaphylaxis occur, the administration of the immunoglobulin should be discontinued immediately and an antidote should be given as noted above.

PRECAUTIONS: *(cont'd)*

CMV-IGIV does not contain a preservative. The vial should be entered only once for administration purposes and the infusion should begin within 6 hours. The infusion schedule should be adhered to closely (see Infusion). Do not use if the solution is turbid.

Pregnancy Category C: Animal reproduction studies have not been conducted with Cytomegalovirus Immune Globulin Intravenous (Human).

It is also not known whether Cytomegalovirus Immune Globulin Intravenous (Human) can cause fetal harm when administered to a pregnant woman or can affect reproduction capacity.

Cytomegalovirus Immune Globulin Intravenous (Human) should be given to a pregnant woman only if clearly needed.

DRUG INTERACTIONS:

Antibodies present in immune globulin preparations may interfere with the immune response to line virus vaccines such as measles, mumps, and rubella; therefore, vaccination with live virus vaccines should be deferred until approximately three months after administration of CMV-IGIV. If such vaccinations were given shortly after CMV-IGIV, a revaccination may be necessary. Admixtures of CMV-IGIV with other drugs have not been evaluated. It is recommended that CMV-IGIV be administered separately from other drugs or medications which the patient may be receiving (See DOSAGE AND ADMINISTRATION.)

ADVERSE REACTIONS:

Minor reactions such as flushing, chills, muscle cramps, back pain, fever, nausea, vomiting, arthralgia, and wheezing were the most frequent adverse reactions observed during the clinical trials of CMV-IGIV. The incidence of these reactions during the clinical trials was less than 5.0% of all infusions and were most often related to infusion rates. A potential side reaction might be hypotension but this has not been observed in over 200 infusions. If a patient develops a minor side effect, slow the rate immediately or temporarily interrupt the infusion.

Severe reactions such as angioneurotic edema and anaphylactic shock, although not observed during clinical trials, are a possibility. Clinical anaphylaxis may occur even when the patient is not known to be sensitized to immune globulin products. A reaction may be related to the rate of infusion; therefore, carefully adhere to the infusion, rates as outlined under DOSAGE AND ADMINISTRATION. If anaphylaxis or drop in blood pressure occurs, discontinue infusion and use antidote such as diphenhydramine and adrenaline.

OVERDOSAGE:

Although little data are available, clinical experience with other immunoglobulin preparations suggests that the major manifestations would be those related to volume overload.

DOSAGE AND ADMINISTRATION:

The maximum recommended total dosage per infusion is 150 mg/kg, administered according to the following schedule:

TABLE 1

Within 72 hours of transplant:	150 mg/kg
2 weeks post transplant:	100 mg/kg
4 weeks post transplant:	100 mg/kg
6 weeks post transplant:	100 mg/kg
8 weeks post transplant:	100 mg/kg
12 weeks post transplant:	50 mg/kg
16 weeks post transplant:	50 mg/kg

Preparation for Administration: Remove the tab portion of the vial cap and clean the rubber stopper with 70% alcohol or equivalent. DO NOT SHAKE VIAL; AVOID FOAMING.

Parenteral drug products should be inspected visually for particulate matter and discoloration prior to administration whenever solution and container permit. Infuse the solution only if it is colorless, free of particulate matter and not turbid.

Infusion: Infusion should begin within 6 hours entering the vial and should be completed within 12 hours of reconstitution. Vital signs should be taken preinfusion, mid-way and post-infusion as well as before any rate increase. CMV-IGIV should be administered through a separate intravenous line using a constant infusion pump (*i.e.*, IVAC pump or equivalent). Pre-dilution of CMV-IGIV before infusion is not recommended. CMV-IGIV should be administered through a separate intravenous line. If this is not possible, CMV-IGIV may be 'piggybacked' into a pre-existing line if that line contains either Sodium Chloride, injection, USP, or one of the following dextrose solutions (with or without NaCl added): 2.5% dextrose in water, 5% dextrose in water, 10% dextrose in water, 20% dextrose in water. If a pre-existing line must be used, the CMV-IGIV should not be diluted more than 1:2 with any of the above-named solutions. Admixtures of CMV-IGIV with any other solutions have not been evaluated. While filters are not necessary, an in-line filter may be used for the infusion of CMV-IGIV.

Initial Dose: Administer intravenously at 15 mg per kg body weight per hour. If no adverse reactions occur after 30 minutes, the rate may be increased to 30 mg/kg/hr; if no adverse reactions occur after a subsequent 30 minutes then the infusion may be increased to 60 mg/kg/hr (volume not to exceed 75 ml/hour). DO NOT EXCEED THIS RATE OF ADMINISTRATION. The patient should be monitored closely during and after each rate change.

Subsequent Doses: Administer at 15 mg/kg/hr for 15 minutes. If no adverse reactions occur, increase to 30 mg/kg/hr for 15 minutes and then increase to a maximum rate of 60 mg/kg/hr (volume not to exceed 75 ml/hour). DO NOT EXCEED THIS RATE OF ADMINISTRATION. The patient should be monitored closely during each rate change.

Potential adverse reactions are: flushing, chills, muscle cramps, back pain, fever, nausea, vomiting, wheezing, drop in blood pressure. Minor adverse reactions have been infusion rate related - if the patient develops a minor side effect (*i.e.*, nausea, back pain, flushing), slow the rate or temporarily interrupt the infusion. If anaphylaxis or drop in blood pressure occurs, discontinue infusion and use antidote such as diphenhydramine and adrenaline.

To prevent the transmission of hepatitis viruses or other infectious agents from one person to another, sterile disposable syringes and needles should be used. The syringes and needles should not be reused.

Storage: CMV-IGIV should be stored between 2°-8°C (35.6°-46.4°F) and used within 6 hours after entering the vial.

REFERENCES:

1. Snydman, D.R., Mclver, J., Leszczynski, J., Cho, S.I., Werner, B.G., Berardi V.P., LoGerfo, F., Heinze-Lacey, B., Grady, G.F. A Pilot Trial of a Novel Cytomegalovirus Immune Globulin in Renal Transplant Recipients. Transplantation 38(5):553-557, 1984. **2.** Horowitz B., Wiebe, M.E., Lippin, A. et al. Inactivation of Viruses in Labile Blood Derivatives. Transfusion 1985;25:516- 522. **3.** Snydman D.R., Werner, B.G. and Heinze-Lacey, B.H., et al. Use of Cytomegalovirus Immune Globulin to Prevent Cytomegalovirus Disease in Renal Transplant Recipients. NEJM 317:1049-1054, 1987. **4.** Snydman, D.R., Werner, B.G. and Tilney, N.L., et al. A Final Analysis of Primary Cytomegalovirus Disease Prevention in Renal Transplant Recipients with a Cytomegalovirus Immune Globulin: Comparison of Randomized and Open-Label Trials. Transplant. Proceed. 23(1): 1357-1360, 1991. **5.** Ho, M., Suwansirikul, S., Dowling, J.N., et al. The Transplanted Kidney as a Source of Cytomegalovirus

REFERENCES: *(cont'd)*

Infection. NEJM 293 (2):1109-1112, 1975. **6.** Werner, B.G., Snydman, D.R., Freeman, R. et al. Cytomegalovirus Immune Globulin for the Prevention of Primary CMV Disease in Renal Transplant Patients: Analysis of Usage Under Treatment of IND Status. Transplant. Proceed.25(1): 1441-1443, 1993

HOW SUPPLIED - EQUIVALENTS NOT AVAILABLE:

Injection, Solution - Intravenous - 2500 mg

1's	$571.25	CYTOGAM, Mass Biol Labs	14362-0119-01
50 ml	$450.81	CYTOGAM, Medimmune	60574-3101-01

DACARBAZINE *(000938)*

CATEGORIES: Antineoplastics; Hodgkin's Disease; Melanoma; Oncologic Drugs; Pregnancy Category C; FDA Approval Pre 1982

BRAND NAMES: *Dacarbazin*; *Dacarbazine DBL*; *Dacarbazine Dome*; *Dacarbazine For Injection*; *Dacatic*; *D.T.I.C.*; *D.T.I.C.-Dome*; *DTIC* (Germany, Canada); *DTIC Dome*; *DTIC-Dome* (England); *Deticene* (France); *Detimedac* (Germany); **Dtic-Dome** *(International brand names outside U.S. in italics)*

FORMULARIES: BC-BS; Medi-Cal; WHO

> WARNING:
> It is recommended that dacarbazine be administered under the supervision of a qualified physician experienced in the use of cancer chemotherapeutic agents.
> 1. Hemopoietic depression is the most common toxicity with dacarbazine (See WARNINGS.)
> 2. Hepatic necrosis has been reported (See WARNINGS.)
> 3. Studies have demonstrated this agent to have a carcinogenic and teratogenic effect when used in animals.
> 4. In treatment of each patient, the physician must weigh carefully the possibility of achieving therapeutic benefit against the risk of toxicity.

DESCRIPTION:

Dacarbazine is a colorless to an ivory colored solid which is light sensitive. Each vial contains 100 mg of dacarbazine, or 200 mg of dacarbazine (the active ingredient), anhydrous citric acid and mannitol. Dacarbazine is reconstituted and administered intravenously (pH 3-4). Dacarbazine is an anticancer agent. Chemically, dacarbazine is 5-(3,3- dimethyl-l-triazeno)-imidazole-4-carboxamide (DTIC).

CLINICAL PHARMACOLOGY:

After IV administration of dacarbazine, the volume of distribution exceeds total body water content in some body tissue, probably the liver. Its disappearance from the plasma is biphasic with initial half- life of 19 minutes and a terminal half-life of 5 hours.[1] In a patient with renal and hepatic dysfunctions, the half-lives were lengthened to 55 minutes and 7.2 hours.[1] The average cumulative excretion of unchanged dacarbazine in the urine is 40% of the injected dose in 6 hours.[1] Dacarbazine is subject to renal tubular secretion rather than glomerular filtration. At therapeutic concentrations, dacarbazine is not appreciably bound to plasma proteins.

In man, dacarbazine is extensively degraded. Besides unchanged dacarbazine, 5-aminoimidazole-4 carboxamide (AIC) is a major metabolite of dacarbazine excreted in the urine. AIC is a major metabolite of dacarbazine excreted on the urine. AIC is not derived endogenously but from the injected dacarbazine, because the administration of radioactive dacarbazine labeled with ^{14}C in the imidazole portion of the molecule (dacarbazine-2-^{14}) gives rise to AIC-2-^{14}C.[1]

Although the exact mechanism of action of dacarbazine is not known, three hypotheses have been offered:

1. inhibition of DNA-synthesis by acting as a purine analog.

2. action as an alkylating agent.

3. interaction with SH groups.

INDICATIONS AND USAGE:

Dacarbazine is indicated in the treatment of metastatic malignant melanoma. In addition, dacarbazine is also indicated for Hodgkin's disease as a second-line therapy when used in combination with other effective agents.

CONTRAINDICATIONS:

Dacarbazine is contraindicated in patients who have demonstrated a hypersensitivity to it in the past.

WARNINGS:

Hemopoietic depression is the most common toxicity with dacarbazine and involves primarily the leukocytes and platelets, although anemia may sometimes occur. Leukopenia and thrombocytopenia may be severe enough to cause death. The possible bone marrow depression requires careful monitoring of white blood cells, red blood cells, and platelet levels. Hemopoietic toxicity may warrant temporary suspension or cessation of therapy with dacarbazine.

Hepatic toxicity, accompanied by hepatic vein thrombosis and hepatocellular necrosis resulting in death, has been reported. The incidence of such reactions has been low; approximately 0.01% of patients treated. This toxicity has been observed mostly when dacarbazine has been administered concomitantly with other anti-neoplastic drugs; however, it has also been reported in some patients treated with dacarbazine alone.

Anaphylaxis can occur following the administration of dacarbazine.

PRECAUTIONS:

Hospitalization is not always necessary but adequate laboratory study capability must be available. Extravasation of the drug subcutaneously during IV administration may result in tissue damage and severe pain. Local pain, burning sensation, and irritation at the site of injection may be relieved by locally applied hot packs.

Carcinogenicity of dacarbazine was studied in rats and mice. Proliferative endocardial lesions, including fibrocarcinomas and sarcomas, were induced by dacarbazine in rats. In mice, administration of dacarbazine resulted in the induction of angiosarcomas of the spleen.

Pregnancy Category C: Dacarbazine has been shown to be teratogenic in rats when given in doses 20 times the human daily dose on day 12 of gestation. Dacarbazine when administered in 10 times the human dose female rats mated to male rats (twice weekly for 9 weeks) did not affect the male libido, although female rats mated to male rats had higher incidence of resorptions than controls. In rabbits, dacarbazine daily dose 7 times the human daily dose

PRECAUTIONS: *(cont'd)*

given on days 6-15 of gestation resulted in fetal skeletal abnormalities. There are no adequate and well controlled studies in pregnant women. Dacarbazine should be used during pregnancy only if the potential benefit justifies the potential risk to the fetus. It is not known whether this drug is excreted in human milk. Because many drugs are excreted in human milk and because the potential for tumorigenicity shown for dacarbazine in animal studies, a decision should be made whether to continue nursing or to discontinue the drug, taking into account the importance of the drug to the mother.

ADVERSE REACTIONS:

Symptoms of anorexia, nausea, and vomiting are the most frequently noted of all toxic reactions. Over 90% of the patients are affected with the initial few doses. The vomiting lasts 1-12 hours and is incompletely and unpredictably palliated with phenobarbital and/or prochlorperazine. Rarely, intractable nausea and vomiting have necessitated discontinuance of therapy with dacarbazine. Rarely, dacarbazine has caused diarrhea. Some helpful suggestions include restricting the patient's oral intake of food for 4-6 hours prior to treatment. The rapid toleration of these symptoms suggests that a central nervous system mechanism may be involved, and usually these symptoms subside after the first 1 or 2 days.

There are a number of minor toxicities that are infrequently noted. Patients have experienced an influenzae-like syndrome of fever to 39° C, myalgias and malaise. These symptoms occur usually after large single doses, may last for several days, and then may occur with successive treatments.

Alopecia has been noted as has facial flushing and facial paresthesia. There have been few reports of significant liver or renal function test abnormalities in man. However, these abnormalities have been observed more frequently in animal studies.

Erythematous and urticarial rashes have been observed infrequently after administration of dacarbazine. Rarely, photosensitivity reactions may occur.

OVERDOSAGE:

Give supportive treatment and monitor blood cell counts.

DOSAGE AND ADMINISTRATION:

Malignant Melanoma: The recommended dosage is 2 to 4.5 mg/kg/day for 10 days. Treatment may be repeated at 4 week intervals. [2].

An alternativee recommended dosage is 250 mg/square meter body surface/day IV for 5 days. Treatment may be repeated every 3 weeks.[3,4]

Hodgkin's Disease: The recommended dosage of dacarbazine in the treatment of Hodgkin's disease is 150 mg/square meter body surface for 5 days, in combination with other effective drugs. Treatment may be repeated every 4 weeks.[5] An alternative recommended dosage is 375 mg/kg square meter body surface on day 1, in combination with other effective drugs, to be repeated every 15 days.[6]

Dacarbazine 100 mg/vial and 200 mg vial are reconstituted with 9.9 ml and 19.7 ml, respectively, of Sterile Water for Injection, USP. The resulting solution contains 10 mg/ml of dacarbazine having a pH of 3.0 to 4.0. The calculated dose of the resulting solution is drawn into a syringe and administered *only* intravenously.

The reconstituted solution may be further diluted with 5% dextrose injection, USP or sodium chloride injection, USP and administered as an IV infusion.

After reconstitution and prior to use, the solution in the vial may be stored at 4°C for up to 72 hours or at normal room conditions (temperature and light) for up to 8 hours. If the reconstituted solution is further diluted in 5% dextrose injection, USP or sodium chloride injection, USP, the resulting solution may be stored at 4°C for up to 24 hours or at normal room conditions for up to 8 hours.

Procedures for proper handling and disposal of anticancer drugs should be considered. Several guidelines on this subject have been published.[7-12] There is no general agreement that all of the procedures recommended in the guidelines are necessary or appropriate.

REFERENCES:

1. Loo, T.J. *et al.* Mechanism of action and pharmacological studies with DTIC (NSC-45388). Cancer Treatment Reports 60: 149-152, 1976. **2.** Nathanson, L. *et al.*:Characteristics of prognosis and response to an imidazole carboxamide in malignant melanoma. Clinical Pharmacology and Therapeutics 12:955-962, 1971. **3.** Costanza, M.E. *et al.*: Therapy of malignant melanoma with an imidazole carboximide and bischloroethyl nitrosourea. Cancer 30: 1457-1461, 1972. **4.** Luce J.K. *et al.*: Clinical Trials with the antitumor agent 5-(3,3-dimethyl-l-triazeno) imidazole-4-carboxamide (NSC-45388). Cancer Chemotherapy Reports 54: 119-124, 1970. **5.** Bonnadonna. G., *et al*: Combined Chemotherapy (MOPP or ABVD)-radiotherapy approach in advanced Hodgkin's disease. Cancer Treatment Reports. 61: 769-777, 1977. **6.** Santoro A., and Bonnadonna, G.: Prolonged disease-free survival in MOPP- resistant Hodgkin's after treatment with adriamycin, bleomycin, vinblastine and dacarbazine (ABVD). Cancer Chemotherapy Pharmocol 2:101- 105, 1979. **7.** Recommendations for the Safe Handling of Parenteral Antineoplastic Drugs. NIH Publication No. 83-2621. For sale by the Superintendent of Documents, U.S. Government Printing Office, Washington D.C. 20402. **8.** AMA Council Report, Guidelines for Handling Parenteral Antineoplastics. JAMA, March 15, 1985. **9.** National Study Commission on Cytotoxic Exposure - Recommendations for Handling Cytotoxic Agents. Available from Louis P. Jeffrey, Sc D. Director of Pharmacy Services, Rhode Island Hospital, 593 Eddy Street, Providence, Rhode Island 02902. **10.** Clinical Oncological Society of Australia: Guidelines and recommendations for the safe handling of antineoplastic agents. Med. J. Australia 1:426-428, 1983. **11.** Jones R.B. *et al:* Safe handling of chemotherapeutic agents: A report from the Mount Sinai Medical Center. Ca-A Cancer Journal for Clinicians Sept./Oct. 258-263, 1983. **12.** American Society of Hospital Pharmacists technical assistance bulletin on handling cytotoxic drugs in hospitals. Am J. Hosp. Pharm 42: 131-137, 1985.

HOW SUPPLIED - EQUIVALENTS NOT AVAILABLE:

Injection, Lyphl-Soln - Intravenous - 10 mg/ml

10 ml	$86.25	Dacarbazine, Fujisawa USA	00469-2270-30
20 ml	$140.63	Dacarbazine, Fujisawa USA	00469-2280-40

Injection, Lyphl-Soln - Intravenous - 100 mg/vial

10 ml	**$165.92**	**DTIC-DOME, Bayer**	**00026-8151-10**
20 ml	**$266.70**	**DTIC-DOME, Bayer**	**00026-8151-20**

DACTINOMYCIN *(000939)*

CATEGORIES: Antibiotics; Antineoplastics; Cancer; Chemotherapy; Choriocarcinoma; Ewing's Sarcoma; Oncologic Drugs; Pain; Rhabdomyosarcoma; Sarcoma; Sarcoma Botryoides; Testicular Carcinoma; Tumors; Uterine Carcinoma; Wilms' Tumor; Pregnancy Category C; FDA Approval Pre 1982

BRAND NAMES: *Ac-De* (Mexico); **Cosmegen**; *Cosmegen, Lyovac* (England); *Cosmogen Lyovac*, *Lyovac* (England)
(International brand names outside U.S. in italics)

FORMULARIES: BC-BS; Medi-Cal; WHO

WARNING:
Dactinomycin is extremely corrosive to soft tissue. If extravasation occurs during intravenous use, severe damage to soft tissues will occur. In at least one instance, this has led to contracture of the arms.
DOSAGE

The dosage of dactinomycin is calculated in micrograms (mcg). The usual adult dosage is 500 micrograms (0.5 mg) daily intravenously for a maximum of five days. The dosage for adults or children should not exceed 15 mcg/kg or 400-600 mcg/square meter of body surface daily intravenously for five days. Calculation of the dosage for obese or edematous patients should be on the basis of surface area in an effort to relate dosage to lean body mass.

DESCRIPTION:

Dactinomycin is one of the actinomycins, a group of antibiotics produced by various species of *Streptomyces*. Dactinomycin is the principal component of the mixture of actinomycins produced by*Streptomyces parvullus*. Unlike other species of*Streptomyces*, this organism yields an essentially pure substance that contains only traces of similar compounds differing in the amino acid content of the peptide side chains.[1] The empirical formula is $C_{62}H_{86}N_{12}O_{16}$.

Dactinomycin is a sterile, yellow lyophilized powder for injection by the intravenous route or by regional perfusion after reconstitution. Each vial contains 0.5 mg (500 mcg) of dactinomycin and 20.0 mg of mannitol.

CLINICAL PHARMACOLOGY:

ACTION

Generally, the actinomycins exert an inhibitory effect on gram-positive and gram-negative bacteria and on some fungi. However, the toxic properties of the actinomycins (including dactinomycin) in relation to antibacterial activity are such as to preclude their use as antibiotics in the treatment of infectious diseases.

Because the actinomycins are cytotoxic, they have an antineoplastic effect that has been demonstrated in experimental animals with various types of tumor implant. This cytotoxic action is the basis for their use in the palliative treatment of certain types of cancer.

PHARMACOKINETICS AND METABOLISM

Results of a study[2] in patients with malignant melanoma indicate that dactinomycin (^{3}H actinomycin D) is minimally metabolized, is concentrated in nucleated cells, and does not penetrate the blood brain barrier. Approximately 30% of the dose was recovered in urine and feces in one week. The terminal plasma half-life for radioactivity was approximately 36 hours.

INDICATIONS AND USAGE:

WILMS' TUMOR[3]

The neoplasm responding most frequently to dactinomycin is Wilms' tumor. With low doses of both dactinomycin and radiotherapy, temporary objective improvement may be as good as and may last longer than with higher doses of each given alone. In the National Wilms' Tumor study, combination therapy with dactinomycin and vincristine together with surgery and radiotherapy, was shown to have significantly improved the prognosis of patients in groups II and III. Dactinomycin and vincristine were given for a total of seven cycles, so maintenance therapy continued for approximately 15 months.[4]

Postoperative radiotherapy in group I patients and optimal combination chemotherapy for those in group IV are unsettled issues. About 70 percent of lung metastases have disappeared with an appropriate combination of radiation, dactinomycin and vincristine.[5]

RHABDOMYOSARCOMA

Temporary regression of the tumor and beneficial subjective results have occurred with dactinomycin in rhabdomyosarcoma which, like most soft tissue sarcomas, is comparatively radio-resistant.

Several groups have reported successful use of cyclophosphamide, vincristine, dactinomycin[6] and doxorubicin hydrochloride in various combinations. Effective combinations have included vincristine and dactinomycin; vincristine, dactinomycin and cyclophosphamide (VAC therapy) and all four drugs in sequence.[7] At present, the most effective treatment for children with inoperable or metastatic rhabdomyosarcoma has been VAC chemotherapy.[8] Two-thirds of these children were doing well without evidence of disease at a median time of three years after diagnosis.[9]

CARCINOMA OF TESTIS AND UTERUS[10]

The sequential use of dactinomycin and methotrexate, along with meticulous monitoring of human chorionic gonadotropin levels until normal, has resulted in survival in the majority of women with metastatic choriocarcinoma.[11] Sequential therapy is used if there is:

1. Stability in gonadotropin titers following two successive courses of an agent.

2. Rising gonadotropin titers during treatment.

3. Severe toxicity preventing adequate therapy.

In patients with nonmetastatic choriocarcinoma, dactinomycin or methotrexate or both, have been used successfully, with or without surgery.[11]

Dactinomycin has been beneficial as a single agent in the treatment of metastatic non-seminomatour testicular carcinoma when used in cycles of 500 mcg/day for five consecutive days, every 6-8 weeks for periods of four months or longer.[12]

OTHER NEOPLASMS

Dactinomycin has been given intravenously or by regional perfusion, either alone or with other antineoplastic compounds or x-ray therapy, in the palliative treatment of Ewing's sarcoma and sarcoma botryoides. For nonmetastatic Ewing's sarcoma, promising results were obtained when dactinomycin (45 mcg/m^2) and cyclophosphamide (1200 mg/m^2) were given sequentially and with radiotherapy over an 18 month period. Those with metastatic disease remain the subject of continued investigation with a more aggressive chemotherapeutic regimen employed initially.[13]

Temporary objective improvement and relief of pain and discomfort have followed the use of dactinomycin usually in conjunction with radiotherapy for sarcoma botryoides.[14] This palliative effect ranges from transitory inhibition of tumor growth to a considerable but temporary regression in tumor size.

DACTINOMYCIN AND RADIATION THERAPY

Much evidence suggests that dactinomycin potentiates the effects of x-ray therapy. The converse also appears likely; i.e., dactinomycin may be more effective when radiation therapy also is given.

With combined dactinomycin-radiation therapy, the normal skin, as well as the buccal and pharyngeal mucosa, shows early erythema. A smaller than usual x-ray dose when given with dactinomycin causes erythema and vesiculation,[7] which progress more rapidly through the stages of tanning and desquamation. Healing may occur in four to six weeks rather than two to three months. Erythema from previous x-ray therapy may be reactivated by dactinomycin alone, even when irradiation occurred many months earlier, and especially when the interval between the two forms of therapy is brief. This potentiation of radiation effect represents a special problem when the irradiation treatment area includes the mucous membrane. When irradiation is directed toward the nasopharynx, the combination may produce severe oropharyngeal mucositis.[13]*Severe reactions may ensue if high doses of both dactinomycin and radiation therapy are used or if the patient is particularly sensitive to such combined therapy.*

INDICATIONS AND USAGE: *(cont'd)*

Because of this potentiating effect, dactinomycin may be tried in radio-sensitive tumors not responding to doses of x-ray therapy that can be tolerated. Objective improvement in tumor size and activity may be observed when lower, better tolerated doses of both types of therapy are employed.

DACTINOMYCIN AND PERFUSION TECHNIC

Dactinomycin alone or with other antineoplastic agents has also been given by the isolation-perfusion technic, either as palliative treatment or as an adjunct to resection of a tumor. Some tumors considered resistant to chemotherapy and radiation therapy may respond when the drug is given by the perfusion technic. Neoplasms in which dactinomycin has been tried by this technic include various types of sarcoma carcinoma and adenocarcinoma.

In some instances tumors regressed, pain was relieved for variable periods, and surgery made possible. On other occasions, however, the outcome has been less favorable. Nevertheless, in selected cases, the drug by perfusion may provide more effective palliation than when given systemically.

Dactinomycin by the isolation-perfusion technic offers certain advantages, provided leakage of the drug through the general circulation into other areas of the body is minimal. By this technic the drug is in continuous contact with the tumor for the duration of treatment. The dose may be increased well over that used by the systemic route, usually without adding to the danger of toxic effects. If the agent is confined to an isolated part, it should not interfere with the patient's defense mechanism. Systemic absorption of toxic product from neoplastic tissue can be minimized by removing the perfusate when the procedure is finished.

CONTRAINDICATIONS:

If dactinomycin is given at or about the time of infection with chicken pox or herpes zoster, a severe generalized disease, which may result in death, may occur.

PRECAUTIONS:

General: Dactinomycin should be administered only under the supervision of a physician who is experienced in the use of cancer chemotherapeutic agents.

This drug is highly toxic and both powder and solution must be handled and administered with care. Inhalation of dust or vapors and contact with skin or mucous membranes especially those of the eyes, must be avoided. Should accidental eye contact occur, copious irrigation with water should be instituted immediately, followed by prompt ophthalmologic consultation. Should accidental skin contact occur, the affected part must be irrigated immediately with copious amounts of water for at least 15 minutes.

As with all antineoplastic agents, dactinomycin is a toxic drug and very careful and frequent observation of the patient for adverse reactions is necessary. These reactions may involve any tissue of the body. The possibility of an anaphylactoid reaction should be borne in mind.

Increased incidence of gastrointestinal toxicity and marrow suppression has been reported when dactinomycin was given with x-ray therapy.

Particular caution is necessary when administering dactinomycin within two months of irradiation for the treatment of right-sided Wilms' tumor, since hepatomegaly and elevated SGOT levels have been noted.[15,16]

Nausea and vomiting due to dactinomycin make it necessary to give this drug intermittently. It is extremely important to observe the patient daily for toxic side effects when multiple chemotherapy is employed, since a full course of therapy occasionally is not tolerated. If stomatitis, diarrhea, or severe hemopoietic depression appear during therapy, these drugs should be discontinued until the patient has recovered.

Recent reports indicate an increased incidence of second primary tumors following treatment with radiation and antineoplastic agents, such as dactinomycin. Multi-modal therapy creates the need for careful, long-term observation of cancer survivors.

Laboratory Tests: Many abnormalities of renal, hepatic, and bone marrow function have been reported in patients with neoplastic disease and receiving dactinomycin. It is advisable to check renal, hepatic, and bone marrow functions frequently.

Drug/Laboratory Test Interactions: It has been reported that dactinomycin may interfere with bioassay procedures for the determination of antibacterial drug levels.[17]

Carcinogenesis, Mutagenesis, and Impairment of Fertility: The International Agency on Research on Cancer has judged that dactinomycin is a positive carcinogen in animals. Local sarcomas were produced in mice and rats after repeated subcutaneous or intraperitoneal injection. Mesenchymal tumors occurred in male F344 rats given intraperitoneal injections of 0.05 mg/kg, 2 to 5 times per week for 18 weeks. The first tumor appeared at 23 weeks.

Dactinomycin has been shown to be mutagenic in a number of test systems*in vitro* and *in vivo* including human fibroblasts and leucocytes, and HELA cells. DNA damage and cytogenetic effects have been demonstrated in the mouse and the rat.

Adequate fertility studies have not been reported.

Pregnancy Category C: Dactinomycin has been shown to cause malformations and embryotoxicity in the rat, rabbit and hamster when given in doses of 50-100 mcg/kg intravenously (3-7 times the maximum recommended human dose). There are no adequate and well-controlled studies in pregnant women. Dactinomycin should be used during pregnancy only if the potential benefit justifies the potential risk to the fetus.

Nursing Mothers: It is not known whether this drug is excreted in human milk. Because many drugs are excreted in human milk and because of the potential for serious adverse reactions in nursing infants from dactinomycin, a decision should be made whether to discontinue nursing or to discontinue the drug, taking into account the importance of the drug to the mother.

Pediatric Use: The greater frequency of toxic effects of dactinomycin in infants suggest that this drug should be given to infants only over the age of 6 to 12 months.

ADVERSE REACTIONS:

Toxic effects (excepting nausea and vomiting) usually do not become apparent until two to four days after a course of therapy is stopped, and may not be maximal before one to two weeks have elapsed. Deaths have been reported. However, adverse reactions are usually reversible on discontinuance of therapy. They include the following:

Miscellaneous: malaise, fatigue, lethargy, fever, myalgia, proctitis, hypocalcemia.

Oral: cheilitis, dysphagia, esophagitis, ulcerative stomatitis, pharyngitis.

Gastrointestinal: anorexia, nausea, vomiting, abdominal pain, diarrhea, gastrointestinal ulceration, liver toxicity including ascites, hepatomegaly, hepatitis, and liver function test abnormalities. Nausea and vomiting, which occur early during the first few hours after administration, may be alleviated by giving antiemetics.

Hematologic: anemia, even to the point of aplastic anemia, agranulocytosis, leukopenia, thrombopenia, pancytopenia, reticulopenia. Platelet and white cell counts should be done *daily* to detect severe hemopoietic depression. If either count markedly decreases, the drug should be withheld to allow marrow recovery. This often takes up to three weeks.

Dermatologic: alopecia, skin eruptions, acne, flare-up of erythema or increased pigmentation of previously irradiated skin.

ADVERSE REACTIONS: *(cont'd)*

Soft tissues: Dactinomycin is extremely corrosive. If extravasation occurs during intravenous use, severe damage to soft tissues will occur. In at least one instance, this has led to contracture of the arms.

OVERDOSAGE:

The intravenous LD_{50} of dactinomycin in the rat is 460 mcg/kg.

DOSAGE AND ADMINISTRATION:

Toxic reactions due to dactinomycin are frequent and may be severe (see ADVERSE REACTIONS), thus limiting in many instances the amount that may be given. However, the severity of toxicity varies markedly and is only partly dependent on the dose employed. The drug must be given in short courses.

INTRAVENOUS USE

The dosage of dactinomycin varies depending on the tolerance of the patient, the size and location of the neoplasm, and the use of other forms of therapy. It may be necessary to decrease the usual dosages suggested below when other chemotherapy or x-ray therapy is used concomitantly or has been used previously.

The dosage for adults or children should not exceed 15 mcg/kg or 400-600 mcg/square meter of body surface daily intravenously for five days.[18,7] Calculation of the dosage for obese or edematous patients should be on the basis of surface area in an effort to relate dosage to lean body mass.

Adults: The usual adult dosage is 500 mcg (0.5 mg) daily intravenously for a maximum of five days.

Children: In children 15 mcg (0.015 mg) per kilogram of body weight is given intravenously daily for five days. An alternative schedule is a total dosage of 2500 mcg (2.5 mg) per square meter of body surface given intravenously over a one week period.

In both adults and children, a second course may be given after at least three weeks have elapsed, provided all signs of toxicity have disappeared.

Reconstitute dactinomycin by adding 1.1 ml of **Sterile Water for Injection (without preservative)** using aseptic precautions. The resulting solution of dactinomycin will contain approximately 500 mcg or 0.5 mg per ml.

Parenteral drug products should be inspected visually for particulate matter and discoloration prior to administration, whenever solution and container permit. When reconstituted, dactinomycin is a clear, gold-colored solution.

Once reconstituted, the solution of dactinomycin can be added to infusion solutions of Dextrose Injection 5 percent or Sodium Chloride Injection either directly or to the tubing of a running intravenous infusion.

Although reconstituted dactinomycin is chemically stable, the product does not contain a preservative and accidental microbial contamination might result. Any unused portion should be discarded. Use of water containing preservatives (benzyl alcohol or parabens) to reconstitute dactinomycin for injection, results in the formation of a precipitate.

Partial removal of dactinomycin from intravenous solutions by cellulose ester membrane filters used in some intravenous in-line filters has been reported.[19]

Since dactinomycin is extremely corrosive to soft tissue precautions for materials of this nature should be observed.

If the drug is given directly into the vein without the use of an infusion, the "two-needle technic" should be used. Reconstitute and withdraw the calculated dose from the vial with one sterile needle. Use another sterile needle for direct injection into the vein.

Discard any unused portion of the dactinomycin solution.

Isolation-Perfusion Technic[20,21,22]

The dosage schedules and the technic itself vary from one investigator to another; the published literature, therefore, should be consulted for details. In general, the following doses are suggested:

50 mcg (0.05 mg) per kilogram of body weight for lower extremity or pelvis.

35 mcg (0.035 mg) per kilogram of body weight for upper extremity.

It may be advisable to use lower doses in obese patients, or when previous chemotherapy or radiation therapy has been employed.

Complications of the perfusion technic are related mainly to the amount of drug that escapes into the systemic circulation and may consist of hemopoietic depression, absorption of toxic products from massive destruction of neoplastic tissue, increased susceptibility to infection, impaired wound healing, and superficial ulceration of the gastric mucosa. Other side effects may include edema of the extremity involved, damage to soft tissues of the perfused area, and (potentially) venous thrombosis.

STORAGE

Protect from light. Store in a dry place below 30°C (86°F); transient temperatures (*i.e.,* for a period not exceeding two weeks) of up to 50°C (122°F) are permissible.

SPECIAL HANDLING

Due to the drug's toxic and mutagenic properties, appropriate precautions including the use of appropriate safety equipment are recommended for the preparation of dactinomycin for parenteral administration. The National Institutes of Health presently recommends that the preparation of injectable antineoplastic drugs should be performed in a Class II laminar flow biological safety cabinet and that personnel preparing drugs of this class should wear surgical gloves and a closed front surgical-type gown with knit cuffs.[23]

REFERENCES:

1. Bullock. E.; Johnson, A. W.: Actinomycin: the structure of actinomycin, D. J. Chem. Soc. Part III: 3280-3285, 1957. **2.** Tattersall, M. H.; et al: Pharmacokinetics of actinomycin D in patients with malignant melanoma, Clin. Pharmacol. Ther. *17:* 701-708, June 1975. **3.** Pochedly, C.: Wilms' tumor III, Special problems in therapy, N.Y. State J. Med. *71:* 1526-1528, June 15, 1971. **4.** D'Angio, G. J.; et al: The treatment of Wilms' tumor: results of the national Wilms' tumor study, Cancer *38:* 633-646, 1976. **5.** Jenkin, R. D.: The treatment of Wilms' tumor, Pediat. Clin. N. Amer. *23:* 147-160, Feb. 1976. **6.** Heyn, R. M.; et al: The role of combined chemotherapy in the treatment of rhabdomyosarcoma in children, Cancer *34:* 2128-2142, 1974. **7.** Ghavimi, F.; et al: Multidisciplinary treatment of embryonal rhabdomyosarcoma in children, Cancer *35:* 677-686, 1975. **8.** Wilbur, J. R.: Treatment of soft tissue sarcomas, Pediat. Clin. N. Amer. *23:*171-181, Feb. 1976. **9.** Wilbur, J. R.; et al: Chemotherapy of sarcomas, Cancer *36:* 765-769, 1975. **10.** Ross, G. T.; Goldstein, D. P.; Hertz, R.; Lipsett, M. B.; Odell, W. D.: Sequential use of methotrexate and actinomycin D in the treatment of metastatic choriocarcinoma and related trophoblastic diseases in women, Amer. J. Obstet. & Gynecol. *93:* 223-229, Sept. 1965. **11.** Piver, M. S.: Chemotherapy for gynecologic malignancies, Drug Therapy*6:* 141-143, 146-147, Oct. 1976. **12.** Merrin, C. E.; Murphy, G. P.: Metastatic testicular carcinoma, N.Y.J. Med. *74:*654-657, Apr. 1974. **13.** Rosen, G.: Management of malignant bone tumors in children and adolescents, Pediat. Clin. N. Amer. *23:*183-213, Feb. 1976. **14.** D'Angio, G. J.; Tefft, M.: Radiation therapy in the management of children with gynecologic cancers, Ann. N. Y. Acad. Sci. *142:* 694-708, May 10, 1967. **15.** McVeagh, P.; Ekert, H.: Hepatotoxicity of chemotherapy following nephrectomy and radiation therapy for right-sided Wilms' tumor, J. Pediat. *87:*627-628, Oct. 1975. **16.** Dayabose, S.; et al: Hepatotoxicity of chemotherapy following nephrectomy and radiation therapy for right-sided Wilms' tumor, J. Pediat. *88:* 898, May 1976 (in Editorial Correspondence). **17.** Wright, D. N.; Matsen, J. M.: Bioassay of antibiotics in body fluids from patients receiving cancer chemotherapeutic agents, Antimicrob. Ag. Chemother. *17:* 417-422, Mar. 1980. **18.** Boctor, Z. N.; et al: Current results from therapy of testicular tumors, Cancer *24:* 870-875, Nov. 1969. **19.** Rusmin, S.; Welton, S.; DeLuca, P.; and DeLuca, P.: The effect of I.V. in-line filtration on the potency of drugs, Am. J. Hosp. Pharm. *34:* 1071-1074, 1977. **20.** Goldstein, D. P.; et al.: Infusion therapy in the treatment of patients with choriocarcinoma and related trophoblastic tumors, Surg. Forum *18:* 426-428, 1967. **21.** Maroulis, G. B.; et al: Arteriography and infusional chemotherapy in localized trophoblastic disease, Obstet. Gynecol.*45:* 397-406, Apr. 1975. **22.** McBride, C. M.: Sarcomas of the limbs, Arch. Surg. *109:* 304-308,

REFERENCES: *(cont'd)*

Aug. 1974. **23.** National Institutes of Health, Division of Safety, in collaboration with Clinical Center pharmacy and nursing staff, and National Cancer Institute; Recommendations for the Safe Handling of Parenteral Antineoplastic Drugs, NIH Publication No. 83-2621.

HOW SUPPLIED - EQUIVALENTS NOT AVAILABLE:

Injection, Solution - Intravenous - 0.5 mg

1's $11.70 COSMEGEN, Merck 00006-3298-22

DALTEPARIN SODIUM *(003197)*

CATEGORIES: Anticoagulants; Anticoagulants/Thrombolytics; Blood Clotting; Blood Formation/Coagulation; Coagulants and Anticoagulants; Coagulopathies; Embolism; Low Molecular Weight Heparin; Pulmonary Embolism; Thrombosis; FDA Class 1S ("Standard Review"); FDA Approved 1994 Dec

BRAND NAMES: **Fragmin**; *Fragmine* (France)
(International brand names outside U.S. in italics)

DESCRIPTION:

For subcutaneous Use Only.

Fragmin (dalteparin sodium injection), is a sterile, low molecular weight heparin for injection. Each syringe contains 2500 (16 mg dalteparin sodium) anti-Factor Xa International units in 0.2 ml (with reference to the W.H.O. First International Low Molecular Weight Heparin Reference Standard). Each syringe also contains water for injection and sodium chloride, when required, to maintain physiologic ionic strength. The pH of the injection is 5.0 to 7.5. Dalteparin is a preservative free and intended for use only as a single dose injection.

Dalteparin sodium is produced through controlled nitrous acid depolymerization of sodium heparin from porcine intestinal mucosa followed by a chromatographic purification process. It is composed of strongly acidic sulphated polysaccharide chains (oligosaccharide, containing 2,5-anhydro-D-mannitol residues as end groups) with an average molecular weight of 5000 and about 90% of the material within the range 20000-9000. The molecular weight distribution is:

<3000 daltons: 3.0 - 15.0%, 3000 to 8000 daltons: 65.0 - 78.0%, >8000 daltons: 14.0 - 26.0%.

CLINICAL PHARMACOLOGY:

Dalteparin is a low molecular weight heparin with antithrombotic properties. It acts by enhancing the inhibition of Factor Xa and thrombin by antithrombin. In man, dalteparin potentiates preferentially the inhibition of coagulation factor Xa, while only slightly affecting clotting time, e.g., activated partial thromboplastin time (APTT).

Pharmacodynamics: Doses of dalteparin of up to 10,000 anti-Factor Xa IU administered subcutaneously as a single dose or two 5,000 IU doses 12 hours apart to healthy subjects do not produce a significant change in platelet aggregation, fibrinolysis, or global clotting tests such as prothrombin time (PT), thrombin time (TT) or APTT. Subcutaneous administration of dalteparin doses of 5,000 IU b.i.d. for seven consecutive days to patients undergoing abdominal surgery did not markedly affect APTT, Platelet Factor (PF4), or lipoprotein lipase.

Pharmacokinetics: Mean peak levels of plasma anti-Factor Xa activity following single subcutaneous doses of 2,500, 5,000 and 10,000 IU were 0.19 ± 0.04, 0.41 ± 0.07 and 0.82 ± 0.10 IU/ml, respectively, and were attained in about 4 hours in most subjects. Absolute bioavailability in healthy volunteers, measured as the anti- Factor Xa activity, was 87 ± 6%. Increasing the dose from 2,500 to 10,000 IU resulted in an overall increase in anti-Factor Xa AUC that was greater than proportional by about one-third. Peak anti-Factor Xa activity increased more or less linearly with dose over the same dose range. There appeared to be no appreciable accumulation of anti-Factor Xa activity with twice-daily dosing of 100 IU/kg subcutaneously for up to 7 days.

The volume of distribution for dalteparin anti-Factor Xa activity was 40 to 60 ml/kg. The mean plasma clearances of dalteparin anti-Factor Xa activity in normal volunteers following single intravenous bolus doses of 30 and 120 anti-Factor Xa IU/kg were 24.6 ± 5.4 and 15.6 ± 2.4 ml/hr/kg, respectively. The corresponding mean disposition half-lives are 1.47 ± 0.3 and 2.5 ± 0.3 hr.

Following intravenous doses of 40 and 60 IU/kg, mean terminal half lives were 2.1 ± 0.3 and 2.3 ± 0.4 hrs, respectively. Longer apparent terminal half-lives (3 to 5 hrs) are observed following subcutaneous dosing, possibly due to delayed absorption. In patients with chronic renal insufficiency requiring hemodialysis, the mean terminal half-life of anti-Factor Xa activity following a single intravenous dose of 5,000 IU dalteparin was 5.7 ± 2.0 hrs, i.e. considerably longer than values observed in healthy volunteers; therefore, greater accumulation can be expected in these patients.

CLINICAL STUDIES:

Clinical Trials: Dalteparin, administered once-daily beginning prior to surgery and continuing for 5 to 10 days after surgery, has been shown to prevent deep vein thrombosis (DVT) in patients at risk for thromboembolic complications (see INDICATIONS AND USAGE and DOSAGE AND ADMINISTRATION). Data from two double-blind randomized controlled clinical trials performed in patients undergoing major abdominal surgery, summarized in TABLE 1 and TABLE 2, show that Dalteparin was superior to placebo and similar to heparin in preventing DVT.

TABLE 1 Abdominal Surgery

Treatment Failures / Dosing Regimen	Treatment Group Fragmin 2500 IU qd	Placebo qd
Number of Patients Treated	102	102
Total Thromboembolic Events (%)	4/91 (4/4)*	16/91 (17.6)
Proximal DVT (%)	0/91 (0)	5/91 (5.5)
Distal DVT (%)	4/91 (4.4)	11/91 (12.1)
PE (%)	0/91 (0)	2/91 (2.2)**

* P-value versus placebo = 0.008
** Both patients also had DVT, 1 proximal and 1 distal

INDICATIONS AND USAGE:

Dalteparin is indicated for prophylaxis against deep vein thrombosis, which may lead to pulmonary embolism, in patients undergoing abdominal surgery who are at risk for thromboembolic complications. Patients at risk include patients who are over 40 years of age, obese, undergoing surgery under general anesthesia lasting longer than 30 minutes or who have additional risk factors such as malignancy or a history of deep vein thrombosis or pulmonary embolism.

TABLE 2 Abdominal Surgery

Treatment Failures / Dosing Regimen	Treatment Group Fragmin 2500 IU qd	Heparin 5000 IU bid
Number of Patients Treated	195	196
Total Thromboembolic Events (%)	7/178 (3.9)*	7/174 (4.0)
Proximal DVT (%)	3/178 (1.7)	4/174 (2.3)
Distal DVT (%)	3/178 (1.7)	3/174 (1.7)
PE (%)	1/178 (0.6)	0/174 (0)

* P-value versus heparin = 0.74

CONTRAINDICATIONS:

Dalteparin is contraindicated in patients with known hypersensitivity to the drug, active major bleeding, or thrombocytopenia associated with positive *in vitro* tests for anti-platelet antibody in the presence of dalteparin.

Patients with known hypersensitivity to heparin or pork products should not be treated with dalteparin.

WARNINGS:

Dalteparin is not intended for intramuscular administration.

Dalteparin cannot be used interchangeably (unit for unit) with unfractionated heparin or other low molecular weight heparins.

Dalteparin should be used with extreme caution in patients with history of heparin-induced thrombocytopenia.

Hemorrhage: Dalteparin, like other anticoagulants, should be used with extreme caution in patients who have an increased risk of hemorrhage, such as those with severe uncontrolled hypertension, bacterial endocarditis, congenital or acquired bleeding disorders, active ulceration and angiodysplastic gastrointestinal disease, hemorrhagic stroke or shortly after brain, spinal or ophthalmological surgery.

As with other anticoagulants, bleeding can occur at any site during therapy with dalteparin. An unexpected drop in hematocrit or blood pressure should lead to a search for a bleeding site.

Thrombocytopenia: Thrombocytopenia with platelet counts of <50,000/mm^3 and <100,000/m/m^3 occurred in <1% and <1%, respectively, of patients undergoing abdominal surgery.

Thrombocytopenia of any degree should be monitored closely. Heparin-induced thrombocytopenia can occur with the administration of dalteparin. The incidence of this complication is unknown at present.

PRECAUTIONS:

General: Dalteparin should not be mixed with other injections or infusions unless specific compatability data are available that support such mixing.

Dalteparin should be used with caution in patients with bleeding diathesis, thrombocytopenia or platelet defects; severe liver or kidney insufficiency, hypertensive or diabetic retinopathy, and recent gastro-intestinal bleeding.

If a thromboembolic event should occur despite dalteparin prophylaxis, dalteparin should be discontinued and appropriate therapy initiated.

Laboratory Tests: Periodic routine complete blood counts, including platelet count, and stool occult blood tests are recommended during the course of treatment with dalteparin. No special monitoring of blood clotting times (*e.g.,* APTT) is needed.

Drug/Laboratory Test Interactions: *Elevations of Serum Transaminases:* Asymptomatic increases in transaminase levels (SGOT/AST and SGPT/ALT) greater than three times the upper limit normal of the laboratory reference range have been reported in 1.7 and 4.3%, respectively, of patients during treatment with dalteparin. Similar significant increases in transaminase levels have also been observed in patients treated with heparin and other low molecular weight heparins. Such elevations are fully reversible and are rarely associated with increases in bilirubin. Since transaminase determinations are important in the differential diagnosis of myocardial infarction, liver disease and pulmonary emboli, elevations that might be caused by drugs like dalteparin should be interpreted with caution.

Carcinogenesis, Mutagenesis, and Impairment of Fertility: Dalteparin sodium has not been tested for its carcinogenic potential in a long-term animal studies. It was not mutagenic in the *in vitro*mouse micronucleus test. Dalteparin sodium at subcutaneous doses up to 1,200 IU/kg (7080 IU/m^2) did not affect the fertility of reproductive performance of male and female rats.

Pregnancy, Teratogenic Effects, Pregnancy Category B: Reproduction studies with dalteparin sodium at intravenous doses up to 2400 IU/kg (14160 IU/m^2) in pregnant rats and 4800 IU/kg (40800 IU/m^2) in pregnant rabbits did not produce any evidence of impaired fertility or harm to the fetuses. There are, however, no adequate and well controlled studies in pregnant women. Because animal reproduction studies are not always predictive of human response, this drug should be used during pregnancy only if clearly needed.

Nursing Mothers: It is not known whether dalteparin sodium is excreted in human milk. Because many drugs are excreted in human milk, caution should be exercised when dalteparin is administered to a nursing mother.

Pediatric Use: Safety and effectiveness in children has not been established.

DRUG INTERACTIONS:

Dalteparin should be used with care in patients receiving oral anticoagulants and/or platelet inhibitors because of increased risk of bleeding.

ADVERSE REACTIONS:

Hemorrhage: The incidence of hemorrhagic complications during dalteparin treatment has been low. The most commonly reported side effect is hematoma at the injection site. The incidence of bleeding may increase with higher dosages.

The following information in TABLE 3A and 3B, summarizes adverse bleeding events that occurred in clinical trials which studied dalteparin 2500 and 5000 IU administered once daily to abdominal surgery patients.

Thrombocytopenia: During clinical trials with dalteparin in thromboprophylaxis, thrombocytopenia, platelet counts of <50,000/mm^3 and <1000,000/mm^3 were reported in <1% and <1%, respectively, of patients given dalteparin and <1% and 1% of patients given heparin.

Other: Pain at injection site was seen in the following percentages of patients involved in clinical trials: 0% for dalteparin 2500 IU qd vs 0.4% for heparin 5000 IU bid; 4.5% for dalteparin 5000 IU qd vs 11.8% for heparin 5000 IU bid; 0% for dalteparin 2500 IU qd vs 0% for placebo and 1.1% for dalteparin 2500 IU qd vs 1.8% for dalteparin 5000 IU qd.

Allergic reactions (*i.e.,* pruritus, rash, fever, injection site reaction, bulleous eruption) and skin necrosis have occurred rarely. A few cases of anaphylactoid reactions have been reported.

TABLE 3A Dalteparin vs. Heparin*				
	Fragmin 2500 IU/24 hr	Heparin 10000 IU/24 hr	Fragmin 5000 IU/24 hr	Heparin 10000 IU/24 hr
Post-Operational Transfusions	8.1% (n=320)	11.3% (n=320)	23.6% (n=369)	18.2% (n=363)
Wound Hematoma	3.4% (n=467)	3.9% (n=467)	2.4% (n=509)	1.2% (n=501)
Reoperation due to Bleeding	0.5% (n=392)	0.8% (n=392)	0.8% (n=509)	0.4% (n=501)
Injection Site Hematoma	0.2% (n=466)	1.1% (n=464)	7.1% (n=508)	9.5% (n=495)

* Fragmin administered once-daily, heparin administered twice daily at a dose of 5000 IU

TABLE 3B				
	Fragmin vs. Placebo		Fragmin vs. Fragmin	
	Fragmin 2500 IU/24 hr	Placebo	Fragmin 2500 IU/24 hr	Fragmin 5000 IU/24 hr
Post-Operationa l Transfusions	11.7% (n=120)	10.9% (n=119)	8.9% (n=1020)	12.3% (n=1016)
Wound Hematoma	2.5% (n=79)	2.6% (n=77)	0.1% (n=1045)	0.4% (n=1041)
Reoperation due to Bleeding	1.3% (n=79)	1.3% (n=78)	0.2% (n=1045)	1.2% (n-1041)
Injection Site Hematoma	4.7% (n=172)	1.1% (n=174)	3.5% (n=1038)	5.4% (n=1039)

OVERDOSAGE:

Symptoms/Treatment: An excessive dosage of dalteparin may lead to hemorrhagic complications. These may generally be stopped by the slow intravenous injection of protamine sulfate (1% solution) at a dose of 1 mg protamine for every 100 anti-Xa IU of dalteparin given. A second infusion of 0.5 mg protamine sulfate per 100 anti-Xa IU of dalteparin may be administered if the APTT measured 2 to 4 hours after the first infusion remains prolonged. Even with these additional doses of protamine, the APTT may remain more prolonged than would usually be found following administration of conventional heparin. In all cases, the anti-Factor Xa activity is never completely neutralized (maximum about 60 to 75%).

Particular care should be taken to avoid overdosage with protamine sulfate. Administration of protamine sulfate can cause severe hypotensive and anaphylactoid reactions. Because fetal reactions, often resembling anaphylaxis, have been reported with protamine sulfate, it should be given only when resuscitation techniques and treatment of anaphylactic shock are readily available. For additional information, consult the labeling of Protamine Sulfate Injection, USP products. A single subcutaneous dose of 100,000 IU/kg of dalteparin to mice caused a mortality of 8% (1/12) whereas 50,000 IU/kg was a non-lethal dose. The observed sign was hematoma at the site of injection.

DOSAGE AND ADMINISTRATION:

In patients undergoing abdominal surgery with a risk of thromboembolic complications, 2500 IU should be administered subcutaneously only, each day, starting 1 to 2 hours prior to surgery and repeated once daily for 5 to 10 days postoperatively (refer to INDICATIONS AND USAGE).

Dosage adjustment and routine monitoring of coagulation parameters are not required if the dosage and administration recommendations specified above are followed.

Administration: Dalteparin is administered by subcutaneous injection. It must not be administered by intramuscular injection.

Subcutaneous injection technique: Patients should be sitting or lying down and dalteparin administered by deep subcutaneous injection. Dalteparin may be injected in a U-shape area around the navel, the upper outer side of the thigh or the upper outer quadrangle of the buttock. The injection site should be varied daily. When the area around the navel or the thigh is used, using the thumb and forefinger, you **must** lift up a fold of skin while giving the injection. The entire length of the needle should be inserted at a 45 to 90 degree angle.

Parental drug products should be inspected visually for particulate matter and discoloration prior to administration, whenever solution and container permit.

HOW SUPPLIED:

Fragmin (dalteparin sodium injection) is available in packs of 10 single dose prefilled syringes in the following strength:

2500 anti-Factor Xa IU/0.2 ml

Each dalteparin prefilled syringe is affixed with a 27 gauge X 1/2 inch needle.

Storage Store at controlled room temperature 20° to 25°C (68° to 77°F).

HOW SUPPLIED - EQUIVALENTS NOT AVAILABLE:

Injection - Subcutaneous - 0.200 ml

10's	$139.50	FRAGMIN, Pharmacia & Upjohn	00013-2406-91
10's	$237.13	FRAGMIN, Pharmacia & Upjohn	00013-2426-91

DANAPAROID SODIUM *(003336)*

CATEGORIES: Antithrombotics; Pulmonary Embolism; Thrombosis; Pregnancy Category B; FDA Approved 1997 Jan

BRAND NAMES: **Orgaran**

DESCRIPTION:

Orgaran injection is a sterile, glycosaminoglycuronan antithrombotic agent. The active components of Orgaran, isolated from the porcine intestinal mucosa, are heparin sulfate (84%), dermatan sulfate (12%), and a small amount of chondroltin sulfate (4%). The average molecular weight is approximately 5500 Daltons.

Orgaran is intended for subcutaneous injection. Each prefilled syringe or ampule contains 750 anti-Xa units in 0.6 ml solution. Orgaran injection is made isotonic with sodium chloride, adjusted to pH 7 with hydrochloric acid, or sodium hydroxide. Orgaran injection contains 0.15% (w/v) sodium sulfite to prevent discoloration of the solution.

CLINICAL PHARMACOLOGY:

PHARMACODYNAMICS

Effect on Coagulation Factors: Danaparoid sodium injection is an antithrombotic agent. Danaparoid sodium prevents fibrin formation in the coagulation pathway via thrombin generation inhibition by anti-Xa and anti-IIa (thrombin) effects. The anti-Xa; anti-IIa activity ratio is greater than 22. Inactivation of factor Xa is mediated by antithrombin-III (AT-III) while factor IIa inactivation is mediated by both AT-III and heparin cofactor II (HC II). Danaparoid sodium has only minor effect on platelet function and platelet aggregability.

Measurements of Hemostasis: Because of its predominant anti-Xa activity, danaparoid sodium injection has little effect on cloning assays (*e.g.,* prothrombin time [PT], partial thromboplastin time [PTT]). Danaparoid sodium has minimal effect on fibrinolytic activity and bleeding time.

PHARMACOKINETICS

The pharmacokinetics of danaparoid sodium injection have been described by monitoring its biological activity (plasma anti-Xa activity) since no specific chemical assay methods are currently available for the components of organ.

By subcutaneous route of administration, danaparoid sodium injection was approximately 100% bioavailable, compared with the same dose administered intravenously. The maximum anti-Xa activity (T_{max}) occurred at approximately two to five hours.

For single subcutaneous doses of 750, 1500, 2250, and 3250 anti-Xa units of danaparoid, the mean peak plasma anti-Xa activities were 102.4, 206.1, 283.9, and 403.4 mU/ml, respectively. The mean value for the terminal half-life ($T_{\frac{1}{2}}$) was about 24 hours and the clearance was 0.36 L/hr. Clearance was affected by body surface area in that the higher body surface area, the faster the clearance. Danaparoid sodium is mainly eliminated via the kidneys. In patients with severely impaired renal function, the half-life elimination of plasma anti-Xa activity may be prolonged, therefore, monitoring such patients carefully is recommended.

CLINICAL STUDIES:

In a European multicenter, double-blind trial, danaparoid sodium injection was compared with placebo in 196 patients undergoing elective hip replacement surgery. The administration of danaparoid sodium for 7 to 14 days post-operatively significantly reduced the overall incidence of DVT to 15% (15/98 patients) compared to the incidence of 57% (56/98 patients) observed with placebo.

TABLE 1 Number of Patients with DVT Intent-To-Treat

	Danaparoid Sodium (N=98)	Placebo (N=98)	p-value*
Proximal; N(%)	8 (8)	26 (27)	0.001
Distal; N(%)	14 (14)	51 (52)	<0.001
Overall; N(%)	15 (15)	56 (57)	<0.001

* A patient may be counted more than once (proximal and/or distal)
* Using the Cochran Mantel-Haenszel test

In a United States multicenter trial, danaparoid sodium was compared with warfarin in 396 patients undergoing elective hip replacement. A significant reduction in the overall incidence of DVT was observed with danaparoid sodium (14.6%; 29/199 patients) compared with warfarin (26.9%; 53/197 patients). p=0.003

TABLE 2 Number (%) of Patients with DVT* Intent-To-Treat

	Danaparoid Sodium (N=199)	Warfarin (N=197)	p-value†
Proximal‡; N (%)	3 (1.5)	8 (4.1)	0.13
Distal§; N (%)	28 (14.1)	49 (24.9)	0.007
Overall¶; N (%)	29 (14.6)	53 (26.9)	0.003

* By positive venogram only
† Using the Cochran Mantel-Haenszel test
‡ Popliteal, lilac, and femoral
§ Calf
¶ A patient may be counted more than once (proximal and distal)

INDICATIONS AND USAGE:

Danaparoid sodium injection is indicated for the prophylaxis of post-operative deep venous thrombosis (DVT), which may lead to pulmonary embolism (PE), in patients undergoing elective hip replacement surgery.

CONTRAINDICATIONS:

Danaparoid sodium injection is contraindicated in the following conditions: severe hemorrhagic diathesis (*e.g.,* hemophilia and idiopathic thrombocytopenic purpura); active major bleeding state, including hemorrhagic stroke in the acute phase; hypersensitivity to danaparoid sodium, type II thrombocytopenia associated with a positive *in vitro* test for antiplatelet antibody in the presence of danaparoid sodium injection. Danaparoid sodium is contraindicated in patients with known hypersensitivity to pork products.

WARNINGS:

General: Danaparoid sodium injection is not intended for intramuscular administration. Since a specific standard for the anti-Xa activity of danaparoid sodium is used, the anti-Xa unit activity of danaparoid sodium is not equivalent to that described for heparin or low molecular weight heparin. Therefore, danaparoid sodium cannot be dosed interchangeably (unit for unit) with either heparin or any low molecular weight heparin.

Miscellaneous: Danaparoid sodium injection contains sodium sulfite which may cause allergic-type reactions, including anaphylactic symptoms and life-threatening or less severe asthmatic episodes in certain susceptible people. The overall prevalence of sulfite sensitivity in the general population is unknown and probably low. Sulfite sensitivity is seen more frequently in asthmatic than in non-asthmatic patients.

Hemorrhage: Hemorrhage can occur at virtually any site in patients receiving danaparoid sodium injection. An unexplained fall in hematocrit and/or fall in blood pressure should lead to serious consideration of a hemorrhagic event. Danaparoid sodium, like anticoagulants, should be used with extreme caution in disease states in which there is increased risk of hemorrhage, such as severe uncontrolled hypertension, acute bacterial endocarditis, congenital or acquired bleeding disorders, active ulcerative and angiodysplastic gastrointestinal disease, non-hemorrhagic stroke, shortly after brain, spinal, or ophthalmological surgery and post-operative indwelling epidural catheter use.

PRECAUTIONS:

General: The risks and benefits of danaparoid sodium injection should be carefully considered before use in patients with severely impaired renal function or hemorrhagic disorders (see DOSAGE AND ADMINISTRATION).

Laboratory Tests: Danaparoid sodium injection has only a small effect on factor IIa (thrombin) activity, therefore, routine coagulation tests (*e.g.,* Prothrombin Time [PT], Activated Partial Thromboplastin Time [APTT], Kaolin Cephalin Clotting Time [KCCT], Whole Blood Clotting Time [WBCT], and Thrombin Time [TT]) are unsuitable for monitoring danaparoid sodium activity at recommended doses.

PRECAUTIONS: *(cont'd)*

Periodic complete blood counts, including platelet count, and stool occult blood tests are recommended during the course of treatment with danaparoid sodium.

Thrombocytopenia: Danaparoid sodium injection shows a low cross-reactivity with antiplatelet antibodies in individuals with Type II heparin-induced thrombocytopenia. No cases of white clot syndrome or cases of type II thrombocytopenia have been reported in clinical studies for the prophylaxis of DVT in patients receiving multiple doses of danaparoid sodium up to 14 days.

Carcinogenesis, Mutagenesis, and Impairment of Fertility: No long term studies in animals have been performed to evaluate the carcinogenic potential of danaparoid sodium injection. Danaparoid sodium was not genotoxic in the Ames test, the *in vitro* CHL/HGPRT forward gene mutation assay, the *in vitro* CHO cell chromosome aberration test, the *in vitro* HeLa cell unscheduled DNA synthesis (UDS) test or the *in vivo* mouse micronucleus test. Danaparoid sodium at intravenous doses of up to 1090 anti-Xa units/kg/day was found to have no effect on fertility or reproductive performance of male and female rats. This dose is 5.9 times the recommended human subcutaneous dose based on body surface area (50 kg body weight and 1.46 m^2 body surface area assumed).

Pregnancy, Teratogenic Effects, Pregnancy Category B: Teratology studies have been performed in pregnant rats at intravenous doses up to 1600 anti-Xa units/kg/day (8.7 times the recommended human dose based on body surface area) and pregnant rabbits at intravenous doses up to 780 anti-Xa units/kg/day (6 times the recommended human dose based on body surface area) and have not revealed evidence of impaired fertility or harm to the fetus due to danaparoid sodium injection. There are, however, no adequate and well-controlled studies in pregnant women. Because animal reproduction studies are not always predictive of human response, this drug should be used during pregnancy only if clearly needed.

Nursing Mothers: It is not known whether danaparoid sodium injection is excreted in breast milk. Because many drugs are excreted in human milk, caution should be exercised when danaparoid sodium is administered to a nursing woman.

Pediatric Use: Safety and effectiveness of danaparoid sodium injection in pediatric patients have not been established.

DRUG INTERACTIONS:

In clinical studies for the prophylaxis of DVT, no clinically significant drug interactions have been noted in the following drugs: digoxin, cloxacillin, ticarcillin, chlorthalidone, and pentobarbital.

Danaparoid sodium injection should be used with caution in patients receiving oral anticoagulants and/or platelet inhibitors. Monitoring of anticoagulant activity of oral anticoagulants by Prothrombin Time and Thrombotest is unreliable within 5 hours after danaparoid sodium injection administration.

ADVERSE REACTIONS:

TABLE 3 summarizes adverse bleeding events that occurred in clinical trials which studied danaparoid sodium injection compared to placebo, warfarin, and others (heparin, heparin/DHE, acetylsalicytic acid, dextran, and low-molecular weight heparins).

TABLE 3 Blood Loss and Transfusions All Patients Treated

Blood Loss and Transfusions	Total N	Danaparoid Sodium	Placebo	Warfarin	Other*
Total (728 Males; 1675 Females)		(N) Mean ± SD	(N) Mean ± SD	(N) Mean ± SD	(N) Mean ± SD
Intraoperative Blood Loss (ml)					
Males	580	(330) 694 ± 555	(27) 586 ± 737	(141) 689 ± 499	(98) 754 ± 661
Females	1259	(686) 486 ± 430	(66) 416 ± 252	(219) 471 ± 306	(288) 530 ± 456
Postoperative Blood Loss (ml)					
Males	580	(318) 954 ± 879	(45) 908 ± 812	(88) 817 ± 585	(129) 1056 ± 1055
Females	1256	(639) 700 ± 778	(122) 715 ± 520	(80) 619 ± 352	(415) 798 ± 779
Transfusions (units PRBCs)					
Males	462	(258) 2.6 ± 1.8	(35) 2.7 ± 1.4	(87) 2.5 ± 1.4	(82) 2.9 ± 2.1
Females	1152	(604) 2.6 ± 1.7	(92) 2.8 ± 1.4	(177) 2.1 ± 1.1	(279) 2.8 ± 2.0

* "Other" includes the following active reference agents: heparin, heparin/DHE, acetylsalicylic acid, dextran, and low-molecular weight heparins.

Total N Total number of patients with available data across all treatment groups.
n The number of patients with available data in each respective treatment group and by gender.

Other: TABLE 4 summarizes adverse events that occurred at a frequency greater than or equal to 2% of patients in clinical trials for the prophylaxis of DVT and PE following elective hip surgery which studied danaparoid sodium injection compared to placebo, warfarin, and others (dextran, heparin/DHE, aspirin).

TABLE 4 Incidence of Adverse Experiences (≥2%), DVT and PE Prophylaxis for Elective Hip Surgery, All Patients Treated

Adverse Experience	Danaparoid Sodium N=645 N(%)	Placebo N=135 N(%)	Warfarin N=243 N(%)	Other N=168 N(%)
Fever	143(22.2)	1(0.7)	138(56.8)	3(1.8)
Nausea	92(14.3)	3(2.2)	78(32.1)	8(4.8)
Constipation	73(11.3)	0(0.0)	70(28.8)	2(1.2)
Injection Site Pain	49(7.6)	4(3.0)	0(0.0)	34(20.2)
Rash	31(4.8)	0(0.0)	18(7.4)	2(1.2)
Pruritis	25(3.9)	1(0.7)	14(5.8)	0(0.0)
Peripheral Edema	21(3.3)	0(0.0)	19(7.8)	4(2.4)
Insomnia	20(3.1)	0(0.0)	32(13.2)	0(0.0)
Vomiting	19(2.9)	3(2.2)	20(8.2)	3(1.8)
Joint Disorder	17(2.6)	0(0.0)	15(6.2)	0(0.0)
Headache	17(2.6)	1(0.7)	13(5.3)	0(0.0)
Urinary Tract Infection	17(2.6)	1(0.7)	5(2.1)	5(3.0)
Edema	17(2.6)	0(0.0)	14(5.8)	2(1.2)
Asthenia	15(2.3)	0(0.0)	10(4.1)	1(0.6)
Dizziness	15(2.3)	0(0.0)	14(5.8)	0(0.0)
Anemia	14(2.2)	3(2.2)	5(2.1)	5(3.0)
Urinary Retention	13(2.0)	0(0.0)	14(5.8)	1(0.6)

ADVERSE REACTIONS: *(cont'd)*

In addition TABLE 5summarizes adverse events that occurred at a frequency greater than or equal to 2% of patients in clinical trials for the prophylaxis of DVT and PE which studied danaparoid sodium injection compared to placebo, warfarin, and others (heparin, heparin sodium, heparin calcium, enoxaparin, dalteparin, dextran, heparin/DHE, aspirin).

TABLE 5 Incidence of Sdverse Experiences (≥2%), DVT and PE Prophylaxis Indication, All Patients Treated

Adverse Experience	Danaparoid Sodium N=2383 N(%)	Placebo N=276 N(%)	Warfarin N=421 N(%)	Other N=1163 N(%)
Injection Site Pain	327(13.7)	53(19.2)	0(0.0)	153(13.2)
Pain	207(8.7)	0(0.0)	202(48.0)	20(1.7)
Fever	173(7.3)	1(0.4)	150(35.6)	21(1.8)
Nausea	98(4.1)	3(1.1)	79(18.8)	13(1.1)
Urinary Tract Infection	96(4.0)	3(1.1)	27(6.4)	65(5.6)
Constipation	83(3.5)	0(0.0)	73(17.3)	3(0.3)
Rash	51(2.1)	0(0.0)	25(5.9)	5(0.4)
Infection	51(2.1)	3(1.1)	0(0.0)	47(4.0)

OVERDOSAGE:

Symptoms/Treatment: Accidental overdosage following administration of danaparoid sodium injection may lead to bleeding complications. The effects of danaparoid sodium on anti-Xa activity cannot be antagonized with any known agent at this time. Although protamine sulfate partially neutralizes the anti-Xa activity of danaparoid and can be safely co-administered, there is no evidence that protamine sulfate is capable of reducing severe non-surgical bleeding during treatment with danaparoid sodium injection. In the event of serious bleeding, danaparoid sodium should be stopped and blood or blood product transfusions should be administered as needed. Withdrawal of danaparoid sodium may be expected to restore the coagulation balance without rebound phenomenon.

Single subcutaneous doses of danaparoid sodium at 3800 anti-Xa units/kg (20.5 times the recommended human dose based on body surface area) and 15200 anti-Xa units/kg (82 times the recommended human dose based on body surface area) were lethal to female and male rats, respectively. Symptoms of acute toxicity after intravenous dosing were respiratory depression, prostration, and twitching.

DOSAGE AND ADMINISTRATION:

Usual Adult Dosage: In patients undergoing hip replacement surgery, the recommended dose of danaparoid sodium injection is 750 anti-Xa units twice daily administered by subcutaneous injection beginning 1-4 hours pre-operatively, and then not sooner than two hours after surgery. Treatment should be continued throughout the period of post-operative care until the risk of deep vein thrombosis has diminished. The average duration of administration in clinical trials was 7 to 10 days, up to 14 days. Patients with serum creatinine ≥2.0 mg/dl should be carefully monitored.

Administration: Orgaran injection is intended for subcutaneous administration and should be administered by intramuscular injection. *Subcutaneous injection technique:* Patients should be lying down and Orgaran injection administered by deep subcutaneous injection using a fine needle (25 to 26 gauge) to minimize tissue trauma. Administration should be alternated between the left and right anterolateral and left and right posterolateral abdominal wall. The whole length of the needle should be introduced into a skin fold held gently between the thumb and forefinger; the skin fold should be held throughout the injection and should neither be pinched nor rubbed afterwards.

Parenteral drug products should be inspected visually for particulate matter and discoloration prior to administration whenever solution and container permit.

HOW SUPPLIED:

Orgaran injection is supplied in ampules containing 0.6 ml (750 anti-Xa units) of danaparoid sodium and in disposable prefilled syringes containing 0.6 ml danaparoid sodium. Each prefilled syringe is affixed with a 25-gauge × 5/8 inch needle.

Storage: Ampules should be stored at temperatures of 2°- 30°C (36°- 86°F). Syringes should be stored at a refrigerated temperature of 2°- 8°C (36° - 46°F). Protect from light.

DANAZOL *(000940)*

CATEGORIES: Androgens; Angioedema; Anterior Pituitary/Hypothalmic Function; Breast Disease; Endometriosis; Gonadotropin Inhibitors; Hormones; Steroids; Infertility*; Pregnancy Category X; FDA Approval Pre 1982
* Indication not approved by the FDA

BRAND NAMES: *Anargil*; *Azol*; *Bonzol* (Japan); *Cyclomen* (Canada); *D-Zol*; *Danatrol* (France); *Danazant*; *Danazol*; *Danazol-Ratiopharm* (Germany); *Danazol Jean Marie*; *Danocil*; *Danokrin*; **Danocrine**; *Danodiol*; *Danogen*; *Danol* (England); *Danotab*; *Danoval*; *Danzocrine*; *Dorink*; *Ectopal*; *Freeborn*; *Gonablok*; *Kendazol* (Mexico); *Ladagol*; *Ladogal*; *Mastodanatrol*; *Nazol*; *Utta*; *Vabon*; *Winobanin* (Germany); *Zoldan-A* (Mexico)
(International brand names outside U.S. in italics)

FORMULARIES: Aetna; BC-BS

WARNING:
Use of danazol in pregnancy is contraindicated. A sensitive test (*e.g.,* beta subunit test if available) capable of determining early pregnancy is recommended immediately prior to start of therapy. Additionally a non-hormonal method of contraception should be used during therapy. If a patient becomes pregnant while taking danazol administration of the drug should be discontinued and the patient should be apprised of the potential risk to the fetus. Exposure to danazol in utero may result in androgenic effects on the female fetus; reports of clitoral hypertrophy, labial fusion, urogenital sinus defect, vaginal atresia, and ambiguous genitalia have been received. (See PRECAUTIONS, Pregnancy, Teratogenic Effects.)
Thromboembolism, thrombotic and thrombophlebitic events including sagittal sinus thrombosis and life-threatening or fetal strokes have been reported.
Experience with long-term therapy with danazol is limited. Peliosis hepatis and benign hepatic adenoma have been observed with long-term use. Peliosis hepatis and benign hepatic adenoma may be silent until

complicated by acute, potentially life-threatening intraabdominal hemorrhage. The physician therefore should be alert to this possibility. Attempts should be made to determine the lowest dose that will provide adequate protection. If the drug was begun at a time of exacerbation of hereditary angioneurotic edema due to trauma, stress or other cause, periodic attempts to decrease or withdraw therapy should be considered.
Danazol has been associated with several cases of benign intracranial hypertension also known as pseudotumor cerebri. Early signs and symptoms of benign intracranial hypertension include papilledema headache, nausea and vomiting, and visual disturbances. Patients with these symptoms should be screened for papilledema and, if present, the patients should be advised to discontinue danazol immediately and be referred to a neurologist for further diagnosis and care.

DESCRIPTION:

Danazol, is a synthetic steroid derived from ethisterone. Chemically, danazol is 17α-Pregna-2,4-dien-20-yno[2,3-*d*]-isoxazol-17-ol

Danocrine Inactive Ingredients: Benzyl Alcohol, Gelatin, Lactose, Magnesium Stearate, Parabens, Sodium Propionate, Starch, Talc. Capsules 50 mg and 200 mg contain D&C Yellow #10, FD&C Red #3. Capsules 100 mg contains D&C Yellow #10, FD&C Yellow #6.

CLINICAL PHARMACOLOGY:

Danazol suppresses the pituitary-ovarian axis. This suppression is probably a combination of depressed hypothalamic-pituitary response to lowered estrogen production, the alteration of sex steroid metabolism, and interaction of danazol with sex hormone receptors. The only other demonstrable hormonal effect is weak androgenic activity. Danazol depresses the output of both follicle-stimulating hormone (FSH) and luteinizing hormone (LH).

Recent evidence suggests a direct inhibitory effect at gonadal sites and a binding of danazol to receptors of gonadal steroids at target organs. In addition, danazol has been shown to significantly decrease IgG, IgM, and IgA levels, as well as phospholipid and IgG isotope autoantibodies in patients with endometriosis and associated elevations of autoantibodies, suggesting this could be another mechanism by which it facilitates regression of the disease.

Bioavailability studies indicate that blood levels do not increase proportionally with increases in the administered dose. When the dose of danazol is doubled the increase in plasma levels is only about 35% to 40%.

Separate single dosing of 100 mg and 200 mg capsules of danazol to female volunteers showed that both he extent of availability and the maximum plasma concentration increased by three-to-four fold, respectively, following a meal (> 30 grams of fat), when compared to the fasted state. Further, food also delayed mean time to peak concentration of danazol by about 30 minutes.

In the treatment of endometriosis, danazol alters the normal and ectopic endometrial tissue so that it becomes inactive and atrophic. Complete resolution of endometrial lesions occurs in the majority of cases.

Changes in vaginal cytology and cervical mucus reflect the suppressive effect of danazol on the pituitary-ovarian axis.

In the treatment of fibrocystic breast disease, danazol usually produces partial to complete disappearance of nodularity and complete relief of pain and tenderness. Changes in the menstrual pattern may occur.

Generally, the pituitary-suppressive action of danazol is reversible. Ovulation and cyclic bleeding usually return within 60 to 90 days when therapy with danazol is discontinued.

In the treatment of hereditary angioedema, danazol at effective doses prevents attacks of the disease characterized by episodic edema of the abdominal viscera, extremities, face, and airway which may be disabling and, if the airway is involved, fatal. In addition, danazol corrects partially or completely the primary biochemical abnormality of hereditary angioedema by increasing the levels of the deficient C1 esterase inhibitor (C1El). As a result of this action the serum levels of the C4 component of the complement system are also increased.

INDICATIONS AND USAGE:

Endometriosis: Danazol is indicated for the treatment of endometriosis amenable to hormonal management.

Fibrocystic Breast Disease: Most cases of symptomatic fibrocystic breast disease may be treated by simple measures (*e.g.,* padded brassieres and analgesics).

In infrequent patients, symptoms of pain and tenderness may be severe enough to warrant treatment by suppression of ovarian function. Danazol is usually effective in decreasing nodularity, pain, and tenderness. It should be stressed to the patient that this treatment is not innocuous in that it involves considerable alterations of hormone levels and that recurrence of symptoms is very common after cessation of therapy.

Hereditary Angioedema: Danazol is indicated for the prevention of attacks of angioedema of all types (cutaneous, abdominal, laryngeal) in males and females.

CONTRAINDICATIONS:

Danazol should not be administered to patients with:

1. Undiagnosed abnormal genital bleeding.

2. Markedly impaired hepatic, renal, or cardiac function.

3. Pregnancy. (See WARNINGS.)

4. Breast feeding.

5. Porphyria-danazol can induce ALA synthetase activity and hence porphyrin metabolism.

WARNINGS:

A temporary alteration of lipoproteins in the form of decreased high density lipoproteins and possibly increased low density lipoproteins has been reported during danazol therapy. These alterations may be marked, and prescribers should consider the potential impact on the risk of atherosclerosis and coronary artery disease in accordance with the potential benefit of the therapy to the patient.

Before initiating therapy of fibrocystic breast disease with danazol, carcinoma of the breast should be excluded. However, nodularity, pain, tenderness due to fibrocystic breast disease may prevent recognition of underlying carcinoma before treatment is begun. Therefore, if any nodule persists or enlarges during treatment, carcinoma should be considered and ruled out.

Patients should be watched closely for signs of androgenic effects some of which may not be reversible even when drug administration is stopped.

PRECAUTIONS:

Because danazol may cause some degree of fluid retention, conditions that might be influenced by this factor, such as epilepsy, migraine, or cardiac or renal dysfunction, require careful observation.

PRECAUTIONS: *(cont'd)*

Since hepatic dysfunction manifested by modest increases in serum transaminase levels has been reported in patients treated with danazol, periodic liver function tests should be performed (see WARNINGS and ADVERSE REACTIONS).

Administration of danazol has been reported to cause exacerbation of the manifestations of acute intermittent porphyria. (see CONTRAINDICATIONS.)

Laboratory Tests: Danazol treatment may interfere with laboratory determinations of testosterone, androstenedione and dehydroepiandrosterone.

Carcinogenesis, Mutagenesis, and Impairment of Fertility: No valid studies have been performed to assess the carcinogenicity of danazol.

Pregnancy, Teratogenic Effects, Pregnancy Category X: (See CONTRAINDICATIONS.) Danazol administered orally to pregnant rats from the 6th through the 15th day of gestation at doses up to 250 mg/kg/day (7-15 times the human dose) did not result in drug-induced embryotoxicity or teratogenicity, nor difference in litter size, viability or weight of offspring compared to controls. In rabbits, the administration of danazol on days 6-18 of gestation at doses of 60 mg/kg/day and above (2-4 times the human dose) resulted in inhibition of fetal development.

Nursing Mothers: (See CONTRAINDICATIONS.)

Pediatric Use: Safety and effectiveness in children have not been established.

DRUG INTERACTIONS:

Prolongation of prothrombin time occurs in patients stabilized on warfarin. Therapy with danazol may cause an increase in carbamazepine in patients taking both drugs.

ADVERSE REACTIONS:

The following events have been reported in association with the use of danazol:

Androgen like effects include weight gain, acne and seborrhea. Mild hirsutism, edema, hair loss, voice change, which may take the form of hoarseness, sore throat or of instability or deepening of pitch, may occur and may persist after cessation of therapy. Hypertrophy of the clitoris is rare.

Other possible endocrine effects include menstrual disturbances in the form of spotting, alteration of the timing of the cycle and amenorrhea. Although cyclical bleeding and ovulation usually return within 60-90 days after discontinuation of therapy with danazol, persistent amenorrhea has occasionally been reported.

Flushing, sweating, vaginal dryness and irritation and reduction in breast size, may reflect lowering of estrogen. Nervousness and emotional liability have been reported. In the male a modest reduction in spermatogenesis may be evident during treatment. Abnormalities in semen volume, viscosity, sperm count, and motility may occur in patients receiving long-term therapy.

Hepatic dysfunction, as evidenced by reversible elevated serum enzymes and/or jaundice, has been reported in patients receiving a daily dosage of danazol of 400 mg or more. It is recommended that patients receiving danazol be monitored for hepatic dysfunction by laboratory tests and clinical observation. Serious hepatic toxicity including cholestatic jaundice, peliosis hepatis, and hepatic adenoma have been reported. (See WARNINGS and PRECAUTIONS.)

Abnormalities is laboratory tests may occur during therapy with danazol including CPK, glucose tolerance, glucagon, thyroid binding globulin, sex hormone binding globulin, other plasma proteins, lipids and lipoproteins.

The following reactions have been reported, a causal relationship to the administration of danazol has neither been confirmed nor refuted;*Allergic:* urticaria, pruritus and rarely, nasal congestion;*Cns Effects:* headache, nervousness and emotional lability, dizziness and fainting, depression, fatigue, sleep disorders, tremor, paresthesias, weakness, visual disturbances, and rarely, benign intracranial hypertension, anxiety, changes in appetite, chills, and rarely convulsions Guillain-Barre syndrome; *Gastrointestinal:* gastroenteritis, nausea, vomiting, constipation, and rarely, pancreatitis; *Musculoskeletal:* muscle cramps or spasms, or pains, joint pain, joint lockup, joint swelling, pain in back, neck, or extremities, and rarely, carpal tunnel syndrome which may be secondary to fluid retention; *Genitourinary:* hematuria, prolonged posttherapy amenorrhea; *Hematologic:* and increase in red cell and platelet count. Reversible erythrocytosis, leukocytosis or polycythemia may be provoked. Eosinophilia, leukopenia and thrombocytopenia have also been noted. *Skin:* rashes (maculopapular, vesicular, papular, purpuric, petechial), and rarely, sun sensitivity, Stevens-Johnson syndrome;*Other:* increased insulin requirements in diabetic patients, change in libido, elevation in blood pressure, and rarely, cataracts, bleeding gums, fever, pelvic pain, nipple discharge.

Malignant liver tumors have been reported in rare instances, after long-term use.

DOSAGE AND ADMINISTRATION:

Endometriosis: In moderate to severe disease, or in patients infertile due to endometriosis, a starting dose of 800 mg given in two divided doses is recommended. Amenorrhea and rapid response to painful symptoms is best achieved at this dosage level. Gradual downward titration to a dose sufficient to maintain amenorrhea may be considered depending upon patient response. For mild cases, an initial daily dose of 200 mg to 400 mg given in two divided doses is recommended and may be adjusted depending on patient response. **Therapy should begin during menstruation. Otherwise, appropriate tests should be performed to ensure that the patient is not pregnant while on therapy with danazol.** (See CONTRAINDICATIONS and WARNINGS.)**It is essential that therapy continue uninterrupted for 3 to 6 months but may be extended to 9 months if necessary.** After termination of therapy, if symptoms recur, treatment can be reinstituted.

Fibrocystic Breast Disease: The total daily dosage of danazol for fibrocystic breast disease ranges from 100 mg to 400 mg given in two divided doses depending upon patient response. **Therapy should begin during menstruation. Otherwise, appropriate tests should be performed to ensure that the patient is not pregnant while on therapy with danazol.** A nonhormonal method of contraception is recommended when danazol is administered at this dose, since ovulation may not be suppressed.

In most instances breast pain and tenderness are significantly relieved by the first month and eliminated in 2 to 3 months. Usually elimination of nodularity requires 4 to 6 months of uninterrupted therapy. Regular menstrual patterns, irregular menstrual patterns, and amenorrhea each occur in approximately one-third of patients treated with 100 mg of danazol. Irregular menstrual patterns and amenorrhea are observed more frequently with higher doses. Clinical studies have demonstrated that 50% of patients may show evidence of recurrence of symptoms within one year. In this event, treatment may be reinstated.

Hereditary Angioedema: The dosage requirements of continuous treatment of hereditary angioedema with danazol should be individualized on the basis of the clinical response of the patient. It is recommended that the patient be started on 200 mg, two or three times a day. After a favorable initial response is obtained in terms of prevention of episodes of edematous attacks, the proper continuing dosage should be determined by decreasing the dosage by 50% or less at intervals of one to threes or longer if frequency of attacks prior to treatment dictates. If an attack occurs, the daily dosage may be increased by up to 200 mg. During the dose adjusting phase, close monitoring of the patient's response is indicated, particularly if the patient has a history of airway involvement.

HOW SUPPLIED - RATED THERAPEUTICALLY EQUIVALENT:

Capsule, Gelatin - Oral - 50 mg

100's	$118.13	DANOCRINE, Sanofi Winthrop	00024-0303-06

Capsule, Gelatin - Oral - 100 mg

100's	$177.26	DANOCRINE, Sanofi Winthrop	00024-0304-06

Capsule, Gelatin - Oral - 200 mg

60's	$200.98	DANOCRINE, Sanofi Winthrop	00024-0305-60
100's	$295.38	DANOCRINE, Sanofi Winthrop	00024-0305-06

HOW SUPPLIED - NOT RATED EQUIVALENT:

Capsule, Gelatin - Oral - 200 mg

100's	$179.99	Danazol, Balan	00304-1930-01
100's	$225.00	Danazol, Genetco	00302-1360-01

DANTROLENE SODIUM *(000944)*

CATEGORIES: Acidosis; Anesthesia; Autonomic Drugs; Cerebral Palsy; Fever; Hyperthermia; Metabolic Acidosis; Muscle Relaxants; Neuromuscular; Skeletal Muscle Hyperactivity; Skeletal Muscle Relaxants; Spasticity; Spinal Cord Injury; Stroke; Tachycardia; FDA Approval Pre 1982

BRAND NAMES: *Danlene*; *Dantamacrin* (Germany); *Dantralen*; **Dantrium**; *Dantrolen*
(International brand names outside U.S. in italics)

FORMULARIES: Aetna; BC-BS; Medi-Cal; PCS

Dantrolene sodium has a potential for hepatotoxicity, and should not be used in conditions other than those recommended. Symptomatic hepatitis (fatal and non-fatal) has been reported at various dose levels of the drug. The incidence reported in patients taking up to 400 mg/day is much lower than in those taking doses of 800 mg or more per day. Even sporadic short courses of these higher dose levels within a treatment regimen markedly increased the risk of serious hepatic injury. Liver dysfunction as evidenced by blood chemical abnormalities alone (liver enzyme elevations) has been observed in patients exposed to dantrolene for varying periods of time. Overt hepatitis has occurred at varying intervals after initiation of therapy, but has been most frequently observed between the third and twelfth month of therapy. The risk of hepatic injury appears to be greater in females, in patients over 35 years of age, and in patients taking other medication(s) in addition to dantrolene. Dantrolene should be used only in conjunction with appropriate monitoring of hepatic function including frequent determination of SGOT or SGPT. If no observable benefit is derived from the administration of dantrolene after a total of 45 days, therapy should be discontinued. The lowest possible effective dose for the individual patient should be prescribed.

DESCRIPTION:

CAPSULES

The chemical formula of dantrolene is hydrated 1-[[[5-(4-nitrophenyl)-2-furanyl]methylene]amino]-2,4-imidazolidinedione sodium salt. It is an orange powder, slightly soluble in water, but due to its slightly acidic nature the solubility increases somewhat in alkaline solution. The anhydrous salt has a molecular weight of 336. The hydrated salt contains approximately 15% water (3-1/2 moles) and has a molecular weight of 399.

Dantrolene is supplied in capsules of 25 mg, 50 mg, and 100 mg.

Inactive Ingredients: Each capsule contains edible black ink, FD&C Yellow No. 6, gelatin, lactose, magnesium stearate, starch, synthetic iron oxide red, synthetic iron oxide yellow talc, and titanium dioxide.

Intravenous Injection: Dantrolene Intravenous is a sterile, non-pyrogenic, lyophilized formulation of dantrolene sodium for injection. Dantrolene Intravenous is supplied in 70 ml vials containing 20 mg dantrolene sodium, 3000 mg mannitol, and sufficient sodium hydroxide to yield a pH of approximately 9.5 when reconstituted with 60 ml sterile water for injection USP (without a bacteriostatic agent).

Dantrolene is classified as a direct-acting skeletal muscle relaxant. Chemically, dantrolene is hydrated 1-[[[5-(4-nitrophenyl)-2-furanyl]methylene]amino]-2,4-imidazolidinedione sodium salt.

The hydrated salt contains approximately 15% water (3-1/2 moles) and has a molecular weight of 399. The anhydrous salt (dantrolene) has a molecular weight of 336.

CLINICAL PHARMACOLOGY:

In isolated nerve-muscle preparation, dantrolene has been shown to produce relaxation by affecting the contractile response of the skeletal muscle at a site beyond the myoneural junction, directly on the muscle itself. In skeletal muscle, dantrolene dissociates the excitation-contraction coupling, probably by interfering with the release of Ca^{++} from the sarcoplasmic reticulum.

Capsules: This effect appears to be more pronounced in fast muscle fibers as compared to slow ones, but generally affects both. A central nervous system effect occurs, with drowsiness, dizziness, and generalized weakness occasionally present. Although dantrolene does not appear to directly affect the CNS, the extent of its indirect effect is unknown. The absorption of dantrolene after oral administration in humans is incomplete and slow but consistent, and dose-related blood levels are obtained. The duration and intensity of skeletal muscle relaxation is related to the dosage and blood levels. The mean biologic half-life of dantrolene in adults is 8.7 hours after a 100-mg dose. Specific metabolic pathways in the degradation and elimination of dantrolene in human subjects have been established. Metabolic patterns are similar in adults and children. In addition to the parent compound, dantrolene, which is found in measurable amounts in blood and urine, the major metabolites noted in body fluids are the 5-hydroxy analog and the acetamido analog. Since dantrolene is probably metabolized by hepatic microsomal enzymes, enhancement of its metabolism by other drugs is possible. However, neither phenobarbital nor diazepam appears to affect dantrolene metabolism.

Clinical experience in the management of fulminant human malignant hyperthermia, as well as experiments conducted in malignant hyperthermia susceptible swine, have revealed that the administration of intravenous dantrolene, combined with indicated supportive measures, is effective in reversing the hypermetabolic process of malignant hyperthermia. Known differences between human and swine malignant hyperthermia are minor.

The prophylactic administration of oral or intravenous dantrolene to malignant hyperthermia susceptible swine will attenuate or prevent the development of signs of malignant hyperthermia in a manner dependent upon the dosage of dantrolene administered and the intensity of the malignant hyperthermia triggering stimulus. Limited clinical experience with the administration of oral dantrolene to patients judged malignant hyperthermia susceptible, when combined with clinical experience in the use of intravenous dantrolene for the treatment of malignant hyperthermia and data derived from the above cited animal model experiments, suggests that oral dantrolene will also attenuate or prevent the development of signs of human malignant hyperthermia, provided that currently accepted practices in the

CLINICAL PHARMACOLOGY: *(cont'd)*

management of such patients are adhered to (see INDICATIONS AND USAGE); intravenous dantrolene should also be available for use should the signs of malignant hyperthermia appear.

Intravenous Injection: The administration of intravenous dantrolene to human volunteers is associated with loss of grip strength and weakness in the legs, as well as subjective CNS complaints (see PRECAUTIONS, Information for the Patient). Information concerning the passage of dantrolene across the blood-brain barrier is not available.

In the anesthetic-induced malignant hyperthermia (MH) syndrome, evidence points to an intrinsic abnormality of skeletal muscle tissue. In affected humans, it has been postulated that "triggering agents" (*e.g.,* general anesthetics and depolarizing neuromuscular blocking agents) produce a change within the cell which results in an elevated myoplasmic calcium. This elevated myoplasmic calcium activates acute cellular catabolic processes that cascade to the MH crisis.

It is hypothesized that the addition of dantrolene to the "triggered" malignant hyperthermic muscle cell reestablishes a normal level of ionized calcium in the myoplasm. Inhibitions of calcium release from the sarcoplasmic reticulum by dantrolene reestablishes the myoplasmic calcium equilibrium, increasing the percentage of bound calcium. In this way, physiologic, metabolic, and biochemical changes associated with the MH crisis may be reversed or attenuated. Experimental results in malignant hyperthermia susceptible (MHS) swine show that prophylactic administration of IV or oral dantrolene prevents or attenuates the vital sign and blood gas changes characteristic of malignant hyperthermia (MH) in a dose related manner. The efficacy of IV dantrolene in the treatment of human and porcine MH crisis, when considered along with prophylactic experiments in MHS swine, lends support to the prophylactic use of oral or IV dantrolene in MHS humans. When prophylactic IV dantrolene is administered as directed, whole blood concentrations remain at a near steady state for 3 or more hours after the infusion is completed. Clinical experience has shown that early vital sign and /or blood gas changes characteristic of MH may appear during or after anesthesia and surgery despite the prophylactic use of dantrolene and adherence to currently accepted patient management practices. These signs are compatible with attenuated MH and respond to the administration of additional IV dantrolene (see DOSAGE AND ADMINISTRATION). The administration of the recommended prophylactic dose of IV dantrolene to healthy volunteers was not associated with clinically significant cardiorespiratory changes.

Specific metabolic pathways for the degradation and elimination of dantrolene in humans have been established. Dantrolene is found in measurable amounts in blood and urine. Its major metabolites in body fluids are 5-hydroxy dantrolene and an acetylamino metabolite of dantrolene. Another metabolite with an unknown structure appears related to the latter. Dantrolene may also undergo hydrolysis and subsequent oxidation forming nitrophenylfuroic acid.

The mean biologic half-life of dantrolene after intravenous administration is variable, between 4 to 8 hours under most experimental conditions. Based on assays of whole blood and plasma, slightly greater amounts of dantrolene are associated with red blood cells than with plasma fraction of blood. Significant amounts of dantrolene are bound to plasma proteins, mostly albumin, and this binding is readily reversible.

Cardiopulmonary depression has not been observed in MHS swine following the administration of up to 7.5 mg/kg/ IV dantrolene. This is twice the amount needed to maximally diminish twitch response to single supramaximal peripheral nerve stimulation (95% inhibition). A transient, inconsistent, depressant effect on gastrointestinal smooth muscle has been observed at high doses.

INDICATIONS AND USAGE:

CAPSULES

In Chronic Spasticity: Dantrolene is indicated in controlling the manifestations of clinical spasticity resulting from upper motor neuron disorders (*e.g.,*spinal cord injury, stroke, cerebral palsy, or multiple sclerosis). It is of particular benefit to the patient whose functional rehabilitation has been retarded by the sequelae of spasticity. Such patients must have presumably reversible spasticity where relief of spasticity will aid in restoring residual function. Dantrolene is not indicated in the treatment of skeletal muscle spasm resulting from rheumatic disorders.

If improvement occurs, it will ordinarily occur within the dosage titration (see DOSAGE AND ADMINISTRATION), and will be manifested by a decrease in the severity of spasticity and the ability to resume a daily function not quite attainable without dantrolene.

Occasionally, subtle but meaningful improvement in spasticity may occur with dantrolene therapy. In such instances, information regarding improvement should be solicited from the patient and those who are in constant daily contact and attendance with him. Brief withdrawal of dantrolene for a period of 2 to 4 days will frequently demonstrate exacerbation of the manifestations of spasticity and may serve to confirm a clinical impression.

A decision to continue the administration of dantrolene on a long-term basis is justified if introduction of the drug into the patient's regimen:

produces a significant reduction in painful and/or disabling spasticity such as clonus, or permits a significant reduction in the intensity and/or degree of nursing care required, or rids the patient of any annoying manifestation of spasticity considered important by the patient himself.

In Malignant Hyperthermia: Oral dantrolene is also indicated preoperatively to prevent or attenuate the development of signs of malignant hyperthermia in known, or strongly suspect, malignant hyperthermia susceptible patients who require anesthesia and/or surgery. Currently accepted clinical practices in the management of such patients must still be adhered to (careful monitoring for early signs of malignant hyperthermia, minimizing exposure to triggering mechanisms and prompt use of intravenous dantrolene sodium and indicated supportive measures should signs of malignant hyperthermia appear); see also the package insert for dantrolene (dantrolene sodium) Intravenous.

Oral dantrolene should be administered following a malignant hyperthermic crisis to prevent recurrence of the signs of malignant hyperthermia.

INTRAVENOUS INJECTION

Dantrolene intravenous is indicated, along with appropriate supportive measures, for the management of the fulminant hypermetabolism of skeletal muscle characteristics of MH crises in patients of all ages. Dantrolene intravenous should be administered by continuous rapid intravenous push as soon as the MH reaction is recognized (*i.e.,* tachycardia, tachypnea, central venous desaturation, hypercarbia, metabolic acidosis, skeletal muscle rigidity, increased utilization of anesthesia circuit carbon dioxide absorber, cyanosis and mottling of the skin, and, in many cases, fever).

Dantrolene intravenous is also indicated preoperatively, and sometimes postoperatively, to prevent or attenuate the development of clinical and laboratory signs of malignant hyperthermia in individuals judged to be malignant hyperthermia susceptible.

CONTRAINDICATIONS:

Capsules: Active hepatic disease, such as hepatitis and cirrhosis, is a contraindication for use of dantrolene. Dantrolene is contraindicated where spasticity is utilized to sustain upright posture and balance in locomotion or whenever spasticity is utilized to obtain or maintain increased function.

Intravenous Injection: None.

WARNINGS:

CAPSULES

It is important to recognize that fatal and non-fatal liver disorders of an idiosyncratic or hypersensitivity type may occur with dantrolene therapy.

At the start of dantrolene therapy, it is desirable to do liver function studies (SGOT, SGPT, alkaline phosphatase, total bilirubin) for a baseline or to establish whether there is pre-existing liver disease. If baseline liver abnormalities exist and are confirmed, there is a clear possibility that the potential for dantrolene hepatotoxicity could be enhanced, although such a possibility has not yet been established.

Liver function studies (*e.g.,* SGOT or SGPT) should be performed at appropriate intervals during dantrolene therapy. If such studies reveal abnormal values, therapy should generally be discontinued. Only where benefits of the drug have been of major importance to the patient, should reinitiation or continuation of therapy be considered. Some patients have revealed a return to normal laboratory values in the face of continued therapy while others have not.

If symptoms compatible with hepatitis, accompanied by abnormalities in liver function tests or jaundice appear, dantrolene should be discontinued. If caused by dantrolene and detected early, the abnormalities in liver function characteristically have reverted to normal when the drug was discontinued.

Dantrolene therapy has been reinstituted in a few patients who have developed clinical and/or laboratory evidence of hepatocellular injury. If such reinstitution of therapy is done, it should be attempted only in patients who clearly need dantrolene and only after previous symptoms and laboratory abnormalities have cleared. The patient should be hospitalized and the drug should be restarted in very small and gradually increasing doses. Laboratory monitoring should be frequent and the drug should be withdrawn immediately if there is any indication of recurrent liver involvement. Some patients have reacted with unmistakable signs of liver abnormality upon administration of a challenge dose, while others have not.

Dantrolene should be used with particular caution in females and in patients over 35 years of age in view of apparent greater likelihood of drug-induced, potentially fatal, hepatocellular disease in these groups.

Long-term safety of dantrolene in humans has not been established. Chronic studies in rats, dogs, and monkeys at dosages greater than 30 mg/kg/day showed growth or weight depression and signs of hepatopathy and possible occlusion nephropathy, all of which were reversible upon cessation of treatment. Sprague-Dawley female rats fed dantrolene sodium for 18 months at dosage levels of 15, 30, and 60 mg/kg/day showed an increased incidence of benign and malignant mammary tumors compared with concurrent controls and, at the highest dosage, an increase in the incidence of hepatic lymphangiomas and hepatic angiosarcomas. These effects were not seen in 2 1/2-year studies in Sprague-Dawley or Fischer 344 rats or in 2-year studies in mice of the HaM/ICR strain. Carcinogenicity in humans cannot be fully excluded, so that this possible risk of chronic administration must be weighed against the benefits of the drug (*i.e.,* after a brief trial) for the individual patient.

Usage In Pregnancy: The safety of dantrolene for use in women who are or who may become pregnant has not been established. Dantrolene should not be used in nursing mothers.

Usage in Children: The long-term safety of dantrolene in children under the age of 5 years has not been established. Because of the possibility that adverse effects of the drug could become apparent only after many years, a benefit-risk consideration of the long-term use of dantrolene is particularly important in pediatric patients.

INTRAVENOUS INJECTION

The use of dantrolene Intravenous in the management of MH crisis is not a substitute for previously known supportive measures. These measures must be individualized, but it will usually be necessary to discontinue the suspect triggering agents, attend to increased oxygen requirements, manage the metabolic acidosis, institute cooling when necessary, monitor urinary output, and monitor electrolyte imbalance.

Since the effects of the disease state and other drugs on the consequences of dantrolene related skeletal muscle weakness, including possible respiratory depression, cannot be predicted, patients who receive IV dantrolene preoperatively should have vital signs monitored.

If patients judged malignant hyperthermia susceptible are administered IV or oral dantrolene preoperatively, anesthetic preparation must still follow a standard MHS regimen, including the avoidance of known triggering agents. Monitoring for early clinical and metabolic signs of MH is indicated because attenuation of MH, rather than prevention, is possible. These signs usually call for the administration of additional IV dantrolene.

PRECAUTIONS:

CAPSULES

Dantrolene should be used with caution in patients with impaired pulmonary function, particularly those with obstructive pulmonary disease, and in patients with severely impaired cardiac function due to myocardial disease. It should be used with caution in patients with a history of previous liver disease or dysfunction (see WARNINGS).

Patients should be cautioned against driving a motor vehicle or participating in hazardous occupations while taking dantrolene. Caution should be exercised in the concomitant administration of tranquilizing agents.

Dantrolene might possibly evoke a photosensitivity reaction; patients should be cautioned about exposure to sunlight while taking it.

INTRAVENOUS INJECTION

General: Care must be taken to prevent extravasation of dantrolene solution into the surrounding tissues due to the high pH of the intravenous formulation.

When mannitol is used for prevention or treatment of late renal complications of MH, the 3 g of mannitol needed to dissolve each 20 mg vial of IV dantrolene should be taken into consideration.

Information for the Patient: Based upon data in human volunteers, it will sometimes be appropriate to tell patients who receive dantrolene Intravenous that decrease in grip strength and weakness of leg muscles, especially walking down stairs, can be expected postoperatively. In addition, symptoms such as "lightheadedness" may be noted. Since some of these symptoms may persist for up to 48 hours, patients must not operate an automobile or engage in other hazardous activity during this time. Caution is also indicated at meals on the day of administration because difficulty swallowing and choking has been reported.

Carcinogenesis, Mutagenesis, and Impairment of Fertility: Studies of dantrolene in animals to evaluate mutagenic potential and the effect on fertility have not been conducted. Sprague-Dawley female rats fed dantrolene for 18 months at dosage levels of 15, 30, and 60 mg/kg/day showed an increased incidence of benign and malignant mammary tumors compared with concurrent controls. At the highest dosage, there was in increase in the incidence of hepatic lymphangiomas and hepatic angiosarcomas. These effects were not seen in 30-month studies in Sprague-Dawley or Fischer-344 rats or in 24-month studies in mice of the HaM/ICR strain. Although the possibility that the drug may be carcinogenic in humans cannot be fully excluded, the risks associated with administration of dantrolene Intravenous in a life-threatening crisis would appear to be minimal.

Pregnancy Category C: Dantrolene has been shown to be embryocidal in the rabbit and has been shown to decrease pup survival in the rat when given at doses seven times the human oral dose. There are no adequate and well controlled studies in pregnant women. Dantrolene Intravenous should be used during pregnancy only if the potential benefit justifies the potential risk to the fetus.

Labor and Delivery: In one uncontrolled study, 100 mg per day of prophylactic of oral dantrolene was administered to term pregnant patients awaiting labor and delivery. Dantrolene readily crossed the placenta, with maternal and fetal whole blood levels approximately equal at delivery; neonatal levels then fell approximately 50% per day for 2 days before declining sharply. No neonatal respiratory and neuromuscular side effects were detected at low dose. More data, at higher doses, are needed before more definitive conclusions can be made.

DRUG INTERACTIONS:

The combination of therapeutic doses of intravenous dantrolene sodium and verapamil in halothane/α-chloralose anesthetized swine has resulted in ventricular fibrillation and cardiovascular collapse in association with marked hyperkalemia. Until the relevance of these findings to humans is established, the combination of dantrolene sodium and verapamil is not recommended during the management of malignant hyperthermia.

CAPSULES

While a definite drug interaction with estrogen therapy has not yet been established, caution should be observed if the two drugs are to be given concomitantly. Hepatotoxicity has occurred more often in women over 35 years of age receiving concomitant estrogen therapy.

There are very rare reports of cardiovascular collapse in patients treated simultaneously with verapamil and dantrolene sodium.

INTRAVENOUS INJECTION

Dantrolene is metabolized by the liver, and it is theoretically possible that its metabolism may be enhanced by drugs known to induce hepatic microsomal enzymes. However, neither phenobarbital nor diazepam appears to affect dantrolene metabolism. Binding to plasma protein is not significantly altered by diazepam, diphenylhydantoin, or phenylbutazone. Binding to plasma proteins is reduced by warfarin and clofibrate and increased by tolbutamide.

ADVERSE REACTIONS:

CAPSULES

The most frequently occurring side effects of dantrolene have been drowsiness, dizziness, weakness, general malaise, fatigue, and diarrhea. These are generally transient, occurring early in treatment, and can often be obviated by beginning with a low dose and increasing dosage gradually until an optimal regimen is established. Diarrhea may be severe and may necessitate temporary withdrawal of dantrolene therapy. If diarrhea recurs upon readministration of dantrolene, therapy should probably be withdrawn permanently.

Other less frequent side effects, listed according to system, are:

Gastrointestinal: Constipation, GI bleeding, anorexia, swallowing difficulty, gastric irritation, abdominal cramps, nausea and/or vomiting.

Hepatobiliary: Hepatitis (see WARNINGS).

Neurologic: Speech disturbance, seizure, headache, light-headedness, visual disturbance, diplopia, alteration of taste, insomnia.

Cardiovascular: Tachycardia, erratic blood pressure, phlebitis, heart failure.

Hematologic: Aplastic anemia, leukopenia, lymphocytic lymphoma.

Psychiatric: Mental depression, mental confusion, increased nervousness.

Urogenital: Increased urinary frequency, crystalluria, hematuria, difficult erection, urinary incontinence and/or nocturia, difficult urination and/or urinary retention.

Integumentary: Abnormal hair growth, acne-like rash, pruritus, urticaria, eczematoid eruption, sweating.

Musculoskeletal: Myalgia, backache.

Respiratory: Feeling of suffocation.

Special Senses: Excessive tearing.

Hypersensitivity: Pleural effusion with pericarditis, anaphylaxis.

Other: Chills and fever.

The published literature has included some reports of dantrolene use in patients with Neuroleptic Malignant Syndrome (NMS). Dantrolene capsules are not included for the treatment of NMS and patients may expire depsite treatment with dantrolene capsules.

INTRAVENOUS INJECTION

There have been occasional reports of death following MH crisis even when treated with IV dantrolene; incidence figures are not available (the pre-dantrolene mortality of MH crisis was approximately 50%). Most of these deaths can be accounted for by late recognition, delayed treatment, inadequate dosage, lack of supportive therapy, intercurrent disease and/or the development of delayed complications such as renal failure or disseminated intravascular coagulopathy. In some cases there are insufficient data to completely rule out therapeutic failure of dantrolene.

There are rare reports of fatality in MH crisis, despite initial satisfactory response to IV dantrolene, which involves patients who could not be weaned from dantrolene after initial treatment.

The following adverse reactions are in approximate order of severity:

There are rare reports of pulmonary edema developing during the treatment of MH crisis in which the diluent volume and mannitol needed to deliver IV dantrolene possibly contributed.

There have been reports of thrombophlebitis following administration of IV dantrolene; actual incidence figures are not available.

There have been rare reports of urticaria and erythema possibly associated with the admission of IV dantrolene. There has been one case of anaphylaxis.

None of the serious reactions occasionally reported with long-term oral dantrolene use, such as hepatitis, seizures, and pleural effusion with pericarditis, have been reasonably associated with short term dantrolene Intravenous therapy.

OVERDOSAGE:

Capsules: For acute overdosage, general supportive measures should be employed along with immediate gastric lavage.

OVERDOSAGE: *(cont'd)*

Intravenous fluids should be administered in fairly large quantities to avert the possibility of crystalluria. An adequate airway should be maintained and artificial resuscitation equipment should be at hand. Electrocardiographic monitoring should be instituted, and the patient carefully observed. To date, no experience has been reported with dialysis and its value in dantrolene overdosage is not known.

Intravenous Injection: Because dantrolene Intravenous must be administered at a low concentration in a large volume of fluid, acute toxicity of dantrolene could not be assessed in animals. In 14-day (subacute) studies, the intravenous formulation of dantrolene was relatively non-toxic to rats at doses of 10 mg/kg/day and 20 mg/kg/day. While 10 mg/kg/day in dogs evoked little toxicity, 20 mg/kg/day for 14 days caused hepatic changes of questionable biologic significance.

No data are available to define the symptomatology of an overdose of dantrolene Intravenous. If an overdose is suspected, treatment is symptomatic and supportive. There is no known antidote.

DOSAGE AND ADMINISTRATION:

CAPSULES

For Use in Chronic Spasticity: Prior to the administration of dantrolene, consideration should be given to the potential response to treatment. A decrease in spasticity sufficient to allow a daily function not otherwise attainable should be the therapeutic goal of treatment with dantrolene. Refer to INDICATIONS AND USAGE section for description of response to be anticipated.

It is important to establish a therapeutic goal (regain and maintain a specific function such as therapeutic exercise program, utilization of braces, transfer maneuvers, etc.) before beginning dantrolene therapy. Dosage should be increased until the maximum performance compatible with the dysfunction due to underlying disease is achieved. No further increase in dosage is then indicated.

Usual Dosage: It is important that the dosage be titrated and individualized for maximum effect. The lowest dose compatible with optimal response is recommended.

In view of the potential for liver damage in long-term dantrolene use, therapy should be stopped if benefits are not evident within 45 days.

Adults: Begin therapy with 25 mg once daily; increase to 25 mg two, three, or four times daily and then by increments of 25 mg up to as high as 100 mg two, three, or four times daily if necessary. As most patients will respond to a dose of 400 mg/day or less, rarely should doses higher than 400 mg/day be used (see BOXED WARNING).

Each dosage level should be maintained for four to seven days to determine the patient's response. The dose should not be increased beyond, and may even have to be reduced to, the amount at which the patient received maximal benefit without adverse effects.

Children: A similar approach should be utilized starting with 0.5 mg/kg of body weight twice daily; this is increased to 0.5 mg/kg three or four times daily and then by increments of 0.5 mg/kg up to as high as 3 mg/kg two, three, or four times daily, if necessary. Doses higher than 100 mg four times daily should not be used in children.

For Malignant Hyperthermia: *Preoperatively:* Administer 4 to 8 mg/kg/day of oral dantrolene in 3 or 4 divided doses for one or two days prior to surgery, with the last dose being given approximately 3 to 4 hours before scheduled surgery with a minimum of water.

This dosage will usually be associated with skeletal muscle weakness and sedation (sleepiness or drowsiness); adjustment can usually be made within the recommended dosage range to avoid incapacitation or excessive gastrointestinal irritation (including nausea and/or vomiting).

Post Crisis Follow-up: Oral dantrolene should also be administered following a malignant hyperthermia crisis, in doses of 4 to 8 mg/kg per day in four divided doses, for a one to three day period to prevent recurrence of the manifestations of malignant hyperthermia.

INTRAVENOUS INJECTION

As soon as the MH reaction is recognized, all anesthetic agents should be discontinued; the administration of 100% oxygen is recommended. Dantrolene Intravenous should be administered by continuous rapid IV push beginning at a minimum dose of 1 mg/kg, and continuing until symptoms subside or the maximum cumulative dose of 10 mg/kg/ has been reached.

If the physiologic and metabolic abnormalities reappear, the regimen may be repeated. It is important to note that administration of dantrolene Intravenous should be continuous until symptoms subside. The effective dose to reverse the crisis is directly dependent upon the individual's degree of susceptibility to MH, the amount of time and exposure to the triggering agent, and the time elapsed between onset of the crisis and the initiation of treatment.

Children's Dose: Experience to date indicates that the dose of dantrolene IV for children is the same as for adults.

Preoperatively: Dantrolene may be administered preoperatively to patients judged MH susceptible as part of the overall patient management to prevent or attenuate the development of clinical and laboratory signs of MH.

The recommended prophylactic dose of dantrolene IV is 2.5 mg/kg, starting approximately 1-1/4 hours before anticipated anesthesia and infused over approximately 1 hour. This dose should prevent or attenuate the development of clinical and laboratory signs of MH provided that the usual precautions, such as avoidance of established MH triggering agents, are followed.

Additional dantrolene Intravenous may be indicated during anesthesia and surgery because of the appearance of early clinical and/or blood gas signs of MH or because of prolonged surgery (see also CLINICAL PHARMACOLOGY, WARNINGS, and PRECAUTIONS). Additional doses must be individualized.

Intravenous dantrolene may be used postoperatively to prevent or attenuate the recurrence of signs of MH when oral dantrolene administration is not practical. The IV dose of dantrolene in the postoperative period must be individualized, starting with 1 mg/kg or more as the clinical situation dictates.

Preparation: Each vial of dantrolene Intravenous should be reconstituted by adding 60 ml of *sterile water for injection USP (without a bacteriostatic agent) and the vial shaken until the solution is clear.* 5% Dextrose Injection USP, 0.9% Sodium Chloride Injection USP, and other acidic solutions are not compatible with dantrolene Intravenous and should not be used. The contents of the vial must be*protected from direct light and used within 6 hours* after reconstitution. Store reconstituted solutions at controlled room temperature (59° to 86°F or 15° to 30°C).

Reconstituted dantrolene Intravenous should *not* be transferred to large glass bottles for prophylactic infusion due to precipitate formation observed with the use of some glass bottles as reservoirs.

For prophylactic infusion, the required number of individual vials of dantrolene IV should be reconstituted as outlined above. The contents of individual vials are then transferred to a larger volume sterile intravenous plastic bag. It is recommended that the prepared infusion be inspected carefully for cloudiness and/or precipitation prior to dispensing and administration. Such solutions should not be used. While stable for 6 hours, it is recommended that the infusion be prepared immediately prior to the anticipated dosage administration.

DOSAGE AND ADMINISTRATION: *(cont'd)*

Parenteral drug products should be inspected visually for particulate matter and discoloration prior to administration.

HOW SUPPLIED:

Capsules: Dantrium is available in:25-mg opaque, orange and tan capsules,50-mg opaque, orange and tan capsules, 100-mg opaque, orange and tan capsules**Avoid excessive heat (over 104° or 40°C).**

Intravenous Injection Dantrium Intravenous is available in vials containing a sterile lyophilized mixture of 20 mg dantrolene sodium, 3000 mg mannitol, and sufficient sodium hydroxide to yield a pH of approximately 9.5 when reconstituted with 60 ml sterile water for injection USP (without a bacteriostatic agent).

Store unreconstituted product at controlled room temperature (59°F to 86°F or 15°C to 30°C) and avoid prolonged exposure to light.

HOW SUPPLIED - EQUIVALENTS NOT AVAILABLE:

Capsule, Gelatin - Oral - 25 mg

100's	$72.17	DANTRIUM, Procter Gamble Pharm	00149-0030-05
100's	$79.31	DANTRIUM, Procter Gamble Pharm	00149-0030-77
500's	$350.03	DANTRIUM, Procter Gamble Pharm	00149-0030-66

Capsule, Gelatin - Oral - 50 mg

100's	$108.12	DANTRIUM, Procter Gamble Pharm	00149-0031-05

Capsule, Gelatin - Oral - 100 mg

100's	$134.46	DANTRIUM, Procter Gamble Pharm	00149-0033-05
100's	$141.42	DANTRIUM, Procter Gamble Pharm	00149-0033-77

Injection, Solution - Intravenous - 20 mg

1's	$55.21	DANTRIUM IV, Procter Gamble Pharm	00149-0734-02

DAPIPRAZOLE HYDROCHLORIDE *(003006)*

CATEGORIES: Alpha-Adrenergic Blocking Agents; EENT Drugs; Eye, Ear, Nose, & Throat Preparations; Mydriasis; Mydiasis, Drug-Induced; Pregnancy Category B; FDA Class 1B ("Modest Therapeutic Advantage"); FDA Approved 1990 Dec

BRAND NAMES: *Glamidolo*; **Rev-Eyes**
(International brand names outside U.S. in italics)

DESCRIPTION:

For ophthalmic use only.

Rev-Eyes (dapiprazole hydrochloride) is an alpha-adrenergic blocking agent.

Dapiprazole hydrochloride is 5,6,7,8-tetrahydro-3-(2-(4-o.tolyl-1-piperazinyl)ethyl)-s-triazolo (4,3-a)pyridine hydrochloride.

Dapiprazole hydrochloride has the empirical formula $C_{19}H_{27}N_5$ HCl and a molecular weight of 361.93.

Dapiprazole hydrochloride is a sterile, white, lyophilized powder soluble in water.

Rev-Eyes (dapiprazole hydrochloride) Eyedrops is a clear, colorless, slightly viscous solution for topical application. Each ml (when reconstituted as directed contains 5 mg of dapiprazole hydrochloride as the active ingredient.

The reconstituted solution has a pH of approximately 6.6 and an osmolarity of approximately 415 mOsm.

The inactive ingredients include: mannitol (2%), sodium chloride, hydroxypropyl methylcellulose (0.4%), edetate sodium (0.01%), sodium phosphate dibasic, sodium phosphate monobasic, water for injection, and benzalkonium chloride (0.01%) as a preservative.

Rev-Eyes Eyedrops, 0.5% is supplied in a kit consisting of one vial of dapiprazole hydrochloride (25 mg), one vial of diluent (5 ml) and one dropper for dispensing.

CLINICAL PHARMACOLOGY:

Dapiprazole acts through blocking the alpha-adrenergic receptors in smooth muscle. Dapiprazole produces miosis through an effect on the dilator muscle of the iris.

Dapiprazole does not have any significant activity on ciliary muscle contraction and, therefore does not induce a significant change in the anterior chamber depth or the thickness of the lens.

Dapiprazole has demonstrated safe and rapid reversal of mydriasis produced by phenylephrine and to a lesser degree tropicamide. In patients with decreased accommodative amplitude due to treatment with tropicamide the miotic effect of dapiprazole may partially increase the accommodative amplitude.

Eye color affects the rate of pupillary constriction. In individuals with brown irides, the rate of pupillary constriction may be slightly slower than in individuals with blue or green irides. Eye color does not appear to affect the final pupil size.

Dapiprazole does not significantly alter intraocular pressure in normotensive or in eyes with elevated intraocular pressure.

INDICATIONS AND USAGE:

Dapiprazole is indicated in the treatment of iatrogenically induced mydriasis produced by adrenergic (phenylephrine) or parasympatholytic (tropicamide) agents. Dapiprazole is not indicated for the reduction of intraocular pressure or in the treatment of open angle glaucoma.

CONTRAINDICATIONS:

Miotics are contraindicated where constriction is undesirable; such as acute iritis, and in those subjects showing hypersensitivity to any component of this preparation.

WARNINGS:

For Topical Ophthalmic Use Only. NOT FOR INJECTION. Do not touch the dropper up to lids or any surface, as this may contaminate the solution. Dapiprazole should not be used in the same patient more frequently than once a week.

PRECAUTIONS:

Information for the Patient: Miosis may cause difficulty in dark adaptation and may reduce the field of vision. Patients should exercise, caution when involved in night driving or other activities in poor illumination.

Carcinogenesis, Mutagenesis, and Impairment of Fertility: Dapiprazole has been shown to significantly increase the incidence of liver tumors in rats after continuous dietary administration for 104 weeks. This effect was found only in male rats treated with the highest dose administered in the study, i.e. 300 mg/kg/day, (80,000 times the human dose) and was not observed in male and female rats at doses of 30 and 100 mg/kg/day and female rats at doses of 300 mg/kg/day.

PRECAUTIONS: *(cont'd)*

Negative results have been reported on the mutagenicity and impairment of fertility studies and dapiprazole.

Pregnancy Category B: Reproduction studies have been preformed in rats and rabbits at doses up to 128.000 (rat) and 27,000 (rabbit) times the human ophthalmic dose and revealed no evidence of impaired fertility or harm to the fetus due to dapiprazole. There are, however, no adequate and well controlled studies in pregnant women. Because animal reproduction studies are not always predictive of human response, this drug should be used during pregnancy only if clearly needed.

Nursing Mothers: It is not known whether this drug is excreted in human milk. Because many drugs are excreted in human milk, caution should be exercised when dapiprazole is administered to a nursing woman.

Pediatric Use: Safety and effectiveness in children has not been established.

ADVERSE REACTIONS:

In controlled studies the most frequent reaction to dapiprazole was conjunctival injection lasting 20 minutes in over 80% of patients. Burning on instillation of dapiprazole was reported in approximately half of all patients. Reactions occurring in 10% to 40% of patients included ptosis, lid erythremia, lid edema, chemosis, itching, punctate keratitis, corneal edema, browache, photophobia and headaches. Other reactions reported less frequently included dryness of eyes, tearing and blurring of vision.

DOSAGE AND ADMINISTRATION:

Two drops followed 5 minutes later by an additional 2 drops applied topically to the conjunctiva of each eye should be administered after the ophthalmic examination to reverse the diagnostic mydriasis. Dapiprazole should not be used in the same patient more frequently than once per week.

Directions for Preparing Eyedrops:

1. Use aseptic technique.

2. Tear of aluminum seals, remove and discard rubber plugs from both drug and diluent vials.

3. Pour diluent into drug vial.

4. Remove dropper assembly from its sterile wrapping and attach to the drug vial.

5. Shake container for several minutes to ensure mixing.

Storage and Stability of Eyedrops: Once the eyedrops have been reconstituted they may be stored at room temperature 15 - 30° C (59 - 86° F) for 21 days. discard any solution that is not clear and colorless.

HOW SUPPLIED - EQUIVALENTS NOT AVAILABLE:

Powder - Topical - 0.5%

5 ml $32.74 REV-EYES, Storz 57706-0761-62

DAPSONE *(000945)*

CATEGORIES: Anti-Infectives; Antimicrobials; Antimycobacterials; Dermatitis; Dermatitis Herpetiformis; Dermatologicals; Laprostatics; Orphan Drugs; Sulfones; Toxoplasmosis; Pregnancy Category C; FDA Approval Pre 1982

BRAND NAMES: *Avlosulfon* (Canada); *Avsulfon*; *Dapson*; *Dapson-Fatol* (Germany); *Dapsone*; *Diaphenylsulfon*; *Disulone*; *Dubronax*; *Protogen* (Japan); *Servidapsone*; *Sulfona*

(International brand names outside U.S. in italics)

FORMULARIES: Aetna; BC-BS; Medi-Cal; PCS; WHO

DESCRIPTION:

Dapsone-USP, 4,4'-diaminodiphenylsulfone (DDS), is a primary treatment for Dermatitis herpetiformis. It is an antibacterial drug for susceptible cases of leprosy. It is a white, odorless crystalline powder, practically insoluble in water and insoluble in fixed and vegetable oils.

Dapsone is issued on prescription in tablets of 25 and 100 mg for oral use.

Jacobus Dapsone Inactive Ingredients: Colloidal silicone dioxide, magnesium stearate, microcrystalline cellulose and corn starch.

CLINICAL PHARMACOLOGY:

Mechanism of Action: The mechanism of action in Dermatitis herpetiformis has not been established. By the kinetic method in mice. Dapsone is bactericidal as well as bacteriostatic against *Mycobacterium leprae.*

Absorption and Excretion: Dapsone, when given orally, is rapidly and almost completely absorbed. About 85 percent of the daily intake is recoverable from the urine mainly in the form of water-soluble metabolites. Excretion of the drug is slow and a constant blood level can be maintained with the usual dosage.

Blood Levels: Detected a few minutes after ingestion, the drug reaches peak concentration in 4-8 hours. Daily administration for at least eight days is necessary to achieve a plateau level. With doses of 200 mg daily, this level averaged 2.3 mcg/ml with a range of 0.1-7.0 mcg/ml. The half-life in the plasma in different individuals varies from ten hours to fifty hours and averages twenty-eight hours. Repeat tests in the same individual are constant. Daily administration (50-100 mg) in leprosy patients will provide blood levels in excess of the usual minimum inhibitory concentration even for patients with a short dapsone half-life.

INDICATIONS AND USAGE:

Dermatitis herpetiformis: (D.H.)

Leprosy: All forms of leprosy except for cases of proven dapsone resistance.

CONTRAINDICATIONS:

Hypersensitivity to dapsone and/or its derivatives.

WARNINGS:

The patient should be warned to respond to the presence of clinical signs such as sore throat, fever, pallor, purpura or jaundice. Deaths associated with the administration of dapsone have been reported from agranulocytosis, aplastic anemia and other blood dyscrasias. Complete blood counts should be done frequently in patients receiving dapsone.

The FDA Dermatology Advisory Committee recommended that, when feasible, counts should be done weekly for the first month, monthly for six months and semi-annually thereafter. If a significant reduction in leucocytes, platelets or hemopoiesis is noted, dapsone should be discontinued and the patient followed intensively. Folic acid antagonists have similar effects and may increase the incidence of hematologic reactions; if co- administered with dapsone the patient should be monitored more frequently. Patients on weekly pyrimethamine and dapsone have developed agranulocytosis during the second and third month of therapy.

Severe anemia should be treated prior to initiation of therapy and hemoglobin monitored. Hemolysis and methemoglobin may be poorly tolerated by patients with severe cardiopulmonary disease.

Carcinogenesis, Mutagenesis: Dapsone has been found carcinogenic (sarcomagenic) for male rats and female mice causing mesenchymal tumors in the spleen and peritoneum, and thyroid carcinoma in female rats. Dapsone is not mutagenic with or without microsomal activation in *S. typhimurium* tester strains 1535, 1537, 1538, 98 or 100.

Cutaneous reactions, especially bullous, include exfoliative dermatitis and are probably one of the most serious, though rare, complications of sulfone therapy. They are directly due to drug sensitization. Such reactions include toxic erythema, erythema multiforme, toxic epidermal necrolysis, morbilliform and scarlatiniform reactions, urticaria and erythema nodosum. If new or toxic dermatologic reactions occur, sulfone therapy must be promptly discontinued and appropriate therapy instituted.

Leprosy reactional states, including cutaneous, are not hypersensitivity reactions to dapsone and do not require discontinuation. See special section.

PRECAUTIONS:

General: Hemolysis and Heinz body formation may be exaggerated in individuals with a glucose-6-phosphate dehydrogenase (G6PD) deficiency, or methemoglobin reductase deficiency, or hemoglobin M. This reaction is frequently dose-related. Dapsone should be given with caution to these patients or if the patient is exposed to other agents or conditions such as infection or diabetic ketosis capable of producing hemolysis. Drugs or chemicals which have produced significant hemolysis in G6PD or methemoglobin reductase deficient patients include dapsone, sulfanilamide, nitrate, aniline, phenylhydrazine, naphthalene, niridazole, nitro-furantoin and 8-amino-antimalarials such as primaquine.

Toxic hepatitis and cholestatic jaundice have been reported early in therapy. Hyperbilirubinemia may occur more often in G6PD deficient patients. When feasible, baseline and subsequent monitoring of liver function is recommended; if abnormal, dapsone should be discontinued until the source of the abnormality is established.

Pregnancy Category C: Animal reproduction studies have not been conducted with dapsone. Extensive, but uncontrolled experience and two published surveys on the use of dapsone in pregnant women have not shown that dapsone increases the risk of fetal abnormalities if administered during all trimesters of pregnancy or affect reproduction capacity. Because of the lack of animal studies or controlled human experience, dapsone should be given to a pregnant woman only if clearly needed. In general, for leprosy, USPHS at Carville recommends maintenance of dapsone. Dapsone has been important for the management of some pregnant D.H. patients.

Nursing Mothers: Dapsone is excreted in breast milk in substantial amounts. Hemolytic reactions can occur in neonates. See section on hemolysis. Because of the potential for tumorigenicity shown for dapsone in animal studies a decision should be made whether to discontinue nursing or discontinue the drug taking into account the importance of the drug to the mother.

Pediatric Use: Children are treated on the same schedule as adults but with correspondingly smaller doses. Dapsone is generally not considered to have an effect on the later growth, development and functional development of the child.

DRUG INTERACTIONS:

Rifampin lowers dapsone levels 7- to 10-fold by accelerating plasma clearance; in leprosy this reduction has not required a change in dosage.

Folic acid antagonists such as pyrimethamine may increase the likelihood of hematologic reactions.

A modest interaction has been reported for patients receiving 100 mg dapsone od in combination with trimethoprim 5 mg/kg q6h. On day 7, the serum dapsone levels averaged 2.1 ± 1.0 mcg/ml in comparison to 1.5 ± 0.5 mcg/ml for dapsone alone. On Day 7, trimethoprim levels averaged 18.4 ± 5.2 mcg/ml in comparison to 12.4 ± 4.5 mcg/ml for patients not receiving dapsone. Thus, there is a mutual interaction between dapsone and trimethoprim in which each raises the level of the other about 1.5 times.

ADVERSE REACTIONS:

In addition to the warnings listed above, the following syndromes and serious reactions have been reported in patients on dapsone.

Hematologic Effects: Dose-related hemolysis is the most common adverse effect and is seen in patients with or without G6PD deficiency. Almost all patients demonstrate the inter-related changes of a loss of 1-2g of hemoglobin, an increase in the reticulocytes (2-12%), a shortened red cell life span and a rise in methemoglobin. G6PD deficient patients have greater responses.

Nervous System Effects: Peripheral neuropathy is a definite but unusual complication of dapsone therapy in non-leprosy patients. Motor loss is predominant. If muscle weakness appears, dapsone should be withdrawn. Recovery on withdrawal is usually substantially complete. The mechanism of recovery is reported by axonal regeneration. Some recovered patients have tolerated retreatment at reduced dosage. In leprosy this complication may be difficult to distinguish from a leprosy reactional state.

Body As A Whole: In addition to the warnings and adverse effects reported above, additional adverse reactions include: nausea, vomiting, abdominal pains, pancreatitis, vertigo, blurred vision, tinnitus, insomnia, fever, headache, psychosis, phototoxicity, pulmonary eosinophilia, tachycardia, albuminuria, the nephrotic syndrome, hypoalbuminemia without proteinuria, renal papillary necrosis, male infertility, drug-induced Lupus erythematosus and an infectious mononucleosis-like syndrome. In general, with the exception of the complications of severe anoxia from overdosage (retinal and optic nerve damage, etc.) these adverse reactions have regressed off drug.

OVERDOSAGE:

Nausea, vomiting, hyperexcitability can appear a few minutes up to 24 hours after ingestion of an overdosage. Methemoglobin induced depression, convulsions or severe cyanosis requires prompt treatment. In normal and methemoglobin reductase deficient patients, methylene blue, 1-2 mg/kg of body weight, given slowly intravenously, is the treatment of choice. The effect is complete in 30 minutes, but may have to be repeated if methemoglobin reaccumulates. For non-emergencies, if treatment is needed, methylene blue may be given orally in doses of 3-5 mg/kg every 4-6 hours. Methylene blue reduction depends on G6PD and should not be given to fully expressed G6PD deficient patients.

DOSAGE AND ADMINISTRATION:

Dermatitis Herpetiformis: The dosage should be individually titrated starting in adults with 50 mg daily and correspondingly smaller doses in children. If full control is not achieved within the range of 50-300 mg daily, higher doses may be tried. Dosage should be reduced to

DOSAGE AND ADMINISTRATION: *(cont'd)*

a minimum maintenance level as soon as possible. In responsive patients there is a prompt reduction in pruritus followed by clearance of skin lesions. There is no effect on the gastrointestinal component of the disease.

Dapsone levels are influenced by acetylation rates. Patients with high acetylation rates, or who are receiving treatment affecting acetylation may require an adjustment in dosage.

A strict gluten free diet is an option for the patient to elect, permitting many to reduce or eliminate the need for dapsone; the average time for dosage reduction is 8 months with a range of 4 months to 2 1/2 years and for dosage elimination 29 months with a range of 6 months to 9 years.

Leprosy: In order to reduce secondary dapsone resistance, the WHO Expert Committee on Leprosy and the USPHS at Carville, LA, recommend that dapsone should be commenced in combination with one or more anti- leprosy drugs. In the multidrug program. Dapsone should be maintained at the full dosage of 100 mg daily without interruption (with corresponding smaller doses for children) and provided to all patients who have sensitive organisms with new or recrudescent disease or who have not yet completed a two year course of dapsone monotherapy. For advice and other drugs, the USPHS at Carville, LA (1-800-642-2477) should be contacted. Before using other drugs, consult appropriate product labeling.

In bacteriologically negative tuberculoid and indeterminate disease, the recommendation is the coadministration of dapsone 100 mg daily with six months of Rifampin 600 mg daily. Under WHO, daily Rifampin may be replaced 600 mg Rifampin monthly, if supervised. The dapsone is continued until all signs of clinical activity are controlled-usually after an additional six months. Then dapsone should be continued for an additional three years for tuberculoid and indeterminate patients and for five years for borderline tuberculoid patients.

In lepromatous and borderline lepromatous patients, the recommendation is the coadministration of dapsone 100 mg daily with two years of Rifampin 600 mg daily. Under WHO daily Rifampin may be replaced by 600 mg Rifampin monthly, if supervised. One may elect the concurrent administration of a third anti-leprosy drug, usually either Clofazamine 50-100 mg daily or Ethionamide 250-500 mg daily. Dapsone 100 mg daily is continued 3-10 years until all signs of clinical activity are controlled with skin scrapings and biopsies negative for one year. Dapsone should then be continued for an additional 10 years for borderline patients and for life for lepromatous patients.

Secondary dapsone resistance should be suspected whenever a lepromatous or borderline lepromatous patient receiving dapsone treatment relapses clinically and bacteriologically, solid staining bacilli being found in the smears taken from the new active lesions. If such cases show no response to regular and supervised dapsone therapy within three to six months or good compliance for the past 3-6 months can be assured, dapsone resistance should be considered confirmed clinically. Determination of drug sensitivity using the mouse footpad method is recommended and, after prior arrangement, is available without charge from the USPHS, Carville, LA. Patients with proven dapsone resistance should be treated with other drugs.

Leprosy Reactional States: Abrupt changes in clinical activity occur in leprosy with any effective treatment and are known as reactional states. The majority can be classified into two groups.

The "Reversal" reaction (Type 1) may occur in borderline or tuberculoid leprosy patients often soon after chemotherapy is started. The mechanism is presumed to result from a reduction in the antigenic load: the patient is able to mount an enhanced delayed hypersensitivity response to residual infection leading to swelling ("Reversal") of existing skin and nerve lesions. If severe, or if neuritis is present, large doses of steroids should always be used. If severe, the patient should be hospitalized. In general, anti-leprosy treatment is continued and therapy to suppress the reaction is indicated such as analgesics, steroids, or surgical decompression of swollen nerve trunks. USPHS, at Carville, LA should be contacted for advice in management.

Erythema nodosum leprosum (ENL) (lepromatous reaction) (Type 2 reaction) occurs mainly in lepromatous patients and small numbers of borderline patients. Approximately 50% of treated patients show this reaction in the first year. The principal clinical features are fever and tender erythematous skin nodules sometimes associated with malaise, neuritis, orchitis, albuminuria, joint swelling, iritis, epistaxis or depression. Skin lesions can become pustular and/or ulcerate. Histologically there is a vasculitis with an intense polymorphonuclear infiltrate. Elevated circulating immune complexes are considered to be mechanism of reaction. If severe, patients should be hospitalized. In general, anti-leprosy treatment is continued. Analgesics, steroids, and other agents available from USPHS, Carville, LA, are used to suppress the reaction.

HOW SUPPLIED:

Dapsone 25 mg, round white scored tablet, debossed "25" above and "102" below the score and on the obverse "Jacobus".

Dapsone 100 mg, round white scored tablet, debossed "100" above and "101" below the score and on the obverse "Jacobus".

Store at controlled room temperature, (59-86°F). Protect from light. Dispense this product in a well-closed child-resistant container.

HOW SUPPLIED - EQUIVALENTS NOT AVAILABLE:

Tablet, Uncoated - Oral - 25 mg

100's $17.10 Dapsone, Jacobus Pharm 49938-0102-01

Tablet, Uncoated - Oral - 100 mg

100's $18.20 Dapsone, Jacobus Pharm 49938-0101-01

DAUNORUBICIN CITRATE LIPOSOME *(003285)*

CATEGORIES: Antibiotics; Antimetabolites; Antineoplastics; Cancer; Cytotoxic Agents; HIV-related Kaposi's Sarcoma; Oncologic Drugs; Pregnancy Category D

BRAND NAMES: **DaunoXome**; *Daunoxome*
(International brand names outside U.S. in italics)

PRIMARY ICD9: 176.9

WARNING:

1. Cardiac function should be monitored regularly in patients receiving Daunorubicin because of the potential risk for cardiac toxicity and congestive heart failure. Cardiac monitoring is advised especially in those patients who have received prior anthracyclines or who have pre-existing cardiac disease.
2. Severe myelosuppression may occur.
3. Daunorubicin should be administered only under the supervision of a physician who is experienced in the use of cancer chemotherapeutic agents.
4. Dosage should be reduced in patients with impaired hepatic function. (See DOSAGE AND ADMINISTRATION)
5. A triad of back pain, flushing, and chest tightness has been reported in 13.8% of the patients (16/116) treated with daunorubicin in the Phase III clinical trial, and in 2.7% of treatment cycles (27/994). This triad generally occurs during the first five minutes of the infusion, subsides with interruption of the infusion, and generally does not recur if the infusion is then resumed at a slower rate.

DESCRIPTION:

Daunorubicin is a sterile, pyrogen-free, preservative-free product in a single use vial for intravenous infusion.

Daunorubicin contains an aqueous solution of the citrate salt of daunorubicin encapsulated within lipid vesicles (liposomes) composed of a lipid bilayer of distearoylphosphatidylcholine and cholesterol (2:1 molar ratio), with a mean diameter of about 45 nm. The lipid to drug weight ratio is 18.7:1 (total lipid:daunorubicin base), equivalent to a 10:5:1 molar ratio of distearoylphosphatidylcholine: cholesterol: daunorubicin. Daunorubicin is an anthracycline antibiotic with antineoplastic activity, originally obtained from *Streptomyces peucetius*. Daunorubicin has a 4-ring anthracycline moiety linked by a glycosidic bond to daunosamine, an amino sugar. Daunorubicin may also be isolated from *Streptomyces coeruleorubidus* and has the following chemical name: (8S- *cis*)-8- acetyl-10- [(3- amino- 2,3,6- trideoxy- α-L- *lyxo*-hexopyranosyl)oxy]- 7,8,9,10-tetrahydro-6,8,11-trihydroxy-1- methoxy-5,12- naphthacenedione hydrochloride.

The diameter of the liposomes in daunorubicin is between 35 and 65 nm.

Note: Liposomal encapsulation can substantially affect a drug's functional properties relative to those of the unencapsulated drug.

In addition, different liposomal drug products may vary from one another in the chemical composition and physical form of the liposomes. Such differences can substantially affect the functional properties of liposomal drug products.

Each vial contains daunorubicin citrate equivalent to 50 mg of daunorubicin base, encapsulated in liposomes consisting of 701 mg distearoylphosphatidylcholine and 171 mg cholesterol. The liposomes encapsulating daunorubicin are dispersed in an aqueous medium containing 2,125 mg sucrose, 94 mg glycine, and 7 mg calcium chloride dihydrate in a total volume of 25 mL/vial. The pH of the dispersion is between 4.9 and 6.0. The liposome dispersion should appear red and translucent.

CLINICAL PHARMACOLOGY:

MECHANISM OF ACTION

Daunorubicin is a liposomal preparation formulated to maximize the selectivity of daunorubicin for solid tumors *in situ*. While in the circulation, the daunorubicin citrate liposome formulation helps to protect the entrapped daunorubicin from chemical and enzymatic degradation, minimizes protein binding, and generally decreases uptake by normal (non-reticuloendothelial system) tissues. The specific mechanism by which daunorubicin citrate liposome is able to deliver daunorubicin to solid tumors *in situ* is not known. However, it is believed to be a function of increased permeability of the tumor neovasculature to some particles in the size range of daunorubicin citrate liposome. In animal studies, daunorubicin has been shown to accumulate in tumors to a greater extent when administered as daunorubicin citrate liposome than when administered as daunorubicin. Once within the tumor environment, daunorubicin is released over time enabling it to exert its antineoplastic activity.

PHARMACOKINETICS

Following intravenous injection of daunorubicin citrate liposome, plasma clearance of daunorubicin shows monoexponential decline. The pharmacokinetic parameter values for total daunorubicin following a single 40 mg/m^2 dose of daunorubicin citrate liposome administered over a 30 - 60 minute period to patients with AIDS-related Kaposi's sarcoma and following a single rapid intravenous, 80 mg/m^2 dose of conventional daunorubicin to patients with disseminated solid malignancies are shown in Table 1.

TABLE 1 Pharmacokinetic Parameters of Daunorubicin Citrate Liposome in AIDS Patients with Kaposi's Sarcoma and Reported Parameters for Conventional Daunorubicin

Parameter (units)	[a]Daunorubicin Citrate Liposome	[b]Conventional Daunorubicin
Plasma Clearance (mL/min)	17.3 ± 6.1	[c]236 ± 181
Volume of Distribution	6.4 ± 1.5	1006 ± 622
Distribution of Half-Life (h)	4.41 ± 2.33	0.77 ± 0.3
Elimination Half-Life (h)	-	55.4 ± 13.7

a N=30; **b** N=4; **c** Calculated

The plasma pharmacokinetics of daunorubicin citrate liposome differ significantly from the results reported for conventional daunorubicin hydrochloride. Daunorubicin citrate liposome has a small steady-state volume of distribution 6.4 L, (probably because it is confined to vascular fluid volume), and clearance of 17 mL/min. These differences in the volume of distribution and clearance result in a higher daunorubicin exposure (in terms of plasma AUC) from daunorubicin citrate liposome than with conventional daunorubicin hydrochloride. The apparent elimination half-life of daunorubicin citrate liposome is 4.4 hours, far shorter than that of daunorubicin, and probably represents a distribution half-life. Although preclinical biodistribution data in animals suggest that daunorubicin citrate liposome crosses the normal blood-brain barrier, it is unknown whether daunorubicin citrate liposome crosses the blood-brain barrier in humans.

Metabolism: Daunorubicinol, the major active metabolite of daunorubicin, was detected at low levels in the plasma following intravenous administration of daunorubicin citrate liposome.

No formal assessments of pharmacokinetic drug-drug interactions between daunorubicin citrate liposome and other agents have been conducted.

Special Populations: The pharmacokinetics of daunorubicin citrate liposome have not been evaluated in women, in different ethnic groups, or in subjects with renal and hepatic insufficiency.

CLINICAL STUDIES:

In an open-label, randomized, controlled clinical study conducted at 13 centers in the U.S.A. and Canada in advanced (25 or more mucocutaneous lesions; the development of 10 or more lesions in a one month period of time; symptomatic visceral involvement; or tumor-associated edema) HIV-related Kaposi's sarcoma, two treatment regimens were compared as first line cytotoxic therapy: daunorubicin citrate liposome 40 mg/m^2 and ABV (doxorubicin (Adriamycin) 10 mg/m^2, bleomycin 15 U, and vincristine 1.0 mg). All drugs were administered intravenously every 2 weeks. Responses were assessed using the AIDS Clinical Trials Group Oncology Committee of the National Institute of Allergy and Infectious Diseases (ACTG) criteria (a response required at least one of any of the following for at least 28 days:

CLINICAL STUDIES: *(cont'd)*

a. 50% reduction in the number; b. 50% reduction in the sums of the products of the largest perpendicular diameters of bidimensionally measurable marker lesions; or c. complete flattening of 50% of all previously raised lesions). Table 2 summarizes the efficacy results.

TABLE 2 Efficacy Data
First Line Cytotoxic Therapy for Advanced Kaposi's Sarcoma

	Daunorubicin Citrate Liposome n=116	ABV n=111
Response Rate	23%*	30%
Duration of Response, Median	110 days**	113 days
Time to Progression. Median	92 days***	105 days
Survival	342 days****	291 days

* The 95% confidence interval for difference in the response rates (ABV - daunorubicin citrate liposome) was [-5%, 18%].
** The hazard ratio (ABV/daunorubicin citrate liposome) for duration of response was 0.80, and the 95% confidence intervals were (0.44, 1.46).
*** The hazard ratio (ABV/daunorubicin citrate liposome) for time to progression was 0.78, and the 95% confidence intervals were (0.57, 1.07).
**** The hazard ratio for mortality (ABV/daunorubicin citrate liposome) was 1.29, and 95% confidence intervals were (0.92, 1.79).

Twenty of the 33 ABV responders responded to therapy by criteria more stringent than flattening of lesions (*i.e.*, shrinkage of lesions and/or reduction in the number of lesions). Eleven of the 27 daunorubicin citrate liposome responders responded to therapy by criteria other than flattening of lesions. Photographic evidence of tumor response to daunorubicin citrate liposome and ABV was comparable across all anatomic sites (*e.g.*, face, oral cavity, trunk, legs, and feet).

INDICATIONS AND USAGE:

Daunorubicin citrate liposome is indicated as a first line cytotoxic therapy for advanced HIV-associated Kaposi's sarcoma. Daunorubicin citrate liposome is not recommended in patients with less than advanced HIV-related Kaposi's sarcoma.

CONTRAINDICATIONS:

Therapy with daunorubicin citrate liposome is contraindicated in patients who have experienced a serious hypersensitivity reaction to previous doses of daunorubicin citrate liposome or to any of its constituents.

WARNINGS:

Daunorubicin citrate liposome is intended for administration under the supervision of a physician who is experienced in the use of cancer chemotherapeutic agents.

The primary toxicity of daunorubicin citrate liposome is myelosuppression, especially of the granulocytic series, which may be severe, with much less marked effects on the platelets and erythroid series. Careful hematologic monitoring is required and since patients with HIV infection are immunocompromised, patients must be observed carefully for evidence of intercurrent or opportunistic infections.

Special attention must be given to the potential cardiac toxicity of daunorubicin citrate liposome, particularly in patients who have received prior anthracyclines or who have pre-existing cardiac disease. Although there is no reliable means of predicting congestive heart failure, cardiomyopathy induced by anthracyclines is usually associated with a decrease of the left ventricular ejection fraction (LVEF). Cardiac function should be evaluated in each patient by means of a history and physical examination before each course of daunorubicin citrate liposome and determination of LVEF should be performed at total cumulative doses of daunorubicin citrate liposome of 320 mg/m^2, 480 mg/m^2 and every 240 mg/m^2 thereafter.

A triad of back pain, flushing, and chest tightness has been reported in 13.8% of the patients (16/116) treated with daunorubicin citrate liposome in the randomized clinical trial and in 2.7% of treatment cycles (27/994). This triad generally occurs during the first five minutes of the infusion, subsides with interruption of the infusion, and generally does not recur if the infusion is then resumed at a slower rate. This combination of symptoms appears to be related to the lipid component of daunorubicin citrate liposome, as a similar set of signs and symptoms has been observed with other liposomal products not containing daunorubicin.

Daunorubicin has been associated with local tissue necrosis at the site of drug extravasation. Although no such local tissue necrosis has been observed with daunorubicin citrate liposome, care should be taken to ensure that there is no extravasation of drug when daunorubicin citrate liposome is administered.

Dosage should be reduced in patients with impaired hepatic function. (See DOSAGE AND ADMINISTRATION)

PREGNANCY CATEGORY D

Daunorubicin citrate liposome can cause fetal harm when administered to a pregnant woman. Daunorubicin citrate liposome was administered to rats on gestation days 6 through 15 at 0.3, 1.0 or 2.0 mg/kg/day, (about 1/20th, 1/6th, or 1/3rd the recommended human dose on a mg/m^2 basis). Daunorubicin citrate liposome produced severe maternal toxicity and embryolethality at 2.0 mg/kg/day and was embryotoxic and caused fetal malformations (anophthalmia, microphthalmia, incomplete ossification) at 0.3 mg/kg/day. Embryotoxicity was characterized by increased embryo-fetal deaths, reduced numbers of litters, and reduced litter sizes.

There are no studies of daunorubicin citrate liposome in pregnant women. If daunorubicin citrate liposome is used during pregnancy, or if the patient becomes pregnant while taking daunorubicin citrate liposome, the patient must be warned of the potential hazard to the fetus. Patients should be advised to avoid becoming pregnant while taking daunorubicin citrate liposome.

PRECAUTIONS:

CARCINOGENESIS, MUTAGENESIS, AND IMPAIRMENT OF FERTILITY

No carcinogenesis, mutagenesis, or impairment of fertility studies were conducted with daunorubicin citrate liposome.

Carcinogenesis: Carcinogenicity and mutagenicity studies have been conducted with daunorubicin, the active component of daunorubicin citrate liposome. A high incidence of mammary tumors was observed about 120 days after a single intravenous dose of 12.5 mg/kg daunorubicin in rats (about 2 times the human dose on a mg/m^2 basis).

Mutagenesis: Daunorubicin was mutagenic *in vitro* tests (Ames assay, V79 hamster cell assay), and clastogenic *in vitro* (CCRF-CEM human lymphoblasts) and *in vivo* (SCE assay in mouse bone marrow) tests.

Impairment of Fertility: Daunorubicin intravenous doses of 0.25 mg/kg/day (about 8 times the human dose on a mg/m^2 basis) in male dogs caused testicular atrophy and total aplasia of spermatocytes in the seminiferous tubules.

PREGNANCY CATEGORY D

See WARNINGS Section.

PRECAUTIONS: *(cont'd)*

PEDIATRIC USE

Safety and effectiveness in pediatric patients have not been established.

GERIATRIC USE

Safety and effectiveness in the elderly have not been established. Special Populations Safety has not been established in patients with pre-existing hepatic or renal dysfunction.

DRUG INTERACTIONS:

In the patient population studied, daunorubicin citrate liposome has been administered to patients receiving a variety of concomitant medications (*e.g.*, antiretroviral agents, antiviral agents, anti-infective agents). Although interactions of daunorubicin citrate liposome with other drugs have not been observed, no systematic studies of interactions have been conducted.

ADVERSE REACTIONS:

Daunorubicin citrate liposome contains daunorubicin, encapsulated within a liposome. Conventional daunorubicin has acute myelosuppression as its dose limiting side effect, with the greatest effect on the granulocytic series. In addition, daunorubicin causes alopecia, and nausea and vomiting in a significant number of patients treated. Extravasation of conventional daunorubicin can cause severe local tissue necrosis. Chronic therapy at total doses above 300 mg/m^2 causes a cumulative-dose-related cardiomyopathy with congestive heart failure.

Administered as daunorubicin citrate liposome, daunorubicin has substantially altered pharmacokinetics and some differences in toxicity. The most important acute toxicity of daunorubicin citrate liposome remains myelosuppression, principally of the granulocytic series, with much less marked effects on the platelets and erythroid series.

In an open-label, randomized, controlled clinical trial conducted in 13 centers in the U.S.A. and Canada in advanced HIV-related Kaposi's sarcoma, two treatment regimens were compared as first line cytotoxic therapy: daunorubicin citrate liposome and ABV (doxorubicin (Adriamycin), bleomycin, and vincristine). All drugs were administered intravenously every 2 weeks. The safety data presented below include ail reported or observed adverse experiences, including those not considered to be drug related. Patients with advanced HIV-associated Kaposi's sarcoma are seriously ill due to their underlying infection and are receiving several concomitant medications including potentially toxic antiviral and antiretroviral agents. The contribution of the study drugs to the adverse experience profile is therefore difficult to establish.

Table 3 summarizes the important safety data.

TABLE 3 Summary of Important Safety Data

	Daunorubicin Citrate Liposome (N=116) % of patients	ABV (N=111) % of patients
Neutropenia (< 1000 $cells/mm^3$)	36%	35%
Neutropenia (< 500 $cells/mm^3$)	15%	5%
Opportunistic Infections/ Illnesses, % of patients	40%	27%
Median time to first Opportunistic Infections/Illnesses	214 days	412 days**
Number of cases with absolute reduction in ejection fraction of 20 - 25%*	3	1
Number of cases removed from therapy due to cardiac causes*	2	0
Alopecia All grades % of patients	8%	36%***
Neuropathy All grades % of patients	13%	41%***

* The denominator is uncertain since there were several instances of missing repeat cardiac evaluations.
** $p = 0.21$
*** $p < 0.001$

A triad of back pain, flushing and chest tightness was reported in 13.8% of the patients (16/116) treated with daunorubicin citrate liposome in the Phase III clinical trial and in 2.7% of treatment cycles (27/994). Most of the episodes were mild to moderate in severity (12% of patients and 2.5% of treatment cycles).

Mild alopecia was reported in 6% of patients treated with daunorubicin citrate liposome and moderate alopecia in 2% of patients. Mild nausea was reported in 35% of daunorubicin citrate liposome patients, moderate nausea in 16% of patients and severe nausea in 3% of patients. For patients treated with daunorubicin citrate liposome, mild vomiting was reported in 10%, moderate in 10%, and severe in 3% of patients. Although grade 3 - 4 injection site inflammation was reported in 2 patients treated with daunorubicin citrate liposome, no instances of local tissue necrosis were observed with extravasation.

Table 4 is a listing of all the mild-moderate and severe adverse events reported on both treatment arms in Protocol 103-09 in 5% of daunorubicin citrate liposome patients.

The following adverse events were reported in 5% of patients treated with daunorubicin citrate liposome, tabulated by body system.

Body As A Whole: Infection site inflammation

Cardiovascular: Hot flushes, hypertension, palpitation, syncope, tachycardia

Digestive: Increased appetite, dysphagia, GI hemorrhage, gastritis, gingival bleeding, hemorrhoids, hepatomegaly, melena, dry mouth, tooth caries

Hemic and Lymphatic: Lymphadenopathy, splenomegaly

Metabolic and Nutritional: Dehydration, thirst

Nervous: Amnesia, anxiety, ataxia, confusion, convulsions, emotional lability, abnormal gait, hallucination, hyperkinesia, hypertonia, meningitis, somnolence, abnormal thinking, tremor

Respiratory: Hemoptysis, hiccups, pulmonary infiltration, increased sputum

Skin: Folliculitis, seborrhea, dry skin

Special Senses: Conjunctivitis, deafness, earache, eye pain, taste perversion, tinnitus

Urogenital: Dysuria, nocturia, polyuria

OVERDOSAGE:

The symptoms of acute overdosage are increased severities of the observed dose-limiting toxicities of therapeutic doses of daunorubicin citrate liposome, myelosuppression (especially granulocytopenia), fatigue, and nausea and vomiting.

DOSAGE AND ADMINISTRATION:

Daunorubicin citrate liposome should be administered intravenously over a 60 minute period at a dose of 40 mg/m^2, with doses repeated every two weeks. Blood counts should be repeated prior to each dose, and therapy withheld if the absolute granulocyte count is less than 750 $cells/mm^3$. Treatment should be continued until there is evidence of progressive disease (*e.g.*,

DOSAGE AND ADMINISTRATION: *(cont'd)*

TABLE 4 Adverse Experiences: Protocol 103–09

	Daunorubicin Citrate Liposome (N=116)		ABV (N=111)	
	Mild Moderate	Severe	Mile Moderate	Severe
Nausea	51%	3%	45%	5%
Fatigue	43%	6%	44%	7%
Fever	42%	5%	49%	5%
Diarrhea	34%	4%	29%	6%
Cough	26%	2%	19%	0%
Dyspnea	23%	3%	17%	3%
Headache	22%	3%	23%	2%
Allergic Reactions	21%	3%	19%	2%
Abdominal Pain	20%	3%	23%	4%
Anorexia	21%	2%	26%	2%
Vomiting	20%	3%	26%	2%
Rigors	19%	0%	23%	0%
Back Pain	16%	0%	8%	0%
Increased Sweating	12%	2%	12%	0%
Neuropathy	12%	1%	38%	3%
Rhinitis	12%	0%	6%	0%
Edema	9%	2%	8%	1%
Chest Pain	9%	1%	7%	0%
Depression	7%	3%	6%	0%
Malaise	9%	1%	11%	0%
Stomatitis	9%	1%	8%	0%
Alopecia	8%	0%	36%	0%
Dizziness	8%	0%	9%	0%
Sinusitis	8%	0%	5%	1%
Arthraigia	7%	0%	6%	0%
Constipation	7%	0%	18%	0%
Myalgia	7%	0%	12%	0%
Pruritus	7%	0%	14%	0%
Insomnia	6%	0%	14%	0%
Influena-like Symptoms	5%	0%	5%	0%
Tenesmus	4%	1%	1%	0%
Abnormal vision	3%	2%	3%	0%

based on best response achieved: new visceral sites of involvement, or progression of visceral disease; development of 10 or more new, cutaneous lesions or a 25% increase in the number of lesions compared to baseline; a change in the character of 25% or more of all previously counted flat lesions to raised; increase in surface area of the indicator lesions), or until other intercurrent complications of HIV disease preclude continuation of therapy.

PATIENTS WITH IMPAIRED HEPATIC AND RENAL FUNCTION

Limited clinical experience exists in treating hepatically and renally impaired patients with daunorubicin citrate liposome.

Therefore, based on experience with daunorubicin HCl, it is recommended that the dosage of daunorubicin citrate liposome be reduced if the bilirubin or creatinine is elevated as follows: Serum bilirubin 1.2 to 3 mg/dL, give 3/4 the normal dose; serum bilirubin or creatinine > 3 mg/dL, give 1/2 the normal dose.

Do not mix daunorubicin citrate liposome with other drugs.

PREPARATION OF SOLUTION

Daunorubicin citrate liposome should be diluted 1:1 with 5% Dextrose Injection (D5W) before administration. Each vial of daunorubicin citrate liposome contains daunorubicin citrate equivalent to 50 mg daunorubicin base, at a concentration of 2 mg/mL. The recommended concentration after dilution is 1 mg daunorubicin/mL of solution.

Use aseptic technique.

Aseptic technique must be strictly observed in all handling, since no preservative or bacteriostatic agent is present in daunorubicin citrate liposome or in the materials recommended for dilution.

Withdraw the calculated volume of daunorubicin citrate liposome from the vial into a sterile syringe, and transfer it into a sterile infusion bag containing an equivalent amount of D5W. Administer diluted daunorubicin citrate liposome immediately. If not used immediately, diluted daunorubicin citrate liposome should be stored refrigerated at 2° - 8°C (36° - 46°F) for a maximum of 6 hours.

Caution: The only fluid which may be mixed with daunorubicin citrate liposome is D5W; daunorubicin citrate liposome must not be mixed with saline, bacteriostatic agents such as benzyl alcohol, or any other solution.

Do not use an in-line filter for the intravenous infusion of daunorubicin citrate liposome.

All parenteral drug products should be inspected visually for particulate matter and discoloration prior to administration, whenever solution and container permit. Daunorubicin citrate liposome is a translucent dispersion of liposomes that scatters light to some degree. Do not use daunorubicin citrate liposome if it appears opaque, or has precipitate or foreign matter present.

Procedures for proper handling and disposal of anticancer drugs should be followed. [1-7]

REFERENCES:

1. Recommendations for the Safe Handling of Parenteral Antineoplastic Drugs. NIH Publication No. 83-2621. For sale by the Superintendent of Documents, US Government Printing Office, Washington, DC 20402. **2.** AMA Council Report, Guidelines for Handling Parenteral Antineoplastics. JAMA 1985; 253 (11): 1590-1592. **3.** National Study Commission on Cytotoxic Exposure - Recommendations for Handling Cytotoxic Agents. Available from Louis P. Jeffrey, Sc.D., Chairman, National Study Commission on Cytotoxic Exposure. Massachusetts College of Pharmacy and Allied Health Sciences, 179 Longwood Avenue, Boston, Massachusetts 02115. **4.** Clinical Oncological Society of Australia, Guidelines and Recommendations for Safe Handling of Antineoplastic Agents. Med. J. Australia 1983; 1:426-428. **5.** Jones RB, et al.; Safe Handling of Chemotherapeutic Agents: A report from the Mount Sinai Medical Center. CA-A Cancer Journal for Clinicians 1983; (Sept/Oct) 258-263. **6.** American Society of Hospital Pharmacists Technical Assistance Bulletin on Handling Cytotoxic and Hazardous Drugs. Am. J. Hosp. Pharm. 1990; 47:1033-1049. **7.** OSHA Work-Practice Guidelines for Personnel Dealing with Cytotoxic (Antineoplastic) Drugs. Am. J. Hosp. Pharm. 1986; 43: 1193-1204.

HOW SUPPLIED:

Daunorubicin is a translucent, red, liposomal dispersion supplied in single use vials, each sealed with a synthetic rubber stopper and aluminum sealing ring with a plastic cap. Daunorubicin provides daunorubicin citrate equivalent to 50 mg of daunorubicin base, at a concentration of 2 mg/mL.

Storage: Store daunorubicin in a refrigerator, 2°-8°C (36°-46°F). Do not freeze. Protect from light.

U.S. PATENT NUMBERS: The United States Patent Numbers applicable to DaunoXome are: 5,441,745; 5,435,989; 5,019,369; 4,946,683; 4,753,788; and additional patents pending.

HOW SUPPLIED - EQUIVALENTS NOT AVAILABLE:

Injectable - Intravenous - 50 mg

50 mg x 1	$268.75	DAUNOXOME, Nexstar	56146-0301-01
50 mg x 4	$1075.00	DAUNOXOME, Nexstar	56146-0301-04
50 mg x 10	$2687.50	DAUNOXOME, Nexstar	56146-0301-00

DAUNORUBICIN HYDROCHLORIDE *(000946)*

CATEGORIES: Acute Nonlymphocytic Leukemia; Antibiotics; Antimetabolites; Antineoplastics; Cancer; Cytotoxic Agents; Leukemia; Oncologic Drugs; Pregnancy Category D; FDA Approval Pre 1982

BRAND NAMES: *Cerubidin*; **Cerubidine**; *Daunoblastin* (Germany); *Daunoblastina*; *Daunomycin* (Japan); *Daunorubicin Hydrochloride for Injection*; *Daunorubicin Hydrochloride Injection* (Australia); *Daunorubicin Injection*; *Rubilem* (Mexico); *Trixilem* (Mexico)

(International brand names outside U.S. in italics)

FORMULARIES: BC-BS; Medi-Cal

WARNING:

1. Daunorubicin HCl must be given into a rapidly flowing intravenous infusion. It must NEVER be given by the intramuscular or subcutaneous route. Severe local tissue necrosis will occur if there is extravasation during administration.
2. Myocardial toxicity manifested in its most severe form by potentially fatal congestive heart failure may be encountered when total cumulative dosage exceeds 550 mg/square m in adults, 300 mg/square m in children more than two years of age, or 10 mg/kg in children less than two years of age. This may occur either during therapy or several months after termination of therapy.
3. Severe myelosuppression occurs when used in therapeutic doses.
4. It is recommended that daunorubicin HCl be administered only by physicians who are experienced in leukemia chemotherapy and in facilities with laboratory and supportive resources adequate to monitor drug tolerance and protect and maintain a patient compromised by drug toxicity. The physician and institution must be capable of responding rapidly and completely to severe hemorrhagic conditions and/or overwhelming infection.
5. Dosage should be reduced in patients with impaired hepatic or renal function.

DESCRIPTION:

Daunorubicin HCl is the hydrochloride salt of an anthracycline cytotoxic antibiotic produced by a strain of*Streptomyces coeruleorubidus*. It is provided as a sterile reddish lyophilized powder in vials for intravenous administration only. Each vial contains 20 mg of base activity (21.4 mg as the hydrochloride salt) and 100 mg of mannitol. It is soluble in water when adequately agitated and produces a reddish solution. It has the following structural formula which may be described with the chemical name of 7-(3-amino-2,3,6-trideoxy- L-lyxohexosyioxy)-9-acetyl-7,8,9,10-tetrahydro-6,9, 11-trihydroxy-4-methoxy-5, 12-naphthacenequinone hydrochloride. Its empirical formula is $C_{27}H_{29}NO_{10}HCl$ with a molecular weight of 563.99. It is a hygroscopic crystalline powder. The pH of a 5 mg/ml aqueous solution is 4.5 to 6.5.

CLINICAL PHARMACOLOGY:

Daunorubicin HCl inhibits the synthesis of nucleic acids; its effect on deoxyribonucleic acid is particularly rapid and marked. Daunorubicin HCl has antimitotic and cytotoxic activity although the precise mode of action is unknown. daunorubicin HCl displays an immunosuppressive effect. It has been shown to inhibit the production of heterohemagglutinins in mice. *In vitro*, it inhibits blast-cell transformation of canine lymphocytes at 0.01 mcg/ml.

Daunorubicin HCl possesses a potent antitumor effect against a wide spectrum of animal tumors either grafted or spontaneous.

Following intravenous injection of daunorubicin HCl, plasma levels of daunorubicin decline rapidly, indicating rapid tissue uptake and concentration. Thereafter, plasma levels decline slowly with a half-life of 18.5 hours. By one hour after drug administration, the predominant plasma species is daunorubicinol, an active metabolite, which disappears with a half-life of 26.7 hours. Further metabolism via reduction cleavage of the glycosidic bond, 4-0 demethylation, and conjugation with both sulfate and glucuronide have been demonstrated. Simple glycosidic cleavage of daunorubicin or daunorubicinol is not a significant metabolic pathway in man. Twenty-five percent of an administered dose of daunorubicin HCl is eliminated in an active form by urinary excretion and an estimated 40% by biliary excretion.

There is no evidence that daunorubicin HCl crosses the blood-brain barrier.

In the treatment of adult acute nonlymphocytic leukemia, daunorubicin HCl, used as a single agent, has produced complete remission rates of 40 to 50%, and in combination with cytarabine, has produced complete remission rates of 53 to 65%.

The addition of daunorubicin HCl to the two-drug induction regimen of vincristine-prednisone in the treatment of childhood acute lymphocytic leukemia does not increase the rate of complete remission. In children receiving identical CNS prophylaxis and maintenance therapy (without consolidation), there is prolongation of complete remission duration (statistically significant, $p < 0.02$) in those children induced with the three-drug (daunorubicin HCl-vincristine-prednisone) regimen as compared to two drugs. There is no evidence of any impact of daunorubicin HCl on the duration of complete remission when a consolidation (intensification) phase is employed as part of a total treatment program.

In adult acute lymphocytic leukemia, in contrast to childhood acute lymphocytic leukemia, daunorubicin HCl during induction significantly increases the rate of complete remission, but not remission duration, compared to that obtained with vincristine, prednisone, and L-asparaginase alone. The use of daunorubicin HCl in combination with vincristine, prednisone, and L-asparaginase has produced complete remission rates of 83% in contrast to a 47% remission in patients not receiving daunorubicin HCl.

INDICATIONS AND USAGE:

Daunorubicin HCl in combination with other approved anticancer drugs is indicated for remission induction in acute nonlymphocytic leukemia (myelogenous, monocytic, erythroid) of adults and for remission induction in acute lymphocytic leukemia of children and adults.

WARNINGS:

Bone Marrow: Daunorubicin HCl is a potent bone-marrow suppressant. Suppression will occur in all patients given a therapeutic dose of this drug. Therapy with daunorubicin HCl should not be started in patients with preexisting drug-induced bone-marrow suppression unless the benefit from such treatment warrants the risk.

Cardiac Effects: Special attention must be given to the potential cardiac toxicity of daunorubicin HCl, particularly in infants and children. Preexisting heart disease and previous therapy with doxorubicin are co-factors of increased risk of daunorubicin HCl-induced cardiac toxicity and the benefit-to-risk ratio of daunorubicin HCl therapy in such patients

WARNINGS: *(cont'd)*

should be weighed before starting daunorubicin HCl. In adults, at total cumulative doses less than 550 mg/m^2, acute congestive heart failure is seldom encountered. However, rare instances of pericarditis-myocarditis, not dose-related, have been reported.

In adults, at cumulative doses exceeding 550 mg/m^2, there is an increased incidence of drug-induced congestive heart failure. Based on prior clinical experience with doxorubicin, this limit appears lower, namely 400 mg/m^2, in patients who received radiation therapy that encompassed the heart.[1]

In infants and children, there appears to be a greater susceptibility to anthracycline-induced cardiotoxicity compared to that in adults, which is more clearly dose-related. However, there is very little risk for children over two years of age in developing daunorubicin HCl-related cardiotoxicity below a cumulative dose of 300 mg/m^2 [2-4] or in children less than two years of age (or < 0.5 m^2 body-surface area) below a cumulative dose of 10 mg/kg. In both children and adults, the total dose of daunorubicin HCl administered should also take into account any previous or concomitant therapy with other potentially cardiotoxic agents or related compounds such as doxorubicin.

There is no absolutely reliable method of predicting the patients in whom acute congestive heart failure will develop as a result of the cardiac toxic effect of daunorubicin HCl. However, certain changes in the electrocardiogram and a decrease in the systolic ejection fraction from pretreatment baseline may help to recognize those patients at greatest risk to develop congestive heart failure. On the basis of the electrocardiogram, a decrease equal to or greater than 30% in limb lead QRS voltage has been associated with a significant risk of drug-induced cardiomyopathy. Therefore, an electrocardiogram and/or determination of systolic ejection fraction should be performed before each course of daunorubicin HCl. In the event that one or the other of these predictive parameters should occur, the benefit of continued therapy must be weighed against the risk of producing cardiac damage.

Early clinical diagnosis of drug-induced congestive heart failure appears to be essential for successful treatment with digitalis, diuretics, sodium restriction, and bed rest.

Evaluation of Hepatic And Renal Function: Significant hepatic or renal impairment can enhance the toxicity of the recommended doses of daunorubicin HCl; therefore, prior to administration, evaluation of hepatic function and renal function using conventional clinical laboratory tests is recommended (see DOSAGE AND ADMINISTRATION.)

Pregnancy: Daunorubicin HCl may cause fetal harm when administered to a pregnant woman because of its teratogenic potential. An increased incidence of fetal abnormalities (parietooccipital cranioschisis, umbilical hernias, or rachischisis) and abortions was reported in rabbits. Decreases in fetal birth weight and postdelivery growth rate were observed in mice. There are no adequate and well-controlled studies in pregnant women. If this drug is used during pregnancy, or if the patient becomes pregnant while taking this drug, the patient should be apprised of the potential hazard to the fetus. Women of childbearing potential should be advised to avoid becoming pregnant.

Extravasation At Injection Site: Extravasation of daunorubicin HCl at the site of intravenous administration can cause severe local tissue necrosis.

PRECAUTIONS:

Therapy with daunorubicin HCl requires close patient observation and frequent complete blood-count determinations. Cardiac, renal, and hepatic function should be evaluated prior to each course of treatment.

Daunorubicin HCl may induce hyperuricemia secondary to rapid lysis of leukemic cells. As a precaution, allopurinol administration is usually begun prior to initiating antileukemic therapy. Blood uric acid levels should be monitored and appropriate therapy initiated in the event that hyperuricemia develops.

Appropriate measures must be taken to control any systemic infection before beginning therapy with daunorubicin HCl.

Daunorubicin HCl may transiently impart a red coloration to the urine after administration, and patients should be advised to expect this.

Carcinogenesis, Mutagenesis, and Impairment of Fertility: Daunorubicin HCl, when injected subcutaneously into mice, causes fibrosarcomas to develop at the injection site. When administered to mice orally or intraperitoneally, no carcinogenic effect was noted after 22 months of observation.

In male dogs at a daily dose of 0.25 mg/kg administered intravenously, testicular atrophy was noted at autopsy. Histologic examination revealed total aplasia of the spermatocyte series in the seminiferous tubules with complete aspermatogenesis.

Pregnancy Category D: See WARNINGS.

ADVERSE REACTIONS:

Dose-limiting toxicity includes myelosuppression and cardiotoxicity (see WARNINGS.) Other reactions include:

Cutaneous: Reversible alopecia occurs in most patients.

Gastrointestinal: Acute nausea and vomiting occur but are usually mild. Antiemetic therapy may be of some help. Mucositis may occur three to seven days after administration. Diarrhea has occasionally been reported.

Local: If extravasation occurs during administration, tissue necrosis can result at the site.

Acute Reactions: Rarely, anaphylactoid reaction, fever, chills, and skin rash can occur.

DOSAGE AND ADMINISTRATION:

Parenteral drug products should be inspected visually for particulate matter and discoloration prior to administration, whenever solution and container permit.

Principles: In order to eradicate the leukemic cells and induce a complete remission, a profound suppression of the bone marrow is usually required. Evaluation of both the peripheral blood and bone marrow are mandatory in the formulation of appropriate treatment plans.

It is recommended that the dosage of daunorubicin HCl be reduced in instances of hepatic or renal impairment. For example, using serum bilirubin and serum creatinine as indicators of liver and kidney function, the following dose modifications are recommended (TABLE 1):

TABLE 1

Serum Bilirubin	Serum Creatinine	Recommended Dose
1.2 to 3.0 mg%		3/4 normal dose
> 3 mg%	>3 mg%	1/2 normal dose

REPRESENTATIVE DOSE SCHEDULES AND COMBINATION FOR THE APPROVED INDICATION OF REMISSION INDUCTION IN ADULT ACUTE NONLYMPHOCYTIC LEUKEMIA

In Combination[6,7]: For patients under age 60, daunorubicin HCl 45 mg/m^2/day IV on days 1, 2, 3 of the first course and on days 1, 2 of subsequent courses AND cytosine arabinoside 100 mg/m^2/day IV infusion daily for 7 days for the first course and for 5 days for subsequent courses.

DOSAGE AND ADMINISTRATION: *(cont'd)*

For patients 60 years of age and above, daunorubicin HCl 30 mg/m^2/day IV on days 1, 2, 3, of the first course and on days 1, 2 of subsequent courses AND cytosine arabinoside 100 mg/m^2/day IV infusion daily for 7 days for the first course and for 5 days for subsequent courses.[7] This daunorubicin HCl dose-reduction is based on a single study and may not be appropriate if optimal supportive care is available.

The attainment of a normal-appearing bone marrow may require up to three courses of induction therapy. Evaluation of the bone marrow following recovery from the previous course of induction therapy determines whether a further course of induction treatment is required.

REPRESENTATIVE DOSE SCHEDULE AND COMBINATION FOR THE APPROVED INDICATION OF REMISSION INDUCTION IN PEDIATRIC ACUTE LYMPHOCYTIC LEUKEMIA

In Combination: Daunorubicin HCl 25 mg/m^2 IV on day 1 every week, vincristine 1.5 mg/m^2 IV on day 1 every week, prednisone 40 mg/m^2 PO daily. Generally, a complete remission will be obtained within four such courses of therapy; however, if after four courses the patient is in partial remission, an additional one or, if necessary, two courses may be given in an effort to obtain a complete remission.

In children less than 2 years of age or below 0.5 m^2 body-surface area, it has been recommended that the daunorubicin HCl dosage calculation should be based on weight (1.0 mg/kg) instead of body-surface area.[15]

REPRESENTATIVE DOSE SCHEDULE AND COMBINATION FOR THE APPROVED INDICATION OF REMISSION INDUCTION IN ADULT ACUTE LYMPHOCYTIC LEUKEMIA

In Combination[8]: Daunorubicin HCl 45 mg/m^2/day IV on days 1,2, and 3 AND vincristine 2 mg IV on days 1,8, and 15; prednisone 40 mg/m^2/day PO on days 1 through 22, then tapered between days 22 to 29; L-asparaginase 500 IU/kg/day x 10 days IV on days 22 through 32.

The contents of a vial should be reconstituted with 4 ml of Sterile Water for Injection, USP, and agitated gently until the material has completely dissolved. The withdrawable vial contents provide 20 mg of daunorubicin activity, with 5 mg of daunorubicin activity per ml. The desired dose is withdrawn into a syringe containing 10 ml to 15 ml of normal saline and then injected into the tubing or sidearm of a rapidly flowing IV infusion of 5 percent glucose or normal saline solution. Daunorubicin HCl should not be administered mixed with other drugs or heparin. The reconstituted solution is stable for 24 hours at room temperature and 48 hours under refrigeration. It should be protected from exposure to sunlight.

Procedures for proper handling and disposal of anticancer drugs should be considered. Several guidelines on this subject have been published.[9-14] There is no general agreement that all of the procedures recommended in the guidelines are necessary or appropriate.

Storage: (+15° to +25° C)

REFERENCES:

1. GILLADOGA AC, MANUEL C, TAN CTC, et al: The cardiotoxicity of Adriamycin and daunomycin in children. Cancer *37:*1070-1078, 1976. **2.** HALZUN JF, WAGNER HR, GAETA JF, et al: Daunorubicin cardiac toxicity in children with acute lymphocytic leukemia. Cancer *33:*545-554, 1974. **3.** VON HOFF DD, ROZENCWEIG M, LAYARD M, et al: Daunomycin-induced cardiotoxicity in children and adults: a review of 110 cases. Am J Med *62:*200-208, 1977. **4.** GOORIN AM, BORROW KM, GOLDMAN A, et al: Congestive heart failure due to Adriamycin cardiotoxicity: its natural history in children. Cancer*47:*2810-2816, 1981. **5.** PRAGA C, BRETTA G, VIGO PL, et al: Adriamycin cardiotoxicity: A survey of 1273 patients. Cancer Treat Rep *63:*827-834, 1979. **6.** RAI KR, HOLLAND JF, GLIDEWELL O, et al: Treatment of acute myelocytic leukemia: a study by Cancer and Leukemia Group B. Blood *58:*1203-1212, 1981. **7.** YATES J, GLIDEWELL O, WIERNIK P, et al: Cytosine arabinoside with daunorubicin or Adriamycin for therapy of acute myelocytic leukemia: a CALGB study. Blood *60:*454-462, 1982. **8.** GOTTLIEB AJ, WEINBERG V, ELLISON RR: Efficacy of daunorubicin in the therapy of adult acute lymphocytic leukemia: a prospective randomized trial by Cancer and Leukemia Group B. Blood *64:*267-274, 1984. **9.** Recommendations for The Safe Handling of Parenteral Antineoplastic Drugs. NIH Publication No. 83-2621. For sale by The Superintendent of Documents, U.S. Government Printing Office, Washington, D.C. 20402. **10.** AMA Council Report. Guidelines for Handling Parenteral Antineoplastics. JAMA, March 15, 1985. **11.** National Study Commission on Cytotoxic Exposure - Recommendations for Handling Cytotoxic Agents. Available from Louis P. Jeffrey, Sc.D., Director of Pharmacy Services, Rhode Island Hospital, 593 Eddy Street, Providence, Rhode Island 02902. **12.** Clinical Oncological Society of Australia: Guidelines and recommendations for safe handling of antineoplastic agents. Med J Australia *1:*426-428, 1983. **13.** JONES RB, et al: Safe handling of chemotherapeutic agents: A report from the Mount Sinai Medical Center, Ca-A Cancer Journal for Clinicians Sept/Oct, 258-263, 1983. **14.** American Society of Hospital Pharmacists technical assistance bulletin on handling cytotoxic drugs in hospitals. Am J Hosp Pharm*42:*131-137, 1985. **15.** SALLAN SE: Personal Communication, 1981.

For How Supplied Information, Contact Wyeth Labs Chiron Thera Specia-Alfort (NDA# 50484 50484 50484)

DEFEROXAMINE MESYLATE *(000947)*

CATEGORIES: Antagonists and Antidotes; Antidotes; Chelating Agents; Heavy Metal Antagonists; Iron Overdose; Thalassemia; Acidosis*; Alzheimer's Disease*; Pregnancy Category C; FDA Approval Pre 1982
* Indication not approved by the FDA

BRAND NAMES: **Desferal**; *Desferin*
(International brand names outside U.S. in italics)

FORMULARIES: WHO

DESCRIPTION:

Deferoxamine mesylate USP, is an iron-chelating agent, available in vials for intramuscular, subcutaneous, and intravenous administration. Each vial contains 500 mg of deferoxamine mesylate USP in sterile, lyophilized form. Deferoxamine mesylate is N-(5-(3-((5- aminopentyl) hydroxycarbamoyl)propionamido)pentyl)-3-((5-(N-hydroxyacetamido)-pentyl) carbamoyl) propionohydroxamic acid monomethanesulfonate (salt).

Deferoxamine mesylate USP is a white to off-white powder. It is freely soluble in water and slightly soluble in methanol. It molecular weight is 656.79.

CLINICAL PHARMACOLOGY:

Deferoxamine chelates iron by forming a stable complex that prevents the iron from entering into further chemical reactions. It readily chelates iron from ferritin and hemosiderin but not readily from transferrin; it does not combine with the iron from cytochromes and hemoglobin. Deferoxamine does not cause any demonstrable increase in the excretion of electrolytes or trace metals. Theoretically, 100 parts by weight of deferoxamine is capable of binding approximately 8.5 parts by weight of ferric iron.

Deferoxamine is metabolized principally by plasma enzymes, but the pathways have not yet been defined. The chelate is readily soluble in water and passes easily through the kidney, giving the urine a characteristic reddish color. Some is also excreted in the feces via the bile.

INDICATIONS AND USAGE:

Deferoxamine is indicated for the treatment of acute iron intoxication and of chronic iron overload due to transfusion-dependent anemia.

INDICATIONS AND USAGE: *(cont'd)*

ACUTE IRON INTOXICATION

Deferoxamine is an adjunct to, and not a substitute for, standard measures used in treating acute iron intoxication, which may include the following: induction of emesis with syrup of ipecac; gastric lavage; suction and maintenance of a clear airway; control of shock with intravenous fluids, blood, oxygen, and vasopressors; and correction of acidosis.

CHRONIC IRON OVERLOAD

Deferoxamine can promote iron excretion in patients with secondary iron overload from multiple transfusions (as may occur in te treatment of some chronic anemias, including thalassemia). Long-term therapy with deferoxamine slows accumulation of hepatic iron and retards or eliminates progression of hepatic fibrosis.

Iron mobilization with deferoxamine is relatively poor in patients under the age of 3 years with relatively little iron overload. The drug should ordinarily not be given to such patients unless significant iron mobilization (*e.g.,* 1 mg or more of iron per day) can be demonstrated.

Deferoxamine is not indicated for the treatment of primary hemochromatosis, since phlebotomy is the method of choice for removing excess iron in this disorder.

CONTRAINDICATIONS:

Deferoxamine is contraindicated in patients with severe renal disease or anuria, since the drug and the iron chelate are excreted primarily by the kidney.

WARNINGS:

Ocular and auditory disturbances have been reported when deferoxamine was administered over prolonged periods of time, at high doses, or in patients with low ferritin levels. The ocular disturbances observed have been blurring of vision; cataracts after prolonged administration in chronic iron overload; decreased visual acuity including visual loss; impaired peripheral, color, and night vision; and retinal pigmentary abnormalities. The auditory abnormalities reported have been tinnitus, and hearing loss including high frequency sensorineural hearing loss. In most cases, both ocular and auditory disturbances were reversible upon immediate cessation of treatment. Slit-lamp examinations performed in patients treated with deferoxamine for acute iron intoxication have not revealed cataracts.

Visual acuity tests, slit-lamp examinations, funduscopy and audiometry are recommended periodically in patients treated for prolonged periods of time. Toxicity is more likely to be reversed if symptoms or test abnormalities are detected early.

PRECAUTIONS:

GENERAL

Flushing of the skin, urticaria, hypotension, and shock have occurred in a few patients when deferoxamine was administered by rapid intravenous infusion. THEREFORE, DEFEROXAMINE SHOULD BE GIVEN INTRAMUSCULARLY OR BY SLOW SUBCUTANEOUS OR INTRAVENOUS INFUSION.

Iron overload increases susceptibility of patients to Yersinia enterocolitica infections. In some rare cases, treatment with deferoxamine had enhanced this susceptibility, resulting in generalized infections by providing this bacteria with a siderophore otherwise missing. In such cases, deferoxamine treatment should be discontinued until the infection is resolved.

In patients undergoing hemodialysis while receiving deferoxamine, there have been rare reports of fungal infections (*i.e.,* mucormycosis) that have sometimes been fatal; however, a casual relationship to the drug has not been established.

INFORMATION FOR THE PATIENT

Patients should be informed that occasionally their urine may show a reddish discoloration.

CARCINOGENESIS, MUTAGENESIS, AND IMPAIRMENT OF FERTILITY

Long-term carcinogenicity studies in animals have not been performed with deferoxamine.

Cytotoxicity may occur, since deferoxamine has been shown to inhibit DNA synthesis *in vitro.*

PREGNANCY CATEGORY C

Delayed ossification in mice and skeletal anomalies in rabbits were observed after deferoxamine was administered in daily doses up to 4.5 times the maximum daily human dose. No adverse effects were observed in similar studies in rats.

There are no adequate and well-controlled studies in pregnant women. Deferoxamine should be used during pregnancy only if the potential benefit justifies the potential risk to the fetus.

NURSING MOTHERS

It is not known whether this drug is excreted in human milk. Because many drugs are excreted in human milk, caution should be exercised when deferoxamine is administered to a nursing woman.

PEDIATRIC USE

Safety and effectiveness in children under the age of 3 years have not been established (see INDICATIONS AND USAGE.)

ADVERSE REACTIONS:

The following adverse reactions have been observed, but there are not enough data to support an estimate of their frequency.

Skin: Localized irritation and pain, swelling and induration, pruritus, erythema, wheal formation.

Hypersensitive Reactions: Generalized erythema (rash), urticaria, anaphylactic reaction.

Cardiovascular: Tachycardia, hypotension, shock.

Digestive: Abdominal discomfort, diarrhea.

Special Senses: Ocular and auditor disturbances (see WARNINGS.)

Other: Dysuria, leg cramps, fever.

OVERDOSAGE:

ACUTE TOXICITY

Intravenous LD_{50}'s (mg/kg): mice, 287; rats, 329.

SIGNS AND SYMPTOMS

Since deferoxamine is available only for parenteral administration, acute poisoning is unlikely to occur. However, tachycardia, hypotension, and gastrointestinal symptoms have occasionally developed in patients who received overdoses of Desferal.

TREATMENT

There is no specific antidote.

Signs and symptoms of overdosage may be eliminated by reducing the dosage.

Deferoxamine is readily dialyzable.

DOSAGE AND ADMINISTRATION:

ACUTE IRON ADMINISTRATION

Intramuscular Administration

This route is preferred and should be used for ALL PATIENTS NOT IN SHOCK.

Dosage: A dose of 1.0 g should be administered initially. This may be followed by 500 mg (one vial) every 4 hours for two doses. Depending upon the clinical response, subsequent doses of 500 mg may be administered every 4-12 hours. The total amount administered should not exceed 6.0 g in 24 hours.

Preparation of Solution: Deferoxamine is dissolved by adding 2 ml os sterile water for injection to each vial, resulting in a solution of 250 mg/ml. The drug should be completely dissolved before the solution is withdrawn. Deferoxamine is then administered intramuscularly. See Note.

Intravenous Administration

THIS ROUTE SHOULD BE USED ONLY FOR PATIENTS IN A STATE OF CARDIOVASCULAR COLLAPSE AND THEN ONLY BY SLOW INFUSION. THE RATE OF INFUSION SHOULD NOT EXCEED 15 MG/KG PER HOUR.

Dosage: An initial dose of 1.0 g should be administered at a rate NOT TO EXCEED 500 mg every 4 hours for two doses. Depending upon the clinical response, subsequent doses of 500 mg may be administered every 4-12 hours. The total amount administered should not exceed 6.0 g in 24 hours.

As soon as the clinical condition of the patient permits, intravenous administration should be discontinued and the drug should be administered intramuscularly.

Preparation of Solution: Deferoxamine is dissolved by adding 2 ml of sterile water for injection to each vial, resulting in a solution of 250 mg/ml. The drug should be completely dissolved before the solution is withdrawn. The solution is then added to physiologic saline, glucose in water, or Ringer's lactate solution and administered at a rate NOT TO EXCEED 15 mg/kg per hour. See Note.

CHRONIC IRON OVERLOAD

The more effective of the following routes of administration must be chosen on an individual basis for each patient.

Intramuscular Administration

A daily dose of 0.5-1.0 g should be administered intramuscularly. In addition, 2.0 g should be administered intravenously with each unit of blood transfused; however, deferoxamine should be administered separately from the blood. The rate of intravenous infusion must not exceed 15 mg/kg per hour.

Subcutaneous Administration

A daily dose of 1.0-2.0 g (20-40 mg/kg per day) should be administered over 8-24 hours, utilizing a small portable pump capable of providing continuous mini-infusion. The duration of infusion must be individualized. In some patients, as much iron will be excreted after a short infusion of 8-12 hours as with the same dose given over 24 hours.

PREPARATION OF SOLUTION FOR SUBCUTANEOUS OR INTRAMUSCULAR ADMINISTRATION

Deferoxamine is dissolved by adding 2.0 ml of sterile water for injection to each vial, resulting in a solution of 250 mg/ml. The drug should be completely dissolved before the solution is withdrawn into the syringe to be used for administration. See Note.

Note: Parenteral drug products should be inspected visually for particulate matter and discoloration prior to administration, whenever solution and container permit.

Deferoxamine reconstituted with sterile water for injection may be stored under sterile conditions and protected from light at room temperature for not longer than 1 week.

Reconstituting deferoxamine in solvents or under conditions other than indicated may result in precipitation. Turbid solutions should not be used.

Do not store above 86°F (30°C).

HOW SUPPLIED - EQUIVALENTS NOT AVAILABLE:

Injection, Solution - Intramuscular; - 500 mg

4's	$39.81	DESFERAL, Novartis	00083-3801-04

DEHYDROCHOLIC ACID *(000951)*

CATEGORIES: Cathartics & Laxatives; Digestants; Gastrointestinal Drugs; FDA Pre 1938 Drugs

BRAND NAMES: Bilidren; *Dehychol; Didrocolo*
(International brand names outside U.S. in italics)

Prescribing information not available at time of publication.

HOW SUPPLIED - EQUIVALENTS NOT AVAILABLE:

Tablet, Uncoated - Oral - 250 mg

100's	$20.30	Dehydrocholic Acid, Goldline Labs	00182-0489-01

DEHYDROCHOLIC ACID; DESOXYCHOLIC; ENZYMES *(000948)*

CATEGORIES: Digestants; Gastrointestinal Drugs; FDA Pre 1938 Drugs

BRAND NAMES: Bilezyme; Chenocol

Prescribing information not available at time of publication.

HOW SUPPLIED - EQUIVALENTS NOT AVAILABLE:

Tablet, Uncoated - Oral

100's	$33.60	CHENOCOL, Lemax	23594-0017-01

DEHYDROCHOLIC ACID; ENZYMES *(000952)*

CATEGORIES: Digestants; Gastrointestinal Drugs; FDA Pre 1938 Drugs

BRAND NAMES: Digestin; Digestozyme; Tolerase; Zymecot

Prescribing information not available at time of publication.

HOW SUPPLIED - EQUIVALENTS NOT AVAILABLE:

Tablet, Coated - Oral

1000's	$59.90	ENZYME-M DUAL COATED, Major Pharms	00904-0596-80

DEHYDROEPIANDROSTERONE *(003258)*

CATEGORIES: Anabolic Steroids; Androgens; Hormones; Pharmaceutical Adjuvants; FDA Unapproved

BRAND NAMES: DHEA; **Prasterone**

Prescribing information not available at time of publication.

HOW SUPPLIED - EQUIVALENTS NOT AVAILABLE:

Powder

125 gm	$751.80	Dehydroepiandrosterone, Elge	58298-0521-01

DELAVIRDINE MESYLATE *(003335)*

CATEGORIES: HIV Infection; Non-Nucleoside Reverse Transcriptase Inh; Pregnancy Category C; FDA Approved 1997 Mar

BRAND NAMES: **Rescriptor**

WARNING:
Delavirdine tablets are indicated for the treatment of HIV-1 infection in combination with appropriate antiretroviral agents when therapy is warranted. This indication is based on surrogate marker changes in clinical studies. Clinical benefit was not demonstrated for delavirdine based on survival or incidence of AIDS-defining clinical events in a completed trial comparing delavirdine plus didanosine with didanosine monotherapy (see CLINICAL STUDIES).
Resistant virus emerges rapidly when delavirdine is administered as monotherapy. Therefore, delavirdine should always be administered in combination with appropriate antiretroviral therapy.

DESCRIPTION:

Rescriptor Tablets contain delavirdine mesylate, a synthetic non-nucleoside reverse transcriptase inhibitor of the human immunodeficiency virus type 1 (HIV-1). The chemical name of delavirdine mesylate is piperazine, 1-[3-[(1-methyl-ethyl)amino]-2pyridinyl]-4-[(5-[(methyl-sulfonyl)amino]-1*H*-indol-2-yl]carbonyl]-monomethanesulfonate. Its molecular formula is $C_{22}H_{28}N_6O_3S{\cdot}CH_4O_3S$ and its molecular weight is 552.68.

Delavirdine mesylate is an odorless white-to-tan crystalline powder. The aqueous solubility of delavirdine free base at 23°C is 2942 mcg/ml at pH 1.0, 295 mcg/ml at pH 2.0, and 0.81 mcg/ml at pH 7.4.

Rescriptor Tablets for oral administration contain 100 mg of delavirdine mesylate (hence forth referred to as delavirdine). Inactive ingredients consist of lactose, microcrystalline cellulose, croscarmellose sodium, colloidal silicon dioxide, magnesium stearate, Opadry YS-1-7000-E White and carnauba wax.

CLINICAL PHARMACOLOGY:

MECHANISM OF ACTION

Delavirdine is a non-nucleoside reverse transcriptase inhibitor (NNRTI) of HIV-1. Delavirdine binds directly to reverse transcriptase (RT) and blocks RNA dependent and DNA dependent DNA polymerase activities. Delavirdine does not compete with template: primer or deoxynucleoside triphosphates. HIV-2 RT and human cellular DNA polymerases α, γ, or Δ are not inhibited by delavirdine. In addition, HIV-1 group O, a group of highly divergent strains that are uncommon in North America, may not be inhibited by delavirdine.

In vitro HIV-1 Susceptibility: *In vitro* anti HIV-1 activity of delavirdine was assessed by infecting cell lines of lymphoblastic and monocytic origin and peripheral blood lymphocytes with laboratory and clinical isolates of HIV-1. IC_{50} and IC_{90} values (50% and 90% inhibitory concentrations) for laboratory isolates (N=5) ranged from 0.005 to 0.030 μM and 0.04 to 0.10 μM, respectively. Mean IC_{50} of clinical isolates (N=74) was 0.038 μM (range 0.001 to 0.69 μM), 73 of 74 clinical isolates had an $IC_{50} \leq 0.18$ μM. The IC_{90} of 24 of these clinical isolates ranged from 0.05 to 0.10 μM. In drug combination studies of delavirdine with zidovudine, didanosine, zalcitabine, lamivudine, interferon-α, and protease inhibitors, additive to synergistic anti-HIV-1 activity was observed in cell culture. The relationship between the *in vitro* susceptibility of HIV-1 RT inhibitors and the inhibition of HIV replication in humans has not been established.

Drug Resistance: Phenotypic analyses of isolates from patients treated with delavirdine as monotherapy showed a 50-fold to 500-fold reduction in sensitivity in 14 of 15 patients by week 8 of therapy. Genotypic analyses of HIV-1 isolates from patients receiving delavirdine plus zidovudine combination therapy (N=19) showed mutations in 16 of 19 isolates by week 24 of therapy. Mutations occurred predominantly at position 103 and less frequently at positions 181 and 236. In a separate study, an average 86-fold increase in the zidovudine sensitivity of patient isolates (N=24) was observed after 24 weeks on delavirdine and zidovudine combination therapy. The clinical relevance of the phenotypic and the genotypic changes associated with delavirdine therapy has not been determined.

Cross-Resistance: Rapid emergence of HIV strains that are cross-resistant to certain NNRTIs has been observed *in vitro*. Mutations at positions 103 and 181 have been associated with resistance to other NNRTIs. Delavirdine may confer cross resistance to other non-nucleoside reverse transcriptase inhibitors when used alone or in combination.

The potential for cross-resistance between delavirdine and protease inhibitors is low because of the different enzyme targets involved. The potential for cross-resistance between NNRTIs and nuceoside analogue RT inhibitors is low because of different sites of binding on the viral RT ard distinct mechanisms of action.

PHARMACOKINETICS

Absorption and Bioavailabitity: Delavirdine is rapidly absorbed following oral administration, with peak plasma concentrations occurring at approximately one hour. Following administration of delavirdine 400 mg three times daily (n=67, HIV-1-infected patients) the mean ± SD steady state peak plasma concentration (C_{max}) was 35 ± 20 μM (range 2 to 100 μM), systemic exposure (AUC) was 180 ± 100 μM · hr (range 5 to 515 μM · hr) and trough concentration (C_{min}) was 15 ± 10 μM (range 0.1 to 45 μM). The single dose bioavailability of delavirdine tablets relative to an oral solution was 85 ± 25% (n=16, non-HIV-infected subjects). The single-dose bioavalability of delavirdine tablets was increased by approximately 20% when a slurry of drug was prepared by allowing delavirdine tablets to disintegrate in water before administration (n=16, non HIV-infected subjects).

Delavirdine may be administered with or without food. Following single-dose administration of delavirdine tablets with a high fat meal (874 kcal, 57 g fat), mean C_{max} was decreased by 60% and mean AUC was decreased by 26%, relative to fasted administration (n=12, non-HIV-infected subjects). In a multiple-dose study, delavirdine was administered every eight hours with food or every eight hours, one hour before or two hours after a meal (n=13, HIV-1-infected patients). Patients remained on their typical diet through out the study; meal content was not standardized. When multiple doses of delavirdine were administered with food, mean C_{max} was reduced by 22% but AUC and C_{min} were not altered.

Distribution: Delavirdine is extensive by bound (approximately 98%) to plasma proteins primarily albumin. The percentage of delavirdine that is protein bound is constant over a delavirdine concentration range of 0.5 to 196 μM. In five HIV-1-infected patients whose total daily dose of delavirdine ranged from 600 to 1200 mg, cerebrospinal fluid concentrations of delavirdine averaged 0.4% ± 0.07% of the corresponding plasma delavirdine concentrations; this represents about 20% of the fraction not bound to plasma proteins. Steady state delavirdine concentrations in saliva (n=5, HIV-1-infected patients who received delavirdine 400 mg three times daily) and semen (n=5, healthy volunteers who received delavirdine 300 mg three times daily) were about 6% and 2%, respectively, of the corresponding plasma delavirdine concentratons collected at the end of a dosing interval.

Pharmacokinetics and Metabolism: Delavirdine is extensively converted to several inactive metabolites. Delavirdine is primarily metabolized by cytochrome P450 3A (CYP3A) but *in vitro* data suggest that delavirdine may also be metabolized by CYP2D6. The major metabolic pathways for delavirdine are N-desalkylation and pyridine hydroxylation. Delavirdine exhibits nonlinear steady-state elmination pharmacokinetics, with apparent oral clearance decreasing by about 22-fold as the total daily dose of delavirdine increases from 60 to 1200 mg/day. In a study of ^{14}C-delavirdine in six healthy volunteers who received multiple doses of delavirdine tablets 300 mg three times daily, approximately 44% of the radio labeled dose was recovered in feces, and approximately 51% of the dose was excreted in urine. Less than 5% of the dose was recovered unchanged in urine. The apparent plasma half-life of delavirdine increases with dose; mean half-life following 400 mg three times daily is 5.8 hours, with a range of 2 to 11 hours.

In vitro and *in vivo* studies have shown that delavirdine reduces CYP3A activity and inhibits its own metabolism. *In vitro* studies have also shown that delavirdine reduces CYP2C9 and CYP2C19 activity. Inhibition of CYP3A by delavirdine is reversible within 1 week after discontinuation of drug.

SPECIAL POPULATIONS

Hepatic or Henal Impairment: The pharmacokinetics of delavirdine in patients with hepatic or renal impairment have not been investigated (see PRECAUTIONS).

Age: The pharmacokinetics of delavirdine have not been studied in patients <16 years or >65 years of age.

Gender: Following administration of delavirdine (400 mg every eight hours), median delavirdine AUC was 31% higher in female patients (n=12) than in male patients (n=55).

Race: No significant differences in the mean trough delavirdine concentrations were observed between different racial or ethnic groups.

CLINICAL STUDIES:

In two of the clinical studies described below (Study 0021, Part 1 and Study 0017) an experimental HIV nucleic acid amplification assay was used to estimate the level of circulating HIV RNA in plasma. In the clinical study ACTG 261, also described below, an approved HIV nucleic acid amplification assay was used.

In general, patients who left the study had lower CD4 cell counts and higher plasma HIV RNA values than patients remaining on study. Therefore, absolute changes from baseline are overstated in all treatment arms, increasingly so at later time points. However, the added effect of delavirdine treatment relative to the control arms does not appear to be signficanty affected by patient dropout.

Study 0021, Part 1: Delavirdine-Zidovudine Dual Therapy Trial: Study 0021, Part 1 was a randomized double blind trial comparing treatment with delavirdine plus zidovudine and zidovudine monotherapy in 718 HIV-1-infected patients (median age 34.3 years [range 17 to 70 years], 19% female, 32 % non-Caucasian). Patients were treatment naive or had received less than 6 months of prior zidovudine therapy. Mean baseline CD4 cell count was 334 cells/mm³ (range 75 to 696 cells/mm³) and mean baseline plasma HIV-1 RNA was 5.25 log_{10} copies/ml. Treatment doses were delavirdine 200 mg, 300 mg, or 400 mg three times daily plus zidovudine 200 mg three times daily or zidovudine monotherapy 200 mg three times daily. No statistically signficant difference in CD4 cell count for the combination of delavirdine plus zidovudine compared with zidovudine monotherapy was observed in a planned analysis at 24 weeks.

Study 0017 Delavirdine-Didanosine Dual Therapy Trial: Study 0017 was a randomized, double-blind trial comparing treatment with delavirdine plus didanosine versus didanosine monotherapy in 1190 HIV-1-infected patients (median age 37.4 years [range 19 to 78 years], 13% female 32% non-Caucasian). Patients had received up to 4 months prior didanosine therapy; there were no restrictions on prior zidovudine use. Mean baseline CD4 cell count was 142 cells/mm³ (range 0 to 541 cells/mm³) and mean baseline plasma HIV-1 RNA was 5.77 log_{10} copies/ml. Treatment doses were delavirdine 400 mg three times daily plus didanosine or didanosine monotherapy. The dose of danosine was adjusted by body weight (<60 kg, 125 mg twice daily; >60 kg, 200 mg twice daily).

An analysis of clinical efficacy end points (death, clinical progression defined as time to AIDS or death) was performed when all patients had completed at least 6 months in the trial. Comparable rates of deaths and AIDS progression between the didanosine monotherapy arm and the combination of delavirdine plus didanosine arm were observed.

ACTG 261: Delavirdine-Zidovudine-Didanosine Multiple Therapy Trial: AIDS Clinical Trials Group (ACTG) Protocol 261 was a randomized trial comparing the following four treatment regimens: delavirdine plus didanosine, delavirdine plus zidovudine, delavirdine plus didanosine and zidovudine, and zidovudine plus didanosine. The study enrolled 544 HIV-1 infected patients (median age 35 years, 18% female and 44% non-Caucasian patients) who were either nucleoside treatment naive or had prior treatment wth zidovudine or didanosine (not both) for less than 6 months. Thirty seven percent reported previous antiretroviral therapy (194 patients with zidovudine and 6 with didanosine). Mean baseline CD4 cell count was 296 cells/mm³ (range 55 to 640 cells/mm³). Median baseline plasma HIV-1 RNA level [available for 229 patients) was 4.45 log_{10} copies/ml (28,260 copies/ml). Treatment doses were delavirdine 400 mg three times daily, zidovudine 200 mg three times daily, and didanosine dose adjusted by body weight (<60 kg, 125 mg twice daily; >60 kg, 200 mg twice daily).

Preliminary results showed no statistically significant difference in CD4 cell count for the three drug combination of delavirdine, zidovudine and didanosine compared with the combination of zidovudine plus didanosine. No statistically significant difference in plasma HIV-1 RNA for the three-drug combination of delavirdine, zidovudine, and didanosine compared with the combination of zidovudine plus didanosine was observed.

INDICATIONS AND USAGE:

Delavirdine tablets are indicated for the treatment of HIV-1 infection in combination with appropriate antiretroviral agents when therapy is warranted. This indication is based on surrogate marker changes in clinical studies. Clinical benefit was not demonstrated for delavirdine based on survival or incidence of AIDS-defining clinical events in a completed trial comparing delavirdine plus danosine with didanosine monotherapy (see CLINICAL STUDIES).

INDICATIONS AND USAGE: *(cont'd)*

Resistant virus emerges rapidly when delavirdine is administered as monotherapy. Therefore delavirdine should always be administered in combination with appropriate antiretroviral therapy.

CONTRAINDICATIONS:

Delavirdine tablets are contraindicated in patients with previously demonstrated clinically signficant hypersensitvity to any of the components of the formulation.

WARNINGS:

Coadministration of delavirdine tablets with certain nonsedating antihistamines, sedative hypnotics, antiarrhythmics, calcium channel blockers, ergot alkaloid preparations, amphetamines, and cisapride, may result in potentially serious and/or life-threatening adverse events due to possible effects of delavirdine on the hepatic metabolism of certain drugs (see DRUG INTERACTIONS).

PRECAUTIONS:

General: Delavirdine is metabolized primarily by the liver. Therefore, caution should be exercised when administering delavirdine tablets to patients with impaired hepatic function.

Resistance/Cross-Resistance: Non-nucleoside reverse transcriptase inhibitors, when used alone or in combination, may confer cross-resistance to other non-nucleoside reverse transcriptase inhibitors.

Skin Rash: Skin rash attributable to delavirdine has occurred in 18% of all patients in combination regimens in phase II and III controlled trials who received delavirdine 400 mg three times daily. Forty-two percent to 50% of patients treated with delavirdine 400 mg three times daily in Studies 0021 and 0017 experienced rash compared with 24% to 32% of patients receiving monotherapy with zidovudine or didanosine, respectively. In Studies 0021 and 0017, 4.3% of patients treated with delavirdine 400 mg three times daily discontinued treatment due to rash.

Dose titration did not signficantly reduce the incidence of rash. Rash was typically diffuse, maculopapular, erythematous, and often pruritic. Skin rash was more common in patients with lower CD4 cell counts and usually occurred within 1 to 3 weeks (median = 11 days) of treatment. Rash classified as severe was observed in 3.6% of patients in Studies 0021 and 0017. In most cases, the duration of the rash was less than 2 weeks and did not reqiuire dose reduction or discontinuation of delavirdine. Most patients were able to resume therapy after rechallenge with delavirdine following a treatment interruption due to rash. The distributon of the rash was mainly on the upper body and proximal arms, with decreasing intensity of the lesions on the neck and face, and progressively less on the rest of the trunk and limbs. Erythema multiforme and Stevens-Johnson syndrome were rarely seen and resolved after withdrawal of delavirdine. Any patient experiencing severe rash or rash accompanied by symptoms such as fever, blistering, oral lesions, conjunctivitis, swelling, muscle or joint aches should discontinue delavirdine and consult a physician. Occurrence of a delavirdine-related rash after 1 month of therapy is uncommon unless prolonged interruption of treatment with delavirdine occurs. Symptomatic relief has been obtained using diphenhydramine hydrochloride, hydroxyzine hydrochloride, and/or topical corticosteroids.

Information for the Patient: Patients should be informed that delavirdine is not a cure for HIV-1 infection and that they may continue to acquire illnesses associated with HIV-1 infection, including opportunistic infections. Treatment with delavirdine has not been shown to reduce the incidence of frequency of such illnesses, and patients should be advised to remain under the care of a physician when using delavirdine.

Patients should be advised that the long-term effects of treatment with delavirdine are unknown at this time. They should be advised that the use of delavirdine has not been shown to reduce the risk of transmission of HIV-1.

Patients should be instructed that the major toxicity of delavirdine is rash and should be advised to promptly notify their physician should rash occur. The majority of rashes associated with delavirdine occur within 1 to 3 weeks after initiating of treatment with delavirdine. The rash normally resolves in 3 to 14 days and may be treated symptomatically while therapy with delavirdine is continued. Any patient experiencing severe rash or rash accompanied by symptoms such as fever, blistering, oral lesions, conjunctivitis, swelling, muscle or joint aches should discontinue medication and consult a physician.

Patients should be informed to take delavirdine every day as prescribed. Patients should not alter the dose of delavirdine without consulting their doctor. If a dose is missed, patients should take the next dose as soon as possible. However, if a dose is skipped, the patient should not double the next dose.

Patients with achlorhydria should take delavirdine with an acidic beverage (*e.g.,* orange or cranberry juice). However, the effect of an acidic beverage on the absorption of delavirdine in patients with achorhydria has not been investigated.

Patients taking both delavirdine and antacids should be advised to take them at least one hour apart.

Because delavirdine may interact with certain drugs, patients should be advised to report to their doctor the use of any prescription or over the counter medications.

Carcinogenesis, Mutagenesis, and Impairment of Fertility Long-term carcinogenicity studies with delavidine in animals have not been completed. A battery of genetic toxicology tests was conducted with delavirdine, including the Ames assay, *in vitro* unscheduled DNA synthesis (UDS) assay, an *in vitro* cytogenetics (chromosome aberration) assay in human peripheral lymphocytes, a mammalian mutation assay in Chinese hamster ovary cells, and the micronucleus test in mice. The results were negative indicating delavirdine is not mutagenic.

Delavirdme at doses of 20, 100 and 200 mg/kg/day did not cause impairment of fertility in rats when males were treated for 70 days and females were treated for 14 days prior to mating.

Pregnancy Category C: Delavirdine has been shown to be teratogenic in rats. Delavirdine caused ventricular septal defects in rats at doses of 50, 100 and 200 mg/kg/day when administered during the period of organogenesis. The lowest dose of delavirdine that caused malformations produced systemic exposures in pregnant rats equal to or lower than the expected human exposure to delavirdine (C_{min}=15 μM) at the recommended dose. Exposure in rats approximately 5-fold higher than the expected human exposure resulted in marked maternal toxicity, embryotoxicity, fetal developmental delay, and reduced pup survival. Additionally, reduced pup survival on postpartum day 0 occurred at an exposure (mean C_{min}) approximately equal to the expected human exposure. Delavirdine was excreted in the milk of lactating rats at a concentration three to five times that of rat plasma.

Delavirdine at doses of 200 and 400 mg/kg/day administered during the period of organogenesis caused maternal toxicity, embryotoxicity and abortions in rabbits. The lowest dose of delavirdine that resulted in these toxic effects produced systemic exposures in pregnant rabbits approximately 6-fold higher than the expected human exposure to delavirdine (C_{min}=15 μM) at the recommended dose. The no observed-adverse effect dose in the pregnant rabbit was 100 mg/kg/day. Various malformations were observed at this dose, but the incidence of such malformations was not statistically significantly different from those observed in the control group. Systemic exposures in pregnant rabbits at a dose of 100 mg/kg/day were lower than those expected in humans at the recommended clinical dose. Malformations were not apparent at 200 and 400 mg/kg/day; however, only a limited number of fetuses were available for examination as a result of maternal and embryo death.

PRECAUTIONS: *(cont'd)*

No adequate and well-controlled studies in pregnant women have been conducted. Delavirdine should be used during pregnancy only if the potential benefit justifies the potential risk to the fetus. Of 7 unplanned pregnancies reported in premarketing clinical studies, 3 were ectopic pregnancics and 3 pregnancies resulted in heathy live births. One infant was born prematurely with a small muscular ventricular septal defect to a patient who received approximately six weeks of treatment with delavirdine and zidovudine early in the course of the pregnancy.

Nursing Mothers: The U.S. Public Health Services Centers for Disease Control and Prevention advises HIV-infected women not to breast-feed to avoid postnatal transmission of HIV to a child who may not yet be infected.

Pediatric Use: Safety and effectiveness of delavirdine in combination with other antiretroviral agents have not been established in HIV-1 infected individuals younger than 16 years of age.

DRUG INTERACTIONS:

GENERAL

Coadministration of delavirdine with certain nonsedating antihistamines, sedative hypnotics, antiarrhythmics, calcium channel blockers, ergot alkaloid preparations, amphetamines, and cisapride, may result in potentially serious and/or life threatening adverse events. Due to the inhibitory effect of delavirdine on CYP3A and CYP2C9, coadministration of delavirdine with drugs primarily metabolized by these liver enzymes may result in increased plasma concentrations. Higher plasma concentrations of these drugs could increase or prolong both therapeutic and adverse effects (TABLE 1). Therefore, appropriate dose adjustments may be necessary for these drugs. Drugs that induce CYP3A may also reduce plasma delavirdine concentrations (TABLE 2). Physicians should consider using alternatives to drugs that induce CYP3A while a patient is taking delavirdine.

ANTACIDS

Doses of an antacid and delavirdine should be separated by at least one hour because the absorption of delavirdine is reduced when coadministered with antacids.

ANTICONVULSANT AGENTS

Phenytoin, Phenobarbital, Carbamazepine: Coadministration of delavirdine with these agents is not recommended, because limited population pharmacokinetic data indicate that a substantial reduction in plasma delavirdine concentrations may result.

ANTIMYCOBACTERIAL AGENTS

Rifabutin: Coadministration of delavirdine and rifabutn is not recommended, because rifabutin substantially decreases plasma delavirdine concentrations and delavirdine increases plasma concentrations of rifabutin.

RIFAMPIN

Delavirdine should not be coadminisitered with rifampin, because rifampin reduces delavirdine systemic exposure (AUC) by almost 100%.

H_2Receptor Antagonists

Cimetidine, Famotidine, Nizatidine and Ranitidine: These agents increase gastric pH and may reduce the absorption of delavirdine. Although the effect of these drugs on delavirdine absorption has not been evaluated, chronic use of these drugs with delavirdine is not recommended.

NUCLEOSIDE ANALOGUE REVERSE TRANSCRIPTASE INHIBITORS

Didanosine: Administration of didanosine and delavirdine should be separated by at least one hour, because coadministration of didanosine and delavirdine resulted in reduced systemic exposure to both drugs by approximately 20%.

PROTEASE INHIBITORS

Indinavir: Due to an increase in indinavir plasma concentrations (preliminary results), a dose reduction of indinavir to 600 mg three times daily should be considered when delavirdine and indinavir are coadministered. Currently, there are no safety and efficacy data available from the use of this combination.

Ritonavir: No studies have been conducted with combination therapy of delavirdine and ritonavir at their recommended doses. Preliminary results indicate there is no evidence of an interaction at doses of delavirdine 400 mg to 600 mg twice daily and ritonavir 300 mg twice daily. Currently, there are no safety and efficacy data available from the use of this combination.

Saquinavir: Saquinavir AUC increased 5-fold when delavirdine (400 mg three times daily) and saquinar (600 mg three times daily) were administered in combination. Currently, there are limited safety and no efficacy data available from the use of this combination. In a small, preliminary study, hepatocellular enzyme elevations occurred in 13% of subjects during the first several weeks of the delavirdine and saquinavir combination (6% grade 3 or 4) hepatocellular enzymes (ALT/AST) should be monitored frequently if this combination is prescribed.

CLINICAL INTERACTION DATA

TABLE 1 Selected Drugs that are Predicted to Have Plasma Concentrations increased by Delavirdine*

HIV protease Inhibitors:	indinavir, saquinavir
Antihistamines:	terfenadine†, astemizole‡
Antimicrobial Agents:	claritromycin, dapsone, rifabutin
Anti-migraine Agents:	ergot derivatives
Benzodiazepines:	alprazolam†, midazolam†, triazolam†
Calcium channel Blockers:	dihydroyridines (*e.g.,* nifedipine)
GI Motility Agents:	cisapride†
Other: quinidine, warfarin	

* This table is not all inclusive.
† See WARNINGS.

TABLE 2 Selected Drugs that are Predicted to Decrease Plasma Delavirdine Concentrations‡§

Anticonvulsants:	carbamazepine, phenobarbital, phenytoin
Antimycobacterial Agents:	rifabutin, rifampin

‡ This table is not all inclusive.
§ See WARNINGS.

Antacids: In a single-dose study in twelve healthy volunteers, simultaneous administration of 300 mg delavirdine with alumina and magnesia oral suspension resulted in a 41 ± 19% reduction in delavirdine AUC.

DRUG INTERACTIONS: *(cont'd)*

Clarithromycin: In a study in six HIV-1-infected patients, coadminstraton of clarithromycin (500 mg twice daily) with delavirdine (300 mg three times daily) resulted in a 44 ± 50% increase in delavirdine AUC. Compared to historical data, clarithromycin AUC was increased by approximately 100% and 14-hydroxyclarithromycin AUC was decreased by 75%.

Didanosine: In a study in nine HIV-1 infected patients, simultaneous administration of didanosine (125 mg or 250 mg twice daily) with delavirdine (400 mg three times daily) for two weeks resulted in an approximately 20% decrease in both didanosine AUC and delavirdine AUC, relative to when administration of delavirdine and didanosine was separated by at least one hour.

Fluconazole: In a study in eight HIV-1-infected patients, coadministration of fluconazole (400 mg once daily) with delavirdine (300 mg three times daily) did not significantly alter the pharmacokinetics of delavirdine. Compared to historical data, fluconazole pharmacokinetics were not altered by delavirdine.

Fluoxetine: Population pharmacokinetic data available for 36 patients suggest that fluoxetine increases trough plasma delavirdine concentrations by about 50%.

Indinavir: Preliminary data (n=14) indicate that delavirdine inhibits the metabolism of indinavir such that coadministration of a 400 mg single dose of indinavir with delavirdine (400 mg three times daily) resulted in indinavir AUC values slightly less than those observed following administration of an 800 mg dose of indinavir alone. Also, coadministration of a 600 mg dose of indinavir with delaviridine (400 mg three times daily) resulted in indinavir AUC values approximately 40% greater than those observed folllowing administration of an 800 mg dose of indinavir alone. Indinavir had no effect on delavirdine pharmacokinetics.

Ketoconazole: Population pharmacokinetic data available for 26 patients suggest that ketoconazole increases trough plasma delavirdine concentrations by about 50%.

Phenytoin, Phenobarbital, and Carbamazepine: Population pharmacokinetic data available for eight patients suggest that coadministration of phenytoin, phenobarbital, or carbamazepine with delavirdine results in a substantial reduction in trough plasma delavirdine concentrations.

Rifabutin: In a study in seven HIV-1-infected patients, coadministration of rifabutin (300 mg once daily) with delavirdine (400 mg three times daily) resulted in an 80 ± 10% decrease in delavirdine AUC. Compared to historical data, rifabutin AUC was increased by at least 100%.

Rifampin: In a study in seven HIV-1 infected patients, coadministration of rifampin (600 mg once daily) with delavirdine (400 mg three times daily) resulted in a 96 ± 4% decrease in delavirdine AUC.

Ritonavir: Preliminary data (n=13) indicate that coadministration of delavirdine (400 mg or 600 mg twice daily) with ritonavir (300 mg twice daily) did not alter ritonavir pharmacokinetics. Coadministration of ritonavir (300 mg twice daily) with delavirdine (400 mg twice daily) did not significantly alter delavirdine pharmacokinetics (n=9). The pharmacokinetic interaction between delavirdine and ritonavir at their recommended doses has not been studied.

Saquinavir: In seven healthy volunteers, coadministration of saquinavir (600 mg three times daily) with delavirdine (400 mg three times daily) resulted in a five-fold increase in saquinavir AUC. In 13 healthy volunteers, coadministration of saquinavir (600 mg three times daily) with delavrdine (400 mg three times daily) resuted in a 15 ± 16% decrease in delavirdine AUC.

Sulfametholazole and Trimethoprim/Sulfamethoxazole (TMP/SMX): Population pharmacokinetic data available for 311 patients suggest that the pharmacokinetics of delavirdine are not affected by sulfamethoxazole or TMP/SMX.

Zidovudine: Zidovudine and delavirdine do not alter one anothers pharmacokinetics.

ADVERSE REACTIONS:

The safety of delavirdine tablets alone and in combination with other therapies has been studied in 1969 patients receiving delavirdine.

Adverse events of moderate or severe intensity reported in ≥2% of patients receiving delavirdine in combination with didanosine or zidovudine in Studies 0017 and 0021 are summarized in TABLE 3. The median duration of treatment in Studies 0017 and 0021 was 34 and 42 weeks (up to 107 weeks for both studies), respectively, at the time of the safety assessment. The most frequently reported drug-related medical event was rash (see PRECAUTIONS, Skin Rash).

TABLE 3 Adverse Events of Moderate or Severe Intensity in ≥2% of Patients Receiving Delavirdine

Body System/ Adverse Event	Study 0017 Didanosine† (n=591)	Delviradine 400 mg tid + Didanosine† (n=594)	Study 0021 Zidovudine 200 mg tid (n=271)	Delaviradine 400 mg tid + Zidovudine 200 mg tid (n=287)
Body as a Whole				
Headache	4.7	5.6	4.8	5.6
Fatigue	2.7	2.9	4.8	5.2
Digestive				
Nausea	3.4	4.9	6.6	10.8
Diarrhea	4.4	4.5	2.2	3.5
Vomiting	1.2	2.4	1.1	2.8
Metabolic and Nutritional				
increased ALT (SGPT)	3.6	5.2	0.7	2.4
increased AST (SGOT)	3.0	4.5	0.7	1.7
Skin				
Rash	3.0	9.8	1.5	12.5
Maculopapular	2.0	6.6	1.1	4.5
Pruritus	1.7	2.2	1.5	3.1

* Includes those adverse events at least possibly related to study drug or of unknown relationship and excludes concurrent HIV conditions.
† Dose adjusted by body weight <60 kg=125 mg bid; ≥60 kg=200 mg bid.

Medical events occurring in less than 2% of patients receiving delavirdine (in combination treatment) in all phase I and III studies, considered possibly related to treatment, and of at least ACTG grade 2 in intensity are listed below by body system.

Body as a Whole: Abdominal cramps, abdominal distention, abdominal pain (generalized or localized), allergic reaction, asthenia, back pain, chest pain, chills, edema (generaized or localized), epidermal cyst, fever, flank pain, flu syndrome, lethargy, lip edema, malaise, neck rigidity, pain (generalized or localized), sebaceous cyst, trauma, and upper respiratory infection.

Cardiovascular System: Bradycardia, migraine, palor, palpitation, postural hypotension, syncope, tachycardia, and vasodilatlon.

ADVERSE REACTIONS: *(cont'd)*

Digestive System: Anorexia, aphthous stomatitis, bloody stool, colitis, constipation, decreased appetite, diarrhea (*Clostridium difficile*) diverticlulits, duodenits, dry mouth, dyspepsia, dysphagia, enteritis, esophagitis, fecal incontinence, flatulence, gagging, gastritis, gastroesophageal reflux, gastrointestinal bleeding, gastrointestinal disorder, gingivitis, gum hemorrhage, increased appetite, increased saliva, increased thirst, mouth ulcer, nonspecific hepatitis, pancreatitis, rectal disorder, sialadenitis, stomatitis, and tongue edema or ulceration.

Hemic and Lymphatic System: Anemia, bruise, ecchymosis, eosinophilia, granulocytosis, neutropenia, pancytopenia, petechia, prolonged partial thrombopastin time, purpura, spleen disorder, and thrombocytopenia.

Metabolic and Nutritional Disorders: Alcohol intolerance, bilirubinemia, hyperkalemia, hyperuricemia, hypocalcemia, hyponatremia, hypophosphatemia, increased gamma glutamyl transpepthree times dailyase, increased lipase, increased serum alkaline phosphatase, increased serum amylase, increased serum creatine phosphokinase, increased serum creatinine, peripheral edema, and weight increase or decrease.

Musculoskeletal System: Arthralgia or arthritis of single and multiple joints, bone disorder, bone pain, leg cramps, muscular weakness, myalgia, tendon disorder, tenosynovitis, and tetany.

Nervous System: Abnormal coordination, agitation, amnesia, anxiety, change in dreams, cognitive impairment, confusion, decreased libido, depressve symptoms, disorentation, dizziness, emotional lability, hallucination, hyperesthesia, hyperreflexia, hypesthesia, impaired concentration, insomnia, manic symptoms, muscle cramp, nervousness, neuropathy, nightmares, nystaginus, paralysis, paranoid symptoms, paresthesia, restlessness, somnolence, tingling, tremor, vertigo and weakness.

Respiratory System: Bronchitis, chest congestion, cough, dyspnea, epistaxis, laryngismus, pharyngitis, rhinitis, and sinusitis.

Skin and Appendages: Angioedema, dermal leukocytoclastic vasculitis, dermatits, desquamation, diaphoresis, dry skin, erythema, erythema multiforme, folliculitis, fungal dermattis, hair loss, nail disorder, petechial rash, seborrhea, skin disorder, skin nodule, Stevens-Johnson syndrome, urticaria, and vesiculobuous rash.

Special Senses: Blepharitis, conjunctivitis, diplopia, dry eyes, ear pain, photophobia, taste perversion and tinnitus.

Urogenital System: Breast enlargement, calculi of the kidney, epididymitis, hematuria, hemospermia impotence, kidney pain, metrorrhagia, nocturia, polyuria, proteinuria, and vaginal moniliasis.

Laboratory Abnormalities: The frequency of clinically important laboratory abnormalities observed during therapy in Studies 0017 and 0021 is summarized in TABLE 4. There was no significant difference in ACTG grades 3 and 4 laboratory abnormalities between treatment groups except a two-fold reduction in neutropenia in the delavirdine plus zidovudine combination group compared with the zidovudine monotherapy group in Study 0021.

TABLE 4 Frequency (%)* of Clinically Important Laboratory Abnormalities

Laboratory Test	Study 0017 Didanosine† (n=591)	Delviradine 400 mg tid + Didanosine† (n=594)	Study 0021 Zidovudine 200 mg tid (n=271)	Delaviradine 400 mg tid + Zidovudine 200 mg tid (n=287)
Neutropenia (ANC <750/mm³)	6.7	5.7	7.7‡	3.5
Anemia (Hgb <7.0 g/dl	0.2	0.7	1.1	1.0
Thrombocytopenia (platelets <50,000/mm³)	1.4	1.5	0.0	0.0
ALT (>5.0 × ULN)	4.6	6.7	3.7	3.8
AST (>5.0 × ULN)	4.9	5.6	3.0	2.1
Bilirubin (>2.5 ULN)	0.7	0.5	0.4	1.0
Amylase (>2.0 ULN)	6.5	5.2	1.1	0.0

* Percentage was based on the number of patients for which data on that laboratory test was available.
† Dose adjusted by body weight <60 kg=125 mg bid; ≥60 kg=200 mg bid.
‡ Significant (P<0.5) delviradine + zidovudine vs zidovudine.
ANC=Absolute neutrophil count; ULN=upper limit of normal.

OVERDOSAGE:

No reports of overdose with delavirdine tablets are available in humans. Several patients have received up to 850 mg three times daily for up to 6 months with no serious drug related medical events.

Management of Overdosage: Treatment of overdosage with delavirdine should consist of general supportive measures, including monitoring of vital signs and observation of the patient's clinical status. There is no specific antidote for overdosage with delavirdine. If indicated, elimination of unabsorbed drug should be achieved by emesis or gastric leavage. Since delavirdine is extensively metabolized by the liver and is highly protein bound, dialysis is unlikely to be beneficial in significant removal of the drug

DOSAGE AND ADMINISTRATION:

The recommended dosage for delavirdine tablets is 400 mg (four 100 mg tablets) three times daily. Delavirdine should be used in combination with appropriate other antiretroviral therapy. The complete prescribing information for other antiretroviral agents should be consulted for information on dosage and administration.

Delavirdine tablets may be dispersed in water prior to consumption. To prepare a dispersion, add four delavirdine tablets to at least 3 ounces of water, allow to stand for a few minutes, and then stir until a uniform dispersion occurs (see CLINICAL PHARMACOLOGY, Absorption and Bioavailability). The dispersion should be consumed promptly. The glass should be rinsed and the rinse swallowed to insure the entire dose is consumed.

Delavirdine tablets may be administered with or without food (see CLINICAL PHARMACOLOGY, Absorption and Bioavailability). Patients with achlorhydria should take delavirdine with an acidic beverage (*e.g.*, orange or cranberry juice). However, the effect of an acidic beverage on the absorption of delavirdine in patients with achhorhydria has not been investigated.

Patients taking both delavirdine and antacids should be advised to take them at east one hour apart.

ANIMAL PHARMACOLOGY:

Toxicities among various organs and organ systems in rats, mice, rabbits, dogs, and monkeys were observed following the administration of delavirdine. Necrotizing vasculitis was the most significant toxicity that occurred in dogs when mean nadir serum concentrations of delavirdine were at least 7-fold higher than the expected human exposure to delavirdine (C_{min}= 15 μM) at the recommended dose. Vasculitis in dogs was not reversible during a 2.5-month recovery period; however, partial resolution of the vascular lesion characterized by reduced inflammation, diminished necrosis, and intitial thickening occurred during this period. Other major target organs included the gastrointestinal tract, endocrine organs, liver, kidneys, bone marrow, lymphoid tissue, lung, and reproductive organs.

HOW SUPPLIED:

Rescriptor tablets are available as 100 mg white, capsule shaped tablets marked with "U 3761".

Store at controlled room temperature 20° to 25°C (68° to 77°F). Keep container tightly closed. Protect from high humdity.

(Pharmacia and Upjohn, 4/97)

DEMECARIUM BROMIDE *(000955)*

CATEGORIES: Antiglaucomatous Agents; Cholinesterase Inhibitors; EENT Drugs; Eye, Ear, Nose, & Throat Preparations; Esotropia; Glaucoma; Iridectomy; Miotics; Ophthalmics; Pregnancy Category X; FDA Approval Pre 1982

BRAND NAMES: **Humorsol**; *Tosmilen* (Japan)
(International brand names outside U.S. in italics)

FORMULARIES: Aetna; Medi-Cal

COST OF THERAPY: $214.32 (Glaucoma; Solution; 0.125 %; 0.2/day; 365 days) vs. Potential Cost of $1,851.63 (Iredectomy)

PRIMARY ICD9: 365.11 (Primary Open-Angle Glaucoma)

DESCRIPTION:

FOR TOPICAL APPLICATION INTO THE CONJUNCTIVAL SAC ONLY

OPHTHALMIC SOLUTION DEMECARIUM BROMIDE IS A STERILE SOLUTION SUPPLIED IN TWO DOSAGE STRENGTHS: 0.125 PERCENT AND 0.25 PERCENT. THE INACTIVE INGREDIENTS ARE SODIUM CHLORIDE AND WATER FOR INJECTION; BENZALKONIUM CHLORIDE 1:5000 IS ADDED AS PRESERVATIVE. DEMECARIUM COMPOUND WITH A MOLECULAR WEIGHT OF 716.60. ITS CHEMICAL NAME IS 3,3'1- (1,10-DECANEDIYLBIS ((METHYLIMINO)-CARBONYLOXY)) BIS (*N,N,N*- TRIMETHYLBENZENAMINIUM) DIBROMIDE. ITS EMPIRICAL FORMULA IS:

$C_{32}H_{52}Br_2N_4O_4$.

CLINICAL PHARMACOLOGY:

Demecarium is a cholinesterase inhibitor with sustained activity. It acts mainly on true (erythrocyte) cholinesterase. Application of demecarium to the eye produces intense miosis and ciliary muscle contraction due to inhibition of cholinesterase, allowing acetylcholine to accumulate at sites of cholinergic transmission. These effects are accompanied by increased capillary permeability of the ciliary body and iris, increased permeability of the blood-aqueous barrier, and vasodilation. Myopia may be induced or, if present, may be augmented by the increased refractive power of the lens that results from the accommodative effect of the drug. Demecarium indirectly produces some of the muscarinic and nicotinic effects of acetylcholine as quantities of the latter accumulate.

INDICATIONS AND USAGE:

Open-angle glaucoma (demecarium should be used in glaucoma only when shorter-acting miotics have proved inadequate).

Conditions obstructing aqueous outflow, such as synechial formation, that are amenable to miotic therapy

Following iridectomy

Accommodative esotropia (accommodative convergent strabismus)

CONTRAINDICATIONS:

Hypersensitivity to any component of this product.

Because of the toxicity of cholinesterase inhibitors in general, demecarium is contraindicated in women who are or who may become pregnant. If this drug is used during pregnancy, or if the patient becomes pregnant while taking this drug, the patient should be apprised of the potential hazard to the fetus.

Because miotics may aggravate inflammation, demecarium should not be used in active uveal inflammation and/or glaucoma associated with iridocyclitis.

WARNINGS:

In patients receiving cholinesterase inhibitors such as demecarium, succinylcholine should be administered with extreme caution before and during general anesthesia.

Because of possible adverse additive effects, demecarium should be administrated only with extreme caution to patients with myasthenia gravis who are receiving systemic anticholinesterase therapy; conversely, extreme caution should be exercised in the use of an anticholinesterase drug for the treatment of myasthenia gravis patients who are already undergoing topical therapy with cholinesterase inhibitors.

PRECAUTIONS:

GENERAL

Gonioscopy is recommended prior to medication with demecarium.

Demecarium should be used with caution in patients with chronic angle-closure (narrow-angle) glaucoma or in patients with narrow angles, because of the possibility of producing pupillary block and increasing angle blockage.

When an intraocular inflammatory process is present, the intensity and persistence of miosis and ciliary muscle contraction that result from anticholinesterase therapy require abstention from, or cautions use of, demecarium.

Systemic effects are infrequent when demecarium is instilled carefully. Compression of the lacrimal duct for several seconds immediately following instillation minimizes drainage into the nasal chamber with its extensive absorption surface. Wash the hands immediately after instillation.

Discontinue demecarium if salivation, urinary incontinence, diarrhea, profuse sweating, muscle weakness, respiratory difficulties, shock, or cardiac irregularities occur.

PRECAUTIONS: *(cont'd)*

Persons receiving cholinesterase inhibitors who are exposed to organophosphate-type insecticides and pesticides (gardeners, organophosphate plant or warehouse workers, farmers, residents of communities which are undergoing insecticide spraying or dusting, etc.) should be warned of the added systemic effects possible from absorption through the respiratory tract or skin. wearing of respiratory masks, frequent washing, and clothing changes may be advisable.

Anticholinesterase drugs should be used with extreme caution, if at all, in patients with marked vagotonia, bronchial asthma, spastic gastrointestinal disturbances, peptic ulcer, pronounced bradycardia and hypotension, recent myocardial infarction, epilepsy, parkinsonism, and other disorders that may respond adversely to vagotonic effects.

After long-term use of demecarium, dilation of blood vessels and resulting greater permeability increase the possibility of hyphema during ophthalmic surgery. Therefore, this drug should be discontinued before surgery.

Despite observance of all precautions and the use of only the recommended dose, there is some evidence that repeated administration may cause depression of the concentration of cholinesterase in the serum and erythrocytes, with resultant systemic effects.

There have been reports of bacterial keratitis associated with the use of multiple dose containers of topical ophthalmic products. These containers had been inadvertently contaminated by patients who, in most cases, had a concurrent corneal disease or a disruption of the ocular epithelial surface. (See Information for the Patient.)

INFORMATION FOR THE PATIENT

Patients should be instructed to avoid allowing the tip of the dispensing container to contact the eye or surrounding structures.

Patients should also be instructed that ocular solutions, if handled improperly, can become contaminated by common bacteria known to cause ocular infections. Serious damage to the eye and subsequent loss of vision may result from using contaminated solutions. (See General.)

Patients should also be advised that if they develop an intercurrent ocular condition (*e.g.*, trauma, ocular surgery or infection), they should immediately seek their physician's advice concerning the continued use of the present multidose container.

CARCINOGENESIS, MUTAGENESIS, AND IMPAIRMENT OF FERTILITY

Long-term studies in animals have not been performed to evaluate the effects of demecarium on fertility or carcinogenic potential.

PREGNANCY CATEGORY X

See CONTRAINDICATIONS.

NURSING MOTHERS

It is not known whether this drug is excreted in human milk. Because of the potential for serious adverse reactions in nursing infants from demecarium, a decision should be made whether to discontinue nursing or to discontinue the drug, taking into account the importance of the drug to the mother.

PEDIATRIC USE

The occurrence of iris cysts is more frequent in children. (See ADVERSE REACTIONS and DOSAGE AND ADMINISTRATION).

Extreme caution should be exercised in children receiving demecarium who may require general anesthesia (see WARNINGS.)

Since demecarium is a potent cholinesterase inhibitor it should be kept out of the reach of children.

DRUG INTERACTIONS:

See WARNINGS regarding possible drug interactions of demecarium with succinylcholine or with other anticholinesterase agents.

ADVERSE REACTIONS:

Stinging, burning, lacrimation, lid muscle twitching, conjunctival and ciliary redness, brow ache, headache, and induced myopia with visual blurring may occur.

Activation of latent iritis or uveitis may occur.

As with all miotic therapy, retinal detachment has been reported occasionally.

Iris cysts may form, enlarge, and obscure vision. Occurrence is more frequent in children. The iris cyst usually shrinks upon discontinuance of the miotic. Rarely, the cyst may rupture or break free into the aqueous. Frequent examination for this occurrence is advised.

Lens opacities have been reported in patients on miotic therapy. Routine slitlamp examinations, including the lens, should accompany prolonged use.

Paradoxical increase in intraocular pressure may follow anticholinesterase instillation. This may be alleviated by pupil-dilating medication.

Prolonged use may cause conjunctival thickening and obstruction of nasolacrimal canals.

Systemic effects, which occur rarely, are suggestive of increased cholinergic activity. Such effects may include nausea, vomiting, abdominal cramps, diarrhea, urinary incontinence, salivation, sweating, difficulty in breathing, bradycardia, or cardiac irregularities. Medical management of systemic effects may be indicated (see Treatment of Adverse Effects.)

TREATMENT OF ADVERSE EFFECTS

If demecarium is taken systemically by accident, or if systemic effects occur after topical application in the eye or from accidental skin contact, administer atropine sulfate parenterally (intravenously if necessary) in a dose (for adults) of 0.4 to 0.6 mg or more. The recommended dosage of atropine in infants and children up to 12 years of age is 0.01 mg/kg repeated every two hours as needed until the desired effect is obtained, or adverse effects of atropine preclude further usage. The maximum single dose should not exceed 0.4 mg.

The use of much larger doses of atropine in treating anticholinesterase intoxication in adults had been reported in the literature. Initially 2 to 6 mg may be given followed by 2 mg every hour or more often, as long as muscarinic effects continue. The greater possibility of atropinization with large doses, particularly in sensitive individuals, should be borne in mind.

Pralidoxime chloride (protopam chloride, Ayerst Laboratories) has been reported to be useful in treating systemic effects due to cholinesterase inhibitors. However, its use is recommended in addition to and not as substitute for atropine.

A short-acting barbiturate is indicated if convulsions occur that are not entirely relieved by atropine. Barbiturate dosage should be carefully adjusted to avoid central respiratory depression. Marked weakness or paralysis of muscles of respiration should be treated promptly by artificial respiration and maintenance of a clear airway.

The oral LD_{50} of demecarium is 2.96 mg/kg in the mouse.

DOSAGE AND ADMINISTRATION:

Demecarium is intended solely for topical use in the conjunctival sac.

As demecarium is an extremely potent drug, the physician should thoroughly familiarize himself with its use and the technic of instillation.

DOSAGE AND ADMINISTRATION: *(cont'd)*

The required dose is applied in the conjunctival sac, with the patient supine, care being taken not to touch the cornea with the tip of the Ocumeter ophthalmic dispenser. *The patient or person administering the medication should apply continuous gentle pressure on the lacrimal duct with the index finger for several seconds immediately following instillation of the drops. This is to prevent drainage overflow of solution into the nasal and pharyngeal spaces, which might cause systemic absorption. Wash the hands immediately after administration.*

DEMECARIUM SHOULD NOT BE USED MORE OFTEN THAN DIRECTED. CAUTION IN NECESSARY TO AVOID OVERDOSAGE.

INITIAL TITRATION AND DOSAGE ADJUSTMENTS WITH DEMECARIUM MUST BE INDIVIDUALIZED TO OBTAIN MAXIMAL THERAPEUTIC EFFECT. THE PATIENT MUST BE CLOSELY OBSERVED DURING THE INITIAL PERIOD. IF THE RESPONSE IS NOT ADEQUATE WITHIN THE FIRST 24 HOURS, OTHER MEASURES SHOULD BE CONSIDERED.

KEEP FREQUENCY OF USE TO A MINIMUM IN ALL PATIENTS, BUT ESPECIALLY IN CHILDREN, TO REDUCE THE CHANCE OF IRIS CYST DEVELOPMENT (SEE ADVERSE REACTIONS.)

GLAUCOMA

For initial therapy with demecarium (0.125 percent or 0.25 percent) place 1 drop (children) or 1 or 2 drops (adults) in the glaucomatous eye. A decrease in intraocular pressure should occur within a few hours. During this period, keep the patient under supervision and make tonometric examinations at least hourly for 3 or 4 hours to be sure that no immediate rise in pressure occurs (see ADVERSE REACTIONS.)

Duration of effect varies with the individual. The usual dosage can vary from as much as 1 or 2 drops twice a day to as little as 1 or 2 drops twice a week. The 0.125 percent strength used twice a day usually results in smooth control of the physiologic diurnal variation in intraocular pressure. This is probably the preferred dosage for most wide (open) angle glaucoma patients.

STRABISMUS

Essentially equal visual acuity of both eyes is a prerequisite to the successful treatment of esotropia with demecarium. For initial evaluation it may be used as a diagnostic aid to determine if an accommodative factor exists. This is especially useful preoperatively in young children and in patients with normal hypermetropic refractive errors. One drop is given daily for 2 weeks, then 1 drop every 2 days for 2 to 3 weeks. If the eyes become straighter, an accommodative factor is demonstrated. This technic may supplement or complement standard testing with atropine and trial with glasses for the accommodative factor.

In esotropia uncomplicated by amblyopia or anisometropia, demecarium may be instilled in both eyes, *not more than 1 drop at a time every day for 2 to 3 weeks,* as too severe a degree of miosis may interfere with vision. Then reduce the dosage to 1 drop every other day for 3 to 4 weeks and reevaluate the patient's status.

Demecarium may be continued in a dosage of 1 drop every 2 days to 1 drop twice a week. (The latter dosage may be maintained for several months.) Evaluate the patient's condition every 4 to 12 weeks. If improvement continues, change the schedule to 1 drop once a week and eventually to a trial without medication. However, if after 4 months, control of the condition sill requires 1 drop every 2 days, therapy with demecarium should be stopped.

Storage: Protect from freezing and excessive heat.

HOW SUPPLIED - EQUIVALENTS NOT AVAILABLE:

Solution - Ophthalmic - 0.125 %

5 ml	$14.68	HUMORSOL, Merck	00006-3255-03

Solution - Ophthalmic - 0.25 %

5 ml	$15.74	HUMORSOL, Merck	00006-3267-03

DEMECLOCYCLINE HYDROCHLORIDE *(000956)*

CATEGORIES: Amebiasis; Amebicides; Anti-Infectives; Antibiotics; Antimicrobials; Conjunctivitis; Granuloma; Granuloma Inguinale; Infections; Lyme Disease; Lymphogranuloma; Pneumonia; Psittacosis; Q Fever; Relapsing Fever; Rheumatic Fever; Rickettsial Disease; Rickettsialpox; Rocky Mountain Fever; Tetracyclines; Tick Fevers; Topical; Typhoid Fever; Typhus; FDA Approval Pre 1982

BRAND NAMES: *Biotercicliin*; *Clortetrin*; **Declomycin**; *Ledermicina* (Mexico); *Ledermycin* (Australia, England, Japan); *Rynabron*
(International brand names outside U.S. in italics)

DESCRIPTION:

Demeclocycline hydrochloride is an antibiotic isolated from a mutant strain of *Streptomyces aureofaciens.* Chemically it is (4S-(4α,4aα,5aα,6β,12aα))-7-Chloro-4-dimethylamino)-1,4,4a,5,5a,6,11, 12a-octahydro-3,6,10,12,12a-pentahydroxy-1,11-dioxo-2-naphthacenecarboxam ide monohydrochloride.

Declomycin contains the following inactive ingredients:

Declomycin Capsules: Benzoin Gum, Blue 1, Colloidal Silicon Dioxide, Corn Starch, FD&C Yellow No. 6, Ethyl Vanillin, Gelatin, Glycerin, Methylparaben, Propenyl Guaethol, Propylene Glycol, Propylparaben, Red 33, Red 40, Terpene Resin, Titanium Dioxide, and other ingredients.

Declomycin Tablets: Alginic Acid, Corn Starch, Ethylcellulose, Hydroxypropyl Methylcellulose, Magnesium Stearate, Red 7, Sorbitol, Titanium Dioxide, Yellow 10 and other ingredients. May also contain Sodium Lauryl Sulfate.

CLINICAL PHARMACOLOGY:

The tetracyclines are primarily bacteriostatic and are thought to exert their antimicrobial effect by the inhibition of protein synthesis. Tetracyclines are active against a wide range of gram-negative and gram-positive organisms. The drugs in the tetracycline class have closely similar antimicrobial spectra, and cross-resistance among them is common. Microorganisms may be considered susceptible if the MIC (minimum inhibitory concentration) is not more than 4 mcg/ml and intermediate if the MIC is 4 12.5 mcg/ml.

Susceptibility plate testing: A tetracycline disc may be used to determine microbial susceptibility to drugs in the tetracycline class. If the Kirby-Bauer method of disc susceptibility testing is used, a 30 mcg tetracycline disc should give a zone of at least 19 mm when tested against a tetracycline-susceptible bacterial strain.

Tetracyclines are readily absorbed and are bound to plasma proteins in varying degrees. They are concentrated by the liver in the bile and excreted in the urine and feces at high concentrations and in a biologically active form.

INDICATIONS AND USAGE:

Demeclocycline HCl demeclocycline hydrochloride is indicated in infections caused by the following microorganisms:

INDICATIONS AND USAGE: *(cont'd)*

Rickettsiae: (Rocky Mountain spotted fever, typhus fever and the typhus group, Q fever, rickettsialpox, tick fevers).

Mycoplasma pneumoniae (PPLO, Eaton agent).

Agents of psittacosis and ornithosis.

Agents of lymphogranuloma venereum and granuloma inguinale.

The spirochetal agent of relapsing fever (*Borrelia recurrentis*).

The following gram-negative microorganisms:

Haemophilus ducreyi (chancroid), *Yersinia pestis and Francisella tularensis,* formerly *Pasteurella pestis* and *Pasteurella tularensis, Bartonella bacilliformis, Bacteroides* species, *Vibrio comma* and *Vibrio fetus, Brucella* species (in conjunction with streptomycin).

Because many strains of the following groups of microorganisms have been shown to be resistant to tetracyclines, culture and susceptibility testing are recommended.

Demeclocycline is indicated for treatment of infections caused by the following gram-negative microorganisms, when bacteriologic testing indicates appropriate susceptibility to the drug:

Escherichia coli, Enterobacter aerogenes (formerly *Aerobacter aerogenes*), *Shigella* species, *Mima* species and *Herellea* species, *Haemophilus influenzae* (respiratory infections), *Klebsiella* species (respiratory and urinary infections).

Declomycin is indicated for treatment of infections caused by the following gram-positive microorganisms when bacteriologic testing indicates appropriate susceptibility to the drug:

Streptococcus species:

Up to 44% of strains of *Streptococcus pyogenes* and 74% of*Streptococcus faecalis* have been found to be resistant to tetracycline drugs. Therefore, tetracyclines should not be used for streptococcal disease unless the organism has been demonstrated to be sensitive.

For upper respiratory infections due to Group A beta-hemolytic streptococci, penicillin is the usual drug of choice, including prophylaxis of rheumatic fever.

Streptococcus pneumoniae,

Staphylococcus aureus, skin and soft tissue infections.

Tetracyclines are not the drugs of choice in the treatment of any type of Staphylococcal infection.

When penicillin is contraindicated, tetracyclines are alternative drugs in the treatment of infections due to:

Neisseria gonorrhoeae,

Treponema pallidum and *Treponema pertenue* (syphilis and yaws),

Listeria monocytogenes,

Clostridium species,

Bacillus anthracis,

Fusobacterium fusiforme (Vincent's infection),

Actinomyces species.

In acute intestinal amebiasis, the tetracyclines may be a useful adjunct to amebicides.

Demeclocycline hydrochloride is indicated in the treatment of trachoma, although the infectious agent is not always eliminated, as judged by immunofluorescence.

Inclusion conjunctivitis may be treated with oral tetracyclines or with a combination of oral and topical agents.

CONTRAINDICATIONS:

This drug is contraindicated in persons who have shown hypersensitivity to any of the tetracyclines.

WARNINGS:

THE USE OF DRUGS OF THE TETRACYCLINE CLASS DURING TOOTH DEVELOPMENT (LAST HALF OF PREGNANCY, INFANCY AND CHILDHOOD TO THE AGE OF 8 YEARS) MAY CAUSE PERMANENT DISCOLORATION OF THE TEETH (YELLOW-GRAY-BROWN). This adverse reaction is more common during long-term use of the drugs but has been observed following repeated short-term courses. Enamel hypoplasia has also been reported. TETRACYCLINE DRUGS, THEREFORE, SHOULD NOT BE USED IN THIS AGE GROUP UNLESS OTHER DRUGS ARE NOT LIKELY TO BE EFFECTIVE OR ARE CONTRAINDICATED. If renal impairment exists, even usual oral or parenteral doses may lead to excessive systemic accumulation of the drug and possible liver toxicity. Under such conditions, lower than usual total doses are indicated and, if therapy is prolonged, serum level determinations of the drug may be advisable.

Phototoxic reactions can occur in individuals taking demeclocycline, and are characterized by severe burn of exposed surfaces resulting from direct exposure of patients to sunlight during therapy with moderate or large doses of demeclocycline. Patients apt to be exposed to direct sunlight or ultraviolet light should be advised that this reaction can occur, and treatment should be discontinued at the first evidence of skin erythema.

The anti-anabolic action of the tetracyclines may cause in increase in BUN. While this is not a problem in those with normal renal function, in patients with significantly impaired function, higher serum levels of tetracycline may lead to azotemia, hyperphosphatemia, and acidosis.

Administration of demeclocycline HCl has resulted in appearance of the diabetes insipidus syndrome (polyuria, polydipsia and weakness) in some patients on long-term therapy. The syndrome has been shown to be nephrogenic, dose-dependent and reversible on discontinuance of therapy.

Usage in Pregnancy: See WARNINGSabout use during tooth development. Results of animal studies indicate that tetracyclines cross the placets, are found in fetal tissues and can have toxic effects on the developing fetus (often related ot retardation of skeletal development). Evidence of embryotoxicity has also been noted in animals treated early in pregnancy.

Usage in Newborns, Infants, and Children: See WARNINGSabout use during tooth development.

All tetracyclines form stable calcium complex in bone forming tissue. A decrease in the fibula growth rate has been observed in prematures given oral tetracycline in doses of 25 mg/kg every six hours. This reaction was shown to be reversible when the drug was discontinued.

Tetracyclines are present in the mild of lactating women who are taking a drug in this class.

PRECAUTIONS:

GENERAL

Pseudotumor cerebri (benign intracranial hypertension) in adults has been associated with the use of tetracyclines. The usual clinical manifestations are headache and blurred vision. Bulging fontanels have been associated with the use of tetracyclines in infants. While both of these conditions and related symptoms usually resolve soon after discontinuation of the tetracyclines, the possibility for permanent sequelae exists.

PRECAUTIONS: *(cont'd)*

As with other antibiotic preparations, use of this drug may result in overgrowth of nonsusceptible organisms, including fungi. If superinfection occurs, the antibiotic should be discontinued and appropriate therapy should be instituted. In venereal diseases when coexistent syphilis is suspected, darkfield examination should be done before treatment is started and the blood serology repeated monthly for at least 4 months.

In long-term therapy, periodic laboratory evaluation of organ systems, including hematopoietic, renal and hepatic studies should be performed.

All infections due to Group A beta-hemolytic streptococci should be treated for at least ten days.

Interpretation of Bacteriologic Studies: Following a course of therapy, persistence for several days in both urine and blood of bacterio-suppressive levels of demeclocycline may interfere with culture studies. These levels should not be considered therapeutic.

DRUG INTERACTIONS:

Because the tetracyclines have been shown to depress plasma prothrombin activity, patients who are on anticoagulant therapy may require downward adjustment of their anticoagulant dosage.

Since bacteriostatic drugs, such as the tetracycline class of antibiotics, may interfere with the bactericidal action of penicillins, it is not advisable to administer these drugs concomitantly.

Concurrent use of tetracyclines with oral contraceptives may render oral contraceptives less effective. Breakthrough bleeding has been reported.

ADVERSE REACTIONS:

Gastrointestinal: Anorexia, nausea, vomiting, diarrhea, glossitis, dysphagia, enterocolitis, pancreatitis, and inflammatory lesions (with monilial overgrowth) in the anogenital region, increases in liver enzymes, and hepatic toxicity has been reported rarely. Rare instances of esophagitis and esophageal ulcerations have been reported in patients taking the tetracycline-class antibiotics in capsule and tablet form. Most of these patients took the medication immediately before going to bed (see DOSAGE AND ADMINISTRATION.)

Skin: Maculopapular and erythematous rashes. Exfoliative dermatitis has been reported but is uncommon. Photosensitivity is discussed above. (See WARNINGS.)

Renal toxicity: Rise in BUN has been reported and is apparently dose related. Nephrogenic diabetes insipidus. (See WARNINGS.)

Hypersensitivity Reactions: Urticaria, angioneurotic edema, anaphylaxis, anaphylactoid purpura, pericarditis and exacerbation of systemic lupus erythematosus.

Blood: Hemolytic anemia, thrombocytopenia, neutropenia and eosinophilia have been reported.

CNS: Pseudotumor cerebri (benign intracranial hypertension) in adults and bulging fontanels in infants (see PRECAUTIONS, General). Dizziness, tinnitus, and visual disturbances have been reported. Myasthenic syndrome has been reported rarely.

Other: When given over prolonged periods, tetracyclines have been reported to produce brown-black microscopic discoloration of thyroid glands. No abnormalities of thyroid function studies are known to occur.

DOSAGE AND ADMINISTRATION:

Therapy should be continued for at least 24 to 48 hours after symptoms and fever have subsided.

Concomitant Therapy: Antacids containing aluminum, calcium, or magnesium impair absorption and should not be given to patients taking oral tetracycline. Foods and some diary products also interfere with absorption. Oral forms of tetracycline should be given one hour before or two hours after meals.

In Patients with Renal Impairment: (See WARNINGS.) Total dosage should be decreased by reduction recommended individual doses and/or by extending time intervals between doses.

In the treatment of streptococcal infections, a therapeutic dose of demeclocycline should be administered for at least ten days.

Adults: *Usual daily dose:* Four divided doses of 150 mg each or two divided doses of 300 mg each.

For Children Above Eight Years of Age: *Usual daily dose:* 3-6 mg per pound body weight per day, depending upon the severity of the disease, divided into two to four doses.

Gonorrhea patients sensitive to penicillin may be treated with demeclocycline administered as an initial oral dose of 600 mg followed by 300 mg every 12 hours for four days to a total of 3 grams.

Store at Controlled Room Temperature 15-30°C (59-86°F).

HOW SUPPLIED - EQUIVALENTS NOT AVAILABLE:

Capsule, Elastic - Oral - 150 mg

100's	$285.30	DECLOMYCIN, Lederle Pharm	00005-9208-23

Tablet, Plain Coated - Oral - 150 mg

100's	$371.14	DECLOMYCIN, Lederle Pharm	00005-9218-23

Tablet, Plain Coated - Oral - 300 mg

48's	$324.15	DECLOMYCIN, Lederle Pharm	00005-9270-29

DESERPIDINE *(000961)*

CATEGORIES: Antihypertensives; Cardiovascular Drugs; Hypertension; Rauwolfia Alkaloids; Renal Drugs; FDA Approval Pre 1982

BRAND NAMES: **Harmonyl**; *Raunormine* (Japan)
(International brand names outside U.S. in italics)

COST OF THERAPY: $128.55 (Schizophrenia; Tablet; 0.25 mg; 2/day; 365 days)

DESCRIPTION:

Deserpidine is a purified rauwolfia alkaloid which occurs as a white to light yellow crystalline powder. Deserpidine is insoluble in water and very slightly soluble in alcohol. Chemically, deserpidine is identified as 17α-methoxy-18β-[(3,4,5-trihydroxybenzoic)oxy]-3β, 20α-yohimban-16β-carboxylic acid methyl ester.

Deserpidine is an oral antihypertensive and antipsychotic agent available as tablets containing 0.25 mg of deserpidine.

Harmonyl Inactive Ingredients: Corn starch, D&C Red No. 36, lactose, magnesium stearate, stearic acid and talc.

CLINICAL PHARMACOLOGY:

The pharmacologic actions of deserpidine are essentially the same as those of other active rauwolfia alkaloids. Deserpidine probably produces its antihypertensive effects through depletion of tissue stores of catecholamines (epinephrine and norepinephrine) from peripheral sites. By contrast, its sedative and tranquilizing properties are thought to be related to depletion of 5-hydroxytryptamine from the brain.

The antihypertensive effect is often accompanied by bradycardia. There is no significant alteration in cardiac output or renal blood flow. The carotid sinus reflex is inhibited, but postural hypotension is rarely seen with the use of conventional doses of deserpidine alone.

Deserpidine, like other rauwolfia alkaloids, is characterized by slow onset of action and sustained effect which may persist following withdrawal of the drug.

Information is limited on the human pharmacokinetics of the rauwolfia alkaloids. Rauwolfia alkaloids appear to be widely distributed in body tissues, especially adipose tissue. They also cross the blood-brain barrier. Rauwolfia alkaloids are extensively metabolized. The unchanged alkaloid and the metabolites are excreted slowly in urine and feces.

INDICATIONS AND USAGE:

Deserpidine is indicated for the treatment of mild essential hypertension. It is also useful as adjunctive therapy with other antihypertensive agents in the move severe forms of hypertension.

The drug is also indicated for the relief of symptoms in agitated psychotic states, e.g., schizophrenia - primarily in those individuals unable to tolerate phenothiazine derivatives or those who also require antihypertensive medication.

CONTRAINDICATIONS:

Deserpidine is contraindicated in patients with known hypersensitivity, history of mental depression especially with suicidal tendencies, active peptic ulcer, and ulcerative colitis. It is also contraindicated in patients receiving electroconvulsive therapy.

WARNINGS:

Deserpidine differs slightly in chemical structure from reserpine, however, its actions, indications, cautions and adverse reactions are common to the class of rauwolfia alkaloids. Reserpine may cause mental depression. Recognition of depression may be difficult because this condition may often be disguised by somatic complaints (Masked Depression). The drug should be discontinued at first signs of depression such as despondency, early morning insomnia, loss of appetite, impotence, or self-deprecation. Drug-induced depression may persist for several months after drug withdrawal and may be severe enough to result in suicide.

PRECAUTIONS:

General: Because rauwolfia preparations increase gastrointestinal motility and secretion, this drug should be used cautiously in patients with a history of peptic ulcer, ulcerative colitis, or gallstones, where biliary colic may be precipitated.

Caution should be exercised when treating hypertensive patients with renal insufficiency since they adjust poorly to lowered blood pressure levels.

Preoperative withdrawal of deserpidine does not assure that circulatory instability will not occur. It is important that the anesthesiologist be aware of the patient's drug intake and consider this in the overall management, since hypotension has occurred in patients receiving rauwolfia preparations. Anticholinergic and/or adrenergic drugs (metaraminol, norepinephrine) have been employed to treat adverse vagocirculatory effects.

Information for the Patient: The patient and his family should be warned of the possibility of depression. If signs of despondency, early morning insomnia, loss of appetite, impotence, or self-deprecation appear the drug should be discontinued and the physician consulted.

Patients who engage in potentially hazardous activities such as operating machinery or driving motor vehicles should be warned about possible central nervous system (CNS) side effects.

The physician should inform patients of other possible side effects and advise patients to take this medication every day as directed.

Concomitant use of alcohol with deserpidine may cause additive CNS depressant effects.

Drug/Laboratory Test Interactions: Rauwolfia alkaloids have been reported to interfere with assay procedures for the determination of urinary 17-hydroxycorticosteroids and 17-ketosteroids.

Carcinogenesis, Mutagenesis, and Impairment of Fertility: No long-term deserpidine data are available concerning the potential for carcinogenicity. Adequate studies for determination of mutagenic potential of deserpidine and its effects on fertility have not been done.

Animal Tumorigenicity: Although, there are no studies demonstrating that deserpidine is an animal tumorigen, it is a prolactin stimulator and structurally related to reserpine. Rodent studies have shown that reserpine is an animal tumorigen, causing an increased incidence of mammary fibroadenomas in female mice, malignant tumors of the seminal vesicles in male mice, and malignant adrenal medullary tumors in male rats. These findings arose in 2 year studies in which the drug was administered in the feed at concentrations of 5 and 10 ppm - about 100 to 300 times the usual human dose. The breast neoplasms are though to be related to reserpine's prolactin-elevating effect. Several other prolactin-elevating drugs have also been associated with an increased incidence of mammary neoplasia in rodents.

The extent to which these findings indicate a risk to humans is uncertain. Tissue culture experiments show that about one-third of human breast tumors are prolactin-dependent *in vitro*, a factor of considerable importance if the use of the drug is contemplated in a patient with previously detected breast cancer. The possibility of an increased risk of breast cancer in reserpine users has been studies extensively; however, no firm conclusion has emerged. Although a few epidemiologic studies have suggested a slightly increased risk (less than twofold in all studies except one) in women who have used reserpine, other studies of generally similar design have not confirmed this. Epidemiologic studies conducted using other drugs (neuroleptic agents) that, like reserpine, increase prolactin levels and, therefore, would be considered rodent mammary carcinogens, have not shown an association between chronic administration of the drug and human mammary tumorigenesis. While long-term clinical observation has not suggested such an association, the available evidence is considered too limited to be conclusive at this time. An association of reserpine intake with pheochromocytoma or tumors of the seminal vesicles has not been explored.

Pregnancy Category C: Animal reproduction studies have not been conducted with deserpidine. It is also not known whether deserpidine can cause fetal harm when administered to a pregnant woman only if clearly needed. *Nonteratogenic Effects:* Rauwolfia alkaloids are known to cross the placental barrier, to enter the fetal circulation, and to appear in cord blood. Increased respiratory secretions, nasal congestion, cyanosis, and anorexia may occur in neonates of rauwolfia alkaloid-treated mothers.

Nursing Mothers: Deserpidine is excreted in human milk. Because of the potential for serious adverse reactions in nursing infants from deserpidine, a decision should be made whether to discontinue nursing or to discontinue the drug, taking into account the importance of the drug to the mother.

PRECAUTIONS: *(cont'd)*

Pediatric Use: Safety and effectiveness in children have not been established.

DRUG INTERACTIONS:

Use deserpidine cautiously with *digitalis* and *quinidine* since cardiac arrhythmias have occurred with rauwolfia preparations.

Hypotensive effects of rauwolfia alkaloids may be enhanced when used concurrently with other *antihypertensive agents, diuretics,* or *phenothiazine derivatives,* therefore, careful titration of dosage is necessary.

Additive CNS-depressant effects can occur when rauwolfia alkaloids are taken concomitantly with other *CNS-depressant agents* or *alcohol.*

Monoamine oxidase inhibitors should be avoided or used with extreme caution.

ADVERSE REACTIONS:

The following adverse reactions have been observed with rauwolfia preparations, but there has not been enough systematic collection of data to support an estimate of their frequency. Consequently, the reactions are categorized by organ system and not frequency.

Body as a Whole: Headache.

Cardiovascular System: Arrhythmias (particularly when used concurrently with digitalis or quinidine), syncope, angina-like symptoms, bradycardia, fluid retention.

Digestive System: Vomiting, diarrhea, nausea, anorexia, dryness of mouth, hypersecretion, increased motility, increased salivation.

Hemic and Lymphatic System: Thrombocytopenic purpura.

Metabolic and Nutritional Disorders: Weight gain.

Musculoskeletal System: Muscular aches.

Nervous System: Rare parkinsonian syndrome and other extrapyramidal tract symptoms, dizziness, paradoxical anxiety, depression, nervousness, nightmares, dull sensorium, drowsiness, decreased libido.

Respiratory System: Asthma in asthmatic patients, dyspnea, epistaxis, nasal congestion.

Special Senses: Deafness, optic atrophy, glaucoma, uveitis, conjunctival injection.

Urogenital System: Nonpuerperal lactation, impotence, dysuria, gynecomastia, breast engorgement.

OVERDOSAGE:

An overdosage of deserpidine is characterized by flushing of the skin, conjunctival injection, and pupillary constriction. Sedation ranging from drowsiness to coma may occur. Hypotension, hypothermia, central respiratory depression and bradycardia may develop in cases of severe overdosage.

Treatment consists of the careful evacuation of stomach contents followed by the usual procedures for the symptomatic management of CNS depressant overdosage. If severe hypotension occurs, it should be treated with a direct acting vasopressor (*e.g.,* norepinephrine). If bradycardia becomes marked, especially with cardiac arrhythmia, consider use of atropine or other anticholinergic drug. Because of prolonged effects of deserpidine, the patient should be closely observed for at least 72 hours.

DOSAGE AND ADMINISTRATION:

Deserpidine is administered orally. For the management of mild essential hypertension in the average patient not receiving other antihypertensive agents, the usual initial adult dose is 0.75 to 1 mg daily. Debilitated and elderly patients may require lower doses. Because 10 to 14 days are required to produce the full effects of the drug, adjustments in the full effects of the drug, adjustments in dosage should not be made more frequently. If the therapeutic response is not adequate, it is generally advisable to add another antihypertensive agent to the regimen. For maintenance, dosage should be reduced. A single daily dose of 0.25 mg of deserpidine may suffice for some patients.

Concomitant use of deserpidine with ganglionic blocking agents, guanethidine, veratrum, hydralazine, methyldopa, chlorthalidone, or thiazides necessitates careful titration of dosage with each agent.

For psychiatric disorders: The average initial oral dose is 0.5 mg daily with a range of 0.125 to 1 mg. Adjust dosage upward or downward according to the patient's response.

HOW SUPPLIED:

Harmonyl tablets (grooved), 0.25 mg are salmon-pink and supplied in bottles of 100.

Recommended Storage: Store at controlled room temperature 59°- 86°F (15°-30°C).

Revised: October, 1991

HOW SUPPLIED - EQUIVALENTS NOT AVAILABLE:

Tablet, Uncoated - Oral - 0.25 mg

100's $17.61 HARMONYL, Abbott 00074-6906-07

DESERPIDINE; HYDROCHLOROTHIAZIDE *(000962)*

CATEGORIES: Antihypertensives; Cardiovascular Drugs; Diuretics; Hypertension; Rauwolfia Alkaloids; Renal Drugs; Thiazides; FDA Approval Pre 1982

BRAND NAMES: **Oreticyl**

Prescribing information not available at time of publication.

HOW SUPPLIED - EQUIVALENTS NOT AVAILABLE:

Tablet, Uncoated - Oral - 0.125 mg/25 mg

100's $24.74 ORETICYL 25, Abbott 00074-6922-01

Tablet, Uncoated - Oral - 0.125 mg/50 mg

100's $38.18 ORETICYL 50, Abbott 00074-6931-01

Tablet, Uncoated - Oral - 0.25 mg/25 mg

100's $34.75 ORETICYL FORTE, Abbott 00074-6927-01

DESERPIDINE; METHYCLOTHIAZIDE *(000963)*

CATEGORIES: Antihypertensives; Cardiovascular Drugs; Diuretics; Hypertension; Rauwolfia Alkaloids; Renal Drugs; Thiazides; FDA Approval Pre 1982

BRAND NAMES: *Dureticyl*; *Enduronil*; **Enduronyl**; Eserdine; Meserpidine
(International brand names outside U.S. in italics)

FORMULARIES: Medi-Cal

WARNING:
This fixed combination drug is not indicated for initial therapy of hypertension. Hypertension requires therapy titrated to the individual patient. If the fixed combination represents the dosage so determined, its use may be more convenient in patient management. The treatment of hypertension is not static, but must be reevaluated as conditions in each patient warrant.

DESCRIPTION:

FOR COMPLETE PRESCRIBING INFORMATION REFER TO THE INDIVIDUAL DRUG MONOGRAPHS (DESERPIDINE; METHYCLOTHIAZIDE).

INDICATIONS AND USAGE:

Enduronyl (methyclothiazide and deserpidine) is indicated in the treatment of mild to moderately severe hypertension (see BOXED WARNING). In many cases Enduronyl alone produces an adequate reduction of blood pressure. In resistant or unusually severe cases Enduronyl also may be supplemented by more potent antihypertensive agents. When administered with Enduronyl, more potent agents can be given at reduced dosage to minimize undesirable side effects.

DOSAGE AND ADMINISTRATION:

Dosage should be determined by individual titration of ingredients (see BOXED WARNING). Dosage of both components should be carefully adjusted to the needs of the individual patient. Since at least ten days to two weeks may elapse before the full effects of the drugs become manifest, the dosage of the drugs should not be adjusted more frequently.

Two tablet strengths, Enduronyl Forte (methyclothiazide 5 mg, deserpidine 0.25 mg) and Enduronyl (methyclothiazide 5 mg, deserpidine 0.5 mg), each grooved, are provided to permit considerable latitude in meeting the dosage requirements of individual patients.

TABLE 1 will help in determining which dose of Enduronyl or Enduronyl Forte best represents the equivalent of the titrated dose.

TABLE 1

Daily Dosage of Enduronyl	Methyclothiazide	Deserpidine
1/2 tablet	2.5 mg	0.125 mg
1 tablet	5.0 mg	0.250 mg
1 1/2 tablets	7.5 mg	0.375 mg
2 tablets	10.0 mg	0.500 mg

Daily Dosage of Enduronyl Forte	Methyclothiazide	Deserpidine
1/2 tablet	2.5 mg	0.250 mg
1 tablet	5.0 mg	0.500 mg
1 1/2 tablets	7.5 mg	0.750 mg
2 tablets	10.0 mg	1.000 mg

The appropriate dose of Enduronyl is administered orally, once daily. The usual adult dosage is one lower-strength Enduronyl tablet daily.

There is no contraindication to combining the administration of Enduronyl with other antihypertensive agents. When other antihypertensive agents are to be added to the regimen, this should be accomplished gradually. Ganglionic blocking agents should be given at only half the usual dose since their effect is potentiated by pretreatment with Enduronyl.

HOW SUPPLIED:

Enduronyl is supplied as monogrammed, grooved, square-shaped tablets in the following dosage sizes and quantities:

Enduronyl (5 mg of methyclothiazide and 0.25 mg of deserpidine) yellow tablets in bottles of 100 and 1000. Also available in ABBO-PAC unit dose packages, 100 tablets, in strips of 10 tablets.

Enduronyl Forte (5 mg of methyclothiazide and 0.5 mg of deserpidine) gray-colored tablets in bottles of 100 and 1000.

*Each component is separately available as Enduron (methyclothiazide) and Harmonyl (deserpidine).

Recommended Storage: Store below 86°F (30°C).

HOW SUPPLIED - EQUIVALENTS NOT AVAILABLE:

Tablet, Uncoated - Oral - 0.25 mg/5 mg

100's $118.05 ENDURONYL, Abbott 00074-6838-01
100's $119.83 ENDURONYL, Abbott 00074-6838-06
1000's $1145.08 ENDURONYL, Abbott 00074-6838-02

Tablet, Uncoated - Oral - 0.5 mg/5 mg

100's $134.91 ENDURONYL FORTE, Abbott 00074-6854-01

DESIPRAMINE HYDROCHLORIDE *(000964)*

CATEGORIES: Antidepressants; Central Nervous System Agents; Depression; Psychostimulants; Psychotherapeutic Agents; Tricyclics; Tricyclic Antidepressants; FDA Approval Pre 1982

BRAND NAMES: *Deprexan*; *Nebril*; **Norpramin**; *Nortimil*; *Perto-Fran*; *Pertofran* (Australia, England, France, Germany); Pertofrane; *Petylyl* (Germany)
(International brand names outside U.S. in italics)

FORMULARIES: Aetna; BC-BS; CIGNA; FHP; Foundation; Humana; Kaiser; Medco; Medi-Cal; PCS; PruCare; United

COST OF THERAPY: $19.63 (Depression; Tablet; 50 mg; 2/day; 90 days) vs. Potential Cost of $2,456.15 (Depression)

PRIMARY ICD9: 311 (Depressive Disorder, Not Elsewhere Classified)

DESCRIPTION:

Desipramine hydrochloride USP tablet form, is an antidepressant drug of the tricyclic type, and is chemically: 5*H*-Dibenz(*b,f*)azepine-5-propanamine, 10,11-dihydro-*N*-methyl-, monohydrochloride

The following inactive ingredients are contained in all Norpramin dosage strengths: acacia, calcium carbonate, corn starch, D&C Red No. 30 and D&C Yellow No. 10 (except 10 mg and 150 mg), FD&C Blue No. 1 (except 50 mg, 75 mg, and 100 mg), hydrogenated soy oil,

DESCRIPTION: *(cont'd)*

iron oxide, light mineral oil, magnesium stearate, mannitol, polyethylene glycol 8000, pregelatinized corn starch, sodium benzoate (except 150 mg), sucrose, talc, titanium dioxide, and other ingredients.

Desipramine hydrochloride USP, capsule form, is a metabolite of imipramine HCl. It is a dibenzazepine derivative, representing the dimethyl analog of imipramine HCl. Chemically it is 10,11-dihydro-5-(3- (methylamino) propyl)-5H-dibenz (b.f.) azepine monohydrochloride, and differs from the parent substance by having only one methyl group on the side chain of nitrogen.

CLINICAL PHARMACOLOGY:

MECHANISM OF ACTION

Available evidence suggests that many depressions have a biochemical basis in the form of a relative deficiency of neurotransmitters such as norepinephrine and serotonin. Norepinephrine deficiency may be associated with relatively low urinary 3-methoxy-4-hydroxyphenyl glycol (MHPG) levels, while serotonin deficiencies may be associated with low spinal fluid levels of 5-hydroxyindoleacetic acid.

While the precise mechanism of action of the tricyclic antidepressants is unknown, a leading theory suggests that they restore normal levels of neurotransmitters by blocking the re-uptake of these substances from the synapse in the central nervous system. Evidence indicates that the secondary amine tricyclic antidepressants, including Desipramine hydrochloride USP, may have greater activity in blocking the re-uptake of norepinephrine. Tertiary amine tricyclic antidepressants, such as amitriptyline, may have greater effect on serotonin re-uptake.

Desipramine hydrochloride is not a monoamine oxidase (MAO) inhibitor and does not act primarily as a central nervous system stimulant. It has been found in some studies to have a more rapid onset of action than imipramine. Earliest therapeutic effects may occasionally be seen in 2 to 5 days, but full treatment benefit usually requires 2 to 3 weeks to obtain.

METABOLISM

Tricyclic antidepressants, such as desipramine hydrochloride, are rapidly absorbed from the gastrointestinal tract. Tricyclic antidepressants or their metabolites are to some extent excreted through the gastric mucosa and reabsorbed from the gastrointestinal tract. Desipramine is metabolized in the liver and approximately 70% is excreted in the urine.

The rate of metabolism of tricyclic antidepressants varies widely from individual to individual, chiefly on a genetically determined basis. Up to a 36-fold difference in plasma level may be noted among individuals taking the same oral dose of desipramine. In general, the elderly metabolize tricyclic antidepressants more slowly than do younger adults.

Certain drugs, particularly the psychostimulants and the phenothiazines, increase plasma levels of concomitantly administered tricyclic antidepressants through competition for the same metabolic enzyme systems. Concurrent administration of cimetidine and tricyclic antidepressants can produce clinically significant increases in the plasma concentrations of the tricyclic antidepressants. Conversely, decreases in plasma levels of the tricyclic antidepressants have been reported upon discontinuation of cimetidine which may result in the loss of the therapeutic efficacy of the tricyclic antidepressant. Other substances, particularly barbiturates and alcohol, induce liver enzyme activity and thereby reduce tricyclic antidepressant plasma levels. Similar effects have been reported with tobacco smoke.

Research on the relationship of plasma level to therapeutic response with the tricyclic antidepressants has produced conflicting results. While some studies report no correlation, many studies cite therapeutic levels for most tricyclics in the range of 50 to 300 nanograms per milliliter. The therapeutic range is different for each tricyclic antidepressant. For desipramine, an optimal range of therapeutic plasma levels has not been established.

INDICATIONS AND USAGE:

Desipramine hydrochloride is indicated for relief of symptoms in various depressive syndromes, especially endogenous depression.

CONTRAINDICATIONS:

Desipramine hydrochloride should not be given in conjunction with, or within 2 weeks of, treatment with an MAO inhibitor drug; hyperpyretic crises, severe convulsions, and death have occurred in patients taking MAO inhibitors and tricyclic antidepressants. When Desipramine hydrochloride is substituted for an MAO inhibitor, at least 2 weeks should elapse between treatments. Desipramine hydrochloride USP should then be started cautiously and should be increased gradually.

The drug is contraindicated in the acute recovery period following myocardial infarction. It should not be used in those who have shown prior hypersensitivity to the drug. Cross-sensitivity between this and other dibenzazepines is a possibility.

WARNINGS:

Extreme caution should be used when this drug is given in the following situations:

a. In patients with cardiovascular disease, because of the possibility of conduction defects, arrhythmias, tachycardias, strokes, and acute myocardial infarction.

b. In patients with a history of urinary retention or glaucoma, because of the anticholinergic properties of the drug.

c. In patients with thyroid disease or those taking thyroid medication, because of the possibility of cardiovascular toxicity, including arrhythmias.

d. In patients with a history of seizure disorder, because this drug has been shown to lower the seizure threshold.

This drug is capable of blocking the antihypertensive effect of guanethidine and similarly acting compounds.

Use In Pregnancy: Safe use of Desipramine hydrochloride during pregnancy and lactation has not been established; therefore, if it is to be given to pregnant patients, nursing mothers, or women of childbearing potential, the possible benefits must be weighed against the possible hazards to mother and child. Animal reproductive studies have been inconclusive.

Usage in Children: Desipramine hydrochloride is not recommended for use in children since safety and effectiveness in the pediatric age group have not been established. (See ADVERSE REACTIONS, Cardiovascular.)

The patient should be cautioned that this drug may impair the mental and/or physical abilities required for the performance of potentially hazardous tasks such as driving a car or operating machinery.

In patients who may use alcohol excessively, it should be borne in mind that the potentiation may increase the danger inherent in any suicide attempt or overdosage.

PRECAUTIONS:

It is important that this drug be dispensed in the least possible quantities to depressed outpatients, since suicide has been accomplished with this class of drug. Ordinary prudence requires that children not have access to this drug or to potent drugs of any kind; if possible, this drug should be dispensed in containers with child-resistant safety closures. Storage of this drug in the home must be supervised responsibly.

PRECAUTIONS: *(cont'd)*

If serious adverse effects occur, dosage should be reduced or treatment should be altered.

Desipramine hydrochloride therapy in patients with manic-depressive illness may induce a hypomanic state after the depressive phase terminates.

The drug may cause exacerbation of psychosis in schizophrenic patients.

Close supervision and careful adjustment of dosage are required when this drug is given concomitantly with anticholinergic or sympathomimetic drugs.

Patients should be warned that while taking this drug their response to alcoholic beverages may be exaggerated.

Clinical experience in the concurrent administration of ECT and antidepressant drugs is limited. Thus, if such treatment is essential, the possibility of increased risk relative to benefits should be considered.

If Desipramine hydrochloride is to be combined with other psychotropic agents such as tranquilizers or sedative/hypnotics, careful consideration should be given to the pharmacology of the agents employed since the sedative effects of Desipramine hydrochloride USP and benzodiazepines (*e.g.,* chlordiazepoxide or diazepam) are additive. Both the sedative and anticholinergic effects of the major tranquilizers are also additive to those of Desipramine hydrochloride USP.

Concurrent administration of cimetidine and tricyclic antidepressants can produce clinically significant increases in the plasma levels of the tricyclic antidepressants (see CLINICAL PHARMACOLOGY, Metabolism.) Conversely, decreases in plasma levels of the tricyclic antidepressants have been reported upon discontinuation of cimetidine which may result in the loss of the therapeutic efficacy of the tricyclic antidepressant.

There have been greater than twofold increases of previously stable plasma levels of tricyclic antidepressants when fluoxetine has been administered in combination with these agents.

This drug should be discontinued as soon as possible prior to elective surgery because of the possible cardiovascular effects. Hypertensive episodes have been observed during surgery in patients taking desipramine hydrochloride.

Both elevation and lowering of blood sugar levels have been reported.

Leukocyte and differential counts should be performed in any patient who develops fever and sore throat during therapy; the drug should be discontinued if there is evidence of pathologic neutrophil depression.

ADVERSE REACTIONS:

Note: Included in the following listing are a few adverse reactions that have not been reported with this specific drug. However, the pharmacologic similarities among the tricyclic antidepressant drugs require that each of the reactions be considered when Desipramine hydrochloride is given.

Cardiovascular: hypotension, hypertension, palpitations, heart block, myocardial infarction, stroke, arrhythmias, premature ventricular contractions, tachycardia, ventricular tachycardia, ventricular fibrillation, sudden death.

There has been a report of an "acute collapse" and "sudden death" in an eight-year old (18 kg) male, treated for two years for hyperactivity. There have been additional reports of sudden death in children. (See WARNINGS, Usage in Children.)

Psychiatric: confusional states (especially in the elderly) with hallucinations, disorientation, delusions; anxiety, restlessness, agitation; insomnia and nightmares; hypomania; exacerbation of psychosis.

Neurologic: numbness, tingling, paresthesias of extremities; incoordination, ataxia, tremors; peripheral neuropathy; extrapyramidal symptoms; seizures; alteration in EEG patterns; tinnitus.

Anticholinergic: dry mouth, and rarely associated sublingual adenitis; blurred vision, disturbance of accommodation, mydriasis, increased intraocular pressure; constipation, paralytic ileus; urinary retention, delayed micturition, dilatation of urinary tract.

Allergic: skin rash, petechiae, urticaria, itching, photosensitization (avoid excessive exposure to sunlight), edema (of face and tongue or general), drug fever, cross sensitivity with other tricyclic drugs.

Hematologic: bone marrow depressions including agranulocytosis, eosinophilia, purpura, thrombocytopenia.

Gastrointestinal: anorexia, nausea and vomiting, epigastric distress, peculiar taste, abdominal cramps, diarrhea, stomatitis, black tongue, hepatitis, jaundice (simulating obstructive), altered liver function, elevated liver function tests, increased pancreatic enzymes.

Endocrine: gynecomastia in the male, breast enlargement and galactorrhea in the female; increased or decreased libido, impotence, painful ejaculation, testicular swelling; elevation or depression of blood sugar levels; syndrome of inappropriate antidiuretic hormone secretion (SIADH).

Other: weight gain or loss; perspiration, flushing; urinary frequency, nocturia; parotid swelling; drowsiness, dizziness, weakness and fatigue, headache; fever; alopecia; elevated alkaline phosphatase.

Withdrawal Symptoms: Though not indicative of addiction, abrupt cessation of treatment after prolonged therapy may produce nausea, headache, and malaise.

OVERDOSAGE:

SIGNS, SYMPTOMS, AND LABORATORY FINDINGS

Signs and symptoms of toxicity with tricyclic antidepressants most often involve the cardiovascular and central nervous systems. Overdosage with this class of drugs has resulted in death. Within a few hours of ingestion, the patient may become agitated, restless, confused, delirious or stuporous, and then comatose. Mydriasis, dry mucous membranes, vomiting, urinary retention, and diminished bowel sounds may occur. Hypotension, shock, respiratory depression, and renal shutdown may ensue. Generalized seizures, both early and later after ingestion, have been reported. Hyperactive reflexes, hyperpyrexia, and muscle rigidity can occur. ECG evidence of impaired conduction and serious disturbances of cardiac rate, rhythm, and output may occur. The duration of the QRS complex on ECG may be a helpful guide to the severity of tricyclic overdose. Physicians should be aware that relapses may occur after apparent recovery.

Oral LD_{50}: The oral LD_{50} of desipramine is 290 mg/kg in male mice and 320 mg/kg in female rats.

TOXIC AND LETHAL DOSES/PLASMA LEVELS

In humans, doses at 10-30 times the usual daily dosage have been considered within the lethal range. The lethal dose for children and geriatric patients would be lower than that for the general adult population. Serious adverse events in general are more frequently associated with plasma levels in excess of 1000 ng/ml.

DIALYSIS

After overdosage, low plasma desipramine concentrations are found because of the drug's large volume of distribution in the body. Forced diuresis and hemodialysis are, therefore, ineffective in removing tricyclic antidepressants.

OVERDOSAGE: *(cont'd)*

TREATMENT

There is no specific antidote for desipramine overdosage, nor are there specific phenomena of diagnostic value characterizing poisoning by the drug.

Because CNS involvement, respiratory depression, and cardiac arrhythmia can occur suddenly, hospitalization and close observation are generally advisable, even when the amount ingested is thought to be small or the initial degree of intoxication appears slight or moderate. Aggressive supportive therapy of cardiac, neurologic, or acid-base disturbances may be necessary.

The initial phase of therapy in a tricyclic antidepressant overdose should be devoted to protection of the patient's airway, stabilization of the vital signs, establishing an intravenous line, obtaining an ECG, and initiating continuous cardiac monitoring, and maintaining renal output. It should be remembered that rapid deterioration of vital signs, seizures, respiratory failure, and ventricular arrhythmias are common during the first twenty-four hours after ingestion.

Ventricular arrhythmias and intraventricular conduction abnormalities may respond to administration of sodium bicarbonate to correct the metabolic acidosis. During alkalinization, the patient's electrolytes and renal function must be closely monitored with frequent laboratory determinations. Arrhythmias may be treated with standard antiarrhythmic therapy (*e.g.*, lidocaine). Physostigmine may be used with caution to reverse severe cardiovascular abnormalities or coma; too rapid administration may result in seizures.

If the patient is hypotensive, supportive measures (*e.g.*, intravenous fluids) should be used. Vasopressor agents may be used with caution if necessary.

If the patient develops seizures, intravenous diazepam may be used. In addition, longer acting anticonvulsants (*e.g.*, barbiturates) may be necessary for repetitive seizures.

Once the patient is stabilized, gastric lavage with a large bore orogastric tube should be used to evacuate the stomach. The physician must be prepared to protect the airway by endotracheal intubation if seizures or loss of consciousness occur prior to completion of the lavage procedure. Because of the potential for rapid onset of life-threatening events, emesis should not be used to empty the stomach. Activated charcoal (as single or repeated doses) in a water slurry should be given by mouth or instilled through the lavage tube.

Additional information regarding treatment of overdosage may be available from poison control centers.

DOSAGE AND ADMINISTRATION:

Tablets: Not recommended for use in children.

Lower dosages are recommended for elderly patients and adolescents. Lower dosages are also recommended for outpatients compared to hospitalized patients, who are closely supervised. Dosage should be initiated at a low level and increased according to clinical response and any evidence of intolerance. Following remission, maintenance medication may be required for a period of time and should be at the lowest dose that will maintain remission.

USUAL ADULT DOSE

The usual adult dose is 100 to 200 mg per day. In more severely ill patients, dosage may be further increased gradually to 300 mg/day if necessary. Dosages above 300 mg/day are not recommended.

Dosage should be initiated at a lower level and increased according to tolerance and clinical response.

Treatment of patients requiring as much as 300 mg should generally be initiated in hospitals, where regular visits by the physician, skilled nursing care, and frequent electrocardiograms (ECG's) are available.

The best available evidence of impending toxicity from very high doses of Desipramine hydrochloride USP is prolongation of the QRS or QT intervals on the ECG. Prolongation of the PR interval is also significant, but less closely correlated with plasma levels. Clinical symptoms of intolerance, especially drowsiness, dizziness, and postural hypotension, should also alert the physician to the need for reduction in dosage. Plasma desipramine measurement would constitute the optimal guide to dosage monitoring.

Initial therapy may be administered in divided doses or a single daily dose.

Maintenance therapy may be given on a once-daily schedule for patient convenience and compliance.

ADOLESCENT AND GERIATRIC DOSE

The usual adolescent and geriatric dose is 25 to 100 mg daily.

Dosage should be initiated at a lower level and increased according to tolerance and clinical response to a usual maximum of 100 mg daily. In more severely ill patients, dosage may be further increased to 150 mg/day. Doses above 150 mg/day are not recommended in these age groups.

Initial therapy may be administered in divided doses or a single daily dose.

Maintenance therapy may be given on a once-daily schedule for patient convenience and compliance.

(Marion Merrell Dow, 11/93)

HOW SUPPLIED - RATED THERAPEUTICALLY EQUIVALENT:

Tablet, Plain Coated - Oral - 10 mg

100's	$15.75	Desipramine Hydrochloride, United Res	00677-1245-01
100's	$25.95	Desipramine HCl, Geneva Pharms	00781-1971-01
100's	**$50.40**	**NORPRAMIN, Hoechst Marion Roussel**	**00068-0007-01**

Tablet, Plain Coated - Oral - 25 mg

100's	$7.14	Desipramine HCl, H.C.F.A. F F P	99999-0964-01
100's	$9.38	Desipramine Hcl, United Res	00677-1198-01
100's	$12.63	Desipramine Hcl, US Trading	56126-0376-11
100's	$16.80	Desipramine Hcl, IDE-Interstate	00814-2300-14
100's	$18.00	Desipramine Hcl, Raway	00686-0489-20
100's	$19.95	Desipramine Hcl, Eon Labs Mfg	00185-0019-01
100's	$23.06	Desipramine Hcl, Major Pharms	00904-1581-61
100's	$23.48	Desipramine Hcl, Qualitest Pharms	00603-3166-21
100's	$23.50	Desipramine Hcl, Sidmak Labs	50111-0436-01
100's	$23.90	NODAMINE, Major Pharms	00904-1570-60
100's	$24.00	Desipramine Hcl, Goldline Labs	00182-1332-01
100's	$25.50	Desipramine HCl, Schein Pharm (US)	00364-2209-01
100's	$26.20	Desipramine Hcl, Martec Pharms	52555-0564-01
100's	$26.72	Desipramine Hcl, HL Moore Drug Exch	00839-7551-06
100's	$26.78	Desipramine HCl, Teva	00093-0325-01
100's	$27.00	Desipramine HCl, Rugby	00536-4881-01
100's	$27.37	Desipramine Hcl, Aligen Independ	00405-4305-01
100's	$27.90	Desipramine HCl, Warner Chilcott	00047-0594-24
100's	$27.95	Desipramine HCl, Geneva Pharms	00781-1972-01
100's	$28.00	Desipramine Hcl, Parmed Pharms	00349-8728-01
100's	$42.00	Desipramine Hcl, Medirex	57480-0318-01
100's	$45.00	Desipramine Hcl, Goldline Labs	00182-1332-89
100's	$46.35	Desipramine Hcl, Vangard Labs	00615-3509-13
100's	$46.36	Desipramine HCl, Geneva Pharms	00781-1972-13

HOW SUPPLIED - RATED THERAPEUTICALLY EQUIVALENT: *(cont'd)*

100's	**$60.60**	**NORPRAMIN, Hoechst Marion Roussel**	**00068-0011-01**
100's	**$65.10**	**NORPRAMIN, Hoechst Marion Roussel**	**00068-0011-61**
500's	$35.70	Desipramine HCl, H.C.F.A. F F P	99999-0964-02
500's	$92.50	Desipramine Hcl, Eon Labs Mfg	00185-0019-05
500's	$101.60	NODAMINE, Major Pharms	00904-1570-40
500's	$122.85	Desipramine HCl, Rugby	00536-4881-05
600's	$170.20	Desipramine Hcl, Medirex	57480-0318-06
1000's	$71.40	Desipramine HCl, H.C.F.A. F F P	99999-0964-03
1000's	$89.99	Desipramine Hcl, Balan	00304-1848-00
1000's	$93.80	Desipramine Hcl, Sidmak Labs	50111-0436-03
1000's	$150.00	Desipramine Hcl, Goldline Labs	00182-1332-10
1000's	$186.40	Desipramine Hcl, Major Pharms	00904-1564-80
1000's	$186.40	Desipramine Hcl, Major Pharms	00904-1570-80
1000's	$189.50	Desipramine Hcl, Eon Labs Mfg	00185-0019-10
1000's	$214.30	Desipramine Hcl, Qualitest Pharms	00603-3166-32
1000's	$214.35	Desipramine HCl, Geneva Pharms	00781-1972-10
1000's	$215.25	Desipramine Hcl, Parmed Pharms	00349-8728-10
1000's	$216.66	Desipramine Hcl, HL Moore Drug Exch	00839-7551-16
1000's	**$445.20**	**NORPRAMIN, Hoechst Marion Roussel**	**00068-0011-10**

Tablet, Plain Coated - Oral - 50 mg

100's	$10.91	Desipramine HCl, H.C.F.A. F F P	99999-0964-04
100's	$14.85	Desipramine Hcl, United Res	00677-1199-01
100's	$17.19	Desipramine Hcl, US Trading	56126-0377-11
100's	$25.28	Desipramine Hcl, IDE-Interstate	00814-2301-14
100's	$30.00	Desipramine Hcl, Raway	00686-0490-20
100's	$36.90	Desipramine Hcl, Talbert Phcy	44514-0495-88
100's	$37.50	Desipramine Hcl, Eon Labs Mfg	00185-0721-01
100's	$42.56	Desipramine Hcl 50, Aligen Independ	00405-4306-01
100's	$43.19	Desipramine Hcl, Major Pharms	00904-1565-61
100's	$43.19	Desipramine Hcl, Major Pharms	00904-1582-61
100's	$47.50	Desipramine Hcl, Major Pharms	00904-1565-60
100's	$47.50	NODAMINE, Major Pharms	00904-1571-60
100's	$48.10	Desipramine Hcl, Qualitest Pharms	00603-3167-21
100's	$48.20	Desipramine Hcl Tabs., 50, Goldline Labs	00182-1333-01
100's	$48.20	Desipramine Hcl, Sidmak Labs	50111-0437-01
100's	$48.83	Desipramine HCl, Schein Pharm (US)	00364-2210-01
100's	$49.53	Desipramine HCl, Teva	00093-0326-01
100's	$49.53	Desipramine Hcl, Medirex	57480-0319-01
100's	$49.65	Desipramine Hcl, Martec Pharms	52555-0565-01
100's	$52.00	Desipramine Hcl, Parmed Pharms	00349-8729-01
100's	$52.72	Desipramine Hcl, HL Moore Drug Exch	00839-7552-06
100's	$59.30	Desipramine HCl, Geneva Pharms	00781-1973-01
100's	$59.35	Desipramine HCl, Warner Chilcott	00047-0595-24
100's	$59.35	Desipramine HCl, Rugby	00536-4882-01
100's	$62.12	Desipramine HCl, Geneva Pharms	00781-1973-13
100's	$63.00	Desipramine Hcl, Goldline Labs	00182-1333-89
100's	$66.15	Desipramine Hcl, Vangard Labs	00615-3510-13
100's	**$113.94**	**NORPRAMIN, Hoechst Marion Roussel**	**00068-0015-01**
100's	**$123.06**	**NORPRAMIN, Hoechst Marion Roussel**	**00068-0015-61**
500's	$54.55	Desipramine HCl, H.C.F.A. F F P	99999-0964-05
500's	$169.30	NODAMINE, Major Pharms	00904-1571-40
500's	$179.95	Desipramine Hcl, Eon Labs Mfg	00185-0721-05
500's	$267.08	Desipramine HCl, Rugby	00536-4882-05
600's	$320.80	Desipramine Hcl, Medirex	57480-0319-06
1000's	$109.10	Desipramine HCl, H.C.F.A. F F P	99999-0964-06
1000's	$119.99	Desipramine Hcl, Balan	00304-1849-00
1000's	$148.50	Desipramine Hcl, Sidmak Labs	50111-0437-03
1000's	$277.20	Desipramine Hcl Tabs., 50, Goldline Labs	00182-1333-10
1000's	$316.00	NODAMINE, Major Pharms	00904-1571-80
1000's	$369.00	Desipramine Hcl, Eon Labs Mfg	00185-0721-10
1000's	$402.80	Desipramine Hcl, Parmed Pharms	00349-8729-10
1000's	$427.53	Desipramine Hcl, HL Moore Drug Exch	00839-7552-16
1000's	$440.81	Desipramine Hcl, Qualitest Pharms	00603-3167-32
1000's	$475.05	Desipramine HCl, Geneva Pharms	00781-1973-10
1000's	**$834.42**	**NORPRAMIN, Hoechst Marion Roussel**	**00068-0015-10**

Tablet, Plain Coated - Oral - 75 mg

100's	$12.42	Desipramine HCl, H.C.F.A. F F P	99999-0964-07
100's	$17.18	Desipramine Hcl, United Res	00677-1210-01
100's	$39.77	Desipramine Hcl, Vangard Labs	00615-3526-13
100's	$45.00	Desipramine Hcl, Eon Labs Mfg	00185-0722-01
100's	$50.00	Desipramine Hcl, Raway	00686-0491-20
100's	$54.15	Desipramine Hcl 75, Aligen Independ	00405-4307-01
100's	$54.88	Desipramine Hcl, Major Pharms	00904-1583-61
100's	$55.25	Desipramine Hcl, Medirex	57480-0320-01
100's	$56.35	Desipramine HCl, Schein Pharm (US)	00364-2243-01
100's	$58.10	Desipramine Hcl., Tabs., 75, Goldline Labs	00182-1335-01
100's	$58.10	Desipramine Hcl, Sidmak Labs	50111-0438-01
100's	$58.15	Desipramine Hcl, Qualitest Pharms	00603-3168-21
100's	$58.30	Desipramine Hcl, Parmed Pharms	00349-8764-01
100's	$59.85	Desipramine Hcl, Martec Pharms	52555-0566-01
100's	$59.90	Desipramine Hcl, Major Pharms	00904-1566-60
100's	$59.90	Desipramine Hcl, Major Pharms	00904-1572-60
100's	$61.15	Desipramine HCl, Teva	00093-0327-01
100's	$62.84	Desipramine Hcl, HL Moore Drug Exch	00839-7553-06
100's	$65.00	Desipramine Hcl, Goldline Labs	00182-1335-89
100's	$72.05	Desipramine HCl, Geneva Pharms	00781-1974-01
100's	$72.10	Desipramine HCl, Warner Chilcott	00047-0596-24
100's	$72.10	Desipramine HCl, Rugby	00536-4883-01
100's	**$145.08**	**NORPRAMIN, Hoechst Marion Roussel**	**00068-0019-01**
500's	$62.10	Desipramine HCl, H.C.F.A. F F P	99999-0964-08
500's	$215.00	Desipramine Hcl, Eon Labs Mfg	00185-0722-05
1000's	$124.20	Desipramine HCl, H.C.F.A. F F P	99999-0964-09
1000's	$171.80	Desipramine Hcl, Sidmak Labs	50111-0438-03

Tablet, Plain Coated - Oral - 100 mg

100's	$40.89	Desipramine HCl, H.C.F.A. F F P	99999-0964-10
100's	$52.50	Desipramine Hcl, Eon Labs Mfg	00185-0736-01
100's	$74.30	Desipramine Hcl, United Res	00677-1211-01
100's	$84.77	Desipramine Hcl 100, HL Moore Drug Exch	00839-7412-06
100's	$100.00	Desipramine Hcl, Goldline Labs	00182-1316-01
100's	$106.74	Desipramine Hcl, Rugby	00536-4958-01
100's	$106.75	Desipramine HCl, Geneva Pharms	00781-1975-01
100's	$110.10	Desipramine HCl, Rugby	00536-4884-01
100's	$110.10	Desipramine Hcl, Major Pharms	00904-1573-60
100's	**$190.56**	**NORPRAMIN, Hoechst Marion Roussel**	**00068-0020-01**
500's	$204.45	Desipramine HCl, H.C.F.A. F F P	99999-0964-11
500's	$249.95	Desipramine Hcl, Eon Labs Mfg	00185-0736-05

Tablet, Plain Coated - Oral - 150 mg

50's	$109.95	Desipramine HCl, Geneva Pharms	00781-1976-50
50's	**$138.06**	**NORPRAMIN, Hoechst Marion Roussel**	**00068-0021-50**

DESMOPRESSIN ACETATE *(000966)*

CATEGORIES: Antidiuretics; Bleeding; Diabetes; Diabetes Insipidus; Enuresis; Hemophilia; Hemostatics; Hormones; Orphan Drugs; Pituitary; Polydipsia; Polyuria; Rhinitis; Von Willebrand's Disease; Pregnancy Category B; FDA Approval Pre 1982

BRAND NAMES: DDAVP; *DDAVP Desmopressin*; *Defirin*; *Desmopressin Nasal Solution* (Japan); *Desmospray* (England); *Minirin* (Australia, France, Germany); *Minirin DDAVP*; *Minirin DDAVP*; *Minirin Nasal Spray* (Australia); *Minrin*; *Minurin*; *Octostim*; Stimate
(International brand names outside U.S. in italics)

FORMULARIES: Aetna; BC-BS; Medi-Cal; WHO

DESCRIPTION:

Desmopressin acetate—nasal spray, rhinal tube, and injection) is an antidiuretic hormone affecting renal water conservation and a synthetic analogue of 8-arginine vasopressin. It is chemically defined as follows:

Empirical formula:$C_{48}H_{74}N_{14}O_{17}S_2$

SCH_2CH_2CO-Tyr-Phe-Gln-Asn-Cys-Pro-D-Arg-Gly-$NH_2 \cdot C_2H_4O_2 \cdot 3H_2O$ 1-(3-mercaptopropionic acid)-8-D-arginine vasopressin monoacetate (salt) trihydrate.

Molecular Weight is 1183.2

NASAL SPRAY/RHINAL TUBE

Desmopressin is provided as a sterile, aqueous solution for intranasal use. Each ml contains:

Desmopressin acetate - 0.1 mg

Chlorobutanol - 5.0 mg

Sodium Chloride - 9.0 mg

Hydrochloric acid to adjust pH to approximately 4.0

The desmopressin nasal spray compression pump delivers 0.1 ml (10 mcg) of desmopressin per spray.

INJECTION

Desmopressin is provided as a sterile, aqueous solution for injection. Each ml contains:

Desmopressin acetate - 4.0 mcg

Sodium Chloride - 9.0 mg

Hydrochloric acid to adjust pH to 4.0

The 10 ml vial contains chlorobutanol as a preservative (5.0 mg/ml).

CLINICAL PHARMACOLOGY:

Desmopressin contains as active substance 1-(3-mercaptopropionic acid)-8-D-arginine vasopressin, which is a synthetic analogue of the natural hormone arginine vasopressin. One ml (0.1 mg) of desmopressin has an antidiuretic activity of about 400 IU; 10 mcg of desmopressin acetate is equivalent to 40 IU.

The biphasic half-lives for desmopressin were 7.8 and 75.5 minutes for the fast and slow phases, compared with 2.5 and 14.5 minutes for lysine vasopressin, another form of the hormone used in this condition. As a result, desmopressin provides a prompt onset of antidiuretic action with a long duration after each administration. 2. The change in structure of arginine vasopressin to desmopressin has resulted in a decreased vasopressor action and decreased actions on visceral smooth muscle relative to the enhanced antidiuretic activity, so that clinically effective antidiuretic doses are usually below threshold levels for effects on vascular or visceral smooth muscle. 3. Desmopressin administered intranasally has an antidiuretic effect about one-tenth that of an equivalent dose administered by injection.

INJECTION ONLY

One ml (4 mcg) of desmopressin acetate solution has an antidiuretic activity of about 16 IU; 1 mcg of desmopressin is equivalent to 4 IU.

Desmopressin has been shown to be more potent than arginine vasopressin in increasing plasma levels of factor VIII activity in patients with hemophilia and von Willebrand's disease Type I.

Dose-response studies were performed in healthy persons, using doses of 0.1 to 0.4 mcg/kg body weight, infused over a 10-minute period. Maximal dose response occurred at 0.3 to 0.4 mcg/kg. The response to desmopressin of factor VIII activity and plasminogen activator is dose-related, with maximal plasma levels of 300 to 400 percent of initial concentrations obtained after infusion of 0.4 mcg/kg body weight. The increase is rapid and evident within 30 minutes, reaching a maximum at a point ranging from 90 minutes to two hours. The factor VII related antigen and ristocetin cofactor activity were also increased to a smaller degree, but still are dose-dependent.

The bioavailability of the subcutaneous route of administration was determined qualitatively using urine output data. The extract fraction of drug absorbed by that route of administration has not been quantitatively determined.

The percentage increase of factor VIII levels in patients with mild hemophilia A and von Willebrand's disease was not significantly different from that observed in normal healthy individuals when treated with 0.3 mcg/kg of desmopressin infused over 10 minutes.

Plasminogen activator activity increases rapidly after desmopressin infusion, but there has been no clinically significant fibrinolysis in patient treated with desmopressin.

The effect of repeated desmopressin administration when doses were given every 12 to 24 hours has generally shown a gradual diminution of the factor VIII activity increase noted with a single dose. The initial response is reproducible in any particular patient if there are 2 or 3 days between administrations.

INDICATIONS AND USAGE:

NASAL SPRAY/RHINAL TUBE

Primary Nocturnal Enuresis

Nasal Spray/Rhinal Tube: Desmopressin is indicated for the management of primary nocturnal enuresis. It may be used alone or adjunctive to behavioral conditioning or other non-pharmacological intervention. It has been shown to be effective in some cases that are refractory to conventional therapies.

CENTRAL CRANIAL DIABETES INSIPIDUS

Nasal Spray/Rhinal Tube/Injection: Desmopressin is indicated as antidiuretic replacement therapy in the management of central cranial diabetes insipidus and for management of the temporary polyuria and polydipsia following head trauma or surgery in the pituitary region. It is ineffective for the treatment of nephrogenic diabetes insipidus.

The use of desmopressin in patients with an established diagnosis will result in a reduction in urinary output with increase in urine osmolality and a decrease in plasma osmolality. This will allow the resumption of a more normal life-style with a decrease in urinary frequency and nocturia.

INDICATIONS AND USAGE: *(cont'd)*

There are reports of an occasional change in response with time, usually greater than 6 months. Some patients may show a decreased responsiveness, others a shortened duration of effect. There is no evidence this effect is due to the development of binding antibodies but may be due to a local inactivation of the peptide.

Patients are selected for therapy by establishing the diagnosis by means of the water deprivation test, the hypertonic saline infusion test, and/or the response to antidiuretic hormone. Continued response to desmopressin can be monitored by urine volume and osmolality.

Desmopressin is also available as a solution for injection when the intranasal route may be compromised. These situations include nasal congestion and blockage, nasal discharge, atrophy of nasal mucosa, and severe atrophic rhinitis. Intranasal delivery may also be inappropriate where there is an impaired level of consciousness. In addition, cranial surgical procedures, such as transsphenoidal hypophysectomy create situations where an alternative route of administration is needed as in cases of nasal packing or recovery from surgery.

HEMOPHILIA A

Injection: Desmopressin injection is indicated for patients with hemophilia A with factor VIII coagulant activity levels greater than 5%.

Desmopressin will often maintain hemostasis in patients with hemophilia A during surgical procedures and postoperatively when administered 30 minutes prior to scheduled procedure.

Desmopressin will also stop bleeding in hemophilia A patients with episodes of spontaneous or trauma-induced injuries such as hemarthroses, intramuscular hematoses or mucosal bleeding.

Desmopressin is not indicated for the treatment of hemophilia A with factor VII coagulant activity levels equal to or less than 5%, or for the treatment of hemophilia B, or in patients who should have factor VIII antibodies.

In certain clinical situations, it may be justified to try desmopressin in patients with factor VIII levels between 2%-5%; however, these patients should be carefully monitored.

VON WILLEBRAND'S DISEASE (TYPE I)

Injection: Desmopressin injection is indicated for patients with mild to moderate classic von Willebrand's disease (Type I) with factor VIII levels greater than 5%. Desmopressin will often maintain hemostasis in patients with mild to moderate von Willebrand's disease during surgical procedure and postoperatively when administered 30 minutes prior to the scheduled procedure.

Desmopressin will usually stop bleeding in mild to moderate von Willebrand's patients with episodes of spontaneous or trauma-induced injuries such as hemarthroses, intramuscular hematoses or mucosal bleeding.

Those von Willebrand's disease patients who are least likely to respond are those with severe homozygous von Willebrand's disease with factor VIII coagulant activity and factor VIII von Willebrand's factor antigen levels less than 1%. Other patients may respond in a variable fashion depending on the type of molecular defect they have. Bleeding time and factor VIII coagulant activity, ristocetin cofactor activity, and von Willebrand's factor antigen should be checked during administration of desmopressin to ensure that adequate levels are being achieved.

Desmopressin is not indicated for the treatment of severe classic von Willebrand's disease (Type I) and when there is evidence of an abnormal molecular form of factor VIII antigen. (See WARNINGS.)

DIABETES INSIPIDUS

Injection: Desmopressin injection is indicated as antidiuretic replacement therapy in the management of central (cranial) diabetes insipidus and for the management of the temporary polyuria and polydipsia following head trauma or surgery in the pituitary region. Desmopressin is ineffective for the treatment of nephrogenic diabetes insipidus.

Desmopressin is also available as an intranasal preparation. However, this means of delivery can be compromised by a variety of factors that can make nasal insufflation ineffective or inappropriate. These include poor intranasal absorption, nasal congestion and blockage, nasal discharge, atrophy of nasal mucosa, and severe atrophic rhinitis. Intranasal delivery may be inappropriate where there is an impaired level of consciousness. In addition, cranial surgical procedures, such as transsphenoidal hypophysectomy, create situations where an alternative route of administration is needed as in cases of nasal packing or recovery from surgery.

CONTRAINDICATIONS:

Known hypersensitivity to desmopressin.

WARNINGS:

NASAL SPRAY/RHINAL TUBE

1. For intranasal use only.

2. In very young and elderly patients in particular, fluid intake should be adjusted in order to decrease the potential occurrence of water intoxication and hyponatremia. Particular attention should be paid to the possibility of the rare occurrence of an extreme decrease in plasma osmolality that may result in seizures which could lead to coma.

INJECTION

Patients who do not have need of antidiuretic hormone and for its diuretic effect, in particularly those who are young or elderly, should be cautioned to ingest only enough fluid to satisfy thirst, in order to decrease the potential occurrence of water intoxication and hyponatremia.

Fluid intake should be adjusted, particularly in very young and elderly patients, in order to decrease the potential occurrence of water intoxication and hyponatremia. Particular attention should be paid to the possibility of the rare occurrence of an extreme decrease in plasma molality that may result in seizures which could lead to coma.

Desmopressin should not be used to treat patients with type IIB von Willebrand's disease since platelet aggregation may be induced.

PRECAUTIONS:

GENERAL

Nasal Spray/Rhinal Tube

Desmopressin at high dosage has infrequently produced a slight elevation of blood pressure, which disappeared with a reduction in dosage. The drug should be used with caution in patients with coronary artery insufficiency and/or hypertensive cardiovascular disease because of possible rise in blood pressure.

Desmopressin should be used with caution in patients with conditions associated with fluid and electrolyte imbalance, such as cystic fibrosis, because these patients are prone to hyponatremia.

Central Cranial Diabetes Insipidus: Since desmopressin is used intranasally, changes in the nasal mucosa such as scarring, edema, or other disease may cause erratic, unreliable absorption in which case desmopressin should not be used. For such situations, desmopressin injection should be considered.

PRECAUTIONS: *(cont'd)*

Primary Nocturnal Enuresis: If changes in the nasal mucosa have occurred, unreliable absorption may result. Desmopressin should be discontinued until the nasal problems resolve.

Injection

For injection use only.

Desmopressin Injection (desmopressin acetate) has infrequently produced changes in blood pressure causing either a slight elevation in blood pressure or a transient fall in blood pressure and a compensatory increase in heart rate. The drug should be used with caution in patients with coronary artery insufficiency and/or hypertensive cardiovascular disease.

Desmopressin Injection should be used with caution in patients with conditions associated with fluid and electrolyte imbalance, such as cystic fibrosis, because these patients are prone to hyponatremia.

There have been rare reports of thrombotic events following desmopressin Injection in patients predisposed to thrombus formation. No causality has been determined, however, the drug should be used with caution in these patients.

Severe allergic reactions have been reported rarely. Fatal anaphylaxis has been reported in one patient who received intravenous desmopressin. It is not known whether antibodies to desmopressin injection are produced after repeated injections.

Hemophilia A: Laboratory tests for assessing patient status include levels of factor VIII coagulant, factor VIII antigen and factor VIII ristocetin cofactor (von Willebrand factor) as well as activated partial thromboplastin time. Factor VIII coagulant agulant activity should be determined before giving desmopressin for hemostasis. If factor VIII coagulant activity is present at less than 5% of normal, desmopressin should not be relied.

von Willebrand's Disease: Laboratory tests doe assessing patient status include levels of factor VIII coagulant activity, factor VIII ristocetin cofactor activity, and factor VIII von Willebrand factor antigen. The skin bleeding time may be helpful in following these patients.

Diabetes Insipidus: Laboratory tests for monitoring the patient include urine volume and osmolality. In some cases, plasma osmolality may be required.

INFORMATION FOR THE PATIENT

Nasal Spray/Rhinal Tube: Patients should be informed that the bottle accurately delivers 50 doses of 10 mcg each. Any solution remaining after 50 doses should be discarded since the amount delivered thereafter may be substantially less than 10 mcg of drug. No attempt should be made to transfer remaining solution to another bottle. Patients should be instructed to read accompanying directions on use of the spray pump carefully before use.

LABORATORY TESTS

Nasal Spray/Rhinal Tube: Laboratory tests for following the patient with central cranial diabetes insipidus or post-surgical or head trauma-related polyuria and polydipsia include urine volume and osmolality. In some cases plasma osmolality may be required. For the healthy patient with primary nocturnal enuresis, serum electrolytes should be checked at least once if therapy is continued beyond 7 days.

CARCINOGENESIS, MUTAGENESIS, AND IMPAIRMENT OF FERTILITY

Teratology studies in rats have shown no abnormalities. No further information is available.

PREGNANCY CATEGORY B

Reproduction studies performed in rats and rabbits with doses up to 12.5 times the human intranasal dose (*i.e.*, about 125 times the total adult human dose given systemically) have revealed no evidence of harm to the fetus due to desmopressin acetate. There are several publications of management of diabetes insipidus in pregnant women with no harm to the fetus reported; however, no controlled studies in pregnant women have been carried out. Published reports stress that, as opposed to preparations containing the natural hormones, desmopressin acetate in antidiuretic doses has no uterotonic action, but the physician will have to weigh possible therapeutic advantages against possible danger in each individual case.

NURSING MOTHERS

Nasal Spray/Rhinal Tube: There have been no controlled studies in nursing mothers. A single study in a post-partum woman demonstrated a marked change in plasma, but little if any change in assayable desmopressin Nasal Spray in breast milk following an intranasal dose of 10 mcg.

Injection: It is not known whether this drug is excreted in human milk. Because of the many drugs are excreted in human milk, caution should be exercised when desmopressin is administered to a nursing woman.

PEDIATRIC USE

Nasal Spray/Rhinal Tube

Primary Nocturnal Enuresis: Desmopressin has been used in childhood nocturnal enuresis. Short-term (4-8 weeks) desmopressin administration has been shown to be safe and modestly effective in children aged 6 years or older with severe childhood nocturnal enuresis. Adequately controlled studies with desmopressin in primary nocturnal enuresis have not been conducted beyond 4-8 weeks. The dose should be individually adjusted to achieve the best results.

Central Cranial Diabetes Insipidus: Desmopressin Nasal Spray has been used in children with diabetes insipidus. Use in infants and children will require careful fluid intake restriction to prevent possible hyponatremia and water intoxication. The dose must be individually adjusted to the patient with attention in the very young to the danger of an extreme decrease in plasma osmolality with resulting convulsions. Dose should start at 0.05 ml or less.

Since the spray cannot deliver less than 0.1 ml (10 mcg), smaller doses should be administered using the rhinal tube delivery system. Do not use the nasal spray in pediatric patients requiring less than 0.1 ml (10 mcg) per dose.

There are reports of an occasional charge in response with time, usually greater than 6 months. Some patients may show a decreased responsiveness, others a shortened duration of effect. There is no evidence this effect is due to the development of binding antibodies but may be due to a local inactivation of the peptide.

Injection

Use in infants and children will require careful fluid intake restriction to prevent possible hyponatremia and water intoxication. *Desmopressin injection should not be used in infants younger than three months* in the treatment of hemophilia A or von Willebrand's disease; safety and effectiveness in children under 12 years of age with diabetes insipidus have not been established.

DRUG INTERACTIONS:

Nasal Spray/Rhinal Tube/Injection: Although the pressor activity of desmopressin is very low compared to the antidiuretic activity, use of large doses of desmopressin with other pressor agents should only be done with careful patient monitoring.

Injection Only: Although the pressor activity of desmopressin is very low compared with the antidiuretic activity, use of the doses as large as 0.3 mcg/kg of desmopressin with other pressor agents should be done only with careful patient monitoring.

Desmopressin has been used with epsilon aminocaproic acid without adverse effects.

ADVERSE REACTIONS:

NASAL SPRAY/RHINAL TUBE

Infrequently, high dosages have produced transient headache and nausea. Nasal congestion, rhinitis and flushing have also been reported occasionally along with mild abdominal cramps. These symptoms disappeared with reduction in dosage. Nosebleed, sore throat, cough and upper respiratory infections have also been reported.

TABLE 1 lists the percent of patients having adverse experiences without regard to relationship to study drug from the pooled pivotal study data for nocturnal enuresis.

TABLE 1

Adverse Reactions	PLACEBO (N=59) %	DDAVP 20 mcg (N=60) %	DDAVP 40 mcg (N=61) %
Body As A Whole			
Abdominal Pain	0	2	2
Asthenia	0	0	2
Chills	0	0	2
Headache	0	2	5
Throat Pain	2	0	0
Nervous System			
Depression	2	0	0
Dizziness	0	0	3
Respiratory System			
Epistaxis	2	3	0
Nostril Pain	0	2	0
Respiratory Infection	2	0	0
Rhinitis	2	8	3
Cardiovascular System			
Vasodilation	2	0	0
Digestive System			
Gastrointestinal Disorder	0	2	0
Nausea	0	0	2
Skin & Appendages			
Leg Rash	2	0	0
Rash	2	0	0
Special Senses			
Conjunctivitis	0	2	0
Edema Eyes	0	2	0
Lachrymation Disorder	0	0	2

INJECTION

Infrequently, desmopressin has produced transient headache, nausea, mild abdominal cramps and vulval pain. These symptoms disappeared with reduction in dosage. Occasionally, injection of desmopressin has produced local erythema, swelling or burning pain. Occasional facial flushing has been reported with the administration of desmopressin.

Desmopressin injection has infrequently produced changes in blood pressure causing either a slight elevation or a transient fall and a compensatory increase in heart rate.

See WARNINGS for the possibility of water intoxication and hyponatremia.

There have been rare reports of thrombotic events (acute cerebrovascular thrombosis, acute myocardial infarction) following desmopressin Injection in patients predisposed to thrombus formulation.

OVERDOSAGE:

See ADVERSE REACTIONS. In case of overdosage, the dose should be reduced, frequency of administration decreased, or the drug withdrawn according to the severity of the condition.

There is no known specific antidote for desmopressin.

An oral LD_{50} has not been established. An intravenous dose of 2 mg/kg in mice demonstrated no effect.

DOSAGE AND ADMINISTRATION:

NASAL SPRAY/RHINAL SPRAY

Primary Nocturnal Enuresis: Dosage should be adjusted according to the individual. The recommended initial dose for those 6 years of age and older is 20 mcg or 0.2 ml solution intranasally at bedtime. Adjustment up to 40 mcg is suggested if the patient does not respond. Some patients may respond to 10 mcg and adjustment to that lower dose may be done if the patient has shown a response to 20 mcg. It is recommended that one-half of the dose be administered per nostril. Adequately controlled studies with desmopressin Nasal Spray in primary nocturnal enuresis have not been conducted beyond 4-8 weeks.

RHINAL SPRAY

Central Cranial Diabetes Insipidus: This drug is administered into the nose through a soft, flexible plastic rhinal tube which has four graduation marks on it that measures 0.2, 0.15, 0.1 and 0.5 ml. Desmopressin rhinal tube dosage must be determined for each individual patient and adjusted according to the diurnal pattern of response. Response should be estimated by two parameters: adequate duration of sleep and adequate, not excessive, water turnover. Patients with nasal congestion and blockage have often responded well to desmopressin Rhinal tube. The usual dosage range in adults is 0.1 to 0.4 nl daily, either as a single dose or divided doses into two or three doses. Most adults require 0.2 ml daily in two divided doses. The morning and evening doses should be separately adjusted for an adequate diurnal rhythm of water turnover. For children aged 3 months to 12 years, the usual dived dosage range is 0.05 to 0.3 ml daily, either as single dose or divided into two doses.

About 1/4 to 1/3 of patients can be controlled by a single dose.

INJECTION

Hemophilia A and von Willebrand's Disease (Type I): DDAVP injection is administered as an IV infusion at a dose of 0.3 mcg desmopressin/kg body weight diluted in sterile physiological saline and infused slowly over 15 to 30 minutes. In adults and children weighing more than 10 kg, 50 ml of diluent is used; in children weighing 10 kg or less, 10 ml of diluent is used. Blood pressure and pulse should be monitored during infusion. If desmopressin injection is used preoperatively, it should be administered 30 minutes prior to the scheduled procedure.

The necessity for repeat administration of desmopressin or use of any blood products for hemostasis should be determined by laboratory response as well as the clinical condition of the patient. The tendency toward tachyphylaxis (lessening of response) with repeated administration given more frequently than every 48 hours should be considered in treating each patient.

Diabetes Insipidus: The formulation is administered subcutaneously by direct IV injection. Desmopressin injection dosage must be administered for each patient and adjusted according to the pattern of response. response should be estimated by two parameters: adequate duration of sleep and adequate, not excessive, water turnover.

DOSAGE AND ADMINISTRATION: *(cont'd)*

The usual dosage range in adults is 0.5 ml (2.0 mcg) to 1 ml (4.0 mcg) daily, administered intravenously or subcutaneously, usually in two divided doses. The morning and evening doses should be separately adjusted for an adequate diurnal rhythm of water turnover. For patients who have been controlled on intranasal desmopressin and who must be switched to the injection form, wither because of poor intranasal absorption or because of the need for surgery, the comparable antidiuretic dose of the injection is about one-tenth the intranasal dose.

Parenteral drug products should be inspected visually for particulate matter and discoloration prior to administration whenever solution and container permit.

HOW SUPPLIED:

Nasal Spray: A 5-ml bottle with spray pump delivering 50 doses of 10 mcg. Also available as 2.5 ml per vial, packaged with two rhinal tube applicators per carton. Keep refrigerated at 2°-8°C (36°-46°F). When traveling, product will maintain stability for up to 3 weeks when stored at room temperature, 22°C(72°F).

Rhinal Tube: 2.5 ml per vial, packaged with two rhinal tube applicators per carton.**KEEP REFRIGERATED AT ABOUT 4°C (39°F).**When traveling—controlled room temperature 22°C (72°F) closed sterile bottles will maintain stability for 3 weeks.

Injection: Desmopressin injection is available as a sterile solution in cartons of ten 1 ml single-dose ampules and in 10 ml multiple-dose vials, each containing 4.0 mcg DDAVP per ml. Keep refrigerated at about

(Nasal Spray: Rhone-Poulenc Rorer); (Rhinal Tube: Rhone-Poulenc Rorer, 12/91, IN-0369D); (Injection: Rhone-Poulenc Rorer, 11/93, IN-4760A)

HOW SUPPLIED - EQUIVALENTS NOT AVAILABLE:

Aerosol, Spray - Nasal - 1.5 mg/ml

2.5 ml	$525.00	STIMATE, Centeon	00053-2453-00

Injection, Solution - Intravenous; Su - 4 mcg/ml

1 ml x 10	$201.85	Desmopressin Acetate, Ferring Labs	55566-5030-01
1 ml x 10	$245.39	DDAVP, Rhone-Poulenc Rorer	00075-2451-01
10 ml	$201.85	Desmopressin Acetate, Ferring Labs	55566-5040-01
10 ml	$248.44	DDAVP, Rhone-Poulenc Rorer	00075-2451-53

Solution - Nasal - 0.1 mg/ml

2.5 ml	$56.19	Desmopressin Acetate, Ferring Labs	55566-5020-01
2.5 ml	$68.28	DDAVP INTRANASAL, Rhone-Poulenc Rorer	00075-2450-01
2.5 ml x 10	$539.50	Desmopressin Acetate, Ferring Labs	55566-5020-02
5.0 ml	$112.01	DDAVP INTRANASAL, Rhone-Poulenc Rorer	00075-2450-02

DESOGESTREL; ETHINYL ESTRADIOL *(003143)*

CATEGORIES: Contraceptives; Hormones; Pregnancy; Pregnancy Category X; FDA Class 1S ("Standard Review"); Sales > $100 Million; FDA Approved 1992 Dec; Top 200 Drugs

BRAND NAMES: **Desogen**; *Desolett*; *Marvelon* (Germany, England, Mexico); *Marvelon 21*; *Marvelon 28* (Australia); *Mercilon*; *Microdiol*; *Novelon*; Ortho-Cept; *Varnoline* (France)
(International brand names outside U.S. in italics)

FORMULARIES: Medi-Cal; PCS

COST OF THERAPY: $266.34 (Contraceptive; Tablet; 0.15 mg/0.03 mg; 1/day; 365 days) vs. Potential Cost of $2,351.94 (Pregnancy)

DESCRIPTION:

The name for desogestrel is (13-ethyl-11- methylene-18,19-dinor-17 alpha-pregn-4-en- 20-yn-17-ol). The name for ethinyl estradiol is (19-nor-17 alpha-pregna-1,3,5 (10)-trien-20-yne-3,17-diol).

Desogen: Desogen 28 tablets provide an oral contraceptive regimen of 21 white round tablets each containing 0.15 mg desogestrel and 0.03 mg ethinyl estradiol. Inactive ingredients include vitamin E, cornstarch, povidone, stearic acid, colloidal silicon dioxide, lactose, hydroxypropyl methylcellulose, polyethylene glycol, titanium dioxide and talc. Desogen 28 also contains 7 green round tablets containing the following inactive ingredients: lactose, corn starch, magnesium stearate, FD&C Blue No. 2 aluminum lake, ferric oxide, hydroxypropyl methylcellulose, polyethylene glycol, titanium dioxide and talc.

Ortho-Cept: Ortho-Cept 21 and Ortho-Cept 28 tablets provide an oral contrceptive regimen of 21 orange round tablets each containing 0.15 mg desogestrel and 0.03 mg ethinyl estradiol. Inactive ingredients include vitamin E, corn starch, povidine, stearic acid, colloidal silicon dioxide, lactose, hydroxypropyl methycellulose, polyethylene glycol, titanium dioxide, talc and ferric oxide. Ortho-Cept 28 also contains 7 green tablets containing the following inactive ingredients: lactose, pregelitanized starch, magnesium stearate, FD&C Blue No. 1 Aluminium Lake, ferric oxide, hydroxypropyl methylcellulose, polyethylene glycol, titanium dioxide and talc.

For prescribing information refer to Ethinyl Estradiol; Norethindrone.

HOW SUPPLIED:

Desogen 28 contains 21 round white tablets and 7 round green tablets in a blister card within a recyclable plastic dispenser. Each white tablet (debossed with "TR/5" on one side and "Organon" on the other side) contains 0.15 mg desogestrel and 0.030 mg ethinyl estradiol. Each green tablet (debossed "KH/2" on one side and "Organon" on the other side) contains inert ingredients.

STORAGE: Store below 86°F (30°C)

HOW SUPPLIED - RATED THERAPEUTICALLY EQUIVALENT:

Tablet, Uncoated - Oral - 0.15 mg/0.03 mg

126 (6 x 21)	$139.74	ORTHO-CEPT 21, Ortho Pharm	00062-1795-15
168 (6 x 28)	**$122.59**	**DESOGEN, Organon**	**00052-0261-06**
168 (6 x 28)	$140.46	ORTHO-CEPT 28, Ortho Pharm	00062-1796-15

DESONIDE *(000967)*

CATEGORIES: Anti-Infectives; Anti-Inflammatory Agents; Dermatitis; Dermatologicals; Dermatoses; EENT Drugs; Eye, Ear, Nose, & Throat Preparations; Otic Preparations; Otologic; Pruritus; Skin/Mucous Membrane Agents; Steroids; Pregnancy Category C; FDA Approval Pre 1982

BRAND NAMES: *Apolar*; *Desonida*; *Desonix*; **Desowen**; *Locapred*; *Reticus*; *Sine Fluor*; *Sterax*; *Topifug*; Tridesilon; *Tridesonit* (France)
(International brand names outside U.S. in italics)

FORMULARIES: Aetna

DESCRIPTION:

Desonide Cream, Ointment and Lotion contain the topical corticosteroid desonide, a non-fluorinated corticosteroid. It has the chemical name: Pregna-1,4-diene-3,20-dione,11,21-dihydroxy-16,17-((1-methylethylidene)bi s(oxy))- (11β-16α)-; the molecular formula: $C_{24}H_{32}O_6$; molecular weight: 416.51;*CAS-638-94-8*.

Each gram of Desonide Cream contains 0.5 mg of desonide microdispersed in a compatible vehicle buffered to the pH range of normal skin. It contains propylene glycol, polysorbate 60, emulsifying wax, isopropyl palmitate, stearic acid, synthetic beeswax, citric acid, sodium hydroxide, and purified water. It is persevered with sorbic acid and potassium sorbate.

Each gram of Desonide Ointment contains 0.5 mg of desonide in a base consisting of mineral oil and polyethylene.

Each gram of Desonide Lotion contains 0.5 mg of desonide in a lotion vehicle consisting of sodium lauryl sulfate, light mineral oil, cetyl alcohol, stearyl paraben, sorbitan monostearate, glyceryl stearate SE, edetate sodium and purified water. May contain citric acid and/or sodium hydroxide for pH adjustment.

CLINICAL PHARMACOLOGY:

Topical corticosteroids share anti-inflammatory, anti-pruritic, and vasoconstrictive actions.

The mechanism of anti-inflammatory activity of the topical corticosteroids is unclear. Various laboratory methods, including vasoconstrictor assay, are used to compare and predict potencies and/or clinical efficacies of the topical corticosteroids. There is some evidence to suggest that a recognizable correlation exists between vasoconstrictor potency and therapeutic efficacy in man.

Pharmacokinetics: The extent of percutaneous absorption of topical corticosteroids is determined by many factors including the vehicle, the integrity of the epidermal barrier, and the use of occlusive dressings.

Topical corticosteroids can be absorbed from normal intact skin. Inflammation and/or other disease processes in the skin increase percutaneous absorption. Occlusive dressing substantially increase the percutaneous absorption of topical corticosteroids. Thus, occlusive dressings may be a valuable therapeutic adjunct for treatment of resistant dermatoses (See DOSAGE AND ADMINISTRATION.)

Once absorbed through the skin, topical corticosteroids are handled through pharmacokinetic pathways similar to systemically administered corticosteroids. Corticosteroids are bound to plasma proteins in varying degrees. Corticosteroids are metabolized primarily in the liver and are then excreted by the kidneys. Some of the topical corticosteroids and their metabolites are also excreted into the bile.

INDICATIONS AND USAGE:

Desonide Cream 0.05%, Ointment 0.05% and Lotion 0.05% are indicated for the relief of the inflammatory and pruritic manifestations of corticosteroid-responsive dermatoses.

CONTRAINDICATIONS:

Topical corticosteroids are contraindicated in those patients with a history of hypersensitivity to any of the components of the preparations.

PRECAUTIONS:

General: Systemic absorption of topical corticosteroids has produced reversible hypothalamic-pituitary-adrenal (HPA) axis suppression manifestations of Cushing's syndrome, hyperglycemia, and glucosuria in some patients.

Conditions which augment systemic absorption include the application of the more potent steroids, use over large surface areas, prolonged use, and the addition of occlusive dressings.

Therefore, patients receiving a large dose of a potent topical steroid applied to a large surface area or under an occlusive dressing should be evaluated periodically for evidence of HPA axis suppression by using the urinary free cortisol and ACTH stimulation tests. If HPA axis suppression is noted, an attempt should be made to withdraw the drug, to reduce the frequency of application, or to substitute a less potent steroid.

Recovery of HPA axis function is generally prompt and complete upon discontinuation of the drug. Infrequently, signs and symptoms of steroid withdrawal may occur requiring supplemental systemic corticosteroids.

Children may absorb proportionally large amounts of topical corticosteroids and thus be more susceptible to systemic toxicity (See PRECAUTIONS, Pediatric Use.)

If irritation develops, topical corticosteroids should be discontinued and appropriate therapy instituted.

In the presence of dermatological infections, the use of an appropriate antifungal or anti-bacterial agent should be instituted. If a favorable response does not occur promptly, the corticosteroid should be discontinued until the infection has been adequately controlled.

Information for the Patient: Patients using topical corticosteroids should severe the following information and instructions:

1. This medication is to be used as directed by the physician. It is for external use only. Avoid contact with the eyes.
2. Patients should be advised not to use this medication for any disorder other than for which it was prescribed.
3. The treated skin area should not be bandaged or otherwise covered or wrapped as to be occlusive unless directed by the physician.
4. Patients should report any signs of local adverse reactions especially under occlusive dressing.
5. Parents of pediatric patients should be advised not to use tight-fitting diapers or plastic pants on a child being treated in the diaper area, as these garments may constitute occlusive dressings.

Laboratory Tests: The following tests may be helpful in evaluating the HPA axis suppression:

Urinary free cortisol test.

ACTH stimulation tests

Carcinogenesis, Mutagenesis, and Impairment of Fertility: Long-term animal studies have not been performed to evaluate the carcinogenic potential or the effect on fertility of topical corticosteroids.

Studies to determine mutagenicity with prednisolone and hydrocortisone have revealed negative results.

Pregnancy Category C: Corticosteroids are generally teratogenic in laboratory animals when administered systemically at relatively low dosage levels. The more potent corticosteroids have been shown to be teratogenic after dermal application in laboratory animals. There are no adequate and well controlled studies in pregnant women on teratogenic effects from topically applied corticosteroids. Therefore, topical corticosteroids should be used during pregnancy only if the potential benefit justifies the potential risk to the fetus. Drug of this class should not be used extensively on pregnant patients, in large amounts or for prolonged periods of time.

PRECAUTIONS: *(cont'd)*

Nursing Mothers: It is not known whether topical administration of corticosteroids could result in sufficient systemic absorption to produce detectable quantities in breast milk. Systemically administered corticosteroids are secreted into breast milk in quantities *not*likely to have a deleterious effect on the infant. Nevertheless, caution should be exercised when topical corticosteroids are administered to a nursing woman.

Pediatric Use: *Pediatric patients may demonstrate greater susceptibility to topical corticosteroids-induced HPA axis suppression and Cushing's syndrome than mature patients because of a larger skin surface area to body weight ratio.*

Hypothalamic-pituitary-adrenal (HPA) axis suppression, Cushing's syndrome, and intracranial hypertension have been reported in children receiving topical corticosteroids. Manifestations of adrenal suppression in children include linear growth retardation, delayed weight gain, low plasma cortisol levels, and absence of response to ACTH simulation. Manifestations of intracranial hypertension include bulging fontanelles, headaches, and bilateral papilledema.

Administration of topical corticosteroids to children should be limited to the least amount compatible with an effective therapeutic regimen. Chronic corticosteroids therapy may interfere with the growth and development of children.

ADVERSE REACTIONS:

The following local adverse reactions are reported infrequently with topical corticosteroids but may occur more frequently with the use of occlusive dressings. These reactions are listed in an approximate decreasing order of occurrence: burning, itching, irritation, dryness, folliculitis, hypertrichosis, acneiform eruptions, hypopigmentation, perioral dermatitis, allergic contact dermatitis, maceration of the skin, secondary infection, skin atrophy, striae, and miliaria.

OVERDOSAGE:

Topically applied corticosteroids can be absorbed in sufficient amounts to produce systemic effects (See PRECAUTIONS.)

DOSAGE AND ADMINISTRATION:

Desonide Cream 0.05%, Ointment 0.05% or Lotion 0.05% should be applied to the affected area as a thin film two or three times daily depending on the severity of the condition. SHAKE LOTION WELL BEFORE USING.

Occlusive dressings may be used for the management of psoriasis or recalcitrant conditions.

If an infection develops, the use of occlusive dressings should be discontinued and appropriate antimicrobial therapy instituted.

Storage Conditions: Store below 86°F (30°C). Avoid freezing.

HOW SUPPLIED - RATED THERAPEUTICALLY EQUIVALENT:

Cream - Topical - 0.05 %

2.3 kg	$454.18	TRIDESILON, Bayer	00026-5561-92
15 gm	$7.96	Desonide, Copley Pharm	38245-0184-70
15 gm	$8.55	Desonide, Qualitest Pharms	00603-7731-74
15 gm	$8.82	Desonide, Geneva Pharms	00781-7230-27
15 gm	$8.95	Desonide, Major Pharms	00904-7724-36
15 gm	$9.05	Desonide, Rugby	00536-7502-20
15 gm	$9.15	Desonide, Goldline Labs	00182-5066-51
15 gm	$9.16	Desonide, H.C.F.A. F F P	99999-0967-02
15 gm	$9.95	Desonide, Taro Pharms (US)	51672-1280-01
15 gm	$10.80	TRIDESILON, Bayer	00026-5561-61
15 gm	$11.33	Desonide, HL Moore Drug Exch	00839-7135-47
15 gm	**$12.94**	**DESOWEN, Galderma**	**00299-5770-15**
60 gm	$22.78	Desonide, Copley Pharm	38245-0184-73
60 gm	$25.06	Desonide, H.C.F.A. F F P	99999-0967-03
60 gm	$25.25	Desonide, Geneva Pharms	00781-7230-35
60 gm	$25.40	Desonide, Rugby	00536-7502-25
60 gm	$25.50	Desonide, Qualitest Pharms	00603-7731-88
60 gm	$25.50	Desonide, Major Pharms	00904-7724-02
60 gm	$25.50	Desonide, Taro Pharms (US)	51672-1280-03
60 gm	$25.60	Desonide, Goldline Labs	00182-5066-52
60 gm	$26.31	Desonide, HL Moore Drug Exch	00839-7135-50
60 gm	$30.93	TRIDESILON, Bayer	00026-5561-62
60 gm	**$33.12**	**DESOWEN, Galderma**	**00299-5770-60**
90 gm	**$35.00**	**DESOWEN, Galderma**	**00299-5770-90**
90 gm	$54.99	Desonide, H.C.F.A. F F P	99999-0967-04
2270 gm	$1386.97	Desonide, H.C.F.A. F F P	99999-0967-01

Ointment - Topical - 0.05 %

15 gm	$9.15	Desonide, Goldline Labs	00182-5115-51
15 gm	$10.80	TRIDESILON, Bayer	00026-5591-61
15 gm	**$12.94**	**DESOWEN, Galderma**	**00299-5775-15**
60 gm	$25.60	Desonide, Goldline Labs	00182-5115-52
60 gm	$30.93	TRIDESILON, Bayer	00026-5591-62
60 gm	**$33.12**	**DESOWEN, Galderma**	**00299-5775-60**

HOW SUPPLIED - NOT RATED EQUIVALENT:

Lotion - Topical - 0.05 %

60 ml	**$23.12**	**DESOWEN, Galderma**	**00299-5765-02**
120 ml	**$33.75**	**DESOWEN, Galderma**	**00299-5765-04**

DESOXIMETASONE *(000968)*

CATEGORIES: Anti-Inflammatory Agents; Dermatologicals; Dermatoses; Pruritus; Skin/Mucous Membrane Agents; Steroids; Topical; Pregnancy Category C; FDA Approval Pre 1982

BRAND NAMES: *Actiderm*; *Desoximethsone*; *Dethasone*; *Esperson* (Asia); *Flubason*; *Ibaril*; *Inerson*; *Stiedex* (England); *Topcort*; *Topicorete*; **Topicort**; *Topicorte* (France); *Topicote*; *Topiderm*; *Topisolon* (Germany)
(International brand names outside U.S. in italics)

FORMULARIES: Aetna; BC-BS

DESCRIPTION:

Desoximetasone emollient cream 0.25%, emollient cream 0.05%, gel 0.05%, and ointment 0.25% contain the active synthetic corticosteroid desoximetasone. The topical corticosteroids constitute a class of primarily synthetic steroids used as anti-inflammatory and anti-pruritic agents. Each gram of desoximetasone emollient cream 0.25% contains 2.5 mg of desoximetasone in an emollient cream consisting of white petrolatum USP, purified water USP, isopropyl myristate NF, lanolin alcohols NF, mineral oil USP, cetostearyl alcohol NF, aluminum stearate, and magnesium stearate.

DESCRIPTION: *(cont'd)*

Each gram of desoximetasone emollient cream 0.05% contains 0.5 mg of desoximetasone in an emollient cream consisting of white petrolatum USP, purified water USP, isopropyl myristate NF, lanolin alcohols NF, mineral oil USP, cetostearyl alcohol NF, aluminum stearate, edetate disodium USP, lactic acid USP, and magnesium stearate.

Each gram of desoximetasone gel 0.05% contains 0.5 mg of desoximetasone in a gel consisting of purified water USP, SD alcohol 40 (20% w/w), isopropyl myristate NF, carbomer 940, trolamine NF, edetate disodium USP, and docusate sodium USP.

Each gram of desoximetasone ointment 0.25% contains 2.5 mg of desoximetasone in a base consisting of white petrolatum USP, propylene glycol USP, sorbitan sesquioleate, beeswax, fatty alcohol citrate, fatty acid pentaerythritol ester, aluminum stearate, citric acid, and butylated hydroxyanisole.

The chemical name of desoximetasone is Pregna-1,4-diene-3,20-dione, 9-fluoro-11,21-dihydroxy-16-methyl-,(11β, 16α)-.

Desoximetasone has the empirical formula $C_{22}H_{29}FO_4$ and a molecular weight of 376.47.

The CAS Registry Number is 382-67-2.

CLINICAL PHARMACOLOGY:

Topical corticosteroids share anti-inflammatory, anti-pruritic and vasoconstrictive actions.

The mechanism of anti-inflammatory activity of the topical corticosteroids is unclear. Various laboratory methods, including vasoconstrictor assays, are used to compare and predict potencies and/or clinical efficacies of the topical corticosteroids. There is some evidence to suggest that a recognizable correlation exists between vasoconstrictor potency and therapeutic efficacy in man.

Pharmacokinetics: The extent of percutaneous absorption of topical corticosteroids is determined by many factors including the vehicle, the integrity of the epidermal barrier, and the use of occlusive dressings.

Topical corticosteroids can be absorbed from normal intact skin. Inflammation and/or other disease processes in the skin increase percutaneous absorption. Occlusive dressings substantially increase the percutaneous absorption of topical corticosteroids. Thus, occlusive dressings may be a valuable therapeutic adjunct for treatment of resistant dermatoses.

Once absorbed through the skin, topical corticosteroids are handled through pharmacokinetic pathways similar to systemically administered corticosteroids. Corticosteroids are bound to plasma proteins in varying degrees. Corticosteroids are metabolized primarily in the liver and are then excreted by the kidneys. Some of the topical corticosteroids and their metabolites are also excreted into the bile.

Pharmacokinetic studies in men with desoximetasone emollient cream 0.25% with tagged desoximetasone showed a total of 5.2% ± 2.9% excretion in urine (4.1% ± 2.3%) and feces (1.1% ± 0.6%) and no detectable level (limit of sensitivity: 0.005 mcg/ml) in the blood when it was applied topically on the back followed by occlusion for 24 hours. Seven days after application, no further radioactivity was detected in urine or feces. The half-life of the material was 15 ± 2 hours (for urine) and 17 ± 2 hours (for feces) between the third and fifth trial day.

Pharmacokinetic studies in men with desoximetasone ointment 0.25% with tagged desoximetasone showed no detectable level (limit of sensitivity: 0.003 mcg/ml) in 1 subject and 0.004 and 0.006 mcg/ml in the remaining 2 subjects in the blood when it was applied topically on the back followed by occlusion for 24 hours. The extent of absorption for the ointment was 7% based on radioactivity recovered from urine and feces. Seven days after application, no further radioactivity was detected in urine or feces. Studies with other similarly structured steroids have shown that predominant metabolite reaction occurs through conjugation to form the glucuronide and sulfate ester.

INDICATIONS AND USAGE:

Desoximetasone emollient cream 0.25%, emollient cream 0.05%, gel 0.05%, and ointment 0.25% are indicated for the relief of the inflammatory and pruritic manifestations of corticosteroid-responsive dermatoses.

CONTRAINDICATIONS:

Topical corticosteroids are contraindicated in those patients with a history of hypersensitivity to any of the components of the preparation.

PRECAUTIONS:

General: Systemic absorption of topical corticosteroids has produced reversible hypothalamic-pituitary-adrenal (HPA) axis suppression, manifestations of Cushing's syndrome, hyperglycemia, and glucosuria in some patients.

Conditions which augment systemic absorption include the application of the more potent steroids, use over large surface areas, prolonged use, and the addition of occlusive dressings.

Therefore, patients receiving a large dose of a potent topical steroid applied to a large surface area or under an occlusive dressing should be evaluated periodically for evidence of HPA axis suppression by using the urinary free cortisol and ACTH stimulation tests. If HPA axis suppression is noted, an attempt should be made to withdraw the drug, to reduce the frequency of application, or to substitute a less potent steroid.

Recovery of HPA axis function is generally prompt and complete upon discontinuation of the drug. Infrequently, signs and symptoms of steroid withdrawal may occur, requiring supplemental systemic corticosteroids.

Pediatric patients may absorb proportionally larger amounts of topical corticosteroids and thus be more susceptible to systemic toxicity (see PRECAUTIONS, Pediatric Use).

If irritation develops, topical corticosteroids should be discontinued and appropriate therapy instituted.

In the presence of dermatological infections, the use of an appropriate antifungal or antibacterial agent should be instituted. If a favorable response does not occur promptly, the corticosteroid should be discontinued until the infection has been adequately controlled.

Information for the Patient: Patients using topical corticosteroids should receive the following information and instructions:

1. This medication is to be used as directed by the physician. It is for external use only. Avoid contact with the eyes.

2. Patients should be advised not to use this medication for any disorder other than for which it was prescribed.

3. The treated skin area should not be bandaged or otherwise covered or wrapped as to be occlusive unless directed by the physician.

4. Patients should report any signs of local adverse reactions especially under occlusive dressing.

5. Parents of pediatric patients should be advised not to use tight-fitting diapers or plastic pants on a child being treated in the diaper area, as these garments may constitute occlusive dressings.

Laboratory Tests: The following tests may be helpful in evaluating the HPA axis suppression:
Urinary free cortisol test

PRECAUTIONS: *(cont'd)*

ACTH stimulation test

Carcinogenesis, Mutagenesis, and Impairment of Fertility: Long-term animal studies have not been performed to evaluate the carcinogenic potential or the effect on fertility of topical corticosteroids.

Studies to determine mutagenicity with prednisolone and hydrocortisone have revealed negative results. Desoximetasone did not show potential for mutagenic activity *in vitro* in the Ames microbial mutagen test with or without metabolic activation.

Pregnancy Category C: Corticosteroids are generally teratogenic in laboratory animals when administered systemically at relatively low dosage levels. The more potent corticosteroids have been shown to be teratogenic after dermal application in laboratory animals.

Desoximetasone has been shown to be teratogenic and embryotoxic in mice, rats, and rabbits when given by subcutaneous or dermal routes of administration in doses 3 to 30 times the human dose of desoximetasone emollient cream 0.25% and ointment 0.25%, or 15 to 150 times the human dose of emollient cream 0.05% and gel 0.05%.

There are no adequate and well-controlled studies in pregnant women on teratogenic effects from topically applied corticosteroids. Therefore, desoximetasone emollient cream 0.25%, emollient cream 0.05%, gel 0.05%, and ointment 0.25% should be used during pregnancy only if the potential benefit justifies the potential risk to the fetus. Drugs of this class should not be used extensively on pregnant patients, in large amounts, or for prolonged periods of time.

Nursing Mothers: It is not known whether topical administration of corticosteroids could result in sufficient systemic absorption to produce detectable quantities in breast milk. Systemically administered corticosteroids are secreted into breast milk in quantities not likely to have a deleterious effect on the infant. Nevertheless, caution should be exercised when topical corticosteroids are administered to a nursing woman.

Pediatric Use: *Pediatric patients may demonstrate greater susceptibility to topical corticosteroid-induced HPA axis suppression and Cushing's syndrome than mature patients because of a larger skin surface area to body weight ratio.*

Hypothalamic-pituitary-adrenal (HPA) axis suppression, Cushing's syndrome, and intracranial hypertension have been reported in pediatric patients receiving topical corticosteroids. Manifestations of adrenal suppression in pediatric patients include linear growth retardation, delayed weight gain, low plasma cortisol levels, and absence of response to ACTH stimulation. Manifestations of intracranial hypertension include bulging fontanelles, headaches, and bilateral papilledema.

Administration of topical corticosteroids to pediatric patients should be limited to the least amount compatible with an effective therapeutic regimen.

Chronic corticosteroid therapy may interfere with the growth and development of pediatric patients. The safety and effectiveness of desoximetasone ointment 0.25% in pediatric patients below the age of 10 have not been established.

ADVERSE REACTIONS:

The following local adverse reactions are reported infrequently with topical corticosteroids, but may occur more frequently with the use of occlusive dressings. These reactions are listed in an approximate decreasing order of occurrence:

TABLE 1 Desoximetasone, Adverse Reactions

Burning	Hypertrichosis	Maceration of the skin
Itching	Acneiform eruptions	Secondary infection
Irritation	Hypopigmentation	Skin atrophy
Dryness	Perioral dermatitis	Striae
Folliculitis	Allergic contact dermatitis	Miliaria

In controlled clinical studies the incidence of adverse reactions was low (0.8%) for desoximetasone emollient cream 0.25% and included burning, folliculitis and folliculo-pustular lesions. The incidence of adverse reactions was also 0.8% for desoximetasone emollient cream 0.05% and included pruritus, erythema, vesiculation and burning sensation. In controlled clinical studies the incidence of adverse reactions was low (0.3%) for desoximetasone ointment 0.25% and consisted of development of comedones at the site of application.

OVERDOSAGE:

Topically applied corticosteroids can be absorbed in sufficient amounts to produce systemic effects (see PRECAUTIONS.)

DOSAGE AND ADMINISTRATION:

Apply a thin film of desoximetasone emollient cream 0.25%, emollient cream 0.05%, gel 0.05% or ointment 0.25% to the affected skin areas twice daily. Rub in gently.

REFERENCES:

1. Stoughton RB, Cornell RC. Review of super-potent topical corticosteroids. *Semin Dermatol.*1987;6(2):72-76. **2.** Data on file, Hoechst-Roussel Pharmaceuticals Inc. **3.** Savin RC, Stoughton RB, Cornell RC, Voorhees JJ, Willis I. Comparative Study of desoximetasone ointment 0.25% versus fluocinonide ointment 0.05% in patients with psoriasis.*Clin Ther.*1985;8(1):118-125. **4.** Willis I, Cornell RC, Penneys NS, Zaias N. Multicenter study comparing 0.05% gel formulations of desoximetasone and fluocinonide in patients with scalp psoriasis. *Clin Ther.*1986;8(3):275-282.

HOW SUPPLIED - RATED THERAPEUTICALLY EQUIVALENT:

Cream - Topical - 0.05 %

15 gm	$7.86	Desoximetasone, H.C.F.A. F F P	99999-0968-01
15 gm	$9.86	Desoximetasone, Taro Pharms (US)	51672-1271-01
15 gm	$9.88	Desoximetasone, Rugby	00536-4228-20
15 gm	$9.90	Desoximetasone.05% Topical, Goldline Labs	00182-5057-51
15 gm	$9.90	Desoximetasone, Geneva Pharms	00781-7185-27
15 gm	$9.90	Desoximetasone, Major Pharms	00904-0765-36
15 gm	**$13.06**	**TOPICORT LP, Hoechst Marion Roussel**	**00039-0012-23**
60 gm	$20.22	Desoximetasone, H.C.F.A. F F P	99999-0968-02
60 gm	$23.55	Desoximetasone, Major Pharms	00904-0765-02
60 gm	$23.58	Desoximetasone, Rugby	00536-4228-25
60 gm	$23.87	Desoximetasone, Taro Pharms (US)	51672-1271-03
60 gm	$23.90	Desoximetasone.05% Topical, Goldline Labs	00182-5057-52
60 gm	$23.90	Desoximetasone, Geneva Pharms	00781-7185-35
60 gm	**$31.60**	**TOPICORT LP, Hoechst Marion Roussel**	**00039-0012-60**

Cream - Topical - 0.25 %

15 gm	$10.25	Desoximetasone, Harber Pharm	51432-0737-10
15 gm	$10.35	Desoximetasone, United Res	00677-1413-40
15 gm	$10.35	Desoximetasone, H.C.F.A. F F P	99999-0968-03
15 gm	$11.85	Desoximetasone, Major Pharms	00904-0764-36
15 gm	$11.90	Desoximetasone, Rugby	00536-4229-20
15 gm	$12.40	Desoximetasone, Qualitest Pharms	00603-7733-74
15 gm	$12.42	Desoximetasone, HL Moore Drug Exch	00839-7665-47
15 gm	$12.45	Desoximetasone 0.25% Topical, Goldline Labs	00182-5054-51
15 gm	$12.49	Desoximetasone, Geneva Pharms	00781-7085-27
15 gm	$13.12	Desoximetasone, Taro Pharms (US)	51672-1270-01
15 gm	**$17.37**	**TOPICORT, EMOLLIENT, Hoechst Marion Roussel**	**00039-0011-23**

HOW SUPPLIED - RATED THERAPEUTICALLY EQUIVALENT: *(cont'd)*

60 gm	$24.50	Desoximetasone, Harber Pharm	51432-0737-17
60 gm	$24.70	Desoximetasone, H.C.F.A. F F P	99999-0968-04
60 gm	$27.48	Desoximetasone, Rugby	00536-4229-25
60 gm	$28.35	Desoximetasone, Major Pharms	00904-0764-02
60 gm	$29.73	Desoximetasone, Qualitest Pharms	00603-7733-88
60 gm	$29.75	Desoximetasone 0.25% Topical, Goldline Labs	00182-5054-52
60 gm	$29.79	Desoximetasone, Geneva Pharms	00781-7085-35
60 gm	$30.24	Desoximetasone, HL Moore Drug Exch	00839-7665-50
60 gm	$31.48	Desoximetasone, Taro Pharms (US)	51672-1270-03
60 gm	$41.40	Desoximetasone, United Res	00677-1413-43
60 gm	**$41.67**	**TOPICORT, EMOLLIENT, Hoechst Marion Roussel**	**00039-0011-60**
120 gm	**$67.62**	**TOPICORT, EMOLLIENT, Hoechst Marion Roussel**	**00039-0011-04**
120 gm	$82.80	Desoximetasone, H.C.F.A. F F P	99999-0968-05

Ointment - Topical - 0.25 %

15 gm	**$17.26**	**TOPICORT, Hoechst Marion Roussel**	**00039-0025-15**
60 gm	**$41.35**	**TOPICORT, Hoechst Marion Roussel**	**00039-0025-60**

HOW SUPPLIED - NOT RATED EQUIVALENT:

Gel - Topical - 0.05 %

15 gm	**$15.09**	**TOPICORT, Hoechst Marion Roussel**	**00039-0014-23**
60 gm	**$36.96**	**TOPICORT, Hoechst Marion Roussel**	**00039-0014-60**

DESOXYRIBONUCLEASE; FIBRINOLYSIN

(000972)

CATEGORIES: Burns; Dermatologicals; Enzymes; Enzymes & Digestants; Fibrinolytic & Proteolytic; Lesions; Mucous Membrane Agents; Skin/Mucous Membrane Agents; Topical; Vaginitis; Wound Care; FDA Pre 1938 Drugs

BRAND NAMES: **Elase**; *Fibrase* (Mexico); *Fibrolan* (Germany); *Parkelase* *(International brand names outside U.S. in italics)*

FORMULARIES: BC-BS

DESCRIPTION:

Desoxyribonuclease with fibrinolysin is a combination of two lytic enzymes, fibrinolysin and desoxyribonuclease, supplied as a lyophilized powder and an ointment. The fibrinolysin component is derived from bovine plasma[1,2] and the desoxyribonuclease is isolated in a purified form from bovine pancreas. The fibrinolysin used in the combination is activated by chloroform.

CLINICAL PHARMACOLOGY:

Combination of these two enzymes is based on the observation that purulent exudates consist largely of fibrinous material and nucleoprotein. Desoxyribonuclease attacks the desoxyribonucleic acid (DNA) and fibrinolysin attacks principally fibrin of blood clots and fibrinous exudates.

The activity of desoxyribonuclease is limited principally to the production of large polynucleotides,[3] which are less likely to be absorbed than the more diffusible protein fractions liberated by certain enzyme preparations obtained from bacteria. The fibrinolytic action of desoxyribonuclease with fibrinolysin is directed mainly against denatured proteins, such as those found in devitalized tissue, while protein elements of living cells remain relatively unaffected.

Desoxyribonuclease with fibrinolysin is a combination of active enzymes. This is an important consideration in treating patients suffering from lesions resulting from impaired circulation.

The enzymatic action of desoxyribonuclease with fibrinolysin helps to produce clean surfaces and thus supports healing in a variety of exudative lesions.

INDICATIONS AND USAGE:

Desoxyribonuclease with fibrinolysin is indicated for topical use as a debriding agent in a variety of inflammatory and infected lesions. These include: (1) general surgical wounds[6-8]; (2) ulcerative lesions[6,7,9]—trophic, decubitus, stasis, arteriosclerotic; (3) second- and third-degree burns[6,7,9]; (4) circumcision and episiotomy[8]. Desoxyribonuclease with fibrinolysin is used intravaginally in: (1) cervicitis[4-6,10]—benign, postpartum, and postconization and (2) vaginitis[6]. Desoxyribonuclease with fibrinolysin is used as an irrigating agent in the following conditions: (1) infected wounds[6,7,9]—abscesses, fistulae, and sinus tracts; (2) otorhinolaryngologic wounds[6]; (3) superficial hematomas[8](except when the hematoma is adjacent to or within adipose tissue).

CONTRAINDICATIONS:

Desoxyribonuclease with fibrinolysin is not recommended for parenteral use since the bovine fibrinolysin may be antigenic.

PRECAUTIONS:

The usual precautions against allergic reactions should be observed, particularly in persons with a history of sensitivity to materials of bovine origin.

To be maximally effective, desoxyribonuclease with fibrinolysin solutions must be freshly prepared before use. The loss in activity is reduced by refrigeration; however, even when stored in a refrigerator, the solution should not be used 24 hours or more after reconstitution.

ADVERSE REACTIONS:

Side effects attributable to the enzymes have not been a problem at the dose and for the indications recommended herein. With higher concentrations, side effects have been minimal, consisting of local hyperemia.

Chills and fever attributable to antigenic action of profibrinolysin activators of bacterial origin are not a problem with desoxyribonuclease with fibrinolysin.

DOSAGE AND ADMINISTRATION:

PREPARATION OF DESOXYRIBONUCLEASE WITH FIBRINOLYSIN SOLUTION

The contents of each vial may be reconstituted with 10 ml of isotonic sodium chloride solution. Higher or lower concentrations can be prepared if desired by varying the amount of the diluent.

Since the conditions for which desoxyribonuclease with fibrinolysin is helpful vary considerably in severity, dosage must be adjusted to the individual case; however, the following general recommendations can be made:

Successful use of enzymatic debridement depends on several factors:

DOSAGE AND ADMINISTRATION: *(cont'd)*

(1) Dense, dry eschar, if present, should be removed surgically before enzymatic debridement is attempted (2) The enzyme must be in constant contact with the substrate (3) Accumulated necrotic debris must be periodically removed(4) The enzyme must be replenished at least once daily (5) Secondary closure or skin grafting must be employed as soon as possible after optimal debridement has been attained. It is further essential that wound-dressing techniques be performed carefully under aseptic conditions and that appropriate systemically acting antibiotics be administered concomitantly if, in the opinion of the physician, they are indicated

General Topical Uses: Local application should be repeated at intervals for as long as enzyme action is desired. Desoxyribonuclease with fibrinolysin solution may be applied topically as a liquid, spray, or wet dressing. Application of a gentle spray of the solution can be accomplished by using a conventional atomizer. A recommended procedure for application of desoxyribonuclease with fibrinolysin using a Wet-to-Dry method is presented in the manufacturer's original package insert. After application, desoxyribonuclease with fibrinolysin, especially in solution, becomes rapidly and progressively less active and is probably exhausted for practical purposes at the end of 24 hours. The dry material for solution is stable at room temperature through the expiration date printed on the package.

Intravaginal Use: In severe cervicitis and vaginitis, the physician may instill 10 ml of the solution intravaginally, wait one or two minutes for the enzyme to disperse and then insert a cotton tampon in the vaginal canal. The tampon should be removed the next day. Continuing therapy should then be instituted with desoxyribonuclease with fibrinolysin ointment (fibrinolysin and desoxyribonuclease combined [bovine] ointment). See desoxyribonuclease with fibrinolysin ointment.

Abscesses, empyema cavities, fistulae, sinus tracts or subcutaneous hematomas: Despite the contraindication against parenteral use, desoxyribonuclease with fibrinolysin has been used in irrigating these specific conditions. The desoxyribonuclease with fibrinolysin solution should be drained and replaced at intervals of six to ten hours to reduce the amount of by-product accumulation and minimize loss of enzyme activity. Traces of blood in the discharge usually indicate active filling in of the cavity.

Storage: Store at no warmer than 30°C (86°F).

REFERENCES:

1. Seegers, W H and Loomis, E C: Science 104:461, 1946. **2.** Loomis, E C, George, C, Jr and Ryder, A: Arch. Biochem, 12:1, 1947. **3.** Smith, J D and Markham, R: Biochem, et Biophys, Acta 8:350, 1952. **4.** Glick, H I, Cavanagh, D and Kiem, I M: Bull Univ. Miami School of Medicine and Jackson Memorial Hospital 15:1, 1961. **5.** Glick, H I, Kiem, I M and Cavanagh, D: Am J Obst & Gynec, 85:112, 1962. **6.** Personal Communications to the Department of Clinical Investigation, Parke, Davis & Company, 1959. **7.** Connell, J F, Jr and Rousselot, L N: Surgery 47:709, 1960. **8.** Margulis, R R, et al: Am J Obst & Gynec 81:840, 1961. **9.** Coon, W W, Wolfman, E F, Jr, Foote, J A and Hodgson, P E: Am J Surg 98:4, 1959. **10.** Friedman, E A, Little, W A and Sachtleben, M R: Am J Obst & Gynec 79:474, 1960. **11.** Christensen, L R: J Clin Invest 28:163, 1949.

HOW SUPPLIED - EQUIVALENTS NOT AVAILABLE:

Ointment - Topical

10 gm	**$15.61**	**ELASE, Fujisawa USA**	**00469-7004-10**
30 gm	**$37.45**	**ELASE, Fujisawa USA**	**00469-7004-30**

Powder - Topical - 15000 unit/25 u

10 ml	**$24.22**	**ELASE, Fujisawa Pharm (US)**	**57317-0030-10**

DEXAMETHASONE *(000974)*

CATEGORIES: Acne; Adrenal Corticosteroids; Adrenal Hyperplasia; Adrenal Insufficiency; Adrenocortical Insufficiency; Airway Obstruction; Allergies; Alopecia; Analgesics; Anemia; Ankylosing Spondylitis; Anti-Inflammatory Agents; Antiarthritics; Antimicrobials; Arthritis; Aspiration Pneumonitis; Asthma; Atopic Dermatitis; Bronchospasm; Bursitis; Cancer; Carditis; Chemotherapy; Chorioretinitis; Choroiditis; Colitis; Conjunctival Inflammation; Conjunctivitis; Corneal Inflammation; Corneal Injury; Corneal Ulcer; Dermatitis; Dermatitis Herpetiformis; Dermatologicals; Diuresis; Drug Hypersensitivity; EENT Drugs; Edema; Enteritis; Epicondylitis; Erythema Multiforme; Eye, Ear, Nose, & Throat Preparations; Glucocorticoids; Gouty Arthritis; Granuloma Annulare; Herpes; Herpes Zoster; Hormones; Hypercalcemia; Iridocyclitis; Keratitis; Laryngeal Edema; Leukemia; Lupus Erythematosus; Lymphoma; Meningitis; Mycosis Fungoides; Nasal Polyps; Nausea and Vomiting; Neoplastic Disease; Nephrotic Syndrome; Ocular Acne; Ocular Infections; Ophthalmics; Osteoarthritis; Pain; Pemphigus; Penicillins; Pneumoconiosis; Pneumonitis; Proteinuria; Pruritus; Psoriasis; Purpura; Retinochoroiditis; Rhinitis; Sarcoidosis; Serum Sickness; Shock; Skin/Mucous Membrane Agents; Spondylitis; Steroids; Synovitis; Synovitis of Osteoarthritis; Tenosynovitis; Thrombocytopenia; Thrombocytopenic Purpura; Thyroiditis; Trichinosis; Tuberculosis; Ulcerative Colitis; Urticaria; Uveitis; FDA Approval Pre 1982

BRAND NAMES: Aeroseb-Dex; *Ak-Dex* (Canada); *Alfalyl*; *Alin* (Mexico); *Artrosone*; *Cetadexon*; *Corotason*; *Corsona*; *Cortidex*; *Cortidexason* (Germany); *Curson*; *Dabu* (Japan); *Danasone*; Decaderm; *Decadran*; **Decadron**; Decarex; Decaspray; *Decdan*; *Decilone*; *Decofluor*; *Dectancyl*; *Deronil* (Canada); *Desalark*; *Dexacortal*; *Dexacortin*; *Dexalocal*; *Dexame* (Japan); *Dexamed*; *Dexametason*; *Dexamethason*; *Dexamonozon* (Germany); *Dexamethasone*; *Dexa-P*; *Dexasone*; *Dexasone S* (Japan); *Dexazone*; *Dexmethsone*; *Dexoclin*; *Dexona*; Dexone; *Dextrasone*; *Dibasona* (Mexico); Dms; *Fortecortin* (Germany); Hexadrol; *Idizone*; *Inflam*; *Isopto*; *Isopto-Dex* (Germany); *Isopto-Maxidex*; *Isopto Maxidex*; *Lebedex*; *Loverine* (Japan); *Lozusu*; Maxidex; *Millicorten*; *Mitason*; Mymethasone; *Oftan-Dexa*; *Oradexon*; *Predni*; *Predni-F* (Germany); *Santenson* (Japan); *Sawasone* (Japan); *Spersadex*; *Taidon*; *Thilodexine*; *Visumetazone*; *Wymesone*

(International brand names outside U.S. in italics)

FORMULARIES: Aetna; BC-BS; FHP; Medi-Cal; PCS; WHO

COST OF THERAPY: $53.32 (Asthma; Tablet; 0.75 mg; 1/day; 365 days)

PRIMARY ICD9: 493.90 (Asthma, Unspecified, Without Mention of Status Asthmaticus)

DESCRIPTION:

Glucocorticoids are adrenocortical steroids, both naturally occurring and synthetic, which are readily absorbed from the gastrointestinal tract.

Dexamethasone, a synthetic adrenocortical steroid, is a white to practically white, odorless, crystalline powder. It is stable in air. It is practically insoluble in water. The molecular weight is 392.47. It is designated chemically as 9-fluoro-11β,17,21-trihydroxy- 16α-methylpregna-1,4-diene-3,20-dione. The empirical formula is $C_{22}H_{29}FO_5$.

DESCRIPTION: *(cont'd)*

Oral Forms: Dexamethasone tablets are supplied in six potencies, 0.25 mg, 0.5 mg, 0.75 mg, 1.5 mg, 4 mg, and 6 mg. Inactive ingredients are calcium phosphate, lactose, magnesium stearate, and starch. Dexamethasone tablets 0.25 mg also contain FD&C yellow 6. Dexamethasone tablets 0.5 mg also contain FD&C Yellow 10 and FD&C Yellow 6. Dexamethasone tablets

0.75 mg also contain FD&C Blue 1. Dexamethasone tablets 1.5 mg also contain FD&C Red 40. Dexamethasone tablets 6 mg also contain FD&C Blue 1 and iron oxide.

Dexamethasone elixir contains 0.5 mg of dexamethasone in each 5 ml. Benzoic acid, 0.1%, is added as a preservative. It also contains alcohol 5%. Inactive ingredients are FD&C Red 40, flavors, glycerin, purified water, and sodium saccharin.

Topical Forms: The topical corticosteroids constitute a class of primarily synthetic steroids used as anti-inflammatory and anti-pruritic agents.

Topical Aerosol Dexamethasone is a topical steroid preparation, each 25 mg of which contains 10 mg of dexamethasone. The inactive ingredients are isopropyl myristate, and isobutane. Each second of spray dispenses approximately 0.75 mg of dexamethasone.

Dexamethasone cream is a topical steroid preparation containing 0.1% of dexamethasone. Each gram contains 1 mg dexamethasone in Estergel, specially formulated vehicle consisting of gelled isopropyl myristate, wood alcohols B.P., refined lanolin alcohol, microcrystalline wax, anhydrous citric acid, and anhydrous sodium phosphate dibasic.

This emollient gel vehicle is anhydrous, lipophilic, hydrophilic, and moisture retentive. The base largely disappears when rubbed on the skin.

CLINICAL PHARMACOLOGY:

ORAL FORMS

Naturally occurring glucocorticoids (hydrocortisone and cortisone), which also have salt-retaining properties, are used as replacement therapy in adrenocortical deficiency states. Their synthetic analogs, including dexamethasone, are primarily used for their potent anti-inflammatory effects in disorders of many organ systems.

Glucocorticoids cause profound and varied metabolic effects. In addition, they modify the body's immune responses to diverse stimuli.

At equipotent anti-inflammatory doses, dexamethasone almost completely lacks the sodium-retaining property of hydrocortisone and closely related derivatives of hydrocortisone.

TOPICAL FORMS

Topical corticosteroids share anti-inflammatory, anti-pruritic, and vasoconstrictive actions.

The mechanism of anti-inflammatory activity of the topical corticosteroids is unclear. Various laboratory methods, including vasoconstrictor assays, are used to compare and predict potencies and/or clinical efficacies of the topical corticosteroids. There is some evidence to suggest that a recognizable correlation exists between vasoconstrictor potency and therapeutic efficacy in man.

Pharmacokinetics

The extent of percutaneous absorption of topical corticosteroids is determined by many factors including the vehicle, the integrity of the epidermal barrier, and the use of occlusive dressings.

Topical corticosteroids can be absorbed from normal intact skin. Inflammation and/or other disease processes in the skin increase percutaneous absorption. Occlusive dressings substantially increase the percutaneous absorption of topical corticosteroids. Thus, occlusive dressings may be a valuable therapeutic adjunct for treatment of resistant dermatoses. (See DOSAGE AND ADMINISTRATION.)

Once absorbed through the skin, topical corticosteroids are handled through pharmacokinetic pathways similar to systemically administered corticosteroids. Corticosteroids are bound to plasma proteins in varying degrees. Corticosteroids are metabolized primarily in the liver and are then excreted by the kidneys. Some of the topical corticosteroids and their metabolites are also excreted into the bile.

INDICATIONS AND USAGE:

ORAL FORMS

Endocrine Disorders: Primary or secondary adrenocortical insufficiency (hydrocortisone or cortisone is the first choice; synthetic analogs may be used in conjunction with mineralocorticoids where applicable; in infancy mineralocorticoid supplementation is of particular importance)

Congenital adrenal hyperplasia; Nonsuppurative thyroiditis;

Hypercalcemia associated with cancer

Rheumatic Disorders: As adjunctive therapy for short-term administration (to tide the patient over an acute episode or exacerbation) in:

Psoriatic arthritis; Rheumatoid arthritis, including juvenile rheumatoid arthritis (selected cases may require low-dose maintenance therapy); Ankylosing spondylitis; Acute and subacute bursitis; Acute nonspecific tenosynovitis; Acute gouty arthritis; Post-traumatic osteoarthritis;

Synovitis of osteoarthritis; Epicondylitis

Collagen Diseases: During an exacerbation or as maintenance therapy in selected cases of—Systemic lupus erythematosus; Acute rheumatic carditis.

Dermatologic Diseases: Pemphigus; Bullous dermatitis herpetiformis; Severe erythema multiforme (Stevens-Johnson syndrome); Exfoliative dermatitis; Mycosis fungoides; Severe psoriasis; Severe seborrheic dermatitis;

Allergic States: Control of severe or incapacitating allergic conditions intractable to adequate trials of conventional treatment: Seasonal or perennial allergic rhinitis; Bronchial asthma; Contact dermatitis; Atopic dermatitis; Serum sickness; Drug hypersensitivity reactions;

Ophthalmic Diseases: Severe acute and chronic allergic and inflammatory processes involving the eye and its adnexa, such as—Allergic conjunctivitis; Keratitis; Allergic corneal marginal ulcers; Herpes zoster ophthalmicus; Iritis and iridocyclitis; Chorioretinitis; Anterior segment inflammation; Diffuse posterior uveitis and choroiditis; Optic neuritis; Sympathetic ophthalmia

Respiratory Diseases: Symptomatic sarcoidosis; Loeffler's syndrome not manageable by other means; Berylliosis; Fulminating or disseminated pulmonary tuberculosis when used concurrently with appropriate antituberculous chemotherapy; Aspiration pneumonitis

Hematologic Disorders: Idiopathic thrombocytopenic purpura in adults; Secondary thrombocytopenia in adults; Acquired (autoimmune) hemolytic anemia; Erythroblastopenic (RBC anemia); Congenital (erythroid) hypoplastic anemia

Neoplastic Disease: For palliative management of: Leukemias and lymphomas in adults; Acute leukemia of childhood

Edematous States: To induce a diuresis or remission of proteinuria in the nephrotic syndrome, without uremia, of the idiopathic type or that due to lupus erythematosus

Gastrointestinal Disease: To tide the patient over a critical period of the disease in: Ulcerative colitis; Regional enteritis

INDICATIONS AND USAGE: *(cont'd)*

Cerebral Edema: associated with primary or metastatic brain tumor, craniotomy, or head injury. Use in cerebral edema is not a substitute for careful neurosurgical evaluation and definitive management such as neurosurgery or other specific therapy.

Miscellaneous: Tuberculous meningitis with subarachnoid block or impending block when used concurrently with appropriate anti-tuberculous chemotherapy, Trichinosis with neurologic or myocardial involvement

Diagnostic testing of adrenocortical hyperfunction

TOPICAL FORMS

Topical dexamethasone is indicated for relief of the inflammatory and pruritic manifestations of corticosteroid-responsive dermatoses.

CONTRAINDICATIONS:

ORAL FORMS

Systemic fungal infections

Hypersensitivity to this drug

TOPICAL FORMS

Topical corticosteroids are contraindicated in those patients with a history of hypersensitivity to any of the components of the preparation.

WARNINGS:

ORAL FORMS

In patients on corticosteroid therapy subjected to unusual stress, increased dosage of rapidly acting corticosteroids before, during, and after the stressful situation is indicated.

Drug-induced secondary adrenocortical insufficiency may result from too rapid withdrawal of corticosteroids and may be minimized by gradual reduction of dosage. This type of relative insufficiency may persist for months after discontinuation of therapy; therefore, in any situation of stress occurring during the period, hormone therapy should be reinstituted. If the patient is receiving steroids already, dosage may have to be increased. Since mineralocorticoid secretion may be impaired, salt and/or a mineralocorticoid should be administered concurrently.

Corticosteroids may mask some signs of infection, and new infections may appear during their use. There may be decreased resistance and inability to localize infection when corticosteroids are used. Moreover, corticosteroids may affect the nitroblue-tetrazolium test for bacterial infection and produce false negative results.

In cerebral malaria, a double-blind trial has shown that the use of corticosteroids is associated with prolongation of come and a higher incidence of pneumonia and gastrointestinal bleeding.

Corticosteroids may activate latent amebiasis. Therefore, it is recommended that latent or active amebiasis be ruled out before initiating corticosteroid therapy in any patient who has spent time in the tropics or any patient with unexplained diarrhea.

Prolonged use of corticosteroids may produce posterior subcapsular cataracts, glaucoma with possible damage to the optic nerves, and may enhance the establishment of secondary ocular infections due to fungi or viruses.

Usage In Pregnancy: Since adequate human reproduction studies have not been done with corticosteroids, use of these drugs in pregnancy or in women of childbearing potential requires that the anticipated benefits be weighed against the possible hazards to the mother and embryo or fetus. Infants born of mothers who have received substantial doses of corticosteroids during pregnancy should be carefully observed for signs of hypoadrenalism.

Corticosteroids appear in breast milk and could suppress growth, interfere with endogenous corticosteroid production, or cause other unwanted effects. Mothers taking pharmacologic doses of corticosteroids should be advised not to nurse.

Average and large doses of hydrocortisone or cortisone can cause elevation of blood pressure, salt and water retention, and increased excretion of potassium. These effects are less likely to occur with the synthetic derivatives except when used in large doses. Dietary salt restriction and potassium supplementation may be necessary. All corticosteroids increase calcium excretion.

Administration of live virus vaccines, including smallpox, is contraindicated in individuals receiving immunosuppressive doses of corticosteroids. If inactivated viral or bacterial vaccines are administered to individuals receiving immunosuppressive doses of corticosteroid the expected serum antibody response may not be obtained. However, immunization procedures may be undertaken in patients who are receiving corticosteroids as replacement therapy, e.g., for Addison's disease.

Patients who are on drugs which suppress the immune system are more susceptible to infections than healthy individuals. Chickenpox and measles, for example, can have a more serious or even fatal course in non-immune children or adults on corticosteroids. In such children or adults who have not had these diseases, particular care should be taken to avoid exposure. The risk of developing a disseminated infection varies among individuals and can be related to the dose, route and duration of corticosteroid administration as well as to the underlying disease. If exposed to chickpox, prophylaxis with varicella zoster immune globulin (VZIG) may be indicated. If chickenpox develops, treatment with antiviral agents may be considered. If exposed to measles, prophylaxis with immune globulin (IG) may be indicated. (See the respective package inserts for VZIG and IG for complete prescribing information.)

The use of dexamethasone tablets or elixir in active tuberculosis should be restricted to those cases of fulminating or disseminated tuberculosis in which the corticosteroid is used for the management of the disease in conjunction with an appropriate antituberculous regimen.

If corticosteroids are indicated in patients with latent tuberculosis or tuberculin reactivity, close observation is necessary as reactivation of the disease may occur. During prolonged corticosteroid therapy, these patients should be receive chemoprophylaxis.

Literature reports suggest an apparent association between corticosteroids' and left ventricular free wall rupture after a recent myocardial infarction; therefore, therapy with corticosteroids should be used with great caution in these patients.

TOPICAL AEROSOL

Avoid spraying in eyes or nose. Contents under pressure. Do not puncture or burn. Keep out of reach of children. Use only as directed. Intentional misuse by deliberately concentrating and inhaling the contents can be harmful or fatal.

Topically applied steroids are absorbed systemically. There may be rare instances in which this absorption results in immunosuppression. Patients who are on drugs which suppress the immune system are more susceptible to infections than healthy individuals.

Chickenpox and measles, for example, can have a more serious or even fatal course in non-immune children (see PRECAUTIONS, Pediatric Use) or adults on corticosteroids. In such children or adults who have not had these diseases, particular care should be taken to avoid exposure. The risk of developing a disseminated infection varies among individuals and can be related to the dose, route, and duration of corticosteroid administration as well as to the underlying disease. If exposed to chickenpox, prophylaxis with varicella zoster immune globulin (VZIG) may be indicated. If chickpox develops, treatment with antiviral agents may

WARNINGS: *(cont'd)*

be considered. If exposed to measles, prophylaxis with immune globulin (IG) may be indicated. (See the respective package inserts for VZIG and IG for complete prescribing information.)

PRECAUTIONS:

ORAL FORMS

Following prolonged therapy, withdrawal of corticosteroids may result in symptoms of the corticosteroid withdrawal syndrome including fever, myalgia, arthralgia, and malaise. This may occur in patients even without evidence of adrenal insufficiency.

There is an enhanced effect of corticosteroids in patients with hypothyroidism and in those with cirrhosis.

Corticosteroids should be used cautiously in patients with ocular herpes simplex because of possible corneal perforation.

The lowest possible dose of corticosteroids should be used to control the condition under treatment, and when reduction in dosage is possible, the reduction should be gradual.

Psychic derangements may appear when corticosteroids are used, ranging from euphoria, insomnia, mood swings, personality changes, and severe depression instability or psychotic tendencies may be aggravated by corticosteroids.

Aspirin should be used cautiously in conjunction with corticosteroids in hypoprothrombinemia.

Steroids should be used with caution in nonspecific ulcerative colitis, if there is a probability of impending perforation, abscess, or other pyogenic infection, diverticulitis, fresh intestinal anastomoses, active or latent peptic ulcer, renal insufficiency, hypertension, osteoporosis, and myasthenia gravis. Signs of peritoneal irritation following gastrointestinal perforation in patients receiving large doses of corticosteroids may be minimal or absent. Fat embolism has been reported as a possible complication of hypercortisonism.

When large doses are given, some authorities advise that corticosteroids be taken with meals and antacids taken between meals to help to prevent peptic ulcer.

Growth and development of infants and children on prolonged corticosteroid therapy should be carefully observed.

Steroids may increase or decrease motility and number of spermatozoa in some patients.

False-negative results in the dexamethasone suppression test (DST) in patients being treated with indomethacin have been reported. Thus, results of the DST should be interpreted with caution in these patients.

The prothrombin time should be checked frequently in patients who are receiving corticosteroids and cumarin anticoagulants at the same time because of reports that corticosteroids have altered the response to these anticoagulants. Studies have shown that the usual effect produced by adding corticosteroids is inhibition of response to coumarins, although there have been some conflicting reports of potentiation not substantiated by studies.

When corticosteroids are administered concomitantly with potassium-depleting diuretics, patients should be observed closely for development of hypokalemia.

TOPICAL FORMS

General: Systemic absorption of topical corticosteroids has produced reversible hypothalamic-pituitary-adrenal (HPA) axis suppression, manifestations of Cushing's syndrome, hyperglycemia, and glycosuria in some patients.

Conditions which augment systemic absorption include the application of the more potent corticosteroids, use over large surface areas, prolonged use, and the addition of occlusive dressings.

Therefore, patients receiving a large dose of a potent topical corticosteroid applied to a large surface area or under an occlusive dressing should be evaluated periodically for evidence of HPA axis suppression by using urinary free cortisol and ACTH stimulation tests. If HPA axis suppression is noted, an attempt should be made to withdraw the drug, to reduce the frequency of application, or to substitute a less potent corticosteroid.

Recovery of HPA axis function is generally prompt and complete upon discontinuation of the drug. Infrequently, signs and symptoms of corticosteroid withdrawal may occur, requiring supplemental systemic corticosteroids.

Children may absorb proportionally larger amounts of topical corticosteroids and thus be more susceptible to systemic toxicity (See PRECAUTIONS, Pediatric Use.)

If irritation develops, topical corticosteroids should be discontinued and appropriate therapy instituted.

In the presence of dermatological infections, the use of an appropriate antifungal or antibacterial agent should be instituted. If a favorable response does not occur promptly, the corticosteroid should be discontinued until the infection has been adequately controlled.

The product is not for ophthalmic use. However, if applied to the eyelids or skin near the eyes, the drug may enter the eyes. In patients with a history of herpes simplex keratitis ocular exposure to corticosteroids may lead to a recurrence. Prolonged ocular exposure may cause steroid glaucoma.

A few individuals may be sensitive to one or more of the components of this product. If any reaction indicating sensitivity is observed, discontinue use.

Generally, occlusive dressings should not be used on weeping or exudative lesions.

If occlusive dressing therapy is used, inspect lesions between dressings for development of infection. If infection develops, the technique should be discontinued and appropriate antimicrobial therapy instituted.

When large areas of the body are covered with an occlusive dressing, thermal homeostasis may be impaired. If elevation of body temperature occurs, use of the occlusive dressing should be discontinued.

Information for the Patient: Patients using topical corticosteroids should receive the following information and instructions:

1. This medication is to be used as directed by the physician. It is for external use only. Avoid contact with the eyes.

2. Patients should be advised not to use this medication for any disorder other than that for which it was prescribed.

3. The treated skin area should not be bandaged or otherwise covered or wrapped so as to be occlusive unless directed by the physician.

4. Patients should report any signs of local adverse reactions, especially under occlusive dressing.

5. Parents of pediatric patients should be advised not to use tight-fitting diapers or plastic pants on a child being treated in the diaper area, as these garments may constitute occlusive dressings.

6. Susceptible patients who are on immunosuppressant doses of corticosteroids should be warned to avoid exposure to chickenpox or measles. Patients should also be advised that if they are exposed, medical advice should be sought without delay.

Laboratory Tests: The following tests may be helpful in evaluating the HPA axis suppression:

Urinary free cortisol test

PRECAUTIONS: *(cont'd)*

ACTH stimulation test

Carcinogenesis, Mutagenesis, and Impairment of Fertility: Long-term animal studies have not been performed to evaluate the carcinogenic potential or the effect on fertility of topical corticosteroids.

Studies to determine mutagenicity with prednisolone and hydrocortisone have revealed negative results.

Pregnancy Category C: Corticosteroids are generally teratogenic in laboratory animals when administered systemically at relatively low dosage levels. The more potent corticosteroids have been shown to be teratogenic after dermal application in laboratory animals. There are no adequate and well-controlled studies in pregnant women on teratogenic effects from topically applied corticosteroids. Therefore, topical corticosteroids should be used during pregnancy only if the potential benefit justifies the potential risk to the fetus. Drugs of this class should not be used extensively on pregnant patients, in large amounts, or for prolonged periods of time.

Nursing Mothers: It is not known whether topical administration of corticosteroids could result in sufficient systemic absorption to produce detectable quantities in breast milk. Systemically administered corticosteroids are secreted into breast milk in quantities *not* likely to have a deleterious effect on the infant. Nevertheless, caution should be exercised when topical corticosteroids are administered to a nursing woman.

Pediatric Use: *Pediatric patients may demonstrate greater susceptibility to topical corticosteroid-induced HPA axis suppression and Cushing's syndrome than mature patients because of a larger skin surface to body weight ratio.*

Hypothalamic-pituitary-adrenal (HPA) axis suppression, Cushing's syndrome, and intracranial hypertension have been reported in children receiving topical corticosteroids. Manifestations of adrenal suppression in children include linear growth retardation, delayed weight gain, low plasma cortisol levels, and absence of response to ACTH stimulation. Manifestations of intracranial hypertension include bulging fontanelles, headaches, and bilateral papilledema.

Administration of topical corticosteroids to children should be limited to the least amount compatible with an effective therapeutic regimen. Chronic corticosteroid therapy may interfere with the growth and development of children.

Topical Aerosol Only

CAUTION: Flammable. Do not use around open flame or while smoking.

DRUG INTERACTIONS:

Phenytoin, phenobarbital, ephedrine, and rifampin may enhance the metabolic clearance of corticosteroids, resulting in decreased blood levels and lessened physiologic activity thus requiring adjustment in corticosteroid dosage. These interactions may interfere with dexamethasone suppression tests which should be interpreted with caution during administration of these drugs.

ADVERSE REACTIONS:

ORAL FORMS

Fluid and Electrolyte Disturbances: Sodium retention; Fluid retention; Congestive heart failure in susceptible patients; Potassium loss; Hypokalemic alkalosis; Hypertension

Musculoskeletal: Muscle weakness; Steroid myopathy; Loss of muscle mass; Osteoporosis; Vertebral compression fractures; Aseptic necrosis of femoral and humeral heads; Pathologic fracture of long bones; Tendon rupture

Gastrointestinal: Peptic ulcer with possible perforation and hemorrhage; Perforation of the small and large bowel, particularly in patients with Inflammatory bowel disease; Pancreatitis; Abdominal distention; Ulcerative esophagitis

Dermatologic: Impaired wound healing; Thin fragile skin; Petechiae and ecchymoses; Erythema; Increased sweating; May suppress reactions to skin tests; Other cutaneous reactions, such as allergic dermatitis, urticaria, angioneurotic edema

Neurologic: Convulsions; Increased intracranial pressure with papilledema (pseudotumor cerebri) usually after treatment; Vertigo; Headache;Psychic disturbances

Endocrine: Menstrual irregularities; Development of cushingoid state; Suppression of growth in children; Secondary adrenocortical and pituitary unresponsiveness, particularly in times of stress,as in trauma, surgery, or illness; Decreased carbohydrate tolerance; Manifestations of latent diabetes mellitus; Increased requirements for insulin or oral hypoglycemic agents in diabetics; Hirsutism

Ophthalmic: Posterior subcapsular cataracts; Increased intraocular pressure; Glaucoma; Exophthalmos

Metabolic: Negative nitrogen balance due to protein catabolism

Cardiovascular: Myocardial rupture following recent myocardial infarction (see WARNINGS)

Other: Hypersensitivity; Thromboembolism; Weight gain; Increased appetite; Nausea; Malaise

TOPICAL FORMS

The following adverse reactions are reported infrequently with topical corticosteroids, but may occur more frequently with the use of occlusive dressings. These reactions are listed in an approximate decreasing order of occurrence: Burning; Itching; Irritation; Dryness; Folliculitis; Hypertrichosis; Acneiform eruptions; Hypopigmentation; Perioral dermatitis; Allergic contact dermatitis; Maceration of the skin; Secondary infection; Skin atrophy; Striae; Miliaria

OVERDOSAGE:

Oral Forms: Reports of acute toxicity and/or death following overdosage of glucocorticoids are rare. In the event of overdosage, no specific antidote is available; treatment is supportive and symptomatic.

The oral LD_{50} of dexamethasone in female mice was 6.5 g/kg.

Topical Forms: Topically applied corticosteroids can be absorbed in sufficient amounts to produce systemic effects (See PRECAUTIONS.)

DOSAGE AND ADMINISTRATION:

ORAL FORMS

FOR ORAL ADMINISTRATION: DOSAGE REQUIREMENTS ARE VARIABLE AND MUST BE INDIVIDUALIZED ON THE BASIS OF THE DISEASE AND THE RESPONSE OF THE PATIENT.

The initial dosage varies from 0.75 to 9 mg a day depending on the disease being treated. In less severe diseases doses lower than 0.75 mg may suffice, while in severe diseases doses higher than 9 mg may be required. The initial dosage should be maintained or adjusted until the patient's response is satisfactory. If satisfactory clinical response does not occur after a reasonable period of time, discontinue dexamethasone tablets or elixir and transfer the patient to other therapy.

After a favorable initial response, the proper maintenance dosage should be determined by decreasing the initial dosage in small amounts to the lowest dosage that maintains an adequate clinical response.

DOSAGE AND ADMINISTRATION: *(cont'd)*

Patients should be observed closely for signs that might require dosage adjustment, including changes in clinical status resulting from remissions or exacerbations of the disease, individual drug responsiveness, and the effect of stress (*e.g.,* surgery, infection, trauma). During stress it may be necessary to increase dosage temporarily.

If the drug is to be stopped after more than a few days of treatment, it usually should be withdrawn gradually.

The following milligram equivalents facilitate changing to dexamethasone from other glucocorticoids (TABLE 1):

TABLE 1

Dexamethasone	Methylprednisolone and Triamcinolone	Prednisolone and Prednisone	Hydrocortisone	Cortisone
0.75 mg=	4 mg=	5 mg=	20 mg=	25 mg

In acute, self-limited allergic disorders or acute exacerbations of chronic allergic disorders , the following dosage schedule combining parenteral and oral therapy is suggested:

Dexamethasone sodium phosphate injection, 4 mg per ml:

First Day: 1 to 2 ml, intramuscularly; dexamethasone tablets, 0.75 mg:

Second Day: 4 tablets in two divided doses

Third Day: 4 tablets in two divided doses

Fourth Day: 2 tablets in two divided doses

Fifth Day: 1 tablet

Sixth Day: 1 tablet

Seventh Day: No treatment

Eighth Day: Follow-up-visit

This schedule is designed to ensure adequate therapy during acute episodes, while minimizing the risk of overdosage in chronic cases.

In cerebral edema, dexamethasone sodium phosphate injection is generally administered initially in a dosage of 10 mg intravenously followed by 4 mg every six hours intramuscularly unit the symptoms of cerebral edema subside. Response is usually noted within 12 to 24 hours and dosage may be reduced after two to four days and gradually discontinued over a period of five to seven days. For palliative management of patients with recurrent or inoperable brain tumors, maintenance therapy with either dexamethasone sodium phosphate injection or dexamethasone tablets in a dosage of two mg two or three times daily may be effective.

Dexamethasone Suppression Tests

Tests for Cushing's syndrome: Give 1.0 mg of dexamethasone orally at 11.00 p.m. Blood is drawn in for plasma cortisol determination at 8.00 a.m. the following morning.

For greater accuracy, give 0.5 mg of dexamethasone orally every 6 hours for 48 hours. Twenty-four hour urine collections are made for determination of 17-hydroxycorticosteroid excretion.

Test to distinguish Cushing's syndrome due to pituitary ACTH excess from Cushing's syndrome due to other causes: Give 2.0 mg of dexamethasone orally 6 hours for 48 hours. Twenty-four hour urine collections are made for determination of 17-hydroxycorticosteroid excretion.

TOPICAL AEROSOL

Patients should be instructed in the correct way to use dexamethasone aerosol spray. The preparation is readily applied, even on hairy areas. It does not have to rubbed into the skin.

Optimal effects will be obtained with dexamethasone aerosol spray when these directions are followed:

1. Keep the affected area clean to reduce the possibility of infection.

2. Shake the container *gently* once or twice each time before using. Hold it about six inches from the area to be treated. Effective medication may be obtained with the container held either upright or inverted, since it is fitted with a special valve that dispenses approximately the same dosage in either position.

3. Spray each four inch square of affected area for one or two seconds three or four times a day, depending on the nature of the condition and the response to therapy.

4. When a favorable response is obtained, reduce dosage gradually and eventually discontinue.

5. Occlusive dressings may be used for the management of psoriasis or recalcitrant conditions.

TOPICAL CREAM

Apply to the affected area as a thin film three or four times daily.

Occlusive dressings may be used for the management of psoriasis or recalcitrant conditions.

Before using this preparation in the ear, clean the aural canal thoroughly and sponge dry. Confirm that the eardrum is intact. With a cotton-tipped applicator, apply a thin coating of the cream to the affected cream to the affected canal area three or four times a day.

(Tablets: Merck, 2/93, 7420545; Elixir: Merck, 3/88, 7412726; Aerosol: Merck, 4/93, 6005319; Cream: Merck, 4/83, 6822406)

HOW SUPPLIED - RATED THERAPEUTICALLY EQUIVALENT:

Elixir - Oral - 0.5 mg/5ml

100 ml	$3.10	Dexamethasone, Raway	00686-0972-33
100 ml	$7.45	Dexameth, Major Pharms	00904-0972-04
100 ml	$7.50	Dexamethasone, Consolidated Midland	00223-6496-01
100 ml	$10.00	Dexamethasone, Schein Pharm (US)	00364-7182-61
100 ml	$11.18	Dexamethasone, H.C.F.A. F F P	99999-0974-01
100 ml	$12.20	Dexamethasone, Morton Grove	60432-0466-00
100 ml	$14.00	Dexamethasone, Alpharma	00472-0972-33
100 ml	**$16.96**	**DECADRON, Merck**	**00006-7622-55**
120 ml	$7.05	HEXADROL, Organon	00052-0793-04
120 ml	$13.41	Dexamethasone, H.C.F.A. F F P	99999-0974-02
240 ml	$9.38	Dexamethasone, Geneva Pharms	00781-6400-46
240 ml	$11.45	Dexamethasone, Harber Pharm	51432-0560-19
240 ml	$11.50	Dexamethasone, HL Moore Drug Exch	00839-7997-66
240 ml	$11.70	Dexamethasone, Qualitest Pharms	00603-1145-56
240 ml	$12.35	Dexamethasone, Goldline Labs	00182-1013-44
240 ml	$12.49	Dexamethasone, HL Moore Drug Exch	00839-6044-66
240 ml	$12.75	Dexamethasone, United Res	00677-0601-42
240 ml	$12.75	Dexamethasone, Geneva Pharms	00781-6400-08
240 ml	$12.95	Dexameth, Major Pharms	00904-0972-09
240 ml	$15.00	Dexamethasone, Schein Pharm (US)	00364-7182-76
240 ml	$16.35	Dexamethasone, Aligen Independ	00405-2625-77
240 ml	$17.50	Dexamethasone, Consolidated Midland	00223-6496-02
240 ml	$23.50	Dexamethasone, Rugby	00536-0452-59
240 ml	$23.50	Dexamethasone, Morton Grove	60432-0466-08

HOW SUPPLIED - RATED THERAPEUTICALLY EQUIVALENT: *(cont'd)*

240 ml	$26.83	Dexamethasone, H.C.F.A. F F P	99999-0974-03
240 ml	$26.95	Dexamethasone, Alpharma	00472-0972-08
240 ml	**$31.62**	**DECADRON, Merck**	**00006-7622-66**
3840 ml	$63.09	Dexamethasone, Rugby	00536-0452-90

Suspension - Ophthalmic - 0.1 %

5 ml	$18.44	MAXIDEX, Alcon-PR	00998-0615-05
15 ml	$31.88	MAXIDEX, Alcon-PR	00998-0615-15

Tablet, Uncoated - Oral - 0.5 mg

100's	$12.01	Dexamethasone, Roxane	00054-4179-25
100's	$14.99	Dexamethasone, Roxane	00054-8179-25
100's	**$51.86**	**DECADRON, Merck**	**00006-0041-68**
1000's	$117.87	Dexamethasone, Roxane	00054-4179-31

Tablet, Uncoated - Oral - 0.75 mg

12's	**$8.16**	**DECADRON, 5-12 PAK, Merck**	**00006-0063-12**
100's	$14.61	Dexamethasone, Roxane	00054-4180-25
100's	$17.22	Dexamethasone, Roxane	00054-8180-25
100's	**$64.84**	**DECADRON, Merck**	**00006-0063-68**

Tablet, Uncoated - Oral - 1.5 mg

50's	**$58.39**	**DECADRON, Merck**	**00006-0095-50**
100's	$27.14	Dexamethasone, Roxane	00054-4182-25
100's	$29.08	Dexamethasone, Roxane	00054-8181-25

Tablet, Uncoated - Oral - 4 mg

50's	**$93.84**	**DECADRON, Merck**	**00006-0097-50**
100's	$56.41	Dexamethasone, Roxane	00054-8175-25
100's	$58.41	Dexamethasone, Roxane	00054-4184-25

HOW SUPPLIED - NOT RATED EQUIVALENT:

Aerosol - Topical - 0.01 %

25 gm	$14.86	DECASPRAY, Merck	00006-7623-25
58 gm	$17.57	AEROSEB-DEX, Allergan	00023-0852-90

Gel - Topical - 0.1 %

30 gm	$19.86	DECADERM, Merck	00006-7631-24

Package - Oral - 0.75 mg/1.5 mg

1's	$5.40	HEXADROL, Organon	00052-0795-14

Solution - Oral - 0.5 mg/.5ml

30 ml	$14.30	DEXAMETHASONE INTENSOL, Roxane	00054-3176-44

Solution - Oral - 0.5 mg/5ml

5 ml x 40	$27.07	Dexamethasone, Roxane	00054-8177-16
20 ml x 40	$34.04	Dexamethasone, Roxane	00054-8168-16
500 ml	$17.56	Dexamethasone, Roxane	00054-3177-63

Tablet, Uncoated - Oral - 0.25 mg

100's	$4.10	Dexamethasone, Par Pharm	49884-0083-01
100's	$4.20	Dexamethasone, Schein Pharm (US)	00364-0397-01
100's	$4.25	Dexamethasone, HL Moore Drug Exch	00839-6019-06
100's	$4.42	Dexamethasone, Aligen Independ	00405-4313-01
100's	$5.20	Dexamethasone, Rugby	00536-3581-01
100's	**$28.85**	**DECADRON, Merck**	**00006-0020-68**
1000's	$40.20	Dexamethasone, Schein Pharm (US)	00364-0397-02
1000's	$41.00	Dexamethasone, Par Pharm	49884-0083-10

Tablet, Uncoated - Oral - 0.5 mg

100's	$5.99	Dexamethasone, Major Pharms	00904-0243-60
100's	$6.40	Dexamethasone, Goldline Labs	00182-1612-01
100's	$6.45	Dexamethasone, Qualitest Pharms	00603-3190-21
100's	$6.50	Dexamethasone, Par Pharm	49884-0084-01
100's	$6.72	Dexamethasone, Aligen Independ	00405-4314-01
100's	$6.75	Dexamethasone, Consolidated Midland	00223-0790-01
100's	$6.82	Dexamethasone, HL Moore Drug Exch	00839-6020-06
100's	$6.85	Dexamethasone, Schein Pharm (US)	00364-0398-01
100's	$7.14	DEXONE, Solvay Pharms	00032-3205-01
100's	$8.95	Dexamethasone, Rugby	00536-3582-01
1000's	$65.00	Dexamethasone, Par Pharm	49884-0084-10

Tablet, Uncoated - Oral - 0.75 mg

12's	$3.50	Dexamethasone, Qualitest Pharms	00603-3191-11
12's	$3.55	Dexamethasone, Major Pharms	00904-0244-12
12's	$5.45	Dexamethasone, Horizon Pharms	60904-0085-27
100's	$6.60	Dexamethasone, United Res	00677-0340-01
100's	$6.65	Dexamethasone, Major Pharms	00904-0244-60
100's	$7.50	Dexamethasone, Goldline Labs	00182-0488-01
100's	$7.50	Dexamethasone, Consolidated Midland	00223-0791-01
100's	$7.50	Dexamethasone, Par Pharm	49884-0085-01
100's	$7.55	Dexamethasone, Qualitest Pharms	00603-3191-21
100's	$7.64	Dexamethasone, Aligen Independ	00405-4315-01
100's	$7.65	Dexamethasone, Martec Pharms	52555-0064-01
100's	$7.75	Dexamethasone, Schein Pharm (US)	00364-0098-01
100's	$7.90	Dexamethasone, HL Moore Drug Exch	00839-1228-06
100's	$10.60	Dexamethasone, Rugby	00536-3583-01
100's	$12.61	DEXONE, Solvay Pharms	00032-3210-01
500's	$37.50	Dexamethasone, Par Pharm	49884-0085-05
1000's	$67.50	Dexamethasone, Consolidated Midland	00223-0791-02
1000's	$75.00	Dexamethasone, Par Pharm	49884-0085-10

Tablet, Uncoated - Oral - 1 mg

100's	$25.51	Dexamethasone, Roxane	00054-4181-25
100's	$25.79	Dexamethasone, Roxane	00054-8174-25

Tablet, Uncoated - Oral - 1.5 mg

50's	$10.40	Dexamethasone, Goldline Labs	00182-1613-19
50's	$10.40	Dexamethasone, Par Pharm	49884-0086-03
100's	$13.50	Dexamethasone, Qualitest Pharms	00603-3192-21
100's	$15.00	Dexamethasone, Consolidated Midland	00223-0792-01
100's	$15.22	Dexamethasone, Schein Pharm (US)	00364-0399-01
100's	$15.90	Dexamethasone, Major Pharms	00904-0245-60
100's	$20.00	Dexamethasone, Par Pharm	49884-0086-01
100's	$25.19	DEXONE, Solvay Pharms	00032-3215-01
500's	$100.00	Dexamethasone, Par Pharm	49884-0086-05
1000's	$197.00	Dexamethasone, Par Pharm	49884-0086-10

Tablet, Uncoated - Oral - 2 mg

100's	$48.76	Dexamethasone, Roxane	00054-8176-25
100's	$49.95	Dexamethasone, Roxane	00054-4183-25

Tablet, Uncoated - Oral - 4 mg

50's	$19.00	Dexamethasone, Goldline Labs	00182-1614-19
50's	$19.00	Dexamethasone, Rugby	00536-3580-06
50's	$19.00	Dexamethasone, Par Pharm	49884-0087-03
100's	$22.54	Dexamethasone, Major Pharms	00904-0246-60

HOW SUPPLIED - NOT RATED EQUIVALENT: *(cont'd)*

100's	$22.55	Dexamethasone, Qualitest Pharms	00603-3194-21
100's	$24.45	Dexamethasone, United Res	00677-0849-01
100's	$32.00	Dexamethasone, Goldline Labs	00182-1614-01
100's	$32.00	Dexamethasone, Par Pharm	49884-0087-01
100's	$32.65	Dexamethasone, Martec Pharms	52555-0066-01
100's	$34.09	Dexamethasone, HL Moore Drug Exch	00839-6734-06
100's	$47.25	HEXADROL, Organon	00052-0798-91
100's	$50.80	HEXADROL, Organon	00052-0798-90
100's	$54.12	DEXONE, Solvay Pharms	00032-3220-01
500's	$160.00	Dexamethasone, Par Pharm	49884-0087-05
1000's	$320.00	Dexamethasone, Par Pharm	49884-0087-10

Tablet, Uncoated - Oral - 6 mg

50's	$31.00	Dexamethasone, Par Pharm	49884-0129-03
100's	$57.00	Dexamethasone, Par Pharm	49884-0129-01
100's	$88.49	Dexamethasone, Roxane	00054-8183-25
100's	$98.88	Dexamethasone, Roxane	00054-4186-25

DEXAMETHASONE ACETATE *(000975)*

CATEGORIES: Adrenal Corticosteroids; Adrenal Hyperplasia; Adrenal Insufficiency; Airway Obstruction; Allergies; Alopecia; Anemia; Ankylosing Spondylitis; Anti-Inflammatory Agents; Antiarthritics; Arteritis; Arthritis; Asthma; Atopic Dermatitis; Bursitis; Cancer; Carditis; Chorioretinitis; Choroiditis; Colitis; Conjunctivitis; Corneal Ulcer; Dermatitis; Dermatitis Herpetiformis; Diagnostic Agents; Diuresis; Drug Hypersensitivity; Epicondylitis; Erythema Multiforme; Erythroblastopenia; Glucocorticoids; Gouty Arthritis; Granuloma Annulare; Herpes; Herpes Zoster; Hormones; Hypercalcemia; Inflammation; Inflammatory Lesions; Iridocyclitis; Keratitis; Laryngeal Edema; Lesions; Leukemia; Lichen Planus; Lichen Simplex Chronicus; Lupus Erythematosus; Lymphoma; Meningitis; Mycosis Fungoides; Necrobiosis Lipoidica; Nephrotic Syndrome; Neuritis; Osteoarthritis; Pain; Pemphigus; Pharmaceutical Adjuvants; Pneumoconiosis; Proteinuria; Psoriasis; Purpura; Retinochoroiditis; Rhinitis; Sarcoidosis; Serum Sickness; Spondylitis; Steroids; Synovitis; Synovitis of Osteoarthritis; Tenosynovitis; Thrombocytopenia; Thyroiditis; Transfusion Reactions; Trichinosis; Tuberculosis; Tumors; Ulcerative Colitis; Urticaria; Uveitis; FDA Approval Pre 1982

BRAND NAMES: Adrenocot L.A.; Dalalone; De-Sone La; Deca-Plex La; *Decadron Depot*; *Decadron I.A.*; **Decadron-La**; Decaject-La; Decapan La; Decarex; Decasone R.P.; Dekasol; Dexacen La-8; Dexacorten-La; Dexasone L.A.; Dexim La; Dexone La; *Fortecortin KS* (Germany); Medidex-La; Or-Dex L.A.; Preladron La; Primethasone; Solurex La
(International brand names outside U.S. in italics)

FORMULARIES: BC-BS

DESCRIPTION:

Dexamethasone Acetate, a synthetic adrenocortical steroid, is a white to practically white, odorless powder. It is a practically insoluble ester of dexamethasone.

Dexamethasone Acetate suspension is present as the monohydrate with the empirical formula:

$C_{24}H_{31}FO_6$-H_2O, and molecular weight, 452.52. Dexamethasone acetate is designated chemically as 21-(acetytaxy)-9-fluoro-11β,17-dihydroxy-16α-methylpregna-1,4-diene -3,20-dione.

Dexamethasone Acetate suspension is a sterile white suspension (pH 5.0 to 7.5) that settles on standing, but is easily resuspended by mild shaking.

Each milliliter contains dexamethasone acetate equivalent to 8 mg dexamethasone. Inactive ingredients per ml: 6.57 mg sodium chloride; 5 mg creatinine; 0.5 mg disodium edetate; 5 mg sodium carboxymethylcellulose: 0.75 mg polysorbate 80; sodium hydroxide to adjust pH; and Water for Injection, as 1 ml, with 9 mg benzyl alcohol, and 1 mg sodium bisulfite added as preservatives.

CLINICAL PHARMACOLOGY:

Dexamethasone Acetate suspension is a long-acting, repository adrenocorticosteroid preparation with a prompt onset of action. It is suitable for intramuscular or local injection, but not when an immediate effect of short duration is desired.

Naturally occurring glucocorticoids (hydrocortisone and cortisone), which also have self-retaining properties, are used as replacement therapy in adrenocortical deficiency states. Their synthetic analogs, including dexamethasone, are primarily used for their potent anti-inflammatory effects in disorders of many organ systems.

Glucocorticoids cause profound and varied metabolic effects. In addition, they modify the body's immune responses to diverse stimuli

At equipotent anti-inflammatory doses, dexamethasone almost completely lacks the sodium-retaining property of hydrocortisone.

INDICATIONS AND USAGE:

BY INTRAMUSCULAR INJECTION WHEN ORAL THERAPY IS NOT FEASIBLE:

Endocrine disorders: Congenital adrenal hyperplasia, Nonsuppurative thyroiditis, Hypercalcemia associated with cancer

Rheumatic disorders: As adjunctive therapy for short-term administration (to tide the patient over an acute episode or exacerbation) in: Post-traumatic osteoarthritis, Synovitis of osteoarthritis, Rheumatoid arthritis, including juvenile rheumatoid arthritis (selected cases may require low-dose maintenance therapy), Acute and subacute bursitis, Epicondylitis, Acute nonspecific tenosynovitis, Acute gouty arthritis, Psoriatic arthritis, Ankylosing spondylitis.

Collagen disease: During an exacerbation or as maintenance therapy in selected cases of: Systemic lupus erythematosus, Acute rheumatic carditis

Dermatologic diseases: Pemphigus, Severe erythema multiforme (Stevens-Johnson syndrome), Exfoliative dermatitis, Bullous dermatitis herpetiformis, Severe seborrheic dermatitis, Severe psoriasis, Mycosis fungoides.

Allergic states:

Control of severe of incapacitating allergic conditions intractable to adequate trails of conventional treatment in Bronchial asthma, Contact dermatitis, Atopic dermatitis, Serum sickness, Seasonal or perennial allergic rhinitis, Drug hypersensitivity reactions, Urticarial transfusion reactions.

Ophthalmic diseases: Severe acute and chronic allergic and inflammatory processes involving the eye, such as:Herpes zoster ophthalmicus; Iritis, Iridocyclitis; Chorioretinitis; Diffuse posterior uveitis and choroiditis; Optic neuritis; Sympathetic ophthalmia; Anterior segment inflammation; Allergic conjunctivitis; Keratitis; Allergic corneal marginal ulcers.

Gastrointestinal diseases: To tide the patient over a critical period of the disease in:Ulcerative colitis (Systemic therapy), Regional arteritis (Systemic therapy).

INDICATIONS AND USAGE: *(cont'd)*

Respiratory diseases: Symptomatic sarcoidosis, Berylliosis, Loeffler's syndrome not manageable by other means, Aspiration pneumonitis.

Hematologic disorders: Acquired (autoimmune) hemolytic anemia Secondary thrombocytopenia in adults, Erythroblastopenia (RBC anemia), Congenital (erythroid) hypoplastic anemia.

Neoplastic diseases: For palliative management of: Leukemias and lymphomas in adults, Acute leukemia of childhood.

Edematous states: To induce diuresis or remission of proteinuria in the nephrotic syndrome, without uremia of the idiopathic type, or that due to lupus erythematosus.

Miscellaneous: Trichinosis with neurologic or myocardial involvement.

BY INTRA-ARTICULAR OR SOFT TISSUE INJECTION AS ADJUNCTIVE THERAPY FOR SHORT-TERM ADMINISTRATION TO TIDE THE PATIENT OVER AN ACUTE EPISODE OR EXACERBATION IN:

Synovitis of osteoarthritis
Rheumatoid arthritis
Acute and subacute bursitis
Acute gouty arthritis
Epicondylitis
Acute nonspecific tenosynovitis
Post-traumatic osteoarthritis.

BY INTRALESIONAL INJECTION IN:

Keroids

Localized hypertrophic, infiltrated, inflammatory lesions of: lichen planus, psoriatic plaques, granuloma annulare, and lichen simplex chronicus (neurodermatitis)

Discoid lupus erythematosus

Necrobiosis lipoidica diabeticorum

Alopecia aerate

May also be useful in cystic tumors of an aponeurosis of tendon (ganglia).

CONTRAINDICATIONS:

Systemic fungal infections

Hypersensitivity to any component of this product.

WARNINGS:

DO NOT INJECT INTRAVENOUSLY

In patients on corticosteroid therapy subjected to any unusual stress, increased dosage of rapidly acting corticosteroids before, during, and after the stressful situation is indicated.

Drug-induced secondary adrenocortical insufficiency may result from too rapid withdrawal of corticosteroids and may be minimized by gradual reduction of dosage. This type of relative insufficiency may persist for months after discontinuation of therapy: therefore, in any situation of stress occurring during that period, hormone therapy should be reinstituted. If the patient is receiving steroids already, dosage may have to be increased. since mineralocorticoid secretion may be impaired, salt and/or a mineralocorticoid should be administered concurrently.

Corticosteroids may mask some signs of infection, and new infections may appear during their used. There may be decreased resistance and inability to localize infection when corticosteroids are used. Moreover, corticosteroids may affect the nitroblue-tetrazolium test for bacterial infection and produce false negative results.

Corticosteroids may activate latent amebiasis. Therefore, it is recommended that latent or active amebiasis be ruled out before initiating corticosteroid therapy in any patient who has spent time in the tropics or any patient with unexplained diarrhea.

Prolonged use of corticosteroids may produce posterior subcapsular cataracts, glaucoma with possible damage to the optic nerves, and may enhance the establishment of secondary ocular infections due to fungi or viruses.

Usage In Pregnancy Since adequate human reproduction studies have not been done with corticosteroids, use of these drugs in pregnancy or in women of childbearing potential requires that the anticipated benefits be weighed against the possible hazards to the mother and embryo or fetus. Infants born of mothers who have received substantial doses of corticosteroids during pregnancy should be carefully observed for signs of hypoadrenalism.

Corticosteroids appear in breast milk and could suppress growth, interfere with endogenous corticosteroid production, or cause other unwanted effects. Mothers taking pharmacologic doses of corticosteroids should be advised not to nurse.

Average and large doses of cortisone or hydrocortisone can cause elevation of blood pressure, salt and water retention, and increased excretion of potassium. These effects are less likely to occur with the synthetic derivatives except when used in large doses. Dietary salt restriction and potassium supplementation may be necessary. All corticosteroids increase calcium excretion.

While on corticosteroid therapy patients should not be vaccinated against smallpox. Other immunization procedures should not be undertaken in patients who are on corticosteroids, especially on high doses, because of possible hazards of neurologic complications and lack of antibody response.

If corticosteroids are indicated in patients, with latent tuberculosis or tuberculin reactivity, close observation is necessary as reactivation of the disease may occur. During prolonged corticosteroid therapy, these patients should receive chemoprophylaxis.

Because rare instances of anaphylactoid reactions have occurred in patients receiving parenteral corticosteroid therapy, appropriate precautionary measures should be taken prior to administration, especially when the patient has a history of allergy to any drug.

Repository adrenocorticosteroid preparations may cause atrophy at the site of injection. To minimize the likelihood and/or severity of atrophy, do not inject subcutaneously, avoid injection into the deltoid muscle, and avoid, repeated intramuscular injections into the same site if possible.

Dosage in children under 12 has not been established.

PRECAUTIONS:

Dexamethasone Acetate suspension is not recommended as initial therapy in acute, life-threatening situations.

This product, like many other steroid formulations, is sensitive to heat. Therefore, if should not be autoclaved when it is desirable to sterilize the exterior of the vial.

Following prolonged therapy, withdrawal of corticosteroids may result in symptoms of the corticosteroid withdrawal syndrome including fever, myalgia, arthralgia, and malaise. This may occur in patients even without evidence of adrenal insufficiency.

There is an enhanced effect of corticosteroids in patients with hypothyroidism and in those with cirrhosis.

Corticosteroids should be used cautiously in patients with ocular herpes simplex for fear of corneal perforation.

Psychic derangements may appear when corticosteroids are used, ranging from euphoria, insomnia, mood swings, personality changes, and severe depression to frank psychotic manifestations. Also, existing emotional instability or psychotic tendencies may be aggravated by corticosteroids.

PRECAUTIONS: *(cont'd)*

Aspirin should be used cautiously in conjunction with corticosteroids in hypoprothrombinemia.

Steroids should be used with caution in nonspecific ulcerative colitis, if there is a probability of impending perforation, abscess or other pyogenic infection, also in diverticulitis, fresh intestinal anastomoses, active or latent peptic ulcer, renal insufficiency, hypertension, osteoporosis, and myasthenia gravis. Fat embolism has been reported as a possible complication of hypercortisonism.

When large doses are given, some authorities advise that antacids be administered between meals to help to prevent peptic ulcer.

Growth and development of infants and children on prolonged corticosteroid therapy should be carefully followed.

Steroids may increase or decrease motility and number of spermatozoa in some patients.

Phenytoin, phenobarbital, ephedrine, and rifampin may enhance the metabolic clearance of corticosteroids, resulting in decreased blood levels and lessened physiologic activity, thus requiring adjustment in corticosteroid dosage.

The prothrombin time should be checked frequently in patients who are receiving corticosteroids and coumarin anticoagulants at the same time because of reports that corticosteroids have altered the response to these anticoagulants. Studies have shown that the usual effect produced by adding corticosteroids is inhibition of response to coumarin, although there have been some conflicting reports of potentiation not substantiated by studies.

When corticosteroids are administered concomitantly with potassium-depleting diuretics, patients-should be observed closely for development of hypokalemia.

Intra-articular injection of a corticosteroid may produce systemic as well as local effects.

Appropriate examination of any joint fluid present is necessary to exclude a septic process.

A marked increase in pain accompanied by local swelling, further restriction of joint motion, fever, and malaise is suggestive of septic arthritis. If this complication occurs and the diagnosis of sepsis is confirmed, appropriate antimicrobial therapy should be instituted.

Injection of a steroid into an infected site is to be avoided.

Corticosteroids should not be injected into unstable joints.

Patients should be impressed strongly with the importance of not overusing joints in which symptomatic benefit has been obtained as long as the inflammatory process remains active.

Frequent intra-articular injection may result in damage to joint-tissues.

ADVERSE REACTIONS:

Fluid and electrolyte disturbances: Sodium retention, Fluid retention, Congestive heart failure in susceptible patients, Potassium loss, Hypokalemic alkalosis, Hypertension.

Musculoskeletal: Muscle weakness, Steroid myopathy, Loss of muscle mass, Osteoporosis, Vertebral compression fractures, Aseptic necrosis of femoral and humeral heads, Pathologic fracture of long bones, Tendon rapture.

Gastrointestinal: Peptic ulcer with possible subsequent perforation and hemorrhage, Pancreatitis, Abdominal distention, Ulcerative esophagitis.

Dermatologic: Impaired wound healing, Thin fragile skin, Petechiae and ecchymoses, Erythema, Increased sweating, May suppress reactions to skin tests, Other cutaneous reactions, such as allergic dermatitis, urticaria, angioneurotic edema

Neurologic: Convulsions, Increased intracranial pressure with papilledema (pseudotumor cerebri) usually after treatment, Vertigo, Headache.

Endocrine: Menstrual irregularities, Development of cushingoid state, Suppression of growth in children, Secondary adrenocortical and pituitary unresponsiveness, particularly in times of stress, as in trauma, surgery, or illness, Decreased carbohydrate tolerance, Manifestations of latent diabetes mellitus, Increased requirements for insulin or oral hypoglycemic agents in diabetics.

Ophthalmic: Posterior subcapsular cataracts, Increased intraocular pressure, Glaucoma, Exophthalmos.

Metabolic: Negative nitrogen balance due to protein catabolism.

Other: Anaphylactoid or hypersensitivity reactions, Thromboembolism, Weight gain, Increased appetite, Nausea, Malaise.

The following *additional* adverse reactions are related to parenteral corticosteroid therapy: Rare instances of blindness associated with intralesional therapy around the face and head;Hyperpigmentation or hypopigmentation; Subcutaneous and cutaneous atrophy; Sterile abscess; Postinjection flare (following intra-articular use); Charcol-like arthropathy; Scarring; Induration; Inflammation; Paresthesia; Delayed pain or soreness; Muscle twitching, ataxia, hiccups, and nystagmus have been reported in low incidence after injection of Dexamethasone Acetate suspension.

DOSAGE AND ADMINISTRATION:

For intramuscular, intralesional, intra-articular, and soft tissue injection.

Dosage Requirements Are Variable and Must Be Individualized on the Basis of the Disease and the Response of the Patient

Dosages in children under 12 has not been established.

Intramuscular Injection: Dosage ranges from 1 to 2 ml, equivalent to 8 to 16 mg of dexamethasone. If further treatment is needed, dosage may be repeated at intervals of 1 to 3 weeks.

Intralesional Injection: The usual dose is 0.1 to 0.2 ml, equivalent to 0.8 to 1.6 mg of dexamethasone, per injection site.

Intra-articular and Soft Tissue Injection: The dose varies, depending on the location and the severity of inflammation. The usual dose is 0.5 to 2 mal, equivalent to 4 to 16 mg of dexamethasone. If further treatment is needed, dosage may be repeated at intervals of 1 to 3 weeks. Frequent intra-articular injection may result in damage to joint tissues.

HOW SUPPLIED - EQUIVALENTS NOT AVAILABLE:

Injection, Susp - Intra-Articular - 8 mg/ml

1 ml	$11.71	DECADRON LA, Merck	00006-7644-01
5 ml	$11.07	Dexamethasone Acetate L.A., Pasadena	00418-4091-31
5 ml	$11.33	Dexamethasone Acetate Suspension, Insource	58441-0115-05
5 ml	$11.50	Dexamethasone Acetate, Consolidated Midland	00223-7390-05
5 ml	$11.94	SOLUREX LA, Hyrex Pharms	00314-0897-75
5 ml	$12.29	Dexamethasone Acetate, McGuff	49072-0155-05
5 ml	$12.90	DE-SONE L A, UAD Labs	00785-8045-05
5 ml	$13.50	ADRENOCOT L.A., C O Truxton	00463-1104-05
5 ml	$17.50	DALALONE L.A., Forest Pharms	00456-1075-05
5 ml	$18.00	Dexamethasone Acetate, United Res	00677-0822-20
5 ml	$18.62	Dexamethasone Acetate, HL Moore Drug Exch	00839-6109-25
5 ml	$20.00	DEXACORTEN-LA, Bolan Pharm	44437-0092-05
5 ml	$22.50	Dexamethasone Acetate, Major Pharms	00904-0906-05
5 ml	$24.45	Dexamethasone Acetate, Goldline Labs	00182-0928-62
5 ml	$27.88	Dexamethasone Acetate, Rugby	00536-4163-65
5 ml	$29.90	Dexamethasone, Geneva Pharms	00781-3008-75

HOW SUPPLIED - EQUIVALENTS NOT AVAILABLE: *(cont'd)*

5 ml	$29.93	Dexamethasone Acetate, Steris Labs	00402-0092-05
5 ml	$32.00	DECAJECT-L.A., Mayrand Pharms	00259-0328-05
5 ml	$32.93	Dexamethasone Acetate, General Inj & Vac	52584-0092-05
5 ml	$32.93	Dexamethasone Acetate, Insource	58441-7644-03
5 ml	$32.93	Dexamethasone Acetate, King Pharms	60793-0108-05
5 ml	$32.95	Dexamethasone Acetate, Schein Pharm (US)	00364-6699-53
5 ml	$47.15	DECADRON LA, Merck	00006-7644-03

Injection, Susp - Intra-Articular - 16 mg/ml

1 ml x 10	$57.00	DALALONE D P, Forest Pharms	00456-1097-41
5 ml	$20.00	DALALONE D P, Forest Pharms	00456-1097-05

Powder

10 gm	$135.20	Dexamethasone Acetate, Paddock Labs	00574-0409-10

DEXAMETHASONE SODIUM PHOSPHATE

(000976)

CATEGORIES: Acne; Acne Rosacea; Adrenal Corticosteroids; Adrenal Hyperplasia; Adrenal Insufficiency; Adrenocortical Insufficiency; Airway Obstruction; Allergies; Alopecia; Alopecia Areata; Anemia; Ankylosing Spondylitis; Anterior Pituitary/Hypothalmic Function; Anti-Inflammatory Agents; Antiarthritics; Antibiotics; Arthritis; Asthma; Atopic Dermatitis; Berylliosis; Bronchospasm; Burns; Bursitis; Cancer; Carditis; Chemotherapy; Chorioretinitis; Choroiditis; Colitis; Conjunctival Inflammation; Conjunctivitis; Corneal Inflammation; Corneal Injury; Corneal Ulcer; Cyclitis; Dermatitis; Dermatitis Herpetiformis; Dermatologicals; Diagnostic Agents; Diuresis; Drug Hypersensitivity; EENT Drugs; Edema; Enteritis; Epicondylitis; Erythema Multiforme; Eye, Ear, Nose, & Throat Preparations; Gouty Arthritis; Granuloma Annulare; Herpes; Herpes Zoster; Hormones; Hypercalcemia; Inflammatory Conditions; Inflammatory Lesions; Iridocyclitis; Keloids; Keratitis; Laryngeal Edema; Lesions; Leukemia; Lichen Planus; Lichen Simplex Chronicus; Lupus Erythematosus; Lymphoma; Meningitis; Mycosis Fungoides; Nasal Polyps; Necrobiosis Lipoidica; Nephrotic Syndrome; Neuritis; Ocular Acne; Ocular Infections; Ophthalmics; Osteoarthritis; Pain; Pemphigus; Pneumoconiosis; Proteinuria; Pruritus; Psoriasis; Purpura; Retinochoroiditis; Rhinitis; Rosacea; Sarcoidosis; Serum Sickness; Shock; Skin/Mucous Membrane Agents; Spondylitis; Synovitis; Synovitis of Osteoarthritis; Tenosynovitis; Thrombocytopenia; Thyroiditis; Transfusion Reactions; Trichinosis; Tuberculosis; Tumors; Ulcerative Colitis; Urticaria; Uveitis; FDA Approval Pre 1982

BRAND NAMES: Adrenocot; Ak-Dex; Baldex; *Cebedex* (France); Dalalone; De-Sone; Deca-Gen; Deca-Plex 10; Decadrol; Decadron; **Decadron Injection**; Decadron Ocumeter; Decadron Ophthalmic Ointment; Decadron Ophthalmic Solution; Decadron Respihaler; Decadron Topical Cream; Decadron Turbinaire; Decagen; Decaject; Decapan; Decarex; Decasone; Dekasol; Dexacen-4; Dexacort Phosphate Turbinaire; Dexacort Respihaler; Dexacorten; Dexair; Dexasol; Dexasone; Dexim; Dexone; Dexotic; Dexsone-E; Dua-Dex S.P.; Hexadrol; I-Methasone; Infa-Dex; *Isoftalmol*; Maxidex; Medidex; Ocu-Dex; Primethasone; Solurex; Spectro-Dex; *Spersadex* (Germany); *Sterodex*; Storz-Dexa
(International brand names outside U.S. in italics)

FORMULARIES: PCS

DESCRIPTION:

Dexamethasone sodium phosphate, a synthetic adrenocortical steroid, is a white or slightly yellow, crystalline powder. It is freely soluble in water and is exceedingly hygroscopic. The molecular weight is 516.41. It is designated chemically as 9-fluoro-11β,17-dihydroxy-16α-methyl-21-(phosphonooxy)pregna-1,4-di ene-3,20-dione disodium salt. The empirical formula is $C_{22}H_{28}FNa_2O_8P$.

Injection: Dexamethasone sodium phosphate injection is a sterile solution (pH 7.0 to 8.5) of dexamethasone sodium phosphate, sealed under nitrogen, and is supplied in two concentrations: 4 mg/ml and 24 mg/ml. The 24 mg/ml concentration offers the advantage of less volume in indications where high doses of corticosteroids by the intravenous route are needed.

Each milliliter of dexamethasone sodium phosphate injection, 4 mg/ml, contains dexamethasone sodium phosphate equivalent to 4 mg dexamethasone phosphate or 3.33 mg dexamethasone. Inactive ingredients per ml: 8 mg creatinine, 10 mg sodium hydroxide to adjust pH, and Water for Injection q.s., with 1 mg sodium bisulfite, 1.5 mg methylparaben, and 0.2 mg propylparaben added as preservatives.

Each milliliter of dexamethasone sodium phosphate injection, 24 mg/ml, contains dexamethasone sodium phosphate equivalent to 24 mg dexamethasone phosphate or 20 mg dexamethasone. Inactive ingredients per ml:8 mg creatinine, 10 mg sodium citrate, 0.5 mg disodium edetate, sodium hydroxide to adjust pH, and Water for Injection q.s., with 1 mg sodium bisulfite, 1.5 mg methylparaben, and 0.2 mg propylparaben added as preservatives.

Ophthalmic Ointment: Sterile Dexamethasone Sodium Phosphate Ophthalmic Ointment is a topical steroid ointment containing dexamethasone sodium phosphate equivalent to 0.5 mg (0.05%) dexamethasone phosphate in each gram. Inactive ingredients: white petrolatum and mineral oil.

Dexamethasone sodium phosphate is an inorganic ester of dexamethasone.

Ophthalmic Solution: Dexamethasone Sodium Phosphate Ophthalmic Solution in the 5 ml Ocumeter ophthalmic dispenser is a topical steroid solution containing dexamethasone sodium phosphate equivalent up to 1 mg (0.1%) dexamethasone phosphate in each milliliter of buffered solution. Inactive ingredients: creatinine, sodium citrate, sodium borate, polysorbate 80, disodium edetate, hydrochloric acid to adjust pH, and water for injection. Sodium bisulfate 0.1%, phenylethanol 0.25% and benzalkonium chloride 0.02% added as preservatives.

Topical Cream: Dexamethasone Sodium Phosphate Topical Cream is a topical steroid preparation.

The topical corticosteroids constitute a class of primarily synthetic steroids used as anti-inflammatory and anti-pruritic agents.

Dexamethasone Sodium Phosphate Topical Cream contains in each gram: dexamethasone sodium phosphate equivalent to 1 mg (0.1%) dexamethasone phosphate in a greaseless bland base. Inactive ingredients: stearyl alcohol, cetyl alcohol, mineral oil, polyoxyl 40 stearate, sorbitol solution, methyl polysilicone emulsion, creatinine, sodium citrate,, disodium edetate, sodium hydroxide to adjust pH, and purified water. Methylparaben, 0.15%, and sorbic acid, 0.1% added as preservatives.

Oral Aerosol: Dexamethasone Sodium Phosphate in Respihaler (Dispenser) is an aerosol for oral inhalation which contains dexamethasone sodium phosphate, an inorganic ester of dexamethasone, a synthetic adrenocortical steroid with basic glucocorticoid actions and effects.

DESCRIPTION: *(cont'd)*

Each Dexamethasone Sodium Phosphate in Respihaler contains an amount sufficient to deliver at least 170 sprays. The metering valve of the aerosol mechanism of the Respihaler dispenses dexamethasone sodium phosphate equivalent to approximately 0.1 mg of dexamethasone phosphate or approximately 0.084 mg of dexamethasone with each activation. On a regimen of 12 inhalations daily, it has been determined that the patient absorbs approximately 0.4-0.6 mg of dexamethasone. The inactive ingredients are the fluorochlorohydrocarbons included as propellants. Alcohol 2%.

Intranasal Aerosol: Dexamethasone Sodium Phosphate in Turbinaire (Dispenser) is an aerosol for intranasal application. The inactive ingredients are fluorochlorohydrocarbons as propellants and alcohol 2%. One cartridge delivers an amount sufficient to ensure delivery of 170 metered sprays, each containing dexamethasone sodium phosphate equivalent to approximate 0.1 mg dexamethasone phosphate or to approximately 0.084 mg dexamethasone. Twelve sprays deliver a theoretical maximum of 1.0 mg dexamethasone.

CLINICAL PHARMACOLOGY:

INJECTION

Dexamethasone Sodium Phosphate Injection has a rapid onset but short duration of action when compared with less soluble preparations. Because of this, it is suitable for the treatment of acute disorders responsive to adrenocortical steroid therapy.

Naturally occurring glucocorticoids (hydrocortisone and cortisone), which also have salt-retaining properties, are used as replacement therapy in adrenocortical deficiency states. Their synthetic analogs, including dexamethasone, are primarily used for their potent anti-inflammatory effects in disorders of many organ systems.

Glucocorticoids cause profound and varied metabolic effects. In addition, they modify the body's immune responses to diverse stimuli.

At equipotent anti-inflammatory doses, dexamethasone almost completely lacks the sodium-retaining property of hydrocortisone and closely related derivatives of hydrocortisone.

OPHTHALMIC OINTMENT

This synthetic corticosteroid causes inhibitions of the inflammatory response to inciting agents of a mechanical, chemical, or immunological nature. No generally accepted explanation of this steroid property has been advanced.

OPHTHALMIC SOLUTION

Dexamethasone sodium phosphate suppresses the inflammatory response to a variety of agents and it probably delays or slows healing. No generally accepted explanation of these steroid properties have been advanced.

TOPICAL CREAM

Topical corticosteroids share anti-inflammatory, anti-pruritic and vasoconstrictive actions.

The mechanism of anti-inflammatory activity of the topical corticosteroids is unclear. Various laboratory methods, including vasoconstrictor assays, are used to compare and predict potencies and/or clinical efficacies of the topical corticosteroids. There is some evidence to suggest that a recognizable correlation exists between vasoconstrictor potency and therapeutic efficacy in man.

Pharmacokinetics

The extent of percutaneous absorption of topical corticosteroids is determined by many factors including the vehicle, the integrity of the epidermal barrier, and the use of occlusive dressings.

Topical corticosteroids can be absorbed from normal intact skin. Inflammation and/or other disease processes in the skin increase percutaneous absorption. Occlusive dressings substantially increase the percutaneous absorption of topical corticosteroids. Thus, occlusive dressings may be a valuable therapeutic adjunct for treatment of resistant dermatoses. (See DOSAGE AND ADMINISTRATION)

Once absorbed through the skin, topical corticosteroids are handled through pharmacokinetic pathways similar to systemically administered corticosteroids. Corticosteroids are bound to plasma proteins in varying degrees. Corticosteroids are metabolized primarily in the liver and are then excreted by the kidneys. Some of the topical corticosteroids and their metabolites are also excreted into the bile.

ORAL AEROSOL

Because of the high water solubility of dexamethasone sodium phosphate, the aerosolized particles dissolve readily in the secretions of the bronchial and bronchiolar mucous membrane.

INTRANASAL AEROSOL

Inhibition of inflammatory response to inciting agents of mechanical, chemical or immunological nature.

INDICATIONS AND USAGE:

INJECTION

By intravenous or intramuscular injection when oral therapy is not feasible:

Endocrine Disorders: Primary or secondary adrenocortical insufficiency (hydrocortisone or cortisone is the drug of choice; synthetic analogs may be used in conjunction with mineralocorticoids where applicable; in infancy, mineralocorticoid supplementation is of particular importance)

Acute adrenocortical insufficiency (hydrocortisone or cortisone is the drug of choice; mineralocorticoid supplementation may be necessary, particularly when synthetic analogs are used)
Preoperatively, and in the event of serious trauma or illness, in patients with known adrenal insufficiency or when adrenocortical reserve is doubtful
Shock unresponsive to conventional therapy if adrenocortical insufficiency exists or is suspected
Congenital adrenal hyperplasia
Nonsuppurative thyroiditis
Hypercalcemia associated with cancer

Rheumatic Disorders: As adjunctive therapy for short-term administration (to tide the patient over an acute episode or exacerbation) in:

Post-traumatic osteoarthritis
Synovitis of osteoarthritis
Rheumatoid arthritis, including juvenile rheumatoid arthritis (selected cases may require low-dose maintenance therapy)
Acute and subacute bursitis
Epicondylitis
Acute nonspecific tenosynovitis
Acute gouty arthritis
Psoriatic arthritis
Ankylosing spondylitis

Collagen Diseases: During an exacerbation or as maintenance therapy in selected cases of:

Systemic lupus erythematosus
Acute rheumatic carditis

Dermatologic Diseases

Pemphigus
Severe erythema multiforme (Stevens-Johnson syndrome)
Exfoliative dermatitis
Bullous dermatitis herpetiformis
Severe seborrheic dermatitis
Severe psoriasis
Mycosis fungoides

INDICATIONS AND USAGE: *(cont'd)*

Allergic States: Control of severe or incapacitating allergic conditions intractable to adequate trials of conventional treatment in:

- Bronchial asthma
- Contact dermatitis
- Atopic dermatitis
- Serum sickness
- Seasonal or perennial allergic rhinitis
- Drug hypersensitivity reactions
- Urticarial transfusion reactions
- Acute noninfectious laryngeal edema (epinephrine is the drug of first choice)

Ophthalmic Diseases: Severe acute and chronic allergic and inflammatory processes involving the eye, such as:

- Herpes zoster ophthalmicus
- Iritis, iridocyclitis
- Chorioretinitis
- Diffuse posterior uveitis and choroiditis
- Optic neuritis
- Sympathetic ophthalmia
- Anterior segment inflammation
- Allergic conjunctivitis
- Keratitis
- Allergic corneal marginal ulcers

Gastrointestinal Diseases: To tide the patient over a critical period of the disease in:

- Ulcerative colitis (Systemic therapy)
- Regional enteritis (Systemic therapy)

Respiratory Diseases

- Symptomatic sarcoidosis
- Berylliosis
- Fulminating or disseminated pulmonary tuberculosis when used concurrently with appropriate antituberculous chemotherapy
- Loeffler's syndrome not manageable by other means
- Aspiration pneumonitis

Hematologic Disorders

- Acquired (autoimmune) hemolytic anemia
- Idiopathic thrombocytopenic purpura in adults (IV only; IM administration is contraindicated)
- Secondary thrombocytopenia in adults
- Erythroblastopenia (RBC anemia)
- Congenital (erythroid) hypoplastic anemia

Neoplastic Diseases: For palliative management of:

- Leukemias and lymphomas in adults
- Acute leukemia of childhood

Edematous States: To induce diuresis or remission of proteinuria in the nephrotic syndrome, without uremia, of the idiopathic type, or that due to lupus erythematosus

Miscellaneous

- Tuberculous meningitis with subarachnoid block or impending block when used concurrently with appropriate antituberculous chemotherapy
- Trichinosis with neurologic or myocardial involvement

Diagnostic testing of adrenocortical hyperfunction

Cerebral Edema: associated with primary or metastatic brain tumor, craniotomy, or head injury. Use in cerebral edema is not a substitute for careful neurosurgical evaluation and definitive management such as neurosurgery or other specific therapy.

By intra-articular or soft tissue injection:

As adjunctive therapy for short-term administration (to tide the patient over an acute episode or exacerbation) in:

- Synovitis of osteoarthritis
- Rheumatoid arthritis
- Acute and subacute bursitis
- Acute gouty arthritis
- Epicondylitis
- Acute nonspecific tenosynovitis
- Post-traumatic osteoarthritis.

By intralesional injection:

- Keloids
- Localized hypertrophic, infiltrated, inflammatory lesions of: lichen planus, psoriatic plaques, granuloma annulare and lichen simplex chronicus (neurodermatitis)
- Discoid lupus erythematosus
- Necrobiosis lipoidica diabeticorum
- Alopecia areata
- May also be useful in cystic tumors of an aponeurosis or tendon (ganglia).

OPHTHALMIC OINTMENT AND SOLUTION

Ophthalmic: Steroid responsive inflammatory conditions of the palpebral and bulbar conjunctiva, cornea, and anterior segment of the globe, such as allergic conjunctivitis, acne rosacea, superficial punctate keratitis, herpes zoster keratitis, iritis, cyclitis, selected infective conjunctivitis, corneal injury from chemical, or thermal burns, or penetration of foreign bodies, when the inherent hazard of steroid use is accepted to obtain an advisable diminution in edema and inflammation; corneal injury from chemical or thermal burns, or penetration of foreign bodies.

OPHTHALMIC SOLUTION ONLY

Otic: Steroid responsive inflammatory conditions of the external auditory meatus, such as allergic otitis externa, selected purulent and nonpurulent infective otitis externa when the hazard of steroid use is accepted to obtain an advisable diminution in edema and inflammation.

TOPICAL CREAM

Dexamethasone Sodium Phosphate Topical Cream is indicated for relief of the inflammatory and pruritic manifestations of corticosteroid-responsive dermatoses.

ORAL AEROSOL

Dexamethasone Sodium Phosphate in Respihaler is indicated for the treatment of bronchial asthma and related corticosteroid responsive bronchospastic states intractable to adequate trial of conventional therapy.

INTRANASAL AEROSOL

Allergic or inflammatory nasal conditions, and nasal polyps (excluding polyps originating within the sinuses).

CONTRAINDICATIONS:

Injection: Systemic fungal infections. (See WARNINGS) regarding amphotericin B, Hypersensitivity to any component of this product, including sulfites (see WARNINGS.)

Ophthalmic Ointment and Ophthalmic Solution: Epithelial herpes simplex keratitis (dendritic keratitis), Acute infectious stages of vaccina, varicella, and many other viral diseases of the cornea and conjunctiva, Mycobacterial infection of the eye, Fungal diseases of ocular or auricular structures, Hypersensitivity to a component of the medication.

Ophthalmic Solution Only: Hypersensitivity to any component of this product, including sulfites (see WARNINGS), Perforation of a drum membrane.

Topical Cream: Topical corticosteroids are contraindicated in those patients with a history of hypersensitivity to any of the components of the preparation.

Oral Aerosol: Systemic fungal infections, Hypersensitivity to any component of this medication, Persistently positive cultures of the sputum for *Candida albicans.*

Intranasal Aerosol: Systemic fungal infections, Hypersensitivity to components, Tuberculous, viral and fungal nasal conditions, ocular herpes simplex.

WARNINGS:

INJECTION

Because rare instances of anaphylactoid reactions have occurred in patients receiving parenteral corticosteroid therapy, appropriate precautionary measures should be taken prior to administration, especially when the patient has a history of allergy to any drug. Anaphylactoid and hypersensitivity reactions have been reported for dexamethasone sodium phosphate injection (see ADVERSE REACTIONS.)

WARNINGS: *(cont'd)*

Dexamethasone sodium phosphate injection contains sodium bisulfite, a sulfite that may cause allergic-type reactions including anaphylactic symptoms and life-threatening or less severe asthmatic episodes in certain susceptible people. The overall prevalence of sulfite sensitivity in the general population is unknown and probably low. Sulfite sensitivity is seen more frequently in asthmatic than in nonasthmatic people.

Corticosteroids may exacerbate systemic fungal infections and therefore should not be used in the presence of such infections unless they are needed to control drug reactions due to amphotericin B. Moreover, there have been cases reported in which concomitant use of amphotericin B and hydrocortisone was followed by cardiac enlargement and congestive failure.

In patients on corticosteroid therapy subjected to any unusual stress, increased dosage of rapidly acting corticosteroids before, during, and after the stressful situation is indicated.

Drug-induced secondary adrenocortical insufficiency may result from too rapid withdrawal of corticosteroids and may be minimized by gradual reduction of dosage. This type of relative insufficiency may persist for months after discontinuation of therapy; therefore, in any situation of stress occurring during that period, hormone therapy should be reinstituted. If the patient is receiving steroids already, dosage may have to be increased. Since mineralocorticoid secretion may be impaired, salt and/or a mineralocorticoid should be administered concurrently.

Corticosteroids may mask some signs of infection, and new infections may appear during their use. There may be decreased resistance and inability to localize infection when corticosteroids are used. Moreover, corticosteroids may affect the nitroblue-tetrazolium test for bacterial infection and produce false negative results.

In cerebral malaria, a double-blind trial has shown that the use of corticosteroids is associated with prolongation of coma and a higher incidence of pneumonia and gastrointestinal bleeding.

Corticosteroids may activate latent amebiasis. Therefore, it is recommended that latent or active amebiasis be ruled out before initiating corticosteroid therapy in any patient who has spent time in the tropics or any patient with unexplained diarrhea.

Prolonged use of corticosteroids may produce posterior subcapsular cataracts, glaucoma with possible damage to the optic nerves, and may enhance the establishment of secondary ocular infections due to fungi or viruses.

Usage In Pregnancy: Since adequate human reproduction studies have not been done with corticosteroids, use of these drugs in pregnancy or in women of childbearing potential requires that the anticipated benefits be weighed against the possible hazards to the mother and embryo or fetus. Infants born of mothers who have received substantial doses of corticosteroids during pregnancy should be carefully observed for signs of hypoadrenalism.

Corticosteroids appear in breast milk and could suppress growth, interfere with endogenous corticosteroid production, or cause other unwanted effects. Mothers taking pharmacologic doses of corticosteroids should be advised not to nurse.

Average and large doses of cortisone or hydrocortisone can cause elevation of blood pressure, salt and water retention, and increased excretion of potassium. These effects are less likely to occur with the synthetic derivatives except when used in large doses. Dietary salt restriction and potassium supplementation may be necessary. All corticosteroids increase calcium excretion.

Administration of live virus vaccines, including smallpox, is contraindicated in individuals receiving immunosuppressive doses of corticosteroids. If inactivated viral or bacterial vaccines are administered to individuals receiving immunosuppressive doses of corticosteroids, the expected serum antibody response may not be obtained. However, immunization procedures may be undertaken in patients who are receiving corticosteroids as replacement therapy, e.g., for Addison's disease.

Patients who are on drugs which suppress the immune system are more susceptible to infection than healthy individuals. Chickenpox and measles, for example, can have a more serious or even fatal course in non-immune children or adults on corticosteroids. In such children or adults who have not had these diseases, particular care should be taken to avoid exposure. The risk of developing a disseminated infection varies among individuals and can be related to the dose, route and duration of corticosteroid administration as well as to the underlying disease. If exposure to chickenpox, prophylaxis with varicella zoster immune globulin (VZIG) may be indicated. If chickenpox develops, treatment with antiviral agents may be considered. If exposed to measles, prophylaxis with immune globulin (IG) may be indicated. See the respective package inserts for VZIG and IG for complete prescribing information.

The use of dexamethasone sodium phosphate injection in active tuberculosis should be restricted to those cases of fulminating or disseminated tuberculosis in which the corticosteroid is used for the management of the disease in conjunction with an appropriate antituberculous regimen.

If corticosteroids are indicated in patients with latent tuberculosis or tuberculin reactivity, close observation is necessary as reactivation of the disease may occur. During prolonged corticosteroid therapy, these patients should receive chemoprophylaxis.

Literature reports suggest an apparent association between use of corticosteroids and left ventricular free wall rupture after a recent myocardial infarction; therefore, therapy with corticosteroids should be used with great caution in these patients.

OPHTHALMIC OINTMENT AND SOLUTION

Prolonged use may result in ocular hypertension and/or glaucoma, with damage to the optic nerve, defects in visual acuity and fields of vision, and posterior subcapsular cataract formation. Prolonged use may suppress the host response and thus increase the hazard of secondary ocular infections. In those diseases causing thinning of the cornea or sclera, perforations have been known to occur with the use of topical corticosteroids. In acute purulent conditions of the eye, corticosteroids may mask infection or enhance existing infection. If these products are used for 10 days or longer, intraocular pressure should be routinely monitored even though it may be difficult in children and uncooperative patients.

Employment of corticosteroid medication in the treatment of herpes simplex other than epithelial herpes simplex keratitis, in which it is contraindicated, requires great caution; periodic slit-lamp microscopy is essential.

OPHTHALMIC SOLUTION ONLY

Dexamethasone sodium phosphate ophthalmic solution contains sodium bisulfate, a sulfite that may cause allergic-type reactions including anaphylactic symptoms and life-threatening or less severe asthmatic episodes in certain susceptible people. The overall prevalence of sulfite sensitivity in the general population is unknown and probably low. Sulfite sensitivity is seen more frequently in asthmatic than nonasthmatic people.

ORAL AND INTRANASAL AEROSOLS

In patients on therapy with Dexamethasone Sodium Phosphate in Respihaler or Turbinaire subjected to unusual stress, increased dosage of rapidly acting corticosteroids before, during, and after the stressful situation is indicated.

Drug-induced secondary adrenocortical insufficiency may result from too rapid withdrawal of corticosteroids and may be minimized by gradual reduction of dosage. This type of relative insufficiency may persist for months after discontinuation of therapy; therefore, in any

WARNINGS: *(cont'd)*

situation of stress occurring during that period, hormone therapy should be reinstituted. If the patient is receiving steroids already, dosage may have to be increased. Since mineralocorticoid secretion may be impaired, salt and/or a mineralocorticoid should be administered concurrently.

Dexamethasone may mask some signs of infection, and new infections may appear during its use. There may be decreased resistance and inability to localize infection when corticosteroids are used. Therefore, patients with bacterial infections should also be given appropriate antibiotic therapy if Dexamethasone Sodium Phosphate in Respihaler or Turbinaire is used. Moreover, dexamethasone may effect the nitroblue-tetrazolium test for bacterial infection and produce false negative results.

Corticosteroids may activate latent amebiasis. Therefore it is recommended that latent or active amebiasis be ruled out before initiating corticosteroid therapy in any patient who has spent time in the tropics or any patients with unexplained diarrhea.

Prolonged use of Dexamethasone Sodium Phosphate in Respihaler or Turbinaire may produce posterior subcapsular cataracts, glaucoma with possible damage to the optic nerves, and may enhance the establishment of secondary ocular infections due to fungi or viruses.

Usage In Pregnancy Since adequate human reproduction studies have not been done with Dexamethasone Sodium Phosphate in Respihaler or Turbinaire, use of this drug in pregnancy or in women of childbearing potential requires that the anticipated benefits be weighed against the possible hazards to the mother and embryo or fetus. Infants born of mothers who have received substantial doses of dexamethasone during pregnancy, should be carefully observed for signs of hypoadrenalism.

Dexamethasone appears in breast milk and could suppress growth, interfere with endogenous corticosteroid production, or cause other unwanted effects. Mothers taking pharmacologic doses of dexamethasone should be advised not to nurse.

Average and large doses of hydrocortisone or cortisone can cause elevation of blood pressure, salt and water retention, and increased excretion of potassium. These effects are less likely to occur with the synthetic derivatives and with Dexamethasone Sodium Phosphate in Respihaler or Turbinaire, except when used in large doses. Dietary salt restriction and potassium supplementation may be necessary. All corticosteroids increase calcium excretion.

Administration of live virus vaccines, including smallpox, is contraindicated in individuals receiving immunosuppressive doses of corticosteroids. If inactivated viral or bacterial vaccines are administered to individuals receiving immunosuppressive doses of corticosteroids, the expected serum antibody response may not be obtained.

Patients who are on drugs which suppress the immune system are more susceptible to infections than healthy individuals. Chickenpox and measles, for example, can have a more serious or even fatal course in non-immune children (see PRECAUTIONS) regarding use of this product in children or adults on corticosteroids. In such children or adults who have not had these diseases, particular care should be taken to avoid exposure. The risk of developing a disseminated infection varies among individuals and can be related to the dose, route and duration of corticosteroid administration as well as to the underlying disease. If exposed to chickenpox, prophylaxis with varicella zoster immune globulin (VZIG) may be indicated. If chickpox develops, treatment with antiviral agents may be considered. If exposed to measles, prophylaxis with immune globulin (IG) may be indicated. See the respective package inserts for VZIG and IG for complete prescribing information.

If Dexamethasone Sodium Phosphate in Respihaler or Turbinaire is indicated in patients with latent tuberculosis or tuberculin reactivity, close observation is necessary as reactivation of the disease may occur. During prolonged therapy with Dexamethasone Sodium Phosphate in Respihaler or Turbinaire, these patients should receive chemoprophylaxis.

Literature reports suggest an apparent association between use of corticosteroids and left ventricular free wall rupture after a recent myocardial infarction; therefore, therapy with corticosteroids should be used with great caution in these patients.

Keep out of reach of children.

ORAL AEROSOL

Rare instances of laryngeal and pharyngeal fungal infections have been observed in patients using Dexamethasone Sodium Phosphate in Respihaler. These have usually responded promptly to discontinuation of therapy and institution of antifungal treatment.

PRECAUTIONS:

GENERAL

Ophthalmic Ointment and Solution: The possibility of persistent fungal infections of the cornea should be considered after prolonged corticosteroid dosing.

There have been reports of bacterial keratitis associated with the use of multiple dose containers of topical ophthalmic products. These containers had been inadvertently contaminated by patients who, in most cases, had a concurrent corneal disease or a disruption of the ocular epithelial surface. See PRECAUTIONS, Information for Patients.

Topical Cream: Systemic absorption of topical corticosteroids has produced reversible hypothalamic-pituitary-adrenal (HPA) axis suppression, manifestations of Cushing's syndrome, hyperglycemia, and glycosuria in some patients.

Conditions which augment systemic absorption include the application of the more potent corticosteroids, use over large surface areas, prolonged use, and the addition of occlusive dressings.

Therefore, patients receiving a large dose of a potent topical corticosteroid applied to a large surface area or under an occlusive dressing should be evaluated periodically for evidence of HPA axis suppression by using urinary free cortisol and ACTH stimulation tests. If HPA axis suppression is noted, an attempt should be made to withdraw the drug, to reduce the frequency of application, or to substitutes a less potent corticosteroid.

Recovery of HPA axis function is generally prompt and complete upon discontinuation of the drug. Infrequently, signs and symptoms of corticosteroid withdrawal may occur, requiring supplemental systemic corticosteroids.

Children may absorb proportionally larger amounts of topical corticosteroids and thus be more susceptible to systemic toxicity (see PRECAUTIONS, Pediatric Use.)

If irritation develops, topical corticosteroids should be discontinued and appropriate therapy instituted.

In the presence of dermatological infections, the use of an appropriate antifungal or antibacterial agent should be instituted. If a favorable response does not occur promptly, the corticosteroid should be discontinued until the infection has been adequately controlled.

This product is not for ophthalmic use. However, if applied to the eyelids or skin near the eyes, the drug may enter the eyes. In patients with a history of herpes simplex keratitis, ocular exposure to corticosteroids may lead to a recurrence. Prolonged ocular exposure may cause steroid glaucoma.

Generally occlusive dressings should not be used on weeping or exudative lesions.

If occlusive dressing therapy is used, inspect lesions between dressings for development of infection.If infection develops, the technique should be discontinued and appropriate antimicrobial therapy instituted.

PRECAUTIONS: *(cont'd)*

When large areas of the body are covered with an occlusive dressing, thermal homeostasis may be impaired. If elevation of body temperature occurs, use of the occlusive dressing should be discontinued.

Injection: This product, like many other steroid formulations, is sensitive to heat. Therefore, it should not be autoclaved when it is desirable to sterilize the exterior of the vial.

Following prolonged therapy, withdrawal of corticosteroids may result in symptoms of the corticosteroid withdrawal syndrome including fever, myalgia, arthralgia, and malaise. This may occur in patients even without evidence of adrenal insufficiency.

There is an enhanced effect of corticosteroids in patients with hypothyroidism and in those with cirrhosis.

Corticosteroids should be used cautiously in patients with ocular herpes simplex for fear of corneal perforation.

The lowest possible dose of corticosteroid should be used to control the condition under treatment, and when reduction in dosage is possible, the reduction must be gradual.

Psychic derangements may appear when corticosteroids are used, ranging from euphoria, insomnia, mood swings, personality changes, and severe depression to frank psychotic manifestations. Also, existing emotional instability or psychotic tendencies may be aggravated by corticosteroids.

Aspirin should be used cautiously in conjunction with corticosteroids in hypoprothrombinemia.

Steroids should be used with caution in nonspecific ulcerative colitis, if there is a probability of impending perforation, abscess, or other pyogenic infection, also in diverticulitis, fresh intestinal anastomoses, active or latent peptic ulcer, renal insufficiency, hypertension, osteoporosis, and myasthenia gravis. Signs of peritoneal irritation following gastrointestinal perforation in patients receiving large doses of corticosteroids may be minimal or absent. Fat embolism has been reported as a possible complication of chickenpox.

When large doses are given, some authorities advise that antacids be administered between meals to help to prevent peptic ulcer.

Growth and development of infants and children on prolonged corticosteroid therapy should be carefully followed.

Steroids may increase or decrease motility and number of spermatozoa in some patients.

False negative results in the dexamethasone suppression test (DST) in patients being treated with indomethacin have been reported. Thus, results of the DST should be interpreted with caution in these patients.

The prothrombin time should be checked frequently in patients who are receiving corticosteroids and coumarin anticoagulants at the same time because of reports that corticosteroids have altered the response to these anticoagulants. Studies have shown that the usual effect produced by adding corticosteroids is inhibition of response to coumarins, although there have been some conflicting reports of potentiation not substantiated by studies.

When corticosteroids are administered concomitantly with potassium-depleting diuretics, patients should be observed closely for development of hypokalemia.

Intra-articular injection of a corticosteroid may produce systemic as well as local effects.

Appropriate examination of any joint fluid present is necessary to exclude a septic process.

A marked increase in pain accompanied by local swelling, further restriction of joint motion, fever, and malaise is suggestive of septic arthritis. If this complication occurs and the diagnosis of sepsis is confirmed, appropriate antimicrobial therapy should be instituted.

Injection of a steroid into an infected site is to be avoided.

Corticosteroids should not be injected into unstable joints.

Patients should be impressed strongly with the importance of not overusing joints in which symptomatic benefit has been obtained as long as the inflammatory process remains active.

Frequent intra-articular injection may result in damage to joint tissues.

The slower rate of absorption by intramuscular administration should be recognized.

INFORMATION FOR PATIENTS

Ophthalmic Ointment and Solution: Patients should be instructed to avoid allowing the tip of the dispensing container to contact the eye or surrounding structures.

Patients should also be instructed that ocular preparations, if handled improperly, can become contaminated by common bacteria known to cause ocular infections. Serious damage to the eye and subsequent loss of vision may result from using contaminated preparations. See PRECAUTIONS, General.

Patients should also be advised that if they develop an intercurrent ocular condition (*e.g.,* trauma, ocular surgery or infection), they should immediately seek their physician's advice concerning the continued use of the present multidose container.

One of the preservatives in Ophthalmic Solution Decadron Phosphate, benzalkonium chloride, may be absorbed by soft contact lenses. Patients wearing soft contact lenses should be instructed to wait at least 15 minutes after instilling Ophthalmic Solution Decadron Phosphate before they insert their lenses.

Topical Cream: Patients using topical corticosteroids should receive the following information and instructions:

1. This medication is to be used as directed by the physician. It is for external use only. Avoid contact with the eyes.

2. Patients should be advised not to use this medication for any disorder other than that for which it was prescribed.

3. The treated skin area should not be bandaged or otherwise covered or wrapped so as to be occlusive unless directed by the physician.

4. Patients should report any signs of local adverse reactions, especially under occlusive dressing.

5. Parents of pediatric patients should be advised not to use tight- fitting diapers or plastic pants on a child being treated in the diaper area, as these garments may constitute occlusive dressings.

6. Susceptible patients who are on immunosuppressant doses of corticosteroids should be warned to avoid exposure to chickenpox or measles. Patients should also be advised that if they are exposed, medical advice should be sought without delay.

Injection: Susceptible patients who are on immunosuppressant doses of corticosteroids should be warned to avoid exposure to chickenpox or measles. Patients should also be advised that if they are exposed, medical advice should be sought without delay.

LABORATORY TESTS

Topical Cream: The following tests may be helpful in evaluating the HPA axis suppression:

Urinary free cortisol test

ACTH stimulation test

CARCINOGENESIS, MUTAGENESIS,IMPAIRMENT OF FERTILITY

Ophthalmic Ointment and Solution: Long-term animal studies have not been performed to evaluate the carcinogenic potential or the effect on fertility of Dexamethasone Sodium Phosphate Ophthalmic Ointment or Solution.

PRECAUTIONS: *(cont'd)*

Topical Cream: Long-term animal studies have not been performed to evaluate the carcinogenic potential or the effect on fertility of topical corticosteroids.

Studies to determine mutagenicity with prednisolone and hydrocortisone have revealed negative results.

PREGNANCY CATEGORY C

Ophthalmic Ointment and Solution: Dexamethasone has been shown to be teratogenic in mice and rabbits following topical ophthalmic application in multiples of the therapeutic dose.

In the mouse, corticosteroids produce fetal resorptions and a specific abnormality, cleft palate. In the rabbit, corticosteroids have produced fetal resorptions and multiple abnormalities involving the head, ears, limbs, palate, etc.

There are no adequate or well-controlled studies in pregnant women. Dexamethasone Sodium Phosphate Ophthalmic Ointment or Solution should be used during pregnancy only if the potential benefit to the mother justifies the potential risk to the embryo or fetus. Infants born of mothers who have received substantial doses of corticosteroids during pregnancy should be observed carefully for signs of hypoadrenalism.

Topical Cream: Corticosteroids are generally teratogenic in laboratory animals when administered systemically at relatively low dosage levels. The more potent corticosteroids have been shown to be teratogenic after dermal application in laboratory animals. There are no adequate and well-controlled studies in pregnant women on teratogenic effects from topically applied corticosteroids. Therefore, topical corticosteroids should be used during pregnancy only if the potential benefit justifies the potential risk to the fetus. Drugs of this class should not be used extensively on pregnant patients, in large amounts, or for prolonged periods of time.

NURSING MOTHERS

Ophthalmic Ointment and Solution: Topically applied steroids are absorbed systemically. Therefore, because of the potential for serious adverse reactions in nursing infants from dexamethasone sodium phosphate, a decision should be made whether to discontinue nursing or to discontinue the drug, taking into account the importance of the drug to the mother.

Topical Cream: It is not known whether topical administration of corticosteroids could result in sufficient systemic absorption to produce detectable quantities in breast milk. Systemically administered corticosteroids are secreted into breast milk in quantities *not* likely to have a deleterious effect on the infant.. Nevertheless, caution should be exercised when topical corticosteroids are administered to a nursing woman.

PEDIATRIC USE

Ophthalmic Ointment and Solution: Safety and effectiveness in children have not been established.

Topical Cream: *Pediatric patients may demonstrate greater susceptibility to topical corticosteroid-induced HPA axis suppression and Cushing's syndrome than mature patients because of a larger skin surface area to body weight ratio.*

Hypothalamic-pituitary-adrenal (HPA) axis suppression, Cushing's syndrome, and intracranial hypertension have been reported in children receiving topical corticosteroids. Manifestations of adrenal suppression in children include linear growth retardation, delayed weight gain, low plasma cortisol levels, and absence of response to ACTH stimulation. Manifestations of intracranial hypertension include bulging fontanelles, headaches, and bilateral papilledema.

Administration of topical corticosteroids to children should be limited to the least amount compatible with an effective therapeutic regimen. Chronic corticosteroid therapy may interfere with the growth and development of children.

ORAL AND INTRANASAL AEROSOLS

Although systemic absorption is low when Dexamethasone Sodium Phosphate in Respihaler or Turbinaire is used in the recommended dosage, adrenal suppression may occur. In addition, other systemic effects of steroid administration must be considered as a possibility.

Following prolonged therapy, withdrawal of corticosteroids may result in symptoms of the corticosteroid withdrawal syndrome including fever, myalgia, arthralgia, and malaise. This may occur in patients even without evidence of adrenal insufficiency.

There is an enhanced effect of dexamethasone in patients with hypothyroidism and in those with cirrhosis.

Dexamethasone Sodium Phosphate in Respihaler or Turbinaire should be used cautiously in patients with ocular herpes simplex for fear of corneal perforation.

The lowest possible dose of Dexamethasone Sodium Phosphate in Respihaler or Turbinaire should be used to control the condition under treatment, and when reduction in dosage is possible, the reduction must be gradual.

Psychic derangements may appear when dexamethasone is used, ranging from euphoria, insomnia, mood swings, personality changes, and severe depression, to frank psychotic manifestations. Also, existing emotional instability or psychotic tendencies may be aggravated.

Aspirin should be used cautiously in conjunction with Dexamethasone Sodium Phosphate in Respihaler or Turbinaire in hypoprothrombinemia.

Dexamethasone Sodium Phosphate in Respihaler or Turbinaire should be used with caution in nonspecific ulcerative colitis, if there is a probability of impending perforation, abscess or other pyogenic infection; also in diverticulitis; fresh intestinal anastomoses; active or latent peptic ulcer; renal insufficiency; hypertension; osteoporosis; and myasthenia gravis. Signs of peritoneal irritation following gastrointestinal perforation in patients receiving large doses of corticosteroids may be minimal or absent. Fat embolism has been reported as a possible complication of chickenpox.

Dexamethasone may increase or decrease motility and number of spermatozoa in some patients.

Phenytoin, phenobarbital, ephedrine and rifampin may enhance the metabolic clearance of dexamethasone, resulting in decreased blood levels and lessened physiologic activity, thus requiring adjustment in dexamethasone dosage.

The prothrombin time should be checked frequently in patients who are receiving Dexamethasone Sodium Phosphate in Respihaler or Turbinaire and coumarin anticoagulants at the same time because of reports that corticosteroids have altered the response to these anticoagulants. Studies have shown that the usual effect produced by adding corticosteroids is inhibition of response to coumarins, although there have been some conflicting reports of potentiation, not substantiated by studies.

When Dexamethasone Sodium Phosphate in Respihaler or Turbinaire is used concurrently with potassium-depleting diuretics, patients should be observed closely for development of hypokalemia.

Since the contents of Dexamethasone Sodium Phosphate in Respihaler and Turbinaire are under pressure, the container should not be broken, stored in extreme heat, or incinerated. It should be stored at a temperature below 120°F.

ORAL AEROSOL ONLY

Dexamethasone Sodium Phosphate in Respihaler is *not* indicated for relief of the occasional mild and isolated attack of asthma which is readily responsive to the immediate, though short-lived, action of epinephrine, isoproterenol, aminophylline, etc., nor should it be employed for the treatment of severe status asthmaticus where intensive measures are required.

PRECAUTIONS: *(cont'd)*

Dexamethasone Sodium Phosphate in Respihaler should be considered only for the following classes of patients: patients not on corticosteroid therapy who have not responded adequately to other treatment; patients already on systemic corticosteroid therapy—in an attempt to reduce or eliminate systemic administration.

Growth and development of infants and children on prolonged therapy with Dexamethasone Sodium Phosphate in Respihaler should be carefully followed.

INTRANASAL AEROSOL ONLY

During local corticosteroid therapy, the possibility of pharyngeal candidiasis should be kept in mind.

Replacement of systemic steroid with Dexamethasone Sodium Phosphate in Turbinaire should be gradual and carefully monitored by the physician.

Because clinical studies have not been done, the use of this product in children under the age of 6 years is not recommended. Growth and development of children 6 years of age or older on prolonged therapy with Dexamethasone Sodium Phosphate in Turbinaire should be carefully followed.

DRUG INTERACTIONS:

Phenytoin, phenobarbital, ephedrine, and rifampin may enhance the metabolic clearance of corticosteroids resulting in decreased blood levels and lessened physiologic activity, thus requiring adjustment in corticosteroid dosage. These interactions may interfere with dexamethasone suppression tests which should be interpreted with caution during administration of these drugs.

ADVERSE REACTIONS:

INJECTION, ORAL AND INTRANASAL AEROSOLS

Fluid and electrolyte disturbances: Sodium retention; Fluid retention; Congestive heart failure in susceptible patients; Potassium loss; Hypokalemic alkalosis; Hypertension

Musculoskeletal: Muscle weakness; Steroid myopathy; Loss of muscle mass; Osteoporosis; Vertebral compression fractures; Aseptic necrosis of femoral and humeral heads; Pathologic fracture of long bones; Tendon rupture

Gastrointestinal: Peptic ulcer with possible subsequent perforation and hemorrhage; Perforation of the small and large bowel, particularly in patients with inflammatory bowel disease; Pancreatitis; Abdominal distention; Ulcerative esophagitis

Dermatologic: Impaired wound healing; Thin fragile skin; Petechiae and ecchymoses; Erythema; Increased sweating; May suppress reactions to skin tests; Burning or tingling, especially in the perineal area (after IV injection); Other cutaneous reactions, such as allergic dermatitis, urticaria, angioneurotic edema

Neurologic: Convulsions; Increased intracranial pressure with papilledema (pseudotumor cerebri) usually after treatment; Vertigo; Headache; Psychic disturbances

Endocrine: Menstrual irregularities; Development of cushingoid state; Suppression of growth in children; Secondary adrenocortical and pituitary unresponsiveness, particularly in times of stress, as in trauma, surgery, or illness; Decreased carbohydrate tolerance; Manifestations of latent diabetes mellitus; Increased requirements for insulin or oral hypoglycemic agents in diabetics; Hirsutism

Ophthalmic: Posterior subcapsular cataracts; increased intraocular pressure; glaucoma; exophthalmos

Metabolic: Negative nitrogen balance due to protein catabolism

Cardiovascular: Myocardial rupture following recent myocardial infarction (see WARNINGS.)

Other: Anaphylactoid or hypersensitivity reactions; thromboembolism; weight gain; increased appetite; nausea; malaise; hiccups

INJECTION ONLY

The following *additional* adverse reactions are related to parenteral corticosteroid therapy:

Rare instances of blindness associated with intralesional therapy around the face and head; Hyperpigmentation or hypopigmentation; Subcutaneous and cutaneous atrophy; Sterile abscess; Postinjection flare (following intra-articular use); Charcot-like arthropathy

ORAL AEROSOL ONLY

Side effects which may occur in patients treated with Dexamethasone Sodium Phosphate in Respihaler include throat irritation, hoarseness, coughing, and laryngeal and pharyngeal fungal infections.

INTRANASAL AEROSOL ONLY

Nasal irritation and dryness are the most common adverse reactions. The following have been reported: headache, lightheadedness, urticaria, nausea, epistaxis, rebound congestion, bronchial asthma, perforation of the nasal septum, and anosmia. Signs of adrenal hypercorticism may occur in some patients, especially with overdosage.

Systemic effects from therapy with Dexamethasone Sodium Phosphate in Turbinaire are less likely to occur than with oral or parenteral corticosteroid therapy because of a lower total dose administered. Nevertheless, patients should be observed for the hormonal effects described above (see ADVERSE REACTIONS) because of absorption of dexamethasone from the nasal mucosa.

OPHTHALMIC OINTMENT AND SOLUTION

Glaucoma with optic nerve damage, visual acuity and field defects, subcapsular cataract formation, secondary ocular infections from pathogens including herpes simplex, perforation of the globe.

Rarely, filtering blebs have been reported when topical steroids have been have been used following cataract surgery.

Rarely, stinging or burning may occur.

TOPICAL CREAM

The following adverse reactions are reported infrequently with topical corticosteroids, but may occur more frequently with the use of occlusive dressings. These reactions are listed in an approximate decreasing order of occurrence:

Burning; Itching; Irritation; Dryness; Folliculitis; Hypertrichosis; Acneiform eruptions; Hypopigmentation; Perioral dermatitis; Allergic contact dermatitis; Maceration of the skin; Secondary infection; Skin atrophy; Striae; Miliaria

OVERDOSAGE:

INJECTION, ORAL AND INTRANASAL AEROSOLS

Reports of acute toxicity and/or death following overdosage of glucocorticoids are rare. In the event of overdosage, no specific antidote is available; treatment is supportive and symptomatic.

The oral LD_{50} of dexamethasone in female mice was 6.5 g/kg. The intravenous LD_{50} of dexamethasone sodium phosphate in female mice was 794 mg/kg.

TOPICAL CREAM

Topically applied corticosteroids can be absorbed in sufficient amounts to produce systemic effects (See PRECAUTIONS.)

OVERDOSAGE: *(cont'd)*

(**Note:** There is no Overdosage information for dexamethasone sodium phosphate ophthalmic ointment or solution).

DOSAGE AND ADMINISTRATION:

INJECTION

Dexamethasone sodium phosphate injection, 4 mg/ml: *For intravenous, intramuscular, intra-articular, intralesional and soft tissue injection.*

Dexamethasone sodium phosphate injection, 24 mg/ml: *For intravenous injection only.*

Dexamethasone sodium phosphate injection can be given directly from the vial, or it can be added to Sodium Chloride Injection or Dextrose Injection and administered by intravenous drip.

Solutions used for intravenous administration or further dilution of this product should be preservative-free when used in the neonate, especially the premature infant.

When it is mixed with an infusion solution, sterile precautions should be observed. Since infusion solutions generally do not contain preservatives, mixtures should be used within 24 hours.

DOSAGE REQUIREMENTS ARE VARIABLE AND MUST BE INDIVIDUALIZED ON THE BASIS OF THE DISEASE AND THE RESPONSE OF THE PATIENT.

INTRAVENOUS AND INTRAMUSCULAR INJECTION

The initial dosage of dexamethasone sodium phosphate injection varies from 0.5 to 9 mg a day depending on the disease being treated. In less severe diseases doses lower than 0.5 mg may suffice, while in severe diseases doses higher than 9 mg may be required.

The initial dosage should be maintained or adjusted until the patient's response is satisfactory. If a satisfactory clinical response does not occur after a reasonable period of time, discontinue dexamethasone sodium phosphate injection and transfer the patient to other therapy.

After a favorable initial response, the proper maintenance dosage should be determined by decreasing the initial dosage in small amounts to the lowest dosage that maintains an adequate clinical response.

Patients should be observed closely for signs that might require dosage adjustment, including changes in clinical status resulting from remissions or exacerbations of the disease, individual drug responsiveness, and the effect of stress (*e.g.,* surgery, infection, trauma). During stress it may be necessary to increase dosage temporarily.

If the drug is to be stopped after more than a few days of treatment, it usually should be withdrawn gradually.

When the intravenous route of administration is used, dosage usually should be the same as the oral dosage. In certain overwhelming, acute, life-threatening situations, however, administration in dosages exceeding the usual dosages may be justified and may be in multiples of the oral dosages. The slower rate of absorption by intramuscular administration should be recognized.

SHOCK

There is a tendency in current medical practice to use high (pharmacologic) doses of corticosteroids for the treatment of unresponsive shock. The following dosages of dexamethasone sodium phosphate injection have been suggested by various authors (TABLE 1):

TABLE 1

Author*	Dosage
Cavanagh[1]	3 mg/kg of body weight per 24 hours by constant intravenous infusion after an initial intravenous injection of 20 mg
Dietzman[2]	2 to 6 mg/kg of body weight as a single intravenous injection
Frank[3]	40 mg initially followed by repeat intravenous injection every 4 to 6 hours while shock persists
Oaks[4]	40 mg initially followed by repeat intravenous injection every 2 to 6 hours while shock persists
Schumer[5]	1 mg/kg of body weight as a single intravenous injection

Administration of high dose corticosteroid therapy should be continued only until the patient's condition has stabilized and usually not longer than 48 to 72 hours.

Although adverse reactions associated with high dose, short term corticosteroid therapy are uncommon, peptic ulceration may occur.

CEREBRAL EDEMA

Dexamethasone sodium phosphate injection is generally administered initially in a dosage of 10 mg intravenously followed by four mg every six hours intramuscularly until the symptoms of cerebral edema subside. Response is usually noted within 12 to 24 hours and dosage may be reduced after two to four days and gradually discontinued over a period of five to seven days. For palliative management of patients with recurrent or inoperable brain tumors, maintenance therapy with two mg two or three times a day may be effective.

ACUTE ALLERGIC DISORDERS

In acute, self-limited allergic disorders or acute exacerbations of chronic allergic disorders, the following dosage schedule combining parenteral and oral therapy is suggested:

Dexamethasone sodium phosphate injection, 4 mg/ml: *first day,* 1 or 2 ml (4 or 8 mg), intramuscularly.

Dexamethasone sodium phosphate tablets, 0.75 mg: *second* and *third* days, 4 tablets in two divided doses each day;*fourth* day, 2 tablets in two divided doses; *fifth* and *sixth* days, 1 tablet each day; *seventh* day, no treatment;*eighth* day, follow-up visit.

This schedule is designed to ensure adequate therapy during acute episodes, while minimizing the risk of overdosage in chronic cases.

INTRA-ARTICULAR, INTRALESIONAL, AND SOFT TISSUE INJECTION

Intra-articular, intralesional, and soft tissue injections are generally employed when the affected joints or areas are limited to one or two sites. Dosage and frequency of injection varies depending on the condition and the site of injection. The usual dose is from 0.2 to 6 mg. The frequency usually ranges from once every three to five days to once every two to three weeks. Frequent intra-articular injection may result in damage to joint tissues (TABLE 2).

TABLE 2

Some of the usual single doses are:

Site of Injection	Amount of Dexamethasone Phosphate (mg)
Large Joints (*e.g.,* Knee)	2 to 4
Small Joints (*e.g.,* Interphalangeal, Temporomandibular)	0.8 to 1
Bursae	2 to 3
Tendon Sheaths	0.4 to 1
Soft Tissue Infiltration	2 to 6
Ganglia	1 to 2

DOSAGE AND ADMINISTRATION: *(cont'd)*

Dexamethasone sodium phosphate injection is particularly recommended for use in conjunction with one of the less soluble, longer-acting steroids for intra-articular and soft tissue injection.

Storage: Sensitive to heat. Do not autoclave. Protect from freezing. Protect from light. Store container in carton until contents have been used.

OPHTHALMIC OINTMENT

The duration of treatment will vary with the type of lesion and may extend from a few days to several weeks, according to therapeutic response. Relapses, more common in chronic active lesions than in self- limited conditions, usually respond to retreatment.

Apply a thin coating of ointment three or four times a day. When a favorable response is observed, reduce the number of daily applications to two, and later to one a day as a maintenance dose if this is sufficient to control symptoms.

Dexamethasone Sodium Phosphate Ophthalmic Ointment is particularly convenient when an eye pad is used. It may also be the preparation of choice for patients in whom therapeutic benefit depends on prolonged contact of the active ingredients with ocular tissues.

OPHTHALMIC SOLUTION

The duration of treatment will vary with the type of lesion and may extend from a few days to several weeks, according to therapeutic response. Relapses, more common in chronic active lesions than in self- limited conditions, usually respond to retreatment.

Eye: Instill one or two drops of solution into the conjunctival sac every hour during the day and every two hours during the night as initial therapy. When a favorable response is observed, reduce dosage to one drop every four hours. Later, further reduction in dosage to one drop three or four times daily may suffice to control symptoms.

Ear: Clean the aural canal thoroughly and sponge dry. Instill the solution directly into the aural canal. A suggested initial dosage is three or four drops two or three times a day. When a favorable response is obtained reduce dosage gradually and eventually discontinue.

If preferred, the aural canal may be packed with a gauze wick saturated with solution. Keep the wick moist with the preparation and remove from the ear after 12 to 24 hours. Treatment may be repeated as often as necessary at the discretion of the physician.

TOPICAL CREAM

Apply to the affected area as a thin film three or four times daily.

Occlusive dressings may be used for the management of psoriasis or recalcitrant conditions.

Before using this preparation in the *ear,* clean the aural canal thoroughly and sponge dry. Confirm that the eardrum is intact. With a cotton-tipped applicator, apply a thin coating of the cream to the affected canal area three or four times a day.

ORAL AEROSOL

Recommended *initial dosage:*

Adults: 3 inhalations 3 or 4 times per day

Children: 2 inhalations 3 or 4 times per day

Maximum Dosage

Adults: 3 inhalations *per dose;*12 inhalations *per day.*

Children: 2 inhalations *per dose;*8 inhalations *per day.*

When a favorable response is attained, the dose may be gradually reduced. In patients on systemic corticosteroids, it is recommended that systemic therapy be reduced or eliminated before reduction of Respihaler dosage is begun. Gradual reduction of systemic corticosteroid therapy must be emphasized to avoid withdrawal symptoms.

Storage: Store at a temperature below 49°C (120°F).

INTRANASAL AEROSOL

DO NOT EXCEED THE RECOMMENDED DOSAGE.

The usual initial dosage of Dexamethasone Sodium Phosphate in Turbinaire is:

Adults: 2 sprays in each nostril 2 or 3 times a day.

Children (6 to 12 years of age): 1 or 2 sprays in each nostril 2 times a day depending on age.

See accompanying instructions on the proper use of Turbinaire.

When improvement occurs the dosage should be gradually reduced. Some patients will be symptom-free on one spray in each nostril 2 times a day. The maximum daily dosage for adults is 12 sprays, and for children, 8 sprays. Therapy should be discontinued as soon as feasible. it may be reinstituted if recurrence of symptoms occurs.

Storage: Store at a temperature below 49°C (120°F).

REFERENCES:

1. Cavanagh, D.; Singh, K. B.: Endotoxin shock in pregnancy and abortion, in: "Corticosteroids in the Treatment of Shock", Schumer, W.; Nyhus, L. M., Editors, Urbana, University of Illinois Press, 1970, pp. 86-96. **2.** Dietzman, R. H.; Ersek R. A.; Bloch, J. M.; Lillehei, R. C.: High-output, low-resistance gram-negative septic shock in man, Angiology *20:* 691-700, Dec. 1969. **3.** Frank, E.: Clinical observations in shock and management (In: Shields, T. F., ed.: Symposium on current concepts and management of shock), J. Maine Med. Ass.*59:* 195-200, Oct. 1968. **4.** Oaks, W. W.; Cohen, H. E.: Endotoxin shock in the geriatric patient, Geriat. *22:* 120-130, Mar. 1967. **5.** Schumer, W.; Nyhus, L. M.: Corticosteroid effect on biochemical parameters of human oligemic shock, Arch. Surg. *100:*405-408, Apr. 1970.(Injection: Merck, 2/93, 7347226); (Ophthalmic Ointment: Merck, 12/91, 7612329); (Ophthalmic Solution: Merck, 10/93, 7261521); (Topical Cream: Merck, 4/93, 6005425); (Oral Aerosol: Merck, 3/93, 7413020)(Intranasal Aerosol: Merck, 3/93, 7413126)

HOW SUPPLIED - RATED THERAPEUTICALLY EQUIVALENT:

Injection, Solution - Intramuscular; - 4 mg/ml

1 ml	$20.63	Dexamethasone Sodium Phosphate, Fujisawa USA	00469-1650-00
1 ml x 25	$11.19	Dexamethasone Sodium Phosphate, Elkins Sinn	00641-0372-25
1 ml x 25	$24.20	HEXADROL PHOSPHATE, Organon	00052-0796-25
1 ml x 25	$27.19	Dexamethasone Sodium Phosphate, Am Regent	00517-4901-25
1 ml x 25	$31.25	Dexamethasone Sodium Phosphate, Consolidated Midland	00223-7407-01
1 ml x 25	$39.10	HEXADROL PHOSPHATE, Organon	00052-0796-26
1 ml x 25	$159.66	DECADRON PHOSPHATE, Merck	00006-7628-66
2.5 ml	$14.03	DECADRON PHOSPHATE, Merck	00006-7628-30
5 ml	$1.05	Dexamethasone Sodium Phosphate, Insource	58441-0126-05
5 ml	$1.20	Dexamethasone Sodium Phosphate, Americal Pharm	54945-0523-51
5 ml	$1.89	Dexamethasone Sodium Phosphate, HL Moore Drug Exch	00839-5160-25
5 ml	$2.28	Dexamethasone Sodium Phosphate, Lannett	00527-0182-65
5 ml	$2.45	Dexamethasone Sodium Phosphate, Goldline Labs	00182-3007-62
5 ml	$2.63	Dexamethasone Sodium Phosphate, IDE-Interstate	00814-2350-38
5 ml	$2.75	Dexamethasone Sodium Phosphate, Consolidated Midland	00223-7404-05
5 ml	$2.79	Dexamethasone Sodium Phosphate, Steris Labs	00402-0807-05
5 ml	$3.00	DEXACORTEN, Bolan Pharm	44437-0807-05
5 ml	$3.20	SOLUREX, Hyrex Pharms	00314-0896-75
5 ml	$3.50	Dexamethasone Sodium Phosphate, United Res	00677-0385-20
5 ml	$4.02	Dexamethasone Sodium Phosphate, Geneva Pharms	00781-3106-75
5 ml	$4.20	ADRENOCOT, C O Truxton	00463-1090-05
5 ml	$4.70	HEXADROL PHOSPHATE, Organon	00052-0796-05
5 ml	$6.00	DALALONE, Forest Pharms	00456-1074-05
5 ml	$6.00	Dexamethasone Sodium Phosphate, Rugby	00536-4151-65

HOW SUPPLIED - RATED THERAPEUTICALLY EQUIVALENT:
(cont'd)

5 ml	$7.30	Dexamethasone Sodium Phosphate, Pasadena	00418-1921-31
5 ml	$7.85	DECAJECT, Mayrand Pharms	00259-0297-05
5 ml	$8.95	SPECTRO DEX INJ 4, Spectrum Scitfc	53268-0106-75
5 ml	$29.46	DECADRON PHOSPHATE, Merck	00006-7628-03
5 ml	$52.19	Dexamethasone Sodium Phosphate, Fujisawa USA	00469-1650-20
5 ml x 1	$1.38	Dexamethasone Sodium Phosphate, Elkins Sinn	00641-2273-41
5 ml x 25	$54.69	Dexamethasone Sodium Phosphate, Am Regent	00517-4905-25
5 ml x 25	$94.40	HEXADROL PHOSPHATE, Organon	00052-0796-27
10 ml	$4.00	Dexamethasone Sodium Phosphate, Consolidated Midland	00223-7408-10
10 ml	$4.20	Dexamethasone Sodium Phosphate, Steris Labs	00402-0807-10
10 ml	$4.95	SOLUREX, Hyrex Pharms	00314-0896-70
10 ml	$5.80	Dexamethasone Sodium Phosphate, Major Pharms	00904-0905-10
10 ml	$13.65	DECAJECT, Mayrand Pharms	00259-0297-10
25 ml	$7.00	Dexamethasone Sodium Phosphate, Consolidated Midland	00223-7406-25
25 ml	$114.34	DECADRON PHOSPHATE, Merck	00006-7628-25
25 x 5 ml	$69.66	Dexamethasone, Schein Pharm (US)	00364-6681-32
30 ml	$2.99	Dexamethasone Sodium Phosphate, Insource	58441-0103-30
30 ml	$3.65	Dexamethasone Sodium Phosphate, Americal Pharm	54945-0523-53
30 ml	$5.39	Dexamethasone Sodium Phosphate, HL Moore Drug Exch	00839-5160-36
30 ml	$5.50	Dexamethasone Sodium Phosphate, Consolidated Midland	00223-7402-30
30 ml	$5.63	Dexamethasone Sodium Phosphate, IDE-Interstate	00814-2350-46
30 ml	$9.00	Dexamethasone Sodium Phosphate, Goldline Labs	00182-3007-66
30 ml	$9.10	Dexamethasone Sodium Phosphate, Steris Labs	00402-0807-30
30 ml	$9.24	Dexamethasone Sodium Phosphate, Major Pharms	00904-0905-30
30 ml	$10.01	Dexamethasone, Schein Pharm (US)	00364-6681-56
30 ml	$10.55	Dexamethasone Sodium Phosphate, Pasadena	00418-1921-30
30 ml	$11.93	SOLUREX, Hyrex Pharms	00314-0896-30
30 ml	$12.50	Dexamethasone Sodium Phosphate, Fujisawa USA	00469-1650-50
30 ml	$13.62	Dexamethasone Sodium Phosphate, Rugby	00536-4151-75
30 ml	$16.66	Dexamethasone Sodium Phosphate, Elkins Sinn	00641-2276-41
30 ml x 25	$195.94	Dexamethasone Sodium Phosphate, Am Regent	00517-4930-25

Injection, Solution - Intramuscular; - 10 mg/ml

1 ml x 25	$58.21	Dexamethasone Sodium Phosphate, Elkins Sinn	00641-0367-25
1 ml x 25	$63.25	HEXADROL PHOSPHATE, Organon	00052-0797-26
10 ml	$12.00	Dexamethasone Sodium Phosphate, Schein Pharm (US)	00364-2360-54
10 ml	$12.00	Dexamethasone Sodium Phosphate, Steris Labs	00402-0661-10
10 ml	$25.25	HEXADROL PHOSPHATE, Organon	00052-0797-10
10 ml x 1	$4.99	Dexamethasone Sodium Phosphate, Gensia Labs	00703-3524-01
10 ml x 1	$15.38	Dexamethasone Sodium Phosphate, Elkins Sinn	00641-2277-41

Injection, Solution - Intravenous - 20 mg/ml

5 ml	$113.51	DECADRON, Merck	00006-7646-03
10 ml	$222.39	DECADRON, Merck	00006-7646-10

Injection, Solution - Intravenous - 24 mg/ml

5 ml	$10.35	Dexamethasone Sodium Phosphate, Rugby	00536-4140-65

Ointment - Ophthalmic - 0.05 %

3.5 gm	$1.30	Dexair, Raway	00686-5640-55
3.5 gm	$2.44	INFA-DEX, Infinity Pharm	58154-0640-55
3.5 gm	$3.02	Dexamethasone Phosphate, HL Moore Drug Exch	00839-6680-43
3.5 gm	$3.12	Dexamethasone Sodium Phosphate, Aligen Independ	00405-0935-08
3.5 gm	$3.36	Dexamethasone Sodium Phosphate, H.C.F.A. F F P	99999-0976-01
3.5 gm	$3.70	Dexamethasone Sodium Phosphate, Goldline Labs	00182-5071-31
3.5 gm	$4.00	Dexamethasone Sodium Phosphate, Major Pharms	00904-3008-38
3.5 gm	$4.29	Dexamethasone Sodium Phosphate, Schein Pharm (US)	00364-2551-70
3.5 gm	$4.90	AK-DEX, Akorn	17478-0278-35
3.5 gm	$4.95	Dexasol, Ocusoft	54799-0526-35
3.5 gm	$5.90	Spectro-Dex, Spectrum Scitfc	53268-0640-55
3.5 gm	$6.34	DECADRON, Merck	00006-7615-04
3.5 gm x 12	$4.29	Dexamethasone Sodium Phosphate, Rugby	00536-6475-91

Solution - Ophthalmic - 0.1 %

	$4.80	ADRENOCOT 0.1%, C O Truxton	00463-1113-05
5 ml	$2.68	Dexamethasone, United Res	00677-0898-20
5 ml	$2.69	Dexamethasone Sodium Phosphate, H.C.F.A. F F P	99999-0976-02
5 ml	$3.08	Dexamethasone Sodium Phosphate, Rugby	00536-0800-65
5 ml	$3.24	Dexamethasone Sodium Phosphate, HL Moore Drug Exch	00839-6663-25
5 ml	$3.53	Dexamethasone Sodium Phosphate, Aligen Independ	00405-6050-05
5 ml	$4.95	Dexasol, Ocusoft	54799-0525-05
5 ml	$5.00	Dexamethasone Sodium Phosphate, Schein Pharm (US)	00364-7237-53
5 ml	$5.00	Dexamethasone Sodium Phosphate, Steris Labs	00402-0748-05
5 ml	$6.20	Dexamethasone Sodium Phosphate, Goldline Labs	00182-7022-62
5 ml	$6.30	AK-DEX, Akorn	17478-0279-10
5 ml	$15.56	DECADRON PHOSPHATE, Merck	00006-7643-03

HOW SUPPLIED - NOT RATED EQUIVALENT:

Aerosol, Spray - Inhalation; Nas - 84 mcg

12.6 gm	$24.79	DECADRON PHOSPHATE TURBINAIRE, Merck	00006-7642-13
12.6 gm	$40.50	DEXACORT PHOSPHATE TURBINAIRE, Medeva Pharms	53014-0201-13
12.6 gm	$40.50	DEXACORT RESPIHALER, Medeva Pharms	53014-0203-13

Cream - Topical - 0.1 %

15 gm	$11.75	DECADRON, Merck	00006-7616-12
30 gm	$17.57	DECADRON, Merck	00006-7616-24

Injection, Solution - Intramuscular; - 40 mg/ml

1 ml x 25	$24.60	Dexamethasone Sodium Phosphate, Gensia Labs	00703-3501-04
5 ml x 25	$41.10	Dexamethasone Sodium Phosphate, Gensia Labs	00703-3513-04

Injection, Solution - Intravenous - 20 mg/ml

5 ml	$24.70	HEXADROL, Organon	00052-0799-06

Injection, Susp - Intra-Articular - 8 mg/ml

5 ml	$24.15	Dexamethasone La, IDE-Interstate	00814-2355-38

Powder

5 gm	$44.30	Dexamethasone Sodium Phosphate, Paddock Labs	00574-0408-05
10 gm	$79.80	Dexamethasone Sodium Phosphate, Paddock Labs	00574-0408-10

Solution - Ophthalmic - 0.1 %

5 ml	$1.87	I-METHASONE, Americal Pharm	54945-0516-10
15 ml	$3.50	Dexamethasone Sodium Phosphate, Consolidated Midland	00223-6488-15

DEXAMETHASONE SODIUM PHOSPHATE; LIDOCAINE HYDROCHLORIDE *(000977)*

CATEGORIES: Acne; Adrenal Corticosteroids; Adrenal Hyperplasia; Adrenal Insufficiency; Airway Obstruction; Allergies; Alopecia; Anemia; Arthritis; Asthma; Bronchospasm; Bursitis; Colitis; Conjunctival Inflammation; Conjunctivitis; Corneal Inflammation; Corneal Injury; Corneal Ulcer; Dermatitis; Diuresis; Edema; Granuloma Annulare; Herpes; Hormones; Hypercalcemia; Laryngeal Edema; Leukemia; Lupus Erythematosus; Lymphoma; Meningitis; Nasal Polyps; Ocular Acne; Osteoarthritis; Pneumoconiosis; Proteinuria; Pruritus; Psoriasis; Purpura; Retinochoroiditis; Rhinitis; Sarcoidosis; Shock; Spondylitis; Tenosynovitis; Thrombocytopenia; Thyroiditis; Trichinosis; Tuberculosis; Urticaria; Uveitis; FDA Approval Pre 1982

BRAND NAMES: **Decadron W Xylocaine**

> **WARNING:**
> For local injection only

DESCRIPTION:

NOT FOR INTRAVENOUS USE

DEXAMETHASONE SODIUM PHOSPHATE IS A WHITE OR SLIGHTLY YELLOW, CRYSTALLINE POWDER. IT IS FREELY SOLUBLE IN WATER AND IS EXCEEDINGLY HYGROSCOPIC. THE MOLECULAR WEIGHT IS 516.41. IT IS DESIGNATED CHEMICALLY AS 9-FLUORO-11, 17-DIHYDROXY-16æ-METHYL-21-(PHOSPHONOOXY) PREGNA-1,4-DIENE-3,20-DIONE DISODIUM SALT. THE EMPIRICAL FORMULA IS $C_{22}H_{28}FNa_2O_8P$.

LIDOCAINE HYDROCHLORIDE IS A WHITE, CRYSTALLINE POWDER THAT IS VERY SOLUBLE IN WATER AND ALCOHOL, SOLUBLE IN CHLOROFORM, AND INSOLUBLE IN ETHER. THE MOLECULAR WEIGHT IS 288.82. IT IS DESIGNATED CHEMICALLY AS 2-(DIETHYLAMINO)-*N*-(2,6-DIMETHYLPHENYL) ACETAMIDE, MONOHYDROCHLORIDE, MONOHYDRATE. THE EMPIRICAL FORMULA IS $C_{14}H_{22}N_2O{\cdot}HCl{\cdot}H_2O$.

DECADRON PHOSPHATE WITH XYLOCAINE (DEXAMETHASONE SODIUM PHOSPHATE-LIDOCAINE HCL) INJECTION IS PROVIDED AS A STERILE SOLUTION (PH 6.5 TO 6.9) SEALED UNDER NITROGEN, FOR THE CONVENIENCE OF PHYSICIANS WHO PREFER TO TREAT PATIENTS WITH SIMULTANEOUS ADMINISTRATION OF A CORTICOSTEROID AND A LOCAL ANESTHETIC.

EACH MILLILITER CONTAINS DEXAMETHASONE SODIUM PHOSPHATE EQUIVALENT TO DEXAMETHASONE PHOSPHATE, 4 MG; AND LIDOCAINE HYDROCHLORIDE, 10 MG. INACTIVE INGREDIENTS PER ML: CITRIC ACID ANHYDROUS, 10 MG; CREATININE, 8 MG; SODIUM BISULFITE, 0.5 MG; DISODIUM EDETATE, 0.5 MG; SODIUM HYDROXIDE TO ADJUST PH; AND WATER FOR INJECTION, Q.S., 1 ML.

METHYLPARABEN, 1.5 MG, AND PROPYLPARABEN, 0.2 MG, ADDED AS PRESERVATIVES.

CLINICAL PHARMACOLOGY:

Dexamethasone sodium phosphate is a synthetic glucocorticoid used primarily for its potent anti-inflammatory effects in disorders of many organ systems. Glucocorticoids cause profound and varied metabolic effects. In addition, they modify the body's immune responses to diverse stimuli.

Lidocaine HCl is a local anesthetic with a rapid onset and moderate duration of action.

Local anesthesia appears within a few minutes after injection of Dexamethasone sodium phosphate with Lidocaine HCl and lasts 45 minutes to one hour. By the time the anesthesia wears off, steroid activity has usually begun. If the anesthesia wears off before full steroid effect appears, there may be some discomfort beginning about an hour after injection and relief of pain may be delayed for a short time.

INDICATIONS AND USAGE:

Acute and subacute bursitis. Acute and subacute nonspecific tenosynovitis.

CONTRAINDICATIONS:

Hypersensitivity to any component of this product, including sulfites (see WARNINGS).

Dexamethasone Sodium Phosphate

Systemic fungal infections

Lidocaine HCl

Patients with known history of hypersensitivity to local anesthetics of the amide type (*e.g.,* mepivacaine, prilocaine)

Severe shock

Heart block

WARNINGS:

Because rare instances of anaphylactoid reactions have occurred in patients receiving parenteral corticosteroid therapy, appropriate precautionary measures should be taken prior to administration, especially when the patient has a history of allergy to any drug. Anaphylactoid and hypersensitivity reactions have been reported for injection dexamethasone sodium phosphate-lidocaine HCl (see ADVERSE REACTIONS.)

Injection dexamethasone sodium phosphate-lidocaine HCl contains sodium bisulfate, a sulfite, a sulfite that may cause allergic-type reactions including anaphylactic symptoms and life-threatening or less severe asthmatic episodes in certain susceptible people. The overall prevalence of sulfite sensitivity in the general population is unknown and probably low. Sulfite insensitivity is seen more frequently in asthmatic than nonasthmatic people.

LIDOCAINE HCL

RESUSCITATIVE EQUIPMENT AND DRUGS SHOULD BE IMMEDIATELY AVAILABLE WHEN ANY LOCAL ANESTHETIC IS USED.

Usage In Pregnancy: The safe use of lidocaine HCl has not been established with respect to adverse effects upon fetal development. Careful consideration should be given to this fact before administering this drug to women of childbearing potential, particularly during early pregnancy.

DEXAMETHASONE SODIUM PHOSPHATE

In patients on corticosteroid therapy subjected to unusual stress, increased dosage of rapidly acting corticosteroids before, during, and after the stressful situation is indicated.

Drug-induced secondary adrenocortical insufficiency may result from too rapid a withdrawal of corticosteroids and may be minimized by gradual reduction of dosage. This type of relative insufficiency may persist for months after discontinuation of therapy: therefore, in

WARNINGS: *(cont'd)*

any situation of stress occurring during that period, hormone therapy should be reinstituted. If the patient is receiving steroids already, dosage may have to be increased. Since mineralocorticoid secretion may be impaired, salt and/or a mineralocorticoid should be administered concurrently.

Corticosteroids may mask some signs of infection, and new infection may appear during their use. There may be decreased resistance and inability to localize infection when corticosteroids are used. Moreover, corticosteroids may affect the nitroblue-tetrazolium test for bacterial infection and produce false negative results.

Corticosteroids may activate latent amebiasis. Therefore, it is recommended that latent or active amebiasis be ruled out before initiating corticosteroid therapy in any patient who has spent time in the tropics or any patient with unexpected diarrhea.

Prolonged use of corticosteroids may produce posterior subcapsular cataracts, glaucoma with possible damage to the optic nerves, and may enhance the establishment of secondary ocular infections due to fungi or viruses.

Usage in Pregnancy: Since adequate human reproduction studies have not been done with corticosteroids, use of these drugs in pregnancy or in women of childbearing potential requires that the anticipated benefits be weighed against the possible hazards to the mother and embryo or fetus. Infants born of mothers who have received substantial doses of corticosteroids during pregnancy should be carefully observed for signs of hypoadrenalism.

Corticosteroids appear in breast milk and could suppress growth, interfere with endogenous corticosteroid production, or cause other unwanted effects. Mothers taking pharmacologic doses of corticosteroids should be advised not to nurse.

Average and large doses of cortisone or hydrocortisone can cause elevation of blood pressure, salt and water retention, and increased excretion of potassium. These effects are less likely to occur with the synthetic derivatives except when used in large doses. Dietary salt restriction and potassium supplementation may be necessary. All corticosteroids increase calcium excretion.

Administration of live virus vaccines, including smallpox, is contraindicated in individuals receiving immunosuppressive doses of corticosteroids. If inactivated viral or bacterial vaccines are administered to individuals receiving immunosuppressive doses of corticosteroids, the expected serum antibody response may not be obtained.

Patients who are on drugs which suppress the immune system are more susceptible to infections than healthy individuals. Chickenpox and measles, for example, can have a more serious or even fatal course in non-immune children or adults on corticosteroids. In such children or adults who have not had these diseases, particular care should be taken to avoid exposure. The risk of developing a disseminated infection varies among individuals and can be related to the dose, route and duration of corticosteroid administration as well as to the underlying disease. If exposed to chickenpox, prophylaxis with varicella zoster immune globulin (VZIG) may by indicated. If chickenpox develops, treatment with antiviral agents may be considered. If exposed to measles, prophylaxis with immune globulin (IG) may be indicated. (See the respective package inserts for VZIG and IG for complete prescribing information.)

If corticosteroids are indicated in patients with latent tuberculosis or tuberculin reactivity, close observation is necessary as reactivation of the disease may occur. During prolonged corticosteroid therapy, these patients should receive chemoprophylaxis.

Literature reports suggest an apparent association between use of corticosteroids and left ventricular free wall rupture after a recent myocardial infarction; therefore, therapy with corticosteroids should be used with great caution in these patients.

PRECAUTIONS:

This product, like many other steroid formulations, is sensitive to heat. Therefore, it should not be autoclaved when it is desirable to sterilize the exterior of the vial.

Therapy with this preparation does not eliminate the need for conventional supportive measures. Although capable of ameliorating symptoms, and even suppressing them completely in some patients, it is not a cure. Neither the hormone nor the anesthetic has any effect on the basic cause of inflammation.

Supportive measures, such as analgesics, pertinent orthopedic procedures, heat or cold, rest, rehabilitation, and physiotherapy must be used as applicable. If physiotherapy is applied immediately following injection, it may cause severe pain.

In some patients, a single injection fully restores mobility. Patients should be strongly impressed with the importance of not overusing the affected part as long as the inflammatory process remains active.

Injection into an infected site is to be avoided.

DEXAMETHASONE SODIUM PHOSPHATE

Following prolonged therapy, withdrawal of corticosteroids may result in symptoms of the corticosteroid withdrawal syndrome including fever, myalgia, arthralgia, and malaise. This may occur in patients even without evidence of adrenal insufficiency.

There is an enhanced effect of corticosteroids in patients with hypothyroidism and in those with cirrhosis.

Corticosteroids should be used cautiously in patients with ocular herpes simplex for fear of corneal perforation.

Psychic derangements may appear when corticosteroids are used, ranging from euphoria, insomnia, mood swings, personality changes and severe depression to frank psychotic manifestations. Also, existing emotional instability or psychotic tendencies my be aggravated by corticosteroids.

Aspirin should be used cautiously in conjunction with corticosteroids in hypoprothrombinemia.

Steroids should be used with caution in non-specific ulcerative colitis, if there is a probability of impending perforation, abscess, or other pyogenic infection, also in diverticulitis, fresh intestinal anastomoses, active or latent peptic ulcer, renal insufficiency, hypertension, osteoporosis, and myasthenia gravis. Signs of peritoneal infection in patients receiving large doses of corticosteroids may be minimal or absent. Fat embolism has been reported as a possible complication of hypercortisonism.

When large doses are given, some authorities advise that antacids be administered between meals to help to prevent peptic ulcer.

Growth and development of infants and children on prolonged corticosteroid therapy should be carefully followed.

Steroids may increase or decrease motility and number of spermatozoa in some patients.

Phenytoin, phenobarbital, ephedrine, and rifampin may enhance the metabolic clearance of corticosteroids, resulting in decreased blood levels and lessened physiologic activity, thus requiring adjustment in corticosteroid dosage.

The prothrombin time should be checked frequently in patients who are receiving corticosteroids and coumarin anticoagulants at the same time because of reports that corticosteroids have altered the response to these anticoagulants. Studies have shown that the usual effect produced by adding corticosteroids is inhibition of response to coumarins, although there have been some conflicting reports of potentiation not substantiated by studies.

PRECAUTIONS: *(cont'd)*

When corticosteroids are administered concomitantly with potassium-depleting diuretics, patients should be observed closely for development of hypokalemia.

LIDOCAINE HYDROCHLORIDE

The safety and effectiveness of lidocaine hydrochloride depend on proper dosage, correct technique, adequate precautions, and readiness for emergencies.

Injection of repeated doses may cause significant increases in blood levels with each repeated dose due to slow accumulation of the drug or its metabolites. Tolerance varies with the status of the patient. Debilitated, elderly patients, acutely ill patients, and children should be given reduced doses commensurate with their age and physical status. INJECTIONS SHOULD BE MADE SLOWLY AND WITH FREQUENT ASPIRATIONS. Aspiration is advisable since it reduces the possibility of intravascular injection, thereby keeping the incidence of side effects and anesthetic failures to a minimum. Consult standard textbooks for specific techniques and precautions for various local anesthetic procedures.

Lidocaine hydrochloride should be used with caution in persons with known drug sensitivities. Patients allergic to para-aminobenzoic acids derivatives (procaine, tetracaine, benzocaine, etc.) have not shown cross sensitivity to lidocaine hydrochloride.

Local anesthetics react with certain metals and cause the release of their respective ions which, if injected, may cause severe local irritation. Adequate precaution should be taken to avoid this type of interaction.

ADVERSE REACTIONS:

DEXAMETHASONE SODIUM PHOSPHATE

Fluid and Electrolyte Disturbances: Sodium retention; fluid retention; congestive heart failure in susceptible patients.; potassium loss; hypokalemic alkalosis; hypertension

Musculoskeletal: Muscle weakness; steroid myopathy; loss of muscle mass; osteoporosis; vertebral compression fractures; aseptic necrosis of femoral and humeral heads; pathologic fracture of long bones; tendon rupture

Gastrointestinal: Peptic ulcer with possible subsequent perforation and hemorrhage; perforation of the small and large bowel, particularly in patients with inflammatory bowel disease; pancreatitis; abdominal distention; ulcerative esophagitis

Dermatologic: Impaired wound healing; thin fragile skin; petechiae and ecchymoses; erythema; increased sweating; may suppress reactions to skin tests; other cutaneous reactions, such as allergic dermatitis, urticaria, angioneurotic edema

Neurologic: Convulsions; Increased intracranial pressure with papilledema (pseudotumor cerebri) usually after treatment; Vertigo; Headache; Psychic disturbances

Endocrine: Menstrual irregularities; Development of cushingoid state; Suppression of growth in children; Secondary adrenocortical and pituitary unresponsiveness, particularly in times of stress, as in trauma, surgery, or illness; Decreased carbohydrate tolerance; Manifestations of latent diabetes mellitus; Increased requirements for insulin or oral hypoglycemic agents in diabetics; Hirsutism

Ophthalmic: Posterior subcapsular cataracts; Increased intraocular pressure; Glaucoma; Exophthalmos

Metabolic: Negative nitrogen balance due to protein catabolism

Cardiovascular: Myocardial rupture following recent myocardial infarction (see WARNINGS)

Other: Anaphylactoid or hypersensitivity reactions; thromboembolism; weight gain; increased appetite; nausea; malaise; hiccups

The following *additional* adverse reactions are related to parenteral corticosteroid therapy:

Rare instances of blindness associated with intralesional therapy around the face and head; hyperpigmentation or hypopigmentation; subcutaneous and cutaneous atrophy; sterile abscess; charcot-like arthropathy

LIDOCAINE HCL

Adverse reactions may result from high plasma levels due to excessive dosage, rapid absorption or inadvertent intravascular injection, or may result from a hypersensitivity, idiosyncrasy or diminished tolerance on the part of the patient. Such reactions are systemic in nature and involve the central nervous system and/or the cardiovascular system.

CNS reactions are excitatory and/or depressant, and may be characterized by nervousness, dizziness, blurred vision, and tremors followed by drowsiness, convulsions, unconsciousness, and possibly respiratory arrest. The excitatory reactions may be very brief or may not occur at all, in which case the first manifestations of toxicity may be drowsiness merging into unconsciousness and respiratory arrest.

Cardiovascular reactions are depressant, and may be characterized by hypotension, myocardial depression, bradycardia and possibly cardiac arrest.

Treatment of a patient with toxic manifestations consists of assuring and maintaining a patent airway and supporting ventilation using oxygen and assisted or controlled respiration as required. This usually will be sufficient in the management of most reactions. Should circulatory depression occur, vasopressors, such as ephedrine or metaraminol, and intravenous fluids may be used. Should a convulsion persist despite oxygen therapy, small increments of an ultra-short acting barbiturate (thiopental or thiamylal) or a short-acting barbiturate (pentobarbital or secobarbital) may be given intravenously.

Allergic reactions are characterized by cutaneous lesions, urticaria, edema or anaphylactoid reactions. The detection of sensitivity by skin testing is of doubtful value.

DOSAGE AND ADMINISTRATION:

For local injection only

NOT FOR INTRAVENOUS USE

DOSAGE AND FREQUENCY OF INJECTION ARE VARIABLE AND MUST BE INDIVIDUALIZED ON THE BASIS OF THE DISEASE AND THE RESPONSE OF THE PATIENT.

Injections should always be made slowly and with frequent aspiration.

The initial dose ranges from 0.1 to 0.75 ml depending on the disease being treated and the size of the area to be injected. Frequency of injection depends on symptomatic response. In some patients, acute conditions are controlled adequately by a single injection. In others, additional injections are required, usually at intervals of four to seven days. If satisfactory clinical response does not occur after a reasonable period of time, discontinue dexamethasone sodium phosphate-lidocaine HCl injection and transfer the patient to other therapy.

Patients should be observed closely for signs that might require dosage adjustment, including changes in clinical status resulting from remissions or exacerbations of the disease, and individual drug responsiveness.

The usual doses are (TABLE 1):

Dexamethasone sodium phosphate-lidocaine HCl may be given undiluted directly from the vial, or it may be diluted with Sterile Water for Injection or Sodium Chloride Injection, using up to five parts of diluent to each part of injection. Dilutions should be used within one hour, since there is a possibility of change in pH, and this may adversely affect the stability or activity of the components.

TABLE 1

	Acute and Subacute Bursitis	Acute and Subacute Nonspecific Tenosynovitis
Amount of injection (ml)	0.5 to 0.75	0.1 to 0.25
Amount of dexamethasone sodium phosphate (mg)	2 to 3	0.4 to 1
Amount of lidocaine hydrochloride (mg)	5 to 7.5	1 to 2.5

HOW SUPPLIED:

Injection Decadron Phosphate with Xylocaine, containing 4 mg dexamethasone phosphate equivalent and 10 mg lidocaine hydrochloride per ml, is a clear, colorless solution.

Storage: Sensitive to heat. Do not autoclave. Protect from freezing.

HOW SUPPLIED - EQUIVALENTS NOT AVAILABLE:

Injection, Solution - Intramuscular; - /10 mg

5 ml $31.71 DECADRON PHOSPHATE WITH XYLOCAINE, Merck 00006-7625-03

DEXAMETHASONE SODIUM PHOSPHATE; NEOMYCIN SULFATE *(000978)*

CATEGORIES: Anti-Infectives; Anti-Inflammatory Agents; Antibacterials; Antibiotics; Burns; Conjunctival Inflammation; Corneal Inflammation; Corneal Injury; Dermatologicals; EENT Drugs; Edema; Eye, Ear, Nose, & Throat Preparations; Inflammatory Conditions; Ocular Infections; Ophthalmic Corticosteroids; Ophthalmics; Pruritus; Skin/Mucous Membrane Agents; Steroids; Uveitis; Pregnancy Category C; FDA Approval Pre 1982

BRAND NAMES: Ak-Neo-Dex; *Angel*; *Colircusi*; *Decadron*; *Decadron Con Neomicina* (Mexico); *Decadron with Neomycin*; *Decaneo*; *Decason*; *Decdan-N Eye ear*; *Delone*; *Dexacort*; *Dexamicina*; *Dexamycin*; *Dexasil*; *Dexaton*; *Dexona Ear Drops*; *Dexona Eye Drops*; *Dexona Eye ear*; *Dexoph*; *Dexoptic-N*; *Dexosyn-N*; *Dextracin*; *Dexylin*; *Eyedex*; *Mycidex*; Neo Dexair; *Neo-Deca*; Neo-Deca-Gen; Neo-Dex; *Neo-Dexacortin*; Neo-Dexair; Neo-Dexide; **Neodecadron**; Neodexameth; *Neomodex*; *Neomodex Ofteno* (Mexico); Neomycin W/Dexamethasone; *Neosulon*; *Sinmesone*; *Soldrin Oftalmico* (Mexico); Storz N-D
(International brand names outside U.S. in italics)

FORMULARIES: BC-BS; FHP; BC-BS; Medi-Cal

DESCRIPTION:

TOPICAL CREAM

Neomycin sulfate-dexamethasone sodium phosphate topical cream is a topical steroid-antibiotic preparation.

Each gram contains: dexamethasone sodium phosphate equivalent to 1 mg (0.1%) dexamethasone phosphate, and neomycin sulfate equivalent to 3.5 mg neomycin base, in a greaseless bland base. Inactive ingredients: stearyl alcohol, cetyl alcohol, mineral oil, polyoxyl 40 stearate, sorbitol solution, methyl polysilicone emulsion, creatinine, disodium edetate, sodium citrate, sodium hydroxide to adjust pH, and purified water. Methylparaben 0.15%, sodium bisulfite 0.18%, and sorbic acid 0.1% added as preservatives.

Dexamethasone sodium phosphate is 9-fluoro-11β, 17-dihydroxy-16α-methyl-21-(phosphonooxy)pregna-1,4-diene-3,20-dione disodium salt. Its empirical formula is $C_{22}H_{28}FNa_2O_8P$.

Dexamethasone sodium phosphate has a molecular weight of 516.41.

Glucocorticoids are adrenocortical steroids, both naturally occurring and synthetic. Dexamethasone is a synthetic analog of naturally occurring glucocorticoids (hydrocortisone and cortisone).

Neomycin sulfate is a mixture of the sulfate salts of neomycin, an antibacterial substance produced by the growth of *Streptomyces fradiae* Waksman (Fam. Streptomycetaceae).

Neomycin is a complex typically containing 8-13% neomycin C, less than 0.2% neomycin A and the rest, neomycin B. The empirical formulas and molecular weights for the three components are: neomycin B, $C_{23}H_{46}N_6O_{13}$, molecular weight 614.65; neomycin C, $C_{23}H_{46}N_6O_{13}$, molecular weight 614.65; neomycin A, (also referred to as neamine), $C_{12}H_{26}N_4O_6$, molecular weight 322.36.

OPHTHALMIC SOLUTION

Neomycin Sulfate-Dexamethasone Sodium Phosphate ophthalmic solution is a topical corticosteroid-antibiotic solution for use in certain disorders of the anterior segment of the eye. Each milliliter of buffered ophthalmic solution contains: dexamethasone sodium phosphate equivalent to 1 mg (0.1%) dexamethasone phosphate, and neomycin sulfate equivalent to 3.5 mg neomycin base. Inactive ingredients: creatinine, sodium citrate, sodium borate, polysorbate 80, disodium edetate, hydrochloric acid to adjust pH to 6.6 - 7.2, and water for injections. Benzalkonium chloride 0.02% and sodium bisulfite 0.1% added as preservatives.

Dexamethasone sodium phosphate is a water soluble, inorganic ester of dexamethasone. Its empirical formula is $C_{22}H_{28}FNa_2O_8P$. It is approximately three thousand times more soluble in water at 25° than hydrocortisone.

Neomycin sulfate is the sulfate salt of neomycin, an antibacterial substance produced by the growth of *Streptomyces fradiae* Waksman (Fam. Streptimycetaceae).

CLINICAL PHARMACOLOGY:

TOPICAL CREAM

Topical corticosteroids share anti-inflammatory, anti-pruritic, and vasoconstrictive actions.

The mechanism of anti-inflammatory activity of the topical corticosteroids is unclear. Various laboratory methods, including vasoconstrictor assays, are used to compare and predict potencies and/or clinical efficacies of the topical corticosteroids. There is some evidence to suggest that a recognizable correlation exists between vasoconstrictor potency and therapeutic efficacy in man.

PHARMACOKINETICS

The extent of percutaneous absorption of topical corticosteroids is determined by many factors including the vehicle, the integrity of the epidermal barrier, and the use of occlusive dressings.

Topical corticosteroids can be absorbed from normal intact skin. Inflammation and/or other disease processes in the skin increase percutaneous absorption. Occlusive dressings substantially increase the percutaneous absorption of topical corticosteroids. Thus, occlusive dressings may be a valuable therapeutic adjunct for treatment of resistant dermatoses. (See DOSAGE AND ADMINISTRATION.)

CLINICAL PHARMACOLOGY: *(cont'd)*

Once absorbed through the skin, topical corticosteroids are handled through pharmacokinetic pathways similar to systemically administered corticosteroids. Corticosteroids are bound to plasma proteins in varying degrees. Corticosteroids are metabolized primarily in the liver and are then excreted by the kidneys. Some of the topical corticosteroids and their metabolites are also excreted into the bile.

The antibiotic component, neomycin, is bactericidal to many gram-positive and gram-negative bacteria.

OPHTHALMIC SOLUTION

Dexamethasone sodium phosphate, a corticosteroid, suppresses the inflammatory response to a variety of agents, and it probably delays or slows healing. Since corticosteroids may inhibit the body's defense mechanism against infection, a concomitant antimicrobial drug may be used when this inhibition is considered to be clinically significant in a particular case.

Neomycin sulfate, the anti-infective component in the combination, is included to provide action against specific organisms susceptible to it. Neomycin sulfate is considered active mainly against gram-negative organisms, except *Bacteroides* spp. and *Pseudomonas aeruginosa*, which are resistant. Gram-positive organisms except for *Staphylococcus aureus* are usually resistant.

When a decision to administer both a corticosteroid and a antimicrobial is made, the administration of such drugs in combination has the advantage of greater patient compliance and convenience, with the added assurance that the appropriate dosage of both drugs is administered, plus assured compatibility of ingredients when both types of drugs are in the same formulation, and, particularly, that the correct volume of drug is delivered and retained.

The relative potency of corticosteroids depends on the molecular structure, concentration, and release from the vehicle.

INDICATIONS AND USAGE:

TOPICAL CREAM

For the treatment of corticosteroid-responsive dermatoses with secondary infection. It has not been demonstrated that this steroid-antibiotic combination provides greater benefit than the steroid component alone after 7 days of treatment. See WARNINGS.

OPHTHALMIC SOLUTION

For steroid-responsive inflammatory ocular conditions for which a corticosteroid is indicated and where bacterial infection or risk of bacterial ocular infection exists.

Ocular steroids are indicated in inflammatory conditions of the palpebral and bulbar conjunctiva, cornea, and anterior segment of the globe where inherent risk of steroid use in certain infective conjunctivides is accepted to obtain a diminution in edema and inflammation. They are also indicated in the chronic anterior uveitis and corneal injury from chemical, radiation, or thermal burns, or penetration of foreign bodies.

The use of a combination drug with an anti-infective component is indicated where the risk of infection is high or where there is an expectation that potentially dangerous numbers of bacteria will be present in the eye.

The particular anti-infective drug in this product is active against the following common bacteria eye pathogens:

Staphylococcus aureus
Escherichia coli
Haemophilus influenzae
*Klebsiella/Enterobacter*species
Neisseria species

The product does not provide adequate coverage against:

Pseudomonas aeruginosa
Serratia marcescens
Streptococci, including *Streptococcus pneumoniae*

CONTRAINDICATIONS:

TOPICAL CREAM

Hypersensitivity to any component of this product, including sulfites (see WARNINGS.)

OPHTHALMIC SOLUTION

Epithelial herpes simplex keratitis (dendritic keratitis), acute infectious stages of vaccina, varicella, and many other viral diseases of the cornea and conjunctiva. Mycobacterial infection of the eye. Fungal diseases of ocular structures. Hypersensitivity to any component of this product, including sulfites (see WARNINGS.)

(Hypersensitivity to the antibiotic component occurs at a higher rate than for other components.)

The use of these combinations is always contraindicated after uncomplicated removal of a corneal foreign body.

WARNINGS:

TOPICAL CREAM

Topical cream neomycin sulfate-dexamethasone sodium phosphate contains sodium bisulfite, a sulfite that may cause allergic-type reactions including anaphylactic symptoms and life-threatening or less severe asthmatic episodes in certain susceptible people. The overall prevalence of sulfite sensitivity in the general population is unknown and probably low. Sulfite sensitivity is seen more frequently in asthmatic than in nonasthmatic people.

Because of the concern of nephrotoxicity and ototoxicity associated with neomycin, this combination product should not be used over a wide area or for extended periods of time.

OPHTHALMIC SOLUTION

Prolonged use may result in glaucoma, with damage to the optic nerve, defects in visual acuity and fields of vision, and posterior subcapsular cataract formation. Prolonged use may suppress the host response and thus increase the hazard of secondary ocular infections. In those diseases causing thinning of the cornea of sclera, perforations have been known to occur with the use of topical corticosteroids. In acute purulent conditions of the eye, corticosteroids may mask infection or enhance existing infection. If these products are used for 10 days or longer, intraocular pressure should be routinely monitored even though it might be more difficult in children and uncooperative patients.

Employment of corticosteroids medication in the treatment of herpes simplex requires great caution: periodic slit-lamp microscopy is recommended.

Any substance (*e.g.,* neomycin sulfate) may occasionally cause cutaneous sensitization. If any reaction indicating such sensitivity is observed, discontinue use.

The Ophthalmic Solution contains sodium bisulfate, a sulfate that may cause allergic-type reactions including anaphylactic symptoms and life-threatening or less severe asthmatic episodes in certain susceptible people. The overall prevalence of sulfite sensitivity in the general population is unknown and probably low. Sulfite sensitivity is seen more frequently in asthmatic than in nonasthmatic people.

PRECAUTIONS:

GENERAL

Topical Cream: Systemic absorption of topical corticosteroids has produced reversible hypothalamic-pituitary-adrenal (HPA) axis suppression, manifestations of Cushing's syndrome, hyperglycemia, and glycosuria in some patients.

Conditions which augment systemic absorption include the application of the more potent corticosteroids, use over large surface areas, prolonged use, and the addition of occlusive dressings.

Therefore, patients receiving a large dose of a potent topical corticosteroid applied to a large surface area or under an occlusive dressing should be evaluated periodically for evidence of HPA axis suppression by using urinary free cortisol and ACTH stimulation tests. If HPA axis suppression is noted, an attempt should be made to withdraw the drug, to reduce the frequency of application, or to substitute a less potent corticosteroid.

Recovery of HPA axis function is generally prompt and complete upon discontinuation of the drug. Infrequently, signs and symptoms of corticosteroid withdrawal may occur, requiring supplemental systemic corticosteroids.

Children may absorb proportionally larger amounts of topical corticosteroids and thus be more susceptible to systemic toxicity (see PRECAUTIONS, Pediatric Use.)

Corticosteroids may mask some signs of infection, and new infections may appear during their use. There may be decreased resistance and inability to localize infection when corticosteroids are used. Therefore, patients with bacterial infections should also be given appropriate antibiotic therapy if topical cream neomycin sulfate-dexamethasone sodium phosphate is used. Moreover, corticosteroids may affect the nitroblue-tetrazolium test for bacterial infections and produce false-negative results.

Corticosteroid therapy exerts its major immunosuppressive effects by impairing the normal function of the T-lymphocyte population and macrophages. When T-cell and/or macrophage function is impaired, latent disease may be activated or there may be an exacerbation of intercurrent infections due to pathogens, including those caused by *Candida*, *Mycobacterium*, Ameba, Toxoplasma, *Strongyloides*, *Pneumocystis*, *Cryptococcus*, Nocardia, etc. Products containing steroids should be used with caution in patients with impaired T-cell function or in patients receiving other immunosuppressive therapy.

In the presence of dermatological infections, the use of an appropriate anti-fungal or antibacterial agent should be instituted. If a favorable response does not occur promptly, the corticosteroid should be discontinued until the infection has been adequately controlled.

If irritation develops, topical corticosteroids should be discontinued and appropriate therapy instituted.

This product is not for ophthalmic use. However, if applied to the eyelids or skin near the eyes, the drug may enter the eyes. In patients with a history of herpes simplex keratitis, ocular exposure to corticosteroids may lead to a recurrence. Prolonged ocular exposure may cause steroid glaucoma.

A few individuals may be sensitive to one or more of the components of this product. Sensitivity to neomycin may occasionally develop, especially when it is applied to abraded skin. If any reaction indicating sensitivity is observed, discontinue use. There are reports in the current medical literature that indicate an increase in the prevalence of persons sensitive to neomycin.

Generally, occlusive dressings should not be used on weeping or exudative lesions.

If the occlusive dressing technique is employed, caution should be exercised with regard to the use of plastic films which are often inflammable and may pose a suffocation hazard for children.

When large areas of the body are covered with an occlusive dressing, thermal homeostasis may be impaired. If elevation of body temperature occurs, use of the occlusive dressing should be discontinued.

Ophthalmic Solution: The initial prescription and renewal of the medication order beyond 20 milliliters should be made by a physician only after examination of the patient with the aid of magnification, such as slit-lamp biomicroscopy and, where appropriate, fluorescein staining.

The possibility of persistent fungal infections of the cornea should be considered after prolonged corticosteroid dosing.

INFORMATION FOR THE PATIENT

Topical Cream: Patients using topical corticosteroids should receive the following information and instructions:

1. This medication is to be used as directed by the physician. It is for external use only. Avoid contact with the eyes.

2. Patients should be advised not to use this medication for any disorder other than that for which it was prescribed.

3. The treated skin area should not be bandaged or otherwise covered or wrapped so as to be occlusive unless directed by the physician.

4. Patients should report any signs of local adverse reactions, especially under occlusive dressing.

5. Parents of pediatric patients should be advised not to use tight-fitting diapers or plastic pants on a child being treated in the diaper area, as these garments may constitute occlusive dressings.

Ophthalmic Solution: One of the preservatives in the ophthalmic solution, benzalkonium chloride, may be absorbed by soft contact lenses. Patients wearing soft contact lenses should be instructed to wait at least 15 minutes after instilling the ophthalmic solution before they insert their lenses.

LABORATORY TESTS

Topical Cream: The following tests may be helpful in evaluating the HPA axis suppression:

Urinary free cortisol test

ACTH stimulation test

CARCINOGENESIS, MUTAGENESIS, AND IMPAIRMENT OF FERTILITY

Topical Cream: Long-term animal studies have not been performed to evaluate the carcinogenic potential or the effect on fertility of topical cream neomycin sulfate-dexamethasone sodium phosphate.

Studies to determine mutagenicity with prednisolone and hydrocortisone have revealed negative results.

PREGNANCY CATEGORY C

Topical Cream: Corticosteroids are generally teratogenic in laboratory animals when administered systemically at relatively low dosage levels. The more potent corticosteroids have been shown to be teratogenic after dermal application in laboratory animals. There are no adequate and well-controlled studies in pregnant women on teratogenic effects from topically applied corticosteroids. Therefore, topical corticosteroids should be used during pregnancy only if the potential benefit justifies the potential risk to the fetus. Drugs of this class should not be used extensively on pregnant patients, in large amounts, or for prolonged periods of time.

PRECAUTIONS: *(cont'd)*

Ophthalmic Solution: Safety of intensive or protracted use of topical steroids during pregnancy has not yet been substantiated.

NURSING MOTHERS

Topical Cream: It is not known whether topical administration of corticosteroids could result in sufficient systemic absorption to produce detectable quantities in breast milk. Systemically administered corticosteroids are secreted into breast milk in quantities *not*likely to have a deleterious effect on the infant. Nevertheless, caution should be exercised when topical corticosteroids are administered to a nursing woman.

PEDIATRIC USE

Topical Cream: *Pediatric patients may demonstrate greater susceptibility to topical corticosteroid-induced HPA axis suppression and Cushing's syndrome than mature patients because of a larger skin surface area to body weight ratio.*

Hypothalamic-pituitary-adrenal (HPA) axis suppression, Cushing's syndrome, and intracranial hypertension have been reported in children receiving topical corticosteroids. Manifestations of adrenal suppression in children include linear growth retardation, delayed weight gain, low plasma cortisol levels, and absence of response to ACTH stimulation. Manifestations of intracranial hypertension include bulging fontanelles, headaches, and bilateral papilledema.

Administration of topical corticosteroids to children should be limited to the least amount compatible with an effective therapeutic regimen. Chronic corticosteroid therapy may interfere with the growth and development of children.

ADVERSE REACTIONS:

TOPICAL CREAM

The following adverse reactions are reported infrequently with topical corticosteroids, but may occur more frequently with the use of occlusive dressings. These reactions are listed in an approximate decreasing order of occurrence:

Burning; Itching; Irritation; Dryness; Folliculitis; Acneiform eruptions; Hypopigmentation; Perioral dermatitis; Allergic contact dermatitis; Maceration of the skin; Secondary infection; Skin atrophy; Striae; Miliaria

Prevalence of neomycin hypersensitivity is increasing. Ototoxicity and nephrotoxicity have been reported with prolonged use or use of large amounts of topical neomycin preparations.

OPHTHALMIC SOLUTION

Adverse reactions have occurred with corticosteroid/anti-infective combination drugs which can be attributed to the corticosteroid component, the anti-infective component, or any other component of this product. Exact incidence figures are not available since no denominator of treated patients is available.

Reactions occurring most often from the presence of the anti-infective ingredients are allergic sensitizations. The reactions due to the corticosteroid component in decreasing order of frequency are: elevation of intraocular pressure (IOP) with possible development of glaucoma, and infrequent optic nerve damage; posterior subcapsular cataract formation; and delayed wound healing.

Secondary Infection: The development of secondary infection has occurred after use of combinations containing corticosteroids and (antimicrobials). Fungal infections of the cornea are particularly prone to develop coincidentally with long-term applications of corticosteroids. The possibility of fungal invasion must be considered in any persistent corneal ulceration where corticosteroid treatment has been used.

Secondary bacterial ocular infection following suppression of host responses also occurs.

OVERDOSAGE:

Topical Cream: Topically applied corticosteroids can be absorbed in sufficient amounts to produce systemic effects (see PRECAUTIONS.)

DOSAGE AND ADMINISTRATION:

TOPICAL CREAM

Apply to the affected area as a thin film three or four times daily.

Before using neomycin sulfate-dexamethasone sodium phosphate in the *ear,* clean the aural canal thoroughly and sponge dry. Confirm that the eardrum is intact. With a cotton-tipped applicator, apply a thin coating of the cream to the affected canal area two or three times a day. When a favorable response is obtained, reduce the number of daily applications to one or two, and eventually discontinue.

OPHTHALMIC SOLUTION

The duration of treatment will vary with the type of lesion and may extend from a few days to several days to several weeks, according to therapeutic response. Relapses, more common in chronic active lesions than in self-limited conditions, usually respond to retreatment.

Instill one or two drops of neomycin sulfate-dexamethasone sodium phosphate ophthalmic solution into the conjunctival sac every hour during the day and every two hours during the night as therapy. When a favorable response is observed, reduce dosage to one drop every four hours. Later, further reduction in dosage to one drop three or four times daily may suffice to control symptoms.

No more than 20 milliliters should be prescribed initially and the prescription should not be refilled without further evaluation as outlined in PRECAUTIONSabove.

STORAGE

Store at 15-30°C (59-86°F).

(Topical Cream: Merck, 10/89, 7612427) (Ophthalmic Solution: Merck, 10/93, 7261323)

HOW SUPPLIED - RATED THERAPEUTICALLY EQUIVALENT:

Solution - Ophthalmic - 0.1 %/3.5 mg/ml

5 ml	$6.38	Neomycin W/Dexamethasone, H.C.F.A. F F P	99999-0978-01
5 ml	$6.75	Neomycin W/Dexamethasone, United Res	00677-1573-20
5 ml	$7.10	Neomycin W/Dexamethasone, Aligen Independ	00405-6090-05
5 ml	$7.90	Neomycin W/Dexamethasone, HL Moore Drug Exch	00839-7111-25
5 ml	$8.10	Neomycin-Dexamethasone, Goldline Labs	00182-1794-62
5 ml	$8.10	Neomycin-Dexamethasone, Steris Labs	00402-0775-05
5 ml	$8.40	AK-NEO-DEX, Akorn	17478-0277-10
5 ml	$8.50	Neo-Dex, Qualitest Pharms	00603-7204-37
5 ml	$8.95	NEO-DEXAMETH, Major Pharms	00904-3007-05
5 ml	$9.50	Neomycin-Dex Ophth Sol, Schein Pharm (US)	00364-0762-53
5 ml	$9.82	Neomycin W/Dexamethasone, Rugby	00536-1905-65
5 ml	**$15.56**	**NEODECADRON, Merck**	**00006-7639-03**

HOW SUPPLIED - NOT RATED EQUIVALENT:

Solution - Ophthalmic - 0.1 %/3.5 mg/ml

5 ml	$8.50	Neomycin W/Dexamethasone, Consolidated Midland	00223-6753-05

DEXAMETHASONE; NEOMYCIN SULFATE; POLYMYXIN B SULFATE *(000979)*

CATEGORIES: Anti-Infectives; Antibiotics; Antihypertensives; Conjunctivitis; Corneal Inflammation; Corneal Injury; EENT Drugs; Edema; Eye, Ear, Nose, & Throat Preparations; Infections; Inflammatory Conditions; Ocular Infections; Ophthalmics; Otic Preparations; Otologic; Steroids; Uveitis; FDA Approval Pre 1982

BRAND NAMES: Ak-Trol; *Aplosyn*; *Cendo Xitrol*; Dex-Ide; Dexacidin; Dexamycin; Dexasporin; Infa-Trol; Infectrol; *Isopto Maxitrol*; Maxigen; **Maxitrol**; *Maxoptic*; Methadex; Neo Polymyxin Dexamethasone; Neomycin Polymyxin Dexameth; Ocu-Trol; *Osatrol*; Poly-Dex; Spectro-Max; Storz N-P-D
(International brand names outside U.S. in italics)

FORMULARIES: Aetna; BC-BS; FHP; Medi-Cal

DESCRIPTION:

Dexamethasone 0.1%, neomycin sulfate, polymyxin B sulfate is a multiple dose anti-infective steroid combination in sterile suspension and sterile ointment forms for topical application.

Established Name: Dexamethasone 0.1%

Chemical Name: Pregna-1,4-diene-3,20-dione,9-fluoro-11,17,21-trihydroxy-16-methyl-, (11β, 16α)-.

The other active ingredients are neomycin sulfate and polymyxin B sulfate.

Each ml of Solution Contains: *Active:* Neomycin sulfate equivalent to neomycin 3.5 mg, polymyxin B sulfate 10,000 units, dexamethasone 0.1%. *Preservative:* Benzalkonium chloride 0.004%. *Vehicle:* Hydroxypropyl methylcellulose 0.5%. *Inactives:* Sodium chloride, polysorbate 20, hydrochloric acid and/or sodium hydroxide (to adjust ph), purified water.

Each Gram of Ointment Contains: *Active:* Neomycin sulfate equivalent to to neomycin 3.5 mg, polymyxin b sulfate 10,000 units, dexamethasone 0.1%. *Preservatives:* Methylparaben 0.05%, propylparaben 0.01%. *Inactives:* White petrolatum, anhydrous liquid lanolin.

CLINICAL PHARMACOLOGY:

Corticoids suppress the inflammatory response to a variety of agents and they probably delay or slow healing. Since corticoids may inhibit the body's defense mechanism against infection, a concomitant antimicrobial drug may be used when this inhibition is considered to be clinically significant in a particular case.

When a decision to administer both a corticoid and an antimicrobial is made, the administration of such drugs in combination has the advantage of greater patient compliance and convenience, with the added assurance that the appropriate dosage of both drugs is administered, plus assured compatibility of ingredients when both types of drugs are in the same formulation and, particularly, that the correct volume of drug is delivered and retained.

The relative potency of corticosteroids depends on the molecular structure, concentration and release from the vehicle.

INDICATIONS AND USAGE:

For steroid-responsive inflammatory ocular conditions for which a corticosteroid is indicated and where bacterial infection or a risk of bacterial ocular infection exists.

Ocular steroids are indicated in inflammatory conditions of the palpebral and bulbar conjunctiva, cornea, and anterior segment of the globe where the inherent risk of steroid use in certain infective conjunctivitises is accepted to obtain a diminution in edema and inflammation. They are also indicated in chronic anterior uveitis and corneal injury from chemical, radiation or thermal burns; or penetration of foreign bodies.

The use of a combination drug with an anti-infective component is indicated where the risk of infection is high or where there is an expectation that potentially dangerous numbers of bacteria will be present in the eye.

The particular anti-infective drug in this product is active against the following common bacterial eye pathogens: *Staphylococcus aureus, Escherichia coli, Haemophilus influenzae, Klebsiella/Enterobacter* species, *Neisseria* species, and *Pseudomonas aeruginosa.*

This product does not provide adequate coverage against: *Serratia marcescens* and Streptococci, including *Streptococcus pneumoniae.*

CONTRAINDICATIONS:

Epithelial herpes simplex keratitis (dendritic keratitis), vaccinia, varicella, and many other viral diseases of the cornea and conjunctiva. Mycobacterial infection of the eye. Fungal diseases of ocular structures. Hypersensitivity to a component of the medication. (Hypersensitivity to the antibiotic component occurs at a higher rate than for other components.)

The use of these combinations is always contraindicated after uncomplicated removal of a corneal foreign body.

WARNINGS:

NOT FOR INJECTION Do not touch dropper or tube tip to any surface, as this may contasminate the contents. Prolonged use may result in glaucoma, with damage to the optic nerve, defects in visual acuity and fields of vision, and posterior subcapsular cataract formation. Prolonged use may suppress the host response and thus increase the hazard of secondary ocular infections. In those diseases causing thinning of the cornea or sclera, perforations have been known to occur with the use of topical steroids. In acute purulent conditions of the eye, steroids may mask infection or enhance existing infection. If these products are used for 10 days or longer, intraocular pressure should be routinely monitored even though it may be difficult in children and uncooperative patients.

Products containing neomycin sulfate may cause cutaneous sensitization.

Employment of steroid medication in the treatment of herpes simplex requires great caution.

PRECAUTIONS:

The initial prescription and renewal of the medication order beyond 20 ml or 8 g should be made by a physician only after examination of the patient with the aid of magnification, such as slit lamp biomicroscopy and, where appropriate, fluorescein staining.

The possibility of persistent fungal infections of the cornea should be considered after prolonged steroid dosing.

ADVERSE REACTIONS:

Adverse reactions have occurred with steroid/anti-infective combination drugs which can be attributed to the steroid component, the anti-infective component, or the combination. Exact incidence figures are not available since no denominator of treated patients is available.

Reactions occurring most often from the presence of the anti-infective ingredient are allergic sensitizations. *The reactions due to the steroid component are:* elevation of intraocular pressure (IOP) with possible development of glaucoma, and infrequent optic nerve damage; posterior subcapsular cataract formation; and delayed wound healing.

ADVERSE REACTIONS: *(cont'd)*

Secondary Infection: The development of secondary infection has occurred after use of combinations containing steroids and antimicrobials. Fungal infections of the cornea are particularly prone to develop coincidentally with long-term applications of steroid. The possibility of fungal invasion must be considered in any persistent corneal ulceration where steroid treatment has been used.

Secondary bacterial ocular infection following suppression of host responses also occurs.

DOSAGE AND ADMINISTRATION:

Dexamethasone 0.1%, Neomycin Sulfate, Polymyxin B Sulfate Suspension: One to two drops topically in the conjunctival sac(s). In severe disease, drops may be used hourly, being tapered to discontinuation as the inflammation subsides. In mild disease, drops may be used up to four to six times daily. *Dexamethasone 0.1%, Neomycin Sulfate, Polymyxin B Sulfate Ointment:* Apply a small amount into the conjunctival sac(s) up to three or four times daily or, may be used adjunctively with drops at bedtime.

Not more than 20 ml or 8 g should be prescribed initially and the prescription should not be refilled without further evaluation as outlined in PRECAUTIONS above.

Storage: Store at 8°-27°C (46°-80°F).

HOW SUPPLIED - RATED THERAPEUTICALLY EQUIVALENT:

Ointment - Ophthalmic - 0.1 %/3.5 mg/10

3.5 gm	$3.25	Dexasporin, Raway	00686-5795-55
3.5 gm	$4.43	Neomycin/Polymyxin/Dexamethasone, H.C.F.A. F F P	99999-0979-01
3.5 gm	$4.44	Infa-Trol Ointment Ophthalmic, Infinity Pharm	58154-0795-55
3.5 gm	$5.40	Dexasporin, Qualitest Pharms	00603-7121-70
3.5 gm	$5.85	DEXASPORIN, HL Moore Drug Exch	00839-6657-43
3.5 gm	$6.45	SPECTRO MAX, Spectrum Scitfc	53268-0795-55
3.5 gm	$7.13	AK-TROL, Akorn	17478-0240-35
3.5 gm	$7.25	Neo/Polymyxin/Dexamethasone, Goldline Labs	00182-5117-31
3.5 gm	$7.25	Neo/Polymyxin/Dexamethasone, Major Pharms	00904-7938-38
3.5 gm	$7.51	Neo/Polymyxin/Dexamethasone, Aligen Independ	00405-1274-08
3.5 gm	$7.59	Neomycin/Polymyxin/Dexamethasone, Fougera	00168-0221-38
3.5 gm	$7.98	DEXACIDIN OPHTHALMIC, Ciba Vision	00058-2255-01
3.5 gm	**$10.00**	**MAXITROL, Alcon**	**00065-0631-37**
3.5 gm	**$20.62**	**MAXITROL, Alcon**	**00065-0631-36**
3.5 gm x 12	$7.18	DEXASPORIN, Rugby	00536-6495-91

Suspension - Ophthalmic - 0.1 %/3.5 mg/10

5 ml	$5.25	Dexa Neo Poly, Harber Pharm	51432-0432-05
5 ml	$6.17	DEXASPORIN, United Res	00677-0900-20
5 ml	$7.18	Neomycin/Polymixin/Dexameth, Aligen Independ	00405-6100-05
5 ml	$7.28	DEXASPORIN, HL Moore Drug Exch	00839-6709-25
5 ml	$7.46	DEXASPORIN, STERILE, Rugby	00536-0830-65
5 ml	$7.50	METHADEX, Major Pharms	00904-3003-05
5 ml	$7.60	Neomycin/Polymyxin/Dexameth, Goldline Labs	00182-7023-62
5 ml	$7.85	POLY-DEX, Ocusoft	54799-0520-05
5 ml	$7.87	Neomycin/Polymyxin/Dexamethasone, Schein Pharm (US)	00364-7394-53
5 ml	$7.87	Neomycin/Polymyxin/Dexamethasone, Steris Labs	00402-0771-05
5 ml	$8.05	Neomycin/Polymyxin/Dexameth, Fougera	00168-0250-03
5 ml	$8.34	DEXACIDIN OPHTHALMIC, Ciba Vision	00058-2250-05
5 ml	$9.00	AK-TROL, Akorn	17478-0239-10
5 ml	**$10.63**	**MAXITROL, Alcon-PR**	**00998-0630-51**
5 ml	**$20.63**	**MAXITROL, Alcon-PR**	**00998-0630-06**

HOW SUPPLIED - NOT RATED EQUIVALENT:

Ointment - Ophthalmic - 0.1 %/3.5 mg/10

3.5 gm	$5.25	Neo/Polymixin/Dexamethasone, Harber Pharm	51432-0860-35

Suspension - Ophthalmic - 0.1 %/3.5 mg/10

5 ml	$3.73	Neo Poly Dex, Logen Pharm	00820-0110-22
5 ml	$3.92	Infa-Trol Ophthalmic Solution, Infinity Pharm	58154-0830-60
5 ml	$6.75	Neomycin/Polymyxin/Dexameth, Consolidated Midland	00223-6754-05
5 ml	$6.95	SPECTRO MAX, Spectrum Scitfc	53268-0830-10

DEXAMETHASONE; TOBRAMYCIN *(000980)*

CATEGORIES: Aminoglycosides; Anti-Infectives; Antibiotics; Antimicrobials; Conjunctivitis; Corneal Inflammation; Corneal Injury; EENT Drugs; Eye, Ear, Nose, & Throat Preparations; Inflammatory Conditions; Ocular Infections; Ophthalmics; Steroids; Uveitis; Pneumonia*; Pregnancy Category C; FDA Approved 1988 Aug
* Indication not approved by the FDA

BRAND NAMES: *Dicon*; **Tobradex**
(International brand names outside U.S. in italics)

FORMULARIES: Aetna; Medi-Cal; PCS

DESCRIPTION:

Tobradex (Tobramycin and Dexamethasone) Ophthalmic Suspension and Ointment are sterile, multiple dose antibiotic and steroid combinations for topical ophthalmic use:

Tobramycin: Empirical Formula: $C_{18}H_{37}N_5O_9$

Chemical Name: *O*-3-Amino-3-deoxy-α-D-glucopyranosyl-(1→4)-*O*-[2,6-diamino-2,3,6-trideoxy-α-D-*ribo*-hexopyransol-(1→6)]-2-deoxy-L-streptamine.

Dexamethasone: *Empirical Formula:* $C_{22}H_{29}FO_5$

Chemical Name: 9-Fluoro-11β,17,21-trihydroxy-16α-methylpregna-1,4-dien-3,20-dione.

Each ml of Tobradex Suspension Contains: *Actives:* Tobramycin 0.3% (3 mg) and dexamethasone 0.1% (1 mg). *Preservative:* Benzalkonium chloride 0.01%. *Inactives:* Tyloxapol, edetate disodium, sodium chloride, hydroxyethyl cellulose, sodium sulfate, sulfuric acid and/or sodium hydroxide (to adjust pH) and purified water.

Each Gram of Tobradex Ointment Contains: *Actives:* Tobramycin 0.3% (3 mg) and dexamethasone 0.1% (1 mg). *Preservative:* Chlorobutanol 0.5%. *Inactives:* Mineral Oil and White Petrolatum.

CLINICAL PHARMACOLOGY:

Corticoids suppress the inflammatory response to a variety of agents and they probably delay or slow healing. Since corticoids may inhibit the body's defense mechanism against infection, a concomitant antimicrobial drug may be used when this inhibition is considered to be clinically significant. Dexamethasone is a potent corticoid.

The antibiotic component in the combination (tobramycin) is included to provide action against susceptible organisms. *In vitro* studies have demonstrated that tobramycin is active against susceptible strains of the following microorganisms:

CLINICAL PHARMACOLOGY: *(cont'd)*

Staphylococci, including *S. aureus* and *S. epidermis* (coagulase-positive and coagulase-negative), including penicillin-resistant strains.

Streptococci, including some of the Group A beta-hemolytic species, some nonhemolytic species, and some *Streptococcus pneumoniae.*

Pseudomonas aeruginosa, Escherichia Coli, Klebsiella pneumoniae, Enterobacter aerogenes, Proteus mirabilis, Morganella morganii most *Proteus vulgaris* strains, *Haemophilus influenzae* and *H. aegyptius, Moraxella lacuna,* and *Acinetobacter calcoaceticus* and some *Neisseria* species.

Bacterial susceptibility studies demonstrate that in some cases microorganisms resistant to gentamicin remain susceptible to tobramycin. No data are available on the extent of systemic absorption from dexamethasone and tobramycin ophthalmic suspension or ointment; however, it is known that some systemic absorption can occur with ocularly applied drugs. If the maximum dose of dexamethasone and tobramycin suspension or ointment is given for the first 48 hours (two drops in each eye every 2 hours) and complete systemic absorption occurs, which is highly unlikely, the daily dose of dexamethasone would be 2.4 mg. The usual physiologic replacement dose id 0.75 mg daily. If dexamethasone and tobramycin ophthalmic suspension is given after the first 48 hours as two drops in each eye every 4 hours, the administered dose of dexamethasone would be 1.2 mg daily.

The administered dose for dexamethasone and tobramycin ophthalmic ointment in both eyes four times daily would be 0.4 mg of dexamethasone daily.

INDICATIONS AND USAGE:

Dexamethasone and tobramycin ophthalmic suspension and ointment are indicated for steroid-responsive inflammatory ocular conditions for which a corticosteroid is indicated and where superficial bacterial ocular infection or a risk of bacterial infection exists.

Ocular steroids are indicated in inflammatory conditions of the palpebral and bulbar conjunctiva, cornea and anterior segment of the globe where the inherent risk of steroid use in certain infective conjunctivides is accepted to obtain a diminution in edema and inflammation. They are also indicated in chronic anterior uveitis and corneal injury from chemical, radiation or thermal burns, or penetration of foreign bodies.

The use of a combination drug with an anti-infective component is indicated where the risk of superficial ocular infection is high or where there is an expectation that potentially dangerous numerous of bacteria will be present in the eye.

The particular anti-infective drug in this product is active against the following common bacterial eye pathogens:

Staphylococci, including *S. aureus* and *S. epidermis* (coagulase-positive and coagulase-negative), including penicillin-resistant strains.

Streptococci, including some of the Group A beta-hemolytic species, some nonhemolytic species, and some *Streptococcus pneumoniae.*

Pseudomonas aeruginosa, Escherichia coli, Klebsiella pneumoniae, Enterobacter aerogenes, Proteus mirabilis, Morganella morganii, most *Proteus vulgaris* strains *Haemophilus influenzae* and *H. aegyptius, Moraxella lacunata, Acinetobacter calcoaceticus* and some *Neisseria* species.

CONTRAINDICATIONS:

Epithelial herpes simplex keratitis (dendritic keratitis), vaccina, varicella, and many other viral diseases of the cornea and conjunctiva. Mycobacterial infection of the eye. Fungal diseases of ocular structures. Hypersensitivity to a component of this medication.

WARNINGS:

NOT FOR INJECTION INTO THE EYE Sensitivity to topically applied aminoglycosides may occur in some patients. If a sensitivity does occur, discontinue use.

Prolonged use of steroids may result in glaucoma, with damage to the optic nerve, defects in visual acuity and fields of vision, and posterior subcapsular cataract formation. Intraocular Pressure should be routinely monitored even though it may be difficult in children and uncooperative patients. Prolonged use may suppress the host response and thus the hazard of secondary ocular infections. In those diseases, causing thinning of the cornea or sclera, perforations have been known to occur with the use of topical steroids. In acute purulent conditions of the eye, steroids may mask infection or enhance existing infection.

PRECAUTIONS:

General: The possibility of fungal infections of the cornea should be considered after long-term steroid dosing. As with other antibiotic preparations, prolonged use may result in overgrowth of nonsusceptible organisms, including fungi. If superinfection occurs, appropriate therapy should be initiated. When multiple prescriptions are required, or whenever clinical judgment dictates, the patient should be examined with the aid of magnification, such as slit lamp biomicroscopy and, where, appropriate, fluorescein staining.

Cross-sensitivity to other aminoglycoside antibiotics may occur, if hypersensitivity develops with this product, discontinue use and institute appropriate therapy.

Information for the Patient: Do not touch dropper or tube tip to any surface as this may contaminate the contents.

Carcinogenesis, Mutagenesis, and Impairment of Fertility: No studies have been conducted to evaluate the carcinogenic or mutagenic potential. No impairment of fertility was noted in studies of subcutaneous tobramycin in rats at doses of 50 and 100 mg/kg/day.

Pregnancy Category C: Corticosteroids have been found to be teratogenic in animal studies. Ocular administration of 0.1% dexamethasone resulted in 15.6% and 32.3% incidence of fetal anomalies in two groups of pregnant rabbits. Fetal growth retardation and increased mortality rates have been observed in rats and rabbits with tobramycin at doses of up to 100 mg/kg/day parenterally and have received no evidence of impaired fertility of harm to the fetus. There are no adequate and well controlled studies in pregnant women. Dexamethasone and tobramycin ophthalmic suspension and ointment should be used during pregnancy only if the potential benefit justifies the potential risk to the fetus.

Nursing Mothers: It is not known whether this drug is excreted in human milk. Because many drugs are excreted in human milk, a decision should be considered to discontinue nursing temporarily while using dexamethasone and tobramycin ophthalmic suspension or ointment.

Pediatric Use: Safety and effectiveness in children have not yet been established.

ADVERSE REACTIONS:

Adverse reactions have occurred with occurred with steroid/anti-infective combination drugs which can be attributed. To the steroid component, the anti-infective component, or the combination. Exact incidence figures are not available. The most frequent adverse reactions to topical ocular tobramycin are hypersensitivity and localized ocular toxicity, including lid itching and swelling, and conjunctival erythema. These reactions occur in less than 4% of patients. Similar reactions may occur with the use of other aminoglycoside antibiotics. Other adverse reactions have not been reported; however; if topical ocular tobramycin is administered concomitantly with systemic aminoglycoside antibiotics, care should be taken to

ADVERSE REACTIONS: *(cont'd)*

monitor the total serum concentration. The reactions due to steroid component are: elevation of intraocular pressure (IOP) with possible development of glaucoma, and infrequent optic nerve damage; posterior subcapsular cataract formation; and delayed wound healing.

Secondary Infection: The development of secondary infection has occurred after use of combinations containing steroids and antimicrobials. Fungal infections of the cornea are particularly prone to develop coincidentally with long-term applications of steroids. The possibility of fungal invasion must be considered in any persistent corneal ulceration where steroid treatment has been used. Secondary bacterial ocular infection following suppression of host responses also occurs.

OVERDOSAGE:

Clinically apparent signs and symptoms of an overdosage of dexamethasone and tobramycin ophthalmic suspension (punctuate keratitis, erythema, increased lacrimation, edema and lid itching) maybe similar to adverse reaction effects seen in some patients.

DOSAGE AND ADMINISTRATION:

Suspension: One or two drops instilled into the conjunctival sac(s) every four to six hours. During the initial 24 to 48 hours, the dosage may be increased to one or two drops every two (2) hours. Frequency should be decreased gradually as warranted by improvement in clinical signs. Care should be taken not to discontinue therapy prematurely.

Not more than 20 ml should be prescribed initially and the prescription should not be refilled without further evaluation as outlined in PRECAUTIONSabove.

Ointment: Apply a small amount (approximately ½ inch ribbon) into the conjunctival sac(s) up to three or four times daily.

How to apply dexamethasone and tobramycin opthalmic ointment:

1. Tilt your head back.

2. Place a finger on your cheek just under your eye and gently pull down until a "V" pocket is formed between your eyeball and your lower lid.

3. Place a small amount (about ½ inch) of dexamethasone and tobramycin ophthalmic ointment in the "V" pocket. Do not let the tip of the tube touch your eye.

4. Look downward before closing your eye.

Not more than 8 g should be prescribed initially and the prescription should not be refilled without further evaluation as outlined in PRECAUTIONSabove.

HOW SUPPLIED:

Suspension Storage: Store at 8° to 27°C (46° to 80°F). Store suspension upright and shake well before using.

Ointment Storage: Store at 8° to 27°C (46° to 80°F).

HOW SUPPLIED - EQUIVALENTS NOT AVAILABLE:

Ointment - Topical - 1 mg/3 mg

3.5 gm	$22.31	TOBRADEX, Alcon	00065-0648-35

Solution - Ophthalmic - 0.3 mg/0.1 %

2.5 ml	$11.06	TOBRADEX, Alcon	00065-0647-25
5 ml	$22.31	TOBRADEX, Alcon	00065-0647-05

DEXBROMPHENIRAMINE; PSEUDOEPHEDRINE *(000982)*

CATEGORIES: Allergies; Antihistamines; Common Cold; Cough Preparations; Nasal Congestion; Respiratory & Allergy Medications; FDA Pre 1938 Drugs

BRAND NAMES: Dexaphen; Dexophed; Disobrom; *Disofrin*; *Disofrol*; Disophrol; *Disophrol Repetabs*; Drexophed; Dri-Rex; *Drixine-D*; *Drixoral* (Canada); *Drixoral Chronosules*; Duomine; Dynobal; Nalfed; *Rinafort*
(International brand names outside U.S. in italics)

Prescribing information not available at time of publication.

HOW SUPPLIED - EQUIVALENTS NOT AVAILABLE:

Tablet, Coated, Sustained Action - Oral - 6 mg/120 mg

100's	$10.75	Dexaphen S. A., Major Pharms	00904-0667-60
100's	$11.40	DUOMINE, IDE-Interstate	00814-2701-14
100's	$15.27	DEXOPHED, H N Norton Co.	50732-0649-01
100's	$15.80	Drexophed, Qualitest Pharms	00603-3505-21
100's	$19.90	DISOBROM, Geneva Pharms	00781-1600-01
100's	$25.00	DISOPHROL, Schering	00085-0340-04
500's	$46.50	DEXAPHEN S. A., Major Pharms	00904-0667-40
500's	$54.15	DUOMINE, IDE-Interstate	00814-2701-28
500's	$67.70	DEXOPHED, H N Norton Co.	50732-0649-05
500's	$74.30	Drexophed, Qualitest Pharms	00603-3505-28
1000's	$122.55	DISOBROM, Geneva Pharms	00781-1600-10
1000's	$122.59	DEXOPHED, H N Norton Co.	50732-0649-10

DEXCHLORPHENIRAMINE MALEATE *(000983)*

CATEGORIES: Alkylamines; Allergic Reactions; Allergies; Anaphylactic Reactions; Anaphylactic Shock; Angioedema; Antihistamines; Common Cold; Conjunctivitis; Respiratory & Allergy Medications; Rhinitis; Urticaria; Pregnancy Category B; FDA Approval Pre 1982

BRAND NAMES: *Delamin*; Dex-Cpm; Dexchlor; *Dexferin*; *Dextromin*; Mylaramine; *Nasamine*; *Polamec*; *Polaramin* (Japan); *Polaramin Prolong Depottab*; *Polaramin Prolongatum*; **Polaramine**; *Polaramine (non-prescription)*; *Polaramine Repetabs* (France); *Polarax*; *Polarist*; *Polaronil* (Germany); *Polazit* (Japan); *Rhiniramine*; *Somin*; *Trenelone*
(International brand names outside U.S. in italics)

FORMULARIES: Aetna; FHP; Medi-Cal

COST OF THERAPY: $47.60 (Rhinitis; Tablet; 2 mg; 4/day; 30 days)

PRIMARY ICD9: 477.9 (Allergic Rhinitis, Cause Unspecified)

DESCRIPTION:

These products contain dexchlorpheniramine maleate, USP, an antihistamine having the formula $C_{16}H_{19}ClN_2.C_4H_4O_4$, and a molecular weight 390.87. Chemically, it is (+)-2-(*p*-Chloro-α-(2-(dimethylamino) ethyl) benzyl) pyridine maleate (1:1).

Tablets contain 2 mg dexchlorpheniramine maleate, USP.

DESCRIPTION: *(cont'd)*

Syrup contains 2 mg dexchlorpheniramine maleate, USP per 5 ml, in a pleasant-tasting vehicle containing 6% alcohol.

Dexchlorpheniramine maleate is a white, odorless, crystalline powder which in aqueous solution has a pH of between 4 and 5. It is freely soluble in water, soluble in alcohol and in chloroform, but only slightly soluble in benzene or ether.

CLINICAL PHARMACOLOGY:

Dexchlorpheniramine maleate is an antihistamine with anticholinergic properties. It is capable of producing a slight to moderate sedative effect. Antihistamines appear to compete with histamine for receptor sites on effector cells and are of value clinically in the prevention and relief of many allergic manifestations.

In vitro and *in vivo* assay of the antihistamine potencies of the optically active isomers of chlorpheniramine demonstrate that the predominant activity is in the dextro-isomer. The dextro-isomer is approximately two times more active than the racemic compound. Since dexchlorpheniramine is the dextro-isomer and active moiety of chlorpheniramine, it can be assumed that experience with chlorpheniramine also applies to dexchlorpheniramine.

Chlorpheniramine maleate 4 mg given to fasting human volunteers produced prompt blood levels after oral administration. Peak blood levels were approximately 7 ng/ml at an average time of 3 hours after administration. The half-life of chlorpheniramine maleate ranged from 20 to 24 hours. Following a single dose of tritium-labeled chlorpheniramine maleate to humans, the drug was found to be extensively metabolized whether given orally or by intravenous administration. The drug and metabolites were primarily excreted in the urine, with 19% of the dose appearing in 24 hours and a total of 34% in 48 hours.

In a study in normal volunteers, a high flow rate of acidic urine resulted in a high excretion rate of chlorpheniramine maleate. Over a concentration range of 0.28 to 1.24 mcg/ml of plasma, chlorpheniramine maleate was 72 to 69% bound to plasma protein, respectively.

INDICATIONS AND USAGE:

Dexchlorpheniramine maleate tablets and syrup are indicated for the treatment of perennial and seasonal allergic rhinitis: vasomotor rhinitis, allergic conjunctivitis, mild, uncomplicated allergic skin manifestations of urticaria and angioedema; amelioration of allergic reactions to blood or plasma; and dermographism. They are also indicated as therapy for anaphylactic reactions adjunctive to epinephrine and other standard measures after the acute manifestations have been controlled.

CONTRAINDICATIONS:

Hypersensitivity to dexchlorpheniramine maleate or other antihistamines of similar chemical structure contraindicates the use of Dexchlorpheniramine maleate tablets or syrup.

Drug products containing Dexchlorpheniramine maleate should not be used in newborn or premature infants because of the possibility of severe reactions, such as convulsions.

Antihistamines *should not* be used to treat lower respiratory tract symptoms. Antihistamines are also contraindicated for use in conjunction with monoamine oxidase inhibitor therapy.

WARNINGS:

Dexchlorpheniramine, as with all antihistamines, should be used with caution in patients with narrow angle glaucoma, stenosing peptic ulcer, pyloroduodenal obstruction, symptomatic prostatic hypertrophy, and bladder neck obstruction.

Overdoses of antihistamines may cause hallucinations, convulsions, or death, especially in infants and children.

Products containing dexchlorpheniramine maleate have additive effects with alcohol and other CNS depressants (hypnotics, sedatives, tranquilizers, etc.) Patients should not engage in activities requiring mental alertness, such as driving a car or operating machinery.

Antihistamines are more likely to cause dizziness, sedation, and hypotension in elderly patients (approximately 60 years or older).

PRECAUTIONS:

General: Dexchlorpheniramine maleate has an atropine-like action and therefore products containing it should be used with caution in patients with: a history of bronchial asthma; increased intraocular pressure; hyperthyroidism; cardiovascular disease; hypertension.

Information for Patients:

1. Dexchlorpheniramine may cause slight to moderate drowsiness.

2. Patients should not engage in activities requiring mental alertness, such as driving or operating machinery.

3. Alcohol or other sedative drugs may enhance the drowsiness caused by antihistamines.

4. Patients should not take Dexchlorpheniramine maleate tablets or syrup in conjunction with a monoamine oxidase inhibitor or oral anticoagulant.

Carcinogenesis, Mutagenesis, and Impairment of Fertility: Although there have been no oncogenic or mutagenic studies on dexchlorpheniramine, 103-week oncogenic study in rats on the racemic mixture, chlorpheniramine, did not produce an increase in the incidence of tumors in the drug-treated groups, as compared with the controls.

An Ames mutagenicity test performed on chlorpheniramine and its nitrosation product was negative. An early study in rats with chlorpheniramine maleate revealed a reduction in fertility in female rats at doses approximately 67 times the human dose. More recent studies in rabbits and rats, using more appropriate methodology and doses up to approximately 50 and 85 times the human dose, showed no reduction in fertility in the animals.

Pregnancy Category B: Reproduction studies have been performed in rabbits and rats at doses up to 50 times and 85 times the human dose, respectively, and have revealed no evidence of harm to the fetus due to chlorpheniramine maleate. (See Impairment of Fertility). There are, however, no adequate and well-controlled studies in pregnant women. Because animal reproduction studies are not always predictive of human response, this drug should be used during the first two trimesters of pregnancy only if clearly needed. Dexchlorpheniramine maleate should not be used in the third trimester of pregnancy because newborn and premature infants may have severe reactions to antihistamines. (See CONTRAINDICATIONS.) *Nonteratogenic Effects:* Studies of chlorpheniramine maleate done in rats revealed a decrease in the postnatal survival rate of pups of animals dosed with 33 and 67 times the human dose.

Nursing Mothers: It is not known whether this drug is excreted in human milk. Because certain other antihistamines are known to be excreted in human milk, and because dexchlorpheniramine maleate is contraindicated in newborn and premature infants, caution should be exercised when it is administered to a nursing woman.

Pediatric Use: Safety and effectiveness in children below the age 2 years have not been established.

DRUG INTERACTIONS:

Dexchlorpheniramine maleate may cause severe hypotension when given in conjunction with a monoamine oxidase inhibitor.

DRUG INTERACTIONS: *(cont'd)*

Alcohol and other sedative drugs will potentiate the sedative effects of dexchlorpheniramine. (See WARNINGS.)

The action of oral anticoagulants may be inhibited by antihistamines.

ADVERSE REACTIONS:

Slight to moderate drowsiness is the most frequent side effect of dexchlorpheniramine maleate. Other possible side effects of antihistamines include:

General: urticaria, drug rash, anaphylactic shock, photosensitivity, excessive perspiration, chills, dryness of mouth, nose, and throat.

Cardiovascular System: headache, palpitations, tachycardia, extrasystoles, hypotension.

Hematologic System: Hemolytic anemia, hypoplastic anemia, thrombocytopenia, agranulocytosis.

Nervous System: sedation, dizziness, vertigo, tinnitus, acute, labyrinthitis, disturbed coordination, fatigue, confusion, restlessness, excitation nervousness, tremor, irritability, insomnia, euphoria, paresthesias, blurred vision, hysteria, neuritis, convulsions.

Gastrointestinal System: epigastric distress, anorexia, nausea, vomiting, diarrhea, constipation.

Genitourinary System: urinary frequency, difficult urination, urinary retention, early menses.

Respiratory System: thickening of bronchial secretions, tightness of chest, wheezing, nasal stuffiness.

OVERDOSAGE:

In the event of overdosage emergency treatment should be started immediately.

Manifestations: Of antihistamine overdosage may vary from central nervous system depression (sedation, apnea, diminished mental alertness, cardiovascular collapse) to stimulation (insomnia, hallucinations, tremors, or convulsions) to death. Other signs and symptoms may be dizziness, tinnitus, ataxia, blurred vision, and hypotension. Stimulation is particularly likely in children, as are atropine-like signs and symptoms (dry mouth; fixed, dilated pupils; flushing; hyperthermia; and gastrointestinal symptoms).

TREATMENT:

The patient should be induced to vomit, even if emesis has occurred spontaneously. Pharmacologic vomiting by the administration of ipecac syrup is a preferred method. However, vomiting should not be induced in patients with impaired consciousness. The action of ipecac is facilitated by physical activity and by the administration of eight to twelve fluid ounces of water. If emesis does not occur within fifteen minutes, the dose of ipecac should be repeated. Precautions against aspiration must be taken, especially in infants and children. Following emesis, any drug remaining, in the stomach may be adsorbed by activated charcoal administered as a slurry with water. If vomiting is unsuccessful or contraindicated, gastric lavage should be performed. Isotonic and one-half isotonic saline are the lavage solutions of choice. Saline cathartics such as milk of magnesium, draw water into the bowel by osmosis and therefore may be valuable for their action in rapid dilution of bowel content. Dialysis is of little value in antihistamine poisoning. After emergency treatment the patient should be continued to be medically monitored.

Treatment of the signs and symptoms of overdosage is symptomatic and supportive. *Stimulants* (analeptic agents) should *not* be used. Vasopressors may be used to treat hypotension. Short-acting barbiturates, diazepam, or paraldehyde may be administered to control seizures. Hyperpyrexia, especially in children, may require treatment with tepid water sponge baths or a hypothermic blanket. Apnea is treated with ventilatory support.

In mice, the oral LD_{50} of dexchlorpheniramine is 258 mg/kg. In humans, the estimated lethal dose of racemic chlorpheniramine is 5 to 10 mg/kg. Thus a dose of 2.5 to 5 mg/kg of dexchlorpheniramine should be similarly regarded.

DOSAGE AND ADMINISTRATION:

DOSAGE SHOULD BE INDIVIDUALIZED ACCORDING TO THE NEEDS AND RESPONSE OF THE PATIENT.

Dexchlorpheniramine Maleate Tablets: *Adults and Children 12 Years of Age and Over:* one tablet every 4 to 6 hours. *Children 6 Through 11 Years:* one-half tablet every 4 to 6 hours. *Children 2 Through 5 Years:* one-quarter tablet every 4 to 6 hours.

Dexchlorpheniramine Maleate Syrup: *Adults and Children 12 Years of Age and Over:* 1 teaspoonful (2 mg) every 4 to 6 hours. *Children 6 Through 11 Years:* one-half teaspoonful (1 mg) every 4 to 6 hours. *Children 2 Through 5 Years:* one-quarter teaspoonful (1/2 mg) every 4 to 6 hours.

Store dexchlorpheniramine maleate tablets and syrup between 2° and 30°C (36°-86°F).

HOW SUPPLIED - RATED THERAPEUTICALLY EQUIVALENT:

Syrup - Oral - 2 mg/5ml

480 ml	$12.77	Dexchlorpheniramine Maleate, H.C.F.A. F F P	99999-0983-01
480 ml	$13.15	Dexchlorpheniramine Maleate, Major Pharms	00904-0624-16
480 ml	$13.33	Dexchlorpheniramine Maleate, Rugby	00536-0460-85
480 ml	$15.00	Dexchlorpheniramine Maleate, Morton Grove	60432-0539-16
480 ml	**$42.08**	**POLARAMINE, Schering**	**00085-0016-05**
3840 ml	$97.00	Dexchlorpheniramine Maleate, Morton Grove	60432-0539-28
3840 ml	$101.90	Dexchlorpheniramine Maleate, Major Pharms	00904-0624-28
3840 ml	$102.14	Dexchlorpheniramine Maleate, H.C.F.A. F F P	99999-0983-02

Tablet, Uncoated - Oral - 2 mg

100's	**$39.67**	**POLARAMINE, Schering**	**00085-0820-03**

HOW SUPPLIED - NOT RATED EQUIVALENT:

Tablet, Coated, Sustained Action - Oral - 4 mg

100's	$13.65	Dexchlorpheniramine Maleate, Major Pharms	00904-0627-61
100's	$29.50	Dexchlorpheniramine Maleate, Pharmacist Choice	54979-0156-01
100's	$31.67	Dexchlorpheniramine Maleate, Aligen Independ	00405-4319-01
100's	$34.50	Dexchlorpheniramine Maleate, Qualitest Pharms	00603-3198-21
100's	$35.90	Dexchlorpheniramine Maleate, HL Moore Drug Exch	00839-6779-06
100's	$37.50	Dexchlor ER, Schein Pharm (US)	00364-0585-01
100's	$37.85	POLADEX T D, Major Pharms	00904-0627-60
100's	$47.85	Dexchlorpheniramine Maleate 4, Rugby	00536-3578-01
100's	$48.00	Dexchlorpheniramine Maleate, Goldline Labs	00182-1014-01
100's	**$67.67**	**POLARAMINE REPETABS, Schering**	**00085-0095-03**
1000's	$70.45	POLADEX T D, Major Pharms	00904-0627-80

Tablet, Coated, Sustained Action - Oral - 6 mg

100's	$16.16	Dexchlorpheniramine Maleate, Major Pharms	00904-0626-61
100's	$40.95	Dexchlorpheniramine Maleate, Pharmacist Choice	54979-0157-01
100's	$44.23	Dexchlorpheniramine Maleate, Aligen Independ	00405-4320-01
100's	$44.25	Dexchlorpheniramine Maleate, Qualitest Pharms	00603-3199-21
100's	$47.51	Dexchlorpheniramine Maleate, HL Moore Drug Exch	00839-6414-06
100's	$50.10	Dexchlorpheniramine Maleate, United Res	00677-0669-01
100's	$50.15	POLADEX T D, Major Pharms	00904-0626-60
100's	$52.25	Dexchlor ER, Schein Pharm (US)	00364-0586-01
100's	$59.95	Dexchlorpheniramine Maleate, Pecos	59879-0504-01

HOW SUPPLIED - NOT RATED EQUIVALENT: *(cont'd)*

100's	$63.90	Dexchlorpheniramine Maleate, Goldline Labs	00182-1015-01
100's	$63.90	Dexchlorpheniramine Maleate, Rugby	00536-3590-01
100's	**$94.58**	**POLARAMINE REPETABS, Schering**	**00085-0148-03**
1000's	$85.35	POLADEX T D, Major Pharms	00904-0626-80
1000's	$368.55	Dexchlorpheniramine Maleate, Pharmacist Choice	54979-0157-10

DEXCHLORPHENIRAMINE; GUAIFENESIN; PSEUDOEPHEDRINE *(000984)*

CATEGORIES: Allergies; Anaphylactic Shock; Angioedema; Antihistamines; Antitussives/Expectorants/Mucolytics; Common Cold; Conjunctivitis; Cough Preparations; Expectorants; Respiratory & Allergy Medications; Rhinitis; Urticaria; Pregnancy Category B; FDA Pre 1938 Drugs

BRAND NAMES: *Demazin Expectorant*; *Polaramin Espett.*; **Polaramine**; *Polaramine Expec* (Mexico); *Polaramine Expectorant*; *Polaramine Expectorante* *(International brand names outside U.S. in italics)*

FORMULARIES: Aetna

DESCRIPTION:

Polaramine Expectorant contains in each 5 ml (one teaspoonful) 2 mg dexchlorpheniramine maleate, USP; 20 mg pseudoephedrine sulfate, USP; and 100 mg guaifenesin, USP.

The inactive ingredients include: alcohol (7.2%), FD&C Red No. 40. FD&C Yellow No. 6, flavors, menthol, propylene glycol, sodium benzoate, sorbitol, sugar, and water.

Dexchlorpheniramine maleate is an antihistamine having the chemical formula, $C_{16}H_{19}ClN_2{\cdot}C_4H_4O_4$ and a molecular weight of 390.87. Chemically, it is (+)-2-[*p*-Chloro-α-[2-(dimethyl-amino)ethyl]benzyl]pyridine maleate (1:1).

Dexchlorpheniramine maleate is a white, odorless, crystalline powder which in aqueous solution has a pH between 4 and 5. It is freely soluble in water, soluble in alcohol and in chloroform, but only slightly soluble in benzene or in ether.

Guaifenesin, an expectorant, is the glyceryl ether of guaiacol having the chemical formula. $C_{10}H_{14}O_4$. It is a white to slightly gray crystalline powder with a molecular weight of 198.22. One gram dissolves in 15 ml of water. The drug is soluble in alcohol, in chloroform, in glycerin, and in propylene glycol. The chemical name is 1.2-Propanediol, 3-(2-methoxyphenoxy)-.

Pseudoephedrine, an adrenergic agent, is one naturally occurring alkaloids obtained from various species of the plant *Ephedra*. The chemical name of pseudoephedrine sulfate is benzenemethanol. α-[1-(methylamino)ethyl]-,[*S*-(*R**,*R**)]-, sulfate (2:1) (salt); it is $(C_{10}H_{15}NO)_2{\cdot}H_2SO_4$. The compound is a white to off-white crystal or powder with a molecular weight of 428.6. It is very soluble in water, freely soluble in alcohol and sparingly in chloroform.

CLINICAL PHARMACOLOGY:

Polaramine Expectorant combines the antihistaminic actions of dexchlorpheniramine maleate with the nasal vasoconstrictive properties of pseudoephedrine sulfate; guaifenesin increases respiratory tract fluid output and eases expectoration.

Dexchlorpheniramine maleate is an antihistamine with anticholinergic properties. It is capable of producing a mild to moderate sedative effect. Antihistamines appear to complete with histamine to receptor sites on effector cells and are of value clinically in the prevention and relief of many allergic manifestations.

In vitro and *in vivo* assays of the antihistamine potencies of the optically active isomers of chlorpheniramine demonstrate that the predominant activity is in the dextro-isomer. The dextro-isomer is approximately two times more active than the racemic compound. Since dexchlorpheniramine, it can be assumed that experience with chlorpheniramine also applies to dexchlorpheniramine.

Chlorpheniramine maleate 4 mg given to fasting human volunteers produced prompt blood levels after oral administration. Peak blood levels were approximately 7 ng/ml at an average time of 3 hours after administration. The half-life of chlorpheniramine maleate ranged from 20 to 24 hours. Following a single dose of tritium-labeled chlorpheniramine maleate to humans, the drug was found to be extensively metabolized whether given orally or by intravenous administration. The drug and metabolites were primarily excreted in the urine, with 19% of the dose appearing in 24 hours and a total of 34% in 48 hours.

In a study in normal volunteers, a high flow rate of acidic urine resulted in a high excretion rate of chlorpheniramine maleate. Over a concentration range of 0.28 to 1.24 mcg/ml of plasma, chlorpheniramine maleate was 72 to 69% bound to plasma protein, respectively.

Guaifenesin increases sputum volume and decreases sputum tenaciousness. It has been claimed that guaifenesin acts reflexly by stimulating receptors in the gastric mucosa which, in turn, stimulate respiratory secretions. This allows ciliary motion and coughing to move the loosened secretions toward the pharynx, thus promoting the expulsion of secretions from the respiratory tract. As a result, unproductive coughs become more productive and less frequent.

Pseudoephedrine sulfate appears to exert its sympathomimetic effect predominantly through indirect means by releasing adrenergic mediators from post-ganglionic nerve terminals. The clinical action is primarily as a nasal decongestant due to vasoconstriction of nasal blood vessels. At recommended doses of other sympathomimetic effects, such as pressor activity and CNS stimulation, are minimal.

It has been reported that excretion of pseudoephedrine was directly related to urinary pH: the more alkaline the urine, the greater the rate of excretion of the drug. Further studies done in rats with ^{14}C-labeled pseudoephedrine revealed that the drug was distributed in the tissues in the following organs in decreasing order of magnitude: kidneys, lungs, spleen, adrenals, liver, intestine, heart, and plasma.

Pseudoephedrine passes through the blood-brain barrier. Wakefulness may occasionally be observed. Fetal-placental transfer and plasma protein binding of pseudoephedrine have not been studied.

The half-life of pseudoephedrine is 5.2 to 8 hours.

INDICATIONS AND USAGE:

Polaramine Expectorant is indicated for relief of coughs and complications associated with allergic disorders and allergic manifestations of respiratory illnesses, such as hay fever and vasomotor rhinitis.

CONTRAINDICATIONS:

Hypersensitivity to dexchlorpheniramine maleate or other antihistamines of similar chemical structure, guaifenesin, or pseudoephedrine contraindicates the use of Polaramine Expectorant.

Drug products containing dexchlorpheniramine maleate should not be used in newborn or premature infants because of the possibility of severe reaction, such as convulsions. Antihistamines *should not* be used to treat lower respiratory tract symptoms. Antihistamines are also contraindicated for use in conjunction with monoamine oxidase (MAO) inhibitor therapy.

CONTRAINDICATIONS: *(cont'd)*

Pseudoephedrine sulfate is contraindicated in patients who have shown hypersensitivity or idiosyncrasy to adrenergic agents, which may be manifested by insomnia, dizziness, weakness, tremor, or arrhythmias. In patients with severe hypertension, severe coronary artery disease, hyperthyroidism, and in those receiving monoamine oxidase (MAO) inhibitor therapy or within 10 days of stopping such treatment, sympathomimetic amines are contraindicated.

WARNINGS:

Dexchlorpheniramine, as with all antihistamines, should be used with caution in patients with narrow angle glaucoma, stenosing peptic ulcer, pyloroduodenal obstruction, symptomatic prostatic hypertrophy, and bladder neck obstruction. Overdosage of antihistamines may cause hallucinations convulsions, or death, especially in infants and children.

Products containing dexchlorpheniramine maleate have additive effects with alcohol and other CNS depressants (hypnotics, sedatives, tranquilizers, etc.). Patients should not engage in activities requiring mental alertness, such as driving a car or operating machinery.

Antihistamines are more likely to cause dizziness, sedation and hypotension in elderly patients (approximately 60 years or older).

In patients with prostatic enlargement, pseudoephedrine may increase difficulty in micturition. In patients with narrow angle glaucoma, it may precipitate angle closure. It should also be used with caution and at a lower dosage in the elderly who are more sensitive to the CNS stimulating effects of the drug which may result in confusion, delirium, hallucinations, and convulsions.

PRECAUTIONS:

General: Dexchlorpheniramine maleate has an atropine-like action and therefore products containing it should be used with caution in patients with: a history of bronchial asthma; increased intraocular pressure; hyperthyroidism; cardiovascular disease; hypertension.

Pseudoephedrine should be used with caution in patients with hypertension, diabetes mellitus, ischemic heart disease, angina, or in patients receiving digitalis.

Information for Patients:

1. Products containing antihistamines may cause drowsiness.

2. Patients should not engage in activities requiring mental alertness such as driving or operating machinery.

3. Alcohol or other sedative drugs may enhance the drowsiness caused by antihistamines.

4. Patients should not take Polaramine Expectorant if they are receiving a monoamine oxidase (MAO) inhibitor or within ten days of stopping such treatment, or if they are receiving oral anticoagulants.

Drug/Laboratory Test Interactions: Guaifenesin has been shown to produce a color interference with certain clinical laboratory determinations of 5-hydroxy-indole-acetic acid (5-HIAA) and vanillylmandelic acid (VMA).

The *in vitro* addition of pseudoephedrine to sera containing the cardiac isoenzyme MB of serum creatine phosphokinase progressively inhibits the activity of the enzyme. The inhibition becomes complete over six hours.

Carcinogenesis, Mutagenesis, and Impairment of Fertility: Although there have been no oncogenic or mutagenic studies on dexchlorpheniramine, a 103-week oncogenic study in rats on the racemate, chlorpheniramine, did not produce an increase in the incidence of tumors in the drug-treated groups as compared with the controls. An Ames mutagenicity test performed on chlorpheniramine and its nitrosation product was negative. An early study in rats with chlorpheniramine maleate revealed a reduction in fertility in female rats at doses approximately 67 times the human dose. More recent studies in rabbits and rats, using more appropriate methodology and doses up to approximately 50 and 85 times the human dose, showed no reduction in fertility in the animals.

Pseudoephedrine and guaifenesin have not been evaluated for oncogenic or mutagenic potential. Their effects on fertility are not known.

Pregnancy Category C: See statements on guaifenesin below. Reproduction studies have been performed in rabbits and rats at doses up to 50 times and 85 times the human dose, respectively, and have revealed no evidence of harm to the fetus due to chlorpheniramine maleate. (See Impairment of Fertility.) Animal reproduction studies have been conducted with guaifenesin. It is also not known whether guaifenesin can cause fetal harm when administered to a pregnant woman or can affect reproduction capacity. Reproduction studies have been done in rats receiving up to 50 times the therapeutic dose and have revealed no evidence of harm to the fetus due to pseudoephedrine. There are, however, no adequate and well-controlled studies of dexchlorpheniramine maleate, guaifenesin, or pseudoephedrine in pregnant women. Because animal reproduction studies are not always predictive of human response. Polaramine Expectorant should be used during the first two trimesters of pregnancy only if clearly needed. Dexchlorpheniramine maleate should no to be used in the third trimester of pregnancy because newborn and premature infants may have severe reactions to antihistamines. (See CONTRAINDICATIONS.)

Nonteratogenic Effects: Studies of chlorpheniramine maleate done in rats revealed a decrease in the postnatal survival rate of pups of animals dosed with 33 and 67 times the human dose.

Nursing Mothers: It is not known whether this drug is excreted in human milk. Because certain antihistamines are known to be excreted in human milk, because dexchlorpheniramine maleate is contraindicated in newborn and premature infants, and because of a report of irritability, excessive crying, and disturbed sleeping patterns in a nursing infant whose mother had taken a product containing an antihistamine and pseudoephedrine, caution should be exercised when Polaramine Expectorant is administered to a nursing woman.

Pediatric Use: Safety and effectiveness in children below the age of 2 years have not been established.

DRUG INTERACTIONS:

Dexchlorpheniramine maleate may cause severe hypotension when given in conjunction with a monoamine oxidase inhibitor.

Alcohol and other sedative drugs will potentiate the sedative effects of dexchlorpheniramine. (See WARNINGS.)

Pseudoephedrine-containing drugs should bot be given to patients treated with monoamine oxidase (MAO) inhibitors or within ten days of stopping such treatment because of the possibility of precipitating a hypertensive crisis, potentially resulting in intracranial hemorrhage, convulsions, coma, and in some cases, death.

Pseudoephedrine should not be used with ganglionic blocking drugs, such as mecamylamine hydrochloride, which potentiates reactions of sympathomimetics. Also, it should not be used with adrenergic blocking drugs, such as guanethidine sulfate or bethanidine, since it antagonizes the hypotensive action of these drugs. Increased ectopic pacemaker activity can occur when pseudoephedrine is used concomitantly with digitalis. Antacids increase the rate of absorption of pseudoephedrine while kaolin decreases it.

ADVERSE REACTIONS:

Dexchlorpheniramine Maleate: Slight to moderate drowsiness is the most frequent side effect of dexchlorpheniramine maleate. Other possible side effects of antihistamines include:

General: urticaria, drug rash, anaphylactic shock, photosensitivity, excessive perspiration, chills, dryness of mouth, nose and throat.

Cardiovascular System: headache, palpitations, tachycardia, extrasystoles, hypotension.

Hematologic System: hemolytic anemia, hypoplastic anemia, thrombocytopenia, agranulocytosis.

Nervous System: sedation, dizziness, vertigo, tinnitus, acute labyrinthitis, disturbed coordination, fatigue, confusion, restlessness, excitation, nervousness, tremor, irritability, insomnia, euphoria, paresthesias, blurred vision. hysteria, neuritis, convulsions.

Gastrointestinal System: epigastric distress, anorexia, nausea, vomiting, diarrhea, constipation.

Genitourinary System: urinary frequency, difficult urination, urinary retention, early menses.

Respiratory System: thickening of bronchial secretions, tightness of chest, wheezing, nasal stuffiness.

Guaifenesin No serious adverse reactions have been reported with guaifenesin. Nausea, gastrointestinal disturbances, and drowsiness have been reported infrequently.

Pseudoephedrine Sulfate Pseudoephedrine, like other sympathomimetic amines, may cause disturbing reactions, such as fear, anxiety, excessive perspiration, tenseness, restlessness, throbbing headache, tremor, weakness, dizziness, nausea, pallor, dysuria, respiratory difficulty, palpitations, tachycardia, and insomnia. Hyperthyroid and hypertensive individuals are particularly susceptible to the untoward and pressor responses of pseudoephedrine, which may also induce angina, hypertension an cardiac arrhythmias. Sympathomimetics have also produced CNS depression and cardiovascular collapse with accompanying hypotension. In psychoneurotic individuals, existing symptoms are often markedly exaggerated by the drug. The elderly are particularly sensitive to the CNS stimulating effects and hallucinations and convulsions have occurred. Symptoms of unusual sensitivity to the effects of pseudoephedrine have been reported in an infant with phenylketonuria.

DRUG ABUSE AND DEPENDENCE:

There is no information to indicate abuse or dependency with dexchlorpheniramine or guaifenesin.

Pseudoephedrine, like other CNS stimulants, has been abused. At elevated dosages, subjects commonly experience an elevation of mood, a sense of increased energy and alertness and decreased appetite. Some individuals become anxious, irritable and loquacious. In addition to the marked euphoria, the user experiences a sense of markedly enhanced physical strength and metal capacity. With continued use, tolerance develops and toxic signs and symptoms appear. Depression may follow rapid withdrawal.

OVERDOSAGE:

In the event of overdosage, emergency treatment should be started immediately.

MANIFESTATIONS

Antihistamine overdosage may vary from central nervous system depression (sedation, apnea, diminished mental alertness, and cardiovascular collapse) to stimulation (insomnia, hallucinations, tremors, or convulsions) to death. Other signs and symptoms may dizziness, tinnitus, ataxia, blurred vision, and hypotension. Stimulation is particularly likely in children, as are atropine-like signs and symptoms (dry mouth; fixed dilated pupils; flushing; hyperthermia; and gastrointestinal symptoms).

In large doses sympathomimetics may give rise to giddiness, headache, nausea, vomiting, sweating, thirst, tachycardia, precordial pain, palpitations, difficulty in micturition, muscular weakness and tenseness, anxiety, restlessness, and insomnia. Many patients can show a full-blown toxic psychosis with delusions and hallucinations. Some may develop cardiac arrhythmias, circulatory collapse, convulsions, coma, and respiratory failure.

TREATMENT

The patient should be induced to vomit, even if emesis has occurred spontaneously. Pharmacologic vomiting by the administration of ipecac syrup is a preferred method. However, vomiting should not be induced in patients with impaired consciousness. The action of ipecac is facilitated by physical activity and by the administration of 8 to 12 fluid ounces of water. If emesis does not occur within 15 minutes, the dose of ipecac should be repeated. Precautions against aspiration must be taken, especially in infants and children. Following emesis, any drug remaining in the stomach may be absorbed by activated charcoal administered as a slurry with water. If vomiting is unsuccessful or contraindicated, gastric lavage should be performed. Isotonic and one-half isotonic saline are the lavage solutions of choice. Saline cathartics, such as milk of magnesia draw water into the bowel by osmosis and therefore may be valuable for their action in rapid dilution of bowel content. Dialysis is of little value in antihistamine poisoning. After emergency treatment, the patient should continue to be medically monitored.

Treatment of the signs and symptoms of overdosage is symptomatic and supportive. *Stimulations* (analeptic agents) should *not* be used. Vasopressors may be used be treat hypotension. Short-acting barbiturates, diazepam, or paraldehyde may be administered to control seizures. Hyperpyrexia, especially in children, may require treatment with tepid water sponge baths or a hypothermic blanket. Apnea is treated with ventilatory support.

In humans, the estimated lethal dose of chlorpheniramine maleate is 5 to 10 mg/kg. Thus a dose of 2.5 to 5 mg/kg of dexchlorpheniramine should be similarly regarded.

The oral LD_{50}s of the active components of Polaramine Expectorant were established in mice as follows:

dexchlorpheniramine 330 ± 71 mg/kg

pseudoephedrine sulfate 300 ± 60 mg/kg

guaifenesin 1200 ± 175 mg/kg

Doses of Polaramine Expectorant up to 32 ml/kg in rats and mice were not lethal to any animal: thus, the LD_{50} could not be determined on the basis of this study.

DOSAGE AND ADMINISTRATION:

Adults and Children 12 Years and Older: One or two teaspoonfuls 3 or 4 times daily.

Children 6 Through 11 Years: One-half to one teaspoonful 3 or 4 times daily.

Children 2 Through 5 Years: One quarter to one-half teaspoonful 3 or 4 times daily.

HOW SUPPLIED:

Polaramine Expectorant, orange-colored liquid: 16 fluid once (473 ml) bottle.

Store between 2° - 30° C (36° - 86° F).

HOW SUPPLIED - EQUIVALENTS NOT AVAILABLE:

Syrup - Oral - 2 mg/100 mg/20

480 ml	$54.25	POLARAMINE EXPECTORANT, Schering	00085-0268-05

DEXFENFLURAMINE HYDROCHLORIDE

(003269)

CATEGORIES: Amphetamines; Anorexients/CNS Stimulants; Appetite Suppressants; Central Nervous System Agents; Obesity; Psychostimulants; Respiratory/Cerebral Stimulant; Weight Loss; FDA Approved 1996 May

BRAND NAMES: *Adifax* (England); *Diomeride* (Mexico); *Dipondal*; *Glypolix*; *Isomeride* (Germany, France); *Isomerin*; *Obesine*; **Redux**; *Siran*
(International brand names outside U.S. in italics)

DESCRIPTION:

Redux (dexfenfluramine hydrochloride capsules), an anti-obesity drug, is a serotonin reuptake inhibitor and releasing agent. Redux is available for oral administration in white, opaque, hard-gelatin capsules. The active ingredient is dexfenfluramine hydrochloride. Each capsule contains 15 mg dexfenfluramine hydrochloride. Inactive ingredients include: lactose, gelatin capsule, corn starch, microcrystalline cellulose, talc, titanium dioxide, magnesium stearate, colloidal silicon dioxide, and edible ink.

Dexfenfluramine hydrochloride, a white to off-white crystalline powder, is designated chemically as (S)-N-ethyl-α-methyl-3-(trifluoromethyl) benzeneethanamine hydrochloride and has a molecular weight of 267.7. Its empirical formula is $C^{12}H^{16}F^{3}N \cdot HCl$. Dexfenfluramine is freely soluble in water, alcohol, chloroform, and methanol The pKa of dexfenfluramine hydrochloride is 10.

CLINICAL PHARMACOLOGY:

PHARMACOLOGIC ACTIONS

The action of dexfenfluramine hydrochloride in treating obesity is primarily via decreased caloric intake associated with increased serotonin levels in brain synapses. Dexfenfluramine hydrochloride is a serotonin reuptake inhibitor and releasing agent. *In vitro* studies have confirmed the dual serotoninergic mechanism of action of dexfenfluramine by demonstrating that the drug inhibits serotonin reuptake by axon terminals and causes the release of serotonin from synaptosomes. In animals, the reduced caloric intake and the loss in body weight elicited by dexfenfluramine is associated with release of serotonin from presynaptic axon terminals in the brain, inhibition of neuronal serotonin reuptake, and, therefore, an increase of serotonin receptor activation. This results in an enhancement of serotoninergic transmission in the centers of feeding behavior, located in the ventro-medial nucleus of the hypothalamus. In rats, enhanced serotoninergic transmission induced by dexfenfluramine selectively suppressed appetite for carbohydrates which resulted in reduction of food consumption when the dietary carbohydrate to protein ratio was high. Unlike amphetamines and other serotonin-active agonists and antagonists, dexfenfluramine neither enhances nor suppresses dopamine-mediated neurotransmission.

In clinical trials, dexfenfluramine treatment in conjunction with a reduced-calorie diet is associated with a reduction in appetite and may slow gastric emptying. These and other actions may contribute to the reduction in caloric consumption associated with dexfenfluramine. In one clinical trial, dexfenfluramine was shown to preferentially decrease carbohydrate consumption at meals and to manage carbohydrate craving between meals by decreasing the consumption of snack foods with a high carbohydrate content in patients who frequently snack on such foods.

PHARMACOKINETICS AND METABOLISM

Systemic Bioavailability: Dexfenfluramine is completely absorbed after oral dosing, with a systemic bioavailability of about 68% because of first pass metabolism by the liver. In studies in which patients received a single 30-mg oral dose of dexfenfluramine, mean peak plasma concentrations of dexfenfluramine ranged between 11 and 41 ng/ml in individual patients after 1.5 to 8.0 hours. The average terminal elimination half-life of plasma dexfenfluramine ranged from 17 to 20 hours, and the average total body clearance of dexfenfluramine was 691.9 ml/min. In man, following doses of 15 mg dexfenfluramine twice a day for 15 days, mean maximal plasma dexfenfluramine concentrations ranging from 15 to 92 ng/ml were observed, and steady-state plasma levels were achieved 8 days after the initial dose. The average steady-state plasma concentrations were somewhat lower than predicted by single-dose pharmacokinetics and the average time to steady-state was longer than the predicted 4 to 5 days. The major active metabolite, d-norfenfluramine, accumulated to maximal plasma concentrations of about 26 ng/ml, with steady-state plasma levels occurring at about 9 days. The *d*-norfenfluramine plasma half-life is estimated to be 32 hours. After reaching steady-state levels, there was no evidence of increasing concentrations of dexfenfluramine or *d*-norfenfluramine in plasma during 12 months of dosing. Following administration of single 30-mg, 40-mg, and 60-mg doses of dexfenfluramine to healthy volunteers, dexfenfluramine C_{max} values of 25 ng/ml, 33 ng/ml, and 51 ng/ml and area-under-the-curve$_{0-t}$ values of 144 ng·hr/ml, 191 ng·hr/ml, and 275 ng·hr/ml, respectively, were found. In a dose response study of dexfenfluramine involving obese patients treated for 12 weeks, dexfenfluramine C_{min} values of 24 ng/ml at a dose of 15 mg twice daily and 58 ng/ml at a dose of 30 mg twice daily were observed. These data suggest that plasma concentrations of dexfenfluramine increase in proportion to the administered dose.

Protein Binding and Distribution: At a dexfenfluramine plasma concentration of 100 ng/ml, 36% is bound to plasma proteins. Dexfenfluramine is distributed into body tissue in non-obese subjects, with a volume of distribution of 839 L.

Metabolism: Dexfenfluramine is metabolized in the liver. The first steps in the metabolism of dexfenfluramine are dealkylation, resulting in formation of the active metabolite, *d*-norfenfluramine and deamination to an inactive *d*-hydroxy derivative. In a study of drug metabolism using radiolabeled dexfenfluramine, levofenfluramine and *d,l*-fenfluramine in two healthy subjects, 92% of the administered radioactivity was found in urine and 1% in feces over 6 days. Fenfluramine accounted for 7% to 19% and norfenfluramine accounted for 4% to 11% of the urine radioactivity. Other metabolites (inactive) included 1-(m-trifluoromethylphenyl)-1,2-propane diol (21 to 38%), m-trifluoromethyl benzoic acid (7 to 22%), m-trifluoromethyl hippuric acid (<1 to 11%), and 1-(m-trifluoromethylphenyl)-propan-2-ol (2 to 4%).

Renal Disease and Liver Disease: Specific studies in patients with renal and hepatic impairment have not been conducted.

Obese Patients: In obese patients who received a single 30-mg dose, a mean peak plasma dexfenfluramine concentration of about 22.3 ng/ml is reached after about 5.2 hours. In a parallel-group, multiple-dose pharmacokinetic study of dexfenfluramine (15 mg twice daily) there were no significant differences in steady-state pharmacokinetic parameters between obese and non-obese subjects.

Age: The pharmacokinetics of a single 30-mg dose of dexfenfluramine in eight elderly patients, ranging from 66 to 83 years of age, have been examined in one study. The mean maximal plasma concentration was 21.8 ng/ml, and ranged from 9.7 to 33.0 ng/ml in individual patients. Time to maximal plasma concentration was about 5 hours and ranged from 3 hours to 10 hours. Area-under-the-curve to infinity was 615 ng·hr/ml and ranged from 16 to 1205 ng·hr/ml. Mean (±SD) steady-state plasma concentrations of dexfenfluramine and *d*-norfenfluramine after six months of treatment (15 mg twice daily) in 18 obese patients over 60 years old were 27.3 (±16.3) ng/ml and 14.0 (±7.4) ng/ml, respectively, compared to values of 24.1 (±15.9) and 15.6 (±11.2), respectively, in 268 patients under 60 years old. In

CLINICAL PHARMACOLOGY: *(cont'd)*

a cohort of these patients followed through 12 months of treatment (15 mg twice daily) mean (±SD) steady-state plasma concentrations of dexfenfluramine and *d*-norfenfluramine in 17 obese patients over 60 years old were 32.9 (±16.8) ng/ml and 18.0 (±8.0) ng/ml, respectively, compared to values of 23.9 (±12.9) and 14.4 (±8.2), respectively, in 186 obese patients under 60 years old.

CLINICAL STUDIES:

Observational epidemiologic studies have established a relationship between obesity and the risks for cardiovascular disease, non-insulin dependent diabetes mellitus (NIDDM), certain forms of cancer, gallstones, certain respiratory disorders, and an increase in overall mortality. These studies suggest that weight loss, if maintained, may produce health benefits for some patients with chronic obesity who may also be at risk for other diseases.

The long-term effects of dexfenfluramine on the morbidity and mortality associated with obesity have not been established. Short-term (<4 months), placebo-controlled, double-blind studies have provided evidence that dexfenfluramine does not adversely affect glycemia, lipid profile, or blood pressure control in obese patients. Some short-term studies have suggested that weight loss with dexfenfluramine may be associated with a reduction in hyperglycemia in obese diabetic patients, a reduction in blood pressure in obese hypertensive patients, and improvement in the lipid profile in obese hyperlipidemic patients.

Dexfenfluramine has been shown to be effective in reducing excess body weight in obese patients. In 16 of 17 double-blind, placebo-controlled trials, of various treatment durations and with different design features, where all patients were on reduced-calorie diets, dexfenfluramine-treated patients lost statistically significantly more weight on average than those treated with placebo. In these studies, weight loss was evident within 4 weeks of initiating treatment, even in some patients where reduced-calorie diet alone had failed to induce a significant weight loss.

In the INDEX study, a one-year, double-blind, placebo-controlled trial of obese patients, dexfenfluramine, in conjunction with a reduced-calorie diet, produced a significant reduction in weight during the first 4 to 6 months. This response was maintained during continuation of therapy (up to 12 months of treatment). The percentage of patients who achieved various levels of weight loss at 1 year are shown in TABLE 1.

TABLE 1 Percentage of Patients Losing Weight at One Year

	≥15% loss		≥10% loss		≥5% loss	
	Dexfenfluramine	Placebo	Dexfenfluramine	Placebo	Dexfenfluramine	Placebo
Completers* (Redux n=297/ Placebo n=262)	29%	16%	52%	30%	72%	50%
All patients** (Redux n=463/ Placebo n=467)	21%	10%	40%	21%	64%	43%

* Data for patients who completed the entire 12-month period of the trial.
** Data for all patients who received study drug and who had any post-baseline measurement; for those patients who discontinued treatment before 12 months, the last observed data is carried forward through the end of the study and analyzed with data from those patients who completed the trial.

Based on another analysis of the INDEX study, among all patients who were treated with dexfenfluramine hydrochloride and identified as initial responders (*i.e.*, lost at least 4 pounds in the first 4 weeks of therapy), 60% went on to lose ≥10% of their initial body weight by the end of 1 year of treatment. Among dexfenfluramine-treated patients, 78% were identified as initial responders. At the end of 1 year, the mean weight loss for the initial responders was 22 pounds, while the non-responders had a mean weight loss of 6 pounds. Among obese patients who had been successful in losing weight by dieting alone (*i.e.*, lost at least 10 pounds in the prior year), the addition of dexfenfluramine to the regimen resulted in the further loss of 26% of initial excess weight, while successful dieters who received placebo lost only 7% of initial excess weight.

INDICATIONS AND USAGE:

Dexfenfluramine is indicated for the management of obesity including weight loss and maintenance of weight loss in patients on a reduced calorie diet. Dexfenfluramine hydrochloride is recommended for obese patients with an initial body mass index ≥30 kg/m^2, or ≥27 kg/m^2 in the presence of other risk factors (*e.g.*, hypertension, diabetes, hyperlipidemia).

The safety and effectiveness of dexfenfluramine beyond 1 year have not been determined at this time.

TABLE 2 is a chart of Body Mass Index (BMI) based on various heights and weights.

BMI is calculated by taking the patient's weight, in kg, divided by the patient's height, in meters, squared. Metric conversions are as follows: pounds ÷ 2.2 = kg; inches x 0.0254 = meters.

TABLE 2 BODY MASS INDEX (BMI), kg/m^2

Weight (pounds)	Height (feet, inches) 5'0"	5'3"	5'6"	5'9"	6'0"	6'3"
140	27	25	23	21	19	18
150	29	27	24	22	20	19
160	31	28	26	24	22	20
170	33	30	28	25	23	21
180	35	32	29	27	25	23
190	37	34	31	28	26	24
200	39	36	32	30	27	25
210	41	37	34	31	29	26
220	43	39	36	33	30	28
230	45	41	37	34	31	29
240	47	43	39	36	33	30
250	49	44	40	37	34	31

Patients with BMI values ≥30 may be candidates for dexfenfluramine therapy.

Patients with BMI values of 27-29 may be candidates for dexfenfluramine therapy if they also have a concomitant risk factor (*e.g.*, hypertension, diabetes, hyperlipidemia).

CONTRAINDICATIONS:

Dexfenfluramine is contraindicated in patients with diagnosed pulmonary hypertension (see WARNINGS). Dexfenfluramine is contraindicated in patients receiving monoamine oxidase inhibitors (see DRUG INTERACTIONS). Dexfenfluramine is contraindicated in patients with hypersensitivity to dexfenfluramine, fenfluramine, or related compounds.

WARNINGS:

PRIMARY PULMONARY HYPERTENSION

A 2-year, international (5 country), case-control (epidemiological) study identified 95 primary pulmonary hypertension (PPH) cases; 20 of these had been exposed to anorexigens in the past, and 9 of the 20 had been exposed to anorexigens for longer than three months. In this study, the use of anorexigens for longer than 3 months was associated with an increase in the risk of developing PPH (odds ratio = 9.1, 95% confidence interval = 2.6-31.5). This increased risk of PPH was concentrated in persons who had used the drugs within the preceding year; there was no significant increase in risk for persons who had taken the drugs more than 1 year ago or for persons who had used these agents for 3 months or less. In the general population, the yearly occurrence of PPH is estimated to be about 1-2 cases per 1,000,000 persons. Therefore, the case-control study indicated an estimated risk associated with the long-term use of anorexigen drugs of about 18 cases per million persons exposed per year. According to the case-control study, obesity itself (body mass index ≥30 kg/m^2) was also associated with an increase of about two-fold in the risk of developing PPH.

PPH is a serious condition; the 4-year survival rate has been reported to be 55%.

The initial symptom of pulmonary hypertension is generally dyspnea. Other initial symptoms include: angina pectoris, syncope, or lower extremity edema. *Patients should be advised to report immediately any deterioration in exercise tolerance. Treatment should be discontinued in patients who develop new, unexplained symptoms of dyspnea, angina pectoris, syncope, or lower extremity edema. These patients should be evaluated for the etiology of these symptoms and the possible presence of pulmonary hypertension.*

NEUROCHEMICAL FINDINGS IN ANIMALS

Dexfenfluramine and its active metabolite *d*-norfenfluramine are believed to reduce food intake through interactions with the serotoninergic neurotransmitter system. In animals, doses of dexfenfluramine that result in brain concentrations approximately 10 times those observed in humans produce prolonged reductions (weeks to months) in brain serotonin concentrations following cessation of dexfenfluramine treatment. These reductions in brain serotonin concentrations are accompanied by correlate observations of diminished visualization of serotoninergic neurons by immunohistochemical techniques and decreased numbers of serotonin transporters. Some investigators have interpreted these results as surrogate indicators of neurotoxicity; others have interpreted these results as an extension of the pharmacology of serotonin reuptake inhibitors. Resolution of differences in the interpretation of the animal findings may occur with further research.

Changes in brain serotonin concentrations following acute, high-dose dexfenfluramine administration have been noted in all animal species and with all routes of drug administration tested. Prolonged reductions in brain serotonin concentrations in rats have been observed following acute, but not escalating, dose regimens. In mice, 2 years of drug administration at a dose producing at least 12 times the human brain level of dexfenfluramine produced no change in brain serotonin concentrations or serotonin transporter number. Changes in brain serotonin concentrations generally have been found to be reversible; however, the dose and brain concentration of dexfenfluramine and *d*-norfenfluramine may affect reversibility. Persistent reductions in brain serotonin concentrations and neuronal serotonin immunoreactivity were observed in three squirrel monkeys 14-17 months after a 4-day, 10 mg/kg/day subcutaneous dose regimen of dexfenfluramine; the effects of lower doses or different dose regimens were not reported in this study. In a separate study, other squirrel monkeys given this high-dose regimen achieved brain concentrations of dexfenfluramine approximately 35 times those of obese patients taking normal therapeutic doses.

Studies employing experimental techniques that are independent of serotonin content (*e.g.*, retrograde transport, silver staining, glial fibrillary acidic protein content) could not detect neuronal damage at doses of dexfenfluramine in animals producing decreased brain serotonin concentrations. The observed neuro-chemical changes were not associated with persistent changes in animal behavior. The relevance of the animal findings to humans is not known.

MISCELLANEOUS

Organic causes of obesity (*e.g.*, hypothyroidism) should be excluded before prescribing dexfenfluramine. Dexfenfluramine should be used with caution in patients with glaucoma.

PRECAUTIONS:

GENERAL

Because of dexfenfluramine's potential to produce mild-to-moderate drowsiness, the patient's individual response should be assessed before engaging in activities requiring alertness. Dexfenfluramine may potentiate the sedative effects of alcohol or other drugs with CNS action.

If the patient develops any symptoms of intolerance, *e.g.*, nausea and vomiting, the dosage should be reduced, or the drug discontinued.

MISUSE POTENTIAL

As with any weight-loss agent, the potential exists for misuse of dexfenfluramine in inappropriate patient populations (*e.g.*, patients with anorexia nervosa or bulimia). See INDICATIONS AND USAGEfor recommended prescribing guidelines.

INFORMATION FOR THE PATIENT

Patients should be informed that false-positive urine drug tests for amphetamines have been observed for up to 24 hours following a 30-mg dose (2 capsules) of dexfenfluramine. See Drug/Laboratory Test Interactions.

COMBINATION THERAPY

The safety and efficacy of dexfenfluramine in combination with other weight-loss agents have not been studied; therefore, concomitant use is not recommended.

USE IN PATIENTS WITH CONCOMITANT ILLNESS

Weight loss has been associated with a reduction in hyperglycemia in obese diabetic patients, a reduction of blood pressure in obese hypertensive patients, and an improvement in the lipid profile in obese hyperlipidemic patients. Therefore, when dexfenfluramine is used for the management of obesity associated with hypertension, diabetes, or dyslipidemia, there may be changes in these conditions and the medications used to treat them should be monitored, and adjusted, if necessary.

DRUG/LABORATORY TEST INTERACTIONS

False-positive urine drug tests for amphetamines by ELISA have been observed for up to 24 hours following a 30-mg dose (2 capsules) of dexfenfluramine. Patients should be informed of this possible false-positive laboratory finding when undergoing urine drug screenings. Gas chromatography/mass spectroscopy can distinguish false-positive urine drug tests caused by dexfenfluramine from true-positive drug tests. See Information for the Patient.

PRECAUTIONS: *(cont'd)*

CARCINOGENESIS, MUTAGENESIS, AND IMPAIRMENT OF FERTILITY

Carcinogenicity studies in rats and mice have not shown a carcinogenic potential for dexfenfluramine at doses up to 12 mg/kg and 27 mg/kg, respectively. These doses are 4.8 and 5.8 times the daily human dose (calculated on a body surface area [mg/m^2] basis). When given to pregnant rats, dexfenfluramine caused a significant reduction in the number of fetuses and live young.

Dexfenfluramine has no detectable mutagenic activity as determined by the Ames test, gene conversion-DNA repair test, evaluation of the clastogenic effect on cultures of human lymphocytes, mouse lymphoma cell mutation test, and the micronucleus test in the mouse.

PREGNANCY

Pregnancy, Teratogenic Effects, Pregnancy Category C: Dexfenfluramine produced dose-related effects on reproduction and fertility in rats. In a three-generation fertility and reproduction study, administration of dexfenfluramine to female rats at 2.5 and 5 times the human daily dose (calculated on a body surface area [mg/m^2] basis) caused significant reductions in body weight and weight gain throughout pregnancy; the number of placental implantations and fetuses was reduced, there was a reduced number of live young, and delayed ossification was seen in the fetuses. No significant treatment-related adverse effects or abnormalities were observed in second- and third-generation rats.

Teratogenicity studies were conducted in rats and rabbits. Neither study showed any treatment-related embryotoxicity or teratogenicity at doses up to 10 times the daily human dose (calculated on a body surface area [mg/m^2] basis). There are no adequate and well-controlled studies of dexfenfluramine in pregnant women. Dexfenfluramine is not recommended for pregnant women.

NURSING MOTHERS

Dexfenfluramine is excreted in rat milk. It is not known whether dexfenfluramine is excreted in human milk. Therefore, dexfenfluramine should not be administered to a nursing woman.

USE IN OTHER POPULATIONS

Pediatric Use: Safety and effectiveness of dexfenfluramine in pediatric patients have not been established.

Geriatric Use: As with all CNS-active medications, caution should be exercised in treating elderly patients with dexfenfluramine. Clinical studies of dexfenfluramine did not include sufficient numbers of patients aged 65 or older to determine whether they respond differently than younger patients. Pharmacokinetics in elderly patients are discussed in CLINICAL PHARMACOLOGY.

DRUG INTERACTIONS:

In patients receiving nonselective monoamine oxidase inhibitors (MAOIs) (*e.g.*, selegiline hydrochloride) in combination with serotoninergic agents (*e.g.*, fluoxetine, fluvoxamine, paroxetine, sertraline, venlafaxine), there have been reports of serious, sometimes fatal, reactions. Because dexfenfluramine is a serotonin releaser and reuptake inhibitor, dexfenfluramine should not be used concomitantly with a MAO inhibitor (see CONTRAINDICATIONS).

At least 14 days should elapse between discontinuation of a MAO inhibitor and initiation of treatment with dexfenfluramine. At least 3 weeks should elapse between discontinuation of dexfenfluramine and initiation of treatment with a MAO inhibitor.

A rare, but serious, constellation of symptoms, termed "serotonin syndrome," has been reported with the concomitant use of selective serotonin reuptake inhibitors (SSRIs) and agents for migraine therapy, such as Imitrex (sumatriptan succinate) and dihydroergotamine. The syndrome requires immediate medical attention and may include one or more of the following symptoms: excitement, hypomania, restlessness, loss of consciousness, confusion, disorientation, anxiety, agitation, motor weakness, myoclonus, tremor, hemiballismus, hyperreflexia, ataxia, dysarthria, incoordination, hyperthermia, shivering, pupillary dilation, diaphoresis, emesis, and tachycardia. Dexfenfluramine should not be administered with other serotoninergic agents. The appropriate interval between administration of these agents and dexfenfluramine has not been established. The use of dexfenfluramine with other CNS-active drugs has not been systematically evaluated; consequently, caution is advised if dexfenfluramine and such drugs are prescribed concurrently.

ADVERSE REACTIONS:

COMMONLY OBSERVED

The most commonly observed, treatment-emergent adverse events associated with the use of dexfenfluramine in double-blind, placebo-controlled clinical trials were diarrhea (17.5%), dry mouth (12.5%), and somnolence (7.1%). These and other commonly observed adverse reactions were generally mild and transient. (Commonly observed is defined as incidence of 5% or greater and incidence in dexfenfluramine group at least twice that of placebo group, as derived from the Table 3 below.)

ASSOCIATED WITH DISCONTINUATION OF TREATMENT

Seven percent of the 1159 patients who received dexfenfluramine in double-blind, placebo-controlled clinical trials discontinued treatment because of an adverse event. The most common adverse events resulting in discontinuation included asthenia, insomnia, headache, and depression. Five percent of the 1138 placebo-treated patients discontinued because of an adverse event.

INCIDENCE IN CONTROLLED CLINICAL TRIALS

The following Table 3 lists treatment-emergent adverse events from several double-blind, placebo-controlled trials that occurred at a frequency of 2% or more among patients treated with dexfenfluramine and occurred at least as frequently as the placebo group, regardless of relationship to study medication.

Patients may experience more than one type of adverse event. Only events that occurred at a frequency of 2% or more in dexfenfluramine-treated patients and were at least as frequent as in placebo-treated patients are included.

OTHER EVENTS OBSERVED IN CONTROLLED CLINICAL TRIALS

The events below are classified within body system categories and enumerated in order of decreasing frequency using the following definitions. Frequent adverse events are those occurring in more than 1/100 patients but were not described above because the frequency in dexfenfluramine-treated patients was less than that in placebo-treated patients or they occurred at a rate less than 2%. Infrequent adverse events are those occurring in 1/100 to 1/1000 patients, while rare adverse events are those occurring in only one patient during placebo-controlled clinical trials.

Body as a Whole:

Frequent: infection, flu syndrome, pain,back pain, fever, allergic reaction.

Infrequent: malaise, neck pain, chest pain, generalized edema, stress, face edema, neoplasm, pelvic pain.

Rare: adenoma, immune system disorder, neck rigidity, suicide attempt.

Cardiovascular System:

Frequent: hypertension, angina pectoris, palpitation, vasodilation, migraine.

ADVERSE REACTIONS: *(cont'd)*

TABLE 3 Treatment-Emergent Adverse Events From Placebo-Controlled Clinical Trials

ADVERSE EVENT	PERCENT OF DEXFENFLURAMINE-TREATED PATIENTS (15 mg twice daily) (n=1159)	PERCENT OF PLACEBO-TREATED PATIENTS (n=1138)
BODY AS A WHOLE		
Headache	16.1	15.5
Asthenia	15.8	10.7
Abdominal Pain	6.7	6.0
Chills	2.9	1.2
Accidental Injury	2.8	2.3
GASTROINTESTINAL SYSTEM		
Diarrhea	17.5	7.3
Vomiting	3.2	2.9
METABOLIC/NUTRITIONAL SYSTEM		
Thirst	2.8	1.1
NERVOUS SYSTEM		
Insomnia	19.9	18.6
Dry Mouth	12.5	5.0
Somnolence	7.1	3.4
Dizziness	5.5	4.0
Depression	4.7	3.6
Vertigo	3.1	1.7
Emotional Liability	3.1	2.7
Abnormal Dreams	2.0	1.4
Thinking Abnormal	2.0	1.1
RESPIRATORY SYSTEM		
Pharyngitis	6.1	5.6
Cough Increased	3.6	3.0
Bronchitis	3.4	1.8
SKIN/APPENDAGES		
Rash	2.3	2.2
UROGENITAL SYSTEM		
Urinary Frequency	2.8	1.1
Polyuria	2.1	1.0

Infrequent: cardiovascular disorder, tachycardia, postural hypotension, hypotension, peripheral vascular disorder, syncope, arrhythmia, extrasystoles, hemorrhage, thrombophlebitis, varicose vein.

Rare: heart block, pulmonary embolus, thrombosis.

Gastrointestinal System:

Frequent: constipation, nausea, dyspepsia, increased appetite, rectal disorder, gastritis, gastroenteritis, flatulence.

Infrequent: colitis, eructation, gastrointestinal hemorrhage, enteritis, peptic ulcer, hepatitis, hepatomegaly.

Rare: appendicitis, cholelithiasis, fecal incontinence, melena, mouth ulceration, pancreatitis, rectal hemorrhage, sialoadenitis.

Endocrine:

Infrequent: goiter, diabetes mellitus, thyroid disorder.

Rare: hypothyroidism.

Hemic and Lymphatic System:

Infrequent: anemia, lymphedema.

Rare: coagulation disorder, lymphadenopathy, polycythemia, thrombocythemia.

Metabolic and nNutritional:

Infrequent: edema, gout, hypoglycemia, hypokalemia.

Rare: hyperglycemia, hyperkalemia, hyperlipemia, hyperuricemia.

Musculoskeletal System:

Frequent: arthralgia, myalgia, arthritis.

Infrequent: leg cramps, joint disorder, bone disorder, tenosynovitis, myasthenia, rheumatoid arthritis.

Rare: bursitis, tetany.

Nervous System:

Frequent: nervousness, anxiety, increased libido, hypertonia, paresthesia.

Infrequent: tremor, amnesia, euphoria, decreased libido, incoordination, neuralgia, speech disorder, ataxia, hypokinesia, sleep disorder, abnormal gait, agitation, confusion, depersonalization, diplopia, hostility, hyperesthesia, hyperkinesia, peripheral neuritis.

Rare: apathy, dementia, hallucinations, hypotonia, neuritis, neurosis, paralysis.

Respiratory System:

Frequent: rhinitis, sinusitis. Infrequent: asthma, dyspnea, epistaxis, laryngitis.

Rare: apnea, hyperventilation.

Skin and Appendages:

Frequent: sweating, alopecia, urticaria, pruritus.

Infrequent: skin disorder, fungal dermatitis, hirsutism, eczema, psoriasis.

Rare: skin hypertrophy.

Special Senses:

Frequent: taste perversion, amblyopia.

Infrequent: abnormal vision, conjunctivitis, eye disorder, glaucoma, tinnitus, vestibular disorder, dry eyes, mydriasis.

Rare: abnormality of accommodation, anisocoria, lacrimation disorder, miosis, parosmia, retinal disorder.

Urogenital System:

Frequent: menstrual disorder, urinary tract infection, nocturia, dysmenorrhea.

Infrequent: amenorrhea, dysuria, oliguria, albuminuria, breast pain, kidney calculus, kidney pain.

Rare: spontaneous abortion, threatened abortion, breast neoplasm, endometrial disorder, female lactation, hematuria, impotence, mastitis, nephritis, prostatic disorder, testis disorder, urinary incontinence, urinary retention, uterine hemorrhage.

In controlled clinical trials, there has been no consistent pattern of laboratory abnormalities in patients treated with dexfenfluramine.

POST-INTRODUCTION REPORTS

Voluntary reports of adverse events temporally associated with dexfenfluramine that have been received since market introduction in countries other than the US, for which the association with the drug is unknown, and which are not included in descriptions of adverse events elsewhere in this labeling, include the following:

ADVERSE REACTIONS: *(cont'd)*

Body as a Whole: anaphylaxis, congenital anomaly, eventration, hypothermia, laryngeal edema, peritonitis, reaction aggravation, retroperitoneal fibrosis, scleroderma, sudden death.

Cardiovascular System: pulmonary hypertension (see WARNINGS), atrial fibrillation, cardiomyopathy, cerebral vasculitis, ECG abnormal, heart arrest, heart failure, myocardial infarction, myocarditis, shock, tachycardia, ventricular fibrillation, ventricular tachycardia.

Digestive System: dysphagia, gastrointestinal disorder, tongue disorder.

Endocrine System: diabetic coma.

Gastrointestinal System: hepatic failure, jaundice, liver damage.

Hemic and Lymphatic System: agranulocytosis, antinuclear antibody present, bone marrow depression, ecchymosis, hemolytic anemia, pancytopenia.

Metabolic and Nutritional: dehydration, elevated lipases, increased prolactin, thyroid disease, weight increase.

Musculoskeletal: myopathy.

Nervous System: antisocial reaction, apathy, cerebellar ataxia, cerebrovascular accident (including cerebral hemorrhage, cerebral infarction, cerebral ischemia and cochlear infarction), choreoathetosis, convulsions, decreased reflexes, delirium, drug dependence, dyslexia, encephalopathy, grand mal convulsions, Guillain-Barre syndrome, hemiplegia, hypoesthesia, manic-depressive psychosis, manic reaction, memory loss, meningism, meningitis, neuropathy, papilledema, paraplegia, personality disorder, reflexes increased, retrobulbar neuritis, schizophrenic reaction, stupor, subdural hematoma, twitch, withdrawal syndrome.

Respiratory System: pulmonary hypertension (see WARNINGS), diffuse interstitial pneumonitis, dyspnea, hiccup, lung edema.

Skin and Appendages: angioedema, bullous eruption, erythema multiforme, lower extremity purpura, purpura annularis telangiectodes, Stevens-Johnson syndrome (erythema multiforme major).

Special Senses: ophthalmoplegia, photophobia, transitory deafness, visual field defects.

Urogenital System: breast enlargement, carcinoma (breast), carcinoma (cervix), ejaculation abnormal, gynecomastia, hypomenorrhea, kidney failure, placenta previa, urinary tract disorder.

ADVERSE EVENTS OCCURRING AFTER DISCONTINUATION

In controlled clinical trials and/or in post-marketing reports, symptoms have been reported within a few days after discontinuation of dexfenfluramine. These include one or more of the following: abdominal pain, anxiety, asthenia, delusion, depression, diarrhea, dizziness, hypertension, insomnia, nausea and vomiting.

DRUG ABUSE AND DEPENDENCE:

CONTROLLED SUBSTANCE CLASS

Dexfenfluramine is a controlled substance in Schedule IV.

ABUSE AND PHYSICAL AND PSYCHOLOGICAL DEPENDENCE

Dexfenfluramine is not an amphetamine or a stimulant. There is no evidence of addictive or drug-seeking behavior in pre-marketing clinical studies. Dexfenfluramine was inactive in rat and monkey self-administration, drug-discrimination, and place-preference models of abuse potential.

OVERDOSAGE:

HUMAN EXPERIENCE

Post-marketing experience in Europe over 10 years (August 1984 through December 1994) in an estimated 10 million patients provided reports of 66 instances of overdose (maximum dose per body mass of 54 mg/kg, maximum total dose of 1800 mg), including eight children 6 years of age or under. Three deaths have occurred in association with dexfenfluramine overdosage. One patient with a history of suicide attempts ingested 1800 mg dexfenfluramine and 20 to 30 capsules of Tranxene (clorazepate), one patient was found dead, assumed to have consumed approximately 1500 mg of dexfenfluramine, and the third patient consumed dexfenfluramine (quantity unknown) and several other drugs in an apparent suicide. The second patient had post-mortem levels of dexfenfluramine of 3300 ng/ml, and positive levels for amphetamines and cannabinoids. The exact causes of death were unknown. In 23 other cases of dexfenfluramine overdose, plasma drug levels were determined; the maximum reported plasma drug level for dexfenfluramine was 778 ng/ml (with *d*-norfenfluramine 37 ng/ml); the maximum *d*-norfenfluramine level was 371 ng/ml (with dexfenfluramine 483 ng/ml).

Symptoms associated with overdosage consisted mainly of agitation, drowsiness, mydriasis, sweating, shivering, nausea, and vomiting. Other symptoms observed with dexfenfluramine overdose and not noted under ADVERSE REACTIONS include cold sensation, excitation, nystagmus, garrulousness, delusions, bladder tenesmus, chattering teeth, abnormal reflexes, facial myoclonus, trismus, tonic-clonic seizures, impairment of consciousness, coma (stage 2-4), sinus bradycardia, repolarization abnormalities, right anterior hemiblock, polypnea, diffuse bronchial rales, and flushing.

ANIMAL EXPERIENCE

Significant acute toxicity occurred at oral doses greater than 40, 70, and 75 mg/kg in rats, mice, and guinea pigs, respectively. A dose of 40 mg/kg is approximately 31 times greater than the effective anorectic dose tn rats.

MANAGEMENT OF OVERDOSE

General supportive measures for oral drug overdose should be instituted. Measures that have been used in dexfenfluramine overdose cases include aspiration of gastric contents, gastric lavage with activated charcoal, osmotic diuresis, forced acid diuresis, and careful monitoring of CNS or respiratory depression. The effectiveness of dialysis is not known. Patients should be followed closely until there is no further evidence of drug-related CNS effects. No specific therapy for dexfenfluramine overdose is known.

DOSAGE AND ADMINISTRATION:

The usual dosage is one 15-mg capsule twice daily, with meals. Doses above 30 mg per day are not recommended.

Analysis of numerous variables has indicated that about 60% of patients who lose at least 4 pounds in the first 4 weeks of treatment with dexfenfluramine in combination with a reduced-calorie diet lose at least 10% of their initial body weight by the end of 1 year of treatment. If a patient has not lost at least 4 pounds in the first 4 weeks of treatment, the physician should consider reevaluation of therapy which may include discontinuation of dexfenfluramine.

The safety and effectiveness of dexfenfluramine beyond 1 year have not been determined at this time.

Infrequently, symptoms (*e.g.,* abdominal pain, anxiety, asthenia, delusion, depression, diarrhea, dizziness, hypertension, insomnia, nausea and vomiting) have occurred within several days following cessation of dexfenfluramine. If the physician notes such symptoms, clinical judgment should guide the treatment, which may include tapering the dose (15 mg once daily) for 2 weeks prior to complete discontinuation.

HOW SUPPLIED:

Redux (dexfenfluramine hydrochloride capsules) 15 mg, is supplied in number 3, white, opaque, hard-gelatin capsules. Each capsule is marked with "Redux" and three black vertical bands.

Storage: Store at room temperature, between 15°C and 30°C (59°F and 86°F).

HOW SUPPLIED - EQUIVALENTS NOT AVAILABLE:

Capsule - Oral - 15 mg

15 mg x 60	$51.00	REDUX, Wyeth Labs	00008-0904-01

DEXPANTHENOL *(000985)*

CATEGORIES: Atony; Flatulence; Gastrointestinal Drugs; Homeostatic & Nutrient; Ileus; Pantothenic/Calcium Panthothenate; Vitamin B Complex; Vitamins; Pregnancy Category C; FDA Pre 1938 Drugs

BRAND NAMES: *Bepanten*; *Bepanthen* (Germany); *Bepanthene* (France); **Ilopan**; *Panthenol* (Germany)

(International brand names outside U.S. in italics)

DESCRIPTION:

Dexpanthenol Injection is a derivative of pantothenic acid, a member of the B complex of vitamins. Dexpanthenol Injection is a sterile aqueous solution indicated for use as a gastrointestinal stimulant. The chemical name is D-(+)-2, 4-dihydroxy-N-(3-hydroxypropyl)-3, 3-dimethylbutylramide.

Each ml contains dexpanthenol 250 mg in distilled water for injection.

CLINICAL PHARMACOLOGY:

Pantothenic acid is a precursor of coenzyme A, which serves as a cofactor for a variety of enzyme-catalyzed reactions involving transfer of acetyl groups. The final step in the synthesis of acetylcholine consists of the choline acetylase transfer of an acetyl group from acetylcoenzyme A to choline. Acetylcholine is the neurohumoral transmitter in the parasympathetic system and as such maintains the normal functions of the intestine. Decrease in acetylcholine content would result in decreased peristalsis and in extreme cases adynamic ileus. The pharmacological mode of action of the drug is unknown. Pharmacokinetic data in humans are

unavailable.

INDICATIONS AND USAGE:

Prophylactic use immediately after major abdominal surgery to minimize the possibility of paralytic ileus. Intestinal atony causing abdominal distention; postoperative or postpartum retention of flatus, or postoperative delay in resumption of intestinal motility; paralytic ileus.

CONTRAINDICATIONS:

There are no known contraindications to the use of Dexpanthenol Injection.

WARNINGS:

There have been rare instances of allergic reactions of unknown cause during the concomitant use of Dexpanthenol Injection with drugs such as antibiotics, narcotics and barbiturates.

Administration of Dexpanthenol Injection directly into the vein is not advised (See DOSAGE AND ADMINISTRATION.)

Dexpanthenol Injection should not be administered within one hour of succinylcholine.

PRECAUTIONS:

General: If any signs of a hypersensitivity reaction appear, Dexpanthenol Injection should be discontinued. If ileus is a secondary consequence of mechanical obstruction, primary attention should be directed to the obstruction. The management of adynamic ileus includes the correction of any fluid and electrolyte imbalance (especially hypokalemia), anemia and hypoproteinemia, treatment of infection, avoidance where possible of drugs which are known to decrease gastrointestinal motility and decompression of the gastrointestinal tract when considerably distended by nasogastric suction or use of a long intestinal tube.

Carcinogenicity, Mutagenicity, Impairment of Fertility: There have been no studies in animals to evaluate the carcinogenic, mutagenic, or impairment of fertility potential of dexpanthenol.

Pregnancy: Category C. Animal reproduction studies have not been conducted with Dexpanthenol Injection. It is also not known whether Dexpanthenol Injection can cause fetal harm when administered to a pregnant woman or can affect reproduction capacity. Dexpanthenol Injection should be given to a pregnant woman only if clearly needed.

Nursing Mothers: It is not known whether this drug is excreted in human milk. Because many drugs are excreted in human milk, caution should be exercised when Dexpanthenol Injection is administered to a nursing woman.

Pediatric Use: Safety and effectiveness in children have not been established.

DRUG INTERACTIONS:

The effects of succinylcholine appeared to have been prolonged in a woman administered dexpanthenol.

ADVERSE REACTIONS:

There have been a few reports of allergic reactions and single reports of several other adverse events in association with the administration of dexpanthenol. A causal relationship is uncertain. One patient experienced itching, tingling, difficulty in breathing. Another patient had red patches of skin. Two patients had generalized dermatitis and one patient urticaria.

One patient experienced temporary respiratory difficulty following administration of Dexpanthenol Injection 5 minutes after succinylcholine was discontinued.

One patient experienced a noticeable but slight drop in blood pressure after administration of dexpanthenol while in the recovery room.

One patient experienced intestinal colic one-half hour after the drug was administered. Two patients vomited following administration and two patients had diarrhea 10 days

post-surgery and after Dexpanthenol Injection. One elderly patient became agitated after administration of the drug.

DOSAGE AND ADMINISTRATION:

Prevention of post-operative adynamic ileus: 250 mg (1 ml) or 500 mg (2 ml) intramuscularly. Repeat in 2 hours and then every 6 hours until all danger of adynamic ileus has passed.

Treatment of adynamic ileus: 500 mg (2 ml) intramuscularly. Repeat in 2 hours and then every 6 hours as needed.

DOSAGE AND ADMINISTRATION: *(cont'd)*

Intravenous administration: Dexpanthenol Injection 2 ml (500 mg) may be mixed with bulk IV solutions such as glucose or Lactated-Ringer's and slowly infused intravenously. Parenteral drug products should be inspected visually for particulate matter and discoloration prior to administration, whenever solution and container permit.

HOW SUPPLIED - EQUIVALENTS NOT AVAILABLE:

Injection, Solution - Intramuscular - 250 mg/ml

2 ml x 25	$131.25	Dexpanthenol, Schein Pharm (US)	00364-2179-48
10 ml	$3.59	Dexpanthenol, McGuff	49072-0161-10
10 ml	$4.50	Dexpanthenol, Steris Labs	00402-0260-10
10 ml	$5.50	Dexpanthenol, Schein Pharm (US)	00364-2179-54
10 ml	$10.05	Dexpanthenol, Pasadena	00418-1250-10

Injection, Solution - Intravenous - 250 mg/ml

2 ml x 25	$101.56	Dexpanthenol, Am Regent	00517-0131-25
2 ml x 25	**$310.56**	**ILOPAN, Savage Labs**	**00281-2356-95**
10 ml	$3.75	Dexpanthenol, Pegasus Med Svs	10974-0260-10
10 ml	$5.00	Dexpanthenol, Consolidated Midland	00223-7414-10
30 ml	$3.60	Dexpanthenol, Americal Pharm	54945-0573-43

DEXRAZOXANE HYDROCHLORIDE *(003242)*

CATEGORIES: Antineoplastics; Breast Carcinoma; Chemotherapy; Chemoprotective Agents; Oncologic Drugs; Orphan Drugs; FDA Class 1P ("Priority Review"); FDA Approved 1995 May

BRAND NAMES: *Razoxin* (England); **Zinecard**
(International brand names outside U.S. in italics)

DESCRIPTION:

Dexrazoxane for injection is a sterile, pyrogen-free lyophilizate intended for intravenous administration. It is a cardioprotective agent for use in conjunction with doxorubicin.

Chemically, dexrazoxane is (*S*)-4,4'-(1-methyl-1,2-ethanediyl)bis-2,6-piperazinedione. The structural formula is $C_{11}H_{16}N_4O_4$. Molecular weight is 268.28.

Dexrazoxane, a potent intracellular chelating agent is a derivative of EDTA. Dexrazoxane is a whitish crystalline powder which melts at 191° to 197°C. It is sparingly soluble in water and 0.1N HCl, slightly soluble in ethanol and methanol and practically insoluble in nonpolar organic solvents. The pk_a is 2.1. Dexrazoxane has an octanol/water partition coefficient of 0.025 and degrades rapidly above a pH of 7.0.

Zinecard is available in 250 mg and 500 mg single use only vials.

Each **250 mg vial** contains dexrazoxane hydrochloride equivalent to 250 mg dexrazoxane. Hydrochloric Acid, NF is added for pH adjustment. When reconstituted as directed with the 25 ml vial of 0.167 Molar (M/6) Sodium Lactate Injection, USP diluent provided, each ml contains: 10 mg dexrazoxane. The pH of the resultant solution is 3.5 to 5.5.

Each **500 mg vial** contains dexrazoxane hydrochloride equivalent to 500 mg dexrazoxane. Hydrochloric Acid, NF is added for pH adjustment. When reconstituted as directed with the 50 ml vial of 0.167 Molar (M/6) Sodium Lactate Injection, USP diluent provided, each ml contains: 10 mg dexrazoxane. The pH of the resultant solution is 3.5 to 5.5.

CLINICAL PHARMACOLOGY:

MECHANISM OF ACTION

The mechanism by which dexrazoxane exerts its cardioprotective activity is not fully understood. Dexrazoxane is a cyclic derivative of EDTA that readily penetrates cell membranes. Results of laboratory studies suggest that dexrazoxane is converted intracellularly to a ring-opened chelating agent that interferes with iron-mediated free radical generation thought to be responsible, in part, for anthracycline-induced cardiomyopathy.

PHARMACOKINETICS

The pharmacokinetics of dexrazoxane have been studied in advanced cancer patients with normal renal and hepatic function. Generally, the pharmacokinetics of dexrazoxane can be adequately described by a two-compartment open model with first-order elimination. Dexrazoxane has been administered as a 15 minute infusion over a dose-range of 60 to 900 mg/m² with 60 mg/m² of doxorubicin, and at a fixed dose of 500 mg/m² with 50 mg/m² doxorubicin. The disposition kinetics of dexrazoxane are dose-independent, as shown by linear relationship between the area under plasma concentration-time curves and administered doses ranging from 60 to 900 mg/m². The mean peak plasma concentration of dexrazoxane was 36.5 mcg/ml at the end of the 15 minute infusion of a 500 mg/m² dose of dexrazoxane administered 15 to 30 minutes prior to the 50 mg/m² doxorubicin dose. The important pharmacokinetic parameters of dexrazoxane are summarized in TABLE 1.

TABLE 1 Dexrazoxane, Clinical Pharmacology
SUMMARY OF MEAN (%CV [a]) DEXRAZOXANE PHARMACOKINETIC PARAMETERS AT A DOSAGE RATIO OF 10:1 OF DEXRAZOXANE: DOXORUBICIN

Dose Doxorubicin (mg/m²)	Dose Zinecard (mg/m²)	Number of Subjects	Elimination Half-life (h)	Plasma Clearance (l/h/m²)	Renal Clearance (l/h/m²)	[b]Volume of Distribution (l/m²)
50	500	10	2.5 (16)	7.88 (18)	3.35 (36)	22.4 (22)
60	600	5	2.1 (29)	6.25 (31)	—	22.0 (55)

[a]Coefficient of variation
[b]Steady-state volume of distribution

Following a rapid distributive phase (-0.2 to 0.3 hours), dexrazoxane reaches post-distributive equilibrium within two to four hours. The estimated steady-state volume of distribution of dexrazoxane suggests its distribution primarily in the total body water (25 l/m²). The mean systemic clearance and steady-state volume of distribution of dexrazoxane in two Asian female patients at 500 mg/m² dexrazoxane along with 50 mg/m² doxorubicin were 15.15 l/h/m² and 36.27 l/m², respectively, but their elimination half-life and renal clearance of dexrazoxane were similar to those of the ten Caucasian patients from the same study. Qualitative metabolism studies with dexrazoxane have confirmed the presence of unchanged drug, a diacid-diamide cleavage product, and two monoacid-monoamide ring products in the urine of animals and man. The metabolite levels were not measured in the pharmacokinetic studies.

Urinary excretion plays an important role in the elimination of dexrazoxane. Forty-two percent of the 500 mg/m² dose of dexrazoxane was excreted in the urine.

Protein Binding: *In vitro* studies have shown that dexrazoxane is not bound to plasma proteins.

Special Populations: The pharmacokinetics of dexrazoxane have not been evaluated in pediatric populations nor in hepatic or renal insufficiency patients.

CLINICAL STUDIES:

The ability of dexrazoxane to prevent/reduce the incidence and severity of doxorubicin-induced cardiomyopathy was demonstrated in three prospectively randomized placebo-controlled studies. In these studies, patients were treated with a doxorubicin-containing regimen and either dexrazoxane or placebo starting with the first course of chemotherapy. There was no restriction on the cumulative dose of doxorubicin. Cardiac function was assessed by measurement of the left ventricular ejection fraction (LVEF), utilizing resting multigated nuclear medicine (MUGA) scans, and by clinical evaluations. Patients receiving dexrazoxane had significantly smaller mean decreases from baseline in LVEF and lower incidences of congestive heart failure than the control group. The difference in decline from baseline in LVEF was evident beginning with a cumulative doxorubicin dose of 150 mg/m² and reached statistical significance in patients who received ≥400 mg/m² of doxorubicin. In addition to evaluating the effect of dexrazoxane on cardiac function, the studies also assessed the effect of the addition of dexrazoxane on the antitumor efficacy of the chemotherapy regimens. In one study (the largest of three breast cancer studies) patients with advanced breast cancer receiving fluorouracil, doxorubicin and cyclophosphamide (FAC) with dexrazoxane had a lower response rate (48% vs 63%; $p=0.007$) and a shorter time to progression than patients who received FAC + placebo, although the survival of patients who did or did not receive dexrazoxane with FAC was similar.

Two of the randomized breast cancer studies evaluating the efficacy and safety of FAC with either dexrazoxane or placebo were amended to allow patients on the placebo arm who had attained a cumulative dose of doxorubicin of 300 mg/m² (six courses of FAC) to receive FAC with open-label dexrazoxane for each subsequent course. This change in design allowed examination of whether there was a cardioprotective effect of dexrazoxane even when it was started after substantial exposure to doxorubicin.

Retrospective historical analyses were then performed to compare the likelihood of heart failure in patients to whom dexrazoxane was added to the FAC regimen after they had received six (6) courses of FAC (and who then continued treatment with FAC therapy) with the heart failure rate in patients who had received six (6) courses of FAC and continued to receive this regimen without added dexrazoxane. These analyses showed that the risk of experiencing a cardiac event at a given cumulative dose of doxorubicin above 300 mg/m² was substantially greater in the 99 patients who did *not* receive dexrazoxane beginning with their seventh course of FAC than in the 102 patients who did receive dexrazoxane.

The Development of Cardiac Events is Shown By:

1. Development of congestive heart failure, defined as having two or more of the following:

a. Cardiomegaly by X-ray

b. Basilar Rales

c. S_3 Gallop

d. Paroxysmal nocturnal dyspnea and/or orthopnea and/or significant dyspnea on exertion.

2. Decline from baseline in LVEF by ≥10% and to below the lower limit of normal for the institution.

3. Decline in LVEF by ≥20% from baseline value.

4. Decline in LVEF to ≥5% below lower limit of normal for the institution.

Because of its cardioprotective effect, dexrazoxane permitted a greater percentage of patients to be treated with extended doxorubicin therapy.

In addition to evaluating the cardioprotective efficacy of dexrazoxane in this setting, the time to tumor progression and survival of these two groups of patients were also compared. There was a similar time to progression in the two groups and survival was at least as long for the group of patients that received dexrazoxane starting with their seventh course, i.e., starting after a cumulative dose of doxorubicin of 300 mg/m². These time to progression and survival data should be interpreted with caution, however, because they are based on comparisons of groups entered sequentially in the studies and are not comparisons of prospectively randomized patients.

INDICATIONS AND USAGE:

Dexrazoxane is indicated for reducing the incidence and severity of cardiomyopathy associated with doxorubicin administration in women with metastatic breast cancer who have received a cumulative doxorubicin dose of 300 mg/m² and who, in their physician's opinion, would benefit from continuing therapy with doxorubicin. It is not recommended for use with the initiation of doxorubicin therapy (see WARNINGS).

CONTRAINDICATIONS:

Dexrazoxane should not be used with chemotherapy regimens that do not contain an anthracycline.

WARNINGS:

Dexrazoxane may add to the myelosuppression caused by chemotherapeutic agents.

There is some evidence that the use of dexrazoxane concurrently with the initiation of fluorouracil, doxorubicin and cyclophosphamide (FAC) therapy interferes with the antitumor efficacy of the regimen, and this use is not recommended. In the largest of three breast cancer trials, patients who received dexrazoxane starting with their first cycle of FAC therapy had a lower response rate (48% vs 63%; $p=0.007$) and shorter time to progression than patients who did not receive dexrazoxane (see CLINICAL STUDIES). Therefore, dexrazoxane should only be used in those patients who have received a cumulative doxorubicin dose of 300 mg/m² and are continuing with doxorubicin therapy.

Although clinical studies have shown that patients receiving FAC with dexrazoxane may receive a higher cumulative dose of doxorubicin before experiencing cardiac toxicity than patients receiving FAC without dexrazoxane, the use of dexrazoxane in patients who have already received a cumulative dose of doxorubicin of 300 mg/m² without dexrazoxane, does not eliminate the potential for anthracycline induced cardiac toxicity. Therefore, cardiac function should be carefully monitored.

Secondary malignancies (primarily acute myeloid leukemia) have been reported in patients treated chronically with oral razoxane. Razoxane is the racemic mixture, of which dexrazoxane is the *S* (+)-enantiomer. In these patients, the total cumulative dose of razoxane ranged from 26 to 480 grams and the duration of treatment was from 42 to 319 weeks. One case of T-cell lymphoma, a case of B-cell lymphoma and six to eight cases of cutaneous basal cell or squamous cell carcinoma have also been reported in patients treated with razoxane.

PRECAUTIONS:

General: Doxorubicin should not be given prior to the intravenous injection of dexrazoxane. Dexrazoxane should be given by slow I.V. push or rapid drip intravenous infusion from a bag. Doxorubicin should be given within 30 minutes after beginning the infusion with dexrazoxane. (See DOSAGE AND ADMINISTRATION.)

As dexrazoxane will always be used with cytotoxic drugs, patients should be monitored closely. While the myelosuppressive effects of dexrazoxane at the recommended dose are mild, additive effects upon the myelosuppressive activity of chemotherapeutic agents may occur.

PRECAUTIONS: *(cont'd)*

Laboratory Tests: As dexrazoxane may add to the myelosuppressive effects of cytotoxic drugs, frequent complete blood counts are recommended. (See ADVERSE REACTIONS.)

Carcinogenesis, Mutagenesis, and Impairment of Fertility: (see WARNINGSfor information on human carcinogenicity) No long-term carcinogenicity studies have been carried out with dexrazoxane in animals. Dexrazoxane was not mutagenic in the Ames test but was found to be clastogenic to human lymphocytes *in vitro* and to mouse bone marrow erythrocytes *in vivo* (micronucleus test).

The possible adverse effects of dexrazoxane on the fertility of humans and experimental animals, male or female, have not been adequately studied. Testicular atrophy was seen with dexrazoxane administration at doses as low as 30 mg/kg weekly for 6 weeks in rats (1/3 the human dose on a mg/m^2 basis) and as low as 20 mg/kg weekly for 13 weeks in dogs (approximately equal to the human dose on a mg/m^2 basis).

Pregnancy Category C: Dexrazoxane was maternotoxic at doses of 2 mg/kg (1/40 the human dose on a mg/m^2 basis) and embryotoxic and teratogenic at 8 mg/kg (approximately 1/10 the human dose on a mg/m^2 basis) when given daily to pregnant rats during the period of organogenesis. Teratogenic effects in the rat included imperforate anus, microphthalmia, and anophthalmia. In offspring allowed to develop to maturity, fertility was impaired in the male and female rats treated *in utero* during organogenesis at 8 mg/kg. In rabbits, doses of 5 mg/kg (approximately 1/10 the human dose on a mg/m^2 basis) daily during the period of organogenesis were maternotoxic and dosages of 20 mg/kg (1/2 the human dose on a mg/m^2 basis) were embryotoxic and teratogenic. Teratogenic effects in the rabbit included several skeletal malformations such as short tail, rib and thoracic malformations, and soft tissue variations including subcutaneous, eye and cardiac hemorrhagic areas, as well as agenesis of the gallbladder and of the intermediate lobe of the lung. There are no adequate and well-controlled studies in pregnant women. Dexrazoxane should be used during pregnancy only if the potential benefit justifies the potential risk to the fetus.

Nursing Mothers: It is not known whether dexrazoxane is excreted in human milk. Because many drugs are excreted in human milk and because of the potential for serious adverse reactions in nursing infants exposed to dexrazoxane, mothers should be advised to discontinue nursing during dexrazoxane therapy.

Pediatric Use: Safety and effectiveness of dexrazoxane in children have not been established.

DRUG INTERACTIONS:

Dexrazoxane does not influence the pharmacokinetics of doxorubicin. There was no significant change in the pharmacokinetics of doxorubicin (50 mg/m^2) and its predominant metabolite, doxorubicinol, in the presence of dexrazoxane (500 mg/m^2) in a crossover study in cancer patients.

ADVERSE REACTIONS:

Dexrazoxane at a dose of 500 mg/m^2 has been administered in combination with FAC in randomized, placebo-controlled, double-blind studies to patients with metastatic breast cancer. The dose of doxorubicin was 50 mg/m^2 in each of the trials. Courses were repeated every three weeks, provided recovery from toxicity had occurred. TABLE 2 below lists the incidence of adverse experiences for patients receiving FAC with either dexrazoxane or placebo in the breast cancer studies. Adverse experiences occurring during courses 1 through 6 are displayed for patients receiving dexrazoxane or placebo with FAC beginning with their first course of therapy (column 1 & 3, respectively). Adverse experiences occurring at course 7 and beyond for patients who received placebo with FAC during the first six courses and who then received either dexrazoxane or placebo with FAC are also displayed (column 2 & 4, respectively).

TABLE 2 Dexrazoxane, Adverse Reactions
PERCENTAGE (%) OF BREAST CANCER PATIENTS WITH ADVERSE EXPERIENCE

ADVERSE EXPERIENCE	FAC + ZINECARD Courses 1-6 N=413	FAC + ZINECARD Courses ≥7 N=102	FAC + PLACEBO Courses 1-6 N=458	FAC + PLACEBO Course ≥7 N=99
Alopecia	94	100	97	98
Nausea	77	51	84	60
Vomiting	59	42	72	49
Fatigue/Malaise	61	48	58	55
Anorexia	42	27	47	38
Stomatitis	34	26	41	28
Fever	34	22	29	18
Infection	23	19	18	21
Diarrhea	21	14	24	7
Pain on Injection	12	13	3	0
Sepsis	17	12	14	9
Neurotoxicity	17	10	13	5
Streaking/Erythema	5	4	4	2
Phlebitis	6	3	3	5
Esophagitis	6	3	7	4
Dysphagia	8	0	10	5
Hemorrhage	2	3	2	1
Extravasation	1	3	1	2
Urticaria	2	2	2	0
Recall Skin Reaction	1	1	2	0

The adverse experiences listed above are likely attributable to the FAC regimen with the exception of pain on injection that was observed mainly on the dexrazoxane arm.

Myelosuppression: Patients receiving FAC with dexrazoxane experienced more severe leucopenia, granulocytopenia and thrombocytopenia at nadir than patients receiving FAC without dexrazoxane, but recovery counts were similar for the two groups of patients.

Hepatic and Renal: Some patients receiving FAC + dexrazoxane or FAC + placebo experienced marked abnormalities in hepatic or renal function test, but the frequency and severity of abnormalities in bilirubin, alkaline phosphatase, BUN, and creatinine were similar for patients receiving FAC with or without dexrazoxane.

OVERDOSAGE:

There have been no instances of drug overdose in the clinical studies sponsored by either Pharmacia Inc. or the National Cancer Institute. The maximum dose administered during the cardioprotective trials was 1000 mg/m^2 every three weeks.

Disposition studies with dexrazoxane have not been conducted in cancer patients undergoing dialysis, but retention of a significant dose fraction (>0.4) of the unchanged drug in the plasma pool, minimal tissue partitioning or binding, and availability of greater than 90% of the systemic drug levels in the unbound form suggest that it could be removed using conventional peritoneal or hemodialysis.

There is no known antidote for dexrazoxane. Instances of suspected overdose should be managed with good supportive care until resolution of myelosuppression and related conditions is complete. Management of overdose should include treatment of infections, fluid regulation, and maintenance of nutritional requirements.

DOSAGE AND ADMINISTRATION:

The recommended dosage ratio of dexrazoxane: DOX is 10:1 (*e.g.,* 500 mg/m^2 dexrazoxane: 50 mg/m^2 DOX). Dexrazoxane must be reconstituted with 0.167 Molar (M/6) Sodium Lactate Injection, USP, to give a concentration of 10 mg dexrazoxane for each ml of sodium lactate. The reconstituted solution should be given by slow I.V. push or rapid drip intravenous infusion from a bag. After completing the infusion of dexrazoxane, and prior to a total elapsed time of 30 minutes (from the beginning of the dexrazoxane infusion), the intravenous injection of doxorubicin should be given.

Incompatibility: Dexrazoxane should not be mixed with other drugs.

Parenteral drug products should be inspected visually for particulate matter and discoloration prior to administration, whenever solution and container permit.

Handling and Disposal: Caution in the handling and preparation of the reconstituted solution must be exercised and the use of gloves is recommended. If dexrazoxane powder or solutions contact the skin or mucosae, immediately wash thoroughly with soap and water.

Procedures normally used for proper handling and disposal of anticancer drugs should be considered for use with dexrazoxane. Several guidelines on this subject have been published.[1-7] There is no general agreement that all of the procedures recommended in the guidelines are necessary or appropriate.

REFERENCES:

1. Recommendations for the Safe Handling of Parenteral Antineoplastic Drugs. NIH Publication No. 83-2621. For sale by the Superintendent of Documents, U.S. Government Printing Office, Washington, DC 20402. **2.** AMA Council Report. Guidelines for Handling Parenteral Antineoplastics JAMA. 1985 March 15. **3.** National Study Commission on Cytotoxic Exposure-Recommendations for Handling Cytotoxic Agents. Available from Louis P. Jeffrey, Sc.D., Chairman, National Study Commission on Cytotoxic Exposure, Massachusetts College of Pharmacy and Allied Health Sciences, 179 Longwood Avenue, Boston, Massachusetts 02115. **4.** Clinical Oncological Society of Australia. Guidelines and Recommendations for Safe Handling of Antineoplastic Agents. Med J Australia. 1983; 1:426-428. **5.** Jones RB. et al. Safe handling of Chemotherapeutic Agents: A report from the Mount Sinai Medical Center. CA-A Cancer Journal for Clinicians. 1983; (Sept/Oct) 258-263. **6.** American Society of Hospital Pharmacists Technical Assistance Bulletin on Handling Cytotoxic and Hazardous Drugs. Am J Hosp Pharm. 1990; 47:1033-1049. **7.** OSHA Work-Practice Guidelines for Personnel Dealing with Cytotoxic (Antineoplastic) Drugs. Am J Hosp Pharm. 1986; 43:1193-1204.

HOW SUPPLIED:

Reconstituted dexrazoxane, when transferred to an empty infusion bag, is stable for 6 hours from the time of reconstitution when stored at controlled room temperature, 15° to 30°C (59° to 86°F) or under refrigeration, 2° to 8°C (36° to 46°F). DISCARD UNUSED SOLUTIONS.

The reconstituted dexrazoxane solution may be diluted with either 0.9% Sodium Chloride Injection, USP or 5.0% Dextrose Injection, USP to a concentration range of 1.3 to 5.0 mg/ml in intravenous infusion bags. The resultant solutions are stable for 6 hours when stored at controlled room temperature, 15° to 30°C (59° to 86°F) or under refrigeration, 2° to 8°C (36° to 46°F). DISCARD UNUSED SOLUTIONS.

Store at controlled room temperature, 15° to 30°C (59° to 86°F). Reconstituted solutions of dexrazoxane are stable for 6 hours at controlled room temperature or under refrigeration, 2° to 8°C (36° to 46°F). DISCARD UNUSED SOLUTIONS.

HOW SUPPLIED - EQUIVALENTS NOT AVAILABLE:

Injection, Solution - Intravenous - 250 mg

1's	$134.38	ZINECARD, Pharmacia & Upjohn	00013-8715-62

Injection, Solution - Intravenous - 500 mg

1's	$268.75	ZINECARD, Pharmacia & Upjohn	00013-8725-89

DEXTRAN *(000987)*

CATEGORIES: Blood Components/Substitutes; Blood Formation/Coagulation; EENT Drugs; Electrolytic, Caloric-Water Balance; Eye, Ear, Nose, & Throat Preparations; Irrigating Solutions; Replacement Solutions; FDA Pre 1938 Drugs

BRAND NAMES: Dextran 70; Dextran 70/Hydroxypropylmethyl; Dextran 75 In Normal Saline; Gentran 75 In Travert 10Pc; Hyskon; Macrodex; Poly-Tears

FORMULARIES: WHO

Prescribing information not available at time of publication.

HOW SUPPLIED - EQUIVALENTS NOT AVAILABLE:

Injection, Solution - Intravenous - 6 %

500 ml	$86.70	6% DEXTRAN & 0.9% SODIUM, Abbott	00074-1505-04
500 ml	$86.70	6% DEXTRAN 75 & 5% DEXTROSE, Abbott	00074-1507-04
500 ml	$1071.60	Dextran 75 In Normal Saline, Abbott	00074-1505-03

Injection, Solution - Intravenous - 32 %

100 ml	$36.67	DEXTRAN 70, Abbott	00074-8085-01

Solution - Ophthalmic

15 ml	$3.75	Poly-Tears, IDE-Interstate	00814-6150-42

DEXTRAN 1 *(000988)*

CATEGORIES: Blood Components/Substitutes; Blood Formation/Coagulation; Electrolytic, Caloric-Water Balance; Replacement Solutions; FDA Pre 1938 Drugs

BRAND NAMES: Promit; *Promiten*
(International brand names outside U.S. in italics)

Prescribing information not available at time of publication.

DEXTRAN; DEXTROSE *(000989)*

CATEGORIES: Blood Components/Substitutes; Blood Formation/Coagulation; Electrolyte Solutions; Electrolytic, Caloric-Water Balance; Homeostatic & Nutrient; Replacement Solutions; FDA Pre 1938 Drugs

BRAND NAMES: Dextran 40 In Dextrose 5Pc; *Dextran 40 Injection*; *Dextran 70 Injection*; Dextran 75 In Dextrose 5%; Dextran 75 In Dextrose 5Pc; Gentran 40; Gentran 40 In D5W; Gentran 40 W/D5W; *Gentran 70*; Lmd 10% W/5% Dextrose; *Lomodex*; *Lomodex-70*; Macrodex; *Macrodex 6%*; *Marodex-D*; *Rheodex-D S*; Rheomacrodex; *Rheomacrodex 10%* (Germany); Rheomacrodex In Dextrose 5%; Rheomacrodex In Dextrose 5Pc
(International brand names outside U.S. in italics)

Prescribing information not available at time of publication.

HOW SUPPLIED - EQUIVALENTS NOT AVAILABLE:

Injection, Solution - Intravenous - 10 gm/5 gm

500 ml	$89.30	DEXTRAN 75 IN DEXTROSE 5%, Abbott	00074-1507-03
500 ml	$99.43	GENTRAN 40 & DEXTROSE, Baxter Hlthcare	00338-0272-03
500 ml	$122.89	10% LMD & 5% DEXTROSE, Abbott	00074-1554-04
500 ml	$123.00	Lmd 10% W/5% Dextrose, Abbott	00074-7418-03
500 ml x 12	$128.21	10% DEXTRAN 40 IN 5% DEXTROSE, McGaw	00264-1962-10

DEXTRAN; SODIUM CHLORIDE *(000990)*

CATEGORIES: Blood Components/Substitutes; Blood Formation/Coagulation; Electrolyte Solutions; Electrolytic, Caloric-Water Balance; Homeostatic & Nutrient; Irrigating Solutions; Replacement Solutions; FDA Pre 1938 Drugs

BRAND NAMES: Dextran 40 In Normal Saline; *Dextran 40 Injection*; Dextran 70 In Normal Saline; *Dextran 70 Injection*; Dextran 75 In Normal Saline; Dextran In Dextrose; *Dextril 70*; Gentran 40; *Gentran 70*; Gentran 40 In Normal Saline; Gentran 75; Gentran 75 In Normal Saline; Hyskon; Lmd 10% W/0.9% Sodium Chloride; *Lomodex*; *Lomodex-70*; Macrodex; *Macrodex 6%* (England); *Macrodex-6%*; Macrodex In Dextrose 5Pc; Macrodex In Normal Saline; Rheomacrodex; *Rheomacrodex 10%* (England, Germany); Rheomacrodex In Normal Saline
(International brand names outside U.S. in italics)

Prescribing information not available at time of publication.

HOW SUPPLIED - EQUIVALENTS NOT AVAILABLE:

Injection, Solution - Intravenous - 6 gm/0.9 gm

500 ml	$73.46	GENTRAN 75 IN SODIUM CHLORIDE, Baxter Hlthcare	00338-0265-03
500 ml x 12	$47.94	6% DEXTRAN 70/0.9% SODIUM CHLORIDE, McGaw	00264-1960-10

Injection, Solution - Intravenous - 10 gm/0.9 gm

500 ml	$99.43	GENTRAN 40 & SODIUM CHLORIDE, Baxter Hlthcare	00338-0270-03
500 ml	$122.89	10% LMD & 0.9% SODIUM, Abbott	00074-1556-04
500 ml	$123.00	Lmd 10% W/0.9% Sodium Chloride, Abbott	00074-7419-03
500 ml x 12	$128.21	10% DEXTRAN 40/0.9% SODIUM CHLORIDE, McGaw	00264-1963-10

DEXTROAMPHETAMINE SULFATE *(000992)*

CATEGORIES: Amphetamines; Anorexients/CNS Stimulants; Appetite Suppressants; Attention Deficit Disorders; Central Nervous System Agents; Narcolepsy; Obesity; Psychostimulants; Respiratory/Cerebral Stimulant; Sympathomimetic Agents; Pregnancy Category C; DEA Class CII; FDA Approval Pre 1982

BRAND NAMES: *Amphaetex*; Das; Dexampex; *Dexamphetamine* (Australia); *Dexamphetamini Sulfas*; *Dexedrina*; **Dexedrine**; *Dexedrine Spansule* (Canada); Ferndex; Oxydess; Spancap No. 1
(International brand names outside U.S. in italics)

FORMULARIES: Aetna; BC-BS; Medi-Cal; PCS

AMPHETAMINES HAVE A HIGH POTENTIAL FOR ABUSE. THEY SHOULD THUS BE TRIED ONLY IN WEIGHT REDUCTION PROGRAMS FOR PATIENTS IN WHOM ALTERNATIVE THERAPY HAS BEEN INEFFECTIVE. ADMINISTRATION OF AMPHETAMINES FOR PROLONGED PERIODS OF TIME IN OBESITY MAY LEAD TO DRUG DEPENDENCE AND MUST BE AVOIDED. PARTICULAR ATTENTION SHOULD BE PAID TO THE POSSIBILITY OF SUBJECTS OBTAINING AMPHETAMINES FOR NON-THERAPEUTIC USE OR DISTRIBUTION TO OTHERS, AND THE DRUGS SHOULD BE PRESCRIBED OR DISPENSED SPARINGLY.

DESCRIPTION:

Dextroamphetamine sulfate is the dextro isomer of the compound *d, l*-amphetamine sulfate, a sympathomimetic amine of the amphetamine group. Chemically, dextroamphetamine is*d*-alpha-methylphenethylamine, and is present in all forms of Dextroamphetamine sulfate as the neutral sulfate.

Sustained Release Capsules: Each sustained release capsule is so prepared that an initial dose is released promptly and the remaining medication is released gradually over a prolonged period.

Each capsule, contains dextroamphetamine sulfate as follows: 5 mg, 10 mg, and 15 mg. Inactive ingredients consist of acacia, benzyl alcohol, calcium sulfate, cetylpyridinium chloride, FD&C Blue No. 1, FD&C Red No. 40, FD&C Yellow No. 5 (tartrazine), FD&C Yellow No. 6, gelatin, glyceryl distearate, glyceryl monostearate, sodium lauryl sulfate, starch, sucrose, wax and trace amounts of other inactive ingredients.

Tablets: Each triangular, orange, scored tablet contains dextroamphetamine sulfate, 5 mg. Inactive ingredients consist of calcium sulfate, FD&C Yellow No. 5 (tartrazine), FD&C Yellow No. 6, gelatin, lactose, mineral oil, starch, stearic acid, sucrose, talc and trace amounts of other inactive ingredients.

CLINICAL PHARMACOLOGY:

Amphetamines are non-catecholamine, sympathomimetic amines with CNS stimulant activity. Peripheral actions include elevations of systolic and diastolic blood pressures and weak bronchodilator and respiratory stimulant action.

There is neither specific evidence which clearly establishes the mechanism whereby amphetamines produce mental and behavioral effects in children, nor conclusive evidence regarding how these effects relate to the condition of the central nervous system.

Drugs of this class used in obesity are commonly known as "anorectics" or "anorexigenics." It has not been established, however, that the action of such drugs in treating obesity is primarily one of appetite suppression. Other central nervous system actions, or metabolic effects, may be involved, for example.

Adult obese subjects instructed in dietary management and treated with "anorectic" drugs lose more weight on the average than those treated with placebo and diet, as determined in relatively short-term clinical trials.

The magnitude of increased weight loss of drug-treated patients over placebo-treated patients is only a fraction of a pound a week. The rate of weight loss is greatest in the first weeks of therapy for both drug and placebo subjects and tends to decrease in succeeding weeks. The origins of the increased weight loss due to the various possible drug effects are not established. The amount of weight loss associated with the use of an "anorectic" drug varies from trial to trial, and the increased weight loss appears to be related in part to variables other than the drug prescribed, such as the physician-investigator, the population treated and the diet prescribed. Studies do not permit conclusions as to the relative importance of the drug and nondrug factors on weight loss.

The natural history of obesity is measured in years, whereas the studies cited are restricted to a few weeks' duration; thus, the total impact of drug-induced weight loss over that of diet alone must be considered clinically limited.

Dextroamphetamine sulfate sustained release capsules are formulated to release the active drug substance *in vivo* in a more gradual fashion than the standard formulation, as demonstrated by blood levels. The formulation has not been shown superior in effectiveness over the same dosage of the standard, noncontrolled-release formulations given in divided doses.

PHARMACOKINETICS

Tablet: The single ingestion of two 5 mg tablets by healthy volunteers produced an average peak dextroamphetamine blood level of 29.2 ng/ml at 2 hours post-administration. The average half-life was 10.25 hours. The average urinary recovery was 45% in 48 hours.

Sustained Release Capsules: Ingestion of a sustained release capsule containing 15 mg radiolabeled dextroamphetamine sulfate by healthy volunteers produced a peak blood level of radioactivity, on the average, at 8 to 10 hours post-administration with peak urinary recovery seen at 12 to 24 hours.

INDICATIONS AND USAGE:

Dextroamphetamine sulfate is indicated:

1. IN NARCOLEPSY.

2. In Attention Deficit Disorder with Hyperactivity: As an integral part of a total treatment program which typically includes other remedial measures (psychological, educational, social) for a stabilizing effect in children with a behavioral syndrome characterized by the following group of developmentally inappropriate symptoms: moderate to severe distractibility, short attention span, hyperactivity, emotional lability, and impulsivity. The diagnosis of this syndrome should not be made with finality when these symptoms are only of comparatively recent origin. Nonlocalizing (soft) neurological signs, learning disability, and abnormal EEG may or may not be present, and a diagnosis of central nervous system dysfunction may or may not be warranted.

CONTRAINDICATIONS:

Advanced arteriosclerosis, symptomatic cardiovascular disease, moderate to severe hypertension, hyperthyroidism, known hypersensitivity or idiosyncrasy to the sympathomimetic amines, glaucoma.

Agitated states.

Patients with a history of drug abuse.

During or within 14 days following the administration of monoamine oxidase inhibitors (hypertensive crises may result).

WARNINGS:

When tolerance to the "anorectic" effect develops, the recommended dose should not be exceeded in an attempt to increase the effect; rather, the drug should be discontinued.

PRECAUTIONS:

General: Caution is to be exercised in prescribing amphetamines for patients with even mild hypertension.

The least amount feasible should be prescribed or dispensed at one time in order to minimize the possibility of overdosage.

These products contain FD&C Yellow No. 5 (tartrazine), which may cause allergic-type reactions (including bronchial asthma) in certain susceptible individuals. Although the overall incidence of FD&C Yellow No. 5 (tartrazine) sensitivity in the general population is low, it is frequently seen in patients who also have aspirin hypersensitivity.

Information for the Patient: Amphetamines may impair the ability of the patient to engage in potentially hazardous activities such as operating machinery or vehicles; the patient should therefore be cautioned accordingly.

DRUG/LABORATORY TEST INTERACTIONS

Amphetamines can cause a significant elevation in plasma corticosteroid levels. This increase is greatest in the evening.

Amphetamines may interfere with urinary steroid determinations.

Carcinogenesis/Mutagenesis: Mutagenicity studies and long-term studies in animals to determine the carcinogenic potential of Dextroamphetamine sulfate have not been performed.

Pregnancy, Teratogenic Effects, Pregnancy Category C: Dextroamphetamine sulfate has been shown to have embryotoxic and teratogenic effects when administered to A/Jax mice and C57BL mice in doses approximately 41 times the maximum human dose. Embryotoxic effects were not seen in New Zealand white rabbits given the drug in doses 7 times the human dose nor in rats given 12.5 times the maximum human dose. There are no adequate and well-controlled studies in pregnant women. Dextroamphetamine sulfate should be used during pregnancy only if the potential benefit justifies the potential risk to the fetus.

Nonteratogenic Effects: Infants born to mothers dependent on amphetamines have an increased risk of premature delivery and low birth weight. Also, these infants may experience symptoms of withdrawal as demonstrated by dysphoria, including agitation, and significant lassitude.

Nursing Mothers: Amphetamines are excreted in human milk. Mothers taking amphetamines should be advised to refrain from nursing.

Pediatric Use: Long-term effects of amphetamines in children have not been well established.

Amphetamines are not recommended for use as anorectic agents in children under 12 years of age, or in children under 3 years of age with Attention Deficit Disorder with Hyperactivity described under INDICATIONS AND USAGE.

Clinical experience suggests that in psychotic children, administration of amphetamines may exacerbate symptoms of behavior disturbance and thought disorder.

Amphetamines have been reported to exacerbate motor and phonic tics and Tourette's syndrome. Therefore, clinical evaluation for tics and Tourette's syndrome in children and their families should precede use of stimulant medications.

Data are inadequate to determine whether chronic administration of amphetamines may be associated with growth inhibition; therefore, growth should be monitored during treatment.

Drug treatment is not indicated in all cases of Attention Deficit Disorder with Hyperactivity and should be considered only in light of the complete history and evaluation of the child.

The decision to prescribe amphetamines should depend on the physician's assessment of the chronicity and severity of the child's symptoms and their appropriateness for his/her age. Prescription should not depend solely on the presence of one or more of the behavioral characteristics.

When these symptoms are associated with acute stress reactions, treatment with amphetamines is usually not indicated.

DRUG INTERACTIONS:

Acidifying Agents: Gastrointestinal acidifying agents (guanethidine, reserpine, glutamic acid HCl, ascorbic acid, fruit juices, etc.) lower absorption of amphetamines. Urinary acidifying agents (ammonium chloride, sodium acid phosphate, etc.) increase the concentration of the ionized species of the amphetamine molecule, thereby increasing urinary excretion. Both groups of agents lower blood levels and efficacy of amphetamines.

Adrenergic Blockers: Adrenergic blockers are inhibited by amphetamines.

Alkalinizing Agents: Gastrointestinal alkalinizing agents (sodium bicarbonate, etc.) increase absorption of amphetamines. Urinary alkalinizing agents (acetazolamide, some thiazides) increase the concentration of the non-ionized species of the amphetamine molecule, thereby decreasing urinary excretion. Both groups of agents increase blood levels and therefore potentiate the actions of amphetamines.

Antidepressants, Tricyclic: Amphetamines may enhance the activity of tricyclic or sympathomimetic agents; d-amphetamine with desipramine or protriptyline and possibly other tricyclics cause striking and sustained increases in the concentration of d-amphetamine in the brain; cardiovascular effects can be potentiated.

MAO Inhibitors: MAOI antidepressants, as well as a metabolite of furazolidone, slow amphetamine metabolism. This slowing potentiates amphetamines, increasing their effect on the release of norepinephrine and other monoamines from adrenergic nerve endings; this can cause headaches and other signs of hypertensive crisis. A variety of neurological toxic effects and malignant hyperpyrexia can occur, sometimes with fatal results.

Antihistamines: Amphetamines may counteract the sedative effect of antihistamines.

Antihypertensives: Amphetamines may antagonize the hypotensive effects of antihypertensives.

Chlorpromazine: Chlorpromazine blocks dopamine and norepinephrine reuptake, thus inhibiting the central stimulant effects of amphetamines, and can be used to treat amphetamine poisoning.

Ethosuximide: Amphetamines may delay intestinal absorption of ethosuximide.

Haloperidol: Haloperidol blocks dopamine and norepinephrine reuptake, thus inhibiting the central stimulant effects of amphetamines.

Lithium Carbonate: The antiobesity and stimulatory effects of amphetamines may be inhibited by lithium carbonate.

Meperidine: Amphetamines potentiate the analgesic effect of meperidine.

Methenamine Therapy: Urinary excretion of amphetamines is increased, and efficacy is reduced, by acidifying agents used in methenamine therapy.

Norepinephrine: Amphetamines enhance the adrenergic effect of norepinephrine.

Phenobarbital: Amphetamines may delay intestinal absorption of phenobarbital; co-administration of phenobarbital may produce a synergistic anticonvulsant action.

Phenytoin: Amphetamines may delay intestinal absorption of phenytoin; co-administration of phenytoin may produce a synergistic anticonvulsant action.

Propoxyphene: In cases of propoxyphene overdosage, amphetamine CNS stimulation is potentiated and fatal convulsions can occur.

Veratrum Alkaloids: Amphetamines inhibit the hypotensive effect of veratrum alkaloids.

ADVERSE REACTIONS:

Cardiovascular: Palpitations, tachycardia, elevation of blood pressure. There have been isolated reports of cardiomyopathy associated with chronic amphetamine use.

Central Nervous System: Psychotic episodes at recommended doses (rare), overstimulation, restlessness, dizziness, insomnia, euphoria, dyskinesia, dysphoria, tremor, headache, exacerbation of motor and phonic tics and Tourette's syndrome.

Gastrointestinal: Dryness of the mouth, unpleasant taste, diarrhea, constipation, other gastrointestinal disturbances. Anorexia and weight loss may occur as undesirable effects when amphetamines are used for other than the anorectic effect.

Allergic: Urticaria.

Endocrine: Impotence, changes in libido.

DRUG ABUSE AND DEPENDENCE:

Dextroamphetamine sulfate is a Schedule II controlled substance.

Amphetamines have been extensively abused. Tolerance, extreme psychological dependence and severe social disability have occurred. There are reports of patients who have increased the dosage to many times that recommended. Abrupt cessation following prolonged high dosage administration results in extreme fatigue and mental depression; changes are also noted on the sleep EEG.

Manifestations of chronic intoxication with amphetamines include severe dermatoses, marked insomnia, irritability, hyperactivity and personality changes. The most severe manifestation of chronic intoxication is psychosis, often clinically indistinguishable from schizophrenia. This is rare with oral amphetamines.

OVERDOSAGE:

Individual patient response to amphetamines varies widely. While toxic symptoms occasionally occur as an idiosyncrasy at doses as low as 2 mg, they are rare with doses of less than 15 mg; 30 mg can produce severe reactions, yet doses of 400 to 500 mg are not necessarily fatal.

In rats, the oral LD_{50} of dextroamphetamine sulfate is 96.8 mg/kg.

Manifestations of acute overdosage with amphetamines include restlessness, tremor, hyperreflexia, rhabdomyolysis, rapid respiration, hyperpyrexia, confusion, assaultiveness, hallucinations, panic states.

Fatigue and depression usually follow the central stimulation.

Cardiovascular effects include arrhythmias, hypertension or hypotension and circulatory collapse. Gastrointestinal symptoms include nausea, vomiting, diarrhea and abdominal cramps. Fatal poisoning is usually preceded by convulsions and coma.

Treatment: Management of acute amphetamine intoxication is largely symptomatic and includes gastric lavage and sedation with a barbiturate. Experience with hemodialysis or peritoneal dialysis is inadequate to permit recommendation in this regard. Acidification of the urine increases amphetamine excretion. If acute, severe hypertension complicates amphetamine overdosage, administration of intravenous phentolamine (Regitine, CIBA) has been suggested. However, a gradual drop in blood pressure will usually result when sufficient sedation has been achieved.

Chlorpromazine antagonizes the central stimulant effects of amphetamines and can be used to treat amphetamine intoxication.

Since much of the sustained release capsule medication is coated for gradual release, therapy directed at reversing the effects of the ingested drug and at supporting the patient should be continued for as long as overdosage symptoms remain. Saline cathartics are useful for hastening the evacuation of pellets that have not already released medication.

DOSAGE AND ADMINISTRATION:

Regardless of indication, amphetamines should be administered at the lowest effective dosage and dosage should be individually adjusted. Late evening doses—particularly with the sustained release capsule form—should be avoided because of the resulting insomnia.

Narcolepsy: Usual dose 5 to 60 mg per day in divided doses, depending on the individual patient response.

Narcolepsy seldom occurs in children under 12 years of age; however, when it does, Dextroamphetamine sulfate may be used. The suggested initial dose for patients aged 6-12 is 5 mg daily; daily dose may be raised in increments of 5 mg at weekly intervals until optimal response is obtained. In patients 12 years of age and older, start with 10 mg daily; daily dosage may be raised in increments of 10 mg at weekly intervals until optimal response is obtained. If bothersome adverse reactions appear (*e.g.*, insomnia or anorexia), dosage should be reduced. Sustained release capsules may be used for once-a-day dosage wherever appropriate. With tablets, give first dose on awakening; additional doses (1 or 2) at intervals of 4 to 6 hours.

Attention Deficit Disorder with Hyperactivity: Not recommended for children under 3 years of age.

In Children From 3 to 5 Years of Age: Start with 2.5 mg daily, by tablet; daily dosage may be raised in increments of 2.5 mg at weekly intervals until optimal response is obtained.

In Children 6 Years of Age and Older: Start with 5 mg once or twice daily; daily dosage may be raised in increments of 5 mg at weekly intervals until optimal response is obtained. Only in rare cases will it be necessary to exceed a total of 40 mg per day.

Sustained release capsules may be used for once-a-day dosage wherever appropriate.

With tablets, give first dose on awakening; additional doses (1 or 2) at intervals of 4 to 6 hours.

Where possible, drug administration should be interrupted occasionally to determine if there is a recurrence of behavioral symptoms sufficient to require continued therapy.

Store at controlled room temperature (15° to 30°C; 59° to 86°F). Dispense in a tight, light-resistant container.

HOW SUPPLIED - RATED THERAPEUTICALLY EQUIVALENT:

Tablet, Uncoated - Oral - 5 mg

100's	$17.58	Dextroamphetamine Sulfate, Rexar	00478-5451-01
100's	$19.13	Dextroamphetamine Sulfate, H.C.F.A. F F P	99999-0992-01
100's	**$19.65**	**DEXEDRINE, SKB Pharms**	**00007-3519-20**
500's	$86.33	Dextroamphetamine Sulfate, Rexar	00478-5451-05
500's	$95.65	Dextroamphetamine Sulfate, H.C.F.A. F F P	99999-0992-02
500's	$147.23	Dexedrine, Rugby	00536-3598-05
1000's	$150.05	Dextroamphetamine Sulfate, Rexar	00478-5451-10
1000's	$191.30	Dextroamphetamine Sulfate, H.C.F.A. F F P	99999-0992-03

Tablet, Uncoated - Oral - 10 mg

100's	$29.80	Dextroamphetamine Sulfate, Rexar	00478-5452-01
500's	$137.28	Dextroamphetamine Sulfate, Rexar	00478-5452-05
1000's	$227.93	Dextroamphetamine Sulfate, Rexar	00478-5452-10

HOW SUPPLIED - NOT RATED EQUIVALENT:

Capsule, Gelatin, Sustained Action - Oral - 5 mg

50's	**$21.30**	**DEXEDRINE, SKB Pharms**	**00007-3512-15**

Capsule, Gelatin, Sustained Action - Oral - 10 mg

50's	**$26.55**	**DEXEDRINE, SKB Pharms**	**00007-3513-15**

Capsule, Gelatin, Sustained Action - Oral - 15 mg

50's	**$33.90**	**DEXEDRINE, SKB Pharms**	**00007-3514-15**

Tablet, Uncoated - Oral - 5 mg

100's	$17.50	DEXTROSTAT, YELLOW, Richwood Pharm	58521-0451-01
500's	$83.27	Dextrostat, Richwood Pharm	58521-0451-05
1000's	$162.62	Dextrostat, Richwood Pharm	58521-0451-10

Tablet, Uncoated - Oral - 10 mg

100's	$31.55	Dextrostat, Richwood Pharm	58521-0452-01
500's	$149.88	Dextrostat, Richwood Pharm	58521-0452-05
1000's	$299.75	Dextrostat, Richwood Pharm	58521-0452-10

DEXTROMETHORPHAN HYDROBROMIDE; GUAIFENESIN *(001000)*

CATEGORIES: Antitussives; Cough Preparations; Expectorants; DEA Class CIII; FDA Pre 1938 Drugs

BRAND NAMES: Aquabid-Dm; Broncot; Fenex Dm; Gani-Tuss-Dm Nr; Guaibid Dm; Guaifenesin Dm; Guaifenesin W/Dextromethorphan; Guiadrine Dm; Humibid Dm; Iofen-Dm Nf; Muco-Fen Dm; Mucobid Dm; Numobid Dx; Pancof Hc; Q-Mibid-Dm; Robafen-Dm; Tusnel; Tussi-Organidin Dm Nr; Tussi-Organidin Dm-S Nr; Tussidin Dm Nr; Tussin Dm

FORMULARIES: Aetna

DESCRIPTION:

Each dark green, scored, sustained-release tablet provides 600 mg guaifenesin and 30 mg dextromethorphan hydrobromide. Inactive ingredients: Dibasic calcium phosphate, stearic acid, FD & C Blue #1 Lake, D & C Yellow #10 Lake, sodium lauryl sulfate, ethylcellulose, magnesium stearate. Chemically, guaifenesin is 3-(2-methoxyphenoxy)-1,2- propanediol.

Dextromethorphan hydrobromide is a salt of the methyl ether of the dextrorotatory isomer of levorphanol, a narcotic analgesic. Chemically, it is 3-methoxy-17-methyl-9α, 13α, 14α-morphinan hydrobromide monohydrate.

CLINICAL PHARMACOLOGY:

Guaifenesin is an expectorant which increases respiratory tract fluid secretions and helps to loosen phlegm and bronchial secretions. By reducing the viscosity of secretions, guaifenesin increases the efficiency of the mucociliary mechanism in removing accumulated secretions from the upper and lower airway. Guaifenesin is readily absorbed from the gastrointestinal tract and is rapidly metabolized and excreted in the urine. Guaifenesin has a plasma half-life of one hour. The major urinary metabolite is β-(2-methoxyphenoxy) lactic acid.

Dextromethorphan is an antitussive agent which, unlike the isomeric levorphanol, has no analgesic or addictive properties. The drug acts centrally and elevates the threshold for coughing. It is about equal to codeine in depressing the cough reflex. In therapeutic dosage, dextromethorphan does not inhibit ciliary activity. Dextromethorphan is rapidly absorbed from the gastrointestinal tract, metabolized by the liver and excreted primarily in the urine.

$C_{18}H_{25}NO°HBr°H_2O$ MW = 370.33

INDICATIONS AND USAGE:

These combination drug tablets are indicated for the temporary relief of coughs associated with upper respiratory tract infections and related conditions such as sinusitis, pharyngitis, and bronchitis, particularly when these conditions are complicated by tenacious mucus and/or mucus plugs and congestion. The product is effective in productive as well as non-productive cough, but is of particular value in dry, non-productive cough which tends to injure the mucous membrane of the air passages.

CONTRAINDICATIONS:

The drug is contraindicated in patients with hypersensitivity to guaifenesin or dextromethorphan and in patients receiving monoamine oxidase inhibitor (MAOI) therapy and for 14 days after stopping MAOI therapy. (See DRUG INTERACTIONS.)

PRECAUTIONS:

General: Before prescribing medication to suppress or modify cough, it is important that the underlying cause of cough is identified, that modification of cough does not increase the risk of clinical or physiological complications, and that appropriate therapy for the primary disease is instituted.

Dextromethorphan should be used with caution in sedated or debilitated patients, and in patients confined to the supine position.

Drug/Laboratory Test Interactions: Guaifenesin may increase renal clearance for urate and thereby lower serum uric acid levels. Guaifenesin may produce an increase in urinary 5-hydroxyindoleacetic acid and may therefore interfere with the interpretation of this test for the diagnosis of carcinoid syndrome. It may also falsely elevate the VMA test for catechols. Administration of this product should be discontinued 48 hours prior to the collection of urine specimens for such tests.

Carcinogenesis, Mutagenesis, and Impairment of Fertility: No data are available on the long-term potential of guaifenesin or of dextromethorphan for carcinogenesis, mutagenesis, or impairment of fertility in animals or humans.

Pregnancy Category C: Animal reproduction studies have not been conducted with these combination drug tablets. It is also not known whether these combination drug tablets can cause fetal harm when administered to a pregnant woman or can affect reproduction capacity. These combination drug tablets should be given to a pregnant woman only if clearly needed.

Nursing Mothers: It is not known whether guaifenesin or dextromethorphan is excreted in human milk. Because many drugs are excreted in human milk, caution should be exercised when this product is administered to a nursing woman and a decision should be made whether to discontinue nursing or to discontinue the drug, taking into account the importance of the drug to the mother.

DRUG INTERACTIONS:

Do not prescribe this product for use in patients that are now taking a prescription MAOI (certain drugs for depression, psychiatric or emotional conditions, or Parkinson's disease), or for 14 days after stopping the MAOI drug therapy.

ADVERSE REACTIONS:

No serious side effects from guaifenesin or dextromethorphan have been reported.

OVERDOSAGE:

Overdosage with guaifenesin is unlikely to produce toxic effects since its toxicity is low. Guaifenesin, when administered by stomach tube to test animals in doses up to 5 grams/kg, produced no signs of toxicity. In severe cases of overdosage, treatment should be aimed at reducing further absorption of the drug. Gastric emptying (Syrup of Ipecac) and/or lavage is recommended as soon as possible after ingestion.

Overdosage with dextromethorphan may produce central excitement and mental confusion. Very high doses may produce respiratory depression. One case of toxic psychosis (hyperactivity, marked visual and auditory hallucinations) after ingestion of a single 300 mg dose of dextromethorphan has been reported.

DOSAGE AND ADMINISTRATION:

Adults and children over 12 years of age: One or two tablets every 12 hours not to exceed 4 tablets in 24 hours. **Children 6 to 12 years:** One tablet every 12 hours not to exceed 2 tablets in 24 hours.**Children 2 to 6 years:** 1/2 tablet every 12 hours not to exceed 1 tablet in 24 hours.

(Adams Laboratories, Inc., 6/94, 304/694)

HOW SUPPLIED - EQUIVALENTS NOT AVAILABLE:

Capsule, Sprinkle - Oral - 15 mg/300 mg

100's	$61.25	HUMIBID DM, SPRINKLE, Medeva Pharms	53014-0034-10

Elixir - Oral - 15 gm/100 mg

1 pt	$7.50	Broncot, C O Truxton	00463-9035-16
480 ml	$46.42	Iofen-Dm Nf, Superior	00144-0638-16

Liquid - Oral - 2 mg/2.5 mg/30

120 ml x 4	$55.33	TUSSI-ORGANIDIN DM-S NR, Wallace Labs	00037-4714-01
178 ml	$6.66	TUSNEL, Llorens Pharm	54859-0502-06
480 ml	$58.03	TUSSI-ORGANIDIN DM NR, Wallace Labs	00037-4714-10
3840 ml	$36.75	ROBAFEN-DM, Major Pharms	00904-0053-28

Liquid - Oral - 100 mg/10 mg/5m

480 ml	$11.50	Guaifenesin Dm, Morton Grove	60432-0048-16
480 ml	$39.95	Gani-Tuss-Dm Nr, Cypress Pharm	60258-0262-16

Tablet, Coated, Sustained Action - Oral - 600 mg/30 mg

100's	$39.14	Guaifenex Dm, Ethex	58177-0213-04
100's	$39.50	Muco-Fen Dm, Wakefield Pharms	59310-0108-10
100's	$41.50	Guaifenesin W/Dextromethorphan, Aligen Independ	00405-4458-01
100's	$41.50	Guiadrine Dm, Pharmacist Choice	54979-0150-01
100's	$41.50	Mucobid Dm, Econolab	55053-0090-01
100's	$41.50	Fenex Dm, Tmk Pharm	59582-0917-01
100's	$42.30	Guaibid Dm, Vintage Pharms	00254-5311-28
100's	$42.30	Q-Mibid-Dm, Qualitest Pharms	00603-5542-21
100's	$42.75	Aquabid-Dm, Alphagen Labs	59743-0054-01
100's	$43.00	Guaifenesin W/Dextromethorphan, Duramed Pharms	51285-0420-02
100's	$43.98	Touro Dm, Dartmouth Pharms	58869-0311-01
100's	$44.03	Guaifenesin Dm, Rugby	00536-5591-01
100's	$44.54	Guiadrine Dm, HL Moore Drug Exch	00839-7897-06
100's	$46.00	Respa-Dm, Respa Pharms	60575-0123-19
100's	$46.35	Guaifenesin W/Dextromethorphan, United Res	00677-1486-01
100's	$50.40	Guaifenesin W/Dextromethorphan, Goldline Labs	00182-1042-01
100's	$75.65	HUMIBID DM, Medeva Pharms	53014-0030-10
100's	$88.00	NUMOBID DX, Teral Labs	51234-0153-90
250's	$89.50	Aquabid-Dm, Alphagen Labs	59743-0054-25
250's	$93.95	Guiadrine Dm, Pharmacist Choice	54979-0150-02

HOW SUPPLIED - EQUIVALENTS NOT AVAILABLE: *(cont'd)*

250's	$99.88	Guaibid Dm, Vintage Pharms	00254-5311-33
250's	$99.88	Q-Bid-Dm, Qualitest Pharms	00603-5542-24
500's	$99.95	Guaifenesin W/Dextromethorphan, Duramed Pharms	51285-0420-04
500's	$190.76	Guaibid Dm, Vintage Pharms	00254-5311-35
500's	$190.76	Q-Bid-Dm, Qualitest Pharms	00603-5542-28
500's	$332.71	HUMIBID DM, Medeva Pharms	53014-0030-50
1000's	$191.00	Guaifenesin W/Dextromethorphan, Duramed Pharms	51285-0420-05

DEXTROMETHORPHAN HYDROBROMIDE; GUAIFENESIN; PHENYLEPHRINE HYDROCHLORIDE *(001002)*

CATEGORIES: Cough Preparations; Expectorants

BRAND NAMES: Albatussin Sr; Giltuss; Numonyl Dx

Prescribing information not available at time of publication.

HOW SUPPLIED - EQUIVALENTS NOT AVAILABLE:

Expectorant - Oral

30 ml	$15.15	NUMONYL DX, Teral Labs	51234-0171-77
120 ml	$15.25	NUMONYL DX, Teral Labs	51234-0172-04

Tablet, Coated, Sustained Action - Oral

100's	$107.00	ALBATUSSIN SR, Alba Pharma	10023-0301-90

DEXTROMETHORPHAN HYDROBROMIDE; GUAIFENESIN; PSEUDOEPHEDRINE *(001003)*

CATEGORIES: Antitussives; Antitussives/Expectorants/Mucolytics; Cough Preparations; Expectorants; Respiratory & Allergy Medications; FDA Pre 1938 Drugs

BRAND NAMES: Broncot; *Dimacol*; Eff Str Cough W/Decongestant; Nasalspan; Noratuss II; Novadyne Dmx; Novagest Dex; Pseudogest; Rolatuss; Ru-Tuss; Ru-Tuss Expectorant; Syn-Rx Dm; *Thymicol*
(International brand names outside U.S. in italics)

DESCRIPTION:

Each Syn-Rx DM 14 Day Treatment Regimen pack of 56 tablets consists of two different drug treatment phases as follows: an **AM Treatment Phase**

comprised of 28 light blue scored controlled-release tablets, each containing 60 mg pseudoephedrine HCl and 600 mg guaifenesin, embossed with "Adams/310"; and **PM Treatment Phase** comprised of 28 yellow scored controlled-release tablets, each containing 30 mg dextromethorphan hydrobromide and 600 mg guaifenesin, embossed with "Adams/309".

This combination drug contains ingredients of three therapeutic classes; nasal decongestant, antitussive, and expectorant.

Pseudoephedrine hydrochloride is a nasal decongestant. Chemically, it is [S-(R*,R*)]-[1-(methylamino)ethyl] benzenemethanol hydrochloride and has a chemical formula of $C_{10}H_{15}NO°HCl$ and it's molecular weight is 201.70.

Dextromethorphan hydrobromide is a salt of the methyl ether of the dextrorotatory isomer of levorphanol, a narcotic analgesic. Chemically, it is 3-methoxy-17-methyl-9α,13α,14α-morphinan hydrobromide monohydrate and has a chemical formula of $C_{18}H_{25}NO{\cdot}HBr{\cdot}H_2O$ and a molecular weight of 370.33.

Guaifenesin is an expectorant. Chemically, it is 3-(2-methoxyphenoxy)-1,2-propanediol and has a chemical formula of $C_{10}H_{14}O_4$ and a molecular weight of 198.22.

Inactive Ingredients: Each light blue AM tablet and yellow PM tablet contains Stearic acid, dibasic calcium phosphate sodium lauryl sulfate, ethylcellulose, magnesium stearate. Each light blue AM tablet also contains FD&C Blue #1 Aluminum Lake. Each yellow PM tablet also contains D & C Yellow #10 Lake.

CLINICAL PHARMACOLOGY:

Pseudoephedrine hydrochloride is an orally indirect acting sympathomimetic amine and exerts a decongestant action on the nasal mucosa. It does this by vasoconstriction which results in reduction of tissue hyperemia, edema, nasal congestion, and an increase in nasal airway patency. In the usual dose it has minimal vasopressor effects. Pseudoephedrine is rapidly and almost completely absorbed from the gastrointestinal tract. It has a plasma half-life of 6 to 8 hours. Alkaline urine is associated with slower elimination of the drug. The drug is distributed to body tissues and fluids, including the central nervous system (CNS). Approximately 50% to 75% of the administered dose is excreted unchanged in the urine; the remainder is apparently metabolized in the liver to inactive compounds by a N-demethylation parahydroxylation and oxidative deamination.

Dextromethorphan is an antitussive agent, which, unlike the isomeric levorphanol, has no analgesic or addictive properties. The drug acts centrally and elevates the threshold for coughing. It is about equal to codeine in depressing the cough reflex. In therapeutic dosage, dextromethorphan does not inhibit ciliary activity. Dextromethorphan is rapidly absorbed from the gastrointestinal tract, metabolized by the liver and excreted primarily in the urine.

Guaifenesin is an expectorant which increases respiratory tract fluid secretions and helps loosen phlegm, bronchial and nasal secretions. By reducing the viscosity of secretions, guaifenesin increases the efficiency of the mucociliary mechanism in removing accumulated secretions from the upper and lower airway. Guaifenesin is readily absorbed from the gastrointestinal tract and is rapidly metabolized and excreted in the urine. Guaifenesin has a plasma half-life of one hour. The major urinary metabolite is β-(2-methoxyphenoxy) lactic acid.

INDICATIONS AND USAGE:

This combination drug is indicated for the temporary relief of nasal congestion and cough associated with respiratory tract infections and related conditions such as sinusitis, bronchitis, and asthma, when these conditions are complicated by tenacious mucus, and/or mucus plugs and congestion. In the treatment of bacterial sinusitis this treatment regimen may be used concomitantly with appropriate antibiotic therapy. The product is effective in productive as well as nonproductive cough, but is of particular value in dry, nonproductive cough which tends to injure the mucous membrane of the air passages.

CONTRAINDICATIONS:

This product is contraindicated in patients with hypersensitivity to guaifenesin, dextromethorphan HBr, and pseudoephedrine HCl, or with hypersensitivity or idiosyncrasy to sympathomimetic amines which may be manifested by insomnia, dizziness, weakness, tremor or arrhythmias.

CONTRAINDICATIONS: *(cont'd)*

Sympathomimetic amines are contraindicated in patients with severe hypertension and severe coronary artery disease.

The product is contraindicated in patients on monoamine oxidase inhibitor (MAOI) therapy and for 14 days after stopping MAOI therapy. (see DRUG INTERACTIONS)

WARNINGS:

Sympathomimetic amines should be used with caution in patients with hypertension, ischemic heart disease, diabetes mellitus. Increased intraocular pressure, hyperthyroidism, or prostatic hypertrophy. Sympathomimetics may produce central nervous system stimulation with convulsions or cardiovascular collapse with accompanying hypotension. **Do not exceed recommended dosage.**

Do not prescribe this product for use in patients that are now taking a prescription MAOI (certain drugs for depression, psychiatric or emotional conditions, or Parkinson's disease), or for 14 days after stopping the MAOI drug therapy.

Hypertensive crises can occur with concurrent use of pseudoephedrine or phenylephrine and monoamine oxidase inhibitors (MAOI), and for 14 days after stopping the MAOI drug therapy, indomethacin, or with beta-blockers and methyldopa. If a hypertensive crisis occurs, these drugs should be discontinued immediately and therapy to lower blood pressure should be instituted. Fever should be managed by means of external cooling.

PRECAUTIONS:

General: Use with caution in patients with diabetes, hypertension, cardiovascular disease and intolerance to ephedrine.

Before prescribing medication to suppress or modify cough, it is important that the underlying cause of cough is identified, that modification of cough does not increase the risk of clinical or physiological complications, and that appropriate therapy for the primary disease is instituted.

Dextromethorphan should be used with caution in sedated or debilitated patients, and in patients confined to the supine position.

Failure of symptoms to completely resolve should alert the patient and physician that further diagnostic studies are indicated.

Pediatric Use: This product is not recommended for use in pediatric patients under 12 years of age.

Use in Elderly: The elderly (60 years and older) are more likely to experience adverse reactions to sympathomimetics. Overdosage of sympathomimetics in this age group may cause hallucinations, convulsions, CNS depression, and death.

Drug/Laboratory Test Interactions: Guaifenesin may increase renal clearance for urate and thereby lower serum uric acid levels. Guaifenesin may produce an increase in urinary 5-hydroxy-indoleacetic and may therefore interfere with the interpretation of this test for the diagnosis of carcinoid syndrome. It may also falsely elevate the VMA test for catechols. Administration of this drug should be discontinued 48 hours prior to the collection of urine specimens for such tests.

Carcinogenesis, Mutagenesis, and Impairment of Fertility: No data are available on the long-term potential of the components of this product for carcinogenesis, mutagenesis, or impairment of fertility in animals or humans.

Pregnancy Category C: Animal reproduction studies have not been conducted with Syn-Rx DM Tablets. It is also not known whether Syn-Rx DM Tablets can cause fetal harm when administered to a pregnant woman or can affect reproduction capacity. Syn-Rx DM Tablets should be given to a pregnant woman only if clearly needed.

Nursing Mothers: Pseudoephedrine is excreted in breast milk. Use of this product by nursing mothers is not recommended because of the higher than usual risk for pediatric patients from sympathomimetic amines.

DRUG INTERACTIONS:

Do not prescribe this product for use in patients that are now taking a monoamine oxidase inhibitor (MAOI) drug (certain drugs for depression, psychiatric or emotional conditions, or Parkinson's disease) or for 14 days after stopping the MAOI drug therapy. Beta-adrenergic blockers and inhibitors (MAOI) may potentiate the pressor effect of pseudoephedrine. Concurrent use of digitalis glycosides may increase the possibility of cardiac arrhythmias. Sympathomimetics may reduce the hypotensive effects of guanethidine, mecamylamine, methyldopa, reserpine and veratrum alkaloids. Concurrent use of tricyclic antidepressants may antagonize the effects of pseudoephedrine.

ADVERSE REACTIONS:

Some individuals may display sympathomimetic amine effects such as tachycardia, palpitations, headache, dizziness or nausea. Sympathomimetics have been associated with certain untoward reactions including, fear, anxiety, nervousness, restlessness, tremor, weakness, pallor, respiratory difficulty, dysuria, insomnia, hallucinations, convulsions, CNS depression, arrhythmias and cardiovascular collapse with hypotension. No serious side effects have been reported with the use of guaifenesin or dextromethorphan HBr.

OVERDOSAGE:

Since this combination drug contains three pharmacologically different compounds, treatment of overdosage should be based upon the symptomatology of the patient as it relates to the individual ingredients. Treatment of acute overdosage would probably be based upon treating the patient for pseudoephedrine toxicity which may manifest itself as excessive CNS stimulation resulting in excitement, tremor, restlessness, and insomnia. Other effects may include tachycardia, hypertension, pallor, mydriasis, hyperglycemia and urinary retention. Severe overdosage may cause tachypnea or hyperpnea, hallucinations, convulsions or delirium, but in some individuals there may be CNS depression with somnolence, stupor or respiratory depression. Arrhythmias (including ventricular fibrillation) may lead to hypotension and circulatory collapse. Severe hypokalemia can occur, probably due to a compartmental shift rather than a depletion of potassium. No organ damage or significant metabolic derangement is associated with pseudoephedrine overdosage. Overdosage with guaifenesin is unlikely to produce toxic effects since toxicity is much lower than that of pseudoephedrine. In severe cases of overdosage, it is recommended to monitor the patient in an intensive care setting.

The LD_{50} of pseudoephedrine (single oral dose) has been reported to be 726 mg/kg in the mouse, 2206 mg/kg in the rat and 1177 mg/kg in the rabbit. The toxic and lethal concentrations in human biologic fluids are not known. Urinary excretion increases with acidification and decreases with alkalinization of the urine. There are few published reports of toxicity due to pseudoephedrine and no case of fatal overdosage has been reported. Guaifenesin, when administered by stomach tube to test animals in doses up to 5 grams/kg, produced signs of toxicity.

Overdosage with dextromethorphan may produce central excitement and mental confusion. Very high doses may produce respiratory depression. One case of toxic psychosis (hyperactivity, marked visual and auditory hallucinations) after ingestion of a single 300 mg dose of dextromethorphan has been reported.

OVERDOSAGE: *(cont'd)*

Since the action of sustained release products may continue for as long as 12 hours, treatment of overdosage should be directed toward reducing further absorption and supporting the patient for at least that length of time. Gastric emptying (Syrup of Ipecac) and/or lavage is recommended as soon as possible after ingestion, even if the patient has vomited spontaneously. Either isotonic or half-isotonic saline may be used for lavage. Administration of an activated charcoal slurry is beneficial after lavage and/or emesis if less than 4 hours have passed since ingestion. Saline cathartics, such as Milk of Magnesia, are useful for hastening the evacuation of unreleased medication.

Adrenergic receptor blocking agents are antidotes to pseudoephedrine. In practice, the most useful is the beta-blocker propranolol which is indicated when there are signs of cardiac toxicity. Theoretically, pseudoephedrine is dialyzable but procedures have not been clinically established.

DOSAGE AND ADMINISTRATION:

Adults and Adolescents Over 12 Years of Age: 1 or 2 light blue AM tablets in the morning and 1 or 2 yellow PM tablets 12 hours later. Repeat AM and PM dosing cycle every 12 hours for 14 days.

Do not crush or chew tablets prior to swallowing.

HOW SUPPLIED:

Syn-Rx DM 14 Day Treatment Regimen, containing 56 controlled-release tablets as follows:

28 light blue elongated and scored AM tablets embossed with "Adams/310", each containing 60 mg pseudoephedrine HCl and 600 mg guaifenesin;

28 yellow elongated and scored PM tablets embossed with "Adams/309", each containing 30 mg dextromethorphan HBr and 600 mg guaifenesin.

Store at controlled room temperature between 15°C and 30°C (59°F-86°F).

Dispense as a complete 14 day pack.

HOW SUPPLIED - EQUIVALENTS NOT AVAILABLE:

Liquid - Oral

90 ml	$4.00	Broncot, C O Truxton	00463-9035-03
120 ml	$3.75	NOVAGEST DEX, Major Pharms	00904-0710-20
120 ml	$3.79	NOVADYNE DMX, H N Norton Co.	50732-0838-04
480 ml	$13.45	Rolatuss, Major Pharms	00904-7627-16
3840 ml	$25.34	PSEUDOGEST, Major Pharms	00904-1517-28

Tablet - Oral - 600 mg/30 mg/60

56's	$35.13	SYN-RX DM, Medeva Pharms	53014-0311-14

DEXTROMETHORPHAN HYDROBROMIDE; IODINATED GLYCEROL *(000994)*

CATEGORIES: Antitussives; Antitussives/Expectorants/Mucolytics; Asthma; Bronchitis; Chronic Bronchitis; Cough Preparations; Croup; Decongestants; Emphysema; Iodide Salts; Mucolytic Agents; Pertussis; Pharyngitis; Respiratory & Allergy Medications; Tracheobronchitis; Pregnancy Category X; DEA Class CV; FDA Pre 1938 Drugs

BRAND NAMES: Bio-Tuss Dm; Biophen-Dm; Equi-Tuss Dm; Genophen-Dm Elixir; Io Tuss-Dm; Iodur-Dm; Iogan-Dm; Iophen Dm; Iophen-Dm; Iotuss-Dm; Myodine Dm; Oridol Dm; Roganidin-Dm; Sil-O-Tuss Dm; Tosmar Dm; Tri-Onex Dm; **Tussi-Organidin Dm**; Tussi-R-Gen Dm; Tusside; Tussidin Dm; Tusso-Dm

FORMULARIES: Aetna; BC-BS

COST OF THERAPY: $53.87 (Asthma; Liquid; 10 mg/30 mg; 30/day; 365 days) vs. Potential Cost of $3,576.99 (DRG 96, Bronchitis & Asthma)

PRIMARY ICD9: 493.90 (Asthma, Unspecified, Without Mention of Status Asthmaticus)

DESCRIPTION:

Iodinated Glycerol with Dextromethorphan Hydrobromide Liquid.

Active Ingredients: *Each 5 mL (one teaspoonful) contains:* Iodinated glycerol 30 mg (Containing 15 mg organically bound iodine), dextromethorphan Hydrobromide USP 10 mg

Inactive Ingredients: Citric Acid, D&C Yellow #10, FD&C Red # 40, Flavor (Natural and Artificial), Glycerin, Propylene Glycol, Purified Water, Sodium Benzoate, Sodium Citrate, Sodium Saccharin, Sorbitol Solution.

(NON-NARCOTIC)

Iodinated glycerol with dextromethorphan hydrobromide is a yellow to amber colored fruit flavored antitussive/mucolytic-expectorant combination available for oral administration as a liquid. *Each 5 mL (teaspoonful) of iodinated glycerol with dextromethorphan hydrobromide contains:* iodinated glycerol 30 mg (15 mg organically bound iodine); and dextromethorphan hydrobromide USP 10 mg. *Other Ingredients:* citric acid, D&C Yellow #10, FD&C Red #40, flavor (natural and artificial), glycerin, propylene glycol, purified water, sodium benzoate, sodium citrate, sodium saccharin, sorbitol solution. Sodium citrate and additional citric acid may be used if necessary to adjust the pH of the product.

CLINICAL PHARMACOLOGY:

Iodinated glycerol with dextromethorphan hydrobromide combines the non-narcotic antitussive action of dextromethorphan with the mucolytic-expectorant action of iodinated glycerol.

INDICATIONS AND USAGE:

Iodinated glycerol with dextromethorphan hydrobromide is indicated for the symptomatic relief of irritating, nonproductive cough associated with respiratory tract conditions such as chronic bronchitis, bronchial asthma, tracheobronchitis, and the common cold; also for the symptomatic relief of cough accompanying other respiratory tract conditions such as laryngitis, pharyngitis, croup pertussis and emphysema. Appropriate therapy should be provided for the primary disease.

CONTRAINDICATIONS:

History of marked sensitivity to inorganic iodides; hypersensitivity to any of the ingredients or related compounds; pregnancy; newborns; and nursing mothers.

The human fetal thyroid begins to concentrate iodine in the 12th to 14th week of gestation and the use of inorganic iodides in pregnant women during this period and thereafter has rarely been reported to induce fetal goiter (with or without hypothyroidism) with the

CONTRAINDICATIONS: *(cont'd)*

potential for airway obstruction. If the patient becomes pregnant while taking iodinated glycerol with dextromethorphan hydrobromide, the drug should be discontinued and the patient should be apprised of the potential risk to the fetus.

WARNINGS:

Discontinue use if rash or other evidence of hypersensitivity appears. Use with caution or avoid use in patients with history or evidence of thyroid disease.

PRECAUTIONS:

General: Iodides have been reported to cause a flare-up of adolescent acne. Children with cystic fibrosis appear to have an exaggerated susceptibility to the goitrogenic effect of iodides. Dermatitis and other reversible manifestations of iodism have been reported with chronic use of inorganic iodides. Although these have not been reported to be a problem clinically with iodinated glycerol formulations, they should be kept in mind in patients receiving these preparations for prolonged periods.

Carcinogenesis, Mutagenesis, and Impairment of Fertility: No long-term animal studies have been performed with iodinated glycerol with dextromethorphan hydrobromide.

Pregnancy, Teratogenic Effects, Pregnancy Category X: (see CONTRAINDICATIONS)

Nursing Mothers: Iodinated glycerol with dextromethorphan hydrobromide should not be administered to a nursing mother.

DRUG INTERACTIONS:

Iodides may potentiate the hypothyroid effect of lithium and other antithyroid drugs.

ADVERSE REACTIONS:

Side effects have been rare, including those which may occur with the individual active ingredients and which may be modified as a result of their combination. Iodinated glycerol; Rare side effects include gastrointestinal irritation, rash, hypersensitivity, thyroid gland enlargement, and acute parotitis, Dextromethorphan; Rarely produces drowsiness or gastrointestinal disturbances.

OVERDOSAGE:

Acute overdose experience with iodinated glycerol has been rare and there have been no reports of any serious problems.

DOSAGE AND ADMINISTRATION:

Adults: 1 to 2 teaspoonfuls every 4 hours.

Children: ½ to 1 teaspoonful every 4 hours.

HOW SUPPLIED - EQUIVALENTS NOT AVAILABLE:

Liquid - Oral - 10 mg/30 mg

5 ml x 40	$17.58	Iodinated Glycerol/Dextromethorphan, Roxane	00054-8396-16
10 ml x 40	$23.90	Iodinated Glycerol/Dextromethorphan, Roxane	00054-8397-16
120 ml	$1.15	Biophen-Dm, Bio Pharm	59741-0131-04
120 ml	$2.65	Iogan-Dm, Hi Tech Pharma	50383-0774-04
120 ml	**$7.79**	**TUSSI-ORGANIDIN DM, Wallace Labs**	**00037-4712-01**
480 ml	$2.45	Biophen-Dm, Bio Pharm	59741-0131-16
480 ml	$7.80	Iogan-Dm, Hi Tech Pharma	50383-0774-16
480 ml	$8.65	TORGANIC-DM, Major Pharms	00904-1549-16
480 ml	$10.15	TUSSI-R-GEN DM, Goldline Labs	00182-1697-40
480 ml	$10.50	Iodinated Glycerol Dm, Geneva Pharms	00781-6303-16
480 ml	$10.75	Iodur-Dm, Aligen Independ	00405-2925-16
480 ml	$12.75	TUSSI-R GEN, Goldline Labs	00182-1656-40
500 ml	$7.07	Iodinated Glycerol/Dextromethorphan, Roxane	00054-3396-63
3785 ml	$82.48	TUSSI-R GEN, Goldline Labs	00182-1656-41
3840 ml	$18.93	Biophen-Dm, Bio Pharm	59741-0131-20
3840 ml	$53.99	Iogan-Dm, Hi Tech Pharma	50383-0774-28
3840 ml	$75.00	TUSSI-R-GEN DM, Goldline Labs	00182-1697-41

DEXTROMETHORPHAN HYDROBROMIDE; PHENYLEPHRINE HYDROCHLORIDE; PYRILAMINE *(001006)*

CATEGORIES: Cough Preparations; Expectorants

BRAND NAMES: Albatussin; Albatussin Nn; Vita-Numonyl

Prescribing information not available at time of publication.

HOW SUPPLIED - EQUIVALENTS NOT AVAILABLE:

Expectorant - Oral

118.3 ml	$14.40	ALBATUSSIN, Alba Pharma	10023-0203-04
120 ml	$14.50	ALBATUSSIN NN, Alba Pharma	10023-0104-04
120 ml	$14.50	VITA-NUMONYL, Teral Labs	51234-0127-04

DEXTROMETHORPHAN HYDROBROMIDE; PHENYLEPHRINE HYDROCHLORIDE; VITAMIN C *(001007)*

CATEGORIES: Cough Preparations; Expectorants

BRAND NAMES: Albatussin Pediatric; Vita-Numonyl

Prescribing information not available at time of publication.

HOW SUPPLIED - EQUIVALENTS NOT AVAILABLE:

Syrup - Oral

30 ml	$14.40	ALBATUSSIN PEDIATRIC, Alba Pharma	10023-0230-70
120 ml	$9.74	VITA-NUMONYL, Teral Labs	51234-0123-04

DEXTROMETHORPHAN HYDROBROMIDE; PROMETHAZINE HYDROCHLORIDE *(000995)*

CATEGORIES: Allergies; Antihistamines; Antitussives; Antitussives/Expectorants/Mucolytics; Common Cold; Cough Preparations; Expectorants; Influenza; Respiratory & Allergy Medications; Rhinitis; Urticaria; Anaphylactic Shock*; Anesthesia*; Angioedema*; Anxiety*; Conjunctivitis*; Nausea*; Pregnancy Category C; FDA Approved 1984 Apr

* Indication not approved by the FDA

BRAND NAMES: Dectuss Dm; *Neo Davenol*; Phen-Tuss Dm; Phenergan W/Dextromethorphan; Pherazine Dm; Promethazine W/Dm; Prothazine

(International brand names outside U.S. in italics)

FORMULARIES: Aetna; BC-BS; FHP; Medi-Cal

COST OF THERAPY: $5.49 (Rhinitis; Syrup; 15 mg/6.25 mg/5ml; 20/day; 30 days)

PRIMARY ICD9: 477.9 (Allergic Rhinitis, Cause Unspecified)

DESCRIPTION:

Each teaspoon (5 ml) of Promethazine Hydrochloride and Dextromethorphan Hydrobromide (abbreviated in this monograph as promethazine DM), contains 6.25 mg promethazine hydrochloride and 15 mg dextromethorphan hydrobromide in a flavored syrup base with a pH between 4.7 and 5.2. Alcohol 7%. The inactive ingredients present are artificial and natural flavors, citric acid, D&C Yellow 10, FD&C Yellow 6, glycerin, saccharin sodium, sodium benzoate, sodium citrate, sodium propionate, water, and other ingredients.

Promethazine hydrochloride is a racemic compound; the empirical formula is $C_{17}H_{20}N_2S{\cdot}HCl$ and its molecular weight is 320.88.

Promethazine hydrochloride, a phenothiazine derivative, is designated chemically as N,N,α-trimethyl-10*H*-phenothiazine-10-ethanamine monohydrochloride.

Promethazine hydrochloride occurs as a white to faint yellow, practically odorless, crystalline powder which slowly oxidizes and turns blue on prolonged exposure to air. It is soluble in water and freely soluble in alcohol.

Dextromethorphan hydrobromide is a salt of the methyl ether of the dextrorotatory isomer of levorphanol, a narcotic analgesic. It is chemically named as 3-methoxy-17-methyl-9α, 13α, 14α-morphinan hydrobromide monohydrate.

Dextromethorphan hydrobromide monohydrate occurs as white crystals, is sparingly soluble in water, and is freely soluble in alcohol. The empirical formula is $C_{18}H_{25}NO{\cdot}HBr{\cdot}H_2O$, and the molecular weight of the monohydrate is 370.33. Dextromethorphan HBr monohydrate is dextrorotatory with a specific rotation of +27.6 degrees in water (20 degrees C, sodium D-line).

CLINICAL PHARMACOLOGY:

PROMETHAZINE

Promethazine is a phenothiazine derivative which differs structurally from the antipsychotic phenothiazines by the presence of a branched side chain and no ring substitution. It is thought that this configuration is responsible for its relative lack (1/10 that of chlorpromazine) of dopaminergic (CNS) action.

Promethazine is an H_1 receptor blocking agent. In addition to its antihistaminic action, it provides clinically useful sedative and antiemetic effects. In therapeutic dosages, promethazine produces no significant effects on the cardiovascular system.

Promethazine is well absorbed from the gastrointestinal tract. Clinical effects are apparent within 20 minutes after oral administration and generally last four to six hours, although they may persist as long as 12 hours. Promethazine is metabolized by the liver to a variety of compounds; the sulfoxides of promethazine and N-demethylpromethazine are the predominant metabolites appearing in the urine.

DEXTROMETHORPHAN

Dextromethorphan is an antitussive agent and, unlike the isomeric levorphanol, it has no analgesic or addictive properties.

The drug acts centrally and elevates the threshold for coughing. It is about equal to codeine in depressing the cough reflex. In therapeutic dosage dextromethorphan does not inhibit ciliary activity.

Dextromethorphan is rapidly absorbed from the gastrointestinal tract and exerts its effect in 15 to 30 minutes. The duration of action after oral administration is approximately three to six hours. Dextromethorphan is metabolized primarily by liver enzymes undergoing O-demethylation, N-demethylation, and partial conjugation with glucuronic acid and sulfate. In humans, (+)-3-hydroxy-N-methylmorphinan, (+)-3-hydroxymorphinan, and traces of unmetabolized drug were found in urine after oral administration.

INDICATIONS AND USAGE:

Promethazine DM is indicated for the temporary relief of coughs and upper respiratory symptoms associated with allergy or the common cold.

CONTRAINDICATIONS:

Promethazine is contraindicated in individuals known to be hypersensitive or to have had an idiosyncratic reaction to promethazine or to other phenothiazines.

Antihistamines are contraindicated for use in the treatment of lower respiratory tract symptoms, including asthma.

Dextromethorphan should not be used in patients receiving a monoamine oxidase inhibitor (MAOI).

WARNINGS:

PROMETHAZINE

Promethazine may cause marked drowsiness. Ambulatory patients should be cautioned against such activities as driving or operating dangerous machinery until it is known that they do not become drowsy or dizzy from promethazine therapy.

The sedative action of promethazine hydrochloride is additive to the sedative effects of central nervous system depressants; therefore, agents such as alcohol, narcotic analgesics, sedatives, hypnotics, and tranquilizers should either be eliminated or given in reduced dosage in the presence of promethazine hydrochloride. When given concomitantly with promethazine hydrochloride, the dose of barbiturates should be reduced by at least one-half, and the dose of analgesic depressants, such as morphine or meperidine, should be reduced by one-quarter to one-half.

Promethazine may lower seizure threshold. This should be taken into consideration when administering to persons with known seizure disorders or when giving in combination with narcotics or local anesthetics which may also affect seizure threshold.

Sedative drugs or CNS depressants should be avoided in patients with a history of sleep apnea.

Antihistamines should be used with caution in patients with narrow-angle glaucoma, stenosing peptic ulcer, pyloroduodenal obstruction, and urinary bladder obstruction due to symptomatic prostatic hypertrophy and narrowing of the bladder neck.

Administration of promethazine has been associated with reported cholestatic jaundice.

WARNINGS: *(cont'd)*

DEXTROMETHORPHAN

Administration of dextromethorphan may be accompanied by histamine release and should be used with caution in atopic children.

PRECAUTIONS:

Animal reproduction studies have not been conducted with the drug combination-promethazine and dextromethorphan. It is not known whether this drug combination can cause fetal harm when administered to a pregnant woman or can affect reproduction capacity. Promethazine DM should be given to a pregnant woman only if clearly needed.

GENERAL

Promethazine should be used cautiously in persons with cardiovascular disease or with impairment of liver function.

Dextromethorphan should be used with caution in sedated patients, in the debilitated, and in patients confined to the supine position.

INFORMATION FOR THE PATIENT

Promethazine DM may cause marked drowsiness or impair the mental and/or physical abilities required for the performance of potentially hazardous tasks, such as driving a vehicle or operating machinery. Ambulatory patients should be told to avoid engaging in such activities until it is known that they do not become drowsy or dizzy from promethazine DM therapy. Children should be supervised to avoid potential harm in bike riding or in other hazardous activities.

The concomitant use of alcohol or other central nervous system depressants, including narcotic analgesics, sedatives, hypnotics, and tranquilizers, may have an additive effect and should be avoided or their dosage reduced.

Patients should be advised to report any involuntary muscle movements or unusual sensitivity to sunlight.

DRUG/LABORATORY TEST INTERACTIONS

The following laboratory tests may be affected in patients who are receiving therapy with promethazine hydrochloride:

PREGNANCY TESTS

Diagnostic pregnancy tests based on immunological reactions between HCG and anti-HCG may result in false-negative or false-positive interpretations.

GLUCOSE TOLERANCE TEST

An increase in blood glucose has been reported in patients receiving promethazine.

CARCINOGENESIS, MUTAGENESIS, IMPAIRMENT OF FERTILITY

Long-term animal studies have not been performed to assess the carcinogenic potential of promethazine or of dextromethorphan. There are no animal or human data concerning the carcinogenicity, mutagenicity, or impairment of fertility with these drugs. Promethazine was nonmutagenic in the *Salmonella* test system of Ames.

PREGNANCY

Pregnancy, Teratogenic Effects, Pregnancy Category C Teratogenic effects have not been demonstrated in rat-feeding studies at doses of 6.25 and 12.5 mg/kg of promethazine. These doses are 8.3 and 16.7 times the maximum recommended total daily dose for a 50-kg subject. Specific studies to test the action of the drug on parturition, lactation, and development of the animal neonate were not done, but a general preliminary study in rats indicated no effect on these parameters. Although antihistamines, including promethazine, have been found to produce fetal mortality in rodents, the pharmacological effects of histamine in the rodent do not parallel those in man. There are no adequate and well-controlled studies of promethazine in pregnant women.

Promethazine DM should be used during pregnancy only if the potential benefit justifies the potential risk to the fetus.

Nonteratogenic Effects Promethazine taken within two weeks of delivery may inhibit platelet aggregation in the newborn.

Labor and Delivery: See Nonteratogenic Effects.

Nursing Mothers: It is not known whether promethazine or dextromethorphan is excreted in human milk. Caution should be exercised when promethazine DM is administered to a nursing woman.

Pediatric Use: This product should not be used in children under 2 years of age because safety for that use has not been established.

DRUG INTERACTIONS:

The sedative action of promethazine is additive to the sedative effects of other central nervous system depressants, including alcohol, narcotic analgesics, sedatives, hypnotics, tricyclic antidepressants, and tranquilizers; therefore, these agents should be avoided or administered in reduced dosage to patients receiving promethazine.

ADVERSE REACTIONS:

PROMETHAZINE

Nervous System: Sedation, sleepiness, occasional blurred vision, dryness of mouth, dizziness; rarely confusion, disorientation, and extrapyramidal symptoms such as oculogyric crisis, torticollis, and tongue protrusion (usually in association with parenteral injection or excessive dosage).

Cardiovascular: Increased or decreased blood pressure.

Dermatologic: Rash, rarely photosensitivity.

Hematologic: Rarely leukopenia, thrombocytopenia; agranulocytosis (1 case).

Gastrointestinal: Nausea and vomiting.

DEXTROMETHORPHAN

Dextromethorphan hydrobromide occasionally causes slight drowsiness, dizziness, and gastrointestinal disturbances.

DRUG ABUSE AND DEPENDENCE:

According to the WHO Expert Committee on Drug Dependence, dextromethorphan could produce very slight psychic dependence but no physical dependence.

OVERDOSAGE:

PROMETHAZINE

Signs and symptoms of overdosage with promethazine range from mild depression of the central nervous system and cardiovascular system to profound hypotension, respiratory depression, and unconsciousness.

Stimulation may be evident, especially in children and geriatric patients. Convulsions may rarely occur. A paradoxical reaction has been reported in children receiving single doses of 75 mg to 125 mg orally, characterized by hyperexcitability and nightmares.

Atropine-like signs and symptoms—dry mouth, fixed, dilated pupils, flushing, as well as gastrointestinal symptoms, may occur.

OVERDOSAGE: *(cont'd)*

DEXTROMETHORPHAN

Dextromethorphan may produce central excitement and mental confusion. Very high doses may produce respiratory depression. One case of toxic psychosis (hyperactivity, marked visual and auditory hallucinations) after ingestion of a single dose of 20 tablets (300 mg) of dextromethorphan has been reported.

TREATMENT

Treatment of overdosage with promethazine DM is essentially symptomatic and supportive. Only in cases of extreme overdosage or individual sensitivity do vital signs including respiration, pulse, blood pressure, temperature, and EKG need to be monitored. Activated charcoal orally or by lavage may be given, or sodium or magnesium sulfate orally as a cathartic. Attention should be given to the reestablishment of adequate respiratory exchange through provision of a patent airway and institution of assisted or controlled ventilation. Diazepam may be used to control convulsions. Acidosis and electrolyte losses should be corrected. The antidotal efficacy of narcotic antagonists to dextromethorphan has not been established; note that any of the depressant effects of promethazine are not reversed by naloxone. Avoid analeptics, which may cause convulsions.

Severe hypotension usually responds to the administration of norepinephrine or phenylephrine. EPINEPHRINE SHOULD NOT BE USED, since its use in a patient with partial adrenergic blockade may further lower the blood pressure.

Limited experience with dialysis indicates that it is not helpful.

DOSAGE AND ADMINISTRATION:

The average effective dose for adults is one teaspoon (5 ml) every 4 to 6 hours, not to exceed 30.0 ml in 24 hours. For children 6 years to under 12 years of age, the dose is one-half to one teaspoon (2.5 to 5.0 ml) every 4 to 6 hours, not to exceed 20.0 ml in 24 hours. For children 2 years to under 6 years of age, the dose is one-quarter to one-half teaspoon (1.25 to 2.5 ml) every 4 to 6 hours, not to exceed 10.0 ml in 24 hours.

Promethazine DM is not recommended for children under 2 years of age.

Keep bottles tightly closed and store at room temperature between 15 and 25°C (59 and 77° F). Protect from light.

Dispense in light-resistant, glass, tight containers.

HOW SUPPLIED - RATED THERAPEUTICALLY EQUIVALENT:

Syrup - Oral - 15 mg/6.25 mg/5

1 pint	$2.61	Promethazine/Dextromethorphan, United Res	00677-0966-33
120 ml	$1.10	Prometh w/Dextromethorphan, H.C.F.A. F F P	99999-0995-02
120 ml	$3.86	Promethazine W/Dm, Morton Grove	60432-0604-04
120 ml	$3.90	Promethazine With Dm, Rugby	00536-1765-97
120 ml	$4.00	PHERAZINE DM SYRUP, Halsey Drug	00879-0516-04
120 ml	$4.24	Prometh w/Dextromethorphan, Alpharma	00472-1630-04
120 ml x 24	$154.54	PHENERGAN W/DEXTROMETHORPHAN, Wyeth Labs	00008-0548-02
180 ml	$1.66	Prometh w/Dextromethorphan, H.C.F.A. F F P	99999-0995-03
240 ml	$2.21	Prometh w/Dextromethorphan, H.C.F.A. F F P	99999-0995-01
473 ml	$18.00	PHEN-TUSS DM, Bergmar Pharm	58173-0034-16
480 ml	$4.42	Prometh w/Dextromethorphan, H.C.F.A. F F P	99999-0995-04
480 ml	$6.40	Promethazine W/Dm, Qualitest Pharms	00603-1579-58
480 ml	$7.36	Prometh DM, Schein Pharm (US)	00364-0734-16
480 ml	$8.10	Prometh w/Dextromethorphan, Goldline Labs	00182-1730-40
480 ml	$9.40	Promethazine W/Dm, Morton Grove	60432-0604-16
480 ml	$10.34	Prometh w/Dextromethorphan, Alpharma	00472-1630-16
480 ml	$10.75	Promethazine With Dm, Rugby	00536-1765-85
480 ml	$10.75	PHERAZINE DM SYRUP, Halsey Drug	00879-0516-16
480 ml	$23.37	PHENERGAN W/DEXTROMETHORPHAN, Wyeth Labs	00008-0548-03
3840 ml	$35.33	Prometh w/Dextromethorphan, H.C.F.A. F F P	99999-0995-05
3840 ml	$39.71	Promethazine With Dm, Rugby	00536-1765-90
3840 ml	$45.60	Prometh w/Dextromethorphan, Alpharma	00472-1630-28
3840 ml	$48.81	Promethazine W/Dm, Qualitest Pharms	00603-1579-60
3840 ml	$53.91	PHERAZINE DM SYRUP, Halsey Drug	00879-0516-28
3840 ml	$59.60	Prometh w/Dextromethorphan, Goldline Labs	00182-1730-41

HOW SUPPLIED - NOT RATED EQUIVALENT:

Syrup - Oral - 15 mg/6.25 mg/5

120 ml	$2.25	Promethazine W/Dm, Major Pharms	00904-1516-20
120 ml	$3.24	Promethazine W/Dm, HL Moore Drug Exch	00839-7062-65
120 ml	$3.25	Promethazine Pediatric, Consolidated Midland	00223-6347-01
120 ml	$3.84	PHENAMETH DM, Major Pharms	00904-1516-00
480 ml	$6.70	Promethazine W/Dm, ESI Lederle	59911-5822-03
480 ml	$7.49	Promethazine W/Dm, HL Moore Drug Exch	00839-7062-69
480 ml	$8.00	Promethazine Pediatric, Consolidated Midland	00223-6347-02
480 ml	$8.00	Promethazine W/Dm, Aligen Independ	00405-3650-16
480 ml	$9.20	PHENAMETH DM, Major Pharms	00904-1516-16
3840 ml	$51.99	Promethazine Pediatric, Consolidated Midland	00223-6347-03
3840 ml	$64.93	PHENAMETH DM, Major Pharms	00904-1516-28

DEXTROMETHORPHAN HYDROBROMIDE; PSEUDOEPHEDRINE *(001009)*

CATEGORIES: Allergies; Antihistamines; Antitussives/Expectorants/Mucolytics; Cough Preparations; Respiratory & Allergy Medications; FDA Pre 1938 Drugs

BRAND NAMES: Tuss-Da

Prescribing information not available at time of publication.

HOW SUPPLIED - EQUIVALENTS NOT AVAILABLE:

Syrup - Oral

120 ml	$6.50	TUSS-DA, Intl Ethical	11584-1026-04

DEXTROTHYROXINE SODIUM *(001024)*

CATEGORIES: Antilipemic Agents; Cardiovascular Drugs; Cholesterol; Heart Disease; Hormones; Hypercholesterolemia; Hyperlipidemia; Hypolipidemics; Nephrotic Syndrome; Thyroid Preparations; Pregnancy Category B; FDA Approval Pre 1982

BRAND NAMES: **Choloxin**; *Dynothel*; *Eulipos* (Germany); *Lisolipin*
(International brand names outside U.S. in italics)

COST OF THERAPY: $539.83 (Hypercholesterolemia; Tablet; 2 mg; 1/day; 365 days)

DESCRIPTION:

Dextrothyroxine sodium, USP is the sodium salt of the dextrorotatory isomer of thyroxine useful in the treatment of hyperlipidemia. It is chemically described as D-3,5,3',5'-tetraiodothyronine sodium salt.

Dextrothyroxine sodium tablets, USP, are available for oral use containing 1, 2, 4, or 6 mg of dextrothyroxine sodium.

Dextrothyroxine sodium tablets contain the following inactive ingredients: Acacia, confectioners' sugar, gelatin, lactose, magnesium stearate, polysorbate 80 (1, 2, and 6 mg tablets only), povidone and talc. The following are the color additives per tablet strength:

Strength (Mg) Color Additive(s): *1 mg:* FD&C Yellow No. 6 (Sunset Yellow), *2 mg:* FD&C Yellow No. 5 (tartrazine), *4 mg:* None, *6 mg:* FD&C Yellow No. 5, (tartrazine) FD&C Blue No. 1

CLINICAL PHARMACOLOGY:

The predominant effect of dextrothyroxine sodium is the reduction of elevated serum cholesterol levels.

Beta lipoprotein and triglyceride fractions may also be reduced from previously elevated levels.

Available evidence indicates that dextrothyroxine sodium stimulates the liver to increase catabolism and excretion of cholesterol and its degradation products via the biliary route into the feces.

Cholesterol synthesis is not inhibited and abnormal metabolic end products do not accumulate in the blood.

INDICATIONS AND USAGE:

Dextrothyroxine sodium may be indicated as an adjunct to diet for the reduction of elevated low density lipoprotein (LDL) cholesterol in patients with primary hypercholesterolemia (Types IIa and IIb)

with no known or suspected heart disease, whose response to diet and other nonpharmacologic measures has been inadequate.

THIS IS NOT AN INNOCUOUS DRUG. STRICT ATTENTION SHOULD BE PAID TO THE INDICATIONS AND CONTRAINDICATIONS. After establishing that the elevation in serum cholesterol represents a primary disorder not due to secondary conditions such as poorly controlled diabetes mellitus, hypothyroidism, the nephrotic syndrome, liver disease, or dysproteinemias, it should be determined that a patient for whom treatment with Dextrothyroxine Sodium is being considered has a persistently elevated LDL cholesterol as the cause of an elevated total serum cholesterol. This may be particularly relevant for patients with elevated total triglycerides or with markedly elevated HDL-C values, where non-LDL lipoprotein fractions may contribute significantly to total cholesterol levels without apparent increase in cardiovascular risk. In most patients, LDL-C may be estimated according to the following equation:

LDL-C = total cholesterol - ((0.16 × triglycerides)

+ HDL-C).

When total triglycerides are greater than 400 mg/dl this equation is less accurate. In such patients, LDL-Cholesterol may be obtained by ultracentrifugation.

IT HAS NOT BEEN CLEARLY ESTABLISHED WHETHER DEXTROTHYROXINE INDUCED LOWERING OF SERUM CHOLESTEROL OR LIPID LEVELS HAS A DETRIMENTAL, BENEFICIAL, OR NO EFFECT ON THE MORBIDITY OR MORTALITY DUE TO ATHEROSCLEROSIS OF CORONARY HEART DISEASE. DEXTROTHYROXINE MAY HAVE A DETRIMENTAL EFFECT ON MORBIDITY AND MORTALITY IN PATIENTS WITH ESTABLISHED CORONARY HEART DISEASE (SEE CONTRAINDICATIONS).

CONTRAINDICATIONS:

The administration of Dextrothyroxine Sodium to euthyroid patients with one or more of the following conditions is contraindicated.

1. Known or suspected organic heart disease, especially coronary artery disease, including angina pectoris; history of myocardial infarction; cardiac arrhythmia or tachycardia, either active or in patients with demonstrated propensity for arrhythmias; rheumatic heart disease; history of congestive heart failure; and decompensated or borderline compensated cardiac status. In a large study, involving men who had had a myocardial infarction, use of the drug was discontinued because of a trend to increased mortality in dextrothyroxine-treated subjects compared with placebo-treated patients.

2. Hypertension (other than mild, labile systolic hypertension.)

3. Pregnancy.

4. Nursing mothers.

5. History of iodism.

6. Safety and effectiveness in children have not been established.

7. In patients with advanced liver or kidney diseases.

WARNINGS:

Drugs with thyroid hormone activity, alone or together with other therapeutic agents, have been used for the treatment of obesity. In euthyroid patients, doses within the range of daily hormonal requirements are ineffective for weight reduction. Larger doses may produce serious or even life threatening manifestations of toxicity, particularly when given in association with sympathomimetic amines such as those used for their anorectic effects. In a large study, in men who have had a myocardial infarction, use of the drug was discontinued because of a trend to increased mortality in dextrothyroxine-treated subjects compared with placebo-treated patients. Even in subjects without known or suspected coronary disease, the potential benefits and risks of using Dextrothyroxine should be carefully considered in patients presenting increased risk of coronary disease because of age, sex, obesity, history of smoking, hypertension and/or other factors increasing the risk of coronary artery disease, such as positive family history of premature coronary artery disease.

DEXTROTHYROXINE MAY POTENTIATE THE EFFECTS OF ANTICOAGULANTS ON PROTHROMBIN TIME. REDUCTIONS OF ANTICOAGULANT BY AS MUCH AS 30% HAVE BEEN REQUIRED IN SOME PATIENTS. CONSEQUENTLY, THE DOSAGE OF ANTICOAGULANTS SHOULD BE REDUCED BY ONE THIRD UPON INITIATION OF DEXTROTHYROXINE THERAPY AND THE DOSAGE SUBSEQUENTLY READJUSTED ON THE BASIS OF PROTHROMBIN TIME. THE PROTHROMBIN TIME OF PATIENTS RECEIVING ANTICOAGULANT THERAPY CONCOMITANTLY

WARNINGS: *(cont'd)*

WITH DEXTROTHYROXINE THERAPY SHOULD BE OBSERVED AS FREQUENTLY AS NECESSARY, AT LEAST WEEKLY DURING THE FIRST FEW WEEKS OF TREATMENT.

In the surgical patient, it is wise to consider withdrawal of the drug two weeks prior to surgery if the use of anticoagulants during surgery is contemplated.

Dextrothyroxine Sodium should not be used with thyroid replacement drugs.

Since the possibility of precipitating cardiac arrhythmias during surgery may be greater in patients treated with thyroid hormones, it may be wise to discontinue Dextrothyroxine Sodium in euthyroid patients at least two weeks prior to an elective operation. Thus during emergency surgery in euthyroid patients, the patients should be carefully observed.

There are reports that dextrothyroxine sodium in diabetic patients is capable of increasing blood sugar levels with a resultant increase in requirements of insulin or oral hypoglycemic agents. Special attention should be paid to parameters necessary for good control of the diabetic state in dextrothyroxine sodium-treated subjects and to dosage requirements of insulin or other antidiabetic drugs. If dextrothyroxine sodium is later withdrawn from patients who had required a dosage increase of insulin or oral hypoglycemic agents during its administration, the dosage of antidiabetic drugs should be reduced and adjusted to maintain good control of the diabetic state.

When impaired liver and/or kidney function are present, the advantages of Dextrothyroxine Sodium therapy must be weighed against the possibility of deleterious results (see CONTRAINDICATIONS.)

PRECAUTIONS:

General: It is expected that patients on Dextrothyroxine Sodium therapy will show increased serum thyroxine levels. These increased serum thyroxine values are evidence of absorption and transport of the drug, and should NOT be interpreted as evidence of hypermetabolism; therefore, they may not be used to determine the effective dose of dextrothyroxine sodium. Thyroxine values in the range of 10% to 25% mcg in dextrothyroxine sodium-treated patients are common.

If signs or symptoms of iodism develop during dextrothyroxine sodium therapy, the drug should be discontinued.

The 2 mg and 6 mg dextrothyroxine sodium tablets contain FD&C Yellow No. 5 (tartrazine) which may cause allergic-type reactions (including bronchial asthma) in certain susceptible individuals.

Although the overall incidence of FD&C Yellow No. 5 (tartrazine) sensitivity in the general population is low, it is frequently seen in patients who also have aspirin hypersensitivity.

Information for the Patient: Patients should receive instruction in appropriate dietary and other nonpharmacologic measures designed to reduce serum cholesterol levels. These include restriction of intake of cholesterol, total calories, and saturated fatty acids, and increasing the ratio of polyunsaturated to saturated fats.

Patients should be instructed to notify physician if any of the following occur: Palpitations, chest pain, diarrhea, excessive sweating, rash or acne, insomnia, headache, increasing nervousness, or visual disturbances.

Carcinogenesis, Mutagenesis, and Impairment of Fertility: Long term studies in animals to evaluate carcinogenic potential have not been performed.

Pregnancy, Teratogenic Effects, Pregnancy Category C: Reproduction studies have been performed in rabbits and rats at doses up to 100 times (mg/kg) the expected maximum daily dose for humans and have revealed no evidence of impaired fertility or harm to the fetus due to dextrothyroxine sodium. There are, however, no adequate and well-controlled studies in pregnant women. Because animal reproduction studies are not always predictive of human response, this drug should be used during pregnancy only if clearly needed.

Women of childbearing age who require drug therapy for hypercholesterolemia should consider use of a bile acid sequestering resin. Since pregnancy may occur despite the use of birth control procedures, administration of dextrothyroxine sodium to women of this age group should be undertaken only after weighing the possible risk to the fetus against the possible benefits to the mother.

Nursing Mothers: It is not known whether dextrothyroxine sodium is excreted in human milk.

Because many drugs are excreted in human milk, caution should be exercised when dextrothyroxine sodium is administered to a nursing woman (see CONTRAINDICATIONS).

Pediatric Use: Safety and effectiveness in children have not been established (see CONTRAINDICATIONS).

DRUG INTERACTIONS:

Dextrothyroxine sodium potentiates the effect of anticoagulants on prothrombin time, thus indicating a decrease in the dosage requirements of the anticoagulants. On the other hand, dosage requirements of antidiabetic drugs have been reported to be increased during dextrothyroxine sodium therapy (see WARNINGS).

ADVERSE REACTIONS:

The side effects attributed to dextrothyroxine sodium therapy are, for the most part, due to increased metabolism, and may be minimized by following the recommended dosage schedule. Adverse effects are least commonly seen in euthyroid patients with no signs or symptoms of organic heart disease.

In the absence of known organic heart disease, some cardiac changes may be precipitated during dextrothyroxine sodium therapy. Angina pectoris, extrasystoles, ectopic beats, supraventricular tachycardia, ECG evidence of ischemic myocardial changes and increase in heart size have all been observed. Myocardial infarctions, both fatal and nonfatal, have occurred, but theses are not unexpected in untreated patients in the age groups studied. It is not known whether any of these infarcts were drug related.

HOWEVER, SHOULD ANY OF THESE SIGNS OR SYMPTOMS DEVELOP, OR OTHER EVIDENCE OF CARDIAC DISEASE APPEAR, DEXTROTHYROXINE IS CONTRAINDICATED AND SHOULD BE DISCONTINUED.

Changes in clinical status that may be related to the metabolic action of the drug include the development of insomnia, nervousness, palpitations, tremors, loss of weight, lid lag, sweating, flushing, hyperthermia, hair loss, diuresis, and menstrual irregularities.

Gastrointestinal complaints during therapy have included dyspepsia, nausea and vomiting, constipation, diarrhea, and decrease in appetite.

Other side effects reported to be associated with dextrothyroxine sodium therapy include the development of headache, changes in libido (increase or decrease), hoarseness, tinnitus, dizziness, peripheral edema, malaise, tiredness, visual disturbances, psychological changes, paresthesia, muscle pain, and various bizarre subjective complaints. Skin rashes, including a few which appeared to be due to iodism, and itching have been attributed to dextrothyroxine sodium by some investigators. Gallstones have been discovered in occasional dextrothyroxine sodium-treated patients and cholestatic jaundice has occurred in one patient, although its relationship to dextrothyroxine sodium therapy was not established.

ADVERSE REACTIONS: *(cont'd)*

In several instances, the previously existing conditions of the patient appeared to continue or progress during the administration of dextrothyroxine sodium. A worsening of peripheral vascular disease, altered sensorium, exophthalmos and retinopathy have been reported.

OVERDOSAGE:

Overdosage with dextrothyroxine sodium may result in signs and symptoms of thyrotoxicosis. The dosage at which such symptoms may appear will depend on the previous thyroid status of the patient, and their individual sensitivity to the drug. Dextrothyroxine sodium is somewhat protein-bound and would not be expected to be appreciably dialyzable. Treatment of overdosage is similar to that of thyrotoxic storm and may include hydration, sedation, and use of beta-adrenergic blocking agents.

DOSAGE AND ADMINISTRATION:

For adult euthyroid hypercholesterolemic patients, the recommended maintenance dose of dextrothyroxine sodium is 4 to 8 mg per day. The initial dose should be 1 to 2 mg daily, to be increased in 1 to 2 mg increments at intervals of not less that one month to a maximal level of 4 to 8 mg daily.

IF SIGNS AND SYMPTOMS OF CARDIAC DISEASE DEVELOP DURING THE TREATMENT PERIOD, THE DRUG SHOULD BE WITHDRAWN.

HOW SUPPLIED - EQUIVALENTS NOT AVAILABLE:

Tablet, Uncoated - Oral - 2 mg

100's $147.90 CHOLOXIN, Knoll Pharms 00048-1250-03

Tablet, Uncoated - Oral - 4 mg

100's $181.70 CHOLOXIN, Knoll Labs 00044-1270-03

DEZOCINE *(003023)*

CATEGORIES: Analgesics; Antipyretics; Central Nervous System Agents; Opiate Agonists (Controlled); Pain; Pregnancy Category C; FDA Class 1C ("Little or No Therapeutic Advantage"); FDA Approved 1989 Dec

BRAND NAMES: **Dalgan**

DESCRIPTION:

Dezocine is a synthetic opioid agonist-antagonist parenteral analgesic of the aminotetralin series. The chemical name is (-)-(5R-(5α, 11α,13S*))-13-amino-5,6,7,8,9,10,11,12-octahydro-5-methyl-5,11-methanobenzocyclo-decen-3-ol.

The molecular weight of the base is 245.4, and the molecular formula is $C_{16}H_{23}NO$. The n-octanol: water partition coefficient of dezocine is 1.7.

Dezocine is available in three concentrations: 5, 10, and 15 mg of dezocine per ml for intravenous or intramuscular administration. Each ml of the 5 mg strength contains 0.15 mg sodium metabisulfite and 7.236 mg lactic acid. Each ml of the 10 mg strength contains 0.15 mg sodium metabisulfite and 9.406 mg lactic acid. Each ml of the 15 mg strength contains 0.075 mg sodium metabisulfite and 11.578 mg lactic acid. Each ml of all three strengths contains 0.3 ml propylene glycol as a preservative and Water for Injection. The pH of dezocine solutions is adjusted to 4.0 with sodium hydroxide.

CLINICAL PHARMACOLOGY:

PHARMACODYNAMICS

Dezocine is a strong opioid analgesic. It analgesic potency, onset, and duration of action in the relief of postoperative pain are comparable to morphine. Pain relief in patients with postoperative pain is clinically evident when steady-state serum levels exceed 5 to 9 ng/ml. The side effects listed under ADVERSE REACTIONS were observed in patients whose average peak levels were less than 45 ng/ml. Peak analgesic effect lags peak serum levels by 20 to 60 minutes (TABLE 1):

TABLE 1 Table of Estimated Pharmacodynamic Parameters Following Intramuscular Dose of dezocine

C(50)est1	5 to 9 ng/ml
C(toxic)est2	45 ng/ml

1 Estimated concentration required to obtain 50% decreased in pain intensity scores in post-operative pain.
2 Estimated concentration above which side effects may be more frequently.

PHARMACOKINETICS

Dezocine is completely and rapidly absorbed following intramuscular injection in normal volunteers, with an average peak serum concentration of 19 ng/ml (range 10 to 38 ng/ml) occurring between 10 and 90 minutes after a 10 mg intramuscular injection. Following a 10 mg intravenous infusion over 5 minuets, the average terminal half-life of dezocine is 2.4 hr (range 1.2 to 7.3 hr). The average volume of distribution (Vss) is 10.1 L/kg (range 4.7 to 20.1 L/kg), and the average total body clearance is 3.3 L/hr/kg (range 1.7 to 7.2 L/hr/kg). There is evidence of nonlinear (dose-dependent) pharmacokinetics at doses above 10 mg: in a study where 5, 10 and 20 mg intravenous doses of dezocine were given (N=12), dose-proportional serum levels were observed after 5 and 10 mg injections, but the area under the serum concentration-time curve for the 20 mg dose was about 25% greater, and the total body clearance was about 20% lower, when compared to the 5 and 10 mg doses. The pharmacokinetic of dezocine following chronic administration (steady-state pharmacokinetics) have not been experimentally determined, but predicted serum levels for 5 and 15 mg intramuscular doses given every 4 hr are presented in the graph.

Approximately two-thirds of a dezocine dose in recovered in the urine with about 1% being excreted as unchanged dezocine and the remainder as the glucuronide conjugate. Protein binding of dezocine has not been studied (TABLE 2):

(For graph showing simulated mean serum concentrations of Dezocine in normal subjects receiving 5 and 15 mg q4h IM doses, please see original package insert).

Hepatic insufficiency did not after total body clearance in one study of 7 patients with cirrhosis. The volume of distribution and consequently the half-life, however, were increased by 30-50% relative to normal volunteers following a 10 mg intravenous dose. It is not known whether the free concentration of dezocine is altered in cirrhotic patients.

The effect of renal insufficiency on dezocine kinetics (urinary elimination) has not been studied. Because the primary elimination of dezocine is through the urine as a glucuronide, however, us in patients with renal disfunction should be done cautiously with reduced doses.

NARCOTIC ANTAGONIST ACTIVITY

Dezocine is a mixed opioid agonist-antagonist analgesic. Its opioid antagonist activity is less than that of nalorphine but greater than that of pentazocine when measured by antagonism of morphine-induced narcosis in rats.

CLINICAL PHARMACOLOGY: *(cont'd)*

TABLE 2 Mean (range) Pharmacokinetic Parameters of Dezocine in Normal Volunteers

		Dose	
IV	5 mg (N=12)	10 mg (N=36)	20 mg (N=12)
Clearance (L/hr/kg)	3.52 (2.1-6.2)	3.33 (1.7-7.2)	2.76 (1.7-4.1)
V_{ss} (L/kg)	10.7 (6.4-15.5)	10.1 (4.7-2 0.1)	8.8 (5.8-13.5)
t1/2 (hr)	1.7 (0.6-4.4)	2.4 (1.2-7.4)	2.4 (1.4-5.2)
IM		(N=24)	
Bioavailability		100%	
C_{max}1 (ng/ml)		10-38	
t_{max}2 (min)		10-90	

1 Peak plasma concentration.
2 Time-to-peak plasma concentration.

EFFECT ON RESPIRATION

Dezocine and morphine produce a similar degree of respiratory depression when given in the usual analgesic doses. The effect is dose dependent and may be reversed by naloxone. As the dose of dezocine is increased, there appears to be an upper limit to the magnitude of the respiratory depression produced by the drug in both animals and healthy human volunteers dezocine, like other mixed agonist-antagonist analgesics, may offer increased safety over pure agonist drugs such as morphine.

CARDIOVASCULAR EFFECTS

Dezocine has not been found to be associated with clinically important adverse effects on cardiac performance. Dalagan has been administered to patients as a 4-minute intravenous infusion at approximately 10 times the usual recommended intravenous dose without causing significant changes in mean systemic artery pressure, mean pulmonary artery pressure, pulmonary capillary wedge pressure, cardiac output, stroke index, and left ventricular stroke work index.

POSTOPERATIVE ANALGESIA

The analgesic efficacy of dezocine was investigated in randomized controlled clinical trials in postoperative general surgical pain (orthopedic, gynecologic and abdominal). The studies were primarily double-blind single-dose, parallel trials in which dezocine in intravenous (IV) doses of 2.5 to 10 mg (85 to 160 patients per treatment group) or intramuscular (IM) doses of 5 to 20 mg (39 to 221 patients per treatment group) was compared to 5 to 10 mg or morphine or 1 mg of IV butorphanol in patients with moderate-to-severe pain at baseline.

The onset of analgesic action was similar for dezocine, morphine, and butorphanol, occurring within 15 minutes of IV and 30 minutes of IM administration of the drug. Dezocine in 10 mg IM doses produced analgesia similar to that produced by 10 mg of IM morphine, while 5 mg of dezocine IV was equivalent to 1 mg of I butorphanol.

The peak analgesic effect and duration of analgesia were comparable for both routes of administration. The time by which approximately half of the patients rededicated was dose related and independent of the route of administration. Half of the patients rededicated within 2 hours after 5 mg of dezocine or 1 mg of butorphanol IV, 3 hours after 10 mg of dezocine or morphine IM, and 4 hours after 15 mg of dezocine IM.

Another measure of the effect of dezocine was the number of patients who did not require remediation during the six hours of the trial. The percentage of patients who did not request additional medication during the trial was 21% after a single dose of 125 mg of dezocine, 15% after 10 mg of dezocine or morphine, and 4% after placebo.

Pain relief was proportional to the dose od dezocine for single doses less than 20 mg. In one study with 39 to 42 patients per treatment group, comparing single doses of 20 or 10 mg of IM dezocine with 10 mg of IM morphine, the patients receiving 20 mg of dezocine did not obtain as much pain relief as that provided by 15 mg of the drug in other studies (the patients who received 10 mg of dezocine or morphine in this study did obtain analgesia comparable to that seen in other trials). These results suggest that the maximally effective dose of dezocine in postoperative pain may be 15 mg due to dezocine's mixed agonist-antagonist pharmacology.

USE IN CHRONIC PAIN STATES

Data on the use of dezocine in chronic pain has been gathered in trials of burn patients (n=16) and cancer pain (n=88). The daily dose of dezocine for most patients with chronic pain has ranged between 20 and 60 mg per day, although doses as large as 90 to 140 per day have been used in 15 patients.

Dezocine has not bee adequately studies in the management of chronic pain. It is not recommended for use in patients who may have developed significant tolerance to opioid drugs from long-term use because of the risk of precipitating acute withdrawal symptoms.

INDICATIONS AND USAGE:

Dezocine is indicated for the management of pain when the use of an opioid analgesic is appropriate (see CLINICAL PHARMACOLOGY).

CONTRAINDICATIONS:

Dezocine should not be administered to patients who have been shown to be hypersensitive to it.

WARNINGS:

CONTAINS SODIUM METABISULFITE, A SULFITE THAT MAY CAUSE ALLERGIC-TYPE REACTIONS INCLUDING ANAPHYLACTIC SYMPTOMS AND LIFE-THREATENING OR LESS SEVERE ASTHMATIC EPISODES IS CERTAIN SUSCEPTIBLE PEOPLE. THE OVERALL PREVALENCE OF SULFITE SENSITIVITY IN THE GENERAL POPULATION IS UNKNOWN AND PROBABLY LOW. SULFITE SENSITIVITY IS SEEN MORE FREQUENTLY IN ASTHMATIC THAN IN NONASTHMATIC PEOPLE.

PATIENTS PHYSICALLY DEPENDENT ON NARCOTICS

Because of its opioid antagonist properties, dezocine is not recommended for patients who are physically dependent on narcotics. Patients who have recently taken substantial amounts of narcotics may experience withdrawal symptoms.

Because of the difficulty in assessing dependence in patients who have previously received substantial amounts of narcotic medication, caution should be used in the administration of dezocine to such patients. To avoid precipitating an acute narcotic abstinence reaction, a sufficient period of withdrawal from opioids should be allowed before dezocine is administered.

PRECAUTIONS:

DEZOCINE IS A STRONG OPIOID ANALGESIC AND, LIKE ALL SUCH DRUGS, IT SHOULD BE ADMINISTERED IN CLINICAL SETTINGS WHERE RESPIRATORY DEPRESSION WILL BE PROMPTLY RECOGNIZED AND APPROPRIATELY MANAGED.

RESPIRATORY DEPRESSION INDUCED BY DEZOCINE CAN BE REVERSED WITH NALOXONE.

Head Injury And Increased Intracranial Pressure: Although there is no clinical experience in patients with head injury, the possible respiratory depressant effect and the potential of strong analgesics to elevate cerebrospinal-fluid pressure (resulting from vasodilatation following CO_2 retention) may be markedly exaggerated in the presence of head injury, intracranial lesions, or a preexisting increase in intracranial pressure. Furthermore, strong analgesics can produce effects that may obscure the clinical course of patients with head injuries. In such patients, dezocine should be used only when essential and with extreme caution.

Use In Chronic Obstructive Pulmonary Disease: Because strong opioids cause some respiration depression, they should be administered only with caution and in low doses to patients with preexisting respiratory depression (*e.g.*, from other medication, uremia, or severe infection), severely limited respiratory reserve, bronchial asthma, obstructive respiratory conditions, or cyanosis. Respiratory depression induced by dezocine can be reversed by naloxone.

Use In Hepatic Or Renal Disease: Dezocine undergoes extensive hepatic metabolism and renal excretion of the glucuronide metabolite (see CLINICAL PHARMACOLOGY). Administration to patients with hepatic or renal dysfunction should be cautious using reduced doses.

Use In Biliary Surgery: Although there is no evidence that dezocine alters the tonic pressure within the common bile duct, therapeutic doses of other opioid analgesics can significantly increase pressure within the common bile duct. Dezocine should be used with caution in such settings.

Use With Other Central Nervous System Depressants: Opioid analgesics, general anesthetics, sedatives, tranquilizers, hypnotics, or other CNS depressants (including alcohol) administered concomitantly with dezocine may have an additive effect. When such combined therapy is contemplated, the dose of one or both agents should be reduced.

Use In Drug Or Alcohol Dependence: Use of dezocine in combination with alcohol and/or other CNS depressant drugs will result in increased risk to the patient dezocine should be used with caution in individuals with active drug or alcohol addiction who are not in a medically controlled environment. Self-administration of any strong opioid may increase the relapse rate in populations recovering from addiction in abstinence-based recovery programs.

Use In Ambulatory Patients: Strong opioid analgesics impair the mental or physical abilities required for the performance of potentially dangerous tasks such as driving a car or operating machinery. Patients who have been given dezocine should not drive or operate dangerous machinery until the effects of the drug are no longer present.

Pregnancy Category: In reproductive studies, dezocine was shown to cause a dose-related suppression of body weight and food consumption of the parenteral generation in rats receiving either intravenous or intramuscular doses. Pup body weight was suppressed in a dose-related fashion. Teratology studies conducted in mice, rats, and rabbits revealed to evidence of teratogenic effects. There are no adequate and well-controlled studies in pregnant women. Dezocine should be used during pregnancy only if the potential benefit justifies the potential risk to the fetus.

Labor and Delivery: Safety to the mother and fetus after dezocine administration during labor is unknown. The drug should be used in labor and delivery only when the physician deems its use essential to the welfare of the mother and infant.

Nursing Mothers: The use of dezocine in mothers nursing infants is not recommended, since it is not known whether this drug is excreted in breast milk.

Pediatric Use: Safety and efficacy in patients under the age of 18 years have not been established.

Use In The Aged: Like all strong, mixed opioid agonist-antagonist analgesics, dezocine has the ability to depress respiration and reduce ventilatory drive to a clinically significant extent. It also has the potential to alter mental status or induce delirium in elderly patients. Dezocine had not undergone sufficient clinical testing in the geriatric population to assess its relative risk compared to other opioid analgesics, but the initial dose of all drugs of this class should be reduced in the geriatric patient and subsequent doses individualized.

ADVERSE REACTIONS:

A total of 2192 patients have received dezocine on an acute or chronic basis in the initial clinical trials of the drug. In nearly all cases, the type and incidence of side effects were those expected of a strong analgesic, and no unforeseen or unusual toxicity was reported. There is, as yet, limited information on the use of dezocine for periods longer than 48 to 72 hours, but there was no evidence of hepatic, hematologic, or renal toxicity in 73 patients who received the drug for periods of time longer than 7 days.

The occurrence of adverse effects with dezocine is based on data obtained from patients treated in both controlled and uncontrolled clinical trials. The adverse effects are listed below by frequency of occurrence within the body system affected.

The frequencies shown reflect the acetal frequency of each adverse effect in patients who received dezocine. There has been no attempt to correct for a placebo effect or to subtract the frequencies reported by placebo-treated patients in controlled trials.

The following adverse reactions were reported at a frequency of 1% or greater:

Gastrointestinal System: Nausea*, vomiting*.

Nervous System: Sedation*, dizziness/vertigo.

Skin: Injection-site reactions*.

(Reactions occurring with a frequency of 1 to <3% are unmarked, while reactions occurring with a frequency of 3 to 9% are marked with an asterisk.*)

The following adverse reactions were reported with a frequency of less than 1% and are probably causally related to the administration of dezocine:

Body as a whole: Sweating, chills, flushing, low hemoglobin, edema.

Cardiovascular system: Hypotension, heart or pulse irregularity, hypertension, chest pain, pallor, thrombophlebitis.

Gastrointestinal system: Dry mouth, constipation, diarrhea, abdominal pain/distress/disorder.

Musculoskeletal system: Cramps/aching/pain.

Nervous system: Anxiety, confusion, crying, delusions, sleep disturbance, headache, delirium, depression.

Respiratory system: Respiratory depression, respiratory symptoms, atelectasis.

Skin: Pruritus, rash, erythema.

Special Senses: Diplopia, slurred speech, blurred vision.

Urogenital system: Urinary frequency, hesitancy, and retention.

The following adverse effects have been reported in less than 1% of the 2192 patients studied, and the association between these events and dezocine administration is unknown. They are being listed to serve as alerting information for the physician.

ADVERSE REACTIONS: *(cont'd)*

Gastrointestinal: Increased alkaline phosphatase and SGOT.

Respiratory system: Hiccups.

Special Senses: Congestion in ears, tinnitus.

There is no information available from postmarketing experience with the drug.

DRUG ABUSE AND DEPENDENCE:

Dezocine has substituted for morphine in abuse-liability testing in animals. It has been identified as a narcotic in abuse-liability testing in experienced drug abusers, but has shown no evidence of abuse in clinical use during drug development. Mixed opioid agonist-antagonists of this type are generally recognized as having less potential for abuse than pure agonists such as morphine or meperidine, but all such drugs have abuse potential in certain individuals, especially those individuals with a prior history of opioid drug abuse or dependence.

Dezocine has a limited capacity to induce physical dependence in animal testing. Increasing tolerance to dezocine or physical dependence on the drug were not seen in clinical trials.

OVERDOSAGE:

CLINICAL PRESENTATION

Although there have been no incidents of overdosage with dezocine during clinical trials, and thus no human experience with the drug, overdosage with dezocine is possible. Based on the preclinical pharmacology of dezocine, overdosage will produce acute respiratory depression, cardiovascular compromise, and delirium. The largest dose of dezocine which has been given to nontolerant healthy volunteers without toxicity has been 30 mg/70 kg.

TREATMENT

The pharmacologic treatment of suspected dezocine overdosage is intravenously administered naloxone. The respiratory and cardiac status of the patient should be evaluated constantly and appropriate supportive measures instituted, such as oxygen, intravenous fluids, vasopressors, and assisted or controlled respiration.

DOSAGE AND ADMINISTRATION:

INTRAMUSCULAR

Although the recommended single dose for an adult is 5 to 20 mg, the majority of patients in clinical trials received an initial dose of 10 mg. Dosage should be adjusted according to the patient's weight, age, severity of pain, physical status, and other medications that the patient may be receiving. dezocine may be repeated every 3 to 6 hours as necessary. The recommended maximum single dose is 20 mg, with a probable upper limit of 120 mg a day based on preclinical pharmacology of the drug. There is insufficient information regarding the risk of chronic use of dezocine to establish limits for the maximum recommended duration of treatment with the drug.

INTRAVENOUS

The recommended range for intravenous administration of dezocine is 2.5 to 10 mg repeated every 2 to 4 hours, with most patients in clinical trials receiving an initial intravenous dose of 5 mg.

SUBCUTANEOUS

Dalagan is not recommended for subcutaneous administration. Repeated injection of dezocine at a single site has been associated with subcutaneous inflammation, vascular irritation, and venous thrombosis in animals. The significance of this finding for patients is unknown, although injection-site reactions occurred in 4% of patients treated with dezocine in clinical trials.

Children And Adolescents: Dezocine is not recommended for patients under 18 years of age.

SAFETY AND HANDLING INSTRUCTIONS

For intramuscular or intravenous injection.

Dezocine is supplied in seated dosage forms and at low concentrations which pose no known risk to health-care workers. Accidental dermal exposure to dezocine should be treated by rinsing the affected area with fresh water.

Dezocine should be stored at room temperature and protected from light. As with all parenteral products, dezocine should be inspected visually for particulate matter and discoloration prior to administration, whenever solution and container permit. Do not use if the solution contains a precipitate.

Dezocine, like other mixed agonist-antagonist opioid analgesics, has low abuse potential in patient populations. However, strong mixed agonist-antagonist drugs have reportedly been associated with abuse and dependence in health-care providers and others with ready access to such drugs. Dezocine should be handled accordingly.

HOW SUPPLIED - EQUIVALENTS NOT AVAILABLE:

Injection, Solution - Intramuscular; - 5 mg/ml

2 ml x 10 (1 ml	$75.34	DALGAN, Astra USA	00186-1529-23
2 ml x 25 (1 ml	$183.43	DALGAN, Astra USA	00186-1520-13

Injection, Solution - Intramuscular; - 10 mg/ml

2 ml x 10 (1 ml	$78.21	DALGAN, Astra USA	00186-1524-23
2 ml x 25 (1 ml	$189.31	DALGAN, Astra USA	00186-1521-13
10 ml x 5	$310.70	DALGAN, Astra USA	00186-1522-12

Injection, Solution - Intramuscular; - 15 mg/ml

2 ml x 10 (1 ml	$80.04	DALGAN, Astra USA	00186-1525-23
2 ml(1 ml fill)	$195.16	DALGAN, Astra USA	00186-1523-13

DIASPORAL; PANCREATIN; PEPSIN *(001028)*

CATEGORIES: Digestants; Gastrointestinal Drugs

BRAND NAMES: Digepepsin

Prescribing information not available at time of publication.

HOW SUPPLIED - EQUIVALENTS NOT AVAILABLE:

Tablet, Uncoated - Oral

60's	$10.88	Digepepsin, Bradley Pharms	00482-0020-06

DIAZEPAM *(001033)*

CATEGORIES: Alcoholism; Analeptics; Anesthesia; Antianxiety Drugs; Anticonvulsants; Anxiety; Anxiolytics, Sedatives, Hypnotic; Athetosis; Benzodiazepines; Central Nervous System Agents; Cerebral Palsy; Convulsions; Delirium; Epilepticus; Inflammation; Muscle Relaxants; Muscles; Neuromuscular; Seizures; Skeletal Muscle Hyperactivity; Skeletal Muscle Relaxants; Spasm; Spasticity; Stiff-Man Syndrome;

Tension; Tetanus; Tranquilizers; Tremor; Insomnia*; DEA Class CIV; Sales > $500 Million; FDA Approval Pre 1982; Top 200 Drugs
* Indication not approved by the FDA

BRAND NAMES: *Alboral* (Mexico); *Aliseum*; *Alupram*; *Amiprol*; *Anlin*; *Ansiolin*; *Antenex* (Australia); *Anxicalm*; *Anxionil*; *Apo-diazepam* (Canada); *Apozepam*; *Armonil*; *Arzepam* (Mexico); *Assival*; *Atensine*; *Azedipamin* (Japan); *Baogin*; *Benzopin*; *Best*; *Betapam*; *Britazepam*; *Calmpose*; *Calmod*; *Caudel*; *Centrazepam*; *Chuansuan*; *Consilium*; D-Val; *Desconet*; *Desloneg*; Di-Tran; *Diaceplex*; *Dialag*; *Dialar* (England); *Diapam*; *Diapax* (Japan); *Diapine*; *Diaquel*; *Diatran*; *Diazemuls* (England); *Diazepam*; *Diazepan*; *Diazepin*; *Dipaz*; *Dipezona*; *Disopam*; *Dizam*; *Doval*; *D-Pam*; *Drenian*; *Ducene* (Australia); *Dupin*; *Eridan*; *Elcion CR*; *Euphorin*; *Euphorin P* (Japan); *Evacalm*; *Gewacalm*; *Gradual*; *Gubex*; *Horizon* (Japan); *Jinpanfan*; *Kratium*; *Kratium 2* ; *Lamra* (Germany); *Lembrol*; *Lovium*; *Mandro*; *Mandro-Zep* (Germany); *Melode*; *Mentalium*; *Meval*; *Nellium*; *Nerozen*; *Neurosedin*; *Nivalen*; *Nixtensyn*; *Noan*; *Notense*; *Novazam* (France); *Novodipam* (Canada); *Ortopsique* (Mexico); *Paceum*; *Pacitran*; *Paralium*; *Parzam*; *Pax*; *Paxate*; *Paxum*; *Pharmadine*; *Placidox 2*; *Placidox 5*; *Placidox 10*; *Plidan*; *Pomin*; *Propam*; *Prozepam*; *Psychopax*; Q-Pam; *Radizepam*; *Relanium*; *Reliver* (Japan); *Rival*; Ro-Azepam; *Saromet*; *Scriptopam*; *Seduxen*; *Servizepam*; *Simasedan*; *Sipam*; *Solis* (England); *Sonacon* (Japan); *Stesolid*; T-Quil; *Tensium*; *Tranquil*; *Tranquirit*; *Trazepam*; *Valaxona*; *Valinter*; *Valitran*; **Valium**; Valrelease; *Valuzepam*; *Vanconin*; *Vatran*; *Vazen*; *Vivol* (Canada); *Winii*; X-O'Spaz; *Zepaxid*; Zetran
(International brand names outside U.S. in italics)

FORMULARIES: Aetna; BC-BS; CIGNA; DoD; FHP; Humana; Foundation; Kaiser; Medco; Medi-Cal; PCS; PruCare; United; WHO

COST OF THERAPY: $4.20 (Anxiety; Tablet; 2 mg; 2/day; 120 days)

DESCRIPTION:

Diazepam is a benzodiazepine derivative developed through original Roche research. Chemically, diazepam is 7-chloro-1,3-dihydro-1- methyl-5-phenyl-2H-1,4-benzodiazepin-2-one. It is a colorless crystalline compound, insoluble in water and has a molecular weight of 284.74.

Tablets: 5-mg tablets contain FD&C Yellow No. 6 and D&C Yellow No. 10 dyes. Diazepam 10-mg tablets contain FD&C Blue No. 1 dye. Diazepam 2-mg tablets contain no dye.

Capsules: Diazepam slow-release capsules provide the actions of diazepam in a slow-release form.

Diazepam slow-release capsule shells contain the following dye system: FD&C Blue No. 1, FD&C Yellow No. 6, and D&C Yellow No. 10.

Injection: Each ml contains 5 mg diazepam compounded with 40% propylene glycol, 10% ethyl alcohol, 5% sodium benzoate and benzoic acid as buffers, and 1.5% benzyl alcohol as preservative.

CLINICAL PHARMACOLOGY:

TABLETS AND INJECTION

In animals, diazepam appears to act on parts of the limbic system, the thalamus and hypothalamus, and induces calming effects. Diazepam, unlike chlorpromazine and reserpine, has no demonstrable peripheral autonomic blocking action, nor does it produce extrapyramidal side effects; however, animals treated with diazepam do have transient ataxia at higher doses. Diazepam was found to have transient cardiovascular depressor effects in dogs. Long-term experiments in rats revealed no disturbances of endocrine function. Injections into animals have produced localized irritation of tissue surrounding injections and some thickening of veins after intravenous use.

TABLETS

Oral LD_{50} of diazepam is 720 mg/kg in mice and 1240 mg/kg in rats. Intraperitoneal administration of 400 mg/kg to a monkey resulted in death on the sixth day.

Reproduction Studies: A series of rat reproduction studies was performed with diazepam in oral doses of 1, 10, 80 and 100 mg/kg. At 100 mg/kg there was a decrease in the number of pregnancies and surviving offspring in these rats. Neonatal survival of rats at doses lower than 100 mg/kg was within normal limits. Several neonates in these rat reproduction studies showed skeletal or other defects. Further studies in rats at doses up to and including 80 mg/kg/day did not reveal teratological effects on the offspring.

In humans, measurable blood levels of diazepam were obtained in maternal and cord blood, indicating placental transfer of the drug.

CAPSULES

The administration of one 15 mg diazepam slow-release capsule results in blood levels of diazepam over a 24-hour period which are comparable to those of 5 mg diazepam tablets given three times daily.

The mean time to maximum plasma diazepam concentrations after administration of 15 mg diazepam slow-release capsules to eleven fasted subjects was 5.3 hours. The harmonic mean half-life of diazepam was 36 hours. The range of average minimum steady-state plasma diazepam concentrations during once-daily administration of 15-mg diazepam slow-release capsules to eleven normal subjects was 196 to 341 ng/ml.

INDICATIONS AND USAGE:

Diazepam is indicated for the management of anxiety disorders or for the short-term relief of the symptoms of anxiety. Anxiety or tension associated with the stress of everyday life usually does not require treatment with an anxiolytic.

In acute alcohol withdrawal, diazepam may be useful in the symptomatic relief of acute agitation, tremor, impending or acute delirium tremens and hallucinosis.

Diazepam is a useful adjunct for the relief of skeletal muscle spasm due to reflex spasm to local pathology (such as inflammation of the muscles or joints, or secondary to trauma); spasticity caused by upper motor neuron disorders (such as cerebral palsy and paraplegia); athetosis; stiff-man syndrome; and tetanus.

Injection: As an adjunct prior to endoscopic procedures if apprehension, anxiety or acute stress reactions are present, and to diminish the patient's recall of the procedures. (See WARNINGS.)

Injectable diazepam is a useful adjunct in status epilepticus and severe recurrent convulsive seizures.

Diazepam is a useful premedication (the IM route is preferred) for relief of anxiety and tension in patients who are to undergo surgical procedures. Intravenously, prior to cardioversion for the relief of anxiety and tension and to diminish the patient's recall of the procedure.

Tablets and Capsules: Oral diazepam may be used adjunctively in convulsive disorders, although it has not proved useful as the sole therapy.

The effectiveness of diazepam in long-term use, that is, more than 4 months, has not been assessed by systematic clinical studies. The physician should periodically reassess the usefulness of the drug for the individual patient.

CONTRAINDICATIONS:

Tablets: Diazepam is contraindicated in patients with a known hypersensitivity to this drug and, because of lack of sufficient clinical experience, in children under 6 months of age. It may be used in patients with open angle glaucoma who are receiving appropriate therapy, but is contraindicated in acute narrow angle glaucoma.

WARNINGS:

TABLETS

Diazepam is not of value in the treatment of psychotic patients and should not be employed in lieu of appropriate treatment. As is true of most preparations containing CNS-acting drugs, patients receiving diazepam should be cautioned against engaging in hazardous occupations requiring complete mental alertness such as operating machinery or driving a motor vehicle.

As with other agents which have anticonvulsant activity, when diazepam is used as an adjunct in treating convulsive disorders, the possibility of an increase in the frequency and/or severity of grand mal seizures may require an increase in the dosage of standard anticonvulsant medication. Abrupt withdrawal of diazepam in such cases may also be associated with a temporary increase in the frequency and/or severity of seizures.

Since diazepam has a central nervous system depressant effect, patients should be advised against the simultaneous ingestion of alcohol and other CNS-depressant drugs during diazepam therapy.

Management of Overdosage: Manifestations of diazepam overdosage include somnolence, confusion, coma and diminished reflexes. Respiration, pulse and blood pressure should be monitored, as in all cases of drug overdosage, although, in general, these effects have been minimal following overdosage. General supportive measures should be employed, along with immediate gastric lavage. Intravenous fluids should be administered and an adequate airway maintained. Hypotension may be combated by the use of levarterenol (Levophed) or metaraminol (Aramine). Dialysis is of limited value. As with the management of intentional overdosage with any drug, it should be borne in mind that multiple agents may have been ingested.

Flumazenil, a specific benzodiazepine-receptor antagonist, is indicated for the complete or partial reversal of the sedative effects of benzodiazepines and may be used in situations when an overdose with benzodiazepine is known or suspected. Prior to the administration of flumazenil, necessary measures should instituted to secure airway,ventilation and intravenous access. Flumazenil is intended as an adjunct to, not as a substitute for, proper management of benzodiazepine overdose. Patients treated with flumazenil should be monitored for re-sedation, raspatory depression and other residual benzodiazepine effects for an appropriate period after treatment. **The prescriber should be aware of a risk of seizure in association with flumazenil treatment, particularly in long-term benzodiazepine user and in cyclic antidepressant overdose.** The complete flumazenil package insert, including CONTRAINDICATIONS, WARNINGS and PRECAUTIONS, should be consulted prior to use.

TABLETS AND INJECTION

Usage in Pregnancy: An increased risk of congenital malformations associated with the use of minor tranquilizers (diazepam, meprobamate and chlordiazepoxide) during the first trimester of pregnancy has been suggested in several studies. Because use of these drugs is rarely a matter of urgency, their use during this period should almost always be avoided. The possibility that a woman of childbearing potential may become pregnant at the time of institution of therapy should be considered. Patients should be advised that if they become pregnant during therapy or intend to become pregnant they should communicate with their physicians about the desirability of discontinuing the drug.

Withdrawal symptoms of the barbiturate type have occurred after the discontinuation of benzodiazepines. (See DRUG ABUSE AND DEPENDENCE.)

INJECTION

When used intravenously, the following procedures should be undertaken to reduce the possibility of venous thrombosis, phlebitis, local irritation, swelling, and, rarely, vascular impairment: the solution should be injected slowly taking at least on minute for each 5 mg (1 ml) given; do not use small veins, such as those on the dorsum of the hand or wrist; extreme care should be taken to avoid intra-arterial administration or extravasation.

Do not mix or dilute diazepam with other solutions or drugs in syringe or infusion flask. If it is not feasible to administer diazepam directly IV, it may be injected slowly through the infusion tubing as close as possible to the vein insertion.

Extreme care must be used in administering injectable diazepam, particularly by the IV route, to the elderly, to very ill patients and to those with limited pulmonary reserve because of the possibility that apnea and/or cardiac arrest may occur. Concomitant use of barbiturates, alcohol, or other central nervous system depressants increases depression with increased risk of apnea. Resuscitative equipment including that necessary to support respiration should be readily available.

When diazepam is used with a narcotic analgesic, the dosage of the narcotic should be reduced by at least one-third and administered in small increments. In some cases the use of a narcotic may not be necessary.

Injectable diazepam should not be administered to patients in shock, coma, or in acute alcoholic intoxication with depression of vital sins. As is true of most CNS-acting drugs, patients receiving diazepam should be cautioned against engaging in hazardous occupations requiring complete mental alertness, such as operating machinery or driving a motor vehicle.

Tonic status epilepticus has been precipitated in patients treated with IV diazepam for petit mal status or petit mal variant status.

In humans, measurable amounts of diazepam were found in maternal and cord blood, indicating placental transfer of the drug. Until additional information is available, diazepam injectable is not recommended for obstetrical use.

Usage in Children: Efficacy and safety of parenteral diazepam has not been established in the neonate (30 days or less of age).

Prolonged central nervous system depression has been observed in neonates, apparently due to inability to biotransform diazepam into inactive metabolites.

In pediatric use, in order to obtain maximum clinical effect with the minimum amount of drug and thus reduce the risk of hazardous side effects, such as apnea, or prolonged periods of somnolence, it is recommended that the drug be given slowly over a three minute period in a dosage not to exceed 0.25 mg/kg. After an interval of 15 to 30 minutes the initial dosage can be safely repeated. If, however, relief of symptoms is not obtained after a third administration, adjunctive therapy appropriate to the condition being treated is recommended.

PRECAUTIONS:

TABLETS, CAPSULES AND INJECTION

If diazepam is to be combined with other psychotropic agents or anticonvulsant drugs, careful consideration should be given to the pharmacology of the agents to be employed - particularly with known compounds which may potentiate the action of diazepam, such as phenothiazines, narcotics, barbiturates, MAO inhibitors and other antidepressants. The usual precautions are indicated for severely depressed patients or those in whom there is any

PRECAUTIONS: *(cont'd)*

evidence of latent depression; particularly the recognition that suicidal tendencies may be present and protective measures may be necessary. The usual precautions in treating patients with impaired renal or hepatic function should be observed.

In elderly and debilitated patients, it is recommended that the dosage be limited to the smallest effective amount to preclude the development of ataxia or oversedation (2 mg to 2.5 mg once or twice daily, initially, to be increased gradually as needed and tolerated).

The clearance of diazepam and certain other benzodiazepines can be delayed in association with cimetidine (Tagamet) administration. The clinical significance of this is unclear.

Information for the Patient: To assure the safe and effective use of benzodiazepines, patients should be informed that, since benzodiazepines may produce psychological and physical dependence, it is advisable that they consult with their physician before either increasing the dose or abruptly discontinuing this drug.

ADDITIONAL INFORMATION FOR INJECTION

Lower doses (usually 2 mg to 5 mg)should be used for elderly and debilitated patients.

The clearance of diazepam and certain other benzodiazepines can be delayed in association with Tagamet (cimetidine administration. The clinical significance of this is unclear.

Although seizures may be brought under control promptly, a significant proportion of patients experience a return to seizure activity presumably due to the short-lived effect of diazepam after IV administration. The physician should be prepared to re-administer the drug. However, diazepam is not recommended for maintenance, and once seizures are brought under control, consideration should be given to the administration of agents useful in longer term control of seizures.

Since an increase in cough reflex and laryngospasm may occur with other peroral endoscopic procedures, the use of a topical anesthetic agent and the availability of necessary countermeasures are recommended.

Until additional information is available, injectable diazepam is not recommended for obstetrical use.

Injectable diazepam has produced hypotension or muscular weakness in some patients particularly when used with narcotics, barbiturates or alcohol.

DRUG INTERACTIONS:

If diazepam is to be combined with other psychotropic agents or anticonvulsant drugs, careful consideration should be given to the pharmacology of the agents to be employed - particularly with known compounds which may potentiate the action of diazepam, such as phenothiazines, narcotics, barbiturates, MAO inhibitors and other antidepressants. The usual precautions are indicated for severely depressed patients or those in whom there is any evidence of latent depression; particularly the recognition that suicidal tendencies may be present and protective measures may be necessary. The usual precautions in treating patients with impaired renal or hepatic function should be observed.

In elderly and debilitated patients, it is recommended that the dosage be limited to the smallest effective amount to preclude the development of ataxia or oversedation (2 mg to 2.5 mg once or twice daily, initially, to be increased gradually as needed and tolerated).

The clearance of diazepam and certain other benzodiazepines can be delayed in association with cimetidine administration. The clinical significance of this is unclear.

ADVERSE REACTIONS:

TABLETS

Side effects most commonly reported were drowsiness, fatigue and ataxia. Infrequently encountered were confusion, constipation, depression, diplopia, dysarthria, headache, hypotension, incontinence, jaundice, changes in libido, nausea, changes in salivation, skin rash, slurred speech, tremor, urinary retention, vertigo and blurred vision. Paradoxical reactions such as acute hyperexcited states, anxiety, hallucinations, increased muscle spasticity, insomnia, rage, sleep disturbances and stimulation have been reported; should these occur, use of the drug should be discontinued.

In peroral endoscopic procedures, coughing, depressed respiration, dyspnea, hyperventilation, laryngospasm and pain in throat or chest have been reported.

Minor changes in EEG patterns, usually low-voltage fast activity, have been observed in patients during and after diazepam therapy and are of no known significance.

Side effects most commonly reported were drowsiness, fatigue and ataxia; venous thrombosis and phlebitis at the site of injection. Other adverse reactions less frequently reported include: *CNS:* confusion, depression, dysarthria, headache, hypoactivity, slurred speech, syncope, tremor, vertigo. *G.I.:* constipation, nausea. *G.U.:* incontinence, changes in libido, urinary retention. *Cardiovascular:* bradycardia, cardiovascular collapse, hypertension. *EENT:* blurred vision, diplopia, nystagmus. *Skin:* urticaria, skin rash. *Other:* hiccups, changes in salivation, neutropenia, jaundice. Paradoxical reactions such as acute hyperexcited states, anxiety,hallucinations, increased muscle spasticity, insomnia, rage, sleep disturbances and stimulation have been reported; should these occur, use of the drug should be discontinued. Minor changes in EEG patterns, usually low-voltage fast activity, have been observed in patients during and after diazepam therapy and are of no known significance.

In peroral endoscopic procedures, depressed respiration, dyspnea, hyperventilation, laryngospasm and pain in throat or chest have been reported.

TABLETS AND INJECTION

Because of isolated reports of neutropenia and jaundice, periodic blood counts and liver function tests are advisable during long-term therapy.

DRUG ABUSE AND DEPENDENCE:

Withdrawal symptoms, similar in character to those noted with barbiturates and alcohol (convulsions, tremor, abdominal and muscle cramps, vomiting and sweating), have occurred following abrupt discontinuance of diazepam. The more severe withdrawal symptoms have usually been limited to those patients who had received excessive doses over an extended period of time. Generally milder withdrawal symptoms (*e.g.,* dysphoria and insomnia) have been reported following abrupt discontinuance of benzodiazepines taken continuously at therapeutic levels for several months. Consequently, after extended therapy, abrupt discontinuation should generally be avoided and a gradual dosage tapering schedule followed. Addiction-prone individuals (such as drug addicts or alcoholics) should be under careful surveillance when receiving diazepam or other psychotropic agents because of the predisposition of such patients to habituation and dependence.

DOSAGE AND ADMINISTRATION:

TABLETS

Dosage should be individualized for maximum beneficial effect. While the usual daily dosages given below will meet the needs of most patients, there will be some who may require higher doses. In such cases dosage should be increased cautiously to avoid adverse effects (See TABLE 1, TABLE 2 and TABLE 3.)

CAPSULES

Whenever oral diazepam 5 mg t.i.d., would be considered the appropriate dosage, one 15 mg diazepam slow-release capsule may be used.

DOSAGE AND ADMINISTRATION: *(cont'd)*

TABLE 1

ADULTS:	**USUAL DAILY DOSE**
Management of Anxiety Disorders and Relief of Symptoms of Anxiety.	Depending upon severity of symptoms-2 mg to 10 mg, 2 to 4 times daily
Symptomatic Relief in Acute Alcohol Withdrawal.	10 mg, 3 or 4 times during the first 24 hours, reducing to 5 mg, 3 or 4 times daily as needed
Adjunctively for Relief of Skeletal Muscle Spasm.	2 mg to 10 mg, 3 or 4 times daily
Adjunctively in Convulsive Disorders.	2 mg to 10 mg, 2 to 4 times daily
Geriatric Patients, or in the presence of debilitating disease.	2 mg to 2.5 mg, 1 or 2 times daily initially; increase gradually as needed and tolerated
Children: Because of varied responses to CNS-acting drugs, initiate therapy with lowest dose and increase as required. Not for use in children under 6 months.	1 mg to 2.5 mg, 3 or 4 times daily initially; increase gradually as needed and tolerated

NOTE: If 1 mg or 2.5 mg is the desired dose, scored diazepam tablets should be used.

Diazepam slow-release 15 mg capsules are recommended for elderly or debilitated patients and children only when it has been determined that 5 mg oral diazepam t.i.d. is the optimum daily dose.

Oral diazepam is not recommended for children under 6 months of age.

TABLE 2

ADULTS:	**USUAL DAILY DOSE**
Management of Anxiety Disorders and Relief of Symptoms of Anxiety.	Depending upon severity of symptoms -1 or 2 (15 to 30 mg) capsules once daily.
Adjunctively for Relief of Skeletal Muscle Spasm.	1 or 2 capsules (15 to 30 mg) once daily.

INJECTION

Dosage should be individualized for maximum beneficial effect. The usual recommended dose in older children and adults ranges from 2 mg to 20 mg IM or IV, depending on the indication and its severity. In some conditions, e.g., tetanus, larger doses may be required. (See dosage for specific indications TABLE 3.) In acute conditions the injection may be repeated within one hour although an interval of 3 to 4 hours is usually satisfactory. Lower doses (usually 2 mg to 5 mg) and slow increase in dosage should be used for elderly or debilitated patients and when other sedative drugs are administered. (See WARNINGS and ADVERSE REACTIONS.)

For dosage in infants above the age of 30 days and children, see the specific indications below (TABLE 3B). When intravenous use is indicated, facilities for respiratory assistance should be readily available.

Intramuscular: Injectable diazepam should be injected deeply into the muscle.

Intravenous Use: (See WARNINGS, particularly for use in children.) The solution should be injected slowly, taking at least one minute for each 5 mg (1 ml) given. Do not use small veins such as those on the dorsum of the hand or wrist. Extreme care should be taken to avoid intra-arterial administration or extravasation.

Do not mix or dilute diazepam with other solutions or drugs in syringe or infusion flask. If it is not feasible to administer diazepam directly IV, it may be injected slowly through the infusion tubing as close as possible to vein insertion.

Once the acute symptomology has been properly controlled with injectable diazepam, the patient may be placed on oral therapy with diazepam if further treatment is required.

MANAGEMENT OF OVERDOSAGE

Manifestations of diazepam overdosage include somnolence, confusion, coma, and diminished reflexes. Respiration, pulse and blood pressure should be monitored, as in all cases of drug overdosage, although, in general, these effects have been minimal. General supportive measures should be employed, along with intravenous fluids, and an adequate airway maintained. Hypotension combated by the use of levarterenol (Levophed) or metaraminol (Aramine). Dialysis is of limited value.

ANIMAL PHARMACOLOGY:

TABLETS AND INJECTION

Oral LD_{50} of diazepam is 720 mg/kg in mice and 1240 mg/kg in rats. Intraperitoneal administration of 400 mg/kg to a monkey resulted in death on the sixth day.

Reproduction Studies: A series of rat reproduction studies was performed with diazepam in oral doses of 1, 10, 80, and 100 mg/kg given for periods ranging from 60-228 days prior to mating. At 100 mg/kg there was a decrease in the number of pregnancies and surviving offspring in these rats. These effects may be attributable to prolonged sedative activity, resulting in lack of interest in mating and lessened maternal nursing and care of the young. Neonatal survival of rats at doses lower than 100 mg/kg was within normal limits. Several neonates, both controls and experimentals, in these rat reproduction studies showed skeletal or other defects. Further studies in rats at doses up to and including 80 mg/kg day did not reveal significant teratological effects in the offspring. Rabbits were maintained on doses of 1, 2, 5 and 8 mg/kg from day 6 through day 18 of gestation. No adverse effects on reproduction and no teratological changes were noted.

PATIENT INFORMATION:

Diazepam is used for the treatment of anxiety, muscle spams, and seizures. Inform your physican if you are pregnant or nursing. Diazepam may cause dizziness and drowsiness; use caution while driving or operating hazardous machinery. Do not take any other sedating drugs or drink alcohol while taking this medication. Diazepam may be habit forming. Withdrawal symptoms may occur after you stop taking it. Diazepam may be taken with or without food.

HOW SUPPLIED - RATED THERAPEUTICALLY EQUIVALENT:

Injection, Solution - Intramuscular; - 5 mg/ml

1 ml x 10	$34.26	Diazepam, Elkins Sinn	00641-6288-11
1 ml x 25	$60.94	Diazepam, Elkins Sinn	00641-0369-25
2 ml	$1.65	Diazepam 5, Abbott	00074-3210-01
2 ml syringe x	$38.18	Diazepam, Elkins Sinn	00641-6287-11
2 ml x 10	$25.88	Diazepam, Elkins Sinn	00641-1408-33
2 ml x 10	$29.21	Diazepam, Lederle Parenterals	00205-2810-95

HOW SUPPLIED - RATED THERAPEUTICALLY EQUIVALENT: *(cont'd)*

TABLE 3A

INDICATION	USUAL ADULT DOSAGE
Moderate Anxiety Disorders and Symptoms of Anxiety	2 mg to 5 mg, IM or IV. Repeat in 3 to 4 hours, if necessary.
Severe Anxiety Disorders and Symptoms of Anxiety	5 mg to 10 mg, IM or IV Repeat in 3 to 4 hours, if necessary.
Acute Alcohol Withdrawal: As an aid in symptomatic relief of acute agitation termor, impending or acute delirium tremens and hallucinosis.	10 mg, IM or IV initially, then 5 mg to 10 mg in 3 to 4 hours, if necessary.
Endoscopic Procedures: Adjunctively, if apprehension, anxiety or acute stress reactions are present prior to endoscopic procedures. Dosage of narcotics should be reduced by at least a third and in some cases may be omitted.	Titrate IV dosage to desired sedative response, such as slurring of speech, with slow administration immediately prior to the procedure. Generally 10 mg or less is adequate, but up to20 mg IV may be given, particularly when concomitant narcotics are omitted. If IV cannot be used, 5 mg to 10 mg IM approximately 30 minutes prior to the procedure.
Muscle Spasm: Associated with local pathology, cerebral palsy, athetosis, stiff-man syndrome or tetanus.	5 mg to 10 mg, IM or IV initially, then 5 mg to 10 mg in 3 to 4 hours, if necessary. For tetanus, larger doses may be required.
Status Epilepticus and Severe Recurrent Convulsive Seizures. In the convulsing patient, the IV route is by far preferred. This injection should be administered slowly. However, if IV administration is impossible, the IM route may be used.	5 mg to 10 mg initially (IV preferred). This injection may be repeated if necessary at 10 to 15 minute intervals up to a maximum dose of 30 mg. If necessary, therapy with diazepam may be repeated in 2 to 4 hours; however, residual active metabolites may persist, and readministration should be made with this consideration. Extreme caution must be exercised with individuals with chronic lung disease or unstable cardiovascular status.
Preoperative Medication: To relieve anxiety and tension. (If atropine, scopolamine or other premedications are desired, they must be administered in separate syringes.)	10 mg, IM (preferred route), before surgery.
Cardioversion: To relieve anxiety and tension and to reduce recall of procedure.	5 mg to 15 mg, IV, within 5 to 10 minutes prior to the procedure.

TABLE 3B

IV administration should be made slowly

INDICATION	DOSAGE RANGE IN CHILDREN
Moderate Anxiety Disorders and Symptoms of Anxiety. Severe Anxiety Disorders and Symptoms of Anxiety Acute Alcohol Withdrawal: As an aid in symptomatic relief of acute agitation termor, impending or acute delirium tremens and hallucinosis. Endoscopic Procedures: Adjunctively, if apprehension, anxiety or acute stress reactions are present prior to endoscopic procedures. Dosage of narcotics should be reduced by at least a third and in some cases may be omitted. See PRECAUTIONS for peroral procedures.	(IV administration should be made slowly)
Muscle Spasm: Associated with local pathology, cerebral palsy, athetosis, stiff-man syndrome or tetanus.	For tetanus in infants over 30 days of age, 1 mg to 2 mg IM or IV, slowly repeated every 3 to 4 hours as necessary. In children 5 years or older, 5 mg to 10 mg repeated every 3 to 4 hours may be required to control tetanus spasms. Respiratory assistance should be available.
Status Epilepticus and Severe Recurrent Convulsive Seizures: In the convulsing patient, the IV route is by far preferred. This injection should be administered slowly. However, if IV administration is impossible, the IM route may be used.	Infants over 30 days of age and children under 5 years, 0.2 mg to 0.5 mg slowly every 2 to 5 minutes up to a maximum of 10 mg (slow IV administration preferred.) Children 5 years or older, 1 mg every 2 to 5 minutes up to a maximum of 10 mg (slow IV administration preferred). Repeat in 2 to 4 hours if necessary. EEG Monitoring of the seizures may be helpful.
Preoperative Medication: To relieve anxiety and tension. (If atropine, scopolamine or other premedications are desired, they must be administered in separate syringes.) Cardioversion: To relieve anxiety and tension and to reduce recall of procedure.	(IV administration should be made slowly)

2 ml x 10	$30.00	Diazepam, Sanofi Winthrop	00024-0376-02
2 ml x 10	$34.38	Diazepam, Elkins Sinn	00641-3201-03
2 ml x 10	$37.69	Diazepam Inj, Lederle Parenterals	00205-2810-46
2 ml x 10	**$40.35**	**VALIUM, Roche Prod**	**00140-1931-06**
2 ml x 10	**$53.34**	**VALIUM, Roche Prod**	**00140-1933-06**
2 ml x 25	$64.06	Diazepam, Elkins Sinn	00641-1408-35
2 ml x 25	$70.31	Diazepam, Elkins Sinn	00641-0371-25
2 ml x 25	$90.00	Diazepam, Schein Pharm (US)	00364-0825-48
10 ml	$6.61	Diazepam 5, Abbott	00074-3213-01
10 ml	$6.90	Diazepam, IDE-Interstate	00814-2399-40
10 ml	$8.09	Diazepam, HL Moore Drug Exch	00839-7190-30
10 ml	$10.00	D-VAL, Dunhall Pharms	00217-6805-08
10 ml	$10.05	Diazepam, Rugby	00536-4200-70
10 ml	$11.25	Diazepam, Goldline Labs	00182-0094-63
10 ml	$11.25	Diazepam, United Res	00677-1088-21
10 ml	$13.35	Diazepam, Steris Labs	00402-0445-10
10 ml	$14.69	Diazepam, Schein Pharm (US)	00364-0825-54
10 ml	**$18.54**	**VALIUM, Roche Prod**	**00140-1932-06**
10 ml x 1	$11.88	Diazepam, Elkins Sinn	00641-2289-41

HOW SUPPLIED - RATED THERAPEUTICALLY EQUIVALENT: *(cont'd)*

10 ml x 10	**$135.17**	**VALIUM, Roche Prod**	**00140-1932-01**
10's	$30.63	Diazepam Inj 5, Elkins Sinn	00641-3200-03

Tablet, Uncoated - Oral - 2 mg

30's	$.62	Diazepam, H.C.F.A. F F P	99999-1033-01
100's	$1.75	Di-Tran, H & H Labs	46703-0084-01
100's	$2.09	Diazepam, United Res	00677-1048-01
100's	$2.09	Diazepam, H.C.F.A. F F P	99999-1033-02
100's	$3.00	Diazepam, Elkins Sinn	00641-4013-86
100's	$3.00	Diazepam, IDE-Interstate	00814-2395-14
100's	$4.85	Diazepam, Geneva Pharms	00781-1482-01
100's	$4.95	VAZEPAM, Major Pharms	00904-3903-60
100's	$5.66	Diazepam, Barr	00555-0163-02
100's	$5.97	Diazepam, Halsey Drug	00879-0546-01
100's	$6.00	Valium, Rugby	00536-3591-01
100's	$7.50	Diazepam, Purepac Pharm	00228-2051-10
100's	$8.40	Diazepam, Zenith Labs	00172-3925-60
100's	$8.40	Diazepam, Goldline Labs	00182-1755-01
100's	$8.51	Diazeapm, HL Moore Drug Exch	00839-7131-06
100's	$8.75	Diazepam, Schein Pharm (US)	00364-0774-01
100's	$8.95	Diazepam, Mylan	00378-0271-01
100's	$8.97	Diazepam, Voluntary Hosp	53258-0604-01
100's	$9.19	Diazepam, Bristol Myers Squibb	00003-0185-50
100's	$10.03	Diazepam, Lederle Pharm	00005-3128-23
100's	$10.03	Diazepam, Aligen Independ	00405-0068-01
100's	$12.00	Diazepam, Voluntary Hosp	53258-0604-13
100's	$17.96	Diazepam, Vangard Labs	00615-1532-47
100's	$24.55	Diazepam, Goldline Labs	00182-1755-89
100's	$25.29	Diazepam, Vangard Labs	00615-1532-13
100's	**$40.35**	**VALIUM, Roche Prod**	**00140-0004-01**
100's	**$42.57**	**VALIUM, Roche Prod**	**00140-0004-49**
500's	$7.50	Di-Tran, H & H Labs	46703-0084-05
500's	$9.45	Diazepam, IDE-Interstate	00814-2395-28
500's	$10.45	Diazepam, United Res	00677-1048-05
500's	$10.45	Diazepam, H.C.F.A. F F P	99999-1033-03
500's	$13.30	Diazepam, Elkins Sinn	00641-4013-88
500's	$17.35	VAZEPAM, Major Pharms	00904-3903-40
500's	$21.20	Valium, Rugby	00536-3591-05
500's	$22.25	Diazepam, Geneva Pharms	00781-1482-05
500's	$23.16	Diazepam, Halsey Drug	00879-0546-05
500's	$23.80	Diazepam, Qualitest Pharms	00603-3216-28
500's	$37.50	Diazepam, Purepac Pharm	00228-2051-50
500's	$39.89	Diazepam, Schein Pharm (US)	00364-0774-05
500's	$39.90	Diazepam, Zenith Labs	00172-3925-70
500's	$39.90	Diazepam, Goldline Labs	00182-1755-05
500's	$39.90	Diazepam, Mylan	00378-0271-05
500's	$40.41	Diazepam, Aligen Independ	00405-0068-02
500's	$41.25	Diazepam, Rugby	00536-3733-05
500's	$45.48	Diazepam, Bristol Myers Squibb	00003-0185-60
500's	$46.40	Diazepam, Lederle Pharm	00005-3128-31
500's	**$200.56**	**VALIUM, Roche Prod**	**00140-0004-14**
750's	$189.40	Diazepam, Glasgow Pharm	60809-0510-55
750's	$189.40	Diazepam, Glasgow Pharm	60809-0510-72
1000's	$20.90	Diazepam, H.C.F.A. F F P	99999-1033-04
1000's	$23.55	Diazepam, Elkins Sinn	00641-4013-89
1000's	$31.01	Diazepam, Barr	00555-0163-05
1000's	$34.76	Diazeapm, HL Moore Drug Exch	00839-7131-16
1000's	$37.60	Diazepam, Halsey Drug	00879-0546-10
1000's	$39.50	Valium, Rugby	00536-3591-10
1000's	$39.59	Diazepam, Schein Pharm (US)	00364-0774-02
1000's	$39.80	Diazepam, Zenith Labs	00172-3925-80
1000's	$39.80	Diazepam, Aligen Independ	00405-0068-03
1000's	$39.90	VAZEPAM, Major Pharms	00904-3903-80
1000's	$75.67	Diazepam, Bristol Myers Squibb	00003-0185-75

Tablet, Uncoated - Oral - 5 mg

30's	$.66	Diazepam, H.C.F.A. F F P	99999-1033-05
30's	$1.08	Diazepam, Talbert Phcy	44514-0955-18
100's	$1.50	Di-Tran, H & H Labs	46703-0085-01
100's	$2.21	Diazepam, United Res	00677-1049-01
100's	$2.21	Diazepam, H.C.F.A. F F P	99999-1033-06
100's	$3.38	Diazepam, IDE-Interstate	00814-2396-14
100's	$3.75	Diazepam, Elkins Sinn	00641-4014-86
100's	$6.85	Diazepam, Major Pharms	00904-3901-60
100's	$6.90	Diazepam, Geneva Pharms	00781-1483-01
100's	$7.92	Diazepam, Barr	00555-0363-02
100's	$8.40	Diazepam, Halsey Drug	00879-0544-01
100's	$9.30	Diazepam, Voluntary Hosp	53258-0605-01
100's	$9.95	Valium, Rugby	00536-3592-01
100's	$10.73	Diazepam, HL Moore Drug Exch	00839-7132-06
100's	$10.76	Diazepam, Purepac Pharm	00228-2052-10
100's	$12.10	Diazepam, Zenith Labs	00172-3926-60
100's	$12.10	Diazepam, Goldline Labs	00182-1756-01
100's	$12.48	Diazepam, Schein Pharm (US)	00364-0775-01
100's	$12.75	Diazepam, Mylan	00378-0345-01
100's	$14.25	Diazepam, Voluntary Hosp	53258-0605-13
100's	$15.96	Diazepam, Lederle Pharm	00005-3129-23
100's	$16.72	Diazepam, Aligen Independ	00405-0069-01
100's	$19.70	Diazepam, Bristol Myers Squibb	00003-0238-50
100's	$22.87	Diazepam, Major Pharms	00904-3901-61
100's	$23.20	Diazepam, Goldline Labs	00182-1756-89
100's	$31.95	Diazepam, Vangard Labs	00615-1533-47
100's	$33.48	Diazepam, Vangard Labs	00615-1533-13
100's	**$62.76**	**VALIUM, Roche Prod**	**00140-0005-01**
100's	**$64.95**	**VALIUM, Roche Prod**	**00140-0005-49**
500's	$6.95	Di-Tran, H & H Labs	46703-0085-05
500's	$10.95	Diazepam, IDE-Interstate	00814-2396-28
500's	$11.05	Diazepam, United Res	00677-1049-05
500's	$11.05	Diazepam, H.C.F.A. F F P	99999-1033-07
500's	$15.00	Diazepam, Elkins Sinn	00641-4014-88
500's	$22.50	Diazepam, Geneva Pharms	00781-1483-05
500's	$24.00	Diazepam, Major Pharms	00904-3901-40
500's	$34.48	Diazepam, Qualitest Pharms	00603-3217-28
500's	$35.19	Diazepam, Halsey Drug	00879-0544-05
500's	$38.95	Valium, Rugby	00536-3592-05
500's	$53.80	Diazepam, Purepac Pharm	00228-2052-50
500's	$57.45	Diazepam, Zenith Labs	00172-3926-70
500's	$57.45	Diazepam, Goldline Labs	00182-1756-05
500's	$57.80	Diazepam, Schein Pharm (US)	00364-0775-05
500's	$57.95	Diazepam, Mylan	00378-0345-05
500's	$73.16	Diazepam, Lederle Pharm	00005-3129-31
500's	$76.20	Diazepam, Aligen Independ	00405-0069-02

HOW SUPPLIED - RATED THERAPEUTICALLY EQUIVALENT:

(cont'd)

500's	$97.84	Diazepam, Bristol Myers Squibb	00003-0238-60
500's	**$312.54**	**VALIUM, Roche Prod**	**00140-0005-14**
720's	$24.20	Diazepam, Rugby	00536-3592-07
750's	$247.50	Diazepam, Glasgow Pharm	60809-0511-55
750's	$247.50	Diazepam, Glasgow Pharm	60809-0511-72
1000's	$22.10	Diazepam, H.C.F.A. F F P	99999-1033-08
1000's	$25.90	Diazepam, Elkins Sinn	00641-4014-89
1000's	$46.78	Diazepam, Barr	00555-0363-05
1000's	$60.10	Diazepam, Major Pharms	00904-3901-80
1000's	$60.20	Diazepam, Halsey Drug	00879-0544-10
1000's	$69.95	X-O'Spaz, Quality Res Pharms	52765-1003-00
1000's	$107.60	Diazepam, Purepac Pharm	00228-2052-96
1000's	$108.35	Diazepam, Aligen Independ	00405-0069-03
1000's	$113.50	Diazepam, Schein Pharm (US)	00364-0775-02
1000's	$113.75	Diazepam, Zenith Labs	00172-3926-80
1000's	$113.75	Diazepam, Goldline Labs	00182-1756-10
1000's	$113.75	Valium, Rugby	00536-3592-10
1000's	$113.79	Diazepam, HL Moore Drug Exch	00839-7132-16
1000's	$193.75	Diazepam, Bristol Myers Squibb	00003-0238-75
1080's	$35.52	Diazepam, Rugby	00536-3592-08

Tablet, Uncoated - Oral - 10 mg

30's	$.73	Diazepam, H.C.F.A. F F P	99999-1033-09
100's	$2.46	Diazepam, United Res	00677-1050-01
100's	$2.46	Diazepam, H.C.F.A. F F P	99999-1033-10
100's	$3.69	Diazepam, Martec Pharms	52555-0437-01
100's	$3.75	Diazepam, IDE-Interstate	00814-2397-14
100's	$10.20	Diazepam, Voluntary Hosp	53258-0606-01
100's	$11.50	Diazepam, Geneva Pharms	00781-1484-01
100's	$11.50	VAZEPAM, Major Pharms	00904-3902-60
100's	$11.61	Diazepam, Barr	00555-0164-02
100's	$12.90	Diazepam, Rugby	00536-3593-01
100's	$16.50	Diazepam, Voluntary Hosp	53258-0606-13
100's	$17.29	Diazepam, Purepac Pharm	00228-2053-10
100's	$17.62	Diazepam, Aligen Independ	00405-0070-01
100's	$19.50	Diazepam, Zenith Labs	00172-3927-60
100's	$19.50	Diazepam, Goldline Labs	00182-1757-01
100's	$19.71	Diazepam, HL Moore Drug Exch	00839-7133-06
100's	$19.75	Diazepam, Schein Pharm (US)	00364-0776-01
100's	$19.95	Diazepam, Mylan	00378-0477-01
100's	$25.25	Diazepam, Lederle Pharm	00005-3130-23
100's	$25.41	Diazepam, Major Pharms	00904-3902-61
100's	$30.21	Diazepam, Bristol Myers Squibb	00003-0245-50
100's	$32.58	Diazepam, Roxane	00054-8206-25
100's	$39.49	Diazepam, Parmed Pharms	00349-8450-01
100's	$42.22	Diazepam, Vangard Labs	00615-1534-47
100's	$43.00	Diazepam, Goldline Labs	00182-1757-89
100's	$44.29	Diazepam, Vangard Labs	00615-1534-13
100's	**$105.72**	**VALIUM, Roche Prod**	**00140-0006-01**
100's	**$107.92**	**VALIUM, Roche Prod**	**00140-0006-49**
500's	$11.93	Diazepam, IDE-Interstate	00814-2397-28
500's	$12.30	Diazepam, United Res	00677-1050-05
500's	$12.30	Diazepam, H.C.F.A. F F P	99999-1033-11
500's	$19.20	Diazepam, Elkins Sinn	00641-4015-88
500's	$40.25	VAZEPAM, Major Pharms	00904-3902-40
500's	$48.00	Diazepam, Geneva Pharms	00781-1484-05
500's	$54.80	Diazepam, Rugby	00536-3593-05
500's	$58.10	Diazepam, Qualitest Pharms	00603-3218-28
500's	$80.22	Diazepam, Aligen Independ	00405-0070-02
500's	$86.45	Diazepam, Purepac Pharm	00228-2053-50
500's	$92.50	Diazepam, Schein Pharm (US)	00364-0776-05
500's	$92.60	Diazepam, Zenith Labs	00172-3927-70
500's	$92.60	Diazepam, Goldline Labs	00182-1757-05
500's	$92.60	Diazepam, Mylan	00378-0477-05
500's	$92.60	Diazepam, HL Moore Drug Exch	00839-7133-12
500's	$123.84	Diazepam, Lederle Pharm	00005-3130-31
500's	$165.48	Diazepam, Bristol Myers Squibb	00003-0245-60
500's	**$527.38**	**VALIUM, Roche Prod**	**00140-0006-14**
720's	$51.21	Diazepam, Rugby	00536-3593-08
1000's	$24.60	Diazepam, H.C.F.A. F F P	99999-1033-12
1000's	$36.30	Diazepam, Elkins Sinn	00641-4015-89
1000's	$70.89	Diazepam, Barr	00555-0164-05
1000's	$102.40	Diazepam, Rugby	00536-3593-10
1000's	$102.70	VAZEPAM, Major Pharms	00904-3902-80
1000's	$141.70	Diazepam, Parmed Pharms	00349-8450-10
1000's	$143.50	Diazepam, Schein Pharm (US)	00364-0776-02
1000's	$183.33	Diazepam, HL Moore Drug Exch	00839-7133-16
1000's	$183.35	Diazepam, Zenith Labs	00172-3927-80
1000's	$183.35	Diazepam, Goldline Labs	00182-1757-10
1000's	$218.33	Diazepam, Bristol Myers Squibb	00003-0245-75
1080's	$69.65	Diazepam, Rugby	00536-3593-11
2500's	$370.75	Diazepam, Parmed Pharms	00349-8450-52

HOW SUPPLIED - NOT RATED EQUIVALENT:

Solution - Oral - 5 mg/ml

30 ml	$21.38	DIAZEPAM INTENSOL, Roxane	00054-3185-44

Solution - Oral - 5 mg/5ml

5 ml x 40	$67.27	Diazepam, Roxane	00054-8207-16
500 ml	$38.79	Diazepam, Roxane	00054-3188-63

Solution - Oral - 10 mg/10ml

10 ml x 40	$94.49	Diazepam, Roxane	00054-8208-16

DIAZOXIDE *(001034)*

CATEGORIES: Antihypertensives; Cardiovascular Drugs; Hypertension; Vasodilating Agents; Pregnancy Category C; FDA Approval Pre 1982

BRAND NAMES: *Eudimine* (England); **Hyperstat**; *Proglicem* (France, Germany); Proglycem
(International brand names outside U.S. in italics)

DESCRIPTION:

Diazoxide IV Injection is a nondiuretic benzothiadiazine antihypertensive agent. Each ampule (20 ml) contains 300 mg diazoxide, USP, in a clear, sterile, colorless aqueous solution; the pH is adjusted to approximately 11.6 with sodium hydroxide.

Diazoxide is 7-chloro-3-methyl-2*H*-1,2,4-benzothiadiazine 1,1-dioxide, with the empirical formula $C_8H_7ClN_2O_2S$, and the molecular weight 230.7. It is a white crystalline powder practically insoluble to sparingly soluble in water.

CLINICAL PHARMACOLOGY:

Diazoxide IV Injection produces a prompt reduction of blood pressure in man by relaxing smooth muscle in the peripheral arterioles. Cardiac output is increased as blood pressure is reduced. Studies in animals demonstrate that coronary blood flow is maintained, while renal blood flow is increased after an initial decrease.

Transient hyperglycemia occurs in the majority of patients treated with diazoxide, but usually requires treatment only in patients with diabetes mellitus. It will respond to the usual management measures, including insulin.

Blood glucose levels should be monitored, especially in patients with diabetes and in those requiring multiple injections of diazoxide. Cataracts have been observed in a few animals receiving repeated daily doses of intravenous diazoxide.

Since diazoxide causes sodium retention, repeated injections may precipitate edema and congestive heart failure. Increased volume of extracellular fluid may be a cause of treatment failure in nonresponsive patients. The increase in fluid volume characteristically responds to diuretic agents if adequate renal function exists. Concurrently administered thiazide diuretics may be expected to potentiate the antihypertensive and hyperuricemic actions of diazoxide. (See DRUG INTERACTIONS.)

Diazoxide is extensively bound to serum protein (>90%). The plasma half-life is 28 ± 8.3 hours; however, the duration of its antihypertensive effect is variable, generally lasting less than 12 hours.

INDICATIONS AND USAGE:

Diazoxide IV Injection is indicated for short-term use in the emergency reduction of blood pressure in severe, nonmalignant and malignant hypertension in hospitalized adults; and in acute severe hypertension in hospitalized children, when prompt and urgent decrease of diastolic pressure is required. Treatment with orally effective antihypertensive agents should not be instituted until blood pressure has stabilized. The use of diazoxide IV Injection for longer than 10 days is not recommended.

Diazoxide IV Injection is ineffective against hypertension due to pheochromocytoma.

CONTRAINDICATIONS:

Diazoxide IV Injection should not be used in the treatment of compensatory hypertension, such as that associated with aortic coarctation or arteriovenous shunt, and should not be used in patients hypersensitive to diazoxide, other thiazides, or other sulfonamide-derived drugs.

WARNINGS:

Rapid Decrease of Blood Pressure: Caution must be observed when reducing severely elevated blood pressure. Diazoxide should only be administered utilizing the new 150-mg minibolus dosage. The use of a 300-mg intravenous dose of diazoxide has been associated with angina and with myocardial and cerebral infarction. One instance of optic nerve infarction was reported when a 100-mmHg reduction in diastolic pressure occurred over ten minutes following a single 300-mg bolus. In one prospective trial conducted in patients with severe hypertension and coexistent coronary artery disease, a 50% incidence of ischemic changes in the electrocardiogram was observed following single 300-mg bolus injection of diazoxide. The desired blood pressure lowering should therefore be achieved over as long a period of time as is compatible with the patient's status. At least several hours and preferably one or two days is tentatively recommended.

Improved safety with equal efficacy can be achieved by administering diazoxide IV Injection as a minibolus dose (1 to 3 mg/kg every 5 to 15 minutes up to a maximum of 150 mg in a single injection) until a diastolic blood pressure below 100 mmHg is achieved. Diazoxide IV Injection should not be administered in a bolus dose of 300 mg since this mode of administration is less predictable and less controllable than the minibolus dosage. If hypotension severe enough to require therapy results from the reduction in blood pressure, it will usually respond to the Trendelenberg maneuver. If necessary, sympathomimetic agents such as dopamine or norepinephrine may be administered.

Special attention is required for patients with diabetes mellitus and those in whom retention of salt and water may present serious problems.

Myocardial Lesions in Animals: Intravenous administration of diazoxide in dogs has induced subendocardial necrosis and papillary muscles. These lesions, which are also produced by other vasodilator drugs (*i.e.,* hydralazine, minoxidil) and by catecholamines, are presumed to be related to anoxia resulting from a combination of reflex tachycardia and decreased perfusion.

PRECAUTIONS:

General: Diazoxide IV Injection is an effective antihypertensive agent requiring close monitoring of the patient's blood pressure at frequent intervals. Its administration may occasionally cause hypotension requiring treatment with sympathomimetic drugs. Therefore, diazoxide IV Injection should be used primarily in the hospital or where adequate facilities exist to treat such untoward responses.

Diazoxide IV Injection should be administered only into a peripheral vein. Because the alkalinity of the solution is irritating to tissue, avoid extravascular injection or leakage. Subcutaneous administration has produced inflammation and pain without subsequent necrosis. If leakage into subcutaneous tissue occurs, the area should be treated with warm compresses and rest.

Diazoxide IV Injection should be used with care in patients who have impaired cerebral or cardiac circulation, that is, patients in whom abrupt reduction in blood pressure might be detrimental or those in whom mild tachycardia or decreased blood perfusion may be deleterious (see WARNINGS) Prolonged hypotension should be avoided so as not to aggravate preexisting renal failure.

Information for the Patient: During and immediately following intravenous injection of diazoxide IV Injection, the patient should remain supine.

Laboratory Tests: Diagnostic laboratory tests necessary to establish the patient's condition and status should be carried out prior to treatment with diazoxide IV Injection. During and following treatment with diazoxide IV Injection, laboratory tests to monitor the effects of treatment with this drug and the patient's condition should be done. Among the tests (not necessarily inclusive) are: hematologic (hematocrit, hemoglobin, white blood cell and platelet counts); metabolic (glucose, uric acid, total protein, albumin,); electrolyte (sodium, potassium) and osmolality; renal function (creatinine urine-protein); electrocardiogram.

Drug/Laboratory Test Interactions: The hyperglycemic and hyperuricemic effects of diazoxide preclude proper assessment of these metabolic states. Increased renin secretion, lgG concentrations and decreased cortisol secretion have also been noted. Diazoxide inhibits glucagon-stimulated insulin release and will cause a false-negative insulin response to glucagon. In the rat, dog, and monkey, diazoxide increased serum free fatty acids and decreased plasma insulin levels.

Carcinogenesis, Mutagenesis, and Impairment of Fertility: No long-term animal dosing study has been done to evaluate the carcinogenic potential of diazoxide. No laboratory studies of mutagenic potential or animal studies of effects on fertility have been done.

PRECAUTIONS: *(cont'd)*

Pregnancy Category C: Diazoxide has been shown to reduce fetal and/or pup survival; and to reduce fetal growth in rats, rabbits, and dogs at daily doses of 30, 21, or 10 mg/kg, respectively. In rats treated at term, diazoxide, at doses of 10 mg/kg and above, prolonged parturition.

The safety of diazoxide IV Injection in pregnancy has not been established.

Nonteratogenic Effects: Diazoxide crosses the placental barrier and appears in cord blood. When given to the mother prior to delivery, the drug may produce fetal or neonatal hyperbilirubinemia, thrombocytopenia, altered carbohydrate metabolism, and possibly other side effects that have occurred in adults.

Labor and Delivery: Diazoxide IV Injection is not indicated for use in pregnancy. Intravenous administration of the drug during labor may cause cessation of uterine contractions, requiring administration of an oxytocic agent.

Nursing Mothers: Information in not available concerning the passage of diazoxide in breast milk. Because many drugs are excreted in human milk and because of the potential for adverse reactions in nursing infants from diazoxide, a decision should be made whether to discontinue nursing or to discontinue the drug, taking into account the importance of the drug to the mother.

Pediatric Use: See INDICATIONS AND USAGE.

DRUG INTERACTIONS:

Diazoxide is highly bound to serum protein. It can be expected to displace other substances which are also bound to protein, such as bilirubin or coumarin and its derivatives, resulting in higher blood levels of these substances.

An undesirable hypotension may result when diazoxide is administered to patients who have received other antihypertensive medication within six hours.

One patient in a clinical study exhibited excessive hypotension after concomitant administration of Diazoxide with hydralazine and methyldopa. An episode of maternal hypotension and fetal bradycardia occurred in hydralazine prior to administration of diazoxide. Neonatal hyperglycemia following intrapartum administration of diazoxide IV Injection has also been reported.

Diazoxide IV Injection should not be administered within six hours of the administration of: hydralazine, reserpine, alphaprodine, methyldopa, beta-blockers, prazosin, minoxidil, the nitrites and other papaverine-like compounds.

Concomitant administration with thiazides or other commonly used diuretics may be expected to potentiate the hyperuricemic and antihypertensive effects of diazoxide.

ADVERSE REACTIONS:

It is reasonable to speculate that the currently recommended minibolus dosing regimen, which has replaced the 300-mg bolus dose in clinical practice, will result in adverse effects which are of similar character but of lesser frequency and severity.

In clinical experience with the rapid bolus administration of 300 mg, the most common adverse reactions reported were: hypotension (7%); nausea and vomiting (4%); dizziness and weakness (2%). Additional adverse reactions reported with bolus administration of 300 mg were as follows:

Cardiovascular: sodium and water retention after repeated injections, especially important in patients with impaired cardiac reserve; hypotension to shock levels; myocardial ischemia, usually transient and manifested by angina, atrial and ventricular arrhythmias, and marked electrocardiographic changes, but occasionally leading to myocardial infarction; optic nerve infarction following too rapid decrease in severely elevated blood pressure; supraventricular tachycardia and palpitation; bradycardia; chest discomfort or nonanginal "tightness in the chest."

Central Nervous System: cerebral ischemia, usually transient but occasionally leading to infarction and manifested by unconsciousness, convulsions, paralysis, confusion, or focal neurological deficit such as numbness of the hands; vasodilative phenomena, such as orthostatic hypotension, sweating, flushing, and generalized or localized sensations of warmth; various transient neurological findings secondary to alteration in regional blood flow to brain, such as headache (sometimes throbbing), dizziness, lightheadedness, sleepiness (also reported as lethargy, somnolence or drowsiness), euphoria or "funny feeling," ringing in the ears and momentary hearing loss, and weakness of short duration; apprehension or anxiety.

Gastrointestinal: rarely, acute pancreatitis; nausea, vomiting and/or abdominal discomfort; anorexia; alteration in taste; parotid swelling; salivation; dry mouth; lacrimation; ileus; constipation and diarrhea.

Other: hyperglycemia in diabetic patients, especially after repeated injections; hyperosmolar coma in an infant; transient hyperglycemia in nondiabetic patients; transient retention of nitrogenous wastes; various respiratory findings secondary to the relaxation of smooth muscle, such as dyspnea, cough and choking sensation; warmth or pain along the injected vein; cellulitis without sloughing and/or phlebitis at the injection site of extravasation; back pain and increased nocturia; hypersensitivity reactions, such as rash, leukopenia and fever; papilledema induced by plasma volume expansion secondary to the administration of diazoxide reported in a patient who had received eleven injections (300 mg/dose) over a 22-day period; malaise and blurred vision; transient cataract in an infant; hirsutism, and decreased libido.

OVERDOSAGE:

Overdosage of diazoxide IV Injection may cause an undesirable hypotension. Usually this can be controlled with the Trendelenberg maneuver. If necessary, sympathomimetic agents, such as dopamine or norepinephrine, may be administered. Failure of blood pressure to rise in response to such agents suggested that the hypotension may have been caused by something other than diazoxide. Excessive hyperglycemia resulting from overdosage will respond to conventional therapy of hyperglycemia.

DOSAGE AND ADMINISTRATION:

Diazoxide IV Injection was originally recommended for use by bolus administration of 300 mg. Recent studies have shown that minibolus administration of Diazoxide IV Injection, i.e., doses of 1 to 3 mg/kg repeated at intervals of 5 to 15 minutes is as effective in reducing blood pressure. Minibolus administration usually provides a more gradual reduction in blood pressure and thus may be expected to reduce the circulatory and neurological risks associated with acute hypotension.

Diazoxide IV Injection is administered undiluted and rapidly by intravenous injections of 1 to 3 mg/kg up to a maximum of 150 mg in a single injection. This dose may be repeated at intervals of 5 to 15 minutes until a satisfactory reduction in blood pressure (diastolic pressure below 100 mmHg) has been achieved.

With the patient recumbent, the calculated dose of diazoxide IV Injection is administered intravenously in 30 seconds or less.

Diazoxide IV Injection should only be given into a peripheral vein. Do not administer it intramuscularly, subcutaneously, or into body cavities. Avoid extravasation of the drug into subcutaneous tissues.

DOSAGE AND ADMINISTRATION: *(cont'd)*

Following the use of diazoxide IV Injection, the blood pressure should be monitored closely until it has stabilized. Thereafter, measurements taken hourly during the balance of the effect should indicate any unusual response. A further decrease in blood pressure 30 minutes or more after injection should be investigated for causes other than the action of diazoxide IV Injection. It is preferable that the patient remain supine for at least one hour after injection. In ambulatory patients, the blood pressure should also be measured with the patient standing before surveillance is ended.

Repeated administration of diazoxide IV Injection at intervals of 4 to 24 hours usually will maintain the blood pressure below pretreatment levels until a regimen of oral antihypertensive medication can be instituted. The interval between injections may be adjusted by the duration of the response to each injection. It is usually unnecessary to continue treatment with diazoxide IV Injection for more than four to five days.

Since repeated administration of diazoxide IV Injection can lead to sodium and water retention, administration of a diuretic may be necessary both for maximal blood pressure reduction and to avoid congestive heart failure. (See CLINICAL PHARMACOLOGY.)

Parenteral drug products should be inspected visually for particulate matter and discoloration prior to administration whenever, solution and container permit.

Protect from light and freezing. Store between 2 and 30°C (36 and 86°F).

HOW SUPPLIED - EQUIVALENTS NOT AVAILABLE:

Injection, Solution - Intravenous - 15 mg/ml

20 ml	$93.33	HYPERSTAT I.V., Schering	00085-0201-05

DIBUCAINE *(001035)*

CATEGORIES: Antipruritics/Local Anesthetics; Pharmaceutical Adjuvants; Skin/Mucous Membrane Agents; FDA Pre 1938 Drugs

FORMULARIES: Aetna

Prescribing information not available at time of publication.

HOW SUPPLIED - EQUIVALENTS NOT AVAILABLE:

Ointment - Topical - 1 %

30 gm	$1.80	Dibucaine, Major Pharms	00904-2646-31

DICHLOROACETIC ACID *(001039)*

CATEGORIES: Dermatologicals; Epistaxis; Keratolytic Agents; Lesions; Skin/Mucous Membrane Agents; FDA Pre 1938 Drugs

DESCRIPTION:

Dichloroacetic acid ($CHC_{12}COOH$) is a clear, colorless liquid (sp. gr. 1.56) supplied full strength ready to use. It does not contain or require a solvent or diluent, is always uniform in potency.

Dichloroacetic acid remains colorless and retains its potency if kept in a tightly closed bottle and not contaminated with dissolved keratin or wooden applicators.

CLINICAL PHARMACOLOGY:

Dichloroacetic acid rapidly penetrates and cauterizes skin, keratin and other tissues. Its cauterizing effect is comparable to that obtained with such methods as electrocautery or freezing.

INDICATIONS AND USAGE:

The lesions for which therapy with dichloroacetic acid is indicated are calluses; hard and soft corns; xanthoma palpebrarum; seborrheic keratoses; ingrown nails; cysts and benign erosion of the cervix including endocervicitis; epistaxis.

CONTRAINDICATIONS:

Topically applied chemical cauterant-keratolytics should not be used for the treatment of malignant or premalignant lesions.

WARNINGS:

Dichloroacetic acid is an extremely powerful keratolytic and cauterant. It should be restricted to those areas where these effects are desired.

DOSAGE AND ADMINISTRATION:

The amount of dichloroacetic acid which should be applied varies with the nature of the lesion. Dense horny lesions such as corns, calluses, require repeated intensive treatment. Lesions of light density such as pedunculated warts, xanthoma palpebrarum, soft corns, seborrheic keratoses, should receive lighter applications. Similarly, the number of treatments necessary will vary depending on the particular lesion being treated.

(Glenwood)

HOW SUPPLIED - EQUIVALENTS NOT AVAILABLE:

Kit

12's	$36.49	BICHLORACETIC ACID, Glenwood	00516-1010-05

Liquid - Topical - 10 ml

10 ml	$44.57	Bichloracetic Acid/Replenishment, Glenwood	00516-1007-11
10 ml	$78.81	Bichloracetic Acid, Treatment Kit, Glenwood	00516-1004-11
75 ml	$110.21	Bichloracetic Acid, Restocking Unit, Glenwood	00516-1006-77

DICHLORODIFLUOROMETHANE; TRICHLOROMONOFLUOROMETHANE *(001040)*

CATEGORIES: Anesthesia; Antipruritics/Local Anesthetics; Local Anesthetics; Skin/Mucous Membrane Agents; Topical Anesthetics; FDA Pre 1938 Drugs

BRAND NAMES: *Derm-Freeze Aerosol*; **Fluori-Methane**
(International brand names outside U.S. in italics)

DESCRIPTION:

This combination drug spray is a vapocoolant intended for topical application.

INDICATIONS AND USAGE:

This combination drug spray is a vapocoolant intended for topical application in the management of myofascial pain, restricted motion, and muscle spasm, and for the control of pain associated with injections.

Clinical conditions that may respond to Spray and Stretch include low back pain (due to muscle spasm), acute stiff neck, torticollis, muscle spasm associated with osteoarthritis, ankle sprain, tight hamstring, masseter muscle spasm, certain types of headache, and referred pain due to trigger points. Relief of pain facilitates early mobilization in restoration of muscle function.

CONTRAINDICATIONS:

This combination drug is contraindicated in individuals with a history of hypersensitivity to dichlorodifluoromethane, and/or trichloromonofluoromethane. This product should not be used on patients having vascular impairment of the extremities.

WARNINGS:

For external use only.

Dichlorodifluoromethane and trichloromonofluoromethane are not classified as carcinogens. Based on animal studies and human experience, these fluorocarbons pose no hazard to man relative to systemic toxicity, carcinogenicity, mutagenicity, or teratogenicity when occupational exposures are below 1000 p.p.m. over an 8 hour time weighted average.

Contents under pressure. Store in a cool place. Do not store above 120°F. Do not store on or near high frequency ultrasound equipment.

PRECAUTIONS:

Care should be taken to minimize inhalation of vapors, especially with application around head or neck. Avoid contact with eyes. This combination drug should not be applied to the point of frost formation.

ADVERSE REACTIONS:

Cutaneous sensitization may occur but appears to be extremely rare. Freezing can occasionally alter pigmentation.

DOSAGE AND ADMINISTRATION:

To apply this combination drug, invert the bottle over the treatment area approximately 12 inches (30 cm.) away from site of application. Open dispenseal spring valve completely, allowing the liquid to flow in a stream from the bottle.

1. SPRAY AND STRETCH TECHNIQUE FOR MYOFASCIAL PAIN

Spray and Stretch technique is a therapeutic system which involves three stages: EVALUATION, SPRAYING, AND STRETCHING.

The therapeutic value of Spray and Stretch becomes most effective when the practitioner has mastered all stages and applies them in proper sequence.

I. EVALUATION

During the evaluation phase the cause of pain is determined as local spasms or an irritated trigger point. The method of applying the spray to a muscle spasm differs slightly from application to a trigger point. A trigger point is a deep hypersensitive localized spot in a muscle which causes a referred pain pattern. With trigger points the source of pain is seldom the site of pain. A trigger point may be detected by a snapping palpation over the muscle, causing the muscle in which the irritated trigger point is situated to "jump."

II. SPRAYING

A. Patient should assume a comfortable position.

B. Take precautions to cover the patient's eyes, nose, mouth, if spraying near face.

C. Hold bottle in an upside down position 12 to 18 inches (30 to 45 cm.) away from the treatment surface allowing the jet stream of vapocoolant to meet the skin at an acute angle to lessen the shock of impact.

D. The spray is directed is parallel sweeps 1.5 to 2 cm. apart.

The rate of spraying is approximately 10 cm/sec. and is continued until the entire muscle has been covered. The number of sweeps is determined by the size of the muscle. In the case of a trigger point, the spray should be applied over the trigger point, through and over the reference zone. In the case of muscle spasm, the spray should be applied from origin to insertion.

III. STRETCHING

During application of the spray, the muscle is passively stretched. Force is gradually increased with successive sweeps, and slack is smoothly taken up as the muscle relaxes, establishing a new stretch length.

Reaching the full normal length of the muscle is necessary to completely inactivate trigger points and relieve pain.

After rewarming, the procedure may be repeated as necessary. Moist heat should be applied for 10 to 15 minutes following treatment.

For lasting benefit, any factors that perpetuate the trigger mechanism must be eliminated.

2. PRE-INJECTION ANESTHESIA

Prepare syringe and have it ready. Spray skin with this combination drug, from a distance of about 12 inches (30 cm.) continuously for 3 to 5 seconds; do not frost the skin. Swab skin with alcohol and quickly introduce the needle with skin taut.

HOW SUPPLIED:

3.5 fl oz (103 ml) amber glass bottle.

Calibrated fine spray and calibrated medium spray.

HOW SUPPLIED - EQUIVALENTS NOT AVAILABLE:

Aerosol, Spray - Topical - 15 %/85 %

4 oz	$187.55	FLUORI-METHANE, Gebauer Chem	00386-0003-04
4 oz	$187.55	FLUORI-METHANE, Gebauer Chem	00386-0003-05

DICHLOROTETRAFLUOROETHANE *(001042)*

CATEGORIES: Anesthesia; Antipruritics/Local Anesthetics; Local Anesthetics; Mucous Membrane Agents; Skin/Mucous Membrane Agents; FDA Pre 1938 Drugs

BRAND NAMES: Frigiderm; Gebauer's 114

Prescribing information not available at time of publication.

HOW SUPPLIED - EQUIVALENTS NOT AVAILABLE:

Aerosol, Spray - Topical - 100 %

8 oz	$195.48	GEBAUERS 114, Gebauer Chem	00386-0006-06

DICHLOROTETRAFLUOROETHANE; ETHYL CHLORIDE *(001043)*

CATEGORIES: Anesthesia; Antipruritics/Local Anesthetics; Local Anesthetics; Skin/Mucous Membrane Agents; Topical Anesthetics; FDA Pre 1938 Drugs

BRAND NAMES: **Fluro-Ethyl**

Prescribing information not available at time of publication.

HOW SUPPLIED - EQUIVALENTS NOT AVAILABLE:

Aerosol, Spray - Topical - 75 %/25 %

9 oz	$209.26	FLURO-ETHYL, Gebauer Chem	00386-0002-09

DICHLORPHENAMIDE *(001044)*

CATEGORIES: Antiglaucomatous Agents; Carbonic Anhydrase Inhibitors; EENT Drugs; Eye, Ear, Nose, & Throat Preparations; Glaucoma; Intraocular Pressure; Ophthalmics; Pregnancy Category C; FDA Approval Pre 1982

BRAND NAMES: *Antidrasi*; **Daranide**; *Defenamida*; *Fenamide*; *Glaucol*; *Glauconide*; *Glaucoral*; *Glaumid*; *Oralcon*; *Oratrol*
(International brand names outside U.S. in italics)

FORMULARIES: Aetna; Medi-Cal

DESCRIPTION:

Dichlorphenamide is an oral carbonic anhydrase inhibitor. Dichlorphenamide, a dichlorinated benzenedisulfonamide, is known chemically as 4,5-dichloro-1,3-benzenedisulfonamide. Its empirical formula is:

$C_6H_6CL_2N_2O_4S_2$

Dichlorphenamide is a white or practically white, crystalline compound with a molecular weight of 305.16. It is very slightly soluble in water, but soluble in sodium hydroxide. Dilute alkaline solution of dichlorphenamide are stable at room temperature.

Dichlorphenamide is supplied as tablets, for oral administration, each containing 50 mg dichlorphenamide. Inactive ingredients are D&C Yellow 10, lactose, magnesium stearate, and starch.

CLINICAL PHARMACOLOGY:

Carbonic anhydrase inhibitors reduce intraocular pressure by partially suppressing the secretion of aqueous humor (inflow), although the mechanism by which they do this is not fully understood. Evidence suggests that HCO_3^- ions are produced in the ciliary body by hydration of carbon dioxide under the influence of carbonic anhydrase and diffuse into the posterior chamber with Na^+ ions. The aqueous fluid contains more Na^+ and HCO_3^- ions than does plasma and consequently is hypertonic. Water is attracted to the posterior chamber by osmosis. Systemic administration of a carbonic anhydrase inhibitor has been shown to inactivate carbonic anhydrase in the ciliary body of the rabbit's eye and to reduce the high concentration of HCO_3^- ions in ocular fluids. As in the case with all carbonic anhydrase inhibitors, dichlorphenamide in high doses causes some decrease in renal blood flow and glomerular filtration rate.

In man, dichlorphenamide begins to act within an hour and maximal effect is observed in two to four hours. The lowered intraocular tension may be maintained for approximately 6 to 12 hours.

INDICATIONS AND USAGE:

For Adjunctive Treatment Of: Chronic simple (open-angle) glaucoma, secondary, glaucoma, and preoperatively in acute angle-closure glaucoma where delay of surgery is desired in order to lower intraocular pressure.

CONTRAINDICATIONS:

Dichlorphenamide is contraindicated in hepatic insufficiency, renal failure, adrenocortical insufficiency, hyperchloremic acidosis, or in conditions in which serum levels of sodium or potassium are depressed. Dichlorphenamide should not be used in patients with severe pulmonary obstruction who are unable to increase their alveolar ventilation since their acidosis may be increased.

Dichlorphenamide is contraindicated in patients who are hypersensitive to this product.

WARNINGS:

Use in Pregnancy: Studies with dichlorphenamide in rate have demonstrated teratogenic effects (skeletal anomalies) at high doses. There is no evidence of these effects in human beings; however, dichlorphenamide should not be used in women of childbearing age or in pregnancy, especially during the first trimester, unless the benefits to be expected outweigh potential adverse effects.

PRECAUTIONS:

Potassium excretion is increased by dichlorphenamide and hypokalemia may develop with brisk diuresis, when severe cirrhosis is present, or during concomitant use of steroids or ACTH.

Interference with adequate oral electrolyte intake will also contribute to hypokalemia. Hypokalemia can sensitize or exaggerate the response of the heart to the toxic effects of digitalis (*e.g.,* increased ventricular irritability). Hypokalemia may be avoided or treated by use of potassium supplements such as foods with a high potassium content. Dichlorphenamide should be used with caution in patients with severe degrees of respiratory acidosis.

ADVERSE REACTIONS:

Certain side effects characteristic of carbonic anhydrase inhibitors may occur with dichlorphenamide. These effects may include gastrointestinal disturbances (anorexia, nausea, and vomiting), loss of weight, constipation, urinary frequency, renal colic, renal calculi, skin eruptions, pruritus, leukopenia, agranulocytosis, thrombocytopenia,headache, weakness, nervousness, globus hystericus, sedation, lassitude, depression, confusion, disorientation, dizziness, ataxia, tremor, tinnitus, and paresthesias of the hands, feet, and tongue.

DOSAGE AND ADMINISTRATION:

Dichlorphenamide is usually most successful when given in conjunction with miotics such as isoflurophate, demecarium bromide, pilocarpine, and physostigmine, or carbachol. In acute angle-closure glaucoma; it may be used together with miotics and osmotic agents in an attempt to reduce intraocular tension rapidly. If this is not quickly relieved, surgery may be mandatory.

DOSAGE AND ADMINISTRATION: *(cont'd)*

Dosage must be adjusted carefully to meet the requirements of the individual patient. A priming dose of 100 to 200 mg of dichlorphenamide (2 to 4 tablets) is suggested for adults, followed by 100 mg (2 tablets) every 12 hours until the desired response has been obtained. The recommended maintenance dosage for adults is 25 to 50 mg (1/2 to 1 tablet) once to three time daily.

HOW SUPPLIED:

Tablets Daranide, 50 mg each, are yellow, round, scored, compressed tablets, coded MSD 49.

HOW SUPPLIED - EQUIVALENTS NOT AVAILABLE:

Tablet, Uncoated - Oral - 50 mg

100's	$50.11	DARANIDE, Merck	00006-0049-68

DICLOFENAC *(001045)*

CATEGORIES: Analgesics; Ankylosing Spondylitis; Anti-Inflammatory Agents; Antiarthritics; Antipyretics; Arthritis; Cataract; Central Nervous System Agents; EENT Drugs; Eye, Ear, Nose, & Throat Preparations; Inflammation; NSAIDS; Nonsteroidal Anti-Inflammatory; Ophthalmics; Osteoarthritis; Pain; Spondylitis; Pregnancy Category B; Sales > $1 Billion; FDA Approved 1988 Jul; Patent Expiration 1993 Jul; Top 200 Drugs

BRAND NAMES: *Abdiflam*; *Abitren*; *Allvoran* (Germany); *Almiral*; *Almiral SR*; *Alonpin* (Japan); *Anfenax*; *Anfenax SR*; *Apo-Diclofenac EC*; *Arcanafenac*; *Arthrifen*; *Artrenac* (Mexico); *Artrites*; *Artrites Retard*; *Betaren*; *Blesin*; *Bolabomin* (Japan); *Calozan*; *Cataflam* (Mexico); *Cataflam Drops*; *Clofec*; *Clofen*; *Clonodifen* (Mexico); *Cordralan*; *Cordralan-N*; *Curinflam*; *Declophen*; *Decrol*; *Depain*; *Diclax*; *Diclax SR*; *Diclo-Basan*; *Diclofenac*; Diclofenac Sodium; *Diclofam*; *Diclofen*; *Diclomax*; *Diclon*; *Diclosian*; *Dicsnal* (Japan); *Difena*; *Difenac* (Japan); *Doflex*; *Doloflam*; *E*; *Ecofenac*; *Fenac* (Australia); *Flexagen*; *Fortfen SR*; *Hizemin* (Japan); *Inflamac*; *Inflanac*; *Klotaren*; *Lidonin*; *Magluphen*; *Monoflam* (Germany); *Naboal* (Japan); *Naclof*; *Nacpot*; *Olfen*; *Oritaren*; *Osteoflam*; *Painstop*; *Panamor*; *Pharmaflam*; *Remethan* (Germany); *Rewodina* (Germany); *Romaril*; *Savismin* (Japan); *Silino*; *Staren*; *Soproxen*; *Taks*; *Toraren*; *Tsudohmin* (Japan); *Valentac*; *Voltalen*; *Voltalen Emulgel*; *Votalen SR*; **Voltaren**; *Voltaren Emulgel* (Australia); *Voltaren Forte*; *Voltaren Ofta* (Germany); *Voltaren Ophta* (Canada); *Voltaren Ophtha*; Voltaren Ophthalmic; *Voltaren Rapid* (Australia); *Voltaren Retard* (Mexico); *Voltaren SR*; *Voltarene* (France); *Voltarol* (England); *Voren*; *Voveran*; *Vurdon*; *Yuren*
(International brand names outside U.S. in italics)

FORMULARIES: Aetna; BC-BS; Foundation; Medi-Cal

COST OF THERAPY: $405.88 (Arthritis; Tablet; 50 mg; 2/day; 365 days)

PRIMARY ICD9: 715.99 (Osteoarthritis, Unspecified, Multiple Sites)

DESCRIPTION:

TABLETS

Diclofenac, as the potassium or sodium salt, is a benzeneacetic acid, monopotassium or monosodium salt.

Diclofenac, as the potassium or sodium salt, is a faintly yellowish white to light beige, virtually odorless, slightly hygroscopic crystalline powder. Molecular weights of the potassium and sodium salts are 334.25 and 318.14, respectively. It is freely soluble in methanol, soluble in ethanol, and practically insoluble in chloroform and in dilute acid. Diclofenac potassium is soluble in water while diclofenac sodium is sparingly soluble in water. The n-octanol/water partition coefficient is, for both diclofenac salts, 13.4 at pH 7.4 and 1545 at pH 5.2. Both salts have a single dissociation constant (pKa) of 4.0 ± 0.2 at 25°C in water.

Diclofenac potassium is available as diclofenac immediate-release tablets of 25 mg and 50 mg for oral administration.

Diclofenac Immediate-Release Inactive Ingredients: Calcium phosphate, colloidal silicon dioxide, iron oxides, magnesium stearate, microcrystalline cellulose, polyethylene glycol, povidone, sodium starch glycolate, starch, sucrose, talc, titanium dioxide

Diclofenac sodium is available as delayed-release (enteric-coated) tablets of 25 mg, 50 mg, and 75 mg for oral administration.

Diclofenac Delayed-Release Inactive Ingredients: Hydroxypropyl methylcellulose, iron oxide,lactose, magnesium stearate, methacrylic acid copolymer, microcrystalline cellulose, polyethylene glycol, povidone, propylene glycol, sodium hydroxide, sodium starch glycolate, talc, titanium dioxide, D&C Yellow No. 10 Aluminum Lake (25-mg tablet only), FD&C Blue No. 1 Aluminum Lake (50-mg tablet only).

OPHTHALMIC SOLUTION

Diclofenac sodium ophthalmic solution, 0.1% solution is a sterile, topical, nonsteroidal, anti-inflammatory product for ophthalmic use. Diclofenac sodium is designated chemically as 2-[(2,6,- dichlorophenyl)amino]benzeneacetic acid, monosodium salt. The empirical formula of diclofenac sodium is $C_{14}H_{10}Cl_2NO_2Na$.

Diclofenac sodium ophthalmic is available as a sterile solution, which contains diclofenac sodium 0.1% (1 mg/ml).

Inactive Ingredients: Boric acid, edetate sodium (1 mg/ml), polyoxyl 35, castor oil, purified water, sorbic acid (2 mg/ml), and tromethamine.

Diclofenac sodium is a faintly yellow-white to light beige, virtually odorless, slightly hygroscopic crystalline powder. It is freely soluble in methanol, sparingly soluble in water, very slightly soluble in acetonitrile, and insoluble in chloroform and in 0.1N hydrochloric acid. Its molecular weight is 318.14.

Diclofenac sodium ophthalmic 0.1% is an iso-osmotic physiologically compatible solution with an osmolality of about 300 mOsmol/1000 g, buffered approximately pH 7.2. Diclofenac Sodium ophthalmic solution has a faint characteristic odor of castor oil.

CLINICAL PHARMACOLOGY:

PHARMACODYNAMICS

Diclofenac, the anion in immediate-release and delayed-release, is a nonsteroidal anti-inflammatory drug (NSAID). In pharmacologic studies, diclofenac has shown anti-inflammatory, analgesic, and antipyretic activity. As with other NSAIDs, its mode of action is not known; its ability to inhibit prostaglandin synthesis, however, may be involved in its anti-inflammatory activity, as well as contribute to its efficacy in relieving pain related to inflammation and primary dysmenorrhea. With regard to its analgesic effect, diclofenac is not a narcotic.

PHARMACOKINETICS

Diclofenac immediate-release tablets and diclofenac delayed-release tablets both contain the same therapeutic moiety, diclofenac. They differ in the cationic portion of the salt (see DESCRIPTION) as well as in their release characteristics. Diclofenac immediate-release tablets are formulated to release diclofenac in the stomach. Conversely, delayed-release (enteric-coated) tablets are in a pharmaceutical formulation that resists dissolution in the low pH of gastric fluid but allows a rapid release of drug in the higher pH-environment in the duodenum. The primary pharmacokinetic difference between the two products is in the pattern of drug release and absorption. For this reason, separate sections are provided below to describe the different absorption profiles of diclofenac immediate-release tablets and delayed-release tablets.

ABSORPTION

Diclofenac Immediate-Release Tablets: Diclofenac is rapidly and completely absorbed from the gastrointestinal tract, with measurable plasma levels being observed, in some fasting volunteers, within 10 minutes of dosing with immediate-release. Peak plasma levels are achieved in approximately 1 hour in fasting normal volunteers, with a range from 0.33 to 2 hours. Only 50% of the absorbed dose of diclofenac from immediate-release is systemically available, due to first pass metabolism. Peak plasma concentrations after oral administration of 25-mg and 50-mg immediate-release tablets were dose-proportional.

The extent of absorption of diclofenac from immediate-release tablets is comparable to that from a buffered solution of diclofenac potassium. After repeated oral administration of immediate-release 50 mg t.i.d., no accumulation of diclofenac in plasma occurred.

The extent of diclofenac absorption is not significantly affected when immediate-release is taken with food. However, the rate of absorption is reduced by food, as indicated by a delay in T_{max} and decrease in C_{max} values by approximately 30%.

Diclofenac Delayed-Release Tablets: Diclofenac is completely absorbed from the gastrointestinal tract after fasting oral administration of delayed-release. Of this, only 50% of the absorbed dose of diclofenac from delayed-release is systemically available, due to first pass metabolism. Peak plasma levels are achieved in 2 hours in fasting normal volunteers, with a range from 1 to 4 hours. The area-under-the-plasma- concentration curve (AUC) is dose-proportional within the range 25 mg to 150 mg. Peak plasma levels are less than dose-proportional and are approximately 1.0, 1.5, and 2.0 mcg/ml for 25-mg, 50-mg, and 75-mg doses, respectively. It should be noted that the administration of several individual delayed-release tablets may not yield equivalent results in peak concentration as the administration of one tablet of a higher strength. This is probably due to the staggered gastric emptying of tablets into the duodenum. After repeated oral administration of delayed-release 50 mg b.i.d., diclofenac did not accumulate in plasma.

When delayed-release is taken with food, there is usually a delay in the onset of absorption of 1 to 4.5 hours, with delays as long as 10 hours in some patients, and a reduction in peak plasma levels of approximately 40%. The extent of absorption, however, is not significantly affected by food intake.

DISTRIBUTION

Plasma concentrations of diclofenac decline from peak levels in a biexponential fashion, with the terminal phase having a half-life of approximately 2 hours. Clearance and volume of distribution are about 350 ml/min and 550 ml/kg, respectively. More than 99% of diclofenac is reversibility bound to human plasma albumin.

A 4-week study, comparing plasma level profiles of diclofenac (delayed-release 50 mg b.i.d. in younger (26-46 years) versus older (66-81 years) adults, did not show different between age groups (10 patients per age group).

As with other NSAIDs, diclofenac diffuses into and out of the synovial fluid. Diffusion into the joint occurs when plasma levels are higher than those in the synovial fluid, after which the process reverses and synovial fluid levels are higher than plasma levels. It is not known whether diffusion into the joint plays a role in the effectiveness of diclofenac.

METABOLISM AND ELIMINATION

Diclofenac is eliminated through metabolism and subsequent urinary and biliary excretion of the glucuronide and the sulfate conjugates of the metabolites. Approximately 65% of the dose is excreted in the urine, and approximately 35% in the bile.

Conjugates of unchanged diclofenac account for 5%-10% of the dose excreted in the urine and for less than 5% excreted in the bile. Little or no unchanged unconjugated drug is excreted. Conjugates of the principal metabolite account for 20%-30% of the dose excreted in the urine and 10%-20% of the dose excreted in the bile. Conjugates of three other metabolites together account for 10%-20%of the dose excreted in the urine and small accounts excreted in the bile. The elimination half-life values for these metabolites are shorter than those for the parent drug. Urinary excretion of an additional metabolite (half-life 80 hours) accounts for only 1.4% of the oral dose. The degree of accumulation of diclofenac metabolites is unknown. Some of the metabolites may have activity.

PATIENTS WITH RENAL AND HEPATIC IMPAIRMENT

To date, no differences in the pharmacokinetics of diclofenac have been detected in studies of patients with renal (50 mg intravenously) or hepatic impairment (100 mg oral solution). In patients with renal impairment (N=5, creatinine clearance 3 to 42 ml/min), AUC values and elimination rates were comparable to those in healthy subjects. In patients with biopsy-confirmed cirrhosis or chronic active hepatitis (variably elevated transaminases and mildly elevated bilirubins, N=10), diclofenac concentrations and urinary elimination values were comparable to those in healthy subjects.

CLINICAL STUDIES:

Diclofenac Immediate-Release Tablets in Analgesia/Primary Dysmenorrhea: The analgesic efficacy of immediate-release was demonstrated in trials of patients with postoperative pain (following gynecologic, oral, and orthopedic surgery), osteoarthritis of the knee, and primarily dysmenorrhea. The effectiveness of immediate-release in studies of pain or primary dysmenorrhea showed that onset of analgesia began, in some patients, as soon as 30 minutes, and relief of pain lasted as long as 8 hours, following single 50-mg or 100-mg doses. Duration of pain relief was judged by the time at which approximately half of the patients needed remedication. The onset and duration of pain relief for either the 50-mg or 100-mg dose was essentially the same, whether patients had moderate or severe pain at baseline.

Immediate-release was studied in single-dose and multiple-dose pain trials. The pain models in single-dose studies were post-dental extraction and post- gynecologic surgery: the efficacy of the 50-mg dose (N=258) and the 100- mg dose (N=255) was comparable to aspirin 650 mg in onset of pain relief, but generally provided a longer duration of analgesia than aspirin. The pain models for multiple-dose trials were post-orthopedic surgery pain as well as pain associated with primary dysmenorrhea: the efficacy of the 50-mg dose (N=101) and the 100-mg dose (N=442), followed by 50 mg every 8 hours, was comparable to naproxen sodium 550 mg followed by 275 mg every 8 hours. In one study of chronic pain, in patients with osteoarthritis (N=196), immediate-release 50 mg t.i.d. was comparable in efficacy to ibuprofen 800 mg t.i.d and Diclofenac delayed-release tablets 50 mg t.i.d.

Diclofenac Delayed-Release Tablets in Osteoarthritis: Delayed-release was evaluated for the management of the signs and symptoms of osteoarthritis of the hip or knee in a total of 633 patients treated for up to 3 months in placebo- and active-controlled clinical trials against aspirin (N=449), and naproxen (N=92). Delayed-release was given both in variable (100-150 mg/day) and fixed (150 mg/day) dosing schedules in either b.i.d. ot t.i.d. dosing regimens. In

CLINICAL STUDIES: *(cont'd)*

these trials, Delayed-release was found to be comparable to 2400 to 3600 mg/day of aspirin or 500 mg/day of naproxen. Delayed-release was effective when administered as either b.i.d. or t.i.d. dosing regimens.

Diclofenac Delayed-Release Tablets in Rheumatoid Arthritis: Delayed-release was evaluated for the management of the signs and symptoms of rheumatoid arthritis in a total of 468 patients treated for up to 3 months in placebo- and active-controlled clinical trials against aspirin (N=290) and ibuprofen (N=74). Delayed-release was given in a fixed (150 or 200 mg/day) dosing schedule as either b.i.d. or t.i.d. dosing regimens. Delayed-release was found to be comparable to 3600 to 4800 mg/day of aspirin, and 2400 mg/day of ibuprofen. Delayed-release was used b.i.d. or t.i.d., administering 150 mg/day in most trials, but 50 mg q.i.d. (200 mg/day) was also studied.

Diclofenac Delayed-Release Tablets in Ankylosing Spondylitis: Delayed-release was evaluated for the management of the signs and symptoms of ankylosing spondylitis in a total of 132 patients in one active-controlled clinical trial against indomethacin (N=130). Both delayed-release and indomethacin patients were started on 25 t.i.d. and were permitted to increase the dose 25 mg/day each week to a maximum dose of 125 mg/day. Delayed-release 75-125 mg/day was found to be comparable to indomethacin 75-125 mg/day.

G.I. Blood Loss/Endoscopy Data: G.I. blood loss and endoscopy studies were performed with delayed-release (enteric-coated) tablets that, unlike immediate-release tablets, do not dissolve in the stomach where the endoscopic lesions are primarily seen; diclofenac immediate-release tablets have not been similarly studied. A repeat-dose endoscopy study, in patients with rheumatoid arthritis or osteoarthritis treated with diclofenac delayed-release tablets 75 mg b.i.d. (N=101), or naproxen (immediate-release tablets) 500 mg b.i.d. (N=103) for 3 months, resulted in a significantly smaller number of patients with an increase in endoscopy score from baseline and a significantly lower mean endoscopy score after treatment in the diclofenac delayed—release treated patients. Two repeat-dose endoscopic studies, in normal volunteers showed that daily doses of diclofenac delayed-release tablets 75 or 100 mg (N=6 and N=14, respectively) for 1 week caused fewer gastric lesions, and those that did occur had lower scores than those observed following daily 500-mg doses of naproxen (immediate-release tablets). In healthy subjects, the daily administration of 150 mg of delayed-release (N=8) for 3 weeks resulted in a mean fecal blood loss less than that observed with 3.0 g of aspirin daily (N=8). In four repeat-dose studies, mean fecal blood loss with 150 mg of delayed-release was also less than that observed with 750 mg of naproxen (N=8 and N=6) or 150 mg of indomethacin (N=8 and N=6). *The clinical significance of these findings is unknown since there is no evidence available to indicate that delayed-release is less likely than other drugs of its class to cause serious gastrointestinal lesions when used in chronic therapy.*

INDIVIDUALIZATION OF DOSAGE

Diclofenac, like other NSAIDs, shows interindividual differences in both pharmacokinetics and clinical response (pharmacodynamics). Consequently, the recommended strategy for initiating therapy is to use a starting dose likely effective for the majority of patients and to adjust dosage thereafter based on observation to diclofenac's beneficial and adverse effects.

In patients weighing less than 60 kg (132 lb), or where the severity of the disease, concomitant medication, or other diseases warrant, the maximum recommended total daily dose of immediate-release or delayed-release should be reduced. Experience with other NSAIDs has shown that starting therapy with maximum doses in patients at increased risk due to renal or hepatic disease, low body weight (<60 kg), advanced age, a known ulcer diathesis, or known sensitivity to NSAID effects, is likely to increase frequency of adverse reactions and is not recommended (see PRECAUTIONS).

Analgesia/Primary Dysmenorrhea: Because of earlier absorption of diclofenac from diclofenac immediate-release tablets, it is the formulation indicated for management of pain an primary dysmenorrhea when prompt onset of pain relief is desired. The results of clinical trials suggest an initial immediate-release dose of 50 mg for pain or for primary dysmenorrhea, followed by doses of 50 mg every 8 hours, as needed. With experience, some patients with recurring pain, such as dysmenorrhea, may find that an initial dose of 100 mg of immediate-release, followed by 50 mg doses, will provide better relief. After the first day, when the maximum recommended dose may be 200 mg, the total daily dose should generally not exceed 150 mg.

Osteoarthritis/Rheumatoid Arthritis/Ankylosing Spondylitis: The usual starting dose of diclofenac delayed-release or diclofenac immediate-release tablets, for patients with osteoarthritis, is 100 to 150 mg/day, using a b.i.d. or t.i.d. dosing regimen. In two variable-dose clinical trials in osteoarthritis, of 266 patients started on 100 mg/day, 176 chose to increase the dose to 150 mg/day. Dosages above 150 mg/day have not been studied in patients with osteoarthritis.

The usual starting dose of diclofenac delayed-release or diclofenac immediate-release tablets for most patients with rheumatoid arthritis is 150 mg/day, using a b.i.d. or t.i.d. dosing regimen. Patients requiring more relief of pain and inflammation may increase the dose to 200 mg/day. In clinical trials, patients receiving 200 mg/day were less likely to drop from the trial due to lack of efficacy than patients receiving 150 mg/day. Dosages above 225 mg/day are not recommended in patients with rheumatoid arthritis because of increased risk of adverse events.

The recommended dose of delayed-release or immediate-release tablets for patients with ankylosing spondylitis is 100 to 125 mg/day, using a q.i.d. dosing regimen (see DOSAGE AND ADMINISTRATION regarding the 125 mg/day dosing regimen). In a variable-dose clinical trial, of 132 patients started on 75 mg/day, 122 chose to increase the dose to 125 mg/day. Dosages above 125 mg/day have not been studied in patients with ankylosing spondylitis.

INDICATIONS AND USAGE:

Tablets: Diclofenac immediate-release or diclofenac delayed-release tablets are indicated for the acute and chronic treatment of signs and symptoms of rheumatoid arthritis, osteoarthritis, ankylosing spondylitis. Only immediate-release is indicated for the management of pain and primary dysmenorrhea, when prompt pain relief is desired, because it is formulated to provide earlier plasma concentrations of diclofenac (see CLINICAL PHARMACOLOGY, Pharmacokinetics and CLINICAL STUDIES).

Ophthalmic Solution: Diclofenca sodium ophthalmic is indicated for the treatment of postoperative inflammation in patients who have undergone cataract extraction.

CONTRAINDICATIONS:

Tablets: Diclofenac in either formulation, immediate-release or delayed-release, is contraindicated in patients with hypersensitivity to diclofenac. Diclofenac should not be given to patients who have experienced asthma, urticaria, or other allergic-type reactions after taking aspirin or other NSAIDs. Severe, rarely fatal, anaphylactic-like reactions to diclofenac have been reported in such patients.

Ophthalmic Solution: Contraindicated in patients concurrently wearing soft contact lenses and in patients who are hypersensitive to any component of the medication. Patients wearing hydrogel soft contact lenses who have received diclofenac ophthalmic concurrently have experienced ocular irritation manifested by redness and burning.

WARNINGS:

GASTROINTESTINAL EFFECTS

Peptic ulceration and gastrointestinal bleeding have been reported in patients receiving diclofenac tablets. Physicians and patients should therefore remain alert for ulceration and bleeding in patients treated chronically with diclofenac even in the absence of previous G.I. tract symptoms. It is recommended that patients be maintained on the lowest dose of diclofenac possible, consistent with achieving a satisfactory therapeutic response.

Risk of G.I. Ulcerations, Bleeding, and Perforation with NSAID Therapy: Serious gastrointestinal toxicity such as bleeding, ulceration, and perforation can occur at any time, with or without warning symptoms, in patients treated chronically with NSAID therapy. Although minor upper gastrointestinal problems, such as dyspepsia, are common, usually developing early in therapy, physicians should remain alert for ulceration and bleeding in patients treated chronically with NSAIDs even in the absence of previous G.I. tract symptoms. In patients observed in clinical trials of several months to 2 years' duration, symptomatic upper G.I. ulcers, gross bleeding, or perforation appear to occur in approximately 1% of patients for 3-6 months, and in about 2%-4% of patients treated for 1 year. Physicians should inform patients about the signs and/or symptoms of serious G.I. toxicity and what steps to take if they occur.

Studies to date have not identified any subset of patients not at risk of developing peptic ulceration and bleeding. Except for a prior history of serious G.I. events and other risk factors known to be associated with peptic ulcer disease, such as alcoholism, smoking,etc., no risk factors (*e.g.,* age, sex) have been associated with increased risk. Elderly or debilitated patients seem to tolerate ulceration or bleeding less well than other individuals, and most spontaneous reports of fatal G.I. events are in this population. Studies to date are inconclusive concerning the relative risk of various NSAIDs in causing such reactions. High doses of any NSAID probably carry a greater risk of these reactions, although controlled clinical trials showing this do not exist in most cases. In considering the use of relatively large doses (within the recommended dosage range), sufficient benefit should be anticipated to offset the potential increased risk of G.I. toxicity.

HEPATIC EFFECTS

As with other NSAIDs, elevations of one or more liver tests may occur during diclofenac therapy. These laboratory abnormalities may progress, may remain unchanged, or may be transient with continued therapy. Borderline elevations (*i.e.,* less than 3 times the ULN (=the Upper Limit of the Normal Range)), or greater elevations of transaminases occurred in about 15% of diclofenac-treated patients. Of the hepatic enzymes, ALT (SGPT) is the one recommended for the monitoring of liver injury.

In clinical trials, meaningful elevations (*i.e.,* more than 3 times the ULN) of AST (SGOT) (ALT was not measured in all studies) occurred in about 2% of approximately 5700 patients at some time during delayed-release treatment. In a large, open, controlled trial, meaningful elevations of ALT and/or AST occurred in about 4% of 3700 patients treated for 2-6 months, including marked elevations (*i.e.,* more than 8 times the ULN) in about 1% of the 3700 patients. In that open-label study, a higher incidence of borderline (less than 3 times the ULN), moderate (3-8 times the ULN), and marked (>8 times the ULN) elevations of ALT or AST was observed in patients receiving diclofenac when compared to other NSAIDs. Transaminase elevations were seen more frequently in patients with osteoarthritis than in those with rheumatoid arthritis (see ADVERSE REACTIONS).

In addition to the enzyme elevations seen in clinical trials, rare cases of severe hepatic reactions, including jaundice and fatal fulminant hepatitis, have been reported.

Physicians should measure transaminases periodically in patients receiving long-term therapy with diclofenac, because severe hepatotoxicity may develop without a prodrome of distinguishing symptoms. The optimum times for making the first and subsequent transaminase measurements are not known. In the largest U.S. trial (open-label) that involved 3700 patients monitored first at 8 weeks and 1200 patients monitored again at 24 weeks, almost all meaningful elevations in transaminases were detected before patients became symptomatic. In 42 of the 51 patients in all trials who developed marked transaminase elevations, abnormal tests occurred during the first 2 months of therapy with diclofenac. Based on this experience, if diclofenac is used chronically, the first transaminase measurement should be made no later than 8 weeks after the start of diclofenac treatment. As with other NSAIDs, if abnormal liver tests persist or worsen, if clinical signs and/or symptoms consistent with liver disease develop, or if systemic manifestations occur (*e.g.,* eosinophilia, rash, etc.), diclofenac should be discontinued.

To minimize the possibility that hepatic injury will become severe between transaminase measurements, physicians should inform patients of the warning signs and symptoms of hepatotoxicity (*e.g.,* nausea, fatigue, lethargy, pruritus, jaundice, right upper quadrant tenderness, and "flu-like" symptoms), and the appropriate action patients should take if these signs and symptoms appear.

PRECAUTIONS:

GENERAL

Diclofenac delayed-release tablets should not be used concomitantly with other diclofenac-containing products since they also circulate in plasma as the diclofenac anion.

Allergic Reactions: As with other NSAIDs, allergic reactions including anaphylaxis have been reported with diclofenac. Specific allergic manifestations consisting of swelling of eyelids, lips, pharynx, and larynx; urticaria; asthma; and bronchospasm, sometimes with a concomitant fall in blood pressure (severe at times) have been observed in clinical trials and/or the marketing experience with diclofenac. Anaphylaxis has rarely been reported from foreign sources; in U.S. clinical trials with diclofenac in over 6000 patients, 1 case of anaphylaxis was reported. In controlled clinical trials, allergic reactions have been observed at an incidence of 0.5%. These reactions can occur without prior exposure to the drug.

Fluid Retention and Edema: Fluid retention and edema have been observed in some patients taking diclofenac. Therefore, as with other NSAIDs, diclofenac should be used with caution in patients with a history of cardiac decompensation, hypertension, or other conditions predisposing to fluid retention.

Renal Effects: As a class, NSAIDs have been associated with renal papillary necrosis and other abnormal renal pathology in long-term administration to animals. In oral diclofenac studies in animals, some evidence of renal toxicity was noted. Isolated incidents of papillary necrosis were observed in a few animals at high doses (20-120 mg/kg) in several baboon subacute studies. In patients treated with diclofenac, rare cases of interstitial nephritis and papillary necrosis have been reported (see ADVERSE REACTIONS).

A second form of renal toxicity, generally associated with NSAIDs, is seen in patients with conditions leading to a reduction in renal blood flow or blood volume, where renal prostaglandins have a supportive role in the maintenance of renal perfusion. In these patients, administration of an NSAID results in a dose-dependent decrease in prostaglandin synthesis and, secondarily, in a reduction of renal blood flow, which may precipitate overt renal failure. Patients at greatest risk of this reaction are those with impaired renal function, heart failure, liver dysfunction, those taking diuretics, and the elderly. Discontinuation of NSAID therapy is typically followed by recovery to the pretreatment state.

Cases of significant renal failure in patients receiving diclofenac have been reported from marketing experience, but were not observed in over 4000 patients in clinical trials during which serum creatinine and BUN values were followed serially. There were only 11 patients

PRECAUTIONS: *(cont'd)*

(0.3%) whose serum creatinine and concurrent serum BUN values were greater than 2.0 mg/dl and 40 mg/dl, respectively, while on diclofenac (mean rise in the 11 patients: creatinine 2.3 mg/dl and BUN 28.4 mg/dl).

Since diclofenac metabolites are eliminated primarily by the kidneys, patients with significantly impaired renal function should be more closely monitored than subjects with normal renal function.

Porphyria: The use diclofenac in patients with hepatic porphyria should be avoided. To date, 1 patient has been described in whom diclofenac probably triggered a clinical attack of porphyria. The postulated mechanism, demonstrated in rats, for causing such attacks by diclofenac, as well as some other NSAIDs, is through stimulation of the porphyrin precursor delta-aminolevulinic acid (ALA).

INFORMATION FOR THE PATIENT

Diclofenac, like other drugs of its class, is not free of side effects. The side effects of these drugs can cause discomfort and, rarely, there are more serious side effects, such as gastrointestinal bleeding, and more rarely, liver toxicity (see WARNINGS, Hepatic Effects), which may result in hospitalization and even fatal outcomes.

NSAIDs are often essential agents in the management of arthritis and have a major role in the management of pain, but they also may be commonly employed for conditions that are less serious.

Physicians may wish to discuss with their patients the potential risks (see WARNINGS, PRECAUTIONS, and ADVERSE REACTIONS) and likely benefits of NSAID treatment, particularly when the drugs are used for less serious conditions where treatment without NSAIDs may represent an acceptable alternative to both the patient and physician.

LABORATORY TESTS

Because serious G.I. tract ulceration and bleeding can occur without warning symptoms, physicians should follow chronically treated patients for the signs and symptoms of ulceration and bleeding and should inform them of the importance of this follow-up (see WARNINGS, Risk of G.I. Ulcerations, Bleeding, and Perforation with NSAID Therapy.) If diclofenac is used chronically, patients should also be instructed to report any signs and symptoms that might be due to hepatotoxicity of diclofenac; these symptoms may become evident between visits when periodic liver laboratory tests are performed (see WARNINGS, Hepatic Effects.)

DRUG/LABORATORY TEST INTERACTIONS

Effect on Blood Coagulation: Diclofenac increases platelet aggregation time but does not affect bleeding time, plasma thrombin clotting time, plasma fibrinogen, or factors V and VII to XII. Statistically significant changes in prothrombin and partial thromboplastin times have been reported in normal volunteers. The mean changes were observed to be less than 1 second in both instances, however, and are unlikely to be clinically important. Diclofenac is a prostaglandin synthetase inhibitor, however, and all drugs that inhibit prostaglandin synthesis interfere with platelet function to some degree; therefore, patients who may be adversely affected by such an action should be carefully observed.

CARCINOGENESIS, MUTAGENESIS, AND IMPAIRMENT OF FERTILITY

Long-term carcinogenicity studies in rats given diclofenac sodium up to 2 mg/kg/day (or 12 mg/m^2/day, approximately the human dose) have revealed no significant increases in tumor incidence. There was a slight increase in benign mammary fibroadenomas in mid-dose-treated (0.5 mg/kg/day or 3 mg/m^2/day) female rats (high-dose females had an excessive mortality), but the increase was not significant for this common rat tumor. A 2-year carcinogenicity study conducted in mice employing diclofenac sodium at doses up to 0.3 mg/kg/day (0.9 mg/m^2/day) in males and 1 mg/kg/day (3 mg/m^2/day) in females did not reveal oncogenic potential. Diclofenac sodium did not show mutagenic activity in *in vitro* point mutation assays in mammalian (mouse lymphoma) and microbial (yeast, Ames) test systems and was nonmutagenic in several mammalian *in vitro* and *in vivo* test, including dominant lethal and male germinal epithelial chromosomal studies in mice, and nucleus anomaly and chromosomal aberration studies in Chinese hamsters. Diclofenac sodium administered to male and female rats at 4 mg/kg/day (24 mg/m^2/day) did not affect fertility.

TERATOGENIC EFFECTS

There are no adequate and well-controlled studies in pregnant women. Diclofenac should be used during pregnancy only if the benefits to the mother justify the potential risk to the fetus.

PREGNANCY CATEGORY B

Reproduction studies have been performed in mice given diclofenac sodium (up to 20 mg/kg/day or 60 mg/m^2/day) and in rats and rabbits given diclofenac sodium (up to 10 mg/kg/day or 60 mg/m^2/day for rats, and 80 mg/m^2/day for rabbits), and have revealed no evidence of teratogenicity despite the induction of maternal toxicity and fetal toxicity. In rats, maternally toxic doses were associated with dystocia, prolonged gestation, reduced fetal weights and growth, and induced fetal survival. Diclofenac has been shown to cross the placental barrier in mice and rats.

LABOR AND DELIVERY

The effects of diclofenac on labor and delivery in pregnant women are unknown. Because of the known effects of prostaglandin-inhibiting drugs on the fetal cardiovascular system (closure of ductus arteriosus), use of diclofenac during late pregnancy should be avoided and, as with other nonsteroidal anti-inflammatory drugs, it is possible to that diclofenac may inhibit uterine contraction.

NURSING MOTHERS

Diclofenac has been found in the milk of nursing mothers. As with other drugs that are excreted in milk, diclofenac is not recommended for use in nursing women.

PEDIATRIC USE

Safety and effectiveness of diclofenac in children have not been established.

GERIATRIC USE

Of the more than 6000 patients treated with diclofenac in U.S. trials, 31% were older than 65 years of age. No overall difference was observed between efficacy, adverse event or pharmacokinetic profiles of older and younger patients. As with any NSAID, the elderly are likely to tolerate adverse reactions less well than younger patients.

DRUG INTERACTIONS:

TABLETS

Aspirin: Concomitant administration of diclofenac and aspirin is not recommended because diclofenac is displaced from its binding sites during the concomitant administration of aspirin, resulting in lower plasma concentrations, peak plasma levels, and AUC levels.

Anticoagulants: While studies have not shown diclofenac to interact with anticoagulant of the warfarin type, caution should be exercised, nonetheless, since interactions have been seen with other NSAIDs. Because prostaglandins play an important role in homeostasis, and NSAIDs affect platelet function as well, concurrent therapy with all NSAIDs, including diclofenac, and warfarin requires close monitoring of patients to be certain that no change in their anticoagulant dosage is required.

Digoxin, Methotrexate, Cyclosporine: Diclofenac, like other NSAIDs, may affect renal prostaglandins and increase the toxicity of certain drugs. Ingestion of diclofenac may increase serum concentrations of digoxin and methotrexate and increase cyclosporine's nephrotoxicity. Patients who begin taking diclofenac or who increase their diclofenac dose or any other

DRUG INTERACTIONS: *(cont'd)*

NSAID while taking digoxin, methotrexate, or cyclosporine may develop toxicity characteristics for these drugs. They should be observed closely, particularly if renal function is impaired. In the case of digoxin, serum levels should be monitored.

Lithium: Diclofenac decreases lithium renal clearance and increases lithium plasma levels. In patients taking diclofenac and lithium concomitantly, lithium toxicity may develop.

Oral Hypoglycemics: Diclofenac does not alter glucose metabolism in normal subjects nor does it alter the effects of oral hypoglycemic agents. There are rare reports, however, from marketing experiences of changes in effects of insulin or oral hypoglycemic agents in the presence of diclofenac that necessitated changes in the doses of such agents. Both hypo- and hyperglycemic effects have been reported. A direct causal relationship has not been established, but physicians should consider the possibility that diclofenac may alter a diabetic patient's response to insulin or oral hypoglycemic agents.

Diuretics: Diclofenac and other NSAIDs can inhibit the activity of diuretics. Concomitant treatment with potassium-sparing diuretics may be associated with increased serum potassium levels.

Other Drugs: In small groups of patients (7-10/interaction study), the concomitant administration of azathioprine, gold chloroquine, D-penicillamine, prednisolone, doxycycline, or digitoxin did not significantly affect the peak levels and AUC values of diclofenac.

PROTEIN BINDING

In vitro, diclofenac interferes minimally or not at all with the protein binding of salicylic acid (20% decrease in binding), tolbutamide, prednisolone (10% decrease in binding), or warfarin. Benzylpenicillin, ampicillin, oxacillin, chlortetracycline, cephalothin, erythromycin, and sulfamethoxazole have no influence *in vitro* on the protein binding of diclofenac in human serum.

ADVERSE REACTIONS:

TABLETS

Adverse reaction information is derived from blinded, controlled and open-label clinical trials, as well as worldwide marketing experience. In the description below, rates of more common events represent clinical study results; rare events are derived principally from marketing experience and publications, and accurate rate estimates are generally not possible.

In a 6-month, double-blind trial comparing diclofenac immediate-release tablets (N=196) vs. diclofenac delayed-release tablets (N=197) vs. ibuprofen (N=197), adverse reactions were similar in nature and frequency. In 718 patients treated for shorter periods, i.e., 2 weeks or less, with diclofenac immediate-release tablets, adverse reactions were reported one-half to one-tenth as frequently as by patients treated for longer periods.

The incidence of common adverse reactions (greater than 1%) is based upon controlled clinical trials in 1543 patients treated up to 13 weeks with diclofenac delayed-release tablets. By far the most common adverse effects were gastrointestinal symptoms, most of them minor, occurring in about 20%, and leading to discontinuation in about 3%, of patients. Peptic ulcer or G.I. bleeding occurred in clinical trials in 0.6% (95% confidence interval: 0.2% to 1%) of approximately 1800 patients during their first 3 months of diclofenac treatment and in 1.6% (95% confidence interval: 0.8% to 2.4%) of approximately 800 patients followed for 1 year.

Gastrointestinal symptoms were followed in frequency by central nervous system side effects such as headache (7%) and dizziness (3%).

Meaningful (exceeding 3 times the Upper Limit of Normal) elevations of ALT (SGPT) or AST (SGOT) occurred at an overall rate of approximately 2% during the first 2 months of delayed-release treatment. Unlike aspirin elevations, which occur more frequently in patients with rheumatoid arthritis, these elevations were more frequently observed in patients with osteoarthritis (2.6%) than in patients with rheumatoid arthritis (0.7%). Marked elevations (exceeding 8 times the ULN) were seen in 1% of patients treated for 2-6 months (see WARNINGS, Hepatic Effects).

The following adverse reactions were reported in patients treated with diclofenac:

Incidence Greater Than 1%-Causal Relationship Probable: (All derived from clinical trials.)

Body as a Whole: Abdominal pain or cramps,* headache,* fluid retention, abdominal distention.

Digestive: Diarrhea,* indigestion,* nausea,* constipation,* flatulence, liver test abnormalities,* PUB, i.e., peptic ulcer, with or without bleeding and/or perforation, or bleeding without ulcer (see above and also WARNINGS).

Nervous System: Dizziness.

Skin and Appendages: Rash, pruritus.

Special Senses: Tinnitus.

*Incidence, 3% to 9% (incidence unmarked reactions is 1%-3%).

Incidence Less Than 1%-Causal Relationship Probable: (The following reactions have been reported in patients taking diclofenac under circumstances that do not permit a clear attribution of the reaction to diclofenac. These reactions are being included as alerting information to physicians. Adverse reactions reported only in *Worldwide Marketing Experience* or in the literature, not seen in clinical trials, are considered rare and are italicized.)

Body as a Whole: Malaise, swelling of lips and tongue, photosensitivity, *anaphylaxis*, anaphylactoid reactions.

Cardiovascular: Hypertension, congestive heart failure.

Digestive: Vomiting, jaundice, melena, aphthous stomatitis, dry mouth and mucous membranes, bloody diarrhea, hepatitis, *hepatic necrosis*, appetite change, pancreatitis with or without concomitant hepatitis, *colitis*.

Hemic and Lymphatic: Hemoglobin disease, leukopenia, thrombocytopenia, *Hemolytic anemia, aplastic anemia, agranulocytosis*, purpura, *allergic purpura*.

Metabolic and Nutritional Disorders: Azotemia.

Nervous System: Insomnia, drowsiness, depression, diplopia, anxiety, irritability, *aseptic meningitis*.

Respiratory: Epistaxis, asthma, laryngeal edema.

Skin and Appendages: Alopecia, urticaria, eczema, dermatitis, *bullous eruption, erythema multiforme major*, angioedema, *Stevens-Johnson syndrome*.

Special Senses: Blurred vision, taste disorder, reversible hearing loss, scotoma.

Urogenital: *Nephrotic syndrome*, proteinuria, *oliguria, interstitial nephritis, papillary necrosis, acute renal failure*.

Incidence Less Than 1%-Causal Relationship Unknown: (Adverse reactions reported only in **Worldwide Marketing Experience** or in the literature, not seen in clinical trials, are considered rare and are italicized.)

Body as a Whole: Chest pain.

Cardiovascular: Palpitations, *flushing*, tachycardia, premature ventricular contractions, myocardial infarction.

Digestive: Esophageal lesions.

Hemic and Lymphatic: *Bruising*.

ADVERSE REACTIONS: *(cont'd)*

Metabolic and Nutritional Disorders: Hypoglycemia, *weight loss.*

Nervous System: Paresthesia, memory disturbance, nightmares, tremor, tic, *abnormal coordination*, convulsions, *disorientation, psychotic reaction.*

Respiratory: Dyspnea, hyperventilation, edema of pharynx.

Skin and Appendages: Excess perspiration, *exfoliative dermatitis.*

Special Senses: Vitreous floaters, night blindness, amblyopia.

Urogenital: Urinary frequency, nocturia, hematuria, impotence, vaginal bleeding.

OVERDOSAGE:

TABLETS

Worldwide reports of overdosage with diclofenac cover 66 cases. In approximately one-half of these reports of overdosage, concomitant medications were also taken. The highest dose of diclofenac was 5.0 g in a 17 year-old male who suffered loss of consciousness, increased intracranial pressure, aspiration pneumonitis, and died 2 days after overdose. The next highest doses of diclofenac were 4.0 g and 3.75 g. The 24 year-old who took 4.0 g and the 28 and 42 year-old females, each of whom took 3.75 g, did not develop any clinically significant signs or symptoms. However, there was a report of a 17 year-old female who experienced vomiting and drowsiness after an overdose of 2.37 g of diclofenac.

Animal LD_{50} values show a wide range of susceptibilities to acute overdosage, with primates being more resistant to acute toxicity than rodents (LD_{50} in mg/kg - rats, 55; dogs, 500; monkeys, 3200).

In case of acute overdosage, it is recommended that the stomach be emptied by vomiting or lavage. Forced diuresis may theoretically be beneficial because the drug is excreted in the urine. The effect of dialysis or hemoperfusion in the elimination of diclofenac (99% protein-bound; see CLINICAL PHARMACOLOGY) remains unproven. In addition to supportive measures, the use of oral activated charcoal may help to reduce the absorption of diclofenac.

DOSAGE AND ADMINISTRATION:

TABLETS

Diclofenac may be administered as 25-mg and 50-mg immediate-release tablets or as 25-mg, 50-mg, and 75-mg diclofenac delayed-release tablets. Regardless of the indication, the dosage of diclofenac should be individualized to the lowest effective dose of immediate-release or delayed-release to minimize adverse effects (see CLINICAL PHARMACOLOGY, Individualization Of Dosage).

Analgesia and Primary Dysmenorrhea: The recommended starting dose of diclofenac immediate-release tablets is 50 mg t.i.d. With experience, physicians may find that in some patients an initial dose of 100 mg of immediate-release, followed by 50-mg doses, will provide better relief. After the first day, when the maximum recommended dose may be 200 mg, the total daily dose should generally not exceed 150 mg.

Osteoarthritis: The recommended dosage is 100-150 mg/day in divided doses, 50 mg b.i.d. or t.i.d. (delayed-release or immediate-release) or 75 mg b.i.d. (delayed-release only). Dosages above 150 mg/day have not been studied in patients with osteoarthritis.

Rheumatoid Arthritis: The recommended dosage is 150-200 mg/day in divided doses, 50 mg t.i.d. or q.i.d. (delayed-release or immediate-release) or 75 mg b.i.d. (delayed-release only). Dosages above 225 mg/day are not recommended in patients with rheumatoid arthritis.

Ankylosing Spondylitis: The recommended dosage is 100-125 mg/day administered as 25 mg q.i.d. with an extra 25-mg dose at bedtime if necessary. Dosages above 125 mg/day have not been studied in patients with ankylosing spondylosis.

OPHTHALMIC SOLUTION

One drop diclofenac ophthalmic should be applied to the affected eye four times daily beginning 24 hours after cataract surgery and continuing throughout the first 2 weeks of the postoperative period.

Store between 59-86°F (15-30°C). Protect from light. *Dispense in original, unopened container only.*

PATIENT INFORMATION:

Diclofenac is a nonsteroidal anti-inflammatory medication. The tablets are used to treat arthritis. The ophthalmic solution is used for the treatment of inflammation following cataract surgery. Notify your physician if you are pregnant or nursing. Do not take diclofenac if you are allergic to aspirin. Take diclofenac tablets with food to avoid stomach upset. This medication may cause dizziness or lightheadedness; use caution while driving or operating hazardous machinery. Do not drink alcohol or take aspirin while taking diclofenac. Notify your physician if you develop severe stomach pain; bloody vomit; or black, tarry, or bloody stools. Diclofenac may cause increased sensitivity to sunlight. Use sunscreens and wear protective clothing until degree of sensitivity is determined. Do not wear contact lenses while using diclofenac eye drops.

HOW SUPPLIED:

Cataflam Tablets 25 mg: Light pink, round, biconvex (imprinted CATAFLAM on one side and 25 on the other side)

Cataflam Tablets 50 mg: Light brown, round, biconvex (imprinted CATAFLAM on one side and 50 on the other side)

Voltaren Delayed-Release Tablet 25 mg: Yellow, biconvex, triangular-shaped (imprinted VOLTAREN 25)

Voltaren Delayed-Released Tablets 50 mg: Light brown, biconvex, triangular-shaped (imprinted VOLTAREN 50)

Voltaren Delayed-Relayed Tablets 75 mg: Light pink, biconvex, triangular-shaped (imprinted VOLTAREN 75)

Do not store above 86°F (30°C). protect from moisture.*Dispense in tight container (USP).*

HOW SUPPLIED - RATED THERAPEUTICALLY EQUIVALENT:

Tablet, Delayed Release - Oral - 25 mg

100's	$51.63	Diclofenac, H.C.F.A. F F P	99999-1045-01

Tablet, Delayed Release - Oral - 50 mg

100's	$85.44	Diclofenac, H.C.F.A. F F P	99999-1045-02

Tablet, Delayed Release - Oral - 75 mg

100's	$96.47	Diclofenac, H.C.F.A. F F P	99999-1045-03

Tablet, Enteric Coated, Sustained Action - Oral - 25 mg

60's	$25.84	Diclofenac Sodium, Geneva Pharms	00781-1285-60
60's	$26.58	Diclofenac Sodium, Roxane	00054-4223-21
60's	**$31.11**	**VOLTAREN, Novartis**	**00028-0258-60**
100's	$43.08	Diclofenac Sodium, Geneva Pharms	00781-1285-01
100's	$44.30	Diclofenac Sodium, Roxane	00054-4223-25
100's	$47.35	Diclofenac Sodium, Geneva Pharms	00781-1285-13
100's	$47.40	Diclofenac Sodium, Roxane	00054-8223-25

HOW SUPPLIED - RATED THERAPEUTICALLY EQUIVALENT: *(cont'd)*

100's	**$51.84**	**VOLTAREN, Novartis**	**00028-0258-01**
100's	**$55.46**	**VOLTAREN, Novartis**	**00028-0258-61**

Tablet, Enteric Coated, Sustained Action - Oral - 50 mg

60's	$51.63	Diclofenac Sodium, Geneva Pharms	00781-1287-60
60's	$51.66	Diclofenac Sodium, Roxane	00054-4221-21
60's	**$60.44**	**VOLTAREN, Novartis**	**00028-0262-60**
100's	$83.75	Diclofenac Sodium, Geneva Pharms	00781-1287-01
100's	$86.13	Diclofenac Sodium, Roxane	00054-4221-25
100's	$91.14	Diclofenac Sodium, Geneva Pharms	00781-1287-13
100's	$92.17	Diclofenac Sodium, Roxane	00054-8221-25
100's	**$100.77**	**VOLTAREN, Novartis**	**00028-0262-01**
100's	**$107.84**	**VOLTAREN, Novartis**	**00028-0262-61**
1000's	$845.58	Diclofenac Sodium, Geneva Pharms	00781-1287-10
1000's	$846.52	Diclofenac Sodium, Roxane	00054-4221-31
1000's	**$990.43**	**VOLTAREN, Novartis**	**00028-0262-10**

Tablet, Enteric Coated, Sustained Action - Oral - 75 mg

60's	$60.84	Diclofenac Sodium, Geneva Pharms	00781-1289-60
60's	$62.58	Diclofenac Sodium, Roxane	00054-4222-21
60's	**$73.23**	**VOLTAREN, Novartis**	**00028-0264-60**
100's	$101.40	Diclofenac Sodium, Geneva Pharms	00781-1289-01
100's	$104.31	Diclofenac Sodium, Roxane	00054-4222-25
100's	$111.50	Diclofenac Sodium, Geneva Pharms	00781-1289-13
100's	$111.63	Diclofenac Sodium, Roxane	00054-8222-25
100's	**$122.04**	**VOLTAREN, Novartis**	**00028-0264-01**
100's	**$130.60**	**VOLTAREN, Novartis**	**00028-0264-61**
1000's	$1014.00	Diclofenac Sodium, Geneva Pharms	00781-1289-10
1000's	$1025.25	Diclofenac Sodium, Roxane	00054-4222-31
1000's	**$1199.55**	**VOLTAREN, Novartis**	**00028-0264-10**

HOW SUPPLIED - NOT RATED EQUIVALENT:

Solution - Ophthalmic - 0.1 %

2.5 ml	**$18.12**	**VOLTAREN OPHTHALMIC, Ciba Vision**	**58768-0100-02**
5 ml	**$28.26**	**VOLTAREN OPHTHALMIC, Ciba Vision**	**58768-0100-05**

Tablet, Uncoated - Oral - 50 mg

100's	$135.20	CATAFLAM, Novartis	00028-0151-01
100's	$144.66	CATAFLAM, Novartis	00028-0151-61

DICLOXACILLIN SODIUM *(001046)*

CATEGORIES: Anti-Infectives; Antibiotics; Antimicrobials; Infections; Penicillins; FDA Approval Pre 1982

BRAND NAMES: *Brispen* (Mexico); *Cervantal*; *Dacocilin*; *Dacocillin*; *Dichlor*; *Dichlor-Stapenor* (Germany); *Diclex*; *Diclo*; *Diclocil*; *Diclocillin*; *Diclocin*; *Diclox*; *Dicloxal*; *Diflor*; Dycill; Dynapen; *H.G. Dicloxacil*; *Maclicine*; *Mediclox*; *Novapen*; *Orbenin*; *Orbenin-d*; **Pathocil**; *Posipen* (Mexico); *Staphcillin*; *Staphcillin A* (Japan); *Ziefmycin*

(International brand names outside U.S. in italics)

FORMULARIES: Aetna; BC-BS; DoD; FHP; Medi-Cal; PCS

COST OF THERAPY: $5.32 (Skin Infections; Capsule; 250 mg; 4/day; 7 days)

DESCRIPTION:

Dicloxacillin sodium is 5-methyl-3-(2,6-dichlorophenyl)-4-isoxazolyl penicillin sodium salt monohydrate, a penicillinase-resistant, acid- resistant, semisynthetic penicillin derived from the penicillin nucleus, 6-aminopenicillanic acid. It is resistant to inactivation by the enzyme penicillinase (beta-lactamase).[1-5]

The structural formula of dicloxacillin sodium is as follows:

$C_{19}H_{16}Cl_2N_3NaO_5{\cdot}H_2O$ 510.32 [CAS-13412-64-1] 4-Thia-1-azabicyclo[3.2.0]heptane-2-carboxylic acid,6-[3-(2,6-dichlorophenyl)-5-methyl-4-isoxazolyl[carbonyl]-amino]-3,3-dimethyl-7-oxo-, monosodium salt, monohydrate, [2S- (2α,5α,6β)]. *Inactive Ingredients:* 250 mg Capsules-FD&C Blue No.2, gelatin, lactose, magnesium stearate, red iron oxide, silicon dioxide, sodium lauryl sulfate, titanium dioxide and yellow iron oxide. 500 mg Capsules-FD&C Blue No. 2, gelatin, magnesium stearate, red iron oxide, silicon dioxide, sodium lauryl sulfate, titanium oxide and yellow iron oxide.

CLINICAL PHARMACOLOGY:

MICROBIOLOGY

Penicillinase-resistant penicillins exert a bactericidal action against penicillin-susceptible microorganisms during the state of multiplication.[6] All penicillins inhibit the biosynthesis of the bacterial cell wall.[3,7]

The drugs in this class are highly resistant to inactivation by staphylococcal penicillinase and are active against penicillinase-producing and nonpenicillinase-producing strains of *Staphylococcus aureus*.The penicillinase-resistant penicillins are active *in vitro* against a variety of other bacteria.[7,3,5,8-17]

SUSCEPTIBILITY TESTING

Quantitative methods of susceptibility testing that require measurements of zone diameters or minimal inhibitory concentrations (MICs) give the most precise estimates of antibiotic susceptibility. One such procedure has been recommended for use with disks to test susceptibility to this class of drugs. Interpretations correlate diameters on the disk test with MIC values.

A penicillinase-resistant class disk may be used to determine microbial susceptibility to cloxacillin, dicloxacillin, methicillin, nafcillin and oxacillin.[18]

Table 1 shows the interpretation of test results for penicillinase-resistant penicillins using the FDA Standard Disk Test Method (formerly Bauer-Kirby-Sherris-Turck method) of disk bacteriological susceptibility testing for staphylococci with a disk containing 5 mcg methicillin sodium.

With this procedure, a report from a laboratory of "susceptible" indicates that the infecting organism is likely to respond to therapy. A report of "resistant" indicates that the infecting organism is not likely to respond to therapy. A report of "intermediate" susceptibility suggests that the organism might be susceptible if high doses of the antibiotic are used, or if the infection is confined to tissues and fluids (*e.g.,* urine) in which high antibiotic levels are attained.

In general, all staphylococci should be tested against the penicillin G disk and against the methicillin disk.[18] Routine methods of antibiotic susceptibility testing may fail to detect strains of organisms resistant to the penicillinase-resistant penicillins. For this reason, the use of large inocula and 48-hour incubation periods may be necessary to obtain accurate susceptibility studies with these antibiotics. Bacterial strains which are resistant to one of the penicillinase-resistant penicillins should be considered resistant to all of the drugs in the

CLINICAL PHARMACOLOGY: *(cont'd)*

class.[3,8]

TABLE 1 STANDARDIZED TEST METHOD OF BACTERIOLOGICAL SUSCEPTIBILITY TESTING USING A CLASS DISK CONTAINING 5 MCG METHICILLIN SODIUM [18]		
Diameter of Zone Indicating "Susceptibility"	**Diameter of Zone Indicating "Intermediate"**	**Diameter of Zone Indicating "Resistant"**
at least 14 mm	10 to 13 mm	less than 10 mm

PHARMACOKINETICS

Methicillin sodium is readily destroyed by gastric acidity and must be administered by intramuscular or intravenous injections.[8,11,17] The isoxazolyl penicillins (cloxacillin and oxacillin) and nafcillin are more acid resistant and may be administered orally.[3,15,16,19,20] Absorption of the isoxazolyl penicillins after oral administration is rapid but incomplete; peak blood levels are achieved in 1 to 1.5 hours.[3,4,19] In one study, after ingestion of a single 500 mg oral dose, peak serum concentrations range from 5 to 7 mcg/ml for oxacillin, from 7.5 to 14.4 mcg/ml for cloxacillin and from 10 to 17 mcg/ml for dicloxacillin. Oral absorption of nafcillin sodium is irregular and wide individual variations in absorption are observed. One hour after ingestion of a single 1 gram oral dose of nafcillin as the sodium salt, the average serum concentration of 1.19 mcg/ml (range 0 to 3.12 mcg/ml) was achieved.[4,20,25]

Oral absorption of cloxacillin, dicloxacillin, oxacillin and nafcillin is delayed when the drugs are administered after meals.[10,14,16,20] Intramuscular injections of nafcillin (1 gram), oxacillin (560 mg) and methicillin sodium (1 gram) produced peak serum levels in 0.5 to 1 hour of 7.61 mcg/ml, 15 mcg/ml and 17 mcg/ml, respectively.[1,8,17,19,25]

Once absorbed, the penicillinase-resistant penicillins bind to serum protein, mainly albumin. The degree of protein binding reported varies with the method of study and the investigator (see TABLE 2.)[3,8]

TABLE 2 PENICILLIN-RESISTANT PENICILLIN PERCENT PROTEIN-BINDING ± SD[8]			
Methicillin	37.3 ± 7.9	Oxacillin	94.2 ± 2.1
Dicloxacillin	97.9 ± 0.6	Nafcillin	89.9 ± 1.5
Cloxacillin	95.2 ± 0.5		

The penicillinase-resistant penicillins vary in the extent to which they are distributed in the body fluids. With normal doses, insignificant concentrations are found in the cerebrospinal fluid and aqueous humor. Methicillin is found in the pericardial and ascitic fluids. All the drugs in this class are found in therapeutic concentrations in the pleural, bile and amniotic fluids.[3,8,22]

The penicillinase-resistant penicillins are rapidly excreted primarily as unchanged drug in the urine by glomerular filtration and active tubular secretion.[3,26] The elimination half-life for methicillin and oxacillin is about 0.5 hour, for nafcillin less than 1 hour and for dicloxacillin about 0.7 hour.[23,26,27] Nonrenal elimination includes hepatic inactivation and excretion in bile.[3,17,27] Renal clearance of methicillin is delayed in premature infants, neonates and patients with renal insufficiency.[8,28]

INDICATIONS AND USAGE:

The penicillinase-resistant penicillins are indicated in the treatment of infections caused by penicillinase-producing staphylococci which have demonstrated susceptibility to the drugs. Cultures and susceptibility tests should be performed initially to determine the causative organisms and their sensitivity to the drug (see CLINICAL PHARMACOLOGY, Susceptibility Testing)[29].

The penicillinase-resistant penicillins may be used to initiate therapy in suspected cases of resistant staphylococcal infections prior to the availability of laboratory test results.[14,29,30] The penicillin-resistant penicillins should not be used in infections caused by organisms susceptible to penicillin G.[16,29,31] If the susceptibility tests indicate that the infection is due to an organism other than a resistant staphylococcus, therapy should not be continued with a penicillinase-resistant penicillin.[30]

CONTRAINDICATIONS:

A history of a hypersensitivity (anaphylactic) reaction to any penicillins is a contraindication.

WARNINGS:

SERIOUS AND OCCASIONALLY FATAL HYPERSENSITIVITY (ANAPHYLACTIC) REACTIONS HAVE BEEN REPORTED IN PATIENTS ON PENICILLIN THERAPY. THESE REACTIONS ARE MORE LIKELY TO OCCUR IN INDIVIDUALS WITH A HISTORY OF PENICILLIN HYPERSENSITIVITY AND/OR A HISTORY OF SENSITIVITY TO MULTIPLE ALLERGENS. THERE HAVE BEEN REPORTS OF INDIVIDUALS WITH A SENSITIVITY TO MULTIPLE ALLERGENS. THERE HAVE BEEN REPORTS OF INDIVIDUALS WITH A HISTORY OF PENICILLIN HYPERSENSITIVITY WHO HAVE BEEN EXPERIENCED SEVERE REACTIONS WHEN TREATED WITH CEPHALOSPORINS. BEFORE INITIATING THERAPY WITH DYCILL, CAREFUL INQUIRY SHOULD BE MADE CONCERNING PREVIOUS HYPERSENSITIVITY REACTIONS TO PENICILLINS, CEPHALOSPORINS, OR OTHER ALLERGENS. IF AN ALLERGIC REACTION OCCURS, DYCILL SHOULD BE DISCONTINUED AND APPROPRIATE THERAPY INSTITUTED. **SERIOUS ANAPHYLACTIC REACTIONS REQUIRE IMMEDIATE EMERGENCY TREATMENT WITH EPINEPHRINE, OXYGEN, INTRAVENOUS STEROIDS, AND AIRWAY MANAGEMENT, INCLUDING INTUBATION, SHOULD ALSO BE ADMINISTERED AS INDICATED.**

Pseudomembranous colitis has been reported with nearly all antibacterial agents, including Dycill, and may range in severity from mild to life-threatening. Therefore, it is important to consider this diagnosis in patients who present with diarrhea subsequent to the administration of antibacterial agents.

Treatment with antibacterial agents alters the normal flora of the colon and may permit overgrowth of clostridia. Studies indicate that a toxin produced by *Clostridium difficile* is one primary cause of "antibiotic-associated colitis."

After the diagnosis of pseudomembranous colitis usually respond to drug discontinuation alone. In moderate to severe cases, consideration should be given to management with fluids and electrolytes, protein supplementation and treatment with an antibacterial drug clinically effective against *C. difficile* colitis.

PRECAUTIONS:

GENERAL

Penicillinase-resistant penicillins should generally not be administered to patients with a history of sensitivity to any penicillin.[30,31,41,42]

Penicillin should be used with caution in individuals with histories of significant allergies and/or asthma.[3] Whenever allergic reactions occur, penicillin should be withdrawn unless, in the opinion of the physician, the condition being treated is life-threatening and amenable

PRECAUTIONS: *(cont'd)*

only to penicillin therapy. The oral route of administration should not be relied upon in patients with severe illness, or with nausea, vomiting, gastric dilation, cardiospasm or intestinal hypermotility. Occasionally patients will not absorb therapeutic amounts of orally administered penicillin.[25]

The use of antibiotics may results in overgrowth of nonsusceptible organisms.[3,32,43] If new infections due to bacteria or fungi occur, the drug should be discontinued and appropriate measures taken.

INFORMATION FOR THE PATIENT

Patients receiving penicillins should be given the following information and instructions by the physician:

1. Patients should be told that penicillin is an antibacterial agent which will work with the body's natural defenses to control certain types of infections. They should be told that the drug should not be taken if they have had an allergic reaction to any form of penicillin previously, and to inform the physician of any allergies or previous allergic reactions to any drugs they may have had[44] (see WARNINGS.)

2. Patients who have previously experienced an anaphylactic reaction to penicillin should be instructed to wear a medical identification tag or bracelet.

3. Because most antibacterial drugs taken by mouth are best absorbed on an empty stomach, patients should be directed, unless circumstances warrant otherwise, to take penicillin 1 hour before meals or 2 hours after eating[36,37] (see CLINICAL PHARMACOLOGY, Pharmacokinetics.)

4. Patients should be told to take the entire course of therapy prescribed, even if fever and other symptoms have stopped (see PRECAUTIONS, General.)

5. If any of the following reactions occur, stop taking your prescription and notify the physician: shortness of breath, wheezing, skin rash, mouth irritation, black tongue, sore throat, nausea, vomiting, diarrhea, fever, swollen joints, or any unusual bleeding or bruising[36] (see ADVERSE REACTIONS.)

6. Do not take any additional medications without physician approval, including nonprescription drugs such as antacids, laxatives or vitamins.[36]

7. Discard and liquid forms of penicillin after 7 days if stored at room temperature or after 14 days if refrigerated.

LABORATORY TESTS

Bacteriologic studies to determine the causative organisms and their susceptibility to the penicillinase-resistant penicillins should be performed (see CLINICAL PHARMACOLOGY, Microbiology). In the treatment of suspected staphylococcal infections, therapy should be changed to another active agent if culture tests fail to demonstrate the presence of staphylococci.[29]

Periodic assessment of organ system function including renal hepatic and hematopoietic should be made during prolonged therapy with the penicillinase-resistant penicillins.[29]

Blood cultures, white blood cell and differential cell counts should be obtained prior to initiation of therapy and at least weekly during therapy with penicillinase-resistant penicillins.[29]

Periodic urinalysis, blood urea nitrogen and creatinine determinations should be performed during therapy with the penicillinase-resistant penicillins and overdosage alterations should be considered if these values become elevated.[29,36] If any impairment of renal function is suspected or known to exist, a reduction in the total dosage should be considered and blood levels monitored to avoid possible neurotoxic reactions[39] (see DOSAGE AND ADMINISTRATION.)

SGOT and SGPT values should be obtained periodically during therapy to monitor for possible liver function abnormalities.[40,41]

CARCINOGENESIS, MUTAGENESIS, AND IMPAIRMENT OF FERTILITY

No long-term animal studies have been conducted with these drugs.

Studies on reproduction (nafcillin) in rats and rabbits reveal no fetal or maternal abnormalities before conception and continuously through weaning (one generation).

PREGNANCY CATEGORY B

Reproduction studies performed in the mouse, rat and rabbit have revealed no evidence of impaired fertility or harm to the fetus due to the penicillinase-resistant penicillins.[45,46] Human experience with the penicillins during pregnancy has not shown any positive evidence of adverse effects on the fetus. There are, however, no adequate or well-controlled studies in pregnant women showing conclusively that harmful effects of these drugs on the fetus can be excluded.[47,48] Because animal reproduction studies are not always predictive of human response, this drug should be used during pregnancy only if clearly needed.

NURSING MOTHERS

Penicillins are excreted in breast milk.[6,49,50] Caution should be exercised when penicillins are administered to a nursing woman.

PEDIATRIC USE

Because of incompletely developed renal function in newborns penicillinase-resistant penicillins (especially methicillin) may not be completely excreted, with abnormally high blood levels resulting.[28] Frequent blood levels are advisable in this group with dosage adjustments when necessary. All newborns treated with penicillins should be monitored closely for clinical and laboratory evidence of toxic or adverse effects[51] (see DOSAGE AND ADMINISTRATION).

DRUG INTERACTIONS:

Tetracycline, a bacteriostatic antibiotic, may antagonize the bactericidal effect of penicillin and concurrent use of these drugs should be avoided.[42,41]

ADVERSE REACTIONS:

Body as a Whole: The reported incidence of allergic reactions to penicillin ranges from 0.7% to 10%[28,34,52-54] (see WARNINGS.) Sensitization is usually the result of treatment but some individuals have had immediate reactions to penicillin when first treated. In such cases, it is thought that the patients may have had prior exposure to the drug via trace amounts present in milk and vaccines.[56]

Two types of allergic reactions to penicillins are noted clinically, immediate and delayed.[52,55,56]

Immediate reactions usually occur within 20 minutes of administration and range in severity from urticaria and pruritus to angioneurotic edema, laryngospasm, bronchospasm, hypotension, vascular collapse and death. Such immediate anaphylactic reactions are very rare (see WARNINGS) and usually occur after parenteral therapy but have occurred in patients receiving oral therapy. Another type of immediate reaction, an accelerated reaction, may occur between 20 minutes and 48 hours after administration and may include urticaria, pruritus and fever. Although laryngeal edema, laryngospasm and hypotension occasionally occur, fatality is uncommon.[34,52,53,55]

Delayed allergic reactions to penicillin therapy usually occur after 48 hours and sometimes as late as 2 to 4 weeks after initiation of therapy.[56] Manifestations of this type of reaction include serum-sickness-like symptoms (*i.e.,* fever, malaise, urticaria, myalgia, arthralgia, ab-

ADVERSE REACTIONS: *(cont'd)*

dominal pain) and various rashes.[20,34,35,53,55] Nausea, vomiting, diarrhea, stomatitis, black or hairy tongue and other symptoms of gastrointestinal irritation may occur, especially during oral penicillin therapy.[3,41]

Nervous System Reactions: Neurotoxic reactions similar to those observed with penicillin G may occur with large intravenous doses of the penicillinase-resistant penicillins, especially with patients with renal insufficiency.[7,39]

Urogenital Reactions: Renal tubular damage and interstitial nephritis have been associated with the administration of methicillin sodium and infrequently with the administration of nafcillin and oxacillin.[8,38,57-61] Manifestations of this reaction may include rash, fever, eosinophilia, hematuria, proteinuria and renal insufficiency. Methicillin-induced nephropathy does not appear to be dose-related and is generally reversible upon prompt discontinuation of therapy.[7,8,57,59]

Metabolic Reactions: Agranulocytosis, neutropenia and bone marrow depression have been associated with the use of methicillin sodium and nafcillin.[14,62-65]

Hepatotoxicity, characterized by fever, nausea and vomiting associated with abnormal liver function tests, mainly elevated SGOT levels, has been associated with the use of oxacillin.[40,41]

DOSAGE AND ADMINISTRATION:

For mild-to-moderate upper-respiratory and localized skin and soft-tissue infections due to sensitive organisms:

Adults and Children Weighing 40 Kg (88 Lbs.) or More: 12.5 mg every 6 hours.

Patients Weighing Less Than 40 Kg (88 Lbs.): 12.5 mg/kg/day in equally divided doses every 6 hours.

For more severe infections such as those of the lower respiratory tract or disseminated infections:

Adults and Children Weighing 40 Kg (88 Lbs.) or More: 250 mg or higher every 6 hours.

Patients Weighing Less Than 40 Kg (88 Lbs.): 25 mg/kg/day or higher in equally divided doses every 6 hours.

Dicloxacillin sodium is best absorbed when taken on an empty stomach, preferably 1 to 2 hours before meals.

Bacteriologic studies to determine the causative organisms and their sensitivity to the penicillinase-resistant penicillins should always be performed. Duration of therapy varies with the type and severity of infection as well as the overall condition of the patient: therefore, it should be determined by the clinical and bacteriological response of the patient. In severe staphylococcal infections, therapy with penicillinase-resistant penicillins should be continued for at least 14 days.[29] Therapy should be continued for at least 48 hours after the patient has become afebrile, asymptomatic, and cultures are negative. The treatment of endocarditis and osteomyelitis may require a longer term of therapy.

Concurrent administration of the penicillinase-resistant penicillins and probenecid increases and prolongs serum penicillin levels. Probenecid decreases the apparent volume of distribution and slows the rate of excretion by competitively inhibiting renal tubular secretion of penicillin.[6,8,21,25,32,66,67] Penicillin-probenecid therapy is generally limited to those infections where very high serum levels of penicillin are necessary.

Oral preparations of the penicillinase-resistant penicillins should not be used as initial therapy in serious, life-threatening infections[16] see PRECAUTIONS, General. Oral therapy with the penicillinase-resistant penicillins may be used to follow up the previous use of a parenteral agent as soon as the clinical condition warrants.[3]

REFERENCES:

1. Douthwaite AH, Trafford JAP: A new style synthetic penicillin.*BMJ.* 1960;2:687-690. **2.** Lane WR: Nafcillin: A comparative*in vitro* trial. *Med J Aust.* 1964;2:499-501. **3.** Marcy SM, Klein JO: The isoxazolyl penicillins: Oxacillin, cloxacillin, and diclocaxillin. *Med Clin North Am.* 1970;54:1127-1143. **4.** Hou JP, Poole JW:β-Lactam antibiotics: Their physicochemical properties and biological activities in relation to structure. *J Pharm Sci.* 1971;60:503-532. **5.** Knox R: A new penicllin (BRL 1241) active against penicillin-resistant staphylococci.*BMJ.*1960;2:690-693. **6.** Prigot A, Froix CJ, Rubin E: Absorption, diffusion, and excretion of a new penicillin, oxacillin.*Antimicrob Agents Chemother.* 1962;1:402-410. **7.** Kucers A, Bennett N: *The Use of Antibiotics*, 2d ed. Philadelphia, J.B. Lippincott Company, 1975. pp 44-70. **8.** Gilbert DN, Sanford JP:Methicillin:Critical appraisal after a decade of experience. *Med Clin North Am.* 1970;54:1113-1125. **9.** Rolinson GN, et al: Bacteriological studies on a new penicillin-BRL 1241. *Lancet.* 1960;2:564-567. **10.** Kislak JW, Eickhoff TC, Finland M: Cloxacillin: Activity *in vitro*, and absorption and urinary excretion in normal young men. *Am J Med Sci.*1965;149:636-646. **11.** Knudsen ET, Rolinson GN: Absorption and excretion of a new antibiotic (BRL 1241). *BMJ.* 1960;2:700-703. **12.** Gravenkemper CF, et al: Dicloxacillin: *In vitro* and pharmacologic comparisons with oxacillin and cloxacillin. *Arch Intern Med.*1965;116:340-345. **13.** Turck M. Ronald A, Petersdorf RG: CLinical studies with cloxacillin: A new antibiotic. *JAMA.* 1965;192:961- 963. **14.** Simon HJ: Current status of methicillin, oxacillin, and cloxacillin. *Antimicrob Agents Chemother.* 1964;1:280-284. **15.** Hammerstrom CF, et al: Clinical, laboratory, and pharmacological studies of dicloxacillin. *Antimicrob Agents Chemother.* 1966;1:69-74. **16.** Dicloxacillin—A new penicillinase-resistant penicillin. *Med Lett Drugs Ther.*1968;10:65-66. **17.** Rolinson GN, Sutherland R: Semisythetic penicillins. *Adv Pharmacol Chemother.* 1973;11:151-220. **18.** Performance Standards for Antimicrobial Disc Suseptibility Tests. National Committee for Clinical Laboratory Standards, 1976, pp 1-11. **19.** Kirby WMM, Rosenfeld LS, Brodie J: Oxacillin: Laboratory and clinical evaluation. *JAMA.*1962;181:739-744. **20.** Eickhoff TC, Kislak JW, Finland M: Clinical evaluation of nafcillin in patients with severe staphylococcal disease. *N. Engl J Med.*1965;272:699-708. **21.** Klein JO, Finland M: Nafcillin—antibacterial action *in vitro* and absorption and excretion in normal young men. *Am J Med Sci.* 1963;246:44-60. **22.** Friend DG: Penicillin therapy-newer semisynthetic penicillins. *Clin Pharmacol Ther.* 1966;7:706-712. **23.** Jackson EA, McLeod DC: Pharmacokinetics and dosing of antimicrobal agents in renal impairment. *Am J Hosp Pharm.*1974;31:36-52. **24.** Barza M. Weinstein L: Pharmacokinetics of the penicillins in man.*Clin Pharmacokinet.*1976;1:297-308. **25.** Whitehouse AC, et al: Blood levels and antistaphyloccal titers produced in human subjects by a penicillinase-resistant penicillin, nafcillin, compared with similar penicillins. *Antimicrob Agents Chemother.* 1962;1:384-392. **26.** Kunin CM: A guide to use of antibiotics in patients with renal disease. *Ann Intern Med.*1967;67:151-158. **27.** Kind AC, et al:Mechanisms responsible for plasma levels of nafcillin lower than those of oxacillin. *Arch Intern Med.*1970;125:685-690. **28.** Weinstein L:Antimicrobial agents. In Goodman LS, Gilman A (eds): *The Pharmacological Basis of Therapeutics,* 5th ed. New York, MacMillan Co., 1975, pp 1130-1158. **29.** KuninCM: Audits of antimicrobial usage—penicillinase-resistant penicllins. *JAMA.*1977;237:1605-1606. **30.** Penicllin G-resistant staphylococcal infections. *Med Lett Drugs Ther.* 1966;8:45-46. **31.** Graham RC:Antibiotics for treatment of infections caused by gram-positive cocci.*Med Clin North Am.*1974;58:505-517. **32.** Douthwaite AH, et al: Methicillin. *BMJ.* 1961;2:6-8. **33.** Stewart GT: Microbiological studies on sodium 6-(2,6-dimethoxybenzamido) penicillante monohydrate (BRL 1241) *in vitro* and in patients. *BMJ.*1960;2:694-699. **34.** Idsoe O. et al: Nature and extent of penicillin side reactions with particular reference to fatalities from anaphylactic shock. *Bull World Health Organ.* 1968;38:159-188. **35.** BunnPA, Milicich S:Laboratory and clinical studies with cloxacillin. *Antimicrob Agents Chemothre.* 1973;1:220-226. **36.** Griffith HW:*Instructions for Patients.* Philadelphia, W.B. Saunders Company, 1975, P 287. **37.** Temkin LA, et al: Communicating information to the ambulant patient. *JAMA.*1975;15:488-493. **38.** Burton JR, et al: Acute interstital nephritis from oxacillin. *Johns Hopkins Med J.* 1974;134:58-61. **39.** Malone AJ, et al: Neurotoxic reaction of oxacillin. *N. Engl. J Med.* 1977;269:453. **40.** Olans RN, Weiner LB: Reversible oxacillin hepatotoxicity. *J. Pediatrics.* 1976;89:835- 838. **41.** Dismukes WE: Oxacillin-induced hepatic dysfunction.*JAMA.* 1973;226:861-863. **42.** Ritschel WA: Therapeutic incompatibilities between penicllin and other antibiotics administered intravenously. *Drug Intell Clin Pharm.* 1969;3:355-356. **43.** Chang TW, Weinstein L: Inhibitory effects of other antibiotics on bacterial morphologic changes induced by penicllin G.*Nature.* 1966;211:763-765. **44.** *Evaluation of Drugs Interactions,*2d ed. Washington, DC, American Pharmaceutical Association, 1976, pp 170-175. **45.** Schardein JL:*Drugs as Teratogens.* Cleveland, Ohio, CRC Press, 1976, pp 156-157, 161-166. **46.** Shepard TH:*Catalog of Teratogenic Agents,* 2 ed. Baltimore. The John Hopkins University Press, 1976, pp 174-175. **47.** Adamsons K, Joelsson I: The effects of pharmacologic agents upon the fetus and newborn. *AM J Obstet Gynecol.*1966;96:437-460. **48.** Saxen I: Associations between oral clefts and drugs taken during pregnancy. *Int J Epidemiol.* 1975;4:37-44. **49.** Greene HJ, Burkhart B. Hobby GL: Excretion of penicillin in human milk following parturition.*J. Obstet Gynecol.*1946;51:732-733. **50.** Drugs in breast milk, *Med Lett Drugs Therapeut.*1974;128:407-419. **51.** McCracken GH: Pharmacological basis for antimicrobial therapy in newborn infants. *Am J Dis Child.*1974;128:407-419. **52.** Westerman G, et al: Adverse reactions to penillicin: A review of treatment. *JAMA.*1966;198:173-174. **53.** Fishman LS Hewitt WL: The natural penicillins.*Med Clin North Am.* 1970;54:1081-1099. **54.** Turck M, Petersdorf RG: The penicllins and their proper use. *In* Kagen BM (ed):*Antimicrobial Therapy*, 2d ed. Philadelphia. W.B. Saunders Company, 1974, pp 16-22. **55.** Ball AP, Gray JA, Murdock JM: Antibacterial drugs today. *Drugs.* 1975;10:9-19. **56.** Isbister JP: Penicillin allergy. A review of the immunological and clinical aspects.*Med J Aust.* 1971;1:1067-1074. **57.** Alexander MR, Ensey R: Methicllin nephritis. *Drug Intell Clin Pharm.* 1974;8:115-117. **58.** Jensen HA, Halveg AB, Saunamaki KI: Permanent impairment of renal function after methicillin nephropathy.*BMJ.*1971;4:406. **59.** Baldwin DS, et al: Renal failure and interstitial nephritis due to penicillin and methicillin. *N Engl J Med.*1968;279:1245-1252. **60.** Parry MF, er al: Nafcillin nephritis, *JAMA.*1973;225:178. **61.** Schrier RW, Bulger RJ, Van Arsdel PP: Nephropathy associated with penicillin and homologues. *Ann Intern Med.*1966;64:116-127. **62.** McElfresh AE,

REFERENCES: *(cont'd)*

Huang NN:Bone marrow depression resulting from the administration of methicllin. *N Engl J Med.*1962;266:246-247. **63.** Sandberg M, Tuazon CU, Sheagren JN: Neutropenia probably resulting from nafcillin. *JAMA.*1975;232:1152-1154. **64.** Markowitz SM, et al: Nafcillin-induced aranulocytosis. *JAMA.* 1975;232:1150-1152. **65.** Levitt BH, et al: Bone marrow depression due to methicillin, a semisynthetic penicillin. *Clin Pharmacol Therapeut.* 1964;5:301-306. **66.** Sabath LD, Psotic B, Finland M: Laboratory studies on methicillin. *Am J Med Sci.* 1962;244:484-500. **67.** Gibaldi M, Schwartz MA: Apparent effect of probenecid on the distribution of penicillins in man.*Clin Pharmacol Therapeut.*1968;9:345-349.

HOW SUPPLIED - RATED THERAPEUTICALLY EQUIVALENT:

Capsule, Gelatin - Oral - 250 mg

40's	$19.95	Dicloxacillin Sodium, Teva	00332-3123-06
100's	$19.00	Dicloxacillin, Raway	00686-0610-20
100's	$19.43	Dicloxacillin, Teva	00332-3123-09
100's	$19.43	Dicloxacillin, United Res	00677-0930-01
100's	$19.43	Dicloxacillin, H.C.F.A. F F P	99999-1046-01
100's	$35.82	Dicloxacillin, Qualitest Pharms	00603-3241-21
100's	$38.07	Dicloxacillin, HL Moore Drug Exch	00839-6178-06
100's	$39.14	Dicloxacillin Sodium, Apothecon	59772-6048-01
100's	$39.25	Dicloxacillin, Rugby	00536-1180-01
100's	$39.75	Dicloxacillin, Geneva Pharms	00781-2220-01
100's	$39.75	Dicloxacillin Sodium, Major Pharms	00904-2647-60
100's	$39.98	Dicloxacillin, Balan	00304-0826-01
100's	$41.60	Dicloxicillin, Lederle Pharm	00005-3135-23
100's	$41.98	Dicloxacillin, Warner Chilcott	00047-0945-24
100's	$42.02	Dicloxacillin, Goldline Labs	00182-1506-01
100's	$42.05	Dicloxacillin, Schein Pharm (US)	00364-0856-01
100's	$42.20	Dicloxacillin Sodium, Aligen Independ	00405-4322-01
100's	$43.05	DYCILL, Beecham	00029-6351-30

Capsule, Gelatin - Oral - 500 mg

50's	$18.71	Dicloxacillin, H.C.F.A. F F P	99999-1046-02
50's	$87.78	DYNAPEN, Mead Johnson	00015-7658-50
100's	$36.00	Dicloxacillin, Raway	00686-0611-20
100's	$37.43	Dicloxacillin, United Res	00677-0931-01
100's	$37.43	Dicloxacillin, H.C.F.A. F F P	99999-1046-03
100's	$42.00	Dicloxacillin Sodium, Raway	00686-3125-09
100's	$60.40	Dicloxacillin Sodium, Harber Pharm	51432-0494-03
100's	$60.50	Dicloxacillin, Qualitest Pharms	00603-3242-21
100's	$66.35	Dicloxacillin, HL Moore Drug Exch	00839-6614-06
100's	$66.95	Dicloxacillin Sodium, Major Pharms	00904-2648-60
100's	$67.45	Dicloxacillin, Geneva Pharms	00781-2225-01
100's	$70.15	Dicloxacillin, Rugby	00536-1190-01
100's	$70.44	Dicloxacillin Sodium, Apothecon	59772-6058-01
100's	$70.50	Dicloxacillin, Schein Pharm (US)	00364-2071-01
100's	$74.11	Dicloxacillin, Lederle Pharm	00005-3136-23
100's	$75.63	Dicloxacillin, Warner Chilcott	00047-0946-24
100's	$75.63	Dicloxacillin, Goldline Labs	00182-1507-01
100's	$75.63	Dicloxacillin, Teva	00332-3125-09
100's	$75.82	Dicloxacillin Sodium, Aligen Independ	00405-4323-01
100's	$76.85	DYCILL, Beecham	00029-6352-30

Powder, Reconstitution - Oral - 62.5 mg/5ml

100 ml	$8.77	DYNAPEN, Mead Johnson	00015-7856-40
200 ml	$15.53	DYNAPEN, Mead Johnson	00015-7856-64

DICUMAROL *(001047)*

CATEGORIES: Anticoagulants; Anticoagulants/Thrombolytics; Atrial Fibrillation; Blood Formation/Coagulation; Coagulants and Anticoagulants; Coronary Occlusion; Embolism; Fibrillation; Pulmonary Embolism; Thrombosis; FDA Approval Pre 1982

BRAND NAMES: *Apekumarol*; *Dicumol*; *Embolin* (Japan)
(International brand names outside U.S. in italics)

DESCRIPTION:

Dicumarol is a coumarin anticoagulant, chemically designated as 3,3'-methylenebis (4-hydroxycoumarin).

Inactive Ingredients: Corn starch, lactose, magnesium stearate and talc.

CLINICAL PHARMACOLOGY:

Dicumarol and other coumarin anticoagulants act by depressing synthesis in the liver of several factors which are known to be active in the coagulation mechanisms in a variety of diseases characterized by thromboembolic phenomena. The resultant *in vivo* effect is a sequential depression of Factors VII, IX, X and II. The degree of depression is dependent upon the dosage administered. Anticoagulants have no direct effect on an established thrombus, nor do they reverse ischemic tissue damage. However, once a thrombosis has occurred, anticoagulant treatment aims to prevent further extension of the formed clot and prevents secondary thromboembolic complications which may result in serious and possible fatal sequelae.

Maximal plasma concentrations are reached in 1 to 9 hours. Approximately 97% is bound to albumin within the plasma. Dicumarol usually induces hypoprothrombinemia in 36 to 48 hours, and its duration of action may persist for 5 to 6 days, thus producing a smooth, long lasting response curve. Little is known of the metabolic pathways involved in the biotransformation of oral anticoagulants in man. However, their metabolites appear to be eliminated principally in the urine.

INDICATIONS AND USAGE:

Dicumarol is indicated for the prophylaxis and treatment of venous thrombosis and its extension, the treatment of atrial fibrillation with embolization, the prophylaxis and treatment of pulmonary embolism, and as an adjunct in the treatment of coronary occlusion.

CONTRAINDICATIONS:

Anticoagulation is contraindicated in any localized or general physical condition or personal circumstance in which the hazard of hemorrhage might be greater than its potential clinical benefits, such as:

Pregnancy: Dicumarol is contraindicated in pregnancy because the drug passes through the placental barrier and may cause, fatal hemorrhage to the fetus in utero. Furthermore, there have been reports of birth malformations in children born to mothers who have been treated with dicumarol during pregnancy. Women of childbearing potential who are candidates for anticoagulant therapy should be carefully evaluated and the indications critically reviewed with the patient. If the patient becomes pregnant while taking this drug, she should be discussed in light of those risks.

Hemorrhagic Tendencies or Blood Dyscrasias: Recent or contemplated surgery of (1) central nervous system; (2) eye; (3) traumatic surgery resulting in large open surfaces.

CONTRAINDICATIONS: *(cont'd)*

Bleeding Tendencies Associated with Active Ulceration or Overt Bleeding Of: (1) gastrointestinal, genitourinary or respiratory tracts; (2) cerebrovascular hemorrhage; (3) aneurysms - cerebral, dissecting aorta; (4) pericarditis and pericardial effusions.

Threatened Abortion: eclampsia and preeclampsia. Inadequate laboratory facilitiesor unsupervised senility, alcoholism, psychosis; or lack of patient cooperation.

Spinal Puncture: and other diagnostic or therapeutic procedures with potential for uncontrollable bleeding.

Miscellaneous: Major regional, lumbar block anesthesia, severe uncontrolled and/or malignant hypertension, subacute bacterial endocarditis, open wounds, visceral carcinoma, vitamin K deficiency, and severe liver or kidney disease.

WARNINGS:

The most serious risks associated with anticoagulant therapy with dicumarol are hemorrhage in any tissue or organ and, less frequently, necrosis and/or gangrene of skin and other tissues. The risk of hemorrhage is related to the level of intensity and the duration of anticoagulant therapy. Hemorrhage and necrosis have in some cases been reported to result in death or permanent disability. Necrosis appears to be associated with local thrombosis and usually appears within a few days of the start of anticoagulant therapy. In severe cases of necrosis, treatment through debridement or amputation of the affected tissue, limb, breast or penis has been reported. Careful diagnosis is required to determine whether necrosis is caused by an underlying disease. Dicumarol therapy should be discontinued when dicumarol is suspected to be the cause of developing necrosis and heparin therapy may be considered for anticoagulation. Although various treatments have been attempted, no treatment for necrosis has been considered uniformly effective. See below for information on predisposing conditions. These and other risks associated with anticoagulant therapy must be weighed against the risk of thrombosis or embolization in untreated cases.

Dicumarol is a potent drug with a half-life of 1 to 2 days; therefore its effects may become more pronounced as daily maintenance doses overlap. It cannot be emphasized too strongly that treatment of each patient is a highly individualized matter. Dosage should be controlled by periodic determinations of prothrombin time or other suitable coagulation tests. Determinations of whole blood clotting and bleeding times are not effective measures for control of therapy. Heparin prolongs the one-stage prothrombin time. Therefore, to obtain a valid prothrombin time when heparin and dicumarol are given together, a period of at least 5 hours should elapse after the last intravenous dose and 24 hours after the last subcutaneous dose of heparin, before blood is drawn.

Caution should be observed when dicumarol is administered in any situation or in the presence of any predisposing condition where added risk of hemorrhage or necrosis is present.

Administration of anticoagulants in the following conditions will be based upon clinical judgement in which the risks of anticoagulant therapy are weighed against the risk of thrombosis or embolization in untreated cases. The following may be associated with these increased risks:

Lactation: Coumarins may pass into the milk of mothers and cause a prothrombinopenic state in the nursing infant.

Mild to Moderate Hepatic or Renal Insufficiency

Infectious Diseases or Disturbances of Intestinal Flora: Sprue, antibiotic therapy.

Trauma: Which may result in internal bleeding.

Surgery or Trauma: Resulting in large exposed raw surfaces.

Indwelling Catheters and/or Drainage Tubes in Any Orifice

Mild to Moderate Hypertension

Known or Suspected Hereditary, Familial or Clinical Deficiency in Protein C: This condition, which should be suspected if there is a history of recurrent episodes of thromboembolic disorders in the patient or in the family, has been associated with an increased risk of developing necrosis following dicumarol administration. Skin necrosis may occur in the absence of protein C deficiency. It has been reported that initiation of anticoagulation therapy with heparin for 4 to 5 days before initiation of therapy with dicumarol may minimize the incidence of this reaction. Dicumarol therapy should be discontinued when dicumarol is suspected to be the cause of developing necrosis and heparin therapy may be considered for anticoagulation.

Miscellaneous: Polycythemia vera, vasculitis, severe diabetes, severe allergic and anaphylactic disorders, active tuberculosis, history of ulcerative disease of the gastrointestinal tract and during the postpartum period.

Patients with congestive heart failure may become more sensitive to dicumarol, thereby requiring more frequent laboratory monitoring, and reduced doses of dicumarol.

Use of anticoagulants with streptokinase or urokinase may be hazardous and caution should be exercised when used concomitantly. (Please note recommendations accompanying these preparations.)

Abrupt cessation of anticoagulant therapy is not generally recommended; taper dose gradually over 3 to 4 weeks.

PRECAUTIONS:

Periodic determination of prothrombin time or other suitable coagulation test is essential.

Numerous factors, alone or in combination, including travel, changes in diet, environment, physical state and medication may influence response of the patient to anticoagulants. It is generally good practice to monitor the patient's response with additional prothrombin time determinations in the period immediately after discharge from the hospital, and whenever other medications are initiated, discontinued or taken haphazardly. The following factors are listed for your reference; however, other factors may also affect the prothrombin response.

The Following Factors Alone or in Combination, May Be Responsible for Increased Prothrombin Time Response:

Endogenous Factors: Carcinoma; collagen disease; congestive heart failure; diarrhea; elevated temperature; hepatic disorders—infectious hepatitis, hyperthyroidism, jaundice; poor nutritional state; vitamin K deficiency—steatorrhea.

Exogenous Factors: Alcohol†; allopurinol; aminosalicylic acid; amiodarone; anabolic steroids; antibiotics; bromelains; chloral hydrate†; chloramphenicol; chlorpropamide; chymotrypsin; cimetidine; cinchophen; clofibrate; dicumarol overdosage; dextran; dextrothyroxine; diazoxide; dietary deficiencies; diflunisal; diuretics†; disulfiram; drugs affecting blood elements; ethacrynic acid; fenoprofen; glucagon; hepatotoxic drugs; ibuprofen; indomethacin; influenza virus vaccine; inhalation anesthetics; mefenamic acid; methyldopa; methylphenidate; methylthiouracil; metronidazole; miconazole; monoamine oxidase inhibitors; nalidixic acid; naproxen; nortriptyline; oxolinic acid; oxyphenbutazone; pentoxifylline; phenylbutazone; phenyramidol; phenytoin; prolonged hot weather; prolonged narcotics; propylthiouracil; pyrazolones; quinidine; quinine; ranitidine†; salicylates; sulfinpyrazone; sulfonamides, long acting; sulindac; thyroid drugs; tolbutamide; triclofos sodium; trimethoprim/sulfamethoxazole; unreliable prothrombin time determinations.

The Following Factors, Alone or in Combination, May Be Responsible for Decreased Prothrombin Time Response:

PRECAUTIONS: *(cont'd)*

Endogenous Factors: Edema; hereditary resistance to coumarin therapy; hyperlipemia; hypothyroidism.

Exogenous Factors: ACTH steroids; alcohol†; antacids; antihistamines; phenobarbital and other barbiturates; carbamazepine; chloral hydrate†; chlordiazepoxide; cholestyramine; dicumarol underdosage; diet high in vitamin K; diuretics†; ethchlorvynol; glutethimide; griseofulvin; haloperidol; meprobamate; oral contraceptives; paraldehyde; primidone; ranitidine†; rifampin; unreliable prothrombin time determinations; vitamin C.

A patient may be exposed to a combination of the above factors, some of which may increase and some decrease his sensitivity to dicumarol. Because the net effect on his prothrombin time response may be unpredictable under these circumstances, more frequent laboratory monitoring is advisable.

Drugs not yet shown to interact or not to interact with coumarins are best regarded with suspicion, and when their administration is started or stopped, the prothrombin time should be determined more often than usual.

Coumarins also affect the action of other drugs. Hypoglycemic agents (chlorpropamide and tolbutamide) and anticonvulsants (phenytoin and phenobarbital) may accumulate in the body as a result of interference with either their metabolism or excretion.

ADVERSE REACTIONS:

Potential adverse reactions to dicumarol may include:

Hemorrhage from any tissue or organ. This is a consequence of the anticoagulant effect. The signs and symptoms will vary according to the location and degree or extent of the bleeding. Therefore, the possibility of hemorrhage should be considered in evaluating the condition of any anticoagulated patient with complaints which do not indicate an obvious diagnosis. Bleeding during anticoagulant therapy does not always correlate with prothrombin activity. (See OVERDOSAGE.)

Adrenal hemorrhage with resultant acute adrenal insufficiency has occurred during anticoagulant therapy. Anticoagulant therapy should be discontinued in patients who develop signs and symptoms compatible with acute adrenal hemorrhage or insufficiency. Plasma cortisol levels should be measured immediately, and vigorous therapy with intravenous corticosteroids should be instituted promptly. Initiation of therapy should not depend upon laboratory confirmation of the diagnosis, since any delay in an acute situation may result in the patient's death.

Ovarian hemorrhage: Reports indicate that a woman receiving short- or long-term therapy with heparin or warfarin sodium may be at risk of developing ovarian hemorrhage at the time of ovulation. Caution should be observed when dicumarol is administered since these compounds have similar actions.

Paralytic ileus and intestinal obstruction have been reported from submucosal or intramural hemorrhage.

Excessive uterine bleeding has occurred but menstrual flow is usually normal.

Bleeding which occurs when the prothrombin time is within the therapeutic range warrants diagnostic investigation since it may unmask a previously unsuspected lesion, e.g., tumor, ulcer, etc.

Necrosis of skin and other tissues. (See WARNINGS.)

Other adverse reactions are infrequent and consist of alopecia, urticaria, dermatitis, fever, nausea, diarrhea, abdominal cramping, a syndrome called "purple toes," hypersensitivity reactions, leukopenia, and vomiting.

Priapism has been associated with anticoagulant administration, however, a causal relationship has not been established.

OVERDOSAGE:

Excessive prothrombinopenia, with or without bleeding, is readily controlled by discontinuing dicumarol, and if necessary, the oral or parenteral administration of vitamin K_1. The appearance of microscopic hematuria, excessive menstrual bleeding, melena, petechiae or oozing from nicks made while shaving are early manifestation of hypoprothrombinemia beyond a safe and satisfactory level.

In excessive prothrombinopenia with mild or no bleeding, omission of one or more doses of dicumarol may suffice; and if necessary, small doses of vitamin K_1 orally, 2 1/2 to 10 mg, will usually correct the problem.

If minor bleeding persists, or progresses to frank bleeding, vitamin K_1 in doses of 5 to 25 mg may be given parenterally. (Please note recommendations accompanying vitamin K preparations prior to use.)

Fresh whole blood transfusions should be considered in cases of severe bleeding or prothrombinopenic states unresponsive to vitamin K_1.

Resumption of dicumarol administration reverses the effect of vitamin K_1, and a therapeutic hypoprothrombinemia level can again be obtained. A hypercoagulable state has been reported to occur following rapid reversal of a prolonged prothrombin time, therefore, caution must be used in determining the need for this vitamin.

DOSAGE AND ADMINISTRATION:

DOSAGE AND LABORATORY CONTROL

The aim of anticoagulant therapy is to impede the coagulation or clotting mechanism to such an extent that avoiding such extensive impairment as might produce spontaneous bleeding. Effective therapeutic levels with minimal complications can best be achieved in cooperative and well-instructed patients, who keep the doctor informed of their status between visits.

The administration and dosage of dicumarol must be individualized for each patient according to the particular patient's sensitivity to the drug as indicated by the prothrombin time. The prothrombin time reflects the depression of vitamin K dependent Factors VII, X and II. These factors, in addition to Factor IX, are affected by coumarin anticoagulants. There are several modifications of the Quick one-stage prothrombin time and the physician should become familiar with the specific method used in his laboratory.

Administration of dicumarol should be gauged according to prothrombin time determinations by a suitable method. The blood prothrombin time should usually be determined daily after the administration of the initial dose until prothrombin time results stabilize in the therapeutic range. Intervals between subsequent prothrombin time determinations should be based upon the physician's judgment of the patient's reliability and response to dicumarol in order to maintain the individual within the therapeutic range. Acceptable intervals for prothrombin time determinations have usually fallen within the range of 1 to 4 weeks. Satisfactory levels for maintenance of therapeutic anticoagulation are 1 1/2 to 2 1/2 times the normal prothrombin time (*e.g.,* 18 to 30 seconds, with a control of 12 seconds).

INDUCTION

The dosage range for the average adult with normal prothrombin activity ranges from 200 to 300 mg the first day.

DOSAGE AND ADMINISTRATION: *(cont'd)*

MAINTENANCE

On subsequent days the dosage ranges from 25 to 200 mg. It is essential that prothrombin time be measured daily while establishing the correct maintenance dose. Once this has been determined, prothrombin times can be checked less frequently. Dicumarol tablets may not be interchangeable with dicumarol capsules. Retitration of the dosage should be considered if the dosage form prescribed is changed.

DURATION OF THERAPY

The duration of therapy in each patient should be individualized. In general, anticoagulant therapy should be continued until the danger of thrombosis and embolism has passed.

TREATMENT DURING DENTISTRY AND SURGERY

The management of patients who undergo dental and surgical procedures requires close liaison between attending physicians, surgeons and dentists. Interruption of anticoagulant therapy may precipitate thromboembolism, and conversely, if anticoagulants are maintained at full doses, some patients may hemorrhage excessively. If it is elected to administer anticoagulants prior to, during, or immediately following dental or surgical procedures, it is recommended that the dosage of dicumarol be adjusted to maintain the prothrombin time at approximately 1 $\frac{1}{2}$ to 2 $\frac{1}{2}$ times the control level. The operative site should be sufficiently limited to permit the effective use of local procedures for hemostasis including absorbable hemostatic agents, sutures, and pressure dressings if necessary. Under these conditions dental and surgical procedures may be performed without undue risk of hemorrhage.

DICUMAROL WITH HEPARIN

Since a delay intervenes between the administration of the initial dose and the therapeutic prolongation of prothrombin time, it may be advisable in emergency situations to administer sodium heparin initially along with dicumarol.

It should be noted that heparin may affect the prothrombin time, and therefore, when patients are receiving both heparin and dicumarol, the blood sample for prothrombin time determination should be drawn just prior to the next heparin dosage, at least 5 hours after the last intravenous injection or 24 hours after the last subcutaneous injection.

†Increased and decreased prothrombin time responses have been reported.

Recommended Storage: Store below 77°F (25°C).

HOW SUPPLIED - EQUIVALENTS NOT AVAILABLE:

Tablet, Uncoated - Oral - 25 mg

100's $9.94 Dicumarol, Abbott 00074-3794-01

DICYCLOMINE HYDROCHLORIDE *(001048)*

CATEGORIES: Anticholinergic Agents; Antimuscarinics/Antispasmodics; Antispasmodics & Anticholinergics; Autonomic Drugs; Gastrointestinal Drugs; Hormones; Irritable Bowel Syndrome; Parasympatholytics; Pregnancy Category B; FDA Approval Pre 1982; Top 200 Drugs

BRAND NAMES: A-Spas; Antispas; *Babyspasmil*; *Balacon* (Japan); Bemot; Benomine; Bentue; **Bentyl**; *Bentylol* (Canada); Bo-Cyclomine; *Clomin*; *Coochil*; *Cyclominol*; Cyclonil; *Dedoxia*; Di-Spaz; Dibent; *Diciclomina*; *Diclomin* (Mexico); *Dicomin*; *Dicyclo*; Dicyclocot; *Formulex* (Canada); *Lomine* (Canada); *Magesan*; *Magesan P* (Japan); *Medicyclomine*; Medispaz-Im; *Merbentyl* (Australia, England); Neoquess; *Nomcramp*; *Nomocramp*; *Notensyl*; *Optimal*; Or-Tyl; *Panakiron* (Japan); Pasmin; *Peristalsinone*; *Protylol*; Quentyl; *Respolimin* (Japan); Shoben; *Spasmoban* (Canada); Spasmoject; *Spasoma*; *Swityl*; *Viscerol*; *Vominox*; *Wintyl*; *Wyovin*
(International brand names outside U.S. in italics)

FORMULARIES: Aetna; BC-BS; CIGNA; DoD; FHP; Humana; Kaiser; Medco; Medi-Cal; PCS; PruCare; United

DESCRIPTION:

Dicyclomine hydrochloride, (abbreviated here as dicyclomine HCl), is an antispasmodic and anticholinergic (antimuscarinic) agent available in the following forms:

1. Dicyclomine HCl capsules for oral use contain 10 mg dicyclomine hydrochloride USP. Dicyclomine HCl 10 mg capsules also contain inactive ingredients: calcium sulfate, corn starch, FD&C Blue No. 1, FD&C Red No. 40, gelatin, lactose, magnesium stearate, pregelatinized corn starch, and titanium dioxide.

2. Dicyclomine HCl tablets for oral use contain 20 mg dicyclomine hydrochloride USP. Dicyclomine HCl 20 mg tablets also contain inactive ingredients: acacia, dibasic calcium phosphate, corn starch, FD&C Blue No. 1, lactose, magnesium stearate, pregelatinized corn starch, and sucrose.

3. Dicyclomine HCl syrup for oral use contains 10 mg dicyclomine hydrochloride USP in each 5 ml (1 teaspoonful). Dicyclomine HCl syrup also contains inactive ingredients: citric acid, D&C Red No. 33, FD&C Blue No. 1, FD&C Red No. 40, FD&C Yellow No. 6, flavors, glucose, methylparaben, propylene glycol, propylparaben, saccharin sodium, and water.

4. Dicyclomine HCl Injection is a sterile, pyrogen-free, aqueous solution for intramuscular injection (NOT FOR INTRAVENOUS USE).

Ampul:2 ml-Each ml contains 10 mg dicyclomine hydrochloride USP in sterile water for injection, made isotonic with sodium chloride.

Vial:10 ml-Each ml contains 10 mg dicyclomine hydrochloride USP in sterile water for injection, made isotonic with sodium chloride. A preservative containing 0.5% chlorobutanol hydrous (chloral derivative) has been added.

Chemically, dicyclomine HCl is (bicyclohexyl)-1-carboxylic acid, 2-(diethylamino)ethyl-ester-, hydrochloride.

Dicyclomine hydrochloride occurs as a fine, white, crystalline, practically odorless powder with a bitter taste. It is soluble in water, freely soluble in alcohol and chloroform, and very slightly soluble in ether.

CLINICAL PHARMACOLOGY:

Dicyclomine relieves smooth muscle spasm of the gastrointestinal tract. Animal studies indicate that this action is achieved via a dual mechanism: (1) a specific anticholinergic effect (antimuscarinic) at the acetylcholine-receptor sites with approximately 1/8 the milligram potency of atropine (*in vitro*, guinea pig ileum); and (2) a direct effect upon smooth muscle (musculotropic) as evidenced by dicyclomine's antagonism of bradykinin- and histamine-induced spasms of the isolated guinea pig ileum. Atropine did not affect responses to these two agonists. *In vivo* studies in cats and dogs showed dicyclomine to be equally potent against acetylcholine (ACh)- or barium chloride ($BaCl_2$)-induced intestinal spasm while atropine was at least 200 times more potent against effects of ACh than $BaCl_2$. Tests for mydriatic effects in mice showed that dicyclomine was approximately 1/500 as potent as atropine; antisialagogue tests in rabbits showed dicyclomine to be 1/300 as potent as atropine.

CLINICAL PHARMACOLOGY: *(cont'd)*

In man, dicyclomine is rapidly absorbed after oral administration, reaching peak values within 60-90 minutes. The principal route of elimination is via the urine (79.5% of the dose). Excretion also occurs in the feces, but to a lesser extent (8.4%). Mean half-life of plasma elimination in one study was determined to be approximately 1.8 hours when plasma concentrations were measured for 9 hours after a single dose. In subsequent studies, plasma concentrations were followed for up to 24 hours after a single dose, showing a secondary phase of elimination with a somewhat longer half-life. Mean volume of distribution for a 20 mg oral dose is approximately 3.65 L/kg suggesting extensive distribution in tissues.

In controlled clinical trials involving over 100 patients who received drug, 82% of patients treated for functional bowel/irritable bowel syndrome with dicyclomine HCl at initial doses of 160 mg daily (40 mg q.i.d.) demonstrated a favorable clinical response compared with 55% treated with placebo. (P<.05). In these trials, most of the side effects were typically anticholinergic in nature (see TABLE 1)and were reported by 61% of the patients.

TABLE 1

Side Effect	Dicyclomine Hydrochloride (40 mg q.i.d.) %	Placebo %
Dry Mouth	33	5
Dizziness	29	2
Blurred Vision	27	2
Nausea	14	6
Light-Headedness	11	3
Drowsiness	9	1
Weakness	7	1
Nervousness	6	2

Nine percent (9%) of patients were discontinued from the drug because of one or more of these side effects (compared with 2% in the placebo group). In 41% of the patients with side effects, side effects disappeared or were tolerated at the 160 mg daily dose without reduction. A dose reduction from 160 mg daily to an average daily dose of 90 mg was required in 46% of the patients with side effects who then continued to experience a favorable clinical response; their side effects either disappeared or were tolerated. (See ADVERSE REACTIONS.)

INDICATIONS AND USAGE:

For the treatment of functional bowel/irritable bowel syndrome.

CONTRAINDICATIONS:

1. Obstructive uropathy

2. Obstructive disease of the gastrointestinal tract

3. Severe ulcerative colitis (See PRECAUTIONS.)

4. Reflux esophagitis

5. Unstable cardiovascular status in acute hemorrhage

6. Glaucoma

7. Myasthenia gravis

8. Evidence of prior hypersensitivity to dicyclomine HCl or other ingredients of these formulations

9. Infants less than 6 months of age (SeeWARNINGS and PRECAUTIONS, Information for Patients.)

10. Nursing Mothers (See WARNINGS and PRECAUTIONS, Information for Patients.)

WARNINGS:

In the presence of a high environmental temperature, heat prostration can occur with drug use (fever and heat stroke due to decreased sweating). If symptoms occur, the drug should be discontinued and supportive measures instituted.

Diarrhea may be an early symptom of incomplete intestinal obstruction, especially in patients with ileostomy or colostomy. In this instance, treatment with this drug would be inappropriate and possibly harmful.

Dicyclomine HCl may produce drowsiness or blurred vision. The patient should be warned not to engage in activities requiring mental alertness, such as operating a motor vehicle or other machinery or performing hazardous work while taking this drug.

Psychosis has been reported in sensitive individuals given anticholinergic drugs. CNS signs and symptoms include confusion, disorientation, short-term memory loss, hallucinations, dysarthria, ataxia, coma, euphoria, decreased anxiety, fatigue, insomnia, agitation and mannerisms, and inappropriate affect. These CNS signs and symptoms usually resolve within 12 to 24 hours after discontinuation of the drug.

There are reports that administration of dicyclomine HCl syrup to infants has been followed by serious respiratory symptoms (dyspnea, shortness of breath, breathlessness, respiratory collapse, apnea, asphyxia), seizures, syncope, pulse rate fluctuations, muscular hypotonia, and coma. Death has been reported. No causal relationship between these effects observed in infants and dicyclomine administration has been established. DICYCLOMINE HCL IS CONTRAINDICATED IN INFANTS LESS THAN 6 MONTHS OF AGE AND IN NURSING MOTHERS. (See CONTRAINDICATIONSand PRECAUTIONS, Nursing Mothers and Pediatric Use.)

Safety and efficacy of dicyclomine HCl in children have not been established.

PRECAUTIONS:

GENERAL

Use with caution in patients with:

1. Autonomic neuropathy

2. Hepatic or renal disease

3. Ulcerative colitis - large doses may suppress intestinal motility to the point of producing a paralytic ileus and the use of this drug may precipitate or aggravate the serious complication of toxic megacolon (See CONTRAINDICATIONS)

4. Hyperthyroidism

5. Hypertension

6. Coronary heart disease

7. Congestive heart failure

8. Cardiac tachyarrhythmia

9. Hiatal hernia (See CONTRAINDICATIONS, reflux esophagitis)

10. Known or suspected prostatic hypertrophy.

Investigate any tachycardia before administration of dicyclomine HCl,since it may increase the heart rate.

With overdosage, a curare-like action may occur (*i.e.,* neuromuscular blockade leading to muscular weakness and possible paralysis).

PRECAUTIONS: *(cont'd)*

INFORMATION FOR THE PATIENT

Dicyclomine HCl may produce drowsiness or blurred vision. The patient should be warned not to engage in activities requiring mental alertness, such as operating a motor vehicle or other machinery or to perform hazardous work while taking this drug.

Dicyclomine HCl is contraindicated in infants less than 6 months of age and in nursing mothers. (See CONTRAINDICATIONS and PRECAUTIONS, Nursing Mothers and Pediatric Use.)

In the presence of a high environmental temperature, heat prostration can occur with drug use (fever and heat stroke due to decreased sweating). If symptoms occur, the drug should be discontinued and a physician contacted.

CARCINOGENESIS, MUTAGENESIS, AND IMPAIRMENT OF FERTILITY

There are no known human data on long-term potential for carcinogenicity or mutagenicity.

Long-term studies in animals to determine carcinogenic potential are not known to have been conducted.

In studies in rats at doses of up to 100 mg/kg/day, dicyclomine HCl produced no deleterious effects on breeding, conception, or parturition.

PREGNANCY, TERATOGENIC EFFECTS, PREGNANCY CATEGORY B

Reproduction studies have been performed in rats and rabbits at doses up to 33 times the maximum recommended human dose based on 160 mg/day (3 mg/kg) and have revealed no evidence of impaired fertility or harm to the fetus due to dicyclomine. Epidemiologic studies in pregnant women with products containing dicyclomine HCl (at doses up to 40 mg/day) have not shown that dicyclomine increases the risk of fetal abnormalities if administered during the first trimester of pregnancy. There are, however, no adequate and well-controlled studies in pregnant women at the recommended doses (80-160 mg day). Because animal reproduction studies are not always predictive of human response, dicyclomine HCl as indicated for functional bowel/irritable bowel syndrome should be used during pregnancy only if clearly needed.

NURSING MOTHERS

Since dicyclomine HCl has been reported to be excreted in human milk, DICYCLOMINE HCL IS CONTRAINDICATED IN NURSING MOTHERS. (See CONTRAINDICATIONS, WARNINGS, PRECAUTIONS, Pediatric Useand ADVERSE REACTIONS.)

PEDIATRIC USE

See CONTRAINDICATIONS, WARNINGS, and PRECAUTIONS, Nursing Mothers. DICYCLOMINE HCL IS CONTRAINDICATED IN INFANTS LESS THAN 6 MONTHS OF AGE.

Safety and effectiveness in children have not been established.

DRUG INTERACTIONS:

The following agents may increase certain actions or side effects of anticholinergic drugs: amantadine, antiarrhythmic agents of Class I (*e.g.*, quinidine), antihistamines, antipsychotic agents (*e.g.*, phenothiazines), benzodiazepines, MAO inhibitors, narcotic analgesics (*e.g.*, meperidine), nitrates and nitrites, sympathomimetic agents, tricyclic antidepressants, and other drugs having anticholinergic activity.

Anticholinergics antagonize the effects of antiglaucoma agents. Anticholinergic drugs in the presence of increased intraocular pressure may be hazardous when taken concurrently with agents such as corticosteroids. (See also CONTRAINDICATIONS.)

Anticholinergic agents may affect gastrointestinal absorption of various drugs, such as slowly dissolving dosage forms of digoxin; increased serum digoxin concentrations may result. Anticholinergic drugs may antagonize the effects of drugs that alter gastrointestinal motility, such as metoclopramide. Because antacids may interfere with the absorption of anticholinergic agents, simultaneous use of these drugs should be avoided.

The inhibiting effects of anticholinergic drugs on gastric hydrochloric acid secretion are antagonized by agents used to treat achlorhydria and those used to test gastric secretion.

ADVERSE REACTIONS:

Controlled clinical trials have provided frequency information for reported adverse effects of dicyclomine HCl listed in a decreasing order of frequency. (See CLINICAL PHARMACOLOGY.)

Not all of the following adverse reactions have been reported with dicyclomine HCl. Adverse reactions are included here that have been reported for pharmacologically similar drugs with anticholinergic/antispasmodic action.

Gastrointestinal: dry mouth, nausea, vomiting, constipation, bloated feeling, abdominal pain, taste loss, anorexia

Central Nervous System: dizziness, light-headedness, tingling, headache, drowsiness, weakness, nervousness, numbness, mental confusion and/or excitement (especially in elderly persons), dyskinesia, lethargy, syncope, speech disturbance, insomnia

Ophthalmologic: blurred vision, diplopia, mydriasis, cycloplegia, increased ocular tension

Dermatologic/Allergic: rash, urticaria, itching, and other dermal manifestations: severe allergic reaction or drug idiosyncrasies including anaphylaxis

Genitourinary: urinary hesitancy, urinary retention

Cardiovascular: tachycardia, palpitations

Respiratory: Dyspnea, apnea, asphyxia (See WARNINGS)

Other: decreased sweating, nasal stuffiness or congestion, sneezing, throat congestion, impotence, suppression of lactation (See PRECAUTIONS, Nursing Mothers)

With the injectable form, there may be a temporary sensation of light-headedness. Some local irritation and focal coagulation necrosis may occur following the IM injection of the drug.

DRUG ABUSE AND DEPENDENCE:

Tolerance, abuse, or dependence with dicyclomine HCl has not been reported.

OVERDOSAGE:

SIGNS AND SYMPTOMS

The signs and symptoms of overdosage are headache; nausea; vomiting; blurred vision; dilated pupils; hot, dry skin; dizziness; dryness of the mouth; difficulty in swallowing; and CNS stimulation. A curare-like action may occur (*i.e.*, neuromuscular blockade leading to muscular weakness and possible paralysis).

The acute oral LD_{50} of the drug is 625 mg/kg in mice.

MINIMUM HUMAN LETHAL DOSE/MAXIMUM HUMAN DOSE RECORDED

The amount of drug in a single dose that is ordinarily associated with symptoms of overdosage or that is likely to be life-threatening, has not been defined. The maximum human oral dose recorded was 600 mg by mouth in a 10 month-old child and approximately 1500 mg in an adult, each of whom survived.

In three of the infants who died following administration of dicyclomine HCl (see WARNINGS), the blood concentrations of drug were 200, 220, and 505 ng/ml, respectively.

OVERDOSAGE: *(cont'd)*

DIALYSIS

It is not known if dicyclomine HCl is dialyzable.

TREATMENT

Treatment should consist of gastric lavage, emetics, and activated charcoal. Sedatives (*e.g.*, short-acting barbiturates, benzodiazepines) may be used for management of overt signs of excitement. If indicated, an appropriate parenteral cholinergic agent may be used as an antidote.

DOSAGE AND ADMINISTRATION:

DOSAGE MUST BE ADJUSTED TO INDIVIDUAL PATIENT NEEDS. (See CLINICAL PHARMACOLOGY.)

ADULTS-ORAL

The only oral dose clearly shown to be effective is 160 mg per day (in 4 equally divided doses). Since this dose is associated with a significant incidence of side effects, it is prudent to begin with 80 mg per day (in 4 equally divided doses). Depending upon the patient's response during the first week of therapy, the dose should be increased to 160 mg per day unless side effects limit dosage escalation.

If efficacy is not achieved within 2 weeks or side effects require doses below 80 mg per day, the drug should be discontinued. Documented safety data are not available for doses above 80 mg daily for periods longer than 2 weeks.

ADULTS - INTRAMUSCULAR INJECTION NOT FOR INTRAVENOUS USE

The intramuscular dosage form is to be used temporarily when the patient cannot take oral medication. Intramuscular injection is about twice as bioavailable as oral dosage forms; consequently, the recommended intramuscular dose is 80 mg daily (in 4 equally divided doses).

Oral dicyclomine HCl should be started as soon as possible and the intramuscular form should not be used for periods longer than 1 or 2 days.

ASPIRATE THE SYRINGE BEFORE INJECTING TO AVOID INTRAVASCULAR INJECTION. SINCE THROMBOSIS MAY OCCUR IF THE DRUG IS INADVERTENTLY INJECTED INTRAVASCULARLY. Parenteral drug products should be inspected visually for particulate matter and discoloration prior to administration, whenever solution and container permit.

Store capsules, tablets and syrup at room temperature, preferably below 86F° (30°C). Protect syrup from excessive heat.

Store injections at room temperature, preferably below 86°F (30°C).

Protect from freezing.

PATIENT INFORMATION:

Dicyclomine is used for the treatment of certain stomach and intestinal disorders. Notify your physician if you are pregnant or nursing. This medication is contraindicated in nursing mothers. Dicyclomine should be taken 30 to 60 minutes before meals. This medication may cause drowsiness; use caution while driving or operating hazardous machinery. Do not take any other sedating drugs or drink alcohol while taking dicyclomine. This medication may decrease the ability of the body to perspire; use caution and avoid overheating. Notify your physician if you develop dry mouth, difficulty urinating, constipation, increased sensitivity to light, skin rash, flushing or eye pain.

HOW SUPPLIED - RATED THERAPEUTICALLY EQUIVALENT:

Capsule, Gelatin - Oral - 10 mg

100's	$3.30	Dicyclomine Hcl, Voluntary Hosp	53258-0405-01
100's	$6.10	Dicyclomine Hcl, Vangard Labs	00615-0327-13
100's	$6.15	Dicyclomine Hcl, Medirex	57480-0380-01
100's	$6.40	Dicyclomine Hcl, Major Pharms	00904-0193-60
100's	$9.14	Dicyclomine Hcl, Major Pharms	00904-0193-61
100's	$12.00	Dicyclomine Hcl, Voluntary Hosp	53258-0405-13
100's	$19.94	Dicyclomine Hcl, Qualitest Pharms	00603-3265-21
100's	$20.95	Dicyclomine, Major Pharms	00904-7896-60
100's	$21.11	Dicyclomine Hcl, Goldline Labs	00182-0519-01
100's	$23.00	Dicyclomine Hcl, Lannett	00527-0586-01
100's	$23.10	DICYCLOMINE HCL, Aligen Independ	00405-4328-01
100's	$23.12	Dicyclomine, Rugby	00536-3367-01
100's	$24.35	Dicyclomine Hcl, HL Moore Drug Exch	00839-5100-06
100's	**$24.84**	**BENTYL, Hoechst Marion Roussel**	**00068-0120-61**
100's	$25.46	Dicyclomine Hcl, United Res	00677-0341-01
250's	$10.15	Dicyclomine Hcl, Major Pharms	00904-0193-70
600's	$78.20	Dicyclomine Hcl, Medirex	57480-0380-06
1000's	$30.90	BENTUE, Macnary	55982-0006-09
1000's	$34.45	Dicyclomine Hcl, Major Pharms	00904-0193-80
1000's	$186.00	Dicyclomine, Major Pharms	00904-7896-80
1000's	$186.20	Dicyclomine Hcl, Aligen Independ	00405-4328-03
1000's	$186.70	Dicyclomine Hcl, Qualitest Pharms	00603-3265-32
1000's	$194.00	Dicyclomine Hcl, Goldline Labs	00182-0519-10
1000's	$194.27	Dicyclomine Hcl, HL Moore Drug Exch	00839-5100-16
1000's	$210.00	Dicyclomine Hcl, Lannett	00527-0586-10
1000's	$210.10	Dicyclomine, Rugby	00536-3367-10

Injection, Solution - Intramuscular - 10 mg/ml

2 ml x 5	**$63.66**	**BENTYL, Hoechst Marion Roussel**	**00068-0809-23**
2 ml x 10	$88.00	PASMIN, Alba Pharma	10023-0114-02
2 ml x 25	$80.00	Dicyclomine HCl, Schein Pharm (US)	00364-6528-48
10 ml	$8.75	Dicyclomine Hcl, Consolidated Midland	00223-7430-10
10 ml	$9.20	Dicyclomine Hcl, Hyrex Pharms	00314-0299-70
10 ml	$9.20	A-Spas, Hyrex Pharms	00314-2501-70
10 ml	$13.00	Dicyclomine Hcl, Steris Labs	00402-0299-10
10 ml	$14.80	Dicyclomine Hcl, Goldline Labs	00182-0708-63
10 ml	$15.50	Dicyclomine HCl, Schein Pharm (US)	00364-6528-54
10 ml	**$40.68**	**BENTYL, Hoechst Marion Roussel**	**00068-0810-61**

Syrup - Oral - 10 mg/5ml

480 ml	$7.00	Dicyclomine Hcl, Rugby	00536-0480-85
480 ml	**$27.66**	**BENTYL, Hoechst Marion Roussel**	**00068-0125-16**
3840 ml	$30.99	Dicyclomine Hcl, Rugby	00536-0480-90

Tablet, Uncoated - Oral - 20 mg

100's	$2.85	Dicyclomine Hcl, Voluntary Hosp	53258-0118-01
100's	$5.25	Dicyclomine Hcl, HL Moore Drug Exch	00839-5047-06
100's	$5.30	Dicyclomine Hcl, Major Pharms	00904-0195-60
100's	$6.00	Dicyclomine Hcl, Medirex	57480-0381-01
100's	$6.25	Dicyclomine Hcl, Consolidated Midland	00223-0795-01
100's	$6.41	Dicyclomine Hcl, Vangard Labs	00615-1516-13
100's	$6.50	Dicyclomine Hcl, United Res	00677-0498-01
100's	$7.99	Dicyclomine Hcl, Major Pharms	00904-0195-61
100's	$10.89	Dicyclomine Hcl, Voluntary Hosp	53258-0118-13
100's	$29.95	Dicyclomine, Rugby	00536-3377-01

HOW SUPPLIED - RATED THERAPEUTICALLY EQUIVALENT:
(cont'd)

100's	**$35.46**	**BENTYL, Hoechst Marion Roussel**	**00068-0123-61**
250's	$8.95	Dicyclomine Hcl, Major Pharms	00904-0195-70
1000's	$24.10	Dicyclomine Hcl, Major Pharms	00904-0195-80
1000's	$25.04	Dicyclomine Hcl, HL Moore Drug Exch	00839-5047-16
1000's	$32.00	Dicyclomine Hcl, United Res	00677-0498-10
1000's	$194.00	Dicyclomine, Rugby	00536-3377-10
6020's	$91.20	Dicyclomine Hcl, Medirex	57480-0381-06

HOW SUPPLIED - NOT RATED EQUIVALENT:
Injection, Solution - Intramuscular - 10 mg/ml

10 ml	$9.50	Dicyclocot, C O Truxton	00463-1104-10

DIDANOSINE *(003060)*

CATEGORIES: AIDS Related Complex; Anti-Infectives; Antivirals; HIV Infection; Nucleoside Analogue Drugs; Viral Agents; Pregnancy Category B; FDA Class 1A ("Important Therapeutic Advantage"); FDA Approved 1991 Oct; Patent Expiration 1995 Sep

BRAND NAMES: DDI; Dideoxyinosine; **Videx**

FORMULARIES: Medi-Cal; PCS

COST OF THERAPY: $1,946.41 (AIDS; Tablet; 100 mg; 4/day; 365 days) vs. Potential Cost of $20,715.13 (HIV)

WARNING:
PANCREATITIS, WHICH HAS BEEN FATAL IN SOME CASES, IS THE MAJOR CLINICAL TOXICITY ASSOCIATED WITH DIDANOSINE THERAPY. PANCREATITIS MUST BE CONSIDERED WHENEVER A PATIENT RECEIVING DIDANOSINE DEVELOPS ABDOMINAL PAIN AND NAUSEA, VOMITING, OR ELEVATED BIOCHEMICAL MARKERS. UNDER THESE CIRCUMSTANCES, DIDANOSINE USE SHOULD BE SUSPENDED UNTIL THE DIAGNOSIS OF PANCREATITIS IS EXCLUDED (SEE WARNINGS.)

DESCRIPTION:

Didanosine, [formerly called dideoxyinosine (ddI)], is a synthetic purine nucleoside analogue active against the Human Immunodeficiency Virus (HIV). Videx Chewable/Dispersible Buffered Tablets are available for oral administration in strengths of 25, 50, 100 or 150 mg of didanosine. Each tablet is buffered with calcium carbonate and magnesium hydroxide. Didanosine tablets also contain aspartame, sorbitol, microcrystalline cellulose, polyplasdone, mandarin orange flavor and magnesium stearate.

Videx Buffered Powder for Oral Solution is supplied for oral administration in single-dose packets containing 100, 167 mg didanosine packets. Packets of each product strength also contain a citrate-phosphate buffer (composed of dibasic sodium phosphate, sodium citrate, and citric acid) and sucrose.

Videx Pediatric Powder for Oral Solution is supplied for oral administration in 4- or 8-ounce glass bottles containing 2 or 4 grams of didanosine, respectively.

The chemical name for didanosine is 2',3'-dideoxyinosine.

Didanosine is a white crystalline powder with the molecular formula $C_{10}H_{12}N_4O_3$ and a molecular weight of 236.2. The aqueous solubility of didanosine at 25°C and pH of approximately 6 is 27.3 mg/ml. Didanosine is unstable in acidic solutions. For example, at pH < 3 and 37°C, 10 percent of didanosine decomposes to hypoxanthine in less than 2 minutes.

CLINICAL PHARMACOLOGY:

MECHANISM OF ACTION

Didanosine is a synthetic nucleoside analogue of the naturally occurring nucleoside deoxyadenosine in which the 3'-hydroxyl(OH) group is replaced by hydrogen. Intracellularly, didanosine is converted by cellular enzymes to the active metabolite, dideoxyadenosine 5'-triphosphate (ddATP). Dideoxyadenosine 5'-triphosphate inhibits the activity of HIV-1 reverse transcriptase both by competing with the natural substrate, deoxyadenosine 5'-triphosphate (dATP), and by its incorporation into viral DNA. The lack of a 3'-OH group in the incorporated nucleoside analogue prevents the formation of the 5' to 3' phosphodiester linkage essential for DNA chain elongation and therefore, the viral DNA growth is terminated.

IN VITRO HIV SUSCEPTIBILITY

The *in vitro* anti-HIV-1 activity of didanosine was evaluated in a variety of HIV-1 infected lymphoblastic cell lines and monocyte/macrophage cell cultures. Didanosine has shown antiviral activity against laboratory and clinical isolates of HIV-1. The concentration of drug necessary to inhibit viral replication by 50 percent (IC_{50}) ranged from 2.5 to 10 μM (1μM = 0.24 μ/ml) in lymphoblastic cell lines and 0.01 to 0.1 μM in monocyte/macrophage cell cultures. The relationship between *in vitro* susceptibility of HIV to didanosine and the inhibition of HIV replication in humans has not been established.

DRUG RESISTANCE

HIV-1 isolates with reduced sensitivity to didanosine have been selected *in vitro* and were also obtained from patients treated with didanosine. Genetic analysis of these isolates showed a predominant mutation at Leu 74 (Leu 74 Val) and another mutation at Met 184 (Met 184 Val) in the Pol gene that encodes for the reverse transcriptase.

CROSS-RESISTANCE

The potential for cross-resistance between reverse transcriptase inhibitors and protease inhibitors is low because of the different enzyme targets involved. Mutations in the reverse transcriptase gene at both codons 74 and 184 are associated with cross-resistance to zalcitabine. Lamivudine-resistant isolates containing only the Met 184 Val mutation have been recovered and these isolates showed a 4- to 8-fold decrease in didanosine sensitivity. HIV-1 isolates with multidrug resistance mutations to zidovudine, didanosine, zalcitabine, stavudine and lamivudine have been reported (2/39 patients) following combination therapy with zidovudine and didanosine for 2 years. Multidrug resistance was dependent on five mutations (Ala 62 Val, Val 75 Ile, Phe 77 Leu, Phe 116 Tyr and Gin 151 Met) in the reverse transcriptase gene. Of these, the mutation at codon position 151 (Q151M) played a significant role in the development of viable virus with a multidrug resistance phenotype.

CLINICAL PHARMACOLOGY: *(cont'd)*

ANIMAL TOXICOLOGY

Evidence of a dose-limiting skeletal muscle toxicity has been observed in mice and rats (but not in dogs) following long-term (greater than 90 days) dosing with didanosine at doses that were approximately 1.2 to 12 times the estimated human exposure. The relationship of this finding to the potential of didanosine to cause myopathy in humans is unclear. However, human myopathy has been associated with administration of other nucleoside analogs.

PHARMACOKINETICS

Didanosine pharmacokinetics were evaluated in 69 patients with AIDS or AIDS-Related Complex. Patients received a 60 minute IV infusion of didanosine once or twice a day for 2 weeks; total daily doses ranged from 0.8 mg/kg to 33 mg/kg. Oral doses equivalent to twice the IV doses were administered for an additional 4 weeks. oral doses were administered as a lyophilized formulation similar in composition to didanosine pediatric powder for oral solution.

Absorption: Although there was significant variability between patients, C_{max} and AUC increased in proportion to dose over the range of doses administered in clinical practice. The absolute bioavailability of didanosine was 33 ± 14% at doses of 7 mg/kg or less. Because didanosine degrades rapidly at acidic pH, didanosine chewable/dispersible tablets and didanosine buffered powder for oral solution contain buffering agents. Didanosine pediatric powder for oral solution must be administered with antacids (see DOSAGE AND ADMINISTRATION.)

Administration of nonmarketed chewable/dispersible buffered didanosine tablets 30 minutes or 1 hour before a meal did not result in any significant changes in bioavailability, compared to administration under fasting conditions (n=10, asymptomatic HIV positive patients). When the tablets were administered 1 or 2 hours after a meal, C_{max} and AUC were decreased by approximately 55% which was comparable to the decreases observed when the formulation was administered immediately after a meal see DOSAGE AND ADMINISTRATION.

Distribution: The steady state volume of distribution following IV administration was 0.81 ± 0.22 L/kg. *In vitro*, didanosine is less than 5 percent bound to human plasma proteins. The concentration of didanosine in cerebrospinal fluid samples (n=5) collected 1 hour after IV infusion averaged 21 percent of the simultaneous plasma concentration.

Elimination: Following IV administration, total clearance was approximately 11.8 ± 3.1 ml/min/kg. Following oral administration, elimination half-life was 1.5 ± 0.6 hours. There was no evidence of accumulation of didanosine after either IV or oral dosing; steady state pharmacokinetic parameters did not differ significantly from values obtained after single dose.

Metabolism: The metabolism of didanosine has not been evaluated in humans. When ^{14}C-radiolabeled didanosine was administered to dogs as a single IV or oral dose, extensive metabolism occurred. The major metabolite identified in the urine, allantoin, represented approximately 61 percent of the administered radiolabel after oral administration. Three putative metabolites tentatively identified in the urine were hypoxanthine, xanthine, and uric acid. A similar metabolic profile was observed in rat plasma after oral administration of ^{14}C-radiolabled didanosine to male and female rats. The metabolic fate of the dideoxyribose moiety, released subsequent to enzymatic or chemical hydrolysis of the glycosidic bond, has not been determined. Based upon data from animal studies, it is presumed that the metabolism of didanosine in humans will occur by the same pathways responsible for the elimination of endogenous purines.

The intracellular half-life of ddATP, the metabolite presumed to be responsible for the antiretroviral activity of didanosine, is reported to be 8 to 24 hours *in vitro*. The half-life of intracellular ddATP *in vivo* has not been measured.

Excretion: Renal clearance was approximately 6.4 ± 2.4 ml/min/kg following either IV or oral administration. Active tubular secretion in addition to glomerular filtration is responsible for the renal elimination of didanosine. Urinary recovery of didanosine after a single dose was 55 ± 17 percent and 20 ± 8 percent of the dose following IV and oral administration, respectively.

SPECIAL POPULATIONS

Renal Impairment: Didanosine pharmacokinetics were compared between HIV positive patients with normal renal function (n=6) and patients with severe renal impairment. Patients with severe renal impairment had creatinine clearances less than 10 ml/min/1.73 m^2 and were maintained on CAPD (n=5) or hemodialysis (n=6). Total body clearance following IV administration was 3.3 ± 0.8 ml/min/kg in patients with severe renal impairment and 13.0 ± 1.6 ml/min/kg in patients with normal renal function. The mean elimination half-life following oral administration of didanosine increased from approximately 1.5 hours in patients with normal renal function to approximately 4 hours in patients with severe renal impairment. The absolute bioavailability of didanosine was not affected in patients with renal impairment. Following oral administration, didanosine was not detectable in peritoneal dialysate fluid; recovery in hemodialysate ranged from 0.6 to 7.4% of the dose over a 3-4 hour dialysis period. Approximately 35% of the didanosine present in the body at the start of dialysis was eliminated during the hemodialysis session (see DOSAGE AND ADMINISTRATION.) The effect of mild to moderate renal impairment on didanosine pharmacokinetics has not been studied.

Hepatic Impairment: The effect of hepatic impairment on didanosine pharmacokinetics has not been studied.

Pediatric Patients: For pharmacokinetic properties of didanosine in pediatric patients, see PRECAUTIONS, Pediatric Use.

CLINICAL STUDIES:

CONTROLLED CLINICAL TRIAL ACTG 175

ACTG 175 was a randomized, double-blind, controlled trial that compared ZDV 200 mg three times a day; Didanosine 200 mg twice daily; ZDV + didanosine; and ZDV + ddC 0.75 mg three times a day. A total of 2467 HIV-infected adults with baseline CD4 counts of 200-500 cells/mm^3 (mean=352) and no prior AIDS- defining event enrolled with the following demographics: male (82%), Caucasian (70%), mean age of 35 years, asymptomatic HIV infection (81%) and prior antiretroviral use (57%, mean duration = 89.5 weeks). The overall mean duration of study treatment was 99 weeks.

Results: The incidence of AIDS-defining events or death is shown in TABLE 1.

CONTROLLED CLINICAL TRIAL ACTG 116A

ACTG 116A was a randomized, double-blind, controlled trial that compared high and recommended doses of didanosine to zidovudine in patients who had received up to 16 weeks of zidovudine therapy. 617 HIV-infected adults enrolled with the following demographics: male (92%), Caucasian (73%), mean age of 36 years, median CD4 cell count of 130 cell/mm^3, symptomatic HIV infection (67%) or AIDS (26%) and median duration of prior antiretroviral use of 8 weeks. The median duration of study treatment was 60 weeks.

Results: In the three treatment groups, the time until development of a first new AIDS-defining event or death was similar. Patients randomized to zidovudine had longer survival times than patients randomized to didanosine recommended dose with mortality rates of 26% and 21% for didanosine recommended dose and zidovudine, respectively.

CLINICAL STUDIES: *(cont'd)*

TABLE 1 First AIDS-Defining Event or Death and Death Only by Study Arm and Antiretoviral Experience

Antiretoviral Experience	Event	Treatment ZDV	Didanosine	ZDV + Didanosine	ZDV + ddC
Overall	n	619	620	613	615
	AIDS/Death	96 (16%)	71 (11%)	65 (11%)	76 (12%)
	Death Only	54 (9%)	29 (5%)	31 (5%)	40 (7%)
Naive	n	269	268	263	267
	AIDS/Death	32 (12%)	23 (9%)	20 (8%)	16 (6%)
	Death Only	18 (7%)	11 (4%)	11 (4%)	9 (3%)
Experienced	n	350	352	350	348
	AIDS/Death	64 (18%)	48 (14%)	45 (13%)	60 (17%)
	Death Only	36 (10%)	18 (5%)	20 (6%)	31 (9%)

CONTROLLED CLINICAL TRIAL ACTG 116B/117

ACTG 116B/117 was a randomized, double-blind, controlled clinical trial that compared high and recommended doses of didanosine to zidovudine in patients who had tolerated four months or greater of prior zidovudine therapy. 913 HIV-infected adults enrolled with the following demographics: male (96%), Caucasian (82%), mean age of 37 years, median CD4 cell count of 95 cells/mm^3, symptomatic HIV infection (60%), or AIDS (30%) and median duration of prior antiretroviral use of 59.4 weeks. The median duration of study treatment was 49.7 weeks.

Results: Subjects randomized to the currently recommended dose of didanosine had a lower rate of progression to a new AIDS-defining event or death compared to those randomized to ZDV (32% vs. 41%, respectively). Survival rates were similar for the two treatment groups.

INDICATIONS AND USAGE:

Didanosine is indicated for the treatment of HIV infection when antiviral therapy is warranted.

This indication is based on the results of four randomized, double-blind controlled clinical trials (see CLINICAL STUDIES) and PRECAUTIONS, Pediatric Use.

The duration of clinical benefit from antiretroviral therapy may be limited. Alteration in antiretroviral therapy should be considered if disease progression occurs while receiving didanosine.

CONTRAINDICATIONS:

Didanosine is contraindicated in patients with previously demonstrated clinically significant hypersensitivity to any of the components of the formulations.

WARNINGS:

Pancreatitis: PANCREATITIS, WHICH HAS BEEN FATAL IN SOME CASES, IS THE MAJOR CLINICAL TOXICITY ASSOCIATED WITH DIDANOSINE THERAPY.PANCREATITIS MUST BE CONSIDERED WHENEVER A PATIENT RECEIVING DIDANOSINE DEVELOPS ABDOMINAL PAIN AND NAUSEA, VOMITING, OR ELEVATED AMYLAPSE OR LIPASE AND DIDANOSINE USE SHOULD BE SUSPENDED UNTIL THE DIAGNOSIS OF PANCREATITIS IS EXCLUDED.

1. When treatment with other drugs known to cause pancreatic toxicity is required (for example, IV pentamidine), suspension of didanosine is recommended.

In patients with risk factors for pancreatitis, such as a history of pancreatitis, alcohol consumption, or elevated triglycerides, didanosine should be used with extreme caution and only if clearly indicated. Patients with advanced HIV infection are at increased risk of pancreatitis and should be followed closely. Patients with renal impairment may be at greater risk for pancreatitis if treated without dose adjustment.

The incidence of pancreatitis rises with increasing doses of didanosine. The incidences of pancreatitis, and the relationship to didanosine dose and zidovudine, for the ACTG 175, 116B/117, and 116A trials are described in TABLE 2.

In phase I studies, the frequency of pancreatitis was dose related and occurred 8/91 (9%) of patients who received <12.5 mg/kg/day and in 21/79 (27%) of patients who received >12.5 mg/kg/day/

In pediatric studies, pancreatitis occurred in 2 of 60 (3%) patients treated at entry doses below 300 mg/m^2/day and in 5 of 38 (13%) patients treated at higher doses. In pediatric doses with symptoms similar to those described above, didanisone use should be suspended until the diagnosis of pancreatitis is excluded.

2. Liver Failure: Hepatitis, which in some instances was fulminant or associated with lactic acidosis, has been reported post-marketing.

3. Retinal Depigmentation and Vision: Retinal changes and optic neuritis have been reported in several pediatric patients who received didanisone at and above the recommended dose. Retinal depigmentation and optic neuritis have been reported in several adult patients. Children receiving didanisone should undergo dilated retinal examination every 6 months or if a change in vision occurs.

Periodic retinal examinations should be considered for adult patients receiving didanosine (see ADVERSE REACTIONS.)

TABLE 2 Percentage of Patients with Pancreatitis (ACTG 175, 116B/117, and 116A Trial Data)

	High Dose Didanosine		Recommended Didanosine Dose			Zidovudine		
	116A	116B/117	175	116A	116B/117	175	116A	116B/117
N	207	311	620	196	298	619	208	304
Pancreatitis	18(9%)*	31(10%)*	7(1%)	14(7%)	17(6%)	1(<1%)	7(3%)	6(2%)

* Two fatalities occurred in this group.

PRECAUTIONS:

GENERAL

Patients receiving didanosine or any other antiretroviral therapy may continue to develop opportunistic infections and other complications of HIV infection and therefore should remain under close clinical observation by physicians experienced in the treatment of patients with associated HIV diseases.

PRECAUTIONS: *(cont'd)*

To avoid a reduction in the bioavailability of didanosine, the drug should be administered at least 30 minutes before a meal.

Patients with Phenylketonuria: Videx Chewable/Dispersible Buffered Tablets contain certain quantities of phenylalanine as indicated in TABLE 3.

TABLE 3

	All Strengths
Phenylalanine per 2-tablet dose	73 mg
Phenylalanine per tablet	36.5 mg

Patients on Sodium-Restricted Diets: Each single-dose packet of Videx contains 1380 mg sodium.

Patients With Renal Impairment: Patients with renal impairment (serum creatinine >1.5 mg/dl or creatinine clearance <60 ml/min) may be at greater risk of toxicity from didanosine due to decreased drug clearance. The clearance of didanosine is reduced in patients with severe renal insufficiency (Clcr 10 ml/min/1.73m^2) (see CLINICAL PHARMACOLOGY.) A dose reduction is recommended in these patients (see DOSAGE AND ADMINISTRATION.) The magnesium content of each buffered tablet of didanosine is 8.6 mEq. This may present an excessive load of magnesium to patients with significant renal impairment, particularly after prolonged dosing.

Patients With Hepatic Impairment: Patients with hepatic impairment may be at greater risk for toxicity related to didanosine treatment due to altered metabolism; a dose reduction may be necessary.

Hyperuricemia: Didanosine has been associated with asymptomatic hyperuricemia; treatment suspension may be necessary if clinical measures aimed at reducing uric acids levels fail.

Diarrhea: Didanosine buffered powder for oral solution was associated with diarrhea in 34 percent of patients in the phase 1 adult studies (See ADVERSE REACTIONS.) If diarrhea develops in a patient receiving didanosine Buffered Powder for Oral Solution, a trial of didanosine Chewable/Dispersible Buffered tablets should be considered.

INFORMATION FOR THE PATIENT

Didanosine is not a cure for HIV infection, and patients may continue to acquire HIV-associated illnesses, including opportunistic infection. Therefore, patients should remain under care of a physician when using didanosine. Patients should be advised that didanosine therapy has not been shown to reduce the risk of transmission of HIV to others through sexual contact or blood contamination.

Patients should be informed that the major toxicity of didanosine is pancreatitis, which has been fatal in some patients. Patients should also be aware that peripheral neuropathy may develop. Patients should be counseled that these toxicities occur with greatest frequency in patients with a history of these events, and that dose modification and/or discontinuation of didanosine may be required if toxicity develops. They should be cautioned about the use of other medications that may exacerbate the didanosine toxicity, including alcohol.

CARCINOGENESIS AND MUTAGENESIS

Lifetime carcinogenicity studies were conducted in mice and rats for 22 and 24 months, respectively. In the mouse study, initial doses of 120, 800, and 1200 mg/kg/day for each sex, were lowered after 8 months to 120, 210, and 210 mg/kg/day for females and 120, 300, and 600 mg/kg/day for males. The two higher doses exceeded the maximally tolerated dose in females and the high dose exceeded in the maximally tolerated dose in males. The low dose in females represented a 0.68-fold maximum human exposure and the intermediate dose in males represented 1.7-fold maximum human exposure. In the rat study, initial doses were 100, 250, and 1000 mg/kg/day, and the high dose was lowered to 500 mg/kg/day after 18 months. The upper dose in male and female rats represented 3-fold maximum human exposure.

Didanosine induced no significant increase in neoplastic lesions in mice or rats at maximally tolerated doses.

No evidence of mutagenicity (with or without metabolic activation) was observed in Ames *Salmonella* mutagenicity assays or in mutagenicity assay conducted with *Escherichia coli* tester strain WP2 uvrA where only a slight increase in revertants was observed with didanosine. In a mammalian cell gene mutation assay conducted in L5178Y/TK+/- mouse lymphoma cells, didanosine was weakly positive both in the absence and presence of metabolic activation at concentrations of approximately 2000 mcg/ml and above. In an *in vitro* cytogenic study performed in cultured human peripheral lymphocytes, high concentrations of didanosine (≥ 500 mcg/ml) elevated the frequency of cells bearing chromosome aberrations. Another *in vitro* mammalian cell chromosome aberration study using Chinese Hamster Lung cells revealed that didanosine produces chromosome aberrations at ≥500 mcg/ml after 48 hours of exposure. However, no significant elevations in the frequency of cells with chromosome aberrations were seen at didanosine concentrations up to 250 mcg/ml. In a BALB/c 3T3 *in vitro* transformation assay, didanosine was considered positive only at concentrations of 3000 mcg/ml and above. no evidence of genotoxicity was observed in rat and mouse micronucleus assays.

The results from the genotoxicity studies suggest that didanosine is not mutagenic at biologically and pharmacologically relevant doses. At significantly elevated doses *in vitro*, the genotoxic effects of didanosine are similar in magnitude to those seen with natural DNA nucleosides.

PREGNANCY, REPRODUCTION AND FERTILITY, PREGNANCY CATEGORY B

Reproduction studies have been performed in rats and rabbits at doses up to 12 and 14.2 times the estimated human exposure (based upon plasma levels), respectively, and have revealed no evidence of impaired fertility or harm to the fetus due to didanosine. At approximately 12 times the estimated human exposure, didanosine was slightly toxic to female rats and their pups during mid and late lactation. These rats showed reduced food intake and body weight gains but the physical and functional development of the offspring was not impaired and there were no major changes in the F2 generation. A study in rats showed that didanosine and/or its metabolites are transferred to the fetus through the placenta. There are no adequate and well-controlled studies in pregnant women. Because animal reproduction studies are not always predictive of human response, this drug should be used during pregnancy only if clearly needed.

NURSING MOTHERS

A study in rats showed that, following oral administration, didanosine and/or its metabolites were excreted into the milk of lactating rats. Although it is not known if didanosine is excreted in human milk, there is the potential for adverse effects from didanosine in nursing infants. Mothers should be instructed to discontinue nursing if they are receiving didanosine. This instruction is consistent with the Centers for Disease Control recommendation that HIV-infected mothers not breast feed their infants to avoid risking potential transmission of HIV infection.

PEDIATRIC USE

Results From Controlled Clinical Trial ACTG 152: ACTG 152 was a randomized, double-blind, controlled trial that compared ZDV 180 mg/m^2 every 6 hours; Didanosine 120 mg/m^2 every 12 hours; and ZDV (120 mg/m^{2}every 6 hours) + didanosine (90 mg/m^2 every 12 hours).

PRECAUTIONS: *(cont'd)*

A total of 831 HIV-infected pediatric patients were enrolled with the following demographics: male (50%), racial minority groups (86%), mean age of 3.8 years (54% were <30 months of age), perinatally acquired infection (90%), naive to antiretroviral treatment (89%). The overall median duration of study treatment was 20 months.

Results: The incidence of clinical progression or death is shown in TABLE 4.

TABLE 4 Clinical Progression or Death and Death Only by Study Arm

Event	ZDV N = 276	Treatment Didanosine N = 281	Didanosine + ZDV N = 274
Disease Progression† or Death	74(27%)	54(19%)	48(18%)
Death Only	31(11%)	20(7%)	23(8%)

† Disease progression was defined as any of the following: weight growth failure, brain growth failure, ≥2 opportunisitic infections or malignancy.

Pharmacokinetic Properties in Pediatric Patients: The pharmacokinetics of didanosine have been evaluated in two pediatric studies. In the first study, 20 patients received a single IV dose ranging from 40 to 90 mg/m^2, and multiple, twice-daily oral doses of 80 to 180 mg/m^2 didanosine. In the second study, 47 patients received a single IV dose, followed by multiple, three-times-daily oral doses ranging from 20 to 180 mg/m^2. The average (+SD) age of the patients enrolled in both studies was 7.5 (+4.9) years, and ranged from 0.7 to 18.9 years. Fourteen patients were older than 12 years of age. In both studies, a lyophilized formulation similar in composition to didanosine pediatric powder for oral solution was administered orally. The C_{max} and AUC values, increased in proportion to dose after IV and oral administration, although a significant variability among patients was noted. Using data from both studies, the average (+SD) elimination half-life after an oral dose was 0.8 (+0.3) hours. Absolute bioavailability averaged 25 (+20) percent after a single dose. Urinary recovery and renal clearance values, obtained only in the first study, averaged 18 (+10) percent and 240 (+90) ml/min/m^2, respectively, after a single oral dose. There was no evidence of accumulation of didanosine after the administration of oral doses for an average of 26 days. The volume of distribution after IV administration averaged 28 (+15) L/m^2. The average total body clearance following a single IV dose was 516 (+184) ml/min/m^2. Total body clearance was independent of age, and was similar to the value obtained in adult patients (446 + 116 ml/min/m^2) administered at doses ranging from 15 to 839 mg/m^2. In cerebrospinal fluid samples collected from 7 patients, at times ranging from 1.5 to 3.5 hr after a single IV or PO dose, the concentration of didanosine (range: 0.04 to 0.12 mcg/ml) corresponded to 12 to 85 percent (average: 46 percent) of the concentration in a simultaneous plasma sample.

DRUG INTERACTIONS:

Coadministration of didanosine with drugs that are known to cause pancreatitis may increase the risk of this toxicity (see WARNINGS) and should be done with extreme caution and only if clearly indicated.Neuropathy has occurred more frequently in patients with a history of neuropathy or neurotoxic drug therapy and these patients may be at increased risk of neuropathy during didanosine therapy (see ADVERSE REACTIONS.)

Drug interaction studies have demonstrated that there are no clinically significant interactions with didanosine and the following: ketoconazole, ranitidine, loperamide, metaclopramide, and rifabutin. Drugs whose absorption can be affected by the level of acidity in the stomach (*e.g.*, ketoconazole, dapsone), should be administered at least 2 hours prior to dosing with didanosine. A study in 4 patients revealed that concomitant administration of ganciclovir does not significantly affect the pharmacokinetics of didanosine. There is no evidence that didanosine potentiates the myelosuppressive effects of ganciclovir or zidovudine.

As with other products containing or mixed with magnesium and/or aluminum antacid components, didanosine chewable/dispersible buffered tablets or didanosine pediatric powder for oral solution should not be administered with a prescription antibiotic containing any form of tetracycline.

Plasma concentrations of some quinolone antibiotics are decreased when administered with antacids containing magnesium or aluminum. Therefore, doses of quinolone antibiotics should not be administered within 2 hours of taking didanosine chewable/dispersible buffered tablets or pediatric powder for oral solution. Concomitant administration of antacids containing magnesium or aluminum with didanosine chewable/dispersible buffered tablets or pediatric powder for oral solution may potentiate adverse effects associated with the antacid components.

ADVERSE REACTIONS:

THE MAJOR TOXICITY OF DIDANOSINE IS PANCREATITIS. OTHER IMPORTANT TOXICITIES INCLUDE LIVER FAILURE AND RETINAL CHANGES (SEE WARNINGS.)

Adults: Clinical adverse events which occurred in at least 5 percent of adult patients in the ACTG 116B/117 or 116A clinical trials are provided in TABLE 5. The types of adverse events reported to occur in the ACTG 175 trial in didanosine-treated patients were generally similar to those events reported in other controlled clinical trials, although the incidence of adverse events was generally lower in all treatment groups in this population with less advanced HIV disease. Adverse events reported to occur in patients treated with didanosine + ZDV combination therapy in the ACTG 175 clinical trials were generally similar to those reported in patients treated with either individual drug.

TABLE 5 Clinical Adverse Events: Cumulative Incidence ≥5% at Didanosine Recommended Dose (ACTG 116B/117 and 116A)

	Percent of Patients			
	Recommended Didanosine Dose		Zidovudine	
Adverse Events	116A N = 197	116B/117 N = 298	116A N = 212	116B/117 N = 304
Diarrhea	19	28	15	21
Neuropathy (all grades)	17	20	14	12
Chills/Fever	9	12	12	11
Rash/Pruritus	7	9	8	5
Abdominal Pain	13	7	8	8
Asthenia	4	7	8	9
Headache	6	7	12	7
Pain	6	7	6	3
Nausea and Vomiting	7	7	14	6
Pancreatitis	7	6	3	2

The cumulative incidences of serious laboratory abnormalities in clinical trials ACTG 116B/117 and 116A are listed in TABLE 6. The types of serious laboratory abnormalities reported in the ACTG 175 trial in didanosine treated patients were generally similar to those reported in other controlled clinical trials. Serious laboratory abnormalities reported in patients treated with didanosine + ZDV combination therapy in the ACTG 175 clinical trial were generally similar to those reported in patients treated with either individual drug.

TABLE 6A ACTG 116B/117 and 116A Clinical Trials: Incidences of Serious Laboratory Abnormalities

	Percent of Patients			
	Recommended Didanosine Dose		Zidovudine	
Lab Tests (Seriously Abnormal Level)	116A N = 197	116B/117 N = 298	116A N = 212	116B/117 N = 304
Hemoglobin (<8.0 g/dl)	6	3	8	5
Leukopenia (<2000/ml)	13	16	26	22
Granulocytopenia (<750/ml)	6	8	19	15

TABLE 6B ACTG 116B/117 and 116A Clinical Trials: Incidences of Serious Laboratory Abnormalities

	Percent of Patients			
	Recommended Videx Dose		Zidovudine	
Lab Tests (Seriously Abnormal Level)	116A N = 197	116B/117 N = 298	116A N = 212	116B/117 N = 304
Thrombocytopenia (<50,000/ml)	2	2	4	3
SGOT (AST)(>5× ULN)	9	7	4	6
SGPT (ALT)(>5× ULN)	9	6	6	6
Alkaline phosphatase (>5× ULN)	4	1	1	1
Bilirubin (>2.6 × ULN)	1	1	1	1
Amylase (≥1.4 × ULN)	17	15	12	5
Uric Acid (>12 mg/dl)	3	2	1	1

Peripheral neuropathy occurs in patients treated with didanosine and the frequency appears to be dose related. In phase 1 studies, neuropathy occurred in 31/91 (34%) patients who received <12.5 mg/kg/day and in 40/79 (51%) patients who received >12.5 mg/kg/day. See TABLE 5 for incidence in controlled trials.

Patients should be monitored for the development of a neuropathy that is usually characterized by numbness, tingling or pain in the feet or hands. Neuropathy has occurred more frequently in patients with a history of neuropathy or neurotoxic drug therapy and these patients may be at increased risk of neuropathy during didanosine therapy.

Other adverse events that have been reported in controlled clinical trials and have been received as part of ongoing surveillance include:

Body as a Whole: anaphylactoid reaction

Digestive Disorders: anorexia, dyspepsia, and flatulence

Exocrine Gland Disorders: sialoadenitis, parotid gland enlargement, dry mouth, and dry eyes

Metabolic Disorders: hypoglycemia and hyperglycemia

Musculoskeletal Disorders: arthralgia and myopathy

Rare cases of rhabdomyolysis associated with didanosine use have been reported. A few of these cases were complicated by acute renal failure, which required hemodialysis.

Retinal depigmentation and optic neuritis have been reported in several adult patients.

Reports of hepatitis, diabetes mellitus, myalgia (with or without increases in creatine phosphokinase), and alopecia have been received post-marketing.

Pediatric Patients: Adverse events reported to occur in the pediatric patients in the ACTG 152 Trial were generally similar to those reported in adults.

In pediatric phase 1 studies, pancreatitis occurred in 2 of 60 (3 percent) patients treated at entry doses below 300 mg/m^2/day and in 5 of 38 (13 percent) patients treated at higher doses.

Retinal changes and optic neuritis have been reported in several pediatric patients who received didanosine at and above the recommended dose.

Serious laboratory abnormalities experienced by the pediatric patients in the ACTG 152 clinical trial are listed in TABLE 7.

TABLE 7 Pediatric Patient Serious Laboratory Abnormalities in ACTG 152 (Cumulative Incidences)

	Percent of Patients		
Lab Tests (Seriously Abnormal Level)	Didanosine N = 281	Didanosine + ZDV N = 274	ZDV N = 276
Hemoglobin (<7.5 g/dl)	5	7	10
Leukopenia (<2000/ml)	<1	<1	1
Granulocytopenia (<500/ml)	11	16	27
Thrombocytopenia (<50,000/ml)	6	7	7
SGOT (AST)(≥5× ULN)	14	10	16
SGPT (ALT)(≥10 × ULN)	5	2	7
Alkaline phosphatase (≥2 × ULN)	7	9	10
Bilirubin (≥2.6 × ULN)	6	3	4
Amylase (≥3.1 × ULN)	5	6	7
Creatine Kinase (≥5.1 × ULN)	6	8	8
Uric Acid (≥3.5 mg/dl)	<1	<1	<1

OVERDOSAGE:

There is no known antidote for didanosine overdosage. In phase 1 studies, in which didanosine was initially administered at doses ten times the currently recommended dose, toxicities included: pancreatitis, peripheral neuropathy, diarrhea, hyperuricemia and hepatic dysfunction. Didanosine is not dialyzable by peritoneal dialysis, although there is some clearance by hemodialysis (see CLINICAL PHARMACOLOGY, Pharmacokinetics.)

DOSAGE AND ADMINISTRATION:

DOSAGE

Adults: The dosing interval should be 12 hours. **All didanosine formulations should be administered at least 30 minutes before a meal. Adult patients should take 2 tablets at each dose so that adequate buffering is provided to prevent gastric acid degradation of didanosine.** The recommended starting dose in adults is dependent on weight as outlined in TABLE 8.

Pediatric Patients: The recommended dosing interval is 12 hours. **All didanosine formulations should be administered at least 30 minutes before a meal.** The recommended dose of didanosine monotherapy in pediatric patients is 120 mg/m^{2}twice daily.

DOSAGE AND ADMINISTRATION: *(cont'd)*

TABLE 8 Adult Dosing

Patient Weight	Didanosine Tablets	Didanosine Buffered Powder
≥ 60 kg	200 mg twice daily	250 mg twice daily
< 60 kg	125 mg twice daily	167 mg twice daily

DOSE ADJUSTMENT

Clinical signs suggestive of pancreatitis should prompt dose suspension and careful evaluation of the possibility of pancreatitis. Only after pancreatitis has been ruled out should dosing be resumed.

Patients who have presented symptoms of neuropathy may tolerate a reduced dose of didanosine after resolution of these symptoms upon drug discontinuation.

Although there are insufficient data to recommend dose adjustment of didanosine in patients with mild or moderate renal impairment, a dose reduction should be considered. In anuric patients requiring dialysis, it is recommended that one fourth of the total daily dose of didanosine be administered once a day (see CLINICAL PHARMACOLOGY.) There are insufficient data to recommend a specific dose adjustment of didanosine in patients with hepatic impairment, but an adjustment in the dose in these patients should also be considered.

METHOD OF PREPARATION

Didanosine Chewable/Dispersible Buffered Tablets

Adult Dosing: Two tablets should be thoroughly chewed, manually crushed, or dispersed in at least 1 ounce of water prior to consumption. To disperse tablets, add 2 tablets to at least 1 ounce of drinking water. Stir until a uniform dispersion forms, and drink the entire dispersion immediately. If additional flavoring is desired, the dispersion may be diluted with one ounce of clear apple juice. Stir the further diluted dispersion just prior to consumption. The dispersion with clear apple juice is stable at room temperature, 62-73°F (17-23°C), for up to one hour.

Didanosine Buffered Powder for Oral Solution

1. Open packet carefully and pour contents into a container with approximately 4 ounces of drinking water. Do not mix with fruit juice or other acid-containing liquid.
2. Stir until the powder completely dissolves (approximately 2 to 3 minutes).
3. Drink the entire solution immediately.

Didanosine Pediatric Powder for Oral Solution

Prior to dispensing, the pharmacist must constitute dry powder with Purified Water, USP, to an initial concentration of 20 mg/ml and immediately mix the resulting solution with antacid to a final concentration of 10 mg/ml as follows:

20 mg/ml Initial Solution: Constitute the product to 20 mg/ml by adding 100 ml or 200 ml of Purified Water, USP to the 2 g or 4 g of didanosine powder, respectively, in the product bottle.

10 mg/ml Final Admixture: 1. Immediately mix one part of the 20 mg/ml initial solution with one part of either Mylanta Double Strength Liquid (Mylanta is a registered trademark of Stuart Pharmaceuticals, Division of ICI Americas, Inc. Mylanta Double Strength, formerly Mylanta II, is distributed by Johnson & Johnson/Merck, Consumer Pharmaceuticals Company, Fort Washington, PA 19034 [USA]), Extra Strength Maalox Plus Suspension, or Maalox TC Suspension (Maalox is a registered trademark of William H. Rorer Inc., Unit of Rhone-Poulenc Rorer) for a final dispensing concentration of 10 mg didanosine per ml. For patient home use, the admixture should be dispensed in appropriately sized, flint-glass bottles with child-resistant closures. This admixture is stable for 30 days under refrigeration, 36° to 46°F (2° to 8°C).

2. Instruct the patient to shake the admixture thoroughly prior to use and to store the tightly closed container in the refrigerator 36° to 46°F (2° to 8°C), up to 30 days.

PATIENT INFORMATION:

Didanosine is used for the treatment of HIV infection. It is not a cure.

Inform your physician if you are pregnant or nursing or if you have kidney or liver disease.

Pancreatitis, in some cases fatal, has been associated with didanosine therapy.

See your physician if you have abdominal pain, or nausea and vomiting.

The powder for solution contains 1380 mg of sodium. If you are on a low sodium diet, consult your physician.

Diarrhea has been associated with the powder for oral solution form of this product.

Patients with phenylketonuria: The tablet form of this product contains phenylalanine.

Take medication at least 30 minutes before meals. Follow mixing and dosing dorections carefully.

HOW SUPPLIED:

Videx (Didanosine) Chewable/Dispersible Buffered Tablets are round, white to light orange/yellow with mottled appearance; orange-flavored, tablets embossed with "VIDEX" on one side and the product strength on the other.

The tablets should be stored in tightly closed bottles at 59° to 86°F (15° to 30°C). If dispersed in water, the dose may be stored at ambient temperature.

Videx (Didanosine) Buffered Powder for Oral Solution is supplied in single-dose, child-resistant foil packets. Each product strength provides a sweetened, buffered solution of didanosine.

The packets should be stored at 59° to 86°F (15° to 30°C). After dissolving in water, the solution may be stored at ambient room temperature for up to 4 hours.

Videx (Didanosine) Pediatric Powder for Oral Solution is supplied in 4- and 8- ounce glass bottles containing 2 g or 4 g of didanosine, respectively.

The bottles of powder should be stored at 59° to 86°F (15° to 30°C). The didanosine admixture may be stored up to 30 days in a refrigerator, 36° to 46°F (2° to 8°C). Discard any unused portion after 30 days.

HANDLING AND DISPOSAL

Spill, Leak and Disposal Procedure: Avoid generating dust during clean-up of powdered products; use wet mop or damp sponge. Clean surface with soap and water as necessary. Containerize larger spills.

There is no single preferred method of disposal of containerized waste. Disposal options include incineration, landfill or sewer as dictated by specific circumstances and relevant national, state and local regulations.

HOW SUPPLIED - EQUIVALENTS NOT AVAILABLE:

Packet - Oral - 167 mg

30's $74.33 VIDEX, Bristol Myers Squibb 00087-6615-43

Packet - Oral - 250 mg

30's $111.26 VIDEX, Bristol Myers Squibb 00087-6616-43

HOW SUPPLIED - EQUIVALENTS NOT AVAILABLE: *(cont'd)*

Powder, Buffered - Oral - 100 mg

30's $44.51 VIDEX, Bristol Myers Squibb 00087-6614-43

Solution - Oral - 20 mg/ml

100 ml $29.66 VIDEX, Bristol Myers Squibb 00087-6632-41

200 ml $59.32 VIDEX, Bristol Myers Squibb 00087-6633-41

Tablet, Buffered Chewable - Oral - 25 mg

60's $22.39 VIDEX, Bristol Myers Squibb 00087-6650-01

Tablet, Buffered Chewable - Oral - 50 mg

60's $41.59 VIDEX, Bristol Myers Squibb 00087-6651-01

Tablet, Buffered Chewable - Oral - 100 mg

60's $79.99 VIDEX, Bristol Myers Squibb 00087-6652-01

Tablet, Buffered Chewable - Oral - 150 mg

60's $197.51 VIDEX, Bristol Myers Squibb 00087-6653-01

Tablet, Chewable - Oral - 25 mg

60's $22.25 VIDEX, Bristol Myers Squibb 00087-6628-43

Tablet, Chewable - Oral - 50 mg

60's $44.51 VIDEX, Bristol Myers Squibb 00087-6624-43

Tablet, Chewable - Oral - 100 mg

60's $89.01 VIDEX, Bristol Myers Squibb 00087-6627-43

Tablet, Chewable - Oral - 150 mg

60's $133.51 VIDEX, Bristol Myers Squibb 00087-6626-43

DIENESTROL *(001050)*

CATEGORIES: Hormones; Kraurosis Vulvae; Skin/Mucous Membrane Agents; Vaginal Preparations; Vaginitis; Pregnancy Category X; FDA Approval Pre 1982

BRAND NAMES: *Cycladiene* (France); *Dienoestrol* (Australia); Dv; Estraguard; *Hormofemin* (England); *Ortho Dienestrol* (Canada); Ortho-Dienestrol; *Ortho Dienoestrol*; *Ortho-Dienoestrol*
(International brand names outside U.S. in italics)

FORMULARIES: Medi-Cal

WARNING:

ESTROGENS HAVE BEEN REPORTED TO INCREASE THE RISK OF ENDOMETRIAL CARCINOMA.

Three independent case control studies have shown an increased risk of endometrial cancer in postmenopausal women exposed to exogenous estrogens for prolonged periods. This risk was independent of the other known risk factors for endometrial cancer. These studies are further supported by the finding that incidence rates of endometrial cancer have increased sharply since 1969 in eight different areas of the United States with population-based cancer reporting systems, an increase which may be related to the rapidly expanding use of estrogens during the last decade.

The three case control studies reported that the risk of endometrial cancer in estrogen users was about 4.5 to 13.9 times greater than in nonusers. The risk appears to depend on both duration of treatment and on estrogen dose. In view of these findings, when estrogens are used for the treatment of menopausal symptoms, the lowest dose that will control symptoms should be utilized and medication should be discontinued as soon as possible. When prolonged treatment is medically indicated, the patient should be reassessed on at least a semiannual basis to determine the need for continued therapy. Although the evidence must be considered preliminary, one study suggests that cyclic administration of low doses of estrogen may carry less risk than continuous administration; it therefore appears prudent to utilize such a regimen.

Close clinical surveillance of all women taking estrogens is important. In all cases of undiagnosed persistent or recurring abnormal vaginal bleeding, adequate diagnostic measures should be undertaken to rule out malignancy. There is no evidence at present that "natural" estrogens are more or less hazardous than "synthetic" estrogens at equiestrogenic doses.

ESTROGENS SHOULD NOT BE USED DURING PREGNANCY.

The use of female sex hormones, both estrogens and progestogens, during early pregnancy may seriously damage the offspring. It has been shown that females exposed in utero to diethylstilbestrol, a non-steroidal estrogen, have an increased risk of developing in later life a form of vaginal or cervical cancer that ordinarily is extremely rare. This risk has been estimated as not greater than 4 per 1000 exposures. Furthermore, a high percentage of such exposed women (from 30 to 90 percent) have been found to have vaginal adenosis, epithelial changes of the vagina and cervix. Although these changes are histologically benign, it is not known whether they are precursors of malignancy. Although similar data are not available with the use of other estrogens, it cannot be presumed they would not induce similar changes. Several reports suggest an association between intrauterine exposure to female sex hormones and congenital anomalies, including congenital heart defects and limb reduction defects. One case control study estimated a 4.7 fold increased risk of limb reduction defects in infants exposed in utero to sex hormones (oral contraceptives, hormone withdrawal tests for pregnancy, or attempted treatment for threatened abortion). Some of these exposures were very short and involved only a few days of treatment. The data suggest that the risk of limb reduction defects in expose fetuses is somewhat less than 1 per 1000.

In the past, female sex hormones have been used during pregnancy in an attempt to treat threatened or habitual abortion. There is considerable evidence that estrogens are ineffective for these indications, and there is no evidence from well controlled studies that progestogens are effective for these uses.

If Dienestrol Cream is used during pregnancy, or if the patient becomes pregnant while using this drug, she should be apprised of the potential risks to the fetus, and the advisability of pregnancy continuation.

DESCRIPTION:

Cream for intravaginal use only.

Active Ingredient: Dienestrol 0.01%.

Dienestrol is a synthetic, non-steroidal estrogen. It is compounded in a cream base suitable for intravaginal use only. The cream base is composed of glyceryl monostearate, peanut oil, glycerin, benzoic acid, glutamic acid, butylated hydroxyanisole, citric acid, sodium hydroxide and water. The pH is approximately 4.3.

4-4'-(Diethylideneethylene) diphenol

CLINICAL PHARMACOLOGY:

Systemic absorption and mode of action of dienestrol are undetermined.

INDICATIONS AND USAGE:

Dienestrol Cream is indicated in the treatment of atrophic vaginitis and kraurosis vulvae.

DIENESTROL CREAM HAS NOT BEEN SHOWN TO BE EFFECTIVE FOR ANY PURPOSE DURING PREGNANCY AND ITS USE MAY CAUSE SEVERE HARM TO THE FETUS (SEE BOXED WARNING)

CONTRAINDICATIONS:

Estrogens may cause fetal harm when administered to a pregnant woman (see BOXED WARNING.) Estrogens are contraindicated in women who are or may become pregnant. If this drug is used during pregnancy, or if the patient becomes pregnant while using this drug, the patient should be apprised of the potential hazard to the fetus.

Estrogens should also not be used in women with any of the following conditions:

1. Known or suspected cancer of the breast.

2. Known or suspected estrogen-dependent neoplasia.

3. Undiagnosed abnormal genital bleeding.

4. Active thrombophlebitis or thromboembolic disorders.

5. A past history of thrombophlebitis, thrombosis, or thromboembolic disorders associated with previous estrogen use.

WARNINGS:

Induction of malignant neoplasms: Long-term continuous administration of natural and synthetic estrogens in certain animal species increases the frequency of carcinomas of the breast, cervix, vagina, and liver. There is now evidence that estrogens increase the risk of carcinoma of the endometrium in humans. (See BOXED WARNING.)

Gall Bladder Disease: A recent study has reported a 2- to 3-fold increase in the risk of surgically confirmed gall bladder disease in women receiving postmenopausal estrogens, similar to the 2-fold increase previously noted in users of oral contraceptives. In the case of oral contraceptives increased risk appeared after two years of use.

Effects Similar To Those Caused By Estrogen-Progestogen Oral Contraceptives: There are several serious adverse effects of oral contraceptives, most of which have not, up to now, been documented as consequences of postmenopausal estrogen therapy. This may reflect the comparatively low doses of estrogen used in postmenopausal women. It would be expected that the larger doses of estrogen used to treat prostatic or breast cancer or postpartum breast engorgement are more likely to result in these adverse effects, and, in fact, it has been shown that there is an increased risk of thrombosis in men receiving estrogens for prostatic cancer and women for postpartum breast engorgement.

Thromboembolic Disease: It is now well established that users of oral contraceptives have an increased risk of various thromboembolic and thrombotic vascular diseases, such as thrombophlebitis, pulmonary embolism, stroke, and myocardial infarction. Cases of retinal thrombosis, mesenteric thrombosis, and optic neuritis have been reported in oral contraceptive users. There is evidence that the risk of several of these adverse reactions is related to the dose of the drug. An increased risk of postsurgery thromboembolic complications has also been reported in users of oral contraceptives. If feasible, estrogen should be discontinued at least 4 weeks before surgery of the type associated with an increased risk of thromboembolism, or during periods of prolonged immobilization.

While an increased rate of thromboembolic and thrombotic disease in postmenopausal users of estrogens has not been found, this does not rule out the possibility that such an increase may be present or that subgroups of women who have underlying risk factor or who are receiving large doses of estrogens may have increased risk. Therefore estrogens should not be used in persons with active thrombophlebitis or thromboembolic disorders, and they should not be used (except in treatment of malignancy) in persons with a history or such disorders in association with estrogen use. They should be used with caution in patients with cerebral vascular or coronary artery disease and only for those in whom estrogens are clearly needed.

Large doses of estrogen (5 mg conjugated estrogens per day), comparable to those used to treat cancer of the prostate and breast, have been shown in a large prospective clinical trial in men to increase the risk of nonfatal myocardial infarction, pulmonary embolism and thrombophlebitis. When estrogen doses of this size are used, any of the thromboembolic and thrombotic adverse effects associated with oral contraceptive use should be considered a clear risk.

Hepatic Adenoma: Benign hepatic adenomas appear to be associated with the use of oral contraceptives. Although benign, and rare, these may rupture and may cause death trough intra-abdominal hemorrhage. Such lesions have not yet been reported in association with other estrogen or progestogen preparations but should be considered in estrogen users having abdominal pain and tenderness, abdominal mass, or hypovolemic shock. Hepatocellular carcinoma has also been reported in women taking estrogen-containing oral contraceptives. The relationship of this malignancy to these drugs is not known at this time.

Elevated Blood Pressure: Increased blood pressure is not uncommon in women using oral contraceptives. There is now a report that this may also occur with the use of estrogens during menopause. Blood pressure should be monitored with estrogen use, especially if high doses are used.

Glucose Tolerance: A worsening of glucose tolerance has been observed in a significant percentage of patient on estrogen-containing oral contraceptives. For this reason, diabetic patients should be carefully observed while receiving estrogen.

Hypercalcemia: Administration of estrogens may lead to severe hypercalcemia in patients with breast cancer and bone metastases. If this occurs, the drug should be stopped and appropriate measures taken to reduce the serum calcium level.

PRECAUTIONS:

General: A complete medical and family history should be taken prior to the initiation of any estrogen therapy. The pretreatment and periodic physical examinations should include special reference to blood pressure, breasts, abdomen, and pelvic organs, and should include a Papanicolaou smear. As a general rule, estrogen should not be prescribed for longer than one year without another physical examination being performed.

PRECAUTIONS: *(cont'd)*

Fluid Retention: Because estrogens may cause some degree of fluid retention, conditions which might be influenced by this factor such as epilepsy, migraine, and cardiac or renal days-function, require careful observation.

Certain patients may develop undesirable manifestations of excessive estrogenic stimulation, such as abnormal or excessive uterine bleeding, mastodynia, etc.

Oral contraceptives appear to be associated with an increased incidence of mental depression. Although it is not clear whether this is due to the estrogenic or progestogenic component of the contraceptive, patients with a history of depression should be carefully observed.

Preexisting uterine leiomyomata may increase in size during estrogen use.

The pathologist should be advised of estrogen therapy when relevant specimens are submitted.

Patients with a past history of jaundice during pregnancy have an increased risk of recurrence of jaundice while receiving estrogen-containing oral contraceptive therapy. If jaundice develops in any patient receiving estrogen, the medication should be discontinued while the cause is investigated.

Estrogens may be poorly metabolized in patients with impaired liver function and they should be administered with caution in such patients.

Because estrogens influence the metabolism of calcium and phosphorus, they should be used with caution in patients with metabolic bone diseases that are associated with hypercalcemia or in patients with renal insufficiency.

Because of the effects of estrogens on epiphyseal closure, they should be used judiciously in young patients in whom bone growth is not complete.

The lowest effective dose appropriate for the specific indication should be utilized. Studies of the addition of a progestin for seven or more days of a cycle estrogen administration have reported a lowered incidence of endometrial hyperplasia, Morphological and biochemical studies of endometrium suggest that 10 to 13 days of progestin are needed to provide maximal maturation of the endometrium and to eliminate any hyperplastic changes. Whether this will provide protection from endometrial carcinoma has not been clearly established. There are possible additional risks which may be associated with the inclusion of progestin in estrogen replacement regimens. The potential risks include adverse effects on carbohydrate and lipid metabolism. The choice of progestin and dosage may be important in minimizing these adverse effects.

Information for the Patient: See text of Patient Package Information which is reproduced below.

Drug/Laboratory Test Interactions: Certain endocrine and liver function tests may be affected by estrogen-containing oral contraceptives. The following similar changes may be expected with larger doses of estrogen:

Increased sulfobromophthalein retention.

Increased prothrombin and factors VII, VIII, IX and X; decreased antithrombin 3; increased norepinephrine-induced platelet aggregability.

Increased thyroid-binding globulin (TBG) leading to increased circulating total thyroid hormone, as measured by PBI, T4 by column, or T4 by radioimmunoassay. Free T3 resin uptake is decreased, reflecting the elevated TBG; free T4 concentration is unaltered.

Impaired glucose tolerance.

Decreased pregnanediol excretion.

Reduced response to metyrapone test.

Reduced serum folate concentration.

Increased serum triglyceride and phospholipid concentration.

Carcinogenesis, Mutagenesis, and Impairment of Fertility: See WARNINGS section for information on carcinogenesis, mutagenesis and impairment of fertility.

Pregnancy Category X: *Teratogenic Effects:* See CONTRAINDICATIONS section.

Nursing Mothers: It is not known whether this drug is excreted in human milk. Because many drugs are excreted in human milk, caution should be exercised when estrogens are administered to a nursing woman.

ADVERSE REACTIONS:

(See WARNINGS regarding induction of neoplasia, adverse effects on the fetus, increased incidence of gall bladder disease, and adverse effects similar to those of oral contraceptives, including thromboembolism.) The following additional adverse reactions have been reported with estrogenic therapy, including oral contraceptives:

Genitourinary system
Increase in size of uterine fibromyomata.
Vaginal candidiasis.
Breakthrough bleeding, spotting, change in menstrual flow.
Dysmenorrhea.
Tenderness, enlargement, secretion.
Cholestatic jaundice.
Nausea, vomiting.
Erythema multiforme.
Erythema nodosum.
Hemorrhagic eruption.
Loss of scalp hair.
Steepening of corneal curvature.
Mental depression.
Headache, migraine, dizziness.
Reduced carbohydrate tolerance.
Aggravation of porphyria.
Edema.
Premenstrual-like syndrome.
Amenorrhea during and after treatment.
Change in cervical eversion and in degree of cervical secretion.
Cystitis-like syndrome. **Breasts**
Gastrointestinal
Abdominal cramps, bloating.
Skin
Hirsutism.
Chloasma or melasma which may persist when drug is discontinued.
Eyes
Intolerance to contact lenses. **CNS**
Chorea.
Miscellaneous
Changes in libido.
Increase or decrease in weight.

OVERDOSAGE:

Numerous reports of ingestion of large doses of estrogen-containing oral contraceptives by young children indicate that serious ill effects do not occur. Overdosage of estrogen may cause nausea, and withdrawal bleeding may occur in females.

DOSAGE AND ADMINISTRATION:

GIVEN CYCLICALLY FOR SHORT TERM USE ONLY

For treatment of atrophic vaginitis, or kraurosis vulvae associated with the menopause.

The lowest dose that will control symptoms should be chosen and medication should be discontinued as promptly as possible.

Attempts to discontinue or taper medication should be made at 3 to 6 month intervals.

The usual dosage range is one or two applicator-full per day for one or two weeks, then gradually reduced to one half initial dosage for a similar period. A maintenance dosage of one applicators-full, one to three times a week, may be used after restoration of the vaginal mucosa has been achieved.

DOSAGE AND ADMINISTRATION: *(cont'd)*

Treated patients with an intact uterus should be monitored closely for signs of endometrial cancer and appropriate diagnostic measures should be taken to rule out malignancy in the event of persistent or recurring abnormal vaginal bleeding.

Store at controlled room temperature.

HOW SUPPLIED - EQUIVALENTS NOT AVAILABLE:

Cream - Vaginal - 0.01 %

78 gm	$22.98	ORTHO-DIENESTROL, Ortho Pharm	00062-5450-00
78 gm	$24.48	ORTHO-DIENESTROL, W/APPLICATOR, Ortho Pharm	00062-5450-77

DIETHYLPROPION HYDROCHLORIDE *(001053)*

CATEGORIES: Amphetamines; Anorexients/CNS Stimulants; Appetite Suppressants; Central Nervous System Agents; Obesity; Psychostimulants; Respiratory/Cerebral Stimulant; Pregnancy Category B; DEA Class CIV; FDA Approval Pre 1982

BRAND NAMES: *Alipid*; *Anorex* (France); *Apisate*; *Atractil*; *Delgamer*; Depletite; Diethylpropion Hcl; *Dietil*; *Dietil Retard*; Dipro; *Dobesin*; Durad; *Linea*; M-Orexic; *Moderatan Diffucap* (France); *Neobes*; *Prefamone*; *Prefamone Chronule* (France); Radtue; *Regenon* (Germany); **Tenuate**; Tenuate Dospan; *Tenuate Retard* (Germany); Tepanil

(International brand names outside U.S. in italics)

DESCRIPTION:

Diethylpropion hydrochloride, (abbreviated here as diethylpropion HCl), is available for oral administration in immediate-release tablets containing 25 mg diethylpropion HCl and in controlled-release tablets containing 75 mg diethylpropion HCl. The inactive ingredients in each immediate-release tablet are: corn starch, lactose, magnesium stearate, pregelatinized corn starch, talc, and tartaric acid. The inactive ingredients in each controlled-release tablet are: carbomer 934P, mannitol, povidone, tartaric acid, zinc stearate. Diethylpropion HCl is a sympathomimetic agent. The chemical name for diethylpropion HCl is 1-phenyl-2-diethylamino-1-propanone HCl.

In diethylpropion HCl controlled-release tablets, diethylpropion HCl is dispersed in a hydrophilic matrix. On exposure to water, the diethylpropion HCl is released at a relatively uniform rate as a result of slow hydration of the matrix. The result is controlled release of the anorectic agent.

CLINICAL PHARMACOLOGY:

Diethylpropion HCl is a sympathomimetic amine with some pharmacologic activity similar to that of the prototype drugs of this class used in obesity, the amphetamines. Actions include some central nervous system stimulation and elevation of blood pressure. Tolerance has been demonstrated with all drugs of this class in which these phenomena have been looked for.

Drugs of this class used in obesity are commonly known as "anorectics" or "anorexigenics." It has not been established, however, that the action of such drugs in treating obesity is primarily one of appetite suppression. For example, other central nervous system actions or metabolic effects may be involved.

Adult obese subjects instructed in dietary management and treated with "anorectic" drugs lose more weight on the average than those treated with placebo and diet, as determined in relatively short-term clinical trials.

The magnitude of increased weight loss of drug-treated patients over placebo-treated patients averages some fraction of a pound a week. However, individual weight loss may vary substantially from patient to patient. The rate of weight loss is greatest in the first weeks of therapy for both drug and placebo subjects and tends to decrease in succeeding weeks. The possible origins of the increased weight loss due to the various drug effects are not established. The amount of weight loss associated with the use of an "anorectic" drug varies from trial to trial, and the increased weight loss appears to be related in part to variables other than the drug prescribed, such as the physician/investigator relationship, the population treated, and the diet prescribed. Studies do not permit conclusions as to the relative importance of the drug and non-drug factors on weight loss.

The natural history of obesity is measured in years, whereas most studies cited are restricted to a few weeks duration; thus, the total impact of drug-induced weight loss over that of diet alone is unknown.

Diethylpropion is rapidly absorbed from the GI tract after oral administration and is extensively metabolized through a complex pathway of biotransformation involving N-dealkylation and reduction. Many of these metabolites are biologically active and may participate in the therapeutic action of diethylpropion HCl or diethylpropion HCl controlled-release. Due to the varying lipid solubilities of these metabolites, their circulating levels are affected by urinary pH. Diethylpropion and/or its active metabolites are believed to cross the blood-brain barrier and the placenta.

Diethylpropion and its metabolites are excreted mainly by the kidney. It has been reported that between 75-106% of the dose is recovered in the urine within 48 hours after dosing. Using a phosphorescence assay that is specific for basic compounds containing a benzoyl group, the plasma half-life of the aminoketone metabolites is estimated to be between 4 to 6 hours.

The controlled-release characteristics of diethylpropion HCl controlled-release have been demonstrated by studies in humans in which plasma levels of diethylpropion-related materials were measured by phosphorescence analysis. Plasma levels obtained with the 75 mg controlled-release formulation administered once daily indicated a more gradual release than the immediate-release formulation (three 25 mg tablets given in a single dose).

Diethylpropion HCl controlled-release has not been shown superior in effectiveness to the same dosage of the immediate-release formulation (one 25 mg tablet three times daily). After administration of a single dose of diethylpropion HCl controlled-release (one 75 mg controlled-release tablet) or diethylpropion HCl solution (75 mg dose) in a crossover study using normal human subjects, the amount of parent compound and its active metabolites recovered in the urine within 48 hours for the two dosage forms were not statistically different.

INDICATIONS AND USAGE:

Diethylpropion HCl and diethylpropion HCl controlled-release are indicated in the management of exogenous obesity as a short-term adjunct (a few weeks) in a regimen of weight reduction based on caloric restriction. The usefulness of agents of this class (see CLINICAL PHARMACOLOGY) should be measured against possible risk factors inherent in their use such as those described below.

CONTRAINDICATIONS:

Advanced arteriosclerosis, hyperthyroidism, known hypersensitivity or idiosyncrasy to the sympathomimetic amines, glaucoma, severe hypertension. (See PRECAUTIONS.)

CONTRAINDICATIONS: *(cont'd)*

Agitated states.

Patients with a history of drug abuse.

During or within 14 days following the administration of monoamine oxidase inhibitors, hypertensive crises may result.

WARNINGS:

If tolerance develops, the recommended dose should not be exceeded in an attempt to increase the effect; rather, the drug should be discontinued. Diethylpropion HCl or diethylpropion HCl controlled-release may impair the ability of the patient to engage in potentially hazardous activities such as operating machinery or driving a motor vehicle; the patient should therefore be cautioned accordingly.

When central nervous system active agents are used, consideration must always be given to the possibility of adverse interactions with alcohol.

PRECAUTIONS:

GENERAL

Caution is to be exercised in prescribing diethylpropion HCl or diethylpropion HCl controlled-release for patients with hypertension or with symptomatic cardiovascular disease, including arrhythmias. Diethylpropion HCl or diethylpropion HCl controlled-release should not be administered to patients with severe hypertension.

Reports suggest that diethylpropion HCl may increase convulsions in some epileptics. Therefore, epileptics receiving diethylpropion HCl or diethylpropion HCl controlled-release should be carefully monitored. Titration of dose or discontinuance of diethylpropion HCl or diethylpropion HCl controlled-release may be necessary.

The least amount feasible should be prescribed or dispensed at one time in order to minimize the possibility of overdosage.

INFORMATION FOR THE PATIENT

The patient should be cautioned about concomitant use of alcohol or other CNS-active drugs and diethylpropion HCl or diethylpropion HCl controlled-release. (See WARNINGS.) The patient should be advised to observe caution when driving or engaging in any potentially hazardous activity.

LABORATORY TESTS

None

CARCINOGENESIS, MUTAGENESIS, AND IMPAIRMENT OF FERTILITY

No long-term animal studies have been done to evaluate diethylpropion HCl for carcinogenicity. Mutagenicity studies have not been conducted. Animal reproduction studies have revealed no evidence of impairment of fertility (see Pregnancy.)

PREGNANCY

Teratogenic Effects: Pregnancy Category B: Reproduction studies have been performed in rats at doses up to 9 times the human dose and have revealed no evidence of impaired fertility or harm to the fetus due to diethylpropion HCl. There are, however, no adequate and well-controlled studies in pregnant women. Because animal reproduction studies are not always predictive of human response, this drug should be used during pregnancy only if clearly needed.

Non-Teratogenic Effects: Abuse with diethylpropion HCl during pregnancy may result in withdrawal symptoms in the human neonate.

NURSING MOTHERS

Since diethylpropion HCl and/or its metabolites have been shown to be excreted in human milk, caution should be exercised when diethylpropion HCl or diethylpropion HCl controlled-release is administered to a nursing woman.

PEDIATRIC USE

Since safety and effectiveness in children below the age of 12 have not been established, diethylpropion HCl or diethylpropion HCl controlled-release is *not* recommended for use in children under 12 years of age.

DRUG INTERACTIONS:

Antidiabetic drug requirements (*i.e.,* insulin) may be altered. Concurrent use with general anesthetics may result in arrhythmias. The pressor effects of diethylpropion and those of other drugs may be additive when the drugs are used concomitantly; conversely, diethylpropion may interfere with antihypertensive drugs (*i.e.,* guanethidine, α-methyldopa). Concurrent use of phenothiazines may antagonize the anorectic effect of diethylpropion.

ADVERSE REACTIONS:

Cardiovascular: Precordial pain, arrhythmia, ECG changes, tachycardia, elevation of blood pressure, palpitation.

Central Nervous System: In a few epileptics an increase in convulsive episodes has been reported; rarely psychotic episodes at recommended doses; dyskinesia, blurred vision, overstimulation, nervousness, restlessness, dizziness, jitteriness, insomnia, anxiety, euphoria, depression, dysphoria, tremor, mydriasis, drowsiness, malaise, headache.

Gastrointestinal: Vomiting, diarrhea, abdominal discomfort, dryness of the mouth, unpleasant taste, nausea, constipation, other gastrointestinal disturbances.

Allergic: Urticaria, rash, ecchymosis, erythema.

Endocrine: Impotence, changes in libido, gynecomastia, menstrual upset.

Hematopoietic System: Bone marrow depression, agranulocytosis, leukopenia.

Miscellaneous: A variety of miscellaneous adverse reactions has been reported by physicians. These include complaints such as dysuria, dyspnea, hair loss, muscle pain, increased sweating, and polyuria.

DRUG ABUSE AND DEPENDENCE:

Diethylpropion HCl and diethylpropion HCl controlled-release are schedule IV controlled substances. Diethylpropion HCl has some chemical and pharmacologic similarities to the amphetamines and other related stimulant drugs that have been extensively abused. There have been reports of subjects becoming psychologically dependent on diethylpropion. The possibility of abuse should be kept in mind when evaluating the desirability of including a drug as part of a weight reduction program. Abuse of amphetamines and related drugs may be associated with varying degrees of psychologic dependence and social dysfunction which, in the case of certain drugs, may be severe. There are reports of patients who have increased the dosage more times than recommended. Abrupt cessation following prolonged high dosage administration results in extreme fatigue and mental depression; changes are also noted on the sleep EEG. Manifestations of chronic intoxication with anorectic drugs include severe dermatoses, marked insomnia, irritability, hyperactivity, and personality changes. The most severe manifestation of chronic intoxication is psychosis, often clinically indistinguishable from schizophrenia.

OVERDOSAGE:

Manifestations of acute overdosage include restlessness, tremor, hyperreflexia, rapid respiration, confusion, assaultiveness, hallucinations, panic states.

Fatigue and depression usually follow the central stimulation.

Cardiovascular effects include arrhythmias, hypertension or hypotension and circulatory collapse. Gastrointestinal symptoms include nausea, vomiting, diarrhea, and abdominal cramps. Overdose of pharmacologically similar compounds has resulted in convulsions, coma and death.

The reported oral LD_{50} for mice is 600 mg/kg, for rats is 250 mg/kg and for dogs is 225 mg/kg.

Management of acute diethylpropion HCl intoxication is largely symptomatic and includes lavage and sedation with a barbiturate. Experience with hemodialysis or peritoneal dialysis is inadequate to permit recommendation in this regard. Intravenous phentolamine has been suggested on pharmacologic grounds for possible acute, severe hypertension, if this complicates diethylpropion HCl or diethylpropion HCl controlled-release overdosage.

DOSAGE AND ADMINISTRATION:

Diethylpropion HCl immediate-release: One immediate-release 25 mg tablet three times daily, one hour before meals, and in midevening if desired to overcome night hunger.

Diethylpropion HCl controlled-release: One controlled-release 75 mg tablet daily, swallowed whole, in midmorning.

Store at room temperature, below 86°F.

HOW SUPPLIED - RATED THERAPEUTICALLY EQUIVALENT:

Tablet, Uncoated - Oral - 25 mg

100's	$4.75	Diethylpropion Hcl, MD Pharm	43567-0518-07
100's	$5.37	Diethylpropion HCl, H.C.F.A. F F P	99999-1053-01
100's	$5.40	Diethylpropion Hcl, IDE-Interstate	00814-2450-14
100's	$6.35	Diethylpropion Hcl, Goldline Labs	00182-1436-01
100's	$8.50	Diethylpropion HCl, Rugby	00536-3702-01
100's	$10.80	Diethylpropion Hydrochloride, Camall	00147-0109-10
100's	$10.80	Diethylpropion HCl, Camall	00147-0237-10
100's	$11.04	Diethylpropion HCl, HL Moore Drug Exch	00839-5109-06
100's	**$38.58**	**TENUATE, Hoechst Marion Roussel**	**00068-0697-61**
500's	$26.85	Diethylpropion HCl, H.C.F.A. F F P	99999-1053-02
500's	$30.00	Diethylpropion Hcl, Camall	00147-0109-05
500's	$30.00	Diethylpropion Hcl, Camall	00147-0237-05
1000's	$19.95	Di-Pro, Calvin Scott	17224-0704-10
1000's	$19.95	Dipro, Calvin Scott	17224-0705-10
1000's	$22.44	Radtue, Macnary	55982-0002-01
1000's	$31.28	Diethylpropion Hcl, IDE-Interstate	00814-2450-30
1000's	$36.00	Diethylpropion Hcl, MD Pharm	43567-0518-12
1000's	$37.50	Diethylpropion Hcl, Rugby	00536-3702-10
1000's	$53.70	Diethylpropion HCl, H.C.F.A. F F P	99999-1053-03
1000's	$67.93	Diethylpropion Hydrochloride, Camall	00147-0109-20
1000's	$67.93	Diethylpropion HCl, Camall	00147-0237-20
1000's	$199.95	Depletite No.2, Quality Res Pharms	52765-1106-00

HOW SUPPLIED - NOT RATED EQUIVALENT:

Tablet, Uncoated, Sustained Action - Oral - 75 mg

100's	$45.88	Diethylpropion Hcl, MD Pharm	43567-0450-07
100's	$61.20	Diethylpropion Hcl, Major Pharms	00904-0618-60
100's	$63.50	Diethylpropion Hcl, Goldline Labs	00182-0870-01
100's	$79.80	Diethylpropion Hcl, United Res	00677-0436-01
100's	$79.85	Diethylpropion Hcl, Qualitest Pharms	00603-3290-21
100's	$88.50	Diethylpropion HCl, Rugby	00536-5673-01
100's	**$96.78**	**TENUATE DOSPAN, Hoechst Marion Roussel**	**00068-0698-61**
250's	$80.50	DURAD 75, Macnary	55982-0008-25
250's	$107.65	Diethylpropion Hcl, Major Pharms	00904-0618-70
250's	$112.32	Diethylpropion Hcl, MD Pharm	43567-0450-10
250's	$158.80	Diethylpropion Hcl, Goldline Labs	00182-0870-02
250's	$189.65	Diethylpropion Hcl, Qualitest Pharms	00603-3290-24
250's	**$235.20**	**TENUATE DOSPAN, Hoechst Marion Roussel**	**00068-0698-62**
1000's	$230.00	DIPRO, Calvin Scott	17224-0702-10

DIETHYLSTILBESTROL *(001054)*

CATEGORIES: Antineoplastics; Breast Carcinoma; Cancer; Estrogens; Hormones; Oncologic Drugs; Prostatic Carcinoma; Pregnancy Category X; FDA Approval Pre 1982

BRAND NAMES: *Boestrol*; *Diaethylstilboestrol*; *Diethyl Stilbestrol*; *Distilbene* (France); *Estimon*; *Oroestron*; Stilbestrol; Stilbetin; *Stilboestrol*
(International brand names outside U.S. in italics)

FORMULARIES: Aetna; BC-BS; Medi-Cal

WARNING:
USE OF ESTROGENS HAS BEEN REPORTED TO INCREASE THE RISK OF ENDOMETRIAL CARCINOMA: Three independent case-control studies have reported an increased risk of endometrial cancer in postmenopausal women exposed to exogenous estrogens for more than 1 year.[1-3] This risk was independent of other known risk factors for endometrial cancer. These studies are further supported by the finding that, since 1969, the incidence rate of endometrial cancer has increased sharply in 8 different areas of the United States which have population-based cancer reporting systems.[4]

The 3 case-control studies reported that the risk of endometrial cancer in estrogen users was about 4.5 to 13.9 times greater than in nonusers. The risk appears to depend on both the duration of treatment[1] and the dose of estrogen.[2] In view of these findings, the lowest dose that will control symptoms should be utilized when estrogens are used for the treatment of menopausal symptoms, and medication should be discontinued as soon as possible. When prolonged treatment is medically indicated, a reassessment should be made on at least a semiannual basis to determine the need for continued therapy. Although the evidence must be considered preliminary, one study suggests that cyclic administration of low doses of estrogen may carry less risk than does continuous administration[3]; it therefore appears prudent to utilize such a regimen.

Close clinical surveillance of all women taking estrogens is important. In all cases of undiagnosed persistent or recurring abnormal vaginal bleeding, adequate diagnostic measures should be undertaken to rule out malignancy.

At present, there is no evidence that "natural" estrogens are more or less hazardous than "synthetic" estrogens at equivalent estrogenic doses.

Estrogens Should Not Be Used During Pregnancy: The use of female sex hormones, both estrogens and progestogens, during early pregnancy may affect the offspring. It has been reported that females exposed in utero to diethylstilbestrol, a nonsteroidal estrogen, may have an increased risk of developing later in life a rare from of vaginal or cervical cancer.[5,6] This risk has been estimated to be 0.14 to 1.4 per 1,000 exposures.[7] Furthermore, from 30% to 90% to of such exposed women have been found to have vaginal adenosis[8-12] and epithelial changes of the vagina and cervix. Although these changes are histologically benign, it is not known whether they are precursors of malignancy. Even though similar data are not available with the use of other estrogens, it cannot be presumed that they would not induced similar changes.

Several reports suggest that there is an association between intrauterine exposure to female sex hormones and congenital anomalies, including congenital heart defects and limb-reduction defects[13-16]. One case-control study[16] estimated a 4.7-fold increased risk of limb-reduction defects in infants exposed in utero to sex hormones (oral contraceptives, hormone withdrawal tests for pregnancy, or attempted treatment for threatened abortion). Some of these exposures were very short and involved only a few days of treatment. The data suggest that the risk of limb-reduction defects in exposed fetuses is somewhat less than 1 per 1,000.

In the past, female sex hormones have been used during pregnancy in an attempt to treat threatened or habitual abortion; however, their efficacy was never conclusively proved or disproved.

If diethylstilbestrol is administered during pregnancy, or if the patient becomes pregnant while taking this drug, she should be apprised of the potential risks to the fetus and of the advisability of pregnancy continuation.

DESCRIPTION:

THIS DRUG PRODUCT SHOULD NOT BE USED AS A POSTCOITAL CONTRACEPTIVE[17]

Diethylstilbestrol is a crystalline synthetic ectogenic substance capable of producing all the pharmacologic and therapeutic responses attributed to natural estrogens. Diethylstilbestrol may be administered orally (in the form of Enseals [enteric-release tablets Lilly] and tablets). Chemically, diethylstilbestrol is α-α'-diethyl-4,4'-stilbenediol.

The Enseals contain corn starch, FD&C Blue No. 2, FD&C Red No. 3, FD&C Yellow No. 6, lactose, magnesium stearate, sucrose, talc, titanium stearate, and talc.

INDICATIONS AND USAGE:

Diethylstilbestrol is indicated in the treatment of:

1. Breast cancer (for palliation only) in appropriately selected women and men with metastatic disease.

2. Prostatic carcinoma—palliative therapy of advanced disease

DIETHYLSTILBESTROL SHOULD NOT BE USED FOR ANY PURPOSE DURING PREGNANCY. ITS USE MAY CAUSE SEVERE HARM TO THE FETUS (SEE BOXED WARNING).

CONTRAINDICATIONS:

Estrogens should not be used in women (or men) with any of the following conditions:

1. Known or suspected cancer of the breast, except in appropriately selected patients being treated for metastatic disease.

2. Known or suspected estrogen-dependent neoplasia.

3. Known or suspected pregnancy (see BOXED WARNING).

4. Undiagnosed abnormalities genital bleeding.

5. Active thrombophlebitis or thromboembolic disorders.

6. A past history of thrombophlebitis, thrombosis, or thromboembolic disorders associated with previous use of estrogen (except when used in treatment of breast or prostatic malignancy).

WARNINGS:

1. Induction of Malignant Neoplasms: In certain animal species, long-term continuous administration of natural and synthetic estrogens increases the frequency of carcinomas of the breast, cervix, vagina, kidney, and liver. There are now reports that prolonged use of estrogens increases the risk of carcinoma of the endometrium in humans. (See BOXED WARNING.) At the present time, there is no satisfactory evidence that administration of estrogens to postmenopausal women increases the risk of cancer of the breast.[18] This possibility, however, has been raised by a recent long-term follow-up of one physician's practice.[19] Because of the animal data, there is a need for caution in prescribing estrogens for women with a family history of breast cancer or for women who have breast nodules, fibrocystic disease, or abnormal mammograms.

2. Gallbladder Disease: A recent study reported a 2 to 3-fold increase in the risk of gallbladder disease occurring in women receiving postmenopausal estrogen therapy,[18] similar to the 2-fold increased risk previously noted in women using oral contraceptives.[20,25] In the case of oral contraceptives, this increased risk appeared after 2 years of use.[25]

3. Effects Similar to Those Caused by Estrogen-Progestogen Oral Contraceptives: There are several serious adverse effects associated with the use of oral contraceptives; however, most of these adverse effects have not as yet been documented as consequences of postmenopausal estrogen therapy. This may reflect the comparatively low doses of estrogen used in postmenopausal women. It would be expected that these adverse effects are more likely to occur following administration of the larger doses of estrogen used for treating prostatic or breast cancer. It has, in fact, been shown that there is an increased risk of thrombosis with the administration of estrogens for prostatic cancer in men and for postpartum breast engorgement in women.[21-24]

a. Thromboembolic Disease: It is now well established that women taking oral contraceptives run an increased risk of various thromboembolic and thrombotic vascular disease, such as thrombophlebitis, pulmonary embolism, stroke, and myocardial infarction.[25-32] Cases of retinal thrombosis, mesenteric thrombosis, and optic neuritis have been reported in users of oral contraceptives. There is evidence that the risk of several of these adverse reactions is related to the dose of the drug.[33,34] An increased risk of postsurgical thromboembolic complications has also been reported in users of oral contraceptives.[35-36] If feasible, estrogen therapy should be discontinued at least 4 weeks before surgery such as that associated with increased risk of thromboembolism, or that requiring periods of prolonged immobilization. Although an increased rate of thromboembolic and thrombotic disease has not been noted in postmenopausal users of estrogen,[18,37] this does not rule out the possibility that such an increase may be

WARNINGS: *(cont'd)*

present or that it exists in subgroups of women who have underlying risk factors or who are receiving relatively large doses of estrogens. Therefore, estrogens should not be used in persons with active thrombophlebitis or thromboembolic disorders, nor should they be used (except in treatment of malignancy) in persons with a history of such disorders associated with estrogen therapy. Estrogens should be administered cautiously to patients with cerebral vascular or coronary artery disease and only when such therapy is clearly needed. In a large prospective clinical trial in men,[38] large doses of estrogen (5 mg of conjugated estrogens per day), comparable to those used to treat cancer of the prostate and breast, have been shown to increase the risk of nonfatal myocardial infarction, pulmonary embolism, and thrombophlebitis. When such large doses of estrogen are used, any of the thromboembolic and thrombotic adverse effects associated with the use of oral contraceptives should be considered a clear risk.

b. Hepatic Adenoma: Benign hepatic adenomas appear to be associated with the use of oral contraceptives.[39-41] Although these adenomas are benign and rare, they may rupture and may cause death by intra-abdominal hemorrhage. Such lesions have not yet been reported in association with the administration of other estrogen or progestogen preparations, but they should be considered when abdominal pain and tenderness, abdominal mass, or hypovolemic shock occurs in persons receiving estrogen therapy. Hepatocellular carcinoma has also been reported in women taking estrogen-containing oral contraceptives.[40] The relationship of this malignancy to these drugs is not known at this time.

c. Elevated Blood Pressure: Increased blood pressure is not uncommon in women taking oral contraceptives. There is now one-report that this may occur with use of estrogens in the menopause,[42] and blood pressure should be monitored during estrogen therapy, especially if high doses are used.

d. Glucose Tolerance: A decrease in glucose tolerance has been observed in a significant percentage of patients on estrogen-containing oral contraceptives. For this reason, diabetic patients should be carefully observed while receiving estrogen.

4. Hypercalcemia: Administration of estrogens may lead to severe hypercalcemia in patients with breast cancer and bone metastases. If this occurs, the drug should be stopped and appropriate measures taken to reduce the serum calcium level.

PRECAUTIONS:

General

1. A complete medical and family history should be taken prior to initiation of any estrogen therapy. In the pretreatment and periodic physical examinations, special consideration should be given to blood pressure, breasts, abdomen, and pelvic organs, and a Papanicolaou smear should be performed. As a general rule, estrogen should not be prescribed for over a year without another physical examination.

2. Fluid Retention: Because estrogens may cause some degree of fluid retention, conditions which might be influenced by this factor, such as epilepsy, migraine, and cardiac or renal dysfunction, require careful observation.

3. Certain patients may develop undesirable manifestations of excessive estrogenic stimulation, such as abnormal or excessive uterine bleeding, mastodynic, etc.

4. Oral contraceptives appear to be associated with an increased incidence of mental depression.[25] Although it is not clear whether this is due to the estrogenic or progestogenic component of the contraceptive agent, patients with a history of depression should be carefully observed.

5. Preexisting uterine leiomyomata may increase in size with administration of estrogens.

6. The pathologist should be advised of estrogen therapy when relevant specimens are submitted.

7. Patients with a past history of jaundice during pregnancy run an increased risk of recurrence of jaundice while receiving estrogen-containing oral contraceptive therapy. If jaundice develops in any patient receiving estrogen, the medication should be discontinued while the cause is investigated.

8. Estrogens may be poorly metabolized in patients with impaired liver function, and they should be administered with caution in such patients.

9. Because estrogens influence the metabolism of calcium and phosphorus, they should be used with caution in patients with metabolic bone diseases associated with hypercalcemia or in patients with renal insufficiency.

10. Because of the effects of estrogens on epiphyseal closure, they should be used judiciously in young patients in whom bone growth is not complete.

11. Certain endocrine and liver function tests may be affected by estrogen-containing oral contraceptives. The following similar changes may be expected with larger doses of estrogen.

a. Increased sulfobromophthalein retention.

b. Increased prothrombin and factors VII, VIII IX, and X; decreased antithrombin 3; increased norepinephrine-induced platelet aggregability.

c. Increased thyroid binding globulin (TBG) leading to increased circulating total thyroid hormone, as measured by PBI, T4 by column, or T4 by radioimmunoassay. Free T3 resin uptake is decreased, reflecting the elevated TBG; free T4 concentration is unaltered.

d. Impaired glucose tolerance.

e. Decreased pregnanediol excretion.

f. Reduced response to metyrapone test.

g. Reduced serum folate concentration.

h. Increased serum triglyceride and phospholipid concentration.

Information for the Patient: *See* text of PATIENT PACKAGE INSERT included below.

Pregnancy Category X: See CONTRAINDICATIONSand BOXED WARNING.

Nursing Mothers: As a general principle, the administration of any drug to nursing mothers should be done only when clearly necessary since many drugs are excreted in human milk.

ADVERSE REACTIONS:

(See WARNINGS regarding induction of neoplasia, adverse effects on the fetus, increased incidence of gallbladder disease, and adverse effects similar to those of oral contraceptives including thromboembolism.) The following additional adverse reactions have been reported with estrogenic therapy, including oral contraceptives:

1. Genitourinary System: Breakthrough bleeding, spotting, change in menstrual flow; dysmenorrhea; premenstrual-like syndrome; amenorrhea during and after treatment; increase in size of uterine fibromyomata; vaginal candidiasis; change in cervical eversion and in degree of cervical secretion; cystitis-like syndrome.

2. Breasts: Tenderness, enlargement, secretion

3. Gastrointestinal: Nausea, vomiting; abdominal cramps, bloating; cholestatic jaundice

4. Skin: Chloasma or melasma, which may persist when drug is discontinued; erythema multiforme; erythema nodosum; hemorrhagic eruption; loss of scalp hair; hirsutism

5. Eyes: Steepening of corneal curvature; Intolerance to contact lenses

6. CNS: Headache, migraine, dizziness; mental depression; chorea

ADVERSE REACTIONS: *(cont'd)*

7. Miscellaneous: Increase or decrease in weight; reduced carbohydrate tolerance; aggravation of porphyria; edema; changes in libido

OVERDOSAGE:

Signs and Symptoms: Symptoms of acute overdose include anorexia, nausea, vomiting, abdominal cramps, and diarrhea. Withdrawal vaginal bleeding may follow large doses.

Chronic toxicity may include salt and water retention, edema, headache, vertigo, leg cramps, gynecomastia, chloasma, and porphyria cutanea tarda. Polydipsia, polyuria, fatigue, and an abnormal glucose tolerance may occur in some patients with preclinical diabetes mellitus.

No information is available on the following: LD_{50}, concentration of diethylstilbestrol in biologic fluids associated with toxicity and/or death, the amount of drug in a single dose usually associated with symptoms of overdosage, or the amount of diethylstilbestrol in a single dose likely to be life threatening.

Treatment: Chronic diethylstilbestrol toxicity should be treated by discontinuing all estrogenic medications and providing supportive care for any symptoms that may be present.

To obtain up-to-date information about the treatment of overdose, a good resource is your certified Regional Poison Control Center. Telephone numbers of certified poison control centers are listed in *Physicians GenRx.* In managing overdosage, consider the possibility of multiple drug overdoses, interaction among drugs, and unusual drug kinetics in your patient.

In treating acute overdose, protect the patient's airway and support ventilation and perfusion. Meticulously monitor and maintain, within acceptable limits, the patient's vital signs, blood gases, serum electrolytes, etc. Absorption of drugs from the gastrointestinal tract may be decreased by giving activated charcoal, which, in many cases, is more effective than emesis or lavage; consider charcoal instead of or in addition to gastric emptying. Repeated doses of charcoal over time may hasten elimination of some drugs that have been absorbed. Safeguard the patient's airway when employing gastric emptying or charcoal.

Forced diuresis, peritoneal dialysis, hemodialysis, or charcoal hemoperfusion have not been established as beneficial for an overdose of diethylstilbestrol.

DOSAGE AND ADMINISTRATION:

GIVEN CHRONICALLY

Inoperable progressing prostatic cancer

1 to 3 mg daily initially, increased in advanced cases; the dosage may later be reduced to an average of 1 mg daily.

Inoperable progressing breast cancer in appropriately selected men and postmenopausal women (see INDICATIONS AND USAGE).

15 mg daily.

Patients with an intact uterus should be closely monitored for signs of endometrial cancer, and appropriate diagnostic measures should be taken to rule out malignancy in the event of persistent or recurring abnormal vaginal bleeding.

REFERENCES:

1. Ziel HK, Finkle WD: Increased risk of endometrial carcinoma among users of conjugated estrogens. *N Engl J Med*1975;293:1167-1170. **2.** Smith DC, Prentic R, Thompson DJ, et al: Association of exogenous estrogen and endometrial carcinoma. *N Engl J Med*1975;293:1164-1167. **3.** Mack TM, Pike MC, Henderson BE, et al: Estrogens and endometrial cancer in a retirement community. *N Engl J Med*1976;294:1262-1267. **4.** Weiss NS, Szekely DR, Austin DF: Increasing incidence of endometrial cancer in the United States. *N Engl J Med*1976;294:1259-1262. **5.** Herbst AL, Ulfelder H, Poskanzer DC: Adenocarcinoma of vagina. *N Engl J Med* 1971;284:878-881. **6.** Greenwald P, Barlow J, Nasca P, et al: Vaginal cancer after maternal treatment with synthetic estrogens.*N Engl J Med*1971;285:390-392. **7.** Herbst AL, Cole P, Colton T, et al: Age-incidence and risk of diethylstilbestrol-related clear cell adenocarcinoma of the vagina and cervix. *Am J Obstet Gynecol* 1977;128:43. **8.** Herbst A, Kurman R, Scully R: Vaginal and cervical abnormalities after exposure to stilbestrol *in utero. Obstet Gynecol* 1972;40:287-298. **9.** Herbst A, Robboy S, Macdonald G, et al: The effects of local progesterone on stilbestrol-associated vaginal adenosis. *Am J Obstet* Gynecol 1974;118:607-615. **10.** Herbst A, Poskanzer D, Robboy S, et al: Prenatal exposure to stilbestrol, a prospective comparison of exposed female offspring with unexposed controls. *N Engl J Med*1975;292:334-339. **11.** Stafl A, Mattingly R, Foley D, et al: Clinical diagnosis of vaginal adenosis. *Obstet Gynecol*1974;43:118-128. **12.** Sherman AI, Goldrath M, Berlin A, et al: Cervical-vaginal adenosis after *in utero* exposure to synthetic estrogens. *Obstet Gynecol*1974;44:531-545. **13.** Gal I, Kirman B, Stern J: Hormonal pregnancy tests and congenital malformation.*Nature* 1967;216:83. **14.** Levy EP, Cohen A, Fraser FC: Hormone treatment during pregnancy and congenital heart defects.*Lancet* 1973;1:611. **15.** Nora J, Nora A: Birth defects and oral contraceptives. *Lancet* 1973:1941-942. **16.** Janerich DT, Piper JM, Glebatis DM: Oral contraceptives and congenital limb-reduction defects. *N Engl J Med* 1974;291:697-700. **17.** Estrogens for oral or parenteral use. *Federal Register* 1975;40-8242. **18.** Boston Collaborative Drug Surveillance Program: Surgically conformed gall bladder disease, venous thromboembolism and breast tumors in relation to post-menopausal estrogen therapy. *N Engl Med*1974;290:15-19. **19.** Hoover R, Gray LA Sr, Cole P, et al: Menopausal estrogens and breast cancer. *N Engl J Med* 1976;295:401-405. **20.** Boston Collaborative Drug Surveillance Program: Oral contraceptives venous thromboembolic disease, surgically confirmed gall bladder disease, and breast tumors.*Lancet* 1973;1:1399-1404. **21.** Daniel D, Campbell GH, Turnbull AO: Puerperal thromboembolism and suppression of lactation.*Lancet* 1967;2:287-289. **22.** The Veterans Administration Cooperative Urological Research Group: Carcinoma of the prostate: Treatment comparisons. *J Urol* 19767;98:516-522. **23.** Baller JC: Thromboembolism and oestrogen therapy. *Lancet*1967;2:560. **24.** Blackard C, Doe R, Mellinger G, et al: Incidence of cardiovascular disease and death in patients receiving diethylstilbestrol for carcinoma of the prostate. *Cancer*1970;26:249-256. **25.** Royal College of General Practitioners: Oral contraception and thromboembolic disease. *J R Coll Gen Pract*1967;13:267-279. **26.** Inman WHW, Vessey MP: Investigation of deaths from pulmonary, coronary and cerebral thrombosis and embolism in women of child-bearing age. *Br Med J* 1968;2:193-199. **27.** Vessey MP, Doll R, Investigation of relation between use of oral contraceptives and thromboembolic disease, a further report, *Br Med J* 1969;2:651-657. **28.** Sartwell PE, Masi AT, Arthes FG, et al: Thromboembolism and oral contraceptives: An epidemiological case control study. *Am J Epidemiol*1969;9:365-380. **29.** Collaborative Group for the Study of Stroke in Young Women: Oral contraception and increased risk of cerebral ischemia or thrombosis. *N Engl J Med* 1973;288:871-873. **30.** Collaborative Group for the Study of Stroke in Young Women: Oral contraceptives and stroke in young women: Associated risk factors.*JAMA* 1975;231:718-722. **31.** Mann JI, Inman WHW: Oral contraceptives and death from myocardial infarction. *Br Med J*1975;2:245-248. **32.** Mann JI, Vessey MP, Thorogood M, et al: Myocardial infarction in young women with special reference to oral contraceptive practice. *Br Med J* 1975;2:241-245. **33.** Inman WHW, Vessey MP, Westerholm B, et al: Thromboembolic disease and the steroidal content of oral content of oral contraceptives, *BrMed J* 1970;2:203-209. **34.** Stolley PD, Tonascia JA, Tockman MS, et al: Thrombosis with low-estrogen oral contraceptives.*Am J Epidemiol* 1975;102:197-208. **35.** Vessey MP, Doll R, Fairbairn AS, et al: Post-operative thromboembolism and the use of the oral contraceptives. *Br Med J*1970;3:123:126. **36.** Greene GR, Sartwell PE: Oral contraceptive use in patients with thromboembolism following surgery, trauma or infection. *Am J PublicHealth* 1972;62:680-685. **37.** Rosenberg L, Armstrong MB, Jick H: Myocardial infarction and estrogen therapy in postmenopausal women. *N Engl J Med*1976;294:1256-1259. **38.** Coronary Drug Project Research Group: The coronary drug project: Initial findings leading to modifications of its research protocol. *JAMA*1970;214:1303-1313. **39.** Baum J, Holtz F, Bookstein JJ, et al: Possible association between benign hepatomas and oral contraceptives.*Lancet*1973;2:926-928. **40.** Mays ET, Christopherson WM, Mahr MM, et al: Hepatic changes in young women ingesting contraceptive steroids, hepatic hemorrhage and primary hepatic tumors. *JAMA*1976;235:730-732. **41.** Edmondson HA, Henderson B, Benton B: Liver cell adenomas associated with the use of oral contraceptives. *N Engl J Med* 1976;294-470-472. **42.** Pfeffer RI, Van Den Noore S: Estrogen use and stroke risk in postmenopausal women. *Am J Epidemiol* 1976;103-545-546.

PATIENT PACKAGE INSERT:

FACTS THAT YOU SHOULD KNOW ABOUT ESTROGENS

Estrogens are female hormones produced by the ovaries. The ovaries produce several different kinds of estrogens. In addition, scientists have been able to develop a variety of synthetic estrogens. As far as we know, all these estrogens have similar properties and, therefore, have much the same usefulness and side effects and involve the same risks. This leaflet is intended to help you understand what estrogens are given for, the possible risks involved in their use, and how to use them as safely as possible.

This leaflet contains the most important information about estrogens. If you want to know more, you may ask your doctor or pharmacist to let you read the package insert prepared for the doctor.

Uses of Estrogen: Estrogens are prescribed by physicians for a number of purposes, and they may be given:

PATIENT PACKAGE INSERT: *(cont'd)*

1. To prevent certain uncomfortable symptoms of estrogen deficiency during a period of adjustment when a woman's ovaries no longer produce estrogen. (All women normally stop producing estrogens, generally between the ages of 45 and 55; this is called the menopause.)

2. To prevent symptoms of estrogen deficiency when a woman's ovaries have been removed surgically before the natural menopause.

3. To prevent pregnancy. (Estrogens are given along with a progestagen, another female hormone; these combinations are called oral contraceptives or birth control pills. Patient information is available to women taking oral contraceptives, and these will not be discussed in this leaflet.)

4. To treat certain cancers in women and men.

NOTE: PREGNANT WOMEN SHOULD NOT TAKE ESTROGENS.

The Use Of Estrogens During The Menopause: All women eventually experience a decrease in estrogen, production during the natural course of life. This usually occurs between the ages of 45 and 55, but it may occur earlier or later. Sometimes, the ovaries may have to be removed by an operation before the natural menopause occurs, thus producing a "surgical menopause."

When the amount of estrogen in the body begins to decrease, many women may develop some of the following typical symptoms: feeling of warmth in the face, neck and chest, or sudden intense episodes of heat and sweating through the body (called "hot flashes" or "hot flushes"). Sometimes these symptoms are quite uncomfortable. A few women may eventually develop changes in the vagina (called "atrophic vaginitis") which cause discomfort, especially during and after intercourse.

Estrogens can be prescribed to treat these symptoms of the menopause. Probably more than half of all women undergoing the menopause have only mild symptoms or none at all and thus do not need estrogens. Some women may require estrogens for only a few months while their bodies adjust to lower estrogen levels, whereas other women will need them for 6 months or longer. In an attempt to avoid overstimulation of the uterus (womb), estrogens are usually given on a cyclic basis each month, that is, 3 weeks of medication followed by 1 week with no medication.

Women sometimes experience nervous symptoms or depression during the menopause. There is no evidence that estrogens are effective for treating such symptoms, and they should not used for this purpose; however, other treatment may be needed.

You may have heard that taking estrogens for a long period of time (years) after the menopause will keep your skin soft and supple and will keep you feeling young. Unfortunately, there is no evidence that this is true, on the other hand, there may be a significant risk involved in the use of such long-term treatment.

1. The Danger Of Estrogens: *Endometrial carcinoma:*There may be an increased risk of *endometrial carcinoma*, a form of cancer of the uterus, if estrogens are used for more than a year after the menopause. The chance of this cancer occurring may be approximately 5 to 10 times greater in women taking estrogen than in those women taking no estrogens. To put this another way, a woman who does not take estrogens after the menopause has 1 chance in 1,000 each year of having cancer of the uterus, whereas a woman who takes estrogens has 5 to 10 chances in 1,000 each year. For this reason, *it is important that estrogens be taken only when needed.* It appears that the longer estrogens are taken, the greater the risk of this cancer, this risk seems to increase when larger doses are taken. For this reason, *it is important to take the lowest dose of estrogen that will control symptoms and to take it only as long as it is needed.* If estrogens are needed for longer periods of time, your doctor will want to reevaluate your need for estrogen at least every 6 months. Women using estrogens should report to their doctors any irregular vaginal bleeding; such bleeding may be of no importance, but it can also be an early warning of cancer of the uterus. If you have vaginal bleeding, you should *not* use estrogens until your doctor has made a diagnosis and has verified that there is no cancer of the uterus. If your uterus has been completely removed (total hysterectomy), there is no danger of endometrial carcinoma occurring.

2. Other Possible Cancers: When given to animals for a long period of time, estrogens have caused development of other tumors, such as tumors of the breast, cervix, vagina, or liver. At present, there is no evidence that there is an increased risk that such tumors will occur in women taking estrogens during the menopause, but there is no way to be sure that there is no risk. One study raises the possibility that the use of estrogens during the menopause may increase the risk that cancer of the breast will develop many years later. This is another reason why estrogens should be used only when clearly needed. While you are taking estrogens, it is important for you to go to your doctor at least once a year for physical examination. Your doctor may also want to make more frequent examinations of your breasts if members of your family have had breast cancer or if you have breast nodules (lumps) or abnormal mammograms (breast x-rays).

3. Gallbladder Disease: Women who use estrogens after the menopause are more likely to develop gallbladder disease than are women who do not use estrogens. Birth control pills have a similar effect.

4. Abnormal Blood Clots: Oral contraceptives increase the risk of blood clots developing in various parts of the body. In rare cases, this can result in a stroke (if the clot is in the brain), a heart attack (a clot in a blood vessel of the heart), or a pulmonary embolus (a clot which forms in the legs or pelvis and then breaks off and travels to the lungs). Any of these can be fatal.

At this time, the use of estrogens during the menopause is not known to cause such blood clots, but this has not been fully studied and could still prove to involve such a risk. If you have blood clots in the legs or lungs or had a heart attack while you were taking estrogens or birth control pills, you should not take estrogens (unless they are being prescribed by your doctor for treating cancer of the breast or prostate). If you have had a stroke or heart attack or if you have angina pectoris, estrogens should be taken with great caution and only if clearly needed (for example, if you have severe symptoms of the menopause).

Special Warning About Pregnancy: You should not take estrogens if you are pregnant, because although the possibility remains small, there may be a greater than usual risk that the developing child may be born with a birth defect. In a female child, there may be an increased risk that cancer of the vagina or cervix will develop later in life (in the teens or 20's). If estrogens have been taken during pregnancy, see your doctor.

Other Effects Of Estrogens: In addition to the serious known risks described above, estrogens have the following side effects and involve the following potential risks:

1. Nausea and Vomiting: The most common side effect of estrogen therapy is nausea. Vomiting occurs less frequently.

2. Effects on the Breasts: Estrogens may cause tenderness or enlargement of the breasts and may cause the breasts to secrete a liquid. These effects are not dangerous.

3. Effects on the Uterus: Estrogens may cause enlargement of benign fibroid tumors of the uterus. Some women will have menstrual bleeding when they stop taking estrogens; however, if bleeding occurs on days when you are still taking estrogens, you should report this to your doctor.

4. Effects on the Liver: On very rare occasions, a few women taking oral contraceptives develop a tumor of the liver which can rupture and bleed into the abdomen. So far, these tumors have not been reported in women taking estrogens during the menopause, but any

PATIENT PACKAGE INSERT: *(cont'd)*

swelling or unusual pain or tenderness in the abdomen should be reported to your doctor immediately. Women with a past history of jaundice (yellowing of the skin and the white parts of the eyes) may have jaundice again when estrogens are administered. If this occurs, stop taking the estrogen and see your doctor.

5. Other Effects: Estrogens may cause excess fluid to be retained in the body. This may worsen some conditions, such an epilepsy, migraine, heart disease, or kidney disease.

Summary

Estrogens have important uses, but there also may be risks involved in their use. Together with your doctor, you must decide whether the risks are acceptable to you in view of the benefits of estrogen therapy. Except when your doctor has prescribed estrogens for treatment of special cases of cancer of the breast or prostate, you should not use estrogens if you have cancer of the breast or uterus, if you are pregnant, if you have undiagnosed abnormal vaginal bleeding or clotting in the legs or lungs, or if you have previously had a stroke, heart attack, angina, or clotting in the legs or lungs.

You can use estrogens as safely as possible by understanding that your doctor will want you to have regular physical examinations while you are taking estrogens, and that he/she will use the smallest dose possible and will try to discontinue the drug as soon as possible. Be alert for signs of trouble, including:

Abnormal bleeding from the vagina.

Pains in the calves or chest, sudden shortness of breath, or coughing up blood (indicating possible clots in the legs, heart, or lungs).

Severe headache, faintness, dizziness, or changes in vision (indicating possible development of clots in the brain or eye).

Lumps in the breast. (You should ask your doctor to show you how you can examine your own breast.)

Jaundice (yellowing of the skin).

Mental depression.

On the basis of his or her assessment of your medical needs, your doctor has prescribed this drug for you. Do not give this drug to anyone else.

HOW SUPPLIED - EQUIVALENTS NOT AVAILABLE:

Tablet, Uncoated - Oral - 1 mg

100's	$9.14	Diethylstilbestrol, Lilly	00002-1052-02
1000's	$77.55	Diethylstilbestrol, Lilly	00002-1052-04

Tablet, Uncoated - Oral - 5 mg

100's	$24.35	Diethylstilbestrol, Lilly	00002-1054-02

DIETHYLSTILBESTROL DIPHOSPHATE

(001055)

CATEGORIES: Antineoplastics; Hormones; Oncologic Drugs; Prostatic Carcinoma; Pregnancy Category X; FDA Approval Pre 1982

BRAND NAMES: **Stilphostrol**

FORMULARIES: Medi-Cal

DESCRIPTION:

Stilphostrol (diethylstilbestrol diphosphate) is available as tablets containing 50 mg diethylstilbestrol diphosphate, colored white to off-white with grey to tan mottling. Inactive ingredients: corn starch, lactose, magnesium stearate and talc. Stilphostrol is also available for intravenous administration as a sterile solution in 5 ml ampules containing 0.25 gram diethylstilbestrol diphosphate as its sodium salt. The solution is clear, colorless to light straw-colored, with a pH of 9.0 to 10.5, and may darken with age and exposure to heat and light.

Diethylstilbestrol diphosphate is a phosphoryiated, nonsteroidal estrogen with the chemical name: Diethylstilbestrol 4,4'-Diphosphoric ester, an empirical formula of $C_{18}H_{22}O_8P_2$.

CLINICAL PHARMACOLOGY:

Putative receptor proteins for estrogens have been detected in estrogen-responsive tissues. Estrogens are first bound to a cytoplasmic receptor protein. Following modification, the estrogen-protein complex is translocated to the nucleus where ultimate binding of the estrogen containing complex occurs. As a result of such binding characteristic metabolic alterations ensue.

In the male patient with androgenic hormone dependent conditions such as metastatic carcinoma of the prostate gland, estrogens counter the androgenic influence by competing for the receptor sites. As a result of treatment with estrogens, metastatic lesions in the bone may also show improvement.

It has been demonstrated in animal studies that diethylstilbestrol diphosphate is rapidly hydrolyzed to diethylstibestrol through phosphatase activity in the blood and tissues.[1] When diethylstilbestrol diphosphate (92 mg/kg body wt.) was injected intravenously into rabbits over a period of 2 to 3 minutes, free diethylstilbestrol appeared in the blood stream as early as 5 minutes after termination of injection, and within 15 minutes had reached a concentration of 16.3 mcg/ml of plasma. This was followed by a rapid decline in concentration, only 1.2 mcg/ml remaining after 2 hours.[1] It is, therefore, expected that the high concentration of serum acid phosphate in patients with prostatic carcinoma will hydrolyse diethylstilbestrol diphosphate to free, active diethylstilbestrol.

Diethylstilbestrol is metabolized by the body in much the same manner as the endogenous hormones. Inactivation of estrogen is carried out mainly in the liver. A certain proportion of the estrogen reaching that organ is excreted into the bile, only to be reabsorbed from the intestine. During this enterohepatic circulation, degradation of estrogen occurs through conversion to less active products, through oxidation to nonestrogenic substances, and through conjugation with sulfuric and glucuronic acids. These water-soluble conjugates are strong acids and are this fully ionized in the body fluids: penetration into cells is therefore limited, and excretion by the kidney is favored because little tubular reabsorption is possible.

INDICATIONS AND USAGE:

Diethylstilbestrol diphosphate is indicated in the treatment of prostatic carcinoma-palliative therapy of advanced disease.

CONTRAINDICATIONS:

Estrogens should not be used in men with any of the following conditions:

1. Known or suspected cancer of the breast except in appropriately selected patients being treated for metastatic disease.
2. Known or suspected estrogen-dependent neoplasia.
3. Active thrombophlebitis or thromboembolic disorders.

CONTRAINDICATIONS: *(cont'd)*

DIETHYLSTILBESTROL DIPHOSPHATE IS NOT INDICATED IN THE TREATMENT OF ANY DISORDER IN WOMEN.

WARNINGS:

1. Induction of Malignant Neoplasms: Long-term continuous administration of natural and synthetic estrogens in certain animal species increases the frequency of carcinomas of the breast, cervix, vagina, and liver.

2. Gallbladder Disease: A study has reported a 2- to 3-fold increase in the risk of surgically confirmed gallbladder disease in women receiving postmenopausal estrogens,[2] similar to a 2-fold increase previously noted in users of oral contraceptives.[3,9]

3. Effects Similar to Those Caused by Estrogen-Progestogen Oral Contraceptives: There are several serious adverse effects of oral contraceptives. It has been shown that there is an increased risk of thrombosis in men receiving estrogens for prostatic cancer and women for postpartum breast engorgement.[4-7]

a. Thromboembolic Disease: It is now well established that users of oral contraceptives have an increased risk of various thromboembolic and thrombotic vascular diseases, such as thrombophlebitis, pulmonary embolism, stroke, and myocardial infarction.[8-16] Cases of retinal thrombosis, mesenteric thrombosis, and optic neuritis have been reported in oral contraceptive users. There is evidence that the risk of several of these adverse reactions is related to the dose of the drug.[17,18] An increased risk of postsurgery thromboembolic complications has also been reported in users of oral contraceptives[19,20] If feasible, estrogen should be discontinued at least 4 weeks before surgery of the type associated with an increased risk of thromboembolism or during periods of prolonged immobilization. Estrogens should not be used in persons with active thrombophlebitis or thromboembolic disorders. They should be used with caution in patients with cerebral vascular or coronary artery disease and only for those in whom estrogens are clearly indicated. Large doses of estrogen (5 mg conjugated estrogens per day), comparable to those used to treat cancer of the prostrate, have been shown in a large prospective clinical trial in men[21] to increase the risk of nonfatal myocardial infarction, pulmonary embolism and thrombophlebitis. When estrogen doses of this size are used, any of the thromboembolic and thrombotic adverse effects associated with oral contraceptive use should be considered a clear risk.

b. Hepatic Adenoma: Benign hepatic adenomas appear to be associated with the use of oral contraceptives.[22-24] Although benign, and rare, these may rupture and may cause death through intra-abdominal hemorrhage. Such lesions have not yet been reported in association with other estrogen or progestogen preparations but should be considered in estrogen users having abdominal pain and tenderness, abdominal mass, or hypovolemic shock. Hepatocellular carcinoma has also been reported in women taking estrogen containing oral contraceptives.[23] The relationship of this malignancy to these drugs is not known at this time.

c. Elevated Blood Pressure: Women using oral contraceptives sometimes experience increased blood pressure which, in most cases, returns to normal on discontinuing the drug. There is now a report that this may occur with use of estrogens in the menopause[25] and blood pressure should be monitored with estrogen use, especially if high doses are used.

d. Glucose Tolerance: A worsening of glucose tolerance has been observed in a significant percentage of patients on estrogen-containing oral contraceptives. For this reason, diabetic patients should be carefully observed while receiving estrogen.

4. Hypercalcemia: Administration of estrogens may lead to severe hypercalcemia in patients with breast cancer and bone metastases. If this occurs, the drug should be stopped and appropriate measures taken to reduce the serum calcium level.

PRECAUTIONS:

General

1. A complete medical and family history should be taken prior to the initiation of any estrogen therapy. The pretreatment and periodic physical examinations should include special reference to blood pressure, breasts, abdomen and pelvic organs. As a general rule, estrogen should not be prescribed for longer than one year without another physical examination being performed.

2. Fluid Retention: Because estrogens may cause some degree of fluid retention, conditions which might be influenced by this factor such as asthma, epilepsy, migraine, and cardiac or renal dysfunction, require careful observation.

3. Certain patients may develop undesirable manifestations of excessive estrogenic stimulation, such as gynecomastia.

4. Oral contraceptives appear to be associated with an increased incidence of mental depression. Although it is not clear whether this is due to the estrogenic or progestogenic component of the contraceptive, patients with a history of depression should be carefully observed.

5. If jaundice develops in any patient receiving estrogen, the medication should be discontinued while the cause is investigated.

6. Estrogens may be poorly metabolized in patients with impaired liver function and they should be administered with caution in such patients.

7. Because estrogens influence the metabolism of calcium and phosphorus, they should be used with caution in patients with metabolic bone diseases that are associated with hypercalcemia or in patients with renal insufficiency.

Information for Patients

1. Diethylstilbestrol diphosphate should not used by women.

2. The following side effects have been reported in patients with Stilphrostrol. If they occur they should be reported promptly to your physician.

Mood changes depression.

Nervousness, dizziness.

Loss of appetite, nausea, vomiting, abdominal cramps, bloating.

Skin rash.

Chest pain and shortness of breath.

Numbness or tingling about the nose or mouth.

Fluid accumulation.

Swelling and tenderness of breasts.

Disturbances of vision.

Frequent or uncomfortable urination.

Painful swelling of extremities.

3. The patients should consult a physician regularly for evaluation of blood pressure and heart rate.

4. Diabetic patients should monitor urines very carefully. Test of blood sugar may be necessary as well.

5. The following clinical problems are associated with the use of diethylstilbestrol diphosphate:

Hepatic cutaneous porphyria

PRECAUTIONS: *(cont'd)*

Erythema nodosum

Erythema multiforme

A significant association has been shown between the use of estrogen containing drugs and the following serious reactions:

1. Thrombophlebitis

2. Pulmonary embolism

3. Cerebral thrombosis

4. There is suggestive evidence that there may be a relationship with coronary thrombosis.

The following adverse reactions are known to have occurred in patients receiving estrogens:

Change in body weight	Loss of scalp hair
Headache	Hemorrhagic eruption
Loss of sex drive	Fatigue
Post injection flare	Backache
Aggravation of migraine headaches	

Drug/Laboratory Test Interactions

1. The pathologist should be advised of estrogen therapy when relevant specimens are submitted.

2. Certain endocrine and liver function tests may be affected by estrogen-containing oral contraceptives. The following similar changes may be expected with larger doses of estrogen.

a. Increased sulfobromophthalein retention.

b. Increased prothrombin and factors VII, VIII, IX and X; decreased antithrombin 3; increased norepinephrine-induced platelet aggregability.

c. Increased thyroid binding globulin (TBG) leading to increased circulating total thyroid hormone, as measured by PBI, T4 by column, or T4 by radioimmunoassay. Free T3 resin uptake is decreased, reflecting the elevated TBG; free T4 concentration is unaltered.

d. Impaired glucose tolerance.

e. Reduced response to metyrapone test.

f. Reduced serum folate concentration.

g. Increased serum triglyceride and phospholipid concentration.

Carcinogenesis, Mutagenesis, Impairment Of Fertility: (see WARNINGS) regarding induction of neoplasia.

Pregnancy Category X: DIETHYLSTILBESTROL DIPHOSPHATE IS NOT INDICATED IN THE TREATMENT OF ANY DISORDER IN WOMEN.

Pediatric Use: Because of the effects of estrogens on epiphyseal closure, they should be used judiciously in young patients in whom bone growth is not complete.

ADVERSE REACTIONS:

(See WARNINGS regarding induction of neoplasia, increased incidence of gallbladder disease, and adverse effects similar to those of oral contraceptives, including thromboembolism.) The following additional adverse reactions have been reported with estrogenic therapy, including oral contraceptives:

1. Breasts: Tenderness, enlargement, secretion

2. Gastrointestinal: Nausea, vomiting, abdominal cramps, bloating; cholestatic jaundice.

3. Skin: Chloasma or melasma which may persist when drug is discontinued; erythema multiforme, erythema nodosum; hemorrhagic eruption; loss of scalp hair; hirsutism.

4. Eyes: Steepening of corneal curvature; intolerance to contact lenses.

5. CNS: Headache, migraine, dizziness, mental depression, chorea.

6. Miscellaneous: Increase or decrease in weight; reduced carbohydrate tolerance; aggravation of porphyria; edema; changes in libido; transient itching and burning sensation in the perineal region.

OVERDOSAGE:

Numerous reports of ingestion of large doses of estrogen-containing oral contraceptives by young children indicate that acute serious ill effects do not occur. Overdosage of estrogen may cause nausea.

DOSAGE AND ADMINISTRATION:

Inoperable, progressing prostatic cancer.

Diethylstilbestrol Diphosphate Tablets 50 mg: Start with one tablet three times a day and increase this dose level to four or more tablets three times a day, depending on the tolerance of the patient. Maximum daily dose not to exceed one gram.

Alternatively, if relief is not obtained with high oral dosages. Diethylstilbestrol diphosphate may be administered intravenously. Diethylstilbestrol diphosphate solution must be diluted before intravenous infusion.

Diethylstilbestrol Diphosphate Ampules 0.25 gram: It is recommended that 0.5 gram (2 ampules) dissolved in approximately 250 ml of normal saline for injection USP, or 5% dextrose for injection USP, be given intravenously the first day, and that each day thereafter one gram (4 ampules) be similarly administered in approximately 250 to 500 ml of normal saline for injection USP, or 5% dextrose for injection USP.

The infusion should be administered slowly (20-30 drops per minute) during the first 10-15 minutes and then the rate of flow adjusted so that the entire amount is given in a period of about one hour. This procedure should be followed for five days or more depending on the response of the patient. Following the first intensive course of therapy. 0-25-0.5 gram (1 or 2 ampules) may be administered in a similar manner once or twice weekly or maintenance obtained with diethylstilbestrol diphosphate tablets.

Stability of Solution: After reconstitution, if storage is desired, the solution should be kept at room temperature and away from direct light. Under these conditions the solution is stable for about 5 days, so long as cloudiness or evidence of a precipitate has not occurred.

REFERENCES:

1. Johnson, W., et al: Proc. Soc. Exp. Biol. Med. 106:327-330, 1961. **2.** Boston Collaborative Drug Surveillance Program N. Eng. J. Med. 290:15-19, 1974. **3.** Boston Collaborative Surveillance Program: Lancet 1:1399-1404, 1973. **4.** Daniel, D.G. et al: Lancet 2:287-289, 1967. **5.** The Veterans Administration Cooperative Urological Research Group: J. Urol. 98:516-522, 1967. **6.** Bailar, J.C.: Lancet 2:560, 1967. **7.** Blackard, C. et al: Cancer 26: 249-256, 1970. **8.** Royal College of General Practitioners: R. Coll. Gen. Pract. 13:267-279, 1967. **9.** Royal College of General Practitioners: Oral Contraceptives and Health, New York, Pitman Corp., 1974. **10.** Inman, W.H.W., et al: Br. Med. J. 2:193-199, 1968. **11.** Vessey, M.P., et al: Br. Med. J. 2:651-657, 1969. **12.** Sartwell, P.E., et al: Am. J. Epidemiol. 90:365-380, 1969. **13.** Collaborative Group for the Study of Stroke in Young Women: N. Eng. J. Med. 288:871-878, 1973. **14.** Collaborative Group for the Study of Stroke in Young Women: J.A.M.A. 231: 718-722, 1975. **15.** Mann, J.I., et al: Br. Med. J. 2:245-248, 1975. **16.** Mann, J.I., et al: Br. Med. J. 2:241-245, 1975. **17.** Inman, W.H.W., et. al: Br. Med. J. 2:203-209, 1970. **18.** Stolley, P.D., et al: Am. J. Epidemiol. 102: 197-208, 1975. **19.** Vessey, M.P., et al: Br. Med. J. 3:123-126, 1970. **20.** Greene, G.R., et al: Am. J. Public Health 62:680-685, 1972. **21.** Coronary Drug Project Research Group: J.A.M.A. 214:1303-1313, 1970. **22.** Baum, J., et al: Lancet 2:926-928, 1973. **23.** Mays, E.T., et al: J.A.M.A. 235:730-732, 1976. **24.** Edmondson, H.A., et al: N. Eng. J. Med. 294:470-472, 1976. **25.** Pfeffer, R.I., et al: Am. J. Epidemiol. 103:445-456, 1976.

HOW SUPPLIED:

Each scored tablet, white to off-white with grey to tan mottling, contains diethylstilbestrol diphosphate 50 mg. Each tablet is identified with: Miles 132.

Each 5 ml ampule contains diethylstilbestrol diphosphate 0.25 gram as a solution of its sodium salt.

Storage: Store at controlled room temperature (59°-86°F), protect from light.

HOW SUPPLIED - EQUIVALENTS NOT AVAILABLE:

Injection, Solution - Intravenous - 250 mg/5ml

5 ml x 20	**$262.89**	**STILPHOSTROL, Bayer**	**00026-8131-20**

Tablet, Uncoated - Oral - 50 mg

50's	**$91.99**	**STILPHOSTROL, Bayer**	**00026-8132-50**

DIFLORASONE DIACETATE *(001057)*

CATEGORIES: Anti-Inflammatory Agents; Dermatitis; Dermatologicals; Dermatoses; Pruritus; Skin/Mucous Membrane Agents; Steroids; Topical; Pregnancy Category C; FDA Approval Pre 1982

BRAND NAMES: *Bexilona*; *Dermonilo*; *Dioderm*; **Florone**; Florone E; Maxiflor; *Murode*; Psorcon; *Soriflor*; *Sparcort*; *Sterodelta*
(International brand names outside U.S. in italics)

FORMULARIES: Aetna; BC-BS

DESCRIPTION:

Not For Ophthalmic Use

Each gram of florone cream and florone ointment contains 0.5 mg diflorasone diacetate in a cream or ointment base.

Chemically, diflorasone diacetate is 6α,9-difluoro-11β,17,21-trihydroxy-16β-methyl-pregna-1,4-diene-3,20-dione17,21-diacetate.

Florone Cream contains diflorasone diacetate in an emulsified and hydrophilic cream base consisting of propylene glycol, stearic acid, polysorbate 60, sorbitan monostearate and monooleate, sorbic acid, citric acid and water. The corticosteroid is formulated as a solution in the vehicle using 15 percent propylene glycol to optimize drug delivery.

Florone Ointment contains diflorasone diacetate in an emollient, occlusive base consisting of polyoxypropylene 15-stearyl ether, stearic acid, lanolin alcohol and white petrolatum.

CLINICAL PHARMACOLOGY:

Topical corticosteroids share anti-inflammatory, antipruritic and vasoconstrictive actions.

The mechanism of anti-inflammatory activity of the topical corticosteroids is unclear. Various laboratory methods, including vasoconstrictor assays, are used to compare and predict potencies and/or clinical efficacies of the topical corticosteroids. There is some evidence to suggest that a recognizable correlation exists between vasoconstrictor potency and therapeutic efficacy in man.

Pharmacokinetics: The extent of percutaneous absorption of topical corticosteroids is determined by many factors including the vehicle, the integrity of the epidermal barrier, and the use of occlusive dressings.

Topical corticosteroids can be absorbed from normal intact skin. Inflammation and/or other disease processes in the skin increase percutaneous absorption. Occlusive dressings substantially increase the percutaneous absorption of topical corticosteroids. Thus, occlusive dressings may be a valuable therapeutic adjunct for treatment of resistant dermatoses. (See DOSAGE AND ADMINISTRATION.)

Once absorbed through the skin, topical corticosteroids are handled through pharmacokinetic pathways similar to systemically administered corticosteroids. Corticosteroids are bound to plasma proteins in varying degrees. They are metabolized primarily in the liver and are then excreted by the kidneys. Some of the topical corticosteroids and their metabolites are also excreted into the bile.

INDICATIONS AND USAGE:

Topical corticosteroids are indicated for relief of the inflammatory and pruritic manifestations of corticosteroid responsive dermatoses.

CONTRAINDICATIONS:

Topical steroids are contraindicated in those patients with a history of hypersensitivity to any of the components of the preparation.

PRECAUTIONS:

General: Systemic absorption of topical corticosteroids has produced reversible hypothalamic-pituitary-adrenal (HPA) axis suppression, manifestations of Cushing's syndrome, hyperglycemia, and glucosuria in some patients.

Conditions which augment systemic absorption include the application of the more potent steroids, use over large surface areas, prolonged use, and the addition of occlusive dressings.

Therefore, patients receiving a large dose of a potent topical steroid applied to a large surface area or under an occlusive dressing should be evaluated periodically for evidence of HPA axis suppression by using the urinary free cortisol and ACTH stimulation tests. If HPA axis suppression is noted, an attempt should be made to withdraw the drug, to reduce the frequency of application, or to substitute a less potent steroid.

Recovery of HPA axis function is generally prompt and complete upon discontinuation of the drug. Infrequently, signs and symptoms of steroid withdrawal may occur, requiring supplemental systemic corticosteroids.

Children may absorb proportionally larger amounts of topical corticosteroids and thus be more susceptible to systemic toxicity. (See PRECAUTIONS, Pediatric Use.)

If irritation develops, topical corticosteroids should be discontinued and appropriate therapy instituted.

In the presence of dermatological infections, the use of an appropriate antifungal or antibacterial agent should be instituted. If a favorable response does not occur promptly, the corticosteroid should be discontinued until the infection has been adequately controlled.

Information for the Patient: Patients using topical corticosteroids should receive the following information and instructions:

1. This medication is to be used as directed by the physician. It is for external use only. Avoid contact with the eyes.

2. Patients should be advised not to use this medication for any disorder other than for which it was prescribed.

3. The treated skin area should not be bandaged or otherwise covered or wrapped as to be occlusive unless directed by the physician.

PRECAUTIONS: *(cont'd)*

4. Patients should report any signs of local adverse reactions especially under occlusive dressing.

5. Parents of pediatric patients should be advised not to use tight-fitting diapers or plastic pants on a child being treated in the diaper area, as these garments may constitute occlusive dressings.

Laboratory Tests: The following tests may be helpful in evaluating the HPA axis suppression:

Urinary free cortisol test

ACTH stimulation test

Carcinogenesis, Mutagenesis, and Impairment of Fertility: Long-term animal studies have not been performed to evaluate the carcinogenic potential or the effect on fertility of topical corticosteroids.

Studies to determine mutagenicity with prednisolone and hydrocortisone have revealed negative results.

Pregnancy Category C: Corticosteroids are generally teratogenic in laboratory animals when administered systemically at relatively low dosage levels. The more potent corticosteroids have been shown to be teratogenic after dermal application in laboratory animals. There are no adequate and well-controlled studies in pregnant women on teratogenic effects from topically applied corticosteroids. Therefore, topical corticosteroids should be used during pregnancy only if the potential benefit justifies the potential risk to the fetus. Drugs of this class should not be used extensively on pregnant patients, in large amounts, or for prolonged periods of time.

Nursing Mothers: It is not known whether topical administration of corticosteroids could result in sufficient systemic absorption to produce detectable quantities in breast milk. Systemically administered corticosteroids are secreted into breast milk in quantities **not** likely to have a deleterious effect on the infant. Nevertheless, caution should be exercised when topical corticosteroids are administered to a nursing woman.

Pediatric Use: *Pediatric patients may demonstrate greater susceptibility to topical corticosteroid-induced HPA axis suppression and Cushing's syndrome than mature patients because of a larger skin surface area to body weight ratio.*

Hypothalamic-pituitary-adrenal (HPA) axis suppression, Cushing's syndrome, and intracranial hypertension have been reported in children receiving topical corticosteroids. Manifestations of adrenal suppression in children include linear growth retardation, delayed weight gain, low plasma cortisol levels, and absence of response to ACTH stimulation. Manifestations of intracranial hypertension include bulging fontanelles, headaches, and bilateral papilledema.

Administration of topical corticosteroids to children should be limited to the least amount compatible with an effective therapeutic regimen. Chronic corticosteroid therapy may interfere with the growth and development of children.

ADVERSE REACTIONS:

The following local adverse reactions have been reported with topical corticosteroids, but may occur more frequently with the use of occlusive dressings. These reactions are listed in approximate decreasing order of occurrence:

1. Burning;
2. Itching;
3. Irritation;
4. Dryness;
5. Folliculitis;
6. Hypertrichosis;
7. Acneiform eruptions;
8. Hypopigmentation;
9. Perioral dermatitis;
10. Allergic contact dermatitis;
11. Maceration of the skin;
12. Secondary infection;
13. Skin atrophy;
14. Striae;
15. Miliaria

OVERDOSAGE:

Topically applied corticosteroids can be absorbed in sufficient amounts to produce systemic effects. (See PRECAUTIONS.)

DOSAGE AND ADMINISTRATION:

Topically corticosteroids should be applied to the affected area as a thin film from one to four times daily depending on the severity of the condition.

Occlusive dressings may be used for the management of psoriasis or recalcitrant conditions.

If an infection develops, the use of occlusive dressings should be discontinued and appropriate antimicrobial therapy initiated.

Store at controlled room temperature 15°-30°C (59°-86°F).

HOW SUPPLIED - EQUIVALENTS NOT AVAILABLE:

Cream - Topical - 0.05 %

15 gm	$17.52	MAXIFLOR, Allergan	00023-0766-15
15 gm	$22.46	PSORCON, Dermik Labs	00066-0069-17
15 gm	**$23.41**	**FLORONE E, Dermik Labs**	**00066-0072-17**
15 gm	**$23.41**	**FLORONE, Dermik Labs**	**00066-0074-17**
30 gm	$24.71	MAXIFLOR, Allergan	00023-0766-30
30 gm	$30.86	PSORCON, Dermik Labs	00066-0069-31
30 gm	**$33.42**	**FLORONE E, Dermik Labs**	**00066-0072-31**
30 gm	**$33.42**	**FLORONE, Dermik Labs**	**00066-0074-31**
60 gm	$40.11	MAXIFLOR, Allergan	00023-0766-60
60 gm	**$56.59**	**FLORONE E, Dermik Labs**	**00066-0072-60**
60 gm	**$56.59**	**FLORONE, Dermik Labs**	**00066-0074-60**
60 gm	$57.16	PSORCON, Dermik Labs	00066-0069-60

Ointment - Topical - 0.05 %

15 gm	**$23.41**	**FLORONE, Dermik Labs**	**00066-0075-17**
15 gm	$24.60	PSORCON, Dermik Labs	00066-0071-17
30 gm	$24.71	MAXIFLOR, Allergan	00023-0770-30
30 gm	**$33.42**	**FLORONE, Dermik Labs**	**00066-0075-31**

HOW SUPPLIED - EQUIVALENTS NOT AVAILABLE: *(cont'd)*

30 gm	$33.80	PSORCON, Dermik Labs	00066-0071-31
60 gm	$40.11	MAXIFLOR, Allergan	00023-0770-60
60 gm	**$56.59**	**FLORONE, Dermik Labs**	**00066-0075-60**
60 gm	$62.55	PSORCON, Dermik Labs	00066-0071-60

DIFLUNISAL *(001058)*

CATEGORIES: Analgesics; Anti-Inflammatory Agents; Antiarthritics; Antipyretics; Arthritis; Central Nervous System Agents; NSAIDS; Nonsteroidal Anti-Inflammatory; Osteoarthritis; Pain; Salicylates; Pregnancy Category C; Sales > $100 Million; FDA Approved 1982 Apr; Patent Expiration 1992 Apr

BRAND NAMES: *Adomal*; *Analeric*; *Ansal*; *Biartac*; *Diflonid*; *Diflunil*; *Diflusal*; *Difuton*; *Dolisal*; **Dolobid**; *Dolobis* (France); *Dolocid*; *Donobid*; *Dopanone*; *Dorbid*; *Dugodol*; *Flovacil*; *Flunidor*; *Fluniget* (Germany); *Fluodonil*; *Flustar*; *Ilacen*; *Noaldol*; *Reuflos*; *Unisal*
(International brand names outside U.S. in italics)

FORMULARIES: Aetna; BC-BS; Medi-Cal

COST OF THERAPY: $425.80 (Arthritis; Tablet; 500 mg; 2/day; 365 days)

PRIMARY ICD9: 715.99 (Osteoarthritis, Unspecified, Multiple Sites)

DESCRIPTION:

Diflunisal is 2',4'-difluoro-4-hydroxy-3-biphenylcarboxylic acid. Its empirical formula is $C_{13}H_8F_2O_3$.

Diflunisal has a molecular weight of 250.20. It is a stable, white, crystalline compound with a melting point of 211°- 213°C. It is practically insoluble in water at neutral or acidic pH. Because it is an organic acid, it dissolves readily in dilute alkali to give a moderately stable solution at room temperature. It is soluble in most organic solvents including ethanol, methanol, and acetone.

Diflunisal is available in 250 mg and 500 mg tablets for oral administration. Tablets Diflunisal contain the following inactive ingredients: cellulose, FD&C Yellow 6, hydroxypropyl cellulose, hydroxypropyl methylcellulose, magnesium stearate, starch, talc, and titanium dioxide.

CLINICAL PHARMACOLOGY:

Action: Diflunisal is a non-steroidal drug with analgesic, anti-inflammatory and antipyretic properties. It is a peripherally-acting non-narcotic analgesic drug. Habituation, tolerance and addiction have not been reported.

Diflunisal is a difluorophenyl derivative of salicylic acid. Chemically, diflunisal differs from aspirin (acetylsalicylic acid) in two respects. The first of these two is the presence of a difluorophenyl substituent at carbon 1. The second difference is the removal of the 0-acetyl group from the carbon 4 position. Diflunisal is not metabolized to salicylic acid, and the fluorine atoms are not displaced from the difluorophenyl ring structure.

The precise mechanism of the analgesic and anti-inflammatory actions of diflunisal is not known. Diflunisal is a prostaglandin synthetase inhibitor. In animals, prostaglandins sensitize afferent nerves and potentiate the action of bradykinin in inducing pain. Since prostaglandins are known to be among the mediators of pain and inflammation, the mode of action of diflunisal may be due to a decrease of prostaglandins in peripheral tissues.

Pharmacokinetics and Metabolism: Diflunisal is rapidly and completely absorbed following oral administration with peak plasma concentrations occurring between 2 to 3 hours. The drug is excreted in the urine as two soluble glucuronide conjugates accounting for about 90% of the administered dose. Little or no diflunisal is excreted in the feces. Diflunisal appears in human milk in concentrations of 2-7% of those in plasma. More than 99% of diflunisal in plasma is bound to proteins.

As is the case with salicylic acid, concentration-dependent pharmacokinetics prevail when Diflunisal is administered; a doubling of dosage produces a greater than doubling of drug accumulation. The effect becomes more apparent with repetitive doses. Following single doses, peak plasma concentrations of 41 ± 11 mcg/ml (mean $\pm$ S.D.) were observed following 250 mg doses, 87 ± 17 mcg/ml were observed following 500 mg and 124 ± 11 mcg/ml following single 1000 mg doses. However, following administration of 250 mg b.i.d., a mean peak level of 56 ± 14 mcg/ml was observed on day 8, while the mean peak level after 500 mg b.i.d. for 11 days was 190 ± 33 mcg/ml. In contrast to salicylic acid which has a plasma half-life of $2\frac{1}{2}$ hours, the plasma half-life of diflunisal is 3 to 4 times longer (8 to 12 hours), because of a difluorophenyl substituent at carbon 1. Because of its long half-life and nonlinear pharmacokinetics, several days are required for diflunisal plasma levels to reach steady state following multiple doses. For this reason, an initial loading dose is necessary to shorten the time to reach steady state levels, and 2 to 3 days of observation are necessary for evaluating changes in treatment regimens if a loading dose is not used.

Studies in baboons to determine passage across the blood-brain barrier have shown that only small quantities of diflunisal, under normal or acidotic conditions are transported into the cerebrospinal fluid (CSF). The ratio of blood/CSF concentrations after intravenous doses of 50 mg/kg or oral doses of 100 mg/kg of diflunisal was 100:1. In contrast, oral doses of 500 mg/kg of aspirin resulted in a blood/CSF ratio of 5:1.

Mild to Moderate Pain: Diflunisal is a peripherally-acting analgesic agent with a long duration of action. Diflunisal produces significant analgesia within 1 hour and maximum analgesia within 2 to 3 hours.

Consistent with its long half-life, clinical effects of diflunisal mirror its pharmacokinetic behavior, which is the basis for recommending a loading dose when instituting therapy. Patients treated with diflunisal, on the first dose, tend to have a slower onset of pain relief when compared with drugs achieving comparable peak effects. However, diflunisal produces longer-lasting responses than the comparative agents.

Comparative single dose clinical studies have established the analgesic efficacy of diflunisal at various dose levels relative to other analgesics. Analgesic effect measurements were derived from hourly evaluations by patients during eight and twelve-hour postdosing observation periods. The following information may serve as a guide for prescribing diflunisal.

Diflunisal 500 mg was comparable in analgesic efficacy to aspirin 650 mg, acetaminophen 600 mg or 650 mg, and acetaminophen 650 mg with propoxyphene napsylate 100 mg. Patients treated with diflunisal had longer lasting responses than the patients treated with the comparative analgesics.

Diflunisal 1000 mg was comparable in analgesic efficacy to acetaminophen 600 mg with codeine 60 mg. Patients treated with diflunisal had longer lasting responses than the patients who received acetaminophen with codeine.

A loading dose of 1000 mg provides faster onset of pain relief, shorter time to peak analgesic effect, and greater peak analgesic effect than an initial 500 mg dose.

In contrast to the comparative analgesics, a significantly greater proportion of patients treated with diflunisal did not remedicate and continued to have a good analgesic effect eight to twelve hours after dosing. Seventy-five percent (75%) of patients treated with diflunisal continued to have a good analgesic response at four hours. When patients having a good analgesic response at four hours were followed, 78% of these patients continued to have a good analgesic response at eight hours and 64% at twelve hours.

Chronic Anti-inflammatory Therapy in Osteoarthritis and Rheumatoid Arthritis: In the controlled, double-blind clinical trials in which diflunisal (500 mg to 1000 mg a day) was compared with anti-inflammatory doses of aspirin (2-4 grams a day), patients treated with diflunisal had a significantly lower incidence of tinnitus and of adverse effects involving the gastrointestinal system than patients treated with aspirin. (See also Effect on Fecal Blood Loss).

Osteoarthritis: The effectiveness of diflunisal for the treatment of osteoarthritis was studied in patients with osteoarthritis of the hip and/or knee. The activity of diflunisal was demonstrated by clinical improvement in the signs and symptoms of disease activity.

In a double-blind multicenter study of 12 weeks' duration in which dosages were adjusted according to patient response, diflunisal, 500 or 750 mg daily, was shown to be comparable in effectiveness to aspirin, 2000 or 3000 mg daily. In open-label extensions of this study to 24 or 48 weeks, diflunisal continued to show similar effectiveness and generally was well tolerated.

Rheumatoid Arthritis: In controlled clinical trials, the effectiveness of diflunisal was established for both acute exacerbations and long-term management of rheumatoid arthritis. The activity of diflunisal was demonstrated by clinical improvement in the signs and symptoms of disease activity.

In a double-blind multicenter study of 12 weeks' duration in which dosages were adjusted according to patient response, diflunisal 500 or 750 mg daily was comparable in effectiveness to aspirin 2600 or 3900 mg daily. In open-label extensions of this study to 52 weeks, diflunisal continued to be effective and was generally well tolerated.

Diflunisal 500, 750, or 1000 mg daily was compared with aspirin 2000, 3000, or 4000 mg daily in a multicenter study of 8 weeks' duration in which dosages were adjusted according to patient response. In this study, diflunisal was comparable in efficacy to aspirin.

In a double-blind multicenter study of 12 weeks' duration in which dosages were adjusted according to patient needs, diflunisal 500 or 750 mg daily and ibuprofen 1600 to 2400 mg daily were comparable in effectiveness and tolerability.

In a double-blind multicenter study of 12 weeks' duration, diflunisal 750 mg daily was comparable in efficacy to naproxen 750 mg daily. The incidence of gastrointestinal adverse effects and tinnitus was comparable for both drugs. This study was extended to 48 weeks on an open-label basis. Diflunisal continued to be effective and generally well tolerated.

In patients with rheumatoid arthritis, diflunisal and gold salts may be used in combination at their usual dosage levels. In clinical studies, diflunisal added to the regimen of gold salts usually resulted in additional symptomatic relief but did not alter the course of the underlying disease.

Antipyretic Activity: Diflunisal is not recommended for use as an antipyretic agent. In single 250 mg, 500 mg, or 750 mg doses, diflunisal produced measurable but not clinically useful decreases in temperature in patients with fever; however, the possibility that it may mask fever in some patients, particularly with chronic or high doses, should be considered.

Uricosuric Effect: In normal volunteers, an increase in the renal clearance of uric acid and a decrease in serum uric acid was observed when diflunisal was administered at 500 mg or 750 mg daily in divided doses. Patients on long-term therapy taking diflunisal at 500 mg to 1000 mg daily in divided doses showed a prompt and consistent reduction across studies in mean serum uric acid levels, which were lowered as much as 1.4 mg%. It is not known whether diflunisal interferes with the activity of other uricosuric agents.

Effect on Platelet Function: As an inhibitor of prostaglandin synthetase, diflunisal has a dose-related effect on platelet function and bleeding time. In normal volunteers, 250 mg b.i.d. for 8 days had no effect on platelet function, and 500 mg b.i.d., the usual recommended dose, had a slight effect. At 1000 mg b.i.d., which exceeds the maximum recommended dosage, however, diflunisal inhibited platelet function. In contrast to aspirin, these effects of diflunisal were reversible, because of the absence of the chemically labile and biologically reactive 0-acetyl group at the carbon 4 position. Bleeding time was not altered by a dose of 250 mg b.i.d., and was only slightly increased at 500 mg b.i.d. At 1000 mg b.i.d., a greater increase occurred, but was not statistically significantly different from the change in the placebo group.

Effect on Fecal Blood Loss: When diflunisal was given to normal volunteers at the usual recommended dose of 500 mg twice daily, fecal blood loss was not significantly different from placebo. Aspirin at 1000 mg four times daily produced the expected increase in fecal blood loss. Diflunisal at 1000 mg twice daily (*NOTE:* exceeds the recommended dosage) caused a statistically significant increase in fecal blood loss, but this increase was only one-half as large as that associated with aspirin 1300 mg twice daily.

Effect on Blood Glucose: Diflunisal did not affect fasting blood sugar in diabetic patients who were receiving tolbutamide or placebo.

INDICATIONS AND USAGE:

Diflunisal is indicated for acute or long-term use for symptomatic treatment of the following:

1. Mild to moderate pain

2. Osteoarthritis

3. Rheumatoid arthritis

CONTRAINDICATIONS:

Patients who are hypersensitive to this product.

Patients in whom acute asthmatic attacks, urticaria, or rhinitis are precipitated by aspirin or other non-steroidal anti-inflammatory drugs.

WARNINGS:

Peptic ulceration and gastrointestinal bleeding have been reported in patients receiving diflunisal. Fatalities have occurred rarely. Gastrointestinal bleeding is associated with higher morbidity and mortality in patients acutely ill with other conditions, the elderly and patients with hemorrhagic disorders. In patients with active gastrointestinal bleeding or an active peptic ulcer, the physician must weigh the benefits of therapy with diflunisal against possible hazards, institute an appropriate ulcer regimen, and carefully monitor the patient's progress. When diflunisal is given to patients with a history of either upper or lower gastrointestinal tract disease, it should be given only after consulting the ADVERSE REACTIONS section and under close supervision.

RISK OF GI ULCERATIONS, BLEEDING AND PERFORATION WITH NSAID THERAPY

Serious gastrointestinal toxicity such as bleeding, ulceration, and perforation, can occur at any time, with or without warning symptoms, in patients treated chronically with NSAID therapy. Although minor upper gastrointestinal problems, such as dyspepsia, are common, usually developing early in therapy, physicians should remain alert for ulceration and bleeding in patients treated chronically with NSAIDs even in the absence of previous GI tract symptoms. In patients observed in clinical trials of several months to two years duration,

WARNINGS: *(cont'd)*

symptomatic upper GI ulcers, gross bleeding or perforation appear to occur in approximately 1% of patients treated for 3-6 months, and in about 2-4% of patients treated for one year. Physicians should inform patients about the signs and/or symptoms of serious GI toxicity and what steps to take if they occur.

Studies to date have not identified any subset of patients not at risk of developing peptic ulceration and bleeding. Except for a prior history of serious GI events and other risk factors known to be associated with peptic ulcer disease, such as alcoholism, smoking, etc., no risk factors (*e.g.,* age, sex) have been associated with increased risk. Elderly or debilitated patients seem to tolerate ulceration or bleeding less well than other individuals and most spontaneous reports of fatal GI events are in this population. Studies to date are inconclusive concerning the relative risk of various NSAIDs in causing such reactions. High doses of any NSAID probably carry a greater risk of these reactions, although controlled clinical trials showing this do not exist in most cases. In considering the use of relatively large doses (within the recommended dosage range), sufficient benefit should be anticipated to offset the potential increased risk of GI toxicity.

PRECAUTIONS:

General: Non-steroidal anti-inflammatory drugs, including diflunisal, may mask the usual signs and symptoms of infection. Therefore, the physician must be continually on the alert for this and should use the drug with extra care in the presence of existing infection.

Although diflunisal has less effect on platelet function and bleeding time than aspirin, at higher doses it is an inhibitor of platelet function; therefore, patients who may be adversely affected should be carefully observed when diflunisal is administered (see CLINICAL PHARMACOLOGY.)

Because of reports of adverse eye findings with agents of this class, it is recommended that patients who develop eye complaints during treatment with diflunisal have ophthalmologic studies.

Peripheral edema has been observed in some patients taking diflunisal. Therefore, as with other drugs in this class, diflunisal should be used with caution in patients with compromised cardiac function, hypertension, or other conditions predisposing to fluid retention.

Acetylsalicylic acid has been associated with Reye syndrome. Because diflunisal is a derivative of salicylic acid, the possibility of its association with Reye syndrome cannot be excluded.

Hypersensitivity Syndrome: A potentially life-threatening, apparent hypersensitivity syndrome has been reported. This multisystem syndrome includes constitutional symptoms (fever, chills), and cutaneous findings (see ADVERSE REACTIONS, Dermatologic.) It may also include involvement of major organs (changes in liver function, jaundice, leukopenia, thrombocytopenia, eosinophilia, disseminated intravascular coagulation, renal impairment, including renal failure), and less specific findings (adenitis, arthralgia, myalgia, arthritis, malaise, anorexia, disorientation). If evidence of hypersensitivity occurs, therapy with diflunisal should be discontinued.

Renal Effects: As with other non-steroidal anti-inflammatory drugs, long term administration of diflunisal to animals has resulted in renal papillary necrosis and other abnormal renal pathology. In humans, there have been reports of acute interstitial nephritis with hematuria and proteinuria and occasionally nephrotic syndrome.

A second form of renal toxicity has been seen in patients with prerenal and renal conditions leading to a reduction in renal blood flow or blood volume, where the renal prostaglandins have a supportive role in the maintenance of renal perfusion. In these patients administration of an NSAID may cause a dose dependent reduction in prostaglandin formation and may precipitate overt renal decompensation. Patients at greatest risk of this reaction are those with conditions such as renal or hepatic dysfunction, diabetes mellitus, advanced age, extracellular volume depletion from any cause, congestive heart failure, septicemia, pyelonephritis, or concomitant use of any nephrotoxic drug. Diflunisal or other NSAIDs should be given with caution and renal function should be monitored in any patient who may have reduced renal reserve. Discontinuation of NSAID therapy is typically followed by recovery to the pretreatment state.

Since diflunisal is eliminated primarily by the kidneys, patients with significantly impaired renal function should be closely monitored; a lower daily dosage should be anticipated to avoid excessive drug accumulation.

Information for the Patient: Diflunisal, like other drugs of its class, is not free of side effects. The side effects of these drugs can cause discomfort and, rarely, there are more serious side effects such as gastrointestinal bleeding, which may result in hospitalization and even fatal outcomes.

NSAIDs (Non-steroidal Anti-inflammatory Drugs) are often essential agents in the management of arthritis and have a major role in the treatment of pain, but they also may be commonly employed for conditions which are less serious.

Physicians may wish to discuss with their patients the potential risks(see WARNINGS, PRECAUTIONS, and ADVERSE REACTIONS) and likely benefits of NSAID treatment, particularly when the drugs are used for less serious conditions where treatment without NSAIDs may represent an acceptable alternative to both the patient and physician.

LABORATORY TESTS

Liver Function Tests: As with other non-steroidal anti-inflammatory drugs, borderline elevations of one or more liver tests may occur in up to 15% of patients. These abnormalities may progress, may remain essentially unchanged, or may be transient with continued therapy. The SGPT (ALT) test is probably the most sensitive indicator of liver dysfunction. Meaningful (3 times the upper limit of normal) elevations of SGPT or SGOT (AST) occurred in controlled clinical trials in less than 1% of patients. A patient with symptoms and/or signs suggesting liver dysfunction, or in whom an abnormal liver test has occurred, should be evaluated for evidence of the development of more severe hepatic reactions while on therapy with diflunisal. Severe hepatic reactions, including jaundice, have been reported with diflunisal as well as with other non-steroidal anti-inflammatory drugs. Although such reactions are rare, if abnormal liver tests persist or worsen, if clinical signs and symptoms consistent with liver disease develop, or if systemic manifestations occur (*e.g.,* eosinophilia, rash, etc.), diflunisal should be discontinued, since liver reactions can be fatal.

Gastrointestinal: Because serious GI tract ulceration and bleeding can occur without warning symptoms, physicians should follow chronically treated patients for the signs and symptoms of ulceration and bleeding and should inform them of the importance of this follow-up (see WARNINGS, Risk of GI Ulcerations, Bleeding and Perforation with NSAID Therapy.)

DRUG/LABORATORY TEST INTERACTIONS

Serum Salicylate Assays: Caution should be used in interpreting the results of serum salicylate assays when diflunisal is present. Salicylate levels have been found to be falsely elevated with some assay methods.

CARCINOGENESIS, MUTAGENESIS, AND IMPAIRMENT OF FERTILITY

Diflunisal did not affect the type or incidence of neoplasia in a 105-week study in the rat given doses up to 40 mg/kg/day (equivalent to approximately 1.3 times the maximum recommended human dose), or in long-term carcinogenic studies in mice given diflunisal at doses up to 80 mg/kg/day (equivalent to approximately 2.7 times the maximum recommended human dose). It was concluded that there was no carcinogenic potential for diflunisal.

Diflunisal passes the placental barrier to a minor degree in the rat. Diflunisal had no mutagenic activity after oral administration in the dominant lethal assay, in the Ames microbial mutagen test or in the V-79 Chinese hamster lung cell assay.

No evidence of impaired fertility was found in reproduction studies in rats at doses up to 50 mg/kg/day.

Pregnancy Category C: A dose of 60 mg/kg/day of diflunisal (equivalent to two times the maximum human dose) was maternotoxic, embryotoxic, and teratogenic in rabbits. In three of six studies in rabbits, evidence of teratogenicity was observed at doses ranging from 40 to 50 mg/kg/day. Teratology studies in mice, at doses up to 45 mg/kg/day, and in rats at doses up to 100 mg/kg/day, revealed no harm to the fetus due to diflunisal. Aspirin and other salicylates have been shown to be teratogenic in a wide variety of species, including the rat and rabbit, at doses ranging from 50 to 400 mg/kg/day (approximately one to eight times the human dose). There are no adequate and well controlled studies with diflunisal in pregnant women. Diflunisal should be used during the first two trimesters of pregnancy only if the potential benefit justifies the potential risk to the fetus. Because of the known effect of drugs of this class on the human fetus (closure of the ductus arteriosus, platelet dysfunction with resultant bleeding, renal dysfunction or failure with oligohydramnios, gastrointestinal bleeding or perforation, and myocardial degenerative changes), use during the third trimester of pregnancy is not recommended.

In rats at a dose of one and one-half times the maximum human dose, there was an increase in the average length of gestation. Similar increases in the length of gestation have been observed with aspirin, indomethacin, and phenylbutazone, and may be related to inhibition of prostaglandin synthetase. Drugs of this class may cause dystocia and delayed parturition in pregnant animals.

Nursing Mothers: Diflunisal is excreted in human milk in concentrations of 2-7% of those in plasma. Because of the potential for serious adverse reactions in nursing infants from diflunisal, a decision should be made whether to discontinue nursing or to discontinue the drug, taking into account the importance of the drug to the mother.

Pediatric Use: The adverse effects observed following diflunisal administration to neonatal animals appear to be species, age, and dose-dependent. At dose levels approximately 3 times the usual human therapeutic dose, both aspirin (200 to 400 mg/kg/day) and diflunisal (80 mg/kg/day) resulted in death, leukocytosis, weight loss, and bilateral cataracts in neonatal (4 to 5-day-old) beagle puppies after 2 to 10 doses. Administration of an 80 mg/kg/day dose of diflunisal to 25-day-old puppies resulted in lower mortality, and did not produce cataracts. In newborn rats, a 400 mg/kg/day dose of aspirin resulted in increased mortality and some cataracts, whereas the effects of diflunisal administration at doses up to 140 mg/kg/day were limited to a decrease in average body weight gain.

Safety and effectiveness in infants and children have not been established, and use of the drug in children below the age of 12 years is not recommended.

DRUG INTERACTIONS:

Oral Anticoagulants: In some normal volunteers, the concomitant administration of diflunisal and warfarin, acenocoumarol, or phenprocoumon resulted in prolongation of prothrombin time. This may occur because diflunisal competitively displaces coumarins from protein binding sites. Accordingly, when diflunisal is administered with oral anticoagulants, the prothrombin time should be closely monitored during and for several days after concomitant drug administration. Adjustment of dosage of oral anticoagulants may be required.

Tolbutamide: In diabetic patients receiving diflunisal and tolbutamide, no significant effects were seen on tolbutamide plasma levels or fasting blood glucose.

Hydrochlorothiazide: In normal volunteers, concomitant administration of diflunisal and hydrochlorothiazide resulted in significantly increased plasma levels of hydrochlorothiazide. Diflunisal decreased the hyperuricemic effect of hydrochlorothiazide.

Furosemide: In normal volunteers, the concomitant administration of diflunisal and furosemide had no effect on the diuretic activity of furosemide. Diflunisal decreased the hyperuricemic effect of furosemide.

Antacids: Concomitant administration of antacids may reduce plasma levels of diflunisal. This effect is small with occasional doses of antacids, but may be clinically significant when antacids are used on a continuous schedule.

Acetaminophen: In normal volunteers, concomitant administration of diflunisal and acetaminophen resulted in an approximate 50% increase in plasma levels of acetaminophen. Acetaminophen had no effect on plasma levels of diflunisal. Since acetaminophen in high doses has been associated with hepatotoxicity, concomitant administration of diflunisal and acetaminophen should be used cautiously, with careful monitoring of patients.

Concomitant administration of diflunisal and acetaminophen in dogs, but not in rats, at approximately 2 times the recommended maximum human therapeutic dose of each (40-52 mg/kg/day of diflunisal/acetaminophen), resulted in greater gastrointestinal toxicity than when either drug was administered alone. The clinical significance of these findings has not been established.

Methotrexate: Caution should be used if diflunisal is administered concomitantly with methotrexate. Non-steroidal anti-inflammatory drugs have been reported to decrease the tubular secretion of methotrexate and to potentiate its toxicity.

Cyclosporine: Administration of non-steroidal anti-inflammatory drugs concomitantly with cyclosporine has been associated with an increase in cyclosporine-induced toxicity, possibly due to decreased synthesis of renal prostacyclin. NSAIDs should be used with caution in patients taking cyclosporine, and renal function should be carefully monitored.

NON-STEROIDAL ANTI-INFLAMMATORY DRUGS

The administration of diflunisal to normal volunteers receiving indomethacin decreased the renal clearance and significantly increased the plasma levels of indomethacin. In some patients the combined use of indomethacin and diflunisal has been associated with fatal gastrointestinal hemorrhage. Therefore, indomethacin and diflunisal should not be used concomitantly.

Since no further clinical data are available about the safety and effectiveness of diflunisal when used in combination with other non-steroidal anti-inflammatory drugs, no recommendation for their concomitant use can be made. The following information was obtained from studies in normal volunteers.

Aspirin: In normal volunteers, a small decrease in diflunisal levels was observed when multiple doses of diflunisal and aspirin were administered concomitantly.

Sulindac: The concomitant administration of diflunisal and sulindac in normal volunteers resulted in lowering of the plasma levels of the active sulindac sulfide metabolite by approximately one-third.

Naproxen: The concomitant administration of diflunisal and naproxen in normal volunteers had no effect on the plasma levels of naproxen, but significantly decreased the urinary excretion of naproxen and its glucuronide metabolite. Naproxen had no effect on plasma levels of diflunisal.

ADVERSE REACTIONS:

The adverse reactions observed in controlled clinical trials encompass observations in 2,427 patients.

Listed below are the adverse reactions reported in the 1,314 of these patients who received treatment in studies of two weeks or longer. Five hundred thirteen patients were treated for at least 24 weeks, 255 patients were treated for at least 48 weeks, and 46 patients were treated for 96 weeks. In general, the adverse reactions listed below were 2 to 14 times less frequent in the 1,113 patients who received short-term treatment for mild to moderate pain.

Incidence Greater Than 1%

Gastrointestinal: The most frequent types of adverse reactions occurring with diflunisal are gastrointestinal: these include nausea*, vomiting, dyspepsia*, gastrointestinal pain*, diarrhea*, constipation, and flatulence.

Psychiatric: Somnolence, insomnia.

Central Nervous System: Dizziness.

Special Senses: Tinnitus.

Dermatologic: Rash*.

Miscellaneous: Headache*, fatigue/tiredness.

Incidence Less Than 1 in 100: The following adverse reactions, occurring less frequently than 1 in 100, were reported in clinical trials or since the drug was marketed. The probability exists of a causal relationship between diflunisal and these adverse reactions.

Dermatologic: Erythema multiforme, exfoliative dermatitis, Stevens-Johnson syndrome, toxic epidermal necrolysis, urticaria, pruritus, sweating, dry mucous membranes, stomatitis, photosensitivity.

Gastrointestinal: Peptic ulcer, gastrointestinal bleeding, anorexia, eructation, gastrointestinal perforation, gastritis. Liver function abnormalities; jaundice, sometimes with fever; cholestasis; hepatitis.

Hematologic: Thrombocytopenia; agranulocytosis; hemolytic anemia.

Genitourinary: Dysuria; renal impairment, including renal failure; interstitial nephritis; hematuria; proteinuria.

Psychiatric: Nervousness, depression, hallucinations, confusion, disorientation.

Central Nervous System: Vertigo; light-headedness; paresthesias.

Special Senses: Transient visual disturbances including blurred vision.

Hypersensitivity Reactions: Acute anaphylactic reaction with bronchospasm; angioedema; flushing. Hypersensitivity vasculitis. Hypersensitivity syndrome (see PRECAUTIONS.)

Miscellaneous: Asthenia, edema.

Causal Relationship Unknown: Other reactions have been reported in clinical trials or since the drug was marketed, but occurred under circumstances where a causal relationship could not be established. However, in these rarely reported events, that possibility cannot be excluded. Therefore, these observations are listed to serve as alerting information to physicians.

Respiratory: Dyspnea.

Cardiovascular: Palpitation, syncope.

Musculoskeletal: Muscle cramps.

Genitourinary: Nephrotic syndrome.

Miscellaneous: Chest pain.

A rare occurrence of fulminant necrotizing fasciitis, particularly in association with Group A β-hemolytic streptococcus, has been described in persons treated with non-steroidal anti-inflammatory agents, including diflunisal, sometimes with fatal outcome (see also PRECAUTIONS, General).

Potential Adverse Effects: In addition, a variety of adverse effects not observed with diflunisal in clinical trials or in marketing experience, but reported with other non-steroidal analgesic/anti-inflammatory agents, should be considered potential adverse effects of diflunisal.

*Incidence between 3% and 9%. Those reactions occurring in 1% to 3% are not marked with an asterisk.

OVERDOSAGE:

Cases of overdosage have occurred and deaths have been reported. Most patients recovered without evidence of permanent sequelae. The most common signs and symptoms observed with overdosage were drowsiness, vomiting, nausea, diarrhea, hyperventilation, tachycardia, sweating, tinnitus, disorientation, stupor and coma. Diminished urine output and cardiorespiratory arrest have also been reported. The lowest dosage of diflunisal at which a death has been reported was 15 grams without the presence of other drugs. In a mixed drug overdose, ingestion of 7.5 grams of diflunisal resulted in death.

In the event of overdosage, the stomach should be emptied by inducing vomiting or by gastric lavage, and the patient carefully observed and given symptomatic and supportive treatment. Because of the high degree of protein binding, hemodialysis may not be effective.

The oral LD_{50} of the drug is 500 mg/kg and 826 mg/kg in female mice and female rats respectively.

DOSAGE AND ADMINISTRATION:

Concentration-dependent pharmacokinetics prevail when diflunisal is administered; a doubling of dosage produces a greater than doubling of drug accumulation. The effect becomes more apparent with repetitive doses.

For mild to moderate pain, an initial dose of 1000 mg followed by 500 mg every 12 hours is recommended for most patients. Following the initial dose, some patients may require 500 mg every 8 hours.

A lower dosage may be appropriate depending on such factors as pain severity, patient response, weight, or advanced age; for example, 500 mg initially, followed by 250 mg every 8-12 hours.

For osteoarthritis and rheumatoid arthritis, the suggested dosage range is 500 mg to 1000 mg daily in two divided doses. The dosage of diflunisal may be increased or decreased according to patient response.

Maintenance doses higher than 1500 mg a day are not recommended.

Diflunisal may be administered with water, milk or meals. Tablets should be swallowed whole, not crushed or chewed.

HOW SUPPLIED - RATED THERAPEUTICALLY EQUIVALENT:

Tablet, Plain Coated - Oral - 250 mg

60's	$46.44	Diflunisal, West Point Pharma	59591-0195-61
60's	$46.66	Diflunisal, Endo Labs	60951-0768-60
60's	$47.85	Diflunisal, Roxane	00054-4210-21
60's	**$57.06**	**DOLOBID, Merck**	**00006-0675-61**
100's	$87.25	Diflunisal, Roxane	00054-8210-25
100's	$98.65	Diflunisal, Major Pharms	00904-7763-61
100's	**$99.78**	**DOLOBID, Merck**	**00006-0675-28**

HOW SUPPLIED - RATED THERAPEUTICALLY EQUIVALENT: *(cont'd)*

500's	$349.94	Diflunisal, West Point Pharma	59591-0195-74
500's	$349.94	Diflunisal, Endo Labs	60951-0768-85

Tablet, Plain Coated - Oral - 500 mg

60's	$58.25	Diflunisal, Teva	00093-0755-06
60's	$58.25	Diflunisal, Aligen Independ	00405-4330-31
60's	$58.25	Diflunisal, HL Moore Drug Exch	00839-7764-05
60's	$58.30	Diflunisal, Goldline Labs	00182-1954-26
60's	$58.33	Diflunisal, West Point Pharma	59591-0196-61
60's	$58.33	Diflunisal, Endo Labs	60951-0769-60
60's	$58.35	Diflunisal, Major Pharms	00904-7764-52
60's	$58.35	Diflunisal, Major Pharms	00904-7808-52
60's	$58.70	Diflunisal, Schein Pharm (US)	00364-2537-06
60's	$59.90	Diflunisal, Roxane	00054-4220-21
60's	$60.25	Diflunisal, Dupont Pharma	00056-0196-60
60's	$65.83	Diflunisal, Rugby	00536-5563-08
60's	**$71.34**	**DOLOBID, Merck**	**00006-0697-61**
100's	$58.33	Diflunisal, United Res	00677-1460-06
100's	$90.29	Diflunisal, Teva	00093-0755-01
100's	$103.05	Diflunisal, Vangard Labs	00615-3586-13
100's	$104.28	Diflunisal, Roxane	00054-8220-25
100's	$104.90	Diflunisal, Goldline Labs	00182-1954-89
100's	$119.85	Diflunisal, Major Pharms	00904-7764-61
500's	$423.48	Diflunisal, Teva	00093-0755-05
500's	$437.47	Diflunisal, West Point Pharma	59591-0196-74
500's	$437.47	Diflunisal, Endo Labs	60951-0769-85

DIGITOXIN *(001060)*

CATEGORIES: Cardiovascular Drugs; Digitalis Glycosides; Fibrillation; Heart Failure; Heart Flutter; Renal Drugs; Tachycardia; Pregnancy Category C; FDA Pre 1938 Drugs

BRAND NAMES: *Coramedan*; **Crystodigin**; *Digicor* (Germany); *Digimed* (Germany); *Digimerck* (Germany); *Digitalin*; *Digitalina*; *Digitaline* (Canada); *Digitaline Nativelle* (France); *Digitoxin* (Japan); *Digitoxin Merck*; *Digitoxin Nyco*; *Digitoxine*; *Digitrin*
(International brand names outside U.S. in italics)

FORMULARIES: Medi-Cal; WHO

DESCRIPTION:

Crystodigin (Digitoxin Tablets, USP, Lilly) is a crystalline-pure single cardiac glycoside obtained from *Digitalis purpurea* and is identical in pharmacologic action with whole-leaf digitalis.

Digitoxin is the most slowly excreted of all digitalis compounds (excretion time is 14 to 21 days). It is most useful in patients with impaired renal function, since excretion and metabolism are independent of renal function.

Crystodigin is noted for its uniform potency, complete absorption, and lack of gastrointestinal irritation. It permits accurate dosage adjustments to produce maximum therapeutic effect smoothly and dependably.

Crystodigin, for oral administration, is available in tablets containing 0.05 mg (0.07 μmol) or 0.1 mg (0.13 μmol) crystalline digitoxin. The tablets also contain corn starch, lactose, magnesium stearate, and povidone. The 0.05 mg tablet also contains FD&C Yellow No. 6, and the 0.1 mg tablet also contains FD&C Red No. 40.

Digitoxin is a cardiotonic glycoside. The chemical name is card-20(22)-enolide,3-[(*O*-2,6-dideoxy-β-D-*ribo*-hexopyranosyl-(1→4)*O*-2,6-dideoxy-β-D-*ribo*-hexopyranosyl)oxy]-14-hydroxy, (3β,5β)-. The empirical formula of digitoxin is $C_{41}H_{64}O_{13}$.

CLINICAL PHARMACOLOGY:

The cellular basis for inotropic effects of digitalis is probably enhancement of excitation-contraction coupling, that process by which chemical energy is converted into mechanical energy when triggered by membrane depolarization. Most evidence relates this process to the entry of calcium ions into the cell during depolarization of the membrane and/or to the release of calcium from intracellular binding sites on the sarcoplasmic reticulum. The free calcium ion mediates the interaction of actin and myosin, resulting in contraction.

The amount of glycoside absorbed depends largely on its polarity, which is a function of the net electronic charge on the molecule. The more nonpolar or lipid soluble, the better is the absorption, because of the greater permeability of lipid membrane of the intestinal mucosa for lipid-soluble substances. The nonpolar, lipophilic digitoxin is completely absorbed. Other glycosides are not as well absorbed.

Nonpolar digitoxin is over 90% bound to tissue proteins. The firm binding of digitoxin to protein is responsible for its long half-life (7 to 9 days).

Digitoxin differs from other commonly used glycosides not only in its firm binding to protein but also because it is metabolized in the liver, with the only active metabolite being digoxin, which represents only a small fraction of the total metabolites. All other metabolites are inert and are probably excreted as such in the urine. The portion of digitoxin that is not metabolized is excreted in the bile to the intestines and recycled to the liver until it is completely metabolized. The portion of digitoxin that is bound to protein is an equilibrium with free digitoxin in the serum. Thus, as more and more of the free digitoxin is metabolized after a single dose, there is proportionately less bound digitoxin.

INDICATIONS AND USAGE:

Digitoxin is indicated in the treatment of heart failure, atrial flutter, atrial fibrillation, and supraventricular tachycardia.

CONTRAINDICATIONS:

If the indications are carefully observed, there are few contraindications to digitalis therapy except toxic response or idiosyncrasy to digitalis, ventricular tachycardia, beriberi, heart disease, and some instances of the hypersensitive carotid sinus syndrome.

Patients already taking digitalis preparations must be given the rapid digitalizing dose of digitoxin or parenteral calcium.

WARNINGS:

Many of the arrhythmias for which digitalis is advised are identical with those reflecting digitalis intoxication. When the possibility of digitalis intoxication cannot be excluded, cardiac glycosides should be withheld temporarily of the clinical situation permits.

The patient with congestive heart failure may complain of nausea and vomiting. Since these symptoms may also be associated with digitalis intoxication, a clinical determination of their cause must be attempted before further administration of the drug.

WARNINGS: *(cont'd)*

Cases of idiopathic hypertrophic subaortic stenosis must be managed with extreme care. Unless cardiac failure is severe, it is doubtful whether digitalis should be employed.

Note: Digitalis glycosides are an important cause of accidental poisoning in children.

PRECAUTIONS:

General: When the risk of digitalis intoxication is great, the use of a short-acting, rapidly eliminated glycoside, such as digoxin, is advisable. Although intoxication cannot always be prevented by the selection of one glycoside over another, certain glycosides may be preferred in patients who have fixed disabilities (*e.g.,* liver impairment, drug tolerance). However, digitoxin can be used in patients with impaired renal function.

Special care must be exercised in elderly patients receiving digitalis, because their body mass tends to be small and renal clearance is likely to be reduced. Frequent electrocardiographic monitoring is important in these patients. In addition, digitalis must be used cautiously in the presence of active heart disease, such as acute myocardial infarction or acute myocarditis. In acute myocardial infarction or acute myocarditis. In patients with acute or unstable chronic atrial fibrillation, digitalis may not normalize the ventricular rate even when the serum concentration exceeds the usual even when the serum concentration exceeds the usual therapeutic level. Although these patients may be less sensitive to the toxic effects of digitalis than are patients with normal sinus rhythm, dosage should not be increased to potentially toxic levels.

Hypokalemia predisposes to digitalis toxicity, and even a moderate decrease in the concentration of serum potassium can precipitate serious arrhythmias.

Impaired liver function may necessitate reduction in dosage of any digitalis preparation, including digitoxin.

Sensitive radioimmunoassay techniques have been developed for measuring serum levels of digitoxin, and these procedures can be instituted in almost any hospital. Serum levels must, however, be evaluated in conjunction with clinical history and the results of the electrocardiogram and other laboratory tests. A therapeutic serum level for one patient may be excessive or inadequate for another patient.

Usage in Pregnancy: Pregnancy Category C: Animal reproduction studies have not been conducted with digitoxin. It is also not known whether this drug can cause fetal harm when administered to a pregnant woman or can affect reproduction capacity. Digitoxin should be given to a pregnant woman only if clearly needed.

Labor and Delivery: No information is available concerning the use of digitoxin in labor and delivery.

Nursing Mothers: It is not known whether this drug is excreted in human breast milk. Because many drugs are excreted in human breast milk, caution should be exercised when digitoxin is administered to a nursing woman.

DRUG INTERACTIONS:

The synthesis of microsomal enzymes that metabolize digitoxin in the liver is subject to stimulation by a number of drugs, such as antihistamines, anticonvulsants, barbiturates, oral hypoglycemic agents, and others.

When digitoxin is the glycoside used for digitalis maintenance, drugs that are liver-microsomal enzyme inducers should not be used at the same time. Phenobarbital, phenylbutazone, and diphenylhydantoin will increase the rate of metabolism of digitoxin. In patients receiving 60 mg of phenobarbital 3 times a day for 12 weeks, the steady-state concentration of digitoxin in plasma fell approximately 50% when the drugs were administered concurrently and returned to previous levels when phenobarbital was discontinued.

When drugs that increase the rate of metabolism of digitoxin in the liver are discontinued, toxicity may occur.

Hypokalemia is most frequently encountered in patients receiving concomitant diuretic therapy, because the most widely used and most effective diuretics (*i.e.,* thiazides and furosemide) increase the urinary loss of potassium. Prescribing a potassium sparing agent (spironolactone or triamterene) together with the potassium-wasting diuretic is a reliable means for maintaining the serum potassium level.

Alternatively, potassium chloride supplements may be prescribed.

Mineralocorticosteroids (*e.g.,* prednisone) and, rarely, certain antibiotics (*e.g.,* amphotericin B) may also cause increased excretion of potassium.

ADVERSE REACTIONS:

Anorexia, nausea, and vomiting have been reported. These effects are central in origin, but following large oral doses, there is also a local emetic action. Abdominal discomfort or pain and diarrhea may also occur.

OVERDOSAGE:

Signs and Symptoms: Symptoms may include alterations in mental status, nausea, vomiting, bradycardia, visual disturbances, heart block, and all known cardiac arrhythmias. Hyperkalemia may be present following acute overdose, whereas hypokalemia is associated with chronic overdose. Peak toxic effects following acute overdose may be delayed up to 12 hours.

Older patients, particularly those coronary insufficiency, are more susceptible to dysrhythmias. Ventricular fibrillation is the most common cause of death from digitalis poisoning. There is insufficient information to accurately determine the minimum toxic or lethal dose in humans. Death from ventricular fibrillation was reported 24 hours after admission in a patient with a plasma concentration of 124 ng/ml shortly before death.

Treatment: To obtain up-to-date information about the treatment of overdose, a good resource is your certified Regional Poison Control Center. Telephone numbers of certified poison control centers are listed in *Physicians GenRx.* In managing overdosage, consider the possibility of multiple drug overdoses, interaction among drugs, and unusual drug kinetics in your patient.

Continuous ECG monitoring is necessary. For any suspected digitoxin-induced dysrhythmia, discontinue the drug. Monitor potassium and digitoxin concentrations. Severe hyperkalemia may require administration of sodium bicarbonate, glucose, and regular insulin.

Protect the patient's airway and support ventilation and perfusion. Meticulously monitor and maintain, within acceptable limits, the patient's vital signs, blood gases, serum electrolytes, etc. Absorption of drugs from the gastrointestinal tract may be decreased by giving activated charcoal, which, in many cases, is more effective than emesis or lavage; consider charcoal instead of or in addition to gastric emptying. Repeated doses of charcoal over time may hasten elimination of some drugs that have been absorbed. Safeguard the patient's airway when employing gastric emptying or charcoal.

Atropine or a pacemaker may be used for bradycardia and heart block. Phenytoin (15 mg/kg), at a rate not to exceed 50 mg/min, may be useful for treating ventricular dysrhythmias and to improve atrioventricular conduction. Lidocaine may also be used, but impaired AV conduction may require a pacemaker. Consider use of digitalis-specific Fab fragments.

Forced diuresis, peritoneal dialysis, hemodialysis, or charcoal hemoperfusion have not been established as beneficial for an overdose of digitoxin.

DOSAGE AND ADMINISTRATION:

ADULTS

Slow Digitalization: 0.2 mg twice daily for a period of 4 days, followed by maintenance dosage.

Rapid Digitalization: Preferably 0.6 mg initially, followed by 0.4 mg and then 0.2 mg at intervals of 4 to 6 hours.

Maintenance Dosage: Ranges from 0.05 to 0.3 mg daily, the most common dose being 0.15 mg daily.

HOW SUPPLIED:

Tablets (scored): 0.05 mg, orange; 0.1 mg pink

Protect from light. Store at controlled room temperature, 59° to 86°F (15° to 30°C).

HOW SUPPLIED - EQUIVALENTS NOT AVAILABLE:

Tablet, Uncoated - Oral - 0.05 mg

100's $2.92 CRYSTODIGIN, Lilly 00002-1075-02

Tablet, Uncoated - Oral - 0.1 mg

100's $5.14 CRYSTODIGIN, Lilly 00002-1060-02

DIGOXIN *(001061)*

CATEGORIES: Anabolic Steroids; Anemia; Antineoplastics; Atrial Fibrillation; Cardiac Output; Cardiovascular Drugs; Congestion; Digitalis Glycosides; Edema; Fibrillation; Heart Failure; Heart Flutter; Hormones; Hyperthyroidism; Oncologic Drugs; Penicillins; Renal Drugs; Renal Function; Tachycardia; Pregnancy Category C; Sales > $100 Million; FDA Approval Pre 1982; Top 200 Drugs

BRAND NAMES: *Cardigox*; *Cardiogoxin*; *Cardioxin*; Cardoxin; *Coragoxine*; *Digacin* (Germany); *Digazolan*; *Digipural*; *Digomal*; *Digon*; *Digosin* (Japan); *Digoxine Navtivelle* (France); *Digoxina-Sandoz*; *Digoxin-Sandoz* (Japan); *Digoxin-Zori*; *Dilanacin*; *Eudigox*; *Fargoxin*; *Grexin*; *Lanacordin*; *Lanacrist*; *Lanicor* (Germany); *Lanorale*; Lanoxicaps; **Lanoxin**; *Lanoxin PG*; *Lenoxicaps*; *Lenoxin* (Germany); *Lifusin*; *Mapluxin* (Mexico); *Natigoxin*; *Novodigal*; *Purgoxin*; *Toloxin*
(International brand names outside U.S. in italics)

FORMULARIES: Aetna; BC-BS; CIGNA; DoD; FHP; Humana; Kaiser; Medco; Medi-Cal; PCS; PruCare; United; WHO

COST OF THERAPY: $27.52 (Heart Failure; Tablet; 0.25 mg; 1/day; 365 days)

DESCRIPTION:

Digoxin is one of the cardiac (or digitalis) glycosides, a closely related group of drugs having in common specific effects on the myocardium. These drugs are found in a number of plants. Digoxin is extracted from the leaves of *Digitalis lanata.* The term "digitalis" is used to designate the whole group. The glycosides are composed of two portions: a sugar and a cardenolide (hence "glycosides").

Digoxin has the molecular formula $C_{41}H_{64}O_{14}$, a molecular weight of 780.95 and melting and decomposition points above 235°C. The drug is practically insoluble in water and in ether; slightly soluble in diluted (50%) alcohol and in chloroform; and freely soluble in pyridine. Digoxin powder is composed of odorless white crystals.

Digoxin has the chemical name: 3β-[(*0*-2, 6-dideoxy-β-*D-ribo*-hexopyranosyl-(1->4)-*0-2,* 6-dideoxy-β-*D-ribo*-hexopyranosyl-(1->4)-2,6- dideoxy-β-*D-ribo*-hexopyranosyl)oxy]-12β, 14-dihydroxy- 5β-card-20(22)-enolide.

Capsules: Digoxin capsules are a stable solution of digoxin enclosed within a soft gelatin capsule for oral use. Each capsule contains the labeled amount of digoxin USP dissolved in a solvent comprised of polyethylene glycol 400 USP, 8 percent ethyl alcohol, propylene glycol USP and purified water USP. Inactive ingredients in the lanoxin capsule shell include FD&C Red No. 40 (0.05 mg capsule), D&C Yellow No. 10 (0.1 mg and 0.2 mg capsules), FD&C Blue No. 1 (0.2 mg capsule), gelatin, glycerin, methylparaben and propylparaben (added as preservatives), purified water and sorbitol. Capsules printed with edible ink.

Tablets: Digoxin tablets with 125 mcg (0.125 mg), 250 mcg (0.25 mg) or 500 mcg (0.5 mg) digoxin USP are intended for oral use. Each lanoxin tablet contains the labeled amount of digoxin USP and the inactive ingredients: 0.125 mg tablet-corn and potato starch, D&C Yellow No. 10, FD&C Yellow No.6, lactose and magnesium stearate; 0.25 mg tablet-corn and potato starch, lactose, magnesium stearate, and steric acid; 0.5 mg tablet-corn and potato starch, D&C Green No. 5 and Yellow No, FD&C Red No. 40, lactose, magnesium stearate, and stearic acid.

Pediatric Elixir: Digoxin pediatric elixir is a stable solution of digoxin specially formulated for oral use in infants and children. Each ml contains 50 mcg (0.05 mg) digoxin USP. Lanoxin lime-flavored elixir contains the inactive ingredients alcohol 10%, methylparaben 0.1% (added as a preservative), citric acid, D&C Green No. 5 and Yellow No. 10, flavor, propylene glycol, sodium phosphate, and sucrose. Each package is supplied with a specially calibrated dropper to facilitate the administration of accurate dosage even in premature infants. Starting at 0.2 ml, this 1 ml dropper is marked in divisions of 0.1 ml, each corresponding to 5 mcg (0.005 mg) digoxin.

Injection: Digoxin injection is a sterile solution of digoxin for intravenous or intramuscular injection. The vehicle contains 40% propylene glycol and 10% alcohol. The injection is buffered to a pH of 6.8 to 7.2 with 0.17% sodium phosphate and 0.08% anhydrous citric acid. Each 2 ml ampule contains 500 mcg (0.5 mg) digoxin (250 mcg [0.25 mg] per ml). Dilution is not required.

Pediatric Injection: Digoxin pediatric injection is a sterile solution of digoxin for intravenous or intramuscular injection. The vehicle contains 40% propylene glycol and 10% alcohol. The injection is buffered to a pH of 6.8 to 7.2 with 0.17% sodium phosphate and 0.08% anhydrous citric acid. Each 1 ml ampule contains 100 mcg (0.1 mg) digoxin. Dilution is not required.

CLINICAL PHARMACOLOGY:

MECHANISM OF ACTION

The influence of digitalis glycosides on the myocardium is dose-related, and involves both a direct action on cardiac muscle and the specialized conduction system, and indirect actions on the cardiovascular system mediated by the autonomic nervous system. The indirect actions mediated by the autonomic nervous system involve a vagomimetic action, which is responsible for the effects of digitalis on the sino-atrial (SA) and atrioventricular (AV) nodes; and also a baroreceptor sensitization which results in increased carotid sinus nerve activity and enhanced sympathetic withdrawal for any given increment in mean arterial pressure. The pharmacologic consequences of these direct and indirect effects are: 1) an increase in the force and velocity of myocardial systolic contraction (positive inotropic action); 2) a slowing of heart rate (negative chronotropic effect); and 3) decreased conduction velocity through the AV node. In higher doses, digitalis increases sympathetic outflow from the central nervous

CLINICAL PHARMACOLOGY: *(cont'd)*

system (CNS) to both cardiac and peripheral sympathetic nerves. This increase in sympathetic activity may be an important factor in digitalis cardiac toxicity. Most of the extracardiac manifestations of digitalis toxicity are also mediated by the CNS.

PHARMACOKINETICS

Note the following data are from studies performed in adults, unless otherwise stated.

Absorption: A comparison of the systemic availability and equivalent doses for digoxin preparations are shown in TABLE 1.

TABLE 1

Product	Absolute Bioavailability	Equivalent Doses (in mg)*		
Digoxin Tablets	60-80%	0.125	0.25	0.5
Digoxin Elixir	70-85%	0.125	0.25	0.5
Digoxin Injection/IM	70-85%	0.125	0.25	0.5
Digoxin Injection/IV	100%	0.1	0.2	0.4
Digoxin Capsules	90-100%	0.1	0.2	0.4

* 1 mg = 1000 mcg

Distribution: Following drug administration, a 6 to 8 hour distribution phase is observed. This is followed by a much more gradual serum concentration decline, which is dependent on digoxin elimination from the body. The peak height and slope of the early portion (absorption/distribution phases) of the serum concentration-time curve are dependent upon the route of administration and the absorption characteristics of the formulation. Clinical evidence indicates that the early high serum concentrations (particularly high for digoxin capsules) do not reflect the concentration of digoxin at its site of action, but that with chronic use, the steady-state post-distribution serum levels are in equilibrium with tissue levels and correlate with pharmacologic effects. In individual patients, these post-distribution serum concentrations are linearly related to maintenance dosage and may be useful in evaluating therapeutic and toxic effects (see DOSAGE AND ADMINISTRATION, Serum Digoxin Concentrations.)

Digoxin is concentrated in tissues and therefore has a large apparent volume of distribution. Digoxin crosses both the blood-brain barrier and the placenta. At delivery, serum digoxin concentration in the newborn is similar to the serum level in the mother. Approximately 20 to 25% of plasma digoxin is bound to protein. Serum digoxin concentrations are not significantly altered by large changes in fat tissue weight, so that its distribution space correlates best with lean (ideal) body weight, not total body weight.

Pharmacologic Response: The approximate times to onset of effect and to peak effect of all the digoxin preparations are given in TABLE 2.

TABLE 2

Product	Time To Onset Of Effect*	Time To Peak Effect*
Digoxin Tablet	0.5-2 hours	2-6 hours
Digoxin Elixir	0.5-2 hours	2-6 hours
Digoxin Injection/IM	0.5-2 hours	2-6 hours
Digoxin Injection/IV	5 to 30 minutes†	1-4 hours
Digoxin Capsules	0.5-2 hours	2-6 hours

* Documented for ventricular response rate in atrial fibrillation, inotropic effect and electrocardiographic changes.
† Depending upon rate of infusion.

Excretion: Elimination of digoxin follows first-order kinetics (that is, the quantity of digoxin eliminated at any time is proportional to the total body content). Following intravenous administration to normal subjects, 50 to 70% of a digoxin dose is excreted unchanged in the urine. Renal excretion of digoxin is proportional to glomerular filtration rate and is largely independent of urine flow. In subjects with normal renal function, digoxin has a half-life of 1.5 to 2.0 days. The half-life in anuric patients is prolonged to 4 to 6 days. Digoxin is not effectively removed from the body by dialysis, exchange transfusion or during cardiopulmonary by-pass because most of the drug is in tissue rather than circulating in the blood.

CAPSULES, TABLETS AND PEDIATRIC ELIXIR

Gastrointestinal absorption of digoxin is a passive process. Absorption of digoxin capsules has been demonstrated to be 90 to 100% complete compared to an identical intravenous dose of digoxin. Absorption of digoxin tablets has been shown demonstrated to be 60 to 80% complete compared to an identical intravenous dose of digoxin (absolute bioavailability). Digoxin pediatric elixir has been demonstrated to be 70 to 85% complete compared to an identical intravenous dose of digoxin. The enhanced absorption from the capsules compared to digoxin tablets and elixir is associated with reduced between-patient and within-patient variability in steady-state serum concentrations. The peak serum concentrations are higher than those observed after tablets. When digoxin tablets or capsules are taken after meals, the rate of absorption is slowed, but the total amount of digoxin absorbed is usually unchanged. When taken with meals high in bran fiber, however, the amount absorbed from an oral dose may be reduced.

In some patients, orally administered digoxin is converted to cardioinactive reduction products (*e.g.,* dihydrodigoxin) by colonic bacteria in the gut. Data suggest that one in ten patients treated with digoxin tablets will degrade 40% or more of the ingested dose. This phenomenon is minimized with digoxin capsules because they are rapidly absorbed in the upper gastrointestinal tract.

INDICATIONS AND USAGE:

HEART FAILURE: The increased cardiac output resulting from the inotropic action of digoxin ameliorates the disturbances characteristic of heart failure (venous congestion, edema, dyspnea, orthopnea and cardiac asthma).

Digoxin is more effective in "low output" (pump) failure than in "high output" heart failure secondary to arteriovenous fistula, anemia, infection or hyperthyroidism.

Digoxin is usually continued after failure is controlled, unless some known precipitating factor is corrected. Studies have shown, however, that even though hemodynamic effects can be demonstrated in almost all patients, corresponding improvement in the signs and symptoms of heart failure is not necessarily apparent. Therefore, in patients in whom digoxin may be difficult to regulate, or in whom the risk of toxicity may be great (*e.g.,* patients with unstable renal function or whose potassium levels tend to fluctuate) a cautious withdrawal of digoxin may be considered. If digoxin is discontinued, the patient should be regularly monitored for clinical evidence of recurrent heart failure.

INDICATIONS AND USAGE: *(cont'd)*

Atrial Fibrillation: Digoxin reduces ventricular rate and thereby improves hemodynamics. Palpitation, precordial distress or weakness are relieved and concomitant congestive failure ameliorated. Digoxin should be continued in doses necessary to maintain the desired ventricular rate.

Atrial Flutter: Digoxin slows the heart and regular sinus rhythm may appear. Frequently the flutter is converted to atrial fibrillation with a controlled ventricular response. Digoxin treatment should be maintained if atrial fibrillation persists. (Electrical cardioversion is often the treatment of choice for atrial flutter. See discussion of cardioversion in PRECAUTIONS.)

Paroxysmal Atrial Tachycardia (PAT): Digoxin may convert PAT to sinus rhythm by slowing conduction through the AV node. If heart failure has ensued or paroxysms recur frequently, digoxin should be continued. In infants, digoxin is usually continued for 3 to 6 months after a single episode of PAT to prevent recurrence.

CONTRAINDICATIONS:

DIGITALIS GLYCOSIDES ARE CONTRAINDICATED IN VENTRICULAR FIBRILLATION.

IN A GIVEN PATIENT, AN UNTOWARD EFFECT REQUIRING PERMANENT DISCONTINUATION OF OTHER DIGITALIS PREPARATIONS USUALLY CONSTITUTES A CONTRAINDICATION TO DIGOXIN. HYPERSENSITIVITY TO DIGOXIN ITSELF IS A CONTRAINDICATION TO ITS USE. ALLERGY TO DIGOXIN, THOUGH RARE, DOES OCCUR. IT MAY NOT EXTEND TO ALL SUCH PREPARATIONS, AND ANOTHER DIGITALIS GLYCOSIDE MAY BE TRIED WITH CAUTION.

WARNINGS:

DIGITALIS ALONE OR WITH OTHER DRUGS HAS BEEN USED IN THE TREATMENT OF OBESITY. THIS USE OF DIGOXIN OR OTHER DIGITALIS GLYCOSIDES IS UNWARRANTED. MOREOVER, SINCE THEY MAY CAUSE POTENTIALLY FATAL ARRHYTHMIAS OR OTHER ADVERSE EFFECTS, THE USE OF THESE DRUGS SOLELY FOR THE TREATMENT OF OBESITY IS DANGEROUS.

ANOREXIA, NAUSEA, VOMITING AND ARRHYTHMIAS MAY ACCOMPANY HEART FAILURE OR MAY BE INDICATIONS OF DIGITALIS INTOXICATION. CLINICAL EVALUATION OF THE CAUSE OF THESE SYMPTOMS SHOULD BE ATTEMPTED BEFORE FURTHER DIGITALIS ADMINISTRATION. IN SUCH CIRCUMSTANCES DETERMINATION OF THE SERUM DIGOXIN CONCENTRATION MAY BE AN AID IN DECIDING WHETHER OR NOT DIGITALIS TOXICITY IS LIKELY TO BE PRESENT. IF THE POSSIBILITY OF DIGITALIS INTOXICATION CANNOT BE EXCLUDED, CARDIAC GLYCOSIDES SHOULD BE TEMPORARILY WITHHELD, IF PERMITTED BY THE CLINICAL SITUATION.

PATIENTS WITH RENAL INSUFFICIENCY REQUIRE SMALLER THAN USUAL MAINTENANCE DOSES OF DIGOXIN (SEE DOSAGE AND ADMINISTRATION.)

HEART FAILURE ACCOMPANYING ACUTE GLOMERULONEPHRITIS REQUIRES EXTREME CARE IN DIGITALIZATION. RELATIVELY LOW LOADING AND MAINTENANCE DOSES AND CONCOMITANT USE OF ANTIHYPERTENSIVE DRUGS MAY BE NECESSARY AND CAREFUL MONITORING IS ESSENTIAL. DIGOXIN SHOULD BE DISCONTINUED AS SOON AS POSSIBLE.

PATIENTS WITH SEVERE CARDITIS, SUCH AS CARDITIS ASSOCIATED WITH RHEUMATIC FEVER OR VIRAL MYOCARDITIS, ARE ESPECIALLY SENSITIVE TO DIGOXIN-INDUCED DISTURBANCES OF RHYTHM.

NEWBORN INFANTS DISPLAY CONSIDERABLE VARIABILITY IN THEIR TOLERANCE TO DIGOXIN. PREMATURE AND IMMATURE INFANTS ARE PARTICULARLY SENSITIVE, AND DOSAGE MUST NOT ONLY BE REDUCED BUT MUST BE INDIVIDUALIZED ACCORDING TO THEIR DEGREE OF MATURITY.

NOTE: DIGITALIS GLYCOSIDES ARE AN IMPORTANT CAUSE OF ACCIDENTAL POISONING IN CHILDREN.

ADDITIONAL INFORMATION FOR CAPSULES

It is recommended that digoxin in soft capsules be administered in divided daily doses to minimize any potential adverse reactions, since peak serum digoxin concentrations resulting from the capsules are approximately twice those after bioequivalent tablet doses (400 mcg of tablets are bioequivalent to 500 mcg of tablets). Studies are underway to determine if there are any increased risks associated with the higher peaks that occur with single daily dosing of soft gelatin capsules.

PRECAUTIONS:

GENERAL: Digoxin toxicity develops more frequently and lasts longer in patients with renal impairment because of the decreased excretion of digoxin. Therefore, it should be anticipated that dosage requirements will be decreased in patients with moderate to severe renal disease (see DOSAGE AND ADMINISTRATION.) Because of the prolonged half-life, a longer period of time is required to achieve an initial or new steady-state concentration in patients with renal impairment than in patients with normal renal function.

In patients with hypokalemia, toxicity may occur despite serum digoxin concentrations within the "normal range," because potassium depletion sensitizes the myocardium to digoxin. Therefore, it is desirable to maintain normal serum potassium levels in patients being treated with digoxin. Hypokalemia may result from diuretic, amphotericin B or corticosteroid therapy, and from dialysis or mechanical suction of gastrointestinal secretions. It may also accompany malnutrition, diarrhea, prolonged vomiting, old age and long-standing heart failure. In general, rapid changes in serum potassium or other electrolytes should be avoided, and intravenous treatment with potassium should be reserved for special circumstances as described below (see OVERDOSAGE, Treatment Of Arrhythmias Produced By Overdosage.)

Calcium, particularly when administered rapidly by the intravenous route, may produce serious arrhythmias in digitalized patients. Hypercalcemia from any cause predisposes the patient to digitalis toxicity. On the other hand, hypocalcemia can nullify the effects of digoxin in humans; thus, digoxin may be ineffective until serum calcium is restored to normal. These interactions are related to the fact that calcium affects contractility and excitability of the heart in a manner similar to digoxin.

Hypomagnesemia may predispose to digitalis toxicity. If low magnesium levels are detected in a patient on digoxin, replacement therapy should be instituted.

Quinidine, verapamil, amiodarone, propafenone, indomethacin, itraconazole, and alprazolam cause a rise in serum digoxin concentration, with the implication that digitalis intoxication may result. This rise appears to be proportional to the dose. The effect is mediated by a reduction in the digoxin clearance and, in the case of quinidine, decreased volume of distribution as well.

Certain antibiotics may increase digoxin absorption in patients who convert digoxin to inactive metabolites in the gut (see CLINICAL PHARMACOLOGY, Pharmacokinetics.) Recent studies have shown that specific colonic bacteria in the lower gastrointestinal tract convert digoxin to cardioinactive reduction products, thereby reducing its bioavailability. Although inactivation of these bacteria by antibiotics is rapid, the serum digoxin concentration will rise at a rate consistent with the elimination half-life of digoxin. The magnitude of

PRECAUTIONS: *(cont'd)*

rise in serum digoxin concentration relates to the extent of bacterial inactivation, and may be as much as two-fold in some cases. This interaction is significantly reduced if digoxin is given as capsules.

Patients with acute myocardial infarction or severe pulmonary disease may be unusually sensitive to digoxin-induced disturbances of rhythm.

Atrial arrhythmias associated with hypermetabolic states (*e.g.,* hyperthyroidism) are particularly resistant to digoxin treatment. Large doses of digoxin are not recommended as the only treatment of these arrhythmias and care must be taken to avoid toxicity if large doses of digoxin are required. In hypothyroidism, the digoxin requirements are reduced. Digoxin responses in patients with compensated thyroid disease are normal.

Reduction of digoxin dosage may be desirable prior to electrical cardioversion to avoid induction of ventricular arrhythmias, but the physician must consider the consequences of rapid increase in ventricular response to atrial fibrillation if digoxin is withheld 1 to 2 days prior to cardioversion. If there is a suspicion that digitalis toxicity exists, elective cardioversion should be delayed. If it is not prudent to delay cardioversion, the energy level selected should be minimal at first and carefully increased in an attempt to avoid precipitating ventricular arrhythmias.

Incomplete AV block, especially in patients with Stokes-Adams attacks, may progress to advanced or complete heart block if digoxin is given.

In some patients with sinus node disease (*i.e.,* Sick Sinus Syndrome), digoxin may worsen sinus bradycardia or sino-atrial block.

In patients with Wolff-Parkinson-White Syndrome and atrial fibrillation, digoxin can enhance transmission of impulses through the accessory pathway. This effect may result in extremely rapid ventricular rates and even ventricular fibrillation.

Digoxin may worsen the outflow obstruction in patients with idiopathic hypertrophic subaortic stenosis (IHSS). Unless cardiac failure is severe, it is doubtful whether digoxin should be employed.

Patients with chronic constrictive pericarditis may fail to respond to digoxin. In addition, slowing of the heart rate by digoxin in some patients may further decrease cardiac output.

Patients with heart failure from amyloid heart disease or constrictive cardiomyopathies respond poorly to treatment with digoxin.

Digoxin is not indicated for the treatment of sinus tachycardia unless it is associated with heart failure.

Digoxin may produce false positive ST-T changes in the electrocardiogram during exercise testing.

Intramuscular injection of digoxin is extremely painful and offers no advantages unless other routes of administration are contraindicated.

Laboratory Tests: Patients receiving digoxin should have their serum electrolytes and renal function (BUN and/or serum creatinine) assessed periodically; the frequency of assessments will depend on the clinical setting. For discussion of serum digoxin concentrations, see DOSAGE AND ADMINISTRATION.

Carcinogenesis, Mutagenesis, Impairment of Fertility: There have been no long-term studies performed in animals to evaluate carcinogenic potential.

Pregnancy, Teratogenic Effects: Pregnancy Category C. Animal reproduction studies have not been conducted with digoxin. It is also not known whether digoxin can cause fetal harm when administered to a pregnant woman or can affect reproduction capacity. Digoxin should be given to a pregnant woman only if clearly needed.

Nursing Mothers: Studies have shown that digoxin concentrations in the mother's serum and milk are similar. However, the estimated daily dose to a nursing infant will be far below the usual infant maintenance dose. Therefore, this amount should have no pharmacologic effect upon the infant. Nevertheless, caution should be exercised when digoxin is administered to a nursing woman.

DRUG INTERACTIONS:

POTASSIUM-DEPLETING **CORTICOSTEROIDS** AND **DIURETICS** MAY BE MAJOR CONTRIBUTING FACTORS TO DIGITALIS TOXICITY. **CALCIUM**, PARTICULARLY IF ADMINISTERED RAPIDLY BY THE INTRAVENOUS ROUTE, MAY PRODUCE SERIOUS ARRHYTHMIAS IN DIGITALIZED PATIENTS. **QUINIDINE, VERAPAMIL, AMIODARONE,** AND **PROPAFENONE** CAUSE A RISE IN SERUM DIGOXIN CONCENTRATION, WITH THE IMPLICATION THAT DIGITALIS INTOXICATION MAY RESULT. CERTAIN **ANTIBIOTICS** INCREASE DIGOXIN ABSORPTION IN PATIENTS WHO INACTIVATE DIGOXIN BY BACTERIAL METABOLISM IN THE LOWER INTESTINE, SO THAT DIGITALIS INTOXICATION MAY RESULT.**PROPANTHELINE** AND **DIPHENOXYLATE**, BY DECREASING GUT MOTILITY, MAY INCREASE DIGOXIN ABSORPTION. **ANTACIDS, KAOLIN-PECTIN, SULFASALAZINE, NEOMYCIN, CHOLESTYRAMINE** AND CERTAIN **ANTICANCER DRUGS** MAY INTERFERE WITH INTESTINAL DIGOXIN ABSORPTION, RESULTING IN UNEXPECTEDLY LOW SERUM CONCENTRATIONS. THERE HAVE BEEN INCONSISTENT REPORTS REGARDING THE EFFECTS OF OTHER DRUGS ON THE SERUM DIGOXIN CONCENTRATION. **THYROID** ADMINISTRATION TO A DIGITALIZED, HYPOTHYROID PATIENT MAY INCREASE THE DOSE REQUIREMENT OF DIGOXIN. CONCOMITANT USE OF DIGOXIN AND **SYMPATHOMIMETICS** INCREASES THE RISK OF CARDIAC ARRHYTHMIAS, BECAUSE BOTH ENHANCE ECTOPIC PACEMAKER ACTIVITY. **SUCCINYLCHOLINE** MAY CAUSE A SUDDEN EXTRUSION OF POTASSIUM FROM MUSCLE CELLS, AND MAY THEREBY CAUSE ARRHYTHMIAS IN DIGITALIZED PATIENTS. ALTHOUGH ADRENERGIC BLOCKERS OR CALCIUM CHANNEL BLOCKERS AND DIGOXIN MAY BE USEFUL IN COMBINATION TO CONTROL ATRIAL FIBRILLATION, THEIR ADDITIVE EFFECTS ON AV NODE CONDUCTION CAN RESULT IN COMPLETE HEART BLOCK.

DUE TO THE CONSIDERABLE VARIABILITY OF THESE INTERACTIONS, DIGOXIN, DOSAGE SHOULD BE CAREFULLY INDIVIDUALIZED WHEN PATIENTS RECEIVE COADMINISTERED MEDICATIONS. FURTHERMORE, CAUTION SHOULD BE EXERCISED WHEN COMBINING DIGOXIN WITH ANY DRUG THAT MAY CAUSE A SIGNIFICANT DETERIORATION IN RENAL FUNCTION, SINCE THIS MAY IMPAIR THE EXCRETION OF DIGOXIN.

ADVERSE REACTIONS:

THE FREQUENCY AND SEVERITY OF ADVERSE REACTIONS TO DIGOXIN DEPEND ON THE DOSE AND ROUTE OF ADMINISTRATION, AS WELL AS ON THE PATIENT'S UNDERLYING DISEASE OR CONCOMITANT THERAPIES (SEE PRECAUTIONS and DOSAGE AND ADMINISTRATION, Serum Digoxin Concentrations. The overall incidence of adverse reactions has been reported as 5 to 20%, with 15 to 20% of them being considered serious (one to four percent of patients receiving digoxin). Evidence suggests that the incidence of toxicity has decreased since the introduction of the serum digoxin assay and improved standardization of digoxin tablets. Cardiac toxicity accounts for about one-half, gastrointestinal disturbances for about one-fourth, and CNS and other toxicity for about one-fourth of these adverse reactions.

ADVERSE REACTIONS: *(cont'd)*

ADULTS

Cardiac: Unifocal or multiform ventricular premature contractions, especially in bigeminal or trigeminal patterns, are the most common arrhythmias associated with digoxin toxicity in adults with heart disease. Ventricular tachycardia may result from digitalis toxicity. Atrioventricular (AV) dissociation, accelerated junctional (nodal) rhythm and atrial tachycardia with block are also common arrhythmias caused by digoxin overdosage.

Excessive slowing of the pulse is a clinical sign of digoxin overdosage. AV block (Wenckebach) of increasing degree may proceed to complete heart block.

Note: The electrocardiogram is fundamental in determining the presence and nature of these cardiac disturbances. Digoxin may also induce other changes in the ECG (*e.g.,* PR prolongation, ST depression), which represent digoxin effect and may or may not be associated with digitalis toxicity.

Gastrointestinal: Anorexia, nausea, vomiting and less commonly diarrhea are common early symptoms of overdosage. However, uncontrolled heart failure may also produce such symptoms. Digitalis toxicity very rarely may cause abdominal pain and hemorrhagic necrosis of the intestines.

CNS: Visual disturbances (blurred or yellow vision), headache, weakness, dizziness, apathy and psychosis can occur.

Other: Gynecomastia is occasionally observed. Maculopapular rash or other skin reactions are rarely observed.

Infants and Children: Toxicity differs from the adult in a number of respects. Anorexia, nausea, vomiting, diarrhea and CNS disturbances may be present but are rare as initial symptoms in infants. Cardiac arrhythmias are more reliable signs of toxicity. Digoxin in children may produce any arrhythmia. The most commonly encountered are conduction disturbances or supraventricular tachyarrhythmias, such as atrial tachycardia with or without block, and junctional (nodal) tachycardia. Ventricular arrhythmias are less common. Sinus bradycardia may also be a sign of impending digoxin intoxication, especially in infants, even in the absence of first degree heart block. Any arrhythmia or alteration in cardiac conduction that develops in a child taking digoxin should initially be assumed to be a consequence of digoxin intoxication.

ADDITIONAL INFORMATION FOR PEDIATRIC ELIXIR AND INJECTION

Cardiac: Conduction disturbances or supraventricular tachyarrhythmias, such as atrioventricular (AV) block (Weckenbach), atrial tachycardia with or without block and junctional (nodal) tachycardia are the most common arrhythmias associated with digoxin toxicity in children. Ventricular arrhythmias, such as unifocal or multiform ventricular premature contractions especially in bigeminal or trigeminal patterns, are less common. Ventricular tachycardia may result from digitalis toxicity. Sinus bradycardia may also be a sign of impending digoxin intoxication, especially in infants, even in the absence of first degree heart block. Any arrhythmias or alteration in cardiac conduction that develops in a child taking digoxin should initially be assumed to be a consequence of digoxin intoxication.

CNS

Visual disturbances (blurred or yellow vision), headache, weakness, dizziness, apathy and psychosis can occur. These may be difficult to recognize in infants and children.

OVERDOSAGE:

TREATMENT OF ARRHYTHMIAS PRODUCED BY OVERDOSAGE

Adults: Digoxin should be discontinued until all signs of toxicity are gone. Discontinuation may be all that is necessary if toxic manifestations are not severe and appear only near the expected time for maximum effect of the drug.

Correction of factors that may contribute to toxicity such as electrolyte disturbances, hypoxia, acid-base disturbances and removal of aggravating agents such as catecholamines, should also be considered. Potassium salts may be indicated, particularly if hypokalemia is present. Potassium administration may be dangerous in the setting of massive digitalis overdosage (see Massive Digitalis Overdosage.) Potassium chloride in divided oral doses totaling 3 to 6 grams of the salt (40 to 80 mEq K+) for adults may be given provided renal function is adequate (see potassium recommendations in Infants and Children.)

When correction of the arrhythmia is urgent and the serum potassium concentration is low or normal, potassium should be administered intravenously in 5% dextrose injection. For adults, a total of 40 to 80 mEq (diluted to a concentration of 40 mEq per 500 ml) may be given at a rate not exceeding 20 mEq per hour, or slower if limited by pain due to local irritation. Additional amounts may be given if the arrhythmia is uncontrolled and potassium well-tolerated. ECG monitoring should be performed to watch for any evidence of potassium toxicity (*e.g.,* peaking of T waves) and to observe the effect on the arrhythmia. The infusion may be stopped when the desired effect is achieved.

Note: Potassium should not be used and may be dangerous in heart block due to digoxin, unless primarily related to supraventricular tachycardia.

Other agents that have been used for the treatment of digoxin intoxication include lidocaine, procainamide, propranolol and phenytoin, although use of the latter must be considered experimental. In advanced heart block, atropine and/or temporary ventricular pacing may be beneficial. Digibind, digoxin Immune Fab (Ovine), can be used to reverse potentially life-threatening digoxin (or digitoxin) intoxication. Improvement in signs and symptoms of digitalis toxicity usually begins within 1/2 hour of Digibind administration. Each 40 mg vial of Digibind will neutralize 0.6 mg of digoxin (which is a usual body store of an adequately digitalized 70 kg patient).

Infants and Children: See Adult section for general recommendations for the treatment of arrhythmias produced by overdosage and for cautions regarding the use of potassium.

If a potassium preparation is used to treat toxicity, it may be given orally in divided doses totaling 1 to 1.5 mEq K+ per kilogram (kg) body weight (1 gram of potassium chloride contains 13.4 mEq K+).

When correction of the arrhythmia with potassium is urgent, approximately 0.5 mEq/kg of potassium per hour may be given intravenously, with careful ECG monitoring. The intravenous solution of potassium should be dilute enough to avoid local irritation; however, especially in infants, care must be taken to avoid intravenous fluid overload.

Massive Digitalis Overdosage: Manifestations of life-threatening toxicity include severe ventricular arrhythmias such as ventricular tachycardia or ventricular fibrillation, or progressive bradyarrhythmias such as severe sinus bradycardia or second or third degree heart block not responsive to atropine. An overdosage of more than 10 mg of digoxin in previously healthy adults or 4 mg in previously healthy children or overdosage resulting in steady-state serum concentrations greater than 10 ng/ml, often results in cardiac arrest.

Severe digitalis intoxication can cause life-threatening elevation in serum potassium concentration by shifting potassium from inside to outside the cell resulting in hyperkalemia. Administration of potassium supplements in the setting of massive intoxication may be hazardous.

Digibind, digoxin Immune Fab (Ovine), may be used at a dose equimolar to digoxin in the body to reverse the effects of ingestion of a massive overdose. The decision to administer Digibind before the onset of toxic manifestations will depend on the likelihood that life-threatening toxicity will occur.

OVERDOSAGE: *(cont'd)*

Patients with massive digitalis ingestion should receive large doses of activated charcoal to prevent absorption and bind digoxin in the gut during enteroenteric recirculation. Emesis or gastric lavage may be indicated especially if ingestion has occurred within 30 minutes of the patient's presentation at the hospital. Emesis should not be induced in patients who are obtunded. If a patient presents more than 2 hours after ingestion or already has toxic manifestations, it may be unsafe to induce vomiting or attempt passage of a gastric tube, because such maneuvers may induce an acute vagal episode that can worsen digitalis-toxic arrhythmias.

DOSAGE AND ADMINISTRATION:

RECOMMENDED DOSAGES ARE AVERAGE VALUES THAT MAY REQUIRE CONSIDERABLE MODIFICATION BECAUSE OF INDIVIDUAL SENSITIVITY OR ASSOCIATED CONDITIONS. DIMINISHED RENAL FUNCTION IS THE MOST IMPORTANT FACTOR REQUIRING MODIFICATION OF RECOMMENDED DOSES.

DUE TO THE MORE COMPLETE ABSORPTION OF DIGOXIN FROM SOFT CAPSULES, RECOMMENDED ORAL DOSES ARE ONLY 80 PERCENT OF THOSE FOR TABLETS, ELIXIR AND IM INJECTION.

IN DECIDING THE DOSE OF DIGOXIN, SEVERAL FACTORS MUST BE CONSIDERED:

1. The disease being treated. Atrial arrhythmias may require larger doses than heart failure.

2. The body weight of the patient. Doses should be calculated based upon lean or ideal body weight.

3. The patient's renal function, preferably evaluated on the basis of creatinine clearance.

4. Age is an important factor in infants and children.

5. Concomitant disease states, drugs or other factors likely to alter the expected clinical response to digoxin (see PRECAUTIONS and DRUG INTERACTIONS).

DIGITALIZATION MAY BE ACCOMPLISHED BY EITHER OF TWO GENERAL APPROACHES THAT VARY IN DOSAGE AND FREQUENCY OF ADMINISTRATION, BUT REACH THE SAME ENDPOINT IN TERMS OF TOTAL AMOUNT OF DIGOXIN ACCUMULATED IN THE BODY.

1. Rapid digitalization may be achieved by administering a loading dose based upon projected peak body digoxin stores, then calculating the maintenance dose as a percentage of the loading dose.

2. More gradual digitalization may be obtained by beginning an appropriate maintenance dose, thus allowing digoxin body stores to accumulate slowly. Steady-state serum digoxin concentrations will be achieved in approximately 5 half-lives of the drug for the individual patient. Depending upon the patient's renal function, this will take between one and three weeks.

CAPSULES

Where compliance is considered a problem, single daily dosing may be appropriate.

Because the significance of the higher peak serum concentrations associated with once daily capsules is not established, divided daily dosing is presently recommended for:

1. Infants and children under 10 years of age;

2. Patients requiring a daily dose of 300 mcg (0.3 mg) or greater;

3. Patients with a previous history of digitalis toxicity;

4. Patients considered likely to become toxic;

5. Patients in whom compliance is not a problem.

INJECTIONS

Parenteral administration of digoxin should be used only when the need for rapid digitalization is urgent or when the drug cannot be taken orally. Intramuscular injection can lead to severe pain at the injection site, thus intravenous administration is preferred. If the drug must be administered by the intramuscular route, it should be injected deep into the muscle followed by massage. No more than 500 mcg (2 ml) should be injected into a single site.

Digoxin injections can be administered undiluted or diluted with a 4-fold greater volume of Sterile Water for Injection, 0.9% Sodium Chloride Injection or 5% Dextrose Injection. The use of less than a 4-fold volume of diluent could lead to the precipitation of the digoxin. Immediate use of the diluted product is recommended.

If tuberculin syringes are used to measure very small doses, one must be aware of the problem of inadvertent overadministration of digoxin. The syringe should not be *flushed* with the parenteral solution after its contents are expelled into an indwelling vascular catheter.

Slow infusion of digoxin injections is preferable to bolus administration. Rapid infusion of digitalis glycosides has been shown to cause systemic and coronary arteriolar constriction, which may be clinically undesirable. Caution is thus advised and digoxin injections should probably be administered over a period of five minutes or longer. Mixing of digoxin injections with other drugs in the same container or simultaneous administration in the same intravenous line is not recommended.

ADULTS

Rapid Digitalization with a Loading Dose: Peak body digoxin stores of 8 to 12 mcg/kg should provide therapeutic effect with minimum risk of toxicity in most patients with heart failure and normal sinus rhythm. Larger stores (10 to 15 mcg/kg) are often required for adequate control of ventricular rate in patients with atrial flutter or fibrillation. Because of altered digoxin distribution and elimination, projected peak body stores for patients with renal insufficiency should be conservative (*i.e.,* 6 to 10 mcg/kg) (see PRECAUTIONS.)

The loading dose should be based on the projected peak body stores and administered in several portions, with roughly half the total given as the first dose. Additional fractions of this planned total dose may be given at 6 to 8 hour intervals, **with careful assessment of clinical response before each additional dose.**

If the patient's clinical response necessitates a change from the calculated dose of digoxin, then calculation of the maintenance dose should be based upon the amount actually given.

Capsules: In previously undigitalized patients, a single initial dose of 400 to 600 mcg (0.4 to 0.6 mg) usually produces a detectable effect in 0.5 to 2 hours that becomes maximal in 2 to 6 hours. Additional doses of 100 to 300 mcg (0.1 to 0.3 mg) may be given cautiously at 6 to 8 hour intervals until clinical evidence of an adequate effect is noted. The usual amount of capsules that a 70 kg patient requires to achieve 8 to 15 mcg/kg peak body stores is 600 to 1000 mcg (0.6 to 1.0 mg).

Tablets: In previously undigitalized patients, a single initial dose of 500 to 700 mcg (0.5 to 0.75 mg) usually produces a detectable effect in 0.5 to 2 hours that becomes maximal in 2 to 6 hours. Additional doses of 125 to 375 mcg (0.125 to 0.375 mg) may be given cautiously at 6 to 8 hour intervals until clinical evidence of an adequate effect is noted. The usual amount that a 70 kg patient requires to achieve 8 to 15 mcg/kg peak body stores is 750 to 1250 mcg (0.75 to 1.25 mg)

Injection: In previously undigitalized patients, a single initial digoxin injection dose of 400 to 600 mcg (0.4 to 0.6 mg) usually produces a detectable effect in 5 to 30 minutes that becomes maximal in 1 to 4 hours. Additional doses of 100 to 300 mcg (0.1 to 0.3 mg) may be given

DOSAGE AND ADMINISTRATION: *(cont'd)*

cautiously at 4 to 8 hour intervals until clinical evidence of an adequate effect is noted. The usual amount of digoxin injection that a 70 kg patient requires to achieve 8 to 15 mcg/kg peak body stores is 600 to 1000 mcg (0.6 to 1.0 mg).

Although peak body stores are mathematically related to loading doses and are utilized to calculate maintenance doses, they do not correlate with measured serum concentrations. This discrepancy is caused by digoxin distribution within the body during the first 6 to 8 hours following a dose. Serum concentrations drawn during this time are usually not interpretable.

The maintenance dose should be based upon the percentage of the peak body stores lost each day through elimination. The formula in TABLE 3 has had wide clinical use.

TABLE 3

Maintenance Dose = [Peak Body Stores (*i.e.,* Loading Dose) × %: Daily: Loss] ÷ 100
Where: % Daily Loss = 14 + Ccr/5

Ccr is creatinine clearance, corrected to 70 kg body weight or 1.73 m^2 body surface area. *For adults,* if only serum creatinine concentrations (Scr) are available, a Ccr (corrected to 70 kg body weight) may be estimated in men as (140-Age)/Scr. For women, this result should be multiplied by 0.85.

Note: This equation cannot be used for estimating creatinine clearance in infants or children.

A common practice involves the use of digoxin injection to achieve rapid digitalization, with conversion to capsules or tablets for maintenance therapy. If patients are switched from IV to oral digoxin formulations, allowances must be made for differences in bioavailability when calculating maintenance dosages (see TABLE 1.)

Adults—Gradual Digitalization with a Maintenance Dose: TABLE 4 and TABLE 5 provide average daily maintenance dose requirements for patients with heart failure based upon lean body weight and renal function:

TABLE 4 Usual Digoxin Capsules Daily Maintenance Dose Requirements (mcg) For Estimated Peak Body Store's of 10 mcg/kg

Corrected Ccr (ml/min per 70 kg)	Lean Body Weight (kg/lbs) 50/ 110	60/ 132	70/ 154	80/ 176	90/ 198	100/ 220	Number of Days Before Steady-State Achieved
0	50	100	100	100	150	150	22
10	100	100	100	150	150	150	19
20	100	100	150	150	150	200	16
30	100	150	150	150	200	200	14
40	100	150	150	200	200	250	13
50	150	150	200	200	250	250	12
60	150	150	200	200	250	300	11
70	150	200	200	250	250	300	10
80	150	200	200	250	300	300	9
90	150	200	250	250	300	350	8
100	200	200	250	300	300	350	7

Example: Based on TABLE 4, a patient in heart failure with an estimated lean body weight of 70 kg and a Ccr of 60 ml/min, should be given 200 mcg (0.2 mg) per day, usually taken as a 100 mcg (0.1 mg) capsule after the morning and evening meals. Steady-state serum concentrations should not be anticipated before 11 days.

TABLE 5 Usual Daily Maintenance Dose Requirements (mcg) For Estimated Peak Body Store's of 10 mcg/kg

Corrected Ccr (ml/min per 70 kg)	Lean Body Weight (kg/lbs) 50/110	60/132	70/154	80/176	90/198	100/220	Number of Days Before Steady-State Achieved
0	63*†	125	125	125	188‡	188	22
10	125	125	125	188	188	188	19
20	125	125	188	188	188	250	16
30	125	188	188	188	250	250	14
40	125	188	188	250	250	250	13
50	188	188	250	250	250	250	12
60	188	188	250	250	250	375	11
70	188	250	250	250	250	375	10
80	188	250	250	250	375	375	9
90	188	250	250	250	375	500	8
100	250	250	250	375	375	500	7

* 63 mcg = 0.063 mg
† 1/2 of 125 mcg tablet or 125 mcg every other day
‡ = 1.5 of 125 mcg tablet

Example: Based on TABLE 5, a patient in heart failure with an estimated lean body weight of 70 kg and a Ccr of 60 ml/min, should be given 250 mcg (0.25 mg) per day, usually taken after the morning meal. Steady-state serum concentrations should not be anticipated before 11 days.

More gradual digitalization can also be accomplished by beginning an appropriate maintenance dose. The range of percentages provided above can be used in calculating this dose for patients with normal renal function. In children with renal disease, digoxin dosing must be carefully titrated based upon desired clinical response.

Long-term use of digoxin is indicated in many children who have been digitalized for acute heart failure, unless the cause is transient. Children with severe congenital heart disease, even after surgery, may require digoxin for prolonged periods.

It cannot be overemphasized that both the adult and pediatric dosage guidelines provided are based upon average patient response and substantial individual variation can be expected. Accordingly, ultimate dosage selection must be based upon clinical assessment of the patient.

SERUM DIGOXIN CONCENTRATIONS

Measurement of serum digoxin concentrations can be helpful to the clinician in determining the state of digitalization and in assigning certain probabilities to the likelihood of digoxin intoxication. Studies in adults considered adequately digitalized (without evidence of toxicity) show that about two-thirds of such patients have serum digoxin levels ranging from 0.8 to 2.0 ng/ml. Patients with atrial fibrillation or atrial flutter require and appear to tolerate higher levels than do patients with other indications. On the other hand, in adult patients with clinical evidence of digoxin toxicity, about two-thirds will have serum digoxin levels greater than 2.0 ng/ml. Thus, whereas levels less than 0.8 ng/ml are infrequently associated with toxicity, levels greater than 2.0 ng/ml are often associated with toxicity. Values in between are not very helpful in deciding whether a certain sign or symptom is more likely caused by digoxin toxicity or by something else. There are rare patients who are unable to tolerate digoxin even at serum concentrations below 0.8 ng/ml. Some researchers suggest that infants and young children tolerate slightly higher serum concentrations than do adults.

DOSAGE AND ADMINISTRATION: *(cont'd)*

To allow adequate time for equilibration of digoxin between serum and tissue, **sampling of serum concentrations for clinical use should be at least 6 to 8 hours after the last dose,** regardless of the route of administration or formulation used. On a twice daily dosing schedule, there will be only minor differences in serum digoxin concentrations whether sampling is done at 8 or 12 hours after a dose. After a single daily dose, the concentration will be 10 to 25% lower when sampled at 24 versus 8 hours, depending upon the patient's renal function. Ideally, sampling for assessment of steady-state concentrations should be done just before the next dose.

If a discrepancy exists between the reported serum concentration and the observed clinical response, the clinician should consider the following possibilities:

1. Analytical problems in the assay procedure.

2. Inappropriate serum sampling time.

3. Administration of a digitalis glycoside other than digoxin.

4. Conditions (described in WARNINGS and PRECAUTIONS) causing an alteration in the sensitivity of the patient to digoxin.

5. The patient falls outside the norm in his response to or handling of digoxin. This decision should only be reached after exclusion of the other possibilities and generally should be confirmed by additional correlations of clinical observations with serum digoxin concentrations.

The serum concentration data should always be interpreted in the overall clinical context and an isolated serum concentration value should not be used alone as a basis for increasing or decreasing digoxin dosage.

Adjustment of Maintenance Dose in Previously Digitalized Patients: Maintenance doses in individual patients on steady-state digoxin can be adjusted upward or downward in proportion to the ratio of the desired versus the measured serum concentration. For example:

Capsules: A patient at steady-state on 100 mcg (0.1 mg) of digoxin capsules per day with a measured serum concentration of 0.7 ng/ml, should have the dose increased to 200 mcg (0.2 mg) per day to achieve a steady-state serum concentration of 1.4 ng/ml,*

Tablets and Pediatric Elixir: A patient at steady-state on 125 mcg (0.125 g) per day with a measured serum concentration of 0.7 ng/ml, should have the dose increased to 250 mcg (0.25 mg) per day to achieve a steady-state serum concentration of 1.4 ng/ml,*

Injection and Pediatric Injection: A patient at steady-state on 100 mcg (0.1 mg) of Digoxin injection per day with a measured serum concentration of 0.7 ng/ml, should have the dose increased to 200 mcg (0.2 mg) per day to achieve a steady state-serum concentration of 1.4 ng/ml,*

***Assuming the serum digoxin concentration measurement is correct, renal function remains stable during this time and the needed adjustment is not the result of a problem with compliance.**

Dosage Adjustment When Changing Preparations: The difference in bioavailability between injectable digoxin, digoxin capsules, tablets, and pediatric elixir must be considered when changing patients from one dosage form to another.

Digoxin injection and capsules of 100 mcg (0.1 mg) and 200 mcg (0.2 mg) are approximately equivalent to 125 mcg (0.125 mg) and 250 mcg (0.25 mg) doses of digoxin tablets and elixir pediatric (see TABLE 1.) Intramuscular injection of digoxin is extremely painful and offers no advantages unless other routes of administration are contraindicated.

INFANTS AND CHILDREN

Digitalization must be individualized. Divided daily dosing is recommended for infants and young children. In these patients, where dosage adjustment is frequent and outside the fixed dosages available, digoxin capsules may not be the formulation of choice. Children over 10 years of age require adult dosages in proportion to their body weight.

In the newborn period, renal clearance of digoxin is diminished and suitable dosage adjustments must be observed. This is especially pronounced in the premature infant. Beyond the immediate newborn period, children generally require proportionally larger doses than adults on the basis of body weight or body surface area.

Rapid Digitalization With a Loading Dose: Digoxin injection pediatric can be used to achieve rapid digitalization, with conversion to an oral formulation for maintenance therapy. If patients are switched from IV to oral digoxin tablets or elixir, allowances must be made for differences in bioavailability when calculating maintenance dosages (see TABLE 1) and dosing tables TABLE 6, TABLE 7, TABLE 8, TABLE 9.

Intramuscular injection of digoxin is extremely painful and offers no advantages unless other routes of administration are contraindicated.

Digitalizing and daily maintenance doses for each age group are given below and should provide therapeutic effect with minimum risk of toxicity in most patients with heart failure and normal sinus rhythm. Larger doses are often required for adequate control of ventricular rate in patients with atrial flutter or fibrillation.

The loading dose should be administered in several portions, with roughly half the total given as the first dose. Additional fractions of this planned total dose may be given at 6 to 8 hour intervals, **with careful assessment of clinical response before each additional dose.** If the patient's clinical response necessitates a change from the calculated dose of digoxin, then calculation of the maintenance dose should be based upon the amount actually given.

TABLE 6 Regular Injection And Capsules Usual Digitalizing and Maintenance Dosages in Children with Normal Renal Function Based on Lean Body Weight

Age	Digitalizing* Dose (mcg/kg)	Daily† Maintenance Dose (mcg/kg)
2-5 Years	25-35	25-35% of the oral or IV loading dose‡
5-10 Years	15-30	
Over 10 Years	8-12	

* IV digitalizing doses are 80% of oral digitizing doses
† Divided daily dosing recommended for children under 10 years of age.
‡ Projected or actual digitalizing dose providing desired clinical response.

TABLE 7 Usual Digitalizing and Maintenance Dosages for in Children with Normal Renal Function Based on Lean Body Weight

Age	Digitalizing* Dose (mcg/kg)	Daily† Maintenance Dose (mcg/kg)
2-5 Years	30-40	25-35% of the oral loading dose‡
5-10 Years	20-35	
Over 10 Years	10-15	

* IV digitalizing doses are the 80% of oral digitalizing doses.
† Divided daily dosing recommended for children under 10 years of age.
‡ Projected or actual digitalizing dose providing desired clinical response.

DOSAGE AND ADMINISTRATION: *(cont'd)*

TABLE 8 Usual Digitalizing and Maintenance Dosages in Children with Normal Renal Function Based on Lean Body Weight

Age	Digitalizing* Dose (mcg/kg)	Daily†IV Maintenance Dose (mcg/kg)
Premature	15 to 25	20 to 30% of IV loading dose
Full-Term	20 to 30	
1 to 24 Months	30 to 50	
2 to 5 Years	25 to 35	
5 to 10 Years	15 to 30	25-35% of the IV loading dose
Over 10 Years	8 to 12	

* IV digitalizing doses are the same as capsules digitalizing doses.
† Divided daily dosing is recommended for children under 10 years of age.
‡ Projected or actual digitalizing dose providing desired clinical response.

TABLE 9 Usual Digitalizing and Maintenance Dosages in Children with Normal Renal Function Based on Lean Body Weight

Age	Digitalizing* Dose (mcg/kg)	Daily† Maintenance Dose (mcg/kg)
Premature	20 to 30	20 to 30% of*oral* loading dose‡
Full-Term	25 to 35	
1 to 24 Months	35 to 60	
2 to 5 Years	30 to 40	
5 to 10 Years	20 to 35	25-35% of the*oral* loading dose‡
Over 10 Years	10 to 15	

* IV digitalizing doses are the same as capsules digitalizing doses.
† Divided daily dosing is recommended for children under 10 years of age.
‡ Projected or actual digitalizing dose providing desired clinical response.

Gradual Digitalization With a Maintenance Dose: More gradual digitalization can also be accomplished by beginning an appropriate maintenance dose. The range of percentages provided above can be used in calculating this dose for patients with normal renal function. In children with renal disease, digoxin dosing must be carefully titrated based upon clinical response.

Long term use of digoxin is indicated in many children who have been digitalized for acute heart failure, unless the cause is transient. Children with severe congenital heart disease, even after surgery, may require digoxin for prolonged periods.

It cannot be overemphasized that both the adult and pediatric dosage guidelines provided are based upon average patient response and substantial individual variation can be expected. Accordingly, ultimate dosage selection must be based upon clinical assessment of the patient.

Adjustment of Maintenance Dose in Previously Digitized Patients: Refer to this section above (Adults).

PEDIATRIC INJECTION

Parenteral administration of digoxin should be used only when the need for rapid digitalization is urgent or when the drug cannot be taken orally. Intramuscular injection can lead to severe pain at the injection site, thus intravenous administration is preferred. If the drug must be administered by the intramuscular route, it should be injected deep into the muscle followed by massage. No more than 200 or 2 ml (pediatric injection) should be injected into a single site.

STORE AT 15 TO 25œC (59 TO 77œF) AND PROTECT FROM LIGHT.

PATIENT INFORMATION:

Digoxin is used for the treatment of congestive heart failure and for irregular heartbeat. Notify your physician if you are pregnant or nursing. Do not stop taking digoxin without talking with your physician. Digoxin may be taken with or without food. It should be taken at approximately the same time each morning. Do not take over-the-counter antacids, cough, cold, allergy or diet medications without notifying your physician and pharmacist. Notify your physician if you develop an irregular heartbeat, trouble breathing, skin rash, nausea, diarrhea, blurred or yellow vision, or unusual weakness or tiredness.

HOW SUPPLIED - RATED THERAPEUTICALLY EQUIVALENT:

Injection, Solution - Intramuscular; - 0.1 mg/ml

1 ml ampul x 10	**$56.63**	**LANOXIN PEDIATRIC, Glaxo Wellcome**	**00173-0262-10**

Injection, Solution - Intramuscular; - 0.25 mg/ml

1 ml x 10	$22.94	Digoxin, Wyeth Labs	00008-0480-02
2 ml ampul x 10	**$23.58**	**LANOXIN, Glaxo Wellcome**	**00173-0260-10**
2 ml ampul x 50	**$96.30**	**LANOXIN, Glaxo Wellcome**	**00173-0260-35**
2 ml x 10	$23.29	Digoxin, Wyeth Labs	00008-0480-01
2 ml x 25	$25.99	Digoxin, Elkins Sinn	00641-1410-35

Tablet, Uncoated - Oral - 0.125 mg

1000's	$31.95	Digoxin, Harber Pharm	51432-0467-06

HOW SUPPLIED - NOT RATED EQUIVALENT:

Capsule, Elastic - Oral - 0.05 mg

100's	$17.04	LANOXICAPS, Glaxo Wellcome	00173-0270-55

Capsule, Elastic - Oral - 0.1 mg

30's	$8.11	LANOXICAPS, Glaxo Wellcome	00173-0272-30
100's	$18.60	LANOXICAPS, Glaxo Wellcome	00173-0272-55

Capsule, Elastic - Oral - 0.2 mg

30's	$9.94	LANOXICAPS, Glaxo Wellcome	00173-0274-30
100's	$21.64	LANOXICAPS, Glaxo Wellcome	00173-0274-55

Elixir - Oral - 0.05 mg/ml

2.5 ml x 40	$41.93	Digoxin, Roxane	00054-8192-16
5 ml x 40	$62.30	Digoxin, Roxane	00054-8193-16
60 ml	$10.40	Digoxin, Roxane	00054-3192-46
60 ml	$14.45	Digoxin, Liquipharm	54198-0148-02
60 ml	**$21.26**	**LANOXIN PEDIATRIC, Glaxo Wellcome**	**00173-0264-27**

Tablet, Uncoated - Oral - 0.125 mg

30's	$2.40	Digoxin, Talbert Phcy	44514-0498-18
30's	**$7.19**	**LANOXIN, Glaxo Wellcome**	**00173-0242-30**
100's	$7.99	Digoxin, Talbert Phcy	44514-0498-88
100's	$9.52	Digoxin, HL Moore Drug Exch	00839-7641-06
100's	$9.57	Digoxin, Rugby	00536-5708-01
100's	$11.00	Digoxin, Voluntary Hosp	53258-0216-13

HOW SUPPLIED - NOT RATED EQUIVALENT: *(cont'd)*

100's	$13.64	Digoxin, Vangard Labs	00615-0547-13
100's	**$14.03**	**LANOXIN, Glaxo Wellcome**	**00173-0242-55**
100's	$15.50	Digoxin, Raway	00686-0547-13
100's	**$19.58**	**LANOXIN, Glaxo Wellcome**	**00173-0242-56**
600's	**$125.40**	**LANOXIN, Medirex**	**57480-0343-06**
750's	$105.00	DIGOXIN, Glasgow Pharm	60809-0155-55
750's	$105.00	DIGOXIN, Glasgow Pharm	60809-0155-72
1000's	$27.95	Digoxin, Parmed Pharms	00349-8716-10
1000's	$31.45	Digoxin, Major Pharms	00904-2061-80
1000's	$34.20	Digoxin, Aligen Independ	00405-4335-03
1000's	$34.20	Digoxin, Qualitest Pharms	00603-3314-32
1000's	$34.20	Digoxin, Halsey Drug	00879-0125-10
1000's	$35.55	Digoxin, IDE-Interstate	00814-2479-30
1000's	$73.54	Digoxin, Rugby	00536-5708-10
1000's	$74.90	Digoxin, Major Pharms	00904-7944-80
1000's	$75.90	Digoxin, Goldline Labs	00182-1336-10
1000's	$88.69	Digoxin, HL Moore Drug Exch	00839-7641-16
1000's	**$107.82**	**LANOXIN, Glaxo Wellcome**	**00173-0242-75**
5000's	$157.05	Digoxin, Halsey Drug	00879-0125-51
5000's	$418.50	Digoxin, HL Moore Drug Exch	00839-7641-20

Tablet, Uncoated - Oral - 0.25 mg

30's	$2.26	Digoxin, Talbert Phcy	44514-0499-18
30's	$2.60	Digoxin, Major Pharms	00904-2058-46
30's	**$7.19**	**LANOXIN, Glaxo Wellcome**	**00173-0249-30**
100's	$7.54	Digoxin (B-W), Talbert Phcy	44514-0499-88
100's	$9.52	Digoxin, HL Moore Drug Exch	00839-1247-06
100's	$9.57	Digoxin, Rugby	00536-5709-01
100's	$11.00	Digoxin, Voluntary Hosp	53258-0217-13
100's	$13.64	Digoxin, Vangard Labs	00615-0518-13
100's	**$14.03**	**LANOXIN, Glaxo Wellcome**	**00173-0249-55**
100's	$16.00	Digoxin, Raway	00686-0518-13
100's	**$19.58**	**LANOXIN, Glaxo Wellcome**	**00173-0249-56**
600's	**$132.00**	**LANOXIN, Medirex**	**57480-0344-06**
750's	$110.00	DIGOXIN, Glasgow Pharm	60809-0156-55
750's	$110.00	DIGOXIN, Glasgow Pharm	60809-0156-72
1000's	$26.25	Digoxin, C O Truxton	00463-6084-10
1000's	$27.60	Digoxin, Aligen Independ	00405-4334-03
1000's	$29.00	Digoxin, Parmed Pharms	00349-8715-10
1000's	$32.75	Digoxin, United Res	00677-0058-10
1000's	$32.80	Digoxin, Major Pharms	00904-2058-80
1000's	$32.95	Digoxin, Harber Pharm	51432-0150-06
1000's	$35.65	Digoxin, Genetco	00302-1850-10
1000's	$35.65	Digoxin, Qualitest Pharms	00603-3313-32
1000's	$35.65	Digoxin, Halsey Drug	00879-0250-10
1000's	$39.45	Digoxin, IDE-Interstate	00814-2480-30
1000's	$73.54	Digoxin, Rugby	00536-5709-10
1000's	$74.90	Digoxin, Major Pharms	00904-7945-80
1000's	$75.90	Digoxin, Goldline Labs	00182-0531-10
1000's	$88.69	Digoxin, HL Moore Drug Exch	00839-1247-16
1000's	**$107.82**	**LANOXIN, Glaxo Wellcome**	**00173-0249-75**
1200's	**$127.27**	**LANOXIN, Glaxo Wellcome**	**00173-0249-01**
5000's	$82.00	Digoxin, Rugby	00536-3740-50
5000's	$163.95	Digoxin, Halsey Drug	00879-0250-51
5000's	$418.50	Digoxin, HL Moore Drug Exch	00839-1247-20
5000's	**$508.84**	**LANOXIN, Glaxo Wellcome**	**00173-0249-80**

Tablet, Uncoated - Oral - 0.5 mg

100's	**$25.00**	**LANOXIN, Glaxo Wellcome**	**00173-0253-55**

DIGOXIN IMMUNE FAB (OVINE) *(001062)*

CATEGORIES: Antagonists and Antidotes; Antidotes; Antiserum; Arrhythmia; Biologicals; Fibrillation; Orphan Drugs; Tachycardia; Pregnancy Category C; FDA Pre 1938 Drugs

BRAND NAMES: **Digibind**; *Digidot* (France); *Digitalis Antidot*; *Digitalis Antidot BM* (Germany); *Digitalis-Antidot BM*; *Digoxin Immune FAB (Ovine) Digibind (International brand names outside U.S. in italics)*

DESCRIPTION:

Digibind, digoxin immune fab (ovine), is a sterile lyophilized powder of antigen binding fragments (Fab) derived from specific antidigoxin antibodies raised in sheep. Production of antibodies specific for digoxin involves conjugation of digoxin as a hapten to human albumin. Sheep are immunized with this material to produce antibodies specific for the antigenic determinants of the digoxin molecule. The antibody is then papain digested and digoxin-specific Fab fragments of the antibody are isolated and purified by affinity chromatography. These antibody fragments have a molecular weight of approximately 50,000.

Each vial, which will bind approximately 0.6 mg of digoxin (or digitoxin), contains 40 mg of digoxin-specific Fab fragments derived from sheep plus 75 mg of sorbitol as a stabilizer and 28 mg of sodium chloride. The vial contains no preservatives.

Digibind is administered by intravenous injection after reconstitution with Sterile Water for Injection (4 ml per vial).

CLINICAL PHARMACOLOGY:

After intravenous injection of digoxin immune fab (ovine) in the baboon, digoxin-specific fab fragments are excreted in the urine with a biological half-life of about 9 to 13 hours.[1] In humans with normal renal function the half-life appears to be 15 to 20 hours.[2] Experimental studies in animals indicate that these antibody fragments have a large volume of distribution in the extracellular space, unlike whole antibody which distributes in a space only about twice the plasma volume.[1] Ordinarily, following administration of digoxin immune fab (ovine), improvement in signs and symptoms of digitalis intoxication begins within one-half hour or less.[2,3,4,5]

The affinity of digoxin immune fab (ovine) for digoxin is in the range of 10^9 to 10^{10} M^{-1}, which is greater than the affinity of digoxin for (sodium, potassium) ATPase, the presumed receptor for its toxic effects. The affinity of igibind for digitoxin is about 10^8 to 10^9 M^{-1}.[5]

Digoxin immune fab (ovine) binds molecules of digoxin, making them unavailable for binding at their site of action on cells in the body. The fab fragment-digoxin complex accumulates in the blood, from which it is excreted by the kidney. The net effect is to shift the equilibrium away from binding of digoxin to its receptors in the body, thereby reversing its effects.

INDICATIONS AND USAGE:

Digoxin immune fab (ovine), is indicated for treatment of potentially life-threatening digoxin intoxication.[3] Although designed specifically to treat life-threatening digoxin overdose, it has also been used successfully to treat life-threatening digitoxin overdose.[3] Since human experience is limited and the consequences of repeated exposures are unknown, digoxin immune fab (ovine) is not indicated for milder cases of digitalis toxicity.

Manifestations of life-threatening toxicity include severe ventricular arrhythmias such as ventricular tachycardia or ventricular fibrillation, or progressive bradyarrhythmias such as severe sinus bradycardia or second or third degree heart block not responsive to atropine.

Ingestion of more than 10 mg of digoxin in previously healthy adults or 4 mg of digoxin in previously healthy children, or ingestion causing steady-state serum concentrations greater than 10 ng/ml, often results in cardiac arrest. Digitalis-induced progressive elevation of the serum potassium concentration also suggests imminent cardiac arrest. If the potassium concentration exceeds 5 mEq/L in the setting of severe digitalis intoxication, digoxin immune fab (ovine) therapy is indicated.

CONTRAINDICATIONS:

There are no known contraindications to the use of digoxin immune fab (ovine).

WARNINGS:

Suicidal ingestion often involves more than one drug; thus, toxicity from other drugs should not be overlooked.

One should consider the possibility of anaphylactic, hypersensitivity or febrile reactions. If an anaphylactoid reaction occurs, the drug infusion should be discontinued and appropriate therapy initiated using aminophylline, oxygen, volume expansion, diphenhydramine, corticosteroids and airway management as indicated. The need for epinephrine should be balanced against its potential risk in the setting of digitalis toxicity.

Since the fab fragment of the antibody lacks the antigenic determinants of the Fc fragment, it should pose less of an immunogenic threat to patients than does an intact immunoglobulin molecule. Patients with known allergies would be particularly at risk, as would individuals who have previously received antibodies or fab fragments raised in sheep. Papain is used to cleave the whole antibody into fab and Fc fragments, and traces of papain or inactivated papain residues may be present in digoxin immune fab (ovine). Patients with allergies to papain, chymopapain, or other papaya extracts also may be particularly at risk.

Skin testing for allergy was performed during the clinical investigation of digoxin immune fab (ovine). Only one patient developed erythema at the site of skin testing, with no accompanying wheal reaction; this individual had no adverse reaction to systemic treatment with digoxin immune fab (ovine). Since allergy testing can delay urgently needed therapy, it is not routinely required before treatment of life-threatening digitalis toxicity with digoxin immune fab (ovine).

Skin testing may be appropriate for high risk individuals, especially patients with known allergies or those previously treated with digoxin immune fab (ovine). The intradermal skin test can be performed by: 1. Diluting 0.1 ml of reconstituted digoxin immune fab (ovine) (10 mg/ml) in 9.9 ml sterile isotonic saline (1:100 dilution, 100 mcg/ml). 2. Injecting 0.1 ml of the 1:100 dilution (10 mcg) intradermally and observing for an urticarial wheal surrounded by a zone of erythema. The test should be read at 20 minutes.

The scratch test procedure is performed by placing one drop of a 1:100 dilution of digoxin immune fab (ovine) on the skin and then making a $\frac{1}{4}$-inch scratch through the drop with a sterile needle. The scratch site is inspected at 20 minutes for an urticarial wheal surrounded by erythema.

If skin testing causes a systemic reaction, a tourniquet should be applied above the site of testing and measures to treat anaphylaxis should be instituted. Further administration of digoxin immune fab (ovine) should be avoided unless its use is absolutely essential, in which case the patient should be pretreated with corticosteroids and diphenhydramine. The physician should be prepared to treat anaphylaxis.

PRECAUTIONS:

GENERAL

Standard therapy for digitalis intoxication includes withdrawal of the drug and correction of factors that may contribute to toxicity, such as electrolyte disturbances, hypoxia, acid-base disturbances and agents such as catecholamines. Also, treatment of arrhythmias may include judicious potassium supplements, lidocaine, phenytoin, procainamide and/or propranolol treatment of sinus bradycardia or atrioventricular block may involve atropine or pacemaker insertion. Massive digitalis intoxication can cause hyperkalemia; administration of potassium supplements in the setting of massive intoxication may be hazardous (see Laboratory Tests). After treatment with digoxin immune fab (ovine), the serum potassium concentration may drop rapidly[2] and must be monitored frequently, especially over the first several hours after digoxin immune fab (ovine) is given (see Laboratory Tests).

The elimination half-life in the setting of renal failure has not been clearly defined. Patients with renal dysfunction have been successfully treated with digoxin immune fab (ovine).[4] There is no evidence to suggest the time-course of therapeutic effect is any different in these patients than in patients with normal renal function, but excretion of the fab fragment-digoxin complex from the body is probably delayed. In patients who are functionally anephric, one would anticipate failure to clear the fab fragment-digoxin complex from the blood by glomerular filtration and renal excretion. Whether failure to eliminate the fab fragment-digoxin complex in severe renal failure can lead to reintoxication following release of newly unbound digoxin into the blood is uncertain. Such patients should be monitored for a prolonged period for possible recurrence of digitalis toxicity.

Patients with intrinsically poor cardiac function may deteriorate from withdrawal of the inotropic action of digoxin. Studies in animals have shown that the reversal of inotropic effect is relatively gradual, occurring over hours. When needed, additional support can be provided by use of intravenous inotropes, such as dopamine or dobutamine, or vasodilators. One must be careful in using catecholamines not to aggravate digitalis toxic rhythm disturbances. Clearly, other types of digitalis glycosides should not be used in this setting.

Redigitalization should be postponed, if possible, until the fab fragments have been eliminated from the body, which may require several days. Patients with impaired renal function may require a week or longer.

LABORATORY TESTS

Digoxin immune fab (ovine) will interfere with digitalis immunoassay measurements.[7] Thus, the standard serum digoxin concentration measurement can be clinically misleading until the fab fragment is eliminated from the body.

Serum digoxin or digitoxin concentration should be obtained before digoxin immune fab (ovine) administration if at all possible. These measurements may be difficult to interpret if drawn soon after the last digitalis dose, since at least 6 to 8 hours are required for equilibration of digoxin between serum and tissue. Patients should be closely monitored, including temperature, blood pressure, electrocardiogram and potassium concentration, during and after administration of digoxin immune fab (ovine). The total serum digoxin

PRECAUTIONS: *(cont'd)*

concentration may rise precipitously following administration of digoxin immune fab (ovine) but this will be almost entirely bound to the fab fragment and therefore not able to react with receptors in the body.

Potassium concentrations should be followed carefully. Severe digitalis intoxication can cause life-threatening elevation in serum potassium concentration by shifting potassium from inside to outside the cell. The elevation in serum potassium concentration can lead to increased renal excretion of potassium. Thus, these patients may have hyperkalemia with a total body deficit of potassium. When the effect of digitalis is reversed by digoxin immune fab (ovine), potassium shifts back inside the cell, with a resulting decline in serum potassium concentration.[4] Hypokalemia may thus develop rapidly. For these reasons, serum potassium concentration should be monitored repeatedly, especially over the first several hours after digoxin immune fab (ovine) is given, and cautiously treated when necessary.

Carcinogenesis, Mutagenesis, and Impairment of Fertility: There have been no long-term studies performed in animals to evaluate carcinogenic potential.

Pregnancy Category C: Animal reproduction studies have not been conducted with digoxin immune fab (ovine). It is also not known whether digoxin immune fab (ovine) can cause fetal harm when administered to a pregnant woman or can affect reproduction capacity. digoxin immune fab (ovine) should be given to a pregnant woman only if clearly needed.

Nursing Mothers: It is not known whether this drug is excreted in human milk. Because many drugs are excreted in human milk, caution should be exercised when digoxin immune fab (ovine) is administered to a nursing woman.

Pediatric Use: Digoxin immune fab (ovine) has been successfully used in infants with no apparent adverse sequelae. As in all other circumstances, use of this drug in infants should be based on careful consideration of the benefits of the drug balanced against the potential risk involved.

ADVERSE REACTIONS:

Allergic reactions to digoxin immune fab (ovine) have been reported rarely. Patients with a history of allergy, especially to antibiotics, appear to be at particular risk (see WARNINGS). In a few instances, low cardiac output states and congestive heart failure could have been exacerbated by withdrawal of the inotropic effects of digitalis. Hypokalemia may occur from re-activation of (sodium, potassium) ATPase (see Laboratory Tests). Patients with atrial fibrillation may develop a rapid ventricular response from withdrawal of the effects of digitalis on the atrioventricular node.[4]

DOSAGE AND ADMINISTRATION:

GENERAL GUIDELINES

The dosage of digoxin immune fab (ovine) varies according to the amount of digoxin (or digitoxin) to be neutralized. The average dose used during clinical testing was 10 vials.

Dosage for Acute Ingestion of Unknown Amount: Twenty (20) vials (800 mg) of digoxin immune fab (ovine) is adequate to treat most life-threatening ingestions in **both adults and children.** However, in children it is important to monitor for volume overload. In general, a large digoxin immune fab (ovine) dose has a faster onset of effect but may enhance the possibility of a febrile reaction. The physician may consider administering 10 vials, observing the patient's response, and following with an additional 10 vials if clinically indicated.

Dosage for Toxicity During Chronic Therapy: For adults, 6 vials (240 mg) usually is adequate to reverse most cases of toxicity. This dose can be used in patients who are in acute distress or for whom a serum digoxin or digitoxin concentration is not available. In infants and small children (≤20 kg) a single vial usually should suffice.

Methods for calculating the dose of digoxin immune fab (ovine) required to neutralize the known or estimated amount of digoxin or digitoxin in the body are given below (see Dosage Calculation).

When determining the dose for digoxin immune fab (ovine), the following guidelines should be considered:

Erroneous calculations may result from inaccurate estimates of the amount of digitalis ingested or absorbed or from nonsteady-state serum digitalis concentrations. Inaccurate serum digitalis concentration measurements are a possible source of error. Most serum digoxin assay kits are designed to measure values less than 5 ng/ml. Dilution of samples is required to obtain accurate measures above 5 ng/ml.

Dosage calculations are based on a steady-state volume of distribution of approximately 6L/kg for digoxin (0.6 L/kg for digitoxin) to convert serum digitalis concentration to the amount of digitalis in the body. The conversion is based on the principle that body load equals drug steady-state serum concentration multiplied by volume of distribution. These volumes are population averages and vary widely among individuals. Many patients may require higher doses for complete neutralization. Doses should ordinarily be rounded up to the next whole vial.

If toxicity has not adequately reversed after several hours or appears to recur, readministration of digoxin immune fab (ovine) at a dose guided by clinical judgment may be required.

Failure to respond to digoxin immune fab (ovine) raises the possibility that the clinical problem is not caused by digitalis intoxication. If there is no response to an adequate dose of digoxin immune fab (ovine), the diagnosis of digitalis toxicity should be questioned.

DOSAGE AND CALCULATION

Acute Ingestion of Known Amount: Each vial of digoxin immune fab (ovine) contains 40 mg of purified digoxin-specific fab fragments which will bind approximately 0.6 mg of digoxin (or digitoxin). Thus one can calculate the total number of vials required by dividing the total digitalis body load in mg by 0.6 mg/vial (see TABLE 1.)

For toxicity from an acute ingestion, total body load in milligrams will be approximately equal to the amount ingested in milligrams for digoxin capsules and digitoxin, or the amount ingested in milligrams multiplied by 0.80 (to account for incomplete absorption) for digoxin tablets.

TABLE 2 gives dosage estimates in number of vials for **adults and children** who have ingested a single large dose of digoxin and for whom the approximate number of tablets or capsules is known. The digoxin immune fab (ovine) dose (in number of vials) represented in TABLE 2 can be approximated using the formula in TABLE 1:

TABLE 1 FORMULA 1

$$\text{Dose (in \# of vials)} = \frac{\text{Total digitalis body load in mg}}{\text{0.6 mg of digitalis bound/vial}}$$

Calculations Based on Steady-State Serum Digoxin Concentrations: TABLE 3 gives dosage estimates in number of vials for **adult patients** for whom a steady-state serum digoxin concentration is known. The digoxin immune fab (ovine) dose (in number of vials) represented in TABLE 2 can be approximated using Formula 2:

FORMULA 2 Dose (in # of vials) = [(Serum digoxin concentration in ng/ml) (weight in kg)] ÷ 100

DOSAGE AND ADMINISTRATION: *(cont'd)*

TABLE 2 Approximate Digoxin Immune Fab (Ovine) Dose for Reversal of a Single Large Digoxin Overdose

Number of Digoxin Tablets or Capsules Ingested*	Digoxin Immune Fab (Ovine) Dose # of Vials
25	9
50	17
75	25
100	34
150	50
200	67

* 0.25 mg tablets with 80% bioavailability or 0.2 mg digoxin capsules with 100% bioavailability.

TABLE 3 Adult Dose Estimate of Digoxin Immune Fab (Ovine) (in # of vials) from Steady-State Serum Digoxin Concentration

Patient Weight (kg)	Serum Digoxin Concentration (ng/ml) 1	2	4	8	12	16	20
40	0.5 V	1 V	2 V	3 V	5 V	7 V	8 V
60	0.5 V	1 V	3 V	5 V	7 V	10 V	12 V
70	1 V	2 V	3 V	6 V	9 V	11 V	14 V
80	1 V	2 V	3 V	7 V	10 V	13 V	16 V
100	1 V	2 V	4 V	8 V	12 V	16 V	20 V

V = vials

TABLE 4 gives dosage estimates in milligrams **for infants and small children** based on the steady-state serum digoxin concentration. The digoxin immune fab (ovine) dose represented in TABLE 4 can be estimated by multiplying the dose (in number of vials) calculated form FORMULA 2 by the amount of digoxin immune fab (ovine) contained in a vial (40 mg/vial) (see FORMULA 3.) Since infants and small children can have much smaller dosage requirements, it is recommended that the 40 mg vial be reconstituted as directed and administered with a tuberculin syringe. For very small doses, a reconstituted vial can be diluted with 36 ml of sterile isotonic saline to achieve a concentration of 1 mg/ml.

FORMULA 3 Dose (in mg) = (Dose (in # of vials)) (40 mg/vial)

TABLE 4 Infants and Small Children: Dose Estimates of Digoxin Immune Fab (Ovine) (in mg) from Steady-State Serum Digoxin Concentration

Patient Weight (Kg)	Serum Digoxin Concentration (ng/ml) 1	2	4	8	12	16	20
1	0.4* mg	1* mg	1.5* mg	3* mg	5 mg	7 mg	8 mg
3	1* mg	3* mg	5 mg	10 mg	15 mg	19 mg	24 mg
5	2* mg	4 mg	8 mg	16 mg	24 mg	32 mg	40 mg
10	4 mg	8 mg	16 mg	32 mg	48 mg	64 mg	80 mg
20	8 mg	16 mg	32 mg	64 mg	96 mg	128 mg	160 mg

* Dilution of reconstituted vial to 1 mg/ml may be desirable.

Calculation Based on Steady-State Digitoxin Concentration: The digoxin immune fab (ovine) dose for digitoxin toxicity can be approximated using the formula (FORMULA 4)

FORMULA 4 Dose (in # of vials) = [(Serum Digitoxin concentration in ng/ml) (weight in kg)] ÷ 1000

If the dose based on ingested amount differs substantially from that calculated from the serum digoxin or digitoxin concentration, it may be preferable to use the higher dose.

Administration:

The contents in each vial to be used should be dissolved with 4 ml of Sterile Water for Injection, by gentle mixing, to give a clear, colorless, approximately isosmotic solution with a protein concentration of 10 mg/ml. Reconstituted product should be used promptly. If it is not used immediately, it may be stored under refrigeration at 2° to 8°C (36° to 46°F) for up to 4 hours. The reconstituted product may be diluted with sterile isotonic saline to a convenient volume. Parenteral drug products should be inspected visually for particulate matter and discoloration prior to administration, whenever solution and container permit.

Digoxin immune fab (ovine), is administered by the intravenous route over 30 minutes. It is recommended that it be infused through a 0.22 micron membrane filter to ensure no undissolved particulate matter is administered. If cardiac arrest is imminent, it can be given as a bolus injection.

Storage: Refrigerate at 2° to 8°C (36° to 46°F). Unreconstituted vials can be stored at up to 30°C (86°F) for a total of 30 days.

REFERENCES:

1. Smith TW, Lloyd BL, Spicer N, Haber E. Immunogenicity and kinetics of distribution and elimination of sheep digoxin-specific IgG and Fab fragments in the rabbit and baboon. *Clin Exp Immunol* 1979; 36:384-396. **2.** Smith TW, Haber E, Yeatman L, Butler VP Jr. Reversal of advanced digoxin intoxication with Fab fragments of digoxin-specific antibodies. *N Engl J Med* 1976; 294:797-800. **3.** Smith TW, Butler VP Jr, Haber E, Fozzard H, Marcus FI, Bremner WF, Schulman IC, Phillips A. Treatment of life-threatening digitalis intoxication with digoxin-specific Fab antibody fragments: Experience in 26 cases. *N Engl J Med* 1982; 307:1357-1362. **4.** Wenger TL, Butler VP Jr, Haber E, Smith TW. Treatment of 63 severely digitalis-toxic patients with digoxin-specific antibody fragments.*JAm Coll Cardiol*1985; 5:118A-123A. **5.** Spiegel A, Marchlinski FE. Time course for reversal of digoxin toxicity with digoxin-specific antibody fragments. *Am Heart J*1985; 109:1397-1399. **6.** Smith TW, Butler VP, Haber E. Characterization of antibodies of high affinity and specificity for the digitalis glycoside digoxin. *Biochemistry* 1970; 9:331-337. **7.** Gibb I, Adams PC, Parnham AJ, Jennings K. Plasma digoxin: Assay anomalies in Fab-treated patients. *Br J Clin Pharmacol* 1983;16:445-447.

HOW SUPPLIED - EQUIVALENTS NOT AVAILABLE:

Injection, Conc-Soln - Intravenous - 40 mg/vial

40 mg $465.08 DIGIBIND, Glaxo Wellcome 00173-0230-44

DIHYDROERGOTAMINE MESYLATE *(001063)*

CATEGORIES: Antimigraine/Other Headaches; Autonomic Drugs; Cephalalgia; Ergot Preparations; Headache; Migraine; Pain; Sympatholytic Agents; FDA Approval Pre 1982

BRAND NAMES: *Adhaegon*; D.H.E.45; **DHE 45**; *Dergiflux* (France); *Dergotamine* (France); *Detemes Retard*; *Dihydergot* (Germany); *Dihydergot Sandoz*; *Dihydroergotamine-Sandoz* (Canada); *Ergont* (Germany); *Ergovasan*; *Ikaran*

(France); *Orstanorm*; *Seglor*; *Seglor Retard*; *Tamik*; *Tenuatina*; *Verladyn* (Germany); *Verteblan*
(International brand names outside U.S. in italics)

DESCRIPTION:

D.H.E. 45 is ergotamine hydrogenated in the 9,10 position as the mesylate salt. D.H.E. 45 is known chemically as ergotaman-3',6',18- trione,9,10 -dihydro -12' -hydroxy-2'-methyl-5'-(phenylmethyl)-, (5'α,10α)-, monomethanesulfonate (salt). It's formula is $C_{33}H_{37}N_5O_5{\cdot}CH_4O_3S$ and it's molecular weight is 679.79.

D.H.E. 45 (dihydroergotamine mesylate) is a clear, colorless solution supplied in sterile ampuls for IV or IM administration containing per ml:

dihydroergotamine mesylate, USP 1 mg
methanesulfonic acid/sodium hydroxide, qs to pH 3.6 ± 0.4
alcohol, USP 6.1% by vol.
glycerin, USP 15% by wt.
water for injection, USP, qs to 1 ml

CLINICAL PHARMACOLOGY:

Dihydroergotamine is an alpha adrenergic blocking agent with a direct stimulating effect on the smooth muscle of peripheral and cranial blood vessels, and produces depression of central vasomotor centers. The compound also has the properties of serotonin antagonism. In comparison to ergotamine, the adrenergic blocking actions are more pronounced, the vasoconstrictive actions somewhat less pronounced, and there is reduced incidence and degree of nausea and vomiting.

Onset of action occurs in 15-30 minutes following intramuscular administration and persists for 3-4 hours.

Repeated dosage at 1 hour intervals up to 3 hours may be required to obtain maximal effect.

INDICATIONS AND USAGE:

Dihydroergotamine mesylate injection, USP therapy is indicated to abort or prevent vascular headache, (*e.g.,* migraine, migraine variants), or so-called "histaminic cephalalgia" when rapid control is desired or when other routes of administration are not feasible.

For best results, treatment should commence at the first symptom or sign of a migraine headache attack.

CONTRAINDICATIONS:

Dihydroergotamine mesylate is contraindicated in patients who previously shown hypersensitivity to ergot alkaloids.

The drug is also contraindicated in patients having conditions predisposing to vasospastic reactions such as known peripheral arterial disease, coronary artery disease (in particular, unstable or vasospastic angina), sepsis, vascular surgery, uncontrolled hypertension, and severely impaired hepatic or renal function.

Dihydroergotamine possess oxytocic properties and, therefore, should not be administered during pregnancy.

Dihydroergotamine should not be used in nursing mothers (see PRECAUTIONS).

Dihydroergotamine should not be used with vasoconstrictors because the combination may result in extreme elevation of blood pressure.

WARNINGS:

Vasospasm: Dihydroergotamine, like other ergot alkaloids, can cause vasospastic reactions, including angina, although it seems to do so less frequently than other ergots. This action appears to be dose related; however, some patients may demonstrate individual sensitivity to the agent.

Vasospastic reactions are manifested by intense arterial vasoconstriction, producing signs and symptoms of peripheral vascular ischemia (*e.g.,* muscle pains, numbness, coldness, and pallor or cyanosis of the digits), angina or unusual syndromes, such as mesenteric ischemia. Because persistent vasospasm can result in gangrene or death, dihydroergotamine mesylate injection, USP, should be discontinued immediately if signs or symptoms of vasoconstriction develop.

PRECAUTIONS:

Information for the Patient: No more than 3 ml intramuscularly or 2 ml intravenously should be injected for any single migraine attack. No more than 6 ml should be injected during an 7-day period.

Dihydroergotamine mesylate injection, USP, should be used only for vascular headaches of the migraine type. It is not effective for other types of headaches and it lacks analgesic properties. Patients should be advised to report to the physician immediately any of the following: numbness or tingling in the fingers and toes, muscle pain in the arms and legs, weakness in the legs, pain in the chest, or temporary speeding or slowing of the heart rate, swelling, or itching.

Pregnancy, Teratogenic Effects, Pregnancy Category X: Animal reproductive (teratogenic) studies in rats, rabbits, and nonhuman primates, employing oral dihydroergotamine mesylate at doses of 1, 3, 10 and 30 mg/kg/day (approximately 12, 36, 120, and 360 times the maximum recommended daily dose based on a 50 kg man) did not produce any evidence of adverse reproductive effects. There are no studies on the placental transfer or teratogenicity of dihydroergotamine mesylate. Ergotamine crosses the placenta in small amounts, although it does not appear to be embryotoxic. However, prolonged vasoconstriction of the uterine vessels and/or increased myometrial tone leading to reduced myometrial and placenta blood flow may contribute to fetal growth retardation in animals. (See CONTRAINDICATIONS.)

Nursing Mothers: Ergot drugs are known to inhibit prolactin. It is likely that dihydroergotamine mesylate is excreted in human milk. It is known that ergotamine is excreted in breast milk and may cause vomiting, diarrhea, weak pulse and unstable blood pressure in nursing infants. Because of the potential for these serious adverse reactions in nursing infants from dihydroergotamine mesylate, nursing should not be undertaken during the use of dihydroergotamine mesylate.

Pediatric Use: Safety and effectiveness of dihydroergotamine mesylate in children have not been established.

DRUG INTERACTIONS:

Vasoconstrictors: Dihydroergotamine mesylate injection, USP, should not be administered with vasoconstrictors or sympathomimetics (pressor agents) because the combination may cause extreme elevation of blood pressure.

Beta Blockers: There have been reports that propanol may potentiate the vasoconstrictive action of ergotamine by blocking the vasodilating property of epinephrine.

Nicotine: Nicotine may provoke vasoconstriction in some patients, predisposing to a greater ischemic response to ergot therapy.

DRUG INTERACTIONS: *(cont'd)*

Macrolide Antibiotics (*e.g.,* Erythromycin): Agents of the ergot alkaloid class, of which dihydroergotamine mesylate injection, USP, is a member, have been shown to interact with antibiotics of the macrolide class, resulting in increased plasma levels of unchanged alkaloids and peripheral vasoconstriction. Vasospastic reactions have been reported with therapeutic doses of ergotamine-containing drugs when coadministered with these antibiotics.

ADVERSE REACTIONS:

Numbness and tingling of fingers and toes, muscle pains in the extremities, weakness in the legs, precordial distress and pain, transient tachycardia or bradycardia, nausea, vomiting, localized edema, itching, and injection site reactions.

In studies with normal volunteers, doses of dihydroergotamine mesylate injection, USP, of 2-3 mg resulted in an increased frequency of headache, leg cramps and soreness, nausea, and vomiting.

There have been reports of pleural and retroperitoneal fibrosis in patients following prolonged use of dihydroergotamine.

DRUG ABUSE AND DEPENDENCE:

Abuse and Dependence: Currently available data have not demonstrated drug abuse and psychological dependence with dihydroergotamine. However, cases of drug abuse and psychological dependence in patients on other forms of ergot therapy have been reported. Thus, due to the chronicity of vascular headaches, it is imperative that patients be advised not to exceed recommended dosages.

OVERDOSAGE:

To date, there have been no reports of acute overdosage with this drug. Due to the risk of vascular spasm, exceeding the recommended doses of dihydroergotamine mesylate injection, USP, is to be avoided. Excessive doses of dihydroergotamine may result in peripheral signs and symptoms of *ergotism.* Treatment includes discontinuance of the drug, local application of warmth to the affected area, the administration of vasodilators, and nursing care to prevent tissue damage.

In general, the symptoms of an acute dihydroergotamine mesylate overdose are similar to those of an ergotamine overdose, although there is less pronounced nausea and vomiting with dihydroergotamine mesylate. The symptoms of an ergotamine overdose include the following: numbness tingling, pain, and cyanosis of the extremities associated with diminished or absent peripheral pulses; respiratory depression; an increase and/or decrease in blood pressure, usually in that order, confusion, delirium, convulsions, and coma: and/or some degree of nausea; vomiting; and abdominal pain.

DOSAGE AND ADMINISTRATION:

Dihydroergotamine mesylate should be administered in a dose of 1 ml intramuscularly at first warning sign of headache, and repeated at 1 hour intervals to a total of 3 ml. Optimal results are obtained by titrating over the course of several headaches to find the minimal effective dose for each patient; this dose should then be employed at onset of subsequent attacks. Where more rapid effect is desired, the intravenous route may be employed to a maximum of 2 ml. Total weekly dosage should not exceed 6 ml.

HOW SUPPLIED:

D.H.E. 45 Injection, USP, is available as a clear colorless, sterile solution in single 1 ml sterile ampuls containing 1 mg of dihydroergotamine mesylate per ml, in packages of 20.

Store and Dispense: To assure constant potency, protect the ampuls from light and heat. Store and dispense below 77°F (25°C), in light-resistant containers. Administer only if clear and colorless.

HOW SUPPLIED - EQUIVALENTS NOT AVAILABLE:

Injection, Solution - Intramuscular; - 1 mg/ml

1 ml x 10 $106.80 D.H.E.45, Novartis 00078-0041-01

DIHYDROTACHYSTEROL *(001065)*

CATEGORIES: Calcium Metabolism; Homeostatic & Nutrient; Hypoparathyroidism; Tetany; Vitamin D; Vitamins; Pregnancy Category C; FDA Pre 1938 Drugs

BRAND NAMES: *A.T.10* (Germany); *AT 10* (Japan); *AT-10*; **DHT**; *Dihydral*; *Dygratyl*; Hytakerol; *Tachyrol*
(International brand names outside U.S. in italics)

FORMULARIES: Aetna; BC-BS; Medi-Cal

DESCRIPTION:

Each tablet contains:
Dihydrotachysterol 0.125 mg, 0.2 mg or 0.4 mg
Each ml Intensol Oral Solution (Concentrate) contains:
Dihydrotachysterol 0.2 mg
Alcohol 20%

Dihydrotachysterol is a synthetic reduction product of tachysterol, a close isomer of vitamin D. Chemically dihydrotachysterol is *9, 10- Secoergosta-5, 7,22-tri-en-3β-ol,* which can be represented by the following structural formula ($C_{28}H_{46}O$; molecular weight 398.65).

Dihydrotachysterol acts as a blood calcium regulator.

DHT Inactive ingredients: The tablets contain butylated hydroxyanisole, FD&C Red No. 3 (0.2 mg only), lactose, magnesium stearate, propyl gallate, starch, and sucrose.

CLINICAL PHARMACOLOGY:

Dihydrotachysterol is hydroxylated in the liver to 25-hydroxydihydrotachysterol, which is the major circulating active form of the drug. It does not undergo further hydroxylation by the kidney and therefore is the analogue of 1,25-dihydroxyvitamin D. Dihydrotachysterol is effective in the elevation of serum calcium by stimulating intestinal calcium absorption and mobilizing bone calcium in the absence of parathyroid hormone and of functioning renal tissue. Dihydrotachysterol also increases renal phosphate excretion. In contrast to parathyroid extract, dihydrotachysterol is active when taken orally, exerts a slow but persistent effect, and may be used for long periods without increasing the dosage or causing tolerance. Dihydrotachysterol is faster-acting than pharmacologic doses of vitamin D and is less persistent after cessation of treatment, thus decreasing the risk of accumulation and of hypercalcemia.

INDICATIONS AND USAGE:

Dihydrotachysterol is indicated for the treatment of acute, chronic, and latent forms of postoperative tetany, idiopathic tetany, and hypoparathyroidism.

CONTRAINDICATIONS:

Contraindicated in patients with hypercalcemia, abnormal sensitivity to the effects of vitamin D, and hypervitaminosis D.

PRECAUTIONS:

General: The difference between therapeutic dose and intoxicating dose may be small in any patient and therefore dosage must be individualized and periodically reevaluated.

In patients with renal osteodystrophy accompanied by hyperphosphatemia, maintenance of a normal serum phosphorus level by dietary phosphate restriction and/or administration of aluminum gels as intestinal phosphate binders is essential to prevent metastatic calcification.

Because of its effect on serum calcium, dihydrotachysterol should be administered to pregnant patients or to patients with renal stones only when, in the judgement of the physician, the potential benefits outweigh the possible hazards.

Laboratory Tests: To prevent hypercalcemia, treatment should always be controlled by regular determinations of blood calcium level, which should be maintained within the normal range.

Pregnancy, Teratogenic Effects, Pregnancy Category C: Animal reproduction studies have shown fetal abnormalities in several species associated with hypervitaminosis D. These are similar to the supravalvular aortic stenosis syndrome described in infants by Black in England (1963). This syndrome was characterized by supravalvular aortic stenosis, elfin facies, and mental retardation.

There are no adequate and well-controlled studies in pregnant women. Dihydrotachysterol should be used during pregnancy only if the potential benefit justifies the potential risk to the fetus.

Nursing Mothers: It is not known whether this drug is excreted in human milk. Because many drugs are excreted in human milk, caution should be exercised when dihydrotachysterol is administered to a nursing woman.

DRUG INTERACTIONS:

Administration of thiazide diuretics to hypoparathyroid patients who are concurrently being treated with dihydrotachysterol may cause hypercalcemia.

OVERDOSAGE:

THE EFFECTS OF DIHYDROTACHYSTEROL CAN PERSIST FOR UP TO ONE MONTH AFTER CESSATION OF TREATMENT.

MANIFESTATIONS: Toxicity associated with dihydrotachysterol is similar to that seen with large doses of vitamin D. Overdosage is manifested by symptoms of hypercalcemia, i.e., weakness, headache, anorexia, nausea, vomiting, abdominal cramps, diarrhea, constipation, vertigo, tinnitus, ataxia, hypotonia, lethargy. depression, amnesia, disorientation, hallucinations, syncope, and coma. Impairment of renal function may result in polyuria, polydipsia, and albuminuria. Widespread calcification of soft tissues, including heart, blood vessels, kidneys, and lungs, can occur. Death can result from cardiovascular or renal failure.

Treatment: Treatment of overdosage consists of withdrawal of dihydrotachysterol, bed rest, liberal intake of fluids, a low-calcium diet, and administration of a laxative. Hypercalcemic crisis with dehydration, stupor, coma, and azotemia requires more vigorous treatment. The first step should be hydration of the patient. Intravenous saline may quickly and significantly increase urinary calcium excretion. A loop diuretic (furosemide or ethacrynic acid) may be given with the saline infusion to further increase renal calcium excretion. Other reported therapeutic measures include dialysis or the administration of citrates, sulfates, phosphates, corticosteroids, EDTA (ethylenediaminetetraacetic acid), and mithramycin via appropriate regimens.

DOSAGE AND ADMINISTRATION:

The dosage depends on the nature and seriousness of the disorder and should be adapted to each individual patient. Serum calcium levels should be maintained between 9 to 10 mg per 100 ml.

The following dosage schedule will serve as a guide:

Initial dose: 0.8 mg to 2.4 mg daily for several days.

Maintenance dose: 0.2 mg to 1.0 mg daily as required for normal serum calcium levels. The average maintenance dose is 0.6 mg daily. The dose may be supplemented with 10 to 15 grams of calcium lactate or gluconate by mouth daily.

HOW SUPPLIED - EQUIVALENTS NOT AVAILABLE:

Capsule, Gelatin - Oral - 0.125 mg

50's	$112.69	HYTAKEROL, Sanofi Winthrop	00024-0792-02

Solution - Oral - 0.2 mg/ml

30 ml	$33.90	DHT, Roxane	00054-3170-44

Tablet, Uncoated - Oral - 0.125 mg

50's	$45.20	DHT, Roxane	00054-4190-19
100's	$95.65	Dihydrotachysterol, Roxane	00054-8172-25

Tablet, Uncoated - Oral - 0.2 mg

10 tab x 10	$104.93	Dihydrotachysterol, Roxane	00054-8182-25
100's	$91.30	DHT, Roxane	00054-4189-25

Tablet, Uncoated - Oral - 0.4 mg

50's	$81.01	DHT, Roxane	00054-4191-19

DILEVALOL *(003222)*

CATEGORIES: Antihypertensives; Beta Adrenergic Blocking Agents; Beta Blockers; Cardiovascular Drugs; Hypertension; FDA Unapproved

BRAND NAMES: **Unicard**

Prescribing information not available at time of publication.

DILTIAZEM HYDROCHLORIDE *(001069)*

CATEGORIES: Angina; Antianginals; Antihypertensives; Arrhythmia; Atrial Fibrillation; Calcium Channel Blockers; Cardiovascular Drugs; Fibrillation; Heart Flutter; Hypertension; Tachycardia; Migraine*; Pregnancy Category C; Sales > $1 Billion; FDA Approved 1982 Nov; Patent Expiration 1992 Nov; Top 200 Drugs
* Indication not approved by the FDA

BRAND NAMES: *Altiazem*; *Altiazem Retard*; *Angiotrofin* (Mexico); *Angiotrofin Retard* (Mexico); *Angizem*; *Apo-diltiazem*; *Britiazem* (England); *Calcicard* (England); *Calnurs* (Japan); *Cardiazem*; *Cardil*; *Cardil Retard*; **Cardizem**; *Cardizem CD* (Australia); *Cardizem Retard*; *Cardizem SR* (Australia); *Carex*; *Cirilen*; *Cirilen AP*; *Clarute*; *Coras* (Australia); *Dazil*; *Deltazen* (France); Dilacor XR; Dilacor Xr; *Diladel*; *Dilatam*; *Dilatam 120*; *Dilatame*; *Dilcard*; *Dilcardia*; *Dilcor*; *Dilem*; *Dilfar*; *Dilgina*; *Dilrene* (France); *Diltahexal* (Germany); *Diltam*; *Diltan*; *Diltan SR*; *Diltelan*; *Diltiasyn*; *Diltikor*; *Diltime*; *Dilzem* (Germany); *Dilzem Retard* (Germany); *Dilzem RR*; *Dilzem SR* (England); *Dilzene*; *Dilzicardin* (Germany); *Dinisor*; *Dinisor Retard*; *DTM*; *Dyalac*; *Gadoserin* (Japan); *Helsibon* (Japan); *Herben*; *Herbesser*; *Herbesser 60*; *Herbesser 90 SR*; *Herbesser 180 SR*; *Hesor*; *Levozem*; *Lytelsen* (Japan); *Masdil*; *Miocardie*; *Myonil*; *Myonil Retard*; *Pazeadin* (Japan); *Presoken* (Mexico); *Tazem*; *Tiadil*; Tiazac; *Tilazem* (Mexico); *Tilazem AS 60*; *Tilazem AS 90*; *Tilazem 90*; *Tildiem* (France, England); *Tildiem CR*; *Tildiem Retard*; *Zilden*; *Ziruvate* (Japan)
(International brand names outside U.S. in italics)

FORMULARIES: Aetna; BC-BS; CIGNA; FHP; Humana; Kaiser; Medco; Medi-Cal; PCS; PruCare; United

COST OF THERAPY: $118.80 (Angina; Tablet; 30 mg; 3/day; 365 days)

DESCRIPTION:

DILTIAZEM HYDROCHLORIDE IS ABBREVIATED HERE AS DILTIAZEM HCL. DILTIAZEM HCL IS A CALCIUM ION INFLUX INHIBITOR (SLOW CHANNEL BLOCKER OR CALCIUM ANTAGONIST). CHEMICALLY, DILTIAZEM HCL IS 1,5-BENZOTHIAZEPIN-4(5H)ONE, 3- (ACETYLOXY)-5-[2-(DIMETHYLAMINO) ETHYL]-2, 3-DIHYDRO-2-(4-METHOXYPHENYL)-, MONOHYDROCHLORIDE, (+)-CIS-.

DILTIAZEM HYDROCHLORIDE IS A WHITE TO OFF-WHITE CRYSTALLINE POWDER WITH A BITTER TASTE. IT IS SOLUBLE IN WATER, METHANOL, AND CHLOROFORM. IT HAS A MOLECULAR WEIGHT OF 450.98.

TABLETS: Each tablet of diltiazem HCl contains 30 mg, 60 mg, 90 mg, or 120 mg diltiazem hydrochloride.

Also contains: D&C Yellow #10, FD&C Yellow #6 (60 mg and 120 mg), or FD&C Blue #1 (30 mg and 90 mg), hydroxypropylcellulose, hydroxypropyl methylcellulose, lactose, magnesium stearate, methylparaben, polyethylene glycol, talc, and other ingredients.

For oral administration.

Sustained Release Capsules: Each Cardizem SR capsule contains either 60 mg, 90 mg, or 120 mg diltiazem hydrochloride.

Also contains: D&C Yellow #10, FD&C Blue #1, FD&C Red #40, FD&C Yellow #6, fumaric acid, povidone, starch, sucrose, talc, titanium dioxide, and other ingredients.

For oral administration.

Once-Daily Capsules: Cardizem CD is formulated as a once-a-day extended release capsule containing either 120 mg, 180 mg, 240 mg, or 300 mg diltiazem hydrochloride.

Also contains: black iron oxide, ethylcellulose, FD&C Blue #1, fumaric acid, gelatin-NF, sucrose, starch, talc, titanium dioxide, white wax and other ingredients.

For oral administration.

Injection: Diltiazem HCl injectable is a clear, colorless, sterile, nonpyrogenic solution. It has a pH range of 3.7 to 4.1.

Diltiazem HCl injectable is for direct intravenous bolus injection and continuous intravenous infusion.

25-mg, 5-ml vial-each sterile vial contains 25 mg diltiazem hydrochloride, 3.75 mg citric acid USP, 3.25 mg sodium citrate dihydrate USP, 357 mg sorbitol solution USP, and water for injection USP up to 5 ml. Sodium hydroxide or hydrochloric acid is used for pH adjustment.

50-mg, 10-ml vial-each sterile vial contains 50 mg diltiazem hydrochloride, 7.5 mg citric acid USP, 6.5 mg sodium citrate dihydrate USP, 714 mg sorbitol solution USP, and water for injection USP up to 10 ml. Sodium hydroxide or hydrochloric acid is used for pH adjustment.

CLINICAL PHARMACOLOGY:

The therapeutic benefits achieved with diltiazem HCl are believed to be related to its ability to inhibit the influx of calcium ions during membrane depolarization of cardiac and vascular smooth muscle.

MECHANISMS OF ACTION

Tablets: Although precise mechanisms of its antianginal actions are still being delineated, diltiazem HCl is believed to act in the following ways:

1. Angina Due to Coronary Artery Spasm: Diltiazem HCl has been shown to be a potent dilator of coronary arteries both epicardial and subendocardial. Spontaneous and ergonovine-induced coronary artery spasm are inhibited by diltiazem HCl.

2. Exertional Angina: Diltiazem HCl has been shown to produce increases in exercise tolerance, probably due to its ability to reduce myocardial oxygen demand. This is accomplished via reductions in heart rate and systemic blood pressure at submaximal and maximal exercise workloads.

Sustained Release Capsules; Hypertension: Diltiazem HCl sustained release capsule produces its antihypertensive effect primarily by relaxation of vascular smooth muscle and the resultant decrease in peripheral vascular resistance. The magnitude of blood pressure reduction is related to the degree of hypertension; thus hypertensive individuals experience an antihypertensive effect, whereas there is only a modest fall in blood pressure in normotensives.

Once-Daily Capsules; Hypertension: Diltiazem HCl once-daily capsule produces its antihypertensive effect primarily by relaxation of vascular smooth muscle and the resultant decrease in peripheral vascular resistance. The magnitude of blood pressure reduction is related to the degree of hypertension; thus hypertensive individuals experience an antihypertensive effect, whereas there is only a modest fall in blood pressure in normotensives.

Angina: Diltiazem HCl once-daily capsule has been shown to produce increases in exercise tolerance, probably due to its ability to reduce myocardial oxygen demand. This is accomplished via reductions in heart rate and systemic blood pressure at submaximal and maximal work loads. Diltiazem has been shown to be a potent dilator of coronary arteries, both epicardial and subendocardial. Spontaneous and ergonovine-induced coronary artery spasm are inhibited by diltiazem.

Tablets and Once-Daily Capsules: In animal models, diltiazem interferes with the slow inward (depolarizing) current in excitable tissue. It causes excitation-contraction uncoupling in various myocardial tissues without changes in the configuration of the action potential. Diltiazem produces relaxation of coronary vascular smooth muscle and dilation of both large and small coronary arteries at drug levels which cause little or no negative inotropic effect. The resultant increases in coronary blood flow (epicardial and subendocardial) occur in ischemic and nonischemic models and are accompanied by dose-dependent decreases in systemic blood pressure and decreases in peripheral resistance.

Injection Diltiazem HCl inhibits the influx of calcium (Ca^{2+}) ions during membrane depolarization of cardiac and vascular smooth muscle. The therapeutic benefits of diltiazem HCl in supraventricular tachycardias are related to its ability to slow AV nodal conduction time and prolong AV nodal refractoriness. Diltiazem HCl exhibits frequency (use) dependent effects on

CLINICAL PHARMACOLOGY: *(cont'd)*

AV nodal conduction such that it may selectively reduce the heart rate during tachycardias involving the AV node with little or no effect on normal AV nodal conduction at normal heart rates.

Diltiazem HCl slows the ventricular rate in patients with a rapid ventricular response during atrial fibrillation or atrial flutter. Diltiazem HCl converts paroxysmal supraventricular tachycardia (PSVT) to normal sinus rhythm by interrupting the reentry circuit in AV nodal reentrant tachycardias and reciprocating tachycardias, e.g., Wolff-Parkinson-White syndrome (WPW).

Diltiazem HCl prolongs the sinus cycle length. It has no effect on the sinus node recovery time or on the sinoatrial conduction time in patients without SA nodal dysfunction. Diltiazem HCl has no significant electrophysiologic effects on tissues in the heart that are fast sodium channel dependent, e.g., His-Purkinje tissue, atrial and ventricular muscle, and extranodal accessory pathways.

Like other calcium channel antagonists, because of its effect on vascular smooth muscle, diltiazem HCl decreases total peripheral resistance resulting in a decrease in both systolic and diastolic blood pressure.

HEMODYNAMIC AND ELECTROPHYSIOLOGIC EFFECTS

Like other calcium antagonists, diltiazem decreases sinoatrial and atrioventricular conduction in isolated tissues and has a negative inotropic effect in isolated preparations. In the intact animal, prolongation of the AH interval can be seen at higher doses.

In man, diltiazem prevents spontaneous and ergonovine-provoked coronary artery spasm. It causes a decrease in peripheral vascular resistance and a modest fall in blood pressure and, in exercise tolerance studies in patients with ischemic heart disease, reduces the heart rate-blood pressure product for any given workload. Studies to date, primarily in patients with good ventricular function, have not revealed evidence of a negative inotropic effect; cardiac output, ejection fraction, and left ventricular end-diastolic pressure have not been affected. Such data have no predictive value with respect to effects in patients with poor ventricular function. There are as yet few data on the interaction of diltiazem and beta-blockers in patients with poor ventricular function. Resting heart rate is usually slightly reduced by diltiazem.

Intravenous diltiazem in doses of 20 mg prolongs AH conduction time and AV node functional and effective refractory periods approximately 20%. In a study involving single oral doses of 300 mg of diltiazem HCl in six normal volunteers, the average maximum PR prolongation was 14% with no instances of greater than first-degree AV block. Diltiazem HCl-associated prolongation of the AH interval is not more pronounced in patients with first-degree heart block. In patients with sick sinus syndrome, diltiazem significantly prolongs sinus cycle length (up to 50% in some cases).

Chronic oral administration of diltiazem HCl in doses of up to 240 mg/day has resulted in small increases in PR interval, but has not usually produced abnormal prolongation.

Additional Information for Sustained Release Capsules: Diltiazem HCl sustained release capsule produces antihypertensive effects both in the supine and standing positions. Postural hypotension is infrequently noted upon suddenly assuming an upright position. No reflex tachycardia is associated with the chronic antihypertensive effects. Diltiazem HCl sustained release capsule decreases vascular resistance, increases cardiac output (by increasing stroke volume), and produces a slight decrease or no change in heart rate. During dynamic exercise, increases in diastolic pressure are inhibited while maximum achievable systolic pressure is usually reduced. Heart rate at maximum exercise does not change or is slightly reduced. Chronic therapy with diltiazem HCl produces no change or an increase in plasma catecholamines. No increased activity of the renin-angiotensin-aldosterone axis has been observed. Diltiazem HCl sustained release capsule reduces the renal and peripheral effects of angiotensin II. Hypertensive animal models respond to diltiazem with reductions in blood pressure and increased urinary output and natriuresis without a change in urinary sodium/potassium ratio.

Additional Information for Once-Daily Capsules: In hypertensive patients, diltiazem HCl once-daily capsule produces antihypertensive effects both in the supine and standing positions. In a double-blind, parallel, dose-response study utilizing doses ranging from 90 to 540 mg once daily, diltiazem HCl once-daily capsule lowered supine diastolic blood pressure in an apparent linear manner over the entire dose range studied. The changes in diastolic blood pressure, measured at trough, for placebo, 90 mg, 180 mg, 360 mg, and 540 mg were -2.9, -4.5, -6.1, -9.5, and -10.5 mm Hg, respectively. Postural hypotension is infrequently noted upon suddenly assuming an upright position. No reflex tachycardia is associated with the chronic antihypertensive effects. Diltiazem HCl once-daily capsule decreases vascular resistance, increases cardiac output (by increasing stroke volume), and produces a slight decrease or no change in heart rate. During dynamic exercise, increases in diastolic pressure are inhibited while maximum achievable systolic pressure is usually reduced. Chronic therapy with diltiazem HCl once-daily capsule produces no change or an increase in plasma catecholamines. No increased activity of the renin-angiotensin-aldosterone axis has been observed. Diltiazem HCl once-daily capsule reduces the renal and peripheral effects of angiotensin II. Hypertensive animal models respond to diltiazem with reductions in blood pressure and increased urinary output and natriuresis without a change in urinary sodium/potassium ratio.

In a double-blind, parallel dose-response study of doses from 60 mg to 480 mg once daily, diltiazem HCl once-daily capsule increased time to termination of exercise in a linear manner over the entire dose range studied. The improvement in time to termination of exercise utilizing a Bruce exercise protocol, measured at trough, for placebo, 60 mg, 120 mg, 240 mg, 360 mg, and 480 mg was 29, 40, 56, 51, 69 and 68 seconds respectively. As doses of diltiazem HCl once-daily capsule were increased, overall angina frequency was decreased. Diltiazem HCl once-daily capsule, 180 mg once daily, or placebo was administered in a double-blind study to patients receiving concomitant treatment with long-acting nitrates and/or beta-blockers. A significant increase in time to termination of exercise and a significant decrease in overall angina frequency was observed. In this trial the overall frequency of adverse events in the diltiazem HCl once-daily capsule treatment group was the same as the placebo group.

Intravenous diltiazem in doses of 20 mg prolongs AH conduction and time and AV node functional and effective refractory periods by approximately 20%. In a study involving single oral doses of 300 mg of diltiazem HCl in six normal volunteers, the average maximum PR prolongation was 14% with no instances of greater than first-degree AV block. Diltiazem-associated prolongation of the AH interval is not more pronounced in patients with first-degree heart block. In patients with sick sinus syndrome, diltiazem significantly prolongs sinus cycle length (up to 50% in some cases).

Chronic oral administration of diltiazem HCl to patients in doses of up to 540 mg/day has resulted in small increases in PR interval, and on occasion produces abnormal prolongation. (See WARNINGS.)

HEMODYNAMICS

Injection: In patients with cardiovascular disease, diltiazem Hydrochloride injectable administered intravenously in single bolus doses, followed in some cases by a continuous infusion, reduced blood pressure, systemic vascular resistance, the rate-pressure product, and coronary vascular resistance and increased coronary blood flow. In a limited number of studies of patients with compromised myocardium (severe congestive heart failure, acute myocardial infarction, hypertrophic cardiomyopathy), administration of intravenous diltiazem produced no significant effect on contractility, left ventricular end diastolic pressure, or pulmonary

CLINICAL PHARMACOLOGY: *(cont'd)*

capillary wedge pressure. The mean ejection fraction and cardiac output/index remained unchanged or increased. Maximal hemodynamic effects usually occurred within 2 to 5 minutes of an injection. However, in rare instances, worsening of congestive heart failure has been reported in patients with preexisting impaired ventricular function.

PHARMACOKINETICS AND METABOLISM

Oral Forms: Diltiazem is well absorbed from the gastrointestinal tract and is subject to an extensive first-pass effect, giving an absolute bioavailability (compared to intravenous dosing) of about 40%. Diltiazem HCl undergoes extensive hepatic metabolism in which 2% to 4% of the unchanged drug appears in the urine. Drugs which induce or inhibit hepatic microsomal enzymes may alter diltiazem disposition.

Total radioactivity measurement following short IV administration in healthy volunteers suggests the presence of other unidentified metabolites, which attain higher concentrations than those of diltiazem and are more slowly eliminated; half-life of total radioactivity is about 20 hours compared to 2 to 5 hours for diltiazem.

In vitro binding studies show diltiazem HCl is 70% to 80% bound to plasma proteins. Competitive *in vitro* ligand binding studies have also shown diltiazem HCl binding is not altered by therapeutic concentrations of digoxin, hydrochlorothiazide, phenylbutazone, propranolol, salicylic acid, or warfarin. The plasma elimination half-life following single or multiple drug administration is approximately 3.0 to 4.5 hours. Desacetyl diltiazem is also present in the plasma at levels of 10% to 20% of the parent drug and is 25% to 50% as potent as a coronary vasodilator as diltiazem. Minimum therapeutic plasma levels of diltiazem HCl appear to be in the range of 50-200 ng/ml. There is a departure from linearity when dose strengths are increased. A study that compared patients with normal hepatic function to patients with cirrhosis found an increase in half-life and a 69% increase in AUC (area-under-the-plasma concentration vs time curve) in the hepatically impaired patients. A single study in nine patients with severely impaired functions showed no difference in the pharmacokinetic profile of diltiazem as compared to patients with normal renal function.

Additional information for Sustained Release Capsules: Diltiazem is absorbed from the capsule formulation to about 92% of a reference solution at steady-state. A single 120-mg dose of the capsule results in detectable plasma levels within two to three hours and peak plasma levels at six to 11 hours. The apparent elimination half-life after single or multiple dosing is five to seven hours. A departure from linearity similar to that observed with the diltiazem tablet is observed. As the dose of diltiazem capsules is increased from a daily dose of 120 mg (60 mg bid) to 240 mg (120 mg bid) daily, there is an increase in the area-under-the-curve of 2.6 times. When the dose is increased from 240 mg to 360 mg daily, there is an increase in the area-under-the-curve of 1.8 times. The average plasma levels of the capsule dosed twice daily at steady-state are equivalent to the tablet dosed four times daily when the same total daily dose is administered.

Additional information for Once-Daily Capsules: When compared to a regimen of diltiazem tablets at steady-state, more than 95% of drug is absorbed from the diltiazem formulation. A single 360-mg dose of the capsule results in detectable plasma levels within 2 hours and peak plasma levels between 10 and 14 hours; absorption occurs throughout the dosing interval. When diltiazem was coadministered with a high fat content breakfast, the extent to diltiazem absorption was not affected. Dose-dumping does not occur. The apparent elimination half-life after single or multiple dosing is 5 to 8 hours. A departure from linearity similar to that seen with diltiazem tablets and diltiazem capsules is observed. As the dose of diltiazem capsules is increased from a daily dose of 120 mg to 240 mg, there is an increase in the area-under-the-curve of 2.7 times. When the dose is increased from 240 mg to 360 mg there is an increase in the area-under-the-curve of 1.6 times.

Injection: Following a single intravenous injection in healthy male volunteers, diltiazem appears to obey linear pharmacokinetics over a dose range of 10.5 to 21.0 mg. The plasma elimination half-life is approximately 3.4 hours. The apparent volume of distribution of diltiazem is approximately 305 L. Diltiazem is extensively metabolized in the liver with a systemic clearance of approximately 65 L/h.

After constant rate intravenous infusion to healthy male volunteers, diltiazem exhibits nonlinear pharmacokinetics over an infusion range of 4.8 to 13.2 mg/h for 24 hours. Over this infusion range, as the dose is increased, systemic clearance decreases from 64 to 48 L/h while the plasma elimination half-life increases from 4.1 to 4.9 hours. The apparent volume of distribution remains unchanged (360 to 391 L). In patients with atrial fibrillation or atrial flutter, diltiazem systemic clearance has been found to be decreased compared to healthy volunteers. In patients administered bolus doses ranging from 2.5 mg to 38.5 mg, systemic clearance averaged 36 L/h. In patients administered continuous infusions at 10 mg/h or 15 mg/h for 24 hours, diltiazem systemic clearance averaged 42 L/h and 31 L/h, respectively.

Based on the results of pharmacokinetic studies in healthy volunteers administered different *oral* diltiazem formulations, constant rate intravenous infusions of diltiazem at 3, 5, 7, and 11 mg/h are predicted to produce steady-state plasma diltiazem concentrations equivalent to 120-, 180-, 240-, and 360-mg total daily oral doses of diltiazem tablets or diltiazem capsules.

After oral administration, diltiazem undergoes extensive metabolism in man by deacetylation, N-demethylation, and O-demethylation via cytochrome P-450 (oxidative metabolism) in addition to conjugation. Metabolites N– monodesmethyl– diltiazem, desacetyldiltiazem, desacetyl-N-monodesmethyldiltiazem, desacetyl-O-desmethyldiltiazem, and desacetyl-N, O-desmethyldiltiazem have been identified in human urine. Following oral administration, 2% to 4% of the unchanged diltiazem appears in the urine. Drugs which induce or inhibit hepatic microsomal enzymes may alter diltiazem disposition.

Following single intravenous injection of diltiazem, however, plasma concentrations of N-monodesmethyldiltiazem and desacetyldiltiazem, two principal metabolites found in plasma after oral administration, are typically not detected. These metabolites are observed, however, following 24 hour constant rate intravenous infusion. Total radioactivity measurement following short IV administration in healthy volunteers suggests the presence of other unidentified metabolites which attain higher concentrations than those of diltiazem and are more slowly eliminated; half-life of total radioactivity is about 20 hours compared to 2 to 5 hours for diltiazem.

Diltiazem is 70% to 80% bound to plasma proteins. In vitro studies suggest $alpha_1$-acid glycoprotein binds approximately 40% of the drug at clinically significant concentrations. Albumin appears to bind approximately 30% of the drug, while other constituents bind the remaining bound fraction. Competitive *in vitro* ligand binding studies have shown that diltiazem binding is not altered by therapeutic concentrations of digoxin, phenytoin, hydrochlorothiazide, indomethacin, phenylbutazone, propranolol, salicylic acid, tolbutamide, or warfarin.

Renal insufficiency, or even end-stage renal disease, does not appear to influence diltiazem disposition following *oral* administration. Liver cirrhosis was shown to reduce diltiazem's apparent *oral* clearance and prolong its half-life.

Additional Information for Injection Pharmacodynamics: The prolongation of PR interval correlated significantly with plasma diltiazem concentration in normal volunteers using the Sigmoidal E_{max} model. Changes in heart rate, systolic blood pressure, and diastolic blood pressure did not correlate with diltiazem plasma concentrations in normal volunteers. Reduction in mean arterial pressure correlated linearly with diltiazem plasma concentration in a group of hypertensive patients.

CLINICAL PHARMACOLOGY: *(cont'd)*

In patients with atrial fibrillation and atrial flutter, a significant correlation was observed between the percent reduction in HR and plasma diltiazem concentration using the Sigmoidal E_{max} model. Based on this relationship, the mean plasma diltiazem concentration required to produce a 20% decrease in heart rate was determined to be 80 ng/ml. Mean plasma diltiazem concentrations of 130 ng/ml and 300 ng/ml were determined to produce reductions in heart rate of 30% and 40%.

CLINICAL STUDIES:

In controlled clinical trials, therapy with antiarrhythmic agents to maintain reduced heart rate in atrial fibrillation or atrial flutter or for prophylaxis of PSVT was generally started within 3 hours after bolus administration of diltiazem HCl injectable. These antiarrhythmic agents were intravenous or oral digoxin, Class I antiarrhythmics (*e.g.,* quinidine, procainamide), calcium channel blockers, and oral beta-blockers.

Experience in the use of antiarrhythmic agents following maintenance infusion of diltiazem HCl injectable is limited. Patients should be dosed on an individual basis and reference should be made to the respective manufacturer's package insert for information relative to dosage and administration.

INDICATIONS AND USAGE:

Oral Forms: Diltiazem tablets, suspended release capsules, and once-daily capsules are indicated for the management of chronic stable angina and angina due to coronary artery spasm. Diltiazem tablets, suspended release capsules, and once-daily capsules are for the treatment of hypertension. It may be used alone or in combination with other antihypertensive medications, such as diuretics.

Injection: Diltiazem Hydrochloride injectable is indicated for the following:

1. Atrial Fibrillation or Atrial Flutter: Temporary control of rapid ventricular rate in atrial fibrillation or atrial flutter. It should not be used in patients with atrial fibrillation or atrial flutter associated with an accessory bypass tract such as in Wolff-Parkinson-White (WPW) syndrome or short PR syndrome.

2. Paroxysmal Supraventricular Tachycardia: Rapid conversion of paroxysmal supraventricular tachycardias (PSVT) to sinus rhythm. This includes AV nodal reentrant tachycardias and reciprocating tachycardias associated with an extranodal accessory pathway such as the WPW syndrome or short PR syndrome. Unless otherwise contraindicated, appropriate vagal maneuvers should be attempted prior to administration of diltiazem HCl injectable.

The use of diltiazem HCl injectable for control of ventricular response in patients with atrial fibrillation or atrial flutter or conversion to sinus rhythm in patients with PSVT should be undertaken with caution when the patient is compromised hemodynamically or is taking other drugs that decrease any or all of the following: peripheral resistance, myocardial filling, myocardial contractility, or electrical impulse propagation in the myocardium.

For either indication and particularly when employing continuous intravenous infusion, the setting should include continuous monitoring of the ECG and frequent measurement of blood pressure. A defibrillator and emergency equipment should be readily available.

In domestic controlled trials in patients with atrial fibrillation or atrial flutter, bolus administration of diltiazem HCl injectable was effective in reducing heart rate by at least 20% in 95% of patients. Diltiazem HCl injectable rarely converts atrial fibrillation or atrial flutter to normal sinus rhythm. Following administration of one or two intravenous bolus doses of diltiazem HCl injectable, response usually occurs within 3 minutes and maximal heart rate reduction generally occurs in 2 to 7 minutes. Heart rate reduction may last from 1 to 3 hours. If hypotension occurs, it is generally short-lived, but may last from 1 to 3 hours. A 24-hour continuous infusion of diltiazem HCl injectable in the treatment of atrial fibrillation or atrial flutter maintained at least a 20% heart rate reduction during the infusion in 83% of patients. Upon discontinuation of infusion, heart rate reduction may last from 0.5 hours to more than 10 hours (median duration 7 hours). Hypotension, if it occurs, may be similarly persistent.

In the controlled clinical trials, 3.2% of patients required some form of intervention (typically, use of intravenous fluids or the Trendelenburg position) for blood pressure support following diltiazem HCl injectable.

In domestic controlled trials, bolus administration of diltiazem HCl injectable was effective in converting PSVT to normal sinus rhythm in 88% of patients within 3 minutes of the first or second bolus dose.

Symptoms associated with the arrhythmia were improved in conjunction with decreased heart rate or conversion to normal sinus rhythm following administration of diltiazem HCl injectable.

CONTRAINDICATIONS:

Oral Forms: Diltiazem HCl is contraindicated in (1) patients with sick sinus syndrome except in the presence of a functioning ventricular pacemaker, (2) patients with second- or third-degree AV block except in the presence of a functioning ventricular pacemaker, (3) patients with hypotension (less than 90 mm Hg systolic), (4) patients who have demonstrated hypersensitivity to the drug, and (5) patients with acute myocardial infarction and pulmonary congestion documented by x-ray on admission.

Injection: diltiazem HCl injectable is contraindicated in:

1. Patients with sick sinus syndrome except in the presence of a functioning ventricular pacemaker.

2. Patients with second- or third-degree AV block except in the presence of a functioning ventricular pacemaker.

3. Patients with severe hypotension or cardiogenic shock.

4. Patients who have demonstrated hypersensitivity to the drug.

5. Intravenous diltiazem and intravenous beta-blockers should not be administered together or in close proximity (within a few hours).

6. Patients with atrial fibrillation or atrial flutter associated with an accessory bypass tract such as in WPW syndrome or short PR syndrome.

7. Patients with ventricular tachycardia. Administration of other calcium channel blockers to patients with wide complex tachycardia (QRS $\geq$ 0.12 seconds) has resulted in hemodynamic deterioration and ventricular fibrillation. It is important that an accurate pretreatment diagnosis distinguish wide complex QRS tachycardia of supraventricular origin from that of ventricular origin prior to administration of diltiazem HCl injectable.

As with other agents which slow AV nodal conduction and do not prolong the refractoriness of the accessory pathway (*e.g.,* verapamil, digoxin), in rare instances patients in atrial fibrillation or atrial flutter associated with an accessory bypass tract may experience a potentially life-threatening increase in heart rate accompanied by hypotension when treated with diltiazem HCl injectable. As such, the initial use of diltiazem HCl injectable should be, if possible, in a setting where monitoring and resuscitation capabilities, including DC cardioversion/defibrillation, are present (see OVERDOSAGE.) Once familiarity of the patient's response is established, use in an office setting may be acceptable.

WARNINGS:

Tablets

1. Cardiac Conduction: Diltiazem HCl prolongs AV node refractory periods without significantly prolonging sinus node recovery time, except in patients with sick sinus syndrome. This effect may rarely result in abnormally slow heart rates (particularly in patients with sick sinus syndrome) or second- or third-degree AV block (six of 1,243 patients for 0.48%). Concomitant use of diltiazem with beta-blockers or digitalis may result in additive effects on cardiac conduction. A patient with Prinzmetal's angina developed periods of asystole (2 to 5 seconds) after a single dose of 60 mg of diltiazem.

2. Congestive Heart Failure: Although diltiazem has a negative inotropic effect in isolated animal tissue preparations, hemodynamic studies in humans with normal ventricular function have not shown a reduction in cardiac index nor consistent negative effects on contractility (dp/dt). Experience with the use of diltiazem HCl alone or in combination with beta-blockers in patients with impaired ventricular function is very limited. Caution should be exercised when using the drug in such patients.

3. Hypotension: Decreases in blood pressure associated with diltiazem HCl therapy may occasionally result in symptomatic hypotension.

4. Acute Hepatic Injury: In rare instances, significant elevations in enzymes such as alkaline phosphatase, LDH, SGOT, SGPT, and other phenomena consistent with acute hepatic injury have been noted. These reactions have been reversible upon discontinuation of drug therapy. The relationship to diltiazem HCl is uncertain in most cases, but probable in some. (See PRECAUTIONS.)

Sustained-Release Capsules

1. Cardiac Conduction: Diltiazem HCl prolongs AV node refractory periods without significantly prolonging sinus node recovery time, except in patients with sick sinus syndrome. This effect may rarely result in abnormally slow heart rates (particularly in patients with sick sinus syndrome) or second- or third-degree AV block (9 of 2,111 patients or 0.43%). Concomitant use of diltiazem with beta-blockers or digitalis may result in additive effects on cardiac conduction. A patient with Prinzmetal's angina developed periods of asystole (2 to 5 seconds) after a single dose of 60 mg of diltiazem.

2. Congestive Heart Failure: Although diltiazem has a negative inotropic effect in isolated animal tissue preparations, hemodynamic studies in humans with normal ventricular function have not shown a reduction in cardiac index nor consistent negative effects on contractility (dp/dt). An acute study of oral diltiazem in patients with impaired ventricular function (ejection fraction 24% $\pm$ 6%) showed improvement in indices of ventricular function without significant decrease in contractile function (dp/dt). Experience with the use of diltiazem hydrochloride in combination with beta-blockers in patients with impaired ventricular function is limited. Caution should be exercised when using this combination.

3. Hypotension: Decreases in blood pressure associated with diltiazem HCl therapy may occasionally result in symptomatic hypotension.

4. Acute Hepatic Injury: Mild elevations of transaminases with and without concomitant elevation in alkaline phosphatase and bilirubin have been observed in clinical studies. Such elevations were usually transient and frequently resolved even with continued diltiazem treatment. In rare instances, significant elevations in enzymes such as alkaline phosphatase, LDH, SGOT, SGPT, and other phenomena consistent with acute hepatic injury have been noted. These reactions tended to occur early after therapy initiation (1 to 8 weeks) and have been reversible upon discontinuation of drug therapy. The relationship to diltiazem HCl is uncertain in some cases, but probable in some. (See PRECAUTIONS.)

Once-Daily Capsules

1. Cardiac Conduction: Diltiazem HCl prolongs AV node refractory periods without significantly prolonging sinus node recovery time, except in patients with sick sinus syndrome. This effect may rarely result in abnormally show heart rates (particularly in patients with sick sinus syndrome) or second- or third-degree AV block (13 of 3,290 patients or 0.40%). Concomitant use of diltiazem with beta-blockers or digitalis may result in additive effects on cardiac conduction. A patient with Prinzmetal's angina developed periods of asystole (2 to 5 seconds) after a single dose of 60 mg of diltiazem.

2. Congestive Heart Failure: Although diltiazem has a negative inotropic effect in isolated animal tissue preparations, hemodynamic studies in humans with normal ventricular function have not shown a reduction in cardiac index nor consistent negative effects on contractility (dp/dt). An acute study of oral diltiazem in patients with impaired ventricular function (ejection fraction 24% $\pm$ 6%) showed improvement in indices of ventricular function without significant decrease in contractile function (dp/dt). Worsening of congestive heart failure has been reported in patients with preexisting impairment of ventricular function. Experience with the use of diltiazem hydrochloride in combination with beta-blockers in patients with impaired ventricular function is limited. Caution should be exercised when using this combination.

3. Hypotension: Decreases in blood pressure associated with diltiazem HCl therapy may occasionally result in symptomatic hypotension.

4. Acute Hepatic Injury: Mild elevations of transaminases with and without concomitant elevation in alkaline phosphatase and bilirubin have been observed in clinical studies. Such elevations were usually transient and frequently resolved even with continued diltiazem treatment. In rare instances, significant elevations in enzymes such as alkaline phosphatase, LDH, SGOT, SGPT, and other phenomena consistent with acute hepatic injury have been noted. These reactions tended to occur early after therapy initiation (1 to 8 weeks) and have been reversible upon discontinuation of drug therapy. The relationship to diltiazem HCl is uncertain in some cases, but probable in some. (See PRECAUTIONS.)

Injection

1. Cardiac Conduction: Diltiazem prolongs AV nodal conduction and refractoriness that may rarely result in second- or third-degree AV block in sinus rhythm. Concomitant use of diltiazem with agents known to affect cardiac conduction may result in additive effects (see DRUG INTERACTIONS.) If high-degree AV block occurs in sinus rhythm, intravenous diltiazem should be discontinued and appropriate supportive measures instituted (see OVERDOSAGE.)

2. Congestive Heart Failure: Although diltiazem has a negative inotropic effect in isolated animal tissue preparations, hemodynamic studies in humans with normal ventricular function and in patients with a compromised myocardium, such as severe CHF, acute MI, and hypertrophic cardiomyopathy, have not shown a reduction in cardiac index nor consistent negative effects on contractility (dp/dt). Administration of oral diltiazem in patients with acute myocardial infarction and pulmonary congestion documented by x-ray on admission is contraindicated. Experience with the use of diltiazem HCl injectable in patients with impaired ventricular function is limited. Caution should be exercised when using the drug in such patients.

3. Hypotension: Decreases in blood pressure associated with diltiazem HCl injectable therapy may occasionally result in symptomatic hypotension (3.2%). The use of intravenous diltiazem for control of ventricular response in patients with supraventricular arrhythmias should be undertaken with caution when the patient is compromised hemodynamically. In addition, caution should be used in patients taking other drugs that decrease peripheral resistance, intravascular volume, myocardial contractility or conduction.

WARNINGS: *(cont'd)*

4. Acute Hepatic Injury: In rare instances, significant elevations in enzymes such as alkaline phosphatase, LDH, SGOT, SGPT, and other phenomena consistent with acute hepatic injury have been noted following oral diltiazem. Therefore, the potential for acute hepatic injury exists following administration of intravenous diltiazem.

5. Ventricular Premature Beats (VPBs): VPBs may be present on conversion of PSVT to sinus rhythm with diltiazem HCl injectable. These VPBs are transient, are typically considered to be benign, and appear to have no clinical significance. Similar ventricular complexes have been noted during cardioversion, other pharmacologic therapy, and during spontaneous conversion of PSVT to sinus rhythm.

PRECAUTIONS:

ORAL FORMS

General: Diltiazem HCl is extensively metabolized by the liver and excreted by the kidneys and in bile. As with any drug given over prolonged periods, laboratory parameters of renal and hepatic function should be monitored at regular intervals. The drug should be used with caution in patients with impaired renal or hepatic function. In subacute and chronic dog and rat studies designed to produce toxicity, high doses of diltiazem were associated with hepatic damage. In special subacute hepatic studies, oral doses of 125 mg/kg and higher in rats were associated with histological changes in the liver which were reversible when the drug was discontinued. In dogs, doses of 20 mg/kg were also associated with hepatic changes; however, these changes were reversible with continued dosing.

Dermatological events (see ADVERSE REACTIONS) may be transient and may disappear despite continued use of diltiazem HCl. However, skin eruptions progressing to erythema multiforme and/or exfoliative dermatitis have also been infrequently reported. Should a dermatologic reaction persist, the drug should be discontinued.

CARCINOGENESIS, MUTAGENESIS, AND IMPAIRMENT OF FERTILITY

Tablets and Sustained-Release Capsules: A 24-month study in rats and a 21-month study in mice showed no evidence of carcinogenicity. There was also no mutagenic response in *in vitro* bacterial tests. No intrinsic effect on fertility was observed in rats.

Once-Daily Capsules: A 24 month study in rats at oral dosage levels of up to 100 mg/kg/day and a 21-month study in mice as oral dosage levels of up to 30 mg/kg/day showed no evidence of carcinogenicity. There was also no mutagenic response *in vitro*or*in vivo* in bacteria. No evidence of impaired fertility was observed in a study performed in male and female rats at oral dosages of up to 100 mg/kg/day.

PREGNANCY CATEGORY C: Reproduction studies have been conducted in mice, rats, and rabbits. Administration of doses ranging from five to ten times greater (on a mg/kg basis) than the daily recommended therapeutic dose has resulted in embryo and fetal lethality. These doses, in some studies, have been reported to cause skeletal abnormalities. In the peri-natal/postnatal studies, there was some reduction in early individual pup weights and survival rates. There was an increased incidence of stillbirths at doses of 20 times the human dose or greater.

There are no well-controlled studies in pregnant women; therefore, use diltiazem HCl in pregnant women only if the potential benefit justifies the potential risk to the fetus.

Nursing Mothers: Diltiazem is excreted in human milk. One report suggests that concentrations in breast milk may approximate serum levels. If use of diltiazem HCl is deemed essential, an alternative method of infant feeding should be instituted.

Pediatric Use: Safety and effectiveness in children have not been established.

INJECTION

General: Diltiazem hydrochloride is extensively metabolized by the liver and excreted by the kidneys and in bile. The drug should be used with caution in patients with impaired renal or hepatic function (see WARNINGS.) High intravenous dosages (4.5 mg/kg tid) administered to dogs resulted in significant bradycardia and alterations in AV conduction. In subacute and chronic dog and rat studies designed to produce toxicity, high oral doses of diltiazem were associated with hepatic damage. In special subacute hepatic studies, oral doses of 125 mg/kg and higher in rats were associated with histological changes in the liver, which were reversible when the drug was discontinued. In dogs, oral doses of 20 mg/kg were also associated with hepatic changes; however, these changes were reversible with continued dosing.

Dermatological events (see ADVERSE REACTIONS) may be transient and may disappear despite continued use of diltiazem HCl. However, skin eruptions progressing to erythema multiforme and/or exfoliative dermatitis have also been infrequently reported. Should a dermatologic reaction persist, the drug should be discontinued.

Carcinogenesis, Mutagenesis, and Impairment of Fertility: A 24-month study in rats at oral dosage levels of up to 100 mg/kg/day, and a 21-month study in mice at oral dosage levels of up to 30 mg/kg/day showed no evidence of carcinogenicity. There was also no mutagenic response *in vitro*or *in vivo*in mammalian cell assays or*in vitro* in bacteria. No evidence of impaired fertility was observed in a study performed in male and female rats at oral dosages of up to 100 mg/kg/day.

Pregnancy Category C: Reproduction studies have been conducted in mice, rats, and rabbits. Administration of doses ranging from five to ten times greater (on a mg/kg basis) than the daily recommended therapeutic dose has resulted in embryo and fetal lethality. These doses, in some studies, have been reported to cause skeletal abnormalities. In the perinatal/postnatal studies there was an increased incidence of stillbirths at doses of 20 times the human dose or greater.

There are no well-controlled studies in pregnant women; therefore, use diltiazem HCl in pregnant women only if the potential benefit justifies the potential risk to the fetus.

Nursing Mothers: Diltiazem is excreted in human milk. One report suggests that concentrations in breast milk may approximate serum levels. If use of diltiazem HCl is deemed essential, an alternative method of infant feeding should be instituted.

Pediatric Use: Safety and effectiveness in children have not been established.

DRUG INTERACTIONS:

Due to the potential for additive effects, caution and careful titration are warranted in patients receiving diltiazem HCl concomitantly with any agents known to affect cardiac contractility and/or conduction. (See WARNINGS.)

Pharmacologic studies indicate that there may be additive effects in prolonging AV conduction when using beta-blockers or digitalis concomitantly with diltiazem HCl. (See WARNINGS.)

As with all drugs, care should be exercised when treating patients with multiple medications. Diltiazem HCl undergoes biotransformation by cytochrome P-450 mixed function oxidase. Coadministration of diltiazem HCl with other agents which follow the same route of biotransformation may result in the competitive inhibition of metabolism. Especially in patients with renal and/or hepatic impairment dosages of similarly metabolized drugs, particularly those of low therapeutic ratio, may require adjustment when starting or stopping concomitantly administered diltiazem to maintain optimum therapeutic blood levels.

Digitalis: Administration of diltiazem HCl with digoxin in 24 healthy male subjects increased plasma digoxin concentrations approximately 20%. Another investigator found no increase in digoxin levels in 12 patients with coronary artery disease. Since there have been conflicting

DRUG INTERACTIONS: *(cont'd)*

results regarding the effect of digoxin levels, it is recommended that digoxin levels be monitored when initiating, adjusting, and discontinuing diltiazem HCl therapy to avoid possible over- or under-digitalization. (See WARNINGS.)

Anesthetics: The depression of cardiac contractility, conductivity, and automaticity as well as the vascular dilation associated with anesthetics may be potentiated by calcium channel blockers. When used concomitantly, anesthetics and calcium blockers should be titrated carefully.

Cyclosporine: A pharmacokinetic interaction between diltiazem and cyclosporine has been observed during studies involving renal and cardiac transplant patients. In renal and cardiac transplant recipients, a reduction of cyclosporine trough dose ranging from 15% to 48% was necessary to maintain concentrations similar to those seen prior to the addition of diltiazem. If these agents are to be administered concurrently, cyclosporine concentrations should be monitored, especially when diltiazem therapy is initiated, adjusted, or discontinued. The effect of cyclosporine on diltiazem plasma concentrations has not been evaluated.

Carbamazepine: Concomitant administration of diltiazem with carbamazepine has been reported to result in elevated serum levels of carbamazepine (40% to 72% increase) resulting in toxicity in some cases. Patients receiving these drugs concurrently should be monitored for a potential drug interaction.

Cimetidine: A study in six healthy volunteers has shown a significant increase in peak diltiazem plasma levels (58%) and area-under-the curve (53%) after a 1-week course of cimetidine at 1200 mg per day and diltiazem 60 mg per day. Ranitidine produced smaller, nonsignificant increases. The effect may be mediated by cimetidine's known inhibition of hepatic cytochrome P-450, the enzyme system probably responsible for the first-pass metabolism of diltiazem. Patients currently receiving diltiazem therapy should be carefully monitored for a change in pharmacological effect when initiating and discontinuing therapy with cimetidine. An adjustment in the diltiazem dose may be warranted.

Propranolol: Oral administration of diltiazem with propranolol in five normal volunteers resulted in increased propranolol levels in all subjects and bioavailability of propanol was increased approximately 50%. *In vitro*, propanolol appears to be displaced from its binding sites by diltiazem.

BETA-BLOCKERS

Oral Forms: Controlled and uncontrolled domestic studies suggest that concomitant use of diltiazem HCl and beta-blockers or digitalis is usually well tolerated. Available data are not sufficient, however, to predict the effects of concomitant treatment, particularly in patients with left ventricular dysfunction or cardiac conduction abnormalities.

Administration of diltiazem HCl concomitantly with propranolol in five normal volunteers resulted in increased propranolol levels in all subjects and bioavailability of propranolol was increased approximately 50%. *In vitro*, propranolol appears to be displaced from its binding sites by diltiazem. If combination therapy is initiated or withdrawn in conjunction with propranolol, an adjustment in the propranolol dose may be warranted. (See WARNINGS.)

Injection: Intravenous diltiazem has been administered to patients on chronic oral beta-blocker therapy. The combination of the two drugs was generally well tolerated without serious adverse effects. If intravenous diltiazem is administered to patients receiving chronic oral beta blocker therapy, the possibility for bradycardia, AV block and/or depression of contractility should be considered (see CONTRAINDICATIONS.)

ADVERSE REACTIONS:

TABLETS

Serious adverse reactions have been rare in studies carried out to date, but it should be recognized that patients with impaired ventricular function and cardiac conduction abnormalities have usually been excluded.

In domestic placebo-controlled angina trials, the incidence of adverse reactions reported during diltiazem HCl therapy was not greater than that reported during placebo therapy.

The following represent occurrences observed in clinical studies of angina patients. In many cases, the relationship to diltiazem HCl has not been established. The most common occurrences from these studies, as well as their frequency of presentation, are edema (2.4%), headache (2.1%), nausea (1.9%), dizziness (1.5%), rash (1.3%), asthenia (1.2%). In addition, the following events were reported infrequently (less than 1%):

Cardiovascular: Angina, arrhythmia, AV block (first degree), AV block (second or third degree - see conduction warning), bradycardia, bundle branch block, congestive heart failure, ECG abnormality, flushing, hypotension, palpitations, syncope, tachycardia, ventricular extrasystoles.

Nervous System: Abnormal dreams, amnesia, depression, gait abnormality, hallucinations, insomnia, nervousness, paresthesia, personality change, somnolence, tremor.

Gastrointestinal: Anorexia, constipation, diarrhea, dysgeusia, dyspepsia, mild elevations of alkaline phosphatase, SGOT, SGPT, and LDH (see WARNINGS), thirst, vomiting, weight increase.

Dermatological: Petechiae, photosensitivity, pruritus, urticaria.

Other: Amblyopia, CPK elevation, dry mouth, dyspnea, epistaxis, eye irritation, hyperglycemia, hyperuricemia, impotence, muscle cramps, nasal congestion, nocturia, osteoarticular pain, polyuria, sexual difficulties, tinnitus.

The following postmarketing events have been reported infrequently in patients receiving diltiazem HCl: alopecia, erythema multiforme, extrapyramidal symptoms, gingival hyperplasia, hemolytic anemia, increased bleeding time, leukopenia, purpura, retinopathy, thrombocytopenia

There have been observed cases of a generalized rash, characterized as leukocytoclastic vasculitis. In addition, events such as myocardial infarction have been observed which are not readily distinguishable from the natural history of the disease in these patients. A definitive cause and effect relationship between these events and diltiazem HCl therapy cannot yet be established. Exfoliative dermatitis (proven by rechallenge) has also been reported.

SUSTAINED RELEASE CAPSULES

Serious adverse reactions have been rare in studies carried out to date, but it should be recognized that patients with impaired ventricular function and cardiac conduction abnormalities have usually been excluded from these studies.

In domestic placebo-controlled trials, the incidence of adverse reactions reported during diltiazem HCl therapy was not greater than that reported during placebo therapy.

The adverse events described in TABLE 1 represent events observed in clinical studies of hypertensive patients receiving either diltiazem HCl tablets or diltiazem HCl sustained release capsules as well as experiences observed in studies of angina and during marketing. The most common events in hypertension studies are shown in a table with rates in placebo patients shown for comparison. Less common events are listed by body system; these include any adverse reactions seen in angina studies that were not observed in hypertension studies. In all hypertensive patients studied (over 900), the most common adverse events were edema (9%), headache (8%), dizziness (6%), asthenia (5%), sinus bradycardia (3%), flushing (3%), and first-degree AV block (3%). Only edema and perhaps bradycardia and dizziness were dose related. The most common events observed in clinical studies (over 2,100 patients) of angina

ADVERSE REACTIONS: *(cont'd)*

patients and hypertensive patients receiving diltiazem HCl tablets or diltiazem HCl sustained release capsules were (*i.e.,* greater than 1%) edema (5.4%), headache (4.5%) dizziness (3.4%), asthenia (2.8%), first-degree AV block (1.8%), flushing (1.7%), nausea (1.6%), bradycardia (1.5%), and rash (1.5%).

TABLE 1 Double Blind Placebo Controlled Hypertension Trials

Adverse Reaction	Diltiazem (n=315) # pts (%)	Placebo (n=211) # pts (%)
headache	38 (12%)	17 (8%)
AV block first degree	24 (7.6%)	4 (1.9%)
dizziness	22 (7%)	6 (2.8%)
edema	19 (6%)	2 (0.9%)
bradycardia	19 (6%)	3 (1.4%)
ECG abnormality	13 (4.1%)	3 (1.4%)
asthenia	10 (3.2%)	1 (0.5%)
constipation	5 (1.6%)	2 (0.9%)
dyspepsia	4 (1.3%)	1 (0.5%)
nausea	4 (1.3%)	2 (0.9%)
palpitations	4 (1.3%)	2 (0.9%)
polyuria	4 (1.3%)	2 (0.9%)
somnolence	4 (1.3%)	-
alk phos increase	3 (1%)	1 (0.5%)
hypotension	3 (1%)	1 (0.5%)
insomnia	3 (1%)	1 (0.5%)
rash	3 (1%)	1 (0.5%)
AV block second degree	2 (0.6%)	-

In addition, the following events were reported infrequently (less than 1%) with diltiazem HCl sustained release capsules or diltiazem HCl tablets or have been observed in angina or hypertension trials:

Cardiovascular: Angina, arrhythmia, second- or third-degree AV block (see conduction warning), bundle branch block, congestive heart failure, syncope, tachycardia, ventricular extrasystoles.

Nervous System: Abnormal dreams, amnesia, depression, gait abnormality, hallucinations, nervousness, paresthesia, personality change, tremor.

Gastrointestinal: Anorexia, constipation, diarrhea, dry mouth, dysgeusia, dyspepsia, mild elevations of SGOT, SGPT, and LDH (see hepatic warnings), somnolence, thirst, tinnitus, vomiting, weight increase.

Dermatological: Petechiae, photosensitivity, pruritus, urticaria.

Other: Amblyopia, CPK increase, dyspnea, epistaxis, eye irritation, hyperglycemia, hyperuricemia, impotence, muscle cramps, nasal congestion, nocturia, osteoarticular pain, polyuria, sexual difficulties, tinnitus.

The following postmarketing events have been reported infrequently in patients receiving diltiazem HCl: alopecia, erythema multiforme, extrapyramidal symptoms, gingival hyperplasia, hemolytic anemia, increased bleeding time, leukopenia, purpura, retinopathy, thrombocytopenia

There have been observed cases of a generalized rash, characterized as leukocytoclastic vasculitis. In addition, events such as myocardial infarction have been observed which are not readily distinguishable from the natural history of the disease in these patients. A definitive cause and effect relationship between these events and diltiazem HCl therapy cannot yet be established. Exfoliative dermatitis (proven by rechallenge) has also been reported.

ONCE-DAILY CAPSULES

Serious adverse reactions have been rare in studies carried out to date, but it should be recognized that patients with impaired ventricular function and cardiac conduction abnormalities have usually been excluded from these studies.

TABLE 2 presents the most common adverse reaction reported in placebo-controlled angina and hypertension trials in patients receiving diltiazem HCl once-daily capsule up to 360 mg with rates in placebo patients shown for comparison.

TABLE 2 Diltiazem HCl Capsule Placebo-Controlled Angina and Hypertension Trials Combined

Adverse Reaction	Diltiazem HCl (n=607)	Placebo (n=301)
Headache	5.4%	5.0%
Bradycardia	3.3%	3.0%
Edema	2.6%	1.3%
Dizziness	3.0%	0.0%
ECG Abnormality	1.6%	1.3%
AV Block First Degree	3.3%	2.3%
Asthenia	1.8%	1.7%

In clinical trials of diltiazem HCl once-daily capsule, diltiazem HCl tablets, and diltiazem HCl sustained release capsules involving over 3200 patients, the most common events (*i.e.,* greater than 1%) were edema (4.6%), headache (4.6%), dizziness (3.5%), asthenia (2.6%), first-degree AV block (2.4%), bradycardia (1.7%), flushing (1.4%), nausea (1.4%), rash (1.2%), and dyspepsia (1.4%).

In addition, the following events were reported infrequently (less than 1%) in angina or hypertension trials:

Cardiovascular: Angina, arrhythmia, AV block (second- or third-degree), bundle branch block, congestive heart failure, ECG abnormalities, hypotension, palpitations, syncope, tachycardia, ventricular extrasystoles.

Nervous System: Abnormal dreams, amnesia, depression, gait abnormality, hallucinations, insomnia, nervousness, paresthesia, personality change, somnolence, tinnitus, tremor.

Gastrointestinal: Anorexia, constipation, diarrhea, dry mouth dysgeusia, mild elevations of SGOT, SGPT, LDH, and alkaline phosphatase(see hepatic warnings), thirst, vomiting, weight increase.

Dermatological: Petechiae, photosensitivity, pruritus, urticaria.

Other: Amblyopia, CPK increase, dyspnea, epistaxis, eye irritation, hyperglycemia, hyperuricemia, impotence, muscle cramps, nasal congestion, nocturia, osteoarticular pain, polyuria, sexual difficulties.

The following postmarketing events have been reported infrequently in patients receiving diltiazem HCl: alopecia, erythema multiforme, exfoliative dermatitis, extrapyramidal symptoms, gingival hyperplasia, hemolytic anemia, increased bleeding time, leukopenia, purpura, retinopathy, thrombocytopenia

In addition, events such as myocardial infarction have been observed which are not readily distinguishable from the natural history of the disease in these patients. A number of well-documented cases of generalized rash, characterized as leukocytoclastic vasculitis, have been reported. However, a definitive cause and effect relationship between these events and diltiazem HCl therapy is yet to be established.

ADVERSE REACTIONS: *(cont'd)*

INJECTION

The following adverse reaction rates are based on the use of Cardizem injectable in over 400 domestic clinical trial patients with atrial fibrillation/flutter or PSVT under double-blind or open-label conditions. Worldwide experience in over 1300 patients was similar.

Adverse events reported in controlled and uncontrolled clinical trials were generally mild and transient. Hypotension was the most commonly reported adverse event during clinical trials. Asymptomatic hypotension occurred in 4.3% of patients. Symptomatic hypotension occurred in 3.2% of patients. When treatment for hypotension was required, it generally consisted of administration of saline or placing the patient in the Trendelenburg position. Other events reported in at least 1% of the diltiazem-treated patients were injection site reactions (*e.g.,* itching, burning) – 3.9%, vasodilation (flushing) – 1.7%, and arrhythmia (junctional rhythm or isorhythmic dissociation) –1.0%.

In addition, the following events were reported infrequently (less than 1%):

Cardiovascular: Atrial flutter, AV block first degree, AV block second degree, bradycardia, chest pain, congestive heart failure, sinus pause, sinus node dysfunction, syncope, ventricular arrhythmia, ventricular fibrillation, ventricular tachycardia.

Dermatologic: Pruritus, sweating.

Gastrointestinal: Constipation, elevated SGOT or alkaline phosphatase, nausea, vomiting.

Nervous system: Dizziness, paresthesia.

Other: Amblyopia, asthenia, dry mouth, dyspnea, edema, headache, hyperuricemia.

Although not observed in clinical trials with diltiazem HCl injectable, the following events associated with oral diltiazem may occur:

Cardiovascular: AV block (third degree), bundle branch, ECH abnormality, palpitations, syncope, tachycardia, ventricular extrasystoles.

Dermatologic: Alopecia, erythema multiforme, exfoliative dermatitis, leukocytoclastic vasculitis, petechiae, photosensitivity, purpura, rash, urticaria.

Gastrointestinal: Anorexia, diarrhea, dysgeusia, dyspepsia, mild elevations of SGPT and LDH, thirst, weight increase.

Nervous System: Abnormal dreams, amnesia, depression, extrapyramidal symptoms, gait abnormality, hallucinations, insomnia, nervousness, personality changes, somnolence, tremor.

Other: CPK elevation, epistaxis, eye irritation, gingival hyperplasia, hemolytic anemia, hyperglycemia, impotence, increased bleeding time, leukopenia, muscle cramps, nasal congestion, nocturia, osteoarticular pain, polyuria, retinopathy, sexual difficulties, thrombocytopenia, tinnitus.

Events such as myocardial infarction have been observed which are not readily distinguishable from the natural history of the disease for the patient.

OVERDOSAGE:

ORAL FORMS

The oral LD_{50}s in mice and rats range from 415 to 740 mg/kg and from 560 to 810 mg/kg, respectively. The intravenous LD_{50}s in these species were 60 and 38 mg/kg, respectively. The oral LD_{50} in dogs is considered to be in excess of 50 mg/kg, while lethality was seen in monkeys at 360 mg/kg.

The toxic dose in man is not known. Due to extensive metabolism, blood levels after a standard dose of diltiazem can vary over tenfold, limiting the usefulness of blood levels in overdose cases.

There have been 29 reports of diltiazem overdose in doses ranging from less than 1 g to 10.8: g. Sixteen of these reports involved multiple drug ingestions.

Twenty-two reports indicated patients had recovered from diltiazem overdose ranging from less than 1 g to 10.8 g. There were seven reports with a fatal outcome; although the amount of diltiazem ingested was unknown, multiple drug ingestions were confirmed in six of the seven reports.

Events observed following diltiazem overdose included bradycardia, hypotension, heart block, and cardiac failure. Most reports of overdose described some supportive medical measure and/or drug treatment. Bradycardia frequently responded favorably to atropine, as did heart block, although cardiac pacing was also frequently utilized to treat heart block. Fluids and vasopressors were used to maintain blood pressure, and in cases of cardiac failure inotropic agents were administered. In addition, some patients received treatment with ventilatory support, gastric lavage, activated charcoal, and/or intravenous calcium. Evidence of the effectiveness of intravenous calcium administration to reverse the pharmacological effects of diltiazem overdose was conflicting.

In the event of overdose or exaggerated response, appropriate supportive measures should be employed in addition to gastrointestinal decontamination. Diltiazem does not appear to be removed by peritoneal or hemodialysis. Based on the known pharmacological effects of diltiazem and/or reported clinical experiences, the following measures may be considered:

Bradycardia: Administer atropine (0.60 to 1.0 mg). If there is no response to vagal blockade, administer isoproterenol cautiously.

High-Degree AV Block: Treat as for bradycardia above. Fixed high-degree AV block should be treated with cardiac pacing.

Cardiac Failure: Administer inotropic agents (isoproterenol, dopamine, or dobutamine) and diuretics.

Hypotension: Vasopressors (*e.g.,* dopamine or levarterenol bitartrate).

Actual treatment and dosage should depend on the severity of the clinical situation and the judgment and experience of the treating physician.

INJECTION

Overdosage experience is limited. In the event of overdosage or an exaggerated response, appropriate supportive measures should be employed. The following measures may be considered:

Bradycardia: Administer atropine (0.60 to 1.0 mg). If there is no response to vagal blockade administer isoproterenol cautiously.

High-degree AV Block: Treat as for bradycardia above. Fixed high-degree AV block should be treated with cardiac pacing.

Cardiac failure: Administer inotropic agents (isoproterenol, dopamine, or dobutamine) and diuretics.

Hypotension: Vasopressors (*e.g.,* dopamine or levarterenol bitartrate).

Actual treatment and dosage should depend on the severity of the clinical situation and the judgment and experience of the treating physician. Diltiazem does not appear to be removed by peritoneal or hemodialysis. The intravenous LD_{50}s in mice and rats were 60 and 38 mg/kg, respectively. The toxic dose in man is not known.

DOSAGE AND ADMINISTRATION:

TABLETS

Exertional Angina Pectoris Due to Atherosclerotic Coronary Artery Disease or Angina Pectoris at Rest Due to Coronary Artery Spasm: Dosage must be adjusted to each patient's needs. Starting with 30 mg four times daily, before meals and at bedtime, dosage should be increased gradually (given in divided doses three or four times daily) at 1- to 2-day intervals until optimum response is obtained. Although individual patients may respond to any dosage level, the average optimum dosage range appears to be 180 to 360 mg/day. There are no available data concerning dosage requirements in patients with impaired renal or hepatic function. If the drug must be used in such patients, titration should be carried out with particular caution.

Concomitant Use with Other Cardiovascular Agents:

1. Sublingual NTG: may be taken as required to abort acute anginal attacks during diltiazem HCl therapy.

2. Prophylactic Nitrate Therapy: Diltiazem HCl may be safely coadministered with short- and long-acting nitrates, but there have been no controlled studies to evaluate the antianginal effectiveness of this combination.

3. Beta-blockers: See WARNINGS and PRECAUTIONS regarding use with beta-blockers.

SUSTAINED-RELEASE CAPSULES

Dosages must be adjusted to each patient's needs, starting with 60 to 120 mg twice daily. Maximum antihypertensive effect is usually observed by 14 days of chronic therapy; therefore, dosage adjustments should be scheduled accordingly. Although individual patients may respond to lower doses, the usual optimum dosage range in clinical trials was 240 to 360 mg/day.

Diltiazem HCl sustained release capsule has an additive antihypertensive effect when used with other antihypertensive agents. Therefore, the dosage of diltiazem HCl sustained release capsule or the concomitant antihypertensives may need to be adjusted when adding one to the other. See WARNINGS and PRECAUTIONS regarding use with beta-blockers.

ONCE-DAILY CAPSULES

Patients controlled on diltiazem alone or in combination with other medications may be switched to diltiazem HCl once-daily capsules at the nearest equivalent total daily dose. Higher doses of diltiazem HCl once-daily capsule may be needed in some patients. Patients should be closely monitored. Subsequent titration to higher or lower doses may be necessary and should be initiated as clinically warranted. There is limited general clinical experience with doses above 360 mg, but doses to 540 mg have been studied in clinical trials. The incidence of side effects increases as the dose increases with first-degree AV block, dizziness and sinus bradycardia bearing the strongest relationship to dose.

Hypertension: Dosage needs to be adjusted by titration to individual patient needs. When used as monotherapy, reasonable starting doses are 180 to 240 mg once daily, although some patients may respond to lower doses. Maximum antihypertensive effects is usually observed by 14 days of chronic therapy; therefore, dosage adjustments should be scheduled accordingly. The usual dosage range studied in clinical trials was 240 to 360 mg once daily. Individual patients may respond to higher doses of up to 480 mg once daily.

Angina: Dosages for the treatment of angina should be adjusted to each patient's needs, starting with a dose of 120 or 180 mg once daily. Individual patients may respond to higher doses of up to 480 mg once daily. When necessary, titration may be carried out over a 7- to 14-day period.

Concomitant Use With Other Cardiovascular Agents

1. Sublingual NTG: may be taken as required to abort acute anginal attacks during diltiazem HCl therapy.

2. Prophylactic Nitrate Therapy: diltiazem HCl once-daily capsule may be safely coadministered with short-and long-acting nitrate.

3. Beta-Blockers: (See WARNINGS and PRECAUTIONS).

4. Antihypertensives: Diltiazem HCl once-daily capsule has an additive antihypertensive effect when used with other antihypertensive agents. Therefore, the dosage of diltiazem HCl once-daily capsule or the concomitant antihypertensives may need to be adjusted when adding one to the other.

INJECTION

Direct Intravenous Single Injections (Bolus): The initial dose of diltiazem HCl injectable should be 0.25 mg/kg actual body weight as a bolus administered over 2 minutes (20 mg is a reasonable dose for the average patient). If response is inadequate, a second dose may be administered after 15 minutes. The second bolus dose of diltiazem HCl injectable should be 0.35 mg/kg actual body weight administered over 2 minutes (25 mg is a reasonable dose for the average patient). Subsequent intravenous bolus doses should be individualized for each patient. Patients with low body weights should be dosed on a mg/kg basis. Some patients may respond to an initial dose of 0.15 mg/kg, although duration of action may be shorter. Experience with this dose is limited.

Continuous Intravenous Infusion For continued reduction of the heart rate (up to 24 hours) in patients with atrial fibrillation or atrial flutter, an intravenous infusion of diltiazem HCl injectable may be administered. Immediately following bolus administration of 20 mg (0.25 mg/kg) or 25 mg (0.35 mg/kg) diltiazem HCl injectable and reduction of heart rate, begin an intravenous infusion of diltiazem HCl injectable. The recommended initial infusion rate of diltiazem HCl injectable is 10 mg/h. Some patients may maintain response to an initial rate of 5 mg/h. The infusion rate may be increased in 5 mg/h increments up to 15 mg/h as needed, if further reduction in heart rate is required. The infusion may be maintained for up to 24 hours.

Diltiazem shows dose-dependent, non-linear pharmacokinetics. Duration of infusion longer than 24 hours and infusion rates greater than 15 mg/h have not been studied. Therefore, infusion duration exceeding 24 hours and infusion rates exceeding 15 mg/h are not recommended.

Dilution: To prepare diltiazem HCl injectable for continuous intravenous infusion aseptically transfer the appropriate quantity (see TABLE 3) of diltiazem HCl injectable to the desired volume of either Normal Saline, D5W, or D5W/0.45% NaCl. Mix thoroughly. Use within 24 hours. Keep refrigerated until use.

TABLE 3 Administration

Diluent Volume	Quantity of Cardizem Injection	Final Concentration	Dose*	Infusion Rate
100 ml	125 mg (25 ml)	1.0 mg/ml	10 mg/h 15 mg/h	10 ml/h 15 ml/h
250 ml	250 mg (50 ml)	0.83 mg/ml	10 mg/h 15 mg/h	12 ml/h 18 ml/h
500 ml	250 mg (50 ml)	0.45 mg/ml	10 mg/h 15 mg/h	22 ml/h 33 ml/h

* 5 mg/h may be appropriate for some patients

DOSAGE AND ADMINISTRATION: *(cont'd)*

Diltiazem HCl injectable was tested for compatibility with three commonly used intravenous fluids at a maximal concentration of 1 mg diltiazem hydrochloride per milliliter. Diltiazem HCl injectable was found to be physically compatible and chemically stable in the following parenteral solutions for at least 24 hours when stored in glass or polyvinylchloride (PVC) bags at controlled room temperature 15-30°C (59-86°F) or under refrigeration 2-8°C (36-46°F).

dextrose (5%) injection USP

sodium chloride (0.9%) injection USP

dextrose (5%) and sodium chloride (0.45%) injection USP.

Because of potential physical incompatibilities, it is recommended that diltiazem HCl injectable not be mixed with any other drugs in the same container.

If possible, diltiazem HCl injectable not be co-infused in the same intravenous line. Physical incompatibilities (precipitate formation or cloudiness) were observed when diltiazem HCl injectable was infused in the same intravenous line with the following drugs: acetazolamide, acyclovir, aminophylline, ampicillin sodium/sulbactam sodium, cefamandole, cefoperazone diazepam, furosemide, hydrocortisone sodium succinate, insulin, (regular: 100 units/ml), methylprednisolone sodium succinate, mezlocillin, nafcillin, phenytoin, rifampin, and sodium bicarbonate.

Parenteral drug products should be inspected visually for particulate matter and discoloration prior to administration whenever solution and container permit.

Transition to Further Antiarrhythmic Therapy. Transition to other antiarrhythmic agents following administration of diltiazem HCl injectable is generally safe. However, reference should be made to the respective agent manufacturer's package insert for information relative to dosage and administration.

PATIENT INFORMATION:

Diltiazem is a calcium channel blocker used for the treatment of high blood pressure and angina (chest pain). Notify your physician if you are pregnant or nursing. Take diltiazem on an empty stomach at approximately the same time each morning. Tablets may be crushed, if needed. Capsules must be swallowed whole; they should not be crushed or chewed. Do not stop taking diltiazem without talking with your physician. This medication may cause dizziness or lightheadedness, use caution while driving or operating hazardous machinery. Avoid sudden changes in posture. Notify your physician if you develop chest pain, difficulty breathing, irregular heartbeat, skin rash, fainting, or swollen ankles.

HOW SUPPLIED:

Oral: Store at controlled room temperature 59-86°F (15-30°C).

Injection: STORE PRODUCT UNDER REFRIGERATION 2-8°C (36 -46°F). DO NOT FREEZE. MAY BE STORED AT ROOM TEMPERATURE FOR UP TO 1 MONTH. DESTROY AFTER 1 MONTH AT ROOM TEMPERATURE.

HOW SUPPLIED - RATED THERAPEUTICALLY EQUIVALENT:

Capsule, Gelatin, Sustained Action - Oral - 60 mg

100's	$69.20	Diltiazem Hcl, Major Pharms	00904-7840-60
100's	$69.60	Diltiazem HCl, Teva	00093-0021-01
100's	$69.93	Diltiazem Hcl, Aligen Independ	00405-4347-01
100's	$77.40	Diltiazem HCl, H.C.F.A. F F P	99999-1069-01
100's	**$81.56**	**CARDIZEM SR, Hoechst Marion Roussel**	**00088-1777-47**
100's	**$91.50**	**CARDIZEM SR, Hoechst Marion Roussel**	**00088-1777-49**

Capsule, Gelatin, Sustained Action - Oral - 90 mg

100's	$79.20	Diltiazem Hcl, Major Pharms	00904-7841-60
100's	$80.01	Diltiazem Hcl, Aligen Independ	00405-4348-01
100's	$80.20	Diltiazem HCl, Teva	00093-0022-01
100's	$84.98	Diltiazem HCl, H.C.F.A. F F P	99999-1069-02
100's	**$93.31**	**CARDIZEM SR, Hoechst Marion Roussel**	**00088-1778-47**
100's	**$104.81**	**CARDIZEM SR, Hoechst Marion Roussel**	**00088-1778-49**

Capsule, Gelatin, Sustained Action - Oral - 120 mg

100's	$103.15	Diltiazem Hcl, Major Pharms	00904-7842-60
100's	$104.21	Diltiazem Hcl, Aligen Independ	00405-4349-01
100's	$104.25	Diltiazem HCl, Teva	00093-0023-01
100's	**$121.56**	**CARDIZEM SR, Hoechst Marion Roussel**	**00088-1779-47**
100's	**$136.44**	**CARDIZEM SR, Hoechst Marion Roussel**	**00088-1779-49**

Tablet, Plain Coated - Oral - 30 mg

30's	$3.25	Diltiazem HCl, H.C.F.A. F F P	99999-1069-03
100's	$10.85	Diltiazem HCl, H.C.F.A. F F P	99999-1069-04
100's	$11.70	Diltiazem, United Res	00677-1451-01
100's	$34.37	Diltiazem Hcl, Aligen Independ	00405-4340-01
100's	$34.37	Diltiazem Hydrochloride, Copley Pharm	38245-0631-10
100's	$34.37	Diltiazem Hcl, West Point Pharma	59591-0071-68
100's	$34.90	Diltiazem, Major Pharms	00904-7707-60
100's	$34.90	Diltiazem, Major Pharms	00904-7714-60
100's	$34.90	Diltiazem Hcl, Martec Pharms	52555-0465-01
100's	$35.35	Diltiazem Hcl, Harber Pharm	51432-0760-03
100's	$35.45	Diltiazem, Lederle Pharm	00005-3333-43
100's	$35.80	Diltiazem HCl, Bristol Myers Squibb	00003-5250-02
100's	$35.96	Diltiazem Hcl, Qualitest Pharms	00603-3319-21
100's	$36.23	Diltiazem HCl, Geneva Pharms	00781-1158-01
100's	$39.50	Diltiazem HCl, Schein Pharm (US)	00364-2541-01
100's	$39.85	Diltiazem Hcl, Zenith Labs	00172-4219-60
100's	$39.85	Diltiazem, Goldline Labs	00182-1937-01
100's	$39.95	Diltiazem, HL Moore Drug Exch	00839-7748-06
100's	$41.08	Diltiazem, Mylan	00378-0023-01
100's	$42.22	Diltiazem HCl, Rugby	00536-3101-01
100's	$42.50	Diltiazem Hcl, Goldline Labs	00182-1937-89
100's	$42.58	Diltiazem Hcl, Major Pharms	00904-7714-61
100's	**$44.31**	**CARDIZEM, Hoechst Marion Roussel**	**00088-1771-47**
100's	$45.15	Diltiazem Hcl, Vangard Labs	00615-3548-13
100's	**$50.13**	**CARDIZEM, Hoechst Marion Roussel**	**00088-1771-49**
500's	$54.25	Diltiazem HCl, H.C.F.A. F F P	99999-1069-05
500's	$170.00	Diltiazem Hcl, Copley Pharm	38245-0631-50
500's	$173.40	Diltiazem Hcl, Martec Pharms	52555-0465-05
500's	$173.95	Diltiazem Hcl, Major Pharms	00904-7714-40
500's	$177.21	Diltiazem HCl, Bristol Myers Squibb	00003-5250-03
500's	$179.48	Diltiazem, HL Moore Drug Exch	00839-7748-12
500's	$182.00	Diltiazem Hcl, Qualitest Pharms	00603-3319-28
500's	$201.87	Diltiazem, Mylan	00378-0023-05
500's	$207.64	Diltiazem HCl, Rugby	00536-3101-05
500's	**$217.81**	**CARDIZEM, Hoechst Marion Roussel**	**00088-1771-55**
750's	$335.62	Diltiazem Hcl, Glasgow Pharm	60809-0123-55
750's	$335.62	Diltiazem Hcl, Glasgow Pharm	60809-0123-72
1000's	$108.50	Diltiazem HCl, H.C.F.A. F F P	99999-1069-06
1000's	$318.97	Diltiazem HCl, Bristol Myers Squibb	00003-5250-04
1000's	$336.82	Diltiazem Hcl, Lederle Pharm	00005-3333-34
1000's	$359.57	Diltiazem Hcl, HL Moore Drug Exch	00839-7748-16
1000's	$384.20	Diltiazem Hcl, Zenith Labs	00172-4219-80

HOW SUPPLIED - RATED THERAPEUTICALLY EQUIVALENT: *(cont'd)*

1000's	$384.20	Diltiazem Hcl, Goldline Labs	00182-1937-10
5000's	$542.50	Diltiazem HCl, H.C.F.A. F F P	99999-1069-07
5000's	**$2178.55**	**CARDIZEM, Hoechst Marion Roussel**	**00088-1771-90**

Tablet, Plain Coated - Oral - 60 mg

30's	$5.06	Diltiazem HCl, H.C.F.A. F F P	99999-1069-08
90's	**$58.94**	**CARDIZEM, Hoechst Marion Roussel**	**00088-1772-42**
100's	$16.89	Diltiazem HCl, H.C.F.A. F F P	99999-1069-09
100's	$18.09	Diltiazem, United Res	00677-1450-01
100's	$53.83	Diltiazem Hcl, Copley Pharm	38245-0662-10
100's	$53.86	Diltiazem Hcl, West Point Pharma	59591-0072-68
100's	$54.50	Diltiazem, Major Pharms	00904-7708-60
100's	$54.50	Diltiazem, Major Pharms	00904-7715-60
100's	$54.85	Diltiazem Hcl, Harber Pharm	51432-0752-03
100's	$55.53	Diltiazem, Lederle Pharm	00005-3334-43
100's	$56.23	Diltiazem Hcl, Aligen Independ	00405-4341-01
100's	$56.23	Diltiazem Hcl, Qualitest Pharms	00603-3320-21
100's	$56.50	Diltiazem HCl, Bristol Myers Squibb	00003-5550-02
100's	$56.77	Diltiazem HCl, Geneva Pharms	00781-1159-01
100's	$56.85	Diltiazem Hcl, Martec Pharms	52555-0466-01
100's	$58.98	Diltiazem, HL Moore Drug Exch	00839-7749-06
100's	$61.00	Diltiazem HCl, Schein Pharm (US)	00364-2542-01
100's	$61.47	Diltiazem Hcl, Major Pharms	00904-7715-61
100's	$62.57	Diltiazem Hcl, Zenith Labs	00172-4220-60
100's	$62.57	Diltiazem, Goldline Labs	00182-1938-01
100's	$64.46	Diltiazem, Mylan	00378-0045-01
100's	$66.30	Diltiazem HCl, Rugby	00536-3102-01
100's	$66.50	Diltiazem Hcl, Goldline Labs	00182-1938-89
100's	**$69.56**	**CARDIZEM, Hoechst Marion Roussel**	**00088-1772-47**
100's	$71.60	Diltiazem Hcl, Vangard Labs	00615-3549-13
100's	**$78.44**	**CARDIZEM, Hoechst Marion Roussel**	**00088-1772-49**
100's UD	$67.63	Diltiazem HCl, U.D., Rugby	00536-3102-21
500's	$84.45	Diltiazem HCl, H.C.F.A. F F P	99999-1069-10
500's	$265.00	Diltiazem Hcl, Copley Pharm	38245-0662-50
500's	$269.25	Diltiazem Hcl, Martec Pharms	52555-0466-05
500's	$271.55	Diltiazem Hcl, Major Pharms	00904-7715-40
500's	$274.80	Diltiazem Hcl, Qualitest Pharms	00603-3320-28
500's	$276.88	Diltiazem HCl, Bristol Myers Squibb	00003-5550-03
500's	$284.51	Diltiazem, HL Moore Drug Exch	00839-7749-12
500's	$316.50	Diltiazem, Mylan	00378-0045-05
500's	$325.52	Diltiazem HCl, Rugby	00536-3102-05
500's	**$341.44**	**CARDIZEM, Hoechst Marion Roussel**	**00088-1772-55**
750's	$525.35	Diltiazem Hcl, Glasgow Pharm	60809-0124-55
750's	$525.35	Diltiazem Hcl, Glasgow Pharm	60809-0124-72
1000's	$168.90	Diltiazem HCl, H.C.F.A. F F P	99999-1069-11
1000's	$498.36	Diltiazem HCl, Bristol Myers Squibb	00003-5550-04
1000's	$527.53	Diltiazem Hcl, Lederle Pharm	00005-3334-34
1000's	$530.82	Diltiazem Hcl, HL Moore Drug Exch	00839-7749-16
1000's	$602.30	Diltiazem Hcl, Zenith Labs	00172-4220-80
1000's	$602.30	Diltiazem Hcl, Goldline Labs	00182-1938-10
5000's	$844.50	Diltiazem HCl, H.C.F.A. F F P	99999-1069-12
5000's	**$3415.75**	**CARDIZEM, Hoechst Marion Roussel**	**00088-1772-90**

Tablet, Plain Coated - Oral - 90 mg

30's	$6.92	Diltiazem HCl, H.C.F.A. F F P	99999-1069-13
90's	**$83.00**	**CARDIZEM, Hoechst Marion Roussel**	**00088-1791-42**
100's	$23.09	Diltiazem, United Res	00677-1449-01
100's	$23.09	Diltiazem HCl, H.C.F.A. F F P	99999-1069-14
100's	$30.92	Diltiazem Hcl, Vangard Labs	00615-3550-13
100's	$75.65	Diltiazem Hcl, Aligen Independ	00405-4342-01
100's	$75.65	Diltiazem Hydrochloride, Copley Pharm	38245-0691-10
100's	$75.70	Diltiazem Hcl, West Point Pharma	59591-0075-68
100's	$76.40	Diltiazem, Major Pharms	00904-7709-60
100's	$76.40	Diltiazem, Major Pharms	00904-7716-60
100's	$76.70	Diltiazem Hcl, Harber Pharm	51432-0756-03
100's	$78.04	Diltiazem, Lederle Pharm	00005-3335-43
100's	$78.40	Diltiazem HCl, Bristol Myers Squibb	00003-5770-02
100's	$78.66	Diltiazem Hcl, Qualitest Pharms	00603-3321-21
100's	$79.25	Diltiazem Hcl, Martec Pharms	52555-0467-01
100's	$79.74	Diltiazem HCl, Geneva Pharms	00781-1174-01
100's	$81.93	Diltiazem, HL Moore Drug Exch	00839-7750-06
100's	$86.29	Diltiazem Hcl, Major Pharms	00904-7716-61
100's	$87.80	Diltiazem HCl, Schein Pharm (US)	00364-2543-01
100's	$87.92	Diltiazem Hcl, Zenith Labs	00172-4221-60
100's	$87.92	Diltiazem, Goldline Labs	00182-1939-01
100's	$90.62	Diltiazem, Mylan	00378-0135-01
100's	$93.23	Diltiazem HCl, Rugby	00536-3103-01
100's	**$97.75**	**CARDIZEM, Hoechst Marion Roussel**	**00088-1791-47**
100's	**$110.44**	**CARDIZEM, Hoechst Marion Roussel**	**00088-1791-49**
500's	$115.45	Diltiazem HCl, H.C.F.A. F F P	99999-1069-15
500's	$372.41	Diltiazem HCl, Bristol Myers Squibb	00003-5770-03
500's	$405.80	Diltiazem, HL Moore Drug Exch	00839-7750-12
500's	$430.43	Diltiazem, Mylan	00378-0135-05
1000's	$230.90	Diltiazem HCl, H.C.F.A. F F P	99999-1069-16
1000's	$737.37	Diltiazem Hcl, HL Moore Drug Exch	00839-7750-16
1000's	$741.37	Diltiazem Hcl, Lederle Pharm	00005-3335-34
5000's	**$4611.60**	**CARDIZEM, Hoechst Marion Roussel**	**00088-1791-90**

Tablet, Plain Coated - Oral - 120 mg

100's	$30.20	Diltiazem HCl, H.C.F.A. F F P	99999-1069-17
100's	$99.00	Diltiazem Hcl, Aligen Independ	00405-4343-01
100's	$99.00	Diltiazem Hydrochloride, Copley Pharm	38245-0720-10
100's	$99.06	Diltiazem, Lederle Pharm	00005-3336-43
100's	$99.06	Diltiazem Hcl, West Point Pharma	59591-0077-68
100's	$99.25	Diltiazem, Major Pharms	00904-7710-60
100's	$99.25	Diltiazem, Major Pharms	00904-7717-60
100's	$99.95	Diltiazem Hcl, Harber Pharm	51432-0757-03
100's	$101.68	Diltiazem HCl, Bristol Myers Squibb	00003-5850-02
100's	$102.50	Diltiazem Hcl, Martec Pharms	52555-0468-01
100's	$104.40	Diltiazem HCl, Geneva Pharms	00781-1175-01
100's	$104.45	Diltiazem Hcl, Major Pharms	00904-7717-61
100's	$105.10	Diltiazem Hcl, Qualitest Pharms	00603-3322-21
100's	$105.64	Diltiazem, HL Moore Drug Exch	00839-7751-06
100's	$115.13	Diltiazem Hcl, Zenith Labs	00172-4222-60
100's	$115.13	Diltiazem, Goldline Labs	00182-1940-01
100's	$115.14	Diltiazem HCl, Schein Pharm (US)	00364-2544-01
100's	$118.62	Diltiazem, Mylan	00378-0525-01
100's	$122.04	Diltiazem HCl, Rugby	00536-3104-01
100's	**$128.00**	**CARDIZEM, Hoechst Marion Roussel**	**00088-1792-47**
100's	**$143.63**	**CARDIZEM, Hoechst Marion Roussel**	**00088-1792-49**
1000's	$302.00	Diltiazem HCl, H.C.F.A. F F P	99999-1069-18
1000's	$941.09	Diltiazem Hcl, Lederle Pharm	00005-3336-34
5000's	**$6034.55**	**CARDIZEM, Hoechst Marion Roussel**	**00088-1792-90**

HOW SUPPLIED - NOT RATED EQUIVALENT:

Capsule, Gelatin, Sustained Action - Oral - 120 mg

30's	**$31.32**	**CARDIZEM CD, Hoechst Marion Roussel**	**00088-1795-30**
90's	**$91.98**	**CARDIZEM CD, Hoechst Marion Roussel**	**00088-1795-42**
100's	$96.48	DILACOR XR, Rhone-Poulenc Rorer	00075-0250-00
100's	**$102.00**	**CARDIZEM CD, Hoechst Marion Roussel**	**00088-1795-49**
1000's	$887.50	DILACOR XR, Rhone-Poulenc Rorer	00075-0250-99
5000's	**$5112.60**	**CARDIZEM CD, Hoechst Marion Roussel**	**00088-1795-90**

Capsule, Gelatin, Sustained Action - Oral - 180 mg

30's	**$38.82**	**CARDIZEM CD, Hoechst Marion Roussel**	**00088-1796-30**
90's	**$111.00**	**CARDIZEM CD, Hoechst Marion Roussel**	**00088-1796-42**
100's	$108.19	DILACOR XR, Rhone-Poulenc Rorer	00075-0251-00
100's	$113.63	DILACOR XR, Rhone-Poulenc Rorer	00075-0251-62
100's	**$122.64**	**CARDIZEM CD, Hoechst Marion Roussel**	**00088-1796-49**
1000's	$995.35	DILACOR XR, Rhone-Poulenc Rorer	00075-0251-99
5000's	**$6170.90**	**CARDIZEM CD, Hoechst Marion Roussel**	**00088-1796-90**

Capsule, Gelatin, Sustained Action - Oral - 240 mg

30's	**$52.62**	**CARDIZEM CD, Hoechst Marion Roussel**	**00088-1797-30**
90's	**$157.50**	**CARDIZEM CD, Hoechst Marion Roussel**	**00088-1797-42**
100's	$116.84	DILACOR XR, Rhone-Poulenc Rorer	00075-0252-00
100's	$122.71	DILACOR XR, Rhone-Poulenc Rorer	00075-0252-62
100's	**$174.30**	**CARDIZEM CD, Hoechst Marion Roussel**	**00088-1797-49**
1000's	$1074.97	DILACOR XR, Rhone-Poulenc Rorer	00075-0252-99
5000's	**$8754.15**	**CARDIZEM CD, Hoechst Marion Roussel**	**00088-1797-90**

Capsule, Gelatin, Sustained Action - Oral - 300 mg

30's	**$68.94**	**CARDIZEM CD, Hoechst Marion Roussel**	**00088-1798-30**
90's	**$204.06**	**CARDIZEM CD, Hoechst Marion Roussel**	**00088-1798-42**
100's	**$224.70**	**CARDIZEM CD, Hoechst Marion Roussel**	**00088-1798-49**

Injection, Solution - Intravenous - 5 mg/ml

5 ml x 6	**$79.32**	**CARDIZEM, Hoechst Marion Roussel**	**00088-1790-32**
10 ml x 6	**$147.00**	**CARDIZEM, Hoechst Marion Roussel**	**00088-1790-33**

DIMENHYDRINATE *(001070)*

CATEGORIES: Antiemetics; Gastrointestinal Drugs; Nausea; Vertigo/Motion Sickness/Vomiting; Vomiting; Pregnancy Category B; FDA Approval Pre 1982

BRAND NAMES: *Amosyt*; *Anautin*; *Andrumin*; *Antimo*; *Apo-Dimenhydrinate* (Canada); *Biodramina*; *Demodenal*; *Denim*; Di-Men; *Dimen* (Germany); *Dimenate*; *Dimeno*; Dimetabs; Dinate; Dommanate; *Dramamine* (Australia, Asia, France, England, Germany, Mexico); **Dramamine Injection**; Dramanate; Dramavance; Dramocen; Dramoject; *Drimen*; Dymenate; *Emes*; *Gravol* (Canada); *Gravol L A* (Canada); *Hydramen*; Hydrate; *Lomarin*; Marmine; *Mendrin*; *Menito*; *Motivan*; *Nauseatol* (Canada); *Nausex*; *Nausicalm* (France); *Novomin*; Or-Dram; Shodram; T-Circ; *Terminol*; *Travelgum*; *Trimin*; *Vertirosan*; *Vomacur* (Germany); *Vomex*; *Vomex A* (Germany); *Vomisin* (Mexico); Wehamine; *Xamamina*
(International brand names outside U.S. in italics)

FORMULARIES: Medi-Cal

DESCRIPTION:

Dimenhydrinate is the 8-chlorotheophylline salt of diphenhydramine. It contains not less than 53% and not more than 55.5% of diphenhydramine, and not less than 44% and not more than 47% of 8-chlorotheophylline, calculated on the dried basis. Chemically it is 8-chlorotheophylline, compound with 2-(diphenylmethoxy)-*N,N*-dimethylethylamine (1:1).

In Sterile Cartridge-Needle Units, each ml contains 50 mg dimenhydrinate, 0.1% edetate disodium, 5% benzyl alcohol, and 50% propylene glycol. Sealed under nitrogen.

CLINICAL PHARMACOLOGY:

While the precise mode of action of dimenhydrinate is not known, it has a depressant action on hyperstimulated labyrinthine function.

INDICATIONS AND USAGE:

Dimenhydrinate injection is indicated for the prevention & treatment of the nausea, vomiting, or vertigo of motion sickness.

CONTRAINDICATIONS:

Neonates and patients with a history of hypersensitivity to dimenhydrinate or its components (diphenhydramine or 8-chlorotheophylline) should not be treated with dimenhydrinate.

WARNINGS:

Caution should be used when dimenhydrinate is given in conjunction with certain antibiotics that may cause ototoxicity, since dimenhydrinate is capable of masking ototoxic symptoms, and an irreversible state may be reached.

This drug may impair the mental and/or physical abilities required for the performance of potentially hazardous tasks, such as driving a vehicle or operating machinery. The concomitant use of alcohol or other central nervous system depressants may have an additive effect. Therefore, patients should be warned accordingly.

Dimenhydrinate should be used with caution in patients having conditions which might be aggravated by anticholinergic therapy (*i.e.,* prostatic hypertrophy, stenosing peptic ulcer, pyloroduodenal obstruction, bladder-neck obstruction, narrow-angle glaucoma, bronchial asthma, or cardiac arrhythmias).

Under no circumstances should intra-arterial injections be given.

USAGE IN CHILDREN

For infants and children, especially, antihistamines in overdosage may cause hallucinations, convulsions, or death.

As in adults, antihistamines may diminish mental alertness in children. In the young child, particularly, they may produce excitation.

PRECAUTIONS:

GENERAL

Drowsiness may be experienced by some patients, especially with high dosage. This effect frequently is not undesirable in conditions for which the drug is used.

INFORMATION FOR THE PATIENT

Because of the potential for drowsiness, patients taking dimenhydrinate should be cautioned against operating automobiles or dangerous machinery. See WARNINGS

PRECAUTIONS: *(cont'd)*

CARCINOGENESIS, MUTAGENESIS, AND IMPAIRMENT OF FERTILITY

Mutagenicity screening tests performed with dimenhydrinate, diphenhydramine, and 8-chlorotheophylline produced positive results in the bacterial systems and negative results in the mammalian systems. There are no human data that indicate dimenhydrinate is a carcinogen or mutagen or that it impairs fertility.

PREGNANCY CATEGORY B

Reproduction studies have been performed in rats at doses up to 20 times the human dose, and in rabbits at doses up to 25 times the human dose (on a mg/kg basis), and have revealed no evidence of impaired fertility or harm to the fetus due to dimenhydrinate. There are no adequate and well-controlled studies in pregnant women. However, clinical studies in pregnant women have not indicated that dimenhydrinate increases the risk of abnormalities when administered in any trimester of pregnancy. It would appear that the possibility of fetal harm is remote when the drug is used during pregnancy. Nevertheless, because the studies in humans cannot rule out the possibility of harm, dimenhydrinate should be used during pregnancy only if clearly needed.

LABOR AND DELIVERY

The safety of dimenhydrinate injection given during labor and delivery has not been established. Reports have indicated dimenhydrinate may have an oxytocic effect. Caution is advised when this effect is unwanted or in situations where it may prove detrimental.

NURSING MOTHERS

Small amounts of dimenhydrinate are excreted in breast milk. Because of the potential for adverse reactions in nursing infants from dimenhydrinate, a decision should be made whether to discontinue nursing or to discontinue the drug, taking into account the importance of the drug to the mother.

ADVERSE REACTIONS:

The most frequent adverse reaction to dimenhydrinate is drowsiness. Dizziness may also occur. Symptoms of dry mouth, nose and throat, blurred vision, difficult or painful urination, headache, anorexia, nervousness, restlessness or insomnia (especially in children), skin rash, thickening of bronchial secretions, tachycardia, epigastric distress, lassitude, excitation, and nausea have been reported.

OVERDOSAGE:

Drowsiness is the usual clinical side effect. Convulsions, coma, and respiratory depression may occur with massive overdosage. No specific antidote is known. If respiratory depression occurs, mechanically assisted respiration should be initiated and oxygen administered. Convulsions should be treated with appropriate doses of diazepam. Phenobarbital (5 to 6 mg/kg) may be given to control convulsions in children.

The oral LD_{50} in mice and rats is 203 mg/kg and 1320 mg/kg, respectively. The intraperitoneal LD_{50} in mice is 149 mg/kg.

DOSAGE AND ADMINISTRATION:

Dimenhydrinate in the injectable form is indicated when the oral form is impractical.

ADULTS

Nausea or vomiting may be expected to be controlled for approximately 4 hours with 50 mg, and prevented by a similar dose every 4 hours. Its administration may be attended by some degree of drowsiness in some patients, and 100 mg every 4 hours may be given in conditions in which drowsiness is not objectionable or is even desirable.

For intramuscular administration, each milliliter (50 mg) of solution is injected as needed, but for intravenous administration, each milliliter (50 mg) of solution must be diluted in 10 ml of 0.9% Sodium Chloride Injection, USP, and injected over a period of 2 minutes.

PEDIATRIC

For intramuscular administration, 1.25 mg/kg of body weight or 37.5 mg/m^2 of body surface area is administered four times daily. The maximum dose should not exceed 300 mg daily.

Parenteral drug products should be inspected visually for particulate matter and discoloration prior to administration, whenever solution and container permit.

Store at room temperature, approx. 25°C (77°F)

Do not use if solution is discolored or contains a precipitate.

HOW SUPPLIED - RATED THERAPEUTICALLY EQUIVALENT:

Injection, Solution - Intramuscular; - 50 mg/ml

1 ml	$2.54	Dimenhydrinate, Steris Labs	00402-0241-01
1 ml x 10	$28.70	Dimenhydrinate, Wyeth Labs	00008-0485-01
1 ml x 25	$82.60	Dimenhydrinate, Schein Pharm (US)	00364-6529-46
10 ml	$1.50	Dimenhydrinate, Lannett	00527-0179-55
10 ml	$4.00	Dimenhydrinate, Consolidated Midland	00223-7475-10
10 ml	$6.00	Dimenhydrinate, C O Truxton	00463-1086-10
10 ml	$6.90	HYDRATE, Hyrex Pharms	00314-0661-70
10 ml	$7.00	Dimenhydrinate, Steris Labs	00402-0241-10
10 ml	$7.12	Dimenhydrinate, Rugby	00536-4430-70
10 ml	$7.13	Dimenhydrinate, United Res	00677-0599-21
10 ml	$10.15	Dimenhydrinate, Schein Pharm (US)	00364-6529-54
10 ml	$11.40	Dimenhydrinate, Goldline Labs	00182-0938-63
10 ml	$15.60	DRAMOJECT, Mayrand Pharms	00259-0298-10
25 x 10 ml	$81.25	Dimenhydrinate, Pasadena	00418-4800-10

HOW SUPPLIED - NOT RATED EQUIVALENT:

Tablet, Uncoated - Oral - 50 mg

100's	$1.92	Dimenhydrinate, Qualitest Pharms	00603-3326-21
100's	$4.20	Dimenhydrinate, Vangard Labs	00615-0525-01
100's	$5.70	Dimenhydrinate, Voluntary Hosp	53258-0119-13
1000's	$12.88	Dimenhydrinate, Qualitest Pharms	00603-3326-32

DIMETHYL SULFOXIDE *(001075)*

CATEGORIES: Cystitis; Blood Formation/Coagulation*; Deficiency Anemias*; Pregnancy Category C; FDA Approval Pre 1982
* Indication not approved by the FDA

BRAND NAMES: **Rimso-50**

DESCRIPTION:

Rimso-50, brand of dimethyl sulfoxide (DMSO) 50% w/w Aqueous Solution for intravesical instillation

Each ml contains 0.54 gm dimethyl sulfoxide

STERILE AND NON-PYROGENIC

Intravesical instillation for the treatment of interstitial cystitis

NOT FOR IM OR IV INJECTION, DO NOT AUTOCLAVE.

DESCRIPTION: *(cont'd)*

Dimethyl sulfoxide has the empirical formula C_2H_6OS.

Dimethyl sulfoxide is a clear, colorless and essentially odorless liquid which is miscible with water and most organic solvents. Other physical characteristics include: molecular weight 78.13, melting point 18.3°C, and a specific gravity of 1.096.

CLINICAL PHARMACOLOGY:

Dimethyl sulfoxide is metabolized in man by oxidation to dimethyl sulfone or by reduction to dimethyl sulfide. Dimethyl sulfoxide and dimethyl sulfone are excreted in the urine and feces. Dimethyl sulfide is eliminated through the breath and skin and is responsible for the characteristic odor from patients on dimethyl sulfoxide medication. Dimethyl sulfone can persist in serum for longer than two weeks after a single intravesical instillation. No residual accumulation of dimethyl sulfoxide has occurred in man or lower animals who have received treatment for protracted periods of time. Following topical application, dimethyl sulfoxide is absorbed and generally distributed in the tissues and body fluids.

INDICATIONS AND USAGE:

Dimethyl sulfoxide is indicated for the symptomatic relief of patients with interstitial cystitis. Dimethyl sulfoxide has not been approved as being safe and effective for any other indication. There is no clinical evidence of effectiveness of dimethyl sulfoxide in the treatment of bacterial infections of the urinary tract.

CONTRAINDICATIONS:

None known.

WARNINGS:

Dimethyl sulfoxide can initiate the liberation of histamine and there has been occasional hypersensitivity reaction with topical administration of dimethyl sulfoxide. This hypersensitivity has been reported in one patient receiving intravesical dimethyl sulfoxide. The physician should be cognizant of this possibility in prescribing dimethyl sulfoxide. If anaphylactoid symptoms develop, appropriate therapy should be instituted.

PRECAUTIONS:

GENERAL

Changes in the refractive index and lens opacities have been seen in monkeys, dogs and rabbits given high doses of dimethyl sulfoxide chronically. Since lens changes were noted in animals, full eye evaluations, including slit lamp examinations, are recommended prior to and periodically during treatment.

Approximately every six months patients receiving dimethyl sulfoxide should have a biochemical screening, particularly liver and renal function tests, and complete blood count.

Intravesical instillation of dimethyl sulfoxide may be harmful to patients with urinary tract malignancy because of dimethyl sulfoxide-induced vasodilation. Some data indicate that dimethyl sulfoxide potentiates other concomitantly administered medications.

PREGNANCY CATEGORY C

Dimethyl sulfoxide caused teratogenic responses in hamsters, rats and mice when administered intraperitoneally at high doses (2.5-12 gm/kg). Oral or topical doses of dimethyl sulfoxide did not cause problems of reproduction in rats, mice and hamsters. Topical doses (5 gm/kg first two days, then 2.5 gm/kg —last eight days) produced terata in rabbits, but in another study, topical doses of 1.1 gm/kg days 3 through 16 of gestation failed to produce any abnormalities. There are no adequate and well controlled studies in pregnant women. Dimethyl sulfoxide should be used during pregnancy only if the potential benefit justifies the potential risk to the fetus.

NURSING MOTHERS

It is not known whether this drug is excreted in human milk. Because many drugs are excreted in human milk, caution should be exercised when dimethyl sulfoxide is administered to a nursing woman.

PEDIATRIC USE

Safety and effectiveness in children have not been established.

ADVERSE REACTIONS:

A garlic-like taste may be noted by the patient within a few minutes after instillation of dimethyl sulfoxide. This taste may last several hours and because of the presence of metabolites, an odor on the breath and skin may remain for 72 hours.

Transient chemical cystitis has been noted following instillation of dimethyl sulfoxide.

The patient may experience moderately severe discomfort on administration. Usually this becomes less prominent with repeated administration.

DRUG ABUSE AND DEPENDENCE:

None known.

OVERDOSAGE:

The oral LD_{50} of dimethyl sulfoxide in the dog is greater than 10 gm/kg. It is improbable that this dosage level could be obtained with intravesical instillation of dimethyl sulfoxide in the patient.

In case of accidental oral ingestion, specific measures should be taken to induce emesis. Additional measures which may be considered are gastric lavage, activated charcoal and forced diuresis.

DOSAGE AND ADMINISTRATION:

Instillation of 50 ml of dimethyl sulfoxide directly into the bladder may be accomplished by catheter or asepto syringe and allowed to remain for 15 minutes. Application of an analgesic lubricant gel such as lidocaine jelly to the urethra is suggested prior to insertion of the catheter to avoid spasm. The medication is expelled by spontaneous voiding. It is recommended that the treatment be repeated every two weeks until maximum symptomatic relief is obtained. Thereafter, time intervals between therapy may be increased appropriately.

Administration of oral analgesic medication or suppositories containing belladonna and opium prior to the instillation of dimethyl sulfoxide can reduce bladder spasm.

In patients with severe interstitial cystitis with very sensitive bladders, the initial treatment, and possibly the second and third (depending on patient response) should be done under anesthesia. (Saddle block has been suggested).

Store at room temperature (59° to 86°F) (15 to 30°C)

HOW SUPPLIED - EQUIVALENTS NOT AVAILABLE:

Irrigation, Solution - Bladder; Intrav - 50 %

50 ml	**$587.50**	**RIMSO-50, Res Inds**	**00433-0433-05**

DINOPROSTONE *(003051)*

CATEGORIES: Abortion; Oxytocics; Prostaglandins; Trophoblastic Disease; Uterine Evacuation; Labor*; Pregnancy Category C; FDA Approval Pre 1982
* Indication not approved by the FDA

BRAND NAMES: Cervidil; *Cerviprime*; *Cerviprost*; *Gravidex*; *Minoprostin E(2)*; *Minprostin E(2)* (Germany); *Prandin E2*; Prepidil; *Primiprost*; *Prostarmon E*; **Prostin E2**; *Prostin E2 Tab*; *Prostin E2 Vaginal Cream*; *Prostin E2 Vaginal Gel*; Prostin E2 Vaginal Suppository; *Prostin VR Pediatric*
(International brand names outside U.S. in italics)

DESCRIPTION:

Dinoprostone vaginal suppository and dinoprostone gel, an oxytocic, contain dinoprostone as the naturally occurring prostaglandin E2 (PGE2).

Its chemical name is (5Z,11α, 13E,15S)-11,15-Dihydroxy-9-oxo- prosta-5, 13-dien-1-oic acid.

The molecular formula is $C_{20}H_{32}O_5$. The molecular weight of dinoprostone is 352.5. Dinoprostone occurs as a white crystalline powder. It has a melting point within the range of 64 to 71°C. Dinoprostone is soluble in ethanol and in 25% ethanol in water. It is soluble in water to the extent of 130 mg/100 ml.

VAGINAL SUPPOSITORY

Each suppository contains 20 mg of dinoprostone in a mixture of glycerides of fatty acids.

CERVICAL GEL

The active constituent of dinoprostone gel is dinoprostone 0.5 mg/3 g (2.5 ml gel); other constituents are colloidal silicon dioxide NF (240 mg/3 g) and triacetin USP (2760 mg/3 g).

CLINICAL PHARMACOLOGY:

VAGINAL SUPPOSITORY

Dinoprostone vaginal suppository administered intravaginally stimulates the myometrium of the gravid uterus to contract in a manner that is similar to the contractions seen in the term uterus during labor. Whether or not this action results from a direct effect of dinoprostone on the myometrium has not been determined with certainty at this time. Nonetheless, the myometrial contractions induced by the vaginal administration of dinoprostone are sufficient to produce evacuation of the products of conception from the uterus in the majority of cases.

Dinoprostone is also capable of stimulating the smooth muscle of the gastrointestinal tract of man. This activity may be responsible for the vomiting and/or diarrhea that is not uncommon when dinoprostone is used to terminate pregnancy.

In laboratory animals, and also in man, large doses of dinoprostone can lower blood pressure, probably as a consequence of its effect on the smooth muscle of the vascular system. With the doses of dinoprostone used for terminating pregnancy this effect has not been clinically significant. In laboratory animals, and also in man, dinoprostone can elevate body temperature. With the clinical doses of dinoprostone used for the termination of pregnancy some patients do exhibit temperature increases.

CERVICAL GEL

Dinoprostone gel administered endocervically may stimulate the myometrium of the gravid uterus to contract in a manner similar to the contractions seen in the term uterus during labor. Whether or not this action results from a direct effect of dinoprostone on the myometrium has not been determined.

Dinoprostone is also capable of stimulating the smooth muscle of the gastrointestinal tract of man. This activity may be responsible for the vomiting and/or diarrhea that is occasionally seen when dinoprostone is used for preinduction cervical ripening.

In laboratory animals, and also in humans, large doses of dinoprostone can lower blood pressure, probably as a consequence of its effect on the smooth muscle of the vascular system. With the doses of dinoprostone used for cervical ripening this effect has not been seen. In laboratory animals, and also in humans, dinoprostone can elevate body temperature; however, with the dosing used for cervical ripening this effect has not been seen.

In addition to an oxytocic effect, there is evidence suggesting that this agent has a local cervical effect in initiating softening, effacement, and dilation. These changes, referred to as cervical ripening, occur spontaneously as the normal pregnancy progresses toward term and allow evacuation of uterine contents by decreasing cervical resistance at the same time that myometrial activity increases. While not completely understood, biochemical changes within the cervix during natural cervical ripening are similar to those following PGE2-induced ripening. Further, it has been shown that these changes can take place independent of myometrial activity; however, it is quite likely that PGE2 administered endocervically produces effacement and softening by combined contraction inducing and cervical ripening properties. There is evidence to suggest that the changes that take place within the cervix are due to collagen degradation resulting from collagenase secretion as a response, at least in part, to PGE2.

Using an unvalidated assay, the following information was determined. When dinoprostone gel was administered endocervically to women undergoing preinduction ripening, results from measurement of plasma levels of the metabolite 13,14-dihydro-15-keto-PGE2 (DHK-PGE2) showed that PGE2 was relatively rapidly absorbed and the T_{max} was 0.5 to 0.75 hours. Plasma mean C_{max} for gel-treated subjects was 433 ± 51 pg/ml versus 137 ± 24 pg/ml for untreated controls. In those subjects in which a clinical response was observed mean C_{max} was 484 ± 57 pg/ml versus 213 ± 69 pg/ml in nonresponders and 219 ± 92 pg/ml in control subjects who had positive clinical progression toward normal labor. These elevated levels in gel-treated subjects appear to be largely a result of absorption of PGE2 from the gel rather than from endogenous sources. PGE2 is completely metabolized in humans. PGE2 is extensively metabolized in the lungs, and the resulting metabolites are further metabolized in the liver and kidney. The major route of elimination of the products of PGE2 metabolism is the kidneys.

INDICATIONS AND USAGE:

VAGINAL SUPPOSITORY

1. Dinoprostone vaginal suppository is indicated for the termination of pregnancy from the 12th through the 20th gestational week as calculated from the first day of the last normal menstrual period.

2. Dinoprostone vaginal suppository is also indicated for evacuation of the uterine contents in the management of missed abortion or intrauterine fetal death up to 28 weeks of gestational age as calculated from the first day of the last normal menstrual period.

3. Dinoprostone vaginal suppository is indicated in the management of nonmetastatic gestational trophoblastic disease (benign hydatidiform mole).

CERVICAL GEL

Dinoprostone gel is indicated for ripening an unfavorable cervix in pregnant women at or near term with a medical or obstetrical need for labor induction.

CONTRAINDICATIONS:

VAGINAL SUPPOSITORY

1. Hypersensitivity to dinoprostone
2. Acute pelvic inflammatory disease
3. Patients with active cardiac, pulmonary, renal, or hepatic disease

CERVICAL GEL

Endocervically administered dinoprostone gel is not recommended for the following:

a. Patients in whom oxytocic drugs are generally contraindicated or where prolonged contractions of the uterus are considered inappropriate, such as:

cases with a history of cesarean section or major uterine surgery
cases in which cephalopelvic disproportion is present
cases in which there is a history of difficult labor and/or traumatic delivery
grand multiparae with six or more previous term pregnancies
cases with non-vertex presentation
cases with hyperactive or hypertonic uterine patterns
cases of fetal distress where delivery is not imminent
in obstetric emergencies where the benefit-to-risk ratio for either fetus or the mother favors surgical intervention.

b. Patients with ruptured membranes.

c. Patients with hypersensitivity to prostaglandins or constituents of the gel.

d. Patients with placenta previa or unexplained vaginal bleeding during this pregnancy

e. Patients for whom vaginal delivery is not indicated, such as vasa previa or active herpes genitalia.

WARNINGS:

FOR HOSPITAL USE ONLY
Dinoprostone, as with other potent oxytocic agents, should be used only with strict adherence to recommended dosages. Dinoprostone should be used by medically trained personnel in a hospital which can provide immediate intensive care and acute surgical facilities.

VAGINAL SUPPOSITORY

Dinoprostone does not appear to directly affect the fetoplacental unit. Therefore, the possibility does exist that the previable fetus aborted by dinoprostone could exhibit transient life signs. Dinoprostone is not indicated if the fetus *in utero* has reached the stage of viability. Dinoprostone should not be considered a feticidal agent.

Evidence from animal studies has suggested that certain prostaglandins may have some teratogenic potential. Therefore, any failed pregnancy termination with dinoprostone should be completed by some other means.

Dinoprostone vaginal suppository should not be used for extemporaneous preparation of any other dosage form.

Neither the dinoprostone vaginal suppository, as dispensed nor any extemporaneous formulation made from the dinoprostone vaginal suppository should be used for cervical ripening or other indication in the patient with term pregnancy.

PRECAUTIONS:

VAGINAL SUPPOSITORY

General: Animal studies lasting several weeks at high doses have shown that prostaglandins of the E and F series can induce proliferation of bone. Such effects have also been noted in newborn infants who have received prostaglandin E1 during prolonged treatment. There is no evidence that short term administration of dinoprostone vaginal suppository can cause similar bone effects.

As in spontaneous abortion, where the process is sometimes incomplete, abortion induced by dinoprostone vaginal suppository may sometimes be incomplete. In such cases, other measures should be taken to assure complete abortion.

In patients with a history of asthma, hypo- or hypertension, cardiovascular disease, renal disease, hepatic disease, anemia, jaundice, diabetes or history of epilepsy, dinoprostone should be used with caution.

Dinoprostone administered by the vaginal route should be used with caution in the presence of cervicitis, infected endocervical lesions, or acute vaginitis.

As with any oxytocic agent, dinoprostone should be used with caution in patients with compromised (scarred) uteri.

Dinoprostone vaginal therapy is associated with transient pyrexia that may be due to its effect on hypothalamic thermoregulation. In the patients studied, temperature elevations in excess of 2°F (1.1°C) were observed in approximately one-half of the patients on the recommended dosage regimen. In all cases, temperature returned to normal on discontinuation of therapy. Differentiation of post-abortion endometritis from drug-induced temperature elevations is difficult, but with increasing clinical exposure and experience with PGE2 vaginal therapy the distinctions become more obviously apparent and are summarized in TABLE 1.

TABLE 1 Dinoprostone Vaginal Suppository

ENDOMETRITIS PYREXIA	PGE2 INDUCED PYREXIA
1. Time of onset: Typically, on third post-abortional day (38°C or higher).	Within 15-45 minutes of suppository administration.
2. Duration: Untreated pyrexia and infection continue and may give rise to other infective pelvic pathology.	Elevations revert to pre-treatment levels within 2-6 hours after discontinuation of therapy or removal of suppository from vagina without any other treatment.
3. Retention: Products of conception are often retained in the cervical os or uterine cavity.	Elevation occurs irrespective of any retained tissue.
4. Histology: Endometrium shows evidence of inflammatory lymphocytic infiltration with areas of necrotic hemorrhagic tissue.	Although the endometrial stroma may be edematous and vascular, there is relative absence of inflammatory reaction.
5. The Uterus: Often remains boggy and soft with tenderness over the fundus, and pain on moving the cervix, on bimanual examination.	Normal uterine involution not tender
6. Discharge: Often associated foul-smelling lochia and leukorrhea.	Lochia normal.

PRECAUTIONS: *(cont'd)*

Cervical Culture: The culture of pathological organisms from the cervix or uterine cavity after abortion does not, of itself, warrant the diagnosis of septic abortion in the absence of clinical evidence of sepsis. It is not uncommon to culture pathogens from cases of recent abortion NOT clinically infected. Persistent positive culture with clear clinical signs of infection are significant in the differential diagnosis.

Blood Count: Leukocytosis and differential white cell counts are not of major clinical importance in distinguishing between the two conditions, since total WBC's may be increased as a result of infection and transient leukocytosis may also be drug induced. In the absence of clinical or bacteriological evidence of intrauterine infection, supportive therapy for drug induced fevers includes the forcing of fluids. As all PGE2-induced fevers have been found to be transient or self-limiting, it is doubtful if any simple empirical measures for temperature reduction are indicated.

LABORATORY TESTS

When a pregnancy diagnosed as missed abortion is electively interrupted with intravaginal administration of dinoprostone, confirmation of intrauterine fetal death should be obtained in respect to a NEGATIVE PREGNANCY TEST for chorionic gonadotropic activity (U.C.G. test or equivalent). When a pregnancy with late fetal intrauterine death is interrupted with intravaginal administration of dinoprostone, confirmation of intrauterine fetal death should be obtained prior to treatment.

CARCINOGENESIS, MUTAGENESIS, AND IMPAIRMENT OF FERTILITY

Carcinogenic bioassay studies have not been conducted in animals with dinoprostone vaginal suppository due to the limited indications for use and short duration of administration. No evidence of mutagenicity was observed in the Micronucleus Test or Ames Assay.

PREGNANCY, TERATOGENIC EFFECTS, PREGNANCY CATEGORY C

Animal studies do not indicate that dinoprostone vaginal suppository is teratogenic, however, it has been shown to be embryotoxic in rats and rabbits and any dose which produces increased uterine tone could put the embryo or fetus at risk. See WARNINGS.

CERVICAL GEL

General: During use, uterine activity, fetal status, and character of the cervix (dilation and effacement) should be carefully monitored either by auscultation or electronic fetal monitoring to detect possible evidence of undesired responses, eg, hypertonus, sustained uterine contractility, or fetal distress. In cases where there is a history of hypertonic uterine contractility or tetanic uterine contractions, it is recommended that uterine activity and the state of the fetus should be continuously monitored. The possibility of uterine rupture should be borne in mind when high-tone myometrial contractions are sustained. Feto-pelvic relationships should be carefully evaluated before use of dinoprostone gel (see CONTRAINDICATIONS).

Caution should be exercised in administration of dinoprostone gel in patients with:

asthma or history of asthma

glaucoma or raised intraocular pressure

Caution should be taken so as not to administer dinoprostone gel above the level of the internal os. Careful vaginal examination will reveal the degree of effacement which will regulate the size of the shielded endocervical catheter to be used. That is, the 20 mm endocervical catheter should be used if no effacement is present, and the 10 mm catheter should be used if the cervix is 50% effaced. Placement of dinoprostone gel into the extra-amniotic space has been associated with uterine hyperstimulation.

As dinoprostone gel is extensively metabolized in the lung, liver, and kidney, and the major route of elimination is the kidney, dinoprostone gel should be used with caution in patients with renal and hepatic dysfunction.

CARCINOGENESIS, MUTAGENESIS, AND IMPAIRMENT OF FERTILITY

Carcinogenic bioassay studies have not been conducted in animals with dinoprostone gel due to the limited indications for use and short duration of administration. No evidence of mutagenicity was observed in the Micronucleus Test or Ames Assay.

PREGNANCY, TERATOGENIC EFFECTS, PREGNANCY CATEGORY C: Prostaglandin E2 produced an increase in skeletal anomalies in rats and rabbits. No effect would be expected clinically, when used as indicated, since dinoprostone gel is administered after the period of organogenesis. Dinoprostone gel has been shown to be embryotoxic in rats and rabbits, and any dose that produces sustained increased uterine tone could put the embryo or fetus at risk. See statements under General Precautions.

DRUG INTERACTIONS:

VAGINAL SUPPOSITORY

Dinoprostone vaginal suppository may augment the activity of other oxytocic drugs. Concomitant use with other oxytocic agents is not recommended.

CERVICAL GEL

Dinoprostone gel may augment the activity of other oxytocic agents and their concomitant use is not recommended. For the sequential use of oxytocin following dinoprostone gel administration, a dosing interval of 6-12 hours is recommended.

ADVERSE REACTIONS:

VAGINAL SUPPOSITORY

The most frequent adverse reactions observed with the use of dinoprostone for abortion are related to its contractile effect on smooth muscle.

In the patients studied, approximately two-thirds experienced vomiting, one-half temperature elevations, two-fifths diarrhea, one-third some nausea, one-tenth headache, and one-tenth shivering and chills.

In addition, approximately one-tenth of the patients studied exhibited transient diastolic blood pressure decreases of greater than 20 mmHg.

Two cases of myocardial infarction following the use of dinoprostone have been reported in patients with a history of cardiovascular disease.

It is not known whether these events were related to the administration of dinoprostone.

Adverse effects in decreasing order of their frequency, observed with the use of dinoprostone, not all of which are clearly drug related include:

Vomiting
Diarrhea
Nausea
Fever
Headache
Chills or shivering
Backache
Joint inflammation or pain new or exacerbated
Flushing or hot flashes
Dizziness
Arthralgia
Vaginal pain
Chest pain
Dyspnea
Endometritis
Uterine rupture
Breast tenderness
Blurred vision
Coughing
Rash
Myalgia
Stiff neck
Dehydration
Tremor
Paresthesia
Hearing impairment
Urine retention
Pharyngitis
Laryngitis
Diaphoresis
Eye pain

ADVERSE REACTIONS: *(cont'd)*

Syncope or fainting sensation
Vaginitis or vulvitis
Weakness
Muscular cramp or pain
Tightness in chest
Nocturnal leg cramps
Wheezing
Cardiac arrhythmia
Skin discoloration
Vaginismus
Tension

CERVICAL GEL

Dinoprostone gel is generally well-tolerated. In controlled trials, in which 1731 women were entered, the following events were reported at an occurrence of ≥ 1% (TABLE 2).

TABLE 2 Dinoprostone Cervical Gel

Adverse Reaction Maternal	PGE2 (N=884) N (%)	Control* (N=847) N (%)
Uterine contractile abnormality	58 (6.6)	34 (4.0)
Any gastrointestinal effect	50 (5.7)	22 (2.6)
Back pain	27 (3.1)	0 (0)
Warm feeling in vagina	13 (1.5)	0 (0)
Fever	12 (1.4)	10 (1.2)
Fetal		
Any fetal heart rate abnormality	150 (17.0)	123 (14.5)
Bradycardia	36 (4.1)	26 (3.1)
Deceleration		
Late	25 (2.8)	18 (2.1)
Variable	38 (4.3)	29 (3.4)
Unspecified	19 (2.1)	19 (2.2)

* placebo gel or no treatment

In addition, in other trials amnionitis and intrauterine fetal sepsis have been associated with extra-amniotic intrauterine administration of PGE2. Uterine rupture has been reported in association with the use of dinoprostone gel intracervically. Additional events reported in the literature, associated by the authors with the use of dinoprostone gel, included premature rupture of membranes, fetal depression (1 min Apgar < 7), and fetal acidosis (umbilical artery pH < 7.15).

DRUG ABUSE AND DEPENDENCE:

CERVICAL GEL

No drug abuse or drug dependence has been seen with the use of dinoprostone gel.

OVERDOSAGE:

CERVICAL GEL

Overdosage with dinoprostone gel may be expressed by uterine hypercontractility and uterine hypertonus. Because of the transient nature of PGE2-induced myometrial hyperstimulation, nonspecific, conservative management was found to be effective in the vast majority of the cases; i.e., maternal position change and administration of oxygen to the mother. β-adrenergic drugs may be used as a treatment of hyperstimulation following the administration of PGE2 for cervical ripening.

DOSAGE AND ADMINISTRATION:

VAGINAL SUPPOSITORY

STORE IN A FREEZER NOT ABOVE -20°C (-4°F) BUT BRING TO ROOM TEMPERATURE JUST PRIOR TO USE.

REMOVE FOIL BEFORE USE.

A suppository containing 20 mg of dinoprostone should be inserted high into the vagina. The patient should remain in the supine position for ten minutes following insertion.

Additional intravaginal administration of each subsequent suppository should be at 3- to 5-hour intervals until abortion occurs. Within the above recommended intervals administration time should be determined by abortifacient progress, uterine contractility response, and by patient tolerance. Continuous administration of the drug for more than 2 days is not recommended.

Storage: Store in a freezer not above -20°c (-4°f).

Dinoprostone vaginal suppository Vaginal Suppositories are available in containers of one suppository each. Each suppository contains 20 mg of dinoprostone in a mixture of glycerides of fatty acids.

CERVICAL GEL

NOTE: USE CAUTION IN HANDLING THIS PRODUCT TO PREVENT CONTACT WITH SKIN. WASH HANDS THOROUGHLY WITH SOAP AND WATER AFTER ADMINISTRATION.

Dinoprostone gel should be brought to room temperature (59 to 86°F; 15 to 30°C) just prior to administration. Do not force the warming process by using a water bath or other source of external heat (*e.g.,* microwave oven).

To prepare the product for use, remove the peel-off seal from the end of the syringe. Then remove the protective end cap (to serve as plunger extension) and insert the protective end cap into the plunger stopper assembly in the barrel of syringe. Choose the appropriate length shielded catheter (10 mm or 20 mm) and aseptically remove the sterile shielded catheter from the package. Careful vaginal examination will reveal the degree of effacement which will regulate the size of the shielded endocervical catheter to be used. That is, the 20 mm endocervical catheter should be used if no effacement is present, and the 10 mm catheter should be used if the cervix is 50% effaced. Firmly attach the catheter hub to the syringe tip as evidenced by a distinct click. Fill the catheter prior to administration to the patient.

To properly administer the product, the patient should be in a dorsal position with the cervix visualized using a speculum. Using sterile technique, introduce the gel with the catheter provided into the cervical canal just below the level of the internal os. Administer the contents of each syringe by gentle expulsion and then remove the catheter. The gel is easily extrudable from the syringe. Use the contents of one syringe for one patient only. No attempt should be made to administer the small amount of gel remaining in the catheter. The syringe, catheter, and any unused package contents should be discarded after use. Following dinoprostone gel administration, the patient should remain in the supine position for at least 15 - 30 minutes to minimize leakage from the cervical canal. If the desired response is obtained from the starting dose of dinoprostone gel, the recommended interval before giving intravenous oxytocin is 6-12 hours. If there is no cervical/uterine response to the initial dose of dinoprostone gel, repeat dosing may be given. The recommended repeat dose is 0.5 mg dinoprostone with a dosing interval of 6 hours. The need for additional dosing and the interval must be determined by the attending physician based on the course of clinical events. The maximum recommended cumulative dose for a 24-hour period is 1.5 mg of dinoprostone (7.5 ml dinoprostone gel).

Storage Dinoprostone gel has a shelf life of 24 months when stored under continuous refrigeration (36 to 46°F; 2 to 8°C).

HOW SUPPLIED - EQUIVALENTS NOT AVAILABLE:

Gel - Vaginal - 0.5 mg/3 gm

3 gm x 5	$490.20	PREPIDIL, Pharmacia & Upjohn	00009-3359-02

Injection, Solution - Vaginal - 0.5 mg/3 gm

1's	$98.04	PREPIDIL, Pharmacia & Upjohn	00009-3359-01

Suppository - Vaginal - 20 mg/supposito

1's	$168.00	CERVIDIL, Forest Pharms	00456-4123-63
5's	**$123.00**	**PROSTIN E2, Pharmacia & Upjohn**	**00009-0827-01**
5's	**$614.99**	**PROSTIN E2 VAGINAL SUPPOSITORY, Pharmacia & Upjohn**	**00009-0827-02**

DIPHENHYDRAMINE HYDROCHLORIDE

(001079)

CATEGORIES: Allergic Reactions; Allergies; Anaphylactic Reactions; Anaphylactic Shock; Angioedema; Antiasthmatics/Bronchodilators; Anticholinergic Agents; Antihistamines; Antiparkinson Agents; Antitussives; Conjunctivitis; Ethanolamines; Dermatographism; Hay Fever; Influenza; Insect Bites; Lacrimation; Motion Sickness; Nasal Congestion; Nausea; Neuromuscular; Parkinsonism; Pharyngitis; Respiratory & Allergy Medications; Rhinitis; Sinus Congestion; Urticaria; Vertigo/Motion Sickness/Vomiting; Extrapyramidal Movement Disorders*; Headache*; Insomnia*; Migraine*; Pruritus*; Pregnancy Category B; FDA Approval Pre 1982
* Indication not approved by the FDA

BRAND NAMES: *Allerdryl* (Canada); Allerdryl 50; Allergia-C; *Allergina*; *Allermin* (Japan); *Amidryl*; Banophen; Beldin; Belix; Ben-A-Vance; Ben-Rex; Bena-D-10; **Benadryl**; *Benadryl Elixir*; *Benadryl N*; Benadryl Steri-Dose; Benahist; *Benamine*; *Benapon*; Bendramine; *Benocten*; Benoject; *Benylin*; Bydramine; *Desentol*; *Diabenyl*; Dibenil; *Dibrondrin* (Germany); *Difenhydramin*; *Dimidril*; *Dimiril*; Diphen; Diphenacen-50; Diphenhist; *Dolestan* (Germany); Dytuss; Fynex; Genahist; *Histergan*; Hydramine; Hydril; Hyrexin; *Insomnal* (Canada); *Menna*; Noradryl; Norafed; Nordryl; *Nytol*; Pharm-A-Dry; *Pheramin-N*; *Resmin* (Japan); *Restamin*; *Sediat* (Germany); Shodryl; Tega Dryl; Truxadryl; Tusstat; Uad Dryl; *Vena* (Japan); *Venasmin* (Japan); Wehdryl
(International brand names outside U.S. in italics)

FORMULARIES: Aetna; BC-BS; DoD; Medi-Cal

COST OF THERAPY: $18.50 (Parkinsonism; Capsule; 25 mg; 3/day; 365 days)

DESCRIPTION:

Diphenhydramine hydrochloride, is an antihistamine drug having the chemical name 2-(Diphenylmethoxy)-N,N-dimethylethylamine hydrochloride and has the empirical formula $C_{17}H_{21}NO\text{·}HCl$. It occurs as a white, crystalline powder and is freely soluble in water and alcohol and has a molecular weight of 291.82.

Each diphenhydramine HCl capsule contains 25 mg or 50 mg diphenhydramine hydrochloride for oral administration.

Each Benadryl 25-mg capsule also contains lactose, NF and magnesium stearate, NF. The capsule shell and/or band contains D&C red No. 28; FD&C blue No. 1; FD&C red No. 3; FD&C red No. 40; gelatin, NF; colloidal silicon dioxide, NF; and sodium lauryl sulfate, NF.

Each Benadryl 50-mg capsule also contains confectioner's sugar, NF and talc, USP. The capsule shell and/or band contains FD&C blue No. 1; FD&C red No. 3; gelatin, NF; glyceryl monooleate; colloidal silicon dioxide, NF; sodium lauryl sulfate, NF; and titanium dioxide, USP.

Each 5 ml of diphenhydramine HCl elixir contains 12.5 mg diphenhydramine HCl with 14% alcohol for oral administration.

Diphenhydramine HCl in the parenteral form is a sterile, pyrogen-free solution available in two concentrations: 10 mg and 50 mg of diphenhydramine hydrochloride per ml. The solutions for parenteral use have been adjusted to a pH between 5.0 and 6.0 either with sodium hydroxide or hydrochloric acid. The multidose Steri-Vials contain 0.1 mg/ml benzethonium chloride as a germicidal agent.

CLINICAL PHARMACOLOGY:

Diphenhydramine HCl is an antihistamine with anticholinergic (drying) and sedative side effects. Antihistamines appear to compete with histamine for cell receptor sites on effector cells.

Diphenhydramine is widely distributed throughout the body, including the CNS.

CAPSULES AND ELIXER

A single oral dose of diphenhydramine HCl is quickly absorbed with maximum activity occurring in approximately one hour. The duration of activity following an average dose of diphenhydramine HCl is from four to six hours. Little, if any, is excreted unchanged in the urine; most appears as the degradation products of metabolic transformation in the liver, which are almost completely excreted within 24 hours.

INJECTION

Diphenhydramine HCl in the injectable form has a rapid onset of action. Detailed information on the pharmacokinetics of diphenhydramine HCl injection is not available.

INDICATIONS AND USAGE:

CAPSULES AND ELIXER

Diphenhydramine HCl in the oral form is effective for the following indications:

Antihistaminic: For allergic conjunctivitis due to foods; mild, uncomplicated allergic skin manifestations of urticaria and angioedema; amelioration of allergic reactions to blood or plasma; dermatographism; as therapy for anaphylactic reactions *adjunctive* to epinephrine and other standard measures after the acute manifestations have been controlled.

Motion sickness: For active and prophylactic treatment of motion sickness.

Antiparkinsonism: For parkinsonism (including drug-induced) in the elderly unable to tolerate more potent agents; mild cases of parkinsonism (including drug-induced) in other age groups; in other cases of parkinsonism (including drug-induced) in combination with centrally acting anticholinergic agents.

INJECTION

Diphenhydramine HCl in the injectable form should only be used when the oral forms are impractical.

CONTRAINDICATIONS:

Use in Newborn or Premature Infants: This drug should *not* be used in newborn or premature infants.

CONTRAINDICATIONS: *(cont'd)*

Use in Nursing Mothers: Because of the higher risk of antihistamines for infants generally, and for newborns and prematures in particular, antihistamine therapy is contraindicated in nursing mothers.

Antihistamines are also contraindicated in the following conditions: Hypersensitivity to diphenhydramine hydrochloride and other antihistamines of similar chemical structure.

INJECTION

Use as a Local Anesthetic: Because of the risk of local necrosis, this drug in the parenteral from should not be used as a local anesthetic.

WARNINGS:

Antihistamines should be used with considerable caution in patients with narrow-angle glaucoma, stenosing peptic ulcer, pyloroduodenal obstruction, symptomatic prostatic hypertrophy, or bladder-neck obstruction.

Usage in Children: In infants and children, especially, antihistamines in *overdosage* may cause hallucinations, convulsions, or death.

As in adults, antihistamines may diminish mental alertness in children. In the young child, particularly, they may produce excitation.

Use in the Elderly (approximately 60 years or older): Antihistamines are more likely to cause dizziness, sedation, and hypotension in elderly patients.

PRECAUTIONS:

GENERAL

Diphenhydramine hydrochloride has an atropine-like action and therefore should be used with caution in patients with a history of lower respiratory disease, including asthma, increased intraocular pressure, hyperthyroidism, cardiovascular disease or hypertension.

INFORMATION FOR THE PATIENT

Patients taking diphenhydramine hydrochloride should be advised that this drug may cause drowsiness and has an additive effect with alcohol.

Patients should be warned about engaging in activities requiring mental alertness such as driving a car or operating appliances, machinery, etc.

CARCINOGENESIS, MUTAGENESIS, AND IMPAIRMENT OF FERTILITY

Long-term studies in animals to determine mutagenic and carcinogenic potential have not been performed.

PREGNANCY CATEGORY B

Reproduction studies have been performed in rats and rabbits at doses up to 5 times the human dose and have revealed no evidence of impaired fertility or harm to the fetus due to diphenhydramine hydrochloride. There are, however, no adequate and well-controlled studies in pregnant women. Because animal reproduction studies are not always predictive of human response, this drug should be used during pregnancy only if clearly needed.

INJECTION

Use with caution in patients with lower respiratory disease including asthma.

DRUG INTERACTIONS:

Diphenhydramine hydrochloride has additive effects with alcohol and other CNS depressants (hypnotics, sedatives, tranquilizers, etc).

MAO inhibitors prolong and intensify the anticholinergic (drying) effects of antihistamines.

ADVERSE REACTIONS:

The most frequent adverse reactions are underscored.

1. General: Urticaria, drug rash, anaphylactic shock, photosensitivity, excessive perspiration, chills, dryness of mouth, nose, and throat.

2. Cardiovascular System: Hypotension, headache, palpitations, tachycardia, extrasystoles

3. Hematologic System: Hemolytic anemia, thrombocytopenia, agranulocytosis

4. Nervous System: Sedation, sleepiness, dizziness, disturbed coordination, fatigue, confusion, restlessness, excitation, nervousness, tremor, irritability, insomnia, euphoria, paresthesia, blurred vision, diplopia, vertigo, tinnitus, acute labyrinthitis, neuritis, convulsions

5. GI System: Epigastric distress, anorexia, nausea, vomiting, diarrhea, constipation

6. GU System: Urinary frequency, difficult urination, urinary retention, early menses

7. Respiratory System: Thickening of bronchial secretions, tightness of chest and wheezing, nasal stuffiness

OVERDOSAGE:

Antihistamine overdosage reactions may vary from central nervous system depression to stimulation. Stimulation is particularly likely in children. Atropine-like signs and symptoms, dry mouth; fixed, dilated pupils; flushing, and gastrointestinal symptoms may also occur.

Stimulants should not be used.

Vasopressors may be used to treat hypotension.

CAPSULES AND ELIXER

If vomiting has not occurred spontaneously the patient should be induced to vomit. This is best done by having him drink a glass of water or milk after which he should be made to gag. Precautions against aspiration must be taken, especially in infants and children.

If vomiting is unsuccessful gastric lavage is indicated within 3 hours after ingestion and even later if large amounts of milk or cream were given beforehand. Isotonic or 1/2 isotonic saline is the lavage solution of choice.

Saline cathartics, as milk of magnesia, by osmosis draw water into the bowel and therefore are valuable for their action in rapid dilution of bowel content.

DOSAGE AND ADMINISTRATION:

DOSAGE SHOULD BE INDIVIDUALIZED ACCORDING TO THE NEEDS AND THE RESPONSE OF THE PATIENT.

CAPSULES

A single oral dose of diphenhydramine hydrochloride is quickly absorbed with maximum activity occurring in approximately one hour. The duration of activity following an average dose of diphenhydramine HCl is from four to six hours.

Adults: 25 to 50 mg three or four times daily.

Children (over 20 lb): 12.5 to 25 mg three to four times daily. Maximum daily dosage not to exceed 300 mg. For physicians who wish to calculate the dose on the basis of body weight or surface area, the recommended dosage is 5 mg/kg/24 hours or 150 mg/m^2/24 hours.

The basis for determining the most effective dosage regimen will be the response of the patient to medication and the condition under treatment.

In motion sickness, full dosage is recommended for prophylactic use, the first dose to be given 30 minutes before exposure to motion and similar doses before meals and upon retiring for the duration of exposure.

DOSAGE AND ADMINISTRATION: *(cont'd)*

ELIXER

A single oral dose of diphenhydramine hydrochloride is quickly absorbed with maximum activity occurring in approximately one hour. The duration of activity following an average dose of diphenhydramine HCl is from four to six hours.

Children (over 20 lb): One to two teaspoonfuls three to four times daily. Maximum daily dosage not to exceed 300 mg.

For physicians who wish to calculate the dose on the basis of body weight or surface area, the recommended dosage is 5 mg/kg/24 hours or 150 mg/m²/24 hours.

Adults: Two to four teaspoonfuls three to four times daily. The basis for determining the most effective dosage regimen will be the response of the patient to medication and the condition under treatment.

In motion sickness, full dosage is recommended for prophylactic use, the first dose to be given 30 minutes before exposure to motion and similar doses before meals and upon retiring for the duration of exposure.

INJECTION

Parenteral drug products should be inspected visually for particulate matter and discoloration prior to administration, whenever solution and container permit.

Children: 5 mg/kg/24 hr or 150 mg/m²/24 hr. Maximum daily dosage is 300 mg. Divide into four doses, administered intravenously or deeply intramuscularly.

Adults: 10 to 50 mg intravenously or deep intramuscularly, 100 mg if required; maximum daily dosage is 400 mg.

Store at controlled room temperature 15-30°C (59-86°F). Protect from moisture, freezing, and light.

(Injection: Parke-Davis, 11/914259G252)

HOW SUPPLIED - RATED THERAPEUTICALLY EQUIVALENT:

Capsule, Gelatin - Oral - 25 mg

24's	$.40	Diphenhydramine HCl, H.C.F.A. F F P	99999-1079-01
24's	$3.00	Diphenhist, Rugby	00536-3594-35
30's	$.50	Diphenhydramine HCl, H.C.F.A. F F P	99999-1079-02
30's	$1.90	Diphenhydramine Hcl, Major Pharms	00904-2055-46
36's	$.60	Diphenhydramine HCl, H.C.F.A. F F P	99999-1079-03
48's	$.81	Diphenhydramine HCl, H.C.F.A. F F P	99999-1079-04
100's	$1.69	Diphenhydramine HCl, H.C.F.A. F F P	99999-1079-05
100's	$2.88	Diphenhydramine HCl, Rugby	00536-3758-01
100's	$3.15	Diphenhydramine Hcl, IDE-Interstate	00814-2550-14
100's	$3.21	Diphenhydramine Hcl, Voluntary Hosp	53258-0231-01
100's	$3.25	Diphenhydramine Hcl, Consolidated Midland	00223-0585-01
100's	$3.75	Diphenhydramine Hcl, Major Pharms	00904-2055-60
100's	$4.52	Diphenhydramine Hcl, Barr	00555-0058-02
100's	$6.14	Diphenhydramine HCl, HL Moore Drug Exch	00839-1278-06
100's	$6.19	Diphenhydramine Hcl, Purepac Pharm	00228-2191-10
100's	$6.30	Diphenhydramine Hcl, Mutual Pharm	53489-0113-01
100's	$6.32	Diphenhydramine Hcl 25, Aligen Independ	00405-4344-01
100's	$6.35	Diphenhydramine Hcl, United Res	00677-0063-01
100's	$6.38	Diphenhist, Rugby	00536-3594-01
100's	$6.50	Diphenhydramine HCl, Geneva Pharms	00781-2458-01
100's	$6.85	Diphenhydramine Hcl, Major Pharms	00904-2055-61
100's	$9.70	Diphenhydramine Hcl, Parmed Pharms	00349-8871-01
100's	$9.95	Diphenydramine Hcl, Medirex	57480-0321-01
100's	$11.16	Diphenhydramine HCl, Geneva Pharms	00781-2458-13
100's	**$21.71**	**BENADRYL, Parke-Davis**	**00071-0471-24**
100's	**$23.33**	**BENADRYL, Parke-Davis**	**00071-0471-40**
250's	$6.98	Diphenhydramine Hcl, IDE-Interstate	00814-2550-22
600's	$69.20	Diphenhydramine Hcl, Medirex	57480-0321-06
1000's	$16.00	TRUX ADRYL, C O Truxton	00463-2022-10
1000's	$16.75	Diphenhydramine Hcl, Goldline Labs	00182-0492-10
1000's	$16.75	Diphenhydramine HCl, Rugby	00536-3758-10
1000's	$16.80	Diphenhydramine Hcl, Qualitest Pharms	00603-3337-32
1000's	$16.90	Diphenhydramine HCl, H.C.F.A. F F P	99999-1079-06
1000's	$17.98	Diphenhydramine Hcl, Balan	00304-0112-00
1000's	$18.50	Diphenhydramine Hcl, Major Pharms	00904-2055-80
1000's	$19.44	Diphenhydramine Hcl, Voluntary Hosp	53258-0406-10
1000's	$22.50	Diphenhydramine Hcl, Consolidated Midland	00223-0585-02
1000's	$22.75	Diphenhydramine Hcl, Dixon Shane	17236-0516-10
1000's	$22.95	Diphenhydramine Hcl, IDE-Interstate	00814-2550-30
1000's	$23.00	Diphenhydramine Hcl, Mutual Pharm	53489-0113-10
1000's	$23.12	Diphenhydramine Hcl 25, Aligen Independ	00405-4344-03
1000's	$24.36	Diphenhydramine Hcl, Schein Pharm (US)	00364-0116-02
1000's	$24.50	Diphenhydramine Hcl, Parmed Pharms	00349-8871-10
1000's	$26.19	Diphenhydramine HCl, HL Moore Drug Exch	00839-1278-16
1000's	$26.60	Diphenhydramine Hcl, United Res	00677-0063-10
1000's	$26.60	Diphenhydramine HCl, Geneva Pharms	00781-2458-10
1000's	$36.34	Diphenhydramine Hcl, Purepac Pharm	00228-2191-96

Capsule, Gelatin - Oral - 50 mg

24's	$.49	Diphenhydramine HCl, H.C.F.A. F F P	99999-1079-07
30's	$.61	Diphenhydramine HCl, H.C.F.A. F F P	99999-1079-08
100's	$1.40	Diphenhydramine Hcl, Anabolic	00722-5105-01
100's	$2.06	Diphenhydramine HCl, H.C.F.A. F F P	99999-1079-09
100's	$3.25	Diphenhydramine Hcl, Consolidated Midland	00223-0586-01
100's	$3.54	Diphenhydramine Hcl, Voluntary Hosp	53258-0407-01
100's	$3.69	Diphenhydramine HCl, Rugby	00536-3762-01
100's	$3.75	Diphenhydramine Hcl, IDE-Interstate	00814-2555-14
100's	$3.95	Diphenhydramine Hcl, Major Pharms	00904-2056-60
100's	$4.50	Diphenhydramine Hcl, Raway	00686-3137-25
100's	$4.83	Diphenhydramine Hcl, Schein Pharm (US)	00364-0117-01
100's	$4.88	Diphenhydramine Hcl, Barr	00555-0059-02
100's	$4.90	Diphenhydramine Hcl, Mutual Pharm	53489-0114-01
100's	$5.34	Diphenhydramine Hcl, Purepac Pharm	00228-2192-10
100's	$6.14	Diphenhydramine HCl, HL Moore Drug Exch	00839-1280-06
100's	$6.70	Diphenhydramine Hcl, United Res	00677-0064-01
100's	$6.95	Diphenhydramine Hcl, Schein Pharm (US)	00364-0117-90
100's	$6.95	Diphenhydramine HCl, Geneva Pharms	00781-2498-01
100's	$6.98	Diphenhydramine Hcl 50, Aligen Independ	00405-4345-01
100's	$7.38	Diphenhydramine Hcl, Voluntary Hosp	53258-0407-13
100's	$10.66	Diphenhydramine Hcl, Vangard Labs	00615-0369-13
100's	$10.85	Diphenhydramine Hcl, Medirex	57480-0322-01
100's	$13.45	Diphenhydramine HCl, Geneva Pharms	00781-2498-13
100's	$18.18	Diphenhydramine Hcl, Parmed Pharms	00349-8872-01
100's	$18.90	Diphenhydramine Hcl, Major Pharms	00904-2056-61
100's	**$29.24**	**BENADRYL KAPSEALS, Parke-Davis**	**00071-0373-24**
250's	$8.25	Diphenhydramine Hcl, IDE-Interstate	00814-2555-22
600's	$84.40	Diphenhydramine Hcl, Medirex	57480-0322-06
750's	$97.50	Diphenhydramine Hcl, Glasgow Pharm	60809-0310-55
750's	$97.50	Diphenhydramine Hcl, Glasgow Pharm	60809-0310-72
1000's	$9.20	Diphenhydramine Hcl, Anabolic	00722-5105-02
1000's	$19.45	Diphenhydramine Hcl, Goldline Labs	00182-0135-10

HOW SUPPLIED - RATED THERAPEUTICALLY EQUIVALENT: *(cont'd)*

1000's	$20.00	TRUX ADRYL, C O Truxton	00463-2023-10
1000's	$20.38	Diphenhydramine HCl, Rugby	00536-3762-10
1000's	$20.60	Diphenhydramine HCl, H.C.F.A. F F P	99999-1079-10
1000's	$21.05	Diphenhydramine Hcl, Major Pharms	00904-2056-80
1000's	$21.69	Diphenhydramine Hcl, Voluntary Hosp	53258-0407-10
1000's	$22.50	Diphenhydramine Hcl, Consolidated Midland	00223-0586-02
1000's	$24.50	Diphenhydramine Hcl, Dixon Shane	17236-0518-10
1000's	$24.55	Diphenhydramine Hcl, Barr	00555-0059-05
1000's	$24.80	Diphenhydramine Hcl, Qualitest Pharms	00603-3338-32
1000's	$25.50	Diphenhydramine Hcl, IDE-Interstate	00814-2555-30
1000's	$26.19	Diphenhydramine HCl, HL Moore Drug Exch	00839-1280-16
1000's	$26.60	Diphenhydramine Hcl, Mutual Pharm	53489-0114-10
1000's	$26.80	Diphenhydramine Hcl, Schein Pharm (US)	00364-0117-02
1000's	$26.95	Bendramine-50, Quality Res Pharms	52765-2252-00
1000's	$27.40	Diphenhydramine Hcl, United Res	00677-0064-10
1000's	$27.40	Diphenhydramine HCl, Geneva Pharms	00781-2498-10
1000's	$27.90	Diphenhydramine Hcl, Parmed Pharms	00349-8872-10
1000's	$32.71	Diphenhydramine Hcl, Purepac Pharm	00228-2192-96
1000's	$41.62	Diphenhydramine Hcl 50, Aligen Independ	00405-4345-03

Elixir - Oral - 12.5 mg/5ml

10 ml x 100	$48.04	Diphenhydramine Hcl, Roxane	00054-8190-04
60 ml	$.36	Diphenhydramine Hcl, H.C.F.A. F F P	99999-1079-13
118 ml	$2.16	HYDRAMINE, HL Moore Drug Exch	00839-5162-65
118.292 ml	$.71	Diphenhydramine Hcl, H.C.F.A. F F P	99999-1079-15
120 ml	$0.60	Tusstat, Century Pharms	00436-0525-04
120 ml	$.73	Diphenhydramine Hcl, H.C.F.A. F F P	99999-1079-14
120 ml	$1.60	Diphenhydramine Hcl, HR Cenci	00556-0061-04
120 ml	$1.95	Bydramine, Major Pharms	00904-1229-20
120 ml	$2.25	Diphenhydramine Hcl, Consolidated Midland	00223-6251-01
120 ml	$3.78	Diphenhist, Rugby	00536-0770-97
120 ml x 24	**$6.21**	**BENADRYL, Parke-Davis**	**00071-2220-17**
180 ml	$1.10	Diphenhydramine Hcl, H.C.F.A. F F P	99999-1079-16
236.584 ml	$1.44	Diphenhydramine Hcl, H.C.F.A. F F P	99999-1079-17
240 ml	$1.46	Diphenhydramine Hcl, H.C.F.A. F F P	99999-1079-18
480 ml	$1.90	Tusstat, Century Pharms	00436-0525-16
480 ml	$1.94	Diphenhydramine Hcl, Lannett	00527-0753-27
480 ml	$2.80	Diphenhydramine Hcl, Lannett	00527-0821-27
480 ml	$2.92	Diphenhydramine Hcl, United Res	00677-1524-33
480 ml	$2.92	Diphenhydramine HCl, H.C.F.A. F F P	99999-1079-12
480 ml	$3.71	Hydramine, HL Moore Drug Exch	00839-5162-69
480 ml	$3.90	DIBENIL, HR Cenci	00556-0061-16
480 ml	$4.50	Diphenhydramine Hcl, Consolidated Midland	00223-6251-02
480 ml	$4.66	Diphenhydramine Hcl, Qualitest Pharms	00603-1175-58
480 ml	$5.67	Diphenhydramine Hcl, Purepac Pharm	00228-2188-16
480 ml	$6.20	BENAPHEN, Major Pharms	00904-1227-16
480 ml	$7.42	Diphenhist, Rugby	00536-0770-85
480 ml	$15.48	Dytuss, Lunsco	10892-0112-65
1920 ml	$11.71	Diphenhydramine Hcl, H.C.F.A. F F P	99999-1079-19
3840 ml	$9.87	Diphenhydramine Hcl, Lannett	00527-0753-28
3840 ml	$11.33	Diphenhydramine Hcl, Harber Pharm	51432-0570-21
3840 ml	$11.44	Tusstat, Century Pharms	00436-0525-28
3840 ml	$15.97	Diphenhydramine Hcl, Lannett	00527-0821-28
3840 ml	$20.64	Hydramine, HL Moore Drug Exch	00839-6122-70
3840 ml	$20.77	Hydramine, HL Moore Drug Exch	00839-5162-70
3840 ml	$21.85	BENAPHEN, Major Pharms	00904-1227-28
3840 ml	$22.08	DIBENIL, HR Cenci	00556-0061-28
3840 ml	$23.42	Diphenhydramine Hcl, H.C.F.A. F F P	99999-1079-11
3840 ml	$24.00	Diphenhydramine Hcl, Consolidated Midland	00223-6251-03
3840 ml	$26.95	Diphenhydramine Hcl, Major Pharms	00904-1230-28
3840 ml	$31.42	Diphenhist, Rugby	00536-0770-90

Injection, Solution - Intramuscular; - 10 mg/ml

5 ml x 10	$82.38	Diphenhydramine Hcl, Fujisawa USA	00469-9085-87
10 ml	$0.84	Diphenhydramine Hcl, Lannett	00527-0200-55
10 ml	**$2.63**	**BENADRYL, Parke-Davis**	**00071-4015-10**
30 ml	$1.48	Diphenhydramine Hcl, Lannett	00527-0200-58
30 ml	$4.25	Diphenhydramine Hcl, Consolidated Midland	00223-7477-30
30 ml	$5.18	Diphenhydramine Hcl, Steris Labs	00402-0826-30
30 ml	$6.00	TRUX- ADRYL, C O Truxton	00463-1080-30
30 ml	**$6.50**	**BENADRYL, Parke-Davis**	**00071-4015-13**
30 ml	$7.51	Diphenhydramine, Schein Pharm (US)	00364-6530-56
30 ml	$7.87	Diphenhydramine Hcl, HL Moore Drug Exch	00839-5569-36
30 ml	$8.85	Diphenhydramine Hcl, IDE-Interstate	00814-2570-46
30 ml x 25	$81.25	Diphenhydramine Hcl, Pasadena	00418-3331-61

Injection, Solution - Intramuscular; - 50 mg/ml

1 ml	$4.35	Diphenhydramine Hcl, Intl Medication	00548-1390-00
1 ml	**$15.24**	**BENADRYL, Parke-Davis**	**00071-4259-03**
1 ml x 10	**$16.80**	**BENADRYL STERI-DOSE, Parke-Davis**	**00071-4259-45**
1 ml x 10	$25.91	DIPHENHYDRAINE HCL, Wyeth Labs	00008-0384-01
1 ml x 25	$15.76	Diphenhydramine Hcl, Elkins Sinn	00641-0376-25
10 ml	$4.49	Diphenhydramine, Balan	00304-1343-56
10 ml	$4.66	Diphenhydramine Injection 50 Mg/Ml, Insource	58441-0117-10
10 ml	$4.75	Diphenhydramine Hcl, Consolidated Midland	00223-7478-10
10 ml	$5.89	Diphenhydramine Hcl Inj, General Inj & Vac	52584-0827-10
10 ml	$6.00	TRUX - ADRYL, C O Truxton	00463-1089-10
10 ml	$6.40	Diphenhydramine Hcl, Major Pharms	00904-0835-10
10 ml	$6.90	HYREXIN, Hyrex Pharms	00314-0673-70
10 ml	$6.90	Diphenhydramine Hcl, Steris Labs	00402-0827-10
10 ml	$8.13	Diphenhydramine Hcl, HL Moore Drug Exch	00839-6305-30
10 ml	**$9.47**	**BENADRYL, Parke-Davis**	**00071-4402-10**
10 ml	$10.00	Diphenhydramine HCl, Schein Pharm (US)	00364-6531-54
10 ml	$11.40	Diphenhydramine Hcl, Goldline Labs	00182-3024-63
10 ml	$12.75	Diphenhydramine HCl, Rugby	00536-4460-70
10 ml	$17.50	BENOJECT-50, Mayrand Pharms	00259-0324-10
10 ml x 25	$90.00	Diphenhydramine Hcl, Pasadena	00418-3341-10

DIPHTHERIA ANTITOXIN *(001086)*

CATEGORIES: Immunologic; Serums, Toxoids and Vaccines; Vaccines; FDA Pre 1938 Drugs

FORMULARIES: WHO

Prescribing information not available at time of publication.

HOW SUPPLIED - EQUIVALENTS NOT AVAILABLE:

Injection, Solution - Intramuscular; - 20000 unit/vial

20000 unt	$341.19	Diphtheria Antitoxin Purified, Connaught Labs	49281-0230-89

DIPHTHERIA TETANUS TOXOIDS *(001087)*

CATEGORIES: Diphtheria; Immunologic; Pertussis; Serums, Toxoids and Vaccines; Tetanus; Toxoids; Vaccines; FDA Pre 1938 Drugs

FORMULARIES: WHO

DESCRIPTION:

The diphtheria toxoid component is prepared by cultivating a suitable strain of *Corynebacterium diphtheriae* on a modified Mueller's casein hydrolysate medium (J. Immunology 37: 103, 1939). The tetanus toxoid component is prepared by cultivating a suitable strain of *Clostridium tetani* on a protein-free semisynthetic medium (Appl. Microbiol. *10:*146, 1962). Formaldehyde is used as the toxoiding (detoxifying) agent for both diphtheria and tetanus toxins. The final product contains no more than 0.02 percent free formaldehyde and contains 0.01 percent thimerosal (mercury derivative) as preservative.

The aluminum content of the final product does not exceed 0.85 mg per 0.5 ml dose.

During processing, hydrochloric acid and sodium hydroxide are used to adjust the pH. Sodium chloride is added to the finished product to control isotonicity.

INDICATIONS AND USAGE:

Diphtheria /tetanus is indicated for active immunization against diphtheria and tetanus in infants and children through 6 years of age. Diphtheria and tetanus toxoids and pertussis vaccine are the preferred agents for primary immunization of infants and children through 6 years of age. However, in instances where the pertussis vaccine component of triple antigen is not tolerated, or where the physician prefers to administer pertussis vaccine as a separate course of injections, this pediatric combination of diphtheria and tetanus toxoids may be used.

CONTRAINDICATIONS:

An acute respiratory infection or other active infection is reason for deferring administration of routine primary immunizing or recall (booster) doses but *not* emergency recall (booster) doses.

Interruption of the recommended schedule with a delay between doses does not interfere with the final immunity achieved, nor does it necessitate starting the series over again, regardless of the length of time elapsed between doses.[1]

PRECAUTIONS:

Only well infants or children should be injected.

If the vial is used, rather than the Sterile Cartridge-Needle Unit, a separate syringe and needle which have been adequately cleaned and sterilized should be used for each patient to prevent transmission of hepatitis B virus and other infectious agents from one person to another.

Individuals receiving therapy with corticosteroids or other immunosuppressive agents (antimetabolites, irradiation, alkylating agents) may not respond optimally to active immunization procedures. Administration of immunizing agents should be deferred in such individuals or repeated thereafter.

Before the injection of any biological, the physician should take all precautions known for prevention of allergic or any other side reactions. This should include: a review of the patient's history regarding possible sensitivity; the ready availability of epinephrine 1:1000 and other appropriate agents used for control of immediate allergic reactions; and a knowledge of the recent literature pertaining to use of the biological concerned.

ADVERSE REACTIONS:

A small area of erythema and induration surrounding the injection site, persisting for a few days, is not unusual.

A nodule may be palpable at the site of injection for a few weeks.

Although both the diphtheria and tetanus toxoid components may evoke local and systemic allergic responses in sensitive individuals, it has been suggested the tetanus toxoid component may be the more common cause.[2,3]

The occurrence of significant local and systemic reactions, following administration of tetanus toxoid, either fluid or adsorbed, is not nearly as rare as once believed.[2-9] Severe systemic reactions, on the other hand, are extremely rare. Over the past several years, published reports from this and foreign countries have appeared describing extensive local reactions which, in some instances, were accompanied by mild-to-moderate systemic responses. A typical reaction of this type, as described in the literature, is manifested by a delayed onset (usually 12 hours or more) of erythema, boggy edema, and induration surrounding the point of injection. Pain and tenderness, if present, are usually not the primary complaints. Frequently, there is itching of the edematous area, and it may resemble a giant "hive." The edema is occasionally extensive: shoulder to elbow or shoulder to wrist. Axillary lymphadenopathy has also been reported. Systemic manifestations have included low-grade fever, malaise, generalized aches and pains, flushing, generalized urticaria or pruritus, tachycardia, and hypotension. The majority of the extensive delayed-type local responses reported in the literature or to the manufacturers have occurred following BOOSTER doses in adults.

Reports have also appeared concerning the occurrence of such reactions in children who have received several doses of tetanus toxoid in the past.[8,9] The increasing incidence of extensive local reactions is one of the reasons why a ten-year interval between ROUTINE booster doses of tetanus toxoid is recommended by the U. S. Public Health Service, American Academy of Pediatrics, American College of Surgeons, and others.[1,10]

Local reactions typical of the type described above have been reported from this and other countries following use of both fluid and adsorbed tetanus toxoids prepared by many different manufacturers. Although their cause is unknown, hypersensitivity to the toxin or bacillary protein of the tetanus organism itself is assumed to be a possibility in some; in others, interreaction between the injected antigen and high levels of preexisting tetanus antibody (antitoxin) from prior booster doses seems to be the most likely cause of the Arthus-type response.

DOSAGE AND ADMINISTRATION:

The basic immunizing course consists of two (primary) doses of 0.5 ml each, given at an interval of 4 to 8 weeks, followed by a third (reinforcing) dose of 0.5 ml 6 to 12 months later. The third (reinforcing) dose is an integral part of the basic immunizing course; basic immunization cannot be considered complete until the third dose has been given. Prolonging the interval between primary immunizing doses, for six months or longer, does not interfere with the final immunity. Injections should be given intramuscularly, preferably into the deltoid or midlateral muscles of the thigh. The same muscle site should not be injected more than once during the course of basic immunization.

If active immunization is initiated during the first year of life, a routine recall (booster) dose of 0.5 ml is indicated at 4 to 6 years of age. Over age 6, the use of Diphtheria/Tetanus (FOR ADULT USE) is recommended for basic immunization and recall (booster) doses.

DOSAGE AND ADMINISTRATION: *(cont'd)*

In event of injury for which tetanus prophylaxis is indicated, an emergency recall (booster) dose of 0.5 ml of the single antigen, tetanus toxoid, should be given:

a. For clean, minor wounds - if more than TEN (10) years have elapsed since the time of administration of the last recall (booster) dose or the last (reinforcing) dose of the basic immunizing series.

b. For all other wounds - if more than FIVE (5) years have elapsed since the time of administration of the last recall (booster) dose or the last (reinforcing) dose of the basic immunizing series.

If emergency tetanus prophylaxis is indicated during the period between the second primary dose and the reinforcing dose, a 0.5 ml dose of the single antigen, tetanus toxoid, should be given. If given before six months have elapsed, it should be counted as a primary dose; if given after six months, it should be regarded as the reinforcing dose.

A 0.5 ml dose of tetanus toxoid *and* an appropriate dose of Tetanus Immune Globulin (Human), given with *separate* syringes and at *different* sites, are indicated at time of injury if:

a. The past immunization history with tetanus toxoid or the date of the last recall (booster) dose is unknown or of questionable validity.

b. The interval since the third (reinforcing) dose of the basic immunizing series or the last recall (booster) dose is more than 10 years; AND a delay of more than 24 hours has occurred between the time of injury and initiation of specific tetanus prophylaxis; AND the injury is of the type that could readily lead to fulminating tetanus (for example - compound fracture; extensive burn; crushing, penetrating, or massively contaminated wound; injury causing interruption or impairment of the local blood supply).

Individuals who have received no prior injections, or only one prior injection of this product or tetanus toxoid, should be given an adequate dose of Tetanus Immune Globulin (Human) at time of injury.

Upon intimate exposure to diphtheria, an emergency recall (booster) dose of 0.5 ml is indicated.[1]

TECHNIC FOR INJECTION

Before injection, the skin over the site to be injected should be cleansed and prepared with a suitable germicide. After insertion of the needle, aspirate to help avoid inadvertent injection into a blood vessel. Expel the antigen slowly and terminate the dose with a small bubble of air (0.1 to 0.2 ml). Do not inject intracutaneously or into superficial subcutaneous structures.

REFERENCES:

1. Report of the Committee on Infectious Diseases, American Academy of Pediatrics (Red Book), 1977. **2.** LEVINE, L., et al.: Adult immunization: Preparation and evaluation of combined fluid tetanus and diphtheria toxoids for adult use. Am. J. Hyg.*73:*20, 1961. **3.** McCOMB, J. and LEVINE, L.: Adult immunization: II. Dosage reduction as a solution to increasing reactions to tetanus toxoid. New Eng. J. Med.*265:*1152, 1961. **4.** EDSALL, G.: Specific prophylaxis of tetanus. JAMA *171:*417, 1959. **5.** KITTLER, F., et al.: Reactions to tetanus toxoid. Southern Med. J.*59:*149, 1966. **6.** EDSALL, G., et al.: Excessive use of tetanus toxoid boosters. JAMA*202:*17, 1967. **7.** FARDON, D.: Unusual reactions to tetanus toxoid. JAMA *199:*125, 1967. **8.** PEEBLES, T., et al.: Tetanus toxoid emergency boosters. A reappraisal. New Eng. J. Med. *280:*575, 1969. **9.** STEIGMAN, A.: Abuse of tetanus toxoid. J. Pediatrics *72:*753, 1968. **10.** Recommendation of the Public Health Advisory Committee on Immunization Practices. Morbidity and Mortality Weekly Report 26 (No. 49): 401, 1977. **11.** GREEN, S. T.: Avoiding needle sticks. Lancet *1(8489):* 1096, 1986.

HOW SUPPLIED - EQUIVALENTS NOT AVAILABLE:

Injection, Susp - Intramuscular

0.5 ml x 10	$25.31	Diphtheria/Tetanus Toxoids Adsorbed, Wyeth Labs	00008-0338-01
0.5 ml x 10	$25.31	Tetanus/Diphtheria Toxoids Adsorbed, Wyeth Labs	00008-0341-01
0.5 ml x 10	$38.28	Tetanus/Diptheria Purogenate, Lederle Pharm	00005-1875-47
5 ml	$13.41	Tetanus/Diphtheria Toxoids Adsorbed, Connaught Labs	49281-0271-83
5 ml	$13.41	Diphtheria/Tetanus Toxoids Adsorbed, Connaught Labs	49281-0275-10
5 ml	$13.64	Diphtheria/Tetanus Toxoids Adsorbed, Wyeth Labs	00008-0338-02
5 ml	$13.64	Tetanus/Diphtheria Toxoids Adsorbed, Wyeth Labs	00008-0341-02
5 ml	$13.88	Diphtheria/Tetanus Toxiods, Lederle Pharm	00005-1858-31
5 ml	$13.88	Tetanus/Diptheria Toxoids, Lederle Pharm	00005-1875-31

DIPHTHERIA; HAEMOPHILUS B; PERTUSSIS; TETANUS *(003159)*

CATEGORIES: Biologicals; Immunologic; Influenza; Serums, Toxoids and Vaccines; Toxoids; Vaccines; Pregnancy Category C; FDA Approved 1993 Mar

BRAND NAMES: **Tetramune**

DESCRIPTION:

Diphtheria and Tetanus Toxoids and Pertussis Vaccine Adsorbed and Haemophilus b Conjugate Vaccine (Diphtheria CRM_{197} Protein Conjugate) (DTP-HbOC), is a sterile combination of Purogenated Diphtheria Toxoid aluminum phosphate-adsorbed, Purogenated Tetanus Toxoid aluminum phosphate-adsorbed, Pertussis Vaccine (DTP, Tri-Immunol, manufactured by Lederle Laboratories Division), and a conjugate of oligosaccharides of the capsular antigen of*Haemophilus influenzae* type b and diphtheria CRM_{197}protein (HbOC, HibTITER, manufactured by Praxis Biologics, Inc.). DTP-HbOC is for intramuscular use only. After shaking, the vaccine is a homogeneous white suspension.

The diphtheria and tetanus toxoids are derived from *Corynebacterium diphtheriae* and *Clostridium tetani,* respectively, which are grown in media according to the method of Mueller and Miller. *C. diphtheriae*is grown in a defined medium containing casamino acids and *C. tetani* in a medium containing beef heart infusion. They are detoxified by use of formaldehyde. The toxoids are refined by the Pillemer alcohol fractionation method and are diluted with a solution containing sodium phosphate monobasic, sodium phosphate dibasic, glycine, and thimerosal (mercury derivative) as a preservative.

Pertussis Vaccine is prepared by growing Phase I *Bordetella pertussis* in a modified Cohen-Wheeler broth containing acid hydrolysate of casein. The *B. pertussis*is inactivated with thimerosal, harvested, and then suspended in a solution containing potassium phosphate monobasic, sodium phosphate dibasic, sodium chloride, and thimerosal (mercury derivative) as a preservative.

The oligosaccharides for the Haemophilus b conjugate component are derived from highly purified capsular polysaccharide, polyribosylribitol phosphate, isolated from *Haemophilus influenzae* type b (Haemophilus b) grown in a chemically defined medium (a mixture of mineral salts, amino acids, and cofactors). The oligosaccharides are purified and sized by diafiltrations through a series of ultrafiltration membranes, and coupled by reductive amination directly to highly purified CRM_{197}. $CRM_{197}$is a nontoxic variant of diphtheria toxin isolated from cultures of *C. diphtheriae*C7 (β 197) grown in casamino acids and yeast extract-based medium. The conjugate is purified through ultrafiltration, ammonium sulfate precipitation, and ion-exchange chromatography to high purity.

The Haemophilus b conjugate component is received as bulk from Praxis Biologics, Inc., and is combined by Lederle Laboratories with the diphtheria and tetanus toxoids and pertussis vaccine adsorbed to produce the final vaccine. As a preservative, thimerosal (mercury deriva-

DESCRIPTION: *(cont'd)*

tive) is added to the combination vaccine to a final concentration of 1:10,000. The aluminum content (from aluminum phosphate adjuvant) of the final product does not exceed 0.85 mg per 0.5 ml dose as determined by assay. The residual-free formaldehyde content by assay is ≤0.02%.

Each single dose of 0.5 ml of DTP-HbOC is formulated to contain 12.5 lf of diphtheria toxoid, 5 lf of tetanus toxoid (both toxoids induce not less than 2 units of antitoxin per ml in the guinea pig potency test), 10 mcg of purified Haemophilus b saccharide, and approximately 25 mcg of CRM_{197} protein. Each 0.5 ml dose of vaccine is formulated to contain less than 16 OPUs of inactivated pertussis cells. The total human immunizing dose (the first three 0.5 ml doses given) contains an estimate of 12 units of pertussis vaccine with an estimate of 4 protective units per single human dose, as determined by the mouse pertussis potency test. The potency for the Haemophilus b conjugate component of DTP-HbOC is determined by gas chromatography assay for total saccharide. Each component of the vaccine—diphtheria, tetanus, pertussis, and Haemophilus b conjugate—meets the required potency standards, and contains no other active ingredients.

CLINICAL PHARMACOLOGY:

Simultaneous immunization against diphtheria, tetanus, and pertussis during infancy and childhood has been a routine practice in the United States since the late 1940's, and immunization against Haemophilus b has been a routine practice since 1985. These immunizations have played a major role in markedly reducing the incidence of cases and deaths from each of these diseases.

Diphtheria is primarily a localized and generalized intoxication caused by diphtheria toxin, an extracellular protein metabolite of toxinogenic strains of *C. diphtheriae.* While the incidence of diphtheria in the US has decreased from over 200,000 cases reported in 1921, before the general use of diphtheria toxoid, to only 15 cases reported from 1980 to 1983, the case fatality rate has remained constant at about 5% to 10%. The highest case fatality rates are in the very young and in the elderly.

Following adequate immunization with diphtheria toxoid, it is thought that protection lasts for at least 10 years.

Antitoxin levels of at least 0.01 antitoxin units/ml are generally regarded as protective. This significantly reduces both the risk of developing diphtheria and the severity of clinical illness. It does not, however, eliminate carriage of *C. diphtheria* in the pharynx or on the skin.

Tetanus is an intoxication manifested primarily by neuromuscular dysfunction caused by a potent exotoxin elaborated by *C. tetani.* The incidence of tetanus in the US has dropped dramatically with the routine use of tetanus toxoid, remaining relatively constant over the last decade at about 90 cases reported annually. Spores of *C. tetani* are ubiquitous, and there is essentially no natural immunity to tetanus toxin.

Thus, universal primary immunization with tetanus toxoid with subsequent maintenance of adequate antitoxin levels, by means of timed boosters, is recommended to protect all age groups. Tetanus toxoid is a highly effective antigen and a completed primary series generally induces serum antitoxin levels of at least 0.01 antitoxin units, a level that has been reported to be protective. It is thought that protection persists for at least 10 years.

The toxoids of tetanus and diphtheria induce neutralizing antibodies to the toxins produced by the infecting organism. In clinical studies with Lederle-produced diphtheria and tetanus toxoids, administered in combination with pertussis vaccine, serum antitoxin levels have been shown to be greater than 0.01 antitoxin units/ml in 97% to 100% of 372 infants following three doses. These levels are generally regarded to be protective.

Pertussis (whooping cough) is a disease of the respiratory tract caused by *B. pertussis.* This gram-negative coccobacillus produces a variety of active components including endotoxin and a number of other substances that have been defined primarily on the basis of their biological activity in animals. These active components have been associated with a number of effects, such as lymphocytosis, leukocytosis, sensitivity to histamine, changes in glucose and/or insulin levels, possible neurological effects and adjuvant activity. The roles of each of the different components in either the pathogenesis of, or immunity to, pertussis is not well understood.

Pertussis (whooping cough) is a highly communicable disease of the respiratory tract. Attack rates of over 90% have been reported in unimmunized household contacts. Since immunization against pertussis (whooping cough) became widespread, the number of reported cases and associated mortality in the US has declined from about 120,000 cases and 1,100 deaths in 1950, to an annual average of about 3,500 cases and 10 fatalities in recent years. Precise data do not exist since bacteriological confirmation of pertussis can be obtained in less than half of the suspected cases. Most reported illness from *B. pertussis* occurs in infants and young children; two thirds of reported deaths occur in children less than 1 year old. Older children and adults, in whom classic signs are often absent, may go undiagnosed and serve as reservoirs of disease.

The potency of the pertussis component of the vaccine is measured and shown to be acceptable in the mouse potency test. Previously, serum agglutinin titers of pertussis vaccines have been correlated with clinical protection in the Medical Research Council trials. The pertussis component induces immunity against pertussis disease in humans.

Haemophilus influenza type b was the most common cause of invasive bacterial disease, including meningitis, in young children in the US prior to licensure of vaccines for this disease. Although nonencapsulated *H. influenzae* are common and six capsular polysaccharide types are known, strains with the type b capsule caused most of the invasive Haemophilus diseases prior to the introduction of Haemophilus b conjugate vaccines.

Prior to routine immunization, Haemophilus b disease occurred primarily in children under 5 years of age. In the US, the incidence of invasive Haemophilus b disease peaked between 6 months and 1 year of age, and approximately 55% of disease occurred between 6 and 18 months of age.The cumulative risk of developing invasive Haemophilus b disease during the first 5 years of life was about 1 in 200 prior to the introduction of Haemophilus b conjugate vaccines. Approximately 60% of cases were meningitis. Cellulitis, epiglottitis, pericarditis, pneumonia, sepsis, or septic arthritis made up the remaining 40%. An estimated 12,000 cases of Haemophilus b meningitis occurred annually prior to the routine use of conjugate vaccines in infants and toddlers.The mortality rate can be 5%, and neurologic sequelae have been observed in up to 38% of survivors.

The incidence of invasive Haemophilus b disease is increased in certain children, such as those who are native Americans, black, or from lower socioeconomic status and those with medical conditions such as asplenia, sickle cell disease, malignancies associated with immunosuppression, and antibody deficiency syndromes.

The protective activity of antibody to Haemophilus b polysaccharide was demonstrated by the efficacy study of Haemophilus b polysaccharide (HbPs) vaccine. Data from passive antibody studies indicate that a preexisting titer of antibody to HbPs of 0.15 mcg/ml correlates with protection. Data from a Finnish field trial in children 18 to 71 months of age indicate that a titer of > 1.0 mcg/ml 3 weeks after vaccination is associated with long-term protection.

Linkage of Haemophilus b saccharides to a protein such as CRM_{197}converts the saccharide (HbO) to a T-dependent (HbOC) antigen, and results in an enhanced antibody response to the saccharide in young infants that primes for an anamnestic response and is predominantly of the IgG class. Laboratory evidence indicates that the native state of the CRM_{197} protein

CLINICAL PHARMACOLOGY: *(cont'd)*

and the use of oligosaccharides in the formulation of HibTITER Haemophilus b Conjugate Vaccine (Diphtheria CRM_{197} Protein Conjugate) (HbOC), enhances its immunogenicity. NO PUBLISHED DATA ARE AVAILABLE TO SUPPORT THE INTERCHANGEABILITY OF HbOC AND OTHER HAEMOPHILUS b CONJUGATE VACCINES WITH ONE ANOTHER FOR PRIMARY IMMUNIZATION.

HbOC was shown to be effective in a large-scale controlled clinical trial in a multiethnic population in northern California carried out between February 1988 and June 1990. It should be noted that DTP was administered simultaneously with HbOC but at a separate site. There were no (0) vaccine failures in infants who received three doses of HbOC and 12 cases of Haemophilus b disease (6 cases of meningitis) in the control group. The estimate of efficacy is 100% (P=.0002) with 95% Confidence Intervals of 68% to 100%. Through the end of 1991, with an additional 49,000 person-years of follow-up, there were still no cases of Haemophilus b disease in fully vaccinated infants less than 2 years of age. Person-years may be defined as the number of individuals receiving the appropriate number of doses times the average number of years of follow-up for all of the individuals. One case of disease has been reported in a 3 1/2-year-old child who did not receive the recommended booster dose.

Evidence of efficacy postlicensure of Haemophilus b conjugate vaccines in the US is indicated by reports of significant reductions (71% to 94%) in Haemophilus b disease that are closely associated with increases in the net doses of Haemophilus b disease that are closely associated with increases in the net doses of Haemophilus b conjugate vaccines distributed. Occasional cases of vaccine failures have, however, been reported to the US Department of Health and Human Services through the Vaccine Adverse Event Reporting System (VAERS) since licensure of Haemophilus b conjugate vaccines.

DTP-HbOC has been given to 6,793 children as part of a series of studies to test the safety and immunogenicity of this combined product when compared to separate administration of DTP and HbOC. The vaccines were given at 2, 4, and 6 months of age or at 15 to 18 months of age. Local reactions and systemic events after vaccination were generally comparable between the groups which received the combination product or separate injections. (It should be noted that comparison of local reactions was done by comparing the combined product to the separate injection site that gave the largest reactions or to the DTP injection site.) Scattered reactions occurred more frequently (P <0.05) in the combination group for some doses (swelling and drowsiness after the first dose; irritability and restless sleep after the second dose; injection site warmth after the third dose; injection site swelling warmth, tenderness, irritability after the toddler dose). Rash was seen more commonly in the separate group. There was no consistent or identifiable pattern to these group differences across studies or doses. The large trial with 6,497 infants receiving DTP-HbOC allowed analysis of rare adverse events, including SIDS (sudden infant death syndrome), hospitalizations, and emergency room visits, following vaccination. No differences were found between the cohorts (see ADVERSE REACTIONS). Taken together the safety studies conducted in infants and in toddlers indicate that this vaccine is safe and that there was no consistent pattern of enhanced adverse events following combined vaccine (DTP-HbOC) as compared to separate injections.

The antibody response to each of the components of DTP-HbOC was measured (n=189) and compared to separate administration of the DTP and HbOC vaccines (n=189). After three doses, the antibody response to DTP-HbOC was equal to or higher for all four components: tetanus (IU/ml), diphtheria (IU/ml), pertussis (microagglutination) and *H. influenzae* b polysaccharide (mcg/lgG/ml as per ELISA). In addition, responses to specific pertussis antigens (*i.e.,* pertussis toxin, FHA, and 69K protein) were found to be as high or higher in the DTP-HbOC product compared to separate administration of DTP. Therefore, the immunogenicity of the combined vaccine is at least as good as the two vaccines given separately.

INDICATIONS AND USAGE:

Diphtheria and Tetanus Toxoids and Pertussis Vaccine Adsorbed and Haemophilus b Conjugate Vaccine (Diphtheria CRM_{197} Protein Conjugate) DTP-HbOC, is indicated for the active immunization of children 2 months of age to 5 years of age for protection against diphtheria, tetanus, pertussis, and Haemophilus b disease when indications for immunization with DTP vaccine and Haemophilus b Conjugate Vaccine coincide. Typically, this is at 2, 4, 6, and 15 months of age. Children who have recovered from culture confirmed pertussis need not receive further doses of a vaccine containing pertussis. However, these children should receive additional doses of Diphtheria and Tetanus Toxoids Adsorbed, for Pediatric Use (DT) as well as Haemophilus b Conjugate Vaccine as appropriate to complete the series.

The American Academy of Pediatrics (AAP) has recommended that children who have experienced invasive Haemophilus b disease when <24 months of age should continue immunization against Haemophilus b, but that children whose disease occurred at ≥24 months need not receive further doses of Haemophilus b Conjugate Vaccine. However, these children should receive additional doses of DTP (or if pertussis is contraindicated, DT should be used) as appropriate to complete the series.

DTP-HbOC is intended for active immunization against diphtheria, tetanus, pertussis, and Haemophilus type b diseases and is not to be used for treatment of actual infection.

DTP-HbOC is not routinely recommended for immunization of persons older than 5 years of age. Under certain circumstances, DTP-HbOC may be used beyond age 5 years. Because DTP-HbOC contains pediatric DTP vaccine, it is not recommended for use beyond the seventh birthday.

As with any vaccine, DTP-HbOC may not protect 100% of individuals receiving the vaccine. If passive immunization is needed, Tetanus Immune Globulin (human TIG) (see DOSAGE AND ADMINISTRATION.)

CONTRAINDICATIONS:

HYPERSENSITIVITY TO ANY COMPONENT OF THE VACCINE, INCLUDING THIMEROSAL, A MERCURY DERIVATIVE, IS A CONTRAINDICATIONS.

IMMUNIZATION SHOULD BE DEFERRED DURING THE COURSE OF ANY FEBRILE ILLNESS OR ACUTE INFECTION. THE IMMUNIZATION PRACTICES ADVISORY COMMITTEE (ACIP) HAS STATED THAT "...MINOR ILLNESSES SUCH AS MILD UPPER RESPIRATORY INFECTIONS WITH OR WITHOUT LOW GRADE FEVER ARE NOT CONTRAINDICATIONS."

IMMUNIZATION WITH DTP-HbOC IS CONTRAINDICATED IF THE CHILD HAS EXPERIENCED ANY EVENT FOLLOWING PREVIOUS IMMUNIZATION WITH A PERTUSSIS-CONTAINING VACCINE, WHICH IS CONSIDERED BY THE AAP OR ACIP TO BE A CONTRAINDICATIONS TO FURTHER DOSES OF PERTUSSIS VACCINE. THESE EVENTS INCLUDE:

AN IMMEDIATE ANAPHYLACTIC REACTION.

ENCEPHALOPATHY OCCURRING WITHIN 7 DAYS FOLLOWING VACCINATION. THIS IS DEFINED AS AN ACUTE, SEVERE CENTRAL-NERVOUS-SYSTEM DISORDER OCCURRING WITHIN 7 DAYS FOLLOWING VACCINATION, AND GENERALLY CONSISTING OF MAJOR ALTERATIONS IN CONSCIOUSNESS, UNRESPONSIVENESS, GENERALIZED OR FOCAL SEIZURES THAT PERSIST MORE THAN A FEW HOURS, WITH A FAILURE TO RECOVER WITHIN 24 HOURS.

CONTRAINDICATIONS: *(cont'd)*

THE OCCURRENCE OF ANY TYPE OF NEUROLOGICAL SYMPTOMS OR SIGNS, INCLUDING ONE OR MORE CONVULSIONS (SEIZURES) FOLLOWING ADMINISTRATION OF DTP-HbOC IS GENERALLY A CONTRAINDICATIONS TO FURTHER USE. ANY DECISION TO ADMINISTER SUBSEQUENT DOSES OF A VACCINE CONTAINING DIPHTHERIA, TETANUS, OR PERTUSSIS ANTIGENS SHOULD BE DELAYED UNTIL THE PATIENT'S NEUROLOGICAL STATUS IS BETTER DEFINED.

THE PRESENCE OF ANY EVOLVING OR CHANGING DISORDER AFFECTING THE CENTRAL NERVOUS SYSTEM IS A CONTRAINDICATIONS TO ADMINISTRATION OF A PERTUSSIS-CONTAINING VACCINE SUCH AS DTP-HbOC REGARDLESS OF WHETHER THE SUSPECTED NEUROLOGICAL DISORDER IS ASSOCIATED WITH OCCURRENCE OF SEIZURE ACTIVITY OF ANY TYPE.

STUDIES HAVE INDICATED THAT A PERSONAL OR FAMILY HISTORY OF SEIZURES IS ASSOCIATED WITH INCREASED FREQUENCY OF SEIZURES FOLLOWING PERTUSSIS IMMUNIZATION.

The ACIP and the AAP recognize certain circumstances in which children with stable central nervous system disorders, including well-controlled seizures or satisfactorily explained single seizures, may receive pertussis vaccine. The ACIP and AAP do not consider a family history of seizures to be a contraindication to pertussis vaccine despite the increased risk of seizures in these individuals.

The decision to administer a pertussis-containing vaccine to children must be made by the physician on an individual basis, with all consideration of all relevant factors, and assessment of potential risks and benefits for that individual. The physician should review the full text of ACIP and AAP guidelines prior to considering vaccination for children. The parent or guardian should be advised of the increased risk involved.

There are no data on whether the prophylactic use of antipyretics can decrease the risk of febrile convulsions. However, data suggest that acetaminophen will reduce the incidence of postvaccination fever.The ACIP and AAP suggest administering acetaminophen at age-appropriate doses at the time of vaccination and every 4 to 6 hours to children at higher risk for seizures than the general population.

DTP-HbOC is not routinely recommended for immunization of persons older than 5 years of age. Under certain circumstances, DTP-HbOC may be used beyond age 5 years. Because DTP-HbOC contains pediatric DTP vaccine, it is not recommended for use beyond the seventh birthday.

ROUTINE IMMUNIZATION SHOULD BE DEFERRED DURING AN OUTBREAK OF POLIOMYELITIS PROVIDING THE PATIENT HAS NOT SUSTAINED AN INJURY THAT INCREASES THE RISK OF TETANUS AND PROVIDING AN OUTBREAK OF DIPHTHERIA OR PERTUSSIS DOES NOT OCCUR SIMULTANEOUSLY.

The clinical judgement of the attending physician should prevail at all times.

WARNINGS:

THE ACIP STATES THAT IF ANY OF THE FOLLOWING EVENTS OCCUR IN TEMPORAL RELATION TO RECEIPT OF DTP, THE DECISION TO GIVE SUBSEQUENT DOSES OF VACCINE CONTAINING THE PERTUSSIS COMPONENT SHOULD BE CAREFULLY CONSIDERED.

TEMPERATURE OF ≥40.5°C (105°F) WITHIN 48 HOURS NOT DUE TO IDENTIFIABLE CAUSE.

COLLAPSE OR SHOCK-LIKE STATE (HYPOTONIC-HYPORESPONSIVE EPISODE) WITHIN 48 HOURS.

PERSISTENT, INCONSOLABLE CRYING LASTING ≥3 HOURS, OCCURRING WITHIN 48 HOURS.

CONVULSIONS WITH OR WITHOUT FEVER OCCURRING WITHIN 3 DAYS.

'ALTHOUGH THESE EVENTS WERE CONSIDERED ABSOLUTE CONTRAINDICATIONS IN PREVIOUS ACIP RECOMMENDATIONS, THERE MAY BE CIRCUMSTANCES, SUCH AS A HIGH INCIDENCE OF PERTUSSIS, IN WHICH THE POTENTIAL BENEFITS OUTWEIGH POSSIBLE RISKS, PARTICULARLY BECAUSE THESE EVENTS ARE NOT ASSOCIATED WITH PERMANENT SEQUELAE.'

IF A CONTRAINDICATIONS TO ANY OF THE COMPONENTS OF THIS COMBINATION VACCINE EXISTS (SEE CONTRAINDICATIONS SECTION), THEN DTP-HbOC SHOULD NOT BE USED. FOR EXAMPLE, IF THERE IS A CONTRAINDICATION AGAINST THE USE OF A PERTUSSIS VACCINE COMPONENT, THAN DIPHTHERIA AND TETANUS TOXOIDS ADSORBED, FOR PEDIATRIC USE (DT) AND HAEMOPHILUS b CONJUGATE VACCINE (DIPHTHERIA CRM_{197} PROTEIN CONJUGATE) HibTITER, AS SEPARATE INJECTIONS, SHOULD BE SUBSTITUTED FOR EACH OF THE REMAINING DOSES.

THE OCCURRENCE OF SUDDEN INFANT DEATH SYNDROME (SIDS) HAS BEEN REPORTED FOLLOWING ADMINISTRATION OF DTP. HOWEVER, A LARGE CASE-CONTROL STUDY IN THE US REVEALED NO CAUSAL RELATIONSHIP BETWEEN RECEIPT OF DTP VACCINE AND SIDS. A RECENT STUDY OF 6,497 INFANTS IN NORTHERN CALIFORNIA FOUND NO INCREASE IN THE RATE OF SIDS AMONG DTP-HbOC RECIPIENTS.

AS WITH ANY INTRAMUSCULAR INJECTION, DTP-HbOC SHOULD BE GIVEN WITH CAUTION TO INFANTS OR CHILDREN WITH THROMBOCYTOPENIA OR ANY COAGULATION DISORDER THAT WOULD CONTRAINDICATE INTRAMUSCULAR INJECTION (SEE DRUG INTERACTIONS).

As reported with Haemophilus b polysaccharide vaccine,, cases of Haemophilus type b disease may occur prior to the onset of the protective effect of this vaccine.

DTP-HbOC WILL NOT PROTECT AGAINST *H. INFLUENZAE* OTHER THAN TYPE b STRAINS. ANTIGENURIA HAS BEEN DETECTED FOLLOWING RECEIPT OF HAEMOPHILUS b CONJUGATE VACCINE AND THEREFORE ANTIGEN DETECTION IN URINE MAY NO HAVE DIAGNOSTIC VALUE IN SUSPECTED HAEMOPHILUS b DISEASE WITHIN 2 WEEKS OF IMMUNIZATION.

PRECAUTIONS:

CARE IS TO BE TAKEN BY THE HEALTH CARE PROVIDER FOR SAFE AND EFFECTIVE USE OF THIS PRODUCT.

1. DTP-HbOC is not routinely recommended for immunization of persons older than 5 years of age. Under certain circumstances, DTP-HbOC may be used beyond age 5 years. Because DTP-HbOC contains pediatric DTP vaccine, it is not recommended for use beyond the seventh birthday.

2. PRIOR TO ADMINISTRATION OF ANY DOSE OF DTP-HbOC, THE PARENT OR GUARDIAN SHOULD BE ASKED ABOUT THE PERSONAL HISTORY, FAMILY HISTORY, AND RECENT HEALTH STATUS. THE HEALTH CARE PROVIDER SHOULD ASCERTAIN PREVIOUS IMMUNIZATION HISTORY, CURRENT HEALTH STATUS, AND OCCURRENCE OF ANY SYMPTOMS AND/OR SIGNS OF AN ADVERSE EVENT AFTER PREVIOUS IMMUNIZATIONS, IN THE CHILD TO BE IMMUNIZED,

PRECAUTIONS: *(cont'd)*

IN ORDER TO DETERMINE THE EXISTENCE OF ANY CONTRAINDICATION TO IMMUNIZATION WITH DTP-HbOC AND TO ALLOW AN ASSESSMENT OF BENEFITS AND RISKS.

3. BEFORE THE INJECTION OF ANY BIOLOGICAL, THE HEALTH CARE PROVIDER SHOULD TAKE ALL PRECAUTIONKNOWN FOR THE PREVENTION OF ALLERGIC OR ANY OTHER SIDE REACTIONS. This should include: a review of the patient's history regarding possible sensitivity; the ready availability of epinephrine 1:1000 and other appropriate agents used for control of immediate allergic reactions; and a knowledge of the recent literature pertaining to use of the biological concerned, including the nature of side effects and adverse reactions that may follow its use.

4. Children with impaired immune responsiveness, whether due to the use of immunosuppressive therapy (including irradiation, corticosteroids, antimetabolites, alkylating agents, and cytotoxic agents), a genetic defect, human immunodeficiency virus (HIV) infection, or other causes, may have a reduced antibody response to active immunization procedures. Deferral of administration of vaccine may be considered in individuals receiving immunosuppressive therapy.Other groups should receive this vaccine according to the usual recommended schedule. (See DRUG INTERACTIONS).

5. This product is not contraindicated based on the presence of human immunodeficiency virus.

6. *Since this product is a suspension containing an adjuvant, shake vigorously to obtain a uniform suspension prior to withdrawing each dose from the multiple dose vial.*

7. A separate sterile syringe and needle or a sterile disposable unit should be used for each individual patient to prevent transmission of infectious agents from one person to another. Needles should be disposed of properly and should not be recapped.

8. Special care should be taken to prevent injection into a blood vessel.

NATIONAL CHILDHOOD VACCINE INJURY ACT

This Act requires that the manufacturer and lot number of the vaccine administered be recorded by the health care provider in the vaccine recipient's permanent medical record (or in a permanent office log or file), along with the date of administration of the vaccine and the name, address, and title of the person administering the vaccine.

The Act further requires the health care provider to report to the Secretary of the Department of Health and Human Services through the Vaccine Adverse Event Reporting System (VAERS) the occurrence following immunization of any event set forth in the Vaccine Injury Table, including: anaphylaxis or anaphylactoid shock within 24 hours; encephalopathy or encephalitis within 7 days; shock collapse or hypotonic-hyporesponsive collapse within 7 days; residual seizure disorder; any acute complication or sequelae (including death) of above events, or any event that would contraindicate further doses of vaccine, according to this DTP-HbOC package insert.

The US Department of Health and Human Services has established VAERS to accept all reports of suspected adverse events after the administration of any vaccine, including but not limited to the reporting of events required by the National Childhood Vaccine Injury Act of 1986.The VAERS toll-free number for VAERS forms and information is 800-822-7967.

INFORMATION FOR THE PATIENT

PRIOR TO ADMINISTRATION OF DTP-HbOC, HEALTH CARE PERSONNEL SHOULD INFORM THE PARENT, GUARDIAN, OR OTHER RESPONSIBLE ADULT OF THE RECOMMENDED IMMUNIZATION SCHEDULE FOR PROTECTION AGAINST DIPHTHERIA, TETANUS, PERTUSSIS, AND HAEMOPHILUS b DISEASE AND THE BENEFITS AND RISKS TO THE CHILD RECEIVING THIS VACCINE. GUIDANCE SHOULD BE PROVIDED ON MEASURES TO BE TAKEN SHOULD ADVERSE EVENTS OCCUR, SUCH AS ANTIPYRETIC MEASURES FOR ELEVATED TEMPERATURES AND THE NEED TO REPORT ADVERSE EVENTS TO THE HEALTH CARE PROVIDER. PARENTS SHOULD BE PROVIDED WITH VACCINE INFORMATION PAMPHLETS AT THE TIME OF EACH VACCINATION, AS STATED IN THE NATIONAL CHILDHOOD VACCINE INJURY ACT.

THE HEALTH CARE PROVIDER SHOULD INFORM THE PATIENT, PARENT, OR GUARDIAN OF THE IMPORTANCE OF COMPLETING THE IMMUNIZATION SERIES.

PATIENTS, PARENTS, OR GUARDIANS SHOULD BE INSTRUCTED TO REPORT ANY SERIOUS ADVERSE REACTIONS TO THEIR HEALTH CARE PROVIDER.

CARCINOGENESIS, MUTAGENESIS, AND IMPAIRMENT OF FERTILITY

DTP-HbOC has not been evaluated for its carcinogenic, mutagenic potential or for impairment of fertility.

PREGNANCY CATEGORY C

Animal reproduction studies have not been conducted with DTP-HbOC. This product is not recommended for use in individuals 7 years of age or older.

PEDIATRIC USE

The safety and effectiveness of DTP-HbOC in children below the age of 6 weeks have not been established.

For immunization of children 7 years of age or older, Tetanus and Diphtheria Toxoids Adsorbed for Adult Use (Td) is recommended. If contraindication to the pertussis component exists, Diphtheria and Tetanus Toxoids Adsorbed, for Pediatric Use (DT) should be substituted in children who have not reached their seventh birthday.

Full protection against the indicated diseases (tetanus, diphtheria, pertussis, and Haemophilus type b disease) is based on a full course of immunization.

DRUG INTERACTIONS:

Children receiving immunosuppressive therapy may have a reduced response to active immunization procedures.

As with other intramuscular injections, DTP-HbOC should be given with caution to children on anticoagulant therapy.

Tetanus Immune Globulin or Diphtheria Antitoxin, if used, should be given in a separate site with a separate needle and syringe.

The AAP recommends that influenza virus vaccine should not be administered within 3 days of immunization with a pertussis-containing vaccine since both vaccines may cause febrile reactions in young children.

Data are not yet available concerning adverse reactions that may occur when DTP-HbOC is given simultaneously with Oral Poliovirus Vaccine (OPV), Measles-Mumps-Rubella (MMR), or Hepatitis B (HB) vaccine at separate sites. Also, data are not available concerning the effects on immune response of OPV, MMR, or HB vaccine when DTP-HbOC is given simultaneously. Clinical studies with DTP-HbOC did however allow for the administration of OPV according to the routine immunization schedule for OPV.

ADVERSE REACTIONS:

The safety of DTP-HbOC has been evaluated in 6,793 children at 2, 4, and 6 months of age or at 15 to 18 months of age in three separate sites. The percent of doses administered associated with injection site reactions within 72 hours, or common systemic within 4 days, is summarized in TABLE 1.

TABLE 1 % of Doses Associated with Symptoms

	Infants‡ (542 doses)	Infants** (7269 doses)	Toddlers (107 doses)
Local*			
Erythema	34	19	40
Pain/Tenderness	21	30	65
Swelling	20	20	43
Warmth	16	—	35
Systemic†			
Fever ≥38.0°C	24	40***	33
Irritability	42	54	49
Drowsiness	26	—	9
Restless sleep	—	28	—
Loss of Appetite	—	4	—
Vomiting	5	2	1
Diarrhea	9	1	10
Rash	3	—	0

* within 72 hours of immunization
** data for this study all collected within 24 hours of immunization (percentages calculated from a range of 7269 to 7500 doses) in the Kaiser Permanente Safety and Immunogenicity Study
*** perceived fever
† within 4 days of immunization
‡ a separate multicenter safety and immunogenicity study, not a subset of the 7269 infant Kaiser study

Based on review of the Kaiser-Permanente Medical Care Program utilization data base of hospitalizations (within 60 days) and emergency room visits (within 30 days of immunization), in 6,497 infants who received DTP-HbOC, the most common reasons for seeking care include: trauma, viral illness, and respiratory illnesses (*e.g.*, upper respiratory infection, otitis media, bronchitis/bronchiolitis, and pneumonia). One child who received DTP-HbOC became transiently pale and tremulous without loss of responsiveness 4 hours after immunization and was hospitalized with a diagnosis of seizure. No other hospital visits for seizure or hypotonic, hyporesponsive episodes were reported within 72 hours of immunization. These results were not different from those observed in 3,935 infants who received DTP and HbOC at separate injection sites.

As with other aluminum-containing vaccines, a nodule may occasionally be palpable at the injection site for several weeks. Although not seen in studies with DTP-HbOC, sterile abscess formation or subcutaneous atrophy at the injection site may also occur.

The following significant adverse events have occurred following administration of DTP vaccines: persistent, inconsolable crying ≥3 hours (1/100 doses), high-pitched, unusual crying (1/1000 doses), fever ≥40.5°C (105°F) (1/330 doses), transient shock-like (hypotonic, hyporesponsive) episode (1/1750 doses), convulsions (1/1750 doses).

The ACIP states: "Although DTP may rarely produce symptoms that some have classified as acute encephalopathy, a causal relation between DTP vaccine and permanent brain damage has been demonstrated. If the vaccine ever causes brain damage, the occurrence of such an event must be exceedingly rare. A similar conclusion has been reached by the Committee on Infectious Diseases of the American Academy of Pediatrics, the Child Neurology Society, the Canadian National Advisory Committee on Immunization, the British Joint Committee on Vaccination and Immunization, the British Pediatric Association, and the Institute of Medicine."

The occurrence of sudden infant death syndrome (SIDS) has been reported following administration of DTP. However, a large case-control study in the US revealed no causal relationship between receipt of DTP vaccine and SIDS. A recent study of 6,497 infants in northern California found no increase in the rate of SIDS among DTP-HbOC recipients.

Onset of infantile spasms has occurred in infants who have recently recieved DTP or DT. Analysis of data from the National Childhood Encephalopathy Study on children with infantile spasms showed that receipt of preparations containing diphtheria, tetanus, and/or pertussis antigens was not causally related to infantile spasms. The incidence of onset of infantile spasms increases at 3 to 9 months of age, the time period in which the second or third doses of DTP are generally given. Therefore, some cases of infantile spasms can be expected to be related by chance alone to recent receipt of vaccines containing DTP.

Bulging fontanel has been reported after DTP immunization, although no cause and effect relationship has been established.

Cardiac effects and respiratory difficulties, including apnea, have been reported rarely following DTP immunization.

Other events that have been reported following administration of vaccines containing diphtheria, tetanus, pertussis, or Haemophilus b antigens include: urticaria, erythema multiforme or other rash, arthralgias, and, more rarely, a severe anaphylactic reaction (*e.g.*, urticaria with swelling of the mouth, difficulty breathing, hypotension, or shock) and neurological complications, such as convulsions, encephalopathy and various mono- and polyneuropathies, including Guillain-Barre syndrome. Permanent neurological disability and death have also been reported rarely in temporal relation to immunization although a causal relationship has not been established.

DOSAGE AND ADMINISTRATION:

FOR INTRAMUSCULAR USE ONLY

For infants beginning at 2 months of age, the immunization series for DTP-HbOC consists of three doses of 0.5 ml each at approximately 2-month intervals, followed by a fourth dose of 0.5 ml at approximately 15 months of age.

DTP-HbOC may be substituted for DTP and HibTITER administered separately, whenever the recommended schedules for use of these two vaccines coincide (see DTP and HibTITER recommended dosage schedules.) However, no published data are available to support the interchangeability of the Haemophilus b conjugate vaccine in DTP-HbOC and HibTITER with other Haemophilus b conjugate vaccines for the primary series. Therefore, it is recommended that the same conjugate vaccine be used throughout the primary series, consistent with the data supporting licensure of the vaccine.

FOR PREVIOUSLY UNVACCINATED OLDER CHILDREN

Immunization schedules should be considered on an individual basis for children not vaccinated according to the recommended schedule. Three doses of a product containing DTP, given at approximately 2 month intervals, are required followed by a fourth dose of a product containing DTP or DTaP approximately 12 months later and a fifth dose of a product containing DTP or DTaP at 4-6 years of age. If the fourth dose of a pertussis-containing vaccine is not given until after the fourth birthday, no further doses of a pertussis-containing vaccine are necessary.

DOSAGE AND ADMINISTRATION: *(cont'd)*

TABLE 2 RECOMMENDED IMMUNIZATION SCHEDULES
For Previously Unvaccinated *Younger*Children

Dose	Age	Immunization
1	2 months	Tetramune
2	4 months	Tetramune
3	6 months	Tetramune
4	15-18 months	Tetramune*
5	4-6 years	DTP or DTaP

* Children 15-18 months of age may receive DTaP plus a Haemophilus b conjugate vaccine as separate injections.

The number of doses of an HbOC-containing product indicated depends on the age that immunization is begun. A child 7-11 months of age should receive 3 doses of a product containing HbOC. A child 12-14 months of age should receive 2 doses of a product containing HbOC. A child 15-59 months of age should receive 1 dose of a product containing HbOC.

As indicated previously, DTP-HbOC may be substituted for DTP and HibTITER administered separately, whenever the recommended schedule for use of these two vaccines coincides.

Preterm infants should be vaccinated with DTP-HbOC according to their chronological age, from birth.

Interruption of the recommended schedules with a delay between doses does not interfere with the final immunity achieved; nor does it necessitate starting the series over again, regardless of the length of time elapsed between doses.

If a contraindication to the pertussis vaccine component occurs, Diphtheria and Tetanus Toxoids Adsorbed, for Pediatric Use (DT) and Haemophilus b Conjugate Vaccine HibTITER, as separate injections, should be substituted for each of the remaining doses.

The use of reduced volume (fractional doses) is not recommended. The effect of such practices on the frequency of serious adverse events and on protection against disease has not been determined.

Shake vigorously to obtain a uniform suspension prior to withdrawing each dose from the multiple dose vial. The vaccine should not be used if it cannot be resuspended.

Parenteral drug products should be inspected visually for particulate matter and discoloration prior to administration whenever solution and container permit. (See DESCRIPTION).

The vaccine should be injected intramuscularly. The preferred sites are the anterolateral aspect of the thigh or the deltoid muscle of the upper arm. The vaccine should not be injected in the gluteal area or areas where there may be a major nerve trunk. Before injection, the skin at the injection site should be cleansed and prepared with a suitable germicide.

After insertion of the needle, aspirate to help avoid inadvertent injection into a blood vessel.

For either primary or booster immunization against tetanus and diphtheria of individuals 7 years of age and older, the use of Tetanus and Diphtheria Toxoids Adsorbed for Adult Use (Td) is recommended.

For passive immunization against tetanus and diphtheria, human TIG, and/or Diphtheria Antitoxin are recommended. A separate syringe and site of injection should be used.

HOW SUPPLIED:

Storage: DO NOT FREEZE. STORE REFRIGERATED, AWAY FROM FREEZER COMPARTMENT, AT 2°C TO 8°C (36° TO 46°F).

HOW SUPPLIED - EQUIVALENTS NOT AVAILABLE:

Injection, Solution - Intramuscular

5 ml $337.20 TETRAMUNE, Lederle Pharm 00005-1960-31

DIPHTHERIA; PERTUSSIS; TETANUS *(001089)*

CATEGORIES: Biologicals; Immunologic; Serums, Toxoids and Vaccines; Toxoids; Vaccines; FDA Approved 1991 Jan

BRAND NAMES: Acel-Imune; **DTP Adsorbed**; Tri-Immunol; Tripedia

FORMULARIES: WHO

DESCRIPTION:

Tripedia, Diphtheria and Tetanus Toxoids and Acellular Pertussis Vaccine Adsorbed, for intramuscular use, is a sterile solution of diphtheria and tetanus toxoids adsorbed, with acellular pertussis vaccine in an isotonic sodium chloride solution containing thimerosal as a preservative and sodium phosphate to control pH. After shaking, the vaccine is a homogenous white suspension.

The acellular pertussis vaccine components are isolated from culture fluids of Phase 1*Bordetella pertussis*grown in a modified Stainer-Scholte medium.[1] After purification by salt precipitation, ultracentrifugation, and ultrafiltration, pertussis toxin (PT) and filamentous hemagglutinin (FHA) are combined to obtain a 1:1 ratio and treated with formaldehyde to inactive PT. Thimerosal (mercury derivative) 1:10,000 is added as a preservative.

Corynebacterium diphtheriae cultures are grown in a modified Mueller and Miller medium. *Clostridium tetani* cultures are grown in a peptone-based medium. Both toxins are detoxified with formaldehyde. The detoxified materials are then separately purified by serial ammonium sulfate fractionation and diafiltration.

The toxoids are adsorbed using aluminum potassium sulfate (alum). The adsorbed diphtheria and tetanus toxoids are combined with acellular pertussis concentrate, and diluted to a final volume using sterile phosphate-buffered physiological saline. Thimerosal (mercury derivative) 1:10,000 is added as a preservative. Each 0.5 ml dose contains, by assay, not more than 0.170 mg of aluminum and not more than 100 mcg (0.02%) of residual formaldehyde. The vaccine contains gelatin and polysorbate 80 (Tween-80) which are used in the production of the pertussis concentrate.

Each 0.5 ml dose is formulated to contain 6.7 Lf units of diphtheria toxoid and 5 Lf units of tetanus toxoid (both toxoids induce at least 2 units of antitoxin per ml in the guinea pig potency test), and 46.8 mcg of pertussis antigens. This is represented in the final vaccine as 23.4 mcg of inactive pertussis toxin (PT—also referred to as lymphocytosis promoting factor or LPF) and 23.4 mcg of filamentous hemagglutinin antigen (FHA).

The potency of the pertussis component is evaluated by measurement, using an ELISA system, of the antibody response to PT and FHA in immunized mice.

DESCRIPTION: *(cont'd)*

Acellular Pertussis Vaccine Concentrate (For Further Manufacturing Use) is produced by The Research Foundation for Microbial Diseases of Osaka University ("BIKEN"), Osaka, Japan under U.S. license, and is combined with diphtheria and tetanus toxoid manufactured by Connaught Laboratories, Inc. The bulk vaccine is prepared by Connaught laboratories Inc. Tripedia is filled, labeled, packaged, and released by Connaught Laboratories, Inc. (CLI).

CLINICAL PHARMACOLOGY:

Simultaneous immunization against diphtheria, tetanus, and pertussis, using a conventional "whole-cell" pertussis DTP vaccine (Diphtheria and Tetanus Toxoids and Pertussis Vaccine Adsorbed—For Pediatric Use), has been a routine practice during infancy and childhood in the United States since the late 1940's. This practice has played a major role in markedly reducing the incidence rates of cases and deaths from each of these diseases.[2]

Tripedia (Diphtheria and Tetanus Toxoids and Acellular Pertussis Vaccine Adsorbed) combines Connaught Laboratories, Inc. diphtheria and tetanus toxoids with purified pertussis antigens (inactivated PT and FHA). These pertussis antigens, produced by the Research Foundation for Microbial Diseases of Osaka University ("BIKEN"), have been used routinely in Japan for approximately ten years[3,4,5,6] and have been under investigational use in Sweden.[1,7,8,9,10] as well as in the United States.[11,12,13,14]

DIPHTHERIA

Corynebacterium diphtheriae may cause both localized and generalized disease. The systemic intoxication is caused by diphtheria exotoxin, an extracellular protein metabolite of toxigenic strains of *C. diphtheriae*. Protection against disease is due to the development of antibody to diphtheria toxin.

At one time, diphtheria was common in the United States. More than 200,000 cases, primarily among children, were reported in 1921. Approximately 5% to 10% of cases were fatal; the highest case-fatality rates were in the very young and the elderly. Reported cases of diphtheria of all types declined from 306 in 1975 to 59 in 1979; most were cutaneous diphtheria reported from a single state. After 1979, cutaneous diphtheria was no longer reportable.[2] From 1980 to 1986, only 18 cases of respiratory diphtheria were reported in the United States; 14 occurred among persons 15 years of age or older.[15,16]

Diphtheria is currently a rare disease in the United States primarily because of the high level of appropriate vaccination among children (97% of children entering school have received ≥ three doses of diphtheria and tetanus toxoids and pertussis vaccine adsorbed (DTP) and because of an apparent reduction in the circulation of toxigenic strains of *Corynebacterium diphtheriae*.[2] Most cases occur among unvaccinated or inadequately vaccinated persons.

Both toxigenic and nontoxigenic strains of *C. diphtheriae* can cause disease, but only strains that produce diphtheria toxin cause severe manifestations, such as myocarditis and neuritis. Diphtheria remains a serious disease, with the highest case fatality rates among infants and the elderly.[2]

Complete immunization significantly reduces the risk of developing diphtheria, and immunized persons who develop disease have milder illness. Protection is thought to last at least 10 years. Immunization does not however, eliminate carriage of *C. diphtheriae* in the pharynx or nose or on the skin.[2]

The efficacy of the CLI's diphtheria toxoid used in Tripedia was determined on the basis of immunogenicity studies, with a comparison to a serological correlate of protection (0.01 antitoxin units/ml) established by the Panel on Review of Bacterial Vaccines & Toxoids.

TETANUS

Tetanus is an intoxication manifested primarily by neuromuscular dysfunction caused by a potent exotoxin elaborated by *Clostridium tetani*.

The occurrence of tetanus in the United States has decreased dramatically from 560 reported cases in 1947 to a record low of 48 reported cases in 1987. Tetanus in the United States in primarily a disease of older adults. Of 99 tetanus patients with complete information reported to the Centers for Disease Control (CDC) during 1987 and 1988, 68% were ≥ 50 years of age, while only six were < 20 years of age. Overall, the case-fatality rate was 21%. The disease continues to occur almost exclusively among persons who are unvaccinated or inadequately vaccinated or whose vaccination or whose vaccination histories are unknown or uncertain.

In 4% of tetanus cases reported during 1987 and 1988, no wound or other condition was implicated. Non-acute skin lesions, such as ulcers, or medical conditions, such as abscesses, were reported in 14% of cases.[2]

Spores of *C. tetani* are ubiquitous. Serological tests indicate that naturally acquired immunity to tetanus toxin does not occur in the United States. Thus, universal primary immunization, with subsequent maintenance of adequate antitoxin levels by means of appropriately timed boosters, is necessary to protect all age groups. Tetanus toxoid is a highly effective antigen, and a completed primary series generally induces protective levels of serum antitoxin that persist for 10 or more years.[2]

The efficacy of the CLI's tetanus toxoid used in tetanus was determined on the basis of immunogenicity studies with a comparison to a serological correlate of protection (0.01 antitoxin units/ml) established by the Panel on Review of Bacterial Vaccines & Toxoids.[17]

PERTUSSIS

Pertussis (whooping cough) is a disease of the respiratory tract caused by *Bordetella pertussis*. This gram-negative coccobacillus produces a variety of biologically active components. One of these components, pertussis toxin (PT), has been associated with a number of effects such as lymphocytosis, sensitivity to histamine, changes in glucose and/or insulin levels, neurological effect, and adjuvant activity.[18] The role of the different components produced by *B. Pertussis* in either the pathogenesis of, or the immunity to, pertussis is not well understood. Immunization with vaccines containing inactivated PT and filamentous hemagglutinin (FHA), have been associated with protection in clinical studies. The pertussis component in tetanus induces immunity against pertussis.[9] The acellular pertussis component, in tetanus, contains not more than 50 endotoxin units/ml.

Pertussis is highly communicable (attack rates of > 90% have been reported among unvaccinated household contacts)[19] and can cause severe disease, particularly among very young children. Of 10,749 patients < 1 year of age reported nationally as having pertussis during the period 1980 to 1989, 69% were hospitalized, 22% had pneumonia, 3.0% had ≥ one seizure, 0.9% had encephalopathy, and 0.6% died.[20]Because of the substantial risks of complications of the disease, completion of a primary series of DTP vaccine early in life is essential.[2]

In older children and adults, including in some instances those previously immunized, infection may result in nonspecific symptoms of bronchitis or an upper respiratory tract infection, and pertussis may not be diagnosed because classic signs, especially the inspiratory whoop, may be absent. Older preschool-aged children and school-aged siblings who are not fully immunized and develop pertussis can be important sources of infection for young infants, the group at highest risk of disease and disease severity.[2]The infected adult is important in the overall transmission of pertussis.

General use of whole-cell pertussis DTP vaccines has resulted in a substantial reduction in cases and deaths from pertussis disease.[23,24]The use of Tripedia as the fourth or fifth dose evokes an antibody response at least as great as Connaught's whole-cell pertussis DTP vaccine following a primary series with commercially available U.S. whole-cell pertussis DTP with respect to PT and FHA antibodies.[1,11,12]

CLINICAL PHARMACOLOGY: *(cont'd)*

Acellular pertussis vaccines have been used in Japan since 1981, mostly in 2-year old children. Evidence for the efficacy of these vaccines, as a group, is demonstrated by the decline of pertussis disease with their routine use in that country.[2,23] In addition, a review of epidemiological studies of the Japanese acellular pertussis vaccines estimated that these vaccines, as a group, were 88%, efficacious in protecting against clinical pertussis on household exposure, with a 95% confidence interval of 79% to 93%.[25]

A large placebo-controlled efficacy trial of two Biken acellular pertussis vaccines was carried out in Sweden in 1986-1987. One of the vaccines contained a Biken two-component acellular pertussis vaccine comparable to that contained in tetanus. In its first phase, the trial in Sweden was a randomized, blinded prospective trial using a standardized case definition and active case ascertainment. In this phase, 1389 children, 5 to 11 months of age, received two doses of the Biken inactivated PT/FHA acellular pertussis vaccine 7 to 13 weeks apart and 954 received a placebo control. During the 15 months of follow-up from 30 days after the second dose, culture-confirmed whooping cough (cough and a positive culture of *Bordetella pertussis*) occurred in 40 placebo and 18 acellular pertussis vaccine recipients. The point estimate of protective efficacy for the vaccine was 69% (95% confidence interval; 47% to 82%) for all cases of culture confirmed pertussis and 80% (95% confidence interval; 59% to 91%) for culture confirmed cases with a cough of over 30 days duration.[9]

A three-year unblinded passive follow-up of vaccine and placebo recipients from above Swedish study has shown a post-trial efficacy of 77% (95% confidence interval; 65% to 85%) for all culture-proven cases of pertussis, and an efficacy of 92% (95% confidence interval; 84% to 96%) for culture-proven cases with a cough of over 30 days duration.[26]

Anti-PT and anti-FHA antibody responses in children enrolled in the trial in Sweden were subsequently compared to responses observed in clinical trials of Tripedia conducted in the U.S. In the U.S. trials, children 15 to 20 months of age who had previously received three doses of licensed whole-cell pertussis DTP and children 4 to 6 years of age who had previously received four doses of licensed whole-cell pertussis DTP were immunized with a single dose of Tripedia. The anti-PT and anti-FHA antibody responses to Tripedia in the U.S. trials were found to be similar to the responses observed in children enrolled in the trial in Sweden.[1] Although in the Swedish efficacy trial immunization with an inactivated PT/FHA vaccine was shown to protect against pertussis, no specific serological correlate or measure of protective immune response was found.[1,9] The role in clinical protection of specific serum antibodies is, therefore, not known at this time.

Additionally, the antibody responses in children immunized with Tripedia were compared to those in children immunized with CLI's licensed whole-cell pertussis DTP vaccine. Immunogenicity data from the clinical trial in the U.S. are summarized in TABLE 1. Anti-PT and anti-FHA responses to Tripedia were significantly higher than those to CLI's whole-cell pertussis DTP vaccine. Serological responses to diphtheria and tetanus antigens, not shown in TABLE 1, were equal to or greater than those produced by CLI's whole-cell pertussis DTP vaccine.[1,11,12]

Clinical experience (immunogenicity) in the United States is summarized in TABLE 1[1,11,12]

TABLE 1 [1,11,12]Comparisonof IgG Antibody to PT and FHA in ELISA Units (EU) and CHO-Cell Neutralization Titers (CHO) Induced by a Single Dose of Either Tripedia or CLI's Whole-Cell Pertussis DTP Vaccine in Children 15 to 20 months of Age* and 4 to 6 years of Age**

Vaccine	Age Group (N=)	PT/GMT† (EU) Pre-	FHA/GMT† (EU) Post-‡
		Vaccination	
Tripedia	15-29 Months (354)	14.5	443.0[b]
CLI's Whole-Cell DTP	15-20 Months (175)	14.5	67.0
Tripedia	4-6 years (211)	14.5	408.0[b]
CLI's Whole-Cell DTP	4-6 Years (65)	15.2	81.0

* All children in the 15- to 20-month group received U.S. licensed while-cell pertussis DTP vaccine for the first three doses of their primary series.
** All children in the 4- to 6-year group received U.S. licensed whole-cell pertussis DTP vaccine for the first four doses in their primary series.
† Geometric mean titer.
‡ Post-vaccination 4 to 6 weeks.
[a]Post-vaccination GMT for the Tripedia group, (4 to 6 year olds), is significantly higher than that of the whole-cell pertussis DTP vaccine group ($P < 0.05$).
[b]Post-vaccination GMT for the tetanus group, at 15 to 20 months and at 4 to 6 years, are significantly higher than those of the matching whole-cell DTP group, ($P<0.001$ in each case).

TABLE 2

Vaccine	Age Group (N=)	FHA/GMT† (EU) Pre-	FHA/GMT† (EU) Post-‡	CHO Pre-	CHO Post-
		Vaccination†		Vaccination†	
Tripedia	15-29 Months (354)	7.0	65.0[b]	25.3	300[b]
CLI's Whole-Cell DTP	15-20 Months (175)	6.0	19.0	24.8	119
Tripedia	4-6 Years (211)	18.9	363.0[b]	23.6	210[a]
CLI's Whole-Cell DTP	4-6 Years (65)	19.2	104.0	27.9	107

A total of 3,700 dose of Tripedia have been administered in the U.S. clinical trials, in children 15-20 months of age and 4-6 years of age. When compared to CLI's whole-cell pertussis DTP vaccine. Tripedia produced fewer and milder local reactions such as erythema, swelling, and tenderness at the injection site: as well as fewer and milder systemic reactions such as fever, irritability, drowsiness, vomiting, anorexia and high-pitched unusual cry.[1] Rates of more serious and infrequent adverse experiences for Tripedia are not known at this time.

INDICATIONS AND USAGE:

Diphtheria and Tetanus Toxoids and Acellular Pertussis Vaccine Adsorbed, tetanus, is indicated as a fourth and/or fifth dose for immunization of children 15 months to 7 years of age (prior to seventh birthday) who have previously been immunized against diphtheria, tetanus and pertussis with three or four doses of whole-cell pertussis DTP vaccine. However, in instances where the pertussis vaccine component is contraindicated, Diphtheria and Tetanus Toxoids Adsorbed (For Pediatric Use) (DT) should be used for each of the remaining doses.

If passive immunization is required. Tetanus Immune Globulin (Human) (TIG) and/or equine Diphtheria Antitoxin should be used.

INDICATIONS AND USAGE: *(cont'd)*

Persons recovering from confirmed pertussis do not need additional doses of DTP but should receive additional doses of DT to complete the series.

Tripedia is not be used for treatment of actual infection.

As with any vaccine, vaccination with tetanus may not protect 100% of susceptible individuals.

THIS VACCINE IS NOT RECOMMENDED FOR USE IN CHILDREN BELOW THE AGE OF 15 MONTHS. THIS VACCINE IS NOT RECOMMENDED FOR USE AS A PRIMARY SERIES IN CHILDREN OF ANY AGE.

CONTRAINDICATIONS:

Hypersensitivity to any component of the vaccine, including thimerosal, a mercury derivative, is a contraindication.

Immunization should be deferred during the course of any febrile illness or acute infection. A minor afebrile illness such a mild upper respiratory infection is not usually reason to defer immunization.

Elective immunization procedures should be deferred during an outbreak of poliomyelitis.[27]

Data on the use of Tripedia in children for whom whole-cell pertussis DTP vaccine is contraindicated are not available. Until such data are available, it would be prudent to consider the Immunization Practices Advisory Committee (ACIP) and American Academy of pediatrics (AAP) contraindication to whole-cell pertussis DTP vaccine to be contraindications to Tripedia.

Immunization with Tripedia is contraindicated if the child has experienced any event following previous immunization with pertussis vaccine (whole-cell DTP or acellular pertussis-containing DTP vaccine), which is considered by the ACIP or AAP to be a contraindication to further doses of pertussis vaccine. The ACIP states that if any of the following events listed in TABLE 3 occur in temporal relation to recipient of DTP, the decision to give subsequent doses of vaccine containing the pertussis component should be carefully considered.

It is a contraindication to use this or any other vaccine after a serious adverse reaction temporally associated with a previous dose, including an anaphylactic reaction.[2]

Encephalopathy not due to an identifiable cause, occurring within 7days of a prior whole-cell pertussis DTP or acellular pertussis DTP immunization and consisting of major alterations of consciousness, unresponsiveness, generalized focal seizures that persist for more than a few hours and failure to recover within 24 hours should be considered a contraindication to further use; this included severe alterations in consciousness with generalized of focal neurologic signs. Even though causation cannot be established, no subsequent doses should be given.[2]

WARNINGS:

This vaccine is not recommended for use in children below the age of 15 months. Efficacy data for Tripedia in infants is not available. although antibody responses to diphtheria, tetanus, and pertussis toxin, and FHA in infants immunized with Tripedia were at least equivalent to those for CLI's whole-cell pertussis DTP vaccine, the role of serum antibodies in protection against pertussis is unknown.

Tripedia is not recommended for immunization on or after the seventh birthday.

If any of the following events occur in temporal relation to receipt of DTP, the decision to give subsequent doses of vaccine containing the pertussis component should be carefully considered. There may be circumstances such as high incidence of pertussis, when the potential benefits outweigh possible risks, particularly since these events are not associated with permanent sequelae.[2]

THE FOLLOWING EVENTS WERE PREVIOUSLY CONSIDERED CONTRAINDICATIONS AND ARE NOW CONSIDERED PRECAUTIONS BY THE ACIP.[2]

Temperature of ≥ 50.5°C (105°F) within 48 hours not due to another identifiable cause. Such a temperature is considered a precaution because of the likelihood that fever following a subsequent dose of DTP vaccine will also be high. Because such febrile reactions are usually attributed to the pertussis component, vaccination with DT should not be discontinued.

Collapse or shock-like state (hypotonic-hyporesponsive episode) within 48 hours. Although these uncommon events have not been recognized to cause death nor to induce permanent neurological sequelae, it is prudent to continue vaccination with DT, omitting the pertussis component.[2]

Persistent, inconsolable crying lasting ≥ 3 hours, occurring within 48 hours of vaccination. Follow-up of infants who have cried inconsolably following DTP vaccination has indicated that this reaction, though unpleasant, is without long-term sequelae and not associated with other reactions of great significance. Inconsolable crying occurs most frequently following the first dose and is less frequently reported following subsequent doses of DTP vaccine.[2]

Convulsions with or without fever occurring within three days. Short-lived convulsions, with or without fever, have not been shown to cause permanent sequelae. Furthermore, the occurrence of prolonged febrile seizures (*i.e.,* status epilepticus-any seizure lasting > 20 minutes or recurrent seizures lasting a total of 30 minutes without the child fully regaining consciousness), irrespective of their cause, involving an otherwise normal child does not substantially increase the risk for subsequent febrile (brief or prolonged) or afebrile seizures. The risk is significantly increased only among those children who are neurologically abnormal before their episodes of status epilepticus.[2]

Tripedia should not be given to children with any coagulation disorder, including thrombocytopenia, that would contraindicate intramuscular injection unless the potential benefit clearly outweighs the risk of administration.

In the opinion of the manufacturer, the use of this vaccine is also contraindicated if the child, siblings, or parents have a history of seizure disorder. Recent studies suggest that infants and children with a history of convulsions in first-degree family members (*i.e.,* siblings and parents) have a 3.2-fold increased risk for neurologic events compared with those without such histories.[2,23,28]

However, the ACIP has concluded that a family history of convulsions in parents and siblings is not a contraindication to pertussis vaccination and that children with such family histories should receive pertussis vaccine according to the recommended schedule.[2,23,28]

Acetaminophen should be given at the time of DTP vaccination and every four hours for 24 hours to reduce the possibility of post-vaccination fever.[2]

Studies have failed to provide evidence to support a causal relation between DTP vaccination and either serious acute neurologic illness or permanent neurologic injury.[2]

Infants and children with recognized possible or potential underlying neurologic conditions seem to be at enhanced risk for the appearance of manifestations of the underlying neurologic disorder within two or three days following vaccination. Whether to administer DTP (or Tripedia) to children with proven or suspected underlying neurologic disorders must be decided on an individual basis. Important considerations include the current local incidence of pertussis, the near absence of diphtheria in the United States and the low risk infection with *C. tentani.*[2]

Only full doses (0.5 ml) of DTP (or Tripedia) vaccine should be given; if a specific contraindication to DTP exists, the vaccine should not be given.[2]

WARNINGS: *(cont'd)*

Controversy regarding the safety of pertussis vaccine during the 1970's led to several studies of the benefits and risks of this vaccination during the 1980's. These epidemiologic analyses clearly indicate that the benefits of the pertussis immunization program outweigh the risks.[2,30]

PRECAUTIONS:

GENERAL

Care is to be taken by the health-care provider for the safe and effective use of this vaccine.

EPINEPHRINE INJECTION (1:1000) MUST BE IMMEDIATELY AVAILABLE SHOULD AN ACUTE ANAPHYLACTIC REACTION OCCUR DUE TO ANY COMPONENT OF THE VACCINE.

Previous immunization history should be ascertained to confirm that at least three doses of whole-cell pertussis DTP vaccine have been given.

Prior to an injection of any vaccine, all known precautions should be taken to prevent adverse reactions. This includes a review of the patient's history with respect to possible sensitivity and any previous adverse reactions to the vaccine or similar vaccines, previous immunization history, current health status (see CONTRAINDICATIONS), and a current knowledge of the literature concerning the use of the vaccine under consideration. Immunosuppressed patients may not respond. Tripedia is not contraindicated based on the presence of HIV infection.[2]

TABLE 3 Contraindications and Precautions to Further DTP (or acellular pertussis) Vaccination

CONTRAINDICATIONS
An immediate anaphylactic reaction. Encephalopathy occurring within 7 days following DTP (or acellular pertussis) vaccination.
PRECAUTIONS
Temperature ≥ 40.5°C (105°F) within 48 hours not due to another identifiable cause Collapse or shock-like state (hypotonic-hyporesponsive episode) within 48 hours Persistent, inconsolable crying lasting ≥ hours, occurring within 48 hours Convulsions with or without fever occurring within 3 days.

Special care should be taken to ensure that the injection does not enter a blood vessel.

A separate syringe and needle or a sterile disposable unit should be used for each patient to prevent transmission of hepatitis or other infectious agents from person to person. Needles should not be recapped and should be disposed of properly.

INFORMATION FOR THE PATIENT

Parents should be fully informed of the benefits and risks of immunization with Tripedia. The health-care provider should provide the Vaccine Information Pamphlets (VIPs) which are required to be given with each immunization.

The physician should inform the parents or guardians about the potential for adverse reactions that have been temporally associated with whole-cell pertussis DTP vaccine and Tripedia administration and obtain informed consent. Parents or guardians should be instructed to report any serious adverse reactions to their health-care provider.

IT IS EXTREMELY IMPORTANT WHEN A CHILD IS RETURNED FOR THE NEXT DOSE IN THE SERIES, THAT THE PARENT SHOULD BE QUESTIONED CONCERNING OCCURRENCE OF ANY SYMPTOMS AND/OR SIGNS OF AN ADVERSE REACTION AFTER THE PREVIOUS DOSE (SEE CONTRAINDICATIONS; ADVERSE REACTIONS).

The health-care provider should inform the parent or guardian the importance of completing the immunization series, unless a contraindication to further immunization exists.

The U.S. Department of Health and Human Services has established a new Vaccine Adverse Event Reporting System (VAERS) to accept all reports of suspected adverse events after the administration of any vaccine, including but not limited to the reporting of events required by the National Childhood Vaccine Injury Act of 1986.[31] The toll-free number for VAERS forms and information is 1-800-822-7967.

The National Vaccine Injury Compensation Program, established by the Childhood Vaccine Injury Act of 1986, requires physicians and other health-care provider who administer vaccines to maintain permanent vaccination records and to report occurrences of certain adverse events to the U.S. Department of health and Human Services. Reportable events include those listed in the Act for each vaccine and events specified in the package insert as contraindications to further doses of the vaccine.[32,33]

CARCINOGENESIS, MUTAGENESIS, AND IMPAIRMENT OF FERTILITY

Tripedia has not been evaluated for its carcinogenic, mutagenic potentials or impairment of fertility.

THE VACCINE IS NOT RECOMMENDED FOR PERSONS 7 YEARS OF AGE AND OLDER.

PEDIATRIC USE

Efficacy data for Tripedia in infants is not available. Although antibody responses to diphtheria, tetanus, and pertussis toxin and FHA in infants immunized with Tripedia were at least equivalent to those for CLI's whole-cell pertussis DTP vaccine, the role of serum antibodies in protection against pertussis is unknown at this time.

Tripedia is not recommended for use in children below 15 months of age. This vaccine is not recommended for use as a primary series in children of any age.

Tripedia is not recommended for individuals over 7 years of age. Tetanus and Diphtheria Toxoids Adsorbed For Adult Use (Td) is to be used in individuals 7 years of age or older. Diphtheria and Tetanus Toxoids and Acellular Pertussis Vaccine Adsorbed, should not be used to immunize children less than 15 months of age.

DRUG INTERACTIONS:

As with other IM injections use with caution in patients on anticoagulant therapy.

Influenza virus vaccine should not be given within three days of the administration of Tripedia.[30]

Immunosuppressive therapies, including irradiation, antimetabolites, alkylating agents, cytotoxic drugs, and corticosteroids (used in great than physiologic doses), may reduce the immune response to vaccines. Although no specific studies with pertussis vaccine are available, if immunosuppressive therapy will be discontinued shortly, it would be reasonable to defer immunization until the patient has been off therapy for at least one month; otherwise the patient should be vaccinated while still on therapy.[2]

If tetanus has been administered to persons receiving immunosuppressive therapy, a recent injection of immune globulin or having an immunodeficiency disorder, an adequate immunologic response may not be obtained.

Tetanus Immune Globulin, or Diphtheria Antitoxin, if used, should be given in a separate site, with a separate needle and syringe.

ADVERSE REACTIONS:

Local adverse reactions which include pain, erythema, heat, edema, and induration, and systemic reactions such as fever, drowsiness, fretfulness, and anorexia may occur following vaccination. TABLE 4 lists the frequency of adverse reactions in 372 children who received Tripedia at 15 to 20 months and 239 children who received Tripedia at 4 to 6 years of age. These children had previously received three or four doses of whole-cell pertussis DTP vaccine at approximately 2, 4, 6, and 18 months of age.[1]

Rarely, an anaphylactic reaction (*i.e.,* hives, swelling of the mouth, difficulty breathing, hypotension, or shock) has been reported after receiving preparations containing diphtheria, tetanus, and/or pertussis antigens.[2]

Arthus-type hypersensitivity reactions, characterized by severe local reactions (generally starting 2 to 8 hours after an injection), may follow receipt of tetanus toxoid. A few cases of peripheral neuropathy have been reported following tetanus toxoid administration, although a causal relationship has not been established.[2]

In the National Childhood Encephalopathy Study (NCES), a large, case-control study in England, children 2 to 35 months of age with serious, acute neurologic disorders such as encephalopathy or complicated convulsion(s), were more likely to have received DTP in the 7 days preceding onset than their age-, sex-, and neighborhood-matched controls. Among children known to be neurologically normal before entering the study, the relative risk (estimated by odds ration) of a neurologic illness occurring within the 7-day period following receipt of DTP dose, compared to children not receiving DTP vaccine in the 7-day period before onset of their illness, was 3.3 ($p < 0.001$).[2]

Within this 7-day period, the risk was significantly increased for immunized children only within 3 days of vaccination (relative risk 4.2, $P < 0.001$). The relative risk for illnesses occurring 4 to 7 days after vaccination was 2.1 ($.05 < p < 0.1$). Serious neurologic illness requiring hospitalization attributable to pertussis vaccine are rare. Final analysis of a comprehensive case-control study has estimated that the risk of such illnesses is 1 in 140,000 doses administered. An earlier analysis had estimated this risk at 1/110,00 doses. In contrast, final analysis of the case control study found that the risk of serious neurologic illness following pertussis disease was 1/11,000 pertussis cases.[34] Repeated evaluations have shown that the benefits of vaccination outweigh the risks, therefore, both the ACIP and the American Academy of Pediatrics continue to recommend the use of DTP vaccine.[2,30]

The methods and results of the NCES have been thoroughly scrutinized since publication of the study. This reassessment by multiple groups has determined that the number of patients was too small and their classification subject to enough uncertainty to preclude drawing valid conclusion about whether a casual relation exists between pertussis vaccine and permanent neurologic damage. Preliminary data from a 10-year follow-up study of some of the children studied in the original NCES study also suggested a relation between symptoms following DTP vaccination and permanent neurologic disability. However, details are not available to evaluate this study adequately, and the same concerns remain about DTP vaccine precipitating initial manifestations of pre-existing neurologic disorders.[2]

Sudden Infant Death Syndrome (SIDS) has occurred in infants following administration of DPT. Large case-control studies of SIDS in the United States have shown that receipt of DTP was not causally related to SIDS.[35,36,37] It should be recognized that the first three primary immunizing doses of DTP are usually administered to infants 2 to 6 months old and that approximately 85% of SIDS cases occur at ages 1 to 6 months, with the peak incidence occurring at 6 weeks to 4 months of age. By chance alone, some cases of SIDS can be expected to be related to recent receipt of DTP.[35] Recent evidence does not indicate a causal relation between DTP vaccine and SIDS.[38]

Onset of infantile spasms has occurred in infants who have recently received DTP or DT. Analysis of data from the NCES on children with infantile spasms showed that receipt of DT or DTP was not causally related to infantile spasms.[39] The incidence of onset of infantile spasms increases at 3 to 9 months of age, the time period in which the second and third doses of DTP are generally given. Therefore, some cases of infantile spasms can be expected to be related by chance alone to recent receipt of DTP.[2]

A bulging fontanelle associated with increased intracranial pressure which occurred within 24 hours following DTP immunization has been reported, although a causal relationship has not been established (TABLE 4).[40,41,42]

TABLE 4
Adverse Events Occurring 24, 48 and 72 Hours Following Diphtheria And Tetanus Toxoids and Acellular Pertussis Vaccine Adsorbed Immunizations Given at 15 to 20 Months and 4 to 6 Years of Age

Event	Frequency 15 to 20 months Reaction % (N=372)			4 to 6 Years Reaction % (n=239)		
	24 hr.	48 hr.	72 hr.	24 hr.	48 hr.	72 hr.
Local						
Erythema	13%	7%	3%	25%	23%	14%
Swelling**	2%	1%	21%	20%	14%	6 %
Tenderness	6%	4%	2%	35%	20%	8%
Mild/Moderate Systemic						
Fever > 101°F	4%	1%	1%	3%	2%	1%
Gastrointestinal						
Diarrhea	3%	3%	2%	0%	0%	0%
Vomiting	2%	1%	0%	1%	1%	0%
Anorexia	6%	4%	3%	5%	3%	1%
Neurological						
Drowsiness	11%	4%	1%	13%	3%	2%
Irritability	15%	9%	5%	10%	7%	5%
High-pitched unusual cry	1%	1%	0%	0%	0%	0%

** Includes all occurrences of swelling.

The following illnesses have been reported as temporally associated with vaccine containing tetanus toxoid: neurological complications[43,44] including cochlear lesion,[45] brachial plexus neuropathies,[45,46] paralysis of the radial nerve,[47] paralysis of the recurrent nerve,[45] accommodation paresis, and EEG disturbances with encephalopathy.[48] In the differential diagnosis of polyradiculoneuropathies following administration of a vaccine containing tetanus toxoid, tetanus toxoid should be considered as a possible etiology.

REPORTING OF ADVERSE EVENTS

Reporting by parents and patients of all adverse events occurring after vaccine administration should be encouraged. Adverse events following immunization with vaccine should be reported by the health-care provider to the U.S. Department of Health and Human Services (DHHS) Vaccine Adverse Event Reporting System (VAERS). Reporting forms and information about reporting requirements or completion of the form can be obtained from VAERS through a toll-free number 1-800-822-7967[31,32,33]

The health-care provider also should report these events to Director of Medical Affairs, Connaught Laboratories, Inc., Route 611, P.O. Box 187, Swiftwater, PA 18370 or call 1-800-822-2463.

DOSAGE AND ADMINISTRATION:

Parenteral drug products should be inspected visually for extraneous particulate matter and/or discoloration prior to administration whenever solution and container permit. If these conditions exist, the vaccine should not be administered.

SHAKE VIAL WELL *before withdrawing each dose.* Inject 0.5 ml Tripedia intramuscularly only. The preferred injection sites are the anterolateral aspect of the thigh and the deltoid muscle of the upper arm. The vaccine should not be injected into the gluteal area or areas where there may be major nerve trunk. During the course of immunizations, injections should not be made more than once at the same site.

The use of reduced volume (fractional doses) is not recommended. The effect of such practices on the frequency of serious adverse events and on protection against disease has not been determined.

Do NOT administer this product subcutaneously. Special care should be taken to ensure that the injection does not enter a blood vessel.

TRIPEDIA IS INDICATED FOR THE FOURTH DOSE OF THE DIPHTHERIA, TETANUS AND PERTUSSIS IMMUNIZATION SERIES. TRIPEDIA MAY BE GIVEN 6 TO 12 MONTHS AFTER THE THIRD DOSE OF WHOLE-CELL PERTUSSIS DTP TO MAINTAIN ADEQUATE IMMUNITY DURING THE PRESCHOOL YEARS. THIS DOSE IN AN INTEGRAL PART OF THE PRIMARY VACCINATING COURSE.

TRIPEDIA IS INDICATED FOR THE FIFTH DOSE OF THE DIPHTHERIA, TETANUS, AND PERTUSSIS IMMUNIZATION SERIES. PRIOR IMMUNIZATIONS MAY CONSIST OF THREE DOSES OF WHOLE-CELL PERTUSSIS DTP AND ONE DOSE OF ACELLULAR PERTUSSIS DTP OR FOUR DOSES OF WHOLE-CELL PERTUSSIS DTP. TRIPEDIA MAY BE GIVEN TO CHILDREN 4 TO 6 YEARS OF AGE. BEFORE ENTERING KINDERGARTEN OR ELEMENTARY SCHOOL (NOT CONSIDERED NECESSARY IF FOURTH PRIMARY VACCINATING DOSE ADMINISTERED AFTER FOURTH BIRTHDAY).

The vial of vaccine should be shaken to ensure a proper suspension of the vaccine prior to use.

The simultaneous administration of DTaP, OPV, and MMR has not been evaluated. However, on the basis of studies using whole-cell DTP, the ACIP does not anticipate any differences in seroconversion rates and rates of side effects from those observed when the vaccines are administered separately. The ACIP recommends the simultaneous administration of all vaccines appropriate to the age and the previous vaccination status of the child., including the special circumstance of simultaneous administration of DTP or DTaP, OPV, HbCV, and MMR at age ≥ 15 months.[51]

STORAGE

Store between 2-8°C (35-46°F). DO NOT FREEZE. Temperature extremes may adversely affect resuspendability of this vaccine.

REFERENCES:

1. Unpublished Data available for Connaught Laboratories, Inc. **2.** Recommendations of the Immunization Practices Advisory Committee (ACIP). Diphtheria, Tetanus, and Pertussis: Recommendations for vaccine use and other preventative measures. MMWR 40: No RR-10, 1991. **3.** Kimura M. et al. Developments in pertussis immunization in Japan. The Lancet:30-32, 1990. **4.** Kimura M. et al. Current epidemiology of pertussis in Japan. Pediatr Infect Dis J 9: 705-709, 1990 **5.** Aoyama T, et al. Efficacy and immunogenicity of acellular pertussis vaccine by manufacturer and patient age. AJDC 143: 655-659. 1989. **6.** Aoyama T. et al. Efficacy of an acellular pertussis vaccine in Japan. J Pediatr 107: 180-183, 1985. **7.** Blennow M. et al. Preliminary data from a clinical trial (phase 2) of an Acellular Pertussis Vaccine, J-NIH-6. Develop Biol Standard 65: 185-190. 1986. **8.** Blennow M. et al. Primary immunization of infants with an Acellular Pertussis Vaccine in a double-blind randomized clinical trial. Pediatr 82: 293-299. 1988. **9.** Kalllings LO et al. Placebo-controlled trial of two Acellular Pertussis Vaccines in Sweden - protective efficacy and adverse events. Lancet: 955-960, 1988. **10.** Storsdaeter J., et al. Mortality and morbidity from invasive bacterial injections during a clinical trial of acellular pertussis vaccines in Sweden. Pediatr Infect Dis J 7: 637-645, 1988. **11.** Bernstein H. et al. Clinical reactions and immunogenicity of the BIKEN Acellular Diphtheria and Tetanus Toxoids and Pertussis Vaccine in 4-through 6-year-old US children. AJDC 146: 556-559, 1992. **12.** Feldman S. et al. Comparison of cellular (B-type) and whole-cell pertussis-components diphtheria-tetanus-pertussis vaccines as the first booster immunization in 15- to 24-month old children. J pediatr. IN PRESS. **13.** Feldmane S. et al. Comparison of two-component acellular and standard whole-cell pertussis vaccines, combined with diphtheria-tetanus toxoids, as the primary immunization series in infants. Southern Medical J. IN PRESS. **14.** Pichichero ME et al. Acellular pertussis vaccination of 2-month old infants in the United States. J Pediatr, Vol 89 No 5, 882-887, 1992. **15.** Mortimer EA, Diphtheria Toxoid, Vaccines. W.B. Saunders Company: P. 35. 1988. **16.** Karzon DT, et al. Diphtheria outbreaks in immunized populations. N Engl J Med 318:41-43, 1988. **17.** Department of Health and Human Services. Food and Drug Administration. Biological Products: Bacterial Vaccines and Toxoids: implementation of Efficacy Review: Proposed Rule. Federal Register Vol. 50 No 240., PP 51002-51117, 1985. **18.** Manclark CR, et al. Pertussis. In: R. Germainier (ed), Bacterial Vaccines Academic Press Inc. NY 69-106. 1984. **19.** Report of the committee on Infectious Diseases. Elk Grove Village, IL, American Academy of Pediatrics, 358-369, 1991. **20.** Fairzo KM et al. Epidemiologic features of pertussis in the United States, 1980-1989. Rev Infect Dise (IN PRESS). **21.** Linnemann CC. et al. Use of pertussis vaccine in an epidemic involving hospital staff. The Lancet 2:540-544, 1975. **22.** Linneman CC et al. Pertussis in the adult. Ann Rev Med 28: 179-185. 1977. **23.** Pertussis. report of the Committee on Infectious Diseases. American Academy of Pediatrics, Evanston, Illinois, 22nd Edition, 1991. **24.** CDC. Pertussis Surveillance - United States, 1986 and 1988. MMWR 39: 57-66, 1990. **25.** Noble GR, et al. Acellular and whole-cell pertussis vaccines in Japan. JAMA 257:1351-1356, 1987. **26.** Olin P. et al. Relative efficacy of two acellular pertussis vaccines during three years of passive surveillance. Vaccine 10:142-144, 1992. **27.** Wilson GS. The Hazards of Immunization. Provocation poliomyelitis. 270-274, 1967. **28.** ACIP. General recommendations on immunization. MMWR 38: 205-227, 1989. **29.** ACIP. Pertussis immunization. Family history of convulsions and use of antipyretics - Supplementary ACIP statement, MMWR 36: 281-282. 1987. **30.** Active immunization procedures. Report of the Committee on Infectious Diseases. AAP, Evanston, IL. 22nd Ed. 1991. **31.** CDC. Vaccine Adverse Event Reporting System - United States. MMWR 39: 730-733. 1990. **32.** CDC. National Childhood Vaccine Injury Act: requirements for permanent vaccination records and for reporting of selected events after vaccinations. MMWR 37: 197-200. 1988. **33.** Food and Drug Administration. New Reporting requirements for vaccine adverse events. FDA Drug Bull 18(2), 16-18, 1988. **34.** Miller D., et al. Pertussis vaccine and whooping cough as risk factors for acute neurological illness and death in young children. **35.** Griffin MR, et al. Risk of sudden infant death syndrome after immunization with the Diphtheria-Tetanus-Pertussis Vaccine. N Engl J Med 618-623, 1988. **36.** Hoffman HJ, et al. Diphtheria-tetanus-pertussis immunization and sudden infant death: Results of the National Institute of Child Health and Human Development Cooperative Epidemiological Study of Sudden Infant Death Syndrome Risk Factors. Pediatr 79: 598-611, 1987. **37.** Walker AM, et al. Diphtheria-tetanus-pertussis immunization and sudden infant death syndrome, Am J Public Health 77:945-951, 1987. **38.** Howson CP, et al. *Adverse Effects of Pertussis and Rubella Vaccines.* National Academy Press, Washington, DC 19991. **39.** Bellman MH, et al. Infantile spasms and pertussis immunization. Lancet 1:1031-1034, 1983. **40.** Jacon J, et al. Increased intracranial pressure after diphtheria, tetanus and pertussis immunization.Am J Dis Child Vol 133:217-218, 1979. **41.** Matthur R, et al. Bulging fontanelle following triple vaccine. Indian Pediatr 18 (6): 417-418, 1981. **42.** Shendurnikar N. et al. Bulging fontanel following DTP vaccine. Indian Pediatr 109: 917-924, 1986. **43.** Rutledge SL, et al. Neurological complications of immunization. J pediatr 109: 917-924, 1986. **44.** Walker AM, et al. Neurologic events following diphtheria-tetanus-pertussis immunization. Pediatr 81: 345-349. 1988. **45.** Wilson GS. The Hazards of Immunization. Allergic manifestations: Post-vaccinal neuritis. 153-156, 1967. **46.** Tsairis P, et al. Natural history of brachial plexus neuropathy. Arch Neurol 27:109-117, 1972. **47.** Blumstein Gl. et al. Peripheral neuropathy following tetanus toxoid administration. JAMA 198: 1030-1031, 1966. **48.** Cody CL. et al. Nature and rates of adverse reactions associated with DTP and DT immunizations in infants and children. Pediatr 68:650-660, 1981. **49.** Schlenska GK. Unusual neurological complications following tetanus toxoid administration. J Neurol 215: 299-302. 1977. **50.** CDC: *Adverse events following immunization.* Surveillance Report No. 3 1985-1986, Issued February 1989. **51.** ACIP. Pertussis Vaccination: Acellular Pertussis Vaccine for reinforcing and booster use - supplementary ACIP statement. MMWR 41: No. RR-1. 1992.(Connaught Labs, 8/92, 17722, T12)

HOW SUPPLIED - EQUIVALENTS NOT AVAILABLE:

Injection, Susp - Intramuscular - 4 unit/0.5ml

5 ml	$111.20	Diptheria/Tetanus/Pertuss Vacc, SKB Pharms	00007-3555-01
5 ml	$194.31	ACEL-IMUNE, Lederle Pharm	00005-1950-31
7.5 ml	$178.20	TRI-IMMUNOL, Lederle Pharm	00005-1948-33
7.5 ml	**$180.09**	**DTP ADSORBED, Connaught Labs**	**49281-0280-84**
7.5 ml	$290.34	TRIPEDIA, ADSORBED, Connaught Labs	49281-0282-15

DIPIVEFRIN HYDROCHLORIDE *(001088)*

CATEGORIES: Antiglaucomatous Agents; Compliance Aids; EENT Drugs; Eye, Ear, Nose, & Throat Preparations; Glaucoma; Intraocular Pressure; Mydriatics; Ophthalmics; Pregnancy Category B; FDA Approval Pre 1982; Patent Expiration 1991 Oct

BRAND NAMES: *D Epifrin* (Germany); *D'Epifrin*; *Diopine* (Mexico); *Diphemin*; Dipivefrin; Dipivefrin Hcl; *Glaucothil* (Germany); *Glaudrops*; **Propine**; *Propine C Cap BID* (Canada); *Propine C Cap QID* (Canada)
(International brand names outside U.S. in italics)

FORMULARIES: Aetna; BC-BS; FHP; PCS

DESCRIPTION:

This solution contains dipivefrin hydrochloride in a sterile, isotonic solution. Dipivefrin HCl is a white, crystalline powder, freely soluble in water.

Empirical Formula: $C_{19}H_{29}O_5N{\cdot}HCl$

Chemical Name: (±)-3.4-Dihydroxy—α—((methylamino) methyl) benzylalcohol 3,4-dipivalate hydrochloride.

Contains: Dipivefrin HCl 0.1% with; benzalkonium chloride 0.005%; edetate disodium; sodium chloride; hydrochloric acid to adjust pH; and purified water.

CLINICAL PHARMACOLOGY:

Dipivefrin HCl is a member of a class of drugs known as prodrugs. Prodrugs are usually not active in themselves and require biotransformation to the parent compound before therapeutic activity is seen. These modifications are undertaken to enhance absorption, decrease side effects and enhance stability and comfort, thus making the parent compound a more useful drug. Enhanced absorption makes the prodrug a more efficient delivery system for the parent drug because less drug will be needed to produce the desired therapeutic response.

Dipivefrin HCl is a prodrug of epinephrine formed by the diesterification of epinephrine and pivalic acid. The addition of pivaloyl groups to the epinephrine molecule enhances its lipophilic character and as a consequence, its penetration into the anterior chamber.

Dipivefrin HCl is converted to epinephrine inside the human eye by enzyme hydrolysis. The liberated epinephrine, an adrenergic agonist, appears to exert its action by decreasing aqueous production and by enhancing outflow facility. The dipivefrin HCl prodrug delivery system is a more efficient way of delivering the therapeutic effects of epinephrine, with fewer side effects than are associated with conventional epinephrine therapy.

The onset of action with one drop of dipivefrin HCl occurs about 30 minutes after treatment, with maximum effect seen at about one hour.

Using a prodrug means that less drug is needed for therapeutic effect since absorption is enhanced with the prodrug. Dipivefrin HCl at 0.1% dipivefrin was judged less irritating than a 1% solution of epinephrine hydrochloride or bitartrate. In addition, only 8 of 455 patients (1.8%) treated with dipivefrin HCl reported discomfort due to photophobia, glare or light sensitivity.

INDICATIONS AND USAGE:

Dipivefrin HCl is indicated as initial therapy for the control of intraocular pressure in chronic open-angle glaucoma. Patients responding inadequately to other antiglaucoma therapy may respond to addition of dipivefrin HCl.

In controlled and open-label studies of glaucoma, dipivefrin HCl demonstrated a statistically significant intraocular pressure-lowering effect. Patients using dipivefrin HCl twice daily in studies with mean durations of 76-146 days experienced mean pressure reductions ranging from 20-24%.

Therapeutic response to dipivefrin HCl twice daily is somewhat less than 2% epinephrine twice daily. Controlled studies showed statistically significant differences in lowering of intraocular pressure between dipivefrin HCl and 2% epinephrine. In controlled studies in patients with a history of epinephrine intolerance, only 3% of patients treated with dipivefrin HCl exhibited intolerance, while 55% of those treated with epinephrine again developed intolerance.

Therapeutic response to dipivefrin HCl twice daily therapy is comparable to 2% pilocarpine 4 times daily. In controlled clinical studies comparing dipivefrin HCl and 2% pilocarpine, there were no statistically significant differences in the maintenance of IOP levels for the two medications. Dipivefrin HCl does not produce miosis or accommodative spasm which cholinergic agents are known to produce. The blurred vision and night blindness often associated with miotic agents are not present with dipivefrin HCl therapy. Patients with cataracts avoid the inability to see around lenticular opacities caused by constricted pupil.

CONTRAINDICATIONS:

Dipivefrin HCl should not be used in patients with narrow angles since any dilation of the pupil may predispose the patient to an attack of angle-closure glaucoma. This product is contraindicated in patients who are hypersensitive to any of its components.

PRECAUTIONS:

Aphakic Patients: Macular edema has been shown to occur in up to 30% of aphakic patients treated with epinephrine. Discontinuation of epinephrine generally results in reversal of the maculopathy.

Pregnancy Category B: Reproduction studies have been performed in rats and rabbits at daily oral doses up to 10 mg/kg body weight (5 mg/kg body weight (5 mg/kg in teratogenicity studies), and have revealed no evidence of impaired fertility or harm to the fetus due to dipivefrin HCl. There are, however, no adequate and well-controlled studies in pregnant women. Because animal reproduction studies are not always predictive of human response, this drug should be used during pregnancy only if clearly needed.

Nursing Mothers: It is not known whether this drug is excreted in human milk. Because many drugs are excreted in human milk, caution should be exercised when dipivefrin HCl is administered to a nursing woman.

Usage in Children: Clinical studies for safety and efficacy in children have not been done.

Animal Studies: Rabbit studies indicated a dose-related incidence of meibomian gland retention cysts following topical administration of both dipivefrin hydrochloride and epinephrine.

ADVERSE REACTIONS:

Cardiovascular Effects: Tachycardia, arrhythmias and hypertension have been reported with ocular administration of epinephrine.

Local Effects: The most frequent side effects reported with dipivefrin HCl alone were injection in 6.5% of patients and burning and stinging in 6%. Follicular conjunctivitis, mydriasis and allergic reactions to dipivefrin HCl have been reported infrequently. Epinephrine therapy can lead to adrenochrome deposits in the conjunctiva and cornea.

DOSAGE AND ADMINISTRATION:

Initial Glaucoma Therapy: The usual dosage of dipivefrin HCl is one drop in the eye(s) every 12 hours.

Replacement with Dipivefrin HCl: When patients are being transferred to dipivefrin HCl from antiglaucoma agents other than epinephrine, on the first day continue the previous medication and add one drop of dipivefrin HCl in each eye every 12 hours. On the following day, discontinue the previously used antiglaucoma agent and continue with dipivefrin HCl.

In transferring patients from conventional epinephrine therapy to dipivefrin HCl, simply discontinue the epinephrine medication and institute the dipivefrin HCl regimen.

Addition of Dipivefrin HCl: When patients on other antiglaucoma agents require additional therapy, add one drop of dipivefrin HCl every 12 hours.

Concomitant Therapy: For difficult to control patients, the addition of dipivefrin HCl to other agents such as pilocarpine, carbachol, echothiophate iodide or acetazolamide has been shown to be effective.

Note: Not for injection.

Note: Store in tight, light-resistant containers.

HOW SUPPLIED - RATED THERAPEUTICALLY EQUIVALENT:

Solution - Ophthalmic; Top - 0.1 %

5 ml	$12.27	Dipivefrin HCl, HL Moore Drug Exch	00839-7952-85
5 ml	$13.25	Dipivefrin HCl, Goldline Labs	00182-7084-62
5 ml	$13.25	Dipivefrin HCl, Qualitest Pharms	00603-7125-37
5 ml	$13.50	Dipivefrin, Falcon Ophthalmics	61314-0235-05
5 ml	$13.65	Dipivefrin HCl, Major Pharms	00904-7943-05
5 ml	$14.07	Dipivefrin HCl, Schein Pharm (US)	00364-3040-53
5 ml	**$15.14**	**PROPINE, Allergan-Amer**	**11980-0260-25**
10 ml	$22.75	Dipivefrin HCl, HL Moore Drug Exch	00839-7952-90
10 ml	$23.70	Dipivefrin HCl, Qualitest Pharms	00603-7125-39
10 ml	$23.75	Dipivefrin HCl, Goldline Labs	00182-7084-63
10 ml	$24.00	Dipivefrin, Falcon Ophthalmics	61314-0235-10
10 ml	$24.75	Dipivefrin HCl, Major Pharms	00904-7943-10
10 ml	$25.31	Dipivefrin HCl, Schein Pharm (US)	00364-3040-54
10 ml	**$27.48**	**PROPINE, Allergan-Amer**	**11980-0260-20**
15 ml	$33.75	Dipivefrin HCl, HL Moore Drug Exch	00839-7952-61
15 ml	$34.75	Dipivefrin HCl, Goldline Labs	00182-7084-64
15 ml	$34.75	Dipivefrin HCl, Qualitest Pharms	00603-7125-41
15 ml	$35.00	Dipivefrin, Falcon Ophthalmics	61314-0235-15
15 ml	$36.40	Dipivefrin HCl, Major Pharms	00904-7943-35
15 ml	$37.21	Dipivefrin HCl, Schein Pharm (US)	00364-3040-72
15 ml	**$40.45**	**PROPINE, Allergan-Amer**	**11980-0260-21**

Solution/Drops - Ophthalmic - 0.1 %

5 ml	$10.95	Dipivefrin Hydrochloride, H.C.F.A. F F P	99999-1088-01
10 ml	$20.25	Dipivefrin Hydrochloride, H.C.F.A. F F P	99999-1088-02
15 ml	$29.92	Dipivefrin Hydrochloride, H.C.F.A. F F P	99999-1088-03

HOW SUPPLIED - NOT RATED EQUIVALENT:

Solution - Ophthalmic; Top - 0.1 %

5 ml	$13.28	Dipivefrin, Caremark	00339-5957-50
10 ml	$23.50	Dipivefrin Hcl, Rugby	00536-6238-70
10 ml	$24.00	Dipivefrin, Caremark	00339-5957-51
15 ml	$35.28	Dipivefrin, Caremark	00339-5957-52

DIPYRIDAMOLE *(001090)*

CATEGORIES: Antianginals; Anticoagulants/Thrombolytics; Blood Formation/Coagulation; Cardiovascular Drugs; Myocardial Perfusion; Platelet Inhibitors; Renal Drugs; Thromboembolism; Vasodilating Agents; Stress Test*; Pregnancy Category B; Sales > $100 Million; FDA Approved 1986 Dec
* Indication not approved by the FDA

BRAND NAMES: *Adezan*; *Adytim*; *Agilease* (Japan); *Agremol*; *Angicor*; *Anginal* (Japan); *Apo-Dipyridamole* (Canada); *Asasantin*; *Atlantin* (Japan); *Atrombin*; *Cardial*; *Cardiwell*; *Cardoxin*; *Cardoxin Forte*; *Centermol*; *Cerebrovase*; *Chilcolan* (Japan); *Cleridium* (France); *Coribon*; *Coronair*; *Coronamole* (Japan); *Coronarine* (France); *Corosan*; *Coroxin*; *Cortab*; *Curantyl N* (Germany); *Depe 75*; *Dilacor*; *Dipramol*; Dipridacot; *Dipymol*; *Dipyridan* (Japan); *Dipyrol*; *Dirinol* (Mexico); *Ethrine*; *Gulliostin* (Japan); *Isephanine* (Japan); *Justpertin* (Japan); *Lodimol* (Mexico); *Mersandien*; *Microbanzol* (Japan); *Miosen*; *Natyl*; *Novodil*; *Nupiron*; *Panachin*; *Parotin*; *Perclodin*; *Perdamol*; *Perisin*; *Permiltin* (Japan); Permole; *Persantin* (Australia, Asia, Europe, Mexico); *Persantin 75* (Mexico); *Persantin 100*; *Persantin Depot*; *Persantin Forte* (Germany); *Persantin PL*; *Persantin PL Prolonguetas* (Mexico); *Persantin Prolonguets*; *Persantin Retard*; *Persantin Retardkapseln*; **Persantine**; *Pertin*; *Piroan* (Japan); *Plato*; *Posanin*; *Powsinchen*; *Prandiol*; *Prexin*; *Procardin*; *Protangix* (France); *Pytazen SR*; *Ridamol*; *Rupenol*; *Sandel*; *Sanpell*; *Solantin*; *Stenocor*; *Stimolcardid*; *Tovincocard*; *Trancocard*; *Trompersantin* (Mexico); *Uginin*; *Vasokor*; *Viscor*
(International brand names outside U.S. in italics)

FORMULARIES: Aetna; BC-BS; FHP; PCS

DESCRIPTION:

Dipyridamole USP tablets is a platelet inhibitor and dipyridamole USP for intravenous injection is a coronary vasodilator chemically described as 2,6-bis-(diethanolamino)-4,8-dipiperidino-pyrimido-(5,4,-d) pyrimidine.

The molecular formula is $C_{24}H_{40}N_8O_4$.

The molecular weight is 504.62.

TABLETS

Dipyridamole is an odorless yellow crystalline powder, having a bitter taste. It is soluble in dilute acids, methanol and chloroform, and practically insoluble in water.

Dipyridamole tablets for oral administration contain:

Persantine Active Ingredient Tablets 25, 50, and 75 mg: dipyridamole USP 25, 50, and 75 mg respectively.

Persantine Inactive Ingredients Tablets 25, 50, and 75 mg: acacia, carnauba wax, corn starch, FD&C blue No. 1 aluminum lake, D&C yellow No. 10 aluminum lake, D&C red No. 30 aluminum lake, lactose, magnesium stearate, polyethylene glycol, povidone, shellac, sodium benzoate, sucrose, talc, titanium dioxide, white wax.

INTRAVENOUS INJECTION

Dipyridamole in solution is an odorless, pale yellow liquid which can be diluted in normal saline and dextrose and water for intravenous administration.

IV dipyridamole as a sterile solution for intravenous administration contains:

DESCRIPTION: *(cont'd)*

Persantine IV Active Ingredient Ampules 2 ml: dipyridamole USP 10 mg; Ampules 10 ml: dipyridamole USP 50 mg; Vial 10 ml: dipyridamole USP 50 mg.

Persantine IV Inactive Ingredients Ampules 2 ml: polyethylene glycol 600 100 mg, tartaric acid 4 mg; Ampules 10 ml: polyethylene glycol 600 500 mg, tartaric acid 20 mg; Vial 10 ml: polyethylene glycol 600 500 mg, tartaric acid 20 mg; pH is adjusted to 2.7 ± 0.5 with hydrochloric acid.

CLINICAL PHARMACOLOGY:

TABLETS

It is believed that platelet reactivity and interaction with prosthetic cardiac valve surfaces, resulting in abnormally shortened platelet survival time, is a significant factor in thromboembolic complications occurring in connection with prosthetic heart valve replacement.

Dipyridamole USP has been found to lengthen abnormally shortened platelet survival time in a dose-dependent manner.

In three randomized controlled clinical trials involving 854 patients who had undergone surgical placement of a prosthetic heart valve, dipyridamole, in combination with warfarin, decreased the incidence of postoperative thromboembolic events by 62 to 91% compared to warfarin treatment alone. The incidence of thromboembolic events in patients receiving the combination of dipyridamole and warfarin ranged from 1.2 to 1.8%. In three additional studies involving 392 patients taking dipyridamole and coumarin-like anticoagulants, the incidence of thromboembolic events ranged from 2.3 to 6.9%.

In these trials, the coumarin anticoagulant was begun between 24 hours and 4 days postoperatively, and the dipyridamole USP was begun between 24 hours and 10 days postoperatively. The length of follow-up in these trials varied from 1 to 2 years.

Dipyridamole does not influence prothrombin time or activity measurements when administered with warfarin.

Mechanism of Action: Dipyridamole is a platelet adhesion inhibitor, although the mechanism of action has not been fully elucidated. The mechanism may relate to inhibition of red blood cell uptake of adenosine, itself an inhibitor of platelet reactivity, phosphodiesterase inhibition leading to increased cyclic-3', 5'-adenosine monophosphate within platelets, and inhibition of thromboxane A_2formation which is a potent stimulator of platelet activation.

Hemodynamics: In dogs intraduodenal doses of dipyridamole of 0.5 to 4.0 mg/kg produced dose-related decreases in systemic and coronary vascular resistance leading to decreases in systemic blood pressure and increases in coronary blood flow. Onset of action was in about 24 minutes and effects persisted for about 3 hours.

Similar effects were observed following IV dipyridamole in doses ranging from 0.025 to 2.0 mg/kg.

In man the same qualitative hemodynamic effects have been observed. However, acute intravenous administration of dipyridamole may worsen regional myocardial perfusion distal to partial occlusion of coronary arteries.

Pharmacokinetics and Metabolism: Following an oral dose of dipyridamole, the average time to peak concentration is about 75 minutes. The decline in plasma concentration following a dose of dipyridamole fits a two-compartment model. The alpha half-life (the initial decline following peak concentration) is approximately 40 minutes. The beta half-life (the terminal decline in plasma concentration) is approximately 10 hours. Dipyridamole is highly bound to plasma proteins. It is metabolized in the liver where it is conjugated as a glucuronide and excreted with the bile.

INTRAVENOUS INJECTION

In a study of 10 patients with angiographically normal or minimally stenosed (less than 25% luminal diameter narrowing) coronary vessels, IV dipyridamole USP in a dose of 0.56 mg/kg infused over 4 minutes resulted in an average five-fold increase in coronary blood flow velocity compared to resting coronary flow velocity (range 3.8 to 7 times resting velocity). The mean time to peak flow velocity was 6.5 minutes from the start of the 4-minute infusion (range 2.5 to 8.7 minutes). Cardiovascular responses to the intravenous administration of dipyridamole when given to patients in the supine position include a mild but significant increase in heart rate of approximately 20% and mild but significant decreases in both systolic and diastolic blood pressure of approximately 2-8%, with vital signs returning to baseline values in approximately 30 minutes.

Mechanism of Action: Dipyridamole is a coronary vasodilator in man. The mechanism of vasodilation has not been fully elucidated, but many result from inhibition of uptake of adenosine, an important mediator of coronary vasodilation. The vasodilatory effects of dipyridamole are abolished by administration of the adenosine receptor antagonist theophylline.

How dipyridamole-induced vasodilation leads to abnormalities in thallium distribution and ventricular function is also uncertain but presumably represents a "steal" phenomenon in which relatively intact vessels dilate, and sustain enhanced flow, leaving reduced pressure and flow across areas of hemodynamically important coronary vascular constriction.

Pharmacokinetics and Metabolism: Plasma dipyridamole concentrations decline in a triexponential fashion following intravenous infusion of dipyridamole, with half-lives averaging 3-12 minutes, 33-62 minutes, and 11.6-15 hours. Two minutes following a 0.568 mg/kg dose of IV dipyridamole administered as a 4-minute infusion, the mean dipyridamole serum concentration is 4.6 ± 1.3 mcg/ml. The average plasma protein binding of dipyridamole is approximately 99%, primarily to α_1-glycoprotein. Dipyridamole is metabolized in the liver to the glucuronic acid conjugate and excreted with the bile. The average total body clearance is 2.3-3.5 ml/min/kg, with an apparent volume of distribution at steady state of 1-2.5 l/kg and a central apparent volume of 3-5 liters.

INDICATIONS AND USAGE:

TABLETS

Dipyridamole USP is indicated as an adjunct to coumarin anticoagulants in the prevention of postoperative thromboembolic complications of cardiac valve replacement.

INTRAVENOUS INJECTION

IV dipyridamole USP is indicated as an alternative to exercise in thallium myocardial perfusion imaging for the evaluation of coronary artery disease in patients who cannot exercise adequately.

In a study of about 1100 patients who underwent coronary arteriography and IV dipyridamole assisted thallium imaging, the results of both tests were interpreted blindly and the sensitivity and specificity of the dipyridamole thallium study in predicting the angiographic outcome were calculated. The sensitivity of the dipyridamole test (true positive dipyridamole divided by the total number of patients with positive angiography) was about 85%. The specificity (true negative divided by the number of patients with negative angiograms) was about 50%.

In a subset of patients who had exercise thallium imaging as well as dipyridamole thallium imaging, sensitivity and specificity of the two tests was almost identical.

CONTRAINDICATIONS:

Tablets: None known.

Intravenous Injection: Hypersensitivity to dipyridamole.

WARNINGS:

INTRAVENOUS INJECTION

Serious adverse reactions associated with the administration of intravenous dipyridamole USP have included cardiac death, fatal and non-fatal myocardial infarction, ventricular fibrillation, symptomatic ventricular tachycardia, stroke, transient cerebral ischemia, seizures, anaphylactoid reaction and bronchospasm. There have been reported cases of asystole, sinus node arrest, sinus node depression and conduction block. Patients with abnormalities of cardiac impulse formation/conduction or severe coronary artery disease may be at increased risk for these events.

In a study of 3911 patients given intravenous dipyridamole as an adjunct to thallium myocardial perfusion imaging, two types of serious adverse events were reported: 1) four cases of myocardial infarction (0.1%), two fatal (0.05%); and two non-fatal (0.05%); and 2) six cases of severe bronchospasm (0.2%). Although the incidence of these serious adverse events was small (0.3%, 10 of 3911), the potential clinical information to be gained through use of intravenous dipyridamole thallium imaging (see INDICATIONS AND USAGE noting the rate of false positive and false negative results) must be weighed against the risk to the patient. Patients with a history of unstable angina may be at a greater risk for severe myocardial ischemia. Patients with a history of asthma may be at a greater risk for bronchospasm during IV dipyridamole use.

When thallium myocardial perfusion imaging is performed with intravenous dipyridamole, parenteral aminophylline should be readily available for relieving adverse events such as bronchospasm or chest pain. Vital signs should be monitored during, and for 10-15 minutes following, the intravenous infusion of dipyridamole and an electrocardiographic tracing should be obtained using at least one chest lead. Should severe chest pain or bronchospasm occur, parenteral aminophylline may be administered by slow intravenous injection (50-100 mg over 30-60 seconds) in doses ranging from 50 to 250 mg. In the case of severe hypotension, the patient should be placed in a supine position with the head tilted down if necessary, before administration of parenteral aminophylline. If 250 mg of aminophylline does not relieve chest pain symptoms within a few minutes, sublingual nitroglycerin may be administered. If chest pain continues despite use of aminophylline and nitroglycerin, the possibility of myocardial infarction should be considered. If the clinical condition of a patient with an adverse event permits a one minute delay in the administration of parenteral aminophylline, thallium-201 may be injected and allowed to circulate for one minute before the injection of aminophylline. This will allow initial thallium perfusion imaging to be performed before reversal of the pharmacologic effects of dipyridamole on the coronary circulation.

PRECAUTIONS:

GENERAL

Tablets: Dipyridamole USP should be used with caution in patients with hypotension since it can produce peripheral vasodilation.

Intravenous Injection: See WARNINGS.

CARCINOGENESIS, MUTAGENESIS, AND IMPAIRMENT OF FERTILITY

Tablets: In a 111 week oral study in mice and in a 128-142 week oral study in rats, dipyridamole USP produced no significant carcinogenic effects at doses of 8, 25 and 75 mg/kg (1, 3.1 and 9.4 times the maximum recommended daily human dose). Mutagenicity testing with dipyridamole was negative. Reproduction studies with dipyridamole revealed no evidence of impaired fertility in rats at dosages up to 60 times the maximum recommended human dose. A significant reduction in number of corpora lutea with consequent reduction in implantations and live fetuses was, however, observed at 155 times the maximum recommended human dose.

Intravenous Injection: In studies in which dipyridamole was administered in the feed at doses of up to 75 mg/kg/day (9.4 times* the maximum recommended daily human oral dose) in mice (up to 128 weeks in males and up to 142 weeks in females) and rats (up to 111 weeks in males and females), there was no evidence of drug related carcinogenesis. Mutagenicity tests of dipyridamole with bacterial and mammalian cell systems were negative. There was no evidence of impaired fertility when dipyridamole was administered to male and female rats at oral doses up to 500 mg/kg/day (63 times* the maximum recommended daily human oral dose). A significant reduction in number of corpora lutea with consequent reduction in implantations and live fetuses was, however, observed at 1250 mg/kg/day.

PREGNANCY, TERATOGENIC EFFECTS, PREGNANCY CATEGORY B

There are, however, no adequate and well-controlled studies in pregnant women. Because animal reproduction studies are not always predictive of human responses, this drug should be used during pregnancy only if clearly needed.

Tablets: Reproduction studies have been performed in mice at doses up to 125 mg/kg (15.6 times the maximum recommended daily human dose), rats at doses up to 1000 mg/kg (125 times the maximum recommended daily human dose) and rabbits at doses up to 40 mg/kg (5 times the maximum recommended daily human dose) and have revealed no evidence of harm to the fetus due to dipyridamole.

Intravenous Injection: Reproduction studies performed in mice and rats at daily oral doses of up to 125 mg/kg (15.6 times* the maximum recommended daily human oral dose) and in rabbits at daily oral doses of up to 20 mg/kg (2.5 times* the maximum recommended daily human oral dose) have revealed no evidence of impaired embryonic development due to dipyridamole.

*Calculation based on assumed body weight of 50 kg.

NURSING MOTHERS

As dipyridamole is excreted in human milk, caution should be exercised when dipyridamole is administered to a nursing woman.

PEDIATRIC USE

Tablets: Safety and effectiveness in children below the age of 12 years has not been established.

Intravenous Injection: Safety and effectiveness in the pediatric population have not been established.

DRUG INTERACTIONS:

INTRAVENOUS INJECTION

Oral maintenance theophylline and other xanthine derivatives such as caffeine may abolish the coronary vasodilation induced by intravenous dipyridamole USP administration. This could lead to a false negative thallium imaging result (see Mechanism of Action.)

Myasthenia gravis patients receiving therapy with cholinesterase inhibitors may experience worsening of their disease in the presence of dipyridamole.

ADVERSE REACTIONS:

TABLETS

Adverse reactions at therapeutic doses are usually minimal and transient. On long-term use of dipyridamole USP, initial side effects usually disappear. The following reactions were reported in two heart valve replacement trials comparing dipyridamole and warfarin therapy to either warfarin alone or warfarin and placebo (TABLE 1):

TABLE 1

	Dipyridamole/ Warfarin (N = 147)	Placebo/ Warfarin (N = 170)
Dizziness	13.6%	8.2%
Abdominal distress	6.1%	3.5%
Headache	2.3%	0.0
Rash	2.3%	1.1%

Other reactions from uncontrolled studies include diarrhea, vomiting, flushing and pruritus. In addition, angina pectoris has been reported rarely and there have been rare reports of liver dysfunction. On those uncommon occasions when adverse reactions have been persistent or intolerable, they have been ceased on withdrawal of the medication.

When dipyridamole USP was administered concomitantly with warfarin, bleeding was no greater in frequency or severity than that observed when warfarin was administered alone.

Adverse reaction information concerning intravenous dipyridamole USP is derived from a study of 3911 patients in which intravenous dipyridamole was used as an adjunct to thallium myocardial perfusion imaging and from spontaneous reports of adverse reactions and the published literature.

Serious adverse events (cardiac death, fatal and non-fatal myocardial infarction, ventricular fibrillation, asystole, sinus node arrest, symptomatic ventricular tachycardia, stroke, transient cerebral ischemia, seizures, anaphylactoid reaction and bronchospasm) are described above (see WARNINGS.)

In the study of 3911 patients, the most frequent adverse reactions were: chest pain/angina pectoris (19.7%), electrocardiographic changes (most commonly ST-T changes) (15.9%), headache (12.2%), and dizziness (11.8%).

Adverse reactions occurring in greater than 1% of the patients in the study are shown in TABLE 2.

TABLE 2

	Incidence (%) of Drug-Related Adverse Events
Chest pain/angina pectoris	19.7
Headache	12.2
Dizziness	11.8
Electrocardiographic Abnormalities/ST-T changes	7.5
Electrocardiographic Abnormalities/Extrasystoles	5.2
Hypotension	4.6
Nausea	4.6
Flushing	3.4
Electrocardiographic Abnormalities/Tachycardia	3.2
Dyspnea	2.6
Pain Unspecified	2.6
Blood Pressure Lability	1.6
Hypertension	1.5
Paresthesia	1.3
Fatigue	1.2

Less common adverse reactions occurring in 1% or less of the patients within the study included:

Cardiovascular System: Electrocardiographic abnormalities unspecified (0.8%), arrhythmia unspecified (0.6%), palpitation (0.3%), ventricular tachycardia (0.2% see WARNINGS), bradycardia (0.2%), myocardial infarction (0.1% see WARNINGS), AV block (0.1%), syncope (0.1%), orthostatic hypotension (0.1%), atrial fibrillation (0.1%, supraventricular tachycardia (0.1%), ventricular arrhythmia unspecified (0.03% see WARNINGS), heart block unspecified (0.03%), cardiomyopathy (0.03%), edema (0.03%).

Central and Peripheral Nervous System: Hypothesia (0.5%), hypertonia (0.3%), nervousness/ anxiety (0.2%), tremor (0.1%), abnormal coordination (0.03%), somnolence (0.03%), dysphonia (0.03%), migraine (0.03%), vertigo (0.03%).

Respiratory System: Pharyngitis (0.3%), bronchospasm (0.2% see WARNINGS), hyperventilation (0.1%), rhinitis (0.1%), coughing (0.03%), pleural pain (0.03%).

Other: Myalgia (0.9%), back pain (0.6%), injection site reaction unspecified (0.4%), diaphoresis (0.4%), asthenia (0.3%), malaise (0.3%), arthralgia (0.3%), injection site pain (0.1%), rigor (0.1%), earache (0.1%), tinnitus (0.1%), vision abnormalities unspecified (0.1%), dysgeusia (0.1%), thirst (0.03%), depersonalization (0.03%), eye pain (0.03%), renal pain (0.03%), perineal pain (0.03%), breast pain (0.03%), intermittent claudication (0.03%), leg cramping (0.03%). In additional postmarketing experience, there have been rare reports of allergic reaction including urticaria, pruritus, dermatitis and rash.

OVERDOSAGE:

TABLETS

Hypotension, if it occurs, is likely to be of short duration, but a vasopressor drug may be used if necessary. The oral LD_{50}in mice is 2, 150 mg/kg. Single oral doses of 6,000 mg/kg in rats and 350 mg/kg in dogs were lethal. Symptoms of acute toxicity included ataxia, decreased locomotion and diarrhea in rodents and emesis, ataxia and depression in dogs. Since dipyridamole USP is highly protein bound, dialysis is not likely to be of benefit.

INTRAVENOUS INJECTION

No cases of overdosage in humans have been reported. It is unlikely that overdosage will occur because of the nature of use (*i.e.,* single intravenous administration in controlled settings). See WARNINGS.

DOSAGE AND ADMINISTRATION:

TABLETS

Adjunctive Use in Prophylaxis of Thromboembolism after Cardiac Valve Replacement. The recommended dose is 75-100 mg four times daily as an adjunct to the usual warfarin therapy. Please note that aspirin is not to be administered concomitantly with coumarin anticoagulants.

Store below 86°F (30°C).

DOSAGE AND ADMINISTRATION: *(cont'd)*

INTRAVENOUS INJECTION

The dose of intravenous dipyridamole USP as an adjunct to thallium myocardial perfusion imaging should be adjusted according to the weight of the patient. The recommended dose is 0.142 mg/kg/minute (0.57 mg/kg total) infused over 4 minutes. Although the maximum tolerated dose has not been determined, clinical experience suggests that a total dose beyond 60 mg is not needed for any patient.

Prior to intravenous administration, IV dipyridamole should be diluted in at least a 1:2 ratio with 0.45% sodium chloride injection, 0.9% sodium chloride injection, or 5% dextrose injection for a total volume of approximately 20 to 50 ml. Infusion of undiluted dipyridamole may cause local irritation.

Thallium-201 should be injected within 5 minutes following the 4-minute infusion of dipyridamole.

Do not mix IV dipyridamole with other drugs in the same syringe or infusion container.

Parenteral drug product should be inspected visually for particulate matter and discoloration prior to administration, whenever solution and container permit.

Store between 15°C (59°F)-25°C (77°F). Protect from direct light. Avoid freezing.

(Tablets - Boehringer Ingelheim Pharmaceuticals, Inc., 10/93, 862020)

(Intravenous Injection - Du Pont Merck Pharmaceutical Co., 4/95, 513113-0495)

HOW SUPPLIED - RATED THERAPEUTICALLY EQUIVALENT:

Tablet, Coated - Oral - 25 mg

100's	$2.25	Dipyridamole, Goldline Labs	00182-1156-01
100's	$2.70	Dipyridamole, H.C.F.A. F F P	99999-1090-01
100's	$2.90	Dipyridamole, Qualitest Pharms	00603-3383-21
100's	$3.23	Dipyridamole, Squibb-Mark	57783-6560-01
100's	$4.48	Dipyridamole, Geneva Pharms	00781-1241-01
100's	$4.60	Dipyridamole, Barr	00555-0252-02
100's	$4.75	Dipyridamole, Consolidated Midland	00223-0837-01
100's	$4.79	Dipyridamole, HL Moore Drug Exch	00839-6327-06
100's	$4.79	Dipyridamole, HL Moore Drug Exch	00839-7918-06
100's	$5.10	Dipyridamole, Martec Pharms	52555-0115-01
100's	$5.20	Dipyridamole, Major Pharms	00904-1083-60
100's	$5.20	Dipyridamole 25 Mg Tablets, Major Pharms	00904-1086-60
100's	$6.00	Dipyridamole, Sidmak Labs	50111-0311-01
100's	$6.27	Dipyridamole, Purepac Pharm	00228-2193-10
100's	$6.27	Dipyridamole, Mova Pharms	55370-0151-07
100's	$6.28	Dipyridamole, Aligen Independ	00405-5350-01
100's	$6.39	Dipyridamole, Major Pharms	00904-1083-61
100's	$6.75	Dipyridamole, Geneva Pharms	00781-1890-01
100's	$6.95	Dipyridamole, Rugby	00536-3570-01
100's	$8.06	Dipyridamole, Schein Pharm (US)	00364-2491-01
100's	$8.10	Dipyridamole 25, Goldline Labs	00182-1568-01
100's	$8.15	Dipyridamole, Aligen Independ	00405-4350-01
100's	$8.56	Dipyridamole, Lederle Pharm	00005-3743-23
100's	$9.80	Dipyridamole, Goldline Labs	00182-1156-89
100's	$10.64	Dipyridamole, Lederle Pharm	00005-3743-60
100's	$15.60	Dipyridamole, Medirex	57480-0323-01
100's	$17.60	Dipyridamole, Goldline Labs	00182-1568-89
100's	$18.26	Dipyridamole, Vangard Labs	00615-1543-13
100's	$19.58	Dipyridamole, Major Pharms	00904-1086-61
100's	**$33.85**	**PERSANTINE, Boehringer Pharms**	**00597-0017-01**
500's	$13.50	Dipyridamole, H.C.F.A. F F P	99999-1090-02
500's	$17.35	Dipyridamole, Barr	00555-0252-04
500's	$33.85	Dipyridamole, Lederle Pharm	00005-3743-31
600's	$90.60	Dipyridamole, Medirex	57480-0323-06
1000's	$13.75	Permole 25, H & H Labs	46703-0044-10
1000's	$17.97	Dipyridamole, Squibb-Mark	57783-6560-03
1000's	$22.40	Dipyridamole, Qualitest Pharms	00603-3383-32
1000's	$27.00	Dipyridamole, H.C.F.A. F F P	99999-1090-03
1000's	$29.01	Dipyridamole, HL Moore Drug Exch	00839-6327-16
1000's	$29.01	Dipyridamole, HL Moore Drug Exch	00839-7918-16
1000's	$29.20	Dipyridamole, Major Pharms	00904-1086-80
1000's	$33.35	Dipyridamole, Barr	00555-0252-05
1000's	$37.10	Dipyridamole, Geneva Pharms	00781-1890-10
1000's	$40.05	Dipyridamole 25, Goldline Labs	00182-1568-10
1000's	$40.19	Dipyridamole, Aligen Independ	00405-4350-03
1000's	$41.22	Dipyridamole, Aligen Independ	00405-5350-03
1000's	$41.50	Dipyridamole, Consolidated Midland	00223-0837-02
1000's	$41.91	Dipyridamole, Purepac Pharm	00228-2193-96
1000's	$41.91	Dipyridamole, Mova Pharms	55370-0151-09
1000's	$41.93	Dipyridamole, Geneva Pharms	00781-1241-10
1000's	$42.20	Dipyridamole, Schein Pharm (US)	00364-2491-02
1000's	$42.25	Dipyridamole, Rugby	00536-3570-10
1000's	$42.25	Dipyridamole, Sidmak Labs	50111-0311-03
2500's	$67.50	Dipyridamole, H.C.F.A. F F P	99999-1090-04

Tablet, Coated - Oral - 50 mg

100's	$4.13	Dipyridamole, H.C.F.A. F F P	99999-1090-05
100's	$6.60	Dipyridamole, Barr	00555-0285-02
100's	$6.95	Dipyridamole, Squibb-Mark	57783-6570-01
100's	$7.10	Dipyridamole, Qualitest Pharms	00603-3384-21
100's	$7.90	Dipyridamole, HL Moore Drug Exch	00839-6494-06
100's	$7.90	Dipyridamole, HL Moore Drug Exch	00839-7919-06
100's	$8.12	Dipyridamole, Martec Pharms	52555-0116-01
100's	$8.50	Dipyridamole, Major Pharms	00904-1085-60
100's	$8.50	Dipyridamole, Major Pharms	00904-1087-60
100's	$9.59	Dipyridamole, Major Pharms	00904-1085-61
100's	$9.66	Dipyridamole, Geneva Pharms	00781-1242-01
100's	$9.90	Dipyridamole, Sidmak Labs	50111-0312-01
100's	$10.34	Dipyridamole, Purepac Pharm	00228-2183-10
100's	$10.34	Dipyridamole, Mova Pharms	55370-0152-07
100's	$10.78	Dipyridamole 50, Goldline Labs	00182-1569-01
100's	$10.82	Dipyridamole, Aligen Independ	00405-4351-01
100's	$10.95	Dipyridamole, Rugby	00536-3619-01
100's	$11.10	Dipyridamole, Schein Pharm (US)	00364-2492-01
100's	$11.25	Dipyridamole, Lederle Pharm	00005-3790-23
100's	$17.17	Dipyridamole, Lederle Pharm	00005-3790-60
100's	$19.23	Dipyridamole, Geneva Pharms	00781-1678-01
100's	$27.25	Dipyridamole, Medirex	57480-0324-01
100's	$30.25	Dipyridamole, Goldline Labs	00182-1569-89
100's	$30.29	Dipyridamole, Major Pharms	00904-1087-61
100's	$31.05	Dipyridamole, Vangard Labs	00615-1573-13
100's	**$54.54**	**PERSANTINE-50, Boehringer Pharms**	**00597-0018-01**
500's	$14.50	Permole 50, H & H Labs	46703-0062-05
500's	$16.80	Dipyridamole, Major Pharms	00904-1085-40
500's	$20.65	Dipyridamole, H.C.F.A. F F P	99999-1090-06
500's	$21.50	Dipyridamole Tablets 50 Mg, Halsey Drug	00879-0479-05
500's	$35.20	Dipyridamole, Rugby	00536-3619-05
500's	$45.80	Dipyradamole, Amer Preferred	53445-1405-05
500's	$50.94	Dipyridamole, Barr	00555-0285-04

HOW SUPPLIED - RATED THERAPEUTICALLY EQUIVALENT:

(cont'd)

500's	$52.60	Dipyridamole, Lederle Pharm	00005-3790-31
600's	$149.20	Dipyridamole, Medirex	57480-0324-06
1000's	$41.30	Dipyridamole, H.C.F.A. F F P	99999-1090-07
1000's	$45.90	Dipyridamole, Squibb-Mark	57783-6570-03
1000's	$48.00	Dipyridamole, Martec Pharms	52555-0116-10
1000's	$49.85	Dipyridamole 50 Mg Tablets, Major Pharms	00904-1087-80
1000's	$51.15	Dipyridamole, Qualitest Pharms	00603-3384-32
1000's	$57.35	Dipyridamole, Barr	00555-0285-05
1000's	$60.08	Dipyridamole, HL Moore Drug Exch	00839-6494-16
1000's	$60.08	Dipyridamole, HL Moore Drug Exch	00839-7919-16
1000's	$62.93	Dipyridamole, Geneva Pharms	00781-1242-10
1000's	$63.35	Dipyridamole, Sidmak Labs	50111-0312-03
1000's	$64.10	Dipyridamole, Geneva Pharms	00781-1678-10
1000's	$75.11	Dipyridamole 50, Goldline Labs	00182-1569-10
1000's	$75.13	Dipyridamole, Schein Pharm (US)	00364-2492-02
1000's	$75.22	Dipyridamole, Aligen Independ	00405-4351-03
1000's	$75.25	Dipyridamole, Rugby	00536-3619-10
1000's	$76.16	Dipyridamole, Purepac Pharm	00228-2183-96
1000's	$76.16	Dipyridamole, Mova Pharms	55370-0152-09
1000's	**$519.19**	**PERSANTINE-50, Boehringer Pharms**	**00597-0018-10**

Tablet, Coated - Oral - 75 mg

100's	$5.93	Dipyridamole, H.C.F.A. F F P	99999-1090-08
100's	$11.19	Dipyridamole, HL Moore Drug Exch	00839-6429-06
100's	$11.19	Dipyridamole, HL Moore Drug Exch	00839-7920-06
100's	$11.25	Dipyridamole, Major Pharms	00904-1084-60
100's	$11.25	Dipyridamole 75 Mg Tablets, Major Pharms	00904-1088-60
100's	$12.22	Dipyridamole, Major Pharms	00904-1084-61
100's	$14.21	Dipyridamole, Geneva Pharms	00781-1243-01
100's	$14.35	Dipyridamole, Sidmak Labs	50111-0313-01
100's	$15.02	Dipyridamole, Purepac Pharm	00228-2185-10
100's	$15.02	Dipyridamole, Mova Pharms	55370-0154-07
100's	$15.10	Dipyridamole, Aligen Independ	00405-5352-01
100's	$18.10	Dipyridamole, Qualitest Pharms	00603-3385-21
100's	$18.50	Dipyridamole, Schein Pharm (US)	00364-2493-01
100's	$18.78	Dipyridamole 75, Goldline Labs	00182-1570-01
100's	$18.78	Dipyridamole, Barr	00555-0286-02
100's	$18.82	Dipyridamole, Aligen Independ	00405-4352-01
100's	$18.95	Dipyridamole, Rugby	00536-3620-01
100's	$19.20	Dipyridamole, United Res	00677-0674-01
100's	$19.20	Dipyridamole, Mutual Pharm	53489-0117-01
100's	$19.23	Dipyridamole, Geneva Pharms	00781-1478-01
100's	$19.25	DIPYRAMIDE, Parmed Pharms	00349-8378-01
100's	$19.88	Dipyridamole, Lederle Pharm	00005-3791-23
100's	$22.98	Dipyridamole, Lederle Pharm	00005-3791-60
100's	$57.25	Dipyridamole, Medirex	57480-0325-01
100's	$61.78	Dipyridamole, Major Pharms	00904-1088-61
100's	$64.00	Dipyridamole, Goldline Labs	00182-1570-89
100's	$67.18	Dipyridamole, Vangard Labs	00615-1574-13
100's	**$72.96**	**PERSANTINE-75, Boehringer Pharms**	**00597-0019-01**
500's	$23.75	Dipyridamole, Major Pharms	00904-1084-40
500's	$29.65	Dipyridamole, H.C.F.A. F F P	99999-1090-09
500's	$56.75	Dipyridamole, Mutual Pharm	53489-0117-05
500's	$59.95	Dipyridamole, Rugby	00536-3620-05
500's	$80.20	Dipyridamole, Barr	00555-0286-04
500's	$82.98	Dipyridamole, Lederle Pharm	00005-3791-31
500's	**$354.78**	**PERSANTINE-75, Boehringer Pharms**	**00597-0019-05**
600's	$203.00	Dipyridamole, Medirex	57480-0325-06
1000's	$59.30	Dipyridamole, HL Moore Drug Exch	00839-6429-16
1000's	$59.30	Dipyridamole, H.C.F.A. F F P	99999-1090-10
1000's	$81.50	Dipyridamole, Major Pharms	00904-1084-80
1000's	$81.50	Dipyridamole, Major Pharms	00904-1088-80
1000's	$88.46	Dipyridamole, Purepac Pharm	00228-2185-96
1000's	$88.46	Dipyridamole, Mova Pharms	55370-0154-09
1000's	$90.44	Dipyridamole, HL Moore Drug Exch	00839-7920-16
1000's	$97.30	Dipyridamole, Qualitest Pharms	00603-3385-32
1000's	$99.65	Dipyridamole, Goldline Labs	00182-1354-10
1000's	$99.65	Dipyridamole, Sidmak Labs	50111-0313-03
1000's	$102.90	Dipyridamole, Geneva Pharms	00781-1243-10
1000's	$104.17	Dipyridamole 75, Goldline Labs	00182-1570-10
1000's	$104.17	Dipyridamole, Barr	00555-0286-05
1000's	$104.28	Dipyridamole, Aligen Independ	00405-4352-03
1000's	$105.00	Dipyridamole, United Res	00677-0674-10
1000's	$105.00	Dipyridamole, Mutual Pharm	53489-0117-10
1000's	$106.00	Dipyridamole, Schein Pharm (US)	00364-2493-02
1000's	$106.00	Dipyridamole, Geneva Pharms	00781-1478-10
1000's	$110.25	Dipyridamole, Rugby	00536-3620-10
1000's	$181.20	Dipyridamole, Parmed Pharms	00349-2354-10
1000's	$181.28	DIPYRAMIDE, Parmed Pharms	00349-8378-10
2500's	$284.00	DIPYRAMIDE, Parmed Pharms	00349-8378-52
5000's	$56.75	Dipyridamole, United Res	00677-0674-05

HOW SUPPLIED - NOT RATED EQUIVALENT:

Injection, Solution - Intravenous - 5 mg/ml

2 ml x 5	**$150.00**	**PERSANTINE I.V., Du Pont Merck**	**00590-0302-21**
10 ml x 5	**$720.00**	**PERSANTINE I.V., E I Dupont De**	**11994-0005-05**

DIRITHROMYCIN *(003229)*

CATEGORIES: Anti-Infectives; Antibiotics; Bronchitis; Erythromycins; Infections; Legionnaire's Disease; Macrolide; Pharyngitis; Pneumonia; FDA Class 1S ("Standard Review"); FDA Approved 1995 Jun

BRAND NAMES: **Dynabac**

DESCRIPTION:

Dynabac (dirithromycin tablets) contain the semi-synthetic macrolide antibiotic dirithromycin for oral administration. It is a pro-drug which is converted non-enzymatically during intestinal absorption into the microbiologically active moiety erythromycylamine.

Chemically, dirithromycin is designated (9*S*)-9-Deoxo-11-deoxy- 9,11-[imino[(1R)-2-(2-methoxyethoxy)-ethylidene]oxy] erythromycin and has the molecular formula $C_{42}H_{78}N_2O_{14}$. Its molecular weight is 835.09.

Chemically, erythromycylamine is designated 9-(*S*)-9-amino-9- deoxoerythromycin and has a molecular formula of $C_{37}H_{70}N_2O_{12}$. Its molecular weight is 743.97.

Dirithromycin is a basic compound. The free base is poorly soluble in water and readily soluble in polar organic solvents. Dirithromycin is hydrolyzed to erythromycylamine in acidic aqueous solutions; hydrolysis is virtually complete within 2 hours.

DESCRIPTION: *(cont'd)*

Dynabac tablets are enteric coated to protect the contents from gastric acid and to permit absorption of the antibiotic in the small intestine. Each enteric-coated tablet contains dirithromycin equivalent to 250 mg and the following inactive ingredients: microcrystalline cellulose, croscarmellose sodium, magnesium carbonate, magnesium stearate, sodium starch glycolate, hydroxypropyl cellulose, hydroxypropyl methylcellulose, polyethylene glycol, propylene glycol, benzyl alcohol, methacrylic acid copolymer, titanium dioxide, triethyl citrate, and talc.

CLINICAL PHARMACOLOGY:

PHARMACOKINETICS

Absorption: Dirithromycin is rapidly absorbed and converted by nonenzymatic hydrolysis to the microbiologically active compound erythromycylamine. The absolute bioavailability of the oral formulation is approximately 10%. The pharmacokinetic parameters of erythromycylamine in plasma after single- and multiple-dose oral administration of two 250-mg dirithromycin tablets once daily for 10 days in 10 fasting healthy subjects (19 to 50 years of age) were as seen in TABLE 1.

TABLE 1

Pharmacokinetic Parameter	Mean (1 S.D.) (n=10 subjects) Day 1		Day 10	
C_{max} (mcg/ml)	0.3	(0.2)	0.4	(0.2)
T_{max} (h)	3.9	(0.9)	4.1	(1.3)
AUC_{0-24}h (mcg·h/ml)	0.9	(0.7)	1.8	(1.1)

Distribution: The protein binding of erythromycylamine ranges from 15% to 30%. Erythromycylamine is widely distributed throughout the body with a mean apparent volume of distribution (V_{Dss}) of 800L (504 to 1041 L).

Rapid distribution of erythromycylamine into tissues and high concentrations within cells results in significantly higher concentrations in tissues than in plasma or serum. There are no data available on cerebrospinal fluid penetration. (TABLE 2)

TABLE 2 Steady-State Tissue Concentrations of Erythromycylamine Following Two 250-mg Tablets (500 mg) of Dirithromycin Given Orally Once Daily

Tissue Ratio	Time After Last Dose (h)	Mean Tissue Concentration (mcg/g or mcg/10^7 cells)	Corresponding Mean Plasma or Serum Concentration	Tissue/Plasma (Serum) (mcg/ml)
Tonsil	14	3.47	0.17	20.4
Healthy lung	12	3.79	0.13	29.2
Pathologic/infected lung	12	3.85	0.13	29.6
Infected bronchial mucosa	12	1.70	0.13	13.1
Alveolar Macrophages	5	0.37	0.35	1.1

High tissue concentrations should not be interpreted to be quantitatively related to clinical efficacy. Erythromycylamine is concentrated in cell lysosomes, which have a low organelle pH at which drug activity is reduced.

Metabolism and Excretion: Erythromycylamine is primarily eliminated in the bile and undergoes little or no hepatic metabolism. Thus, the primary route of elimination is fecal/hepatic with 81% to 97% of the dose eliminated in this manner. Approximately 2% of the administered dose is eliminated through the kidney, mainly within the first 36 hours following drug administration.

The mean plasma half-life of erythromycylamine was estimated to be about 8 h (2 to 36 h), while a mean urinary terminal elimination half-life of about 44 h (16 to 65 h) and a mean apparent total body clearance of approximately 23 l/h (20 to 32 l/h) were observed in patients with normal renal function.

Food Effect on Absorption: Dirithromycin tablets should be administered with food or within an hour of having eaten. The effect of food on the bioavailability of dirithromycin was evaluated following oral administration of two 250-mg dirithromycin tablets 1 or 4 hours before food and immediately after a standard breakfast. Results obtained indicated a slight increase in the absorption of erythromycylamine when dirithromycin tablets were administered after food, while a significant decrease in C_{max} (33%) and AUC (31%) occurred when administered 1 hour before food. The effects of high and low fat meals on the bioavailability of dirithromycin were also investigated. The results showed that the amount of dietary fat had little or no effect on the bioavailability of dirithromycin.

SPECIAL POPULATIONS

Hepatic Insufficiency: In patients with mild (Child's Grade A) hepatic impairment, mean peak serum concentration, AUC, and volume of distribution increased somewhat with multiple-dose administration; however, based on the magnitude of these changes, no dosage adjustment should be necessary in patients with mildly impaired hepatic function. The pharmacokinetics of dirithromycin in patients with moderate or severe impairment in hepatic function (Child's Grade B or greater) have not been studied.

Renal Insufficiency: The mean peak plasma concentration (C_{max}) and AUC tended to increase as creatinine clearance decreased; however, based on data available to date, no dosage adjustment should be necessary in patients with impaired renal function, including dialysis patients.

Geriatric Patients: In a multiple-dose study in which 19 healthy elderly subjects (65 to 83 years of age) were given two 250-mg dirithromycin tablets every day for 10 days, C_{max} and AUC tended to increase with age; however, neither C_{max} nor AUC was statistically or clinically significantly altered with age. Therefore, based on these pharmacokinetic results, no dosage adjustment should be necessary in elderly patients.

MICROBIOLOGY

Erythromycylamine, the microbiologically active product of dirithromycin hydrolysis, exerts its activity by binding to the 50S ribosomal subunits of susceptible microorganisms resulting in inhibition of protein synthesis.

Dirithromycin/Erythromycylamine has been shown to be active against most strains of the following microorganisms both *in vitro* and in clinical infections as described in the INDICATIONS AND USAGE section:

Gram-positive aerobes: *Staphylococcus aureus* (methicillin-susceptible strains only), *Streptococcus pneumoniae, Streptococcus pyogenes*

Gram-negative aerobes: *Legionella pneumophila, Moraxella catarrhalis*

Other bacteria: *Mycoplasma pneumoniae*

The following *in vitro* data are available, **but their clinical significance is unknown**. Dirithromycin exhibits *in vitro* minimum inhibitory concentrations (MIC's) of 2 mcg/ml or less against most (≥90%) strains of the following microorganisms; however, the safety and effectiveness of dirithromycin in treating clinical infections due to these microorganisms have not been established in adequate and well-controlled clinical trials.

Gram-Positive Aerobes: *Listeria monocytogenes,* Streptococci, groups C, F, and G, *Streptococcus agalactiae,* Viridans group streptococci

CLINICAL PHARMACOLOGY: *(cont'd)*

Gram-Negative Aerobes: *Bordetella pertussis*

Anaerobic bacteria: *Propionibacterium acnes*

Note: Microorganisms that are resistant to other macrolides are cross-resistant to dirithromycin/erythromycylamine. Enterococci and most strains of methicillin-resistant staphylococci are resistant to macrolides. In addition, due to the lack of standardized methodology and interpretive criteria, it is impossible at present to determine if strains of *Haemophilus* are susceptible or are resistant to dirithromycin/erythromycylamine.

SUSCEPTIBILITY TESTING

Dilution Techniques: Quantitative methods are used to determine antimicrobial minimum inhibitory concentrations (MIC's). These MIC's provide estimates of the susceptibility of bacteria to antimicrobial compounds. The MIC's should be determined using a standardized procedure. Standardized procedures are based on a dilution method[1,2] (broth, agar, or microdilution) or equivalent with standardized inoculum concentrations and standardized concentrations of dirithromycin powder. The MIC values should be interpreted according to the criteria found in TABLE 3.

TABLE 3

MIC (mcg/ml)	Interpretation
≤2	Susceptible (S)
4	Intermediate (I)
≥8	Resistant (R)

A report of "Susceptible" indicates that the pathogen is likely to be inhibited if the antimicrobial compound in blood reaches the concentrations usually achievable. A report of "Intermediate" indicates that the result should be considered equivocal, and, if the microorganism is not fully susceptible to alternative, clinically feasible drugs, the test should be repeated. This category implies possible clinical applicability in body sites where the drug is physiologically concentrated or in situations where high dosage of drug can be used. This category also provides a buffer zone which prevents small uncontrolled technical factors from causing major discrepancies in interpretation. A report of "Resistant" indicates that the pathogen is not likely to be inhibited if the antimicrobial compound in the blood reaches the concentrations usually achievable; other therapy should be selected.

Standardized susceptibility test procedures require the use of laboratory control microorganisms to control the technical aspects of the laboratory procedures. Standard dirithromycin powder should provide the following MIC values: (TABLE 4)

TABLE 4

Microorganism	MIC (mcg/ml)
S. aureus ATCC 29213	1.0 to 4.0

Diffusion Techniques: Quantitative methods that require measurement of zone diameters also provide reproducible estimates of the susceptibility of bacteria to antimicrobial compounds. One such standardized procedure[3] requires the use of standardized inoculum concentrations. This procedure uses paper disks impregnated with 15-mcg dirithromycin to test the susceptibility of microorganisms to dirithromycin.

Reports from the laboratory providing results of the standard single-disk susceptibility test with a 15-mcg dirithromycin disk should be interpreted according to the criteria found in TABLE 5.

TABLE 5

Zone Diameter (mm)	Interpretation
≥19	Susceptible (S)
16 to 18	Intermediate (I)
≤15	Resistant (R)

Interpretation should be as stated above for results using dilution techniques. Interpretation involves correlation of the diameter obtained in the disk test with the MIC for dirithromycin.

As with standardized dilution techniques, diffusion methods require the use of laboratory control microorganisms that are used to control the technical aspects of the laboratory procedures. For the diffusion technique, the 15-mcg dirithromycin disk should provide the following zone diameters in this laboratory test quality control stain: (TABLE 6)

TABLE 6

Microorganism	Zone Diameter (mm)
S. aureus ATCC 25923	18 to 26

INDICATIONS AND USAGE:

Dirithromycin is indicated for the treatment of individuals age 12 years and older with mild-to-moderate infections caused by susceptible strains of the designated microorganisms in the specific conditions listed below. **Dirithromycin should not be used in patients with known, suspected, or potential bacteremias as serum levels are inadequate to provide antibacterial coverage of the blood stream.**

Acute Bacterial Exacerbations of Chronic Bronchitis: due to *Moraxella catarrhalis* or *Streptococcus pneumoniae.*

Note: Because the safety and efficacy of dirithromycin in the treatment of respiratory disease secondary to *H. influenzae* have not been demonstrated, dirithromycin is NOT indicated for the empiric treatment of acute bacterial exacerbations of chronic or secondary bacterial infection of acute bronchitis. Infections known, suspected, or considered potentially to be caused by *Haemophilus* species should be treated by an antibacterial agent indicated for such treatment.

Secondary Bacterial Infection of Acute Bronchitis: due to *Moraxella catarrhalis* or *Streptococcus pneumoniae.* (See INDICATIONS AND USAGE, Note.)

Community-Acquired Pneumonia: due to *Legionella pneumophila, Mycoplasma pneumoniae,* or *Streptococcus pneumoniae.*

Pharyngitis/Tonsillitis: due to *Streptococcus pyogenes.*

Note: The usual drug of choice in the treatment and prevention of streptococcal infections and the prophylaxis of rheumatic fever is penicillin. Dirithromycin generally is effective in the eradication of *S. pyogenes* from the nasopharynx; however, data establishing the efficacy of dirithromycin in the subsequent prevention of rheumatic fever are not available at present.

Uncomplicated Skin and Skin Structure Infections: due to *Staphylococcus aureus* (methicillin-susceptible strains). (Abscesses usually require surgical drainage.)

INDICATIONS AND USAGE: *(cont'd)*

Note: Because the safety and efficacy of dirithromycin in the treatment of uncomplicated skin and skin structure infections due to *S. pyogenes* have not been demonstrated, dirithromycin is NOT indicated for the empiric treatment of uncomplicated skin and skin structure infections. Infections known, suspected, or potentially caused by *S. pyogenes* should be treated with an antibacterial agent indicated for such treatment.

CONTRAINDICATIONS:

Dirithromycin is contraindicated in patients with known hypersensitivity to dirithromycin, erythromycin, or any other macrolide antibiotic.

WARNINGS:

In a prospective study involving 6 healthy male volunteers, dirithromycin did not affect the metabolism of terfenadine. These six volunteers received terfenadine alone (60 mg twice daily) for 8 days, followed by terfenadine in combination with dirithromycin (500 mg once daily) for 10 days. (Both drugs were thus dosed to steady state.) The pharmacokinetics of terfenadine and its acid metabolite and the electrocardiographic QT_c interval were measured during both periods: with terfenadine alone, and with terfenadine plus dirithromycin. In five men, terfenadine levels were undetectable (<5 ng/ml) throughout the study; in one man, the $C_{max}$of terfenadine was 8.1 ng/ml with terfenadine alone and 7.2 ng/ml with terfenadine plus dirithromycin. The mean C_{max}, $T_{max}$and AUC of the acid metabolite of terfenadine were not significantly changed. The mean QT_cinterval (msec) was 369 with terfenadine alone and 367 with terfenadine plus dirithromycin.

Serious cardiac dysrhythmias, some resulting in death, have occurred in patients receiving terfenadine concomitantly with other macrolide antibiotics. In addition, most macrolides are contraindicated in patients receiving terfenadine therapy who have pre-existing cardiac abnormalities (arrhythmia, bradycardia, QT_c interval prolongation, ischemic heart disease, congestive heart failure, etc.) or electrolyte disturbances. Until further use data are available, it is prudent to monitor the terfenadine levels when dirithromycin and terfenadine are coadministered.

Dirithromycin should not be used in patients with known, suspected, or potential bacteremias as serum levels are inadequate to provide antibacterial coverage of the blood stream.

Pseudomembranous colitis has been reported with nearly all antibacterial agents, including dirithromycin, and may range in severity from mild to life-threatening. Therefore, it is important to consider this diagnosis in patients who present with diarrhea subsequent to the administration of antibacterial agents.

Treatment with antibacterial agents alters the normal flora of the colon and may permit overgrowth of clostridia. Studies indicate that a toxin produced by *Clostridium difficile* is a primary cause of "antibiotic-associated colitis."

After the diagnosis of pseudomembranous colitis has been established, therapeutic measures should be initiated. Mild cases of pseudomembranous colitis usually respond to discontinuation of the drug alone. In moderate-to-severe cases, consideration should be given to management with fluids and electrolytes, protein supplementation, and treatment with an antibacterial drug clinically effective against *C. difficile* colitis.

PRECAUTIONS:

Hepatic Insufficiency: Because dirithromycin/erythromycylamine is principally eliminated via the liver and because no data exist regarding the safety of administering dirithromycin to patients with Child's Grade B or greater hepatic impairment, dirithromycin should be administered to such patients only when absolutely necessary. No dosage adjustment should be necessary in patients with mildly impaired hepatic function. (See CLINICAL PHARMACOLOGY.)

Information for the Patient: Dirithromycin tablets should be taken with food or within one hour of having eaten. They should not be cut, chewed, or crushed.

Carcinogenesis, Mutagenesis, and Impairment of Fertility: Lifetime studies in animals to evaluate carcinogenic potential have not been performed with dirithromycin.

No mutagenic potential was demonstrated when dirithromycin was used in standard tests of genotoxicity, which included the following bacterial mutation tests *in vitro* and *in vivo* mammalian systems:

Bacterial Reverse-Mutation Test (Ames test); DNA repair (UDS) in rat hepatocytes; Chinese hamster lung fibroblast (V79) test; Micronucleus test in mice; Sister-chromatid exchange —human lymphocytes; Sister-chromatid exchange—Chinese hamsters; Mouse Lymphoma Assay

In rats, fertility and reproductive performance were not affected when dirithromycin was administered at doses up to 21 times the maximum recommended human dose on a mg/m^2 basis.

Pregnancy, Teratogenic Effects, Pregnancy Category C: Teratology studies conducted in rats at doses up to 21 times the maximum recommended human dose on a mg/m^2 basis and in rabbits at doses up to 4 times the maximum recommended human dose on a mg/m^2 basis have revealed no evidence of impaired fertility or harm to the fetus due to dirithromycin administration. An additional teratology study in CD-1 mice demonstrated that fetal weight was significantly depressed at the 1000 mg/kg dose (8 times the maximum recommended human dose on a mg/m^2 basis), and there was an increased occurrence of incomplete ossification among these fetuses—a manifestation of retarded development. This decrease in ossification was also seen in rats given 1000 mg/kg/day for 2 weeks prior to mating, throughout the mating period, and throughout gestation.

There are no adequate and well-controlled studies in pregnant women. Dirithromycin should be used during pregnancy only if the potential benefit justifies the potential risk to the fetus.

Labor and Delivery: Dirithromycin has not been studied for use during labor and delivery. Treatment with dirithromycin should be given during labor and delivery only if clearly needed.

Nursing Mothers: It is not known whether either dirithromycin or erythromycylamine is excreted in human milk. It is known that dirithromycin is excreted in the milk of lactating rodents and that other drugs of this class are excreted in human milk. Because many drugs are excreted in human milk, caution should be exercised when dirithromycin is administered to a nursing woman.

Pediatric Use: Safety and effectiveness in infants and children less than 12 years of age have not been established.

Geriatric Use: In a clinical pharmacology study, 19 healthy geriatric volunteers (65 to 83 years of age) with normal renal and hepatic function had no statistically significant differences in AUC or C_{max} when compared with 10 healthy adult volunteers (19 to 50 years of age). In clinical trials in geriatric patients who received the usual recommended adult dose (500 mg q.d. P.O.), clinical efficacy and safety were comparable with results in non-geriatric adult patients.

DRUG INTERACTIONS:

Terfenadine: See WARNINGS.

Theophylline: Following co-administration of two 250-mg dirithromycin tablets administered once daily with 200-mg theophylline tablets administered twice daily for 10 days to 14 healthy subjects, the steady-state plasma concentration of theophylline was not significantly altered. In general, most patients treated with dirithromycin who are receiving concomitant theophylline therapy *may*not require empiric adjustment of theophylline dosage or monitoring of theophylline plasma concentrations. However, theophylline plasma concentrations should be monitored, with dosage adjustment as appropriate, in patients whose pulmonary disease requires maintaining a given theophylline plasma concentration for optimal pulmonary function or in patients with theophylline concentrations at the higher end of the therapeutic range.

Antacids or H_2 receptor antagonists: When dirithromycin is administered immediately following antacids or H_2-receptor antagonists, the absorption of dirithromycin is slightly enhanced.

The following drug interactions have been reported with erythromycin products. It is presently not known whether these same drug interactions occur with dirithromycin. **Until further data are available regarding the potential interaction of dirithromycin with these compounds, caution should be used during coadministration.**

Triazolam: Erythromycin has been reported to decrease the clearance of triazolam and, thus, may increase the pharmacologic effect of triazolam.

Digoxin: Concomitant administration of erythromycin and digoxin has been reported to result in elevated digoxin serum levels.

Anticoagulants: There have been reports of increased anticoagulant effects when erythromycin and oral anticoagulants were used concomitantly. Increased anticoagulation effects due to a drug interaction with erythromycin may be more pronounced in the elderly.

Ergotamine: Concurrent use of erythromycin and ergotamine or dihydroergotamine has been associated in some patients with acute ergot toxicity characterized by severe peripheral vasospasm and dysesthesia.

Other drugs: Drug interactions have been reported with concomitant administration of erythromycin and other medications, including cyclosporine, hexobarbital, carbamazepine, alfentanil, disopyramide, phenytoin, bromocriptine, valproate, astemizole, and lovastatin.

ADVERSE REACTIONS:

In clinical trials, 3299 patients were treated with dirithromycin 500 mg q.d. P.O. for approximately 7 to 14 days. There were no deaths or permanent disabilities thought related directly to drug toxicity. Eighty-seven (2.6%) patients discontinued medication due to adverse reactions. Thirty-five (40%) of the 87 patients who discontinued therapy did so because of nausea or abdominal pain.

The following adverse clinical and laboratory reactions were reported during the dirithromycin clinical trials conducted in North America (n=1894 patients). (See TABLE 7 and TABLE 8).

TABLE 7 Adverse Clinical Reactions (Incidence equal to or greater than 1%) Clinical Trials - North America

Adverse Reactions	Dirithromycin	Erythromycin
Abdominal pain	9.7%	7.5%
Headache	8.6%	8.2%
Nausea	8.3%	7.5%
Diarrhea	7.7%	7.3%
Vomiting	3.0%	2.8%
Dyspepsia	2.6%	2.1%
Dizziness/vertigo	2.3%	2.3%
Pain (non-specific)	2.2%	1.6%
Asthenia	2.0%	1.9%
Gastrointestinal disorder	1.6%	1.4%
Increased Cough	1.5%	2.6%
Flatulence	1.5%	1.5%
Rash	1.4%	2.6%
Dyspnea	1.2%	1.2%
Pruritus/Urticaria	1.2%	1.0%
Insomnia	1.0%	0.7%

Adverse reactions occurring during the clinical trials with dirithromycin with an incidence of less than 1% but greater than 0.1% included the following (listed alphabetically):

Abnormal stools, allergic reaction (not further defined), amblyopia, anorexia, anxiety, constipation, dehydration, depression, dry mouth, dysmenorrhea, edema, epistaxis, eye disorder (not further defined), fever, flu syndrome, gastritis, gastroenteritis, hemoptysis, hyperventilation, malaise, mouth ulceration, myalgia, neck pain, nervousness, palpitation, paraesthesia, peripheral edema, somnolence, sweating, syncope, taste perversion, thirst, tinnitus, tremor, urinary frequency, vaginal moniliasis, vaginitis, vasodilatation.

TABLE 8 Adverse Laboratory Reactions (Incidence equal to or greater than 1%) Clinical Trials - North America

Adverse Reactions	Dirithromycin	Erythromycin
Platelet count*increased*	3.8%	4.8%
Potassium*increased*	2.6%	0.0%
Bicarbonate*decreased*	1.4%	2.0%
CPK*increased*	1.2%	0.9%
Eosinophils*increased*	1.2%	0.6%
Seg Neutrophils*increased*	1.2%	1.3%

Adverse laboratory reactions occurring during the clinical trials with dirithromycin with an incidence of less than 1% but greater than 0.1% included the following (listed alphabetically):

Decreased: Albumin, chloride, hematocrit, hemoglobin, seg neutrophils, phosphorus, platelet count, and total protein.

Increased: Alkaline phosphatase, ALT, AST, bands, basophils, total bilirubin, creatinine, GGT, leukocyte count, lymphocytes, monocytes, phosphorous, and uric acid.

Macrolide-Class Adverse Reactions: Although not observed in patients treated with dirithromycin in clinical trials, the following adverse reactions and altered laboratory test results have been reported in patients treated with macrolide antibiotics: Bullous fixed eruptions or serious allergic reactions, including anaphylaxis, have been reported. A few cases of transient deafness have been reported with high doses of oral erythromycin. Rarely, cholestatic hepatitis has been reported. In individuals with prolonged QT intervals, erythromycin has been associated, rarely, with the production of ventricular arrhythmias, including ventricular tachycardia and torsade de pointes.

OVERDOSAGE:

The toxic symptoms following an overdose of a macrolide antibiotic may include nausea, vomiting, epigastric distress, and diarrhea. Forced diuresis, peritoneal dialysis, hemodialysis, or hemoperfusion have not been established as beneficial for an overdose of dirithromycin. Hemodialysis has been shown to be ineffective in hastening the elimination of erythromycylamine from plasma in patients with chronic renal failure.

DOSAGE AND ADMINISTRATION:

Dirithromycin should be administered with food or within 1 hour of having eaten. (See CLINICAL PHARMACOLOGY, Food Effect on Absorption.) **Dirithromycin tablets should not be cut, crushed, or chewed.**

TABLE 9 Recommended Dosage Schedule for Dirithromycin (12 years of age and older)

Infection (Mild to Moderate Severity)	Dose	Frequency	Duration (days)
Acute Bacterial Exacerbations of Chronic Bronchitis due to*Moraxella catarrhalis* or *Streptococcus pneumoniae*	500 mg	q day	7
NOT FOR EMPIRIC THERAPY(See INDICATIONS AND USAGE)			
Secondary Bacterial Infection of Acute Bronchitis due to*M. catarrhalis* or *S. pneumoniae*	500 mg	q day	7
NOT FOR EMPIRIC THERAPY(See INDICATIONS AND USAGE)			
Community-Acquired Pneumonia due to*Legionella pneumophila, Mycoplasma* pneumoniae, or *S. pneumoniae*	500 mg	q day	14
Pharyngitis/Tonsillitis due to*Streptococcus pyogenes*	500 mg	q day	10
Uncomplicated Skin and Skin Structure Infections due to*Staphylococcus aureus* (methicillinsusceptible)	500 mg	q day	7
NOT FOR EMPIRIC THERAPY(See INDICATIONS AND USAGE)			

ANIMAL PHARMACOLOGY:

Toxicology: Cardiac and skeletal muscle lesions occurred in rats in studies up to three months by the intravenous route and in six-month studies in the rat and the dog by the oral route. While no target organ toxicity was identified in three-month oral studies, both cardiac and skeletal muscles were identified as target tissues after one-month intravenous studies in rats. Histologic changes from oral dosing occurred only after more than four months of treatment in rats and after six months in dogs. These findings were associated with high tissue-to-plasma concentration ratios of antimicrobial activity. The extensive drug uptake by tissues was reversible upon termination of treatment. Lesions in cardiac and skeletal muscle also were reversed upon termination of treatment. Dirithromycin and/or its microbiologically active metabolite appeared to accumulate in tissues with time. Despite the drug uptake in rat tissues at high multiples (approximately 14 times the anticipated clinical dose in mg/m^2), there were no lesions in this species until oral treatment was extended beyond four months.

REFERENCES:

1. National Committee for Clinical Laboratory Standards. Methods for Dilution Antimicrobial Susceptibility Tests for Bacteria that Grow Aerobically—Third Edition; Approved Standard NCCLS Document M7-A3, Vol. 13, No. 25, NCCLS, Villanova, PA, December 1993 **2.** National Committee for Clinical Laboratory Standards. Methods for Antimicrobial Susceptibility Testing of Anaerobic Bacteria—Third Edition; Approved Standard NCCLS Document M11-A3, Vol. 13, No. 26, NCCLS, Villanova, PA, December 1993 **3.** National Committee for Clinical Laboratory Standards. Performance Standards for Antimicrobial Disk Susceptibility Tests—Fifth Edition; Approved Standard NCCLS Document M2-A5, Vol. 13, No. 24, NCCLS, Villanova, PA, December 1993

HOW SUPPLIED:

Dynabac Tablets: enteric-coated, elliptical-shaped, white, 250 mg.

Store at controlled room temperature, 15° to 30°C (59° to 86°F).

HOW SUPPLIED - EQUIVALENTS NOT AVAILABLE:

Tablet, Enteric Coated - Oral - 250 mg

60's $112.50 DYNABAC, Bock Pharma 00563-0490-60

DISOPYRAMIDE PHOSPHATE *(001093)*

CATEGORIES: Antianginals; Antiarrhythmic Agents; Arrhythmia; Cardiovascular Drugs; Renal Drugs; Tachycardia; Pregnancy Category C; FDA Approval Pre 1982

BRAND NAMES: *Dicorantyl*; *Dimodan* (Mexico); *Dimodan Retard*; *Dirythmin SA* (England); *Dirytmin*; *Dirytmin Depottab*; *Diso Durules*; *Disofarin* (Mexico); *Disonorm* (Germany); *Durbis*; *Durbis Retard*; *Isorythm* (France); *Lispine* (Japan); **Norpace**; Norpace CR; *Norpace Retard*; *Norpaso*; *Pyramide*; *Regubeat*; *Rhythmodan*; *Ritmodan*; *Ritmoforine*; *Rythmical*; *Rythmodan* (Australia, England, France, Canada, Japan); *Rythmodan Retard*; *Rythmodan LA* (Canada); *Rythmodul* (Germany); *Rytmilen*
(International brand names outside U.S. in italics)

FORMULARIES: Aetna; BC-BS; FHP

COST OF THERAPY: $174.17 (Arrhythmia; Capsule; 150 mg; 4/day; 365 days)

DESCRIPTION:

Disopyramide phosphate is an antiarrhythmic drug available for oral administration in immediate-release and controlled-release capsules containing 100 mg or 150 mg of disopyramide base, present as the phosphate. The base content of the phosphate salt is 77.6%.

Disopyramide phosphate is freely soluble in water, and the free base (pKa 10.4) has an aqueous solubility of 1 mg/ml. The chloroform:water partition coefficient of the base is 3.1 at pH 7.2.

Disopyramide phosphate is a racemic mixture of *d*- and *l*-isomers. This drug is not chemically related to other antiarrhythmic drugs.

Disopyramide phosphate controlled-release capsules are designed to afford a gradual and consistent release of disopyramide. Thus, for maintenance therapy, disopyramide phosphate controlled-release provides the benefit of less-frequent dosing (every 12 hours) as compared with the every-6-hour dosage schedule of immediate-release disopyramide phosphate capsules.

Inactive ingredients of Norpace include corn starch, edible ink, FD&C Red No. 3, FD&C Yellow No. 6, gelatin, lactose, talc, and titanium dioxide; the 150 mg capsule also contains FD&C Blue No. 1.

Inactive ingredients of Norpace CR include corn starch, D&C Yellow No. 10, edible ink, ethylcellulose, FD&C Blue No. 1, gelatin, shellac, sucrose, talc, and titanium dioxide, the 150 mg capsule also contains FD&C Red No. 3 and FD&C Yellow No. 6.

CLINICAL PHARMACOLOGY:

MECHANISMS OF ACTION

Disopyramide phosphate is a Type 1 antiarrhythmic drug (*i.e.,* similar to procainamide and quinidine). *In animal studies* disopyramide phosphate decreases the rate of diastolic depolarization (phase 4) in cells with augmented automaticity, decreases the upstroke velocity (phase 0) and increases the action potential duration of normal cardiac cells, decreases the disparity in refractoriness between infarcted and adjacent normally perfused myocardium, and has no effect on alpha- or beta-adrenergic receptors.

ELECTROPHYSIOLOGY

In man, disopyramide phosphate at therapeutic plasma levels shortens the sinus node recovery time, lengthens the effective refractory period of the atrium, and has a minimal effect on the effective refractory period of the AV node. Little effect has been shown on AV-nodal and His-Purkinje conduction times or QRS duration. However, prolongation of conduction in accessory pathways occurs.

HEMODYNAMICS

At recommended oral doses, disopyramide phosphate rarely produces significant alterations of blood pressure in patients without congestive heart failure (see WARNINGS.) With intravenous disopyramide phosphate, either increases in systolic/diastolic or decreases in systolic blood pressure have been reported, depending on the infusion rate and the patient population. Intravenous disopyramide phosphate may cause cardiac depression with an approximate mean 10% reduction of cardiac output, which is more pronounced in patients with cardiac dysfunction.

ANTICHOLINERGIC ACTIVITY

The *in vitro* anticholinergic activity of disopyramide phosphate is approximately 0.06% that of atropine; however, the usual dose for disopyramide phosphate is 150 mg every 6 hours and for disopyramide phosphate controlled-release 300 mg every 12 hours, compared to 0.4 to 0.6 mg for atropine (see WARNINGSand ADVERSE REACTIONS for anticholinergic side effects.)

PHARMACOKINETICS

Following oral administration of immediate-release disopyramide phosphate, disopyramide phosphate is rapidly and almost completely absorbed, and peak plasma levels are usually attained within 2 hours. The usual therapeutic plasma levels of disopyramide base are 2 to 4 mcg/ml, and at these concentrations protein binding varies from 50% to 65%. Because of concentration-dependent protein binding, it is difficult to predict the concentration of the free drug when total drug is measured.

The mean plasma half-life of disopyramide in healthy humans is 6.7 hours (range of 4 to 10 hours). In six patients with impaired renal function (creatinine clearance less than 40 ml/min), disopyramide half-life values were 8 to 18 hours.

After the oral administration of 200 mg of disopyramide to 10 cardiac patients with borderline to moderate heart failure, the time to peak serum concentration of 2.3 ± 1.5 hours (mean ± SD) was increased, and the mean peak serum concentration of 4.8 ± 1.6 mcg/ml was higher than in healthy volunteers. After intravenous administration in these same patients, the mean elimination half-life was 9.7 ± 4.2 hours range in healthy volunteers of 4.4 to 7.8 hours). In a second study of the oral administration of disopyramide to 7 patients with heart disease, including left ventricular dysfunction, the mean plasma half-life was slightly prolonged to 7.8 ± 1.9 hours (range of 5 to 9.5 hours).

In healthy men, about 50% of a given dose of disopyramide is excreted in the urine as the unchanged drug, about 20% as the mono-N-dealkylated metabolite, and 10% as the other metabolites. The plasma concentration of the major metabolite is approximately one tenth that of disopyramide. Altering the urinary pH in man does not affect the plasma half-life of disopyramide.

In a crossover study in healthy subjects, the bioavailability of disopyramide from disopyramide phosphate controlled-release capsules was similar to that from the immediate-release capsules. With a single 300 mg oral dose, peak disopyramide plasma concentrations of 3.23 ± 0.75 mcg/ml (mean ± SD) at 2.5 ± 2.3 hours were obtained with two 150 mg immediate-release capsules and 2.22 ± 0.47 mcg/ml at 4.9 ± 1.4 hours with two 150 mg disopyramide phosphate controlled-release capsules. The elimination half-life of disopyramide was 8.31 ± 1.83 hours with the immediate-release capsules and 11.65 ± 4.72 hours with disopyramide phosphate controlled-release capsules. The amount of disopyramide and mono-N-dealkylated metabolite excreted in the urine in 48 hours was 128 and 48 mg, respectively, with the immediate-release capsules, and 112 and 33 mg, respectively, with disopyramide phosphate controlled-release capsules. The differences in the urinary excretion of either constituent were not statistically significant.

Following multiple doses, steady-state plasma levels of between 2 and 4 mcg/ml were attained following either 150 mg every-6-hour dosing with immediate-release capsules or 300 mg every-12-hour dosing with disopyramide phosphate controlled-release capsules.

INDICATIONS AND USAGE:

Disopyramide phosphate and disopyramide phosphate controlled-release are indicated for the treatment of documented ventricular arrhythmias, such as sustained ventricular tachycardia, that, in the judgment of the physician, are life-threatening. Because of the proarrhythmic effects of disopyramide phosphate and disopyramide phosphate controlled-release, their use with lesser arrhythmias is generally not recommended. Treatment of patients with asymptomatic ventricular premature contractions should be avoided.

Initiation of disopyramide phosphate or disopyramide phosphate controlled-release treatment, as with other antiarrhythmic agents used to treat life-threatening arrhythmias, should be carried out in the hospital. Disopyramide phosphate controlled-release should not be used initially if rapid establishment of disopyramide plasma levels is desired.

Antiarrhythmic drugs have not been shown to enhance survival in patients with ventricular arrhythmias.

CONTRAINDICATIONS:

Disopyramide phosphate and disopyramide phosphate controlled-release are contraindicated in the presence of cardiogenic shock, preexisting second- or third-degree AV block (if no pacemaker is present), congenital Q-T prolongation, or known hypersensitivity to the drug.

WARNINGS:

MORTALITY

In the National Heart, Lung and Blood Institute's Cardiac Arrhythmia Suppression Trial (CAST), a long-term, multi-centered, randomized, double-blind study in patients with asymptomatic non-life-threatening ventricular arrhythmias who had had myocardial infarctions more than 6 days but less than 2 years previously, an excessive mortality or non-fatal cardiac arrest rate was seen in patients treated with encainide or flecainide (56/730) compared with that seen in patients assigned to matched placebo-treated groups (22/725). The average duration of treatment with encainide or flecainide in this study was 10 months.

The applicability of these results to other populations (*e.g.,* those without recent myocardial infarctions) or to other antiarrhythmic drugs is uncertain, but at present it is prudent to consider any antiarrhythmic agent to have a significant risk in patients with structural heart disease.

NEGATIVE INOTROPIC PROPERTIES

WARNINGS: *(cont'd)*

Heart Failure/Hypotension

Disopyramide phosphate or disopyramide phosphate controlled-release may cause or worsen congestive heart failure or produce severe hypotension as a consequence of its negative inotropic properties. Hypotension has been observed primarily in patients with primary cardiomyopathy or inadequately compensated congestive heart failure. Disopyramide phosphate or disopyramide phosphate controlled-release should not be used in patients with uncompensated or marginally compensated congestive heart failure or hypotension unless the congestive heart failure or hypotension is secondary to cardiac arrhythmia. Patients with a history of heart failure may be treated with disopyramide phosphate or disopyramide phosphate controlled-release, but careful attention must be given to the maintenance of cardiac function, including optimal digitalization. If hypotension occurs or congestive heart failure worsens, disopyramide phosphate or disopyramide phosphate controlled-release should be discontinued and, if necessary, restarted at a lower dosage only after adequate cardiac compensation has been established.

QRS Widening

Although it is unusual, significant widening (greater than 25%) of the QRS complex may occur during disopyramide phosphate or disopyramide phosphate controlled-release administration; in such cases disopyramide phosphate or disopyramide phosphate controlled-release should be discontinued.

Q-T Prolongation

As with other Type 1 antiarrhythmic drugs, prolongation of the Q-T interval (corrected) and worsening of the arrhythmia, including ventricular tachycardia and ventricular fibrillation, may occur. Patients who have evidenced prolongation of the Q-T interval in response to quinidine may be at particular risk. As with other Type 1A antiarrhythmics, disopyramide phosphate has been associated with torsade de pointes.

If a Q-T prolongation of greater than 25% is observed and if ectopy continues, the patient should be monitored closely, and consideration be given to discontinuing disopyramide phosphate or disopyramide phosphate controlled-release.

Hypoglycemia

In rare instances significant lowering of blood glucose values has been reported during disopyramide phosphate administration. The physician should be alert to this possibility, especially in patients with congestive heart failure, chronic malnutrition, hepatic, renal or other diseases, or drugs (*e.g.,* beta adrenoceptor blockers, alcohol) which could compromise preservation of the normal glucoregulatory mechanisms in the absence of food. In these patients the blood glucose levels should be carefully followed.

Concomitant Antiarrhythmic Therapy

The concomitant use of disopyramide phosphate or disopyramide phosphate controlled-release with other Type 1 antiarrhythmic agents (such as quinidine or procainamide) and/or propranolol should be reserved for patients with life-threatening arrhythmias who are demonstratably unresponsive to single-agent antiarrhythmic therapy. Such use may produce serious negative inotropic effects, or may excessively prolong conduction. This should be considered particularly in patients with any degree of cardiac decompensation or those with a prior history thereof. Patients receiving more than one antiarrhythmic drug must be carefully monitored.

Heart Block

If first-degree heart block develops in a patient receiving disopyramide phosphate or disopyramide phosphate controlled-release, the dosage should be reduced. If the block persists despite reduction of dosage, continuation of the drug must depend upon weighing the benefit being obtained against the risk of higher degrees of heart block. Development of second- or third-degree AV block or unifascicular, bifascicular, or trifascicular block requires discontinuation of disopyramide phosphate or disopyramide phosphate controlled-release therapy, unless the ventricular rate is adequately controlled by a temporary or implanted ventricular pacemaker.

Anticholinergic Activity

Because of its anticholinergic activity, disopyramide phosphate should not be used in patients with glaucoma, myasthenia gravis, or urinary retention unless adequate overriding measures are taken; these consist of the topical application of potent miotics (*e.g.,* pilocarpine) for patients with glaucoma, and catheter drainage or operative relief for patients with urinary retention. Urinary retention may occur in patients of either sex as a consequence of disopyramide phosphate or disopyramide phosphate controlled-release administration, but males with benign prostatic hypertrophy are at particular risk. In patients with a family history of glaucoma, intraocular pressure should be measured before initiating disopyramide phosphate or disopyramide phosphate controlled-release therapy. Disopyramide phosphate should be used with special care in patients with myasthenia gravis since its anticholinergic properties could precipitate a myasthenic crisis in such patients.

PRECAUTIONS:

GENERAL

Atrial Tachyarrhythmias

Patients with atrial flutter or fibrillation should be digitalized prior to disopyramide phosphate or disopyramide phosphate controlled-release administration to ensure that drug-induced enhancement of AV conduction does not result in an increase of ventricular rate beyond physiologically acceptable limits.

Conduction Abnormalities

Care should be taken when prescribing disopyramide phosphate or disopyramide phosphate controlled-release for patients with sick sinus syndrome (bradycardia-tachycardia syndrome), Wolff-Parkinson-White syndrome (WPW), or bundle branch block. The effect of disopyramide phosphate in these conditions is uncertain at present.

Cardiomyopathy

Patients with myocarditis or other cardiomyopathy may develop significant hypotension in response to the usual dosage of disopyramide phosphate, probably due to cardiodepressant mechanisms. Therefore, a loading dose of disopyramide phosphate should not be given to such patients, and initial dosage and subsequent dosage adjustments should be made under close supervision (see DOSAGE AND ADMINISTRATION.)

Renal Impairment

More than 50% of disopyramide is excreted in the urine unchanged. Therefore disopyramide phosphate dosage should be reduced in patients with impaired renal function (see DOSAGE AND ADMINISTRATION.) The electrocardiogram should be carefully monitored for prolongation of PR interval, evidence of QRS widening, or other signs of overdosage (see OVERDOSAGE.)

Disopyramide phosphate controlled-release is not recommended for patients with severe renal insufficiency (creatinine clearance 40 ml/min or less).

Hepatic Impairment

Hepatic impairment also causes an increase in the plasma half-life of disopyramide. Dosage should be reduced for patients with such impairment. The electrocardiogram should be carefully monitored for signs of overdosage (see OVERDOSAGE.)

Patients with cardiac dysfunction have a higher potential for hepatic impairment; this should be considered when administering disopyramide phosphate or disopyramide phosphate controlled-release.

PRECAUTIONS: *(cont'd)*

Potassium Imbalance

Antiarrhythmic drugs may be ineffective in patients with hypokalemia, and their toxic effects may be enhanced in patients with hyperkalemia. Therefore, potassium abnormalities should be corrected before starting disopyramide phosphate or disopyramide phosphate controlled-release therapy.

CARCINOGENESIS, MUTAGENESIS, AND IMPAIRMENT OF FERTILITY

Eighteen months of disopyramide phosphate administration to rats, at oral doses up to 400 mg/kg/day (about 30 times the usual daily human dose of 600 mg/day, assuming a patient weight of at least 50 kg), revealed no evidence of carcinogenic potential. An evaluation of mutagenic potential by Ames test was negative. Disopyramide phosphate, at doses up to 250 mg/kg/day, did not adversely affect fertility of rats.

PREGNANCY, TERATOGENIC EFFECTS, PREGNANCY CATEGORY C

Disopyramide phosphate was associated with decreased numbers of implantation sites and decreased growth and survival of pups when administered to pregnant rats at 250 mg/kg/day (20 or more times the usual daily human dose of 12 mg/kg, assuming a patient weight of at least 50 kg), a level at which weight gain and food consumption of dams were also reduced. Increased resorption rates were reported in rabbits at 60 mg/kg/day (5 or more times the usual daily human dose). Effects on implantation, pup growth, and survival were not evaluated in rabbits. There are no adequate and well-controlled studies in pregnant women. Disopyramide phosphate or disopyramide phosphate controlled-release should be used during pregnancy only if the potential benefit justifies the potential risk to the fetus.

Nonteratogenic Effects: Disopyramide phosphate has been reported to stimulate contractions of the pregnant uterus. Disopyramide has been found in human fetal blood.

LABOR AND DELIVERY

It is not known whether the use of disopyramide phosphate or disopyramide phosphate controlled-release during labor or delivery has immediate or delayed adverse effects on the fetus, or whether it prolongs the duration of labor or increases the need for forceps delivery or other obstetric intervention.

NURSING MOTHERS

Studies in rats have shown that the concentration of disopyramide and its metabolites is between one and three times greater in milk than it is in plasma. Following oral administration, disopyramide has been detected in human milk at a concentration not exceeding that in plasma. Because of the potential for serious adverse reactions in nursing infants from disopyramide phosphate or disopyramide phosphate controlled-release, a decision should be made whether to discontinue nursing or to discontinue the drug, taking into account the importance of the drug to the mother.

DRUG INTERACTIONS:

If phenytoin or other hepatic enzyme inducers are taken concurrently with disopyramide phosphate or disopyramide phosphate controlled-release, lower plasma levels of disopyramide may occur. Monitoring of disopyramide plasma levels is recommended in such concurrent use to avoid ineffective therapy. Other antiarrhythmic drugs (*e.g.,* quinidine, procainamide, lidocaine, propranolol) have occasionally been used concurrently with disopyramide phosphate. Excessive widening of the QRS complex and/or prolongation of the Q-T interval may occur in these situations (see WARNINGS.) In healthy subjects, no significant drug-drug interaction was observed when disopyramide phosphate was coadministered with either propranolol or diazepam. Concomitant administration of disopyramide phosphate and quinidine resulted in slight increases in plasma disopyramide levels and slight decreases in plasma quinidine levels. disopyramide phosphate does not increase serum digoxin levels.

Until data on possible interactions between verapamil and disopyramide phosphate are obtained, disopyramide should not be administered within 48 hours before or 24 hours after verapamil administration.

ADVERSE REACTIONS:

The adverse reactions which were reported in disopyramide phosphate clinical trials encompass observations in 1,500 patients, including 90 patients studied for at least 4 years. The most serious adverse reactions are hypotension and congestive heart failure. The most common adverse reactions, which are dose dependent, are associated with the anticholinergic properties of the drug. These may be transitory, but may be persistent or can be severe. Urinary retention is the most serious anticholinergic effect.

The following reactions were reported in 10% to 40% of patients:

Anticholinergic: dry mouth (32%), urinary hesitancy (14%), constipation (11%)

The following reactions were reported in 3% to 9% of patients:

Anticholinergic: blurred vision, dry nose/eyes/throat

Genitourinary: urinary retention, urinary frequency and urgency

Gastrointestinal: nausea, pain/bloating/gas

General: dizziness, general fatigue/muscle weakness, headache, malaise, aches/pains

The following reactions were reported in 1% to 3% of patients:

Genitourinary: impotence

Cardiovascular: hypotension with or without congestive heart failure, increased congestive heart failure (see WARNINGS), cardiac conduction disturbances (see WARNINGS), edema/weight gain, shortness of breath, syncope, chest pain

Gastrointestinal: anorexia, diarrhea, vomiting

Dermatologic: generalized rash/dermatoses, itching

Central nervous system: nervousness

Other: hypokalemia, elevated cholesterol/triglycerides

The Following Reactions Were Reported In Less Than 1%: Depression, insomnia, dysuria, numbness/tingling, elevated liver enzymes, AV block, elevated BUN, elevated creatinine, decreased hemoglobin/hematocrit

Hypoglycemia has been reported in association with disopyramide phosphate administration (see WARNINGS.)

Infrequent occurrences of reversible cholestatic jaundice, fever, and respiratory difficulty have been reported in association with disopyramide therapy, as have rare instances of thrombocytopenia, reversible agranulocytosis, and gynecomastia. Some cases of LE (lupus erythematosus) symptoms have been reported; most cases occurred in patients who had been switched to disopyramide from procainamide following the development of LE symptoms. Rarely, acute psychosis has been reported following disopyramide phosphate therapy, with prompt return to normal mental status when therapy was stopped. The physician should be aware of these possible reactions and should discontinue disopyramide phosphate or disopyramide phosphate controlled-release therapy promptly if they occur.

OVERDOSAGE:

SYMPTOMS

Deliberate or accidental overdosage of oral disopyramide may be followed by apnea, loss of consciousness, cardiac arrhythmias, and loss of spontaneous respiration. Death has occurred following overdosage.

Toxic plasma levels of disopyramide produce excessive widening of the QRS complex and Q-T interval, worsening of congestive heart failure, hypotension, varying kinds and degrees of conduction disturbance, bradycardia, and finally asystole. Obvious anticholinergic effects are also observed.

The approximate oral LD_{50} of disopyramide phosphate is 580 and 700 mg/kg for rats and mice, respectively.

TREATMENT

Experience indicates that prompt and vigorous treatment of overdosage is necessary, even in the absence of symptoms. Such treatment may be lifesaving. No specific antidote for disopyramide phosphate has been identified. Treatment should be symptomatic and may include induction of emesis or gastric lavage, administration of a cathartic followed by activated charcoal by mouth or stomach tube, intravenous administration of isoproterenol and dopamine, insertion of an intraaortic balloon for counterpulsation, and mechanically assisted ventilation. Hemodialysis or, preferably, hemoperfusion with charcoal may be employed to lower serum concentration of the drug.

The electrocardiogram should be monitored, and supportive therapy with cardiac glycosides and diuretics should be given as required.

If progressive AV block should develop, endocardial pacing should be implemented. In case of any impaired renal function, measures to increase the glomerular filtration rate may reduce the toxicity (disopyramide is excreted primarily by the kidney).

The anticholinergic effects can be reversed with neostigmine at the discretion of the physician.

Altering the urinary pH in humans does not affect the plasma half-life or the amount of disopyramide excreted in the urine.

DOSAGE AND ADMINISTRATION:

The dosage of disopyramide phosphate or disopyramide phosphate controlled-release must be individualized for each patient on the basis of response and tolerance. The usual adult dosage of disopyramide phosphate or disopyramide phosphate controlled-release is 400 to 800 mg per day given in divided doses. The recommended dosage for most adults is 600 mg/day given in divided doses (either 150 mg every 6 hours for immediate-release disopyramide phosphate or 300 mg every 12 hours for disopyramide phosphate controlled-release). For patients whose body weight is less than 110 pounds (50 kg), the recommended dosage is 400 mg/day given in divided doses (either 100 mg every 6 hours for immediate-release disopyramide phosphate or 200 mg every 12 hours for disopyramide phosphate controlled-release).

For patients with cardiomyopathy or possible cardiac decompensation, a loading dose, as discussed below, should not be given, and initial dosage should be limited to 100 mg of immediate-release disopyramide phosphate every 6 to 8 hours. Subsequent dosage adjustments should be made gradually, with close monitoring for the possible development of hypotension and/or congestive heart failure (see WARNINGS.)

For patients with moderate renal insufficiency (creatinine clearance greater than 40 ml/min) or hepatic insufficiency, the recommended dosage is 400 mg/day given in divided doses (either 100 mg every 6 hours for immediate-release disopyramide phosphate or 200 mg every 12 hours for disopyramide phosphate controlled-release).

For patients with severe renal insufficiency (C_{cr}40 ml/min or less), the recommended dosage regimen of immediate-release disopyramide phosphate is 100 mg at intervals shown in TABLE 1, with or without an initial loading dose of 150 mg.

TABLE 1 IMMEDIATE-RELEASE DISOPYRAMIDE PHOSPHATE DOSAGE INTERVAL FOR PATIENTS WITH RENAL INSUFFICIENCY

Creatinine clearance (ml/min)	40-30	30-15	less than 15
Approximate maintenance-dosing interval	q 8 hr	q 12 hr	q 24 hr

TABLE 1 dosing schedules are for disopyramide phosphate immediate-release capsules; disopyramide phosphate controlled-release is not recommended for patients with severe renal insufficiency.

For patients in whom rapid control of ventricular arrhythmia is essential, an initial loading dose of 300 mg of immediate-release disopyramide phosphate (200 mg for patients whose body weight is less than 110 pounds) is recommended, followed by the appropriate maintenance dosage. Therapeutic effects are usually attained 30 minutes to 3 hours after administration of a 300 mg loading dose. If there is no response or evidence of toxicity within 6 hours of the loading dose, 200 mg of immediate-release disopyramide phosphate every 6 hours may be prescribed instead of the usual 150 mg. If there is no response to this dosage within 48 hours, either disopyramide phosphate should then be discontinued or the physician should consider hospitalizing the patient for careful monitoring while subsequent immediate-release disopyramide phosphate doses of 250 mg or 300 mg every 6 hours are given. A limited number of patients with severe refractory ventricular tachycardia have tolerated daily doses of disopyramide phosphate up to 1600 mg per day (400 mg every 6 hours), resulting in disopyramide plasma levels up to 9 mcg/ml. If such treatment is warranted, it is essential that patients be hospitalized for close evaluation and continuous monitoring.

Disopyramide phosphate should not be used initially if rapid establishment of disopyramide plasma levels is desired.

TRANSFERRING TO DISOPYRAMIDE PHOSPHATE OR DISOPYRAMIDE PHOSPHATE CONTROLLED-RELEASE

The following dosage schedule based on theoretical considerations rather than experimental data is suggested for transferring patients with normal renal function from either quinidine sulfate or procainamide therapy (Type 1 antiarrhythmic agents) to disopyramide phosphate or disopyramide phosphate controlled-release therapy:

Disopyramide phosphate or disopyramide phosphate controlled-release should be started using the regular maintenance schedule without a **loading dose** 6 to 12 hours after the last dose of quinidine sulfate or 3 to 6 hours after the last dose of procainamide.

In patients in whom withdrawal of quinidine sulfate or procainamide is likely to produce life-threatening arrhythmias, the physician should consider hospitalization of the patient. When transferring a patient from immediate-release disopyramide phosphate to disopyramide phosphate controlled-release, the maintenance schedule of disopyramide phosphate controlled-release may be started 6 hours after the last dose of immediate-release disopyramide phosphate.

PEDIATRIC DOSAGE

Controlled clinical studies have not been conducted in pediatric patients; however, the following suggested dosage table is based on published clinical experience.

DOSAGE AND ADMINISTRATION: *(cont'd)*

Total daily dosage should be divided and equal doses administered orally every 6 hours or at intervals according to individual patient needs. Disopyramide plasma levels and therapeutic response must be monitored closely. Patients should be hospitalized during the initial treatment period, and dose titration should start at the lower end of the ranges provided in TABLE 2.

TABLE 2 SUGGESTED TOTAL DAILY DOSAGE*

Age (years)	Disopyramide (mg/kg body weight/day)
Under 1	10 to 30
1 to 4	10 to 20
4 to 12	10 to 15
12 to 18	6 to 15

*(From TABLE 2) Dosage is expressed in milligrams of disopyramide base. Since disopyramide phosphate 100 mg capsules contain 100 mg of disopyramide base, the pharmacist can readily prepare a 1 mg/ml to 10 mg/ml liquid suspension by adding the entire contents of disopyramide phosphate capsules to cherry syrup, NF. The resulting suspension, when refrigerated, is stable for one month and should be thoroughly shaken before the measurement of each dose. The suspension should be dispensed in an amber glass bottle with a child-resistant closure.

Disopyramide phosphate controlled-release capsules should not be used to prepare the above suspension.

Store below 86°F (30°C).

HOW SUPPLIED - RATED THERAPEUTICALLY EQUIVALENT:

Capsule, Gelatin - Oral - 100 mg

100's	$10.43	Disopyramide, United Res	00677-1020-01
100's	$10.43	Disopyramide, H.C.F.A. F F P	99999-1093-01
100's	$12.38	Disopyramide, US Trading	56126-0330-11
100's	$20.18	Disopyramide, Teva	00332-3127-09
100's	$22.30	Disopyramide Phosphate, Aligen Independ	00405-4357-01
100's	$22.88	Disopyramide, HL Moore Drug Exch	00839-7091-06
100's	$22.89	Disopyramide Phosphate, Caremark	00339-5681-12
100's	$22.95	Disopyramide, Goldline Labs	00182-1743-01
100's	$23.60	Disopyramide, Qualitest Pharms	00603-3408-21
100's	$23.95	Disopyramide, Rugby	00536-3595-01
100's	$23.95	Disopyramide Phosphate, Major Pharms	00904-2482-60
100's	$24.10	Disopyramide, Schein Pharm (US)	00364-0739-01
100's	$35.44	Disopyramide, Schein Pharm (US)	00364-0739-90
100's	**$54.55**	**NORPACE, Searle**	**00025-2752-31**
100's	**$57.11**	**NORPACE, Searle**	**00025-2752-34**
500's	$52.15	Disopyramide, HL Moore Drug Exch	00839-7091-12
500's	$52.15	Disopyramide, H.C.F.A. F F P	99999-1093-02
500's	$95.90	Disopyramide, Teva	00332-3127-13
500's	$116.70	Disopyramide Phosphate, Major Pharms	00904-2482-40
500's	$117.08	Disopyramide, Schein Pharm (US)	00364-0739-05
500's	$132.54	Disopyramide, Lederle Pharm	00005-3156-31
1000's	$104.30	Disopyramide, H.C.F.A. F F P	99999-1093-03
1000's	**$502.95**	**NORPACE, Searle**	**00025-2752-52**

Capsule, Gelatin - Oral - 150 mg

100's	$11.93	Disopyramide, United Res	00677-1021-01
100's	$11.93	Disopyramide, H.C.F.A. F F P	99999-1093-04
100's	$23.84	Disopyramide, Teva	00332-3129-09
100's	$26.35	Disopyramide Phosphate, Aligen Independ	00405-4358-01
100's	$27.48	Disopyramide Phosphate, Caremark	00339-5683-12
100's	$27.66	Disopyramide, HL Moore Drug Exch	00839-7092-06
100's	$28.09	Disopyramide, Schein Pharm (US)	00364-0740-01
100's	$28.40	Disopyramide, Qualitest Pharms	00603-3409-21
100's	$28.50	Disopyramide, Goldline Labs	00182-1744-01
100's	$28.69	Disopyramide, Rugby	00536-3596-01
100's	$28.75	Disopyramide Phosphate, Major Pharms	00904-2483-60
100's	$32.93	Disopyramide Phosphate, Major Pharms	00904-2483-61
100's	$42.53	Disopyramide, Schein Pharm (US)	00364-0740-90
100's	**$64.43**	**NORPACE, Searle**	**00025-2762-31**
100's	**$67.02**	**NORPACE, Searle**	**00025-2762-34**
500's	$59.31	Disopyramide, Rugby	00536-3597-05
500's	$59.65	Disopyramide, H.C.F.A. F F P	99999-1093-05
500's	$113.29	Disopyramide, Teva	00332-3129-13
500's	$131.21	Disopyramide, HL Moore Drug Exch	00839-7092-12
500's	$131.25	Disopyramide Phosphate, Major Pharms	00904-2483-40
500's	$137.81	Disopyramide, Schein Pharm (US)	00364-0740-05
1000's	$119.30	Disopyramide, H.C.F.A. F F P	99999-1093-06

Capsule, Gelatin, Sustained Action - Oral - 100 mg

100's	$53.10	Disopyramide, Major Pharms	00904-2488-60
100's	$57.56	Disopyramide Phosphate, Caremark	00339-5845-12
100's	$57.56	Disopyramide, Ethex	58177-0003-04
100's	**$65.69**	**NORPACE CR, Searle**	**00025-2732-31**
100's	**$68.78**	**NORPACE CR, Searle**	**00025-2732-34**
500's	**$312.20**	**NORPACE CR, Searle**	**00025-2732-51**

Capsule, Gelatin, Sustained Action - Oral - 150 mg

100's	$39.75	Disopyramide, Genetco	00302-2303-01
100's	$54.50	Disopyramide, Harber Pharm	51432-0168-03
100's	$62.94	Disopyramide Phosphate, Caremark	00339-5884-12
100's	$64.58	Disopyramide, Caremark	00339-5684-12
100's	$66.30	Disopyramide, Major Pharms	00904-2489-60
100's	$68.03	Disopyramide, Ethex	58177-0002-04
100's	**$77.64**	**NORPACE CR, Searle**	**00025-2742-31**
100's	**$80.73**	**NORPACE CR, Searle**	**00025-2742-34**
500's	**$368.85**	**NORPACE CR, Searle**	**00025-2742-51**

DISULFIRAM *(001094)*

CATEGORIES: Alcoholism; Central Nervous System Agents; FDA Approval Pre 1982

BRAND NAMES: *Antabus* (Germany); **Antabuse**; *Antadict*; *Aversan*; *Busetal*; *Disulfram*; *Esperal* (France); *Nocbin* (Japan); *Refusal*; *Tetmosol*; *Tetradin* *(International brand names outside U.S. in italics)*

FORMULARIES: BC-BS; FHP; Medi-Cal

> **WARNING:**
> Disulfiram should NEVER be administered to a patient when he is in a state of alcohol intoxication, or without his full knowledge.
> The physician should instruct relatives accordingly.

DESCRIPTION:

Chemical Name: bis(diethylthiocarbamoyl) disulfide.

Disulfiram occurs as a white-to-off-white, odorless, and almost tasteless powder, soluble in water to the extent of about 20 mg in 100 ml, and in alcohol to the extent of about 3.8 g in 100 ml.

Disulfiram contains these inactive ingredients: magnesium aluminum silicate; magnesium stearate, NF; povidone, USP; starch, NF.

CLINICAL PHARMACOLOGY:

Disulfiram produces a sensitivity to alcohol which results in a highly unpleasant reaction when the patient under treatment ingests even small amounts of alcohol.

Disulfiram blocks the oxidation of alcohol at the acetaldehyde stage. During alcohol metabolism following disulfiram intake, the concentration of acetaldehyde occurring in the blood may be 5- to 10-times higher than that found during metabolism of the same amount of alcohol alone.

Accumulation of acetaldehyde in the blood produces a complex of highly unpleasant symptoms referred to hereinafter as the disulfiram-alcohol reaction. This reaction, which is proportional to the dosage of both disulfiram and alcohol, will persist as long as alcohol is being metabolized. Disulfiram does not appear to influence the rate of alcohol elimination from the body.

Disulfiram is absorbed slowly from the gastrointestinal tract and eliminated slowly from the body. One (or even two) weeks after a patient has taken his last dose of Disulfiram, ingestion of alcohol may produce unpleasant symptoms.

Prolonged administration of disulfiram does not produce tolerance; the longer a patient remains on therapy, the more exquisitely sensitive he becomes to alcohol.

INDICATIONS AND USAGE:

Disulfiram is an aid in the management of selected chronic alcoholic patients who *want* to remain in a state of enforced sobriety so that supportive and psychotherapeutic treatment may be applied to best advantage. (Used alone, without proper motivation and supportive therapy, disulfiram is not a cure for alcoholism, and it is unlikely that it will have more than a brief effect on the drinking pattern of the chronic alcoholic.)

CONTRAINDICATIONS:

Patients who are receiving or have recently received metronidazole, paraldehyde, alcohol, or alcohol-containing preparations, e.g., cough syrups, tonics and the like, should not be given disulfiram.

Disulfiram is contraindicated in the presence of severe myocardial disease or coronary occlusion, psychoses, and hypersensitivity to disulfiram or to other thiuram derivatives used in pesticides and rubber vulcanization.

WARNINGS:

> **Disulfiram should NEVER be administered to a patient when he is in a state of alcohol intoxication, or without his full knowledge.**
> **The physician should instruct relatives accordingly.**

The patient must be fully informed of the disulfiram-alcohol reaction. He must be strongly cautioned against surreptitious drinking while taking the drug, and he must be fully aware of possible consequences. He should be warned to avoid alcohol in disguised form, i.e., in sauces, vinegars, cough mixtures, and even aftershave lotions and back rubs. He should also be warned that reactions may occur with alcohol up to 14 days after ingesting.

THE DISULFIRAM-ALCOHOL REACTION

Disulfiram plus alcohol, even small amounts, produces flushing, throbbing in head and neck, throbbing headache, respiratory difficulty, nausea, copious vomiting, sweating, thirst, chest pain, palpitation, dyspnea, hyperventilation, tachycardia, hypotension, syncope, marked uneasiness, weakness, vertigo, blurred vision, and confusion. In severe reactions there may be respiratory depression, cardiovascular collapse, arrhythmias, myocardial infarction, acute congestive heart failure, unconsciousness, convulsions, and death.

The intensity of the reaction varies with each individual but is generally proportional to the amounts of disulfiram and alcohol ingested. Mild reactions may occur in the sensitive individual when the blood alcohol concentration is increased to as little as 5 to 10 mg per 100 ml. Symptoms are fully developed at 50 mg per 100 ml, and unconsciousness usually results when the blood alcohol level reaches 125 to 150 mg.

The duration of the reaction varies from 30 to 60 minutes, to several hours in the more severe cases, or as long as there is alcohol in the blood.

CONCOMITANT CONDITIONS

Because of the possibility of an accidental disulfiram-alcohol reaction, should be used with extreme caution in patients with any of the following conditions: diabetes mellitus, hypothyroidism, epilepsy, cerebral damage, chronic and acute nephritis, hepatic cirrhosis or insufficiency.

USAGE IN PREGNANCY

The safe use of this drug in pregnancy has not been established. Therefore, disulfiram should be used during pregnancy only when, in the judgment of the physician, the probable benefits outweigh the possible risks.

PRECAUTIONS:

Patients with a history of rubber contact dermatitis should be evaluated for hypersensitivity to thiuram derivatives before receiving (see CONTRAINDICATIONS.)

It is suggested that every patient under treatment carry *an Identification Card* stating that he is receiving disulfiram and describing the symptoms most likely to occur as a result of the disulfiram-alcohol reaction. In addition, this card should indicate the physician or institution to be contacted in an emergency. (Cards may be obtained from Ayerst Laboratories upon request.)

Alcoholism may accompany or be followed by dependence on narcotics or sedatives. Barbiturates and disulfiram have been administered concurrently without untoward effects; the possibility of initiating a new abuse should be considered.

Baseline and follow-up transaminase tests (10 to 14 days) are suggested to detect any hepatic dysfunction that may result with therapy. In addition, a complete blood count and a sequential multiple analysis-12 (SMA-12) test should be made every six months.

PRECAUTIONS: *(cont'd)*

Patients taking disulfiram tablets should not be exposed to ethylene dibromide or its vapors. This precaution is based on preliminary results of animal research currently in progress that suggest a toxic interaction between inhaled ethylene dibromide and ingested disulfiram resulting in a higher incidence of tumors and mortality in rats. A correlation between this finding and humans, however, has not been demonstrated.

DRUG INTERACTIONS:

Disulfiram appears to decrease the rate at which certain drugs are metabolized and therefore may increase the blood levels and the possibility of clinical toxicity of drugs given concomitantly.

DISULFIRAM SHOULD BE USED WITH CAUTION IN THOSE PATIENTS RECEIVING PHENYTOIN AND ITS CONGENERS, SINCE THE CONCOMITANT ADMINISTRATION OF THESE TWO DRUGS CAN LEAD TO PHENYTOIN INTOXICATION. PRIOR TO ADMINISTERING DISULFIRAM TO A PATIENT ON PHENYTOIN THERAPY, A BASELINE PHENYTOIN SERUM LEVEL SHOULD BE OBTAINED. SUBSEQUENT TO INITIATION OF DISULFIRAM THERAPY, SERUM LEVELS ON PHENYTOIN SHOULD BE DETERMINED ON DIFFERENT DAYS FOR EVIDENCE OF AN INCREASE OR FOR A CONTINUING RISE IN LEVELS. INCREASED PHENYTOIN LEVELS SHOULD BE TREATED WITH APPROPRIATE DOSAGE ADJUSTMENT.

It may be necessary to adjust the dosage of oral anticoagulants upon beginning or stopping disulfiram, since disulfiram may prolong prothrombin time.

Patients taking isoniazid when disulfiram is given should be observed for the appearance of unsteady gait or marked changes in mental status; the disulfiram should be discontinued if such signs appear.

In rats, simultaneous ingestion of disulfiram and nitrite in the diet for 78 weeks has been reported to cause tumors, and it has been suggested that disulfiram may react with nitrites in the rat stomach to form a nitrosamine, which is tumorigenic. Disulfiram alone in the rats' diet did not lead to such tumors. The relevance of this finding to humans is not known at this time.

ADVERSE REACTIONS:

(See CONTRAINDICATIONS, WARNINGS and PRECAUTIONS)

OPTIC NEURITIS, PERIPHERAL NEURITIS, AND POLYNEURITIS MAY OCCUR FOLLOWING ADMINISTRATION OF DISULFIRAM.

Multiple cases of both cholestatic and fulminant hepatitis have been reported to be associated with administration of disulfiram.

Occasional skin eruptions are, as a rule, readily controlled by concomitant administration of an antihistaminic drug.

In a small number of patients, a transient mild drowsiness, fatigability, impotence, headache, acneform eruptions, allergic dermatitis, or a metallic or garlic-like after-taste may be experienced during the first two weeks of therapy. These complaints usually disappear spontaneously with the continuation of therapy, or with reduced dosage.

Psychotic reactions have been noted, attributable in most cases to high dosage, combined toxicity (with metronidazole or isoniazid), or to the unmasking of underlying psychoses in patients stressed by the withdrawal of alcohol.

DOSAGE AND ADMINISTRATION:

Disulfiram should never be administered until the patient has abstained from alcohol for at least 12 hours.

INITIAL DOSAGE SCHEDULE

In the first phase of treatment, a *maximum*of 500 mg daily is given in a single dose for one to two weeks. Although usually taken in the morning, disulfiram may be taken on retiring by patients who experience a sedative effect. Alternatively, to minimize, or eliminate, the sedative effect, disulfiram dosage may be adjusted downward.

MAINTENANCE REGIMEN

The average maintenance dose is 250 mg daily (range, 125 to 500 mg); it should not exceed 500 mg daily.

NOTE: Occasionally patients, while seemingly on adequate maintenance doses of disulfiram, report that they are able to drink alcoholic beverages with impunity and without any symptomatology. All appearances to the contrary, such patients must be presumed to be disposing of their tablets in some manner without actually taking them. Until such patients have been observed reliably taking their daily tablets (preferably crushed and well mixed with liquid), it cannot be concluded that disulfiram is ineffective.

DURATION OF THERAPY

The daily, uninterrupted administration of disulfiram must be continued until the patient is fully recovered socially and a basis for permanent self-control is established. Depending on the individual patient, maintenance therapy may be required for months, or even years.

TRIAL WITH ALCOHOL

During early experience with disulfiram, it was thought advisable for each patient to have at least one supervised alcohol-drug reaction. More recently, the test reaction has been largely abandoned. Furthermore, such a test reaction should never be administered to a patient over 50 years of age. A clear, detailed, and convincing description of the reaction is felt to be sufficient in most cases.

However, where a test reaction is deemed necessary, the suggested procedure is as follows:

After the first one to two weeks' therapy with 500 mg daily, a drink of 15 ml (1/2 oz) of 100 proof whiskey, or equivalent, is taken slowly. This test dose of alcoholic beverage may be repeated once only, so that the total dose does not exceed 30 ml (1 oz) of whiskey. Once a reaction develops, no more alcohol should be consumed. Such tests should be carried out only when the patient is hospitalized, or comparable supervision and facilities, including oxygen, are available.

MANAGEMENT OF DISULFIRAM-ALCOHOL REACTION

In severe reactions, whether caused by an excessive test dose or by the patient's unsupervised ingestion of alcohol, supportive measures to restore blood pressure and treat shock should be instituted. Other recommendations include: oxygen, carbogen (95% oxygen and 5% carbon dioxide), vitamin C intravenously in massive doses (1 g), and ephedrine sulfate. Antihistamines have also been used intravenously. Potassium levels should be monitored, particularly in patients on digitalis, since hypokalemia has been reported.

HOW SUPPLIED - EQUIVALENTS NOT AVAILABLE:

Tablet, Uncoated - Oral - 250 mg

100's	$7.43	Disulfiram, Rugby	00536-3767-01
100's	$7.65	Disulfiram, Major Pharms	00904-1180-60
100's	$7.90	Disulfiram, Geneva Pharms	00781-1060-01
100's	$7.91	Disulfiram, Qualitest Pharms	00603-3431-21
100's	$8.05	Disulfiram, United Res	00677-1001-01
100's	$8.09	Disulfiram, HL Moore Drug Exch	00839-1286-06
100's	$8.30	Disulfiram, Goldline Labs	00182-0532-01

HOW SUPPLIED - EQUIVALENTS NOT AVAILABLE: *(cont'd)*

100's	$8.30	Disulfiram, Sidmak Labs	50111-0331-01
100's	$11.24	Disulfiram, Aligen Independ	00405-4363-01
100's	$16.10	Disulfiram, Major Pharms	00904-1180-61
100's	**$73.79**	**ANTABUSE, Ayerst**	**00046-0809-81**
1000's	$60.80	Disulfiram, Sidmak Labs	50111-0331-03

Tablet, Uncoated - Oral - 500 mg

50's	$6.30	Disulfiram, Major Pharms	00904-1181-51
50's	$19.15	Disulfiram, Rugby	00536-3768-06
50's	**$44.50**	**ANTABUSE, Ayerst**	**00046-0810-50**
100's	$11.95	Disulfiram, Major Pharms	00904-1181-60
100's	$19.12	Disulfiram, Goldline Labs	00182-0533-01
100's	$19.12	Disulfiram, Sidmak Labs	50111-0332-01
500's	$48.13	Disulfiram, Rugby	00536-3768-05

DIVALPROEX SODIUM *(001096)*

CATEGORIES: Anticonvulsants; Antidepressants; Antiepileptics; Antimanic Agents; Bipolar Disorder; Central Nervous System Agents; Convulsions; Depression; Epilepsy; Mania; Neuromuscular; Seizures; Migraine; Pregnancy Category D; FDA Approved 1983 Mar; Top 200 Drugs

BRAND NAMES: **Depakote**; Depakote Sprinkle; *Epival* (Canada)
(International brand names outside U.S. in italics)

FORMULARIES: Aetna; BC-BS; CIGNA; FHP; Humana; Kaiser; Medco; Medi-Cal; PCS; PruCare; United

COST OF THERAPY: $818.18 (Epilepsy; Tablet; 500 mg; 2/day; 365 days)

WARNING:
HEPATIC FAILURE RESULTING IN FATALITIES HAS OCCURRED IN PATIENTS RECEIVING VALPROIC ACID AND ITS DERIVATIVES. EXPERIENCE HAS INDICATED THAT CHILDREN UNDER THE AGE OF TWO YEARS ARE AT A CONSIDERABLY INCREASED RISK OF DEVELOPING FATAL HEPATOTOXICITY, ESPECIALLY THOSE ON MULTIPLE ANTICONVULSANTS, THOSE WITH CONGENITAL METABOLIC DISORDERS, THOSE WITH SEVERE SEIZURE DISORDERS ACCOMPANIED BY MENTAL RETARDATION, AND THOSE WITH ORGANIC BRAIN DISEASE. WHEN DIVALPROEX SODIUM IS USED IN THIS PATIENT GROUP, IT SHOULD BE USED WITH EXTREME CAUTION AND AS A SOLE AGENT. THE BENEFITS OF THERAPY SHOULD BE WEIGHED AGAINST THE RISKS. ABOVE THIS AGE GROUP, EXPERIENCE IN EPILEPSY HAS INDICATED THAT THE INCIDENCE OF FATAL HEPATOTOXICITY DECREASES CONSIDERABLY IN PROGRESSIVELY OLDER PATIENT GROUPS.
THESE INCIDENTS USUALLY HAVE OCCURRED DURING THE FIRST SIX MONTHS OF TREATMENT. SERIOUS OR FATAL HEPATOTOXICITY MAY BE PRECEDED BY NON-SPECIFIC SYMPTOMS SUCH AS MALAISE, WEAKNESS, LETHARGY, FACIAL EDEMA, ANOREXIA AND VOMITING. IN PATIENTS WITH EPILEPSY, A LOSS OF SEIZURE CONTROL MAY ALSO OCCUR. PATIENTS SHOULD BE MONITORED CLOSELY FOR APPEARANCE OF THESE SYMPTOMS. LIVER FUNCTION TESTS SHOULD BE PERFORMED PRIOR TO THERAPY AND AT FREQUENT INTERVALS THEREAFTER, ESPECIALLY DURING THE FIRST SIX MONTHS.
Teratogenicity: VALPROATE CAN PRODUCE TERATOGENIC EFFECTS SUCH AS NEURAL TUBE DEFECTS (*E.G.*, SPINA BIFIDA), ACCORDINGLY, THE USE OF DIVALPROEX SODIUM IN WOMEN OF CHILDBEARING POTENTIAL REQUIRES THAT THE BENEFITS OF ITS USE BE WEIGHED AGAINST THE RISK OF INJURY TO THE FETUS. THIS IS ESPECIALLY IMPORTANT WHEN THE TREATMENT OF A SPONTANEOUSLY REVERSIBLE CONDITION NOT ORDINARILY ASSOCIATED WITH PERMANENT INJURY OR RISK OF DEATH (*E.G.*, MIGRAINE) IS CONTEMPLATED. SEE Information for the Patient.

DESCRIPTION:

Divalproex sodium is a stable co-ordination compound comprised of sodium valproate and valproic acid in a 1:1 molar relationship and formed during the partial neutralization of valproic acid with 0.5 equivalent of sodium hydroxide. Chemically it is designated as sodium hydrogen bis(2-propylpentanoate).

Divalproex sodium occurs as a white powder with a characteristic odor.

Depakote tablets and Sprinkle capsules are antiepileptics for oral administration. Depakote Sprinkle capsules contain specially coated particles of divalproex sodium equivalent to 125 mg of valproic acid in a hard gelatin capsule. Depakote tablets are supplied in three dosage strengths containing divalproex sodium equivalent to 125 mg, 250 mg or 500 mg of valproic acid.

INACTIVE INGREDIENTS

125 mg Sprinkle capsules: cellulosic polymers, D&C Red No. 28, FD&C Blue No. 1, gelatin, iron oxide, magnesium stearate, silica gel, titanium dioxide and triethyl citrate.

Depakote tablets: cellulosic polymers, diacetylated monoglycerides, povidone, pregelatinized starch (contains corn starch), silica gel, talc, titanium dioxide and vanillin.

In addition, individual tablets contain: *125 mg tablets:* FD&C Blue No. 1 and FD&C Red No. 40.*250 mg tablets:* FD&C Yellow No. 6 and iron oxide. *500 mg tablets:* D&C Red No. 30, FD&C Blue No. 2, and iron oxide.

CLINICAL PHARMACOLOGY:

PHARMACODYNAMICS

Divalproex sodium dissociates to the valproate ion in the gastrointestinal tract. The mechanisms by which valproate exerts its therapeutic effects have not been established. It has been suggested that its activity in epilepsy is related to increased brain concentrations of gamma-aminobutyric acid (GABA).

PHARMACOKINETICS

Absorption/Bioavailability: Equivalent oral doses of divalproex sodium products and valproic acid capsules deliver equivalent quantities of valproate ion systemically. Although the rate of valproate ion absorption may vary with the formulation administered (liquid, solid, or sprinkle), the conditions of use (*e.g.*, fasting or postprandial) and the method of administration

CLINICAL PHARMACOLOGY: *(cont'd)*

(*e.g.*, whether the contents of the capsule are sprinkled on food or the capsule is taken intact), these differences should be of minor clinical importance under the steady state conditions achieved in chronic use in the treatment of epilepsy.

However, it is possible that differences among the various valproate products in T_{max} and C_{max} could be important upon initiation of treatment. For example, in single dose studies, the effect of feeding had a greater influence on the rate of absorption of the tablet (increase in T_{max} from 4 to 8 hours) than on the absorption of the sprinkle capsules (increase in T_{max} from 3.3 to 4.8)

While the absorption rate from the G.I. tract and fluctuation in valproate plasma concentrations vary with dosing regimen and formulation, the efficacy of valproate as an anticonvulsant in chronic use is unlikely to be affected. Experience employing dosing regimens from once-a-day to four-times-a-day, as well as studies in primate epilepsy models involving constant rate infusion, indicate that total daily systemic bioavailability (extent of absorption) is the primary determinant of seizure control and that differences in the ratios of plasma peak to trough concentrations between valproate formulations are inconsequential from a practical clinical standpoint. Whether or not rate of absorption influences the efficacy of valproate as an antimanic or antimigraine agent is unknown.

Co-administration of oral valproate products with food and substitution among the various divalproex sodium and valproic acid formulations should cause no clinical problems in the management of patients with epilepsy. (See DOSAGE AND ADMINISTRATION.) Nonetheless, any changes in dosage administration, or the addition or discontinuance of concomitant drugs should ordinarily be accompanied by close monitoring of clinical status and valproate plasma concentrations.

Distribution: *Protein Binding:* The plasma protein binding of valproate is concentration dependent and the free fraction increases from approximately 10% at 40 mcg/ml to 18.5% at 130 mcg/ml. Protein binding of valproate is reduced in the elderly, in patients with chronic hepatic diseases, in patients with renal impairment, and in the presence of other drugs (*e.g.*, aspirin). Conversely, valproate may displace certain protein-bound drugs (*e.g.*, phenytoin, carbamazepine, warfarin, and tolbutamide). (See DRUG INTERACTIONS for more detailed information on the pharmacokinetic interactions of valproate with other drugs.)

CNS Distribution: Valproate concentrations in cerebrospinal fluid (CSF) approximate unbound concentrations in plasma (about 10% of total concentration).

Metabolism: Valproate is metabolized almost entirely by the liver. In adult patients on monotherapy, 30-50% of an administered dose appears in urine as a glucuronide conjugate. Mitochondrial β-oxidation is the other major metabolic pathway, typically accounting for over 40% of the dose. Usually less than 15-20% of the dose is eliminated by other oxidative mechanisms. Less than 3% of an administered dose is excreted unchanged in urine.

The relationship between dose and total valproate concentration is nonlinear; concentration does not increase proportionally with the dose, but rather, increases to a lesser extent due to saturable plasma protein binding. The kinetics of unbound drug are linear.

Elimination: Mean plasma clearance and volume of distribution for total valproate are 0.56 $L/hr/1.73\ m^2$ and 11 $L/1.73\ m^2$, respectively. Mean plasma clearance and volume of distribution for free valproate are 4.6 $L/hr/1.73\ m^2$ and 92 $L/hr/1.73\ m^2$. Mean terminal half-life for valproate monotherapy ranged from 9 to 16 hours following oral dosing regimens of 250 to 1000 mg.

The estimates cited apply primarily to patients who are not taking drugs that affect hepatic metabolizing enzyme systems. For example, patients taking enzyme-inducing antiepileptic drugs (carbamazepine, phenytoin, and phenobarbital) will clear valproate more rapidly. Because of these changes in valproate clearance, monitoring of antiepileptic concentrations should be intensified whenever concomitant antiepileptics are introduced or withdrawn.

Special Populations: *Effect of Age: Neonates:* Children within the first two months of life have a markedly decreased ability to eliminate valproate compared to older children and adults. This is a result of reduced clearance (perhaps due to delay in development of glucuronosyl transferase and other enzyme systems involved in valproate elimination) as well as increased volume of distribution (in part due to decreased plasma protein binding). For example, in one study, the half-life in children under ten days ranged from 10 to 67 hours compared to a range of 7 to 13 hours in children greater than 2 months. *Children:* Pediatric patients (*i.e.*, between 3 months and 10 years) have 50% higher clearances expressed on weight (*i.e.*, ml/min/kg) than do adults. Over the age of 10 years, children have pharmacokinetic parameters that approximate those of adults. *Elderly:* The capacity of elderly patients (age range: 69 to 89 years) to eliminate valproate has been shown to be reduced compared to younger adults (age range: 22 to 26 years). Intrinsic clearance is reduced by 39%; the free fraction is increased by 44%. Accordingly, the initial dosage should be reduced in the elderly. (See DOSAGE AND ADMINISTRATION)

Effect of Gender: There are no differences in the body surface area adjusted unbound clearance between males and females (4.8 ± 0.17 and 4.7 ± 0.07 L/hr per $1.73m^2$, respectively).

Effect of Race: The effects of race on the kinetics of valproate have not been studied.

Effect of Disease: *Liver Disease:* See BOXED WARNING, CONTRAINDICATIONS, and WARNINGS. Liver disease impairs the capacity to eliminate valproate. In one study, the clearance of free valproate was decreased by 50% in 7 patients with cirrhosis and by 16% in 4 patients with acute hepatitis, compared with 6 healthy subjects. In that study, the half-life of valproate was increased from 12 to 18 hours. Liver disease is also associated with decreased albumin concentrations and larger unbound fractions (2 to 2.6 fold increases) of valproate. Accordingly, monitoring of total concentrations may be misleading since free concentrations may be substantially elevated in patients with hepatic disease whereas total concentrations may appear to be normal. *Renal Disease:* A slight reduction (27%) in the unbound clearance of valproate has been reported in patients with renal failure (creatinine clearance < 10 ml/minute); however, hemodialysis typically reduces valproate concentrations by about 20%. Therefore, no dosage adjustment appears to be necessary in patients with renal failure. Protein binding in these patients is substantially reduced; thus, monitoring total concentrations may be misleading.

PLASMA LEVELS AND CLINICAL EFFECT

The relationship between plasma concentration and clinical response is not well documented. One contributing factor is the nonlinear, concentration dependent protein binding of valproate which affects the clearance of the drug. Thus, monitoring of total serum valproate cannot provide a reliable index of the bioactive valproate species.

For example, because the plasma protein binding of valproate is concentration dependent, the free fraction increases from approximately 10% at 40 mcg/ml to 18.5% at 130 mcg/ml. Higher than expected free fractions occur in the elderly, in hyperlipidemic patients, and in patients with hepatic and renal diseases.

Epilepsy: The therapeutic range in epilepsy is commonly considered to be 50 to 100 mcg/ml of total valproate, although some patients may be controlled with lower or higher plasma concentrations.

Mania: In placebo-controlled trials of acute mania, patients were dosed to clinical response with trough plasma concentrations between 50 and 125 mcg/ml (See DOSAGE AND ADMINISTRATION.)

CLINICAL STUDIES:

MANIA

The effectiveness of divalproex sodium for the treatment of acute mania was demonstrated in two 3-week, placebo controlled, parallel group studies.

Study 1: The first study enrolled adult patients who met DSM-III-R criteria for Bipolar Disorder and who were hospitalized for acute mania. In addition, they had a history of failing to respond to or not tolerating previous lithium carbonate treatment. Divalproex sodium was initiated at a dose of 250 mg three times daily and adjusted to achieve serum valproate concentrations in a range of 50-100 mcg/ml by day 7. Mean divalproex sodium doses for completers in this study were 1118, 1525, and 2402 mg/day at days 7,14, and 21, respectively. Patients were assessed on the Young Mania Rating Scale (YMRS; score ranges from 0-60), an augmented Brief Psychiatric Rating Scale (BPRS-A), and the Global Assessment Scale (GAS). Baseline score and change from baseline in the week 3 endpoint (last-observation-carry-forward) analysis can be seen in TABLE 1.

TABLE 1 Study 1

Group	Baseline[1]	YMRS Total Score BL to Wk3[2]	Difference[3]
Placebo	28.8	+0.2	
Divalproex Sodium	28.5	−9.5	9.7
Group	**Baseline[1]**	**BPRS-A Total Score BL to Wk3[2]**	**Difference[3]**
Placebo	76.2	+1.8	
Divalproex Sodium	76.4	−17.0	18.8
Group	**Baseline[1]**	**GAS Total Score BL to Wk3[2]**	**Difference[3]**
Placebo	31.8	0.0	
Divalproex Sodium	30.3	+18.1	18.1

1 Mean score at baseline
2 Change from baseline to week 3 (LOCF)
3 Difference in change from baseline to week 3 endpoint (LOCF) between divalproex sodium and placebo

Divalproex Sodium was statistically significantly superior to placebo on all three measures of outcome.

Study 2: The second study enrolled adult patients who met Research Diagnostic Criteria for manic disorder and who were hospitalized for acute mania. Divalproex sodium was initiated at a dose of 250 mg three times daily and adjusted within a dose range of 750-2500 mg/day to achieve serum valproate concentrations in a range of 40-150 mcg/ml. Mean divalproex sodium doses for completers in this study were 1116, 1683, and 2006 mg/day at days 7, 14, and 21, respectively. Study 2 also included a lithium group for which lithium doses for completers were 1312, 1869, and 1984 mg/day at days 7, 14, and 21, respectively. Patients were assessed on the Manic Rating Scale (MRS; score ranges from 11-63), and the primary outcome measures were the total MRS score, and scores for two subscales of the MRS (*i.e.*, the Manic Syndrome Scale (MSS) and the Behavior and Ideation Scale (BIS)) Baseline scores and change from baseline in the week 3 endpoint (last-observation-carry-forward) analysis can be seen in TABLE 2.

TABLE 2 Study 2

Group	Baseline[1]	MRS Total Score BL to Day 21[2]	Difference[3]
Placebo	38.9	−4.4	
Lithium	37.9	−10.5	6.1
Divalproex Sodium	38.1	−9.5	5.1
Group	**Baseline[1]**	**MSS Total Score BL to Day 21[2]**	**Difference[3]**
Placebo	18.9	−2.5	
Lithium	18.5	−6.2	3.7
Divalproex Sodium	18.9	−6.0	3.5
Group	**Baseline[1]**	**BIS Total Score BL to Day 21[2]**	**Difference[3]**
Placebo	16.4	−1.4	
Lithium	16.0	−3.8	2.4
Divalproex Sodium	15.7	−3.2	1.8

1 Mean score at baseline
2 Change from baseline to day 21 (LOCF)
3 Difference in change from baseline to day 21 endpoint (LOCF) between divalproex sodium, lithium, and placebo

Divalproex sodium was statistically significantly superior to placebo on all three measures of outcome. An exploratory analysis for age and gender effects on outcome did not suggest any differential responsiveness on the basis of age or gender.

A comparison of the percentage of patients showing ≥ 30% reduction in the symptom score from baseline in each treatment group, separated by study is shown on the original patient package insert.

MIGRAINE

The results of two multicenter, double-blind, placebo-controlled clinical trials established the effectiveness of divalproex sodium in the prophylactic treatment of migraine headache.

Both studies employed essentially identical designs and recruited patients with a history of migraine with or without aura (of at least 6 months in duration) who were experiencing at least 2 migraine headaches a month during the 3 months prior to enrollment. Patients with cluster headaches were excluded. Women of childbearing potential were excluded entirely from one study, but were permitted in the other if they were deemed to be practicing an effective method of contraception.

In each study following a 4-week single-blind placebo baseline period, patients were randomized, under double blind conditions, to divalproex sodium or placebo for a 12-week treatment phase, comprised of a 4-week dose titration period followed by an 8-week maintenance period. Treatment outcome was assessed on the basis of 4-week migraine headache rates during the treatment phase.

In the first study, a total of 107 patients (24 M, 83 F), ranging in age from 26 to 73 were randomized 2:1, divalproex sodium to placebo. Ninety patients completed the 8-week maintenance period. Drug dose titration, using 250 mg tablets, was individualized at the investigator's discretion. Adjustments were guided by actual/sham trough total serum valproate levels in order to maintain the study blind. In patients on divalproex sodium doses ranged from 500 to 2500 mg a day. Doses over 500 mg were given in three divided doses. The mean dose during the treatment phase was 1087 mg/day resulting in a mean trough total valproate level of 72.5 mcg/ml, with a range of 31 to 133 mg/ml.

CLINICAL STUDIES: *(cont'd)*

The mean 4–week migraine headache rate during the treatment phase was 5.7 in the placebo group compared to 3.5 in the divalproex sodium group. These rates were significantly different.

In the second study, a total of 176 patients (19 males and 157 females), ranging in age from 17 to 76 years, were randomized equally to one of three divalproex sodium dose groups (500, 1000, or 1500 mg/day) or placebo. The treatments were given in two divided doses. One hundred thirty-seven patients completed the 8–week maintenance period. Efficacy was to be determined by a comparison of the 4–week migraine headache rate in the combined 1000/1500 mg/day group and placebo group.

The initial dose was 250 mg daily. The regimen was advanced by 250 mg every 4 days (8 days for 500 mg/day group), until the randomized dose was achieved. The mean trough total valproate levels during the treatment phase were 39.6, 62.5, and 72.5 mcg/ml in the divalproex sodium 500, 1000, and 1500 mg/day groups, respectively.

The mean 4–week migraine headache rates during the treatment phase, adjusted for differences in baseline rates, were 4.5 in the placebo group, compared to 3.3, 3.0, and 3.3 in the divalproex sodium 500, 1000, and 1500 mg/day groups, respectively, based on intent-to-treat results. Migraine headache rates in the combined divalproex sodium 1000/1500 mg group were significantly lower than in the placebo group.

EPILEPSY

The efficacy of divalproex sodium to reduce the incidence of complex partial seizures (CPS) that occur in isolation or in association with other seizure types was established in two controlled trials.

In one, a multiclinic, placebo controlled study employing an add-on design, 144 patients who continued to suffer eight or more CPS per 8 weeks during an 8 week period of monotherapy with doses of either carbamazepine or phenytoin sufficient to assure plasma concentrations within the "therapeutic range" were randomized to receive, in addition to their original antiepilepsy drug (AED), either divalproex sodium, or placebo. Randomized patients were to be followed for a total of 16 weeks. TABLE 3 presents the findings.

TABLE 3 Adjunctive Therapy Study

Add-On Treatment	Median Incidence of CPS Per 8 Weeks: Number of Patients	Baseline Incidence	Experimental Incidence
Divalproex Sodium	75	16.0	8.9*
Placebo	69	14.5	11.5

* Reduction from baseline statistically signigicantly greater for divalproex sodium than placebo at $p \leq 0.05$ level.

Figure 3 (available on manufacturer's original package insert) presents the proportion of patients whose percentage reduction from baseline in complex partial seizure rates was at least as great as those found in the adjunctive therapy study. A positive percent reduction indicates an improvement (*i.e.*, a decrease in seizure frequency), while a negative percent reduction indicates worsening. Thus, in a display of this type, the curve for an effective treatment is shifted to the left of the curve for placebo. Figure 3 shows that the proportion of patients achieving any particular level of improvement was treated with divalproex sodium had a ≥ 50% reduction in partial complex seizure rate compared to 23% of patients treated with placebo.

The second study assessed the capacity of divalproex sodium to reduce the incidence of CPS when administered as the sole AED. The study compared the incidence of CPS among patients randomized to either a high or low dose treatment arm. Patients qualified for entry into the randomized comparison phase of this study only if 1) they continued to experience 2 or more CPS per 4 weeks during an 8 to 12 week long period of monotherapy with adequate doses of an AED (*i.e.*, phenytoin, carbamazepine, phenobarbital, or primidone) and 2) they made a successful transition over a two week interval to divalproex sodium. Patients entering the randomized phase were then brought to their assigned target dose, gradually tapered off their concomitant AED and followed for an interval as long as 22 weeks. Less than 50% of the patients randomized, however, completed the study. In patients converted to divalproex sodium monotherapy, the mean total valproate concentrations during monotherapy were 71 and 123 mcg/ml in the low dose and high dose groups, respectively.

TABLE 4 presents the findings for all patients randomized who had at least one post-randomization assessment.

TABLE 4 Monotherapy Therapy Study

Treatment	Median Incidence of CPS Per 8 Weeks: Number of Patients	Baseline Incidence	Randomized Phase Incidence
High Dose Divalproex Sodium	131	13.2	10.7*
Low Dose Divalproex Sodium	134	14.2	13.8

* Reduction from baseline statistically significantly greater for high dose than low dose at $p \leq 0.05$ level.

Figure 4 (graphic available on the manufacturer's original package insert) presents the proportion of patients whose percentage reduction from baseline in complex partial seizure rates was at least as great as that indicated in the monotherapy study. A positive percent reduction indicates an improvement (*i.e.*, a decrease in seizure frequency), while a negative percent reduction indicates worsening. Thus, in a display of this type, the curve for a more effective treatment is shifted to the left of the curve for a less effective treatment. This figure shows that the proportion of patients achieving any particular level of reduction was consistently higher for high dose divalproex sodium than for low dose divalproex sodium. For example, when switching from carbamazepine, phenytoin, phenobarbital, or primidone monotherapy to high dose divalproex sodium monotherapy, 63% of patients experienced no change or a reduction in complex partial seizure rates compared to 54% of patients receiving low dose divalproex sodium.

INDICATIONS AND USAGE:

MANIA

Divalproex sodium is indicated for the treatment of the manic episodes associated with bipolar disorder. A manic episode is a distinct period of abnormally and persistently elevated, expansive, or irritable mood. Typical symptoms of mania include pressure of speech, motor hyperactivity, reduced need for sleep, flight of ideas, grandiosity, poor judgement, aggressiveness, and possible hostility.

The efficacy of divalproex sodium was established in 3-week trials with patients meeting DSM-III-R criteria for bipolar disorder who were hospitalized for acute mania (See CLINICAL STUDIES.)

The safety and effectiveness of divalproex sodium for long-term use in mania (*i.e.*, more than 3 weeks) has not been systematically evaluated in controlled clinical trials. Therefore, physicians who elect to use divalproex sodium for extended periods of time should continually re-evaluate the long term usefulness of the drug for the individual patient.

INDICATIONS AND USAGE: *(cont'd)*

EPILEPSY

Divalproex sodium is indicated as monotherapy and adjunctive therapy in the treatment of patients with complex partial seizures that occur either in isolation or in association with other types of seizures. Divalproex sodium is also indicated for use as sole and adjunctive therapy in the treatment of simple complex absence seizures, and adjunctively in patients with multiple seizure types that include absence seizures.

Simple absence is defined as very brief clouding of the sensorium or loss of consciousness, accompanied by certain generalized epileptic discharges without other detectable clinical signs. Complex absence is the term used when other signs are also present.

MIGRAINE

Divalproex sodium is indicated for the prophylaxis of migraine headaches. There is no evidence that divalproex sodium is useful in the acute treatment of migraine headaches. Because valproic acid may be a hazard to the fetus, divalproex sodium should be considered for women of childbearing potential only after this risk has been thoroughly discussed with the patient and weighed against the potential benefits of treatment (see WARNINGS, Usage in Pregnancy and Information for the Patient).

See WARNINGS) FOR STATEMENT REGARDING FATAL HEPATIC DYSFUNCTION.

CONTRAINDICATIONS:

DIVALPROEX SODIUM SHOULD NOT BE ADMINISTERED TO PATIENTS WITH HEPATIC DISEASE OR SIGNIFICANT DYSFUNCTION.

Divalproex sodium is contraindicated in patients with known hypersensitivity to the drug.

WARNINGS:

Hepatic failure resulting in fatalities has occurred in patients receiving valproic acid. These incidents usually have occurred during the first six months of treatment. Serious or fatal hepatotoxicity may be preceded by non-specific symptoms such as loss of seizure control, malaise, weakness, lethargy, facial edema, anorexia and vomiting. In patients with epilepsy, a loss of seizure control may also occur. Patients should be monitored closely for appearance of these symptoms. Liver function tests should be performed prior to therapy and at frequent intervals thereafter, especially during the first six months. However, physicians should not rely totally on serum biochemistry since these tests may not be abnormal in all instances, but should also consider the results of careful interim medical history and physical examination.

Caution should be observed when administering divalproex sodium products to patients with a prior history of hepatic disease. Patients on multiple anticonvulsants, children, those with congenital metabolic disorders, those with severe seizure disorders accompanied by mental retardation, and those with organic brain disease may be at particular risk. Experience has indicated that children under the age of two years are at a considerably increased risk of developing fatal hepatotoxicity, especially those with the aforementioned conditions. When divalproex sodium is used in this patient group, it should be used with extreme caution and as a sole agent. The benefits of therapy should be weighed against the risks. Above this age group, experience in epilepsy has indicated that the incidence of fatal hepatotoxicity decreases considerably in progressively older patient groups.

The drug should be discontinued immediately in the presence of significant hepatic dysfunction, suspected or apparent. In some cases, hepatic dysfunction has progressed in spite of discontinuation of drug.

The frequency of adverse effects (particularly elevated liver enzymes and thrombocytopenia (see PRECAUTIONS) may be dose-related. In a clinical trial of divalproex sodium as monotherapy in patients with epilepsy, 34/126 patients (27%) receiving approximately 50 mg/kg/day on average, had at least one value of platelets $\leq 75 \times 10^9/L$. Approximately half of these patients had treatment discontinued, with return of platelet counts to normal. In the remaining patients, platelet counts normalized with continued treatment. In this study, the probability of thrombocytopenia appeared to increase significantly at total valproate concentrations of ≥135 mcg/ml (males). The therapeutic benefit which may accompany the higher doses should therefore be weighed against the possibility of a greater incidence of adverse effects.

USAGE IN PREGNANCY

ACCORDING TO PUBLISHED AND UNPUBLISHED REPORTS, VALPROIC ACID MAY PRODUCE TERATOGENIC EFFECTS IN THE OFFSPRING OF HUMAN FEMALES RECEIVING THE DRUG DURING PREGNANCY.

THERE ARE MULTIPLE REPORTS IN THE CLINICAL LITERATURE WHICH INDICATE THAT THE USE OF ANTIEPILEPTIC DRUGS DURING PREGNANCY RESULTS IN AN INCREASED INCIDENCE OF BIRTH DEFECTS IN THE OFFSPRING. ALTHOUGH DATA ARE MORE EXTENSIVE WITH RESPECT TO TRIMETHADIONE, PARAMETHADIONE, PHENYTOIN, AND PHENOBARBITAL, REPORTS INDICATE A POSSIBLE SIMILAR ASSOCIATION WITH THE USE OF OTHER ANTIEPILEPTIC DRUGS.

THE INCIDENCE OF NEURAL TUBE DEFECTS IN THE FETUS MAY BE INCREASED IN MOTHERS RECEIVING VALPROATE DURING THE FIRST TRIMESTER OF PREGNANCY. THE CENTERS FOR DISEASE CONTROL (CDC) HAS ESTIMATED THE RISK OF VALPROIC ACID EXPOSED WOMEN HAVING CHILDREN WITH SPINA BIFIDA TO BE APPROXIMATELY 1 TO 2%.[1].

OTHER CONGENITAL ANOMALIES (*E.G.*, CRANIOFACIAL DEFECTS, CARDIOVASCULAR MALFORMATIONS AND ANOMALIES INVOLVING VARIOUS BODY SYSTEMS), COMPATIBLE AND INCOMPATIBLE WITH LIFE, HAVE BEEN REPORTED. SUFFICIENT DATA TO DETERMINE THE INCIDENCE OF THESE CONGENITAL ANOMALIES IS NOT AVAILABLE.

THE HIGHER INCIDENCE OF CONGENITAL ANOMALIES IN ANTIEPILEPTIC DRUG-TREATED WOMEN WITH SEIZURE DISORDERS CANNOT BE REGARDED AS A CAUSE AND EFFECT RELATIONSHIP. THERE ARE INTRINSIC METHODOLOGIC PROBLEMS IN OBTAINING ADEQUATE DATA ON DRUG TERATOGENICITY IN HUMANS; GENETIC FACTORS OR THE EPILEPTIC CONDITION ITSELF, MAY BE MORE IMPORTANT THAN DRUG THERAPY IN CONTRIBUTING TO CONGENITAL ANOMALIES.

PATIENTS TAKING VALPROATE MAY DEVELOP CLOTTING ABNORMALITIES. A PATIENT WHO HAD LOW FIBRINOGEN WHEN TAKING MULTIPLE ANTICONVULSANTS INCLUDING VALPROATE GAVE BIRTH TO AN INFANT WITH AFIBRINOGENEMIA WHO SUBSEQUENTLY DIED OF HEMORRHAGE. IF VALPROATE IS USED IN PREGNANCY, THE CLOTTING PARAMETERS SHOULD BE MONITORED CAREFULLY.

HEPATIC FAILURE, RESULTING IN THE DEATH OF A NEWBORN AND OF AN INFANT, HAVE BEEN REPORTED FOLLOWING THE USE OF VALPROATE DURING PREGNANCY.

Animal studies also have demonstrated valproate-induced teratogenicity. Increased frequencies of malformation, as well as intrauterine growth retardation and death, have been observed in mice, rats, rabbits, and monkeys following prenatal exposure to valproate. Malformations of the skeletal system are the most common structural abnormalities produced in experimental animals, but neural tube closure defects have been seen in mice exposed to

WARNINGS: *(cont'd)*

maternal plasma valproate concentrations exceeding 230 mcg/ml (2.3 times the upper limit of the human therapeutic range) during susceptible periods of embryonic development. Administration of an oral dose of 200 mg/kg/day or greater to pregnant rats during organogenesis produced malformations (skeletal, cardiac, and urogenital) and growth retardation in the offspring. These doses resulted in peak maternal plasma valproate levels of approximately 340 mcg/ml or greater (3.4 times the upper limit of the human therapeutic range or greater). Behavioral deficits have been reported in the offspring of rats given a dose of 200 mg/kg/day throughout most of the pregnancy. An oral dose of 350 mg/kg/day (approximately 2 times the maximum human daily dose on a mg/m^{2}basis) produced skeletal and visceral malformations in rabbits exposed during organogenesis. Skeletal malformations, growth retardation, and death were observed in rhesus monkeys following administration of an oral dose of 200 mg/kg/day during organogenesis. This dose resulted in peak maternal plasma valproate levels of approximately 280 mcg/ml (2.8 times the upper limit of the human therapeutic range).

The prescribing physician will wish to weigh the benefits of therapy against the risks in treating or counseling women of childbearing potential. If this drug is used during pregnancy, or if the patient becomes pregnant while taking this drug, the patient should be apprised of the potential hazard to the fetus.

Antiepileptic drugs should not be discontinued abruptly in patients in whom the drug is administered to prevent major seizures because of the strong possibility of precipitating status epilepticus with attendant hypoxia and threat to life. In individual cases where the severity and frequency of the seizure disorder are such that the removal of medication does not pose a serious threat to the patient, discontinuation of the drug may be considered prior to and during pregnancy, although it cannot be said with any confidence that even minor seizures do not pose some hazard to the developing embryo or fetus.

Tests to detect neural tube and other defects using current accepted procedures should be considered a part of routine prenatal care in childbearing women receiving valproate.

PRECAUTIONS:

HEPATIC DYSFUNCTION

See BOXED WARNING, CONTRAINDICATIONS and WARNINGS.

GENERAL

Because of reports of thrombocytopenia, inhibition of the secondary phase of platelet aggregation, and abnormal coagulation parameters (*e.g.,* low fibrinogen), platelet counts and coagulation tests are recommended before initiating therapy and at periodic intervals. It is recommended that patients receiving divalproex sodium be monitored for platelet count and coagulation parameters prior to planned surgery. In a clinical trial of divalproex sodium as monotherapy in patients with epilepsy, 34/126 patients (27%) receiving approximately 50 mg/kg/day on average, had at least one value of platelets $\leq 75 \times 10^9$ /L. Approximately half of these patients had treatment discontinued, with return of platelet counts to normal. In the remaining patients, platelet counts normalized with continued treatment. In this study, the probability of thrombocytopenia appeared to increase significantly at total valproate concentrations of $\geq$ 110 mcg/ml (females) or $\geq$ 135 mcg/ml (males). Evidence of hemorrhage, bruising or a disorder of hemostasis/coagulation is an indication for reduction of the dosage or withdrawal of therapy.

Hyperammonemia with or without lethargy or coma has been reported and may be present in the absence of abnormal liver function tests. Asymptomatic elevations of ammonia are more common and when present require more frequent monitoring. If clinically significant symptoms occur, divalproex sodium therapy should be modified or discontinued.

Since divalproex sodium may interact with concurrently administered drugs which are capable of enzyme induction, periodic plasma concentration determinations of valproate and concomitant drugs are recommended during the early course of therapy. (See DRUG INTERACTIONS.)

Valproate is partially eliminated in the urine as a keto-metabolite which may lead to a false interpretation of the urine ketone test.

There have been reports of altered thyroid function tests associated with valproate. The clinical significance of these is unknown.

Suicidal ideation may be a manifestation of certain psychiatric disorders, and may persist until significant remission of symptoms occurs. Close supervision of high risk patients should accompany initial drug therapy.

INFORMATION FOR PATIENTS

Since divalproex sodium products may produce CNS depression, especially when combined with another CNS depressant (*e.g.,* alcohol), patients should be advised not to engage in hazardous activities, such as driving an automobile or operating dangerous machinery, until it is known that they do not become drowsy from the drug.

Migraine Patients: Since divalproex sodium has been associated with certain types of birth defects, female patients of child-bearing age considering the use of divalproex sodium for the prevention of migraine should be advised to read the Patient Information Leaflet, which appears as the last section of the labeling.

CARCINOGENESIS, MUTAGENESIS, IMPAIRMENT OF FERTILITY

Carcinogenesis: Valproic acid was administered to Sprague Dawley rats and ICR (HA/ICR) mice at doses of 0, 80 and 170 mg/kg/day (approximately 10 to 50% of the maximum human daily dose on a mg/m^{2}basis) for two years. A variety of neoplasms were observed in both species. The chief findings were a statistically significant increase in the incidence of subcutaneous fibrosarcomas in high dose male rats receiving valproic acid and a statistically significant dose-related trend for benign pulmonary adenomas in male mice receiving valproic acid. The significance of these findings for humans is unknown.

Mutagenesis: Valproate was not mutagenic in an *in vitro* bacterial assay (Ames test), did not produce dominant lethal effects in mice, and did not increase chromosome aberration frequency in an *in vivo* cytogenic study in rats. Increased frequencies of sister chromatid exchange (SCE) have been reported in a study of epileptic children taking valproate, but this association was not observed in another study conducted in adults. There is some evidence that increased SCE frequencies may be associated with epilepsy. The biological significance of increase in SCE frequency is not known.

Impairment of Fertility: Chronic toxicity studies in juvenile and adult rats and dogs demonstrated reduced spermatogenesis and testicular atrophy at doses of 400 mg/kg/day or greater in rats (approximately equivalent to or greater than the maximum human daily dose on a mg/m^2 basis) and 150 mg/kg/day in dogs (approximately 1.4 times the maximum human daily dose or greater on a mg/kg/day basis). Segment I fertility studies in rats have shown doses up to 350 mg/kg/day for 60 days to have no effect on fertility. THE EFFECT OF VALPROATE ON TESTICULAR DEVELOPMENT AND ON SPERM PRODUCTION AND FERTILITY IN HUMANS IS UNKNOWN.

Pregnancy Category D: See WARNINGS.

Nursing Mothers: Valproate is excreted in breast milk. Concentrations in breast milk have been reported to be 1-10% of serum concentrations. It is not known what effect this would have on a nursing infant. Caution should be exercised when divalproex sodium is administered to a nursing woman.

PRECAUTIONS: *(cont'd)*

PEDIATRIC

Experience has indicated that children under the age of two years are at a considerably increased risk of developing fatal hepatotoxicity, especially those with the aforementioned conditions (See BOXED WARNING). When divalproex sodium is used in this patient group, it should be used with extreme caution and as a sole agent. The benefits of therapy should be weighed against the risks. Above the age of 2 years, experience in epilepsy has indicated that the incidence of fatal hepatotoxicity decreases considerably in progressively older patient groups.

Younger children, especially those receiving enzyme-inducing drugs, will require larger maintenance doses to attain targeted total and unbound valproic acid concentrations.

The variability in free fraction limits the clinical usefulness of monitoring total serum valproic acid concentrations. Interpretation of valproic acid concentrations in children should include consideration of factors that affect hepatic metabolism and protein binding.

The safety and effectiveness of divalproex sodium for the treatment of acute mania has not been studied in individuals below the age of 18 years.

The safety and effectiveness of divalproex sodium for the prophylaxis of migraines has not been studied in individuals below the age of 16 years.

The basic toxicology and pathologic manifestations of valproate sodium in neonatal (4-day old) and juvenile (14-day old) rats are similar to those seen in young adult rats. However, additional findings, including renal alterations in juvenile rats and renal alterations and retinal dysplasia in neonatal rats, have been reported. These findings occurred at 240 mg/kg/day, a dosage approximately equivalent to the human maximum recommended daily dose on a mg/m^2 basis. They were not seen at 90 mg/kg, or 40% of the maximum human daily dose on a mg/m^2 basis.

GERIATRIC

No patients above the age of 65 years were enrolled in double-blind prospective clinical trials of mania associated with bipolar illness. In a case review study of 583 patients, 72 patients (12%) were greater than 65 years of age. A higher percentage of patients above 65 years of age reported accidental injury, infection, pain, somnolence, and tremor. Discontinuation of valproate was occasionally associated with the latter two events. It is not clear whether these events indicate additional risk or whether they result from preexisting medical illness and concomitant medication use among these patients.

There is insufficient information available to discern the safety and effectiveness of divalproex sodium for the prophylaxis of migraines in patients over 65.

DRUG INTERACTIONS:

EFFECTS OF CO-ADMINISTERED DRUGS ON VALPROATE CLEARANCE

Drugs that effect the level of expression of hepatic enzymes, particularly those that elevate levels of glucuronosyl transferases, may increase the clearance of valproate. For example, phenytoin, carbamazepine, and phenobarbital (or primidone) can double the clearance of valproate. Thus, patients on monotherapy will generally have longer half-lives and higher concentrations than patients receiving polytherapy with antiepilepsy drugs.

In contrast, drugs that are inhibitors of cytochrome P450 isozymes (*e.g.,* antidepressants) may be expected to have little effect on valproate clearance because cytochrome P450 microsomal mediated oxidation is a relatively minor secondary metabolic pathway compared to glucuronidation and beta-oxidation.

Because of these changes in valproate clearance, monitoring of valproate and concomitant drug concentrations should be increased whenever enzyme inducing drugs are introduced or withdrawn

The following list provides information about the potential for an influence of several commonly prescribed medications on valproate pharmacokinetics. The list is not exhaustive, nor could it be, since new interactions are continuously being reported.

Drugs for which a potentially important interaction has been observed:

Aspirin: A study involving the co-administration of aspirin at antipyretic doses (11 to 16 mg/kg) with valproate to pediatric patients (n=6) revealed a decrease in protein binding and an inhibition of metabolism of valproate. Valproate free fraction was increased 4-fold in the presence of aspirin compared to valproate alone. The β-oxidation pathway consisting of 2-E-valproic acid, 3-OH-valproic acid, and 3-keto valproic acid was decreased from 25% of total metabolites excreted on valproate alone to 8.3% in the presence of aspirin. Caution should be observed if valproate and aspirin are to be co-administered.

Felbamate: A study involving the co-administration of 1200 mg/day of felbamate with valproate to patients with epilepsy (n=10) revealed an increase in mean valproate peak concentration by 35% (from 86 to 115 mcg/ml) compared to valproate alone. Increasing the felbamate dose to 2400 mg/day increased the mean valproate peak concentration to 133 mcg/ml (another 16% increase). A decrease in valproate dosage may be necessary when felbamate therapy is initiated.

Rifampin: A study involving the administration of a single dose of valproate (7 mg/kg) 36 hours after 5 nights of daily dosing with rifampin (600 mg) revealed a 40% increase in the oral clearance of valproate. Valproate dosage adjustment may be necessary when it is co-administered with rifampin.

Drugs for which either no interaction or a likely clinically unimportant interaction has been observed:

Antacids: A study involving the co-administration of valproate 500 mg with commonly administered antacids (Maalox, Trisogel, and Titralac—160 mEq doses) did not reveal any effect on the extent of absorption of valproate.

Chlorpromazine: A study involving the administration of 100 to 300 mg/day of chlorpromazine to schizophrenic patients already receiving valproate (200 mg twice daily) received a 15% increase in trough plasma levels of valproate.

Haloperidol: A study involving the administration of 6 to 10 mg/day of haloperidol to schizophrenic patients already receiving valproate (200 mg twice daily) revealed no significant changes in valproate trough plasma levels.

Cimetidine and Ranitidine: Cimetidine and ranitidine do not affect the clearance of valproate.

EFFECTS OF VALPROATE ON OTHER DRUGS

Valproate has been found to be a weak inhibitor of some P450 isozymes, epoxide hydrase, and glucuronyl tranferases.

The following list provides information about the potential for an influence of valproate co-administration on the pharmacokinetics or pharmacodynamics of several commonly prescribed medications. The list is not exhaustive, since new interactions are continuously being reported.

Drugs for which a potentially important valproate interaction has been observed:

Carbamazepine/carbamazepine-10,11-Epoxide: Serum levels of carbamazepine (CBZ) decreased 17% while that of carbamazepine -10,11-epoxide (CBZ-E) increased by 45% upon co-administration of valproate and CBZ to epileptic patients.

Clonazepam: The concomitant use of valproic acid and clonazepam may induce absence status in patients with a history of absence type seizures.

DRUG INTERACTIONS: *(cont'd)*

Diazepam: Valproate displaces diazepam from its plasma albumin binding sites and inhibits its metabolism. Co-administration of valproate (1500 mg daily) increased the free fraction of diazepam (10 mg) by 90% in healthy volunteers (n=6). Plasma clearance and volume of distribution for free diazepam were reduced by 25% and 20%, respectively, in the presence of valproate. The elimination half-life of diazepam remained unchanged upon addition of valproate.

Ethosuximide: Valproate inhibits the metabolism of ethosuximide. Administration of a single ethosuximide dose of 500 mg with valproate (800 to 1600 mg/day) to healthy volunteers (n=6) was accompanied by a 25% increase in elimination half-life of ethosuximide and a 15% decrease in its total clearance as compared to ethosuximide alone. Patients receiving valproate and ethosuximide, especially along with other anticonvulsants, should be monitored for alterations in serum concentrations of both drugs.

Lamotrigine: In a steady-state study involving 10 healthy volunteers, the elimination half-life of lamotrigine increased from 26 to 70 hours with valproate co-administration (a 165% increase). The dose of lamotrigine should be reduced when co-administered with valproate.

Phenobarbital: Valproate was found to inhibit the metabolism of phenobarbital. Co-administration of valproate (250 mg twice daily for 14 days) with phenobarbital to normal subjects (n=6) resulted in a 50% increase in half-life and a 30% decrease in plasma clearance of phenobarbital (60 mg single dose). The fraction of phenobarbital dose excreted unchanged increased by 50% in presence of valproate. There is evidence for severe CNS depression, with or without significant elevations of barbiturate or valproate serum concentrations. All patients receiving concomitant barbituate therapy should be closely monitored for neurologic toxicity. Serum barbituate concentrations should be obtained, if possible, and the barbituate dosage decreased, if appropriate.

Primidone: which is metabolized to a barbituate, may be involved in a similar interaction with valproate.

Phenytoin: Valproate displaces phenytoin from its plasma albumin binding sites and inhibits its hepatic metabolism. Co-administration of valproate (400 mg three times daily) with phenytoin (250 mg) in normal volunteers (n=7) was associated with a 60% increase in the free fraction of phenytoin. Total plasma clearance and apparent volume of distribution of phenytoin increased 30% in the presence of valproate. Both the clearance and apparent volume of distribution of free phenytoin were reduced by 25%. In patients with epilepsy, there have been reports of breakthrough seizures occurring with the combination of valproate and phenytoin. The dosage of phenytoin should be adjusted as required by the clinical situation.

Tolbutamide: From *in vitro* experiments, the unbound fraction of tolbutamide was increased from 20% to 50% when added to plasma samples taken from patients treated with valproate. The clinical relevance of this displacement is unknown.

Warfarin: In an *in vitro* study, valproate increased the unbound fraction of warfarin by up to 32.6%. The therapeutic relevance of this is unknown: however, coagulation tests should be monitored if divalproex sodium therapy is instituted in patients taking anticoagulants.

Zidovudine: In six patients who were seropositive for HIV, the clearance of zidovudine (100 mg every 8 hours) was decreased by 38% after administration of valproate (250 or 500 mg every 8 hours); the half-life of zidovudine was unaffected.

Drugs for which either no interaction or a likely clinically unimportant interaction has been observed:

Acetaminophen: Valproate had no effect on any of the pharmacokinetic parameters of acetaminophen when it was concurrently administered to three epileptic patients.

Amitriptyline/Nortriptyline: Administration of a single oral 50 mg dose of amitriptyline to 15 normal volunteers (10 males and 5 females) who received valproate (500 mg twice daily) resulted in a 21% decrease in plasma clearance of amitriptyline and a 34% decrease in the net clearance of nortriptyline.

Clozapine: In psychotic patients (n=11), no interaction was observed when valproate was co-administered with clozapine.

Lithium: Co-administration of valproate (500 mg twice daily) and lithium carbonate (300 mg twice daily) to normal male volunteers (n=16) had no effect on the steady-state kinetics of lithium.

Lorazepam: Concomitant administration of valproate (500 mg BID) and lorazepam (1 mg twice daily) in normal male volunteers (n=9) was accompanied by a 17% decrease in the plasma clearance of lorazepam.

Oral Contraceptive Steroids: Administration of a single dose of ethinyloestradiol (50 mcg)/ levonorgestrel (250 mcg) to 6 women on valproate (200 mg twice daily) therapy for 2 months did not reveal any pharmacokinetic interaction.

ADVERSE REACTIONS:

MANIA

The incidence of treatment-emergent events has been ascertained based on combined data from two placebo-controlled clinical trials of divalproex sodium in the treatment of manic episodes associated with bipolar disorder. The adverse events were usually mild or moderate in intensity, but sometimes were serious enough to interrupt treatment. In clinical trials, the rates of premature termination due to intolerance were not statistically different between placebo, divalproex sodium, and lithium carbonate. A total of 4%, 8%, and 11% of patients discontinued therapy due to intolerance in the placebo, divalproex sodium, and lithium carbonate groups, respectively.

TABLE 5 summarizes those adverse events reported for patients in these trials where the incidence rate in divalproex sodium-treated group was greater than 5% and greater than the placebo incidence, or where the incidence in the divalproex sodium-treated group was statistically greater than the placebo group. Vomiting was the only event that was reported by significantly ($p \leq 0.05$) more patients receiving divalproex sodium compared to placebo.

TABLE 5 Adverse Events Reported by > 5% of Divalproex Sodium-Treated Patients During Placebo-Controlled Trials of Acute Mania [1]

Adverse Event	Divalproex Sodium (n=89)	Placebo (n=97)
Nausea	22%	15%
Somnolence	19%	12%
Dizziness	12%	4%
Vomiting	12%	3%
Accidental Injury	11%	5%
Asthenia	10%	7%
Abdominal Pain	9%	8%
Dyspepsia	9%	8%
Rash	6%	3%

[1]The following adverse events occured at an equal or greater incidence for placebo than for divalproex sodium: back pain, headache, pain (unspecified), constipation, diarrhea, tremor, and pharyngitis.

ADVERSE REACTIONS: *(cont'd)*

The following additional adverse events were reported by greater than 1% but not more than 5% of the 89 divalproex sodium-treated patients in controlled clinical trials:

Body as a Whole: Chest pain, chills, chills and fever, cyst, fever, infection, neck pain, neck rigidity

Cardiovascular System: Hypertension, hypotension, palpitations, postural hypotension, tachycardia, vascular anomaly, vasodialation

Digestive System: Anorexia, fecal incontinence, flatulence gastroenteritis, glossitis, periodontal abscess

Hemic and Lymphatic System: Ecchymosis

Metabolic and Nutritional Disorders: Edema, peripheral edema

Musculoskeletal System: Arthralgia, arthrosis, leg cramps, twitching

Nervous System: Abnormal dreams, abnormal gait, agitation, ataxia, catatonic reaction, confusion, depression, diplopia, dysarthria, hallucinations, hypertonia, hypokinesia, insomnia, paresthesia, reflexes increased, tardive dyskinesia, thinking abnormalities, vertigo

Respiratory System: Dyspnea, rhinitis

Skin and Appendages: Alopecia, discoid lupus erythematosis, dry skin, furunculosis, masculopapular rash, seborrhea

Special Senses: Abnormal vision, amblyopia, conjunctivitis, deafness, dry eyes, ear disorder, ear pain, tinnitus

Urogenital System: Dysmenorrhea, dysuria, urinary incontinence.

MIGRAINE

Based on two placebo-controlled clinical trials and their long term extension, divalproex sodium was generally well tolerated with most adverse events rated as mild to moderate in severity. Of the 202 patients exposed to divalproex sodium in the placebo-controlled trials, 17% discontinued for intolerance. This is compared to a rate of 5% for the 81 placebo patients. Including the long term extension study, the adverse events reported as the primary reason for discontinuation by ≥ 1% of 248 divalproex sodium-treated patients were alopecia (6%), nausea and/or vomiting (5%), weight gain (2%), tremor (2%), somnolence (1%), elevated SGOT and/or SGPT (1%), and depression (1%).

TABLE 6 includes those adverse events reported for patients in the placebo-controlled trials where the incidence rate in the divalproex sodium-treated group was greater than 5% and was greater than that for placebo patients.

TABLE 6 Adverse Events Reported by >5% of Divalproex Sodium-Treated Patients During Migraine Placebo-Controlled Trials With a Greater Incidence Than Patients Taking Placebo [1]

Body System Event	Divalproex Sodium (N=202)	Placebo (N=81)
Gastrointestinal System		
Nausea	31%	10%
Dyspepsia	13%	9%
Diarrhea	12%	7%
Vomiting	11%	1%
Abdominal pain	9%	4%
Increased appetite	6%	4%
Nervous System		
Asthenia	20%	9%
Somnolence	17%	5%
Dizziness	12%	6%
Tremor	9%	0%
Other		
Weight gain	8%	2%
Back pain	8%	6%
Alopecia	7%	1%

[1]The following adverse events occurred in at least 5% of divalproex sodium-treated patients and at an equal or greater incidence for placebo than for divalproex sodium: flu syndrome, and pharyngitis.

The following additional adverse events were reported by greater than 1% but not more than 5% of the 202 divalproex sodium-treated patients in the controlled clinical trials:

Body as a Whole: Accidental injury, allergic reaction, chest pain, chills, face edema, fever, malaise, and neck pain.

Cardiovascular System: Vasodilation.

Digestive System: Anorexia, constipation, dry mouth, flatulence, gastrointestinal disorder (unspecified), and stomatitis.

Hemic and Lymphatic System: Ecchymosis.

Metabolic and Nutritional Disorders: Peripheral edema, SGOT increase, and SGPT increase.

Musculoskeletal System: Leg cramps and myalgia.

Nervous System: Abnormal dreams, amnesia, confusion, depression, emotional liability, insomnia, nervousness, paresthesia, speech disorder, thinking abnormalities, and vertigo.

Respiratory System: Cough increased, dyspnea, rhinitis, and sinusitis.

Skin and Appendages: Pruritus and rash.

Special Senses: Conjunctivitis, ear disorder, taste perversion, and tinnitus.

Urogenital System: Cystitis, metrorrhagia, and vaginal hemorrhage.

EPILEPSY

Based on a placebo controlled trial of adjunctive therapy for treatment of complex partial seizures, divalproex sodium was generally well tolerated with most adverse events rated as mild to moderate in severity. Intolerance was the primary reason for discontinuation in the divalproex sodium-treated patients (6%), compared to 1% of the placebo-treated patients.

TABLE 7 lists treatment-emergent adverse events which were reported by ≥5% of divalproex sodium-treated patients and for which the incidence was greater than in the placebo group, in the placebo-controlled trial of adjunctive therapy for treatment of complex partial seizures. Since patients were also treated with other antiepilepsy drugs, it is not possible, in most cases, to determine whether the following adverse events can be ascribed to divalproex sodium alone, or the combination of divalproex sodium and other antiepilepsy drugs.

TABLE 8 lists treatment-emergent adverse events which were reported by ≥5% of patients in the high dose divalproex sodium group, and for which the incidence was greater than in the low dose group, in a controlled trial of divalproex sodium monotherapy treatment of complex partial seizures. Since patients were being titrated off another antiepilepsy drug during the first portion of the trial, it is not possible, in many cases, to determine whether the following adverse events can be ascribed to divalproex sodium alone, or the combination of divalproex sodium and other antiepilepsy drugs.

The following additional adverse events were reported by greater than 1% but less than 5% of the 358 patients treated with divalproex sodium in the controlled trials of complex partial seizures:

Body as a Whole: Back pain, chest pain, malaise

ADVERSE REACTIONS: *(cont'd)*

TABLE 7 Adverse Events Reported by ≥5% of Patients Treated with Divalproex Sodium During Placebo-Controlled Trial of Adjunctive Therapy for Complex Partial Seizures

Body System/Event	Divalproex Sodium (%) (n=77)	Placebo (%) (n=70)
Body As A Whole		
Headache	31	21
Asthenia	27	7
Fever	6	4
Gastrointestinal System		
Nausea	48	14
Vomiting	27	7
Abdominal Pain	23	6
Diarrhea	13	6
Anorexia	12	0
Dyspepsia	8	4
Constipation	5	1
Nervous System		
Somnolence	27	11
Tremor	25	6
Dizziness	25	13
Diplopia	16	9
Amblyopia/Blurred Vision	12	9
Ataxia	8	1
Nystagmus	8	1
Emotional Lability	6	4
Thinking Abnormal	6	0
Amnesia	5	1
Respiratory System		
Flu Syndrome	12	9
Infection	12	6
Bronchitis	5	1
Rhinitis	5	4
Other		
Alopecia	6	1
Weight Loss	6	0

TABLE 8 Adverse Events Reported by ≥5% of Patients in the High Dose Group in the Controlled Trial of Divalproex Sodium Monotherapy for Complex Partial Seizures[1]

Body System/Event	High Dose (%) (n=131)	Low Dose (%) (n=134)
Body As A Whole		
Asthenia	21	10
Digestive System		
Nausea	34	26
Diarrhea	23	19
Vomiting	23	15
Abdominal Pain	12	9
Anorexia	11	4
Dyspepsia	11	10
Hemic/Lymphatic System		
Thrombocytopenia	24	1
Ecchymosis	5	4
Metabolic/Nutritional		
Weight Gain	9	4
Peripheral Edema	8	3
Nervous System		
Tremor	57	19
Somnolence	30	18
Dizziness	18	13
Insomnia	15	9
Nervousness	11	7
Amnesia	7	4
Nystagmus	7	1
Depression	5	4
Respiratory System		
Infection	20	13
Pharyngitis	8	2
Dyspnea	5	1
Skin and Appendages		
Alopecia	24	13
Special Senses		
Amblyopia/Blurred Vision	8	4
Tinnitus	7	1

1 Headache was the only adverse that occurred in ≥5% of patients in the high dose group and at equal or greater incidence in the low dose group.

Cardiovascular System: Tachycardia, hypertension, palpitation

Digestive System: Increased appetite, flatulence, hematemesis, eructation, pancreatitis, periodontal abscess

Hemic and Lymphatic System: Petechia

Metabolic and Nutritional Disorders: SGOT increased, SGPT increased

Musculoskeletal System: Myalgia, twitching, arthralgia, leg cramps, myasthenia

Nervous System: Anxiety, confusion, speech disorder, abnormal gait, paresthesia, hypertonia, incoordination, abnormal dreams, personality disorder

Respiratory System: Sinusitis, cough increased, pneumonia, epistaxis

Skin and Appendages: Rash, pruritus, dry skin

Special Senses: Taste perversion, abnormal vision, ear disorder, deafness, otitis media

Urogenital System: Urinary incontinence, vaginitis, dysmenorrhea, amenorrhea, urinary frequency

OTHER PATIENT POPULATIONS

Adverse reactions that have been reported with valproate from epilepsy trials, spontaneous reports, and other sources are listed below by body system.

Gastrointestinal: The most commonly reported side effects at the initiation of therapy are nausea, vomiting and indigestion. These effects are usually transient and rarely require discontinuation of therapy. Diarrhea, abdominal cramps and constipation have been reported. Both anorexia with some weight loss and increased appetite with weight gain have also been reported. The administration of delayed-release divalproex sodium may result in reduction of gastrointestinal side effects in some patients.

CNS Effects: Sedative effects have occurred in patients receiving valproate alone but occur most often in patients receiving combination therapy. Sedation usually abates upon reduction of other antiepileptic medication. Tremor (may be dose-related), hallucinations, ataxia, headache, nystagmus, diplopia, asterixis, "spots before eyes," dysarthria, dizziness, confusion

ADVERSE REACTIONS: *(cont'd)*

hypesthesia, vertigo, and incoordination. Rare cases of coma have occurred in patients receiving valproate alone or in conjunction with phenobarbital. In rare instances encephalopathy with fever has developed shortly after the introduction of valproate monotherapy without evidence of hepatic dysfunction or inappropriate plasma levels, all patients recovered after the drug was withdrawn. Several reports have noted reversible cerebral atrophy and dementia in association with valproate therapy.

Dermatologic: Transient hair loss, skin rash, photosensitivity, generalized pruritus and erythema multiforme, and Stevens-Johnson syndrome. Rare cases of toxic epidermal necrolysis have been reported including a fatal case in a six month old infant taking valproate and several other concomitant medications. An additional case of toxic epidermal necrosis resulting in death was reported in a 35 year old patient with AIDS taking several concomitant medications and had with a history of multiple cutaneous drug reactions.

Psychiatric: Emotional upset, depression, psychosis, aggression, hyperactivity and behavioral deterioration.

Musculoskeletal: Weakness.

Hematologic: Thrombocytopenia and inhibition of the secondary phase of platelet aggregation may be reflected in altered bleeding time, petechiae, bruising, hematoma formation and frank hemorrhage (see General and DRUG INTERACTIONS). Relative lymphocytosis, macrocytosis, hypofibrinogenemia, leukopenia, eosinophilia, anemia including macrocytic with or without folate deficiency, bone marrow suppression, pancytopenia, aplastic anemia, and acute intermittent porphyria.

Hepatic: Minor elevations of transaminases (*e.g.,* SGOT and SGPT) and LDH are frequent and appear to be dose-related. Occasionally, laboratory test results include increases in serum bilirubin and abnormal changes in other liver function tests. These results may reflect potentially serious hepatotoxicity (see WARNINGS).

Endocrine: Irregular menses, secondary amenorrhea, breast enlargement, galactorrhea, and parotid gland swelling. Abnormal thyroid function tests (see PRECAUTIONS).

Pancreatic: Acute pancreatitis including fatalities.

Metabolic: Hyperammonemia (see PRECAUTIONS), hyponatremia, and inappropriate ADH secretion. There have been rare reports on Fanconi's syndrome occurring chiefly in children. Decreased carnitine concentrations have been reported although the clinical relevance is undetermined. Hyperglycemia has occurred and was associated with a fatal outcome in a patient with preexistent nonketotic hyperglycinemia.

Genitourinary: Enuresis and urinary tract infection.

Special Senses: Hearing loss, either reversible or irreversible, has been reported; however, a cause and effect relationship has not been established. Ear pain has also been reported.

Other: Edema of the extremities, lupus erythematosus, bone pain, cough increased, pneumonia, otitis media, bradycardia, cutaneous vasculitis, and fever

OVERDOSAGE:

Overdosage with valproate may result in somnolence, heart block, and deep coma. Fatalities have been reported; however, patients have recovered from valproate levels as high as 2120 mcg/ml.

In overdose situations, the fraction of drug not bound to protein is high and hemodialysis or tandem hemodialysis plus hemoperfusion may result in significant removal of the drug. The benefit of gastric lavage or emesis will vary with the time since ingestion. General supportive measures should be applied with particular attention to the maintenance of adequate urinary output.

Naloxone has been reported to reverse the CNS depressant effects of valproate overdosage. Because naloxone could theoretically also reverse the antiepileptic effects of valproate, it should be used with caution in patients with epilepsy.

DOSAGE AND ADMINISTRATION:

MANIA

Divalproex sodium tablets are administered orally. The recommended initial dose is 750 mg daily in divided doses. The dose should be increased as rapidly as possible to achieve the lowest therapeutic dose which produces the desired clinical effect or the desired range of plasma concentrations. In placebo-controlled clinical trials of acute mania, patients were dosed to a clinical response with a trough plasma concentration between 50 and 125 mcg/ml. Maximum concentrations were generally achieved within 14 days. The maximum recommended dose is 60 mg/kg/day.

There is no body of evidence available from controlled trials to guide a clinician in the longer term management of a patient who improves during divalproex sodium treatment of an acute manic episode. While it is generally agreed that pharmacological treatment beyond an acute response in mania is desirable, both for maintenance of the initial response and for prevention of new manic episodes, there are no systematically obtained data to support the benefits of divalproex sodium in such longer-term treatment. Although there are no efficacy data that specifically address longer-term antimanic treatment with divalproex sodium, the safety of divalproex sodium in long-term use is supported by data from record reviews involving approximately 360 patients treated with divalproex sodium for greater than three months.

EPILEPSY

Divalproex sodium tablets are administered orally. Divalproex sodium has been studied as monotherapy and adjunctive therapy in complex partial seizures, and in simple and complex absence seizures in adults and adolescents. As the divalproex sodium dosage is titrated upward, concentrations of phenobarbital, carbamazepine, and/or phenytoin may be affected (see DRUG INTERACTIONS).

Complex Partial Seizures: For adults and children 10 years of age and older.

Monotherapy (Initial Therapy): Divalproex sodium has not been systematically studied as initial therapy. Patients should initiate therapy at 10 to 15 mg/kg/day. The dosage should be increased by 5 to 10 mg/kg/week to achieve optimal clinical response. Ordinarily, optimal clinical response is achieved at daily doses below 60 mg/kg/day. If unsatisfactory clinical response has not been achieved, plasma levels should be measured to determine whether or not they are in the usually accepted therapeutic range (50 to 100mcg/ml). No recommendation regarding the safety of valproate for use at doses above 60 mg/kg/day can be made.

The probability of thromocytopenia increases significantly at total trough valproate plasma concentrations above 100 mcg/ml in females and 135 mcg/ml in males. The benefit of improved seizure control with higher doses should be weighed against the possibility of a greater incidence of adverse reactions.

Conversion to Monotherapy: Patients should initiate therapy at 10 to 15 mg/kg/day. The dosage should be increased by 5 to 10 mg/kg/week to achieve optimal clinical response. Ordinarily, optimal clinical response is achieved at daily doses below 60 mg/kg/day. If satisfactory clinical response has not been achieved, plasma levels should be measured to determine whether or not they are in the usually accepted therapeutic range (50-100 mcg/ml). No recommendation regarding the safety of valproate for use at doses above 60 mg/kg/day can be made. Concomitant antiepilepsy drug (AED) dosage can ordinarily be reduced by approximately 25% every 2 weeks. This reduction may be started at initiation of divalproex sodium therapy, or delayed by 1 to 2 weeks if there is a concern that seizures are likely to

DOSAGE AND ADMINISTRATION: *(cont'd)*

occur with a reduction. The speed and duration of withdrawal of the concomitant AED can be highly variable, and patients should be monitored closely during his period for increased seizure frequency.

Adjunctive Therapy: Divalproex sodium may be added to the patient's regimen at a dosage of 10 to 15 mg/kg/day. The dosage may be increased by 5 to 10 mg/kg/week to achieve optimal clinical response. Ordinarily, optimal clinical response is achieved at daily doses below 60 mg/kg/day. If satisfactory clinical response has not been achieved, plasma levels should be measured to determine whether or not they are in the usually accepted therapeutic range (50 to 100 mcg/ml). No recommendation regarding the safety of valproate for the use at doses above 60 mg/kg/day can be made. If the total daily dose exceeds 250 mg, it should be given in divided doses.

In a study of adjunctive therapy for complex partial seizures in which patients were receiving either carbamazepine or phenytoin in addition to divalproex sodium, no adjustment of carbamazepine or phenytoin dosage was needed (see CLINICAL STUDIES.) However, since valproate may interact with these or other concurrently administered AEDs as well as other drugs (see DRUG INTERACTIONS), periodic plasma concentration determinations of concomitant AEDs are recommended during the early course of therapy (see DRUG INTERACTIONS.)

Simple and Complex Absence Seizures: The recommended initial dose is 15 mg/kg/day, increasing at one week intervals by 5 to 10 mg/kg/day until seizures are controlled or side effects preclude further increases. The maximum recommended dosage is 60 mg/kg/day. If the total daily dose exceeds 250 mg, it should be given in divided doses.

A good correlation has not been established between daily dose, serum concentrations, and therapeutic effect. However, therapeutic valproate serum concentrations for most patients with absence seizures is considered to range from 50 to 100 mcg/ml. Some patients may be controlled with lower or higher serum concentrations (see CLINICAL PHARMACOLOGY.)

As the divalproex sodium dosage is titrated upward, blood concentrations of phenobarbital and/or phenytoin may be affected (see PRECAUTIONS.)

Antiepilepsy drugs should not be abruptly discontinued in patients in whom the drug is administered to prevent major seizures because of the strong possibility of precipitating status elipticus with attendant hypoxia and threat to life.

In epileptic patients previously receiving divalproex sodium (valproic acid) therapy, divalproex sodium tablets should be initiated at the same daily dose and dosing schedule.

After the patient is stabilized on divalproex sodium tablets, a dosing schedule of two or three times daily may be elected in selected patients.

MIGRAINE

Divalproex sodium tablets are administered orally. The recommended starting dose is 250 mg twice daily. Some patients may benefit from doses up to 1000 mg/day. In the clinical trials, there was no evidence that higher doses led to greater efficacy.

GENERAL DOSING ADVICE

Dosing in Elderly Patients: Due to a decrease in unbound clearance of valproate, the starting dose should be reduced; the ultimate therapeutic dose should be achieved on the basis of clinical response.

Dose-Related Adverse Events: The frequency of adverse effected (particularly elevated liver enzymes and thrombocytopenia) may be dose-related. The probability of thrombocytopenia appears to increase significantly at total valproate concentrations of ≥110 mcg/ml (females) or ≥135 mcg/ml (males) (see PRECAUTIONS). The benefit of improved therapeutic effect with higher doses should be weighed against the possibility of a greater incidence of adverse reactions.

G.I. Irritation: Patients who experience G.I. irritation may benefit from administration of the drug with food or by slowly building up the dose from an initial low level.

REFERENCES:

1. Centers for Disease Control, Valproate: A New Cause of Birth Defects - Report from Italy and Follow-up from France, *Morbidity and Mortality Weekly Report* 32(33):438-439, August 26, 1983. 2. Wilder, BJ, et al, Gastrointestinal Tolerance of Divalproex Sodium, *Neurology* 33:808-811, June 1983. 3. Wilder, BJ, et al, Twice-Daily Dosing of Valproate with Divalproex, *Clin Pharmacol Ther* 34(4): 501-504, 1983.

PATIENT PACKAGE INSERT:

IMPORTANT INFORMATION FOR WOMEN WHO COULD BECOME PREGNANT, ABOUT THE USE OF DIVALPROEX SODIUM TABLETS FOR TREATMENT OF MIGRAINE

Please read this information carefully before you take divalproex sodium tablets. The following provides a summary of important information about taking divalproex sodium for migraine to women who could become pregnant. Divalproex sodium is also prescribed for uses other than those discussed here. If you have any questions or concerns, or want more information about divalproex sodium, contact your doctor or pharmacist.

Information For Women Who Could Become Pregnant: Divalproex sodium is used to prevent or reduce the number of migraines you experience. Divalproex sodium can be obtained only by prescription from your doctor. The decision to use divalproex sodium for the prevention of migraine is one that you and your doctor should make together, taking into account your individual needs and medical condition.

Before using divalproex sodium, women who can become pregnant should consider the fact that **Divalproex has been associated with birth defects, in particular, with spina bifida and other defects related to failure of the spinal canal to close normally. Although the incidence is unknown in migraine patients treated with divalproex sodium, approximately 1 to 2% of children born to women with epilepsy taking divalproex sodium in the first 12 weeks of pregnancy had these defects (based on data from the Centers for Disease Control and Prevention, and U.S. agency based in Atlanta). The incidence in the general population is 0.1 to 0.2%.**

Information For Women Who Are Planning to Get Pregnant: Women taking divalproex sodium for the prevention of migraine who are planning to get pregnant should discuss with their doctor temporarily stopping divalproex sodium, before and during their pregnancy.

Information For Women Who Become Pregnant While Taking Divalproex Sodium If you become pregnant while taking divalproex sodium for the prevention of migraine, you should contact your doctor immediately.

Other Important Information About Divalproex Sodium Tablets Divalproex sodium tablets should be taken exactly as it is prescribed by your doctor to get the most benefits from divalproex sodium and reduce the risk of side effects.

If you have taken more than the prescribed dose of divalproex sodium, contact your hospital emergency room or local poison center immediately.

This medication was prescribed for your particular condition. Do not use it for another condition or give the drug to others.

Facts About Birth Defects: It is important to know that birth defects may occur even in children of individuals not taking any medications or without any additional risk factors.

Facts About Migraine: About 23 million Americans suffer from migraine headaches. About 75% of migraine sufferers are women. A migraine is described as a throbbing headache that gets worse with activity. Migraine may also include nausea and/or vomiting as well as

PATIENT PACKAGE INSERT: *(cont'd)*

sensitivity to light and sound. Migraine usually happens about once a month, but some people may have them as often as once or twice a week. Often, the symptoms from a migraine can cause people to miss work or school. If you have frequent migraines, or if acute treatment is not working for you, your doctor may prescribe a preventative therapy. Preventative (prophylactic) treatment is used to prevent attacks and reduce the frequency and severity of headache events.

This summary provides important information about the use of divalproex sodium for migraine to women who could become pregnant. If you would like more information about the other potential risks and benefits of divalproex sodium, ask your doctor or pharmacist to let you read the professional labeling and then discuss it with them. If you have any questions or concerns about taking divalproex sodium, you should discuss them with your doctor.

PATIENT INFORMATION:

Divalproex sodium is used in the treatment of epilepsy, mania, and other conditions. Do not use if you are pregnant, nursing, or have liver disease. Avoid alcohol and other depressants. Inform your doctor if you are taking any other medications, including over-the-counter drugs. Divalproex Sodium may cause drowsiness. Use caution while driving or operating hazardous machinery. In addition, divalproex sodium may cause nausea, sleepiness, dizziness, vomiting, weakness, or stomach pain. Notify your doctor or pharmacist if these occur.

HOW SUPPLIED:

Depakote tablets are available as 125 mg tablets (salmon pink), 250 mg tablets (peach), and 500 mg tablets (lavender).

Recommended Storage: Store capsules below 77°F (25°C). Store tablets below 86°F (30°C)

HOW SUPPLIED - EQUIVALENTS NOT AVAILABLE:

Capsule, Enteric Coated - Oral - 125 mg

100's	$31.11	DEPAKOTE SPRINKLE 125, Abbott	00074-6114-13
100's	$32.89	DEPAKOTE SPRINKLE 125, Abbott	00074-6114-11

Tablet, Enteric Coated - Oral - 125 mg

100's	$30.95	DEPAKOTE, Abbott	00074-6212-13
100's	$32.73	DEPAKOTE, Abbott	00074-6212-11

Tablet, Enteric Coated - Oral - 250 mg

100's	$60.76	DEPAKOTE, Abbott	00074-6214-13
100's	$62.55	DEPAKOTE, Abbott	00074-6214-11
500's	$303.82	DEPAKOTE, Abbott	00074-6214-53

Tablet, Enteric Coated - Oral - 500 mg

100's	$112.08	DEPAKOTE, Abbott	00074-6215-13
100's	$113.86	DEPAKOTE, Abbott	00074-6215-11
500's	$560.38	DEPAKOTE, Abbott	00074-6215-53

DOBUTAMINE HYDROCHLORIDE *(001099)*

CATEGORIES: Atrial Fibrillation; Autonomic Drugs; Cardiac Decompression; Cardiovascular Drugs; Fibrillation; Inotropic Agents; Sympathomimetic Agents; Hypotension/Shock*; Sales > $100 Million; FDA Approval Pre 1982; Patent Expiration 1993 Oct

* Indication not approved by the FDA

BRAND NAMES: *Cardiject*; *Dobril*; *Dobuject* (Mexico); *Dobutamin Giulini* (Germany); *Dobutamin Hexal* (Germany); Dobutamine Hcl In Dextrose; Dobutamine Hcl W/Dextrose; *Dobutamin-Ratiopharm* (Germany); **Dobutrex**; *Inotrex*; *Oxiken* (Mexico); *Tobrex*

(International brand names outside U.S. in italics)

COST OF THERAPY: $7.50 (Cardiac Decompression; Injection; 12.5 mg/ml; 20/day; 1 days)

DESCRIPTION:

Dobutamine in 5% Dextrose Injection is a sterile, nonpyrogenic, prediluted solution of dobutamine hydrochloride and dextrose in water for injection. It is administered by intravenous infusion.

Each 100 ml contains dobutamine hydrochloride equivalent to 50 mg, 100 mg, 200 mg, or 400 mg of dobutamine; dextrose, hydrous 5 g in water for injection, with sodium metabisulfite 25 mg and edetate disodium, dihydrate 10 mg added as stabilizers; osmolar concentration, respectively, 260, 263, 270, or 284 mOsmol/liter (calc.). The pH is 3.0 (2.5 to 5.5). May contain hydrochloric acid and/or sodium hydroxide for pH adjustment. Dobutamine in 5% Dextrose Injection is oxygen sensitive.

Dobutamine Hydrochloride, USP is chemically designated (±)-4-[2-[[3-(p-hydroxyphenyl)-1-methylpropyl]amino]ethyl]-pyrocatechol hydrochloride. It is a synthetic catecholamine.

Dextrose, USP is chemically designated D-glucose monohydrate ($C_{16}H_{12}O_6 \cdot H_2O$), a hexose sugar freely soluble in water.

Water for Injection, USP is chemically designated H_2O.

The flexible plastic container is fabricated from a specially formulated nonplasticized, thermoplastic co-polyester (CR3). Water can permeate from inside the container into the overwrap but not in amounts sufficient to affect the solution significantly. Solutions inside the plastic container also can leach out certain of its chemical components in very small amounts before the expiration period has attained. However, the safety of the plastic has been confirmed by tests in animals according to USP biological standards for plastic containers.

CLINICAL PHARMACOLOGY:

Dobutamine is a direct-acting inotropic agent whose primary activity results from stimulation of the β-receptors of the heart while producing comparatively mild chronotropic, hypertensive, arrhythmogenic, and vasodilative effects. It does not cause the release of endogenous norepinephrine, as does dopamine. In animal studies, dobutamine produces less increase in heart rate and less decrease in peripheral vascular resistance for a given inotropic effect than does isoproterenol.

In patients with depressed cardiac function, both dobutamine and isoproterenol increase the cardiac output to a similar degree. In the case of dobutamine, this increase is usually not accompanied by marked increases in heart rate (although tachycardia is occasionally observed), and the cardiac stroke volume is usually increased. In contrast, isoproterenol increases the cardiac index primarily by increasing the heart rate while stroke volume changes little or declines.

Facilitation of atrioventricular conduction has been observed in human electrophysiologic studies and in patients with atrial fibrillation.

Systemic vascular resistance is usually decreased with administration of dobutamine. Occasionally, minimum vasoconstriction has been observed.

CLINICAL PHARMACOLOGY: *(cont'd)*

Most clinical experience with dobutamine is short-term-not more than several hours in duration. In the limited number of patients who were studied for 24, 48, and 72 hours, a persistent increase in cardiac output occurred in some, whereas output returned toward baseline values in others.

The onset of action of dobutamine in 5% dextrose injection is within 1 or 2 minutes; however, as much as 10 minutes may be required to obtain the peak effect of a particular infusion rate.

The plasma half-life of dobutamine in humans is 2 minutes. The principal routes of metabolism are methylation of the catechol and conjugation. In human urine, the major excretion products are the conjugates of dobutamine and 3-O-methyl dobutamine. The 3-O-methyl derivative of dobutamine is inactive.

Alteration of synaptic concentrations of catecholamines with either reserpine or tricyclic antidepressants does not alter the actions of dobutamine in animals, which indicates that the actions of dobutamine are not dependent on presynaptic mechanisms.

INDICATIONS AND USAGE:

Dobutamine in 5% Dextrose Injection is indicated when parenteral therapy is necessary for inotropic support in the short-term treatment of adults with cardiac decompensation due to depressed contractility resulting either from organic heart disease or from cardiac surgical procedures.

In patients who have atrial fibrillation with rapid ventricular response, a digitalis preparation should be used prior to institution of therapy with dobutamine.

CONTRAINDICATIONS:

Dobutamine in 5% Dextrose Injection is contraindicated in patients with idiopathic hypertrophic subaortic stenosis and in patients who have shown previous manifestations of hypersensitivity to dobutamine.

Dextrose solutions without electrolytes should not be administered simultaneously blood through the same infusion set because of the possibility that pseudoagglutination of red cells may occur.

WARNINGS:

1. Increase in Heart Rate or Blood Pressure: Dobutamine hydrochloride may cause a marked increase in heart rate or blood pressure, especially systolic pressure. Approximately 10% of patients in clinical studies have had rate increases of 30 beats/minute or more, and about 7.5% have had a 50-mm Hg or greater increase in systolic pressure. Usually, reduction of dosage promptly reverses these effects. Because dobutamine facilitates atrioventricular conduction, patients with a trial fibrillation are at risk of developing rapid ventricular response. Patients with preexisting hypertension appear to face an increased risk of developing an exaggerated pressor response.

2. Ectopic Activity: Dobutamine may precipitate or exacerbate ventricular ectopic activity, but it rarely has caused ventricular tachycardia.

3. Hypersensitivity: Reactions suggestive of hypersensitivity associated with administration of dobutamine in 5% Dextrose Injection, including skin rash, fever, eosinophilia, and bronchospasm, have been reported occasionally. Addictive medications should not be delivered via this solution.

4. Dobutamine in 5% Dextrose Injection contains sodium bisulfite, a sulfite that may cause allergic-type reactions, including anaphylactic symptoms and life-threatening or less severe asthmatic episodes in certain susceptible people. The overall prevalence of sulfite sensitivity in the general population is unknown and probably low. Sulfite sensitivity is seen more frequently in asthmatic than in nonasthmatic people.

PRECAUTIONS:

1. During the administration of Dobutamine in 5% Dextrose Injection Solution, as with any adrenergic agent, ECG and blood pressure should be continuously monitored. In addition, pulmonary wedge pressure and cardiac output should be monitored whenever possible to aid in the safe and effective infusion of Dobutamine in 5% Dextrose Injection.

2. Hypovolemia should be corrected with suitable volume expanders before treatment with Dobutamine in 5% Dextrose Injection is instituted.

3. Animal studies indicated that dobutamine may be ineffective if the patient has recently received a β-blocking drug. In such a case, peripheral vascular resistance may increase.

4. No improvement may be observed in the presence of marked mechanical obstruction, such as severe valvular aortic stenosis.

5. Dobutamine, like other β-agonists, can produced a mild reduction in serum potassium concentration, rarely to hypokalemic levels. Accordingly, consideration should be given to monitoring serum potassium.

6. Excess administration of potassium-free solutions may result in significant hypokalemia. The intravenous administration of these solutions can cause fluid and/or solute overloading resulting in dilution of serum electrolyte concentrations, overhydration, congested states or pulmonary edema.

7. Avoid bolus administration of the drug. (See DOSAGE AND ADMINISTRATION) Clinical evaluation and periodic laboratory determinations are necessary to monitor changes in fluid balance, electrolyte concentrations and acid-base balance during prolonged parenteral therapy or whenever the condition of the patient warrants such elevation. Solutions containing dextrose should be used with caution in patients with known subclinical or overt diabetes mellitus.

8. Dobutamine in 5% Dextrose Injection may exhibit a pink color that, if present, will increase with time. This color change is due to slight oxidation of the drug, but there is no significant loss of potency during the time of administration. Do not administer unless solution is clear and container is undamaged. Discard unused portion.

Usage Following Acute Myocardial Infarction: Clinical experience with dobutamine following myocardial infarction has been insufficient to establish the safety of drug for this use. There is concern that any agent that increases contractile force and heart rate may increase the size of an infarction by intensifying ischemia, but it is not known whether dobutamine does so.

Carcinogenesis, Mutagenesis, and Impairment of Fertility: Studies to evaluate the carcinogenic or mutagenic potential of dobutamine or the potential of the drug to affect fertility adversely have not been performed.

Pregnancy Category B: Reproduction studies performed in rats and rabbits have revealed no evidence of harm to the fetus due to dobutamine. The drug, however, has not been administered to pregnant women and should be used only when the expected benefits clearly outweigh the potential risks to the fetus.

Pediatric Use: The safety and effectiveness of Dobutamine in 5% Dextrose Injection for use in children have not been studied.

DRUG INTERACTIONS:

There was no evidence of drug interactions in clinical studies in which dobutamine hydrochloride was administered concurrently with other drugs, including digitalis preparations, furosemide, spironolactone, lidocaine, glyceryl trinitrate, isosorbide dinitrate, morphine, atropine, heparin, protamine, potassium chloride, folic acid, and acetaminophen. Preliminary studies indicate that the concomitant use of dobutamine and nitroprusside results in a higher cardiac output and, usually, a lower pulmonary wedge pressure than when either drug is used alone.

ADVERSE REACTIONS:

Increased Heart Rate, Blood Pressure, and Ventricular Ectopic Activity: A 10- to 20-mm increase in systolic blood pressure and an increase in heart rate of 5 to 15 beats/minute have been noted in most patients (see WARNINGS regarding exaggerated chronotropic and pressor effects). Approximately 5% of patients have had increased premature ventricular beats during infusions. These effects are dose related.

Hypotension: Precipitous decreases in blood pressure have occasionally been described in association with dobutamine therapy. Decreasing the dose or discontinuing the infusion typically results in rapid return of blood pressure to baseline values. In rare cases, however, intervention may be required and reversibility may not be immediate.

Reactions at Sites of Intravenous Infusion: Phlebitis has occasionally been reported. Local inflammatory changes have been described following inadvertent infiltration.

Miscellaneous Uncommon Effects: The following adverse effects have been reported in 1% to 3% of patients: nausea, headache, anginal pain, nonspecific chest pain, palpitations, and shortness of breath.

Administration of dobutamine, like other catecholamines, can produce a mild reduction in serum potassium concentrations, rarely to hypokalemic levels (see PRECAUTIONS.)

Longer-Term Safety: Infusions of up to 72 hours have revealed no adverse effects other than those seen with shorter infusions.

OVERDOSAGE:

Overdoses of dobutamine have been reported rarely. The following is provided to serve as a guide if such an overdose is encountered.

Signs and Symptoms: Toxicity from dobutamine hydrochloride is usually due to excessive cardiac β-receptor stimulation. The duration of action of Dobutamine hydrochloride is generally short ($T_{1/2}$ = 2 minutes) because it is rapidly metabolized by catechol-O-methyltransferase. The symptoms of toxicity may include anorexia, nausea, vomiting, tremor, anxiety, palpitations, headache, shortness of breath, and anginal and nonspecific chest pain. The positive inotropic and chronotropic effects of Dobutamine on the myocardium may cause hypertension, tachyarrhythmias, myocardial ischemia, and ventricular fibrillation. Hypotension may result from vasodilation.

If the product is ingested, unpredictable absorption may occur from the mouth and the gastrointestinal tract.

Treatment: To obtain up-to-date information about the treatment of overdose, a good resource is your certified Regional Poison Control Center. Telephone numbers of certified poison control centers are listed in the *Physicians GenRx*. In managing overdosage, consider the possibility of multiple drug overdosage, interaction among drugs, and unusual drug kinetics in your patient.

The initial actions to be taken in a dobutamine hydrochloride overdose are discontinuing administration, establishing an airway, and ensuring oxygenation and ventilation. Resuscitative measures should be initiated promptly. Severe ventricular tachyarrhythmias may be successfully treated with propranolol or lidocaine. Hypertension usually responds to a reduction in dose or discontinuation of therapy.

Protect the patient's airway and support ventilation and perfusion. If needed, meticulously monitor and maintain, within acceptable limits, the patient's vital signs, blood gases, serum electrolytes, etc. Absorption of drugs from the gastrointestinal tract may be decreased by giving activated charcoal, which, in many cases, is more effective than emesis or lavage; consider charcoal instead of or in addition to gastric emptying. Repeated doses of charcoal over time may hasten elimination of some drugs that have been absorbed. Safeguard the patient's airway when employing gastric emptying or charcoal.

Forced diuresis, peritoneal dialysis, hemodialysis, or charcoal hemoperfusion have not been established as beneficial for an overdose of dobutamine hydrochloride.

DOSAGE AND ADMINISTRATION:

Do NOT add sodium bicarbonate or other alkalinizing substance, since dobutamine is inactivated in alkaline solution. Dobutamine in 5% Dextrose Injection is administered only intravenously via a suitable catheter or needle infusion. The less concentrated 0.5 mg/ml solution may be preferred when fluid expansion is not a problem. The more concentrated 1 mg/ml, 2 mg/ml, or 4 mg/ml solutions may be preferred in patients with fluid retention or when a slower rate of infusion is desired.

Recommended Dosage: The rate of infusion needed to increase cardiac output usually ranged from 2.5 to 15 mcg/kg/min. On rare occasions, infusion rates up to 40 mcg/kg/min have been required to obtain the desired effect.

Rate of Administration: When administering dobutamine (or any potent medication) by continuous intravenous infusion, it is advisable to use a precision volume control IV set.

Each patient must be individually titrated to the desired hemodynamic response to dobutamine. The rate of administration and the duration of therapy should be adjusted according to the patient's response as determined by heart rate, presence of ectopic activity, blood pressure, urine flow, and, whenever possible, measurement of central venous or pulmonary wedge pressure and cardiac output.

As with all potent intravenously administered drugs, care should be taken to control the rate of infusion so as to avoid inadvertent administration of a bolus of the drug.

Parenteral drug products should be visually inspected for particulate matter and discoloration prior to administration, whenever solution and container permit (see PRECAUTIONSand TABLE 1 throughTABLE 4.

TABLE 1 Dobutamine Infusion Rate (ml/hr) Chart Using 500 mcg/ml Concentration

	Patient Body Weight (kg)									
*	30	40	50	60	70	80	90	100	110	120
2.5	9	12	15	18	21	24	27	30	33	36
5	18	24	30	36	42	48	54	60	66	72
7.5	27	36	45	54	63	72	81	90	99	108
10	36	48	60	72	84	96	108	120	132	144
12.5	45	60	75	90	105	120	135	150	165	180
15	54	72	90	108	126	144	162	180	198	216
17.5	63	84	105	126	147	168	189	210	231	252

*Infusion rate (mcg/kg/min)

DOSAGE AND ADMINISTRATION: *(cont'd)*

TABLE 2 Dobutamine Infusion Rate (ml/hr) Chart Using 1000 mcg/ml Concentration

	Patient Body Weight (kg)									
*	30	40	50	60	70	80	90	100	110	120
2.5	4.5	6	7.5	9	10.5	12	13.5	15	16.5	18
5	9	12	15	18	21	24	27	30	33	36
7.5	13.5	18	22.5	27	31.5	36	40.5	45	49.5	54
10	18	24	30	36	42	48	54	60	66	72
12.5	22.5	30	37.5	45	52.5	60	67.5	75	82.5	90
15	27	36	45	54	63	72	81	90	99	108
17.5	31.5	42	52.5	63	73.5	84	94.5	105	115.5	126

*Infusion rate (mcg/kg/min)

TABLE 3A Dobutamine Infusion Rate (ml/hr) Chart Using 2000 mcg/ml Concentration

	Patient Body Weight (kg)				
Infusion rate (mcg/kg/min)	30	40	50	60	70
2.5	2.25	3	3.75	4.5	5.25
5	4.5	6	7.5	9	10.5
7.5	6.75	9	11.25	13.5	15.75
10	9	12	15	18	21
12.5	11.25	15	18.75	22.5	26.25
15	13.5	18	22.5	27	31.5
17.5	15.75	21	26.25	31.5	36.75

TABLE 3B Dobutamine Infusion Rate (ml/hr) Chart Using 2000 mcg/ml Concentration

	Patient Body Weight (kg)				
Infusion rate (mcg/kg/min)	80	90	100	110	120
2.5	6	6.75	7.5	8.25	9
5	12	13.5	15	16.5	18
7.5	18	20.25	22.5	24.75	27
10	24	27	30	33	36
12.5	30	33.75	37.5	41.25	45
15	36	40.5	45	49.5	54
17.5	42	47.25	52.5	57.75	63

TABLE 4A Dobutamine Infusion Rate (ml/hr) Chart Using 4000 mcg/ml Concentration

	Patient Body Weight (kg)				
Infusion rate (mcg/kg/min)	30	40	50	60	70
2.5	1.125	1.5	1.875	2.25	2.625
5	2.25	3	3.75	4.5	5.25
7.5	3.375	4.5	5.625	6.75	7.875
10	4.5	6	7.5	9	10.5
12.5	5.625	7.5	9.375	11.25	13.125
15	6.75	9	11.25	13.5	15.75
17.5	7.875	10.5	13.125	15.75	18.375

TABLE 4B Dobutamine in 5% Dextrose Injection, Adverse Reactions Dobutamine Infusion Rate (ml/hr) Chart Using 4000 mcg/ml Concentration

	Patient Body Weight (kg)				
Infusion rate (mcg/kg/min)	80	90	100	110	120
2.5	3	3.375	3.75	4.125	4.5
5	6	6.75	7.5	8.25	9
7.5	9	10.125	11.25	12.375	13.5
10	12	13.5	15	16.5	18
12.5	15	16.875	18.75	20.625	22.5
15	18	20.25	22.5	24.75	27
17.5	21	23.625	26.25	28.875	31.5

INSTRUCTIONS FOR USE

To Open: Tear outer wrap at notch and remove solution container. Some opacity of the plastic due to moisture absorption during the sterilization process may be observed. This is normal and does not affect the solution quality or safety. The opacity will diminish gradually.

PREPARATION FOR ADMINISTRATION (USE ASEPTIC TECHNIQUE)

1. Close flow control clamp of administration set.

2. Remove cover from outlet port at bottom of container.

3. Insert piercing pin of administration set into port with a twisting motion until the set is firmly seated. **Note:** See full directions on administration set carton.

4. Suspend container from hanger.

5. Squeeze and release drip chamber to establish proper fluid level in chamber.

6. Open flow control clamp and clear air from set. Close clamp.

7. Attach set to venipuncture device. If device is not indwelling, prime and make venipuncture.

8. Regulate rate of administration with flow control clamp.

WARNING: Do not use flexible container in series connections.

HOW SUPPLIED:

Dobutamine in 5% Dextrose Injection is supplied in 250 and 500 ml LifeCare flexible containers.

Exposure of pharmaceutical products to heat should be minimized.

Avoid excessive heat. Protect from freezing. It is recommended that the product be stored at room temperature (25°C); however, brief exposure up to 40°C does not adversely affect the product.

(Abbott Laboratories, 06-9106-R3-Rev. 7/94)

HOW SUPPLIED - RATED THERAPEUTICALLY EQUIVALENT:

Injection, Dry-Soln - Intravenous - 12.5 mg/ml

20 ml	$7.50	Dobutamine Hydrochloride, Astra USA	00186-1931-01
20 ml	$21.00	DOBUTAMINE HYDROCHLORIDE, Bedford Labs	55390-0560-20
20 ml	$43.15	Dobutamine Hcl, Schein Pharm (US)	00364-3031-55
20 ml	$44.52	Dobutamine Hydrochloride, Abbott	00074-2344-02
20 ml	$47.06	Dobutamine Hydrochloride, Abbott	00074-2344-01

HOW SUPPLIED - RATED THERAPEUTICALLY EQUIVALENT: *(cont'd)*

20 ml	$47.56	Dobutamine Hydrochloride, Gensia Labs	00703-1815-03
20 ml x 1	**$12.00**	**DOBUTREX, Lilly**	**00002-7175-01**
20 ml x 10	$75.00	Dobutamine Hydrochloride, Astra USA	00186-1931-03
20 ml x 10	**$120.00**	**DOBUTREX, Lilly**	**00002-7175-10**
20 ml x 10	$125.00	Dobutamine Hydrochloride, Sanofi Winthrop	00024-0593-01

Injection, Dry-Soln - Intravenous - 500 mcg/ml

250 ml x 12	$724.17	DOBUTAMINE HCL W/DEXTROSE, Abbott	00074-2345-32
250 ml x 12	$838.74	DOBUTAMINE HCL W/DEXTROSE, Abbott	00074-2345-34
500 ml	$49.72	DOBUTAMINE HCL IN DEXTROSE, Baxter Hlthcare	00338-1071-03

Injection, Dry-Soln - Intravenous - 1000 mcg/ml

250 ml	$49.72	DOBUTAMINE HCL IN DEXTROSE, Baxter Hlthcare	00338-1073-02
250 ml x 12	$800.55	DOBUTAMINE HCL W/DEXTROSE, Abbott	00074-2346-32
500 ml	$86.07	DOBUTAMINE HCL IN DEXTROSE, Baxter Hlthcare	00338-1073-03
500 ml x 12	$1518.90	DOBUTAMINE HCL W/DEXTROSE, Abbott	00074-2346-34

Injection, Dry-Soln - Intravenous - 2000 mcg/ml

250 ml	$86.07	DOBUTAMINE HCL IN DEXTROSE, Baxter Hlthcare	00338-1075-02
250 ml x 12	$1480.71	DOBUTAMINE HCL W/DEXTROSE, Abbott	00074-2347-32

Injection, Dry-Soln - Intravenous - 4000 mcg/ml

250 ml	$145.42	DOBUTAMINE HCL IN DEXTROSE, Baxter Hlthcare	00338-1077-02
250 ml	$1601.13	Dobutamine HCl In Dextrose, Abbott	00074-3724-32

HOW SUPPLIED - NOT RATED EQUIVALENT:

Injection, Dry-Soln - Intravenous - 500 mcg/ml

500 ml x 12	$379.38	Dobutamine Hcl In Dextrose, Lilly	00002-7497-01

Injection, Dry-Soln - Intravenous - 1000 mcg/ml

250 ml x 18	$544.32	Dobutamine Hcl In Dextrose, Lilly	00002-7496-01
500 ml x 12	$673.92	Dobutamine Hcl In Dextrose, Lilly	00002-7499-01

Injection, Dry-Soln - Intravenous - 2000 mcg/ml

250 ml x 18	$984.96	Dobutamine Hcl In Dextrose, Lilly	00002-7498-01

Injection, Dry-Soln - Intravenous - 4000 mcg/ml

250 ml x 18	$1795.01	Dobutamine Hcl In Dextrose, Lilly	00002-7500-01

DOCETAXEL *(003205)*

CATEGORIES: Antineoplastics; Breast Carcinoma; Cancer; Chemotherapy; Oncologic Drugs; Tumors; FDA Approved 1996 May

BRAND NAMES: **Taxotere**

WARNING:

Docetaxel for Injection Concentrate should be administered under the supervision of a qualified physician experienced in the use of antineoplastic agents. Appropriate management of complications is possible only when adequate diagnostic and treatment facilities are readily available.

The incidence of treatment-related mortality associated with docetaxel therapy is increased in patients with abnormal liver function and in patients receiving higher doses (see WARNINGS).

Docetaxel should generally not be given to patients with bilirubin > upper limit of normal (ULN), or to patients with SGOT and/or SGPT > 1.5 x ULN concomitant with alkaline phosphatase > 2.5 x ULN. Patients with elevations of bilirubin or abnormalities of transaminase concurrent with alkaline phosphatase are at increased risk for the development of grade 4 neutropenia, febrile neutropenia, infections, severe thrombocytopenia, severe stomatitis, severe skin toxicity, and toxic death. Patients with isolated elevations of transaminase > 1.5 x ULN also had a higher rate of febrile neutropenia grade 4 but did not have an increased incidence of toxic death. Bilirubin, SGOT or SGPT, and alkaline phosphatase values should be obtained prior to each cycle of docetaxel therapy and reviewed by the treating physician.

Docetaxel therapy should not be given to patients with neutrophil counts of < 1500 cells/mm^3. In order to monitor the occurrence of neutropenia, which may be severe and result in infection, frequent blood cell counts should be performed on all patients receiving docetaxel.

Severe hypersensitivity reactions characterized by hypotension and/or bronchospasm, or generalized rash/erythema occurred in 0.9% of patients who received the recommended dexamethasone premedication. Hypersensitivity reactions requiring discontinuation of the docetaxel infusion were reported in five patients who did not receive premedication. These reactions resolved after discontinuation of the infusion and the administration of appropriate therapy. Docetaxel must not be given to patients who have a history of severe hypersensitivity reactions to docetaxel or to other drugs formulated with polysorbate 80.

Severe fluid retention occurred in 6% of patients despite use of a 5-day dexamethasone premedication regimen. It was characterized by one or more of the following events: poorly tolerated peripheral edema, generalized edema, pleural effusion requiring urgent drainage, dyspnea at rest, cardiac tamponade, or pronounced abdominal distention (due to ascites).

DESCRIPTION:

Docetaxel is an antineoplastic agent belonging to the taxoid family. It is prepared by semisynthesis beginning with a precursor extracted from the renewable needle biomass of yew plants. The chemical name for docetaxel is (2R,3S)-N-carboxy-3-phenylisoserine,N-*tert*-butyl ester,13-ester with 5β-20-epoxy-1,2α, 4,7β,10β,13α -hexahydroxytax-11 -en-9-one 4-acetate 2-benzoate, trihydrate.

Docetaxel is a white to almost-white powder with an empirical formula of $C_{43}H_{53}NO_{14} \cdot 3H_2O$, and a molecular weight of 861.9. It is highly lipophilic and practically insoluble in water. Docetaxel for Injection Concentrate is a clear yellow to brownish-yellow viscous solution. Taxotere is sterile, non-pyrogenic, and is available in single-dose vials containing 20 mg (0.5 mL) or 80 mg (2.0 mL) docetaxel (anhydrous). Each mL contains 40 mg docetaxel (anhydrous) and 1040 mg polysorbate 80. Taxotere for Injection Concentrate requires dilution

DESCRIPTION: *(cont'd)*

prior to use. A sterile, non-pyrogenic, single-dose diluent is supplied for that purpose. The diluent for docetaxel contains 13% ethanol in Water for Injection, and is supplied in 1.5 mL (to be used with 20 mg docetaxel for Injection Concentrate) and 6.0 mL (to be used with 80 mg docetaxel for Injection Concentrate) vials.

CLINICAL PHARMACOLOGY:

Docetaxel is an antineoplastic agent that acts by disrupting the microtubular network in cells that is essential for mitotic and interphase cellular functions. Docetaxel binds to free tubulin and promotes the assembly of tubulin into stable microtubules while simultaneously inhibiting their disassembly. This leads to the production of microtubule bundles without normal function and to the stabilization of microtubules, which results in the inhibition of mitosis in cells. Docetaxel's binding to microtubules does not alter the number of protofilaments in the bound microtubules, a feature which differs from most spindle poisons currently in clinical use.

HUMAN PHARMACOKINETICS

The pharmacokinetics of docetaxel have been evaluated in cancer patients after administration of 20 - 115 mg/m^2 in phase I studies. The area under the curve (AUC) was dose proportional following doses of 70 - 115 mg/m^{2}with infusion times of one to two hours. Docetaxel's pharmacokinetic profile is consistent with a three-compartment pharmacokinetic model, with half-lives for the α, β, and γ phases of 4 min, 36 min, and 11.1 hr, respectively. The initial rapid decline represents distribution to the peripheral compartments and the late (terminal) phase is due, in part, to a relatively slow efflux of docetaxel from the peripheral compartment. Mean values for total body clearance and steady state volume of distribution were 21 L/h/m^2 and 113 L, respectively. Mean total body clearance for Japanese patients dosed at the range of 10-90 mg/m^2 was similar to that of European/American populations dosed at 100 mg/m^2, suggesting no significant difference in the elimination of docetaxel in the two populations.

A study of ^{14}C-docetaxel was conducted in three cancer patients. Docetaxel was eliminated in both the urine and feces following oxidative metabolism of the tert-butyl ester group, but fecal excretion was the main elimination route. Within seven days, urinary and fecal excretion accounted for approximately 6% and 75% of the administered radioactivity, respectively. About 80% of the radioactivity recovered in feces is excreted during the first 48 hours as one major and 3 minor metabolites with very small amounts (less than 8%) of unchanged drug. Based on *in vitro* studies, isoenzymes of the cytochrome P4503A (CYP 3A) subfamily appear to be involved in docetaxel metabolism.

A population pharmacokinetic analysis was carried out after docetaxel treatment of 535 patients dosed at 100 mg/m^2. Pharmacokinetic parameters estimated by this analysis were very close to those estimated from phase I studies. The pharmacokinetics of docetaxel were not influenced by age or gender and docetaxel total body clearance was not modified by pretreatment with dexamethasone. In patients with clinical chemistry data suggestive of mild to moderate liver function impairment (SGOT and/or SGPT > 1.5 times the upper limit of normal (ULN) concomitant with alkaline phosphatase > 2.5 times ULN), total body clearance was lowered by an average of 27%, resulting in a 38% increase in systemic exposure (AUC). This average, however, includes a substantial range and there is, at present, no measurement that would allow recommendation for dose adjustment in such patients. Patients with combined abnormalities of transaminase and alkaline phosphatase should, in general, not be treated with docetaxel.

In vitro studies showed that docetaxel is about 94% protein bound, mainly to α_1-acid glycoprotein, albumin, and lipoproteins. In three cancer patients, the*in vitro* binding to plasma proteins was found to be approximately 97%. Dexamethasone does not affect the protein binding of docetaxel.

CLINICAL STUDIES:

The efficacy and safety of docetaxel has been evaluated in advanced breast carcinoma patients in independent clinical studies at doses of 100, 75, and 60 mg/m^2.

Safety and Efficacy at 100 mg/m^2: The safety and efficacy of docetaxel have been evaluated in three phase II studies which were conducted in a total of 134 patients with anthracycline-resistant, locally advanced or metastatic breast carcinoma. Anthracycline resistance was defined as progressive disease on anthracyclines for advanced disease or relapse on anthracycline adjuvant therapy. In these studies, docetaxel was administered at a 100 mg/m^2 dose given as a one-hour infusion every 3 weeks.

The overall response rate (ORR) considering all patients (intent-to-treat) was 41% and the complete response (CR) was 2%. The median survival time was 43 weeks. In the evaluable patients (see TABLE 1), the ORR was 47% and the CR was 2.8%. Overall response rates (ORR), duration of response, and time to progression are shown in TABLE 1.

TABLE 1 Efficacy of Docetaxel In Anthracycline-Resistant Breast Cancer Patients Treated At 100 mg/m^2

Overall Response Rates		**(95% C.I.)**
Intent-to-Treat Patients (n=34)	41%	(33-49)
Evaluable Patients (n=106)*	47%	(38-57)
Response Rate in Patients with Visceral Involvement		
Intent-to-Treat Patients (n=95)	37%	
Evaluable Patients (n=76)*	43%	
Median Response Duration**	6 months	(2.1-17.5)
Median Time to Progression**	4 months	(0.2-17.5)
Median Survival**	10 months	(0.2-24.6+)
1 Year Survival**	43%	

* Evaluable patients include those meeting the study eligibility requirements and having received at least two cycles of docetaxel unless disease progression occurred earlier.
** Intent-to-treat population.

For the 134 anthracycline-resistant breast cancer patients who received docetaxel, 127 had normal LFTs (see TABLE 2 for definition) at baseline, and 7 had elevated LFTs at baseline. Patients with elevated LFTs at baseline had an increased incidence of thrombocytopenia, infection, febrile neutropenia, and death considered at least possibly treatment related. TABLE 2 shows the incidence of important hematologic adverse events during the study.

TABLE 3shows important non-hematologic adverse events for the anthracycline-resistant breast cancer patients with normal and elevated LFTs at baseline.

Safety at 75 mg/m^2: Docetaxel at a dose of 75 mg/m^2 every 3 weeks has been evaluated in two phase II studies in 55 previously untreated patients with normal liver function and locally advanced or metastatic breast carcinoma. TABLE 4 shows the important hematologic adverse events in these studies

TABLE 5 shows the important non-hematologic adverse events at 75 mg/m^2.

CLINICAL STUDIES: *(cont'd)*

TABLE 2 Hematologic Adverse Events In Anthracycline-Resistant Breast Cancer Patients Treated At 100 mg/m^2 With Normal Or Elevated Baseline Liver Function Tests

Adverse Event		Normal LFTs* at Baseline n=127	Elevated LFTs** at Baseline n=7
Neutropenia			
Any	<2000 cells/mm^3	99.2	100
Grade 4	<500 cells/mm^3	94.5	100
Thrombocytopenia			
Any	<100,000 cells/mm^3	11.8	71.4
Grade 4	<20,000 cells/mm^3	0	14.3
Anemia	<11 g/dL	98.4	85.7
Infection* **			
Any		25.2	71.4
Grade 3 and 4		7.1	57.1
Febrile Neutropenia******			
By Patient		22.0	42.9
By Course		4.0	14.3
Septic Death		0.8	14.3
Non-Septic Death		0	14.3

* Normal LFTs: ≤ 1.5 times ULN or alkaline phosphatast ≤ 2.5 times ULN or isolated elevations of transaminases or alkaline phosphatase up to 5 times ULN.
** Elevated LFTs: SGOT and/or SGPT > 1.5 times ULN concurrent with alkaline phosphatase > 2.5 times ULN.
*** Incidence of infection requiring hospitalization and/or intravenous antibiotics was 13.4% (n=17) among the 127 patients with normal LFTs at baseline. There were two patients with grade 2, one with grade 3, and fourteen with grade 4 neutropenia.
**** Febrile Neutropenia: ANC grade 4 with fever > 38° C with IV antibiotics and/or hospitalization.

TABLE 3 Non-Hematologic Adverse Events In Anthracycline-Resistant Breast Cancer Patients Treated At 100 mg/m^2 With Normal Or Elevated Baseline Liver Function Tests

Adverse Event		Normal LFTs* at Baseline n=127 %	Elevated LFTs** at Baseline n=7 %
Acute Hypersensitivity Reaction Regardless of Premedication			
	Any	11.8	0
	Severe	0	0
Fluid Retention*** Regardless of Type of Premedication			
	Any	56.7	57.1
	Severe	9.4	14.3
With Recommended Premediction		n=29	n=3
	Any	41.4	66.6
	Severe	3.4	33.3
Neurosensory			
	Any	66.1	42.9
	Severe	7.1	0
Myalgia		35.4	57.1
Cutaneous			
	Any	62.2	57.1
	Severe	10.2	14.3
Asthenia			
	Any	80.3	42.9
	Severe	22.8	28.6
Stomatitis			
	Any	55.9	71.4
	Severe	8.7	57.1

* Normal LFTs: Transaminases ≤ 1.5 times ULN or alkaline phosphatase ≤ 2.5 times ULN or isolated elevations of transaminases or alkaline phosphatase up to 5 times ULN.
** Elevated Liver Function: SGOT and/or SGPT > 1.5 times ULN concurrent with alkaline phosphatase > 2.5 times ULN.
*** Fluid Retention includes (by COSTART): edema (peripheral, localized, generalized, lymphedema, pulmonary edema, and edema otherwise not specified) and effusion (pleural, pericardial, and ascites).

TABLE 4 Hematologic Adverse Events in 55 Breast Cancer Patients Treated with 75 mg/m^2

Adverse Event			%
Neutropenia			
	Any	<2000 cells/mm^3	98.1
	Grade 4	<500 cells/mm^3	80.0
Thrombocytopenia			
	Any	<100,000 cells/mm^3	5.5
	Grade 4	<20,000 cells/mm^3	0
Anemia		<11 g/dL	89.1
Infection			
	Any		21.8
	Grade 3 and 4		0
Febrile Neutropenia*			
	By Patient		1.8
Septic Death			0
Non-Septic Death			0

* Febrile Neutropenia: ANC grade 4 with fever > 38° C with IV antibiotics and/or hospitalization.

Safety and Efficacy at 60 mg/m^2: The safety and efficacy of docetaxel have been evaluated in three phase II Japanese studies in 174 patients (3 patients had elevated LFTs) who had received prior chemotherapy for locally advanced or metastatic breast carcinoma; 26 patients had progression of disease as best response to prior anthracycline treatment. In the 26 patients who had progression of disease as best response to prior anthracycline treatment, the ORR was 34.6% (95% C.I.: 17.2 - 55.7) and the CR was 3.8%. The median duration of response was 4 months.

TABLE 6 shows important hematologic adverse events for the Japanese breast cancer trials.

CLINICAL STUDIES: *(cont'd)*

TABLE 5 Non-Hematologic Adverse Events In 55 Breast Cancer Patients Treated With 75 mg/m²

Adverse Event		%
Acute Hypersensitivity Reaction*		
	Any	29.1
	Severe	1.8
Fluid Retention**		
	Any	69.1
	Severe	10.9
Neurosensory		
	Any	38.2
	Severe	1.8
Myalgia		
	Any	12.7
	Severe	1.8
Cutaneous		
	Any	47.3
	Severe	1.8
Asthenia		
	Any	63.6
	Severe	7.3
Stomatitis		
	Any	30.9
	Severe	3.6

* Regardless of premedication.
** Without recommended premedication.

TABLE 6 Hematologic Adverse Events In 174 Breast Cancer Patients Treated With 60 mg/m² Who Had Received Prior Chemotherapy In Trials Conducted In Japan

Adverse Event			%
Neutropenia			
	Any	<2000 cells/mm³	95.4
	Grade 4	<500 cells/mm³	74.9
Thrombocytopenia			
	Any	<100,000 cells/mm³	14.4
	Grade 4	<20,000 cells/mm³	1.1
Anemia		<11 g/dL	64.9
Infection			
	Any		1.1
	Grade 3 and 4		0
Febrile Neutropenia*			
	By Patient		0
Septic Death			1.1
Non-Septic Death			0

* Febrile Neutropenia: ANC grade 3/4 concomitant with fever > 38.1° C.

TABLE 7 shows important non-hematologic adverse events for the Japanese breast cancer trials; the incidence of severe non-hematologic toxicity in patients dosed at 60 mg/m² is negligible.

TABLE 7 Non-Hematologic Adverse Events in 174 Breast Cancer Patients Treated With 60 mg/m² Who Had Received Prior Chemotherapy In Trials Conducted In Japan

Adverse Event		%
Acute Hypersensitivity Reaction		
	Any	0.6
	Severe	0
Fluid Retention*		
	Any	12.6
	Severe	0
Neurosensory		
	Any	19.5
	Severe	0
Cutaneous		
	Any	30.5
	Severe	0
Myalgia		
	Any	3.4
	Severe	0
Asthenia		
	Any	65.5
	Severe	0
Stomatitis		
	Any	19.0
	Severe	0.6

* without premedication

INDICATIONS AND USAGE:

Docetaxel for Injection Concentrate is indicated for the treatment of patients with locally advanced or metastatic breast cancer who have progressed during anthracycline-based therapy or have relapsed during anthracycline-based adjuvant therapy.

CONTRAINDICATIONS:

Docetaxel is contraindicated in patients who have a history of severe hypersensitivity reactions to docetaxel or to other drugs formulated with polysorbate 80. Docetaxel should not be used in patients with neutrophil counts of < 1500 cells/mm³.

WARNINGS:

Docetaxel for Injection Concentrate should be administered under the supervision of a qualified physician experienced in the use of antineoplastic agents. Appropriate management of complications is possible only when adequate diagnostic and treatment facilities are readily available.

Toxic Deaths: Docetaxel administered at 100 mg/m² was associated with deaths considered possibly or probably related to treatment in 2.4% (34/1435) of patients with normal liver function and in 11% (6/55) of patients with abnormal liver function (SGOT and/or SGPT > 1.5 times ULN together with AP > 2.5 times ULN). Among patients dosed at 60 mg/m², mortality related to treatment occurred in 0.6% (3/481) of patients with normal liver function, and in 3 of 7 patients with abnormal liver function. Approximately half of these deaths occurred during the first cycle. Sepsis accounted for the majority of the deaths.

WARNINGS: *(cont'd)*

Premedication Regimen: Although the optimal premedication regimen is not defined, all patients should be premedicated with oral corticosteroids such as dexamethasone 16 mg per day (*e.g.,* 8 mg BID) for 5 days starting 1 day prior to docetaxel to reduce the severity of fluid retention and hypersensitivity reactions (see DOSAGE AND ADMINISTRATION).

Hypersensitivity Reactions: Patients should be observed closely for hypersensitivity reactions, especially during the first and second infusions. Severe hypersensitivity reactions characterized by hypotension and/or bronchospasm, or generalized rash/erythema occurred in 0.9% of patients who received the recommended premedication. Hypersensitivity reactions requiring discontinuation of the docetaxel infusion were reported in 5 out of 1260 patients who did not receive premedication. Patients with a history of severe hypersensitivity reactions should not be rechallenged with docetaxel.

Hematologic Effects: Neutropenia (less than 2000 neutrophils/mm³) occurs in virtually all patients given 60 - 100 mg/m² of docetaxel and grade 4 neutropenia (less than 500 cells/mm³) occurs in nearly all patients given 100 mg/m² and 75 - 80% of patients given 60 - 75 mg/m². Frequent monitoring of blood counts is, therefore, essential so that dose can be adjusted. Docetaxel should not be administered to patients with neutrophils < 1500 cells/mm³.

Febrile neutropenia occurred in about 12% of patients given 100 mg/m² but was very uncommon in patients given 60 - 75 mg/m². Hematologic responses, febrile reactions and infections, and rates of septic death for different regimens are dose related and are described in CLINICAL STUDIES.

Three breast cancer patients with severe liver impairment (bilirubin > 1.7 times ULN) developed fatal gastrointestinal bleeding associated with severe drug-induced thrombocytopenia.

Hepatic Impairment: See BOXED WARNING.

Fluid Retention: See BOXED WARNING.

Use in Pregnancy: Docetaxel can cause fetal harm when administered to pregnant women. Studies in both rats and rabbits at doses ≥ 0.3 and 0.03 mg/kg/day, respectively (about 1/50 and 1/300 the daily maximum recommended human dose on a mg/m² basis), administered during the period of organogenesis, have shown that docetaxel is embryotoxic and fetotoxic (characterized by intrauterine mortality, increased resorption, reduced fetal weight, and fetal ossification delay). The doses indicated above also caused maternal toxicity.

There are no adequate and well-controlled studies in pregnant women using docetaxel. If docetaxel is used during pregnancy, or if the patient becomes pregnant while receiving this drug, the patient should be apprised of the potential hazard to the fetus or potential risk for loss of the pregnancy. Women of childbearing potential should be advised to avoid becoming pregnant during therapy with docetaxel.

PRECAUTIONS:

General: Responding patients may not experience an improvement in performance status on therapy and may experience worsening. The relationship between changes in performance status, response to therapy and treatment-related side effects has not been established.

Hematologic Effects: In order to monitor the occurrence of myelotoxicity, it is recommended that frequent peripheral blood cell counts be performed on all patients receiving docetaxel. Patients should not be retreated with subsequent cycles of docetaxel until neutrophils recover to a level > 1500 cells/mm³ and platelets recover to a level > 100,000 cells/mm³.

A 25% reduction in the dose of docetaxel is recommended during subsequent cycles following severe neutropenia (< 500 cells/mm³) lasting 7 days or more, febrile neutropenia, or a grade 4 infection in a docetaxel cycle (see DOSAGE AND ADMINISTRATION).

Hypersensitivity Reactions: Hypersensitivity reactions may occur within a few minutes following initiation of a docetaxel infusion. If minor reactions such as flushing or localized skin reactions occur, interruption of therapy is not required. More severe reactions, however, require the immediate discontinuation of docetaxel and aggressive therapy. All patients should be premedicated with an oral corticosteroid prior to the initiation of the infusion of docetaxel (see WARNINGS, Premedication Regimen).

Cutaneous: Localized erythema of the extremities with edema followed by desquamation has been observed. In case of severe skin toxicity, an adjustment in dosage is recommended (see DOSAGE AND ADMINISTRATION). The discontinuation rate due to skin toxicity was 1.7%.

Fluid Retention: Severe fluid retention has been reported following docetaxel therapy (see BOXED WARNING and ADVERSE REACTIONS). Patients should be premedicated with oral corticosteroids prior to each docetaxel administration to reduce the incidence and severity of fluid retention (see DOSAGE AND ADMINISTRATION). Patients with pre-existing effusions should be closely monitored from the first dose for the possible exacerbation of the effusions.

In patients who received the recommended premedication, moderate fluid retention occurred in 17.4% with severe fluid retention in 6% and a 1.7% discontinuation rate. Fluid retention was completely, but sometimes slowly, reversible following discontinuation of docetaxel (median of 29 weeks). The median cumulative dose to onset of moderate or severe fluid retention was 705 mg/m² in patients receiving premedication. Patients developing peripheral edema may be treated with standard measures, *e.g.,* salt restriction, oral diuretic(s).

Neurologic: Severe neurosensory symptoms (paresthesia, dysesthesia, pain) were observed among 7% of 134 patients with anthracycline-resistant breast cancer. When these occur, dosage must be adjusted. If symptoms persist, treatment should be discontinued (see DOSAGE AND ADMINISTRATION). Patients who experienced neurotoxicity in clinical trials and for whom follow-up information on the complete resolution of the event was available had spontaneous reversal of symptoms within a median of 9 weeks from onset (range: 0 to 106 weeks) and only about 3.8% of patients required discontinuation due to neurotoxicity. Peripheral motor neuropathy mainly manifested as distal extremity weakness occurred in 13.4% (7.1% severe) of the 127 anthracycline-resistant breast cancer patients with normal LFTs. No neuromotor toxicity was reported in the 7 patients with elevated LFTs.

Asthenia: Severe asthenia has been reported in 11.1% of the patients but has led to treatment discontinuation in only 2.6% of the patients. Severe asthenia was reported in 23% of 134 patients with anthracycline-resistant breast cancer and 5.5% of the 786 cycles received. Symptoms of fatigue and weakness may last a few days up to several weeks and may be associated with deterioration of performance status in patients with progressive disease.

Carcinogenicity, Mutagenicity, Impairment of Fertility: No studies have been conducted to assess the carcinogenic potential of docetaxel. Docetaxel has been shown to be clastogenic in the *in vitro* chromosome aberration test in CHO-K_1 cells and in the *in vivo* micronucleus test in the mouse, but it did not induce mutagenicity in the Ames test, or the CHO/HGPRT gene mutation assays. Docetaxel produced no impairment of fertility in rats when administered in multiple IV doses of up to 0.3 mg/kg (about 1/50 the recommended human dose on a mg/m² basis), but decreased testicular weights were reported. This correlates with findings of a 10-cycle toxicity study (dosing once every 21 days for 6 months) in rats and dogs in which testicular atrophy or degeneration was observed at IV doses of 5 mg/kg in rats and 0.375 mg/kg in dogs (about 1/3 and 1/15 the recommended human dose on a mg/m² basis, respectively). An increased frequency of dosing in rats produced similar effects at lower dose levels.

Pregnancy Category D: See WARNINGS.

PRECAUTIONS: *(cont'd)*

Nursing Mothers: It is not known whether docetaxel is excreted in human milk. Because many drugs are excreted in human milk, and because of the potential for serious adverse reactions in nursing infants from docetaxel, mothers should discontinue nursing prior to taking the drug.

Pediatric Use: The safety and effectiveness of docetaxel in pediatric patients have not been established.

DRUG INTERACTIONS:

There have been no formal clinical studies to evaluate the drug interactions of docetaxel with other medications. *In vitro* studies have shown that the metabolism of docetaxel may be modified by the concomitant administration of compounds that induce, inhibit or are metabolized by cytochrome P450 3A4, such as cyclosporine, terfenadine, ketoconazole, erythromycin, and troleandomycin. Caution should be exercised with these drugs when treating patients receiving docetaxel as there is a potential for a significant interaction.

ADVERSE REACTIONS:

There were 1495 patients enrolled in 37 clinical trials conducted in North America and Europe (624 breast carcinoma patients and 866 patients with other tumor types) who received docetaxel at an initial dose of 100 mg/m² every 3 weeks. Five patients were not evaluable for toxicity since they discontinued docetaxel treatment due to acute hypersensitivity reactions with the first infusion. At least 95% of these patients did not receive hematopoietic support. The following Table 8 lists adverse reactions that occurred in at least 5% of 1435 patients with normal liver function tests at baseline (Normal LFTs: Transaminases ≤ 1.5 times ULN or alkaline phosphatase ≤ 2.5 times ULN or isolated elevations of transaminases or alkaline phosphatase up to 5 times ULN) as well as all deaths and adverse reactions in patients with abnormal liver function tests. These reactions were considered possibly or probably related to docetaxel. The safety profile is generally similar in patients receiving docetaxel for the treatment of breast carcinoma or for other tumor types.

TABLE 8 Summary Of Adverse Events In Patients Receiving Docetaxel At 100 mg/m²

Adverse Event		Normal LFTs* at Baseline n=1435 %	Elevated LFTs** at Baseline n=55 %
Hematologic			
Neutropenia	<2000 cells/mm³	96.3	96.0
	<500 cells/mm³	76.0	86.0
Leukopenia	<4000 cells/mm³	96.5	98.1
	<1000 cells/mm³	31.0	44.2
Thrombocytopenia	<100,000 cells/mm³	7.5	27.3
Anemia	<11 g/dL	89.5	92.7
	<8 g/dL	8.4	30.9
Febrile Neutropenia		11.8	26.4
Septic Death		1.8	3.6
Non-Septic Death		0.6	7.3
Infections			
	Any	21.7	32.7
	Severe	5.6	16.4
Fevere in absence of Infection			
	Any	30.2	50.9
	Severe	1.7	9.1
Hypersensitivity Reactions			
with recommended premedication		n=229	n=6
	Any	15.7	0
	Severe	0.9	0
Fluid Retention			
with recommended premedication		n=229	n=6
	Any	48.5	66.7
	Severe	5.2	33.3
Neurosensory			
	Any	53.7	41.8
	Severe	3.9	0
Neuromotor (principally distal extremity weakness)			
	Any	13.4	5.5
	Severe	3.7	1.8
Cutaneous			
	Any	58.5	61.8
	Severe	5.6	10.9
Nail Changes			
	Any	28.2	18.2
	Severe	2.6	4.6
Gastrointestinal			
	Nausea	40.4	40.0
	Diarrhea	40.3	32.7
	Vomiting	24.0	25.5
Alopecia		80.0	61.8
Asthenia			
	Any	61.5	54.5
	Severe	11.1	23.6
Stomatitis			
	Any	42.3	47.3
	Severe	5.3	14.5
Myalgia			
	Any	19.4	18.2
	Severe	1.4	1.9
Arthralgia		8.6	7.3
Infusion Site Reactions		5.6	3.6

* Normal LFTs: Transaminases ≤ 1.5 times ULN or alkaline phosphatase ≤ 2.5 times ULN or isolated elevations of transaminases or alkaline phosphatase up to 5 times ULN.
** Elevated LFTs: SGOT and/or SGPT > 1.5 times ULN concurrent with alkaline phosphatase > 2.5 times ULN.

Hematologic: Bone marrow suppression was the major dose-limiting toxicity of docetaxel. Neutropenia is reversible and not cumulative. The median day to nadir was 8 days, while the median duration of severe neutropenia (< 500 cells/mm³) was 7 days. Among patients with normal liver function treated with docetaxel, severe neutropenia occurred in 76% and lasted for more than 7 days in 4.3% of cycles. Anemia was reported in 89.5% of patients, with severe cases being reported in 8.4% of the patients (see WARNINGSsection).

Febrile neutropenia (< 500 cells/mm³ with fever > 38° C with IV antibiotics and/or hospitalization) occurred in 11.8% of the patients with normal liver function (3% of the cycles). Infectious episodes occurred in 21.7% of the patients (6.2% of the cycles) and were fatal in 1.6% of those treated with docetaxel (1.4% in breast cancer patients).

ADVERSE REACTIONS: *(cont'd)*

Thrombocytopenia (< 100,000 cells/mm³) occurred in 7.5% of the patients with normal liver function. Bleeding episodes were reported in 2.3% of the patients. A fatal gastrointestinal hemorrhage associated with thrombocytopenia was reported in one patient. Three breast cancer patients with severe liver impairment (bilirubin > 1.7 times ULN) developed fatal gastrointestinal bleeding associated with severe drug-induced thrombocytopenia.

Hypersensitivity Reactions: Hypersensitivity reactions requiring discontinuation of the docetaxel infusion were reported in 5 patients of 1260 who did not receive premedication. Severe hypersensitivity reactions characterized by hypotension and/or bronchospasm, or generalized rash/erythema have been observed in only 0.9% of patients with normal liver function receiving the recommended premedication regimen and none of these patients had to discontinue therapy.

Minor events, including flushing, rash with or without pruritus, chest tightness, back pain, dyspnea, drug fever, or chills, have been reported and resolved after discontinuing the infusion and appropriate therapy (see WARNINGS).

Fluid Retention (see BOXED WARNING): Events such as edema and weight gain and, less frequently, pleural effusion, pericardial effusion or ascites have been described. Among 229 patients with normal liver function receiving the recommended pretreatment, severe fluid retention was observed in 6%, causing treatment discontinuation in 1.7%. When it occurs, peripheral edema usually starts at the lower extremities and may become generalized with a median weight gain of 2 kg. Fluid retention is cumulative in incidence and severity. The median cumulative dose to onset of moderate or severe fluid retention was 705 mg/m². Fluid retention was completely reversible, resolving a median of 29 weeks (range: 0 to 42+ weeks) from the last docetaxel infusion.

Cutaneous: Reversible cutaneous reactions characterized by a rash including localized eruptions, mainly on the feet and/or hands, but also on the arms, face or thorax, usually associated with pruritus, have been observed. Eruptions generally occurred within one week after docetaxel infusion, recovered before the next infusion and were not disabling. Severe symptoms, such as eruptions followed by desquamation, occurred in 5.6% of the patients and rarely led to interruption or discontinuation of docetaxel treatment. Alopecia occurred in 80% of patients, and it was severe in 61.8% of patients.

Severe nail disorders occurred in 2.6% of the patients. These reactions were characterized by hypo- or hyperpigmentation, and occasionally by onycholysis (in 0.8% of patients) and pain.

Neurologic: Neurosensory symptoms characterized by paresthesia, dysesthesia or pain (including burning sensation) have been reported in patients receiving docetaxel. Severe reactions were observed in 3.9%.

Neuromotor events characterized mainly by weakness have been reported and were severe in 3.7% of the patients.

Gastrointestinal: Gastrointestinal reactions (nausea, and/or vomiting, and/or diarrhea) were generally mild to moderate and severe reactions occurred in 8.2% of the patients. Stomatitis was reported in 42.3% of patients receiving docetaxel. Severe reactions were observed in 5.3% of patients.

Cardiovascular: Hypotension occurred in 3.6% of the patients; 3.4% required treatment. Clinically meaningful events such as heart failure, sinus tachycardia, atrial flutter, dysrhythmia, unstable angina, pulmonary edema, and hypertension occurred rarely.

Infusion Site Reactions: Infusion site reactions were generally mild and consisted of hyperpigmentation, inflammation, redness or dryness of the skin, phlebitis, extravasation, or swelling of the vein.

Hepatic: In patients with normal LFTs at baseline, bilirubin values greater than the ULN occurred in 8.9% of patients. Increases in SGOT or SGPT > 1.5 times the ULN, or alkaline phosphatase > 2.5 times ULN, were observed in 18.1% and 7.6% of patients, respectively. During the study, increases in SGOT and/or SGPT > 1.5 times ULN concomitant with alkaline phosphatase > 2.5 times ULN occurred in 4.5% of patients with normal LFTs at baseline. (Whether these changes were related to the drug or underlying disease has not been established.)

Ongoing Evaluation: The following serious adverse events of uncertain relationship to docetaxel have been reported:

Body as a whole: abdominal pain, diffuse pain, chest pain

Cardiovascular: atrial fibrillation, deep vein thrombosis, ECG abnormalities, thrombophlebitis, pulmonary embolism, syncope, tachycardia

Digestive: constipation, duodenal ulcer, esophagitis, gastrointestinal hemorrhage, intestinal obstruction, ileus

Nervous: confusion

Respiratory: dyspnea, acute pulmonary edema, acute respiratory distress syndrome

Urogenital: renal insufficiency

OVERDOSAGE:

There is no known antidote for docetaxel overdosage. In case of overdosage, the patient should be kept in a specialized unit where vital functions can be closely monitored. Anticipated complications of overdosage include: bone marrow suppression, peripheral neurotoxicity, and mucositis.

There were two reports of overdose. One patient received 150 mg/m² and the other received 200 mg/m² as one-hour infusions. Both patients experienced severe neutropenia, mild asthenia, cutaneous reactions, and mild paresthesia, and recovered without incident.

In mice, lethality was observed following single i.v. doses that were ≥ 154 mg/kg (about 4.5 times the recommended human dose on a mg/m² basis); neurotoxicity associated with paralysis, non-extension of hind limbs and myelin degeneration was observed in mice at 48 mg/kg (about 1.5 times the recommended human dose on a mg/m² basis). In male and female rats, lethality was observed at a dose of 20 mg/kg, (comparable to the recommended human dose on a mg/m² basis) and was associated with abnormal mitosis and necrosis of multiple organs.

DOSAGE AND ADMINISTRATION:

For treatment of patients with locally advanced or metastatic carcinoma of the breast after progression during anthracycline-based therapy for metastatic disease or relapse during anthracycline-based adjuvant therapy, the recommended dose of docetaxel is 60 - 100 mg/m² administered intravenously over 1 hour every three weeks.

Premedication Regimen: All patients should be premedicated with oral corticosteroids such as dexamethasone 16 mg per day (*e.g.*, 8 mg twice daily) for 5 days starting 1 day prior to docetaxel administration in order to reduce the incidence and severity of fluid retention as well as the severity of hypersensitivity reactions (see WARNINGS and PRECAUTIONS).

Dosage Adjustments During Treatment: Patients who are dosed initially at 100 mg/m² and who experience either febrile neutropenia, neutrophils < 500 cells/mm³ for more than one week, severe or cumulative cutaneous reactions, or severe peripheral neuropathy during docetaxel therapy should have the dosage adjusted from 100 mg/m² to 75 mg/m². If the patient continues to experience these reactions, the dosage should either be decreased from 75 mg/m² to 55 mg/m² or the treatment should be discontinued. Conversely, patients who are

DOSAGE AND ADMINISTRATION: *(cont'd)*

dosed initially at 60 mg/m^2 and who do not experience febrile neutropenia, neutrophils < 500 cells/mm^3 for more than one week, severe or cumulative cutaneous reactions, or severe peripheral neuropathy during docetaxel therapy may tolerate higher doses.

Special Populations

Hepatic Impairment: Patients with bilirubin > ULN should generally not receive docetaxel. Also, patients with SGOT and/or SGPT > 1.5 x ULN concomitant with alkaline phosphatase > 2.5 x ULN should generally not receive docetaxel.

Children: The safety and effectiveness of docetaxel in pediatric patients below the age of 16 years have not been established.

Elderly: No dosage adjustments are required for use in elderly.

Docetaxel is a cytotoxic anticancer drug and, as with other potentially toxic compounds, caution should be exercised when handling and preparing docetaxel solutions. The use of gloves is recommended. Please refer to Handling and Disposal.

If docetaxel concentrate, premix solution, or infusion solution should come into contact with the skin, immediately and thoroughly wash with soap and water.

If docetaxel concentrate, premix solution, or infusion solution should come into contact with mucosa, immediately and thoroughly wash with water.

Docetaxel for Injection Concentrate requires dilution prior to administration. Please follow the preparation instructions provided below. Note: Both the docetaxel for Injection Concentrate and the diluent vials contain an overfill.

A. Preparation of the Premix Solution

1. Remove the appropriate number of vials of docetaxel for Injection Concentrate and diluent from the refrigerator. Allow the vials to stand at room temperature for approximately 5 minutes.

2. Aseptically withdraw the entire contents of the diluent vial into a syringe and transfer it to the vial of docetaxel for Injection Concentrate. Infection regarding fill volumes is listed below:

Strength	Vial Content	Diluent Vial
Docetaxel 20 mg	23.6 mg/0.59 ml	1.83 ml
Docetaxel 80 mg	94.4 mg/2.36 ml	7.33 ml
This will assure a final premix concentration of 10 mg docetaxel/mL		

3. Gently rotate each premix solution vial for approximately 15 seconds to assure full mixture of the concentrate and diluent.

4. The docetaxel premix solution (10 mg docetaxel/mL) should be clear; however, there may be some foam on top of the solution due to the polysorbate 80. Allow the premix solution to stand for a few minutes to allow any foam to dissipate. It is not required that all foam dissipate prior to continuing the preparation process.

B. Preparation of the Infusion Solution

1. Aseptically withdraw the required amount of docetaxel premix solution (10 mg docetaxel mL) with a calibrated syringe and inject the required volume of premix solution into a 250 mL infusion bag or bottle of either 0.9% Sodium Chloride solution or 5% Dextrose solution to produce a final concentration of 0.3 to 0.9 mg/ml. If a dose greater than 240 mg of docetaxel is required, use a larger volume of the infusion vehicle so that a concentration of 0.9 mg/ml docetaxel is not exceeded.

2. Thoroughly mix the infusion by manual rotation.

3. As with all parenteral products, docetaxel should be inspected visually for particulate matter or discoloration prior to administration whenever the solution and container permit. If the docetaxel for Injection premix solution or infusion solution is not clear or appears to have precipitation, the solution should be discarded.

Docetaxel infusion solution should be administered intravenously as a one-hour infusion under ambient room temperature and lighting conditions.

Contact of the undiluted concentrate with plasticized PVC equipment or devices used to prepare solutions for infusion is not recommended. In order to minimize patient exposure to the plasticizer DEHP (di-2-ethylexyl phthalate), which may be leached from PVC infusion bags or sets, diluted docetaxel solution should be stored in bottles (glass, polypropylene) or plastic bags (polypropylene, polyolefin) and administered through polyethylene-lined administration sets.

Stability: Unopened vials of docetaxel are stable until the expiration date indicated on the package when stored refrigerated, 2° to 8° C (36° to 46° F), and protected from bright light. Freezing does not adversely affect the product.

REFERENCES:

1. OSHA Work-Practice Guidelines for Personnel Dealing with Cytotoxic (Antineoplastic) Drugs. Am J Hosp Pharm. 1986; 43(5): 1193-1204. **2.** American Society of Hospital Pharmacists Technical Assistance Bulletin on Handling Cytotoxic and Hazardous Drugs. Am J Hosp Pharm. 1990; 47(95): 1033-1049. **3.** AMA Council Report. Guidelines for Handling Parenteral Antineoplastics. JAMA. 1985; 253(11): 1590-1592. **4.** Oncology Nursing Society Clinical Practice Committee. Cancer Chemotherapy Guidelines. Module II - Recommendations of Nursing Practice in the Acute Care Setting. ONS. 1988; 2-14.

HOW SUPPLIED:

Taxotere for Injection Concentrate is supplied in a single-dose vial as a sterile, pyrogen-free, non-aqueous, viscous solution with an accompanying sterile, non-pyrogenic, diluent (13% ethanol in Water for Injection) vial. The following strengths are available:

80 mg Concentrate for Infusion: 80 mg docetaxel in 2 mL polysorbate 80 (Fill: 94.4 mg docetaxel in 0.59 mL polysorbate 80) and diluent for Taxotere 80 mg. 13% (w/w) ethanol in Water for Injection (Fill: 7.33 mL). Both items are in a blister pack in one carton.

20 mg Concentrate for Infusion: 20 mg docetaxel in 0.5 ml polysorbate 80 (Fill: 23.6 docetaxel in 0.59 mL polysorbate 80) and diluent for Taxotere 20 mg. 13% (w/w) ethanol in Water for Injection (Fill: 1.83 mL). Both items are in a blister pack in one carton.

Storage: Store refrigerated, 2° to 8° C (36° to 46° F). Retain in the original package to protect from bright light. Taxotere premix solution (10 mg Taxotere/ml) and fully prepared Taxotere infusion solution (in either 0.9% Sodium Chloride solution or 5% Dextrose solution) should be used as soon as possible after preparation. However, the premix solution is stable for 8 hours either at room temperature, 15° to 25° C (59° to 77° F), or stored refrigerated, 2° to 8° C (36° to 46° F).

Handling and Disposal: Procedures for proper handling and disposal of anticancer drugs should be considered. Several guidelines on this subject have been published[1-4]. There is no general agreement that all of the procedures recommended in the guidelines are necessary or appropriate.

HOW SUPPLIED - EQUIVALENTS NOT AVAILABLE:

Injectable - Intravenous - 20 mg

20 mg vial x 1	$248.00	TAXOTERE, Rhone-Poulenc Rorer	00075-8001-20

HOW SUPPLIED - EQUIVALENTS NOT AVAILABLE: *(cont'd)*

Injection - Intravenous - 80 mg

80 mg vial x 1	$992.00	TAXOTERE, Rhone-Poulenc Rorer	00075-8001-80

DOCUSATE SODIUM; FERROUS FUMARATE; FOLIC ACID; MULTIVITAMINS *(001119)*

CATEGORIES: Antianemia Drugs; Blood Formation/Coagulation; Homeostatic & Nutrient; Iron Preparations; Multivitamins; Vitamins; FDA Pre 1938 Drugs

BRAND NAMES: Hemaferrin; Hem Fe; Maternal 90; Mynate 90 Plus; Nephron Fa; Prenatal + 90; Prenatal Mr 90; Prenatal Plus 90; **Tabron**

Prescribing information not available at time of publication.

HOW SUPPLIED - EQUIVALENTS NOT AVAILABLE:

Tablet, Coated, Sustained Action - Oral

100's	$10.74	Mynate 90 Plus, ME Pharm	58607-0103-90
100's	$15.72	Equi-Natal 90, Equipharm	57779-0110-04
100's	$16.21	Prenatal Mr 90, Ethex	58177-0212-04
100's	$17.05	Prenatal + 90, Qualitest Pharms	00603-5355-21
100's	$18.00	Prenatal Plus 90, Goldline Labs	00182-4453-01
100's	$18.90	Obnate 90, Econolab	55053-0840-01
100's	$19.00	Maternal 90, Pecos	59879-0102-01
100's	$19.90	Elemental Iron-90, Aligen Independ	00405-4382-01
100's	$20.25	Prenatal Plus 90, Major Pharms	00904-7762-60
500's	$81.05	Prenatal Mr 90 Fe, Ethex	58177-0212-08

Tablet, Plain Coated - Oral

100's	$14.00	RENAL VITAMINS PLUS IRON, Vitaline	54022-1333-01
100's	$18.75	Nephron Fa, Nephro-Tech	59528-4456-01

DONEPEZIL HYDROCHLORIDE *(003311)*

CATEGORIES: Alzheimer's Disease; Autonomic Drugs; Central Nervous System Agents; Cholinesterase Inhibitors; Cholinomimetric; Dementia; FDA Approved 1996 Nov; FDA Class 1P ('Priority Review'); Neuromuscular; Parasympathomimetic Agents

BRAND NAMES: **Aricept**

DESCRIPTION:

Donepezil hydrochloride is a reversible inhibitor of the enzyme acetylcholinesterase, known chemically as (±)-2,3-dihydro-5,6-dimethoxy-2-1 [[1-(phenylmethyl)-4-piperidinyl]methyl]-1*H*-inden-1-one hydrochloride. Donepezil hydrochloride is commonly referred to in the pharmacological literature as E2020. It has an empirical formula of $C_{24}H_{29}NO_3HCl$ and a molecular weight of 415.96. Donepezil hydrochloride is a white crystalline powder and is freely soluble in chloroform, soluble in water and in glacial acetic acid, slightly soluble in ethanol and in acetonitrile and practically insoluble in ethyl acetate and in n-hexane.

Aricept is available for oral administration in film-coated tablets containing 5 or 10 mg of donepezil hydrochloride. Inactive ingredients are lactose monohydrate, corn starch, microcrystalline cellulose, hydroxypropyl cellulose, and magnesium stearate. The film coating contains talc, polyethylene glycol, hydroxypropyl methylcellulose and titanium dioxide. Additionally, the 10 mg tablet contains yellow iron oxide (synthetic) as a coloring agent.

CLINICAL PHARMACOLOGY:

Current theories on the pathogenesis of the cognitive signs and symptoms of Alzheimer's Disease attribute some of them to a deficiency of cholinergic neurotransmission. Donepezil hydrochloride is postulated to exert its therapeutic effect by enhancing cholinergic function. This is accomplished by increasing the concentration of acetylcholine through reversible inhibition of its hydrolysis by acetylcholinesterase. If this proposed mechanism of action is correct, donepezil's effect may lessen as the disease process advances and fewer cholinergic neurons remain functionally intact. There is no evidence that donepezil alters the course of the underlying dementing process.

PHARMACOKINETICS

Donepezil is well absorbed with a relative oral bioavailability of 100% and reaches peak plasma concentrations in 3 to 4 hours. Pharmacokinetics are linear over a dose range of 1-10 mg given once daily. Neither food nor time of administration (morning vs. evening dose) influences the rate or extent of absorption. The elimination half life of donepezil is about 70 hours and the mean apparent plasma clearance (Cl/F) is 0.13 L/hr/kg. Following multiple dose administration, donepezil accumulates in plasma by 4-7 fold and steady state is reached within 15 days. The steady state volume of distribution is 12 L/kg. Donepezil is approximately 96% bound to human plasma proteins, mainly to albumins (about 75%) and $alpha_1$ -acid glycoprotein (about 21%) over the concentration range of 2 - 1000 ng/ml.

Donepezil is both excreted in the urine intact and extensively metabolized to four major metabolites, two of which are known to be active, and a number of minor metabolites, not all of which have been identified. Donepezil is metabolized by CYP 450 isoenzymes 2D6 and 3A4 and undergoes glucuronidation. Following administration of ^{14}C-labeled donepezil, plasma radioactivity, expressed as a percent of the administered dose, was present primarily as intact donepezil (53%) and as 6-O-desmethyl donepezil (11%), which has been reported to inhibit AChE to the same extent as donepezil *in vitro* and was found in plasma at concentrations equal to about 20% of donepezil. Approximately 57% and 15% of the total radioactivity was recovered in urine and feces, respectively, over a period of 10 days, while 28% remained unrecovered, with about 17% of the donepezil dose recovered in the urine as unchanged drug.

SPECIAL POPULATIONS

Hepatic Disease: In a study of 10 patients with stable alcoholic cirrhosis, the clearance of donepezil HCl was decreased by 20% relative to 10 healthy age and sex matched subjects.

Renal Disease: In a study of 4 patients with moderate to severe renal impairment (Cl_{cr} <22 ml/min/1.73 m^2) the clearance of donepezil HCl did not differ from 4 age and sex matched healthy subjects.

Age: No formal pharmacokinetic study was conducted to examine age related differences in the pharmacokinetics of donepezil HCl. However, mean plasma donepezil HCl concentrations measured during therapeutic drug monitoring of elderly patients with Alzheimer's Disease are comparable to those observed in young healthy volunteers.

Gender and Race: No specific pharmacokinetic study was conducted to investigate the effects of gender and race on the disposition of donepezil HCl. However, retrospective pharmacokinetic analysis indicates that gender and race (Japanese and Caucasians) did not affect the clearance of donepezil HCl.

CLINICAL STUDIES:

The effectiveness of donepezil HCl as a treatment for Alzheimer's Disease is demonstrated by the results of two randomized, double-blind, placebo-controlled clinical investigations in patients with Alzheimer's Disease (diagnosed by NINCDS and DSM III-R criteria, Mini-Mental State Examination ≤10 and ≤26 and Clinical Dementia Rating of 1 or 2). The mean age of patients participating in donepezil HCl trials was 73 years with a range of 50 to 94. Approximately 62% of patients were women and 38% were men. The racial distribution was white 95%, black 3% and other races 2%.

Study Outcome Measures: In each study, the effectiveness of treatment with donepezil HCl was evaluated using a dual outcome assessment strategy.

The ability of donepezil HCl to improve cognitive performance was assessed with the cognitive subscale of the Alzheimer's Disease Assessment Scale (ADAS-cog), a multi-item instrument that has been extensively validated in longitudinal cohorts of Alzheimer's Disease patients. The ADAS-cog examines selected aspects of cognitive performance including elements of memory, orientation, attention, reasoning, language and praxis. The ADAS-cog scoring range is from 0 to 70, with higher scores indicating greater cognitive impairment. Elderly normal adults may score as low as 0 or 1, but it is not unusual for non-demented adults to score slightly higher.

The patients recruited as participants in each study had mean scores on the Alzheimer's Disease Assessment Scale (ADAS-cog) of approximately 26 units, with a range from 4 to 61. Experience gained in longitudinal studies of ambulatory patients with mild to moderate Alzheimer's Disease suggest that they gain 6 to 12 units a year on the ADAS-cog. However, lesser degrees of change are seen in patients with very mild or very advanced disease because the ADAS-cog is not uniformly sensitive to change over the course of the disease. The annualized rate of decline in the placebo patients participating in donepezil HCl trials was approximately 2 to 4 units per year.

The ability of donepezil HCl to produce an overall clinical effect was assessed using a Clinician's Interview Based Impression of Change that required the use of care giver information, the CIBIC plus. The CIBIC plus is not a single instrument and is not a standardized instrument like the ADAS-cog. Clinical trials for investigational drugs have used a variety of CIBIC formats, each different in terms of depth and structure. As such, results from a CIBIC plus reflect clinical experience from the trial or trials in which it was used and can not be compared directly with the results of CIBIC plus evaluations from other clinical trials. The CIBIC plus used in donepezil HCl trials was a semi-structured instrument that was intended to examine four major areas of patient function: General, Cognitive, Behavioral and Activities of Daily Living. It represents the assessment of a skilled clinician based upon his/her observations at an interview with the patient, in combination with information supplied by a caregiver familiar with the behavior of the patient over the interval rated. The CIBIC plus is scored as a seven point categorical rating, ranging from a score of 1, indicating "markedly improved", to a score of 4, indicating "no change" to a score of 7, indicating "markedly worse". The CIBIC plus has not been systematically compared directly to assessments not using information from caregivers (CIBIC) or other global methods.

THIRTY-WEEK STUDY

In a study of 30 weeks duration, 473 patients were randomized to receive single daily doses of placebo, 5 mg/day or 10 mg/day of donepezil HCl. The 30-week study was divided into a 24-week double-blind active treatment phase followed by a 6-week single-blind placebo washout period. The study was designed to compare 5 mg/day or 10 mg/day fixed doses of donepezil HCl to placebo. However, to reduce the likelihood of cholinergic effects, the 10 mg/day treatment was started following an initial 7-day treatment with 5 mg/day doses.

Effects on the ADAS-cog: After 24 weeks of treatment, the mean differences in the ADAS-cog change scores for donepezil HCl treated patients compared to the patients on placebo were 2.8 and 3.1 units for the 5 mg/day and 10 mg/day treatments, respectively. These differences were stastically significant. While the treatment effect size may appear to be slightly greater for the 10 mg/day treatment, there was no statistically significant difference between the two active treatments.

Following 6 weeks of placebo washout, scores on the ADAS-cog for both the donepezil HCl treatment groups were indistinguishable from those patients who had received only placebo for 30 weeks. This suggests that the beneficial effects of donepezil HCl abate over 6 weeks following discontinuation of treatment and do not represent a change in the underlying disease. There was no evidence of a rebound effect 6 weeks after abrupt discontinuation of therapy.

Patients assigned to placebo and donepezil HCl had a wide range of improvement responses, but the active treatment groups were more likely to show the greater improvements.

Effects on the CIBIC plus: The mean drug-placebo differences for the three treatment groups of patients who completed 24 weeks of treatment were 0.35 units and 0.39 units for 5 mg/day and 10 mg/day of donepezil HCl, respectively. These differences were statistically significant. There was no statistically significant difference between the two active treatments.

FIFTEEN-WEEK STUDY

In a study of 15 weeks duration, patients were randomized to receive single daily doses of placebo or either 5 mg/day or 10 mg/day of donepezil HCl for 12 weeks, followed by a 3-week placebo washout period. As in the 30-week study, to avoid acute cholinergic effects, the 10 mg/day treatment followed an initial 7 day treatment with 5 mg/day doses.

Effects on the ADAS-Cog: After 12 weeks of treatment, the differences in mean ADAS-cog change scores for the donepezil HCl treated patients compared to the patients on placebo were 2.7 and 3.0 units each, for the 5 and 10 mg/day donepezil HCl treatment groups respectively. These differences were statistically significant. The effect size for the 10 mg/day group may appear to be slightly larger than that for 5 mg/day. However, the differences between active treatments were not statistically significant.

Following 3 weeks of placebo washout, scores on the ADAS-cog for both the donepezil HCl treatment groups increased, indicating that discontinuation of donepezil HCl resulted in a loss of its treatment effect. The duration of this placebo washout period was not sufficient to characterize the rate of loss of the treatment effect, but, the 30 week study (see Thirty Week Study) demonstrated that treatment effects associated with the use of donepezil HCl abate within 6 weeks of treatment discontinuation.

As observed in the 30-week study, patients assigned to either placebo or to donepezil HCl have a wide range of responses, but the donepezil HCl treated patients are more likely to show the greater improvements in cognitive performance.

Effects on the CIBIC plus: The differences in mean CIBIC plus scores for donepezil HCl treated patients compared to the patients on placebo at Week 12 were 0.36 and 0.38 units for the 5 mg/day and 10 mg/day treatment groups, respectively. These differences were statistically significant.

In both studies, patient age, sex and race were not found to predict the clinical outcome of donepezil HCl treatment.

INDICATIONS AND USAGE:

Donepezil HCl is indicated for the treatment of mild to moderate dementia of the Alzheimer's type.

CONTRAINDICATIONS:

Donepezil HCl is contraindicated in patients with known hypersensitivity to donepezil hydrochloride or to piperidine derivatives.

WARNINGS:

Anesthesia: Donepezil HCl, as a cholinesterase inhibitor, is likely to exaggerate succinylcholine-type muscle relaxation during anesthesia.

Cardiovascular Conditions: Because of their pharmacological action, cholinesterase inhibitors may have vagotonic effects on heart rate (*e.g.,* bradycardia). The potential for this action may be particularly important to patients with "sick sinus syndrome" or other supraventricular cardiac conduction conditions. Syncopal episodes have been reported in association with the use of donepezil HCl.

Gastrointestinal Conditions: Through their primary action, cholinesterase inhibitors may be expected to increase gastric acid secretion due to increased cholinergic activity. Therefore, patients should be monitored closely for symptoms of active or occult gastrointestinal bleeding, especially those at increased risk for developing ulcers (*e.g.,* those with a history of ulcer disease or those receiving concurrent nonsteroidal anti-inflammatory drugs (NSAIDS)). Clinical studies of donepezil HCl have shown no increase, relative to placebo, in the incidence of either peptic ulcer disease or gastrointestinal bleeding.

Donepezil HCl, as a predictable consequence of its pharmacological properties, has been shown to produce diarrhea, nausea and vomiting. These effects, when they occur, appear more frequently with the 10 mg/day dose than with the 5 mg/day dose. In most cases, these effects have been mild and transient, sometimes lasting one to three weeks, and have resolved during continued use of donepezil HCl.

Genitourinary: Although not observed in clinical trials of donepezil HCl, cholinomimetics may cause bladder outflow obstruction.

Neurological Conditions: *Seizures:* Cholinomimetics are believed to have some potential to cause generalized convulsions. However, seizure also may be a manifestation of Alzheimer's Disease.

Pulmonary Conditions: Because of their cholinomimetic actions, cholinesterase inhibitors should be prescribed with care to patients with a history of asthma or obstructive pulmonary disease.

PRECAUTIONS:

Drug-Drug Interactions: See DRUG INTERACTIONS.

Carcinogenesis, Mutagenesis, and Impairment of Fertility: Carcinogenicity studies of donepezil have not been completed.

Donepezil was not mutagenic in the Ames reverse mutation assay in bacteria. In the chromosome aberration test in cultures of Chinese hamster lung (CHL) cells, some clastogenic effects were observed. Donepezil was not clastogenic in the *in vivo* mouse micronucleus test.

Donepezil had no effect on fertility in rats at doses up to 10 mg/kg/day (approximately 8 times the maximum recommended human dose on a mg/m^2 basis).

Pregnancy Category C: Teratology studies conducted in pregnant rats at doses up to 16 mg/kg/day (approximately 13 times the maximum recommended human dose on a mg/m^2 basis) and in pregnant rabbits at doses up to 10 mg/kg/day (approximately 16 times the maximum recommended human dose on a mg/m^2 basis) did not disclose any evidence for a teratogenic potential of donepezil. However, in a study in which pregnant rats were given up to 10 mg/kg/day (approximately 8 times the maximum recommended human dose on a mg/m^{2}basis) from day 17 of gestation through day 20 postpartum, there was a slight increase in still births and a slight decrease in pup survival through day 4 postpartum at this dose; the next lower dose tested was 3 mg/kg/day. There are no adequate or well-controlled studies in pregnant women. Donepezil HCl should be used during pregnancy only if the potential benefit justifies the potential risk to the fetus.

Nursing Mothers: It is not known whether donepezil is excreted in human breast milk. Donepezil HCl has no indication for use in nursing mothers.

Pediatric Use: There are no adequate and well-controlled trials to document the safety and efficacy of donepezil HCl in any illness occurring in children.

DRUG INTERACTIONS:

Drugs Highly Bound to Plasma Proteins: Drug displacement studies have been performed *in vitro* between this highly bound drug (96%) and other drugs such as furosemide, digoxin, and warfarin. Donepezil HCl at concentrations of 0.3-10 mcg/ml did not affect the binding of furosemide (5 mcg/ml), digoxin (2 ng/ml), and warfarin (3 mcg/ml) to human albumin. Similarly, the binding of donepezil HCl to human albumin was not affected by furosemide, digoxin and warfarin.

Effect of Donepezil HCl on the Metabolism of Other Drugs: No *in vivo* clinical trials have investigated the effect of donepezil HCl on the clearance of drugs metabolized by CYP 3A4 (*e.g.,* cisapride, terfenadine) or by CYP 2D6 (*e.g.,* imipramine). However, *in vitro* studies show a low rate of binding to these enzymes (mean about 50-130 μM), that, given the therapeutic plasma concentrations of donepezil (164 nM), indicates little likelihood of interference.

Whether donepezil HCl has any potential for enzyme induction is not known.

Formal pharmacokinetic studies evaluated the potential of donepezil HCl for interaction with theophylline, cimetidine, warfarin and digoxin. No significant effects on the pharmacokinetics of these drugs were observed.

Effect of Other Drugs on the Metabolism of Donepezil HCl: Ketoconazole and quinidine, inhibitors of CYP 450, 3A4 and 2D6, respectively, inhibit donepezil metabolism *in vitro.* Whether there is a clinical effect of these inhibitors is not known. Inducers of CYP 2D6 and CYP 3A4 (*e.g.,* phenytoin, carbamazepine, dexamethasone, rifampin, and phenobarbital) could increase the rate of elimination of donepezil HCl.

Formal pharmacokinetic studies demonstrated that the metabolism of donepezil HCl is not significantly affected by concurrent administration of digoxin or cimetidine.

Use with Anticholinergics: Because of their mechanism of action, cholinesterase inhibitors have the potential to interfere with the activity of anticholinergic medications.

Use with Cholinomimetics and Other Cholinesterase Inhibitors: A synergistic effect may be expected when cholinesterase inhibitors are given concurrently with succinylcholine, similar neuromuscular blocking agents or cholinergic agonists such as bethanechol.

ADVERSE REACTIONS:

ADVERSE EVENTS LEADING TO DISCONTINUATION

The rates of discontinuation from controlled clinical trials of donepezil HCl due to adverse events for the donepezil HCl 5 mg/day treatment groups were comparable to those of placebo-treatment groups at approximately 5%. The rate of discontinuation of patients who received 7-day escalations from 5 mg/day to 10 mg/day, was higher at 13%.

The most common adverse events leading to discontinuation, defined as those occurring in at least 2% of patients and at twice the incidence seen in placebo patients, are in TABLE 1.

ADVERSE REACTIONS: *(cont'd)*

TABLE 1 Most Frequent Adverse Events Leading to Withdrawl from Controlled Clinical Trials by Dose Group

Dose Group	Placebo	5 mg/ day Donepezil HCl	10 mg/ day Donepezil HCl
Patients Randomized	**355**	**350**	**315**
Event / % Discontinuing			
Nausea	1%	1%	3%
Diarrhea	0%	<1%	3%
Vomiting	<1%	<1%	2%

MOST FREQUENT ADVERSE CLINICAL EVENTS SEEN IN ASSOCIATION WITH THE USE OF DONEPEZIL HCL

The most common adverse events, defined as those occurring at a frequency of at least 5% in patients receiving 10 mg/day and twice the placebo rate, are largely predicted by donepezil HCl's cholinomimetic effects. These include nausea, diarrhea, insomnia, vomiting, muscle cramp. Fatigue and anorexia. These adverse events were often of mild intensity and transient, resolving during continued donepezil HCl treatment without the need for dose modification.

There is evidence to suggest that the frequency of these common adverse events may be affected by the rate of titration. An open-label study was conducted with 269 patients who received placebo in the 15 and 30-week studies. These patients were titrated to a dose of 10 mg/day over a 6-week period. The rates of common adverse events were lower than those seen in patients titrated to 10 mg/day over one week in the controlled clinical trials and were comparable to those seen in patients on 5 mg/day.

See TABLE 2 for a comparison of the most common adverse events following one and six week titration regimens.

TABLE 2 Comparison of Rates of Adverse Events in Patients Titrated to 10 mg/day Over 1 to 6 Weeks

Titration:	None		1 Week	6 Weeks
Adverse Event	**Placebo**	**5 mg/day**	**10 mg/day**	**10 mg/day**
	(n=315) %	(n=311) %	(n=315) %	(n=269) %
Nausea	6	5	19	6
Diarrhea	5	8	15	9
Insomnia	6	6	14	6
Fatigue	3	4	8	3
Vomiting	3	3	8	5
Muscle Cramps	2	6	8	3
Anorexia	2	3	7	3

ADVERSE EVENTS REPORTED IN CONTROLLED TRIALS

The events cited reflect experience gained under closely monitored conditions of clinical trials in a highly selected patient population. In actual clinical practice or in other clinical trials, these frequency estimates may not apply, as the conditions of use, reporting behavior, and the kinds of patients treated may differ. TABLE 3 lists treatment emergent signs and symptoms that were reported in at least 2% of patients in placebo-controlled trials who received donepezil HCl and for which the rate of occurrence was greater for donepezil HCl assigned than placebo assigned patients. In general, adverse events occurred more frequently in female patients and with advancing age.

TABLE 3 Adverse Events Reported in Controlled Clinical Trials in at Least 2% of Patients Receiving Donepezil HCl and at Higher Frequency Than Placebo-treated Patients

Body System/ Adverse Event	Placebo (n=355)	Donepezil HCl (n=747)
Percent of Patients with any Adverse Event	**72**	**74**
Body as a Whole		
Headache	9	10
Pain, various locations	8	9
Accident	6	7
Fatigue	3	5
Cardiovascular System		
Syncope	1	2
Digestive System		
Nausea	6	11
Diarrhea	5	10
Vomiting	3	5
Anorexia	2	4
Hemic and Lymphatic System		
Ecchymosis	3	4
Metabolic and Nutritional Systems		
Weight Decrease	1	3
Musculoskeletal System		
Muscle Cramps	2	6
Arthritis	1	2
Nervous System		
Insomnia	6	9
Dizziness	6	8
Depression	<1	3
Abnormal Dreams	0	3
Somnolence	<1	2
Urogenital System		
Frequent Urination	1	2

OTHER ADVERSE EVENTS OBSERVED DURING CLINICAL TRIALS

Donepezil HCl has been administered to over 1700 individuals during clinical trials worldwide. Approximately 1200 of these patients have been treated for at least 3 months and more than 1000 patients have been treated for at least 6 months. Controlled and uncontrolled trials in the United States included approximately 900 patients. In regards to the highest dose of 10 mg/day, this population includes 650 patients treated for 3 months, 475 patients treated for 6 months and 116 patients treated for over 1 year. The range of patient exposure is from 1 to 1214 days.

Treatment emergent signs and symptoms that occurred during 3 controlled clinical trials and two open label trials in the United States were recorded as adverse events by the clinical investigators using terminology of their own choosing. To provide an overall estimate of the proportion of individuals having similar types of events, the events were grouped into a smaller number of standardized categories using a modified COSTART dictionary and event frequencies were calculated across all studies. These categories are used in the listing below. The frequencies represent the proportion of 900 patients from these trials who experienced that event while receiving donepezil HCl. All adverse events occurring at least twice are included, except for those already listed in TABLE 2 or TABLE 3, COSTART terms too general to be informative, or events less likely to be drug caused. Events are classified by body system and listed using the following definitions: *frequent adverse events* - those occurring in at least 1/100 patients; *infrequent adverse events* - those occurring in 1/100 to 1/

ADVERSE REACTIONS: *(cont'd)*

1000 patients. These adverse events are not necessarily related to donepezil HCl treatment and in most cases were observed at a similar frequency in placebo treated patients in the controlled studies. No important additional adverse events were seen in studies conducted outside the United States.

Body as a Whole: *Frequent:*influenza, chest pain, toothache; *Infrequent:*fever, edema face, periorbital edema, hernia hiatal, abscess, cellulitis, chills, generalized coldness, head fullness, listlessness.

Cardiovascular System: *Frequent:*hypertension, vasodilation, atrial fibrillation, hot flashes, hypotension; *Infrequent:*angina pectoris, postural hypotension, myocardial infarction, AV block (first degree), congestive heart failure, arteritis, bradycardia, peripheral vascular disease, supraventricular tachycardia, deep vein thrombosis.

Digestive System: *Frequent:* fecal incontinence, gastrointestinal bleeding, bloating, epigastric pain; *Infrequent:*eructation, gingivitis, increased appetite, flatulence, periodontal abscess, cholelithiasis, diverticulitis, drooling, dry mouth, fever sore, gastritis, irritable colon, tongue edema, epigastric distress, gastroenteritis, increased transaminases, hemorrhoids, ileus, increased thirst, jaundice, melena, polydypsia, duodenal ulcer, stomach ulcer.

Endocrine System: *Infrequent:*diabetes mellitus, goiter.

Hemic and Lymphatic System: *Infrequent:*anemia, thrombocythemia, thrombocytopenia, eosinophilia, erythrocytopenia.

Metabolic and Nutritional Disorders: *Frequent:*dehydration; *Infrequent:* gout, hypokalemia, increased creatine kinase, hyperglycemia, weight increase, increased lactate dehydrogenase.

Musculoskeletal System: *Frequent:*bone fracture; *Infrequent:* muscle weakness, muscle fasciculation.

Nervous System: *Frequent:*delusions, tremor, irritability, paresthesia, aggression, vertigo, ataxia, increased libido, restlessness, abnormal crying, nervousness, aphasia; *Infrequent:*cerebrovascular accident, intracranial hemorrhage, transient ischemic attack, emotional lability, neuralgia, coldness (localized), muscle spasm, dysphoria, gait abnormality, hypertonia, hypokinesia, neurodermatitis, numbness (localized), paranoia, dysarthria, dysphasia, hostility, decreased libido, melancholia, emotional withdrawal, nystagmus, pacing.

Respiratory System: *Frequent:*dyspnea, sore throat, bronchitis; *Infrequent:*epistaxis, post nasal drip, pneumonia, hyperventilation, pulmonary congestion, wheezing, hypoxia, pharyngitis, pleurisy, pulmonary collapse, sleep apnea, snoring.

Skin and Appendages: *Frequent:* pruritis, diaphoresis, urticaria; *Infrequent:*dermatitis, erythema, skin discoloration, hyperkeratosis, alopecia, fungal dermatitis, herpes zoster, hirsutism, skin striae, night sweats, skin ulcer.

Special Senses: *Frequent:*cataract, eye irritation, vision blurred; *Infrequent:*dry eyes, glaucoma, earache, tinnitus, blepharitis, decreased hearing, retinal hemorrhage, otitis externa, otitis media, bad taste, conjunctival hemorrhage, ear buzzing, motion sickness, spots before eyes.

Urogenital System: *Frequent:*urinary incontinence, nocturia; *Infrequent:*dysuria, hematuria, urinary urgency, metrorrhagia, cystitis, enuresis, prostate hypertrophy, pyelonephritis, inability to empty bladder, breast fibroadenosis, fibrocystic breast, mastitis, pyuria, renal failure, vaginitis.

OVERDOSAGE:

Because strategies for the management of overdose are continually evolving, it is advisable to contact a Poison Control Center to determine the latest recommendations for the management of an overdose of any drug.

As in any case of overdose, general supportive measures should be utilized. Overdosage with cholinesterase inhibitors can result in cholinergic crisis characterized by severe nausea, vomiting, salivation, sweating, bradycardia, hypotension, respiratory depression, collapse and convulsions. Increasing muscle weakness is a possibility and may result in death if respiratory muscles are involved. Tertiary anticholinergics such as atropine may be used as an antidote for donepezil HCl overdosage. Intravenous atropine sulfate titrated to effect is recommended: an initial dose of 1.0 to 2.0 mg IV with subsequent doses based upon clinical response. Atypical responses in blood pressure and heart rate have been reported with other cholinomimetics when co-administered with quaternary anticholinergics such as glycopyrrolate. It is not known whether donepezil HCl and/or its metabolites can be removed by dialysis (hemodialysis, peritoneal dialysis, or hemofiltration).

Dose-related signs of toxicity in animals included reduced spontaneous movement, prone position, staggering gait, lacrimation, clonic convulsions, depressed respiration, salivation, miosis, tremors, fasciculation and lower body surface temperature.

DOSAGE AND ADMINISTRATION:

The dosages of donepezil HCl shown to be effective in controlled clinical trials are 5 mg and 10 mg administered once per day.

The higher dose of 10 mg did not provide a statistically significantly greater clinical benefit than 5 mg. There is a suggestion, however, based upon order of group mean scores and dose trend analyses of data from these clinical trials, that a daily dose of 10 mg of donepezil HCl might provide additional benefit for some patients. Accordingly, whether or not to employ a dose of 10 mg is a matter of prescriber and patient preference.

Evidence from the controlled trials indicates that the 10 mg dose, with a one week titration, is likely to be associated with a higher incidence of cholinergic adverse events than the 5 mg dose. In open label trials using a 6 week titration, the frequency of these same adverse events was similar between the 5 mg and 10 mg dose groups. Therefore, because steady state is not achieved for 15 days and because the incidence of untoward effects may be influenced by the rate of dose escalation, treatment with a dose of 10 mg should not be contemplated until patients have been on a daily dose of 5 mg for 4 to 6 weeks.

Donepezil HCl should be taken in the evening, just prior to retiring. Donepezil HCl can be taken with or without food.

PATIENT INFORMATION:

Donepezil is used for the treatment of mild to moderate symptoms of Alzheimer's Disease.

Inform your physician if you are taking any other medications, or have heart, gastrointestinal, genitourinary, pulmonary or neurological conditions.

Inform your physician if you are pregnant or nursing.

May cause nausea, diarrhea, insomnia, vomiting, muscular cramps, fatigue or anorexia.

Take in the evening, just prior to bedtime. Donepezil may be taken without regard to meals.

HOW SUPPLIED:

Aricept is supplied as film-coated, round tablets containing either 5 mg or 10 mg of donepezil hydrochloride.

The 5 mg tablets are white. The strength, in mg (5), is debossed on one side and the medication code number (E 245) is debossed on the other side.

The 10 mg tablets are yellow and have the strength debossed on one side (10) and the medication code (E 246) on the other side.

DOPAMINE HYDROCHLORIDE *(001108)*

CATEGORIES: Autonomic Drugs; Cardiac Output; Cardiovascular Drugs; Heart Failure; Hypotension/Shock; Myocardial Infarction; Renal Failure; Septicemia; Sympathomimetic Agents; Vasopressors; Pregnancy Category C; FDA Approval Pre 1982

BRAND NAMES: *Cardiopal*; *Cardiosteril* (Germany); *Docard*; *Dopamed*; *Dopamex*; *Dopamin*; *Dopamin AWD* (Germany); *Dopamin Braun*; *Dopamin Guilini* (Germany); *Dopamin Leopold*; *Dopamin Natterman* (Germany); *Dopamina* ; *Dopamine* (France); Dopamine HCl; Dopamine HCl Additive Syringe; Dopamine HCl Univer Addit; *Dopamine Injection*; *Dopaminex*; *Dopaminum*; *Dopinga*; *Dopmin*; *Dopramin*; *Drynalken* (Mexico); *Dynatra*; *Dynos*; *Giludop*; *Inopin*; *Inotropin* (Mexico); **Intropin**; *Intropin IV*; *Revimine* (Canada); *Uramin*
(International brand names outside U.S. in italics)

FORMULARIES: WHO

> WARNING:
> NOT FOR DIRECT INTRAVENOUS INJECTION. MUST BE DILUTED BEFORE USE.

DESCRIPTION:

Dopamine hydrochloride injection is a clear, practically colorless, aqueous, additive solution for intravenous infusion after dilution. Each mL contains either 40 mg, 80 mg, or 160 mg dopamine HCl, USP (equivalent to 32.3 mg, 64.6 mg, and 129.2 mg dopamine base, respectively) in Water for Injection, USP containing 1% sodium metabisulfite, NF as an antioxidant. Hydrochloric acid or sodium hydroxide added to adjust pH when necessary. The solution is sterile and nonpyrogenic. The pH is 2.5 - 5.0. Dopamine HCl, a naturally occurring catecholamine, is an inotropic vasopressor agent. Its chemical name is 3,4, dihydroxyphenethylamine hydrochloride.

Empirical Formula: C_8H_{11}·HCl

Molecular Weight: 189.64

Dopamine HCl is sensitive to alkalis, iron salts and oxidizing agents.**Dopamine HCl must be diluted in an appropriate, sterile parenteral solution** (see DOSAGE AND ADMINISTRATION) **before intravenous administration.**

CLINICAL PHARMACOLOGY:

Dopamine is a natural catecholamine formed by the decarboxylation of 3,4-dihydroxyphenylalanine (DOPA). It is a precursor to norepinephrine in noradrenergic nerves and is also a neurotransmitter in certain areas of the central nervous system, especially in the nigrostriatal tract, and in a few peripheral sympathetic nerves.

Dopamine produces positive chronotropic and inotropic effects on the myocardium, resulting in increased heart rate and cardiac contractility. This is accomplished directly by exerting an agonist action on beta-adrenoceptors and indirectly by causing release of norepinephrine from storage sites in sympathetic nerve endings.

Dopamine's onset of action occurs within five minutes of intravenous administration, and with dopamine's plasma half-life of about two minutes, the duration of action is less than ten minutes. However, if monoamine oxidase (MAO) inhibitors are present, the duration may increase to one hour. The drug is widely distributed in the body but does not cross the blood-brain barrier to a significant extent. Dopamine is metabolized in the liver, kidney and plasma by MAO and catechol-O- methyltransferase to the inactive compounds homovanillic acid (HVA) and 3,4-dihydroxyphenylacetic acid. About 25% of the dose is taken up into specialized neurosecretory vesicles (the adrenergic nerve terminals), where it is hydroxylated to form norepinephrine. It has been reported that about 80% of the drug is excreted in the urine within 24 hours, primarily as HVA and its sulfate and glucuronide conjugates and as 3,4-dihydroxyphenylacetic acid. A very small portion is excreted unchanged.

The predominant effects of dopamine are dose-related, although it should be noted that actual response of an individual patient will largely depend on the clinical status of the patient at the time the drug is administered. At low rates of infusion (0.5-2 mcg/kg/min) dopamine causes vasodilation that is presumed to be due to a specific agonist action on dopamine receptors (distinct from alpha- and beta-adrenoceptors) in the renal, mesenteric, coronary and intracerebral vascular beds. At these dopamine receptors, haloperidol is an antagonist. The vasodilation in these vascular beds is accompanied by increased glomerular filtration rate, renal blood flow, sodium excretion and urine flow. Hypotension sometimes occurs. An increase in urinary output produced by dopamine is usually not associated with a decrease in osmolality of the urine.

At intermediate rates of infusion (2-10 mcg/kg/min), dopamine acts to stimulate the $beta_1$-adrenoceptors, resulting in improved myocardial contractility, increased SA rate and enhanced impulse conduction in the heart. There is little, if any, stimulation of the $beta_2$-adrenoceptors (peripheral vasodilation). Dopamine causes less increase in myocardial oxygen consumption than isoproterenol, and its use is not usually associated with a tachyarrhythmia. Clinical studies indicate that it usually increases systolic and pulse pressure with either no effect or a slight increase in diastolic pressure. Blood flow to the peripheral vascular beds may decrease while mesenteric flow increases due to increased cardiac output. At low and intermediate doses, total peripheral resistance (which would be raised by alpha activity) is usually unchanged.

At higher rates of infusion (10-20 mcg/kg/min), there is some effect on alpha-adrenoceptors, with consequent vasoconstrictor effects and a rise in blood pressure. The vasoconstrictor effects are first seen in the skeletal muscle vascular beds, but with increasing doses, they are also evident in the renal and mesenteric vessels. At very high rates of infusion (above 20 mcg/kg/min), stimulation of alpha-adrenoceptors predominates and vasoconstriction may compromise the circulation of the limbs and override the dopaminergic effects of dopamine, reversing renal dilation and natruresis.

INDICATIONS AND USAGE:

Dopamine HCl Injection is indicated for the correction of hemodynamic imbalances present in the shock syndrome due to myocardial infarction, trauma, endotoxic septicemia, open-heart surgery, renal failure and chronic cardiac decompensation as in congestive failure.

Where appropriate, restoration of blood volume with a suitable plasma expander or whole blood should be instituted or completed prior to administration of dopamine HCl.

Patients most likely to respond adequately to dopamine HCl are those in whom physiological parameters, such as urine flow, myocardial function and blood pressure, have not undergone profound deterioration. Multiclinic trials indicate that the shorter the time interval between onset of signs and symptoms and initiation of therapy with volume correction and dopamine HCl, the better the prognosis.

INDICATIONS AND USAGE: *(cont'd)*

POOR PERFUSION OF VITAL ORGANS

Urine flow appears to be one of the better diagnostic signs by which adequacy of vital organ perfusion can be monitored. Nevertheless, the physician should also observe the patient for signs of reversal of confusion or reversal of comatose condition. Loss of pallor, increase in toe temperature and/or adequacy of nail bed capillary filling may also be used as indices of adequate dosage. Clinical studies have shown that when dopamine HCl is administered before urine flow has diminished to levels approximately 0.3 ml/minute, prognosis is more favorable. Nevertheless, in a number of oliguric or anuric patients, administration of dopamine HCl has resulted in an increase in urine flow which, in some cases, reached normal levels. Dopamine HCl may also increase urine flow in patients whose output is within normal limits and thus may be of value in reducing the degree of preexisting fluid accumulation. It should be noted that at doses above those optimal for the individual patient, urine flow may decrease, necessitating reduction of dosage.

Concurrent administration of dopamine HCl and diuretic agents may produce an additive or potentiating effect.

LOW CARDIAC OUTPUT

Increased cardiac output is related to dopamine's direct inotropic effect on the myocardium. Increased cardiac output at low or moderate doses appears to be related to a favorable prognosis. Increase in cardiac output has been associated with either static or decreased systemic vascular resistance (SVR). Static or decreased SVR associated with low or moderate movements in cardiac output is believed to be a reflection of differential effects on specific vascular beds with increased resistance in peripheral beds (*e.g.,* femoral) and concomitant decreases in mesenteric and renal vascular beds. Redistribution of blood flow parallels these changes so that an increase in cardiac output is accompanied by an increase in mesenteric and renal blood flow. In many instances the renal fraction of the total cardiac output has been found to increase. The increase in cardiac output produced by dopamine is not associated with substantial decreases in systemic vascular resistance as may occur with isoproterenol.

HYPOTENSION

Hypotension due to inadequate cardiac output can be managed by administration of low to moderate doses of dopamine HCl, which have little effect on SVR. At high therapeutic doses, dopamine's alpha-adrenergic activity becomes more prominent and thus may correct hypotension due to diminished SVR. As in the case of other circulatory decompensation states, prognosis is better in patients whose blood pressure and urine flow have not undergone profound deterioration. Therefore, it is suggested that the physician administer dopamine HCl as soon as a definite trend toward decreased systolic and diastolic pressure becomes evident.

CONTRAINDICATIONS:

Dopamine HCl should not be used in patients with pheochromocytoma.

WARNINGS:

Dopamine HCl should not be administered to patients with uncorrected tachyarrhythmias or ventricular fibrillation.

Do **NOT** add dopamine HCl to any alkaline diluent solution since the drug is inactivated in alkaline solution.

Patients who have been receiving MAO inhibitors prior to the administration of dopamine HCl will require substantially reduced dosage. Dopamine is metabolized by MAO, and inhibition of this enzyme prolongs and potentiates the effect of dopamine HCl. The starting dose in such patients should be reduced to at least one-tenth (1/10) of the usual dose.

Contains sodium bisulfite, a sulfite that may cause allergic-type reactions including anaphylactic symptoms and life-threatening or less severe asthmatic episodes in certain susceptible people. The overall prevalence of sulfite sensitivity in the general population is unknown and probably low. Sulfite sensitivity is seen more frequently in asthmatic than in nonasthmatic people.

PRECAUTIONS:

GENERAL

Careful monitoring required: Close monitoring of the following indices - urine flow, cardiac output and blood pressure - during dopamine infusion is necessary as in the case of any adrenergic agent.

Avoid hypovolemia: Prior to treatment with dopamine HCl, hypovolemia should be fully corrected, if possible, with either whole blood or plasma as indicated.

Decreased pulse pressure: If a disproportionate increase in diastolic blood pressure (*i.e.,* a marked decrease in pulse pressure) is observed in patients receiving dopamine HCl, the infusion rate should be decreased and the patient observed carefully for further evidence of predominant vasoconstrictor activity, unless such an effect is desired.

Extravasation: Dopamine HCl should be infused into a large vein whenever possible to prevent the possibility of extravasation into tissue adjacent to the infusion site. Extravasation may cause necrosis and sloughing of surrounding tissue. Large veins of the antecubital fossa are preferred to veins in the dorsum of the hand or ankle. Less suitable infusion sites should be used only if the patient's condition requires immediate attention. The physician should switch to more suitable sites as rapidly as possible. The infusion site should be continuously monitored for free flow.

Occlusive vascular disease: Patients with a history of occlusive vascular disease (for example, atherosclerosis, arterial embolism, Raynaud's disease, cold injury, diabetic endarteritis and Buerger's disease) should be closely monitored for any change in color or temperature of the skin in the extremities. If a change in skin color or temperature occurs and is thought to be the result of compromised circulation to the extremities, the benefits of continued Dopamine HCl infusion should be weighed against the risk of possible necrosis. This condition may be reversed by either decreasing the rate of infusion or discontinuing the infusion.

> IMPORTANT
> **Antidote for Peripheral Ischemia:** To prevent sloughing and necrosis in ischemic areas, the area should be infiltrated as soon as possible with 10 to 15 ml of saline solution containing from 5 to 10 mg of phentolamine mesylate, an adrenergic-blocking agent. A syringe with a fine hypodermic needle should be used, and the solution liberally infiltrated throughout the ischemic area. Sympathetic blockade with phentolamine causes immediate and conspicuous local hyperemic changes if the area is infiltrated within 12 hours. Therefore, PHENTOLAMINE SHOULD BE GIVEN AS SOON AS POSSIBLE after the extravasation is noted.

CARCINOGENESIS, MUTAGENESIS, AND IMPAIRMENT OF FERTILITY

Long-term studies in animals have not been performed to evaluate carcinogenic potential.

PRECAUTIONS: *(cont'd)*

PREGNANCY CATEGORY C

Animal studies have revealed no evidence of teratogenic effects from dopamine HCl. In one study, administration of dopamine HCl to pregnant rats resulted in a decreased survival rate of the newborn and a potential for cataract formation in the survivors. There are no adequate and well- controlled studies in pregnant women. Dopamine HCl should be used during pregnancy only if the potential benefit justifies the potential risk to the fetus.

LABOR AND DELIVERY

Information on labor and delivery is unknown.

NURSING MOTHERS

It is not known whether this drug is excreted in human milk. Because many drugs are excreted in human milk, caution should be exercised when dopamine HCl is administered to a nursing mother.

PEDIATRIC USE

Safety and effectiveness in children have not been established. However, peripheral gangrene has been reported in neonates and children.

DRUG INTERACTIONS:

Avoid cyclopropane or halogenated hydrocarbon anesthetics: Cyclopropane or halogenated hydrocarbon anesthetics increase cardiac autonomic irritability and therefore may sensitize the myocardium to the action of certain intravenously administered catecholamines. This interaction appears to be related both to pressor activity and the beta adrenergic stimulating properties of these catecholamines. Therefore, as with certain other catecholamines, and because of the theoretical arrhythmogenic potential, Dopamine should be used with EXTREME CAUTION in patients inhaling cyclopropane or halogenated hydrocarbon anesthetics.

(See also WARNINGS).

ADVERSE REACTIONS:

The most frequent adverse reactions observed in clinical evaluation of dopamine HCl included ectopic beats, nausea, vomiting, tachycardia, anginal pain, palpitation, dyspnea, headache, hypotension, and vasoconstriction. Other adverse reactions which have been reported infrequently were aberrant conduction, bradycardia, piloerection, widened QRS complex, azotemia, and elevated blood pressure.

OVERDOSAGE:

In case of accidental overdosage, as evidenced by excessive blood pressure elevation, reduce rate of administration or temporarily discontinue dopamine HCl until patient's condition stabilizes. Since the duration of action in dopamine HCl is quite short, no additional remedial measures are usually necessary. If these measures fail to stabilize the patient's condition, use of the short-acting alpha-adrenergic blocking agent phentolamine should be considered.

DOSAGE AND ADMINISTRATION:

WARNING: This is a potent drug. It must be diluted before administration to patient.

SUGGESTED DILUTION

Transfer contents of one or more ampuls or vials by aseptic technique to either a 250 ml or 500 ml bottle of one of the following sterile intravenous solutions:

1. Sodium Chloride Injection, USP

2. Dextrose (5%) Injection, USP

3. Dextrose (5%) and Sodium Chloride (0.9%) Injection, USP

4. 5% Dextrose in 0.45% Sodium Chloride Solution

5. Dextrose (5%) in Lactated Ringer's Injection

6. Sodium Lactate (1/6 Molar) Injection, USP

7. Lactated Ringer's Injection, USP

Dopamine HCl has been found to be stable for a minimum of 24 hours after dilution in the sterile intravenous solutions listed above. However, as with all intravenous admixtures, dilution should be made just prior to administration.

Do **NOT** add dopamine HCl to 5% Sodium Bicarbonate or other alkaline intravenous solution since the drug is inactivated in alkaline solution.

RATE OF ADMINISTRATION

Dopamine HCl, after dilution, is administered intravenously through a suitable intravenous catheter or needle. An IV drip chamber or other suitable metering device is essential for controlling the rate of flow in drops/minute. Each patient must be individually titrated to the desired hemodynamic and/or renal response with dopamine HCl. In titrating to the desired increase in systolic blood pressure, the optimum dosage rate for renal response may be exceeded, thus necessitating a reduction in rate after the hemodynamic condition is stabilized.

Administration at rates greater than 50 mcg/kg/minute has been safely used in advanced circulatory decompensation states. If unnecessary fluid expansion is of concern, adjustment of drug concentration may be preferred over increasing the flow rate of a less concentrated dilution.

SUGGESTED REGIMEN

1. When appropriate, increase blood volume with whole blood or plasma until central venous pressure is 10-15 cm H_2O or pulmonary wedge pressure is 14-18 mm Hg.

2. Begin administration of diluted solution at doses of 2-5 mcg/kg/minute of dopamine HCl in patients who are likely to respond to modest increments of heart force and renal perfusion.

In more seriously ill patients, begin administration of diluted solution at doses of 5 mcg/kg/minute and increase gradually using 5 to 10 mcg/kg/minute increments up to 20-50 mcg/kg/minute as needed. If doses of dopamine HCl in excess of 50 mcg/kg/minute are required, it is suggested that urine output be checked frequently. Should urine flow begin to decrease in the absence of hypotension, reduction of dopamine HCl dosage should be considered. Multiclinic trials have shown that more than 50% of the patients were satisfactorily maintained on doses of dopamine HCl less than 20 mcg/kg/minute. In patients who do not respond to these doses with adequate arterial pressures or urine flow, additional increments of dopamine HCl may be employed in an effort to produce an appropriate arterial pressure and central perfusion.

3. Treatment of all patients requires constant evaluation of therapy in terms of the blood volume, augmentation of myocardial contractility and distribution of peripheral perfusion. Dosage of dopamine HCl should be adjusted according to the patient's response, with particular attention to diminution of established urine flow rate, increasing tachycardia or development of new dysrhythmias as indices for decreasing or temporarily suspending the dosage.

4. As with all potent intravenously administered drugs, care should be taken to control the rate of administration so as to avoid inadvertent administration of a bolus of drug.

Parenteral drug products should be inspected visually for particulate matter and discoloration prior to administration, whenever solution and container permit.

DOSAGE AND ADMINISTRATION: *(cont'd)*

Store at controlled room temperature 15-30°C (59-86°F).

WARNING: NOT FOR DIRECT INTRAVENOUS INJECTION. MUST BE DILUTED BEFORE USE.

(Dupont, 6227-2/Rev.Aug., 1992)

HOW SUPPLIED - RATED THERAPEUTICALLY EQUIVALENT:

Injection, Conc-Soln - Intravenous - 40 mg/ml

5 ml	$9.42	Dopamine Hcl, Abbott	00074-5820-01
5 ml	$11.04	Dopamine Hcl Inj., Abbott	00074-5809-01
5 ml	$11.22	Dopamine Hcl, Abbott	00074-5820-10
5 ml	$13.34	Dopamine HCl, Abbott	00074-5819-16
5 ml	$73.44	Dopamine Hcl, Solopak Labs	39769-0009-05
5 ml	$92.19	Dopamine Hcl, Fujisawa USA	00469-1330-20
5 ml x 10	$71.25	Dopamine Hcl, Astra USA	00186-0638-01
5 ml x 10	$75.13	Dopamine Hcl, Fujisawa USA	00469-9092-87
5 ml x 25	$37.50	Dopamine Hcl, Elkins Sinn	00641-1416-35
5 ml x 25	$48.13	Dopamine Hcl, Elkins Sinn	00641-0112-25
5 ml x 25	$54.69	Dopamine HCl, Am Regent	00517-1805-25
10 ml	$14.16	Dopamine Hcl, Intl Medication	00548-6137-00
10 ml	$15.65	Dopamine Hcl, Abbott	00074-9106-01
10 ml	$18.67	Dopamine Hcl, Abbott	00074-9104-01
10 ml	$22.24	Dopamine Hcl, Abbott	00074-9104-20
10 ml	$24.69	Dopamine HCl Additive Syringe, Abbott	00074-9105-18
10 ml x 10	$141.50	Dopamine Hcl, Fujisawa USA	00469-9093-87
10 ml x 10	$146.30	Dopamine Hcl, Astra USA	00186-0639-01
20 ml	$23.50	Dopamine Hcl, Intl Medication	00548-6135-00

Injection, Conc-Soln - Intravenous - 80 mg/ml

5 ml	$140.63	Dopamine Hcl Inj 80, Solopak Labs	39769-0010-05
5 ml	$170.63	Dopamine Hcl, Fujisawa USA	00469-1340-20
5 ml x 10	$118.75	Dopamine Hcl, Astra USA	00186-0641-01
5 ml x 25	$72.00	Dopamine Hcl, Consolidated Midland	00223-7486-05
5 ml x 25	$75.00	Dopamine Hcl 400, Elkins Sinn	00641-1413-35
5 ml x 25	$88.50	Dopamine Hcl, Gensia Labs	00703-1613-04
5 ml x 25	$102.19	Dopamine Hcl, Am Regent	00517-1905-25
5 ml x 25	$181.25	Dopamine Hcl, Consolidated Midland	00223-7487-05
10 ml	$35.87	Dopamine Hcl 800, Abbott	00074-4265-01
10 ml	$39.53	Dopamine Hcl Univer Addit, Abbott	00074-4266-18
250 ml	$18.26	Dopamine Hcl, Abbott	00074-7808-02
250 ml	$19.10	Dopamine Hcl In 5% Dextrose, Abbott	00074-4141-02
500 ml	$25.61	Dopamine Hcl, Abbott	00074-7808-03
500 ml	$30.08	Dopamine Hcl In 5% Dextrose, Abbott	00074-4141-03

Injection, Conc-Soln - Intravenous - 80 mg/100ml

250 ml	$19.30	Dopamine HCl, Baxter Hlthcare	00338-1005-02
250 ml	$20.54	DOPAMINE HCL IN 5% DEXTROSE, Abbott	00074-7808-22
250 ml x 12	$19.68	Dopamine HCl In 5% Dextrose Injecti, McGaw	00264-5144-20
500 ml	$28.38	Dopamine HCl, Baxter Hlthcare	00338-1005-03
500 ml	$28.81	DOPAMINE HCL IN 5% DEXTROSE, Abbott	00074-7808-24
500 ml x 12	$27.73	Dopamine HCl In 5% Dextrose Injecti, McGaw	00264-5144-10

Injection, Conc-Soln - Intravenous - 160 mg/ml

5 ml	$378.44	Dopamine Hcl, Fujisawa USA	00469-1350-20
5 ml x 10	$157.11	Dopamine Hcl, Astra USA	00186-0642-01
5 ml x 25	$203.44	Dopamine Hcl, Am Regent	00517-1305-25
250 ml	$30.08	Dopamine Hcl In 5% Dextrose Inj., Abbott	00074-4142-02
500 ml	$45.73	Dopamine Hcl In 5% Dextrose Inj., Abbott	00074-4142-03

Injection, Conc-Soln - Intravenous - 160 mg/100ml

250 ml	$26.89	Dopamine Hcl, Abbott	00074-7809-02
250 ml	$28.38	Dopamine HCl, Baxter Hlthcare	00338-1007-02
250 ml	$30.23	DOPAMINE HCL IN 5% DEXTROSE, Abbott	00074-7809-22
250 ml x 12	$27.73	Dopamine HCl In 5% Dextrose Injecti, McGaw	00264-5148-20
500 ml	$38.93	Dopamine Hcl, Abbott	00074-7809-03
500 ml	$43.14	Dopamine HCl 400, Baxter Hlthcare	00338-1007-03
500 ml	$43.78	DOPAMINE HCL IN 5% DEXTROSE, Abbott	00074-7809-24
500 ml x 12	$43.82	Dopamine HCl In 5% Dextrose Injecti, McGaw	00264-5148-10

Injection, Conc-Soln - Intravenous - 320 mg/100ml

250 ml	$39.77	Dopamine Hcl, Abbott	00074-7810-02
250 ml	$43.14	Dopamine HCl 800, Baxter Hlthcare	00338-1009-02
250 ml	$44.72	DOPAMINE HCL IN 5% DEXTROSE, Abbott	00074-7810-22
250 ml	$45.73	Dopamine Hcl In 5% Dextrose, Abbott	00074-4155-02
250 ml x 12	$43.82	Dopamine HCl In 5% Dextrose Injecti, McGaw	00264-5149-20

HOW SUPPLIED - NOT RATED EQUIVALENT:

Injection, Conc-Soln - Intravenous - 40 mg/ml

5 ml x 10	$31.50	Dopamine Hcl, Voluntary Hosp	53258-9092-08
5 ml x 25	$49.80	Dopamine Hcl, Gensia Labs	00703-1603-04
5 ml x 25	$81.25	Dopamine Hcl, Consolidated Midland	00223-7484-05
5 ml x 25	$142.00	Dopamine Hcl, Consolidated Midland	00223-7485-05
10 ml x 10	$44.70	Dopamine Hcl, Voluntary Hosp	53258-9093-08

DORNASE ALFA *(003180)*

CATEGORIES: Biologicals; Cough Preparations; Cystic Fibrosis; Enzymes & Digestants; Respiratory & Allergy Medications; Respiratory Tract Infections; Bronchiectasis*; Lung Surfactant*; FDA Class 1P ("Priority Review"); Recombinant DNA Origin; Sales > $100 Million; FDA Approved 1993 Dec

* Indication not approved by the FDA

BRAND NAMES: Deoxyribonuclease; DNase; **Pulmozyme**

FORMULARIES: Medi-Cal

DESCRIPTION:

Pulmozyme (dornase alfa) Inhalation Solution is a sterile, clear, colorless, highly purified solution of recombinant human deoxyribonuclease I (rhDNase), an enzyme which selectively cleaves DNA. The protein is produced by genetically engineered Chinese Hamster Ovary (CHO) cells containing DNA encoding for the native human protein, deoxyribonuclease I (DNase). The product is purified by tangential flow filtration and column chromatography. The purified glycoprotein contains 260 amino acids with an approximate molecular weight of 37,000 daltons (1). The primary amino acid sequence is identical to that of the native human enzyme.

Dornase Alfa is administered by inhalation of an aerosol mist produced by a compressed air driven nebulizer system (see CLINICAL STUDIES). Each Dornase Alfa single-use ampule will deliver 2.5 ml of the solution to the nebulizer bowl. The aqueous solution contains 1.0 mg/ml dornase alfa, 0.15 mg/ml calcium chloride dihydrate and 8.77 mg/ml sodium chloride. The solution contains no preservative. The nominal pH of the solution is 6.3.

CLINICAL PHARMACOLOGY:

General: In cystic fibrosis (CF) patients, retention of viscous purulent secretions in the airways contributes both to reduced pulmonary function and to exacerbations of infection (2,3).

Purulent pulmonary secretions contain very high concentrations of extracellular DNA released by degenerating leukocytes that accumulate in response to infection (4). *In vitro*, Dornase Alfa hydrolyzes the DNA in sputum of CF patients and reduces sputum viscoelasticity (1).

Pharmacokinetics: When 2.5 mg Dornase Alfa was administered by inhalation to eighteen CF patients, mean sputum concentrations of 3 mcg/ml DNase were measurable within 15 minutes. Mean sputum concentrations declined to an average of 0.6 mcg/ml two hours following inhalation. Inhalation of up to 10 mg TID of Dornase Alfa by 4 CF patients for six consecutive days, did not result in a significant elevation of serum concentrations of DNase above normal endogenous levels (5,6). After administration of up to 2.5 mg of Dornase Alfa twice daily for six months to 321 CF patients, no accumulation of serum DNase was noted.

CLINICAL STUDIES:

Dornase Alfa has been evaluated in a large, randomized, placebo-controlled trial of clinically stable cystic fibrosis patients, 5 years of age and older, with baseline forced vital capacity (FVC) greater than or equal to 40% of predicted and receiving standard therapies for cystic fibrosis (7). Patients were treated with placebo (325 patients), 2.5 mg of Dornase Alfa once a day (322 patients), or 2.5 mg of Dornase Alfa twice a day (321 patients) for six months administered via a Hudson T Up-draft II nebulizer with a Pulmo-Aide compressor.

Both doses of Dornase Alfa resulted in significant reductions compared with the placebo group in the number of patients experiencing respiratory tract infections requiring use of parenteral antibiotics. Administration of Dornase Alfa reduced the relative risk of developing a respiratory tract infection by 27% and 29% for the 2.5 mg daily dose and the 2.5 mg twice daily dose, respectively (see TABLE 1.) The data suggest that the effects of Dornase Alfa on respiratory tract infections in older patients (>21 years) may be smaller than in younger patients, and that twice daily dosing may be required in the older patients. Patients with baseline FVC>85% may also benefit from twice a day dosing (see TABLE 1.) The reduced risk of respiratory infection observed in Dornase Alfa treated patients did not directly correlate with improvement in FEV_1, during the initial two weeks of therapy.

Within 8 days of the start of treatment with Dornase Alfa, mean FEV_1 increased 7.9% in those treated once a day and 9.0% in those treated twice a day compared to the baseline values. The mean FEV_1 observed during long-term therapy increased 5.8% from baseline at the 2.5 mg daily dose level and 5.6% from baseline at the 2.5 mg twice daily dose level. Placebo recipients did not show significant mean changes in pulmonary function testing.

For patients 5 years of age or older, with baseline FVC greater than or equal to 40%, administration of Dornase Alfa decreased the incidence of occurrence of first respiratory tract infection requiring parenteral antibiotics, and improved mean FEV_1, regardless of age or baseline FVC.

TABLE 1 Incidence of First Respiratory Tract Infection Requiring Parenteral Antibiotics in a Controlled Trial

	Placebo N=325	2.5 mg QD N=332	2.5 mg BID N=321
Percent of Patients Infected	43%	34%	33%
Relative Risk (vs placebo)		0.73	0.71
p-value (vs placebo)		0.015	0.007
Subgroup by Age and Baseline FVC:			
Age	(N)	(N)	(N)
5-20 years	42% (201)	25% (199)	28% (184)
21 years and older	44% (124)	48% (123)	39% (137)
Baseline FVC			
40-85% Predicted	54% (194)	41% (201)	44% (203)
>85% Predicted	27% (131)	21% (121)	14% (118)

Dornase Alfa did not produce a pulmonary function benefit in short-term usage in patients with FVC less than 40% of predicted. Studies are in progress to assess the impact of chronic use on pulmonary function and infection risk in this population.

Clinical trials have indicated that Dornase Alfa therapy can be continued or initiated during an acute respiratory exacerbation.

Short-term dose ranging studies demonstrated that doses in excess of 2.5 mg bid did not provide further improvement in FEV_1. Patients who have received drug on a cyclical regimen (*i.e.,* administration of Dornase Alfa 10 mg BID for 14 days, followed by a 14 day wash out period) showed rapid improvement in FEV_1 with the initiation of each cycle and a return to baseline with each Dornase Alfa withdrawal.

INDICATIONS AND USAGE:

Daily administration of Dornase Alfa in conjunction with standard therapies is indicated in the management of cystic fibrosis patients to reduce the frequency of respiratory infections requiring parenteral antibiotics and to improve pulmonary function. Safety and efficacy of daily administration have not been demonstrated in patients under the age of 5 years, or with FVC<40% of predicted, or for longer than twelve months.

CONTRAINDICATIONS:

Dornase Alfa is contraindicated in patients with known hypersensitivity to dornase alfa, Chinese Hamster Ovary cell products, or any component of the product.

WARNINGS:

None.

PRECAUTIONS:

GENERAL

Dornase Alfa should be used in conjunction with standard therapies for CF.

INFORMATION FOR THE PATIENT

Dornase Alfa must be stored in the refrigerator at 2-8°C (36-46°F) and protected from strong light. It should be kept refrigerated during transport and should not be exposed to room temperatures for a total time of 24 hours. The solution should be discarded if it is cloudy or discolored. Dornase Alfa contains no preservative and, once opened, the entire ampule must be used or discarded. Patients should be instructed in the proper use and maintenance of the nebulizer and compressor system used in its delivery.

Dornase Alfa should not be diluted or mixed with other drugs in the nebulizer. Mixing of Dornase Alfa with other drugs could lead to adverse physicochemical and/or functional changes in Dornase Alfa or the admixed compound.

PRECAUTIONS: *(cont'd)*

CARCINOGENESIS, MUTAGENESIS, AND IMPAIRMENT OF FERTILITY

Carcinogenesis: A two year inhalation (head-only) toxicity study of Dornase Alfa in rats to assess oncogenic potential is in progress.

Mutagenesis: Ames tests using six different tester strains of bacteria (4 of S. typhimurium and 2 of E. coli) at concentrations up to 5000 mcg/plate, a cytogenic assay using human peripheral blood lymphocytes at concentrations up to 2000 mcg/plate, and a mouse lymphoma assay at concentrations up to 1000 mcg/plate, with and without metabolic activation, revealed no evidence of mutagenesis potential. Dornase Alfa was tested in a micronucleus (*in vivo*) assay for its potential to produce chromosome damage in bone marrow cells of mice following a bolus intravenous dose of 10 mg/kg on two consecutive days. No evidence of chromosomal damage was noted.

Impairment of Fertility: In studies with rats receiving up to 10 mg/kg/day, a dose representing systemic exposures greater than 600 times that expected following the recommended human dose, fertility and reproductive performance of both males and females was not affected.

PREGNANCY CATEGORY B

Reproduction studies have been performed in rats and rabbits with intravenous doses up to 10 mg/kg/day, representing systemic exposures greater than 600 times that expected following the recommended human dose. These studies have revealed no evidence of impaired fertility, harm to the fetus, or effects on development due to Dornase Alfa. There are, however, no adequate and well-controlled studies in pregnant women. Because animal reproductive studies are not always predictive of the human response, this drug should be used during pregnancy only if clearly needed.

NURSING MOTHERS

It is not known whether the drug is excreted in human milk. Because many drugs are excreted in human milk, caution should be exercised when Dornase Alfa is administered to a nursing woman.

PEDIATRIC USE

Safety and effectiveness of Dornase Alfa in children under the age of 5 years has not been studied.

DRUG INTERACTIONS:

Clinical trials have indicated that Pulmozyme (dornase alfa) can be effectively and safely used in conjunction with standard cystic fibrosis therapies including oral, inhaled and parenteral antibiotics, bronchodilators, enzyme supplements, vitamins, oral and inhaled corticosteroids, and analgesics. No formal drug interaction studies have been performed.

ADVERSE REACTIONS:

Patients have been exposed to Dornase Alfa for up to 12 months in clinical trials. In a large, randomized, placebo-controlled clinical trial, over 600 patients received Dornase Alfa once or twice daily for six months; most adverse events were not more common on Dornase Alfa than on placebo and probably reflected the sequelae of the underlying lung disease. In most cases events that were increased were mild, transient in nature, and did not require alterations in dosing. Few patients experienced adverse events resulting in permanent discontinuation from Dornase Alfa, and the discontinuation rate was similar for placebo (2%) and Dornase Alfa (3%).

Events that were more frequent in Dornase Alfa treated patients than in placebo treated patients are listed in TABLE 2.

TABLE 2 Adverse Events Reported in a Controlled Trial

Adverse Event	Placebo n=325	Pulmozyme QD n=322	Pulmozyme BID n=321
Voice alteration	7%	12%	16%
Pharyngitis	33%	36%	40%
Laryngitis	1%	3%	4%
Rash	7%	10%	12%
Chest pain	16%	18%	21%
Conjunctivitis	2%	4%	5%

EVENTS OBSERVED AT SIMILAR RATES IN DORNASE ALFA AND PLACEBO TREATED PATIENTS

Body as a Whole: Abdominal pain, Asthenia, Fever, Flu syndrome, Malaise, Sepsis

Digestive System: Intestinal Obstruction, Gall Bladder disease, Liver disease, Pancreatic disease

Metabolic Nutritional System: Diabetes Mellitus, Hypoxia, Weight Loss

Respiratory System: Apnea, Bronchiectasis, Bronchitis, Change in Sputum, Cough Increase, Dyspnea, Hemoptysis, Lung Function Decrease, Nasal Polyps, Pneumonia, Pneumothorax, Rhinitis, Sinusitis, Sputum Increase, Wheeze

Mortality rates observed in a controlled trial were similar for the placebo (1%) and Pulmozyme (dornase alfa) (1%). Causes of death were consistent with progression of cystic fibrosis and included apnea, cardiac arrest, cardiopulmonary arrest, cor pulmonale, heart failure, massive hemoptysis, pneumonia, pneumothorax, and respiratory failure.

Allergic Reactions: There have been no reports of anaphylaxis attributed to the administration of Dornase Alfa to date. Skin rash and urticaria have been observed, and were mild and transient in nature. Within all of the studies, a small percentage (average of 2-4%) of patients treated with Dornase Alfa developed serum antibodies to Dornase Alfa. None of these patients developed anaphylaxis, and the clinical significance of serum antibodies to Dornase Alfa is unknown.

OVERDOSAGE:

Single-dose inhalation studies in rats and monkeys at doses up to 180-times higher than doses routinely used in clinical studies are well tolerated. Single dose oral administration of Dornase Alfa in doses up to 200 mg/kg are also well tolerated by rats.

Cystic fibrosis patients have received up to 20 mg BID for up to 6 days and 10 mg BID intermittently (2 weeks on/2 weeks off drug) for 168 days. These doses were well tolerated.

DOSAGE AND ADMINISTRATION:

The recommended dose for use in most cystic fibrosis patients is one 2.5 mg single-use ampule inhaled once daily using a recommended nebulizer. Some patients may benefit from twice daily administration (see TABLE 1). Clinical trials have been performed with the following nebulizers and compressors: the disposable jet nebulizer Hudson T Up-draft II and disposable jet nebulizer Marquest Acorn II in conjunction with a Pulmo-Aide compressor, and the reusable PARI LC Jet+ nebulizer, in conjunction with the PARI PRONEB compressor. Safety and efficacy have been demonstrated only with these recommended nebulizer systems. No clinical data are currently available that support the safety and efficacy of administration of Dornase Alfa with other nebulizer systems. That patient should follow the manufacturer's instructions on the use and maintenance of the equipment.

DOSAGE AND ADMINISTRATION: *(cont'd)*

Dornase Alfa should not be diluted or mixed with other drugs in the nebulizer. Mixing of Dornase Alfa with other drugs could lead to adverse physiochemical and/or functional changes in Dornase Alfa or the admixed compound.

REFERENCES:

1. Shak S, Capon DJ, Hellmiss R, Marsters SA, Baker CL. Recombinant human DNase I reduces the viscosity of cystic fibrosis sputum. Proc Natl Acad Sci USA 1990;87:9188-92. **2.** Boat TF. Cystic Fibrosis. In: Murray JF, Nadel JA, editors. Textbook of respiratory medicine. Philadelphia: Saunders WB, 1988;1:1126-52. **3.** Collins FS. Cystic Fibrosis: molecular biology and therapeutic implications. Science 1992;256:774-9. **4.** Potter JL, Spector S, Matthews LW, Lemm J. Studies of pulmonary secretions. Amer Rev of Respiratory Disease 1969;99:909-15. **5.** Hubbard RC, McElvaney NG, Birrer P, Shak S, Robinson WW, Jolley C, et al. A preliminary study of aerosolized recombinant human deoxyribonuclease I in the treatment of cystic fibrosis. New Eng J Med 1992;326:812-5. **6.** Aitken ML, Burke W, McDonald G, Shak S, Montgomery AB, Smith A. Recombinant human DNase inhalation in normal subjects and patients with cystic fibrosis. JAMA 1992;267(14):1947-51. **7.** Fuchs HJ, Borowitz D, Christianson D, Morris E, Nash M, Ramsey B, et al. Aerosolized recombinant human DNase reduces pulmonary exacerbations and improves pulmonary function in patients with cystic fibrosis. Presented by Mary Ellen Wohl, M.D. at the 36th Annual Conference on Chest Disease, Intermountain Thoracic Society, January 26, 1993.

HOW SUPPLIED:

Dornase Alfa Inhalation Solution is supplied in single-use ampules. Each ampule delivers 2.5 ml of a sterile, clear, colorless, aqueous solution containing 1.0 mg/ml dornase alfa, 0.15 mg/ml calcium chloride dihydrate and 8.77 mg/ml sodium chloride with no preservative. The nominal pH of the solution is 6.3.

Pulmozyme is Supplied In:

14 unit cartons, containing 14 single-use ampules in single- unit foil pouches.

30 unit cartons containing 5 foil pouches of 6 single-use ampules.

Storage: Dornase Alfa should be stored under refrigeration (2- 8°C/36-46°F). Ampules should be protected from light. Do not use beyond the expiration date stamped on the ampule. Unused ampules should be stored in their protective foil pouch under refrigeration.

HOW SUPPLIED - EQUIVALENTS NOT AVAILABLE:

Solution - Inhalation - 1 mg/ml

2.5 ml x 14	$453.60	PULMOZYME, Genentech	50242-0100-38
2.5 ml x 30	$972.00	PULMOZYME, Genentech	50242-0100-40

DORZOLAMIDE HYDROCHLORIDE *(003235)*

CATEGORIES: Antiglaucomatous Agents; Carbonic Anhydrase Inhibitors; EENT Drugs; Eye, Ear, Nose, & Throat Preparations; Glaucoma; Intraocular Pressure; Ocular Hypertension; Ophthalmics; FDA Class 1P ("Priority Review"); FDA Approved 1994 Dec; Top 200 Drugs; Top 200 Drugs

BRAND NAMES: **Trusopt**

FORMULARIES: PCS

COST OF THERAPY: $459.90 (Glaucoma; Solution; 2 %; 0.3/day; 365 days)

PRIMARY ICD9: 365.11 (Primary Open-Angle Glaucoma)

DESCRIPTION:

Trusopt (Dorzolamide Hydrochloride Ophthalmic Solution) is a carbonic anhydrase inhibitor formulated for topical ophthalmic use.

Dorzolamide hydrochloride is described chemically as: (4*S-trans*)- 4-(ethylamino)-5,6-dihydro-6-methyl-4*H*-thieno[2,3-*b*]thiopyran-2-sulfonamide 7,7-dioxide monohydrochloride. Dorzolamide hydrochloride is optically active. Its empirical formula is $C_{10}H_{16}N_2O_4S_3{\cdot}HCl$.

Dorzolamide hydrochloride has a molecular weight of 360.9 and a melting point of about 275°C. It is a white to off-white, crystalline powder, which is soluble in water and slightly soluble in methanol and ethanol.

Trusopt Sterile Ophthalmic Solution is supplied as a sterile, isotonic, buffered, slightly viscous, aqueous solution of dorzolamide hydrochloride. The pH of the solution is approximately 5.6. Each ml of Trusopt 2% contains 20 mg dorzolamide (22.3 mg of dorzolamide hydrochloride). Inactive ingredients are hydroxyethyl cellulose, mannitol, sodium citrate dihydrate, sodium hydroxide (to adjust pH) and water for injection. Benzalkonium chloride 0.0075% is added as a preservative.

CLINICAL PHARMACOLOGY:

MECHANISM OF ACTION

Carbonic anhydrase (CA) is an enzyme found in many tissues of the body including the eye. It catalyzes the reversible reaction involving the hydration of carbon dioxide and the dehydration of carbonic acid. In humans, carbonic anhydrase exists as a number of isoenzymes, the most active being carbonic anhydrase II (CA-II), found primarily in red blood cells (RBCs), but also in other tissues. Inhibition of carbonic anhydrase in the ciliary processes of the eye decreases aqueous humor secretion, presumably by slowing the formation of bicarbonate ions with subsequent reduction in sodium and fluid transport. The result is a reduction in intraocular pressure (IOP).

Trusopt Ophthalmic Solution contains dorzolamide hydrochloride, an inhibitor of human carbonic anhydrase II. Following topical ocular administration, Trusopt reduces elevated intraocular pressure. Elevated intraocular pressure is a major risk factor in the pathogenesis of optic nerve damage and glaucomatous visual field loss.

PHARMACOKINETICS/PHARMACODYNAMICS

When topically applied, dorzolamide reaches the systemic circulation. To assess the potential for systemic carbonic anhydrase inhibition following topical administration, drug and metabolite concentrations in RBCs and plasma and carbonic anhydrase inhibition in RBCs were measured.

Dorzolamide accumulates in RBCs during chronic dosing as a result of binding to CA-II. The parent drug forms a single N-desethyl metabolite, which inhibits CA-II less potently than the parent drug but also inhibits CA-1. The metabolite also accumulates in RBCs where it binds primarily to CA-1. Plasma concentrations of dorzolamide and metabolite are generally below the assay limit of quantitation (15nM). Dorzolamide binds moderately to plasma proteins (approximately 33%). Dorzolamide is primarily excreted unchanged in the urine; the metabolite also excreted in urine. After dosing is stopped, dorzolamide washes out of RBCs nonlinearly, resulting in a rapid decline of drug concentration initially, followed by a slower elimination phase with a half-life of about four months.

To simulate the systemic exposure after long-term topical ocular administration, dorzolamide was given orally to eight healthy subjects for up to 20 weeks. The oral dose of 2 mg b.i.d. closely approximates the amount of drug delivered by topical ocular administration of Trusopt 2% t.i.d. Steady state was reached within 8 weeks. The inhibition of CA-II and total carbonic anhydrase activities was below the degree of inhibition anticipated to be necessary for a pharmacological effect on renal function and respiration in healthy individuals.

CLINICAL STUDIES:

The efficacy of Trusopt was demonstrated in clinical studies in the treatment of elevated intraocular pressure in patients with glaucoma or ocular hypertension (baseline IOP ≥ 23 mmHg). The IOP-lowering effect of Trusopt was approximately 3 to 5 mmHg throughout the day and this was consistent in clinical studies of up to one year duration.

The efficacy of Trusopt when dosed less frequently than three times a day (alone or in combination with other products) has not been established.

INDICATIONS AND USAGE:

Trusopt Ophthalmic Solution is indicated in the treatment of elevated intraocular pressure in patients with ocular hypertension or open-angle glaucoma.

CONTRAINDICATIONS:

Trusopt is contraindicated in patients who are hypersensitive to any component of this product.

WARNINGS:

Trusopt is a sulfonamide and although administered topically is absorbed systemically. Therefore, the same types of adverse reactions that are attributable to sulfonamides may occur with topical administration with Trusopt. Fatalities have occurred, although rarely, due to severe reactions to sulfonamides including Stevens-Johnson syndrome, toxic epidermal necrolysis, fulminant hepatic necrosis, agranulocytosis, aplastic anemia, and other blood dyscrasias. Sensitization may recur when a sulfonamide is readministered irrespective of the route of administration. If signs of serious reactions or hypersensitivity occur, discontinue the use of this preparation.

PRECAUTIONS:

GENERAL

Carbonic anhydrase activity has been observed in both the cytoplasm and around the plasma membranes of the corneal endothelium. The effect of continued administration of Trusopt on the corneal endothelium has not been fully evaluated.

The management of patients with acute angle-closure glaucoma requires therapeutic interventions in addition to ocular hypotensive agents. Trusopt has not been studied in patients with acute angle-closure glaucoma.

Trusopt has not been studied in patients with severe renal impairment (CrCl < 30 ml/min). Because Trusopt and its metabolite are excreted predominantly by the kidney, Trusopt is not recommended in such patients.

Trusopt has not been studied in patients with hepatic impairment and should therefore be used with caution in such patients.

In clinical studies, local ocular adverse effects, primarily conjunctivitis and lid reactions, were reported with chronic administration of Trusopt. Many of these reactions had the clinical appearance and course of an allergic-type reaction that resolved upon discontinuation of drug therapy. If such reactions are observed, Trusopt should be discontinued and the patient evaluated before considering restarting the drug. (See ADVERSE REACTIONS.)

There is a potential for an additive effect on the known systemic effects of carbonic anhydrase inhibition in patients receiving an oral carbonic anhydrase inhibitor and Trusopt. The concomitant administration of Trusopt and oral carbonic anhydrase inhibitors is not recommended.

There have been reports of bacterial keratitis associated with the use of multiple dose containers of topical ophthalmic products. These containers had been inadvertently contaminated by patients who, in most cases, had a concurrent corneal disease or a disruption of the ocular epithelial surface.

The preservative in Trusopt Ophthalmic Solution, benzalkonium chloride, may be absorbed by soft contact lenses. Trusopt should not be administered while wearing soft contact lenses.

INFORMATION FOR THE PATIENT

Trusopt is a sulfonamide and although administered topically is absorbed systemically. Therefore the same types of administration. Patients should be advised that if serious or unusual reactions or signs of hypersensitivity occur, they should discontinue the use of the product (see WARNINGS.)

Patients should be advised that if they develop any ocular reactions, particularly conjunctivitis and lid reactions, they should discontinue use and seek their physician's advice.

Patients should be instructed to avoid allowing the tip of the dispensing container to contact the eye or surrounding structures.

Patients should also be instructed that ocular solutions, if handled improperly or if the tip of the dispensing container contacts the eye or surrounding structures, can become contaminated by common bacteria known to cause ocular infections. Serious damage to the eye and subsequent loss of vision may result from using contaminated solutions.

Patients also should be advised that if they develop an intercurrent ocular condition (*e.g.*, trauma, ocular surgery or infection), they should immediately seek their physician's advice concerning the continued use of the present multidose container.

If more than one topical ophthalmic drug is being used, the drugs should be administered at least ten minutes apart.

CARCINOGENESIS, MUTAGENESIS, AND IMPAIRMENT OF FERTILITY

In a two-year study of dorzolamide hydrochloride administrated orally to male and female Sprague-Dawley rats, urinary bladder papillomas were seen in male rats in the highest dosage group of 20 mg/kg/day (250 times the recommended human ophthalmic dose). Papillomas were not seen in rats given oral doses equivalent to approximately 12 times the recommended human ophthalmic dose. No treatment-related tumors were seen in a 21- month study in female and male mice given oral doses up to 75 mg/kg/day (~900 times the recommended human ophthalmic dose).

The increased incidence of urinary bladder papillomas seen in the high-dose male rats is a class-effect of carbonic anhydrase inhibitors in rats. Rats are particularly prone to developing papillomas in response to foreign bodies, compounds causing crystalluria, and diverse sodium salts.

No changes in bladder urothelium were seen in dogs given oral dorzolamide hydrochloride for one year at 2 mg/kg/day (25 times the recommended human ophthalmic dose) or monkeys dosed topically to the eye at 0.4 mg/kg/day (~5 times the recommended human ophthalmic dose) for one year.

The following tests for mutagenic potential were negative: (1) *in vivo* (mouse) cytogenetic assay; (2) *in vitro* chromosomal aberration assay; (3) alkaline elution assay; (4) V-79 assay; and (5) Ames test.

In reproduction studies of dorzolamide hydrochloride in rats, there were no adverse effects on the reproductive capacity of males or females at doses up to 188 or 94 times, respectively, the recommended human ophthalmic dose.

PRECAUTIONS: *(cont'd)*

PREGNANCY, TERATOGENIC EFFECTS, PREGNANCY CATEGORY C

Developmental toxicity studies dorzolamide hydrochloride in rabbits at oral doses of ≥ 2.5 mg/kg/day (31 times the recommended human ophthalmic dose) revealed malformations of vertebral bodies. These malformations occurred at doses that caused metabolic acidosis with decreased body weight gain in dams and decreased fetal weights. No treatment-related malformations were seen at 1.0 mg/kg/day (13 times the recommended human ophthalmic dose). There were no treatment-related fetal malformations in developmental toxicity studies with dorzolamide hydrochloride in rats at oral doses up to 10 mg/kg/day (125 times the recommended human ophthalmic dose). There are no adequate and well- controlled studies in pregnant women. Trusopt should be used during pregnancy only if the potential benefit justifies the potential risk to the fetus.

NURSING MOTHERS

In a study of dorzolamide hydrochloride in lactating rats, decreases in body weight gain of 5 to 7% in offspring at an oral dose of 7.5 mg/kg/day (94 times the recommended human ophthalmic dose) were seen during lactation. A slight delay in postnatal development (incisor eruption, vaginal canalization and eye openings), secondary to lower fetal body weight, was noted.

It is not known whether this drug is excreted in human milk. Because many drugs are excreted in human milk and because of the potential for serious adverse reactions in nursing infants from Trusopt, a decision should be made whether to discontinue nursing or to discontinue the drug, taking into account the importance of the drug to the mother.

PEDIATRIC USE

Safety and effectiveness in children have not been established.

GERIATRIC USE

Of the total number of patients in clinical studies of Trusopt, 44% were 65 years of age and over, while 10% were 75 years of age and over. No overall differences in effectiveness or safety were observed between patients and younger patients, but greater sensitivity of some older individuals to the product cannot be ruled out.

DRUG INTERACTIONS:

Although acid-base and electrolyte disturbances were not reported in the clinical trials with Trusopt, these disturbances have been reported with oral carbonic anhydrase inhibitors and have, in some instances, resulted in drug interactions (*e.g.,* toxicity associated with high-dose salicylate therapy). Therefore, the potential for such drug interactions should be considered in patients receiving Trusopt.

ADVERSE REACTIONS:

In clinical studies, the most frequent adverse events associated with Trusopt were ocular burning, stinging, or discomfort immediately following ocular administration (approximately one-third of patients). Approximately one-quarter of patients noted a bitter taste following administration. Superficial punctate keratitis occurred in 10-15% of patients and signs and symptoms of ocular allergic reaction in approximately 10%. Events occurring in approximately 1-5% of patients were blurred vision, tearing, dryness, and photophobia. Other ocular events and systemic events were reported infrequently, including headache, nausea, asthenia/fatigue; and, rarely, skin rashes, urolithiasis, and iridocyclitis.

OVERDOSAGE:

Although no human data are available, electrolyte imbalance, development of an acidotic state, and possible central nervous system effects may occur. Serum electrolyte levels (particularly potassium) and blood pH levels should be monitored.

Significant lethality was observed in female rats and mice after single oral doses of dorzolamide hydrochloride 1927 mg/kg and 1320 mg/kg, respectively.

DOSAGE AND ADMINISTRATION:

The dose is one drop Trusopt Ophthalmic Solution in the affected eye(s) three times daily.

Trusopt may be used concomitantly with other topical ophthalmic drug products to lower intraocular pressure. If more than one topical ophthalmic drug is being used, the drugs should be administered at least ten minutes apart.

PATIENT INFORMATION:

Dorzolamide HCl is any eye drop used to treat increased pressure in the eye. For the drops to most effective, proper instillation into the eye is important. Your pharmacist or physician can instruct you. This drug may produce allergic reactions in those with sulfa allergies. Allergies can developed after several exposures and any signs of allergy (itchy watery eyes, rash, difficulty breathing in severe cases) should be reported to a healthcare professional immediately. This eye drop does contain a preservative (benzalkonium chloride) to which some may be sensitive. It should not be used by those wearing contact lenses. With all eyedrops, care should be taken to avoid touching the tip of the dropper to the eye or surrounding skin. This could cause contamination of the medication and result in a serious eye infection. Potentially contaminated solutions should be replaced. If you are using more than one eyedrop medication, wait ten minutes between each medication. Some patients will experience burning, itching or discomfort after instilling the eyedrops, and fewer will experience a bitter taste in their mouth. Talk to your pharmacist or physician if you are concerned about eye discomfort.

HOW SUPPLIED:

Trusopt Ophthalmic Solution is a slightly opalescent, nearly colorless slightly viscous solution.

No. 3519 - Trusopt Ophthalmic Solution 2% is supplied in Ocumeter, a white, opaque, plastic ophthalmic dispenser with a controlled drop tip as follows: 5 mL; 10 mL; 3 X 5 mL.

Storage: Store Trusopt Ophthalmic Solution at 15-30°C (59- 86°F). Protect from light.

HOW SUPPLIED - EQUIVALENTS NOT AVAILABLE:

Solution - Ophthalmic - 2 %

5 ml	**$21.00**	**TRUSOPT, Merck**	**00006-3519-03**
5 ml x 3	**$63.00**	**TRUSOPT, Merck**	**00006-3519-34**
10 ml	**$42.00**	**TRUSOPT, Merck**	**00006-3519-10**

DOXACURIUM CHLORIDE *(003028)*

CATEGORIES: Anesthesia; Autonomic Drugs; Endotracheal Intubation; Muscle Relaxants; Neuromuscular; Neuromuscular Blocking Agents; Non-Depolarizing Muscle Relaxants; Skeletal Muscle Relaxants; Pregnancy Category C; FDA Class 1C ("Little or No Therapeutic Advantage"); FDA Approved 1991 Mar

BRAND NAMES: **Nuromax**

This drug should be administered only by adequately trained individuals familiar with its actions, characteristics, and hazards.

DESCRIPTION:

Doxacurium chloride is a long-acting, nondepolarizing skeletal muscle relaxant for intravenous administration. Doxacurium chloride is [1α,2β(1'*S**.2'*R**)]-2.2'-[(1,4-dioxo-1,4-butanediyl)bis(oxy-3,1-propanediyl)]bis[1,2,3,4-tetrahydro-6,7,8- trimethoxy-2-methyl-1-[(3,4,5-trimethoxyphenyl)methyl]isoquinolinium]dichloride (meso form). The molecular formula is $C_{56}H_{78}Cl_2N_2O_{16}$ and the molecular weight is 1106.14. The compound does not partition into the 1-octanol phase of a distilled water/1-octanol system, *i.e.,* the n-octanol:water partition coefficient is 0.

Doxacurium chloride is a mixture of three *trans, trans* stereoisomers, a *dl* pair [(1*R*, 1'*R*, 2*S*, 2'*S*) and (1*S*, 1'*S*, 2*R*, 2'*R*)] and a meso form (1*R*, 1'*S*, 2*S*, 2'*R*).

Nuromax Injection is a sterile, non-pyrogenic aqueous solution (pH 3.9 to 5.0) containing doxacurium chloride equivalent to 1 mg/ml doxacurium in Water for Injection. Hydrochloric acid may have been added to adjust pH. Doxacurium chloride injection contains 0.9% w/v benzyl alcohol.

CLINICAL PHARMACOLOGY:

Doxacurium chloride binds competitively to cholinergic receptors on the motor end-plate to antagonize the action of acetylcholine, resulting in a block of neuromuscular transmission. This action is antagonized by acetylcholinesterase inhibitors, such as neostigmine.

Pharmacodynamics: Doxacurium chloride is approximately 2.5 to 3 times more potent than pancuronium and 10 to 12 times more potent than metocurine. Doxacurium chloride in doses of 1.5 to 2 x ED_{95} has a clinical duration of action (range and variability) similar to that of equipotent doses of pancuronium and metocurine (historic data and limited comparison). The average ED_{95} (dose required to produce 95% suppression of the adductor pollicis muscle twitch response to ulnar nerve stimulation) of doxacurium chloride is 0.025 mg/kg (range: 0.020 to 0.033) in adults receiving balanced anesthesia.

The onset and clinically effective duration (time from injection to 25% recovery) of doxacurium chloride administered alone or after succinylcholine during stable balanced anesthesia are shown in TABLE 1.

TABLE 1 Pharmacodynamic Dose Response* Balanced Anesthesia

	Initial Nuromax Dose (mg/kg)		
	0.025† (n=34)	**0.05 (n=27)**	**0.08 (n=9)**
Time to Maximum Block (min)	9.3 (5.4-16)	5.2 (2.5-13)	3.5 (2.4-5)
Clinical Duration (min) (Time to 25% Recovery)	55 (9-145)	100 (39-232)	160 (110-338)

* Values shown are means (range).
† Doxacurium chloride administered after 10% to 100% recovery from an intubating dose of succinylcholine.

Initial doses of 0.05 mg/kg (2 x ED_{95}) and 0.08 mg/kg (3 x ED_{95}) doxacurium chloride administered during the induction of thiopental-narcotic anesthesia produced good-to-excellent conditions for tracheal intubation in 5 minutes (13 of 15 cases studied) and 4 minutes (8 of 9 cases studied) (which are before maximum block), respectively.

As with other long-acting agents, the clinical duration of neuromuscular block associated with doxacurium chloride shows considerable interpatient variability. An analysis of 390 cases in U.S. clinical trials utilizing a variety of premedications, varying lengths of surgery, and various anesthetic agents, indicates that approximately two-thirds of the patients had clinical durations within 30 minutes of the duration predicted by dose (based on mg/kg actual body weight). Patients ≥60 years old are approximately twice as likely to experience prolonged clinical duration (30 minutes longer than predicted) than patients < 60 years old; thus, care should be used in older patients when prolonged recovery is undesirable (see PRECAUTIONS, Geriatric Use and Individualization of Dosages.) In addition, obese patients (patients weighing ≥30% more than ideal body weight for height) were almost twice as likely to experience prolonged clinical duration than non-obese patients; therefore, dosing should be based on ideal body weight (IBW) for obese patients (see CLINICAL PHARMACOLOGY,.)

The mean time for spontaneous T_1 recovery from 25% to 50% of control following initial doses of doxacurium chloride is approximately 26 minutes (range: 7 to 104, n=253) during balanced anesthesia. The mean time for spontaneous T_1 recovery from 25% to 75% is 54 minutes (range: 14 to 184, n=184).

Most patients receiving doxacurium chloride in clinical trials required pharmacologic reversal prior to full spontaneous recovery from neuromuscular block (see OVERDOSAGE, Antagonism of Neuromuscular Block); therefore, relatively few data are available on the time from injection to 95% spontaneous recovery of the twitch response. As with other long-acting neuromuscular blocking agents, doxacurium chloride may be associated with prolonged times to full spontaneous recovery. Following an initial dose of 0.025 mg/kg doxacurium chloride, some patients may require as long as 4 hours to exhibit full spontaneous recovery.

Cumulative neuromuscular blocking effects are not associated with repeated administration of maintenance doses of doxacurium chloride at 25% T_1 recovery. As with initial doses, however, the duration of action following maintenance doses of doxacurium chloride may vary considerably among patients.

The doxacurium chloride ED_{95} for children 2 to 12 years of age receiving halothane anesthesia is approximately 0.03 mg/kg. Children require higher doxacurium chloride doses on a mg/kg basis than adults to achieve comparable levels of block. The onset time and duration of block are shorter in children than adults. During halothane anesthesia, doses of 0.03 mg/kg and 0.05 mg/kg doxacurium chloride produce maximum block in approximately 7 and 4 minutes, respectively. The duration of clinically effective block is approximately 30 minutes after an initial dose of 0.03 mg/kg and approximately 45 minutes after 0.05 mg/kg. Doxacurium chloride has not been studied in children below the age of 2 years.

The neuromuscular block produced by doxacurium chloride may be antagonized by anticholinesterase agents. As with other nondepolarizing neuromuscular blocking agents, the more profound the neuromuscular block at reversal, the longer the time and the greater the dose of anticholinesterase required for recovery of neuromuscular function.

Hemodynamics: Administration of doxacurium chloride doses up to and including 0.08 mg/kg (~3 x ED_{95}) over 5 to 15 seconds to healthy adult patients during stable state balanced anesthesia and to patients with serious cardiovascular disease undergoing coronary artery bypass grafting, cardiac valvular repair, or vascular repair produced no dose-related effects on mean arterial blood pressure (MAP) or heart rate (HR).

No dose-related changes in MAP and HR were observed following administration of up to 0.05 mg/kg doxacurium chloride over 5 to 15 seconds in 2- to 12-year-old children receiving halothane anesthesia.

CLINICAL PHARMACOLOGY: *(cont'd)*

Doses of 0.03 to 0.08 mg/kg (1.2 to 3 x ED_{95}) were not associated with dose-dependent changes in mean plasma histamine concentration. Clinical experience with more than 1,000 patients indicates that adverse experiences typically associated with histamine release (*e.g.,* bronchospasm, hypotension, tachycardia, cutaneous flushing, urticaria,*etc.*) are very rare following the administration of doxacurium chloride (see ADVERSE REACTIONS.)

Pharmacokinetics: Pharmacokinetic and pharmacodynamic results from a study of 24 healthy young adult patients and 8 healthy elderly patients are summarized in TABLE 2. The pharmacokinetics are linear over the dosage range tested (*i.e.,* plasma concentrations are approximately proportional to dose). The pharmacokinetics of doxacurium chloride are similar in healthy young adult and elderly patients. Some healthy elderly patients tend to be more sensitive to the neuromuscular blocking effects of doxacurium chloride than healthy young adult patients receiving the same dose. The time to maximum block is longer in elderly patients than in young adult patients (11.2 minutes versus 7.7 minutes at 0.025 mg/kg doxacurium chloride). In addition, the clinically effective durations of block are more variable and tend to be longer in healthy elderly patients than in healthy young adult patients receiving the same dose.

TABLE 2 Pharmacokinetic and Pharmacodynamic Parameters [1] of Doxacurium Chloride in Young Adult and Elderly Patients (Isoflurane Anesthesia)

Parameter	Healthy Young Adult Patients (22 to 49 yrs) 0.25 mg/kg (n=8)	0.05 mg/kg (n=8)	0.08 mg/kg (n=8)	Healthy Elderly Patients (67 to 72 yrs) 0.025 mg/kg (n=8)
$t_{1/2}$ elimination (min)	86 (25-171)	123 (61-163)	98 (47-163)	96 (50-114)
Volume of Distribution at Steady State (L/kg)	0.15 (0.10-0.21)	0.24 (0.13-0.30)	0.22 (0.16-0.33)	0.22 (0.14-0.40)
Plasma Clearance (ml/min/kg)	2.22 (1.02-3.95)	2.62 (1.21-5.70)	2.53 (1.88-3.38)	2.47 (1.58-3.60)
Maximum Block (%)	97 (88-100)	100 (100-100)	100 (100-100)	96 (90-100)
Clinically Effective Duration of Block[2] (min)	68 (35-90)	91 (47-132)	177 (74-268)	97 (36-179)

[1]Values shown are means (range).
[2]Time from injection to 25% recovery of the control twitch height.

TABLE 3 summarizes the pharmacokinetic and pharmacodynamic results from a study of 9 healthy young adult patients, 8 patients with end-stage kidney disease undergoing kidney transplantation, and 7 patients with end-stage liver disease undergoing liver transplantation. The results suggest that a longer $t_{\frac{1}{2}}$ can be expected in patients with end-stage kidney disease; in addition, these patients may be more sensitive to the neuromuscular blocking effects of doxacurium chloride. The time to maximum block was slightly longer and the clinically effective duration of block was prolonged in patients with end-stage kidney disease.

TABLE 3 Pharmacokinetic and Pharmacodynamic Parameters [1] of Doxacurium Chloride in Healthy Patients and in Patients Undergoing Kidney or Liver Transplantation (Isoflurane Anesthesia)

Parameter 0.015 mg/kg	Healthy Young Adult Patients 0.015 mg/kg (n=9)	Kidney Transplant Patients 0.015 mg/kg (n=8)	Liver Transplant Patients (n=7)
$t_{1/2}$ elimination (min)	99 (48-193)	221 (84-592)	115 (69-148)
Volume of Distribution at Steady State (L/kg)	0.22 (0.11-0.43)	0.27 (0.17-0.55)	0.29 (0.17-0.35)
Plasma Clearance (ml/min/kg)	2.66 (1.35-6.66)	1.23 (0.48-2.40)	2.30 (1.96-3.05)
Maximum Block (%)	86 (59-100)	98 (95-100)	70 (0-100)
Clinically Effective Duration of Block (min)	36 (19-80)	80 (29-133)	52 (20-91)

[1]Values shown are means (range).

No data are available from patients with liver disease not requiring transplantation. There are no significant alterations in the pharmacokinetics of doxacurium chloride in liver transplant patients. Sensitivity to the neuromuscular blocking effects of doxacurium chloride was highly variable in patients undergoing liver transplantation. Three of 7 patients developed ≤50% block, indicating that a reduced sensitivity to doxacurium chloride may occur in such patients. In those patients who developed >50% neuromuscular block, the time to maximum block and the clinically effective duration tended to be longer than in healthy young adult patients (see CLINICAL PHARMACOLOGY, Individualization of Dosages.)

Consecutively administered maintenance doses of 0.005 mg/kg doxacurium chloride, each given at 25% T_1 recovery following the preceding dose, do not result in a progressive increase in the plasma concentration of doxacurium or a progressive increase in the depth or duration of block produced by each dose.

Doxacurium chloride is not metabolized *in vitro* in fresh human plasma. Plasma protein binding of doxacurium chloride is approximately 30% in human plasma.

In vivo data from humans suggest that doxacurium chloride is not metabolized and that the major elimination pathway is excretion of unchanged drug in urine and bile. In studies of healthy adult patients, 24% to 38% of an administered dose was recovered as parent drug in urine over 6 to 12 hours after dosing. High bile concentrations of doxacurium chloride (relative to plasma) have been found 35 to 90 minutes after administration. The overall extent of biliary excretion is unknown. The data derived from analysis of human urine and bile are

CLINICAL PHARMACOLOGY: *(cont'd)*

consistent with data from *in vivo* studies in the rat, cat, and dog, which indicate that all of an administered dose of doxacurium chloride is recovered as parent drug in the urine and bile of these species.

Individualization of Dosages: In elderly patients or patients who have impaired renal function, the potential for a prolongation of block may be reduced by decreasing the initial doxacurium chloride dose and by titrating the dose to achieve the desired depth of block. In obese patients (patients weighing ≥30% more than ideal body weight for height), the doxacurium chloride dose should be determined using the patient's ideal body weight (IBW), according to the formulae in TABLE 4.

TABLE 4

Men: IBW in kg = [106 + (6 × inches in height above 5 feet] ÷ 2.2
Women: IBW in kg = [100 + (5 × inches in height above 5 feet] ÷ 2.2

Dosage requirements for patients with severe liver disease are variable; some patients may require a higher than normal initial doxacurium chloride dose to achieve clinically effective block. Once adequate block is established, the clinical duration of block may be prolonged in such patients relative to patients with normal liver function.

As with pancuronium, metocurine, and vecuronium, resistance to doxacurium chloride, manifested by a reduced intensity and/or shortened duration of block, must be considered when doxacurium chloride is selected for use in patients receiving phenytoin or carbamazepine (see DRUG INTERACTIONS).

As with other nondepolarizing neuromuscular blocking agents, a reduction in dosage of doxacurium chloride must be considered in cachectic or debilitated patients, in patients with neuromuscular diseases, severe electrolyte abnormalities, or carcinomatosis, and in other patients in whom potentiation of neuromuscular block or difficulty with reversal is anticipated. Increased doses of doxacurium chloride may be required in burn patients (see PRECAUTIONS).

INDICATIONS AND USAGE:

Doxacurium chloride is a long-acting neuromuscular blocking agent, indicated to provide skeletal muscle relaxation as an adjunct to general anesthesia, for endotracheal intubation or to facilitate mechanical ventilation.

CONTRAINDICATIONS:

Doxacurium chloride is contraindicated in patients known to have hypersensitivity to it.

WARNINGS:

DOXACURIUM CHLORIDE SHOULD BE ADMINISTERED IN CAREFULLY ADJUSTED DOSAGE BY OR UNDER THE SUPERVISION OF EXPERIENCED CLINICIANS WHO ARE FAMILIAR WITH THE DRUG'S ACTIONS AND THE POSSIBLE COMPLICATIONS OF ITS USE. THE DRUG SHOULD NOT BE ADMINISTERED UNLESS FACILITIES FOR INTUBATION, ARTIFICIAL RESPIRATION, OXYGEN THERAPY, AND AN ANTAGONIST ARE WITHIN IMMEDIATE REACH. IT IS RECOMMENDED THAT CLINICIANS ADMINISTERING LONG-ACTING NEUROMUSCULAR BLOCKING AGENTS SUCH AS DOXACURIUM CHLORIDE EMPLOY A PERIPHERAL NERVE STIMULATOR TO MONITOR DRUG RESPONSE, NEED FOR ADDITIONAL RELAXANTS, AND ADEQUACY OF SPONTANEOUS RECOVERY OR ANTAGONISM.

DOXACURIUM CHLORIDE HAS NO KNOWN EFFECT ON CONSCIOUSNESS, PAIN, THRESHOLD, OR CEREBRATION. TO AVOID DISTRESS TO THE PATIENT, NEUROMUSCULAR BLOCK SHOULD NOT BE INDUCED BEFORE UNCONSCIOUSNESS.

Doxacurium chloride injection is acidic (pH 3.9 to 5.0) and may not be compatible with alkaline solutions having a pH greater than 8.5 (*e.g.,* barbiturate solutions).

Doxacurium chloride injection contains benzyl alcohol. In newborn infants, benzyl alcohol has been associated with an increased incidence of neurological and other complications which are sometimes fatal. (See PRECAUTIONS, Pediatric Use.)

PRECAUTIONS:

General: Doxacurium chloride has no clinically significant effects on heart rate; therefore, doxacurium chloride will not counteract the bradycardia produced by many anesthetic agents or by vagal stimulation.

Neuromuscular blocking agents may have a profound effect in patients with neuromuscular diseases (*e.g.,* myasthenia gravis and the myasthenic syndrome). In these and other conditions in which prolonged neuromuscular block is a possibility (*e.g.,* carcinomatosis), the use of a peripheral nerve stimulator and a small test dose of doxacurium chloride is recommended to assess the level of neuromuscular block and to monitor dosage requirements. Shorter acting muscle relaxants than doxacurium chloride may be more suitable for these patients.

Resistance to nondepolarizing neuromuscular blocking agents may develop in patients with burns depending upon the time elapsed since the injury and the size of the burn. Doxacurium chloride has not been studied in patients with burns.

Acid-base and/or serum electrolyte abnormalities may potentiate or antagonize the action of neuromuscular blocking agents. The action of neuromuscular blocking agents may be enhanced by magnesium salts administered for the management of toxemia of pregnancy.

Doxacurium chloride has not been studied in patients with asthma.

No data are available to support the use of doxacurium chloride by intramuscular injection.

Renal and Hepatic Disease: Doxacurium chloride has been studied in patients with end-stage kidney (n=8) or liver (n=7) disease undergoing transplantation procedures (see CLINICAL PHARMACOLOGY). The possibility of prolonged neuromuscular block in patients undergoing renal transplantation and the possibility of a variable onset and duration of neuromuscular block in patients undergoing liver transplantation must be considered when doxacurium chloride is used in such patients.

Obesity: Administration of doxacurium chloride on the basis of actual body weight is associated with a prolonged duration of action in obese patients (patients weighing ≥ 30% more than ideal body weight for height) (see CLINICAL PHARMACOLOGY). Therefore, the dose of doxacurium chloride should be based upon ideal body weight in obese patients (see Individualization of Dosages.)

Malignant Hyperthermia (MH): In a study of MH-susceptible pigs, doxacurium chloride did not trigger MH. Doxacurium chloride has not been studied in MH-susceptible patients. Since MH can develop in the absence of established triggering agents, the clinician should be prepared to recognize and treat MH in any patient scheduled for general anesthesia.

Long-Term Use in the Intensive Care Unit (ICU): Information on the use of doxacurium chloride in the ICU is limited. In a double-blind randomized study, 17 patients received doxacurium chloride by intermittent bolus injection for a mean of 2.7 ± 0.5 days (range 0.8 to 6.8 days) to facilitate mechanical ventilation. No evidence of tachyphylaxis, accumulation, or prolonged recovery was observed. The adverse experiences in patients receiving doxacurium chloride were consistent in type, severity, and frequency to those expected in a

PRECAUTIONS: *(cont'd)*

critically ill patient population. Since many ICU patients have and/or renal failure, a prolonged duration of block should be anticipated in these patients after administration of doxacurium chloride.

WHENEVER THE USE OF DOXACURIUM CHLORIDE OR ANY NEUROMUSCULAR BLOCKING AGENT IS CONTEMPLATED IN THE ICU. IT IS RECOMMENDED THAT NEUROMUSCULAR TRANSMISSION BE MONITORED CONTINUOUSLY DURING ADMINISTRATION WITH THE HELP OF A NERVE STIMULATOR. ADDITIONAL DOSES OF DOXACURIUM CHLORIDE OR ANY OTHER NEUROMUSCULAR BLOCKING AGENT SHOULD NOT BE GIVEN BEFORE THERE IS A DEFINITE RESPONSE TO T_1, OR TO THE FIRST TWITCH. IF NO RESPONSE IS ELICITED, BOLUS ADMINISTRATION SHOULD BE DELAYED UNTIL A RESPONSE RETURNS.

Carcinogenesis, Mutagenesis, and Impairment of Fertility: Carcinogenesis and fertility studies have not been performed. Doxacurium chloride was evaluated in a battery of four short-term mutagenicity tests. It was non-mutagenic in the Ames Salmonella assay, in the mouse lymphoma assay, and in the human lymphocyte assay. In the *in vivo* rat bone marrow cytogenetic assay, statistically significant increases in the incidence of structural abnormalities, relative to vehicle controls, were observed in male rats dosed with 0.1 mg/kg (0.625 mg/m^2) doxacurium chloride and sacrificed at 6 hours, but not at 24 or 48 hours, and in female rats dosed with 0.2 mg/kg (1.25 mg/m^2) doxacurium chloride and sacrificed at 24 hours, but not at 6 or 48 hours. There was no increase in structural abnormalities in either male or female rats given 0.3 mg/kg (1.875 mg/m^2) doxacurium chloride and sacrificed at 6, 24, or 48 hours. Thus, the incidence of abnormalities in the *in vivo* rat bone marrow cytogenetic assay was not dose-dependent and, therefore, the likelihood that the observed abnormalities were treatment-related or clinically significant is low.

Pregnancy, Teratogenic Effects, Pregnancy Category C: Teratology testing in nonventilated, pregnant rats and mice treated subcutaneously with maximum subparalyzing doses of doxacurium chloride revealed no maternal or fetal toxicity or teratogenic effects. There are no adequate and well-controlled studies of doxacurium chloride in pregnant women. Because animal studies are not always predictive of human response and the doses used were subparalyzing, doxacurium chloride should be used during pregnancy only if the potential benefit justifies the potential risk to the fetus.

Labor and Delivery: The use of doxacurium chloride during labor, vaginal delivery, or cesarean section has not been studied. It is not known whether doxacurium chloride administered to the mother has immediate or delayed effects on the fetus. The duration of action of doxacurium chloride exceeds the usual duration of operative obstetrics (cesarean section). Therefore, doxacurium chloride is not recommended for use in patients undergoing C-section.

Nursing Mothers: It is not known whether doxacurium chloride is excreted in human milk. Because many drugs are excreted in human milk, caution should be exercised following doxacurium chloride administration to a nursing woman.

Pediatric Use: Doxacurium chloride has not been studied in children below the age of 2 years. See CLINICAL PHARMACOLOGY and DOSAGE AND ADMINISTRATION for clinical experience and recommendations for use in children 2 to 12 years of age.

Geriatric Use: Doxacurium chloride has been used in elderly patients, including patients with significant cardiovascular disease. In elderly patients the onset of maximum block is slower and the duration of neuromuscular block produced by doxacurium chloride is more variable and, in some cases, longer than in young adult patients (see Individualization of Dosages.)

DRUG INTERACTIONS:

Prior administration of succinylcholine has no clinically important effect on the neuromuscular blocking action of doxacurium chloride.

The use of doxacurium chloride before succinylcholine to attenuate some of the side effects of succinylcholine has not been studied.

There are no clinical data on concomitant use of doxacurium chloride and other nondepolarizing neuromuscular blocking agents.

Isoflurane, enflurane and halothane decrease the $ED_{50}$of doxacurium chloride by 30% to 45%. These agents may also prolong the clinically effective duration of action by up to 25%.

Other drugs which may enhance the neuromuscular blocking action of nondepolarizing agents such as doxacurium chloride include certain antibiotics (*e.g.,* aminoglycosides, tetracyclines, bacitracin, polymyxins, lincomycin, clindamycin, colistin, and sodium colistimethate), magnesium salts, lithium, local anesthetics, procainamide, and quinidine.

As with some other nondepolarizing neuromuscular blocking agents, the time of onset of neuromuscular block induced by doxacurium chloride is lengthened and the duration of block is shortened in patients receiving phenytoin or carbamazepine.

ADVERSE REACTIONS:

The most frequent adverse effect of nondepolarizing blocking agents as a class consists of an extension of the pharmacological action beyond the time needed for surgery and anesthesia. This effect may vary from skeletal muscle weakness to profound and prolonged skeletal muscle paralysis resulting in respiratory insufficiency and apnea which require manual or mechanical ventilation until recovery is judged to be clinically adequate (see OVERDOSAGE). Inadequate reversal of neuromuscular block from doxacurium chloride is possible, as with all nondepolarizing agents. Prolonged neuromuscular block and inadequate reversal may lead to postoperative complications.

Observed in Clinical Trials: Adverse experiences were uncommon among the 1034 surgical patients and volunteers who received doxacurium chloride and other drugs in U.S. clinical studies in the course of a wide variety of procedures conducted during balanced or inhalational anesthesia. The following adverse experiences were reported in patients administered doxacurium chloride (all events judged by investigators during the clinical trials to have a possible causal relationship):

Incidence Greater than 1%: None

Incidence Less than 1%

Cardiovascular*: hypotension, †flushing,†ventricular fibrillation, myocardial infarction

Respiratory: bronchospasm, wheezing

Dermatological: urticaria, injection site reaction

Special Senses: diplopia

Nonspecific: difficult neuromuscular block reversal, prolonged drug effect, fever

* Reports of ventricular fibrillation (n=1) and myocardial infarction (n=1) were limited to ASA Class 3-4 patients undergoing cardiac surgery (n=142).

† 0.3% incidence. All other reactions unmarked were ≤ 0.1%.

OVERDOSAGE:

Overdosage with neuromuscular blocking agents may result in neuromuscular block beyond the time needed for surgery and anesthesia. The primary treatment is maintenance of a patent airway and controlled ventilation until recovery of normal neuromuscular function is assured. Once evidence of recovery from neuromuscular block is observed, further recovery may be facilitated by administration of an anticholinesterase agent (*e.g.,* neostigmine, edrophonium) in conjunction with an appropriate anticholinergic agent (see OVERDOSAGE, Antagonism of Neuromuscular Block).

Antagonism of Neuromuscular Block: ANTAGONISTS (SUCH AS NEOSTIGMINE) SHOULD NOT BE ADMINISTERED PRIOR TO THE DEMONSTRATION OF SOME SPONTANEOUS RECOVERY FROM NEUROMUSCULAR BLOCK. THE USE OF A NERVE STIMULATOR TO DOCUMENT RECOVERY AND ANTAGONISM OF NEUROMUSCULAR BLOCK IS RECOMMENDED. T_4/T_1 SHOULD BE > ZERO BEFORE ANTAGONISM IS ATTEMPTED.

In an analysis of patients in whom antagonism of neuromuscular block was evaluated following administration of single doses of neostigmine averaging 0.06 mg/kg (range: 0.05 to 0.075) administered at approximately 25% T_1 spontaneous recovery during balanced anesthesia, 71% of patients exhibited $T_4/T_1 \geq 0.7$ before monitoring was discontinued. For these patients, the mean time to $T_4/T_1 \geq 0.7$ was 19 minutes (range: 7 to 55). As with other long-acting nondepolarizing neuromuscular blocking agents, the time for recovery of neuromuscular function following administration of neostigmine is dependent upon the level of residual neuromuscular block at the time of attempted reversal; longer recovery times than those cited above may be anticipated when neostigmine is administered at more profound levels of block (*i.e.,* at < 25% T_1 recovery).

Patients should be evaluated for adequate clinical evidence of antagonism, e.g., 5-second head lift, and grip strength. Ventilation must be supported until no longer required. As with other neuromuscular blocking agents, physicians should be alert to the possibility that the action of the drugs used to antagonize neuromuscular block may wear off before the effects of doxacurium chloride on the neuromuscular junction have declined sufficiently.

Antagonism may be delayed in the presence of debilitation, carcinomatosis, and the concomitant use of certain broad spectrum antibiotics, or anesthetic agents and other drugs which enhance neuromuscular block or separately cause respiratory depression (see DRUG INTERACTIONS). Under such circumstances the management is the same as that of prolonged neuromuscular block.

In clinical trials, a dose of 1 mg/kg edrophonium was not as effective as a dose of 0.06 mg/kg neostigmine in antagonizing moderate to deep levels of neuromuscular block (*i.e.,* < 60% T_1 recovery). Therefore, the use of 1 mg/kg edrophonium is not recommended for reversal from moderate to deep levels of block. The use of pyridostigmine has not been studied.

DOSAGE AND ADMINISTRATION:

NUROMAX SHOULD ONLY BE ADMINISTERED INTRAVENOUSLY.

DOXACURIUM CHLORIDE, LIKE OTHER LONG-ACTING NEUROMUSCULAR BLOCKING AGENTS, DISPLAYS VARIABILITY IN THE DURATION OF ITS EFFECT. THE POTENTIAL FOR A PROLONGED CLINICAL DURATION OF NEUROMUSCULAR BLOCK MUST BE CONSIDERED WHEN DOXACURIUM CHLORIDE IS SELECTED FOR ADMINISTRATION. THE DOSAGE INFORMATION PROVIDED BELOW IS INTENDED AS A GUIDE ONLY. DOSES SHOULD BE INDIVIDUALIZED (SEE Individualization of Dosages). Factors that may warrant dosage adjustment include: advancing age, the presence of kidney or liver disease, or obesity (patients weighing ≥ 30% more than ideal body weight for height). The use of a peripheral nerve stimulator will permit the most advantageous use of doxacurium chloride, minimize the possibility of overdosage or underdosage, and assist in the evaluation of recovery.

PARENTERAL DRUG PRODUCTS SHOULD BE INSPECTED VISUALLY FOR PARTICULATE MATTER AND DISCOLORATION PRIOR TO ADMINISTRATION WHENEVER SOLUTION AND CONTAINER PERMIT.

ADULTS

Initial Doses: When administered as a component of a thiopental/narcotic induction-intubation paradigm as well as for production of long-duration neuromuscular block during surgery, 0.05 mg/kg (2 x ED_{95}) doxacurium chloride produces good-to-excellent conditions for tracheal intubation in 5 minutes in approximately 90% of patients. Lower doses of doxacurium chloride may result in a longer time for development of satisfactory intubation conditions. Clinically effective neuromuscular block may be expected to last approximately 100 minutes on average (range: 39 to 232) following 0.05 mg/kg doxacurium chloride administered to patients receiving balanced anesthesia.

An initial doxacurium chloride dose of 0.08 mg/kg (3 x ED_{95}) should be reserved for instances in which a need for very prolonged neuromuscular block is anticipated. In approximately 90% of patients, good-to-excellent intubation conditions may be expected in 4 minutes after this dose; however, clinically effective block may be expected to persist for as long as 160 minutes or more (range: 110 to 338) (see CLINICAL PHARMACOLOGY.)

If doxacurium chloride is administered during steady-state isoflurane, enflurane, or halothane anesthesia, reduction of the doxacurium chloride dose by one-third should be considered.

When succinylcholine is administered to facilitate tracheal intubation in patients receiving balanced anesthesia, an initial dose of 0.025 mg/kg (ED_{95}) doxacurium chloride provides about 60 minutes (range: 9 to 145) of clinically effective neuromuscular block for surgery. For a longer duration of action, a larger initial dose may be administered.

Maintenance Doses: Maintenance dosing will generally be required about 60 minutes after an initial dose of 0.025 mg/kg doxacurium chloride or 100 minutes after an initial dose of 0.05 mg/kg doxacurium chloride during balanced anesthesia. Repeated maintenance doses administered at 25% T_1 recovery may be expected to be required at relatively regular intervals in each patient. The interval may vary considerably between patients. Maintenance doses of 0.005 and 0.01 mg/kg doxacurium chloride each provide an average 30 minutes (range: 9 to 57) and 45 minutes (range: 14 to 108), respectively, of additional clinically effective neuromuscular block. For shorter or longer desired durations, smaller or larger maintenance doses may be administered.

CHILDREN

When administered during halothane anesthesia, an initial dose of 0.03 mg/kg (ED_{95}) produces maximum neuromuscular block in about 7 minutes (range: 5 to 11) and clinically effective block for an average of 30 minutes (range: 12 to 54). Under halothane anesthesia, 0.05 mg/kg produces maximum block in about 4 minutes (range: 2 to 10) and clinically effective block for 45 minutes (range: 30 to 80). Maintenance doses are generally required more frequently in children than in adults. Because of the potentiating effect of halothane seen in adults, a higher dose of doxacurium chloride may be required in children receiving balanced anesthesia than in children receiving halothane anesthesia to achieve a comparable onset and duration of neuromuscular block. Doxacurium chloride has not been studied in children below the age of 2 years.

Compatibility: Y-site Administration: Doxacurium chloride injection may not be compatible with alkaline solutions with a pH greater than 8.5 (*e.g.,* barbiturate solutions).

Doxacurium chloride is compatible with:

5% Dextrose Injection USP

0.9% Sodium chloride injection USP

5% Dextrose and 0.9% Sodium chloride injection USP

Lactated Ringer's Injection USP

DOSAGE AND ADMINISTRATION: *(cont'd)*

5% Dextrose and Lactated Ringer's Injection

Sufenta (sufentanil citrate) injection, diluted as directed

Alfentan (Alfentanil hydrochloride) Injection, diluted as directed

Sublimaze (fentanyl citrate) Injection, diluted as directed

Dilution Stability: Doxacurium chloride diluted up to 1:10 in 5% Dextrose Injection USP or 0.9% Sodium Chloride Injection USP has been shown to be physically and chemically stable when stored in polypropylene syringes at 5° to 25°C (41° to 77°F), for up to 24 hours. Since dilution diminishes the preservative effectiveness of benzyl alcohol, aseptic techniques should be used to prepare the diluted product. Immediate use of the diluted doxacurium chloride should be discarded after 8 hours.

HOW SUPPLIED:

Nuromax Injection, 1 mg doxacurium in each ml.

5 ml Multiple Dose vials containing 0.9% w/v benzyl alcohol as a preservative (see WARNINGS.)

Storage: Store doxacurium chloride injection at room temperature of 15° to 25°C (59° to 77°F). DO NOT FREEZE.

HOW SUPPLIED - EQUIVALENTS NOT AVAILABLE:

Injection, Solution - Intravenous - 1 mg/ml

5 ml x 10 $181.02 NUROMAX, Glaxo Wellcome 00173-0763-44

DOXAPRAM HYDROCHLORIDE *(001110)*

CATEGORIES: Analeptics; Anesthesia; Apnea; CNS Depression; Central Nervous System Agents; Pulmonary Disease; Respiratory Depression; Respiratory Insufficiency; Respiratory Stimulants; Respiratory/Cerebral Stimulant; Stimulants; Pregnancy Category B; FDA Approval Pre 1982

BRAND NAMES: **Dopram**; *Doxapram*
(International brand names outside U.S. in italics)

DESCRIPTION:

Dopram Injectable (Doxapram Hydrochloride Injection, USP) is a clear, colorless, sterile, non-pyrogenic, aqueous solution with pH 3.5-5.0, for intravenous administration.

Each 1 ml Contains: Doxapram Hydrochloride, USP 20 mg, Benzyl Alcohol, NF (as preservative) 0.9%, and Water for Injection, USP q.s.

Due to its benzyl alcohol content, Dopram Injectable should not be used in newborns.

Dopram Injectable is a respiratory stimulant.

Doxapram hydrochloride is a white to off-white, crystalline powder, sparingly soluble in water, alcohol and chloroform.

Its chemical structure is 1-ethyl-4-(2-(4-morpholinyl)ethyl)-3,3-diphenyl-2-pyrrolidinone monohydrochloride, monohydrate.

CLINICAL PHARMACOLOGY:

Doxapram hydrochloride produces respiratory stimulation mediated through the peripheral carotid chemoreceptors. As the dosage level is increased, the central respiratory centers in the medulla are stimulated with progressive stimulation of other parts of the brain and spinal cord.

The onset of respiratory stimulation following the recommended single intravenous injection of doxapram hydrochloride usually occurs in 20-40 seconds with peak effect at 1-2 minutes. The duration of effect may vary from 5-12 minutes.

The respiratory stimulant action is manifested by an increase in tidal volume associated with a slight increase in respiratory rate.

A pressor response may result following doxapram administration. Provided there is no impairment of cardiac function, the pressor effect is more marked in hypovolemic than in normovolemic states. The pressor response is due to the improved cardiac output rather than peripheral vasoconstriction. Following doxapram administration, an increased release of catecholamines has been noted.

Although opiate induced respiratory depression is antagonized by doxapram, the analgesic effect is not affected.

INDICATIONS AND USAGE:

Postanesthesia: When the possibility of airway obstruction and/or hypoxia have been eliminated, doxapram may be used to stimulate respiration in patients with drug-induced post-anesthesia respiratory depression or apnea other than that due to muscle relaxant drugs.

To pharmacologically stimulate deep breathing in the so-called "stir-up" regimen in the postoperative patient. (Simultaneous administration of oxygen is desirable.)

Drug-Induced Central Nervous System Depression: Exercising care to prevent vomiting and aspiration, doxapram may be used to stimulate respiration, hasten arousal, and to encourage the return of laryngopharyngeal reflexes in patients with mild to moderate respiratory and CNS depression due to drug overdosage.

Chronic Pulmonary Disease Associated With Acute Hypercapnia: Doxapram is indicated as a temporary measure in hospitalized patients with acute respiratory insufficiency superimposed on chronic obstructive pulmonary disease. Its use should be for a short period of time (approximately 2 hours) as an aid in the prevention of elevation of arterial CO_2 tension during the administration of oxygen. It should not be used in conjunction with mechanical ventilation.

CONTRAINDICATIONS:

Due to its benzyl alcohol content, Dopram Injectable should not be used in newborns.

Doxapram should not be used in patients with epilepsy or other convulsive disorders.

Doxapram is contraindicated in patients with mechanical disorders of ventilation such as mechanical obstruction, muscle paresis, flail chest, pneumothorax, acute bronchial asthma, pulmonary fibrosis or other conditions resulting in restriction of chest wall, muscles of respiration or alveolar expansion.

Doxapram is contraindicated in patients with evidence of head injury or cerebral vascular accident and in those with significant cardiovascular impairment, severe hypertension, or known hypersensitivity to the drug.

WARNINGS:

In Postanesthetic Use: Doxapram is neither an antagonist to muscle relaxant drugs nor a specific narcotic antagonist. Adequacy of airway and oxygenation must be assured prior to doxapram administration.

WARNINGS: *(cont'd)*

Doxapram should be administered with great care and only under careful supervision to patients with hypermetabolic states such as hyperthyroidism or pheochromocytoma.

Since narcosis may recur after stimulation with doxapram, care should be taken to maintain close observation until the patient has been fully alert for 1/2 to 1 hour.

In Drug-Induced Cns And Respiratory Depression: Doxapram alone may not stimulate adequate spontaneous breathing or provide sufficient arousal in patients who are **severely** depressed either due to respiratory failure or to CNS depressant drugs, but should be used as an adjunct to established supportive measures and resuscitative techniques.

In Chronic Obstructive Pulmonary Disease: Because of the associated increased work of breathing, do not increase the rate of infusion of doxapram in severely ill patients in an attempt to lower pCO_2.

Doxapram should not be used in conjunction with mechanical ventilation.

PRECAUTIONS:

GENERAL

An adequate airway is essential.

Recommended dosages of doxapram should be employed and maximum total dosages should not be exceeded. In order to avoid side effects, it is advisable to use the minimum effective dosage.

Monitoring of the blood pressure and deep tendon reflexes is recommended to prevent overdosage.

Vascular extravasation or use of a single injection site over an extended period should be avoided since either may lead to thrombophlebitis or local skin irritation.

Rapid infusion may result in hemolysis.

Lowered pCO_2 induced by hyperventilation produces cerebral vasoconstriction and slowing of the cerebral circulation. This should be taken into consideration on an individual basis.

Intravenous short-acting barbiturates, oxygen and resuscitative equipment should be readily available to manage overdosage manifested by excessive central nervous system stimulation. Slow administration of the drug and careful observation of the patient during administration and for some time subsequently are advisable. These precautions are to assure that the protective reflexes have been restored and to prevent possible post-hyperventilation hypoventilation.

Doxapram should be administered cautiously to patients receiving sympathomimetic or monoamine oxidase inhibiting drugs, since an additive pressor effect may occur.

Blood pressure increases are generally modest but significant increases have been noted in some patients. Because of this doxapram is not recommended for use in severe hypertension (see CONTRAINDICATIONS.)

If sudden hypotension or dyspnea develops, doxapram should be stopped.

IN POSTANESTHETIC USE

The same consideration to pre-existing disease states should be exercised as in non-anesthetized individuals. See Contraindications and Warnings covering use in hypertension, asthma, disturbances of respiratory mechanics including airway obstruction, CNS disorders including increased cerebrospinal fluid pressure, convulsive disorders, acute agitation, and profound metabolic disorders.

See DRUG INTERACTIONS.

IN CHRONIC OBSTRUCTIVE PULMONARY DISEASE

Arrhythmias seen in some patients in acute respiratory failure secondary to chronic obstructive pulmonary disease are probably the result of hypoxia. Doxapram should be used with caution in these patients.

Arterial blood gases should be drawn prior to the initiation of doxapram infusion and oxygen administration, then at least every 1/2 hour. Doxapram administration does not diminish the need for careful monitoring of the patient or the need for supplemental oxygen in patients with acute respiratory failure. Doxapram should be stopped if the arterial blood gases deteriorate, and mechanical ventilation initiated.

CARCINOGENESIS, MUTAGENESIS, AND IMPAIRMENT OF FERTILITY

No carcinogenic or mutagenic studies have been performed using doxapram. Doxapram did not adversely affect the breeding performance of rats.

PREGNANCY CATEGORY B

Reproduction studies have been performed in rats at doses up to 1.6 times the human dose and have revealed no evidence of impaired fertility or harm to the fetus due to doxapram. There are, however, no adequate and well-controlled studies in pregnant women. Since the animals in the reproduction studies were dosed by the IM and oral routes and animal reproduction studies, in general, are not always predictive of human response, this drug should be used during pregnancy only if clearly needed.

NURSING MOTHERS

It is not known whether this drug is excreted in human milk. Because many drugs are excreted in human milk, caution should be exercised when doxapram hydrochloride is administered to a nursing mother.

PEDIATRIC USE

The use of the preservative benzyl alcohol in the newborn has been associated with metabolic, CNS, respiratory, circulatory, and renal dysfunction. Safety and effectiveness in children below the age of 12 years have not been established.

DRUG INTERACTIONS:

Administration of doxapram to patients who are receiving sympathomimetic or monoamine oxidase inhibiting drugs may result in an additive pressor effect. (See PRECAUTIONS.)

In patients who have received muscle relaxants doxapram may temporarily mask the residual effects of muscle relaxant drugs.

In patients who have received anesthetics known to sensitize the myocardium to catecholamines, such as halothane, cyclopropane and enflurane, initiation of doxapram therapy should be delayed for at least 10 minutes following discontinuance of anesthesia, since an increase in epinephrine release has been noted with doxapram.

ADVERSE REACTIONS:

The following adverse reactions have been reported:

Central And Autonomic Nervous Systems: Pyrexia, flushing, sweating; pruritus and paresthesia, such as a feeling of warmth, burning, or hot sensation, especially in the area of genitalia and perineum; apprehension, disorientation, pupillary dilatation, headache, dizziness, hyperactivity, involuntary movements, muscle spasticity, increased deep tendon reflexes, clonus, bilateral Babinski, and convulsions.

Respiratory: Dyspnea, cough, tachypnea, laryngospasm, bronchospasm, hiccough, and rebound hypoventilation.

Cardiovascular: Phlebitis, variations in heart rate, lowered T-waves, arrhythmias, chest pain, tightness in chest. A mild to moderate increase in blood pressure is commonly noted and may be of concern in patients with severe cardiovascular diseases.

ADVERSE REACTIONS: *(cont'd)*

Gastrointestinal: Nausea, vomiting, diarrhea, desire to defecate.

Genitourinary: Stimulation of urinary bladder with spontaneous voiding; urinary retention.

Laboratory Determinations: A decrease in hemoglobin, hematocrit, or red blood cell count has been observed in postoperative patients. In the presence of pre-existing leukopenia, a further decrease in WBC has been observed following anesthesia and treatment with doxapram hydrochloride. Elevation of BUN and albuminuria have also been observed. As some of the patients cited above had received multiple drugs concomitantly, a cause and effect relationship could not be determined.

OVERDOSAGE:

Signs and Symptoms: Symptoms of overdosage are extensions of the pharmacologic effects of the drug. Excessive pressor effect, tachycardia, skeletal muscle hyperactivity, and enhanced deep tendon reflexes may be early signs of overdosage. Therefore, the blood pressure, pulse rate and deep tendon reflexes should be evaluated periodically and the dosage or infusion rate adjusted accordingly.

Convulsive seizures are unlikely at recommended dosages. In unanesthetized animals, the convulsant dose is 70 times greater than the respiratory stimulant dose. Intravenous LD_{50} values in the mouse and rat were approximately 75 mg/kg and in the cat and dog were 40-80 mg/kg.

Except for management of chronic obstructive pulmonary disease associated with acute hypercapnia, the maximum recommended dosage is 3 GRAMS/24 HOURS. (See DOSAGE AND ADMINISTRATION.)

Management of Overdose: There is no specific antidote for doxapram. Management should be symptomatic. Short-acting intravenous barbiturates, oxygen and resuscitative equipment should be used as needed for supportive treatment.

There is no evidence that doxapram is dialyzable; further, the half-life of doxapram makes it unlikely that dialysis would be appropriate in managing overdose with this drug.

DOSAGE AND ADMINISTRATION:

Doxapram hydrochloride is compatible with 5% and 10% dextrose in water or normal saline. ADMIXTURE OF DOXAPRAM WITH ALKALINE SOLUTIONS SUCH AS 2.5% THIOPENTAL SODIUM, BICARBONATE, OR AMINOPHYLLINE WILL RESULT IN PRECIPITATION OR GAS FORMATION.

In Postanesthetic Use: *By IV Injection:* See TABLE 1.

Slow administration of the drug and careful observation of the patient during administration and for some time subsequently are advisable.

TABLE 1 dosage For Postanesthetic Use.-IV

IV Administration	Recommended dosage mg/kg	mg/lb	Maximum dose per single injection mg/kg	mg/lb	Maximum total dose mg/kg	mg/lb
Single Injection	0.5-1.0	0.25-0.5	1.5	0.70	1.5	0.70
Repeat Injections (5 min. intervals)	0.5-1.0	0.25-0.5	1.5	0.70	2.0	1.0
Infusion	0.5-1.0	0.25-0.5	-	-	4.0	2.0

By Infusion: The solution is prepared by adding 250 mg of doxapram (12.5 ml) to 250 ml of dextrose or saline solution. The infusion is initiated at a rate of approximately 5 mg/minute until a satisfactory respiratory response is observed, and maintained at a rate of 1-3mg/minute. The rate of infusion should be adjusted to sustain the desired level of respiratory stimulation with a minimum of side effects. The recommended total dosage by infusion is 4 mg/kg (2.0 mg/lb), or approximately 300 mg for the average adult.

In The Management Of Drug-Induced CNS Depression.) See TABLE 2.

TABLE 2 Dosage for drug-induced CNS depression.

Level of Depression	Method One Priming dose single/repeat IV injection mg/kg	mg/lb	Method Two Rate of intermittent IV infusion mg/kg/hr	mg/lb/hr
Mild*	1.0	0.5	1.0-2.0	0.5-1.0
Moderate†	2.0	1.0	2.0-3.0	1.0-1.5

* Mild Depression Class 0: Asleep, but can be aroused and can answer questions. Class 1: Comatose, will withdraw from painful stimuli, reflexes intact.

† Moderate Depression Class 2: Comatose, will not withdraw from painful stimuli, reflexes intact. Class 3: Comatose, reflexes absent, no depression of circulation or respiration

METHOD ONE

Using Single and/or Repeat Single IV *Injections*:

Give priming dose of 1.0 mg/lb (2.0 mg/kg) body weight and repeat in 5 minutes.

Repeat same dose q1-2h until patient wakens. Watch for relapse into unconsciousness or development of respiratory depression, since Dopram does not affect the metabolism of CNS-depressant drugs.

If relapse occurs, resume injections q1-2h until arousal is sustained, or total maximum daily dose (3 grams) is given. Allow patient to sleep until 24 hours have elapsed from first injection of Dopram, using assisted or automatic respiration if necessary.

Repeat procedure the following day until patient breathes spontaneously and sustains desired level of consciousness, or until maximum dosage (3 grams) is given.

Repetitive doses should be administered only to patients who have shown response to the initial dose.

Failure to respond appropriately indicates the need for neurologic evaluation for a possible central nervous system source of sustained coma.

METHOD TWO

By Intermittent IV *Infusion*:

Give priming dose as in Method One.

If patient wakens, watch for relapse; if no response, continue general supportive treatment for 1-2 hours and repeat Dopram. If some respiratory stimulation occurs, prepare IV infusion by adding 250 mg of Dopram (12.5 ml) to 250 ml of saline or dextrose solution.Deliver at rate of 1-3 mg/min (60-180 ml/hr) according to size of patient and depth of coma. Discontinue Dopram if patient begins to waken or at end of 2 hours.

Continue supportive treatment for 1/2 to 2 hours and repeat Step b.

Do not exceed 3 grams/day.

DOSAGE AND ADMINISTRATION: *(cont'd)*

Chronic Obstructive Pulmonary Disease Associated With Acute Hypercapnia: One vial of doxapram (400 mg) should be mixed with 180 ml of dextrose or saline solution (concentration of 2.0 mg/ml). The infusion should be started at 1-2 mg/minute (1/2-1 ml/minute); if indicated, increase to a maximum of 3 mg/minute. Arterial blood gases should be determined prior to the onset of doxapram's administration and at least every half hour during the two hours of infusion to insure against the insidious development of CO_2-RETENTION AND ACIDOSIS. Alteration of oxygen concentration or flow rate may necessitate adjustment in the rate of doxapram infusion.

Predictable blood gas patterns are more readily established with a continuous infusion of doxapram. If the blood gases show evidence of deterioration, the infusion of doxapram should be discontinued.

ADDITIONAL INFUSIONS BEYOND THE SINGLE MAXIMUM TWO HOUR ADMINISTRATION PERIOD ARE NOT RECOMMENDED. Parenteral drug products should be inspected visually for particulate matter and discoloration prior to administration, whenever solution and container permit.

Store at Controlled Room Temperature, Between 15° and 30° (59° and 86°F).

HOW SUPPLIED - RATED THERAPEUTICALLY EQUIVALENT:

Injection, Solution - Intravenous - 20 mg/ml

20 ml	$38.48	Doxapram Hcl, Schein Pharm (US)	00364-3021-55
20 ml	**$42.75**	**DOPRAM, AH Robins**	**00031-4849-83**

DOXAZOSIN MESYLATE *(003007)*

CATEGORIES: Alpha Adrenergic Receptor Inhibitors; Alpha Blockers; Antihypertensives; Benign Prostatic Hyperplasia; Cardiovascular Drugs; Hypertension; Prostate Enlargement; Pregnancy Category B; FDA Class 1C ("Little or No Therapeutic Advantage"); Sales > $100 Million; FDA Approved 1990 Nov; Top 200 Drugs

BRAND NAMES: *Alfadil*; *Cardoxan*; *Cardular* (Germany); **Cardura**; *Carduran*; *Dedralen*; *Diblocin* (Germany); *Doxaben*; *Kaltensif*; *Supressin*
(International brand names outside U.S. in italics)

FORMULARIES: Aetna; BC-BS; CIGNA; FHP; Humana; Medi-Cal; WellPoint; WHO; PCS

COST OF THERAPY: $282.10 (Hypertension; Tablet; 1 mg; 1/day; 365 days)

PRIMARY ICD9: 401.1 (Essential Hypertension, Benign)

DESCRIPTION:

Doxazosin mesylate is a quinazoline compound that is a selective inhibitor of the $alpha_1$ subtype of alpha adrenergic receptors. The chemical name of doxazosin mesylate is 1-(4-amino-6,7-dimethoxy-2-quinazolinyl)-4-(1,4-benzodioxan-2-ylcarbonyl) piperazine methanesulfonate. The empirical formula for doxazosin mesylate is $C_{23}H_{25}N_5O_5{\cdot}CH_4O_3S$ and the molecular weight is 547.6.

Doxazosin mesylate is freely soluble in dimethylsulfoxide, soluble in dimethylformamide, slightly soluble in methanol, ethanol, and water (0.8% at 25°C), and very slightly soluble in acetone and methylene chloride. Cardura is available as colored tablets for oral use and contains 1 mg (white), 2 mg (yellow), 4 mg (orange) and 8 mg (green) of doxazosin as the free base.

The inactive ingredients for all tablets are: microcrystalline cellulose, lactose, sodium starch glycolate, magnesium stearate and sodium lauryl sulfate. The 2 mg tablet contains D & C yellow 10 and FD & C yellow 6; the 4 mg tablet contains FD & C yellow 6; the 8 mg tablet contains FD & C blue 10 and D & C yellow 10.

CLINICAL PHARMACOLOGY:

PHARMACODYNAMICS

Benign Prostatic Hyperplasia (BPH): Benign prostatic hyperplasia (BPH) is a common cause of urinary outflow obstruction in aging males. Severe BPH may lead to urinary retention and renal damage. A static and a dynamic component contribute to the symptoms and reduced urinary flow rate associated with BPH. The static component is related to an increase in prostate size caused, in part, by a proliferation of smooth muscle cells in the prostatic stroma. However, the severity of BPH symptoms and the degree of urethral obstruction do not correlate well with the size of the prostate. The dynamic component of BPH is associated with an increase in smooth muscle tone in the prostate and bladder neck. The degree of tone in this area is mediated by the $alpha_1$ adrenoceptor, which is present in high density in the prostatic stroma, prostatic capsule and bladder neck. Blockade of the $alpha_1$ receptor decreases urethral resistance and may relieve the obstruction and BPH symptoms. In the human prostate, doxazosin mesylate antagonizes phenylephrine ($alpha_1$ agonist)-induced contractions, *in vitro*, and binds with high affinity to the $alpha_1$ adrenoceptor. The receptor subtype is thought to be the predominant functional type in the prostate. Doxazosin mesylate acts within 1-2 weeks to decrease the severity of BPH symptoms and improve urinary flow rate. Since $alpha_1$ adrenoceptors are of low density in the urinary bladder (apart from the bladder neck). Doxazosin mesylate should maintain bladder contractility.

Hypertension: The mechanism of action of doxazosin mesylate is selective blockade of the $alpha_1$(postjunctional subtype of adrenergic receptors. Studies in normal human subjects have shown that doxazosin competitively antagonized the pressor effects of phenylephrine (an $alpha_1$agonist) and the systolic pressor effect of norepinephrine. Doxazosin and prazosin have similar abilities to antagonize phenylephrine. The antihypertensive effect of doxazosin mesylate results from a decrease in systemic vascular resistance. The parent compound doxazosin is primarily responsible for the antihypertensive activity. The low plasma concentrations of known active and inactive metabolites of doxazosin (2-piperazinyl, 6' - and 7'-hydroxy and 6- and 7-0-desmethyl compounds) compared to parent drug indicate that the contribution of even the most potent compound (6'-hydroxy) to the antihypertensive effect of doxazosin in man is probably small. The 6'- and 7 '-hydroxy metabolites have demonstrated antioxidant properties at concentrations of 5 μM, *in vitro*.

Administration of doxazosin mesylate results in a reduction in systemic vascular resistance. In patients with hypertension there is little change in cardiac output. Maximum reductions in blood pressure usually occur 2-6 hours after dosing and are associated with a small increase in standing heart rate. Like other $alpha_1$-adrenergic blocking agents, doxazosin has a greater effect on blood pressure and heart rate in the standing position.

In a pooled analysis of placebo-controlled hypertension studies with about 300 hypertensive patients per treatment group, doxazosin, at doses of 1-16 mg given once daily, lowered blood pressure at 24 hours by about 10/8 mmHg compared to placebo in the standing position and about 9/5 mmHg in the supine position. Peak blood pressure effects (1-6 hours) were larger by about 50-75% (*i.e.*, trough values were about 55-70% of peak effect), with the larger peak-trough differences seen in systolic pressures. There was no apparent difference in the blood pressure response of Caucasians and blacks or of patients above and below age 65. In these predominantly normocholesterolemic patients doxazosin produced small reductions in total

CLINICAL PHARMACOLOGY: *(cont'd)*

serum cholesterol (2-3%), LDL cholesterol (4%), and a similarly small increase in HDL/total cholesterol ratio (4%). The clinical significance of these findings is uncertain. In the same patient population, patients receiving doxazosin mesylate gained a mean of 0.6 kg compared to a mean loss of 0.1 kg for placebo patients.

PHARMACOKINETICS

After oral administration of therapeutic doses, peak plasma levels of doxazosin mesylate occur at about 2-3 hours. Bioavailability is approximately 65% reflecting first pass metabolism of doxazosin by the liver. The effect of food on the pharmacokinetics of doxazosin mesylate was examined in a crossover study with twelve hypertensive subjects. Reductions of 18% in mean maximum plasma concentration and 12% in the area under the concentration-time curve occurred when doxazosin mesylate was administered with food. Neither of these differences was statistically or clinically significant.

Doxazosin mesylate is extensively metabolized in the liver, mainly by O- demethylation of the quinazoline nucleus or hydroxylation of the benzodioxan moiety. Although several active metabolites of doxazosin have been identified, the pharmacokinetics of these metabolites have not been characterized. In a study of two subjects administered radiolabelled doxazosin 2 mg orally and 1 mg intravenously on two separate occasions, approximately 63% of the dose was eliminated in the feces and 9% of the dose was found in the urine. On average only 4.8% of the dose was excreted as unchanged drug in the feces and only a trace of the total radioactivity in the urine was attributed to unchanged drug. At the plasma concentrations achieved by therapeutic doses approximately 98% of the circulating drug is bound to plasma proteins.

Plasma elimination of doxazosin is biphasic, with a terminal elimination half-life of about 22 hours. Steady-state studies in hypertensive patients given doxazosin doses of 2-16 mg once daily showed linear kinetics and dose proportionality. In two studies, following the administration of 2 mg orally once daily, the mean accumulation ratios (steady-state AUC vs first dose AUC) were 1.2 and 1.7. Enterohepatic recycling is suggested by secondary peaking of plasma doxazosin concentrations.

In a crossover study in 24 normotensive subjects, the pharmacokinetics and safety of doxazosin were shown to be similar with morning and evening dosing regimens. The area under the curve after morning dosing was, however, 11% less than that after evening dosing and the time to peak concentration after evening dosing occurred significantly later than after morning dosing (5.6 hr vs. 3.5 hr).

The pharmacokinetics of doxazosin mesylate in young (<65 years) and elderly (≥ 65 years) subjects were similar for plasma half-life values and oral clearance. Pharmacokinetic studies in elderly patients and patients with renal impairment have shown no significant alterations compared to younger patients with normal renal function. There have, however, been no studies of patients with liver impairment, and there are only limited data on the effects of drugs known to influence hepatic metabolism [*e.g.*, cimetidine (see PRECAUTIONS)]. Use of doxazosin in patients with altered liver function should be undertaken with particular caution, if at all, as excretion is almost wholly hepatic.

In two placebo-controlled studies, of normotensive and hypertensive BPH patients, in which doxazosin was administered in the morning and the titration interval was two weeks and one week, respectively, trough plasma concentrations of doxazosin mesylate were similar in the two populations. Linear kinetics and dose proportionality were observed.

CLINICAL STUDIES:

The efficacy of doxazosin mesylate was evaluated extensively in over 900 patients with BPH in double-blind, placebo-controlled trials. Doxazosin mesylate treatment was superior to placebo in improving patient symptoms and urinary flow rate. Significant relief with doxazosin mesylate was seen as early as one week into the treatment regimen, with doxazosin mesylate treated patients (N=173) showing a significant (p<0.01) increase in maximum flow rate of 0.8 ml/sec compared to a decrease of 0.5 ml/sec in the placebo group (N=41). In long term studies improvement was maintained for up to 2 years of treatment. In 66- 71% of patients, improvements above baseline were seen in both symptoms and maximum urinary flow rate.

In three placebo-controlled studies of 14-16 weeks duration obstructive symptoms (hesitation, intermittency, dribbling, weak urinary stream, incomplete emptying of the bladder) and irritative symptoms (nocturia, daytime frequency, urgency, burning) of BPH were evaluated at each visit by patient-assessed symptom questionnaires. The bothersomeness of symptoms was measured with a modified Boyarsky questionnaire. Symptom severity/frequency was assessed using a modified Boyarsky questionnaire or an AUA-based questionnaire. Uroflowmetric evaluations were performed at times of peak (2-6 hours post-dose) and/or trough (24 hours post-dose) plasma concentrations of doxazosin mesylate.

The results form the three placebo-controlled studies (N=609) showing significant efficacy with 4 mg and 8 mg doxazosin are summarized in TABLE 1. In all three studies, doxazosin mesylate resulted in statistically significant relief of obstructive and irritative symptoms compared to placebo. Statistically significant improvements of 2.3-3.3 ml/sec in maximum flow rate seen with doxazosin mesylate in Studies 1 and 2, compared to 0.1-0.7 ml/sec with placebo.

In one fixed dose study (study 2) doxazosin mesylate therapy (4-8 mg, once daily) resulted in a significant and sustained improvement in maximum urinary flow rate of 2.3-3.3 ml/sec (TABLE 1) compared to placebo (0.1 ml/sec). In this study, the only study in which weekly evaluations were made, significant improvement with doxazosin mesylate vs. placebo was seen after one week. The proportion of patients who responded with a maximum flow rate improvement of ≥ 3 ml/sec was significantly larger with doxazosin mesylate (34- 42%) than placebo (13-17%). A significantly greater improvement was also seen in average flow rate with doxazosin mesylate (1.6 ml/sec) than with placebo (0.2 ml/sec).

In BPH patients (N=450) treated for up to 2 years in open-label studies. Doxazosin mesylate therapy resulted in significant improvement above baseline in urinary flow rates and BPH symptoms. The significant effects of doxazosin mesylate were maintained over the entire treatment period.

Although blockade of alpha-1 adrenoceptors also lowers blood pressure in hypertensive patients with increased peripheral vascular resistance. Doxazosin mesylate treatment of normotensive men with BPH did not result in a clinically significant blood pressure lowering effect (TABLE 2). The proportion of normotensive patients with a sitting systolic blood pressure less than 90 mmHg and/or diastolic blood pressure less than 60 mmHg at any time during treatment with doxazosin mesylate 1-8 mg once daily was 6.7% with doxazosin and not significantly different (statistically) from that with placebo (5%).

INDICATIONS AND USAGE:

Benign Prostatic Hyperplasia (BPH): Doxazosin mesylate is indicated for the treatment of both the urinary outflow obstruction and obstructive and irritative symptoms associated with BPH: obstructive symptoms (hesitation, intermittency, dribbling, weak urinary stream, incomplete emptying of the bladder) and irritative symptoms (nocturia, daytime frequency, urgency, burning). Doxazosin mesylate may be used in all BPH patients whether hypertensive or normotensive. In patients with hypertension and BPH, both conditions were effectively treated with doxazosin mesylate monotherapy. Doxazosin mesylate provides rapid improvement in symptoms and urinary flow rate in 66-71% of patients. Sustained improvements with doxazosin mesylate were seen in patients treated for up to 14 weeks in double-blind studies and up to 2 years in open-label studies.

TABLE 1 Summary Of Effectiveness Data In Placebo-Controlled Trials

	Symptom Score[a]			Maximum Flow Rate (ml/sec)		
	N	Mean Baseline	Mean[b] Change	N	Mean Baseline	Mean[c] Change
Study 1 (Titration To Maximum Dose Of 8 Mg)[A]						
Placebo	47	15.6	-2.3	41	9.7	+0.7
Doxazosin mesylate	49	14.5	-4.9**	41	9.8	+2.9**
Study 2 (Titration to fixed dose-14 weeks)[d]						
Placebo	37	20.7	-2.5	30	10.6	+0.1
Doxazosin mesylate 4 mg	38	21.2	-5.0**	32	9.8	+2.3*
Doxazosin mesylate 8 mg	42	19.9	-4.2*	36	10.5	+3.3**
Study 3 (Titration to fixed dose-12 weeks)						
Placebo	47	14.9	-4.7	44	9.9	+2.1
Doxazosin mesylate 4 mg	46	16.6	-6.1*	46	9.6	+2.6

[a]AUA questionnaire (range 0-30) in studies 1 and 3. Modified Boyarsky Questionnaire (range 7-39) in study 2.
[b]Change is to endpoint.
[c]Change is to fixed-dose efficacy phase, 22-26 hours post-dose for studies 1 and 3 and 2-6 hours post-dose for study 2.
[d]Study in hypertensives with BPH.
[e]36 patients received a dose of 8 mg doxazosin mesylate*.
* p < 0.05 (0.01) compared to placebo mean change.
** p < 0.05 (0.01) compared to placebo mean change.

TABLE 2 Mean Changes in Blood Pressure from Baseline to the Mean of the Final Efficacy Phase in Normotensives (Diastolic BP/90 mmHg) in Two Double-blind, Placebo-controlled U.S. Studies with Doxazosin mesylate 1-8 mg once daily

BP (mmHg)	Placebo (N=85) Baseline	Change	Doxazosin mesylate (N=183) Baseline	Change
Sitting				
Systolic	128.4	-1.4	128.8	-4.9*
Diastolic	79.2	1.2	79.6	-2.4*
Standing				
Systolic	128.5	-0.6	128.5	5.3*
Diastolic	80.5	0.7	80.4	-2.6*

* p = 0.05 compared to placebo.

Hypertension: Doxazosin mesylate is also indicated for the treatment of hypertension. Doxazosin mesylate may be used alone or in combination with diuretics, beta-adrenergic blocking agents, calcium channel blockers or angiotensin-converting enzyme inhibitors.

CONTRAINDICATIONS:

Doxazosin mesylate is contraindicated in patients with a known sensitivity to quinazolines (*e.g.*, prazosin, terazosin).

WARNINGS:

Syncope and 'First-dose' Effect: Doxazosin, like other alpha- adrenergic blocking agents, can cause marked hypotension, especially in the upright position, with syncope and other postural symptoms such as dizziness. Marked orthostatic effects are most common with the first dose but can also occur when there is a dosage increase, or if therapy is interrupted for more than a few days. To decrease the likelihood of excessive hypotension and syncope, it is essential that treatment be initiated with the 1 mg dose. The 2, 4, and 8 mg tablets are not for initial therapy. Dosage should then be adjusted slowly (see DOSAGE AND ADMINISTRATION)**with evaluations and increases in dose every two weeks to the recommended dose. Additional antihypertensive agents should be added with caution.**

Patients being titrated with doxazosin should be cautioned to avoid situations where injury could result should syncope occur, during both the day and night.

In an early investigational study of the safety and tolerance of increasing daily doses of doxazosin in normotensives beginning at 1 mg/day, only 2 of 6 subjects could tolerate more than 2 mg/day without experiencing symptomatic postural hypotension. In another study of 24 healthy normotensive male subjects receiving initial doses of 2 mg/day of doxazosin, seven (29%) of the subjects experienced symptomatic postural hypotension between 0.5 and 6 hours after the first dose necessitating termination of the study. In this study 2 of the normotensive subjects experienced syncope. Subsequent trials in hypertensive patients always began doxazosin dosing at 1 mg/day resulting in a 4% incidence of postural side effects at 1 mg/day with no cases of syncope.

In multiple dose clinical trials in hypertension involving over 1500 hypertensive patients with dose titration every one to two weeks, syncope was reported in 0.7% of patients. None of these events occurred at the starting dose of 1 mg and 1.2% (8/664) occurred at 16 mg/day.

In placebo-controlled, clinical trials in BPH, 3 out of 665 patients (0.5%) taking doxazosin reported syncope. Two of the patients were taking 1 mg doxazosin, while one patient was taking 2 mg doxazosin when syncope occurred. In the open-label, long-term extension follow-up of approximately 450 BPH patients, there were 3 reports of syncope (0.7%). One patient was taking 2 mg, one patient was taking 8 mg and one patient was taking 12 mg when syncope occurred. In a clinical pharmacology study, one subject receiving 2 mg experienced syncope.

If syncope occurs, the patient should be placed in a recumbent position and treated supportively as necessary.

PRECAUTIONS:

GENERAL

Prostate Cancer: Carcinoma of the prostate causes many of the symptoms associated with BPH and the two disorders frequently co- exist. Carcinoma of the prostate should therefore be ruled out prior to commencing therapy with doxazosin mesylate.

PRECAUTIONS: *(cont'd)*

Orthostatic Hypotension: While syncope is the most severe orthostatic effect of doxazosin mesylate, other symptoms of lowered blood pressure, such as dizziness, lightheadedness, or vertigo can occur, especially at initiation of therapy or at the time of dose increases.

Hypertension: These symptoms were common in clinical trials in hypertension, occurring in up to 23% of all patients treated and causing discontinuation of therapy in about 2%.

In placebo-controlled titration trials in hypertension, orthostatic effects were minimized by beginning therapy at 1 mg per day and titrating every two weeks to 2, 4, or 8 mg per day. There was an increased frequency of orthostatic effects in patients given 8 mg or more, 10%, compared to 5% at 1-4 mg and 3% in the placebo group.

Benign Prostatic Hyperplasia: In placebo-controlled trials in BPH, the incidence of orthostatic hypotension with doxazosin was 0.3% and did not increase with increasing dosage (to 8 mg/day). The incidence of discontinuations due to hypotensive or orthostatic symptoms was 3.3% with doxazosin and 1% with placebo. The titration interval in these studies was one to two weeks.

Patients in occupations in which orthostatic hypotension could be dangerous should be treated with particular caution. As alpha-antagonists can cause orthostatic effects, it is important to evaluate standing blood pressure two minutes after standing and patients should be advised to exercise care when arising from a supine or sitting position.

If hypotension occurs, the patient should be placed in the supine position and, if this measure is inadequate, volume expansion with intravenous fluids or vasopressor therapy may be used. A transient hypotensive response is not a contraindication to further doses of doxazosin mesylate.

INFORMATION FOR THE PATIENT

Patients should be made aware of the possibility of syncopal and orthostatic symptoms, especially at the initiation of therapy, and urged to avoid driving or hazardous tasks for 24 hours after the first dose, after a dosage increase, and after interruption of therapy when treatment is resumed. They should be cautioned to avoid situations where injury could result should syncope occur during initiation of doxazosin therapy. They should also be advised of the need to sit or lie down when symptoms of lowered blood pressure occur, although these symptoms are not always orthostatic, and to be careful when rising from a sitting or lying position. If dizziness, lightheadedness, or palpitations are bothersome they should be reported to the physician, so that dose adjustment can be considered. Patients should also be told that drowsiness or somnolence can occur with doxazosin mesylate or any selective alpha-adrenoceptor antagonist, requiring caution in people who must drive or operate heavy machinery.

DRUG/LABORATORY TEST INTERACTIONS

Doxazosin mesylate does not affect the plasma concentration of prostate specific antigen in patients treated for up to 3 years. Both doxazosin, an $alpha_1$ inhibitor, and finasteride, a 5-alpha reductase inhibitor, are highly protein bound and hepatically metabolized. There is no definitive controlled clinical experience on the concomitant use of $alpha_1$ inhibitors and 5-alpha reductase inhibitors at this time.

Impaired Liver Function: Doxazosin mesylate should be administered with caution to patients with evidence of impaired hepatic function or to patients receiving drugs known to influence hepatic metabolism (see CLINICAL PHARMACOLOGY). There is no controlled clinical experience with doxazosin mesylate in patients with these conditions.

Leukopenia/Neutropenia: Analysis of hematologic data from hypertensive patients receiving doxazosin mesylate in controlled hypertension clinical trials showed that the mean WBC (N=474) and mean neutrophil counts (N=419) were decreased by 2.4% and 1.0% respectively, compared to placebo, a phenomenon seen with other alpha blocking drugs. In BPH patients the incidence of clinically significant WBC abnormalities was 0.4% (2/459) with doxazosin mesylate and 0% (0/147) with placebo, with no statistically significant difference between the two treatment groups. A search through a data base of 2400 hypertensive patients and 665 BPH patients revealed 4 hypertensives in which drug-related neutropenia could not be ruled out and one BPH patient in which drug related leukopenia could not be ruled out. Two hypertensives had a single low value on the last day of treatment. Two hypertensives had stable, non-progressive neutrophil counts in the $1000/mm^3$ range over periods of 20 and 40 weeks. One BPH patient had a decrease from WBC count of $4800/mm^3$ to $2700/mm^3$ at the end of the study; there was no evidence of clinical impairment. In cases where follow-up was available the WBCs and neutrophil counts returned to normal after discontinuation of doxazosin mesylate. No patients became symptomatic as a result of the low WBC or neutrophil counts.

Cardiac Toxicity in Animals: An increased incidence of myocardial necrosis or fibrosis was displayed by Sprague-Dawley rats after 6 months of dietary administration at concentrations calculated to provide 80 mg doxazosin/kg/day and after 12 months of dietary administration at concentrations calculated to provide 40 mg doxazosin/kg/day (AUC exposure in rats 8 times the human AUC exposure with a 12 mg/day therapeutic dose). Myocardial fibrosis was observed in both rats and mice treated in the same manner with 40 mg doxazosin/kg/day for 18 months (exposure 8 times human AUC exposure in rats and somewhat equivalent to human C_{max} exposure in mice). No cardiotoxicity was observed at lower doses (up to 10 or 20 mg/kg/day, depending on the study) in either species. These lesions were not observed after 12 months of oral dosing in dogs at maximum doses of 20 mg/kg/day [maximum plasma concentrations (C_{max}) in dogs 14 times the C_{max} exposure in humans receiving a 12 mg/day therapeutic dose] and in Wistar rats at doses of 100 mg/kg/day (C_{max} exposures 15 times human C_{max} exposure with a 12 mg/day therapeutic dose). There is no evidence that similar lesions occur in humans.

CARCINOGENESIS, MUTAGENESIS, AND IMPAIRMENT OF FERTILITY

Chronic dietary administration (up to 24 months) of doxazosin mesylate at maximally tolerated concentrations (highest dose 40 mg/kg/day: 8 times human AUC exposure) revealed no evidence of carcinogenicity in rats. There was no evidence of carcinogenicity in a similarly conducted 18 month oral study in mice. The mouse study, however, was compromised by the failure to use a maximally tolerated dose of doxazosin.

Mutagenicity studies revealed no drug- or metabolite-related effects at either chromosomal or subchromosomal levels.

Studies in rats showed reduced fertility in males treated with doxazosin at oral doses of 20 (but not 5 or 10) mg/kg/day, about 4 times the AUC exposures obtained with a 12 mg/day human dose. This effect was reversible within two weeks of drug withdrawal. There have been no reports of any effects of doxazosin on male fertility in humans.

PREGNANCY, TERATOGENIC EFFECTS, PREGNANCY CATEGORY C

Studies in pregnant rabbits and rats at daily oral doses of up to 41 and 20 mg/kg, respectively (plasma drug concentrations 10 and 4 times human C_{max} and AUC exposures with a 12 mg/day therapeutic dose), have revealed no evidence of harm to the fetus. A dosage regimen of 82 mg/kg/day in the rabbit was associated with reduced fetal survival. There are no adequate and well-controlled studies in pregnant women. Because animal reproduction studies are not always predictive of human response, doxazosin mesylate should be used during pregnancy only if clearly needed.

Radioactivity was found to cross the placenta following oral administration of labelled doxazosin to pregnant rats.

PRECAUTIONS: *(cont'd)*

Nonteratogenic Effects: In peri-postnatal studies in rats, postnatal development at maternal doses of 40 or 50 mg/kg/day of doxazosin (8 times human AUC exposure with a 12 mg/day therapeutic dose) was delayed as evidenced by slower body weight gain and a slightly later appearance of anatomical features and reflexes.

NURSING MOTHERS

Studies in lactating rats given a single oral dose of 1 mg/kg of [2-^{14}C]-doxazosin mesylate indicate that doxazosin accumulates in rat breast milk with a maximum concentration about 20 times greater than the maternal plasma concentration. It is not known whether this drug is excreted in human milk. Because many drugs are excreted in human milk, caution should be exercised when doxazosin mesylate is administered to a nursing mother.

PEDIATRIC USE

The safety and effectiveness of doxazosin mesylate as an antihypertensive agent have not been established in children.

GERIATRIC USE

The safety and effectiveness profile of doxazosin mesylate in BPH was similar in the elderly (age $\geq$ 65 years) and younger (age < 65 years) patients.

DRUG INTERACTIONS:

Most (98%) of plasma doxazosin is protein bound. *In vitro* data in human plasma indicate that doxazosin mesylate has no effect on protein binding of digoxin, warfarin, phenytoin or indomethacin. There is no information on the effect of other highly plasma protein bound drugs on doxazosin binding. Doxazosin mesylate has been administered without any evidence of an adverse drug interaction to patients receiving thiazide diuretics, beta-blocking agents, and nonsteroidal anti-inflammatory drugs. In a placebo-controlled trial in normal volunteers, the administration of a single 1 mg dose of doxazosin on day 1 of a four-day regimen of oral cimetidine (400 mg twice daily) resulted in a 10% increase in mean AUC of doxazosin (p=0.006), and a slight but not statistically significant increase in mean C_{max} and mean half-life of doxazosin. The clinical significance of this increase in doxazosin AUC is unknown.

In clinical trials, doxazosin mesylate tablets have been administered to patients on a variety of concomitant medications; while no formal interaction studies have been conducted, no interactions were observed. Doxazosin mesylate tablets have been used with the following drugs or drug classes:

Analgesic/Anti-Inflammatory Agents (*e.g.,* acetaminophen, aspirin, codeine and codeine combinations, ibuprofen, indomethacin)

Antibiotics (*e.g.,* erythromycin, trimethoprim and sulfamethoxazole, amoxicillin)

Antihistamines (*e.g.,* chlorpheniramine)

Cardiovascular Agents (*e.g.,* atenolol, hydrochlorothiazide, propranolol)

Corticosteroids

Gastrointestinal Agents (*e.g.,* antacids)

Hypoglycemics and Endocrine Drugs

Sedatives and Tranquilizers (*e.g.,* diazepam)

Cold and Flu Remedies

ADVERSE REACTIONS:

Benign Prostatic Hyperplasia: The incidence of adverse events has been ascertained from worldwide clinical trials in 965 BPH patients. The incidence rates presented in TABLE 3 are based on combined data from seven placebo-controlled trials involving once daily administration of doxazosin mesylate in doses of 1-16 mg in hypertensives and 0.5-8 mg in normotensives. The adverse events when the incidence in the doxazosin mesylate group was at least 1% are summarized in TABLE 3. No significant difference in the incidence of adverse events compared to placebo was seen except for dizziness, fatigue, hypotension, edema and dyspnea. Dizziness and dyspnea appeared to be dose-related.

TABLE 3 Adverse Reactions During Placebo-Controlled Studies Benign Prostatic Hyperplasia

Body System	Doxazosin mesylate (N=665)	Placebo (N=300)
Body As A Whole		
Back pain	1.8%	2.0%
Chest pain	1.2%	0.7%
Fatigue	8.0%	1.7%
Headache	9.9%	9.0%
Influenza-like symptoms	1.1%	1.0%
Pain	2.0%	1.0%
Cardiovascular System		
Hypertension	1.7%	0.0%
Palpitation	1.2%	0.3%
Digestive System		
Abdominal Pain	2.4%	2.0%
Diarrhea	2.3%	2.0%
Dyspepsia	1.7%	1.7%
Nausea	1.5%	0.7%
Metabolic And Nutritional Disorders		
Edema	0.7%	2.7%
Nervous System		
Dizziness†	15.6%*	9.0%
Mouth Dry	1.4%	0.3%
Somnolence	3.0%	1.0%
Respiratory System		
Dyspnea	2.6%*	0.3%
Respiratory Disorder	1.1%	0.7%
Special Senses		
Vision Abnormal	1.4%	0.7%
Urogenital System		
Impotence	1.1%	1.0%
Urinary Tract Infection	1.4%	2.3%
Skin & Appendages		
Sweating Increased	1.1%	1.0%
Psychiatric Disorders		
Anxiety	1.1%	0.3%
Insomnia	1.2%	0.3%

* $p \leq 0.05$ for treatment differences.
† includes vertigo.

In these placebo-controlled studies of 665 doxazosin mesylate patients, treated for a mean of 85 days, additional adverse reactions have been reported. These are less than 1% and not distinguishable from those that occurred in the placebo group.

Adverse Reactions With An Incidence Of Less Than 1% But Of Clinical Interest Are (Doxazosin Mesylate Vs. Placebo):

ADVERSE REACTIONS: *(cont'd)*

Cardiovascular System: angina pectoris (0.6% vs. 0.7%), postural hypotension (0.3% vs. 0.3%), syncope (0.5% vs. 0.0%), tachycardia (0.9% vs. 0.0%).

Urogenital System: dysuria (0.5% vs. 1.3%)

Psychiatric Disorders: libido decreased (0.8% vs. 0.3%)

The safety profile in patients treated for up to three years was similar to that in the placebo-controlled studies.

The majority of adverse experiences with doxazosin mesylate were mild.

Hypertension: Doxazosin mesylate has been administered to approximately 4000 hypertensive patients, of whom 1679 were included in the hypertension clinical development program. In that program, minor adverse effects were frequent, but led to discontinuation of treatment in only 7% of patients. In placebo-controlled studies adverse effects occurred in 49% and 40% of patients in the doxazosin and placebo groups, respectively, and led to discontinuation in 2% of patients in each group. The major reasons for discontinuation were postural effects (2%), edema, malaise/fatigue, and some heart rate disturbance, each about 0.7%.

In controlled hypertension clinical trials directly comparing doxazosin mesylate to placebo there was no significant difference in the incidence of side effects, except for dizziness (including postural), weight gain, somnolence and fatigue/malaise. Postural effects and edema appeared to be dose related. The prevalence rates presented below are based on combined data from placebo-controlled studies involving once daily administration of doxazosin at doses ranging from 1-16 mg. TABLE 4 summarizes those adverse experiences (possibly/probably related) reported for patients in these hypertension studies where the prevalence rate in the doxazosin group was at least 0.5% or where the reaction is of particular interest.

TABLE 4 Adverse Reactions During Placebo-Controlled Studies

	Hypertension	
	Doxazosin (N=339)	Placebo (N=336)
Cardiovascular System		
Dizziness	19%	9%
Vertigo	2%	1%
Postural Hypotension	0.3%	0%
Edema	4%	3%
Palpitation	2%	3%
Arrhythmia	1%	0%
Hypotension	1%	0%
Tachycardia	0.3%	1%
Peripheral Ischemia	0.3%	0%
Skin Appendages		
Rash	1%	1%
Pruritus	1%	1%
Musculoskeletal System		
Arthralgia/Arthritis	1%	0%
Muscle Weakness	1%	0%
Myalgia	1%	0%
Central & Peripheral N.S.		
Headache	14%	16%
Paresthesia	1%	1%
Kinetic Disorders	1%	0%
Ataxia	1%	1%
Hypertonia	1%	0%
Muscle Cramps	1%	0%
Autonomic		
Mouth Dry	2%	2%
Flushing	1%	0%
Special Senses		
Vision Abnormal	2%	1%
Conjunctivitis/Eye Pain	1%	1%
Tinnitus	1%	0.3%
Psychiatric		
Somnolence	5%	1%
Nervousness	2%	2%
Depression	1%	1%
Insomnia	1%	1%
Sexual Dysfunction	2%	1%
Gastrointestinal		
Nausea	3%	4%
Diarrhea	2%	3%
Constipation	1%	1%
Dyspepsia	1%	1%
Flatulence	1%	1%
Abdominal Pain	0%	2%
Vomiting	0%	1%
Respiratory		
Rhinitis	3%	1%
Dyspnea	1%	1%
Epistaxis	1%	0%
Urinary		
Polyuria	2%	0%
Urinary Incontinence	1%	0%
Micturition Frequency	0%	2%
General		
Fatigue/Malaise	12%	6%
Chest Pain	2%	2%
Asthenia	1%	1%
Face Edema	1%	0%
Pain	2%	2%

Additional adverse reactions have been reported, but these are, in general, not distinguishable from symptoms that might have occurred in the absence of exposure to doxazosin. The following adverse reactions occurred with a frequency of between 0.5% and 1%: syncope, hypoesthesia, increased sweating, agitation, increased weight.

The following additional adverse reactions were reported by <0.5% of 3960 patients who received doxazosin in controlled or open, short- or long-term clinical studies, including international studies.

Cardiovascular System: angina pectoris, myocardial infarction, cerebrovascular accident

Autonomic Nervous System: pallor

Metabolic: thirst, gout, hypokalemia

Hematopoietic: lymphadenopathy, purpura

Reproductive System: breast pain

Skin Disorders: alopecia, dry skin, eczema

Central Nervous System: paresis, tremor, twitching, confusion, migraine, impaired concentration

Psychiatric: paroniria, amnesia, emotional lability, abnormal thinking, depersonalization

Special Senses: parosmia, earache, taste perversion, photophobia, abnormal lacrimation

ADVERSE REACTIONS: *(cont'd)*

Gastrointestinal System: increased appetite, anorexia, fecal incontinence, gastroenteritis

Respiratory System: bronchospasm, sinusitis, coughing, pharyngitis

Urinary System: renal calculus

General Body System: hot flushes, back pain, infection, fever/rigors, decreased weight, influenza-like symptoms.

Doxazosin mesylate has not been associated with any clinically significant changes in routine biochemical tests. No clinically relevant adverse effects were noted on serum potassium, serum glucose, uric acid, blood urea nitrogen, creatinine or liver function tests. Doxazosin mesylate has been associated with decreases in white blood cell counts (See PRECAUTIONS).

OVERDOSAGE:

Experience with doxazosin mesylate overdosage is limited. Two adolescents who each intentionally ingested 40 mg doxazosin mesylate with diclofenac or paracetamol, were treated with gastric lavage with activated charcoal and made full recoveries. A two year-old child who accidentally ingested 4 mg doxazosin mesylate was treated with gastric lavage and remained normotensive during the five hour emergency room observation period. A six-month old child accidentally received a crushed 1 mg tablet of doxazosin mesylate and was reported to have been drowsy. A 32 year old female with chronic renal failure, epilepsy and depression intentionally ingested 60 mg doxazosin mesylate (blood level 0.9 mcg/ml; normal values in hypertensives=0.02 mcg/ml); death was attributed to a grand mal seizure resulting from hypotension. A 39 year- old female who ingested 70 mg doxazosin mesylate, alcohol and Dalmane (flurazepam) developed hypotension which responded to fluid therapy.

The oral LD_{50} of doxazosin is greater than 1000 mg/kg in mice and rats. The most likely manifestation of overdosage would be hypotension, for which the usual treatment would be intravenous infusion of fluid. As doxazosin is highly protein bound, dialysis would not be indicated.

DOSAGE AND ADMINISTRATION:

Dosage Must Be Individualized: The initial dosage of doxazosin mesylate in patients with hypertension and/or BPH is 1 mg given once daily in the a.m. or p.m. This starting dose is intended to minimize the frequency of postural hypotension and first dose syncope associated with doxazosin mesylate. Postural effects are most likely to occur between 2 and 6 hours after a dose. Therefore blood pressure measurements should be taken during this time period after the first dose and with each increase in dose. If doxazosin mesylate administration is discontinued for several days, therapy should be restarted using the initial dosing regimen.

Benign Prostatic Hyperplasia 1-8 Mg Once Daily: The initial dosage of doxazosin mesylate is 1 mg, given once daily in the a.m. or p.m. Depending on the individual patient's urodynamics and BPH symptomatology, dosage may then be increased to 2 mg and thereafter to 4 mg and 8 mg once daily, the maximum recommended dose for BPH. The recommended titration interval is 1-2 weeks. Blood pressure should be evaluated routinely in these patients.

Hypertension 1-16 Mg Once Daily: The initial dosage of doxazosin mesylate is 1 mg given once daily. Depending on the individual patient's standing blood pressure response (based on measurements taken at 2-6 hours post-dose and 24 hours post-dose), dosage may then be increased to 2 mg and thereafter if necessary to 4 mg, 8 mg and 16 mg to achieve the desired reduction in blood pressure. **Increases in dose beyond 4 mg increase the likelihood of excessive postural effects including syncope, postural dizziness/vertigo and postural hypotension. At a titrated dose of 16 mg once daily the frequency of postural effects is about 12% compared to 3% for placebo.**

PATIENT INFORMATION:

Doxazosin mesylate is known as an alpha-blocker. It is used to treat high blood pressure and is also used to treat enlarged prostate glands in men who experience difficulty urinating. This medication causes lightheadedness and dizziness with the first dose. It is important not to drive or partake in tasks where getting dizzy would be dangerous. For this reason, it is advised that the first dose be taken in the evening at home. You should be careful getting up after lying down or sitting. Fatigue and headache are the most common side effects. If you get dizzy or feel faint, sit or lie down. This effect disappears after the first 24 hours of therapy. If you are taking this medication for high blood pressure, it is important to have your blood pressure checked regularly.

HOW SUPPLIED:

Cardura is available as colored tablets for oral administration. Each tablet contains doxazosin mesylate equivalent to 1 mg (white), 2 mg (yellow), 4 mg (orange), or 8 mg (green) of the active constituent, doxazosin.

Cardura Tablets are available as 1 mg (white), 2 mg (yellow), 4 mg (orange), and 8 mg (green) scored tablets.

Recommended Storage: Store below 86°F (30°C).

HOW SUPPLIED - EQUIVALENTS NOT AVAILABLE:

Tablet - Oral - 2.5 mg

100's	$93.60	PROAMATINE, Roberts Labs	54092-0003-01

Tablet, Uncoated - Oral - 1 mg

100's	**$77.29**	**CARDURA, Roerig**	**00049-2750-66**
100's	**$79.60**	**CARDURA, Roerig**	**00049-2750-41**

Tablet, Uncoated - Oral - 2 mg

100's	**$77.29**	**CARDURA, Roerig**	**00049-2760-66**
100's	**$79.60**	**CARDURA, Roerig**	**00049-2760-41**

Tablet, Uncoated - Oral - 4 mg

100's	**$81.14**	**CARDURA, Roerig**	**00049-2770-66**
100's	**$83.57**	**CARDURA, Roerig**	**00049-2770-41**

Tablet, Uncoated - Oral - 8 mg

100's	**$85.20**	**CARDURA, Roerig**	**00049-2780-66**
100's	**$87.75**	**CARDURA, Roerig**	**00049-2780-41**

DOXEPIN HYDROCHLORIDE *(001111)*

CATEGORIES: Alcoholism; Antianxiety Drugs; Antidepressants; Antipruritics/Local Anesthetics; Anxiety; Central Nervous System Agents; Depression; Dermatitis; Mania; Pruritus; Psychotherapeutic Agents; Psychotic Disorders; Sedatives/Hypnotics; Skin/Mucous Membrane Agents; Tension; Tranquilizers; Tricyclics; Tricyclic Antidepressants; FDA Approval Pre 1982

BRAND NAMES: Adapin; *Alopam*; *Anten*; *Aponal* (Germany); *Deptran*; *Doneurin* (Germany); *Doxal*; *Doxecan*; *Doxetar*; *Doxin*; *Gilex*; *Mareen* (Germany); *Quitaxon* (France); **Sinequan**; *Sinquan* (Germany); *Sinquane*; *Spectra*; *Triadapin* (Canada); Xepin; Zonalon
(International brand names outside U.S. in italics)

FORMULARIES: Aetna; BC-BS; FHP; PCS

COST OF THERAPY: $8.03 (Depression; Capsule; 75 mg; 1/day; 90 days)

PRIMARY ICD9: 311 (Depressive Disorder, Not Elsewhere Classified)

DESCRIPTION:

CAPSULES AND ORAL CONCENTRATE

Doxepin hydrochloride (abbreviated here as doxepin HCl), is one of a class of psychotherapeutic agents known as dibenzoxepin tricyclic compounds. The molecular formula of the compound is $C_{19}H_{21}NO{\cdot}HCl$ having a molecular weight of 316. It is a white crystalline solid readily soluble in water, lower alcohols and chloroform.

Inert ingredients for the capsule formulations are: hard gelatin capsules (which may contain Blue 1, Red 3, Red 40, Yellow 10, and other inert ingredients); magnesium stearate; sodium lauryl sulfate; starch.

Inert ingredients for the Sinequan oral concentrate formulation are: glycerin; methylparaben; peppermint oil; propylparaben; water.

CHEMISTRY

Doxepin HCl is a dibenzoxepin derivative and is the first of a family of tricyclic psychotherapeutic agents. Specifically, it is an isomeric mixture of: 1-Propanamine, 3-dibenz(*b,e*)oxepin-11 (6*H*)ylidene-*N,N*-dimethyl-, hydrochloride.

TOPICAL CREAM

Doxepin HCl cream is a topical antipruritic cream. Each gram contains: 50 mg of doxepin HCl (equivalent to 44.3 mg of doxepin).

Doxepin HCl is one of a class of agents known as dibenzoxepin tricyclic compounds. It is an isomeric mixture of N,N- Dimethyldibenz(*b,e*)oxepin-$\Delta^{11(6H),\gamma}$-propylamine HCl.

Doxepin HCl has an empirical formula of $C_{19}H_{21}NO{\cdot}HCl$ and a molecular weight of 316.

The base is a cream of pH 3.5 to 5.5 that includes the inactive ingredients: sorbitol, cetyl alcohol, isopropyl myristate, glyceryl stearate, PEG-100 stearate, petrolatum, benzyl alcohol, titanium dioxide, and purified water.

CLINICAL PHARMACOLOGY:

CAPSULES AND ORAL CONCENTRATE

The mechanism of action of doxepin HCl is not definitely known. It is not a central nervous system stimulant nor a monoamine oxidase inhibitor. The current hypothesis is that the clinical effects are due, at least in part, to influences on the adrenergic activity at the synapses so that deactivation of norepinephrine by reuptake into the nerve terminals is prevented. Animal studies suggest that doxepin HCl does not appreciably antagonize the antihypertensive action of guanethidine. In animal studies anticholinergic, antiserotonin and antihistamine effects on smooth muscle have been demonstrated. At higher than usual clinical doses, norepinephrine response was potentiated in animals. This effect was not demonstrated in humans.

At clinical dosages up to 150 mg per day, doxepin HCl can be given to man concomitantly with guanethidine and related compounds without blocking the antihypertensive effect. At dosages above 150 mg per day blocking of the antihypertensive effect of these compounds has been reported.

Doxepin HCl is virtually devoid of euphoria as a side effect. Characteristic of this type of compound, doxepin HCl has not been demonstrated to produce the physical tolerance or psychological dependence associated with addictive compounds.

TOPICAL CREAM

The exact mechanism by which doxepin exerts its antipruritic effect is unknown. Doxepin HCl does have potent H1 and potent H2 receptor blocking actions. Histamine-blocking drugs appear to compete at histamine receptor sites and inhibit the biological activation of histamine receptors. In addition, doxepin produces drowsiness in significant numbers of patients. Sedation may have an effect on certain pruritic symptoms. In 19 pruritic eczema patients treated with Zonalon cream, plasma doxepin concentrations ranged from nondetectable to 47 ng/ml from percutaneous absorption. Target therapeutic plasma levels of oral doxepin HCl for the treatment of depression range from 30 to 150 ng/ml.

Once absorbed into the systemic circulation, doxepin undergoes hepatic metabolism that results in conversion to pharmacologically-active desmethyldoxepin. Further glucuronidation results in urinary excretion of the parent drug and its metabolites. Desmethyldoxepin has a half life reportedly that ranges from 28 to 52 hours and is not affected by multiple dosing. Plasma levels of both doxepin and desmethyldoxepin are highly variable and are poorly correlated with dosage. Wide distribution occurs in body tissues including lungs, heart, brain, and liver. Renal disease, genetic factors, age, and other medications affect the metabolism and subsequent elimination of doxepin. (See DRUG INTERACTIONS.)

INDICATIONS AND USAGE:

CAPSULES AND ORAL CONCENTRATE

Doxepin HCl is recommended for the treatment of:

1. Psychoneurotic patients with depression and/or anxiety.

2. Depression and/or anxiety associated with alcoholism (not to be taken concomitantly with alcohol).

3. Depression and/or anxiety associated with organic disease (the possibility of drug interaction should be considered if the patient is receiving other drugs concomitantly).

4. Psychotic depressive disorders with associated anxiety including involutional depression and manic-depressive disorders.

The target symptoms of psychoneurosis that respond particularly well to doxepin HCl include anxiety, tension, depression, somatic symptoms and concerns, sleep disturbances, guilt, lack of energy, fear, apprehension and worry.

Clinical experience has shown that doxepin HCl is safe and well tolerated even in the elderly patient. Owing to lack of clinical experience in the pediatric population, doxepin HCl is not recommended for use in children under 12 years of age.

TOPICAL CREAM

Zonalon cream is indicated for the short-term (up to 8 days) management of moderate pruritus in adult patients with the following forms of eczematous dermatitis; atopic dermatitis and lichen simplex chronicus.(See DOSAGE AND ADMINISTRATION.)

CONTRAINDICATIONS:

CAPSULES AND ORAL CONCENTRATE

Doxepin HCl is contraindicated in individuals who have shown hypersensitivity to the drug. Possibility of cross sensitivity with other dibenzoxepines should be kept in mind.

CONTRAINDICATIONS: *(cont'd)*

Doxepin HCl is contraindicated in patients with glaucoma or a tendency to urinary retention. These disorders should be ruled out, particularly in older patients.

TOPICAL CREAM

Because doxepin HCl has an anticholinergic effect and because significant plasma levels of doxepin are detectable after topical doxepin HCl cream application, the use of doxepin HCl cream is contraindicated in patients with untreated narrow angle glaucoma or a tendency to urinary retention.

Doxepin HCl cream is contraindicated in individuals who have shown previous sensitivity to any of its components.

WARNINGS:

CAPSULES AND ORAL CONCENTRATE

The once-a-day dosage regimen of doxepin HCl in patients with intercurrent illness or patients taking other medications should be carefully adjusted. This is especially important in patients receiving other medications with anticholinergic effects.

USAGE IN GERIATRICS

The use of doxepin HCl on a once-a-day dosage regimen in geriatric patients should be adjusted carefully based on the patient's condition.

USAGE IN PREGNANCY

Reproduction studies have been performed in rats, rabbits, monkeys and dogs and there was no evidence of harm to the animal fetus. The relevance to humans is not known. Since there is no experience in pregnant women who have received this drug, safety in pregnancy has not been established. There has been a report of apnea and drowsiness occurring in a nursing infant whose mother was taking doxepin HCl.

USAGE IN CHILDREN

The use of doxepin HCl in children under 12 years of age is not recommended because safe conditions for its use have not been established.

TOPICAL CREAM

Drowsiness occurs in over 20% of patients treated with doxepin HCl cream, especially in patients receiving treatment to greater than 10% of their body surface area. Patients should be warned of this possibility and cautioned against driving a motor vehicle or operating hazardous machinery while being treated with doxepin HCl cream.

Patients should also be warned that the effects of alcoholic beverages can be potentiated when using doxepin HCl cream.

If excessive drowsiness occurs it may be necessary to reduce the number of applications, the amount of cream applied, and/or the percentage of body surface area treated, or discontinue the drug.

Keep this product away from the eyes.

PRECAUTIONS:

CAPSULES AND ORAL CONCENTRATE

Since drowsiness may occur with the use of this drug, patients should be warned of the possibility and cautioned against driving a car or operating dangerous machinery while taking the drug. Patients should also be cautioned that their response to alcohol may be potentiated.

Since suicide is an inherent risk in any depressed patient and may remain so until significant improvement has occurred, patients should be closely supervised during the early course of therapy. Prescriptions should be written for the smallest feasible amount.

Should increased symptoms of psychosis or shift to manic symptomatology occur, it may be necessary to reduce dosage or add a major tranquilizer to the dosage regimen.

TOPICAL CREAM

Carcinogenesis, Mutagenesis, and Impairment of Fertility: Carcinogenesis, mutagenesis, and impairment of fertility studies have not been conducted with doxepin HCl.

Pregnancy Category B: Teratology studies have been performed in rats and rabbits at oral doses up to 8 times the topical human dose (based on a mg/kg basis) and have revealed no evidence of impaired fertility or harm to the fetus due to doxepin. There are, however, no adequate and well-controlled studies in pregnant women. Because animal reproduction studies are not always predictive of human response, this drug should be used during pregnancy only if clearly needed.

Nursing Mothers: Doxepin is excreted in human milk after oral administration. There have been no studies conducted to date to determine if doxepin is excreted in human milk after topical administration;; however, it is known that significant systemic levels of doxepin are obtained after topical administration. It is therefore possible that doxepin could be secreted in human milk following topical administration.

One case has been reported of apnea and drowsiness in a nursing infant whose mother was taking an oral dosage form of doxepin HCl.

Because of the potential for serious adverse reactions in nursing infants from doxepin, a decision should be made whether to discontinue nursing or to discontinue taking the drug, taking into account the importance of the drug to the mother.

Pediatric Use: Safety and effectiveness of doxepin HCl cream in children have not been established.

CAPSULES, ORAL CONCENTRATE, AND CREAM

Drugs Metabolized by $P_{450}11D_6$

A subset (3% to 10%) of the population has reduced activity of certain drug metabolizing enzymes such as the cytochrome P_{450}isozyme $P_{450}11D_6$. Such individuals are referred to as "poor metabolizers" of drug such as debrisoquine, dextromethorphan, and the tricyclic antidepressants. These individuals may have higher than expected plasma concentrations of tricyclic antidepressant when given usual doses. In addition, certain drugs that are metabolized by this isozyme, including many antidepressants (tricyclic antidepressants, selective serotonin reuptake inhibitors, and others), may inhibit the activity of this isozyme, and thus may make normal metabolizers resemble poor metabolizers with regard to concomitant therapy with other drugs metabolized by this enzyme system, leading to drug interactions.

Concomitant use of tricyclic antidepressants with other drugs metabolized by cytochrome $P_{450}11D_6$ may require lower doses than usually prescribed for either the tricyclic antidepressant or the other drug. Therefore, co-administration of tricyclic antidepressants with other drugs that are metabolized by this isoenzyme, including other antidepressants, phenothiazines, carbamazepine, and Type 1C antiarrhythmics (*e.g.*, propafenone, flecainide and encainide), or that inhibit this enzyme (*e.g.*, quinidine), should be approached with caution. Concomitant use of doxepin HCl cream with drugs metabolized by cytochrome $P_{450}11D_6$has not been formally studied.

DRUG INTERACTIONS:

CAPSULES, ORAL CONCENTRATE, AND CREAM

MAO Inhibitors: Serious side effects and even death have been reported following the concomitant use of certain drugs with MAO inhibitors. Therefore, MAO inhibitors should be discontinued at least two weeks prior to the cautious initiation of therapy with doxepin HCl. The exact length of time may vary and is dependent upon the particular MAO inhibitor being used, the length of time it has been administered, and the dosage involved.

Cimetidine: Cimetidine has been reported to produce clinically significant fluctuations in steady-state serum concentrations of various tricyclic antidepressants. Serious anticholinergic symptoms (*i.e.*, severe dry mouth, urinary retention and blurred vision) have been associated with elevations in the serum levels of tricyclic antidepressant when cimetidine therapy is initiated. Additionally, higher than expected tricyclic antidepressant levels have been observed when they are begun in patients already taking cimetidine. In patients who have been reported to be well controlled on tricyclic antidepressants receiving concurrent cimetidine therapy, discontinuation of cimetidine has been reported to decrease established steady-state serum tricyclic antidepressant levels and compromise their therapeutic effects.

CAPSULES AND ORAL CONCENTRATE

Alcohol: It should be borne in mind that alcohol ingestion may increase the danger inherent in any intentional or unintentional doxepin HCl overdosage. This is especially important in patients who may use alcohol excessively.

Tolazamide: A case of severe hypoglycemia has been reported in a type II diabetic patient maintained on tolazamide (1 gm/day) 11 days after the addition of doxepin (75 mg/day).

Topical Cream: Studies have not been performed examining drug interactions with Zonalon cream. However, data are available regarding potentially significant drug interactions regarding doxepin. As plasma levels of doxepin similar to therapeutic ranges for antidepressant therapy can be obtained following topical application of doxepin HCl cream, it would not be unexpected for the following drug interactions to be possible following topical doxepin HCl cream application.

CREAM

Alcohol: Alcohol ingestion may exacerbate the potential sedative effects of doxepin HCl cream.

ADVERSE REACTIONS:

CAPSULES AND ORAL CONCENTRATE

NOTE: Some of the adverse reactions noted below have not been specifically reported with doxepin HCl use. However, due to the close pharmacological similarities among the tricyclics, the reactions should be considered when prescribing doxepin HCl.

Anticholinergic Effects: Dry mouth, blurred vision, constipation, and urinary retention have been reported. If they do not subside with continued therapy, or become severe, it may be necessary to reduce the dosage.

Central Nervous System Effects: Drowsiness is the most commonly noticed side effect. This tends to disappear as therapy is continued. Other infrequently reported CNS side effects are confusion, disorientation, hallucinations, numbness, paresthesias, ataxia, extrapyramidal symptoms, seizures, tardive dyskinesia, and tremor.

Cardiovascular: Cardiovascular effects including hypotension, hypertension, and tachycardia have been reported occasionally.

Allergic: Skin rash, edema, photosensitization, and pruritus have occasionally occurred.

Hematologic: Eosinophilia has been reported in a few patients. There have been occasional reports of bone marrow depression manifesting as agranulocytosis, leukopenia, thrombocytopenia, and purpura.

Gastrointestinal: Nausea, vomiting, indigestion, taste disturbances, diarrhea, anorexia, and aphthous stomatitis have been reported. (See anticholinergic effects.)

Endocrine: Raised or lowered libido, testicular swelling, gynecomastia in males, enlargement of breasts and galactorrhea in the female, raising or lowering of blood sugar levels, and syndrome of inappropriate antidiuretic hormone secretion have been reported with tricyclic administration.

Other: Dizziness, tinnitus, weight gain, sweating, chills, fatigue, weakness, flushing, jaundice, alopecia, headache, exacerbation of asthma, and hyperpyrexia (in association with chlorpromazine) have been occasionally observed as adverse effects.

Withdrawal Symptoms: The possibility of development of withdrawal symptoms upon abrupt cessation of treatment after prolonged doxepin HCl administration should be borne in mind. These are not indicative of addiction and gradual withdrawal of medication should not cause these symptoms.

TOPICAL CREAM CONTROLLED CLINICAL TRIALS

Systemic Adverse Effects: In controlled clinical trials of patients treated with doxepin HCl cream, the most common systemic adverse effect reported was drowsiness. Drowsiness occurred in 22% of patients treated with doxepin HCl cream (and 2% of patients treated with placebo cream) and resulted in the premature discontinuation of the drug in approximately 5% of patients treated.

Other systemic adverse effects reports in approximately 1 to 10% of these patients included:

Dry mouth, dry lips, thirst, headache, fatigue, dizziness, emotional changes, and taste changes.

Other systemic adverse effects reported in less than 1% of these patients included:

Nausea, anxiety, and fever.

Local Site Adverse Effects: In controlled clinical trials of patients treated with doxepin HCl cream, the most common local site adverse effect reported was burning and/or stinging at the site of application. These occurred in approximately 21% of these patients. Most of these reactions were categorized as "mild"; however, approximately 25% of patients who reported burning and/or stinging reported the reaction as "severe." Four patients treated with doxepin HCl cream withdrew from the study because of the burning and/or stinging.

Other local site adverse effects reported in approximately 1 to 10% of these patients included:

Pruritus exacerbation, eczema exacerbation, dryness and tightness to skin, paresthesias, and edema.

Other local site adverse effects reported in less than 1% of these patients included:

Irritation, tingling, scaling, and cracking.

OVERDOSAGE:

CAPSULES, ORAL CONCENTRATE, AND CREAMS

A. Signs and Symptoms

1. Mild: Drowsiness, stupor, blurred vision, excessive dryness of mouth.

2. Severe: Respiratory depression, hypotension, coma, convulsions, cardiac arrhythmias and tachycardias.

Also: urinary retention (bladder atony), decreased gastrointestinal motility (paralytic ileus), hyperthermia (or hypothermia), hypertension, dilated pupils, hyperactive reflexes.

B. Management and Treatment

OVERDOSAGE: *(cont'd)*

1. Mild: Observation and supportive therapy is all that is usually necessary.

2. Severe: Medical management of severe doxepin HCl overdosage consists of aggressive supportive therapy. Arrhythmias should be treated with the appropriate antiarrhythmic agent. It has been reported that many of the cardiovascular and CNS symptoms of tricyclic antidepressant poisoning in adults may be reversed by the slow intravenous administration of 1 mg to 3 mg of physostigmine salicylate. Because physostigmine is rapidly metabolized, the dosage should be repeated as required. Convulsions may respond to standard anticonvulsant therapy, however, barbiturates may potentiate any respiratory depression. Dialysis and forced diuresis generally are not of value in the management of overdosage due to high tissue and protein binding of doxepin HCl.

CAPSULES AND ORAL CONCENTRATE

Management and Treatment: *Severe:* If the patient is conscious, gastric lavage, with appropriate precautions to prevent pulmonary aspiration, should be performed even though doxepin HCl is rapidly absorbed. The use of activated charcoal has been recommended, as has been continuous gastric lavage with saline for 24 hours or more. An adequate airway should be established in comatose patients and assisted ventilation used if necessary. EKG monitoring may be required for several days, since relapse after apparent recovery has been reported.

TOPICAL CREAM

Management and Treatment: *Mild:* It may be necessary to reduce the percent of body surface area treated or the frequency of application or apply a thinner layer of cream.

Severe: Medical management of severe doxepin overdosage consists of aggressive supportive therapy. The area covered with doxepin HCl cream should be thoroughly washed. An adequate airway should be established in comatose patients and assisted ventilation used if necessary. EKG monitoring may be required for several days, because relapse after apparent recovery has been reported with oral doxepin HCl.

DOSAGE AND ADMINISTRATION:

CAPSULES AND ORAL CONCENTRATE

For most patients with illness of mild to moderate severity, a starting daily dose of 75 mg is recommended. Dosage may subsequently be increased or decreased at appropriate intervals and according to individual response. The usual optimum dose range is 75 mg/day to 150 mg/day.

In more severely ill patients higher doses may be required with subsequent gradual increase to 300 mg/day if necessary. Additional therapeutic effect is rarely to be obtained by exceeding a dose of 300 mg/day.

In patients with very mild symptomatology or emotional symptoms accompanying organic disease, lower doses may suffice. Some of these patients have been controlled on doses as low as 25-50 mg/day.

The total daily dosage of doxepin HCl may be given on a divided or once-a-day dosage schedule. If the once-a-day schedule is employed the maximum recommended dose is 150 mg/day. This dose may be given at bedtime. **The 150 mg capsule strength is intended for maintenance therapy only and is not recommended for initiation of treatment.**

Antianxiety effect is apparent before the antidepressant effect. Optimal antidepressant effect may not be evident for two to three weeks.

TOPICAL CREAM

A thin film of doxepin HCl cream should be applied four times each day with at least a 3 to 4 hour interval between applications. There are no data to establish the safety and effectiveness of doxepin HCl cream when used for greater than 8 days. Chronic use beyond eight days may result in higher systemic levels.

Clinical experience has shown that **drowsiness is significantly more common in patients applying doxepin HCl cream to over 10% of body surface area;** therefore, patients with greater than 10% of body surface area affected should be particularly cautioned concerning possible drowsiness and other systemic adverse effects of doxepin. If excessive drowsiness occurs it may be necessary to do one or more of the following: reduce the body surface area treated, reduce the number of applications per day, reduce the amount of cream applied, or discontinue the drug.

Occlusive dressings may increase the absorption of most topical drugs; therefore, occlusive dressings with doxepin HCl cream should not be utilized.

HOW SUPPLIED:

TOPICAL CREAM

Zonalon cream is available in 30 g aluminum tubes. Store at or below 27°C (80°F).

(Topical Cream: GenDerm, 1/94, 126861)

HOW SUPPLIED - RATED THERAPEUTICALLY EQUIVALENT:

Capsule - Oral - 10 mg

100's	$13.75	Doxepin Hcl, Duramed Pharms	51285-0910-02
1000's	$134.50	Doxepin Hcl, Duramed Pharms	51285-0910-05

Capsule - Oral - 25 mg

100's	$14.05	Doxepin Hcl, Duramed Pharms	51285-0911-02
100's	$137.50	Doxepin Hcl, Duramed Pharms	51285-0911-05

Capsule - Oral - 50 mg

100's	$19.60	Doxepin Hcl, Duramed Pharms	51285-0912-02
1000's	$193.00	Doxepin Hcl, Duramed Pharms	51285-0912-05

Capsule, Gelatin - Oral - 10 mg

100's	$3.98	Doxepin Hcl, United Res	00677-1101-01
100's	$3.98	Doxepin HCl, H.C.F.A. F F P	99999-1111-01
100's	$6.41	Doxepin Hcl, US Trading	56126-0345-11
100's	$9.05	Doxepin Hcl, Qualitest Pharms	00603-3455-21
100's	$10.48	Doxepin Hcl, Lederle Pharm	00005-3183-23
100's	$10.50	Doxepin Hcl, Major Pharms	00904-1260-60
100's	$11.50	Doxepin HCl, Schein Pharm (US)	00364-2113-01
100's	$11.95	Doxepin HCl, Rugby	00536-4563-01
100's	$12.20	Doxepin Hcl, Aligen Independ	00405-4369-01
100's	$12.90	Doxepin Hcl, Royce	51875-0309-01
100's	$12.95	Doxepin Hcl, Goldline Labs	00182-1325-01
100's	$12.95	Doxepin Hcl, Par Pharm	49884-0217-01
100's	$12.95	Doxepin Hcl, Martec Pharms	52555-0294-01
100's	$13.56	Doxepin Hcl, HL Moore Drug Exch	00839-7892-06
100's	$13.95	Doxepin Hcl, Mylan	00378-1049-01
100's	$13.95	Doxepin HCl, Geneva Pharms	00781-2800-01
100's	$14.70	Doxepin Hcl, Voluntary Hosp	53258-0411-01
100's	$22.20	DOXEPIN HCL, Voluntary Hosp	53258-0411-13
100's	$24.70	Doxepin Hcl, Goldline Labs	00182-1325-89
100's	$24.70	Doxepin HCl, Schein Pharm (US)	00364-2113-90
100's	$25.75	Doxepin HCl, Geneva Pharms	00781-2800-13
100's	$25.77	Doxepin Hcl, Vangard Labs	00615-0395-13
100's	$25.86	Doxepin Hcl, Major Pharms	00904-1260-61
100's	$28.31	ADAPIN, Lotus Biochem	59417-0356-71

HOW SUPPLIED - RATED THERAPEUTICALLY EQUIVALENT:
(cont'd)

100's	**$33.87**	**SINEQUAN, Roerig**	**00049-5340-66**
500's	$19.90	Doxepin HCl, H.C.F.A. F F P	99999-1111-02
500's	$64.50	Doxepin Hcl, Par Pharm	49884-0217-05
1000's	$39.80	Doxepin HCl, H.C.F.A. F F P	99999-1111-03
1000's	$45.50	Doxepin Hcl, Elkins Sinn	00641-4500-89
1000's	$49.50	Doxepin HCl, Rugby	00536-4563-10
1000's	$80.43	Doxepin Hcl, Qualitest Pharms	00603-3455-32
1000's	$80.55	Doxepin Hcl 10 Mg Capsules, Major Pharms	00904-1260-80
1000's	$115.20	Doxepin Hcl, Royce	51875-0309-04
1000's	$125.62	Doxepin Hcl, Par Pharm	49884-0217-10
1000's	$131.89	Doxepin Hcl, HL Moore Drug Exch	00839-7892-16
1000's	$133.95	Doxepin Hcl, Mylan	00378-1049-10
1000's	**$295.59**	**SINEQUAN, Roerig**	**00049-5340-82**

Capsule, Gelatin - Oral - 25 mg

90's	**$34.09**	**SINEQUAN, Roerig Pfizer**	**00662-5350-68**
100's	$4.43	Doxepin Hcl, United Res	00677-1102-01
100's	$4.43	Doxepin HCl, H.C.F.A. F F P	99999-1111-04
100's	$7.77	Doxepin Hcl, US Trading	56126-0346-11
100's	$10.50	Doxepin Hcl, Mova Pharms	55370-0530-07
100's	$11.60	Doxepin Hcl, Qualitest Pharms	00603-3456-21
100's	$12.95	Doxepin Hcl, Major Pharms	00904-1261-60
100's	$13.14	Doxepin Hcl, Lederle Pharm	00005-3184-23
100's	$13.20	Doxepin HCl, Schein Pharm (US)	00364-2114-01
100's	$13.20	Doxepin Hcl, Aligen Independ	00405-4370-01
100's	$13.25	Doxepin Hcl, Goldline Labs	00182-1326-01
100's	$13.25	Doxepin HCl, Rugby	00536-4564-01
100's	$13.25	Doxepin Hcl, Par Pharm	49884-0218-01
100's	$13.25	Doxepin Hcl, Royce	51875-0310-01
100's	$13.30	Doxepin Hcl, Martec Pharms	52555-0295-01
100's	$13.49	Doxepin Hcl, HL Moore Drug Exch	00839-7221-06
100's	$13.91	Doxepin Hcl, HL Moore Drug Exch	00839-7893-06
100's	$14.25	Doxepin Hcl, Mylan	00378-3125-01
100's	$14.25	Doxepin Hcl, Geneva Pharms	00781-2801-01
100's	$14.85	Doxepin Hcl, Voluntary Hosp	53258-0412-01
100's	$22.47	DOXEPIN HCL, Voluntary Hosp	53258-0412-13
100's	$27.00	Doxepin HCl, Schein Pharm (US)	00364-2114-90
100's	$31.10	Doxepin Hcl, Goldline Labs	00182-1326-89
100's	$31.71	Doxepin Hcl, Vangard Labs	00615-0396-13
100's	$31.71	Doxepin HCl, Geneva Pharms	00781-2801-13
100's	$36.51	ADAPIN, Lotus Biochem	59417-0357-71
100's	$38.26	Doxepin Hcl, Major Pharms	00904-1261-61
100's	**$43.68**	**SINEQUAN, Roerig**	**00049-5350-66**
360's	$35.53	Doxepin Hcl, Rugby	00536-3728-07
500's	$22.15	Doxepin HCl, H.C.F.A. F F P	99999-1111-05
500's	$66.25	Doxepin Hcl, Par Pharm	49884-0218-05
1000's	$44.30	Doxepin HCl, H.C.F.A. F F P	99999-1111-06
1000's	$59.90	Doxepin Hcl, Elkins Sinn	00641-4501-89
1000's	$89.50	Doxepin Hcl, Major Pharms	00904-1261-80
1000's	$99.84	Doxepin HCl, Schein Pharm (US)	00364-2114-02
1000's	$110.91	Doxepin Hcl, Qualitest Pharms	00603-3456-32
1000's	$115.50	Doxepin HCl, Rugby	00536-4564-10
1000's	$120.05	Doxepin Hcl, Royce	51875-0310-04
1000's	$128.53	Doxepin Hcl, Par Pharm	49884-0218-10
1000's	$128.90	Doxepin Hcl, Aligen Independ	00405-4370-03
1000's	$141.35	Doxepin Hcl, HL Moore Drug Exch	00839-7221-16
1000's	$141.35	Doxepin Hcl, HL Moore Drug Exch	00839-7893-16
1000's	$142.95	Doxepin HCl, Geneva Pharms	00781-2801-10
1000's	$143.95	Doxepin Hcl, Mylan	00378-3125-10
1000's	**$380.93**	**SINEQUAN, Roerig**	**00049-5350-82**
5000's	$221.50	Doxepin HCl, H.C.F.A. F F P	99999-1111-07
5000's	**$1866.65**	**SINEQUAN, Roerig**	**00049-5350-94**

Capsule, Gelatin - Oral - 50 mg

30's	$1.98	Doxepin HCl, H.C.F.A. F F P	99999-1111-08
90's	**$46.85**	**SINEQUAN, Roerig Pfizer**	**00662-5360-68**
100's	$6.60	Doxepin Hcl, United Res	00677-1103-01
100's	$6.60	Doxepin HCl, H.C.F.A. F F P	99999-1111-09
100's	$9.23	Doxepin Hcl, US Trading	56126-0347-11
100's	$14.75	Doxepin Hcl, Mova Pharms	55370-0531-07
100's	$16.61	Doxepin Hcl, Qualitest Pharms	00603-3457-21
100's	$18.25	Doxepin Hcl, Major Pharms	00904-1262-60
100's	$18.42	Doxepin Hcl, Lederle Pharm	00005-3185-23
100's	$18.82	Doxepin HCl, Schein Pharm (US)	00364-2115-01
100's	$18.90	Doxepin Hcl, Goldline Labs	00182-1327-01
100's	$18.90	Doxepin Hcl, Par Pharm	49884-0219-01
100's	$18.94	Doxepin Hcl 50, Aligen Independ	00405-4371-01
100's	$19.02	Doxepin Hcl, Royce	51875-0311-01
100's	$19.10	Doxepin Hcl, Martec Pharms	52555-0296-01
100's	$19.24	Doxepin Hcl, HL Moore Drug Exch	00839-7894-06
100's	$19.25	Doxepin Hcl, Rugby	00536-4565-01
100's	$19.95	Doxepin Hcl, Mylan	00378-4250-01
100's	$20.85	Doxepin Hcl, Voluntary Hosp	53258-0413-01
100's	$32.10	DOXEPIN HCL, Voluntary Hosp	53258-0413-13
100's	$43.40	Doxepin Hcl, Goldline Labs	00182-1327-89
100's	$43.50	Doxepin HCl, Schein Pharm (US)	00364-2115-90
100's	$43.87	Doxepin Hcl, Vangard Labs	00615-0397-13
100's	$46.76	Doxepin Hcl, Major Pharms	00904-1262-61
100's	$51.42	ADAPIN, Lotus Biochem	59417-0358-71
100's	**$57.67**	**SINEQUAN, Roerig Pfizer**	**00662-5360-41**
100's	**$61.49**	**SINEQUAN, Roerig**	**00049-5360-66**
360's	$46.92	Doxepin Hcl, Rugby	00536-3729-07
500's	$33.00	Doxepin HCl, H.C.F.A. F F P	99999-1111-10
500's	$94.50	Doxepin Hcl, Par Pharm	49884-0219-05
1000's	$66.00	Doxepin HCl, H.C.F.A. F F P	99999-1111-11
1000's	$87.70	Doxepin Hcl, Elkins Sinn	00641-4502-89
1000's	$100.67	Doxepin Hcl, Qualitest Pharms	00603-3457-32
1000's	$138.50	Doxepin Hcl, Major Pharms	00904-1262-80
1000's	$143.00	Doxepin HCl, Schein Pharm (US)	00364-2115-02
1000's	$163.50	Doxepin HCl, Rugby	00536-4565-10
1000's	$176.00	Doxepin Hcl, Royce	51875-0311-04
1000's	$183.33	Doxepin Hcl, Par Pharm	49884-0219-10
1000's	$183.52	Doxepin Hcl 50, Aligen Independ	00405-4371-03
1000's	$203.11	Doxepin Hcl, HL Moore Drug Exch	00839-7222-16
1000's	$203.11	Doxepin Hcl, HL Moore Drug Exch	00839-7894-16
1000's	$203.95	Doxepin Hcl, Mylan	00378-4250-10
1000's	**$536.59**	**SINEQUAN, Roerig**	**00049-5360-82**
5000's	$330.00	Doxepin HCl, H.C.F.A. F F P	99999-1111-12
5000's	**$2629.10**	**SINEQUAN, Roerig**	**00049-5360-94**

Capsule, Gelatin - Oral - 75 mg

100's	$8.93	Doxepin Hcl, United Res	00677-1104-01
100's	$8.93	Doxepin HCl, H.C.F.A. F F P	99999-1111-13
100's	$11.85	Doxepin Hcl, US Trading	56126-0348-11

HOW SUPPLIED - RATED THERAPEUTICALLY EQUIVALENT:
(cont'd)

100's	$19.12	Doxepin Hcl, Qualitest Pharms	00603-3458-21
100's	$21.25	Doxepin Hcl, Elkins Sinn	00641-4503-86
100's	$29.00	Doxepin, Major Pharms	00904-1263-60
100's	$32.50	Doxepin HCl, Rugby	00536-3737-01
100's	$33.17	Doxepin HCl, Schein Pharm (US)	00364-2116-01
100's	$35.75	Doxepin Hcl, Goldline Labs	00182-1328-01
100's	$35.75	Doxepin Hcl, Par Pharm	49884-0220-01
100's	$35.80	Doxepin Hcl, Martec Pharms	52555-0331-01
100's	$35.82	Doxepin Hcl 75, Aligen Independ	00405-4372-01
100's	$35.88	Doxepin Hcl, Voluntary Hosp	53258-0414-01
100's	$41.24	Doxepin Hcl, HL Moore Drug Exch	00839-7895-06
100's	$41.95	Doxepin Hcl, Mylan	00378-5375-01
100's	$53.34	DOXEPIN HCL, Voluntary Hosp	53258-0414-13
100's	$59.00	Doxepin HCl, Schein Pharm (US)	00364-2116-90
100's	$69.60	Doxepin Hcl, Goldline Labs	00182-1328-89
100's	$70.64	Doxepin Hcl, Vangard Labs	00615-0398-13
100's	$73.31	Doxepin, Major Pharms	00904-1263-61
100's	$85.27	ADAPIN, Lotus Biochem	59417-0361-71
100's	**$96.47**	**SINEQUAN, Roerig Pfizer**	**00662-5390-41**
100's	**$101.97**	**SINEQUAN, Roerig**	**00049-5390-66**
500's	$44.65	Doxepin HCl, H.C.F.A. F F P	99999-1111-14
500's	$101.25	Doxepin HCl, Rugby	00536-3737-05
500's	$178.75	Doxepin Hcl, Par Pharm	49884-0220-05
1000's	$89.30	Doxepin HCl, H.C.F.A. F F P	99999-1111-15
1000's	$134.91	Doxepin Hcl, Qualitest Pharms	00603-3458-32
1000's	$155.60	Doxepin Hcl, Elkins Sinn	00641-4503-89
1000's	$346.78	Doxepin Hcl, Par Pharm	49884-0220-10
1000's	$364.10	Doxepin Hcl, HL Moore Drug Exch	00839-7895-16
1000's	$365.95	Doxepin Hcl, Mylan	00378-5375-10
1000's	**$927.47**	**SINEQUAN, Roerig**	**00049-5390-82**

Capsule, Gelatin - Oral - 100 mg

100's	$11.25	Doxepin Hcl, United Res	00677-1105-01
100's	$11.25	Doxepin HCl, H.C.F.A. F F P	99999-1111-16
100's	$14.42	Doxepin Hcl, US Trading	56126-0349-11
100's	$28.85	Doxepin Hcl, Mova Pharms	55370-0532-07
100's	$29.96	Doxepin Hcl, Qualitest Pharms	00603-3459-21
100's	$33.61	Doxepin Hcl, Lederle Pharm	00005-3187-23
100's	$37.08	Doxepin HCl, Schein Pharm (US)	00364-2117-01
100's	$39.50	Doxepin Hcl, Major Pharms	00904-1264-60
100's	$41.07	Doxepin Hcl, Voluntary Hosp	53258-0415-01
100's	$42.05	Doxepin Hcl, Goldline Labs	00182-1329-01
100's	$42.05	Doxepin Hcl, Par Pharm	49884-0221-01
100's	$42.30	Doxepin Hcl, Martec Pharms	52555-0332-01
100's	$42.32	Doxepin Hcl 100, Aligen Independ	00405-4373-01
100's	$42.65	Doxepin Hcl, HL Moore Drug Exch	00839-7224-06
100's	$42.65	Doxepin Hcl, HL Moore Drug Exch	00839-7896-06
100's	$43.95	Doxepin Hcl, Mylan	00378-6410-01
100's	$43.95	Doxepin HCl, Rugby	00536-4566-01
100's	$54.60	Doxepin HCl, Schein Pharm (US)	00364-2117-90
100's	$65.10	DOXEPIN HCL, Voluntary Hosp	53258-0415-13
100's	$77.70	Doxepin Hcl, Goldline Labs	00182-1329-89
100's	$77.83	Doxepin Hcl, Vangard Labs	00615-0399-13
100's	$82.37	Doxepin Hcl, Major Pharms	00904-1264-61
100's	$92.96	ADAPIN, Lotus Biochem	59417-0359-71
100's	**$111.17**	**SINEQUAN, Roerig**	**00049-5380-66**
500's	$56.25	Doxepin HCl, H.C.F.A. F F P	99999-1111-17
500's	$210.25	Doxepin Hcl, Par Pharm	49884-0221-05
1000's	$112.50	Doxepin HCl, H.C.F.A. F F P	99999-1111-18
1000's	$193.75	Doxepin HCl, Rugby	00536-4566-10
1000's	$407.89	Doxepin Hcl, Par Pharm	49884-0221-10
1000's	$428.22	Doxepin Hcl, HL Moore Drug Exch	00839-7896-16
1000's	$429.95	Doxepin Hcl, Mylan	00378-6410-10
1000's	**$982.13**	**SINEQUAN, Roerig**	**00049-5380-82**

Capsule, Gelatin - Oral - 150 mg

50's	$14.96	Doxepin HCl, H.C.F.A. F F P	99999-1111-19
50's	$25.30	Doxepin Hcl, Lederle Pharm	00005-3188-18
50's	$33.50	Doxepin Hydrochloride, Par Pharm	49884-0222-03
50's	$77.18	ADAPIN, Lotus Biochem	59417-0370-65
50's	**$92.30**	**SINEQUAN, Roerig**	**00049-5370-50**
100's	$29.93	Doxepin HCl, H.C.F.A. F F P	99999-1111-20
100's	$31.48	Doxepin Hcl, Vangard Labs	00615-1301-13
100's	$36.47	Doxepin Hcl, US Trading	56126-0401-11
100's	$48.10	Doxepin Hcl, Qualitest Pharms	00603-3460-21
100's	$52.45	Doxepin Hcl, Major Pharms	00904-1265-60
100's	$55.50	Doxepin Hcl, Goldline Labs	00182-1878-01
100's	$55.50	Doxepin Hcl, Par Pharm	49884-0222-01
100's	$55.61	Doxepin HCl, Schein Pharm (US)	00364-2525-01
100's	$58.25	Doxepin Hydrochloride Capsules 150 Mg, HL Moore Drug Exch	00839-7509-06
100's	$58.42	Doxepin Hcl, Aligen Independ	00405-4374-01
100's	$59.85	Doxepin Hcl, Martec Pharms	52555-0322-01
100's	$59.93	Doxepin HCl, Rugby	00536-3738-01
100's	**$164.26**	**SINEQUAN, Roerig Pfizer**	**00662-5370-41**
500's	$149.65	Doxepin HCl, H.C.F.A. F F P	99999-1111-21
500's	$277.50	Doxepin Hcl, Par Pharm	49884-0222-05
500's	**$839.97**	**SINEQUAN, Roerig**	**00049-5370-73**

Concentrate - Oral - 10 mg/ml

120 ml	$12.50	Doxepin Hcl, Harber Pharm	51432-0531-18
120 ml	$13.00	Doxepin Hcl, Raway	00686-0612-14
120 ml	$13.00	Doxepin Hcl, Copley Pharm	38245-0612-14
120 ml	$14.90	Doxepin Hcl, HL Moore Drug Exch	00839-7470-65
120 ml	$15.20	Doxepin Hcl, Aligen Independ	00405-2680-76
120 ml	$16.00	Doxepin Hcl, Goldline Labs	00182-6043-71
120 ml	$16.14	Doxepin HCl Concentrate, Schein Pharm (US)	00364-2278-77
120 ml	$16.34	Doxepin HCl, H.C.F.A. F F P	99999-1111-22
120 ml	$16.35	Doxepin HCl, Warner Chilcott	00047-2623-35
120 ml	$16.35	Doxepin HCl Concentrate, Rugby	00536-0685-97
120 ml	$18.25	Doxepin Hcl, Morton Grove	60432-0651-04
120 ml	$20.00	Doxepin Hcl, Geneva Pharms	00781-6420-04
120 ml	**$26.13**	**SINEQUAN, Roerig**	**00049-5100-47**

HOW SUPPLIED - NOT RATED EQUIVALENT:

Cream - Topical - 5 %

30 gm	$20.78	ZONALON, Genderm Corp	29936-0523-30
30 gm	$20.78	ZONALON, Genderm	52761-0523-30

DOXORUBICIN HYDROCHLORIDE *(001112)*

CATEGORIES: Antibiotics; Antineoplastics; Bladder Carcinoma; Breast Carcinoma; Cancer; Cytotoxic Agents; Leukemia; Lymphoma; Neuroblastoma; Oncologic Drugs; Ovarian Carcinoma; Sarcoma; Stomach Carcinoma; Thyroid Carcinoma; Tumors; Wilms' Tumor; Melanoma*; Renal Carcinoma*; Sales > $100 Million; FDA Approval Pre 1982
* Indication not approved by the FDA

BRAND NAMES: *Adiblastine*; *Adriablastina*; *Adriablastine*; *Adriablatina*; *Adriacin*; **Adriamycin**; Adriamycin Rdf; *Adriblastina*; *Adriblatina*; Doxorubicin Hcl; *Farmablastina*; Rubex
(International brand names outside U.S. in italics)

FORMULARIES: BC-BS; Medi-Cal; WHO

COST OF THERAPY: $3,775.85 (Ovarian Carcinoma; Injection; 2 mg/ml; 2.38/day; 182 days) vs. Potential Cost of $10,302.00 (Ovarian Malig.)

1. Severe local tissue necrosis will occur if there is extravasation during administration (See DOSAGE AND ADMINISTRATION.) Doxorubicin must not be given by the intramuscular or subcutaneous route.

2. Myocardial toxicity manifested in its most severe form by potentially fatal congestive heart failure may occur either during therapy or months to years after termination of therapy. The probability of developing impaired myocardial function based on a combined index of signs, symptoms and decline in left ventricular ejection fraction (LVEF) is estimated to be 1 to 2% at a total cumulative dose of 300 mg/m^2 of doxorubicin, 3 to 5% at a dose of 400 mg/m^2, 5 to 8% at 450 mg/m^2 and 6 to 20% at 500mg/m^2.The risk of developing CHF increases rapidly with increasing total cumulative doses of doxorubicin in excess of 450 mg/m2. This toxicity may occur at lower cumulative doses in patients with prior mediastinal irradiation or on concurrent cyclophosphamide therapy or with pre-existing heart disease.

3. Dosage should be reduced in patients with impaired hepatic function.

4. Severe myelosuppression may occur.

5. Doxorubicin should be administered only under the supervision of a physician who is experienced in the use of cancer chemotherapeutic agents.

* Data on file at Pharmacia Adria

DESCRIPTION:

Doxorubicin is a cytotoxic anthracycline antibiotic isolated from cultures of *Streptomyces peucetius* var. *caesius.*

Doxorubicin consists of a naphthacenequinone nucleus linked through a glycosidic bond at ring atom 7 to an amino sugar, daunosamine.

Chemically, doxorubicin hydrochloride is:

5,12-Naphthacenedione, 10-[(3-amino-2,3,6-trideoxy-α-L-*lyxo*-hexopyranosyl)oxy]-7,8,9,10-tetrahydro-6,8,11-trihydroxy-8- (hydroxylacetyl)-1-methoxy-, hydrochloride (8*S-cis*)-.

$C_{27}H_{29}NO_{11}$·HCl M.W.—579.99

Doxorubicin binds to nucleic acids, presumably by specific intercalation of the planar anthracycline nucleus with the DNA double helix. The anthracycline ring is lipophilic, but the saturated end of the ring system contains abundant hydroxyl groups adjacent to the amino sugar, producing a hydrophilic center. The molecule is amphoteric, containing acidic functions in the ring phenolic groups and a basic function in the sugar amino group. It binds to cell membranes as well as plasma proteins.

Doxorubicin hydrochloride for injection a sterile red-orange lyophilized powder for intravenous use only, is available in 10, 20, and 50 mg single dose vials and a 150 mg multidose vial.

Each 10 mg single dose vial contains 10 mg of doxorubicin HCl, 50 mg of lactose, NF (hydrous), and 1 mg of methylparaben, NF (added to enhance dissolution) as a sterile red-orange lyophilized powder.

Each Adriamycin 20 mg single dose vial contains 20 mg of doxorubicin HCl, 100 mg of lactose, NF (hydrous), and 2 mg of methylparaben, NF (added to enhance dissolution) as a sterile red-orange lyophilized powder.

Each Adriamycin 50 mg single dose vial contains 50 mg of doxorubicin HCl, 250 mg of lactose, NF (hydrous), and 5 mg of methylparaben, NF (added to enhance dissolution) as a sterile red-orange lyophilized powder.

Each Adriamycin 150 mg multidose vial contains 150 mg of doxorubicin HCl, 750 mg of lactose, NF (hydrous), and 15 mg of methylparaben, NF (added to enhance dissolution) as a sterile red-orange lyophilized powder.

Adriamycin Injection is a sterile parenteral, isotonic solution for intravenous use only, containing no preservative, available in 5 ml (10 mg), 10 ml (20 mg), 25 ml (50 mg), and 37.5 ml (75 mg) single dose vials and a 100 ml (200 mg) multidose vial.Each ml contains doxorubicin HCl 2 mg, and the following inactive ingredients: sodium chloride 0.9% and water for injection q.s. Hydrochloric acid is used to adjust the pH to a target pH of 3.0.

CLINICAL PHARMACOLOGY:

The cytotoxic effect of doxorubicin on malignant cells and its toxic effects on various organs are thought to be related to nucleotide base intercalation and cell membrane lipid binding activities of doxorubicin. Intercalation inhibits nucleotide replication and action of DNA and RNA polymerases. The interaction of doxorubicin with topoisomerase II to form DNA-cleavable complexes appears to be an important mechanism of doxorubicin cytocidal activity. Doxorubicin cellular membrane binding may effect a variety of cellular functions. Enzymatic electron reduction of doxorubicin by a variety of oxidases, reductases, and dehydrogenases generate highly reactive species including the hydroxyl free radical OH·. Free radical formation has been implicated in doxorubicin cardiotoxicity by means of Cu (II) and Fe (III) reduction at the cellular level.

Animal studies have shown activity in a spectrum of experimental tumors, immunosuppression, carcinogenic properties in rodents, induction of a variety of toxic effects, including delayed and progressive cardiac toxicity, myelosuppression in all species and atrophy to testes in rats and dogs.

Pharmacokinetic studies, determined in patients with various types of tumors undergoing either single or multi-agent therapy have shown that doxorubicin follows a multiphasic disposition after intravenous injection. The initial distributive half-life of approximately 5.0 minutes suggests rapid tissue uptake of doxorubicin, while its slow elimination from tissues is reflected by a terminal half-life of 20 to 48 hours. Steady-state distribution volumes exceed 20 to 30 l/kg and are indicative of extensive drug uptake into tissues. Plasma clearance is in the range of 8 to 20 ml/min/kg and is predominantly by metabolism and biliary excretion. Approximately 40% of the dose appears in the bile in 5 days, while only 5 to 12% of the drug and its metabolites appear in the urine during the same period. Binding of doxorubicin and its major metabolite, doxorubicinol to plasma proteins is about 74 to 76% and is independent of plasma concentration of doxorubicin up to 2 μM. Enzymatic reduction at the 7 position and cleavage of the daunosamine sugar yields aglycones which are accompanied by free radical formation, the local production of which may contribute to the cardiotoxic activity of doxorubicin. Disposition of doxorubicinol (DOX-OL) in patients is formation rate limited. The terminal half-life of DOX-OL is similar to doxorubicin. The relative exposure of DOX-OL, compared to doxorubicin ranges between 0.4 to 0.6. In urine, <3% of the dose was recovered as DOX-OL over 7 days. The literature contains no information regarding gender-related differences in the pharmacokinetics of doxorubicin and doxorubicinol.

In four patients, dose-dependent pharmacokinetics have been shown for doxorubicin in the dose range of 30 to 70 mg/m^2. Systemic clearance of doxorubicin is *significantly* reduced in obese women with ideal body weight greater than 130%. There was a significant reduction in clearance without any change in volume of distribution in obese patients when compared with normal patients with less than 115% ideal body weight. The clearance of doxorubicin and doxorubicinol was also reduced in patients with impaired hepatic function. Doxorubicin was excreted in the milk of one lactating patient, with peak milk concentration at 24 hours after treatment being approximately 4.4-fold greater than the *corresponding plasma concentration.* Doxorubicin was detectable in the milk up to 72 hours after therapy with 70 mg/m^2 of doxorubicin given as a 15 minute intravenous infusion and 100 mg/m^2 of cisplatin as a 26 hour intravenous infusion. The peak concentration of doxorubicinol in milk at 24 hours was 0.2 μM and AUC up to 24 hours was 16.5 μM/hr while the AUC for doxorubicin was 9.9 μM/hr.

Doxorubicin does not cross the blood brain barrier.

INDICATIONS AND USAGE:

Doxorubicin HCl has been used successfully to produce regression in disseminated neoplastic conditions such as acute lymphoblastic leukemia, acute myeloblastic leukemia, Wilms' tumor, neuroblastoma, soft tissue and bone sarcomas, breast carcinoma, ovarian carcinoma, transitional cell bladder carcinoma, thyroid carcinoma, gastric carcinoma, Hodgkin's disease, malignant lymphoma, and bronchogenic carcinoma in which the small cell histologic type is the most responsive compared to other cell types.

CONTRAINDICATIONS:

Doxorubicin therapy should not be started in patients who have marked myelosuppression induced by previous treatment with other antitumor agents or by radiotherapy. Doxorubicin treatment is contraindicated in patients who received previous treatment with complete cumulative doses of doxorubicin, daunorubicin, idarubicin, and/or other anthracyclines and anthracenes.

WARNINGS:

Special attention must be given to the cardiotoxicity induced by doxorubicin. Irreversible myocardial toxicity, manifested in its most severe form by life-threatening and potentially fatal congestive heart failure, may occur either during therapy or months to years after termination of therapy. The probability of developing impaired myocardial function, based on a combined index of signs, symptoms and decline in left ventricular ejection fraction (LVEF) is estimated to be 1 to 2% at a total cumulative dose of 300 mg/m^2 of doxorubicin, 3 to 5% at a dose of 400 mg/m^2, 5 to 8% at a dose of 450 mg/m^2 and 6 to 20% at a dose of 500 mg/m^2 given in a schedule of a bolus injection once every 3 weeks (data on file at Pharmacia Adria). In a retrospective review by Von Hoff et al, the probability of developing congestive heart failure was reported to be 5/168 (3%) at a cumulative dose of 430 mg/m^2 of doxorubicin, 8/110 (7%) at 575 mg/m^{2}and 3/14 (21%) at 728 mg/m^2. The cumulative incidence of CHF was 2.2%. In a prospective study of doxorubicin in combination with cyclophosphamide, fluorouracil and/or vincristine in patients with breast cancer or small cell lung cancer, the cumulative incidence of congestive heart failure was 5 to 6%. The probability of CHF at various cumulative doses of doxorubicin was 1.5% at 300 mg/m^2, 4.9% at 400 mg/m^2, 7.7% at 450 mg/m^2 and 20.5% at 500 mg/m^2.

Cardiotoxicity may occur at lower doses in patients with prior mediastinal irradiation, concurrent cyclophosphamide therapy and advanced age. Data also suggest that pre-existing heart disease is a co-factor for increased risk of doxorubicin cardiotoxicity. In such cases, cardiac toxicity may occur at doses lower than the respective recommended cumulative dose of doxorubicin. Studies have suggested that concomitant administration of doxorubicin and calcium channel entry blockers may increase the risk of doxorubicin cardiotoxicity. The total dose of doxorubicin administered to the individual patient should also take into account previous or concomitant therapy with related compounds such as daunorubicin, idarubicin and mitoxantrone. Cardiomyopathy and/or congestive heart failure may be encountered several months or years after discontinuation of doxorubicin therapy.

The risk of congestive heart failure and other acute manifestations of doxorubicin cardiotoxicity in children may be as much or lower than in adults. Children appear to be at particular risk for developing delayed cardiac toxicity in that doxorubicin-induced cardiomyopathy impairs myocardial growth as children mature, subsequently leading to possible development of congestive heart failure during early adulthood. As many as 40% of children may have subclinical cardiac dysfunction and 5 to 10% of children may develop congestive heart failure on long term follow-up. This late cardiac toxicity may be related to the dose of doxorubicin. The longer the length of follow-up the greater the increase in the detection rate.

Treatment of doxorubicin-induced congestive heart failure includes the use of digitalis, diuretics, after load reducers such as angiotensin I converting enzyme (ACE) inhibitors, low salt diet, and bed rest. Such intervention may relieve symptoms and improve the functional status of the patient.

Monitoring Cardiac Function: In adult patients severe cardiac toxicity may occur precipitously without antecedent ECG changes. Cardiomyopathy induced by anthracyclines is usually associated with very characteristic histopathologic changes on an endomyocardial biopsy (EM biopsy), and a decrease of left ventricular ejection fraction (LVEF), as measured by multi-gated radionuclide angiography (MUGA scans) and/or echocardiogram (ECHO), from pretreatment baseline values. However, it has not been demonstrated that monitoring of the ejection fraction will predict when individual patients are approaching their maximally tolerated cumulative dose of doxorubicin. Cardiac function should be carefully monitored during treatment to minimize the risk of cardiac toxicity. A baseline cardiac evaluation with an ECG, LVEF, and/or an (ECHO) is recommended especially in patients with risk factors for increased cardiac toxicity (pre-existing heart disease, mediastinal irradiation, or concurrent cyclophosphamide therapy). Subsequent evaluations should be obtained at a cumulative dose of doxorubicin of at least 400 mg/m^2 and periodically thereafter during the course of therapy. Children are at increased risk for developing delayed cardiotoxicity following doxorubicin administration and therefore a follow-up cardiac evaluation is recommended periodically to monitor for this delayed cardiotoxicity.

In adults, a 10% decline in LVEF to below the lower limit of normal or an absolute LVEF of 45%, or a 20% decline in LVEF at any level is indicative of deterioration in cardiac function. In children, deterioration in cardiac function during or after the completion of therapy with doxorubicin is indicated by a drop in fractional shortening (FS) by an absolute value of ≥10 percentile units or below 29%, and a decline in LVEF of 10 percentile units or an LVEF below 55%. In general, if test results indicate deterioration in cardiac function associated with doxorubicin, the benefit of continued therapy should be carefully evaluated against the risk of producing irreversible cardiac damage.

WARNINGS: *(cont'd)*

Acute life-threatening arrhythmias have been reported to occur during or within a few hours after doxorubicin administration.

There is a high incidence of bone marrow depression, primarily of leukocytes, requiring careful hematologic monitoring. With the recommended dose schedule, leukopenia is usually transient, reaching its nadir 10-14 days after treatment with recovery usually occurring by the 21st day. White blood cell counts as low as 1000 $mm/^3$ are to be expected during treatment with appropriate doses of doxorubicin. Red blood cell and platelet levels should also be monitored since they may be depressed. Hematologic toxicity may require dose reduction or suspension or delay of doxorubicin therapy. Persistent severe myelosuppression may result in superinfection or hemorrhage.

Doxorubicin may potentiate the toxicity of other anticancer therapies. Exacerbation of cyclophosphamide-induced hemorrhagic cystitis and enhancement of the hepatotoxicity of 6-mercaptopurine have been reported. Radiation-induced toxicity to the myocardium, mucosae, skin and liver have been reported to be increased by the administration of doxorubicin.

Since metabolism and excretion of doxorubicin occurs predominantly by the hepatobiliary route, toxicity to recommended doses of doxorubicin can be enhanced by hepatic impairment; therefore, prior to the individual dosing, evaluation of hepatic function is recommended using conventional laboratory tests such as SGOT, SGPT, alkaline phosphatase and bilirubin. (See DOSAGE AND ADMINISTRATION.)

Necrotizing colitis manifested by typhlitis (cecal inflammation), bloody stools and severe and sometimes fatal infections have been associated with a combination of doxorubicin given by IV push daily for 3 days and cytarabine given by continuous infusion daily for 7 or more days.

On intravenous administration of doxorubicin, extravasation may occur with or without an accompanying stinging or burning sensation, even if blood returns well on aspiration of the infusion needle (See DOSAGE AND ADMINISTRATION.) If any signs or symptoms of extravasation have occurred, the injection or infusion should be immediately terminated and restarted in another vein.

Pregnancy Category D—Safe use of doxorubicin in pregnancy has not been established. Doxorubicin is embryotoxic and teratogenic in rats and embryotoxic and abortifacient in rabbits. There are no adequate and well-controlled studies in pregnant women. If doxorubicin is to be used during pregnancy, or if the patient becomes pregnant during therapy, the patient should be apprised of the potential hazard to the fetus. Women of childbearing age should be advised to avoid becoming pregnant.

PRECAUTIONS:

General: Doxorubicin is not an antimicrobial agent.

Information for the Patient: Doxorubicin HCl impart a red coloration to the urine for 1 to 2 days after administration, and patients should be advised to expect this during active therapy.

Laboratory Tests: Initial treatment with doxorubicin requires observation of the patient and periodic monitoring of complete blood counts, hepatic function tests, and radionuclide left ventricular ejection fraction (See WARNINGS.)

Like other cytotoxic drugs, doxorubicin may induce "tumor lysis syndrome" and hyperuricemia in patients with rapidly growing tumors. Appropriate supportive and pharmacologic measures may prevent or alleviate this complication.

Carcinogenesis, Mutagenesis, and Impairment of Fertility: Formal long- term carcinogenicity studies have not been conducted with doxorubicin. Doxorubicin and related compounds have been shown to have mutagenic and carcinogenic properties when tested in experimental models (including bacterial systems, mammalian cells in culture, and female Sprague-Dawley rats).

The possible adverse effect on fertility in males and females in humans or experimental animals have not been adequately evaluated. Testicular atrophy was observed in rats and dogs.

A variant of chemotherapy-related acute non-lymphocytic leukemia has been reported to occur infrequently a few years after multiple drug treatment of some neoplasms, which sometimes included doxorubicin. The exact role of doxorubicin has not been elucidated.

Pregnancy Category D: (See WARNINGS.)

Nursing Mothers: Because of the potential for serious adverse reactions in nursing infants from doxorubicin, mothers should be advised to discontinue nursing during doxorubicin therapy.

DRUG INTERACTIONS:

Literature contain the following drug interactions with doxorubicin in humans: cyclosporine (Sandimmune) may induce coma and/or seizures; phenobarbital increases the elimination of doxorubicin; phenytoin levels may be decreased by doxorubicin; streptozocin (Zanosar) may inhibit the hepatic metabolism; and administration of live vaccines to immunosuppressed patients, including those undergoing cytotoxic chemotherapy, may be hazardous. Information on other potential drug interactions may be found in the literature.

ADVERSE REACTIONS:

Dose-limiting toxicities of therapy are myelosuppression and cardiotoxicity. Other reactions reported are:

Cardiotoxicity: (See WARNINGS.)

Cutaneous: Reversible complete alopecia occurs in most cases. Hyperpigmentation of nailbeds and dermal crease, primarily in children, and onycholysis have been reported in a few cases. Recall of skin reaction due to prior radiotherapy has occurred with doxorubicin administration.

Gastrointestinal: Acute nausea and vomiting occurs frequently and may be severe. This may be alleviated by antiemetic therapy. Mucositis (stomatitis and esophagitis) may occur 5 to 10 days after administration. The effect may be severe leading to ulceration and represents a site of origin for severe infections. The dosage regimen consisting of administration of doxorubicin on three successive days results in greater incidence and severity of mucositis. Ulceration and necrosis of the colon, especially the cecum, may occur leading to bleeding or severe infections which can be fatal. This reaction has been reported in patients with acute non-lymphocytic leukemia treated with a 3-day course of doxorubicin combined with cytarabine. Anorexia and diarrhea have been occasionally reported.

Vascular: Phlebosclerosis has been reported especially when small veins are used or a single vein is used for repeated administration. Facial flushing may occur if the injection is given too rapidly.

Local: Severe cellulitis, vesication and tissue necrosis will occur if extravasation of doxorubicin occurs during administration. Erythematous streaking along the vein proximal to the site of injection had been reported (See DOSAGE AND ADMINISTRATION.)

Hematologic: The occurrence of secondary acute myeloid leukemia with or without a preleukemic phase has been reported rarely in patients concurrently treated with doxorubicin in association with DNA-damaging antineoplastic agents. Such cases could have a short (1-3 years) latency period.

ADVERSE REACTIONS: *(cont'd)*

Hypersensitivity: Fever, chills and urticaria have been reported occasionally. Anaphylaxis may occur. A case of apparent cross sensitivity to lincomycin has been reported.

Other: Conjunctivitis and lacrimation occur rarely.

OVERDOSAGE:

Acute overdosage with doxorubicin enhances the toxic effect of mucositis, leukopenia and thrombocytopenia. Treatment of acute overdosage consists of treatment of the severely myelosuppressed patient with hospitalization, antimicrobials, platelet transfusions and symptomatic treatment of mucositis. Use of hemopoietic growth factor (G-CSF, GM-CSF) may be considered.

The 150 mg Doxorubicin HCl and the 100 ml (2 mg/ml) Doxorubicin HCl vials are packaged as multiple dose vials and caution should be exercised to prevent inadvertent overdosage.

Cumulative dosage with doxorubicin increases the risk of cardiomyopathy and resultant congestive heart failure (See WARNINGS). Treatment consists of vigorous management of congestive heart failure with digitalis preparations, diuretics, and after-load reducers such as ACE inhibitors.

DOSAGE AND ADMINISTRATION:

Care in the administration of doxorubicin HCl will reduce the chance of perivenous infiltration (See WARNINGS.) It may also decrease the chance of local reactions such as urticaria and erythematous streaking. On intravenous administration of doxorubicin, extravasation may occur with or without an accompanying burning or stinging sensation, even if blood returns well on aspiration of the infusion needle. If any signs or symptoms of extravasation have occurred, the injection or infusion should be immediately terminated and restarted in another vein. If extravasation is suspected, intermittent application of ice to the site for 15 min. q.i.d. x 3 days may be useful. The benefit of local administration of drugs has not been clearly established. Because of the progressive nature of extravasation reactions, close observation and plastic surgery consultation is recommended. Blistering, ulceration, and/or persistent pain are indications for wide excision surgery, followed by split-thickness skin grafting.[1]

The most commonly used dose schedule when used as a single agent is 60 to 75 mg/m^2 as a single intravenous injection administered at 21-day intervals. The lower dosage should be given to patients with inadequate marrow reserves due to old age, or prior therapy, or neoplastic marrow infiltration. Doxorubicin HCl have been used concurrently with other approved chemotherapeutic agents. Evidence is available that in some types of neoplastic disease combination chemotherapy is superior to single agents. The benefits and risks of such therapy continue to be elucidated. When used in combination with other chemotherapy drugs, the most commonly used dosage of doxorubicin is 40 to 60 mg/m^2 given as a single intravenous injection every 21 to 28 days. Doxorubicin dosage must be reduced in case of hyperbilirubinemia as follows (TABLE 1):

TABLE 1 Doxorubicin Hydrochloride, Dosage and Administration

Plasma bilirubin concentration (mg/dl)	Dosage reduction (%)
1.2 - 3.0	50
3.1 - 5.0	75

Reconstitution Directions: Doxorubicin HCl 10 mg, 20 mg, 50 mg, and 150 mg vials should be reconstituted with 5 ml, 10 ml, 25 ml, and 75 ml, respectively, of Sodium Chloride Injection, USP (0.9%), to give a final concentration of 2 mg/ml of doxorubicin hydrochloride. An appropriate volume of air should be withdrawn from the vial during reconstitution to avoid excessive pressure buildup. Bacteriostatic diluents are not recommended.

After adding the diluent, the vial should be shaken and the contents allowed to dissolve. The reconstituted solution is stable for 7 days at room temperature and under normal room light (100 foot-candles) and 15 days under refrigeration (2°-8°C). It should be protected from exposure to sunlight. Discard any of the unused solution from the 10 mg, 20 mg, and 50 mg single dose vials. Unused solutions of the multiple dose vial remaining beyond the recommended storage times should be discarded.

It is recommended that doxorubicin HCl be slowly administered into the tubing of a freely running intravenous infusion of Sodium Chloride Injection, USP, or 5% Dextrose Injection, USP. The tubing should be attached to a Butterfly needle inserted preferably into a large vein. If possible, avoid veins over joints or in extremities with compromised venous or lymphatic drainage. The rate of administration is dependent on the size of the vein and the dosage. However, the dose should be administered in not less than 3 to 5 minutes. Local erythematous streaking along the vein as well as facial flushing may be indicative of too rapid an administration. A burning or stinging sensation may be indicative of perivenous infiltration and the infusion should be immediately terminated and restarted in another vein. Perivenous infiltration may occur painlessly.

Doxorubicin should not be mixed with heparin or fluorouracil since it has been reported that these drugs are incompatible to the extent that a precipitate may form. Until specific compatibility data are available, it is not recommended that doxorubicin be mixed with other drugs.

Parenteral drug products should be inspected visually for particulate matter and discoloration prior to administration, whenever solution and container permit.

Handling and Disposal: Skin reactions associated with doxorubicin have been reported. Skin accidentally exposed to doxorubicin should be rinsed copiously with soap and warm water, and if the eyes are involved, standard irrigation techniques should be used immediately. The use of goggles, gloves, and protective gowns is recommended during preparation and administration of the drug.

Procedures for proper handling and disposal of anti-cancer drugs should be considered. Several guidelines on this subject have been published.[2-8] There is no general agreement that all the procedures recommended in the guidelines are necessary or appropriate.

REFERENCES:

1. Rudolph R., Larson DL: Etiology and Treatment of Chemotherapeutic Agent Extravasation Injuries: A Review J. Clin Oncol 5:1116-1126, 1987. **2.** Recommendations for the Safe Handling of Parenteral Antineoplastic Drugs. NIH Publication No. 83-2621. For sale by the Superintendent of Documents, US Government Printing Office, Washington, DC 20402. **3.** AMA Council Report, Guidelines for Handling Parenteral Antineoplastics, JAMA. 1985; 253 (11): 1590-1592. **4.** National Study Commission on Cytotoxic Exposure- Recommendations for Handling Cytotoxic Agents. Available from Louis P. Jeffrey, Sc.D., Chairman, National Study Commission on Cytotoxic Exposure, Massachusetts College of Pharmacy and Allied Health Sciences, 179 Longwood Avenue, Boston, Massachusetts 02115. **5.** Clinical Oncological Society of. Australia. Guidelines and Recommendations for Safe Handling of Antineoplastic Agents. Med J Australia. 1983; 1:426-428. **6.** Jones RB, et al: Safe Handling of Chemotherapeutic Agents: A Report from the Mount Sinai Medical Center. Ca - A Cancer Journal for Clinicians. 1983; (Sept/Oct) 258-263. **7.** American Society of Hospital Pharmacists Technical Assistance Bulletin on Handling Cytotoxic and Hazardous Drugs. Am J Hosp Pharm. 1990; 47:1033-1049. **8.** OSHA Work-Practice Guidelines for Personnel Dealing with Cytotoxic (Antineoplastic) Drugs. Am J Hosp Pharm. 1986; 43:1193-1204.

HOW SUPPLIED:

Doxorubicin hydrochloride for injection, USP) is available as follows:

10 mg single dose vial, 10 vial packs

20 mg single dose vial, 10 vial packs

HOW SUPPLIED: *(cont'd)*

50 mg single dose vial, single packs

Store at controlled room temperature, 15° to 30°C (59° to 86°F). Protect from light. Retain in carton until time of use. Contains no preservative. Discard unused portion.

MULTIDOSE VIAL: 150 mg multidose vial, single packs

Store at controlled room temperature, 15° to 30°C (59° to 86°F). Protect from light. Retain in carton until time of use.

RECONSTITUTED SOLUTION STABILITY: After adding the diluent, the vial should be shaken and the contents allowed to dissolve. The reconstituted solution is stable for 7 days at room temperature and under normal room light (100 foot-candles) and 15 days under refrigeration (2° to 8°C). It should be protected from exposure to sunlight. Discard any unused solution from the 10 mg, 20 mg and 50 mg single dose vials. Unused solutions of the multiple dose vial remaining beyond the recommended storage times should be discarded.

Doxorubicin hydrochloride injection

SINGLE DOSE VIALS:

Sterile single use only, contains no preservative.

10 mg vial, 2 mg/ml, 5 ml, 10 vial packs

20 mg vial, 2 mg/ml, 10 ml, 10 vial packs

50 mg vial, 2 mg/ml, 25 ml, single vial packs

75 mg vial, 2 mg/ml, 37.5 ml, single vial packs

Store under refrigeration, 2° to 8°C (36° to 46°F). Protect from light. Retain in carton until time of use. Discard unused portion.

MULTIDOSE VIAL:

Sterile multidose vial, contains no preservative.

200 mg, 2 mg/ml, 100 ml, multidose vial, single vial packs

Store under refrigeration, 2° to 8°C (36° to 46°F). Protect from light. Retain in carton until contents are used.

HOW SUPPLIED - RATED THERAPEUTICALLY EQUIVALENT:

Injection, Lyphl-Soln - Intravenous - 10 mg/vial

1's	$42.06	RUBEX, Immunex	58406-0511-01
5 ml	**$48.31**	**ADRIAMYCIN-PFS, Pharmacia & Upjohn**	**00013-1136-91**
10 mg	$207.25	Doxorubicin Hcl, Astra USA	00186-1530-13
10mg x 10	**$46.00**	**ADRIAMYCIN RDF 10, Pharmacia & Upjohn**	**00013-1086-91**

Injection, Lyphl-Soln - Intravenous - 20 mg/vial

1's	**$92.00**	**ADRIAMYCIN RDF, Pharmacia & Upjohn**	**00013-1096-94**
10 ml	**$96.63**	**ADRIAMYCIN-PFS, Pharmacia & Upjohn**	**00013-1146-91**
20 mg	$200.00	Doxorubicin Hcl, Astra USA	00186-1575-12
20 mg x 10	**$92.00**	**ADRIAMYCIN RDF 20, Pharmacia & Upjohn**	**00013-1096-91**

Injection, Lyphl-Soln - Intravenous - 50 mg/vial

1's	$189.26	RUBEX, Immunex	58406-0512-01
25 ml	**$241.56**	**ADRIAMYCIN-PFS, Pharmacia & Upjohn**	**00013-1156-79**
50 mg	$103.00	Doxorubicin Hcl, Astra USA	00186-1531-01
50 mg	$189.26	RUBEX 50, Mead Johnson	00015-3352-22
50 mg	**$230.00**	**ADRIAMYCIN RDF 50, Pharmacia & Upjohn**	**00013-1106-79**

Injection, Lyphl-Soln - Intravenous - 75 mg/vial

37.5 ml	**$362.35**	**ADRIAMYCIN-PFS, Pharmacia & Upjohn**	**00013-1176-87**

Injection, Solution - Intravenous - 2 mg/ml

5 ml	$44.47	DOXORUBICIN HCL, Gensia Labs	00703-5043-03
10 ml	**$96.63**	**ADRIAMYCIN-PFS, Pharmacia & Upjohn**	**00013-1146-94**
25 ml	$295.75	DOXORUBICIN HCL, Gensia Labs	00703-5046-01
100 ml	$871.70	DOXORUBICIN HCL, Gensia Labs	00703-5040-01

Injection, Solution - Intravenous - 200 mg

100 ml	**$946.94**	**ADRIAMYCIN PFS, Pharmacia & Upjohn**	**00013-1166-83**

HOW SUPPLIED - NOT RATED EQUIVALENT:

Injection, Lyphl-Soln - Intravenous - 150 mg

150 mg x 1	**$676.19**	**ADRIAMYCIN RDF, Pharmacia & Upjohn**	**00013-1116-83**

Injection, Solution - Intravenous - 100 mg/vial

1's	$378.52	RUBEX, Immunex	58406-0513-01
100 mg	$378.52	RUBEX 100, Mead Johnson	00015-3353-22

DOXORUBICIN, LIPOSOMAL *(003276)*

CATEGORIES: AIDS Related Complex; Antineoplastics; Cytotoxic Agents; HIV Infection; Kaposi's Sarcoma; Oncologic Drugs; Orphan Drugs; Recombinant DNA Origin; FDA Approved 1995 Nov

BRAND NAMES: *ADM*; *A.D. Mycin*; *Adriablastin*; *Adriablastina*; *Adriablastina R.D.*; *Adriacin* (Japan); *Adriamycin* (Australia, England); *Adriamycin P.F.S.*; *Adriamycin PFS* (Canada); *Adriamycin RD*; *Adriamycin R.D.F.*; *Adriamycin RDF* (Canada); *Adriblastin* (Germany); *Adriblastine* (France); *Adriblastina*; *Adrim*; *Adrubicin*; **Doxil**; *Doxolem* (Mexico); *Doxorubin*; *Doxorubicin*; *Doxorubicin Meiji*; *Farmablastina*; *Pallagicin*
(International brand names outside U.S. in italics)

WARNING:
Experience with doxorubicin HCl liposome injection at high cumulative doses is too limited to have established its effect on the myocardium. It should therefore be assumed that doxorubicin will have myocardial toxicity similar to conventional formulations of doxorubicin HCl. With these formulations of doxorubicin HCl, serious irreversible myocardial toxicity leading to congestive heart failure often unresponsive to cardiac supportive therapy may be encountered as the total dosage of doxorubicin HCl approaches 550 mg/m^2. Prior use of other anthracyclines or anthracenediones will reduce the total dose of doxorubicin HCl that can be given without cardiac toxicity. Cardiac toxicity also may occur at lower cumulative doses in patients with prior mediastinal irradiation or who are receiving concurrent cyclophosphamide therapy. Doxorubicin HCl should be administered to patients with a history of cardiovascular disease only when the benefit outweighs the risk to the patient.
Acute infusion-associated reactions (flushing, shortness of breath, facial swelling, headache, chills, back pain, tightness in the chest or throat, and/or hypotension) have occurred in about 7% of patients treated with doxorubicin HCl. In most patients, these reactions resolve over the course of several hours to a day once the infusion is terminated. In some patients, the reaction resolves by slowing the infusion rate. (See WARNINGS, Infusion Reactions.)
Severe myelosuppression may occur.
Dosage should be reduced in patients with impaired hepatic function. (See DOSAGE AND ADMINISTRATION.)
Doxorubicin HCl should be administered only under the supervision of a physician who is experienced in the use of cancer chemotherapeutic agents.

DESCRIPTION:

Doxorubicin hydrochloride encapsulated in Stealth liposomes for intravenous administration.

Note: Liposomal encapsulation can substantially affect a drug's functional properties relative to those of the unencapsulated drug.

In addition, different liposomal drug products may vary from one another in the chemical composition and physical form of the liposomes. Such differences can substantially affect the functional properties of liposomal drug products.

Doxorubicin is a cytotoxic anthracycline antibiotic isolated from *Streptomyces peucetius* var. *caesius*.

Doxorubicin HCl, which is the established name for (8*S*,10*S*)-10-[(3-amino-2, 3, 6-trideoxy-α-L-*lyxo*-hexopyranosyl)oxy]-8-glycolyl-7, 8, 9, 10-tetrahydro-6, 8, 11-trihydroxy-1-methoxy-5, 12-naphthacenedione hydrochloride.

The molecular formula of the drug is $C_{27}H_{29}NO_{11}\cdot HCl$; its molecular weight is 579.99.

Doxorubicin HCl is provided as a sterile, translucent, red liposomal dispersion in 10-ml glass, single use vials. Each vial contains 20 mg doxorubicin HCl at a concentration of 2 mg/mL and a pH of 6.5. The Stealth liposome carriers are composed of N-(carbamoyl-methoxypolyethylene glycol 2000)-1,2-distearoyl-sn-glycero-3-phosphoethanolamine sodium salt (MPEG-DSPE), 3.19 mg/ml; fully hydrogenated soy phosphatidylcholine (HSPC), 9.58 mg/ml; and cholesterol, 3.19 mg/ml. Each ml also contains ammonium sulfate, approximately 2 mg; histidine as a buffer; hydrochloric acid and/or sodium hydroxide for pH control; and sucrose to maintain isotonicity. Greater than 90% of the drug is encapsulated in the Stealth liposomes.

CLINICAL PHARMACOLOGY:

MECHANISM OF ACTION

The active ingredient of doxorubicin HCl liposome injection is doxorubicin HCl. The mechanism of action of doxorubicin HCl is thought to be related to its ability to bind DNA and inhibit nucleic acid synthesis. Cell structure studies have demonstrated rapid cell penetration and perinuclear chromatin binding, rapid inhibition of mitotic activity and nucleic acid synthesis, and induction of mutagenesis and chromosomal aberrations.

Doxorubicin HCl is encapsulated in long-circulating Stealth liposomes. Liposomes are microscopic vesicles composed of a phospholipid bilayer that are capable of encapsulating active drugs. The Stealth liposomes of doxorubicin HCl liposome are formulated with surface-bound methoxypolyethylene glycol (MPEG), a process often referred to as pegylation, to protect liposomes from detection by the mononuclear phagocyte system (MPS) and to increase blood circulation time.

Stealth liposomes have a half-life of approximately 55 hours in humans. They are stable in blood, and direct measurement of liposomal doxorubicin shows that at least 90% of the drug (the assay used cannot quantify less than 5-10% free doxorubicin) remains liposome-encapsulated during circulation.

It is hypothesized that because of their small size (ca. 100 nm) and persistence in the circulation the pegylated doxorubicin HCl liposomes are able to penetrate the altered and often compromised vasculature of tumors. This hypothesis is supported by studies using colloidal gold-containing Stealth liposomes, which can be visualized microscopically. Evidence of penetration of Stealth liposomes from blood vessels and their entry and accumulation in tumors has been seen in mice with C-26 colon carcinoma tumors and in transgenic mice with Kaposi's sarcoma-like lesions. Once the Stealth liposomes distribute to the tissue compartment, the encapsulated doxorubicin HCl becomes available. The exact mechanism of release is not understood.

PHARMACOKINETICS

The plasma pharmacokinetics of doxorubicin HCl liposome were evaluated in 42 patients with AIDS-related Kaposi's sarcoma (KS) who received single doses of 10 or 20 mg/m^2 administered by a 30-minute infusion. Twenty-three of these patients received single doses of both 10 and 20 mg/m^2 with a 3-week wash-out period between doses. The pharmacokinetic parameter values of doxorubicin HCl liposome, given for total doxorubicin (most liposomally bound), are presented in TABLE 1.

TABLE 1 Pharmacokinetic Parameters of Doxorubicin in AIDS Patients with Kaposi's Sarcoma

Parameter	Dose 10mg/m^2	10mg/m^2
Peak Plasma Concentration (mcg/mL)	4.12 ± 0.215	8.34 ± 0.49
Plasma Clearance (L/h/m^2)	0.056 ± 0.01	0.041 ± 0.004
Steady-State Volume of Distribution (L/m^2)	2.83 ± 0.145	2.72 ± 0.120
AUC (mcg/mL·h)	277 ± 32.9	590 ± 58.7
First Phase ([lgr]$_1$) Half-Life (h)	4.7 ± 1.1	5.2 ± 1.4
Second Phase ([lgr]$_2$) Half-Life (h)	52.3 ± 5.6	55.0 ± 4.8

n=23
Mean ± Standard Error

Doxorubicin displayed linear pharmacokinetics. Disposition occurred in two phases after doxorubicin HCl liposome administration, with a relatively short first phase (-5 hours) and a prolonged second phase (-55 hours) that accounted for the majority of the area under the curve (AUC).

Distribution: In contrast to the pharmacokinetics of doxorubicin, which display a large volume of distribution ranging from 700 to 1100 L/m^2, the steady state volume of distribution of doxorubicin HCl liposome indicated that doxorubicin HCl liposome was confined mostly to the vascular fluid volume. Plasma protein binding of doxorubicin HCl liposome has not been determined; however, the plasma protein binding of doxorubicin is approximately 70%.

Metabolism: Doxorubicinol, the major metabolite of doxorubicin, was detected at very low levels (range: 0.8 to 26.2 ng/ml) in the plasma of patients who received 10 or 20 mg/m^2 doxorubicin HCl liposome.

Excretion: The plasma clearance of doxorubicin HCl liposome was slow, with a mean clearance value of 0.041 L/h/m^{2}at a dose of 20 mg/m^2. This is in contrast to doxorubicin, which displays a plasma clearance value ranging from 24 to 35 L/h/m^2.

CLINICAL PHARMACOLOGY: *(cont'd)*

Because of its slower clearance, the AUC of doxorubicin HCl liposome, primarily representing the circulation of liposome-encapsulated doxorubicin, is approximately two to three orders of magnitude larger than the AUC for a similar dose of conventional doxorubicin HCl as reported in the literature.

Special Populations: The pharmacokinetics of doxorubicin HCl liposome have not been separately evaluated in women, in members of different ethnic groups, or in individuals with renal or hepatic insufficiency.

Drug-Drug Interactions: Although the patient population for the current indication is on various antiviral medications, the drug-drug interactions between doxorubicin HCl liposome and the antiviral drugs have not been evaluated.

TISSUE DISTRIBUTION

Kaposi's sarcoma lesions and normal skin biopsies were obtained at 48 and 96 hours postinfusion of 20 mg/m^2 doxorubicin HCl liposome in 11 patients. The concentration of doxorubicin HCl liposome in KS lesions was a median of 19 (range, 3-53) times higher than in normal skin at 48 hours posttreatment; however, this was not corrected for likely differences in blood content between KS lesions and normal skin. The corrected ratio may lie between 1 and 22 times. Thus, higher concentrations of doxorubicin HCl liposome are delivered to KS lesions than to normal skin.

CLINICAL STUDIES:

AIDS-RELATED KAPOSI'S SARCOMA

Doxorubicin HCl liposome was studied in an open-label, single-arm, multicenter study utilizing doxorubicin HCl liposome at 20 mg/m^2 by intravenous infusion every three weeks generally until progression or intolerance occurred. In an interim analysis, the treatment history of 383 patients were reviewed, and a cohort of 77 patients was retrospectively identified as having disease progression on prior systemic combination chemotherapy (at least 2 cycles of a regimen containing at least two of three treatments: bleomycin, vincristine or vinblastine, or doxorubicin) or as being intolerant to such therapy. Forty-nine of the 77 (64%) patients had received prior doxorubicin HCl.

These 77 patients were predominantly white, homosexual males with a median CD4 count of 10 cells/mm3. Their age ranged from 24 to 54 years, with a mean age of 38 years. Using the ACTG staging criteria,1 78% of the patients were at poor risk for tumor burden, 96% at poor risk for immune system, and 58% at poor risk for systemic illness at baseline. Their mean Karnofsky status score was 74%. All 77 patients had cutaneous or subcutaneous lesions, 40% also had oral lesions, 26% pulmonary lesions, and 14% of patients had lesions of the stomach/intestine. The majority of these patients had disease progression on prior systemic combination chemotherapy.

The median time on study for these 77 patients was 155 days and ranged from 1 to 456 days. The median cumulative dose was 154 mg/m^2 and ranged from 20 to 620 mg/m^2.

Two analyses of tumor response were used to evaluate the effectiveness of doxorubicin HCl liposome: one analysis based on investigator assessment of changes in lesions over the entire body, and one analysis based on changes in indicator lesions.

INVESTIGATOR ASSESSMENT

Investigator response was based on modified ACTG criteria.[1] Partial response was defined as no new lesions, sites of disease, or worsening edema; flattening of $\geq$ 50% of previously raised lesions or area of indicator lesions decreasing by $\geq$ 50%; and response lasting at least 21 days with no prior progression.

INDICATOR LESION ASSESSMENT

A retrospectively defined analysis was conducted based on assessment of the response of up to five prospectively identified representative indicator lesions. A partial response was defined as flattening of $\geq$ 50% of previously raised indicator lesions, or > 50% decrease in the area of indicator lesions and lasting at least 21 days with no prior progression.

Only patients with adequate documentation of baseline status and follow-up assessments were considered evaluable for response. Patients who received concomitant KS treatment during study, who completed local radiotherapy to sites encompassing one or more of the indicator lesions within two months of study entry, who had less than four indicator lesions, or who had less than three raised indicator lesions at baseline (the latter applies solely to indicator lesion assessment) were considered nonevaluable for response. Of the 77 patients who had disease progression on prior systemic combination chemotherapy or who were intolerant to such therapy, 34 were evaluable for investigator assessment and 42 were evaluable for indicator lesion assessment. Response is summarized in TABLE 2.

TABLE 2 Response in Refractory [a]AIDS-KS

Investigator Assessment	All Evaluable Patients (n=34)	Evaluable Patients Who Received Prior Doxorubicin (n=20)
Response[b]		
Partial(PR)	27%	30%
Stable	29%	40%
Progression	44%	30%
Duration of PR (days)		
Median	73	89
Range	42+ - 210+	42+ - 210+
Time to PR (days)		
Median	43	53
Range	15 - 133	15 - 109
Indicator Lesion Assessment	**All Evaluable Patients (n=42)**	**Evaluable Patients Who Received Prior Doxorubicin (n=23)**
Response[b]		
Partial (PR)	48%	52%
Stable	26%	30%
Progression	26%	17%
Duration of PR (days)		
Median	71	79
Range	15 - 109	15 - 109

a Patients with disease that progressed on prior combination chemotherapy or who were intolerant to such therapy.
b There were no complete responses in this population.

CLINICAL BENEFIT

Clinical benefit (*e.g.,* decreased pain, disfigurement, pulmonary or gastrointestinal symptoms) was not well evaluated in the open studies carried out to date. A controlled trial with double-blinded assessment of clinical endpoints is ongoing.

INDICATIONS AND USAGE:

Doxorubicin HCl liposome injection is indicated for the treatment of AIDS-related Kaposi's sarcoma in patients with disease that has progressed on prior combination chemotherapy or in patients who are intolerant to such therapy.

CONTRAINDICATIONS:

Doxorubicin HCl liposome injection is contraindicated in patients who have a history of hypersensitivity reactions to a conventional formulation of doxorubicin HCl or the components of doxorubicin HCl liposome.

WARNINGS:

CARDIAC TOXICITY

Experience with doxorubicin HCl liposome injection is limited in evaluating cardiac risk. Therefore, warnings related to the use of conventional formulation doxorubicin HCl should be observed.

Special attention must be given to the cardiac toxicity exhibited by doxorubicin HCl. Although uncommon, acute left ventricular failure has occurred, particularly in patients who have received total dosage of the drug exceeding the currently recommended limit of 550 mg/m^2. This limit appears to be lower (400 mg/m^2) in patients who received radiotherapy to the mediastinal area or concomitant therapy with other potentially cardiotoxic agents such as cyclophosphamide.

Caution should be observed in patients who have received other anthracyclines. The total dose of doxorubicin HCl administered to the individual patient should also take into account any previous or concomitant therapy with related compounds such as daunorubicin. Congestive heart failure and/or cardiomyopathy may be encountered after discontinuation of therapy. Patients with a history of cardiovascular disease should be administered doxorubicin HCl liposome only when the potential benefit of treatment outweighs the risk.

The long-term cardiac effects of doxorubicin HCl liposome in patients relative to the conventional formulation of doxorubicin HCl have not been adequately evaluated.

Cardiac function should be carefully monitored in patients treated with doxorubicin HCl liposome. The most definitive test for anthracycline myocardial injury is endomyocardial biopsy. Other methods such as echocardiography or gated radionuclide scans have been used to monitor cardiac function during anthracycline therapy. Any of these methods should be employed to monitor potential cardiac toxicity during doxorubicin HCl liposome therapy. If these test results indicate possible cardiac injury associated with doxorubicin HCl liposome therapy, the benefit of continued therapy must be carefully weighed against the risk of myocardial injury. (See ADVERSE REACTIONS, Cardiac Events.)

MYELOSUPPRESSION

The majority of experience with doxorubicin HCl liposome has been in AIDS-KS patients who present with baseline myelosuppression due to such factors as their HIV disease or numerous concomitant medications. In this population, myelosuppression appears to be the dose-limiting adverse event. Leukopenia is the most common adverse event (about 60%) experienced in this population; anemia (about 20%) and thrombocytopenia (about 10%) can also be expected.

Because of the potential for bone marrow suppression, careful hematologic monitoring is required during use of doxorubicin HCl liposome, including white blood cell and platelet counts and Hgb/Hct. With the recommended dosage schedule, leukopenia is usually transient. Hematologic toxicity may require dose reduction or suspension or delay of doxorubicin HCl liposome therapy. Persistent severe myelosuppression may result in superinfection or hemorrhage.

Doxorubicin HCl liposome may potentiate the toxicity of other anticancer therapies. In particular, hematologic toxicity may be more severe when doxorubicin HCl liposome is administered in combination with other agents that cause bone marrow suppression. Patients treated with doxorubicin HCl liposome may require G-CSF (or GM-CSF) to support their blood counts. (See ADVERSE REACTIONS, Hematologic.)

INFUSION REACTIONS

Acute infusion-associated reactions characterized by flushing, shortness of breath, facial swelling, headache, chills, back pain, tightness in the chest and throat, and/or hypotension have occurred in approximately 6.8% of patients treated with doxorubicin HCl liposome. The reaction appears to occur with the first infusion and does not appear to occur with later infusions if not present initially. In most patients, these reactions resolve over the course of several hours to a day once the infusion is terminated. In some patients, the reaction resolves by slowing the rate of infusion. Similar reactions have not been reported with conventional doxorubicin and they presumably represent a reaction to the doxorubicin HCl liposome liposomes or one of its surface components.

Many patients were able to tolerate further infusions without complications, however, six patients were terminated from doxorubicin HCl liposome therapy because of an infusion reaction.

PALMAR-PLANTAR ERYTHRODYSESTHESIA

Among 705 patients with AIDS-related Kaposi's sarcoma treated with doxorubicin HCl liposome, 24 (3.4%) developed palmar-plantar skin eruptions characterized by swelling, pain, erythema and, for some patients, desquamation of the skin on the hands and the feet (palmar-plantar erythrodysesthesia). The syndrome was generally seen after six or more weeks of treatment but may occur earlier. The incidence of this reaction may be higher when doxorubicin HCl liposome is administered at doses that are higher or at intervals that are shorter than those recommended. In most patients, the reaction is mild and resolves in one to two weeks so that prolonged delay of therapy need not occur (see DOSAGE AND ADMINISTRATION). The reaction can be severe and debilitating in some patients, however, and may require discontinuation of treatment.

PREGNANCY CATEGORY D

Doxorubicin HCl liposome can cause fetal harm when administered to a pregnant woman. Doxorubicin HCl liposome is embryotoxic at doses of 1 mg/kg/day (about 1/3 the recommended human dose on a mg/m2 basis) in rats. Doxorubicin HCl liposome is embryotoxic and abortifacient at 0.5 mg/kg/day (about 1/4 the recommended human dose on a mg/m2 basis) in rabbits. Embryotoxicity was characterized by increased embryo-fetal deaths and reduced live litter sizes.

There are no adequate and well-controlled studies in pregnant women. If doxorubicin HCl liposome is to be used during pregnancy, or if the patient becomes pregnant during therapy, the patient should be apprised of the potential hazard to the fetus. Women of childbearing potential should be advised to avoid pregnancy.

TOXICITY POTENTIATION

The doxorubicin in doxorubicin HCl liposome may potentiate the toxicity of other anticancer therapies. Exacerbation of cyclophosphamide-induced hemorrhagic cystitis and enhancement of the hepatotoxicity of 6-mercaptopurine have been reported with the conventional formulation of doxorubicin HCl. Radiation-induced toxicity to the myocardium, mucosae, skin and liver have been reported to be increased by the administration of doxorubicin HCl.

INJECTION SITE EFFECTS

Doxorubicin HCl liposome should be considered an irritant and precautions should be taken to avoid extravasation. On intravenous administration of doxorubicin HCl liposome, extravasation may occur with or without an accompanying stinging or burning sensation and even if blood returns well on aspiration of the infusion needle (see DOSAGE AND ADMINISTRATION). If any signs or symptoms of extravasation have occurred, the infusion should be immediately terminated and restarted in another vein. The application of ice over the site

WARNINGS: *(cont'd)*

of extravasation for approximately 30 minutes may be helpful in alleviating the local reaction. **Doxorubicin HCl liposome must not be given by the intramuscular or subcutaneous route.**

In studies with rabbits, lesions that were induced by subcutaneous injection of doxorubicin HCl liposome were minor and reversible compared to more severe and irreversible lesions and tissue necrosis that were induced after subcutaneous injection of conventional doxorubicin HCl.

HEPATIC IMPAIRMENT

The pharmacokinetics of doxorubicin HCl liposome have not been studied in patients with hepatic impairment. Doxorubicin is known to be eliminated in large part by the liver. Thus doxorubicin HCl liposome dosage should be reduced in patients with impaired hepatic function. (See DOSAGE AND ADMINISTRATION.) Prior to doxorubicin HCl liposome administration, evaluation of hepatic function is recommended using conventional clinical laboratory tests such as SGOT, SGPT, alkaline phosphatase and bilirubin. (See DOSAGE AND ADMINISTRATION.)

PRECAUTIONS:

LABORATORY TESTS

Complete blood counts, including platelet counts, should be obtained frequently and at a minimum prior to each dose of doxorubicin HCl liposome.

CARCINOGENESIS, MUTAGENESIS, AND IMPAIRMENT OF FERTILITY

Although no studies have been conducted with doxorubicin HCl liposome, doxorubicin HCl and related compounds have been shown to have mutagenic and carcinogenic properties when tested in experimental models.

Stealth liposomes without drug are negative when tested in Ames, mouse lymphoma and chromosomal aberration assays *in vitro*, and mammalian micronucleus assay *in vivo*.

The possible adverse effects on fertility in males and females in humans or experimental animals have not been adequately evaluated. However, doxorubicin HCl liposome resulted in mild to moderate ovarian and testicular atrophy in mice after a single dose of 36 mg/kg (about 5 times the recommended human dose on a mg/m^2 basis). Decreased testicular weights and hypospermia were present in rats after repeat doses of ≥ 0.25 mg/kg/day (about 1/13 the recommended human dose on a mg/m^{2}basis), and diffuse degeneration of the seminiferous tubules and a marked decrease in spermatogenesis were observed in dogs after repeat doses of 1 mg/kg/day (equivalent to the recommended human dose on a mg/m^{2}basis).

PREGNANCY

Pregnancy Category D: (See WARNINGS.)

NURSING MOTHERS

It is not known whether this drug is excreted in human milk. Because many drugs are excreted in human milk and because of the potential for serious adverse reactions in nursing infants from doxorubicin HCl liposome, mothers should discontinue nursing prior to taking this drug.

PEDIATRIC USE

The safety and effectiveness of doxorubicin HCl liposome in pediatric patients have not been established.

RADIATION THERAPY

Recall of skin reaction due to prior radiotherapy has occurred with doxorubicin HCl liposome administration.

DRUG INTERACTIONS:

No formal drug interaction studies have been conducted with doxorubicin HCl liposome. Until specific compatibility data are available, it is not recommended that doxorubicin HCl liposome be mixed with other drugs. Doxorubicin HCl liposomes may interact with drugs known to interact with the conventional formulation of doxorubicin HCl.

ADVERSE REACTIONS:

Information on adverse events is based on the experience reported in 753 patients with AIDS-related KS enrolled in four studies. The majority of patients were treated with 20 mg/m^2 of doxorubicin HCl liposome injection every two to three weeks. The median time on study was 127 days and ranged from 1 to 811 days. The median cumulative dose was 120 mg/m^2 and ranged from 3.3 to 798.6 mg/m^2.

Twenty-six patients (3.0%) received cumulative doses of greater than 450 mg/m^2.

Of these 753 patients, 61.2% were considered poor risk for KS tumor burden, 91.5% poor for immune system, and 46.9% for systemic illness; 36.2% were poor risk for all three categories. Patients' median CD4 count was 21.0 cells/mm^3, with 50.8% of patients having less than 50 cells/mm^3. The mean absolute neutrophil count at study entry was approximately 3000 cells/mm^3.

Patients received a variety of potentially myelotoxic drugs in combination with doxorubicin HCl liposome. Of the 693 patients with concomitant medication information, 58.7% were on one or more antiretroviral medications; 34.9% patients were on zidovudine (AZT), 20.8% on didanosine (ddI), 16.5% on zalcitabine (ddC), and 9.5% on stavudine (D4T). A total of 85.1% patients were on PCP prophylaxis, most (54.4%) on sulfamethoxazole/trimethoprim. Eighty-five percent of patients were receiving antifungal medications, primarily fluconazole (75.8%). Seventy-two percent of patients were receiving antivirals, 56.3% acyclovir, 29% ganciclovir, and 16% foscarnet. In addition, 47.8% patients received colony stimulating factors (sargramostim/filgrastim) sometime during their course of treatment.

Of the 753 patients enrolled in the doxorubicin HCl liposome clinical trials, adverse event information was available for 705 patients. In many instances it was difficult to determine whether adverse events resulted from doxorubicin HCl liposome, from concomitant therapy, or from the patients' underlying disease(s).

HEMATOLOGIC

Neutropenia (<1000 neutrophils/mm3) occurred in 49% of patients on study with 13% of patients having at least one episode of ANC < 500 cells/mm^3.

Sepsis occurred in 5% of patients; for 0.7% of patients the event was considered possibly or probably related to doxorubicin HCl liposome. Ten patients developed sepsis in the setting of neutropenia. Eleven patients (1.6%) discontinued study because of bone marrow suppression or neutropenia.

Opportunistic infections occurred in 355 patients (50.4%), most commonly candidiasis (23.5%), cytomegalovirus (20.1%), herpes simplex (10.5%), *Pneumocystis carinii* pneumonia (9.2%), and mycobacterium avium (8.4%). Four patients (0.6%) discontinued doxorubicin HCl liposome therapy because of opportunistic infection.

INFUSION-RELATED REACTIONS (SEE WARNINGS)

Six patients (0.9%) discontinued doxorubicin HCl liposome therapy because of infusion reactions.

PALMAR-PLANTAR ERYTHRODYSESTHESIA

Three patients (0.4%) discontinued doxorubicin HCl liposome therapy because of palmar-plantar erythrodysesthesia. (See WARNINGS.)

ADVERSE REACTIONS: *(cont'd)*

CARDIAC EVENTS

Sixty-eight (9.6%) patients experienced cardiac-related adverse events. In 30 patients (4.3%), the event was thought to be possibly or probably related to doxorubicin HCl liposome. Nine cases of possibly or probably related cardiomyopathy and/or congestive heart failure were reported. Seven (1.0%) of the possibly or probably related cardiac events were severe. These severe events included arrhythmia (nonspecific), cardiomyopathy, heart failure, pericardial effusion, and tachycardia. Three patients discontinued study due to cardiac events.

RADIATION THERAPY

Recall of skin reaction due to prior radiotherapy has occurred with doxorubicin HCl liposome administration.

Eighty-three percent of the patients reported adverse events that were considered to be possibly or probably related to the treatment with doxorubicin HCl liposome. These adverse events are provided below. TABLE 3 shows all events occurring in ≥ 5% in the overall treated population that were considered by investigators at least possibly related to doxorubicin HCl liposome. Rates are also given for the subset of refractory/intolerant patients. Adverse reactions only infrequently (5%) led to discontinuation of treatment. Those that did so included bone marrow suppression, cardiac adverse events, infusion-related reactions, toxoplasmosis, palmar-plantar erythrodysesthesia, pneumonia, cough/dyspnea, fatigue, optic neuritis, progression of a non-KS tumor, allergy to penicillin, and unspecified reasons.

TABLE 3 Probably and Possibly Drug-Related Adverse Events Reported in ≥ 5% of Treated Patients

	Refractory or Intolerant AIDS-KS Patients	Total AIDS-KS Patients
Number of Patients	77	705
Number of Patients Reporting Adverse Events	57 (74.0%)	586 (83.1%)
Adverse Event		
Neutropenia (ANC <100/mm^3)	34 (44.2%)	352 (49.9%)
Anemia	5 (6.5%)	137 (19.4%)
Nausea	14 (18.2%)	119 (16.9%)
Asthenia	5 (6.5%)	70 (9.9%)
Hypochromic Anemia	4 (5.2%)	69 (9.8%)
Thrombocytopenia	5 (6.5%)	65 (9.2%)
Fever	6 (7.8%)	64 (9.1%)
Alopecia	7 (9.1%)	63 (8.9%)
Alkaline Phosphate Increase	1 (1.3%)	55 (7.8%)
Vomiting	6 (7.8%)	55 (7.8%)
Diarrhea	4 (5.2%)	55 (7.8%)
Stomatitis	4 (5.2%)	48 (6.8%)
Oral Moniliasis	1 (1.3%)	39 (5.5%)

Incidence 1% to 5% (Possibly or Probably Related)

Body as a Whole: headache, back pain, infection, allergic reaction, chills.

Cardiovascular: chest pain, hypotension, tachycardia.

Cutaneous: Herpes simplex, rash, itching.

Digestive System: mouth ulceration, glossitis, constipation, aphthous stomatitis, anorexia, dysphagia, abdominal pain.

Hematologic: hemolysis, increased prothrombin time.

Metabolic/Nutritional: SGPT increase, weight loss, hypocalcemia, hyperbilirubinemia, hyperglycemia.

Other: dyspnea, albuminuria, pneumonia, retinitis, emotional lability, dizziness. somnolence.

Incidence Less Than 1% (Possibly or Probably Related)

Body As A Whole: face edema, cellulitis, sepsis, abscess, radiation injury, flu syndrome, moniliasis, hypothermia, injection site hemorrhage, injection site pain, cryptococcosis, ascites.

Cardiovascular System: thrombophlebitis, cardiomyopathy, pericardial effusion, hemorrhage, palpitation, syncope, bundle branch block, congestive heart failure, cardiomegaly, heart arrest, migraine, thrombosis, ventricular arrhythmia.

Digestive System: dyspepsia, cholestatic jaundice, gastritis, gingivitis, ulcerative proctitis, colitis, esophageal ulcer, esophagitis, gastrointestinal hemorrhage, hepatic failure, leukoplakia of mouth, pancreatitis, ulcerative stomatitis, hepatitis, hepatosplenomegaly, increased appetite, jaundice, sclerosing cholangitis, tenesmus, fecal impaction.

Endocrine System: diabetes mellitus.

Hemic and Lymphatic System: eosinophilia, lymphadenopathy, lymphangitis, lymphedema, petechia, thromboplastin decrease.

Metabolic/Nutritional Disorders: lactic dehydrogenase increase, hypernatremia, creatinine increase, BUN increase, dehydration, edema, hypercalcemia, hyperkalemia, hyperlipemia, hyperuricemia, hypoglycemia, hypokalemia, hypolipemia, hypomagnesemia, hyponatremia, hypophosphatemia, hypoproteinemia, ketosis, weight gain.

Musculoskeletal System: myalgia, arthralgia, bone pain, myositis.

Nervous System: paresthesia, insomnia, peripheral neuritis, depression, neuropathy, anxiety, convulsion, hypotonia, acute brain syndrome, confusion, hemiplegia, hypertonia, hypokinesia, vertigo.

Respiratory System: pleural effusion, asthma, bronchitis, cough increase, hyperventilation, pharyngitis, pneumothorax, rhinitis, sinusitis.

Skin and Appendages: maculopapular rash, skin ulcer, exfoliative dermatitis, skin discoloration, herpes zoster, cutaneous moniliasis, erythema multiforme, erythema nodosum, furunculosis, psoriasis, pustular rash, skin necrosis, urticaria, vesiculobullous rash.

Special Senses: otitis media, taste perversion, abnormal vision, blindness, conjunctivitis, eye pain, optic neuritis, tinnitus, visual field defect.

Urogenital System: hematuria, balanitis, cystitis, dysuria, genital edema, glycosuria, kidney failure.

OVERDOSAGE:

Acute overdosage with doxorubicin HCl causes increases in mucositis, leukopenia,and thrombocytopenia.

Treatment of acute overdosage consists of treatment of the severely myelosuppressed patient with hospitalization, antibiotics, platelet and granulocyte transfusions, and symptomatic treatment of mucositis.

DOSAGE AND ADMINISTRATION:

AIDS-KS PATIENTS

Doxorubicin HCl liposome injection should be administered intravenously at a dose of 20 mg/m^2 (doxorubicin HCl equivalent) over 30 minutes, once every three weeks, for as long as patients respond satisfactorily and tolerate treatment.

Do not administer as a bolus injection or an undiluted solution. Rapid infusion may increase the risk of infusion-related reactions. (See WARNINGS, Infusion Reactions.)

DOSAGE AND ADMINISTRATION: *(cont'd)*

Each vial contains 20 mg doxorubicin HCl at a concentration of 2 mg/mL.

Doxorubicin HCl liposome should be considered an irritant and precautions should be taken to avoid extravasation. On intravenous administration of doxorubicin HCl liposome, extravasation may occur with or without an accompanying stinging or burning sensation and even if blood returns well on aspiration of the infusion needle. If any signs or symptoms of extravasation have occurred the infusion should be immediately terminated and restarted in another vein. The application of ice over the site of extravasation for approximately 30 minutes may be helpful in alleviating the local reaction. **Doxorubicin HCl liposome must not be given by the intramuscular or subcutaneous route.**

DOSE MODIFICATIONS

The dose modifications shown in the TABLES 4, 5, and 6 below are recommended for managing possible adverse events.

TABLE 4 Palmar-Plantar Erythodysesthesia

Toxicity Grade	Symptoms	Weeks Since Last Dose	
0	no symptoms	Redose at 3-week interval	Redose at 3-week interval
1	mild erythema, swelling, or desquamation not interfering with daily activities	Redose unless patient has experienced a previous Grade 3 or 4 skin toxicity in which case wait an additional week	Redose at 25% dose reduction; return to 3-week interval
2	erytherma, desquamation, or swelling interfering with, but not precluding normal physical activities; small blisters or ulcerations less than 2cm in diameter	Wait an additional week	Redose at 50% dose reduction; return to a 3-week interval
3	blistering, ulceration, or swelling interfering with walking or normal daily activities; cannot wear regular clothing	Wait an additional week	Discontinue Doxorubicin HCl Liposome Injection
4	diffuse or local process causing infectous complications, or a bed ridden state or hospitalization		

TABLE 5 Hematological Toxicity

Grade	ANC (cells/mm³)	Platelets (cells/mm³)	Modification
1	1500 - 1900	75,000 - 150,000	None
2	1000 - <1500	50,000 - <75,000	None
3	500 - 999	25,000 - <50,000	Wait until ANC ≥ 1,000 and/or platelets ≥ 50,000 then redose at 25% dose reduction
4	<500	<25,000	Wait until ANC ≥ 1,000 and/or platelets ≥ 50,000 then redose at 50% dose reduction

TABLE 6 Stomatitis

Grade	Symptoms	Modification
1	Painless ulcers, erythema, or mild soreness	None
2	Painful erythema, or ulcers, but can eat	Wait one week and if symptoms improve redose at 100% dose
3	Painful erythema, edema or ulcers, and cannot eat	Wait one week and if symptoms improve redose at 25% dose reduction
4	Requires parental or enteral support	Wait one week and if symptoms improve redose at 50% dose reduction

PATIENTS WITH IMPAIRED HEPATIC FUNCTION

Limited clinical experience exists in treating hepatically impaired patients with doxorubicin HCl liposome.

Therefore, based on experience with doxorubicin HCl, it is recommended that doxorubicin HCl liposome dosage be reduced if the bilirubin is elevated as follows: Serum bilirubin 1.2 to 3.0 mg/dL, give 1/2 normal dose; >3 mg/dL, give 1/4 normal dose.

PREPARATION FOR INTRAVENOUS ADMINISTRATION

The appropriate dose of doxorubicin HCl liposome, up to a maximum of 90 mg, must be diluted in 250 mL of 5% Dextrose Injection, USP prior to administration. Aseptic technique must be strictly observed since no preservative or bacteriostatic agent is present in doxorubicin HCl liposome. Diluted doxorubicin HCl liposome should be refrigerated at 2°C to 8°C (36°F to 46°F) and administered within 24 hours.

Do not use with in-line filters.

Do not mix with other drugs.

Do not use with any diluent other than 5% Dextrose Injection.

Do not use any bacteriostatic agent, such as benzyl alcohol.

Doxorubicin HCl liposome is not a clear solution but a translucent, red liposomal dispersion. **Parenteral drug products should be inspected visually for particulate matter and discoloration prior to administration, whenever solution and container permit. Do not use if a precipitate or foreign matter is present.**

STORAGE AND STABILITY

Refrigerate unopened vials of doxorubicin HCl liposome at 2°C to 8°C (36°F to 46°F). Avoid freezing. Prolonged freezing may adversely affect liposomal drug products; however, short-term freezing (less than 1 month) does not appear to have a deleterious effect on doxorubicin HCl liposome.

PROCEDURE FOR PROPER HANDLING AND DISPOSAL

Caution should be exercised in the handling and preparation of doxorubicin HCl liposome.

The use of gloves is required.

If doxorubicin HCl liposome comes into contact with skin or mucosa, immediately wash thoroughly with soap and water.

DOSAGE AND ADMINISTRATION: *(cont'd)*

Doxorubicin HCl liposome should be considered an irritant and precautions should be taken to avoid extravasation. On intravenous administration of doxorubicin HCl liposome, extravasation may occur with or without an accompanying stinging or burning sensation and even if blood returns well on aspiration of the infusion needle. If any signs or symptoms of extravasation have occurred, the infusion should be immediately terminated and restarted in another vein. Doxorubicin HCl liposome must not be given by the intramuscular or subcutaneous route.

Doxorubicin HCl liposome should be handled and disposed of in a manner consistent with other anticancer drugs. Several guidelines on this subject exist 2-8 although there is no general agreement that all of the procedures listed in these guidelines are appropriate or necessary.

HOW SUPPLIED:

Doxorubicin HCl liposome injection is supplied as a sterile, translucent, red liposomal dispersion in 10 mL glass, single use vials.

Each vial contains 20 mg doxorubicin HCl at a concentration of 2 mg/mL.

Refrigerate at 2-8°C. Avoid freezing. Prolonged freezing may adversely affect liposomal drug products: however, short-term freezing (less than 1 month) does not appear to have a deleterious effect on doxorubicin HCl liposome.

Available as individually cartoned vials in packages of six.

REFERENCES:

1. Krown et al. Kaposi's sarcoma in the acquired immune deficiency syndrome: A proposal for uniform evaluation, response, and staging criteria. J Clin Oncol. 1989; 7(9):1201-1207. **2.** Recommendations for the safe handling of cytotoxic drugs. NIH Publication No. 92-2621. US Government Printing Office, Washington, DC 20402. **3.** OSHA Work-Practice guidelines for personnel dealing with cytotoxic (antineoplastic) drugs. Am J Hosp Pharm. 1986; 43:1193-1204. **4.** American Society of Hospital Pharmacists Technical Assistance Bulletin on Handling Cytotoxic and Hazardous Drugs. Am J Hosp Pharm. 1985; 42:131-137. **5.** National Study Commission on Cytotoxic Exposure—Recommendations for Handling Cytotoxic Agents. Available from Louis P. Jeffrey, Sc. D., Chairman, National Study Commission on Cytotoxic Exposure, Massachusetts College of Pharmacy and Allied Health Sciences, 179 Longwood Avenue, Boston, Massachusetts 02115. **6.** AMA Council Report. Guidelines for handling parenteral antineoplastics. JAMA 1985; 253(11):1590-1592. **7.** Clinical Oncologic Society of Australia: Guidelines and recommendations for safe handling of antineoplastic agents. Med. J. Australia 1983; 1: 426-428. **8.** Jones RB, et al. Safe handling of chemotherapeutic agents: a report from the Mount Sinai Medical Center. Ca-A Cancer Journal for Clinicians. 1983; Sept/Oct:258-263.

DOXYCYCLINE *(001113)*

CATEGORIES: Acne; Actinomycosis; Amebiasis; Amebicides; Anthrax; Anti-Infectives; Antiarthritics; Antibiotics; Antimicrobials; Brucellosis; Chancroid; Chlamydia; Cholera; Conjunctivitis; Gonorrhea; Granuloma; Granuloma Inguinale; Infections; Listeriosis; Lyme Disease; Lymphogranuloma; Malaria; Pain; Penicillins; Plague; Pneumonia; Psittacosis; Q Fever; Relapsing Fever; Respiratory Tract Infections; Rickettsial Disease; Rickettsialpox; Rocky Mountain Fever; Skin/Mucous Membrane Agents; Syphilis; Tetracyclines; Tick Fevers; Trachoma; Tularemia; Typhoid Fever; Typhus; Urethritis; Urinary Tract Infections; Vincent's Infection; Yaws; Sales > $100 Million; Pregnancy Category D; FDA Approval Pre 1982; Top 200 Drugs

BRAND NAMES: Ak-Ramycin; Ak-Ratabs; *Asidoxyn*; *Azudoxat* (Germany); *Bactidox* (Germany); *Banndoclin*; *Basedillin* (Japan); *Bassado*; *Biocolyn*; *Biodoxi*; *Bronmycin*; *Cendox*; *Cloran*; *Cyclidox*; *Dagracycline*; *Deoxymykoin*; Dermateque; *Doinmycin*; *Doryx* (Australia); *Dosil*; *Dotur*; *Doxaciclin* (Japan); *Doxalin*; *Doxat*; *Doximed*; *Doximycin*; *Doxin*; *Doxine*; *Doxi-Sergo*; *Doxt*; Doxy; *Doxy-1*; Doxy-100; Doxychel; *Doxyclin*; *Doxycline*; *Doxycycline*; Doxycycline Hyclate; Doxycycline Monohydrate; Doxygen; *Doxylag*; *Doxylin* (Australia); *Doxymycin*; *Dumoxin*; *Duracyclin*; *Esdoxin* (Japan); *Gewacyclin*; *Granudoxy*; *Ibimycin*; *Idocyklin*; *Interdoxin*; *Lexcycline*; *Lydox*; *Magdrin* (Japan); *Medomycin*; *Miraclin*; *Monocin*; Monodox; *Paldomycin* (Japan); *Probracin*; *Radox*; *Remycin*; Ro-Doxy; *Roximycin* (Japan); *Servidoxyne*; *Siadocin*; *Siclidon*; *Sigadoxin* (Germany); *Supracyclin*; *Tenutan*; *Tetradox*; *Texomycin*; *Tolexine* (France); *Torymycin*; *Tsurupioxin* (Japan); *Unidox*; *Unidoxy*; *Vibrabiotic*; *Vibradox*; *Vibracina*; *Vibramicina* (Mexico); **Vibramycin**; Vibramycin Calcium; Vibramycin Hyclate; Vibramycin IV; Vibramycin Monohydrate; *Vibramycin-N*; *Vibramycine* (France); *Vibra-S*; *Vibra-Tabs* (Australia, Canada); *Vibraveineuse* (France); *Vibravends*; *Vibravenos* (Germany); *Vibravenos SF*; *Viradoxyl-N*; *Vivocycline*; *Wanmycin*; *Withamycin*; *Xidox*; *Zadorin*
(International brand names outside U.S. in italics)

FORMULARIES: Aetna; BC-BS; DoD; FHP; PCS; WHO

DESCRIPTION:

Doxycycline is a broad-spectrum antibiotic synthetically derived from oxytetracycline and is available as doxycycline monohydrate; doxycycline hyclate; doxycycline hydrochloride hemiethanolate hemihydrate; and doxycycline calcium for oral administration. It is also available as doxycycline hyclate for intravenous use as well as coated hyclate pellets.

The molecular formula of doxycycline monohydrate is $C_{22}H_{24}N_2O_8{\cdot}H_2O$ and a molecular weight of 462.46. The chemical designation for doxycycline is 4-(Dimethylamino)-1, 4, 4a, 5, 5a, 6, 11, 12a-octahydro-3,5,10,12,12a-pentahydroxy-6-methyl-1, 11-dioxo-2-naphthacenecarboxamide monohydrate. The molecular formula for doxycycline hydrochloride hemiethanolate hemihydrate is $(C_{22}H_{24}N_2O_8{\cdot}HCl)_2{\cdot}C_2H_6O{\cdot}H_2O$ and the molecular weight is 1025.89. Doxycycline is a light-yellow crystalline powder. Doxycycline hyclate is soluble in water, while doxycycline monohydrate is very slightly soluble in water.

Doxycycline has a high degree of lipoid solubility and a low affinity for calcium binding. It is highly stable in normal human serum. Doxycycline will not degrade into an epianhydro form.

Inert ingredients in the syrup formulation are: apple flavor; butylparaben; calcium chloride; carmine; glycerin; hydrochloric acid; magnesium aluminum silicate; povidone; propylene glycol; propylparaben; raspberry flavor; simethicone emulsion; sodium hydroxide; sodium metabisulfite; sorbitol solution; water.

Inert ingredients in the capsule formulations are: hard gelatin capsules (which may contain Blue 1 and other inert ingredients); magnesium stearate; microcrystalline cellulose; sodium lauryl sulfate.

Inert ingredients for the oral suspension formulation are: carboxymethylcellulose sodium; Blue 1; methylparaben; microcrystalline cellulose; propylparaben; raspberry flavor; Red 28; simethicone emulsion; sucrose.

Inert ingredients for the tablet formulation are: ethylcellulose; hydroxypropyl methylcellulose; magnesium stearate; microcrystalline cellulose; propylene glycol; sodium lauryl sulfate; talc; titanium dioxide; Yellow 6 Lake.

Inert ingredients for the coated pellets are lactose, NF; microcrystalline cellulose, NF; povidone, USP. Each shell and/or band contains FD and C blue No. 1; FD and C yellow No. 6, D and C yellow No. 10; gelatin NF: silicon dioxide; sodium laurel sulfate, NF; titanium dioxide, USP.

CLINICAL PHARMACOLOGY:

Tetracyclines are readily absorbed and are bound to plasma proteins in varying degree. They are concentrated by the liver in the bile, and excreted in the urine and feces at high concentrations and in a biologically active form. Doxycycline is virtually completely absorbed after oral administration.

Following a 200 mg dose, normal adult volunteers averaged peak serum levels of 2.6 mg/ml of doxycycline at 2 hours decreasing to 1.45 mg/ml at 24 hours. Excretion of doxycycline by the kidney is about 40%/72 hours in individuals with normal function (creatinine clearance about 75 ml/min.) This percentage excretion may fall as low as 1-5%/72 hours in individuals with severe renal insufficiency (creatinine clearance below 10 ml/min.). Studies have shown no significant difference in serum half-life of doxycycline (range 18-22 hours) in individuals with normal and severely impaired renal function.

Hemodialysis does not alter serum half-life.

Results of animal studies indicate that tetracyclines cross the placenta and are found in fetal tissues.

MICROBIOLOGY

The tetracyclines are primarily bacteriostatic and are thought to exert their antimicrobial effect by the inhibition of protein synthesis. The tetracyclines, including doxycycline, have a similar antimicrobial spectrum of activity against a wide range of gram-positive and gram-negative organisms. Cross-resistance of these organisms to tetracyclines is common.

Gram-Negative Bacteria

Neisseria gonorrhoeae
Calymmatobacterium granulomatis
Haemophilus ducreyi
Haemophilus influenzae
Yersinia pestis (formerly *Pasteurella pestis*)
Francisella tularensis (formerly *Pasteurella tularensis*)
Vibrio cholera (formerly *Vibrio comma*)
Bartonella bacilliformis
Brucella

Because many strains of the following groups of gram-negative microorganisms have been shown to be resistant to tetracyclines, culture and susceptibility testing are recommended:

Escherichia coli
Klebsiella species
Enterobacter aerogenes, Shigella species
Acinetobacter species (formerly *Mima* species and *Herellea* species)
Bacteroides species

GRAM-POSITIVE BACTERIA

Because many strains of the following groups of gram-positive microorganisms have been shown to be resistant to tetracycline, culture and susceptibility testing are recommended. Up to 44 percent of strains of *Streptococcus pyogenes* and 74 percent of*Streptococcus faecalis* have been found to be resistant to tetracycline drugs. Therefore, tetracycline should not be used for streptococcal disease unless the organism has been demonstrated to be susceptible.

Streptococcus pyogenes
Streptococcus pneumoniae
Enterococcus group (*Streptococcus faecalis* and *Streptococcus faecium).*Alpha-hemolytic streptococci (viridans group).

Other Microorganisms

Rickettsiae
Clostridium species
Chlamydia psittaci
Fusobacterium fusiforme
Chlamydia trachomatis
Actinomyces species
Mycoplasma pneumoniae
Bacillus anthracis
Ureaplasma urealyticum
Propionbacterium acnes
Borrelia recurrentis
Entamoeba species
Treponema pallidum
Balantidium coli
Treponema pertenue
Plasmodium falciparum

Doxycycline has been found to be active against the asexual erythrocytic forms of *plasmodium falciparum* but not against the gametocytes of *P.falciparum.* The precise mechanism of action of the drug is not known.

Susceptibility Tests: *Diffusion Techniques:* Quantitative methods that require measurement of zone diameters give the precise estimate of the susceptibility of bacteria to antimicrobial agents. One such standard procedure[1] which has been recommended for use with disks to test susceptibility of organisms to doxycycline, uses the 30 mcg tetracycline-class disk or the 30-mcg doxycycline disk. Interpretation involves the correlation of the diameter obtained in the disk test with the minimum inhibitory concentration (MIC) for tetracycline or doxycycline, respectively.

Reports from the laboratory giving results of the standard single-disk susceptibility test with a 30-mcg tetracycline-class disk or the 30-mcg doxycycline disk should be interpreted according to the criteria in TABLE 1.

TABLE 1

Zone Diameter (mm) tetracycline	doxycycline	Interpretation
≥19	≥16	Susceptible
15-18	13-15	Intermediate
≥14	≤12	Resistant

A report of "Susceptible" indicates that the pathogen is likely lo be inhibited by generally achievable blood levels. A report of "Intermediate" suggests that the organism would be susceptible if a high dosage is used or if the infection is confined to tissues and fluids in which high antimicrobial levels are attained. A report of "Resistant" indicates that achievable concentrations are unlikely to be inhibitory, and other therapy should be selected.

Standardized procedures require the use of laboratory control organisms. The 30-mcg tetracycline-class disk or the 30-mcg doxycycline disk should give the zone diameters in TABLE 2.

CLINICAL PHARMACOLOGY: *(cont'd)*

TABLE 2

Organism	Zone Diameter (mm) tetracycline	doxycycline
E. coli ATCC 25922	18-25	18-24
S. aureus ATCC 25923	19-28	23-29

Dilution Techniques: Use a standardized dilution method[2] (broth, agar, microdilution) or equivalent with tetracycline powder. The MIC values obtained should be interpreted according to the criteria found in TABLE 3.

TABLE 3

MIC (mcg/ml)	Interpretation
≤4	Susceptible
8	Intermediate
≥16	Resistant

As with standard diffusion techniques, dilution methods require the use of laboratory control organisms. Standard tetracycline powder should provide the MIC values found in TABLE 4.

TABLE 4

Organism	MIC (mcg/ml)
E. coli ATCC 25922	1.0-4.0
S. aureus ATCC 29213	0.25-1.0
E. faecalis ATCC 29212	8-32
P. aeruginosa ATCC 27853	8-32

Additional Information For IV: The drugs in the tetracycline class have closely similar antimicrobial spectra, and cross resistance among them is common. Microorganisms may be considered susceptible to doxycycline (likely to respond to doxycycline therapy) if the minimum inhibitory concentration (MIC) is not more than 40 mcg/ml. Microorganisms may be considered intermediate (harboring partial resistance) if the MIC is 4.0 to 12.5 mcg/ml and resistant (not likely to respond to therapy) if the MIC is greater than 12.5 mcg/ml.

Susceptibility Plate Testing: If the Kirby-Bauer method of disk susceptibility testing is used, a 30 mcg doxycycline disk should give a zone of at least 16 mm when tested against a doxycycline-susceptible bacterial strain. A tetracycline disk may be used to determine microbial susceptibility. If the Kirby-Bauer method of disk susceptibility is used, a 30 mcg tetracycline disk should give a zone of at least 19 mm when tested against a tetracycline-susceptible bacterial strain.

Following a single 100 mg dose administered in a concentration of 0.4 mg/ml in a one-hour infusion, normal adult volunteers average a peak of 2.5 mcg/ml, while 200 mg of a concentration of 0.4 mg/ml administered over two hours averaged a peak of 3.6 mcg/ml.

INDICATIONS AND USAGE:

Doxycycline Is Indicated For The Treatment Of The Following Infections:

Rocky mountain spotted fever, typhus fever and the typhus group, Q fever, rickettsialpox, and tick fevers caused by Rickettsiae.

Respiratory tract infections caused by *Mycoplasma pneumoniae.*

Lymphogranuloma venereum caused by *Chlamydia trachomatis.*

Psittacosis (ornithosis) caused by *Chlamydia psittaci.*

Trachoma caused by *Chlamydia trachomatis,* although the infectious agent is not always eliminated as judged by immunofluorescence.

Inclusion conjunctivitis caused by *Chlamydia trachomatis.*

Uncomplicated urethral, endocervical or rectal infections in adults caused by *Chlamydia trachomatis.*

Nongonococcal urethritis caused by *Ureaplasma urealyticum.*

Relapsing fever due to *Borrelia recurrentis.*

Doxycycline Is Also Indicated For The Treatment Of Infections Caused By The Following Gram-Negative Microorganisms:

Chancroid caused by *Haemophilus ducreyi.*

Plague due to *Yersinia pestis* (formerly *Pasteurella pestis).*

Tularemia due to *Francisella tularensis* (formerly *Pasteurella tularensis).*

Cholera caused by *Vibrio cholerae* (formerly *Vibrio comma).*

Campylobacter fetus infections caused by *Campylobacter fetus* (formerly *Vibrio fetus).*

Brucellosis due to *Brucella* species (in conjunction with streptomycin).

Bartonellosis due to *Bartonella bacilliformis.*

Granuloma inguinale caused by *Calymmatobacterium granulomatis.*

Prophylaxis: Doxycycline is indicated for the prophylaxis of malaria due to*Plasmodium falciparum*in short term travelers (4 months) to areas with chloroquine and/or pyrimethamine-sulfadoxine resistant strains. See DOSAGE AND ADMINISTRATION and Information for the Patient.

Because many strains of the following groups of microorganisms have been shown to be resistant to doxycycline, culture and susceptibility testing are recommended.

Doxycycline Is Indicated For Treatment Of Infections Caused By The Following Gram-Negative Microorganisms, When Bacteriologic Testing Indicates Appropriate Susceptibility To The Drug:

Escherichia coli.

Enterobacter aerogenes (formerly *Aerobacter aerogenes).*

Shigella species.

Acinetobacter species (formerly *Mima* species and *Herellea* species).

Respiratory tract infections caused by *Haemophilus influenzae.*

Respiratory tract and urinary tract infections caused by *Klebsiella* species.

Doxycycline Is Indicated For Treatment Of Infections Caused By The Following Gram-Positive Microorganisms When Bacteriologic Testing Indicates Appropriate Susceptibility To The Drug:

Upper respiratory tract infections caused by *Streptococcus pneumoniae* (formerly *Diplococcus pneumoniae).*

When Penicillin Is Contraindicated, Doxycycline Is An Alternative Drug In The Treatment Of The Following Infections:

Uncomplicated gonorrhea caused by *Neisseria gonorrhoeae.*

Syphilis caused by *Treponema pallidum.*

Yaws caused by *Treponema pertenue.*

INDICATIONS AND USAGE: *(cont'd)*

Listeriosis due to *Listeria monocytogenes*.

Anthrax due to *Bacillus anthracis*.

Vincent's infection caused by *Fusobacterium fusiforme*.

Actinomycosis caused by *Actinomyces israelii*.

Infections caused by *Clostridium* species.

In acute intestinal amebiasis, doxycycline may be a useful adjunct to amebicides.

In severe acne, doxycycline may be useful adjunctive therapy.

CONTRAINDICATIONS:

This drug is contraindicated in persons who have shown hypersensitivity to any of the tetracyclines.

WARNINGS:

THE USE OF DRUGS OF THE TETRACYCLINE CLASS DURING TOOTH DEVELOPMENT (LAST HALF OF PREGNANCY, INFANCY AND CHILDHOOD TO THE AGE OF 8 YEARS) MAY CAUSE PERMANENT DISCOLORATION OF THE TEETH (YELLOW-GRAY-BROWN). THIS ADVERSE REACTION IS MORE COMMON DURING LONG-TERM USE OF THE DRUGS, BUT IT HAS BEEN OBSERVED FOLLOWING REPEATED SHORT-TERM COURSES. ENAMEL HYPOPLASIA HAS ALSO BEEN REPORTED. TETRACYCLINE DRUGS, THEREFORE, SHOULD NOT BE USED IN THIS AGE GROUP UNLESS OTHER DRUGS ARE NOT LIKELY TO BE EFFECTIVE OR ARE CONTRAINDICATED.

All tetracyclines form a stable calcium complex in any bone-forming tissue. A decrease in fibula growth rate has been observed in prematures given oral tetracycline in doses of 25 mg/kg every 6 hours. This reaction was shown to be reversible when the drug was discontinued.

Results of animal studies indicate that tetracyclines cross the placenta, are found in fetal tissues, and can have toxic effects on the developing fetus (often related to retardation of skeletal development). Evidence of embryotoxicity has also been noted in animals treated early in pregnancy. If any tetracycline is used during pregnancy or if the patient becomes pregnant while taking this drug, the patient should be apprised of the potential hazard to the fetus.

The antianabolic action of the tetracyclines may cause an increase in BUN. Studies to date indicate that this does not occur with the use of doxycycline in patients with impaired renal function.

Photosensitivity manifested by an exaggerated sunburn reaction has been observed in some individuals taking tetracyclines. Patients apt to be exposed to direct sunlight or ultraviolet light should be advised that this reaction can occur with tetracycline drugs, and treatment should be discontinued at the first evidence of skin erythema.

Doxycycline syrup contains sodium metabisulfite, a sulfite that may cause allergic-type reactions including anaphylactic symptoms and life-threatening or less severe asthmatic episodes in certain susceptible people. The overall prevalence of sulfite sensitivity in the general population is unknown and probably low. Sulfite sensitivity is seen more frequently in asthmatic than in non-asthmatic people.

Additional information for IV: There have been no studies done with doxycycline hyclate IV and pregnant patients. It should not be used in pregnant women unless,in the judgement of the physician, it is essential for the welfare of the patient.

The use of doxycycline hyclate IV in children under 8 years is not recommended because safe conditions for its use have not been established.

PRECAUTIONS:

GENERAL

As with other antibiotic preparations, use of this drug may result in overgrowth of nonsusceptible organisms, including fungi. If superinfection occurs, the antibiotic should be discontinued and appropriate therapy instituted.

Bulging fontanels in infants and benign intracranial hypertension in adults have been reported in individuals receiving tetracyclines. These conditions disappeared when the drug was discontinued.

Incision and drainage or other surgical procedures should be performed in conjunction with antibiotic therapy, when indicated.

Doxycycline others substantial but not complete suppression of the asexual blood stages of *Plasmodium* strains.

Doxycycline does not suppress *P. falciparums* sexual blood stage gamocytes. Subjects completing this prophylactic regimen may still transmit the infection to mosquitoes outside endemic areas.

INFORMATION FOR THE PATIENT

Patients Taking Doxycycline For Malaria Prophylaxis Should Be Advised:

that no present-day antimalarial agent, including doxycycline, guarantees protection against malaria.

to avoid being bitten by mosquitoes by using personal protective measures that help avoid contact with mosquitoes, especially from dusk to dawn (*e.g.,* staying in well-screened areas, using mosquito nets, covering the body with clothing, and using an effective insect repellent.

that doxycycline prophylaxis:

should begin 1-2 days before travel to the malarious area.

should be continued daily while in the malarious area and after leaving the malarious area.

should be continued for 4 further weeks to avoid development of malaria after returning from an endemic area.

—should not exceed 4 months.

All Patients Taking Doxycycline Should Be Advised:

to avoid excessive sunlight or artificial ultraviolet light while receiving doxycycline and to discontinue therapy if phototoxicity (*e.g.,* skin eruption, etc.) occurs. Sunscreen or sunblock should be considered (See WARNINGS.)

to drink fluids liberally along with doxycycline to reduce the risk of esophageal irritation and ulceration. (See ADVERSE REACTIONS.)

that the absorption of tetracyclines is reduced when taken with foods, especially those which contain calcium. However, the absorption of doxycycline is not markedly influenced by simultaneous ingestion of food or milk. (See DRUG INTERACTIONS.)

that the absorption of tetracyclines is reduced when taking bismuth subsalicylate (see DRUG INTERACTIONS).

that the use of doxycycline might increase the incidence of vaginal candidiasis.

LABORATORY TESTS

In venereal disease, when co-existent syphilis is suspected, dark field examinations should be done before treatment is started and the blood serology repeated monthly for at least 4 months.

PRECAUTIONS: *(cont'd)*

In long-term therapy, periodic laboratory evaluation of organ systems, including hematopoietic, renal, and hepatic studies, should be performed.

DRUG/LABORATORY TEST INTERACTIONS

False elevations of urinary catecholamine levels may occur due to interference with the fluorescence test.

CARCINOGENESIS, MUTAGENESIS, AND IMPAIRMENT OF FERTILITY

Long-term studies in animals to evaluate carcinogenic potential of doxycycline have not been conducted. However, there has been evidence of oncogenic activity in rats in studies with the related antibiotics, oxytetracycline (adrenal and pituitary tumors), and minocycline (thyroid tumors).

Likewise, although mutagenicity studies of doxycycline have not been conducted, positive results *in vitro* mammalian cell assays have been reported for related antibiotics (tetracycline, oxytetracycline).

Doxycycline administered orally at dosage levels as high as 250 mg/kg/day had no apparent effect on the fertility of female rats. Effect on male fertility has not been studied.

PREGNANCY, TERATOGENIC EFFECTS, PREGNANCY CATEGORY D

See WARNINGS.

Nonteratogenic Effects: See WARNINGS.

LABOR AND DELIVERY

The effect of tetracyclines on labor and delivery is unknown.

NURSING MOTHERS

Tetracyclines are excreted in human milk. Because of the potential for serious adverse reactions in nursing infants from doxycycline, a decision should be made whether to discontinue nursing or to discontinue the drug, taking into account the importance of the drug to the mother. (See WARNINGS.)

PEDIATRIC USE

See WARNINGS and DOSAGE AND ADMINISTRATION.

DRUG INTERACTIONS:

Because tetracyclines have been shown to depress plasma prothrombin activity, patients who are on anticoagulant therapy may require downward adjustment of their anticoagulant dosage.

Since bacteriostatic drugs may interfere with the bactericidal action of penicillin, it is advisable to avoid giving tetracyclines in conjunction with penicillin.

Absorption of tetracyclines is impaired by antacids containing aluminum, calcium, or magnesium, and iron-containing preparations.

Absorption of tetracycline is impaired by bismuth subsalicylate.

Barbiturates, carbamazepine, and phenytoin decrease the half-life of doxycycline.

The concurrent use of tetracycline and Penthrane (methoxyflurane) has been reported to result in fatal renal toxicity.

Concurrent use of tetracycline may render oral contraceptives less effective.

ADVERSE REACTIONS:

Due to oral doxycycline's virtually complete absorption, side effects of the lower bowel, particularly diarrhea, have been infrequent. The following adverse reactions have been observed in patients receiving tetracyclines:

Gastrointestinal: anorexia, nausea, vomiting, diarrhea, glossitis, dysphagia, enterocolitis, and inflammatory lesions (with monilial overgrowth) in the anogenital region. Hepatotoxicity has been reported rarely. These reactions have been caused by both the oral and parenteral administration of tetracyclines. Rare instances of esophagitis and esophageal ulcerations have been reported in patients receiving capsule and tablet forms of the drugs in the tetracycline class. Most of these patients took medications immediately before going to bed. (See DOSAGE AND ADMINISTRATION.)

Skin: maculopapular and erythematous rashes. Exfoliative dermatitis has been reported but is uncommon. Photosensitivity is discussed above. (See WARNINGS.)

Renal toxicity: rise in BUN has been reported and is apparently dose related. (See WARNINGS.)

Hypersensitivity reactions: urticaria, angioneurotic edema, anaphylaxis, anaphylactoid purpura, serum sickness, pericarditis, and exacerbation of systemic lupus erythematosus.

Blood: Hemolytic anemia, thrombocytopenia, neutropenia, and eosinophilia have been reported.

Other: bulging fontanels in infants and intracranial hypertension in adults. See General.

When given over prolonged periods, tetracyclines have been reported to produce brown-black microscopic discoloration of the thyroid gland. No abnormalities of thyroid function studies are known to occur.

OVERDOSAGE:

In case of overdosage, discontinue medication, treat symptomatically, and institute supportive measures. Dialysis does not alter serum half-life and thus would not be of benefit in treating cases of overdosage.

DOSAGE AND ADMINISTRATION:

SYRUP, CAPSULES, ORAL SUSPENSION, AND TABLETS

THE USUAL DOSAGE AND FREQUENCY OF ADMINISTRATION OF DOXYCYCLINE DIFFERS FROM THAT OF THE OTHER TETRACYCLINES. EXCEEDING THE RECOMMENDED DOSAGE MAY RESULT IN AN INCREASED INCIDENCE OF SIDE EFFECTS.

Adults: The usual dose of oral doxycycline is 200 mg on the first day of treatment (administered 100 mg every 12 hours) followed by a maintenance dose of 100 mg/day. The maintenance dose may be administered as a single dose or as 50 mg every 12 hours.

In the management of more severe infections (particularly chronic infections of the urinary tract), 100 mg every 12 hours is recommended.

For Children Above Eight Years Of Age: The recommended dosage schedule for children weighing 100 pounds or less is 2 mg/lb of body weight divided into two doses on the first day of treatment, followed by 1 mg/lb of body weight given as a single daily dose or divided into two doses, on subsequent days. For more severe infections up to 2 mg/lb of body weight may be used. For children over 100 lb the usual adult dose should be used.

The therapeutic antibacterial serum activity will usually persist for 24 hours following recommended dosage.

When used in streptococcal infections, therapy should be continued for 10 days.

Administration of adequate amounts of fluid along with capsule and tablet forms of drugs in the tetracycline class is recommended to wash down the drugs and reduce the risk of esophageal irritation and ulceration. (See ADVERSE REACTIONS.)

DOSAGE AND ADMINISTRATION: *(cont'd)*

If gastric irritation occurs, it is recommended that doxycycline be given with food or milk. The absorption of doxycycline is not markedly influenced by simultaneous ingestion of food or milk.

Studies to date have indicated that administration of doxycycline at the usual recommended doses does not lead to excessive accumulation of the antibiotic in patients with renal impairment.

Uncomplicated Gonococcal Infections In Adults (Except Anorectal Infections In Men): 100 mg, by mouth, twice a day for 7 days. As an alternate single visit dose, administer 300 mg stat followed in one hour by a second 300 mg dose. The dose may be administered with food, including milk or carbonated beverage, as required.

Uncomplicated urethral, endocervical, or rectal infection in adults caused by *Chlamydia trachomatis:* 100 mg by mouth twice a day for 7 days.

Nongonococcal urethritis (NGU) caused by *C. trachomatis or U.urealyticum:*100 mg by mouth twice a day for 7 days.

Syphilis-Early: Patients who are allergic to penicillin should be treated with doxycycline 100 mg by mouth twice a day for 2 weeks. Syphilis of more than one year's duration: Patients who are allergic to penicillin should be treated with doxycycline 100 mg by mouth twice a day for 4 weeks.

Acute epididymo-orchitis caused by *N. gonorrhoeae:* 100 mg, by mouth, twice a day for at least 10 days.

Acute epididymo-orchitis caused by *C. trachomatis:* 100 mg, by mouth, twice a day for at least 10 days.

For Prophylaxis Of Malaria: For adults, the recommended dose is 100 mg daily. For children over 8 years of age, the recommended dose is 2 mg/kg given once daily up to the adult dose. Prophylaxis should begin 1-2 days before travel to the malarious area and for 4 weeks after the traveler leaves the malarious area.

All products are to be stored below 86°F (30°C) and dispensed in tight, light-resistant containers (USP). The unit dose packs should also be stored in a dry place.

IV

Note: Rapid administration is to be avoided. Parenteral therapy is indicated only when oral therapy is not indicated. Oral therapy should be instituted as soon as possible. If IV therapy is given over prolonged periods of time, thrombophlebitis may result.

THE USUAL DOSAGE AND FREQUENCY OF ADMINISTRATION OF DOXYCYCLINE IV (100-200 MG/DAY) DIFFERS FROM THAT OF THE OTHER TETRACYCLINES (1-2 G/DAY). EXCEEDING THE RECOMMENDED DOSAGE MAY RESULT IN AN INCREASED INCIDENCE OF SIDE EFFECTS.

Studies to date have indicated that doxycycline at the usual recommended doses does not lead to excessive accumulation of the antibiotic inpatients with renal impairment.

Adults: The usual dosage of doxycycline IV is 200 mg on the first day of treatment administered in one or two infusions. Subsequent daily dosage is 100 to 200 mg depending upon the severity of infection, with 200 mg administered in one or two infusions.

In the treatment of primary and secondary syphilis, the recommended dosage is 300 mg daily for at least 10 days.

For Children Above Eight Years Of Age: The recommended dosage schedule for children weighing 100 pounds or less is 2 mg/lb of body weight on the first day of treatment, administered in one or two infusions, depending on the severity of the infection. For children over 100 pounds the usual dose should be used (see WARNINGS, Usage in Children.)

General: The duration of infusion may vary with the dose (100-200 mg per day), but it is usually one to four hours. A recommended minimum infusion time for 100 mg of a 0.5 mg/ml solution is one hour. Therapy should be continued for at least 24-48 hours after the symptoms and fever have subsided. The therapeutic antibacterial serum activity will usually persist for 24 hours following recommended dosage.

IV solutions should not be injected intramuscularly or subcutaneously. Caution should be taken to avoid the inadvertent introduction of the IV solution into the adjacent soft tissue.

PREPARATION OF SOLUTION

To prepare a solution containing 10 mg/ml, the contents of the vial should be reconstituted with 10 ml (for the 100 mg/vial container) or 20 ml (for the 200 mg/vial container) of Sterile Water for Injection or any of the ten IV infusion solutions listed below. Each 100 mg of doxycycline (*i.e.,* withdraw entire solution from the 100 mg vial) is further diluted with 100 ml to 1000 ml of the IV solutions listed below. Each 200 mg of doxycycline (*i.e.,* withdraw entire solution from the 200 mg vial) is further diluted with 200 to 2000 ml of the following IV solutions:

1. Sodium Chloride Injection, USP

2. 5% Dextrose Injection, USP

3. Ringer's Injection, USP

4. Invert Sugar, 10% in Water

5. Lactated Ringer's Injection, USP

6. Dextrose 5% in Lactated Ringer's

7. Normosol-M in D5-W (Abbott)

8. Normosol-R in D5-W (Abbott)

9. Plasma-Lyte 56 in 5% Dextrose (Travenol)

10. Plasma-Lyte 148 in 5% Dextrose (Travenol)

This will result in desired concentrations of 0.1 to 1.0 mg/ml. Concentrations lower than 0.1 mg/ml or higher than 1.0 mg/ml are not recommended.

STABILITY

Doxycycline IV is stable for 48 hours in solution when diluted with Sodium Chloride Injection, USP, or 5% Dextrose Injection, USP, to concentrations between 1.0 mg/ml and 0.1 mg/ml and stored at 25°C. Doxycycline IV in these solutions is stable under fluorescent light for 48 hours, but must be protected from direct sunlight during storage and infusion. Reconstituted solutions (1.0 to 0.1 mg/ml) may be stored up to 72 hours prior to start of infusion if refrigerated and protected from sunlight and artificial light. Infusion must then be completed within 12 hours. Solutions must be used within these time periods or discarded.

Doxycycline IV, when diluted with Ringer's Injection, USP or Invert Sugar, 10% in water, or Normosol-M in D5-W (Abbott) or Normosol-R in D5-W (Abbott), or Plasma-Lyte 56 in 5% Dextrose (Travenol), or Plasma-Lyte 148 in 5% Dextrose (Travenol) to a concentration between 1.0 mg/ml and 0.1 mg/ml, must be completely infused in 12 hours after reconstitution to ensure adequate stability. During infusion, the solution must be protected from direct sunlight. Reconstituted solutions (1.0 to 0.1 mg/ml) may be stored up to 72 hours prior to start of infusion if refrigerated and protected from sun and artificial light. Infusion must then be completed within 12 hours. Solutions must be used within these time periods or be discarded.

DOSAGE AND ADMINISTRATION: *(cont'd)*

When diluted with Lactated Ringer's Injection, USP, or Dextrose 5% in Lactated Ringer's, infusion of the solution (ca. 1.0 mg/ml) or lower concentrations (not less than 0.1 mg.ml) must be completed within six hours after reconstitution to ensure adequate stability. During infusion, the solution must be protected from direct sunlight. Solutions must be used within this period or discarded.

Solutions of doxycycline hyclate for injection at a concentration of 10 mg/ml in Sterile Water for Injection, when frozen immediately after reconstitution are stable for 8 weeks when stored at -20°C. If the product is warmed, care should be taken to avoid heating it after the thawing is complete. Once thawed the solution should not be refrozen.

ANIMAL PHARMACOLOGY:

Hyperpigmentation of the thyroid has been produced by members of the tetracycline class in the following species: in rats by oxytetracycline, doxycycline, tetracycline PO_4, and methacycline; in minipigs by doxycycline, minocycline, tetracycline PO_4, and methacycline; in dogs by doxycycline and minocycline; in monkeys by minocycline.

Minocycline, tetracycline PO_4, methacycline, doxycycline, tetracycline base, oxytetracycline HCl, and tetracycline HCl were goitrogenic in rats fed a low iodine diet. This goitrogenic effect was accompanied by high radioactive iodine uptake. Administration of minocycline also produced a large goiter with high radioiodine uptake in rats fed a relatively high iodine diet.

Treatment of various animal species with this class of drugs has also resulted in the induction of thyroid hyperplasia in the following: in rats and dogs (minocycline); in chickens (chlortetracycline); and in rats and mice (oxytetracycline). Adrenal gland hyperplasia has been observed in goats and rats treated with oxytetracycline.

REFERENCES:

1. National Committee for Clinical Laboratory Standards,*Performance Standards for Antimicrobial Disk Susceptibility Tests,* Fourth Edition. Approved Standard NCCLS Document M2-A4, Vol. 10, No. 7 NCCLS, Villanova, PA, April 1990. **2.** National Committee for Clinical Laboratory Standards,*Methods for Dilution Antimicrobial Susceptibility Tests for Bacteria that Grow Aerobically,* Second Edition. Approved Standard NCCLS Document M7-A2, Vol. 10, No. 8 NCCLS, Villanova, PA, April 1990.(Syrup, Capsules, Oral Suspension, and Tablets: Pfizer, 4/93, 69-1680-00-5)(IV: Roerig, 3/91, 70-1940-00-2)

PATIENT INFORMATION:

Doxycycline is a tetracycline antibiotic used to treat infections. This antibiotic should not be used by pregnant women or by children under 8 years of age.

Notify your physician if you are nursing.

Shake the suspension well before each use.

Do not take this medication if it has expired; outdated doxycycline may be toxic.

Take at regular intervals and complete the entire course of therapy.

This medication may be taken with or without meals.

Do not take antacids, laxatives, dairy products, or iron-containing products within two to three hours of taking doxycycline.

Doxycycline may cause increased sensitivity to sunlight.

Use sunscreens and wear protective clothing until degree of sensitivity is determined.

This antibiotic may decrease the effectiveness of birth control pills; use another form of birth control while taking this medication.

HOW SUPPLIED - RATED THERAPEUTICALLY EQUIVALENT:

Capsule, Gelatin - Oral - 50 mg

50's	$2.88	DOXYCHEL HYCLATE, Rachelle Labs	00196-0552-02
50's	$4.88	Doxycycline Hyclate Cap 50, Genetco	00302-2350-48
50's	$6.30	Doxycycline Hyclate, IDE-Interstate	00814-2663-08
50's	$7.45	Doxycycline Hyclate, Qualitest Pharms	00603-3480-19
50's	$8.02	Doxycycline Hyclate, Geneva Pharms	00781-2525-50
50's	$8.25	Doxycycline Hyclate, Voluntary Hosp	53258-0422-04
50's	$9.00	Doxycycline Hyclate, West Ward Pharm	00143-3141-50
50's	$9.50	Doxy-D, Dunhall Pharms	00217-0804-50
50's	$10.70	Doxycycline Hyclate, Major Pharms	00904-0427-51
50's	$11.74	Doxycycline Hyclate, Warner Chilcott	00047-0829-19
50's	$11.90	Doxycycline Hyclate, United Res	00677-0598-02
50's	$11.90	Doxycycline Hyclate, Mutual Pharm	53489-0118-02
50's	$11.95	Doxycycline Hyclate, Rugby	00536-0280-06
50's	$12.50	Doxycycline Hyclate, Zenith Labs	00172-2984-48
50's	$12.50	Doxycyline Hyclate, Goldline Labs	00182-1090-19
50's	$12.50	Doxycycline Hyclate, Mylan	00378-0145-89
50's	$12.60	Doxycycline Hyclate, Schein Pharm (US)	00364-2032-50
50's	$12.60	Doxycycline Hyclate, Halsey Drug	00879-0525-50
50's	$13.23	Doxycycline Hyclate, HL Moore Drug Exch	00839-1288-04
50's	$14.65	Doxycycline Hyclate, Martec Pharms	52555-0433-00
50's	$15.93	Doxycycline Hyclate, Aligen Independ	00405-4378-50
50's	$25.51	Doxycycline Hyclate, Lederle Pharm	00005-3767-18
50's	$28.95	Doxycycline Hyclate, Parmed Pharms	00349-1007-50
50's	$37.25	Doxycycline Hyclate, Teva	00093-0642-53
50's	$37.36	Doxycycline Hyclate, Bristol Myers Squibb	00003-8708-01
50's	$37.36	Doxycycline Hyclate, Bristol Myers Squibb	00003-8709-01
50's	$85.65	VIBRAMYCIN HYCLATE, Pfizer Labs	00069-0940-50
100's	$7.00	Doxychel Hyclate, Rachelle Labs	00196-0552-04
100's	$19.20	Doxycycline Hcl, Raway	00686-0148-20
100's	$26.58	Doxycycline Hyclate, Voluntary Hosp	53258-0422-13
100's	$51.53	Doxycycline Hyclate, Schein Pharm (US)	00364-2032-90
500's	$75.50	Doxycycline Hyclate, Halsey Drug	00879-0525-05
500's	$78.60	Doxycycline Hyclate, Mutual Pharm	53489-0118-05
500's	$108.50	Doxycycline Hyclate, Zenith Labs	00172-2984-70

Capsule, Gelatin - Oral - 100 mg

20's	$4.40	Doxycycline Hyclate, Major Pharms	00904-0428-95
50's	$8.35	Doxycycline Hyclate, Qualitest Pharms	00603-3481-19
50's	$8.70	Doxycycline, IDE-Interstate	00814-2665-08
50's	$9.68	Doxycycline Hyclate, Geneva Pharms	00781-2522-50
50's	$12.69	Doxycycline Hyclate, Voluntary Hosp	53258-0416-04
50's	$17.50	Doxycycline Hyclate, Major Pharms	00904-0428-51
50's	$17.95	Doxycycline Hyclate, West Ward Pharm	00143-3142-50
50's	$18.40	Doxycycline Hyclate, Warner Chilcott	00047-0830-19
50's	$19.20	Doxycycline Hyclate, United Res	00677-0562-02
50's	$19.20	Doxycycline Hyclate, Mutual Pharm	53489-0119-02
50's	$19.95	DOXY-CAPS, Edwards Pharms	00485-0041-50
50's	$21.65	Doxycycline Hyclate, Martec Pharms	52555-0434-00
50's	$23.50	Doxycycline Hyclate, Schein Pharm (US)	00364-2033-50
50's	$23.95	Doxycycline Hyclate, Zenith Labs	00172-2985-48
50's	$23.95	Doxycycline Hyclate, Goldline Labs	00182-1035-19
50's	$23.95	Doxycycline Hyclate, Mylan	00378-0148-89
50's	$24.05	Doxycycline Hyclate, Halsey Drug	00879-0526-50
50's	$24.82	Doxycycline Hyclate, Aligen Independ	00405-4377-50
50's	$25.25	Doxycycline Hyclate, HL Moore Drug Exch	00839-1289-04
50's	$29.65	Doxycycline Hyclate, Parmed Pharms	00349-1008-50

HOW SUPPLIED - RATED THERAPEUTICALLY EQUIVALENT: *(cont'd)*

50's	$29.85	Doxycycline Hyclate, Lederle Pharm	00005-3768-18
50's	$67.10	Doxycycline Hyclate, Teva	00093-0653-53
50's	$67.10	Doxycycline Hyclate, Rugby	00536-0230-06
50's	$67.14	Doxycycline Hyclate, Bristol Myers Squibb	00003-0814-05
50's	$92.92	Doxycycline Hyclate, H.C.F.A. F F P	99999-1113-01
50's	$102.50	Doxycycline, Major Pharms	00904-0429-51
50's	$153.97	VIBRAMYCIN HYCLATE, Pfizer Labs	00069-0950-50
100's	$12.02	Doxycycline Hyclate, US Trading	56126-0019-11
100's	$20.00	Doxycycline Hcl, Raway	00686-0522-20
100's	$29.70	Doxycycline Hyclate, Voluntary Hosp	53258-0416-13
100's	$32.82	Doxycycline Hyclate, Major Pharms	00904-0428-61
100's	$39.00	Doxycycline Hyclate, West Ward Pharm	00143-3142-25
100's	$111.43	Doxycycline Hyclate, Schein Pharm (US)	00364-2033-90
100's	$121.90	Doxycycline Hyclate, Goldline Labs	00182-1035-89
100's	$123.13	Doxycycline Hyclate, Vangard Labs	00615-0385-13
100's	$309.12	VIBRAMYCIN HYCLATE, Pfizer Labs	00069-0950-41
200's	$76.25	Doxycycline Hyclate, Rugby	00536-0230-32
200's	$371.70	Doxycycline Hyclate, H.C.F.A. F F P	99999-1113-02
500's	$69.95	Doxycycline Hyclate, Balan	00304-0118-05
500's	$75.00	Doxycycline Hyclate, West Ward Pharm	00143-3142-05
500's	$80.63	Doxycycline, IDE-Interstate	00814-2665-28
500's	$82.95	Doxycycline Hyclate, Geneva Pharms	00781-2522-05
500's	$94.25	Doxycycline Hyclate, Major Pharms	00904-0428-40
500's	$140.11	Doxycycline Hyclate, Qualitest Pharms	00603-3481-28
500's	$149.00	Doxycycline Hyclate, United Res	00677-0562-05
500's	$149.00	Doxycycline Hyclate, Mutual Pharm	53489-0119-05
500's	$185.20	Doxycycline Hyclate, Martec Pharms	52555-0434-05
500's	$198.00	Doxycycline Hyclate, Aligen Independ	00405-4377-02
500's	$204.50	Doxycycline Hyclate, Warner Chilcott	00047-0830-30
500's	$204.50	Doxycycline Hyclate, Zenith Labs	00172-2985-70
500's	$204.50	Doxycycline Hyclate, Goldline Labs	00182-1035-05
500's	$210.50	Doxycycline Hyclate, Parmed Pharms	00349-1008-05
500's	$215.18	Doxycycline Hyclate, Schein Pharm (US)	00364-2033-05
500's	$215.55	Doxycycline Hyclate, Mylan	00378-0148-05
500's	$216.50	Doxycycline Hyclate, Halsey Drug	00879-0526-05
500's	$227.33	Doxycycline Hyclate, HL Moore Drug Exch	00839-1289-12
500's	$269.48	Doxycycline Hyclate, Lederle Pharm	00005-3768-31
500's	$580.00	Doxycycline Hyclate, Teva	00093-0653-05
500's	$580.00	Doxycycline Hyclate, Rugby	00536-0230-05
500's	$581.65	Doxycycline Hyclate, Bristol Myers Squibb	00003-0814-01
500's	$929.25	Doxycycline Hyclate, H.C.F.A. F F P	99999-1113-03
500's	$1333.29	VIBRAMYCIN HYCLATE, Pfizer Labs	00069-0950-73

Capsule, Gelatin, Coated Pellets - Oral - 100 mg

50's	$86.32	Doxycycline Hyclate, Warner Chilcott	00047-0091-19
50's	$86.32	Doxycycline Hyclate, Harber Pharm	51432-0643-01
50's	$90.00	Doxycycline Hyclate, Sidmak Labs	50111-0377-05
50's	$92.50	Doxycycline, United Res	00677-1409-02
50's	$92.92	Doxycycline Hyclate, H.C.F.A. F F P	99999-1113-04
50's	$93.79	Doxycycline Hyclate, Purepac Pharm	00228-2598-07
50's	$128.04	DORYX, Parke-Davis	00071-0838-19

Injection, Solution - Intravenous - 100 mg/vial

1's	$16.70	Doxycycline Hyclate, Elkins Sinn	00641-2292-41
5's	$88.72	VIBRAMYCIN IV, Roerig	00049-0960-77
20 ml	$73.75	Doxy 100, Fujisawa USA	00469-1300-30

Injection, Solution - Intravenous - 200 mg/vial

1's	$33.69	Doxy-200, Fujisawa USA	00469-1640-40

Powder, Reconstitution - Oral - 25 mg/5ml

60 ml	$9.39	VIBRAMYCIN, Pfizer Labs	00069-0970-65

Tablet, Plain Coated - Oral - 100 mg

50's	$5.62	Doxycycline Hyclate, United Res	00677-0799-02
50's	$5.62	Doxycycline Hyclate, Geneva Pharms	00781-1075-50
50's	$5.62	Doxycycline Hyclate, H.C.F.A. F F P	99999-1113-05
50's	$10.43	Doxycycline Hyclate, IDE-Interstate	00814-2660-08
50's	$17.50	Doxycycline Hyclate, Major Pharms	00904-0430-51
50's	$17.70	Doxycycline Hyclate, Mova Pharms	55370-0814-05
50's	$17.78	Doxycycline Hyclate, Warner Chilcott	00047-0813-19
50's	$18.45	Doxycycline Hyclate, Qualitest Pharms	00603-3482-19
50's	$19.20	Doxycycline Hyclate, Mutual Pharm	53489-0120-02
50's	$19.39	Doxycycline Hyclate, Schein Pharm (US)	00364-2063-50
50's	$21.65	Doxycycline Hyclate, Martec Pharms	52555-0229-00
50's	$22.75	Doxycycline Hyclate, Teva	00093-0750-53
50's	$22.95	Doxycycline Hyclate, Zenith Labs	00172-3626-48
50's	$22.95	Doxycycline Hyclate, Goldline Labs	00182-1535-19
50's	$22.95	Doxycycline Hyclate, Mylan	00378-0167-89
50's	$24.05	Doxycycline Hyclate, Halsey Drug	00879-0725-50
50's	$24.99	Doxycycline Hyclate, Purepac Pharm	00228-2187-05
50's	$25.01	Doxycycline Hyclate, Aligen Independ	00405-4379-50
50's	$25.25	Doxycycline Hyclate, HL Moore Drug Exch	00839-6641-04
50's	$28.95	Doxycycline Hyclate, Parmed Pharms	00349-1100-50
50's	$29.85	Doxycycline Hyclate, Lederle Pharm	00005-3116-18
50's	$29.85	Doxycycline Hyclate, Rugby	00536-0340-06
50's	$67.14	Doxycyline Hyclate, Bristol Myers Squibb	00003-0812-40
50's	$98.35	BIO-TAB, Universal Labs	52906-1001-01
50's	$153.97	VIBRA-TABS, Pfizer Labs	00069-0990-50
100's	$19.00	Doxycycline Hcl, Raway	00686-0554-20
100's	$32.82	Doxycycline Hyclate, Major Pharms	00904-0430-61
100's	$111.75	Doxycycline Hyclate, Schein Pharm (US)	00364-2063-90
100's	$121.90	Doxycycline Hyclate, Goldline Labs	00182-1535-89
100's	$309.12	VIBRA-TABS, Pfizer Labs	00069-0990-41
200's	$22.50	Doxycycline Hyclate, H.C.F.A. F F P	99999-1113-06
200's	$31.44	Doxycycline Hyclate, Rugby	00536-0340-32
500's	$56.25	Doxycycline Hyclate, Zenith Labs	00172-3626-70
500's	$56.25	Doxycycline Hyclate, Parmed Pharms	00349-1100-05
500's	$56.25	Doxycycline Hyclate, United Res	00677-0799-05
500's	$56.25	Doxycycline Hyclate, Geneva Pharms	00781-1075-05
500's	$56.25	Doxycycline Hyclate, H.C.F.A. F F P	99999-1113-07
500's	$63.75	Doxycycline Hyclate, Major Pharms	00904-0430-40
500's	$140.55	Doxycycline Hyclate, Goldline Labs	00182-1535-05
500's	$142.40	Doxycycline Hyclate, Qualitest Pharms	00603-3482-28
500's	$149.00	Doxycycline Hyclate, Mutual Pharm	53489-0120-05
500's	$176.63	Doxycycline Hyclate, Schein Pharm (US)	00364-2063-05
500's	$184.22	Doxycycline Hyclate, Aligen Independ	00405-4379-02
500's	$185.20	Doxycycline Hyclate, Martec Pharms	52555-0229-05
500's	$204.50	Doxycycline Hyclate, Warner Chilcott	00047-0813-30
500's	$204.50	Doxycycline Hyclate, Teva	00093-0750-05
500's	$206.55	Doxycycline Hyclate, Mylan	00378-0167-05
500's	$216.50	Doxycycline Hyclate, Halsey Drug	00879-0725-05
500's	$227.33	Doxycycline Hyclate, HL Moore Drug Exch	00839-6641-12
500's	$269.48	Doxycycline Hyclate, Lederle Pharm	00005-3116-31

HOW SUPPLIED - RATED THERAPEUTICALLY EQUIVALENT: *(cont'd)*

500's	$269.48	Doxycycline Hyclate, Rugby	00536-0340-05
500's	$338.70	Doxycycline Hyclate, Amer Preferred	53445-1535-05
500's	$581.65	Doxycyline Hyclate, Bristol Myers Squibb	00003-0812-60
500's	$1333.29	VIBRA-TABS, Pfizer Labs	00069-0990-73

HOW SUPPLIED - NOT RATED EQUIVALENT:

Capsule, Gelatin - Oral - 50 mg

100's	$98.64	MONODOX, Oclassen Pharms	55515-0260-06

Capsule, Gelatin - Oral - 100 mg

50's	$18.70	Doxycycline Hyclate, Mova Pharms	55370-0813-05
50's	$80.52	MONODOX, Oclassen Pharms	55515-0259-04
250's	$387.00	MONODOX, Oclassen Pharms	55515-0259-07
500's	$147.80	Doxycycline Hyclate, Mova Pharms	55370-0813-08

Solution - Topical - 0.05%

25 ml	$18.72	CORMAX, Oclassen Pharms	55515-0430-25
50 ml	$36.02	CORMAX, Oclassen Pharms	55515-0430-50

Syrup - Oral - 50 mg/5ml

480 ml	**$142.48**	**VIBRAMYCIN CALCIUM, Pfizer Labs**	**00069-0971-93**

DRONABINOL *(001116)*

CATEGORIES: AIDS Related Complex; Anorexia; Antiemetics; Cancer; Chemotherapy; Gastrointestinal Drugs; Marijuana; Nausea; Nausea and Vomiting; Orphan Drugs; Vomiting; Motion Sickness*; Vertigo/Motion Sickness/Vomiting*; Weight Loss*; Pregnancy Category B; DEA Class CII; FDA Approved 1985 May
* Indication not approved by the FDA

BRAND NAMES: Marezine; **Marinol**

DESCRIPTION:

Dronabinol is a cannabinoid designated chemically as (6a*R-trans*)-6a,7,8,10a-tetrahydro-6,6,9-trimethyl-3-pentyl-6*H*-dibenzo(*b,d*)pyran-1-ol.

Empirical Formula: $C_{21}H_{30}O_2$ (molecular weight = 314.7)

Dronabinol, delta-9-tetrahydrocannabinol (delta-9-THC), is naturally occurring and has been extracted from *Cannabis sativa* L. (marijuana).

Dronabinol is also chemically synthesized and is a light-yellow resinous oil that is sticky at room temperature and hardens upon refrigeration. Dronabinol is insoluble in water and is formulated in sesame oil. It has a pK_a of 10.6 and an octanol-water partition coefficient: 6,000:1 at pH 7.

Capsules For Oral Administration: Marinol is supplied as round, soft gelatin capsules containing either 2.5 mg, 5 mg, or 10 mg dronabinol. Each Marinol capsule is formulated with the following inactive ingredients: sesame oil, gelatin, glycerin, methylparaben, propylparaben, and titanium dioxide.

CLINICAL PHARMACOLOGY:

Dronabinol is an orally active cannabinoid which, like other cannabinoids, has complex effects on the central nervous system (CNS), including central sympathomimetic activity. Cannabinoid receptors have been discovered in neural tissues. These receptors may play a role in mediating the effects of dronabinol and other cannabinoids.

PHARMACODYNAMICS

Dronabinol-induced sympathomimetic activity may result in tachycardia and/or conjunctival injection. Its effects on blood pressure are inconsistent, but occasional subjects have experienced orthostatic hypotension and/or syncope upon abrupt standing.

Dronabinol also demonstrates reversible effects on appetite, mood, cognition, memory, and perception. These phenomena appear to be dose related, increasing in frequency with higher dosages, and subject to great interpatient variability.

After oral administration, dronabinol has an onset of action of approximately 0.5 to 1 hours and peak effect at 2 to 4 hours. Duration of action for psychoactive effects is 4 to 6 hours, but the appetite stimulant effect of dronabinol may continue for 24 hours or longer after administration.

Tachyplaxis and tolerance develop to some of the pharmacologic effects of dronabinol and other cannabinoids with chronic use, suggesting an indirect effect on sympathetic neurons. In a study of the pharmacodynamics of chronic dronabinol exposure, healthy male volunteers (N=12) received 210 mg/day dronabinol, administered orally in divided doses; for 16 days. An initial tachycardia induced by dronabinol was replaced successively by normal sinus rhythm and then bradycardia. A decrease in supine blood pressure, made worse by standing, was also observed initially. These volunteers developed tolerance to the cardiovascular and subjective adverse CNS effects of dronabinol within 12 days of treatment initiation.

Tachyplaxis and tolerance do not, however, appear to develop to the appetite stimulant effect of dronabinol. In studies involving patients with Acquired Immune Deficiency Syndrome (AIDS), the appetite stimulant effect of dronabinol has been sustained for up to five months in clinical trials, at dosages ranging from 2.5 mg/day to 20 mg/day.

PHARMACOKINETICS

Absorption and Distribution: Dronabinol is almost completely absorbed (90 to 95 %) after single oral doses. Due to the combined effects of first—pass hepatic metabolism and high lipid solubility, only 10 to 20% of the administered dose reaches the systemic circulation. Dronabinol has a large apparent volume of distribution, approximately 10 l/kg, because of its lipid solubility. The plasma protein binding of dronabinol and its metabolites is approximately 97%.

The elimination phase of dronabinol can be described using a two compartment model with an initial (alpha) half-life of about 4 hours and a terminal (beta) half-life of 25 to 36 hours. Because of its large volume of distribution, dronabinol and its metabolites may be excreted at low levels for prolonged periods of time.

Metabolism: Dronabinol undergoes extensive first-pass hepatic metabolism, primarily by microsomal hydroxylation, yielding both active and inactive metabolites. Dronabinol and its principal active metabolite, 11-OH-delta-9-THC, are present in approximately equal concentrations in plasma. Concentrations of both parent drug and metabolite peak at approximately 2 to 4 hours after oral dosing and decline over several days. Values for clearance average about 0.2 l/kg/hr, but are highly variable due to the complexity of cannabinoid distribution.

Elimination: Dronabinol and its biotransformation products are excreted in both feces and urine. Biliary excretion is the major route of elimination with about half of a radiolabeled oral dose being recovered from the feces within 72 hours as contrasted with 10 to 15% recovered from urine. Less than 5% of an oral dose is recovered unchanged in the feces.

Following single dose administration, low levels of dronabinol metabolites have been detected for more than 5 weeks in the urine and feces.

CLINICAL PHARMACOLOGY: *(cont'd)*

In a study of dronabinol involving AIDS patients, urinary cannabinoid/creatinine concentration ratios were studied biweekly over a six week period. The urinary cannabinoid/creatinine ratio was closely correlated with dose. No increase in the cannabinoid/creatinine ratio was observed after the first two weeks of treatment, indicating that steady- state cannabinoid levels had been reached. This conclusion is consistent with prediction based on the observed terminal half-life of dronabinol.

Special Populations: The pharmacokinetic profile of dronabinol has not been investigated in either pediatric or geriatric patients.

CLINICAL STUDIES:

APPETITE STIMULATION

The appetite stimulant effect of dronabinol in the treatment of AIDS-related anorexia associated with weight loss was studied in a randomized, double-blind, placebo-controlled study involving 139 patients. The initial dosage of dronabinol in all patients was 5 mg/day, administered in doses of 2.5 mg one hour before lunch and one hour before supper. In pilot studies, early morning administration of dronabinol appeared to have been associated with an increased frequency of adverse experiences, as compared to dosing later in the day. The effect of dronabinol on appetite, weight, mood, and nausea was measured at scheduled intervals during the six-week treatment period. Side effects (feeling high, dizziness, confusion, somnolence) occurred in 13 of 72 patients (18%) at this dosage level and the dosage was reduced to 2.5 mg/day, administered as a single dose at supper or bedtime.

As compared to placebo, dronabinol treatment resulted in a statistically significant improvement in appetite as measured by visual analog scale (For a graphic representation, please refer to the manufacturer's original package insert). Trends toward improved body weight and mood, and decreases in nausea were also seen.

After completing the 6-week study, patients were allowed to continue treatment with dronabinol in an open-label study, in which there was a sustained improvement in appetite.

ANTIEMETIC

dronabinol (dronabinol) treatment of chemotherapy-induced emesis was evaluated in 454 patients with cancer, who received a total of 750 courses of treatment of various malignancies. The antiemetic efficacy of dronabinol was greatest in patients receiving cytotoxic therapy with MOPP for Hodgkin's and non-Hodgkin's lymphomas. Dronabinol dosages ranged from 2.5 mg/day to 40 mg/day, administered in equally divided doses every four to six hours (four times daily). As indicated in the following table (TABLE 1), escalating the dronabinol dose above 7 mg/m^2 increased the frequency of adverse experiences, with no additional antiemetic benefit.

TABLE 1 Dronabinol Dose: Response Frequency and Adverse Experiences*
(N=750 Treatment Courses)

	Response Frequency (%)			Adverse Events Frequency (%)		
Marinol Dose	**Complete**	**Partial**	**Poor**	**Complete**	**Partial**	**Poor**
< 7 mg/m^2	36	32	32	23	65	12
> 7 mg/m^2	33	31	36	13	58	28

* Nondysphoric events consisted of drowsiness, tachycardia etc.

Combination antiemetic therapy with dronabinol and a phenothiazine (prochlorperazine) may result in synergistic or additive antiemetic effects and attenuate the toxicities associated with each of the agents.

INDIVIDUALIZATION OF DOSES

The pharmacologic effects of dronabinol are dose-related and subject to considerable interpatient variability. Therefore, dosage individualization is critical in achieving the maximum benefit of dronabinol treatment.

APPETITE STIMULATION

In the clinical trials, the majority of patients were treated with 5 mg/day dronabinol, although the dosages ranged from 2.5 to 20 mg/day.

For An Adult:

1. Begin with 2.5 mg before lunch and 2.5 mg before supper. If CNS symptoms (feeling high, dizziness, confusion, somnolence) do occur, they usually resolve in 1 to 3 days with continued dosage.

2. If CNS symptoms are severe or persistent, reduce the dose to 2.5 mg before supper. If symptoms continue to be a problem, taking the single dose in the evening or at bedtime may reduce their severity.

3. When adverse effects are absent or minimal and further therapeutic effect is desired, increase the dose to 2.5 mg before lunch and 5 mg before supper or 5 and 5 mg. Although most patients respond to 2.5 mg twice daily, 10 mg twice daily has been tolerated in about half of the patients in appetite stimulation studies.

The pharmacologic effects of dronabinol are reversible upon treatment cessation.

ANTIEMETIC

Most patients respond to 5 mg three or four times daily. Dosage may be escalated during a chemotherapy cycle or at subsequent cycles, based upon initial results. Therapy should be initiated at the lowest recommended dosage and titrated to clinical response. Administration of dronabinol with phenothiazines, such as prochlorperazine, has resulted in improved efficacy as compared to either drug alone, without additional toxicity.

PEDIATRICS

Dronabinol is not recommended for AIDS-related anorexia in pediatric patients because it has not been studied in this population. The pediatric dosage for the treatment of chemotherapy-induced emesis is the same as in adults. Caution is recommended in prescribing dronabinol in children because of the psychoactive effects.

GERIATRICS

Caution is advised in prescribing dronabinol in elderly patients because they are generally more sensitive to the psychoactive effects of drugs. In antiemetic studies, no difference in tolerance or efficacy was apparent in patients > 55 years old.

INDICATIONS AND USAGE:

Dronabinol Is Indicated For The Treatment Of:

1. Anorexia associated with weight loss in patients with AIDS

2. Nausea and vomiting associated with cancer chemotherapy in patients who have failed to respond adequately to conventional antiemetic treatments.

CONTRAINDICATIONS:

Dronabinol is contraindicated in any patient who has a history of hypersensitivity to any cannabinoid or sesame oil.

WARNINGS:

Dronabinol is a medication with a potential for abuse. Physicians and pharmacists should use the same care in prescribing and accounting for dronabinol as they would with morphine or other drugs controlled under Schedule II (CII) of the Controlled Substances Act. Because of the risk of diversion, it is recommended that prescriptions be limited to the amount necessary for the period between clinic visits.

Patients receiving treatment with dronabinol should be specifically warned not to drive, operate machinery, or engage in any hazardous activity until it is established that they are able to tolerate the drug and to perform such tasks safely.

PRECAUTIONS:

GENERAL

The risk/benefit ratio of Dronabinol use should be carefully evaluated in patients with the following medical conditions because of individual variation in response and tolerance to the effects of dronabinol.

Dronabinol should be used with caution in patients with cardiac disorders because of occasional hypotension, possible hypertension, syncope, or tachycardia (see CLINICAL PHARMACOLOGY).

Dronabinol should be used with caution in patients with a history of substance abuse, including alcohol abuse or dependence, because they may be more prone to abuse dronabinol as well. Multiple substance abuse is common, and marijuana, which contains the same active compound, is a frequently abused substance.

Dronabinol should be used with caution and careful psychiatric monitoring in patients with mania, depression, or schizophrenia because dronabinol may exacerbate these illnesses.

Dronabinol should be used with caution in patients receiving concomitant therapy with sedatives, hypnotics, or other psychoactive drugs because of the potential for additive or synergistic CNS effects.

Dronabinol should be used with caution in pregnant patients, nursing mothers, or pediatric patients because it has not been studied in these patient populations.

Dronabinol should be used with caution for treatment of anorexia and weight loss in elderly patients with AIDS because they may be more sensitive to the psychoactive effects and because its use in these patients has not been studied.

INFORMATION FOR THE PATIENT

Patients receiving treatment with Dronabinol should be alerted to the potential for additive central nevous system depression if dronabinol is used concomitantly with alcohol or other CNS depressants such as benzodiazepines and barbiturates.

Patients receiving treatment with dronabinol should be specifically warned not to drive, operate machinery, or engage in any hazardous activity until it is established that they are able to tolerate the drug and to performe such tasks safely.

Patients using dronabinol should be advised of possible changes in mood and other adverse behavioral effects of the drug so as to avoid panic in the event of such manifestations. Patients should remain under the supervision of a responsible adult during initial use of dronabinol and following dosage adjustments.

CARCINOGENESIS, MUTAGENESIS, AND IMPAIRMENT OF FERTILITY

Carcinogenicity studies have not been performed with dronabinol. Mutagenicity testing of dronabinol was negative in an Ames test. In a long-term study (77 days) in rats, oral administration of dronabinol at doses of 30 to 150 mg/m^2, equivalent to 0.3 to 1.5 times maximum recommended human dose (MRHD) of 90 mg/m^2/day in cancer patients or 2 to 10 times MRHD of 15 mg/m^2/day in AIDS patients, reduced ventral prostate, seminal vesicle; and epididymal weights and caused a decrease in seminal fluid volume. Decreases in spermatogenesis, number of developing germ cells, and number of Leydig cells in the testis were also observed. However, sperm count, mating success, and testosterone levels were not affected. The significance of these animal findings in humans is not known.

PREGNANCY CATEGORY C

Reproduction studies with dronabinol have been performed in mice at 15 to 450 mg/m^2, equivalent to 0.2 to 5 times maximum recommended human dose (MRHD) of 90 mg/m^2/day in cancer patients or 1 to 30 times MRHD of 15 mg/m^2/day in AIDS patients, and in rats at 74 to 295 mg/m^2 (equivalent to 0.8 to 3 times MRHD of 90 mg/m^2 in cancer patients or 5 to 20 times MRHD of 15 mg/m^2/day in AIDS patients). These studies have revealed no evidence of teratogenicity due to dronabinol. At these dosages in mice and rats, dronabinol decreased maternal weight gain and number of viable pups and increased fetal mortality and early resorptions. Such effects were dose dependent and less apparent at lower doses which produced less maternal toxicity. There are no adequate and well-controlled studies in pregnant women. Dronabinol should be used only if the potential benefit justifies the potential risk to the fetus.

NURSING MOTHERS

Use of dronabinol is not recommended in nursing mothers since, in addition to the secretion of HIV virus in breast milk, dronabinol is concentrated in and secreted in human breast milk and is absorbed by the nursing baby.

DRUG INTERACTIONS:

In studies involving patients with AIDS and/or cancer, dronabinol has been co-administered with a variety of medications (*e.g.*, cytotoxic agents, anti-infective agents, sedatives, or opioid analgesics) without resulting in any clinically significant drug/drug interactions. Although no drug/drug interactions were discovered during the clinical trials of dronabinol, cannabinoids may interact with other medication through both metabolic and pharmacodynamic mechanisms. Dronabinol is highly protein bound to plasma proteins, and therefore, might displace other protein-bound drugs. Although this displacement has not been confirmed *in vivo*, practitioners should monitor patients for a change in dosage requirements when administering dronabinol to patients receiving other highly protein-bound drugs. Published reports of drug/drug interactions involving cannabinoids are summarized in TABLE 2.

ADVERSE REACTIONS:

Adverse experiences information summarized in the tables below was derived from well-controlled clinical trials conducted in the US and US territories involving 474 patients exposed to dronabinol. Studies of AIDS-related weight loss included 157 patients receiving dronabinol at a dose of 2.5 mg twice daily and 67 receiving placebo. Studies of nausea and vomiting related to cancer chemotherapy included 317 patients receiving dronabinol and 68 receiving placebo.

A cannabinoid dose-related "high" (easy laughing, elation and heightened awareness) has been reported by patients receiving dronabinol in both the antiemetic (24%) and the lower dose appetite stimulant clinical trials (8%) (see CLINICAL STUDIES).

The most frequently reported adverse experiences in patients with AIDS during placebo-controlled clinical trials involved the CNS and were reported by 33% of patients receiving dronabinol. The frequency of adverse experiences did not correlate with the duration of therapy.

ADVERSE REACTIONS: *(cont'd)*

TABLE 2

Concomitant Drug	Clinical Effect(s)
Amphetamines, cocaine, other sympathomimetic agents	Additive hypertension, tachycardia ,possibly cardiotoxicity
Atropine, scopolamine, antihistamines, other anticholinergic agents	Additive or super-additive tachycardia, drowsiness
Amitriptyline, amoxapine, desipramine, other tricyclic antidepressants	Additive tachycardia, hypertension, drowsiness
Barbiturates, benzodiazepine ethanol, lithium, opioids, buspirone, antihistamines, muscle relaxants, other CNS depressants	Additive drowsiness and CNS depression
Disulfiram	A reversible hypomanic reaction was reported in a 28 y/o man who smoked marijuana; confirmed by dechallenge and rechallenge.
Fluoxetine	A 21 y/o female with depression and bulimia receiving 20 mg/day fluoxetine X 4 weeks became hypomanic after smoking marijuana; symptoms resolved after 4 days.
Antipyrine, barbiturates	Decreased clearance of these agents, presumably via competitive inhibition of metabolism
Theophylline	Increased theophylline metabolism reported with smoking of marijuana; effect similar to that following smoking tobacco

PROBABLY CAUSALLY RELATED: INCIDENCE GREATER THAN 1%

Rates derived from clinical trials in AIDS-related anorexia (n=157) and chemotherapy-related nausea (n=317). Rates were generally higher in the anti-emetic use (given in parenthesis).

Body as a whole: Asthenia.

Cardiovascular: Palpitations, tachycardia, vasodilation.

Digestive: Nausea*, vomiting*.

Nervous system: (Amnesia), (ataxia), confusion, depersonalization, dizziness*, euphoria* (24%), (hallucination), paranoid reaction*, somnolence*, thinking abnormal.

Special Senses: Vision difficulties.

* Incidence of events 3% to 10%.

PROBABLY CAUSALLY RELATED: INCIDENCE LESS THAN 1%

Event rates derived from clinical trials in AIDs-related anorexia (n=157) and chemotherapy-related nausea (n=317).

Cardiovascular: Conjunctivitis*, hypotension*.

Digestive: Diarrhea*, fecal incontinence

Musculoskeletal: Myalgias.

Nervous system: Depression, emotional ability, nightmares, speech difficulties, tinnitus.

Respiratory: Cough, rhinitis, sinusitis.

Skin and appendages: Flushing*.

* Incidence of events 0.3% to 1%.

CAUSAL RELATIONSHIP UNKNOWN: INCIDENCE LESS THAN 1%

The clinical significance of the association of these events with dronabinol treatment is unknown, but they are reported as alerting information for the clinician.

Body as a whole: Headache.

Digestive: Anorexia, hepatic enzyme elevation.

Nervous system: Anxiety/nervousness, tremors.

Skin and appendages: Sweating.

DRUG ABUSE AND DEPENDENCE:

Dronabinol is one of the psychoactive compounds present in cannabis and is abusable and controlled schedule II (CII) under the Controlled Substances Act. Both psychological and physiological dependence have been noted in healthy individuals receiving dronabinol, but addiction is uncommon and has only been seen after prolonged high dose administration.

Chronic abuse of cannabis has been associated with decrements in motivation, cognition, judgment, and perception. The etiology of these impairments is unknown but may be associated with the complex process of addiction rather than an isolated effect of the drug. No such decrements in psychological, social, or neurological status have been associated with the administration of dronabinol for therapeutic purposes.

In an open-label study in patients with AIDS who received dronabinol for up to five months, no abuse, diversion, or systematic change in personality or social functioning were observed despite the inclusion of a substantial number of patients with a past history of drug abuse.

An abstinence syndrome has been reported after the abrupt discontinuation of dronabinol in volunteers receiving dosage of 210 mg/day for 12 to 16 consecutive days. Within 12 hours after discontinuation, these volunteers manifested symptoms such as irritability, insomnia, and restlessness. By approximately 24 hours post-dronabinol discontinuation, withdrawal symptoms intensified to include "hot flashes," sweating, rhinorrhea, loose stools, hiccoughs, and anorexia.

These withdrawal symptoms gradually dissipated over the next 48 hours. Electroencephalographic changes consistent with the effects of drug withdrawal (hyperexcitation) were recorded in patients after abrupt dechallenge. Patients also complained of disturbed sleep for several weeks after discontinuing therapy with high dosages of dronabinol.

OVERDOSAGE:

Signs and Symptoms: Signs and symptoms following MILD dronabinol intoxication include drowsiness, euphoria, heightened sensory awareness, alerted time perception, reddened conjunctiva, dry mouth and tachycardia; following MODERATE intoxication include memory impairment, depersonalization, mood alteration, urinary retention, and reduced bowel motility; and following SEVERE intoxication include decreased motor coordination, lethargy, slurred speech, and postural hypotension. Apprehensive patients may experience panic reactions and seizures may occur in patients with existing seizure disorders.

The estimated lethal human dose of intravenous dronabinol is 30 mg/kg (2100 mg/70 kg). Significant CNS symptoms in antiemetic studies followed oral doses of 0.4 mg/kg (28 mg/70 kg) of dronabinol.

Management of Overdose: A potentially serious oral ingestion, if recent, should be managed with gut decontamination. In unconscious patients with a secure airway, instill activated charcoal (30 to 100 g in adults, 1 to 2 g/kg in infants) via a nasogastric tube. A saline cathartic or sorbitol may be added to the first dose of activated charcoal. Patients experiencing depressive, hallucinatory or psychotic reactions should be placed in a quiet area and

OVERDOSAGE: *(cont'd)*

offered reassurance. Benzodiazepines (5 to 10 mg diazepam*po*) may be used for treatment of extreme agitation. Hypotension usually responds to Trendelenburg position and IV fluids. Pressors are rarely required.

DOSAGE AND ADMINISTRATION:

APPETITE STIMULATION

Initially, 2.5 mg dronabinol should be administered orally twice daily (b.i.d.), before lunch and supper. For patients unable to tolerate this 5 mg/day dosage of dronabinol, the dosage can be reduced to 2.5 mg/day, administered as a single dose in the evening or at bedtime. If clinically indicated and in the absence of significant adverse effects, the dosage may be gradually increased to a maximum of 20 mg/day dronabinol, administered in divided oral doses. Caution should be exercised in escalating the dosage of dronabinol because of the increased frequency of dose-related adverse experiences at higher dosages (see PRECAUTIONS.)

ANTIEMETIC

Dronabinol is best administered at an initial dose of 5 mg/m^2, given 1 to 3 hours prior to the administration of chemotherapy, then every 2 to 4 hours after chemotherapy is given, for a total of 4 to 6 doses/day. Should the 5 mg/m^2 dose prove to be ineffective, and in the absence of significant side effects, the dose may be escalated by 2.5 mg/m^2 increments to a maximum of 15 mg/m^2 per dose. Caution should be exercised in dose escalation, however, as the incidence of disturbing psychiatric symptoms increases significantly at maximum dose (see PRECAUTIONS.)

SAFETY AND HANDLING

Dronabinol should be packaged in a well-closed container and stored in a cool environment between 8 and 15° C (46 and 59°F). Protect from freezing. No particular hazard to health care workers handling the capsules has been identified.

Access to abusable drugs such as dronabinol presents an occupational hazard for addiction in the health care industry. Routine procedures for handling controlled substances developed to protect the public may not be adequate to protect health care workers. Implementation of more effective accounting procedures and measures to appropriately restrict access to drugs of this class may minimize the risk of self-administration by health-care providers.**DEA Order Form Required**

PATIENT PACKAGE INSERT:

YOUR DOCTOR HAS PRESCRIBED THIS DRUG FOR YOUR USE ONLY. DO NOT LET ANYONE ELSE USE IT.

KEEP THIS MEDICINE OUT OF THE REACH OF CHILDREN AND PETS. If a child puts a capsule in their mouth or swallows dronabinol, take the medicine away from the child and contact a poison control center immediately, or contact a doctor immediately.

Do not drive a car or operate machinery until you know how dronabinol affects you. While taking dronabinol, do not drink alcohol, smoke marijuana, or take other drugs that have an effect on the central nervous system (such as sedatives or hypnotic). Unless advised by your doctor, do not use dronabinol if you are pregnant or nursing.

INTRODUCTION

This leaflet provides a summary of information about dronabinol. Please read it and keep it with your medicines in case you need to look at it again. Ask your doctor, nurse, or pharmacist if you have any questions.

Dronabinol contains dronabinol (THC), which occurs naturally, and has been extracted from *Cannabis sativa* L. (marijuana).

PRECAUTIONS

Be Sure To Tell Your Doctor If You Have Had Any Of The Following:

Heart disease

Current of past drug abuse

Current or past alcohol abuse

Mental health problems (mania, depression, schizophrenia)

Allergies to drugs

If you become pregnant while taking dronabinol, stop using it until you have talked to your doctor.

Dronabinol can dangerously interact with alcohol and with other dugs that have an effect on the central nervous system (such as Valium, Librium, Xanax, Seconal, Nembutal, or phenobarbital).

Do not drive or operate machinery until you are sure how dronabinol affects you and you are able to perform safely.

You may experience changes in mood or have other effects when first taking dronabinol. Be sure that there is a responsible person nearby when you first take dronabinol or when there is an adjustment in your dose.

Tell your doctor if you are taking any other prescription or nonprescription medicines.

Do not smoke marijuana while using dronabinol. This can cause an overdose.

INFORMATION ABOUT USING DRONABINOL

Introduction

Eating a nutritionally balanced diet is fundamental for all stages of life. For persons living with Human Immunodeficiency Virus (HIV), it's especially important to ensure an adequate diet to maintain an ideal weight and good nutritional status. There is some indication that optimal nutrition can help maintain the integrity of the immune system, and an adequate diet will allow your to allow you to better withstand the diseases associated with an AIDS diagnosis.

Many conditions, frequently interrelated, may cause a loss of appetite. Chewing and swallowing may become difficult or painful, due to inflammation or sores in your mouth and throat.

You may experience intermittent diarrhea or overall physical discomfort associated with AIDS. Sometimes, shopping for food and preparing adequate meals may drain your energy and your desire to eat. Mental depression also may result in a loss of your appetite, or you simply may grow increasingly frustrated with repeated eating problems.

A loss of appetite may occur at various time during illness associated with HIV infection. It often leads to the selection of an inadequate diet. Because a poor nutrient intake can result in weight loss and malnutrition, its important to learn to recognize and handle a temporary loss of your appetite.

Your doctor may prescribe an appetite stimulant such as dronabinol. Dronabinol should be taken exactly as directed by your doctor, and as indicated on the prescription label. You will most likely start therapy by taking one white capsule (2.5 mg) of dronabinol twice daily, before lunch and supper. Your doctor may adjust your dronabinol dosage if needed to maximize its effect or to decrease any side effects.

If you miss a dose, take it as soon as you remember. However, if it is almost time for your next dose, skip the missed dose and go back to your regular dosing schedules. **Do not double your dose.** Dronabinol must be swallowed whole to work effectively. Do not crush or chew the capsules.

PATIENT PACKAGE INSERT: *(cont'd)*

It is important not to take sedatives, hypnotics, other mind altering substances, or alcohol, while taking dronabinol without notifying your healthcare givers (physician, pharmacists and nurses). Do not drive or attempt other activities requiring full alertness while taking dronabinol. Your doctor will advise when you may resume these activities.

Your doctor and the pharmacist should be made aware of any other prescription medications or over-the-counter products you may be taking, as they could affect the way you respond to dronabinol.

Your doctor must write a new prescription each time you need more dronabinol. It is important to call your doctor before you take your last capsules. You should also give your pharmacist a few days notice of your need for more dronabinol.

Remember to keep this and all other medication out of the reach of children.

Increasing your appetite is only the first step in improving your nutritional status. How, what and when you eat are also very important.

How to eat

The purpose of consuming an adequate diet, even at times when you don't feel like eating, is to maintain an ideal weight and good nutritional status. Key to an adequate diet for HIV-infected individuals are foods dense in calories and nutrients. In other words, when you find it difficult to eat, make the most of what you do consume by selecting foods that provide many calories or nutrients in each mouthful.

Try some of the following ideas to boost your food intake. Keep in mind the foods you previously may have limited in your diet, especially those higher in fat, now can provide a significant source of calories. Enjoy an ice cream sundae frequently.

Cool or cold foods can dull pain from mouth and throat sores; popsicles may even numb your mouth prior to eating a larger meal. The cooler temperatures also diminish the aroma of unappetizing food.

Blend one cup of nonfat dry milk powder with one quart of whole milk. refrigerate and use "double-strength" milk for all traditional uses (puddings, cereal, shakes, soups).

Foods with a softer consistency, such as applesauce, may aid in swallowing. Creamed sauces or gravies also moisten food to encourage swallowing. Creating an appetizing meal involves more than just food. Try to eat in a pleasant atmosphere - sit in a comfortable chair, use a tablecloth and china, invite a friend to share your meal.

What to eat

Planning ahead is one of the most effective ways to deal with a loss of appetite. Stock up on staple foods, particularly those high in calories and protein, so they're available when you need them. Include favorite foods on your shopping list. Also consider these protein and nutrient dense foods:

Nonfat dry milk powder
Powdered breakfast drinks
Peanut butter and jelly
Pudding cups
"Trail mix" (dried fruit, nuts, cereals)
Creamed soups
Canned (or frozen) fruit in heavy syrup
Canned tuna, chicken or other sandwich spreads
Boxed macaroni and cheese

In addition to staples, refrigerated and frozen foods contribute important nutrients to an adequate diet. Several key choices, high in protein and calories, are listed below:

Yogurt
Cheeses
Cold cuts, beef and poultry
Cottage cheese
Ice cream and sherbet
Popsicles or pudding pops
Hard cooked eggs or pasteurized eggs*

*Raw or undercooked eggs pose danger of *Salmonella.*

The compromised immune function of persons with AIDS places them at greater than average risk from *Salmonella* infection.

Commercial food supplements are also available to boost your caloric and nutrient intake. Offered in a variety of flavors and textures, these products supply a concentrated source of calories and protein. You may want to ask your treatment provider for information about supplements. You may also request a referral to a registered dietitian who can provide individualized dietary recommendations to you.

When to eat

"Nutritious" meals can be eaten three times a day, but frequent, small snacks or meals can help you consume the calories and protein you need without feeling full from a large meal. Eat when you feel hungry, using modern technology, including your microwave, to quickly prepare a nutritious snack or meal.

Storage Instructions

The best place to store dronabinol is in the refrigerator. Be careful that the capsules don't freeze. Heat or moisture may cause your dronabinol to break down or stick together, so keep your medicine away from heat and direct light, and potentially damp places like in the bathroom or near the kitchen sink.

If You Are Taking Medicines

Dronabinol use may change the effect of other medicines. It is important to tell your doctor about all the medicines you are taking including all non-prescription medication.

What to Watch For (Adverse Effects)

You should not smoke marijuana while using dronabinol. It is possible to get too much dronabinol (an overdose), especially if you use dronabinol and smoke marijuana at the same time. Signs of a minor overdose would include drowsiness, euphoria, heightened sensory awareness, altered time perception, red eyes, dry mouth and rapid heart rate (tachycardia). Moderate overdosage would produce memory problems, depersonalization, mood alteration, urinary retention, and constipation. Severe overdosage would lead to decreased motor coordination, lethargy, slurred speech, and dizziness when standing up too fast (postural hypotension).

An overdose may cause you to faint.

If You Have Problems in the First Few Days

When you first use dronabinol your body is more sensitive and you may experience dizziness, confusion, sleepiness, or a high feeling. These symptoms usually go away in 1 to 3 days with continued dosage, If these symptoms are troublesome or persist, notify your doctor at once. Your doctor may then reduce the dose to one capsule before supper, or later in the evening, or even at bedtime.

PATIENT PACKAGE INSERT: *(cont'd)*

What to Do When Problems Occur **IF YOU NOTICE ANY WORRISOME SYMPTOMS OR PROBLEMS, STOP THE DRONABINOL AND CALL YOUR DOCTOR AT ONCE.**

(Roxane, 12/92, 4056050, 122)

(Patient Information, Roxane, 3/93, 47076640 033)

HOW SUPPLIED - EQUIVALENTS NOT AVAILABLE:

Capsule, Elastic - Oral - 2.5 mg

25's	$48.51	MARINOL, Roxane	00054-8541-11
25's	$81.61	MARINOL, Roxane	00054-2601-11
60's	$186.58	MARINOL, Roxane	00054-2601-21
100's	$289.98	MARINOL, Roxane	00054-2601-25

Capsule, Elastic - Oral - 5 mg

25's	$95.63	MARINOL, Roxane	00054-8542-11
25's	$160.89	MARINOL, Roxane	00054-2602-11
100's	$570.24	MARINOL, Roxane	00054-2602-25

Capsule, Elastic - Oral - 10 mg

25's	$189.00	MARINOL, Roxane	00054-8543-11
25's	$321.78	MARINOL, Roxane	00054-2603-11

DROPERIDOL *(001117)*

CATEGORIES: Analeptics; Anesthesia; Anxiety; Butyrophenones; Central Nervous System Agents; Nausea; Nausea and Vomiting; Psychotherapeutic Agents; Tranquilizers; Vomiting; Sedatives*; Pregnancy Category C; FDA Approval Pre 1982

* Indication not approved by the FDA

BRAND NAMES: *Dehidrobenzoperidol*; *Dehydrobenzperidol* (Germany, Mexico); *Droleptan* (Australia, England, France); *Droperidol*; *Inapsin*; **Inapsine**; *Sintodian* *(International brand names outside U.S. in italics)*

DESCRIPTION:

FOR INTRAVENOUS OR INTRAMUSCULAR USE ONLY

Droperidol is a neuroleptic (tranquilizer) agent available in ampules and vials. Each milliliter contains 2.5 mg of droperidol in an aqueous solution adjusted to pH 3.4 ± 0.4 with lactic acid. Droperidol in 10 ml multidose vials also contains 1.8 mg of methylparaben and 0.2 mg propylparaben per ml. Droperidol is chemically identified as 1-(1-[3-(p- fluorobenzoyl) propyl]-1,2,3,6-tetrahydro-4-pyridyl) -2-benzimidazolinone with a molecular weight of 379.43.

Droperidol injection is a sterile, non-pyrogenic aqueous solution for intravenous or intramuscular injection.

CLINICAL PHARMACOLOGY:

Droperidol produces marked tranquilization and sedation. It allays apprehension and provides a state or mental detachment and indifference while maintaining a state of reflex alertness.

Droperidol produces an antiemetic effect as evidenced by the antagonism of apomorphine in dogs. It lowers the incidence of nausea and vomiting during surgical procedures and provides antiemetic protection in the postoperative period.

Droperidol potentiates other CNS depressants. It produces mild alpha-adrenergic blockade, peripheral vascular dilatation and reduction of the pressor effect of epinephrine. It can produce hypotension and decreased peripheral vascular resistance and may decrease pulmonary arterial pressure (particularly if it is abnormally high). It may reduce the incidence of epinephrine-induced arrhythmias but it does not prevent other cardiac arrhythmias.

The onset of action of single intramuscular and intravenous doses is from three to ten minutes following administration, although the peak effect may not be apparent for up to thirty minutes. The duration of the tranquilizing and sedative effects generally is two to four hours, although alteration of alertness may persist for as long as twelve hours.

INDICATIONS AND USAGE:

Droperidol injection is indicated:

to produce tranquilization and to reduce the incidence of nausea and vomiting in surgical and diagnostic procedures.

for premedication, induction, and as an adjunct in the maintenance of general and regional anesthesia.

in neuroleptanalgesia in which droperidol is given concurrently with an opioid analgesic, such as fentanyl citrate injection, to aid in producing tranquility and decreasing anxiety and pain.

CONTRAINDICATIONS:

Droperidol injection is contraindicated in patients with known hypersensitivity to the drug.

WARNINGS:

FLUIDS AND OTHER COUNTER MEASURES TO MANAGE HYPOTENSION SHOULD BE READILY AVAILABLE.

As with other CNS depressant drugs, patients who have received droperidol should have appropriate surveillance.

It is recommended that opioids, when required, initially be used in reduced doses.

As with other neuroleptic agents, very rare reports of neuroleptic malignant syndrome (altered consciousness, muscle rigidity and autonomic instability) have occurred in patients who have received droperidol.

Since it may be difficult to distinguish neuroleptic malignant syndrome from malignant hyperpyrexia in the perioperative period, prompt treatment with dantrolene should be considered if increases in temperature, heart rate or carbon dioxide production occur.

Cases of sudden death have been reported following use of droperidol at high doses (generally 25 mg or greater) in patients at risk for cardiac dysrhythmia due to anoxia, hypercarbia, severe electrolyte disturbances, or alcohol withdrawal. While these reports do not establish the cause of such death, QT prolongation after droperidol administration has been reported and there is at least one case of nonfatal torsade de pointes confirmed by rechallenge.

Because of these reports, droperidol is not recommended in the treatment of alcohol withdrawal or in other clinical situations where high doses are likely to be needed in patients at risk for dysrhythmia.

PRECAUTIONS:

General: The initial dose of droperidol should be appropriately reduced in elderly, debilitated and other poor-risk patients. The effect of the initial dose should be considered in determining incremental doses.

PRECAUTIONS: *(cont'd)*

Certain forms of conduction anesthesia, such as spinal anesthesia and some peridural anesthetics, can alter respiration by blocking intercostal nerves and can cause peripheral vasodilatation and hypotension because of sympathetic blockade. Through other mechanisms (see CLINICAL PHARMACOLOGY), droperidol can also alter circulation. Therefore, when droperidol is used to supplement these forms of anesthesia, the anesthetist should be familiar with the physiological alterations involved, and be prepared to manage them in the patients elected for these forms of anesthesia.

If hypotension occurs, the possibility of hypovolemia should be considered and managed with appropriate parenteral fluid therapy. Repositioning the patient to improve venous return to the heart should be considered when operative conditions permit. It should be noted that in spinal and peridural anesthesia, tilting the patient into a head-down position may result in a higher level of anesthesia than is desirable, as well as impair venous return to the heart. Care should be exercised in moving and positioning of patients because of a possibility of orthostatic hypotension. If volume expansion with fluids plus these other countermeasures do not correct the hypotension, then the administration of pressor agents other than epinephrine should be considered. Epinephrine may paradoxically decrease the blood pressure in patients treated with droperidol due to the alpha-adrenergic blocking action of droperidol.

Since droperidol may decrease pulmonary arterial pressure, this fact should be considered by those who conduct diagnostic or surgical procedures where interpretation of pulmonary arterial pressure measurements might determine final management of the patient.

Vital signs should be monitored routinely.

When the EEG is used for postoperative monitoring, it may be found the EEG pattern returns to normal slowly.

Impaired Hepatic or Renal Function: Droperidol should be administered with caution to patients with liver and kidney dysfunction because of the importance of these organs in the metabolism and excretion of drugs.

Carcinogenesis, Mutagenesis, and Impairment of Fertility: No carcinogenicity studies have been carried out with droperidol. The micronucleus test in female rats revealed no mutagenic effects in single oral doses as high as 160 mg/kg. An oral study in rats (Segment I) revealed no impairment of fertility in either males of females at 0.63, 2.5 and 10 mg/kg doses (approximately 2, 9 and 36 times maximum recommended human IV/IM dosage).

Pregnancy Category C: Droperidol administered intravenously has been shown to cause a slight increase in mortality of the newborn rat at 4.4 times the upper human dose. At 44 times the upper human dose, mortality rate was comparable to that for control animals. Following intramuscular administration, increased mortality of the offspring at 1.8 times the upper human dose is attributed to CNS depression in the dams who neglected to remove placentae from their offspring. Droperidol has not been shown to be teratogenic in animals. There are no adequate and well-controlled studies in pregnant women. Droperidol should be used during pregnancy only if the potential benefit justifies the potential risk to the fetus.

Labor and Delivery: There are insufficient data to support the use of droperidol in labor and delivery. Therefore, such use is not recommended.

Nursing Mothers: It is not known whether droperidol is excreted in human milk. Because many drugs are excreted in human milk, caution should be exercised when droperidol is administered to a nursing mother.

Pediatric Use: The safety of droperidol in children younger than two years of age has not been established.

DRUG INTERACTIONS:

Other CNS depressant drugs (*e.g.,* barbiturates, tranquilizers, opioids and general anesthetics) have additive or potentiating effects with droperidol. When patients have received such drugs, the dose of droperidol required will be less than usual. Following the administration of droperidol, the dose of other CNS depressant drugs should be reduced.

ADVERSE REACTIONS:

The most common somatic adverse reactions reported to occur with droperidol are mild to moderate hypotension and tachycardia, but these effects usually subside without treatment. If hypotension occurs and is severe or persists, the possibility of hypovolemia should be considered and managed with appropriate parenteral fluid therapy.

The most common behavioral adverse effects of droperidol include dysphoria, postoperative drowsiness, restlessness, hyperactivity and anxiety, which can either be the result of an inadequate dosage (lack of adequate treatment effect) or of an adverse drug reaction (part of the symptom complex of akathisia).

Care should be taken to search for extrapyramidal signs and symptoms (dystonia, akathisia, oculogyric crisis) to differentiate these different clinical conditions. When extrapyramidal symptoms are the cause, they can usually be controlled with anticholinergic agents.

Postoperative hallucinatory episodes (sometimes associated with transient periods of mental depression) have also been reported.

Other less common adverse reactions include anaphylaxis, dizziness, chills and/or shivering, laryngospasm, and bronchospasm.

Elevated blood pressure, with or without pre-existing hypertension, has been reported following administration of droperidol combined with fentanyl citrate injection of other parenteral analgesics. This might be due to unexplained alterations in sympathetic activity following large doses; however, it is also frequently attributed to anesthetic or surgical stimulation during light anesthesia.

OVERDOSAGE:

Signs and Symptoms: The manifestations of droperidol overdosage are an extension of its pharmacologic actions.

Treatment: In the presence of hypoventilation or apnea, oxygen should be administered and respiration should be assisted or controlled as indicated. A patient airway must be maintained; an oropharyngeal airway or endotracheal tube might be indicated. The patient should be carefully observed for 24 hours; body warmth and adequate fluid intake should be maintained. If hypotension occurs and is severe or persists, the possibility of hypovolemia should be considered and managed with appropriate parenteral fluid therapy. (See PRECAUTIONS.)

If significant extrapyramidal reactions occur in the context of an overdose, an anticholinergic should be administered.

The intravenous LD_{50} of droperidol is 20-43 mg/kg in mice; 30 mg/kg in rats; 25 mg/kg in dogs and 11-13 mg/kg in rabbits. The intramuscular LD_{50} of droperidol is 195 mg/kg in mice; 104-110 mg/kg in rats; 97 mg/kg in rabbits and 200 mg/kg in guinea pigs.

DOSAGE AND ADMINISTRATION:

Dosage Should Be Individualized: Some of the factors to be considered in determining the dose are age, body weight, physical status, underlying pathological condition, use of other drugs, type of anesthesia to be used, and the surgical procedure involved.

Vital signs should be monitored routinely.

DOSAGE AND ADMINISTRATION: *(cont'd)*

USUAL ADULT DOSAGE

I. Premedication: (to be appropriately modified in the elderly, debilitated and those who have received other depressant drugs) 2.5 to 10 mg (1 to 4 ml) may be administered intramuscularly 30 to 60 minutes preoperatively.

II. Adjunct to General Anesthesia: *Induction:* 2.5 mg (1 ml) per 20 to 25 pounds may be administered (usually intravenously) along with analgesic and/or general anesthetic. Smaller doses may be adequate. The total amount of droperidol administered should be titrated to obtain the desired effect based on the individual patient's response. *Maintenance:* 1.25 to 2.5 mg (0.5 to 1 ml) usually intravenously.

III. Use Without A General Anesthetic In Diagnostic Procedures: Administer the usual IM premedication 2.5 to 10 mg (1 to 4 ml) 30 to 60 minutes before the procedure. Additional 1.25 to 2.5 mg (0.5 to 1 ml) amounts of droperidol may be administered, usually intravenously. *Note:* When droperidol is used in certain procedures, such as bronchoscopy, appropriate topical anesthesia is still necessary.

IV. Adjunct To Regional Anesthesia: 2.5 to 5 mg (1 to 2 ml) may be administered intramuscularly or slowly intravenously when additional sedation is required.

USUAL CHILDREN'S DOSAGE

For children two to 12 years of age, a reduced dose as low as 1 to 1.5 mg (0.4 to 0.6 ml) per 20 to 25 pounds is recommended for premedication or for induction of anesthesia.

See WARNINGS and PRECAUTIONS for use of droperidol with other CNS depressants and in patients with altered response.

Parenteral drug products should be inspected visually for particulate matter and discoloration prior to administration, whenever solution and container permit. If such abnormalities are observed, the drug should not be administered.

Storage: Store at controlled room temperature 15°C- 30°C (59°F-86°F). Protect from light.

HOW SUPPLIED - RATED THERAPEUTICALLY EQUIVALENT:

Injection, Solution - Intramuscular; - 2.5 mg/ml

2 ml	$7.03	Droperidol 2.5, Abbott	00074-1187-01
2 ml	$34.38	Droperidol, Solopak Labs	39769-0123-02
2 ml x 10	$31.56	Droperidol, Astra USA	00186-1220-03
2 ml x 10	$36.88	Droperidol, Astra USA	00186-1226-13
2 ml x 10	$42.50	Droperidol, Am Regent	00517-9702-10
5 ml x 10	$54.00	Droperidol, Astra USA	00186-1221-03
5 ml x 10	$61.25	Droperidol, Astra USA	00186-1227-13
5 ml x 10	$75.00	Droperidol, Am Regent	00517-9705-10
10 ml x 5	$51.50	Droperidol, Astra USA	00186-1224-12
10 ml x 10	$118.75	Droperidol, Am Regent	00517-9710-10

DROPERIDOL; FENTANYL CITRATE *(001118)*

CATEGORIES: Analeptics; Analgesics; Anesthesia; Antipyretics; Butyrophenones; Central Nervous System Agents; Narcotics, Synthetics & Combinations; Opiate Agonists (Controlled); Pain; Psychotherapeutic Agents; Tranquilizers; Anxiety*; Pregnancy Category C; DEA Class CII; FDA Approval Pre 1982
* Indication not approved by the FDA

BRAND NAMES: Fentanyl W/Droperidol; **Innovar**; *Thalamonal* (England)
(International brand names outside U.S. in italics)

> **WARNING:**
> The two components of fentanyl citrate and droperidol injection, fentanyl citrate and droperidol, have different pharmacologic actions. Before administering fentanyl citrate and droperidol injection, the user should become familiar with the special properties of each drug, particularly the widely differing durations of action.

DESCRIPTION:

Fentanyl citrate and droperidol injection contains a potent opioid analgesic (fentanyl citrate) and a neuroleptic (tranquilizer) agent (droperidol). Each ml contains (in a 1:50 ratio) fentanyl citrate equivalent to 50 mcg of fentanyl base and 2.5 mg of droperidol in a solution adjusted to pH 3.5 ± 0.3 with lactic acid.

Fentanyl citrate is chemically identified as N-(1-phenethyl-4-piperidyl) propionanilide citrate (1:1).

Droperidol is chemically identified as 1-[1-[3-(p-fluorobenzoyl) propyl]-1,2,3,6-tetrahydro-4-pyridyl]-2-benzimidazolinone.

Fentanyl citrate and droperidol injection is a sterile, preservative free aqueous solution for intravenous or intramuscular injection.

CLINICAL PHARMACOLOGY:

Fentanyl citrate and droperidol injection is a combination drug containing an opioid analgesic, fentanyl citrate, and a neuroleptic (major tranquilizer), droperidol. The combined effect, sometimes referred to as neuroleptanalgesia, is characterized by general quiescence, reduced motor activity, and profound analgesia; complete loss of consciousness usually does not occur from use of fentanyl citrate and droperidol injection alone. The incidence of early postoperative pain and emesis may be reduced.

Fentanyl citrate is an opioid analgesic. A dose of 100 mcg (0.1 mg) (2.0 ml), is approximately equivalent in analgesic activity to 10 mg of morphine or 75 mg of meperidine. The principal actions of therapeutic value are analgesia and sedation. Alterations in respiratory rate and alveolar ventilation, associated with opioid analgesics, may last longer than the analgesic effect. As the dose of opioid is increased, the decrease in pulmonary exchange becomes greater. Large doses may produce apnea. Fentanyl citrate appears to have less emetic activity than either morphine or meperidine. Histamine assays and skin wheal testing in man indicate that clinically significant histamine release rarely occurs with fentanyl citrate. Assays in man show no clinically significant histamine release in dosages up to 50 mcg/kg (0.05 mg/kg) (1 ml/kg).

The pharmacokinetics of fentanyl citrate can be described as a three—compartment model, with a distribution time of 1.7 minutes, redistribution of 13 minutes and a terminal elimination half-life of 219 minutes. The volume of distribution for fentanyl citrate is 4 L/kg.

Fentanyl citrate plasma protein binding capacity increases with increasing ionization of the drug. Alterations in pH may affect its distribution between plasma and the central nervous system. It accumulates in skeletal muscle and fat, and is released slowly into the blood. Fentanyl citrate, which is primarily transformed in the liver, demonstrates a high first pass clearance and releases approximately 75% of an intravenous dose in urine, mostly as metabolites with less than 10% representing the unchanged drug.

Approximately 9% of the dose is recovered in the feces, primarily as metabolites.

CLINICAL PHARMACOLOGY: *(cont'd)*

The onset of action of fentanyl citrate is almost immediate when the drug is given intravenously; however, the maximal analgesic and respiratory depressant effect may not be noted for several minutes. The usual duration of action of the analgesic effect is 30 to 60 minutes after a single intravenous dose of up to 100 mcg (0.1 mg) (2.0 ml). Following intramuscular administration, the onset of action is from seven to eight minutes, and the duration of action is one to two hours. As with longer acting opioid analgesics, the duration of the respiratory depressant effect of fentanyl may be longer than the analgesic effect. The following observations have been reported concerning altered respiratory response to CO_2 stimulation following administration of fentanyl citrate to man:

Diminished sensitivity to CO_2 stimulation may persist longer than depression of respiratory rate. (Altered sensitivity to CO_2 stimulation has been demonstrated for up to four hours following a single dose of 600 mcg (0.6 mg) (12 ml) fentanyl citrate to healthy volunteers). Fentanyl frequently slows the respiratory rate, duration and degree of respiratory depression being dose related.

The peak respiratory depressant effect of a single intravenous dose of fentanyl citrate is noted 5 to 15 minutes following injection. See also WARNINGS and PRECAUTIONS concerning respiratory depression.

Droperidol produces marked tranquilization and sedation. Droperidol allays apprehension and provides a state of mental detachment and indifference while maintaining a state of reflex alertness.

Droperidol also produces an antiemetic effect as evidenced by the antagonism of apomorphine in dogs. It lowers the incidence of nausea and vomiting during surgical procedures and provides antiemetic protection in the postoperative period.

Droperidol potentiates other CNS depressants. It produces mild alpha-adrenergic blockade, peripheral vascular dilatation and reduction of then pressor effect of epinephrine. It can produce hypotension and decreased peripheral vascular resistance and may decrease pulmonary arterial pressure (particularly if it is abnormally high.) It may reduce the incidence of epinephrine-induced arrhythmias, but does not prevent other cardiac arrhythmias.

The onset of action of single intramuscular and intravenous doses of droperidol is from three to ten minutes following administration, although the peak effect may not be apparent for up to thirty minutes.The duration of the tranquilizing and sedative effect generally is two to four hours, although alteration of consciousness may persist for as long as twelve hours. This is in contrast to the much shorter duration of fentanyl.

INDICATIONS AND USAGE:

Fentanyl citrate and droperidol injection is indicated to produce tranquilization and analgesia for surgical and diagnostic procedures. It may be used as an anesthetic premedication, as an adjunct to the induction of anesthesia, and as an adjunct in the maintenance of general and regional anesthesia. If the supplementation of analgesia is necessary, fentanyl citrate injection alone rather than the combination drug, fentanyl citrate and droperidol injection, should usually be used, see DOSAGE AND ADMINISTRATION.

CONTRAINDICATIONS:

Fentanyl citrate and droperidol injection is contraindicated in patients with known hypersensitivity to either component.

WARNINGS:

FENTANYL CITRATE AND DROPERIDOL INJECTION SHOULD BE ADMINISTERED ONLY BY PERSONS SPECIFICALLY TRAINED IN THE USE OF INTRAVENOUS ANESTHETICS AND MANAGEMENT OF THE RESPIRATORY EFFECTS OF POTENT OPIOIDS.

AN OPIOID ANTAGONIST, RESUSCITATIVE AND INTUBATION EQUIPMENT AND OXYGEN SHOULD BE READILY AVAILABLE.

See also discussion of opioid antagonists in PRECAUTIONS and OVERDOSAGE sections.

Fluids and other counter measures to manage hypotension should also be available.

The respiratory depressant effect of opioids persists longer than the measured analgesic effect. When used with fentanyl citrate and droperidol injection, the total dose of all opioid analgesics administered should be considered by the practitioner before ordering opioid analgesics during recovery from anesthesia. It is recommended that opioids, when required, be used in reduced doses initially, as low as 1/4 to 1/3 those usually recommended.

Fentanyl citrate and droperidol injection may cause muscle rigidity, particularly involving the muscles of respiration. This effect is due to the fentanyl citrate component and is related to the dose and speed of injection. Its incidence can be reduced by the use of slow intravenous injection. Once the effect occurs, it is managed by the use of assisted or controlled respiration and, if necessary, by a neuromuscular blocking agent compatible with the patient's condition.

Head Injuries and Increased Intracranial Pressure: Fentanyl citrate and droperidol injection should be used with caution in patients who may be particularly susceptible to respiratory depression such as comatose patients who may have a head injury or a brain tumor. In addition, this product may obscure the clinical course of patients with head injury.

As with other neuroleptic agents, very rare reports of neuroleptic malignant syndrome (altered consciousness, muscle rigidity and autonomic instability) have occurred in patients who have received the droperidol component of this drug.

Since it may be difficult to distinguish neuroleptic malignant syndrome from malignant hyperthermia in the peri-operative period, prompt treatment with an appropriate treatment (such as dantrolene) should be considered in cases where increases in temperature, heart rate or carbon dioxide production occur.

Cases of sudden death have been reported following use of droperidol at high doses (generally 25 mg or greater) in patients at risk for cardiac dysrhythmia due to anoxia, hypercarbia, electrolyte disturbances, or alcohol withdrawal. While these reports do not establish the cause of death, QT prolongation after administration of the droperidol component of this drug has been reported and there is at least one case of torsades de pointes which was confirmed by re-challenge.

Because of these reports, this drug is not recommended in the treatment of alcohol withdrawal syndromes or in other clinical situations where high doses are likely to be needed in patients at risk for dysrhythmia.

PRECAUTIONS:

GENERAL

The initial dose of fentanyl citrate and droperidol injection should be appropriately reduced in elderly, debilitated and other poor-risk patients. The effect of the initial dose should be considered in determining incremental doses.

Certain forms of conduction anesthesia, such as spinal anesthesia and some peridural anesthetics, can alter respiration by blocking intercostal nerves and can cause peripheral vasodilation and hypotension because of sympathetic blockade. Through other mechanism (see CLINICAL PHARMACOLOGY) fentanyl citrate and droperidol can also depress respiration and blood pressure. Therefore, when this combination product is used to supplement these forms of anesthesia, the anesthetist should be familiar with the physiological alterations involved, and be prepared to manage them in the patients selected for these forms of anesthesia.

The droperidol component of this product may decrease pulmonary arterial pressure. This fact should be considered by those who conduct diagnostic or surgical procedures where interpretation of pulmonary arterial pressure measurements might determine final management of the patient.

Vital signs should be monitored routinely.

When the EEG is used for postoperative monitoring, it may be found that the EEG pattern returns to normal slowly.

Hypotension: If hypotension occurs, the possibility of hypovolemia should be considered and managed with appropriate parental fluid therapy. Repositioning the patient to improve venous return to the heart should be considered when operative conditions permit. It should be noted that in spinal and peridural anesthesia, tilting the patient into a head down position may result in a higher level of anesthesia than is desirable, as well as impair venous return to the heart. Care should be exercised in the moving a positioning of patients because of a possibility of orthostatic hypotension. If volume expansion with fluids plus these other countermeasures do not correct the hypotension, then the administration of pressor agents other than epinephrine should be considered. Epinephrine may paradoxically decrease the blood pressure in patients treated with fentanyl citrate and droperidol injection due to the alpha-adrenergic blocking action of droperidol.

Impaired Respiration: Fentanyl citrate and droperidol injection and fentanyl citrate injection should be used with caution in patients with chronic obstructive pulmonary disease, patients with decreased respiratory reserve and others with potentially compromised ventilation. In such patients opioids may additionally decrease respiratory drive and increase airway resistance. During anesthesia, this can be managed by assisted or controlled respiration. Respiratory depression caused by opioid analgesics can be reversed by opioid antagonists. Appropriate surveillance should be maintained because the duration of respiratory depression of doses of fentanyl citrate (as fentanyl citrate injection or fentanyl citrate and droperidol injection) employed during anesthesia may be longer than the duration of the opioid antagonist action. Consult individual prescribing information (nalorphine and naloxone) before employing opioid antagonists.

Impaired Hepatic or Renal Function: This combination product should be administered with caution to patients with liver and kidney dysfunction because of the importance of these organs in the metabolism and excretion of drugs.

Cardiovascular Effects: The fentanyl citrate component may produce bradycardia, which may be treated with atropine. Fentanyl citrate and droperidol injection should be used with caution in patients with cardiac bradyarrhythmias.

Carcinogenesis, Mutagenesis, and Impairment of Fertility: No carcinogenicity studies have been conducted with fentanyl citrate and droperidol injection or its components, fentanyl citrate and droperidol. A subcutaneous study of the combination product in female rats revealed no impairment of fertility at doses 9 times the upper human dose. An intravenous study revealed no effect on fertility at 2 times the upper human dose (highest dosage level tested).

Pregnancy Category C: Fentanyl citrate and droperidol injection had no embryotoxic effects in rats at intravenous doses approximately 2 times the upper human dose. A subcutaneous study of this product in female rats showed increased fetal resorptions at 18 times the upper human dose. No teratogenic effects were revealed at 36 times the upper human dose. In rabbits, increased resorptions and decreased litter size were found at intravenous doses approximately 2 times the upper human dose. Maternal mortality occurred at 7 times the upper human dose.

This product has not been shown to be teratogenic in animals. There are no adequate and well-controlled studies in pregnant women. Fentanyl citrate and droperidol injection should be used during pregnancy only if the potential benefit justifies the potential risk to the fetus.

Labor and Delivery: There are insufficient data to support the use of this product in labor and delivery. Therefore, such use is not recommended.

Nursing Mothers: It is not known whether fentanyl citrate or droperidol are excreted in human milk. Because many drugs are excreted in human milk, caution should be exercised when this product is administered to a nursing woman.

Pediatric Use: The safety and efficacy of fentanyl citrate and droperidol injection in children under two years of age has not been established.

DRUG INTERACTIONS:

Other CNS depressant drugs (*e.g.,* barbiturates, tranquilizers, opioids and general anesthetics) have additive or potentiating effects with fentanyl citrate and droperidol injection. When patients have received such drugs, the dose of this combination product required will be less than usual. Following the administration of fentanyl citrate and droperidol injection, the dose of other CNS depressant drugs should be reduced.

ADVERSE REACTIONS:

The most common serious adverse reactions reported to occur with fentanyl citrate and droperidol injection are respiratory depression, apnea and muscular rigidity. If these remain untreated, respiratory arrest, circulatory depression or cardiac arrest could occur. Mild to moderate hypotension and tachycardia also occur, but these effects usually subside without treatment. If hypotension occurs and is severe or persists, the possibility of hypovolemia should be considered and managed with appropriate parenteral fluid therapy.

The most common behavioral adverse effects of this drug include dysphoria, postoperative drowsiness, restlessness, hyperactivity and anxiety, many of which can either be the result of an inadequate dosage (lack of adequate treatment effect) or of an adverse drug reaction (part of the symptom complex of akathisia).

Care should be taken to search for extrapyramidal signs and symptoms (dystonia, akathisia, oculogyric crisis) to differentiate these different clinical conditions. When extrapyramidal symptoms are the cause, they can usually be controlled with anticholinergic agents.

Postoperative hallucinatory episodes (sometimes associated with transient periods of mental depression) have also been reported.

Other less common reported adverse reactions include anaphylaxis, dizziness, chills and/or shivering, twitching, blurred vision, laryngospasm, bronchospasm, bradycardia, nausea and emesis, diaphoresis, and emergence delirium.

DRUG ABUSE AND DEPENDENCE:

The fentanyl citrate component of fentanyl citrate and droperidol injection is a Schedule II opioid that can produce drug dependence of the morphine type and, therefore, has the potential for being abused.

OVERDOSAGE:

Signs and Symptoms: The manifestations of fentanyl citrate and droperidol injection overdosage are an extension of its pharmacologic actions.

OVERDOSAGE: *(cont'd)*

Treatment: In the presence of hypoventilation or apnea, oxygen should be administered and respiration should be assisted or controlled as indicated. A patent airway must be maintained; an oropharyngeal airway or endotracheal tube might be indicated. If depressed respiration is associated with muscular rigidity, an intravenous neuromuscular blocking agent might be required to facilitate assisted or controlled respiration. The patient should be carefully observed for 24 hours; body warmth and adequate fluid intake should be maintained. If hypotension occurs and is severe or persists, the possibility of hypovolemia should be considered and managed with appropriate parental fluid therapy (see PRECAUTIONS). A specific opioid antagonist such as nalorphine or naloxone should be available for use as indicated to manage respiratory depression caused by the opioid component, fentanyl citrate. This does not preclude the use of more immediate countermeasures. The duration of respiratory depression following overdosage of fentanyl citrate may be longer than the duration of opioid antagonist action. Consult the package inserts of the individual opioid antagonists for details about use.

If significant extrapyramidal reactions occur in the context of an overdose, an anticholinergic should be administered.

The LD_{50} values after intravenous administration were 4.1-5.27 mg/kg for the rat and the rabbit and 17 mg/kg or more for the mouse and the dog. After intramuscular administration LD_{50}determinations were 6.7-14.5 mg/kg for the rabbit and 75 mg/kg for the mouse.

DOSAGE AND ADMINISTRATION:

Dosage Should Be Individualized: Some of the factors to be considered in determining dose are age, body weight, physical status, underlying pathological condition, use of other drugs, the type of anesthesia to be used and the surgical procedure involved.

Vital signs should be monitored routinely.

Most patients who have received fentanyl citrate and droperidol injection do not require opioid analgesics during the immediate postoperative period. It is recommended that opioid analgesics, when required, be used initially in reduced doses, as low as 1/4 to 1/3 those usually recommended.

USUAL ADULT DOSAGE

I. Premedication: (to be appropriately modified in the elderly, debilitated and those who have received other depressant drugs)— 0.5 to 2 ml may be administered **intramuscularly**45 to 60 minutes prior to surgery with or without atropine.

II. Adjunct to General Anesthesia: *Induction:* 1 ml per 20 to 25 pounds of body weight may be slowly administered intravenously. Smaller doses may be adequate. The total amount of fentanyl citrate and droperidol injection administered should be carefully titrated to obtain the desired effect based on the individual patient's response. There are several methods of administration of fentanyl citrate and droperidol injection for induction of anesthesia. *Intravenous Injection:*To allow for the variable needs of patients this product may be administered intravenously in fractional parts of the calculated dose. With the onset of somnolence, the general anesthetic may be administered. *Intravenous Drip:*10 ml of fentanyl citrate and droperidol injection are added to 250 ml of dextrose injection 5% and the drip given rapidly until the onset of somnolence. At that time, the drip may be either slowed or stopped and the general anesthetic administered. *Maintenance:*Fentanyl citrate and droperidol injection is not indicated as the sole agent for the maintenance of surgical anesthesia. It is customarily used in combination with other measures such as nitrous oxide-oxygen, other inhalation anesthetics and/or topical or regional anesthesia. To prevent the possibility of excessive accumulation of the relatively long-acting droperidol component, fentanyl citrate injection, alone should be used in increments of 25 to 50 mcg (0.025 to 0.05 mg) (0.5 to 1 ml) for the maintenance of analgesia in patients initially given fentanyl citrate and droperidol injection as an adjunct to general anesthesia. (See fentanyl citrate injection package insert for additional prescribing information.) However, in prolonged operations, additional 0.5 to 1 ml amounts of this combination product may be administered with caution intravenously if changes in the patient's condition indicate lightening of tranquilization and analgesia.

III. Use Without a General Anesthetic in Diagnostic Procedures: Administer the usual intramuscular premedication (0.5 to 2 ml) 45 to 60 minutes before the procedure. To prevent the possibility of excessive accumulation of the relatively long-acting droperidol component, fentanyl citrate injection alone should be used in increments of 25 to 50 mcg. (0.025 to 0.05 mg) (0.5 to 1 ml) for the maintenance of analgesia in patients initially given fentanyl citrate and droperidol injection. See fentanyl citrate injection package insert for additional information. However, in prolonged operations, additional 0.5 to 1 ml amounts of this combination product may be administered with caution intravenously if changes in the patient's condition indicate lightening of tranquilization and analgesia. *Note:* When fentanyl citrate and droperidol injection is used in certain procedures such as bronchoscopy, appropriate topical anesthesia is still necessary.

IV. Adjunct to Regional Anesthesia: 1 to 2 ml may be administered intramuscularly or slowly intravenously when additional sedation and analgesia are required.

USUAL CHILDREN'S DOSAGE

For premedication and as an adjunct to general anesthesia in children over 2 years of age (see PRECAUTIONS):

I. Premedication: 0.25 ml per 20 lbs. body weight administered **intramuscularly** 45 to 60 minutes prior to surgery with or without atropine.

II. Adjunct to General Anesthesia: The total combined dose for induction and maintenance averages 0.5 ml per 20 lbs. body weight. Following induction with fentanyl citrate and droperidol injection, fentanyl citrate injection alone in a dose of 1/4 to 1/3 that recommended in the adult dosage section should usually be used when indicated to avoid the possibility of excessive accumulation of droperidol. However, in prolonged operations, additional increments of this combination product may be administered with caution when changes in the patient's condition indicate lightening of tranquilization and analgesia.

See WARNINGS and PRECAUTIONS for use of fentanyl citrate and droperidol injection with other CNS depressants, and in patients with altered response.

Parenteral drug products should be inspected visually for particulate matter and discoloration prior to administration, whenever solution and container permit. If such abnormalities are observed, the drug should not be administered.

(FOR INTRAVENOUS USE BY HOSPITAL PERSONNEL SPECIFICALLY TRAINED IN THE USE OF OPIOID ANALGESICS.)

Storage: Store at controlled room temperature 15°- 30°C (59°-86°F). Protect from light.

HOW SUPPLIED - RATED THERAPEUTICALLY EQUIVALENT:

Injection, Solution - Intramuscular; - 2.5 mg/0.05 mg

2 ml	$159.60	Fentanyl W/Droperidol, Abbott	00074-1186-12
2 ml x 10	$99.38	Fentanyl Citrate & Droperidol, Astra USA	00186-1230-03
2 ml x 10	$105.63	Fentanyl Citrate & Droperidol, Astra USA	00186-1232-13
5 ml x 10	$164.38	Fentanyl Citrate & Droperidol, Astra USA	00186-1233-13
5 ml x 10	$165.63	Fentanyl Citrate & Droperidol, Astra USA	00186-1231-03

DYCLONINE HYDROCHLORIDE *(001121)*

CATEGORIES: Analgesics; Anesthesia; Antipruritics/Local Anesthetics; EENT Drugs; Eye, Ear, Nose, & Throat Preparations; Gag Reflex; Lesions; Local Anesthetics; Pain; Skin/Mucous Membrane Agents; Stomatitis; Topical Analgesics; Pregnancy Category C; FDA Approval Pre 1982

BRAND NAMES: **Dyclone**

FORMULARIES: Aetna

DESCRIPTION:

Dyclonine Hydrochloride 0.5% and 1% Topical Solutions contain a local anesthetic agent and are administered topically. See INDICATIONS AND USAGE for specific uses.

Dyclonine HCl 0.5% and 1% Topical Solutions contain dyclonine HCl, which is chemically designated as 4'-butoxy-3-piperi-dinopropiophenone HCl. Dyclonine HCl is a white crystalline powder that is sparingly soluble in water.

COMPOSITION OF DYCLONINE HCL 0.5% AND 1% TOPICAL SOLUTIONS

Each ml of 0.5% Solution contains dyclonine HCl, 5 mg.

Each ml of 1% Solution contains dyclonine HCl, 10 mg.

Both solutions also contain chlorbutanol hydrous and sodium chloride, and the pH is adjusted to 3.0-5.0 by means of hydrochloric acid.

CLINICAL PHARMACOLOGY:

Dyclonine HCl topical solutions effect surface anesthesia when applied topically to mucous membranes. Effective anesthesia varies with different patients, but usually occurs from 2 to 10 minutes after application and persists for approximately 30 minutes.

INDICATIONS AND USAGE:

Dyclonine HCl topical solutions are indicated for anesthetizing accessible mucous membranes (*e.g.,* the mouth, pharynx, larynx, trachea, esophagus, and urethra) prior to various endoscopic procedures.

Dyclonine HCl topical solutions 0.5% may also be used to block the gag reflex, to relieve the pain of oral ulcers of stomatitis and to relieve pain associated with ano-genital lesions.

CONTRAINDICATIONS:

Dyclonine is contraindicated in patents known to be hypersensitive (allergic) to the local anesthetic or to other components of dyclonine HCl topical solutions.

WARNINGS:

IN ORDER TO MANAGE POSSIBLE ADVERSE REACTIONS, RESUSCITATIVE EQUIPMENT, OXYGEN AND OTHER RESUSCITATIVE DRUGS SHOULD BE IMMEDIATELY AVAILABLE WHENEVER LOCAL ANESTHETIC AGENTS, SUCH AS DYCLONINE, ARE ADMINISTERED TO MUCOUS MEMBRANES.

Dyclonine HCl topical solutions should not be injected into tissue or used in the eyes because of highly irritant properties.

Dyclonine HCl topical solutions should be used with extreme caution in the presence of sepsis or severely traumatized mucosa in the area of application since under such conditions there is the potential for rapid systemic absorption.

PRECAUTIONS:

General: The safety and effectiveness of dyclonine depend on proper dosage, correct technique, adequate precautions, and readiness for emergencies (See WARNINGS and ADVERSE REACTIONS). The lowest dosage that results in effective anesthesia should be used to avoid high plasma levels and serious adverse effects. Repeated doses of dyclonine may cause significant increases in blood levels with each repeated dose because of slow accumulation of the drug or its metabolites. Tolerance to elevated blood levels varies with the status of the patient. Debilitated, elderly patients, acutely ill patients, and children should be given reduced doses commensurate with their age, weight and physical condition. Dyclonine should also be used with caution in patients with severe shock or heart block.

Dyclonine HCl topical solutions should be used with caution in persons with known drug sensitivities.

Information for the Patient: When topical anesthetics are used in the mouth or throat, the patient should be aware that the production of topical anesthesia may impair swallowing and thus enhance the danger of aspiration. For this reason, food should not be ingested for 60 minutes following use of local anesthetic preparations in the mouth or throat area. This is particularly important in children because of their frequency of eating.

Numbness of the tongue or buccal mucosa may increase the danger of biting trauma. When dyclonine HCl 0.5% topical solution is used to relieve the pain of oral ulcers or stomatitis which interferes with eating, patients should be warned about the risk of biting trauma before they accept this treatment; caution should be exercised in selecting food and eating. Following other uses in the mouth and throat area, food and/or chewing gum should not be used while the area is anesthetized.

Drug/Laboratory Test Interactions Dyclonine HCl topical solutions should not be used in cystoscopic procedures following intravenous pyelography because an iodine precipitate occurs which interferes with visualization.

Carcinogenesis, Mutagenesis, and Impairment of Fertility Studies of dyclonine in animals to evaluate the carcinogenic and mutagenic potential or the effect on fertility have not been conducted.

Pregnancy, Teratogenic Effects, Pregnancy Category C: Animal reproduction studies have not been conducted with dyclonine. It is also not known whether dyclonine can cause fetal harm when administered to a pregnant woman or can affect reproduction capacity. General consideration should be given to this fact before administering dyclonine to women of childbearing potential, especially during early pregnancy when maximum organogenesis takes place.

Nursing Mothers: It is not known whether this drug is excreted in human milk. Because many drugs are excreted in human milk, caution should be exercised when dyclonine is administered to a nursing woman.

Pediatric Use: Safety and effectiveness in children under the age of 12 have not been established.

ADVERSE REACTIONS:

Adverse experiences following the administration of dyclonine are similar in nature to those observed with other local anesthetic agents. These adverse experiences are, in general, dose-related and may result from high plasma levels caused by excessive dosage or rapid absorption, or may result from a hypersensitivity, idiosyncrasy or diminished tolerance on the part of the patient. Serious adverse experiences are generally systemic in nature. The following types are those most commonly reported:

ADVERSE REACTIONS: *(cont'd)*

Central Nervous System: CNS manifestations are excitatory and/or depressant and may be characterized by lightheadedness, nervousness, apprehension, euphoria, confusion, dizziness, drowsiness, tinnitus, blurred or double vision, vomiting, sensations of heat, cold or numbness, twitching, tremors, convulsions, unconsciousness, respiratory depression and arrest. The excitatory manifestations may be very brief or may not occur at all, in which case the first manifestation of toxicity may be drowsiness merging into unconsciousness and respiratory arrest.

Drowsiness following the administration of dyclonine is usually an early sign of a high blood level of the drug and may occur as a consequence of rapid absorption.

Cardiovascular System: Cardiovascular manifestations are usually depressant and are characterized by bradycardia, hypotension, and cardiovascular collapse, which may lead to cardiac arrest.

Allergic: Allergic reactions are characterized by cutaneous lesions, urticaria, edema or anaphylactoid reactions. Allergic reactions may occur as a result of sensitivity either to the local anesthetic agent or to the other ingredients used in this formulation. Allergic reactions, if they occur, should be managed by conventional means. The detection of sensitivity by skin testing is of doubtful value. Local reactions include irritation, stinging, urethritis with and without bleeding.

OVERDOSAGE:

Acute emergencies from local anesthetics are generally related to high plasma levels encountered during therapeutic use of local anesthetics.(See ADVERSE REACTIONS, WARNINGS, and PRECAUTIONS).

Management Of Local Anesthetic Emergencies: The first consideration is prevention, best accomplished by careful and constant monitoring of cardiovascular and respiratory vital signs and respiratory vital signs and the patients'state of consciousness after each local anesthetic administration.

The first step in the management of convulsions consists of immediate attention to the maintenance of a patent airway and assisted or controlled ventilation with oxygen and a delivery system capable of permitting immediate positive airway pressure by mask. Immediately after the institution of these ventilatory measures, the adequacy of the circulation should be evaluated, keeping in mind that drugs used to treat convulsions sometimes depress the circulation when administered intravenously. Should convulsions persist despite adequate respiratory support, and if the status of the circulation permits, small increments of an ultrashort acting barbiturate (such as thiopental or thiamylal) or a benzodiazepine (such as diazepam) may be administered intravenously. The clinician should be familiar, prior to use of local anesthetics, with these anticonvulsant drugs. Supportive treatment of circulatory depression may require administration of intravenous fluids and, when appropriate, a vasopressor as directed by the clinical situation (*e.g.,* ephedrine).

If not treated immediately, both convulsions and cardiovascular depression can result in hypoxia, acidosis, bradycardia, arrhythmias and cardiac arrest. If cardiac arrest should occur, standard cardiopulmonary resuscitative measures should be instituted.

The median lethal dose (LD_{50}) of dyclonine HCl administered orally to female rats is 176 mg/kg and 90 mg/kg in female mice. Intraperitoneally the LD_{50} in female rats in 31 mg/kg and 43 mg/kg in female mice.

DOSAGE AND ADMINISTRATION:

As with all local anesthetics, the dosage varies and depends upon the area to be anesthetized, vascularity of the tissues, individual tolerance and the technique of anesthesia. The lowest dosage needed to provide effective anesthesia should be administered.

A maximum dose of 30 ml of 1% dyclonine HCl topical solutions (300 mg of dyclonine HCl) may be used, although satisfactory anesthesia is usually produced within the range of 4 to 20 ml. For specific techniques and procedures refer to standard textbooks.

Although as much as 300 mg of dyclonine HCl (as a 1% solution) have been tolerated, this dosage as a 0.5% solution has not been administered primarily because satisfactory anesthesia in endoscopic procedures can usually be produced by lesser amounts. For specific techniques for endoscopic procedures refer to standard textbooks.

Proctology: Apply pledgets of cotton or sponges moistened with the dyclonine HCl topical solution 0.5% to postoperative wounds for the relief of discomfort and pain.

Gynecology: Apply dyclonine HCl topical solution 0.5% as wet compresses or as a spray to relieve the discomfort of episiotomy or perineorrhaphy wounds.

Oncology-Radiology: Apply dyclonine HCl topical solution 0.5% as a rinse or swab to inflamed or ulcerated mucous membrane of the mouth caused by anti-neoplastic chemotherapy or radiation therapy. In lesions of the esophagus, 5-15 ml of the anesthetic may be swallowed to relieve pain and allow more comfortable deglutition.

Otorhinolaryngology: To suppress the gag reflex and to facilitate examination of the posterior pharynx or larynx, apply dyclonine HCl topical solution 0.5% as a spray or gargle.

Dyclonine HCl topical 0.5% may be applied as a rinse or swab to relieve the discomfort of aphthous stomatitis, hepatic stomatitis, or other painful oral lesions.

Dentistry: Dyclonine HCl topical 0.5% solution is useful to suppress the gag reflex in the positioning of x-ray films, making prosthetic impressions, and doing surgical procedures in the molar areas. It is also useful as a preinjection mucous membrane anesthetic or applied to the gums prior to scaling (prophylaxis). The anesthetic can be applied as a mouthwash or gargle and the excess spit out.

Store at controlled room temperature: 15-30°C (59-86°F).

HOW SUPPLIED - EQUIVALENTS NOT AVAILABLE:

Solution - Topical - 0.5 %

30 ml	$27.60	DYCLONE, Astra USA	00186-3001-67

Solution - Topical - 1 %

30 ml	$37.19	DYCLONE, Astra USA	00186-3002-67

DYPHYLLINE *(001122)*

CATEGORIES: Airway Obstruction; Antiasthmatics/Bronchodilators; Asthma; Bronchial Dilators; Bronchitis; Bronchospasm; Chronic Bronchitis; Emphysema; Respiratory & Allergy Medications; Respiratory Muscle Relaxant; Smooth Muscle Relaxants; Xanthine Derivatives; FDA Approval Pre 1982

BRAND NAMES: *Difilina*; *Difillin*; **Dilor**; *Diprophyllin* (Germany); *Diprophylline*; *Diprophyllinum*; Droxine; *Dyasthmol*; Dyflex; *Glyfyllin*; *Isophyllen*; *Katasma*; Lufyllin; *Neothyllin*; Neothylline; *Neufil*; *Neutraphylline*; *Protophylline* (Canada); *Silbephylline*; Thylline
(International brand names outside U.S. in italics)

COST OF THERAPY: $388.36 (Asthma; Tablet; 400 mg; 8/day; 365 days)

PRIMARY ICD9: 493.90 (Asthma, Unspecified, Without Mention of Status Asthmaticus)

DESCRIPTION:

Dyphylline (7-(2,3-dihydroxypropyl) theophylline) ($C_{10}H_{14}N_4O_4$) is a white, extremely bitter, amorphous solid, freely soluble in water and soluble to the extent of 2 g in 100 ml alcohol.

Tablets: Each blue, scored tablet contains dyphylline (dihydroxypropyl theophylline) 200 or 400 mg and the following inactive ingredients: colloidal silicon dioxide, corn starch, food starch, povidone, sodium lauryl sulfate, stearic acid and artificial coloring.

Elixir: Each tablespoon (15 ml) of Dyphylline elixir contains dyphylline 160 mg and alcohol USP 18% in a mint flavored base containing the following: citric acid, glycerin, saccharin sodium, sorbitol, sucrose, artificial coloring and flavorings. Methylparaben and propylparaben added as preservatives.

Injection: Dyphylline is chemically dihydroxypropyl theophylline, an alkylated theophylline molecule. Single dose ampules: Each 2 ml ampule contains dyphylline 500 mg (250 mg/ml) in water for injection USP, with sodium hydroxide NF to adjust pH.

CLINICAL PHARMACOLOGY:

As a xanthine derivative, dyphylline possesses the peripheral vasodilator and bronchodilator actions characteristic of theophylline. It has diuretic and myocardial stimulant effects, and is effective orally. Dyphylline may show fewer side effects than aminophylline, but its blood levels and possibly its activity are also lower.

The injectable preparation is for IM use only, and is indicated for treatment of an acute asthma attack.

INDICATIONS AND USAGE:

For relief of acute bronchial asthma and for reversible bronchospasm associated with chronic bronchitis and emphysema.

CONTRAINDICATIONS:

In individuals who have shown hypersensitivity to any of its components; dyphylline should not be administered concurrently with other xanthine preparations.

WARNINGS:

Status asthmaticus is a medical emergency. Excessive doses may be expected to be toxic. In children treated with dyphylline elixir, the alcoholic vehicle of the drug product poses a truly significant factor of drug dependence including all three components of tolerance, physical dependence and compulsive abuse.

Usage in Pregnancy: Safe use in pregnancy has not been established relative to possible adverse effects on fetal development. Therefore, dyphylline should not be used in pregnant women unless, in the judgement of the physician, the potential benefits outweigh the possible hazards.

PRECAUTIONS:

Use with caution in patients with severe cardiac disease, hypertension, hyperthyroidism, or acute myocardial injury. Particular caution in dose administration must be exercised in patients with peptic ulcers, since the condition may be exacerbated. Chronic oral administration in high doses (500 to 1,000 mg) is usually associated with gastrointestinal irritation.

Great caution should be used in giving dyphylline to patients in congestive heart failure. Such patients have shown markedly prolonged blood level curves which have persisted for long periods following discontinuation of the drug.

DRUG INTERACTIONS:

Toxic synergism with ephedrine and other sympathomimetic bronchodilator drugs may occur.

Recent controlled studies suggest that the addition of ephedrine to adequate dosage regimens of dyphylline produces no increase in effectiveness over that of dyphylline alone, but does produce an increase in toxic effects.

ADVERSE REACTIONS:

Note: Included in this listing which follows are a few adverse reactions which may not have been reported with this specific drug. However, pharmacological similarities among the xanthine drugs require that each of the reactions be considered when dyphylline is administered.

The most consistent adverse reactions are:

Gastrointestinal irritation: nausea, vomiting, and epigastric pain, generally preceded by headache, hematemesis, diarrhea.

Central nervous system stimulation: irritability, restlessness, insomnia, reflex hyperexcitability, muscle twitching, clonic and tonic generalized convulsions, agitation.

Cardiovascular: palpitation, tachycardia, extra systoles, flushing, marked hypotension, and circulatory failure.

Respiratory: tachypnea, respiratory arrest.

Renal: albuminuria, increased excretion of renal tubule and red blood cells.

Others: fever, dehydration.

OVERDOSAGE:

Signs and Symptoms

In Infants And Small Children: agitation, headache, hyperreflexia, fasciculations, and clonic and tonic convulsions.

In Adults: nervousness, insomnia, nausea, vomiting, tachycardia, and extra systoles.

Therapy

Discontinue drug immediately.

No specific treatment.

Ipecac syrup for oral ingestion.

Avoid sympathomimetics.

Supportive treatment for hypotension, seizure, arrhythmias and dehydration.

Sedatives such as short acting barbiturates will help control central nervous system stimulation.

Restore the acid-base with lactate or bicarbonate.

Oxygen and antibiotics provide supportive treatment as indicated.

DOSAGE AND ADMINISTRATION:

Pulmonary functional measurements before and after a period of treatment allow an objective assessment of whether or not therapy should be continued in patients with chronic bronchitis and emphysema.

DOSAGE AND ADMINISTRATION: *(cont'd)*

TABLETS

When administered orally it produces less nausea than aminophylline and other alkaline theophylline compounds. Absorption orally appears to be faster on an empty stomach; preferably the drug is to be given at six hour intervals.

Adults: *Usual Adult Dose:* 15 mg/kg every 6 hours up to 4 times a day. The dosage should be individualized by titration to the condition and response of the patient.

INJECTION

The injectable product is for IM use only and is to be injected very slowly. Preferably the drug is to be given at six hour intervals.

Adults: *Usual Adult Dose:* 500 mg, may be injected intramuscularly very slowly; and may be repeated if necessary.

Children: 14 mg/kg/24 hours; 0.45 g/kg/24 hours.

Store the injectable drug at room temperature. Excess cold may cause the injectable product to precipitate. DO NOT USE if precipitate is present, but clear solution can be achieved by autoclaving for 10 minutes at 250°F.

ELIXIR

When administered orally it produces less nausea than aminophylline and other alkaline theophylline compounds. Absorption orally appears to be faster on an empty stomach; preferably the drug is to be given at six hour intervals.

Adults: *Usual Adult Dose:* 15 mg/kg every 6 hours up to 4 times a day. The dosage should be individualized by titration to the condition to the condition and response of the patient.

Children: Dyphylline elixir dosage is based on the adult dose of 15 mg/kg every 6 hours.

20 - 40 lbs = 9 to 18 kg = 0.75 to 1.5 tablespoons every 6 hours.

40 - 60 lbs = 18 to 27 kg = 1.5 to 2.5 tablespoons every 6 hours.

60 - 80 lbs = 27 to 36 kg = 2.5 to 3.25 tablespoons very 6 hours.

80 - 100 lbs = 36 to 45 kg = 3.25 to 4.0 tablespoons every 6 hours.

HOW SUPPLIED - EQUIVALENTS NOT AVAILABLE:

Elixir - Oral - 100 mg/15ml

480 ml	$29.88	Dyphylline, Lunsco	10892-0150-65
480 ml	$61.74	LUFYLLIN, Wallace Labs	00037-0515-68
3840 ml	$465.52	LUFYLLIN, Wallace Labs	00037-0515-69

Elixir - Oral - 160 mg/5ml

480 ml	**$32.28**	**DILOR, Savage Labs**	**00281-1118-74**

Injection, Solution - Intramuscular - 250 mg/ml

2 ml x 6	**$26.85**	**DILOR, Savage Labs**	**00281-1112-31**
2 ml x 25	$368.76	LUFYLLIN, Wallace Labs	00037-0537-01

Tablet, Uncoated - Oral - 200 mg

100's	$11.95	LUFENESIN, Major Pharms	00904-1556-60
100's	$13.78	NEOTHYLLINE, Teva	00093-0030-01
100's	**$29.96**	**DILOR, Savage Labs**	**00281-1115-53**
100's	**$45.26**	**DILOR, Savage Labs**	**00281-1115-63**
100's	$98.56	LUFYLLIN, Wallace Labs	00037-0521-92
100's	$1097.93	LUFYLLIN, Wallace Labs	00037-0521-85
1000's	**$250.91**	**DILOR, Savage Labs**	**00281-1115-57**
1000's	$948.02	LUFYLLIN, Wallace Labs	00037-0521-97
5000's	$4612.30	LUFYLLIN, Wallace Labs	00037-0521-98

Tablet, Uncoated - Oral - 400 mg

100's	$13.30	LUFENESIN, Major Pharms	00904-1557-60
100's	$16.86	NEOTHYLLINE, Teva	00093-0037-01
100's	**$43.65**	**DILOR-400, Savage Labs**	**00281-1116-53**
100's	**$68.92**	**DILOR-400, Savage Labs**	**00281-1116-63**
100's	$144.74	LUFYLLIN-400, Wallace Labs	00037-0731-92
1000's	**$325.62**	**DILOR-400, Savage Labs**	**00281-1116-57**
1000's	$1306.75	LUFYLLIN-400, Wallace Labs	00037-0731-97
2500's	$3266.90	Lufyllin-400, Wallace Labs	00037-0731-99

DYPHYLLINE; EPHEDRINE; GUAIFENESIN; PHENOBARBITAL *(001123)*

CATEGORIES: Antiasthmatics/Bronchodilators; DESI Drugs; Respiratory & Allergy Medications; Respiratory Muscle Relaxant; Smooth Muscle Relaxants; FDA Pre 1938 Drugs

BRAND NAMES: Lufyllin-Epg

Prescribing information not available at time of publication.

HOW SUPPLIED - EQUIVALENTS NOT AVAILABLE:

Elixir - Oral - 100 mg/16 mg/20

480 ml	$125.20	LUFYLLIN-EPG, Wallace Labs	00037-0565-68

Tablet, Uncoated - Oral - 100 mg/16 mg/20

100's	$166.32	LUFYLLIN-EPG, Wallace Labs	00037-0561-92

DYPHYLLINE; GUAIFENESIN *(001124)*

CATEGORIES: Airway Obstruction; Antiasthmatics/Bronchodilators; Asthma; Bronchial Dilators; Bronchospasm; Decongestants; Respiratory & Allergy Medications; Respiratory Muscle Relaxant; Smooth Muscle Relaxants; Xanthine Derivatives; Pregnancy Category C; FDA Pre 1938 Drugs

BRAND NAMES: Difil-G; Dilex-G; Dilor-G; Dy-G Liquid; Dyfilin Gg; Dyflex-G; Dyline G.G.; Dyphyl Gg; Dyphylline Gg; Emfaseem; Lufenesin-G; **Lufyllin-Gg**; Neothylline Gg; Nuphyll-Gg; Panfil G; Thylline Gg

COST OF THERAPY: $284.70 (Asthma; Tablet; 200 mg/200 mg; 8/day; 365 days) vs. Potential Cost of $3,576.99 (Bronchitis & Asthma)

Prescribing information not available at time of publication.

HOW SUPPLIED - RATED THERAPEUTICALLY EQUIVALENT:

Elixir - Oral - 100 mg/100 mg

480 ml	$13.00	DYPHYLLINE-GG, Harber Pharm	51432-0578-20

HOW SUPPLIED - NOT RATED EQUIVALENT:

Elixir - Oral - 100 mg/100 mg

480 ml	$10.95	Dyphylline-Gg, Consolidated Midland	00223-6136-01
480 ml	$12.50	Dyphylline And Guaifenesin Liquid, Mikart	46672-0614-16
480 ml	$13.24	Dyphylline-Gg, Silarx Pharms	54838-0513-08
480 ml	$13.24	Dyphylline-Gg, Silarx Pharms	54838-0513-80
480 ml	$13.50	Dyphyl Gg, H N Norton Co.	50732-0897-16
480 ml	$14.10	DYPHYLLINE GG, Goldline Labs	00182-1375-40
480 ml	$14.15	Dyphlline Gg, Rugby	00536-0690-85
480 ml	$15.00	Dyphylline Gg, Hi Tech Pharma	50383-0806-16
480 ml	$15.30	Dyphylline Gg, Qualitest Pharms	00603-1190-58
480 ml	$15.75	DYPHYLLINE GG, Alpharma	00472-1238-16
480 ml	$16.94	DILEX-G, Poly Pharms	50991-0200-16
480 ml	$25.68	Dy-G Liquid, Cypress Pharm	60258-0371-16
480 ml	$29.66	DILOR-G, Savage Labs	00281-1127-74
480 ml	**$86.02**	**LUFYLLIN-GG, Wallace Labs**	**00037-0545-68**
3840 ml	$97.19	Dyphyl Gg, H N Norton Co.	50732-0897-28
3840 ml	**$659.94**	**LUFYLLIN-GG, Wallace Labs**	**00037-0545-69**

Tablet, Uncoated - Oral - 200 mg/200 mg

100's	$9.75	DYFLEX TABLETS, Embrex Economed	38130-0066-01
100's	$14.28	DYFLEX-G, Embrex Economed	38130-0012-01
100's	**$15.75**	**Lufyllin-Gg, Alphagen Labs**	**59743-0006-01**
100's	$15.80	DYPHYLLINE GG, United Res	00677-1037-01
100's	$16.45	LUFENESIN-GG, Major Pharms	00904-1558-60
100's	$16.94	DILEX-G, Poly Pharms	50991-0400-01
100's	$17.50	Dyphylline & Guaifenesin, Econolab	55053-0522-01
100's	$39.03	DILOR-G, Savage Labs	00281-1124-53
100's	$59.46	DILOR-G, Savage Labs	00281-1124-63
100's	**$147.26**	**LUFYLLIN-GG, Wallace Labs**	**00037-0541-92**
100's	**$1603.98**	**LUFYLLIN-GG, Wallace Labs**	**00037-0541-85**
1000's	$84.75	DYFLEX TABLETS, Embrex Economed	38130-0066-10
1000's	$107.70	DYFLEX-G, Embrex Economed	38130-0012-10
1000's	$135.00	Dilex-G, Poly Pharms	50991-0400-05
1000's	$344.47	DILOR-G, Savage Labs	00281-1124-57
1000's	**$1424.64**	**LUFYLLIN-GG, Wallace Labs**	**00037-0541-97**
3000's	**$4149.69**	**LUFYLLIN-GG, Wallace Labs**	**00037-0541-96**

ECHOTHIOPHATE IODIDE *(001126)*

CATEGORIES: Cataract; Cholinesterase Inhibitors; EENT Drugs; Esotropia; Eye, Ear, Nose, & Throat Preparations; Glaucoma; Miotics; Ophthalmics; Pregnancy Category C; FDA Approval Pre 1982

BRAND NAMES: *Phospholine*; **Phospholine Iodide**; *Phospholine Jodide*; *Phospholin-jodid* (Germany)
(International brand names outside U.S. in italics)

FORMULARIES: Aetna; BC-BS; FHP; Medi-Cal

COST OF THERAPY: $344.26 (Glaucoma; Solution; 0.03 %; 0.2/day; 365 days)

PRIMARY ICD9: 365.11 (Primary Open-Angle Glaucoma)

DESCRIPTION:

Chemical name: (2-mercaptoethyl) trimethylammonium iodide O,O- diethyl phosphorothioate

Echothiophate iodide occurs as a white, crystalline, water-soluble, hygroscopic solid having a slight mercaptan-like odor. When freeze-dried in the presence of potassium acetate, the mixture appears as a white amorphous deposit on the walls of the bottle.

Each package contains materials for dispensing 5 ml of eyedrops: (1) bottle containing sterile echothiophate iodide in one of four potencies (1.5 mg (0.03%), 3 mg (0.06%), 6.25 mg (0.125%), or 12.5 mg (0.25%)) as indicated on the label, with 40 mg potassium acetate in each case. Sodium hydroxide or acetic acid may have been incorporated to adjust pH during manufacturing. (2) a 5 ml bottle of sterile diluent containing chlorobutanol (chloral derivative), 0.55%; mannitol, 1.2%; boric acid, 0.06%; and exsiccated sodium phosphate, 0.026%. (3) sterilized dropper.

CLINICAL PHARMACOLOGY:

Echothiophate iodide is a long-acting cholinesterase inhibitor for topical use which enhances the effect of endogenously liberated acetylcholine in iris, ciliary muscle, and other parasympathetically innervated structures of the eye. It thereby causes miosis, increase in facility of outflow of aqueous humor, fall in intraocular pressure, and potentiation of accommodation.

Echothiophate iodide will depress both plasma and erythrocyte cholinesterase levels in most patients after a few weeks of eyedrop therapy.

INDICATIONS AND USAGE:

GLAUCOMA

Chronic open-angle glaucoma. Subacute or chronic angle-closure glaucoma after iridectomy or where surgery is refused or contraindicated. Certain non-uveitic secondary types of glaucoma, especially glaucoma following cataract surgery.

ACCOMMODATIVE ESOTROPIA

Concomitant esotropias with a significant accommodative component.

CONTRAINDICATIONS:

Active uveal inflammation.

Most cases of angle-closure glaucoma, due to the possibility of increasing angle block.

Hypersensitivity to the active or inactive ingredients.

WARNINGS:

Succinylcholine should be administered only with great caution, if at all, prior to or during general anesthesia to patients receiving anticholinesterase medication because of possible respiratory or cardiovascular collapse.

Caution should be observed in treating glaucoma with echothiophate iodide in patients who are at the same time undergoing treatment with systemic anticholinesterase medications for myasthenia gravis, because of possible adverse additive effects.

See DRUG INTERACTIONS for further information.

PRECAUTIONS:

GENERAL

Gonioscopy is recommended prior to initiation of therapy. Routine examination to detect lens opacity should accompany clinical use of echothiophate iodide.

Where there is a quiescent uveitis or a history of this condition, anticholinesterase therapy should be avoided or used cautiously because of the intense and persistent miosis and ciliary muscle contraction that may occur.

PRECAUTIONS: *(cont'd)*

While systemic effects are infrequent, proper use of the drug requires digital compression of the nasolacrimal ducts for a minute or two following instillation to minimize drainage into the nasal chamber with its extensive absorption area. To prevent possible skin absorption, hands should be washed following instillation.

Temporary discontinuance of medication is necessary if cardiac irregularities occur.

Anticholinesterase drugs should be used with extreme caution, if at all, in patients with marked vagotonia, bronchial asthma, spastic gastrointestinal disturbances, peptic ulcer, pronounced bradycardia and hypotension, recent myocardial infarction, epilepsy, parkinsonism, and other disorders that may respond adversely to vagotonic effects.

Anticholinesterase drugs should be employed prior to ophthalmic surgery only as a considered risk because of the possible occurrence of hyphema.

Echothiophate iodide should be used with great caution, if at all, where there is a prior history of retinal detachment.

Temporary discontinuance of medication is necessary if salivation, urinary incontinence, diarrhea, profuse sweating, muscle weakness, or respiratory difficulties occur.

Patients receiving echothiophate iodide who are exposed to carbamate- or organophosphate-type insecticides and pesticides (professional gardeners, farmers, workers in plants manufacturing or formulating such products, etc.) should be warned of the additive systemic effects possible from absorption of the pesticide through the respiratory tract or skin. During periods of exposure to such pesticides, the wearing of respiratory masks, and frequent washing and clothing changes may be advisable.

CARCINOGENESIS, MUTAGENESIS, AND IMPAIRMENT OF FERTILITY

No data is available regarding carcinogenesis, mutagenesis, and impairment of fertility.

PREGNANCY, TERATOGENIC EFFECTS, PREGNANCY CATEGORY C

Animal reproduction studies have not been conducted with echothiophate iodide. It is also not known whether echothiophate iodide can cause fetal harm when administered to a pregnant woman or can affect reproduction capacity. Echothiophate iodide should be given to a pregnant woman only if clearly needed.

NURSING MOTHERS

Because of the potential for serious adverse reactions in nursing infants from echothiophate iodide, a decision should be made whether to discontinue nursing or to discontinue the drug, taking into account the importance of the drug to the mother.

DRUG INTERACTIONS:

Echothiophate iodide potentiates other cholinesterase inhibitors such as succinylcholine or organophosphate and carbamate insecticides. Patients undergoing systemic anticholinesterase treatment should be warned of the possible additive effects of echothiophate iodide.

ADVERSE REACTIONS:

Although the relationship, if any, of retinal detachment to the administration of echothiophate iodide has not been established, retinal detachment has been reported in a few cases during the use of echothiophate iodide in adult patients without a previous history of this disorder.

Stinging, burning, lacrimation, lid muscle twitching, conjunctival and ciliary redness, browache, induced myopia with visual blurring may occur.

Activation of latent iritis or uveitis may occur.

Iris cysts may form, and if treatment is continued, may enlarge and obscure vision. This occurrence is more frequent in children. The cysts usually shrink upon discontinuance of the medication, reduction in strength of the drops or frequency of instillation. Rarely, they may rupture or break free into the aqueous. Regular examinations are advisable when the drug is being prescribed for the treatment of accommodative esotropia.

Prolonged use may cause conjunctival thickening, obstruction of nasolacrimal canals.

Lens opacities occurring in patients under treatment for glaucoma with echothiophate iodide have been reported and similar changes have been produced experimentally in normal monkeys. Routine examinations should accompany clinical use of the drug.

Paradoxical increase in intraocular pressure may follow anticholinesterase instillation. This may be alleviated by prescribing a sympathomimetic mydriatic such as phenylephrine.

Cardiac irregularities.

DOSAGE AND ADMINISTRATION:

Directions for Preparing Eyedrops

1. Use aseptic technique.
2. Tear off aluminum seals, and remove and discard rubber plugs from both drug and diluent containers.
3. Pour diluent into drug container.
4. Remove dropper assembly from its sterile wrapping. Holding dropper assembly by the screw cap and, WITHOUT COMPRESSING RUBBER BULB, insert into drug container and screw down tightly.
5. Shake for several seconds to ensure mixing.
6. Do not cover nor obliterate instructions to patient regarding storage of eyedrops.

GLAUCOMA

Selection of Therapy: The *medication prescribed* should be that which will control the intraocular pressure around-the-clock with the least risk of side effects or adverse reactions. "Tonometric glaucoma" (ocular hypertension without other evidence of the disease) is frequently not treated with any medication, and echothiophate iodide is certainly not recommended for this condition. In early chronic simple glaucoma with field loss or disc changes, pilocarpine is generally used for initial therapy and can be recommended so long as control is thereby maintained over the 24 hours of the day.

When this is not the case, echothiophate iodide 0.03% may be effective and probably has no greater potential for side effects. If this dosage is inadequate, epinephrine and a carbonic anhydrase inhibitor may be added to the regimen. When still more effective medication is required, the higher strengths of echothiophate iodide may be prescribe with the recognition that the control of the intraocular pressure should have priority regardless of potential side effects. In secondary glaucoma following cataract surgery, the higher strengths of the drug are frequently needed and are ordinarily very well tolerated.

The *dosage regimen* prescribed should call for the lowest concentration that will control the intraocular pressure around-the-clock. Where tonometry around-the-clock is not feasible, it is suggested that appointments for tension-taking be made at different times of the day so that inadequate control may be more readily detected. Two doses a day are preferred to one in order to maintain as smooth a diurnal tension curve as possible, although a single dose per day or every other day has been used with satisfactory results. Because of the long duration

DOSAGE AND ADMINISTRATION: *(cont'd)*

of action of the drug, it is never necessary or desirable to exceed a schedule of twice a day. The daily dose or one of the two daily doses should always be instilled just before retiring to avoid inconvenience due to the miosis.

Early Chronic Simple Glaucoma: Echothiophate iodide (echothiophate iodide) 0.03% instilled twice a day, just before retiring and in the morning, may be prescribed advantageously for cases of early chronic simple glaucoma that are not controlled around-the-clock with other less potent agents. Because of prolonged action, control during the night and early morning hours may then sometimes be obtained. A change in therapy is indicated if, at any time, the tension fails to remain at an acceptable level on this regimen.

Advanced Chronic Simple Glaucoma and Glaucoma Secondary to Cataract Surgery: These cases may respond satisfactorily to echothiophate iodide 0.03% twice a day as above. When the patient is being transferred to echothiophate iodide) because of unsatisfactory control with pilocarpine, carbachol, epinephrine, etc., one of the higher strengths, 0.06%, 0.125%, or 0.25% will usually be needed. In this case, a brief trial with the 0.03% eyedrops will be advantageous in that the higher strengths will then be more easily tolerated.

Concomitant Therapy: Echothiophate iodide may be used concomitantly with epinephrine, a carbonic anhydrase inhibitor, or both.

Technique: Good technique in the administration of echothiophate iodide requires that finger pressure at the inner canthus should be exerted for a minute or two following instillation of the eyedrops, to minimize drainage into the nose and throat. Excess solution around the eye should be removed with tissue and any medication on the hands should be rinsed off.

ACCOMMODATIVE ESOTROPIA (PEDIATRIC USE)

In Diagnosis: One drop of 0.125% may be instilled once a day in both eyes on retiring, for a period of two or three weeks. If the esotropia is accommodative, a favorable response will usually be noted which may begin within a few hours.

In Treatment: Echothiophate iodide (echothiophate iodide) is prescribed at the lowest concentration and frequency which gives satisfactory results. After the initial period of treatment for diagnostic purposes, the schedule may be reduced to 0.125% every other day or 0.06% every day. These dosages can often be gradually lowered as treatment progresses. The 0.03% strength has proven to be effective in some cases. The maximum usually recommended dosage is 0.125% once a day, although more intensive therapy has been used for short periods.

Technique: See DOSAGE AND ADMINISTRATION, Glaucoma.

Duration of Treatment: In diagnosis, only a short period is required and little time will be lost in instituting other procedures if the esotropia proves to be unresponsive. In therapy, there is no definite limit so long as the drug is well tolerated. However, if the eyedrops, with or without eyeglasses, are gradually withdrawn after about a year or two and deviation recurs, surgery should be considered. As with other miotics, tolerance may occasionally develop after prolonged use. In such cases, a rest period will restore the original activity of the drug.

Store at room temperature (approximately 25°C).

HOW SUPPLIED - EQUIVALENTS NOT AVAILABLE:

Solution - Ophthalmic - 0.03 %

5 ml	$23.58	PHOSPHOLINE IODIDE, Ayerst	00046-1062-05

Solution - Ophthalmic - 0.06 %

5 ml	$24.70	PHOSPHOLINE IODIDE, Ayerst	00046-1064-05

Solution - Ophthalmic - 0.125 %

5 ml	$27.71	PHOSPHOLINE IODIDE, Ayerst	00046-1065-05

Solution - Ophthalmic - 0.25 %

5 ml	$31.23	PHOSPHOLINE IODIDE, Ayerst	00046-1066-05

ECONAZOLE NITRATE *(001127)*

CATEGORIES: Anti-Infectives; Antibacterials; Antibiotics; Antifungals; Candidiasis; Dermatologicals; Fungal Agents; Skin/Mucous Membrane Agents; Tinea Corporis; Tinea Cruris; Tinea Pedis; Tinea Versicolor; Topical; Pregnancy Category C; FDA Approved 1982 Dec

BRAND NAMES: *Amicel*; *Bismultin*; *Dermazole*; *Ecanol*; *Eco*; *Econ*; *Ecostatin* (Australia, England, Canada); *Ecotam*; *Ecreme*; *Epi-Pevaryl* (Germany); *Fungazol*; *Micolis*; *Micos*; *Micostyl* (Mexico); *Palavale* (Japan); *Penicomb*; *Pevaryl* (Europe); **Spectazole**
(International brand names outside U.S. in italics)

FORMULARIES: Aetna; BC-BS; Medi-Cal

COST OF THERAPY: $12.37 (Tinea Pedis; Cream; 1 %; 1/day; 28 days)

DESCRIPTION:

Econazole Nitrate Cream contains the antifungal agent, econazole nitrate 1%, in a water-miscible base consisting of pegoxol 7 stearate, peglicol 5 oleate, mineral oil, benzoic acid, butylated hydroxyanisole, and purified water. The white to off-white soft cream is for topical use only.

Chemically, econazole nitrate is 1-(2-((4-chlorophenyl)methoxy)-2-(2,4-dichlorophenyl)ethyl)-1H-imidazole mononitrate.

CLINICAL PHARMACOLOGY:

After topical application to the skin of normal subjects, systemic absorption of econazole nitrate is extremely low. Although most of the applied drug remains on the skin surface, drug concentrations were found in the stratum corneum which, by far, exceeded the minimum inhibitory concentration for dermatophytes. Inhibitory concentrations were achieved in the epidermis and as deep as the middle region of the dermis. Less that 1% of the applied dose was recovered in the urine and feces.

Microbiology: In *in vitro* studies, econazole nitrate exhibits broad-spectrum antifungal activity against the dermatophytes, *Trichophyton rubrum, Trichophyton mentagrophytes, Trichophyton tonsurans, Microsporum canis, Microsporum audouini, Microsporum gypseum*, and *Epidermophyton floccosum*, the yeasts, *Candida albicans* and *Pityrosporum orbiculare* (the organism responsible for tinea versicolor), and certain gram positive bacteria.

INDICATIONS AND USAGE:

Econazole Nitrate Cream is indicated for topical application in the treatment of tinea pedis, tinea cruris, and tinea corporis caused by *Trichophyton rubrum, Trichophyton mentagrophytes, Trichophyton tonsurans, Microsporum canis, Microsporum audouini, Microsporum gypseum*, and *Epidermophyton floccosum*, in the treatment of cutaneous candidiasis, and in the treatment of tinea versicolor.

CONTRAINDICATIONS:

Econazole Nitrate Cream is contraindicated in individuals who have shown hypersensitivity to any of its ingredients.

WARNINGS:

Econazole Nitrate is not for ophthalmic use.

PRECAUTIONS:

General: If a reaction suggesting sensitivity or chemical irritation should occur, use of the medication should be discontinued.

For external use only. Avoid introduction of Econazole Nitrate Cream into the eyes.

Carcinogenicity Studies: Long-term animal studies to determine carcinogenic potential have not been performed.

Fertility (Reproduction): Oral administration of econazole nitrate in rats has been reported to produce prolonged gestation. Intravaginal administration in humans has not shown prolonged gestation or other adverse reproductive effects attributable to econazole nitrate therapy.

Pregnancy Category C Econazole nitrate has not been shown to be teratogenic when administered orally to mice, rabbits or rats. Fetotoxic or embryotoxic effects were observed in Segment I oral studies with rats receiving 10 to 40 times the human dermal dose. Similar effects were observed in Segment II of Segment III studies with mice, rabbits and/or rats receiving oral doses 80 or 40 times the human dermal dose.

Econazole should be used in the first trimester of pregnancy only when the physician considers it essential to the welfare of the patient. The drug should be used during the second and third trimesters of pregnancy only if clearly needed.

Nursing Mothers: It is not known whether econazole nitrate is excreted in human milk. Following oral administration of econazole nitrate to lactating rats, econazole and/or metabolites were excreted in milk and were found in nursing pups. Also, in lactating rats receiving large oral doses (40 to 80 times the human dermal dose), there was a reduction in post partum viability of pups and survival to weaning; however, at these high doses, maternal toxicity was present and may have been a contributing factor. Caution should be exercised when econazole nitrate is administered to a nursing woman.

ADVERSE REACTIONS:

During clinical trials, approximately 3% of patients treated with econazole nitrate 1% cream reported side effects thought possibly to be due to the drug, consisting mainly of burning itching, stinging and erythema. One case of pruritic rash has also been reported.

OVERDOSAGE:

Overdosage of econazole nitrate in humans has not been reported to date. In mice, rats, guinea pigs and dogs, the oral LD 50 values were found to be 462, 668, 272 and > 160 mg/kg respectively.

DOSAGE AND ADMINISTRATION:

Sufficient Econazole Nitrate Cream should be applied to cover affected areas once daily in patients with tinea pedis, tinea cruris, tinea corporis, and tinea versicolor, and twice daily (morning and evening) in patients with cutaneous candidiasis.

Early relief of symptoms is experienced by the majority of patients and clinical improvement may be seen fairly soon after treatment is begun; however, candidal infections and tinea cruris and corporis should be treated for two weeks and tinea pedis for one month in order to reduce the possibility of recurrence. If a patient shows no clinical improvement after the treatment period, the diagnosis should be redetermined. Patients with tinea versicolor usually exhibit clinical and mycological clearing after two weeks of treatment.

Store Econazole Nitrate Cream below 86°F.

HOW SUPPLIED - EQUIVALENTS NOT AVAILABLE:

Cream - Topical - 1 %

15 gm	$11.46	SPECTAZOLE, Ortho Pharm	00062-5460-02
30 gm	$19.44	SPECTAZOLE, Ortho Pharm	00062-5460-01
85 gm	$37.56	SPECTAZOLE, Ortho Pharm	00062-5460-03

EDETATE CALCIUM DISODIUM *(001128)*

CATEGORIES: Antagonists and Antidotes; Antidotes; Chelating Agents; Heavy Metal Antagonists; Poisoning; FDA Approval Pre 1982

BRAND NAMES: **Calcium Disodium Versenate**; *Calcitetracemate Disodique L'Arguenon* (France); *Ledclair* (England); *Natriumkalcium Edetat*; Sodium Calcium Edetate

(International brand names outside U.S. in italics)

FORMULARIES: WHO

> **WARNING:**
> Calcium Disodium Versenate is capable of producing toxic effects which can be fatal. In young children, the intravenous route may be fatal and, therefore, is not recommended. Lead encephalopathy is relatively rare in adults, but occurs more often in children in whom it may be incipient and thus overlooked. The mortality rate in these children has been high. Patients with lead encephalopathy and cerebral edema may experience a lethal increase in intracranial pressure following intravenous infusion; the intramuscular route is preferred for these patients. In cases where the intravenous route is necessary, avoid rapid infusion. The dosage schedule should be followed and at no time should be recommended daily dose be exceeded.

DESCRIPTION:

Calcium Disodium Versenate (edetate calcium disodium injection, USP) is a sterile, injectable, chelating agent in concentrated solution for intravenous infusion or intramuscular injection. Each 5 ml ampul contains 1000 mg of edetate calcium disodium (equivalent to 200 mg/ml) in water for injection. Chemically, this product is called ((N,N',-1,2- ethanediylbis(N-(carboxymethyl)-glycinato))(4-)-N,N',O,O',$O^{N}O^{N'}$)-, disodium, hydrate, (OC-6-21)- Calciate(2-). Molecular weight 374.27 (anhydrous)

CLINICAL PHARMACOLOGY:

The pharmacologic effects of edetate calcium disodium are due to the formation of chelates with divalent and trivalent metals. A stable chelate will form with any metal that has the ability to displace calcium from the molecule, a feature shared by lead, zinc, cadmium, manganese, iron and mercury. The amounts of manganese and iron mobilized are not significant. Copper[1] is not mobilized and mercury is unavailable for chelation because it is too tightly bound to body ligands or it is stored in inaccessible body compartments. The excretion of calcium by the body is not increased following intravenous administration of edetate calcium disodium, but the excretion of zinc is considerably increased.[1]

Edetate calcium disodium is poorly absorbed from the gastrointestinal tract. In blood, all the drug is found in the plasma. Edetate calcium disodium does not appear to penetrate cells; it is distributed primarily in the extracellular fluid with only about 5% of the plasma concentration found in spinal fluid.

The half life of edetate calcium disodium is 20 to 60 minutes. It is excreted primarily by the kidney, with about 50% excreted in one hour and over 95% within 24 hours.[2] Almost none of the compound is metabolized.

The primary source of lead chelated by Calcium Disodium Versenate is from bone; subsequently, soft-tissue lead is redistributed to bone when chelation is stopped.[3,4] There is also some reduction in kidney lead levels following chelation therapy.

It has been shown in animals that following a single dose of Calcium Disodium Versenate urinary lead output increases, blood lead concentration decreases, but brain lead is significantly increased due to internal redistribution of lead.[5] (See WARNINGS.) These data are in agreement with the recent results of others in experimental animals showing that after a five day course of treatment there is no net reduction in brain lead.[6]

INDICATIONS AND USAGE:

Edetate calcium disodium is indicated for the reduction of blood levels and depot stores of lead in lead poisoning (acute and chronic) and lead encephalopathy, in both children and adults.

Chelation therapy should not replace effective measures to eliminate or reduce further exposure to lead.

CONTRAINDICATIONS:

Edetate calcium disodium should not be given during periods of anuria, nor to patients with active renal disease or hepatitis.

WARNINGS:

See BOXED WARNING.

PRECAUTIONS:

GENERAL

Edetate calcium disodium may produce the same renal damage as lead poisoning, such as proteinuria and microscopic hematuria. Treatment- induced nephrotoxicity is dose-dependent and may be reduced by assuring adequate diuresis before therapy begins. Urine flow must be monitored throughout therapy which must be stopped if anuria or severe oliguria develop. The proximal tubule hydropic degeneration usually recovers upon cessation of therapy. Edetate calcium disodium must be used in reduced doses in patients with pre-existing mild renal disease.

Patients should be monitored for cardiac rhythm irregularities and other ECG changes during intravenous therapy.

INFORMATION FOR THE PATIENT

Patients should be instructed to immediately inform their physician if urine output stops for a period of 12 hours.

LABORATORY TESTS

Urinalysis and urine sediment, renal and hepatic function and serum electrolyte levels should be checked before each course of therapy and then be monitored daily during therapy in severe cases, and in less serious cases after the second and fifth day of therapy. Therapy must be discontinued at the first sign of renal toxicity. The presence of large renal epithelial cells or increasing number of red blood cells in urinary sediment or greater proteinuria call for immediate stopping of edetate calcium disodium administration. Alkaline phosphatase values are frequently depressed (possibly due to decreased serum zinc levels), but return to normal within 48 hours after cessation of therapy. Elevated erythrocyte protoporphyrin levels (>35 mcg/dl of whole blood) indicate the need to perform a venous blood lead determination. If the whole blood lead concentration is between 25-55 mcg/dl a mobilization test can be considered.[7,8] (See Diagnostic Test.) An elevation of urinary coproporphyrin (adults: >250 mcg/day; children under 80 lbs:>75 mcg/day) and elevation of urinary delta aminolevulinic acid (ALA) (adults:>4 mg/day; children:>3 $mg/m^2/day$) are associated with blood lead levels >40 mcg/dl. Urinary coproporphyrin may be falsely negative in terminal patients and in severely iron-depleted children who are not regenerating heme.[9] In growing children long bone x-rays showing lead lines and abdominal x-rays showing radio-opaque material in the abdomen may be of help in estimating the level of exposure to lead.

CARCINOGENESIS, MUTAGENESIS, AND IMPAIRMENT OF FERTILITY

Long term animal studies have not been conducted with edetate calcium disodium to evaluate its carcinogenic potential, mutagenic potential or its effect on fertility.

PREGNANCY

Category B: One reproduction study was performed in rats at doses up to 13 times the human dose and revealed no evidence of impaired fertility or harm to the fetus due to Calcium Disodium Versenate.[10]Another reproduction study performed in rats at doses up to about 25 to 40 times the human dose revealed evidence of fetal malformations due to Calcium Disodium Versenate, which were prevented by simultaneous supplementation of dietary zinc.[11] There are, however, no adequate and well-controlled studies in pregnant women. Because animal reproduction studies are not always predictive of human response, this drug should be used during pregnancy only if clearly needed.

LABOR AND DELIVERY

Calcium Disodium Versenate has no recognized use during labor and delivery, and its effects during these processes are unknown.

NURSING MOTHERS

It is not known whether this drug is excreted in human milk. Because many drugs are excreted in human milk, caution should be exercised when Calcium Disodium Versenate is administered to a nursing women.

PEDIATRIC USE

Since lead poisoning occurs in children and adults but is frequently more severe in children, Calcium Disodium Versenate is used in patients of all ages.

DRUG INTERACTIONS:

There is no known drug interference with standard clinical laboratory tests. Steroids enhance the renal toxicity of edetate calcium disodium in animals.[7] Edetate calcium disodium interferes with the action of zinc insulin preparations by chelating the zinc.[7]

ADVERSE REACTIONS:

The following adverse effects have been associated with the use of edetate calcium disodium:

Body as a Whole: pain at intramuscular injection site, fever, chills, malaise, fatigue, myalgia, arthralgia.

Cardiovascular: hypotension, cardiac rhythm irregularities.

Renal: acute necrosis of proximal tubules (which may result in fatal nephrosis), infrequent changes in distal tubules and glomeruli.

Urinary: glycosuria, proteinuria, microscopic hematuria and large epithelial cells in urinary sediment.

Nervous System: tremors, headache, numbness, tingling.

Gastrointestinal: cheilosis, nausea, vomiting, anorexia, excessive thirst.

Hepatic: mild increases in SGOT and SGPT are common, and return to normal within 48 hours after cessation of therapy.

Immunogenic: histamine-like reactions (sneezing, nasal congestion, lacrimation), rash.

Hematopoietic: transient bone morrow depression, anemia.

Metabolic: zinc deficiency, hypercalcemia.

OVERDOSAGE:

Symptoms: Inadvertent administration of 5 times the recommended dose, infused intravenously over a 24 hour period, to an asymptomatic 16 month old patient with a blood lead content of 56 mcg/dl did not cause any ill effects. Edetate calcium disodium can aggravate the symptoms of severe lead poisoning, therefore, most toxic effects (cerebral edema, renal tubular necrosis) appear to be associated with lead poisoning. Because of cerebral edema, a therapeutic dose may be lethal to an adult or a child with lead encephalopathy. Higher dosage of edetate calcium disodium may produce a more severe zinc deficiency.

Treatment: Cerebral edema should be treated with repeated doses of mannitol. Steroids enhance the renal toxicity of edetate calcium disodium in animals and, therefore, are no longer recommended.[7] Zinc levels must be monitored. Good urinary output must be maintained because diuresis will enhance drug elimination. It is not known if edetate calcium disodium is dialyzable.

DOSAGE AND ADMINISTRATION:

When a source for the lead intoxication has been identified, the patient should be removed from the source, if possible.

The recommended dose of Calcium Disodium Versenate for asymptomatic adults and children whose blood lead level is <70 mcg/dl but >20 mcg/dl (World Health Organization recommended upper allowable level) is 1000 mg/m^2/day whether given intravenously or intramuscularly.

For adults with lead nephropathy, the following dosage regimen has been suggested: 500 mg/m^2 every 24 hours for 5 days for patients with serum creatinine levels of 2-3 mg/dl, every 48 hours for 3 doses for patients with creatinine levels of 3-4 mg/dl, and once weekly for patients with creatinine levels above 4 mg/dl. These regimens may be repeated at one month intervals.[12]

Calcium Disodium Versenate, used alone, may aggravate symptoms in patients with very high blood lead levels. When the blood lead level is >70 mcg/dl or clinical symptoms consistent with lead poisoning are present, it is recommended that Calcium Disodium Versenate be used in conjunction with BAL (dimercaprol). Please consult published protocols and specialized references for dosage recommendations of combination therapy.[14-18]

Therapy of lead poisoning in adults and children with Calcium Disodium Versenate is continued over a period of five days. Therapy is then interrupted for 2 to 4 days to allow redistribution of the lead and to prevent severe depletion of zinc and other essential metals. Two courses of treatment are usually employed; however, it depends on severity of the lead toxicity and the patient's tolerance of the drug.

Calcium Disodium Versenate is equally effective whether administered intravenously or intramuscularly. The intramuscular route is used for all patients with overt lead encephalopathy and this route is exclusively recommended for young children.

Acutely ill individuals may be dehydrated from vomiting. Since edetate calcium disodium is excreted almost exclusively in the urine, it is very important to establish urine flow with intravenous fluid administration before the first dose of the chelating agent is given; however, excessive fluid must be avoided in patients with encephalopathy. Once urine flow is established, further intravenous fluid is restricted to basal water and electrolyte requirements. Administration of Calcium Disodium Versenate should be stopped whenever there is cessation of urine flow in order to avoid unduly high tissue levels of the drug. Edetate calcium disodium must be used in reduced doses in patients with pre-existing mild renal disease.

Intravenous Administration: Add to total daily dose of Calcium Disodium Versenate (1000 mg/m^2/day) to 250-500 ml of 5% dextrose or 0.9% sodium chloride injection. The total daily dose should be infused over a period of 8-12 hours. Calcium Disodium Versenate injection is incompatible with 10% dextrose, 10% invert sugar in 0.9% sodium chloride, lactate Ringer's, Ringer's, one-sixth molar sodium lactate injections, and with injectable amphotericin B and hydralazine hydrochloride.

Intramuscular Administration: The total daily dosage (1000 mg/m^2/day) should be divided into equal doses spaced 8-12 hours apart. Lidocaine or procaine should be added to the Calcium Disodium Versenate injection to minimize pain at the injection site. The final lidocaine or procaine concentration of 5 mg/ml (0.5%) can be obtained as follows: 0.25 ml of 10% lidocaine solution per 5 ml (entire content of ampul) concentrated Calcium Disodium Versenate; 1 ml of 1% lidocaine or procaine solution per ml of concentrated Calcium Disodium Versenate. When used alone, regardless of method of administration, Calcium Disodium Versenate should not be given at doses larger than those recommended.

Diagnostic Test: Several methods have been described for lead mobilization tests using edetate calcium disodium to assess body stores.[7,9,12,13,18]

These procedures have advantages and disadvantages that should be reviewed in current references. Edetate calcium disodium mobilization tests should not be performed in symptomatic patients and in patients with blood lead levels above 55 mcg/dl for whom appropriate therapy is indicated.

Parenteral drugs should be inspected visually for particulate matter and discoloration prior to administration, whenever solution and container permit.

Store at controlled room temperature 15°-30°C (59°-86°F).

REFERENCES:

1. Thomas DJ, Chisolm JJ. Lead, zinc and copper decorporation during calcium disodium ethylenediamine tetraacetate treatment of lead- poisoned children. J Pharmacol Exp Therapeu 1986; 239:829-835. **2.** The Pharmacological Basis of Therapeutics, 7th edition, Goodman and Gilman, editors. MacMillan Publishing Company, New York, 1985, pp. 1619-1622. **3.** Hammond PB, Aronson AL, Olson WC. The mechanism of mobilization of lead by ethylenediaminetetraacetate. J Pharmacol Exp Therapeu 1967; 157:196-206. **4.** Van de Vyver FL, D'Haese PC, Visser WJ, et al. Bone lead in dialysis patients. Kidney Intl 1988; 33:601-607. **5.** Cory-Slecta DA, Weiss B, Cox C. Mobilization and redistribution of lead over the course of calcium disodium ethylenediamine tetraacetate chelation therapy. J Pharmacol Exp Therapeu 1987; 243:804-813. **6.** Chisolm JJ. Mobilization of lead by calcium disodium edetate. Am J Dis Child 1987; 141:1256-1257. **7.** Drug Evaluations, 6th Edition, American Medical Association, Saunders, Philadelphia, 1986, pp. 1637-1639. **8.** Centers for Disease Control: Preventing lead poisoning in young children. Atlanta, GA, Department of Health and Human Services,

REFERENCES: *(cont'd)*

1985 Jan. **9.** Finberg L, Rajagopal V. Diagnosis and treatment of lead poisoning in children. J Family Med 1985 April: 3-12. **10.** Schardein JL, Sakowski R, Petrere J, et al. Teratogenesis studies with EDTA and its salts in rats. Toxicol Appl Pharmacol 1981; 61:423- 428. **11.** Swenerton H, Hurley LS. Teratogenic effects of a chelating agent and their prevention by zinc. Science 1971; 173:62-64. **12.** American Hospital Formulary Service, Drug Information, 1988, pp. 1695-1698. **13.** Markowitz ME, Rosen JF. Assessment of lead stores in children: Validation of an 8-hour $CaNa_2EDTA$ (Calcium Disodium Versenate) provocative test. J Pediatrics 1984; 104:337-341. **14.** Piomelli S, Rosen JF, Chisolm JJ, et al. Management of childhood lead poisoning. J Pediatrics 1984; 105:523-532. **15.** Sachs HK Blanksma LA, Murray EF, et al. Ambulatory treatment of lead poisoning: Report of 1,155 cases. Pediatrics 1970; 46:389. **16.** Chisolm JJ. The use of chelating agents in the treatment of acute and chronic lead intoxication in childhood. J Pediatrics 1968; 73:1. **17.** Coffin R, Phillips JL, Staples WI, et al. Treatment of lead encephalopathy in children. J Pediatrics 1966; 69:198-206. **18.** Chisolm JJ. Increased lead absorption and acute lead poisoning. Current Pediatric Therapy 12, Gillis and Kagan, editors, WB Saunders, Philadelphia, 1986, pp. 667-671.

HOW SUPPLIED - EQUIVALENTS NOT AVAILABLE:

Injection, Solution - Intravenous - 200 mg/ml

5 ml x 6 $189.78 CALCIUM DISODIUM VERSENATE, 3M Pharms 00089-0510-06

EDETATE DISODIUM *(001129)*

CATEGORIES: Antagonists and Antidotes; Antidotes; Arrhythmia; Calcium Metabolism; Heavy Metal Antagonists; Homeostatic & Nutrient; Hypercalcemia; Ophthalmics; Toxicity, Digitalis; Atherosclerosis*; Chelating Agents*; Pregnancy Category C; FDA Approval Pre 1982

* Indication not approved by the FDA

BRAND NAMES: Chealamide; Disodium Edetate; Disotate; EDTA; **Endrate**; Sodium Versenate; *Tracemate* (France)

(International brand names outside U.S. in italics)

FOR INTRAVENOUS INFUSION ONLY AFTER DILUTION

THE USE OF THIS DRUG IN ANY PARTICULAR PATIENT IS RECOMMENDED ONLY WHEN THE SEVERITY OF THE CLINICAL CONDITION JUSTIFIES THE AGGRESSIVE MEASURES ASSOCIATED WITH THIS TYPE OF THERAPY.

DESCRIPTION:

Edetate disodium injection is a sterile, nonpyrogenic, concentrated solution of edetate disodium in water for injection which as a result of a pH adjustment with sodium hydroxide contains varying amounts of disodium and trisodium salts. After dilution, it is administered by intravenous infusion.

Each milliliter (ml) contains edetate disodium, anhydrous 150 mg. The pH is 7.0 (approx.) adjusted with sodium hydroxide.

Edetate disodium is classified as a clinical chelating agent for emergency lowing of serum calcium in hypercalcemia.

The solution contains no bacteriostat, antimicrobial agent or buffer (except for pH adjustment) and is intended only for use (after dilution) as a single dose infusion. When smaller doses are required, the unused portion should be discarded.

Edetate disodium is chemically designated disodium (ethylenedinitrilo) tetraacetate dihydrate, a white crystalline powder soluble in water. It is also described as the disodium salt of ethylenediamine tetraacetic acid (EDTA).

CLINICAL PHARMACOLOGY:

Edetate disodium injection forms chelates with the cations of calcium and many divalent and trivalent metals. Because of its affinity for calcium, edetate disodium will produce a lowering of the serum calcium level during intravenous infusion. Slow infusion over a protracted period may cause mobilization of extracirculatory calcium stores. Edetate disodium exerts a negative inotropic effect upon the heart.

After intravenous administration, the chelate formed is excreted in the urine with 50% appearing in 1 hour and over 95% in 24 hours.

Edetate disodium likewise forms chelates with other polyvalent metals and produces increases in urinary excretion of magnesium, zinc and other trace elements. It does not form a chelate with potassium but may reduce the serum level and increase urinary loss of potassium.

INDICATIONS AND USAGE:

Edetate disodium injection is indicated in selected patients for the emergency treatment of hypercalcemia and for the control of ventricular arrhythmias associated with digitalis toxicity.

CONTRAINDICATIONS:

Edetate disodium injection is contraindicated in anuric patients. It is not indicated for the treatment of generalized arteriosclerosis associated with advancing age.

WARNINGS:

See BOXED WARNING.

Rapid intravenous infusion or attainment of high serum concentration of edetate disodium may cause a precipitous drop in the serum calcium level and may result in fatality. Toxicity appears to be dependent upon both total dosage and speed of administration. The rate of administration and dosage should not exceed that indicated in DOSAGE AND ADMINISTRATION.

Because of its irritant effect on the tissues and because of the danger of serious side effects if administered in the undiluted form, Edetate disodium injection, should be diluted before infusion. See DOSAGE AND ADMINISTRATION.

PRECAUTIONS:

Alter the infusion of edetate disodium, the patient should remain in bed for a short time because of the possibility of postural hypotension.

The possibility of an adverse effect on myocardial contractility should be considered when administering the drug to patients with heart disease. Caution is dictated in the use of this drug in patients with limited cardiac reserve or incipient congestive failure.

Edetate disodium injection therapy should be used with caution in patients with clinical or subclinical potassium deficiency states. In such cases it is advisable to perform serum potassium blood levels for possible hypokalemia and to monitor ECG changes.

The possibility of hypomagnesemia should be kept in mind during prolonged therapy.

Treatment with edetate disodium has been shown to cause a lowering of blood sugar and insulin requirements in patients with diabetes who are treated with insulin.

Do not use unless solution is clear and container is intact. Discard unused portion.

LABORATORY TESTS

Renal excretory function should be assessed prior to treatment. Periodic BUN and creatinine determinations and daily urinalysis should be performed on patients receiving this drug.

PRECAUTIONS: *(cont'd)*

Because of the possibility of inducing an electrolyte imbalance during treatment with edetate disodium, appropriate laboratory determinations and studies to evaluate the status of cardiac function should be performed. Repetition of these tests is recommended as often as clinically indicated, particularly in patients with ventricular arrhythmia and those with a history of seizure disorders or intracranial lesions. If clinical evidence suggests any disturbance of liver function during treatment, appropriate laboratory determinations should be performed and withdrawal of the drug may be required.

DRUG/LABORATORY TEST INTERACTIONS

The oxalate method of determining serum calcium tends to give low readings in the presence of edetate disodium; modification of this method, as by acidifying the sample or use of a different method may be required for accuracy. The least interference will be noted immediately before a subsequent dose is administered.

CARCINOGENESIS, MUTAGENESIS, AND IMPAIRMENT OF FERTILITY

Definitive statements cannot be made due to insufficient data and conflicting information.

PREGNANCY CATEGORY C

Animal reproduction studies have not been conducted with Edetate Disodium injection. It is also not known whether Edetate Disodium injection can cause fetal harm when administered to a pregnant woman or can affect reproduction capacity. Edetate Disodium injection should be given to a pregnant woman only if clearly needed.

NURSING MOTHERS

The safety of this product in nursing mothers has not been established.

DRUG INTERACTIONS:

Additives may be incompatible with the reconstituted (diluted) solution required for intravenous infusion. Consult with pharmacist, if available. When introducing additives, use aseptic technique, mix thoroughly and do not store.

ADVERSE REACTIONS:

Gastrointestinal symptoms such as nausea, vomiting and diarrhea are fairly common following administration of this drug. Transient symptoms such as circumoral paresthesia, numbness and headache and a transient drop in systolic and diastolic blood pressure may occur. Thrombophlebitis, febrile reactions, hyperuricemia, anemia, exfoliative dermatitis and other toxic skin and mucous membrane reactions have been reported.

Nephrotoxicity and damage to the reticuloendothelial system with hemorrhagic tendencies have been reported with excessive dosages.

OVERDOSAGE:

Because of the possibility that Edetate disodium injection may produce a precipitous drop in the serum calcium level, a source of calcium replacement suitable for intravenous administration (such as calcium gluconate) should be instantly available at the bedside before edetate disodium is administered. Extreme caution is dictated in the use of intravenous calcium in the treatment of tetany, especially in digitalized patients because the action of the drug and the replacement of calcium ions may produce a reversal of the desired digitalis effect.

DOSAGE AND ADMINISTRATION:

Edetate disodium injection is administered by intravenous infusion only after dilution.

For Adults: The recommended daily dosage is 50 mg/kg of body weight to maximum dose of 3 g in 24 hours. The dose, calculated by body weight, should be diluted in 500 ml of 5% Dextrose injection, USP or 0.9% Sodium chloride injection, USP. The intravenous infusion should be regulated so that three or more hours are required for completion and the cardiac reserve of the patient is not exceeded. A suggested regimen includes five consecutive daily doses followed by two days without medication, with repeated courses as necessary to a total of 15 doses.

For Children: The recommended daily dosage is 40 mg/kg (1 g per 25 kg) of body weight. The dose, calculated by body weight, should be diluted in a sufficient volume of 5% Dextrose injection, USP or 0.9% Sodium chloride injection, USP to bring the final concentration of edetate disodium to not more than 3%. The intravenous infusion should be regulated so that three or more hours are required for completion and the cardiac reserve of the patient is not exceeded. The maximum dose is 70 mg/kg per 24-hour period.

Parenteral drug products should be inspected visually for particulate matter and discoloration prior to administration, whenever solution and container permit. See PRECAUTIONS.

Storage: Exposure of pharmaceutical products to heat should be minimized. Avoid excessive heat. Protect from freezing. It is recommended that the product be stored at room temperature (25°C); however, brief exposure up to 40°C does not adversely affect the product.

HOW SUPPLIED - RATED THERAPEUTICALLY EQUIVALENT:

Injection, Solution - Intravenous - 150 mg/ml

20 ml	$3.05	Edetate Disodium, McGuff	49072-0177-20
20 ml	$4.15	Disodium Edetate, Pegasus Med Svs	10974-0079-20
20 ml	$5.50	Edetate Disodium, Hyrex Pharms	00314-0277-20
20 ml	$6.25	Edetate Disodium, Consolidated Midland	00223-7494-20
20 ml	$10.00	DISOTATE, Forest Pharms	00456-0724-17
20 ml	$18.70	Edetate Disodium, Steris Labs	00402-0277-20
20 ml	$20.57	Edetate Disodium, Schein Pharm (US)	00364-2485-55
20 ml	**$26.70**	**ENDRATE, Abbott**	**00074-6940-03**
20 ml x 25	$118.75	Disodium Edetate (EDTA), Pasadena	00418-0351-20

EDROPHONIUM CHLORIDE *(001130)*

CATEGORIES: Antiarrhythmic Agents; Autonomic Drugs; Cholinesterase Inhibitors; Diagnostic Agents; Myasthenia Gravis; Neuromuscular; Parasympathomimetic Agents; Renal Drugs; Respiratory Depression; FDA Approval Pre 1982

BRAND NAMES: Enlon; Reversol; **Tensilon**

DESCRIPTION:

Edrophonium chloride is a short and rapid-acting cholinergic drug. Chemically, edrophonium chloride is ethyl(*m*-hydroxyphenyl)dimethyl-ammonium chloride.

Each ml contains, in a sterile solution, 10 mg edrophonium chloride compounded with 0.45% phenol and 0.2% sodium sulfite as an antioxidant, buffered with sodium citrate and citric acid, and pH adjusted to approximately 5.4.

Edrophonium chloride is intended for IV and IM use.

CLINICAL PHARMACOLOGY:

Edrophonium chloride is an anticholinesterase drug. Its pharmacological action is due primarily to the inhibition or inactivation of acetylcholinesterase at sites of cholinergic transmission. Its effect is manifest within 30 to 60 seconds after injection and lasts an average of 10 minutes.

INDICATIONS AND USAGE:

Edrophonium chloride is recommended for the differential diagnosis of myasthenia gravis and as an adjunct in the evaluation of treatment requirements in this disease. It may also be used for evaluating emergency treatment in myasthenic crises. Because of its brief duration of action, it is not recommended for maintenance therapy in myasthenia gravis.

Edrophonium chloride is also useful whenever a curare antagonist is needed to reverse the neuromuscular block produced by curare, tubocurarine, gallamine triethiodide or dimethyl-tubocurarine. It is not effective against decamethonium bromide and succinylcholine chloride. It may be used adjunctively in the treatment of respiratory depression caused by curare overdosage.

CONTRAINDICATIONS:

Known hypersensitivity to anticholinesterase agents; intestinal and urinary obstructions of mechanical type.

WARNINGS:

Whenever anticholinesterase drugs are used for testing, a syringe containing 1 mg of atropine sulfate should be immediately available to be given in aliquots intravenously to counteract severe cholinergic reactions which may occur in the hypersensitive individual, whether he is normal or myasthenic. Edrophonium chloride should be used with caution in patients with bronchial asthma or cardiac dysrhythmias. The transient bradycardia which sometimes occurs can be relieved by atropine sulfate. Isolated instances of cardiac and respiratory arrest following administration of edrophonium chloride have been reported. It is postulated that these are vagotonic effects.

Edrophonium chloride solution contains sodium sulfite, a sulfite that may cause allergic-type reactions, including anaphylactic symptoms and life-threatening or less severe asthmatic episodes in certain susceptible people. The overall prevalence of sulfite sensitivity in the general population is unknown and probably low. Sulfite sensitivity is seen more frequently in asthmatic than in non-asthmatic people.

Usage in Pregnancy: The safety of edrophonium chloride during pregnancy or lactation in humans has not been established. Therefore, use of edrophonium chloride in women who may become pregnant requires weighing the drug's potential benefits against its possible hazards to mother and child.

PRECAUTIONS:

Patients may develop "anticholinesterase insensitivity" for brief or prolonged periods. During these periods the patients should be carefully monitored and may need respiratory assistance. Dosages of anticholinesterase drugs should be reduced or withheld until patients again become sensitive to them.

DRUG INTERACTIONS:

Care should be given when administering this drug to patients with symptoms of myasthenic weakness who are also on anticholinesterase drugs. Since symptoms of anticholinesterase overdose (cholinergic crisis) may mimic underdosage (myasthenic weakness), their condition may be worsened by the use of this drug. (See OVERDOSAGE for treatment.)

ADVERSE REACTIONS:

Careful observation should be made for severe cholinergic reactions in the hyperreactive individual. The myasthenic patient in crisis who is being tested with edrophonium chloride should be observed for bradycardia or cardiac standstill and cholinergic reactions if an overdose is given. The following reactions common to anticholinesterase agents may occur, although not all of these reactions have been reported with the administration of edrophonium chloride, probably because of its short duration of action and limited indications:

Eye: Increased lacrimation, pupillary constriction, spasm of accommodation, diplopia, conjunctival hyperemia.

CNS: Convulsions, dysarthria, dysphonia, dysphagia.

Respiratory: Increased tracheobronchial secretions, laryngospasm, bronchiolar constriction, paralysis of muscles of respiration, central respiratory paralysis.

Cardiac: Arrhythmias (especially bradycardia), fall in cardiac output leading to hypotension.

G.I. : Increased salivary, gastric and intestinal secretion, nausea, vomiting, increased peristalsis, diarrhea, abdominal cramps.

Skeletal Muscle: Weakness, fasciculations.

Miscellaneous: Increased urinary frequency and incontinence, diaphoresis.

OVERDOSAGE:

With drugs of this type, muscarine-like symptoms (nausea, vomiting, diarrhea, sweating, increased bronchial and salivary secretions and bradycardia) often appear with overdosage (cholinergic crisis). An important complication that can arise is obstruction of the airway by bronchial secretions. These may be managed with suction (especially if tracheostomy has been performed) and by the use of atropine. Many experts have advocated a wide range of dosages of atropine (for Edrophonium chloride, see atropine dosage below), but if there are copious secretions, up to 1.2 mg intravenously may be given initially and repeated every 20 minutes until secretions are controlled. Signs of atropine overdosage such as dry mouth, flush and tachycardia should be avoided as tenacious secretions and bronchial plugs may form. A total dose of atropine of 5 to 10 mg or even more may be required. The following steps should be taken in the management of overdosage of edrophonium chloride:

1. Adequate respiratory exchange should be maintained by assuring an open airway, and the use of assisted respiration augmented by oxygen.

2. Cardiac function should be monitored until complete stabilization has been achieved.

3. Atropine sulfate in doses of 0.4 to 0.5 mg should be administered intravenously. This may be repeated every 3 to 10 minutes. Because of the short duration of action of edrophonium chloride the total dose required will seldom exceed 2 mg.

4. Pralidoxime chloride (a cholinesterase reactivator) may be given intravenously at the rate of 50 to 100 mg per minute; usually the total dose does not exceed 1000 mg. Extreme caution should be exercised in the use of pralidoxime chloride when the cholinergic symptoms are induced by double-bond phosphorous anticholinesterase drugs.[9]

5. If convulsions or shock is present, appropriate measures should be instituted.

DOSAGE AND ADMINISTRATION:

Edrophonium chloride Test in the Differential Diagnosis of Myasthenia Gravis:[1-8]

Intravenous Dosage (Adults): A tuberculin syringe containing 1 ml (10 mg) of edrophonium chloride is prepared with an intravenous needle, and 0.2 ml (2 mg) is injected intravenously within 15 to 30 seconds. The needle is left in situ. Only if no reaction occurs after 45 seconds is the remaining 0.8 ml (8 mg) injected. If a cholinergic reaction (muscarinic side effects, skeletal muscle fasciculations and increased muscle weakness) occurs after injection of 0.2 ml (2 mg), the test is discontinued and atropine sulfate 0.4 mg to 0.5 mg is administered intravenously. After one-half hour the test may be repeated.

DOSAGE AND ADMINISTRATION: *(cont'd)*

Intramuscular Dosage (Adults): In adults with inaccessible veins, dosage for intramuscular injection is 1 ml (10 mg) of edrophonium chloride. Subjects who demonstrate hyperreactivity to this injection (cholinergic reaction), should be retested after one-half hour with 0.2 ml (2 mg) of edrophonium chloride intramuscularly to rule out false-negative reactions.

Dosage (Children): The intravenous testing dose of edrophonium chloride in children weighing up to 75 lbs is 0.1 ml (1 mg): above this weight, the dose is 0.2 ml (2 mg). If there is no response after 45 seconds, it may be titrated up to 0.5 ml (5 mg) in children under 75 lbs, given in increments of 0.1 ml (1 mg) every 30 to 45 seconds and up to 1 ml (10 mg) in heavier children. In infants, the recommended dose is 0.05 ml (0.5 mg). Because of technical difficulty with intravenous injection in children, the intramuscular route may be used. In children weighing up to 75 lbs, 0.2 ml (2 mg) is injected intramuscularly. In children weighing more than 75 lbs, 0.5 ml (5 mg) is injected intramuscularly. All signs which would appear with the intravenous test appear with the intramuscular test except that there is a delay of two to ten minutes before a reaction is noted.

Edrophonium chloride Test for Evaluation of Treatment Requirements in Myasthenia Gravis: The recommended dose is 0.1 ml to 0.2 ml (1 mg to 2 mg) of edrophonium chloride, administered intravenously one hour after oral intake of the drug being used in treatment.[1-5] Response will be myasthenic in the undertreated patient, adequate in the controlled patient, and cholinergic in the overtreated patient. Responses to edrophonium chloride in myasthenic and nonmyasthenic individuals are summarized in the following chart (TABLE 1):

TABLE 1 Edrophonium chloride, DOSAGE AND ADMINISTRATION

	Myasthenic*	Adequate†	Cholinergic‡
Muscle Strength (ptosis, diplopia, dysphonia, dysphagia, dysarthria, respiration, limb strength)	Increased	No change	Decreased
Fasciculations (orbicularis oculi, facial muscles, limb muscles)	Absent	Present or absent	Present or absent
Side reactions (lacrimation, diaphoresis, salivation, abdominal cramps, nausea, vomiting, diarrhea)	Absent	Minimal	Severe

*** Myasthenic Response**-occurs in untreated myasthenics and may serve to establish diagnosis; in patients under treatment, indicates that therapy is inadequate.
† Adequate Response-observed in treated patients when therapy is stabilized; a typical response in normal individuals. In addition to this response in nonmyasthenics, the phenomenon of forced lid closure is often observed in psychoneurotics.[1]
‡ Cholinergic Response-seen in myasthenics who have been overtreated with anticholinesterase drugs.

Edrophonium Chloride Test in Crisis: The term crisis is applied to the myasthenic whenever severe respiratory distress with objective ventilatory inadequacy occurs and the response to medication is not predictable. This state may be secondary to a sudden increase in severity of myasthenia gravis (myasthenic crisis), or to overtreatment with anticholinesterase drugs (cholinergic crisis).

When a patient is apneic, controlled ventilation must be secured immediately in order to avoid cardiac arrest and irreversible central nervous system damage. No attempt is made to test with edrophonium chloride until respiratory exchange is adequate.

Dosage used at this time is most important: If the patient is cholinergic, edrophonium chloride will cause increased oropharyngeal secretions and further weakness in the muscles of respiration. If the crisis is myasthenic, the test clearly improves respiration and the patient can be treated with longer-acting intravenous anticholinesterase medication. When the test is performed, there should not be more than 0.2 ml (2 mg) edrophonium chloride in the syringe. An intravenous dose of 0.1 ml (1 mg) is given initially. The patient's heart action is carefully observed. If, after an interval of one minute, this dose does not further impair the patient, the remaining 0.1 ml (1 mg) can be injected. If no clear improvement of respiration occurs after 0.2 ml (2 mg) dose, it is usually wisest to discontinue all anticholinesterase drug therapy and secure controlled ventilation by tracheostomy with assisted respiration.[5]

For Use as a Curare Antagonist: Edrophonium chloride should be administered by intravenous injection in 1 ml (10 mg) doses given slowly over a period of 30 to 45 seconds so that the onset of cholinergic reaction can be detected. This dosage may be repeated whenever necessary. The maximal dose for any one patient should be 4 ml (40 mg). Because of its brief effect, edrophonium chloride should not be given prior to the administration of curare, tubocurarine, gallamine triethiodide or dimethyl-tubocurarine; it should be used at the time when its effect is needed. When given to counteract curare overdosage, the effect of each dose on the respiration should be carefully observed before it is repeated, and assisted ventilation should always be employed.

Parenteral drug products should be inspected visually for particulate matter and discoloration prior to administration, whenever solution and container permit.

REFERENCES:

1. Osserman KE, Kaplan LI, *JAMA*, 1952;150:265. 2. Osserman KE, Kaplan LI., Besson, G. *J. Mt. Sinai Hosp*1953;20:165. 3. Osserman KE Kaplan, LI. Arch. Neurol. & Psychiatr 1953;71:385. 4. Osserman KE, Teng P. *JAMA* 1956;160:153. 5. Osserman KE, Genkins, G.*Ann NY Acad Sci*1966;135:312. 6. Tether JE, *Second International Symposium Proceedings, Myasthenia Gravis*, 1961, p.444. 7. Tether JE, in HF Conn:*Current Therapy*1960, Philadelphia, WB Saunders Co, p. 551. 8. Tether, JE, in HF Conn: *Current Therapy* 1965, Philadelphia, WB Saunders Co, p.556. 9. Grob D. Johns RJ.*JAMA*, 1958;166:1855.

HOW SUPPLIED - RATED THERAPEUTICALLY EQUIVALENT:

Injection, Solution - Intramuscular; - 10 mg/ml

1 ml	**$42.50**	**TENSILON, ICN Pharms**	**00187-3200-10**
10 ml	**$192.31**	**TENSILON, ICN Pharms**	**00187-3200-20**
10 ml x 25	$198.00	REVERSOL, Organon	00052-0466-34
15 ml	$12.86	ENLON, Ohmeda Pharm	10019-0873-15

EFLORNITHINE HYDROCHLORIDE *(003008)*

CATEGORIES: Antiprotozoals; Orphan Drugs; Trypanosomiasis - Brucei Gambiense; AIDS Related Complex*; Pneumocystis Carinii Pneumonia*; Pregnancy Category C; FDA Class 1A ("Important Therapeutic Advantage"); FDA Approved 1990 Nov

* Indication not approved by the FDA

BRAND NAMES: **Ornidyl**

FORMULARIES: WHO

DESCRIPTION:

CONCENTRATE MUST BE DILUTED BEFORE USE

Eflornithine hydrochloride is an antiprotozoal agent for intravenous injection. Its activity has been attributed to inhibition of the enzyme ornithine decarboxylase.

DESCRIPTION: *(cont'd)*

The chemical name for eflornithine hydrochloride is 2-(difluoromethyl)-DL-ornithine monohydrochloride monohydrate. Its molecular formula as the monohydrate is $C_6H_{12}F_2N_2O_2{\cdot}HCl{\cdot}H_2O$,and its molecular weight is 236.65.

Eflornithine hydrochloride is a white to off-white odorless crystalline powder. It is freely soluble in water and sparingly soluble in ethanol.

Eflornithine is available as a sterile concentrate containing 200 mg/ml eflornithine hydrochloride as the monohydrate. **DILUTION IS REQUIRED** (see DOSAGE AND ADMINISTRATION.)

CLINICAL PHARMACOLOGY:

Following intravenous administration of eflornithine hydrochloride to human, approximately 80% of the administered dose is excreted unchanged in the urine within 24 hours, and the terminal plasma elimination half-life is approximately 3 hours. Eflornithine's excretion through the kidney approximates that of creatinine clearance. In renally-impaired patients, dosing adjustments are necessary to compensate for the slower excretion of the drug (See DOSAGE AND ADMINISTRATION.) When only serum creatine is available, the following formula (Cockcroft's equation) may be used to estimate creatinine clearance. The serum creatinine should represent a steady state of renal function:

TABLE 1 Creatinine clearance (ml/min)

Males: [Weight (kg) × 140 - age (yrs)] ÷ [72 × serum creatinine (mg/dl)]
Females: 0.85 × the above value

Eflornithine hydrochloride does not bind significantly to human plasma proteins. It crosses the blood-brain barrier and produces cerebrospinal fluid blood ratios between 0.13 and 0.51 (studies in 5 patients).

MICROBIOLOGY

Eflornithine hydrochloride differs form other currently available antiprotozoal drugs in both structure and mode of action. It is aspecific, enzyme-activated, irreversible inhibitor of ornithine decarboxylase. In all mammalian and many non-mammalian cells, decarboxylation of ornithine by ornithine decarboxylase is an obligatory step in the biosynthesis of polyamines such as putrescine, spermidine and spermine, which are ubiquitous in living cells and thought to play important roles in cell division and differentiation.

The following *in vitro* and *in vivo* data are available, but their clinical significance is unknown.

In tissue culture, eflornithine hydrochloride inhibits the growth of*Trypanosoma brucei brucei*. This effect is reversed by the addition of the polyamine putrescine to the culture medium.

Eflornithine hydrochloride has been shown to be active in the treatment of African trypanosomal infections in various animal models, including*Trypanosoma brucei gambiense* infection in a monkey model.

INDICATIONS AND USAGE:

Eflornithine is indicated for the treatment of meningoencephalitic stage of *Trypanosoma brucei gambiense* infection (sleeping sickness). Extended follow-up of patients is required to assure adequate further therapy should relapse occur (see PRECAUTIONS.)

CONTRAINDICATIONS:

None known.

WARNINGS:

Eflornithine hydrochloride has been reported to cause clinically significant thrombocytopenia, anemia,and leukopenia.

Eflornithine hydrochloride has also been temporally associated with seizures, an adverse event that can also be caused by the underlying disease. Seizures occurred in approximately 8% of patients treated with IV eflornithine hydrochloride in clinical trials. The etiology of the seizures (intrinsic meningoencephalitis or drug or combination) has not been determined. Physicians should be aware of the potential for seizure activity in patients treated with eflornithine hydrochloride.

Occasional hearing impairment has been reported in some other studies using eflornithine hydrochloride. When feasible, it is recommended that serial audiograms be obtained.

Since approximately 80% of the intravenous dose of eflornithine hydrochloride is eliminated unchanged in the urine, caution should be exercised in patients with renal impairment (see CLINICAL PHARMACOLOGY.)

Due to limited data on the risk of relapse after eflornithine therapy for Stage II *gambiense* trypanosomiasis, physicians are advised to follow their patients for at least 24 months to assure further therapy should relapses occur.

PRECAUTIONS:

GENERAL

The safe and effective use of eflornithine demands thorough knowledge of the natural history of trypanosomiasis due to *T.b.gambiense* and of the condition of the patient. The most frequent, serious, toxic effect of eflornithine hydrochloride is myelosuppression, which may be unavoidable if successful treatment is to be completed. Decisions to modify dosage or to interrupt or cease treatment, the severity of the observed adverse event(s), and the availability of support facilities.

Anemia (hemoglobin < 10 g/100 ml or a decrease of ≥ 2 g/dl hemoglobin during treatment of hematocrit < 35% or a decrease of >5% in hematocrit during treatment) occurred in about 55% of monitored patients, but was generally found to be reversible upon stopping treatment. It should be noted that many of these patients were chronically anemic prior to the start of therapy.

Leukopenia (≤ 4,00 WBC/mm^3) occurred in about 37% of the patients monitored. The minimum value usually occurred within 8 days of the start of eflornithine hydrochloride therapy, and the condition usually resolved after discontinuation of therapy.

Thrombocytopenia (< 100,000/mm^3) developed in approximately 14% of the patients receiving intravenous eflornithine hydrochloride in clinical trials. In these patients, thrombocytopenia was reversible with interruption of or after completion of eflornithine hydrochloride therapy.

Because of the incidence of myelosuppression, physicians are advised to monitor hematologic profiles prior to therapy, twice weekly during therapy, and at least weekly after therapy until the patient's hematologic profile status returns to baseline.

LABORATORY TESTS

Complete blood counts, including platelet counts, should be performed before treatment, twice weekly during therapy, and weekly after completion of therapy until hematologic values return to baseline levels.

PRECAUTIONS: *(cont'd)*

CARCINOGENESIS, MUTAGENESIS, AND IMPAIRMENT OF FERTILITY

Long-term studies in animals have not been performed to evaluate the carcinogenic potential of eflornithine hydrochloride.

In *in vitro* studies using *Salmonella* and two strains of *Saccharomyces*, eflornithine hydrochloride did not induce mutagenic changes.

Impaired fertility and decreased spermatogenic effects in rats and rabbits were observed at doses equivalent to one-half the recommended human dose and in mice at approximately twice the human dose.

PREGNANCY CATEGORY C:

Teratogenic Effects: Eflornithine hydrochloride has been shown to be contragestational in rats, rabbits, and mice when given, respectively, in doses 0.5, 0.5, and 2 times the human dose. There are no adequate and well-controlled studies in pregnant women. Eflornithine hydrochloride should be used during pregnancy only if the potential benefit justifies the potential risk to the fetus.

Nonteratogenic Effects: In postnatal studies, retarded development was reported in rat pups receiving slightly higher than the human dose.

NURSING MOTHERS

It is not known whether this drug is excreted in human milk. Because many drugs are excreted in human milk, and because of the potential for serious adverse reactions in nursing infants from eflornithine hydrochloride, a decision should be made whether to discontinue nursing or to discontinue the drug to the mother.

PEDIATRIC USE

Safety and effectiveness in children have not been established.

DRUG INTERACTIONS:

No data are available.

ADVERSE REACTIONS:

Adverse reaction data are available from clinical trials of eflornithine hydrochloride for the treatment of Stage II trypanosomiasis due to *T.b. gambiense*. The most frequently reported adverse events, whether thought to be drug related or not, were: anemia (55%), leukopenia (37%), thrombocytopenia (14%), diarrhea (9%), and seizures (8%). Hearing impairment was not reported in these patients treated for trypanosomiasis; however, other reports indicate that hearing impairment may occur in 5% of patients.

Four percent (4%) of patients died during therapy or shortly after completion of treatment. It could not be established whether these deaths were caused by underlying disease or the use of eflornithine.

Other adverse events reported included: Vomiting (5%), alopecia (3%), abdominal pain (2%), anorexia (2%), headache (2%), asthenia (2%), facial edema (2%), eosinophilia (2%), and dizziness (1%).

OVERDOSAGE:

In mice, oral doses of 5 g/kg did not produce death in any animal. When given intraperitoneally at a dose of 3 g/kg, moderate CNS depression was observed after 4 hours. No deaths were reported in this study.

In rats, oral doses of 5 g/kg did not produce death in any animal. When administered intraperitoneally at a dose of 3 g/kg, moderate CNS depression was observed after 2 hours. Convulsions were observed in 3 out of 10 rats, and of these, 2 out of 10 died within 3 hours following receipt of the drug.

No information is available on the effects of overdosage in humans.

DOSAGE AND ADMINISTRATION:

The dosage of eflornithine for the treatment of *T.b. gambiense* sleeping sickness is 100 mg/kg/dose (46 mg/lb/dose) administered every 6 hours by intravenous infusion for 14 days. **THE INFUSION SHOULD BE ADMINISTERED OVER A MINIMUM OF 45 CONSECUTIVE MINUTES.** Other drugs should not be administered intravenously during the infusion of Eflornithine.

PREPARATION FOR INTRAVENOUS ADMINISTRATION

Eflornithine for injection concentrate is hypertonic and must be diluted with Sterile Water for Injection, USP, before infusion.

Solutions within 10% of plasma tonicity can be produced using 1 part eflornithine for injection concentrate to 4 parts Sterile Water for injection, USP, by volume as described below.

Using strict aseptic technique, withdraw the entire contents of each 100 ml vial. Inject 25 ml of Eflornithine for Injection Concentrate into each of four IV diluent bags, each of which contains 100 ml of sterile water, USP. The eflornithine concentration following dilution will be 40 mg/ml (5000 mg of eflornithine in 125 ml total volume). The diluted drug must be used within 24 hours of preparation. Bags containing diluted eflornithine should be stored at 4°C (39°F) to minimize the risk of microbial proliferation.

PARENTERAL DRUG PRODUCTS SHOULD BE INSPECTED VISUALLY FOR PARTICULATE MATTER AND DISCOLORATION PRIOR TO ADMINISTRATION, WHENEVER SOLUTION AND CONTAINER PERMIT.

Store vial at room temperature, preferably below 30°C (86°F). Protect from freezing and light.

HOW SUPPLIED - EQUIVALENTS NOT AVAILABLE:

Injection, Solution - Intravenous - 200 mg/ml

100 ml	$0.00	ORNIDYL, Hoechst Marion Roussel	00088-0851-35

ELECTROLYTES *(001133)*

CATEGORIES: Cathartics & Laxatives; EENT Drugs; Electrolyte Solutions; Electrolytic, Caloric-Water Balance; Eye, Ear, Nose, & Throat Preparations; Gastrointestinal Drugs; Homeostatic & Nutrient; Nutrition, Enteral/Parenteral; Replacement Solutions; Vitamins; FDA Pre 1938 Drugs

BRAND NAMES: Genlyte-20; Hyperlyte; Intralyte; Isolyte; Lypholyte; Nutrilyte; Paralyte; Pharmalyte; Saliv-Aid; Tpn Electrolytes; Tracelyte

FORMULARIES: PCS

Prescribing information not available at time of publication.

HOW SUPPLIED - RATED THERAPEUTICALLY EQUIVALENT:

Injection, Solution - Intravenous

500 ml	$24.65	ISOLYTE S, McGaw	00264-7703-10
1000 ml x 12	$26.73	ISOLYTE S, McGaw	00264-7703-00

HOW SUPPLIED - NOT RATED EQUIVALENT:

Injection, Solution - Intravenous

20 ml	$12.24	TPN ELECTROLYTES, Abbott	00074-5882-19
20 ml x 25	$93.75	NUTRILYTE II, Am Regent	00517-2020-25
20 ml x 25	$109.38	NUTRILYTE, Am Regent	00517-3120-25
25 ml	$5.40	HYPERLYTE R, McGaw	00264-3000-62
25 ml	$6.24	HYPERLYTE, McGaw	00264-3001-12
25 ml	$6.32	HYPERLYTE, Gensia Labs	00703-5300-04
25 ml	$6.32	HYPERLYTE R, Gensia Labs	00703-5310-04
25 ml	$7.10	HYPERLYTE, McGaw	00264-5300-04
25 ml	$7.10	HYPERLYTE R, McGaw	00264-5310-04
25 ml x 25	$99.00	GENLYTE-20, Gensia Labs	00703-5430-04
25 ml x 25	$105.00	GENLYTE-40, Gensia Labs	00703-5420-04
100 ml	$24.68	TPN Electrolytes, Abbott	00074-3296-06
100 ml	$25.45	TPN Electrolytes II, Abbott	00074-3297-06
100 ml	$25.45	TPN Electrolytes III, Abbott	00074-3298-06
100 ml x 25	$375.00	NUTRILYTE II, Am Regent	00517-2000-25
100 ml x 25	$562.50	NUTRILYTE, Am Regent	00517-3100-25
100 ml x 40	$749.00	LYPHOLYTE-II, Fujisawa USA	00469-1460-61
100 ml x 40	$905.00	LYPHOLYTE, Fujisawa USA	00469-0900-61
200 ml x 20	$696.72	LYPHOLYTE-II, Fujisawa USA	00469-1460-65
200 ml x 20	$799.00	LYPHOLYTE, Fujisawa USA	00469-0900-65
500 ml	$21.76	ISOLYTE S, PH 7.4, McGaw	00264-7707-10
500 ml x 12	$12.13	ISOLYTE S, McGaw	00264-1307-10
1000 ml	$26.77	ISOLYTE S, PH 7.4, McGaw	00264-7707-00
1000 ml x 6	$11.96	ISOLYTE S, EXTRACELLULAR REPLACEMENT, McGaw	00264-1303-00
1000 ml x 6	$13.57	ISOLYTE E, EXTRACELLULAR REPLACEMENT, McGaw	00264-1300-00
1000 ml x 6	$14.90	ISOLYTE S, McGaw	00264-1307-00
1000 ml x 6	$31.88	ISOLYTE H/900 CAL-HIGH, McGaw	00264-1318-00
1000 ml x 12	$19.41	ISOLYTE E, McGaw	00264-7700-00

ELECTROLYTES; FRUCTOSE *(001132)*

CATEGORIES: Caloric Agents; Electrolyte Solutions; Electrolytic, Caloric-Water Balance; Homeostatic & Nutrient; Replacement Solutions; FDA Pre 1938 Drugs

BRAND NAMES: Isolyte M/Fructose

Prescribing information not available at time of publication.

HOW SUPPLIED - EQUIVALENTS NOT AVAILABLE:

Injection, Solution - Intravenous

1000 ml	$16.39	5% TRAVERT, & ELECTROLYTES NO. 2, Baxter Hlthcare	00338-0236-04
1000 ml	$20.17	10 % TRAVERT, & ELECTROLYTE NO 2, Baxter Hlthcare	00338-0250-04
1000 ml x 6	$45.00	ISOLYTE M W/ 5% FRUCTOSE, McGaw	00264-1323-00

ELECTROLYTES; MULTIMINERALS *(001135)*

CATEGORIES: Electrolyte Solutions; Electrolytic, Caloric-Water Balance; Homeostatic & Nutrient; Irrigating Solutions; Replacement Solutions; Vitamins; FDA Pre 1938 Drugs

BRAND NAMES: Hyperlyte; Intralyte; Lypholyte; Multilyte-20; Multiple Electrolyte Additive; Normosol-M; Normosol-R; Physiolyte; Physiosol; Plasma-Lyte; Tis-U-Sol; Tpn Electrolytes; Tracelyte

Prescribing information not available at time of publication.

HOW SUPPLIED - RATED THERAPEUTICALLY EQUIVALENT:

Injection, Solution - Intravenous

500 ml	$13.69	PLASMA-LYTE 148, Baxter Hlthcare	00338-0179-03
500 ml	$17.63	PLASMA-LYTE A, Baxter Hlthcare	00338-0221-03
1000 ml	$13.11	TIS-U-SOL, Baxter Hlthcare	00338-0189-44
1000 ml	$15.67	PLASMA-LYTE 148, Baxter Hlthcare	00338-0179-04
1000 ml	$16.67	IRRIGATING, Baxter Hlthcare	00338-0286-04
1000 ml	$21.26	PLASMA-LYTE A, Baxter Hlthcare	00338-0221-04
1000 ml	$22.73	TIS-U-SOL, Baxter Hlthcare	00338-0190-04

HOW SUPPLIED - NOT RATED EQUIVALENT:

Injection, Solution - Intravenous

20 ml	$7.47	TPN ELECTROLYTES, Abbott	00074-5779-01
20 ml	$7.71	TPN ELECTROLYTES II, Abbott	00074-3236-01
20 ml	$7.71	TPN ELECTROLYTES III, Abbott	00074-3844-01
20 ml	$7.92	TPN ELECTROLYTES II, Abbott	00074-3237-01
20 ml	$7.92	TPN ELECTROLYTES III, Abbott	00074-3845-01
20 ml	$9.54	TPN ELECTROLYTES, Abbott	00074-5881-01
20 ml	$10.68	TPN ELECTROLYTES III, Abbott	00074-3846-01
20 ml	$11.32	TPN ELECTROLYTES II, Abbott	00074-3238-01
20 ml	$122.81	LYPHOLYTE-II, Fujisawa USA	00469-1460-40
20 ml	$145.63	LYPHOLYTE, Fujisawa USA	00469-0900-40
20 ml	$258.13	TRACELYTE, Fujisawa USA	00469-0800-40
20 ml	$258.13	TRACELYTE-II, Fujisawa USA	00469-1470-40
25 ml	$5.40	HYPERLYTE, McGaw	00264-3001-62
40 ml	$230.93	TRACELYTE WITH DOUBLE ELECTROLYTES, Fujisawa USA	00469-1550-60
40 ml	$230.93	TRACELYTE II/DOUBLE ELECTROLYTES, Fujisawa USA	00469-1570-60
40 ml	$249.37	LYPHOLYTE-II, Fujisawa USA	00469-1460-60
40 ml	$283.43	LYPHOLYTE, Fujisawa USA	00469-0900-60
50 ml	$7.84	MULTIPLE ELECTROLYTE ADDITIVE STERILE SO, Intl Medication	00548-6220-00
50 ml	$7.84	HIGH ACETATE MULTIPLE ELECTROLYTE ADDITI, Intl Medication	00548-6221-00
250 ml	$20.53	PHYSIOSOL, Abbott	00074-6141-02
250 ml x 12	$30.67	SUPER-VIAL HYPERLYTE, McGaw	00264-1943-20
500 ml	$11.95	NORMOSOL-R, Abbott	00074-1567-03
500 ml	$15.20	NORMOSOL-R PH 7.4, Abbott	00074-1570-03
500 ml	$16.96	NORMOSOL-R, Abbott	00074-7967-03
500 ml	$20.53	PHYSIOSOL, Abbott	00074-6141-03
500 ml	$21.83	NORMOSOL-R PH 7.4, Abbott	00074-7670-03
1000 ml	$14.01	NORMOSOL-R, Abbott	00074-1567-05
1000 ml	$16.33	PLASMA-LYTE 56, Baxter Hlthcare	00338-0168-04
1000 ml	$16.62	PLASMA-LYTE, Baxter Hlthcare	00338-0177-04
1000 ml	$19.40	NORMOSOL-R, Abbott	00074-7967-09
1000 ml	$23.86	PHYSIOSOL, Abbott	00074-6141-09
1000 ml	$26.35	NORMOSOL-R PH 7.4, Abbott	00074-7670-09

HOW SUPPLIED - NOT RATED EQUIVALENT: *(cont'd)*

1000 ml	$28.03	NORMOSOL-R PH 7.4, Abbott	00074-1570-05
1000 ml	$33.90	NORMOSOL-M 900 CAL, Abbott	00074-1566-05
1000 ml x 10	$23.52	PHYSIOLYTE, McGaw	00264-2205-00

ELECTROLYTES; TROMETHAMINE *(001136)*

CATEGORIES: Alkalinizing Agents; Electrolyte Solutions; Electrolytic, Caloric-Water Balance; Homeostatic & Nutrient; FDA Pre 1938 Drugs

BRAND NAMES: Tham-E

Prescribing information not available at time of publication.

HOW SUPPLIED - EQUIVALENTS NOT AVAILABLE:

Injection, Dry-Soln - Intravenous - 0.37 gm/1.75 gm

36 gm	$132.36	THAM-E, Abbott	00074-1591-01

ENALAPRIL MALEATE *(001138)*

CATEGORIES: ACE Inhibitors; Angiotensin Converting Enzyme Inhibitors; Antihypertensives; Cardiovascular Drugs; Congestive Heart Failure; Heart Failure; Hypertension; Renal Drugs; Pregnancy Category C; Sales > $1 Billion; FDA Approved 1985 Dec; Patent Expiration 2000 Feb; Top 200 Drugs

BRAND NAMES: *Acetensil*; *Alphrin*; *Amprace* (Australia); *Analept*; *Controlvas*; *Converten*; *Convertin*; *Enaladil* (Mexico); *Enalapril* (Germany); *Enaloc*; *Enapren*; *Enaprin*; *Enaril*; *Envas*; *Glioten* (Mexico); *Hytrol*; *Innovace* (England); *Innovade*; *Inoprilat*; *Invoril*; *Lapril*; *Lipraken* (Mexico); *Lotrial*; *Minipril*; *Naprilene*; *Naritec*; *Nuril*; *Pres* (Germany); *Pril*; *Renavace* (Japan); *Renitec* (Australia, France, Mexico); *Reniten*; *Tenace*; *Unipril*; **Vasotec**; *Xanef* (Germany)
(International brand names outside U.S. in italics)

FORMULARIES: Aetna; BC-BS; CIGNA; FHP; Humana; Kaiser; Medco; Medi-Cal; PruCare; United

COST OF THERAPY: $346.75 (Hypertension; Tablet; 5 mg; 1/day; 365 days)

PRIMARY ICD9: 401.1 (Essential Hypertension, Benign)

> WARNING:
> When used in pregnancy during the second and third trimesters, ACE inhibitors can cause injury and even death to the developing fetus. When pregnancy is detected, enalapril should be discontinued as soon as possible. See WARNINGS, Fetal/Neonatal Morbidity and Mortality.

DESCRIPTION:

Vasotec is the maleate salt of enalapril, the ethyl ester of a long-acting angiotensin converting enzyme inhibitor, enalaprilat. Enalapril maleate is chemically described as (*S*)-1-[*N*-[1-(ethoxycarbonyl) -3-phenylpropyl]-L-alanyl] -L-proline, (*Z*)-2-butenedioate salt (1:1). Its empirical formula is $C_{20}H_{28}N_2O_5{\cdot}C_4H_4O_4$.

Enalapril maleate is a white to off-white, crystalline powder with a molecular weight of 492.53. It is sparingly soluble in water, soluble in ethanol, and freely soluble in methanol.

Enalapril is a pro-drug; following oral administration, it is bioactivated by hydrolysis of the ethyl ester to enalaprilat, which is the active angiotensin converting enzyme inhibitor.

Enalapril maleate is supplied as 2.5 mg, 5 mg, 10 mg, and 20 mg tablets for oral administration. In addition to the active ingredient enalapril maleate, each tablet contains the following inactive ingredients: lactose, magnesium stearate, starch, and other ingredients. The 2.5 mg, 10 mg and 20 mg tablets also contain iron oxides.

Enalapril IV is a sterile aqueous solution for intravenous administration. Enalaprilat is an angiotensin converting enzyme inhibitor. It is chemically described as (*S*)-1-(*N*-1(- carboxy-3-phenylpropyl)-L-alanyl)-L-proline dihydrate. Its empirical formula is $C_{18}H_{24}N_2O_5{\cdot}2H_2O$.

Enalaprilat is a white to off-white, crystalline powder with a molecular weight of 384.43. It is sparingly soluble in methanol and slightly soluble in water.

Each milliliter of enalapril IV contains 1.25 mg enalaprilat (anhydrous equivalent); sodium chloride to adjust tonicity; sodium hydroxide to adjust pH; water for injection, q.s.; with benzyl alcohol, 9 mg, added as a preservative.

CLINICAL PHARMACOLOGY:

Enalaprilat, an angiotensin-converting enzyme (ACE) inhibitor when administered intravenously, is the active metabolite of the orally administered pro-drug, enalapril maleate. Enalapril is poorly absorbed orally.

MECHANISM OF ACTION

Intravenous enalaprilat, or oral enalapril, after hydrolysis to enalaprilat, inhibits angiotensin-converting enzyme (ACE) in human subjects and animals. ACE is a peptidyl dipeptidase that catalyzes the conversion of angiotensin I to the vasoconstrictor substance, angiotensin II. Angiotensin II also stimulates aldosterone secretion by the adrenal cortex. The beneficial effects of enalapril in hypertension and heart failure appear to result primarily from suppression of the renin-angiotensin-aldosterone system. Inhibition of ACE results in decreased plasma angiotensin II, which leads to decreased vasopressor activity and to decreased aldosterone secretion. Although the latter decrease is small, it results in small increases of serum potassium. In hypertensive patients treated with enalapril alone for up to 48 weeks, mean increases in serum potassium of approximately 0.2 mEq/L were observed. In patients treated with enalapril plus a thiazide diuretic, there was essentially no change in serum potassium. (See PRECAUTIONS.) Removal of angiotensin II negative feedback on renin secretion leads to increased plasma renin activity.

ACE is identical to kininase, an enzyme that degrades bradykinin. Whether increased levels of bradykinin, a potent vasodepressor peptide, play a role in the therapeutic effects of enalapril remains to be elucidated.

While the mechanism through which enalapril lowers blood pressure is believed to be primarily suppression of the renin-angiotensin-aldosterone system, enalapril is antihypertensive even in patients with low-renin hypertension. Although enalapril was antihypertensive in all races studied, black hypertensive patients (usually a low-renin hypertensive population) has a smaller average response to enalapril monotherapy than non-black patients.

PHARMACOKINETICS AND METABOLISM

Tablets: Following oral administration of enalapril, peak serum concentrations of enalapril occur within about one hour. Based on urinary recovery, the extent of absorption of enalapril is approximately 60 percent. Enalapril absorption is not influenced by the presence of food in the gastrointestinal tract. Following absorption, enalapril is hydrolyzed to enalaprilat, which is a more potent angiotensin converting enzyme inhibitor than enalapril; enalaprilat is poorly absorbed when administered orally. Peak serum concentrations of enalaprilat occur three to four hours after an oral dose of enalapril maleate. Excretion of enalapril is primarily renal. Approximately 94 percent of the dose is recovered in the urine and feces as enalaprilat or enalapril. The principal components in urine are enalaprilat, accounting for about 40 percent of the dose, and intact enalapril. There is no evidence of metabolites of enalapril, other than enalaprilat.

IV Injection: Following intravenous administration of a single dose, the serum concentration profile of enalaprilat is polyexponential with a prolonged terminal phase, apparently representing a small fraction of the administered dose that has been bound to ACE. The amount bound does not increase with dose, indicating a saturable site of binding. The effective half-life for accumulation of enalaprilat, as determined from oral administration of multiple doses of enalapril maleate, is approximately 11 hours. Excretion of enalaprilat is primarily renal with more than 90 percent of an administered dose recovered in the urine as unchanged drug within 24 hours. Enalaprilat is poorly absorbed following oral administration.

The serum concentration profile of enalaprilat exhibits a prolonged terminal phase, apparently representing a small fraction of the administered dose that has been bound to ACE. The amount bound does not increase with dose, indicating a saturable site of binding. The effective half-life for accumulation of enalaprilat following multiple doses of enalapril maleate is 11 hours.

The disposition of enalapril and enalaprilat in patients with renal insufficiency is similar to that in patients with normal renal function until the glomerular filtration rate is 30 ml/min or less. With glomerular filtration rate ≤30 ml/min, peak and trough enalaprilat levels increase, time to peak concentration increases and time to steady state may be delayed. The effective half-life of enalaprilat following multiple doses of enalapril maleate is prolonged at this level of renal insufficiency. (See DOSAGE AND ADMINISTRATION.) Enalaprilat is dialyzable at the rate of 62 ml/min.

Studies in dogs indicate that enalapril crosses the blood-brain barrier poorly, if at all; enalaprilat does not enter the brain. Multiple doses of enalapril maleate in rats do not result in accumulation in any tissues. Milk of lactating rats contains radioactivity following administration of ^{14}C enalapril maleate. Radioactivity was found to cross the placenta following administration of labeled drug to pregnant hamsters.

PHARMACODYNAMICS

Hypertension: Administration of enalapril to patients with hypertension of severity ranging from mild to severe results in a reduction of both supine and standing blood pressure usually with no orthostatic component. Symptomatic postural hypotension is therefore infrequent, although it might be anticipated in volume-depleted patients.(See WARNINGS.)

In most patients studied, after oral administration of a single dose of enalapril, onset of antihypertensive activity was seen at one hour with peak reduction of blood pressure achieved by four to six hours.

At recommended doses, antihypertensive effects have been maintained for at least 24 hours. In some patients the effects may diminish toward the end of the dosing interval (see DOSAGE AND ADMINISTRATION.)

In some patients achievement of optimal blood pressure reduction may require several weeks of therapy.

The antihypertensive effects of enalapril have continued during long term therapy. Abrupt withdrawal of enalapril has not been associated with a rapid increase in blood pressure.

CLINICAL STUDIES:

In hemodynamic studies in patients with essential hypertension, blood pressure reduction was accompanied by a reduction in peripheral arterial resistance with an increase in cardiac output and little or no change in heart rate. Following administration of enalapril, there is an increase in renal blood flow; glomerular filtration rate is usually unchanged. The effects appear to be similar in patients with renovascular hypertension.

When given together with thiazide-type diuretics, the blood pressure lowering effects of enalapril are approximately additive.

In a clinical pharmacology study, indomethacin or sulindac was administered to hypertensive patients receiving enalapril. In this study there was no evidence of a blunting of the antihypertensive action of enalapril.

Heart Failure: In trials in patients treated with digitalis and diuretics, treatment with enalapril resulted in decreased systemic vascular resistance, blood pressure, pulmonary capillary wedge pressure and heart size, and increased cardiac output and exercise tolerance. Heart rate was unchanged or slightly reduced, and mean ejection fraction was unchanged or increased. There was a beneficial effect on severity of heart failure as measured by the New York Heart Association (NYHA) classification and on symptoms of dyspnea and fatigue. Hemodynamic effects were observed after the first dose, and appeared to be maintained in uncontrolled studies lasting as long as four months. Effects on exercise tolerance, heart size, and severity and symptoms of heart failure were observed in placebo-controlled studies lasting from eight weeks to over one year.

Heart Failure, Mortality Trials: In a multicenter, placebo-controlled clinical trial, 2569 patients with all degrees of symptomatic heart failure and ejection fraction ≤35 percent were randomized to placebo or enalapril and followed for up to 55 months (SOLVD Treatment). Use of enalapril was associated with an 11 percent reduction in all-cause mortality and a 30 percent reduction in hospitalization for heart failure. Diseases that excluded patients from enrollment in the study included severe stable angina (>2 attacks/day), hemodynamically significant valvular or outflow tract obstruction, renal failure (creatinine >2.5 mg/dl), cerebral vascular disease (*e.g.,* significant carotid artery disease), advanced pulmonary disease, malignancies, active myocarditis and constrictive pericarditis. The mortality benefit associated with enalapril does not appear to depend upon digitalis being present.

A second multicenter trial used the SOLVD protocol for study of asymptomatic or minimally symptomatic patients. SOLVD-Prevention patients, who had left ventricular ejection fraction ≤35% and no history of symptomatic heart failure, were randomized to placebo (n=2117) or enalapril (n=2111) and followed for up to 5 years. The majority of patients in the SOLVD-Prevention trial had a history of ischemic heart disease. A history of myocardial infarction was present in 80 percent of patients, current angina pectoris in 34 percent, and a history of hypertension in 37 percent. No statistically significant mortality effect was demonstrated in the population. Enalapril-treated subjects had 32% fewer first hospitalizations for heart failure, and 32% fewer total heart failure hospitalizations. Compared to placebo, 32 percent fewer patients receiving enalapril developed symptoms of overt heart failure. Hospitalizations for cardiovascular reasons were also reduced. There was an insignificant reduction in hospitalizations for any cause in the enalapril treatment group (for enalapril vs. placebo, respectively, 1166vs.1201 first hospitalizations, 2649 vs. 2840 total hospitalizations), although the study was not powered to look for such an effect.

The SOLVD-Prevention trial was not designed to determine whether treatment of asymptomatic patients with low ejection fraction would be superior, with respect to preventing hospitalization, to closer follow-up and use of enalapril at the earliest sign of heart failure. However, under the conditions of follow-up in the SOLVD-Prevention trial (every 4 months

CLINICAL STUDIES: *(cont'd)*

at the study clinic; personal physician as needed), 68% of patients on placebo who were hospitalized for heart failure had no prior symptoms recorded which would have signaled initiation of treatment.

The SOLVD-Prevention trial was also not designed to show whether enalapril modified the progression of underlying heart disease.

In another multicenter, placebo-controlled trial (CONSENSUS) limited to patients with NYHA Class IV congestive heart failure and radiographic evidence of cardiomegaly, use of enalapril was associated with improved survival. The results are shown in TABLE 1.

TABLE 1

	Survival (%)	
	Six Months	**One Year**
Vasotec (n = 127)	74	64
Placebo (n = 126)	56	48

In both CONSENSUS and SOLVD-Treatment trials, patients were also usually receiving digitalis, diuretics or both.

Enalapril IV results in reduction of both supine and standing systolic and diastolic blood pressure, usually with no orthostatic component. Symptomatic postural hypotension is therefore infrequent, although it might be anticipated in volume-depleted patients (see WARNINGS). The onset of action usually occurs within fifteen minutes of administration with the maximum effect occurring within one to four hours. The abrupt withdrawal of enalaprilat has not been associated with a rapid increase in blood pressure.

The duration of hemodynamic effects appears to be dose-related. However, for the recommended dose, the duration of action in most patients is approximately six hours.

Following administration of enalapril, there is an increase in renal blood flow; glomerular filtration rate is usually unchanged. The effects appear to be similar in patients with renovascular hypertension.

INDICATIONS AND USAGE:

HYPERTENSION: *Tablets:* Enalapril is indicated for the treatment of hypertension.

Enalapril is effective alone or in combination with other antihypertensive agents, especially thiazide-type diuretics. The blood pressure lowering effects of enalapril and thiazides are approximately additive.

Heart Failure: Enalapril is indicated for the treatment of symptomatic congestive heart failure, usually in combination with diuretics and digitalis. In these patients enalapril improves symptoms, increases survival, and decreases the frequency of hospitalization (see CLINICAL STUDIES, Heart Failure, Mortality Trials for details and limitations of survival trials).

Asymptomatic Left Ventricular Dysfunction: In clinically stable asymptomatic patients with left ventricular dysfunction (ejection fraction ≤35 percent), enalapril decreases the rate of development of overt heart failure and decreases the incidence of hospitalization for heart failure. (see CLINICAL STUDIES, Heart Failure, Mortality Trials for details and limitations of survival trials).

In using enalapril consideration should be given to the fact that another angiotensin converting enzyme inhibitor, captopril, has caused agranulocytosis, particularly in patients with renal impairment or collagen vascular disease, and that available data are insufficient to show that enalapril does not have a similar risk. (See WARNINGS.)

IV INJECTION

Enalapril IV is indicated for the treatment of hypertension when oral therapy is not practical.

Enalapril IV has been studied with only one other antihypertensive agent, furosemide, which showed approximately additive effects on blood pressure. Enalapril, the pro-drug of enalaprilat, has been used extensively with a variety of other antihypertensive agents, without apparent difficulty except for occasional hypotension.

CONTRAINDICATIONS:

TABLETS AND IV INJECTION

Enalapril and enalapril IV are contraindicated in patients who are hypersensitive to this product and in patients with a history of angioedema related to previous treatment with an angiotensin converting enzyme inhibitor.

WARNINGS:

Anaphylactoid and Possibly Related Reactions: Presumably because angiotensin-converting enzyme inhibitors affect the metabolism of eicosanoids and polypeptides, including endogenous bradykinin, patients receiving ACE inhibitors (including enalapril) may be subject to a variety of adverse reactions, some of them serious.

Angioedema: Angioedema of the face, extremities, lips, tongue, glottis and/or larynx has been reported in patients treated with angiotensin converting enzyme inhibitors, including enalapril. In such cases enalapril or enalapril IV should be promptly discontinued and appropriate therapy and monitoring should be provided until complete and sustained resolution of signs and symptoms has occurred. In instances where swelling has been confined to the face and lips the condition has generally resolved without treatment, although antihistamines have been useful in relieving symptoms. Angioedema associated with laryngeal edema may be fatal. **Where there is involvement of the tongue, glottis or larynx, likely to cause airway obstruction, appropriate therapy, e.g., subcutaneous epinephrine solution 1:1000 (0.3 ml to 0.5 ml) and/or measures necessary to ensure a patent airway, should be promptly provided.** (See ADVERSE REACTIONS.)

Patients with a history of angioedema unrelated to ACE inhibitor therapy may not be at increased risk of angioedema while receiving an ACE inhibitor (see CONTRAINDICATIONS).

Anaphylactoid Reactions During Desensitization: Two patients undergoing desensitizing treatment with hymenoptera venom while receiving ACE inhibitors sustained life-threatening anaphylactoid reactions. In the same patients, these reactions were avoided when ACE inhibitors were temporarily withheld, but they reappeared upon inadvertent rechallenge.

Anaphylactoid Reactions During Membrane Exposure: Anaphylactoid reactions have been reported in patients dialyzed with high-flux membranes and treated concomitantly with an ACE inhibitor. Anaphylactoid reactions have also been reported in patients undergoing low-density lipoprotein apheresis with dextran sulfate absorption (a procedure dependent upon devices not approved in the United States).

Hypotension: Excessive hypotension is rare in uncomplicated hypertensive patients treated with enalapril alone. Patients with heart failure given enalapril commonly have some reduction in blood pressure, especially with the first dose, but discontinuation of therapy for continuing symptomatic hypotension usually is not necessary when dosing instructions are followed; caution should be observed when initiating therapy. (See DOSAGE AND ADMINISTRATION.) Patients at risk for excessive hypotension, sometimes associated with oliguria and/or progressive azotemia, and rarely with acute renal failure and/or death, include those with the following conditions or characteristics: heart failure, hyponatremia, high dose

WARNINGS: *(cont'd)*

diuretic therapy, recent intensive diuresis or increase in diuretic dose, renal dialysis, or severe volume and/or salt depletion of any etiology. It may be advisable to eliminate the diuretic (except in patients with heart failure), reduce the diuretic dose or increase salt intake cautiously before initiating therapy with enalapril or enalapril IV in patients at risk for excessive hypotension who are able to tolerate such adjustments. (See DRUG INTERACTIONS) and ADVERSE REACTIONS.) In patients at risk for excessive hypotension, therapy should be started under very close medical supervision and such patients should be followed closely for the first two weeks of treatment and whenever the dose of enalapril and/or diuretic is increased. Similar considerations may apply to patients with ischemic heart or cerebrovascular disease, in whom an excessive fall in blood pressure could result in a myocardial infarction or cerebrovascular accident.

If excessive hypotension occurs, the patient should be placed in the supine position and, if necessary, receive an intravenous infusion of normal saline. A transient hypotensive response is not a contraindication to further doses of enalapril, which usually can be given without difficulty once the blood pressure has stabilized and/or has increased after volume expansion. If symptomatic hypotension develops, a dose reduction or discontinuation of enalapril or concomitant diuretic may be necessary.

Neutropenia/Agranulocytosis: Another angiotensin converting enzyme inhibitor, captopril, has been shown to cause agranulocytosis and bone marrow depression, rarely in uncomplicated patients but more frequently in patients with renal impairment especially if they also have a collagen vascular disease. Available data from clinical trials of enalapril are insufficient to show that enalapril does not cause agranulocytosis at similar rates. Marketing experience has revealed several cases of neutropenia or agranulocytosis in which a causal relationship to enalapril cannot be excluded. Periodic monitoring of white blood cell counts in patients with collagen vascular disease and renal disease should be considered.

Hepatic Failure: Rarely, ACE inhibitors have been associated with a syndrome that starts with cholestatic jaundice and progresses to fulminant hepatic necrosis, and (sometimes) death. The mechanism of this syndrome is not understood. Patients receiving ACE inhibitors who develop jaundice or marked elevations of hepatic enzymes should discontinue the ACE inhibitor and receive appropriate medical follow-up.

Fetal/Neonatal Morbidity and Mortality: ACE inhibitors can cause fetal and neonatal morbidity and death when administered to pregnant women. Several dozen cases have been reported in the world literature. When pregnancy is detected, ACE inhibitors should be discontinued as soon as possible.

The use of ACE inhibitors during the second and third trimesters of pregnancy has been associated with fetal and neonatal injury, including hypotension, neonatal skull hypoplasia, anuria, reversible or irreversible renal failure, and death. Oligohydramnios has also been reported, presumably resulting from decreased fetal renal function; oligohydramnios in this setting has been associated with fetal limb contractures, craniofacial deformation, and hypoplastic lung development. Prematurity, intrauterine growth retardation, and patent ductus arteriosus have also been reported, although it is not clear whether these occurrences were due to the ACE-inhibitor exposure.

These adverse effects do not appear to have resulted from intrauterine ACE-inhibitor exposure that has been limited to the first trimester. Mothers whose embryos and fetuses are exposed to ACE inhibitors only during the first trimester should be so informed. Nonetheless, when patients become pregnant, physicians should make every effort to discontinue the use of enalapril as soon as possible.

Rarely (probably less often than once in every thousand pregnancies), no alternative to ACE inhibitors will be found. In these rare cases, the mothers should be apprised of the potential hazards to their fetuses, and serial ultrasound examinations should be performed to assess the intraamniotic environment.

If oligohydramnios is observed, enalapril or enalapril IV should be discontinued unless it is considered lifesaving for the mother. Contraction stress testing (CST), a non-stress test (NST), or biophysical profiling (BPP) may be appropriate, depending upon the week of pregnancy. Patients and physicians should be aware, however, that oligohydramnios may not appear until after the fetus has sustained irreversible injury.

Infants with histories of *in utero* exposure to ACE inhibitors should be closely observed for hypotension, oliguria, and hyperkalemia. If oliguria occurs, attention should be directed toward support of blood pressure and renal perfusion. Exchange transfusion or dialysis may be required as means of reversing hypotension and/or substituting for disordered renal function. Enalapril, which crosses the placenta, has been removed from neonatal circulation by peritoneal dialysis with some clinical benefit, and theoretically may be removed by exchange transfusion, although there is no experience with the latter procedure.

No teratogenic effects of enalapril were seen in studies of pregnant rats, and rabbits. On a mg/kg basis, the doses used were up to 333 times (in rats), and 50 times (in rabbits) the maximum recommended human dose.

PRECAUTIONS:

GENERAL

Impaired Renal Function: As a consequence of inhibiting the renin-angiotensin-aldosterone system, changes in renal function may be anticipated in susceptible individuals. In patients with severe heart failure whose renal function may depend on the activity of the renin-angiotensin-aldosterone system, treatment with angiotensin converting enzyme inhibitors, including enalapril or enalaprilat, may be associated with oliguria and/or progressive azotemia and rarely with acute renal failure and/or death.

In clinical studies in hypertensive patients with unilateral or bilateral renal artery stenosis, increases in blood urea nitrogen and serum creatinine were observed in 20 percent of patients. These increases were almost always reversible upon discontinuation of enalapril and/or diuretic therapy. In such patients renal function should be monitored during the first few weeks of therapy.

Some patients with hypertension or heart failure with no apparent pre-existing renal vascular disease have developed increases in blood urea and serum creatinine, usually minor and transient, especially when enalapril or enalapril IV has been given concomitantly with a diuretic. This is more likely to occur in patients with pre-existing renal impairment. Dosage reduction and/or discontinuation of the diuretic and/or enalapril or enalapril IV may be required.

Evaluation of patients with hypertension or heart failure should always include assessment of renal function. (See DOSAGE AND ADMINISTRATION.)

Hyperkalemia: Elevated serum potassium (greater than 5.7 mEq/L) was observed in approximately one percent of hypertensive patients in clinical trials. In most cases these were isolated values which resolved despite continued therapy. Hyperkalemia was a cause of discontinuation of therapy in 0.28 percent of hypertensive patients. In clinical trials in heart failure, hyperkalemia was observed in 3.8 percent of patients but was not a cause for discontinuation.

Risk factors for the development of hyperkalemia include renal insufficiency, diabetes mellitus, and the concomitant use of potassium-sparing diuretics, potassium supplements and/or potassium-containing salt substitutes, which should be used cautiously, if at all, with enalapril or enalapril IV. (See DRUG INTERACTIONS.)

PRECAUTIONS: *(cont'd)*

Cough: Cough has been reported with the use of ACE inhibitors. Characteristically, the cough is nonproductive, persistent and resolves after discontinuation of therapy. ACE inhibitor-induced cough should be considered as part of the differential diagnosis of cough.

Surgery/Anesthesia: In patients undergoing major surgery or during anesthesia with agents that produce hypotension, enalapril may block angiotensin II formation secondary to compensatory renin release. If hypotension occurs and is considered to be due to this mechanism, it can be corrected by volume expansion.

INFORMATION FOR THE PATIENT

Angioedema: Angioedema, including laryngeal edema, may occur especially following the first dose of enalapril. Patients should be so advised and told to report immediately any signs or symptoms suggesting angioedema (swelling of face, extremities, eyes, lips, tongue, difficulty in swallowing or breathing) and to take no more drug until they have consulted with the prescribing physician.

Hypotension: Patients should be cautioned to report light-headedness, especially during the first few days of therapy. If actual syncope occurs, the patients should be told to discontinue the drug until they have consulted with the prescribing physician.

All patients should be cautioned that excessive perspiration and dehydration may lead to an excessive fall in blood pressure because of reduction in fluid volume. Other causes of volume depletion such as vomiting or diarrhea may also lead to a fall in blood pressure; patients should be advised to consult with the physician.

Hyperkalemia: Patients should be told not to use salt substitutes containing potassium without consulting their physician.

Neutropenia: Patients should be told to report promptly any indication of infection (*e.g.*, sore throat, fever) which may be a sign of neutropenia.

Pregnancy: Female patients of childbearing age should be told about the consequences of second- and third-trimester exposure to ACE inhibitors, and they should also be told that these consequences do not appear to have resulted from intrauterine ACE-inhibitor exposure that has been limited to the first trimester. These patients should be asked to report pregnancies to their physicians as soon as possible.

NOTE: As with many other drugs, certain advice to patients being treated with enalapril is warranted. This information is intended to aid in the safe and effective use of this medication. It is not a disclosure of all possible adverse or intended effects.

CARCINOGENESIS, MUTAGENESIS, AND IMPAIRMENT OF FERTILITY

There was no evidence of a tumorigenic effect when enalapril was administered for 106 weeks to rats at doses up to 90 mg/kg/day (150 times** the maximum daily human dose). Enalapril has also been administered for 94 weeks to male and female mice at doses up to 90 and 180 mg/kg/day, respectively, (150 and 300 times** the maximum daily dose for humans) and showed no evidence of carcinogenicity.

Neither enalapril maleate nor the active diacid was mutagenic in the Ames microbial mutagen test with or without metabolic activation. Enalapril was also negative in the following genotoxicity studies: rec-assay, reverse mutation assay with *E. coli*, sister chromatid exchange with cultured mammalian cells, and the micronucleus test with mice, as well as in an *in vivo* cytogenic study using mouse bone marrow.

There were no adverse effects on reproductive performance in male and female rats treated with 10 to 90 mg/kg/day of enalapril.

Carcinogenicity studies have not been done with enalapril IV.

PREGNANCY CATEGORY C (FIRST TRIMESTER) AND PREGNANCY CATEGORY D (SECOND AND THIRD TRIMESTERS). SEE WARNINGS, Fetal/Neonatal Morbidity and Mortality.

NURSING MOTHERS

Enalapril and enalaprilat are detected in human milk in trace amounts. Caution should be exercised when enalapril or enalapril IV is given to a nursing mother.

PEDIATRIC USE

Safety and effectiveness in children have not been established.

DRUG INTERACTIONS:

Hypotension: Patients on Diuretic Therapy: Patients on diuretics and especially those in whom diuretic therapy was recently instituted, may occasionally experience an excessive reduction of blood pressure after initiation of therapy with enalapril or enalaprilat. The possibility of hypotensive effects with enalapril or enalaprilat can be minimized by either discontinuing the diuretic or increasing the salt intake prior to initiation of treatment with enalapril or enalaprilat. If it is necessary to continue the diuretic, provide close medical supervision after the initial dose for at least two hours and until blood pressure has stabilized for at least an additional hour. (See WARNINGS) and DOSAGE AND ADMINISTRATION.

Agents Causing Renin Release: The antihypertensive effect of enalapril and enalapril IV is augmented by antihypertensive agents that cause renin release (*e.g.*, diuretics).

Other Cardiovascular Agents: Enalapril and enalapril IV have been used concomitantly with beta adrenergic-blocking agents, methyldopa, nitrates, calcium-blocking agents, hydralazine, prazosin and digoxin without evidence of clinically significant adverse interactions.

Enalapril IV has been used concomitantly with digitalis without evidence of clinically significant adverse reactions.

Agents Increasing Serum Potassium: Enalapril and enalapril IV attenuate potassium loss caused by thiazide-type diuretics. Potassium-sparing diuretics (*e.g.*, spironolactone, triamterene, or amiloride), potassium supplements, or potassium-containing salt substitutes may lead to significant increases in serum potassium. Therefore, if concomitant use of these agents is indicated because of demonstrated hypokalemia, they should be used with caution and with frequent monitoring of serum potassium. Potassium sparing agents should generally not be used in patients with heart failure receiving enalapril.

Lithium: Lithium toxicity has been reported in patients receiving lithium concomitantly with drugs which cause elimination of sodium, including ACE inhibitors. A few cases of lithium toxicity have been reported in patients receiving concomitant enalapril/enalapril IV and lithium and were reversible upon discontinuation of both drugs. It is recommended that serum lithium levels be monitored frequently if enalapril is administered concomitantly with lithium.

ADVERSE REACTIONS:

TABLETS

Enalapril has been evaluated for safety in more than 10,000 patients, including over 1000 patients treated for one year or more. Enalapril has been found to be generally well tolerated in controlled clinical trials involving 2987 patients.

For the most part, adverse experiences were mild and transient in nature. In clinical trials, discontinuation of therapy due to clinical adverse experiences was required in 3.3 percent of patients with hypertension and in 5.7 percent of patients with heart failure. The frequency of adverse experiences was not related to total daily dosage within the usual dosage ranges. In patients with hypertension the overall percentage of patients treated with enalapril reporting adverse experiences was comparable to placebo.

HYPERTENSION

Adverse experiences occurring in greater than one percent of patients with hypertension treated with enalapril in controlled clinical trials are shown in TABLE 2. In patients treated with enalapril, the maximum duration of therapy was three years; in placebo treated patients the maximum duration of therapy was 12 weeks.

TABLE 2

	Vasotec (n=2314) Incidence (discontinuation)	Placebo (n=230) Incidence
Body as a Whole		
Fatigue	3.0 (<0.1)	2.6
Orthostatic Effects	1.2 (<0.1)	0.0
Asthenia	1.1 (0.1)	0.9
Digestive		
Diarrhea	1.4 (<0.1)	1.7
Nausea	1.4 (0.2)	1.7
Nervous/Psychiatric		
Headache	5.2 (0.3)	9.1
Dizziness	4.3 (0.4)	4.3
Respiratory		
Cough	1.3 (0.1)	0.9
Skin		
Rash	1.4 (0.4)	0.4

HEART FAILURE

Adverse experiences occurring in greater than one percent of patients with heart failure treated with enalapril are shown in TABLE 3. The incidences represent the experiences from both controlled and uncontrolled clinical trials (maximum duration of therapy was approximately one year). In the placebo treated patients, the incidences reported are from the controlled trials (maximum duration of therapy is 12 weeks). The percentage of patients with severe heart failure (NYHA Class IV) was 29 percent and 43 percent for patients treated with enalapril and placebo, respectively.

TABLE 3

	Vasotec (n=673) Incidence (discontinuation)	Placebo (n=339) Incidence
Body as a Whole		
Orthostatic Effects	2.2 (0.1)	0.3
Syncope	2.2 (0.1)	0.9
Chest Pain	2.1 (0.0)	2.1
Fatigue	1.8 (0.0)	1.8
Abdominal Pain	1.6 (0.4)	2.1
Asthenia	1.6 (0.1)	0.3
Cardiovascular		
Hypotension	6.7 (1.9)	0.6
Orthostatic Hypotension	1.6 (0.1)	0.3
Angina Pectoris	1.5 (0.1)	1.8
Myocardial Infarction	1.2 (0.3)	1.8
Digestive		
Diarrhea	2.1 (0.1)	1.2
Nausea	1.3 (0.1)	0.6
Vomiting	1.3 (0.0)	0.9
Nervous/Psychiatric		
Dizziness	7.9 (0.6)	0.6
Headache	1.8 (0.1)	0.9
Vertigo	1.6 (0.1)	1.2
Respiratory		
Cough	2.2 (0.0)	0.6
Bronchitis	1.3 (0.0)	0.9
Dyspnea	1.3 (0.1)	0.4
Pneumonia	1.0 (0.0)	2.4
Skin		
Rash	1.3 (0.0)	2.4
Urogenital		
Urinary Tract Infection	1.3 (0.0)	2.4

Other serious clinical adverse experiences occurring since the drug was marketed or adverse experiences occurring in 0.5 to 1.0 percent of patients with hypertension or heart failure in clinical trials are listed below and, within each category, are in order of decreasing severity.

Since enalapril is converted to enalaprilat, those adverse experiences associated with enalapril might also be expected to occur with enalapril IV.

Body as a Whole: Anaphylactoid reactions (see PRECAUTIONS, Hemodialysis Patients).

Cardiovascular: Cardiac arrest; myocardial infarction or cerebrovascular accident, possibly secondary to excessive hypotension in high risk patients (see WARNINGS, Hypotension); pulmonary embolism and infarction; pulmonary edema; rhythm disturbances including atrial tachycardia and bradycardia; atrial fibrillation; palpitation.

Digestive: Ileus, pancreatitis, hepatitis (hepatocellular (proven on rechallenge) or cholestatic jaundice), melena, anorexia, dyspepsia, constipation, glossitis, stomatitis, dry mouth.

Musculoskeletal: Muscle cramps.

Nervous/Psychiatric: Depression, confusion, ataxia, somnolence, insomnia, nervousness, peripheral neuropathy (*e.g.*, paresthesia, dysesthesia).

Respiratory: Bronchospasm, rhinorrhea, sore throat and hoarseness, asthma, upper respiratory infection, pulmonary infiltrates

Skin: Exfoliative dermatitis, toxic epidermal necrolysis, Stevens-Johnson syndrome, herpes zoster, erythema multiforme, urticaria, pruritus, alopecia, flushing, diaphoresis, photosensitivity.

Special Senses: Blurred vision, taste alteration, anosmia, tinnitus, conjunctivitis, dry eyes, tearing.

Urogenital: Renal failure, oliguria, renal dysfunction (see PRECAUTIONS) and DOSAGE AND ADMINISTRATION, flank pain, gynecomastia, impotence.

Miscellaneous: A symptom complex has been reported which may include a positive ANA, an elevated erythrocyte sedimentation rate, arthralgia/arthritis, myalgia, fever, serositis, vasculitis, leukocytosis, eosinophilia, photosensitivity, rash and other dermatologic manifestations.

Angioedema: Angioedema has been reported in patients receiving enalapril (0.2 percent). Angioedema associated with laryngeal edema may be fatal. If angioedema of the face, extremities, lips, tongue, glottis and/or larynx occurs, treatment with enalapril should be discontinued and appropriate therapy instituted immediately. (See WARNINGS.)

ADVERSE REACTIONS: *(cont'd)*

Hypotension: In the hypertensive patients, hypotension occurred in 0.9 percent syncope occurred in 0.5 percent of patients following the initial dose or during extended therapy. Hypotension or syncope was a cause for discontinuation of therapy in 0.1 percent of hypertensive patients. In heart failure patients, hypotension occurred in 6.7 percent and syncope occurred in 2.2 percent of patients. Hypotension or syncope was a cause for discontinuation of therapy in 1.9 percent of patients with heart failure. (See WARNINGS.)

Fetal/Neonatal Morbidity and Mortality: See WARNINGS, Fetal/Neonatal Morbidity and Mortality.

Cough: See PRECAUTIONS, Cough.

CLINICAL LABORATORY TEST FINDINGS

Serum Electrolytes: Hyperkalemia (see PRECAUTIONS, hyponatremia).

Creatinine, Blood Urea Nitrogen: In controlled clinical trials minor increases in blood urea nitrogen and serum creatinine, reversible upon discontinuation of therapy, were observed in about 0.2 percent of patients with essential hypertension treated with enalapril alone. Increases are more likely to occur in patients receiving concomitant diuretics or in patients with renal artery stenosis. (See PRECAUTIONS.) In patients with heart failure who were also receiving diuretics with or without digitalis increases in blood urea nitrogen or serum creatinine, usually reversible upon discontinuation of enalapril and/or other concomitant diuretic therapy, were observed in about 11 percent of patients. Increases in blood urea nitrogen or creatinine were a cause for discontinuation in 1.2 percent of patients.

Hematology: Small decreases in hemoglobin and hematocrit (mean decreases of approximately 0.3 g percent and 1.0 vol percent, respectively) occur frequently in either hypertension or congestive heart failure patients treated with enalapril but are rarely of clinical importance unless another cause of anemia coexists. In clinical trials, less than 0.1 percent of patients discontinued therapy due to anemia. Hemolytic anemia, including cases of hemolysis in patients with G-6-PD deficiency, has been reported; a causal relationship to enalapril has not been established.

Liver Function Tests: Elevations of liver enzymes and/or serum bilirubin have occurred (see WARNINGS, Hepatic Failure).

OVERDOSAGE:

TABLETS

In clinical studies, some hypertensive patients received a maximum dose of 80 mg of enalaprilat intravenously over a fifteen month period. At this high dose, no adverse effects beyond those as associated with the recommended dosages were observed.

Limited data are available in regard to overdosage in humans.

The oral LD_{50} of enalapril is 2000 mg/kg in mice and rats.

The intravenous LD_{50} of enalaprilat is 3740-5890 mg/kg in female mice.

The most likely manifestation of overdosage would be hypotension, for which the usual treatment would be intravenous infusion of normal saline solution.

Enalaprilat may be removed from general circulation by hemodialysis and has been removed from neonatal circulation by peritoneal dialysis.

DOSAGE AND ADMINISTRATION:

TABLETS

Hypertension: In patients who are currently being treated with a diuretic, symptomatic hypotension occasionally may occur following the initial dose of enalapril. The diuretic should, if possible, be discontinued for two to three days before beginning therapy with enalapril to reduce the likelihood of hypotension. (See WARNINGS.) If the patient's blood pressure is not controlled with enalapril alone, diuretic therapy may be resumed.

If the diuretic cannot be discontinued an initial dose of 2.5 mg should be used under medical supervision for at least two hours and until blood pressure has stabilized for at least an additional hour. (See WARNINGS and DRUG INTERACTIONS.)

The recommended initial dose in patients not on diuretics is 5 mg once a day. Dosage should be adjusted according to blood pressure response. The usual dosage range is 10 to 40 mg per day administered in a single dose or two divided doses. In some patients treated once daily, the antihypertensive effect may diminish toward the end of the dosing interval. In such patient an increase in dosage or twice daily administration should be considered. If blood pressure is not controlled with enalapril alone, a diuretic may be added.

Concomitant administration of enalapril with potassium supplements, potassium salt substitutes, or potassium-sparing diuretics may lead to increases of serum potassium (see PRECAUTIONS).

Dosage Adjustment in Hypertensive Patients with Renal Impairment: The usual dose of enalapril is recommended for patients with a creatinine clearance >30 ml/min (serum creatinine of up to approximately 3 mg/dl). For patients with creatinine clearance ≤30 ml/min (serum creatinine ≥3 mg/dl), the first dose is 2.5 mg once daily. The dosage may be titrated upward until blood pressure is controlled or to a maximum of 40 mg daily (TABLE 4).

TABLE 4

Renal Status	Creatinine-Clearance ml/min	Initial Dose mg/day
Normal Renal Function	>80 ml/min	5 mg
Mild Impairment	≤80 >30 ml/min	5 mg
Moderate to Severe Impairment	≤30 ml/min	2.5 mg
Dialysis Patients*	—	2.5 mg on dialysis days**

* See PRECAUTIONS, Hemodialysis Patients
** Dosage on non-dialysis days should be adjusted depending on the blood pressure response.

Heart Failure: Enalapril is indicated for the treatment of symptomatic heart failure, usually in combination with diuretics and digitalis. In the placebo-controlled studies that demonstrated improved survival, patients were titrated as tolerated up to 40 mg, administered in two divided doses.

The recommended starting dose is 2.5 mg. The recommended dosing range is 2.5 to 20 mg given twice a day. Doses should be titrated upward, as tolerated, over a period of a few days or weeks. The maximum daily dose administered in clinical trials was 40 mg in divided doses.

After the initial dose of enalapril, the patient should be observed under medical supervision for at least two hours and until blood pressure has stabilized for at least an additional hour. (See WARNINGS) and DRUG INTERACTIONS. If possible, the dose of any concomitant diuretic should be reduced which may diminish the likelihood of hypotension. The appearance of hypotension after the initial dose of enalapril does not preclude subsequent careful dose titration with the drug, following effective management of the hypotension.

DOSAGE AND ADMINISTRATION: *(cont'd)*

Asymptomatic Left Ventricular Dysfunction: In the trial that demonstrated efficacy, patients were started on 2.5 mg twice daily and were titrated as tolerated to the targeted daily dose of 20 mg (in divided doses).

After the initial dose of enalapril, the patient should be observed under medical supervision for at least two hours and until blood pressure has stabilized for at least an additional hour. (See WARNINGS) and DRUG INTERACTIONS. If possible, the dose of any concomitant diuretic should be reduced which may diminish the likelihood of hypotension. The appearance of hypotension after the initial dose of enalapril does not preclude subsequent careful dose titration with the drug, following effective management of the hypotension.

Dosage Adjustment in Patients with Heart Failure and Renal Impairment or Hyponatremia: In patients with heart failure who have hyponatremia (serum sodium less than 130 mEq/L) or with serum creatinine greater than 1.6 mg/dl, therapy should be initiated at 2.5 mg daily under close medical supervision. See DOSAGE AND ADMINISTRATION, Heart Failure, WARNINGS, and DRUG INTERACTIONS. The dose may be increased to 2.5 mg twice daily, then 5 mg twice daily. And higher as needed, usually at intervals of four days or more if at the time of dosage adjustment there is not excessive hypotension or significant deterioration of renal function. The maximum daily dose is 40 mg.

IV

Intravenous Administration Only. The dose in hypertension is 1.25 mg every six hours administered intravenously over a five minute period. A clinical response is usually seen within 15 minutes. Peak effects after the first dose may not occur for up to four hours after dosing. The peak effects of the second and subsequent doses may exceed those of the first.

No dosage regimen for enalapril IV has been clearly demonstrated to be more effective in treating hypertension than 1.25 mg every six hours. However, in controlled clinical studies in hypertension, doses as high as 5 mg every six hours were well tolerated for up to 36 hours. There has been inadequate experience with doses greater than 20 mg per day.

In studies of patients with hypertension, enalapril IV has not been administered for periods longer than 48 hours. In other studies, patients have received enalapril IV for as long as seven days.

The dose for patients being converted to enalapril IV from oral therapy for hypertension with enalapril maleate is 1.25 mg every six hours. For conversion from intravenous to oral therapy, the recommended initial dose of Tablets enalapril is 5 mg once a day with subsequent dosage adjustments as necessary.

PATIENTS ON DIURETIC THERAPY

For patients on diuretic therapy the recommended starting dose for hypertension is 0.625 mg administered intravenously over a five minute period; also see below, Patients at Risk of Excessive Hypotension. A clinical response is usually seen within 15 minutes. Peak effects after the first dose may not occur for up to four hours after dosing, although most of the effect is usually apparent within the first hour. If after one hour there is an inadequate clinical response, the 0.625 dose may be repeated. Additional doses of 1.25 mg may be administered at six hour intervals.

For conversion from intravenous to oral therapy, the recommended initial dose of Tablets enalapril for patients who have responded to 0.625 mg of enalaprilat every six hours is 2.5 mg once a day with subsequent dosage adjustment as necessary.

DOSAGE ADJUSTMENT IN RENAL IMPAIRMENT

The usual dosage of 1.25 mg of enalaprilat every six hours is recommended for patients with a creatinine clearance >30 ml/min (serum creatinine of up to approximately 3 mg/dl). For patients with creatinine clearance ≤ 30 ml/min (serum creatinine ≥3 mg/dl), the initial dose is 0.625 mg. (See WARNINGS.)

If after one hour there is an inadequate clinical response, the 0.625 mg dose may be repeated. Additional doses of 1.25 mg may be administered at six hour intervals.

For dialysis patients, Patients at Risk of Excessive Hypotension.

For conversion from intravenous to oral therapy, the recommended initial dose of Tablets is 5 mg once a day for patients with creatinine clearance >30 ml and 2.5 mg once a day for patients with creatinine clearance ≤30 ml/min. Dosage should then be adjusted according to blood pressure response.

PATIENTS AT RISK OF EXCESSIVE HYPOTENSION

Hypertensive patients at risk of excessive hypotension include those with the following concurrent conditions or characteristics: heart failure, hyponatremia, high doses of diuretic therapy, recent intensive diuresis or increase in diuretic dose, renal dialysis, or severe volume and/or salt depletion of any etiology (see WARNINGS.) Single doses of enalaprilat as low as 0.2 mg have produced excessive hypotension in normotensive patients with these diagnoses. Because of the potential for an extreme hypotensive response in these patients, therapy should be started under very close medical supervision. The starting dose should be no greater than 0.625 mg administered intravenously over a period of no less than five minutes and preferably longer (up to one hour).

Patients should be followed closely whenever the dose of enalaprilat is adjusted and/or diuretic is increased.

ADMINISTRATION

Enalapril IV should be administered as a slow intravenous infusion, as indicated above. It may be administered as provided or diluted with up to 50 ml of a compatible diluent.

Parenteral drug products should be inspected visually for particulate matter and discoloration prior to use whenever solution and container permit.

COMPATIBILITY AND STABILITY

Vasotec IV as supplied and mixed with the following intravenous diluent has been found to maintain full activity for 24 hours at room temperature:

5 percent Dextrose Injection

0.9 percent Sodium Chloride Injection

0.9 percent Sodium Chloride Injection in 5 percent Dextrose

5 percent Dextrose in Lactated Ringer's Injection

McGaw Isolyte E

PATIENT INFORMATION:

Enalapril is an angiotensin-converting enzyme (ACE) inhibitor used for the treatment of high blood pressure or heart failure. Notify your physician if you are pregnant or nursing. The use of enalapril during months four through nine of pregnancy may permanently injure or cause the death of the developing fetus. Avoid using potassium containing salt substitutes without notifying your physician. Enalapril may be taken with or without food. Dizziness, lightheadedness or fainting may occur after the first dose or during the first week of therapy. Avoid sudden changes in posture. A persistent dry cough or taste alterations may occur while taking enalapril. Notify your physician if these become bothersome. Notify your physician if you develop trouble swallowing or breathing; swelling of the face, lips, or tongue; irregular heartbeat; rash, hives or severe itching; unexplained fever; or easy bruising.

HOW SUPPLIED:

No. 3411-Tablets VASOTEC, 2.5 mg, are yellow, biconvex barrel shaped, scored compressed tables with code MSD 14 on one side and Vasotec on the other.

No. 3412-Tablets VASOTEC, 5 mg, are white, barrel shaped, scored, compressed tables, with code MSD 712 on one side and Vasotec on the other.

No. 3413-Tablets VASOTEC, 10 mg, are salmon, barrel shaped, compressed tablets, with code MSD 713 on one side and VASOTEC on the other.

No. 3414-Tablets VASOTEC, 20 mg, are peach, barrel shaped, compressed tablets, with code MSD 714 on one side and VASOTEC on the other.

STORAGE

Tablets: Store below 30°C (86°F) and avoid transient temperatures above 50°C (122°F). Keep container tightly closed. Protect from moisture.

Dispense in a tight container, if product package is subdivided.

Injection: Store below 30°C (86°F)

HOW SUPPLIED - EQUIVALENTS NOT AVAILABLE:

Tablet, Uncoated - Oral - 2.5 mg

100's	$74.78	VASOTEC, Merck	00006-0014-68
100's	$78.71	VASOTEC, Merck	00006-0014-28
1000's	$747.86	VASOTEC, Merck	00006-0014-82
1080's	$807.74	VASOTEC, 90 X 12, Merck	00006-0014-94
2160's	$1615.51	VASOTEC, 180 X 12, Merck	00006-0014-98
10000's	$7478.60	VASOTEC, Merck	00006-0014-87

Tablet, Uncoated - Oral - 5 mg

100's	$95.00	VASOTEC, Merck	00006-0712-68
100's	$98.96	VASOTEC, Merck	00006-0712-28
1000's	$950.13	VASOTEC, Merck	00006-0712-82
1080's	$1026.28	VASOTEC, 90 X 12, Merck	00006-0712-94
2160's	$2052.58	VASOTEC, 180 X 12, Merck	00006-0712-98
4000's	$3800.60	VASOTEC, Merck	00006-0712-81
10000's	$9501.50	VASOTEC, Merck	00006-0712-87

Tablet, Uncoated - Oral - 10 mg

100's	$99.75	VASOTEC, Merck	00006-0713-68
100's	$103.70	VASOTEC, Merck	00006-0713-28
1000's	$997.68	VASOTEC, Merck	00006-0713-82
1080's	$1077.65	VASOTEC, 90 X 12, Merck	00006-0713-94
2160's	$2155.31	VASOTEC, 180 X 12, Merck	00006-0713-98
4000's	$3990.72	VASOTEC, Merck	00006-0713-81
10000's	$9976.80	VASOTEC, Merck	00006-0713-87

Tablet, Uncoated - Oral - 20 mg

100's	$141.90	VASOTEC, Merck	00006-0714-68
100's	$145.88	VASOTEC, Merck	00006-0714-28
1000's	$1419.11	VASOTEC, Merck	00006-0714-82
1080's	$1532.81	VASOTEC, 90 X 12, Merck	00006-0714-94
10000's	$13171.25	VASOTEC, Merck	00006-0714-87

ENALAPRIL MALEATE; FELODIPINE *(003325)*

CATEGORIES: ACE Inhibitors; Angiotensin Converting Enzyme Inhibitors; Antihypertensives; Cardiovascular Drugs; Congestive Heart Failure; Calcium Channel Blockers; Heart Failure; Hypertension; Pregnancy Category C, 1st Trimester; Pregnancy Category D, 2nd & 3rd Trimesters

BRAND NAMES: **Lexxel**

USE IN PREGNANCY

When used in pregnancy during the second and third trimesters, ACE inhibitors can cause injury and even death to the developing fetus. When pregnancy is detected, this product should be discontinued as soon as possible. (See WARNINGS, Fetal/Neonatal Morbidity and Mortality).

DESCRIPTION:

Lexxel is a combination product, consisting of an outer layer of enalapril maleate surrounding a core tablet of an extended-release felodipine formulation.

See Enalalpril Maleate, DESCRIPTION and Felopdipine, DESCRIPTION.

CLINICAL PHARMACOLOGY:

MECHANISM OF ACTION

The two components of enalapril maleate/felodipine have complementary antihypertensive actions. Enalapril is a pro-drug; following oral administration, it is bioactivated by hydrolysis of the ethyl ester to enalaprilat, which is the active angiotensin converting enzyme (ACE) inhibitor. Enalaprilat inhibits angiotensin-converting enzyme in humans and animals. ACE is a peptidyl dipeptidase that catalyzes the conversion of angiotensin I to the vasoconstrictor substance, angiotensin II. Angiotensin II also stimulates aldosterone secretion by the adrenal cortex. The beneficial effects of enalapril in hypertension appear to result primarily from suppression of the renin-angiotensin-aldosterone system.

Inhibition of ACE results in decreased plasma angiotensin II, which leads to decreased vasopressor activity and to decreased aldosterone secretion. Although the latter decrease is small, it results in small increases of serum potassium. In hypertensive patients treated with enalapril maleate alone for up to 48 weeks, mean increases in serum potassium of approximately 0.2 mEq/L were observed. In patients treated with enalapril maleate plus a thiazide diuretic, there was essentially no change in serum potassium. (See PRECAUTIONS.) Removal of angiotensin II negative feedback on renin secretion leads to increased plasma renin activity.

ACE is identical to kininase, an enzyme that degrades bradykinin. Whether increased levels of bradykinin, a potent vasodepressor peptide, play a role in the therapeutic effects of enalapril maleate remains to be elucidated.

While the mechanism through which enalapril lowers blood pressure is believed to be primarily suppression of the renin-angiotensin-aldosterone system, enalapril is antihypertensive even in patients with low-renin hypertension. Although enalapril was antihypertensive in all races studied, black hypertensive patients (usually a low-renin hypertensive population) had a smaller average response to enalapril monotherapy than non-black patients.

Felodipine is a dihydropyridine calcium channel blocker that reduces the influx of Ca^{++} by an effect on the voltage dependent L-channels in vascular smooth muscle and cultured rabbit atrial cells and blocks potassium-induced contracture of the rat portal vein.

Pharmacologic studies show that the effects of felodipine on contractile processes are selective, with greater effects on vascular smooth muscle than cardiac muscle. Negative inotropic effects can be detected *in vitro*, but such effects have not been seen in intact animals.

CLINICAL PHARMACOLOGY: *(cont'd)*

The consequences of vasodilation produced by felodipine include a modest, short-lived reflex increase in heart rate. A mild diuretic effect is seen in several animal species and man. but most of the effects of felodipine are accounted for by its effects on peripheral vascular resistance.

PHARMACOKINETICS AND METABOLISM

Concomitant administration of enalapril and felodipine as an extended-release formulation has little effect on the bioavailability of either compound. The rate and extent of absorption of enalapril from the combination is not significantly different from that of enalapril (see Enalapril Maleate, CLINICAL PHARMACOLOGY). The rate and extent of absorption of felodipine from the combination has not been directly compared to the extended-release formulation of felodipine (see Felodipine, CLINICAL PHARMACOLOGY).

Following oral administration of enalapril maleate/felodipine, peak concentrations of enalapril occur within about one hour. Enalapril is hydrolyzed to enalaprilat, which is a more potent angiotensin converting enzyme inhibitor than enalapril. Peak serum concentrations of enalaprilat occur about three hours after an oral dose of enalapril maleate/felodipine. Based on urinary recovery, the extent of absorption of enalapril is approximately 60 percent.

Peak concentrations of the isomers of felodipine are generally seen at 3-6 hours after administration of enalapril maleate/felodipine. Following oral administration, felodipine is almost completely absorbed and undergoes extensive first-pass metabolism; the systemic bioavailability of felodipine extended release is approximately 20 percent.

When enalapril maleate/felodipine is taken with food with a high fat content, some of the pharmacokinetics of its components are changed. Although the $AUC_{(0-48\ hr)}$ of felodipine is not changed, the peak concentration of its isomers is almost doubled and the trough concentration is approximately halved. The bioavailability of enalapril, as measured by total urinary recovery of enalaprilat, is slightly reduced. As with other dihydropyridine calcium channel blockers, the bioavailability of felodipine was increased when taken with grapefruit juice, compared to when taken with water or orange juice.

The systemic plasma clearance of felodipine in young healthy subjects is about 0.8 L/min and the apparent volume of distribution is 10 L/kg. Approximately 99% of felodipine is bound to plasma proteins.

Following administration of ^{14}C-labeled intravenous or immediate-release oral felodipine in man, about 70 percent of the dose of radioactivity was recovered in urine and 10 percent in the feces. A negligible amount of intact felodipine was recovered in the urine and feces (<0.5%). Six metabolites, which account for 23 percent of the oral dose, have been identified; none has significant vasodilating activity. Following oral administration of the immediate-release formulation, the plasma levels of felodipine declined polyexponentially with a mean terminal half-life of 11 to 16 hours.

Excretion of enalaprilat and enalapril is primarily renal. Approximately 94% of the dose is recovered in the urine and feces as enalaprilat or enalapril. The principal components in urine are enalaprilat, accounting for about 40 percent of the dose, and intact enalapril. There is no evidence of metabolites of enalapril, other than enalaprilat. The serum concentration profile of enalaprilat exhibits a prolonged terminal phase, apparently representing a small fraction of the administered dose that has been bound to ACE. The amount bound does not increase with dose, indicating a saturable site of binding. The effective half-life for accumulation of enalaprilat following multiple doses of enalapril maleate is 11 hours.

The disposition of enalapril and enalaprilat in patients with renal insufficiency is similar to that in patients with normal renal function until the glomerular filtration rate is reduced to 30 ml/min or less. With glomerular filtration rate ≤30 ml/min, peak and trough enalaprilat levels increase, time to peak concentration increases, and time to steady state may be delayed. The effective half-life of enalaprilat following multiple doses of enalapril maleate is prolonged at this level of renal insufficiency. Enalaprilat is dialyzable at a rate of 62 ml/min.

Plasma concentrations of felodipine, after a single dose and at steady state, increase with age. Mean clearance of felodipine in elderly hypertensives (mean age 74) was only 45 percent of that for young volunteers (mean age 26). At steady state, the mean AUC for young patients was 39 percent of that for the elderly. Data for intermediate age ranges suggest that the AUCs fall between the extremes of the young and the elderly.

In patients with hepatic disease, the clearance of felodipine was reduced to about 60 percent of that seen in normal young volunteers.

Blood Brain Barrier and Blood Placental Barrier: Animal studies have shown that felodipine crosses the blood brain barrier. The plasma to brain concentration ratio of felodipine is about 20:1. Felodipine crosses the placenta. Fetal plasma levels of felodipine are similar to maternal plasma levels. Studies in dogs indicate that enalapril crosses the blood brain barrier poorly, if at all; enalaprilat does not enter the brain. Multiple doses of enalapril maleate in rats do not result in accumulation in any tissues. Milk of lactating rats contains radioactivity following administration of ^{14}C enalapril maleate. Radioactivity was found to cross the placenta following administration of labeled drug to pregnant hamsters.

PHARMACODYNAMICS

Administration of enalapril maleate to patients with hypertension of severity ranging from mild to severe results in a reduction of both supine and standing blood pressure, usually with no orthostatic component. Symptomatic postural hypotension is infrequent with enalapril alone, although it might be anticipated in volume-depleted patients. (See WARNINGS) In most patients studied, after oral administration of a single dose of enalapril, onset of antihypertensive activity was seen at one hour, with peak reduction of blood pressure achieved by four to six hours. At recommended doses, antihypertensive effects have been maintained for at least 24 hours. In some patients the effects may diminish toward the end of the dosing interval.

In most patients, achievement of optimal blood pressure reduction may require several weeks of therapy. The antihypertensive effects of enalapril have continued during long term therapy. Abrupt withdrawal of enalapril has not been associated with a rapid increase in blood pressure. In hemodynamic studies in patients with essential hypertension, blood pressure reduction was accompanied by a reduction in peripheral arterial resistance with an increase in cardiac out-put and little or no change in heart rate. Following administration of enalapril maleate. there is an increase in renal blood flow; glomerular filtration rate is usually unchanged. The effects appear to be similar in patients with renovascular hypertension.

In a clinical pharmacology study, indomethacin or sulindac was administered to hypertensive patients receiving enalapril. In this study there was no evidence of a blunting of the antihypertensive action of enalapril.

The effect of felodipine on blood pressure is principally a consequence of a dose-related decrease in peripheral vascular resistance. Blood pressure response following administration of felodipine extended release to hypertensive patients is correlated with dose and plasma concentrations of felodipine. A reduction in blood pressure generally occurs within two to five hours. During chronic administration, substantial blood pressure control lasts for 24 hours with trough reductions in diastolic blood pressure approximately 40-50 percent of peak reductions. A reflex increase in heart rate frequently occurs during the first week of therapy: this increase attenuates over time. Heart rate increases of 5-10 beats per minute may be seen during chronic dosing. The increase is inhibited by beta-blocking agents.

CLINICAL PHARMACOLOGY: *(cont'd)*

Felodipine has no significant effect on cardiac conduction (P-R, P-Q and H-V intervals). In clinical trials in hypertensive patients without clinical evidence of left ventricular dysfunction, no symptoms suggestive of a negative inotropic effect were noted; however, none would be expected in this population.

In an 8-week, fixed-dose, parallel-group, double-blind study, 707 hypertensive patients were randomized among all possible combinations of enalapril (0, 5, or 20 mg), and extended-release felodipine (0, 2.5, 5, or 10 mg), both taken once daily. Each of the non-placebo combinations was significantly more effective than placebo in reducing seated systolic and diastolic blood pressure at peak (three to five hours after dosing) and trough (24 hours after dosing). Enalapril and felodipine contributed additively to the effect, so that each active combination was significantly more effective than either of its component monotherapies. Most of the drug effect seen at peak was still present at trough. The efficacy of combination therapy relative to monotherapy was not significantly affected by race, sex, or age.

During chronic dosing with enalapril maleate/felodipine, the maximum reduction in blood pressure is generally achieved after one to two weeks. The antihypertensive effects of enalapril maleate/felodipine have continued during chronic therapy for at least one year.

INDICATIONS AND USAGE:

Enalapril maleate/felodipine is indicated for the treatment of hypertension.

This fixed combination drug is not indicated for the initial therapy of hypertension. (See DOSAGE AND ADMINISTRATION).

In using enalapril maleate/felodipine, consideration should be given to the fact that another angiotensin converting enzyme inhibitor, captopril, has caused agranulocytosis, particularly in patients with renal impairment or collagen vascular disease, and that available data are insufficient to show that enalapril does not have a similar risk. (See WARNINGS, Neutropenia/Agranulocytosis).

In considering use of enalapril maleate/felodipine, it should be noted that black patients receiving ACE inhibitors have been reported to have a higher incidence of angioedema compared to non-blacks. (See Enalapril Maleate, WARNINGS, Angioedema).

CONTRAINDICATIONS:

Enalapril maleate/felodipine is contraindicated in patients who are hypersensitive to any component of this product. Because of the enalapril component, this drug is contraindicated in patients with a history of angioedema related to previous treatment with an angiotensin converting enzyme inhibitor.

WARNINGS:

Anaphylactoid and Possibly Related Reactions: See Enalapril Maleate, WARNINGS.

Angioedema: See Enalapril Maleate, WARNINGS.

Anaphylactoid Reactions During Desensitization: See Enalapril Maleate, WARNINGS.

Anaphylactoid Reactions During Membrane Exposure: See Enalapril Maleate, WARNINGS.

Hypotension: See Enalapril Maleate, WARNINGS. Felodipine, like other calcium channel blockers, may occasionally precipitate significant hypotension and rarely syncope. It may lead to reflex tachycardia which in susceptible individuals may precipitate angina pectoris. See ADVERSE REACTIONS.

Neutropenia/Agranulocytosis: See Enalapril Maleate, WARNINGS.

Hepatic Failure: See Enalapril Maleate, WARNINGS.

Fetal/Neonatal Morbidity and Mortality: See Enalapril Maleate, WARNINGS.

In rats administered the combination of enalapril and felodipine (enalapril [E]=1.9-felodipine [F]=2.5 mg/kg/day), an increased incidence of fetuses with dilated renal pelvis/ureter was observed. However, there was no evidence of this effect in the offspring postweaning. In mice, with doses of E=23, F=30 mg/kg/day or greater, there was an increased incidence of both early and late *in utero* deaths. Other than a transient and slight decrease in body weight gain in the first generation offspring, there were no adverse effects in offspring with regard to sexual maturation, behavioral developement, fertility or fecundity.

Enalapril-felodipine given to pregnant mice (enalapril 20.8, felodipine 27 mg/kg/day) and rats (enalapril=17.3, felodipine=22.5 mg/kg/day) produced plasma levels (C_{max} and AUC values) of enalapril/enalaprilat that were 76 to 418-fold greater and plasma levels of felodipine that were 151 to 433-fold greater than those expected in humans (non-pregnant) at the dose to be used in humans.

PRECAUTIONS:

GENERAL

See Enalapril Maleate, PRECAUTIONS, General, Impaired Renal Function, Hyperkalemia, Cough, and Surgery/Anesthesia.

See Felodipine, PRECAUTIONS, Elderly Patients or Patients with Impaired Renal Liver Function and Peripheral Edema.

INFORMATION FOR THE PATIENT

See Enalapril Maleate, PRECAUTIONS, Information for the Patient.

Gingival Hyperplasia: Patients should be told that mild gingival hyperplasia (gum swelling) as been reported. Good dental hygiene decreases its incidence and severity.

Note: As with many other drugs, certain advice to patients being treated with this drug is warranted. This information is intended to aid in the safe and effective use of this medication. It is not a disclousure of all possible adverse or intended effects.

CARCINOGENESIS, MUTAGENESIS, AND IMPAIRMENT OF FERTILITY

No long-term carcinogenicity tests have been performed with the combination. Enalapril-felodipine was not mutagenic with or without metabolic activation *in vitro* in the Ames microbial mutation assay, the V-79 mammalian cell forward mutation assay, the alkaline elution assay with rat hepatocytes or the CHO mammalian cell cytogenetics assay. An *in vivo* mouse bone marrow cytogenetics assay was also negative.

In rats given enalapril-felodipine, there was no effect on fertility in males at doses up to 6.9/9 mg/kg/day, and in females at doses up to 17.3/22.5 mg/kg/day.

There was no evidence of a tumorgenic effect when enalapril was admistered for 106 weeks to male and female rats at doses up to 90 mg/kg/day or for 94 weeks to male and female mice at doses up to 90 and 180 mg/kg/day, respectively. These doses are 26 times (in rats and female mice) and 13 times (in male mice) the maximum recommended human daily dose (MRHDD) when compared on a body surface area basis.

See also Enalapril Maleate, PRECAUTIONS, Carcinogenesis, Mutagenesis, and Impairment of Fertility.

There were no adverse effects on reproductive performance of male and female rats treated with up to 90 mg/kg/day of enalapril (26 times the MRHDD when compared on a body surface area basis).

See also Felodipine, PRECAUTIONS, Carcinogenesis, Mutagenesis, and Impairment of Fertility.

PRECAUTIONS: *(cont'd)*

PREGNANCY

Pregnancy Categories C (first trimester) and D (second and third trimesters). See Enalapril Maleate, WARNINGS, Fetal/Neonatal Morbidity and Mortality.

See also Felodipine, PRECAUTIONS, Pregnancy, Teratogenic and Nonteratogenic Effects.

NURSING MOTHERS

Enalapril and enaprilat are dectected in human breast milk. It is not known whether felodipine administered as monotherapy is secreted in human milk; studies of the combination of enalapril and felodipine in rats indicate that felodipine concentrates in milk to a level almost ten-fold that found in plasma. Because of the potential for serious adverse reactions from enalapril and felopdipine in the infant, a decision should be made either to discontinue nursing or to discontinue the drug, taking into account the importance of the drug to the mother. Therefore caution should be exercised when this drug is given to a nursing mother.

PEDIATRIC USE

Safety and effectiveness in pediatric patients have not been established.

DRUG INTERACTIONS:

See Enalapril Maleate, DRUG INTERACTIONS for interactions concerning the following:

Hypotension	Agents Increasing Serum Potassium
Agents Causing Renin Release	Lithium

See Felodipine, DRUG INTERACTIONS for interactions concerning the following:

Betablocking Agents	Anticonvulsants
Cimetidine	Other Concomitant Therapy
Digixon	

ADVERSE REACTIONS:

In a factorial study, combinations of enalapril at doses of 0, 5 and 20 mg and felodipine extended release at doses of 0, 2.5,5, and 10 mg were evaluated for safety in more than 700 patients with hypertension. In addition more than 500 patients received various combinations of enalapril (5 or 10 mg) and felodipine extended release (2.5, 5 or 10 mg) with or without hydrochlorothiazide (12.5 mg) in an open-labeled study up to 52 weeks (mean 33 weeks.) Adverse events were similar to those described with the individual components.

In general, treatment with enalapril maleate-felodipine extended release was well tolerated and adverse events were mild and transient in nature. In the placebo-controlled, double-blind trial, discontinuation of therapy due to adverse events considered related (possibly, probably, or definately) occurred in 2.8 percent vs 1.3 percent of patients treated with the combination or placebo, respectively. The most frequent observed clinical adverse events considered related to treatment with the combination were headache, edema or swelling, and dizziness.

Clinical adverse events related (possibly, probably, or definitely) to treatment with enalapril maleate-felodipine extended release that occurred with an incidence of one percent or greater with the combination during the placebo-controlled, double-blind trial are compared to individual components and placebo in TABLE 1.

TABLE 1 Percent of Patients with Adverse Events in the Double-Blind Trial (Percent discontinution shown in parentheses)

Body System/ Adverse Event	Enalapril* Felodipine† N=319	Enalapril* N=133	Felodipine† N=176	Placebo N=79
Body as a Whole				
Edema/ swelling	4.1 (0.3)	2.3 (0.0)	10.8 (1.7)	1.3 (0.0)
Asthenia/ fatigue	1.9 (0.0)	2.3 (0.8)	0.6 (0.6)	3.8 (0.0)
Nervous/ Psychiatric				
Headache	10.3 (0.6)	3.8 (0.0)	10.2 (1.1)	7.6 (1.3)
Dizziness	4.4 (0.3)	1.5 (0.0)	2.8 (0.6)	0.0 (0.0)
Respiratory				
Cough	2.2 (0.6)	2.3 (0.0)	0.6 (0.0)	0.0 (0.0)
Skin				
Flushing	1.6 (0.3)	0.0 (0.0)	2.3 (1.1)	0.0 (0.0)

* Combination of dose of 5 and 20 mg daily.
† Combination of dose of 2.5, 5 and 10 mg daily.

Other clinical adverse events considered related (possibly, probably, or definitely) to treatment with enalapril maleate-felodipine extended release that occurred with an incidence of less than one percent in the placebo-controlled, double-blind trial are listed. These events are in order of decreasing frequency within each category. *Body as a Whole:* Syncope, facial edema, orthostatic effects, chest pain; *Cardiovascular:* Palpitation, hypotension, bradycardia, premature ventricular contraction, increased blood pressure; *Digestive:* Dry mouth, constipation, dyspepsia, flatulence, acid regurgitation, vomiting, diarrhea, nausea, anal/rectal pain; *Metabolic:* Gout; *Musculoskeletal:* Neck pain, joint swelling; *Nervous/Psychiatric:* Insomnia, nervousness, somnolence, ataxia, agitation, paresthesia, tremor; *Respiratory:* Dyspnea, respiratory congestion, pharyngeal discomfort, dry throat; *Skin:* Rash, angioedema, pruritus, alopecia, dry skin; *Special Senses:* Increased intraocular pressure; *Urogenital:* Impotence, hot flashes.

Other frequently reported adverse events were seen in clinical trials with enalapril-feldodipine extended release (causal relationship unknown). These included:*Body as a Whole:* Abdominal pain, fever; *Digestive:* Dental pain;*Metabolic:* Increased ALT and AST, hyperglycemia; *Musculoskeletal:* Back pain, myalgia, foot pain, knee pain, shoulder pain, tendonitis; *Respiratory:* Upper respiratory infection, sinusitis, pharyngitis, bronchitis, nasal congestion, influenza, sinus disorder; *Special Senses:* Conjunctivitis; *Urogenital:* Proteinuria, pyuria, urinary tract infection.

Enalapril Maleate: For other adverse events that have been reported with enalapril, without regard to causality see Enalapril Maleate, ADVERSE REACTIONS.

Felodipine: For other adverse events that have been reported with felodipine, without regard to causality see Felodipine, ADVERSE REACTIONS.

LABORATORY TESTS

In controlled clinical trials with enalapril-felodipine extended release, clinically important changes in standard laboratory parameters associated with administration of enalapril maleate/felodipine were rare. No changes peculiar to the combination treatment were observed.

Serum Electrolytes: See Felodipine, PRECAUTIONS.

Creatinine: Minor reversible increases in serum creatinine were observed in patients treated with enalapril maleate/felodipine. Increases in creatinine are more likely to occur in patients with renal insufficiency or those pretreated with a diuretic and based on experience with other ACE inhibitors, would be expected to be especially likely in patients with renal artery stenosis (see PRECAUTIONS).

Other: Minor reversible increases or decreases in serum potassium were infrequently observed in patients treated with enalapril maleate/felodipine: rarely were these measurements outside the normal range.

OVERDOSAGE:

Limited data are available in regard to enalapril overdosage in humans. In a suicide atempt, one patient took 150 mg felodipine together with 15 tablets each of atenolol and spironolactone and 20 tablets of nitrazepam The patient's blood pressure and heart rate were normal on admission to hospital, he subsequently recovered without significant sequelae.

Human overdoses with any combination of enalapril and felodipine extended release have not been reported.

Single oral doses of enalapril above 1000 mg/kg and ≥1775 mg/kg were associated with lethality in mice and rats, respectively. Oral doses of felodipine at 240 mg/kg and 264 mg/kg in male and female mice, respectively, and 2390 mg/kg and 2250 mg/kg in male and female rats, respectively, caused significant lethality.

In interaction studies on the acute oral toxicity of the combination in mice, pretreatment with felodipine (50 mg/kg) for one hour led to an increase in mortality at doses of enalapril maleate that exceeded 1000 mg/kg. Significant lethality with felodipine was not increased by pretreatment of mice for one hour with 1O0 mg/kg of enalapril maleate.

Treatment: To obtain up-to-date information about the treatment of overdose, consult your Regional Poison-Control Center. Telephone numbers of certified poison control centers are listed in Physicians GenRx. In managing overdose, consider the possibilities of multiple drug overdoses, drug-drug interactions, and unusual drug kinetics in your patient. The most likely effect of overdose with enalapril maleate/felodipine is vasodilation, with consequent hypotension and tachycardia. Repletion of central fluid volume (Trendelenburg positioning, infusion of crystalloids) may be sufficient therapy, but pressor agents (norepinephrine or high-dose dopamine) may be required.

Enalaprilat may be removed from general circulation by hemodialysis at a rate of 62 ml/min and has been removed from neonatal circulation by peritoneal dialysis. It has not been established whether felodipine can be removed from the circulation by hemodialysis.

DOSAGE AND ADMINISTRATION:

Enalapril maleate/felodipine is an effective treatment for hypertension. This fixed combination drug is not indicated for initial therapy of hypertension.

The recommended initial dose of enalapril maleate for hypertension in patients not receiving diuretics is 5 mg once a day. The usual dosage range of enalapril maleate for hypertension is 10-40 mg per day administered in a single dose or two divided doses. In some patients treated once daily with enalapril, the antihypertensive effect may diminish toward the end of the dosing interval. In such patients, an increase in dosage or twice daily administration should be considered. The recommended initial dose of felodipine extended release is 5 mg once a day with a usual dosage range of 2.5 mg-10 mg once a day. In elderly or hepatically impaired patients, the recommended initial dose of felodipine is 2.5 mg. When enalapril maleate/felodipine is taken with food, the peak concentration of felodipine is almost doubled. and the trough (24-hour) concentration is approximately halved (see CLINICAL PHARMACOLOGY, Pharmacokinetics and Metabolism).

In clinical trials of enalapril-felodipine extended release combination therapy using enalapril doses of 5-20 mg and felodipine extended release doses of 2.5-10 mg once daily, the antihypertensive effects increased with increasing doses of each component in all patient groups.

The hazards (see WARNINGS and ADVERSE REACTIONS) of enalapril are generally independent of dose; those of felodipine are a mixture of dose-dependent phenomena (primarily peripheral edema) and dose-independent phenomena, the former much more common than the latter. Therapy with any combination of enalapril and felodipine will thus be associated with both sets of dose-independent hazards.

Rarely, the dose-independent hazards associated with enalapril or felodipine are serious. To minimize dose-independent hazards, it is usually appropriate to begin therapy with enalapril maleate/felodipine only after a patient has failed to achieve the desired antihypertensive effect with one or the other monotherapy.

Replacement Therapy: Although the felodipine component of enalapril maleate/felodipine has not been shown to be bioequivalent to the available extended-release felodipine, patients receiving enalapril and felodipine from separate tablets once a day may instead wish to receive the tablets of enalapril maleate/felodipine containing the same component doses.

Therapy Guided By Clinical Effect: A patient whose blood pressure is not adequately controlled with felodipine or enalapril monotherapy may be switched to combination therapy with an initial dose of one tablet daily. If blood pressure control is inadequate after a week or two, the dose may be increased to two tablets daily. If control remains unsatisfactory, consider addition of a thiazide diuretic.

Use in Patients with Metabolic Impairments: Regimens of therapy with enalapril maleate/felodipine need not be adjusted for renal function as long as the patient's creatinine clearance is >30 ml/min/ 1.73m^2 (serum creatinine roughly ≤3 mg/dl or 265 μmol/L). In patients with more severe renal impairment, the recommended initial dose of enalapril is 2.5 mg.

Enalapril maleate/felodipine should be swallowed whole and not divided, crushed or chewed.

HOW SUPPLIED:

No. 3661 Tablets Lexxel, 5-5 are white, round/biconvex shaped, film-coated tablets, coded LEXXEL 1, 5-5 on one side and no markings on the other. Each tablet contains 5 mg of enalapril maleate and 5 mg of felodipine as an extended release formulation.

Storage: Store at 25°C (77°F); excursions permitted between 15°C and 30°C (59°F and 86°F). Keep container tightly closed. Protect from moisture and light. Dispense in a tight container, if product package is subdivided.

HOW SUPPLIED - EQUIVALENTS NOT AVAILABLE:

Tablets, Film-Coated - Oral - 5 mg/5 mg

30's	$36.00	LEXXEL, Astra Merck	61113-0001-31
100's	$120.00	LEXXEL, Astra Merck	61113-0001-68
100's UD	$126.00	LEXXEL, Astra Merck	61113-0001-28

ENALAPRIL MALEATE; HYDROCHLOROTHIAZIDE *(001139)*

CATEGORIES: ACE Inhibitors; Angiotensin Converting Enzyme Inhibitors; Antihypertensives; Cardiovascular Drugs; Diuretics; Hypertension; Renal Drugs; Thiazides; Pregnancy Category C; FDA Approved 1986 Oct

BRAND NAMES: *Acesistem*; *Angiozide*; *Co-Renitec* (France, Mexico); *Co-Reniten*; *Gliotenzide* (Mexico); *Corenitec*; *Innozide* (England); *Lotrial D*; *Pres Plus* (Germany); *Renacor* (Germany); *Renidur*; **Vaseretic**; *Vasoretic*
(International brand names outside U.S. in italics)

FORMULARIES: Aetna; BC-BS; Medi-Cal

COST OF THERAPY: $405.44 (Hypertension; Tablet; 10 mg/25 mg; 1/day; 365 days)

PRIMARY ICD9: 401.1 (Essential Hypertension, Benign)

DESCRIPTION:

Vaseretic (Enalapril Maleate-Hydrochlorothiazide) combines an angiotensin converting enzyme inhibitor, enalapril maleate, and a diuretic, hydrochlorothiazide.

FOR COMPLETE PRESCRIBING INFORMATION, REFER TO THE INDIVIDUAL MONOGRAPHS (ENALAPRIL MALEATE; HYCROCHLOROTHIAZIDE).

INDICATIONS AND USAGE:

Vaseretic is indicated for the treatment of hypertension in patients for whom combination therapy is appropriate.

This fixed dose combination is not indicated for initial therapy. Patients already receiving a diuretic when enalapril is initiated, or given a diuretic and enalapril simultaneously, can develop symptomatic hypotension. In the initial titration of the individual entities, it is important, if possible, to stop the diuretic for several days before starting enalapril or, if this is not possible, begin enalapril at a low initial dose(see DOSAGE AND ADMINISTRATION). This fixed dose combination is not suitable for titration but may be substituted for the individual components if the titrated doses are the same as those in the combination.

In using Vaseretic, consideration should be given to the fact that another angiotensin converting enzyme inhibitor, captopril, has caused agranulocytosis, particularly in patients with renal impairment or collagen vascular disease, and that available data are insufficient to show that enalapril does not have a similar risk.

DOSAGE AND ADMINISTRATION:

DOSAGE MUST BE INDIVIDUALIZED. THE FIXED COMBINATION IS NOT FOR INITIAL THERAPY. THE DOSE OF 'VASERETIC' SHOULD BE DETERMINED BY THE TITRATION OF THE INDIVIDUAL COMPONENTS.

Once the patient has been successfully titrated with the individual components as described below, Vaseretic (one or two 10-25 tablets once daily) may be substituted if the titrated doses are the same as those in the fixed combination. (See INDICATIONS AND USAGE.)

Patients usually do not require doses in excess of 50 mg of hydrochlorothiazide daily; when combined with other antihypertensive agents. Therefore, since each tablet of Vaseretic includes 25 mg of hydrochlorothiazide, the daily dosage of Vaseretic should not exceed two tablets. If further blood pressure control is indicated, additional doses of enalapril or other non-diuretic antihypertensive agents should be considered.

For enalapril monotherapy the recommended initial dose in patients not on diuretics is 5 mg of enalapril once a day. Dosage should be adjusted according to blood pressure response. The usual dosage range of enalapril is 10 to 40 mg per day administered in a single dose or two divided doses. In some patients treated once daily, the antihypertensive effects may diminish toward the end of the dosing interval. In such patients, an increase in dosage or twice daily administration should be considered. If blood pressure is not controlled with enalapril alone, a diuretic may be added.

In patients who are currently being treated with a diuretic, symptomatic hypotension occasionally may occur following the initial dose of enalapril. The diuretic should, if possible, be discontinued for two to three days before beginning therapy with enalapril to reduce the likelihood of hypotension. If the patient's blood pressure is not controlled with enalapril alone, diuretic therapy may be resumed.

If the diuretic cannot be discontinued an initial dose of 2.5 mg of enalapril should be used under medical supervision for at least two hours and until blood pressure has stabilized for at least an additional hour.

Concomitant administration of Vaseretic with potassium supplements, potassium salt substitutes, or potassium sparing agents may lead to increases of serum potassium.

Dosage Adjustment in Renal Impairment: The usual dose of Vaseretic is recommended for patients with a creatinine clearance >30 ml/min (serum creatinine of up to approximately 3 mg/dl).

When concomitant diuretic therapy is required in patients with severe renal impairment, a loop diuretic, rather than a thiazide diuretic is preferred for use with enalapril; therefore, for patients with severe renal dysfunction the enalapril maleate-hydrochlorothiazide combination tablet is not recommended.

HOW SUPPLIED:

Tablets Vaseretic 10-25, are rust, squared capsule-shaped, compressed tablets, coded MSD 720 on one side and Vaseretic on the other. Each tablet contains 10 mg of enalapril maleate and 25 mg of hydrochlorothiazide.

Storage: Store below 30°C (86°F) and avoid transient temperatures above 50°C (122°F). Keep container tightly closed. Protect from moisture. Dispense in a tight container, if product package is subdivided.

HOW SUPPLIED - EQUIVALENTS NOT AVAILABLE:

Tablet, Uncoated - Oral - 10 mg/25 mg

100's	$111.08	VASERETIC, Merck	00006-0720-68

ENALAPRILAT *(001140)*

CATEGORIES: ACE Inhibitors; Angiotensin Converting Enzyme Inhibitors; Antihypertensives; Cardiovascular Drugs; Heart Failure; Hypertension; Renal Drugs; Pregnancy Category C; Sales > $100 Million; FDA Approved 1988 Feb

BRAND NAMES: **Vasotec-IV**

DESCRIPTION:

.For Full Prescribing Information, Please Refer to Enalapril Maleate.

HOW SUPPLIED - EQUIVALENTS NOT AVAILABLE:

Injection, Solution - Intravenous - 1.25 mg/ml

1 ml	$13.34	VASOTEC IV, Merck	00006-3508-01
2 ml	$26.70	VASOTEC IV, Merck	00006-3508-04

ENCAINIDE HYDROCHLORIDE *(001141)*

CATEGORIES: Antiarrhythmic Agents; Arrhythmia; Cardiovascular Drugs; Tachycardia; Pregnancy Category B; FDA Approved 1986 Dec

BRAND NAMES: **Enkaid**

COST OF THERAPY: $698.50 (Arrhythmia; Capsule; 25 mg; 3/day; 365 days) vs. Potential Cost of $3,462.83 (Arrhythmia)

DESCRIPTION:

.Product voluntarily withdrawn but still available on limited basis.

HOW SUPPLIED - EQUIVALENTS NOT AVAILABLE:

Capsule, Gelatin - Oral - 25 mg

100's	$63.79	ENKAID, Bristol Myers Squibb	00087-0732-41
100's	$66.97	ENKAID, Bristol Myers Squibb	00087-0732-42
500's	$303.01	ENKAID, Bristol Myers Squibb	00087-0732-43

Capsule, Gelatin - Oral - 35 mg

100's	$95.71	ENKAID, Bristol Myers Squibb	00087-0734-41
100's	$100.48	ENKAID, Bristol Myers Squibb	00087-0734-42
500's	$454.57	ENKAID, Bristol Myers Squibb	00087-0734-43

Capsule, Gelatin - Oral - 50 mg

100's	$127.60	ENKAID, Bristol Myers Squibb	00087-0735-41
100's	$133.97	ENKAID, Bristol Myers Squibb	00087-0735-42

ENOXACIN *(003103)*

CATEGORIES: Anti-Infectives; Antibacterials; Antibiotics; Cystitis; Fluoroquinolones; Gonorrhea; Quinolones; Sexually Transmitted Diseases; Urinary Tract Infections; FDA Class 1C ("Little or No Therapeutic Advantage"); FDA Approved 1991 Dec

BRAND NAMES: *Abenox*; *Bactidan*; *B-Mack*; *Comprecin* (England, Mexico); *Enoxacine* (France); *Enoxen*; *Enoxor* (Germany, France); *Flumark* (Japan); *Gyramid* (Germany); **Penetrex**
(International brand names outside U.S. in italics)

COST OF THERAPY: $2.84 (Gonorrhea; Tablet; 400 mg; 1/day; 1 days)

DESCRIPTION:

Penetrex (enoxacin) is a broad-spectrum azafluoroquinolone antibacterial agent for oral administration. Enoxacin is 1-ethyl-6-fluoro-1,4-dihydro-4-oxo-7-(1-piperazinyl)-1,8-naphthyridine-3-carboxylic acid sesquihydrate.

Its empirical formula is $C_{15}H_{17}N_4O_3F$°1 1/2 H_2O, and its molecular weight is 320.32 (anhydrous). Enoxacin is an ivory-to-slightly yellow powder. In dilute aqueous solution, it is unstable in strong sunlight.

Penetrex is available in 200-mg and 400-mg film-coated tablets. Each "200" and "400" Penetrex tablet contains enoxacin sesquihydrate equivalent to 200 mg and 400 mg of anhydrous enoxacin, respectively. Each Penetrex 200-mg and 400-mg tablet contains the following inactive ingredients: cellulose microcrystalline NF, colloidal silicon dioxide NF, croscarmellose sodium NF, FD&C Blue No. 2 aluminum lake, hydroxypropyl cellulose NF, hydroxypropyl methylcellulose, magnesium stearate USP, polyethylene glycol, simethicone, sorbic acid, stearate emulsifiers, and titanium dioxide.

CLINICAL PHARMACOLOGY:

Following oral administration to healthy subjects, peak plasma enoxacin concentrations were achieved within 1 to 3 hours. Absolute oral bioavailability of enoxacin is approximately 90%. Maximum plasma concentrations of enoxacin average 0.93 mcg/mL and 2.0 mcg/mL after single 200-mg and 400-mg doses, respectively. Enoxacin plasma half-life is 3 to 6 hours. Enoxacin is excreted primarily via the kidney. After a single dose, greater than 40% was recovered in urine by 48 hours as unchanged drug. In elderly patients, the mean peak enoxacin plasma concentration was 50% higher than that in young adult volunteers receiving comparable single doses of enoxacin. This appears to correspond to age-associated reduction of renal function in the elderly population. Five metabolites of enoxacin have been identified in human urine and account for 15% to 20% of the administered dose.

Enoxacin diffuses into cervix, fallopian tube, and myometrium at levels approximately 1-2 times those achieved in plasma, and into kidney and prostate at levels approximately 2-4 times those achieved in plasma. Studies have not been conducted to assess the penetration of enoxacin into human cerebrospinal fluid.

Enoxacin is approximately 40% bound to plasma proteins in healthy subjects and is approximately 14% bound to plasma proteins in patients with impaired renal function.

The effect of food on the absorption of enoxacin from the tablet formulation has not been studied. Some isozymes of the cytochrome P-450 hepatic microsomal enzyme system are inhibited by enoxacin. This inhibition results in significant drug/drug interactions with theophylline and caffeine. Enoxacin interferes with the metabolism of theophylline, resulting in a dose-related decrease in theophylline clearance. Elevated serum theophylline concentrations may increase the risk of theophylline-related adverse reactions (see DRUG INTERACTIONS).

Clearance of enoxacin is reduced in patients with impaired renal function (creatinine clearance ≤30 ml/min/1.73 M^2), and dosage adjustment is necessary (see DOSAGE AND ADMINISTRATION).

Microbiology: Enoxacin is an inhibitor of the bacterial enzyme DNA gyrase and is a bactericidal agent. Enoxacin may be active against pathogens resistant to drugs that act by different mechanisms.

Enoxacin has been shown to be active against most strains of the following organisms both *in vitro* and in clinical infections (see INDICATIONS AND USAGE):

Gram-Positive Aerobes: *staphylococcus epidermidis, staphylococcus saprophyticus.*

Gram-Negative Aerobes: *Enterobacter cloacae, Escherichia coli, Klebsiella pneumoniae, Neisseria gonorrhoeae, Proteus mirabilis, Pseudomonas aeruginosa.*

The following *in vitro* data are available but their clinical significance is unknown.

In addition, enoxacin exhibits *in vitro* minimum inhibitory concentrations (MICs) of 2.0 mcg/ml or less against most strains of the following organisms; however, the safety and effectiveness of enoxacin in treating clinical infections due to these organisms have not been established in adequate and well-controlled trials.

Gram-Negative Aerobes: *Aeromonas hydrophila, Citrobacter diversus, Citrobacter freundii, Citrobacter koseri, Enterobacter aerogenes, Haemophilus ducreyi, Klebsiella oxytoca, Klebsiella ozaenae, Morganella morganii, Proteus vulgaris, Providencia stuartii, Providencia alcalifaciens, Serratia marcescens, Serratia proteomaculans (formerly S. liquefaciens).*

Many strains of *Streptococcus* species and anaerobes are usually resistant to enoxacin.

The activity of enoxacin against *Treponema pallidum* has not been evaluated; however, other quinolones are not active against *T. pallidum* (see WARNINGS).

Cross-resistance with other quinolones has been demonstrated.

The addition of human serum has no effect on the *in vitro* MIC values; however, enoxacin activity is decreased in acidic (pH 5.5) environments.

CLINICAL PHARMACOLOGY: *(cont'd)*

SUSCEPTIBILITY TESTING

Diffusion Techniques: Quantitative methods that require measurement of zone diameters give the most precise estimate of susceptibility of bacteria to antimicrobial agents. One such standardized procedure that has been recommended for use with disks to test susceptibility of organisms to enoxacin uses the 10-mcg enoxacin disk.

Interpretation involves the correlation of the diameter obtained in the disk test with the minimum inhibitory concentration (MIC) for enoxacin.

Reports from the laboratory giving results of the standard single-disk susceptibility test with a 10-mcg enoxacin disk should be interpreted according to the criteria found in TABLE 1.

TABLE 1
Susceptibility Testing, Diffusion Techniques

Zone Diameter (mm)	Interpretation
≥ 18	(S) Susceptible
15-17	(MS) Moderately susceptible
≤ 14	(R) Resistant

A report of "susceptible" indicates that the pathogen is likely to be inhibited by generally achievable blood concentrations. A report of "moderately susceptible" suggests that the organism would be susceptible if high dosage is used or if the infection is confined to tissues or fluids in which high antimicrobial levels are attained. A report of "resistant" indicates that achievable drug concentrations are unlikely to be inhibitory, and other therapy should be selected.

Standardized susceptibility test procedures require the use of laboratory control organisms. The 10-mcg enoxacin disk should give the zone diameters found in TABLE 2.

TABLE 2
Susceptibility Testing, Diffusion Techniques

Organism	Zone Diameter (mm)
Escherichia coli (ATCC 25922)	28-36
Neisseria gonorrhoeae (ATCC 49226)	43-51
Pseudomonas aeruginosa (ATCC 27853)	22-28
Staphylococcus aureus (ATCC 25923)	22-28

Other quinolone antibacterial disks should not be substituted when performing susceptibility tests for enoxacin because of spectrum differences. The 10-mcg enoxacin disk should be used for all *in vitro* testing of isolates for enoxacin susceptibility using diffusion techniques.

Dilution Techniques: Use a standardized dilution method[2](broth, agar, or microdilution) or equivalent with enoxacin powder. The MIC values obtained should be interpreted according to the criteria found in TABLE 3.

TABLE 3
Susceptibility Testing, Dilution Techniques

MIC (mcg/ml)	Interpretation
≤ 2	(S) Susceptible
4	(MS) Moderately susceptible
≥ 8	(R) Resistant

As with standard diffusion methods, dilution procedures require the use of laboratory control organisms. Standard enoxacin powder should give the MIC values found in TABLE 4.

TABLE 4 Susceptibility Testing, Dilution Techniques

Organism	MIC (mcg/ml)
Enterococcus faecalis (ATCC 29212)	2-16
Escherichia coli (ATCC 25922)	0.06-0.25
Neisseria gonorrhoeae (ATCC 49226)	0.015-0.06
Pseudomonas aeruginosa (ATCC 27853)	2-8
Staphylococcus aureus (ATCC 29213	0.5-2

INDICATIONS AND USAGE:

Enoxacin is indicated for the treatment of adults (≥18 years of age) with the following infections caused by susceptible strains of the designated microorganisms:

Sexually Transmitted Diseases: (See WARNINGS.) **Uncomplicated urethral or cervical gonorrhea** due to *neisseria gonorrhoeae.*

Urinary Tract: Uncomplicated urinary tract infections (cystitis) due to *Escherichia coli, Staphylococcus epidermidis*, or Staphylococcus saprophyticus*.*

Complicated Urinary Tract Infections due to *Escherichia coli, Klebsiella pneumoniae, Proteus mirabilis, Pseudomonas aeruginosa, Staphylococcus epidermidis, or Enterobacter cloacae*.*

*Efficacy for this organism in this organ system at the recommended dose was studied in fewer than ten infections. The dosage regimens for complicated and uncomplicated urinary tract infections are different (see DOSAGE AND ADMINISTRATION).

Penicillinase production should have no effect on enoxacin activity.

Appropriate culture and susceptibility tests should be performed before treatment in order to isolate and identify organisms causing the infection and to determine their susceptibility to enoxacin. Therapy with enoxacin may be initiated while awaiting the results of these studies; therapy should be adjusted if necessary once the results are known. Culture and susceptibility testing performed periodically during therapy will provide information not only on the therapeutic effect of the antimicrobial agent but also on the possible emergence of bacterial resistance.

CONTRAINDICATIONS:

Enoxacin is contraindicated for individuals with a history of hypersensitivity to enoxacin or to any of the other members of the quinolone class of antimicrobial agents.

WARNINGS:

THE SAFETY AND EFFECTIVENESS OF ENOXACIN IN CHILDREN, ADOLESCENTS (UNDER THE AGE OF 18 YEARS), PREGNANT WOMEN, AND LACTATING WOMEN HAVE NOT BEEN ESTABLISHED. See Pregnancy, Teratogenic Effects, Pregnancy Category C, Nursing Mothers, and Pediatric Use. Enoxacin has been shown to cause arthropathy in immature rats and dogs when given in oral doses approximately 1.5 and 3.8 times, respectively, the highest human clinical dose based on a mg/m^2basis after a four-week dosage regimen. Gross and histopathological examination of the weight-bearing joints of the dogs revealed lesions of the cartilage. Other quinolones also produce erosions of cartilage of weight-bearing joints and other signs of arthropathy in immature animals of various species (see ANIMAL PHARMACOLOGY.)

WARNINGS: *(cont'd)*

Enoxacin Has Not Been Shown To Be Effective In The Treatment Of Syphilis. Antimicrobial agents used in high doses for short periods of time to treat gonorrhea may mask or delay the symptoms of incubating syphilis. All patients with gonorrhea should have a serologic test for syphilis at the time of diagnosis. Patients treated with enoxacin should have a follow-up serologic test for syphilis after 3 months.

Serious and occasionally fatal hypersensitivity (anaphylactoid or anaphylactic) reactions, some following the first dose, have been reported in patients receiving quinolone therapy. Some reactions were accompanied by cardiovascular collapse, loss of consciousness, tingling, pharyngeal or facial edema, dyspnea, urticaria, or itching. Only a few patients had a history of previous hypersensitivity reactions. Serious hypersensitivity reactions have also been reported following treatment with enoxacin. If an allergic reaction to enoxacin occurs, discontinue the drug. Serious acute hypersensitivity reactions may require immediate treatment with epinephrine. Oxygen, intravenous fluids, antihistamines, corticosteroids, pressor amines, and airway management, including intubation, should be administered as indicated.

Convulsions and abnormal electroencephalograms have been reported in some patients receiving enoxacin. Convulsions, increased intracranial pressure, and/or toxic psychoses have also been reported in patients receiving other drugs in this class. Quinolones may also cause central nervous system (CNS) stimulation which may lead to tremors, restlessness, lightheadedness, confusion, or hallucinations. If these reactions occur in patients receiving enoxacin, the drug should be discontinued and appropriate measures instituted. Enoxacin, as well as other quinolones, should be used with caution in patients with known or suspected CNS disorders, such as severe cerebral arteriosclerosis, epilepsy, and other factors that predispose to seizures (see ADVERSE REACTIONS).

Pseudomembranous colitis has been reported with nearly all antibacterial agents, including enoxacin, and may range in severity from mild to life-threatening. Therefore, it is important to consider this diagnosis in patients who present with diarrhea subsequent to the administration of antibacterial agents.

Treatment with broad-spectrum antibacterial agents alters the normal flora of the colon and may permit overgrowth of clostridia. Studies indicate that a toxin produced by *clostridium difficile* is a primary cause of "antibiotic-associated colitis."

After the diagnosis of pseudomembranous colitis has been established, therapeutic measures should be initiated.

Mild cases of pseudomembranous colitis usually respond to discontinuation of the drug alone. In moderate to severe cases, consideration should be given to management with fluids and electrolytes, protein supplementation, and treatment with an antibacterial drug clinically effective against *C. difficile* colitis.

Enoxacin is a potent inhibitor of the hepatic microsomal enzyme system resulting in significant drug/drug interactions with theophylline and caffeine (see DRUG INTERACTIONS).

PRECAUTIONS:

General: Alteration of the dosage regimen is necessary for patients with impaired renal function (creatinine clearance ≤30 ml/min/1.73 m^2) (see DOSAGE AND ADMINISTRATION).

Moderate-to-severe phototoxicity reactions have been observed in patients exposed to direct sunlight while receiving enoxacin or some other drugs in this class. Excessive sunlight should be avoided. Therapy should be discontinued if phototoxicity occurs.

Ophthalmologic abnormalities, including cataracts and multiple punctate lenticular opacities, have been noted in patients undergoing treatment with enoxacin, as well as with some other quinolones, but have also been observed in patients receiving placebo in comparative trials. In clinical trials using multiple-dose therapy, ophthalmic tissue levels of enoxacin and other quinolones were significantly higher than respective plasma concentrations. The causal relationship, if any, of quinolones to lenticular abnormalities has not been established.

Decreased spermatogenesis and subsequent decreased fertility were noted in rats and dogs treated with doses of enoxacin that produced plasma levels in the animals three times higher than those produced in humans at the recommended therapeutic dosage. The potential for enoxacin to affect spermatogenesis in male patients is unknown.

Information for the Patient: Patients should be advised:

not to take magnesium-, aluminum-, or calcium-containing antacids, bismuth subsalicylate, products containing iron, or multivitamins containing zinc for 8 hours prior to enoxacin or for 2 hours after enoxacin administration (see DRUG INTERACTIONS);

to drink fluids liberally;

to avoid consumption of caffeine-containing products (certain drugs, coffee, tea, chocolate, certain carbonated beverages during enoxacin therapy (see DRUG INTERACTIONS);

that enoxacin may cause dizziness and lightheadedness and, therefore, patients should know how they react to enoxacin before they operate an automobile or machinery or engage in activities requiring mental alertness and coordination;

that enoxacin may be associated with hypersensitivity reaction, even following the first dose, and to discontinue the drug at the first sign of a skin rash or other allergic reaction;

to avoid undue exposure to excessive sunlight while receiving enoxacin and to discontinue therapy if phototoxicity occurs.

Carcinogenesis, Mutagenesis, and Impairment of Fertility: Long-term studies in animals to determine the carcinogenic potential of enoxacin have not been conducted.

Genetic toxicology test included *in vitro* mutagenicity and cytogenetic assays and *in vitro* cytogenetic and micronucleus tests. Enoxacin did not induce point mutations in bacterial cells or mitotic gene conversion in yeast cells, with or without metabolic activation. Enoxacin did not induce sister chromatid exchanges or structural chromosomal aberrations in mammalian cells *in vitro*, with or without metabolic activation. In addition, enoxacin did not chromosomal aberrations in mice.

There was a minimal, dose-related, statistically significant increase in micronuclei at high doses in mice. The significance of these findings, in the absence of effects in other test systems, is not established.

Enoxacin produced no consistent effects on fertility and reproductive parameters in female rats given oral doses of enoxacin at levels up to 1000 mg/kg. Decreased spermatogenesis and subsequent impaired fertility was noted in male rats given oral doses of 1000 mg/kg. This dose is approximately 13-fold greater than the highest human clinical daily oral dose of 16 mg/kg, assuming a 50 kg person and based on a mg/m^{2}basis.

Pregnancy, Teratogenic Effects, Pregnancy Category C: Studies with enoxacin given orally to mice and rats have shown no evidence of teratogenic potential. The intravenous infusion of enoxacin into pregnant rabbits at doses of 10 to 50 mg/kg caused dose-related maternal toxicity (venous irritation, body weight loss, and reduced food intake) and, at 50 mg/kg, fetal toxicity (increased post-implantation loss and stunted fetuses).

At 50 mg/kg, the incidence of fetal malformations was significantly increased in the presence of overt maternal and fetal toxicity. There are no adequate and well-controlled studies in pregnant women. Enoxacin should be used during pregnancy only if the potential benefit justifies the potential risk to the fetus (see WARNINGS.)

PRECAUTIONS: *(cont'd)*

Nursing Mothers: it is not known whether enoxacin is excreted in human milk. Enoxacin is excreted in the milk of lactating rats. Because drugs of this class are excreted in human milk and because of the potential for serious adverse reactions from enoxacin in nursing infants, a decision should be made whether to discontinue nursing or to discontinue the drug, taking into account the importance of the drug to the mother.

Pediatric Use: Safety and effectiveness in children and adolescents below the age of 18 years have not been established. Enoxacin causes arthropathy in juvenile animals (see WARNINGS and ANIMAL PHARMACOLOGY).

Geriatric Use: In multiple-dose clinical trials of enoxacin, elderly patients (≥65 years of age) experienced significantly more overall adverse events than patients under 65 years of age. However, the incidence of drug-related adverse reactions was comparable between age groups.

DRUG INTERACTIONS:

Bismuth: Bismuth subsalicylate, given concomitantly with enoxacin or 60 minutes following enoxacin administration, decreased enoxacin bioavailability by approximately 25%. Thus, concomitant administration of enoxacin and bismuth subsalicylate should be avoided.

Caffeine: Enoxacin is a potent inhibitor of the cytochrome P-450 isozymes responsible for the metabolism of methylxanthine. In a multiple-dose study, enoxacin caused a dose-related increase in the mean elimination half-life of caffeine, thereby decreasing the clearance of caffeine by up to 80% and leading to a five-fold increase in the AUC and the half-life of caffeine. Trough plasma enoxacin levels were also 20% higher when caffeine and enoxacin were administered concomitantly. Caffeine-related adverse effects have occurred in patients consuming caffeine while on therapy with enoxacin (see WARNINGS).

Cyclosporine: Elevated serum levels of cyclosporine have been reported with concomitant use of cyclosporine with other members of the quinolone class.

Digoxin: Enoxacin may raise serum digoxin levels in some individuals. If signs and symptoms suggestive of digoxin toxicity occur when enoxacin and digoxin are given concomitantly, physicians are advised to obtain serum digoxin levels and adjust digoxin doses appropriately.

Nonsteroidal anti-inflammatory agents: Seizures have been reported in patients taking enoxacin concomitantly with the nonsteroidal anti-inflammatory drug fenbufen. Animal studies also suggest an increased potential for seizures when these two drugs are given concomitantly. Fenbufen is not approved in the United States at this time.

Sucralfate and antacids: Quinolones form chelates with metal cations. Therefore, administration of quinolones with antacids containing calcium, magnesium or aluminum; with sucralfate; with divalent or trivalent cations such as iron; or with multivitamins containing zinc may substantially interfere with drug absorption and result in insufficient plasma and tissue quinolone concentrations. Antacids containing aluminum hydroxide and magnesium hydroxide reduce the oral absorption of enoxacin by 75%. The oral bioavailability of enoxacin is reduced by 60% with coadministration of ranitidine. These agents should not be taken for 8 hours before or for 2 hours after enoxacin administration.

Theophylline: Enoxacin is a potent inhibitor of the cytochrome P-450 isozymes responsible for the metabolism of methylxanthine. Enoxacin interferes with the metabolism of theophylline resulting in a 42% to 74% dose-related decrease in theophylline clearance and a subsequent 260% to 350% increase in serum theophylline levels. Theophylline-related adverse effects have occurred in patients when theophylline and enoxacin were coadministered (see WARNINGS).

Warfarin: Quinolones, including enoxacin, decrease the clearance of R-warfarin, the less active isomer of racemic warfarin. Enoxacin does not affect the clearance of the active S-isomer, and changes in clotting time have not been observed when enoxacin and warfarin were coadministered. Nevertheless, the prothrombin time or other suitable coagulation test should be monitored when warfarin or its derivatives and enoxacin are given concomitantly.

ADVERSE REACTIONS:

Single-Dose Studies: During clinical trials, approximately 9% of patients treated with a single dose of 400 mg of enoxacin for uncomplicated urethral or endocervical gonorrhea reported adverse events.

The most frequently reported events in single-dose trials, without regard to drug relationship, were nausea and vomiting (2%). Events that occurred in less than 1% of patients are listed below.

Central Nervous System: headache, dizziness, somnolence;

Gastrointestinal: abdominal pain;

Gynecologic: vaginal moniliasis;

Skin/Hypersensitivity: rash;

Laboratory Abnormalities: increased AST (SGOT), decreased hemoglobin, decreased hematocrit, eosinophilia, leukocytosis, leukopenia, thrombocytosis, increased urinary protein, increased alkaline phosphatase, increased ALT (SGPT), increased bilirubin, hyperkalemia.

Multiple-Dose Studies: The incidence of adverse events reported by patients in multiple-dose clinical trials, without regard to drug relationship, was 23%. The incidence of drug-related adverse reactions in multiple-dose clinical trials was 16%. Among patients receiving multiple-dose therapy, enoxacin was discontinued because of an adverse event in 3.8% of patients.

The following events were considered likely to be drug-related in patients receiving multiple doses of enoxacin in clinical trials: nausea and/or vomiting 6%, dizziness 2%, headache 1%, abdominal pain 1%, diarrhea 1%, dyspepsia 1%.

The most frequently reported events in all multiple-dose clinical trials, without regard to drug relationship, were as follows: nausea and/or vomiting 8%, dizziness and/or vertigo 3%, headache 2%, diarrhea 2%, abdominal pain 2%, insomnia 1%, rash 1%, nervousness and/or anxiety 1%, unusual taste 1%, pruritus 1%.

Additional events that occurred in less than 1% of patients but >0.1% of patients are listed below:

Body as a Whole: Asthenia, fatigue, fever, malaise, back pain, chest pain, edema, chills;

Gastrointestinal: flatulence, constipation, dry mouth/throat, stomatitis, anorexia, gastritis, bloody stools;

Central Nervous System: somnolence, tremor, convulsions, paresthesia, confusion, agitation, depression, syncope, myoclonus, depersonalization, hypertonia;

Skin/Hypersensitivity: photosensitivity reaction, urticaria, hyperhidrosis, mycotic infection, erythema multiforme, toxic epidermal necrolysis, Stevens-Johnson syndrome;

Special Senses: tinnitus, conjunctivitis, visual disturbances including amblyopia;

Musculoskeletal: myalgia, arthralgia;

Cardiovascular: palpitations, tachycardia, vasodilation,

Respiratory: dyspnea, cough, epistaxis;

Hemic and Lymphatic: purpura;

Urogenital: vaginal moniliasis, vaginitis, urinary incontinence, renal failure.

The following adverse events occurred in less than 0.1% of patients in multiple-dose clinical trials but were considered significant: pseudomembranous colitis, hyperkinesia, amnesia, ataxia, hypotonia, psychosis, emotional lability, hallucination, schizophrenic reaction.

Laboratory Changes: The following laboratory abnormalities appeared in ≥1.0% of patients receiving multiple doses of enoxacin: elevated AST (SGOT), elevated ALT (SGPT). It is not known whether these abnormalities were caused by the drug or the underlying conditions.
Worldwide Post-Marketing Experience: The most frequent spontaneously-reported adverse events in the worldwide post-marketing experience with multiple- and single-dose enoxacin use have been rashes, seizures/convulsions, and photosensitivity reactions; however, there is no evidence that the incidences of these events were larger than those observed in the clinical trials population.
Quinolone-Class Adverse Reactions: Although not reported in completed clinical studies with enoxacin, a variety of adverse events have been reported with other quinolones.
Clinical Adverse Events Include: erythema nodosum, hepatic necrosis, possible exacerbation of myasthenia gravis, nystagmus, intestinal perforation, hyperpigmentation, interstitial nephritis, polyuria, urinary retention, renal calculi, cardiopulmonary arrest, cerebral thrombosis, and laryngeal or pulmonary edema.
Laboratory Adverse Events Include: agranulocytosis, elevation of serum triglycerides and/or serum cholesterol, prolongation of the prothrombin time, candiduria, and crystalluria.

OVERDOSAGE:

In the event of acute overdosage, the stomach should be emptied by inducing vomiting or by gastric lavage and the patient carefully observed and given supportive treatment. Enoxacin is poorly removed (<5% over 4 hours) by hemodialysis.

DOSAGE AND ADMINISTRATION:

Enoxacin should be taken at least one hour before or at least two hours after a meal. See INDICATIONS AND USAGE for information on appropriate pathogens and patient populations.

SEXUALLY TRANSMITTED DISEASES

Uncomplicated urethral or cervical gonorrhea: 400 mg single dose

URINARY TRACT INFECTIONS

Uncomplicated urinary tract infections: 200 mg every 12 hours for 7 days
Complicated urinary tract infections: 400 mg every 12 hours for 14 days
Dosage Adjustment for Renal Impairment: Dosage should be adjusted in patients with a creatinine clearance value of 30 ml/min/1.73 m² or less. After a normal initial dose, the dosing interval should be adjusted as indicated in TABLE 5.

TABLE 5

Creatinine Clearance	Dosage Adjustment	Dosage Interval
>30 ml/min/1.73 m²	None	12 hours
≤30 ml/min/1.73 m²	½ recommended dose	12 hours

When only the serum creatinine is known, the following formula may be used to estimate creatinine clearance: Men: Creatinine clearance (ml/min) = Weight (kg) x (140-age) divided by 72 x serum creatinine (mg/dl); Women: 0.85 x the value calculated for men.
The serum creatinine should represent a steady state of renal function.
Dosage adjustment is not necessary in elderly patients with normal renal function, but dose should be adjusted according to the previous guidelines in elderly patients with compromised renal function.

ANIMAL PHARMACOLOGY:

Enoxacin and other members of the quinolone class have been shown to cause arthropathy in immature animals of most species tested (see WARNINGS.)

REFERENCES:

National Committee for Clinical Laboratory Standards, Performance Standards for Antimicrobial Disk Susceptibility Tests-Fourth Edition. Approved Standard NCCLS Document M2-A4, Vol. 10, No. 7, NCCLS, Villanova, PA, 1990. 2. National Committee for Clinical Laboratory Standards, Methods for Dilution Antimicrobial Susceptibility Tests for Bacteria that Grow Aerobically-Second Edition. Approved Standard NCCLS Document M7-A2, Vol. 10, No. 8, NCCLS. Villanova, PA, 1990.

HOW SUPPLIED

200 mg tablet is light blue and marked "rPr" and "5100". The 400 mg tablet is dark blue and marked "rPR and "5140".

HOW SUPPLIED-EQUIVALENTS NOT AVAILABLE

Tablet, Uncoated - Oral - 200 mg

50's	$142.19	PENETREX, Rhone-Poulence Rorer	00075-5100-50

Tablet, Uncoated - Oral - 400 mg

50's	$142.19	PENETREX, Rhone-Poulenc Rorer	00075-5140-50

ENOXAPARIN SODIUM *(003160)*

CATEGORIES: Abdominal Surgery, Anticoagulants, Anticoagulants/Thrombolytics, Blood Clotting, Blood Formation/Coagulation, Coagulants and Anticoagulants, Coagulopathies, Colorectal Surgery, Embolism, Hip Replacement Surgery, Knee Replacement Surgery, Low Molecular Weight Heparin, Pulmonary Embolism, Thrombosis, Pregnancy Category B, FDA Class 1P ("Priority Review"), FDA Approved 1993 Mar
BRAND NAMES: Clexan; Clexane; Clexane 40; Heparin, Low Weight; Klexane (Canada); Lovenox (International names outside U.S. in italics)

DESCRIPTION:

Enoxaparin sodium is a sterile, low molecular weight heparin for injection. Prefilled syringes contain 30 mg enoxaparin sodium per 0.3 ml Water for Injection or 40 mg enoxaparin sodium per 0.4 ml Water for Injection (see DOSAGE AND ADMINISTRATION and HOW SUPPLIED).The approximate anti-Factor Xa activity per syringe is 1000 IU per every 10 mg of drug (with reference to the W.H.O. First International Low Molecular Weight Heparin Reference Standard). Nitrogen is used in the headspace to inhibit oxidation. The pH of the injection is 5.5 - 7.5. The solution is preservative-free and intended for use only as a single-dose-injection.
Enoxaparin is obtained by alkaline degradation of heparin benzyl ester derived from porcine intestinal mucosa. Its structure is characterized by a 2-O-sulfo-4-enepyranosuronic acid group at the non-reducing end and a 2-N,6-O-disulfo-D-glucosamine at the reducing end of the chain. The substance is the sodium salt. The average molecular weight is about 4500. The molecular weight distribution is: <2000 daltons ≤20%, 2000 to 8000 daltons ≥68%, >8000 daltons ≤15%

CLINICAL PHARMACOLOGY:

Enoxaparin is a low molecular weight heparin which has antithrombotic properties. In man enoxaparin is characterized by a higher ratio of anti-Factor Xa to anti-Factor IIa activity (3.35 ± 0.89) than unfractioned heparin (1.22 ± 0.13). Following the administration of a single subcutaneous dose of up to 90 mg of enoxaparin to healthy subjects, no appreciable change was observed in fibrinogen level and other parameters of fibrinolysis. At the recommended doses, single injections of enoxaparin do not significantly influence platelet aggregation or affect global clotting tests (*i.e.*, prothrombin time [PT] or activated partial thromboplastin time [APTT]).

PHARMACODYNAMICS

Maximum anti-Factor Xa and antithrombin (anti-Factor IIa) activities occur 3 to 5 hours after subcutaneous injection of enoxaparin. Mean peak anti-FactorXa activity was 0.16 IU/ml (1.58 mcg/ml) and 0.38 IU/ml (3.83 mcg/ml) afterthe 20 mg and the 40 mg clinically tested doses, respectively. Mean absolute bioavailability of enoxaparin based on anti- Factor Xa activity is 92% inhealthy volunteers. The volume of distribution of anti-Factor Xa activity is about 6 L. Following IV dosing, the total body clearance of enoxaparin is 25 ml/min. Elimination half-life based on anti-Factor Xa activity was about 4.5 hours after subcutaneous administration. Following a 40 mg dose significant anti- Factor Xa activity persists in plasma for about 12 hours. There appears to be no appreciable increase in anti-Factor Xa activity after dosing for 3 days in young healthy subjects. Clearance and C_{max} for anti- Factor Xa values following single and multiple s.c. dosing in elderly subjects and subjects with renal failure were close to those observed in normal subjects. An increase of 25% in the area under anti-Factor Xa activity versus time curve was observed following once daily dosing in healthy elderly subjects for 10 days. The kinetics of anti-Factor Xa activity in anuric patients undergoingdialysis are similar to those in historical control normal subjects following IV dosing.
The decline of anti-Factor Xa activity with time was parallel to the decay curve of plasma total radioactivity (^{99m}Tc) in healthy volunteers. Following intravenous dosing of enoxaparin labeled with the gamma-emitter, ^{99m} Tc, 40% of radioactivity and 8-20% of anti- Factor Xa activity were recovered in urine in 24 hours.

CLINICAL STUDIES:

Hip Or Knee Replacement Surgery: Enoxaparin has been shown to prevent postoperative deep vein thrombosis (DVT) following hip or knee replacement surgery.
In a double-blind study, enoxaparin 30 mg every 12 hours sc was compared to placebo. Provided that hemostasis was established, treatment was initiated within 12-24 hours post surgery and was continued for 10-14 days post-operatively (TABLE 1).

TABLE 1 Efficacy of Enoxaparin in Hip Replacement Surgery

Treatment Failures	Enoxaparin 30 mg q12h (n=50)	Placebo q12h n=50
Total DVT	5 (10%)*	23 (46%)
Proximal DVT	1 (2%)†	11 (22%)
*p value versus placebo = 0.0002; †p value versus placebo = 0.0134		

A double-blind, multicenter study compared three dosing regimens of enoxaparin in hip replacement patients. Treatment was initiated within two days post-surgery and was continued for 7-11 days post-operatively TABLE 2).

TABLE 2 Efficacy of Enoxaparin in Hip Replacement Surgery

Treatment Failures	10 mg QD (n=161)	30mg q12h (n=208)	40mg QD n=(199)
Total DVT	40 (25%)	22 (11%)*	199 (100%)†
Proximal DVT	17 (11%)	8 (4%)	9 (5%)
*p value versus enoxaparin 10 mg QD = 0.0008; †p value versus enoxaparin 10 mg QD = 0.0168			

In a double blind study with 99 patients undergoing knee replacement surgery, enoxaparin 30 mg every 12 hours sc was compared to placebo. Provided that hemostasis was established, treatment was initiated 12-24 hours post-operatively and was continued up to 15 days post-operatively. The incidence of post-operative proximal and total deep vein thrombosis was significantly lower for enoxaparin compared to placebo.

TABLE 3 Efficacy of Enoxaparin in Knee Replacement Surgery

	Treatment Group	
Treatment Failures	Enoxaparin 30 mg q12h (n=47)	Placebo q12h (n=52)
Total DVT	5 (11%)* (95% CI: 1-21%)	32 (62%) (95% CI: 47-76%)
Proximal DVT	0 (0%)† (95% Upper CL: 5%)	7 (13%) (95% CI: 3-24%)
*p value versus placebo = 0.0001; CI=Confidence Interval; †p value versus placebo = 0.013; CL=Confidence Limit		

Additionally, in an open-label, parallel group, randomized clinical study in patients undergoing elective knee replacement surgery, enoxaparin sodium injection 30 mg every 12 hours sc was compared to unfractioned heparin 500 U every 8 hours sc. Treatment was intitiated post-operatively and continued up to 14 days. The incidence of deep vein thrombosis was significantly lower for enoxaparin to heparin.
Abdominal Surgery: In a double-blind, parallel group study of 1115 patients undergoing elective cancer surgery of the gastrointestinal, urological, or gynecological tract, enoxaparin 40 mg sc administered once-daily, beginning 2 hours prior to surgery and continuing for a maximum of 12 days after surgery, was compared to heparin 5000 U every 8 hours sc in preventing deep vein thrombosis (DVT). The data are provided in TABLE 4.

TABLE 4 Efficacy of Enoxaparin in Abdominal Surgery for Cancer

Treatment Failures	Enoxaparin 40 mg QD (n=555)	Heparin 5000 U q8h (n=560)
Total VTE[1]	56 (10.1%) (95% CI[2]: 8-13%)	63 (11.3%) (95% CI: 9-14%)
DVT Only	54 (9.7%) (95% CI: 7-12%)	61 (10.9%) (95% CI: 8-13%)
[1]VTE=Venous thromboembolic events which include DVT, PE, and death considered to be thromboembolic in origin. [2]CI=Confidence Interval		

In a second double-blind, parallel group study, enoxaparin 40 mg sc once-daily was compared to heparin 5000 U every 8 hours sc in 1347 patients undergoing colorectal surgery (one third with cancer). Treatment was initiated approximately 2 hours prior to surgery and continued for approximately 7-10 days post-operatively. The data are provided in TABLE 5.

TABLE 5 Efficacy in Enoxaparin in Colorectal Surgery

Treatment Failures	Enoxaparin 40 mg QD (n=673)	Heparin 5000 U/q8h (n=674)
Total VTE[1]	48 (7.1%) (95% CI[2]: 5-9%)	45 (6.7%) (95% CI: 5-9%)
DVT Only	47 (7.0%) (95% CI: 5-9%)	44 (6.5%) (95% CI: 5-8%)
[1]VTE=Venous thromboembolic events which include DVT, PE, and death considered to be thromboembolic in origin. [2]CI=Confidence Interval		

INDICATIONS AND USUAGE:

Enoxaparin is for the prevention of deep vein thrombosis, which may lead to pulmonary embolism: (1) in patients undergoing hip or knee replacement therapy (2) in patients undergoing abdominal surgery who are at risk for thromboembolic complications (patients at risk included patients who are over 40 years of age, obese, undergoing surgery under general anesthesis lasting longer than 30 minutes or who have abdominal risk factors such as malignancy or a history of deep venous thrombosis or pulmonary embolism).

CONTRAINDICATIONS:

Enoxaparin is contraindicated in patients with active major bleeding, in patients with thrombocytopenia associated with a positive *in vitro* test for anti-platelet antibody in the presence of enoxaparin,or in patients with hypersensitivity to enoxaparin.
Patients with known hypersensitivity to heparin or pork products should not be treated with enoxaparin.

WARNINGS:

Enoxaparin cannot be used interchangeably (unit for unit) with unfractioned heparin or other low molecular weight heparins as they differ in their manufacturing process, molecular weight distribution, anti-Xa and anti-IIe activities, units and dosage. Special attention and compliance with the instructions for use specific to each proprietary medical product is therefore required.

Enoxaparin should be used with extreme caution in patients with history of heparin-induced thrombocytopenia.

Hemorrhage: Enoxaparin, like other anticoagulants, should be used with extreme caution in conditions with increased risk of hemorrhage, such as bacterial endocarditis, congenital or acquired bleeding disorders, active ulceration and angiodysplastic gastrointestinal disease, hemorrhagic stroke or shortly after brain, spinal or ophthalmological surgery, or in patients treated concomitantly with platelet inhibitors. Bleeding can occur at any site during therapy with enoxaparin. An unexplained fall in hematocrit or blood pressure should lead to a search for a bleeding site.

Neuraxial Anesthesia and Post-operative Indwelling Edipural Catheter Use: *Spinal/Epidural Anesthesia*: As with other anticoagulants, there have been rare cases of neuraxial/epidural hemotomas reported with the current use of enoxaparin and spinal/epidural anesthesia resulting in long-term or permanent paralysis. The risk of these rare events may be higher with use of post-operative indwelling epidural catheters.

Thrombocytopenia: Thrombocytopenia can occur with the administration of enoxaparin. Moderate thrombocytopenia (platelet counts between 100,000/mm³ and 50,000mm³) occurred at a rate of 1.8% in patients given enoxaparin, 1.7% in patients given heparin, and 1.7% in patients given placebo following surgery in clinical trials.

Platelet counts less than 50,000/mm³ occurred at a rate of 0.1% in patients given enoxaparin, 0.4% in patients given heparin, and 0% in patients given placebo in the same trials.

Thrombocytopenia of any degree should be monitored closely. If the platelet count falls below 100,000/mm³, enoxaparin should be discontinued. Rare cases of thrombocytopenia with thrombosis have also been observed in clinical practice. The rate of incidence of this complication is unknown at present.

PRECAUTIONS:

GENERAL

Enoxaparin should not be mixed with other injection or infusions. Enoxaparin should be used with care in patients with a bleeding diathesis, uncontrolled arterial hypertension or a history of recent gastrointestinal ulceration and hemorrhage. Elderly patients and patients with renal insufficiency may show delayed elimination of enoxaparin. Enoxaparin should be used with care in these patients. If thromboembolic events occur despite enoxaparin prophylaxis, enoxaparin should be discontinued and appropriate therapy initiated.

LABORATORY TESTS

Periodic complete blood counts, including platelet count, and stool occult blood test are recommended during the course of treatment with enoxaparin.

Elevations of Serum Transaminases: Asymptomatic increases in asparate AST [SGOT] and alanine ALT [SGPT] aminotranferase levels greater than three times the upper limit of normal of the laboratory reference range have been reported in up to 3.9% and 5% of patients respectively, during treatment with enoxaparin. Similar significant increases in transaminase levels have also been observed in patients and normal volunteers treated with heparin and other low molecular weight heparin. Such elevations are fully reversible and are rarely associated with increases in bilirubin. Since aminotransaminase determinations are important in the differential diagnosis of myocardial infarction, liver disease, and pulmonary emboli, elevations that might be caused by drugs like enoxaparin should be interpreted with caution.

CARCINOGENESIS, MUTAGENESIS AND IMPAIRMENT OF FERTILITY

No long- term studies in animals have been performed to evaluate carcinogenic potential of enoxaparin. Enoxaparin was not mutagenic in *in vitro* tests, including the Ames test, mouse lymphoma cell forward mutation test, and human lymphocyte chromosomal aberration test and the *in vitro* rat bone marrow chromosomal aberration test. Enoxaparin was found to have no effect on fertility or reproductive performance of male and female rats at subcutaneous doses up to 20 mg/kg/day or 141 mg/m²/day. The maximum received human dose in clinical trials was 1.5 mg/kg/day or 48.4 mg/m²/day.

PREGNANCY CATEGORY B

Teratogenic Effects: Teratology studies have been conducted in rats and rabbits at subcutaneous doses of enoxaparin up to 30 mg/kg/day or 211 mg/m²/day and 410 mg/m²/day, respectively. The maximum received human dose in clinical trials was 1.5 mg/kg/day or 48.4 mg/m²/day. There was no evidence of teratogenic effects or fetotoxicity due to enoxaparin. There are, however, no adequate and well-controlled studies in pregnant women. Because animal reproduction studies are not always predictive of human response, this drug should be used during pregnancy only if clearly needed.

Non-teratogenic Effects: See WARNINGS.

NURSING MOTHERS

It is not known whether this drug is excreted in human milk. Because many drugs are excreted in human milk, caution should be exercised when enoxaparin is administered to nursing women.

PEDIATRIC USE

Safety and effectiveness of enoxaparin in pediatric patients has not been established.

DRUG INTERACTIONS:

Enoxaparin should be used with care in patients receiving oral anticoagulants, and/or platelet inhibitors.

ADVERSE REACTIONS:

Hemorrhage: The incidence of hemorrhagic complications during enoxaparin treatment has been low. The following rates of major bleeding events have been reported during clinical trials.

TABLE 6 Major Bleeding Episodes in Hip or Knee Replacement Surgery

	Enoxaparin 30 mg q12h	Heparin 15,000 U/24h	Placebo
Hip Replacement Surgery	n=786 31 (4%)	n=541 32 (6%)	n=50 2 (4%)
Knee Replacement Surgery	n=294 3 (1%)	n=225 3 (1%)	n=65 2 (3%)

*Bleeding complications were considered major: (1) if the hemorrhage caused a significant clinical event, or (2) if accompanied by a hemoglobin decrease ≥2 g/dl or transfusion of 2 or more units of blood products. Retroperitoneal and intracranial hemorrhages were always considered major.

TABLE 7 Major Bleeding Episodes in Abdominal and Colorectal Surgery

	Enoxaparin 400 mg QD	Heparin 5000 U q8h
Abdominal Surgery	n=555 23 (4%)	n=541 16 (3%)
Colorectal Surgery	n=673 28 (4%)	n=674 21 (3%)

*Bleeding complications were considered major: (1) if the hemorrhage caused a significant clinical event, or (2) if accompanied by a hemoglobin decrease ≥2 g/dl or transfusion of 2 or more units of blood products. Retroperitoneal and intracranial hemorrhages were always considered major.

Thrombocytopenia: See WARNINGS.

Local Reactions: Mild local irritation, pain, hematoma, ecchymosis and erythema may follow subcutaneous injection of enoxaparin.

Enoxaparin is not intended for intramuscular administration.

Other: Other adverse effects that were thought to be possibly or probably related to treatment with enoxaparin, heparin or placebo in clinical trials, and that occurred at a rate of at least 2% in the enoxaparin group, are shown in TABLE 8 and TABLE 9.

TABLE 8 Adverse Events Occurring at ≥ 2% Incidence in Enoxaparin Treated Patients Undergoing Hip or Knee Replacement Surgery (Excluding Unrelated Adverse Events)

	Enoxaparin 30 mg q12h (n=1080)		Heparin 15,000 U/24h (n=766)		Placebo (n=115)	
Adverse Event	Severe	Total	Severe	Total	Severe	Total
Fever	<1%	5%	<1%	4%	0%	3%
Hemorrhage	<1%	4%	1%	4%	0%	3%
Nausea	<1%	3%	<1%	2%	0%	2%
Hypochromic anemia	<1%	2%	2%	5%	<1%	7%
Edema	<1%	2%	<1%	2%	0%	2%
Peripheral edema	<1%	3%	<1%	4%	0%	3%

TABLE 9 Adverse Events Occurring at ≥2% Incidence in Enoxaparin Treated Patients Undergoing Abdominal or Colorectal Surgery (Excluding Unrelated Adverse Events)

Adverse	Enoxaparin 40 mg qd (n=1228)		Heparin 5000 U q8h (n=1234)	
Event	Severe	Total	Severe	Total
Hemorrhage	<1%	7%	<1%	6%
Anemia	<1%	3%	<1%	3%
Ecchymosis	0%	3%	0%	3%

Ongoing Safety Surveillance: There have been rare reports of neuraxial hematoma formation with concurrent use of enoxaparin and spinal/epidural anesthesia, and post-operative indwelling catheters. These events resulted in varying degrees of neurologic injuries including long-term or permanent paralysis.

Other reports include: skin necrosis at the injection site, inflammatory nodules at the injection site, purpura, systemic allergic reactions, and thrombocythemia.

OVERDOSAGE:

Symptoms/Treatment: Accidental overdosage following administration of enoxaparin may lead to hemorrhagic complications. This may be largely neutralized by the slow intravenous injection of protamine sulfate (1% solution). The dose of protamine sulfate should be equal to the dose of enoxaparin injected: 1 mg protamine sulfate should be administered to neutralize 1 mg enoxaparin. A second infusion of 0.5 mg/mg protamine sulfate may be administered if the APTT measured 2 to 4 hours after the first infusion remains prolonged. However, even with higher doses of protamine, the APTT may remain more prolonged than under normal conditions found following administration of conventional heparin. In all cases, the anti-Factor Xa activity is never completely neutralized (maximum about 60%). Particular care should be taken to avoid overdosage with protamine sulfate. Administration of protamine sulfate can cause severe hypotensive and anaphylactoid reactions. Because fatal reactions, often resembling anaphylaxis, have been reported with protamine sulfate, it should be given only when resuscitation techniques and treatment of anaphylactic shock are readily available. For additional information consult the Protamine Sulfate monograph. A single subcutaneous dose of 46.4 mg/kg enoxaparin was lethal to rats. The symptoms of acute toxicity were ataxia, decreased motility, dyspnea, cyanosis,and coma.

DOSAGE AND ADMINISTRATION:

All patients should be screened prior to prophylactic administration of enoxaparin to rule out a bleedingdisorder. There is usually no need for daily monitoring of coagulation parameters in patients with normal presurgical values.

ADULT DOSAGE

Hip or Knee Replacement Surgery: In patients undergoing hip replacement, the recommended dose of enoxaparin is **30 mg twice daily** administered by subcutaneous injection. Provided that hemostasis has been established, the initial dose should be given 12-24 hours post-operatively. Up to 14 days administration has been well tolerated in controlled clinical trials. The average duration of administration is 7 to 10 days.

Abdominal Surgery: In patients undergoing abdominal surgery who are at risk for thromboembolic complications, the recommended dose of enoxaparin is **40 mg once daily** administered by subcutaneous injection with the initial dose given 2 hours prior to surgery. The usual duration of administration is 7 to 10 days; up to 12 days administration has been well tolerated in clinical trials.

Administration: Enoxaparin injection is a clear colorless to pale-yellow sterile solution and was with other parenteral drug products should be inspected visually for particulate matter and discoloration prior to administration.

Enoxaparin is administered by subcutaneous injection. It must **not** be administered by intramuscular injection.

Subcutaneous Injection Technique: Patients should be lying down and enoxaparin administered by deep subcutaneous injection. To avoid the loss of drug when using prefilled syringes, do not expel the air bubble from the syringe before injection. Administration should be alternated between the left and right anterolateral and left and right posterolateral abdominal wall. The whole length of the needle should be introduced into a skin fold held between the thumb and forefinger; the skin fold should be held throughout the injection. To minimize bruising, do not rub the injection site after completion of the injection.

HOW SUPPLIED:

Lovenox Injection is available in packs of 10 prefilled syringes. Each Lovenox prefilled syringe is affixed with a 27 gauge x 1/2 inch needle the label color for the 30 mg/0.3 ml strength is blue (hip or knee replacement). The label color for the 40 mg/0.4 ml strength is yellow (abdominal surgery).

Lovenox Injection should be stored at or below 25°C. Do not freeze.

HOW SUPPLIED- EQUIVALENTS NOT AVAILABLE:

Injection, Solution – Subcutaneous – 30 mg/0.3 ml

0.3 ml x 10 $155.34 LOVENOX, Rhone-Poulenc Rorer 00075-0624-30

ENZYMES; HYOSCYAMINE SULFATE; PHENYLTOLOXAMINE *(001145)*

CATEGORIES: Abdominal Distress; Antispasmodics & Anticholinergics; Diarrhea; Digestants; Enzymes & Digestants; Flatulence; Gastrointestinal Drugs; Pregnancy Category C; FDA Pre 1938 Drugs

BRAND NAMES: Amylase, Cellulase, Lipase, **Kutrase**, Protease

FORMULARIES: BC-BS; Omnicare; PruCare

DESCRIPTION:

Kutrase Capsules contain four standardized digestive enzymes: lipase,amylase, protease, cellulase, and hyoscyamine sulfate USP and phenyltoloxamine citrate. Lipase, amylase, protease and cellulase are derived from fungal, plant and animal sources and are oral digestive enzyme supplements. Hyoscyamine sulfate USP is one of the principal anticholinergic/antispasmodic components of belladonna alkaloids. Phenyltoloxamine citrate is a non-barbiturate sedative. Each capsule contains: lipase - 1,200 USP Units; amylase - 30 mg; protease – 6 mg; cellulase – 2 mg.

DESCRIPTION: *(cont'd)*

hyoscyamine sulfate USP - 0.0625 mg

phenyltoloxamine citrate - 15 mg

Each capsule also contains as inactive ingredients: D&C yellow #10, ethylcellulose, FD&C green #3, FD&C yellow #6, gelatin, lactose, magnesium stearate, titanium dioxide, vanillin, and other ingredients.

CLINICAL PHARMACOLOGY:

Diminution of secretions from exocrine glands is often a result of the normal aging process. Kutrase provides a balanced combination of natural proteolytic, amylolytic, cellulolytic and lipolytic enzymes to enhance digestion of proteins, starch and fat in the gastrointestinal tract. These enzymes do not exert any systemic pharmacologic effects. Kutrase should be considered an enzyme supplement and not an enzyme replacement therapy. Enzymes in Kutrase are basically derived from fungal and plant sources and possess a broad spectrum of pH activity. Enzymes are promptly released from the capsule and are bioavailable for digestion of food in the stomach and intestines. Hyoscyamine sulfate provides a potent spasmolytic effect in reducing gastrointestinal hypermotility and intestinal spasm. A mild sedative effect is provided by phenyltoloxamine citrate.

INDICATIONS AND USAGE:

Kutrase is indicated for the relief of the symptoms of functional indigestion devoid of organic pathology commonly referred to as nervous indigestion and colloquially as "butterflies". The symptoms are bloating, gas, and fullness.

CONTRAINDICATIONS:

Glaucoma, obstructive uropathy, obstructive disease of the gastrointestinal tract (as in achalasia, pyloroduodenal stenosis), paralytic ileus, intestinal atony of the elderly or debilitated patients; unstable cardiovascular status in acute hemorrhage; serve ulcerative colitis; toxic megacolon complicating ulcerative colitis; myasthenia gravis, or a hypersensitivity to any of the ingredients.

WARNINGS:

Do not administer to patients who are allergic to pork products. In the presence of high environmental temperature, heat prostration can occur with drug use (fever and heat stroke due to decreased sweating). Diarrhea may be an early symptom of incomplete intestinal obstruction, especially in patients with ileostomy or colostomy. In this instance, treatment with this drug would be inappropriate. Kutrase may produce drowsiness or blurred vision. In this event, the patient should be warned not to engage in activities requiring mental alertness such as operating a motor vehicle or other machinery or to perform hazardous work while taking this drug.

PRECAUTIONS:

General: Use with caution in patients with autonomic neuropathy, hyperthyroidism, coronary heart disease, congestive heart failure, cardiac arrhythmias, and hypertension. Investigate any tachycardia before giving any anticholinergic drug since they may increase the heart rate. Use with caution in patients with hiatal hernia associated with reflux esophagitis.

Information for Patients: If capsules are opened, avoid inhalation of the powder. Sensitive individuals may experience allergic reactions.

Carcinogenesis, Mutagenesis, Impairment of Fertility: Long-term studies in animals have not been performed to evaluate the carcinogenic, mutagenic or impairment of fertility potential of Kutrase.

Pregnancy-Pregnancy Category C: Animal reproduction studies have not been conducted with Kutrase. It is also not known whether Kutrase can cause fetal harm when administered to a pregnant woman or can affect reproduction capacity. Kutrase should be given to a pregnant woman only if clearly needed.

Nursing Mothers: Hyoscyamine sulfate is excreted in human milk. It is not known whether the enzymes or phenyltoloxamine citrate are excreted in human milk. Caution should be exercised when Kutrase is administered to a nursing woman.

ADVERSE REACTIONS:

Occasionally a slight looseness of the stools may be noticed. If so, dosage should be reduced. Finely powered pancreatic enzyme may be irritating to the mucous membranes and respiratory tract. Inhalation of the airborne powder may precipitate an asthma attack in sensitive individuals. Other adverse reactions may include dryness of the mouth; urinary hesitancy and retention; blurred vision; tachycardia; palpitations; mydriasis; cycloplegia; increased ocular tension; headache; nervousness; drowsiness; weakness; suppression of lactation, allergic reactions or drug idiosyncrasies, urticaria and other dermal manifestations and decreased sweating.

OVERDOSAGE:

The signs and symptoms of overdose are headache, nausea, vomiting, blurred vision, dilated pupils, hot dry skin, dizziness, dryness of the mouth, difficulty in swallowing.

Measures to be taken are immediate lavage of the stomach and injection of physostigmine 0.5 to 2 mg intravenously and repeated as necessary up to a total of 5 mg. Fever may be treated symptomatically. Excitement to a degree which demands attention may be managed with sodium thiopental 2% solution given slowly intravenously. In the event of paralysis of the respiratory muscles, artificial respiration should be instituted.

DOSAGE AND ADMINISTRATION:

1 or 2 capsules taken with each meal or snack. Dosage may be adjusted according to the conditions and severity of symptoms to assure symptomatic control with a minimum of adverse effects.

Store at controlled room temperature 15-30°C (59-86°F). Protect from high humidity.

(Schwarz Pharma, PC0203E, 2/94)

HOW SUPPLIED - EQUIVALENTS NOT AVAILABLE:

Capsule, Gelatin - Oral - 30 mg/2 mg/0.06

100's	$45.45	KUTRASE, Schwarz Pharma (US)	00091-3475-01

ENZYMES; PHENOBARBITAL; SODIUM BICARBONATE *(001147)*

CATEGORIES: Antacids and Adsorbents; Gastrointestinal Drugs; DEA Class CIV; FDA Pre 1938 Drugs

BRAND NAMES: Truxaphen

Prescribing information not available at time of publication.

HOW SUPPLIED - EQUIVALENTS NOT AVAILABLE:

Tablet, Coated - Oral - 8.1 mg/8.1 mg/1

1000's	$22.00	TRUXAPHEN, C O Truxton	00463-6239-10

EPHEDRINE *(001149)*

CATEGORIES: Antiasthmatics/Bronchodilators; Autonomic Drugs; Hypotension/Shock; Nasal Congestion; Renal Drugs; Respiratory & Allergy Medications; Sympathomimetic Agents; Sympathomimetics, Beta Agonist; Urinary Incontinence*; FDA Pre 1938 Drugs

* Indication not approved by the FDA

BRAND NAMES: Ephedrine Sulfate

FORMULARIES: Aetna; Medi-Cal

Prescribing information not available at time of publication.

HOW SUPPLIED - RATED THERAPEUTICALLY EQUIVALENT:

Injection, Solution - Intramuscular; - 50 mg/ml

1 ml x 25	$31.56	Ephedrine Sulfate, UDL	51079-0705-45

HOW SUPPLIED - NOT RATED EQUIVALENT:

Capsule, Gelatin - Oral - 24.3 mg

100's	$4.50	Ephedrine Sulfate, Major Pharms	00904-2074-60
100's	$6.40	Ephedrine Sulfate, United Res	00677-0066-01
1000's	$19.50	Ephedrine Sulfate, C O Truxton	00463-2010-10
1000's	$21.59	Ephedrin Sulfate, HL Moore Drug Exch	00839-5042-16
1000's	$23.70	Ephedrine Sulfate, United Res	00677-0066-10

Injection, Solution - Intramuscular; - 5 mg/ml

10 ml x 10	$121.25	Ephedrine Sulfate, Fujisawa USA	00469-9090-87

Injection, Solution - Intramuscular; - 25 mg/ml

1 ml x 6	$10.15	Ephedrine Sulfate, Lilly	00002-1631-16

Injection, Solution - Intramuscular; - 50 mg/ml

ml x 25	$24.00	Ephedrine Sulfate, Bedford Labs	55390-0875-01
1 ml	$1.53	Ephedrine Sulfate, Abbott	00074-3073-03
1 ml	$99.00	Ephedrine Sulfate Inj. 50Mg/Ml, Jordan Pharms	58196-0010-11
1 ml x 6	$11.17	Ephedrine Sulfate, Lilly	00002-1603-16
1 ml x 25	$26.25	Ephedrine, Jordan Pharms	58196-0020-39

Powder

30 gm	$14.29	Ephedrine Sulfate, Mallinckrodt	00406-4967-34

EPHEDRINE HYDROCHLORIDE; PHENOBARBITAL; THEOPHYLLINE ANHYDROUS *(001151)*

CATEGORIES: Airway Obstruction; Allergies; Antiasthmatics/Bronchodilators; Asthma; Bronchial Dilators; Bronchitis; DESI Drugs; Respiratory & Allergy Medications; Respiratory Muscle Relaxant; Smooth Muscle Relaxants; Sympathomimetic Agents; Xanthine Derivatives; FDA Pre 1938 Drugs

BRAND NAMES: Azma-Aid; *Sedral*; *Tedral*; *Tedral AS*; **Tedral Sa**; *Tedral SA*; *Tedralan* (France); Theocord; Theodrine; Theofed; Theofedral; Theophed; Theotal
(International brand names outside U.S. in italics)

DESCRIPTION:

(Note: To avoid confusion, the brand name of this drug has been left in the monograph).

Tedral Suspension: Each 5 ml teaspoonful of suspension contains 65 mg theophylline (59.1 mg anhydrous), 12 mg ephedrine hydrochloride, and 4 mg phenobarbital. (**Warning** - May be habit forming.) Also contains: benzoic acid, USP; D&C Yellow No. 10; FD&C Yellow No. 6; flavors; saccharin sodium, NF; sugar, invert; tragacanth, USP; water, potable.

Tedral Elixir: Each 5 ml teaspoonful contains 32.5 mg theophylline (29.5 mg anhydrous), 6 mg ephedrine hydrochloride, and 2 mg phenobarbital. (**Warning** - May be habit forming.) The alcohol content is 15%. Also contains: D&C Green No. 5 and Red No. 33; FD&C Red No. 40; flavors; propylene glycol, USP; saccharin sodium, NF; sorbitol solution, USP; water, purified, USP.

CLINICAL PHARMACOLOGY:

Tedral combines theophylline and ephedrine - widely accepted oral bronchodilators, with differing modes of action - with the sedative phenobarbital.

From experimental evidence,[1] it appears that a combination of a sympathomimetic and methylxanthine is more effective than either drug alone in inhibiting the release of bronchoconstricting mediators (histamine and slow-reacting substance of anaphylaxis) produced by antigen-antibody (IgE) interaction on sensitive cells. The β-adrenergic stimulation by the sympathomimetics produces cyclic 3'5'-adenosine monophosphate (cAMP), and the degradation of cAMP by the specific enzyme, phosphodiesterase, is inhibited by methylxanthines. Thus, at present, the principal action of the Tedral formulations in the relief or prevention of bronchoconstriction appears to be involved with the cAMP system.

Phenobarbital is incorporated to counteract possible stimulation by ephedrine and to provide a mild, long-acting sedative for the apprehensive asthmatic patient.

Tedral Suspension and Tedral Elixir are convenient formulations for children and other persons who may have difficulty in swallowing tablets.

INDICATIONS AND USAGE:

Tedral Suspension and Tedral Elixir are indicated for the symptomatic relief of bronchial asthma, asthmatic bronchitis, and other bronchospastic disorders. They may also be used prophylactically to abort or minimize asthmatic attacks and are of value in managing occasional, seasonal or perennial asthma.

Tedral Suspension and Tedral Elixir are convenient for persons who may have difficulty in swallowing tablets.

These Tedral formulations are adjuncts in the total management of the asthmatic patient. Acute or severe asthmatic attacks may necessitate supplemental therapy with other drugs by inhalation or other parenteral routes.

CONTRAINDICATIONS:

Sensitivity to any of the ingredients; porphyria.

WARNINGS:

Drowsiness may occur. Phenobarbital may be habit forming.

PRECAUTIONS:

Use with caution in the presence of cardiovascular disease, severe hypertension, hyperthyroidism, prostatic hypertrophy, or glaucoma.

INFORMATION FOR THE PATIENT:

As with any drug, if you are pregnant or nursing a baby, seek the advice of a health professional before using this product.

Keep this and all drugs out of the reach of children. In case of accidental overdose, seek professional assistance or contact a poison control center immediately.

ADVERSE REACTIONS:

Mild epigastric distress, palpitation, tremulousness, insomnia, difficulty of micturition, and CNS stimulation have been reported.

DOSAGE AND ADMINISTRATION:

TEDRAL TABLETS

Adults-one tablet on arising and one tablet 12 hours later. Tablets should not be chewed.

TEDRAL SUSPENSION

SHAKE BOTTLE WELL.

Adults-two to four teaspoonfuls every 4 hours.

Children-one teaspoonful per 60 lb body weight, every 4-6 hours.

Should be given to children under 2 years of age only with extreme caution.

TEDRAL ELIXIR

Children-one teaspoonful per 30 lb body weight, every 4-6 hours.

Should be given to children under 2 years of age only with extreme caution.

Adults-one to two tablespoonfuls every 4 hours.

Store between 15-30°C (59-86°F).

REFERENCES:

1.Koopman WJ, Orange RP, Austen KF: *J Immunol* 105:1096, November 1970.

HOW SUPPLIED - RATED THERAPEUTICALLY EQUIVALENT:

Tablet, Soluble - Oral - 40 mg/25 mg/180

1000's	$100.50	TEP, Harber Pharm	51432-0450-06

HOW SUPPLIED - NOT RATED EQUIVALENT:

Tablet, Soluble - Oral - 40 mg/25 mg/180

100's	$14.20	THEOTAL, Major Pharms	00904-0774-60
100's	$14.30	Theophenyllin, HL Moore Drug Exch	00839-5111-06
100's	**$70.42**	**TEDRAL SA, Parke-Davis**	**00071-0231-24**
1000's	$120.45	THEOTAL, Major Pharms	00904-0774-80
1000's	$120.49	Theophenyllin, HL Moore Drug Exch	00839-5111-16

EPHEDRINE HYDROCHLORIDE; POTASSIUM IODIDE; PHENOBARBITAL; THEOPHYLLINE

(001160)

CATEGORIES: Airway Obstruction; Antiasthmatics/Bronchodilators; Asthma; Bronchial Dilators; Bronchitis; Bronchospasm; DESI Drugs; Decongestants; Iodide Salts; Mucolytic Agents; Pulmonary Emphysema; Respiratory & Allergy Medications; Respiratory Muscle Relaxant; Smooth Muscle Relaxants; Sympathomimetic Agents; Xanthine Derivatives; Pregnancy Category X; FDA Pre 1938 Drugs

BRAND NAMES: **Quadrinal**

Prescribing information not available at time of publication.

HOW SUPPLIED - EQUIVALENTS NOT AVAILABLE:

Tablet, Uncoated - Oral - 24 mg/24 mg/320

100's	**$39.90**	**QUADRINAL, Knoll Labs**	**00044-4520-02**

EPHEDRINE SULFATE; HYDROXYZINE HYDROCHLORIDE; THEOPHYLLINE *(001152)*

CATEGORIES: Antiasthmatics/Bronchodilators; Bronchial Dilators; Bronchospasm; Common Cold; DESI Drugs; Respiratory & Allergy Medications; Respiratory Muscle Relaxant; Smooth Muscle Relaxants; Sympathomimetic Agents; Xanthine Derivatives; FDA Pre 1938 Drugs

BRAND NAMES: Ami Rax; Hydrophed; Hydroxphed; Hydroxy Compound; Hydroxyephed; Lyrizine; **Marax**; *Marex*; Martabs; Moxy Compound; T.E.H.; Theomax Df; Theozine; Therax

(International brand names outside U.S. in italics)

DESCRIPTION:

(Note: This monograph pertains to the tablet as well as the syrup forms).

Each Tablet Contains:

Ephedrine Sulfate 25 mg

Theophylline 130 mg

Hydroxyzine HCl 10 mg

Inert ingredients are: alginic acid; magnesium stearate; precipitated calcium carbonate; sodium lauryl sulfate.

Each Teaspoon of syrup (5 ml) contains:

Ephedrine Sulfate 6.25 mg

Theophylline 32.50 mg

Hydroxyzine HCl 2.5 mg

Alcohol (Ethyl Alcohol) 5% v/v

Inert ingredients are: alcohol; cherry flavor, hydrochloric acid, sodium benzoate; special flavor compound; sucrose; water.

CLINICAL PHARMACOLOGY:

The action of ephedrine as a vasoconstrictor is well known. It is therefore of significant benefit in symptomatic relief of the congestion occurring in bronchial asthma. As a bronchodilator, it has a slower onset but longer duration of action than does epinephrine, which, in contrast to ephedrine, is not effective upon oral administration.

The diverse actions of theophylline-bronchospasmolytic, cardiovascular, and diuretic -are well established, and make it a particularly useful drug in the treatment of bronchial asthma, both in the acute attack and in the prophylactic therapy of the disease.

Atarax (hydroxyzine HCl) modifies the central stimulatory action of ephedrine preventing excessive excitation in patients on Ephedrine sulfate, theophylline, hydroxyzine HCl therapy.

In animal studies Atarax has demonstrated antiserotonin activity and antispasmodic potency of a nonspecific nature.

Additional information for the syrup: The syrup produces an expectorant action wherein the tenacity of sputum is decreased and the ease of expectoration is increased.

INDICATIONS AND USAGE:

Based on a review of this drug by the National Academy of Sciences-National Research Council and/or other information, FDA has classified the indications as follows: "Possibly" Effective: For controlling bronchospastic disorders. Final classification of the less than effective indication requires further investigation.

CONTRAINDICATIONS:

Because of the ephedrine, Ephedrine sulfate, theophylline, hydroxyzine HCl is contraindicated in cardiovascular disease, hyperthyroidism, and hypertension. This drug is contraindicated in individuals who have shown hypersensitivity to the drug or its components.

Hydroxyzine, when administered to the pregnant mouse, rat, and rabbit induced fetal abnormalities in the rat at doses substantially above the human therapeutic range. Clinical data in human beings are inadequate to establish safety in early pregnancy. Until such data are available, hydroxyzine is contraindicated in early pregnancy.

PRECAUTIONS:

Because of the ephedrine component this drug should be used with caution in elderly males or those with known prostatic hypertrophy.

The potentiating action of hydroxyzine, although mild, must be taken into consideration when the drug is used in conjunction with central nervous system depressants; and when other central nervous system depressants are administered concomitantly with hydroxyzine their dosage should be reduced. Patients should be cautioned that hydroxyzine can increase the effect of alcohol.

Patients should be warned-because of the hydroxyzine component-of the possibility of drowsiness occurring and cautioned against driving a car or operating dangerous machinery while taking this drug.

ADVERSE REACTIONS:

With large doses of ephedrine, excitation, tremulousness, insomnia, nervousness, palpitation, tachycardia, precordial pain, cardiac arrhythmias, vertigo, dryness of the nose and throat, headache, sweating, and warmth may occur. Because ephedrine is a sympathomimetic agent some patients may develop vesical sphincter spasm and resultant urinary hesitation, and occasionally acute urinary retention. This should be borne in mind when administering preparations containing ephedrine to elderly males or those with known prostatic hypertrophy. At the recommended dose for Ephedrine sulfate, theophylline, hydroxyzine HCl, a side effect occasionally reported is palpitation, and this can be controlled with dosage adjustment, additional amounts of concurrently administered Atarax (hydroxyzine HCl), or discontinuation of the medication. When ephedrine is given three or more times daily patients may develop tolerance after several weeks of therapy.

Theophylline when given on an empty stomach frequently causes gastric irritation accompanied by upper abdominal discomfort, nausea, and vomiting. Administration of the medication after meals will serve to minimize this side effect. Theophylline may cause diuresis and cardiac stimulation. The amount of Atarax present in Ephedrine sulfate, theophylline, hydroxyzine HCl has not resulted in disturbing side effects. When used alone specifically as a tranquilizer in the normal dosage range (25 to 50 mg three or four times a day), side effects are infrequent; even at these higher doses, no serious side effects have been reported and confirmed to date. Those which do occasionally occur when Atarax is used alone are drowsiness, xerostomia and, at extremely high doses, involuntary motor activity, unsteadiness of gait, neuromuscular weakness, all of which may be controlled by reduction of the dosage or discontinuation of the medication.

With the relatively low dose of Atarax in Ephedrine sulfate, theophylline, hydroxyzine HCl, these effects are not likely to occur. In addition, the ataractic action of Atarax may modify the cardiac stimulatory action of ephedrine, and concurrently, increasing the amount of Atarax may control or abolish this undesirable effect of ephedrine.

DOSAGE AND ADMINISTRATION:

The dosage of Ephedrine sulfate, theophylline, hydroxyzine HCl should be adjusted according to the severity of complaints, and the patient's individual toleration.

TABLETS: In general, an adult dose of 1 tablet, 2 to 4 times daily, should be sufficient. Some patients are controlled adequately with 1/2 to 1 tablet at bedtime. The time interval between doses should not be shorter than four hours.

The dosage for children over 5 years of age and for adults who are sensitive to ephedrine, is one-half the usual adult dose. Clinical experience to date has been confined to ages above 5 years.

Syrup: Dosage for children 2 to 5 years of age is 1/2 to 1 teaspoon (2.5-5 ml), 3 to 4 times daily. Not recommended for children under 2 years of age.

HOW SUPPLIED - RATED THERAPEUTICALLY EQUIVALENT:

Tablet, Uncoated - Oral - 25 mg/10 mg/130

1000's	$14.47	Hydroxyzine Compound, Harber Pharm	51432-0222-06

HOW SUPPLIED - NOT RATED EQUIVALENT:

Syrup - Oral - 6.25 mg/2.5 mg/

480 ml	$8.09	HYDROPHED D.F., Rugby	00536-0970-85
480 ml	$10.50	Hydroxyzine Compound, Consolidated Midland	00223-6526-01
480 ml	$10.50	MOXY COMPOUND D.F., Major Pharms	00904-0720-16
480 ml	$11.55	THEOMAX DF SYRUP, Alpharma	00472-1552-16
480 ml	**$33.34**	**MARAX-DF, Roerig**	**00049-2550-93**
3840 ml	$33.75	HYDROPHED, Rugby	00536-0970-90
3840 ml	$52.45	MOXY COMPOUND D.F., Major Pharms	00904-0720-28
3840 ml	$59.48	Hydroxyzine Compound, Consolidated Midland	00223-6526-02

Tablet, Uncoated - Oral - 25 mg/10 mg/130

100's	$8.95	T.E.H., Geneva Pharms	00781-1988-01

HOW SUPPLIED - NOT RATED EQUIVALENT: *(cont'd)*

100's	$20.00	HYDROXYZINE COMPOUND, Consolidated Midland	00223-1074-01
100's	$30.23	HYDROPHED, Rugby	00536-3906-01
100's	$31.20	Hydroxyzine Compound, Goldline Labs	00182-1344-01
100's	$31.93	Hydroxyzine Compound, HL Moore Drug Exch	00839-6216-06
100's	$32.65	MOXY COMPOUND, Major Pharms	00904-0623-60
100's	$32.81	Hydroxy Compound, Qualitest Pharms	00603-3948-21
100's	**$34.47**	**MARAX, Roerig**	**00049-2540-66**
500's	$41.95	T.E.H., Geneva Pharms	00781-1988-05
500's	$132.35	Hydroxyzine Compound, Goldline Labs	00182-1344-05
500's	**$183.45**	**MARAX, Roerig**	**00049-2540-73**
1000's	$24.90	MOXY COMPOUND, Major Pharms	00904-0623-80
1000's	$26.19	HYDROPHED, Rugby	00536-3906-10
1000's	$102.00	Hydroxyzine Compound, Consolidated Midland	00223-1074-02
1000's	$269.87	Hydroxyzine Compound, HL Moore Drug Exch	00839-6216-16

EPHEDRINE; GUAIFENESIN *(001155)*

CATEGORIES: Antitussives/Expectorants/Mucolytics; Autonomic Drugs; Cough Preparations; Expectorants; Respiratory & Allergy Medications; Sympathomimetic Agents; FDA Pre 1938 Drugs

BRAND NAMES: **Broncholate**; Ephex Sr

Prescribing information not available at time of publication.

HOW SUPPLIED - EQUIVALENTS NOT AVAILABLE:

Syrup - Oral - 6.25 mg/100 mg

480 ml	**$12.28**	**BRONCHOLATE SYRUP, Bock Pharma**	**00563-0280-16**

Tablet, Coated, Sustained Action - Oral - 600 mg/37.5 mg

40's	$38.00	EPHEX SR, Teral Labs	51234-0150-40
100's	$90.00	EPHEX SR, Teral Labs	51234-0150-90

EPHEDRINE; GUAIFENESIN; PHENOBARBITAL; THEOPHYLLINE *(001156)*

CATEGORIES: Antiasthmatics/Bronchodilators; DESI Drugs; Expectorants; Respiratory & Allergy Medications; Respiratory Muscle Relaxant; Smooth Muscle Relaxants; FDA Pre 1938 Drugs

BRAND NAMES: Guiaphed; Mudrane GG

Prescribing information not available at time of publication.

HOW SUPPLIED - EQUIVALENTS NOT AVAILABLE:

Elixir - Oral - 4 mg/26 mg/2.5

480 ml	$24.00	MUDRANE GG, ECR Pharms	00095-0053-16

Tablet, Uncoated - Oral - 130 mg/16 mg/10

100's	$24.00	MUDRANE GG, ECR Pharms	00095-0051-01

EPHEDRINE; GUAIFENESIN; THEOPHYLLINE *(001158)*

CATEGORIES: DESI Drugs; Respiratory Muscle Relaxant; Smooth Muscle Relaxants

BRAND NAMES: Guiaphed

Prescribing information not available at time of publication.

HOW SUPPLIED - EQUIVALENTS NOT AVAILABLE:

Elixir - Oral

480 ml	$15.50	Guiaphed, Consolidated Midland	00223-6513-01

EPHEDRINE; POTASSIUM IODIDE *(001162)*

CATEGORIES: Antitussives/Expectorants/Mucolytics; Autonomic Drugs; Expectorants; Respiratory & Allergy Medications; Sympathomimetic Agents; FDA Pre 1938 Drugs

BRAND NAMES: **Kie**

Prescribing information not available at time of publication.

HOW SUPPLIED - EQUIVALENTS NOT AVAILABLE:

Syrup - Oral - 8 mg/150 mg

480 ml	**$17.57**	**KIE, Laser**	**00277-0110-02**
3840 ml	**$129.25**	**KIE, Laser**	**00277-0110-03**

EPINEPHRINE *(001166)*

CATEGORIES: Allergic Reactions; Allergies; Anaphylactic Reactions; Anaphylactic Shock; Antiasthmatics/Bronchodilators; Asthma; Autonomic Drugs; Bronchospasm; Cardiac Arrest; Cycloplegics/Mydriatics; EENT Drugs; Eye, Ear, Nose, & Throat Preparations; Glaucoma; Hay Fever; Heart Block; Hemostatics; Hypotension/Shock; Insect Bites; Insect Sting Emergency Kits; Mydriatics; Nasal Congestion; Ophthalmics; Respiratory & Allergy Medications; Respiratory Depression; Respiratory Distress; Rhinitis; Serum Sickness; Shock Emergency Kits; Sinusitis; Sympathomimetic Agents; Sympathomimetics, Beta Agonist; Syncope; Urticaria; Uterine Contractions; Vasoconstrictors; Pregnancy Category C; FDA Approval Pre 1982

BRAND NAMES: *Adrenalin* (Canada); Adrenalin Chloride; *Adrenalina*; *Adrenalina Nuovo*; *Adrenalina Sintetica*; *Adrenaline*; *Adrenaline Injection* (Australia); *Adrenaline Aguettant* (France); *Adrenalini Bitarticas*; Ana-Guard; *Bosmin*; Epifrin; **Epipen**; *Epipen Junior*; *Epipen Jr. 0.15mg Adrenaline Auto-Injector*; *Eppy* (France, Germany); *Eppy "N"*; *Eppystabil* ; Glaucon; *Isopto Epinal*; *L-Adrenalin*; *Isopto-Epinal*; Philip; Racepinephrine; *Simplene* (England); *Suprarenin*; Sus-Phrine; *Weimer Adrenaline* *(International brand names outside U.S. in italics)*

FORMULARIES: Aetna; BC-BS; FHP; Medi-Cal; WHO

COST OF THERAPY: $64.18 (Glaucoma; Solution; 1 %; 0.1/day; 365 days) vs. Potential Cost of $1,851.63 (Iredectomy)

PRIMARY ICD9: 365.11 (Primary Open-Angle Glaucoma)

DESCRIPTION:

Injection: A sterile solution intended for subcutaneous or intramuscular injection. When diluted, it may also be administered intracardially or intravenously. Each milliliter contains 1 mg Epinephrine as the hydrochloride dissolved in Water for Injection, USP, with sodium chloride added for isotonicity. The ampoules contain not more than 0.1% sodium bisulfite as an antioxidant, and the air in the ampoule has been displaced by nitrogen. The Steri-Vials contain 0.5% Chloretone (chlorobutanol) (chloroform derivative) as a preservative and not more than 0.15% sodium bisulfite as an antioxidant. Epinephrine is the active principle of the adrenal medulla, chemically described as (—)-3,4-Dihydroxy-α-((methylamino) methyl) benzyl alcohol.

Ophthalmic Solution: Epinephrine sterile ophthalmic solution is a topical sympathomimetic agent for ophthalmic use.

Chemical Name: 1,2-Benzenediol, 4-(1-hydroxy-2-(methyl-amino)ethyl)- (R)-

Contains: Epinephrine, USP - 0.5%, 1%, 2%

with benzalkonium chloride; sodium metabisulfite; edetate disodium; hydrochloric acid; and purified water.

CLINICAL PHARMACOLOGY:

Injection: Epinephrine is a sympathomimetic drug. It activates an adrenergic receptive mechanism on effector cells and imitates all actions of the sympathetic nervous system except those on the arteries of the face and sweat glands. Epinephrine acts on both alpha and beta receptors and is the most potent alpha receptor activator.

Ophthalmic Solution: Epinephrine is an adrenergic agonist that stimulates α- and β-adrenergic receptors. The capacity of Epinephrine to decrease the aqueous inflow in open-angle glaucoma has been well documented. Studies have also shown that prolonged topical Epinephrine therapy offers significant improvement in the coefficient of aqueous outflow.

Epinephrine ophthalmic solution is effective alone in reducing intraocular pressure and is particularly useful in combination with miotics or beta-adrenergic blocking agents for the difficult-to-control patients. The addition of Epinephrine ophthalmic solution to the patient's regimen often provides better control of intraocular pressure than the original ingredient alone.

INDICATIONS AND USAGE:

Injection: In general, the most common uses of epinephrine are to relieve respiratory distress due to bronchospasm, to provide rapid relief of hypersensitivity reactions to drugs and other allergens, and to prolong the action of infiltration anesthetics. Its cardiac effects may be of use in restoring cardiac rhythm in cardiac arrest due to various causes, but it is not used in cardiac failure or in hemorrhagic, traumatic, or cardiogenic shock.

Epinephrine is used as a hemostatic agent. It is also used in treating mucosal congestion of hay fever, rhinitis, and acute sinusitis; to relieve bronchial asthmatic paroxysms; in syncope due to complete heart block or carotid sinus hypersensitivity; for symptomatic relief of serum sickness, urticaria, angioneurotic edema; for resuscitation in cardiac arrest following anesthetic accidents; in simple (open angle) glaucoma; for relaxation of uterine musculature and to inhibit uterine contractions. Epinephrine Injection can be utilized to prolong the action of intraspinal and local anesthetics (see CONTRAINDICATIONS.)

Ophthalmic Solution: Epinephrine ophthalmic solution is indicated for the treatment of chronic simple glaucoma.

CONTRAINDICATIONS:

Injection: Epinephrine is contraindicated in narrow angle (congestive) glaucoma, shock, during general anesthesia with halogenated hydrocarbons or cyclopropane and in individuals with organic brain damage. Epinephrine is also contraindicated with local anesthesia of certain areas, e.g., fingers, toes, because of the danger of vasoconstriction producing sloughing of tissue; in labor because it may delay the second stage; in cardiac dilatation and coronary insufficiency.

Ophthalmic Solution: Epinephrine ophthalmic solution should not be used in patients who have had an attack of narrow-angle glaucoma, since dilation of the pupil may trigger an acute attack. Do not use if hypersensitive to any ingredient.

WARNINGS:

Injection: Administer with caution to elderly people, to those with cardiovascular disease, hypertension, diabetes or hyperthyroidism; in psychoneurotic individuals; and in pregnancy.

Patients with long-standing bronchial asthma and emphysema who have developed degenerative heart disease should be administered the drug with extreme caution.

Overdosage or inadvertent intravenous injection of epinephrine may cause cerebrovascular hemorrhage resulting from the sharp rise in blood pressure.

Fatalities may also result from pulmonary edema because of the peripheral constriction and cardiac stimulation produced. Rapidly acting vasodilators such as nitrites, or alpha blocking agents may counteract the marked pressor effects of epinephrine.

Epinephrine is the preferred treatment for serious allergic or other emergency situations even though this product contains sodium bisulfite, a sulfite that may in other products cause allergic-type reactions including anaphylactic symptoms or life-threatening or less severe asthmatic episodes in certain susceptible persons. The alternatives to using epinephrine in a life-threatening situation may not be satisfactory. The presence of a sulfite in this product should not deter administration of the drug for treatment of serious allergic or other emergency situations.

Ophthalmic Solution:

1. Epinephrine ophthalmic solution should be used with caution in patients with a narrow-angle, since dilation of the pupil may trigger an acute attack of narrow-angle glaucoma.

2. Use with caution in patients with hypersensitive cardiovascular disease or coronary artery disease.

3. Epinephrine has been reported to produce reversible macular edema in some aphakic patients and should be used with caution in these patients.

Contains sodium metabisulfite, a sulfite agent that may cause allergic-type reactions including anaphylactic symptoms and life-threatening or less severe asthmatic episodes in certain susceptible people. The overall prevalence of sulfite sensitivity in the general population is unknown and probably low. Sulfite sensitivity is seen more frequently in asthmatic than in nonasthmatic people.

PRECAUTIONS:

GENERAL

Injection: Epinephrine injection should be protected from exposure to light. Do not remove ampoules or vials from carton until ready to use. The solution should not be used if it is pinkish or darker than slightly yellow or if it contains a precipitate.

Epinephrine is readily destroyed by alkalies and oxidizing agents. In the latter category are oxygen, chlorine, bromine, iodine, permanganates, chromates, nitrites and salts of easily reducible metals, especially iron.

Ophthalmic Solution: Epinephrine in any form is relatively uncomfortable upon instillation. However, discomfort lessens as the concentration of epinephrine decreases. Epinephrine ophthalmic solution is not for injection.

USAGE IN PREGNANCY: PREGNANCY CATEGORY C

Epinephrine has been shown to be teratogenic in rats when given in doses about 25 times the human dose. There are no adequate and well-controlled studies in pregnant women. Epinephrine should be used during pregnancy only if the potential benefit justifies the potential risk to the fetus.

CARCINOGENESIS, MUTAGENESIS AND IMPAIRMENT OF FERTILITY

No studies have been conducted in animals or in humans to evaluate the potential of these effects.

PEDIATRIC USE

Safety and effectiveness in children has not been established.

DRUG INTERACTIONS:

Injection: Use of epinephrine with excessive doses of digitalis, mercurial diuretics, or other drugs that sensitize the heart to arrhythmias is not recommended. Anginal pain may be induced when coronary insufficiency is present.

The effects of epinephrine may be potentiated by tricyclic antidepressants; certain antihistamines, e.g., diphenhydramine, tripelennamine, d-chlorpheniramine; and sodium l-thyroxine.

ADVERSE REACTIONS:

Injection: Transient and minor side effects of anxiety, headache, fear and palpitations often occur with therapeutic doses, especially in hyperthyroid individuals. Repeated local injections can result in necrosis at sites of injection from vascular constriction. "Epinephrine- fastness" can occur with prolonged use.

Ophthalmic Solution: Undesirable reactions to topical epinephrine include eye pain or ache, browache, headache, conjunctival hyperemia and allergic lid reactions.

Adrenochrome deposits in the conjunctiva and cornea after prolonged epinephrine therapy have been reported to produce reversible macular edema is some aphakic patients.

OVERDOSAGE:

Ophthalmic Solution: Accidental ingestion will not cause problems because pharmacologically active concentrations of epinephrine cannot be achieved orally in man. Should accidental overdosage in the eye(s) occur, flush eye(s) with water or normal saline.

DOSAGE AND ADMINISTRATION:

Injection: Parenteral drug products should be inspected visually for particulate matter and discoloration whenever solution and container permit.

Subcutaneously or intramuscularly: 0.2 to 1 ml (mg). Start with a small dose and increase if required.

Note: The subcutaneous is the preferred route of administration. If given intramuscularly, injection into the buttocks should be avoided.

For bronchial asthma and certain allergic manifestations, e.g., angioedema, urticaria, serum sickness, anaphylactic shock, use epinephrine subcutaneously. For bronchial asthma in pediatric patients, administer 0.01 mg/kg or 0.3 mg/m^2 to a maximum of 0.5 mg subcutaneously, repeated every four hours if required.

For cardiac resuscitation: A dose of 0.5 ml (0.5 mg) diluted to 10 ml with sodium chloride injection can be administered intravenously or intracardially to restore myocardial contractility. External cardiac massage should follow intracardial administration to permit the drug to enter coronary circulation. The drug should be used secondarily to unsuccessful attempts with physical or electromechanical methods.

Ophthalmologic use (for producing conjunctival decongestion, to control hemorrhage, produce mydriasis and reduce intraocular pressure): use a concentration of 1:10,000 (0.1 mg/ml) to 1: 1,000 (1 mg/ml).

Intraspinal use (Amp 88): Usual dose is 0.2 to 0.4 ml (0.2 to 0.4 mg) added to anesthetic spinal fluid mixture (may prolong anesthetic action by limiting absorption). For use with local anesthetic—Epinephrine 1:100,000 (0.01 mg/ml) to 1:20,000 (0.05 mg/ml) is the usual concentration employed with local anesthetics.

Ophthalmic Solution: The usual dosage is 1 drop in the affected eye(s) once or twice daily. However, the dosage should be adjusted to meet the needs of the individual patients. This is made easier with Epinephrine ophthalmic solution available in four strengths.

Injection Storage: Store between 15 and 25°C (59 and 77°F).

Protect from light and freezing.

Solution Storage: Protect from light and excessive heat. If the solution discolors or a precipitate forms, it should be discarded.

(Allergan, PR-7253 30-2/J)

HOW SUPPLIED - RATED THERAPEUTICALLY EQUIVALENT:

Solution - Ophthalmic - 1/2 %

15 ml	$27.66	EPIFRIN 1/2%, Allergan-Amer	11980-0119-15

HOW SUPPLIED - NOT RATED EQUIVALENT:

Injection, Solution - Intramuscular - 0.15mg/ 0.3ml

1's	$24.60	EPIPEN, JR AUTOINJECTOR, Ctr Labs	00268-0302-01

Injection, Solution - Intramuscular - 0.3 mg/ml

1's	$24.60	EPIPEN, AUTO-INJECTOR, Ctr Labs	00268-0301-01

Injection, Solution - Intramuscular; - 0.1 mg/ml

3 ml	$4.77	Epinephrine, Intl Medication	00548-1046-00
10 ml	$5.25	Epinephrine Injetion 1, Intl Medication	00548-2016-00
10 ml	$12.28	EPINEPHRINE, Abbott	00074-4921-18
10 ml	$13.09	Epinephrine, Abbott	00074-4921-23
10 ml	$13.38	Epinephrine, Intl Medication	00548-3016-00
10 ml	$13.61	EPINEPHRINE, Abbott	00074-4921-34
10 ml	$13.78	EPINEPHRINE, Abbott	00074-4901-18
10 ml x 10	$72.33	Epinephrine, Astra USA	00186-0653-01
10 ml x 10	$72.63	Epinephrine, Fujisawa USA	00469-9423-77
10 ml x 10	$81.75	Epinephrine, Fujisawa USA	00469-9423-87

HOW SUPPLIED - NOT RATED EQUIVALENT: *(cont'd)*

Injection, Solution - Intramuscular; - 1 mg/ml

1 ml	$0.91	Epinephrine 1:1000, Abbott	00074-7241-01
1 ml	$4.35	Epinephrine, Intl Medication	00548-1071-00
1 ml	$14.46	ADRENALIN CHLORIDE, Parke-Davis	00071-4188-03
1 ml	$15.00	ANA-GUARD, Miles Spokane	00118-9984-01
1 ml x 6	$90.00	ANA-GUARD, Miles Spokane	00118-9984-06
1 ml x 25	$11.25	Epinephrine, Elkins Sinn	00641-1420-35
1 ml x 25	$12.19	Epinephrine, Am Regent	00517-1061-25
1 ml x 25	$20.00	Epinephrine, Consolidated Midland	00223-7520-05
1 ml x 25	$109.38	Epinephrine, Am Regent	00517-1071-25
1 ml x 100	$48.75	Epinephrine, Am Regent	00517-1061-71
1 ml x 100	$60.00	Epinephrine, Consolidated Midland	00223-7520-01
30 ml	$9.25	Epinephrine, Am Regent	00517-1130-01
30 ml	$9.82	ADRENALIN CHLORIDE, Parke-Davis	00071-4011-13

Injection, Solution - Intravenous - 5 mg/ml

0.3 ml x 12	$33.86	SUS-PHRINE, Berlex Labs	50419-0137-12

Injection, Susp - Subcutaneous - 0.5 %

0.3 ml x 10	$51.35	SUS-PHRINE, Forest Pharms	00456-0664-39
0.3 ml x 25	$124.00	SUS-PHRINE, Forest Pharms	00456-0664-34
5.0 ml	$35.68	SUS-PHRINE, Forest Pharms	00456-0664-05

Solution - Inhalation - 1 %

7.5 ml	$13.19	ADRENALIN CHLORIDE, Parke-Davis	00071-3014-09

Solution - Ophthalmic; Top - 1 %

15 ml	$29.66	EPIFRIN, Allergan-Amer	11980-0122-15

Solution - Ophthalmic; Top - 2 %

15 ml	$32.46	EPIFRIN, Allergan-Amer	11980-0058-15

EPINEPHRINE BITARTRATE; ETIDOCAINE HYDROCHLORIDE *(001168)*

CATEGORIES: Anesthesia; Caudal; Epidural; Injectable Anesthetics; Local Anesthetics; Retrobulbar Anesthetics; Pregnancy Category B; FDA Approval Pre 1982; Patent Expiration 1992 Jan

BRAND NAMES: **Duranest w Epinephrine**; *Duranest 1% Adrenaline* (France)
(International brand names outside U.S. in italics)

Prescribing information not available at time of publication.

HOW SUPPLIED - EQUIVALENTS NOT AVAILABLE:

Injection, Solution - Epidural - 1 %

30 ml	$19.52	DURANEST, WITH EPINEPHRINE, Astra USA	00186-0825-01

Injection, Solution - Epidural - 1.5 %

1.8 ml x 100	$62.50	DURANEST 1.5%/EPINEPHRINE, Astra USA	00186-0840-14
20 ml	$20.90	DURANEST, WITH EPINEPHRINE, Astra USA	00186-0836-03

EPINEPHRINE BITARTRATE; PRILOCAINE HYDROCHLORIDE *(003121)*

CATEGORIES: Anesthesia; Dental; FDA Approval Pre 1982

BRAND NAMES: **Citanest Forte**; *Citanest Adrenalin*
(International brand names outside U.S. in italics)

DESCRIPTION:

For Complete Prescribing Information See: PRILOCAINE HYDROCHLORIDE

EPINEPHRINE HYDROCHLORIDE *(001170)*

CATEGORIES: Antiasthmatics/Bronchodilators; Antiglaucomatous Agents; Autonomic Drugs; Cycloplegics/Mydriatics; EENT Drugs; Eye, Ear, Nose, & Throat Preparations; Glaucoma; Hypotension/Shock; Mydriatics; Nasal Congestion; Ophthalmics; Renal Drugs; Respiratory & Allergy Medications; Sympathomimetic Agents; Sympathomimetics, Beta Agonist; Pregnancy Category C; FDA Pre 1938 Drugs

BRAND NAMES: Ana-Guard; Epifrin; **Glaucon**

Prescribing information not available at time of publication.

HOW SUPPLIED - EQUIVALENTS NOT AVAILABLE:

Injection, Solution - Intramuscular; - 1 mg/ml

1 ml x 10	$23.40	Epinephrine, Wyeth Labs	00008-0263-01
10 ml	$4.88	Epinephrine, Intl Medication	00548-1016-00
10 ml	$6.80	Epinephrine, Intl Medication	00548-1014-00
30 ml	$1.00	Epinephrine Hcl, Lannett	00527-0172-58

Powder

30 gm	$14.56	Ephedrine Hcl, Mallinckrodt	00406-4965-34

Solution - Nasal - 1 mg/ml

1 oz	$9.82	Adrenalin Chloride, Parke-Davis	00071-3003-13

Solution - Ophthalmic - 2 %

10 ml	**$19.38**	**GLAUCON, Alcon-PR**	**00998-0250-10**

Solution - Ophthalmic; Top - 1 %

10 ml	**$17.81**	**GLAUCON, Alcon-PR**	**00998-0249-10**

EPINEPHRINE; LIDOCAINE HYDROCHLORIDE *(001171)*

CATEGORIES: Anesthesia; Antiarrhythmic Agents; Local Anesthetics; Renal Drugs; FDA Approved 1985 Jan

BRAND NAMES: Alphacaine HCl w Epinephrine; Lidocaton; Lignospan; Norocaine; Octocaine; *Xylanaest Mit Epinephrin*; *Xylocain Adrenalin*; *Xylocain-Adrenalin*; *Xylocain-Epinephrin*; *Xylocaine with Adrenaline* (Australia); *Xylocaine w Adrenaline*; **Xylocaine w Epinephrine**
(International brand names outside U.S. in italics)

DESCRIPTION:

.For Full Prescribing Information, See "LIDOCAINE HYDROCHLORIDE".

HOW SUPPLIED - RATED THERAPEUTICALLY EQUIVALENT:

Injection, Solution - Buccal; Dental; - 20 mcg/20 mg

1.8 ml x 100	$35.00	XYLOCAINE 2%/EPINEPHRINE 1:50000, Astra USA	00186-0180-14

Injection, Solution - Caudal Block; I - 5 mcg/10 mg

30 ml x 5	$49.22	XYLOCAINE 1%/EPINEPHRINE 1:200000, Astra USA	00186-0260-02
30 ml x 5	$54.05	XYLOCAINE 1%/EPINEPHRINE 1:200000, Astra USA	00186-0260-92

Injection, Solution - Caudal Block; I - 5 mcg/15 mg

5 ml x 10	$21.45	XYLOCAINE 1.5%/EPINEPHRINE 1:200000, Astra USA	00186-0265-03
30 ml x 5	$53.27	XYLOCAINE 1.5%/EPINEPHRINE 1:200000, Astra USA	00186-0265-02
30 ml x 5	$58.15	XYLOCAINE 1.5%/EPINEPHRINE 1:200000, Astra USA	00186-0265-92

Injection, Solution - Caudal Block; M - 5 mcg/15 mg

30 ml	$10.44	1.5% LIDOCAINE/EPINEPHRINE 1:200000, Abbott	00074-3181-01

Injection, Solution - Dental; Infiltr - 10 mcg/20 mg

1.8 ml cartridg	$35.00	XYLOCAINE 2%/EPINEPHRINE 1:100000, Astra USA	00186-0175-14
10 ml x 5	$11.54	XYLOCAINE 2%/EPINEPHRINE 1:100000, Astra USA	00186-0125-12
20 ml	$2.71	XYLOCAINE 2%/EPINEPHRINE 1:100000, Astra USA	00186-0125-01

Injection, Solution - Epidural - 0.005 mg/10 mg

5 ml x 10	$21.56	XYLOCAINE 1 %/EPINEPHRINE, Astra USA	00186-0114-13
10 ml x 5	$25.98	XYLOCAINE 1 %/EPINEPHRINE, Astra USA	00186-0114-12
30 ml	$9.17	XYLOCAINE 1%/EPINEPHRINE, Astra USA	00186-0114-01
30 ml x 5	$46.44	XYLOCAINE 1%/EPINEPHRINE, Astra USA	00186-0114-91

Injection, Solution - Epidural - 5 mcg/10 mg

30 ml	$9.51	LIDOCAINE/EPINEPHRINE, Abbott	00074-3179-01

Injection, Solution - Epidural - 5 mcg/15 mg

5 ml x 10	$26.98	XYLOCAINE 1.5%/EPINEPHRINE, Astra USA	00186-0117-13
10 ml x 5	$29.33	XYLOCAINE 1.5%/EPINEPHRINE, Astra USA	00186-0117-12
15 ml	$3.76	1.5% LIDOCAINE HCL & EPINEPHRINE, Abbott	00074-1209-01
30 ml	$10.62	XYLOCAINE 1.5%/EPINEPHRINE, Astra USA	00186-0117-01
30 ml	$10.75	LIDOCAINE HCL & EPINEPHRINE, Abbott	00074-3180-02
30 ml x 5	$52.74	XYLOCAINE 1.5%/EPINEPHRINE, Astra USA	00186-0117-91

Injection, Solution - Epidural - 10 mcg/10 mg

20 ml	$2.53	LIDOCAINE/EPINEPHRINE, Abbott	00074-3178-01
50 ml	$4.28	LIDOCAINE/EPINEPHRINE, Abbott	00074-3178-03

Injection, Solution - Epidural - 10 mcg/20 mg

20 ml	$2.70	LIDOCAINE/EPINEPHRINE, Abbott	00074-3182-01
30 ml	$4.41	LIDOCAINE/EPINEPHRINE, Abbott	00074-3182-02
50 ml	$5.05	LIDOCAINE/EPINEPHRINE, Abbott	00074-3182-03

Injection, Solution - Epidural; Infil - 0.001 %/1 %

5 ml	$5.30	Lidocaine Hcl With Epinephrine, Intl Medication	00548-1113-00

Injection, Solution - Epidural; Infil - 5 mcg/20 mg

5 ml x 10	$24.80	XYLOCAINE 2%/EPINEPHRINE 1:200000, Astra USA	00186-0122-13
5 x 20 ml	$57.43	XYLOCAINE 2%/EPINEPHRINE 1:200000, Astra USA	00186-0250-02
10 ml x 5	$34.24	XYLOCAINE 2%,WITH EPINEPH 1:200000, Astra USA	00186-0122-12
20 ml	$11.80	XYLOCAINE 2%/EPINEPHRINE 1:200000, Astra USA	00186-0122-01
20 ml x 5	$58.94	XYLOCAINE 2%/EPINEPHRINE 1:200000, Astra USA	00186-0122-91

Injection, Solution - Infiltration - 0.01 mg/10 mg

30 ml x 25	$32.49	Lidocaine Hcl With Epinephrine, Elkins Sinn	00641-2415-45

Injection, Solution - Infiltration - 0.01 mg/20 mg

30 ml x 25	$35.00	Lidocaine Hcl With Epinephrine, Elkins Sinn	00641-2425-45

Injection, Solution - Infiltration; S - 1 %

10 ml x 5	$10.19	XYLOCAINE, WITH EPINEPHRINE 1:100000, Astra USA	00186-0115-12
20 ml	$2.55	XYLOCAINE, WITH EPINEPHRINE 1:100000, Astra USA	00186-0115-01

Injection, Solution - Infiltration; S - 5 mcg/5 mg

50 ml	$4.29	XYLOCAINE 0.5%/EPINEPHRINE 1:200000, Astra USA	00186-0140-01

Injection, Solution - Infiltration; S - 10 mcg/10 mg

50 ml	$4.39	XYLOCAINE 1%/EPINEPHRINE 1:100000, Astra USA	00186-0150-01

Injection, Solution - Infiltration; S - 10 mcg/20 mg

50 ml	$4.99	XYLOCAINE 2%/EPINEPHRINE 1:100000, Astra USA	00186-0160-01

Injection, Solution - Intravenous - 0.5 mg/0.0005 m

50 ml	$4.50	Lidocaine Hcl W/Epinephrine, Abbott	00074-3177-01

Injection, Solution - Intravenous - 1 mg/0.001 mg

30 ml	$4.28	Lidocaine Hcl W/Epinephrine, Abbott	00074-3178-02

Injection, Solution - Intravenous - 1.5 mg/0.0005 m

5 ml	$4.75	LIDOCAINE HCL W/EPINEPHRINE, Abbott	00074-2528-01

Injection, Solution - Intravenous - 2 mg/0.0005 mg

20 ml	$11.41	Lidocaine Hcl W/Epinephrine, Abbott	00074-3183-01

EPINEPHRINE; PILOCARPINE *(001172)*

CATEGORIES: EENT Drugs; Eye, Ear, Nose, & Throat Preparations; Glaucoma; Miotics; Ophthalmics; FDA Pre 1938 Drugs

BRAND NAMES: **E-Pilo**; *Epilo*; P1E1
(International brand names outside U.S. in italics)

FORMULARIES: Aetna; Medi-Cal

Prescribing information not available at time of publication.

HOW SUPPLIED - EQUIVALENTS NOT AVAILABLE:

Solution - Ophthalmic - 10 mg/10 mg

10 ml	**$13.38**	**E-PILO-1 OPHTHALMIC, Ciba Vision**	**00058-2344-10**
15 ml	$17.81	P1E1, Alcon-PR	00998-0365-15

Solution - Ophthalmic - 10 mg/20 mg

10 ml	**$13.62**	**E-PILO-2 OPHTHALMIC, Ciba Vision**	**00058-2345-10**
15 ml	$17.81	P2E1, Alcon-PR	00998-0366-15

Solution - Ophthalmic - 10 mg/30 mg

15 ml	$18.75	P3E1, Alcon-PR	00998-0367-15

Solution - Ophthalmic - 10 mg/40 mg

10 ml	**$14.70**	**E-PILO-4 OPHTHALMIC, Ciba Vision**	**00058-2355-10**
15 ml	$19.69	P4E1, Alcon-PR	00998-0368-15

Solution - Ophthalmic - 10 mg/60 mg

10 ml	**$15.18**	**E-PILO-6 OPHTHALMIC, Ciba Vision**	**00058-2357-10**
15 ml	$20.63	P6E1, Alcon-PR	00998-0369-15

EPINEPHRYL BORATE *(001169)*

CATEGORIES: Antiglaucomatous Agents; EENT Drugs; Eye, Ear, Nose, & Throat Preparations; Glaucoma; Mydriatics; Ophthalmics; Pregnancy Category C; FDA Pre 1938 Drugs

BRAND NAMES: *Epiboran*; *Epiboran Ofteno* (Mexico); Epinal; *Epista* (Japan); *Eppy N*; **Eppy N**; *Isopto*
(International brand names outside U.S. in italics)

FORMULARIES: Medi-Cal

COST OF THERAPY: (Glaucoma; Solution; 1 %; 0.2/day; 365 days) (DRG 38)

PRIMARY ICD9: 365.11 (Primary Open-Angle Glaucoma)

DESCRIPTION:

A sterile ophthalmic solution of Epinephryl Borate in two strengths.

Established name:

Epinephryl Borate

CHEMICAL NAMES:

1,3,2-Benzodioxaborole-5-methanol, 2-hydroxy-*a*-((methylamino)methyl)-,(*R*)-.

(—)-3,4-Dihydroxy-*a*-((methylamino)methyl)benzyl alcohol, cyclic 3,4-ester with boric acid.

Each ml contains: Active: Epinephryl Borate equivalent to Epinephrine 0.5%, or 1.0%. Preservative: Benzalkonium Chloride 0.01%. Inactive: Ascorbic Acid, Acetylcysteine, Boric Acid, Sodium Carbonate (to adjust pH), Purified Water.

CLINICAL PHARMACOLOGY:

Lowers intraocular pressure by reducing the production of aqueous and increasing the facility of outflow.

INDICATIONS AND USAGE:

For the control of simple (open angle) glaucoma; may be used in combination with miotics, beta blockers, hyperosmotic agents, or carbonic anhydrase inhibitors when indicated.

CONTRAINDICATIONS:

Do not use in narrow or shallow angle (angle closure) glaucoma. Contraindicated in those persons who have shown hypersensitivity to any component of this preparation.

WARNINGS:

For topical use only — not for injection. To avoid inducing angle closure glaucoma, an estimation of the depth of the angle of the anterior chamber should be made. Use with caution in individuals with history of hyperthyroidism, hypertension, organic cardiac disease and long-standing bronchial asthma.

PRECAUTIONS:

Do not use this preparation on soft contact lenses. Patient should immediately report any decrease in visual acuity. If a general anesthetic is to be used, consult the anesthesiologist. Patient should not use if solution is brown.

ADVERSE REACTIONS:

Systemic side effects such as headache, palpitation, faintness, tachycardia, and extrasystoles may occur. Prolonged use may be associated with conjunctival or corneal pigmentation. Following prolonged administration, ocular irritation (hypersensitivity) may develop in a significant number of patients. Severe side effects such as hypertension and cardiac arrhythmia have been reported. Maculopathy with associated decrease in visual acuity may occur in the aphakic eye; in this event, administration should be discontinued promptly.

DOSAGE AND ADMINISTRATION:

Usual dosage is one drop topically in the eye(s) twice daily for the control of glaucoma.

Storage: Store bottle in upright position with the dropper tightly sealed. Protect from excessive heat and light. Store below 75°F in a dark place.

HOW SUPPLIED - EQUIVALENTS NOT AVAILABLE:

Solution - Ophthalmic - 0.5 %

7.5 ml	$15.00	EPINAL, Alcon	00065-0265-07

Solution - Ophthalmic - 1 %

7.5 ml	$15.62	EPINAL, Alcon	00065-0264-07

EPOETIN ALFA *(001173)*

CATEGORIES: AIDS Related Complex; Anemia; Antianemia Drugs; Blood Formation/Coagulation; Chemotherapy; Deficiency Anemias; Erythropoisis Enhancers; Gastrointestinal Bleeding; Hematopoietic Agents; Hemolysis; HIV Infection; Orphan Drugs; Renal Drugs; Renal Failure; Pregnancy Category C; Recombinant DNA Origin; Sales > $500 Million; FDA Approved 1989 Jun; Patent Expiration 2004 Dec

BRAND NAMES: E.P.O.; **Epogen**; *Epoxitin*; Eprex; *Erypo* (Germany); Erythropoietin; Procrit
(International brand names outside U.S. in italics)

FORMULARIES: Aetna; BC-BS; Medi-Cal

DESCRIPTION:

Erythropoietin is a glycoprotein which stimulates red blood cell production. It is produced in the kidney and stimulates the division and differentiation of committed erythroid progenitors in the bone marrow. Epogen, a 165 amino acid glycoprotein manufactured by recombinant DNA technology, has the same biological effects as endogenous erythropoietin.[1]It has a molecular weight of 30,400 daltons and is produced by mammalian cells into which the human erythropoietin gene has been introduced. The product contains the identical amino acid sequence of isolated natural erythropoietin.

Epogen is formulated as a sterile, colorless liquid in an isotonic sodium chloride/sodium citrate buffered solution for intravenous (IV) or subcutaneous (SC) administration.

Epogen Single-Dose, Preservative-Free Vial: Each 1 ml of solution contains 2000, 3000, 4000 or 10,000 Units of epoetin alfa, 2.5 mg albumin (Human), 5.8 mg sodium citrate, 5.8 mg sodium chloride, and 0.06 mg citric acid in Water for Injection, USP (pH 6.9 ± 0.3). This formulation contains no preservative.

Epogen Multidose, Preserved Vial: 2 ml (20,000 Units, 10,000 Units/ml).

Each 1 ml of solution contains 10,000 Units of epoetin alfa, 2.5 mg albumin (Human), 1.3 mg sodium citrate, 8.2 mg sodium chloride, 0.11 mg citric acid, and 1% benzyl alcohol as preservative in Water for Injection, USP (pH 6.1 ± 0.3).

Epogen Multidose, Preserved Vial: 1 ml (20,000 Units/ml). Each 1 ml of solution contains 20,000 Units of epoetin alfa, 2.5 mg albumin (human), 1.3 mg sodium citrate, 8.2 mg chloride, 0.11 mg citric acid, and 1% benzyl alcohol as preservative in Water for Injection, USP (pH 6.1 ± 0.3).

CLINICAL PHARMACOLOGY:

Chronic Renal Failure Patients: Endogenous production of erythropoietin is normally regulated by the level of tissue oxygenation. Hypoxia and anemia generally increase the production of erythropoietin, which in turn stimulates erythropoiesis.[2] In normal subjects, plasma erythropoietin levels range from 0.01 to 0.03 Units/ml,[2,3]and increase up to 100- to 1000-fold during hypoxia or anemia.[2,3] In contrast, in patients with chronic renal failure (CRF), production of erythropoietin is impaired, and this erythropoietin deficiency is the primary cause of their anemia.[3,4]

Chronic renal failure is the clinical situation in which there is a progressive and usually irreversible decline in kidney function. Such patients may manifest the sequelae of renal dysfunction, including anemia, but do not necessarily require regular dialysis. Patients with end-stage renal disease (ESRD) are those patients with CRF who require regular dialysis or kidney transplantation for survival.

Epoetin alfa has been shown to stimulate erythropoiesis in anemic patients with CRF, including both patients on dialysis and those who do not require regular dialysis.[4-13] The first evidence of a response to the three times weekly administration of epoetin alfa is an increase in the reticulocyte count within 10 days, followed by increases in the red cell count, hemoglobin, and hematocrit, usually within 2-6 weeks.[4,5] *Because of the length of time required for erythropoiesis — several days for erythroid progenitors to mature and be released into the circulation — a clinically significant increase in hematocrit is usually not observed in less than 2 weeks and may require up to 6 weeks in some patients.* Once the hematocrit reaches the target range (30-36%), that level can be sustained by epoetin alfa therapy in the absence of iron deficiency and concurrent illnesses.

The rate of hematocrit increase varies between patients and is dependent upon the dose of epoetin alfa, within a therapeutic range of approximately 50-300 Units/kg three times weekly[4] A greater biologic response is not observed at doses exceeding 300 Units/kg three times weekly[6] Other factors affecting the rate and extent of response include availability of iron stores, the baseline hematocrit, and the presence of concurrent medical problems.

Zidovudine-treated HIV-infected Patients: Responsiveness to epoetin alfa in HIV-infected patients is dependent upon the endogenous serum erythropoietin level prior to treatment. Patients with endogenous serum erythropoietin levels ≤ 500 mUnits/ml, and who are receiving a dose of zidovudine ≤ 4200 mg/week, may respond to epoetin alfa therapy. Patients with endogenous serum erythropoietin levels > 500 mUnits/ml do not appear to respond to epoetin alfa therapy. In a series of four clinical trials involving 255 patients, 60% to 80% of HIV-infected patients treated with zidovudine had endogenous serum erythropoietin levels ≤ 500 mUnits/ml.

Response to epoetin alfa in zidovudine-treated HIV-infected patients is manifested by reduced transfusion requirements and increased hematocrit.

Cancer Patients on Chemotherapy: Anemia in cancer patients may be related to the disease itself or the effect of concomitantly administered chemotherapeutic agents. Epoetin alfa has been shown to increase hematocrit and decrease transfusion requirements after the first month of therapy (months 2 and 3), in anemic cancer patients undergoing chemotherapy.

A series of clinical trials enrolled 131 anemic cancer patients who were receiving cyclic cisplatin- or non cisplatin-containing chemotherapy. Endogenous baseline serum erythropoietin levels varied among patients in these trials with approximately 75% (N=83/110) having endogenous serum erythropoietin levels ≤ 132 mUnits/ml, and approximately 4% (N=4/110) of patients having endogenous serum erythropoietin levels > 500 mUnits/ml. In general, patients with lower baseline serum erythropoietin levels responded more vigorously to epoetin alfa than patients with higher baseline erythropoietin levels. Although no specific serum erythropoietin level can be stipulated above which patients would be unlikely to respond to epoetin alfa therapy, treatment of patients with grossly elevated serum erythropoietin levels (*e.g.*, > 200 mUnits/ml) is not recommended.

Pharmacokinetics: Intravenously administered Epoetin alfa is eliminated at a rate consistent with first order kinetics with a circulating half-life ranging from approximately 4 to 13 hours in patients with CRF. Within the therapeutic dose range, detectable levels of plasma erythropoietin are maintained for at least 24 hours.[7] After subcutaneous administration of epoetin alfa to patients with CRF, peak serum levels are achieved within 5- 24 hours after administration and decline slowly thereafter. There is no apparent difference in half-life between patients not on dialysis whose serum creatinine levels were greater than 3, and patients maintained on dialysis.

In normal volunteers, the half-life of intravenously administered epoetin alfa is approximately 20% shorter than the half-life in CRF patients. The pharmacokinetics of epoetin alfa have not been studied in HIV-infected patients.

CLINICAL STUDIES:

RESPONSE TO EPOETIN ALFA

Chronic Renal Failure Patients: Response to epoetin alfa was consistent across all studies. In the presence of adequate iron stores (see PRECAUTIONS, Therapy Iron Evaluation), the time to reach the target hematocrit is a function of the baseline hematocrit and the rate of hematocrit rise.

CLINICAL STUDIES: *(cont'd)*

The rate of increase in hematocrit is dependent upon the dose of epoetin alfa administered and individual patient variation. In clinical trials at starting doses of 50-150 Units/kg three times weekly, patients responded with an average rate of hematocrit rise as shown in TABLE 1.

TABLE 1

Starting Dose (three times weekly, IV)	Hematocrit Increase Points/Day	Points/2 Weeks
50 Units/kg	0.11	1.5
100 Units/kg	0.18	2.5
150 Units/kg	0.25	3.5

Over this dose range, approximately 95% of all patients responded with a clinically significant increase in hematocrit, and by the end of approximately 2 months of therapy virtually all patients were transfusion-independent. Changes in the quality of life of epoetin alfa-treated patients were assessed as part of a Phase III clinical trial.[5,8] Once the target hematocrit (32-38%) was achieved, statistically significant improvements were demonstrated for most quality of life parameters measured, including energy and activity level, functional ability, sleep and eating behavior, health status, satisfaction with health, sex life, well-being, psychological effect, life satisfaction, and happiness. Patients also reported improvement in their disease symptoms. They showed a statistically significant increase in exercise capacity (VO_2 max), energy, and strength with a significant reduction in aching, dizziness, anxiety, shortness of breath, muscle weakness, and leg cramps.[8,14]

Patients on Dialysis: Thirteen clinical studies were conducted, involving intravenous administration to a total of 1010 anemic patients on dialysis for 986 patient-years of epoetin alfa therapy. In the three largest of these clinical trials, the median maintenance dose necessary to maintain the hematocrit between 30-36% was approximately 75 Units/kg (three times weekly). In the U.S. multicenter Phase III study, approximately 65% of the patients required doses of 100 Units/kg three times weekly, or less, to maintain their hematocrit at approximately 35%. Almost 10% of patients required a dose of 25 Units/kg, or less, and approximately 10% required a dose of more than 200 Units/kg three times weekly to maintain their hematocrit at this level.

A multicenter unit dose study was also conducted in 119 patients receiving peritoneal dialysis who self-administered epoetin alfa subcutaneously for approximately 109 patient-years of experience. Patients responded to epoetin alfa administered subcutaneously in a manner similar to patients receiving intravenous administration.[18]

Patients with CRF Not Requiring Dialysis: Four clinical trials were conducted in patients with CRF not on dialysis involving 181 epoetin alfa-treated patients for approximately 67 patient-years of experience. These patients responded to epoetin alfa therapy in a manner similar to that observed in patients on dialysis. Patients with CRF not on dialysis demonstrated a dose-dependent and sustained increase in hematocrit when epoetin alfa was administered by either an intravenous or subcutaneous route, with similar rates of rise of hematocrit when epoetin alfa was administered by either route. Moreover, epoetin alfa doses of 75-150 Units/kg *per week* have been shown to maintain hematocrits of 36-38% for up to 6 months. Correcting the anemia of progressive renal failure will allow patients to remain active even though their renal function continues to decrease.[19-21]

Zidovudine-treated HIV-infected Patients: Epoetin alfa has been studied in four placebo-controlled trials enrolling 297 anemic (hematocrit < 30%) HIV-infected (AIDS) patients receiving concomitant therapy with zidovudine (all patients were treated with epoetin alfa manufactured by Amgen Inc.). In the subgroup of patients (89/125 epoetin alfa and 88/130 placebo) with prestudy endogenous serum erythropoietin levels ≤ 500 mUnits/ml. Epoetin alfa reduced the mean cumulative number of units of blood transfused per patient by approximately 40% as compared to the placebo group.[22] Among those patients who required transfusions at baseline, 43% of epoetin alfa-treated patients versus 18% of placebo-treated patients were transfusion-independent during the second and third months of therapy. Epoetin alfa therapy also resulted in significant increases in hematocrit in comparison to placebo. When examining the results according to the weekly dose of zidovudine received during month 3 of therapy, there was a statistically significant ($p < 0.003$) reduction in transfusion requirements in epoetin alfa-treated patients (n=51) compared to placebo treated patients (n=54) whose mean weekly zidovudine dose was ≤ 4200 mg/week.[22]

Approximately 17% of the patients with endogenous serum erythropoietin levels ≤ 500 mUnits/ml receiving epoetin alfa in doses from 100-200 Units/kg three times weekly (three times weekly) achieved a hematocrit of 38% without administration of transfusions or significant reduction in zidovudine dose. In the subgroup of patients whose prestudy endogenous serum erythropoietin levels were > 500 mUnits/ml, epoetin alfa therapy did not reduce transfusion requirements or increase hematocrit, compared to the corresponding responses in placebo-treated patients. In a six month open label epoetin alfa study, patients responded with decreased transfusion requirements and sustained increases in hematocrit and hemoglobin with doses of epoetin alfa up to 300 Units/kg three times weekly[21-23]

Responsiveness to epoetin alfa therapy may be blunted by intercurrent infectious/inflammatory episodes and by an increase in zidovudine dosage. Consequently, the dose of epoetin alfa must be titrated based on these factors to maintain the desired erythropoietic response.

Cancer Patients on Chemotherapy Epoetin alfa has been studied in a series of placebo-controlled, double-blind trials in a total of 131 anemic cancer patients. Within this group, 72 patients were treated with concomitant non cisplatin-containing chemotherapy regimens and 59 patients were treated with concomitant cisplatin-containing chemotherapy regimens. Patients were randomized to epoetin alfa 150 Units/kg or placebo subcutaneously three times weekly for 12 weeks.

Epoetin alfa therapy was associated with a significantly ($p < 0.008$) greater hematocrit response than in the corresponding placebo-treated patients (see TABLE 2).[22]

TABLE 2 Hematocrit (%): Mean Change From Baseline To Final Value*

Study	Epoetin alfa	Placebo
Chemotherapy	7.6	1.3
Cisplatin	6.9	0.6

* Significantly higher in Epoetin alfa patients than in placebo patients ($p < 0.008$)

In the two types of chemotherapy studies (utilizing an epoetin alfa dose of 150 Units/kg three times weekly), the mean number of units of blood transfused per patient after the first month of therapy was significantly ($p < 0.02$) lower in epoetin alfa-treated patients (0.71 units in months 2, 3) than in corresponding placebo-treated patients (1.84 units in Months 2, 3). Moreover, the proportion of patients transfused during months 2 and 3 of therapy combined was significantly ($p < 0.03$) lower in the epoetin alfa-treated patients than in the corresponding placebo-treated patients (22% versus 43%).[22]

Comparable intensity of chemotherapy in the epoetin alfa and placebo groups in the chemotherapy trials was suggested by a similar area under the neutrophil time curve in epoetin alfa- and placebo-treated patients as well as by a similar proportion of patients in epoetin alfa- and placebo-treated groups whose absolute neutrophil counts fell below 1,000

CLINICAL STUDIES: *(cont'd)*

cells/mcl. Available evidence suggests that patients with lymphoid and solid cancers respond equivalently to epoetin alfa therapy, and that patients with or without tumor infiltration of the bone marrow respond equivalently to epoetin alfa therapy.

Surgery Patients: Epoetin alfa has been studied in placebo-controlled, double-blind trial enrolling 316 patients scheduled for major, elective orthopedic hip or knee surgery who were expected to require ≥2 units of blood and who were not able or willing to participate in an autologous blood donation program. Based on previous studies which demonstrated that pretreatment hemoglobin is a predictor of risk of receiving transfusion,[16, 24] patients were stratified into one of three groups based on their pretreatment hemoglobin [≤10(n=2), >10 to ≤13 (n=96), and >13 to ≤15 g/dl (n=218)] and then randomly assigned to receive 300 Units/kg epoetin alfa, 100 Units/kg epoetin alfa or placebo by subcutaneous injection for 10 days before surgery, on the day of surgery, and for four days after surgery.[14] All patients received oral iron and a low-dose post-operative warfarin regimen.[14]

Treatment with epoetin alfa 300 Units/kg significantly (p=0.024) reduced the risk of allogeneic transfusion in patients with a pretreatment hemoglobin of >10 to ≤13 g/dl; 5/31 (16%) of epoetin alfa 300 Units/kg, 6/26 (23%) of epoetin alfa 100 Units/kg, and 13/29 (45%) of placebo treated patients were transfused.[14] There was no significant difference in the number of patients transfused between epoetin alfa (9% 300 Units/kg, 6% 100 Units/kg and placebo (13%) in the >13 to ≤15 g/dl hemoglobin stratum. There were too few patients in the ≤10 g/dl group to determine if epoetin alfa is useful in this hemoglobin strata. In the >10 to ≤13 g/dl pretreatment stratum, the mean number of units transfused per epoetin alfa treated patient (0.45 units blood for 300 Units/kg, 0.42 units blood for 100 Units/kg) was less than the mean transfused per placebo-treated patient (1.14 units) (overall p=0.028). In addition, mean hemoglobin, hematocrit and reticulocyte counts increased significantly during the presurgery period in patients treated with epoetin alfa.[14]

Epoetin alfa was also studied in an open-label, parallel-group trial enrolling 145 subjects with a pretreatment hemoglobin level of ≥10 to ≤13 g/dl who were scheduled for major orthopedic hip or knee surgery and who were not participating in an autologous program.[15] Subjects were randomly assigned to receive one of two SC dosing regimens of epoetin alfa (600 Units/kg once weekly for three weeks prior to surgery and on the day of surgery, or 300 Units/kg once daily for 10 days prior to surgery, and on the day of surgery, and for 4 days after surgery). All subjects received oral iron and appropriate pharmacological anticoagulation therapy.

From pretreatment to presurgery, the mean increase in hemoglobin in the 600 Units/kg weekly group (1.44 g/dl) was greater than observed in the 300 Units/kg daily group.[15] The mean increase in absolute reticulocyte count was smaller in the weekly group ($0.11 \times 10^6/mm^3$) compared to the daily group ($0.17 \times 10^6/mm^3$). Mean hemoglobin levels were similar for the two treatment groups throughout the postsurgical period.

The erythropoietic response observed in both treatment groups resulted in similar transfusion rates [11/69 (16%) in the 600 Units/kg weekly group and 14/71 (20%) in the 300 Units/kg daily group.][15] The mean number of units transfused per subject was approximately 0.3 units in both treatment groups.

INDICATIONS AND USAGE:

Treatment of Anemia of Chronic Renal Failure Patients: Epoetin alfa is indicated in the treatment of anemia associated with chronic renal failure, including patients on dialysis (end-stage renal disease) and patients not on dialysis. Epoetin alfa is indicated to elevate or maintain the red blood cell level (as manifested by the hematocrit or hemoglobin determinations) and to decrease the need for transfusions in these patients.

Non-dialysis patients with symptomatic anemia considered for therapy should have a hematocrit less than 30%.

Epoetin alfa is not intended for patients who require immediate correction of severe anemia. Epoetin alfa may obviate the need for maintenance transfusions but is not a substitute for emergency transfusion.

Prior to initiation of therapy, the patient's iron stores should be evaluated. Transferrin saturation should be at least 20% and ferritin at least 100 ng/ml. Blood pressure should be adequately controlled prior to initiation of epoetin alfa therapy, and must be closely monitored and controlled during therapy.

Epoetin alfa should be administered under the guidance of a qualified physician (see DOSAGE AND ADMINISTRATION.)

Treatment of Anemia in Zidovudine-treated HIV-infected Patients: Epoetin alfa is indicated for the treatment of anemia related to therapy with zidovudine in HIV-infected patients. Epoetin alfa is indicated to elevate or maintain the red blood cell level (as manifested by the hematocrit or hemoglobin determinations) and to decrease the need for transfusions in these patients. Epoetin alfa is not indicated for the treatment of anemia in HIV-infected patients due to other factors such as iron or folate deficiencies, hemolysis or gastrointestinal bleeding, which should be managed appropriately.

Epoetin alfa, at a dose of 100 Units/kg three times per week, is effective in decreasing the transfusion requirement and increasing the red blood cell level of anemic, HIV-infected patients treated with zidovudine, when the endogenous serum erythropoietin level is ≤ 500 mUnits/ml and when patients are receiving a dose of zidovudine ≤ 4200 mg/week.

Treatment of Anemia in Cancer Patients on Chemotherapy: Epoetin alfa is indicated for the treatment of anemia in patients with non-myeloid malignancies where anemia is due to the effect of concomitantly administered chemotherapy. Epoetin alfa is indicated to decrease the need for transfusions in patients who will be receiving concomitant chemotherapy for a minimum of 2 months. Epoetin alfa is not indicated for the treatment of anemia in cancer patients due to other factors such as iron or folate deficiencies, hemolysis or gastrointestinal bleeding which should be managed appropriately.

Reduction of Allogeneic Blood Transfusion in Surgery Patients: Epoetin alfa is indicated for the treatment of anemic patients (hemoglobin >10 to ≤13 g/dl) scheduled to undergo elective, noncardiac, nonvascular surgery to reduce the need for allogeneic blood transfusions.[14-16] Epoetin alfa is indicated for patients at high risk for perioperative transfusions with significant, anticipated blood loss. Epoetin alfa is not indicated for anemic patients who are willing to donate autologous blood. The safety of the perioperative use of epoetin alfa has been studied only in patients who are receiving anticoagulant prophylaxis.

CONTRAINDICATIONS:

Epoetin alfa is contraindicated in patients with:

1. Uncontrolled hypertension.

2. Known hypersensitivity to mammalian cell-derived products.

3. Known hypersensitivity to albumin (human).

WARNINGS:

PEDIATRIC USE

The multidose preserved formulation contains benzyl alcohol. Benzyl alcohol has been reported to be associated with and increased incidence of neurological and other complications in premature infants which are sometimes fatal. The safety and effectiveness of epoetin alfa in pediatric patients have not been established.

WARNINGS: *(cont'd)*

THROMBOTIC EVENTS AND INCREASED MORTALITY

A randomized, prospective trial of 1265 hemodialysis patients with clinically evident cardiac disease (ischemic heart disease or congestive heart failure) was conducted in which patients were assigned to epoetin alfa treatment targeted to a maintenance hematocrit of either 42 ± 3% or 30 ± 3%. Increased mortality was observed in 634 patients randomized to a target hematocrit of 42% [221 deaths (35% mortality)] compared to 631 patients targeted to remain at a hematocrit of 30% [185 deaths (29%mortality)]. The reason for increased mortality observed in these studies is unknown, however the incidence of non-fatal myocardial infarctions (3.1% vs 2.3%), vascular access thromboses (39% vs 29%), and all other thrombotic events (22% vs 18%) were also higher in the group randomized to achieve a hematocrit of 42%.

Increased mortality was also observed in a randomized placebo-controlled study of epoetin alfa in patients who did not have CRF who were undergoing coronary artery bypass surgery (7 deaths in 126 patients randomized to epoetin alfa versus no deaths among 56 patients receiving placebo). Four of these deaths occurred during the period of study drug administration and all 4 deaths were associated with thrombotic events. While the extent of the population affected in unknown, in patients at risk of thrombosis, the anticipated benefits of epoetin alfa treatment should be weighed against the potential for increased risks associated with therapy.

CHRONIC RENAL FAILURE PATIENTS

Hypertension: Patients with uncontrolled hypertension should not be treated with epoetin alfa; blood pressure should be controlled adequately before initiation of therapy. Up to 80% of patients with CRF have a history of hypertension.[25] Although there does not appear to be any direct pressor effects of epoetin alfa, blood pressure may rise during epoetin alfa therapy. During the early phase of treatment when the hematocrit is increasing, approximately 25% of patients on dialysis may require initiation of, or increases in, antihypertensive therapy. Hypertensive encephalopathy and seizures have been observed in patients with CRF treated with epoetin alfa.

Special care should be taken to closely monitor and aggressively control blood pressure in epoetin alfa-treated patients. Patients should be advised as to the importance of compliance with antihypertensive therapy and dietary restrictions. If blood pressure is difficult to control by initiation of appropriate measures, the hematocrit may be reduced by decreasing or withholding the dose of epoetin alfa. A clinically significant decrease in hematocrit may not be observed for several weeks.

It is recommended that the dose of epoetin alfa be decreased if the hematocrit increase exceeds 4 points in any two-week period, because of the possible association of excessive rate of rise of hematocrit with an exacerbation of hypertension.

In CRF patients on hemodialysis with clinically evident ischemic heart disease or congestive heart failure, the hematocrit should be managed carefully, not to exceed 36% (see WARNINGS, Thrombotic Events).

Seizures: Seizures have occurred in patients with CRF participating in epoetin alfa clinical trials.

In patients on dialysis, there was a higher incidence of seizures during the first 90 days of therapy (occurring in approximately 2.5% of patients) as compared with later time points.

Given the potential for an increased risk of seizures during the first 90 days of therapy, blood pressure and the presence of premonitory neurologic symptoms should be monitored closely. Patients should be cautioned to avoid potentially hazardous activities such as driving or operating heavy machinery during this period.

While the relationship between seizures and the rate of rise of hematocrit is uncertain, *it is recommended that the dose of epoetin alfa be decreased if the hematocrit increase exceeds 4 points in any two-week period.*

Thrombotic Events: During hemodialysis, patients treated with epoetin alfa may require increased anticoagulation with heparin to prevent clotting of the artificial kidney (see ADVERSE REACTIONSfor more information about thrombotic events).

Other thrombotic events (*e.g.,* myocardial infarction, cerebrovascular accident, transient ischemic attack) have occurred in clinical trials at an annualized rate of less than 0.04 events per patient year of epoetin alfa therapy. These trials were conducted in patients with CRF (whether on dialysis or not) in whom the target hematocrit was 32% to 40%. However, the risk of thrombotic events, including vascular access thrombosis, was significantly increased in patients with ischemic heart disease or congestive heart failure receiving epoetin alfa therapy with the goal of reaching a normal hematocrit (42%) as compared to a target hematocrit of 30%. Patients with pre-existing cardiovascular disease should be monitored closely.

Zidovudine-treated HIV-infected Patients: In contrast to CRF patients, epoetin alfa therapy has not been linked to exacerbation of hypertension, seizures, and thrombotic events in HIV-infected patients.

PRECAUTIONS:

GENERAL

The parenteral administration of any biologic product should be attended by appropriate precautions in case allergic or other untoward reactions occur (see CONTRAINDICATIONS.) In clinical trials, while transient rashes were occasionally observed concurrently with epoetin alfa therapy, no serious allergic or anaphylactic reactions were reported. See ADVERSE REACTIONSfor more information regarding allergic reactions.

The safety and efficacy of epoetin alfa therapy have not been established in patients with a known history of a seizure disorder or underlying hematologic disease (*e.g.,* sickle cell anemia, myelodysplastic syndromes, or hypercoagulable disorders).

In some female patients, menses have resumed following epoetin alfa therapy; the possibility of pregnancy should be discussed and the need for contraception evaluated.

Hematology: Exacerbation of porphyria has been observed rarely in epoetin alfa-treated patients with CRF. However, epoetin alfa has not caused increased urinary excretion of porphyrin metabolites in normal volunteers, even in the presence of a rapid erythropoietic response. Nevertheless, epoetin alfa should be used with caution in patients with known porphyria.

In preclinical studies in dogs and rats, but not in monkeys, epoetin alfa therapy was associated with subclinical bone marrow fibrosis. Bone marrow fibrosis is a known complication of CRF in humans and may be related to secondary hyperparathyroidism or unknown factors. The incidence of bone marrow fibrosis was not increased in a study of patients on dialysis who were treated with epoetin alfa for 12-19 months, compared to the incidence of bone marrow fibrosis in a matched group of patients who had not been treated with epoetin alfa.

Hematocrit in CRF patients should be measured twice a week; zidovudine-treated HIV-infected and cancer patients should have hematocrit measured once a week until hematocrit has been stabilized, and measured periodically thereafter.

Delayed or Diminished Response: If the patient fails to respond or to maintain a response to doses within the recommended dosing range, the following etiologies should be considered and evaluated:

PRECAUTIONS: *(cont'd)*

1. **Iron deficiency:** Virtually all patients will eventually require supplemental iron therapy (see Iron Evaluation.)
2. Underlying infectious, inflammatory, or malignant processes.
3. Occult blood loss.
4. Underlying hematologic disease (*i.e.,* thalassemia, refractory anemia, or other myelodysplastic disorders).
5. **Vitamin deficiencies:** folic acid or vitamin B12.
6. Hemolysis.
7. Aluminum intoxication.
8. Osteitis fibrosa cystica.

Iron Evaluation: During epoetin alfa therapy, absolute or functional iron deficiency may develop. Functional iron deficiency, with normal ferritin levels but low transferrin saturation, is presumably due to the inability to mobilize iron stores rapidly enough to support increased erythropoiesis. Transferrin saturation should be at least 20% and ferritin should be at least 100 ng/ml.

Prior to and during epoetin alfa therapy, the patient's iron status, including transferrin saturation (serum iron divided by iron binding capacity) and serum ferritin, should be evaluated. Virtually all patients will eventually require supplemental iron to increase or maintain transferrin saturation to levels which will adequately support epoetin alfa-stimulated erythropoiesis. All surgery patients being treated with epoetin alfa should receive adeqate iron supplementation throughout the course of therapy in oder to support erythropoesis and avoid depletion of iron stores.

Carcinogenesis, Mutagenesis, and Impairment of Fertility

Carcinogenic potential of epoetin alfa has not been evaluated. Epoetin alfa does not induce bacterial gene mutation (Ames Test), chromosomal aberrations in mammalian cells, micronuclei in mice, or gene mutation at the HGPRT locus. In female rats treated intravenously with epoetin alfa, there was a trend for slightly increased fetal wastage at doses of 100 and 500 Units/kg.

Pregnancy: Pregnancy Category C

Epoetin alfa has been shown to have adverse effects in rats when given in doses five times the human dose. There are no adequate and well-controlled studies in pregnant women. Epoetin alfa should be used during pregnancy only if potential benefit justifies the potential risk to the fetus.

In studies in female rats, there were decreases in body weight gain, delays in appearance of abdominal hair, delayed eyelid opening, delayed ossification, and decreases in the number of caudal vertebrae in the F1 fetuses of the 500 Units/kg group. In female rats treated intravenously, there was a trend for slightly increased fetal wastage at doses of 100 and 500 Units/kg. Epoetin alfa has not shown any adverse effect at doses as high as 500 Units/kg in pregnant rabbits (from day 6 to 18 of gestation).

Nursing Mothers

Postnatal observations of the live offspring (F1 generation) of female rats treated with epoetin alfa during gestation and lactation revealed no effect of epoetin alfa at doses of up to 500 Units/kg. There were, however, decreases in body weight gain, delays in appearance of abdominal hair, eyelid opening, and decreases in the number of caudal vertebrae in the F1 fetuses of the 500 Units/kg group. There were no epoetin alfa-related effects on the F2 generation fetuses.

It in not known whether epoetin alfa is excreted in human milk. Because many drugs are excreted in human milk, caution should be exercised when epoetin alfa is administered to a nursing woman.

Pediatric Use

The safety and effectiveness of epoetin alfa in children have not been established (see WARNINGS.)

CHRONIC RENAL FAILURE PATIENTS

Patients with CRF Not Requiring Dialysis: Blood pressure and hematocrit should be monitored no less frequently than for patients maintained on dialysis. Renal function and fluid and electrolyte balance should be closely monitored, as an improved sense of well-being may obscure the need to initiate dialysis in some patients.

Hematology: Sufficient time should be allowed to determine a patient's responsiveness to a dosage of epoetin alfa before adjusting the dose. Because of the time required for erythropoiesis and the red cell half-life, an interval of 2-6 weeks may occur between the time of a dose adjustment (initiation, increase, decrease, or discontinuation) and a significant change in hematocrit.

In order to avoid reaching the suggested target hematocrit too rapidly, or exceeding the suggested target range (hematocrit of 30-36%), the guidelines for dose and frequency of dose adjustments (see DOSAGE AND ADMINISTRATION) should be followed.

For patients who respond to epoetin alfa with a rapid increase in hematocrit (*e.g.,* more than 4 points in any two-week period), the dose of epoetin alfa should be reduced because of the possible association of excessive rate of rise of hematocrit with an exacerbation of hypertension.

The elevated bleeding time characteristic of CRF decreases toward normal after correction of anemia in epoetin alfa-treated patients. Reduction of bleeding time also occurs after correction of anemia by transfusion.

Laboratory Monitoring: The hematocrit should be determined twice a week until it has stabilized in the suggested target range and the maintenance dose has been established. After any dose adjustment, the hematocrit should also be determined twice weekly for at least 2-6 weeks until it has been determined that the hematocrit has stabilized in response to the dose change. The hematocrit should then be monitored at regular intervals.

A complete blood count with differential and platelet count should be performed regularly. During clinical trials, modest increases were seen in platelets and while blood cell counts. While these changes were statistically significant, they were not clinically significant and the values remained within normal ranges.

In patients with CRF, serum chemistry values [including blood urea nitrogen (BUN), uric acid, creatinine, phosphorus, and potassium] should be monitored regularly. During clinical trials in patients on dialysis, modest increases were seen in BUN, creatinine, phosphorus, and potassium. In some patients with CRF not on dialysis, treated with epoetin alfa, modest increases in serum uric acid and phosphorus were observed. While changes were statistically significant, the values remained within the ranges normally seen in patients with CRF.

Diet: As the hematocrit increases and patients experience an improved sense of well-being and quality of life, the importance of compliance with dietary and dialysis prescriptions should be reinforced. In particular, hyperkalemia is not uncommon in patients with CRF. In U.S. studies in patients on dialysis, hyperkalemia has occurred at an annualized rate of approximately 0.11 episodes per patient-year of epoetin alfa therapy, often in association with poor compliance to medication, dietary, and/or dialysis prescriptions.

PRECAUTIONS: *(cont'd)*

Dialysis Management: Therapy with epoetin alfa results in an increase in hematocrit and a decrease in plasma volume which could affect dialysis efficiency. In studies to date, the resulting increase in hematocrit did not appear to adversely affect dialyzer function[9,10] or the efficiency of high flux hemodialysis.[11]During hemodialysis, patients treated with epoetin alfa may require increased anticoagulation with heparin to prevent clotting of the artificial kidney.

Patients who are marginally dialyzed may require adjustments in their dialysis prescription. As with all patients on dialysis, the serum chemistry values [including blood urea nitrogen (BUN), creatinine, phosphorus, and potassium] in epoetin alfa-treated patients should be monitored regularly to assure the adequacy of the dialysis prescription.

Information for the Patient: In those situations in which the physician determines that a home dialysis patient can safely and effectively self-administer epoetin alfa, the patient should be instructed as to the proper dosage and administration. Home dialysis patients should be referred to the full "Information for Home Dialysis Patients" section; it is not a disclosure of all possible effects. Patients should be informed of the signs and symptoms of allergic drug reaction and advised of appropriate actions. If home use is prescribed for a home dialysis patient, the patient should be thoroughly instructed in the importance of proper disposal and cautioned against the reuse of needles, syringes, or drug product. A puncture-resistant container for the disposal of used syringes and needles should be available to the patient. The full container should be disposed of according to the directions provided by the physician.

Renal Function: In patients with CRF not on dialysis, renal function and fluid and electrolyte balance should be closely monitored, as an improved sense of well-being may obscure the need to initiate dialysis in some patients. In patients with CRF not on dialysis, placebo-controlled studies of progression of renal dysfunction over periods of greater than one year have not been completed. In shorter term trials in patients with CRF not on dialysis, changes in creatinine and creatinine clearance were not significantly different in epoetin alfa-treated patients, compared with placebo-treated patients. Analysis of the slope of 1/serum creatinine versus time plots in these patients indicates no significant change in the slope after the initiation of epoetin alfa therapy.

ZIDOVUDINE-TREATED HIV-INFECTED PATIENTS

Hypertension: Exacerbation of hypertension has not been observed in zidovudine-treated HIV-infected patients treated with epoetin alfa. However, epoetin alfa should be withheld in these patients if pre-existing hypertension is uncontrolled, and should not be started until blood pressure is controlled. In double-blind studies, a single seizure has been experienced by an epoetin alfa-treated patient.[19]

CANCER PATIENTS ON CHEMOTHERAPY

Hypertension: Hypertension, associated with a significant increase in hematocrit, has been noted rarely in epoetin alfa-treated cancer patients. Nevertheless, blood pressure in epoetin alfa-treated patients should be monitored carefully, particularly in patients with an underlying history of hypertension or cardiovascular disease.

Seizures: In double-blind, placebo-controlled trials, 3.2% (n=2/63) of epoetin alfa-treated patients and 2.9% (n=2/68) of placebo-treated patients had seizures. Seizures in 1.6% (n=1/63) of epoetin alfa-treated patients occurred in the context of a significant increase in blood pressure and hematocrit from baseline values. However, both epoetin alfa- treated patients also had underlying CNS pathology which may have been related to seizure activity.

Thrombotic Events: In double-blind, placebo-controlled trials, 3.2% (n=2/63) of epoetin alfa-treated patients and 11.8% (n=8/68) of placebo-treated patients had thrombotic events (*e.g.,* pulmonary embolism, cerebrovascular accident).

Growth Factor Potential: Epoetin alfa is a growth factor that primarily stimulates red cell production. However, the possibility that epoetin alfa can act as a growth factor for any tumor type, particularly myeloid malignancies, cannot be excluded.

SURGERY PATIENTS

Thrombotic/Vascular Events: In perioperative clinical trials with orthopedic patients, the overall incidence of thrombotic/vascular events was similar in epoetin alfa and placebo-treated patients who had a pretreatment hemoglobin of >10 to ≤13 g/dl. In patients with a hemoglobin of >13 g/dl treated with 300 Units/kg of epoetin alfa, and he possibility that epoetin alfa treatment may be associated with an increased risk of postoperative thrombotic/vascular events cannot be excluded.[14-16]

In one study in which epoetin alfa was administered in the perioperative period to patients undergoing coronary artery bypass graft surgery, there were seven deaths in the group treated with epoetin alfa (n=126) and no deaths in the placebo-treated group. Among the seven deaths in the patients treated with epoetin alfa, four were at the time of therapy (between study day 2 and 8). The four deaths at the time of therapy (3%) were associated with thrombotic/vascular events. A causative role in epoetin alfa cannot be excluded (see WARNINGS).

Hypertension: Blood pressure may rise in the perioperative period in patients being treated with epoetin alfa. Therefore, blood pressure should be monitored carefully.

DRUG INTERACTIONS:

No evidence of interaction of epoetin alfa with other drugs was observed in the course of clinical trials.

ADVERSE REACTIONS:

CHRONIC RENAL FAILURE PATIENTS

Epoetin alfa is generally well-tolerated. The adverse events reported are frequent sequelae of CRF and are not necessarily attributable to epoetin alfa therapy. In double-blind, placebo-controlled studies involving over 300 patients with CRF, the events reported in greater than 5% of epoetin alfa-treated patients during the blinded phase can be seen in TABLE 3.

TABLE 3

Event	Percent of Patients Reporting Event: Epoetin alfa -Treated Patients (N=200)	Placebo-Treated Patients (N=135)
Hypertension	24%	19%
Headache	16%	12%
Arthralgias	11%	6%
Nausea	11%	9%
Edema	9%	10%
Fatigue	9%	14%
Diarrhea	9%	6%
Vomiting	8%	5%
Chest Pain	7%	9%
Skin reaction (administration site)	7%	12%
Asthenia	7%	12%
Dizziness	7%	13%
Clotted access	7%	2%

Significant adverse events of concern in patients with CRF treated in double-blind, placebo-controlled trials occurred in patients during the blinded phase of the studies as seen in TABLE 4.

ADVERSE REACTIONS: *(cont'd)*

TABLE 4

Seizure	1.1%	1.1%
CVA/TIA	0.4%	0.6%
MI	0.4%	1.1%
Death	0	1.7%

In the U.S. epoetin alfa studies in patients on dialysis (over 567 patients), the incidence (number of events per patient-year) of the most frequently reported adverse events were: hypertension (0.75), headache (0.40), tachycardia (0.31), nausea/vomiting (0.26), clotted vascular access (0.25), shortness of breath (0.14), hyperkalemia (0.11), and diarrhea (0.11). Other reported events occurred at a rate of less than 0.10 events per patient per year.

Events reported to have occurred within several hours of administration of epoetin alfa were rare, mild, and transient, and included injection site stinging in dialysis patients and flu-like symptoms such as arthralgias and myalgias.

In all studies analyzed to date, epoetin alfa administration was generally well-tolerated, irrespective of the route of administration.

Hypertension: Increases in blood pressure have been reported in clinical trials, often during the first 90 days of therapy. On occasion, hypertensive encephalopathy and seizures have been observed in patients with CRF treated with epoetin alfa. When data from all patients in the U.S. Phase III multicenter trial were analyzed, there was an apparent trend of more reports of hypertensive adverse events in patients on dialysis with a faster rate of rise of hematocrit (greater than 4 hematocrit points in any two-week period). However, in a double-blind, placebo-controlled trial, hypertensive adverse events were not reported at an increased rate in the epoetin alfa-treated group (150 units/kg three times weekly) relative to the placebo group.

Seizures: There have been 47 seizures in 1010 patients on dialysis treated with epoetin alfa in clinical trials, with an exposure of 986 patient-years for a rate of approximately 0.048 events per patient-year. However, there appeared to be a higher rate of seizures during the first 90 days of therapy (occurring in approximately 2.5% of patients) when compared to subsequent 90-day periods. The baseline incidence of seizures in the untreated dialysis population is difficult to determine; it appears to be in the range of 5-10% per patient-year.[26-28]

Thrombotic Events: In clinical trials where the maintenance hematocrit was 35 ± 3% on epoetin alfa, clotting of the vascular access (A-V- shunt) has occurred at an annualized rate of about 0.25 events per patient-year, and other thrombotic events (*e.g.,* myocardial infarction, cerebrovascular accident, transient ischemic attack, and pulmonary embolism) occurred at a rate of less than 0.04 events per patient-year. In a separate study of 1111 untreated dialysis patients, clotting of the vascular access occurred at a rate of 0.50 events per-patient-year. However, in CRF patients on hemodialysis who also had clinically evident ischemic heart disease or congestive heart failure, the risk of A-V shunt thrombosis was higher (39% vs 29%), p<0.001), and myocardial infarctions, vascular ischemic events, and venous thrombosis were increased, in patients targeted to a hematocrit of 42 ± 3% compared to those maintained at 30 ± 3% (see WARNINGS).

In patients treated with commercial epoetin alfa, there have been rare reports of serious or unusual thrombo-embolic events including migratory thrombophlebitis, microvascular thrombosis, pulmonary embolus, and thrombosis of the retinal artery, and temporal and renal veins. A causal relationship has not been established.

Allergic Reactions: There have been no reports of serious allergic reactions or anaphylaxis associated with epoetin alfa administration during clinical trials. Skin rashes and urticaria have been observed rarely and when reported have generally been mild and transient in nature.

There have been rare reports of potentially serious allergic reactions including urticaria with associated respiratory symptoms or circumoral edema or urticaria alone. Most reactions occurred in situations where a causal relationship could not be established. Symptoms recurred with rechallenge in a few instances, suggesting that allergic reactivity may occasionally be associated with epoetin alfa therapy.

There has been no evidence for development of antibodies to erythropoietin in patients tested to date, including those receiving epoetin alfa for over 4 years. Nevertheless, if an anaphylactoid reaction occurs, epoetin alfa should be immediately discontinued and appropriate therapy initiated.

ZIDOVUDINE-TREATED HIV-INFECTED PATIENTS

Adverse events reported in clinical trials with epoetin alfa in zidovudine-treated HIV-infected patients were consistent with the progression of HIV infection. In double-blind, placebo-controlled studies of three-months duration involving approximately 300 zidovudine-treated HIV-infected patients, adverse events with an incidence of ≥ 10% in either epoetin alfa-treated patients or placebo-treated patients as seen in TABLE 5.

TABLE 5 Epoetin alfa, Adverse Reactions

Event	Percent of Patients Reporting Event Epoetin alfa -Treated Patients (N=144)	Placebo-Treated Patients (N=153)
Pyrexia	38%	29%
Fatigue	25%	31%
Headache	19%	14%
Cough	18%	14%
Diarrhea	16%	18%
Rash	16%	8%
Congestion, Respiratory	15%	10%
Nausea	15%	12%
Shortness of Breath	14%	13%
Asthenia	11%	14%
Skin Reaction, Medication Site	10%	7%
Dizziness	9%	10%

There were no statistically significant differences between treatment groups in the incidence of the above events.

In the 297 patients studied, epoetin alfa was not associated with significant increases in opportunistic infections or mortality.[22] In 71 patients from this group treated with epoetin alfa at 150 Units/kg three times weekly, serum p24 antigen levels did not appear to increase.[25] Preliminary data showed no enhancement of HIV replication in infected cell lines *in vitro.*[19]

Peripheral white blood cell and platelet counts are unchanged following epoetin alfa therapy.

Allergic Reactions: Two zidovudine-treated HIV-infected patients had urticarial reactions within 48 hours of their first exposure to study medication. One patient was treated with epoetin alfa and one was treated with placebo (epoetin alfa vehicle alone). Both patients had positive immediate skin tests against their study medication with a negative saline control. The basis for this apparent pre-existing hypersensitivity to components of the epoetin alfa formulation is unknown, but may be related to HIV-induced immunosuppression or prior exposure to blood products.

ADVERSE REACTIONS: *(cont'd)*

Seizures: In double-blind and open label trials of epoetin alfa in zidovudine-treated HIV-infected patients, ten patients have experienced seizures.[22] In general, these seizures appear to be related to underlying pathology such as meningitis or cerebral neoplasms, not epoetin alfa therapy.

CANCER PATIENTS ON CHEMOTHERAPY

Adverse experiences reported in clinical trials with epoetin alfa in cancer patients were consistent with the underlying disease state. In double-blind, placebo-controlled studies of up to 3 months duration involving 131 cancer patients, adverse events with an incidence > 10% in either epoetin alfa-treated or placebo-treated patients can be seen in TABLE 6.

TABLE 6 Percent of Patients Reporting Event

Event	Percent of Patients Reporting Epoetin alfa-Treated Patients (n=63)	Placebo-Treated Patients (n=68)
Pyrexia	29%*	19%
Diarrhea	21%*	7%
Nausea	17%†	32%
Vomiting	17%	15%
Edema	17%‡	1%
Asthenia	13%	16%
Fatigue	13%	15%
Shortness of Breath	13%	9%
Paresthesia	11%	6%
Upper Respiratory Infection	11%	4%
Dizziness	5%	12%
Trunk Pain	3%§	16%

*p=0.041, †p=0.069, ‡p=0.0016, d§p=0.017

Although some statistically significant differences between epoetin alfa- and placebo-treated patients were noted, the overall safety profile of epoetin alfa appeared to be consistent with the disease process of advanced cancer. During double-blind and subsequent open-label therapy in which patients (N=72 for total epoetin alfa exposure) were treated for up to 32 weeks with doses as high as 927 Units/kg, the adverse experience profile of epoetin alfa was consistent with the progression of advanced cancer.

Based on comparable survival data and on the percentage of epoetin alfa- and placebo-treated patients who discontinued therapy due to death, disease progression, or adverse experiences (22% and 13%, respectively; p=0.25), the clinical outcome in the epoetin alfa- and placebo-treated patients appeared to be similar. Available data from animal tumor models and measurement of proliferation of solid tumor cells from clinical biopsy specimens in response to epoetin alfa suggest that epoetin alfa does not potentiate tumor growth. Nevertheless, as a growth factor, the possibility that epoetin alfa may potentiate growth of some tumors, particularly myeloid tumors, cannot be excluded. A randomized controlled Phase IV study is currently ongoing to further evaluate this issue.

The mean peripheral white blood cell count was unchanged following epoetin alfa therapy compared to the corresponding value in the placebo-treated group.

SURGERY PATIENTS

Adverse events with an incidence of ≥10% are shown in TABLE 7.

TABLE 7 Percent of Patients Reporting Event

Event	Patients Treated With : Epoetin alfa 300 U/kg (n=112)*	Epoetin alfa 100 U/kg (n=101)*	Placebo (n=103)*	Epoetin alfa 600 U/kg (n=73)†	Epoetin alfa 300 U/kg (n=72)†
Pyrexia	51%	50%	60%	47%	42%
Nausea	48%	43%	45%	45%	58%
Constipation	43%	42%	43%	51%	53%
Skin reaction, Medication site	25%	19%	22%	26%	29%
Vomiting	22%	12%	14%	21%	29%
Skin pain	18%	18%	17%	5%	4%
Pruritis	16%	16%	14%	14%	22%
Insomnia	13%	16%	13%	21%	18%
Headache	13%	11%	9%	10%	19%
Dizziness	12%	9%	12%	11%	21%
Urinary tract infection	12%	3%	11%	11%	8%
Hypertension	10%	11%	10%	5%	10%
Diarrhea	10%	7%	12%	10%	6%
Deep venous thrombosis	10%	3%	5%	0%‡	0%‡
Dyspepsia	9%	11%	6%	7%	8%
Anxiety	7%	2%	11%	11%	4%
Edema	6%	11%	8%	11%	7%

* Study including patients undergoing orthopedic surgery treated with epoetin alfa or placebo for 15 days
† Study including patients undergoing orthopedic surgery treated with epoetin alfa 600 Units/kg weekly x 4 or 300 Units/kg daily x 15
‡ Determined by clinical symptoms

Thrombotic/Vascular Events: In three double-blind, placebo-controlled orthopedic surgery studies, the rate of deep venous thrombosis (DVT) was similar among epoetin alfa and placebo-treated patients in the recommended population of patients with a pretreatment hemoglobin of >10 to ≤13 g/dl.[14, 16, 24]

However, in 2 of 3 orthopedic surgery studies the overall rate (all pretreatment hemoglobin groups combined) of DVTs detected by postoperative ultrasonography and /or surveillance venography was higher in the group treated with epoetin alfa than in the placebo-treated group (11% vs 6%). This finding was attributable to the difference in DVT rates observed in the subgroup of patients with pretreatment hemoglobin > 13 g/dl. However, the incidence of DVTs was within the range of that reported in the literature for orthopedic surgery patients.

In the orthopedic surgery study of patients with pretreatment hemoglobin of >10 to ≤13 g/dl which compared two dosing regimens (600 Units/kg weekly x 4 and 300 Units/kg daily x 15), 4 subjects in the 600 Units/kg weekly epoetin alfa group (5%) and no subjects in the 300 Units/kg daily group had a thrombotic vascular event during the study period.[15]

In a study examining the use of epoetin alfa in 182 patients scheduled for coronary artery bypass graft surgery 23% of patients treated with epoetin alfa and 29% treated with placebo experienced thrombotic/vascular events. There were 4 deaths among the epoetin alfa-treated patients that were associated with a thrombotic/vascular event. A causative role of epoetin alfa cannot be excluded (see WARNINGS).

OVERDOSAGE:

The maximum amount of epoetin alfa that can be safely administered in single or multiple doses has not been determined. Doses of up to 1500 Units/kg three times weekly for 3-4 weeks have been administered without any direct toxic effects of epoetin alfa itself.[6] Therapy with epoetin alfa can result in polycythemia if the hematocrit is not carefully monitored and the dose appropriately adjusted. If the suggested target range is exceeded, epoetin alfa may be temporarily withheld until the hematocrit returns to the suggested target range; epoetin alfa therapy may then be resumed using a lower dose (see DOSAGE AND ADMINISTRATION.) If polycythemia is of concern, phlebotomy may be indicated to decrease the hematocrit.

DOSAGE AND ADMINISTRATION:

CHRONIC RENAL FAILURE PATIENTS

Starting doses of epoetin alfa over the range of 50-100 Units/kg three times weekly (three times weekly) have been shown to be safe and effective in increasing hematocrit and eliminating transfusion dependency in patients with CRF (see CLINICAL STUDIES). The dose of epoetin alfa should be reduced as the hematocrit approaches 36% or increases by more than 4 points in any 2-week period. The dosage of epoetin alfa must be individualized to maintain the hematocrit within the suggested target range. At the physician's discretion, the suggested target hematocrit range may be expanded to achieve maximal patient benefit.

Epoetin alfa may be given either as an intravenous or subcutaneous injection. In patients on hemodialysis, epoetin alfa usually has been administered as an IV bolus three times weekly While the administration of epoetin alfa is independent of the dialysis procedure, epoetin alfa may be administered into the venous line at the end of the dialysis procedure to obviate the need for additional venous access. In patients with CRF not on dialysis, epoetin alfa may be given either as an IV or subcutaneous injection.

Patients who have been judged competent by their physicians to self-administer epoetin alfa without medical or other supervision may give themselves either an IV or SC injection. TABLE 7 provides general therapeutic guidelines for patients with CRF.

TABLE 7

Starting Dose:	50-100 Units/kg T.I.W.; IV or subcutaneous
Reduce Dose When:	1. Hct. approaches 36% or, 2. Hct. increases > 4 points in any 2-week period
Increase Dose If:	Hct. does not increase by 5-6 points after 8 weeks of therapy, and hct. is below suggested target range.
Maintenance Dose:	Individually titrate
Suggested Target Hct. Range:	30-36%

During therapy, hematological parameters should be monitored regularly (see Laboratory Monitoring.)

Pre-Therapy Iron Evaluation: Prior to and during epoetin alfa therapy, the patient's iron stores, including transferrin saturation (serum iron divided by iron binding capacity) and serum ferritin, should be evaluated. Transferrin saturation should be at least 20%, and ferritin should be at least 100 ng/ml. Virtually all patients will eventually require supplemental iron to increase or maintain transferrin saturation to levels that will adequately support epoetin alfa-stimulated erythropoiesis.

Dose Adjustment: Following epoetin alfa therapy, a period of time is required for erythroid progenitors to mature and be released into circulation resulting in an eventual increase in hematocrit. Additionally, red blood cell survival time affects hematocrit and may vary due to uremia. As a result, the time required to elicit a clinically significant change in hematocrit (increase or decrease) following any dose adjustment may be at 2-6 weeks.

Dose adjustment should not be made more frequently than once a month, unless clinically indicated. After any dose adjustment, the hematocrit should be determined twice weekly for at least 2-6 weeks (see Laboratory Monitoring.)

If the hematocrit is increasing and approaching 36%, the dose should be reduced to maintain the suggested target hematocrit range. If the reduced dose does not stop the rise in hematocrit, and it exceeds 36%, doses should be temporarily withheld until the hematocrit begins to decrease, at which point therapy should be reinitiated at a lower dose.

At any time, if the hematocrit increases by more than 4 points in a 2-week period, the dose should be immediately decreased. After the dose reduction, the hematocrit should be monitored twice weekly for 2-6 weeks, and further dose adjustments should be made as outlined in Maintenance Dose.

If a hematocrit increase of 5-6 points is not achieved after an 8-week period and iron stores are adequate (see Delayed or Diminished Response), the dose of epoetin alfa may be incrementally increased. Further increases may be made at 4-6 week intervals until the desired response is attained.

Maintenance Dose: The maintenance dose must be individualized for each patient on dialysis. In the U.S. Phase III multicenter trial in patients on hemodialysis, the median maintenance dose was 75 Units/kg three times weekly, with a range from 12.5 to 525 Units/kg three times weekly Almost 10% of the patients required a dose of 25 Units/kg, or less, and approximately 10% of the patients required more than 200 Units/kg three times weekly to maintain their hematocrit in the suggested target range.

If the hematocrit remains below, or falls below, the suggested target range, iron stores should be re-evaluated. If the transferrin saturation is less than 20%, supplemental iron should be administered. If the transferrin saturation is greater than 20%, the dose of epoetin alfa may be increased. Such dose increases should not be made more frequently than once a month, unless clinically indicated, as the response time of the hematocrit to a dose increase can be 2-6 weeks. Hematocrit should be measured twice weekly for 2-6 weeks following dose increases. In patients with CRF not on dialysis, the maintenance dose must also be individualized. Epoetin alfa doses of 75-150 Units/kg per week have been shown to maintain hematocrits of 36-38% for up to 6 months.

Delayed or Diminished Response: Over 95% of patients with CRF responded with clinically significant increases in hematocrit, and virtually all patients were transfusion-independent within approximately 2 months of initiation of epoetin alfa therapy.

If a patient fails to respond or maintain a response, other etiologies should be considered and evaluated as clinically indicated. See PRECAUTIONSfor discussion of delayed or diminished response.

ZIDOVUDINE-TREATED HIV-INFECTED PATIENTS

Prior to beginning epoetin alfa, it is recommended that the endogenous serum erythropoietin level be determined (prior to transfusion). Available evidence suggests that patients receiving zidovudine with endogenous serum erythropoietin levels > 500 mUnits/ml are unlikely to respond to therapy with epoetin alfa.

Starting Dose: For patients with serum erythropoietin levels ≤ 500 mUnits/ml who are receiving a dose of zidovudine ≤ 4200 mg/week, the recommended starting dose of epoetin alfa is 100 Units/kg as an intravenous or subcutaneous injection three times weekly (three times weekly) for 8 weeks.

DOSAGE AND ADMINISTRATION: *(cont'd)*

Increase Dose: During the dose adjustment phase of therapy, the hematocrit should be monitored weekly. If the response is not satisfactory in terms of reducing transfusion requirements or increasing hematocrit after 8 weeks of therapy, the dose of epoetin alfa can be increased by 50-100 Units/kg three times weekly Response should be evaluated every 4-8 weeks thereafter and the dose adjusted accordingly by 50-100 Units/kg increments three times weekly If patients have not responded satisfactorily to an epoetin alfa dose of 300 Units/kg three times weekly, it is unlikely that they will respond to higher doses of epoetin alfa.

Maintenance Dose: After attainment of the desired response (*i.e.,* reduced transfusion requirements or increased hematocrit), the dose of epoetin alfa should be titrated to maintain the response based on factors such as variations in zidovudine dose and the presence of intercurrent infectious or inflammatory episodes. If the hematocrit exceeds 40%, the dose should be discontinued until the hematocrit drops to 36%. The dose should be reduced by 25% when treatment is resumed and then titrated to maintain the desired hematocrit.

CANCER PATIENTS ON CHEMOTHERAPY

Baseline endogenous serum erythropoietin levels varied among patients in these trials with approximately 75% (N=83/110) having endogenous serum erythropoietin levels < 132 mUnits/ml, and approximately 4% (N=4/110) of patients having endogenous serum erythropoietin levels > 500 mUnits/ml. In general, patients with lower baseline serum erythropoietin levels responded more vigorously to epoetin alfa than patients with higher erythropoietin levels. Although no specific serum erythropoietin level can be stipulated above which patients would be unlikely to respond to epoetin alfa therapy, treatment of patients with grossly elevated serum erythropoietin levels (*e.g.,* > 200 mUnits/ml) is not recommended. The hematocrit should be monitored on a weekly basis in patients receiving epoetin alfa therapy until hematocrit becomes stable.

Starting Dose: The recommended starting dose of epoetin alfa is 150 Units/kg subcutaneously three times weekly

Dose Adjustment: If the response is not satisfactory in terms of reducing transfusion requirements or increasing hematocrit after 8 weeks of therapy, the dose of epoetin alfa can be increased up to 300 Units/kg three times weekly If patients have not responded satisfactorily to an epoetin alfa dose of 300 Units/kg three times weekly, it is unlikely that they will respond to higher doses of epoetin alfa. If the hematocrit exceeds 40%, the dose of epoetin alfa should be withheld until the hematocrit falls to 36%. The dose of epoetin alfa should be reduced by 25% when treatment is resumed and titrated to maintain the desired hematocrit. If the initial dose of epoetin alfa includes a very rapid hematocrit response (*e.g.,* an increase of more than 4 percentage points in any 2 week period), the dose of epoetin alfa should be reduced.

SURGERY PATIENTS

Prior to initializing treatment with epoetin alfa, a hemoglobin should be obtained to establish that it is >10 to ≤13 g/dl.[14] The recommended dose of epoetin alfa is 300 Units/kg/day subcutaneously for 10 days before surgery, on the day of surgery, and for 4 days after surgery.

An alternate dose schedule is 600 Units/kg epoetin alfa subcutaneously in once weekly doses (21, 14, and 7 days before surgery) plus a fourth dose on the day of surgery.[15]

All patients should receive adequate iron supplementation. Iron supplementation should be initiated no later than the beginning of treatment with epoetin alfa and should continue throughout the course of therapy.

PREPARATION AND ADMINISTRATION OF EPOETIN ALFA

1. Do not shake. It is not necessary to shake epoetin alfa. Prolonged vigorous shaking may denature any glycoprotein, rendering it biologically inactive.

2. Parenteral drug products should be inspected visually for particulate matter and discoloration prior to administration. Do not use any vials exhibiting particulate matter or discoloration.

3. Using aseptic techniques, attach a sterile needle to a sterile syringe. Remove the flip top from the vial containing epoetin alfa, and wipe the septum with a disinfectant. Insert the needle into the vial, and withdraw into the syringe an appropriate volume of solution.

4. Single-dose 1 ml vial contains no preservative. Use one dose per vial; do not re-enter the vial. Discard unused portions.

Multidose 2 ml vial contains preservative. Store at 2 to 8°C after initial entry and between doses. Discard 21 days after initial entry.

5. Do not dilute or administer in conjunction with other drug solutions. However, at the time of subcutaneous administration, preservative-free epoetin alfa from single-use vials may be admixed in a syringe with bacteriostatic 0.9% sodium chloride injection, USP, with benzyl alcohol 0.9% (bacteriostatic saline) at a 1:1 ratio using aseptic technique. The benzyl alcohol in the bacteriostatic saline acts as a local anesthetic which may ameliorate subcutaneous injection site discomfort.

REFERENCES:

1. Egrie JC, Strickland TW, Lane J, *et al.* (1986). "Characterization and Biological Effects of Recombinant Human Erythropoietin." *Immunobiol.* 72:213-224. **2.** Graber SE and Krantz SB (1978). "Erythropoietin and the Control of Red Cell Production." *Ann Rev Med.* 29:51-66. **3.** Eschbach JW and Adamson JW (1985). "Anemia of End-Stage Renal Disease (ESRD)." *Kidney Intl.*28:1-5. **4.** Eschbach JW, Egrie JC, Downing MR, *et al.* (1987). "Correction of the Anemia of End-Stage Renal Disease with Recombinant Human Erythropoietin." *NEJM.*316: 73-78. **5.** Eschbach JW, Abdulhadi MH, Browne JK, *et al.* (1989). "Recombinant Human Erythropoietin in Anemic Patients with End-Stage Renal Disease."*Ann Intern Med.*111:12. **6.** Eschbach JW, Egrie JC, Downing MR, *et al.* (1989). "The Use of Recombinant Human Erythropoietin (r-HuEPO): Effect in End-Stage Renal Disease (ESRD)." *Prevention of Chronic Uremia* (Friedman, Beyer, DeSanto, Giordano, eds.), Field and Wood Inc., Philadelphia, PA, pp 148-155. **7.** Egrie JC, Eschbach JW, McGuire T, and Adamson JW (1988). "Pharmacokinetics of Recombinant Human Erythropoietin (r-HuEPO) Administered to Hemodialysis (HD) Patients." *Kidney Intl.* 33:262. **8.** Evans RW, Radar B, Manninen DL, *et al.* (1990). "The Quality of Life of Hemodialysis Recipients Treated with Recombinant Human Erythropoietin." *JAMA.*263:6. **9.** Paganini E, Garcia J, Ellis P, *et al.* (1988)."Clinical Sequelae of Correction of Anemia with Recombinant Human Erythropoietin (r-HuEPO); Urea Kinetics, Dialyzer Function and Reuse."*Am J Kid Dis.* 11:16. **10.** Delano BG, Lundin AP, Golansky R, *et al.* (1988). "Dialyzer Urea and Creatinine Clearances Not Significantly Changed in r-HuEPO Treated Maintenance Hemodialysis (MD) Patients." *Kidney Intl.* 33:219. **11.** Stivelman J, Van Wyck D, and Ogden D (1988). "Use of Recombinant Erythropoietin (r-HuEPO) with High Flux Dialysis (HFD) Does Not Worsen Azotemia or Shorten Access Survival." *Kidney Intl.*33:239. **12.** Lim VS, DeGowin RL, Zavala D, *et al.* (1989). "Recombinant Human Erythropoietin Treatment in Pre-Dialysis Patients: A Double-Blind Placebo Controlled Trial." *Ann Int Med.*110:108-114. **13.** Stone WJ, Graber SE, Krantz SB, *et al.* (1988). "Treatment of the Anemia of Pre- Dialysis Patients with Recombinant Human Erythropoietin: A Randomized, Placebo-Controlled Trial." *Am J Med Sci.* 296:171-179. **14.** deAndrade JR and Jove M (1996) "Baseline Hemoglobin as a Predictor of Risk of Transfusion and Response to Epoetin Alfa in Orthopedic Surgery Patients" *Am J of Orthoped.*;25 (8):533-542. **15.** Goldberg MA and McCutchen JW. (1996) "Safety and Efficacy Comparison Study of Two Dosing Regimens of Epoetin Alfa in Patients Undergoing Major Orthopedic Surgery" *Am J of Orthoped.*25 (8):544-552. **16.** Faris PM and Ritter MA (1996). "The effects of Recombinant Human Erythropoietin on Perioperative Transfusion Requirements in Patients Having a Major Orhtopedic Operation." *J. Bone and Joint Surgery.* 78-A:62-72. **17.** Lundin AP, Akerman MJH, Chesler RM, *et al.* (1991). "Exercise in Hemodialysis Patients after Treatment with Recombinant Human Erythropoietin." *Nephron.*58:315-319. **18.** Amgen Inc., Data on file **19.** Eschbach JW, Kelly MR, Galey NR, *et al.* (1989). "Treatment of the Anemia of Progressive Renal Failure with Recombinant Human Erythropoietin." *NEJM.*321:158-163. **20.** The US Recombinant Human Erythropoietin Predialysis Study Group (1991). "Double-Blind, Placebo-Controlled Study of the Therapeutic Use of Recombinant Human Erythropoietin for Anemia Associated with Chronic Renal Failure in Predialysis Patients." *Am J Kid Dis.*18(1):50-59. **21.** Danna RP, Rudnick SA, and Abels RI (1990). "Erythropoietin Therapy for the Anemia Associated with AIDS and AIDS Therapy and Cancer."*Erythropoietin in Clinical Applications - An International Perspective* (MB Garnick, ed.), Marcel Dekker, New York, NY, pp 301- 324. **22.** Ortho Biologics, Inc., Data on file **23.** Fischl M, Galpin JE, Levine JD, *et al.* (1990). "Recombinant Human Erythropoietin for Patients with AIDS Treated with Zidovudine."*NEJM.* 322:1488-1493. **24.** Laupacis A. (1993) "Effectiveness of Perioperative Recombinant Human Erythropoietin in Elective Hip Replacement." *Lancet.* 341:1228-1232. **25.** Kerr DN (1979) "Chronic Renal Failure." *Cecil Textbook of Medicine* (Beeson PB, McDermott W, Wyngaarden JB, eds.), W.B. Saunders, Philadelphia, PA, pp 1351-1367. **26.** Raskin NH and Fishman RA (1976). "Neurologic Disorders in Renal Failure (First

REFERENCES: *(cont'd)*

of Two Parts).' *NEJM.* 294:143-148. **27.** Raskin NH and Fishman RA (1976). 'Neurologic Disorder in Renal Failure (Second of Two Parts).' *NEJM.* 294:204-210. **28.** Messing RO and Simon RP (1986). 'Seizures as a Manifestation of Systemic Disease.' *Neurologic Clinics.*4:563-584.

PATIENT PACKAGE INSERT:

WHAT IS EPOETIN ALFA AND HOW DOES IT WORK?

Epoetin alfa is a copy of human erythropoietin, a hormone produced primarily by healthy kidneys. Epoetin alfa replaces the erythropoietin that the failed kidneys can no longer produce, and signals the bone marrow to make the oxygen-carrying red blood cells once again. Epoetin alfa is produced in mammalian cells that have been genetically altered by the addition of a gene for the natural substance erythropoietin.

HOW SHOULD I TAKE EPOETIN ALFA?

In those situations where your doctor has determined that you, as a home dialysis patient, can self-administer epoetin alfa, you will receive instruction on how much epoetin alfa to use, how to inject it, how often you should inject it, and how you should dispose of the unused portions of each vial.

You will be instructed to monitor your blood pressure carefully everyday and to report any changes outside of the guidelines that your doctor has given you. When a number of red blood cells increases, your blood pressure can also increase, so your doctor may prescribe some new or additional blood pressure medication. Be sure to follow your doctor's orders. You may also be instructed to have certain laboratory tests, such as additional hematocrit or iron level measurements, done more frequently. You may be asked to report these tests to your doctor or dialysis center. Also, your doctor may prescribe additional iron for you to take. Be sure to comply with your doctor's orders.

Continue to check your access, as your doctor has shown you, to make sure it is working. Be sure to let your health care professional know right away if there is a problem.

ALLERGY TO EPOETIN ALFA

Patients occasionally experience redness, swelling, or itching at the site of injection of epoetin alfa. This may indicate an allergy to the components of epoetin alfa, or it may indicate a local reaction. If you have a local reaction, consult your doctor. A potentially more serious reaction would be a generalized allergy to epoetin alfa, which could cause a rash over the whole body, shortness of breath, wheezing, reduction in blood pressure, fast pulse, or sweating. Severe cases of generalized allergy may be life-threatening. If you think you are having a generalized allergic reaction, stop taking epoetin alfa and notify a doctor or emergency medical personnel immediately.

HOW WILL I KNOW IF EPOETIN ALFA IS WORKING?

The effectiveness of epoetin alfa is measured by the increase in hematocrit (the amount of red blood cells in the blood) that results from epoetin alfa therapy. The rise in hematocrit is not immediate. It usually takes about 2 to 6 weeks before the hematocrit starts to rise. The amount of time it takes, and the dose of epoetin alfa that is needed to make the hematocrit increase, varies from patient to patient.

WHAT IS THE MOST IMPORTANT INFORMATION I SHOULD KNOW ABOUT EPOETIN ALFA AND CHRONIC RENAL FAILURE?

Epoetin alfa has been prescribed for you by your doctor because you:

1. Have anemia due to your kidney disease.

2. Are able to dialyze at home.

3. Have been determined to be able to administer epoetin alfa without direct medical or other supervision.

A lack of energy or feeling of tiredness is the major symptom of anemia. Additional symptoms include shortness of breath, chest pain, and feeling cold all the time. The reason for these symptoms is that there is a lack of red blood cells. Red blood cells carry oxygen, which is important for all of the body's functions. When there are fewer red blood cells, the body does not get all the oxygen it needs.

Kidneys remove toxins from the blood; they also measure the amount of oxygen in the blood. If there is not enough oxygen, the kidneys will produce a hormone called erythropoietin. Erythropoietin is released into the bloodstream and travels to the bone marrow where red blood cells are made. Erythropoietin signals the bone marrow to make more oxygen-carrying red blood cells.

As the kidneys fail, they stop cleansing toxins from your body. They also make less erythropoietin than they should. Therefore, the bone marrow does not receive a strong-enough signal to make the oxygen-carrying red blood cells. Fewer red blood cells are produced so the muscles, brain, and other parts of the body do not get the oxygen they need to function properly.

Most patients treated with epoetin alfa no longer need blood transfusions. However, certain medical conditions, or unexpected blood loss, may result in the need for a transfusion.

WHAT DO I NEED TO KNOW IF I AM GIVING MYSELF EPOETIN ALFA INJECTIONS?

When you receive your epoetin alfa from the dialysis center, doctor's office or home dialysis supplier, always check to see that:

1. The name Epogen appears on the carton and vial label.

2. You will be able to use epoetin alfa before the expiration date stamped on the package.

The epoetin alfa solution in the vial should always be clear and colorless. Do not use epoetin alfa if the contents of the vial appear discolored or cloudy, or if the vial appears to contain lumps, flakes, or particles. In addition, if the vial has been shaken vigorously, the solution may appear to be frothy and should not be used. Therefore, care should be taken not to shake the epoetin alfa vial vigorously before use.

Single Use Vials -S: If you have been prescribed epogen vials for single use, your vial will have a capital 'S' with a number next to it identifying the concentration of epoetin alfa in the vial, printed in a colored dot on the front left side of the label (for example, 'S2' identifies a single use vial with 2000 Units/ml). Single use means the vial cannot be used more than once, and any unused portion of the vial should be discarded as directed by your doctor or dialysis center.

Mulitdose Use Vials -M: If you have been prescribed epogen multidose vials, your vial will have a capital 'M' with a number under it identifying the concentration of epoetin alfa in the vial, printed in a colored dot on the front left side of the label (for example, 'M10' identifies a Multidose vial with 10,000 Units/ml). Multidose epogen can be used to inject multiple doses as prescribed by your doctor, and may be stored in the refrigerator (but not the freezing compartment) between doses for up to 21 days. Follow your doctor's or dialysis center's instructions on what to do with the used vials.

HOW SHOULD I STORE EPOETIN ALFA?

Epoetin alfa should be stored in the refrigerator, but not in the freezing compartment. DO not let the vial freeze and do not leave it in direct sunlight. Do not use a vial of epoetin alfa that as been frozen or after the expiration date that is stamped on the label. If you have any questions about the safety of a vial of epoetin alfa that has been subjected to temperature extremes, be sure to check with your dialysis unit staff.

PATIENT PACKAGE INSERT: *(cont'd)*

ALWAYS USE THE CORRECT SYRINGE

Your doctor has instructed you on how to give yourself the correct dosage of epoetin alfa. This dosage will usually be measured in Units per milliliter or CCs. It is important to use a syringe that is marked in tenths of milliliters (for example, 0.2 ml or CC). Failure to use the proper syringe can lead to a mistake in dosage, and you may receive too much or too little epoetin alfa. Too little epoetin alfa may not be effective in increasing your hematocrit, and too much epoetin alfa may lead to a hematocrit that is too high. Only use disposable syringes and needles as they do not require sterilization; they should be used once and disposed of as instructed by your doctor.

IMPORTANT: TO HELP AVOID CONTAMINATION AND POSSIBLE INFECTION, FOLLOW THESE INSTRUCTIONS EXACTLY.

PREPARING THE DOSE

1. Wash your hands thoroughly with soap and water before preparing the medication.

2. Check the date on the epoetin alfa vial to be sure that the drug has not expired.

3. Remove the vial of epoetin alfa from the refrigerator and allow it to reach room temperature. Unless you are using a mulitdose vial, each epoetin alfa vial is designed to be used only once. It is not necessary to shake epoetin alfa. Prolonged vigorous shaking may damage the product. Assemble the other supplies you will need for your injection.

4. Hemodialysis patients should wipe off the venous port of the hemodialysis tubing with an antiseptic swab. Peritoneal dialysis patients should cleanse the skin with an antiseptic swab where the injection is to be made.

5. Flip off the red protective cap but do not remove the gray rubber stopper. Wipe the top of the gray rubber stopper with an antiseptic swab.

6. Using a syringe and needle designed for subcutaneous injection, draw air into the syringe by pulling back on the plunger. The amount of air should be equal to your epoetin alfa dose.

7. Carefully remove the needle cover. Put the needle through the gray rubber stopper of the epoetin alfa vial.

8. Push the plunger in to discharge air into the vial. The air injected into the vial will allow epoetin alfa to be easily withdrawn into the syringe.

9. Turn the vial and syringe upside down in one hand. Be sure the tip of the needle is in the epoetin alfa solution. Your other hand will be free to move the plunger. Draw back on the plunger slowly to draw the correct dose of epoetin alfa into the syringe.

10. Check for air bubbles. The air is harmless, but too large an air bubble will reduce the epoetin alfa dose. To remove air bubbles, gently tap the syringe to move the air bubbles to the top of the syringe, then use the plunger to push the solution and the air back into the vial. Then remeasure your correct dose of epoetin alfa.

11. Double check your dose. Remove the needle from the vial. Do not lay the syringe down or allow the needle to touch anything.

INJECTING THE DOSE

Patients on home hemodialysis using the intravenous injection route:

1. Insert the needle of the syringe into the previously cleansed venous port and inject the epoetin alfa.

2. Remove the syringe and dispose of the whole unit. **Use the disposable syringe only once.**Dispose of syringes and needles as directed by your doctor, by following these simple steps:

Place all used needles and syringes in a hard plastic container with a screw-on-cap, or a metal container with a plastic lid, such as a coffee can properly labeled as to content. If a metal container is used, cut a hole in the plastic lid and tape the lid to the metal container. If a hard-plastic container is used, always screw the cap on tightly after each use. When the container is full, tape around the cap or lid, and dispose of according to your doctor's instructions.

Do not use glass or clear plastic containers, or any container that will be recycled or returned to a store.

Always store the container out of the reach of children.

Please check with your doctor, nurse, or pharmacist for other suggestions. There may be special state and local laws that they will discuss with you.

Patients on home peritoneal dialysis or home hemodialysis using the subcutaneous route:

1. With one hand, stabilize the previously cleansed skin by spreading it or by pinching up a large area with your free hand.

2. Hold the syringe with the other hand, as you would a pencil. Double check that the correct amount of epoetin alfa is in the syringe. Insert the needle straight into the skin (90 degree angle). Pull the plunger back slightly. If blood comes into the syringe, do not inject epoetin alfa, as the needle has entered a blood vessel; withdraw the syringe and inject at a different site. Inject the epoetin alfa by pushing the plunger all the way down.

3. Hold an antiseptic swab near the needle and pull the needle straight out of the skin. Press the antiseptic swab over the injection site for several seconds.

4. Use the disposable syringe only once. Dispose of syringes and needles as directed by your doctor, by following these simple steps:

Place all used needles and syringes in a hard plastic container with a screw-on-cap, or a metal container with a plastic lid, such as a coffee can properly labeled as to content. If a metal container is used, cut a small hole in the plastic lid and tape the lid to the metal container. If a hard-plastic container is used, always screw the cap on tightly after each use. When the container is full, tape around the cap or lid, and dispose of according to your doctor's instructions.

Do not use glass or clear plastic containers, or any container that will be recycled or returned to a store.

Always store the container out of the reach of children.

Please check with your doctor, nurse, or pharmacist for other suggestions. There may be special state and local laws that they will discuss with you.

5. Always change the site for each injection as directed. Occasionally a problem may develop at the injection site. If you notice a lump, swelling, or bruising that doesn't go away, contact your physician. You may wish to record the site just used so that you can keep track.

USAGE IN PREGNANCY

If you are pregnant or nursing a baby, consult your doctor before using epoetin alfa.

IMPORTANT NOTES

Since you are a home dialysis patient and your doctor allows you to self-administer epoetin alfa, please note the following:

1. Always follow the instructions of your doctor concerning dosage and administration of epoetin alfa. Do not change the dose or instructions for administration of epoetin alfa without consulting your doctor.

2. Your doctor will tell you what to do if you miss a dose of epoetin alfa. Always keep a spare syringe and needle on hand.

PATIENT PACKAGE INSERT: *(cont'd)*

3. Always consult your doctor if you notice anything unusual about your condition or your use of epoetin alfa.

HOW SUPPLIED:

Storage: Store at 2° to 8°C (36° to 46°F). Do not freeze or shake.

HOW SUPPLIED - EQUIVALENTS NOT AVAILABLE:

Injection, Solution - Intravenous; Su - 2,000 unit/ml

1 ml vials x 10	**$240.00**	**EPOGEN 2000 UNT/ML, Amgen**	**55513-0126-10**
1 ml x 6	$144.00	Procrit, Ortho Biotech	59676-0302-01
1 ml x 25	$600.00	Procrit, Ortho Biotech	59676-0302-02

Injection, Solution - Intravenous; Su - 3,000 unit/ml

1 ml vials x 10	**$360.00**	**EPOGEN 3000 UNT/ML, Amgen**	**55513-0267-10**
1 ml x 6	$216.00	Procrit, Ortho Biotech	59676-0303-01
1 ml x 25	$900.00	Procrit, Ortho Biotech	59676-0303-02

Injection, Solution - Intravenous; Su - 4,000 unit/ml

1 ml vials x 10	**$480.00**	**EPOGEN 4000 UNT/ML, Amgen**	**55513-0148-10**
1 ml x 6	$288.00	Procrit, Ortho Biotech	59676-0304-01
1 ml x 25	$1200.00	Procrit, Ortho Biotech	59676-0304-02

Injection, Solution - Intravenous; Su - 10,000 unit/ml

1 ml vials x 10	**$1200.00**	**EPOGEN 10000 UNT/ML, Amgen**	**55513-0144-10**
1 ml x 6	$684.00	Procrit, Ortho Biotech	59676-0310-01
1 ml x 25	$2850.00	Procrit, Ortho Biotech	59676-0310-02
2 ml	$228.00	Procrit, Ortho Biotech	59676-0312-01
2 ml x 10	**$2400.00**	**Epogen, Amgen**	**55513-0283-10**

EPOETIN BETA *(003223)*

CATEGORIES: Anemia; Antianemia Drugs; Blood Formation/Coagulation; Deficiency Anemias; Erythropoisis Enhancers; Hematopoietic Agents; Hemolysis; Orphan Drugs; Renal Drugs; Renal Failure; Recombinant DNA Origin; FDA Unapproved

BRAND NAMES: **Marogen**; *Recormon* (Europe)
(International brand names outside U.S. in italics)

Prescribing information not available at time of publication.

EPOPROSTENOL SODIUM *(003248)*

CATEGORIES: Orphan Drugs; Pulmonary Hypertension; FDA Class 1P ("Priority Review"); FDA Approved 1995 Sep

BRAND NAMES: **Flolan**

DESCRIPTION:

Flolan (epoprostenol sodium) for Injection is a sterile sodium salt formulated for intravenous administration. Each vial of Flolan contains epoprostenol sodium equivalent to either 0.5 mg (500,000 ng) or 1.5 mg (1,500,000 ng) epoprostenol, 3.76 mg glycine, 2.93 mg sodium chloride, and 50 mg mannitol. Sodium hydroxide may have been added to adjust pH.

Epoprostenol (PGI_2, PGX, prostacyclin), a metabolite of arachidonic acid, is a naturally occurring prostaglandin with potent vasodilatory activity and inhibitory activity of platelet aggregation.

Epoprostenol is (5*Z*,9α,11α,13*E*,15*S*)-6,9-epoxy- 11,15-dihydroxyprosta-5,13-dien-1-oic acid.

Epoprostenol sodium has a molecular weight of 374.45 and a molecular formula of $C_{20}H_{31}NaO_5$.

Flolan is a white to off-white powder that must be reconstituted with STERILE DILUENT for Flolan. STERILE DILUENT for Flolan is supplied in 50 ml glass vials containing 94 mg glycine, 73.5 mg sodium chloride, sodium hydroxide (added to adjust pH), and Water for Injection, USP.

The reconstituted solution of Flolan has a pH of 10.2 to 10.8 and is increasingly unstable at a lower pH.

CLINICAL PHARMACOLOGY:

General: Epoprostenol has two major pharmacological actions: (1) direct vasodilation of pulmonary and systemic arterial vascular beds, and (2) inhibition of platelet aggregation. In animals, the vasodilatory effects reduce right and left ventricular afterload and increase cardiac output and stroke volume. The effect of epoprostenol on heart rate in animals varies with dose. At low doses, there is vagally mediated bradycardia, but at higher doses, epoprostenol causes reflex tachycardia in response to direct vasodilation and hypotension. No major effects on cardiac conduction have been observed. Additional pharmacologic effects of epoprostenol in animals include bronchodilation, inhibition of gastric acid secretion, and decreased gastric emptying.

Pharmacokinetics: Epoprostenol is rapidly hydrolyzed at neutral pH in blood and is also subject to enzymatic degradation. Animal studies using tritium-labelled epoprostenol have indicated a high clearance (93 ml/min/kg), a small volume of distribution (357 ml/kg), and a short half- life (2.7 minutes). During infusions in animals, steady-state plasma concentrations of tritium-labelled epoprostenol were reached within 15 minutes and were proportional to infusion rates.

No available chemical assay is sufficiently sensitive and specific to assess the *in vivo* human pharmacokinetics of epoprostenol. The*in vitro* half-life of epoprostenol in human blood at 37°C and pH 7.4 is approximately 6 minutes; the *in vivo* half-life of epoprostenol in man is therefore expected to be no greater than 6 minutes. The *in vitro* pharmacologic half-life of epoprostenol in human plasma, based on inhibition of platelet aggregation, was similar for males (n = 954) and females (n = 1024).

Tritium-labelled epoprostenol has been administered to humans in order to identify the metabolic products of epoprostenol. Epoprostenol is metabolized to two primary metabolites: 6-keto-$PGF_{1\alpha}$ (formed by spontaneous degradation) and 6,15-diketo-13,14-dihydro- $PGF_{1\alpha}$ (enzymatically formed), both of which have pharmacological activity orders of magnitude less than epoprostenol in animal test systems. The recovery of radioactivity in urine and feces over a one-week period was 82% and 4% of the administered dose, respectively. Fourteen additional minor metabolites have been isolated from urine, indicating that epoprostenol is extensively metabolized in man.

CLINICAL STUDIES:

CLINICAL TRIALS IN PRIMARY PULMONARY HYPERTENSION (PPH):

Hemodynamic Effects: Acute intravenous infusions of epoprostenol sodium for up to 15 minutes in patients with secondary and primary pulmonary hypertension produce dose-related increases in cardiac index (CI) and stroke volume (SV), and dose-related decreases in pulmonary vascular resistance (PVR), total pulmonary resistance (TPR), and mean systemic arterial pressure (SAPm). The effects of epoprostenol sodium on mean pulmonary artery pressure (PAPm) in patients with PPH were variable and minor.

Chronic continuous infusions of epoprostenol sodium in patients with PPH were studied in two prospective, open, randomized trials of 8 and 12 weeks duration comparing epoprostenol sodium plus standard therapy to standard therapy alone. Dosage of epoprostenol sodium was determined as described in DOSAGE AND ADMINISTRATIONand averaged 9.2 ng/kg/min at study end. Standard therapy varied among patients and included some or all of the following: anticoagulants in essentially all patients; oral vasodilators, diuretics, and digoxin in one-half to two-thirds of patients; and supplemental oxygen in about half the patients. Except for two New York Heart Association (NYHA) functional Class II patients, all patients were either functional Class III or Class IV. As results were similar in the two studies, the pooled results are described. Chronic hemodynamic effects were generally similar to acute effects. CI, SV, and arterial oxygen saturation were increased, and PAPm, right atrial pressure (RAP), TPR, and systemic vascular resistance (SVR) were decreased in patients who received epoprostenol sodium chronically compared to those who did not. TABLE 1 illustrates the treatment-related hemodynamic changes in these patients after 8 or 12 weeks of treatment.

TABLE 1 Hemodynamics During Chronic Administration of Epoprostenol Sodium

Hemodynamic Parameter	Baseline		Mean change from baseline at end of treatment period*	
	Flolan (n = 52)	Standard Therapy (n = 54)	Flolan (n = 48)	Standard Therapy (n = 41)
CI ($L/min/m^2$)	2.0	2.0	0.3**	-0.1
PAPm (mm Hg)	60	60	-5**	1
PVR (Wood U)	16	17	-4*	1
SAPm (mm Hg)	89	91	-4	-3
SV (ml/beat)	44	43	6**	-1
TPR (Wood U)	20	21	-5**	1

* At 8 weeks: Flolan n = 10; Standard Therapy n = 11. At 12 weeks: Flolan n = 38; Standard Therapy n = 30.
** Denotes statistically significant change between Flolan and Standard Therapy groups.
CI = cardiac index
PAPm = mean pulmonary arterial pressure
PVR = pulmonary vascular resistance
SAPm = mean systemic arterial pressure
SV = stroke volume
TPR = total pulmonary resistance.

These hemodynamic improvements appeared to persist when epoprostenol sodium was administered for at least 36 months in an open, non-randomized study.

Clinical Effects: Exercise capacity, as measured by the 6-minute walk test, improved significantly in patients receiving continuous intravenous epoprostenol sodium plus standard therapy for 8 or 12 weeks compared to those receiving standard therapy alone. Improvements were apparent as early as the first week of therapy. Increases in exercise capacity were accompanied by significant improvement in dyspnea and fatigue, as measured by the Congestive Heart Failure Questionnaire and the Dyspnea Fatigue Index.

Survival was improved in NYHA functional Class III and Class IV PPH patients treated with epoprostenol sodium for 12 weeks in a multicenter, open, randomized, parallel study. At the end of the treatment period, 8 of 40 patients receiving standard therapy alone died, whereas none of the 41 patients receiving epoprostenol sodium died (*P* = 0.003).

INDICATIONS AND USAGE:

Epoprostenol sodium is indicated for the long-term intravenous treatment of primary pulmonary hypertension in NYHA Class III and Class IV patients (see CLINICAL STUDIES.)

CONTRAINDICATIONS:

A large study evaluating the effect of epoprostenol sodium on survival in NYHA Class III and IV patients with CHF due to severe left ventricular systolic dysfunction was terminated after an interim analysis of 471 patients revealed a higher mortality in patients receiving epoprostenol sodium plus standard therapy than in those receiving standard therapy alone. The chronic use of epoprostenol sodium in patients with CHF due to severe left ventricular systolic dysfunction is therefore contraindicated.

Epoprostenol sodium is also contraindicated in patients with known hypersensitivity to the drug or to structurally-related compounds.

WARNINGS:

Epoprostenol sodium must be reconstituted only as directed using STERILE DILUENT for epoprostenol sodium. Epoprostenol sodium must not be reconstituted or mixed with any other parenteral medications or solutions prior to or during administration.

Abrupt Withdrawal: Abrupt withdrawal (including interruptions in drug delivery) or sudden large reductions in dosage of epoprostenol sodium may result in symptoms associated with rebound pulmonary hypertension, including dyspnea, dizziness, and asthenia. In clinical trials, one Class III PPH patient's death was judged attributable to the interruption of epoprostenol sodium. Abrupt withdrawal should be avoided.

Pulmonary Edema: Some patients with primary pulmonary hypertension have developed pulmonary edema during dose ranging, which may be associated with pulmonary veno-occlusive disease. Epoprostenol sodium should not be used chronically in patients who develop pulmonary edema during dose ranging.

Sepsis: See ADVERSE REACTIONS: Adverse Events Attributable to the Drug Delivery System.

PRECAUTIONS:

General: Epoprostenol sodium should be used only by clinicians experienced in the diagnosis and treatment of PPH. The diagnosis of PPH should be carefully established by standard clinical tests to exclude secondary causes of pulmonary hypertension.

Epoprostenol sodium is a potent pulmonary and systemic vasodilator. Dose ranging with epoprostenol sodium must be performed in a setting with adequate personnel and equipment for physiologic monitoring and emergency care. Although dose ranging in clinical trials was performed during right heart catheterization employing a pulmonary artery catheter, in uncontrolled studies utilizing epoprostenol sodium, acute dose ranging was performed without cardiac catheterization. The risk of cardiac catheterization in patients with PPH should be carefully weighted against the potential benefits. During acute dose ranging, asymptomatic

PRECAUTIONS: *(cont'd)*

increases in pulmonary artery pressure coincident with increases in cardiac output occurred rarely. In such cases, dose reduction should be considered, but such an increase does not imply that chronic treatment is contraindicated.

During chronic use, epoprostenol sodium is delivered continuously on an ambulatory basis through a permanent indwelling central venous catheter. Unless contraindicated, anticoagulant therapy should be administered to PPH patients receiving epoprostenol sodium to reduce the risk of pulmonary thromboembolism or systemic embolism through a patent foramen ovale. In order to reduce the risk of infection, aseptic technique must be used in the reconstitution and administration of epoprostenol sodium as well as in routine catheter care. Because epoprostenol sodium is metabolized rapidly, even brief interruptions in the delivery of epoprostenol sodium may result in symptoms associated with rebound pulmonary hypertension including dyspnea, dizziness, and asthenia. The decision to initiate therapy with epoprostenol sodium should be based upon the understanding that there is a high likelihood that intravenous therapy with epoprostenol sodium will be needed for prolonged periods, possibly years, and the patient's ability to accept and care for a permanent intravenous catheter and infusion pump should be carefully considered.

Based on clinical trials, the acute hemodynamic response to epoprostenol sodium did not correlate well with improvement in exercise tolerance or survival during chronic use of epoprostenol sodium. Dosage of epoprostenol sodium during chronic use should be adjusted at the first sign of recurrence or worsening of symptoms attributable to PPH or the occurrence of adverse events associated with epoprostenol sodium (see DOSAGE AND ADMINISTRATION). Following dosage adjustments, standing and supine blood pressure and heart rate should be monitored closely for several hours.

Information for Patients: Patients receiving epoprostenol sodium should receive the following information: **Epoprostenol sodium must be reconstituted only with STERILE DILUENT for epoprostenol sodium.** Epoprostenol sodium is infused continuously through a permanent indwelling central venous catheter via a small, portable infusion pump. Thus, therapy with epoprostenol sodium requires commitment by the patient to drug reconstitution, drug administration, and care of the permanent central venous catheter. Sterile technique must be adhered to in preparing the drug and in the care of the catheter, and even brief interruptions in the delivery of epoprostenol sodium may result in rapid symptomatic deterioration. The decision to receive epoprostenol sodium for PPH should be based upon the understanding that there is a high likelihood that therapy with epoprostenol sodium will be needed for prolonged periods, possibly years, and the patient's ability to accept and care for a permanent intravenous catheter and infusion pump should be carefully considered.

Carcinogenesis, Mutagenesis, Impairment of Fertility: Long-term studies in animals have not been performed to evaluate carcinogenic potential. A micronucleus test in rats revealed no evidence of mutagenicity. The Ames test and DNA elution tests were also negative, although the instability of epoprostenol makes the significance of these tests uncertain. Fertility was not impaired in rats given epoprostenol sodium by subcutaneous injection at doses up to 100 mcg/kg/day, [600 mcg/m^2/day, 2.5 times the recommended human dose (4.6 ng/kg/min or 245.1 mcg/m^2/day, I.v.) based on body surface area].

Pregnancy: Pregnancy Category B. Reproductive studies have been performed in pregnant rats and rabbits at doses up to 100 mcg/kg/day (600 mcg/m^2/day in rats, 2.5 times the recommended human dose, and 1180 mcg/m^2/day in rabbits, 4.8 times the recommended human dose based on body surface area) and have revealed no evidence of impaired fertility or harm to the fetus due to epoprostenol sodium. There are, however, no adequate and well-controlled studies in pregnant women. Because animal reproduction studies are not always predictive of human response, this drug should be used during pregnancy only if clearly needed.

Labor and Delivery: The use of epoprostenol sodium during labor, vaginal delivery, or caesarean section has not been adequately studied in humans.

Nursing Mothers: It is not known whether this drug is excreted in human milk. Because many drugs are excreted in human milk, caution should be exercised when epoprostenol sodium is administered to a nursing woman.

Pediatric Use: Safety and effectiveness in pediatric patients have not been established.

Geriatric Use: Clinical studies of epoprostenol sodium did not include sufficient numbers of patients aged 65 and over to determine whether they respond differently from younger patients. In general, dose selection for an elderly patient should be cautious, reflecting the greater frequency of decreased hepatic, renal, or cardiac function and of concomitant disease or other drug therapy.

DRUG INTERACTIONS:

Additional reductions in blood pressure may occur when epoprostenol sodium is administered with diuretics, antihypertensive agents, or other vasodilators. When other anti-platelet agents or anticoagulants are used concomitantly, there is the potential for epoprostenol sodium to increase the risk of bleeding. However, patients receiving epoprostenol sodium infusions in clinical trials were maintained on anticoagulants without evidence of increased bleeding. In clinical trials, epoprostenol sodium was used with digoxin, diuretics, anticoagulants, oral vasodilators, and supplemental oxygen.

ADVERSE REACTIONS:

During clinical trials, adverse events were classified as follows: (1) adverse events during acute dose ranging, (2) adverse events during chronic dosing, and (3) adverse events associated with the drug delivery system.

Adverse Events During Acute Dose Ranging: During acute dose ranging, epoprostenol sodium was administered in 2 ng/kg/min increments until the patients developed symptomatic intolerance. The most common adverse events and the adverse events that limited further increases in dose were generally related to the major pharmacologic effect of epoprostenol sodium, vasodilation. The most common dose-limiting adverse events (occurring in ≥1% of patients) were nausea, vomiting, headache, hypotension, and flushing, but also include chest pain, anxiety, dizziness, bradycardia, dyspnea, abdominal pain, musculoskeletal pain, and tachycardia. TABLE 2 lists the adverse events reported during acute dose ranging in decreasing order of frequency.

Adverse Events During Chronic Administration: Interpretation of adverse events is complicated by the clinical features of PPH, which are similar to some of the pharmacologic effects of epoprostenol sodium (*e.g.,* dizziness, syncope). Adverse events probably related to the underlying disease include dyspnea, fatigue, chest pain, right ventricular failure, and pallor. Several adverse events, on the other hand, can clearly be attributed to epoprostenol sodium. These include headache, jaw pain, flushing, diarrhea, nausea and vomiting, flu-like symptoms, and anxiety/nervousness. In an effort to separate the adverse effects of the drug from the adverse effects of the underlying disease, TABLE 3 lists adverse events that occurred at a rate at least 10% different in the two groups in controlled trials.

Thrombocytopenia has been reported during uncontrolled clinical trials in patients receiving epoprostenol sodium.

TABLE 4 lists additional adverse events reported in PPH patients receiving epoprostenol sodium plus standard therapy or standard therapy alone during controlled clinical trials.

ADVERSE REACTIONS: *(cont'd)*

TABLE 2 Adverse Events During Acute Dose Ranging

Adverse Events Occurring in ≥1% of Patients	Flolan (% of patients) (n = 391)
Flushing	58
Headache	49
Nausea/Vomiting	32
Hypotension	16
Anxiety, nervousness, agitation	11
Chest pain	11
Dizziness	8
Bradycardia	5
Abdominal pain	5
Musculoskeletal pain	3
Dyspnea	2
Back pain	2
Sweating	1
Dyspepsia	1
Hypesthesia/Paresthesia	1
Tachycardia	1

TABLE 3 Adverse Events Regardless of Attribution Occurring with ≥10% Difference Between Epoprostenol Sodium and Standard Therapy Alone

Adverse Event	Flolan % (n = 52)	Standard therapy % (n = 54)
Occurrence More Common with Flolan		
GENERAL		
Chills/Fever/Sepsis/Flu-like symptoms	25	11
CARDIOVASCULAR		
Tachycardia	35	24
Flushing	42	2
GASTROINTESTINAL		
Diarrhea	37	6
Nausea/Vomiting	67	48
MUSCULOSKELETAL		
Jaw Pain	54	0
Myalgia	44	31
Non-specific musculoskeletal pain	35	15
NEUROLOGICAL		
Anxiety/nervousness/tremor	21	9
Dizziness	83	70
Headache	83	33
Hypesthesia, Hyperesthesia, Paresthesia	12	2
Occurrence More Common With Standard Therapy		
CARDIOVASCULAR		
Heart failure	31	52
Syncope	13	24
Shock	0	13
RESPIRATORY		
Hypoxia	25	37

TABLE 4 Adverse Events Regardless of Attribution Occurring with <10% Difference Between Epoprostenol Sodium and Standard Therapy

Adverse Event	Flolan % (n = 52)	Standard therapy % (n = 54)
GENERAL		
Asthenia	87	81
CARDIOVASCULAR		
Angina pectoris	19	20
Arrhythmia	27	20
Bradycardia	15	9
Supraventricular tachycardia	8	0
Pallor	21	30
Cyanosis	31	39
Palpitation	63	61
Cerebrovascular accident	4	0
Hemorrhage	19	11
Hypotension	27	31
Myocardial ischemia	2	6
GASTROINTESTINAL		
Abdominal pain	27	31
Anorexia	25	30
Ascites	12	17
Constipation	6	2
METABOLIC		
Edema	60	63
Hypokalemia	6	4
Weight reduction	27	24
Weight gain	6	4
MUSCULOSKELETAL		
Arthralgia	6	0
Bone pain	0	4
Chest pain	67	65
NEUROLOGICAL		
Confusion	6	11
Convulsion	4	0
Depression	37	44
Insomnia	4	4
RESPIRATORY		
Cough Increase	38	46
Dyspnea	90	85
Epistaxis	4	2
Pleural effusion	4	2
DERMATOLOGIC		
Pruritus	4	0
Rash	10	13
Sweating	15	20
SPECIAL SENSES		
Amblyopia	8	4
Vision abnormality	4	0

Adverse Events Attributable to the Drug Delivery System: Chronic infusions of epoprostenol sodium are delivered using a small, portable infusion pump through an indwelling central venous catheter. During controlled trials of up to 12 weeks duration, 21% of patients reported a local infection and 13% of patients reported pain at the injection site. During long-term fol-

ADVERSE REACTIONS: *(cont'd)*

low-up, sepsis was reported at least once in 14% of patients and occurred at a rate of 0.32 infections per patient per year in patients treated with epoprostenol sodium. This rate was higher than reported in patients using chronic indwelling central venous catheters to administer parenteral nutrition, but lower than reported in oncology patients using these catheters. Malfunctions in the delivery system resulting in an inadvertent bolus of or a reduction in epoprostenol sodium were associated with symptoms related to excess or insufficient epoprostenol sodium, respectively (see ADVERSE REACTIONS, Adverse Events During Chronic Administration.)

OVERDOSAGE:

Signs and symptoms of excessive doses of epoprostenol sodium during clinical trials are the expected dose-limiting pharmacologic effects of epoprostenol sodium, including flushing, headache, hypotension, tachycardia, nausea, vomiting, and diarrhea. Treatment will ordinarily require dose reduction of epoprostenol sodium.

One patient with secondary pulmonary hypertension accidentally received 50 ml of an unspecified concentration of epoprostenol sodium. The patient vomited and became unconscious with an initially unrecordable blood pressure. Epoprostenol sodium was discontinued and the patient regained consciousness within seconds. No fatal events have been reported following overdosage of epoprostenol sodium.

Single intravenous doses of epoprostenol sodium at 10 and 50 mg/kg (2,703 and 27,027 times the recommended acute phase human dose based on body surface area) were lethal to mice and rats, respectively. Symptoms of acute toxicity were hypoactivity, ataxia, loss of righting reflex, deep slow breathing, and hypothermia.

DOSAGE AND ADMINISTRATION:

Important Note: Epoprostenol sodium must be reconstituted only with STERILE DILUENT for epoprostenol sodium. Reconstituted solutions of epoprostenol sodium must not be diluted or administered with other parenteral solutions or medications(see WARNINGS.)

Dosage: *Acute Dose Ranging:* The initial chronic infusion rate of epoprostenol sodium is determined by an acute dose-ranging procedure. During controlled clinical trials, this procedure was performed during cardiac catheterization (see PRECAUTIONS), but in subsequent uncontrolled clinical trials, acute dose ranging was performed without cardiac catheterization. In either case, the infusion rate is initiated at 2 ng/kg/min and increased in increments of 2 ng/kg/min every 15 minutes or longer until dose-limiting pharmacologic effects are elicited. The most common dose-limiting pharmacologic effects (occurring in ≥1% of patients) during dose ranging are nausea, vomiting, headache, hypotension, and flushing, but also include chest pain, anxiety, dizziness, bradycardia, dyspnea, abdominal pain, musculoskeletal pain, and tachycardia. During acute dose ranging in clinical trials, the mean maximum dose which did not elicit dose-limiting pharmacologic effects was 8.6 ± 0.3 ng/kg/min.

Continuous Chronic Infusion: Chronic continuous infusion of epoprostenol sodium should be administered through a central venous catheter. Temporary peripheral intravenous infusions may be used until central access is established. Chronic infusions of epoprostenol sodium should be initiated at 4 ng/kg/min less than the maximum-tolerated infusion rate determined during acute dose ranging. If the maximum-tolerated infusion rate is less than 5 ng/kg/min, the chronic infusion should be started at one-half the maximum-tolerated infusion rate. During clinical trials, the mean initial chronic infusion rate was 5 ng/kg/min.

Dosage Adjustments: Changes in the chronic infusion rate should be based on persistence, recurrence, or worsening of the patient's symptoms of PPH and the occurrence of adverse events due to excessive doses of epoprostenol sodium. In general, increases in dose from the initial chronic dose should be expected. In the controlled 12-week trial, for example, the dose increased from a mean starting dose of 5.2 mcg/kg/min (4 mcg/kg/min less than the new tolerated dose) to 9.2 mcg/kg/min by the end of week 12, just 1.6 mcg/kg/min less than the mean non-tolerated dose.

Increments in dose should be considered if symptoms of PPH persist or recur after improving. The infusion should be increased by 1 to 2 ng/kg/min increments at intervals sufficient to allow assessment of clinical response; these intervals should be at least 15 minutes. Following establishment of a new chronic infusion rate, the patient should be observed, and standing and supine blood pressure and heart rate monitored for several hours to ensure that the new dose is tolerated.

During chronic infusion, the occurrence of dose-related pharmacological events similar to those observed during acute dose ranging may necessitate a decrease in infusion rate, but the adverse events may occasionally resolve without dosage adjustment. Dosage decreases should be made gradually in 2 ng/kg/min decrements every 15 minutes or longer until the dose-limiting effects resolve. Abrupt withdrawal of epoprostenol sodium or sudden large reductions in infusion rates should be avoided. Except in life-threatening situations (*e.g.,* unconsciousness, collapse, etc.), infusion rates of epoprostenol sodium should be adjusted only under the direction of a physician.

In patients receiving lung transplants, doses of epoprostenol sodium were tapered after the initiation of cardiopulmonary bypass.

Administration: Epoprostenol sodium is administered by continuous intravenous infusion via a central venous catheter using an ambulatory infusion pump. During dose-ranging, epoprostenol sodium may be administered peripherally.

The ambulatory infusion pump used to administer epoprostenol sodium should: (1) be small and lightweight, (2) be able to adjust infusion rates in 2 ng/kg/min increments, (3) have occlusion, end of infusion, and low battery alarms, (4) be accurate to ±6% of the programmed rate, and (5) be positive pressure driven (continuous or pulsatile) with intervals between pulses not exceeding 3 minutes at infusion rates used to deliver epoprostenol sodium. The reservoir should be made of polyvinyl chloride, polypropylene, or glass. Infusion pumps used in clinical trials were the CADD-1 HFX 5100 (Pharmacia Deltec), Walk-Med 410 C (Medfusion, Inc.), and the Auto Syringe AS2F (Baxter Health Care).

To avoid potential interruptions in drug delivery, the patient should have access to a backup infusion pump and intravenous infusion sets. A multi-lumen catheter should be considered if other intravenous therapies are routinely administered.

To facilitate extended use at ambient temperatures exceeding 25°C (77°F), a cold pouch with frozen gel packs was used in clinical trials (see DOSAGE AND ADMINISTRATION, Storage and Stability). The cold pouches and gel packs used in clinical trials were obtained from Palco Labs, Palto Alto, California. Any cold pouch used must be capable of maintaining the temperature of reconstituted epoprostenol sodium between 2° and 8°C for 12 hours.

Reconstitution: Epoprostenol sodium is only stable when reconstituted with STERILE DILUENT for epoprostenol sodium. Epoprostenol sodium must not be reconstituted or mixed with any other parenteral medications or solutions prior to or during administration.

A concentration for the solution of epoprostenol sodium for acute dose ranging or chronic therapy should be selected which is compatible with the infusion pump being used with respect to minimum and maximum flow rates, reservoir capacity, and the infusion pump criteria listed above. Epoprostenol sodium, when administered chronically, should be prepared in a drug delivery reservoir appropriate for the infusion pump with a total reservoir

DOSAGE AND ADMINISTRATION: *(cont'd)*

volume of at least 100 ml. Epoprostenol sodium should be prepared using 2 vials of STERILE DILUENT for epoprostenol sodium for use during a 24-hour period. TABLE 5 gives directions for preparing several different concentrations of epoprostenol sodium:

TABLE 5

To make 100 ml of solution with final Concentration of: ng/ml	Directions:
3,000 ng/ml	Dissolve contents of one 0.5 mg vial with 5 ml of STERILE DILUENT for Flolan. Withdraw 3 ml and add to sufficient STERILE DILUENT for Flolan to make a total of 100 ml.
5,000 ng/ml	Dissolve contents of one 0.5 mg vial with 5 ml of STERILE DILUENT for Flolan. Withdraw entire vial contents and add sufficient STERILE DILUENT for Flolan to make a total of 100 ml.
10,000 ng/ml	Dissolve contents of two 0.5 mg vials each with 5 ml of STERILE DILUENT for Flolan. Withdraw entire vial contents and add sufficient STERILE DILUENT for Flolan to make a total of 100 ml.
15,000 ng/ml*	Dissolve contents of one 1.5 mg vial with 5 ml of STERILE DILUENT for Flolan. Withdraw entire vial contents and add sufficient STERILE DILUENT for Flolan to make a total of 100 ml.

* Higher concentrations may be required for patients who receive Flolan long-term.

More than one solution strength may be required to accommodate the range of infusions anticipated during acute dose-ranging. Generally, 3,000 ng/ml and 10,000 ng/ml are satisfactory concentrations to deliver between 2 to 16 ng/kg/min in adults. Infusion rates may be calculated using the following formula (TABLE 6):

TABLE 6

$$\text{Infusion Rate (ml/hr)} = \frac{[\text{Dose (ng/kg/min)} \times \text{Weight (kg)} \times 60 \text{ min/hr}]}{\text{Final Concentration (ng/ml)}}$$

TABLES 7 through 10 provide infusion delivery rates for doses up to 16 ng/kg/min based upon patient weight, drug delivery rate, and concentration of the solution of epoprostenol sodium to be used. These tables may be used to select the most appropriate concentration of epoprostenol sodium that will result in an infusion rate between the minimum and maximum flow rates of the infusion pump and which will allow the desired duration of infusion from a given reservoir volume. Higher infusion rates, and therefore, more concentrated solutions may be necessary with long-term administration of epoprostenol sodium.

TABLE 7 Infusion Rates for Epoprostenol Sodium at a Concentration of 3,000 ng/ml

Patient Weight (kg)	Dose or Drug Delivery Rate (ng/kg/min) Infusion Delivery Rate (ml/hr)							
	2	4	6	8	10	12	14	16
10	—	—	1.2	1.6	2.0	2.4	2.8	3.2
20	—	1.6	2.4	3.2	4.0	4.8	5.6	6.4
30	1.2	2.4	3.6	4.8	6.0	7.2	8.4	9.6
40	1.6	3.2	4.8	6.4	8.0	9.6	11.2	12.8
50	2.0	4.0	6.0	8.0	10.0	12.0	14.0	16.0
60	2.4	4.8	7.2	9.6	12.0	14.4	16.8	19.2
70	2.8	5.6	8.4	11.2	14.0	16.8	19.6	22.4
80	3.2	6.4	9.6	12.8	16.0	19.2	22.4	25.6
90	3.6	7.2	10.8	14.4	18.0	21.6	25.2	28.8
100	4.0	8.0	12.0	16.0	20.0	24.0	28.0	32.0

TABLE 8 Infusion Rates for Epoprostenol Sodium at a Concentration of 5,000 ng/ml

Patient Weight (kg)	Dose or Drug Delivery Rate (ng/kg/min) Infusion Delivery Rate (ml/hr)							
	2	4	6	8	10	12	14	16
10	—	—	—	1.0	1.2	1.4	1.7	1.9
20	—	1.0	1.4	1.9	2.4	2.9	3.4	3.8
30	—	1.4	2.2	2.9	3.6	4.3	5.0	5.8
40	1.0	1.9	2.9	3.8	4.8	5.8	6.7	7.7
50	1.2	2.4	3.6	4.8	6.0	7.2	8.4	9.6
60	1.4	2.9	4.3	5.8	7.2	8.6	10.1	11.5
70	1.7	3.4	5.0	6.7	8.4	10.1	11.8	13.4
80	1.9	3.8	5.8	7.7	9.6	11.5	13.4	15.4
90	2.2	4.3	6.5	8.6	10.8	13.0	15.1	17.3
100	2.4	4.8	7.2	9.6	12.0	14.4	16.8	19.2

TABLE 9 Infusion Rates for Epoprostenol Sodium at a Concentration of 10,000 ng/ml

Patient Weight (kg)	Dose or Drug Delivery Rate (ng/kg/min) Infusion Delivery Rate (ml/hr)						
	4	6	8	10	12	14	16
20	—	—	1.0	1.2	1.4	1.7	1.9
30	—	1.1	1.4	1.8	2.2	2.5	2.9
40	1.0	1.4	1.9	2.4	2.9	3.4	3.8
50	1.2	1.8	2.4	3.0	3.6	4.2	4.8
60	1.4	2.2	2.9	3.6	4.3	5.0	5.8
70	1.7	2.5	3.4	4.2	5.0	5.9	6.7
80	1.9	2.9	3.8	4.8	5.8	6.7	7.7
90	2.2	3.2	4.3	5.4	6.5	7.6	8.6
100	2.4	3.6	4.8	6.0	7.2	8.4	9.6

TABLE 10 Infusion Rates for Epoprostenol Sodium at a Concentration of 15,000 ng/ml

Patient Weight (kg)	Dose or Drug Delivery Rate (ng/kg/min) Infusion Delivery Rate (ml/hr)						
	4	6	8	10	12	14	16
30	—	—	1.0	1.2	1.4	1.7	1.9
40	—	1.0	1.3	1.6	1.9	2.2	2.6
50	—	1.2	1.6	2.0	2.4	2.8	3.2
60	1.0	1.4	1.9	2.4	2.9	3.4	3.8
70	1.1	1.7	2.2	2.8	3.4	3.9	4.5
80	1.3	1.9	2.6	3.2	3.8	4.5	5.1
90	1.4	2.2	2.9	3.6	4.3	5.0	5.8
100	1.6	2.4	3.2	4.0	4.8	5.6	6.4

DOSAGE AND ADMINISTRATION: *(cont'd)*

Storage and Stability: Unopened vials of epoprostenol sodium are stable until the date indicated on the package when stored at 15° to 25°C (59° to 77°F) and protected from light in the carton. Unopened vials of STERILE DILUENT for epoprostenol sodium are stable until the date indicated on the package when stored at 15° to 25°C (59° to 77°F).

Prior to use, reconstituted solutions of epoprostenol sodium must be protected from light and must be refrigerated at 2° to 8°C (36° to 46°F) of not used immediately. **Do not freeze reconstituted solutions of epoprostenol sodium. Discard any reconstituted solution that has been frozen. Discard any reconstituted solution if it has been refrigerated for more than 48 hours.**

During use, a single reservoir of reconstituted solution of epoprostenol sodium can be administered at room temperature for a total duration of 8 hours, or it can be used with a cold pouch and administered up to 24 hours with the use of two frozen 6-oz gel packs in a cold pouch. When stored or in use, reconstituted epoprostenol sodium must be insulated from temperatures greater than 25°C (77°F) and less than 0°C (32°F), and must not be exposed to direct sunlight.

Use at Room Temperature: Prior to use at room temperature, 15° to 25°C (59° to 77°F), reconstituted solutions of epoprostenol sodium may be stored refrigerated at 2° to 8°C (36° to 46°F) for no longer than 40 hours. When administered at room temperature, reconstituted solutions may be used for no longer than 8 hours. This 48-hour period allows the patient to reconstitute a 2-day supply (200 ml) of epoprostenol sodium. Each 100 ml daily supply may be divided into three equal portions. Two of the portions are stored refrigerated at 2° to 8°C (36° to 46°F) until they are used.

Use with a Cold Pouch: Prior to infusion with the use of a cold pouch, solutions may be stored refrigerated at 2° to 8°C (36° to 46°F) for up to 24 hours. When a cold pouch is employed during the infusion, reconstituted solutions of epoprostenol sodium may be used for no longer than 24 hours. The gel packs should be changed every 12 hours. Reconstituted solutions may be kept at 2° to 8°C (36° to 46°F), either in refrigerated storage or in a cold pouch or a combination of the two, for no more than 48 hours.

Parenteral drug products should be inspected visually for particulate matter and discoloration prior to administration whenever solution and container permit. If either occurs, epoprostenol sodium should not be administered.

HOW SUPPLIED:

Flolan for Injection is supplied as a sterile freeze-dried powder in 17 ml flint glass vials with gray butyl rubber closures, individually packaged in a carton.

Store the vials of Flolan at 15° to 25°C (59° to 77°F). Protect from light.

The STERILE DILUENT for Flolan is supplied in 50 ml flint glass vials with fluororesin faced butyl rubber closures.

Store the vials of STERILE DILUENT for Flolan at 15° to 25°C (59° to 77°F). DO NOT FREEZE.

(Burroughs Wellcome Co., 10/6/95, THZZ/94/0030, 103/W5)

HOW SUPPLIED - EQUIVALENTS NOT AVAILABLE:

Injection - Intravenous - 0.5 mg

12's $189.36 FLOLAN, Glaxo Wellcome 00173-0517-00

Injection - Intravenous - 1.5 mg

12's $31.56 FLOLAN, Glaxo Wellcome 00173-0519-00

ERGOCALCIFEROL *(001174)*

CATEGORIES: Calcium Metabolism; Homeostatic & Nutrient; Hypoparathyroidism; Hypophosphatemia; Rickets; Vitamin D; Vitamins; Pregnancy Category C; FDA Approval Pre 1982

BRAND NAMES: *Biocatines D2 masiva*; Calciferol; *Chocola-D*; *Chocola D* (Japan); **Deltalin**; Drisdol; *Etalpha*; *Kalciferol Olie*; *One-Alpha*; *Ostelin*; *Ostoforte* (Canada); *Radiostol*; *Radiostol Forte* (Canada); *Raquiferol*; *Sterogyl*; *Sterogyl-15* (France); *Sterogyl 15*; *Uvesterol D* (France); *Vigantol* (Germany); Vitamin D; *Vitaminol* *(International brand names outside U.S. in italics)*

FORMULARIES: Aetna; BC-BS; FHP; Humana; Kaiser; PruCare; United; WHO

DESCRIPTION:

Ergocalciferol USP, is a synthetic calcium regulator for oral administration.

Ergocalciferol is a white, colorless crystal insoluble in water, soluble in organic solvents, and slightly soluble in vegetable oils. It is affected by air and by light. Ergosterol or provitamin D2 is found in plants and yeast and has no antirachitic activity.

There are more than 10 substances belonging to a group of steroid compounds, classified as having vitamin D or antirachitic activity.

One USP unit of vitamin D2 is equivalent to 1 International Unit (IU), and 1 mcg of vitamin D2 is equal to 40 IU or USP units.

Ergocalciferol, also called vitamin D2 is 9, 10-secoergosta-5, 7, 10(19), 22-tetraen-3-ol, (3-beta, 5Z, 7E, -22E); ($C_{28}H_{44}O$) with a molecular weight of 396.65.

Each Ergocalciferol capsule for oral administration, contains ergocalciferol (activated ergosterol), 1.25 mg (3.15 mmol) (50,000 USP units vitamin D). In addition, each capsule contains the following inactive ingredients: butylated hydroxyanisole, caramel, corn oil, cottonseed oil, ethyl vanillin, gelatin, glycerin, methylparaben, peppermint oil, propylparaben, and purified water.

CLINICAL PHARMACOLOGY:

The *in vivo* synthesis of the major biologically active metabolites of vitamin D occurs in two steps. The first hydroxylation of ergocalciferol takes place in the liver (to 25-hydroxyvitamin D) & the second in the kidneys (to 1,25-dihydroxyvitamin D). Vitamin D metabolites promote the active absorption of calcium and phosphorus by the small intestine, thus elevating serum calcium and phosphate levels sufficiently to permit bone mineralization. Vitamin D metabolites also mobilize calcium and phosphate from bone and probably increase the reabsorption of calcium and perhaps also of phosphate by the renal tubules.

There is a time lag of 10 to 24 hours between the administration of vitamin D and the initiation of its action in the body due to the necessity of synthesis of the active metabolites in the liver and kidneys. Parathyroid hormone is responsible for the regulation of this metabolism in the kidneys.

INDICATIONS AND USAGE:

Ergocalciferol is indicated for use in the treatment of hypoparathyroidism, refractory rickets (also known as vitamin D-resistant rickets), and familial hypophosphatemia.

CONTRAINDICATIONS:

Ergocalciferol is contraindicated in patients with hypercalcemia, malabsorption syndrome, abnormal sensitivity to the toxic effects of vitamin D and hypervitaminosis D.

WARNINGS:

Hypersensitivity to vitamin D may be one etiologic factor in infants with idiopathic hypercalcemia. In these cases, vitamin D must be strictly restricted.

Keep this product out of the reach of children.

PRECAUTIONS:

General: Vitamin D administration from fortified foods, dietary supplements, self-administered and prescription drug sources should be evaluated.

Therapeutic dosage should be readjusted as soon as there is clinical improvement. Dosage levels must be individualized, and great care should be exercised to prevent serious toxic effects. IN VITAMIN D-RESISTANT RICKETS, THE RANGE BETWEEN THERAPEUTIC AND TOXIC DOSES IS NARROW. When high therapeutic doses are used, progress should be followed with frequent blood calcium determinations.

In the treatment of hypoparathyroidism, intravenous calcium, parathyroid hormone, and/or dihydrotachysterol may be required.

Maintenance of a normal serum phosphorus level by dietary phosphate restriction and/or administration of aluminum gels as intestinal phosphate binders in those patients with hyperphosphatemia as frequently seen in renal osteodystrophy is essential to prevent metastatic calcification.

Adequate dietary calcium is necessary for clinical response to vitamin D therapy.

Protect from light.

Carcinogenesis, Mutagenesis, and Impairment of Fertility: No long-term animal studies have been performed to evaluate the drug's potential in these areas.

Pregnancy Category C: Animal reproduction studies have shown fetal abnormalities in several species associated with hypervitaminosis D. These are similar to the supravalvular aortic stenosis syndrome described in infants by Black in England (1963). This syndrome was characterized by supravalvular aortic stenosis, elfin facies, and mental retardation. For the protection of the fetus, therefore, the use of vitamin D in excess of the recommended dietary allowance during normal pregnancy should be avoided unless, in the judgment of the physician, potential benefits in a specific, unique case outweigh the significant hazards involved. The safety in excess of 400 USP units of vitamin D daily during pregnancy has not been established.

Nursing Mothers: Caution should be exercised when Ergocalciferol is administered to a nursing woman. In a mother given large doses of vitamin D, 25- hydroxycholecalciferol appeared in the milk and caused hypercalcemia in her child. Monitoring of the infant's serum calcium concentration is required in that case (Goldberg, 1972).

Pediatric Use: Pediatric doses must be individualized (See DOSAGE AND ADMINISTRATION.)

DRUG INTERACTIONS:

Mineral oil interferes with the absorption of fat-soluble vitamins, including vitamin D preparations.

Administration of thiazide diuretics to hypoparathyroid patients who are concurrently being treated with Ergocalciferol may cause hypercalcemia.

ADVERSE REACTIONS:

Hypervitaminosis D is characterized by effects on the following organ system:

Renal: Impairment of renal function with polyuria, nocturia, polydipsia, hypercalciuria, reversible azotemia, hypertension, nephrocalcinosis, generalized vascular calcification, or irreversible renal insufficiency that may result in death.

CNS: Mental retardation.

Soft Tissues: Widespread calcification of the soft tissues, including the heart, blood vessels, renal tubules, and lungs.

Skeletal: Bone demineralization (osteoporosis) in adults occurs concomitantly.

Decline in the average rate of linear growth and increased mineralization of bones in infants and children (dwarfism), vague aches, stiffness, and weakness.

Gastrointestinal: Nausea, anorexia, constipation.

Metabolic: Mild acidosis, anemia, weight loss.

OVERDOSAGE:

THE EFFECTS OF ADMINISTERED VITAMIN D CAN PERSIST FOR 2 OR MORE MONTHS AFTER CESSATION OF TREATMENT.

Hypervitaminosis D is characterized by:

1. Hypercalcemia with anorexia, nausea, weakness, weight loss, vague aches and stiffness, constipation, mental retardation, anemia, and mild acidosis.

2. Impairment of renal function with polyuria, nocturia, polydipsia, hypercalciuria, reversible azotemia, hypertension, nephrocalcinosis, generalized vascular calcification, or irreversible renal insufficiency that may result in death.

3. Widespread calcification of the soft tissues, including the heart, blood vessels, renal tubules, and lungs. Bone demineralization (osteoporosis) in adults occurs concomitantly.

4. Decline in the average rate of linear growth and increased mineralization of bones in infants and children (dwarfism).

The treatment of hypervitaminosis D with hypercalcemia consists in immediate withdrawal of the vitamin, a low-calcium diet, generous intake of fluids, along with symptomatic and supportive treatment. Hypercalcemic crisis with dehydration, stupor, coma, and azotemia requires more vigorous treatment. The first step should be hydration of the patient. Intravenous saline may quickly and significantly increase urinary calcium excretion. A loop diuretic (furosemide or ethacrynic acid) may be given with the saline infusion to further increase renal calcium excretion. Other reported therapeutic measures include dialysis or the administration of citrates, sulfates, phosphates, corticosteroids, EDTA (ethylenediaminetetraacetic acid), and mithramycin via appropriate regimens. With appropriate therapy, recovery is the usual outcome when no permanent damage has occurred. Deaths via renal or cardiovascular failure have been reported.

The median lethal dose in animals is unknown. The toxic oral dose of ergocalciferol in the dog is 4 mg/kg.

To obtain up-to-date information about the treatment of overdose, a good resource is your certified Regional Poison Control Center. Telephone numbers of certified poison control centers are listed in the *Physicians GenRx*. In managing overdosage, consider the possibility of multiple drug overdoses, interaction among drugs, and unusual drug kinetics in your patient.

DOSAGE AND ADMINISTRATION:

THE RANGE BETWEEN THERAPEUTIC AND TOXIC DOSES IS NARROW.

Vitamin D-Resistant Rickets: 12,000 to 500,000 USP units daily.

Hypoparathyroidism: 50,000 to 200,000 USP units daily concomitantly with calcium lactate 4 g, administered 6 times/day.

DOSAGE MUST BE INDIVIDUALIZED UNDER CLOSE MEDICAL SUPERVISION.

Calcium intake should be adequate. Blood calcium and phosphorus determinations must be made every 2 weeks, or more frequently if necessary.

The bones should be x-rayed every month until the condition is corrected and stabilized.

Store at controlled room temperature, 15° to 30°C (59° to 86°F). Keep tightly closed. Dispense in a tight, light-resistant container.

HOW SUPPLIED - RATED THERAPEUTICALLY EQUIVALENT:

Capsule - Oral - 50,000 iu

100's	$5.78	Ergocalciferol, H.C.F.A. F F P	99999-1174-01

Capsule, Elastic - Oral - 50,000 unit

50's	$48.28	DRISDOL, Sanofi Winthrop	00024-0392-02
100's	$2.90	VITAMIN D, Lannett	00527-0512-01
100's	$4.70	Vitamin D, Dixon Shane	17236-0644-01
100's	$5.78	VITAMIN D, United Res	00677-0765-01
100's	$6.15	Vitamin-D, Major Pharms	00904-0291-60
100's	$7.48	Vitamin D, Rugby	00536-4783-01
100's	$8.03	Vitamin D, HL Moore Drug Exch	00839-5254-06
100's	**$11.56**	**DELTALIN, Lilly**	**00002-0260-02**
100's	$12.00	Vitamin D, Consolidated Midland	00223-1970-01
100's	$12.00	VITAMIN D, Consolidated Midland	00223-1971-01
500's	$9.60	VITAMIN D, Lannett	00527-0512-05
1000's	$17.40	VITAMIN D, Lannett	00527-0512-10
1000's	$33.90	Vitamin D, Dixon Shane	17236-0644-10

HOW SUPPLIED - NOT RATED EQUIVALENT:

Injection, Solution - Intramuscular - 12.5 mg/ml

1 ml x 5	$78.66	CALCIFEROL IN OIL, Schwarz Pharma (US)	00091-1150-05

Tablet, Plain Coated - Oral - 50,000 unit

100's	$37.56	CALCIFEROL, Schwarz Pharma (US)	00091-3150-01

ERGOLOID MESYLATES *(001175)*

CATEGORIES: Alzheimer's Disease; Antimigraine/Other Headaches; Autonomic Drugs; Central Nervous System Agents; Cerebral Metabolic Enhancer; Cholinergics; Dementia; Hormones; Renal Drugs; Sympatholytic Agents; Vascular Disorders, Cerebral/Peripheral; Relaxants/Stimulants, Uterine*; Sales > $100 Million; FDA Approval Pre 1982; Patent Expiration 1996 Dec

* Indication not approved by the FDA

BRAND NAMES: *Alizon* (Japan); Alkergot; *Cebralest*; *Cereloid*; *Circanol*; *Cirloid*; *Codergine*; *Coergot*; *Coristin*; *DCCK*; Deapril-St; *Dulcion*; *Erdergine*; *Ergagin*; *Ergodose*; *Ergohydrin*; *Ergomed*; *Ergotika*; *Ergoxin*; *Epos* (Japan); Gerimal; *Headgen*; Hybalergine; *Hyceral*; *Hydergin*; *Hydergina*; **Hydergine**; Hydro-Ergoloid; Hydrogenat; Hydrogin; *Hymed*; Niloric; *Progeril*; *Redergin*; *Scamin*; Uni-Gine; *Vasculin*; *Vasian*; *Vasolax* (Japan)

(International brand names outside U.S. in italics)

FORMULARIES: Medi-Cal

DESCRIPTION:

Note: This monograph contains complete prescribing information for the tablets (oral), tablets (sublingual), and liquid capsule forms of Ergoloid Mesylates.

All forms of this drug contains (1 mg) contain Ergoloid Mesylates, USP as follows: dihydroergocornine mesylate 0.333 mg, dihydroergocristine mesylate 0.333 mg and dihydroergocryptine (di-hydro-alpha-ergocryptine and dihydro-beta-ergocryptine in the proportion of 2:1) mesylate 0.333 mg, representing a total of 1 mg.

Tablet Inactive ingredients: *1 mg, Oral Tablets:* lactose, povidone, starch, stearic acid, and talc. *1 mg, Sublingual Tablets:* gelatin, mannitol, starch, stearic acid, and sucrose. *Liquid Capsules:* ascorbic acid, gelatin, glycerin, methylparaben, polyethylene glycol, propylparaben, propylene glycol, sorbitol, and titanium dioxide.

Ergoloid Mesylates sublingual tablet 0.5 mg, each contains ergoloid mesylates, USP as follows: dihydroergocornine mesylate 0.167 mg, dihydrocristine mesylate 0.167 mg, and dihydroergocryptine (dihydro- alpha-ergocryptine and dihydro-beta-ergocryptine in the proportion of 2: 1) mesylate 0.167 mg, representing a total of 0.5 mg. *Inactive Ingredients:* gelatin, mannitol, starch, stearic acid, and sucrose.

Ergoloid Mesylates liquid 1 mg/mL , each mL contains ergoloid mesylates, USP as follows: dihydroergocornine mesylate 0.333, dihydroergocristine mesylate 0.333 mg and dihydroergocryptine (dihydro- alpha-ergocryptine and dihydro-beta-ergocryptine in the proportion of 2: 1) mesylate 0.333 mg, representing a total of 1 mg; alcohol, 28.5% by volume. *Inactive Ingredients:* alcohol, glycerin, propylene glycol, and purified water.

CLINICAL PHARMACOLOGY:

There is no specific evidence which clearly establishes the mechanism by which ergoloid mesylate preparations produce mental effects, nor is there conclusive evidence that the drug particularly affects cerebral arteriosclerosis or cerebrovascular insufficiency.

PHARMACOKINETIC PROPERTIES

Pharmacokinetic studies have been performed in normal volunteers with the help of radiolabeled drug as well as employing a specific radioimmunoassay technique. From the urinary excretion quotient of orally and intravenously administered tritium-labelled ergoloid mesylates the absorption of ergoloid was calculated to be 25%. Following oral administration, peak levels of 0.5 ng Eq/mL/mg were achieved within 1.5-3 hr. Bioavailability studies with the specific radioimmunoassay confirm that ergoloid is rapidly absorbed from the gastrointestinal tract, with mean peak levels of 0.05-0.13 ng/mL/mg (with extremes of 0.03 and 0.18 ng/mL/mg) achieved within 0.6-1.3 hr. (with extremes of 0.4 and 2.8 hrs.) The finding of lower peak levels of ergoloid compared to the total drug- metabolite composite is consistent with a considerable first pass liver metabolism, with less than 50% of the therapeutic moiety reaching the systemic circulation. The elimination of radioactivity, representing ergoloid plus metabolites bearing the radiolabel, was biphasic with half-lives of 4 and 13 hr. The mean half-life of unchange ergoloid in plasma is about 2.6-5.1 hr; after 3 half-lives ergoloid plasma levels are less than 10% of radioactivity levels, and by 24 hr no ergoloid is detectable.

Bioequivalence studies were performed comparing Ergoloid Mesylates oral tablets (administered orally) with Ergoloid Mesylates sublingual tablets (administered sublingually), Ergoloid Mesylates oral tablets with Ergoloid Mesylates liquid and Ergoloid Mesylates oral tablets with LC liquid capsules. The oral tablet, sublingual tablet and liquid capsule oral forms were

CLINICAL PHARMACOLOGY: *(cont'd)*

shown to be bioequivalent. Within the bioequivalence limits, the liquid capsule showed a statistically significant (12%) greater bioavailability than the oral tablet. In the study comparing the oral tablet and liquid forms, both forms tested showed and equivalent rate of absorption and an equivalent peak plasma concentrations (C_{max}).

INDICATIONS AND USAGE:

A proportion of individuals over sixty who manifest signs and symptoms of an idiopathic decline in mental capacity (*i.e.,* cognitive and interpersonal skills, mood, self-care, apparent motivation) can experience some symptomatic relief upon treatment with ergoloid mesylates preparations. The identity of the specific trait(s) or condition(s), if any, which would usefully predict a response to ergoloid mesylates therapy is not known. It appears, however, that those individuals who do respond come from groups of patients who would be considered clinically to suffer from some ill-defined process related to aging or to have some underlying dementing condition (*i.e.,* primary progressive dementia, Alzheimer's dementia, senile onset, multi-infarct dementia).

Before prescribing ergoloid mesylates therapy, the physician should exclude the possibility that the patient's signs and symptoms arise from a potentially reversible and treatable condition. Particular care should be taken to exclude delirium and dementiform illness secondary to systemic disease, primary neurological disease or primary disturbance of mood.

Ergoloid mesylates preparations are not indicated in the treatment of acute or chronic psychosis, regardless of etiology (see CONTRAINDICATIONS).

The decision to use Ergoloid mesylates therapy in the treatment of an individual with a symptomatic decline in mental capacity of unknown etiology should be continually reviewed since the presenting clinical picture may subsequently evolve sufficiently to allow a specific diagnosis and a specific alternative treatment. In addition, continued clinical evaluation is required to determine whether any initial benefit conferred by ergoloid mesylates therapy persists with time.

The efficacy of ergoloid mesylates therapy was evaluated using a special rating scale known as the SCAG (Sandoz-Clinical Assessment Geriatric). The specific items on this scale on which modest but statistically significant changes were observed at the end of twelve weeks include: mental alertness, confusion, recent memory, orientation, emotional lability, self-care, depression, anxiety/fears, cooperation, sociability, appetite, dizziness, fatigue, bothersome(ness), and an overall impression clinical status.

CONTRAINDICATIONS:

Ergoloid mesylates preparations are contraindicated in individuals who have previously shown hypersensitivity to the drug. Ergoloid mesylates preparations are also contraindicated in patients who have psychosis, acute or chronic, regardless of etiology.

PRECAUTIONS:

Practitioners are advised that because the target symptoms are of unknown etiology, careful diagnosis should be attempted before prescribing Ergoloid Mesylates preparations.

ADVERSE REACTIONS:

Ergoloid mesylates preparations have not been found to produce serious side effects. Some sublingual irritation with the sublingual tablets, transient nausea, and gastric disturbances have been reported. Ergoloid mesylates preparations do not possess the vasoconstrictor properties of the natural ergot alkaloids.

DOSAGE AND ADMINISTRATION:

1 mg three times a day.

Alleviation of symptoms is usually gradual and results may not be observed for 3-4 weeks.

HOW SUPPLIED:

Hydergine tablets (for oral use): *1 mg:* Round, white, engraved "HYDERGINE 1" on one side, "S" (contained within a triangle) on other side.

Hydergine sublingual tablets: *1 mg:* Oval, white, engraved "HYDERGINE" on one side, "78-77" on other side. *0.5 mg:* Round, white, engraved "HYDERGINE 0.5" on one side, "S" (contained within a triangle) on other side.

Hydergine liquid: *1 mg/ml:* Supplied with an accompanying dropper graduated to deliver 1 mg.

Hydergine LC liquid capsules: *1 mg:* Oblong, off-white, branded "HYDERGINE LC 1 mg" on one side, "S" (contained within a triangle) on other side.

(Encapsulated by R. P. Scherrer, N.A., Clearwater, FL 33518)

HOW SUPPLIED - RATED THERAPEUTICALLY EQUIVALENT:

Tablet, Sublingual - Sublingual - 0.5 mg

100's	$4.91	GERIMAL 0.5, Rugby	00536-3859-01
100's	$12.22	Ergoloid Mesylates, Schein Pharm (US)	00364-0415-01
100's	$15.75	HYDROLOID-G, Major Pharms	00904-0661-60
100's	$18.33	Ergoloid Mesylates, H.C.F.A. F F P	99999-1175-01

Tablet, Sublingual - Sublingual - 1 mg

100's	$8.89	HYDROGENATED ERGOT ALKA, HL Moore Drug Exch	00839-6229-06
100's	$9.57	Ergoloid Mesylates, H.C.F.A. F F P	99999-1175-02
100's	$11.00	UNI-GINE, United Res	00677-0566-01
100's	$12.73	Ergoloid Mesylates, Schein Pharm (US)	00364-0446-01
100's	$13.50	Ergoloid Mesylates, US Trading	56126-0252-11
100's	$14.25	GERIMAL 1.0, Rugby	00536-3857-01
100's	$16.45	Ergoloid Mesylates, Zenith Labs	00172-2959-60
100's	$16.45	Ergoloid Mesylates, Goldline Labs	00182-1059-01
100's	$16.45	HYDROLOID, Major Pharms	00904-0662-60
100's	$29.25	Ergoloid Mesylates, Voluntary Hosp	53258-0120-13
100's	$32.31	Ergoloid Mesylates, Major Pharms	00904-0336-61
100's	$54.87	Ergoloid Mesylates, Martec Pharms	52555-0504-01
100's	**$73.98**	**HYDERGINE, Novartis**	**00078-0070-06**
500's	$45.50	GERIMAL 1.0, Rugby	00536-3857-05
500's	$47.85	Ergoloid Mesylates, H.C.F.A. F F P	99999-1175-03
500's	$59.95	H E A 1 Mg Oral, H & H Labs	46703-0047-05
500's	$263.25	Ergoloid Mesylates, Martec Pharms	52555-0504-05
500's	**$285.18**	**HYDERGINE, Novartis**	**00078-0070-18**
1000's	$95.70	Ergoloid Mesylates, H.C.F.A. F F P	99999-1175-04
1000's	$96.25	Ergoloid Mesylates, Zenith Labs	00172-2959-80
1000's	$96.25	Ergoloid Mesylates, Goldline Labs	00182-1059-10
1000's	**$618.00**	**HYDERGINE, Novartis**	**00078-0077-09**

Tablet, Uncoated - Oral - 1 mg

100's	$9.57	Ergoloid Mesylates, H.C.F.A. F F P	99999-1175-05
100's	$13.88	UNI-GINE, United Res	00677-0782-01
100's	$13.88	Ergoloid Mesylates, Mutual Pharm	53489-0281-01
100's	$14.90	Ergoloid Mesylates, Squibb-Mark	57783-6630-01
100's	$18.30	Ergoloid Mesylates, Schein Pharm (US)	00364-0622-01

HOW SUPPLIED - RATED THERAPEUTICALLY EQUIVALENT: *(cont'd)*

100's	$18.50	Ergoloid Mesylates, Major Pharms	00904-0336-60
100's	$19.44	Ergoloid Mesylates, HL Moore Drug Exch	00839-6606-06
100's	$20.40	Ergoloid Mesylates, Goldline Labs	00182-1518-01
100's	$20.40	Ergoloid Mesylates, Qualitest Pharms	00603-3527-21
100's	$20.80	Ergoloid Mesylates, Aligen Independ	00405-4384-01
100's	$21.40	GERIMAL, Rugby	00536-3856-01
100's	**$71.58**	**HYDERGINE, Novartis**	**00078-0070-05**
500's	$47.85	Ergoloid Mesylates, H.C.F.A. F F P	99999-1175-06
500's	$60.00	Ergoloid Mesylates, Squibb-Mark	57783-6630-02
500's	$69.40	UNI-GINE, United Res	00677-0782-05
500's	$71.00	Ergoloid Mesylates, Schein Pharm (US)	00364-0622-05
500's	$71.50	Ergoloid Mesylates, Mutual Pharm	53489-0281-05
500's	$74.95	Ergoloid Mesylates, Major Pharms	00904-0336-40
500's	$76.20	Ergoloid Mesylates, Aligen Independ	00405-4384-02
500's	$91.80	Ergoloid Mesylates, Goldline Labs	00182-1518-05
500's	**$341.76**	**HYDERGINE, Novartis**	**00078-0070-08**
1000's	$95.70	Ergoloid Mesylates, H.C.F.A. F F P	99999-1175-07
1000's	$119.00	Ergoloid Mesylates, Squibb-Mark	57783-6630-03
1000's	$148.00	Ergoloid Mesylates, Mutual Pharm	53489-0281-10
1000's	$157.30	Ergoloid Mesylates, Goldline Labs	00182-1518-10
1000's	$162.50	Ergoloid Mesylates, HL Moore Drug Exch	00839-6606-16
1000's	$162.75	GERIMAL, Rugby	00536-3856-10

HOW SUPPLIED - NOT RATED EQUIVALENT:

Capsule, Elastic - Oral - 1 mg

100's	**$75.30**	**HYDERGINE LC, Novartis**	**00078-0101-05**
100's	**$79.92**	**HYDERGINE LC, Novartis**	**00078-0101-06**
500's	**$323.82**	**HYDERGINE LC, Novartis**	**00078-0101-18**
500's	**$367.20**	**HYDERGINE LC, Novartis**	**00078-0101-08**

Liquid - Oral - 1 mg

100 ml	**$58.92**	**HYDERGINE, Novartis**	**00078-0100-36**

Tablet, Sublingual - Sublingual - 0.5 mg

100's	$4.75	Ergoloid Mesylates, Consolidated Midland	00223-0895-01
100's	$7.15	Ergoloid Mesylates, Raway	00686-2944-13
100's	$7.50	Ergoloid Mesylates, Squibb-Mark	57783-6610-01

Tablet, Sublingual - Sublingual - 1 mg

100's	$9.40	Ergoloid Mesylates, Squibb-Mark	57783-6620-01
100's	$11.10	Ergoloid Mesylates, Mova Pharms	55370-0512-07
100's	$15.10	Ergoloid Mesylates, Raway	00686-2946-13
100's	$16.00	Ergoloid Mesylates, Raway	00686-2982-13
100's	$21.95	Ergoloid Mesylates, Amer Preferred	53445-1518-01
1000's	$69.00	Ergoloid Mesylates, Squibb-Mark	57783-6620-03
1000's	$96.25	Ergoloid Mesylates, Mova Pharms	55370-0512-09

ERGONOVINE MALEATE *(001176)*

CATEGORIES: Hormones; Oxytocics; Relaxants/Stimulants, Uterine; Migraine*; FDA Pre 1938 Drugs
* Indication not approved by the FDA

BRAND NAMES: *Cryovinal*; Ergometrine; *Ergometrine Lek*; *Ergometron*; *Ergotrate* (Mexico); **Ergotrate Maleate**; *Ergovin*; *Ryegostin* (Japan); *UL Ergometrine*
(International brand names outside U.S. in italics)

FORMULARIES: Aetna; BC-BS; FHP; Medi-Cal; WHO

Prescribing information not available at time of publication.

HOW SUPPLIED - EQUIVALENTS NOT AVAILABLE:

Injection, Solution - Intravenous - 0.2 mg/ml

1 ml x 6	**$13.23**	**ERGOTRATE MALEATE, Lilly**	**00002-1629-16**
1 ml x 25	**$118.50**	**ERGOTRATE MALEATE, Bedford Labs**	**55390-0502-01**
1 ml x 100	**$160.30**	**ERGOTRATE MALEATE, Lilly**	**00002-1629-02**

Tablet, Uncoated - Oral - 0.2 mg

100's	**$24.57**	**ERGOTRATE MALEATE, Lilly**	**00002-1036-02**
100's	**$28.76**	**ERGOTRATE MALEATE, Lilly**	**00002-1036-33**
1000's	**$215.06**	**ERGOTRATE MALEATE, Lilly**	**00002-1036-04**

ERGOTAMINE TARTRATE *(001177)*

CATEGORIES: Antimigraine/Other Headaches; Autonomic Drugs; Cephalalgia; Ergot Preparations; Headache; Migraine; Pain; Sympatholytic Agents; Pregnancy Category X; FDA Approval Pre 1982

BRAND NAMES: *Clavigrenin Akut* (Germany); *Ergate*; *Ergo-Kranit* (Germany); *Ergo Sanol* (Germany); *Ergodryl Mono*; Ergomar; **Ergostat**; *Ergotamin Medihaler* (Germany); *Lingraine* (England); *Medihaler-Ergotamine*; *Medihaler Ergotamine* (England, Canada); Wigrettes
(International brand names outside U.S. in italics)

FORMULARIES: Aetna; BC-BS; Medi-Cal; WHO

DESCRIPTION:

Each Ergotamine Tartrate sublingual tablet contains 2 mg ergotamine tartrate, USP. Also contains hydroxypropyl cellulose, NF; FD & C yellow No. 6 Al lake; lactose, NF; magnesium stearate, NF; mannitol, USP; artificial peppermint flavor; pregelatinized starch, NF; saccharin, NF; saccharin sodium, USP; and corn starch, NF.

Pharmacological Category: Vasoconstrictor, uterine stimulant, alpha adrenoreceptor antagonist.

Therapeutic Class: Antimigraine.

Chemical Name: Ergotaman-3',6',18-trione, 12'-hydroxy-2'-methyl-5'-(phenylmethyl)-(5'*a*)-,(*R*-(*R**,*R**))-2,3-dihydroxybutanedioate (2:1) (salt).

Molecular weight: 1313.43

CLINICAL PHARMACOLOGY:

The pharmacological properties of ergotamine are extremely complex; some of its actions are unrelated to each other, and even mutually antagonistic. The drug has partial agonist and/or antagonist activity against tryptaminergic, dopaminergic and alpha adrenergic receptors depending upon their site, and it is a highly active uterine stimulant. It causes constriction of peripheral and cranial blood vessels and produces depression of central vasomotor centers. The pain of a migraine attack is believed to be due to greatly increased amplitude of pulsations in the cranial arteries, especially the meningeal branches of the external carotid artery. Ergotamine reduces extracranial blood flow, causes a decline in the amplitude of pulsation in the cranial arteries, and decreases hyperperfusion of the territory of the basilar artery. It does not reduce cerebral hemispheric blood flow. Long-term usage has established the fact that ergotamine tartrate is effective in controlling up to 70% of acute migraine attacks, so that it is now considered specific for the treatment of this headache syndrome. Ergotamine produces constriction of both arteries and veins. In doses used in the treatment of vascular headaches, ergotamine usually produces only small increases in blood pressure, but it does increase peripheral resistance and decrease blood flow in various organs. Small doses of the drug increase the force and frequency of uterine contraction; larger doses increase the resting tone of the uterus also. The gravid uterus is particularly sensitive to these effects of ergotamine. Although specific teratogenic effects attributable to ergotamine have not been found, the fetus suffers if ergotamine is given to the mother. Retarded fetal growth and an increase in intrauterine death and resorption have been seen in animals. These are thought to result from ergotamine-induced increases in uterine motility and vasoconstriction in the placental vascular bed.

The bioavailability of sublingually administered ergotamine has not been determined.

Ergotamine is metabolized in the liver by largely undefined pathways, and 90% of the metabolites are excreted in the bile. The unmetabolized drug is erratically secreted in the saliva, and only traces of unmetabolized drug appear in the urine and feces. Ergotamine is secreted into breast milk. The elimination half-life of ergotamine from plasma is about 2 hours, but the drug may be stored in some tissues, which would account for its long-lasting therapeutic and toxic actions.

INDICATIONS AND USAGE:

Ergotamine tartrate is indicated as therapy to abort or prevent vascular headache, e.g., migraine, migraine variants, or so called "histaminic cephalalgia".

CONTRAINDICATIONS:

Ergotamine is contraindicated in peripheral vascular disease (thromboangiitis obliterans, luetic arteritis, severe arteriosclerosis, thrombophlebitis, Raynaud's disease), coronary heart disease, hypertension, impaired hepatic or renal function, severe pruritus, and sepsis. It is also contraindicated in patients who are hypersensitive to any of its components. Ergotamine may cause fetal harm when administered to a pregnant woman by virtue of its powerful uterine stimulant actions. It is contraindicated in women who are, or may become, pregnant.

PRECAUTIONS:

General: Although signs and symptoms of ergotism rarely develop even after long-term intermittent use of ergotamine, care should be exercised to remain within the limits of recommended dosage.

Carcinogenesis: No studies have been performed to investigate ergotamine tartrate for carcinogenic effects.

Pregnancy: Pregnancy Category X - See CONTRAINDICATIONS section.

Nursing Mothers: Ergotamine is secreted into human milk. It can reach the breast-fed infant by this route and exert pharmacologic effects in it. Caution should be exercised when ergotamine is administered to a nursing woman. Excessive dosing or prolonged administration of ergotamine may inhibit lactation.

DRUG INTERACTIONS:

The effects of ergotamine tartrate may be potentiated by triacetyloleandomycin which inhibits the metabolism of ergotamine. The pressor effects of ergotamine and other vasoconstrictor drugs can combine to cause dangerous hypertension.

ADVERSE REACTIONS:

Nausea and vomiting occur in up to 10% of patients after ingestion of therapeutic doses of ergotamine. Weakness of the legs and pain in limb muscles are also frequent complaints. Numbness and tingling of the fingers and toes, precordial pain, transient changes in heart rate and localized edema and itching may also occur, particularly in patients who are sensitive to the drug.

DRUG ABUSE AND DEPENDENCE:

Patients who take ergotamine for extended periods of time may become dependent upon it and require progressively increasing doses for relief of vascular headaches, and for prevention of dysphoric effects which follow withdrawal of the drug.

OVERDOSAGE:

Overdosage with ergotamine causes nausea, vomiting, weakness of the legs, pain in limb muscles, numbness and tingling of the fingers and toes, precordial pain, tachycardia or bradycardia, hypertension or hypotension and localized edema and itching together with signs and symptoms of ischemia due to vasoconstriction of peripheral arteries and arterioles. The feet and hands become cold, pale and numb. Muscle pain occurs while walking and later at rest also. Gangrene may ensue. Confusion, depression, drowsiness, and convulsions are occasional signs of ergotamine toxicity. Overdosage is particularly likely to occur in patients with sepsis or impaired renal or hepatic function. Patients with peripheral vascular disease are especially at risk of developing peripheral ischemia following treatment with ergotamine. Some cases of ergotamine poisoning have been reported in patients who have taken less than 5 mg of the drug. Usually, however, toxicity is seen at doses of ergotamine tartrate in excess of about 15 mg in 24 hours or 40 mg in a few days.

Treatment of ergotamine overdosage consists of the withdrawal of the drug followed by symptomatic measures including attempts to maintain an adequate circulation in the affected parts. Anticoagulant drugs, low molecular weight dextran and potent vasodilator drugs may all be beneficial. Intravenous infusion of sodium nitroprusside has also been reported to be successful. Vasodilators must be used with special care in the presence of hypotension.

Nausea and vomiting may be relieved by atropine or antiemetic compounds of the phenothiazine group. Ergotamine is dialyzable.

DOSAGE AND ADMINISTRATION:

All efforts should be made to initiate therapy as soon as possible after the first symptoms of the attack are noted, because success is proportional to rapidity of treatment, and lower dosages will be effective. At the first sign of an attack or to relieve the symptoms of the full-blown attack, one sublingual tablet (2 mg) is placed under the tongue. Another sublingual tablet (2 mg) should be placed under the tongue at half-hourly intervals thereafter, if necessary, for a total of three tablets (6 mg). Dosage must not exceed three tablets (6 mg) in any 24-hour period. Limit dosage to not more than five tablets (10 mg) in any one week.

Store at controlled room temperature 15-30°C (59-86°F). Protect from moisture and light.

HOW SUPPLIED - RATED THERAPEUTICALLY EQUIVALENT:

Tablet, Sublingual - Sublingual - 2 mg

20's	$71.80	ERGOMAR, Lotus Biochem	59417-0120-20
24 foil wrapped	**$17.72**	**ERGOSTAT, Parke-Davis**	**00071-0111-13**

ERYTHROMYCIN *(001179)*

CATEGORIES: Acne; Acne Vulgaris; Amebiasis; Anti-Infectives; Antibacterials; Antibiotics; Antimicrobials; Chlamydia; Conjunctivitis; Dental; Dermatologicals; EENT Drugs; Endocarditis; Erythromycins; Eye, Ear, Nose, & Throat Preparations; Inflammatory Disease; Legionnaire's Disease; Lincosamides/Macrolides; Ocular Infections; Ophthalmics; Otitis Media; Pelvic Inflammatory Disease; Penicillins; Pertussis; Pharmaceutical Adjuvants; Pharyngitis; Pneumonia; Respiratory Tract Infections; Rheumatic Fever; Skin Infections; Skin/Mucous Membrane Agents; Stenosis; Streptococcal Infection; Sulfonamides; Syphilis; Topical; Pregnancy Category B; Sales > $500 Million; FDA Approval Pre 1982; Top 200 Drugs

BRAND NAMES: A T S; *Abboticin*; *Abboticine* (France); *Abomacetin* (Japan); *Acneryne*; *Acnesol*; *Acnetrim*; Ak-Mycin; *Akne Cordes Losung* (Germany); *Aknederm Ery Gel* (Germany); Akne-Mycin; *Aknemycin* (Germany); C-Solve-2; Del-Mycin; *Derimer*; *Deripril*; *Dumotrycin*; E-Base; *E-Mycin* (Canada); ETS; Emgel; *Emu-V* (Australia); *Emu-Ve*; *Emuvin*; *Endoeritrin*; *Erecin*; *Erimycin-T*; *Erisone*; *Eritomicina*; *Eritrocina*; *Eritromicina*; *Ermycin*; *Erpathrocin*; *Ery-B*; *Eryc* (Australia); *Eryc-125* (Canada); *Eryc-250* (Canada); *Erycen* (England); Erycette; *Erycin*; *Erycinum*; *Eryderm* (Mexico); *Erydermer* (Germany); *Ery-Diolan*; Erygel; *Eryhexal* (Germany); *Erymax*; *Ery-maxin*; *Erysafe*; *Ery-Tab*; *Erytab*; *Erythrocin*; *Erythroderm*; *Erythromid* (England, Canada); *Erythromid DS* (England); *Erythromycin*; Erythromycin Base; *Erythropen*; *Erythro-Teva*; *Erytop* (Germany); Erytra-Derm; *Erytrarco*; Erytro; *Erytrociclin*; *Etromycin*; *Ilocap*; *Ilosone*; *Iloticina*; **Ilotycin**; *Ilotycin T.S.*; *Latotryd* (Mexico); *Lederpax* (Mexico); *Mephamycin*; *Mercina*; *Monomycin* (Germany); *Oftamolets*; *Oftalmolosa Cusi Eritromicina*; PCE; *Paediathrocin* (Germany); *Pantoderm*; *Pantodrin*; *Pantomicina*; *Pharyngocin* (Germany); *Proterytrin*; *Retcin*; *Robimycin*; Romycin; *Roug-mycin*; *Sans-acne* (Canada, Mexico); *Skid Gel E* (Germany); Spectro-Erythromycin; Staticin; *Stiemicyn* (Mexico); *Stiemycin* (England); *Stimycine* (France); T-Stat; *Zalig*
(International brand names outside U.S. in italics)

FORMULARIES: Aetna; BC-BS; CIGNA; DoD; FHP; Foundation; Humana; Kaiser; Medco; Medi-Cal; PCS; PruCare; United; WHO

COST OF THERAPY: $3.39 (Skin Infections; Tablet; 250 mg; 4/day; 7 days) vs. Potential Cost of $3,022.62 (Skin Disorders)

DESCRIPTION:

Erythromycin is produced by a strain of *Streptomyces erythraeus* and belongs to the macrolide group of antibiotics. It is basic and readily forms salts with acids but it is the base which is microbiologically active.

Erythromycin base is (3*R**, 4*S**, 5*S**, 6*R**, 7*R**, 9*R**, 11*R**, 12*R**, 13*S**, 14*R**)-4-((2,6-Dideoxy-3-C-methyl-3-*O*-methyl-α-L- *ribo*- hexopyranosyl) -oxy) -14- ethyl-7,12,13- trihydroxy - 3,5,7,9,11,13-hexa methyl-6- ((3,4,6-trideoxy-3-(dimethylamino)-β-D-*xylo*- hexopyran osyl) oxy)oxacyclotetradecane-2,10-dione.

The base is white to off-white crystals or powder slightly soluble in water, soluble in alcohol, in chloroform, and in ether. Erythromycin delayed-release tablets are specially enteric-coated to protect the contents from the inactivating effects of gastric acidity and to permit efficient absorption of the antibiotic in the small intesting.

Erythromycin Delayed-Release Capsules contain enteric-coated pellets of erythromycin base for oral administration. Each Erythromycin delayed-release capsules, USP contains 250 milligrams of erythromycin base. Also contains: croscarmellose sodium, NF; nonpareil seeds; povidone, USP: FD&C Yellow No. 6 Aluminum Lake and other ingredients. The capsule shell contains gelatin, NF; titanium dioxide, USP; FD&C Yellow No. 6.

Topical: Erythromycin topical solution contains 20 mg of erythromycin base in a vehicle consisting of alcohol USP (66%), propylene glycol USP, and citric acid USP to adjust pH.

CLINICAL PHARMACOLOGY:

Orally administered erythromycin base and its salts are readily absorbed in the microbiologically active form. Interindividual variations in the absorption of erythromycin are, however, observed, and some patients do not achieve acceptable serum levels. Erythromycin is largely bound to plasma proteins, and the freely dissociating bound fraction after administration of erythromycin base represents 90% of the total erythromycin absorbed. After absorption, erythromycin diffuses readily into most body fluids. In the absence of meningeal inflammation, low concentrations are normally achieved in the spinal fluid, but the passage of the drug across the blood-brain barrier increases in meningitis. Erythromycin is excreted in breast milk. The drug crosses the placental barrier, but fetal plasma levels are low. Erythromycin is not removed by peritoneal dialysis or hemodialysis.

In the presence of normal hepatic function erythromycin is concentrated in the liver and is excreted in the bile; the effect of hepatic dysfunction on biliary excretion of erythromycin is not known. After oral administration, less than 5% of the administered dose can be recovered in the active form in the urine.

The enteric coating of pellets in Erythromycin delayed-release capsules, USP protects the erythromycin base from inactivation by gastric acidity. Because of their small size and enteric coating, the pellets readily pass intact from the stomach to the small intestine and dissolve efficiently to allow absorption of erythromycin in a uniform manner. After administration of a single dose of a 250-mg Erythromycin delayed-release capsules, USP, peak serum levels in the range of 1.13 to 1.68 mcg/ml are attained in approximately 3 hours and decline to 0.30-0.42 mcg/ml in 6 hours. Optimal conditions for stability in the presence of gastric secretion and for complete absorption are attained when Erythromycin delayed-release capsules, USP is taken on an empty stomach.

Microbiology: Erythromycin acts by inhibition of protein synthesis by binding 50 S ribosomal subunits of susceptible organisms. It does not affect nucleic acid synthesis. Antagonism has been demonstrated *in vitro* between erythromycin, clindamycin, lincomycin, and chloramphenicol. Many strains of *Haemophilus influenzae*are resistant to erythromycin alone, but are susceptible to erythromycin and sulfonamides together. Staphylococci resistant to erythromycin may emerge during a course of erythromycin therapy. Specimens should be obtained for culture and susceptibility testing.

Erythromycin is usually active against the following organisms *in vitro* and in clinical infections:

Streptococcus pyogenes (group A Beta-hemolytic streptococci)
Alpha-hemolytic streptococci (viridans group)
Staphylococcus aureus (Resistant organisms may emerge during treatment.)

CLINICAL PHARMACOLOGY: *(cont'd)*

Streptococcus pneumoniae
Mycoplasma pneumoniae
Treponema pallidum
Corynebacterium diphtheriae
Corynebacterium minutissimum
Entamoeba histolytica
Listeria monocytogenes
Neisseria gonorrhoeae
Bordetella pertussis
Legionella pneumophila (agent of Legionnaires' disease)
Ureaplasma urealyticum
Chlamydia trachomatis

Susceptibility Testing: Quantitative methods that require measurement of zone diameters give the most precise estimates of antibiotic susceptibility. One such standardized single disc procedure has been recommended for use with discs to test susceptibility to erythromycin.[1]

Interpretation involves correlation of the zone diameters obtained in the disc test with minimal inhibitory concentration (MIC) values for erythromycin.

Reports from the laboratory giving results of the standardized single-disc susceptibility test using a 15-mcg erythromycin disc should be interpreted according to the following criteria:

Susceptible organisms produce zones of 18 mm or greater indicating hat the tested organism is likely to respond to therapy.

Resistant organisms produce zones of 13 mm or less, indicating that other therapy should be selected.

Organisms of intermediate susceptibility produce zones of 14 to 17 mm. The "intermediate" category provides a "buffer zone" which should prevent small, uncontrolled technical factors from causing major discrepancies in interpretations; thus when a zone diameter falls within the "intermediate" range, the results may be considered equivocal. If alternate drugs are not available, confirmation by dilution tests may be indicated.

Standardized procedures require the use of control organisms. The 15-mcg erythromycin disc should give some diameter between 22 and 30 mm for *S aureus* ATCC 25923 control strain.

A bacterial isolate may be considered susceptible if the MIC value[2] for erythromycin is not more than 2 mcg/ml. Organisms are considered resistant if the MIC is 8 mcg/ml or higher.

The MIC of erythromycin for *S. aureus* ATCC 29213 control strain should be between 0.12 and 0.5 mcg/ml.

Topical: Although the mechanism by which this form acts in reducing inflammatory lesions of acne vulgaris is unknown, it is presumably due to its antibiotic actions.

INDICATIONS AND USAGE:

ERYTHROMYCIN DELAYED-RELEASE CAPSULES

Erythromycin delayed-release capsules, USP is indicated in the treatment of infections caused by susceptible strains of the designated microorganisms in the diseases listed below:

Upper Respiratory Tract Infection: Upper respiratory tract infections of mild to moderate degree caused by *Streptococcus pyogenes* (group A beta-hemolytic streptococci); *Streptococcus pneumoniae (Diplococcus pneumoniae); Haemophilus influenzae* (when used concomitantly with adequate doses of sulfonamides, since many strains of *H influenzae* are not susceptible at the erythromycin concentrations ordinarily achieved). See appropriate sulfonamide labeling for prescribing information.

Lower Respiratory Tract Infection: Lower respiratory tract infections of mild to moderate severity caused by *Streptococcus pyogenes* (group A beta-hemolytic streptococci);*Streptococcus pneumoniae (Diplococcus pneumoniae).*

Respiratory Tract Infection: Respiratory tract infections due to *Mycoplasma pneumoniae.*

Pertussis: Pertussis (whooping cough) caused by *Bordetella pertussis.* Erythromycin is effective in eliminating the organism from the nasopharynx of infected individuals, rendering them noninfectious. Some clinical studies suggest that erythromycin may be helpful in the prophylaxis of pertussis in exposed susceptible individuals.

Diphtheria: As an adjunct to antitoxin in infections due to *Corynebacterium diphtheriae*, to prevent establishment of carriers and to eradicate the organism in carriers.

Erythrasma: In the treatment of infections due to *Corynebacterium minutissimum.*

Intestinal Amebiasis: Intestinal amebiasis caused by *Entamoeba histolytica* (oral erythromycins only). Extraenteric amebiasis requires treatment with other agents.

Acute Pelvic Inflammatory Disease: Acute pelvic inflammatory disease caused by *Neisseria gonorrhoeae.* Erythromycin lactobionate for injection, USP followed by erythromycin base orally, as an alternative drug in treatment of acute inflammatory disease caused by *N gonorrhoeae* in female patients with a history of sensitivity to penicillin. Before treatment of gonorrhoeae, patients who are suspected of also having syphilis should have a microscopic examination for *Treponema pallidum* (by immunofluorescence or dark field) before receiving erythromycin and monthly serologic tests for a minimum of 4 months thereafter.

Infection: Infections due to *Listeria monocytogenes, Moraxella (Branhamella) catahalis.*

Skin And Soft Tissue Infection: Skin and soft tissue infections of mild to moderate severity caused by *Streptococcus pyogenes*and *Staphylococcus aureus* (resistant staphylococci may emerge during treatment).

Primary Syphilis: Primary syphilis caused by *Treponema pallidum.* Erythromycin (oral forms only) is an alternate choice of treatment for primary syphilis in patients allergic to the penicillins. In treatment of primary syphilis, spinal fluid should be examined before treatment and as part of the follow-up after therapy.

Erythromycins are indicated for treatment of the following infections caused by *Chlamydia trachomatis*:*conjunctivitis of the newborn, pneumonia of infancy, urogenital infections during pregnancy. When tetracyclines are contraindicated or not tolerated, erythromycin is indicated for the treatment of uncomplicated urethral, endocervical, or rectal infections in adults due to Chlamydia trachomatis.*[4]

Nongonococcal Urethritis: Erythromycin is indicated for the treatment of nongonococcal urethritis caused by *Ureaplasma urealyticum* when tetracyclines are contraindicated or not tolerated.[4]

Legionnaires' Disease: Legionnaires' disease caused by *Legionella pneumophila.* Although no controlled clinical efficacy studies have been conducted, *in vitro* and limited preliminary clinical data suggest that erythromycin may be effective in treating Legionnaires' disease.

Therapy with erythromycin should be monitored by bacteriological studies and by clinical response (see CLINICAL PHARMACOLOGY, Microbiology.)

Prevention of Initial Attacks of Rheumatic Fever: Penicillin is considered by the American Heart Association to be the drug of choice in the prevention of initial attacks of rheumatic fever (treatment of group A beta-hemolytic streptococcal infections of the upper respiratory tract).[5] Erythromycin is indicated for the treatment of penicillin-allergic patients. The therapeutic dose should be administered for 10 days.

INDICATIONS AND USAGE: *(cont'd)*

Prevention of Recurrent Attacks of Rheumatic Fever: Penicillin or sulfonamides are considered by the American Heart Association to be the drug of choice in the prevention of recurrent attacks of rheumatic fever. In patients allergic to penicillin and sulfonamides, oral erythromycin is recommended by the American Heart Association in the long-term prophylaxis of streptoccal pharyngitis (for the prevention of recurrent attacks of rheumatic fever).[5]

Prevention of Bacterial Endocarditis: Although no controlled clinical efficacy trials have been conducted, oral erythromycin has been recommended by the American Heart Association for the prevention of bacterial endocarditis in penicillin-allergic patients with most congenital cardiac malformations, rheumatic or other acquired valvular dysfunction, idiopathic hypertrophic, subaortic stenosis (HSS), previous history of bacterial endocarditis and mitral valve prolapse with insufficiency when they undergo dental procedures and surgical procedures of the upper respiratory tract.[5]

TOPICAL

Indicated for the topical control of acne vulgaris.

CONTRAINDICATIONS:

Erythromycin is contraindicated in patients with known hypersensitivity to this antibiotic.

WARNINGS:

There have been reports of hepatic dysfunction, with or without jaundice, occurring in patients receiving oral erythromycin products.

Pseudomembranous colitis has been reported with nearly all antibacterial agents, including erythromycin, and may range from severity from mild to life-threatening. Therefore, it is important to consider the diagnosis in patients who present with diarrhea subsequent to the administration of antibacterial agents.

Treatment with antibacterial agents alters the normal flora of the colon and may permit overgrowth of clostridia. Studies indicate that a toxin produced by *Clostridium difficile* is a primary cause of "antibiotic-associated colitis."

After diagnosis of pseudomembranous colitis has been established, therapeutic measures should be initiated. Mild cases of pseudomembranous colitis usually respond to discontinuation of thr drug alonw. In moderate to severe cases, consideration should be given to management with fluids and electrolytes, protein supplementation and treatment with an antibacterial drug effective against *Clostridium difficile.*

Rhabdomyolysis with or without renal impairment has been reported in seriously ill patients receiving erythromycin concomitantly with lovastatin. Therefore, patients receiving concomitant lavastatin and erythromycin should be monitored carefully for creatine kinase (CK) and serum transaminase levels.

PRECAUTIONS:

GENERAL

Delayed Release Capsules: Erythromycin is principally excreted by the liver. Caution should be exercised when erythromycin is administered to patients with impaired hepatic function (see CLINICAL PHARMACOLOGY) and WARNINGS.

Prolonged or repeated use of erythromycin may result in an overgrowth of nonsusceptible bacteria or fungi. If superinfection occurs, erythromycin should be discontinued and appropriate therapy instituted.

When indicated, incision and drainage or other surgical procedures should be performed in conjunction with antibiotic therapy.

Topical: The use of antibiotic agents may be associated with the overgrowth of antibiotic-resistant organisms. If this occurs, administration of the drug should be discontinued and appropriate measures taken.

INFORMATION FOR THE PATIENT

Topical: This form of Erythromycin is for external use only and should be kept away from the eyes, nose, mouth, and other mucous membranes. Concomitant topical acne therapy should be used with caution because a cumulative irritant effect may occur, especially with the use of peeling, desquamating, or abrasive agents.

LABORATORY TESTS

Delayed Release Capsules: Erythromycin may interfere with AGT (SGOT) determinations if azonefast violet B or diphenylhydrazine colormetric determinations are used. Erythromycin interferes with the fluorometric determination of urinary catecholamines.

CARCINOGENESIS, MUTAGENESIS AND IMPAIRMENT OF FERTILITY

Long-term (20-month) oral studies conducted in rats with erythromycin base did not provide evidence of tumorigenicity. Mutagenicity studies have not been conducted. There was no apparent effect on male or female fertility in rats fed erythromycin (base) at levels up to 0.25 percent of diet.

PREGNANCY CATEGORY B

Delayed Release Capsules: There is no evidence of teratogenicity or any other adverse effect on reproduction in female rats fed erythromycin base (up to 0.25 percent of diet) prior to and during mating, during gestation, and through weaning of two successive litters. There are, however, no adequate and well-controlled studies in pregnant women. Because animal reproduction studies are not always predictive of human response, this drug should be used during pregnancy only if clearly needed. Erythromycin has been reported to cross the placental barrier in humans, but fetal plasma levels are generally low.

Topical: Animal reproduction studies have not been conducted with this drug. It is also not known whether erythromycin can cause fetal harm when administered to a pregnant woman or can affect reproduction capacity. Erythromycin should be given to a pregnant women only when clearly needed.

LABOR AND DELIVERY

The effect of erythromycin on labor and delivery is unknown.

NURSING MOTHERS

Delayed Release Capsules: Erythromycin is excreted in breast milk; therefore, caution should be exercised when erythromycin is administered to a nursing woman.

PEDIATRIC USE

Delayed Release Capsules: See INDICATIONS AND USAGEand DOSAGE AND ADMINISTRATION.

DRUG INTERACTIONS:

Erythromycin use in patients who are receiving high doses of theophylline may be associated with an increase of serum theophylline levels and potential theophylline toxicity. In cases of theophylline toxicity and/or elevated serum theophylline levels, the dose of theophylline should be reduced while the patient is receiving concomitant erythromycin therapy.

Concomitant administration of erythromycin and digoxin has been reported to result in elevated digoxin serum levels.

There have been reports of increased anticoagulant effects when erythromycin and oral anticoagulants were used concomitantly.

DRUG INTERACTIONS: *(cont'd)*

Concurrent use of erythromycin and ergotamine or dihydroergotamine has been associated in some patients with acute ergot toxicity characterized by severe vasospasm and dysesthesia.

Erythromycin has been reported to decrease the clearance of triazolam and thus may increase the pharmacologic effect of triazolam.

The use of erythromycin in patients concurrently taking drugs metabolized by the cytochrome P450 system may be associated with elevations in serum levels of these other drugs. There have been reports of interactions of erythromycin with carbamazepine, cyclosporine, hexobarbital, phenytoin, alfentanil, disopyramide, lovastin and bromocriptine. Serum concentrations of drugs metabolized by the cytochrome P450 system should be monitored closely in patients concurrently receiving erythromycin.

Erythromycin significantly alters metabolism of terfenadine when taken concomitantly. Rare cases of serious cardiovascular adverse events, including death, cardiac arrest, torsades de pointes, and other ventricular arrhythmias, have been observed (see CONTRAINDICATIONS.)

ADVERSE REACTIONS:

ERYTHROMYCIN DELAYED-RELEASE CAPSULES, USP

The most frequent side effects of oral erythromycin preparations are gastrointestinal and are dose-related. They include nausea, vomiting, abdominal pain, diarrhea and anorexia. Symptoms of hepatic dysfunction and/or abnormal liver function test results may occur (see WARNINGS.)

Rarely, erythromycin has been associate with production of ventricular arrhythmias, including ventricular tachycardia and torsades de pointes, in individuals with prolonged QT interval. there have been isolated reports of other cardiovascular symptoms such as chest pain, dizziness, and palpitations; however,a cause and effect has not been established.

Pseudomembranous colitis has been rarely reported in association with erythromycin therapy.

Allergic reactions ranging from urticaria and mild eruptions to anaphylaxis have occurred. Skin reactions ranging from mild eruptions to erythema multiforme, Stevens-Johnson syndrome, and toxic epidermal necrolysis have been reported rarely.

There have been isolated reports of transient central nervous system sideeffects including confusion, allucinations, seizures, and vertigo; however a cause and effect has not been established.

There have been isolated reports of reversible hearing loss occurring chiefly in patients with renal insufficiency and in patients receiving high doses of erythromycin.

TOPICAL

Adverse conditions reported with the use of erythromycin topical solutions include dryness, tenderness, pruritus, desquamation, erythema, oiliness, and burning sensation. Irritation of the eyes has also been reported. A case of generalized urticarial reaction, possibly related to the drug, which required the use of systemic steroid therapy has been reported.

Of a total of 90 patients exposed to this form during clinical effectiveness studied, 17 experienced some type of adverse effect. These included dry skin, scaly skin, pruritis, irritation of the eye, and burning sensation.

OVERDOSAGE:

In case of overdosage, erythromycin should be discontinued. Overdosage should be handled with the prompt elimination of unabsorbed drug and all other appropriate measures.

Erythromycin is not removed by peritoneal dialysis or hemodialysis.

DOSAGE AND ADMINISTRATION:

ERYTHROMYCIN DELAYED-RELEASE CAPSULES

Erythromycin delayed-release capsules, USP are well absorbed and may be given without regard to meals. Optimum blood levels are obtained in a fasting state (administration at least one half hour and preferably two hours before or after a meal); however, blood levels obtained upon administration of enteric-coated erythromycin products in the presence of food are still above minimal inhibitory concentrations (MICs) of most organisms for which erythromycin is indicated.

Adults: The usual dose is 250 mg every 6 hours taken one hour before meals. If twice-a-day dosage is desired, the recommended dose is 500 mg every 12 hours. The 333 mg tablet is recommended is dosage is desired every 8 hours. Dosage may be increased up to 4 grams per day, according to the severity of the infection. Twice-a-day dosing is not recommended when doses larger than 1 gram daily are administered.

Children: Age, weight, and severity of the infection are important factors in determining the proper dosage. The usual dosage is 30 to 50 mg/kg/day in divided doses. For the treatment of more severe infections, this dose may be doubled but should not exceed 4 mg per day.

Streptococcal Infections: A therapeutic dosage of oral erythromycin should be administered for at least 10 days. For continuous prophylaxis against recurrences of streptococcal infections in persons with a history of rheumatic heart disease, the dose is 250 mg twice a day. The American Heart Assocation suggests a dosage of 250 mg of erythromycin orally, twice a day in long-term prophylaxis of streptoccal upper respiratory tract infections for the prevention of recurring attacks of rheumatic fever in patients allergic to penicillin and sulfonamides.[4]

For the prevention of bacterial endocarditis in penicillin-allergic patients with valvular heart disease who are to undergo dental procedures or surgical procedures of the upper respiratory tract, the adult dose is 1 gram orally (20 mg/kg for children) one hour prior to the procedure and then 500 mg (10 mg/kg for children) orally 6 hours later[3] (see INDICATIONS AND USAGE.)

Primary Syphilis: 30-40 grams given in divided doses over a period of 10-15 days.

Intestinal Amebiasis: 250 mg four times daily for 10 to 14 days for adults; 30 to 50 mg/kg/day in divided doses for 10 to 14 days for children.

Legionnaires' Disease: Although optimal doses have not been established, doses utilized in reported clinical data were those recommended above (1 to 4 grams daily in divided doses).

For conjunctivitis of the newborn caused by *Chlamydia trachomatis:* *Oral erytromycin suspension 50 mg/kg/day in 4 divided doses for at least 2 weeks.*[2]

For pneumonia of infancy caused by *Chlamydia trachomatis:* *Although the optimal duration of therapy has not been established, the recommended therapy is oral erythromycin suspension 50 mg/kg/day in 4 divided doses for at least 3 weeks.*[2]

Urogenital infections during pregnancy due to *Chlamydia trachomatis:* *Although the optimal dose and duration of therapy have not been established, the suggested treatment is erythromycin 500 mg, by mouth, 4 times a day on an empty stomach for at least 7 days. For women who cannot tolerate this regimen, a decreased dose of 250 mg, by mouth, 4 times a day should be used for at least 14 days.*[4]

For adults with uncomplicated urethral, endocervical, or rectal infections caused by *Chlamydia trachomatis* in whom tetracyclines are contraindicated or not tolerated: 500 mg, by mouth, 4 times a day for at least 7 days.[4]

Pertussis: Although optimum dosage and duration of therapy have not been established, doses of erythromycin utilized in reported clinical studies were 40-50 mg/kg/day, given in divided doses for 5 to 14 days.

DOSAGE AND ADMINISTRATION: *(cont'd)*

Nongonococcal urethritis due to *Ureaplasma urealyticum*:

When tetracycline is contraindicated or not tolerated: 500 mg of erythromycin, orally, four times daily for at least 7 days[4].

Acute pelvic inflammatory disease due to *N gonorrhoeae*:*500 mg IV of erythromycin lactobionate for injection, USP every 6 hours for 3 days followed by 250 mg of erythromycin, orally every 6 hours for 7 days.*

TOPICAL

Erythromycin topical solution should be applied to the affected area twice a day after the skin is thoroughly washed with warm water and soap and patted dry. Moisten the applicator or a pad with the solution, then rub over the affected area. Acne lesions of the face, neck, shoulder, chest, and back may be treated in this manner.

Storage Conditions: Store at a room temperature below 30°C (86°F).

REFERENCES:

1. Approved Standard ASM-2 "Performance Standards for Antimicrobial Disc Susceptibility Test." National Committee for Clinical Laboratory Standards, 771 East Lancaster Avenue, Villanova, PA 19085. 2. Ericson, H.M. and Sherris, J.C.: "Antibiotic Sensitivity Testing Report of an International Collaborative Study." *Acta Pathologica et Microbiologica Scandinavica*, Section B, Supp. 217, 1971, pp. 1-90. 3. CDC Sexually Transmitted Diseases Treatment Guidelines 1985. 4. Committee on Rheumatic Fever and Infective Endocarditis of the Council on Cardiovascular Disease of the Young: Prevention of Rheumatic Fever, Circulation 70(6): 1118A-1122A, December 1984. 5. Committee on Rheumatic Fever and Infective Endocarditis of the Council on Cardiovascular Disease of the Young: Prevention of Bacterial Endocarditis, Circulation 70(6): 1123A-1127A, December 1984.

PATIENT INFORMATION:

Erythromycin is an antibiotic for the treatment of infection. Topical erythromycin may be used to treat acne. Take at regular intervals and complete the entire course of therapy. Notify your physician if you are pregnant or nursing. Notify your physician if you develop severe abdominal pain, yellowing of the skin or eyes, rash, dark urine, or pale stools. May cause nausea, vomiting, or diarrhea; notify your physician if these occur. Erythromycin should be taken on an empty stomach with a full glass of water; may be taken with food if GI upset occurs.

HOW SUPPLIED - RATED THERAPEUTICALLY EQUIVALENT:

Capsule, Gelatin, Sustained Action - Oral - 250 mg

40's	$14.81	ERYC, Parke-Davis	00071-0696-16
100's	$19.13	Erythromycin, United Res	00677-1381-01
100's	$19.13	Erythromycin, H.C.F.A. F F P	99999-1179-01
100's	$24.23	Erythromycin Delayed-Release, HL Moore Drug Exch	00839-7602-06
100's	$24.32	Erythromycin, Abbott	00074-6301-13
100's	$25.25	Erythromycin Base, Major Pharms	00904-7743-60
100's	$26.65	Erythromycin Delayed-Release, Barr	00555-0584-02
100's	$26.72	Erythromycin Base, Purepac Pharm	00228-2553-10
100's	$27.00	Erythromycin Delayed-Release 250, Goldline Labs	00182-1398-01
100's	$27.88	Erythromycin Base, Rugby	00536-0368-01
100's	$28.05	Erythromycin Base, Aligen Independ	00405-4399-01
100's	$28.80	Erythromycin, Qualitest Pharms	00603-3548-21
100's	$30.65	Erythromycin Base, Parmed Pharms	00349-8974-01
100's	$38.53	ERYC, Parke-Davis	00071-0696-40
100's	$42.88	ERYC, Parke-Davis	00071-0696-24
100's	$45.69	Erythromycin, Voluntary Hosp	53258-6301-76
100's	$114.68	Erythromycin Delayed-Release, HL Moore Drug Exch	00839-7602-12
250's	$122.92	Erythromycin Base, Purepac Pharm	00228-2553-50
500's	$95.65	Erythromycin, H.C.F.A. F F P	99999-1179-02
500's	$114.20	Erythromycin Base, Major Pharms	00904-7743-40
500's	$118.54	Erythromycin, Abbott	00074-6301-53
500's	$120.00	Erythromycin Delayed-Release 250, Goldline Labs	00182-1398-05
500's	$122.90	Erythromycin Delayed-Release, Barr	00555-0584-04
500's	$124.60	Erythromycin, Qualitest Pharms	00603-3548-28
500's	$128.63	Erythromycin Base, Rugby	00536-0368-05
500's	$129.37	Erythromycin Base, Aligen Independ	00405-4399-02
500's	$133.95	Erythromycin Base, Parmed Pharms	00349-8974-05

Gel - Topical - 2 %

27 gm	$19.94	EMGEL, Glaxo Wellcome	00173-0440-01
30 gm	$13.25	Erythromycin Base, Harber Pharm	51432-0817-11
30 gm	$13.27	Erythromycin Base, Qualitest Pharms	00603-7735-78
30 gm	$15.73	Erythromycin, H.C.F.A. F F P	99999-1179-04
30 gm	$16.50	Erythromycin Base, Glades Pharms	59366-2462-03
30 gm	$16.70	A/T/S ACNE TOPICAL GEL, Hoechst Marion Roussel	00039-0116-30
30 gm	$18.36	ERYGEL, Allergan	00023-4312-30
50 gm	$30.40	EMGEL, Glaxo Wellcome	00173-0440-02
60 gm	$24.89	Erythromycin Base, Qualitest Pharms	00603-7735-88
60 gm	$24.90	Erythromycin Base, Harber Pharm	51432-0817-17
60 gm	$27.99	Erythromycin Base, Glades Pharms	59366-2462-05
60 gm	$29.98	Erythromycin, H.C.F.A. F F P	99999-1179-06
60 gm	$34.51	ERYGEL, Allergan	00023-4312-60

Ointment - Ophthalmic - 0.5 %

3.5 gm	$1.87	Erythromycin, H.C.F.A. F F P	99999-1179-08
3.5 gm	$4.70	ROMYCIN, Ocusoft	54799-0513-35

Ointment - Ophthalmic - 5 mg/gm

1 gm x 24	**$112.31**	**ILOTYCIN, Dista**	**00777-1863-52**
1 gm x 50	$208.50	Erythromycin, Fougera	00168-0070-11
3.5 gm	$1.89	Erythromycin, Logen Pharm	00820-0106-65
3.5 gm	$2.20	Erythromycin, Harber Pharm	51432-0717-30
3.5 gm	$2.35	Erythromycin, United Res	00677-1017-18
3.5 gm	$3.20	SPECTRO ERYTHROMYCIN, Spectrum Scitfc	53268-0910-55
3.5 gm	$4.00	Erythromycin, Major Pharms	00904-7926-38
3.5 gm	$4.15	Erythromycin, Aligen Independ	00405-0945-08
3.5 gm	$4.35	Erythromycin, Rugby	00536-6530-91
3.5 gm	$4.39	Erythromycin, HL Moore Drug Exch	00839-6767-43
3.5 gm	$4.40	Erythromycin, Qualitest Pharms	00603-7137-70
3.5 gm	$4.43	Erythromycin Ophthalmic, Fougera	00168-0070-38
3.5 gm	**$5.00**	**ILOTYCIN, Dista**	**00777-1863-17**
3.5 gm x 24	$106.32	Erythromycin, Fougera	00168-0070-39

Solution - Topical - 1.5 %

60 ml	$5.25	Erythromycin, Major Pharms	00904-2844-03
60 ml	$6.25	Erythromycin, Consolidated Midland	00223-6145-01
60 ml	$21.41	STATICIN, Westwood Squibb	00072-8000-60

Solution - Topical - 2 %

59 ml	$7.50	Erythromycin 2% Topical, Goldline Labs	00182-1561-43
60 ml	$3.50	Erythromycin, Raway	00686-1244-02
60 ml	$3.90	Erythromycin Base, United Res	00677-1402-25
60 ml	$3.90	Erythromycin, H.C.F.A. F F P	99999-1179-10
60 ml	$3.95	Erythromycin, Raway	00686-0386-46
60 ml	$4.32	Erythromycin Topical, Clay Park Labs	45802-0038-46
60 ml	$4.80	Erythromycin, Consolidated Midland	00223-6146-01
60 ml	$4.93	AKNE-MYCIN, Ctr Labs Hermal	48017-9211-05

HOW SUPPLIED - RATED THERAPEUTICALLY EQUIVALENT: *(cont'd)*

60 ml	$4.95	C-SOLVE-2, Syosset Labs	47854-0668-20
60 ml	$5.22	Erythromycin 2% Topical, Schein Pharm (US)	00364-2073-58
60 ml	$5.25	Erythromycin, Aligen Independ	00405-2825-56
60 ml	$5.30	Erythromycin, Qualitest Pharms	00603-7737-52
60 ml	$5.30	Erythromycin, Harber Pharm	51432-0587-17
60 ml	$5.80	Erythromycin, Major Pharms	00904-2845-03
60 ml	$6.20	Erythromycin, Morton Grove	60432-0671-60
60 ml	$6.88	Erythromycin, Alpharma	00472-1244-92
60 ml	$6.95	Erythromycin, Rugby	00536-0292-96
60 ml	$6.95	Erythromycin Topical, HL Moore Drug Exch	00839-7023-64
60 ml	$7.05	ERYTHRA-DERM, Paddock Labs	00574-0014-02
60 ml	$7.49	Erythromycin, Geneva Pharms	00781-7013-61
60 ml	$15.84	ERYDERM, Abbott	00074-2698-02
60 ml	$16.40	A/T/S ACNE TOPICAL, Hoechst Marion Roussel	00039-0016-60
60 ml	$16.55	T-STAT, Westwood Squibb	00072-8300-60
60 ml	$17.47	THERAMYCIN-2, Medicis	99207-0550-02
60 ml	$17.86	ERYMAX, Allergan	00023-0540-02
120 ml	$31.56	ERYMAX, Allergan	00023-0540-04

Swab, Medicated - Topical - 2 %

60 pledget	$19.68	ERYCETTE, Ortho Pharm	00062-1185-01
60's	$18.59	T-STAT, Westwood Squibb	00072-8303-60

Tablet, Enteric Coated, Sustained Action - Oral - 250 mg

30's	$7.13	ERY-TAB, Abbott	00074-6304-30
40's	$8.91	ERY-TAB, Abbott	00074-6304-40
40's	$9.85	E-MYCIN DELAYED RELEASE, Boots Pharm	00524-0207-99
100's	$12.12	Erythromycin, Voluntary Hosp	53258-6304-76
100's	$13.09	Erythromycin, Voluntary Hosp	53258-0121-13
100's	$13.45	E-MYCIN DELAYED RELEASE, Boots Pharm	00524-0207-21
100's	$14.19	Erythromycin, Voluntary Hosp	53258-6304-77
100's	$23.75	ERY-TAB, Abbott	00074-6304-13
100's	$25.05	E-MYCIN DELAYED RELEASE, Boots Pharm	00524-0207-01
100's	$26.13	ERY-TAB, Abbott	00074-6304-11
500's	$112.81	ERY-TAB, Abbott	00074-6304-53
500's	$119.60	E-MYCIN DELAYED RELEASE, Boots Pharm	00524-0207-05

Tablet, Enteric Coated, Sustained Action - Oral - 333 mg

30's	$10.34	Erythromycin, H.C.F.A. F F P	99999-1179-12
30's	$11.92	ERY-TAB, Abbott	00074-6320-30
100's	$16.71	Erythromycin, Voluntary Hosp	53258-6320-76
100's	$18.90	Erythromycin, Voluntary Hosp	53258-6320-77
100's	$31.04	Erythromycin, HL Moore Drug Exch	00839-7656-06
100's	$33.74	Erythromycin Delayed-Release, HL Moore Drug Exch	00839-7660-06
100's	$34.49	Erythromycin, H.C.F.A. F F P	99999-1179-13
100's	$34.97	ERY-TAB, Abbott	00074-6320-13
100's	$35.22	Erythromycin Base, Aligen Independ	00405-4398-01
100's	$35.80	E-MYCIN DELAYED RELEASE, Boots Pharm	00524-0208-21
100's	$37.35	ERY-TAB, Abbott	00074-6320-11
500's	$99.89	Erythromycin, HL Moore Drug Exch	00839-7656-12
500's	$162.82	Erythromycin Base, Aligen Independ	00405-4398-02
500's	$166.12	ERY-TAB, Abbott	00074-6320-53
500's	$172.45	Erythromycin, H.C.F.A. F F P	99999-1179-14

Tablet, Enteric Coated, Sustained Action - Oral - 500 mg

100's	$17.95	Erythromycin, Harber Pharm	51432-0173-03
100's	$31.50	E-BASE ERYTHOMYCIN, DELAYED-RELEASE, Parmed Pharms	00349-8016-01
100's	$34.65	Erythromycin, Voluntary Hosp	53258-6321-76
100's	$37.17	Erythromycin, Voluntary Hosp	53258-6321-77
100's	$40.10	ERY-TAB, Abbott	00074-6321-13
100's	$42.48	ERY-TAB, Abbott	00074-6321-11

HOW SUPPLIED - NOT RATED EQUIVALENT:

Ointment - Ophthalmic - 5 mg/gm

3.5 gm	$4.35	Erythromycin, Goldline Labs	00182-5116-31

Ointment - Topical - 2 %

25 g	$19.94	AKNE-MYCIN, Ctr Labs Hermal	48017-3501-01

Powder

10 gm	$9.45	Erythromycin, Paddock Labs	00574-0410-10
25 gm	$17.50	Erythromycin, Paddock Labs	00574-0410-25
100 gm	$57.60	Erythromycin, Paddock Labs	00574-0410-01

Swab, Medicated - Topical - 2 %

60's	$16.00	Erytro, Goldline Labs	00182-5097-26

Tablet, Plain Coated - Oral - 250 mg

100's	$13.95	Erythromycin Base, Abbott	00074-6326-13
100's	$16.33	Erythromycin Base, Abbott	00074-6326-11
500's	$66.27	Erythromycin, Abbott	00074-6326-53

Tablet, Plain Coated - Oral - 333 mg

60's	$70.20	PCE, Abbott	00074-6290-60

Tablet, Plain Coated - Oral - 500 mg

100's	$25.60	Erythromycin Base, Abbott	00074-6227-13
100's	$154.29	PCE, Abbott	00074-3389-13

ERYTHROMYCIN ESTOLATE *(001180)*

CATEGORIES: Amebiasis; Anti-Infectives; Antibiotics; Antimicrobials; Chlamydia; Conjunctivitis; Dental; Endocarditis; Erythrasma; Erythromycins; Heart Disease; Infections; Legionnaire's Disease; Lincosamides/Macrolides; Otitis Media; Pharyngitis; Pneumonia; Rheumatic Fever; Syphilis; FDA Approval Pre 1982

BRAND NAMES: *Adco-Erythromycin*; *Althrocin*; *Betamycin*; *Derimicina*; *Dyna-Erythromycin*; *EM Cap*; *E-Mycin*; *Elate I.D.*; *Eltocin*; *Emu-K*; *Eribus*; *Erisone*; *Erisuspen*; *Eritrin*; *Eritro-Quim* (Mexico); *Eroate*; *Eromycin*; *Ery*; *Erysil*; *Erythro*; *Erythro-P*; Erythrozone; *Estomycin*; **Ilosone**; *Infectomycin* (Germany); *Irose*; *Latocin*; *Lauricin* (Mexico); *Lauritran* (Mexico); *Neo Iloticina*; *Novorythro* (Canada); *Procephal*; *Purmycin*; *Taimoxin* (Japan); *Thromycin*; *Ulosina*
(International brand names outside U.S. in italics)

FORMULARIES: Aetna; BC-BS

WARNING:
Hepatic dysfunction with or without jaundice has occurred, chiefly in adults, in association with erythromycin estolate administration. It may be accompanied by malaise, nausea vomiting, abdominal colic and fever. In some instances, severe abdominal pain may simulate an abdominal

surgical emergency.
If the above findings occur, discontinue erythromycin estolate promptly.
Erythromycin estolate is contraindicated for patients with a known history of sensitivity to this drug and for those with pre-existing liver disease.

DESCRIPTION:

Erythromycin is produced by a strain of *Streptomyces erythraeus* and belongs to the macrolide group of antibiotics. It is basic and readily forms salts with acids. The base, the stearate salt and the esters are poorly soluble in water and are suitable for oral administration.

Erythromycin estolate is the lauryl sulfate salt of the propionyl ester of erythromycin.

The capsules contain 250 mg (0.237 mmol) erythromycin estolate. They also contain FD&C Red No. 3, FD&C Yellow No. 6, gelatin, iron oxides, magnesium stearate, mineral oil, silica gel, talc, titanium dioxide, and other inactive ingredients.

The tablets contain 500 mg (0.473 mmol) erythromycin estolate. They also contain cornstarch, magnesium stearate, providone, titanium dioxide, and other inactive ingredients.

The suspensions contain 125 mg (0.118 mmol) or 250 mg (0.237 mmol) of erythromycin estolate per 5 ml. The suspensions also contain butylparaben, carboxymethylcellulose, cellulose, citric acid, edetate calcium disodium, flavors, methylparaben, propylparaben, silicone, sodium chloride, sodium citrate, sodium citrate, sodium lauryl sulfate, sucrose, and water. The 125-mg suspension also contains FD&C Yellow No. 6. The 250-mg suspension also contains FD&C Red No. 40.

CLINICAL PHARMACOLOGY:

Erythromycin inhibits protein synthesis without affecting nucleic acid synthesis. Some strains of *Hemophilus influenzae* and staphylococci have demonstrated resistance to erythromycin. Some strains of *H. influenzae* that are resistant *in vitro* to erythromycin alone are susceptible to erythromycin and sulfonamides used concomitantly. Culture and susceptibility testing should be done. If the Bauer-Kirby method of disk susceptibility testing is used, a 15-mcg erythromycin disc should give a zone diameter of at lest 18 mm when tested against an erythromycin-susceptible organism.

Orally administered erythromycin estolate is readily and reliably absorbed. Because of acid stability, serum levels are comparable whether the estolate is taken in the fasting state or after food. After a single 250-mg dose, blood concentrations average 0.29, 1.2 and 1.2 mcg/ml respectively at 2, 4, and 6 hours. Following a 500-mg dose, blood concentrations average 3, 1.9 and 0.7 mcg/ml respectively at 2, 6, and 12 hours.

After oral administration, serum antibiotic levels consist of erythromycin base and propionyl erythromycin ester. The propionyl ester continuously hydrolyzes to the base form of erythromycin to maintain an equilibrium ratio of approximately 20% base and 80% ester in the serum.

After absorption, erythromycin diffuses readily into most body fluids. In the absence of meningeal inflammation, low concentrations are normally achieved in the spinal fluid, but passage of the drug across the blood-brain barrier increases in meningitis. In the presence of normal hepatic function, erythromycin is concentrated in the liver and excreted in the bile; the effect of hepatic dysfunction on excretion of erythromycin by the liver into the bile is not known. After oral administration, less than 5% of the administered dose can be recovered as the active form in the urine.

Erythromycin crosses the placental barrier, but fetal plasma levels are low.

INDICATIONS AND USAGE:

Streptococcus pyogenes (Group A β-Hemolytic): Upper and lower respiratory tract, skin and soft-tissue infections of mild to moderate severity.

Injectable penicillin G benzathine is considered by the American Heart Association to be the drug of choice in the treatment and prevention of streptococcal pharyngitis and in long-term prophylaxis of rheumatic fever.

When oral medication is preferred for these conditions penicillin G or V or erythromycin is the alternate drug of choice.

The importance of the patient's strict adherence to the prescribed dosage regimen must be stressed when oral medication is given. A therapeutic dose should be administered for at least 10 days.

α-Hemolytic Streptococci **(viridans group):** Although no controlled clinical efficacy trials have been conducted, oral erythromycin has been suggested by the American Heart Association and American Dental Association for use in a regimen for prophylaxis against bacterial endocarditis in patients hypersensitive to penicillin who have congenital and/or rheumatic or other acquired valvular heart disease when they undergo dental procedures and surgical procedures of the upper respiratory tract.[1] Erythromycin is not suitable prior to genitourinary or gastrointestinal tract surgery.

Note: When selecting antibiotics for the prevention of bacterial endocarditis, the physician or dentist should read the full joint statement of the American Heart Association and the American Dental Association.[1]

Staphylococcus aureus: Acute infections of skin and soft tissue that are mild to moderately severe. Resistance may develop during treatment.

Streptococcus pneumoniae: Infections of the upper respiratory tract (*e.g.,* otitis media, pharyngitis) and lower respiratory tract (*e.g.,* pneumonia) of mild to moderate severity.

Mycoplasma pneumoniae: In the treatment of respiratory tract infection due to this organism.

H. influenzae: May be used concomitantly with adequate doses of sulfonamides in treating upper respiratory tract infections of mild to moderate severity. Not all strains of this organism are susceptible at the erythromycin concentrations ordinarily achieved (see appropriate sulfonamide labeling for prescribing information.)

Treponema pallidum: Erythromycin is an alternate choice of treatment for primary syphilis in penicillin-allergic patients. In primary syphilis, spinal fluid examination should be done before treatment and as part of follow-up after therapy.

Corynebacterium diphtheriae: As an adjunct to antitoxin, to prevent establishment of carriers, and to eradicate the organism in carriers.

Corynebacterium minutissimum: In the treatment of erythrasma.

Entamoeba histolytica: In the treatment of intestinal amebiasis only. Extraenteric amebiasis requires treatment with other agents.

Listeria monocytogenes: Infections due to this organism.

Bordetella pertussis: Erythromycin is effective in eliminating the organism from the nasopharynx of infected individuals, rendering them noninfectious. Some clinical studies suggest that erythromycin may be helpful in the prophylaxis of pertussis in exposed susceptible individuals.

Legionnaires' Disease: Although no controlled clinical efficacy studies have been conducted, *in vitro* and limited preliminary clinical data suggest that erythromycin may be effective in treating Legionnaires' disease.

INDICATIONS AND USAGE: *(cont'd)*

Chlamydia trachomatis: Erythromycins are indicated for treatment of the following infections caused by *C. trachomatis*: conjunctivitis of the newborn, pneumonia of infancy, urogenital infections during pregnancy (see PRECAUTIONS). When tetracyclines are contraindicated or not tolerated, erythromycin is indicated for the treatment of adults with uncomplicated urethral, endocervical, or rectal infections due to *C. trachomatis*.[2]

CONTRAINDICATIONS:

Erythromycin is contraindicated in patients with known hypersensitivity to this antibiotic.

Erythromycin is contraindicated in patients taking terfenadine (see DRUG INTERACTIONS).

WARNINGS:

(See BOXED WARNING.) The administration of erythromycin estolate has been associated with the infrequent occurrence of cholestatic hepatitis. Laboratory findings have been characterized by abnormal hepatic function test values, peripheral eosinophilia and leukocytosis. Symptoms may include malaise, nausea, vomiting, abdominal cramps, and fever. Jaundice may or may not be present. In some instances, severe abdominal pain may simulate the pain of biliary colic, pancreatitis, perforated ulcer, or an acute abdominal surgical problem. In other instances, clinical symptoms and results of liver function tests have resembled findings in extrahepatic obstructive jaundice.

Initial symptoms have developed in some cases after a few days of treatment but generally have followed 1 or 2 weeks of continuous therapy. Symptoms reappear promptly, usually within 48 hours after the drug is readministered to sensitive patients. The syndrome seems to result from a form of sensitization, occurs chiefly in adults, and has been reversible when medication is discontinued.

Pseudomembranous colitis has been reported with virtually all broad-spectrum antibiotic (including macrolides, semisynthetic penicillins, and cephalosporins); therefore, it is important to consider its diagnosis in patients who develop diarrhea in association with the use of antibiotics. Such colitis may range in severity from mild to life threatening.

Treatment with broad-spectrum antibiotic alters the normal flora of the colon and may permit overgrowth of clostridia. Studies indicate that a toxin produced by *Clostridium difficile* is a primary cause of antibiotic-associated colitis.

Mild cases of pseudomembranous colitis usually respond to drug discontinuance alone. In moderate to severe cases, management should include sigmoidoscopy, appropriate bacteriologic studies, and fluid, electrolyte, and protein supplementation. When colitis does not improve after the drug has been discontinued, or when it is severe, oral vancomycin is the drug of choice for antibiotic-associated pseudomembranous colitis caused by *C. difficile*. Other causes of colitis should be ruled out.

PRECAUTIONS:

GENERAL:

Since erythromycin is excreted principally by the liver, caution should be exercised in administering the antibiotic to patients with impaired hepatic function.

Surgical procedures should be performed when indicated.

The antibacterial activity of erythromycin is markedly greater in alkaline than in neutral or acid media, and several investigators have recommended concomitant administration of urinary alkalinizing agents, such as sodium bicarbonate or acetazolamide (Diamox), when erythromycin is prescribed for treatment of urinary infections.

LABORATORY TESTS:

There are reports that erythromycin interferes in some clinical laboratory tests and causes aberrant results. For example, evidence has been published indicating that high SGOT values recorded for some patients receiving erythromycin estolate may be artifacts and may not necessarily reflect changes in liver function.

PREGNANCY: PREGNANCY CATEGORY B:

Reproduction studies have been performed in rats, mice, and rabbits using erythromycin and its various salts and esters at doses several times the usual human dose. No evidence of impaired fertility or harm to the fetus that appeared to be related to erythromycin was reported in these studies. There are, however, no adequate and well-controlled studies in pregnant women. Because animal reproductive studies are not always predictive of human response, this drug should be used during pregnancy only if clearly needed.

NURSING MOTHERS:

Erythromycin is excreted in breast milk. Caution should be exercised when erythromycin is administered to a nursing woman.

PEDIATRIC USE:

See INDICATIONS AND USAGE and DOSAGE AND ADMINISTRATION.

DRUG INTERACTIONS:

Erythromycin has been reported to significantly alter the metabolism of the nonsedating antihistamine terfenadine or astemizole, when taken concomitantly. Rare cases of serious cardiovascular adverse events, including electrocardiographic QT/QT_c interval prolongation, cardiac arrest, torsades de pointes, and other ventricular arrhythmias, have been observed (see CONTRAINDICATIONS). In addition, rare reports of death have also been reported with concomitant administration of terfenadine and erythromycin.

Since probenecid inhibits tubular reabsorption of erythromycin in animals, it prolongs maintenance of plasma levels.

Erythromycin and lincomycin or clindamycin may under some conditions be antagonistic. Lincomycin or clindamycin therapy should be avoided in treatment of infections due to erythromycin-resistant organisms.

Erythromycin use in patients who are receiving high doses of theophylline may be associated with an increase in serum theophylline levels and potential theophylline toxicity. In case of theophylline toxicity and/or elevated serum theophylline levels, the dose of theophylline should be reduced while the patient is receiving concomitant erythromycin therapy.

Concomitant administration of erythromycin and digoxin has been reported to result in elevated digoxin serum levels.

There have been reported of increased anticoagulant effects when erythromycin and oral anticoagulants were used concomitantly. Increased anticoagulation effects due to this interaction may be more pronounced in the elderly.

Concurrent use of erythromycin and ergotamine or dihydroergotamine has been associated in some patients with acute ergot toxicity characterized by severe peripheral vasospasm and dysesthesia.

Erythromycin has been reported to decrease the clearance of triazolam and midazolam and thus may increase the pharmacologic effect of these benzodiazepines.

The use of erythromycin in patients concurrently taking drugs metabolized by the cytochrome P-450 system may be associated with elevations in serum concentrations of these other drugs. Elevated serum concentrations of the following drugs have been reported when administered concurrently with erythromycin: carbamazepine, cyclosporine, hexobarbital, phenytoin, alfen-

DRUG INTERACTIONS: *(cont'd)*

tanil, disopyramide, lovastatin, bromocriptine, and valproate. Serum concentrations of these an other drugs metabolized by the cytochrome P-450 system should be monitored closely in patients concurrently receiving erythromycin.

ADVERSE REACTIONS:

The most frequent side-effects of erythromycin preparations are gastrointestinal (*e.g.*, abdominal cramping and discomfort) and are dose related. Nausea, vomiting, and diarrhea occur infrequently with usual oral doses.

During prolonged or repeated therapy, there is a possibility of overgrowth of nonsusceptible bacteria or fungi. If such infections arise, the drug should be discontinued and appropriate therapy instituted.

Mild allergic reactions, such as urticaria and other skin rashes, have occurred. Serious allergic reactions, including anaphylaxis have been reported.

There have been isolated reports of hearing loss and/or tinnitus in patients receiving erythromycin. The ototoxic effect of the drug is usually reversible with drug discontinuance; however, in rare instances involving intravenous administration, the ototoxic effect has been irreversible. Ototoxic effects occur chiefly in patients with renal or hepatic insufficiency and in patients receiving high doses of erythromycin.

Rarely, erythromycin has been associated with the production of ventricular arrhythmias, including ventricular tachycardia and torsades de pointes, in individuals with prolonged QT intervals.

OVERDOSAGE:

SIGNS AND SYMPTOMS

Symptoms of oral overdose or erythromycin estolate may include nausea, vomiting, epigastric distress and the diarrhea are dose related. Reversible mild acute pancreatitis has been reported. Hearing loss, with or without tinnitus and vertigo, may occur, especially in patients with renal or hepatic insufficiency.

TREATMENT

To obtain up-to-date information about the treatment of overdose, a good resource is your certified regional poison control center. Telephone numbers of certified poison control centers are listed in *Physicians GenRx*. In managing overdosage, consider the possibility of multiple drug overdoses, interactions among drugs, and unusual drug kinetics in your patient.

Unless 5 times the normal single dose of erythromycin estolate has been ingested, gastrointestinal decontamination should not be necessary. An accidental ingestion of erythromycin should not be predicted to have minimal toxicity unless there is a good approximation of how much was ingested and unless only a single medication was involved.

Protect the patient's airway and support ventilation and perfusion. Meticulously monitor and maintain, within acceptable limits, the patient's vital signs, blood gases, serum electrolytes, etc. Absorption of drugs from the gastrointestinal tract may be decreased by giving activated charcoal, which, in many cases is more effective than emesis or lavage; consider charcoal instead of or in addition to gastric emptying. Repeated doses of charcoal over time may hasten elimination of some drugs that have been absorbed. Safeguard the patient's airway when employing gastric emptying or charcoal.

Forced diuresis, peritoneal dialysis, hemodialysis, or charcoal hemoperfusion have not been established as beneficial for an overdosage of erythromycin estolate.

DOSAGE AND ADMINISTRATION:

Adults: The usual dosage is 250 mg every 6 hours. This may be increased up to 4 g/day or more according to the severity of the infection.

Children: Age, weight and severity of the infection are important factors in determining the proper dosage. The usual regimen is 30 to 50 mg per kg per day in divided doses. For more severe infections, this dosage may be doubled.

If administration is desired on a twice-a-day schedule in either adults or children, 1/2 of the total daily dose may be given every 12 hours.

Twice-a-day dosing is not recommended when doses larger than 1 g daily are administered.

Streptococcal Infections: For the treatment of streptococcal pharyngitis and tonsillitis, the usual dosage range is 20 to 50 mg/kg/day in divided doses (TABLE 1).

TABLE 1

Body Weight	Total Daily Dose
10 kg or less (less than 25 lb)	250 mg
11-18 kg (25-40 lb)	375 mg
18-25 kg (40-55 lb)	500 mg
25-36 kg (40-55 lb)	750 mg
36 kg or more (more than 80 lb)	1,000 mg (adult dose)

In the treatment of group A β-hemolytic streptococcal infections, a therapeutic dosage of erythromycin should be administered for at least 10 days. In continuous prophylaxis of streptococcal infections in persons with a history of rheumatic heart disease, the dosage is 250 mg twice a day.

For prophylaxis against bacterial endocarditis[1] in penicillin-allergic patients with congenital heart disease or rheumatic or other acquired valvular heart disease when undergoing dental procedures or surgical procedures of the upper respiratory tract, the dosage schedule for adults is 1 g (20 mg/kg for children) orally 1 hour before the procedure, and then 500 mg (10 mg/kg for children) orally 6 hours later.

Primary Syphilis: A regimen of 20 g of erythromycin estolate in divided doses over a period of ten days has been shown to be effective in treatment of primary syphilis.

Dysenteric Amebiasis: Dosage for adults is 250 mg 4 times daily for 10 to 14 days; for children, 30 to 50 mg/kg/day in divided doses for ten to fourteen days.

Pertussis: Although optimum dosage and duration have not been established, the dosage of erythromycin utilized in reported clinical studies was 40 to 50 mg/kg/day, given in divided doses for 5 to 14 days.

Legionnaires' Disease: Although optimum doses have not been established, doses utilized in reported clinical data were those recommended above (1 to 4 g erythromycin estolate daily in divided doses.)

Conjunctivitis of the Newborn Caused by *C. trachomatis*: Oral erythromycin suspension 50 mg/kg/day in 4 divided doses for at least 2 weeks.[2]

Pneumonia of Infancy Caused by *C. trachomatis*: Although the optimal duration of therapy has not been established the recommended therapy is oral erythromycin suspension, 50 mg/kg/day in 4 divided doses for at least 3 weeks.[2]

Urogenital Infections During Pregnancy Due to *C. trachomatis*: Although the optimum dose and duration of therapy have not been established, the suggested treatment is erythromycin 500 mg orally 4 times a day for at least 7 days. For women who cannot tolerate this regimen, a decreased dose of 250 mg, by mouth, 4 times a day should be used for at least 14 days.[2]

DOSAGE AND ADMINISTRATION: *(cont'd)*

For adults with uncomplicated urethral, endocervical, or rectal infections caused by *C. trachomatis* in whom tetracyclines are contraindicated or not tolerated: 500 mg orally 4 times a day for at least 7 days.[2]

Storage: Store at controlled room temperature, 59° to 86°F (15° to 30°C)

Suspension: Shake well before using. Refrigerate to maintain optimum taste.

REFERENCES:

1. American Heart Association: Prevention of bacterial endocarditis. *Circulation* 1984;70:1123A. 2. Sexually Transmitted Diseases Treatment Guidelines 1982. Centers for Disease Control, Morbidity and Mortality Weekly Report, US Department of Health and Human Services, Atlanta, 1982;31(suppl):355

HOW SUPPLIED - RATED THERAPEUTICALLY EQUIVALENT:

Capsule, Gelatin - Oral - 250 mg

100's	**$22.92**	**ILOSONE, Dista**	**00777-0809-02**
100's	$22.92	Erythromycin Estolate, H.C.F.A. F F P	99999-1180-01
100's	$27.70	Erythromycin Estolate, United Res	00677-0653-01
100's	$27.75	Erythromycin Estolate, Geneva Pharms	00781-2070-01
100's	$28.55	Erythromycin Estolate, Rugby	00536-0322-01
100's	$31.30	Erythromycin Estolate, Schein Pharm (US)	00364-0530-01
100's	$31.38	Erythromycin Estolate, Barr	00555-0230-02
100's	$31.40	Erythromycin Estolate, Qualitest Pharms	00603-3551-21
100's	**$41.61**	**ILOSONE, Dista**	**00777-0809-33**
100's	$43.32	Erythromycin Estolate, Aligen Independ	00405-4401-01
100's	$48.70	Erythromycin Estolate, Major Pharms	00904-2468-60

Suspension - Oral - 125 mg/5ml

100 ml	**$7.65**	**ILOSONE, Dista**	**00777-2315-48**
480 ml	$20.83	Erythromycin Estolate, Lederle Pharm	00005-3119-65
480 ml	$23.50	Erythromycin Estolate, Harber Pharm	51432-0581-20
480 ml	$23.88	Erthromycin Estolate, HL Moore Drug Exch	00839-6713-69
480 ml	**$24.57**	**ILOSONE, Dista**	**00777-2315-05**
480 ml	$24.57	Erythromycin Estolate, H.C.F.A. F F P	99999-1180-02
480 ml	$26.40	Erythromycin Estolate, Major Pharms	00904-2470-16
480 ml	$27.50	Erythromycin Estolate, Consolidated Midland	00223-6140-01
480 ml	$28.60	Erythromycin Estolate, Goldline Labs	00182-1560-40
480 ml	$28.60	Erythromycin Estolate, Alpharma	00472-0977-16
480 ml	$31.05	Erythromycin Estolate, Rugby	00536-0335-85
480 ml	$31.50	Erythromycin Estolate, Schein Pharm (US)	00364-2078-16
480 ml	$31.95	Erythromycin Estolate, Qualitest Pharms	00603-1202-58

Suspension - Oral - 250 mg/5ml

100 ml	**$8.58**	**ILOSONE, Dista**	**00777-2317-48**
100 ml	$8.58	Erythromycin Estolate, H.C.F.A. F F P	99999-1180-03
480 ml	$41.10	Erythromycin Estolate, Harber Pharm	51432-0591-20
480 ml	**$41.18**	**ILOSONE, Dista**	**00777-2317-05**
480 ml	$41.18	Erythromycin Estolate, H.C.F.A. F F P	99999-1180-04
480 ml	$41.90	Erythromycin Estolate, Major Pharms	00904-2471-16
480 ml	$42.50	Erythromycin Estolate, Consolidated Midland	00223-6141-01
480 ml	$47.30	Erythromycin Estolate, Alpharma	00472-0979-16
480 ml	$52.45	ERTHROMYCIN ESTOLATE, HL Moore Drug Exch	00839-6714-69
480 ml	$55.25	Erythromycin Estolate, Rugby	00536-0337-85
480 ml	$56.85	Erythromycin Estolate, Qualitest Pharms	00603-1203-58
480 ml	$60.40	Erythromycin Estolate, Schein Pharm (US)	00364-2079-16
480 ml	$60.60	Erythromycin Estolate, Goldline Labs	00182-1567-40

HOW SUPPLIED - NOT RATED EQUIVALENT:

Tablet, Coated - Oral - 500 mg

50's	**$44.39**	**ILOSONE, Dista**	**00777-2126-50**

ERYTHROMYCIN ETHYLSUCCINATE *(001182)*

CATEGORIES: Amebiasis; Anti-Infectives; Antibiotics; Antimicrobials; Chlamydia; Dental; Endocarditis; Erythrasma; Erythromycins; Fever; Heart Disease; Hemophilus; Legionnaire's Disease; Ocular Infections; Ophthalmics; Otitis Media; Penicillins; Pertussis; Pharyngitis; Pneumonia; Respiratory Tract Infections; Rheumatic Fever; Sulfonamides; Syphilis; Urethritis; Sales > $100 Million; FDA Approval Pre 1982

BRAND NAMES: *Abboticin Novum*; *Abboticine* (France); *Alphatrocin*; *Ambamida*; *Anamycin*; *Apo-Erythro-ES* (Canada); *Baknyl*; *Bannthrocin*; *E-Mycin*; E-Mycin E; *E.E.S.*; **EES**; *EES-200* (Canada); *EES-400* (Canada); *EES 400*; *EES Granules*; *ERA*; *ERA I.M.*; *ESE*; *Ebalin*; *Econoped* (Germany); *Ericin*; *Eriecu*; *Eritrazon*; *Eritrobiotic*; *Eritrocina*; *Eritrolag*; *Eritrowel* (Mexico); *Ermysin*; *Erotab*; *Ery* (France); *Ery-Maxin*; Eryped; *Eryped 400*; *Eryromycen* (Japan); *Eryson*; *Erysrocin*; Erythro; *Erythro-DS* (Japan); *Erythrocin* (Germany); *Erythrocin ES 500*; *Erythrocin I.M.*; *Erythrocine* (France); *Erythrodar*; *Erythrogenat TS* (Germany); *Erythrogram* (France); *Erythromycin-Ratiopharm TS*; *Erythroped* (England); *Erytran*; *Erytro*; *Esinol* (Japan); *Esmycin* (Japan); *Ethiocin*; *Etromycin*; *Macrocin*; *Malocin*; *Mercina*; *Minotin* (Japan); *Monomycin*; *Monomycina*; *Oritromin*; *Paediathrocin* (Germany); *Pamycin*; *Panjomicina*; *Pantomicina* (Mexico); *Pantomucol*; *Pantopenil*; Pediamycin; *Pediamicina*; *Pentate* (Japan); *Proterytrin*; *Ranthrocin*; Ro-Mycin; *Servitrocin*; *Succin*; Wyamycin E

(International brand names outside U.S. in italics)

FORMULARIES: Aetna; BC-BS; Medi-Cal; PCS

COST OF THERAPY: $7.46 (Infections; Tablet; 400 mg; 4/day; 10 days) vs. Potential Cost of $7,048.46 (Respiratory Infections)

PRIMARY ICD9: 136.9 (Unspecified Infections And Parasitic Diseases)

DESCRIPTION:

Erythromycin is produced by a strain of *Streptomyces erythraeus* and belongs to the macrolide group of antibiotics. It is basic and readily forms salts with acids. The base, the stearate salt, and the esters are poorly soluble in water. Erythromycin ethylsuccinate is an ester of erythromycin suitable for oral administration.

The granules are intended for reconstitution with water. When reconstituted, they are palatable cherry-flavored suspensions.

The pleasant tasting, fruit-flavored liquids are supplied ready for administration.

Granules and ready-made suspensions are intended primarily for pediatric use but can also be used in adults.

The Filmtab tablets are intended primarily for adults or older children.

Inactive Ingredients E.E.S. 200 Liquid: FD&C Red No. 40, methylparaben, polysorbate 60, propylparaben, sodium citrate, sucrose, water, xanthan gum and natural and artificial flavors.

DESCRIPTION: *(cont'd)*

E.E.S 400 Liquid: D&C Yellow No. 10, FD&C Yellow No. 6, methylparaben, polysorbate 60, propylparaben, sodium citrate, sucrose, water, xanthan gum and natural and artificial flavors.

E.E.S. Granules: Citric acid, FD&C Red No. 3, magnesium aluminum silicate, sodium carboxymethylcellulose, sodium citrate, sucrose and artificial flavor.

E.E.S. 400 Filmtab Tablets: Cellulosic polymers, confectioner's sugar (contains corn starch), corn starch, D&C Red No. 30, D&C Yellow No. 10, FD&C Red No. 40, magnesium stearate, polacrilin potassium, polyethylene glycol, propylene glycol, sodium citrate, sorbic acid, sorbitan monooleate, titanium dioxide and vitamin E.

CLINICAL PHARMACOLOGY:

Microbiology Biochemical tests demonstrate that erythromycin inhibits protein synthesis of the pathogen without directly affecting nucleic acid synthesis. Antagonism has been demonstrated between clindamycin and erythromycin.

NOTE: Many strains of *Hemophilus influenzae* are resistant to erythromycin alone, but are susceptible to erythromycin and sulfonamides together. Staphylococci resistant to erythromycin may emerge during a course of erythromycin therapy. Culture and susceptibility testing should be performed.

Disc Susceptibility Tests Quantitative methods that require measurement of zone diameters give the most precise estimates of antibiotic susceptibility. One recommended procedure (21 CFR section 460.1) uses erythromycin class discs for testing susceptibility; interpretations correlate zone diameters of this disc test with MIC values for erythromycin. With this procedure, a report from the laboratory of "susceptible" indicates that the infecting organism is likely to respond to therapy. A report of "resistant" indicates, that the infective organism is not likely to respond to therapy. A report of "intermediate susceptibility" suggests that the organism would be susceptible if higher doses were used.

Erythromycin binds to the 50 S ribosomal subunits of susceptible bacteria and suppresses protein synthesis.

Orally administered erythromycin ethylsuccinate suspensions and Filmtab tablets are readily and reliably absorbed. Comparable serum levels of erythromycin are achieved in the fasting and nonfasting states.

Erythromycin diffuses readily into most body fluids. Only low concentrations are normally achieved in the spinal fluid, but passage of the drug across the blood-brain barrier increases in meningitis. In the presence of normal hepatic function, erythromycin is concentrated in the liver and excreted in the bile; the effect of hepatic dysfunction on excretion of erythromycin by the liver into the bile is not known. Less than 5 percent of the orally administered dose of erythromycin is excreted in active form in the urine.

Erythromycin crosses the placental barrier and is excreted in breast milk.

INDICATIONS AND USAGE:

Streptococcus pyogenes(Group A beta hemolytic streptococcus): Upper and lower respiratory tract, skin, and soft tissue infections of mild to moderate severity.

Injectable benzathine penicillin G is considered by the American Heart Association to be the drug of choice in the treatment and prevention of streptococcal pharyngitis and in long-term prophylaxis of rheumatic fever.

When oral medication is preferred for treatment of the above conditions, penicillin G, V, or erythromycin are alternate drugs of choice.

When oral medication is given, the importance of strict adherence by the patient to the prescribed dosage regimen must be stressed. A therapeutic dose should be administered for at least 10 days.

Alpha-hemolytic streptococci (viridans group): Although no controlled clinical efficacy trials have been conducted, oral erythromycin has been suggested by the American Heart Association and American Dental Association for use in a regimen for prophylaxis against bacterial endocarditis in patients hypersensitive to penicillin who have congenital heart disease, or rheumatic or other acquired valvular heart disease when they undergo dental procedures and surgical procedures of the upper respiratory tract.[1] Erythromycin is not suitable prior to genitourinary or gastrointestinal tract surgery. NOTE: When selecting antibiotics for the prevention of bacterial endocarditis the physician or dentist should read the full joint statement of the American Heart Association and the American Dental Association.[1]

Staphylococcus aureus:Acute infections of skin and soft tissue of mild to moderate severity. Resistant organisms may emerge during treatment.

Streptococcus pneumoniae (Diplococcus pneumoniae):Upper respiratory tract infections (e.g., otitis media, pharyngitis) and lower respiratory tract infections (*e.g.,* pneumonia) of mild to moderate degree.

Mycoplasma pneumoniae(Eaton agent, PPLO): For respiratory infections due to this organism.

Hemophilus influenzae:For upper respiratory tract infections of mild to moderate severity when used concomitantly with adequate doses of sulfonamides. (See sulfonamide labeling for appropriate prescribing information.)The concomitant use of the sulfonamides is necessary since not all strains of Hemophilus influenzae are susceptible to erythromycin at the concentrations of the antibiotic achieved with usual therapeutic doses.

Chlamydia trachomatis:For the treatment of urethritis in adult males due to Chlamydia trachomatis.

Ureaplasma urealyticum:For the treatment of urethritis in adult males due to Ureaplasma urealyticum.

Treponema pallidum:Erythromycin is an alternate choice of treatment for primary syphilis in patients allergic to the penicillins. In treatment of primary syphilis, spinal fluid examinations should be done before treatment and as part of follow-up after therapy.

Corynebacterium diphtheriae:As an adjunct to antitoxin, to prevent establishment of carriers, and to eradicate the organism in carriers.

Corynebacterium minutissimum:For the treatment of erythrasma.

Entamoeba histolytica:In the treatment of intestinal amebiasis only. Extraenteric amebiasis requires treatment with other agents.

Listeria monocytogenes:Infections due to this organism.

Bordetella pertussis:Erythromycin is effective in eliminating the organism from the nasopharynx of infected individuals, rendering them non-infectious. Some clinical studies suggests that erythromycin may be helpful in the prophylaxis of pertussis in exposed susceptible individuals.

Legionnaires' Disease: Although no controlled clinical efficacy studies have been conducted, *in vitro* and limited preliminary clinical data suggest that erythromycin may be effective in treating Legionnaires' Disease.

CONTRAINDICATIONS:

Erythromycin is contraindicated in patients with known hypersensitivity to this antibiotic.

WARNINGS:

There have been reports of hepatic dysfunction with or without jaundice, occurring in patients receiving oral erythromycin products.

PRECAUTIONS:

General: Erythromycin is principally excreted by the liver. Caution should be exercised when erythromycin is administered to patients with impaired hepatic function. (See CLINICAL PHARMACOLOGY and WARNINGS).

Prolonged or repeated use of erythromycin may result in an overgrowth of nonsusceptible bacteria or fungi. If superinfection occurs, erythromycin should be discontinued and appropriate therapy instituted.

When indicated, incision and drainage or other surgical procedures should be performed in conjunction with antibiotic therapy.

Laboratory Tests: Erythromycin interferes with the fluorometric determination of urinary catecholamines.

Carcinogenesis, Mutagenesis, and Impairment of Fertility: Long-term (2-year) oral studies conducted in rats with erythromycin base did not provide evidence of tumorigenicity. Mutagenicity studies have not been conducted. There was no apparent effect on male or female fertility in rats fed erythromycin (base) at levels up to 0.25 percent of diet.

Pregnancy Category B: There is no evidence of teratogenicity or any other adverse effect on reproduction in female rats fed erythromycin base (up to 0.25 percent of diet) prior to and during mating, during gestation, and through weaning of two successive litters. There are, however, no adequate and well-controlled studies in pregnant women. Because animal reproduction studies are not always predictive of human response, this drug should be used during pregnancy only if clearly needed. Erythromycin has been reported to cross the placental barrier in humans, but fetal plasma levels are generally low.

Labor and Delivery: The effect of erythromycin on labor and delivery is unknown.

Nursing Mothers: Erythromycin is excreted in breast milk, therefore, caution should be exercised when erythromycin is administered to a nursing woman.

Pediatric Use: See INDICATIONS AND USAGE and DOSAGE AND ADMINISTRATION.

DRUG INTERACTIONS:

Erythromycin use in patients who are receiving high doses of theophylline may be associated with an increase in serum theophylline levels and potential theophylline toxicity. In case of theophylline toxicity and/or elevated serum theophylline levels, the dose of theophylline should be reduced while the patient is receiving concomitant erythromycin therapy.

Concomitant administration of erythromycin and digoxin has been reported to result in elevated digoxin serum levels.

There have been reports of increased anticoagulant effects when erythromycin and oral anticoagulants were used concomitantly.

Concurrent use of erythromycin and ergotamine or dihydroergotamine has been associated in some patients with acute ergot toxicity characterized by severe peripheral vasospasm and dysesthesia.

Erythromycin has been reported to decrease the clearance of triazolam and thus may increase the pharmacologic effect of triazolam.

The use of erythromycin in patients concurrently taking drugs metabolized by the cytochrome P450 system may be associated with elevations in serum erythromycin with carbamazepine, cyclosporine, hexobarbital and phenytoin. Serum concentrations of drugs metabolized by the cytochrome P450 system should be monitored closely in patients concurrently receiving erythromycin.

Troleandomycin significantly alters the metabolism of terfenadine when taken concomitantly; therefore, observe caution when erythromycin and terfenadine are used concurrently.

Patients receiving concomitant lovastatin and erythromycin should be carefully monitored; cases of rhabdomyolysis have been reported in seriously ill patients.

ADVERSE REACTIONS:

The most frequent side effects of oral erythromycin preparations are gastrointestinal and are dose-related. They include nausea, vomiting, abdominal pain, diarrhea and anorexia. Symptoms of hepatic dysfunction and/or abnormal liver function test results may occur (see WARNINGS.) Pseudomembranous colitis has been rarely reported in association with erythromycin therapy.

There have been isolated reports of transient central nervous system side effects including confusion, hallucinations, seizures, and vertigo; however, a cause and effect relationship has not been established.

Occasional case reports of cardiac arrhythmias such as ventricular tachycardia have been documented in patients receiving erythromycin therapy. There have been isolated reports of other cardiovascular symptoms such as chest pain, dizziness, and palpitations; however, a cause and effect relationship has not been established.

Allergic reactions ranging from urticaria and mild skin eruptions to anaphylaxis have occurred.

There have been isolated reports of reversible hearing loss occurring chiefly in patients with renal insufficiency and in patients receiving high doses of erythromycin.

OVERDOSAGE:

In case of overdosage, erythromycin should be discontinued. Overdosage should be handled with the prompt elimination of unabsorbed drug and all other appropriate measures.

Erythromycin is not removed by peritoneal dialysis or hemodialysis.

DOSAGE AND ADMINISTRATION:

Erythromycin ethylsuccinate suspensions and Filmtab tablets may be administered without regard to meals.

Children: Age, weight, and severity of the infection are important factors in determining the proper dosage. In mild to moderate infections the usual dosage of erythromycin ethylsuccinate for children is 30 to 50 mg/kg/day in equally divided doses every 6 hours. For more severe infections this dosage may be doubled. If twice-a-day dosage is desired, one-half of the total daily dose may be given every 12 hours. Doses may also be given three times daily by administering one-third of the total daily dose every 8 hours.

The following dosage schedule (TABLE 1) is suggested for mild to moderate infections:

TABLE 1

Body Weight	Total Daily Dose
Under 10 lbs	30-50 mg/kg/day 15-25 mg/lb/day
10 to 15 lbs	200 mg
16 to 25 lbs	400 mg
26 to 50 lbs	800 mg
51 to 100 lbs	1200 mg
Over 100 lbs	1600 mg

DOSAGE AND ADMINISTRATION: *(cont'd)*

Adults: 400 mg erythromycin ethylsuccinate every 6 hours is the usual dose. Dosage may be increased up to 4 g per day according to the severity of the infection. If twice-a-day dosage is desired, one-half of the total daily dose may be given every 12 hours. Doses may also be given three times daily by administering one-third of the total daily dose every 8 hours.

For adult dosage calculation, use a ratio of 400 mg of erythromycin activity as the ethylsuccinate to 250 mg of erythromycin activity as the stearate, base or estolate.

In the treatment of streptococcal infections, a therapeutic dosage of erythromycin ethylsuccinate should be administered for at least 10 days. In continuous prophylaxis against recurrences of streptococcal infections in persons with a history of rheumatic heart disease, the usual dosage is 400 mg twice a day.

For prophylaxis against bacterial endocarditis[1] in patients with congenital heart disease, or rheumatic or other acquired valvular heart disease when undergoing dental procedures or surgical procedures of the upper respiratory tract, give 1.6 g (20 mg/kg for children) orally 1-1/2 to 2 hours before the procedure, and then, 800 mg (10 mg/kg for children) orally every 6 hours for 8 doses.

For treatment of urethritis due to *C. trachomatis* or *U. urealyticum*: 800 mg three times a day for 7 days.

For treatment of primary syphilis: Adults: 48 to 64 g given in divided doses over a period of 10 to 15 days.

For intestinal amebiasis: Adults: 400 mg four times daily for 10 to 14 days. Children: 30 to 50 mg/kg/day in divided doses for 10 to 14 days.

For use in pertussis : Although optimal dosage and duration have not been established, doses of erythromycin utilized in reported clinical studies were 40 to 50 mg/kg/day, given in divided doses for 5 to 14 days.

For treatment of Legionnaires' Disease: Although optimal doses have not been established, doses utilized in reported clinical data were those recommended above (1.6 to 4 g daily in divided doses).

Recommended storage: Store tablets and granules (prior to mixing) below 86°F (30°C).

REFERENCES:

1. American Heart Association. 1977. Prevention of bacterial endocarditis. Circulation 56: 139A-143A.

HOW SUPPLIED - RATED THERAPEUTICALLY EQUIVALENT:

Granule, Reconstitution - Oral - 200 mg/5ml

5 ml	$0.74	ERYPED, Abbott	00074-6302-05
100 ml	$5.14	Erythromycin Ethylsuccinate, Aligen Independ	00405-2730-60
100 ml	$7.01	Erythromycin Ethylsuccinate, Barr	00555-0215-22
100 ml	$7.41	Erthromycin Ethylsuccinate, HL Moore Drug Exch	00839-6362-73
100 ml	$7.70	ERYPED, Abbott	00074-6302-13
100 ml	$7.91	E.E.S., Abbott	00074-6369-02
100 ml	$8.18	Erythromycin Ethylsuccinate, Rugby	00536-0318-82
100 ml	$8.24	Erythromycin Ethylsuccinate, H.C.F.A. F F P	99999-1182-02
100 ml	$8.65	Erythromycin Ethylsuccinate, Major Pharms	00904-2653-04
200 ml	$9.29	Erythromycin Ethylsuccinate, Parmed Pharms	00349-8806-02
200 ml	$9.95	Erythromycin Ethylsuccinate, Aligen Independ	00405-2730-70
200 ml	$12.95	Erythromycin Ethylsuccinate, Barr	00555-0215-23
200 ml	$14.02	ERYPED, Abbott	00074-6302-53
200 ml	$14.07	Erythromycin Ethylsuccinate, HL Moore Drug Exch	00839-6362-78
200 ml	$14.43	E.E.S., Abbott	00074-6369-10
200 ml	$15.64	Erythromycin Ethylsuccinate, H.C.F.A. F F P	99999-1182-04
200 ml	$16.30	Erythromycin Ethylsuccinate, Major Pharms	00904-2653-08

Powder, Reconstitution - Oral - 200 mg/5ml

100 ml	$7.80	Erythromycin Ethylsuccinate, Goldline Labs	00182-1530-70
200 ml	$13.90	Erythromycin Ethylsuccinate, Goldline Labs	00182-1530-73

Suspension - Oral - 200 mg/5ml

100 ml	$3.95	Erythromycin Ethylsuccinate, Harber Pharm	51432-0693-14
100 ml	$4.50	E.E.S. 200, Abbott	00074-6306-13
100 ml	$6.95	Erythromycin Ethylsuccinate, Consolidated Midland	00223-6142-10
200 ml	$5.69	Erythromycin Ethylsuccinate, H.C.F.A. F F P	99999-1182-08
480 ml	$11.90	Erythromycin Ethylsuccinate, H.C.F.A. F F P	99999-1182-09
480 ml	$13.00	Erythromycin Ethylsuccinate, Logen Pharm	00820-0117-38
480 ml	$14.90	Erythromycin Ethylsuccinate, Raway	00686-0971-16
480 ml	$16.67	Erythromycin Ethylsuccinate, Lederle Pharm	00005-3706-65
480 ml	$17.50	Erythromycin Ethylsuccinate, Harber Pharm	51432-0582-20
480 ml	$19.00	Erythromycin, Goldline Labs	00182-1371-40
480 ml	$19.04	Erythromycin Ethylsuccinate, Alpharma	00472-0971-16
480 ml	$19.59	Erythromycin Ethylsuccinate, Abbott	00074-3747-16
480 ml	$19.59	EES 200, Abbott	00074-6306-16
480 ml	$19.85	Erythromycin Ethylsuccinate, Qualitest Pharms	00603-1206-58
480 ml	$20.95	Erythromycin Ethylsuccinate, Major Pharms	00904-2462-16
480 ml	$21.47	Erythromycin Ethylsuccinate, HL Moore Drug Exch	00839-6482-69
480 ml	$22.00	Erythromycin Ethylsuccinate, Schein Pharm (US)	00364-2067-16
480 ml	$23.50	Erythromycin Ethylsuccinate, Consolidated Midland	00223-6142-01
480 ml	$23.50	Erythromycin Ethylsuccinate, Rugby	00536-0360-85

Suspension - Oral - 400 mg/5ml

100 ml	$8.09	EES 400, Abbott	00074-6373-13
100 ml	$10.95	Erythromycin Ethylsuccinate, Consolidated Midland	00223-6143-10
480 ml	$20.92	Erythromycin Ethylsuccinate, H.C.F.A. F F P	99999-1182-11
480 ml	$22.45	Erythromycin Ethylsuccinate, Logen Pharm	00820-0118-38
480 ml	$23.00	Erythromycin Ethylsuccinate, Raway	00686-0974-16
480 ml	$30.60	Erythromycin Ethylsuccinate, Lederle Pharm	00005-3732-65
480 ml	$31.95	Erythromycin Ethylsuccinate, Harber Pharm	51432-0584-20
480 ml	$33.39	Erythromycin Ethylsuccinate, Alpharma	00472-0974-16
480 ml	$34.63	Erythromycin Ethylsuccinate, HL Moore Drug Exch	00839-6568-69
480 ml	$34.90	Erythromycin Ethylsuccinate, Qualitest Pharms	00603-1207-58
480 ml	$36.49	Erythromycin Ethylsuccinate, Abbott	00074-3748-16
480 ml	$36.49	EES 400, Abbott	00074-6373-16
480 ml	$37.45	Erythromycin Ethylsuccinate, Goldline Labs	00182-1773-40
480 ml	$38.99	Erythromycin Ethylsuccinate, Schein Pharm (US)	00364-2070-16
480 ml	$39.75	Erythromycin Ethylsuccinate, Major Pharms	00904-2463-16
480 ml	$42.50	Erythromycin Ethylsuccinate, Consolidated Midland	00223-6143-01
480 ml	$42.50	Erythromycin Ethylsuccinate, Rugby	00536-0371-85

Tablet, Chewable - Oral - 200 mg

40's	$19.64	ERYPED, Abbott	00074-6314-40

Tablet, Plain Coated - Oral - 400 mg

100's	$18.66	Erythromycin Ethylsuccinate, US Trading	56126-0387-11
100's	$19.59	Erythromycin Ethylsuccinate, Lederle Pharm	00005-3061-23
100's	$21.92	ERYTHROMYCIN ETHYLSUCCINATE, Abbott	00074-2589-13
100's	$21.92	EES 400, Abbott	00074-5729-13
100's	$22.43	Erythromycin Ethylsuccinate, H.C.F.A. F F P	99999-1182-12
100's	$24.30	EES 400, Abbott	00074-5729-11
100's	$25.75	Erythromycin Ethylsuccinate, Qualitest Pharms	00603-3552-21
100's	$25.77	Erythromycin Ethylsuccinate, HL Moore Drug Exch	00839-6588-06
100's	$26.45	Erythromycin Ethylsuccinate, Goldline Labs	00182-1489-01

HOW SUPPLIED - RATED THERAPEUTICALLY EQUIVALENT: *(cont'd)*

100's	$26.95	Erythromicin Ethylsuccinate, Mylan	00378-6400-01
100's	$30.87	Erythromycin Ethylsuccinate, Voluntary Hosp	53258-5729-76
100's	$33.09	Erythromycin Ethylsuccinate, Voluntary Hosp	53258-5729-77
500's	$94.70	Erythromycin Ethylsuccinate, Lederle Pharm	00005-3061-31
500's	$104.12	Erythromycin Ethylsuccinate, Abbott	00074-2589-53
500's	$104.12	EES 400, Abbott	00074-5729-53
500's	$109.40	Erythromycin Ethylsuccinate, Goldline Labs	00182-1489-05
500's	$112.15	Erythromycin Ethylsuccinate, H.C.F.A. F F P	99999-1182-13
500's	$120.61	Erythromycin Ethylsuccinate, Qualitest Pharms	00603-3552-28
500's	$120.95	Erythromycin Ethylsuccinate, Mylan	00378-6400-05
500's	$143.10	Erythromycin Ethylsuccinate, HL Moore Drug Exch	00839-6588-12
1000's	$189.57	EES 400, Abbott	00074-5729-19
1000's	$224.30	Erythromycin Ethylsuccinate, H.C.F.A. F F P	99999-1182-14

HOW SUPPLIED - NOT RATED EQUIVALENT:

Drops - Oral - 200 mg/5ml

50 ml	$6.21	ERYPED DROPS, Abbott	00074-6303-50

Powder, Reconstitution - Oral - 400 mg/5ml

5 ml	$1.08	ERYPED, Abbott	00074-6305-05
60 ml	$7.78	ERYPED, Abbott	00074-6305-60
100 ml	$11.85	ERYPED, Abbott	00074-6305-13
200 ml	$21.62	ERYPED, Abbott	00074-6305-53

ERYTHROMYCIN ETHYLSUCCINATE; SULFISOXAZOLE ACETYL *(001181)*

CATEGORIES: Anti-Infectives; Antibiotics; Antimicrobials; Erythromycins; Hemophilus; Lincosamides/Macrolides; Otic Preparations; Otitis Media; Otologic; Sulfonamides; FDA Approved 1989 Sep

BRAND NAMES: Erythromycin W/Sulfisoxazole; Eryzole; Ilosone Sulfa; **Pediazole**; Sulfimycin

FORMULARIES: Aetna; BC-BS; CIGNA; FHP; Foundation; Humana; Kaiser; Medco; Medi-Cal; PruCare; United

DESCRIPTION:

This product is a combination of erythromycin ethylsuccinate, USP and sulfisoxazole acetyl, USP. When reconstituted with water as directed on the label, the granules form a white, strawberry-banana flavor suspension that provides the equivalent of 200 mg of erythromycin activity and the equivalent of 600 mg of sulfisoxazole per teaspoonful (5 ml).

Erythromycin is produced by a strain of *Sa erythraea* and belongs to the macrolide group of antibiotics. It is basic and readily forms salts and esters. Erythromycin ethylsuccinate is the 2'-ethylsuccinyl ester of erythromycin. It is essentially a tasteless form of the antibiotic suitable for oral administration, particularly in suspension dosage forms. The chemical name is erythromycin 2'-(ethylsuccinate).

Sulfisoxazole acetyl or N^1-acetyl sulfisoxazole is an ester of sulfisoxazole. Chemically, sulfisoxazole is N-(3,4-Dimethyl-5-isoxazolyl)-N-sulfanilylacetamide.

Inactive Ingredients: Citric acid, magnesium aluminum silicate, poloxamer, sodium carboxymethylcellulose, sodium citrate, sucrose, and artificial flavoring.

CLINICAL PHARMACOLOGY:

Orally administered erythromycin ethylsuccinate suspensions are readily and reliably absorbed. Erythromycin ethylsuccinate products have demonstrated rapid and consistent absorption in both fasting and nonfasting conditions. Higher serum concentrations are obtained when these products are given with food. Bioavailability data are available from Ross Products Division. Erythromycin is largely bound to plasma proteins. After absorption, erythromycin diffuses readily into most body fluids. In the absence of meningeal inflammation, low concentrations are normally achieved in the spinal fluid, but the passage of the drug across the blood-brain barrier increases in meningitis. Erythromycin crosses the placental barrier and is excreted in human milk. Erythromycin is not removed by peritoneal dialysis or hemodialysis.

In the presence of normal hepatic function, erythromycin is concentrated in the liver and is excreted in the bile; the effect of hepatic dysfunction on biliary excretion of erythromycin is not known. After oral administration, less than 5% of the administered dose can be recovered in the active form in the urine.

Wide variation in blood levels may result following identical doses of sulfonamide. Blood levels should be measured in patients receiving these drugs for serious infections. Free sulfonamide blood levels of 50 to 150 mcg/ml may be considered therapeutically effective for most infections, with blood levels of 120 to 150 mcg/ml being optimal for serious infections. The maximum sulfonamide level should be 200 mcg/ml, because adverse reactions occur more frequently above this concentration.

Following oral administration, sulfisoxazole is rapidly and completely absorbed; the small intestine is the major site of absorption, but some of the drug is absorbed from the stomach. Sulfonamides are present in the blood as free, conjugated (acetylated and possibly other forms), and protein-bound forms. The amount present as "free" drug is considered to be the therapeutically active form. Approximately 85% of a dose of sulfisoxazole is bound to plasma proteins, primarily to albumin; 65% to 72% of the unbound portion is in the nonacetylated form.

Maximum plasma concentrations of intact sulfisoxazole following a single 2-g oral dose of sulfisoxazole to healthy adult volunteers ranged from 127 to 211 mcg/ml (mean, 169 mcg/ml), and the time of peak plasma concentration ranged from 1 to 4 hours (mean, 2.5 hours). The elimination half-life of sulfisoxazole ranged from 4.6 hours to 7.8 hours after oral administration. The elimination of sulfisoxazole has been shown to be slower in elderly subjects (63 to 75 years) with diminished renal function (creatine clearance 37 to 68 ml/min).[1] After multiple- dose oral administration of 500 mg q.i.d. to healthy volunteers, the average steady-state plasma concentrations of intact sulfisoxazole ranged from 49.9 to 88.8 mcg/ml (mean, 63.4 mcg/ml).[2]

Sulfisoxazole and its acetylated metabolites are excreted primarily by the kidneys through glomerular filtration. Concentrations of sulfisoxazole are considerably higher in the urine than in the blood. The mean urinary recovery following oral administration of sulfisoxazole is 97% within 48 hours; 52% of this is intact drug, and the remainder is the N^4-acetylated metabolite.

Sulfisoxazole is distributed only in extracellular body fluids. it is excreted in human milk. It readily crosses the placental barrier. In healthy subjects, cerebrospinal fluid concentrations of sulfisoxazole vary; in patients with meningitis, however, concentrations of free drug in cerebrospinal fluid as high as 94 mcg/ml have been reported.

MICROBIOLOGY

The drug has been formulated to contain sulfisoxazole for concomitant use with erythromycin.

CLINICAL PHARMACOLOGY: *(cont'd)*

Erythromycin acts by inhibition of protein synthesis by binding 50 S ribosomal subunits of susceptible organisms. It does not affect nucleic acid synthesis. Antagonism has been demonstrated *in vitro* between erythromycin and clindamycin, lincomycin, and chloramphenicol.

The sulfonamides are bacteriostatic agents, and the spectrum of activity is similar for all. Sulfonamides inhibit bacterial synthesis of dihydrofolic acid by preventing the condensation of the pteridine with*para*-aminobenzoic acid through competitive inhibition of the enzyme dihydropteroate synthetase. Resistant strains have altered dihydropterase synthetase with reduced affinity for sulfonamides or produce increased quantities of *para*-aminobenzoic acid.

SUSCEPTIBILITY TESTING

Quantitative methods that require measurement of zone diameter give the most precise estimates of the susceptibility of bacteria to antimicrobial agents. One such standardized single-disc procedure[3]has been recommended for use with discs to test susceptibility to erythromycin and sulfisoxazole. Interpretation involves correlation of the zone diameters obtained in the disc test with minimal inhibitory concentration (MIC) values for erythromycin.

If the standardized procedure of disc susceptibility is used, a 15-mcg erythromycin disc should give a zone diameter of at least 18 mm when tested against an erythromycin-susceptible bacterial strain and a 250-300 mcg sulfisoxazole disc should give a zone diameter of at least 17 mm when tested against a sulfisoxazole-susceptible bacterial strain.

In vitro sulfonamide susceptibility tests are not always reliable because media containing excessive amounts of thymidine are capable of reversing the inhibitory effect of sulfonamides, which may result in false resistant reports. The tests must be carefully coordinated with bacteriological and clinical responses. When the patient is already taking sulfonamides, follow-up cultures should have aminobenzoic acid added to the isolation media but not to subsequent susceptibility test media.

INDICATIONS AND USAGE:

For treatment of ACUTE OTITIS MEDIA in children that is caused by susceptible strains of *Hemophilus influenzae.*

CONTRAINDICATIONS:

Patients with a known hypersensitivity to either of its components, children younger than 2 months of age, pregnant women *at term*, and mothers nursing infants less than 2 months of age.

Use in pregnant women at term, in children less than 2 months of age, and in mothers nursing infants less than 2 months of age is contraindicated because sulfonamides may promote kernicterus in the newborn by displacing bilirubin from plasma proteins.

Erythromycin is contraindicated in patients taking terfenadine (See DRUG INTERACTIONS.)

WARNINGS:

FATALITIES ASSOCIATED WITH THE ADMINISTRATION OF SULFONAMIDES, ALTHOUGH RARE, HAVE OCCURRED DUE TO SEVERE REACTIONS INCLUDING STEVENS-JOHNSON SYNDROME, TOXIC EPIDERMAL NECROLYSIS, FULMINANT HEPATIC NECROSIS, AGRANULOCYTOSIS, APLASTIC ANEMIA, AND OTHER BLOOD DYSCRASIAS.

SULFONAMIDES, INCLUDING SULFONAMIDE-CONTAINING PRODUCTS SUCH AS PEDIAZOLE, SHOULD BE DISCONTINUED AT THE FIRST APPEARANCE OF SKIN RASH OR ANY SIGN OF ADVERSE REACTION. In rare instances, a skin rash may be followed by a more severe reaction, such as Stevens-Johnson syndrome, toxic epidermal necrolysis, hepatic necrosis, and serious blood disorders. (See PRECAUTIONS.)

Clinical signs such as sore throat, fever, pallor, rash, purpura, or jaundice may be early indications of serious reactions.

There have been reports of hepatic dysfunction, with or without jaundice, occurring in patients receiving oral erythromycin products.

Cough, shortness of breath, and pulmonary infiltrates are hypersensitivity reactions of the respiratory tract that have been reported in association with sulfonamide treatment.

The sulfonamides should not be used for the treatment of group A beta-hemolytic streptococcal infections. In an established infection, they will not eradicate the streptococcus, and, therefore, will not prevent sequelae such as rheumatic fever.

Pseudomembranous colitis has been reported with nearly all antibacterial agents, including this drug, and may range in severity from mild to life-threatening. Therefore, it is important to consider this diagnosis in patients who present with diarrhea subsequent to the administration of antibacterial agents.

Treatment with antibacterial agents alters the normal flora of the colon and may permit overgrowth of clostridia. Studies indicate that a toxin produced by *Clostridium difficile* is one primary cause of "antibiotic-associated colitis."

After diagnosis of pseudomembranous colitis has been established, therapeutic measures should be initiated. Mild cases of pseudomembranous colitis usually respond to drug discontinuation alone. In moderate to severe cases, consideration should be given to management with fluids and electrolytes, protein supplementation, and treatment with an antibacterial drug clinically effective against *Clostridium difficile* colitis.

There have been reports suggesting that erythromycin does not reach the fetus in adequate concentration to prevent congenital syphilis. Infants born to women treated during pregnancy with erythromycin for early syphilis should be treated with an appropriate penicillin regimen.

Rhabdomyolysis with or without renal impairment has been reported in seriously ill patients receiving erythromycin concomitantly with lovastatin. Therefore, patients receiving concomitant lovastatin and erythromycin should be carefully monitored for creatine kinase (CK) and serum transaminase levels. (See prescribing informtion for lovastatin.)

PRECAUTIONS:

General: Erythromycin is principally excreted by the liver. Caution should be exercised in administering the antibiotic to patients with impaired hepatic function. (See CLINICAL PHARMACOLOGY and WARNINGS.)

Prolonged or repeated use of erythromycin may result in an overgrowth of nonsusceptible bacteria or fungi. If superinfection occurs, erythromycin should be discontinued and appropriate therapy instituted.

There have been reports that erythromycin may aggravate the weakness of patients with myasthenia gravis.

When indicated, incision and drainage or other surgical procedures should be performed in conjunction with antibiotic therapy.

Sulfonamides should be given with caution to patients with impaired renal or hepatic function and to those with severe allergy or bronchial asthma. In glucose-6-phosphate dehydrogenase-deficient individuals, hemolysis may occur; this reaction is frequently dose-related.

Information for the Patient: Patients should maintain an adequate fluid intake to prevent crystalluria and stone formation.

PRECAUTIONS: *(cont'd)*

Laboratory Tests: Complete blood counts should be done frequently in patients receiving sulfonamides. If a significant reduction in the count of any formed blood element is noted, the drug should be discontinued. Urinalysis with careful microscopic examination and renal function tests should be performed during therapy, particularly for those patients with impaired renal function. Blood levels should be measured in patients receiving a sulfonamide for serious infections. (See INDICATIONS AND USAGE.)

Drug/Laboratory Test Interactions: Erythromycin interferes with the fluorometric determination of urinary catecholamines.

CARCINOGENESIS, MUTAGENESIS, AND IMPAIRMENT OF FERTILITY

Carcinogenesis: The drug has not undergone adequate trials relating to carcinogenicity; each component, however, has been evaluated separately. Long-term (21 month) oral studies conducted in rats with erythromycin ethylsuccinate did not provide evidence of tumorigenicity. Sulfisoxazole was not carcinogenic in either sex when administered to mice by gavage for 103 weeks at dosages up to approximately 18 times the recommended human dose or to rats at 4 times the human dose. Rats appear to be especially susceptible to the goitrogenic effects of sulfonamides, and long-term administration of sulfonamides has resulted in thyroid malignancies in this species.

Mutagenesis: There are no studies available that adequately evaluate the mutagenic potential of the drug or either of its components. However, sulfisoxazole was not observed to be mutagenic in *E. coli* Sd-4-73 when tested in the absence of a metabolic activating system. There was no apparent effect on male or female fertility in rats fed erythromycin (base) at levels up to 0.25% of diet.

Impairment of Fertility: The drug has not undergone adequate trials relating to impairment of fertility. In a reproduction study in rats given 7 times the human dose per day of sulfisoxazole, no effects were observed regarding mating behavior, conception rate or fertility index (percent pregnant).

Pregnancy: Teratogenic Effects. Pregnancy Category C. At dosages 7 times the human daily dose, sulfisoxazole was not teratogenic in either rats or rabbits. However, in two other teratogenicity studies, cleft palates developed in both rats and mice after administration of 5 to 9 times the human therapeutic dose of sulfisoxazole.

There is no evidence of teratogenicity or any other adverse effect on reproduction in female rats fed erythromycin base (up to 0.25% of diet) prior to and during mating, during gestation, and through weaning of two successive litters. There are, however, no adequate and well-controlled studies in pregnant women. Because animal reproduction studies are not always predictive of human response, this drug should be used during pregnancy only if clearly needed. Erythromycin has been reported to cross the placental barrier in humans, but fetal plasma levels are generally low.

There are no adequate or well-controlled studies of the drug in either laboratory animals or in pregnant women. It is not known whether the drug can cause fetal harm when administered to a pregnant woman prior to term or can affect reproduction capacity. The drug should be used during pregnancy only if potential benefit justifies potential risk to the fetus.

Nonteratogenic Effects: Kernicterus may occur in the newborn as a result of treatment of a pregnant woman *at term*with sulfonamides. (See CONTRAINDICATIONS.)

Labor and Delivery: The effects of erythromycin and sulfisoxazole on labor and delivery are unknown.

Nursing Mothers: Both erythromycin and sulfisoxazole are excreted in human milk. **Because of the potential for the development of kernicterus in neonates due to the displacement of bilirubin from plasma proteins by sulfisoxazole, a decision should be made whether to discontinue nursing or discontinue the drug, taking into account the importance of the drug to the mother.** (See CONTRAINDICATIONS.)

Pediatric Use: See INDICATIONS AND USAGE and DOSAGE AND ADMINISTRATION sections. Not for use in children under 2 months of age.(See CONTRAINDICATIONS.)

DRUG INTERACTIONS:

Erythromycin use in patients who are receiving high doses of theophylline may be associated with an increase of serum theophylline levels and potential theophylline toxicity. In case of theophylline toxicity and/or elevated serum theophylline levels, the dose of theophylline should be reduced while the patient is receiving concomitant erythromycin therapy.

Concomitant administration of erythromycin and digoxin has been reported to result in elevated digoxin serum levels.

There have been reports of increased anticoagulant effects when erythromycin and oral anticoagulants were used concomitantly. Increased anticoagulation effects due to this drug may be more pronounced in the elderly.

Concurrent use of erythromycin and ergotamine or dihydroergotamine has been associated in some patients with acute ergot toxicity characterized by severe peripheral vasospasm and dysesthesia.

Erythromycin has been reported to decrease the clearance of triazolam and midazolam and thus may increase the pharmacologic effect of these benzodiazepines.

The use of erythromycin in patients concurrently taking drugs metabolized by the cytochrome P450 system may be associated with elevations of serum levels of these other drugs. There have been reports of interactions of erythromycin with carbamazepine, cyclosporine, hexobarbital, phenytoin, alfentanil, disopyramide, lovastatin, and bromocriptine. Serum concentrations of drugs metabolized by the cytochrome P450 system should be monitored closely in patients concurrently receiving erythromycin.

Erythromycin significantly alters the metabolism of terfenadine when taken concomitantly. Rare cases of serious cardiovascular adverse events, including death, cardiac arrest, torsades de pointes, and other ventricular arrhythmias, have been observed (See CONTRAINDICATIONS.)

It has been reported that sulfisoxazole may prolong the prothrombin time in patients who are receiving the anticoagulant warfarin. This interaction should be kept in mind when the drug is given to patients already on the anticoagulant therapy, and the coagulation time should be reassessed.

It has been proposed that sulfisoxazole competes with thiopental for plasma protein binding. In one study involving 48 patients, intravenous sulfisoxazole resulted in a decrease in the amount of thiopental required for anesthesia and in a shortening of the awakening time. it is not known whether chronic oral doses of sulfisoxazole have a similar effect. Until more is known about this interaction, physicians should be aware that patients receiving sulfisoxazole might require less thiopental for anesthesia.

Sulfonamides can displace methotrexate from plasma protein binding sites, thus increasing free methotrexate concentrations. Studies in man have shown sulfisoxazole infusions to decrease plasma protein-bound methotrexate by one fourth.

Sulfisoxazole can also potentiate the blood-sugar-lowering activity of sulfonylureas.

ADVERSE REACTIONS:

Erythromycin ethylsuccinate: The most frequent side effects of oral erythromycin preparations are gastrointestinal and are dose-related. They include nausea, vomiting, abdominal pain, diarrhea and anorexia. Symptoms of hepatic dysfunction and/or abnormal liver-function test results may occur (see WARNINGS.) Pseudomembranous colitis has been rarely reported in association with erythromycin therapy.

Allergic reactions ranging from urticaria and mild skin eruptions to anaphylaxis have occurred.

There have been isolated reports of reversible hearing loss occurring chiefly in patients with renal insufficiency and in patients receiving high doses of erythromycin.

Onset of pseudomembranous colitis symptoms may occur during or after antibiotic treatment. (See WARNINGS.)

Sulfisoxazole acetyl: Included in this listing that follows are adverse reactions that have been reported with other sulfonamide products; pharmacologic similarities require that each of the reactions be considered with the drug's administration.

Allergic/Dermatologic: Anaphylaxis, erythema multiforme (Stevens- Johnson syndrome), toxic epidermal necrolysis (Lyell's syndrome), exfoliative dermatitis, angioedema, arteritis, vasculitis, allergic myocarditis, serum sickness, rash, urticaria, pruritus, photosensitivity, and conjunctival and scleral injection. In addition, periarteritis nodosa and systemic lupus erythematosus has been reported. (See WARNINGS.)

Cardiovascular: Tachycardia, palpitations, syncope, and cyanosis.

Rarely, erythromycin has been associated with the production of ventricular arrhythmias, including ventricular tachycardia and torsade de pointes, in individuals with prolonged QT intervals.

Endocrine: The sulfonamides bear certain chemical similarities to some goitrogens, diuretics (acetazolamide and the thiazides) and oral hypoglycemic agents. Cross-sensitivity may exist with these agents. Developments of goiter, diuresis, and hypoglycemia have occurred rarely in patients receiving sulfonamides.

Gastrointestinal: Hepatitis, hepatocellular necrosis, jaundice, pseudomembranous colitis, nausea, emesis, anorexia, abdominal pain, diarrhea, gastrointestinal hemorrhage, melena, flatulence, glossitis, stomatitis, salivary gland enlargement, and pancreatitis. Onset of pseudomembranous colitis symptoms may occur during or after treatment with sulfisoxazole, a component of this drug. (See WARNINGS.)

The sulfisoxazole acetyl component of this drug has been reported to cause increased elevation of liver-associated enzymes in patients with hepatitis.

Genitourinary: Crystalluria, hematuria, BUN and creatinine elevations, nephritis, and toxic nephrosis with oliguria and anuria. Acute renal failure and urinary retention have also been reported.

The frequency of renal complications, commonly associated with some sulfonamides, is lower in patients receiving the more soluble sulfonamides such as sulfisoxazole.

Hematologic: Leukopenia, agranulocytosis, aplastic anemia, thrombocytopenia, purpura, hemolytic anemia, eosinophilia, clotting disorders including hypoprothrombinemia and hypofibrinogenemia, sulfhemoglobinemia, and methemoglobinemia.

Neurologic: Headache, dizziness, peripheral neuritis, paresthesia, convulsions, tinnitus, vertigo, ataxia, and intracranial hypertension.

Psychiatric: Psychosis, hallucinations, disorientation, depression, and anxiety.

Respiratory: Cough, shortness of breath, and pulmonary infiltrates. (See WARNINGS.)

Vascular: Angioedema, arteritis, and vasculitis.

Miscellaneous: Edema (including periorbital), pyrexia, drowsiness, weakness, fatigue, lassitude, rigors, flushing, hearing loss, insomnia, and pneumonitis.

OVERDOSAGE:

No information is available on a specific result of overdose with this drug. Overdosage of erythromycin should be handled with prompt elimination of unabsorbed drug and all other appropriate measures. Erythromycin is not removed by peritoneal dialysis or hemodialysis.

The amount of a single dose of sulfisoxazole that is either associated with symptoms of overdosage or is likely to be life-threatening has not been reported. Signs and symptoms of overdosage reported with sulfonamides include anorexia, colic, nausea, vomiting, dizziness, headache, drowsiness and unconsciousness. Pyrexia, hematuria and crystalluria may be noted. Blood dyscrasias and jaundice are potential late manifestations of overdosage.

General principles of treatment include the immediate discontinuation of the drug, instituting gastric lavage or emesis, forcing oral fluids, and administering intravenous fluids if urine output is low and renal function is normal. The patient should be monitored with blood counts and appropriate blood chemistries, including electrolytes. If the patient becomes cyanotic, the possibility of methemoglobinemia should be considered and, if present, the condition should be treated appropriately with intravenous 1% methylene blue. If a significant blood dyscrasia or jaundice occurs, specific therapy should be instituted for these complications. Peritoneal dialysis is not effective, and hemodialysis is only moderately effective in removing sulfonamides.

The acute toxicity of sulfisoxazole in animals is as follows (TABLE 1):

TABLE 1

Species	$LD_{50} \pm$ S.E.·(mg/kg)
mouse	5700 ± 235
rat	> 10,000
rabbits	> 2,000

DOSAGE AND ADMINISTRATION:

THIS DRUG SHOULD NOT BE ADMINISTERED TO INFANTS UNDER 2 MONTHS OF AGE BECAUSE OF CONTRAINDICATIONS OF SYSTEMIC SULFONAMIDES IN THIS AGE GROUP.

For Acute Otitis Media in Children: The dose of erythromycin ethylsuccinate w/ Sulfisoxazole Acetyl can be calculated based on the erythromycin component (50 mg/kg/day) or the sulfisoxazole component (150 mg/kg/day to a maximum of 6 g/day). The total daily dose of erythromycin ethylsuccinate w/ Sulfisoxazole Acetyl should be administered in equally divided doses three or four times a day for 10 days. Erythromycin ethylsuccinate w/ Sulfisoxazole Acetyl may be administered without regard to meals.

The following approximate dosage schedules are recommended for using erythromycin ethylsuccinate w/ sulfisoxazole acetyl:

Children: Two months of age or older (TABLE 2):

Recommended storage: Before mixing, store below 86°F (30°C).

TABLE 2A

Weight	FOUR-TIMES-A-DAY SCHEDULE Dose — every 6 hours
Less than 8 kg (<18 lbs)	Adjust dosage by body weight
8 kg (18 lbs)	1/2 teaspoonful (2.5 ml)
16 kg (35 lbs)	1 teaspoonful (5 ml)
24 kg (53 lbs)	1 1/2 teaspoonfuls (7.5 ml)
Over 32 kg (over 70 lbs)	2 teaspoonfuls (10 ml)

TABLE 2B

Weight	THREE-TIMES-A-DAY SCHEDULE Dose - every 8 hours
Less than 6 kg (<13 lbs)	Adjust dosage by body weight
6 kg (13 lbs)	1/2 teaspoonful (2.5 ml)
12 kg (26 lbs)	1 teaspoonful (5 ml)
18 kg (40 lbs)	1 1/2 teaspoonfuls (7.5 ml)
24 kg (53 lbs)	2 teaspoonfuls (10 ml)
Over 30 kg (over 65 lbs)	2 1/2 teaspoonfuls (12.5 ml)

REFERENCES:

1. Biovert A, Barbeau G, Belanger PM: Pharmacokinetics of sulfisoxazole in young and elderly subjects. *Gerontology*1984; 30:125-131. **2.** Oie S, Gambertoglio JG, Fleckenstein L: Comparison of the disposition of total and unbound sulfisoxazole after single and multiple dosing. *J Pharmacokinet Biopharm* 1982; 10:157-172. **3.** National Committee for Clinical Laboratory Standards:*Performance Standards for Antimicrobial Disk Susceptibility Tests*, ed 4. Approved Standard NCCLS Document M2-A4, Vol 10, No. 7. Villanova, Pa:NCCLS, 1990.

HOW SUPPLIED - RATED THERAPEUTICALLY EQUIVALENT:

Granule - Oral - 200 mg/600 mg/5

100 ml	$8.93	Erythromycin Ethylsuccinate; Sulfisoxazo, H.C.F.A. F F P	99999-1181-01
150 ml	$12.75	Erythromycin Ethylsuccinate; Sulfisoxazo, H.C.F.A. F F P	99999-1181-02
200 ml	$16.48	Erythromycin Ethylsuccinate; Sulfisoxazo, H.C.F.A. F F P	99999-1181-03

Granule, Reconstitution - Oral - 200 mg/600 mg/5

100 ml	$8.93	Erythromycin/Sulfisoxazole, United Res	00677-1303-27
100 ml	$9.75	Erythromycin/Sulfisoxazole, Harber Pharm	51432-0826-14
100 ml	$11.00	Erythromycin/Sulfisoxazole, HL Moore Drug Exch	00839-7514-73
100 ml	$11.00	ERYZOLE, Alra Labs	51641-0111-64
100 ml	$11.60	Erythromycin W/Sulfisoxazole, Qualitest Pharms	00603-6563-64
100 ml	$11.83	Erythromycin/Sulfisoxazole Acetyl, Schein Pharm (US)	00364-2319-61
100 ml	$11.93	Erythromycin/Sulfisoxazole, Goldline Labs	00182-7063-70
100 ml	$11.93	Erythromycin W/Sulfisoxazole, Aligen Independ	00405-2735-60
100 ml	$11.95	Erythromycin/Sulfisoxazole, Major Pharms	00904-2475-04
100 ml	$11.97	E.E.S./ SULFISOXAZOLE ACETYL, Lederle Pharm	00005-3700-46
100 ml	$12.45	Erythromycin W/Sulfisoxazole, Warner Chilcott	00047-2545-17
100 ml	$12.50	Erythromycin/Sulfisoxazole, Geneva Pharms	00781-7043-46
100 ml	$12.70	Erythromycin/Sulfisoxazole, Barr	00555-0445-22
100 ml	$13.65	Erythromycin/Sulfisoxazole, Rugby	00536-0050-82
100 ml	**$16.65**	**PEDIAZOLE, Abbott**	**00074-8030-13**
150 ml	$13.39	Erythromycin/Sulfisoxazole, United Res	00677-1303-28
150 ml	$15.75	Erythromycin/Sulfisoxazole, Harber Pharm	51432-0826-15
150 ml	$16.13	ERYZOLE, Alra Labs	51641-0111-66
150 ml	$17.30	Erythromycin/Sulfisoxazole, Major Pharms	00904-2475-07
150 ml	$17.40	Erythromycin W/Sulfisoxazole, Qualitest Pharms	00603-6563-66
150 ml	$17.70	Erythromycin/Sulfisoxazole Acetyl, Schein Pharm (US)	00364-2319-62
150 ml	$17.74	E.E.S./ SULFISOXAZOLE ACETYL, Lederle Pharm	00005-3700-49
150 ml	$17.76	Erythromycin/Sulfisoxazole, Goldline Labs	00182-7063-72
150 ml	$17.80	Erythromycin W/Sulfisoxazole, Aligen Independ	00405-2735-78
150 ml	$17.81	Erythromycin/Sulfisoxazole, HL Moore Drug Exch	00839-7514-75
150 ml	$18.25	Erythromycin/Sulfisoxazole, Rugby	00536-0050-74
150 ml	$18.50	Erythromycin/Sulfisoxazole, Geneva Pharms	00781-7043-55
150 ml	$18.55	Erythromycin W/Sulfisoxazole, Warner Chilcott	00047-2545-18
150 ml	$18.80	Erythromycin/Sulfisoxazole, Barr	00555-0445-21
150 ml	**$24.73**	**PEDIAZOLE, Abbott**	**00074-8030-43**
200 ml	$17.86	Erythromycin/Sulfisoxazole, United Res	00677-1303-29
200 ml	$21.25	ERYZOLE, Alra Labs	51641-0111-68
200 ml	$23.15	Erythromycin W/Sulfisoxazole, Qualitest Pharms	00603-6563-68
200 ml	$23.25	Erythromycin/Sulfisoxazole, Major Pharms	00904-2475-08
200 ml	$23.30	Erythromycin/Sulfisoxazole Acetyl, Schein Pharm (US)	00364-2319-63
200 ml	$23.33	Erythromycin/Sulfisoxazole, Goldline Labs	00182-7063-73
200 ml	$24.04	E.E.S./ SULFISOXAZOLE ACETYL, Lederle Pharm	00005-3700-60
200 ml	$24.50	Erythromycin/Sulfisoxazole, Geneva Pharms	00781-7043-48
200 ml	$24.53	Erythromycin W/Sulfisoxazole, Warner Chilcott	00047-2545-20
200 ml	$24.65	Erythromycin/Sulfisoxazole, Rugby	00536-0050-84
200 ml	$24.78	Erythromycin/Sulfisoxazole, Barr	00555-0445-23
200 ml	$25.37	Erythromycin/Sulfisoxazole, HL Moore Drug Exch	00839-7514-78
200 ml	**$32.48**	**PEDIAZOLE, Abbott**	**00074-8030-53**
250 ml	**$39.98**	**PEDIAZOLE, Abbott**	**00074-8030-73**

Powder, Reconstitution - Oral - 200 mg/600 mg/5

100 ml	$12.77	Erythromycin W/Sulfisoxazole, Abbott	00074-7156-13
100 ml	$12.79	Erythromycin/Sulfisoxazole, Parmed Pharms	00349-8835-01
150 ml	$18.88	Erythromycin W/Sulfisoxazole, Abbott	00074-7156-43
150 ml	$18.91	Erythromycin/Sulfisoxazole, Parmed Pharms	00349-8835-05
200 ml	$24.82	Erythromycin W/Sulfisoxazole, Abbott	00074-7156-53
200 ml	$24.83	Erythromycin/Sulfisoxazole, Parmed Pharms	00349-8835-02

Suspension - Oral - 200 mg/600 mg/5

100 ml	$9.38	SULFIMYCIN, Rugby	00536-0050-52
150 ml	$13.69	SULFIMYCIN, Rugby	00536-0059-74

ERYTHROMYCIN GLUCEPTATE *(001183)*

CATEGORIES: Anti-Infectives; Antibiotics; Antimicrobials; Endocarditis; Gonorrhea; Infections; Inflammatory Disease; Legionnaire's Disease; Lincosamides/Macrolides; Otitis Media; Pelvic Inflammatory Disease; Pharyngitis; Pneumonia; Respiratory Tract Infections; Rheumatic Fever; Skin Infections; Syphilis; FDA Approval Pre 1982

BRAND NAMES: *Ilotycin* (Canada); **Ilotycin Gluceptate**
(International brand names outside U.S. in italics)

DESCRIPTION:

Erythromycin is produced by a strain of *Streptomyces erythraeus* and belongs to the macrolide group of antibiotics. It is basic and readily forms a salt when combined with an acid.

CLINICAL PHARMACOLOGY:

Erythromycin inhibits protein synthesis without affecting nucleic acid synthesis. Some strains of *Haemophilus influenzae* and staphylococci have demonstrated resistance to erythromycin. Culture and susceptibility testing should be done. If the Bauer-Kirby method of disk susceptibility testing is used, a 15-mcg erythromycin disk should give a zone diameter of at least 18 mm when tested against an erythromycin susceptible organism.

Intravenous injection of 200 mg of erythromycin produces peak serum levels of 3 to 4 mcg/ml at 1 hour and 0.5 mcg/ml at 6 hours.

Erythromycin diffuses readily into the body fluids. Only low concentrations are normally achieved in the spinal fluid, but passage of the drug across the blood-brain barrier increases in meningitis. In the presence of normal hepatic function, erythromycin is concentrated in the liver and excreted in the bile; the effect of hepatic dysfunction on excretion of erythromycin by the liver into the bile is not known. From 12% to 15% of intravenously administered erythromycin is excreted in active form in the urine.

Erythromycin crosses the placental barrier, but fetal plasma levels are low.

INDICATIONS AND USAGE:

Streptococcus pyogenes (group A β-hemolytic): Upper and lower respiratory tract, skin and soft-tissue infections of mild to moderate severity.

Injectable penicillin G benzathine is considered by the American Heart Association to be the drug of choice in the treatment and prevention of streptococcal pharyngitis and in long-term prophylaxis of rheumatic fever.

Staphylococcus aureus: Acute infections of skin and soft tissue that are mild to moderately severe. Resistance may develop during treatment.

Streptococcus pneumoniae: Infections of the upper respiratory tract (*e.g.*, otitis media and pharyngitis) and lower respiratory tract (*e.g.*, pneumonia) of mild to moderate severity.

Mycoplasma pneumoniae: In the treatment of respiratory tract infections due to this organism.

H. influenzae: May be used concomitantly with adequate doses of sulfonamides in treating upper respiratory tract infections of mild to moderate severity. Not all strains of this organism are susceptible at the erythromycin concentrations ordinarily achieved (see appropriate sulfonamide labeling for prescribing information.)

Corynebacterium diphtheriae: As an adjunct to antitoxin.

Listeria monocytogenes: Infections due to this organism.

Neisseria gonorrhoeae: In female patients with a history of sensitivity to penicillin, a parenteral erythromycin (such as the gluceptate) may be administered in conjunction with an oral erythromycin as alternate therapy in acute pelvic inflammatory disease caused by *N. gonorrhoeae*. In the treatment of gonorrhea, patients suspected of having concomitant syphilis should have microscopic examinations (by immunofluorescence or dark-field) before receiving erythromycin and monthly serologic tests for a minimum of 4 months.

Legionnaires' Disease: Although no controlled clinical efficacy studies have been conducted, in vitro and limited preliminary clinical data suggest that erythromycin may be effective in treating Legionnaires' disease.

CONTRAINDICATIONS:

Intravenous erythromycin is contraindicated in patients with known hypersensitivity to this antibiotic.

Erythromycin is contraindicated in patients taking terfenadine (see DRUG INTERACTIONS).

WARNINGS:

Usage in Pregnancy: Safety of this drug for use during pregnancy has not been established.

Pseudomembranous colitis has been reported with virtually all broad-spectrum antibiotics (including macrolides, semisynthetic penicillins, and cephalosporins); therefore, it is important to consider its diagnosis in patients who develop diarrhea in association with the use of antibiotics. Such colitis may range in severity from mild to life threatening.

Treatment with broad-spectrum antibiotics alters the normal flora of the colon and may permit overgrowth of clostridia. Studies indicate that a toxin produced by *Clostridium difficile*is one primary cause of antibiotic-associated colitis.

Mild cases of pseudomembranous colitis usually respond to drug discontinuance along. In moderate to severe cases, management should include sigmoidoscopy, appropriate bacteriologic studies, and fluid, electrolyte, and protein supplementation. When the colitis does not improve after the drug has been discontinued, or when it is severe, oral vancomycin is the drug of choice for antibiotic-associated pseudomembranous colitis produced by *C. difficile.* Other causes of colitis should be ruled out.

PRECAUTIONS:

Surgical procedures should be performed when indicated.

Side effects following the use of intravenous erythromycin are rare. Occasional venous irritation has been encountered, but if the injection is given slowly, in dilute solution, preferably by continuous intravenous infusion over 20 to 60 minutes, pain and vessel trauma are minimized.

Since erythromycin is excreted principally by the liver, caution should be exercised in administering the antibiotic to patients with impaired hepatic function.

DRUG INTERACTIONS:

Erythromycin significantly alters the metabolism of terfenadine when taken concomitantly. Rare cases of serious cardiovascular adverse events, including death, cardiac arrest, torsades de pointes, and other ventricular arrhythmias have been observed (see CONTRAINDICATIONS).

Erythromycin use in patients who are receiving high doses of theophylline may be associated with an increase in serum theophylline levels and potential theophylline toxicity. In case of theophylline toxicity and/or elevated serum theophylline levels, the dose of theophylline should be reduced while the patient is receiving concomitant erythromycin therapy.

Concomitant administration of erythromycin and digoxin has been reported to result in elevated digoxin serum levels.

There have been reports of increased anticoagulant effects when erythromycin and oral anticoagulants were used concomitantly. Increased anticoagulation effects due to this drug interaction may be more pronounced in the elderly.

Concurrent use of erythromycin and ergotamine or dihydroergotamine has been associated in some patients with acute ergot toxicity characterized by severe peripheral vasospasm and dysesthesia.

Erythromycin has been reported to decrease the clearance of triazolam and midazolam thus may increase the pharmacologic effect of these benzodiazepines.

DRUG INTERACTIONS: *(cont'd)*

The use of erythromycin in patients concurrently taking drugs metabolized by the cytochrome P-450 system may be associated with elevations in serum concentrations of these other drugs. Elevated serum concentrations of the following drugs have been reported when administered concurrently with erythromycin: carbamazepine, cyclosporine, hexobarbital, phenytoin, alfentanil, disopyramide, lovastatin, and bromocriptine. Serum concentrations of these and other drugs metabolized by the cytochrome P-450 system should be monitored closely in patients concurrently receiving erythromycin.

ADVERSE REACTIONS:

Allergic reactions, ranging from urticaria and mild skin eruptions to anaphylaxis, have occurred with intravenously administered erythromycin.

During prolonged or repeated therapy, there is a possibility of overgrowth of nonsusceptible bacteria or fungi. If such infections arise, the drug should be discontinued and appropriate therapy instituted.

Variations in liver function have been observed following daily doses at high levels or after prolonged therapy. Hepatic function tests should be performed when such therapy is given.

Reversible hearing loss associated with the intravenous infusion of 4 g/day or more of erythromycin has been reported rarely.

Rarely, erythromycin has been associated with the production of ventricular arrhythmias, including ventricular tachycardia and torsade des pointes, in individuals with prolonged QT intervals.

OVERDOSAGE:

SIGNS AND SYMPTOMS

Experience with overdosage of erythromycin gluceptate is limited. Alterations in liver function tests and reversible hearing loss are possible, especially in patients with renal insufficiency.

TREATMENT

To obtain up-to-date information about the treatment of overdose, a good resource is your certified Regional Poison Control Center. telephone numbers of certified poison control centers are listed in *Physician's GenR$_X$ (PGR$_X$)*. In managing overdosage, consider the possibility of multiple drug overdoses, interaction among drugs, and unusual drug kinetics in your patient.

Protect the patient's airway and support ventilation and perfusion. Meticulously monitor and maintain, within acceptable limits, the patient's vital signs, blood gases, serum electrolytes, etc.

Forced diuresis, peritoneal dialysis, hemodialysis, or charcoal hemoperfusion have been established as beneficial for an overdose of erythromycin gluceptate.

DOSAGE AND ADMINISTRATION:

Prepare the initial solution of Ilotycin Gluceptate by (1) adding at least 20 ml of Sterile Water for Injection to the 1-g vial of Ilotycin Gluceptate and (2) shaking the vial until all of the drug is dissolved.**It is important that the product be diluted only with Sterile Water for Injection without preservatives.**

After reconstitution, the sterile solution should be stored in a refrigerator and used within 7 days.

When all of the drug is dissolved, the solution may then be added to 0.9% Sodium Chloride Injection or to 5% Dextrose in Water to give 1 g per liter for slow, continuous infusion. IV fluid admixtures with a pH below 5.5 tend to lose potency rapidly. Therefore, such solutions should be administered completely within 4 hours after dilution.

If the period of administration is prolonged, the pH of the infusion fluid should be buffered to neutrality with a sterile agent such as Neut (Sodium Bicarbonate 4% Additive Solution, Abbott) or Buff™(Phosphate-Carbonate Buffer, Travenol). For administration of the antibiotic in 500 or 1,000 ml of 5% Dextrose in Water, add 1 ampoule of full-strength Buff or 5 ml of Neut; for administration of the antibiotic in the same volumes of 0.9% Sodium Chloride Injection, and 1 ampoule of half-strength Buff of 5 ml of Neut. These solutions should be completely administered within 24 hours after dilution.

If the medication is to be given in 100 to 250 ml of fluid by a volume control set such as Metriset (McGaw), Volu-Trole "B" (Cutter), Soluset (Abbott), or Buretrol (Baxter-Travenol), the IV fluid should be buffered in its primary container before being added to the volumetric administration set.

If the medication is to be given by intermittent injection, one fourth of the total daily dose can be given in 20 to 60 minutes by slow intravenous injection of 250 to 500 mg in 100 to 250 ml of 0.9% Sodium Chloride Injection or 5% Dextrose in Water. Injection should be sufficiently slow to avoid pain along the vein.

The recommended IV dosage for severe infections in adults and children is 15 to 20 mg/kg of body weight/day. Higher doses (up to 4 g/day) may be given in very severe infections. Continuous infusion is preferable, but administration in divided doses at intervals of no more than every 6 hours is also effective.

For treatment of acute pelvic inflammatory disease caused by *N. gonorrhoeae*, administer 500 mg Ilotycin Gluceptate intravenously every 6 hours for at least 3 days, followed by 250 mg oral erythromycin every 6 hours for 7 days.

Patients receiving intravenous erythromycin should be transferred to the oral dosage form as soon as possible.

For Treatment of Legionnaires' Disease: Although optimum doses have not been established, doses utilized in reported clinical data were those recommended above (1 to 4 g daily in divided doses).

STORAGE

Prior to reconstitution, store at controlled room temperature, 59 to 86°F(15 to 30°C).

HOW SUPPLIED - EQUIVALENTS NOT AVAILABLE:

Injection, Dry-Soln - Intravenous - 1 gm/ampul

50 ml $22.45 ILOTYCIN GLUCEPATE, Dista 00777-1441-01

ERYTHROMYCIN LACTOBIONATE *(001184)*

CATEGORIES: Anti-Infectives; Antibiotics; Antimicrobials; Dental; Endocarditis; Erythrasma; Erythromycins; Gonorrhea; Hemophilus; Infections; Inflammatory Disease; Legionnaire's Disease; Lincosamides/Macrolides; Oncologic Drugs; Otitis Media; Pelvic Inflammatory Disease; Perioperative Prophylaxis; Pharyngitis; Pneumonia; Respiratory Tract Infections; Rheumatic Fever; Sulfonamides; Syphilis; Pregnancy Category B; FDA Approval Pre 1982

Erythromycin Lactobionate

BRAND NAMES: *Abboticin*; *ERA IV*; *Erycinum* (Germany); **Erythrocin**; *Erythrocin I.V.* (Germany); *Erythrocin I V* ; *Erythrocin Lactobionate*; *Erythrocine* (France); *Erythromycin Lactobionate*; *Pantomicina*
(International brand names outside U.S. in italics)

FORMULARIES: BC-BS

DESCRIPTION:

Erythromycin is produced by a strain of *Streptomyces erythraeus* and belongs to the macrolide group of antibiotics. It is basic and readily forms with salts and acids.

Erythromycin Lactobionate (for injection) is a soluble salt of Erythromycin for IV administration.

CLINICAL PHARMACOLOGY:

MICROBIOLOGY

Biochemical tests demonstrate that Erythromycin inhibits protein synthesis of the pathogen without directly affecting nucleic acid synthesis. Antagonism has been demonstrated between clindamycin and Erythromycin.

NOTE: Many strains of *Hemophilus influenzae* are resistant to Erythromycin alone, but are susceptible to Erythromycin and Sulfonamides together. Staphylococci resistant to Erythromycin may emerge during a course of Erythromycin therapy. Culture and susceptibility testing should be performed.

DISC SUSCEPTIBILITY TESTS

Quantitative methods that require measurements of zone diameters give the most precise estimate of antibiotic susceptibility. One recommended procedure (21 CFR section 460.1) uses Erythromycin class disc tests with MIC values for Erythromycin. With this procedure, a report from the laboratory of "susceptible" indicates that the infecting organism is not likely to respond to therapy. A report of "intermediate susceptible" suggests that the organism would be susceptible if higher doses were used.

Erythromycin binds to the 50 s ribosomal subunits of susceptible bacteria and suppresses protein synthesis.

IV infusion of 500 mg Erythromycin Lactobionate at a constant rate over 1 hour in fasting adults produced a mean serum Erythromycin level of approximately 7 mcg/ml/ at 20 minutes, 10 mcg/ml/ at 1 hour, 2.6 mcg/ml at 2.5 hours, and 1 mcg/ml at 6 hours.

Erythromycin diffuses readily into most body fluids. Only low concentrations are normally achieved in the spinal fluid, but passage of the drug across the blood-brain barrier increases in meningitis. In the presence of normal hepatic function, Erythromycin is concentrated in the liver and excreted in the bile; the effect of hepatic dysfunction on excretion of Erythromycin by the liver into the bile is not known. From 12 to 15 percent of IV administered Erythromycin is excreted in the active form in the urine.

Erythromycin crosses the placental barrier and is excreted in human breast milk.

INDICATIONS AND USAGE:

Erythromycin Lactobionate for injection is indicated in the treatment of patients where oral administration is not possible or where the severity of the infection requires immediate high serum levels of Erythromycin Intravenous therapy should be replaced by oral administration at the appropriate time.

Streptococcus pyogenes (Group A beta hemolytic streptococcus): Upper and lower respiratory tract, and soft tissue infections of mild to moderate severity.

Injectable benzathine penicillin G is considered by the American Heart Association to be the drug of choice in the treatment and prevention of streptococcal pharyngitis and in long-term prophylaxis of rheumatic fever.

When oral medication is preferred for treatment of the above conditions, penicillin G,V, or Erythromycin are alternate drugs of choice.

Alpha-hemolytic streptococci (viridans group): Short-term prophylaxis of bacterial endocarditis prior to dental or other operative procedures in patients with a history of rheumatic fever or congenital heart diseases who are hypersensitive to penicillin. (Erythromycin is not suitable prior to genitourinary surgery where the organisms likely to lead to bacteremia are gram-negative bacilli or the enterococcus group of streptococci).

Staphylococcus aureus: Acute infections of skin and soft tissue of mild to moderate severity. Resistant organisms may emerge during treatment.

Streptococcus pneumoniae (Diplococcus pneumoniae): For upper respiratory tract infections (*e.g.*, otitis media, pharyngitis) and lower respiratory tract infections (*e.g.*, pneumonia) of mild to moderate severity.

Mycoplasma pneumonia (Eaton agent, PPLO): For respiratory infections due to this organism.

Hemophilus influenzae: For upper respiratory tract infections of mild to moderate severity when used concomitantly with adequate doses of sulfonamides (See sulfonamide labeling for appropriate prescribing information.) The concomitant use of sulfonamides is necessary since not all strains of *Hemophilus influenzae* are susceptible to Erythromycin at the concentrations of the antibiotic achieved with usual therapeutic doses.

Corynebacterium diphtheriae: As an adjunct to antitoxin to prevent the establishment of carriers and to eradicate the organism in carriers.

Corynebacterium minutissimum: In the treatment of erythrasma.

Listeria monocytogenes: Infections due to this organism.

Neisseria gonorrhoeae: Erythromycin Lactobionate IV in conjunction with Erythromycin Stearate or base orally, as an alternative drug in treatment of acute pelvic inflammatory disease caused by *N. gonorrhoeae* in female patients with a history of sensitivity to penicillin. Before treatment of gonorrhea in female patients who are suspected of also having syphilis should have a microscopic examination for *T. pallidum* (by immunofluorescence on dark-field) before receiving Erythromycin and monthly serotologic tests for a minimum of 4 months.

Legionnaire's Disease: Although no controlled clinical efficacy studies have been conducted, *in vitro* and limited preliminary clinical data suggests that Erythromycin may be effective in treating Legionnaire's Disease.

CONTRAINDICATIONS:

Erythromycin is contraindicated in patients with known hypersensitivity to this antibiotic.

PRECAUTIONS:

Since Erythromycin is principally excreted by the liver, caution should be administered to patients with impaired hepatic function.

Prolonged or repeated use of Erythromycin may result in an overgrowth of non-susceptible bacteria or fungi. If superinfection occurs, Erythromycin should be discontinued and appropriate therapy instituted.

Areas of localized infection may require surgical drainage in addition to antibiotic therapy.

PRECAUTIONS: *(cont'd)*

Recent data from studies of Erythromycin reveal that its use in patients who are receiving high doses of theophylline may be associated with an increase of serum theophylline levels and potential theophylline toxicity and/or elevated serum theophylline levels, the dose of theophylline should be reduced while the patient is receiving concomitant erythromycin therapy.

Usage During Pregnancy And Lactation: The safety of Erythromycin for use during pregnancy has not been established.

Erythromycin crosses the placental barrier. Erythromycin also appears in breast milk.

ADVERSE REACTIONS:

Side effects following the use of IV Erythromycin are rare. Occasional venous irritation has been encountered but if the infusion is given slowly, in dilute solution, preferably by continuous IV infusion or intermittent infusion in no less than 20 to 60 minutes, pain and vessel trauma are minimized.

Allergic reactions, ranging from urticaria and mild skin eruptions to anaphylaxis, have occurred with IV administered Erythromycin.

Reversible hearing loss associated with the IV infusion of 4 or more grams per day of Erythromycin has been reported rarely.

DOSAGE AND ADMINISTRATION:

To reconstitute add 10 ml of Sterile Water for Injection, USP, to the 500 mg vial or 20 ml to the 1 gram vial. Use only Sterile Water for Injection, USP, to dissolve Erythromycin Lactobionate IV. Use of other diluents may cause precipitations during reconstitution. Do not use diluents containing preservatives or inorganic salts. After reconstitution, each ml contains 50 mg of Erythromycin activity (500 mg in 10 ml or 1,000 mg in 20 ml). The initial solution is stable at refrigerator temperature for 2 weeks, or for 24 hours at room temperature.

Prior to IV administration, the initial Erythromycin Lactobionate solution prepared with Sterile Water for Injection, USP. i.e. without preservatives is added to Sodium Chloride Injection, USP or Lactated Ringers's Injection, USP, or Normosol-R solutions. It may also be used with the following solutions to which Nuet (4% sodium bicarbonate) is first added to raise the pH (Add 5 ml of Nuet to each 500 or 1,000 ml of solution used. Five ml of Neut contains approximately 2.4 mEq of Na+ and HCO_3-.):

5% Dextrose Injection

5% Dextrose and Lactated Ringer's Injection

5% Dextrose and 0.9% Sodium Chloride Injection

Normosol-M and 5% Dextrose Injection

Normosol-R and 5% Dextrose Injection

The final diluted solution of Erythromycin Lactobionate should be completely administered within 8 hours since it is not suitable for storage (contact Abbott Laboratories. Dept. 498 for additional stability data).

Acidic solutions of Erythromycin Lactobionate are unstable and lose their potency rapidly. A pH of at least 5.5 is desirable for the final diluted solution of Erythromycin Lactobionate. No drug or chemical agent should be added to an Erythromycin Lactobionate IV fluid admixture unless its effect on the chemical and physical stability of the solution has first determined.

For the treatment of severe infections in adults and children, the recommended IV dose of Erythromycin Lactobionate is 15 to 20 mg/kg/day. Higher doses up to 4 g/day may be given for very severe infections.

Continuous infusion of Erythromycin Lactobionate is preferable; however intermittent infusion at intervals not greater than every 6 hours is also effective. IV Erythromycin should be replaced by oral Erythromycin Lactobionate soon as possible.

For slow continuous infusion: the final diluted solution of Erythromycin Lactobionate is prepared to give a concentration of 1 g per liter.

For intermittent infusion (for administration of one fourth the total daily dose of Erythromycin Lactobionate by IV infusion in 20 to 60 minutes at intervals not greater than 6 hours): The final diluted solution of Erythromycin Lactobionate is prepared to give a concentration of 250 to 500 mg in 100 to 250 ml. Infusion should be sufficient slow to avoid pain along the vein.

For treatment of acute pelvic inflammatory disease caused by *N. gonorrhea*, in female patients hypersensitive to penicillins, administer 500 mg Erythromycin Lactobionate every 6 hours for 3 days, followed by 250 mg erythromycin stearate or base every 6 hours for 7 days.

For treatment of Legionnaires Disease: Although optimal doses have not been established, doses utilized in reported clinical data were those recommended above (1 to 4 g daily in divided doses).

HOW SUPPLIED - RATED THERAPEUTICALLY EQUIVALENT:

Injection, Lyphl-Soln - Intravenous - 1 gm/vial

1 gm	**$18.20**	**ERYTHROCIN LACTOBIONATE I.V., Abbott**	**00074-6481-01**
1 gm	**$18.94**	**ERYTHROCIN LACTOBIONATE IV, Abbott**	**00074-6342-05**
1 gm	**$19.44**	**ERYTHROCIN LACTOBIONATE -I.V., Abbott**	**00074-6478-44**
1's	$120.00	Erythromycin Lactobionate, Pasadena	00418-2309-41
20 ml x 5	$47.23	Erythromycin Lactobionate, Lederle Parenterals	00205-2849-02
25's	$289.69	Erythromycin Lactobionate, Elkins Sinn	00641-2309-45
30 ml	$236.88	Sterile Erythromycin Lactobionate, Fujisawa USA	00469-1670-50

Injection, Lyphl-Soln - Intravenous - 500 mg/vial

1's	$65.00	Erythromycin Lactobionate, Pasadena	00418-2304-41
10 ml x 5	$25.40	Erythromycin Lactobionate, Lederle Parenterals	00205-2848-56
20 ml	$134.38	Erythromycin Lactobionate 500, Fujisawa USA	00469-1660-40
25's	$156.25	Erythromycin Lactobionate, Elkins Sinn	00641-2304-45
100 ml	$6.71	Erythromycin Lactobionate, Elkins Sinn	00641-2313-41
100 ml	$28.13	Sterile Erythromycin Lactobionate, Fujisawa USA	00469-1663-00
500 mg	**$10.07**	**ERYTHROCIN LACTOBIONATE-I.V., Abbott**	**00074-6482-01**
500 mg	**$10.45**	**ERYTHROCIN LACTOBIONATE IV, Abbott**	**00074-6365-02**
500 mg	**$10.72**	**ERYTHROCIN PIGGYBACK, Abbott**	**00074-6483-01**
500 mg	**$10.93**	**ERYTHROCIN LACTOBIONATE I.V., Abbott**	**00074-6476-44**
500mg	**$11.15**	**ERYTHROCIN PIGGYBACK, Abbott**	**00074-6368-13**

Kit - Intravenous - 1 gm

1's	**$28.95**	**ERYTHROCIN LACTOBIONATE, Abbott**	**00074-3246-01**

Kit - Intravenous - 500 mg

1's	**$21.22**	**ERYTHROCIN LACTOBIONATE, Abbott**	**00074-3247-01**

ERYTHROMYCIN STEARATE *(001185)*

CATEGORIES: Amebiasis; Anti-Infectives; Antibiotics; Antimicrobials; Chlamydia; Conjunctivitis; Dental; Endocarditis; Erythrasma; Erythromycins; Fever; Gonorrhea; Hemophilus; Infections; Inflammatory Disease; Legionnaire's Disease; Lincosamides/Macrolides; Otitis Media; Pelvic Inflammatory Disease; Penicillins; Pharyngitis; Pneumonia; Rheumatic Fever; Stenosis; Streptococcal Infection; Sulfonamides; Syphilis; Tonsillitis; FDA Approval Pre 1982; Top 200 Drugs

BRAND NAMES: *Abboticin*; *Apo-Erythro-S* (Canada); *Arsitrocin*; *Baknyl*; *Bannthrocin*; *Birithrocin*; *Cusimicina*; *Doranol*; *Ebalin*; *Elocin*; *Emestid*; *Emtrocin*; *Emu-V E*; *ERA*; *Eribus* (Mexico); *Eriecu*; *Erimit*; *Erimycin*; *Eritrobiotic*; *Eritrocina*; *Eritrolag*; *Eritromicina*; *Ermycin*; *Eromel*; *Erotab*; *Erycin*; *Erymid*; *Erymycin AF*; Erypar; *Erystac*; *Erythrocin* (Australia, England, Germany, Canada); **Erythrocin Stearate**; *Erythrocine*; Erythrocot; *Erythrogenat* (Germany); *Erythromil* (Europe); *Erythromycin* (Germany); *Erythromycine*; *Erythromycinum*; *Erythro-Teva*; Ethril; *Etocin*; *Galentromicina* (Mexico); *Latocin*; *Malocin*; *Mercina*; My-E; *Novorythro* (Canada); *Pantomicina* (Mexico); *Pantomucol*; *Pocin*; *Protomicina*; *Rubimycin*; *Rythocin*; *Servitrocin*; *Tomcin*; *Urycin*; Wintrocin; Wyamycin S
(International brand names outside U.S. in italics)

FORMULARIES: Aetna; BC-BS; CIGNA; FHP; Humana; Kaiser; Medco; Medi-Cal; PruCare; United

COST OF THERAPY: $3.60 (Infections; Tablet; 250 mg; 4/day; 10 days)

PRIMARY ICD9: 136.9 (Unspecified Infections And Parasitic Diseases)

DESCRIPTION:

Erythromycin is produced by a strain of *Streptomyces erythraeus* and belongs to the macrolide group of antibiotics. It is basic and readily forms salts with acids. The base, the stearate salt, and the esters are poorly soluble in water, and are suitable for oral administration.

Abbott Erythrocin Stearate Filmtab tablets (erythromycin stearate tablets, USP) contain the stearate salt of the antibiotic in a unique film coating. *Inactive Ingredients 250 mg tablet:* Cellulosic polymers, corn starch, D&C Red No. 7, polacrilin potassium, polyethylene glycol, povidone, propylene glycol, sodium carboxymethylcellulose, sodium citrate, sorbic acid, sorbitan monooleate and titanium dioxide. *500 mg tablet:* Cellulosic polymers, corn starch, FD&C Red No. 3, magnesium hydroxide, polacrilin potassium, povidone, propylene glycol, sorbitan monooleate, titanium dioxide and vanillin.

CLINICAL PHARMACOLOGY:

Microbiology: Biochemical tests demonstrate that erythromycin inhibits protein synthesis of the pathogen without directly affecting nucleic acid synthesis. Antagonism has been demonstrated between clindamycin and erythromycin.

Note: Many strains of *Hemophilus influenzae* are resistant to erythromycin alone, but are susceptible to erythromycin and sulfonamides together. Staphylococci resistant to erythromycin may emerge during a course of erythromycin therapy. Culture and susceptibility testing should be performed.

Disc Susceptibility Tests: Quantitative methods that require measurement of zone diameters give the most precise estimates of antibiotic susceptibility. One recommended procedure (21 CFR section 460.1) uses erythromycin class discs for testing susceptibility; interpretations correlate zone diameters of this disc test with MIC values for erythromycin. With this procedure, a report from the laboratory of "susceptible" indicates that the infecting organism is likely to respond to therapy. A report of "resistant" indicates that the infective organism is not likely to respond to therapy. A report of "intermediate susceptibility" suggests that the organism would be susceptible if higher doses were used.

Erythromycin binds to the 50 S ribosomal subunits of susceptible bacteria and suppresses protein synthesis.

Orally administered erythrocin stearate tablets are readily and reliably absorbed. Optimal serum levels of erythromycin are reached when the drug is taken in the fasting state or immediately before meals.

Erythromycin diffuses readily into most body fluids. Only low concentrations are normally achieved in the spinal fluid, but passage of the drug across the blood-brain barrier increases in meningitis. In the presence of normal hepatic function, erythromycin is concentrated in the liver and excreted in the bile; the effect of hepatic dysfunction on excretion of erythromycin by the liver into the bile is not known. Less than 5 percent of the orally administered dose of erythromycin is excreted in active form in the urine.

Erythromycin crosses the placental barrier and is excreted in breast milk.

INDICATIONS AND USAGE:

Streptococcus pyogenes (Group A beta hemolytic streptococcus): Upper and lower respiratory tract, skin, and soft tissue infections of mild to moderate severity.

Injectable benzathine penicillin G is considered by the American Heart Association to be the drug of choice in the treatment and prevention of streptococcal pharyngitis and in long-term prophylaxis of rheumatic fever.

When oral medication is preferred for treatment of the above conditions, penicillin G, V, or erythromycin are alternate drugs of choice.

When oral medication is given, the importance of strict adherence by the patient to the prescribed dosage regimen must be stressed. A therapeutic dose should be administered for at least 10 days.

Alpha-hemolytic streptococci (viridans group): Although no controlled clinical efficacy trials have been conducted, oral erythromycin has been suggested by the American Heart Association and American Dental Association for use in a regimen for prophylaxis against bacterial endocarditis in patients hypersensitive to penicillin who have congenital heart disease, or rheumatic or other acquired valvular heart disease when they undergo dental procedures and surgical procedures of the upper respiratory tract.[1]Erythromycin is not suitable prior to genitourinary or gastrointestinal tract surgery. NOTE: When selecting antibiotics for the prevention of bacterial endocarditis the physician or dentist should read the full joint statement of the American Heart Association and the American Dental Association.[1]

*Staphylococcus aureus:*Acute infections of skin and soft tissue of mild to moderate severity. Resistant organisms may emerge during treatment.

*Streptococcus pneumoniae (Diplococcus pneumoniae):*Upper respiratory tract infections (*e.g.,* otitis media, pharyngitis) and lower respiratory tract infections (*e.g.,* pneumonia) of mild to moderate degree.

Mycoplasma pneumoniae (Eaton agent, PPLO): For respiratory infections due to this organism.

INDICATIONS AND USAGE: *(cont'd)*

*Hemophilus influenzae:*For upper respiratory tract infections of mild to moderate severity when used concomitantly with adequate doses of sulfonamides. (See sulfonamide labeling for appropriate prescribing information.)The concomitant use of the sulfonamides is necessary since not all strains of *Hemophilus influenzae* are susceptible to erythromycin at the concentrations of the antibiotic achieved with usual therapeutic doses.

*Chlamydia trachomatis:*Erythromycin is indicated for treatment of the following infections caused by *Chlamydia trachomatis:* conjunctivitis of the newborn, pneumonia of infancy and urogenital infections during pregnancy. When tetracyclines are contraindicated or not tolerated, erythromycin is indicated for the treatment of uncomplicated urethral, endocervical, or rectal infections in adults due to Chlamydia trachomatis.[2]

*Treponema pallidum:*Erythromycin is an alternate choice of treatment for primary syphilis in patients allergic to the penicillins. In treatment of primary syphilis, spinal fluid examinations should be done before treatment and as part of follow-up after therapy.

*Corynebacterium diphtheriae:*As an adjunct to antitoxin, to prevent establishment of carriers, and to eradicate the organism in carriers.

*Corynebacterium minutissimum:*For the treatment of erythrasma.

*Entamoeba histolytica:*In the treatment of intestinal amebiasis only. Extra-enteric amebiasis requires treatment with other agents.

*Listeria monocytogenes:*Infections due to this organism.

*Neisseria gonorrhoeae:*Erythrocin Lactobionate-IV (erythromycin lactobionate for injection) in conjunction with erythromycin stearate orally, as an alternative drug in treatment of acute pelvic inflammatory disease caused by *N. gonorrhoeae* in female patients with a history of sensitivity to penicillin. Before treatment of gonorrhea, patients who are suspected of also having syphilis should have a microscopic examination for *T. pallidum* (by immunofluorescence or darkfield) before receiving erythromycin, and monthly serologic tests for a minimum of 4 months.

*Bordetella pertussis:*Erythromycin is effective in eliminating the organism from the nasopharynx of infected individuals, rendering them non-infectious. Some clinical studies suggests that erythromycin may be helpful in the prophylaxis of pertussis in exposed susceptible individuals.

*Legionnaires' Disease:*Although no controlled clinical efficacy studies have been conducted, *in vitro* and limited preliminary clinical data suggest that erythromycin may be effective in treating Legionnaires' Disease.

CONTRAINDICATIONS:

Erythromycin is contraindicated in patients with known hypersensitivity to this antibiotic.

WARNINGS:

There have been reports of hepatic dysfunction with or without jaundice, occurring in patients receiving oral erythromycin products.

PRECAUTIONS:

General: Erythromycin is principally excreted by the liver. Caution should be exercised when erythromycin is administered to patients with impaired hepatic function. (See CLINICAL PHARMACOLOGY and WARNINGS.)

Prolonged or repeated use of erythromycin may result in an overgrowth of nonsusceptible bacteria or fungi. If superinfection occurs, erythromycin should be discontinued and appropriate therapy instituted.

When indicated, incision and drainage or other surgical procedures should be performed in conjunction with antibiotic therapy.

Laboratory Tests: Erythromycin interferes with the fluorometric determination of urinary catecholamines.

Carcinogenesis, Mutagenesis, and Impairment of Fertility: Long-term (2-year) oral studies conducted in rats with erythromycin base did not provide evidence of tumorigenicity. Mutagenicity studies have not been conducted. There was no apparent effect on male or female fertility in rats fed erythromycin (base) at levels up to 0.25 percent of diet.

Pregnancy Category B: There is no evidence of teratogenicity or any other adverse effect on reproduction in female rats fed erythromycin base (up to 0.25 percent of diet) prior to and during mating, during gestation, and through weaning of two successive litters. There are, however, no adequate and well-controlled studies in pregnant women. Because animal reproduction studies are not always predictive of human response, this drug should be used during pregnancy only if clearly needed. Erythromycin has been reported to cross the placental barrier in humans, but fetal plasma levels are generally low.

Labor and Delivery: The effect of erythromycin on labor and delivery is unknown.

Nursing Mothers: Erythromycin is excreted in breast milk, therefore, caution should be exercised when erythromycin is administered to a nursing woman.

Pediatric Use: See INDICATIONS AND USAGE and DOSAGE AND ADMINISTRATION.

DRUG INTERACTIONS:

Erythromycin use in patients who are receiving high doses of theophylline may be associated with an increase in serum theophylline levels and potential theophylline toxicity. In case of theophylline toxicity and/or elevated serum theophylline levels, the dose of theophylline should be reduced while the patient is receiving concomitant erythromycin therapy.

Concomitant administration of erythromycin and digoxin has been reported to result in elevated digoxin serum levels.

There have been reports of increased anticoagulant effects when erythromycin and oral anticoagulants were used concomitantly.

Concurrent use of erythromycin and ergotamine or dihydroergotamine has been associated in some patients with acute ergot toxicity characterized by severe peripheral vasospasm and dysesthesia.

Erythromycin has been reported to decrease the clearance of triazolam and thus may increase the pharmacologic effect of triazolam.

The use of erythromycin in patients concurrently taking drugs metabolized by the cytochrome P450 system may be associated with elevations in serum erythromycin with carbamazepine, cyclosporine, hexobarbital and phenytoin. Serum concentrations of drugs metabolized by the cytochrome P450 system should be monitored closely in patients concurrently receiving erythromycin.

Troleandomycin significantly alters the metabolism of terfenadine when taken concomitantly; therefore, observe caution when erythromycin and terfenadine are used concurrently.

Patients receiving concomitant lovastatin and erythromycin should be carefully monitored; cases of rhabdomyolysis have been reported in seriously ill patients.

ADVERSE REACTIONS:

The most frequent side effects of oral erythromycin preparations are gastrointestinal and are dose-related. They include nausea, vomiting, abdominal pain, diarrhea and anorexia. Symptoms of hepatic dysfunction and/or abnormal liver function test results may occur (see WARNINGS.) Pseudomembranous colitis has been rarely reported in association with erythromycin therapy.

There have been isolated reports of transient central nervous system side effects including confusion, hallucinations, seizures, and vertigo; however, a cause and effect relationship has not been established.

Occasional case reports of cardiac arrhythmias such as ventricular tachycardia have been documented in patients receiving erythromycin therapy. There have been isolated reports of other cardiovascular symptoms such as chest pain, dizziness, and palpitations; however, a cause and effect relationship has not been established.

Allergic reactions ranging from urticaria and mild skin eruptions to anaphylaxis have occurred.

There have been isolated reports of reversible hearing loss occurring chiefly in patients with renal insufficiency and in patients receiving high doses of erythromycin.

OVERDOSAGE:

In case of overdosage, erythromycin should be discontinued. Overdosage should be handled with the prompt elimination of unabsorbed drug and all other appropriate measures.

Erythromycin is not removed by peritoneal dialysis or hemodialysis.

DOSAGE AND ADMINISTRATION:

Optimal serum levels of erythromycin are reached when erythrocin stearate (erythromycin stearate) is taken in the fasting state or immediately before meals.

Adults: The usual adult dosage is 250 mg every 6 hours; or 500 mg every 12 hours, taken in the fasting state or immediately before meals. Up to 4 g per day may be administered, depending upon the severity of the infection.

Children: Age, weight, and severity of the infection are important factors in determining the proper dosage. For the treatment of mild to moderate infections, the usual dosage is 30 to 50 mg/kg/day in 3 or 4 divided doses. When dosage is desired on a twice-a-day schedule, one-half of the total daily dose may be taken every 12 hours in the fasting state or immediately before meals. For the treatment of more severe infections the total daily dose may be doubled.

In the treatment of streptococcal infections, a therapeutic dosage of erythromycin should be administered for at least 10 days. In continuous prophylaxis of streptococcal infections in persons with a history of rheumatic heart disease, the dose is 250 mg twice a day.

For prophylaxis against bacterial endocarditis[1] in patients with congenital heart disease, or rheumatic or other acquired valvular heart disease when undergoing dental procedures or surgical procedures of the upper respiratory tract, give 1 g (20 mg/kg for children) orally 1 1/2 to 2 hours before the procedure, and then, 500 mg (10 mg/kg for children) orally every 6 hours for 8 doses.

For conjunctivitis of the newborn caused by *Chlamydia trachomatis*: Oral erythromycin suspension 50 mg/kg/day in 4 divided doses for at least 2 weeks.[2]

For Pneumonia Of Infancy Caused By *Chlamydia Trachomatis*: Although the optimal duration of therapy has not been established, the recommended therapy is oral erythromycin suspension 50 mg/kg/day in 4 divided doses for at least 3 weeks.[2]

For Urogenital Infections During Pregnancy Due To *Chlamydia Trachomatis*: Although the optimal dose and duration of therapy have not been established, the suggested treatment is erythromycin 500 mg, by mouth, 4 times a day on an empty stomach for at least 7 days. For women who cannot tolerate this regimen, a decreased dose of 250 mg, by mouth, 4 times a day should be used for at least 14 days.[2]

For Adults With Uncomplicated Urethral, Endocervical, Or Rectal Infections Caused By *Chlamydia Trachomatis* In Whom Tetracyclines Are Contraindicated Or Not Tolerated: 500 mg, by mouth, 4 times a day for at least 7 days.[2]

For Treatment Of Primary Syphilis : 30 to 40 g given in divided doses over a period of 10 to 15 days.

For Treatment Of Acute Pelvic Inflammatory Disease Caused By *N. Gonorrhoeae*:500 mg Erythrocin Lactobionate-IV (erythromycin lactobionate for injection) every 6 hours for 3 days, followed by 250 mg erythrocin stearate every 6 hours for 7 days.

For Intestinal Amebiasis: *Adults:* 250 mg four times daily for 10 to 14 days. *Children:* 30 to 50 mg/kg/day in divided doses for 10 to 14 days.

For Use In Pertussis: Although optimal dosage and duration have not been established, doses of erythromycin utilized in reported clinical studies were 40 to 50 mg/kg/day, given in divided doses for 5 to 14 days.

For Treatment Of Legionnaires' Disease: Although optimal doses have not been established, doses utilized in reported clinical data were 1 to 4 g daily in divided doses.

Storage: Store below 86°F (30°C).

REFERENCES:

1. American Heart Association. 1977. Prevention of bacterial endocarditis. Circulation 56: 139A-143A. 2. CDC Sexually Transmitted Diseases Treatment Guidelines 1982.

PATIENT INFORMATION:

Erythromycin stearate is an antibiotic for the treatment of infection. Take at regular intervals and complete the entire course of therapy. Notify your physician if you are pregnant or nursing. Notify your physician if you develop severe abdominal pain, yellowing of the skin or eyes, rash, dark urine, or pale stools. May cause nausea, vomiting, or diarrhea; notify your physician if these occur. Erythromycin Stearate should be taken on an empty stomach with a full glass of water; may be taken with food if GI upset occurs.

HOW SUPPLIED - RATED THERAPEUTICALLY EQUIVALENT:

Tablet, Plain Coated - Oral - 250 mg

40's	**$5.59**	**ERYTHROCIN STEARATE, Abbott**	**00074-6346-41**
40's	$5.70	Erythromycin Stearate, H.C.F.A. F F P	99999-1185-01
100's	$9.00	Erythrocot, C O Truxton	00463-5012-01
100's	$12.44	Erythromycin Stearate, US Trading	56126-0397-11
100's	$13.72	Erythromycin Stearate, Lederle Pharm	00005-3250-60
100's	**$13.75**	**ERYTHROCIN STEARATE, Abbott**	**00074-6346-20**
100's	$14.19	Erythromycin Stearate, Voluntary Hosp	53258-6346-76
100's	$14.25	Erythromycin Stearate, H.C.F.A. F F P	99999-1185-02
100's	$15.50	Erythromycin Stearate, Schein Pharm (US)	00364-2005-01
100's	$15.50	Erythromycin Stearate, Major Pharms	00904-2458-60
100's	$15.85	Erythromycin Stearate, Goldline Labs	00182-0538-01
100's	**$16.13**	**ERYTHROCIN STEARATE, Abbott**	**00074-6346-38**
100's	$16.86	MY-E ERTHOMYCIN STEARATE, Seneca Pharms	47028-0013-01
100's	$18.16	Erythromycin Stearate, HL Moore Drug Exch	00839-5079-06
100's	$18.25	Erythromycin Stearate, Mylan	00378-0106-01
100's	$18.75	Erythromycin Stearate, Voluntary Hosp	53258-6346-77

HOW SUPPLIED - RATED THERAPEUTICALLY EQUIVALENT: *(cont'd)*

500's	$48.69	Erythromycin Stearate, Lederle Pharm	00005-3250-31
500's	$50.75	Erythromycin Stearate, H & H Labs	46703-0018-05
500's	$57.50	Erythromycin Stearate, Major Pharms	00904-2458-40
500's	$60.00	Erythromycin Stearate, Goldline Labs	00182-0538-05
500's	**$65.31**	**ERYTHROCIN STEARATE, Abbott**	**00074-6346-53**
500's	$71.10	Erythromycin Stearate, Barr	00555-0013-04
500's	$71.25	Erythromycin Stearate, H.C.F.A. F F P	99999-1185-03
500's	$71.30	Erythromycin Stearate, Qualitest Pharms	00603-3553-28
500's	$71.95	Erythromycin Stearate, Mylan	00378-0106-05
500's	$123.20	Erythromycin Stearate, Aligen Independ	00405-4412-02
1000's	$81.00	Erythrocot, C O Truxton	00463-5012-10
1000's	**$126.70**	**ERYTHROCIN STEARATE, Abbott**	**00074-6346-19**
1000's	$133.58	Erythromycin Stearate, HL Moore Drug Exch	00839-5079-16
1000's	$140.00	Erythromycin Stearate, Zenith Labs	00172-2458-80
1000's	$142.50	Erythromycin Stearate, H.C.F.A. F F P	99999-1185-04

Tablet, Plain Coated - Oral - 500 mg

100's	$21.96	Erythromycin Stearate, US Trading	56126-0391-11
100's	$21.97	Erythromycin Stearate, Lederle Pharm	00005-3251-23
100's	$22.68	Erythromycin Stearate, Lederle Pharm	00005-3251-60
100's	$23.25	Erythromycin Stearate, H.C.F.A. F F P	99999-1185-05
100's	$24.28	Erythromycin Stearte, Barr	00555-0219-02
100's	**$24.85**	**ERYTHROCIN STEARATE, Abbott**	**00074-6316-13**
100's	$25.60	Erythromycin Stearate, Major Pharms	00904-2459-60
100's	$26.00	Erythromycin Stearate, Goldline Labs	00182-0539-01
100's	$28.80	Erythromycin Stearate, Qualitest Pharms	00603-3554-21
100's	$28.90	Erythromycin Stearate, Zenith Labs	00172-2823-60
100's	$28.95	Erythromycin Stearate, Mylan	00378-0107-01
100's	$35.76	Erythromycin Stearate, Voluntary Hosp	53258-6316-76
100's	$40.84	Erythromycin Stearate, HL Moore Drug Exch	00839-5185-06
500's	$104.65	Erythromycin Stearate, Major Pharms	00904-2459-40
500's	$116.25	Erythromycin Stearate, H.C.F.A. F F P	99999-1185-06
500's	$122.85	Erythromycin Stearate, Barr	00555-0219-04

ESMOLOL HYDROCHLORIDE *(001186)*

CATEGORIES: Antiarrhythmic Agents; Atrial Fibrillation; Beta Adrenergic Blocking Agents; Beta Blockers; Cardiovascular Drugs; Fibrillation; Heart Flutter; Hypertension; Renal Drugs; Tachycardia; Angina*; Pregnancy Category C; FDA Approved 1986 Dec

* Indication not approved by the FDA

BRAND NAMES: **Brevibloc**

DESCRIPTION:

NOT FOR DIRECT INTRAVENOUS INJECTION. AMPUL MUST BE DILUTED PRIOR TO ITS INFUSION—SEE DOSAGE AND ADMINISTRATION.

Brevibloc (esmolol HCl) is a beta$_1$-selective (cardioselective) adrenergic receptor blocking agent with a very short duration of action (elimination half-life is approximately 9 minutes). Esmolol HCl is:

(±)-Methyl p-[2-hydroxy-3-(isopropylamino) propoxy] hydrocinnamate hydrochloride.

Esmolol HCl has the empirical formula $C_{16}H_{26}NO_4Cl$ and a molecular weight of 331.8. It has one asymmetric center and exists as an enantiomeric pair.

Esmolol HCl is a white to off-white crystalline powder. It is a relatively hydrophilic compound which is very soluble in water and freely soluble in alcohol. Its partition coefficient (octanol/water) at pH 7.0 is 0.42 compared to 17.0 for propranolol.

Brevibloc Injection is a clear, colorless to light yellow, sterile, nonpyrogenic solution.

2.5 g, 10 ml Ampul: Each ml contains 250 mg esmolol HCl in 25% Propylene Glycol, USP, 25% Alcohol, USP and Water for Injection, USP; buffered with 17.0 mg Sodium Acetate, USP, and 0.00715 ml Glacial Acetic Acid, USP. Sodium hydroxide and/or hydrochloric acid added, as necessary, to adjust pH to 3.5-5.5.

100 mg, 10 ml Single Dose Vial: Each ml contains 10 mg esmolol HCl and Water for Injection, USP; buffered with 2.8 mg Sodium Acetate, USP, and 0.546 mg Glacial Acetic Acid, USP. Sodium hydroxide and/or hydrochloric acid added, as necessary, to adjust pH to 4.5-5.5.

CLINICAL PHARMACOLOGY:

Brevibloc (esmolol HCl) is a beta$_1$-selective (cardioselective) adrenergic receptor blocking agent with rapid onset, a very short duration of action, and no significant intrinsic sympathomimetic or membrane stabilizing activity at therapeutic dosages. Its elimination half-life after intravenous infusion is approximately 9 minutes. Brevibloc inhibits the beta$_1$ receptors located chiefly in cardiac muscle, but this preferential effect is not absolute and at higher doses it begins to inhibit beta$_2$ receptors located chiefly in the bronchial and vascular musculature.

Pharmacokinetics and Metabolism: Brevibloc (esmolol HCl) is rapidly metabolized by hydrolysis of the ester linkage, chiefly by the esterases in the cytosol of red blood cells and not by plasma cholinesterases or red cell membrane acetylcholinesterase. Total body clearance in man was found to be about 20 l/kg/hr, which is greater than cardiac output; thus the metabolism of Brevibloc is not limited by the rate of blood flow to metabolizing tissues such as the liver or affected by hepatic or renal blood flow. Brevibloc has a rapid distribution half-life of about 2 minutes and an elimination half-life of about 9 minutes.

Using an appropriate loading dose, steady-state blood levels of Brevibloc for dosages from 50-300 mcg/kg/min (0.05-0.3 mg/kg/min) are obtained within five minutes. (Steady-state is reached in about 30 minutes without the loading dose.) Steady-state blood levels of Brevibloc increase linearly over this dosage range and elimination kinetics are dose-independent over this range. Steady-state blood levels are maintained during infusion but decrease rapidly after termination of the infusion. Because of its short half-life, blood levels of Brevibloc can be rapidly altered by increasing or decreasing the infusion rate and rapidly eliminated by discontinuing the infusion.

Consistent with the high rate of blood-based metabolism of Brevibloc, less than 2% of the drug is excreted unchanged in the urine. Within 24 hours of the end of infusion, approximately 73-88% of the dosage has been accounted for in the urine as the acid metabolite of Brevibloc.

Metabolism of Brevibloc results in the formation of the corresponding free acid and methanol. The acid metabolite has been shown in animals to have about 1/1500th the activity of esmolol and in normal volunteers its blood levels do not correspond to the level of beta-blockade. The acid metabolite has an elimination half-life of about 3.7 hours and is excreted in the urine with a clearance approximately equivalent to the glomerular filtration rate. Excretion of the acid metabolite is significantly decreased in patients with renal disease, with the elimination half-life increased to about ten-fold that of normals, and plasma levels considerably elevated.

CLINICAL PHARMACOLOGY: *(cont'd)*

Methanol blood levels, monitored in subjects receiving Brevibloc for up to 6 hours at 300 mcg/kg/min (0.3 mg/kg/min) and 24 hours at 150 mcg/kg/min (0.15 mg/kg/min), approximated endogenous levels and were less than 2% of levels usually associated with methanol toxicity.

Brevibloc has been shown to be 55% bound to human plasma protein, while the acid metabolite is only 10% bound.

Pharmacodynamics: Clinical pharmacology studies in normal volunteers have confirmed the beta blocking activity of Brevibloc (esmolol HCl), showing reduction in heart rate at rest and during exercise, and attenuation of isoproterenol-induced increases in heart rate. Blood levels of Brevibloc have been shown to correlate with extent of beta blockade. After termination of infusion, substantial recovery from beta blockade is observed in 10-20 minutes.

In human electrophysiology studies, Brevibloc produced effects typical of a beta blocker: a decrease in the heart rate, increase in sinus cycle length, prolongation of the sinus node recovery time, prolongation of the AH interval during normal sinus rhythm and during atrial pacing, and an increase in antegrade Wenckebach cycle length.

In patients undergoing radionuclide angiography, Brevibloc, at dosages of 200 mcg/kg/min (0.2 mg/kg/min), produced reductions in heart rate, systolic blood pressure, rate pressure product, left and right ventricular ejection fraction and cardiac index at rest, which were similar in magnitude to those produced by intravenous propranolol (4 mg). During exercise, Brevibloc produced reductions in heart rate, rate pressure product and cardiac index which were also similar to those produced by propranolol, but produced a significantly larger fall in systolic blood pressure. In patients undergoing cardiac catheterization, the maximum therapeutic dose of 300 mcg/kg/min (0.3 mg/kg/min) of Brevibloc produced similar effects, and, in addition, there were small, clinically insignificant, increases in the left ventricular end diastolic pressure and pulmonary capillary wedge pressure. At thirty minutes after the discontinuation of Brevibloc infusion, all of the hemodynamic parameters had returned to pretreatment levels.

The relative cardioselectivity of Brevibloc was demonstrated in 10 mildly asthmatic patients. Infusions of Brevibloc [100, 200 and 300 mcg/kg/min (0.1, 0.2 and 0.3 mg/kg/min)] produced no significant increases in specific airway resistance compared to placebo. At 300 mcg/kg/min (0.3 mg/kg/min), Brevibloc produced slightly enhanced bronchomotor sensitivity to dry air stimulus. These effects were not clinically significant, and Brevibloc was well tolerated by all patients. Six of the patients also received intravenous propranolol, and at a dosage of 1 mg, two experienced significant, symptomatic bronchospasm requiring bronchodilator treatment. One other propranolol-treated patient also experienced dry air-induced bronchospasm. No adverse pulmonary effects were observed in patients with COPD who received therapeutic dosages of Brevibloc for treatment of supraventricular tachycardia (51 patients) or in perioperative settings (32 patients).

Supraventricular Tachycardia: In two multicenter, randomized, double-blind, controlled comparisons of Brevibloc (esmolol HCl) with placebo and propranolol, maintenance doses of 50 to 300 mcg/kg/min (0.05 to 0.3 mg/kg/min) of Brevibloc were found to be more effective than placebo and about as effective as propranolol, 3-6 mg given by bolus injections, in the treatment of supraventricular tachycardia, principally atrial fibrillation and atrial flutter. The majority of these patients developed their arrhythmias postoperatively. About 60-70% of the patients treated with Brevibloc had a desired therapeutic effect (either a 20% reduction in heart rate, a decrease in heart rate to less than 100 bpm, or, rarely, conversion to NSR) and about 95% of those who responded did so at a dosage of 200 mcg/kg/min (0.2 mg/kg/min) or less. The average effective dosage of Brevibloc was approximately 100-115 mcg/kg/min (0.1-0.115 mg/kg/min) in the two studies. Other multicenter baseline-controlled studies gave essentially similar results. In the comparison with propranolol, about 50% of patients in both the Brevibloc and propranolol groups were on concomitant digoxin. Response rates were slightly higher with both beta-blockers in the digoxin-treated patients.

In all studies significant decreases of blood pressure occurred in 20-50% of patients, identified either as adverse reaction reports by investigators, or by observation of systolic pressure less than 90 mmHg or diastolic pressure less than 50 mmHg. The hypotension was symptomatic (mainly diaphoresis or dizziness) in about 12% of patients, and therapy was discontinued in about 11% of patients, about half of whom were symptomatic. In comparison to propranolol, hypotension was about three times as frequent with Brevibloc, 53% vs. 17%. The hypotension was rapidly reversible with decreased infusion rate or after discontinuation of therapy with Brevibloc. For both Brevibloc and propranolol, hypotension was reported less frequently in patients receiving concomitant digoxin.

INDICATIONS AND USAGE:

Supraventricular Tachycardia: Brevibloc (esmolol HCl) is indicated for the rapid control of ventricular rate in patients with atrial fibrillation or atrial flutter in perioperative, postoperative, or other emergent circumstances where short term control of ventricular rate with a short-acting agent is desirable. Brevibloc is also indicated in noncompensatory sinus tachycardia where, in the physician's judgement, the rapid heart rate requires specific intervention. Brevibloc is not intended for use in chronic settings where transfer to another agent is anticipated.

Intraoperative and Postoperative Tachycardia and/or Hypertension: Brevibloc (esmolol HCl) is indicated for the treatment of tachycardia and hypertension that occur during induction and tracheal intubation, during surgery, on emergence from anesthesia, and in the postoperative period, when in the physician's judgment such specific intervention is considered indicated.

Use of Brevibloc to prevent such events is not recommended.

CONTRAINDICATIONS:

Brevibloc (esmolol HCl) is contraindicated in patients with sinus bradycardia, heart block greater than first degree, cardiogenic shock or overt heart failure (see WARNINGS.)

WARNINGS:

Hypotension: In clinical trials 20-50% of patients treated with Brevibloc (esmolol HCl) have experienced hypotension, generally defined as systolic pressure less than 90 mmHg and/or diastolic pressure less than 50 mmHg. About 12% of the patients have been symptomatic (mainly diaphoresis or dizziness). Hypotension can occur at any dose but is dose-related so that doses beyond 200 mcg/kg/min (0.2 mg/kg/min) are not recommended. Patients should be closely monitored, especially if pretreatment blood pressure is low. Decrease of dose or termination of infusion reverses hypotension, usually within 30 minutes.

Cardiac Failure: Sympathetic stimulation is necessary in supporting circulatory function in congestive heart failure, and beta blockade carries the potential hazard of further depressing myocardial contractility and precipitating more severe failure. Continued depression of the myocardium with beta blocking agents over a period of time can, in some cases, lead to cardiac failure. At the first sign or symptom of impending cardiac failure, Brevibloc should be withdrawn. Although withdrawal may be sufficient because of the short elimination half-life of Brevibloc, specific treatment may also be considered (See OVERDOSAGE.) The use of Brevibloc for control of ventricular response in patients with supraventricular arrhythmias should be undertaken with caution when the patient is compromised hemodynamically or is taking other drugs that decrease any or all of the following: peripheral resistance, myocardial

WARNINGS: *(cont'd)*

filling, myocardial contractility, or electrical impulse propagation in the myocardium. Despite the rapid onset and offset of Brevibloc's effects, several cases of death have been reported in complex clinical states where Brevibloc was presumably being used to control ventricular rate.

Intraoperative and Postoperative Tachycardia and/or Hypertension: Brevibloc (esmolol HCl) should not be used as the treatment for hypertension in patients in whom the increased blood pressure is primarily due to the vasoconstriction associated with hypothermia.

Bronchospastic Diseases: PATIENTS WITH BRONCHOSPASTIC DISEASES SHOULD, IN GENERAL, NOT RECEIVE BETA BLOCKERS. Because of its relative $beta_1$ selectivity and titratability, Brevibloc (esmolol HCl) may be used with caution in patients with bronchospastic diseases. However, since $beta_1$ selectivity is not absolute, Brevibloc should be carefully titrated to obtain the lowest possible effective dose. In the event of bronchospasm, the infusion should be terminated immediately; a $beta_2$ stimulating agent may be administered if conditions warrant but should be used with particular caution as patients already have rapid ventricular rates.

Diabetes Mellitus and Hypoglycemia: Brevibloc (esmolol HCl) should be used with caution in diabetic patients requiring a beta blocking agent. Beta blockers may mask tachycardia occurring with hypoglycemia, but other manifestations such as dizziness and sweating may not be significantly affected.

PRECAUTIONS:

General: Infusion concentrations of 20 mg/ml were associated with more serious venous irritation, including thrombophlebitis, than concentrations of 10 mg/ml. Extravasation of 20 mg/ml may lead to a serious local reaction and possible skin necrosis. Concentrations greater than 10 mg/ml or infusion into small veins or through a butterfly catheter should be avoided.

Because the acid metabolite of Brevibloc is primarily excreted unchanged by the kidney, Brevibloc (esmolol HCl) should be administered with caution to patients with impaired renal function. The elimination half-life of the acid metabolite was prolonged ten-fold and the plasma level was considerably elevated in patients with end-stage renal disease.

Care should be taken in the intravenous administration of Brevibloc as sloughing of the skin and necrosis have been reported in association with infiltration and extravasation of intravenous infusions.

Carcinogenesis, Mutagenesis, and Impairment of Fertility: Because of its short term usage no carcinogenicity, mutagenicity or reproductive performance studies have been conducted with Brevibloc (esmolol HCl).

Pregnancy Category C: Teratogenicity studies in rats at intravenous dosages of Brevibloc (esmolol HCl) up to 3000 mcg/kg/min (3 mg/kg/min) (ten times the maximum human maintenance dosage) for 30 minutes daily produced no evidence of maternal toxicity, embryotoxicity or teratogenicity, while a dosage of 10,000 mcg/kg/min (10 mg/kg/min) produced maternal toxicity and lethality. In rabbits, intravenous dosages up to 1000 mcg/kg/min (1 mg/kg/min) for 30 minutes daily produced no evidence of maternal toxicity, embryotoxicity or teratogenicity, while 2500 mcg/kg/min (2.5 mg/kg/min) produced minimal maternal toxicity and increased fetal resorptions.

Although there are no adequate and well-controlled studies in pregnant women. Brevibloc should be used during pregnancy only if the potential benefit justifies the potential risk to the fetus.

Nursing Mothers: It is not known whether Brevibloc (esmolol HCl) is excreted in human milk, however, caution should be exercised when Brevibloc is administered to a nursing woman.

Pediatric Use: The safety and effectiveness of Brevibloc in children have not been established.

DRUG INTERACTIONS:

Catecholamine-depleting drugs, e.g., reserpine, may have an additive effect when given with beta blocking agents. Patients treated concurrently with Brevibloc (esmolol HCl) and a catecholamine depletor should therefore be closely observed for evidence of hypotension or marked bradycardia, which may result in vertigo, syncope, or postural hypotension.

A study of interaction between Brevibloc and warfarin showed that concomitant administration of Brevibloc and warfarin does not alter warfarin plasma levels. Brevibloc concentrations were equivocally higher when given with warfarin, but this is not likely to be clinically important.

When digoxin and Brevibloc were concomitantly administered intravenously to normal volunteers, there was a 10-20% increase in digoxin blood levels at some time points. Digoxin did not affect Brevibloc pharmacokinetics. When intravenous morphine and Brevibloc were concomitantly administered in normal subjects, no effect on morphine blood levels was seen, but Brevibloc steady-state blood levels were increased by 46% in the presence of morphine. No other pharmacokinetic parameters were changed.

The effect of Brevibloc on the duration of succinylcholine-induced neuromuscular blockade was studied in patients undergoing surgery. The onset of neuromuscular blockade by succinylcholine was unaffected by Brevibloc, but the duration of neuromuscular blockade was prolonged from 5 minutes to 8 minutes.

Although the interactions observed in these studies do not appear to be of major clinical importance, Brevibloc should be titrated with caution in patients being treated concurrently with digoxin, morphine, succinylcholine or warfarin.

While taking beta-blockers, patients with a history of severe anaphylactic reaction to a variety of allergens may be more reactive to repeated challenge, either accidental, diagnostic, or therapeutic. Such patients may be unresponsive to the usual doses of epinephrine used to treat allergic reaction.

Caution should be exercised when considering the use of Brevibloc and Verapamil in patients with depressed myocardial function. Fatal cardiac arrests have occurred in patients receiving both drugs. Additionally, Brevibloc should not be used to control supraventricular tachycardia in the presence of agents which are vasoconstrictive and inotropic such as dopamine, epinephrine, and norepinephrine because of the danger of blocking cardiac contractility when systemic vascular resistance is high.

ADVERSE REACTIONS:

The following adverse reaction rates are based on use of Brevibloc (esmolol HCl) in clinical trials involving 369 patients with supraventricular tachycardia and over 600 intraoperative and postoperative patients enrolled in clinical trials. Most adverse effects observed in controlled clinical trial settings have been mild and transient. The most important adverse effect has been hypotension (see WARNINGS.) Deaths have been reported in post-marketing experience occurring during complex clinical states where Brevibloc was presumably being used simply to control ventricular rate (see WARNINGS, Cardiac Failure.)

Cardiovascular: Symptomatic hypotension (diaphoresis, dizziness) occurred in 12% of patients, and therapy was discontinued in about 11%, about half of whom were symptomatic. Asymptomatic hypotension occurred in about 25% of patients. Hypotension resolved during Brevibloc (esmolol HCl) infusion in 63% of these patients and within 30 minutes after discontinuation of infusion in 80% of the remaining patients. Diaphoresis accompanied hypotension in 10% of patients. Peripheral ischemia occurred in approximately 1% of patients. Pallor, flushing, bradycardia (heart rate less than 50 beats per minute), chest pain,

ADVERSE REACTIONS: *(cont'd)*

syncope, pulmonary edema and heart block have each been reported in less than 1% of patients. In two patients without supraventricular tachycardia but with serious coronary artery disease (post inferior myocardial infarction or unstable angina), severe bradycardia/sinus pause/asystole has developed, reversible in both cases with discontinuation of treatment.

Central Nervous System: Dizziness has occurred in 3% of patients; somnolence in 3%, confusion, headache, and agitation in about 2%, and fatigue in about 1% of patients. Paresthesia, asthenia, depression, abnormal thinking, anxiety, anorexia, and lightheadedness were reported in less than 1% of patients. Seizures were also reported in less than 1% of patients, with one death.

Respiratory: Bronchospasm, wheezing, dyspnea, nasal congestion, rhonchi, and rales have each been reported in less than 1% of patients.

Gastrointestinal : Nausea was reported in 7% of patients. Vomiting has occurred in about 1% of patients. Dyspepsia, constipation, dry mouth, and abdominal discomfort have each occurred in less than 1% of patients. Taste perversion has also been reported.

Skin (Infusion Site): Infusion site reactions including inflammation and induration were reported in about 8% of patients. Edema, erythema, skin discoloration, burning at the infusion site, thrombophlebitis, and local skin necrosis from extravasation have each occurred in less than 1% of patients.

Miscellaneous: Each of the following has been reported in less than 1% of patients: Urinary retention, speech disorder, abnormal vision, midscapular pain, rigors, and fever.

OVERDOSAGE:

Acute Toxicity: A few cases of massive accidental overdosage of Brevibloc (esmolol HCl) have occurred due to errors in dilution. These intravenous bolus doses of Brevibloc of 5000-6250 mcg/kg (5-6.25 mg/kg) over 1-2 minutes have produced hypotension, bradycardia, drowsiness and loss of consciousness. The effects have resolved within 10 minutes, in some cases with administration of a pressor agent.

Because of its approximately 9-minute elimination half-life, the first step in the management of toxicity should be to discontinue the Brevibloc infusion. Then, based on the observed clinical effects, the following general measures should also be considered:

Bradycardia: Intravenous administration of atropine or another anticholinergic drug.

Bronchospasm: Intravenous administration of a beta$_2$stimulating agent and/or a theophylline derivative.

Cardiac Failure: Intravenous administration of a diuretic and/or digitalis glycoside. In shock resulting from inadequate cardiac contractility, intravenous administration of dopamine, dobutamine, isoproterenol, or amrinone may be considered.

Symptomatic Hypotension: Intravenous administration of fluids and/or pressor agents.

DOSAGE AND ADMINISTRATION:

2.5 g AMPUL: THE 2.5 g AMPUL IS NOT FOR DIRECT INTRAVENOUS INJECTION. THIS DOSAGE FORM IS A CONCENTRATED, POTENT DRUG WHICH MUST BE DILUTED PRIOR TO ITS INFUSION. BREVIBLOC SHOULD NOT BE ADMIXED WITH SODIUM BICARBONATE. BREVIBLOC SHOULD NOT BE MIXED WITH OTHER DRUGS PRIOR TO DILUTION IN A SUITABLE INTRAVENOUS FLUID. (See Compatibility.)

Dilution: Aseptically prepare a 10 mg/ml infusion, by adding two 2.5 g ampuls to a 500 ml container, or one 2.5 g ampul to a 250 ml container, of a compatible intravenous solution listed below. (Remove overage prior to dilution as appropriate.) This yields a final concentration of 10 mg/ml. The diluted solution is stable for at least 24 hours at room temperature. Note: Concentrations of Brevibloc (esmolol HCl) greater than 10 mg/ml are likely to produce irritation on continued infusion (see PRECAUTIONS.) Brevibloc has, however, been well tolerated when administered via a central vein.

100 mg VIAL: This dosage form is prediluted to provide a ready-to-use 10 mg/ml concentration recommended for Brevibloc intravenous administration. It may be used to administer the appropriate Brevibloc (esmolol HCl) loading dosage infusions by hand-held syringe while the maintenance infusion is being prepared.

When using the 100 mg vial, a loading dose of 0.5 mg/kg/min for a 70 kg patient would be 3.5 ml.

Supraventricular Tachycardia: In the treatment of supraventricular tachycardia, responses to Brevibloc (esmolol HCl) usually (over 95%) occur within the range of 50 to 200 mcg/kg/min (0.05 to 0.2 mg/kg/min). The average effective dosage is approximately 100 mcg/kg/min (0.1 mg/kg/min) although dosages as low as 25 mcg/kg/min (0.025 mg/kg/min) have been adequate in some patients. Dosages as high as 300 mcg/kg/min (0.3 mg/kg/min) have been used, but these provide little added effect and an increased rate of adverse effects, and are not recommended. Dosage of Brevibloc in supraventricular tachycardia must be individualized by titration in which each step consists of a loading dosage followed by a maintenance dosage.

To initiate treatment of a patient with supraventricular tachycardia, administer a loading infusion of 500 mcg/kg/min (0.5 mg/kg/min) over one minute followed by a four-minute maintenance infusion of 50 mcg/kg/min (0.05 mg/kg/min). If an adequate therapeutic effect is observed over the five minutes of drug administration, maintain the maintenance infusion dosage with periodic adjustments up or down as needed. If an adequate therapeutic effect is not observed, the same loading dosage is repeated over one minute followed by an increased maintenance rate infusion of 100 mcg/kg/min (0.1 mg/kg/min).

Continue titration procedure as above, repeating the original loading infusion of 500 mcg/kg/min (0.5 mg/kg/min) over 1 minute, but increasing the maintenance infusion rate over the subsequent four minutes by 50 mcg/kg/min (0.05 mg/kg/min) increments. As the desired heart rate or blood pressure is approached, omit subsequent loading doses and titrate the maintenance dosage up or down to endpoint. Also, if desired, increase the interval between steps from 5 to 10 minutes (TABLE 1).

This specific dosage regimen has not been studied intraoperatively and, because of the time required for titration, may not be optimal for intraoperative use.

The safety of dosages above 300 mcg/kg/min (0.3 mg/kg/min) has not been studied.

In the event of an adverse reaction, the dosage of Brevibloc may be reduced or discontinued. If a local infusion site reaction develops, an alternate infusion site should be used and caution should be taken to prevent extravasation. The use of butterfly needles should be avoided.

Abrupt cessation of Brevibloc in patients has not been reported to produce the withdrawal effects which may occur with abrupt withdrawal of beta blockers following chronic use in coronary artery disease (CAD) patients. However, caution should still be used in abruptly discontinuing infusions of Brevibloc in CAD patients.

After achieving an adequate control of the heart rate and a stable clinical status in patients with supraventricular tachycardia, transition to alternative antiarrhythmic agents such as propranolol, digoxin, or verapamil, may be accomplished. A recommended guideline for such a transition is given below but the physician should carefully consider the labeling instructions for the alternative agent selected (TABLE 2):

The dosage of Brevibloc (esmolol HCl) should be reduced as follows:

DOSAGE AND ADMINISTRATION: *(cont'd)*

TABLE 1

Time (minutes)	Loading Dose (over 1 minute) mcg/kg/min	mg/kg/min	Maintenance Dosage (over 4 minutes) mcg/kg/min	mg/kg/min
0-1	500	0.5		
1-5			50	0.05
5-6	500	0.5		
6-10			100	0.1
10-11	500	0.5		
11-15			150	0.15
15-16	•	•		
16-20			*200	*0.2
20-(24 hrs.)			Maintenance dose titrated to heart rate or other clinical endpoint.	

* As the desired heart rate or endpoint is approached, the loading infusion may be omitted and the maintenance infusion titrated to 300 mcg/kg/min (0.3 mg/kg/min) or downward as appropriate. Maintenance dosages above 200 mcg/kg/min (0.2 mg/kg/min) have not been shown to have significantly increased benefits. The interval between titration steps may be increased.

TABLE 2

Alternative Agent	Dosage
Propranolol hydrochloride	10-20 mg q 4-6 hrs
Digoxin	0.125-0.5 mg q 6 h (p.o. or i.v.)
Verapamil	80 mg q 6 hrs

1. Thirty minutes following the first dose of the alternative agent, reduce the infusion rate of Brevibloc by one-half (50%).

2. Following the second dose of the alternative agent, monitor the patient's response and if satisfactory control is maintained for the first hour, discontinue Brevibloc.

The use of infusions of Brevibloc up to 24 hours has been well documented; in addition, limited data from 24-48 hrs (N=48) indicate that Brevibloc is well tolerated up to 48 hours.

Inoperative and Postoperative Tachycardia and/or Hypertension: In the intraoperative and postoperative settings it is not always advisable to slowly titrate the dose of Brevibloc (esmolol HCl) to a therapeutic effect. Therefore, two dosing options are presented: immediate control dosing and a gradual control when the physician has time to titrate.

1. Immediate Control: For intraoperative treatment of tachycardia and/or hypertension give an 80 mg approximately 1 mg/kg) bolus dose over 30 seconds followed by a 150 mcg/kg/min infusion, if necessary. Adjust the infusion rate as required up to 300 mcg/kg/min to maintain desired heart rate and/or blood pressure.

2. Gradual Control: For postoperative tachycardia and hypertension, the dosing schedule is the same as that used in supraventricular tachycardia. To initiate treatment, administer a loading dosage infusion of 500 mcg/kg/min of Brevibloc for one minute followed by a four-minute maintenance infusion of 50 mcg/kg/min. If an adequate therapeutic effect is not observed within five minutes, repeat the same loading dosage and follow with a maintenance infusion increased to 100 mcg/kg/mon (see Supraventricular Tachycardia).

Note: Higher doses (250-300 mcg/kg/min) may be required for adequate control of blood pressure than those required for the treatment of atrial fibrillation, flutter and sinus tachycardia. One third of the postoperative hypertensive patients required these higher doses.

Compatibility with Commonly Used Intravenous Fluids: Brevibloc (esmolol HCl) Injection was tested for compatibility with ten commonly used intravenous fluids at a final concentration of 10 mg esmolol HCl per ml. Brevibloc Injection was found to be compatible with the following solutions and was stable for at least 24 hours at controlled room temperature or under refrigeration:

Dextrose (5%) Injection, USP

Dextrose (5%) in Lactated Ringer's Injection

Dextrose (5%) in Ringer's Injection

Dextrose (5%) and Sodium Chloride (0.45%) Injection, USP

Dextrose (5%) and Sodium Chloride (0.9%) Injection, USP

Lactated Ringer's Injection, USP

Potassium Chloride (40 mEq/liter) in Dextrose (5%) Injection, USP

Sodium Chloride (0.45%) Injection, USP

Sodium Chloride (0.9%) Injection, USP

Brevibloc Injection was NOT compatible with Sodium Bicarbonate (5%) Injection, USP.

Note: Parenteral drug products should be inspected visually for particulate matter and discoloration prior to administration, whenever solution and container permit.

STORE AT CONTROLLED ROOM TEMPERATURE (59-86°F, 15-30°C). Freezing does not adversely affect the product, but exposure to elevated temperatures should be avoided.

HOW SUPPLIED - EQUIVALENTS NOT AVAILABLE:

Injection, Solution - Intravenous - 2.5 gm/10ml

10 ml x 10 $70.50 BREVIBLOC, Ohmeda Pharm 10019-0025-18

Injection, Solution - Intravenous - 100 mg/ml

10 ml x 20 $14.88 BREVIBLOC, Ohmeda Pharm 10019-0015-71

ESTAZOLAM *(003009)*

CATEGORIES: Anxiolytics, Sedatives, Hypnotic; Benzodiazepines; Central Nervous System Agents; Insomnia; Pregnancy Category X; DEA Class CIV; FDA Class 1C ("Little or No Therapeutic Advantage"); FDA Approved 1990 Dec

BRAND NAMES: *Domnamid*; *Esilgan*; *Eurodin* (Japan); *Evrodin*; *Kainever*; *Nuctalon* (France); *Nuctulon*; **Prosom**; *Tasedan* (Mexico)
(International brand names outside U.S. in italics)

FORMULARIES: Aetna; BC-BS

COST OF THERAPY: $6.19 (Insomnia; Tablet; 1 mg; 1/day; 7 days)

DESCRIPTION:

Estazolam, a triazolobenzodiazepine derivative, is an oral hypnotic agent. Estazolam occurs as a fine, white, odorless powder that is soluble in alcohol and practically insoluble in water. The chemical name for estazolam is 8-chloro-6-phenyl-4H-s-triazolo(4,3- a) (1,4)benzodiazepine. The empirical formula is $C_{16}H_{11}ClN_4$.

Estazolam tablets are scored and contain either 1 mg or 2 mg of estazolam.

DESCRIPTION: *(cont'd)*

Inactive Ingredients: *1 mg tablets:* corn starch, lactose and stearic acid. *2 mg tablets:* corn starch, iron oxide, lactose and stearic acid.

CLINICAL PHARMACOLOGY:

Pharmacokinetics: Estazolam tables have been found to be equivalent in absorption to an orally administered solution of estazolam. Independent of concentration, estazolam in plasma is 93% protein bound.

In healthy subjects who received up to three times the recommended dose of estazolam, peak estazolam plasma concentrations occurred within two hours after dosing (range 0.5 to 6.0 hours) and were proportional to the administered dose, suggesting linear pharmacokinetics over the dosage range tested.

The range of estimates for the elimination half-life of estazolam varied from 10 to 24 hours. The clearance of benzodiazepines is accelerated in smokers compared to nonsmokers and there is evidence that this occurs with estazolam. This decrease in half-life, presumably due to enzyme induction by smoking, is consistent with other drugs with similar hepatic clearance characteristics. In all subjects, and at all doses, the mean elimination half-life appeared to be independent of the dose.

In a small study (N=8), using various doses in older subjects (59 to 68 years), peak estazolam concentrations were found to be similar to those observed in younger subjects with a mean elimination half-life of 18.4 hours (range 13.5 to 34.6 hours).

Estazolam is extensively metabolized and the metabolites are excreted primarily in the urine. Less than 5% of a 2 mg dose of estazolam is excreted unchanged in the urine with only 4% of the dose appearing in the feces. 4'-hydroxy estazolam is the major metabolite in plasma with concentrations approaching 12% of those of the parent eight hours after administration. While it and the lesser metabolite, 1-oxo-estazolam have some pharmacologic activity, their low potencies and low concentrations preclude any significant contribution to the hypnotic effect of estazolam.

Postulated Relationship Between Elimination Rate Of Benzodiazepine Hypnotics And Their Profile Of Common Untoward Effects: The type and duration of hypnotic effects and the profile of unwanted effects during administration of benzodiazepine drugs may be influenced by the biologic half-life of administered drug and any active metabolites formed. When half-lives are long, drug or metabolites may accumulate during periods of nightly administration and be associated with impairments of cognitive and/or motor performance during waking hours; the possibility of interaction with other psychoactive drugs or alcohol will be enhanced. In contrast, if half-lives are short, drug and metabolites will be cleared before the next dose is ingested, and carry-over effects related to excessive sedation or CNS depression should be minimal or absent. However, during nightly use for an extended period, pharmacodynamic tolerance or adaptation to some effects of benzodiazepine hypnotics may develop. If the drug has a short elimination half-life, it is possible that a relative deficiency of the drug or its active metabolites (*i.e.,* in relationship to the receptor site) may occur at some point in the interval between each night's use. This sequence of events may account for two clinical findings reported to occur after several weeks of nightly use of rapidly eliminated benzodiazepine hypnotics, namely, increased wakefulness during the last third of the night, and the appearance of increased signs of daytime anxiety in selected patients.

Controlled Trials Supporting Efficacy: In three 7-night, double- blind, parallel-group trials comparing estazolam 1 and/or 2 mg with placebo in adult outpatients with chronic insomnia, estazolam 2 mg was consistently superior to placebo on subjective measures of sleep induction (latency) and sleep maintenance (duration, number of awakenings, depth and quality of sleep) in all three studies; estazolam 1 mg was similarly superior to placebo on all measures of sleep maintenance, however, it significantly improved sleep induction in only one of two studies utilizing the 1 mg dose. In a similarly designed trial comparing estazolam 0.5 mg and 1 mg with placebo in geriatric outpatients with chronic insomnia, only the 1 mg estazolam dose was consistently superior to placebo on sleep induction (latency) and on only one measure of sleep maintenance (*i.e.,* duration of sleep).

In a single-night, double-blind, parallel-group trial comparing estazolam 2 mg and placebo in patients admitted for elective surgery and requiring sleep medications, estazolam was superior to placebo on subjective measures of sleep induction and maintenance.

In a 12-week, double-blind, parallel-group trial including a comparison of estazolam 2 mg and placebo in adult outpatients with chronic insomnia, estazolam was superior to placebo on subjective measures of sleep induction (latency) and maintenance (duration, number of awakenings, total wake time during sleep) at week 2, but resulted in persistent improvement over 12 weeks only for sleep duration and total wake time during sleep. Following withdrawal at week 12, rebound insomnia was seen at the first withdrawal week, but there was no difference between drug and placebo by the second withdrawal week in all parameters except for latency, for which normalization did not occur until the fourth withdrawal week.

Adult outpatients with chronic insomnia were evaluated in a sleep laboratory trial comparing 4 doses of estazolam (0.25, 0.50, 1.0 and 2.0 mg) and placebo, each administered for 2 nights in a crossover design. The higher estazolam doses were superior to placebo on most EEG measures of sleep induction and maintenance, especially at the 2 mg dose, but only for sleep duration on subjective measures of sleep.

INDICATIONS AND USAGE:

Estazolam is indicated for the short-term management of insomnia characterized by difficulty in falling asleep, frequent nocturnal awakenings, and/or early morning awakenings. Both outpatient studies and a sleep laboratory study have shown that estazolam administered at bedtime improved sleep induction and sleep maintenance (see CLINICAL PHARMACOLOGY).

Because insomnia is often transient and intermittent, the prolonged administration of estazolam is generally not necessary nor recommended. Since insomnia may be a symptom of several other disorders, the possibility that the complaint may be related to a condition for which there is a more specific treatment should be considered.

There is evidence to support the ability of estazolam to enhance the duration and quality of sleep for intervals up to 12 weeks (See CLINICAL PHARMACOLOGY.)

CONTRAINDICATIONS:

Benzodiazepines may cause fetal damage when administered during pregnancy. An increased risk of congenital malformations associated with the use of diazepam and chlordiazepoxide during the first trimester of pregnancy has been suggested in several studies.

Transplacental distribution has resulted in neonatal CNS depression and also withdrawal phenomena following the ingestion of therapeutic doses of a benzodiazepine hypnotic during the last weeks of pregnancy.

Estazolam is contraindicated in pregnant women. If there is a likelihood of the patient becoming pregnant while receiving estazolam she should be warned of the potential risk to the fetus. Patients should be instructed to discontinue the drug prior to becoming pregnant. The possibility that a woman of childbearing potential may be pregnant at the time of institution of therapy should be considered.

WARNINGS:

Estazolam, like other benzodiazepines, has CNS-depressant effects. For this reason, patients should be cautioned against engaging in hazardous occupations requiring complete mental alertness such as operating machinery or driving a motor vehicle after ingesting the drug, including potential impairment of the performance of such activities that may occur the day following ingestion of estazolam. Patients should also be cautioned about possible combined effects with alcohol and other CNS-depressant drugs.

As with all benzodiazepines, amnesia, paradoxical reactions (*e.g.,* excitement, agitation, etc..), and other adverse behavioral effects may occur unpredictably.

There have been reports of withdrawal signs and symptoms of the type associated with withdrawal from CNS depressant drugs following the rapid decrease or the abrupt discontinuation of benzodiazepines. (See DRUG ABUSE AND DEPENDENCE.)

PRECAUTIONS:

GENERAL

Impaired motor and/or cognitive performance attributable to the accumulation of benzodiazepines and their active metabolites following several days of repeated use at their recommended doses is a concern in certain vulnerable patients (*e.g.,* those especially sensitive to the effects of benzodiazepines or those with a reduced capacity to metabolize and eliminate them). (See DOSAGE AND ADMINISTRATION.)

Elderly or debilitated patients and those with impaired renal or hepatic function should be cautioned about these risks and advised to monitor themselves for signs of excessive sedation or impaired conditions.

Estazolam appears to cause dose-related respiratory depression that is ordinarily not clinically relevant at recommended doses in patients with normal respiratory function. However, patients with compromised respiratory function may be at risk and should be monitored appropriately. As a class, benzodiazepines have the capacity to depress respiratory drive; there are insufficient data available, however, to characterize their relative potency in depressing respiratory drive at clinically recommended doses.

As with other benzodiazepines, estazolam should be administered with caution to patients exhibiting signs or symptoms of depression. Suicidal tendencies may be present in such patients and protective measures may be required. Intentional overdosage is more common in this group of patients; therefore, the least amount of drug that is feasible should be prescribed for the patient at any one time.

INFORMATION FOR THE PATIENT

To assure the safe and effective use of estazolam, the following information and instructions should be given to patients:

1. Inform your physician about any alcohol consumption and medicine you are taking now, including drugs you may buy without a prescription. Alcohol should not be used during treatment with hypnotics.

2. Inform your physician if you are planning to become pregnant, if you are pregnant, or if you become pregnant while you are taking this medicine.

3. You should not take this medicine if you are nursing as the drug may be excreted in breast milk.

4. Until you experience how this medicine affects you, do not drive a car, operate potentially dangerous machinery, or engage in hazardous occupations requiring complete mental alertness after taking this medicine.

5. Since benzodiazepines may produce psychological and physical dependence, you should not increase the dose before consulting with your physician. In addition, since the abrupt discontinuation of estazolam may be associated with a temporary worsening of sleep, you should consult your physician before abruptly discontinuing doses of 2 mg per night or more.

LABORATORY TESTS

Laboratory tests are not ordinarily required otherwise healthy patients. When treatment with estazolam tablets is protracted, periodic blood counts, urinalysis, and blood chemistry analyses are advisable.

CARCINOGENESIS, MUTAGENESIS, AND IMPAIRMENT OF FERTILITY

Two-year carcinogenicity studies were conducted in mice and rats at dietary doses of 0.8, 3, 10 mg/kg/day and 0.5, 2, and 10 mg/kg/day, respectively. Evidence of tumorigenicity was not observed in either study. Hyperplastic liver nodules were increased in female mice given the mid and high dose levels. The significance of such nodules in mice is not known at this time.

In vitro and *in vivo* mutagenicity tests including the Ames test, DNA repair in B. subtilis, *in vivo* cytogenetics in mice and rats, and the dominant lethal test in mice did not show a mutagenic potential for estazolam.

Fertility in male and female rats was not affected by doses up to 30 times the usual recommended human dose.

PREGNANCY CATEGORY X

Teratogenic Effects: (See CONTRAINDICATIONS.)

Non-Teratogenic Effects: The child born of a mother who is taking benzodiazepines may be at some risk for withdrawal symptoms from the drug during the postnatal period. Neonatal flaccidity has been reported in an infant born of a mother who received benzodiazepines during pregnancy.

LABOR AND DELIVERY

Estazolam has no established use in labor or delivery.

NURSING MOTHERS

Human studies have not been conducted; however, studies in lactating rats indicate that estazolam and/or its metabolites are secreted in the milk. The use of estazolam in nursing mothers is not recommended.

PEDIATRIC USE

Safety and effectiveness in children below the age of 18 have not been established.

GERIATRIC USE

Approximately 18% of individuals participating in the premarketing clinical trials of estazolam were 60 years of age or older. Overall, the adverse event profile did not differ substantively from that observed in younger individuals. Care should be exercised when prescribing benzodiazepines to small or debilitated elderly patients (See DOSAGE AND ADMINISTRATION.)

DRUG INTERACTIONS:

If estazolam is given concomitantly with other drugs acting on the central nervous system, careful consideration should be given to the pharmacology of the agents to be employed. The action of the benzodiazepines may be potentiated by anticonvulsants, antihistamines, alcohol, barbiturates, monoamine oxidase inhibitors, narcotics, phenothiazines, psychotropic medications, or other drugs that produce CNS depression. Smokers have an increased clearance of benzodiazepines as compared to nonsmokers; this was seen in studies with estazolam (See CLINICAL PHARMACOLOGY.)

ADVERSE REACTIONS:

Commonly Observed: The most commonly observed adverse events associated with the use of estazolam and not seen at an equivalent incidence among placebo treated patients were somnolence, hypokinesia, dizziness and abnormal coordination.

Associated with Discontinuation of Treatment: Approximately 3% of 1277 patients who received estazolam in US premarketing clinical trials discontinued treatment because of an adverse clinical event.

The only event commonly associated with discontinuation, accounting for 1.3% of the total, was somnolence.

Incidence in Controlled Clinical Trials: The table enumerates adverse events that occurred at an incidence of 1% or greater among patients with insomnia who received estazolam in 7-night, placebo- controlled trials. Events reported by investigators were classified into standard dictionary (COSTART) terms for the purpose of establishing event frequencies. Event frequencies reported were not corrected for the occurrence of these events at baseline. The frequencies were obtained from data pooled across 6 studies: estazolam, N=685; placebo, N=433. The prescriber should be aware that these figures cannot be used to predict the incidence of side effects in the course of usual medical practice, in which patient characteristics and other factors differ from those that prevailed in these 6 clinical trials. Similarly, the cited frequencies cannot be compared with figures obtained from other clinical investigators involving related drug products and uses, since each group of drug trials is conducted under a different set of conditions. However, the cited figures provide the physician with a basis of estimating the relative contribution of drug and nondrug factors to the incidence of side effects in the population studied.

TABLE 1 Incidence Of Adverse Experiences In Placebo-Controlled Clinical Studies

Body System/Adverse Event*	(Percentage of Patients Reporting) Estazolam (N = 685)	Placebo (N = 433)
Body as a Whole		
Headache	16	27
Asthenia	11	8
Malaise	5	5
Lower extremity pain	3	2
Back pain	2	2
Body Pain	2	2
Abdominal pain	1	2
Chest pain	1	1
Digestive System		
Nausea	4	5
Dyspepsia	2	2
Musculoskeletal System		
Stiffness	1	—
Nervous System		
Somnolence	42	27
Hypokinesia	8	4
Nervousness	8	11
Dizziness	7	3
Coordination abnormal	4	1
Hangover	3	2
Confusion	2	—
Depression	2	3
Dream abnormal	2	2
Thinking abnormal	2	1
Respiratory System		
Cold Symptoms	3	5
Pharyngitis	1	2
Skin and Appendages		
Pruritus	1	—

* Events reported by at least 1% of estazolam patients are included

Other Adverse Events: During clinical trials conducted by Abbott, some of which were not placebo-controlled, estazolam was administered to approximately 1300 patients. Untoward events associated with this exposure were recorded by clinical investigators using terminology of their own choosing. To provide a meaningful estimate of the proportion of individuals experiencing adverse events, similar types of untoward events must be grouped into a smaller number of standardized event categories. In the tabulations that follow, a standard COSTART dictionary terminology has been used to classify reported adverse events. The frequencies presented, therefore, represent the proportion of the 1277 individuals exposed to estazolam who experienced an event of the type cited on at least one occasion while receiving estazolam. All reported events are included except those already listed in the previous table, those COSTART terms so general as to be uninformative, and those events where a drug cause was remote. Events are further classified within body system categories and enumerated in order of decreasing frequency using the following definitions: frequent adverse events are defined as those occurring on one or more occasions in at least 1/100 patients; infrequent adverse events are those occurring in 1/100 to 1/1000 patients; rare events are those occurring in less than 1/1000 patients. It is important to emphasize that, although the events reported did occur during treatment with estazolam, they were not necessarily caused by it.

Body as a Whole: Infrequent: allergic reaction, chills, fever, neck pain, upper extremity pain; Rare: edema, jaw pain, swollen breast.

Cardiovascular System: Infrequent: flushing, palpitation; Rare: Arrhythmia, syncope.

Digestive System: Frequent: constipation, dry mouth; Infrequent: decreased appetite, flatulence, gastritis, increased appetite, vomiting; Rare: enterocolitis, melena, ulceration of the mouth.

Endocrine System: Rare: thyroid nodule.

Hematologic and Lymphatic System: Rare: leukopenia, purpura, swollen lymph nodes.

Metabolic/Nutritional Disorders: Infrequent: thirst; Rare: increased SGOT, weight gain, weight loss.

Musculoskeletal System: Infrequent: arthritis, muscle spasm, myalgia; Rare: arthralgia.

Nervous System: Frequent: anxiety; Infrequent: agitation, amnesia, apathy, emotional lability, euphoria, hostility, paresthesia, seizure, sleep disorder, stupor, twitch; Rare: ataxia, circumoral paresthesia, decreased libido, decreased reflexes, hallucinations, neuritis, nystagmus, tremor.

Minor changes in EEG patterns, usually low-voltage fast activity, have been observed in patients during estazolam therapy or withdrawal and are of no known clinical significance.

Respiratory System: *Infrequent:* asthma, cough, dyspnea, rhinitis, sinusitis, *Rare:* epistaxis, hyperventilation, laryngitis.

Skin and Appendages: *Infrequent:* rash, sweating, urticaria; *Rare:* acne, dry skin.

Special Senses: *Infrequent:* abnormal vision, ear pain, eye irritation, eye pain, eye swelling, perverse taste, photophobia, tinnitus; *Rare:* decreased hearing, diplopia, scotomata.

Urogenital System: *Infrequent:* frequent urination, menstrual cramps, urinary hesitancy, urinary urgency, vaginal discharge/itching; *Rare:* hematuria, nocturia, oliguria, penile discharge, urinary incontinence.

ADVERSE REACTIONS: *(cont'd)*

Postintroduction Reports: Voluntary reports from non-U.S. postmarketing experience of estazolam have included rare occurrences of the following events: photosensitivity; agranulocytosis. Because of the uncontrolled nature of these spontaneous reports, a casual relationship to estazolam treatment has not been determined.

DRUG ABUSE AND DEPENDENCE:

Controlled Substance: Withdrawal symptoms similar in character to those noted with sedatives/hypnotics and alcohol have occurred following the abrupt discontinuation of drugs in the benzodiazepine class. The symptoms can range from mild dysphoria and insomnia to a major syndrome which may include abdominal and muscle cramps, vomiting, sweating, tremors, and convulsions.

Although withdrawal symptoms are more commonly noted after the discontinuation of higher than therapeutic doses of benzodiazepines, a proportion of patients taking doses of benzodiazepines chronically at therapeutic doses may become physically dependent upon them. Available data, however, cannot provide a reliable estimate of the incidence of dependency or the relationship of the dependency to dose and duration of treatment. There is some evidence to suggest that gradual reduction of dosage will attenuate or eliminate some withdrawal phenomena. In most instances, withdrawal phenomena are relatively mild and transient; however, life-threatening events (*e.g.,* seizures, delirium, etc..) have been reported.

Gradual withdrawal is the preferred course for any patient taking benzodiazepines for a prolonged period. Patients with a history of seizures, regardless of their concomitant anti-seizure drug therapy, should not be withdrawn abruptly from benzodiazepines. Individuals with a history of addiction to, or abuse of, drugs or alcohol should be under careful surveillance when receiving benzodiazepines because of the risk to such patients of habituation and dependence.

OVERDOSAGE:

As with other benzodiazepines, experience with estazolam indicates that manifestations of overdosage include somnolence, respiratory depression, confusion, impaired coordination, slurred speech, and ultimately, coma. Patients have recovered from overdosage as high as 40 mg. As in the management of intentional overdose with any drug, it should be borne in mind that multiple agents may have been taken. Gastric evacuation either by the induction of emesis, lavage, or both, should be performed immediately. Maintenance of adequate ventilation is essential. General supportive care, including frequent monitoring of the vital signs and close observation of the patient, is indicated. Fluids should be administered intravenously to maintain blood pressure and encourage diuresis. The value of dialysis in treatment of benzodiazepine overdose has not been determined. The physician may wish to consider contacting a Poison Control Center for up-to-date information on the management of hypnotic drug product overdose.

DOSAGE AND ADMINISTRATION:

The recommended initial dose for adults is 1 mg at bedtime; however, some patients may need a 2 mg dose. In healthy elderly patients 1 mg is also the appropriate starting dose, but increases should be initiated with particular care. In small or debilitated older patients, a starting dose of 0.5 mg, while only marginally effective in the overall elderly population, should be considered.

Store below 86°F (30°C).

HOW SUPPLIED - EQUIVALENTS NOT AVAILABLE:

Tablet, Uncoated - Oral - 1 mg

100's	$88.54	PROSOM, Abbott	00074-3735-13
100's	$90.32	PROSOM, Abbott	00074-3735-11

Tablet, Uncoated - Oral - 2 mg

100's	$98.63	PROSOM 2, Abbott	00074-3736-13
100's	$100.42	PROSOM 2, Abbott	00074-3736-11

ESTRADIOL *(001188)*

CATEGORIES: Antineoplastics; Dermatologicals; Estrogens; Hormones; Hypogonadism; Kraurosis Vulvae; Menopause; Osteoporosis; Ovarian Failure; Skin/Mucous Membrane Agents; Vaginitis; Breast Carcinoma*; Prostatic Carcinoma*; Pregnancy Category X; Sales > $100 Million; FDA Approval Pre 1982; Top 200 Drugs
* Indication not approved by the FDA

BRAND NAMES: Climara; Estrace; *Estracomb TTS*; **Estraderm**; *Estraderm TTS* (France, England, Germany); *Estrofem* (France); *Femtran*; *Ginedisc* (Mexico); *Oesclim* (France); *Oestradiol Berco* (Germany); *Progynon*; *Progynova*; *Systen* (Mexico); Vivelle; *Zumenon* (England)
(International brand names outside U.S. in italics)

FORMULARIES: Aetna; BC-BS; Medi-Cal; PCS

COST OF THERAPY: $73.14 (Osteoporosis; Tablet; 0.5 mg; 1/day; 300 days)

WARNING:

1. Estrogens Have Been Reported To Increase The Risk Of Endometrial Carcinoma In Postmenopausal Women:Close clinical surveillance of all women taking estrogens is important. Adequate diagnostic measures, including endometrial sampling when indicated, should be undertaken to rule out malignancy in all cases of undiagnosed persistent or recurring abnormal vaginal bleeding. There is no evidence that "natural" estrogens are more or less hazardous than "synthetic" estrogens at equiestrogenic doses.

2. Estrogens Should Not Be Used During Pregnancy:There is no indication for estrogen therapy during pregnancy or during the immediate postpartum period. Estrogens are ineffective for the prevention or treatment of threatened or habitual abortion. Estrogens are not indicated for the prevention of postpartum breast engorgement.

Estrogen therapy during pregnancy is associated with an increased risk of congenital defects in the reproductive organs of the fetus, and possibly other birth defects. Studies of women who received diethylstilbestrol (DES) during pregnancy have shown that female offspring have an increased risk of vaginal adenosis, squamous cell dysplasia of the uterine cervix, and clear cell vaginal cancer later in life; male offspring have an increased risk of urogenital abnormalities and possibly testicular cancer later in life. The 1985 DES Task Force concluded that the use of DES

> during pregnancy is associated with a subsequent increased risk of breast cancer in the mothers, although a causal relationship remains unproven and the observed level of excess risk is similar to that for a number of other breast cancer risk factors.

DESCRIPTION:

Estradiol USP (17β-estradiol) is a white, crystalline powder, chemically described as estra-1,3,5(10)-triene-3,17β-diol. It has an empirical formula of $C_{18}H_{24}O_2$ and molecular weight of 272.37.

TRANSDERMAL SYSTEM

The estradiol transdermal system is designed to release 17β-estradiol through a rate-limiting membrane continuously upon application to intact skin.

Two systems are available to provide nominal *in vivo* delivery of 0.05 or 0.1 mg of estradiol per day via skin of average permeability (interindividual variation in skin permeability is approximately 20%) Each corresponding system having a contact surface area of 10 or 20 cm^2 contains 4 or 8 mg of estradiol USP and 0.3 or 0.6 ml of alcohol USP, respectively. The composition of the systems per unit area is identical.

The estradiol transdermal system comprises four layers. Proceeding from the visible surface toward the surface attached to the skin, these layers are (1) a transparent polyester film, (2) a drug reservoir of estradiol USP and alcohol USP gelled with hydroxypropyl cellulose, (3) an ethylene-vinyl acetate copolymer membrane, and (4) an adhesive formulation of light mineral oil and polyisobutylene. A protective liner (5) of siliconized polyethylene terephthalate film is attached to the adhesive surface and must be removed before the system can be used.

The active component of the system is estradiol. The remaining components of the system are pharmacologically inactive. Alcohol is also released from the system during use.

VAGINAL CREAM

Estradiol vaginal cream contains 0.1 mg estradiol per gram in a nonliquefying base containing purified water, propylene glycol, stearyl alcohol, white ceresin wax, glyceryl monostearate, hydroxypropyl methylcellulose, 2208 4000 cps, sodium lauryl sulfate, methylparaben, edetate disodium and *tertiary*-butylhydroquinone.

TABLETS

Estradiol tablets for oral administration contain 0.5, 1 or 2 mg of micronized estradiol per tablet.

Estradiol tablets, 0.5 mg, contain the following inactive ingredients: acacia, dibasic calcium phosphate, lactose hydrous, magnesium stearate, colloidal silicon dioxide, starch (corn), and talc.

Estradiol tablets, 1 mg, contain the following inactive ingredients: acacia, D&C Red No. 27 (aluminum lake), dibasic calcium phosphate, FD&C Blue No. 1 (aluminum lake), lactose hydrous, magnesium stearate, colloidal silicon dioxide, starch (corn), and talc.

Estradiol tablets, 2 mg, contain the following inactive ingredients: acacia, dibasic calcium phosphate, FD&C Blue No. 1 (aluminum lake), FD&C Yellow No. 5 (tartrazine) (aluminum lake), lactose hydrous, magnesium stearate, colloidal silicon dioxide, starch (corn), and talc.

CLINICAL PHARMACOLOGY:

TRANSDERMAL SYSTEM

The estradiol transdermal system releases estradiol, the major estrogenic hormone secreted by the human ovary. Estradiol transdermal system provides systemic estrogen replacement therapy. Among numerous effects, estradiol is largely responsible for the development and maintenance of the female reproductive system and of secondary sexual characteristics. It promotes growth and development of the vagina, uterus, fallopian tubes, and breasts. Indirectly, estradiol contributes to the shaping of the skeleton, to the maintenance of tone and elasticity of urogenital structures, to changes in the epiphyses of the long bones that allow for the pubertal growth spurt and its termination, to the growth of axillary and pubic hair, and to the pigmentation of the nipples and genitals.

In the anovulatory cycle estrogen is the primary determinant in the onset of menstruation. Estradiol also affects the release of pituitary gonadotropins.

Loss of ovarian estradiol secretion after menopause can result in instability of thermoregulation, causing hot flushes associated with sleep disturbance and excessive sweating, and urogenital atrophy, causing dyspareunia and urinary incontinence. Estradiol replacement therapy alleviates many of these symptoms of estradiol deficiency in the menopausal woman.

Orally administered estradiol is rapidly metabolized by the liver to estrone and its conjugates, giving rise to higher circulating levels of estrone than estradiol. In contrast, the skin metabolized estradiol only to a small extent. Therefore, transdermal administration produces therapeutic serum levels of estradiol with lower circulating levels of estrone and estrone conjugates, and requires smaller total doses than does oral therapy. Because estradiol has a short half-life (≈1 hour), transdermal administration of estradiol allows a in blood levels after an estradiol transdermal system is removed, e.g. in a cycling regimen.

In a study transdermally using estradiol, 0.1 mg daily, plasma levels increased by 66 pg/ml resulting in an average plasma level of 73 pg/ml. There were no significant increases in the concentration of renin substrate or other hepatic proteins (sex-hormone-binding globulin, thyroxine-binding globulin and corticosteroid-binding globulin).

PHARMACOKINETICS

Administration of estradiol transdermal system produces mean serum concentrations of estradiol comparable to those produced by daily oral administration estradiol at about 20 times the daily transdermal dose. In single-application studies in 14 postmenopausal women using estradiol transdermal systems that provided 0.05 and 0.1 mg of exogenous estradiol per day, these systems produced increased blood levels within 4 hours and maintained respective mean serum estradiol concentrations of 32 and 67 pg/ml above baseline over the application period. At the same time, increases in estrone serum concentration averaged only 9 and 27 pg/ml above baseline, respectively. Serum concentrations of estradiol and estrone returned to preapplication levels within 24 hours after removal of the system. The estimated daily urinary output of estradiol conjugates increased 5 to 10 times the baseline values and returned to near baseline within 2 day after removal of the system.

By comparison, estradiol (2 mg per day) administered orally to postmenopausal women resulted in increases in mean serum concentration 59 pg/ml of estradiol and 302 pg/ml of estrone above baseline on the third consecutive day dosing. Urinary output of estradiol conjugates after oral administration increased to about 100 times the baseline values and did not approach baseline until 7-8 days after the last dose.

In a 3 week multiple-application study of 14 postmenopausal women in which estradiol transdermal systems 0.05 was applied twice weekly, the mean increments in steady-state serum concentration were 30 pg/ml for estradiol and 12 pg/ml for estrone. Urinary output of estradiol conjugates returned to baseline within 3 days after removal of the last (6th) indicating little or no estrogen accumulation in the body.

VAGINAL CREAM AND TABLETS

Estrogen drug products act by regulating the transcription of a limited number of genes. Estrogens diffuse through cell membranes, distribute themselves throughout the cell, and bind to and activate the nuclear estrogen receptor, a DNA-binding protein which is found in estro-

CLINICAL PHARMACOLOGY: *(cont'd)*

gen-responsive tissues. The activated estrogen receptor binds to specific DNA sequences, or hormone-response elements, which enhance the transcription of adjacent genes and in turn lead to the observed effects. Estrogen receptors have been identified in tissues of the reproductive tract, breast, pituitary, hypothalamus, liver, and bone of women.

Estrogens are important in the development and maintenance of the female reproductive system and secondary sex characteristics. By a direct action, they cause growth and development of the uterus, fallopian tubes, and vagina. With other hormones, such as pituitary hormones and progesterone, they cause enlargement of the breasts through promotion of ductal growth, stromal development, and the accretion of fat. Estrogens are intricately involved with other hormones, especially progesterone, in the processes of the ovulatory menstrual cycle and pregnancy, and affect the release of pituitary gonadotropins. They also contribute to the shaping of the skeleton, maintenance of tone and elasticity of urogenital structures, changes in the epiphyses of the long bones that allow for the pubertal growth spurt and its termination, and pigmentation of the nipples and genitals.

Estrogens occur naturally in several forms. The primary source of estrogen in normally cycling adult women is the ovarian follicle, which secretes 70 to 500 micrograms of estradiol daily, depending on the phase of the menstrual cycle. This is converted primarily to estrone, which circulates in roughly equal proportion to estradiol, and to small amounts of estriol. After menopause, most endogenous estrogen is produced by conversion of androstenedione, secreted by the adrenal cortex, to estrone by peripheral tissues. Thus, estrone—especially in its sulfate form—is the most abundant circulating estrogen in postmenopausal women. Although circulating estrogens exist in a dynamic equilibrium of metabolic interconversions, estradiol is the principal intracellular human estrogen and is substantially more potent than estrone or estriol at the receptor.

Estrogens used in therapy are well absorbed through the skin, mucous membranes, and gastrointestinal tract. When applied for a local action, absorption is usually sufficient to cause systemic effects. When conjugated with aryl and alkyl groups for parenteral administration, the rate of absorption of oily preparations is slowed with a prolonged duration of action, such that a single intramuscular injection of estradiol valerate or estradiol cypionate is absorbed over several weeks.

Administered estrogens and their esters are handled within the body essentially the same as endogenous hormones. Metabolic conversion of estrogens occurs primarily in the liver (first pass effect), but also at local target tissue sites. Complex metabolic processes result in a dynamic equilibrium of circulating conjugated and unconjugated estrogenic forms which are continually interconverted, especially between estrone and estradiol and between esterified and unesterified forms. Although naturally-occurring estrogens circulate in the blood largely bound to sex hormone-binding globulin and albumin, only unbound estrogens enter target tissue cells. A significant proportion of the circulating estrogen exists as sulfate conjugates, especially estrone sulfate, which serves as a circulating reservoir for the formation of more active estrogenic species. A certain proportion of the estrogen is excreted into the bile and then reabsorbed from the intestine. During this enterohepatic recirculation, estrogens are desulfated and resulfated and undergo degradation through conversion to less active estrogens (estriol and other estrogens), oxidation to nonestrogenic substances (catecholestrogens, which interact with catecholamine metabolism, especially in the central nervous system), and conjugation with glucuronic acids (which are then rapidly excreted in the urine).

When given orally, naturally-occurring estrogens and their esters are extensively metabolized (first pass effect) and circulate primarily as estrone sulfate, with smaller amounts of other conjugated and unconjugated estrogenic species. This results in limited oral potency. By contrast, synthetic estrogens, such as ethinyl estradiol and the nonsteroidal estrogens, are degraded very slowly in the liver and other tissues, which results in their high intrinsic potency. Estrogen drug products administered by non-oral routes are not subject to first-pass metabolism, but also undergo significant hepatic uptake, metabolism, and enterohepatic recycling.

INDICATIONS AND USAGE:

TRANSDERMAL SYSTEM

Estradiol transdermal system is indicated for the treatment of the following: moderate-to-severe vasomotor symptoms associated with menopause; female hypogonadism; female castration; primary ovarian failure; atrophic conditions caused by deficient endogenous estrogen production, such as atrophic vaginitis and kraurosis vulvae; and prevention of osteoporosis (loss of bone mass).

Estrogen replacement therapy is the most effective single modality for the prevention of postmenopausal osteoporosis in women. Case-controlled studies have shown a reduction of approximately 60% in the incidence of hip and wrist fractures in women who began estrogen replacement therapy within a few years of menopause. A recent, well-controlled, double-blind, prospective trial conducted at the Mayo Clinic has demonstrated that treatment with estradiol transdermal system prevents bone loss in postmenopausal women at a dosage of 0.05 mg per day.

Treatment with estradiol transdermal system 0.05 mg showed full maintenance of bone density with slight (0.8%), but not significant, increase. Placebo treatment resulted in a significant loss of more than 6% below baseline vertebral bone mass. Patients using either estradiol transdermal system 0.1 mg, or 0.05 mg, had significantly greater bone densities than those using placebo.

Other studies suggest that estrogen replacement therapy reduces the rate of vertebral fracture.

Peak bone mass is reached at age 30 to 35 and can best be maximized by adequate calcium intake and exercise during the adolescent and early adult years. Early menopause is one of the best predictors for the development of osteoporosis. White women are at higher risk for osteoporosis than white men, black women are at higher risk than black men, and thin women are at higher risk than obese women. Cigarette smoking may be an additional risk factor. Calcium deficiency has been implicated in the pathogenesis of this disease. Therefore, when not contraindicated, a calcium intake of 1000-1500 mg/day either by diet or supplements is recommended for postmenopausal women.

Immobilization and prolonged bedrest produce rapid bone loss, while weight-bearing exercise has been shown to both reduce bone loss and to increase bone mass. The optimal type and amount of physical activity that might lower the risk for osteoporosis have not been established.

VAGINAL CREAM

Estradiol vaginal cream is indicated in the treatment of vulval and vaginal atrophy.

TABLETS

Estradiol tablets are indicated in the:

1. Treatment of moderate to severe vasomotor symptoms associated with the menopause. There is no adequate evidence that estrogens are effective for nervous symptoms or depression which might occur during menopause and they should not be used to treat these conditions.

2. Treatment of vulval and vaginal atrophy.

3. Treatment of hypoestrogenism due to hypogonadism, castration or primary ovarian failure.

4. Treatment of breast cancer (for palliation only) in appropriately selected women and men with metastatic disease.

INDICATIONS AND USAGE: *(cont'd)*

5. Treatment of advanced androgen-dependent carcinoma of the prostate (for palliation only).
6. Prevention of osteoporosis.

Since estrogen administration is associated with risk, selection of patients should ideally be based on prospective identification of risk factors for developing osteoporosis. Unfortunately, there is no certain way to identify those women who will develop osteoporotic fractures. Most prospective studies of efficacy for this indication have been carried out in white menopausal women, without stratification by other risk factors, and tend to show a universally salutary effect on bone. Thus, patient selection must be individualized based on the balance of risks and benefits. A more favorable risk/benefit ratio exists in a hysterectomized woman because she has no risk of endometrial cancer (see BOXED WARNING.)

Estrogen replacement therapy reduces bone resorption and retards or halts postmenopausal bone loss. Case-control studies have shown an approximately 60 percent reduction in hip and waist fractures in women whose estrogen replacement was begun within a few years of menopause. Studies also suggest that estrogen reduces the rate of vertebral fractures. Even when started as late as 6 years after menopause, estrogen prevents further loss of bone mass for as long as the treatment is continued. The results of a two-year, randomized, placebo-controlled, double-blind, dose-ranging study have shown that treatment with 0.5 mg estradiol daily for 23 days (of a 28 day cycle) prevents vertebral bone mass loss in postmenopausal women. When estrogen therapy is discontinued, bone mass declines at a rate comparable to the immediate postmenopausal period. There is no evidence that estrogen replacement therapy restores bone mass to premenopausal levels.

At skeletal maturity there are sex and race differences in both the total amount of bone present and its density, in favor of men and blacks. Thus, women are at higher risk than men because they start with less bone mass and, for several years following natural or induced menopause, the rate of bone mass decline is accelerated. White and Asian women are at higher risk than black women.

Early menopause is one of the strongest predictors for the development of osteoporosis. In addition, other factors affecting the skeleton which are associated with osteoporosis include genetic factors (small build, family history), and endocrine factors (nulliparity, thyrotoxicosis, hyperparathyroidism, Cushing's syndrome, hyperprolactinemia, Type I diabetes), lifestyle (cigarette smoking, alcohol abuse, sedentary exercise habits) and nutrition (below average body weight, dietary calcium intake).

The mainstays of prevention and management of osteoporosis are estrogen, adequate lifetime calcium intake, and exercise. Postmenopausal women absorb dietary calcium less efficiently than premenopausal women and require an average of 1500 mg/day of elemental calcium to remain in neutral calcium balance. By comparison, premenopausal women require about 1000 mg/day and the average calcium intake in the USA is 400-600 mg/day. Therefore, when not contraindicated, calcium supplementation may be helpful.

Weight-bearing exercise and nutrition may be important adjuncts to the prevention and management of osteoporosis. Immobilization and prolonged bed rest produce rapid bone loss, while weight-bearing exercise has been shown both to reduce bone loss and to increase bone mass. The optimal type and amount of physical activity that would prevent osteoporosis have not been established, however in two studies, an hour of walking and running exercise twice or three times weekly significantly increased lumbar spine bone mass.

CONTRAINDICATIONS:

Estrogens should not be used in women or men with any of the following conditions:

1. Known or suspected pregnancy (see BOXED WARNING). Estrogens may cause fetal harm when administered to a pregnant woman.
2. Undiagnosed abnormal genital bleeding.
3. Known or suspected cancer of the breast except in appropriately selected patients being treated for metastatic disease.
4. Known or suspected estrogen-dependent neoplasia.
5. Active thrombophlebitis or thromboembolic disorders.

WARNINGS:

1. Induction Of Malignant Neoplasms.

Endometrial Cancer. The reported endometrial cancer risk among unopposed estrogen users is about 2- to 12-fold greater than in non-users, and appears dependent on duration of treatment and on estrogen dose. Most studies show no significant increased risk associated with use of estrogens for less than one year. The greatest risk appears associated with prolonged use—with increased risks of 15- to 24-fold for five to ten years or more. In three studies, persistence of risk was demonstrated for 8 to over 15 years after cessation of estrogen treatment. In one study a significant decrease in the incidence of endometrial cancer occurred six months after estrogen withdrawal. Concurrent progestin therapy may offset this risk but the overall health impact in postmenopausal women is not known (see PRECAUTIONS.)

Breast Cancer: While the majority of studies have not shown an increased risk of breast cancer in women who have ever used estrogen replacement therapy, some have reported a moderately increased risk (relative risks of 1.3-2.0) in those taking higher doses or those taking lower doses for prolonged periods of time, especially in excess of 10 years. Other studies have not shown this relationship.

Congenital Lesions With Malignant Potential: Estrogen therapy during pregnancy is associated with an increased risk of fetal congenital reproductive tract disorders, and possibly other birth defects. Studies of women who have received DES during pregnancy have shown that female offspring have an increased risk of vaginal adenosis, squamous cell dysplasia of the uterine cervix, and clear cell vaginal cancer later in life; male offspring have an increased risk of urogenital abnormalities and possibly testicular cancer later in life. Although some of these changes are benign, others are precursors of malignancy.

2. Gallbladder Disease: Two studies have reported a 2- to 4-fold increase in the risk of gallbladder disease requiring surgery in women receiving postmenopausal estrogens.

3. Cardiovascular Disease: Large doses of estrogen (5 mg conjugated estrogens per day), comparable to those used to treat cancer of the prostate and breast, have been shown in a large prospective clinical trial in men to increase the risks of nonfatal myocardial infarction, pulmonary embolism, and thrombophlebitis. These risks cannot necessarily be extrapolated from men to women. However, to avoid the theoretical cardiovascular risk to women caused by high estrogen doses, the dose for estrogen replacement therapy should not exceed the lowest effective dose.

4. Elevated Blood Pressure: Occasional blood pressure increases during estrogen replacement therapy have been attributed to idiosyncratic reactions to estrogens. More often, blood pressure has remained the same or has dropped. One study showed that postmenopausal estrogen users have higher blood pressure than nonusers. Two other studies showed slightly lower blood pressure among estrogen users compared to nonusers. Postmenopausal estrogen use does not increase the risk of stroke. Nonetheless, blood pressure should be monitored at regular intervals with estrogen use.

5. Hypercalcemia: Administration of estrogens may lead to severe hypercalcemia in patients with breast cancer and bone metastases. If this occurs, the drug should be stopped and appropriate measures taken to reduce the serum calcium level.

WARNINGS: *(cont'd)*

TRANSDERMAL SYSTEM

Effects Similar to Those Caused by Estrogen-Progestogen Oral Contraceptives: There are several serious adverse effects of oral contraceptives and other high-dose oral estrogen treatments, most of which have not, up to now, been documented as consequences of postmenopausal estrogen replacement therapy. This may reflect the comparatively low doses of estrogen used in postmenopausal women.

Thromboembolic Disease: It is now well established that users of oral contraceptives have an increased risk of various thromboembolic and thrombotic vascular disease, such as thrombophlebitis, pulmonary embolism, stroke, and myocardial infarction. Cases of retinal thrombosis, mesenteric thrombosis, and optic neuritis have been reported in oral contraceptive users. There is evidence that the risk of several of these adverse reactions is related to the dose of the drug. An increased risk of postsurgery thromboembolic complications has also been reported in users of oral contraceptives. If feasible, estrogen should be discontinued at least 4 weeks before surgery of the type associated with an increased risk of thromboembolism, or during periods of prolonged immobilization.

While an increased rate of thromboembolic and thrombotic disease in postmenopausal users of estrogens has not been found, this does not rule out the possibility that such an increase may be present or that subgroups of women who have underlying risk factors or who are receiving relatively large doses of estrogens may have increased risk. Therefore, estrogens should not be used in persons with active thrombophlebitis or thromboembolic disorders, and they should not be used in persons with a history of such disorders in association with estrogen use. They should be used with caution in patients with cerebral vascular or coronary artery disease and only for those in whom estrogens are clearly needed.

Large doses of estrogen (5 mg conjugated estrogens per day), comparable to those used to treat cancer of the prostate and breast, have been shown in a large prospective clinical trial in men to increase the risk of nonfatal myocardial infarction, pulmonary embolism, and thrombophlebitis. When estrogen doses of this size are used, any of the thromboembolic and thrombotic adverse effects associated with oral contraceptive use should be considered a clear risk.

Hepatic Adenoma: Benign hepatic adenomas have been associated with the use of oral contraceptives. Although benign and rare, these tumors may rupture and cause death from intra-abdominal hemorrhage. Such lesions have not yet been reported in association with other estrogen or progestogen preparations, but they should be considered if abdominal pain and tenderness, abdominal mass, or hypovolemic shock occurs in patients receiving estrogen. Hepatocellular carcinoma has also been reported in women taking estrogen-containing oral contraceptives. The causal relationship of this malignancy to these drugs is not known.

Glucose Tolerance: A worsening of glucose tolerance has been observed in a significant percentage of patients on estrogen-containing oral contraceptives. For this reason, diabetic patients should be carefully observed while receiving estrogen.

VAGINAL CREAM AND TABLETS

Cardiovascular Disease: Large doses of estrogen (5 mg conjugated estrogens per day), comparable to those used to treat cancer of the prostate and breast, have been shown in a large prospective clinical trial in men to increase the risks of nonfatal myocardial infarction, pulmonary embolism, and thrombophlebitis. These risks cannot necessarily be extrapolated from men to women. However, to avoid the theoretical cardiovascular risk to women caused by high estrogen doses, the dose for estrogen replacement therapy should not exceed the lowest effective dose.

PRECAUTIONS:

GENERAL

Addition Of A Progestin: Studies of the addition of a progestin for 7 or more days of a cycle of estrogen administration have reported a lowered incidence of endometrial hyperplasia. Morphological and biochemical studies of endometrium suggest that 12 to 13 days of progestin are needed to provide maximal maturation of the endometrium and to eliminate any hyperplastic changes. Whether this will provide protection from endometrial carcinoma has not been clearly established. There are possible additional risks that may be associated with the inclusion of progestin in estrogen replacement regimens. The potential risks include adverse effects on carbohydrate and lipid metabolism. The choice of progestin and dosage may be important in minimizing these adverse effects.

Physical Examination: A complete medical and family history should be taken prior to the initiation of any estrogen therapy. The pretreatment and periodic physical examinations should include special reference to blood pressure, breasts, abdomen, and pelvic organs, and should include a Papanicolaou smear. As a general rule, estrogen should not be prescribed for longer than one year without reexamining the patient.

Fluid Retention: Because estrogens may cause some degree of fluid retention, conditions which might be exacerbated by this factor, such as asthma, epilepsy, migraine, and cardiac or renal dysfunction, require careful observation.

Uterine Bleeding And Mastodynia: Certain patients may develop undesirable manifestations of estrogenic stimulation, such as abnormal uterine bleeding and mastodynia.

Impaired Liver Function: Estrogens may be poorly metabolized in patients with impaired liver function and should be administered with caution.

Transdermal System

Prolonged administration of unopposed estrogen therapy has been reported to increase the risk of endometrial hyperplasia in some patients. Estrogens should be used with caution in patients who have or have had endometriosis.

Oral contraceptives, appear to be associated with an increased incidence of mental depression. Although it is not clear whether this is due to the ectogenic or progestogenic component of the contraceptive, patients with a history of depression should be carefully observed.

Preexisting uterine leiomyomata may increase in size during prolonged estrogen use. If this occurs, estrogen therapy should be discontinued while the cause is investigated.

In patients with a history of jaundice during pregnancy, there is an increased risk that jaundice will recur with the use of estrogen-containing oral contraceptives. If jaundice develops in any patient receiving estrogen, the medication should be discontinued while the cause is investigated.

Because the prolonged use of estrogens influences the metabolism of calcium and phosphorus, estrogens should be used with caution in patients with metabolic bone diseases associated with hypercalcemia and in patients with renal insufficiency.

Vaginal Cream and Tablets

Hypercoagulability: Some studies have shown that women taking estrogen replacement therapy have hypercoagulability, primarily related to decreased antithrombin activity. This effect appears dose- and duration-dependent and is less pronounced than that associated with oral contraceptive use. Also, postmenopausal women tend to have increased coagulation parameters at baseline compared to premenopausal women. There is some suggestion that low dose postmenopausal mestranol may increase the risk of thromboembolism, although the majority of studies (of primarily conjugated estrogens users) report no such increase. There is insufficient information on hypercoagulability in women who have had previous thromboembolic disease.

PRECAUTIONS: *(cont'd)*

Familial Hyperlipoproteinemia: Estrogen therapy may be associated with massive elevations of plasma triglycerides leading to pancreatitis and other complications in patients with familial defects of lipoprotein metabolism.

Tablets

Estradiol tablets USP, 2 mg, contain FD&C Yellow No. 5 (tartrazine) which may cause allergic-type reactions (including bronchial asthma) in certain susceptible individuals. Although the overall incidence of FD&C Yellow No. 5 (tartrazine) sensitivity in the general population is low, it is frequently seen in patients who also have aspirin hypersensitivity.

INFORMATION FOR THE PATIENT

See PATIENT PACKAGE INSERT.

DRUG/LABORATORY TEST INTERACTIONS

Accelerated prothrombin time, partial thromboplastin time, and platelet aggregation time; increased platelet count; increased factors II, VII antigen, VIII antigen, VIII coagulant activity, IX, X, XII, VII-X complex, II-VII-X complex, and beta-thromboglobulin; decreased levels of anti-factor Xa and antithrombin III, decreased antithrombin III activity; increased levels of fibrinogen and fibrinogen activity; increased plasminogen antigen and activity.

Increased thyroid-binding globulin (TBG) leading to increased circulating total thyroid hormone, as measured by protein-bound iodine (PBI), T4 levels (by column or by radioimmunoassay) or T3 levels by radioimmunoassay. T3 resin uptake is decreased, reflecting the elevated TBG. Free T4 and free T3 concentrations are unaltered.

Other binding proteins may be elevated in serum, (*i.e.,* corticosteroid binding globulin (CBG), sex hormone-binding globulin (SHBG)), leading to increased circulating corticosteroids and sex steroids, respectively. Free or biologically active hormone concentrations are unchanged. Other plasma proteins may be increased (angiotensinogen/renin substrate, alpha-1-antitrypsin, ceruloplasmin).

Increased plasma HDL and HDL-2 subfraction concentrations, reduced LDL cholesterol concentration, increased triglycerides levels.

Impaired glucose tolerance.

Reduced response to metyrapone test.

Reduced serum folate concentration.

LABORATORY TESTS

Vaginal Cream and Tablets: Estrogen administration should generally be guided by clinical response at the smallest dose, rather than laboratory monitoring, for relief of symptoms for those indications in which symptoms are observable. For prevention of osteoporosis, however, see DOSAGE AND ADMINISTRATION.

CARCINOGENESIS, MUTAGENESIS, AND IMPAIRMENT OF FERTILITY

Long term continuous administration of natural and synthetic estrogens in certain animal species increases the frequency of carcinomas of the breast, uterus, cervix, vagina, testis, and liver. See (CONTRAINDICATIONS and WARNINGS).

PREGNANCY CATEGORY X

Estrogens should not be used during pregnancy. See (CONTRAINDICATIONS and BOXED WARNING).

NURSING MOTHERS

As a general principle, the administration of any drug to nursing mothers should be done only when clearly necessary since many drugs are excreted in human milk.

Vaginal Cream and Tablets: Estrogen administration to nursing mothers has been shown to decrease the quantity and quality of the milk.

ADVERSE REACTIONS:

TRANSDERMAL SYSTEM

See WARNINGS and BOXED WARNING regarding potential adverse effects on the fetus, induction of malignant neoplasms, increased incidence of gallbladder disease, and adverse effects similar to those of oral contraceptives, including thromboembolism.

The most commonly reported adverse reaction to estradiol transdermal system in clinical trials was redness and irritation at the application site. This occurred in about 17% of the women treated and caused approximately 2% to discontinue therapy. Reports of rash have been rare.

The following additional adverse reactions have been reported with estrogenic therapy, including oral contraceptives:

Genitourinary System: Breakthrough bleeding, spotting, change in menstrual flow; increase in size of uterine fibromyomata; change in cervical erosion and amount of cervical secretion.

Endocrine: Breast tenderness, breast enlargement.

Gastrointestinal: Nausea, vomiting; abdominal cramps, bloating; cholestatic jaundice have been observed with oral estrogen therapy.

Eyes: Steepening of corneal curvature; intolerance to contact lenses.

Central Nervous System: Headache, migraine, dizziness.

Miscellaneous: Change in weight, edema, change in libido.

VAGINAL CREAM AND TABLETS

The following additional adverse reactions have been reported with estrogen therapy (see WARNINGS regarding induction of neoplasia, adverse effects on the fetus, increased incidence of gallbladder disease, cardiovascular disease, elevated blood pressure, and hypercalcemia).

Genitourinary system: Changes in vaginal bleeding pattern and abnormal withdrawal bleeding or flow; breakthrough bleeding, spotting. Increase in size of uterine leiomyomata. Vaginal candidiasis. Change in amount of cervical secretion.

Breasts: Tenderness, enlargement.

Gastrointestinal: Nausea, vomiting. Abdominal cramps, bloating. Cholestatic jaundice. Increased incidence of gallbladder disease.

Skin: Chloasma or melasma which may persist when drug is discontinued. Erythema multiforme. Erythema nodosum. Hemorrhagic eruption. Loss of scalp hair. Hirsutism.

Eyes: Steepening of corneal curvature. Intolerance to contact lenses.

Central Nervous System: Headache, migraine, dizziness. Mental depression. Chorea.

Miscellaneous: Increase or decrease in weight. Reduced carbohydrate tolerance. Aggravation of porphyria. Edema. Changes in libido.

OVERDOSAGE:

Serious ill effects have not been reported following acute ingestion of large doses of estrogen-containing oral contraceptives by young children. Overdosage of estrogen may cause nausea and vomiting, and withdrawal bleeding may occur in females.

DOSAGE AND ADMINISTRATION:

TRANSDERMAL SYSTEM

The adhesive side of the estradiol transdermal system should be placed on a clean, dry area of the skin on the trunk of the body (including the buttocks and abdomen). *Estradiol transdermal system should not be applied to the breasts.* The sites of application must be rotated, with an interval of at least 1 week allowed between applications to a particular site. The area selected should not be oily, damaged, or irritated. The waistline should be avoided, since tight clothing may rub the system off. The system should be applied immediately after opening the pouch and removing the protective liner. The system should be pressed firmly in place with the palm of the hand for about 10 seconds, making sure there is good contact, especially around the edges. In the unlikely event that a system should fall off, the same system may be reapplied. If necessary, a new system may be applied. In either case, the original treatment schedule should be continued.

INITIATION OF THERAPY

Treatment of menopausal symptoms is usually initiated with estradiol transdermal system 0.05 mg applied to the skin twice weekly. The dosage should be adjusted as necessary to control of symptoms. The lowest dosage necessary for the control of symptoms should be used, especially in women with an intact uterus. Attempts to taper or discontinue the medication should be made at 3-to 6-month intervals.

Prophylactic therapy with estradiol transdermal system to prevent postmenopausal bone loss should be initiated with the 0.05 mg/day dosage as soon as possible after menopause. The dosage may be adjusted if necessary to control concurrent menopausal symptoms. Discontinuation of estrogen replacement therapy may reestablish the natural rate of bone loss.

In women not currently taking oral estrogens, treatment with estradiol transdermal system may be initiated at once. In women who are currently taking oral estrogen, treatment with estradiol transdermal system should be initiated 1 week after withdrawal of oral hormone replacement therapy, or sooner if menopausal symptoms reappear in less than 1 week.

THERAPEUTIC REGIMEN

Estradiol transdermal system therapy may be given continuously in patients who do not have an intact uterus. In those patients with an intact uterus, estradiol transdermal system may be given on a cycle schedule (*e.g.,* 3 weeks on drug followed by 1 week off drug).

Do not store above 86°F (30°C)

Do not store unpouched. Apply immediately upon removal from the protective pouch.

VAGINAL CREAM

For treatment of vulval and vaginal atrophy associated with the menopause, the lowest dose and regimen that will control symptoms should be chosen and medication should be discontinued as promptly as possible.

Attempts to discontinue or taper medication should be made at 3-month to 6-month intervals.

Usual Dosage: The usual dosage range is 2 to 4 g (marked on the applicator) daily for one or two weeks, then gradually reduced to one half initial dosage for a similar period. A maintenance dosage of 1 g, one to three times a week, may be used after restoration of the vaginal mucosa has been achieved.

NOTE: The number of doses per tube will vary with dosage requirements and patient handling.

Patients with intact uteri should be monitored closely for signs of endometrial cancer and appropriate diagnostic measures should be taken to rule out malignancy in the event of persistent or recurring abnormal vaginal bleeding.

Store at room temperature. Protect from temperatures in excess of 40°C (104°F).

TABLETS

For Treatment Of Moderate To Severe Vasomotor Symptoms, Vulval And Vaginal Atrophy Associated With The Menopause, The Lowest Dose And Regimen That Will Control Symptoms Should Be Chosen And Medication Should Be Discontinued As Promptly As Possible: Attempts to discontinue or taper medication should be made at 3-month to 6-month intervals.

The usual initial dosage range is 1 to 2 mg daily of estradiol adjusted as necessary to control presenting symptoms. The minimal effective dose for maintenance therapy should be determined by titration. Administration should be cyclic (*e.g.,* 3 weeks on and 1 week off).

For Treatment Of Female Hypoestrogenism Due To Hypogonadism, Castration, Or Primary Ovarian Failure: Treatment is usually initiated with a dose of 1 to 2 mg daily of estradiol, adjusted as necessary to control presenting symptoms; the minimal effective dose for maintenance therapy should be determined by titration.

For Treatment Of Breast Cancer, For Palliation Only, In Appropriately Selected Women And Men With Metastatic Disease: Suggested dosage is 10 mg three times daily for a period of at least three months.

For Treatment Of Advanced Androgen-Dependent Carcinoma Of The Prostate, For Palliation Only: Suggested dosage is 1 to 2 mg three times daily. The effectiveness of therapy can be judged by phosphatase determinations as well as by symptomatic improvement of the patient.

For The Prevention Of Osteoporosis: Therapy with estradiol tablets to prevent postmenopausal bone loss should be initiated as soon as possible after menopause. A daily dosage of 0.5 mg should be administered cyclically (*i.e.,* 23 days on and 5 days off). The dosage may be adjusted if necessary to control concurrent menopausal symptoms. Discontinuation of estrogen replacement therapy may re-establish the natural rate of bone loss.

PATIENT PACKAGE INSERT:

NOTE: The number of doses per tube of estradiol vaginal cream will vary with dosage requirements and patient handling.

This leaflet describes when and how to use estrogens, and the risks and benefits of estrogen treatment.

Estrogens have important benefits but also some risks. You must decide, with your doctor, whether the risks to you of estrogen use are acceptable because of their benefits. If you use estrogens, check with your doctor to be sure you are using the lowest possible dose that works, and that you don't use them longer than necessary. How long you need to use estrogens will depend on the reason for use.

1. Estrogens Increase The Risk Of Cancer Of The Uterus In Women Who Have Had Their Menopause ("Change Of Life"): If you are using any estrogen-containing drug, it is important to visit your doctor regularly and report any unusual vaginal bleeding right away. Vaginal bleeding after menopause may be a warning sign of uterine cancer. Your doctor should evaluate any unusual vaginal bleeding to find out the cause.
2. Estrogens Should Not Be Used During Pregnancy:Estrogens do not prevent miscarriage (spontaneous abortion) and are not needed in the days following childbirth. If you take estrogens during pregnancy, your unborn child has a greater than usual chance of having birth defects. The risk of developing these defects is small, but clearly larger than the risk in children whose mothers did not take estrogens during pregnancy. These

PATIENT PACKAGE INSERT: *(cont'd)*

birth defects may affect the baby's urinary system and sex organs. Daughters born to mothers who took DES (an estrogen drug) have a higher than usual chance of developing cancer of the vagina or cervix when they become teenagers or young adults. Sons may have a higher than usual chance of developing cancer of the testicles when they become teenagers or young adults.

USES OF ESTROGEN

Not Every Estrogen Drug Is Approved For Every Use Listed In This Section: If you want to know which of these possible uses are approved for the medicine prescribed for you, ask your doctor or pharmacist to show you the professional labeling. You can also look up the specific estrogen in a book called "Physicians GenRx", which is available in many book stores and public libraries. Generic drugs carry virtually the same labeling information as their name brand versions.)

To Reduce Moderate or Severe Menopausal Symptoms: Estrogens are hormones made by the ovaries of normal women. Between ages 45 and 55, the ovaries normally stop making estrogens. This leads to a drop in body estrogen levels which causes the "change of life" or menopause (the end of monthly menstrual periods). If both ovaries are removed during an operation before natural menopause takes place, the sudden drop in estrogen levels causes "surgical menopause."

When the estrogen levels begin dropping, some women develop very uncomfortable symptoms, such as feelings of warmth in the face, neck and chest, or sudden intense episodes of heat and sweating ("hot flashes or "hot flushes"). Using estrogen drugs can help the body adjust to lower estrogen levels and reduce these symptoms. Most women have only mild menopausal symptoms or none at all and do not need to use estrogen drugs for these symptoms. Others may need to take estrogens for a few months while their bodies adjust to lower estrogen levels. The majority of women do not need estrogen replacement for longer than six months for these symptoms.

To Treat Vulval And Vaginal Atrophy: (itching, burning, dryness in or around the vagina, difficulty or burning on urination) associated with menopause.

To treat certain conditions in which a young woman's ovaries do not produce enough estrogen naturally.

To treat certain types of abnormal vaginal bleeding due to hormonal imbalance when your doctor has found no serious cause of the bleeding.

To treat certain cancers in special situations, in men and women.

To prevent thinning of bones.

Osteoporosis is a thinning of the bones that makes them weaker and allows them to break more easily. The bones of the spine, wrists and hips break most often in osteoporosis. Both men and women start to lose bone mass after about age 40, but women lose bone mass faster after the menopause. Using estrogens after the menopause slows down bone thinning and prevent bones from breaking. Lifelong adequate calcium intake, either in the diet (such as dairy products) or by calcium supplements (to reach a total daily intake of 1000 milligrams per day before menopause or 1500 milligrams per day after menopause), may help to prevent osteoporosis. Regular weight-bearing exercise (like walking and running for an hour, two or three times a week) may also help to prevent osteoporosis. Before you change your calcium intake or exercise habits, it is important to discuss these lifestyle changes with your doctor to find out if they are safe for you.

Since estrogen use has some risks, only women who are likely to develop osteoporosis should use estrogens for prevention. Women who are likely to develop osteoporosis often have the following characteristics: white or Asian race, slim, cigarette smokers, and a family history of osteoporosis in a mother, sister, or aunt. Women who have relatively early menopause, often because their ovaries were removed during an operation ("surgical menopause") are more likely to develop osteoporosis than women whose menopause happens at the average age.

WHO SHOULD NOT USE ESTROGENS

Estrogens should not be used:

During Pregnancy: (see BOXED WARNING) If you think you may be pregnant, do not use any form of estrogen-containing drug. Using estrogens while you are pregnant may cause your unborn child to have birth defects. Estrogens do not prevent miscarriage.

If You Have Unusual Vaginal Bleeding Which Has Not Been Evaluated By Your Doctor: (see BOXED WARNING.) Unusual vaginal bleeding can be a warning sign of cancer of the uterus, especially if it happens after menopause. Your doctor must find out the cause of the bleeding so that he or she can recommend the proper treatment. Taking estrogens without visiting your doctor can cause you serious harm if your vaginal bleeding is caused by cancer of the uterus.

If You Have Had Cancer: Since estrogens increase the risk of certain types of cancer, you should not use estrogens if you have ever had cancer of the breast or uterus, unless your doctor recommends that the drug may help in cancer treatment. (For certain patients with breast or prostate cancer, estrogens may help.)

If You Have Any Circulation Problems: Estrogen drugs should not be used except in unusually special situations in which your doctor judges that you need estrogen therapy so much that the risks are acceptable. Men and women with abnormal blood clotting conditions should avoid estrogen use (see Dangers of Estrogens),.

When They Do Not Work: During menopause, some women develop nervous symptoms or depression.Estrogens do not relieve these symptoms. You may have heard that taking estrogens for years after menopause will keep your skin soft and supple and keep you feeling young. There is no evidence for these claims and such long-term estrogen use may have serious risks.

After Childbirth Or When Breastfeeding A Baby: Estrogens should not be used to try to stop the breasts from filling with milk after a baby is born. Such treatment may increase the risk of developing blood clots (see Dangers of Estrogens),.

If you are breastfeeding, you should avoid using any drugs because many drugs pass through to the baby in the milk. While nursing a baby, you should take drugs only on the advice of your health care provider.

DANGERS OF ESTROGENS

Cancer Of The Uterus: Your risk of developing cancer of the uterus gets higher the longer you use estrogens and the larger doses you use. One study showed that after women stop taking estrogens, this higher cancer risk quickly returns to the usual level of risk (as if you had never used estrogen therapy). Three other studies showed that the cancer risk stayed high for 8 to more than 15 years after stopping estrogen treatment. Because of this risk, **IT IS IMPORTANT TO TAKE THE LOWEST DOSE THAT WORKS AND TO TAKE IT ONLY AS LONG AS YOU NEED IT.**

Using progestin therapy together with estrogen therapy may reduce the higher risk of uterine cancer related to estrogen use (but see OTHER INFORMATION, below).

If you have had your uterus removed (total hysterectomy), there is no danger of developing cancer of the uterus.

PATIENT PACKAGE INSERT: *(cont'd)*

Cancer Of The Breast: Most studies have not shown a higher risk of breast cancer in women who have ever used estrogens. However, some studies have reported that breast cancer developed more often (up to twice the usual rate) in women who used estrogens for long periods of time (especially more than 10 years), or who used higher doses for shorter time periods.

Regular breast examinations by a health professional and monthly self-examination are recommended for all women.

Gallbladder Disease: Women who use estrogens after menopause are more likely to develop gallbladder disease needing surgery than women who do not use estrogens.

Abnormal Blood Clotting: Taking estrogens may cause changes in your blood clotting system. These changes allow the blood to clot more easily, possibly allowing clots to form in your bloodstream. If blood clots do form in your bloodstream, they can cut off the blood supply to vital organs, causing serious problems. These problems may include a stroke (by cutting off blood to the brain), a heart attack (by cutting off blood to the heart), a pulmonary embolus (by cutting off blood to the lungs), or other problems. Any of these conditions may cause death or serious long term disability. However, most studies of low dose estrogen usage by women do not show an increased risk of these complications.

SIDE EFFECTS

In addition to the risks listed above, the following side effects have been reported with estrogen use:

Nausea and vomiting.

Breast tenderness or enlargement.

Enlargement of benign tumors ("fibroids") of the uterus.

Retention of excess fluid. This may make some conditions worsen, such as asthma, epilepsy, migraine, heart disease, or kidney disease.

A spotty darkening of the skin, particularly of the face.

REDUCING RISK OF ESTROGEN USE

If you use estrogens, you can reduce your risks by doing these things:

See Your Doctor Regularly: While you are using estrogens, it is important to visit your doctor at least once a year for a check-up. If you develop vaginal bleeding while taking estrogens, you may need further evaluation. If members of your family have had breast cancer or if you have ever had breast lumps or an abnormal mammogram (breast x-ray), you may need to have more frequent breast examinations.

Reassess Your Need For Estrogens: You and your doctor should reevaluate whether or not you still need estrogens at least every six months.

Be Alert For Signs Of Trouble: If any of these warning signals (or any other unusual symptoms) happen while you are using estrogens, call your doctor immediately:

Abnormal bleeding from the vagina (possible uterine cancer)

Pains in the calves or chest, sudden shortness of breath, or coughing blood (possible clot in the legs, heart or lungs)

Severe headache or vomiting, dizziness, faintness, changes in vision or speech, weakness or numbness of an arm or leg (possible clot in the brain or eye)

Breast lumps (possible breast cancer; ask your doctor or health professional to show you how to examine your breasts monthly)

Yellowing of the skin or eyes (possible liver problem)

Pain, swelling, or tenderness in the abdomen (possible gallbladder problem)

OTHER INFORMATION

Some doctors may choose to prescribe a progestin, a different hormonal drug, for you to take together with your estrogen treatment. Progestins lower your risk of developing endometrial hyperplasia (a possible pre-cancerous condition of the uterus) while using estrogens. Taking estrogens and progestins together may also protect you from the higher risk of uterine cancer, but this has not been clearly established. Combined use of progestin and estrogen treatment may have additional risks, however, the possible risks include unhealthy effects on blood fats (especially a lowering of HDL cholesterol, the "good" blood fat which protects against heart disease risk), unhealthy effects on blood sugar (which might worsen a diabetic condition), and a possible further increase in the breast cancer risk which may be associated with long-term estrogen use. The type of progestin drug used and its dosage schedule may be important in minimizing these effects.

Your doctor has prescribed this drug for you and you alone. Do not give the drug to anyone else.

If you will be taking calcium supplements as part of the treatment to help prevent osteoporosis, check with your doctor about how much to take.

Keep this and all drugs out of the reach of children. In case of overdose, call your doctor, hospital or poison control center immediately.

This leaflet provides a summary of the most important information about estrogens. If you want more information, ask your doctor or pharmacist to show you the professional labeling. The professional labeling is also published in a book called "Physicians GenRx," which is available in book stores and public libraries. Generic drugs carry virtually the same labeling information as their name brand versions.

HOW SUPPLIED:

Estrace 0.5 mg: round, white scored tablets imprinted with 021 and MJ on one side.

Estrace 1 mg: round, lavender scored tablets imprinted with 755 and MJ on one side.

Estrace 2 mg: round, turquoise scored tablets imprinted with 756 and MJ on one side.

Store at controlled room temperature 15°-30°C (59°-86°F).

HOW SUPPLIED - RATED THERAPEUTICALLY EQUIVALENT:

Tablet, Uncoated - Oral - 0.5 mg

100's	$25.63	ESTRACE, Bristol Myers Squibb	00087-0021-41

Tablet, Uncoated - Oral - 1 mg

100's	$34.15	ESTRACE, Bristol Myers Squibb	00087-0755-01
500's	$162.23	Estrace, Bristol Myers Squibb	00087-0755-48

Tablet, Uncoated - Oral - 2 mg

100's	$49.86	ESTRACE, Bristol Myers Squibb	00087-0756-01
500's	$236.82	Estrace, Bristol Myers Squibb	00087-0756-48

HOW SUPPLIED - NOT RATED EQUIVALENT:

Cream - Vaginal - 0.01 %

42.5 gm	$26.70	ESTRACE, Bristol Myers Squibb	00087-0754-42

Film, Continuous Release - Percutaneous - 0.05 mg/day

4's	$19.10	CLIMARA, Berlex Labs	50419-0451-04
24's	**$50.96**	**ESTRADERM, Novartis**	**00083-2310-24**
48's	**$105.04**	**ESTRADERM, Novartis**	**00083-2310-62**

HOW SUPPLIED - NOT RATED EQUIVALENT: *(cont'd)*

Film, Continuous Release - Percutaneous - 0.1 mg/day

4's	$19.10	CLIMARA, Berlex Labs	50419-0452-04
24's	$55.54	ESTRADERM, Novartis	00083-2320-24
48's	$114.50	ESTRADERM, Novartis	00083-2320-62

ESTRADIOL CYPIONATE *(001189)*

CATEGORIES: Estrogen; Estrogens; Hormones; Hypogonadism; Menopause; Pregnancy Category X; FDA Approval Pre 1982

BRAND NAMES: D-Est 5; Depgynogen; Depo-Estradiol; *Depofemin*; Depogen; Dura-Estrin; E-Cypionate; Esdinate; Estra-C; Estro-Cyp; Estro-L.A.; Estro-Span C; Estrofem; Estroject-L.A.; Estronol-La

(International brand names outside U.S. in italics)

WARNING:

1. ESTROGENS HAVE BEEN REPORTED TO INCREASE THE RISK OF ENDOMETRIAL CARCINOMA.

Three independent case control studies have shown an increased risk of endometrial cancer in postmenopausal women exposed to exogenous estrogens for prolonged periods. This risk was independent of the other known risk factors for endometrial cancer. These studies are further supported by the finding that incidence rates of endometrial cancer have increased sharply since 1969 in eight different areas of the United States with population based cancer reporting systems, an increase which may be related to the rapidly expanding use of estrogens during the last decade.

The three case control studies reported that the risk of endometrial cancer in estrogen users was about 4.5 to 13.9 times greater than in nonusers. The risk appears to depend on both duration of treatment and on estrogen dose. In view of these findings, when estrogens are used for the treatment of menopausal symptoms, the lowest dose that will control symptoms should be utilized and medication should be discontinued as soon as possible. When prolonged treatment is medically indicated, the patient should be reassessed on at least a semiannual basis to determine the need for continued therapy. Although the evidence must be considered preliminary, one study suggests that cyclic administration of low doses of estrogen may carry less risk than continuous administration, it therefore appears prudent to utilize such a regimen.

Close clinical surveillance of all women taking estrogens is important. In all cases of undiagnosed persistent or recurring abnormal vaginal bleeding, adequate diagnostic measures should be undertaken to rule out malignancy.

There is no evidence at present that "natural" estrogens are more or less hazardous than "synthetic" estrogens at equiestrogenic doses.

2. ESTROGENS SHOULD NOT BE USED DURING PREGNANCY.

The use of female sex hormones, both estrogens and progestagens, during early pregnancy may have adverse effects on the offspring. An association has been reported between *in utero* exposure of the female fetus to diethylstilbestrol (and other nonsteroidal estrogens) and increased risk of the postpubertal development of an ordinarily extremely rare form of vaginal or cervical cancer. The risk has been estimated as not greater than 4 per 1000 exposures. Furthermore, a high percentage of such exposed women (from 30 to 90 percent) have been found to have vaginal adenosis, epithelial changes of the vagina and cervix. Although these changes are histologically benign, it is not known whether they are precursors of malignancy. Although similar data are not available with the use of other estrogens, it cannot be presumed they would not induce similar changes.

Several reports suggest an association between intrauterine exposure to female sex hormones and congenital anomalies, including congenital heart defects and limb reduction defects. One case control study estimated a 4.7 fold increased risk of limb reduction defects in infants exposed *in utero* to sex hormones (oral contraceptives, hormone withdrawal tests for pregnancy, or attempted treatment for threatened abortion). Some of these exposures were very short and involved only a few days of treatment. The data suggest that the risk of limb reduction defects in exposed fetuses is somewhat less than 1 per 1000.

Female sex hormones have been used during pregnancy in an attempt to treat threatened or habitual abortion. There is now considerable literature to the effect that both estrogens and progestagens are ineffective for these indications.

If estradiol cypionate sterile solution is used during pregnancy, or if the patient becomes pregnant while taking this drug, she should be apprised of the potential risks to the fetus, and the advisability of pregnancy continuation.

DESCRIPTION:

DEPO-Estradiol Sterile Solution contains estradiol cypionate which is available in two concentrations for intramuscular use. Each ml contains:

1 mg/ml - 1 mg estradiol cypionate, 5.4 mg chlorobutanol anhydrous (chloral derivative) added as preservative; in 916 mg cottonseed oil.

5 mg/ml - 5 mg estradiol cypionate, 5.4 mg chlorobutanol anhydrous (chloral derivative) added as preservative; in 913 mg cottonseed oil.

WARNING: Chlorobutanol may be habit forming.

DEPO-Estradiol contains an oil soluble ester of estradiol 17 beta. The chemical name for estradiol cypionate is estradiol 17- cyclopentanepropionate.

CLINICAL PHARMACOLOGY:

Estradiol cypionate provides estradiol 17 beta, the most potent of the naturally occurring estrogens, in the form of a highly fat- soluble derivative with prolonged estrogenic effect.

Comparative clinical studies have demonstrated that estradiol cypionate produces estrogenic effects that are qualitatively the same as those produced by other estradiol esters. In menopausal women, the average duration of estrogenic effect (as measured by vaginal smear) following a single injection of 5 mg of estradiol cypionate was found to be approximately 3 to 4 weeks. Relief of vasomotor symptoms was observed to occur within 1 to 5 days and to be maintained for 1 to 8 weeks, with an average of approximately 5 weeks.

INDICATIONS AND USAGE:

DEPO-Estradiol Sterile Solution is indicated in the treatment of:

1. Moderate to severe VASOMOTOR symptoms associated with the menopause. (There is no evidence that estrogens are effective for nervous symptoms or depression which might occur during menopause, and they should not be used to treat these conditions.)

2. Female hypogonadism

ESTRADIOL CYPIONATE HAS NOT BEEN SHOWN TO BE EFFECTIVE FOR ANY PURPOSE DURING PREGNANCY AND ITS USE MAY CAUSE SEVERE HARM TO THE FETUS. See BOXED WARNING.

CONTRAINDICATIONS:

Estrogens should not be used in women (or men) with any of the following conditions:

1. Known or suspected cancer of breast

2. Known or suspected estrogen-dependent neoplasia

3. Known or suspected pregnancy. See BOXED WARNING

4. Undiagnosed abnormal genital bleeding

5. Active thrombophlebitis or thromboembolic disorders

6. Presence of or a history of thrombophlebitis, thrombosis, or thromboembolic disorders associated with previous estrogen use.

WARNINGS:

Induction of malignant neoplasms: Long-term continuous administration of natural and synthetic estrogens in certain animal species increases the frequency of carcinomas of the breast, cervix, vagina, and liver. There is now evidence that estrogens increase the risk of carcinoma of the endometrium in humans. See BOXED WARNING. At the present time there is no satisfactory evidence that estrogens given to postmenopausal women increase the risk of cancer of the breast, although a recent long-term follow-up of a single physician's practice has raised this possibility. Because of the animal data, there is a need for caution in prescribing estrogens for women with a strong family history of breast cancer or who have breast nodules, fibrocystic disease, or abnormal mammograms.

Gall bladder disease: A recent study has reported a 2- to 3- fold increase in the risk of surgically confirmed gall bladder disease in women receiving postmenopausal estrogens, similar to the 2-fold increase previously noted in users of oral contraceptives. In the case of oral contraceptives the increased risk appeared after two years of use.

Effects similar to those caused by estrogen-progestogen oral contraceptives. There are several serious adverse effects of oral contraceptives, most of which have not, up to now, been documented as consequences of postmenopausal estrogen therapy. This may reflect the comparatively low doses of estrogen used in postmenopausal women. It would be expected that the larger doses of estrogen used to treat prostatic or breast cancer or postpartum breast engorgement are more likely to result in these adverse effects, and, in fact, it has been shown that there is an increased risk of thrombosis in men receiving estrogens for prostatic cancer and women for postpartum breast engorgement.

Thromboembolic Disease: It is now well established that users of oral contraceptives have an increased risk of various thromboembolic and thrombotic vascular diseases, such as thrombophlebitis, pulmonary embolism, stroke, and myocardial infarction. Cases of retinal thrombosis, mesenteric thrombosis, and optic neuritis have been reported in oral contraceptive users. There is evidence that the risk of several of these adverse reactions is related to the dose of the drug. An increased risk of thromboembolic complications following surgery has also been reported in users of oral contraceptives. If feasible, estrogen should be discontinued at least 4 weeks before surgery of the type associated with an increased risk of thromboembolism, or during periods of prolonged immobilization. While an increased rate of thromboembolic and thrombotic disease in postmenopausal users of estrogens has not been found, this does not rule out the possibility that such an increase may be present or that subgroups of women who have underlying risk factors or who are receiving relatively large doses of estrogens may have increased risk. Therefore, estrogens should not be used in persons with active thrombophlebitis or thromboembolic disorders, and they should not be used (except in treatment of malignancy) in persons with a history of such disorders in association with estrogen use. They should be used with caution in patients with cerebral vascular or coronary artery disease and only for those in whom estrogens are clearly needed. Large doses of estrogen (5 mg conjugated estrogens per day), comparable to those used to treat cancer of the prostate and breast, have been shown in a large prospective clinical trial in men to increase the risk of nonfatal myocardial infarction, pulmonary embolism and thrombophlebitis. When estrogen doses of this size are used, any of the thromboembolic and thrombotic adverse effects associated with oral contraceptive use should be considered a clear risk.

Hepatic Adenoma: Benign hepatic adenomas appear to be associated with the use of oral contraceptives. Although benign, and rare, these may rupture and may cause death through intra-abdominal hemorrhage. Such lesions have not yet been reported in association with other estrogen or progestogen preparations but should be considered in estrogen users having abdominal pain and tenderness, abdominal mass,m or hypovolemic shock. Hepatocellular carcinoma has also been reported in women taking estrogen-containing oral contraceptives. The relationship of this malignancy to these drugs is not known at this time.

Elevated Blood Pressure: Increased blood pressure. Increased blood pressure is not uncommon in women using oral contraceptives. There is now a report that this may occur with use of estrogens in the menopause and blood pressure should be monitored with estrogen use, especially if high doses are used.

PRECAUTIONS:

General: A complete medical and family history should be taken prior to the initiation of any estrogen therapy. The pretreatment and periodic physical examinations should include special reference to blood pressure, breasts, abdomen, and pelvic organs, and should include a Papanicolaou smear. As a general rule, estrogen should not be prescribed for longer than 6 months without another physical examination being performed.

Because estrogens may cause some degree of fluid retention, conditions which might be influenced by this factor such as epilepsy, migraine, and cardiac or renal dysfunction, require careful observation.

Certain patients may develop undesirable manifestations of excessive estrogenic stimulation, such as abnormal or excessive uterine bleeding or mastodynia.

Oral contraceptives appear to be associated with an increased incidence of mental depression. Although it is not clear whether this is due to the estrogenic or progestagenic component of the contraceptive, patients with a history of depression should be carefully observed.

Uterine leiomyomata may increase in size during estrogen use.

The pathologist should be advised of estrogen therapy when relevant specimens are submitted.

PRECAUTIONS: *(cont'd)*

Patients with a history of jaundice during pregnancy have an increased risk of recurrence of jaundice while receiving estrogen- containing oral contraceptive therapy. If jaundice develops in any patient receiving estrogen, the medications should be discontinued while the cause is investigated.

Estrogens may be poorly metabolized in patients with impaired liver function and the should be administered with caution in such patients.

Because estrogens influence the metabolism of calcium and phosphorus, they should be used with caution in patients with metabolic bone diseases that are associated with hypercalcemia or in patients with renal insufficiency.

Because of the effects of estrogens on epiphyseal closure, they should be used judiciously in young patients in whom bone growth is not complete.

Laboratory Tests: Certain endocrine and liver function tests may be affected by estrogen-containing oral contraceptives. The following similar changes may be expected with larger doses of estrogen:

a. Increased sulfobromophthalein retention.

b. Increased prothrombin and factors, VII, VIII, IX, and X; decreased antithrombin 3; increased norepinephrine-induced platelet aggregability.

c. Increased thyroid binding globulin (TBG) leading to increased circulating total thyroid hormone, as measured by PBI, T4 by column, or T4 by radioimmunoassay. Free T3 resin uptake is decreased, reflecting the elevated TBG; free T4 concentration is unaltered.

d. Impaired glucose tolerance.

e. Decreased pregnanediol excretion.

f. Reduced response to metyrapone test.

g. Reduced serum folate concentration.

h. Increased serum triglyceride and phospholipid concentration.

Glucose Tolerance: A worsening of glucose tolerance has been observed in a significant percentage of patients on estrogen- containing oral contraceptives. For this reason, diabetic patients should be carefully observed while receiving estrogen.

Hypercalcemia: Administration of estrogens may lead to severe hypercalcemia in patients with breast cancer and bone metastases. If this occurs, the drug should be stopped and appropriate measures taken to reduce the serum calcium level.

Carcinogenesis, Mutagenesis, and Impairment of Fertility: See WARNINGS for information on carcinogenesis and mutagenesis.

Pregnancy: Pregnancy Category X. See CONTRAINDICATIONS and BOXED WARNING.

Nursing Mothers: As a general principle, the administration of any drug to nursing mothers should be done only when clearly necessary since many drugs are excreted in human milk.

Pediatric Use: Safety and effectiveness in children have not been established.

In Menopausal Use: The lowest effective dose appropriate for the specific indication should be utilized. Studies of the addition of a progestin for seven or more days of a cycle of estrogen administration have reported a lowered incidence of endometrial hyperplasia. Morphological and biochemical studies of endometrium suggest that 10 to 13 days of progestin are needed to provide maximal maturation of the endometrium and to eliminate any hyperplastic changes. Whether this will provide protection from endometrial carcinoma has not been clearly established. There are possible additional risks which may be associated with the inclusion of progestin in estrogen replacement regimens. The potential risks include adverse effects on carbohydrate and lipid metabolism. The choice of progestin and dosage may be important in minimizing these adverse effects.

ADVERSE REACTIONS:

See WARNINGS regarding induction of neoplasia, adverse effects on the fetus, increased incidence of gall bladder disease, and adverse effects similar to those of oral contraceptives, including thromboembolism. The following additional adverse reactions have been reported with estrogenic therapy, including oral contraceptives:

Genitourinary System: Breakthrough bleeding, spotting, change in menstrual flow, Dysmenorrhea, Premenstrual-like syndrome, Amenorrhea during and after treatment, Increase in size of uterine fibromyomata, Vaginal candidiasis, Change in cervical eversion and in degree of cervical secretion, Cystitis-like syndrome

Breasts: Tenderness, enlargement, secretion

Gastrointestinal: Nausea, vomiting, Abdominal cramps, bloating, Cholestatic jaundice

Skin: Chloasma or melasma which may persist when drug is discontinued, Erythema multiforme, Erythema nodosum, Hemorrhagic eruption, Loss of scalp hair

Eyes: Steepening of corneal curvature, Intolerance to contact lenses

CNS: Headache, migraine, dizziness, Mental depression,Chorea

Miscellaneous: Increase or decrease in weight, Reduced carbohydrate tolerance, Aggravation of porphyria, Edema, Changes in libido

DRUG ABUSE AND DEPENDENCE:

Chlorobutanol anhydrous (chloral derivative) added as a preservative may be habit forming.

OVERDOSAGE:

Overdosage of estrogen may cause nausea, withdrawal bleeding in females, and mastodynia in females and males.

DOSAGE AND ADMINISTRATION:

Parenteral drug products should be inspected visually for particulate matter and discoloration prior to administration whenever solution and container permit.

Warming and shaking the vial should redissolve any crystals that may have formed during storage at temperatures lower than recommended.

ESTRADIOL CYPIONATE STERILE SOLUTION IS FOR INTRAMUSCULAR USE ONLY.

Short-Term Cyclic Use For Treatment of Moderate to Severe Vasomotor Symptoms Associated With the Menopause. The lowest dose that will control symptoms should be chosen and medication discontinued as promptly as possible. Attempts to discontinue or taper medication should be made at 3 to 6 month intervals. The usual dosage range is 1 to 5 mg injected every 3 to 4 weeks.

Cyclic Use For the Treatment of Hypogonadism. 1.5 to 2.0 mg injected at monthly intervals.

Treated patients with an intact uterus should be monitored closely for signs of endometrial cancer and appropriate diagnostic measures should be taken to rule out malignancy in the event of persistent or recurring abnormal vaginal bleeding.

WARNING: Chlorobutanol may be habit forming.

HOW SUPPLIED - RATED THERAPEUTICALLY EQUIVALENT:

Injection, Solution - Intramuscular - 5 mg/ml

5 ml	$14.80	DEPO-ESTRADIOL CYPIONATE, Pharmacia & Upjohn	00009-0271-01
10 ml	$4.99	Estradiol Cypionate, McGuff	49072-0215-10
10 ml	$5.30	ESTROFEM, Pasadena	00418-6541-41
10 ml	$5.95	ESTRO-LA, AF Hauser	52637-0332-10
10 ml	$6.50	Estradiol Cypionate, Consolidated Midland	00223-7602-10
10 ml	$7.59	Estradiol Cypionate, HL Moore Drug Exch	00839-5575-30
10 ml	$7.61	Estradiol Cypionate, Steris Labs	00402-0254-10
10 ml	$8.25	Estradiol Cypionate, IDE-Interstate	00814-3020-40
10 ml	$9.00	ESTRA-C, Bolan Pharm	44437-0254-10
10 ml	$9.02	DEPOGEN, Hyrex Pharms	00314-0855-70
10 ml	$10.00	DEPGYNOGEN, Forest Pharms	00456-1021-10
10 ml	$10.85	Estradiol Cypionate, Goldline Labs	00182-0662-63
10 ml	$11.25	Estradiol Cypionate, Rugby	00536-6851-70
10 ml	$11.49	Estradiol Cypionate, Schein Pharm (US)	00364-6608-54

ESTRADIOL CYPIONATE; TESTOSTERONE CYPIONATE *(001190)*

CATEGORIES: Anabolic Steroids; Androgens; Antineoplastics; Hormones; Menopause; Steroids; Pregnancy Category X; DEA Class CIII; FDA Approval Pre 1982

BRAND NAMES: Bionate 50-2; Depandrogyn; Depatesogen; **Depo-Testadiol**; Depotestogen; Duo-Cyp; Duo-Span; Duratestrin; Menoject-L.A.; Pan Estra Test; T-E Cypionate; Tes-Est-Cyp; Testosterone w Estradiol; Tripole-S

FORMULARIES: Medi-Cal

WARNING:
ESTROGENS HAVE BEEN REPORTED IN INCREASE THE RISK OF ENDOMETRIAL CARCINOMA IN POSTMENOPAUSAL WOMEN.
Close clinical surveillance of all women taking estrogens is important. Adequate diagnostic measures, including endometrial sampling when indicated, should be undertaken to rule out malignancy in all cases of undiagnosed persistent or recurring abnormal vaginal bleeding. There is no evidence that "natural" estrogens are more or less hazardous than "synthetic" estrogens at equi-estrogenic doses.
ESTROGENS SHOULD NOT BE USED DURING PREGNANCY.
There is no indication for estrogen therapy during pregnancy or during the immediate postpartum period. Estrogens are ineffective for the prevention or treatment of threatened or habitual abortion. Estrogens are not indicated for the prevention of postpartum breast engorgement.
Estrogen therapy during pregnancy is associated with an increased risk of congenital defects in the reproductive organs of the fetus, and possibly over birth defects. Studies of women who received diethylstilbestrol (DES) during pregnancy have shown that female offspring have an increased risk of vaginal adenosis, squamous cell dysplasia of the uterine cervix and clear cell vaginal cancer later in life; male offspring have an increased risk of urogenital abnormalities and possibly testicular cancer later in life. The 1985 DES Task Force concluded that use of DES during pregnancy is associated with a subsequent increased risk of breast cancer in the mothers, although a casual relationship remains unproven and the observed level of excess risk is similar to that for a number of other breast cancer risk factors.

DESCRIPTION:

The Sterile Solution contains the androgenic testosterone cypionate and the estrogenic hormone, estradiol cypionate formulated for intramuscular administration only.

Each ml of the Sterile Solution contains:

Testosterone... 50 mg

Estradiol cypionate... 2 mg

Cottonseed oil... 874 mg

Chlorobutanol Anhydrous(chloral derivative)added as preservative... 5.4 mg

WARNING - Chlorobutanol may be habit forming.

The chemical name for testosterone cypionate is androst 4-ene-3-one, 17- (3-cyclopentyl-1-oxopropoxy)-, (17β)-. Its molecular weight is $C_{27}H_{40}O_3$, and the molecular weight is 412.61.

The chemical name for estradiol cypionate is Estra-1,3,5(10)-triene-3,17-diol,(17β)-,17-cyclopentanepropriate. Its molecular formula is $C_{26}H_{36}O_3$, and the molecular weight is 396.57.

CLINICAL PHARMACOLOGY:

The pharmacologic characteristics of the two components of the Sterile Solution (testosterone cypionate-estradiol cypionate) are indicated below:

Testosterone Cypionate: Androgen is responsible for the normal growth and development of the male sex organs and for the maintenance of secondary male characteristics. Androgens also cause retention of nitrogen, sodium, potassium, phosphorus, and decreased urinary excretion of calcium. Androgens have been reported to increase protein anabolism. Androgens have been reported to stimulate the production of red blood cells by enhancing the production or erythropoietic stimulating factor. Androgens also have a negative feedback relationship to pituitary luteinizing hormone (LH).

The half-life of testosterone cypionate when injected intramuscularly is approximately 8 days.

Estradiol Cypionate: Estrogen drug products act by regulating the transcription of a limited number of genes. Estrogens diffuse through cell membranes, distribute themselves through the cell, and bind to and activate the nuclear estrogen receptor, a DNA-binding protein which is found in estrogen-responsive tissues. The activated estrogen receptor binds to specific DNA sequences, or hormone-response elements, which enhance the transcription of adjacent genes and in turn lead to the observed effects. Estrogen receptors have been identified in tissues of the reproductive tract, breast, pituitary, hypothalamus, liver, and bone of women.

Estrogens are important in the development and maintenance of the female reproductive system and secondary sex characteristics. By a direct action, they cause growth and development of the uterus. Fallopian tubes, and vagina. With other hormones, such as pituitary hormones and progesterone, they cause enlargement of the breasts through promotion of ductal growth, stromal development, and the accretion of fat. Estrogens are intricately involved with other hormones, especially progesterone, in the processes of the ovulatory menstrual cycle and pregnancy, and affect the release of pituitary gonadotropins. They also

CLINICAL PHARMACOLOGY: *(cont'd)*

contribute to the shaping of the skeleton, maintenance of tone and elasticity of urogenital structures, changes in the epiphyses of the long bones that allow for the pubertal growth spurt and its termination, and pigmentation of the nipples and genitals.

Estrogens occur naturally in several forms. The primary source of estrogen in normally cycling adult women in the ovarian follicle, which secretes 70 to 500 mcg of estradiol daily, depending on the phase of the menstrual cycle. This is converted primarily to estrone, which circulates in roughly equal proportion to estradiol, and to small amounts of estriol. After menopause, most endogenous estrogen is produced by conversion of androstenedione, secreted by the adrenal cortex, to estrone by peripheral tissues. Thus, estrone — especially in its sulfate ester form — is the most abundant circulating estrogen in postmenopausal women. Although circulating estrogens exist in a dynamic equilibrium of metabolic interconversions, estradiol is the principal intracellular human estrogen and is substantially more potent than estrone or estradiol at the receptor.

Estrogens used in therapy are well absorbed through the skin, mucous membranes, and gastrointestinal tract. When conjugated with aryl and alkyl groups for parenteral administration, the rate of absorption of oily preparations is slowed with a prolonged duration of action, such that a single intramuscular injection of estradiol valerate or estradiol cypionate is absorbed over several weeks.

Administered estrogens and their esters are handled within the body essentially the same as the endogenous hormones. Metabolic conversion of estrogens occurs primarily in the liver (first pass effect), but also at local target tissue sites. Complex metabolic processes result in a dynamic equilibrium of circulating conjugated and unconjugated estrogenic forms which are continually interconverted, especially between estrone and estradiol and between esterified and unesterified forms. Although naturally-occurring estrogens circulate in the blood largely bound to sex hormone-binding globulin and albumin, only unbound estrogens enter target tissue cells. A significant proportion of the circulating estrogen exists as sulfate conjugates, especially estrone sulfate, which serves as a circulating reservoir for the formation of more active estrogenic species. A certain proportion of the estrogen is excreted into the bile and then reabsorbed from the intestine. During this enterohepatic recirculation, estrogens are desulfated and resulfated and undergo degradation through conversion to less active estrogens (estriol and other estrogens), oxidation to nonestrogenic substances (catecholestrogens, which interact with catecholamine metabolism, especially in the central nervous system), and conjugation with glucuronic acids (which are then rapidly excreted in the urine.

When given orally, naturally-occurring estrogens and their esters are extensively metabolized (first pass effect) and circulate primarily as estrone sulfate, with smaller amounts of other conjugated and unconjugated estrogenic species. This results in limited oral potency. By contrast, synthetic estrogens, such as ethinyl estradiol and the nonsteroidal estrogens are degraded very slowly in the liver and other tissues, which results in their high intrinsic potency. Estrogen drug products administered by non-oral routes are not subject to first-pass metabolism, but also undergo significant hepatic uptake, metabolism, and enterohepatic recycling.

The half-life of estradiol cypionate when injected and intramuscularly is approximately 5 days.

INDICATIONS AND USAGE:

This Sterile Solution (testosterone cypionate-estradiol cypionate) is indicated in the treatment of moderate to severe vasomotor symptoms associated with the menopause. There is no adequate evidence that estrogens are effective for nervous symptoms or depression which might occur during menopause and they should not be used to treat these conditions.

CONTRAINDICATIONS:

1. Known or suspected pregnancy (see BOXED WARNING.) Estrogens may cause fetal harm when administered to a pregnant woman.
2. Undiagnosed abnormal genital bleeding.
3. Known or suspected cancer of the breast except in appropriately selected patients being treated for metastatic disease.
4. Known or suspected estrogen-dependent neoplasia.
5. Active thrombophlebitis or thromboembolic disorders.

WARNINGS:

INDUCTION OF MALIGNANT NEOPLASMS

Endometrial cancer: The reported endometrial cancer risk among unopposed estrogen users was about 2 to12 fold greater than in non-users, and appears dependent on duration of treatment and on estrogen dose. Most studies show no significant increased risk associated with the use of estrogens for less than one year. The greatest risk appears associated with prolonged use with increased risks of 15- to 24-fold for five to ten years or more. In three studies, persistence of risk was demonstrated for 8 to over 15 years after cessation of estrogen treatment. In one study a significant decrease in the incidence of endometrial cancer occurred six months after estrogen withdrawal. Concurrent progestin therapy may offset this risk but the overall health impact in postmenopausal women is not known (see PRECAUTIONS.)

Breast cancer: While the majority of studies have not shown an increased risk of breast cancer in women who have ever used estrogen replacement therapy, some have reported a moderately increased risk (relative risk of 1.3-2.0) in those taking higher doses or those taking lower doses for prolonged periods of time, especially in excess of 10 years. Other studies have not shown this relationship.

Congenital lesions with malignant potential: Estrogen therapy during pregnancy is associated with an increased risk of fetal congenital reproductive tract disorders, and possibly other birth defects. Studies of women who received DES during pregnancy have shown that female offspring have an increased risk of vaginal adenosis, squamous cell dysplasia of the uterine cervix, and clear cell vaginal cancer later in life. Although some of these changes are benign, other are precursors of malignancy.

Gallbladder disease: Two studies have reported a 2- to 4-fold increase in the risk of gallbladder disease requiring surgery in women receiving postmenopausal estrogens.

Cardiovascular disease: Large doses of estrogen (5 mg conjugated estrogens per day), comparable to those used to treat cancer of the prostate and breast, have been shown in a large prospective clinical trial in men to increase the risks of nonfatal myocardial infarction, pulmonary embolism, and thrombophlebitis. These risks cannot necessarily be extrapolated from men to women. However, to avoid the theoretical cardiovascular risk to women caused by high estrogen doses, the dose for estrogen replacement therapy should not exceed the lowest effective dose.

Elevated blood pressure: Occasional blood pressure increases during estrogen replacement therapy have been attributed to idiosyncratic reactions to estrogens. More often, blood pressure has remained the same or has dropped. One study showed that postmenopausal estrogen users have higher blood pressure than nonusers. Two other studies showed slightly lower blood pressure among estrogen users compared to nonusers. Postmenopausal estrogen use does not increase the risk of stroke. Nonetheless, blood pressure should be monitored at regular intervals with estrogen use.

WARNINGS: *(cont'd)*

Hypercalcemia: Administration of estrogens may lead to severe hypercalcemia in patients with breast cancer and bone metastases. If this occurs, the drug should be stopped and appropriate measures taken to reduce the serum calcium level.

Virilization: Female patients on androgen therapy should be watched closely for signs of virilization. Some effects such as voice changes may not be reversible even when the drug is stopped.

Liver disease: Androgens have been associated with the development of peliosis hepatitis, cholestatic hepatitis, jaundice and hepatocellular carcinoma. Peliosis hepatitis can be a life-threatening or fatal complication. If cholestatic hepatitis with jaundice appears, the androgen should be discontinued.

Edema: Edema with or without congestive heart failure, may occur in patients, receiving androgens. This may be a serious complication in patients with preexisting cardiac, renal or hepatic disease. Diuretic therapy may be required if edema occurs.

PRECAUTIONS:

A. GENERAL

1. Addition of a progestin: Studies of the addition of a progestin for seven or more days of a cycle of estrogen administration have reported a lowered incidence of endometrial hyperplasia which would otherwise be induced by estrogen treatment. Morphological and biochemical studies of endometrium suggest that 10 to 14 days of progestin are needed to provide maximal maturation of the endometrium and to eliminate any hyperplastic changes. There are possible additional risks which may be associated with the inclusion of progestins in estrogen replacement regimens. These include: (1) adverse effects on lipoprotein metabolism (lowering HDL and raising LDL) which may diminish the possible cardioprotective effect of estrogen therapy, (See PRECAUTIONS D.4.),; (2) impairment of glucose tolerance; and (3) possible enhancement of mitotic activity in breast epithelial tissue (although few epidemiological data are available to address this point). The choice of progestin, its dose, and its regimen may be important in minimizing these adverse effects, but these issues remain to be clarified.

2. Physical examination: A complete medical and family history should be taken prior to the initiation of any estrogen therapy. The pretreatment and periodic physical examinations should include special reference to blood pressure, breasts, abdomen, and pelvic organs, and should include a Papanicolaou smear. As a general rule, estrogen should not be prescribed for longer than one year without reexamining the patient.

3. Hypercoagulability: Some studies have shown that women taking estrogen replacement therapy have hypercoagulability, primarily related to decreased antithrombin activity. This effect appears dose- and duration-dependent and is less pronounced than that associated with oral contraceptive use. Also, post-menopausal women tend to have increased coagulation parameters at baseline compared to premenopausal women. There is some suggestion that low dose estrogens may increase the risk of thromboembolism. Patients with a past history of such disease may be at a higher risk. The likelihood of thromboembolism has been reported to be increased when pharmacologic doses of estrogen are used to treat breast or prostatic cancer.

4. Familial hyperlipoproteinemia: Estrogen therapy may be associated with massive elevations of plasma triglycerides leading to pancreatitis and other complications in patients with familial defects of lipoprotein metabolism.

5. Fluid retention: Because estrogens may cause some degree of fluid retention, conditions which might be exacerbated by this factor, such as asthma, epilepsy, migraine, and cardiac or renal dysfunction require careful observation.

6. Uterine bleeding and mastodynia: Certain patients may develop undesirable manifestations of estrogenic stimulation, such as abnormal uterine bleeding and mastodynia.

7. Impaired liver function: Estrogens may be poorly metabolized in patients with impaired liver function and should be administered with caution.

8. Because estrogens and/or androgens influence the metabolism of calcium and phosphorus, they should be used with caution in patients with metabolic bone diseases that are associated with hypercalcemia or in patients with renal insufficiency.

9. Androgen may increase sensitivity to oral anticoagulants. Dosage of the anticoagulant may require reduction in order to maintain a satisfactory therapeutic hypoprothrombinemia.

10. Serum cholesterol and/or bilirubin may increase during androgen therapy.

11. In diabetic patients the metabolic effect of androgens may result in reduction of insulin requirements.

B. INFORMATION FOR THE PATIENT

See PATIENT PACKAGE INSERT.

C. LABORATORY TESTS

Estrogen administration should generally be guided by clinical response at the smallest dose, rather than laboratory monitoring, for relief of symptoms for those indications in which symptoms are observable.

D. DRUG/LABORATORY TEST INTERACTIONS

1. Accelerated prothrombin time, partial thromboplastin time, and platelet aggregation time; increased platelet count; increased factors II, VII antigen, VII antigen, VIII coagulant activity, IX, X, XII, VII-X complex, II-VII-X complex, and beta-thromboglobulin; decreased levels of anti-factor Xa and antithrombin III, decreased antithrombin III activity; increased levels of fibrinogen and fibrinogen activity; increased plasminogen antigen and activity.
2. Increased thyroid-binding globulin (TBG) leading to increased circulating total thyroid hormone, as measured by protein-bound iodine (PBI), T4 levels (by column or radioimmunoassay) or T3 levels by radioimmunoassay. T3 resin uptake is decreased, reflecting the elevated TBG. Free T4 and free T3 concentrations are unaltered. The PBI may decrease during androgen therapy without clinical significance.
3. Other binding proteins may be elevated in serum, i.e., corticosteroid binding globulin (CBG), sex-hormone binding globulin (SHBG), leading to increased circulating corticosteroids and sex steroids respectively. Free or biologically active hormone concentrations are unchanged. Other plasma proteins may be increased (angiotensinogen/renin substrate, alpha-1-antitrypsin, ceruloplasmin).
4. Increased plasma HDL and HDL-2 subfraction concentrations, reduced LDL cholesterol concentration, increased triglycerides levels.
5. Impaired glucose tolerance.
6. Reduced response to metyrapone test.
7. Reduced serum folate concentration.
8. The concomitant administration of an androgen, as in the case of the Sterile Solution, may alter the estrogen effect on many of the above values.

E. CARCINOGENESIS, MUTAGENESIS, AND IMPAIRMENT OF FERTILITY

Long term continuous administration of natural and synthetic estrogens in certain animal species increases the frequency of carcinomas of the breast, urterus, cervix, vagina, testis, and liver. See CONTRAINDICATIONS and WARNINGS.

PRECAUTIONS: *(cont'd)*

F. PREGNANCY CATEGORY X

Estrogens should not be used during pregnancy. See CONTRAINDICATIONS and BOXED WARNING.

G. LABOR AND DELIVERY

There is no reason why this drug should be administered during labor and delivery.

H. NURSING MOTHERS

As a general principle, the administration of any drug to nursing mothers should be done only when clearly necessary since many drugs are excreted in human milk. In addition, estrogen administration to nursing mothers has been shown to decrease the quantity and quality of the milk.

I. HEMOGLOBIN AND HEMATOCRIT

An increase in red blood count, hemoglobin and hematocrit may occur in patients receiving large doses of androgen. Hemoglobin and hematocrit should be checked periodically for polycythemia in patients who are receiving high doses of androgens.

ADVERSE REACTIONS:

The following additional adverse reactions have been reported with estrogen therapy (see WARNINGS regarding induction of neoplasia, adverse effects on the fetus, increased incidence of gallbladder disease, cardiovascular disease, elevated blood pressure, and hypercalcemia).

1. Genitourinary System: Changes in vaginal bleeding pattern and abnormal withdrawal bleeding or flow; breakthrough bleeding, spotting. Increase in size of uterine leiomyomata. Vaginal candidiasis. Change in amount of cervical secretion.

2. Breasts: Tenderness, enlargement.

3. Gastrointestinal: Nausea, vomiting. Abdominal cramps, bloating. Cholestatic jaundice. Increased incidence of gallbladder disease.

4. Skin: Chloasma or melasma that may persist when drug is discontinued. Erythema multiforme. Erythema nodosum. Hemorrhagic eruption. Loss of scalp hair. Hirsutism.

5. Eyes: Steepening of corneal curvature. Intolerance to contact lenses.

6. Central Nervous System Headache, migraine, dizziness. Mental depression. Chorea.

7. Miscellaneous: Increase or decrease in weight. Reduced carbohydrate tolerance. Aggravation of porphyria. Edema. Changes in libido.

Additional adverse reactions which have occurred with injectable androgen therapy alone include acne; hypersensitivity, including skin manifestations and anaphylactoid reactions; virilization; hypercalcemia (especially in immobilized patients); and local irritation.

DRUG ABUSE AND DEPENDENCE:

Chlorobutanol anhydrous (chloral derivative) added as a preservative may be habit forming.

OVERDOSAGE:

Serious ill effects have not been reported following acute ingestion of large doses of estrogen-containing oral contraceptives by young children. Overdosage of estrogen may cause nausea and vomiting, and withdrawal bleeding may occur in females. The accidental injection of a large dose of the Sterile Solution (testosterone cypionate-estradiol cypionate) could produce androgenic or estrogenic effects, none of which would be expected to be life threatening.

DOSAGE AND ADMINISTRATION:

Parenteral drug products should be inspected visually for particulate matter and discoloration prior to administration whenever solution and container permit.

Warming and shaking the vial should redissolve any crystals that may have formed during storage at temperatures lower than recommended.

The Sterile Solution *(testosterone cypionate-estradiol cypionate) is for intramuscular use only.*

1. Short-term cyclic use is for treatment of moderate to severe vasomotor symptoms associated with the menopause. The lowest dose and regimen that will control symptoms should be chosen and medication should be discontinued as promptly as possible.

Attempts to discontinue or taper medication should be made at 3 to 6 month intervals. The usual dosage is 1 ml injected at 4-week intervals.

PATIENT PACKAGE INSERT:

The Sterile Solution contains an estrogen (estradiol cypionate) a female hormone, and an androgen (testosterone cypionate) a male hormone. This leaflet describes when and how to use estrogens, and the risks and benefits of estrogen treatment.

Estrogens have important benefits but also some risks. You must decide, with your doctor, whether the risks to you of estrogen use are acceptable because of their benefits. If you use estrogens, check with your doctor to be sure you are using the lowest possible dose that works, and that you don't use them longer than necessary. How long you need to use estrogens will depend upon the reason for use.

ESTROGENS INCREASE THE RISK OF CANCER OF THE UTERUS IN WOMEN WHO HAVE HAD THEIR MENOPAUSE ("CHANGE OF LIFE").

If you use any estrogen-containing drug, it is important to visit your doctor regularly and report any unusual vaginal bleeding right away. Vaginal bleeding after menopause may be a warning sign of uterine cancer. Your doctor should evaluate any unusual vaginal bleeding to find out the cause.

ESTROGENS SHOULD NOT BE USED DURING PREGNANCY.

Estrogens do not prevent miscarriage (spontaneous abortion) and are not needed in the days following childbirth. If you take estrogens during pregnancy, your unborn child has a greater than usual chance of having birth defects. The risk of developing developing these defects is small, but clearly larger than the risk in children whose mothers did not take estrogens during pregnancy. These birth defects may affect the baby's urinary system and sex organs. Daughters born to mothers who took DES (an estrogen drug) have a higher than usual chance of developing cancer of the vagina or cervix when they become teenagers or young adults. Sons may have a higher than usual chance of developing cancer of the testicles when they become teenagers or young adults.

Uses of Estrogen: (Not every estrogen drug product is approved for every use listed in this section. If you want to know which of these possible uses are approved for the medicine prescribed for you, ask your doctor or pharmacist to show you the professional labeling. Generic drugs carry virtually the same labeling information as their brand name counterparts.)

PATIENT PACKAGE INSERT: *(cont'd)*

To reduce moderate or severe menopausal symptoms: Estrogens are hormones made by the ovaries of normal adult women. Between ages 45 and 55, the ovaries normally stop making estrogens. This leads to a drop in body estrogen levels which causes the "change of life" or menopause (the end of monthly menstrual periods). If both ovaries are removed during an operation before natural menopause takes place, the sudden drop in estrogen levels causes "surgical menopause".

When the estrogen levels begin dropping, some women develop very uncomfortable symptoms, such as feelings of warmth in the face, neck and chest or sudden intense episodes of heat and sweating ("hot flashes" or "hot flushes"). Using estrogen drugs can help the body adjust to lower estrogen levels and reduce these symptoms. Most women have only mild menopausal symptoms or none at all and do not need to use estrogen drugs for these symptoms. Others may need to take estrogens for a few months while their bodies adjust to lower estrogen levels. The majority of women do not need estrogen replacement for longer than six months for these symptoms.

To treat vulvar and vaginal atrophy: (itching, burning, dryness in or around the vagina, difficulty or burning on urination) associated with menopause.

To treat certain conditions in which a young women's ovaries do not produce enough estrogen naturally: To treat certain types of abnormal vaginal bleeding due to hormonal imbalance when your doctor has found no serious cause of the bleeding.

TO TREAT CERTAIN CANCERS IN SPECIAL SITUATIONS, IN MEN AND WOMEN

To prevent thinning of bones: Osteoporosis is a thinning of the bones that makes them weaker and allows them to break more easily. The bones of the spine, wrists and hips break most often in osteoporosis. Both men and women start to lose bone mass after about age 40, but women lose bone mass faster after the menopause. Using estrogens after the menopause slows down bone thinning and may prevent bones from breaking. Lifelong adequate calcium intake, wether in the diet (such as dairy products) or calcium supplements (to reach a total daily intake of 1000 milligrams per day before menopause or 1500 milligrams per day after menopause), may help to prevent osteoporosis. Regular weight-bearing exercise (like walking and running for an hour, two or three times a week) may also help to prevent osteoporosis. Before you change your calcium intake or exercise habits, it is important to discuss these lifestyle changes with your doctor to find out if they are safe for you.

Since estrogen use has some risks, only women who are likely to develop osteoporosis should use estrogens for prevention. Women, who are likely to develop osteoporosis often have the following characteristics: white or Asian race, slim, cigarette smokers, and a family history of osteoporosis in a mother, sister, or aunt. Women who have relatively early menopause, often because their ovaries were removed during an operation ("surgical menopause"), are more likely to develop osteoporosis than women whose menopause happens at the average age.

WHO SHOULD NOT USE ESTROGENS Estrogens should not be used:

During pregnancy (see BOXED WARNING.) If you think you may be pregnant, do not use any form of estrogen-containing drug. Using estrogens while you are pregnant may cause your unborn child to develop birth defects. Estrogens do not prevent miscarriages.

If you have unusual vaginal bleeding which has not been evaluated by your doctor (see BOXED WARNING.) Unusual vaginal bleeding can be a warning sign of cancer of the uterus, especially if it happens after menopause. Your doctor must find out the cause of the bleeding so that he or she can recommend the proper treatment. Taking estrogens without visiting your doctor can lead to serious harm if your vaginal bleeding is caused by cancer of the uterus.

If you have had cancer: Since estrogens increase the risk of certain types of cancer, you should generally not take estrogens if you have ever had cancer of the breast, uterus, unless your doctor recommends that the drug may help in the cancer treatment. (For certain patients with breast or prostate cancer, estrogens may help.)

If you have any circulation problems: Estrogen therapy should not be used except in unusually special situations in which your doctor judges that you need estrogen therapy so much that the risks are acceptable. Men and women with abnormal blood clotting conditions should avoid estrogen use see PATIENT PACKAGE INSERT, Dangers of Estrogens,.

When they do not work . During menopause, some women develop nervous symptoms or depression. Estrogens do not relieve these symptoms. You may have heard that taking estrogens for years after menopause will keep your skin soft and supple and keep you feeling young. There is no evidence for these claims and such long-term estrogen use may have serious risks.

After childbirth or when breast feeding a baby: Estrogens should not be used to try to stop the breasts from filling with milk after a baby is born. Such treatment may increase the risk of developing blood clots PATIENT PACKAGE INSERT, Dangers of Estrogens,.

If you are breast feeding, you should avoid using any drugs because many drugs pass through to the baby in the milk. While nursing a baby, you should take drugs only on the advice of your health care provider.

DANGERS OF ESTROGENS

Cancer of the uterus: Your risk of developing cancer of the uterus gets higher the longer you use estrogens, and the larger doses you use. One study showed that after women stop taking estrogens, this higher cancer risk quickly returns to the usual risk (as if you had never used estrogen therapy). Three other studies showed that cancer risk stayed high for 8 to more than 15 years after stopping estrogen treatment. Because of this risk, IT IS IMPORTANT TO TAKE THE LOWEST DOSE THAT WORKS AND TO TAKE IT ONLY AS LONG AS YOU NEED IT.

Using progestin therapy together with estrogen therapy may reduce the higher risk of uterine cancer related to estrogen use see PATIENT PACKAGE INSERT, Other Information.

If you have had your uterus removed (total hysterectomy), there is no danger of developing cancer of the uterus.

Cancer of the breast: Most studies have not shown a higher risk of breast cancer in women who have ever used estrogens. However, some studies have reported that breast cancer developed more often (up to twice the usual rate) in women who used estrogens for long periods of time (especially more than 10 years), or who used higher doses of estrogens for shorter time periods.

Regular breast examinations by a health professional and monthly self-examination are recommended for all women.

Gall bladder disease: Women who use estrogens after menopause are more likely to develop gall bladder disease needing surgery than women who do not use estrogens.

Abnormal blood clotting: Taking estrogens may cause changes in your blood clotting system. These changes allow the blood to clot more easily, possibly allowing clots to form in your blood stream. If blood clots do form in your bloodstream, they can cut off blood supply to vital organs, causing serious problems. These problems may include a stroke (by cutting off blood to the brain), a heart attack (by cutting of blood to the heart), a pulmonary embolus (by cutting off blood to the lungs), or other problems. Any of these conditions may cause death or serious long-term disability. However, most studies of low dose estrogen usage by women do not show an increased risk of these complications.

PATIENT PACKAGE INSERT: *(cont'd)*

Side Effects: In addition to the risks listed above, the following side effects have been reported with estrogen use: Nausea and vomiting, Breast tenderness or enlargement, Enlargement of benign tumors ("fibroids") of the uterus, Retention of excess fluid. This may make some conditions worsen, such as asthma, epilepsy, migraine, heart disease, or kidney disease, A spotty darkening of the skin, particularly on the face.

Reducing Risk Of Estrogen Use: If you use estrogens, you can reduce your risks by doing these things:

See your doctor regularly: While you are using estrogens, it is important to visit your doctor at least once a year for a check-up. If you develop vaginal bleeding while taking estrogens, you may need further evaluation. If members of your family have had breast cancer or f you have ever had breast lumps or an abnormal mammogram (breast X-ray), you may need to have more frequent breast examinations.

Reassess your need for estrogens: You and your doctor should reevaluate whether or not you still need estrogens at least every six months.

Be alert for signs of trouble: If any of these warning signals (or any other unusual symptoms) happen while you are using estrogens, call your doctor immediately:

1. Abnormal bleeding from the vagina (possible uterine cancer).

2. Pains in the calves or chest, sudden shortness of breath, or coughing blood (possible clot in the legs, heart or lungs).

3. Severe headache or vomiting, dizziness, faintness, changes in vision or speech, weakness, or numbness of an arm or leg (possible clot in the brain or eye).

4. Breast lumps (possible breast cancer; ask your doctor or health professional to show you how to examine your breasts monthly).

5. Yellowing of the skin or eyes (possible liver problem).

6. Pain or tenderness in the upper abdomen (possible gall bladder problem).

Other Information: Some doctors may choose to prescribe a progestin, a different hormonal drug, for you to take together with your estrogen treatment. Progestins lower your risk of developing endometrial hyperplasia (a possible pre-cancerous condition of the uterus) while using estrogens. Taking estrogens and progestins together may also protect you from the higher risk of uterine cancer, but this has not been clearly established. Combined use of progestin and estrogen treatment may have additional risks, however. The possible risks include unhealthy effects on blood fats (especially a lowering of HDL cholesterol, the "good" blood fat which protects against heart disease risk), unhealthy effects on blood sugar (which might worsen a diabetic condition), and a possible further increase in the breast cancer risk which may be associated with long term estrogen use. The type of progestin drug used and its dosage schedule may be important in minimizing these effects.

Your doctor has prescribed this drug for you and you alone. Do not give the drug to anyone else.

If you will be taking calcium supplements as part of the treatment to help prevent osteoporosis, check with your doctor about how much to take.

Keep this and all drugs out of the reach of children. In case of overdose, call your doctor, hospital or poison control center immediately.

This leaflet provides a summary of the most important information about estrogens. If you want more information, ask you doctor or pharmacist to show you the professional labeling. Generic drugs carry virtually the same labeling information as their brand name versions.

HOW SUPPLIED - RATED THERAPEUTICALLY EQUIVALENT:

Injection, Solution - Intramuscular - 2 mg/50 mg/ml

10 ml	$9.10	ANDROFEM, Pasadena	00418-6571-41
10 ml	$10.71	Testosterone Cypionate/Estradiol, Steris Labs	00402-0257-10
10 ml	$10.90	DEPOTESTOGEN, Hyrex Pharms	00314-0875-70
10 ml	$11.55	Testosterone Cypionate/Estradiol, IDE-Interstate	00814-7737-40
10 ml	$13.00	DEPANDROGYN, Forest Pharms	00456-1020-10
10 ml	$14.70	TEST-ESTRO-CYPIONATE, Rugby	00536-9470-70
10 ml	$16.56	DE-COMBEROL, Schein Pharm (US)	00364-6611-54
10 ml	**$26.17**	**DEPO-TESTADIOL, Pharmacia & Upjohn**	**00009-0253-02**

ESTRADIOL VALERATE *(001191)*

CATEGORIES: Estrogen; Estrogens; Hormones; Hypogonadism; Infertility; Kraurosis Vulvae; Ovarian Failure; Prostatic Carcinoma; Vaginitis; FDA Approval Pre 1982

BRAND NAMES: Deladiol-40; Delestrogen; Diol L.A.; Dioval; Dura-Estradiol; Duragen; Esdival; Estone L.A.-20; Estra-L; Estra-V; Estro-Span; Feminate; Gynogen L.A.; *Gynokadin* (Germany); L.A.E.; Lanestrin; Medidiol 10; Menaval; Pan-Estra La 40; *Primogyn Depot*; *Progynon*; *Progynon Amp Depot*; *Progynon Depot* (Germany); *Progynon-Depot*; *Progynova* (Australia, England, France); *Progynova 21* (Germany); Repository Hormone; Valergen; Valesco

(International brand names outside U.S. in italics)

1. Estrogens have been reported to increase the risk of endometrial carcinoma.

Three independent case control studies have shown an increased risk of endometrial cancer in postmenopausal women exposed to exogenous estrogens for prolonged periods.[1-3] This risk was independent of the other known risk factors for endometrial cancer. These studies are further supported by the finding that incidence rates of endometrial cancer have increased sharply since 1969 in eight different areas of the United States with population-based cancer reporting systems, an increase which may be related to the rapidly expanding use of estrogens during the last decade.[4]

The three case control studies reported that the risk of endometrial cancer in estrogen users was about 4.5 to 13.9 times greater than in nonusers. The risk appears to depend on both duration of treatment[1] and on estrogen dose.[3] In view of these findings, when estrogens are used for the treatment of menopausal symptoms, the lowest dose that will control symptoms should be utilized and medication should be discontinued as soon as possible. When prolonged treatment is medically indicated, the patient should be reassed on at least a semiannual basis to determine the need for continued therapy. Although the evidence must be considered preliminary, one study suggests that cyclic administration of low doses of estrogen may carry less risk than continuous administration;[3] it therefore appears prudent to utilize such a regimen.

Close clinical surveillance of all women taking estrogens is important. In all cases of undiagnosed persistent or recurring abnormal vaginal bleeding, adequate diagnostic measures should be undertaken to rule out malignancy.

There is no evidence at present that "natural" estrogens are more or less hazardous than "synthetic" estrogens at equiestrogenic doses.

2. Estrogens should not be used during pregnancy.

The use of femal sex hormones, both estrogens and progestogens, during early pregnancy may seriously damage the offspring. An association has been reported between *in utero* exposure of the femal fetus to diethylstilbestrol, a nonsteroidal estrogen, and an increased risk of the postpubertal development of an ordinarily extremely rare form of vaginal or cervical cancer.[5,6] This risk has recently been estimated to be in the range 0.14 to 1.4 per 1000 exposed females, consistent with a previous risk estimate of not greater than 4 per 1000 exposures.[7] Furthermore, a high percentage of such exposed women (from 30 to 90 percent) have been found to have vaginal adenosis.[8-12] With epithelial changes of the vagina and cervix. Although these changes are histologically benign. It is not known whether they are precursors of malignancy. Although similar data are not available with the use of other estrogens, it cannot be presumed they would not induce similar changes.

Several reports suggest an association between intrauterine exposure to female sex hormones and congenital anomalies, including congenital heart defects and limb reduction defects.[13-16] One case control study[16] estimated a 4.7-fold increased risk of limb reduction defects in infants exposed *in utero* to sex hormones (oral contraceptives, hormone withdrawal test for pregnancy, or attempted treatment for threatened abortion). Some of these exposures were very short and involved only a few days of treatment. The data suggest that the risk of limb reduction defects in exposed fetuses is somewhat less than 1 per 1000.

In the past, female sex hormones have been used during pregnancy in an attempt to treat threatened or habitual abortion. There is now considerable literature to the effect that estrogens are ineffective for these indications, and the data are not now considered adequate to support the conclusion that progestogens are effective for these uses.

If estradiol valerate is used during pregnancy or if the patient becomes pregnant while taking this drug, she should be apprised of the potential risks to the fetus and the advisability of pregnancy continuation.

DESCRIPTION:

Estradiol Valerate Injection contains estradiol valerate, a long-acting estrogen in sterile oil solutions for intramuscular use. These solutions are clear, colorless to pale yellow. Formulations (per ml): 10 mg estradiol valerate in a vehicle containing 5 mg chlorobutanol (chloral derivative/preservative) and sesame oil; 20 mg estradiol valerate in a vehicle containing 224 mg benzyl benzoate, 20 mg benzyl alcohol (preservative), and castor oil; 40 mg estradiol valerate in a vehicle containing 447 mg benzyl benzoate, 20 mg benzyl alcohol, and castor oil.

Estradiol valerate is designated chemically as estra-1,3,5(10)-triene-3,17-dio(17β)-, 17-pentanoate.

CLINICAL PHARMACOLOGY:

Estradiol valerate is a hormone with a potent and prolonged estrogenic effect. In estrogen responsive tissues (female genital organs, breasts, hypothalamus, pituitary), estrogen binds to tissue-specific receptor proteins in the cytoplasm. The resulting estrogen-protein complex penetrates the nuclear membrane and ultimately binds to materials in the cell nucleus. Such binding activates increased synthesis of DNA, RNA, and various proteins that in turn effect characteristic changes in irresponsive tissues. Estradiol valerate promotes the growth of the endometrium; promotes thickening, stratification, and cornification of the vagina; causes growth of mammary gland ducts; and inhibits the anterior pituitary gland. These effects occur soon after administration and last for approximately two to three weeks after a single intramuscular injection.

About 80 percent of estradiol is reported to be bound to sex hormone binding globulin; most of the remainder is loosely bound to albumin and about two percent is unbound. Estradiol is metabolized to a relatively inactive form in the liver and then excreted in the urine and the bile.

INDICATIONS AND USAGE:

Estradiol Valerate Injection is indicated in the treatment of moderate to severe *vasomotor* symptoms associated with the menopause. (There is no evidence that estrogens are effective for nervous symptoms or depression which might occur during menopause, and they should not be used to treat these conditions.) It is also indicated for the treatment of atrophic vaginitis, kraurosis vulvae, female hypogonadism, female castration, and primary ovarian failure. Estradiol Valerate injection may also be used for the palliative therapy of inoperable, progressing prostatic carcinoma.

ESTRADIOL VALERATE INJECTION HAS NOT BEEN SHOWN TO BE EFFECTIVE FOR ANY PURPOSE DURING PREGNANCY, AND ITS USE MAY CAUSE SEVERE HARM TO THE FETUS (SEE BOXED WARNING.)

CONTRAINDICATIONS:

Estrogens should not be used in women (or men) with any of the following conditions.

1. Known or suspected cancer of the breast except in appropriately selected patients being treated for metastatic disease.

2. Known or suspected estrogen-dependent neoplasia (e.g.. genital malignancy).

3. Known or suspected pregnancy (see BOXED WARNING.)

4. Undiagnosed abnormal genital bleeding.

5. Active thrombophlebitis or thromboembolic disorders.

6. A past history of thrombophlebitis, thrombosis, or thromboembolic disorders associated with previous estrogen use (except when used in treatment of breast or prostatic malignancy).

7. A history of hypersensitivity to estradiol valerate.

WARNINGS:

INDUCTION OF MALIGNANT NEOPLASMS

Long-term continuous administration of natural and synthetic estrogens in certain animal species increase the frequency of carcinomas of the breast, cervix, vagina, and liver. There is now evidence that estrogens increase the risk of carcinoma of the endometrium in humans (see BOXED WARNING.)

At the present time there is no satisfactory evidence that estrogens given to postmenopausal women increase the risk of cancer of the breast, although a recent long-term follow-up of a single physician's practice has raised this possibility. Because of the animal data, there is a need for caution in prescribing estrogens for women with a strong family history of breast cancer or who have breast nodules, fibrocystic disease, or abnormal mammograms.

GALLBLADDER DISEASE

A recent study has reported a 2- to 3-fold increase in the risk of surgically confirmed gallbladder disease in women receiving postmenopausal estrogens, similar to the 2-fold increase previously noted in users of oral contraceptives. In the case of oral contraceptives the increased risk appeared after two years of use.

EFFECTS SIMILAR TO THOSE CAUSED BY ESTROGEN-PROGESTOGEN ORAL CONTRACEPTIVES

There are several serious adverse effects of oral contraceptives, most of which have not, up to now, been documented as consequences of postmenopausal estrogen therapy. This may reflect the comparatively low doses of estrogen used in postmenopausal women. It would be expected that the larger doses of estrogen used to treat prostatic or breast cancer are more likely to result in these adverse effects, and, in fact, it has been shown that there is an increased risk of thrombosis in men receiving estrogens for prostatic cancer.

WARNINGS: *(cont'd)*

Thromboembolic Disease: It is now well established that users of oral contraceptives have an increased risk of various thromboembolic and thrombotic vascular diseases, such as thrombophlebitis, pulmonary embolism, stroke, and myocardial infarction. Cases of retinal thrombosis, mesenteric thrombosis, and optic neuritis have been reported in oral contraceptive users. There is evidence that the risk of several of these adverse reactions is related to the dose of the drug. An increased risk of post surgery thromboembolic complications has also been reported in users of oral contraceptives. If feasible, estrogen should be discontinued at least four weeks before surgery of the type associated with an increased risk of thromboembolism or during periods of prolonged immobilization.

While an increased rate of thromboembolic and thrombotic disease in postmenopausal users of estrogens has not been found, this does not rule out the possibility that such an increase may be present or that subgroups of women who have underlying risk factors or who are receiving relatively large doses of estrogens may have increased risk. Therefore, estrogens should not be used in persons with active thrombophlebitis or thromboembolic disorders, and they should not be used (except in treatment of malignancy)in persons with a history of such disorders in association with estrogen use. They should be used with caution in patients with cerebral vascular or coronary artery disease and only for those in whom estrogens are clearly needed.

Large doses of estrogen (5 mg conjugated estrogens per day), comparable to those used to treat cancer of the prostrate and breast, have been shown in a large prospective clinical trial in men to increase the risk of nonfatal myocardial infarction, pulmonary embolism, and thrombophlebitis. When estrogen doses of this size are used, any of the thromboembolic and thrombotic adverse effects associated with oral contraceptive use should be considered a clear risk.

Hepatic adenoma: Benign hepatic adenomas appear to be associated with the use of oral contraceptives. Although benign, and rare, these may rupture and may cause death through intra-abdominal hemorrhage. Such lesions have not yet been reported in association with other estrogen or progestogen preparations but should be considered in estrogen users having abdominal pain and tenderness, abdominal mass, or hypovolemic shock. Hepatocellular carcinoma has also been reported in women taking estrogen-containing oral contraceptives. The relationship of this malignancy to these drugs is not known at this time.

Elevated blood pressure: Increased blood pressure is not uncommon in women using oral contraceptives. There is now a report that this may occur with use of estrogens in the menopause, and blood pressure should be monitored with estrogen use, especially if high doses are used.

Glucose tolerance: A worsening of glucose tolerance has been observed in a significant percentage of patients on estrogen-containing oral contraceptives. For this reason, diabetic patients should be carefully observed while receiving estrogen.

HYPERCALCEMIA

Administration of estrogens may lead to severe hypercalcemia in patients with breast cancer and bone metastases. If this occurs, the drug should be stopped and appropriate measures taken to reduce the serum calcium level.

PRECAUTIONS:

GENERAL

1. A complete medical and family history should be taken prior to any estrogen therapy. The pretreatment and periodic physical examination should include special reference to blood pressure, breasts, abdomen, and pelvic organs and should include a Papanicolaou smear. As a general rule, estrogen should not be prescribed for longer than one year without another physical examination being performed.

2. Fluid retention: Because estrogens may cause some degree of fluid retention, conditions which might be influenced by this factor, such as epilepsy, migraine, and cardiac or renal dysfunction, require careful observation.

3. Certain patients may develop undesirable manifestations of excessive estrogenic stimulation, such as abnormal or excessive uterine bleeding, mastodynia, etc.

4. Oral contraceptives appear to be associated with an increased incidence of mental depression. Although it is not clear whether this is due to the estrogenic or progestogenic component of the contraceptive, patients with history of depression or other psychic abnormality should be carefully observed.

5. Preexisting uterine leiomyomata may increase in size during estrogen use.

6. The pathologist should be advised of estrogen therapy when relevant specimens are submitted.

7. Patients with a past history of jaundice during pregnancy have an increased risk of recurrence of jaundice while receiving estrogen-containing oral contraceptive therapy. If jaundice develops in any patient receiving estrogen, the medication should be discontinued while the cause is investigated.

8. Estrogens may be poorly metabolized in patients with impaired liver function, and they should be administered with caution in such patients.

9. Because estrogens influence the metabolism of calcium and phosphorus, they should be used with caution in patients with metabolic bone disease that are associated with hypercalcemia or in patients with renal insufficiency.

10. The lowest effective dose appropriate for the specific indication should be utilized. Studies of the addition of a progestin for seven or more days of a cycle of estrogen administration have reported a lowered incidence of endometrial hyperplasia. Morphological and biochemical studies of endometrium suggest that 10 to 13 days or progestin are needed to provide maximal maturation of the endometrium and to eliminate any hyperplastic changes. Whether this will provide protection from endometrial carcinoma has not been clearly established. There are possible additional risks which may be associated with the inclusion of progestin in estrogen replacement regimens. The potential risks include adverse effects on carbohydrate and lipid metabolism. The choice of progestin and dosage may be important in minimizing these adverse effects.

INFORMATION FOR THE PATIENT

A Patient information Sheet is available for this product. See text following PHYSICIAN REFERENCES.

LABORATORY TESTS

The following procedures may be helpful in monitoring the patient's response to therapy: physical examination at least every 6 to 12 months with special attention given to breast and pelvic organs, Papanicolaou test, and hepatic function determinations.

DRUG/LABORATORY TEST INTERACTIONS

Certain endocrine and liver function tests may be affected by estrogen-containing oral contraceptives. The following similar changes may be expected with larger doses of estrogen:

1. Increased sulfobromophthalein retention.

2. Increased prothrombin and factors VII, VIII, IX, and X; decreased antithrombin 3; increased norepinephrine-induced platelet aggregability.

3. Increased thyroid binding globulin (TBG) leading to increased circulating total thyroid hormone, as measured by PBI, T_4 by column, or T_4 by radioimmunoassay. Free T_3 resin uptake is decreased, reflecting the elevated TBG; free T_4 concentration is unaltered.

PRECAUTIONS: *(cont'd)*

4. Impaired glucose tolerance.

5. Decreased pregnanediol excretion..

6. Reduced response to metyrapone test.

7. Reduced serum folate concentration.

8. Increased serum triglyceride and phospholipid concentration.

CARCINOGENESIS, MUTAGENESIS, AND IMPAIRMENT OF FERTILITY

In long-term studies in animals, continuous administration of estrogens increased the frequency of certain carcinomas (See WARNINGS.) There is evidence that estrogens increase the risk of endometrial carcinoma in postmenopausal women (see BOXED WARNING.) Long-term studies in animals have not been performed to evaluate mutagenic potential or impairment of fertility in males or females.

PREGNANCY CATEGORY X

See CONTRAINDICATIONS and BOXED WARNING.

NURSING MOTHERS

As a general principle, the administration of any drug to nursing mothers should be done only when clearly necessary since many drug including estrogens are excreted in human milk.

PEDIATRIC USE

Safety and effectiveness in children have not been established. Because of the effects of estrogens on epiphyseal closure, they should be used judiciously in young patients in whom bone growth is not complete.

DRUG INTERACTIONS:

Estrogens reduce the effect of oral anticoagulants; monitor prothrombin levels and increase anticoagulant dosage accordingly. Rifampin an anticonvulsant drug may decrease the effect of estrogens by accelerating estrogen metabolism. Estrogens may increase the number of toxic reactions to tricyclic antidepressants.

ADVERSE REACTIONS:

(See WARNINGS Regarding induction of neoplasia, adverse effects on the fetus, increased incidence of gallbladder disease, and adverse effects similar to those of oral contraceptives, including thromboembolism.) The following additional adverse reactions have been reported with estrogenic therapy, including oral contraceptives:

1. Genitourinary System: Breakthrough bleeding; spotting; change in menstrual flow; dysmenorrhea; premenstrual-like syndrome; amenorrhea during and after treatment; increase in size of uterine fibromyomata; vaginal candidiasis; change in cervical eversion and in degree of cervical secretion; cystitis-like syndrome.

2. Breasts: Tenderness; enlargement; secretion.

3. Gastrointestinal: Nausea; vomiting; abdominal cramps; bloating; cholestatic jaundice.

4. Skin: Chloasma or melasma which may persist when drug is discontinued; erythema multiforme; erythema nodosum; hemorrhagic eruption; loss of scalp hair; hirsutism; localized dermatitis.

5. Eyes: Steepening of corneal curvature; intolerance to contact lenses.

6. CNS: Headache; migraine; dizziness; mental depression; chorea; convulsions.

7. Miscellaneous: Increase or decrease in weight; reduced carbohydrate tolerance; aggravation of porphyria; edema; changes in libido; pain at the site of injection; sterile abscess; postinjection flare.

OVERDOSAGE:

Numerous reports of ingestion of large doses of estrogen-containing oral contraceptives by young children indicate that serious ill effects do not occur. Overdosage of estrogen may cause nausea, and withdrawal bleeding may occur in females.

DOSAGE AND ADMINISTRATION:

Care should be taken to inject deeply into the upper, outer quadrant of the gluteal muscle following the usual precautions for intramuscular administration. By virtue of the low viscosity of the vehicles, the various preparations of Estradiol Valerate injections may be administered with a small gauge needle. Since the 40 mg potency provides a high concentration in a small volume, particular care should be observed to administer the full dose.

Estradiol Valerate should be visually inspected for particulate matter and color prior to administration; the solution is clear, colorless to pale yellow. Storage at low temperatures may result in the separation of some crystalline material which redissolves readily on warming.

Note: A dry needle and syringe should be used. Use of a wet needle or syringe may cause the solution to become cloudy; however, this does not affect the potency of the material.

CYCLIC REGIMENS

For Short-Term Use Only: For the treatment of moderate to severe *vasomotor* symptoms, atrophic vaginitis, or kraurosis vulvae associated with the menopause. ***Given Cyclically:***For the treatment of female hypogonadism, female castration, or primary ovarian failure.

The dosage for each of the above indications is 10 to 20 mg Estradiol Valerate injection every four weeks.

If in the physician's judgement a patient requires cyclic estrogen-progesterone therapy, 10 to 20 mg Estradiol Valerate injection may be given as an initial injection followed two weeks later by 250 mg Hydroxyprogesterone Caproate injection, USP and 5 mg Estradiol Valerate injection. Four weeks after the initial injection, the cycle may be repeated starting with 10 to 20 mg Estradiol Valerate injection.

The lowest dose that will control symptoms should be chosen, and medication should be discontinued as promptly as possible.

Attempts to discontinue or taper medication should be made at three- to six-month intervals.

Treated patients with an intact uterus should be monitored closely for signs of endometrial cancer, and appropriate diagnostic measures should be taken to rule out malignancy in the event of persistent or recurring abnormal vaginal bleeding.

CHRONIC REGIMEN

For the palliative treatment of inoperable, progressing prostatic carcinoma, the usual dosage is 30 mg or more administered every one or two weeks.

Storage: Store at room temperature.

HOW SUPPLIED - RATED THERAPEUTICALLY EQUIVALENT:

Injection, Solution - Intramuscular - 10 mg/ml

5 ml	$33.16	DELESTROGEN, Bristol Myers Squibb	00003-0330-50
10 ml	$4.17	Estradiol Valerate, HL Moore Drug Exch	00839-5580-30
10 ml	$6.95	Estradiol Valerate, Consolidated Midland	00223-7605-10
10 ml	$7.45	Estradiol Valerate, Major Pharms	00904-2909-10
10 ml	$8.40	VALERGEN, Hyrex Pharms	00314-0780-70
10 ml	$10.80	DIOL L A, C O Truxton	00463-1027-10

HOW SUPPLIED - RATED THERAPEUTICALLY EQUIVALENT: *(cont'd)*

Injection, Solution - Intramuscular - 20 mg/ml

1 ml	$16.31	DELESTROGEN, Bristol Myers Squibb	00003-0343-16
5 ml	$46.73	DELESTROGEN, Bristol Myers Squibb	00003-0343-50
10 ml	$6.39	Estradiol Valerate, McGuff	49072-0217-10
10 ml	$8.95	Estradiol Valerate, Major Pharms	00904-2910-10
10 ml	$9.10	ESTRA-L 20, Pasadena	00418-0451-41
10 ml	$9.30	Estradiol Valerate, Steris Labs	00402-0027-10
10 ml	$9.75	Estradiol Valerate, Consolidated Midland	00223-7606-10
10 ml	$10.00	ESTRA-V-20, Bolan Pharm	44437-0424-70
10 ml	$14.25	GYNOGEN LA, Forest Pharms	00456-0784-10
10 ml	$15.04	VALERGEN, Hyrex Pharms	00314-0782-70
10 ml	$18.63	Estradiol Valerate, Schein Pharm (US)	00364-6613-54
10 ml	$19.40	Estradiol Valerate, Goldline Labs	00182-1805-63

Injection, Solution - Intramuscular - 40 mg/ml

5 ml	$77.53	DELESTROGEN, Bristol Myers Squibb	00003-0251-50
10 ml	$12.50	Estradiol Valerate, Consolidated Midland	00223-7607-10
10 ml	$12.60	Estradiol Valerate, Major Pharms	00904-2911-10
10 ml	$12.66	Estradiol Valerate, Steris Labs	00402-0244-10
10 ml	$12.95	ESTRA-L 40, Pasadena	00418-0461-41
10 ml	$14.89	Estradiol Valerate, Schein Pharm (US)	00364-6614-54
10 ml	$19.00	ESTRA-V-40, Bolan Pharm	44437-0444-70
10 ml	$24.20	Estradiol Valerate, Hyrex Pharms	00314-0781-70
10 ml	$25.09	VALERGEN, Hyrex Pharms	00314-0784-70

ESTRADIOL VALERATE; TESTOSTERONE ENANTHATE *(001192)*

CATEGORIES: Anabolic Steroids; Androgens; Breast Engorgement; Hormones; Pregnancy Category X; DEA Class CIII; FDA Approval Pre 1982

BRAND NAMES: Andrest 90-4; Andro-Estro 90-4; Androgyn L.A.; **Deladumone**; Delatestadiol; Dep-Androgyn; Depotestogen; *Disemone*; Ditate-Ds; Duogen L.A.; Dura-Dumone; *Primodian Depot* (Germany); Teev; Testaval 90 4; Testradiol L.A.; Valertest

(International brand names outside U.S. in italics)

WARNING:

1. ESTROGENS HAVE BEEN REPORTED TO INCREASE THE RISK OF ENDOMETRIAL CARCINOMA.Three independent case control studies have shown an increased risk of endometrial cancer in postmenopausal women exposed to exogenous estrogens for prolonged periods. This risk was independent of the other known risk factors for endometrial cancer. These studies are further supported by the finding that incidence rates of endometrial cancer have increased sharply since 1969 in eight different areas of the United States with population-based cancer reporting systems, an increase which may be related to the rapidly expanding use of estrogens during the last decade.

The three case control studies reported that the risk of endometrial cancer in estrogen users was about 4.5 to 13.9 times greater than in nonusers. The risk appears to depend on both duration of treatment and on estrogen dose. In view of these findings, when estrogens are used for the treatment of menopausal symptoms, the lowest dose that will control symptoms should be utilized and medication should be discontinued as soon as possible. When prolonged treatment is medically indicated, the patient should be reassessed on at least a semiannual basis to determine the need for continued therapy. Although the evidence must be considered preliminary, one study suggests that cyclic administration of low doses of estrogen may carry less risk than continuous administration; it therefore appears prudent to utilize such a regimen.

Close clinical surveillance of all women taking estrogens is important. In all cases of undiagnosed persistent or recurring abnormal vaginal bleeding, adequate diagnostic measures should be undertaken to rule out malignancy.

There is no evidence at present that "natural" estrogens are more or less hazardous than "synthetic" estrogens at equiestrogenic doses.

2. ESTROGENS SHOULD NOT BE USED DURING PREGNANCY.

The use of female sex hormones, both estrogens and progestogens, during early pregnancy may seriously damage the offspring. An association has been reported between In Utero exposure of the female fetus to diethylstilbestrol, a nonsteroidal estrogen, and an increased risk of the post-pubertal development of an ordinarily extremely rare form of vaginal or cervical cancer. This risk has recently been estimated to be in the range of 0.14 to 1.4 per 1000 exposed females, consistent with a previous risk estimate of not greater than 4 per 1000 exposures. Furthermore, a high percentage of such exposed women (from 30 to 90 percent) have been found to have vaginal adenosis, epithelial changes of the vagina and cervix. Although these changes are histologically benign, it is not known whether they are precursors of malignancy. Although similar data are not available with the use of other estrogens, it cannot be presumed they would not induce similar changes.

Several reports suggest an association between intrauterine exposure to female sex hormones and congenital anomalies, including congenital heart defects and limb reduction defects. One case control study estimated a 4.7-fold increased risk of limb reduction defects in infants exposed In Utero to sex hormones (oral contraceptives, hormone withdrawal tests for pregnancy or attempted treatment for threatened abortion). Some of these exposures were very short and involved only a few days of treatment. The data suggest that the risk of limb reduction defects in exposed fetuses is somewhat less than 1 per 1000.

In the past, female sex hormones have been used during pregnancy in an attempt to treat threatened or habitual abortion. There is now considerable literature to the effect that estrogens are ineffective for these indications, and the data are not now considered adequate to support the conclusion that progestogens are effective for these uses.

If this drug is used during pregnancy, or if the patient becomes pregnant while taking this drug, she should be apprised of the potential risks to the fetus and the advisability of pregnancy continuation.

DESCRIPTION:

Testosterone Enanthate and Estradiol Valerate Injection is a sterile, long-acting androgen-estrogen preparation for intramuscular administration providing a precisely balanced combination of the naturally-occurring testicular and follicular hormones in ester form dissolved in a vehicle of sesame oil. Each 2 mL Unimatic single dose syringe contains 360 mg testosterone enanthate and 16 mg estradiol valerate per 2 mL (180 mg testosterone enanthate and 8 mg estradiol valerate per mL) with 2% (w/v) benzyl alcohol as a preservative.

The chemical names of testosterone enanthate and estradiol valerate are androst-4-en-3-one, 17-((1-oxoheptyl)oxy)-, (17-beta)- and estra-1,3,5(10)-triene-3,17-diol(17-beta)-, 17-pentanoate, respectively.

CLINICAL PHARMACOLOGY:

Estradiol Valerate with Testosterone Enanthate is a long-acting androgen-estrogen preparation which combines the action of two potent hormonal agents, testosterone enanthate and estradiol valerate. Estradiol Valerate with Testosterone Enanthate inhibits the release of lactogenic hormone.

INDICATIONS AND USAGE:

Testosterone Enanthate and Estradiol Valerate Injection is indicated for the prevention of postpartum breast engorgement. Although estrogens have been widely used for the prevention of postpartum breast engorgement, controlled studies have demonstrated that the incidence of significant painful engorgement in patients not receiving such hormonal therapy is low and usually responsive to appropriate analgesic or other supportive therapy. Consequently, the benefit to be derived from estrogen therapy for this indication must be carefully weighed against the potential increased risk of puerperal thromboembolism associated with the use of large doses of estrogens.

THIS DRUG HAS NOT BEEN SHOWN TO BE EFFECTIVE FOR ANY PURPOSE DURING PREGNANCY AND ITS USE MAY CAUSE SEVERE HARM TO THE FETUS (SEE BOXED WARNING).

CONTRAINDICATIONS:

Estrogens should not be used in women (or men) with any of the following conditions:

1. Known or suspected cancer of the breast except in appropriately selected patients being treated for metastatic disease.

2. Known or suspected estrogen-dependent neoplasia (*e.g.,* genital malignancy).

3. Known or suspected pregnancy (See BOXED WARNING.)

4. Undiagnosed abnormal genital bleeding.

5. Active thrombophlebitis or thromboembolic disorders.

6. A past history of thrombophlebitis, thrombosis, or thromboembolic disorders associated with previous estrogen use (except when used in treatment of breast or prostatic malignancy).

7. A history of hypersensitivity to estradiol valerate or testosterone enanthate.

WARNINGS:

See BOXED WARNING.

INDUCTION OF MALIGNANT NEOPLASMS

Long-term continuous administration of natural and synthetic estrogens in certain animal species increases the frequency of carcinomas of the breast, cervix, vagina, and liver. There is now evidence that estrogens increase the risk of carcinoma of the endometrium in humans.

At the present time there is no satisfactory evidence that estrogens given to postmenopausal women increase the risk of cancer of the breast, although a recent long-term follow-up of a single physician's practice has raised this possibility. Because of the animal data, there is a need for caution in prescribing estrogens for women with a strong family history of breast cancer or who have breast nodules, fibrocystic disease, or abnormal mammograms.

GALLBLADDER DISEASE

A recent study has reported a 2- to 3-fold increase in the risk of surgically confirmed gallbladder disease in women receiving postmenopausal estrogens, similar to the 2-fold increase previously noted in users of oral contraceptives. In the case of oral contraceptives the increased risk appeared after two years of use.

EFFECTS SIMILAR TO THOSE CAUSED BY ESTROGEN-PROGESTOGEN ORAL CONTRACEPTIVES

There are several serious adverse effects of oral contraceptives, most of which have not, up to now, been documented as consequences of postmenopausal estrogen therapy. This may reflect the comparatively low doses of estrogen used in postmenopausal women. It would be expected that the larger doses of estrogen used to treat prostatic or breast cancer or postpartum breast engorgement are more likely to result in these adverse effects, and, in fact, it has been shown that there is an increased risk of thrombosis in men receiving estrogens for prostatic cancer and women for postpartum breast engorgement.

Thromboembolic Disease: It is now well established that users of oral contraceptives have an increased risk of various thromboembolic and thrombotic vascular diseases, such as thrombophlebitis, pulmonary embolism, stroke, and myocardial infarction. Cases of retinal thrombosis, mesenteric thrombosis, and optic neuritis have been reported in oral contraceptive users. There is evidence that the risk of several of these adverse reactions is related to the dose of the drug. An increased risk of postsurgery thromboembolic complications has also been reported in users of oral contraceptives. If feasible, estrogen should be discontinued at least four weeks before surgery of the type associated with an increased risk of thromboembolism, or during periods of prolonged immobilization.

While an increased rate of thromboembolic and thrombotic disease in postmenopausal users of estrogens has not been found, this does not rule out the possibility that such an increase may be present or that subgroups of women who have underlying risk factors or who are receiving relatively large doses of estrogens may have increased risk. Therefore, estrogens should not be used in persons with active thrombophlebitis or thromboembolic disorders, and they should not be used (except in treatment of malignancy) in persons with a history of such disorders in association with estrogen use. They should be used with caution in patients with cerebral vascular or coronary artery disease and only for those in whom estrogens are clearly needed.

Large doses of estrogen (5 mg conjugated estrogens per day), comparable to those used to treat cancer of the prostate and breast, have been shown in a large prospective clinical trial in men to increase the risk of nonfatal myocardial infarction, pulmonary embolism, and thrombophlebitis. When estrogen doses of this size are used, any of the thromboembolic and thrombotic adverse effects associated with oral contraceptive use should be considered a clear risk.

WARNINGS: *(cont'd)*

Hepatic Adenoma: Benign hepatic adenomas appear to be associated with the use of oral contraceptives. Although benign, and rare, these may rupture and may cause death through intraabdominal hemorrhage. Such lesions have not yet been reported in association with other estrogen or progestogen preparations but should be considered in estrogen users having abdominal pain and tenderness, abdominal mass, or hypovolemic shock. Hepatocellular carcinoma has also been reported in women taking estrogen-containing oral contraceptives. The relationship of this malignancy to these drugs is not known at this time.

Elevated Blood Pressure: Increased blood pressure is not uncommon in women using oral contraceptives. There is now a report that this may occur with use of estrogens in the menopause, and blood pressure should be monitored with estrogen use, especially if high doses are used.

Glucose Tolerance: A worsening of glucose tolerance has been observed in a significant percentage of patients on estrogen-containing oral contraceptives. For this reason, diabetic patients should be carefully observed while receiving estrogen.

HYPERCALCEMIA

Administration of estrogens may lead to severe hypercalcemia in patients with breast cancer and bone metastases. If this occurs, the drug should be stopped and appropriate measures taken to reduce the serum calcium level.

PRECAUTIONS:

GENERAL

A complete medical and family history should be taken prior to the initiation of any estrogen therapy. The pretreatment and periodic physical examinations should include special reference to blood pressure, breasts, abdomen, and pelvic organs and should include a Papanicolaou smear. As a general rule, estrogen should not be prescribed for longer than one year without another physical examination being performed.

Fluid retention: Because estrogens may cause some degree of fluid retention, conditions which might be influenced by this factor such as epilepsy, migraine, asthma, and cardiac or renal dysfunction, require careful observation.

Certain patients may develop undesirable manifestations of excessive estrogenic stimulation, such as abnormal or excessive uterine bleeding, mastodynia, etc.

Oral contraceptives appear to be associated with an increased incidence of mental depression. Although it is not clear whether this is due to the estrogenic or progestogenic component of the contraceptive, patients with a history of depression or other psychic abnormality should be carefully observed.

Preexisting uterine leiomyomata may increase in size during estrogen use.

The pathologist should be advised of estrogen therapy when relevant specimens are submitted.

Patients with a past history of jaundice during pregnancy have an increased risk of recurrence of jaundice while receiving estrogen-containing oral contraceptive therapy. If jaundice develops in any patient receiving estrogen, the medication should be discontinued while the cause is investigated.

Estrogens may be poorly metabolized in patients with impaired liver function, and they should be administered with caution in such patients.

Because estrogens influence the metabolism of calcium and phosphorus, they should be used with caution in patients with metabolic bone diseases that are associated with hypercalcemia or in patients with renal insufficiency.

Because of the effects of estrogens on epiphyseal closure, they should be used judiciously in young patients in whom bone growth is not complete.

Certain endocrine and liver function tests may be affected by estrogen-containing oral contraceptives. The following similar changes may be expected with larger doses of estrogen:

a. Increased sulfobromophthalein retention.

b. Increased prothrombin and factors VII, VIII, IX, and X; decreased antithrombin 3; increased norepinephrine-induced platelet aggregability.

c. Increased thyroid binding globulin (TBG) leading to increased circulating total thyroid hormone, as measured by PBI, T4 by column, or T4 by radioimmunoassay. Free T3 resin uptake is decreased, reflecting the elevated TBG; free T4 concentration is unaltered.

d. Impaired glucose tolerance.

e. Decreased pregnanediol excretion.

f. Reduced response to metyrapone test.

g. Reduced serum folate concentration.

h. Increased serum triglyceride and phospholipid concentration.

PREGNANCY CATEGORY X

See CONTRAINDICATIONS and BOXED WARNING.

NURSING MOTHERS

As a general principle, the administration of any drug to nursing mothers should be done only when clearly necessary since many drugs are excreted in human milk.

ADVERSE REACTIONS:

(See WARNINGS regarding induction of neoplasia, adverse effects on the fetus, increased incidence of gallbladder disease and adverse effects similar to those of oral contraceptives, including thromboembolism.) The following additional adverse reactions have been reported with estrogenic therapy, including oral contraceptives:

Genitourinary System: breakthrough bleeding; spotting; change in menstrual flow; dysmenorrhea; premenstrual-like syndrome; amenorrhea during and after treatment; increase in size of uterine fibromyomata; vaginal candidiasis; change in cervical eversion and in degree of cervical secretion; cystitis-like syndrome.

Breasts: tenderness; enlargement; secretion.

Gastrointestinal: nausea; vomiting; abdominal cramps; bloating; cholestatic jaundice.

Skin: chloasma or melasma which may persist when drug is discontinued; erythema multiforme; erythema nodosum; hemorrhagic eruption; loss of scalp hair; hirsutism; localized dermatitis.

Eyes: steepening of corneal curvature; intolerance to contact lenses.

CNS: headache; migraine; dizziness; mental depression; chorea; convulsions.

Miscellaneous: increase or decrease in weight; reduced carbohydrate tolerance; aggravation of porphyria; edema; changes in libido; pain at the site of injection; sterile abscess; postinjection flare.

In addition to the adverse reactions above, the following reactions may occur with androgen-estrogen therapy: virilization, manifested by changes in the voice (hoarseness or deepening), and acne.

OVERDOSAGE:

Numerous reports of ingestion of large doses of estrogen-containing oral contraceptives by young children indicate that serious ill effects do not occur. Overdosage of estrogen may cause nausea, and withdrawal bleeding may occur in females.

DOSAGE AND ADMINISTRATION:

GIVEN ONCE

For the prevention of postpartum breast engorgement, 2 mL of Estradiol Valerate with Testosterone Enanthate should be given as a single intramuscular injection. It appears that the optimal time for administration of Estradiol Valerate with Testosterone Enanthate is just prior to the onset of the second stage of labor because the percentage of favorable results has been shown to decline when the dose is administered at a later time. It is worthwhile noting, however, that the preparation has been successfully used from the early first stage of labor to as late as 10 hours after expulsion of the placenta. A second injection is not recommended.

Care should be taken to inject Estradiol Valerate with Testosterone Enanthate deeply into the upper, outer quadrant of the gluteal muscle following the usual precautions for intramuscular administration.

Because of the viscosity of the preparation, and since Estradiol Valerate with Testosterone Enanthate provides a high concentration in a small volume, particular care should be taken to administer the full dose. A slow, steady pressure on the syringe plunger is recommended.

Treated patients with an intact uterus should be monitored closely for signs of endometrial cancer and appropriate diagnostic measures should be taken to rule out malignancy in the event of persistent or recurring abnormal vaginal bleeding.

Store at room temperature.

HOW SUPPLIED - RATED THERAPEUTICALLY EQUIVALENT:

Injection, Solution - Intramuscular - 4 mg/90 mg/ml

5 ml	**$26.87**	**DELADUMONE, Bristol Myers Squibb**	**00003-0385-30**
10 ml	$13.75	Testosterone W/Estradiol, Goldline Labs	00182-3069-63
10 ml	$16.07	VALERTEST NO. 1, Hyrex Pharms	00314-0786-70

HOW SUPPLIED - NOT RATED EQUIVALENT:

Injection, Solution - Intramuscular - 4 mg/90 mg/ml

10 ml	$8.00	Delatestadiol, Dunhall Pharms	00217-6807-08
10 ml	$10.50	TESTRADIOL L A, C O Truxton	00463-1085-10
10 ml	$10.75	Testosterone Enanthate/Estradiol, Steris Labs	00402-0360-10
10 ml	$10.78	Estra- Testin, Pasadena	00418-0501-41
10 ml	$18.85	Testosterone W/Estradiol, Goldline Labs	00182-3073-63

Injection, Solution - Intramuscular - 8 mg/180 mg

2 ml	**$30.52**	**DELADUMONE OB, Bristol Myers Squibb**	**00003-0364-20**
2 ml	**$33.58**	**DELADUMONE OB, Bristol Myers Squibb**	**00003-0364-16**
2 ml x 10	$75.00	Testosterone W/Estradiol, Consolidated Midland	00223-8611-10

ESTRAMUSTINE PHOSPHATE SODIUM

(001195)

CATEGORIES: Antineoplastics; Cytotoxic Agents; Nitrogen Mustard Derivatives; Oncologic Drugs; Prostatic Carcinoma; FDA Approval Pre 1982

BRAND NAMES: *Cellmustin* (Germany); **Emcyt**; *Estracyt* (Australia, Europe, Japan) *(International brand names outside U.S. in italics)*

FORMULARIES: BC-BS; Medi-Cal

DESCRIPTION:

Estramustine phosphate sodium, an antineoplastic agent, is an off-white powder readily soluble in water. Emcyt is available as white opaque capsules, each containing estramustine phosphate sodium as the disodium salt monohydrate equivalent to 140 mg estramustine phosphate, for oral administration. Each capsule also contains magnesium stearate, silicon dioxide, sodium lauryl sulfate and talc. Gelatin capsule shells contain the following pigment: titanium dioxide.

Chemically, estramustine phosphate sodium is estra-1,3,5 (10)-triene-3, 17-diol(17β)-,3-(bis(2-chloroethyl)carbamate) 17-(dihydrogen phosphate), disodium salt, monohydrate. It is also referred to as estradiol 3-(bis(2-chloroethyl)carbamate) 17-(dihydrogen phosphate), disodium salt, monohydrate.

Estramustine phosphate sodium has an empiric formula of $C_{23}H_{30}Cl_2NNa_2O_6P{\cdot}H_2O$, a calculated molecular weight of 582.4.

CLINICAL PHARMACOLOGY:

Estramustine phosphate is a molecule combining estradiol and nornitrogen mustard by a carbamate link. The molecule is phosphorylated to make it water soluble.

Estramustine phosphate taken orally is readily dephosphorylated during absorption, and the major metabolites in plasma are estramustine, the estrone analog, estradiol and estrone.

Prolonged treatment with estramustine phosphate produces elevated total plasma concentrations, of estradiol that fall within ranges similar to the elevated estradiol levels found in prostatic cancer patients given conventional estradiol therapy. Estrogenic effects, as demonstrated by changes in circulating levels of steroids and pituitary hormones, are similar in patients treated with either estramustine phosphate or conventional estradiol.

The metabolic urinary patterns of the estradiol moiety of estramustine phosphate and estradiol itself are very similar, although the metabolites derived from estramustine phosphate are excreted at a slower rate.

INDICATIONS AND USAGE:

Emcyt is indicated in the palliative treatment of patients with metastatic and/or progressive carcinoma of the prostate.

CONTRAINDICATIONS:

Emcyt should not be used in patients with any of the following conditions:

1) Known hypersensitivity to either estradiol or to nitrogen mustard.

2) Active thrombophlebitis or thromboembolic disorders, except in those cases where the actual tumor mass is the cause of the thromboembolic phenomenon and the physician feels the benefits of therapy may outweigh the risks.

WARNINGS:

It has been shown that there is an increased risk of thrombosis, including nonfatal myocardial infarction, in men receiving estrogens for prostatic cancer. Emcyt should be used with caution in patients with a history of thrombophlebitis, thrombosis or thromboembolic disorders, especially if they were associated with estrogen therapy. Caution should also be used in patients with cerebral vascular or coronary artery disease.

Glucose Tolerance: Because glucose tolerance may be decreased, diabetic patients should be carefully observed while receiving Emcyt.

Elevated Blood Pressure: Because hypertension may occur, blood pressure should be monitored periodically.

PRECAUTIONS:

GENERAL

Fluid Retention: Exacerbation of preexisting or incipient peripheral edema or congestive heart disease has been seen in some patients receiving Emcyt therapy. Other conditions which might be influenced by fluid retention, such as epilepsy, migraine or renal dysfunction, require careful observation.

Emcyt may be poorly metabolized in patients with impaired liver function and should be administered with caution in such patients.

Because Emcyt may influence the metabolism of calcium and phosphorus, it should be used with caution in patients with metabolic bone diseases that are associated with hypercalcemia or in patients with renal insufficiency.

INFORMATION FOR THE PATIENT

Because of the possibility of mutagenic effects, patients should be advised to use contraceptive measures.

LABORATORY TESTS

Certain endocrine and liver function tests may be affected by estrogen-containing drugs. Abnormalities of hepatic enzymes and of bilirubin have occurred in patients receiving Emcyt, but have seldom been severe enough to require cessation of therapy. Such tests should be done at appropriate intervals during therapy and repeated after the drug has been withdrawn for two months.

FOOD/DRUG INTERACTION

Milk, milk products and calcium-rich foods or drugs may impair the absorption of Emcyt.

CARCINOGENESIS, MUTAGENESIS, IMPAIRMENT OF FERTILITY

Long-term continuous administration of estrogens in certain animal species increases the frequency of carcinomas of the breast and liver. Compounds structurally similar to Emcyt are carcinogenic in mice. Carcinogenic studies of Emcyt have not been conducted in man. Although testing by the Ames method failed to demonstrate mutagenicity for estramustine phosphate sodium, it is known that both estradiol and nitrogen mustard are mutagenic. For this reason and because some patients who had been impotent while on estrogen therapy have regained potency while taking Emcyt, the patient should be advised to use contraceptive measures.

ADVERSE REACTIONS:

In a randomized, double-blind trial comparing therapy with Emcyt in 93 patients (11.5 to 15.9 mg/kg/day) or diethylstilbestrol (DES) in 93 patients (3.0 mg/day), the following adverse effects were reported (TABLE 1):

OVERDOSAGE:

Although there has been no experience with overdosage to date, it is reasonable to expect that such episodes may produce pronounced manifestations of the known adverse reactions. In the event of overdosage, the gastric contents should be evacuated by gastric lavage and symptomatic therapy should be initiated. Hematologic and hepatic parameters should be monitored for at least six weeks after overdosage of Emcyt.

DOSAGE AND ADMINISTRATION:

The recommended daily dose is 14 mg per kg of body weight (*i.e.,* one 140 mg capsule for each 10 kg or 22 lb of body weight), given in 3 or 4 divided doses. Most patients in studies in the United States have been treated at a dosage range of 10 to 16 mg per kg per day.

Patients should be instructed to take Emcyt at least one hour before or two hours after meals. Emcyt should be swallowed with water. Milk, milk products and calcium-rich foods or drugs (such as calcium-containing antacids) must not be taken simultaneously with Emcyt.

Patients should be treated for 30 to 90 days before the physician determines the possible benefits of continued therapy. Therapy should be continued as long as the favorable response lasts. Some patients have been maintained on therapy for more than three years at doses ranging from 10 to 16 mg per kg of body weight per day.

Procedures for proper handling and disposal of anticancer drugs should be considered. Several guidelines on this subject have been published.[1-6] There is no general agreement that all of the procedures recommended in the guidelines are necessary or appropriate.

NOTE: Emcyt should be stored in the refrigerator at 36 to 46°F (2 to 8°C).

REFERENCES:

1. Recommendations for the safe handling of parenteral antineoplastic drugs. Washington, DC, U.S. Government Printing Office (NIH Publication No. 83-2621). **2.** AMA Council Report. Guidelines for handling parenteral antineoplastics. *JAMA 253*:1590-1592, Mar 15, 1985. **3.** National Study Commission on Cytotoxic Exposure: Recommendations for handling cytotoxic agents. Available from Louis P. Jeffrey, ScD, Director of Pharmacy Services, Rhode Island Hospital, 593 Eddy Street, Providence, Rhode Island 02902. **4.** Clinical Oncological Society of Australia: Guidelines and recommendations for safe handling of antineoplastic agents. *Med J Aust 1*: 426-428, Apr 30, 1983. **5.** Jones RB, Frank R, Mass T: Safe handling of chemotherapeutic agents: a report from the Mount Sinai Medical Center.*CA 33*:258-263, Sept-Oct 1983. **6.** ASHP technical assistance bulletin on handling cytotoxic drugs in hospitals. *Am J Hosp Pharm 42*:131-137, Jan 1985.

HOW SUPPLIED - EQUIVALENTS NOT AVAILABLE:

Capsule, Gelatin - Oral - 140 mg

100's	**$291.81**	**EMCYT, Pharmacia & Upjohn**	00013-0132-02

ESTROGENIC SUBSTANCES *(001196)*

CATEGORIES: Antineoplastics; Estrogen; Estrogens; Hormones; Oncologic Drugs; FDA Pre 1938 Drugs

BRAND NAMES: Aquest; Estroject-2; Estrone; Genostrin; Gynogen; Kestrin; Lanestrin; Primestrin; Theelin; Unigen; Wehgen

Prescribing information not available at time of publication.

HOW SUPPLIED - EQUIVALENTS NOT AVAILABLE:

Injection, Solution - Intramuscular - 2 mg/ml

10 ml	$5.50	Estrone, Consolidated Midland	00223-7660-10
10 ml	$6.30	Estrogenic Substance, Pasadena	00418-0181-41

HOW SUPPLIED - EQUIVALENTS NOT AVAILABLE: *(cont'd)*

TABLE 1 Estramustine Phosphate Sodium, Adverse Reactions

	EMCYT n = 93	**DES n = 93**
Cardiovascular-Respiratory		
Cardiac Arrest	0	2
Cerebrovascular Accident	2	0
Myocardial Infarction	3	1
Thrombophlebitis	3	7
Pulmonary Emboli	2	5
Congestive Heart Failure	3	2
Edema	19	17
Dyspnea	11	3
Leg Cramps	8	11
Upper Respiratory Discharge	1	1
Hoarseness	1	0
Gastrointestinal		
Nausea	15	8
Diarrhea	12	11
Minor Gastrointestinal Upset	11	6
Anorexia	4	3
Flatulence	2	0
Vomiting	1	1
Gastrointestinal Bleeding	1	0
Burning Throat	1	0
Thirst	1	0
Integumentary		
Rash	1	4
Pruritus	2	2
Dry Skin	2	0
Pigment Changes	0	3
Easy Bruising	3	0
Flushing	1	0
Night Sweats	0	1
Fingertip—Peeling Skin	1	0
Thinning Hair	1	1
Breast Changes		
Tenderness	66	64
Enlargement		
Mild	60	54
Moderate	10	16
Marked	0	5
Miscellaneous		
Lethargy Alone	4	3
Depression	0	2
Emotional Lability	2	0
Insomnia	3	0
Headache	1	1
Anxiety	1	0
Chest Pain	1	1
Hot Flashes	0	1
Pain in Eyes	0	1
Tearing of Eyes	1	1
Tinnitus	0	1
Laboratory Abnormalities		
Hematologic		
Leukopenia	4	2
Thrombopenia	1	2
Hepatic		
Bilirubin Alone	1	5
Bilirubin and LDH	0	1
Bilirubin and SGOT	2	1
Bilirubin, LDH and SGOT	2	0
LDH and/or SGOT	31	28
Miscellaneous		
Hypercalcemia—Transient	0	1

10 ml	$6.50	Estrogenic Substance, Consolidated Midland	00223-7620-10
10 ml	$10.00	AQUEST, Dunhall Pharms	00217-6802-08
10 ml	$15.85	Estrone, Goldline Labs	00182-3027-63

Injection, Solution - Intramuscular - 5 mg/ml

10 ml	$5.75	Estrone, Consolidated Midland	00223-7670-10
10 ml	$15.45	ESTRONE, Rugby	00536-5602-70

ESTROGENS, CONJUGATED *(001197)*

CATEGORIES: Antineoplastics; Breast Carcinoma; Cancer; Hemostatics; Hormonal Imbalance; Hormones; Kraurosis Vulvae; Menopause; Oncologic Drugs; Osteoporosis; Ovarian Failure; Prostatic Carcinoma; Skin/Mucous Membrane Agents; Urethritis; Uterine Bleeding; Vaginal Preparations; Vaginitis; Colon Carcinoma*; Urinary Incontinence*; Rectal Carcinoma*; Pregnancy Category X; Sales > $500 Million; FDA Approval Pre 1982; Top 200 Drugs
* Indication not approved by the FDA

BRAND NAMES: *Ayerogen*; *Ayerogen Crema Vaginal*; *Azumon*; *C.E.S.* (Canada); *Climarest* (Germany); Conjugated Estrogens; *Conjugen*; *Dagynil*; *Emopremarin*; *Equigyne*; *Equin*; *Femavit* (Germany); *Hyphorin* (Japan); Mannest; Menopak-E; *Menpoz*; *Neo-Menovar*; *Oestro-Feminal* (Germany); Ovest; *Premaril*; **Premarin**; *Premarin Crema V* (Mexico); *Premarin Creme* (Australia); *Premarin Vaginal Creme*; *Premarina*; *Presomen* (Germany); *Prevagin-Premaril*; *Romeda* (Japan); *Sefac* (Japan); *Srogen*; *Sukingpo*; *Transannon* (Germany)
(International brand names outside U.S. in italics)

FORMULARIES: Aetna; BC-BS; CIGNA; DoD; FHP; Humana; Kaiser; Medco; Medi-Cal; PCS; PruCare; United

COST OF THERAPY: $107.99 (Osteoporosis; Tablet; 0.625 mg; 0.75/day; 365 days)

WARNING:
TABLETS
ESTROGENS HAVE BEEN REPORTED TO INCREASE THE RISK OF ENDOMETRIAL CARCINOMA IN POSTMENOPAUSAL WOMEN. Close clinical surveillance of all women taking estrogens is important. Adequate diagnostic measures, including endometrial sampling when indicated, should be undertaken to rule out malignancy in all cases of undiagnosed persistent or recurring abnormal vaginal bleeding. There is currently no evidence that "natural" estrogens are more or less hazardous

than "synthetic" estrogens at equiestrogenic doses.
ESTROGENS SHOULD NOT BE USED DURING PREGNANCY. Estrogen therapy during pregnancy is associated with an increased risk of congenital defects in the reproductive organs of the male and female fetus, an increased risk of vaginal adenosis, squamous cell dysplasia of the uterine cervix, and vaginal cancer in the female later in life. The 1985 DES Task Force concluded that women who used DES during their pregnancies may subsequently experience an increased risk of breast cancer. However, a causal relationship is still unproven, and the observed level of risk is similar to that for a number of other breast-cancer risk factors. There is no indication for estrogen therapy during pregnancy. Estrogens are ineffective for the prevention or treatment of threatened or habitual abortion.
INJECTION AND VAGINAL CREAM
ESTROGENS HAVE BEEN REPORTED TO INCREASE THE RISK OF ENDOMETRIAL CARCINOMA. Three independent, case-controlled studies have reported an increased risk of endometrial cancer in postmenopausal women exposed to exogenous estrogens for more than one year.[1-3] This risk was independent of the other known risk factors for endometrial cancer. These studies are further supported by the finding that incidence rates of endometrial cancer have increased sharply since 1969 in eight different areas of the United States with population-based cancer-reporting systems, an increase which may be related to the rapidly expanding use of estrogens during the last decade.[4] The three case-controlled studies reported that the risk of endometrial cancer in estrogen users was about 4.5 to 13.9 times greater than in nonusers. The risk appears to depend on both duration of treatment1 and on estrogen dose.[3]In view of these findings, when estrogens are used for the treatment of menopausal symptoms, the lowest dose that will control symptoms should be utilized and medication should be discontinued as soon as possible. When prolonged treatment is medically indicated, the patient should be reassessed, on at least a semiannual basis, to determine the need for continued therapy. Although the evidence must be considered preliminary, one study suggests that cyclic administration of low doses of estrogen may carry less risk than continuous administration.[3] It therefore appears prudent to utilize such a regimen. Close clinical surveillance of all women taking estrogens is important. In all cases of undiagnosed persistent or recurring abnormal vaginal bleeding, adequate diagnostic measures should be undertaken to rule out malignancy. There is no evidence at present that "natural" estrogens are more or less hazardous than "synthetic" estrogens at equiestrogenic doses.
ESTROGENS SHOULD NOT BE USED DURING PREGNANCY. The use of female sex hormones, both estrogens and progestogens, during early pregnancy may seriously damage the offspring. It has been shown that females exposed in utero to diethylstilbestrol, a nonsteroidal estrogen, have an increased risk of developing, in later life, a form of vaginal or cervical cancer that is ordinarily extremely rare.[5,6] This risk has been estimated as not greater than 4 per 1,000 exposures.[7] Furthermore, a high percentage of such exposed women (from 30% to 90%) have been found to have vaginal adenosis,8-12 epithelial changes of the vagina and cervix. Although these changes are histologically benign, it is not known whether they are precursors of malignancy. Although similar data are not available with the use of other estrogens, it cannot be presumed they would not induce similar changes. Several reports suggest an association between intrauterine exposure to female sex hormones and congenital anomalies, including congenital heart defects and limb-reduction defects. 13-16 One case-controlled study 16 estimated a 4.7-fold increased risk of limb-reduction defects in infants exposed in utero to sex hormones (oral contraceptives, hormone withdrawal tests for pregnancy, or attempted treatment for threatened abortion). Some of these exposures were very short and involved only a few days of treatment. The data suggest that the risk of limb-reduction defects in exposed fetuses is somewhat less than 1 per 1,000. In the past, female sex hormones have been used during pregnancy in an attempt to treat threatened or habitual abortion. There is considerable evidence that estrogens are ineffective for these indications, and there is no evidence from well-controlled studies that progestogens are effective for these uses. If Premarin (conjugated estrogens, USP) is used during pregnancy, or if the patient becomes pregnant while taking this drug, she should be apprised of the potential risks to the fetus, and the advisability of pregnancy continuation.

DESCRIPTION:

TABLETS

Premarin (conjugated estrogens tablets, USP) for oral administration contains a mixture of estrogens obtained exclusively from natural sources, occurring as the sodium salts of water-soluble estrogen sulfates blended to represent the average composition of material derived from pregnant mares' urine. It contains estrone, equilin, and 17 α-dihydroequilin, together with smaller amounts of 17 α-estradiol, equilenin, and 17 α-dihydroequilenin as salts of their sulfate esters. Tablets for oral administration are available in 0.3 mg, 0.625 mg, 0.9 mg, 1.25 mg, and 2.5 mg strengths of conjugated estrogens.

Premarin Tablets contain the following inactive ingredients: calcium phosphate tribasic, calcium sulfate anhydrous (white tablet), calcium sulfate, carnauba wax, cellulose, glyceryl monooleate, lactose, magnesium stearate, methylcellulose, pharmaceutical glaze, polyethylene glycol, stearic acid, sucrose, talc, titanium dioxide.

0.3 mg Tablets Also Contain: D&C Yellow No. 10, FD&C Blue No. 1, FD&C Blue No. 2, FD&C Yellow No. 6;

0.625 mg Tablets Also Contain: FD&C Blue No. 2, D&C Red No. 27, FD&C Red No. 40;

0.9 mg Tablets Also Contain: D&C Red No. 6, D&C Red No. 7;

1.25 mg Tablets Also Contain: Black iron oxide, D&C Yellow No. 10, FD&C Yellow No. 6;

2.5 mg Tablets Also Contain: FD&C Blue No. 2, D&C Red No. 7.

INJECTION

Each Secule vial contains 25 mg of conjugated estrogens, USP, in a sterile lyophilized cake which also contains lactose 200 mg, sodium citrate 12.2 mg, and simethicone 0.2 mg. The pH is adjusted with sodium hydroxide or hydrochloric acid. A sterile diluent (5 ml) containing 2% benzyl alcohol in sterile water is provided for reconstitution. The reconstituted solution is suitable for intravenous or intramuscular injection.

DESCRIPTION: *(cont'd)*

Premarin (conjugated estrogens, USP) is a mixture of estrogens, obtained exclusively from natural sources, occurring as the sodium salts of water-soluble estrogen sulfates blended to represent the average composition of material derived from pregnant mares' urine. It contains estrone, equilin, and 17 α-dihydroequilin, together with smaller amounts of 17 α-estradiol, equilenin, and 17 α-dihydroequilenin as salts of their sulfate esters.

VAGINAL CREAM

Each gram of Premarin (conjugated estrogens) Vaginal Cream contains 0.625 mg conjugated estrogens, USP, in a nonliquefying base containing cetyl esters wax, cetyl alcohol, white wax, glyceryl monostearate, propylene glycol monostearate, methyl stearate, benzyl alcohol, sodium lauryl sulfate, glycerin, and mineral oil. Premarin Vaginal Cream is applied intravaginally.

Premarin (conjugated estrogens) is a mixture of estrogens obtained exclusively from natural sources, occurring as the sodium salts of water-soluble estrogen sulfates blended to represent the average composition of material derived from pregnant mares' urine. It contains estrone, equilin, and 17 α-dihydroequilin, together with smaller amounts of 17 α-estradiol, equilenin, and 17 α-dihydroequilenin as salts of their sulfate esters.

CLINICAL PHARMACOLOGY:

Estrogens are important in the development and maintenance of the female reproductive system and secondary sex characteristics. They promote growth and development of the vagina, uterus, and fallopian tubes, and enlargement of the breasts. Indirectly, they contribute to the shaping of the skeleton, maintenance of tone and elasticity of urogenital structures, changes in the epiphyses of the long bones that allow for the pubertal growth spurt and its termination, growth of axillary and pubic hair, and pigmentation of the nipples and genitals. Decline of estrogenic activity at the end of the menstrual cycle can bring on menstruation, although the cessation of progesterone secretion is the most important factor in the mature ovulatory cycle. However, in the preovulatory or nonovulatory cycle, estrogen is the primary determinant in the onset of menstruation. Estrogens also affect the release of pituitary gonadotropins.

The pharmacologic effects of conjugated estrogens are similar to those of endogenous estrogens. The tablets are soluble in water and are well absorbed from the gastrointestinal tract. The injection is soluble in water and may be administered by intravenous or intramuscular injection. The cream is soluble in water and may be absorbed from mucosal surfaces after local administration.

In responsive tissues (female genital organs, breasts, hypothalamus, pituitary) estrogens enter the cell and are transported into the nucleus. As a result of estrogen action, specific RNA and protein synthesis occurs.

Metabolism and inactivation occur primarily in the liver. Some estrogens are excreted into the bile; however, they are reabsorbed from the intestine and returned to the liver through the portal venous system. Water-soluble estrogen conjugates are strongly acidic and, therefore, ionized in body fluids, which favor excretion through the kidneys since tubular reabsorption is minimal.

INDICATIONS AND USAGE:

TABLETS

Conjugated estrogens tablets are indicated in the treatment of:

1. Moderate to severe vasomotor symptoms associated with the menopause. There is no adequate evidence that estrogens are effective for nervous symptoms or depression which might occur during menopause and they should not be used to treat these conditions.
2. Atrophic vaginitis.
3. Osteoporosis (loss of bone mass). The mainstays of prevention and management of osteoporosis are estrogen and calcium; exercise and nutrition may be important adjuncts. Estrogen replacement therapy is the most effective single modality for the prevention of osteoporosis in women. Estrogen reduces bone resorption and retards or halts postmenopausal bone loss. Case-controlled studies have shown an approximately 60-percent reduction in hip and wrist fractures in women whose estrogen replacement was begun within a few years of menopause. Studies also suggest that estrogen reduces the rate of vertebral fractures. Even when started as late as 6 years after menopause, estrogen prevents further loss of bone mass but does not restore it to premenopausal levels. The lowest effective dose for prevention and treatment of osteoporosis should be utilized. (See DOSAGE AND ADMINISTRATION.) Women are at higher risk than men because they have less bone mass, and for several years following natural or induced menopause, the rate of bone mass decline is accelerated. Early menopause is one of the strongest predictors for the development of osteoporosis. White women are at higher risk than black women, and white men are at higher risk than black men. Women who are underweight also have osteoporosis more often than overweight women. Cigarette smoking may be an additional factor in increasing risk. Calcium deficiency has been implicated in the pathogenesis of this disease. Therefore, when not contraindicated, it is recommended that postmenopausal women receive an elemental calcium intake of 1000 to 1500 mg/day. Immobilization and prolonged bed rest produce rapid bone loss, while weight-bearing exercise has been shown both to reduce bone loss and to increase bone mass. The optimal type and amount of physical activity that would prevent osteoporosis have not been established.
4. Hypoestrogenism due to hypogonadism, castration, or primary ovarian failure.
5. Breast cancer (for palliation only) in appropriately selected women and men with metastatic disease.
6. Advanced androgen-dependent carcinoma of the prostate (for palliation only).

INJECTION

Intravenous conjugated estrogens are indicated in the treatment of abnormal uterine bleeding due to hormonal imbalance in the absence of organic pathology.

VAGINAL CREAM

Conjugated estrogens vaginal cream is indicated in the treatment of atrophic vaginitis and kraurosis vulvae.

Conjugated estrogens vaginal cream HAS NOT BEEN SHOWN TO BE EFFECTIVE FOR ANY PURPOSE DURING PREGNANCY AND ITS USE MAY CAUSE SEVERE HARM TO THE FETUS (See BOXED WARNING.)

CONTRAINDICATIONS:

TABLETS

Estrogens should not be used in women (or men) with any of the following conditions:

1. Known or suspected pregnancy (see BOXED WARNING.) Estrogen may cause fetal harm when administered to a pregnant woman.
2. Known or suspected cancer of the breast except in appropriately selected patients being treated for metastatic disease.
3. Known or suspected estrogen-dependent neoplasia.
4. Undiagnosed abnormal genital bleeding.
5. Active thrombophlebitis or thromboembolic disorders.

CONTRAINDICATIONS: *(cont'd)*

6. Women on estrogen replacement therapy have not been reported to have an increased risk of thrombophlebitis and/or thromboembolic disease. However, there is insufficient information regarding women who have had previous thromboembolic disease.

Conjugated estrogens tablets should not be used in patients hypersensitive to their ingredients.

INJECTION AND VAGINAL CREAM

Estrogens should not be used in women with any of the following conditions:

1. Known or suspected cancer of the breast, except in appropriately selected patients being treated for metastatic disease.

2. Known or suspected estrogen-dependent neoplasia.

3. Known or suspected pregnancy (see BOXED WARNING.)

4. Undiagnosed abnormal genital bleeding.

5. Active thrombophlebitis or thromboembolic disorders.

6. A past history of thrombophlebitis, thrombosis, or thromboembolic disorders associated with previous estrogen use (except when used in treatment of breast malignancy).

Conjugated estrogens vaginal cream should not be used in patients hypersensitive to its ingredients.

WARNINGS:

TABLETS

1. Induction Of Malignant Neoplasms: Some studies have suggested a possible increased incidence of breast cancer in those women on estrogen therapy taking higher doses for prolonged periods of time. The majority of studies, however, have not shown an association with the usual doses used for estrogen replacement therapy. Women on this therapy should have regular breast examinations and should be instructed in breast self-examination. The reported endometrial cancer risk among estrogen users was about 4-fold or greater than in nonusers and appears dependent on duration of treatment and on estrogen dose. There is no significant increased risk associated with the use of estrogens for less than one year. The greatest risk appears associated with prolonged use—five years or more. In one study, persistence of risk was demonstrated for 10 years after cessation of estrogen treatment. In another study, a significant decrease in the incidence of endometrial cancer occurred six months after estrogen withdrawal. Estrogen therapy during pregnancy is associated with an increased risk of fetal congenital reproductive-tract disorders. In females there is an increased risk of vaginal adenosis, squamous cell dysplasia of the cervix, and cancer later in life; in the male, urogenital abnormalities. Although some of these changes are benign, it is not known whether they are precursors of malignancy.

2. Gallbladder Disease: A recent study has reported a 2.5-fold increase in the risk of surgically confirmed gallbladder disease in women receiving postmenopausal estrogens.

3. Cardiovascular Disease: Large doses of estrogen (5 mg conjugated estrogens per day), comparable to those used to treat cancer of the prostate and breast, have been shown in a large prospective clinical trial in men to increase the risk of nonfatal myocardial infarction, pulmonary embolism, and thrombophlebitis. It cannot necessarily be extrapolated from men to women. However, to avoid the theoretical cardiovascular risk caused by high estrogen doses, the doses for estrogen replacement therapy should not exceed the recommended dose.

4. Elevated Blood Pressure: There is no evidence that this may occur with use of estrogens in the menopause. However, blood pressure should be monitored with estrogen use, especially if high doses are used.

5. Hypercalcemia: Administration of estrogens may lead to severe hypercalcemia in patients with breast cancer and bone metastases. If this occurs, the drug should be stopped and appropriate measures taken to reduce the serum calcium level.

INJECTION AND VAGINAL CREAM

1. Induction Of Malignant Neoplasms: Long-term, continuous administration of natural and synthetic estrogens in certain animal species increases the frequency of carcinomas of the breast, cervix, vagina, and liver. There are now reports that estrogens increase the risk of carcinoma of the endometrium in humans (see BOXED WARNING.) At the present time there is no satisfactory evidence that estrogens given to postmenopausal women increase the risk of cancer of the breast,[17]although a recent long-term follow-up of a single physician's practice has raised this possibility.[18] Because of the animal data, there is a need for caution in prescribing estrogens for women with a strong family history of breast cancer, or who have breast nodules, fibrocystic disease, or abnormal mammograms.

2. Gallbladder Disease: A recent study has reported a 2- to 3-fold increase in the risk of surgically confirmed gallbladder disease in women receiving postmenopausal estrogens,[17] similar to the 2-fold increase previously noted in users of oral contraceptives.[19,24a]

3. Effects Similar To Those Caused By Estrogen-Progestogen Oral Contraceptives: There are several serious adverse effects of oral contraceptives, most of which have not, up to now, been documented as consequences of postmenopausal estrogen therapy. This may reflect the comparatively low doses of estrogen used in postmenopausal women. It would be expected that the larger doses of estrogen used to treat prostatic or breast cancer are more likely to result in these adverse effects, and, in fact, it has been shown that there is an increased risk of thrombosis in men receiving estrogens for prostatic cancer.[20-23]

a. Thromboembolic Disease: It is now well established that users of oral contraceptives have an increased risk of various thromboembolic and thrombotic vascular diseases, such as thrombophlebitis, pulmonary embolism, stroke, and myocardial infarction.[24-31]Cases of retinal thrombosis, mesenteric thrombosis, and optic neuritis have been reported in oral-contraceptive users. There is evidence that the risk of several of these adverse reactions is related to the dose of the drug.[32,33] An increased risk of postsurgery thromboembolic complications has also been reported in users of oral contraceptives.[34,35] If feasible, estrogen should be discontinued at least 4 weeks before surgery of the type associated with an increased risk of thromboembolism, or during periods of prolonged immobilization. While an increased rate of thromboembolic and thrombotic disease in postmenopausal users of estrogens has not been found,[17-24,25-36]this does not rule out the possibility that such an increase may be present, or that subgroups of women who have underlying risk factors, or who are receiving relatively large doses of estrogens, may have increased risk. Therefore, estrogens should not be used in persons with active thrombophlebitis or thromboembolic disorders, and they should not be used (expect in treatment of malignancy) in persons with a history of such disorders in association with estrogen use. They should be used with caution in patients with cerebral vascular or coronary artery disease and only for those in whom estrogens are clearly needed. Large doses of estrogen (5 mg conjugated estrogens per day), comparable to those used to treat cancer of the prostate and breast, have been shown in a large prospective clinical trial in men[37] to increase the risk of nonfatal myocardial infarction, pulmonary embolism, and thrombophlebitis. When estrogen doses of this size are used, any of the thromboembolic and thrombotic adverse effects associated with oral-contraceptive use should be considered a clear risk.

b. Hepatic Adenoma: Benign hepatic adenomas appear to be associated with the use of oral contraceptives.[38-40] Although benign, and rare, these may rupture and may cause death through intra-abdominal hemorrhage. Such lesions have not yet been reported in association with other estrogen or progestogen preparations but should be considered in estrogen users having abdominal pain and tenderness, abdominal mass, or hypovolemic shock. Hepatocellular carcinoma has also been reported in women taking estrogen-containing oral contraceptives.[39]The relationship of this malignancy to these drugs is not known at this time.

c. Elevated Blood Pressure: Women using oral contraceptives sometimes experience increased blood pressure which, in most cases, returns to normal on discontinuing the drug. There is now a report that this may occur with use of estrogens in the menopause[41] and blood pressure should be monitored with estrogen use, especially if high doses are used.

d. Glucose Tolerance: A worsening of glucose tolerance has been observed in a significant percentage of patients on estrogen-containing oral contraceptives. For this reason, diabetic patients should be carefully observed while receiving estrogen.

4. Hypercalcemia: Administration of estrogens may lead to severe hypercalcemia in patients with breast cancer and bone metastases. If this occurs, the drug should be stopped and appropriate measures taken to reduce the serum calcium level.

PRECAUTIONS:

TABLETS

General

Addition of a progestin: Studies of the addition of a progestin for seven or more days of a cycle of estrogen administration have reported a lowered incidence of endometrial hyperplasia. Morphological and biochemical studies of endometrium suggest that 10 to 13 days of progestin are needed to provide maximal maturation of the endometrium and to eliminate any hyperplastic changes. Whether this will provide protection from endometrial carcinoma has not been clearly established. There are possible additional risks which may be associated with the inclusion of progestin in estrogen replacement regimens. The potential risks include adverse effects on carbohydrate and lipid metabolism. The choice of progestin and dosage may be important in minimizing these adverse effects.

Physical Examination: A complete medical and family history should be taken prior to the initiation of any estrogen therapy. The pretreatment and periodic physical examinations should include special reference to blood pressure, breasts, abdomen, and pelvic organs, and should include a Papanicolaou smear. As a general rule, estrogen should not be prescribed for longer than one year without another physical examination being performed.

Familial Hyperlipoproteinemia: Estrogen therapy may be associated with massive elevations of plasma triglycerides leading to pancreatitis and other complications in patients with familial defects of lipoprotein metabolism.

Fluid Retention: Because estrogens may cause some degree of fluid retention, conditions which might be influenced by this factor, such as asthma, epilepsy, migraine, and cardiac or renal dysfunction, require careful observation.

Uterine Bleeding and Mastodynia: Certain patients may develop undesirable manifestations of estrogenic stimulation, such as abnormal uterine bleeding and mastodynia.

Uterine Fibroids: Preexisting uterine leiomyomata may increase in size during prolonged high-dose estrogen use.

Impaired Liver Function: Estrogens may be poorly metabolized in patients with impaired liver function and should be administered with caution.

Hypercalcemia and Renal Insufficiency: Prolonged use of estrogens can alter the metabolism of calcium and phosphorus. Estrogens should be used with caution in patients with metabolic bone disease.

Information for the Patient

See text of PATIENT PACKAGE INSERTwhich appears before the HOW SUPPLIED section.

Laboratory Tests

Clinical response at the smallest dose should generally be the guide to estrogen administration for relief of symptoms for those indications in which symptoms are observable. However, for prevention and treatment of osteoporosis see DOSAGE AND ADMINISTRATION. Tests used to measure adequacy of estrogen replacement therapy include serum estrone and estradiol levels and suppression of serum gonadotrophin levels.

Drug/Laboratory Test Interactions

Some of these drug/laboratory test interactions have been observed only with estrogen-progestin combinations (oral contraceptives):

1. Increased prothrombin and factors VII, VIII, IX and X; decreased antithrombin 3; increased norepinephrine-induced platelet aggregability, decreased fibrinolysis.

2. Increased thyroid-binding globulin (TBG) leading to increased circulating total thyroid hormone, as measured by T4 levels determined either by column or by radioimmunoassay. Free T3 resin uptake is decreased, reflecting the elevated TBG; free T4 concentration is unaltered.

3. Impaired glucose tolerance.

4. Reduced response to metyrapone test.

5. Reduced serum folate concentration.

Mutagenesis And Carcinogenesis

Long-term continuous administration of natural and synthetic estrogens in certain animal species increases the frequency of carcinomas of the breast, cervix, vagina, and liver.

Pregnancy Category X

Estrogens should not be used during pregnancy. See CONTRAINDICATIONSand BOXED WARNING.

Nursing Mothers

As a general principle, the administration of any drug to nursing mothers should be done only when clearly necessary since many drugs are excreted in human milk.

INJECTION AND VAGINAL CREAM

General: A complete medical and family history should be taken prior to the initiation of any estrogen therapy. The pretreatment and periodic physical examinations should include special reference to blood pressure, breasts, abdomen, and pelvic organs, and should include a Papanicolaou smear. As a general rule, estrogens should not be prescribed for longer than one year without another physical examination being performed.

Fluid Retention: Because estrogens may cause some degree of fluid retention, conditions which might be influenced by this factor, such as asthma, epilepsy, migraine, and cardiac or renal dysfunction, require careful observation.

Familial Hyperlipoprotenemia: Estrogen therapy may be associated with massive elevations of plasma triglycerides leading to pancreatitis and other complications in patients with familial defects of lipoprotein metabolism.

Certain patients may develop undesirable manifestations of excessive estrogenic stimulation, such as abnormal or excessive uterine bleeding, mastodynia, etc.

Vaginal Cream: Prolonged administration of unopposed estrogen therapy has been reported to increase the risk of endometrial hyperplasia in some patients.

PRECAUTIONS: *(cont'd)*

Oral contraceptives appear to be associated with an increased incidence of mental depression.[24a]Although it is not clear whether this is due to the estrogenic or progestogenic component of the contraceptive, patients with a history of depression should be carefully observed.

Preexisting uterine leiomyomata may increase in size during estrogen use.

The pathologist should be advised of estrogen therapy when relevant specimens are submitted.

Patients with a past history of jaundice during pregnancy have an increased risk of recurrence of jaundice while receiving estrogen-containing oral-contraceptive therapy. If jaundice develops in any patient receiving estrogen, the medication should be discontinued while the cause is investigated.

Estrogens may be poorly metabolized in patients with impaired liver function and should be administered with caution in such patients.

Because estrogens influence the metabolism of calcium and phosphorus, they should be used with caution in patients with metabolic bone diseases that are associated with hypercalcemia or in patients with renal insufficiency.

Because of the effects of estrogens on epiphyseal closure, they should be used judiciously in young patients in whom bone growth is not yet complete.

Vaginal Cream: *Concomitant Progestin Use:* The lowest effective dose appropriate for the specific indication should be utilized. Studies of the addition of a progestin for 7 or more days of a cycle of estrogen administration have reported a lowered incidence of endometrial hyperplasia. Morphological and biochemical studies of the endometrium suggest that 10 to 13 days of progestin are needed to provide maximal maturation of the endometrium and to eliminate any hyperplastic changes. Whether this will provide protection from endometrial carcinoma has not been clearly established. There are possible additional risks which may be associated with the inclusion of a progestin in estrogen replacement regimens. If concomitant progestin therapy is used, potential risks may include adverse effects on carbohydrate and lipid metabolism. The choice of progestin and dosage may be important in minimizing these adverse effects.

Information for the Patient: See PATIENT PACKAGE INSERT.

Drug/Laboratory Tests Interactions: Certain endocrine and liver function tests may be affected by estrogen-containing oral contraceptives. The following similar changes may be expected with larger doses of estrogen:

Increased sulfobromophthalein retention.

Increased prothrombin and factors VII, VIII, IX, and X; decreased antithrombin 3; increased norepinephrine-induced platelet aggregability.

Increased thyroid binding globulin (TBG) leading to increased circulating total thyroid hormone, as measured by PBI, $T_4$by column, or T_4 by radioimmunoassay. Free T_3 resin uptake is decreased, reflecting the elevated TBG; free T_4 concentration is unaltered.

Impaired glucose tolerance.

Decreased pregnanediol excretion.

Reduced response to metyrapone test.

Reduced serum folate concentration.

Increased serum triglyceride and phospholipid concentration.

Carcinogenesis, Mutagenesis, and Impairment of Fertility: See WARNINGSfor information on carcinogenesis.

Pregnancy Category X (See CONTRAINDICATIONSand BOXED WARNING.)

Nursing Mothers: It is not known whether this drug is excreted in human milk. Because many drugs are excreted in human milk and because of the potential for serious adverse reactions in nursing infants from estrogens, a decision should be made whether to discontinue nursing or to discontinue the drug, taking into account the importance of the drug to the mother.

Pediatric Use: Safety and effectiveness in children have not been established.

INJECTION

Certain endocrine and liver function tests may be affected by estrogen-containing oral contraceptives. The following similar changes may be expected with larger doses of estrogen:

Increased sulfobromophthalein retention.

Increased prothrombin and factors VII, VIII, IX, and X; decreased antithrombin 3; increased norepinephrine-induced platelet aggregability.

Increased thyroid binding globulin (TBG) leading to increased circulating total thyroid hormone, as measured by PBI, T4 by column, or T4 by radioimmunoassay. Free T3 resin uptake is decreased, reflecting the elevated TBG; free T4 concentration is unaltered.

Impaired glucose tolerance.

Decreased pregnanediol excretion.

Reduced response to metyrapone test.

Reduced serum folate concentration.

Increased serum triglyceride and phospholipid concentration.

ADVERSE REACTIONS:

TABLETS

See WARNINGS regarding induction of neoplasia, adverse effects on the fetus, increased incidence of gallbladder disease. The following additional adverse reactions have been reported with estrogen therapy.

Genitourinary system: Changes in vaginal bleeding pattern and abnormal withdrawal bleeding or flow. Breakthrough bleeding, spotting. Increase in size of uterine fibromyomata. Vaginal candidiasis. Change in amount of cervical secretion.

Breasts: Tenderness, enlargement.

Gastrointestinal: Nausea, vomiting; abdominal cramps, bloating; cholestatic jaundice.

Skin: Chloasma or melasma that may persist when drug is discontinued; erythema multiforme; erythema nodosum; hemorrhagic eruption; loss of scalp hair; hirsutism.

Eyes: Steepening of corneal curvature; intolerance of contact lenses.

CNS: Headache, migraine, dizziness; mental depression; chorea.

Miscellaneous: Increase or decrease in weight; reduced carbohydrate tolerance; aggravation of porphyria; edema; changes in libido.

INJECTION AND VAGINAL CREAM

See WARNINGS regarding induction of neoplasia, adverse effects on the fetus, increased incidence of gallbladder disease, and adverse effects similar to those of oral contraceptives, including thromboembolism. The following additional adverse reactions have been reported with estrogenic therapy, including oral contraceptives:

Genitourinary system: Breakthrough bleeding, spotting, change in menstrual flow; dysmenorrhea; premenstrual-like syndrome; amenorrhea during and after treatment; increase in size of uterine fibromyomata; vaginal candidiasis; change in cervical erosion and in degree of cervical secretion; cystitis-like syndrome.

ADVERSE REACTIONS: *(cont'd)*

Breasts: Tenderness, enlargement, secretion.

Gastrointestinal: Nausea, vomiting, abdominal cramps, bloating; cholestatic jaundice, pancreatitis.

Skin: Chloasma or melasma which may persist when drug is discontinued; erythema multiforme; erythema nodosum; hemorrhagic eruption; loss of scalp hair; hirsutism.

Eyes: Steepening of corneal curvature; intolerance to contact lenses.

CNS: Headache, migraine, dizziness; mental depression; chorea.

Miscellaneous: Increase or decrease in weight; reduced carbohydrate tolerance; aggravation of porphyria; edema; changes in libido.

OVERDOSAGE:

ACUTE OVERDOSAGE

Tablets: Numerous reports of ingestion of large doses of estrogen-containing oral contraceptives by young children indicate that acute serious ill effects do not occur. Overdosage of estrogen may cause nausea and vomiting.

Injection and Vaginal Cream: Numerous reports of ingestion of large doses of estrogen-containing oral contraceptives by young children indicate that acute serious ill effects do not occur. Overdosage of estrogens may cause nausea, and withdrawal bleeding may occur in females.

DOSAGE AND ADMINISTRATION:

TABLETS

For treatment of moderate to severe vasomotor symptoms and atrophic vaginitis associated with the menopause. The lowest dose that will control symptoms should be chosen, and medication should be discontinued as promptly as possible.

Attempts to discontinue or taper medication should be made at 3-month to 6-month intervals.

Usual Dosage Ranges: Vasomotor symptoms—1.25 mg daily. If the patient has not menstruated within the last two months or more, cyclic administration is started arbitrarily. If the patient is menstruating, cyclic (*e.g.,* three weeks on and one week off) administration is started on day 5 of bleeding.

Atrophic Vaginitis: 0.3 mg to 1.25 mg or more daily, depending upon the tissue response of the individual patient. Administer cyclically.

Hypoestrogenism Due To

Female Hypogonadism: 2.5 mg to 7.5 mg daily, in divided doses for 20 days, followed by a rest period of 10 days' duration. If bleeding does not occur by the end of this period, the same dosage schedule is repeated. The number of courses of estrogen therapy necessary to produce bleeding may vary depending on the responsiveness of the endometrium.

If bleeding occurs before the end of the 10-day period, begin a 20-day estrogen-progestin cyclic regimen with conjugated estrogens, 2.5 mg to 7.5 mg daily in divided doses, for 20 days. During the last five days of estrogen therapy, give an oral progestin. If bleeding occurs before this regimen is concluded, therapy is discontinued and may be resumed on the fifth day of bleeding.

Female Castration Or Primary Ovarian Failure: 1.25 mg daily, cyclically. Adjust dosage, upward or downward, according to severity of symptoms and response of the patient. For maintenance, adjust dosage to lowest level that will provide effective control.

Osteoporosis (Loss Of Bone Mass): 0.625 mg daily. Administration should be cyclic (*e.g.,* three weeks on and one week off).

Advanced Androgen-Dependent Carcinoma Of The Prostate, For Palliation Only

1.25 mg to 2.5 mg three times daily. The effectiveness of therapy can be judged by phosphatase determinations as well as by symptomatic improvement of the patient.

Breast cancer (for palliation only) in appropriately selected women and men with metastatic disease. Suggested dosage is 10 mg three times daily for a period of at least three months.

Treated patients with an intact uterus should be monitored closely for signs of endometrial cancer, and appropriate diagnostic measures should be taken to rule out malignancy in the event of persistent or recurring abnormal vaginal bleeding.

Store at room temperature (approximately 25° C)

Dispense in a well-closed container as defined in the USP

INJECTION

Abnormal Uterine Bleeding Due To Hormonal Imbalance: One 25 mg injection, intravenously or intramuscularly. Intravenous use is preferred since more rapid response can be expected from this mode of administration.

Repeat in 6 to 12 hours if necessary. The use of conjugated estrogens intravenous for injection does not preclude the advisability of other appropriate measures.

The usual precautionary measures governing intravenous administration should be adhered to. Injection should be made SLOWLY to obviate the occurrence of flushes.

Infusion of conjugated estrogens intravenous for injection with other agents is not generally recommended. In emergencies, however, when an infusion has already been started it may be expedient to make the injection into the tubing just distal to the infusion needle. If so used, compatibility of solutions must be considered.

Compatibility of solutions: Conjugated estrogens intravenous is compatible with normal saline, dextrose, and invert sugar solutions. IT IS NOT COMPATIBLE WITH PROTEIN HYDROLYSATE, ASCORBIC ACID, OR ANY SOLUTION WITH AN ACID pH.

Treated patients with an intact uterus should be monitored closely for signs of endometrial cancer, and appropriate diagnostic measures should be taken to rule out malignancy in the event of persistent or recurring abnormal vaginal bleeding.

DIRECTIONS FOR STORAGE AND RECONSTITUTION

Storage Before Reconstitution: Store package in refrigerator, 2°-8° C (36°-46° F).

To Reconstitute: First withdraw air from Secule vial so as to facilitate introduction of sterile diluent. Then, flow the sterile diluent slowly against side of Secule vial and agitate gently. DO NOT SHAKE VIOLENTLY.

Storage After Reconstitution: It is common practice to utilize the reconstituted solution within a few hours. If it is necessary to keep the reconstituted solution for more than a few hours, store the reconstituted solution under refrigeration (2°-8° C). Under these conditions, the solution is stable for 60 days, and is suitable for use unless darkening or precipitation occurs.

VAGINAL CREAM

Given Cyclically For Short-Term Use Only: For treatment of atrophic vaginitis, or kraurosis vulvae.

The lowest dose that will control symptoms should be chosen and medication should be discontinued as promptly as possible.

Administration should be cyclic (*e.g.,* three weeks on and one week off).

Attempts to discontinue or taper medication should be made at three- to six-month intervals.

DOSAGE AND ADMINISTRATION: *(cont'd)*

Usual Dosage Range: 1/2 to 2 g daily, intravaginally, depending on the severity of the condition. Treated patients with an intact uterus should be monitored closely for signs of endometrial cancer, and appropriate diagnostic measures should be taken to rule out malignancy in the event of persistent or recurring abnormal vaginal bleeding.

Instructions For Use Of Gentle Measure Applicator:

1. Remove cap from tube.

2. Screw nozzle end of applicator onto tube.

3. *Gently* squeeze tube from the *bottom* to force sufficient cream into the barrel to provide the prescribed dose. Use the marked stopping points on the applicator as a guideline to measure the correct dose.

4. Unscrew applicator from tube.

5. Lie on back with knees drawn up. To deliver medication, gently insert applicator deeply into vagina and press plunger downward to its original position.

TO CLEANSE: Pull plunger to remove it from barrel. Wash with mild soap and warm water.**Do not boil or use hot water.**

Store at room temperature (approximately 25° C).

REFERENCES:

1. Ziel, H.K. et al: N. Engl. J. Med. *293:*1167-1170, 1975. **2.** Smith, D.C. et al: N. Engl. J. Med. *293:*1164- 1167, 1975. **3.** Mack, T.M. et al: N. Engl. J. Med.*294:*1262-1267, 1976. **4.** Weiss, N.S. et al: N. Engl. J. Med. *294:*1259-1262, 1976. **5.** Herbst, A.L. et al: N. Engl. J. Med. *284:*878-881, 1971. **6.** Greenwald, P. et al: N. Engl. J. Med. *285:*390-392, 1971. **7.** Lanier, A. et al: Mayo Clin. Proc. *48:*793-799, 1973. **8.** Herbst, A. et al: Obstet. Gynecol. *40:*287-298, 1972. **9.** Herbst, A. et al: Am. J. Obstet. Gynecol. *118:*607-615, 1974. **10.** Herbst, A. et al: N. Engl. J. Med. *292:*334-339, 1975. **11.** Stafl, A. et al: Obstet. Gynecol. *43:*118-128, 1974. **12.** Sherman, A.I. et al: Obstet. Gynecol. *44:*531-545, 1974. **13.** Gal, I. et al: Nature *216:*83, 1967. **14.** Levy, E.P. et al: Lancet *1:*611, 1973. **15.** Nora, J. et al: Lancet*1:*941-942, 1973. **16.** Janerich, D.T. et al: N. Engl. J. Med. *291:*697-700, 1974. **17.** Boston Collaborative Drug Surveillance Program: N. Engl. J. Med. *290:*15-19, 1974. **18.** Hoover, R. et al: N. Engl. J. Med. *295:*401-405, 1976. **19.** Boston Collaborative Drug Surveillance Program: Lancet.*1:*1399-1404, 1973. **20.** Daniel, D.G. et al: Lancet*2:*287-289, 1967. **21.** The Veterans Administration Cooperative Urological Research Group: J. Urol. *98:*516-522, 1967. **22.** Bailar, J.C.: Lancet *2:*560, 1967. **23.** Blackard, C. et al: Cancer *26:*249-256, 1970. **24.** Royal College of General Practitioners: J.R. Coll. Gen. Pract. *13:*267- 279, 1967. **24a.**Royal College of General Practitioners: Oral Contraceptives and Health, New York, Pitman Corp., 1974. **25.** Inman, W.H.W. et al: Br. Med. J. *2:*193-199, 1968. **26.** Vessey, M.P. et al: Br. Med. J. *2:*651-657, 1969. **27.** Sartwell, P.E. et al: Am. J. Epidemiol. *90:*365-380, 1969. **28.** Collaborative Group for the Study of Stroke in Young Women: N. Engl. J. Med. *288:*871-878, 1973. **29.** Collaborative Group for the Study of Stroke in Young Women: J.A.M.A. *231:*718-722, 1975. **30.** Mann, J.I. et al: Br. Med. J. *2:*245-248, 1975. **31.** Mann, J.I. et al: Br. Med. J. *2:*241-245, 1975. **32.** Inman, W.H.W. et al: Br. Med. J. *2:*203-209, 1970. **33.** Stolley, P.D. et al: Am. J. Epidemiol. *102:*197-208, 1975. **34.** Vessey, M.P. et al: Br. Med. J. *3:*123-126, 1970. **35.** Greene, G.R. et al: Am. J. Public Health*62:*680-685, 1972. **36.** Rosenberg, L. et al: N. Engl. J. Med. *294:*1256-1259, 1976. **37.** Coronary Drug Project Research Group: J.A.M.A. *214:*1303-1313, 1970. **38.** Baum, J. et al: Lancet *2:*926-928, 1973. **39.** Mays, E.T. et al: J.A.M.A. *235:*730-732, 1976. **40.** Edmondson, H.A. et al: N. Engl. J. Med. *294:*470-472, 1976. **41.** Pfeffer, R.I. et al: Am. J. Epidemiol. *103:*445-456, 1976.

PATIENT PACKAGE INSERT:

WHAT YOU SHOULD KNOW ABOUT ESTROGENS

Estrogens are female hormones produced by the ovaries. The ovaries make several different kinds of estrogens. In addition, scientists have been able to make a variety of synthetic estrogens. As far as we know, all these estrogens have similar properties and, therefore, much the same usefulness, side effects, and risks. This leaflet is intended to help you understand what estrogens are used for, the risks involved in their use, and how to use them as safely as possible.

This leaflet includes the most important information about estrogens, but not all the information. If you want to know more, you should ask your doctor for more information, or you can ask your doctor or pharmacist to let you read the package insert prepared for the doctor.

USES OF ESTROGEN

THERE IS NO PROPER USE OF ESTROGENS IN A PREGNANT WOMAN.

Estrogens are prescribed by doctors for a number of purposes, including:

1. To provide estrogen during a period of adjustment when a woman's ovaries stop producing a majority of her estrogens, in order to prevent certain uncomfortable symptoms of estrogen deficiency. (With the menopause, which generally occurs between the ages of 45 and 55, women produce a much smaller amount of estrogens.)

2. To prevent symptoms of estrogen deficiency when a woman's ovaries have been removed surgically before the natural menopause.

3. To prevent pregnancy. (Estrogens are given along with a progestogen, another female hormone; these combinations are called oral contraceptives, or birth-control pills. Patient labeling is available to women taking oral contraceptives and they will not be discussed in this leaflet.)

4. To treat certain cancers in women and men.

ESTROGENS IN THE MENOPAUSE

In the natural course of their lives, all women eventually experience a decrease in estrogen production. This usually occurs between ages 45 and 55, but may occur earlier or later. Sometimes the ovaries may need to be removed before natural menopause by an operation, producing a "surgical menopause."

When the amount of estrogen in the blood begins to decrease, many women may develop typical symptoms: feelings of warmth in the face, neck, and chest, or sudden intense episodes of heat and sweating throughout the body (called "hot flashes" or "hot flushes"). These symptoms are sometimes very uncomfortable. Some women may also develop changes in the vagina (called "atrophic vaginitis") that cause discomfort, especially during and after intercourse.

Estrogens can be prescribed to treat these symptoms of the menopause. It is estimated that considerably more than half of all women undergoing the menopause have only mild symptoms or no symptoms at all and, there fore, do not need estrogens. Other women may need estrogens for a few months, while their bodies adjust to lower estrogen levels. Sometimes the need will be for periods longer than six months. In an attempt to avoid overstimulation of the uterus (womb), estrogens are usually given cyclically during each month of use, such as three weeks of pills followed by one week without pills.

Sometimes women experience nervous symptoms or depression during menopause. There is no evidence that estrogens are effective for such symptoms without associated vasomotor symptoms. In the absence of vasomotor symptoms, estrogens should not be used to treat nervous symptoms, although other treatment may be needed.

You may have heard that taking estrogens for long periods (years) after the menopause will keep your skin soft and supple and keep you feeling young. There is no evidence that this is so, however, and such long-term treatment carries important risks.

THE DANGERS OF ESTROGENS

Endometrial Cancer: There are reports that if estrogens are used in the postmenopausal period for more than a year, there is an increased risk of endometrial cancer (cancer of the lining of the uterus). Women taking estrogens have roughly 5- to 1 0-times as great a chance of getting this cancer as women who take no estrogens. To put this another way, while a postmenopausal woman not taking estrogens has 1 chance in 1,000 each year of getting endometrial cancer, a woman taking estrogens has 5 to 10 chances in 1,000 each year. For this reason it is important to take estrogens only when they are really needed. The risk of this cancer is greater the longer estrogens are used and when larger doses are taken. Therefore, you should

PATIENT PACKAGE INSERT: *(cont'd)*

not take more estrogen than your doctor prescribes. It is important to take the lowest dose of estrogen that will control symptoms and to take it only as long as it is needed. If estrogens are needed for longer periods of time, your doctor will want to reevaluate your need for estrogens at least every six months. Women using estrogens should report any vaginal bleeding to their doctors; such bleeding may be of no importance, but it can be an early warning of endometrial cancer. If you have undiagnosed vaginal bleeding, you should not use estrogens until a diagnosis is made and you are certain there is no endometrial cancer. Note: If you have had your uterus removed (total hysterectomy), there is no danger of developing endometrial cancer.

Other Possible Cancers: Estrogens can cause development of other tumors in animals, such as tumors of the breast, cervix, vagina, or liver, when given for a long time. At present there is no good evidence that women using estrogens in the menopause have an increased risk of such tumors, but there is no way yet to be sure they do not; and one study raises the possibility that use of estrogens in the menopause may increase the risk of breast cancer many years later This is a further reason to use estrogens only when clearly needed. While you are taking estrogens, it is important that you go to your doctor at least once a year for a physical examination. Also, if members of your family have had breast cancers, or if you have breast nodules, or abnormal mammograms (breast X rays), your doctor may wish to carry out more frequent examinations of your breasts.

Gallbladder Disease: Women who use estrogens after menopause are more likely to develop gallbladder disease needing surgery than women who do not use estrogens. Birth-control pills have a similar effect.

Abnormal Blood Clotting: Oral contraceptives increase the risk of blood clotting in various parts of the body. This can result in a stroke (if the clot is in the brain), a heart attack (a clot in a blood vessel of the heart), or a pulmonary embolus (a clot which forms in the legs or pelvis, then breaks off and travels to the lungs). Any of these can be fatal. At this time, use of estrogens in the menopause is not known to cause such blood clotting, but this has not been fully studied and there could still prove to be such a risk. It is recommended that if you have had clotting in the legs or lungs, or a heart attack or stroke, while you were using estrogens or birth-control pills, you should not use estrogens (unless they are being used to treat cancer of the breast or prostate). If you have had a stroke or heart attack, or if you have angina pectoris, estrogens should be used with great caution and only if clearly needed for example, if you have severe symptoms of the menopause).

SPECIAL WARNING ABOUT PREGNANCY

You should not receive estrogen if you are pregnant. If this should occur, there is a greater than usual chance that the developing child will be born with a birth defect, although the possibility remains fairly small. A female child may have an increased risk of developing cancer of the vagina or cervix later in life (in the teens or twenties). Every possible effort should be made to avoid exposure to estrogens during pregnancy. If exposure occurs, see your doctor.

OTHER EFFECTS OF ESTROGENS

In addition to the serious known risks of estrogens described above, estrogens have the following side effects and potential risks:

Nausea And Vomiting: The most common side effect of estrogen therapy is nausea. Vomiting is less common.

Effects On Breasts: Estrogens may cause breast tenderness or enlargement and may cause the breasts to secrete a liquid. These effects are not dangerous.

Effects On The Uterus: Estrogens may cause benign fibroid tumors of the uterus to get larger.

Effects On Liver: Women taking oral contraceptives develop, on rare occasions, a tumor of the liver which can rupture and bleed into the abdomen and may cause death. So far, these tumors have not been reported in women using estrogens in the menopause, but you should report any swelling or unusual pain or tenderness in the abdomen to your doctor immediately. Women with a past history of jaundice (yellowing of the skin and white parts of the eyes) may get jaundice again during estrogen use. If this occurs, stop taking estrogens and see your doctor.

Other Effects: Estrogens may cause excess fluid to be retained in the body. This may make some conditions worse, such as asthma, epilepsy, migraine, heart disease, or kidney disease.

SUMMARY

Estrogens have important uses, but they have serious risks as well. You must decide, with your doctor, whether the risks are acceptable to you in view of the benefits of treatment. Except where your doctor has prescribed estrogens for use in special cases of cancer of the breast or prostate, you should not use estrogens if you have cancer of the breast or uterus, are pregnant, have undiagnosed abnormal vaginal bleeding, clotting in the legs or lungs, or have had a stroke, heart attack or angina, or clotting in the legs or lungs in the past while you were taking estrogens.

You can use estrogens as safely as possible by understanding that your doctor will require regular physical examinations while you are taking them, will try to discontinue the drug as soon as possible, and will use the smallest dose possible. Be alert for signs of trouble including:

Abnormal bleeding from the vagina.

Pains in the calves or chest, sudden shortness of breath, or coughing blood.

Severe headache, dizziness, faintness, or changes in vision.

Breast lumps (you should ask your doctor how to examine your own breasts).

Jaundice (yellowing of the skin).

Mental depression.

Your doctor has prescribed this drug for you and you alone. Do not give the drug to anyone.

HOW SUPPLIED:

TABLETS

Premarin (conjugated estrogens tablets, USP): each oval purple tablet contains 2.5 mg, each oval yellow tablet contains 1.25 mg, each oval white tablet contains 0.625 mg, each oval maroon tablet contains 0.625 mg, each oval green tablet contains 0.3 mg, each oval white (dye-free) tablet contains 0.625 mg. The appearance on these tablets is a trademark of Wyeth-Ayerst Laboratories.

INJECTION

Each package provides: (1) One Secule vial containing 25 mg of conjugated estrogens, USP, for injection (also lactose 200 mg, sodium citrate 12.2 mg, and simethicone 0.2 mg). The pH is adjusted with sodium hydroxide or hydrochloric acid. (2) One 5 ml ampul sterile diluent with 2% benzyl alcohol in sterile water.

Premarin Intravenous (conjugated estrogens, USP) for injection is prepared by cryodesiccation.

Secule—Registered trademark to designate a vial containing an injectable preparation in dry form.

VAGINAL CREAM

Premarin (conjugated estrogens) Vaginal Cream: Each gram contains 0.625 mg conjugated estrogens, USP.

HOW SUPPLIED: *(cont'd)*

Combination package: Each contains Net Wt. 1 1/2 oz (42.5 g) tube with one plastic applicator calibrated in 1/2 g increments to a maximum of 2 g.
Refill Package: Each contains Net Wt. 1 1/2 oz (42.5 g) tube.

HOW SUPPLIED - EQUIVALENTS NOT AVAILABLE:

Cream - Topical; Vagina - 0.625 mg/gm

45 gm	$29.15	PREMARIN, Ayerst	00046-0872-01
45 gm	$32.46	PREMARIN, Ayerst	00046-0872-93

Injection, Lyphl-Soln - Intramuscular; - 25 mg/5ml

5 ml	$32.11	PREMARIN 25, Ayerst	00046-0749-05
30 ml	$3.00	LANESTRIN, Lannett	00527-0119-58

Tablet, Sugar Coated - Oral - 0.3 mg

100's	$28.31	PREMARIN, Ayerst	00046-0868-81
1000's	$273.05	PREMARIN, Ayerst	00046-0868-91

Tablet, Sugar Coated - Oral - 0.625 mg

100's	$39.45	PREMARIN, Ayerst	00046-0867-81
100's	$39.45	PREMARIN, Ayerst	00046-3867-81
100's	$42.41	PREMARIN, Ayerst	00046-0867-99
1000's	$380.20	PREMARIN, Ayerst	00046-0867-91
5000's	$1854.50	PREMARIN, Ayerst	00046-0867-95

Tablet, Sugar Coated - Oral - 0.9 mg

100's	$46.73	PREMARIN, Ayerst	00046-0864-81

Tablet, Sugar Coated - Oral - 1.25 mg

100's	$53.99	PREMARIN, Ayerst	00046-0866-81
100's	$56.68	PREMARIN, Ayerst	00046-0866-99
1000's	$520.48	PREMARIN, Ayerst	00046-0866-91
5000's	$2538.85	PREMARIN, Ayerst	00046-0866-95

Tablet, Sugar Coated - Oral - 2.5 mg

100's	$93.49	PREMARIN 2.5, Ayerst	00046-0865-81
1000's	$901.77	PREMARIN 2.5, Ayerst	00046-0865-91

ESTROGENS, CONJUGATED; MEDROXYPROGESTERONE ACETATE *(003239)*

CATEGORIES: Hormonal Imbalance; Hormones; Menopause; Osteoporosis; Ovarian Failure; Progestins; Pregnancy Category X; FDA Approved 1994 Dec; Top 200 Drugs

BRAND NAMES: *Menoprem Continuous* (Australia); *Premaril Plus*; Premarin MPA; *Premarin Pak* (Mexico); Premphase; **Prempro**; *Provette Continuous*
(International brand names outside U.S. in italics)

FORMULARIES: PCS

> **WARNING:**
> ESTROGENS HAVE BEEN REPORTED TO INCREASE THE RISK OF ENDOMETRIAL CARCINOMA IN POSTMENOPAUSAL WOMEN. THIS FINDING REFERS TO ESTROGENS GIVEN WITHOUT PROGESTIN.
> Progestins taken with estrogen drugs significantly reduce but do not eliminate this risk. Close clinical surveillance of all women taking estrogens is important. Adequate diagnostic measures, including endometrial sampling when indicated, should be undertaken to rule out malignancy in all cases of undiagnosed persistent or recurring abnormal vaginal bleeding. There is no evidence that "natural" estrogens are more or less hazardous than "synthetic" estrogens at equiestrogenic doses.
> ESTROGENS/PROGESTINS SHOULD NOT BE USED DURING PREGNANCY.
> There is no indication for estrogen therapy during pregnancy or during the immediate postpartum period. Estrogen therapy during pregnancy os associated with an increased risk of congenital defects in the reproductive organs of the fetus, and possibly other birth defects. Estrogens are not indicated for the prevention of partum breast enlargement.
> Studies of women who received diethylstilbestrol (DES) during pregnancy have shown that female offspring have an increased risk of vaginal adenosis, squamous cell dysplasia of the uterine cervix, and clear cell vaginal cancer later in life. The 1985 DES Task Force concluded that use of DES during pregnancy is associated with subsequent increased risk of breast cancer in the mothers, although a casual relationship remains unproven and the observed level of excess risk is similar to that for a number of other breast cancer risk factors.
> Several reports also suggest an association between intrauterine exposure to progestational drugs in the first trimester of pregnancy and genital abnormalities in male and female fetuses. The risk of hypospadias, 5 to 8 per 1000 male births in the general population, may be approximately doubled with exposure to these drugs. There are insufficient data to quantify the risk to exposed female fetuses; some of these drugs induce mild virilization of the external genitalia of the female fetus. If the patient is exposed to Prempro/Premphase (conjugated estrogens/medroxyprogesterone acetate) during pregnancy, or if she becomes pregnant while taking these drugs, she should be apprised of the potential risk to the fetus.
> Estrogens are ineffective for the prevention or treatment of threatened or habitual abortion. There is no adequate evidence that progestational agents are effective in preventing habitual abortion when such drugs are given during the first trimester of pregnancy. Furthermore, in the vast majority of women, the cause of abortion is a defective ovum, which progestational agents could not be expected to influence. In addition, the use of progestational agents with their uterine-relaxant properties, in patients with fertilized defective ova, may cause a delay in spontaneous abortion.

DESCRIPTION:

Prempro therapy consists of two separate tablets: Premarin brand of conjugated estrogens 0.625 mg tablets, and Cycrin brand of medroxyprogesterone acetate (MPA), 2.5 mg tablets, for oral administration.

DESCRIPTION: *(cont'd)*

Premarin is a mixture of sodium estrone sulfate and sodium equilin sulfate. It contains as concomitant components sodium sulfate conjugates 17α-estradiol and 17α-estradiol and 17β-dihydroequilin. Each tablet for oral administration contains 0.625 mg of conjugated estrogens and the following inactive ingredients: calcium phosphate tribasic, calcium sulfate, carnauba wax, cellulose, glycerol monooleate, lactose, magnesium stearate, methylcellulose, pharmaceutical glaze, polyethylene glycol, stearic acid, titanium dioxide, FD&C Blue No. 2, D&C Red No. 27, FD&C Red No. 40.

Cycrin contains medroxyprogesterone acetate, a derivative of progesterone. It is white to off-white, odorless, crystalline powder, stable in air, melting between 200° C and 210° C. It is freely soluble in chloroform, soluble in acetone and in dioxane, sparingly soluble in alcohol and in methanol, slightly soluble in ether, and insoluble in water. The chemical name for MPA is pregn-4-ene-3,20-dione, 17-(acetyloxy)-6-methyl-, (6α)-, Cycrin is available in tablet form for oral administration and is given in combination with Premarin at a dose of 2.5 mg. Each white, oval tablet contains 2.5 mg of MPA and the following inactive ingredients: lactose, magnesium stearate, methylcellulose, microcrystalline cellulose.

Premphase therapy consists of two separate tablets: Premarin brand of conjugated estrogens, 0.625 mg tablets which are taken orally for 28 days, and Cycrin brand of medroxyprogesterone acetate (MPA), 5.0 mg tablets which are taken orally with a Premarin tablet on days 15 through 28.

Premarin is a mixture of sodium estrone sulfate and sodium equilin sulfate. It contains as concomitant components sodium sulfate conjugates 17α-dihydroequilin, 17α-estradiol and 17β-dihydroequilin. Each tablet for oral administration contains 0.625 mg of conjugated estrogens and the following inactive ingredients: calcium phosphate tribasic, calcium sulfate, carnauba wax, cellulose, glycerol monooleate, lactose, magnesium stearate, methylcellulose, pharmaceutical glaze, polyethylene glycol, stearic acid, sucrose, titanium dioxide, FD&C Blue No. 2, D&C Red No.27, FD&C Red No. 40.

Cycrin contains medroxyprogesterone acetate, a derivative of progesterone. It is a white to off-white, odorless crystalline powder, stable in air, melting between 200° C and 210° C. It is freely soluble in chloroform, soluble in acetone and in dioxane, sparingly soluble in alcohol and in methanol, slightly soluble in ether and insoluble in water. The chemical name for MPA is pregn-4-ene-3,20-dione, 17-(acetyloxy)-6-methyl-, (6α)-. Cycrin is available in tablet form for oral administration. Each light-purple, oval tablet contains 5.0 mg of MPA and the following inactive ingredients; lactose, magnesium stearate, methylcellulose, microcrystalline cellulose, D&C Red No. 30 and FD&C Blue No. 1.

CLINICAL PHARMACOLOGY:

Estrogens are important in the development and maintenance of the female reproductive system and secondary sex characteristics. By a direct action, they cause growth and development of the uterus, fallopian tubes, and vagina. With other hormones, such as pituitary hormones and progesterone, they cause enlargement of the breasts through promotion of ductal growth, stromal development, and the accretion of fat.

Estrogens are intricately involved with other hormones, especially progesterone, in the processes of the ovulatory menstrual cycle and pregnancy and affect the release of pituitary gonadotropins. They also contribute to the shaping of the skeleton, maintenance of tone and elasticity of urogenital structures, changes in the epiphyses of the long bones that allow for the pubertal growth spurt and its termination, and pigmentation of the nipples and genitals.

The use of unopposed estrogen therapy has been associated with an increased risk of endometrial hyperplasia, a possible precursor of endometrial adenocarcinoma. The results of clinical studies indicate that the addition of a progestin to an estrogen replacement regimen for more than 10 days per cycle reduces the incidence of endometrial hyperplasia and the attendant risk of adenocarcinoma in women with intact uteri. The addition of a progestin to an estrogen replacement regimen has not been shown to interfere with the efficacy of estrogen replacement therapy for its approved indications. Data from a large clinical trial indicate that MPA administered in the recommended dose to women receiving Premarin 0.625 mg reduces the incidence of hyperplastic changes and hence reduces the risk of developing adenocarcinoma. This is the clinical rationale for Prempro/Premphase.

The following table summarizes the incidence of endometrial hyperplasia after 1 year treatment with the combined regimens. (TABLE 1).

TABLE 1 Incidence Of Endometrial Hyperplasia After One Year Of Treatment

	Dose Groups	
Patient	**PREMPRO 0.625 mg/2.5 mg**	**Premarin 0.625 mg**
Total number of patients	279	283
No. (%) of patients with biopsies •all focal and non-focal hyperplasia	2(<1)*	57 (20)
•excluding focal cystic hyperplasia	2(<1)*	25 (8)

* Significant (p<0.001) in comparison with Premarin alone (0.625 mg).

Information Regarding Lipid Effects: The results of a clinical trial conducted in a 97% Caucasian population at low risk fore cardiovascular disease show that Prempro/Premphase increases HDL-C and the HDL_2-C subfraction significantly less than Premarin alone, but lower after 1 year of treatment than at baseline, the HDL/Total Cholesterol ratio showed a significantly smaller rise with Prempro than with Premarin alone.

The following table summarizes the incidence of endometrial hyperplasia after 1 year of treatment with the combined regimens. (TABLE 2)

TABLE 2 Mean Percent Change From Baseline Lipid Profile Values After One Year

	Dose Groups	
Lipid Parameter	**PREMPRO 0.625 mg/2.5 mg**	**Premarin 0.625 mg**
Total Cholesterol	-4.7*,†	0.2
HDL/Total Cholesterol ratio	9.1*,†	14.2*
HDL-C	3.5*,†	14.1*
HDL_2-C	34.7*,†	70.8*
LDL-C	-10.3*,†	-7.7*
Triglycerides	24.1*,†	39.4*

* Significantly ($p \leq 0.05$) different from baseline value.
†Significantly ($p \leq 0.05$) different from Premarin alone.

The pharmacologic effects of the administered conjugated estrogens are similar to those of endogenous estrogens. In responsive tissue (female genital organs, breasts, hypothalamus, pituitary) estrogens enter the cell and are transported into the nucleus. As a result of the estrogen action, specific RNA and protein synthesis occurs.

Androgenic and anabolic effects of MPA have been noted, but the drug is apparently devoid of significant estrogenic activity. Parenterally administered MPA inhibits gonadotropin production, which in turn prevents follicular maturation and ovulation, although available data

CLINICAL PHARMACOLOGY: *(cont'd)*

indicate that this does not occur when the usually recommended oral dosage is given as single daily doses. MPA may achieve its beneficial effect on the endometrium in part by decreasing nuclear estradiol receptors and suppression of epithelial DNA synthesis in endometrial tissue.

PHARMACOKINETICS

Absorption: Conjugated estrogens are soluble in water and are well absorbed from the gastrointestinal tract after release from the drug formulation. However, Prempro/Premphase contains a modified-release formulation of conjugated estrogens that slowly releases estrogens over several hours. Maximum plasma concentrations of the various conjugated and unconjugated estrogens are attained within 4 to 10 hours after dose administration. MPA is rapidly absorbed from the gastrointestinal tract, and maximum MPA plasma concentrations are attained within 2 to 4 hours after dose administration.

Distribution: The conjugated estrogens bind mainly to albumin, but the unconjugated estrogens bind to both albumin and sex-hormone-binding globulin (SHBG). The apparent terminal-phase disposition half-life ($t_{1/2}$) of the various estrogens is prolonged by the slow absorption from Prempro/Premphase and ranges from 10 to 24 hours. MPA is approximately 90% bound to plasma proteins but does not bind to SHBG. MPA has a $t_{1/2}$ of 24 to 36 hours.

Metabolism: Metabolism and inactivation of estrogens occur primarily in the liver. Some estrogens are excreted into the bile; however, they are reabsorbed from the intestine and returned to the liver through the portal venous system. Metabolism and elimination of MPA occurs primarily in the liver via hydroxylation, with subsequent conjugation and elimination in the urine.

Excretion: Water-soluble estrogen conjugates are strongly acidic and are ionized in body fluids, which favor excretion through the kidneys since tubular reabsorption is minimal. Most metabolites of MPA are excreted as glucuronide conjugates with only minor amounts excreted as sulfates.

Drug-Drug Interactions: Coadministration of conjugated estrogens with MPA does not affect the pharmacokinetic profile of MPA; similarly, MPA does not affect the pharmacokinetic profile of the conjugated or unconjugated estrogens.

Food-Drug Interactions: Administration with food does not affect the pharmacokinetic profile of the conjugated or unconjugated estrogen. Administration with food approximately doubles MPA $C_{max}$and increases MPA AUC by approximately 30%.

TABLE 3 Pharmacokinetic Parameters For Premarin And Medroxyprogesterone Acetate

Drug	C_{max} (pg/ml)	t_{max} (h)	$t_{1/2}$ (h)	AUC (pg°h/ml)
Profile of Unconjugated Estrogens Following a Dose of 2 X 0.625 mg				
estrone	181	8.4	28.2	5981
baseline-adjusted estrone	161	8.4	16.6	3731
equilin	76	7.0	11.2	1277
Profile of Conjugated Estrogens Following a Dose of 2 X 0.625 mg				
total estrone	7.0	7.6	17.0	132
baseline-adjusted total estrone	6.8	7.6	13.0	114
total equilin	5.2	5.7	10.3	68
Pharmacokinetic Profile of MPA Following a Dose of 2 X 2.5 mg				
medroxyprogesterone acetate	1.7	2.7	35.3	2.5

INDICATIONS AND USAGE:

Prempro/Premphase therapy (Premarin brand conjugated estrogens and Cycrin brand of medroxyprogesterone acetate) is indicated in women with an intact uterus for the:

1. Treatment of moderate to severe vasomotor symptoms associated with the menopause. There is no adequate evidence that estrogens are effective for nervous symptoms or depression which might occur during menopause and they should not be used to treat these conditions.

2. Treatment of vulvar and vaginal atrophy.

3. Prevention of osteoporosis.

Since estrogen administration is associated with risks as well as benefits, selection of patients should ideally be based on prospective identification of risk factors for developing osteoporosis. Unfortunately, there is no certain way to identify those women who will develop osteoporotic fractures. Most prospective studies of efficacy for this indication have been carried out in white menopausal women, without stratification by other risk factors, and tend to show a universally salutary effect on bone. Thus, patient selection must be individualized based on the balance of risks and benefits.

Estrogen replacement therapy reduces bone resorption and retards or halts postmenopausal bone loss. Case-control studies have shown an approximately 60% reduction in hip and wrist fractures in women whose estrogen replacement was begun within a few years of menopause. Studies also suggest that estrogen reduces the rate of vertebral fractures. Even when started as late as 6 years after menopause, estrogen may prevent further loss of bone mass for as long as the treatment is continued. When estrogen therapy is discontinued, bone mass declines at a rate comparable to that in the immediate postmenopausal period. There is no evidence that estrogen replacement therapy restores bone mass to premenopausal levels.

At skeletal maturity there are sex and race differences in both the total amount of bone present and its destiny, in favor of men and blacks. Thus, women are at higher risk than men because they start with less bone mass and for several years following natural or induced menopause, the rate of bone mass declined is accelerated. White and Asian women are at higher risk than black women.

Early menopause is one of the strongest predictors for the development of osteoporosis. In addition, other factors affecting the skeleton which are associated with osteoporosis include genetic factors (small build, family history), endocrine factors (nulliparity, thyrotoxicosis, hyperparathyroidism, Cushing's syndrome, hyperprolactinemia, type I diabetes), life-style (cigarette smoking, alcohol abuse, sedentary exercise habits), and nutrition (below average body weight, dietary calcium intake).

The mainstays of prevention of osteoporosis are estrogen, an adequate lifetime calcium intake, and exercise. Postmenopausal women absorb dietary calcium less efficiently than premenopausal women and require an average of 1500 mg/day of elemental calcium to remain in neutral calcium balance. By comparison, premenopausal women require about 1000 mg/day and the average calcium intake in the USA is 400-600 mg/day. Therefore, when not contraindicated, calcium supplementation may be helpful.

Weight-bearing exercise and nutrition may be important adjuncts to the prevention and management of osteoporosis. Immobilization and prolonged bed rest produce rapid bone loss, while weight-bearing exercise has been shown both to reduce bone less and to increase bone mass. The optimal type and amount of physical activity that would prevent osteoporosis have not been established; however, in two studies an hour of walking and running exercises two or three times weekly significantly increased lumbar spine bone mass.

CONTRAINDICATIONS:

Estrogens/progestins combined should not be used in women under any of the following conditions or circumstances:

1. Known or suspected pregnancy, including use for missed abortion or as a diagnostic test for pregnancy (see BOXED WARNING.) Estrogen or progestin may cause fetal harm when administered to a pregnant woman.

2. Known or suspected cancer of the breast.

3. Known or suspected estrogen-dependent neoplasia.

4. Undiagnosed abnormal genital bleeding.

5. Active or past history of thrombophlebitis, thromboembolic disorders, or stroke.

6. Liver dysfunction or disease.

Prempro/Premphase therapy should not be used in patients hypersensitive to the ingredients contained in Premarin or Cycrin.

WARNINGS:

ALL WARNINGS BELOW PERTAIN TO THE USE OF THIS COMBINATION PRODUCT.

Based on experience with estrogens and/or progestins:

INDUCTION OF MALIGNANT NEOPLASMS

Breast cancer: Some studies have reported a moderately increased risk of breast cancer (relative risk of 1.3 to 2.0) in those women of estrogen replacement therapy taking higher doses, or in those taking lower doses for prolonged periods of time, especially in excess of 10 years. The majority of studies, however, have not shown an association in women who have ever used estrogen replacement therapy.

The effect of added progestin on the risk of breast cancer in unknown, although a moderately increased risk in those taking combination estrogen/progestin therapy has been reported. Other studies have not shown this relationship. In a one year clinical trials of Prempro/Premphase and Premarin alone, 5 new cases of breast cancer were detected among 1377 women who received the combination treatments, while no new cases were detected among 347 women who received Premarin alone. The overall incidence of breast cancer in this clinical trial does not exceed that expected in the general population.

Women on hormone replacement therapy should have regular breast examinations and should be instructed in breast self-examination, and women over the age of 50 should have regular mammograms.

Endometrial cancer: The reported endometrial cancer risk among users unopposed estrogen was about 2- to 12-fold or greater than in nonusers and appears dependent on duration of treatment and on estrogen dose. There is no significant increased risk associated with use of estrogens for less than one year. The greatest risk appears associated with prolonged use, with increased risks of 15- to 24-fold for five years or more. In one study, a significant decrease in the incidence of endometrial cancer occurred six months after estrogen withdrawal.

A large clinical trial has demonstrated that when MPA is administered with Premarin, there is a markedly reduced incidence of endometrial hyperplasia, a possible precursor of endometrial cancer. Endometrial hyperplasia has been reported in a large clinical trial to occur at a rate of approximately 1% or less with Prempro/Premphase. Studies have also demonstrated a reduced risk of endometrial cancer when a progestin is administered with estrogen replacement therapy. In the large clinical trial described above, only a single case of endometrial cancer was reported to occur among women taking combination Premarin/MPA therapy.

Clinical surveillance of all women taking estrogen/progestin combinations is important. Adequate diagnostic measures, including endometrial sampling when indicated, should be undertaken to rule out malignancy in all cases of undiagnosed persistent or recurring abnormal vaginal bleeding.

CARDIOVASCULAR DISEASE

Large doses of estrogens (5 mg conjugated estrogens per day), comparable to those used to treat cancer of the prostate and breast, have been shown in large prospective clinical trial in men to increase the risk of nonfatal myocardial infarction, pulmonary embolism, and thrombophlebitis. These risks cannot necessarily be extrapolated from men to women or from unopposed estrogen to combination estrogen/progestin therapy. However, to avoid the theoretical cardiovascular risk to women caused by high estrogen doses, the dose for estrogen replacement therapy should not exceed the lowest effective dose.

EFFECTS DURING PREGNANCY

Use in pregnancy is not recommended. See BOXED WARNING.

GALLBLADDER DISEASE

Two studies have reported a 2- to 4-fold increase in the risk of surgically confirmed gallbladder disease in women receiving postmenopausal estrogens. In a large clinical trial, 5 of 1029 subjects taking Premarin/Cycrin at doses comparable to Prempro/Premphase developed cholecystitis with cholelithiasis that required cholecystectomy.

ELEVATED BLOOD PRESSURE

Occasional blood pressure increases during estrogen replacement therapy have been attributed to idiosyncratic reactions to estrogens. More often, blood pressure has remained the same or has dropped. One study showed that postmenopausal estrogen users have higher blood pressure than nonusers. In a large clinical trial, transient elevations from baseline of 40 mm Hg or more systolic and 20 mm Hg or more diastolic were reported in less than 2% and 4% of postmenopausal subjects, respectively. Two other studies showed slightly lower blood pressure among estrogen users compared to nonusers. Postmenopausal estrogen use does not increase the risk of stroke. Nonetheless, blood pressure should be monitored at regular intervals with estrogen use.

HYPERCALCEMIA

Administration of estrogens may lead to severe hypercalcemia in patients with breast cancer and bone metastases. If this occurs, the drugs should be stopped and appropriate measures taken to reduce the serum calcium level.

THROMBOEMBOLIC DISORDERS

The physician should be alert to the earliest manifestations of thrombotic disorders (thrombophlebitis, cerebrovascular disorders, pulmonary embolism, and retinal thrombosis). Should any of these occur or be suspected, the drugs should be discontinued immediately.

VISUAL ABNORMALITIES

Discontinue medication pending examination if there is sudden partial or complete loss of vision, or a sudden onset of proptosis, diplopia, or migraine. If examinations reveals papilledema or retinal vascular lesions, medication should be withdrawn.

PRECAUTIONS:

Based on experience with estrogens and/or progestins:

Cardiovascular risk: A casual relationship between estrogen replacement therapy and reduction of cardiovascular disease in postmenopausal women has not been proven. Furthermore, the effect of added progestins on this putative benefit is not yet known.

PRECAUTIONS: *(cont'd)*

In recent years many published studies have suggested that there may be a cause-effect relationship between postmenopausal oral estrogen replacement therapy *without added progestins* and a decrease in cardiovascular disease in women. Although most of the observational studies which assessed this statistical association have reported a 20% to 50% reduction in coronary heart disease risk and associated mortality in estrogen takers, the following should be considered when interpreting these reports.

Because only one of these studies was randomized and it was too small to yield statistically significant results, all relevant studies were subject to selection bias. Thus, the apparently reduced risk of coronary artery disease cannot be attributed with certainty to estrogen replacement therapy. It may instead have been caused by life-style and medical characteristics of the women studied with the result that healthier women were selected for estrogen therapy. In general, treated women were of higher socioeconomic and educational status, more slender, more physically active, more likely to have undergone surgical menopause, and less likely to have diabetes than the untreated women. Although some studies attempted to control for these selection factors, it is common for properly designed randomized trials to fail to confirm benefits suggested by less rigorous study designs. Thus, ongoing and future large-scale randomized trials may fail to confirm this apparent benefit.

Current medical practice often includes the use of concomitant progestin therapy in women with intact uteri. While the effects of added progestins on the risk of ischemic heart disease are not known, medroxyprogesterone acetate at the dose in Prempro/Premphase attenuates much of the favorable effect of conjugated estrogens on LDL levels (see CLINICAL PHARMACOLOGY).

While the effects of added progestins on the risk of breast cancer are also unknown, available epidemiologic evidence suggests that progestins do not reduce, and may enhance, the moderately increased breast cancer risk that had been reported with prolonged estrogen replacement therapy (see WARNINGS).

The safety data regarding Prempro/Premphase were obtained from clinical trials and epidemiologic studies of postmenopausal Caucasian women, who were at generally low risk for cardiovascular disease and higher than average risk for osteoporosis. The safety profile of Prempro/Premphase derived from these study demographic composition. When considering prescribing Prempro/Premphase, physicians are advised to weigh the potential benefits and risks of therapy as applicable to each individual patient.

Use in hysterectomized women: Existing data do not support the use of the combination of estrogen and progestin in postmenopausal women without a uterus. There are possible risks which may be associated with the inclusion of progestin in estrogen, replacement regimens. The potential risks include some deterioration in glucose tolerance, as reported in a large clinical trial of Prempro/Premphase, and adverse effects on lipid metabolism as compared to the lipid effects of Premarin alone (see CLINICAL PHARMACOLOGY).

Physical examination: A complete medical and family history should be taken prior to the initiation of any estrogen/progestin therapy. The pretreatment and periodic physical examinations should include special reference to blood pressure, breasts, abdomen, and pelvic organs, and should include a Papanicolaou smear. As a general rule, estrogen should not be prescribed for longer than one year without another physical examination being performed.

Fluid retention: Because estrogens/progestins may cause some degree of fluid retention, conditions which might be influenced by this factor, such as asthma, epilepsy, migraine, and cardiac or renal dysfunction, require careful observation.

Uterine bleeding: Certain patients may develop abnormal uterine bleeding. In cases of undiagnosed abnormal bleeding, adequate diagnostic measures are indicated. (See WARNINGS.)

The pathologist should be advised of estrogen/progestin therapy when relevant specimens are submitted.

BASED ON EXPERIENCE WITH ESTROGENS

Familial Hyperlipoproteinemia: Estrogen therapy may be associated with massive elevations of plasma triglycerides leading to pancreatitis and other complications in patients with familial defects of lipoprotein metabolism.

Hypercoagulability: Some studies have shown that women taking estrogen replacement therapy have hypercoagulability primarily related to decreased antithrombin activity. This effect appears dose- and duration-dependent and is less pronounced than that associated with oral contraceptive use. Also, postmenopausal women tend to have changes in levels of coagulation parameters at baseline compared to premenopausal women, although the majority of studies (of primarily conjugated estrogens users) report no such increase. There is insufficient information on hypercoagulability in women who have had previous thromboembolic disease. In a large clinical trial of Prempro/Premphase, factors VII and X concentrations and plasminogen activity increased by 20%, 13%, and 14% over baseline, respectively, and antithrombin III activity decreased approximately 5% from baseline.

Mastodynia: Certain patients may develop undesirable manifestations of estrogenic stimulation such as mastodynia. In a large clinical trial of Prempro/Premphase, approximately one third of the subjects reported breast pain during treatment with Prempro/Premphase, versus 12% for Premarin alone.

BASED ON EXPERIENCE WITH PROGESTINS

Lipoprotein Metabolism: See CLINICAL PHARMACOLOGY.

Impaired Glucose Tolerance: See Use in hysterectomized women, above.

Depression: Patients who have a history of depression should be observed and the drugs discontinued if the depression recurs to a serious degree.

INFORMATION FOR THE PATIENT

(See PATIENT PACKAGE INSERT.)

DRUG/LABORATORY TEST INTERACTIONS

1. Accelerated prothrombin time, partial thromboplastin time, and platelet aggregation time; increased platelet count; increased factors II, VII antigen, VIII coagulant activity, IX, X, XII, VII-X complex, II- VII-X complex, and beta-thromboglobulin; decreased levels of anti-factor Xa and antithrombin III decreased antithrombin III activity; increased levels of fibrinogen and fibrinogen activity; increased plasminogen antigen and activity.

2. Increased thyroid-binding globulin (TBG) leading to increased circulating total thyroid hormone, as measured by protein-bound iodine (PBI), T_4 levels (by column or by radioimmunoassay) or T_3 by radioimmunoassay. T_3 resin uptake is decreased, reflecting the elevated TBG. Free T_4 and free T_3 concentrations are unaltered.

3. Other binding proteins may be elevated in serum, i.e., corticosteroid binding globulin (CBG), sex hormone-binding globulin (SHBG), leading to increased circulating corticosteroids and sex steroids respectively. Free or biologically active hormone concentrations are unchanged. Other plasma proteins may be increased (angiotensinogen/renin substrated, alpha-1-antitrypsin, ceruloplasmin).

4. Increased plasma HDL and HDL-2 subfraction concentrations, reduced LDL cholesterol concentration, increased triglycerides levels.

5. Impaired glucose tolerance. For this reason, diabetic patients should be carefully observed while receiving estrogen/progestin therapy.

6. Reduced response to metyrapone test.

PRECAUTIONS: *(cont'd)*

7. Reduced serum folate concentration.

8. Aminoglutethimide administered concomitantly with MPA may significantly depress the bioavailability of MPA.

MUTAGENESIS AND CARCINOGENESIS

In a two-year oral study in which female rats were exposed to dosages of up to 5000 mcg/kg/day in their diets (50 times higher-based on AUC values-than the level observed experimentally in women taking 10 mg of MPA), a dose-related increase in pancreatic islet cell tumors (adenomas and carcinomas) occurred. Pancreatic tumor incidence increased at 1000 and 5000 mcg/kg/day, but not at 200 mcg/kg/day.

A decreased incidence of spontaneous mammary gland tumors was observed in all three MPA-treated groups, compared to controls, in the two-year rat study. The mechanism for the decreased incidence of mammary gland tumors observed in the MPA-treated rats may be linked to the significant decrease in serum prolactin concentration observed in rats.

Beagle dogs treated with MPA developed mammary nodules, some of which were malignant. Although nodules occasionally appeared in control animals, they are intermittent in nature, whereas the nodules in the drug-treated animals were larger, more numerous, persistent, and there were some breast malignancies with metastases. It is known that progestogens stimulate synthesis and release growth hormone in dogs. The growth hormone, along progestogen, stimulates mammary growth and tumors. In contrast, growth hormone in humans is not increased, nor does growth hormone have any significant mammotrophic role. Therefore, the MPA-induced increase of mammary tumors in dogs probably has no significance to humans. No pancreatic tumors occurred in dogs.

PREGNANCY CATEGORY X

Estrogens/progestins should not be used during pregnancy. (See CONTRAINDICATIONS) and BOXED WARNING.

NURSING MOTHERS

As a general principle, the administration of any drug to nursing mothers should be done only when clearly necessary since many drugs are excreted in human milk. Estrogen administration to nursing mothers has been shown to decrease the quantity and quality of the milk. Detectable amounts of progestin have been identified in the milk of mothers receiving the drug. The effect of this on the nursing infant has not been determined.

ADVERSE REACTIONS:

(See WARNINGS regarding induction of neoplasia, adverse effects on the fetus, increased incidence of gallbladder disease, elevated blood pressure, thromboembolic disorders, cardiovascular disease, visual abnormalities, and hypercalcemia and PRECAUTIONSfor cardiovascular disease.)

The following adverse reactions have been reported with estrogen and/or progestin therapy:

Genitourinary System: Changes in vaginal bleeding pattern and abnormal withdrawal bleeding or flow, break through bleeding, spotting, change in amount of cervical secretion, premenstrual-like syndrome, cystitis-like syndrome, increase in size of uterine leiomyomata, vaginal candidiasis, amenorrhea, changes in cervical erosion.

Breasts: Tenderness, enlargement, galactorrhea.

Gastrointestinal: Nausea, cholestatic jaundice, changes in appetite, vomiting, abdominal cramps, bloating, increased incidence of gallbladder disease.

Skin: Chloasma or melasma that may persist when drug is discontinued, erythema multiforme, erythema nodosum, hemorrhagic eruption, loss of scalp hair, hirsutism, itching, urticaria, pruritus, generalized rash, rash (allergic) with and without pruritus acne.

Cardiovascular: In susceptible individuals, change in blood pressure, thrombophlebitis, pulmonary embolism, cerebral thrombosis and embolism.

CNS: Headache, dizziness, mental depression, nervousness, migraine, chorea, insomnia, somnolence.

Eyes: Neuro-ocular lesions (*e.g.,* retinal thrombosis and optic neuritis). Steepening of corneal curvature, intolerance of contact lenses.

Miscellaneous: Increase or decrease in weight, edema, changes in libido, fatigue, backache, reduced carbohydrate tolerance, aggravation of porphyria, pyrexia, anaphylactoid reactions, anaphylaxis.

OVERDOSAGE:

Acute Overdosage: Serious ill effects have not been reported following acute ingestion of large doses of estrogen/progestin-containing oral contraceptives by young children. Overdosage may cause nausea and vomiting, and withdrawal bleeding may occur in females.

DOSAGE AND ADMINISTRATION:

Prempro: Prempro therapy consists of two separate tablets to be taken together, once daily.

1. For treatment of moderate to severe vasomotor symptoms and vulvar and vaginal atrophy associated with menopause-Prempro 0.625 mg/2.5 mg daily. Patients should be reevaluated at 3-month to 6-month intervals to determine if treatment for symptoms is still necessary.

2. For prevention of osteoporosis-Prempro 0.625 mg/2.5 mg daily. Treated patients with an intact uterus should be monitored closely for signs of endometrial cancer, and appropriate diagnostic measures should be taken to rule out malignancy in the event of persistent or recurring abnormal vaginal bleeding.

Premphase: Premphase therapy consists of two separate tablets: one maroon tablet taken daily for 28 days and one light-purple tablet taken with a maroon tablet on days 15 through 28.

1. For treatment of moderate to severe vasomotor symptoms and vulvar and vaginal atrophy associated with menopause. Patients should be reevaluated at 3-month to 6-month intervals to determine if treatment for symptoms is still necessary.

2. For prevention of osteoporosis. Treated patients with an intact uterus should be monitored closely for signs of endometrial cancer, and appropriate diagnostic measures should be taken to rule out malignancy in the event of persistent or recurring abnormal vaginal bleeding.

PATIENT PACKAGE INSERT:

ESTROGENS INCREASE THE RISK OF CANCER OF THE UTERUS IN WOMEN WHO HAVE HAD THEIR MENOPAUSE ("CHANGE OF LIFE"). THIS FINDING REFERS TO ESTROGENS GIVEN WITHOUT PROGESTIN.

Progestin drugs taken with estrogen-containing drugs significantly reduce but do not eliminate this risk. If you use any estrogen-containing drug, it is important to visit your doctor regularly and report any unusual vaginal bleeding right away. Vaginal bleeding after menopause may be a warning sign of uterine cancer.

Your doctor should evaluate any unusual vaginal bleeding to find the cause.

ESTROGENS/PROGESTINS SHOULD NOT BE USED DURING

PATIENT PACKAGE INSERT: *(cont'd)*

PREGNANCY.

Estrogens and progestins do not prevent miscarriage (spontaneous abortion) and are not needed in the days following childbirth. If you take estrogens during pregnancy your unborn child has a greater than usual chance of having birth defects. The risk of developing these defects is small, but clearly larger than the risk of children whose mother did not take estrogens during pregnancy. These birth defects may affect the baby's urinary system and sex organs. Daughters born to mothers who took DES (an estrogen drug) have a higher than usual chance of developing cancer of the vagina or cervix when they become teenagers or young adults. Sons may have a higher than usual chance of developing cancer of the testicles when they become teenagers or young adults.

There is an increased risk of birth defects in children whose mothers take this drug during the first four months of pregnancy. Several reports suggest an association between mothers who take these drugs in the first trimester of pregnancy and genital abnormalities in male and female babies. The risk to the male baby is the possibility of being born with a condition in which the opening of the penis is on the underside and rather than the tip of the penis (hypospadias). Hypospadias occurs in about 5 to 8 per 1,000 male births and is about doubled with exposure to these drugs. There is not enough information to quantify the risk to exposed female fetuses. However, enlargement of the clitoris and fusion of the labia may occur, although rarely.

Therefore, since drugs of this type may include mild masculinization of the external genitalia of the female fetus, as well as hypospadias in the male fetus, it is wise to avoid using the drug during the first trimester of pregnancy. These drugs have been used as a test for pregnancy, but such use is no longer considered safe because of possible damage to a developing baby. Also, more rapid methods for testing for pregnancy are now available. If you take Prempro/Premphase and later find you were pregnant when you took it, be sure to discuss this with your doctor as soon as possible.

Your doctor has prescribed Prempro/Premphase, a combination of two hormones, an estrogen and a progestin. This leaflet describes the major benefits and risks of your treatment, as well as how and when treatment should be taken.

Prempro/Premphase replaces the hormones in your body which naturally decrease at menopause. The hormone combination you will be taking has been shown to provide the benefits of estrogen replacement therapy while lowering the frequency of a possible precancerous condition of the uterine lining. This therapy is not intended for women who have had a hysterectomy (surgical removal of the uterus).

Estrogens have several important uses but also some risks. You must decide, with your doctor, whether the risks of estrogens are acceptable when weighed against their benefits. The length of treatment with estrogens can vary from woman to woman. Check with your doctor to make sure you are using the lowest possible effective dose.

With Prempro/Premphase therapy several menstrual-like bleeding patterns may occur. These may range from absence of bleeding to irregular bleeding. if bleeding occurs, it is frequently light spotting or moderate menstrual-like bleeding, but it may be heavy. If you experience vaginal bleeding while taking Prempro/Premphase, you should discuss your bleeding pattern with your doctor and set up an appropriate schedule for follow-up care.

USE OF ESTROGEN

To Reduce Moderate To Severe Menopausal Symptoms: Estrogens are hormones produced by the ovaries of normal women. When a woman is between the ages of 45 and 55, the ovaries normally stop making estrogens. This leads to a drop in body estrogen levels that causes the "change of life" or menopause (the end of monthly menstrual periods). A sudden drop in estrogen levels also occurs if both ovaries are removed during an operation before natural menopause takes place. This is referred to as "surgical menopause."

When the estrogen levels begin dropping, some women develop very uncomfortable symptoms, such as feelings of warmth in the face, neck, and chest, or sudden intense episodes of heat and sweating ("hot flashes" or hot flushes"). Using estrogen drugs can help the body adjust to lower estrogen levels and reduce these symptoms. In some women the symptoms are mild; in others they can be severe. These symptoms may last only for a few months or longer. Taking Prempro/Premphase can alleviate these symptoms. If you are not taking hormones for other reasons, such as the prevention of osteoporosis, you should take Prempro/Premphase only as long as you need it for relief from your menopausal symptoms.

To Prevent Thinning Of Bones: Osteoporosis is a thinning of the bones that makes them weaker and allows them to break more easily. The bones of the spine, wrists, and hips break most often in osteoporosis. Both men and women start to loss bone mass after about age 40, but women lose bone mass faster after the menopause. Using estrogens after the menopause slows down bone thinning and may prevent bones from breaking. Lifelong adequate calcium intake, either from diet (such as dairy products) or from calcium supplements (to reach a total daily intake of 1000 milligrams per day before menopause or 1500 milligrams per day after menopause), may help to prevent osteoporosis. Regular weight-bearing exercise (like walking and running for an hour, two or three time a week) may also help to prevent osteoporosis. Before you change your calcium intake or exercise habits, it is important to discuss these life-style changes with your doctor to find out if they are safe for you.

Since estrogen use has some risks, only women who are likely to develop osteoporosis should use estrogens for prevention. Women who are likely to develop osteoporosis often have the following characteristics:

White or Asian race

Small, slim body frame

Cigarette-smoking habit

Family history of osteoporosis (in a mother, sister, or aunt)

Early menopause with natural or because of surgical removal of ovaries ("surgical menopause")

To Treat Vulvar And Vaginal Atrophy: (itching burning, dryness in or around the vagina, difficulty or burning on urination) associated with menopause.

WHO SHOULD NOT USE ESTROGENS

During Pregnancy: (see BOXED WARNING.) If you think you may be pregnant, do not use any form of estrogen-containing drug. Using estrogens while you are pregnant may cause your unborn child to have birth defects. Estrogens do not prevent miscarriage.

If You Have Unusual Vaginal Bleeding Which Has Not Been Evaluated By Your Doctor: (see BOXED WARNING) Unusual vaginal bleeding can be a warning sign of cancer of the uterus, especially if it happens after menopause. Your doctor must find out the cause of the bleeding so that he or she can recommend the proper treatment. Taking estrogens without visiting your doctor can cause you serious harm if your vaginal bleeding is caused by cancer of the uterus.

PATIENT PACKAGE INSERT: *(cont'd)*

If You Have Had Cancer: Since estrogens increase the risk of certain types of cancer, you should not use estrogens if you have ever had cancer of the breast or uterus.

If You Have Any Circulation Problems: Estrogen drugs should not be used except in unusually special situations in which your doctor decides that you need estrogen use (see PATIENT PACKAGE INSERT, Risks of Estrogens and/or Progestins).

When They Do Not Work: During menopause, some women develop nervous symptoms or depression. Estrogens do not relieve these symptoms. You may have heard that taking estrogens for years after menopause will keep your skin soft and supple and keep you feeling young. There is no evidence for these claims and such long-term estrogen use may have serious risks.

After Childbirth Or When Breast-Feeding A Baby: Estrogen should not be used to try to stop the breast from filling with milk after a baby is born. Such treatment may increase the risk of developing blood clots(see PATIENT PACKAGE INSERT, Risks of Estrogens and/or Progestins).

If you are breast-feeding, you should avoid using any drugs because many drugs pass through to the baby in the milk. While nursing a baby, you should take drugs only on the advice of your health-care provider.

RISKS OF ESTROGENS AND/OR PROGESTINS

Cancer Of The Uterus: The risk of cancer of the uterus increases when estrogens are used alone, the longer they are used, and when larger doses are taken. There is a higher risk of cancer of the uterus of you are over-weight, diabetic, or have high blood pressure. The hormone combination you will be taking contains estrogen and progestin. This combination has been shown to provide the benefits of estrogen replacement therapy for the **Uses of Estrogen**, while reducing the risk of a precancerous condition of the uterine lining (see PATIENT PACKAGE INSERT, Other Information).

However, additional risks may be associated with the inclusion of a progestin in estrogen treatment. The possible risks include unfavorable effects on blood fats and sugars, and a possible increase in breast cancer risk (see PATIENT PACKAGE INSERT, Cancer Of The Breast). Usually, the smaller the dose and the shorter the duration of treatment, the more these effects are minimized. Check with your doctor to make sure you are using the lowest effective dose and only for as long as you need it.

If you have had your uterus removed, there is no risk of developing cancer of the uterus and no benefit to be gained by using a combination estrogen/progestin product.

Cancer Of The Breast: Most studies have not shown a higher risk of breast cancer in women who have ever used estrogens. However, some studies have reported that breast cancer developed more often (up to twice the usual rate) in women who used estrogens for long periods of time especially more than 10 years), or who used high doses for shorter time periods. The effects of added progestin on the risk of breast cancer are unknown. Some studies have reported a somewhat increased risk, even higher than the possible risk associated with estrogens alone. Others have not. Regular breast examinations by a health professional and monthly self-examination ar recommended for all women. Regular mammograms are recommended for all women over 50 years of age.

Gallbladder Disease: Women who use estrogens after menopause are more likely to develop gallbladder disease needing surgery than woman who do not use estrogens.

Abnormal Blood Clotting: Taking estrogens may cause changes in your blood clotting system. These changes allow the blood to clot more easily, possibly allowing clots to form in your bloodstream. If blood clots do form in your bloodstream, they can cut off the blood supply to vital organs causing serious problems. These problems may include a stroke (by cutting off blood to the brain), a heart attack (by cutting off blood to the heart), a pulmonary embolus (by cutting off blood to the lungs), or other problems. Any of these conditions may cause death or serious long-term disability. However, most studies of low-dose estrogen use by women do not show an increased risk of these complications.

Excess Calcium In The Blood: Taking estrogens may lead to severe hypercalcemia in women with breast and/or bone cancer.

During Pregnancy: There is an increased risk of birth defects in children whose mothers take this drug during the first four months of pregnancy. Several reports suggest an association between mothers who take these drugs in the first trimester of pregnancy and genital abnormalities in male and female babies. The risk to the male baby is the possibility of being born with a condition in which the opening of the penis is on the underside rather than the tip of the penis (hypospadias). Hypospadias occurs in about 5 to 8 1,000 male births and is about doubled with exposure to these drugs. There is not enough information to quantify the risk to exposed female fetuses. However, enlargement of the clitoris and fusion of the labia may occur, although rarely.

Therefore, since drugs of this type may induce mild masculinization of the external genitalia of the female fetus, as well as hypospadias in the male fetus, it is wise to avoid using the drug during the first trimester if pregnancy. These drugs have been used as a test for pregnancy, but such use is no longer considered safe because of possible damage to a developing baby. Also, more rapid methods for testing for pregnancy are now available. If you take Prempro/Premphase and later find you were pregnant when you took it, be sure to discuss this with your doctor as soon as possible.

Side Effects with Estrogens and/or Progestins: In addition to the risks listed above, the following side effects have been reported with estrogen and/or progestin use:

Nausea, vomiting, pain, cramps, swelling, or tenderness in the abdomen.

Yellowing of the skin and/or whites of the eyes.

Breast tenderness or enlargement.

Enlargement of benign tumors ("fibroids") of the uterus.

Irregular bleeding or spotting.

Change in amount of cervical secretion.

Vaginal yeast infections.

Retention of excess fluid. This may make some conditions worsen, such as asthma, epilepsy, migraine, heart disease, or kidney disease.

A spotty darkening of the skin, particularly on the face; reddening of the skin; skin rashes.

Worsening of porphyria.

Headache migraines, dizziness, faintness, or changes in vision (including intolerance to contact lenses).

Mental depression.

Involuntary muscle spasms.

Hair loss or abnormal hairiness.

Increase or decrease in weight.

Changes in sex drive.

Possible changes in the blood sugar.

REDUCING THE RISKS OF ESTROGEN/PROGESTIN USE

If you decide to take an estrogen/progestin combination, you can reduce your risks by carefully monitoring your treatment.

PATIENT PACKAGE INSERT: *(cont'd)*

See Your Doctor Regularly: While you are taking Prempro/Premphase, it is important to visit your doctor at least once a year for a checkup. If you develop vaginal bleeding while taking estrogens, you may need further evaluation. If members of your family have had breast cancer or if you have ever had breast lumps or an abnormal mammogram (breast x-ray), you may need to have more frequent breast examinations.

Reassess Your Need For Treatment: You and your doctor should reevaluate whether or not you still need estrogens at least every six months.

Be Alert For Signs Or Troubles: If any of these warning signals (or any other unusual symptoms) happen while you are using estrogen/progestin, call your doctor immediately:

Abnormal bleeding from the vagina (possible uterine abnormality).

Pains in the calves or chest, a sudden shortness of breath or coughing blood (indicates possible clots in the legs, heart, or lungs).

Severe headache or vomiting, dizziness, faintness, or changes in vision or speech, weakness or numbness of an arm or leg (indicating possible clots in the brain or eye).

Breast lumps (possibly breast cancer; ask your doctor or health professional to show you how to examine your breasts monthly).

Yellowing of the skin and/or whites of the eyes (possible liver problems).

Pain, swelling, or tenderness in the abdomen (possible gallbladder problem).

OTHER INFORMATION

Estrogens increase the risk of developing a condition (endometrial hyperplasia) that may lead to cancer of the lining of the uterus. Taking progestins, another hormonal drug, with estrogens lowers the risk of developing in this condition. Therefore, since your uterus has not been removed, your doctor has prescribed Prempro/Premphase, which includes both a progestin and estrogens.

You should know, however, that taking estrogens *with* progestins may have unhealthy effects on blood sugar, which might make a diabetic condition worse. Additional risks include possible further increase in breast cancer risk which may be associated with long-term estrogen use.

Some research has shown that estrogens taken *without* progestins may protect women against developing heart disease. However, this is not certain. The protection shown may have been caused by the characteristics of the estrogen-treated women and not by the estrogen treatment itself. In general, treated women were slimmer, more physically active, and were less likely to have diabetes than the untreated women. These characteristics are known to protect against heart disease.

You are cautioned to discuss very carefully with your doctor or health-care provider all the possible risks and benefits of long-term estrogen and progestin treatment as they affect you personally.

Your doctor has prescribed this drug for you and you alone. Do not give the drug to anyone else.

If you will be taking calcium supplements as part of the treatment to help prevent osteoporosis, check with your doctor about the amounts recommended.

Keep this and all drugs out of the reach of children. In case of overdose, call your doctor, hospital, or poison control center immediately.

This leaflet provides the most important information about Prempro/Premphase. If you want to read more, ask your doctor or pharmacist to let you read the professional labeling.

HOW SUPPLIED:

Prempro: Prempro therapy consists of two separate tablets (one maroon tablet and one white tablet) to be taken together once daily.

Each carton contains 2 blister cards. Each blister card contains 14 oval, maroon tablets containing 0.625 mg of Premarin brand of conjugated estrogens for oral administration and 14 white, oval tablets with a score debossed on one side and opposing "C's" debossed on the reverse side which contain 2.5 mg of Cycrin brand medroxyprogesterone acetate.

The appearance of Premarin Tablets is a trademark of Wyeth-Ayerst Laboratories. The appearance of medroxyprogesterone acetate tablets is a registered trademark.

Storage: Store at room temperature 15° C-25° C (59° F-77° F).

Premphase: Premphase therapy consists of two separate tablets: one maroon tablet taken daily for 28 days and one light-purple tablet taken with a maroon tablet on days 15 through 28.

Each carton contains 2 blister cards. One blister card contains 14 oval, maroon tablets containing 0.625 mg of Premarin brand conjugated estrogens for oral administration. The second blister card contains 14 oval, maroon tablets which contain 0.625 mg of Premarin brand conjugated estrogens for oral administration and 14 light-purple, oval tablets with "CYCRIN" and a score debossed on one side and opposing "C's" debossed on the reverse side which contain 5.0 mg of Cycrin brand of medroxyprogesterone acetate for oral administration.

The appearance of Premarin Tablets is a trademark of Wyeth-Ayerst Laboratories. The appearance of medroxyprogesterone acetate tablets is a registered trademark.

Storage: Store at room temperature 15° C-25° C (59° F-77° F).

HOW SUPPLIED - EQUIVALENTS NOT AVAILABLE:

Tablet, Uncoated - Oral - 0.625 mg/2.5 mg

168's $50.40 PREMPRO, Ayerst 00046-2572-02

Tablet, Uncoated - Oral - 0.625 mg/5 mg

126's $46.20 PREMPHASE, Ayerst 00046-2570-02

ESTROGENS, CONJUGATED; MEPROBAMATE *(001198)*

CATEGORIES: Antianxiety Drugs; Anxiety; Hormones; Menopause; Tension; Tranquilizers; Pregnancy Category X; FDA Approval Pre 1982

BRAND NAMES: Milprem; **PMB**

WARNING:

1. ESTROGENS HAVE BEEN REPORTED TO INCREASE THE RISK OF ENDOMETRIAL CARCINOMA.

Three independent, case-controlled studies have reported an increased risk of endometrial cancer in postmenopausal women exposed to exogenous estrogens for more than one year. This risk was independent of the other known risk factors for endometrial cancer. These studies are further supported by the finding that incidence rates of endometrial cancer have increased sharply since 1969 in eight different areas of the United States with population- based cancer-reporting systems, an increase which may be related to the rapidly expanding use of estrogens during the last decade.

The three case-controlled studies reported that the risk of endometrial cancer in estrogen users was about 4.5 to 13.9 times greater than in nonusers. The risk appears to depend on both duration of treatment and on estrogen dose. In view of these findings, when estrogens are used for the treatment of menopausal symptoms, the lowest dose that will control symptoms should be utilized and medication should be discontinued as soon as possible. When prolonged treatment is medically indicated, the patient should be reassessed on at least a semiannual basis to determine the need for continued therapy. Although the evidence must be considered preliminary, one study suggests that cyclic administration of low doses of estrogen may carry less risk than continuous administration. It, therefore, appears prudent to utilize such a regimen.

Close clinical surveillance of all women taking estrogens is important. In all cases of undiagnosed persistent or recurring abnormal vaginal bleeding, adequate diagnostic measures should be undertaken to rule out malignancy.

There is no evidence at present that "natural" estrogens are more or less hazardous than "synthetic" estrogens at equiestrogenic doses.

2. ESTROGENS SHOULD NOT BE USED DURING PREGNANCY.

The use of female sex hormones, both estrogens and progestogens, during early pregnancy may seriously damage the offspring. It has been shown that females exposed *in utero* to diethylstilbestrol, a nonsteroidal estrogen, have an increased risk of developing in later life a form of vaginal or cervical cancer that is ordinarily extremely rare. This risk has been estimated as not greater than 4 per 1,000 exposures. Furthermore, a high percentage of such exposed women (from 30% to 90%) have been found to have vaginal adenosis, epithelial changes of the vagina and cervix. Although these changes are histologically benign, it is not known whether they are precursors of malignancy. Although similar data are not available with the use of other estrogens, it cannot be presumed they would not induce similar changes.

Several reports suggest an association between intrauterine exposure to female sex hormones and congenital anomalies, including congenital heart defects and limb-reduction defects. One case-controlled study estimated a 4.7-fold increased risk of limb-reduction defects in infants exposed *in utero* to sex hormones (oral contraceptives, hormone withdrawal tests for pregnancy, or attempted treatment for threatened abortion). Some of these exposures were very short and involved only a few days of treatment. The data suggest that the risk of limb-reduction defects in exposed fetuses is somewhat less than 1 per 1,000.

In the past, female sex hormones have been used during pregnancy in an attempt to treat threatened or habitual abortion. There is considerable evidence that estrogens are ineffective for these indications, and there is no evidence from well-controlled studies that progestogens are effective for these users.

If PMB is used during pregnancy, or if the patient becomes pregnant while taking this drug, she should be apprised of the potential risks to the fetus,and the advisability of pregnancy continuation.

3. THIS FIXED-COMBINATION DRUG IS NOT INDICATED FOR INITIAL THERAPY.

In cases where estrogen given alone has not alleviated anxiety and tension existing as part of the menopausal symptom complex, therapy may then consist of separate administration of estrogen and meprobamate in order to determine the appropriate dosage of each drug for the patient. If this fixed combination represents the dosage so determined, its use may be more convenient in patient management. The treatment of such patients is not static but must be reevaluated as conditions in each patient warrant.

DESCRIPTION:

PMB is a combination of Premarin (conjugated estrogens, USP) and meprobamate, USP, a tranquilizing agent, in tablet form for oral administration.

Premarin (conjugated estrogens, USP) is a mixture of estrogens, obtained exclusively from natural sources, occurring as the sodium salts of water-soluble estrogen sulfates blended to represent the average composition of material derived from pregnant mares' urine. It contains estrone, equilin, and 17 α-dihydroequilin together, with smaller amounts of 17 α-estradiol, equilenin, and 17 α-dihydroequilenin as salts of their sulfate esters.

Meprobamate, USP, is the dicarbamic acid ester of 2-methyl-2-*n*- propyl-1, 3-propanediol.

PMB 200: Each tablet contains 0.45 mg of Premarin (conjugated estrogens, USP) and 200 mg Meprobamate, USP.

PMB 400: Each tablet contains 0.45 mg of Premarin (conjugated estrogens, USP) and 400 mg Meprobamate, USP.

PMB Tablets contain the following inactive ingredients: calcium phosphate, calcium sulfate, carnauba wax, cellulose, lactose, magnesium stearate, methylcellulose, pharmaceutical glaze, sucrose, talc, titanium dioxide.

PMB 200 Tablets also contain: D&C Yellow No. 10, FD&C Blue No. 1, FD&C Yellow No. 6;

PMB 400 Tablets also contain: FD&C Blue No. 2, D&C Red No. 7, D&C Red No. 27.

CLINICAL PHARMACOLOGY:

Estrogens are important in the development and maintenance of the female reproductive system and secondary sex characteristics. They promote growth and development of the vagina, uterus, and fallopian tubes and enlargement of the breasts. Indirectly, they contribute to the shaping of the skeleton, maintenance of tone and elasticity of urogenital structures, changes in the epiphyses of the long bones that allow for the pubertal growth spurt and its termination, growth of axillary and pubic hair, and pigmentation of the nipples and genitals. Decline of estrogenic activity at the end of the menstrual cycle can bring on menstruation, although the cessation of progesterone secretion is the most important factor in the mature ovulatory cycle. However, in the preovulatory or nonovulatory cycle, estrogen is the primary determinant in the onset of menstruation. Estrogens also affect the release of pituitary gonadotropins.

The pharmacologic effects of conjugated estrogens are similar to those of endogenous estrogens. They are soluble in water and are well absorbed from the gastrointestinal tract.

CLINICAL PHARMACOLOGY: *(cont'd)*

In responsive tissues (female genital organs, breasts, hypothalamus, pituitary) estrogens enter the cell and are transported into the nucleus. As a result of estrogen action, specific RNA and protein synthesis occurs.

Metabolism and inactivation occur primarily in the liver. Some estrogens are excreted into the bile; however, they are reabsorbed from the intestine and returned to the liver through the portal venous system. Water-soluble estrogen conjugates are strongly acidic and are ionized in body fluids, which favor excretion through the kidneys since tubular reabsorption is minimal.

Meprobamate is used clinically for the reduction of anxiety and tension. The precise mechanism(s) of its action is not known. It is well absorbed from the gastrointestinal tract and has a physiologic half-life of about 10 hours. It is excreted in the urine primarily as hydroxymeprobamate and as a glucuronide.

The combination of Premarin with meprobamate as provided in PMB relieves the underlying estrogen deficiency and affords tranquilizing activity to ameliorate the anxiety and tension not due to estrogen deficiency.

INDICATIONS AND USAGE:

For the treatment of moderate-to-severe vasomotor symptoms of the menopause when anxiety and tension are part of the symptom complex and only in those cases in which the use of estrogens alone has not resulted in alleviation of such symptoms. PMB HAS NOT BEEN SHOWN TO BE EFFECTIVE FOR ANY PURPOSE DURING PREGNANCY, AND ITS USE MAY CAUSE SEVERE HARM TO THE FETUS (SEE BOXED WARNING).

CONTRAINDICATIONS:

Estrogens should not be used in women with any of the following conditions:

1. Known or suspected cancer of the breast except in appropriately selected patients being treated for metastatic disease.

2. Known or suspected estrogen-dependent neoplasia.

3. Known or suspected pregnancy (see BOXED WARNING).

4. Undiagnosed abnormal genital bleeding.

5. Active thrombophlebitis or thromboembolic disorders.

6. A past history of thrombophlebitis, thrombosis, or thromboembolic disorders associated with previous estrogen use.

Meprobamate should not be used in patients with the following conditions:

1. A history of allergic or idiosyncratic reactions to meprobamate or related compounds such as carisoprodol, mebutamate, tybamate, or carbromal.

2. Acute intermittent porphyria.

WARNINGS:

USAGE IN PREGNANCY AND LACTATION

An increased risk of congenital malformations associated with the use of minor tranquilizers (meprobamate, chlordiazepoxide, and diazepam) during the first trimester of pregnancy has been suggested in several studies. Because use of these drugs is rarely a matter of urgency, their use during this period should almost always be avoided. The possibility that a woman of childbearing potential may be pregnant at the time of institution of therapy should be considered. Patients should be advised that if they become pregnant during therapy or intend to become pregnant they should communicate with their physicians about the desirability of discontinuing the drug.

Meprobamate passes the placental barrier. It is present both in umbilical cord blood at or near maternal plasma levels and in breast milk of lactating mothers at concentrations two to four times that of maternal plasma. When use of meprobamate is contemplated in breast-feeding patients, the drug's higher concentrations in breast milk as compared to maternal plasma levels should be considered.

USAGE IN CHILDREN

PMB is not intended for use in children.

ASSOCIATED WITH ESTROGEN ADMINISTRATION

INDUCTION OF MALIGNANT NEOPLASMS

Estrogens have been reported to increase the risk of endometrial carcinoma. (See BOXED WARNING.) However, a recent, large, case-controlled study indicated no increase in risk of breast cancer in postmenopausal women.

GALLBLADDER DISEASE

A recent study has reported a 2- to 3- fold increase in the risk of surgically confirmed gallbladder disease in women receiving postmenopausal estrogens, similar to the 2-fold increase previously noted in users of oral contraceptives.

EFFECTS SIMILAR TO THOSE CAUSED BY ESTROGEN-PROGESTOGEN ORAL CONTRACEPTIVES

There are several serious adverse effects of oral contraceptives, most of which have not, up to now, been documented as consequences of postmenopausal estrogen therapy. This may reflect the comparatively low doses of estrogen used in postmenopausal women. It would be expected that the larger doses of estrogen used to treat prostatic or breast cancer, or postpartum breast engorgement, are more likely to result in these adverse effects, and, in fact, it has been shown that there is an increased risk of thrombosis in men receiving estrogens for prostatic cancer and women for postpartum breast engorgement.

Thromboembolic Disease: It is now well established that users of oral contraceptives have an increased risk of various thromboembolic and thrombotic vascular diseases, such as thrombophlebitis, pulmonary embolism, stroke, and myocardial infarction. Cases of retinal thrombosis, mesenteric thrombosis, and optic neuritis have been reported in oral-contraceptive users. There is evidence that the risk of several of these adverse reactions is related to the dose of the drug. An increased risk of postsurgery thromboembolic complications has also been reported in users of oral contraceptives. If feasible, estrogen should be discontinued at least 4 weeks before surgery of the type associated with an increased risk of thromboembolism, or during periods of prolonged immobilization.

While an increased rate of thromboembolic and thrombotic disease in postmenopausal users of estrogens has not been found, this does not rule out the possibility that such an increase may be present or that subgroups of women who have underlying risk factors or who are receiving relatively large doses of estrogens may have increased risk. Therefore, estrogens should not be used in persons with active thrombophlebitis or thromboembolic disorders, and they should not be used (except in treatment of malignancy) in persons with a history of such disorders in association with estrogen use. They should be used with caution in patients with cerebral-vascular or coronary-artery disease and only for those in whom estrogens are clearly needed.

Large doses of estrogen (5 mg conjugated estrogens per day), comparable to those used to treat cancer of the prostate and breast, have been shown in a large prospective clinical trial in men to increase the risk of nonfatal myocardial infarction, pulmonary embolism, and

WARNINGS: *(cont'd)*

thrombophlebitis. When estrogen doses of this size are used, any of the thromboembolic and thrombotic adverse effects associated with oral-contraceptive use should be considered a clear risk.

Hepatic Adenoma: Benign hepatic adenomas appear to be associated with the use of oral contraceptives. Although benign, and rare, these may rupture and may cause death through intra-abdominal hemorrhage. Such lesions have not yet been reported in association with other estrogen or progestogen preparations but should be considered in estrogen users having abdominal pain and tenderness, abdominal mass, or hypovolemic shock. Hepatocellular carcinoma has also been reported in women taking estrogen-containing oral contraceptives. The relationship of this malignancy to these drugs is not known at this time.

Elevated Blood Pressure: Women using oral contraceptives sometimes experience increased blood pressure which, in most cases, returns to normal on discontinuing the drug. There is now a report that this may occur with use of estrogens in the menopause, and blood pressure should be monitored with estrogen use, especially if high doses are used.

Glucose Tolerance: A worsening of glucose tolerance has been observed in a significant percentage of patients on estrogen-containing oral contraceptives. For this reason, diabetic patients should be carefully observed while receiving estrogens.

HYPERCALCEMIA

Administration of estrogens may lead to severe hypercalcemia in patients with breast cancer and bone metastases. If this occurs, the drug should be stopped and appropriate measures taken to reduce the serum calcium level.

ASSOCIATED WITH MEPROBAMATE ADMINISTRATION

Drug Dependence: Physical dependence, psychological dependence, and abuse have occurred. When chronic intoxication from prolonged use occurs, it usually involves ingestion of greater than recommended doses and is manifested by ataxia, slurred speech, and vertigo. Therefore, careful supervision of dose and amounts prescribed is advised, as well as avoidance of prolonged administration, especially for alcoholics and other patients with a known propensity for taking excessive quantities of drugs.

Sudden withdrawal of the drug after prolonged and excessive use may precipitate recurrence of preexisting symptoms, such as anxiety, anorexia, or insomnia, or withdrawal reactions, such as vomiting, ataxia, tremors, muscle twitching, confusional states, hallucinosis, and, rarely, convulsive seizures. Such seizures are more likely to occur in persons with central nervous system damage or preexistent or latent convulsive disorders. Onset of withdrawal symptoms occurs usually within 12 to 48 hours after discontinuation of meprobamate; symptoms usually cease within the next 12 to 48 hours.

When excessive dosage has continued for weeks or months, dosage should be reduced gradually over a period of one or two weeks, rather than abruptly stopped. Alternatively, a short-acting barbiturate may be substituted, then gradually withdrawn.

Potentially Hazardous Tasks: Patients should be warned that this drug may impair the mental and/or physical abilities required for the performance of potentially hazardous tasks, such as driving a motor vehicle or operating machinery.

Additive Effects: Since the effects of meprobamate and alcohol or meprobamate and other CNS depressants or psychotropic drugs may be additive, appropriate caution should be exercised with patients who take more than one of these agents simultaneously.

PRECAUTIONS:

GENERAL

Associated with Estrogens

1. A complete medical and family history should be taken prior to the initiation of any estrogen therapy. The pretreatment and periodic physical examinations should include special reference to blood pressure, breasts, abdomen, and pelvic organs and should include a Papanicolaou smear. As a general rule, estrogen should not be prescribed for longer than one year without another physical examination being performed.

2. Fluid retention: Because estrogens may cause some degree of fluid retention, conditions which might be influenced by this factor, such as asthma, epilepsy, migraine, and cardiac or renal dysfunction, require careful observation.

3. Certain patients may develop undesirable manifestations of excessive estrogenic stimulation, such as abnormal or excessive uterine bleeding, mastodynia, etc.

4. Prolonged administration of unopposed estrogen therapy has been reported to increase the risk of endometrial hyperplasia in some patients.

5. Oral contraceptives appear to be associated with an increased incidence of mental depression. Although it is not clear whether this is due to the estrogenic or progestogenic component of the contraceptive, patients with a history of depression should be carefully observed.

6. Preexisting uterine leiomyomata may increase in size during estrogen use.

7. The pathologist should be advised of estrogen therapy when relevant specimens are submitted.

8. Patients with a past history of jaundice during pregnancy have an increased risk of recurrence of jaundice while receiving estrogen-containing oral-contraceptive therapy. If jaundice develops in any patient receiving estrogen, the medication should be discontinued while the cause is investigated.

9. Estrogens may be poorly metabolized in patients with impaired liver function and should be administered with caution in such patients.

10. Because estrogens influence the metabolism of calcium and phosphorus, they should be used with caution in patients with metabolic bone diseases that are associated with hypercalcemia or in patients with renal insufficiency.

11. Because of the effects of estrogens on epiphyseal closure, they should be used judiciously in young patients in whom bone growth is not yet complete.

Concomitant Progestin Use

The lowest effective dose appropriate for the specific indication should be utilized. Studies of the addition of a progestin for 7 or more days of a cycle of estrogen administration have reported a lowered incidence of endometrial hyperplasia. Morphological and biochemical studies of the endometrium suggest that 10 to 13 days of progestin are needed to provide maximal maturation of the endometrium and to eliminate any hyperplastic changes. Whether this will provide protection from endometrial carcinoma has not been clearly established. There are possible additional risks which may be associated with the inclusion of progestin in estrogen- replacement regimens. If concomitant progestin therapy is used, potential risks may include adverse effects on carbohydrate and lipid metabolism. The choice of progestin and dosage may be important in minimizing these adverse effects.

Associated with Meprobamate

1. The lowest effective dose should be administered, particularly to debilitated patients, in order to preclude oversedation.

2. The possibility of suicide attempts should be considered, and the least amount of drug feasible should be dispensed at any one time.

PRECAUTIONS: *(cont'd)*

3. Meprobamate is metabolized in the liver and excreted by the kidney; to avoid its excess accumulation, caution should be exercised in administration to patients with compromised liver or kidney function.

4. Meprobamate occasionally may precipitate seizures in epileptic patients.

DRUG/LABORATORY TEST INTERACTIONS Certain endocrine and liver-function tests may be affected by estrogen-containing oral contraceptives. The following similar changes may be expected with larger doses of estrogen.

a. Increased sulfobromophthalein retention.

b. Increased prothrombin and factors VII, VIII, IX, and X; decreased antithrombin 3; increased norepinephrine-induced platelet aggregability.

c. Increased thyroid binding globulin (TBG) leading to increased circulating total thyroid hormone, as measured by PBI, T_4 by column or T_4 by radioimmunoassay. Free T_3 resin uptake is decreased, reflecting the elevated TBG; free T_4 concentration is unaltered.

d. Impaired glucose tolerance.

e. Decreased pregnanediol excretion.

f. Reduced response to metyrapone test.

g. Reduced serum folate concentration.

h. Increased serum triglyceride and phospholipid concentration.

MUTAGENESIS AND CARCINOGENESIS

Long-term, continuous administration of natural and synthetic estrogens in certain animal species increases the frequency of carcinomas of the breast, cervix, vagina, and liver. However, in a recent, large, case- controlled study of post-menopausal women, there was no increase in risk of breast cancer with use of conjugated estrogens.

PREGNANCY CATEGORY X

See CONTRAINDICATIONS and BOXED WARNING.

NURSING MOTHERS

Because of the potential for serious adverse reactions in nursing infants from PMB, a decision should be made whether to discontinue nursing or to discontinue the drug, taking into account the importance of the drug to the mother. See WARNINGS for information on use in pregnancy and lactation.

PEDIATRIC USE

Safety and effectiveness in children have not been established.

ADVERSE REACTIONS:

ASSOCIATED WITH ESTROGEN ADMINISTRATION

(See WARNINGS regarding induction of neoplasia, adverse effects on the fetus, increased incidence of gallbladder disease, and adverse effects similar to those of oral contraceptives, including thromboembolism.) The following additional adverse reactions have been reported with estrogenic therapy, including oral contraceptives:

1. Genitourinary System: Breakthrough bleeding, spotting, change in menstrual flow; dysmenorrhea; premenstrual-like syndrome; amenorrhea during and after treatment; increase in size of uterine fibromyomata; vaginal candidiasis; change in cervical erosion and in degree of cervical secretion; cystitis-like syndrome.

2. Breasts: Tenderness, enlargement, secretion.

3. Gastrointestinal: Nausea, vomiting, abdominal cramps, bloating, cholestatic jaundice.

4. Skin: Chloasma or melasma which may persist when drug is discontinued; erythema multiforme; erythema nodosum, hemorrhagic eruption, loss of scalp hair, hirsutism.

5. Eyes: Steepening of corneal curvature; intolerance to contact lenses.

6. CNS: Headache, migraine, dizziness; mental depression; chorea.

7. Miscellaneous: Increase or decrease in weight; reduced carbohydrate tolerance; aggravation of porphyria, edema; changes in libido.

THE FOLLOWING HAVE BEEN REPORTED WITH MEPROBAMATE THERAPY

1. Central Nervous System: Drowsiness, ataxia, dizziness, slurred speech, headache, vertigo, weakness, paresthesias, impairment of visual accommodation, euphoria, overstimulation, paradoxical excitement, fast EEG activity.

2. Gastrointestinal: Nausea, vomiting, diarrhea.

3. Cardiovascular: Palpitations, tachycardia, various forms of arrhythmia, transient ECG changes, syncope; also hypotensive crises (including one fatal case).

4. Allergic or Idiosyncratic: Allergic or idiosyncratic reactions are usually seen within the period of the first to fourth dose in patients having had no previous contact with the drug. Milder reactions are characterized by an itchy, urticarial, or erythematous maculopapular rash which may be generalized or confined to the groin. Other reactions have included leukopenia, acute nonthrombocytopenic purpura, petechiae, ecchymoses, eosinophilia, peripheral edema, adenopathy, fever, fixed-drug eruption with cross reaction to carisoprodol, and cross sensitivity between meprobamate/mebutamate and meprobamate/carbromal.

More severe hypersensitivity reactions, rarely reported, include hyperpyrexia, chills, angioneurotic edema, bronchospasm, oliguria, and anuria. Also, anaphylaxis, erythema multiforme, exfoliative dermatitis, stomatitis, proctitis, Stevens-Johnson syndrome, and bullous dermatitis, including one fatal case of the latter following administration of meprobamate in combination with prednisolone.

In case of allergic or idiosyncratic reactions to meprobamate, discontinue the drug and initiate appropriate symptomatic therapy, which may include epinephrine, antihistamines, and in severe cases corticosteroids. In evaluating possible allergic reactions, also consider allergy to excipients (information on excipients is available to physicians on request).

5. Hematologic: See ADVERSE REACTIONS, Allergic or Idiosyncratic Agranulocytosis and aplastic anemia have been reported, although no causal relationship has been established. These cases rarely were fatal. Rare cases of thrombocytopenic purpura have been reported.

6. Other: Exacerbation of porphyric symptoms.

OVERDOSAGE:

Acute Overdosage (Estrogen Alone): Numerous reports of ingestion of large doses of estrogen-containing oral contraceptives by young children indicate that acute serious ill effects do not occur. Overdosage of estrogens may cause nausea, and withdrawal bleeding may occur in females.

Acute Simple Overdosage (Meprobamate Alone): Death has been reported with ingestion of as little as 12 grams meprobamate and survival with as much as 40 grams.

Blood Levels: 0.5 to 2.0 mg% represents the usual blood-level range of meprobamate after therapeutic doses. The level may occasionally be as high as 3.0 mg%. 3 to 10 mg% usually corresponds to findings of mild-to-moderate symptoms of overdosage, such as stupor or light coma. 10 to 20 mg% usually corresponds to deeper coma, requiring more intensive treatment. Some fatalities occur. At levels greater than 20 mg%, more fatalities than survivals can be expected.

OVERDOSAGE: *(cont'd)*

ACUTE COMBINED (ALCOHOL OR OTHER CNS DEPRESSANTS OR PSYCHOTROPIC DRUGS)

Overdosage: Since effects can be additive, a history of ingestion of a low dose of meprobamate plus any of these compounds (or of a relatively low blood or tissue level) cannot be used as a prognostic indicator.

In cases where excessive doses have been taken, sleep ensues rapidly and blood pressure, pulse, and respiratory rates are reduced to basal levels. Any drug remaining in the stomach should be removed and symptomatic therapy given. Should respiration or blood pressure become compromised, respiratory assistance, central nervous system stimulants, and pressor agents should be administered cautiously as indicated. Meprobamate is metabolized in the liver and excreted by the kidney. Diuresis, osmotic (mannitol) diuresis, peritoneal dialysis, and hemodialysis have been used successfully. Careful monitoring of urinary output is necessary, and caution should be taken to avoid overhydration. Relapse and death, after initial recovery, have been attributed to incomplete gastric emptying and delayed absorption. Meprobamate can be measured in biological fluids by two methods: colorimetric and gas chromatographic.

DOSAGE AND ADMINISTRATION:

GIVEN CYCLICALLY FOR SHORT-TERM USE ONLY

For the treatment of moderate-to-severe *vasomotor* symptoms of the menopause when anxiety and tension are part of the symptom complex and only in those cases in which the use of estrogens alone has not resulted in alleviation of such symptoms.

The lowest dose that will control symptoms should be chosen, and medication should be discontinued as promptly as possible. The usual dosage of conjugated estrogens is 1.25 milligrams daily. The usual dosage of meprobamate is 1200 to 1600 milligrams daily.

Administration should be cyclic (*e.g.,* three weeks on and one week off).

Attempts to discontinue or taper medication should be made at three- to six-month intervals.

PMB 200 & PMB 400

The usual dosage is one tablet of either strength three times daily administered cyclically. Use of meprobamate during the rest period should be considered for those patients who may require continuing medication with tranquilizer. After the first few cycles of therapy, the patient's need for continuing the use of the meprobamate component should be reevaluated.

Daily dosage should be adjusted to individual requirements. The daily dosage should not exceed 6 tablets of PMB 200 per day or 4 tablets of PMB 400 per day.

Treated patients with an intact uterus should be monitored closely for signs of endometrial cancer, and appropriate diagnostic measures should be taken to rule out malignancy in the event of persistent or recurring abnormal vaginal bleeding.

Store at room temperature (approximately 25°C).

HOW SUPPLIED - EQUIVALENTS NOT AVAILABLE:

Tablet, Coated - Oral - 0.45 mg/200 mg

60's	$56.35	PMB-200, Ayerst	00046-0880-60

Tablet, Coated - Oral - 0.45 mg/400 mg

60's	$66.79	PMB-400, Ayerst	00046-0881-60
100's	$158.28	MILPREM-400, Wallace Labs	00037-5401-01

ESTROGENS, CONJUGATED; METHYLTESTOSTERONE *(001199)*

CATEGORIES: Anabolic Steroids; Androgens; Hormones; Menopause; Pregnancy Category X; DEA Class CIII; FDA Pre 1938 Drugs

BRAND NAMES: **Premarin w Methyltestosterone**

FORMULARIES: Medi-Cal

WARNING:
1. ESTROGENS HAVE BEEN REPORTED TO INCREASE THE RISK OF ENDOMETRIAL CARCINOMA. Three independent, case-controlled studies have reported an increased risk of endometrial cancer in postmenopausal women exposed to exogenous estrogens for more than one year. This risk was independent of the other known risk factors for endometrial cancer. These studies are further supported by the finding that incidence rates of endometrial cancer have increased sharply since 1969 in eight different areas of the United States with population-based cancer-reporting systems, an increase which may be related to the rapidly expanding use of estrogens during the last decade.

The three case-controlled studies reported that the risk of endometrial cancer in estrogen users was about 4.5 to 13.9 times greater than in nonusers. The risk appears to depend on both duration of treatment and on estrogen dose. In view of these findings, when estrogens are used for the treatment of menopausal symptoms, the lowest dose that will control symptoms should be utilized and medication should be discontinued as soon as possible. When prolonged treatment is medically indicated, the patient should be reassessed, on at least a semi-annual basis, to determine the need for continued therapy. Although the evidence must be considered preliminary, one study suggests that cyclic administration of low doses of estrogen may carry less risk than continuous administration. It, therefore, appears prudent to utilize such a regimen.

Close clinical surveillance of all women taking estrogens is important. In all cases of undiagnosed persistent or recurring abnormal vaginal bleeding, adequate diagnostic measures should be under-taken to rule out malignancy.

There is no evidence at present that "natural" estrogens are more or less hazardous than "synthetic" estrogens at equi-estrogenic doses.

2. ESTROGENS SHOULD NOT BE USED DURING PREGNANCY. The use of female sex hormones, both estrogens and progestogens, during early pregnancy may seriously damage the offspring. It has been shown that females exposed IN UTERO to diethylstilbestrol, a nonsteroidal estrogen, have an increased risk of developing, in later life, a form of vaginal or cervical cancer that is ordinarily extremely rare. This risk has been estimated as not greater than 4 per 1,000 exposures.7 Furthermore, a high percentage of such exposed women (from 30% to 90%) have been found to have vaginal adenosis, epithelial changes of the vagina and cervix. Although these changes are histologically benign, it is not known whether they are precursors of malignancy. Although similar data are not

available with the use of other estrogens, it cannot be presumed they would not induce similar changes.

Several reports suggest an association between intrauterine exposure to female sex hormones and congenital anomalies, including congenital heart defects and limb-reduction defects. One case-controlled study estimated a 4.7-fold increased risk of limb-reduction defects in infants exposed IN UTERO to sex hormones (oral contraceptives, hormone withdrawal tests for pregnancy, or attempted treatment for threatened abortion). Some of these exposures were very short and involved only a few days of treatment. The data suggest that the risk of limb-reduction defects in exposed fetuses is somewhat less than 1 per 1,000.

In the past, female sex hormones have been used during pregnancy in an attempt to treat threatened or habitual abortion. There is considerable evidence that estrogens are ineffective for these indications, and there is no evidence from well-controlled studies that progestogens are effective for these uses.

If Premarin with methyltestosterone is used during pregnancy, or if the patient becomes pregnant while taking this drug, she should be apprised of the potential risks to the fetus, and the advisability of pregnancy continuation.

DESCRIPTION:

Premarin with methyltestosterone is provided in tablets for oral administration.

Premarin (conjugated estrogens, USP) is a mixture of estrogens, obtained exclusively from natural sources, occurring as the sodium salts of water-soluble estrogen sulfates blended to represent the average composition of material derived from pregnant mares' urine. It contains estrone, equilin, and 17 α-dihydroequilin, together, with smaller amounts of 17 α-estradiol, equilenin, and 17 α-dihydroequilenin as salts of their sulfate esters.

Methyltestosterone is an androgen.

Androgens are derivatives of cyclopentane-perhydrophenanthene. Endogenous androgens are C-19 steroids with a side chain at C-17, and with two angular methyl groups. Testosterone is the primary endogenous androgen. Fluoxymesterone and methyltestosterone are synthetic derivatives of testosterone.

Methyltestosterone is a white to light-yellow crystalline substance that is virtually insoluble in water but soluble in organic solvents. It is stable in air but decomposes in light.

Premarin with methyltestosterone tablets contain the following inactive ingredients: calcium phosphate tribasic, calcium sulfate, carnauba wax, cellulose, glyceryl monooleate, guar gum, lactose, magnesium stearate, methylcellulose, pharmaceutical glaze, polyethylene glycol, stearic acid, sucrose, talc, titanium dioxide.

1.25 mg Premarin with 10.0 mg methyltestosterone tablets also contain: D&C Yellow #10, FD&C Yellow #6.

CLINICAL PHARMACOLOGY:

ESTROGENS

Estrogens are important in the development and maintenance of the female reproductive system and secondary sex characteristics. They promote growth and development of the vagina, uterus, and fallopian tubes, and enlargement of the breasts. Indirectly, they contribute to the shaping of the skeleton, maintenance of tone and elasticity of urogenital structures; changes in the epiphyses of the long bones that allow for the pubertal growth spurt and its termination, growth of axillary and pubic hair, and pigmentation of the nipples and genitals. Decline of estrogenic activity at the end of the menstrual cycle can bring on menstruation, although the cessation of progesterone secretion is the most important factor in the mature ovulatory cycle. However, in the preovulatory or non-ovulatory cycle, estrogen is the primary determinant in the onset of menstruation. Estrogens also affect the release of pituitary gonadotropins.

The pharmacologic effects of conjugated estrogens are similar to those of endogenous estrogens. They are soluble in water and are well absorbed from the gastrointestinal tract.

In responsive tissues (female genital organs, breasts, hypothalamus, pituitary) estrogens enter the cell and are transported into the nucleus. As a result of estrogen action, specific RNA and protein synthesis occurs.

Estrogen Pharmacokinetics

Metabolism and inactivation occur primarily in the liver. Some estrogens are excreted into the bile; however, they are reabsorbed from the intestine and returned to the liver through the portal venous system. Water-soluble estrogen conjugates are strongly acidic and are ionized in body fluids, which favor excretion through the kidneys since tubular reabsorption is minimal.

ANDROGENS

Endogenous androgens are responsible for the normal growth and development of the male sex organs and for maintenance of secondary sex characteristics. These effects include the growth and maturation of prostate, seminal vesicles, penis, and scrotum; the development of male hair distribution, such as beard, pubic, chest, and axillary hair, laryngeal enlargement, vocal chord thickening, alterations in body musculature, and fat distribution. Drugs in this class also cause retention of nitrogen, sodium, potassium, phosphorus, and decreased urinary excretion of calcium. Androgens have been reported to increase protein anabolism and decrease protein catabolism. Nitrogen balance is improved only when there is sufficient intake of calories and protein.

Androgens are responsible for the growth spurt of adolescence and for the eventual termination of linear growth which is brought about by fusion of the epiphyseal growth centers. In children, exogenous androgens accelerate linear growth rates but may cause a disproportionate advancement in bone maturation. Use over long periods may result in fusion of the epiphyseal growth centers and termination of growth process. Androgens have been reported to stimulate the production of red blood cells by enhancing the production of erythropoietic stimulating factor.

Androgen Pharmacokinetics

Testosterone given orally is metabolized by the gut, and 44% is cleared by the liver in the first pass. Oral doses as high as 400 mg per day are needed to achieve clinically effective blood levels for full replacement therapy. The synthetic androgens (methyltestosterone and fluoxymesterone) are less extensively metabolized by the liver and have longer half-lives. They are more suitable than testosterone for oral administration. Testosterone in plasma is 98% bound to a specific testosterone-estradiol binding globulin, and about 2% is free. Generally, the amount of this sex-hormone-binding globulin in the plasma will determine the distribution of testosterone between free and bound forms, and the free testosterone concentration will determine its half-life.

About 90% of a dose of testosterone is excreted in the urine as glucuronic and sulfuric acid conjugates of testosterone and its metabolites; about 6% of a dose is excreted in the feces, mostly in the unconjugated form. Inactivation of testosterone occurs primarily in the liver.

CLINICAL PHARMACOLOGY: *(cont'd)*

Testosterone is metabolized to various 17-keto steroids through two different pathways. There are considerable variations of the half- life to testosterone as reported in the literature, ranging from 10 to 100 minutes.

In many tissues the activity of testosterone appears to depend on reduction to dihydrotestosterone, which binds to cytosol receptor proteins. The steroid-receptor complex is transported to the nucleus where it initiates transcription events and cellular changes related to androgen action.

INDICATIONS AND USAGE:

Premarin (conjugated estrogens, USP) with Methyltestosterone is indicated in the treatment of:

Moderate-to-severe *vasomotor* symptoms associated with the menopause in those patients not improved by estrogens alone. (There is no evidence that estrogens are effective for nervous symptoms or depression without associated vasomotor symptoms, and they should not be used to treat such conditions.)

PREMARIN WITH METHYLTESTOSTERONE HAS NOT BEEN SHOWN TO BE EFFECTIVE FOR ANY PURPOSE DURING PREGNANCY, AND ITS USE MAY CAUSE SEVERE HARM TO THE FETUS (SEE BOXED WARNING).

CONTRAINDICATIONS:

Estrogens should not be used in women with any of the following conditions:

1. Known or suspected cancer of the breast, except in appropriately selected patients being treated for metastatic disease.

2. Known or suspected estrogen-dependent neoplasia.

3. Known or suspected pregnancy (see BOXED WARNING).

4. Undiagnosed abnormal genital bleeding.

5. Active thrombophlebitis or thromboembolic disorders.

6. A past history of thrombophlebitis, thrombosis, or thromboembolic disorders associated with previous estrogen use (except when used in treatment of breast malignancy).

Methyltestosterone should not be used in:

1. The presence of severe liver damage.

2. Pregnancy and in breast-feeding mothers because of the possibility of masculinization of the female fetus or breast-fed infant.

WARNINGS:

ASSOCIATED WITH ESTROGENS

Induction Of Malignant Neoplasms

Long-term, continuous administration of natural and synthetic estrogens in certain animal species increases the frequency of carcinomas of the breast, cervix, vagina, and liver. There are now reports that estrogens increase the risk of carcinoma of the endometrium in humans (see BOXED WARNING).

At the present time there is no satisfactory evidence that estrogens given to postmenopausal women increase the risk of cancer of the breast, although a recent, long-term follow-up of a single physician's practice has raised this possibility. Because of the animal data, there is a need for caution in prescribing estrogens for women with a strong family history of breast cancer or who have breast nodules, fibrocystic disease, or abnormal mammograms.

Gallbladder Disease

A recent study has reported a 2- to 3-fold increase in the risk of surgically confirmed gallbladder disease in women receiving postmenopausal estrogens, similar to the 2-fold increase previously noted in users of oral contraceptives.

Effects Similar To Those Caused By Estrogen-Progestogen Oral Contraceptives

There are several serious adverse effects of oral contraceptives, most of which have not, up to now, been documented as consequences of postmenopausal estrogen therapy. This may reflect the comparatively low doses of estrogen used in postmenopausal women. It would be expected that the larger doses of estrogen used to treat prostatic or breast cancer are more likely to result in these adverse effects, and, in fact, it has been shown that there is an increased risk of thrombosis in men receiving estrogens for prostatic cancer.

a. Thromboembolic Disease: It is now well established that users of oral contraceptives have an increased risk of various thromboembolic and thrombotic vascular diseases, such as thrombophlebitis, pulmonary embolism, stroke, and myocardial infarction. Cases of retinal thrombosis, mesenteric thrombosis, and optic neuritis have been reported in oral-contraceptive users. There is evidence that the risk of several of these adverse reactions is related to the dose of the drug. An increased risk of postsurgery thromboembolic complications has also been reported in users of oral contraceptives. If feasible, estrogen should be discontinued at least 4 weeks before surgery of the type associated with an increased risk of thromboembolism, or during periods of prolonged immobilization.

While an increased rate of thromboembolic and thrombotic disease in postmenopausal users of estrogens has not been found, this does not rule out the possibility that such an increase may be present or that subgroups of women who have underlying risk factors or who are receiving relatively large doses of estrogens may have increased risk. Therefore, estrogens should not be used in persons with active thrombophlebitis or thromboembolic disorders, and they should not be used (except in treatment of malignancy) in persons with a history of such disorders in association with estrogen use. They should be used with caution in patients with cerebral-vascular or coronary-artery disease and only for those in whom estrogens are clearly needed.

Large doses of estrogen (5 mg conjugated estrogens per day), comparable to those used to treat cancer of the prostate and breast, have been shown in a large prospective clinical trial in men to increase the risk of nonfatal myocardial infarction, pulmonary embolism, and thrombophlebitis. When estrogen doses of this size are used, any of the thromboembolic and thrombotic adverse effects associated with oral-contraceptive use should be considered a clear risk.

b. Hepatic Adenoma: Benign hepatic adenomas appear to be associated with the use of oral contraceptives. Although benign, and rare, these may rupture and may cause death through intra-abdominal hemorrhage. Such lesions have not yet been reported in association with other estrogen or progestogen preparations but should be considered in estrogen users having abdominal pain and tenderness, abdominal mass, or hypovolemic shock. Hepatocellular carcinoma has also been reported in women taking estrogen-containing oral contraceptives. The relationship of this malignancy to these drugs is not known at this time.

c. Elevated Blood Pressure: Women using oral contraceptives sometimes experience increased blood pressure which, in most cases, returns to normal on discontinuing the drug. There is now a report that this may occur with use of estrogens in the menopause, and blood pressure should be monitored with estrogen use, especially if high doses are used.

d. Glucose Tolerance: A worsening of glucose tolerance has been observed in a significant percentage of patients on estrogen-containing oral contraceptives. For this reason, diabetic patients should be carefully observed while receiving estrogens.

WARNINGS: *(cont'd)*

Hypercalcemia

Administration of estrogens may lead to severe hypercalcemia in patients with breast cancer and bone metastases. If this occurs, the drug should be stopped and appropriate measures taken to reduce the serum calcium level.

ASSOCIATED WITH METHYLTESTOSTERONE

In patients with breast cancer, androgen therapy may cause hypercalcemia by stimulating osteolysis. In this case, the drug should be discontinued.

Prolonged use of high doses of androgens has been associated with the development of peliosis hepatis and hepatic neoplasms including hepatocellular carcinoma. See PRECAUTIONS, Carcinogenesis. Peliosis hepatis can be a life, threatening or fatal complication.

Cholestatic hepatitis and jaundice occur with 17-alpha-alkylandrogens at a relatively low dose. If cholestatic hepatitis with jaundice appears or if liver-function tests become abnormal, the androgen should be discontinued and the etiology should be determined. Drug-induced jaundice is reversible when the medication is discontinued.

Edema with or without congestive heart failure may be a serious complication in patients with preexisting cardiac, renal, or hepatic disease. In addition to discontinuation of the drug, diuretic therapy may be required.

PRECAUTIONS:

ASSOCIATED WITH ESTROGENS

General

1. Addition of a progestin: Studies of the addition of a progestin for 7 or more days of a cycle of estrogen administration have reported a lowered incidence of endometrial hyperplasia. Morphological and biochemical studies of the endometrium suggest that 10 to 13 days of progestin are needed to provide maximal maturation of the endometrium and to eliminate any hyperplastic changes. Whether this will provide protection from endometrial carcinoma has not been clearly established. There are possible additional risks which may be associated with the inclusion of progestin in estrogen-replacement regimens. The potential risks include adverse effects on carbohydrate and lipid metabolism. The choice of progestin and dosage may be important in minimizing these adverse effects.

2. Physical examination: A complete medical and family history should be taken prior to the initiation of any estrogen therapy. The pretreatment and periodic physical examinations should include special reference to blood pressure, breasts, abdomen, and pelvic organs and should include a Papanicolaou smear. As a general rule, estrogen should not be prescribed for longer than one year without another physical examination being performed.

3. Fluid retention: Because estrogens may cause some degree of fluid retention, conditions which might be influenced by this factor, such as asthma, epilepsy, migraine, and cardiac or renal dysfunction, require careful observation.

4. Certain patients may develop undesirable manifestations of excessive estrogenic stimulation, such as abnormal or excessive uterine bleeding, mastodynia, etc.

5. Prolonged administration of unopposed estrogen therapy has been reported to increase the risk of endometrial hyperplasia in some patients.

6. Oral contraceptives appear to be associated with an increased incidence of mental depression. Although it is not clear whether this is due to the estrogenic or progestogenic component of the contraceptive, patients with a history of depression should be carefully observed.

7. Preexisting uterine leiomyomata may increase in size during estrogen use.

8. The pathologist should be advised of estrogen therapy when relevant specimens are submitted.

9. Patients with a past history of jaundice during pregnancy have an increased risk of recurrence of jaundice while receiving estrogen-containing oral-contraceptive therapy. If jaundice develops in any patient receiving estrogen, the medication should be discontinued while the cause is investigated.

10. Estrogens may be poorly metabolized in patients with impaired liver function and should be administered with caution in such patients.

11. Because estrogens influence the metabolism of calcium and phosphorus, they should be used with caution in patients with metabolic bone diseases that are associated with hypercalcemia or in patients with renal insufficiency.

12. Because of the effects of estrogens on epiphyseal closure, they should be used judiciously in young patients in whom bone growth is not yet complete.

13. Certain endocrine and liver-function tests may be affected by estrogen-containing oral contraceptives. The following similar changes may be expected with larger doses of estrogen:

a. Increased sulfobromophthalein retention.

b. Increased prothrombin and factors VII, VIII, IX, and X; decreased antithrombin 3; increased norepinephrine-induced platelet aggregability.

c. Increased thyroid-binding globulin (TBG) leading to increased circulating total thyroid hormone, as measured by PBI, T_4 by column or T_4 by radioimmunoassay. Free T_3 resin uptake is decreased, reflecting the elevated TBG; free T_4 concentration is unaltered.

d. Impaired glucose tolerance.

e. Decreased pregnanediol excretion.

f. Reduced response to metyrapone test.

g. Reduced serum folate concentration.

h. Increased serum triglyceride and phospholipid concentration.

Information for the Patient

See Estrogens, Conjugated, PATIENT PACKAGE INSERT

Pregnancy Category X

See CONTRAINDICATIONS and BOXED WARNING.

Nursing Mothers

As a general principle, the administration of any drug to nursing mothers should be done only when clearly necessary since many drugs are excreted in human milk.

ASSOCIATED WITH METHYL TESTOSTERONE

General

1. Women should be observed for signs of virilization (deepening of the voice, hirsutism, acne, clitoromegaly, and menstrual irregularities). Discontinuation of drug therapy at the time of evidence of mild virilism is necessary to prevent irreversible virilization. Such virilization is usual following androgen use at high doses.

2. Prolonged dosage of androgen may result in sodium and fluid retention. This may present a problem, especially in patients with compromised cardiac reserve or renal disease.

3. Hypersensitivity may occur rarely.

4. PBI may be decreased in patients taking androgens.

5. Hypercalcemia may occur. If this does occur, the drug should be discontinued.

PRECAUTIONS: *(cont'd)*

Information for the Patient

The physician should instruct patients to report any of the following side effects of androgens:

Women: Hoarseness, acne, changes in menstrual periods, or more hair on the face.

All Patients: Any nausea, vomiting, changes in skin color, or ankle swelling.

Laboratory Tests

1. Women with disseminated breast carcinoma should have frequent determination of urine and serum calcium levels during the course of androgen therapy (see WARNINGS).

2. Because of the hepatotoxicity associated with the use of 17-alpha-alkylated androgens, liver-function tests should be obtained periodically.

3. Hemoglobin and hematocrit should be checked periodically for polycythemia in patients who are receiving high doses of androgens.

Drug/Laboratory Test Interactions

Androgens may decrease levels of thyroxine-binding globulin, resulting in decreased total T_4 serum levels and increased resin uptake of T_3 and T_4. Free thyroid hormone levels remain unchanged, however, and there is no clinical evidence of thyroid dysfunction.

Carcinogenesis

Animal Data: Testosterone has been tested by subcutaneous injection and implantation in mice and rats. The implant induced cervical-uterine tumors in mice, which metastasized in some cases. There is suggestive evidence that injection of testosterone into some strains of female mice increases their susceptibility to hepatoma. Testosterone is also known to increase the number of tumors and decrease the degree of differentiation of chemically induced carcinomas of the liver in rats.

Human Data: There are rare reports of hepatocellular carcinoma in patients receiving long-term therapy with androgens in high doses. Withdrawal of the drugs did not lead to regression of the tumors in all cases.

Geriatric patients treated with androgens may be at an increased risk for the development of prostatic hypertrophy and prostatic carcinoma.

Pregnancy, Teratogenic Effects, Pregnancy Category X

See CONTRAINDICATIONS.

Nursing Mothers

It is not known whether androgens are excreted in human milk. Because many drugs are excreted in human milk and because of the potential for serious adverse reactions in nursing infants from estrogens, a decision should be made whether to discontinue nursing or to discontinue the drug, taking into account the importance of the drug to the mother.

DRUG INTERACTIONS:

1. Anticoagulants: C-17 substituted derivatives of testosterone, such as methandrostenolone, have been reported to decrease the anticoagulant requirements of patients receiving oral anticoagulants. Patients receiving oral-anticoagulant therapy require close monitoring, especially when androgens are started or stopped.

2. Oxyphenbutazone: Concurrent administration of oxyphenbutazone and androgens may result in elevated serum levels of oxyphenbutazone.

3. Insulin: In diabetic patients the metabolic effects of androgens may decrease blood glucose and insulin requirements.

ADVERSE REACTIONS:

ASSOCIATED WITH ESTROGENS

(See WARNINGS regarding induction of neoplasia, adverse effects on the fetus, increased incidence of gallbladder disease, and adverse effects similar to those of oral contraceptives, including thromboembolism.) The following additional adverse reactions have been reported with estrogenic therapy, including oral contraceptives:

1. Genitourinary System: Breakthrough bleeding, spotting, change in menstrual flow; dysmenorrhea; premenstrual-like syndrome; amenorrhea during and after treatment; increase in size of uterine fibromyomata; vaginal candidiasis; change in cervical erosion and in degree of cervical secretion; cystitis-like syndrome.

2. Breasts: Tenderness, enlargement, secretion.

3. Gastrointestinal: Nausea, vomiting, abdominal cramps, bloating; cholestatic jaundice.

4. Skin: Chloasma or melasma which may persist when drug is discontinued; erythema multiforme; erythema nodosum; hemorrhagic eruption; loss of scalp hair; hirsutism.

5. Eyes: Steepening of corneal curvature; intolerance to contact lenses.

6. CNS: Headache, migraine, dizziness; mental depression; chorea.

7. Miscellaneous: Increase or decrease in weight; reduced carbohydrate tolerance; aggravation of porphyria; edema; changes in libido.

ASSOCIATED WITH METHYLTESTOSTERONE

Endocrine and Urogenital

1. Female: The most common side effects of androgen therapy are amenorrhea and other menstrual irregularities, inhibition of gonadotropin secretion, and virilization, including deepening of the voice and clitoral enlargement. The latter usually is not reversible after androgens are discontinued. When administered to a pregnant woman, androgens cause virilization of external genitalia of the female fetus.

2. Skin and Appendages: Hirsutism, male pattern of baldness, and acne.

3. Fluid and Electrolyte Disturbances: Retention of sodium, chloride, water, potassium, calcium, and inorganic phosphates.

4. Gastrointestinal: Nausea, cholestatic jaundice, alterations in liver- function tests, rarely hepatocellular neoplasms, and peliosis hepatis (see WARNINGS).

5. Hematologic: Suppression of clotting factors II, V, VII, and X, bleeding in patients on concomitant anticoagulant therapy, and polycythemia.

6. Nervous System: Increased or decreased libido, headache, anxiety, depression, and generalized paresthesia.

7. Metabolic: Increased serum cholesterol.

8. Miscellaneous: Inflammation and pain at the site of intramuscular injection or subcutaneous implantation of testosterone-containing pellets, stomatitis with buccal preparations, and rarely anaphylactoid reactions.

OVERDOSAGE:

Numerous reports of ingestion of large doses of estrogen-containing oral contraceptives by young children indicate that acute serious ill effects do not occur. Overdosage of estrogens may cause nausea, and withdrawal bleeding may occur in females.

There have been no reports of acute overdosage with the androgens.

DOSAGE AND ADMINISTRATION:

Given Cyclically For Short-Term Use Only

For treatment of moderate-to-severe *vasomotor* symptoms associated with the menopause in patients not improved by estrogen alone.

The lowest dose that will control symptoms should be chosen, and medication should be discontinued as promptly as possible.

Administration should be cyclic (*e.g.*, three weeks on and one week off).

Attempts to discontinue or taper medication should be made at 3- to 6-month intervals.

Usual Dosage Range: 1.25 mg conjugated estrogens, USP, and 10.0 mg methyltestosterone (1 yellow tablet, No. 879, or 2 white tablets, No. 878) daily and cyclically.

Treated patients with an intact uterus should be monitored closely for signs of endometrial cancer, and appropriate diagnostic measures should be taken to rule out malignancy in the event of persistent or recurring abnormal vaginal bleeding.

Store at room temperature (approximately 25°C).

The appearance of these tablets is a trademark of Ayerst Laboratories.

HOW SUPPLIED - EQUIVALENTS NOT AVAILABLE:

Tablet, Coated - Oral - 0.625 mg/5 mg

100's	$79.44	PREMARIN W/METHYLTESTOSTERONE, Ayerst	00046-0878-81

Tablet, Coated - Oral - 1.25 mg/10 mg

100's	$133.64	PREMARIN WITH METHYLTESTOSTERONE, Ayerst	00046-0879-81

ESTROGENS, ESTERIFIED *(001200)*

CATEGORIES: Antineoplastics; Breast Carcinoma; Cancer; Endometrial Carcinoma; Hormones; Hypogonadism; Kraurosis Vulvae; Menopause; Oncologic Drugs; Ovarian Failure; Prostatic Carcinoma; Vaginitis; Pregnancy Category X; FDA Approval Pre 1982

BRAND NAMES: Amnestrogen; Esterified Estrogens; **Estratab**; Evex; Femogen; Menest; *Neo-Estrone* (Canada)
(International brand names outside U.S. in italics)

FORMULARIES: Aetna; FHP; Medi-Cal

WARNING:

1. ESTROGENS HAVE BEEN REPORTED TO INCREASE THE RISK OF ENDOMETRIAL CARCINOMA: Three independent case control studies have shown an increased risk of endometrial cancer in postmenopausal women exposed to exogenous estrogens for prolonged periods.(1-3) This risk was independent of the other known risk factors for endometrial cancer. These studies are further supported by the finding that incidence rates of endometrial cancer have increased sharply since 1969 in eight different areas of the U.S. with population-based cancer reporting systems, an increase which may be related to the rapidly expanding use of estrogens during the last decade.[4] The three case control studies reported that the risk of endometrial cancer in estrogen users was about 4.5 to 13.9 times greater than in nonusers. The risk appears to depend on both duration of treatment and estrogen dose.[3] In view of these findings, when estrogens are used for the treatment of menopausal symptoms, the lowest dose that will control symptoms should be utilized and medication should be discontinued as soon as possible. When prolonged treatment is medically indicated, the patient should be reassessed on at least a semiannual basis to determine the need for continued therapy. Although the evidence must be considered preliminary, one study suggests that cyclic administration of low doses of estrogen may carry less risk than continuous administration(3); it therefore appears prudent to utilize such a regimen. Close clinical surveillance of all women taking estrogens is important. In all cases of undiagnosed persistent or recurring abnormal vaginal bleeding, adequate diagnostic measures should be undertaken to rule out malignancy. There is no evidence at present that "natural" estrogens are more or less hazardous than "synthetic" estrogens at equiestrogenic doses.

2. ESTROGENS SHOULD NOT BE USED DURING PREGNANCY: The use of female sex hormones, both estrogens and progestogens, during early pregnancy may seriously damage the offspring. It has been shown that females exposed in utero to diethylstilbestrol, a non-steroidal estrogen, have an increased risk of developing in later life a form of vaginal or cervical cancer that is ordinarily extremely rare.[5,6] The risk has been estimated as not greater than 4 per 1000 exposures.[7] Furthermore, a high percentage of such exposed women (from 30 to 90 percent) have been found to have vaginal adenosis,[8-12] epithelial changes of the vagina and cervix. Although these changes are histologically benign, it is not known whether they are precursors of malignancy. Although similar data are not available with the use of other estrogens, it cannot be presumed they would not induce similar changes. Several reports suggest an association between intrauterine exposure to female sex hormones and congenital anomalies, including congenital heart defects and limb reduction defects. (13-16) One case control study estimated a 4.7 fold increased risk of limb reduction defects in infants exposed in utero to sex hormones (oral contraceptives, hormone withdrawal tests for pregnancy, or attempted treatment for threatened abortion). Some of these exposures were very short and involved only a few days of treatment. The data suggest that the risk of limb reduction defects in exposed fetuses is somewhat less than 1 per 1000. In the past, female sex hormones have been used during pregnancy in an attempt to treat threatened or habitual abortion. There is considerable evidence that estrogens are ineffective for these indications, and there is no evidence from well controlled studies that progestogens are effective for these uses. If esterified estrogens is used during pregnancy, or if the patient becomes pregnant while taking this drug, she should be apprised of the potential risks to the fetus, and the advisability of pregnancy continuation.

DESCRIPTION:

Esterified estrogens, USP is a mixture of the sodium salts of the sulfate esters of the estrogenic substances, principally estrone, that are of the type excreted by pregnant mares. Esterified estrogens contain not less than 75 percent and not more than 85 percent of sodium estrone sulfate, and not less than 6 percent and not more than 15 percent of sodium equilin sulfate, in such proportion that the total of these two components is not less than 90 percent.

Estratab Inactive Ingredients: Acacia, calcium carbonate, carnauba wax, carboxymethylcellulose sodium, citric acid, collodial silicon dioxide, diacetylated monoglyceride, gelatin, lactose, magnesium stearate, methylparaben, microcrystalline cellulose, pharmaceutical glaze, povidone, propylparaben, shellac, sodium benzoate, sodium bicarbonate, sorbic acid, sucrose, corn starch, talc, titanium dioxide and tribasic calcium phosphate. The 0.3 mg tablet coating contains FD&C Blue #1 Lake; the 0.625 mg tablet coating contains D&C Yellow #10 Lake, FD&C yellow #6 Lake and FD&C Blue #2 Lake; the 1.25 mg tablet coating contains FD&C Yellow #6 Lake and the 2.5 mg tablet coating contains FD&C Red #40 Lake and FD&C Blue #2 Lake. In addition the tablet imprinting ink for the 0.3 mg, 0.625 mg and the 1.25 mg tablets contain black iron oxide, FD&C Blue #2 Lake, FD&C Red #40 Lake and FD&C Yellow #6 Lake. Thew 2.5 mg imprinting ink contains Soya lecithin, Dimethyl Polysiloxane, pharmaceutical Shellac and Titanium dioxide.

CLINICAL PHARMACOLOGY:

Estrogens are important in the development and maintenance of the female reproductive system and secondary sex characteristics. They promote growth and development of the vagina, uterus, and fallopian tubes, and enlargement of the breasts. Indirectly, they contribute to the shaping of the skeleton, maintenance of tone and elasticity of urogenital structures, changes in the epiphyses of the long bones that allow for the pubertal growth spurt and its termination, growth of axillary and pubic hair, and pigmentation of the nipples and genitals. Decline of estrogenic activity at the end of the menstrual cycle can bring on menstruation, although the cessation of progesterone secretion is the most important factor in the mature ovulatory cycle. However, in the preovulatory or nonovulatory cycle, estrogen is the primary determinant in the onset of menstruation. Estrogens also affect the release of pituitary gonadotropins. The pharmacologic effects of esterified estrogens are similar to those of endogenous estrogens. They are soluble in water and are well absorbed from the gastrointestinal tract.

In responsive tissues (female genital organs, breasts, hypothalamus, pituitary) estrogens enter the cell and are transported into the nucleus. As a result of estrogen action, specific RNA and protein synthesis occurs.

Metabolism and inactivation occur primarily in the liver. Some estrogens are excreted into the bile; however they are reabsorbed from the intestine and returned to the liver through the portal venous system. Water soluble estrogen conjugates are strongly acidic and are ionized in body fluids, which favor excretion through the kidneys since tubular reabsorption is minimal.

INDICATIONS AND USAGE:

Esterified estrogens is indicated in the treatment of:

1. Moderate to severe *vasomotor* symptoms associated with the menopause. (There is no evidence that estrogens are effective for nervous symptoms or depression which might occur during menopause, and they should not be used to treat these conditions.)

2. Atrophic vaginitis.

3. Kraurosis vulvae.

4. Female hypogonadism.

5. Female castration.

6. Primary ovarian failure.

7. Breast cancer (for palliation only) in appropriately selected women and men with metastatic disease.

8. Prostatic carcinoma - palliative therapy of advanced disease.

ESTERIFIED ESTROGENS HAVE NOT BEEN SHOWN TO BE EFFECTIVE FOR ANY PURPOSE DURING PREGNANCY AND ITS USE MAY CAUSE SEVERE HARM TO THE FETUS (SEE BOXED WARNING).

CONTRAINDICATIONS:

Estrogens should not be used in women (or men) with any of the following conditions:

1. Known or suspected cancer of the breast except in appropriately selected patients being treated for metastatic disease.

2. Known or suspected estrogen-dependent neoplasia.

3. Known or suspected pregnancy (See BOXED WARNING.)

4. Undiagnosed abnormal genital bleeding.

5. Active thrombophlebitis or thromboembolic disorders.

6. A past history of thrombophlebitis, thrombosis, or thromboembolic disorders associated with previous estrogen use (except when used in treatment of breast or prostatic malignancy).

WARNINGS:

INDUCTION OF MALIGNANT NEOPLASMS

Long term continuous administration of natural and synthetic estrogens in certain animal species increases the frequency of carcinomas of the breast, cervix, vagina, and liver. There is now evidence that estrogens increase the risk of carcinoma of the endometrium in humans. (See BOXED WARNING.)

At the present time there is no satisfactory evidence that estrogens given to postmenopausal women increase the risk of cancer of the breast[18] although a recent long-term follow up of a single physician's practice has raised this possibility.[18A] Because of the animal data, there is a need for caution in prescribing estrogens for women with a strong family history of breast cancer or who have breast nodules, fibrocystic disease, or abnormal mammograms.

GALL BLADDER DISEASE

A recent study has reported a 2- to 3-fold increase in the risk of surgically confirmed gall bladder disease in women receiving postmenopausal estrogens,[18] similar to the 2-fold increase previously noted in users of oral contraceptives.[19-24] In the case of oral contraceptives the increased risk appeared after 2 years of use.[24]

EFFECTS SIMILAR TO THOSE CAUSED BY ESTROGEN-PROGESTOGEN ORAL CONTRACEPTIVES

There are several serious adverse effects of oral contraceptives, most of which have not, up to now, been documented as consequences of postmenopausal estrogen therapy. This may reflect the comparatively low doses of estrogen used in postmenopausal women. It would be expected that the larger doses of estrogen used to treat prostatic or breast cancer or postpartum breast engorgement are more likely to result in these adverse effects, and, in fact, it has been shown that there is an increased risk of thrombosis in men receiving estrogens for prostatic cancer and women for postpartum breast engorgement.[20-23]

Thromboembolic Disease: It is now well established that users of oral contraceptives have an increased risk of various thromboembolic and thrombotic vascular diseases, such as thrombophlebitis, pulmonary embolism, stroke, and myocardial infarction.[24-31] Cases of retinal

WARNINGS: *(cont'd)*

thrombosis, mesenteric thrombosis, and optic neuritis have been reported in oral contraceptive users. There is evidence that the risk of several of these adverse reactions is related to the dose of the drug.[32-33] An increased risk of post-surgery thromboembolic complications has also been reported in users of oral contraceptives.[34, 35] If feasible, estrogens should be discontinued at least 4 weeks before surgery of the type associated with an increased risk of thromboembolism, or during periods of prolonged immobilization. While an increased rate of thromboembolic and thrombotic disease in postmenopausal users of estrogens has not been found,[18-36] this does not rule out the possibility that such an increase may be present or that subgroups of women who have underlying risk factors or who are receiving relatively large doses of estrogens may have increased risk.

Therefore estrogens should not be used in persons with active thrombophlebitis or thromboembolic disorders, and they should not be used (except in treatment of malignancy) in persons with a history of such disorders in association with estrogen use. They should be used with caution in patients with cerebral vascular or coronary artery disease and only for those in whom estrogens are clearly needed.

Large doses of estrogens (5 mg esterified estrogens per day), comparable to those used to treat cancer of the prostate and breast have been shown in a large prospective clinical trial in men[37] to increase the risk of nonfat myocardial infarction, pulmonary embolism and thrombophlebitis. When estrogen doses of this size are used, any of the thromboembolic and thrombotic adverse effects associated with oral contraceptive use should be considered a clear risk.

Hepatic Adenoma: Benign hepatic adenomas appear to be associated with the use of oral contraceptives.[38-40] Although benign and rare, these may rupture and may cause death through intra- abdominal hemorrhage. Such lesions have not yet been reported in association with other estrogen or progesterone preparations but should be considered in estrogen users having abdominal pain and tenderness, abdominal mass, or hypovolemic shock. Hepatocellular carcinoma has also been reported in women taking estrogen-containing oral contraceptives.[39] The relationship of this malignancy to these drugs is not known at this time.

Elevated Blood Pressure: Increased blood pressure is not uncommon in women using oral contraceptives. There is now a report that this may occur with the use of estrogens in the menopause[41] and blood pressure blood pressure should be monitored with estrogen use, especially if high doses are used.

Glucose Tolerance: A worsening of glucose tolerance has been observed in a significant percentage of patients on estrogen-containing oral contraceptives. For this reason, diabetic patients should be carefully observed while receiving estrogen.

HYPERCALCEMIA

Administration of estrogens may lead to severe hypercalcemia in patients with breast cancer and bone metastases. If this occurs, the drug should be stopped and appropriate measures taken to reduce the serum calcium level.

PRECAUTIONS:

GENERAL

1. A complete medical and family history should be taken prior to the initiation of any estrogen therapy. The pre-treatment and periodic physical examinations should include special reference to blood pressure, breast, abdomen, and pelvic organs, and should include a Papanicolaou smear. As a general rule, estrogen should not be prescribed for longer than one year without another physical examination being performed.

2. Fluid retention-Because estrogens may cause some degree of fluid retention, conditions which might be influenced by this factor, such as epilepsy, migraine, and cardiac or renal dysfunction, require careful observation.

3. Certain patients may develop undesirable manifestations of excessive estrogenic stimulation, such as abnormal or excessive uterine bleeding, mastodynia, etc.

4. Oral contraceptives appear to be associated with an increased incidence of mental depression.[24]Although it is not clear whether this is due to the estrogenic or progestagenic component of the contraceptive, patients with a history of depression should be carefully observed.

5. Pre-existing uterine leiomyomata may increase in size during estrogen use.

6. The pathologist should be advised of estrogen therapy when relevant specimens are submitted.

7. Patients with a past history of jaundice during pregnancy have an increased risk of reoccurrence of jaundice while receiving estrogen- containing oral contraceptive therapy. If jaundice develops in any patient receiving estrogen, the medication should be discontinued while the cause is investigated.

8. Estrogens may be poorly metabolized in patients with impaired liver function and they should be administered with caution in such patients.

9. Because estrogens influence the metabolism of calcium and phosphorus, they should be used with caution in patients with metabolic bone diseases that are associated with hypercalcemia or in patients with renal insufficiency.

10. Because of the effects of estrogens on epiphyseal closure, they should be used judiciously in young patients in whom bone growth is not complete.

11. The lowest effective dose appropriate for the specific indication should be utilized. Studies of the addition of a progestin for seven or more days of a cycle of estrogen administration have reported a lower incidence of endometrial hyperplasia. Morphological and biochemical studies of endometrium suggest that 10 to 13 days of progestin are needed to provide maximal maturation of the endometrium and to eliminate any hyperplastic changes. Whether this will provide protection from endometrial carcinoma has not been clearly established. There are possible additional risks which may be associated with the inclusion of progestin in estrogen replacement regimens. The potential risks include adverse effects on carbohydrate and lipid metabolism. The choice of progestin and dosage may be important in minimizing these adverse effects.

12. Certain endocrine and liver function tests may be affected by estrogen-containing oral contraceptives. The following similar changes may be expected with larger doses of estrogen:

a. Increased sulfobromophthalein retention.

b. Increased prothrombin and factors VII, VIII, IX, and X; decreased antithrombin 3; increased norepinephrine-induced platelet agreeability.

c. Increased thyroid binding globulin (TBG) leading to increased circulating total thyroid hormone, as measured by PBI, T4 by column, or T4 by radioimmunoassay. Free T3 resin uptake is decreased, reflecting the elevated TBG; free T4 concentration is unaltered.

d. Impaired glucose tolerance.

e. Decreased pregnanediol excretion.

f. Reduced response to metyrapone test.

g. Reduced serum folate concentration.

h. Increased serum triglyceride and phospholipid concentration.

PREGNANCY CATEGORY X

See CONTRAINDICATIONS and BOXED WARNING.

PRECAUTIONS: *(cont'd)*

NURSING MOTHERS

As a general principle, the administration of any drug to nursing mothers should be done only when clearly necessary since many drugs are excreted in human milk.

ADVERSE REACTIONS:

(See WARNINGS regarding induction of neoplasia, adverse effects on the fetus, increased incidence of gall bladder disease, and adverse effects similar to those of oral contraceptives, including thromboembolism). The following additional adverse reactions have been reported with estrogenic therapy, including oral contraceptives:

Genitourinary system: Breakthrough bleeding, spotting, change in menstrual flow, Dysmenorrhea, Premenstrual-like syndrome, Amenorrhea during increase in size of uterine fibromyomata, Vaginal candidiasis, Change in cervical eversion and in degree of cervical secretion, Cystitis-like syndrome.

Breasts: Tenderness, enlargement, secretion.

Gastrointestinal: Nausea, vomiting, abdominal cramps, bloating, Cholestatic jaundice.

Skin: Chloasma or melasma which may persist when drug is discontinued, Hemorrhagic eruption, Loss of scalp hair, Hirsutism.

Eyes: Steepening of corneal curvature, Intolerance to contact lenses.

CNS: Headache, migraine, dizziness, Mental depression, Chorea.

Miscellaneous: Increase or decrease in weight, Reduced carbohydrate tolerance, Aggravation of porphyria, Edema, Changes in libido.

OVERDOSAGE:

Numerous reports of ingestion of large doses of estrogen-containing oral contraceptives by young children indicate that serious ill effects do not occur. Overdosage of estrogen may cause nausea, and withdrawal bleeding may occur in females.

DOSAGE AND ADMINISTRATION:

GIVEN CYCLICALLY FOR SHORT TERM USE ONLY

For treatment of moderate to severe *vasomotor symptoms, atrophic vaginitis,* or *kraurosis vulvae* associated with the menopause.

The lowest dose that will control symptoms should be chosen and medication should be discontinued as promptly as possible.

Administration should be cyclic (*e.g.,* 3 weeks on and 1 week off).

Attempts to discontinue or taper medication should be made at 3 to 6 month intervals.

Usual Dosage Ranges

Vasomotor symptoms - 1.25 mg daily. If the patient has not menstruated within the last two months or more, cyclic administration is started arbitrarily. If the patient is menstruating, cyclic administration is started on day 5 of bleeding.

Atrophic vaginitis and kraurosis vulvae - 0.3 mg to 1.25 mg or more daily, depending upon the tissue response to the individual patient. Administer cyclically.

GIVEN CYCLICALLY

Female hypogonadism; female castration; primary ovarian failure.

Usual Dosage Ranges

Female Hypogonadism: 2.5 to 7.5 mg daily, in divided doses for 20 days, followed by a rest period of 10 days' duration. If bleeding does not occur by the end of this period, the same dosage schedule is repeated. The number of courses of estrogen therapy necessary to produce bleeding may vary depending on responsiveness of the endometrium.

If bleeding occurs before the end of the 10 day period, begin a 20 day estrogen-progestin cyclic regimen with esterified estrogen tablets, 2.5 to 7.5 mg daily in divided doses, for 20 days. During the last 5 days of estrogen therapy, give an oral progestin. If bleeding occurs before this regimen is concluded, therapy is discontinued and may be resumed on the fifth day of bleeding.

Female Castration And Primary Ovarian Failure: 1.25 mg daily, cyclically. Adult dosage upward or downward according to severity of symptoms and response of the patient. For maintenance, adjust dosage to lowest level that will provide effective control.

GIVEN CHRONICALLY

Inoperable progressing prostate cancer-1.25 to 2.5 mg three times daily. The effectiveness of therapy can be judged by phosphatase determinations as well as by symptomatic improvement of the patient.

Inoperable progressing breast cancer in appropriately selected men and postmenopausal women (see INDICATIONS AND USAGE). Suggested dosage is 10 mg three times daily for a period of at least 3 months.

Treated patients with an intact uterus should be monitored closely for a signs of endometrial cancer and appropriate diagnostic measures should be taken to rule out malignancy in the event of persistent or recurring abnormal vaginal bleeding.

(For reference materials, please see Estrogens, Conjugated, REFERENCES)

HOW SUPPLIED - EQUIVALENTS NOT AVAILABLE:

Tablet, Sugar Coated - Oral - 0.3 mg

100's	$12.20	MENEST, Beecham	00029-2800-30
100's	**$21.63**	**ESTRATAB, Solvay Pharms**	**00032-1014-01**

Tablet, Sugar Coated - Oral - 0.625 mg

100's	$17.25	MENEST, Beecham	00029-2810-30
100's	**$30.13**	**ESTRATAB, Solvay Pharms**	**00032-1022-01**
1000's	**$295.27**	**ESTRATAB, Solvay Pharms**	**00032-1022-10**

Tablet, Sugar Coated - Oral - 1.25 mg

100's	$29.05	MENEST, Beecham	00029-2820-30

Tablet, Sugar Coated - Oral - 2.5 mg

50's	$27.05	MENEST, Beecham	00029-2830-29
100's	**$71.40**	**ESTRATAB, Solvay Pharms**	**00032-1025-01**

ESTROGENS, ESTERIFIED; METHYLTESTOSTERONE *(001201)*

CATEGORIES: Anabolic Steroids; Androgens; Antineoplastics; Hormones; Menopause; Oncologic Drugs; Pregnancy Category X; DEA Class CIII; FDA Pre 1938 Drugs

BRAND NAMES: **Estratest**

FORMULARIES: Aetna; BC-BS

Prescribing information not available at time of publication.

HOW SUPPLIED - EQUIVALENTS NOT AVAILABLE:

Tablet, Sugar Coated - Oral - 0.625 mg/1.25 m

100's	$66.84	ESTRATEST H.S., Solvay Pharms	00032-1023-01

Tablet, Sugar Coated - Oral - 1.25 mg/2.5 mg

100's	$83.22	ESTRATEST, Solvay Pharms	00032-1026-01
1000's	$815.35	ESTRATEST, Solvay Pharms	00032-1026-10

ESTRONE *(001202)*

CATEGORIES: Antineoplastics; Hypogonadism; Hormones; Kraurosis Vulvae; Menopause; Hypogonadism; Oncologic Drugs; Prostatic Carcinoma; Ovarian Failure; Vaginitis; Pregnancy Category X; FDA Approval Pre 1982

BRAND NAMES: Bestrone; Estro-A; Estronol; Kestrone 5; *Kolpon Pessaries*; *Oestrilin*; Propagon-S; Theelin; Theogen
(International brand names outside U.S. in italics)

WARNING:
1. Estrogens have been reported to increase the risk ratio for endometrial carcinoma.
Three independent case control studies reported an increased risk ratio for endometrial cancer in postmenopausal women exposed to exogenous estrogens for prolonged periods.[1-3] This risk was independent of the other known risk factors. These studies are further supported by the finding that incidence rates of endometrial cancer have increased sharply since 1969 in eight different areas of the United States with population-based cancer reporting systems, an increase which may be related to the rapidly expanding use of estrogens during the last decade. [4]
The three case control studies reported that the risk ratio for endometrial cancer in estrogen users was about 4.5 to 13.9 times greater than in nonusers. The risk ratio appeared to depend on both duration of treatment[1] and on estrogen dose.[3] In view of these reports, when estrogens are used for the treatment of menopausal symptoms, the lowest dose that will control symptoms should be utilized and medication should be discontinued as soon as possible. When prolonged treatment is medically indicated, the patient should be reassessed on at least a semiannual basis to determine the need for continued therapy. Although the evidence must be considered preliminary, the results of one study suggest that cyclic administration of low doses of estrogen may carry less risk than continuous administration;[3] it, therefore, appears prudent to utilize such a regimen.
Close clinical surveillance of all women taking estrogens is important. In all cases of undiagnosed persistent or recurring abnormal vaginal bleeding, adequate diagnostic measures should be undertaken to rule out malignancy.
There is no evidence at present that "natural" estrogens are more or less hazardous than "synthetic" estrogens at equivalent estrogenic doses.
2. Sterile Estrone Suspension, USP should not be used during pregnancy.
The use of estrogens during early pregnancy may seriously damage the offspring. An association has been reported between in utero exposure of the female fetus to nonsteroidal estrogens (*e.g.,*diethylstilbestrol) and an increased risk of the postpubertal development of a form of vaginal or cervical cancer that is ordinarily regarded as extremely rare.[5,6] This risk has recently been estimated to be in the range of 0.14 to 1.4 per 1000 exposed
* females,[7] consistent with a previous risk estimate* of not * greater than 4 per 1000 exposures.[8]Furthermore,a high percentage of females exposed in utero (from 30 to 90 percent) have been found to have vaginal adenosis,[9-13] epithelial changes of the vagina and cervix. Although these changes are histologically benign, it is not known whether they are precursors of adenocarcinoma.
Several reports suggest an association between fetal exposure to female sex hormones and congenital anomalies, including congenital heart defects and limb-reduction defects.[14-17]
In the past, female sex hormones have been used during pregnancy in an attempt to treat threatened or habitual abortion. There is considerable literature reporting that estrogens are ineffective for these indications. Sterile estrone suspension, USP has not been indicated for these uses and should not be used during pregnancy.
If estrone is used during pregnancy, or if the patient becomes pregnant while taking this drug, she should be apprised of the potential risks to the fetus, and the advisability of pregnancy continuation.

DESCRIPTION:

Estrone is one of the three main estrogens of man and was the first to be isolated chemically in a pure crystalline form.

Estrone is 3-hydroxyestra-1,3,5(10)-trien-17-one.

Sterile estrone suspension, USP is a sterile suspension of estrone in isotonic sodium chloride solution for intramuscular administration and is available in a concentration of 2 mg per ml. Benzethonium chloride, 0.1 mg per ml, and benzyl alcohol, 2%, added as preservatives.

CLINICAL PHARMACOLOGY:

Estrone is a naturally-occurring estrogenic hormone and, as such, acts to produce the physiological and pharmacological effects characteristic of estrogens.

The structure of estrone is closely related to that of estradiol, and free interconversion between estrone and estradiol takes place in the liver.

The estrogenic activity of 0.1 mcg of crystalline estrone constitutes the international unit (IU) of estrogenic activity. Accordingly, 1 mg of estrone is equivalent to 10,000 international units of estrogenic activity.

Inactivation of estrogen in the body is carried out mainly in the liver with a certain proportion excreted into the bile and reabsorbed from the intestine. During this enterohepatic circulation, degradation of estrogen occurs through conversion to less active products such as estriol and numerous other estrogens, through oxidation to nonestrogenic substances, and through conjugation with sulfuric and glucuronic acids. Since these water soluble conjugates are strong acids and are fully ionized in the body fluids, penetration into cells is therefore limited, and excretion by the kidney is favored.

INDICATIONS AND USAGE:

Estrone Aqueous Suspension is indicated in the treatment of

1. Moderate to severe *vasomotor* symptoms associated with the menopause. (There is no evidence that estrogens are effective for nervous symptoms or depression which might occur during menopause, and they should not be used to treat these conditions.)
2. Atrophic vaginitis
3. Kraurosis vulvae
4. Female hypogonadism
5. Female castration
6. Primary ovarian failure
7. Prostatic carcinoma—palliative therapy of advanced disease

Estrone is not indicated for use during pregnancy and its use during pregnancy may cause severe harm to the fetus (See BOXED WARNING.)

CONTRAINDICATIONS:

Estrone Aqueous Suspension should not be used in women (or men) with any of the following conditions:

1. Known or suspected cancer of the breast except in appropriately selected patients being treated for metastatic disease
2. Known or suspected estrogen-dependent neoplasia
3. Known or suspected pregnancy (See BOXED WARNING)
4. Undiagnosed abnormal genital bleeding
5. Active thrombophlebitis or thromboembolic disorders
6. A past history of thrombophlebitis, thrombosis, or thromboembolic disorders (except when used in treatment of breast or prostatic malignancy)

WARNINGS:

INDUCTION OF MALIGNANT NEOPLASMS

Long-term continuous administration of natural and synthetic estrogens in certain animal species has been reported to increase the frequency of carcinomas of the breast, cervix, vagina, and liver. There is now evidence that estrogens increase the risk of carcinoma of the endometrium in humans. (See BOXED WARNING.)

At the present time there is no satisfactory evidence that estrogens given to postmenopausal women increase the risk of cancer of the breast,[18] although a recent long-term follow-up of a single physician's practice has raised this possibility.[19]

Because of the animal data, there is a need for caution in prescribing estrogens for women with a strong family history of breast cancer or who have breast nodules, fibrocystic disease, or abnormal mammograms.

GALLBLADDER DISEASE

A recent study has reported a 2- to 3-fold increase in the risk of surgically confirmed gallbladder disease in women receiving postmenopausal estrogens,[18] similar to the 2-fold increase previously reported in users of oral contraceptives.20 In the case of oral contraceptives the increased risk appeared after two years of use.[21]

EFFECTS SIMILAR TO THOSE CAUSED BY ESTROGEN-PROGESTOGEN ORAL CONTRACEPTIVES

There are several serious adverse effects of oral contraceptives, most of which have not been documented as consequences of postmenopausal estrogen therapy. This may reflect the comparatively low doses of estrogen used in postmenopausal women. It would be expected that the larger doses of estrogen used to treat prostatic or breast cancer or postpartum breast engorgement are more likely to result in these adverse effects, and, in fact, it has been shown that there is an increased risk of thrombosis in men receiving estrogens for prostatic cancer and women for postpartum breast engorgement.[22-25]

Thromboembolic Disease: It is now established that users of oral contraceptives have an increased risk of various thromboembolic and thrombotic vascular diseases, such as thrombophlebitis, pulmonary embolism, stroke, and myocardial infarction.[21,26,33] Cases of retinal thrombosis, mesenteric thrombosis, and optic neuritis have been reported in oral contraceptive users. There is evidence that the risk of several of these adverse reactions is related to the dose of the drug.[34,35] An increased risk of postsurgery thromboembolic complications has also been reported in users of oral contraceptives.[36,37] If feasible, estrogen should be discontinued at least 4 weeks before surgery of the type associated with an increased risk of thromboembolism, or during periods of prolonged immobilization.

While an increased rate of thromboembolic and thrombotic disease in postmenopausal users of estrogens has not been found,[18,38]this does not rule out the possibility that such an increase may be present or that subgroups of women who have underlying risk factors or who are receiving relatively large doses of estrogens may have increased risk. Therefore, estrogens should not be used in persons with active thrombophlebitis or thromboembolic disorders, and they should not be used (except in the treatment of malignancy) in persons with a history of such disorders. They should be used with caution in patients with cerebral vascular or coronary artery disease and only for those in whom estrogens are clearly needed.

Doses of estrogen (5 mg conjugated estrogens per day), comparable to those used to treat cancer of the prostate and breast, have been shown in a large prospective clinical trial in men[39] to increase the risk of nonfatal myocardial infarction, pulmonary embolism and thrombophlebitis. When estrogen doses of this size are used, any of the thromboembolic and thrombotic adverse effects apparently associated with oral contraceptive use should be considered a clear risk.

Hepatic Adenoma: Benign hepatic adenomas appear to be associated with the use of oral contraceptives.[40-42]Although benign, and rare, these may rupture and may cause death through intra-abdominal hemorrhage. Such lesions have not yet been reported in association with other estrogen or progestogen preparations but should be considered in estrogen users having abdominal pain and tenderness, abdominal mass, or hypovolemic shock. Hepatocellular carcinoma has also been reported in women taking estrogen-containing oral contraceptives.[41] The relationship of this malignancy to these drugs is not known at this time.

Elevated Blood Pressure: Increased blood pressure is not uncommon in women using oral contraceptives. There is now a report that this may occur with the use of estrogens in the menopause[43]and blood pressure should be monitored with estrogen use, especially if high doses are used.

Glucose Tolerance: A decrease in glucose tolerance has been observed in a significant percentage of patients on estrogen-containing oral contraceptives. For this reason, diabetic patients should be carefully observed while receiving estrogen.

HYPERCALCEMIA

Administration of estrogens may lead to severe hypercalcemia in patients with breast cancer and bone metastases. If this occurs, the drug should be stopped and appropriate measures taken to reduce the serum calcium level.

PRECAUTIONS:

GENERAL

1. A complete medical and family history should be taken prior to the initiation of any estrogen therapy. The pretreatment and periodic physical examinations should include special reference to blood pressure, breasts, abdomen, and pelvic organs, and should include a Papanicolaou smear. As a general rule, estrogen should not be prescribed for longer than one year without another physical examination being performed.

2. Fluid retention—Because estrogens may cause some degree of fluid retention, conditions which might be influenced by this factor, such as epilepsy, migraine, and cardiac or renal dysfunction, require careful observation.

3. Certain patients may develop undesirable manifestations of excessive estrogenic stimulation, such as abnormal or excessive uterine bleeding, mastodynia, etc.

4. Oral contraceptives have been reported to be associated with an increased incidence of mental depression.[21,26] Although it is not clear whether this is due either to the estrogenic or progestogenic component of the contraceptive, patients with a history of depression should be carefully observed.

5. Preexisting uterine leiomyoma may increase in size during estrogen use.

6. The pathologist should be advised of estrogen therapy when relevant specimens are submitted.

7. Patients with a past history of jaundice during pregnancy have an increased risk of recurrence of jaundice while receiving estrogen-containing oral contraceptive therapy. If jaundice develops in any patient receiving estrogen, the medication should be discontinued while the cause is investigated.

8. Estrogens may be poorly metabolized in patients with impaired liver function and they should be administered with caution in such patients.

9. Because estrogens influence the metabolism of calcium and phosphorus, they should be used with caution in patients with metabolic bone diseases that are associated with hypercalcemia or in patients with renal insufficiency.

10. Because of the effects of estrogens on epiphyseal closure, they should be used judiciously in young patients in whom bone growth is not complete.

CONCOMITANT PROGESTIN USE

The lowest effective dose appropriate for the specific indication should be utilized. Studies of the addition of a progestin for seven or more days of a cycle of estrogen administration have reported a lowered incidence of endometrial hyperplasia. Morphological and biochemical studies of endometrium suggest that 10 to 13 days of progestin are needed to provide maximal maturation of the endometrium and to eliminate any hyperplastic changes. Whether this will provide protection from endometrial carcinoma has not been clearly established. There are possible additional risks which may be associated with the inclusion of progestin in estrogen replacement regimens. The potential risks include adverse effects on carbohydrate and lipid metabolism. The choice of progestin and dosage may be important in minimizing these adverse effects.

INFORMATION FOR THE PATIENT

See text of Patient Package Insertwhich appears after the reference section.

DRUG/LABORATORY TEST INTERACTIONS

Certain endocrine and liver function tests may be affected by estrogen-containing oral contraceptives. The following similar changes may be expected with larger doses of estrogen:

a. Increased sulfobromophthalein retention.

b. Increased prothrombin and factors VII, VIII, IX, and X; decreased antithrombin 3; increased norepinephrine-induced platelet aggregability.

c. Increased thyroid binding globulin (TBG) leading to increased circulating total thyroid hormone, as measured by PBI, T4 by column, or T4 by radioimmunoassay. Free T3 resin uptake is decreased, reflecting the elevated TBG; free T4 concentration is unaltered.

d. Impaired glucose tolerance.

e. Decreased pregnanediol excretion.

f. Reduced response to metyrapone test.

g. Reduced serum folate concentration.

h. Increased serum triglyceride and phospholipid concentration.

CARCINOGENESIS, MUTAGENESIS, IMPAIRMENT OF FERTILITY

See WARNINGS including BOXED WARNING.

PREGNANCY CATEGORY X

See CONTRAINDICATIONS and BOXED WARNING.

NURSING MOTHERS

Because of the potential for serious adverse reactions in nursing infants from estrogens, a decision should be made whether to discontinue nursing or to discontinue the drug, taking into account the importance of the drug to the mother.

PEDIATRIC USE

Safety and effectiveness in children have not been established.

ADVERSE REACTIONS:

(See WARNINGS regarding induction of neoplasia, adverse effects on the fetus, increased incidence of gallbladder disease, and adverse effects similar to those of oral contraceptives, including thromboembolism.) The following additional adverse reactions have been reported with estrogenic therapy, including oral contraceptives:

Genitourinary System: breakthrough bleeding, spotting, change in menstrual flow, dysmenorrhea, premenstrual-like syndrome, amenorrhea during and after treatment, increase in size of uterine fibromyomata, vaginal candidiasis, change in cervical eversion and in degree of cervical secretion, cystitis-like syndrome.

Breasts: tenderness, enlargement, secretion

Gastrointestinal: nausea, vomiting; abdominal cramps, bloating; cholestatic jaundice.

Skin: chloasma or melasma which may persist when drug is discontinued;erythema multiforme; erythema nodosum; hemorrhagic eruption; loss of scalp hair; hirsutism.

Eyes: steepening of corneal curvature, intolerance to contact lenses

CNS: headache, migraine, dizziness; mental depression; chorea.

Miscellaneous: increase or decrease in weight, reduced carbohydrate tolerance, aggravation of porphyria, edema, changes in libido.

OVERDOSAGE:

Numerous reports of ingestion of large doses of estrogen-containing oral contraceptives by young children indicate that serious ill effects do not occur. Overdosage of estrogen may cause nausea, and withdrawal bleeding may occur in females.

DOSAGE AND ADMINISTRATION:

GIVEN CYCLICALLY FOR SHORT TERM USE ONLY

For treatment of moderate to severe *vasomotor* symptoms, atrophic vaginitis, or kraurosis vulvae associated with the menopause.

The lowest dose that will control symptoms should be chosen and medication should be discontinued as promptly as possible.

Administration should be cyclic (*e.g.*3 weeks on and 1 week off).

Attempts to discontinue or taper medication should be made at 3 to 6 month intervals.

The usual dosage range is 0.1 mg to 0.5 mg of estrone two or three times weekly.

GIVEN CYCLICALLY

Female hypogonadism.

Female castration.

Primary ovarian failure.

Initial relief of symptoms may be achieved through the administration of 0.1 mg to 1 mg of estrone weekly in single or divided dosage. Some patients may require 0.5 mg to 2 mg weekly.

GIVEN CHRONICALLY

Inoperable progressing prostatic cancer.

For palliation in prostatic cancer, estrone may be employed at a dosage level of 2 mg to 4 mg two or three times weekly. If a response to estrogen therapy is going to occur, it should be apparent within 3 months of the beginning of therapy. If a response does occur, the hormone should be continued until the disease is again progressive.

STORAGE

Store the multiple-dose vials of Estrone Aqueous Suspension in an upright position at room temperature. Do not freeze. Improper storage may cause agglomeration (clumping), adherence of the product to vial walls, or the formation of large crystals which settle rapidly. Do not use the preparation if agglomerates, adherents or large crystals are apparent.

REFERENCES:

1. Ziel, H. K., and W. D. Finkle, "Increased Risk of Endometrial Carcinoma Among Users of Conjugated Estrogens," *New England Journal of Medicine*, 293:1167-1170, 1975. **2.** Smith, D. C., R. Prentic, D. J. Thompson, and W. L. Hermann, "Association of Exogenous Estrogen and Endometrial Carcinoma," *New England Journal of Medicine*, 293:1164-1167, 1975. **3.** Mack, T. M., M. C. Pike, B. E. Henderson, R. I. Pfeffer, V. R. Gerkins, M. Arthur, and S. E. Brown, "Estrogens and Endometrial Cancer in a Retirement Community," *New England Journal of Medicine*,294:1262-1267, 1976. **4.** Weiss, N. S., D. R. Szekely and D. F. Austin, "Increasing Incidence of Endometrial Cancer in the United States," *New England Journal of Medicine*, 294:1259-1262, 1976. **5.** Herbst, A. L., H. Ulfelder and D. C. Poskanzer, "Adenocarcinoma of Vagina," *New England Journal of Medicine*, 284: 878-881, 1971. **6.** Greenwald, P., J. Barlow, P.Nasca, and W. Burnett, "Vaginal Cancer after Maternal Treatment with Synthetic Estrogens," *New England Journal of Medicine*, 285:390-392, 1971. **7.** Herbst, A. L., Cole, P., Colton, T., et al, "Latency Period and Incidence Aspects of DES-Related Clear Cell Adenocarcinoma of the Vagina and Cervix." *Am. J. Obstet. Gynecol,* In Press. **8.** Lanier, A., K. Noller, D. Decker, L. Elveback, and L. Kurland, "Cancer and Stilbestrol. A Follow-up of 1719 Persons Exposed to Estrogens in Utero and Born 1943-1959." *Mayo Clinic Proceedings,* 48:793-799, 1973. **9.** Herbst, A., R. Kurman, and R. Scully, "Vaginal and Cervical Abnormalities After Exposure to Stilbestrol In Utero." *Obstetrics and Gynecology*, 40:287-298, 1972. **10.** Herbst, A., S. Robboy, G. Macdonald, and R. Scully, "The Effects of Local Progesterone on Stilbestrol-Associated Vaginal Adenosis,"*American Journal of Obstetrics and Gynecology*, 118:607-615, 1974. **11.** Herbst, A., R. Poskanzer, S. Robboy, L. Friedlander, and R. Scully, "Prenatal Exposure to Stilbestrol. A Prospective Comparison of Exposed Female Offspring with Unexposed Controls," *New England Journal of Medicine*, 292:334-339, 1975. **12.** Stafl, A., R. Mattingly, D. Foley, and W. Fetherston, "Clinical Diagnosis of Vaginal Adenosis," *Obstetrics and Gynecology,*43:118-128, 1974. **13.** Sherman, A. I., M. Goldrath, A. Berlin, V. Vakhariya, F. Banooni, W. Michaels, P. Goodman, S. Brown, "Cervical-Vaginal Adenosis After *In Utero* Exposure to Synthetic Estrogens," *Obstetrics and Gynecology,*44:531-545, 1974. **14.** Gal, I., B. Kirman, and J. Stern, "Hormone Pregnancy Tests and Congenital Malformation," *Nature*, 216:83, 1967. **15.** Levy, E. P., A. Cohen, and F. C. Fraser, "Hormone Treatment During Pregnancy and Congenital Heart Defects," *Lancet*, 1:611, 1973. **16.** Nora, J. and A. Nora, "Birth Defects and Oral Contraceptives,"*Lancet*, 1:941-942, 1973. **17.** Janerich, D. T., J. M. Piper, and D. M. Glebatis, "Oral Contraceptives and Congenital Limb Reduction Defects," *New England Journal of Medicine*, 291:697-700, 1974. **18.** Boston Collaborative Drug Surveillance Program, "Surgically Confirmed Gall Bladder Disease, Venous Thromboembolism and Breast Tumors in Relation to Post-Menopausal Estrogen Therapy," *New England Journal of Medicine*, 290:15-19, 1974. **19.** Hoover, R., L. A. Gray, Sr., P. Cole, and B. MacMahon, "Menopausal Estrogens and Breast Cancer," *New England Journal of Medicine,*295:401-405, 1976. **20.** Boston Collaborative Drug Surveillance Program, "Oral Contraceptives and Venous Thromboembolic Disease, Surgically Confirmed Gall Bladder Disease, and Breast Tumors," *Lancet*, 1:1399-1404, 1973. **21.** Royal College of General Practitioners, "Oral Contraception and Thromboembolic Disease," *Journal of the Royal College of General Practitioners*, 13:267-279, 1967. **22.** Daniel, D., G. H. Campbell, and A. C. Turnbull, "Puerperal Thromboembolism and Suppression of Lactation," *Lancet*, 2:287-289, 1967. **23.** The Veterans Administration Cooperative Urological Research Group, "Carcinoma of the Prostate: Treatment Comparisons," *Journal of Urology*, 98:516-522, 1967. **24.** Bailar, J. C. "Thromboembolism and Oestrogen Therapy,"*Lancet*, 2:560, 1967. **25.** Blackard, C., R. Doe, G. Mellinger, and D. Byar, "Incidence of Cardiovascular Disease and Death in Patients Receiving Diethylstilbestrol for Carcinoma of the Prostate," *Cancer*, 26:249-256, 1970. **26.** Oral contraceptives and health—an interim report from the oral contraception study of the Royal College of General Practitioners. Pitman, London and New York, 1974. **27.** Inman, W. H. W. and M. P. Vessey, "Investigation of Deaths from Pulmonary Coronary and Cerebral Thrombosis and Embolism in Women of Child Bearing Age, *British Medical Journal*, 2:193-199, 1968. **28.** Vessey M. P. and R. Doll, "Investigation of Relation Between Use of Oral Contraceptives and Thromboembolic Disease, A Further Report,"*British Medical Journal*, 2:651-657, 1969. **29.** Sartwell P.E., A. T. Masi, F.G. Arthes, G. R. Greene and H. E. Smith, "Thromboembolism and Oral Contraceptives: An Epidemiological Case Control Study," *American Journal of Epidemiology*, 90:365-380, 1969. **30.** Collaborative Group for the Study of Stroke in Young Women, "Oral Contraception and Increased Risk of Cerebral Ischemia or Thrombosis,"*New England Journal of Medicine,*288:871-878, 1973. **31.** Collaborative Group for the Study of Stroke in Young Women, "Oral Contraceptives and Stroke in Young Women: Associated Risk Factors,"*Journal of the American Medical Association,* 231:718-722, 1975. **32.** Mann, J. I. and W. H. W. Inman, "Oral Contraceptives and Death from Myocardial Infarction," *British Medical Journal,* 2:245-248, 1975. **33.** Mann, J. I., M. P. Vessey, M. Thorogood, and R. Doll, "Myocardial Infarction in Young Women with Special Reference to Oral Contraceptive Practice," *British Medical Journal*, 2:241-245, 1975. **34.** Inman, W. H. W., M. P. Vessey, B. Westerholm, and A. Engelund, "Thromboembolic Disease and the Steroidal Content of Oral Contraceptives," *British Medical Journal,*2:203-209, 1970. **35.** Stolley, P.D., J. A. Tonascia, M. S. Tockman, P.E. Sartwell, A. H. Rutledge, and M. P. Jacobs, "Thrombosis with Low Estrogen Oral Contraceptives," *American Journal of Epidemiology,* 102:197-208, 1975. **36.** Vessey, M. P., R. Doll, A. S. Fairbairn, and G. Glober, "Post-Operative Thromboembolism and the Use of Oral Contraceptives,"*British Medical Journal*, 3:123-126, 1970. **37.** Greene, G. R. and P.E. Sartwell, "Oral Contraceptive Use in Patients with Thromboembolism Following Surgery, Trauma or Infection,"*American Journal of Public Health*, 62:680-685, 1972. **38.** Rosenberg L., M. B. Armstrong and H. Jick, "Myocardial Infarction and Estrogen Therapy in Postmenopausal Women," *New England Journal of Medicine*, 294:1256-1259, 1976. **39.** Coronary Drug Project Research Group, "The Coronary Drug Project: Initial Findings Leading to Modifications of its Research Protocol,"*Journal of the American Medical Association*, 214: 1303-1313, 1970. **40.** Baum, J., F. Holtz, J. J. Bookstein and E. W. Klein, "Possible Association Between Benign Hepatomas and Oral Contraceptives,"*Lancet,* 2:926-928, 1973. **41.** Mays, E. T., W. M. Christopherson, M. M. Mahr, and H. C. Williams, "Hepatic Changes in Young Women Ingesting Contraceptive Steroids, Hepatic Hemorrhage and Primary Hepatic Tumors," *Journal of the American Medical Association,* 235:730-732, 1976. **42.** Edmondson, H. A., B. Henderson, and B. Benton, "Liver Cell Adenomas Associated with the Use of Oral Contraceptives," *New England Journal of Medicine*, 294:470-472, 1976. **43.** Pfeffer, R. I. and S. Van Den Noore, "Estrogen Use and Stroke Risk in Postmenopausal Women." *American Journal of Epidemiology*, 103:445-456, 1976.

PATIENT PACKAGE INSERT:

See the Patient Package Insert for Estrogens, Conjugated for more patient information regarding the use of estrogens.

ESTROGENS TO PREVENT SWELLING OF THE BREASTS AFTER PREGNANCY

If you do not breast feed your baby after delivery your breasts may fill up with milk and become painful and engorged. This usually begins about 3 to 4 days after delivery and may last for a few days to up to a week or more. Sometimes the discomfort is severe but usually it is not and can be controlled by pain relieving drugs such as asprin and by binding the breasts up tightly. Estrogens can be used to try to prevent the breasts from filling up. While this treatment is sometimes less sucessful, in many cases the breasts fill up to some degree in spite of treatment. The dose of estrogens needed to prevent pain and swelling of the breasts is much larger than the dose needed to treat symptoms of the menopause and this may increase your chances of developing blood clots in the legs or lungs. Therefore its important that you discuss the beneefits and the risks of estrogen use with your doctor if you have decided not to breast feed your baby.

HOW SUPPLIED - EQUIVALENTS NOT AVAILABLE:

Injection, Susp - Intramuscular - 2 mg/ml

10 ml	$4.95	ESTRO-A, AF Hauser	52637-0313-10
10 ml	$5.85	Estrone, United Res	00677-0273-21
10 ml	$25.56	ESTROGENIC SUBSTANCE, Ayerst	00046-0567-10

Injection, Susp - Intramuscular - 5 mg/ml

10 ml	$5.85	Estrone, Pasadena	00418-0301-10
10 ml	$9.95	KESTRONE, Hyrex Pharms	00314-0644-70
10 ml	$10.48	Estrone Aqueous, HL Moore Drug Exch	00839-5585-30
10 ml	$12.10	Sterile Estrone, United Res	00677-0274-21
10 ml	$12.75	Estrone Aqueous, IDE-Interstate	00814-3050-40
10 ml	$13.00	Sterile Estrone, Steris Labs	00402-0041-10
10 ml	$16.21	Sterile Estrone, Schein Pharm (US)	00364-6601-54

ESTROPIPATE *(001204)*

CATEGORIES: Antineoplastics; Estrogen Deficiency; Estrogens; Hormones; Hypogonadism; Kraurosis Vulvae; Menopause; Oncologic Drugs; Osteoporosis; Ovarian Failure; Skin/Mucous Membrane Agents; Vaginal Preparations; Vaginitis; Pregnancy Category X; FDA Approval Pre 1982

BRAND NAMES: *Harmogen* (England); *Harmonet*; **Ogen**; Ortho-Est; *Sultrex* *(International brand names outside U.S. in italics)*

FORMULARIES: Aetna; BC-BS; PCS

1. ESTROGENS HAVE BEEN REPORTED TO INCREASE THE RISK OF ENDOMETRIAL CARCINOMA IN POSTMENOPAUSAL WOMEN.

Close clinical surveillance of all women taking estrogens is important. Adequate diagnostic measures, including endometrial sampling when indicated, should be undertaken to rule out malignancy in all cases of undiagnosed persistent or recurring abnormal vaginal bleeding. There is no evidence that "natural" estrogens are more or less hazardous than "synthetic" estrogens at equi-estrogenic doses.

2. ESTROGENS SHOULD NOT BE USED DURING PREGNANCY. There is no indication for estrogen therapy during pregnancy or during the immediate postpartum period. Estrogens are ineffective for the prevention or treatment of threatened, or habitual abortion. Estrogens are not indicated for the prevention of postpartum breast engorgement.

Estrogen therapy during pregnancy is associated with an increased risk of congenital defects in the reproductive organs of the fetus, and possibly other birth defects. Studies of women who received diethylstilbestrol (DES) during pregnancy have shown that female offspring have an increased risk of vaginal adenosis, squamous cell dysplasia of the uterine cervix, and clear cell vaginal cancer later in life; male offspring have an increased risk of urogenital abnormalities and possibly testicular cancer later in life. The 1985 DES Task Force concluded that use of DES during pregnancy is associated with a subsequent increased risk of breast cancer in the mothers, although a causal relationship remains unproven and the observed level of excess risk is similar to that for a number of other breast cancer risk factors.

DESCRIPTION:

Tablets and Vaginal Cream: Estropipate tablets, (formerly piperazine estrone sulfate), is a natural estrogenic substance prepared from purified crystalline estrone, solubilized as the sulfate and stabilized with piperazine. It is appreciably soluble in water and has almost no odor or taste - properties which are ideally suited for oral administration. The amount of piperazine in Estropipate is not sufficient to exert a pharmacological action. Its addition ensures solubility, stability, and uniform potency of the estrone sulfate. Chemically estropipate, molecular weight: 436.56, is represented by estra-1,3,5(10)-trien-17-one,3-(sulfooxy)-, compound with piperazine (1:1).

Tablets: Estropipate is available as tablets for oral administration containing either 0.75 mg (Estropipate.625), 1.5 mg (Estropipate 1.25) or 3 mg (Estropipate 2.5) estropipate. (Calculated as sodium estrone sulfate 0.625 mg, 1.25 mg, and 2.5 mg, respectively).

Inactive Ingredients: *Each tablet may contain:* Colloidal silicon dioxide, dibasic potassium phosphate, hydrogenated vegetable oil wax, hydroxypropyl cellulose, lactose, magnesium stearate, microcrystalline cellulose, sodium starch glycolate and tromethamine. *Estropipate.625 tablet also contains:* D&C Yellow No. 10 and FD&C Yellow No 6. *Ogen 1.25 tablet also contains:* FD&C Yellow No. 6. *Ogen 2.5 tablet also contains:* FD&C Blue No 2.

Vaginal Cream: Each gram ofEstropipateVaginal Cream contains 1.5 mg estropipate in a base composed of the following ingredients: glycerin, mineral oil, glyceryl monostearate, polyethylene glycol ether complex of higher fatty alcohols, cetyl alcohol, anhydrous lanolin, sodium biosphate, cis-N-(3-chloroallyl) hexaminimum chloride, propylparaben, methylparaben, piperazine hexahydrate, citric acid and water.

CLINICAL PHARMACOLOGY:

TABLETS

Estrogen drug products act by regulating the transcription of a limited number of genes. Estrogens diffuse through cell membranes, distribute themselves throughout the cell, and bind to and activate the nuclear estrogen receptor, a DNA-binding protein which is found in estrogen responsive tissues. The activated estrogen receptor binds to specific DNA sequences, or hormone-response elements, which enhance the transcription of adjacent genes and in turn lead to the observed effects. Estrogen receptors have been identified in tissues of the reproductive tract, breast, pituitary, hypothalamus, liver, and bone of women.

Estrogens are important in the development and maintenance of the female reproductive system and secondary sex characteristics. By a direct action, they cause growth and development of the uterus. Fallopian tubes, and vagina. With other hormones, such as pituitary hormones and progesterone, they cause enlargement of the breasts through promotion of ductal growth, stromal development, and the accretion of fat. Estrogens are intricately involved with other hormones, especially progesterone, in the processes of the ovulatory menstrual cycle and pregnancy, and affect the release of pituitary gonadotropins. They also contribute to the shaping of the skeleton, maintenance of tone and elasticity of urogenital structures, changes in the epiphyses of the long bones that allow for the pubertal growth spurt and its termination, and pigmentation of the nipples and genitals.

Estrogens occur naturally in several forms. The primary source of estrogen in normally cycling adult women is the ovarian follicle, which secretes 70 to 500 micrograms of estradiol daily, depending on the phase of the menstrual cycle. This is converted primarily to estrone, which circulates in roughly equal proportion to estradiol, and to small amounts of estriol. After menopause, most endogenous estrogen is produced by conversion of androstenedione, secreted by the adrenal cortex, to estrone by peripheral tissues. Thus, estrone - especially in its sulfate ester form - is the most abundant circulating estrogen in postmenopausal women. Although circulating estrogens exist in a dynamic equilibrium of metabolic interconversions, estradiol is the principal intracellular human estrogen and is substantially more potent than estrone or estriol at the receptor.

Estrogens used in therapy are well absorbed through the skin, mucous membranes, and gastrointestinal tract. When applied for a local action, absorption is usually sufficient to cause systemic effects. When applied for a local action, absorption is usually sufficient to cause

CLINICAL PHARMACOLOGY: *(cont'd)*

systemic effects. When conjugated with aryl and alkyl groups for parenteral administration, the rate of absorption of oily preparations is slowed with a prolonged duration of action, such that a single intramuscular injection of estradiol valerate or estradiol cypionate is absorbed over several weeks.

Administered estrogens and their esters are handled within the body essentially the same as the endogenous hormones. Metabolic conversion of estrogens occurs primarily in the liver (first pass effect), but also at local target tissue sites. Complex metabolic processes result in a dynamic equilibrium of circulating conjugated and unconjugated estrogenic forms which are continually interconverted, especially between estrone and estradiol and between esterified and unesterified forms. Although naturally-occurring estrogens circulate in the blood largely bound to sex hormone-binding globulin and albumin, only unbound estrogens enter target tissue cells. A significant proportion of the circulating estrogen exists as sulfate conjugates, especially estrone sulfate, which serves as a circulating reservoir for the formation of more active estrogenic species. A certain proportion of the estrogen is excreted into the bile and then reabsorbed from the intestine. During this enterohepatic recirculation, estrogens are desulfated and resulfated and undergo degradation through conversion to less active estrogens (estriol and other estrogens), oxidation to nonestrogenic substances (catecholestrogens, which interact with catecholamine metabolism, especially in the central nervous system), and conjugation with glucuronic acids (which are then rapidly excreted in the urine).

When given orally, naturally-occurring estrogens and their esters are extensively metabolized (first pass effect) and circulate primarily as estrone sulfate, with smaller amounts of other conjugated and unconjugated estrogenic species. This results in limited oral potency. By contrast, synthetic estrogens, such as ethinyl estradiol and the nonsteroidal estrogens, are degraded very slowly in the liver and other tissues, which results in their high intrinsic potency. Estrogen drug products administered by non-oral routes are not subject to first-pass metabolism, but also undergo significant hepatic uptake, metabolism, and enterohepatic recycling.

INDICATIONS AND USAGE:

TABLETS

Estrogen drug products are indicated in the:

1. Treatment of moderate to severe vasomotor symptoms associated with the menopause. There is no adequate evidence that estrogens are effective for nervous symptoms or depression which might occur during menopause and they should not be used to treat these conditions.

2. Treatment of vulval and vaginal atrophy.

3. Treatment of hypoestrogenism due to hypogonadism, castration or primary ovarian failure.

4. Prevention of osteoporosis.

Since estrogen administration is associated with risk, selection of patients should ideally be based on prospective identification of risk factors for developing osteoporosis. Unfortunately, there is no certain way to identify those women who will develop osteoporotic fractures. Most prospective studies of efficacy for this indication have been carried out in white menopausal women, without stratification by other risk factors, and must be individualized based on the balance of risks and benefits. A more favorable risk/benefit ratio exists in a hysterectomized woman because she has no risk of endometrial cancer (see BOXED WARNING.)

Estrogen replacement therapy reduces bone resorption and retards or halts postmenopausal bone loss. Case-control studies have shown an approximately 60 percent reduction in hip and wrist fractures in women whose estrogen replacement has begun within a few years of menopause. Studies also suggest that estrogen reduces the rate of vertebral fractures. Even when started as late as 6 years after menopause, estrogen prevents further loss of bone mass for as long as the treatment is continued. The results of a double-blind, placebo-controlled two-year study have shown that treatment with one tablet ofEstropipate.625 daily for 25 days (of a 31-day cycle per month) prevents vertebral bone mass loss in postmenopausal women. When estrogen therapy is discontinued, bone mass declines at a rate comparable to the immediate postmenopausal period. There is no evidence that estrogen replacement therapy restores bone mass to premenopausal levels.

At skeletal maturity there are sex and race differences in both the total amount of bone present and its density, in favor of men and blacks. Thus, women are at higher risk than men because they start with less bone mass and, for several years following natural or induced menopause, the rate of bone mass decline is accelerated. White and Asian women are at higher risk than black women.

Early menopause is one of the strongest predictors for the development of osteoporosis. In addition, other factors affecting the skeleton which are associated with osteoporosis include genetic factors (small build, family history), endocrine factors (nulliparity, thyrotoxicosis, hyperparathyroidism, Cushing's syndrome, hyperprolactinemia, Type I diabetes), lifestyle (cigarette smoking, alcohol abuse, sedentary exercise habits) and nutrition (below average body weight, dietary calcium intake).

The mainstays of prevention and management of osteoporosis are estrogen, an adequate lifetime calcium intake, and exercise. Postmenopausal women absorb dietary calcium less efficiently than premenopausal women and require an average of 1500 mg/day of elemental calcium to remain in neutral calcium balance. By comparison, premenopausal women require about 1000 mg/day and the average calcium intake in the USA is 400-600 mg/day. Therefore, when not contraindicated, calcium supplementation may be helpful.

Weight-bearing exercise and nutrition may be important adjuncts to the prevention and management of osteoporosis. Immobilization and prolonged bed rest produce rapid bone loss, while weight-bearing exercise has been shown both to reduce bone loss and increase bone mass. The optimal type and amount of physical activity that would prevent osteoporosis have not been established, however in two studies an hour of walking and running exercises twice or three times weekly significantly increased lumbar spine bone mass.

VAGINAL CREAM

The cyclic administration ofEstropipateVaginal Cream is indicated for the treatment of atrophic vaginitis or kraurosis vulvae. (See DOSAGE AND ADMINISTRATION.)

OGEN VAGINAL CREAM HAS NOT BEEN TESTED FOR EFFICACY FOR ANY PURPOSE DURING PREGNANCY. SINCE ITS EFFECT UPON THE FETUS IS UNKNOWN, IT CANNOT BE RECOMMENDED FOR ANY CONDITION DURING PREGNANCY (SEE BOXED WARNING).

CONTRAINDICATIONS:

TABLETS

Estrogens should not be used in individuals with any of the following conditions:

1. Known or suspected pregnancy (see BOXED WARNING.) Estrogens may cause fetal harm when administered to a pregnant woman.

2. Undiagnosed abnormal genital bleeding.

3. Known or suspected cancer of the breast except in appropriately selected patients being treated for metastatic disease.

4. Known or suspected estrogen-dependent neoplasia.

CONTRAINDICATIONS: *(cont'd)*

5. Active thrombophlebitis or thromboembolic disorders.

WARNINGS:

TABLETS

Induction of Malignant Neoplasms

Endometrial Cancer: The reported endometrial cancer risk among unopposed estrogen users is about 2 to 12 fold greater than in nonusers, and appears dependent on duration of treatment and on estrogen dose. Most studies show no significant increased risk associated with the use of estrogens for less than one year. The greatest risk appears associated with prolonged use - with increased risks of 15 to 24-fold for five to ten years or more. In three studies, persistence of risk was demonstrated for 8 to over 15 years after cessation of estrogen treatment. In one study a significant decrease in the incidence of endometrial cancer occurred six months after estrogen withdrawal. Concurrent progestin therapy may offset this risk but the overall health impact in postmenopausal women is not known (see PRECAUTIONS.)

Breast Cancer: While the majority of studies have not shown an increased risk of breast cancer in women who have ever used estrogen replacement therapy, some have reported a moderately increased risk (relative risks of 1.3-2.0) in those taking higher doses or those taking lower doses for prolonged periods of time, especially in excess of 10 years. Other studies have not shown this relationship.

Congenital Lesions with Malignant Potential: Estrogen therapy during pregnancy is associated with an increased risk of fetal congenital reproductive tract disorders, and possibly other birth defects. Studies of women who received DES during pregnancy have shown that female offspring have an increased risk of vaginal adenosis, squamous cell dysplasia of the uterine cervix, and clear cell vaginal cancer later in life; male offspring have an increased risk of urogenital abnormalities and possibly testicular cancer later in life. Although some of these changes are benign, others are precursors of malignancy.

Gallbladder Disease

Two studies have reported a 2- to 4-fold increase in the risk of gallbladder disease requiring surgery in women receiving postmenopausal estrogens.

Cardiovascular Disease

Large doses of estrogen (5 mg conjugated estrogens per day), comparable to those used to treat cancer of the prostate and breast, have been shown in a large prospective clinical trial in men to increase the risks of nonfatal myocardial infarction, pulmonary embolism, and thrombophlebitis. These risks cannot necessarily be extrapolated from men to women. However, to avoid the theoretical cardiovascular risk to women caused by high estrogen doses, the dose for estrogen replacement therapy should not exceed the lowest effective dose.

Elevated Blood Pressure

Occasional blood pressure increases during estrogen replacement therapy have been attributed to idiosyncratic reactions to estrogens. More often, blood pressure has remained the same or has dropped. One study showed that postmenopausal estrogen users have higher blood pressure than nonusers. Two other studies showed slightly lower blood pressure among estrogen users compared to nonusers. Postmenopausal estrogen use does not increase the risk of stroke. Nonetheless, blood pressure should be monitored at regular intervals with estrogen use.

Hypercalcemia

Administration of estrogens may lead to severe hypercalcemia in patients with breast cancer and bone metastases. If this occurs, the drug should be stopped and appropriate measures taken to reduce the serum calcium level.

PRECAUTIONS:

TABLETS

General

Addition of a Progestin: Studies of the addition of a progestin for seven or more days of a cycle of estrogen administration have reported a lowered incidence of endometrial hyperplasia which would otherwise be induced by estrogen treatment. Morphological and biochemical studies of endometrium suggest that 10 to 14 days of progestin are needed to provide maximal maturation of the endometrium and to eliminate any hyperplastic changes. There are possible additional risks which may be associated with the inclusion of progestins in estrogen replacement regimens. These include: (1) adverse effects on lipoprotein metabolism (lowering HDL and raising LDL) which may diminish the possible cardioprotective effect of estrogen therapy (see PRECAUTIONS), (2) impairment of glucose tolerance; and (3) possible enhancement of miotic activity in breast epithelial tissue (although few epidemiological data are available to address this point). The choice of progestin, its dose, and its regimen may be important in minimizing these adverse effects, but these issues remain to be clarified.

Physical Examination: A complete medical and family history should be taken prior to the initiation of any estrogen therapy. The pretreatment and periodic physical examinations should include special reference to blood pressure, breasts, abdomen, and pelvic organs, and should include a Papanicolaou smear. As a general rule,, estrogen should not be prescribed for longer than one year without reexamining the patient.

Hypercoagulability: Some studies have shown that women taking estrogen replacement therapy have hypercoagulability, primarily related to decreased antithrombin activity. This effect appears dose- and duration-dependent and is less pronounced than that associated with oral contraceptive use. Also, postmenopausal women tend to have increased coagulation parameters at baseline compared to premenopausal women. There is some suggestion that low dose postmenopausal mestranol may increase the risk of thromboembolism, although the majority of studies (of primarily conjugated estrogens users) report no such increase. There is insufficient information on hypercoagulability in women who have had previous thromboembolic disease.

Familial Hyperlipoproteinemia: Estrogen therapy may be associated with massive elevations of plasma triglycerides leading to pancreatitis and other complications in patients with familial defects of lipoprotein metabolism.

Fluid Retention: Because estrogens may cause some degree of fluid retention, conditions which might be exacerbated by this factor, such as asthma, epilepsy, migraine, and cardiac or renal dysfunction, require careful observation.

Uterine Bleeding And Mastodynia: Certain patients may develop undesirable manifestations of estrogenic stimulation, such as abnormal uterine bleeding and mastodynia.

Impaired Liver Function: Estrogen may be poorly metabolized in patients with impaired liver function and should be administered with caution.

Information for the Patient

See PATIENT PACKAGE INSERT.

Laboratory Tests

Estrogen administration should generally be guided by clinical response at the smallest dose, rather than laboratory monitoring, for relief of symptoms for those indications in which symptoms are observable. For prevention and treatment of osteoporosis, however, see DOSAGE AND ADMINISTRATION.

PRECAUTIONS: *(cont'd)*

Drug/Laboratory Test Interactions

Accelerated prothrombin time, partial thromboplastin time, and platelet aggregation time; increased platelet count; increased factors II, VII antigen, VIII antigen, VIII coagulant activity, IX,X, XII, VII-X complex, II-VII-X complex, and beta-thromboglobulin; decreased levels of anti-factor Xa and antithrombin III, decreased antithrombin III activity; increased levels of fibrinogen and fibrinogen activity; increased plasminogen antigen and activity.

Increased thyroid-binding globulin (TBG) leading to increased circulating total thyroid hormone, as measured by protein-bound iodine (PBI), T4 levels (by column or by radioimmunoassay) or T3 levels by radioimmunoassay. T3 resin uptake is decreased, reflecting the elevated TBG. Free T4 and free T3 concentrations are unaltered.

Other binding proteins may be elevated in serum, i.e., corticosteroid binding globulin (CBG), sex hormone-binding globulin (SHBG), leading to increased circulating corticosteroids and sex steroids respectively. Free or biologically active hormone concentrations are unchanged. Other plasma proteins may be increased (angiotensinogen/renin substrate, alpha-1- antitrypsin, ceruloplasmin).

Increased plasma HDL and HDL-2 subfraction concentrations, reduced LDL cholesterol concentration, increased triglycerides levels.

Impaired glucose intolerance.

Reduced response to metyrapone test.

Reduced serum folate concentration.

Carcinogenesis, Mutagenesis, and Impairment of Fertility

Long term continuous administration of natural and synthetic estrogens in certain animal species increases the frequency of carcinomas of the breast, uterus, cervix, testis, and liver. See CONTRAINDICATIONS and WARNINGS.

Pregnancy Category X

Estrogens should not be used during pregnancy. See CONTRAINDICATIONS and BOXED WARNING.

Nursing Mothers

As a general principle, the administration of any drug to nursing mothers should be done only when clearly necessary since many drugs are excreted in human milk. In addition, estrogen administration to nursing mothers has been shown to decrease the quantity and quality of the milk.

ADVERSE REACTIONS:

TABLETS

The following additional adverse reactions have been reported with estrogen therapy (see WARNINGS regarding induction of neoplasia, adverse effects on the fetus, increased incidence of gallbladder disease, cardiovascular disease, elevated blood pressure, and hypercalcemia).

Genitourinary System: Changes in vaginal bleeding pattern and abnormal withdrawal bleeding or flow, Breakthrough bleeding, SpottingIncrease in size of uterine leiomyomata, Vaginal candidiasis, Change in amount of cervical secretion

Breast: Tenderness, Enlargement

Gastrointestinal: Nausea; Vomiting; Abdominal cramps; Bloating; Cholestatic jaundice; Increased incidence of gallbladder disease

Skin: Chloasma or melasma that may persist when drug is discontinued; Erythema multiforme; Erythema nodosum; Hemorrhagic eruption; Loss of scalp hair; Hirsutism

Eyes: Steepening of corneal curvature; Intolerance to contact lenses

Central Nervous System: Headache; Migraine; Dizziness; Mental depression; Chorea

Miscellaneous: Increase or decrease in weight; Reduced carbohydrate tolerance; Aggravation of porphyria; Edema; Changes in libido

OVERDOSAGE:

Tablets: Serious ill effects have not been reported following acute ingestion of large doses of estrogen-containing oral contraceptives by young children. Overdosage of estrogen may cause nausea and vomiting, and withdrawal bleeding may occur in females.

DOSAGE AND ADMINISTRATION:

TABLETS

For treatment of moderate to severe vasomotor symptoms, vulval and vaginal atrophy associated with the menopause, the lowest dose and regimen that will control symptoms should be chosen and medication should be discontinued as promptly as possible.

Attempts to discontinue or taper medication should be made at 3-month to 6-month intervals.

Usual Dosage Ranges

Vasomotor Symptoms: One Estropipate 625 (0.75) mg estropipate) tablet to two Estropipate 2.5 (3 mg estropipate) tablets per day. The lowest dose that will control symptoms should be chosen. If the patient has not menstruated within the last two weeks or more, cyclic administration is started arbitrarily. If the patient is menstruating, cyclic administration is started on day 5 of bleeding.

Vulval And Vaginal Atrophy: One Estropipate 625 (0.75 mg estropipate) tablet to two Estropipate 2.5 (3 mg estropipate) tablets daily, depending upon the tissue response of the individual patient. The lowest dose that will control symptoms should be chosen. Administer cyclically.

For treatment of female hypoestrogenism due to hypogonadism, castration, or primary ovarian failure.

Usual Dosage Ranges

Female Hypogonadism: A daily dose of one Estropipate 1.25 (1.5 mg estropipate) tablet to three Estropipate 2.5 (3 mg estropipate) tablets may be given for the first three weeks of a theoretical cycle, followed by a rest period of eight to ten days. The lowest dose that will control symptoms should be chosen. If bleeding does not occur by the end of this period, the same dosage schedule is repeated. The number of courses of estrogen therapy necessary to produce bleeding may vary depending on the responsiveness of the endometrium. If satisfactory withdrawal bleeding does not occur, an oral progestogen may be given in addition to estrogen during the third week of the cycle.

Female Castration Or Primary Ovarian Failure: A daily dose of one Estropipate 1.25 (1.5 mg estropipate) tablet to three Estropipate 2.5 (3 mg estropipate) tablets may be given for the first three weeks of a theoretical cycle, followed by a rest period of eight to ten days. Adjust dosage upward or downward according to severity of symptoms and response of the patient. For maintenance, adjust dosage to lowest level that will provide effective control.

Treated patients with an intact uterus should be monitored closely for signs of endometrial cancer and appropriate diagnostic measures should be taken to rule out malignancy in the event of persistent or recurring abnormal vaginal bleeding.

For the prevention of osteoporosis. A daily dose of one Estropipate.625 (0.75 mg estropipate) tablet for 25 days of a 31-day cycle per month.

DOSAGE AND ADMINISTRATION: *(cont'd)*

Recommended storage: Store below 77°F (25°C).

VAGINAL CREAM

To Be Administered Cyclically For Short-Term Use Only: For treatment of atrophic vaginitis or kraurosis vulvae. The lowest dose that will control symptoms should be chosen and medication should be discontinued as promptly as possible. Administration should be cyclic (*e.g.,* three weeks on and one week off). Attempts to discontinue or taper medication should be made at three to six-month intervals. Treated patients with an intact uterus should be monitored closely for signs of endometrial cancer and appropriate diagnostic measures should be taken to rule out malignancy in the event of persistent or recurring abnormal vaginal bleeding. Usual dosage: Intravaginally, 2 to 4 grams of Estropipate Vaginal Cream daily, depending upon the severity of the condition.

The following instructions for use are intended for the patient and are printed on the carton label for Estropipate Vaginal Cream:

1. Remove cap from tube.

2. Make sure plunger of applicator is all the way into the barrel.

3. Screw nozzle end of applicator onto the tube.

4. Squeeze tube to force sufficient cream into applicator so that number on plunger indicating prescribed dose is level with top of barrel.

5. Unscrew applicator from tube and replace cap on tube.

6. To deliver medication, insert end of applicator into vagina and push plunger all the way down.

Between uses, pull plunger out of barrel and wash applicator in wash soapy water. DO NOT PUT APPLICATOR IN HOT OR BOILING WATER.

PATIENT PACKAGE INSERT:

Introduction: Estrogens have important benefits but also some risks. You must decide, with your doctor, whether the risks to you of estrogen use are acceptable because of their benefits. If you use estrogens, check with your doctor to be sure you are using the lowest possible dose that works, and that you don't use them longer than necessary. How long you need to use estrogens will depend on the reason for use.

WARNING: ESTROGENS INCREASE THE RISK OF CANCER OF THE UTERUS IN WOMEN WHO HAVE HAD THEIR MENOPAUSE ("CHANGE OF LIFE").
If you use any estrogen-containing drug, it is important to visit your doctor regularly and report any unusual vaginal bleeding right away. Vaginal bleeding after menopause may be a warning sign of uterine cancer. Your doctor should evaluate any unusual vaginal bleeding to find out the cause.
ESTROGENS SHOULD NOT BE USED DURING PREGNANCY.
Estrogens do not prevent miscarriage (spontaneous abortion) and not needed in the days following childbirth. If you take estrogens during pregnancy, your unborn child has a greater than usual chance of having birth defects. The risk of developing these defects is small, but clearly larger than the risk in children whose mothers did not take estrogens during pregnancy. These birth defects may affect the baby's urinary system and sex organs. Daughters born to mothers who took DES (an estrogen drug) have a higher than usual chance of developing cancer of the vagina or cervix when they become teenagers or young adults. Sons may have a higher than usual chance of developing cancer of the testicles when they become teenagers or young adults.

USES OF ESTROGEN

(Not every estrogen drug is approved for every use listed in this section. If you want to know which of these possible uses are approved for the medicine prescribed for you, ask your doctor or pharmacist to show you the professional labeling. Generic drugs carry virtually the same labeling information as their brand name versions.)

† **To reduce moderate or severe menopausal symptoms:** Estrogens are hormones made by the ovaries of normal women. Between ages of 45 to 55, the ovaries normally stop making estrogens. This leads to a drop in body estrogen levels which causes the "change in life" or menopause (the end of monthly menstrual periods). If both ovaries are removed during an operation before natural menopause takes place, the sudden drop in estrogen levels causes "surgical menopause."

When the estrogen levels begin dropping, some women develop very uncomfortable symptoms, such as feelings of warmth in the face, neck, chest, or sudden intense episodes of heat and sweating ("hot flashes" or "hot flushes"). Using estrogen drugs can help the body adjust to lower estrogen levels and reduce these symptoms. Most women have only mild menopausal symptoms or none at all and do not need to use estrogen drugs for these symptoms. Others may need to take estrogens for a few months while their bodies adjust to lower estrogen levels. The majority of women do not need estrogen replacement for longer than six months for these symptoms.

† **To treat vulval and vaginal atrophy:** (itching, burning, dryness in or around the vagina, difficulty or burning on urination) associated with menopause.

†**To treat certain conditions in which a young woman's ovaries do not produce enough estrogen naturally**.

† **To treat certain types of abnormal vaginal bleeding due to hormonal imbalance when your doctor has found no serious cause of the bleeding.**

† **To treat certain cancers in special situations, in men and women.**

TO PREVENT THINNING OF BONES

Osteoporosis is a thinning of the bones that makes them weaker and allows them to break more easily. The bones of the spine, wrists and hips break most often in osteoporosis. Both men and women start to lose bone mass after about age 40, but women lose bone mass faster after the menopause. Using estrogens after the menopause slows down bone thinning and may prevent bones from breaking. Lifelong adequate calcium intake, either in the diet (such as dairy products) or by calcium supplements (to reach a total daily intake of 1000 milligrams per day before menopause or 1500 milligrams per day after menopause), may help to prevent osteoporosis. Regular weight-bearing exercise (like walking and running) for an hour, two to three times a week) may also help to prevent osteoporosis. Before you change your calcium intake or exercise habits, it is important to discuss these lifestyle changes with your doctor to find out if they are safe for you.

Since estrogen use has some risks, only women who are likely to develop osteoporosis should use estrogens for prevention. Women who are likely to develop osteoporosis often have the following characteristics: white or Asian race, slim, cigarette smokers, and a family history of osteoporosis in a mother, sister or aunt. Women who have relatively early menopause, often because their ovaries were removed during an operation ("surgical menopause"), are more likely to develop osteoporosis than women whose menopause happens at the average age.

PATIENT PACKAGE INSERT: *(cont'd)*

WHO SHOULD NOT USE ESTROGENS

Estrogens should not be used:

† **During pregnancy:** (see BOXED WARNING.) f you think you may be pregnant, do not use any form of estrogen- containing drug. Using estrogens while you are pregnant may cause your unborn child to have birth defects. Estrogens do not prevent miscarriage.

†**If you have unusual vaginal bleeding which has not been evaluated by your doctor:** (see BOXED WARNING.) nusual vaginal bleeding can be a warning sign of cancer of the uterus, especially if it happens after menopause. Your doctor must find out the cause of the bleeding so that he or she can recommend the proper treatment. Taking estrogens without visiting your doctor can cause you serious harm if your vaginal bleeding is caused by cancer of the uterus.

† **If you have had cancer:** Since estrogens increase the risk of certain types of cancer, you should not use estrogens if you have ever had cancer of the breast or uterus, unless your doctor recommends that the drug may help in the cancer treatment. (For certain patients with breast or prostate cancer, estrogens may help.)

† **If you have any circulation problems:** Estrogen drugs should not be used except in unusually special situations in which your doctor judges that you need estrogen therapy so much that the risks are acceptable. Men and women with abnormal blood clotting conditions should avoid estrogen use (see Dangers of Estrogens.)

† **When they do not work:** During menopause, some women develop nervous symptoms or depression. Estrogens do not relieve these symptoms. You may have heard that taking estrogens for years after menopause will keep your skin soft and supple and keep you feeling young. There is no evidence for these claims and such long-term estrogen use may have serious risks.

† **After childbirth or when breastfeeding a baby:** strogens should not be used to try to stop the breasts from filling with milk after a baby is born. Such treatment may increase the risk of developing blood clots (see Dangers of Estrogens,).

If you are breastfeeding, you should avoid using any drugs because many drugs pass through to the baby in the milk.While nursing a baby, you should take drugs only on the advice of your health care provider.

DANGERS OF ESTROGENS

Cancer of the uterus: Your risk of developing cancer of the uterus gets higher the longer you use estrogens and the larger doses you use. One study showed that after women stop taking estrogens, this higher cancer risk quickly returns to the usual level of risk (as if you had never used estrogen therapy). Three other studies showed that the cancer risk stayed high for 8 to more than 15 years after stopping estrogen treatment. **Because of this risk, IT IS IMPORTANT TO TAKE THE LOWEST DOSE THAT WORKS AND TO TAKE IT ONLY AS LONG AS YOU NEED IT.**

Using progestin therapy together with estrogen therapy together with estrogen therapy may reduce the higher risk of uterine cancer related to estrogen use (but see Other Information, below).

If you have had your uterus removed (total hysterectomy), there is no danger of developing cancer of the uterus.

† **Cancer of the Breast:** Most studies have not shown a higher risk of breast cancer in women who have ever used estrogens. However, some studies have reported that breast cancer developed more often (up to twice the usual rate) in women who used estrogens for long periods of time (especially more than 10 years), or who used higher doses for shorter time periods.

Regular breast examinations by a health professional and monthly self-examination are recommended for all women.

† **Gallbladder Disease:** Women who use estrogens after menopause are more likely to develop gallbladder disease needing surgery than women who do not use estrogens.

† **Abnormal blood clotting:** Taking estrogens may cause changes in your blood clotting system. These changes allow the blood to clot more easily, possibly allowing clots to form in your bloodstream. If blood clots do form in your bloodstream, they can cut off the blood supply to vital organs, causing serious problems. These problems may include a stroke (by cutting off blood to the brain), a heart attack (by cutting off blood to the heart), a pulmonary embolus (by cutting off blood to the lungs), or other problems. Any of these conditions may cause death or serious long term disability. However, most studies of low dose estrogen usage by women do not show an increased risk of these complications.

SIDE EFFECTS

In addition to the risks listed above, the following side effects have been reported with estrogen use:

Nausea and vomiting

Breast tenderness of enlargement

Enlargement of benign tumors ("fibroids") of the uterus

Retention of excess fluid. This may make some conditions worsen, such as asthma, epilepsy, migraine, heart disease, or kidney disease.

A spotty darkening of the skin, particularly on the face

REDUCING RISK OF ESTROGEN USE

If you use estrogens, you can reduce your risks by doing these things:

†**See your doctor regularly:** While you are using estrogens, it is important to visit your doctor at least once a year for a check-up. If you develop vaginal bleeding while taking estrogens, you may need further evaluation. If members of your family have had breast cancer or if you have breast lumps or an abnormal mammogram (breast x-ray), you may need to have more frequent breast examinations.

†**Reassess your need for estrogens:** You and your doctor should reevaluate whether or not you still need estrogens at least every six months.

† **Be alert for signs of trouble:** If any of these warning signals (or any other unusual symptoms) happen while you are using estrogens, call your doctor immediately:

Abnormal bleeding from the vagina (possible uterine cancer).

Pains in the calves or chest, sudden shortness of breath, or coughing blood (possible clot in the legs, heart, or lungs).

Severe headache or vomiting, dizziness, faintness, changes in vision or speech, weakness or numbness of an arm or leg (possible clot in the brain or eye).

Breast lumps (possible breast cancer; ask your doctor or health professional to show how to examine your breasts monthly).

Yellowing of the skin or eyes (possible liver problem).

Pain, swelling, or tenderness in the abdomen (possible gallbladder problem).

OTHER INFORMATION

Some doctors may choose to prescribe a progestin, a different hormonal drug, for you to take together with your estrogen treatment. Progestins lower your risk of developing endometrial hyperplasia (a possible pre- cancerous condition of the uterus) while using estrogens. Taking estrogens and progestins together may also protect you from the higher risk of uterine cancer, but this has not been clearly established. Combined use of progestin and estrogen treatment

PATIENT PACKAGE INSERT: *(cont'd)*

may have additional risks, however. The possible risks include unhealthy effects on blood fats (especially a lowering of HDL cholesterol, the "good" blood fat which protects against heart disease risk), unhealthy effects on blood sugar (which might worsen a diabetic condition), and a possible further increase in the breast cancer risk which may be associated with long-term estrogen use. The type of progestin drug used and its dosage schedule may be important in minimizing these effects.

Your doctor has prescribed this drug for you and you alone. Do not give the drug to anyone else.

If you will be taking calcium supplements as part of the treatment to help osteoporosis, check with your doctor about how much to take.

Keep this and other drugs out of the reach of children. In case of overdose, call your doctor, hospital or poison control center immediately.

This leaflet provides a summary of the most important information about estrogens. If you want more information, ask your doctor or pharmacist to show you the professional labeling. The professional labeling is also published in a book called the "Physicians GenRx," which is available in book stores and public libraries. Generic drugs carry virtually the same labeling information as their brand name versions.

Recommended storage: Store below 77°F (25°C).

HOW SUPPLIED:

TABLETS

Ogen (estropipate tablets, USP) is supplied as: Estropipate 625 (0.75 mg estropipate), yellow tablets; Estropipate 1.25 (1.5 mg estropipate), peach- colored tablets; Estropipate 2.5 (3 mg estropipate), blue tablets.

VAGINAL CREAM

Ogen (estropipate vaginal cream, USP), 1.5 mg estropipate per gram, is available in packages containing a 1 1/2 oz (42.5 gm) tube with one plastic applicator calibrated at 1, 2, 3, and 4 gm levels.

HOW SUPPLIED - RATED THERAPEUTICALLY EQUIVALENT:

Tablet - Oral - 0.75 mg

100's	$40.90	Estropipate, Duramed Pharms	51285-0875-02

Tablet - Oral - 1.5 mg

100's	$57.14	Estropipate, Duramed Pharms	51285-0876-02

Tablet, Uncoated - Oral - 0.625 mg

100's	$34.66	Ortho-Est, Ortho Pharm	00062-1801-01
100's	$38.45	Estropipate, Goldline Labs	00182-1976-01
100's	$41.28	Estropipate, Watson Labs	52544-0414-01
100's	$43.00	Estropipate, United Res	00677-1508-01
100's	$43.05	ESTROPIPATE, Aligen Independ	00405-4413-01
100's	$43.12	Estropipate, Qualitest Pharms	00603-3559-21
100's	$43.15	Estropipate, Schein Pharm (US)	00364-2600-01
100's	$45.95	Estropipate, Warner Chilcott	00047-0124-24
100's	$46.05	Estropipate, Rugby	00536-3560-01
100's	**$53.22**	**OGEN, Pharmacia & Upjohn**	**00009-3772-01**
100's	**$53.22**	**OGEN, Abbott**	**00074-3943-04**

Tablet, Uncoated - Oral - 1.25 mg

100's	$47.40	Ortho-Est, Ortho Pharm	00062-1800-01
100's	$57.67	Estropipate, Watson Labs	52544-0415-01
100's	$60.14	ESTROPIPATE, Aligen Independ	00405-4414-01
100's	$60.35	Estropipate, Qualitest Pharms	00603-3560-21
100's	$61.07	Estropipate, Goldline Labs	00182-1977-01
100's	$62.00	Estropipate, Schein Pharm (US)	00364-2601-01
100's	$64.00	Estropipate, Warner Chilcott	00047-0126-24
100's	$64.17	Estropipate, United Res	00677-1509-01
100's	$64.46	Estropipate, Rugby	00536-3561-01
100's	**$74.35**	**OGEN, Pharmacia & Upjohn**	**00009-3773-01**
100's	**$74.35**	**OGEN, Abbott**	**00074-3946-04**

Tablet, Uncoated - Oral - 2.5 mg

100's	$100.35	Estropipate, Qualitest Pharms	00603-3561-21
100's	$100.39	Estropipate, Watson Labs	52544-0416-01
100's	$105.76	Estropipate, Warner Chilcott	00047-0128-24
100's	$106.30	Estropipate, Goldline Labs	00182-1978-01
100's	**$129.40**	**OGEN, Pharmacia & Upjohn**	**00009-3774-01**
100's	**$129.40**	**OGEN, Abbott**	**00074-3951-04**

Tablet, Uncoated - Oral - 3 mg

100's	$109.40	Estropipate, H.C.F.A. F F P	99999-1204-01

HOW SUPPLIED - NOT RATED EQUIVALENT:

Cream - Vaginal - 1.5 mg/gm

42.5 gm	**$39.14**	**OGEN, Pharmacia & Upjohn**	**00009-3776-01**
45 gm	**$39.14**	**OGEN, Abbott**	**00074-2467-42**

Tablet, Uncoated - Oral - 0.625 mg

100's	$42.80	Estropipate, Caremark	00339-5981-12

Tablet, Uncoated - Oral - 1.25 mg

100's	$61.19	Estropipate, Caremark	00339-5983-12

Tablet, Uncoated - Oral - 2.5 mg

100's	$105.06	Estropipate, Caremark	00339-5985-12
100's	$111.97	Estropipate, Rugby	00536-5691-01

ETHACRYNIC ACID *(001205)*

CATEGORIES: Antihypertensives; Antitussives/Expectorants/Mucolytics; Cardiovascular Drugs; Cirrhosis; Congestive Heart Failure; Diuresis; Diuretics; Edema; Electrolytic, Caloric-Water Balance; Ethacrynate Sodium; Heart Disease; Heart Failure; Loop Diuretics; Nephrotic Syndrome; Renal Drugs; Glaucoma*; Pregnancy Category B; FDA Approval Pre 1982
* Indication not approved by the FDA

BRAND NAMES: *Edecril*; **Edecrin**; Edecrin Sodium; *Edecrina*; *Hydromedin* (Germany); *Reomax*; Sodium Edecrin
(International brand names outside U.S. in italics)

FORMULARIES: Aetna; Medi-Cal

COST OF THERAPY: $310.68 (Edema; Tablet; 50 mg; 2/day; 365 days)

DESCRIPTION:

Ethacrynic acid is a potent diuretic which, if given in excessive amounts, may lead to profound diuresis with water and electrolyte depletion. Therefore, careful medical supervision is required, and dose and dose schedule must be adjusted to the individual patient's needs (see DOSAGE AND ADMINISTRATION.)

Ethacrynic acid is an unsaturated ketone derivative of an anyloxyacetic acid. It is designated chemically as (2,3-dichloro-4-(2-methylenebutyryl)phenoxy) acetic acid. Ethacrynic acid is a white, or practically white, crystalline powder, very slightly soluble in water, but soluble in most organic solvents such as alcohols, chloroform, and benzene. Its empirical formula is $C_{13}H_{11}Cl_2NaO_4$.

Ethacrynate sodium, the sodium salt of ethacrynic acid, is soluble in water at 25°C to the extent of about 7 percent. Solutions of the sodium salt are relatively stable at about pH 7 at room temperature for short periods, but as the pH or temperature increases the solutions are less stable. its empirical formula is $C_{13}H_{11}Cl_2NaO_4$.

Edecrin is supplied as 25 mg and 50 mg tablets for oral use. Each tablet contains the following inactive ingredients: colloidal silicon dioxide, lactose, magnesium stearate, starch and talc. The 50 mg tablet also contains D&C Yellow 10, FD&C Blue 1 and FD&C Yellow 6. Intravenous Sodium Edecrin (Ethacrynate Sodium) is a sterile freeze-dried powder and is supplied in a vial containing: Ethacrynate sodium equivalent to ethacrynic acid: 50.0 mg

Inactive ingredients: Mannitol: 62.5 mg

CLINICAL PHARMACOLOGY:

PHARMACOKINETICS AND METABOLISM

Ethacrynic acid acts on the ascending limb of the loop of Henle and on the proximal and distal tubules. Urinary output is usually dose dependent and related to the magnitude of fluid accumulation. Water and electrolyte excretion may be increased several times over that observed with thiazide diuretics, since ethacrynic acid inhibits reabsorption of a much greater proportion of filtered sodium than most other diuretic agents. Therefore, ethacrynic acid is effective in many patients who have significant degrees of renal insufficiency (see WARNINGS concerning deafness). Ethacrynic acid has little or no effect on glomerular filtration or on renal blood flow, except following pronounced reductions in plasma volume when associated with rapid diuresis.

The electrolyte excretion pattern of ethacrynic acid varies from that of the thiazides and mercurial diuretics. Initial sodium and chloride excretion is usually substantial and chloride loss excretion is usually substantial and chloride loss exceeds that of sodium. With prolonged administration, chloride excretion declines, and potassium and hydrogen ion excretion may increase. Ethacrynic acid is effective whether or not there is clinical acidosis or alkalosis.

Although ethacrynic acid, in carefully controlled studies in animals and experimental subjects, produces a more favorable sodium/potassium excretion ratio than the thiazides, in patients with increased diuresis excessive amounts of potassium may be excreted.

Onset of action is rapid, usually within 30 minutes after an oral dose of ethacrynic acid or within 5 minutes after an intravenous injection of sodium ethacrynic acid (ethacrynate sodium). After oral use, diuresis peaks in about 2 hours and lasts about 6 to 8 hours.

The sulfhydryl binding propensity of ethacrynic acid differs somewhat from that of the organomercurials; its mode of action is not by carbonic anhydrase inhibition.

Ethacrynic acid does not cross the blood-brain barrier.

INDICATIONS AND USAGE:

Ethacrynic acid is indicated for treatment of edema when an agent with greater diuretic potential than those commonly employed is required.

1. Treatment of the edema associated with congestive heart failure, cirrhosis of the liver, and renal disease, including the nephrotic syndrome.

2. Short-term management of ascites due to malignancy, idiopathic edema, and lymphedema.

3. Short-term management of hospitalized pediatric patients, other than infants, with congenital heart disease or the nephrotic syndrome.

4. Intravenous administration of sodium ethacrynic acid is indicated when a rapid onset of diuresis is desired, *e.g.*, in acute pulmonary edema, or when gastrointestinal absorption is impaired or oral medication is not practicable.

CONTRAINDICATIONS:

All diuretics, including ethacrynic acid, are contraindicated in anuria. If increasing electrolyte imbalance, azotemia, and/or oliguria occur during treatment of severe, progressive renal disease, the diuretic should be discontinued.

In a few patients this diuretic has produced severe, watery diarrhea. If this occurs, it should be discontinued and not readministered.

Until further experience in infants is accumulated, therapy with oral and parenteral ethacrynic acid is contraindicated.

Hypersensitivity to any component of this product.

WARNINGS:

The effects of ethacrynic acid on electrolytes are related to its renal pharmacologic activity and are dose dependent. The possibility of profound electrolyte and water loss may be avoided by weighing the patient throughout the treatment period, by careful adjustment of dosage, by initiating treatment with small doses, and by using the drug on an intermittent schedule when possible. When excessive electrolyte loss occurs, the dosage should be reduced or the drug temporarily withdrawn.

Initiation of diuretic therapy with ethacrynic acid in the cirrhotic patient with ascites is best carried out in the hospital. When maintenance therapy has been established, the individual can be satisfactorily followed as an outpatient.

Ethacrynic acid should be given with caution to patients with advanced cirrhosis of the liver, particularly those with a history of previous episodes of electrolyte imbalance of hepatic encephalopathy. Like other diuretics it may precipitate hepatic coma and death.

Too vigorous a diuresis, as evidenced by rapid and excessive weight loss, may induce an acute hypotensive episode. In elderly cardiac patients, rapid contraction of plasma volume and the resultant hemoconcentration should be avoided to prevent the development of thromboembolic episodes, such as cerebral vascular thromboses and pulmonary emboli which may be fatal. Excessive loss of potassium in patients receiving digitalis glycosides may precipitate digitalis toxicity. Care should also be exercised in patients receiving potassium-depleting steroids.

A number of possibly drug-related deaths have occurred in critically ill patients refractory to other diuretics. These generally have fallen into two categories: (1) patients with severe myocardial disease who have been receiving digitalis and presumably developed acute hypokalemia with fatal arrhythmia; (2) patients with severity decompensated hepatic cirrhosis with ascites, with or without accompanying encephalopathy, who were in electrolyte imbalance and died because of intensification of the electrolyte defect.

WARNINGS: *(cont'd)*

Deafness, tinnitus, and vertigo with a sense of fullness in the ears have occurred, most frequently in patients with severe impairment of renal function. These symptoms have been associated most often with intravenous administration and with doses in excess of those recommended. The deafness has usually been reversible and of short duration (one to 24 hours). However, in some patients the hearing loss has been permanent. A number of these patients were also receiving drugs known to be ototoxic. Ethacrynic acid may increase the ototoxic potential of other drugs.

PRECAUTIONS:

General: Weakness, muscle cramps, paresthesias, thirst, anorexia, and signs of hyponatremia, hypokalemia, and/or hypochloremic alkalosis may occur following vigorous or excessive diuresis and these may be accentuated by rigid salt restriction. Rarely tetany has been reported following vigorous diuresis. *During therapy with ethacrynic acid, liberalization of salt intake and supplementary potassium chloride are often necessary.*

When a metabolic alkalosis may be anticipated, e.g., in cirrhosis with ascites, the use of potassium chloride with or a potassium-sparing agent before and during therapy with ethacrynic acid may mitigate or prevent the hypokalemia.

Loop diuretics have been shown to increase the urinary excretion of magnesium; this may result in hypomagnesemia.

The safety and efficacy of ethacrynic acid in hypertension have not been established. However, the dosage of coadministered antihypertensive agents may require adjustment.

Orthostatic hypotension may occur in patients receiving other antihypertensive agents when given ethacrynic acid.

Ethacrynic acid has little or no effect on glomerular filtration or on renal blood flow, except following pronounced reductions in plasma volume when associated with rapid diuresis. A transient increase in serum urea nitrogen may occur. Usually, this readily reversible when the drug is discontinued.

As with other diuretics used in the treatment of renal edema, hypoproteinemia may reduce responsiveness to ethacrynic acid and the use of salt-poor albumin should be considered.

A number of drugs, including ethacrynic acid, have been shown to displace warfarin from plasma protein; a reduction in the usual anticoagulant dosage may be required in patients receiving both drugs.

Ethacrynic acid may increase the risk of gastric hemorrhage associated with corticosteroid treatment.

Laboratory Tests: Frequent serum electrolyte, CO_2 and BUN determinations should be performed early in therapy and periodically thereafter during active diuresis. Any electrolyte abnormalities should be corrected or the drug temporarily withdrawn.

Increases in blood glucose and alterations in glucose tolerance tests have been observed in patients receiving ethacrynic acid.

Carcinogenesis, Mutagenesis, and Impairment of Fertility: There was no evidence of a tumorigenic effect in a 79-week oral toxicity study in rats at doses up to 45 times the human dose.

Ethacrynic acid had no effect on fertility in a two-litter study in rats or a two-generation study in mice at 10 times the human dose.

Pregnancy Category B: Reproduction studies in the mouse and rabbit at doses up to 50 times the human dose showed no evidence of external abnormalities of the fetus due to ethacrynic acid.

In a two-litter study in the dog and rat, oral doses of 5 or 20 mg/kg/day (2 1/2 or 10 times the human dose), respectively, did not interfere with pregnancy or with growth and development of the pups. Although there was reduction in the mean body weights of the fetuses in a teratogenic study in the rat at a dose level of 100 mg/kg/day (50 times the human dose), there was no effect on mortality or postnatal development. Functional and morphologic abnormalities were not observed.

There are, however, no adequate and well-controlled studies in pregnant women. Since animal reproduction studies are not always predictive of human response, ethacrynic acid should be used during pregnancy only if clearly needed.

Nursing Mothers: It is not known whether or not this drug is excreted in human milk. Because many drugs are excreted in human milk and because of the potential for serious adverse reactions from ethacrynic acid, a decision should be made whether to discontinue nursing or to discontinue the drug, taking into account the importance of the drug to the mother.

Pediatric Use: For information on oral use in pediatrics, other than infants, see INDICATIONS AND USAGE and DOSAGE AND ADMINISTRATION.

Safety and effectiveness in infants have not been established (see CONTRAINDICATIONS.)

Safety and effectiveness of intravenous use in children have not been established (see DOSAGE AND ADMINISTRATION, Intravenous Use.)

ADVERSE REACTIONS:

Gastrointestinal: Anorexia, malaise, abdominal discomfort or pain, dysphagia, nausea, vomiting, and diarrhea have occurred. These are more frequent with large doses or after one to three months of continuous therapy. A few patients have had sudden onset of watery, profuse diarrhea. Discontinue ethacrynic acid if diarrhea is severe and do not give it again. Gastrointestinal bleeding has been reported in some patients. Rarely, acute pancreatitis has been reported.

Metabolic: Reversible hyperuricemia and acute gout have been reported. Acute symptomatic hypoglycemia with convulsions occurred in two uremic patients who received doses above those recommended. Hyperglycemia has been reported. Rarely, jaundice and abnormal liver function tests have been reported in seriously ill patients receiving multiple drug therapy, including ethacrynic acid.

Hematologic: Agranulocytosis or severe neutropenia has been reported in a few critically ill patients also receiving agents known to produce this effect. Thrombocytopenia has been reported rarely. Henoch-Schonlein purpura has been reported rarely in patients with rheumatic heart disease receiving multiple drug therapy, including ethacrynic acid.

Special Senses: (see WARNINGS) Deafness, tinnitus and vertigo with a sense of fullness in the ears, and blurred vision have occurred.

Central Nervous System: Headache, fatigue, apprehension, confusion.

Miscellaneous: Skin rash, fever, chills, hematuria.

Sodium ethacrynic acid occasionally has caused local irritation and pain after intravenous use.

OVERDOSAGE:

Overdosage may lead to excessive diuresis with electrolyte depletion and dehydration.

In the event of overdosage, symptomatic and supportive measures should be employed. Emesis should be induced or gastric lavage performed. Correct dehydration, electrolyte imbalance, hepatic coma, and hypotension by established procedures. If required, give oxygen or artificial respiration for respiratory impairment.

OVERDOSAGE: *(cont'd)*

In the mouse, the oral LD_{50} of ethacrynic acid in 627 mg/kg and the intravenous LD_{50} of ethacrynate sodium is 175 mg/kg.

DOSAGE AND ADMINISTRATION:

Dosage must be regulated carefully to prevent a more rapid or substantial loss of fluid or electrolyte than is indicated or necessary. The magnitude of diuresis and natriuresis is largely dependent on the degree of fluid accumulation present in the patient. Similarly, the extent of potassium excretion is determined in large measure by the presence and magnitude of aldosteronism.

ORAL USE

Ethacrynic acid is available for oral use as 25 mg and 50 mg tablets.

DOSAGE: TO INITIATE DIURESIS

In Adults: The smallest dose required to produce gradual weight loss (about 1 to 2 pounds per day) is recommended. Onset of diuresis usually occurs at 50 to 100 mg for adults. After diuresis has been achieved, the minimally effective dose (usually from 50 to 200 mg daily) may be given on a continuous or intermittent dosage schedule. Dosage adjustments are usually in 25 to 50 mg increments to avoid derangement of water and electrolyte excretion.

The patient should be weighed under standard conditions before and during the institution of diuretic therapy with this compound. Small alterations in dose should effectively prevent a massive diuretic response. The following schedule may be helpful in determining the smallest effective dose.

Day 1-50 mg (single dose) after a meal

Day 2-50 mg twice daily after meals, if necessary

Day 3-100 mg in the morning and 50 to 100 mg following the afternoon or evening meal, depending upon response to the morning dose

A few patients may require initial and maintenance doses as high as 200 mg twice daily. These higher doses, which should be achieved gradually, are most required in patients with severe, refractory edema.

In Children: (excluding infants, See CONTRAINDICATIONS) the initial dose should be 25 mg. Careful stepwise increments in dosage of 25 mg should be made to achieve effective maintenance.

MAINTENANCE THERAPY

It is usually possible to reduce the dosage and frequency of administration once dry weight has been achieved.

Ethacrynic acid may be given intermittently after an effective diuresis is obtained with the regimen outlined above. Dosage may be on an alternate daily schedule or more prolonged periods of diuretic therapy may be interspersed with rest periods. Such an intermittent dosage schedule allows time for correction of any electrolyte imbalance and may provide a more efficient diuretic response.

The chloruretic effect of this agent may give rise to retention of bicarbonate and a metabolic alkalosis. This may be corrected by giving chloride (ammonium chloride or arginine chloride). Ammonium chloride should not be given to cirrhotic patients.

Ethacrynic acid has had additive effects when used with other diuretics. For example, a patient who is on maintenance dosage of an oral diuretic may required additional intermittent diuretic therapy, such as an organomercurial, for the maintenance of basal weight. The intermittent use of ethacrynic acid orally may eliminate the need or injections of organomercurials. Small doses of ethacrynic acid may be added to existing diuretic regimens to maintain basal weight. This drug may potentiate the action of carbonic anhydrase inhibitors, with augmentation of natriuresis and kaliuresis. Therefore, when adding ethacrynic acid the initial dose and changes of dose should be in 25 mg increments, to avoid electrolyte depletion. Rarely patients who failed to respond to ethacrynic acid have responded to older established agents.

While many patients do not require supplemental potassium, the use of potassium chloride or potassium-sparing agents, or both, during treatment with ethacrynic acid is advisable, especially in cirrhotic or nephrotic patients,and in patients receiving digitalis.

Salt liberalization usually prevents the development of hyponatremia and hypochloremia. During treatment with ethacrynic acid, salt may be liberalized to a greater extent than with other diuretics. Cirrhotic patients however, usually require at least moderate salt restriction concomitant with diuretic therapy.

INTRAVENOUS USE

Intravenous sodium ethacrynic acid is to intravenous use when oral intake is impractical or in urgent conditions, such as acute pulmonary edema.

The usual intravenous dose for the average sized adult is 50 mg, or 0.5 to 1.0 mg per kg of body weight. Usually only one dose has been necessary; occasionally a second dose at a new injection site to avoid possible thrombophlebitis, may be required. A single intravenous dose not exceeding 100 mg has been used in critical situations.

Insufficient pediatric experience precludes recommendation for this age group.

To reconstitute the dry material, add 50 ml of 5 percent Dextrose Injection or Sodium Chloride Injection to the vial. Occasionally, some 5 percent Dextrose Injection solutions may have a low pH (below 5). The resulting solution with such a diluent may be hazy or opalescent. Intravenous use of such a solution is not recommended. Inspect the vial containing intravenous sodium ethacrynic acid for particulate matter and discoloration before use.

The solution may be given slowly through the tubing of a running infusion or by direct intravenous injection over a period of several minutes. Do not mix this solution with whole blood or its derivatives. Discard unused reconstituted solution after 24 hours.

HOW SUPPLIED - EQUIVALENTS NOT AVAILABLE:

Injection, Solution - Intravenous - 50 mg

1's	$19.05	EDECRIN SODIUM, Merck	00006-3330-50

Tablet, Uncoated - Oral - 25 mg

100's	$29.86	EDECRIN, Merck	00006-0065-68

Tablet, Uncoated - Oral - 50 mg

100's	$42.56	EDECRIN, Merck	00006-0090-68

ETHAMBUTOL HYDROCHLORIDE *(001206)*

CATEGORIES: Anti-Infectives; Antimicrobials; Antimycobacterials; Antituberculosis Agents; Pulmonary Disease; Respiratory Tract Infections; Tuberculosis; FDA Approval Pre 1982

BRAND NAMES: *Afimocil*; *Althocin*; *Ambutol*; *Apo-Ethambutol*; *Asiabutol*; *Blomison*; *Carnotol*; *Cidanbutol*; *Clobutol*; *Combutol*; *Conbutol*; *Corsabutol*; *Coxytol*; *Danbutol*; *Dexambutol* (France); *EMB* (Germany); *ET 800*; *Ebutol* (Japan); *Esan-*

butol (Japan); *Etapiam*; *Etibi* (Canada); *Etinol*; *Interbutol*; **Myambutol**; *Mycobutol*; *Mycrol*; *Odetol*; *Sintiabutol*; *Stambutol*; *Tambutol*; *Tibitol*; *Tibutol*
(International brand names outside U.S. in italics)

FORMULARIES: Aetna; BC-BS; FHP; Medi-Cal; PCS; WHO

COST OF THERAPY: $571.50 (Tuberculosis; Tablet; 400 mg; 2/day; 180 days)

PRIMARY ICD9: 011.93 (Pulmonary Tuberculosis, Unspecified, Tubercle Bacilli Found)

DESCRIPTION:

Ethambutol hydrochloride is an oral chemotherapeutic agent which is specifically effective against actively growing microorganisms of the genus *Mycobacterium*, including *M. tuberculosis*.

Myambutol 100 and 400 mg tablets contain the following inactive ingredients: Gelatin, Hydroxypropyl Methylcellulose, Magnesium Stearate, Sodium Lauryl Sulfate, Sorbitol, Stearic Acid, Sucrose, Titanium Dioxide and other ingredients.

CLINICAL PHARMACOLOGY:

Ethambutol HCl following a single oral dose of 25 mg/kg of body weight, attains a peak of 2 to 5 micrograms/ml in serum 2 to 4 hours after administration. When the drug is administered daily for longer periods of time at this dose, serum levels are similar. The serum level of ethambutol HCl falls to undetectable levels by 24 hours after the last dose except in some patients with abnormal renal function. The intracellular concentrations of erythrocytes reach peak values approximately twice those of plasma and maintain this ratio throughout the 24 hours.

During the 24-hour period following oral administration of ethambutol HCl approximately 50 percent of the initial dose is excreted unchanged in the urine, while an additional 8 to 15 percent appears in the form of metabolites. The main path of metabolism appears to be an initial oxidation of the alcohol to an aldehydic intermediate, followed by conversion to a dicarboxylic acid. From 20 to 22 percent of the initial dose is excreted in the feces as unchanged drug. No drug accumulation has been observed with consecutive single daily doses of 25 mg/kg in patients with normal kidney function, although marked accumulation has been demonstrated in patients with renal insufficiency.

Ethambutol HCl diffuses into actively growing *mycobacterium* cells such as tubercle bacilli. Ethambutol HCl appears to inhibit the synthesis of one or more metabolites, thus causing impairment of cell metabolism, arrest of multiplication, and cell death. No cross resistance with other available antimycobacterial agents has been demonstrated.

Ethambutol HCl has been shown to be effective against strains of *Mycobacterium tuberculosis* but does not seem to be active against fungi, viruses, or other bacteria. *Mycobacterium tuberculosis* strains previously unexposed to ethambutol HCl have been uniformly sensitive to concentrations of 8 or less micrograms/ml, depending on the nature of the culture media. When ethambutol HCl has been used alone for treatment of tuberculosis, tubercle bacilli from these patients have developed resistance to ethambutol HCl ethambutol hydrochloride by *in vitro* susceptibility tests; the development of resistance has been unpredictable and appears to occur in a step-like manner. No cross resistance between ethambutol HCl and other antituberculous drugs has been reported. Ethambutol HCl has reduced the incidence of the emergence of mycobacterial resistance to isoniazid when both drugs have been used concurrently.

An agar diffusion microbiologic assay, based upon inhibition of *Mycobacterium smegmatis* (ATCC 607) may be used to determine concentrations of ethambutol HCl in serum and urine. This technique has not been published, but further information can be obtained upon inquiry to Lederle Laboratories.

INDICATIONS AND USAGE:

Ethambutol HCl is indicated for the treatment of pulmonary tuberculosis. It should not be used as the sole antituberculous drug, but should be used in conjunction with at least one other antituberculous drug. Selection of the companion drug should be based on clinical experience, considerations of comparative safety and appropriate *in vitro* susceptibility studies. In patients who have not received previous antituberculous therapy, i.e., initial treatment, the most frequently used regimens have been the following:

Ethambutol HCl plus isoniazid

Ethambutol HCl pus isoniazid plus streptomycin.

In patients who have received previous antituberculous therapy, mycobacterial resistance to other drugs used in initial therapy is frequent. Consequently, in such retreatment patients, ethambutol HCl should be combined with at least one of the second line drugs not previously administered to the patient and to which bacterial susceptibility has been indicated by appropriate *in vitro* studies. Antituberculous drugs used with ethambutol HCl have included cycloserine, ethionamide, pyrazinamide, viomycin and other drugs. Isoniazid, aminosalicylic acid, and streptomycin have also been used in multiple drug regimens. Alternating drug regimens have also been utilized.

CONTRAINDICATIONS:

Ethambutol HCl is contraindicated in patients who are known to be hypersensitive to this drug. It is also contraindicated with known optic neuritis unless clinical judgement determines that it may be used.

PRECAUTIONS:

The effects of combinations of ethambutol HCl ethambutol hydrochloride with other antituberculous drugs on the fetus is not known. While administration of this drug to pregnant human patients has produced no detectable effect upon the fetus, the possible teratogenic potential in women capable of bearing children should be weighed carefully against the benefits of therapy. There are published reports of five women who received the drug during pregnancy without apparent adverse effect upon the fetus.

Ethambutol HCl is not recommended for use in children under thirteen years of age since safe conditions for use have not been established.

Patients with decreased renal function need the dosage reduced as determined by serum levels of ethambutol HCl, since the main path of excretion of this drug is by the kidneys.

Because this drug may have adverse effects on vision, physical examination should include ophthalmoscopy, finger perimetry and testing of color discrimination. In patients with visual defects such as cataracts, recurrent inflammatory conditions of the eye, optic neuritis, and diabetic retinopathy, the evaluation of changes in visual acuity is more difficult, and care should be taken to be sure the variations in vision are not due to the underlying disease conditions. In such patients, consideration should be given to relationship between benefits expected and possible visual deterioration since evaluation of visual changes is difficult. (For recommended procedures, see next paragraphs under Adverse Reactions.)

As with any potent drug, periodic assessment of organ system functions, including renal, hepatic, and hematopoietic, should be made during long-term therapy.

ADVERSE REACTIONS:

Ethambutol HCl may produce decreases in visual acuity which appear to be due to optic neuritis and to be related to dose and duration of treatment. The effects are generally reversible when administration of the drug is discontinued promptly. In rare cases recovery may be delayed for up to one year or more and effect may possibly be irreversible in these cases.

Patients should be advised to report promptly to their physician any change of visual acuity.

The change in visual acuity may be unilateral or bilateral and hence *each eye must be tested separately and both eyes tested together.* Testing of visual acuity should be performed before beginning ethambutol HCl therapy and periodically during drug administration, except that it should be done monthly when a patient is on a dosage of more than 15 mg per kilogram per day. Snellen eye charts are recommended for testing of visual acuity. Studies have shown that there are definite fluctuations of one or two lines of the Snellen chart in the visual acuity of many tuberculous patients *not* receiving ethambutol HCl.

TABLE 1 may be useful in interpreting possible changes in visual acuity attributable to ethambutol HCl.

TABLE 1

Initial Snellen Reading	Reading Indicating Significant Decrease	Significant Number of Lines	Decrease Number of Points
20/13	20/25	3	12
20/15	20/25	2	10
20/20	20/30	2	10
20/25	20/40	2	15
20/30	20/50	2	20
20/40	20/70	2	30
20/50	20/70	1	20

In general changes in visual acuity less than those indicated under "Significant Number of Lines" and "Decrease-Number of Points", may be due to chance variation, limitations of the testing method or physiologic variability. Conversely, changes in visual acuity equaling or exceeding those under "Significant Number of Lines" and "Decrease-Number of Points" indicate need for retesting and careful evaluation of the patient's visual status. If careful evaluation confirm the magnitude of visual change and fails to reveal another cause, ethambutol HCl should be discontinued and the patient reevaluated at frequent intervals. Progressive decreases in visual acuity during therapy must be considered to be due to ethambutol HCl.

If corrective glasses are used prior to treatment, these must be worn during visual acuity testing. During 1 to 2 years of therapy, a refractive error may develop which must be corrected in order to obtain accurate test results. Testing the visual acuity through a pinhole eliminates refractive error. Patients developing visual abnormality during ethambutol HCl treatment may show subjective visual symptoms before, or simultaneously with, the demonstration of decreases in visual acuity, and other subjective eye symptoms.

Recovery of visual acuity generally occurs over a period of weeks to months after the drug has been discontinued. Patients have then received ethambutol HCl ethambutol hydrochloride again without recurrence of loss of visual acuity.

Other adverse reactions reported include: anaphylactoid reactions, dermatitis pruritus and joint pain; anorexia, nausea, vomiting, gastrointestinal upset, abdominal pain; fever, malaise, headache, and dizziness; mental confusion, disorientation and possible hallucinations. Numbness and tingling of the extremities due to peripheral neuritis have been reported infrequently.

Elevated serum uric acid levels occur and precipitation of acute gout has been reported. Transient impairment of liver function as indicated by normal liver function tests is not an unusual finding. Since ethambutol HCl is recommended for therapy in conjunction with one or more other antituberculous drugs, these changes may be related to the concurrent therapy.

DOSAGE AND ADMINISTRATION:

Ethambutol HCl should not be used alone, in initial treatment or in retreatment. Ethambutol HCl should be administered on a once every 24-hour basis only. Absorption is not significantly altered by administration with food. Therapy in general, should be continued until bacteriological conversion has become permanent and maximal improvement has occurred.

Ethambutol HCl is not recommended for use in children under thirteen years of age since safe conditions for use have not been established.

Initial Treatment: In patients who have not received previous antituberculous therapy, administer ethambutol HCl 15 mg per kilogram (7 mg per pound) of body weight, as a single oral dose once every 24 hours. In the more recent studies, isoniazid has been administered concurrently in a single, daily, oral dose.

Retreatment: In patients who have received previous antituberculous therapy, administer ethambutol HCl 25 mg per kilogram (11 mg per pound) of body weight, as a single oral dose once every 24 hours. Concurrently administer at least one other antituberculous drug to which the organisms have been demonstrated to be susceptible by appropriate *in vitro* tests. Suitable drugs usually consist of those not previously used in the treatment of the patient. After 60 days of ethambutol HCl administration, decrease the dose to 15 mg per kilogram (7 mg per pound) of body weight, and administer as a single oral dose once every 24 hours.

During the period when a patient is on a daily dose of 25 mg/kg, monthly eye examinations are advised.

See TABLES 2 and 3 for easy selection of proper weight-dose tablet(s).

TABLE 2 Weight-Dose Table
15 mg/kg (7 mg/lb) Schedule

Weight Range		Daily Dose
Pounds	Kilograms	In mg
Under 85 lbs.	Under 37 kg	500
85-94.5	37-43	600
95-109.5	43-50	700
110-124.5	50-57	800
125-139.5	57-64	900
140-154.5	64-71	1000
155-169.5	71-79	1100
170-184.5	79-84	1200
185-199.5	84-90	1300
200-214.5	90-97	1400
215 and Over	Over 97	1500

Store at Controlled Room Temperature 15-30°C (59-86°F).

TABLE 3 25 mg/kg (11 mg/lb) Schedule

Under 85 lbs.	Under 38 kg	900
85-92.5	38-42	1000
93-101.5	42-45.5	1100
102-109.5	45.5-50	1200
110-118.5	50-54	1300
119-128.5	54-58	1400
129-136.5	58-62	1500
137-146.5	62-67	1600
147-155.5	67-71	1700
156-164.5	71-75	1800
165-173.5	75-79	1900
174-182.5	79-83	2000
183-191.5	83-87	2100
192-199.5	87-91	2200
200-209.5	91-95	2300
210-218.5	95-99	2400
219 and Over	Over 99	2500

ANIMAL PHARMACOLOGY:

Toxicological studies in dogs on high prolonged doses produced evidence of myocardial damage and failure, and depigmentation of the tapetum lucidum of the eyes, the significance of which is not known. Degenerative changes in the central nervous system, apparently not dose-related, have also been noted in dogs receiving ethambutol hydrochloride over a prolonged period.

In the rhesus monkey, neurological signs appeared after treatment with doses given daily over a period of several months. These were correlated with specific serum levels of ethambutol hydrochloride and with definite neuroanatomical changes in the central nervous system. Focal interstitial carditis was also noted in monkeys which received ethambutol hydrochloride in high doses for a prolonged period.

When pregnant mice or rabbits were treated with high doses of ethambutol hydrochloride, fetal mortality was slightly but not significantly ($P>0.05$) increased. Female rats treated with ethambutol hydrochloride displayed slight but insignificant ($P>0.05$) decreases in fertility and litter size.

In fetuses born of mice treated with high doses of ethambutol HCl during pregnancy, a low incidence of cleft palate, exencephaly and abnormality of the vertebral column were observed. Minor abnormalities of the cervical vertebra were seen in the newborn of rats treated with high doses of ethambutol hydrochloride during pregnancy. Rabbits receiving high doses of ethambutol HCl during pregnancy gave birth to two fetuses with monophthalmia, one with a shortened right forearm accompanied by bilateral wrist-joint contracture and one with hare lip and cleft palate.

HOW SUPPLIED - EQUIVALENTS NOT AVAILABLE:

Tablet, Uncoated - Oral - 100 mg

100's	$47.45	MYAMBUTOL, Lederle Pharm	00005-5015-23

Tablet, Uncoated - Oral - 400 mg

10 (2 x 5)	$164.43	MYAMBUTOL, Lederle Pharm	00005-5084-60
100's	$158.75	MYAMBUTOL, Lederle Pharm	00005-5084-62
1000's	$1460.60	MYAMBUTOL, Lederle Pharm	00005-5084-34

ETHANOLAMINE OLEATE *(001207)*

CATEGORIES: Bleeding; Blood Formation/Coagulation; Cardiovascular Drugs; Hemostatics; Orphan Drugs; Sclerosing Agents; Pregnancy Category C; FDA Approved 1988 Dec

BRAND NAMES: **Ethamolin**; *Ethanolamine Oleate*
(International brand names outside U.S. in italics)

DESCRIPTION:

Ethamolin (ethanolamine oleate) Injection is a mild sclerosing agent. Chemically it is $C_{17}H_{33}COOH{\cdot}NH_2CH_2CH_2OH$.

The empirical formula is $C_{20}H_{41}NO_3$, representing a molecular weight of 343.55.

Ethamolin Injection consists of ethanolamine, a basic substance, which when combined with oleic acid forms a clear, straw to pale yellow colored, deliquescent oleate. The pH ranges from 8.0 to 9.0.

Ethamolin Injection is a sterile, apyrogenic, aqueous solution containing in each ml approximately 50 mg ethanolamine oleate with benzyl alcohol 2% by volume as preservative.

CLINICAL PHARMACOLOGY:

When injected intravenously, Ethamolin Injection acts primarily by irritation of the intimal endothelium of the vein and produces a sterile dose-related inflammatory response. This results in fibrosis and occlusion of the vein. Ethamolin Injection also rapidly diffuses through the venous wall and produces a dose-related extravascular inflammatory reaction.

The oleic acid component of the Ethamolin injection is responsible for the inflammatory response, and may also activate coagulation *in vivo* by release of tissue factor and activation of Hageman factor. The ethanolamine component, however, may inhibit fibrin clot formation by chelating calcium, so that a procoagulant action of Ethamolin has not been demonstrated.

After injection, Ethamolin disappears from the injection site within five minutes via the portal vein. When volumes larger than 20 ml are injected, some Ethamolin also flows into the azygos vein through the periesophageal vein. In human autopsy studies it was found that within four days after injection there is neutrophil infiltration of the esophageal wall and hemorrhage within six days. Granulation tissue is first seem at ten days, red thrombi obliterating the varices by twenty days, and sclerosis of the varices by two and a half months. The time course of these findings suggests that sclerosis of esophageal varices will be a delayed rather than an immediate effect of the drug.

The minimum lethal dose of Ethamolin Injection administered intravenously to rabbits is 130 mg/kg.

In dogs, Ethamolin (ethanolamine oleate) injected into the right atrium at a dose of 1 ml/kg over one minute has been shown to increase intravascular lung water. The maximum recommended human dose is 20 ml, or 0.4 ml/kg for a 50-kg person. The concentration of Ethamolin reaching the lung in human treatment will be less than in the dog studies, but pleural effusions, pulmonary edema, pulmonary infiltration, and pneumonitis have been reported in clinical trials, and minimizing the total per session dose, especially in patients with concomitant cardiopulmonary disease, is recommended (see PRECAUTIONS.)

INDICATIONS AND USAGE:

Ethamolin Injection is indicated for the treatment of patients with esophageal varices that recently bled, to prevent rebleeding.

INDICATIONS AND USAGE: *(cont'd)*

Ethamolin is not indicated for the treatment of patients with esophageal varices that have not bled. There is no evidence that treatment of this population decreases the likelihood of bleeding.

Sclerotherapy with Ethamolin has no beneficial effect upon portal hypertension, the cause of esophageal varices, so that recanalization and collateralization may occur, necessitating reinjection.

CONTRAINDICATIONS:

Ethamolin Injection should not be administered to subjects with a known hypersensitivity to ethanolamine, oleic acid, or ethanolamine oleate.

WARNINGS:

Ethamolin Injection should be used in pregnant women only when clearly needed (see PRECAUTIONS.)

The practice of injecting varicosities of the leg with Ethamolin Injection is not supported by adequately controlled clinical trials. Therefore, such use is not recommended.

PRECAUTIONS:

Fatal anaphylactic shock was reported following injection of a larger than normal volume of Ethamolin Injection into a male who had a known allergic disposition. Although there are only three known reports of anaphylaxis, the possibility of an anaphylactic reaction should be kept in mind, and the physician should be prepared to treat it appropriately. In extreme emergencies, 0.25 ml of a 1:1000 intravenous solution of epinephrine (0.25 mg) should be used and allergic reactions should be controlled with antihistamines.

Acute renal failure with spontaneous recovery followed injection of 15 to 20 ml of Ethamolin Injection in two women.

The physician should bear in mind that severe injection necrosis may result from direct injection of sclerosing agents, especially if excessive volumes are used. At least one fatal case of extensive esophageal necrosis and death has been reported. The drug should be administered by physicians who are familiar with an acceptable injection technique.

Patients in Child Class C are more likely to develop esophageal ulceration than those in Classes A and B. Complications of ulceration, necrosis, and delayed esophageal perforation appear to occur more frequently when Ethamolin (ethanolamine oleate) Injection is injected submucosally. This route is not recommended.

In patients with concomitant cardiorespiratory disease, careful monitoring and minimization of the total dose per session is recommended.

Fatal aspiration pneumonia has occurred in elderly patients undergoing esophageal variceal sclerotherapy with Ethamolin Injection. This adverse event appears to be procedure-related rather than drug-related, but as aspiration of blood and/or stomach contents is not uncommon in patients with bleeding esophageal varices, special precautions should be taken to prevent its occurrence, especially in the elderly and critically ill subjects.

PREGNANCY, TERATOGENIC EFFECTS, PREGNANCY CATEGORY C

Animal reproduction studies have not been conducted with Ethamolin Injection. It is also not known whether Ethamolin Injection can cause fetal harm when administered to a pregnant woman or can affect reproduction capacity.

Ethamolin Injection should be given to a pregnant woman only if clearly needed.

NURSING MOTHERS

It is not known whether this drug is excreted in human milk. Because many drugs are excreted in human milk, caution should be exercised when Ethamolin Injection is administered to a nursing woman.

PEDIATRIC USE

Safety and effectiveness in children have not been established.

ADVERSE REACTIONS:

The reported frequency of complications/adverse events per injection session was 13%. The most common complications were pleural effusion/infiltration (2.1%), esophageal ulcer (2.1%), pyrexia (1.8%), retrosternal pain (1.6%), esophageal stricture (1.3%), and pneumonia (1.2%).

Other adverse local esophageal reactions have also been reported at rates of 0.1 to 0.4%, including esophagitis, tearing of the esophagus, sloughing of the mucosa overlying the injected varix, ulceration, stricture, necrosis, periesophageal abscess and perforation (see PRECAUTIONS.) These complications appear to be dependent upon the dose and the patient's clinical state.

Bacteremia has been observed in patients following injection of esophageal varices with Ethamolin. Pyrexia and retrosternal pain are not infrequently observed during the post-injection period. Fetal aspiration pneumonia has occurred in patients with esophageal varices who underwent Ethamolin Injection sclerotherapy (see PRECAUTIONS.) Anaphylactic shock and acute renal failure with spontaneous recovery have occurred (see PRECAUTIONS.) A case of disseminated intravascular coagulation has been reported.

Spinal cord paralysis due to occlusion of the anterior spinal artery has been reported in one child eight hours after Ethamolin sclerotherapy.

OVERDOSAGE:

Overdosage of Ethamolin Injection can result in severe intramural necrosis of the esophagus. Complications resulting from such overdosage have resulted in death.

DOSAGE AND ADMINISTRATION:

Local Ethamolin (ethanolamine oleate) Injection sclerotherapy of esophageal varices should be performed by physicians who are familiar with an acceptable technique. The usual intravenous dose is 1.5 to 5 ml per varix. The maximum total dose per treatment session should not exceed 20 ml. Patients with significant liver dysfunction (Child Class C) or concomitant cardiopulmonary disease should usually receive less than the recommended maximum dose. Submucosal injections are not recommended as they are reportedly more likely to result in ulceration at the site of injection.

To obliterate the varix, injections may be made at the time of the acute bleeding episode and then after one week, six weeks, three months, and six months as indicated.

NOTE: Parenteral drug products should be inspected visually for particulate matter and discoloration before administration whenever solution and container permit.

Store at Controlled Room Temperature, 15-30°C (59-86°F). Protect from light.

(Reed & Carnrick, 7/92, 4790020004)

HOW SUPPLIED - EQUIVALENTS NOT AVAILABLE:

Injection, Solution - Intravenous - 5 %

2 ml x 10	$229.51	ETHAMOLIN, Reed & Carnrick	00021-4790-06

ETHAVERINE HYDROCHLORIDE *(001208)*

CATEGORIES: Analeptics; Anesthesia; Antispasmodics; Antispasmodics & Anticholinergics; Cardiovascular Drugs; Peripheral Vasodilators; Renal Drugs; Urinary Tract Infections; Vascular Disorders, Cerebral/Peripheral; Vasodilating Agents; Vertigo/Motion Sickness/Vomiting; FDA Pre 1938 Drugs

BRAND NAMES: *Etaverol*; Ethaquin; **Ethatab**; Ethavex-100; *Ethavin*; Isovex; Rothav
(International brand names outside U.S. in italics)

DESCRIPTION:

Each tablet contains Ethaverine Hydrochloride 100 mg, D&C Yellow No. 6, D&C Yellow No. 10, FD&C Yellow No. 6, and other ingredients.

CLINICAL PHARMACOLOGY:

Ethaverine Hydrochloride acts directly on the smooth muscle cells without involving the autonomic nervous system or its receptors. It produces smooth muscle relaxation, particularly where spasm exists, affecting the larger blood vessels, especially systemic, peripheral, and pulmonary vessels, and smooth muscle of the intestines, biliary tree, and ureters.

INDICATIONS AND USAGE:

In peripheral and cerebral vascular insufficiency associated with arterial spasm; also useful as a smooth muscle spasmolytic in spastic conditions of the gastrointestinal and genitourinary tracts.

CONTRAINDICATIONS:

The use of Ethaverine Hydrochloride is contraindicated in the presence of complete atrioventricular dissociation.

PRECAUTIONS:

As with all vasodilators, Ethaverine Hydrochloride should be administered with caution to all patients with glaucoma. The safety of ethaverine hydrochloride during pregnancy or lactation has not been established; therefore, it should not be used in pregnant women or in women of childbearing age unless, in the judgment of the physician, its use is deemed essential to the welfare of the patient.

ADVERSE REACTIONS:

Even though the incidence of adverse reactions as reported in the literature is very low, it is possible for a patient to evidence nausea; anorexia; abdominal distress, including diarrhea; dryness of the throat; hypotension; malaise; lassitude; drowsiness; flushing; sweating; vertigo; respiratory depression; cardiac depression; cardiac arrhythmia; and headache.

If these adverse reactions occur, reduce dosage or discontinue medication.

DOSAGE AND ADMINISTRATION:

In mild or moderate disease, the usual dosage for adults is one tablet three times a day. In more difficult cases, dosage may be increased to two tablets three times a day. It is most effective given early in the course of the vascular disorder. Because of the chronic nature of the disease, long-term therapy is required.

HOW SUPPLIED - EQUIVALENTS NOT AVAILABLE:

Tablet, Uncoated - Oral - 100 mg

100's	$9.75	Ethaverine Hcl, Major Pharms	00904-2213-60
100's	$10.73	Ethaverine Hcl, Sidmak Labs	50111-0336-01
100's	$14.28	ETHAVEX-100, Embrex Economed	38130-0011-01
100's	$57.84	ETHAQUIN, Ascher	00225-0250-15
500's	$282.00	ETHAQUIN, Ascher	00225-0250-20
1000's	$107.70	ETHAVEX-100, Embrex Economed	38130-0011-10
1000's	$549.48	ETHAQUIN, Ascher	00225-0250-25

ETHCHLORVYNOL *(001213)*

CATEGORIES: Anxiolytics, Sedatives, Hypnotic; Central Nervous System Agents; Hypnotics; Insomnia; Sedatives/Hypnotics; Pregnancy Category C; DEA Class CIV; FDA Approval Pre 1982

BRAND NAMES: *Arvynol* (Japan); *Nostel* (Japan); **Placidyl**
(International brand names outside U.S. in italics)

COST OF THERAPY: $9.06 (Insomnia; Capsule; 500 mg; 1/day; 7 days) vs. Potential Cost of $3,628.44 (Psychoses)

DESCRIPTION:

Ethchlorvynol is a tertiary carbinol. It is chemically designated as 1-chloro-3-ethyl-1-penten-4-yl-3-ol. Ethchlorvynol occurs as a liquid which is immiscible with water and miscible with most organic solvents.

Ethchlorvynol is an oral hypnotic available in capsule form containing either 200 mg, 500 mg or 750 mg of ethchlorvynol.

INACTIVE INGREDIENTS

200 mg capsule: FD&C Red No. 40, gelatin, glycerin, methylparaben, polyethylene glycol, propylparaben, sorbitol and titanium dioxide.

500 mg capsule: FD&C Red No. 40, gelatin, glycerin, iron oxide, methylparaben polyethylene glycol, propylparaben, sorbitol and titanium dioxide.

750 mg capsule: FD&C Blue No. 1, FD&C Yellow No. 5 (tartrazine), FD&C Yellow No. 6, gelatin, glycerin, iron oxide, methylparaben, polyethylene glycol, propylparaben, sorbitol and titanium dioxide.

CLINICAL PHARMACOLOGY:

The usual hypnotic dose of ethchlorvynol induces sleep within 15 minutes to one hour. The duration of the hypnotic effect is about five hours. The mechanism of action is unknown.

Ethchlorvynol is rapidly absorbed from the gastrointestinal tract with peak plasma concentrations usually occurring within two hours after a single oral fasting dose. Plasma concentrations required for hypnotic effects are unknown. The plasma half-life ($t_{1/2},\beta$) of the parent compound is approximately ten to twenty hours. Studies with ^{14}C-Ethchlorvynol have demonstrated that within 24 hours, 33% of a single 500 mg dose is excreted in the urine mostly as metabolites. The major plasma and urinary metabolite is the secondary alcohol of ethchlorvynol. The free and conjugated forms of this metabolite in the urine account for about 40% of the dose. Other minor metabolites have been identified as the primary alcohol and a secondary alcohol with an altered acetylene group. Studies with ^{14}C-Ethchlorvynol in animals indicate that the parent compound and its metabolites undergo extensive enterohepatic recirculation.

Distribution studies indicate that there is extensive tissue localization of ethchlorvynol, particularly in adipose tissue. Ethchlorvynol and/or its metabolites have also been detected in liver, kidneys, spleen, brain, bile and cerebrospinal fluid.

INDICATIONS AND USAGE:

Ethchlorvynol is indicated as short-term hypnotic therapy for periods up to one week in duration for the management of insomnia. If retreatment becomes necessary, after drug-free intervals of one or more weeks, it should only be undertaken upon further evaluation of the patient.

CONTRAINDICATIONS:

Ethchlorvynol is contraindicated in patients with known hypersensitivity to the drug and in patients with porphyria.

WARNINGS:

ETHCHLORVYNOL SHOULD BE ADMINISTERED WITH CAUTION TO MENTALLY DEPRESSED PATIENTS WITH OR WITHOUT SUICIDAL TENDENCIES. IT SHOULD ALSO BE ADMINISTERED WITH CAUTION TO THOSE WHO HAVE A PSYCHOLOGICAL POTENTIAL FOR DRUG DEPENDENCE. THE LEAST AMOUNT OF DRUG THAT IS FEASIBLE SHOULD BE PRESCRIBED FOR THESE PATIENTS.

PSYCHOLOGICAL AND PHYSICAL DEPENDENCE

PROLONGED USE OF ETHCHLORVYNOL MAY RESULT IN TOLERANCE AND PSYCHOLOGICAL AND PHYSICAL DEPENDENCE. PROLONGED ADMINISTRATION OF THE DRUG IS NOT RECOMMENDED. (See DRUG ABUSE AND DEPENDENCE.)

PRECAUTIONS:

General: Elderly or debilitated patients should receive the smallest effective amount of ethchlorvynol.

Caution should be exercised when treating patients with impaired hepatic or renal function.

Patients who exhibit unpredictable behavior, or paradoxical restlessness or excitement in response to barbiturates or alcohol may react in this manner to ethchlorvynol.

Ethchlorvynol should not be used for the management of insomnia in the presence of pain unless insomnia persists after pain is controlled with analgesics.

The 750 mg dosage strength of ethchlorvynol contains FD&C Yellow No. 5 (tartrazine) which may cause allergic-type reactions (including bronchial asthma) in certain susceptible individuals. Although the overall incidence of FD&C Yellow No. 5 (tartrazine) sensitivity in the general population is low, it is frequently seen in patients who also have aspirin hypersensitivity.

Information for Patients: The use of ethchlorvynol carries with it an associated risk of psychological and/or physical dependence. The patient should be warned against increasing the dose of the drug without consulting a physician.

Patients should be advised that, for the duration of the effect of ethchlorvynol, mental and/or physical abilities required for the performance of potentially hazardous tasks such as the operation of dangerous machinery including motor vehicles, may be impaired.

Patients should be cautioned to avoid the concomitant use of ethchlorvynol with alcohol, barbiturates, other CNS depressants, or MAO inhibitors.

Carcinogenesis: A study in mice receiving oral doses of ethchlorvynol up to 7 times the maximum human daily dose for 22 to 24 months produced equivocal results. When compared to controls, a statistically significant increase in total lung tumors was found in female mice given the high dose of ethchlorvynol. However, the 48% incidence is not substantially higher than the high value (39%) reported for the historical laboratory controls.

No evidence of carcinogenic potential was observed in rats given ethchlorvynol at 5 to 15 times the maximum human daily dose for up to 2 years.

Pregnancy Category C: *Teratogenic:* Ethchlorvynol has been associated with a higher percentage of stillbirths and a lower survival rate of progeny among rats given 40 mg/kg/day. There are no adequate and well-controlled studies in pregnant women. Therefore, ethchlorvynol is not recommended for use during the first and second trimesters of pregnancy. Ethchlorvynol should be used during pregnancy only if the potential benefit justifies the potential risk to the fetus. *Non-teratogenic:* Clinical experience has indicated that ethchlorvynol taken during the third trimester of pregnancy may produce CNS depression and transient withdrawal symptoms in the newborn. These symptoms resemble congenital narcotic withdrawal symptoms (See DRUG ABUSE AND DEPENDENCE.)

Nursing Mothers: It is not known whether this drug is excreted in breast milk. Because many drugs are excreted in human milk and because of the potential for serious adverse reactions in nursing infants from ethchlorvynol, a decision should be made whether to discontinue nursing or to discontinue the drug, taking into account the importance of the drug to the mother.

Pediatric Use: Ethchlorvynol is not recommended for use in children since its safety and effectiveness in the pediatric age group has not been determined.

DRUG INTERACTIONS:

The concomitant use of ethchlorvynol with alcohol, barbiturates, other CNS depressants, or MAC inhibitors may produce exaggerated depressant effects.

Ethchlorvynol may cause a decreased prothrombin time response to coumarin anticoagulants; therefore, the dosage of these drugs may require adjustment when therapy with ethchlorvynol is initiated and after it is discontinued.

Transient delirium has been reported with the concomitant use of ethchlorvynol and amitriptyline; therefore, ethchlorvynol should be administered with caution to patients receiving tricyclic antidepressants.

ADVERSE REACTIONS:

Adverse effects in decreasing order of severity within each of the following categories are:

Hypersensitivity: cholestatic jaundice, urticaria and rash.

Hematologic: thrombocytopenia—one case of fatal immune thrombocytopenia due to ethchlorvynol has been reported.

Gastrointestinal: vomiting, gastric upset, nausea and aftertaste.

Neurologic: dizziness and facial numbness.

Miscellaneous: blurred vision, hypotension and mild "hangover".

The following idiosyncratic responses have been reported occasionally: syncope without marked hypotension, profound muscular weakness, hysteria, marked excitement, prolonged hypnosis and mild stimulation.

ADVERSE REACTIONS: *(cont'd)*

Transient ataxia, and giddiness have occurred in patients in whom absorption of the drug is especially rapid. These effects can sometimes be controlled by giving ethchlorvynol with food.

(See DRUG ABUSE AND DEPENDENCE for the signs and symptoms of chronic intoxication.)

DRUG ABUSE AND DEPENDENCE:

Ethchlorvynol is subject to control by the Federal Controlled Substances Act under DEA schedule IV.

Abuse: Pulmonary edema of rapid onset has resulted from the IV abuse of ethchlorvynol.

Dependence: Signs and symptoms of intoxication have been reported with the prolonged use of doses as low as 1 g/day. Signs and symptoms of chronic intoxication may include incoordination, tremors, ataxia, confusion, slurred speech, hyperreflexia, diplopia, and generalized muscle weakness. Toxic amblyopia, scotoma, nystagmus, and peripheral neuropathy have also been reported with prolonged use of ethchlorvynol; these symptoms are usually reversible.

Severe withdrawal symptoms similar to those seen during barbiturate and alcohol withdrawal have been reported following abrupt discontinuance of prolonged use of ethchlorvynol. These symptoms may appear as late as nine days after sudden withdrawal of the drug. Signs and symptoms of ethchlorvynol withdrawal may include convulsions, delirium hallucinations, schizoid reaction, perceptual distortions, memory loss, ataxia, insomnia, slurring of speech, unusual anxiety, irritability, agitation, and tremors. Other signs and symptoms may include anorexia, nausea, vomiting, weakness, dizziness, sweating, muscle twitching, and weight loss.

Management of a patient who manifests withdrawal symptoms from ethchlorvynol involves readministration of the drug to approximately the same level of chronic intoxication which existed before the abrupt discontinuance. (Phenobarbital may be substituted for ethchlorvynol.) A gradual, stepwise reduction of dosage may then be made over a period of days or weeks. A phenothiazine compound may be used in addition to this regimen for those patients who exhibit psychotic symptoms during the withdrawal period. The patient undergoing withdrawal from ethchlorvynol must be hospitalized or closely observed, and given general supportive care as indicated.

In one report an infant born to a mother who received 500 mg ethchlorvynol at bedtime daily throughout the third trimester, exhibited withdrawal symptoms on the second day of life. The symptoms included episodic jitteriness, hyperactivity, restlessness, irritability, disturbed sleep and hunger. The neonate responded to a single oral dose of phenobarbital (3 mg/kg). The withdrawal symptoms gradually decreased and completely disappeared by the tenth day of life.

OVERDOSAGE:

Acute intoxication is characterized by prolonged deep coma, severe respiratory depression, hypothermia, hypotension, and relative bradycardia. Nystagmus and pancytopenia resulting from acute ethchlorvynol overdose have been reported.

Although death has occurred following the ingestion of 6 g of ethchlorvynol, there have been reports of patients who have survived overdoses of 50 g and more with intensive care. Fatal blood concentrations usually range from 20 to 50 mcg/ml.[1] Because large amounts of ethchlorvynol are taken up by adipose tissue, the blood concentration is an unreliable indicator of the magnitude of overdosage.

Management of acute ethchlorvynol intoxication is similar to that of acute barbiturate intoxication.[2] Gastric evacuation should be performed immediately. (In the unconscious patient, gastric lavage should be preceded by tracheal intubation with a cuffed tube.) Supportive care (assisted ventilation, frequent and careful monitoring of vital signs, control of blood pressure) is essential. Emphasis should be placed on pulmonary care and monitoring of blood gases. Hemoperfusion utilizing the Amberlite column technique has been reported in the literature to be the most effective method in the management of acute ethchlorvynol overdosage.[3] In addition, hemodialysis and peritoneal dialysis have each been reported to be of some value. (Aqueous and oil dialysates have been used. Forced diuresis with maintenance of a high urinary output has also been reported of some value.)

(See DRUG ABUSE AND DEPENDENCE for the signs and symptoms of chronic intoxication.)

DOSAGE AND ADMINISTRATION:

The usual adult hypnotic dose of ethchlorvynol is 500 mg taken orally at bedtime. A dose of 750 mg may be required for patients whose sleep response to a 500 mg capsule is inadequate, or for patients being changed from barbiturates or other nonbarbiturate hypnotics. Up to 1000 mg may be given as a single bedtime dose when insomnia is unusually severe. A single supplemental dose of 200 mg may be given to reinstitute sleep in patients who may awaken after the original bedtime dose of 500 or 750 mg.

For patients whose insomnia is characterized only by untimely awakening during the early morning hours, a single dose of 200 mg taken upon awakening may be adequate for relief.

The smallest effective dose of ethchlorvynol should be given to elderly or debilitated patients.

Ethchlorvynol should not be prescribed for periods exceeding one week. (See DRUG ABUSE AND DEPENDENCE.)

Recommended storage: 59°-77°F (15°-25°C).

REFERENCES:

1. AMA Dept. of Drugs. *AMA Drug Evaluations*, Massachusetts: Publishing Sciences Group, Inc., 1980. **2.** Khantzian, E.J., McKenna, G.J., Acute Toxic and Withdrawal Reactions Associated with Drug Use and Abuse, *Annals of Internal Medicine*, 90:361-372, 1979. **3.** Lynn, R.I., et al., Resin Hemoperfusion for Treatment of Ethchlorvynol Overdose, *Annals of Internal Medicine*, 91:549-553, 1979.

HOW SUPPLIED - RATED THERAPEUTICALLY EQUIVALENT:

Capsule, Gelatin - Oral - 200 mg

100's	**$105.07**	**PLACIDYL, Abbott**	**00074-6661-08**

Capsule, Gelatin - Oral - 500 mg

100's	**$129.44**	**PLACIDYL, Abbott**	**00074-6685-15**
100's	**$131.22**	**PLACIDYL, Abbott**	**00074-6685-10**

Capsule, Gelatin - Oral - 750 mg

100's	$66.50	Ethchlorvynol, Major Pharms	00904-3391-60
100's	**$171.78**	**PLACIDYL, Abbott**	**00074-6630-01**

ETHINYL ESTRADIOL *(001216)*

CATEGORIES: Antineoplastics; Breast Carcinoma; Cancer; Estrogens; Hormones; Hypogonadism; Menopause; Oncologic Drugs; Prostatic Carcinoma; Pregnancy Category X; FDA Approval Pre 1982

BRAND NAMES: *Estigyn*; **Estinyl**; *Estinyl Oestradiol* (France); *Esto*; *Ethinylestradiolum*; *Etinilestradiolo*; Feminone; *Ginormon*; *Lynoral*; *Mikrofollin*; *Progynon C* (Germany)
(International brand names outside U.S. in italics)

FORMULARIES: Aetna; BC-BS; FHP; Medi-Cal; WHO

1. ESTROGENS HAVE BEEN REPORTED TO INCREASE THE RISK RATIO OF ENDOMETRIAL CARCINOMA.

Three independent case control studies have reported an increased risk ratio of endometrial cancer in postmenopausal women exposed to exogenous estrogens for prolonged periods. This risk ratio was independent of the other risk factors for endometrial cancer. These studies are further supported by the report that incidence rates of endometrial cancer have increased sharply since 1969 in eight different areas of the United States with population-based cancer reporting systems, an increase which may be related to the rapidly expanding use of estrogens during the last decade.

The three case control studies reported that the risk ratio of endometrial cancer in estrogen users was about 4.5 to 13.9 times greater than in nonusers. The risk ratio appears to depend on both duration of treatment and on estrogen dose. In view of these reports, when estrogens are used for the treatment of menopausal symptoms, the lowest dose that will control symptoms should be utilized and medication should be discontinued as soon as possible. When prolonged treatment is medically indicated, the patient should be reassessed on at least a semi-annual basis to determine the need for continued therapy. Although the evidence must be considered preliminary, one study suggests that cyclic administration of low doses of estrogen may carry less risk than continuous administration, it therefore appears prudent to utilize such a regimen.

Close clinical surveillance of all women taking estrogens is important. In all cases of undiagnosed persistent of recurring abnormal vaginal bleeding, adequate diagnostic measures should be undertaken to rule out malignancy.

There is no evidence at present that "natural" estrogens are more or less hazardous than "synthetic" estrogens at equiestrogenic doses.

2. ESTROGENS SHOULD NOT BE USED DURING PREGNANCY.

The use of estrogens during early pregnancy may seriously damage the offspring. It has been reported that females exposed in utero to diethylstilbestrol, a nonsteroidal estrogen, may have an increased risk of developing in later life a form of vaginal or cervical cancer that is ordinarily extremely rare. This risk has been estimated statistically as not greater than 4 per 1000 exposures. In certain studies, a high percentage of such exposed women (from 30% to 90%) have been found to have vaginal adenosis, epithelial changes of the vagina and cervix. Although these changes are histologically benign, it is not known whether they are precursors of malignancy. Although similar data are not available with the use of other estrogens, it cannot be presumed they would not induce similar changes. Exposure to diethylstilbestrol has also been associated with adverse effects on reproductive performance, including increased rates of spontaneous abortion, ectopic pregnancy, premature deliveries, and perinatal deaths.

Several reports suggest an association between intrauterine fetal exposure to female sex hormones and congenital anomalies, including congenital heart defects and limb reduction defects. One case control study estimated a 4.7-fold increased risk of limb reduction defects in infants exposed in utero to sex hormones (oral contraceptives, hormone withdrawal tests for pregnancy, or attempted treatment for threatened abortion). Some of these exposures were very short and involved only a few days of treatment. The data suggests that the risk of limb reduction defects in exposed fetuses is somewhat less than 1 per 1000.

In the past, estrogens have been used during pregnancy in an attempt to treat threatened of habitual abortion. There is considerable evidence that estrogens are ineffective for these indications.

If ethinyl estradiol is used during pregnancy, or if the patient becomes pregnant while taking this drug, she should be apprised of the potential risks to the fetus, and the advisability of pregnancy continuation.

DESCRIPTION:

Estinyl contains ethinyl estradiol, USP, a potent synthetic estrogen, having the chemical name 19-Nor-17α-pregna-1,3,5(10)-trien-20-yne-3,17-diol; the chemical formula $C_{20}H_{24}O_2$; a molecular weight of 296.41.

Ethinyl estradiol is a white to creamy white, odorless, crystalline powder. It is insoluble in water, soluble in alcohol, chloroform, either, and vegetable oils.

Biologically, estrogens may be defined as compounds capable of stimulating, female secondary sex characteristics. Chemically, there are different groups of estrogens, depending on whether they are natural or synthetic, steroidal or non-steroidal. Natural human estrogens are ultimately formed from either androstenedione of testosterone as immediate precursors. Ethinyl estradiol is a synthetic, steroidal estrogen.

Ethinyl estradiol, for oral administration, is available in tablets containing 0.02, 0.05, or 0.5 mg ethinyl estradiol, USP.

The inactive ingredients for ethinyl estradiol 0.02 mg include: acacia, butylparaben, calcium phosphate, calcium sulfate, carnauba wax, corn starch, FD&C Blue No. 2 Al Lake, FD&C Yellow No. 5, FD&C Yellow No. 5 Al Lake, FD&C Yellow No. 6 Al Lake, gelatin, lactose, magnesium stearate, potato starch, sodium phosphate, sugar, and white wax. May contain talc.

The inactive ingredients for ethinyl estradiol 0.05 mg include, acacia, butylparaben, calcium phosphate, calcium sulfate, carnauba wax, corn starch, FD&C Blue No. 1, FD&C Red No. 3, gelatin, lactose, magnesium stearate, potato starch, sodium phosphate, and white wax. May also contain talc.

The inactive ingredients for ethinyl estradiol 0.5 mg include: corn starch, FD&C Yellow No. 6, lactose, magnesium stearate and sodium phosphate.

CLINICAL PHARMACOLOGY:

Ethinyl estradiol is synthetic derivative of the natural estrogen, estradiol.

Ethinyl estradiol, like estradiol, promotes growth of the endometrium and thickening, stratification and cornification of the vagina. It causes growth of the ducts of the mammary glands, but inhibits lactation. It also inhibits the anterior pituitary and causes capillary dilatation, fluid retention, and protein anabolism.

Estradiol is the major estrogen in premenopausal women, with up to 100 to 600 mcg being secreted daily by the ovary. Natural estrogens are poorly effective when given by mouth. Apparently this is due to rapid clearance of the endogenous hormone from blood, along with a "first-pass-effect" after oral administration. The addition of a 17-alpha-ethinyl group to estradiol increases potency and enhances oral activity by impeding hepatic degradation. The oral efficacy of ethinyl estradiol is related to slower elimination than estradiol from the

CLINICAL PHARMACOLOGY: *(cont'd)*

circulation. A part of ingested ethinyl estradiol is excreted in glucuronide form via urine in animals and in man, but also extensive metabolism of the steroid nucleus occurs. The major metabolism takes place mainly in the liver. Large amounts of ethinyl estradiol metabolites are excreted via human bite, much similar to what has been reported for estradiol. However, unlike, ethinyl estradiol metabolites do not exclusively leave via urine. Urinary recovery is much less than that of estradiol and substantial amounts of ethinyl estradiol metabolites appear in human feces. Quantitatively, the major metabolic pathway for ethinyl estradiol, both in rats and in humans, is aromatic hydroxylation, as it is for the natural estrogens.

Rapid and complete absorption follows oral intake of ethinyl estradiol. Elimination of ethinyl estradiol from plasma proceeds slower than that of estradiol. After oral administration, an initial peak occurs in plasma at 2 to 3 hours, with a secondary peak at about 12 hours after dosing; the second peak is interpreted as evidence for extensive enterohepatic circulation of ethinyl estradiol.

INDICATIONS AND USAGE:

Ethinyl estradiol are indicated in the treatment of: 1) Moderate to severe *vasomotor* symptoms associated with the menopause. (There is no evidence that estrogens are effective for nervous symptoms or depression which might occur during menopause, and they should not be used to treat these conditions.) 2) Female hypogonadism. 3) Prostatic carcinoma-palliative therapy of advanced disease. 4) Breast cancer (for palliation only) in appropriately selected women; such as those who are more than 5 years postmenopausal with progressing inoperable or radiation-resistant disease.

ETHINYL ESTRADIOL HAS NOT BEEN SHOWN TO BE EFFECTIVE FOR ANY PURPOSE DURING PREGNANCY AND ITS USE MAY CAUSE SEVERE HARM TO THE FETUS (SEE BOXED WARNING.)

The lowest effective dose appropriate for the specific indication should be used. Studies of the addition of a progestin for seven or more days or a cycle of estrogen administration have reported a lowered incidence of endometrial hyperplasia. Morphological and biochemical studies of endometrium suggest that 10 to 13 days or progestin are needed to provide maximal maturation of the endometrium and to eliminate any hyperplastic changes. Whether this will provide protection from endometrial carcinoma has not been clearly established. There are possible additional risks which may be associated with the inclusion of progestin in estrogen replacement regimens. The potential risks include adverse effects on carbohydrate and lipid metabolism. The choice of progestin and dosage may be important in minimizing these adverse effects.

CONTRAINDICATIONS:

Estrogens should not be used in women (or men) with any of the following conditions:

1. Known or suspected cancer of the breast except in appropriately selected patients being treated for metastatic disease.

2. Known or suspected estrogen-dependent neoplasia.

3. Known or suspected pregnancy (see BOXED WARNING.)

4. Undiagnosed abnormal genital bleeding.

5. Active thrombophlebitis or thromboembolic disorders.

6. A past history of thrombophlebitis, thrombosis, or thromboembolic disorders associated with previous estrogen use (except when used in treatment of breast or prostatic malignancy).

WARNINGS:

INDUCTION OF MALIGNANT NEOPLASMS

Long-term continuous administration of natural and synthetic estrogens in certain animal species increases the frequency of carcinomas of the breast, cervix, vagina, and liver. There is now evidence that estrogens increase the risk of carcinoma of the endometrium in humans. (See BOXED WARNING.)

At the present time there is no satisfactory evidence that estrogens given to postmenopausal women increase the risk of cancer of the breast, although a recent long-term follow-up of a single physician's practice has raised this possibility. Because of the animal data, there is a need for caution in prescribing estrogens for women with a strong family history of breast cancer or who have breast nodules, fibrocystic disease, or abnormal mammograms.

Estrogens have been reported to be associated with carcinoma of the male breast and suspicious lesions in males receiving estrogen therapy should be investigated accordingly.

GALLBLADDER DISEASE

A recent study has reported a 2- to 3-fold increase in the risk of surgically confirmed gallbladder disease in women receiving postmenopausal estrogens, similar to the 2-fold increase previously noted in users of oral contraceptives. In the case of oral contraceptives, the increased risk appeared after two years of use.

EFFECTS SIMILAR TO THOSE CAUSED BY ESTROGEN-PROGESTOGEN ORAL CONTRACEPTIVES

There are several serious adverse effects of oral contraceptives, most of which have not, up to now, been documented as consequences of postmenopausal estrogen therapy. This may reflect the comparatively low doses of estrogen used in postmenopausal women. It would be expected that the larger doses of estrogen used to treat prostatic or breast cancer are more likely to result in these adverse effects, and, in fact, it has been shown that there is an increased risk of thrombosis in men receiving estrogens for prostatic cancer.

Thromboembolic Disease: It is now well established that users of oral contraceptives have an increased risk of various thromboembolic and thrombolic vascular diseases, such as thrombophlebitis, pulmonary embolism, stroke, and myocardial infarction. Cases of retinal thrombosis, mesenteric thrombosis, and optic neuritis have been reported in oral contraceptive users. There is evidence that the risk of several of these adverse reactions is related to the dose of the drug. An increased risk of postsurgery thromboembolic complications has also been reported in users of oral contraceptives. If feasible, estrogen should be discontinued at least 4 weeks before surgery of the type associated with an increased risk of thromboembolism, or during periods of immobilization.

While an increased rate of thromboembolic and thrombotic disease in postmenopausal users of estrogen has not been found, this does not rule out the possibility that such an increase may be present or that subgroups of women who have underlying risk factors or who are receiving relatively large doses of estrogens may have increased risk. Therefore, estrogens should not be used in persons with active thrombophlebitis or thromboembolic disorders, and they should not be used (except in treatment of malignancy) in persons with a history of such disorders in association with estrogen use. They should be used with caution in patients with cerebral vascular or coronary artery disease and only for those in whom estrogens are clearly needed.

Large doses of estrogen (5 mg conjugated estrogens per day), comparable to those used to treat cancer of the prostate and breast, have been shown in a large prospective clinical trial in men to increase the risk of nonfatal myocardial infarction, pulmonary embolism and thrombophlebitis. When estrogen doses of this size are used, any of the thromboembolic and thrombotic adverse effects associated with oral contraceptive use should be considered a clear risk.

WARNINGS: *(cont'd)*

Hepatic Adenoma: Benign hepatic adenomas appear to be associated with the use of oral contraceptives. Although benign, and rate, these may rupture and may cause death through intra-abdominal hemorrhage. Such lesions have not yet been reported in association with other estrogen or progestogen preparations, but should be considered in estrogen users having abdominal pain and tenderness, abdominal mass, or hypovolemic shock. Hepatocellular carcinoma has also been reported in women taking estrogen-containing oral contraceptives. The relationship of this malignancy to these drugs is not known at this time.

Elevated Blood Pressure: Increased blood pressure is not uncommon in women using oral contraceptives. There is now a report that this may occur with use of estrogens in the menopause and blood pressure should be monitored with estrogen use, especially if high doses are used.

Glucose Tolerance: A worsening or glucose tolerance has been observed in a significant percentage of patients on estrogen-containing oral contraceptives. For this reason, diabetic patients should be carefully observed while receiving estrogen.

HYPERCALCEMIA

Administration of estrogens may lead to severe hypercalcemia in patients with breast cancer and bone metastases. If this occurs, the drug should be stooped and appropriate measures taken to reduce the serum calcium level.

PRECAUTIONS:

GENERAL

1. A complete medical and family history should be taken prior to the initiation of any estrogen therapy. The pretreatment and periodic physical examinations should include special reference to blood pressure, breasts, abdomen, and pelvic organs, and should include a Papanicolaou smear. As a general rule, estrogen should not be prescribed for longer than one year without another physical examination being performed.

2. Fluid retention-Because estrogens may cause some degree of fluid retention, conditions which might be influenced by this factor, such as epilepsy, migraine, and cardiac or renal dysfunction, require careful observation.

3. Certain patients may develop undesirable manifestations of excessive estrogenic stimulation, such as abnormal or excessive uterine bleeding, mastodynia, etc.

4. Oral contraceptives appear to be associated with an increased incidence of mental depression. Although it is not clear whether this is due to the estrogenic or progestogenic component of the contraceptive, patients with a history of depression should be carefully observed.

5. Preexisting uterine leiomyomata may increase in size during estrogen use.

6. The pathologist should be advised of estrogen therapy when relevant specimens are submitted.

7. Patients with a past history of jaundice during pregnancy have an increased risk of recurrence of jaundice while receiving estrogen-containing oral contraceptive therapy. If jaundice develops in any patient receiving estrogen, the medication should be discontinued while the cause is investigated.

8. Estrogens may be poorly metabolized in patients with impaired liver function and they should be administered with caution in such patients.

9. Because estrogens influence the metabolism or calcium an phosphorus, they should be used with caution in patients with metabolic bone diseases that are associated with hypercalcemia or in patients with renal insufficiency.

10. Because of the effects of estrogens on epiphyseal closure, they should be used judiciously in young patients in whom bone growth is not complete.

11. Ethinyl estradiol, 0.02 mg, contain FD&C Yellow No. 5 (tartrazine) which may cause allergic-type reactions (including bronchial asthma) in certain susceptible individuals. Although the overall incidence of FD&C Yellow No. 5 (tartrazine) sensitivity in the general population is low, it is frequently seen in patients who also have aspirin hypersensitivity.

CARCINOGENESIS, MUTAGENESIS, AND IMPAIRMENT OF FERTILITY

See BOXED WARNING.

PREGNANCY CATEGORY X

See CONTRAINDICATIONS and BOXED WARNING.

NURSING MOTHERS

Because of the potential for tumorigenicity shown for ethinyl estradiol in animal and human studies, a decision should be made whether to discontinue nursing or to discontinue the drug, taking into account the importance of the drug to the mother.

PEDIATRIC USE

Safety and effectiveness in children have not been established.

DRUG INTERACTIONS:

Certain endocrine and liver function tests may be affected by estrogen-containing oral contraceptives. The following similar changes may be expected with large doses of estrogen:

Increased sulfobromophthalein retention; increased prothrombin and factors VII, VIII, IX, and X; decreased antithrombin 3; increased norepinephrine-induced platelet aggregation; increased thyroid binding globulin (TBG) leading to increased circulating total thyroid hormone, as measured by PBI, T_4 by column, or T_4 by radioimmunoassay. Free T_3 resin uptake is decrease, reflecting the elevated TBG; free T_4 concentration is unaltered; impaired glucose tolerance; decreased pregnanetriol excretion; reduced response to metyrapone test; reduced serum folate concentration; increased serum triglyceride and phospholipid concentration.

ADVERSE REACTIONS:

(See WARNINGS regarding induction of neoplasia, adverse effects on the fetus, increased incidence of gallbladder disease, and adverse effects similar to those oral contraceptives, including thromboembolism). The following additional adverse reactions have been reported with estrogenic therapy, including oral contraceptives:

Genitourinary System: Breakthrough bleeding, spotting, change in menstrual flow; dysmenorrhea; premenstrual-lie syndrome; amenorrhea during and after treatment; increase in sizes of uterine fibromyomata; vaginal candidiasis; change in cervical eversion and in degree of cervical secretion; cystitis-like syndrome.

Breasts: Tenderness, enlargement, secretion.

Gastrointestinal: Nausea, vomiting; abdominal cramps, bloating; cholestatic jaundice.

Skin: Chloasma or melasma which may persist when drug is discontinued; erythema multiforme; erythema nodosum; hemorrhagic eruption; loss of scalp hair; hirsutism.

Eyes: Steeping of corneal curvature; intolerance to contact lenses.

CNS: Headache, migraine, dizziness; mental depression; chorea.

Miscellaneous: Increase or decrease in weight; reduced carbohydrate tolerance; aggravation of porphyria; edema; changes in libido.

OVERDOSAGE:

Numerous reports of ingestion of large doses of estrogen-containing oral contraceptives by young children indicate that serious ill effects do not occur. Overdosage of estrogen may cause nausea, and withdrawal bleeding may occur in females.

DOSAGE AND ADMINISTRATION:

1. Given cyclically for short-term use only: For treatment of moderate to severe vasomotor symptoms associated with the menopause. The lowest dose that will control symptoms should be chosen and medication should be discontinued as promptly as possible. Administration should be cyclic (*e.g.,* 3 weeks on a 1 week off). Attempts to discontinue or taper medication should be made at 3- to 6-month intervals. The usual dosage range is one 0.02 mg or 0.05 mg tablet daily. In some instances, the effective dose may be as low as one 0.02 mg tablet every other day. A useful dosage schedule for early menopause, while spontaneous menstruation continues, is 0.05 mg once a day for twenty-one days and then a rest period for seven days. For the initial treatment of the late menopause, the same regimen is indicated with the 0.02 mg Estinyl Tablet for the first few cycles, after which the 0.05 mg dosage may be substituted. In more severe cases, such as those due to surgical and roentgenologic castration, one 0.05 mg tablet may be administered three times daily at the start of treatment. With adequate clinical improvement, usually obtainable in a few weeks, the dosage may be reduced to one 0.05 mg tablet daily and the patient continued thereafter on a maintenance dosage as in the average case.

2. Given Cyclically, Female Hypogonadism: One 0.05 mg tablet is given one to three times daily during the first 2 weeks of a theoretical menstrual cycle. This is followed by progesterone during the last half of the arbitrary cycle. This regimen is continued for 3 to 6 months. The patients is then allowed to go untreated for two months to determine whether or not she can maintain the cycle without hormonal therapy. If not, additional courses of therapy may be prescribed.

3. Given Chronically, Inoperable Progressing Prostatic Cancer: From three 0.05 mg to four 0.05 mg tablets may be administered daily for palliation.

Inoperable Progressing Breast Cancer In Appropriately Selected Postmenopausal Women: (see INDICATIONS AND USAGE) Two 0.05 mg tablets three times daily for palliation.

Treated patients with an intact uterus should be monitored closely for signs of endometrial cancer and appropriate diagnostic measures should be taken to rule out malignancy in the event of persistent or recurring abnormal vaginal bleeding.

Store between 2° and 30°C (36° and 86°F).

REFERENCES:

HOW SUPPLIED - EQUIVALENTS NOT AVAILABLE:

Tablet, Coated - Oral - 0.02 mg

100's	$30.41	ESTINYL, Schering	00085-0298-03
250's	$71.50	ESTINYL, Schering	00085-0298-06

Tablet, Coated - Oral - 0.05 mg

100's	$51.25	ESTINYL, Schering	00085-0070-03
250's	$119.58	ESTINYL, Schering	00085-0070-06

Tablet, Coated - Oral - 0.5 mg

100's	$103.57	ESTINYL, Schering	00085-0150-03

ETHINYL ESTRADIOL; ETHYNODIOL DIACETATE *(001217)*

CATEGORIES: Contraceptives; Hormones; Pregnancy; Progesterone; Progestogen & Estrogen Combinations; Pregnancy Category X; Sales > $100 Million; FDA Approval Pre 1982; Top 200 Drugs

BRAND NAMES: *Conova*; **Demulen**; *Demulen 50* (Canada); *Metrulen*; *Neovulen*; *Ovulen*; *Ovulen 1 50*; *Ovulen 50*
(International brand names outside U.S. in italics)

FORMULARIES: Aetna; FHP; Foundation; Medi-Cal

COST OF THERAPY: $303.07 (Contraceptive; Tablet; 35 mcg/1 mg; 1/day; 365 days) vs. Potential Cost of $2,351.94 (Pregnancy)

DESCRIPTION:

The chemical name for ethyndiol diacetate is 19-nor-17α-pregn-4-en-20-yne-3β,17-diol diacetate, and for ethinyl estradiol it is 19-nor- 17α-pregna-1,3,5 (10)-trien-20-yne-3,17-diol.

Demulen 1/35-21 and Demulen 1/35-28: Each white tablet contains 1 mg of ethynodiol diacetate and 35 mcg of ethinyl estradiol, and the inactive ingredients include calcium acetate, calcium phosphate, corn starch, hydrogenated castor oil, and povidone. Each blue tablet in the Demulen 1/35-28 package is a placebo containing no active ingredients, and the inactive ingredients include calcium sulfate, corn starch, FD&C Blue No. 1 Lake, magnesium stearate, and sucrose.

Demulen 1/50-21 and Demulen 1/50-28: Each white tablet contains 1 mg of ethynodiol diacetate and 50 mcg of ethinyl estradiol, and the inactive ingredients include calcium acetate, calcium phosphate, corn starch, hydrogenated castor oil, and povidone. Each pink tablet in the Demulen 1/50-28 package is a placebo containing no active ingredients, and the inactive ingredients include calcium sulfate, corn starch, FD&C Red No. 3, FD&C Yellow No. 6, magnesium stearate, and sucrose.

For prescribing information refer to Ethinyl Estradiol; Norethindrone.

HOW SUPPLIED:

Demulen 1/35: Each white Demulen 1/35 tablet is round in shape, with a debossed SEARLE on one side and 151 and design on the other side, and contains 1 mg of ethynodiol diacetate and 35 mcg of ethinyl estradiol. (Blue placebo tablets have a debossed SEARLE on one side and a "P" on the other side.)

Demulen 1/50: Each white Demulen 1/50 tablet is round in shape, with a debossed SEARLE on one side and 71 on the other side, and contains 1 mg of ethynodiol diacetate and 50 mcg of ethinyl estradiol. (Blue placebo tablets have a debossed SEARLE on one side and a "P" on the other side.)

HOW SUPPLIED - RATED THERAPEUTICALLY EQUIVALENT:

Tablet, Uncoated - Oral - 35 mcg/1 mg

126 (6 x 21)	$145.31	DEMULEN 1/35-21, Searle	00025-0151-07
168 (6 x 28)	$146.78	DEMULEN 1/35-28, Searle	00025-0161-09
504 (24 x 21)	$552.33	DEMULEN 1/35-21, Searle	00025-0151-24
672 (24 x 28)	$558.00	DEMULEN 1/35-28, Searle	00025-0161-24

HOW SUPPLIED - RATED THERAPEUTICALLY EQUIVALENT: *(cont'd)*

Tablet, Uncoated - Oral - 50 mcg/1 mg

6 X 28	$163.53	DEMULEN 1/50-28, Searle	00025-0081-09
126 (6 x 21)	$162.02	DEMULEN 1/50-21, Searle	00025-0071-07
504 (24 x 21)	$562.48	DEMULEN 1/50-21, Searle	00025-0071-24
672 (24 x 28)	$567.91	DEMULEN 1/50-28, Searle	00025-0081-24

ETHINYL ESTRADIOL; FERROUS FUMARATE; NORETHINDRONE ACETATE *(001221)*

CATEGORIES: Contraceptives; Hormones; Pregnancy; Pregnancy Category X; FDA Approval Pre 1982; Top 200 Drugs

BRAND NAMES: Estrostep Fe; **Loestrin Fe**; Loestrin Fe 1.5/30; Loestrin Fe 1/20; Norlestrin Fe; Norquest Fe

FORMULARIES: Aetna; PCS

COST OF THERAPY: $57.57 (Contraceptive; Tablet; 20 mcg/75 mg/1 mg; 1/day; 365 days) vs. Potential Cost of $2,351.94 (Pregnancy)

DESCRIPTION:

The name for norethindrone is [(17 alpha)-17 (acetylox)-19-norpregna-4-en-20-yn-3-one] and the name for ethinyl estradiol is [(17 alpha)-19-norpregna-1,3,5(10)-trien-20-yne-3,17-diol].

Loestrin Fe: Each white tablet contains norethindrone acetate (17 alpha-ethinyl-19-nortestosterone acetate), 1 mg; ethinyl estradiol (17 alpha-ethinyl-1,3,5(10)-estratriene-3, 17 beta-diol), 20 mcg. Also contains acacia, NF; lactose, NF; magnesium stearate, NF; starch, NF; confectioner's sugar, NF; talc, USP.

Each green tablet contains norethindrone acetate (17 alpha-ethinyl-19-nortestosterone acetate), 1.5 mg; ethinyl estradiol (17 alpha-ethinyl-1,3,5(10)-estratriene-3, 17 beta-diol), 30 mcg. Also contains acacia, NF; lactose, NF; magnesium stearate, NF; starch, NF; confectioner's sugar, NF; talc, USP; D&C yellow No. 10; FD&C yellow No. 6; FD&C blue No. 1.

Each brown tablet contains microcrystalline cellulose, NF; ferrous fumarate, USP; magnesium stearate, NF; povidone, USP; sodium starch glycolate, NF; sucrose with modified dextrins.

Loestrin Fe is a progestogen-estrogen combination.

Loestrin Fe 1/20 and 1.5/30: Each provides a continuous dosage regimen consisting of 21 oral contraceptive tablets and seven ferrous fumarate tablets. The ferrous fumarate tablets are present to facilitate ease of drug administration via a 28-day regimen and do not serve any therapeutic purpose.

Estrostep Fe: Each triangular tablet contains 1 mg norethindrone acetate and 20 mcg ethinyl estradiol; each white square tablet contains 1 mg norethindrone acetate and 30 mcg ethinyl estradiol; each white round tablets contains 1 mg norethindrone acetate and 35 mcg ethinyl estradiol; each brown tablet contains 75 mg ferrous fumarate.

Each Estrostep Fe tablet dispenser contains 5 white triangular tablets, seven white square tablets, nine white round tablets and seven brown tablets. These tablets are to be taken in the following order: one triangular tablet each day for five days, then one square tablet each day for seven days; followed by one round tablet each day for nine days, and then one brown tablet each day for seven days.

For prescribing information refer to Ethinyl Estradiol; Norethindrone.

HOW SUPPLIED - EQUIVALENTS NOT AVAILABLE:

Tablet, Uncoated - Oral - 20 mcg/75 mg/1

28's	$21.52	ESTROSTEP FE, Parke-Davis	00071-0928-47
840 (30 x 28)	$132.51	LOESTRIN FE 1/20, Parke-Davis	00071-0913-47
840 (30 x 28)	$795.06	LOESTRIN FE 1/20, Parke-Davis	00071-0913-15

Tablet, Uncoated - Oral - 30 mcg/75 mg/1.

140 (5 x 28)	$132.51	LOESTRIN FE 1.5/30, Parke-Davis	00071-0917-47
840 (30 x 28)	$795.06	LOESTRIN FE 1.5/30, Parke-Davis	00071-0917-15

ETHINYL ESTRADIOL; LEVONORGESTREL *(001219)*

CATEGORIES: Contraceptives; Contraceptives, Emergency*; Hormones; Pregnancy; Progestogen & Estrogen Combinations; Pregnancy Category X; Sales > $100 Million; FDA Approved 1982 May; Top 200 Drugs
* Indication not approved by the FDA

BRAND NAMES: *Anna*; *Gynatrol*; Levlen; *Levlen ED* (Australia); Levora-21; Levora-28; *Logynon*; *Logynon ED* (Australia); *Microgest ED*; *Microgyn*; *Microgynon* (Mexico); *Microgynon CD* (Mexico); *Microgynon 21* (Germany); *Microgynon 28* (Germany); *Microgynon 30* (Australia, England); *Microgynon 30 ED* (Australia); *Minigynon*; *Minidril* (France); *Minivlar 30*; *Monofeme 28* (Australia); *Neogynon 21* (Germany); *Nordet* (Mexico); *Nordette*; *Nordette 21* (Australia); *Nordette 28* (Australia); *Ovoplex 30-150*; *Ovral-Lo*; *Ovranette* (England); *Rigevidon 21+7*; *Stediril 30* (Germany); *Triagynon*; *Triciclor*; *Trifeme 28* (Australia); *Trigoa* (Germany); *Trigynon*; Tri-Levlen; Tri-Levlen 21; *Trinordiol* (England, France, Germany, Mexico); *Trinordiol 21* (Germany); *Trinordiol 28*; Triphasil; *Triphasil 21* (Australia, Canada); *Triphasil 28* (Australia, Canada); *Triquilar* (Australia, Germany, Mexico); *Triquilar ED* (Australia)
(International brand names outside U.S. in italics)

FORMULARIES: Aetna; BC-BS; CIGNA; DoD; FHP; Foundation; Humana; Kaiser; Medco; Medi-Cal; PCS; PruCare; United; WHO

COST OF THERAPY: $255.62 (Contraceptive; Tablet; 0.03 mg/0.05 mg; 1/day; 365 days) vs. Potential Cost of $2,351.94 (Pregnancy)

DESCRIPTION:

Triphasil: Each Triphasil cycle of 21 tablets consists of three differen drug phases as follows: Phase 1 comprised of 6 brown tablets, each containing 0.050 mg of levonorgestrel, a totally synthetic progestogen, and 0.030 mg of ethinyl estradiol; phase 2 comprised of 5 white tablets, each containing 0.075 mg levongestrel and 0.040 mg ethinyl estradiol; phase 3 comprised of 10 light-yellow tablets, each containing 0.125 mg levongestrel and 0.030 mg ethinyl estradiol. The inactive ingredients present are calcium carbonate, glycerin, iron oxides, lactose, magnesium stearate, methylparaben, polyethylene glycol, povidone, propylparaben, sodium benzoate, starch, sucrose, talc, and titanium dioxide.

DESCRIPTION: *(cont'd)*

Nordette: Each Nordette tablet contains 0.15 mg of levongestrel, a totally synthetic progestogen, and 0.03 mg of ethinyl estradiol. The inactive ingredients present are cellulose, FD&C yellow 6, lactose, magnesium stearate, and polacrillin potassium. The tablets are round, light orange and marked with "WYETH" and "75".

For prescribing information refer to Ethinyl Estradiol; Norethindrone.

FDA RECOMMENDED DOSAGE GUIDELINES FOR POSTCOITAL EMERGENCY CONTRACEPTION

The FDA has declared oral contraceptives safe and effective for emergency contraception. Vomiting, sometimes severe enough to prevent the pills from working, and nausea are potential side effects. The dosing regimens for ethinyl estradiol/levonorgestrel can be taken within 72 hours of unprotected intercourse with a follow-up dose of the same number of pills 12 hours after the first dose:

Levlen: Four light orange tablets

Nordette: Four light orange tablets

Triphasil: Four yellow tablets

Tri-Levlen: Four yellow tablets

HOW SUPPLIED - RATED THERAPEUTICALLY EQUIVALENT:

Tablet, Uncoated - Oral - 0.03 mg/0.15 mg

63 (3 x 21)	$66.12	LEVLEN 21, Berlex Labs	50419-0410-21
84 (3 x 28)	$66.12	LEVLEN 28, Berlex Labs	50419-0411-28
126 (6 x 21)	$159.15	NORDETTE 21, Wyeth Labs	00008-0075-01
168 (6 x 28)	$161.15	NORDETTE 28, Wyeth Labs	00008-2533-02

HOW SUPPLIED - NOT RATED EQUIVALENT:

Tablet, Uncoated - Oral - 0.03 mg/0.05 mg

63 (3 x 21)	$61.68	TRI-LEVLEN 21, Berlex Labs	50419-0432-03
63 (3 x 21)	$77.25	TRIPHASIL 21, Wyeth Labs	00008-2535-01
84 (3 x 28)	$61.68	TRI-LEVLEN 28, Berlex Labs	50419-0433-03
84 (3 x 28)	$78.17	TRIPHASIL 28, Wyeth Labs	00008-2536-01
126 (6 x 21)	$117.66	Tri-Levlen 21, Berlex Labs	50419-0432-06
168 (6 x 28)	$117.66	TRI-LEVLEN 28, Berlex Labs	50419-0433-06

Tablet, Uncoated - Oral - 0.03 mg/0.15 mg

126 (6 x 21)	$88.99	Levora 21, Hamilton Pharma	60322-0145-21
168 (6 x 28)	$88.99	Levora 28, Hamilton Pharma	60322-0147-28

ETHINYL ESTRADIOL; NORETHINDRONE

(001220)

CATEGORIES: Contraceptives; Hormones; Ovarian Carcinoma; Pregnancy; Progestogen; Progestogen & Estrogen Combinations; Pregnancy Category X; Sales > $500 Million; Top 200 Drugs; FDA Approval Pre 1982

BRAND NAMES: *Anovlar*, *Anovulatorio*; Brevicon; *Brevinor* (Australia); *Brevinor 21*; *Brevinor 28* (Australia); *Brevinor-1 21*; *Brevinor-1 28* (Australia); *Ciclovulan*; *Estrinor*, Genora; Jenest-28; Loestrin; Micronor; *Milli*; *Minovlar*; Modicon; N.E.E.; Nelova; *Neocon* (England); *Nodiol*; Norcept-E; Norethin; *Norimin* (England); Norinyl; Norlestrin; *Orlest*; *Ortho 7 7 7* (Canada); *Ortho 1 35* (Canada); *Ortho-Novin 1 50* (England); **Ortho-Novum**; Ortho-Novum 7 7 7; *Ortho-Novum 1 35* (France); *Ortho-Novum 1 50* (Germany); Ovcon; *Ovysmen*; *Ovysmen 0.5 35* (Germany); *Ovysmen 1 35* (Germany); *Synphase*; *Synphasic 28* (Australia); *Triella* (France); Tri-Norinyl; *Trinovum* (Mexico, Germany, England); *Trinovum 21*
(International brand names outside U.S. in italics)

FORMULARIES: Aetna; BC-BS; CIGNA; DoD; FHP; Foundation; Humana; Kaiser; Medco; Medi-Cal; PruCare; United; WHO; PCS

COST OF THERAPY: $146.86 (Contraceptive; Tablet; 0.035 mg/0.5 mg; 1/day; 365 days)

WARNING:
Patients should be counseled that this product does not protect against HIV infection (AIDS) and other sexually transmitted diseases.

DESCRIPTION:

The chemical name for norethindrone is 17-hydroxy-19-nor-17α-pregn-4-en-20-yn-3-one, for ethinyl estradiol is 19-nor-17α-pregna-1,3,5(10)- trien -20-yne-3,17-diol, and for mestranol is 3-methoxy-19-nor-17α- pregna-1,3,5 (10)-trien-20-yn-17-ol.

Each of the following products is a combination oral contraceptive containing the progestational compound norethindrone and the estrogenic compound ethinyl estradiol:

Ortho-Novum 7/7/7: Each white tablet contains 0.5 mg of norethindrone and 0.035 mg of ethinyl estradiol. Inactive ingredients include lactose, magnesium stearate and pregelatinized starch. Each light peach tablet contains 0.75 mg of norethindrone and 0.035 mg of ethinyl estradiol. Inactive ingredients include FD&C Yellow No. 6 lactose, magnesium stearate and pregelatinized starch. Each peach tablet contains 1 mg of norethindrone and 0.035 of ethinyl estradiol. Inactive ingredients include FD&C Yellow No. 6, lactose, magnesium stearate and pregelatinized starch. Each green tablet in the Ortho-Novum 7/7/7 28 package contains only inert ingredients, as follows: D&C Yellow No. 10 Aluminum Lake, FD&C Blue No.2 Aluminum Lake lactose, magnesium stearate, microcrystalline cellulose and pregelatinized starch.

Ortho-Novum 10/11: Each white tablet contains 0.5 mg of norethindrone and 0.035 mg of ethinyl estradiol. inactive ingredients include lactose, magnesium stearate and pregelatinized starch. Each peach tablet contains 1 mg norethindrone and 0.035 ethinyl estradiol. Inactive ingredients include FD&C Yellow No. 6, lactose, magnesium stearate and pregelatinized starch. Each green tablet in the Ortho-Novum 10/11 28 package contains only inert ingredients, as listed under green tablets in Ortho-Novum 7/7/7 28.

Ortho-Novum 1/35: Each peach tablet contains 1 mg of norethindrone and 0.035 mg of ethinyl estradiol. Inactive ingredients include FD&C Yellow No. 6, lactose, magnesium stearate and pregelatinized starch. Each green tablet in the Ortho-Novum 1/35 28 package contains only inert ingredients, as listed under green tablets in Ortho-Novum 7/7/7 28.

Modicon: Each white tablet contains 0.5 mg of norethindrone and 0.035 mg of ethinyl estradiol. Inactive ingredients include lactose, magnesium stearate and pregelatinized starch. Each green tablet in the Modicon 28 package contains only inert ingredients, as listed under green tablets in Ortho- Novum 7/7/7 28.

CLINICAL PHARMACOLOGY:

Combination Oral Contraceptives: Combination oral contraceptives act by suppression of gonadotropins. Although the primary mechanism of this action is inhibition of ovulation, other alterations include changes in the cervical mucus (which increase the difficulty of sperm entry into the uterus) and the endometrium (which may reduce the likelihood of implantation).

Progestin-Only Oral Contraceptives: The primary mechanism through which norethindrone prevents conception is not known, but progestogen-only contraceptives are known to alter the cervical mucus, exert a progestational effect on the endometrium, interfering with implantation, and, in some patients, suppress ovulation.

INDICATIONS AND USAGE:

Oral contraceptives are indicated for the prevention of pregnancy in women who elect to use the products as a method of contraception.

Oral contraceptives are highly effective. TABLE 1 lists the typical accidental pregnancy rates for users of combination oral contraceptives and other methods of contraception. The efficacy of these contraceptive methods, except sterilization, depends upon the reliability upon the reliability with which they are used. Correct and consistent use of methods can result in lower failure rates.

TABLE 1 Lowest Expected and Typical Failure Rates During the First Year of Continuous Use of a Method
% of Women Experiencing an Accidental Pregnancy in the First Year of Continuous Use

Method	Lowest Expected*	Typical**
No contraception	(85)	(85)
Oral contraceptives		3
combined	0.1	N/A‡
progestin only	0.5	N/A‡
Diaphragm with spermicidal cream or jelly	6	18
Spermicides alone (foam, creams, gels, jellies, vaginal suppositories and vaginal film)	6	21
Vaginal Sponge		
nulliparous	9	18
parous	20	36
Implant (6 capsules)	0.09	0.09
Injection: depot medroxyprogesterone acetate	0.3	0.3
IUD		
progesterone T	1.5	2.0
copper T 380 A	0.6	0.8
LN g 20	0.1	0.1
Condom without spermicides		
female	5	21
male	3	12
Cervical Cap with spermacidal cream or jelly	2	12
nulliparous	9	18
parous	26	36
Periodic abstinence (all methods)	1-9	20
Withdrawl	4	19
Female sterilization	0.4	0.4
Male sterilization	0.10	0.15

* The authors' best guess of the percentage of women expected to experience an accidental pregnancy among couples who initiate a method (not necessarily for the first time) and who use it consistently and correctly during first year if they do not stop for any other reason.
† This term represents "typical" couples who initiate a method (not necessarily for the first time), who experience an accidental pregnancy during the first year if they do not stop use for any other reason.
‡ N/A - Data not available
Adapted from RA Hatcher et al, Reference 7.

CONTRAINDICATIONS:

Oral contraceptives should not be used in women who have the following combinations:

Thrombophlebitis or thromboembolic disorders

A past history of deep vein thrombophlebitis or thromboembolic disorders

Cerebral vascular of coronary artery disease

Known or suspected carcinoma of the breast

Carcinoma of the endometrium or other known or suspected estrogen- dependent neoplasia

Undiagnosed abnormal genital bleeding

Cholestatic jaundice of pregnancy or jaundice with prior pill use

Hepatic adenomas or carcinomas

Known or suspected pregnancy

WARNINGS:

Cigarette smoking increases the risk of serious cardiovascular side effects from oral conceptive use. This risk increases with age and with heavy smoking (15 or more cigarettes per day) and is quite marked in women over 35 years of age. Women who use oral contraceptives should be strongly advised not to smoke.

The use of oral contraceptives is associated with increased risks of several serious conditions including myocardial infarction, thromboembolism, stroke, hepatic neoplasia and gallbladder disease, although the risk of serious morbidity or mortality is very small in healthy women with out underlying risk factors. The risk of morbidity and mortality increases significantly in the presence of other underlying risk factors such as hypertension, hyperlipidemias, hypercholesterolemia, obesity and diabetes.

Practitioners prescribing oral should be familiar with the following information relating to these risks.

The information contained in this package insert is principally based on studies carried out in patients who used oral contraceptives with higher formulations of estrogens and progestogens than those in common use today. The effect of long-term use of oral contraceptives with lower formulations of both estrogens and progestogens remains to be determined.

Throughout this labeling, epidemiological studies reported are of two types: retrospective or case control studies and prospective or cohort studies. Case control studies provide a measure of the relative risk of a disease, namely, a *ratio* of the incidence of a disease among oral contraceptive users to that among non-users. The relative risk does not provide information on the actual clinical occurrence of a disease. Cohort studies provide a measure of attributable risk, which is the *difference* in the incidence of disease between oral contraceptive users and non-users. The attributable risk does provide information about the actual occurrence of a disease in the population (adapted from references 8 and 9 with the author's permission). For further information, the reader is referred to a text on epidemiological methods.

WARNINGS: *(cont'd)*

THROMBOEMBOLIC DISORDERS AND VASCULAR PROBLEMS

Myocardial Infarction: An increased risk of myocardial infarction has been attributed to oral contraceptive use. This risk is primarily in smokers or women with other underlying risk factors for coronary artery disease such as hypertension, hypercholesterolemia, morbid obesity and diabetes. The relative risk of heart attack for current oral contraceptive users has been estimated to be 2 to 6.[10-16] The risk is very low under the age of 30.

Smoking in combination with oral contraceptive use has been shown to contribute substantially to the incidence of myocardial infarctions in women in their mid-thirties or older with smoking accounting for the majority of excess cases.[17] Mortality rates associated with circulatory disease have been shown to increase substantially in smokers over the age of 35 and non-smokers over the age of 40 among women who use oral contraceptives.

Oral contraceptives may compound the effects of well-known risk factors such as hypertension, diabetes, hyperlipidemias, age and obesity.[19] In particular, some progestogens are known to decrease HDL cholesterol and cause glucose intolerance, while estrogens may create a state of hyperinsulinism.[20-24] Oral contraceptives have been shown to increase blood pressure among users (see Elevated Blood Pressure). Similar effects on risk factors have been associated with an increased risk of heart disease. Oral contraceptives must be used with caution in women with cardiovascular disease risk factors.

Thromboembolism: An increased risk of thromboembolic and thrombotic disease associated with the use of oral contraceptives is well established. Case control studies have found the relative risk of users compared to nonusers to be 3 for the first episode of superficial venous thrombosis, 4 to 11 for deep vein thrombosis or pulmonary embolism, and 1.5 to 6 for women with predisposing conditions for venous thromboembolic disease.[9,10,25-30] Cohort studies have shown the relative risk to be somewhat lower, about 3 for new cases and about 4.5 for new cases requiring hospitalization.[31] The risk of thromboembolic disease due to oral contraceptives is not related to length of use and disappears after pill use is stopped.[8]

A two- to four-fold increase in relative risk of postoperative thromboembolic complications has been reported with the use of oral contraceptives.[15,32] The relative risk of venous thrombosis in women who have predisposing conditions is twice that of women without such medical conditions.[15,32] If feasible, oral contraceptives should be discontinued at least 4 weeks prior to and for 2 weeks after elective surgery of a type associated with an increase in risk of thromboembolism and during and following prolonged immobilization. Since the immediate postpartum period is also associated with an increased risk of thromboembolism, oral contraceptives should be started no earlier than 4 to 6 weeks after delivery in women who elect not to breast feed.

Cerebrovascular Diseases: Oral contraceptives have been shown to increase in both the relative and attributable risks of cerebrovascular events (thrombotic and hemorrhagic strokes) although, in general, the risk is greatest among older (>35 years), hypertensive women who also smoke. Hypertension was found to be a risk factor for both users and nonusers for both types of strokes while smoking interacted to increase the risk of stroke.[33-35]

In a large study, the relative risk of thrombotic strokes has been shown to range from 3 for normotensive users to 14 for users with severe hypertension.[36] The relative risk of hemorrhagic stroke is reported to be 1.2 for non-smokers who used oral contraceptives, 2.6 for smokers who did not use oral contraceptives, 7.6 for smokers who used oral contraceptives, 1.8 for normotensive users and 25.7 for users with severe hypertension.[36] The attributable risk also is greater in older women.[9]

Dose-Related Risk of Vascular Disease From Oral Contraceptives: A positive association has been observed between the amount of estrogen and progestogen in oral contraceptives and the risk of vascular disease.[37-39] A decline in serum high density lipoproteins (HDL) has been reported with many progestational agents.[20-22] A decline in serum high density lipoproteins has been associated with an increased incidence of ischemic heart disease. Because estrogens increase HDL cholesterol, the net effect of an oral contraceptive depends on a balance achieved between doses of estrogen and progestogen and the nature of the progestin used in the contraceptives. The amount and activity of both hormones should be considered in the choice of an oral contraceptive.

Minimizing exposure to estrogen and progestogen is in keeping with good principles of therapeutics. For any particular oral contraceptive, the dosage regimen prescribed should be one which contains the least amount of estrogen and progestogen that is compatible with the needs of the individual patient. New acceptors of oral contraceptive agents should be started on preparations containing the lowest dose of estrogen which produces satisfactory results for the patient.

Persistence of Risk of Vascular Disease: There are two studies which have shown persistence of risk of vascular disease for ever-users of oral contraceptives. In a study in the United States, the risk of developing myocardial infarction after discontinuing oral contraceptives persists for at least 9 years for women 40-49 who had used oral contraceptives for 5 or more years, but this increased risk was not demonstrated in other age groups.[14] In another study in Great Britain, the risk of cerebrovascular disease persisted for at least 6 years after discontinuation of oral contraceptives, although excess risk was very small.[40] However, both studies were performed with oral contraceptive formulations containing 50 mcg or higher of estrogens.

ESTIMATES OF MORTALITY FROM CONTRACEPTIVE USE

One study gathered data from a variety of sources which have estimated the mortality rate associated with different methods of contraception at different ages (see TABLE 2). These estimates include the combined risk of death associated with contraceptive methods plus the risk attributable to pregnancy in the event of method failure. Each method of contraception has its specific benefits and risks. The study concluded that with the exception of oral contraceptive users 35 and older who smoke and 40 and older who do not smoke, mortality associated with all methods of birth control is low and below that associated with childbirth. The observation of an increase in risk of mortality with age for oral contraceptive users is based on data gathered in the 1970's but not reported until 1983.[41] However, current clinical practice involves the use of lower estrogen dose formulations combined with careful restriction of oral contraceptive use to women who do not have the various risk factors listed in this labeling.

Because of these changes in practice and, also, because of some limited new data which suggest that the risk of cardiovascular disease with the use of oral contraceptives may now be less than previously observed (Porter JB, Hunter J, Jick H, et al. Oral contraceptives and nonfatal vascular disease. Obset Gynecol 1985;66:1-4; and Porter JB, Hershel J, Walker AM. Mortality among oral contraceptive users. Obset Gunecol 1987;70:29-32), the Fertility and Maternal Health Drugs Advisory Committee was asked to review the topic in 1989. The Committee concluded that although cardiovascular disease risks may be increased with oral contraceptive use after age 40 in healthy non-smoking women (even with the newer low-dose formulations), there are greater potential health risks associated with pregnancy in older women and with the alternative surgical and medical procedures which may be necessary if such women do not have access to effective and acceptable means of contraception.

Therefore, the Committee recommended that the benefits of oral contraceptive use by healthy non-smoking women over 40 may outweigh the possible risks. Of course, older women, as all women w

WARNINGS: *(cont'd)*

TABLE 2 Annual Number of Birth-Related or Method-Related Deaths Associated with Control of Fertility Per 100,000 Non-Sterile Women, by Fertility Control Method According to Age

Method of control and outcome	15-19	20-24	25-29	30-34	35-39	40-44
No fertility controls methods*	7.0	7.4	9.1	14.8	25.7	28.2
Oral contraceptives non-smoker†	0.3	0.5	0.9	1.9	13.8	31.6
Oral contraceptives smoker†	2.2	3.4	6.6	13.5	51.1	117.2
IUD†	0.8	0.8	1.0	1.0	1.4	1.4
Condom*	1.1	1.6	0.7	0.2	0.3	0.4
Diaphragm/Spermicide*	1.9	1.2	1.2	1.3	2.2	2.8
Periodic abstinence*	2.5	1.6	1.6	1.7	2.9	3.6

* Deaths are birth-related
† Deaths are method-related
Adapted from H.W. Ory, reference 41.

CARCINOMA OF REPRODUCTIVE ORGANS

Numerous epidemiological studies have been performed or the incidence of breast, endometrial, ovarian and cervical cancer in women using oral contraceptives. Most of the studies on breast cancer and oral contraceptive use report that the use of oral contraceptives is not associated with an increase in the risk of developing breast cancer.[42,44,89] Some studies have reported an increased risk of developing breast cancer in certain subgroups of oral contraceptive users, but the findings reported in these studies are not consistent.[43,45-49,85-88]

Some studies suggest that oral contraceptive use has been associated with an increase in risk of cervical intraepithelial neoplasia in some populations of women.[51-54] However, there continues to be controversy about the extent to which such findings may be due to differences in sexual behavior and other factors.

In spite of many studies of the relationship between oral conraceptive use and breast and cervical cancers, a cause and effect relationship has not been established.

HEPATIC NEOPLASIA

Benign hepatic adenomas are associated with oral contraceptive use, although the incidence of benign tumors is rare in the United States. Indirect calculations have estimated the attributable risk to be in the range of 3.3 cases/100,000 for users, a risk that increases after 4 or more years of use.[55] Rupture of rare, benign, hepatic adenomas may cause death through intra-abdominal hemorrhage.[56,57]

Studies from Britain have shown an increased risk of developing hepatocellular carcinoma[58-60] in long-term (>8 years) oral contraceptive users. However, these cancers are extremely rare in the U.S. and the attributable risk (the excess incidence) of liver cancers in oral contraceptive users approaches less than one per million users.

OCULAR LESIONS

There have been clinical case reports of retinal thrombosis associated with the use of oral contraceptives. Oral contraceptives should be discontinued if there is unexplained partial or complete loss of vision; onset of proptosis or diplopia; papilledema; or retinal vascular lesions. Appropriate diagnostic and therapeutic measures should be undertaken immediately.

ORAL CONTRACEPTIVE USE BEFORE OR DURING EARLY PREGNANCY

Extensive epidemiological studies have revealed no increased risk of birth defects in women who have used oral contraceptives prior to pregnancy.[61-63] Studies also do not suggest a teratogenic effect, particularly insofar as cardiac anomalies and limb reduction defects are concerned,[61,62,64,65] when taken inadvertently during early pregnancy.

The administration of oral contraceptives to induce withdrawal bleeding should not be used as a test for pregnancy. Oral contraceptives should not be used during pregnancy to treat threatened or habitual abortion.

It is recommended that for any patient who has missed 2 consecutive periods, (or after 45 days from the last menstrual period if the progestogen-only oral contraceptives are used) pregnancy should be ruled out before continuing oral contraceptive use. If the patient has not adhered to the prescribed schedule, the possibility of pregnancy should be considered at the time of the first missed period or upon missing one Micronor Tablet. Oral contraceptive use should be discontinued if pregnancy is confirmed.

GALLBLADDER DISEASE

Earlier studies have reported an increased lifetime relative risk of gallbladder surgery in users of oral contraceptives and estrogens.[66-67] More recent studies, however, have shown that the relative risk of developing gallbladder disease among oral contraceptive users may be minimal.[68-70] The recent findings of minimal risk may be related to the use of oral contraceptive formulations containing lower hormonal doses of estrogens and progestogens.

CARBOHYDRATE AND LIPID METABOLIC EFFECTS

Oral contraceptives have been shown to cause a glucose intolerance in a significant percentage of users.[23] Oral contraceptives containing greater than 75 mcg of estrogens cause hyperinsulinism, while loer doses of estrogen cause less glucose intolerance.[71] Progestogens increase insulin secretion and create insulin resistance, this effect varying with different progestational agents.[23,72] However, in the non-diabetic woman, oral contraceptives appear to have no effect on fasting blood glucose.[73] Because of these demonstrated effects, prediabetic and diabetic women should be carefully observed while taking oral contraceptives.

A small proportion of women will have persistent hypertriglyceridemia while on the pill. As discussed earlier (see WARNINGS, Myocardial Infarction and Dose Related Risk of Vascular Disease), changes in serum triglycerides and lipoprotein levels have been reported in oral contraceptive users.

ELEVATED BLOOD PRESSURE

An increase in blood pressure has been reported in women taking oral contraceptives[74] and this increase is more likely in older oral contraceptive users[75] and with extended duration of use.[74] Data from the Royal College of General Practitioners[18] and subsequent randomized trials have shown that the incidence of hypertension increases with increasing concentrations of progestogens.

Women with a history of hypertension or hypertension-related diseases, or renal disease[76] should be encouraged to use another method of contraception. If women elect to use oral contraceptives, they should be monitored closely and if significant elevation of blood pressure occurs, oral contraceptives should be discontinued. For most women, elevated blood pressure will return to normal after stopping oral contraceptives and there is no difference in the occurrence of hypertension between former and never users.[74,76,77]

HEADACHE

The onset or exacerbation of migraine or development of headache with a new pattern which is recurrent, persistent or severe requires discontinuation of oral contraceptives and evaluation of the cause.

WARNINGS: *(cont'd)*

BLEEDING IRREGULARITIES

Breakthrough bleeding and spotting are sometimes encountered in patients on oral contraceptives, especially during the first 3 months of use. Non-hormonal causes should be considered and adequate diagnostic measures taken to rule out malignancy or pregnancy in the event of breakthrough bleeding, as in the case of any abnormal vaginal bleeding. If pathology has been excluded, time or a change to another formulation may solve the problem. In the event of amenorrhea, pregnancy should be ruled out.

An alteration in menstrual patterns is likely to occur in women using progestogen-only contraceptives. The amount and duration of flow, cycle length, breakthrough bleeding, spotting and amenorrhea will probably be quite variable. Bleeding irregularities occur more frequently with the use of progestogen-only oral contraceptives than with the combinations and the dropout rate due to such conditions is higher.

Some women may encounter post-pill amenorrhea or oligomenorrhea, especially when such a condition was preexistent.

ECTOPIC PREGNANCY

Ectopic as well as intrauterine pregnancy may occur in contraceptive failures. However, in progestogen-only oral contraceptive failures, the ratio of ectopic to intrauterine pregnancies is higher than in women who are not receiving contraceptives, since the drugs are more effective in preventing intrauterine than ectopic pregnancies.

ADDITIONAL INFORMATION FOR PROGESTEN ONLY CONTRACEPTIVES

Mascululinization of the female fetus has occurred who progestogens have been used in pregnant women.

Some beagle dogs treated with medroxyprogesterone acetate developed mammary nodules. Although nodules occasionally appeared in control animals they were intermittent in nature, whereas nodules in treated animals were larger and more numerous, and they persisted. There is no general agreement as to whether the nodules are benign or malignant. Their significance with respect to humans has not been estableised.

PRECAUTIONS:

Patients should be counseled that this product does not protect against HIV infection (AIDS) and other sexually transmitted diseases.

PHYSICAL EXAMINATION AND FOLLOW-UP

It is good medical practice for all women to have annual history and physical examinations, including women using oral contraceptives. The physical examination, however, may be deferred until after initiation of oral contraceptives if requested by the women and judged appropriate by the clinician. The physical examination should include special reference to blood pressure, breasts, abdomen and pelvic organs, including cervical cytology, and relevant laboratory tests. In case of undiagnosed, persistent or recurrent abnormal vaginal bleeding, appropriate measures should be conducted to rule out malignancy. Women with a strong family history of breast cancer or who have breast nodules should be monitored with particular care.

LIPID DISORDERS

Women who are being treated for hyperlipidemia should be followed closely if they elect to use oral contraceptives. Some progestogens may elevate LDL levels and may render the control of hyperlipidemias more difficult.

LIVER FUNCTION

If jaundice develops in any woman receiving such drugs, the medication should be discontinued. Steroid hormones may be poorly metabolized in patients with impaired liver function.

FLUID RETENTION

Oral contraceptives may cause some degree of fluid retention. They should be prescribed with caution, and only with careful monitoring, in patients with conditions which might be aggravated by fluid retention.

EMOTIONAL DISORDERS

Women with a history of depression should be carefully observed and the drug discontinued if depression recurs to a serious degree.

CONTACT LENSES

Contact lens wearers who develop visual changes or changes in lens tolerance should be assessed by an ophthalmologist.

INTERACTIONS WITH LABORATORY TESTS

Certain endocrine and liver function tests and blood components may be affected by oral contraceptives:

a. Increased prothrombin and factors VII, VIII, IX, and X; decreased antithrombin 3; increased norepinephrine-induced platelet aggregability.

b. Increased thyroid binding globulins (TBG) leading to increased circulating total thyroid hormone, as measured by protein-bound iodine (PBI), T_4 by column or by radioimmunoassay. Free T_3 resin uptake is decreased, reflecting the elevated TBG. Free T_4 concentration is unaltered.

c. Other binding proteins may be elevated in serum.

d. Sex-binding globulins are increased and result in elevated levels of total circulating sex steroids and corticoids; however, free or biologically active levels remain unchanged.

e. Triglycerides may be increased.

f. Glucose tolerance may be decreased.

g. Serum folate levels may be depressed by oral contraceptive therapy. This may be of clinical significance if a woman becomes pregnant shortly after discontinuing oral contraceptives.

CARCINOGENESIS

See WARNINGS.

PREGNANCY CATEGORY X

See CONTRAINDICATIONS and WARNINGS.

NURSING MOTHERS

Small amounts of oral contraceptive steroids have been identified in the milk of nursing mothers, and a few adverse effects on the child have been reported, including jaundice and breast enlargement. In addition, oral contraceptives given in the postpartum period may interfere with lactation by decreasing the quantity and quality of breast milk. If possible, the nursing mother should be advised not to use oral contraceptives but to use other forms of contraception until she has completely weaned her child.

INFORMATION FOR THE PATIENT

See PATIENT PACKAGE INSERT.

SEXUALLY TRANSMITTED DISEASES

Patients should be counseled that this product does not protect against HIV infection (AIDS) and their sexually transmitted diseases.

DRUG INTERACTIONS:

Reduced efficacy and increased incidence of breakthrough bleeding and menstrual irregularities have been associated with concomitant use of rifampin. A similar association though less marked, has been suggested with barbiturates, phenylbutazone, phenytoin sodium, and possibly with griseofulvin, ampicillin and tetracyclines.[78]

ADVERSE REACTIONS:

An increased risk of the following serious adverse reactions has been associated with the use of oral contraceptives (see WARNINGS):

Thrombophlebitis	Cerebral thrombosis
Arterial thromboembolism	Hypertension
Pulmonary embolism	Gallbladder disease
Myocardial infarction	Hepatic adenomas, carcinomas or benign liver tumors
Cerebral hemorrhage	

There is evidence of an association between the following conditions and the use of oral contraceptives, although additional confirmatory studies are needed:

Mesenteric thrombosis	Retinal thrombosis

The following adverse reactions have been reported in patients receiving oral contraceptives and are believed to be drug-related:

Nausea
Vomiting
Gastrointestinal symptoms (such as abdominal cramps and bloating)
Breakthrough bleeding
Spotting
Change in menstrual flow
Amenorrhea
Temporary infertility after discontinuation of treatment
Edema
Melasma which may persist
Breast changes; tenderness, enlargement, secretion
Change in weight (increase or decrease)
Change in cervical erosion and secretion
Diminution in lactation when given immediately postpartum
Cholestatic jaundice
Migraine
Rash (allergic)
Mental depression
Reduced tolerance to carbohydrates
Vaginal candidiasis
Change in corneal curvature (steepening)
Intolerance to contact lenses

The following adverse reactions have been reported in users of oral contraceptives and the association has been neither confirmed nor refuted:

Pre-menstrual syndrome	Erythema nodosum
Cataracts	Hemorrhagic eruption
Changes in appetite	Vaginitis
Cystitis-like syndrome	Porphyria
Headache	Impaired renal function
Nervousness	Hemolytic uremic syndrome
Dizziness	Budd Chiari syndrome
Hirsutism	Acne
Loss of scalp hair	Changes in libido
Erythema multiforme	Colitis

OVERDOSAGE:

Serious ill effects have not been reported following acute ingestion of large doses of oral contraceptives by young children. Overdosage may cause nausea, and withdrawal bleeding may occur in females.

DOSAGE AND ADMINISTRATION:

To achieve maximum contraceptive effectiveness, tablets must be taken exactly as directed and at intervals not exceeding 24 hours.

The patient should be instructed to use an additional method of protection until after the first week of administration in the initial cycle when utilizing the Sunday-Start Regimen. Most dispensors are preset for Sunday Start. Day 1 Start is also available.

The possibility of ovulation and conception prior to initiation of use should be considered.

21-DAY REGIMEN (SUNDAY START)

The first tablet should be taken on the first Sunday after menstruation begins. If period begins on Sunday, the first tablet is taken on the same day. One tablet is taken daily for 21 days. For subsequent cycles, no tablets are taken for 7 days, then a tablet is taken the next day (Sunday). For the first cycle of a Sunday Start regimen, another method of contraception should be used until after the first 7 consecutive days of administration.

21-DAY REGIMEN (DAY 1 START)

The initial cycle of therapy is one tablet administered daily from the 1st day through 21st day of the menstrual cycle, counting the first day of menstrual flow as "Day 1". For subsequent cycles, no tablets are taken for 7 days, then a new course is started of one tablet a day for 21 days. The dosage regimen then continues with 7 days of no medication, followed by 21 days of medication, instituting a three-weeks- on, one-week-off dosage regimen.

28-DAY REGIMEN (SUNDAY START)

The fist tablet should be taken on the first Sunday after menstruation begins. If period begins on Sunday, the first tablet should be taken that day. Take one active tablet daily for 21 days followed by one green placebo tablet daily for 7 days. After 28 tablets have been taken, a new course is started the next (Sunday). For the first cycle of a Sunday Start regimen, another method of contraception should be used until after the first 7 consecutive days of administration.

28-DAY REGIMEN (DAY 1 START)

The first initial cycle of therapy is one active tablet administered daily from the 1st through the 21st day of the menstrual cycle, counting the first day of menstrual flow as "Day 1" followed by one green tablet daily for 7 days. Tablets are taken without interruption for 28 days. After 28 tablets have been taken, a new course is started the next day.

The use of Ortho-Novum 7/7/7, Ortho-Novum 10/11, Ortho-Novum 1/35, Modicon and Ortho-Novum 1/50 for contraception may be initiated 4 weeks postpartum in women who elect not to breast feed. When the tablets are administered during the postpartum period, the increased risk of thromboembolic disease associated with the postpartum period must be

DOSAGE AND ADMINISTRATION: *(cont'd)*

considered. See CONTRAINDICATIONS and WARNINGS, Thromboembolic diseases. See also PRECAUTIONS, Nursing Mothers. The possibility of ovulation and conception prior to initiation of medication should considered.

See Discussion of Dose, Related Risk of Vascular Disease from Oral Contraceptives.

NORETHINDRONE (CONTINUOUS REGIMEN)

Norethindrone is administered on a continuous daily dosage regimen starting on the first day of menstruation (*i.e.,*one tablet each day) every day of the year. Tablets should be taken at the same time each day and continued daily. The patient should be advised that if prolonged bleeding occurs she should consult her physician.

The use of norethindrone for contraception may be initiated postpartum (see WARNINGS). When norethindrone is administered during postpartum period, the increased risk of thromboembolic disease associated with the postpartum period must be considered. See CONTRAINDICATIONSand WARNINGS concerning thromboembolic disease.

If the patient misses one tablet, norethindrone should be discontinued immediately and a method or nonhormonal contraception should be used until menses has appeared or pregnancy has been excluded.

Alternatively, if the patient has taken the tablets correctly, and if menses does not appear when expected, a nonhormonal method of contraception should be substituted until an appropriate diagnostic procedure is performed to rule out pregnancy.

ADDITIONAL INSTRUCTIONS FOR ALL DOSING REGIMENS

Breakthrough bleeding, spotting and amenorrhea are frequent reasons for patients discontinuing oral contraceptives. In breakthrough bleeding, as in all cases of irregular bleeding from the vagina, nonfunctional causes should be borne in mind. In undiagnosed persistent or recurrent abnormal bleeding from the vagina, adequate diagnostic measures are indicated to rule out pregnancy or malignancy. If pathology has been excluded, time or a change to another formulation may solve the problem. Changing to an oral contraceptive with a higher estrogen content, while potentially useful in minimizing menstrual irregularity, should be done only if necessary since this may increase the risk of thromboembolic disease.

SPECIAL NOTES ON ADMINISTRATION

Menstruation usually begins two or three days, but may begin as late as the fourth or fifth day, after discontinuing medication. If spotting occurs while on the usual regimen of ont tablet daily, the patient should continue medication without interruption.

If the patient forgets to take one or more active tablets, the following is suggested:

One tablet missed:

take tablet as soon as remembered

take next tablet at the regular time

Two consecutive tablets are missed (week one or week two):

take two tablets as soon as remembered

take two tablets the next day

use another birth control method for seven days following the missed tablets

Two consecutive tablets are missed (week three):

take one tablet daily until Sunday

discard remaining tablets

start a new pack of tablets immediately (Sunday)

use another birth control method for seven days following the missed tablets

Three or more consecutive tablets are missed:

take one tablet daily until Sunday

discard remaining tablets

start a new pack of tablets immediately (Sunday)

use another birth control method for seven days following the missed tablets

The possibility of ovulation increases with each sucessive day that scheduled tablets are missed. While there is little likelihood of ovulation occurring if only one tablet is missed, the possibility of spotting or bleeding is increased. This is particularly likely if two or more consecutive tablets are missed.

In rare cases of bleeding which resembles menstruation, the patinet should be advised to discontinue medication and then begin taking tablets from a new tablet dispenser on the next Sunday. Persistent bleeding which is not controlled by this method indicates the need for reexaminstion of the patient, at which time nonfunctional causes should be considered.

Use of Oral contraceptives in the event of a missed menstrual period:

1. If the patient has not adhered to the prescribed schedule, the possibility of pregnancy should be considered after the first missed period (or upon missing one Micronor Tablet) and oral contraceptive use should be withheld until pregnancy is ruled out.

2. If the patient has adhered to the prescribed regimen and misses two consecutive periods (or after 45 days from the last menstrual period if the progestogen-only oral contraceptives are used), pregnancy should be ruled out before continuing the contraceptive regimen.

Non-Contraceptive Health Benefits: The following non-contraceptive health benefits related to the use of oral contraceptives are supported by epidemiological studies which largely utilized oral contraceptive formulations containing estrogen doses exceeding 0.035 mg of ethinyl estradiol or 0.05 mg of mestranol.[79-84]

Effects on menses:

Increased menstrual cycle regularity

Decreased blood loss and decreased incidence of iron deficiency anemia

Decreased incidence of dysmenorrhea

Effects related to inhibition of ovulation:

Decreased incidence of functional ovarian cysts

Decreased incidence of ectopic pregnancies

Effects from long-term use:

Decreased incidence of fibroadenomas and fibrocystic disease of the breast

Decreased incidence of acute pelvic inflammatory disease

Decreased incidence of endometrial cancer

Decreased incidence of ovarian cancer

FDA RECOMMENDED DOSAGE GUIDELINES FOR POSTCOITAL EMERGENCY CONTRACEPTION

See Ethinyl Estradiol; Levonorgestrel and Ethinyl Estradiol; Norgestrel

REFERENCES:

1. Back DJ, Breckenridge AM, Crawford FE, McIver M, Orme ML'E, Rowe PH, Smith E: Kinetics of norethindrone in women II. Single-dose kinetics. Clin Pharmacol Ther 1978;24:448-453. **2.** Hulnpel M, Nieuweboer B, Wendt H and Speck U: Investigations of pharmacokinetics of ethinyloestradiol to specific consideration of a possible first-pass effect in women Contraception 1979;19:421-432. **3.** Back DJ, Breckenridge AM, Crawford FE, Maclver M, Orme ML'E, Rowe PH and Watts MJ say. An investigation of the pharmacokinetics of ethinylestradiol in women using radioimmunoassay. Contraception 1979;20:263-273. **4.** Hammond GL, L¨ahteenm¨aki PLA, L¨ahteenm¨aki P and Luukkainen T. Distribution and percentages of non-protein bound contraceptive steroids in human serum. J Steroid Biochem 1982;17:375-380. **5.** Fotherby K. Pharmacokinetics

REFERENCES: *(cont'd)*

and metabolism of progestins in humans in Pharmacology of the contraceptive steroids, Goldzieher JW, Fotherby K (eds), Raven Press Ltd., New York 1994, 99-126. **6.** Goldzieher JW, Pharmacokinetics and metabolism of ethynyl estrogens in Pharmacology of the contraceptive steroids, Goldzieher JW, Fotherby K (eds), Raven Press Ltd., New York 1994, 127-151. **7.** Hatcher RA, et al. 1994. Contraceptive Technology, Sixteenth Edition, New York. Irvington Publishers. **8.** Stadel BV, Oral contraceptives and cardiovascular disease. (Pt.1). N Engl J Med 1981; 305:612-618. **9.** Stadel BV, Oral contraceptives and cardiovascular disease. (Pt.2). N Engl J Med 1981; 305:672-677. **10.** Adam SA, Thorogood M. oral contraception and myocardial infarction revisited: the effects of new preparations and prescribing patterns. Br J Obstet Gynaecol 1981; 88-838-845. **11.** Mann Jl, Inman WH Oral contraceptives and death from myocardial infarction. Br Med J 1975; 2(5965):245-248. **12.** Mann Jl, Vessey MP, Thorogood M, Doll R. Myocardial infarction in young women with special reference to oral contraceptive practice. Br Med J 1975; 2(5956):241-245. **13.** Royal College of General Practitioners' Oral Contraception Study: Further analyses of mortality in oral contraceptive users. Lancet 1981; 1:541-546. **14.** Slone D, Shapiro S, Kaufman DW, Rosenburg L, Miettinen OS, Stolley PD. Risk of myocardial infarction in relation to current and discontinued use of oral contraceptives. N Engl J Med 1981;305:420-424. **15.** Vessey MP. Female hormones and vascular disease - an epidemiological overview. Br J Fam Plann 1980 6(Supplement):1-12. **16.** Russell-Briefel RG, Ezzati TM, Fulwood R, Perlman JA, Murphy RS. Cardiovascular risk status and oral contraceptive use, United States, 1976-80. Prevent Med 1986; 15; 352-362. **17.** Goldbaum GM, Kendrick JS, Hogelin GC, Gentry EM. The relative impact of smoking and oral contraceptive use on women in the United States. JAMA 1987; 258:1339-1342. **18.** Layde PM, Beral V. Further analyses of mortality in oral contraceptive users; Royal College of General Practitioners' Oral Contraception Study. (Table 5) Lancet 1981; 1:541-546. **19.** Knopp RH, Arteriosclerosis risk: the roles of oral contraceptives and postmenopausal estrogens. J Reprod Med 1986; 31(9) (Supplement): 913-921. **20.** Krauss RM Roy S, Mishell DR, Casagrande J, Pike MC. Effects of two low-dose oral contraceptives on serum lipids and lipoproteins: Differential changes in high-density lipoproteins subclasses. Am J Obstet 1983; 145:446-452. **21.** Wahl P, Walden C. Knopp R, Hoover J. Wallace R, Heiss G, Rifkind B. Effect of estrogen/progestin potency on lipid/lipoprotein cholesterol. N Engl J Med 1983; 308:862-867. **22.** Wynn V, Niththyananthan R. The effect of progestin is combined oral contraceptives on serum lipids with special reference to high density lipoproteins. Am J Obstet Gynecol 1982; 142:766-771. **23.** Wynn V, Godsland I. Effects of oral contraceptives on carbohydrate metabolism. J Reprod Med 1986; 31(9) (Supplement):892-897. **24.** LaRosa JC. Atherosclerotic risk factors in cardiovascular disease. J Reprod Med 1986; 31(9) (Supplement):906-912. **25.** Inman WH, Vessey MP. Investigation of death from pulmonary, coronary, and cerebral thrombosis and embolism in women of children bearing age. Br Med J 1968; 2:(5599):193-199. **26.** Maguire MG, Tonascia J, Sartwell PE Stolley PD, Tockman MS. Increased risk of thrombosis due to oral contraceptives: a further report. Am J Epidemiol 1979; 110(2):188-195. **27.** Petitti DB, Wingerd J, Pellegrin F, Ramacharan S. Risk of vascular disease in women: smoking, oral contraceptives, noncontraceptive estrogens, and others factors. JAMA 1979; 242:1150-1154. **28.** Vessey MP Doll R. Investigation of relation between use of oral contraceptives and thromboembolic disease. Br Med J 1968; 2 (5599):199- 205. **29.** Vessey MP, Doll R. Investigation of relation between use of oral contraceptives and thromboembolic disease. A further report. Br Med J 1969; 2(5658):651-657. **30.** Porter JB, Hunter JR, Danielson DA, Jick H, Stergachis A. Oral contraceptives and non-fatal vascular disease-recent experience. Obstet Gynecol 1982; 59(3):299-302. **31.** Vessey M. Doll R, Peto R, Johnson B, Wiggins P. A long-term follow-up study of women using different methods of contraception: an interim report. J. Biosocial Sci 1976;8:393-427. **32.** Royal College of General Practitioners: Oral Contraceptives, venous thrombosis, and varicose veins. J Royal Coll Gen Pract 1978; 28:393-399. **33.** Collaborative Group for the Study of Stroke in Young Women: Oral Contraception and increased risk of cerebral ischemia or thrombosis. N Engl J Med 1973; 228:871-878. **34.** Petitti DB, Wingerd J. Use of oral contraceptives, cigarette smoking, and risk of subarachnoid hemorrhage. Lancet 1978; 2:234-236. **35.** Inman WH, Oral contraceptives and fatal subarachnoid hemorrhage. Br Med J 1979:2(6203):1468-1470. **36.** Collaborative Group for the Study of Stroke in Young Women: Oral Contraceptives and stroke in young women: associated risk factors. JAMA 1975; 231:718-722. **37.** Inman WH, Vessey MP, Westerholm, Engelund A. Thromboembolic disease and the steroidal content of oral contraceptives. A report to the Committee on Safety of Drugs. Br Med J 1970; 2:203-209. **38.** Meade TW, Greenberg G, Thompson SG. Progestogens and cardiovascular reactions associated with oral contraceptives and a comparison of the safety of 50- and 35-mcg oestrogen preparations. Br Med J 1980; 280(6224):1157-1161. **39.** Kay CR. Progestogens and arterial disease-evidence from the Royal College of General Practitioners' Study. Am J Obstet Gynecol 1982; 142:762-765. **40.** Royal College of General Practitioners: Incidence of arterial disease among oral contraceptive users. J Royal Coll Gen Pract 1983; 33:75-82. **41.** Ory HW. Mortality associated with fertility and fertility control: 1983. Family Planning Perspectives 1983;15:50-56. **42.** The Cancer and Steroid Hormone Study of the Centers for Disease Control and the National Institute of Child Health and Human Development: Oral contraceptive use and the risk of breast cancer. N Engl J Med 1986; 315:405-411. **43.** Pike MC, Henderson BE, Krailo MD, Duke A, Roy S. Breast cancer in young women and use of oral contraceptives: possible modifying effect of formulation and age at use. Lancet 1983; 2:926-929. **44.** Paul C, Skegg DG, Spears GFS, Kaldor JM. Oral contraceptives and breast cancer: A national study. Br Med J 1986; 293-723-725. **45.** Miller DR. Rosenberg L, Kaufman DW, Schottenfeld D, Stolley PD, Shapiro S. Breast cancer risk in relation to early oral contraceptive use. Obstet Gynecol 1986; 68: 863-868. **46.** Olson H, Olson KL Moller TR, Ranstam J, Holm P. Oral contraceptive use and breast cancer in young women in Sweden (letter). Lancet 1985; 2:748-749. **47.** McPherson K, Vessey M, Neil A, Doll R, Jones L, Roberts M. Early contraceptive use and breast cancer: Results of another case-control study. Br J Cancer 1987; 56:653-660. **48.** Higgins GR, Zucker PF. Oral contraceptives and neoplasia; 1987 update. Fertil Steril 1987; 47: 733-761. **49.** McPherson K, Drife JO. The pill and breast cancer: why the uncertainty? Br Med J 1986; 293:709-710. **50.** Shapiro S. Oral contraceptives - time to take stock N Engl J Med 1987; 315:450-451. **51.** Ory H, Naib Z, Conger SB, Hatcher RA, Tyler CW. Contraceptive choice and prevalence of cervical dysplasia and carcinoma in situ. Am J Obstet Gynecol 1976; 124:573-577. **52.** Vessey MP, Lawless M, McPherson K, Yeates D. Neoplasia of the cervix uteri and contraception: a possible adverse effect of the pill. Lancet 1983; 2:930. **53.** Brinton LA, Huggins GR, Lehman HF, Malli K. Savitz DA, Trapido E, Rosenthal J, Hoover R. Long term use of oral contraceptives and risk of invasive cervical cancer. Int J Cancer 1986; 38:339-344. **54.** WHO Collaborative Study of Neoplasia and Steroid Contraceptives: Invasive cervical cancer and combined oral contraceptives. Br Med J 1985; 290:961-965. **55.** Rooks JB, Ory HW, Ishak KG, Strauss LT, Greenspan JR, Hill AP, Tyler CW. Epidemiology of hepatocellular adenoma: the role of oral contraceptive use. JAMA 1979; 242:644-648. **56.** Bein NN, Goldsmith HS. Recurrent massive hemorrhage from benign hepatic tumors secondary to oral contraceptives. Br J Surg 1977; 64:433-435. **57.** Klatskin G. Hepatic tumors: possible relationship to use of oral contraceptives. Gastroenterology 1977; 73:386-394. **58.** Henderson BE, Preston-Martin S, Edmondson HA, Peters RL, Pike MC. Hepatocellular carcinoma and oral contraceptives. Br J Cancer 1983; 48:437-440. **59.** Neuberger J, Forman D, Doll R, Williams R Oral contraceptives. Br J Cancer 1986; 292:1355-1357. **60.** Forman D, Vincent TJ, Doll R Cancer of the liver and oral contraceptives. Br Med J 1986; 292-1357-1361. **61.** Harlap S, Eldor J. Births following oral contraceptive failures. Obstet Gynecol 1980; 55:447-452. **62.** Savolainen E, Saksela E, Sakelsa E, Saxen L. Teratogenic hazards of oral contraceptives analyzed in a national malformation register. Am J Obstet Gynecol 1981; 140:521-524. **63.** Janerich DT, Piper JM, Glebatis DM. oral contraceptives and birth defects. Am J Epidemiol 1980; 112:73-79. **64.** Ferencz C, Matanoski GM, Wilson PD, Rubin JD, Neill CA, Gutberlet R. Maternal hormone therapy and congenital heart disease. Teratology 1980; 21:225-239. **65.** Rothman KJ, Fyler DC, Goldblatt A, Kreidberg MB. Exogenous hormones and other drug exposures of children with congenital heart disease. Am J Epidemiol 1979; 109:433-439. **66.** Boston Collaborative Drug Surveillance Program: Oral contraceptives and venous thromboembolic disease, surgically confirmed gallbladder disease, and breast tumors. Lancet 1973; 1:1399-1404. **67.** Royal College of General Practitioners: Oral contraceptives and health. New York, Pittman 1974. **68.** Layde PM, Vessey MP, Yeates D. Risk of gallbladder disease: a cohort study of young women attending family planning clinics. J Epidemiol Community Health 1982; 36:274-278. **69.** Rome Group for Epidemiology and Prevention of Cholelithiasis (GREPCO): Prevalence of gallstone disease in an Italian adult female population. Am J Epidemiol 1984; 119:796-805. **70.** Storm BL, Tamragouri RT, Morse ML, Lazar EL, West SL, Stolley PD Jones JK. Oral contraceptives and other risk factors for gallbladder disease. Clin Pharmacol Ther 1986; 39:335-341. **71.** Wynn V. Adams PW, Godsland IF, Melrose J, Niththyananthan R, Oakley NW, Seedj A. Comparison of effects of different combined oral contraceptive formulations on carbohydrate and lipid metabolism. Lancet 1979; 1:1045-1049. **72.** Wynn V. Effect of progesterone and progestins on carbohydrate metabolism. In: Progesterone and Progestin. Bardin CW, Milgrom E, Mauvis-Jarvis P. eds. New York, Raven Press 1983; pp. 395-410. **73.** Perlman JA, Roussell-Briefel RG, Ezzati TM, Lieberknecht G. Oral glucose tolerance and the potency of oral contraceptive progestogens. J Chronic Dis 1985; 38:857-864. **74.** Royal College of General Practitioners' Oral Contraception Study: Effect on hypertension and benign breast disease of progestogen component in combined oral contraceptives. Lancet 1977; 1:624. **75.** Fisch IR, Frank J. Oral contraceptives and blood pressure. JAMA 1977; 237:2499- 2503. **76.** Laragh AJ. Oral contraceptive induced hypertension— nine years later. Am J obstet Gynecol 1976; 126:141-147. **77.** Ramcharan S, Peritz E, Pellegrin FA, Williams WT. Incidence of hypertension in the Walnut Creek Contraceptive Drug Study cohort: In Pharmacology of steroid contraceptive drugs. Garattini S, Berendes HW. Eds. New York, Raven Press, 1977; pp. 277-288 (Monographs of the Mario Negri Institute for Pharmacological Research Milan). **78.** Stockley I. Interactions with oral contraceptives. J Pharm 1976; 216:140-143. **79.** The Cancer and Steroid Hormone Study of the Centers for Disease Control and the National Institute of Child Health and Human Development: Oral contraceptive use and risk of ovarian cancer. JAMA 1983; 249:1596-1599. **80.** The Cancer and Steroid Hormone Study of the Centers for Disease Control and the National Institute of Child Health and Human Development: Combination oral contraceptive use and the risk of endometrial cancer. JAMA 1987; 257:796-800. **81.** Ory HW Functional ovarian cysts and oral contraceptives: negative association confirmed surgically. JAMA 1974; 228:68-69. **82.** Ory HW, Cole P, MacMahon B, Hoover R. Oral contraceptives and reduced risk of benign breast disease. N Engl J Med 1976; 294:419-422. **83.** Ory HW, The noncontraceptive health benefits from oral contraceptive use. Fam Plann Perspect 1982; 14:182-184. **84.** Ory HW, Forrest RR, JD, Lincoln R. Making choices: Evaluating the health risks and benefits of birth control methods. New York, The Alan Guttmacher Institute, 1983; p.1. **85.** Miller DR, Rosenberg L, Kaufman DW, Stolley P, Warshauer ME, Shapiro S. Breast cancer before age 45 and oral contraceptive use: New Findings. Am J Epidemiol 1989; 129:269-280. **86.** Kay CR, Hannaford PC. Breast cancer and the pill - A further report from the Royal College Of General Practitioners' Oral Contraception Study. Br J Cancer 1988; 58:675-680. **87.** Stadel BV, Lai S, Schlesselman JJ, Murray P. Oral contraceptives and premenopausal breast cancer in nulliparous women. Contraception 1988; 38:287-299. **88.** The UK National Case-Control Study Group, Oral contraceptive use and breast cancer risk in young women. Lancet 1989; 1:973-982.

PATIENT PACKAGE INSERT:

BRIEF SUMMARY

This product (like all other contraceptives) is intended to prevent pregnancy. it does not protect against hiv infection (aids) and other sexually transmitted diseases.

Oral contraceptives, also known as "birth control pills" or "the pill", are taken to prevent pregnancy, and when taken correctly, have a failure rate of about 1% per year when used without missing any pills. The typical failure rate of large numbers of pill users is less than

CLINICAL PHARMACOLOGY: *(cont'd)*

3% per year when women who miss pills are included. For most women, oral contraceptives are also free of serious or unpleasant side effects. However, forgetting to take pills considerably increases the chances of pregnancy.

For the majority of women, oral contraceptives can be taken safely. But there are some women who are at high risk of developing certain serious diseases that can be life-threatening or may cause temporary or permanent disability. The risks associated with taking oral contraceptives increase significantly if you:

Smoke

Have high blood pressure, diabetes, high cholesterol

Have or have had clotting disorders, heart attack, stroke, angina pectoris, cancer of the breast or sex organs, jaundice or malignant or benign liver tumors

Although cardiovascular disease risks may be increased with oral contraceptive use after age 40 in healthy, non-smoking women (even with newer low-dose formulations), there are also greater potential health risks associated with pregnancy in older women.

You should not take the pill if you suspect you are pregnant or have unexplained vaginal bleeding.

Cigarette smoking increases the risk of serious cardiovascular side effects from oral contraceptive use. This risk increases with age and with heavy smoking (15 or more cigarettes per day) and is quite marked in women over 35 years of age. Women who use oral contraceptives are strongly advised not to smoke.

Most side effects of the pill are not serious. The most common such effects are nausea, vomiting, bleeding between menstrual periods, weight gain, breast tenderness, headache, and difficulty wearing contact lenses. These side effects, especially nausea, vomiting and breakthrough bleeding, may subside within the first three months of use.

The serious side effects of the pill occur very infrequently, especially if you are in good health and are young. However, you should know that the following medical conditions have been associated with or made worse by the pill:

1. Blood clots in the legs (thrombophlebitis), lungs (pulmonary embolism), stoppage or rupture of a blood vessel in the brain (stroke), blockage of blood vessels in the heart (heart attack or angina pectoris), or other organs of the body. As mentioned above, smoking increases the risk of heart attacks and strokes and subsequent serious medical consequences.

2. Liver tumors, which may rupture and cause severe bleeding. A possible but not definite association has been found with the pill and liver cancer. However, liver cancers are extremely rare. The chance of developing liver cancer from using the pill is thus even rarer.

3. High blood pressure, although blood pressure usually returns to normal when the pill is stopped.

The symptoms associated with these serious side effects are discussed in the detailed leaflet given to you with your supply of pills. Notify your doctor or health care professional if you notice any unusual physical disturbances while taking the pill. In addition, drugs such as rifampin, as well as some anticonvulsants and some antibiotics may decrease oral contraceptive effectiveness.

Most of the studies to date on breast cancer and pill use have found no increase in the risk of developing breast cancer although some studies have reported an increased risk of developing cancer in certain groups of women. However, some studies have found an increase in the risk of developing cancer of the cervix in women taking the pill, but this finding may be related to differences in sexual behavior or other factors not related to use of the pill. Therefore, there is insufficient evidence to rule out the possibility that the pill may cause cancer of the breast or cervix.

Taking the combination pill provides some important non-contraceptive benefits. These include less painful menstruation, less menstrual blood loss and anemia, fewer pelvic infections, and fewer cancers of the ovary and the lining of the uterus.

Be sure to discuss any medical condition you may have with your health care provider. Your health care provider will take a medical and family history and examine you before prescribing oral contraceptives. The physical examination may be delayed to another time if you request it and your health care provider believes that it is a good medical practice to postpone it. You should be reexamined at least once a year while taking oral contraceptives. The detailed patient information labeling gives you further information which you should read and discuss with your health care provider.

DETAILED PATIENT LABELING

This product (like all oral contraceptives) is intended to prevent pregnancy. it does not protect against transmission of HIV (AIDS) and other sexually transmitted diseases such as chlamydia, genital herpes, genital warts, gonorrhea, hepatitis B, and syphilis.

What You Should Know About Oral Contraceptives: Any woman who considers using oral contraceptives (the "birth control pill" or "the pill") should understand the benefits and risks of using this form of birth control. This patient labeling will give you much of the information you will need to make this decision and will also help you determine if you are at risk of developing any of the serious side effects of the pill. It will tell you how to use the pill properly so that it will be as effective as possible. However, this labeling is not a replacement for a careful discussion between you and your health care provider. You should discuss the information provided in this labeling with him or her, both when you first start taking the pill and during your revisits. You should also follow your doctor's or clinic's advice with regard to regular check-ups while you are on the pill.

Effectiveness of Oral Contraceptives: Oral contraceptives or "birth control pills" or "the pill" are used to prevent pregnancy and are more effective than other non-surgical methods of birth control. When they are taken correctly, the chance of becoming pregnant is less than 1% (1 pregnancy per 100 women per year of use) when used perfectly, without missing any pills. Typical failure rates are actually 3% per year. The chance of becoming pregnant increases with each missed pill during a menstrual cycle.

In comparison, typical failure rates for other nonsurgical methods of birth control during the first year of use are as follows:

Implant (6 capsules): <1%	Male Sterilization: <1%
Injection: <1%	Cervical Cap: 18 to 36%
IUD: <1% to 2%	Condom alone (male): 12%
Diaphragm with spermicides: 18%	Condom alone (female): 21%
Spermicides alone: 21%	Periodic abstinence: 20%
Vaginal Sponge: 18 to 36%	Withdrawal: 19%
Female Sterilization: <1%	No method: 85%

CLINICAL PHARMACOLOGY: *(cont'd)*

Who Should Not Take Oral Contraceptives

Cigarette smoking increases the risk of serious cardiovascular side effects from oral contraceptive use. This risk increases with age and with heavy smoking (15 or more cigarettes per day) and is quite marked in women over 35 years of age. Women who use oral contraceptives are strongly advised not to smoke.

Some women should not use the pill. For example, you should not take the pill if you are pregnant or think you may be pregnant. You should also not use the pill if you have any of the following conditions:

A history of heart attack or stroke

Blood clots in the legs (thrombophlebitis), lungs (pulmonary embolism), or eyes

A history of blood clots in the deep veins of your legs

Chest pain (angina pectoris)

Known or suspected breast cancer or cancer of the lining of the uterus, cervix or vagina

Unexplained vaginal bleeding (until a diagnosis is reached by your doctor)

Yellowing of the whites of the eyes or of the skin (jaundice) during pregnancy or during previous use of the pill

Liver tumor (benign or cancerous)

Known or suspected pregnancy

Tell your health care provider if you have ever had any of these conditions. Your health care provider can recommend another method of birth control.

Other Considerations Before Taking Oral Contraceptives: Tell your doctor or clinic if you have:

Breast nodules, fibrocystic disease of the breast, an abnormal breast x-ray or mammogram

Diabetes

Elevated cholesterol or triglycerides

High blood pressure

Migraine or other headaches or epilepsy

Mental depression

Gallbladder, heart or kidney disease

History of scanty or irregular menstrual periods

Women with any of these conditions should be checked often by their doctor or clinic if they choose to use oral contraceptives.

Also, be sure to inform your doctor or clinic if you smoke or are on any medications.

Risks Of Taking Oral Contraceptives

Risk Of Developing Blood Clots: Blood clots and blockage of blood vessels are one of the most serious side effects of taking oral contraceptive; in particular, a clot in the leg can cause thrombophlebitis, and a clot that travels to the lungs can cause a sudden blocking of the vessel carrying blood to the lungs. Rarely, clots occur in the blood vessels of the eye and may cause blindness, double vision, or impaired vision.

If you take oral contraceptives and need elective surgery, need to stay in bed for a prolonged illness or have recently delivered a baby, you may be at risk of developing blood clots. You should consult your doctor or clinic about stopping oral contraceptives three to four weeks before surgery and not taking oral contraceptives for two weeks after surgery or during bed rest. You should also not take oral contraceptives soon after delivery of a baby. It is advisable to wait for at least four weeks after delivery if you are not breast feeding or four weeks after a second trimester abortion. If you are breast feeding, you should wait until you have weaned your child before using the pill. See also General Precautions, While Breast Feeding.

The risk of circulatory disease in oral contraceptive users may be higher in users of high dose pills and may be greater with longer duration of oral contraceptive use. In addition, some of these increased risks may continue for a number of years after stopping oral contraceptives. The risk of abnormal blood clotting increases with age in both users and nonusers of oral contraceptives, but the increased risk from the oral contraceptive appears to be present at all ages. For women aged 20 to 44 it is estimated that about 1 in 2,000 using oral contraceptives will be hospitalized each year because of abnormal clotting. Among non-sers in the same age group, about 1 in 20,000 would be hospitalized each year. For oral contraceptive users in general, it has been estimated that in women between the ages of 15 and 34 the risk of death due to a circulatory disorder is about 1 in 12,000 per year, whereas for non-users the rate is about 1 in 50,000 per year. In the age group 35 to 44, the risk is estimated to be about 1 in 2,500 per year for oral contraceptive users and about 1 in 10,000 per year for non-users.

Heart Attacks And Strokes: Oral contraceptives may increase the tendency to develop strokes (stoppage or rupture of blood vessels in the brain) and angina pectoris and heart attacks (blockage of blood vessels in the heart). Any of these conditions can cause death or serious disability.

Smoking greatly increases the possibility of suffering heart attacks and strokes. Furthermore, smoking and the use of oral contraceptives greatly increase the chances of developing and dying of heart disease.

Gallbladder Disease: Oral contraceptive users probably have a greater risk than non-users of having gallbladder disease, although this risk may be related to pills containing high doses of estrogens.

Liver Tumors: In rare cases, oral contraceptives can cause benign but dangerous liver tumors. These benign liver tumors can rupture and cause fatal internal bleeding. In addition, a possible but not definite association has been found with the pill and liver cancers in two studies, in which a few women who developed these very rare cancers were found to have used oral contraceptives for long periods. However, liver cancers are rare. The chancee of developing liver cancer from using the pill is thus even rarer.

Cancer Of The Reproductive Organs And Breasts: There is, at present, no confirmed evidence that oral contraceptive use increases the risk of deleopling cancer of the reproductive organs. Studies to date of women taking the pill have reported conflicting findings on whether pill use increases the risk of develloping cancer of the breast or cervix. Most of the studies on breast cancer and pill use have found no overall increase in the risk of developing breast cancer although some studies have reported an increased risk of developing breast cancer in certain groups of women. Women who use oral contraceptives and have a strong family history of breast cancer or who have breast nodules or abnormal mammograms should be closelt follwed by their doctors.

Some studies have found an increase in the incidence of cancer of the cervix in women who use oral contraceptives. However, this finding may be related to factors other than the use of oral contraceptives.

Estimated Risk Of Death From A Birth Control Method Or Pregnancy

All methods of birth control and pregnancy are associated with a risk of developing certain diseases which may lead to disability or death. An estimate of the number of deaths associated with different methods of birth control and pregnancy has been calculated and is shown in TABLE 2.

PATIENT PACKAGE INSERT: *(cont'd)*

In TABLE 2, the risk of death from any birth control method is less than the risk of childbirth, except for oral contraceptive users over the age of 35 who smoke and pill users over the age of 40 even if they do not smoke. It can be seen in the table that for women aged 15 to 39, the risk of death was highest with pregnancy (7-26 deaths per 100,000 women, depending on age). Among pill users who do not smoke, the risk of death is always lower than that associated with pregnancy for any age group, although over the age of 40, the risk increases to 32 deaths per 100,000 women, compared to 28 associated with pregnancy at that age. However, for pill users who smoke and are over the age of 35, the estimated number of deaths exceeds those for other methods of birth control. If a woman is over the age of 40 and smokes, her estimated risk of death is four times higher (117/100,000 women) than the estimated risk associated with pregnancy (28/100,000 women) in that age group.

The suggestion that women over 40 who do not smoke should not take oral contraceptives is based on information from older higher-dose pills and on less selective use of pills than is practiced today. An Advisory Committee of the FDA discussed this issue in 1989 and recommended that the benefits of low-dose oral contraceptive use by healthy, non-smoking women over 40 years of age may outweigh the possible risks. However, all women, especially older women, are cautioned to use the lowest dose pill that is effective.

Warning Signals: If any of these adverse effects occur while you are taking oral contraceptives, call your doctor or clinic immediately:

Sharp chest pain, coughing of blood, or sudden shortness of breath (indicating a possible clot in the lung)

Pain in the calf (indicating a possible clot in the leg)

Crushing chest pain or heaviness in the chest (indicating a possible heart attack)

Sudden severe headache or vomiting, dizziness or fainting, disturbances of vision or speech, weakness, or numbness in an arm or leg (indicating a possible stroke)

Sudden partial or complete loss of vision (indicating a possible clot in the eye)

Breast lumps (indicating possible breast cancer or fibrocystic disease of the breast; ask your doctor or health care provider to show you how to examine your breasts)

Severe pain or tenderness in the stomach area (indicating a possibly ruptured liver tumor)

Difficulty in sleeping, weakness, lack of energy, fatigue, or change in mood (possibly indicating severe depression)

Jaundice or a yellowing of the skin or eyeballs, accompanied frequently by fever, fatigue, loss of appetite, dark colored urine, or light colored bowel movements (indicating possible liver problems)

Side Effects Of Oral Contraceptives

1. Vaginal Bleeding: Irregular vaginal bleeding or spotting may occur while you are taking the pills. Irregular bleeding may vary from slight staining between menstrual periods to breakthrough bleeding which is a flow much like a regular period. Irregular bleeding occurs most often during the first few months of oral contraceptive use, but may also occur after you have been taking the pill for some time. Such bleeding may be temporary and usually does not indicate any serious problems. It is important to continue taking your pills on schedule. If the bleeding occurs in more than one cycle or lasts more than a few days, talk to your doctor or health care provider.

2. Contact Lenses: If you wear contact lenses and notice a change in vision or an inability to wear your lenses, contact your doctor or clinic.

3. Fluid Retention: Oral contraceptives may cause edema (fluid retention) with swelling of the fingers or ankles and may raise your blood pressure. If you experience fluid retention, contact your doctor or health care provider.

4. Melasma: A spotty darkening of the skin is possible, particularly of the face.

5. Other Side Effects: Other side effects may include change in appetite, headache, nervousness, depression, dizziness, loss of scalp hair, rash, and vaginal infections.

If any of these side effects bother you, call your doctor or health care provider.

General Precautions

Missed Periods And Use Of Oral Contraceptives Before Or During Early Pregnancy: There may be times when you may not menstruate regularly after you have completed taking a cycle of pills. If you have taken your pills regularly and miss one menstrual period, continue taking your pills for the next cycle but be sure to inform your doctor or health care provider before doing so. If you have not taken the pills daily as instructed and missed a menstrual period or if you have missed two consecutive menstrual periods, you may be pregnant. Check with your health care provider immediately to determine whether you are pregnant. Do not continue to take oral contraceptives until you are sure you are not pregnant, but continue to use another method of contraception.

There is no conclusive evidence that oral contraceptive use is associated with an increase in birth defects, when taken inadvertently during early pregnancy. Previously, a few studies had reported that oral contraceptives might be associated with birth defects, but these studies have not been confirmed. Nevertheless, oral contraceptives or any other drugs should not be used during pregnancy unless clearly necessary and prescribed by your doctor. You should check with your doctor or clinic about risks to your unborn child of any medication taken during pregnancy.

While Breast Feeding: If you are breast feeding, consult your doctor or clinic before starting oral contraceptives. Some of the drug will be passed on to the child in the milk. A few adverse effects on the child have been reported, including yellowing of the skin (jaundice) and breast enlargement. In addition, oral contraceptives may decrease the amount and quality of your milk. If possible, do not use oral contraceptives while breast feeding. You should use another method of contraception since breast feeding provides only partial protection from becoming pregnant and this partial protection decreases significantly as you breast feed for longer periods of time. You should consider starting oral contraceptives only after you have weaned your child completely.

Laboratory Tests: If you are scheduled for any laboratory tests, tell your doctor you are taking birth control pills. Certain blood tests may be affected by birth control pills.

Drug Interactions: Certain drugs may interact with birth control pills to make them less effective in preventing pregnancy or cause an increase in breakthrough bleeding. Such drugs include rifampin, drugs used for epilepsy such as barbiturates (for example, phenobarbital), phenytoin (Dilantin is one brand of this drug), phenylbutazone (Butazolidin is one brand), and possibly certain antibiotics. You may need to use additional contraception when you take drugs which can make oral contraceptives less effective.

INSTRUCTIONS TO THE PATIENT

These are general instructions. Package configuartions and pill colors vary from product to product.

This product (like all oral contraceptives) is intended to prevent pregnancy. it does not protect against transmission of HIV (AIDS) and other sexually transmitted diseases such as chlamydia, genital herpes, genital warts, gonorrhea, hepatitis B, and syphilis.

How To Take The Pill-Important Points To Remember

Before You Start Taking Your Pills:

1. Be Sure To Read These Directions: Before you start taking your pills. Anytime you are not sure what to do.

PATIENT PACKAGE INSERT: *(cont'd)*

2. The right way to take the pill is to take one pill every day at the same time. If you miss pills you could get pregnant. This includes starting the pack late. The more pills you miss, the more likely you are to get pregnant.

3. Many women have spotting or light bleeding, or may feel sick to their stomach during the first 1-3 packs of pills. If you do have spotting or light bleeding or feel sick to your stomach, do not stop taking the pill. The problem will usually go away. If it doesn't go away, check with your doctor or clinic.

4. Missing pills can also cause spotting or light bleeding , even when you make up these missed pills. On the days you take 2 pills to make up for missed pills, you could also feel a little sick to your stomach.

5. If you have vomiting or diarrhea, for any reason, or if you take some medicines, including some antibiotics, your pills may not work as well. Use a back-up method (such as condoms, foam, or sponge) until you check with your doctor or clinic.

6. If you have trouble remembering to take the pill, talk to your doctor or clinic about how to make pill-taking easier or about using another method of birth control.

7. If you have any questions or are unsure about the information in this leaflet, call your doctor or clinic.

Before You Start Taking Your Pills:

1. Decide what time of day you want to take your pill. It is important to take it about the same time every day.

2. Look at your pill pack to see if it has 21 or 28 pills:

The **21-pill pack** has 21 "active" pills (with hormones) to take for 3 weeks, followed by 1 week without pills.

The **28-pill pack** has 21 "active" pills (with hormones) to take for 3 weeks, followed by 1 week of reminder pills (without hormones).

3. Also find:

A) Where on the pack to start taking pills,

B) In what order to take the pills (follow the arrows) and

C) The week numbers printed on the pack.

4. Be sure you have ready at all times:

Another kind of birth control (such as condoms or foam) to use as a back-up in case you miss pills.

An extra full pill pack.

When To Start The First Pack Of Pills:

You may have a choice of which day to start taking your first pack of pills. Decide with your doctor or clinic which is the best day for you. Pick a time of day which will be easy to remember.

Day 1 Start:

1. Pick the day label strip that starts with the first day of your period (this is the day you start bleeding or spotting, even if it is almost midnight when the bleeding begins).

2. Place this day label strip in the cycle tablet dispenser over the area that has the days of the week (starting with Sunday) imprinted in the plastic. Note: If the first day of your period is a Sunday, you can skip steps #1 AND #2. Note: If the first day of your period is a Sunday, you can skip steps and #2.

3. Take the first "active" [white] pill of the first pack during the first 24 hours of your period.

4. You will not need to use a back-up method of birth control, since you are starting the pill at the beginning of your period.

Sunday Start:

1. Take the first "active" pill of the first pack on the Sunday after your period starts, even if you are still bleeding. If your period begins on Sunday, start the pack that same day.

2. Use another method of birth control as a back-up method if you have sex anytime from the Sunday you start your first pack until the next Sunday (7 days). Condoms or foam are good back-up methods of birth control.

What To Do During The Month:

1. Take one pill at the same time every day until the pack is empty. Do not skip pills even if you are spotting or bleeding between monthly periods or feel sick to your stomach (nausea). Do not skip pills even if you do not have sex very often.

2. When You Finish A Pack Or Switch Your Brand Of Pills:

21 pills: Wait 7 days to start the next pack. You will probably have your period during that week. Be sure that no more than 7 days pass between 21-day packs.

28 pills: Start the next pack on the day after your last "reminder" pill. Do not wait any days between packs.

What To Do If You Miss Pills:

If you **MISS 1** "active" pill:

1. Take it as soon as you remember. Take the next pill at your regular time. This means you take 2 pills in 1 day.

2. You do not need to use a back-up birth control method if you have sex.

If you **MISS 2** "active" pills in a row in **WEEK I OR WEEK 2** of your pack:

1. Take 2 pills on the day you remember and 2 pills the next day.

2. Then take 1 pill a day until you finish the pack.

3. You COULD GET PREGNANT if you have sex in the **7 days** after you miss pills. You MUST use another birth control method (such as condoms or foam) as a back-up method of birth control until you have taken an "active" pill every day for 7 days.

If you **MISS 2** "active" pills in a row in the **3RD WEEK:**

1a. If you are a Day 1 Starter: THROW OUT the rest of the pill pack and start a new pack that same day.

1b. If you are a Sunday Starter:

Keep taking 1 pill every day until Sunday.

On Sunday, THROW OUT the rest of the pack and start a new pack of pills that same day.

2. You may not have your period this month but this is expected. However, if you miss your period 2 months in a row, call your doctor or clinic because you might be pregnant.

3. You COULD GET PREGNANT if you have sex in the **7 days** after you miss pills. You MUST use another birth control method (such as condoms or foam) as a back-up method of birth control until you have taken an "active" pill every day for 7 days.

If you **MISS 3 OR MORE** "active" pills in a row (during the first 3 weeks).

1a. If you are a Day 1 Starter: THROW OUT the rest of the pill pack and start a new pack that same day.

1b. If you are a Sunday Starter:

Keep taking 1 pill every day until Sunday.

On Sunday, THROW OUT the rest of the pack and start a new pack of pills that same day.

PATIENT PACKAGE INSERT: *(cont'd)*

2. You may not have your period this month but this is expected. However, if you miss your period 2 months in a row, call your doctor or clinic because you might be pregnant.

3. You COULD GET PREGNANT if you have sex in the **7 days** after you miss pills. You MUST use another birth control method (such as condoms or foam) as a back-up method of birth control until you have taken an "active" pill every day for 7 days.

A Reminder For Those On 28-Day Packs:

If you forget any of the 7 "reminder" pills in Week 4:

THROW AWAY the pills you missed.

Keep taking 1 pill each day until the pack is empty.

You do not need a back-up method.

Finally, If You Are Still Not Sure What To Do About The Pills You Have Missed:

Use a back-up method anytime you have sex.

Keep taking one "active" pill each day until you can reach your doctor or clinic.

Pregnancy Due To Pill Failure: The incidence of pill failure resulting in a pregnancy is approximately 1% (*i.e.*, one pregnancy per 100 women per year) if taken every day as directed, but more typical failure rates are about 3%. If failure does occur, the risk to the fetus is minimal.

Pregnancy After Stopping The Pill: There may be some delay in becoming pregnant after you stop using oral contraceptives, especially if you had irregular menstrual cycles before you used oral contraceptives. It may be advisable to postpone conception until you begin menstruating regularly once you have stopped taking the pill and desire pregnancy.

There does not appear to be any increase in birth defects in newborn babies when pregnancy occurs soon after stopping the pill.

Overdosage: Serious ill effects have not been reported following ingestion of large doses of oral contraceptives by young children. Overdosage may cause nausea and withdrawal bleeding in females. In case of overdosage, contact your health care provider or pharmacist.

Other Information: Your doctor or clinic will take a medical and family history and examine you before prescribing oral contraceptives. The physical examination may be delayed to another time if you request it and your health care provider believes it is a good medical practice to postpone it. You should be reexamined at least once a year. Be sure to inform your health care provider if there is a family history of any of the conditions listed previously in this leaflet. Be sure to keep all appointments with your health care provider because this is a time to determine if there are early signs of side effects of oral contraceptive use.

Do not use the drug for any condition other than the one for which it was prescribed. This drug has been prescribed specifically for you; do not give it to others who may want birth control pills.

Health Benefits From Oral Contraceptives

In addition to preventing pregnancy, use of combination oral contraceptives may provide certain benefits. They are:

Menstrual cycles may become more regular

Blood flow during menstruation may be lighter and less iron may be lost. Therefore, anemia due to iron deficiency is less likely to occur.

Pain or other symptoms during menstruation may be encountered less frequently.

Ectopic (tubal) pregnancy may occur less frequently.

Noncancerous cysts or lumps in the breast may occur less frequently.

Acute pelvic inflammatory disease may occur less frequently.

Oral contraceptive use may provide some protection against developing two forms of cancer: cancer of the ovaries and cancer of the lining of the uterus.

If you want more information about birth control pills, ask your doctor, clinic or pharmacist. They have a more technical leaflet called the "Professional Labeling", which you may wish to read.

Remembering to take tablets according to schedule is stressed because of its importance in providing you the greatest degree of protection.

Missed Menstrual Periods for Both Dosage Regimens

At times there may be no menstrual period after a cycle of pills. Therefore, if you miss one menstrual period but have taken the pills exactly as you were supposed to, continue as usual into the next cycle. If you have not taken the pills correctly and miss a menstrual period, you may be pregnant and should stop taking oral contraceptives until your doctor or health care provider determines whether or not you are pregnant. Until you can get to your doctor, use another method of contraception. If two consecutive menstrual periods are missed, you should stop taking pills until it is determined whether or not you are pregnant. Although there does not appear to be any increase in birth deffects in newborn babies, if you become pregnant while using oral contraceptives, you should discuss the situation with your doctor or health care provider.

Periodic Examination: Your doctor or health care provider will take a complete medical and family history before prescribing oral contraceptives. At that time and about once a year thereafter, he or she will generally examine your blood pressure, breasts, abdomen, and pelvic organs (including a Papanicolanou smear [*i.e.*, test for cancer]).

(Parke-Davis, 96/10)

HOW SUPPLIED - RATED THERAPEUTICALLY EQUIVALENT:

Tablet, Uncoated - Oral - 0.035 mg/0.5 &

126 (6 x 21)	**$152.16**	**ORTHO-NOVUM 10/11 21, Ortho Pharm**	**00062-1770-15**
168 (6 x 28)	$83.80	Nelova, Warner Chilcott	00047-0944-35
168 (6 x 28)	**$153.12**	**ORTHO-NOVUM 10/11 28, Ortho Pharm**	**00062-1771-15**

Tablet, Uncoated - Oral - 0.035 mg/0.5 mg

21's	$8.45	Norethindrone/Ethin Estradiol, H.C.F.A. F F P	99999-1220-01
28's	$11.27	Norethindrone/Ethin Estradiol, H.C.F.A. F F P	99999-1220-02
28's	$23.28	MODICON 28, Ortho Pharm	00062-1714-20
63 (3 x 21)	$69.52	BREVICON 21, Syntex FP	42987-0108-13
84 (3 x 28)	$57.60	Genora, Rugby	00536-4057-48
84 (3 x 28)	$69.52	BREVICON 28, Syntex FP	42987-0110-14
126 (6 x 21)	$152.16	MODICON 21, Ortho Pharm	00062-1712-15
168 (6 x 28)	$90.30	Nelova, Warner Chilcott	00047-0926-35
168 (6 x 28)	$110.29	JENEST 28, Organon	00052-0269-06
168 (6 x 28)	$153.12	MODICON 28, Ortho Pharm	00062-1714-15
672 (24 x 28)	$539.26	BREVICON 28, Syntex FP	42987-0110-61

Tablet, Uncoated - Oral - 0.035 mg/1 mg

21's	$8.03	Norethindrone/Ethin Estradiol, H.C.F.A. F F P	99999-1220-03
28's	$10.71	Norethindrone/Ethin Estradiol, H.C.F.A. F F P	99999-1220-04
63 (3 x 21)	$52.50	Genora, Rugby	00536-4058-44
126 (6 x 21)	$72.00	Norethin 1/35, Roberts Labs	54092-0071-21
126 (6 x 21)	$90.30	Nelova, Warner Chilcott	00047-0930-11
126 (6 x 21)	$134.79	NORINYL 1/35 21, Syntex FP	42987-0109-23
126 (6 x 21)	**$138.84**	**ORTHO-NOVUM 1/35 21, Ortho Pharm**	**00062-1760-15**
168 (6 x 28)	$72.00	Norethin 1/35E, Roberts Labs	54092-0071-28
168 (6 x 28)	$90.30	Nelova, Warner Chilcott	00047-0927-35

HOW SUPPLIED - RATED THERAPEUTICALLY EQUIVALENT: *(cont'd)*

168 (6 x 28)	$105.00	Genora 1/35 28, Rugby	00536-4055-48
168 (6 x 28)	$133.34	NORINYL 1/35 28, Syntex FP	42987-0111-28
168 (6 x 28)	$134.79	NORINYL 1/35 28, Syntex FP	42987-0111-24
168 (6 x 28)	**$139.62**	**ORTHO-NOVUM 1/35 28, Ortho Pharm**	**00062-1761-15**
672 (24 x 28)	$539.26	NORINYL 1/35 28, Syntex FP	42987-0111-61

HOW SUPPLIED - NOT RATED EQUIVALENT:

Tablet, Uncoated - Oral - 0.035 mg/0.4 mg

126 (6 x 21)	$152.19	OVCON-35 21, Bristol Myers Squibb	00087-0583-42
168 (6 x 28)	$152.19	OVCON-35 28, Bristol Myers Squibb	00087-0578-41

Tablet, Uncoated - Oral - 0.035 mg/0.5, 0

126 (6 x 21)	**$139.74**	**ORTHO-NOVUM 7/7/7 21, Ortho Pharm**	**00062-1780-15**
168 (6 x 28)	**$140.46**	**ORTHO-NOVUM 7/7/7 28, Ortho Pharm**	**00062-1781-15**
252 (12 x 21)	**$277.08**	**ORTHO-NOVUM 7/7/7 21, Ortho Pharm**	**00062-1780-22**
336 (12 x 28)	**$278.76**	**ORTHO-NOVUM 7/7/7 28, Ortho Pharm**	**00062-1781-22**

Tablet, Uncoated - Oral - 0.035 mg/0.5 &

126 (6 x 21)	$128.16	TRI-NORINYL 21, Syntex FP	42987-0114-27
126 (6 x 21)	$129.56	TRI-NORINYL 21, Syntex FP	42987-0114-23
168 (6 x 28)	$128.16	TRI-NORINYL 28, Syntex FP	42987-0115-28
168 (6 x 28)	$129.56	TRI-NORINYL 28, Syntex FP	42987-0115-24
672 (24 x 28)	$549.41	TRI-NORINYL 28, Syntex FP	42987-0115-61

Tablet, Uncoated - Oral - 0.05 mg/1 mg

21 x 6	$158.29	OVCON-50, Bristol Myers Squibb	00087-0584-42
28 x 6	$167.93	OVCON-50 28, Bristol Myers Squibb	00087-0579-41

ETHINYL ESTRADIOL; NORETHINDRONE ACETATE *(003315)*

CATEGORIES: Contraceptives; Hormones; Ovarian Carcinoma; Pregnancy; Progestogen; Progestogen & Estrogen Combinations; Pregnancy Category X; Sales > $500 Million; Top 200 Drugs; FDA Approval Pre 1982

BRAND NAMES: Loestrin 21; Estrostep 21; Norlestrin 21; Norelestrin 28

DESCRIPTION:

These products are progestogen-estrogen combinations.

The chemical name for norethindrone is (17alpha-ethinyl-19-nortestosterone acetate). The name for ethinyl estradiol is (17 alpha-ethinyl-1,3,5(10)-estratriene-3,17 beta-diol)

Loestrin: Each white tablet contains norethindrone acetate (17 alpha-ethinyl-19-nortestosterone acetate), 1 mg; ethinyl estradiol (17 alpha-ethinyl-1,3,5(10)-estratriene-3, 17 beta-diol), 20 mcg. Also contains acacia, NF; lactose, NF; magnesium stearate, NF; starch, NF; confectioner's sugar, NF; talc, USP.

Each green tablet contains norethindrone acetate (17 alpha-ethinyl-19-nortestosterone acetate), 1.5 mg; ethinyl estradiol (17 alpha-ethinyl-1,3,5(10)-estratriene-3, 17 beta-diol), 30 mcg. Also contains acacia, NF; lactose, NF; magnesium stearate, NF; starch, NF; confectioner's sugar, NF; talc, USP; D&C yellow No. 10; FD&C yellow No. 6; FD&C blue No. 1.

Norlestrin: Each yellow tablet contains norethindrone acetate 1 mg; ethinyl estradiol 50 mcg. Also contains acacia, NF; lactose, NF; magnesium stearate, NF; starch, NF; confectioner's sugar, NF; talc, USP; D&C yellow No. 10; FD&C yellow No. 6.

Each pink tablet contains norethindrone acetate 2.5 mg; ethinyl estradiol 50 mcg. Also contains acacia, NF; lactose, NF; magnesium stearate, NF; starch, NF; confectioner's sugar, NF; talc, USP; FD&C red No. 40.

Each brown tablet contains microcrystalline cellulose, NF; ferrous fumarate, USP; magnesium stearate, NF; povidone, USP; sodium starch glycolate, NF; sucrose with modified dextrins.

Each white tablet contains magnesium stearate, NF and sucrose with modified dextrins.

Estrostep: Each white triangular tablet contains 1 mg norethindrone acetate and 20 mcg ethinyl estradiol; each white square tablet contains 1 mg norethindrone acetate and 30 mcg ethinyl estradiol; each white round tablet contains 1 mg norethindrone acetate and 35 mcg ethinyl estradiol.

Each Estrostep Fe tablet dispenser contains 5 white triangular tablets, seven white square tablets, nine white round tablets and seven brown tablets. These tablets are to be taken in the following order: one triangular tablet each day for five days, followed by one square tablet each day for seven days; and then one round tablet each day for nine days.

For prescribing information refer to Ethinyl Estradiol; Norethindrone.

HOW SUPPLIED - EQUIVALENTS NOT AVAILABLE:

Tablet, Uncoated - Oral - 0.02 mg/1 mg

105 (5 x 21)	$132.52	LOESTRIN 1/20 21, Parke-Davis	00071-0915-47

Tablet, Uncoated - Oral - 0.03 mg/1.5 mg

105 (5 x 21)	$132.52	LOESTRIN 1.5/30 21, Parke-Davis	00071-0916-47
630 (30 x 21)	$795.05	LOESTRIN 1.5/30 21, Parke-Davis	00071-0916-15

ETHINYL ESTRADIOL; NORGESTIMATE *(003270)*

CATEGORIES: Acne Vulgaris; Contraceptives; Hormones; Pregnancy; Progestogen & Estrogen Combinations; Pregnancy Category X; FDA Approved 1989 Dec

BRAND NAMES: *Cilest* (Germany, England, France, Mexico); **Ortho Cyclen**; Ortho Cyclen 21; Ortho Cyclen 28; Ortho Tri-Cyclen; Ortho Tri-Cyclen 21; Ortho Tri-Cyclen 28

(International brand names outside U.S. in italics)

FORMULARIES: PCS

DESCRIPTION:

The chemical name for norgestimate is (18, 19-Dinor-17-pregn-4-en-20-yn-3-one, 17-(acetyloxy)-13-ethyl-oxime, (17α)-(+)-). The chemical name for ethinyl estradiol is (19-nor-17α-pregna,1,3,5(10)-trien-20-yne-3, 17-diol).

Ortho Cyclen: Each blue tablet contains 0.250 mg of the progestational compound norgestimate and 0.035 mg of the estrogenic compound, ethinyl estradiol. Inactive ingredients include FD&C Blue No. 2 Aluminum Lake, lactose, magnesium stearate, and pregelitanized starch.

Each green tablet in the Ortho Cyclen 28 package contains only inert ingredients, as follows: D&C Yellow No. 10 Aluminum Lake, FD&C Blue No. 2 Aluminum Lake, lactose, magnesium stearate, microcrystalline cellulose and pregelitanized starch.

DESCRIPTION: *(cont'd)*

Ortho Tri-Cyclen: Each white tablet contains 0.180 mg of the progestational compound norgestimate and 0.035 mg of the estrogenic compound, ethinyl estradiol. Inactive ingredients include lactose, magnesium stearate, and pregelitanized starch.

Each light blue tablet contains 0.215 mg of the progestational compound norgestimate and 0.035 mg of the estrogenic compound, ethinyl estradiol. Inactive ingredients include FD&C Blue No. 2 Aluminum Lake, lactose, magnesium stearate, and pregelitanized starch.

Each blue tablet contains 0.250 mg of the progestational compound norgestimate and 0.035 mg of the estrogenic compound, ethinyl estradiol. Inactive ingredients include FD&C Blue No. 2 Aluminum Lake, lactose, magnesium stearate, and pregelitanized starch.

Each green tablet in the Ortho Cyclen 28 package contains only inert ingredients, as follows: D&C Yellow No. 10 Aluminum Lake, FD&C Blue No. 2 Aluminum Lake, lactose, magnesium stearate, microcrystalline cellulose and pregelitanized starch.

For contraceptive prescribing information refer to Ethinyl Estradiol; Norethindrone.

HOW SUPPLIED - EQUIVALENTS NOT AVAILABLE:

Tablet, Uncoated - Oral - 0.035 mg/0.18,

126 (6 x 21)	$139.74	ORTHO TRI-CYCLEN 21, Ortho Pharm	00062-1902-15
168 (6 x 28)	$140.46	ORTHO TRI-CYCLEN 28, Ortho Pharm	00062-1903-15

Tablet, Uncoated - Oral - 0.035 mg/0.25 m

126 (6 x 21)	$139.74	ORTHO-CYCLEN 21, Ortho Pharm	00062-1900-15
168 (6 x 28)	$140.46	ORTHO-CYCLEN 28, Ortho Pharm	00062-1901-15

ETHINYL ESTRADIOL; NORGESTREL *(001222)*

CATEGORIES: Contraceptives; Contraceptives, Emergency*; Hormones; Pregnancy; Progestogen & Estrogen Combinations; Abortion*; Pregnancy Category X; Sales > $100 Million; FDA Approval Pre 1982; Top 200 Drugs
* Indication not approved by the FDA

BRAND NAMES: *Cilest*; *Daphiron*; *Duoluton* (Germany, Mexico, Japan); *Eugynon* (Mexico); *Eugynon 21* (Germany); *Eugynon 28* (Germany); *Eugynon 30*; *Femenal*; **Lo Ovral**; *Min-Ovral* (Canada); *Ovral* (Mexico, Canada); *Planovar* (Japan); *Stediril* (Germany, France)
(International brand names outside U.S. in italics)

FORMULARIES: Aetna; BC-BS; DoD; Medi-Cal; PCS

COST OF THERAPY: $362.65 (Contraceptive; Tablet; 0.03 mg/0.3 mg; 1/day; 365 days) vs. Potential Cost of $2,351.94 (Pregnancy)

DESCRIPTION:

Ovral-28: 21 white Ovral-28 tablets, each containing 0.5 mg of norgestrel (*dl*-13-beta-ethyl-17-alpha-ethinyl-17-beta-hydroxygon-4-en-3-one), a totally synthetic progestogen, and 0.05 mg of ethinyl estradiol (19-nor-17α-pregna-1,3,5 (10)-trien-20-yne-3,17-diol), and 7 pink inert tablets. The inactive ingredients present are cellulose, D&C Red 30, lactose, magnesium stearate, and polacrilin potassium.

Lo/Ovral-28: 21 white Lo/Ovral-28 tablets, each containing 0.3 mg of norgestrel (*dl*-13-beta-ethyl-17-alpha-ethinyl-17-beta-hydroxygon-4-en-3-one), a totally synthetic progestogen, and 0.03 mg of ethinyl estradiol (19-nor-17α-pregna-1,3,5 (10)-trien-20-yne-3,17- diol), and 7 pink inert tablets. The inactive ingredients present are cellulose, lactose, magnesium stearate, and polacrilin potassium.

For prescribing information refer to Ethinyl Estradiol; Norethindrone.

FDA RECOMMENDED DOSAGE GUIDELINES FOR POSTCOITAL EMERGENCY CONTRACEPTION

The FDA has declared oral contraceptives safe and effective for emergency contraception. Vomiting, sometimes severe enough to prevent the pills from working, and nausea are potential side effects. The dosing regimens for ethinyl estradiol/norgestrel can be taken within 72 hours of unprotected intercourse with a follow-up dose of the same number of pills 12 hours after the first dose:

Ovral: Two white tablets

Lo/Ovral: Four white tablets

HOW SUPPLIED - EQUIVALENTS NOT AVAILABLE:

Tablet, Uncoated - Oral - 0.03 mg/0.3 mg

126 (6 x 21)	**$164.92**	**LO/OVRAL, Wyeth Labs**	**00008-0078-01**
168 (6 x 28)	**$166.92**	**LO/OVRAL 28, Wyeth Labs**	**00008-2514-02**

Tablet, Uncoated - Oral - 0.05 mg/0.5 mg

21's	$32.90	OVRAL, Wyeth Labs	00008-0056-02
126 (6 x 21)	$252.72	OVRAL, Wyeth Labs	00008-0056-01
168 (6 x 28)	$255.54	OVRAL 28, Wyeth Labs	00008-2511-02

ETHIODIZED OIL *(001223)*

CATEGORIES: Diagnostic Agents; Hysterosalpingography; Iodine Deficiency; Lymphography; Roentgenography; FDA Approval Pre 1982

BRAND NAMES: **Ethiodol**

DESCRIPTION:

Ethiodized oil injection contains 37% iodine in organic combination with the ethyl esters of the fatty acids of poppyseed oil. Ethiodized Oil is a straw to amber colored, oily fluid, which because of simplified molecular structure, possesses a greatly reduced viscosity (1.280 specific gravity at 15 deg. C yield viscosity of 0.5 - 1.0 poise). This high fluidity provides a new flexibility for radiographic exploration.

INDICATIONS AND USAGE:

Ethiodized Oil is indicated for use in the radiographic exploration for hysterosalpingography and lymphography. Not recommended for bronchography.

HYSTEROSALPINGOGRAPHY

1. In detecting patency or non-patency of the tubes.
2. In the determination and localization of occlusion of the tubes.
3. In the visualization and orientation of the uterine cavity, including internal os.
4. In the diagnosis of intra-uterine tumors.
5. In demonstrating other abnormalities of the uterine and tubal cavities (uterine subinvolution, infantile uterus, tubal kinks).
6. In the diagnosis and localization of ectopic pregnancy.
7. As an aid in the diagnosis of abdominal pregnancy.

INDICATIONS AND USAGE: *(cont'd)*

8. In checking the results of plastic operations on the tubes.
9. In determining whether a tube or the uterus in the region of the pelvic mass is or is not an integral part of the mass.
10. As an indication for hysterectomy for fibroids in preference to myomectomy in cases in which the tubes can be shown to be occluded.

GENERAL INDICATIONS FOR LYMPHOGRAPHY

The intralymphatic injection of Ethiodized Oil permits study of the dynamics of the lymphatic system and radiographic demonstration of lymph vessels and lymph nodes. Following cannulization and injection of a lymphatic in the lower extremity, the nodes in the inguinal, external iliac, common iliac and para-aortic areas, as well as the thoracic duct and supraclavicular nodes, are roentgenographically visualized. When the injection is made in a lymphatic of the hand, the axillary and supraclavicular nodes are demonstrated. Ethiodized Oil (ethiodized oil injection) lymphography has been found useful in the detection and evaluation of abnormalities of the lymphatic system and as a guide to lymph node dissection. When radiation therapy is indicated, more accurate placement of the ports is achieved. The delayed elimination of ethiodol (ethiodized oil injection) makes possible assessment of response to either chemotherapeutic or radiotherapeutic treatment.

SPECIFIC INDICATIONS FOR LYMPHOGRAPHY

1. The evaluation of edema of the extremities in situations where neoplasia is suspect.
2. The detection and evaluation of the nature and extent of neoplastic diseases which involve the lymphatic system and as a corollary in a differential diagnosis of intra-abdominal masses.
3. The determination of abnormalities in the thoracic duct, such as manifested by chylothorax and chyloperitoneum.
4. The evaluation of surgical, chemotherapeutic and radiation treatment of neoplastic diseases.
5. As a guide to lymph node dissection.
6. More accurate portal placement in the radiation therapy of lymphomata and carcinoma.

CONTRAINDICATIONS:

Ethiodized Oil is contraindicated in patients hypersensitive to it. Ethiodized Oil should not be injected intrathecally or intravascularly.

Hysterosalpingography is contraindicated in intrauterine pregnancy, acute pelvic inflammatory disease, in the presence of intrauterine bleeding or within 30 days of curettage or conization.

Lymphography is contraindicated in patients with a right to left cardiac shunt, in patients with advanced pulmonary disease, especially those with alveolar-capillary block, and in patients who have had radiotherapy to the lungs.

WARNINGS:

Ethiodized Oil is not intended for use in bronchography and, therefore, is not to be introduced into the bronchial tree. A history of sensitivity to iodine or to other contrast materials is not an absolute contraindication to Ethiodized Oil, but calls for extreme caution. Since iodine-containing contrast materials may alter the results of certain thyroid function tests, such tests, if indicated, should be performed prior to the administration of this drug. Safety in pregnancy has not been established.

LYMPHOGRAPHY

The use of intralymphatic Ethiodized Oil presents a significant hazard in patients with pre-existing pulmonary disease characterized by a decrease in pulmonary diffusing capacity and/or pulmonary blood flow. A few fatalities have been noted in such patients. With reference to this potential complication, recent studies indicate a significant decrease in both pulmonary difusing capacity and pulmonary capillary blood flow following Ethiodized Oil lymphography without appreciable concomitant clinical manifestations. Also, care should be exercised in patients with other types of pulmonary diseases in view of the more frequent incidence of overt pulmonary complications such as pulmonary infarction, in these groups. However, it is to be noted that pulmonary infarction, although rare, has occurred in patients without evidence of pre-existing pulmonary disease.

The safety of intralymphatic Ethiodized Oil has not been established in pregnant women, and accordingly, its use should be restricted to such situations were it is deemed necessary.

PRECAUTIONS:

HYSTEROSALPINGOGRAPHY

Pulmonary embolization of the contrast material may occur if hysterosalpingography is performed under conditions which may lead to intravasation of the contrast materials. These conditions include uterine bleeding, recent curettage or conization and injection of the contrast material under excessive pressure.

Facilities for emergency treatment of hypersensitivity reactions should be immediately available.

LYMPHOGRAPHY

Although subclinical pulmonary embolization occurs in a majority of patients following Ethiodized Oil lymphography, clinical evidence of such embolization is infrequent and is usually of a transient nature. Such clinical manifestations are usually immediate, but may be delayed from a few hours to days. It would appear that it is advantageous to use the smallest volume of Ethiodized Oil necessary for radiographic visualization. For this reason, and to prevent inadequate venous administration, radiographic monitoring of patients is recommended during the injection of Ethiodized Oil.

The timing and choice of anesthesia following Ethiodized Oil injection may be influenced by consideration of the above noted decrease in pulmonary and capillary blood flow and diffusing capacity. It should be noted that although an average of 2 to 3 days was required for complete reversibility for such tests, an occasional patient required up to 12 days to return to baseline values.

PBI determination or thyroid uptake studies should be carried out prior to the lymphographic procedure because interference with these tests may be anticipated for as long as one year. In the presence of known iodine sensitivity, Ethiodized Oil lymphography should be carried out with greatest precaution.

ADVERSE REACTIONS:

HYSTEROSALPINGOGRAPHY

Hypersensitivity reactions, foreign body reactions and exacerbation of pelvic inflammatory disease, although infrequent, have been reported. Transient abdominal pain may occur following injection.

LYMPHOGRAPHY

The occasional observation of pulmonary Ethiodized Oil embolization (infarction) several hours after injection has been reported. This was noticed more frequently when excessive amounts of Ethiodized Oil (ethiodized oil injection) have been injected, in the presence of marked lymphatic obstruction or through accidental intravenous injection. Radiologic manifestations are fine, granular, stippling throughout both lung fields. The clinical symptoms

ADVERSE REACTIONS: *(cont'd)*

usually noted have been mild, consisting of moderate temperature elevation, dyspnea, and cough. However, severe acute symptoms developed in two patients both of whom were severely ill and required extensive care. Fuchs experienced 1 severe and 3 minor complications in a series of 20 bilateral procedures. Two are described by the author as cardiovascular collapse occurring at two hours respectively following the completion of the procedure. It was postulated that minute emboli may have been causative. Recovery was rapid and complete in both instances.

The occurrence of pulmonary invasion may be minimized if radiographic confirmation of intralymphatic (rather than venous) injection is secured, and the procedure discontinued when the medium becomes visible in the thoracic duct or the presence of lymphatic obstruction is noticed.

While rare, other side effects reported include transient fever, lymphangitis, iodism (headache, soreness of mouth and pharynx, coryza and skin rash), allergic dermatitis, and lipogranuloma formation. Delayed wound healing at the site of incision and secondary infection are occasionally seen, and can be prevented or minimized by adhering to a strict sterile technique.

Transient edema or temporary exacerbation of preexisting lymphedema, as well as thrombophlebitis have also been reported.

In the extremely rare presence of concomitant lymphatic and inferior vena cava obstruction the contrast medium may be shunted partially to the liver, resulting in hepatic embolization. Also, when accidental intravenous administration of Ethiodized Oil results in a considerable amount of this medium entering the circulation, embolization other than pulmonary may occur as reported in 2 cases. Both cases developed a transient, psychotic like manifestation, which in all probability stemmed from the entrance of fine oil droplets into the cerebral circulation. Recovery was uneventful and complete without evidence of neurological sequelae.

DOSAGE AND ADMINISTRATION:

HYSTEROSALPINGOGRAPHY

The hysterosalpingogram is preferably taken during the patient's preovulatory phase (as determined from her basal body temperature record) and not less than two days after cessation of her menstrual flow. It has been frequently observed that some bleeding will occur during or after the onset of pregnancy which cannot be distinguished by the patient from a normal menstrual period. In such cases a basal body temperature record will reveal a sustained high temperature phase, and thus enable an operator to avoid hysterosalpingography when a pregnancy may exist. Salpingography should not be performed if the blood is exuding from the cervical os (which occasionally occurs without the patient being aware of it) or if any gross evidence of endocervicitis exists.

Careful aseptic technique should be employed as for any operative procedure in which the uterus is entered. A self-retaining cannula should be used thereby permitting removal of the vaginal speculum so that the outline of the cervical canal may be seen in the film. The use of a radio-opaque aluminum speculum may be employed in patients where a lacerated or patulous cervix does not permit the use of a retaining cannula.

The radio-opaque agent is introduced under pressure and preferably with fluoroscopic control. A preliminary film is exposed and a skiagram is made after the injection of 5 ml of the agent. The pressure is raised to 80-90 mm Hg. In cases of normal bilateral tubal patency, the pressure falls immediately to below 60 mm Hg. The wet film may be viewed immediately and if both tubes are seen to "fill," the apparatus is removed and the procedure is finished, except for the 24-hour follow-up to establish whether or not "spill" into the peritoneal cavity had occurred.

If both tubes do not "fill," further increments of 2 ml of the agent are injected and successive films exposed until tubal patency is established or until the patient's limit of tolerance to discomfort is reached. It may be observed in cases of unilateral tubal patency that the pressure does not fall below 90 mm Hg. and may rise to above 100 mm Hg. before it begins to fall. Few patients will complain of discomfort at pressures under 200 mm Hg.

In an occasional patient, abdominal pains may occur. Such pains may be the result of tubal torsion, or possibly due to too rapid a rate of instillation or excessive pressure, or both. The condition is usually only transitory, lasting one to two hours at most, and may be relieved by the administration of any of the commonly used analgesics.

LYMPHOGRAPHY

This method applies for both the upper and lower extremities. A lymphatic vessel is selected for cannulization.

The patient should be comfortably arranged in a supine position on a portable stretcher or an x-ray table. When available, a radiolucent pad will add to the patient's comfort during the one to two hours required for completion of the examination. It is important that the patient be in a cooperative state. Premedication might be advisable in the unusually apprehensive patient.

In the unusually restless patient, the extremities should be immobilized during the entire procedure to prevent displacement of the needle. Thomas splits have been satisfactorily employed for the legs and simple arms boards for the upper extremities.

The cut-down and injection instruments and materials include the following: Sterile pediatric cut-down set.

Sterile towels for draping, sponges, etc.

Local anesthetic, such as procaine hydrochloride, and a syringe.

Bactericidal painting solution.

20 ml syringe containing 15 ml of Ethiodized Oil with an 18" catheter to which is affixed a 27 or 30 gauge needle. (If bilateral lymphography is scheduled, two syringes should be prepared.)

A manually driven or motorized unit (a pressure regulated pump) to provide for slow injection.

Under local infiltration anesthesia, a transverse, curvilinear or longitudinal small skin incision should be made near the ankle or wrist (just lateral and distal to the first metatarsal head on the dorsum of the foot, or just above the "snuff-box" in the dorsum of the hand).

Upon superficial dissection (but not penetrating the subcutaneous layer of tissue) lymph vessels will be noted in the immediate subcutaneous tissue, while larger lymph vessel trunks are found in the extrafascial plane. The deeper lymph trunks will be easier to cannulate.

One lymph vessel is then exposed, avoiding circumferential dissection. The less manipulation performed, the better the results that will be obtained. The lymphatic, thus isolated, is then cannulated with a 27 or 30 gauge 5/8" needle, depending on the size of the lymphatic selected for injection. It is rarely possible to cannulate with a needle greater than 27 gauge. Insertion of the needle through the skin flap before cannulating the lymphatics serves to reduce movement of the needle within the vessel. Additional security of the needle in the lymphatic is obtained by strapping, with sterile tape, the polyethylene tubing to the patient's foot.

The injection should be started at a slow rate, i.e., 0.1 ml to 0.2 ml per minute. Radiographic monitoring either by fluoroscopy or serial radiographs after 1 ml to 2 ml has been injected, will confirm the proper intralymphatic placement of the needle, and rule out accidental intravenous injection or extravasation of the medium by perforation or rupture of the

DOSAGE AND ADMINISTRATION: *(cont'd)*

lymphatic. Monitoring will also permit prompt termination of the procedure in the event that lymphatic blockage is present. In such situations, continuation of the injection will result in unnecessary introduction of contrast material into the venous system via the lymphovenous communication channels. If the injection is satisfactory, approximately 6 to 8 ml, are then injected.

However, as soon as it becomes radiographically evident that Ethiodized Oil (ethiodized oil injection) has entered the thoracic duct, the procedure should be terminated to minimize entry of the contrast material into the sub-clavian vein. Two to four ml of Ethiodized Oil injected into the upper extremity will suffice to demonstrate the axillary and supraclavicular nodes. In penile lymphography approximately 2 to 3 ml Ethiodized Oil is required. In infants and children, a minimum of 1 ml to a maximum of 6 ml should be employed.

The rate of speed at which the contrast material may be introduced varies and is dependent upon the receptivity of the lymphatics in the individual patient. If the injection is proceeding at too rapid a rate extravasation will be noted and the patient may refer to pain in the foot, leg or arm.

At the completion of the injection, anteroposterior roentgenograms are obtained of the legs or arms, thighs, pelvis, abdomen and chest (dorsal spine technique). Lateral or oblique views as well as laminograms are obtained when indicated. Follow-up films at 24 or 48 hours provide better demonstration of lymph nodes and permit more concise evaluation of nodal architecture.

As a general rule, the smallest possible amount of Ethiodized Oil should be employed according to the anatomical area to be visualized.

Therefore, and to prevent inadvertent venous administration, fluoroscopic monitoring or serial radiographic guidance of patients is recommended during the injection of Ethiodized Oil.

Average dose in the adult patient for unilateral lymphography of the upper extremities is 2 to 4 ml; of lower extremities 6 to 8 ml; of penile lymphography 2 to 3 ml, of cervical lymphography 1 to 2 ml.

In the pediatric patient, a minimum of 1 ml to a maximum of 6 ml may be employed according to the anatomical area to be visualized.

Summary Of Steps To Avoid Complications In Lymphography

1. Contraindicate patients:

A. With a known hypersensitivity to Ethiodized Oil.

B. With a right to left cardiac shunt.

C. With advanced pulmonary disease, especially those with alveolar-capillary block. Pulmonary gas diffusion studies should be done if in doubt.

D. Who have had radiation therapy to the lungs.

2. Contraindicate Relatively:

A. Patients having markedly advanced neoplastic disease with expected lymphatic obstruction.

B. Patients having undergone previous surgery interrupting the lymphatic system.

C. Patients having had deep radiation therapy to the examined area. If in these relatively contraindicated cases lymphography is still necessary, a smaller dose of oily contrast medium with protracted injection time with less pressure and careful monitoring is required.

3. Skin testing should be done on all patients before submitting them to lymphography. Be aware of possible hypersensitivity to local anesthetics and skin disinfectants. Careful history taking is important.

4. Technique of Cannulation: Extravasation is to be avoided and/or detected early. The injection site should be included on the "scout film" or observed under image amplification fluoroscopy. The needle tip must remain visible in the incision wound.

5. Oily Contrast Materials: Once opened, vials should be discarded. Vials of ethiodol should not be used if the color has darkened. The average dose for each foot in an adult is 5-6 ml; one-half as much for the upper extremity. The amount for children should be determined by careful monitoring. It should stay below 0.25 ml/kg.

6. Injection pressure should be regulated to deliver the average dose in less than 1 1/4 hours. Continuous monitoring helps to determine the speed most appropriate for each individual.

7. Scout Roentgenograms: If scout roentgenograms are used for monitoring, they should be developed and viewed immediately in order to apply corrective measures when needed. e.g., discontinuation of the study when one sees intravenous injection or lymphatic-venous anastomosis. Reduction of injection-speed is needed if evidence of collateral circulation occurs or if the higher abdominal-aortic nodes do not opacify in spite of usual injection pressure. This is highly suggestive of lymphatic obstruction. Scout roentgenograms should be taken more frequently in such cases.

8. Surgical Technique: Strict aseptic surgical technique is followed including the wearing of a face mask. Before suturing the incision wound, the remnants of the lymphatic vessels and loose tissue are removed and the wound well washed with saline to remove any possible oil. In case of reflux type lymphedema, the cannulated large lymphatic vessel may have to be closed by catgut to avoid development of a lymphocyst. The patient is instructed to elevate the legs as often as possible to promote healing. the sutures are removed from the feet on the 10th day, and on the 5th or 6th from the hands.

HOW SUPPLIED - EQUIVALENTS NOT AVAILABLE:

Injection, Solution - Misc - 37 %

10 ml x 2 $72.26 ETHIODOL, Savage Labs 00281-7062-37

ETHIONAMIDE *(001224)*

CATEGORIES: Anti-Infectives; Antimicrobials; Antimycobacterials; Antituberculosis Agents; Tuberculosis; FDA Approval Pre 1982

BRAND NAMES: *Ethatyl*; *Etiocidan*; *Myobid-250*; **Trecator-Sc**; *Tubermin* (Japan) *(International brand names outside U.S. in italics)*

COST OF THERAPY: $642.56 (Tuberculosis; Tablet; 250 mg; 2/day; 180 days)

PRIMARY ICD9: 011.93 (Pulmonary Tuberculosis, Unspecified, Tubercle Bacilli Found)

DESCRIPTION:

Trecator-SC (ethionamide) is used in the treatment of tuberculosis. The chemical name for ethionamide is 2-ethyl-thioisonicotinamide.

Ethionamide is a yellow, crystalline, nonhygroscopic compound with a faint-to-moderate sulfide odor. It is practically insoluble in water and ether but soluble in methanol and ethanol. It melts at about 162°C and is stable at ordinary temperatures and humidities.

DESCRIPTION: *(cont'd)*

Trecator-SC tablets contain 250 mg of ethionamide. The inactive ingredients present are acacia, calcium carbonate, carnauba wax, confectioners sugar, FD&C Yellow 6, gelatin, lactose, magnesium stearate, methylcellulose, pharmaceutical glaze, polacrilin potassium, povidone, sodium benzoate, sucrose, talc, titanium dioxide, and white wax.

CLINICAL PHARMACOLOGY:

Bacteriostatic against *Mycobacterium tuberculosis.*

INDICATIONS AND USAGE:

Failure after adequate treatment with primary drugs (*i.e.,* isoniazid, streptomycin, aminosalicylic acid) in any form of active tuberculosis. Ethionamide should only be given with other effective antituberculous agents.

CONTRAINDICATIONS:

Severe hypersensitivity.

Severe hepatic damage.

WARNINGS:

USE IN PREGNANCY

Teratogenic effects have been demonstrated in animals (rabbits, rats) receiving doses in excess of those recommended in humans. Use of the drug should be avoided during pregnancy or in women of childbearing potential unless the benefits outweigh its possible hazard.

USE IN CHILDREN

Optimum dosage for children has not been established. This, however, does not preclude use of the drug when its use is crucial to therapy.

PRECAUTIONS:

Pretreatment examinations should include *in vitro* susceptibility tests of recent cultures of *M. tuberculosis* from the patient as measured against ethionamide and the usual primary antituberculous drugs.

Determinations of serum transaminase (SGOT, SGPT) should be made prior to and every 2 to 4 weeks during therapy.

In patients with diabetes mellitus, management may be more difficult and hepatitis occurs more frequently.

Ethionamide may intensify the adverse effects of the other antituberculous drugs administered concomitantly. Convulsions have been reported, and special care should be taken, particularly when ethionamide is administered with cycloserine.

ADVERSE REACTIONS:

The most common side effect is gastrointestinal intolerance.

Other adverse effects similar to those seen with isoniazid have been reported: peripheral neuritis, optic neuritis, psychic disturbances (including mental depression), postural hypotension, skin rashes, thrombocytopenia, pellagralike syndrome, jaundice and/or hepatitis, increased difficulty in management of diabetes mellitus, stomatitis, gynecomastia, and impotence.

DOSAGE AND ADMINISTRATION:

Ethionamide should be administered with at least one other effective antituberculous drug.

Average Adult Dose: 0.5 gram to 1.0 gram/day in divided doses.

Concomitant administration of pyridoxine is recommended.

Keep tightly closed.

Dispense in tight container.

HOW SUPPLIED - EQUIVALENTS NOT AVAILABLE:

Tablet, Sugar Coated - Oral - 250 mg

100's $178.49 TRECATOR SC, Wyeth Labs 00008-4130-01

ETHOSUXIMIDE *(001226)*

CATEGORIES: Anticonvulsants; Central Nervous System Agents; Convulsions; Epilepsy; Neuromuscular; Seizures; Succinimide Anticonvulsants; FDA Approval Pre 1982

BRAND NAMES: *Emeside* (England); *Ethosuximide*; *Ethymal*; *Etosuximida*; *Petinamid*; *Petinimid* (Germany); *Petnidan* (Germany); *Pyknolepsinum* (Germany); *Simatin*; *Suximal*; *Suxinutin* (Germany); *Thosutin*; *Zarondan*; **Zarontin** *(International brand names outside U.S. in italics)*

FORMULARIES: Aetna; BC-BS; FHP; Medi-Cal; PCS; WHO

DESCRIPTION:

Zarontin (ethosuximide) is an anticonvulsant succinimide, chemically designated as alpha-ethyl-alpha-methyl-succinimide.

Each Zarontin capsule contains 250 mg ethosuximide, USP. Also contains: polyethylene glycol 400, NF. The capsule contains D&C yellow No. 10; FD&C red No. 3; gelatin, NF; glycerin, USP; and sorbitol.

CLINICAL PHARMACOLOGY:

Ethosuximide suppresses the paroxysmal three cycle per second spike and wave activity associated with lapses of consciousness which is common in absence (petit mal) seizures. The frequency of epileptiform attacks is reduced, apparently by depression of the motor cortex and elevation of the threshold of the central nervous system to convulsive stimuli.

INDICATIONS AND USAGE:

Zarontin is indicated for the control of absence (petit mal) epilepsy.

CONTRAINDICATIONS:

Ethosuximide should not be used in patients with a history of hypersensitivity to succinimides.

WARNINGS:

Blood dyscrasias, including some with fatal outcome, have been reported to be associated with the use of ethosuximide; therefore, periodic blood counts should be performed. Should signs and/or symptoms of infection (*e.g.,* sore throat, fever) develop, blood counts should be considered at that point.

WARNINGS: *(cont'd)*

Ethosuximide is capable of producing morphological and functional changes in the animal liver. In humans, abnormal liver and renal function studies have been reported.

Ethosuximide should be administered with extreme caution to patients with known liver or renal disease. Periodic urinalysis and liver function studies are advised for all patients receiving the drug.

Cases of systemic lupus erythematosus have been reported with the use of ethosuximide. The physician should be alert to this possibility.

Usage in Pregnancy: Reports suggest an association between the use of anticonvulsant drugs by women with epilepsy and an elevated incidence of birth defects in children born to these women. Data are more extensive with respect to phenytoin and phenobarbital, but these are also the most commonly prescribed anticonvulsants; less systematic or anecdotal reports suggest a possible similar association with the use of all known anticonvulsant drugs.

The reports suggesting an elevated incidence of birth defects in children of drug-treated epileptic women cannot be regarded as adequate to prove a definite cause and effect relationship. There are intrinsic methodological problems in obtaining adequate data on drug teratogenicity in humans; the possibility also exists that other factors, e.g., genetic factors or the epileptic condition itself, may be more important than drug therapy in leading to birth defects. The great majority of mothers on anticonvulsant medication deliver normal infants. It is important to note that anticonvulsant drugs should not be discontinued in patients in whom the drug is administered to prevent major seizures because of the strong possibility of precipitating status epilepticus with attendant hypoxia and threat to life. In individual cases where the severity and frequency of the seizure disorder are such that the removal of medication does not pose a serious threat to the patient, discontinuation of the drug may be considered prior to and during pregnancy, although it cannot be said with any confidence that even minor seizures do not pose some hazard to the developing embryo or fetus.

The prescribing physician will wish to weigh these considerations in treating or counseling epileptic women of childbearing potential.

PRECAUTIONS:

GENERAL:

Ethosuximide, when used alone in mixed types of epilepsy, may increase the frequency of grand mal seizures in some patients.

As with other anticonvulsants, it is important to proceed slowly when increasing or decreasing dosage, as well as when adding or eliminating other medication. Abrupt withdrawal of anticonvulsant medication may precipitate absence (petit mal) status.

INFORMATION FOR THE PATIENT:

Ethosuximide may impair the mental and/or physical abilities required for the performance of potentially hazardous tasks, such as driving a motor vehicle or other such activity requiring alertness; therefore, the patient should be cautioned accordingly.

Patients taking ethosuximide should be advised of the importance of adhering strictly to the prescribed dosage regimen.

Patients should be instructed to promptly contact their physician if they develop signs and/or symptoms (*e.g.,* sore throat, fever) suggesting an infection.

PREGNANCY:

See WARNINGS.

DRUG INTERACTIONS:

Since Zarontin (ethosuximide) may interact with concurrently administered antiepileptic drugs, periodic serum level determinations of these drugs may be necessary (*e.g.,* ethosuximide may elevate phenytoin serum levels and valproic acid has been reported to both increase and decrease ethosuximide levels).

ADVERSE REACTIONS:

Gastrointestinal System: Gastrointestinal symptoms occur frequently and include anorexia, vague gastric upset, nausea and vomiting, cramps, epigastric and abdominal pain, weight loss, and diarrhea. There have been reports of gum hypertrophy and swelling of the tongue.

Hemopoietic System: Hemopoietic complications associated with the administration of ethosuximide have included leukopenia, agranulocytosis, pancytopenia, with or without bone marrow suppression, and eosinophilia.

Nervous System: Neurologic and sensory reactions reported during therapy with ethosuximide have included drowsiness, headache, dizziness, euphoria, hiccups, irritability, hyperactivity, lethargy, fatigue, and ataxia. Psychiatric or psychological aberrations associated with ethosuximide administration have included disturbances of sleep, night terrors, inability to concentrate, and aggressiveness. These effects may be noted particularly in patients who have previously exhibited psychological abnormalities. There have been rare reports of paranoid psychosis, increased libido, and increased state of depression with overt suicidal intentions.

Integumentary System: Dermatologic manifestations which have occurred with the administration of ethosuximide have included urticaria, Stevens-Johnson syndrome, systemic lupus erythematosus, pruritic erythematous rashes, and hirsutism.

Special Senses: Myopia.

Genitourinary System: Vaginal bleeding, microscopic hematuria.

OVERDOSAGE:

Acute overdoses may produce nausea, vomiting, and CNS depression including coma with respiratory depression. A relationship between ethosuximide toxicity and its plasma levels has not been established. The therapeutic range of serum levels is 40 mcg/ml to 100 mcg/ml, although levels as high as 150 mcg/ml have been reported without signs of toxicity.

TREATMENT:

Treatment should include emesis (unless the patient is or could rapidly become obtunded, comatose, or convulsing) or gastric lavage, activated charcoal, cathartics and general supportive measures. Hemodialysis may be useful to treat ethosuximide overdose. Forced diuresis and exchange transfusions are ineffective.

DOSAGE AND ADMINISTRATION:

Zarontin is administered by the oral route. The *initial* dose for patients 3 to 6 years of age is one capsule (250 mg) per day; for patients 6 years of age and older, 2 capsules (500 mg) per day. The dose thereafter must be individualized according to the patient's response. Dosage should be increased by small increments. One useful method is to increase the daily dose by 250 mg every four to seven days until control is achieved with minimal side effects. Dosages exceeding 1.5 g daily, in divided doses, should be administered only under the strictest supervision of the physician. The *optimal* dose for most children is 20 mg/kg/day. This dose has given average plasma levels within the accepted therapeutic range of 40 to 100 mcg/ml. Subsequent dose schedules can be based on effectiveness and plasma level determinations.

Zarontin may be administered in combination with other anticonvulsants when other forms of epilepsy coexist with absence (petit mal). The*optimal* dose for most children is 20 mg/kg/day.

DOSAGE AND ADMINISTRATION: *(cont'd)*

Store below 30°C (86°F).

HOW SUPPLIED - RATED THERAPEUTICALLY EQUIVALENT:

Syrup - Oral - 250 mg

480 ml	$63.20	Ethosuximide, Copley Pharm	38245-0660-07
480 ml	**$79.21**	**ZARONTIN, Parke-Davis**	**00071-2418-23**

HOW SUPPLIED - NOT RATED EQUIVALENT:

Capsule, Gelatin - Oral - 250 mg

100's	**$75.30**	**ZARONTIN, Parke-Davis**	**00071-0237-24**

ETHOTOIN *(001227)*

CATEGORIES: Anticonvulsants; Central Nervous System Agents; Convulsions; Epilepsy; Hydantoin Anticonvulsants; Neuromuscular; Seizures; Tonic-Clonic Seizures; Pregnancy Category C; FDA Approval Pre 1982

BRAND NAMES: *Accenon (Japan)*; **Peganone**
(International brand names outside U.S. in italics)

DESCRIPTION:

Peganone (ethotoin tablets, USP) is an oral antiepileptic of the hydantoin series and is chemically identified as 3-ethyl-5-phenyl-2,4-imidazolidinedione.

Peganone tablets are available in two dosage strengths of 250 mg and 500 mg respectively.

INACTIVE INGREDIENTS

250 mg and 500 mg tablets: Acacia, lactose, sodium carboxymethylcellulose, stearic acid and talc.

CLINICAL PHARMACOLOGY:

Ethotoin exerts an antiepileptic effect without causing general central nervous system depression. The mechanism of action is probably very similar to that of phenytoin. The latter drug appears to stabilize rather than to raise the normal seizure threshold, and to prevent the spread of seizure activity rather than to abolish the primary focus of seizure discharges.

In laboratory animals, the drug was found effective against electroshock convulsions, & to a lesser extent, against complex partial (psychomotor) and pentylenetetrazol-induced seizures.

In mice, the duration of antiepileptic activity was prolonged by hepatic injury but not by bilateral nephrectomy; the drug is apparently biotransformed by the liver.

Ethotoin is fairly rapidly absorbed; the extent of oral absorption is not known. The drug exhibits saturable metabolism with respect to the formation of N-deethyl and p-hydroxyl-ethotoin, the major metabolites. Where plasma concentrations are below about 8 mcg/ml, the elimination half-life of ethotoin is in the range of 3 to 9 hours. A study comparing single doses of 500 mg, 1000 mg, and 1500 mg of ethotoin demonstrated that ethotoin, and to a lesser extent 5-phenylhydantoin, a major metabolite, exhibits substantial nonlinear kinetics. The degree of nonlinearity with multiple dosing may be increased over that seen after a single dose, given the likelihood of plasma accumulation based on a reported elimination half-life of 6 to 9 hours and a dosing interval of 4 to 6 hours. Experience suggests that therapeutic plasma concentrations fall in the range of 15 to 50 mcg/ml; however, this range is not as extensively documented as those quoted for other antiepileptics.

INDICATIONS AND USAGE:

Ethotoin is indicated for the control of tonic-clonic (grand mal) and complex partial (psychomotor) seizures.

CONTRAINDICATIONS:

Ethotoin is contraindicated in patients with hepatic abnormalities or hematologic disorders.

WARNINGS:

USAGE DURING PREGNANCY—THERE ARE MULTIPLE REPORTS IN THE CLINICAL LITERATURE WHICH INDICATE THAT THE USE OF ANTIEPILEPTIC DRUGS DURING PREGNANCY RESULTS IN AN INCREASED INCIDENCE OF BIRTH DEFECTS IN THE OFFSPRING. ALTHOUGH DATA ARE MORE EXTENSIVE WITH RESPECT TO TRIMETHADIONE, PARAMETHADIONE, PHENYTOIN, AND PHENOBARBITAL, REPORTS INDICATE A POSSIBLE SIMILAR ASSOCIATION WITH THE USE OF OTHER ANTIEPILEPTIC DRUGS. THEREFORE, ANTIEPILEPTIC DRUGS SHOULD BE ADMINISTERED TO WOMEN OF CHILD-BEARING POTENTIAL ONLY IF THEY ARE CLEARLY SHOWN TO BE ESSENTIAL IN THE MANAGEMENT OF THEIR SEIZURES.

ANTIEPILEPTIC DRUGS SHOULD NOT BE DISCONTINUED IN PATIENTS IN WHOM THE DRUG IS ADMINISTERED TO PREVENT MAJOR SEIZURES BECAUSE OF THE STRONG POSSIBILITY OF PRECIPITATING STATUS EPILEPTICUS WITH ATTENDANT HYPOXIA AND RISK TO BOTH MOTHER AND THE UNBORN CHILD. CONSIDERATION SHOULD, HOWEVER, BE GIVEN TO DISCONTINUATION OF ANTIEPILEPTICS PRIOR TO AND DURING PREGNANCY WHEN THE NATURE, FREQUENCY AND SEVERITY OF THE SEIZURES DO NOT POSE A SERIOUS THREAT TO THE PATIENT. IT IS NOT, HOWEVER, KNOWN WHETHER EVEN MINOR SEIZURES CONSTITUTE SOME RISK TO THE DEVELOPING EMBRYO FETUS.

REPORTS HAVE SUGGESTED THAT THE MATERNAL INGESTION OF ANTIEPILEPTIC DRUGS, PARTICULARLY BARBITURATES, IS ASSOCIATED WITH A NEONATAL COAGULATION DEFECT THAT MAY CAUSE BLEEDING DURING THE EARLY (USUALLY WITHIN 24 HOURS OF BIRTH) NEONATAL PERIOD. THE POSSIBILITY OF THE OCCURRENCE OF THIS DEFECT WITH THE USE OF PEGANONE SHOULD BE KEPT IN MIND. THE DEFECT IS CHARACTERIZED BY DECREASED LEVELS OF VITAMIN K-DEPENDENT CLOTTING FACTORS, AND PROLONGATION OF EITHER THE PROTHROMBIN TIME OR THE PARTIAL THROMBOPLASTIN TIME, OR BOTH. IT HAS BEEN SUGGESTED THAT VITAMIN K BE GIVEN PROPHYLACTICALLY TO THE MOTHER ONE MONTH PRIOR TO AND DURING DELIVERY, AND TO THE INFANT, INTRAVENOUSLY, IMMEDIATELY AFTER BIRTH. THE PHYSICIAN SHOULD WEIGH THESE CONSIDERATIONS IN TREATMENT AND COUNSELING OF EPILEPTIC WOMEN OF CHILD-BEARING POTENTIAL.

PRECAUTIONS:

General: Blood dyscrasias have been reported in patients receiving Peganone. Although the etiologic role of Peganone has not been definitely established, physicians should be alert for general malaise, sore throat and other symptoms indicative of possible blood dyscrasia.

PRECAUTIONS: *(cont'd)*

There is some evidence suggesting that hydantoin-like compounds may interfere with folic acid metabolism, precipitating a megaloblastic anemia. If this should occur during gestation, folic acid therapy should be considered.

Information for the Patient: Patients should be advised to report immediately such signs and symptoms as sore throat, fever, malaise, easy bruising, petechiae, epistaxis, or others that may be indicative of an infection or bleeding tendency.

Laboratory Tests: Liver function tests should be performed if clinical evidence suggests the possibility of hepatic dysfunction. Signs of liver damage are indication for withdrawal of the drug.

It is recommended that blood counts and urinalyses be performed when therapy is begun and at monthly intervals for several months thereafter. As in patients receiving other hydantoin compounds and other antiepileptic drugs, blood dyscrasias have been reported in patients receiving ethotoin. Marked depression of the blood count is indication for withdrawal of the drug.

Carcinogenesis: No data are available on long-term potential for carcinogenicity in animals or humans.

Pregnancy Category C: See WARNINGS.

Nursing Mothers: Ethotoin is excreted in breast milk. Because of the potential for serious adverse reactions in nursing infants from ethotoin, a decision should be made whether to discontinue nursing or to discontinue the drug, taking into account the importance of the drug to the mother.

DRUG INTERACTIONS:

Peganone used in combination with other drugs known to adversely affect the hematopoietic system should be avoided if possible.

Considerable caution should be exercised if Peganone is administered concurrently with *Phenurone (phenacemide)* since paranoid symptoms have been reported during therapy with this combination.

A two-way interaction between the hydantoin antiepileptic, *phenytoin* , and the *coumarin anticoagulants* has been suggested. Presumably, phenytoin acts as a stimulator of coumarin metabolism and has been reported to cause decreased serum levels of the coumarin anticoagulants and increased prothrombin-proconvertin concentrations. Conversely, the coumarin anticoagulants have been reported to increase the serum levels and prolong the serum half-life of phenytoin by inhibiting its metabolism. Although there is no documentation of such, a similar interaction between ethotoin and the coumarin anticoagulants may occur. Caution is therefore advised when administering Peganone to patients receiving coumarin anticoagulants.

ADVERSE REACTIONS:

Adverse reactions associated with Peganone, in decreasing order of severity, are:

Isolated cases of lymphadenopathy and systemic lupus erythematosus have been reported in patients taking hydantoin compounds, and lymphadenopathy has occurred with Peganone. Withdrawal of therapy has resulted in remission of the clinical and pathological findings. Therefore, if a lymphoma-like syndrome develops, the drug should be withdrawn and the patient should be closely observed for regression of signs and symptoms before treatment is resumed.

Ataxia and gum hypertrophy have occurred only rarely-usually only in patients receiving an additional hydantoin derivative. It is of interest to note that ataxia and gum hypertrophy have subsided in patients receiving other hydantoins when ethotoin was given as a substitute antiepileptic.

Occasionally, vomiting or nausea after ingestion of Peganone has been reported, but if the drug is administered after meals, the incidence of gastric distress is reduced. Other side effects have included chest pain, nystagmus, diplopia, fever, dizziness, diarrhea, headache, insomnia, fatigue, numbness, and skin rash.

OVERDOSAGE:

Symptoms of acute overdosage include drowsiness, visual disturbance, nausea and ataxia. Coma is possible at very high dosage.

Treatment should be begun by inducing emesis; gastric lavage may be considered as an alternative. General supportive measures will be necessary. A careful evaluation of blood-forming organs should be made following recovery.

DOSAGE AND ADMINISTRATION:

Ethotoin is administered orally in 4 to 6 divided doses daily. The drug should be taken after food, and doses should be spaced as evenly as practicable. Initial dosage should be conservative. For adults, the initial daily dose should be 1 g or less, with subsequent gradual dosage increases over a period of several days. The optimum dosage must be determined on the basis of individual response. The usual adult maintenance dose is 2 to 3 g daily. Less than 2 g daily has been found ineffective in most adults.

Pediatric dosage depends upon the age and weight of the patient. The initial dose should not exceed 750 mg daily. The usual maintenance dose in children ranges from 500 mg to 1 g daily, although occasionally 2 or (rarely) 3 g daily may be necessary.

If a patient is receiving another antiepileptic drug, it should not be discontinued when Peganone therapy is begun. The dosage of the other drug should be reduced gradually as that of Peganone is increased. Peganone may eventually replace the other drug or the optimal dosage of both antiepileptics may be established.

Peganone is compatible with all commonly employed antiepileptic medications with the possible exception of Phenurone (phenacemide). In tonic-clonic (grand mal) seizures, use of the drug with phenobarbital may be beneficial. Peganone may be used in combination with drugs such as Tridione (trimethadione) or Paradione (paramethadione), as an adjunct in those patients with absence (petit mal) associated with tonic-clonic (grand mal).

HOW SUPPLIED:

Peganone (ethotoin tablets, USP) grooved, white tablets are supplied in two dosage strengths: 250 mg, bottles of 100 (NDC 0074-6902-01); 500 mg, bottles of 100 (NDC 0074-6905-04).

Recommended storage: Store below 77°F (25°C).

HOW SUPPLIED - EQUIVALENTS NOT AVAILABLE:

Tablet, Uncoated - Oral - 250 mg

100's	**$41.28**	**PEGANONE, Abbott**	**00074-6902-01**

Tablet, Uncoated - Oral - 500 mg

100's	**$77.47**	**PEGANONE, Abbott**	**00074-6905-04**

ETHYL CHLORIDE *(001228)*

CATEGORIES: Anesthesia; Antipruritics/Local Anesthetics; Local Anesthetics; Skin/Mucous Membrane Agents; FDA Pre 1938 Drugs

DESCRIPTION:

Ethyl Chloride (Chloroethane) is a colorless, **flammable**, volatile liquid. Its boiling point is between 12° and 13°C, causing it to vaporize at room temperature when applied from its special glass or metal container.

INDICATIONS AND USAGE:

Ethyl Chloride is a vapocoolant intended for topical application to control pain associated with minor surgical procedures (such as lancing boils, or incision and drainage of small abscesses), athletic injuries, injections, and for treatment of myofascial pain, restricted motion, and muscle spasm.

CONTRAINDICATIONS:

Ethyl Chloride is contraindicated in individuals with a history of hypersensitivity to it.

WARNINGS:

For external use only.

Skin absorption of Ethyl Chloride can occur; no cases of chronic poisoning have been reported. Ethyl Chloride is known as a liver and kidney toxin; long term exposure may cause liver or kidney damage.

Contents under pressure. Store in a cool place. Do not store above 120°F.

Do not store or near high frequency ultrasound equipment.

Warning: This product contains a chemical known to the State of California to cause cancer.

PRECAUTIONS:

Inhalation of Ethyl Chloride should be avoided as it may produce narcotic and general anesthetic effects, and may produce deep anesthesia or fatal coma with respiratory or cardiac arrest. Ethyl Chloride is **flammable** and should never be used in the presence of an open flame, or electrical cautery equipment. When used to produce local freezing of tissues, adjacent skin areas should be protected by application of petrolatum. The thawing process may be painful, and freezing may lower local resistance to infection and delay healing.

ADVERSE REACTIONS:

Cutaneous sensitization may occur, but appears to be extremely rare. Freezing can occasionally alter pigmentation.

DOSAGE AND ADMINISTRATION:

To apply Ethyl Chloride from metal tube, invert nozzle 12 inches (30 cm.) above the treatment area. Open adjustable dispensing valve until the spray flows freely.

To apply Ethyl Chloride from amber bottle with dispenseal valve, invert over the treatment area approximately 12 inches (30 cm.) away from site of application. Open dispenseal spring valve completely allowing Ethyl Chloride to flow in a stream from the bottle.

The dispenseal spring cap is available in four calibrations:

1. FINE: under.005 inch spray

2. MEDIUM: 005 to.008 inch spray

3. COARSE: 008 to.011 inch spray

4. Spra-Pak Nozzle: provides a mist like spray for surface cooling of a large skin area.

TOPICAL ANESTHESIA IN MINOR SURGERY

The operative site should be cleansed with a suitable antiseptic. Apply petrolatum to protect the adjacent area. Spray Ethyl Chloride for a few seconds to the point of frost formation, when the tissue becomes white. Avoid prolonged spraying of skin beyond this state. The anesthetic action of Ethyl Chloride rarely lasts more than a few seconds to a minute. Quickly swab operative site with antiseptic and promptly make incision. Reapply as needed.

SPORTS INJURIES

The pain of bruises, contusions, abrasions, swelling, and minor sprains may be controlled with Ethyl Chloride.

Spray affected area for a few seconds until the tissue begins to frost and turn white. Avoid spraying of skin beyond this state. Use as you would ice. The amount of cooling depends on the dosage. The smallest dose needed to produce the desired effect should be used. Dosage varies with the nozzle size and duration of application.

Determine the extent of injury (fracture, sprain, etc.) The anesthetic effect of Ethyl Chloride rarely lasts more than a few seconds to a minute. This time interval is usually sufficient to help reduce or relieve the initial trauma of the injury.

FOR PRE-INJECTION ANESTHESIA

Prepare syringe and have it ready. Spray skin with Ethyl Chloride from a distance of about 12 inches (30 cm) continuously for 3 to 5 seconds; do not frost skin. Swab skin with alcohol and quickly introduce needle with skin taut.

SPRAY AND STRETCH TECHNIQUE FOR MYOFASCIAL PAIN

Ethyl Chloride may be used as a counterirritant in the management of myofascial pain, restricted motion, and muscle spasm. Clinical conditions that may respond to Ethyl Chloride include low back pain (due to muscle spasm), acute stiff neck, torticollis, acute bursitis of the shoulder, muscle spasm associated with osteoarthritis, tight hamstring, sprained ankle, masseter muscle spasm, certain types of headaches, and referred pain due to irritated trigger point. Relief of pain facilitates early mobilization in restoration of muscle function. The Spray and Stretch technique is a therapeutic system which involves three stages: EVALUATION, SPRAYING AND STRETCHING.

The therapeutic value of Spray and Stretch becomes most effective when the practitioner has mastered all stages and applies them in the proper sequence.

I. Evaluation: During the evaluation phase the cause of pain is determined as local spasms or an irritated trigger point. The method of applying the spray to a muscle spasm differs slightly from application to a trigger point. A trigger point is a deep hypersensitive localized spot in a muscle which causes a referred pain pattern. With trigger points the source of pain is seldom the site of the pain. A trigger point may be detected by a snapping palpation over the muscle causing the muscle in which the irritated trigger point is situated to "jump."

II. Spraying:

A. Patient should assume a comfortable position.

B. Take precautions to cover the patient's eyes, nose, mouth, if spraying near face.

C. Hold bottle in an upside down position 12 to 18 inches (30-45 cm.) away from the treatment surface allowing the jet stream of vapocoolant to meet the skin at an acute angle to lessen the shock of impact. The rate of spraying is approximately 10 cm./sec. and is continued until the entire muscle has been covered. The number of sweeps is determined by the size of the muscle. In the case of a trigger point, the spray should be applied over the trigger point through and over the reference zone. In case of muscle spasm, the spray should be applied from origin to insertion.

DOSAGE AND ADMINISTRATION: *(cont'd)*

III. Stretching: During application of the spray, the muscle is passively stretched. Force is gradually increased with successive sweeps, and the slack is smoothly taken up as the muscle relaxes, establishing a new stretch length. Reaching the full normal length of the muscle is necessary to completely inactivate trigger points and relieve pain. After rewarming, the procedure may be repeated as necessary. Moist heat should be applied for 10 to 15 minutes following treatment. For lasting benefit, any factors that perpetuate the trigger mechanism must be eliminated.

HOW SUPPLIED:

100 gram metal tube

4 ounce amber glass bottle: Fine Spray; Medium Spray; Coarse Spray

3.5 ounce amber glass bottle: "Spra-Pak"

*For more information about this product contact Gebauer Company.

HOW SUPPLIED - EQUIVALENTS NOT AVAILABLE:

Aerosol, Spray - Topical - 100 %

3.5 oz	$119.28	GEBAUERS ETHYL CHLORIDE, Gebauer Chem	00386-0001-01
4 oz	$116.28	GEBAUERS ETHYL CHLORIDE, Gebauer Chem	00386-0001-02
4 oz	$116.28	GEBAUERS ETHYL CHLORIDE, Gebauer Chem	00386-0001-03
4 oz	$116.28	GEBAUERS ETHYL CHLORIDE, Gebauer Chem	00386-0001-04
120 ml	$9.17	Ethyl Chloride, HL Moore Drug Exch	00839-6046-65

ETIDOCAINE HYDROCHLORIDE *(001233)*

CATEGORIES: Anesthesia; Caudal; Epidural; Injectable Anesthetics; Local Anesthetics; Retrobulbar Anesthetics; Pregnancy Category B; FDA Approval Pre 1982; Patent Expiration 1992 Jan

BRAND NAMES: **Duranest**

DESCRIPTION:

Duranest (Etidocaine Hydrochloride, abbreviated here as Etidocaine HCl) Injections are sterile aqueous solutions that contain a local anesthetic agent and are administered parenterally by injection. See INDICATIONS AND USAGE for specific uses. The specific quantitative composition of each available solution is shown in TABLE 1.

Duranest Injections contain Etidocaine HCl, which is chemically designated as butanamide, N-(2,6-dimethylphenyl)-2-(ethylpropylamine)-, monohydrochloride.

Epinephrine is (-)-3, 4-Dihydroxy-α-((methylamino) methyl) benzyl alcohol.

The pKa of Etidocaine (7.74) is similar to that of lidocaine (7.86). However, Etidocaine possesses a greater degree of lipid solubility and protein binding capacity that does lidocaine. Duranest Injections are sterile and, except for the 1.5% concentration, are available with or without epinephrine 1:200,000. Single dose containers of Duranest Injection without epinephrine may be reautoclaved if necessary.

TABLE 1 Composition of Available Solutions

Duranest (Etidocaine HCl) Concentration %	Product Identification Epinephrine Dilution (as the bitartrate)	pH
1.0	None	4.0-5.0
1.0	1:200,000	3.0-4.5
1.5	1:200,000	3.0-4.5

Sodium Chloride (mg/ml)	Formula Single Dose Vilas/Dental Cartridge Sodium metabisulfite (mg/ml)	Citric Acid (mg/ml)
7.1	None	-
7.1	0.5	0.2
6.2	0.5	0.2

NOTE: pH of all solutions adjusted with sodium hydroxide and/or hydrochloric acid. Duranest dental cartridges are only available as 1.5% solution with epinephrine. 1:200,000. Filled under nitrogen.

CLINICAL PHARMACOLOGY:

MECHANISM OF ACTION

Etidocaine stabilizes the neuronal membrane by inhibiting the ionic fluxes required for the initiation and conduction of impulses, thereby effecting local anesthetic action.

Onset and Duration of Action: *In vivo* animal studies have shown that Etidocaine has a rapid onset (3-5 minutes) and prolonged duration of action (5 - 10 hours). Based on comparative clinical studies of lidocaine and Etidocaine, the anesthetic properties of Etidocaine in man may be characterized as follows: Initial onset of sensory analgesia and motor blockage is rapid (usually 3 - 5 minutes) and similar to that produced by lidocaine. Duration of sensory analgesia is 1.5 to 2 times longer than that of lidocaine by the peridural route. The difference in analgesic duration between Etidocaine and lidocaine may be even greater following peripheral nerve blockade than following central neural block. Duration of analgesia in excess of 9 hours is not infrequent when Etidocaine is used for peripheral nerve blocks such as brachial plexus blockade. Etidocaine produces a profound degree of motor blockade and abdominal muscle relaxation when used for peridural analgesia.

HEMODYNAMICS

Excessive blood levels may cause changes in cardiac output, total peripheral resistance, and mean arterial pressure. With central neural blockade these changes may be attributable to block of autonomic fibers, a direct depressant effect of the local anesthetic agent on various components of the cardiovascular system, and/or the beta-adrenergic receptor stimulating action of epinephrine when present. The net effect is normally a modest hypotension when the recommended dosages are not exceeded.

PHARMACOKINETICS AND METABOLISM

Information derived from diverse formulations, concentrations and usages reveals that Etidocaine is completely absorbed following parenteral administration, its rate of absorption depending, for example, upon such factors as the site of administration and the presence or absence of a vasoconstrictor agent. Except for intravenous administration, the highest blood levels are obtained following intercostal nerve block and the lowest after subcutaneous administration.

The plasma binding of Etidocaine is dependent on drug concentration, and the fraction bound decreases with increasing concentration. At 0.5-1.0 mcg/ml, 95% is bound to plasma protein.

CLINICAL PHARMACOLOGY: *(cont'd)*

Etidocaine crosses the blood-brain an placental barriers, presumably by passive diffusion.

Etidocaine is metabolized rapidly by the liver, and metabolites and unchanged drug are excreted by the kidney. Biotransformation includes oxidative N-dealkylation, ring hydroxylation, cleavage of the amide linkage, and conjugation. To date, approximately 20 metabolites of Etidocaine have been found in the urine. The percent of dose excreted as unchanged drug is less than 10%.

The mean elimination half-life of Etidocaine following a bolus intravenous injection is about 2.5 hours. Because of the rapid rate at which Etidocaine is metabolized, any condition that affects liver function may alter Etidocaine kinetics. Renal dysfunction may not affect Etidocaine kinetics but may increase the accumulation of metabolites.

Factors such as acidosis and the concomitant use of CNS stimulants and depressants affect the CNS levels of Etidocaine required to produce overt systemic effects. In the rhesus monkey arterial blood levels of 4.5 mcg/ml have been shown to be threshold for convulsive activity.

INDICATIONS AND USAGE:

Etidocaine HCl solutions are indicated for infiltration anesthesia, peripheral nerve blocks (*e.g.,* brachial plexus, intercostal, retrobulbar, ulnar, inferior alveolar), and central neural block (*i.e.,* lumbar or caudal epidural blocks).

CONTRAINDICATIONS:

Etidocaine is contraindicated in patients with a known history of hypersensitivity to local anesthetics of the amide type.

WARNINGS:

ETIDOCAINE HCl INJECTIONS FOR INFILTRATION AND NERVE BLOCK SHOULD BE EMPLOYED ONLY BY CLINICIANS WHO ARE WELL VERSED IN DIAGNOSIS AND MANAGEMENT OF DOSE-RELATED TOXICITY AND OTHER ACUTE EMERGENCIES THAT MIGHT ARISE FROM THE BLOCK TO BE EMPLOYED AND THEN ONLY AFTER ENSURING THE *IMMEDIATE* AVAILABILITY OF OXYGEN, OTHER RESUSCITATIVE DRUGS, CARDIOPULMONARY EQUIPMENT, AND THE PERSONNEL NEEDED FOR PROPER MANAGEMENT OF TOXIC REACTIONS AND RELATED EMERGENCIES (see also ADVERSE REACTIONS and PRECAUTIONS). DELAY IN PROPER MANAGEMENT OF DOSE-RELATED TOXICITY, UNDERVENTILATION FROM ANY CAUSE AND/OR ALTERED SENSITIVITY MAY LEAD TO THE DEVELOPMENT OF ACIDOSIS, CARDIAC ARREST AND, POSSIBLY, DEATH.

To avoid intravascular injection, aspiration should be performed before the local anesthetic solution is injected. The needle must be repositioned until no return of blood can be elicited by aspiration. Note, however, that the absence of blood in the syringe does not guarantee that intravascular injection has been avoided.

Local anesthetic solutions containing antimicrobial preservatives (*e.g.,* methylparaben) should not be used for epidural anesthesia because the safety of these agents has not been established with regard to intrathecal injection, either intentional or accidental.

Vasopressor agents administered for the treatment of hypotension related to caudal or other epidural blocks should not be used in the presence of ergot-type oxytocic drugs, since severe persistent hypertension and even rupture of cerebral blood vessels may occur.

Etidocaine HCl with epinephrine solutions contain sodium metabisulfite, a sulfite that may cause allergic-type reactions including anaphylactic symptoms and life-threatening or less severe asthmatic episodes in certain susceptible people. The overall prevalence of sulfate sensitivity in the general population is unknown and probably low. Sulfite sensitivity is seen more frequently in asthmatic than in nonasthmatic people.

PRECAUTIONS:

GENERAL

The safety and effectiveness of Etidocaine depend on proper dosage, correct technique, adequate precautions, and precautions, and readiness for emergencies. Standard textbooks should be consulted for specific techniques and precautions for various regional anesthetic procedures. Resuscitative equipment, oxygen, and other resuscitative drugs should be available for immediate use. (See WARNINGS and ADVERSE REACTIONS.) The lowest dosage that results in effective anesthesia should be used to avoid high plasma levels and serious adverse effects. Syringe aspirations should also be performed before and during each supplemental injection when using indwelling catheter techniques. During the administration of epidural anesthesia, it is recommended that a test dose be administered initially and that the patient be monitored for central nervous system toxicity and cardiovascular toxicity, as well as for signs of unintended intrathecal administration, before proceeding. When clinical conditions permit, consideration should be given to employing local anesthetic solutions that contain epinephrine for the test dose because circulatory changes compatible with epinephrine may also serve as a warning sign of unintended intravascular injection. An intravascular injection is still possible even if aspirations for blood are negative. Repeated doses of Etidocaine may cause significant increases in blood levels with each repeated dose because of slow accumulation of the drug or its metabolites. Tolerance to elevated blood levels varies with the status of the patient. Debilitated, elderly patients, acutely ill patients, and children should be given reduced doses commensurate with their age and physical condition.

Etidocaine should also be used with caution in patients with severe shock or heart block.

Lumbar and caudal epidural anesthesia should be used with extreme caution in persons with the following conditions: existing neurological disease, spinal deformities, septicemia, and severe hypertension.

Local anesthetic solutions containing a vasoconstrictor should be used cautiously and in carefully circumscribed quantities in areas of the body supplied by end arteries or having otherwise compromised blood supply. Patients with peripheral vascular disease and those with hypertensive vascular disease may exhibit exaggerated vasoconstrictor response. Ischemic injury or necrosis may result. Preparations containing a vasoconstrictor should be used with caution in patients during or following the administration of potent general anesthetic agents, since cardiac arrhythmias may occur under such conditions.

Careful and constant monitoring of cardiovascular and respiratory (adequacy of ventilation) vital signs and the patient's state of consciousness should be accomplished after each local anesthetic injection. It should be kept in mind at such times that restlessness, anxiety, tinnitus, dizziness, blurred vision, tremors, depression or drowsiness may be early warning signs of central nervous system toxicity.

Since amide-type local anesthetics are metabolized by the liver, Etidocaine HCl Injections should be used with caution in patients with hepatic disease.

Patients with severe hepatic disease, because of their inability to metabolize local anesthetics normally, are at greater risk of developing toxic plasma concentrations. Etidocaine HCl Injection should also be used with caution in patients with impaired cardiovascular function since they may be less able to compensate for functional changes associated with the prolongation of A-V conduction produced by these drugs.

PRECAUTIONS: *(cont'd)*

Many drugs used during the conduct of anesthesia are considered potential triggering agents for familiar malignant hyperthermia. Since it is not known whether amide-type local anesthetics may trigger this reaction and since the need for supplemental general anesthesia cannot be predicted in advance, it is suggested that a standard protocol for the management of malignant hyperthermia should be available. Early unexplained signs of tachycardia, tachypnea, labile blood pressure and metabolic acidosis may precede temperature elevation. Successful outcome is dependent on early diagnosis, prompt discontinuance of the suspect triggering agent(s) and institution of treatment, including oxygen therapy, indicated supportive measures and dantrolene (consult dantrolene sodium intravenous package insert before using).

Etidocaine should be used with caution in persons with known drug sensitivities. Patients allergic to para-aminobenzoic acid derivatives (procaine, tetracaine, benzocaine, etc.) have not shown cross sensitivity to Etidocaine.

Use in the Head and Neck Area: Small doses of local anesthetics injected into the head and neck area, including retrobulbar, dental and stellate ganglion blocks, may produce adverse reactions similar to systemic toxicity seen with unintentional intravascular injections of larger doses. The injection procedures require the utmost care. Confusion, convulsions, respiratory depression and/or respiratory arrest, and cardiovascular stimulation or depression have been reported. These reactions may be due to intra-arterial injection of the local anesthetic with retrograde flow to the cerebral circulation. They may also be due to puncture of the dural sheath of the optic nerve during retrobulbar block with diffusion of any local anesthetic along the subdural space to the midbrain. Patients receiving these blocks should have their circulation and respiration monitored and be constantly observed. Resuscitative equipment and personnel for treating adverse reactions should be immediately available. Dosage recommendations should not be exceeded. See DOSAGE AND ADMINISTRATION.)

Use in Ophthalmic Surgery: When local anesthetic injections are employed for retrobulbar block, lack of corneal sensation should not be relied upon to determine whether or not the patient is ready for surgery. This is because complete lack of corneal sensation usually precedes clinically acceptable external ocular muscle akinesia.

Use in Dentistry: Because of the long duration of anesthesia, when Duranest 1.5% with epinephrine is used for dental injections, patients should be cautioned about the possibility of inadvertent trauma to tongue, lips and buccal mucosa and advised not to chew solid foods or test the anesthetized area by biting or probing.

INFORMATION FOR THE PATIENT

When appropriate, patients should be informed in advance that they may experience temporary loss of sensation and motor activity, usually in the lower half of the body, following proper administration of epidural anesthesia.

DRUG LABORATORY TEST INTERACTIONS

The intramuscular injection of Etidocaine may result in an increase in creatine phosphokinase levels. Thus, the use of this enzyme determination, without isoenzyme separation, as a diagnostic test for the presence of acute myocardial infarction may be compromised by the intramuscular injection of Etidocaine.

CARCINOGENESIS, MUTAGENESIS, AND IMPAIRMENT OF FERTILITY

Studies of Etidocaine in animals to evaluate the carcinogenic and mutagenic potential have not been conducted. Studies in rats at 1.7 times the maximum recommended human dose have revealed no impairment of fertility.

USE IN PREGNANCY: TERATOGENIC EFFECTS. PREGNANCY CATEGORY B.

Reproduction studies have been performed in rats and rabbits at doses up to 1.7 times the human dose and have revealed no evidence of harm to the fetus caused by Etidocaine. There are, however, no adequate and well-controlled studies in pregnant women. Animal reproduction studies are not always predictive of human response. General consideration should be given to this fact before administering Etidocaine to woman of childbearing potential, especially during early pregnancy when maximum organogenesis takes place.

LABOR AND DELIVERY

Local anesthetics rapidly cross the placenta and when used for epidural, paracervical, pudendal or caudal block anesthesia, can cause varying degrees of maternal, fetal and neonatal toxicity. (See CLINICAL PHARMACOLOGY, Pharmacokinetics.) The incidence and degree toxicity depend upon the procedure performed, the type and amount of drug used, and the technique of drug administration. Adverse reactions in the parturient, fetus and neonate involve allegations of the central nervous system, peripheral vascular tone and cardiac function.

Maternal hypotension has resulted from regional anesthesia. Local anesthetics produce vasodilation by blocking sympathetic nerves. Elevating the patient's legs and positioning her on her left side will help prevent decreases in blood pressure. The fetal heart rate also should be monitored continuously and electronic fetal monitoring is highly advisable.

Epidural anesthesia may alter the forces of parturition through changes in uterine contractility or maternal expulsive efforts. Because Etidocaine HCl Injection may produce profound motor block, it is not recommended for epidural anesthesia in normal delivery. Etidocaine HCl Injection is, however, recommended for epidural anesthesia when caesarean section is to be performed.

The use of some local anesthetic drug products during labor and delivery may be followed by diminished muscle strength and tone for the first day or two of life. The long-term significance of these observations is unknown.

Fetal bradycardia may occur in 20 to 30 percent of patients receiving paracervical nerve block anesthesia with the amide-type local anesthetics and may be associated with fetal acidosis. Fetal heart rate should always be monitored during paracervical anesthesia. The physician should weigh the possible advantages against risks when considering paracervical block in prematurity, toxemia of pregnancy, and fetal distress. Careful adherence to recommended dosage is of the utmost importance in obstetrical paracervical block. Failure to achieve adequate analgesia with recommended doses should arouse suspicion of intravascular or fetal intracranial injection. Cases compatible with unintended fetal intracranial injection of local anesthetic solution have been reported following intended paracervical or pudendal block or both. Babies so affected present with unexplained neonatal depression at birth, which correlates with high local anesthetic serum levels, and often manifest seizures within six hours. Prompt use of supportive measures combined with forced urinary excretion of the local anesthetic has been used successfully to manage this complication. Case reports of maternal convulsions and cardiovascular collapse following use of some local anesthetics for paracervical block in early pregnancy (as anesthesia for elective abortion) suggest that systemic absorption under these circumstances may be rapid. There are inadequate data in support of safe and effective use of Etidocaine for obstetrical or non-obstetrical paracervical block, therefore, such use is not recommended.

NURSING MOTHERS

It is not known whether this drug is excreted in human milk. Because many drugs are excreted in human milk, caution should be exercised when Etidocaine is administered to a nursing woman.

PEDIATRIC USE

No information is currently available on appropriate pediatric doses.

DRUG INTERACTIONS:

The administration of local anesthetic solutions containing epinephrine or norepinephrine to patients receiving monoamine oxidase inhibitors, tricyclic antidepressants or phenothiazines may produce severe, prolonged hypotension or hypertension or hypertension. Concurrent use of these agents should generally be avoided. In situations when concurrent therapy is necessary, careful patient monitoring is essential.

Concurrent administration of vasopressor drugs (for the treatment of hypotension related to epidural blocks) and ergot-type oxytocic drugs may cause severe, persistent hypertension or cerebrovascular accidents.

ADVERSE REACTIONS:

Systemic: Adverse experiences following the administration of Etidocaine are similar in nature to those observed with other amide local anesthetic agents. These adverse experiences are, in general, dose- related and may result from high plasma levels caused by excessive dosage, rapid absorption or unintended intravascular injection, or may result from a hypersensitivity, idiosyncrasy or diminished tolerance on the part of the patient. Serious adverse experiences are generally systemic in nature. The following types are those most commonly reported:

Central Nervous System: CNS manifestations are excitatory and/or depressant and may be characterized by light-headedness, nervousness, apprehension, euphoria, confusion, dizziness, drowsiness, tinnitus, blurred or double vision, vomiting, sensations of heat, cold or numbness, twitching, tremors, convulsions, unconsciousness, respiratory depression and arrest. The excitatory manifestations may be very brief or may not occur at all, in which case the first manifestation of toxicity may be drowsiness merging into unconsciousness and respiratory arrest. Drowsiness following the administration of Etidocaine is usually an early sign of a high blood level of the drug and may occur as a consequence of rapid absorption.

Cardiovascular System: Cardiovascular manifestations are usually depressant and are characterized by bradycardia, hypotension, and cardiovascular collapse, which may lead to cardiac arrest.

Allergic: Allergic reactions are characterized by cutaneous lesions, urticaria, edema or anaphylactoid reactions. Allergic reactions may occur as a result of sensitivity either to local anesthetic agents or to the methylparaben used as a preservative in multiple dose vials. The detection of sensitivity by skin testing is of doubtful value.

Neurologic: The incidences of adverse reactions associated with the use of local anesthetics may be related to the total dose of local anesthetic administered and are also dependent upon the particular drug used, the route of administration and the physical status of the patient.

In the practice of caudal or lumbar epidural block, occasional unintentional penetration of the subarachnoid space by the catheter may occur. Subsequent adverse effects may depend partially on the amount of drug administered subdurally. These may include spinal block of varying magnitude (including total spinal block), hypotension secondary to spinal block, loss of bladder and bowel control, and loss of perineal sensation and sexual function. Persistent motor, sensory and/or autonomic (sphincter control) deficit of some lower spinal segments with slow recovery (several months) or incomplete recovery have been reported in rare instances when caudal or lumbar epidural block has been attempted. Backache and headache have also been noted following use of these anesthetic procedures.

OVERDOSAGE:

Acute emergencies from local anesthetics are generally related to high plasma levels encountered during therapeutic use of local anesthetics or to unintended subarachnoid injection of local anesthetic solution (see ADVERSE REACTIONS, WARNINGS, and PRECAUTIONS).

Management of Local Anesthetic Emergencies: The first consideration is prevention, best accomplished by careful and constant monitoring of cardiovascular and respiratory vital signs and the patient's state of consciousness after each local anesthetic injection. At the first sign of change, oxygen should be administered.

The first step in the management of convulsions, as well as underventilation or apnea dur to unintentional subarachnoid injection of drug solution, consists of immediate attention to the maintenance of a patent airway and assisted or controlled ventilation with oxygen and a delivery system capable of permitting immediate positive airway pressure by mask. Immediately after the institution of these ventilatory measures, the adequacy of the circulation should be evaluated, keeping in mind that drugs used to treat convulsions sometimes depress the circulation when administered intravenously. Should convulsions persist despite adequate respiratory support, and if the status of the circulation permits, small increments of an ultra-short acting barbiturate (such as thiopental or thiamylal) or a benzodiazepine (may be administered intravenously. The clinician should be familiar, prior to use of local anesthetics, with these anticonvulsant drugs. Supportive treatment of circulatory depression may require administration of intravenous fluids and, when appropriate, a vasopressor as directed by the clinical situation (*e.g.*, ephedrine).

If not treated immediately, both convulsions and cardiovascular depression can result in hypoxia, acidosis, bradycardia, arrhythmias and cardiac arrest. Underventilation or apnea due to unintentional subarachnoid injection of local anesthetic solution may produce these same signs and also lead to cardiac arrest if ventilatory support is not instituted. If cardiac arrest should occur, standard cardiopulmonary resuscitative measures should be instituted.

Endotracheal intubation, employing drugs and techniques familiar to the clinician, may be indicated, after initial administration of oxygen by mask, if difficulty is encountered in the maintenance of a patent airway or if prolonged ventilatory support (assisted or controlled) is indicated.

Dialysis is of negligible value in the treatment of acute overdosage with Etidocaine.

The intravenous $LD_{50}$of Etidocaine HCl in female mice is 7.6 (6.6 - 8.5) mg/kg and the subcutaneous $LD_{50}$is 112 (96 - 166) mg/kg.

DOSAGE AND ADMINISTRATION:

As with all local anesthetic agents, the dose of Etidocaine HCl Injection to be employed will depend upon the area to be anesthetized, the vascularity of the tissues, the number of neuronal segments to be blocked, the type of regional anesthetic technique, and the physical condition and tolerance of the individual patient.

The maximum dose to be employed as a single injection should be determined on the basis of the status of the patient and the type of regional anesthetic technique to be performed. Although single injections of 450 mg have been employed for regional anesthesia without adverse effects, at present it is strongly recommended that the maximal dose as a single injection should not exceed 400 mg (approximately 8.0 mg/kg or 3.6 mg/lb based on a 50 kg person) with epinephrine 1:200,000 and 300 mg (approximately 6 mg/kg and 2.7 mg/lb based on a 50 kg person) without epinephrine. Because Etidocaine has been shown to disappear quite rapidly from blood, toxicity is influenced by rapidity of administration, and therefore, slow injection in vascular areas is highly recommended. Incremental doses of Etidocaine HCl Injection may be repeated at 2 - 3 hour intervals.

Caudal and Lumbar Epidural Block: As a precaution against the adverse experiences sometimes observed following unintentional penetration of the subarachnoid space, a test dose of 2-5 ml should be administered at least 5 minutes prior to injecting the total volume required for a lumbar or caudal epidural block. The test dose should be repeated if the patient is moved in a manner that may have displaced the catheter. Epinephrine, if contained in the test dose (10-15 mcg have been suggested), may serve as a warning of unintentional intravascular injection. If injected into a blood vessel, this amount of epinephrine is likely to produce a transient "epinephrine response" within 45 seconds, consisting of an increase in heart rate and systolic blood pressure, circumoral pallor, palpitations and nervousness in the unsedated patient. The sedated patient may exhibit only a pulse rate increase of 20 or more beats per minute for 15 or more seconds. Patients on beta-blockers may not manifest changes in heart rate, but blood pressure monitoring can detect an evanescent rise in systolic blood pressure. Adequate time should be allowed for onset of anesthesia after administration of each test dose. The rapid injection of a large volume of Etidocaine HCl Injection through the catheter should be avoided, and when feasible, fractional doses should be administered.

In the event of the known injection of a large volume of local anesthetic solution into the subarachnoid space after suitable resuscitation and if the catheter is in place, consider attempting the recovery of drug by draining a moderate amount of cerebrospinal fluid (such as 10 ml) through the epidural catheter.

USE IN DENTISTRY

When used for local anesthesia in dental procedures the dosage of Etidocaine HCl Injection depends on the physical status of the patient, the area of the oral cavity to be anesthetized, the vascularity of the oral tissues, and the technique of anesthesia. The least volume of solution that results in effective local anesthesia should be administered. For specific techniques and procedures of local anesthesia in the oral cavity, refer to standard textbooks.

Dosage requirements should be determined on an individual basis. In maxillary infiltration and/or inferior alveolar nerve block, initial dosages of 1.0 - 5.0 ml (1/2 - 2 1/2 cartridges) of Etidocaine HCl Injection 1.5% with epinephrine 1:200,000 are usually effective.

Aspiration is recommended since it reduces the possibility of intravascular injection, thereby keeping the incidence of side effects and anesthetic failures to a minimum.

The following dosage recommendations are intended as guides for the use of Etidocaine HCl Injection in the average adult patient. As indicated previously, the dosage should be reduced for elderly or debilitated patients or patients with severe renal disease.

NOTE

Parenteral drug products should be inspected visually for particulate matter and discoloration prior to administration whenever the solution and container permit. The Injection is not to be used if its color is pinkish or darker than slightly yellow or if it contains a precipitate (TABLE 2):

TABLE 2 Dosage Recommendations

Procedure	Etidocaine HCl with epinephrine 1:200,000 Conc. (%)	Vol. (ml)	Total Dose (mg)
Peripheral Nerve Block	1.0	5 - 40	50 - 400
Central Neural Block			
Lumbar Peridural			
Intraabdominal or Pelvic Surgery	1.0	10 - 30	100 - 300
Lower Limb Surgery or Caesarean Section	1.5	10 - 20	150 - 300
Caudal	1.0	10 - 30	100 - 300
Retrobulbar	1.0 or 1.5	2 - 4	20 - 60
Maxillary Infiltration and/or inferior Alveolar Nerve Block	1.5	1 - 5	15 - 75

Store at controlled room temperature 15-30° C (59-86°F).

HOW SUPPLIED - EQUIVALENTS NOT AVAILABLE:

Injection, Solution - Epidural - 1 %

30 ml $17.95 DURANEST, Astra USA 00186-0820-01

ETIDRONATE DISODIUM *(001234)*

CATEGORIES: Biphosphonates; Bone Metabolism Regulators; Calcium Metabolism; Calcium Preparations; Heterotopic Ossification Agents; Homeostatic & Nutrient; Hypercalcemia; Hypercalcemic Agents; Orphan Drugs; Paget's Disease; Pain; Spinal Cord Injury; Osteoporosis*; Pregnancy Category B; FDA Approval Pre 1982; Patent Expiration 1996 Dec

* Indication not approved by the FDA

BRAND NAMES: *Didronate*; **Didronel**; *Difosfen*; *Dinol*; *Diphos* (Germany); *Osteum* *(International brand names outside U.S. in italics)*

FORMULARIES: Aetna; BC-BS

COST OF THERAPY: $660.59 (Paget's Disease; Tablet; 400 mg; 1/day; 182 days)

DESCRIPTION:

TABLETS

Didronel tablets contain either 200 mg or 400 mg of etidronate disodium, the disodium salt of (1-hydroxyethylidene) diphosphonic acid, for oral administration. This compound, also known as EHDP, regulates bone metabolism. It is a white powder, highly soluble in water, with a molecular weight of 250.

Didronel Inactive Ingredients: Each tablet contains magnesium stearate, microcrystalline cellulose, and starch.

IV INFUSION

Dilute Before Use. Etidronate disodium IV infusion is a clear, colorless, sterile solution of etidronate disodium, the disodium salt of (1-hydroxyethylidene) diphosphonic acid. Each 6-ml ampule contains a 5% solution of 300 mg etidronate disodium in water for injection for slow intravenous infusion.

Etidronate disodium is a white powder, highly soluble in water, with a molecular weight of 250.

CLINICAL PHARMACOLOGY:

TABLETS

Etidronate disodium acts primarily on bone. It can inhibit the formation, growth & dissolution of hydroxyapatite crystals and their amorphous precursors by chemisorption to calcium phosphate surfaces. Inhibition of crystal resorption occurs at lower doses than are required to inhibit crystal growth. Both effects increase as the dose increases.

Etidronate disodium is not metabolized. The amount of drug absorbed after an oral dose is approximately 3%. In normal subjects, plasma half-life ($t_{1/2}$) of etidronate, based on noncompartmental pharmacokinetics is one to six hours. Within 24 hours, approximately half the absorbed dose is excreted in urine; the remainder is distributed to bone compartments from

CLINICAL PHARMACOLOGY: *(cont'd)*

which it is slowly eliminated. Animal studies have yielded bone clearance estimates up to 165 days. In humans, the residence time on bone may vary due to such factors as specific metabolic condition and bone type. Unabsorbed drug is excreted intact in the feces. Preclinical studies indicate etidronate disodium does not cross the blood-brain barrier.

Etidronate disodium therapy does not adversely affect serum levels of parathyroid hormone or calcium.

Paget's Disease: Paget's disease of bone (osteitis deformans) is an idiopathic, progressive disease characterized by abnormal and accelerated bone metabolism in one or more bones. Signs and symptoms may include bone pain and/or deformity, neurologic disorders, elevated cardiac output and other vascular disorders, and increased serum alkaline phosphatase and/or urinary hydroxyproline levels. Bone fractures are common in patients with Paget's disease.

Etidronate disodium slows accelerated bone turnover (resorption and accretion) in pagetic lesions and, to a lesser extent, in normal bone. This has been demonstrated histologically, scintigraphically, biochemically, and through calcium kinetic and balance studies. Reduced bone turnover is often accompanied by symptomatic improvement, including reduced bone pain. Also, the incidence of pagetic fractures may be reduced, and elevated cardiac output and other vascular disorders may be improved by etidronate disodium therapy.

Heterotopic Ossification: Heterotopic ossification, also referred to as myositis ossificans (circumscripta, progressiva or traumatica), ectopic calcification, periarticular ossification, or paraosteoarthropathy, is characterized by metaplastic osteogenesis. It usually presents with signs of localized inflammation or pain, elevated skin temperature, and redness. When tissues near joints are involved, functional loss may also be present.

Heterotopic ossification may occur for no known reason as in myositis ossificans progressiva or may follow a wide variety of surgical, occupational, and sports trauma (*e.g.*, hip arthroplasty, spinal cord injury, head injury, burns, and severe thigh bruises). Heterotopic ossification has also been observed in non-traumatic conditions (*e.g.*, infections of the central nervous system, peripheral neuropathy, tetanus, biliary cirrhosis, Peyronie's disease, as well as in association with a variety of benign and malignant neoplasms).

Clinical trials have demonstrated the efficacy of etidronate disodium in heterotopic ossification following total hip replacement, or due to spinal cord injury.

Heterotopic Ossification Complicating Total Hip Replacement: typically develops radiographically 3-8 weeks postoperatively in the pericapsular area of the affected hip joint. The overall incidence is about 50%; about one-third of these cases are clinically significant.

Heterotopic Ossification Due to Spinal Cord Injury: typically develops radiographically 1-4 months after injury. It occurs below the level of injury, usually at major joints. The overall incidence is about 40%; about one-half of these cases are clinically significant.

Etidronate disodium chemisorbs to calcium hydroxyapatite crystals and their amorphous precursors, blocking the aggregation, growth and mineralization of these crystals. This is thought to be the mechanism by which etidronate disodium prevents or retards heterotopic ossification. There is no evidence etidronate disodium affects mature heterotopic bone.

IV INFUSION

Etidronate disodium acts primarily on bone. Its major pharmacologic action is the reduction of normal and abnormal bone resorption. Secondarily, it reduces bone formation since bone formation is coupled to resorption. This reduces bone turnover, but the reduction of bone turnover, *per se*, is not the important action in the reduction of hypercalcemia.

Etidronate disodium's reduction of abnormal bone resorption is responsible for its therapeutic benefit in hypercalcemia. The antiresorptive action of etidronate disodium has been demonstrated under a variety of conditions, although the exact mechanism(s) is not fully understood. It may be related to the drug's inhibition of hydroxyapatite crystal dissolution and/or its action or bone resorbing cells. The number of osteoclasts in active bone turnover sites is substantially reduced after Didronel therapy is administered. Etidronate disodium also can inhibit the formation and growth hydroxyapatite crystals and their amorphous precursors at concentrations in excess of those required to inhibit crystal dissolution.

Etidronate disodium is not metabolized. A large fraction of the infused dose is excreted rapidly and unchanged in the urine. The mean residence time in the exchangeable pool is approximately 8.7 ± 1.0 hours. The mean volume of distribution at steady-state in normal humans is 1370 ± 203 ml/kg while the plasma half-life (t1/2) is 6.0 ± 0.7 hours. In these same subjects, nonrenal clearance from exchangeable pool amounts to 30-50% of the infused dose. This is a nonrenal clearance is considered to be due to uptake of the drug by bone; subsequently the drug is slowly eliminated through bone turnover. The half-life of the dose on bone is in excess of 90 days.

Hyperphosphatemia, which is often observed in association with oral etidronate disodium medication at doses of 10-20 mg/kg/day, occurs less frequently. In association with intravenous medication of patients with hypercalcemia of malignancy.

Hyperphosphatemia is apparently due to increased tubular reabsorption of phosphate by the kidney. No adverse effects have been associated with etidronate disodium-related hyperphosphatemia and its occurrence is not a contraindication to therapy. Serum phosphate elevations usually return to normal 2-4 weeks after medication is discontinued.

The responsiveness of animal tumors susceptible to four commonly employed classes or subclasses of chemotherapeutic agents, antitumor antibiotics (doxorubicin), a classic alkylating agent (cyclophosphamide), a nitrosourea (carmustine), and a pyrimidine antagonist (5-fluorouracil), were not adversely altered by the concurrent administration of intravenous etidronate disodium.

Hypercalcemia of Malignancy: Hypercalcemia of malignancy is usually related to increased bone resorption associated with the presence of neoplastic tissue. It occurs in 8 to 20% of patients with malignant disease. Whereas hypercalcemia is more often seen in patients with demonstrable osteolytic, osteoblastic, or mixed metastatic tumors in bone, discrete skeletal lesions cannot be demonstrated in at least 30% of patients.

Patients with certain types of neoplasms, such as carcinoma of the breast, bronchogenic carcinoma, renal cell carcinoma cancers of the head and neck, lymphomas, and multiple myeloma, are especially prone to developing hypercalcemia.

As hypercalcemia of malignancy evolves, the renal tubules develop a diminished capacity to concentrate urine. The resultant polyuria and nocturia decrease the extracellular fluid volume. This decrease may be aggravated by vomiting and reduced fluid intake. Thus, the ability of the kidney to eliminate excess calcium is compromised. Renal impairment can eventually cause nitrogen retention, acidosis, renal failure, and further decrease in excretion of calcium. Etidronate disodium IV infusion, by inhibiting excessive bone resorption, interrupts this process. Salt loading and use of "high ceiling" or "loop" diuretics may be used to promote calcium excretion, because the rate of renal calcium excretion is directly related to the rate of sodium excretion.

The physiologic derangements induced by excessive serum calcium are due to increased levels of ionized calcium. The pathophysiologic effects of excessive serum calcium are heightened by reductions in serum albumin which normally binds a fraction (about 40%) of the total serum calcium. In patients with hypercalcemia of malignancy, serum albumin is often reduced and this tends to mask the magnitude of the increase in the level of ionized calcium. By reducing the flow of calcium from resorbing bone, Etidronate disodium IV infusion effectively reduces total and ionized serum calcium.

CLINICAL PHARMACOLOGY: *(cont'd)*

In the principal clinical study of etidronate disodium for hypercalcemia of malignancy, patients with elevated calcium levels (10.1-17.4 mg/dl) were treated simultaneously with daily administrations of intravenous etidronate disodium over a 3-day period and up to 3000 ml of saline and 80 mg of loop diuretic. The response to treatment for these patients was compared with that from patients treated with saline and loop diuretic. The response to treatment for these patients was compared with that from patients treated with saline and loop diuretics alone. In terms of total serum calcium changes, 88% of patients treated with etidronate disodium IV infusion as described, had reductions of serum calcium of 1 mg/dl or more. Total serum calcium returned to normal in 63% of patients within 7 days compared to 33% of patients treated with hydration alone.

Reductions in urinary calcium excretion, which accompany reductions in excessive bone resorption, became apparent after 24 hours. This was accompanied or followed by maximum decreases in serum calcium which were observed, most frequently, 72 hours after the first infusion.

The physiologically important component of serum calcium is the ionized portion. In most institutions, this cannot be measured directly. It is important to recognize that factors influencing the ratio of free and bound calcium such as serum proteins, particularly albumin, may complicate the interpretation of total serum calcium measurements. If indicated, a corrected serum calcium value should be calculated using an established algorithm.

When total serum calcium values are adjusted for serum albumin levels, there was a return to normocalcemia in 24% of etidronate disodium-treated patients and in 7% of patients treated with saline infusion. Eighty-seven percent of patients receiving Didronel and 67% of patients on saline had albumin-adjusted serum calcium levels returned to normal or reduced by at least 1 mg/dl.

In the above mentioned study, a second course of etidronate disodium IV infusion was tried in a small number of patients who had a recurrence of hypercalcemia following an initial response to a 3-day infusion of the drug. All patients who received a second 3-day course of etidronate disodium IV infusion showed a decrease of total serum calcium of at least one 1 mg/dl. Normalization of total serum calcium occurred in 11 out of 14 patients.

Etidronate disodium IV infusion does not appear to alter renal tubular reabsorption of calcium, and does not affect hypercalcemia in patients with hyperparathyroidism where increased calcium reabsorption may be a factor in the hypercalcemia.

Limited clinical study results suggest that continuation of etidronate disodium therapy with oral tablets may maintain clinically acceptable serum calcium levels and prolong normocalcemia.

INDICATIONS AND USAGE:

TABLETS

Paget's Disease: Etidronate disodium is indicated for the treatment of symptomatic Paget's disease of bone. Etidronate disodium therapy usually arrests or significantly impedes the disease process as evidenced by:

Symptomatic relief, including decreased pain and/or increased mobility (experienced by 3 out of 5 patients).

Reductions in serum alkaline phosphatase and urinary hydroxyproline levels (30% or more in 4 out of 5 patients).

Histomorphometry showing reduced numbers of osteoclasts and osteoblasts, and more lamellar bone formation.

Bone scans showing reduced radionuclide uptake at pagetic lesions.

In addition, reductions in pagetically elevated cardiac output and skin temperature have been observed in some patients.

In many patients, the disease process will be suppressed for a period of at least one year following cessation of therapy. The upper limit of this period has not been determined.

The effects of the etidronate disodium treatment in patients with asymptomatic Paget's disease have not been studied. However, etidronate disodium treatment of such patients may be warranted if extensive involvement threatens irreversible neurologic damage, major joints, or major weight-bearing bones.

Heterotopic Ossification: Etidronate disodium is indicated in the prevention and treatment of heterotopic ossification following total hip replacement or due to spinal cord injury.

Etidronate disodium reduces the incidence of clinically important heterotopic bone by about two-thirds. Among those patients who form heterotopic bone, etidronate disodium retards the progression of immature lesions and reduces the severity by at least half. Follow-up data (at least nine months posttherapy) suggest these benefits persist.

In Total Hip Replacement Patients: Etidronate disodium does not promote loosening of the prosthesis or impede trochanteric reattachment.

In Spinal Cord Injury Patients: Etidronate disodium does not inhibit fracture healing or stabilization of the spine.

IV INFUSION

Etidronate disodium IV infusion, together with achievement and maintenance of adequate hydration, is indicated for the treatment of hypercalcemia of malignancy inadequately managed by dietary modification and/or oral hydration.

In the treatment of hypercalcemia of malignancy, it is important to initiate rehydration with saline together with "high ceiling" or "loop" diuretics if indicated to restore urine output. This also is intended to increase the renal excretion of calcium and initiate a reduction in serum calcium. Since increased bone resorption is usually the underlying cause of an increased flux of calcium into the vascular compartment concurrent therapy with etidronate disodium IV infusion is recommended as soon as there is a restoration of urine output. Since etidronate disodium is excreted by the kidney, it is important to know that renal function is adequate to handle not only the increased fluid load but also the excretion of the drug itself. (See WARNINGS.)

Etidronate disodium IV infusion is also indicated for the treatment of hypercalcemia of malignancy which persists after adequate hydration has been restored. Patients with and without metastases and with a variety of tumors have been responsive to treatment with etidronate disodium IV infusion. Adequate hydration of patients should be maintained, but in aged patients and in those with cardiac failure, care must be taken to avoid overhydration.

CONTRAINDICATIONS:

Tablets: Etidronate disodium tablets are contraindicated in patients with known hypersensitivity to etidronate disodium or in patients with clinically overt osteomalacia.

IV Infusion: In patients with Class Dc and higher renal functional impairment (serum creatinine greater than 5.0 mg/dl) Didronel IV infusion should be withheld.

WARNINGS:

TABLETS

In Paget's Patients: the response to therapy may be of slow onset and continue for months after etidronate disodium therapy is discontinued. Dosage should not be increased prematurely. A 90-day drug-free interval should be provided between courses of therapy.

WARNINGS: *(cont'd)*

Heterotopic Ossification: No specific warnings.

IV INFUSION

Occasional mild to moderate abnormalities in renal function (elevated BUN and/or serum creatinine) have been observed when etidronate disodium IV infusion was given as directed to patients with hypercalcemia of malignancy. These changes were reversible or remained stable, without worsening, after completion of the course of etidronate disodium IV infusion. In some patients with pre-existing renal impairment or in those who had received potentially nephrotoxic drugs, further depression of renal function was sometimes seen. This suggests that etidronate disodium IV infusion may produce or aggravate the depression of renal function in approximately 8 of 203 treatment courses when used to treat hypercalcemia of malignancy. Therefore, it is recommended that appropriate monitoring of renal function with serum creatinine and/or BUN be carried out with etidronate disodium IV infusion treatment.

The effects of etidronate disodium IV infusion administration on renal function in patients with serum creatinine greater than 2.5 mg/dl (Class Cc and higher, classification of Renal Functional Impairment. Council on the kidney in Cardiovascular Disease, American Heart Association, Ann. Int. Med. 75:251-52, 1971) has not been systematically examined in controlled trials.

Since etidronate disodium is excreted by the kidney, it is important to know that renal function is adequate to handle not only the increased fluid load but also the excretion of the drug itself. Since these capacities are impaired in patients with underlying renal disease and since experience with etidronate disodium IV infusion in patients with serum creatinine > 2.5 mg/dl is limited, the use of etidronate disodium IV infusion in such patients should occur only after a careful assessment of renal status or potential risks and potential benefits. (See WARNINGS.)

Reduction of the dose of etidronate disodium IV infusion, if used at all, may be advisable in Class Cc renal function impairment (serum creatinine 2.5 to 4.9 mg/dl); and, etidronate disodium IV infusion be used only if the potential benefit of hypercalcemia correction will substantially exceed the potential for worsening of renal function. In patients with Class Dc and higher renal functional impairment (serum creatinine greater than 5.0 mg/dl) etidronate disodium IV infusion should be withheld.

PRECAUTIONS:

GENERAL

Tablets: Patients should maintain an adequate nutritional status, particularly an adequate intake of calcium and vitamin D.

Therapy has been withheld from some patients with enterocolitis since diarrhea may be experienced, particularly at higher doses.

Etidronate disodium is not metabolized and is excreted intact via the kidney. Hyperphosphatemia may occur at doses of 10-20 mg/kg/day, apparently as a result of drug-related increases in tubular reabsorption of phosphate. Serum phosphate levels generally return to normal 2-4 weeks post-therapy. There is no experience to specifically guide treatment in patients with impaired renal function. Etidronate disodium dosage should be reduced when reductions in glomerular filtration rates are present. Patients with renal impairment should be closely monitored. In approximately 10% of patients in clinical trials of etidronate disodium IV infusion (etidronate disodium) for hypercalcemia of malignancy, occasional, mild-to-moderate abnormalities in renal function (increases of >0.5 mg/dl serum creatinine) were observed during or immediately after treatment.

Etidronate disodium suppresses bone turnover, and may retard mineralization of osteoid laid down during the bone accretion process. These effects are dose and time dependent. Osteoid, which may accumulate noticeably at doses of 10-20 mg/kg/day, mineralizes normally post-therapy. In patients with fractures, especially of long bones, it may be advisable to delay or interrupt treatment until callus is evident.

In Paget's Patients: treatment regimens exceeding the recommended (see DOSAGE AND ADMINISTRATION) daily maximum dose of 20 mg/kg or continuous administration of medication for periods greater than 6 months may be associated with an increased risk of fracture.

Long bones predominantly affected by lytic lesions, particularly in those patients unresponsive to etidronate disodium therapy, may be especially prone to fracture. Patients with predominantly lytic lesions should be monitored radiographically and biochemically to permit termination of etidronate disodium in those patients unresponsive to treatment.

IV Infusion: Hypercalcemia may cause or exacerbate impaired renal function. In clinical trials, while elevations of serum creatine or blood urea nitrogen were seen in patients with hypercalcemia of malignancy prior to treatment with etidronate disodium IV infusion, these measurements improved in some patients or remained unchanged in most patients. Nevertheless, elevations in serum creatinine during treatment with etidronate disodium IV infusion have been observed in approximately 10% of patients.

Rare cases of acute renal failure have been reported in association with the use of etidronate disodium IV infusion (See WARNINGS.) Concomitant use of non-steroidal anti-inflammatory drugs and diuretics in these patients may have contributed to the renal failure.

In animal preclinical studies, administration of etidronate disodium IV infusion in amounts or at rates in excess of those recommended produced transient hypocalcemia or induced proximal renal tubular damage.

In the principal clinical of etidronate disodium IV infusion, 33 of 185 patients (18%) treated one or more times with etidronate disodium IV infusion had serum calcium values below the lower limits of normal. When adjusted for levels of reduced serum albumin, less than 1% of the 185 patients are estimated to have hypocalcemic ionized serum calcium levels. No adverse effects have been traced to hypocalcemia.

The hypercalcemia of hyperparathyroidism is refractory to etidronate disodium IV infusion. It is possible for this disease to coexist in patients with malignancy.

CARCINOGENESIS, MUTAGENESIS, AND IMPAIRMENT OF FERTILITY

Tablets and IV Infusion: Long-term studies in rats have indicated that etidronate disodium is not carcinogenic.

PREGNANCY, TERATOGENIC EFFECTS, PREGNANCY CATEGORY C

Tablets: In teratology and developmental toxicity studies conducted in rats and rabbits treated with dosages of up to 100 mg/kg (5-20 times the clinical dose), no adverse or teratogenic effects have been observed in the offspring. Etidronate disodium has been shown to cause skeletal abnormalities in rats when given at oral dose levels of 300 mg/kg (15-60 times the human dose). Other effects on the offspring (including decreased live births) are at dosages that cause significant toxicity in the parent generation and are 25 to 200 times the human dose. The skeletal effects are thought to be the result of the pharmacological effects of the drug on bone.

There are no adequate and well-controlled studies in pregnant women. Etidronate disodium-Didronel should be used during pregnancy only if the potential benefit justifies the potential risk to the fetus.

PRECAUTIONS: *(cont'd)*

IV Infusion: Animal reproduction studies have not been conducted with etidronate disodium. It is also not known whether etidronate disodium IV infusion can cause fetal harm when administered to a pregnant woman or can affect reproduction capacity. Etidronate disodium IV infusion should be given to a pregnant woman only if clearly needed.

NURSING MOTHERS

It is not known whether this drug is excreted in human milk. Because many drugs are excreted in human milk, caution should be exercised when etidronate disodium tablets or etidronate disodium IV infusion is administered to a nursing woman.

PEDIATRIC USE

Tablets: Safety and effectiveness in children have not been established. Children have been treated with etidronate disodium, at doses recommended for adults, to prevent heterotopic ossifications or soft tissue calcifications. A rachitic syndrome has been reported infrequently at doses of 10 mg/kg/day and more for prolonged periods approaching or exceeding a year. The epiphyseal radiologic changes associated with retarded mineralization of new osteoid and cartilage, and occasional symptoms reported, have been reversible when medication is discontinued.

IV Infusion: Safety and effectiveness in children have not been established.

ADVERSE REACTIONS:

TABLETS

The incidence of gastrointestinal complaints (diarrhea, nausea) is the same for etidronate disodium at 5 mg/kg/day as for placebo, about 1 patient in 15. At 10-20 mg/kg/day the incidence may increase to 2 or 3 in 10. These complaints are often alleviated by dividing the total daily dose.

In Paget's Patients: Increased or recurrent bone pain at pagetic sites, and/or the onset of pain at previously asymptomatic sites has been reported. At 5 mg/kg/day about 1 patient in 10 (versus 1 in 15 in the placebo group) report these phenomena. At higher doses the incidence rises to about 2 in 10. When therapy continues, pain resolves in some patients but persists in others.

Heterotopic Ossification: No specific adverse reactions.

Worldwide Postmarketing Experience: The worldwide postmarketing experience for etidronate disodium reflects its use in the following indications: Paget's disease, heterotopic ossification, hypercalcemia of malignancy. It also reflects the use of etidronate disodium for osteoporosis where approved in some overseas countries. Other adverse events that have been reported and were thought to be possibly related to etidronate disodium include the following: alopecia; arthropathies, including arthralgia and arthritis; bone fracture; esophagitis; glossitis; hypersensitivity reactions, including angioedema, follicular eruption, macular rash, maculopapular rash pruritus, a single case of Stevens-Johnson syndrome, and urticaria; osteomalacia; neuro-psychiatric events, including amnesia, confusion, depression, and hallucination; and paresthesias.

In patients receiving etidronate disodium, there have been rare reports of agranulocytosis, pancytopenia, and a report of leukopenia with recurrence on rechallenge. In addition, exacerbation of existing peptic ulcer disease has been reported in a few patients. In one patient, perforation also occurred.

IV INFUSION

Hypercalcemia of malignancy is frequently associated with abnormal elevations of serum creatinine and BUN. One- third of the patients participating in multiclinic trials had such elevations before receiving etidronate disodium IV infusion. In these trials, the elevations of BUN or serum creatinine improved in some patients, or remained unchanged in most patients; however, in approximately 10% of patients, occasional mild to moderate abnormalities in renal function (increases of > 0.5 mg/dl serum creatinine) were observed during or immediately after treatment. The possibility that etidronate disodium IV infusion contributed to these changes cannot be excluded (see WARNINGS.)

Of patients who participated in the controlled hypercalcemia trials, 10 of 221 (5%) treatment courses reported a metallic or altered taste, or loss of taste, which usually disappeared within hours, during and/or shortly after etidronate disodium IV infusion. A few patients with Paget's Disease of none have reported allergic skin rashes in association with oral etidronate disodium medication.

OVERDOSAGE:

TABLETS

Clinical experience with acute etidronate disodium overdosage is extremely limited. Decreases in serum calcium following substantial overdosage may be expected in some patients. Signs and symptoms of hypocalcemia also may occur in some of these patients. Some patients may develop vomiting. In one event, and 18-year-old female who ingested an estimated single dose of 4,000-6,000 mg (67-100 mg/kg) of etidronate disodium was reported to be mildly hypocalcemic (7.52 mg/dl) and experienced paresthesia of the fingers. Hypocalcemia resolved 6 hours after lavage and treatment with intravenous calcium gluconate. A 92-year-old female who accidentally received 1,600 mg of etidronate disodium per day for 3.5 days experienced marked diarrhea and required treatment for electrolyte imbalance. Orally administered etidronate disodium may cause hematologic abnormalities in some patients (see ADVERSE REACTIONS.)

Etidronate disodium suppresses bone turnover and may retard mineralization of osteoid laid down during the bone accretion process. These effects are dose and time dependent. Osteoid which may accumulate noticeably at doses of 10-20 mg/kg/day of chronic, continuous dosing mineralizes normally posttherapy.

Prolonged continuous treatment (chronic overdose) has been reported to cause nephrotic syndrome and fracture.

Gastric lavage may remove unabsorbed drug. Standard procedures for treating hypocalcemia, including the administration of Ca++ intravenously, would be expected to restore physiologic amounts of ionized calcium and relieve signs and symptoms of hypocalcemia. Such treatment has been effective.

IV INFUSION

Rapid intravenous administration of etidronate disodium at doses above 27 mg/kg has produced ECG changes and bleeding problems in animals. These abnormalities are probably related to marked and/or rapid decreases in ionized calcium levels in blood and tissue fluids. They are thought to be due to chelation of calcium by massive amounts of the diphosphate. These abnormalities have been shown to be reversible in animal studies by the administration of ionizable calcium salts.

Similar problems are not expected to occur in human treated with etidronate disodium IV infusion used as recommended (see DOSAGE AND ADMINISTRATION.) Moreover, signs and symptoms of hypocalcemia such as paresthesias and carpopedal spasms have not been reported. The chelation effects of the diphosphonate, should they occur in man, should be reversible with intravenous administration of calcium gluconate.

Administration of intravenous etidronate disodium at doses and possibly at rates in excess of those recommended has been reported to be associated with renal insufficiency.

DOSAGE AND ADMINISTRATION:

Tablets: Etidronate disodium should be taken as a single, oral dose. However, should gastrointestinal discomfort occur, the dose may be divided. To maximize absorption, patients should avoid taking the following items within two hours of dosing:

Food, especially food high in calcium, such as milk or milk products.

Vitamins with mineral supplements or antacids which are high in metals such as calcium, iron, magnesium or aluminum.

Paget's Disease: Initial Treatment Regimens: 5-10 mg/kg/day, not to exceed 6 months, or 11-20 mg/kg/day, not to exceed 3 months.

The recommended initial dose is 5 mg/kg/day for a period not to exceed six months. Doses above 10 mg/kg/day should be reserved for when 1) lower doses are ineffective or 2) there is an overriding need to suppress rapid bone turnover (especially when irreversible neurologic damage is possible) or reduce elevated cardiac output. Doses in excess of 20 mg/kg/day are not recommended.

Retreatment Guidelines: Retreatment should be initiated only after 1) a etidronate disodium-free period of at least 90 days and 2) there is biochemical, symptomatic or other evidence of active disease process. It is advisable to monitor patients every 3-6 months although some patients may go drug free for extended periods. Retreatment regimens are the same as for initial treatment. For most patients the original dose will be adequate for retreatment. If not, consideration should be given to increasing the dose within the recommended guidelines.

Heterotopic Ossification: The following treatment regimens have been shown to be effective:

Total Hip Replacement Patients: 20 mg/kg/day for 1 month before and 3 months after surgery (4 months total).

Spinal Cord Injured Patients: 20 mg/kg/day for 2 weeks followed by 10 mg/kg/day for 10 weeks (12 weeks total). Etidronate disodium therapy should begin as soon as medically feasible following the injury, preferably prior to evidence of heterotopic ossification. Retreatment has not been studied.

IV INFUSION

The recommended dose of etidronate disodium IV infusion is 7.5 mg/kg body weight/day for three successive days. **This daily dose must be diluted in at least 250 ml of sterile normal saline.** Stability studies show that diluted solution stored at controlled room temperature (59°F to 86°F or 15°C to 30°C) shows no loss of drug for a 48-hour period.

THE DILUTED DOSE OF ETIDRONATE DISODIUM IV INFUSION SHOULD BE ADMINISTERED INTRAVENOUSLY OVER A PERIOD OF AT LEAST 2 HOURS. Etidronate disodium IV infusion may be added to volumes of fluid greater than 250 ml when this is convenient.

REGARDLESS OF THE VOLUME OF SOLUTION IN WHICH DIDRONEL IV INFUSION IS DILUTED. SLOW INFUSION IS IMPORTANT TO SAFETY. The minimum infusion time of two hours at the recommended dose, or smaller doses, should be observed. The usual course of treatment is one infusion of 7.5 mg/kg body weight/day on each of 3 consecutive days but some patients have been treated for up to 7 days. When patients are treated for more than 3 days, there may be an increased possibility of producing hypocalcemia.

Retreatment with etidronate disodium IV infusion may be appropriate if hypercalcemia recurs. There should be at least a seven-day interval between courses of treatment with etidronate disodium IV infusion. The dose and manner of retreatment is the same as that for initial treatment. Retreatment for more than three days has not been adequately studied. The safety and efficacy of more than two courses of therapy with etidronate disodium IV infusion have not been studied. In the presence of renal impairment, reduction of the dose may be advisable.

Parenteral drug products should be inspected visually for particulate matter and discoloration prior to administration whenever solution and container permit.

MORE INFORMATION ON ETIDRONATE DISODIUM ORAL TABLETS

Etidronate disodium tablets may be started on the day following the last dose of Didronel IV infusion. The recommended oral dose of etidronate disodium for patients who have had hypercalcemia is 20 mg/kg body weight/day for 30 days. If serum calcium levels remain normal or at clinically acceptable levels, treatment may be extended. Treatment for more than 90 days has not been adequately studied and is not recommended. Please consult the package insert pertaining to oral etidronate disodium tablets for additional prescribing information.

HOW SUPPLIED:

TABLETS

Didronel is available as 200-mg, white, rectangular tablets with "P & G" on one face and "402" on the other.

400-mg, white, scored, capsule-shaped tablets with "N E" on one face and "406" on the other.

Avoid excessive heat (over 104°F or 40°C).

IV INFUSION

Didronel IV Infusion is supplied in 6 ml ampules as a 5% solution containing 300 mg etidronate disodium.

Avoid excessive heat (over 104°F to 40°C) for undiluted product.

(Proctor & Gamble, Tablets, 7/94)

(MGI Pharma, Inc. IV Infusion, 1/93)

HOW SUPPLIED - EQUIVALENTS NOT AVAILABLE:

Injection, Solution - Intravenous - 300 mg/6ml

6 ml x 6 $381.60 DIDRONEL, MGI Pharma 58063-0457-01

Tablet, Uncoated - Oral - 200 mg

60's $108.89 DIDRONEL, Procter Gamble Pharm 00149-0405-60

Tablet, Uncoated - Oral - 400 mg

60's $217.78 DIDRONEL, Procter Gamble Pharm 00149-0406-60

ETODOLAC *(003029)*

CATEGORIES: Analgesics; Antipyretics; Central Nervous System Agents; NSAIDS; Nonsteroidal Anti-Inflammatory; Osteoarthritis; Pain; Pregnancy Category C; FDA Class 1C ("Little or No Therapeutic Advantage"); Sales > $100 Million; FDA Approved 1991 Jan; Top 200 Drugs

BRAND NAMES: *Antilak*; *Ecridoxan*; *Edine*; *Edolan*; *Elderin*; *Entrang*; **Lodine**; *Lodine Retard* (Mexico); *Lonine*; *Tedolan*; Ultradol; *Zedolac*
(International brand names outside U.S. in italics)

FORMULARIES: Aetna; BC-BS

DESCRIPTION:

Lodine is a pyranocarboxylic acid, chemically designated as (±) 1,8-diethyl-1,3,4,9-tetrahydropyrano-[3,4-b]indole-1-acetic acid. Lodine is a racemic mixture of R- and S-etodolac.

The empirical formula for etodolac is $C_{17}H_{21}NO_3$. The molecular weight of the base is 287.37. It has a pKa of 4.65 and an n-octanol:water partition coefficient of 11.4 at pH 7.4. Etodolac is a white crystalline compound, insoluble in water but soluble in alcohols, chloroform, dimethyl sulfoxide, and aqueous polyethylene glycol.

The inactive ingredients present in the capsules are cellulose, gelatin, iron oxides, lactose, magnesium stearate, povidone, sodium lauryl sulfate, sodium starch glycolate, and titanium dioxide.

The inactive ingredients present in the tablets are cellulose, FD&C Yellow #10, FD&C Blue #2, FD&C Yellow #6, hydroxypropyl methylcellulose, lactose, magnesium stearate, polyethylene glycol, polysorbate 80, povidone, sodium starch glycolate, and titanium dioxide.

Lodine is available in 200 and 300 mg capsules and 400 mg tablets for oral administration.

CLINICAL PHARMACOLOGY:

Etodolac is a nonsteroidal anti-inflammatory drug (NSAID) that exhibits anti-inflammatory, analgesic, and antipyretic activities in animal models. The mechanism of action of etodolac, like that of other NSAIDs, is not known but is believed to be associated with the inhibition of prostaglandin biosynthesis.

Etodolac is a racemic mixture of R- and S-etodolac. As with other NSAIDs, it has been demonstrated in animals that the S-form is biologically active and the R-form is not. Both enantiomers are stable and there is no R-to-S conversion *in vivo*.

PHARMACODYNAMICS

Analgesia was demonstrable by 1/2 hour following single doses of 200 to 400 mg etodolac, with the peak effect occurring in 1 to 2 hours. The analgesic effect generally lasts for 4 to 6 hours (with some patients maintaining analgesia up to 8 to 12 hours; see CLINICAL STUDIES, Analgesia and Osteoarthritis).

PHARMACOKINETICS

The pharmacokinetics of etodolac have been evaluated in 267 normal subjects, 44 elderly patients (>65 years old), 19 patients with renal failure (creatinine clearance 37 to 88 ml/min), 9 patients on hemodialysis, and 10 patients with compensated hepatic cirrhosis. Etodolac is well absorbed and had a relative bioavailability of 100% when 200 mg capsules were compared with a solution of etodolac. Based on mass balance studies, the systemic availability of Lodine is at least 80%, and etodolac does not undergo significant first-pass metabolism following oral administration. The dose-proportionality based on AUC (the area under the plasma concentration-time curve) is linear following doses up to 600 mg every 12 hours. Peak concentrations are dose-proportional for both total and free etodolac following doses up to 400 mg very 12 hours, but following a 600 mg dose, the peak is about 20% higher than predicted on the basis of lower doses. Etodolac plasma concentrations, after multiple-dose administration, are slightly higher than after single doses, as predicted, indicating no change in pharmacokinetics with multiple-dose use. Etodolac is more than 99% bound to plasma proteins. The free fraction is less than 1% and is independent of etodolac total concentration over the dose range studied.

Etodolac, when administered orally, exhibits characteristics which are well described by a two-compartment model with first-order absorption. Mean (±1 SD) peak plasma concentrations range from approximately 14±4 to 37±9 mcg/ml after 200 to 600 mg single doses and are reached in 80±30 minutes. The mean plasma clearance of etodolac is 47 (±16) ml/h/kg, and terminal disposition half-life is 7.3 (±4.0) hours (see TABLE 1 for Summary of Pharmacokinetic Parameters).

As with many drugs which are hepatically metabolized and not dosed on a mg/kg basis, the intersubject variability of etodolac plasma levels, achieved after recommended doses, is substantial.

TABLE 1 Table of Etodolac Steady-State Pharmacokinetic Parameters (n = 267)

Kinetic Parameters	Scientific Notation (units)	Mean (24) SD ±
Extent of oral absorption (bioavailability)	F (%)	≥ 80
Peak concentration time	t_{max} (h)	1.7 ± 1.3
Oral-dose clearance	Cl/F (ml/h/kg)	47 ± 16
Central compartment volume	V_c/F (ml/kg)	132 ± 47
Steady-state volume	V_{ss}/F (ml/kg)	362 ± 129
Distribution half-life	$T_{1/2,}$ α (h)	0.71 ± 0.50
Terminal half-life	$T_{1/2,}$ β (h)	7.3 ± 4.0

Etodolac is extensively metabolized in the liver, with renal elimination of etodolac and its metabolites being the primary route of excretion. Approximately 72% of the administered dose is recovered in the urine as the following, indicated as % of the administered dose (TABLE 2):

TABLE 2

Etodolac, unchanged	1%
Etodolac, glucuronide	13%
Hydroxylated metabolites (6-, 7-, and 8-OH)	5%
Hydroxylated metabolite glucuronides	20%
Unidentified metabolites	33%

Fecal excretion accounted for 16% of the dose. Therefore, enterohepatic circulation, if present, is not extensive.

The extent of absorption of etodolac is not affected when etodolac is administered after a meal or with an antacid. Food intake, however, reduces the peak concentration reached by approximately one half and increases the time-to-peak concentration by 1.4 to 3.8 hours. Coadministration with an antacid decreases the peak concentration reached by about 15 to 20%, with no measurable effect on time-to-peak.

In studies in the elderly, age was found to have no effect on etodolac $t_{1/2}$ or protein binding, and there was no drug accumulation. Etodolac clearance was reduced by about 15%. Because the reduction in clearance is small, no dosage adjustment is generally necessary in the elderly on the basis of pharmacokinetics. The elderly may need dosage adjustment, however, on the basis of body size (see GERIATRIC POPULATION), and they may be more sensitive to antiprostaglandin effects than younger patients (see PRECAUTIONS).

In studies of the effects of mild-to-moderate renal impairment, no significant differences in the disposition of total and free etodolac were observed. In patients undergoing hemodialysis, there was a 50% greater apparent clearance of total etodolac, due to a 50% greater unbound fraction. Free etodolac clearance was not altered, indicating the importance of protein binding in etodolac's disposition. Nevertheless, etodolac is not dialyzable. No dosage adjustment of etodolac is generally required in patients with mild-to-moderate renal impairment;

CLINICAL PHARMACOLOGY: *(cont'd)*

however, etodolac should be used with caution in such patients because, as with other NSAIDs, it may further decrease renal function in some patients with impaired renal function (see PRECAUTIONS).

In patients with compensated hepatic cirrhosis, the disposition of total and free etodolac is not altered. Although no dosage adjustment is generally required in this patient population, etodolac clearance is dependent on hepatic function and could be reduced in patients with severe hepatic failure.

Special Studies: Etodolac was compared with other NSAIDs in inducing gastrointestinal (GI) microbleeding. Etodolac 1200 mg/day caused less GI blood loss than ibuprofen 2400 mg/day, indomethacin 200 mg/day, or naproxen 750 mg/day. Etodolac was also compared with piroxicam 20 mg/day in two studies; piroxicam caused more blood loss than Lodine in one of these studies but not the other.

Etodolac was also compared to other NSAIDs in GI endoscopic studies. Endoscopic scores in studies of 12 healthy subjects following 1 week of etodolac 1200 mg/day showed significantly fewer GI mucosal erosions with etodolac than with aspirin 3900 mg/day. In another study performed in healthy males 18 to 41 years of age, 12 subjects treated with etodolac 1000 mg/day for one week had lower endoscopic scores than 12 subjects treated with indomethacin 200 mg/day, naproxen 1000 mg/day, or ibuprofen 2400 mg/day. Another endoscopic study comparing effects of etodolac 1000 mg/day with piroxicam 20 mg/day, each administered to 12 normal volunteers for one month, yielded equivocal results, with both treatments showing higher scores than the 12-subject placebo-treated group.

The clinical significance of these findings is unknown.

Osteoarthritis: The use of etodolac in managing the signs and symptoms of osteoarthritis of the hip or knee was assessed in double-blind, randomized, controlled clinical trials in 341 patients. In patients with osteoarthritis of the knee, etodolac, in doses of 600 to 1000 mg/day, was better than placebo in 2 studies. The clinical trials in osteoarthritis used b.i.d. dosage regimens. The initial dosing recommendation for etodolac in patients with osteoarthritis is t.i.d. administration, due to etodolac's pharmacokinetic profile (see Pharmacokinetics and Individualization of Dosages.)

Rheumatoid Arthritis: Etodolac is not recommended for the treatment of patients with rheumatoid arthritis because in controlled clinical trials, although etodolac treatment was sometimes better than placebo treatment, it was generally not as effective as treatment with other marketed NSAIDs.

Individualization of Dosages: Etodolac, like other NSAIDs, shows considerable interindividual variation in response. Consequently, the recommended strategy for initiating therapy is to use a starting dose likely to be effective for the majority of patients and to adjust dosage thereafter based on observations of etodolac's beneficial and adverse effects.

The effectiveness of etodolac in otherwise healthy, young to middle-aged adults in acute pain studies showed symptom relief to last approximately 5 to 6 hours following single 400 mg doses and 4 to 5 hours following 200 mg doses as judged by the time by which approximately half of the patients needed remedication. In dental-extraction studies, hourly comparisons were made of the number of placebo-treated patients versus the number of etodolac-treated patients who needed to be remedicated. In theses studies, the 200 mg etodolac group had significantly fewer patients who needed remedication up to 6 hours than the placebo group, while the 400 mg etodolac group had significantly fewer patients who required remedication for up to 12 hours.

These results suggest an initial etodolac dose of 400 mg for acute pain followed by doses of 200 to 400 mg every 6 to 8 hours, as needed, not to exceed a maximum daily dose of 1200 mg. If a patient taking 400 mg doses has adequate pain relief that does not last 8 hours, then 300 mg every 6 hours (q.i.d.) is a reasonable schedule to try. As with all NSAIDs, if symptoms are still not adequately controlled by recommended doses, another analgesic should be tried.

In osteoarthritis, the recommended starting dose of etodolac is 800 to 1200 mg/day in divided doses: 400 mg t.i.d. or b.i.d. or 300 mg q.i.d. or t.i.d. which is derived from pharmacokinetic and single-dose analgesic trial data. In controlled clinical trials in patients with osteoarthritis, total daily doses of 600 to 1000 mg of etodolac were successfully given on a b.i.d. schedule. In one study, some patients were apparently adequately treated with as little as 200 mg etodolac b.i.d. The pharmacokinetic profile of etodolac and the results of single-dose analgesia studies suggest, however, that the drug may provide greater benefit when given on a t.i.d. schedule. As with other NSAIDs, the lowest dose and longest dosing interval should be sought for each patient. Therefore, after observing the response to initial therapy with etodolac, the dose and frequency should be adjusted to suit individual patient's needs. The recommended total daily dose of etodolac is 600 to 1200 mg/day given in divided doses: 400 mg t.i.d. or b.i.d.; 300 mg q.i.d., t.i.d., or b.i.d.; 200 mg q.i.d. or t.i.d.

Total daily doses of etodolac above 20 mg/kg/day have not been studied. Therefore, in patients weighing less than 60 kg (132 lbs), or where the severity of the disease, concomitant medications, or other diseases warrant, the maximum recommended total daily dose of 1200 mg should be reduced (see PRECAUTIONS.)

CLINICAL STUDIES:

Analgesia: Controlled clinical trials in analgesia were single-dose, randomized, double-blind, parallel studies in 3 pain models (dental extractions, post-general surgery, and post-episiotomy pain). In these studies, there were patients treated with placebo, 2 or more doses of etodolac, and varying combinations of aspirin, acetaminophen with codeine (oral surgery only), or zomepirac. The analgesic effective dose for etodolac established in these acute pain models was 200 to 400 mg. The onset of analgesia occurred approximately 30 minutes after oral administration and was comparable for etodolac (200 to 400 mg), aspirin (650 mg), acetaminophen with codeine (600 mg + 60 mg), and zomepirac (100 mg). The peak analgesic effect was between 1 to 2 hours. Duration of relief averaged 4 to 5 hours for 200 mg of etodolac and 5 to 6 hours for 400 mg of etodolac as measured by when approximately half of the patients required remedication. However, in some studies there were still statistically significant differences between the degree of pain relief experienced by patients treated with 200 and 400 mg of etodolac and placebo-treated patients at 8 hours.

INDICATIONS AND USAGE:

Etodolac is indicated for acute and long-term use in the management of signs and symptoms of osteoarthritis. Etodolac is also indicated for the management of pain.

CONTRAINDICATIONS:

Etodolac is contraindicated in patients who have previously shown hypersensitivity to it. Etodolac should not be given to patients in whom etodolac, aspirin, or other NSAIDs induce asthma, rhinitis, urticaria, or other allergic reactions. Fatal asthmatic reactions have been reported in such patients receiving NSAIDs.

WARNINGS:

RISK OF GASTROINTESTINAL (GI) ULCERATION, BLEEDING, AND PERFORATION WITH NONSTEROIDAL ANTI-INFLAMMATORY DRUG THERAPY

WARNINGS: *(cont'd)*

Serious GI toxicity, such as bleeding, ulceration, and perforation, can occur at any time, with or without warning symptoms, in patients treated chronically with NSAIDs. Although minor upper GI problems, such as dyspepsia, are common, usually developing early in therapy, physicians should remain alert for ulceration and bleeding in patients treated chronically with NSAIDs even in the absence of previous GI-tract symptoms. In patients observed in clinical trials of such agents for several months to 2 years' duration, symptomatic upper GI ulcers, gross bleeding, or perforation appear to occur in approximately 1% of patients treated for 3 to 6 months and in about 2% to 4% of patients treated for 1 year. Physicians should inform patients about the signs and/or symptoms of serious GI toxicity and what steps to take if they occur.

Studies to date have not identified any subset of patients not at risk of developing peptic ulceration and bleeding. Except for a prior history of serious GI events and other risk factors known to be associated with peptic ulcer disease, such as alcoholism, smoking, etc., no risk factors (*e.g.,* age, sex) have been associated with increased risk. Elderly or debilitated patients seem to tolerate ulceration or bleeding less well than other individuals, and most spontaneous reports of fatal GI events are in this population. Studies to date are inconclusive concerning the relative risk of various NSAIDs in causing such reactions. High doses of any NSAID probably carry a greater risk of these reactions, although controlled clinical trials showing this do not exist in most cases. In considering the use of relatively large doses (within the recommended dosage range), sufficient benefit should be anticipated to offset the potential increased risk of GI toxicity.

PRECAUTIONS:

GENERAL

Renal Effects: As with other NSAIDs, long-term administration of etodolac to rats has resulted in renal papillary necrosis and other renal medullary changes. Renal pelvic transitional epithelial hyperplasia, a spontaneous change occurring with variable frequency, was observed with increased frequency in treated males rats in a 2-year chronic study. The cause-effect relationship to etodolac has not been established.

A second form of renal toxicity encountered with etodolac, as with other NSAIDs, is seen in patients with conditions in which renal prostaglandins have a supportive role in the maintenance of renal perfusion. In these patients, administration of a nonsteroidal anti-inflammatory drug may cause a dose-dependent reduction in prostaglandin formation and, secondarily, in renal blood flow, which may precipitate overt renal decompensation. Patients at greatest risk of this reaction are those with impaired renal function, heart failure, liver dysfunction, those taking diuretics, and the elderly. Discontinuation of nonsteroidal anti-inflammatory drug therapy is usually followed by recovery to the pretreatment state.

Etodolac metabolites are eliminated primarily by the kidneys. The extent to which the inactive glucuronide metabolites may accumulate in patients with renal failure has not been studied. As with other drugs whose metabolites are excreted by the kidney, the possibility that adverse reactions (not listed in ADVERSE REACTIONS) may be attributable to these metabolites should be considered.

Hepatic Effects: As with all NSAIDs, borderline elevations of one or more liver tests may occur in up to 15% of patients. These abnormalities may disappear, remain essentially unchanged, or progress with continued therapy. Meaningful elevations of ALT or AST (approximately three or more times the upper limit of normal) have been reported in approximately 1% of patients in clinical trials with etodolac. A patient with symptoms and/or signs suggesting liver dysfunction, or in whom an abnormal liver test has occurred, should be evaluated for evidence of the development of a more severe hepatic reaction while on therapy with etodolac. Although such reactions are rare, if abnormal liver tests persist or worsen, if clinical signs and symptoms consistent with liver disease develop, or if systemic manifestations occur (*e.g.,* eosinophilia, rash, etc.), etodolac should be discontinued.

Hematological Effects: Anemia is sometimes seen in patients receiving etodolac or other NSAIDs. This may be due to fluid retention, gastrointestinal blood loss, or an incompletely described effect upon erythropoiesis. Patients on long-term treatment with NSAIDs, including etodolac, should have their hemoglobin or hematocrit checked if they develop signs or symptoms of anemia.

All drugs which inhibit the biosynthesis of prostaglandins may interfere to some extent with platelet function and vascular responses to bleeding. Patients receiving Lodine who may be adversely affected by such actions should be carefully observed.

Fluid Retention and Edema: Fluid retention and edema have been observed in some patients taking etodolac. Therefore, as with other NSAIDs, etodolac should be used with caution in patients with fluid retention, hypertension, or heart failure.

Information for the Patient: Etodolac, like other NSAIDs (Nonsteroidal Anti-Inflammatory Drugs), is not free of side effects. The side effects of these drugs can cause discomfort and, rarely, there may be serious side effects, such as GI bleeding, that may result in hospitalization and even fatal outcomes.

NSAIDs are often essential agents in the management of arthritis and have a major role in the treatment of pain, but they also may be commonly employed for conditions that are less serious.

Physicians may wish to discuss with their patients the potential risks (see WARNINGS, PRECAUTIONS, and ADVERSE REACTIONS) and likely benefits of etodolac treatment, particularly when it may be used for less serious conditions in which treatment without etodolac may represent an acceptable alternative to both the patient and physician.

LABORATORY TESTS

Because serious GI-tract ulceration and bleeding can occur without warning symptoms, physicians should observe chronically treated patients for the signs and symptoms of ulceration and bleeding and should inform them of the importance of this follow-up (see RISK OF GI ULCERATION, BLEEDING, AND PERFORATION WITH NSAID THERAPY.)

DRUG/LABORATORY TEST INTERACTIONS

The urine of patients who take Lodine can give a false-positive reaction for urinary bilirubin (urobilin) due to the presence of phenolic metabolites of etodolac. Diagnostic dip-stick methodology, used to detect ketone bodies in urine, has resulted in false-positive findings in some patients treated with etodolac. Generally, this phenomenon has not been associated with other clinically significant events. No dose-relationship has been observed.

Etodolac treatment is associated with a small decrease in serum uric acid levels. In clinical trials, mean decreases of 1 to 2 mg/dl were observed in arthritic patients receiving etodolac (600 mg to 1000 mg/day) after 4 weeks of therapy. These levels then remained stable for up to one year of therapy.

CARCINOGENESIS, MUTAGENESIS, AND IMPAIRMENT OF FERTILITY

No carcinogenic effect of etodolac was observed in mice or rats receiving oral doses of 15 mg/kg/day (45 to 89 mg/m^2, respectively) or less for periods of 2 years or 18 months, respectively. Etodolac was not mutagenic in *in vitro* tests performed with S. typhimurium and mouse lymphoma cells as well as in an *in vivo* mouse micronucleus test. However, data from the *in vitro* human peripheral lymphocyte test showed an increase ($p = 0.06$) in the number of gaps (3.0 to 5.3% unstained regions in the chromatid without dislocation) among the etodolac-treated cultures (50 to 200 mcg/ml) compared to negative controls (2.0%); no other

PRECAUTIONS: *(cont'd)*

difference was noted between the controls and drug-treated groups. Etodolac showed no impairment of fertility in male and female rats up to oral doses of 16 mg/kg (94 mg/m^2). However, reduced implantation of fertilized eggs occurred in the 8 mg/kg group.

TERATOGENIC EFFECTS: PREGNANCY CATEGORY C

In teratology studies, isolated occurrences of alterations in limb development were found and included polydactyly, oligodactyly, syndactyly, and unossified phalanges in rats and oligodactyly and synostosis of metatarsals in rabbits. These were observed at dose levels (2 to 14 mg/kg/day) close to human clinical doses. However, the frequency and the dosage group distribution of these findings in initial or repeated studies did not establish a clear drug or dose-responsive relationship.

There are no adequate or well-controlled studies in pregnant women. Etodolac should be used during pregnancy only if the potential benefits justify the potential risk to the fetus. Because of the known effects of NSAIDs on parturition and on the human fetal cardiovascular system with respect to closure of the ductus arteriosus, use during late pregnancy should be avoided.

LABOR AND DELIVERY

In rat studies with etodolac, as with other drugs known to inhibit prostaglandin synthesis, an increased incidence of dystocia, delayed parturition, and decreased pup survival occurred. The effects of etodolac on labor and delivery in pregnant women are unknown.

NURSING MOTHERS

Caution should be exercised if etodolac is administered to a nursing woman, because many drugs are excreted in human milk. It is not known whether etodolac is excreted in human milk.

PEDIATRIC USE

Safety and effectiveness in pediatric patients have not been established.

GERIATRIC POPULATION

In patients 65 years and older, no substantial differences in the pharmacokinetics or the side-effect profile of etodolac were seen compared with the general population. Therefore, no dosage adjustment is generally necessary in the elderly. As with any NSAID, however, caution should be exercised in treating the elderly, and when individualizing their dosage, extra care should be taken when increasing the dose because the elderly seem to tolerate NSAID side effects less well than younger patients (see Pharmacokinetics).

DRUG INTERACTIONS:

Antacids: The concomitant administration of antacids has no apparent effect on the extent of absorption of etodolac. However, antacids can decrease the peak concentration reached by 15 to 20% but have no detectable effect on the time-to-peak.

Aspirin: When etodolac is administered with aspirin, its protein binding is reduced, although the clearance of free etodolac is not altered. The clinical significance of this interaction is not known; however, as with other NSAIDs, concomitant administration of etodolac and aspirin is not generally recommended because of the potential of increased adverse effects.

Warfarin: Short-term pharmacokinetic studies have demonstrated that concomitant administration of warfarin and etodolac results in reduced protein binding of warfarin, but there was no change in the clearance of free warfarin. There was no significant difference in the pharmacodynamic effect of warfarin administered alone and warfarin administered with etodolac as measured by prothrombin time. Thus, concomitant therapy with warfarin and etodolac should not require dosage adjustment of either drug. However, following US market introduction of etodolac, there have been a few spontaneous reports of prolonged prothrombin times in etodolac-treated patients receiving concomitant warfarin therapy. Caution should be exercised because interactions have been seen with other NSAIDs.

Phenytoin: Etodolac has no apparent pharmacokinetic interaction when administered with phenytoin.

Glyburide: Etodolac has no apparent pharmacokinetic or pharmacodynamic interaction when administered with glyburide.

Diuretics: Etodolac has no apparent pharmacokinetic interaction when administered with furosemide or hydrochlorothiazide; nor does etodolac attenuate the diuretic response of either of these drugs in normal volunteers. Etodolac and other NSAIDs, nevertheless, should be used with caution in patients receiving diuretics, who have cardiac, renal, or hepatic failure (see Renal Effects.)

Cyclosporine, Digoxin, Lithium, Methotrexate: Etodolac, like other NSAIDs, through effects on renal prostaglandins, may cause changes in the elimination of these drugs leading to elevated serum levels of digoxin, lithium, and methotrexate and increased toxicity. Nephrotoxicity associated with cyclosporine may also be enhanced. Patients receiving these drugs who are given etodolac, or any other NSAID, and particularly those patients with altered renal function, should be observed for the development of the specific toxicities of these drugs.

Protein Binding: Data from *in vitro* studies, using peak serum concentrations at reported therapeutic doses in humans, show that the etodolac free fraction is not significantly altered by acetaminophen, ibuprofen, indomethacin, naproxen, piroxicam, chlorpropamide, glipizide, glyburide, phenytoin, and probenecid. In contrast, phenylbutazone causes an increase (by about 80%) in the free fraction of etodolac. Although *in vivo* studies have not been done to see if etodolac clearance is changed by coadministration of phenylbutazone, it is not recommended that they be coadministered.

ADVERSE REACTIONS:

Adverse-reaction information for etodolac was derived from 2,629 arthritic patients treated with etodolac in double-blind and open-label clinical trials of 4 to 320 weeks in duration and worldwide postmarketing surveillance studies in approximately 60,000 patients.

In clinical trials, most adverse reactions were mild and transient. The discontinuation rate in controlled clinical trials, because of adverse events, was 9% for patients treated with etodolac.

New patient complaints (with an incidence greater than or equal to 1%) are listed below by body system. The incidences were determined from clinical trials involving 465 patients with osteoarthritis treated with 300 to 500 mg of etodolac b.i.d. (*i.e.,* 600 to 1000 mg per day).

Incidence Greater Than or Equal to 1%: Probably Causally Related

Body as a whole: Chills and fever.

Digestive system: Dyspepsia (10%), abdominal pain*, diarrhea*, flatulence*, nausea*, constipation, gastritis, melena, vomiting.

Nervous system: Asthenia/malaise*, dizziness*, depression, nervousness.

Skin and appendages: Pruritus, rash.

Special senses: Blurred vision, tinnitus.

Urogenital system: Dysuria, urinary frequency.

*DRUG-RELATED PATIENT COMPLAINTS OCCURRING IN 3 TO 9% OF PATIENTS TREATED WITH ETODOLAC. DRUG-RELATED PATIENT COMPLAINTS OCCURRING IN FEWER THAN 3%, BUT MORE THAN 1%, ARE UNMARKED.

ADVERSE REACTIONS: *(cont'd)*

Incidence Less Than 1%: Probably Causally Related (Adverse reactions reported only in worldwide postmarketing experience, not seen in clinical trials, are considered rarer and are italicized):

Body As A Whole: *allergic reaction, anaphylactoid reaction.*

Cardiovascular System: Hypertension, congestive heart failure, flushing, palpitations, syncope, *vasculitis (including necrotizing and allergic).*

Digestive System: Thirst, dry mouth, ulcerative stomatitis, anorexia, eructation, elevated liver enzymes, *cholestatic hepatitis,* hepatitis, *cholestatic jaundice, jaundice,* PUB, (*i.e.,*peptic ulcer with or without bleeding and/or perforation), *intestinal ulceration, pancreatitis.*

Hemic and Lymphatic System: Ecchymosis, anemia, thrombocytopenia, bleeding time increased, *agranulocytosis, hemolytic anemia,neutropenia, pancytopenia.*

Metabolic and Nutritional: Edema, serum creatinine increase, *hyperglycemia in previously controlled diabetic patients.*

Nervous System: Insomnia, somnolence.

Respiratory System: Asthma.

Skin and Appendages: Angioedema, sweating, urticaria, vesiculobullous rash, *cutaneous vasculitis with purpura, Stevens-Johnson syndrome,* hyperpigmentation, *erythema multiforme.*

Special Senses: Photophobia, transient visual disturbances.

Urogenital System: *Elevated BUN, renal failure, renal insufficiency, renal papillary necrosis.*

Incidence Less Than 1%: Causal Relationship Unknown (Medical events occurring under circumstances where causal relationship to etodolac is uncertain. These reactions are listed as alerting information for physicians):

Body As A Whole: Infection.

Cardiovascular System: Arrhythmias, myocardial infarction.

Digestive System: Esophagitis with or without stricture or cardiospasm, colitis.

Hemic and Lymphatic System: Leukopenia.

Metabolic and Nutritional: Change in weight.

Nervous System: Paresthesia, confusion.

Respiratory System: Bronchitis, dyspnea, pharyngitis, rhinitis, sinusitis.

Skin and Appendages: Maculopapular rash, alopecia, skin peeling, photosensitivity.

Special Senses: Conjunctivitis, deafness, taste perversion.

Urogenital System: Cystitis, hematuria, leukorrhea, renal calculus, interstitial nephritis, uterine bleeding irregularities.

DRUG ABUSE AND DEPENDENCE:

Etodolac is a non-narcotic drug. Several predictive animal studies indicated that etodolac has no addiction potential in humans.

OVERDOSAGE:

Symptoms following acute NSAID overdose are usually limited to lethargy, drowsiness, nausea, vomiting, and epigastric pain which are generally reversible with supportive care. Gastrointestinal bleeding can occur and coma has occurred following massive ibuprofen or mefenamic-acid overdose. Hypertension, acute renal failure, and respiratory depression may occur but are rare. Anaphylactoid reactions have been reported with therapeutic ingestion of NSAIDs, and may occur following overdose.

Patients should be managed by symptomatic and supportive care following an NSAID overdose. There are no specific antidotes. Gut decontamination may be indicated in patients seen within 4 hours of ingestion with symptoms or following a large overdose (5 to 10 times the usual dose). This should be accomplished via emesis and/or activated charcoal (60 to 100 g in adults, 1 to 2 g/kg in children) with an osmotic cathartic. Forced diuresis, alkalinization of the urine, hemodialysis, or hemoperfusion would probably not be useful due to etodolac's high protein binding.

There have been infrequent reports of etodolac overdose. In one case of intentional etodolac overdosage (Human Toxicol. 1988;7:203-4, a 53-year-old female ingested from 15 to 46 two-hundred mg etodolac capsules (3 to 8.6 grams). Plasma etodolac concentrations were measured frequently over the next 4 days. At 5 hours after ingestion (3 hours after gastric lavage) the plasma etodolac level was 22 mcg/ml. These plasma levels and her subsequent recovery with no signs or symptoms of etodolac toxicity were consistent with systemic absorption of 600 to 800 mg. Her laboratory tests on admission showed a prolonged prothrombin time and a false-positive urine bilirubin (attributed to the phenolic etodolac metabolites).

DOSAGE AND ADMINISTRATION:

Analgesia: The recommended dose of etodolac for acute pain is 200 to 400 mg every 6 to 8 hours, as needed, not to exceed a total daily dose of 1200 mg. For patients weighing 60 kg or less, the total daily dose of etodolac should not exceed 20 mg/kg. For more details see Individualization of Dosages.

Osteoarthritis: The recommended dose of etodolac for the management of the signs and symptoms of osteoarthritis is initially 800 to 1200 mg/day in divided doses, followed by dosage adjustment within the range of 600 to 1200 mg/day given in divided doses: 400 mg t.i.d. or b.i.d.; 300 mg q.i.d., t.i.d., or b.i.d.; 200 mg q.i.d. or t.i.d. The total daily dose of etodolac should not exceed 1200 mg. For patients weighing 60 kg or less, the total daily dose of etodolac should not exceed 20 mg/kg. For more details see Individualization of Dosages.

PATIENT INFORMATION:

Etodolac is a non-steroidal anti-inflammatory (NSAID) drug used to treat arthritis and mild to moderate pain. Etodolac should not be used by those who are allergic to aspirin or other NSAIDs. This class of medications has been associated with ulcer and bleeding in the stomach. This is often relieved by taking the medication with food. Water retention may also occur and you should report any swelling of the feet or difficulty breathing to your physician immediately. This medication can be taken with or without food, however, food often alleviates stomach irritation.

HOW SUPPLIED:

Lodine is available as: 200 mg capsules (light gray with one wide red band with Lodine 200/white with two narrow red bands). 300 mg capsules (light gray with one wide red band with Lodine 300/light gray with two narrow red bands)

Store at controlled room temperature, 20°-25° C (68°-77° F), protected from moisture.

Lodine Tablets 400 mg tablets (yellow-orange, oval, film-coated tablet, debossed Lodine 400 on one side)

Store at controlled room temperature, 20°-25° C (68°-77° F).

HOW SUPPLIED - EQUIVALENTS NOT AVAILABLE:

Capsule, Gelatin - Oral - 200 mg

100's	$108.50	LODINE, Ayerst	00046-0738-81
100's	$113.61	LODINE, Ayerst	00046-0738-99

HOW SUPPLIED - EQUIVALENTS NOT AVAILABLE: *(cont'd)*

Capsule, Gelatin - Oral - 300 mg

100's	$122.89	LODINE 300, Ayerst	00046-0739-81
100's	$127.90	LODINE 300, Ayerst	00046-0739-99

Tablet, Uncoated - Oral - 400 mg

100's	$129.89	LODINE, Ayerst	00046-0761-81
100's	$132.34	LODINE, Ayerst	00046-0761-99

ETOMIDATE *(001235)*

CATEGORIES: Anesthesia; Anxiolytics, Sedatives, Hypnotic; Central Nervous System Agents; General Anesthetics; Hypnotics; Pregnancy Category C; FDA Approved 1982 Sep; Patent Expiration 1992 Sep

BRAND NAMES: **Amidate**; *Hypnomidat*; *Hypnomidate* (Germany, England, France, Mexico); *Radenarcon* (Germany)
(International brand names outside U.S. in italics)

DESCRIPTION:

Etomidate is a sterile, nonpyrogenic solution. Each milliliter contains etomidate, 2 mg, propylene glycol 35% v/v.

It is intended for the induction of general anesthesia by intravenous injection.

The drug etomidate is chemically identified as (R)-(+)-ethyl-1-(1- phenylethyl) -1H-imidazole-5-carboxylate.

CLINICAL PHARMACOLOGY:

Etomidate is a hypnotic drug without analgesic activity. Intravenous injection of etomidate produces hypnosis characterized by a rapid onset of action, usually within one minute. Duration of hypnosis is dose dependent but relatively brief, usually three to five minutes when an average dose of 0.3 mg/kg is employed. Immediate recovery from anesthesia (as assessed by awakening time, time needed to follow simple commands and time to perform simple tests after anesthesia as well as they were performed before anesthesia), based upon data derived from short operative procedures where intravenous etomidate was used for both induction and maintenance of anesthesia, is about as rapid as, or slightly faster than, immediate recovery after similar use of thiopental. These same data revealed that the immediate recovery period will usually be shortened in adult patients by the intravenous administration of approximately 0.1 mg of intravenous fentanyl, one or two minutes before induction of anesthesia, probably because less etomidate is generally required under these circumstances (consult the package insert for fentanyl before using).

The most characteristic effect of intravenous etomidate on the respiratory system is a slight elevation in arterial carbon dioxide tension ($PaCO_2$). See ADVERSE REACTIONS.

Reduced cortisol plasma levels have been reported with induction doses of 0.3 mg/kg etomidate. These persist for approximately 6 to 8 hours and appear to be unresponsive to ACTH administration.

The intravenous administration of up to 0.6 mg/kg of etomidate to patients with severe cardiovascular disease has little or no effect on myocardial metabolism, cardiac output, peripheral circulation or pulmonary circulation. The hemodynamic effects of etomidate have in most cases been qualitatively similar to those of thiopental sodium, except that the heart rate tended to increase by a moderate amount following administration of thiopental under conditions where there was little or no change in heart rate following administration of etomidate. There are insufficient data concerning use of etomidate in patients with recent severe trauma or hypovolemia to predict cardiovascular response under such circumstances.

Clinical experience and special studies to date suggest that standard doses of intravenous etomidate ordinarily neither elevate plasma histamine nor cause signs of histamine release.

Limited clinical experience, as well as animal studies, suggests that inadvertent intra-arterial injection of etomidate, unlike thiobarbiturates, will not usually be followed by necrosis of tissue distal to the injection site. Intra-arterial injection of etomidate is, however, not recommended.

Etomidate induction is associated with a transient 20-30% decrease in cerebral blood flow. This reduction in blood flow appears to be uniform in the absence of intracranial space occupying lesions. As with other intravenous induction agents, reduction in cerebral oxygen utilization is roughly proportional to the reduction in cerebral blood flow. In patients with and without intracranial space occupying lesions, etomidate induction is usually followed by a moderate lowering of intracranial pressure, lasting several minutes. All of these studies provided for avoidance of hypercapnia. Information concerning regional cerebral perfusion in patients with intracranial space occupying lesions is too limited to permit definitive conclusions.

Preliminary data suggests that etomidate will usually lower intraocular pressure moderately.

Etomidate is rapidly metabolized in the liver. Minimal hypnotic plasma levels of unchanged drug are equal to or higher than 0.23 mcg/ml; they decrease rapidly up to 30 minutes following injection and thereafter more slowly with a half-life value of about 75 minutes. Approximately 75% of the administered dose is excreted in the urine during the first day after injection. The chief metabolite is R-(+)-1-(1-phenylethyl)-1H-imidazole-5-carboxylic acid, resulting from hydrolysis of etomidate, and accounts for about 80% of the urinary excretion. Limited pharmacokinetic data in patients with cirrhosis and esophageal varices suggest that the volume of distribution and elimination half-life of etomidate are approximately double that seen in healthy subjects.

Reduced plasma cortisol and aldosterone levels have been reported following induction doses of etomidate. These results persist for approximately 6-8 hours and appear to be unresponsive to ACTH stimulation. This probably represents blockage of 11 beta- hydroxylation within the adrenal cortex.

INDICATIONS AND USAGE:

Etomidate is indicated by intravenous injection for the induction of general anesthesia. When considering use of etomidate, the usefulness of its hemodynamic properties (See CLINICAL PHARMACOLOGY) should be weighed against the high frequency of transient skeletal muscle movements (See ADVERSE REACTIONS.)

Intravenous etomidate is also indicated for the supplementation of subpotent anesthetic agents, such as nitrous oxide in oxygen, during maintenance of anesthesia for short operative procedures such as dilation and curettage or cervical conization.

CONTRAINDICATIONS:

Etomidate is contraindicated in patients who have shown hypersensitivity to it.

WARNINGS:

INTRAVENOUS ETOMIDATE SHOULD BE ADMINISTERED ONLY BY PERSONS TRAINED IN THE ADMINISTRATION OF GENERAL ANESTHETICS AND IN THE MANAGEMENT OF COMPLICATIONS ENCOUNTERED DURING THE CONDUCT OF GENERAL ANESTHESIA.

WARNINGS: *(cont'd)*

BECAUSE OF THE HAZARDS OF PROLONGED SUPPRESSION OF ENDOGENOUS CORTISOL AND ALDOSTERONE PRODUCTION, THIS FORMULATION IS NOT INTENDED FOR ADMINISTRATION BY PROLONGED INFUSION.

PRECAUTIONS:

GENERAL

Do not administer unless solution is clear and container is undamaged. Discard unused portion (see DOSAGE AND ADMINISTRATION.)

CARCINOGENESIS, MUTAGENESIS, AND IMPAIRMENT OF FERTILITY

No carcinogenesis or mutagenesis studies have been carried out on etomidate. The results of reproduction studies showed no impairment of fertility in male and female rats when etomidate was given prior to pregnancy at 0.31, 1.25 and 5 mg/kg (approximately 1 x, 4 x and 16 x human dosage).

PEDIATRIC USE

There are inadequate data to make dosage recommendations for induction of anesthesia in patients below the age of ten (10) years; therefore, such use is not recommended (see DOSAGE AND ADMINISTRATION.)

PREGNANCY CATEGORY C

Etomidate has been shown to have an embryocidal effect in rats when given in doses 1 and 4 times the human dose. There are no adequate and well-controlled studies in pregnant women. Etomidate should be used during pregnancy only if the potential benefit justifies the potential risks to the fetus. Etomidate has not been shown to be teratogenic in animals. Reproduction studies with etomidate have been shown to:

(a) Decrease pup survival at 0.3 and 5 mg/kg in rats (approximately 1 x and 16 x human dosage) and at 1.5 and 4.5 mg/kg in rabbits (approximately 5 x and 15 x human dosage). No clear dose-related pattern was observed.

(b) Increase slightly the number of stillborn fetuses in rats at 0.3 and 1.25 mg/kg (approximately 1 x and 4 x human dosage).

(c) Cause maternal toxicity with deaths of 6/20 rats at 5 mg/kg (approximately 16 x human dosage) and 6/20 rabbits at 4.5 mg/kg (approximately 15 x human dosage).

LABOR AND DELIVERY

There are insufficient data to support use of intravenous etomidate in obstetrics, including Cesarean section deliveries. Therefore, such use is not recommended.

NURSING MOTHERS

It is not known whether this drug is excreted in human milk. Because many drugs are excreted in human milk, caution should be exercised when etomidate is administered to a nursing mother.

PLASMA CORTISOL LEVELS

Induction doses of etomidate have been associated with reduction in plasma cortisol and aldosterone concentrations (see CLINICAL PHARMACOLOGY.) These have not been associated with changes in vital signs or evidence of increased mortality; however, where concern exists for patients undergoing severe stress, exogenous replacement should be considered.

ADVERSE REACTIONS:

The most frequent adverse reactions associated with use of intravenous etomidate are transient venous pain on injection and transient skeletal muscle movements, including myoclonus:

1. Transient venous pain was observed immediately following intravenous injection of etomidate in about 20% of the patients, with considerable difference in the reported incidence (1.2% to 42%). This pain is usually described as mild to moderate in severity but it is occasionally judged disturbing. The observation of venous pain is not associated with a more than usual incidence of thrombosis or thrombophlebitis at the injection site. Pain also appears to be less frequently noted when larger, more proximal arm veins are employed and it appears to be more frequently noted when smaller, more distal, hand or wrist veins are employed.

2. Transient skeletal muscle movements were noted following use of intravenous etomidate in about 32% of the patients, with considerable difference in the reported incidence (22.7% to 63%). Most of these observations were judged mild to moderate in severity but some were judged disturbing. The incidence of disturbing movements was less when 0.1 mg of fentanyl was given immediately before induction. These movements have been classified as myoclonic in the majority of cases (74%), but averting movements (7%), tonic movements (10%), and eye movements (9%) have also been reported. No exact classification is available, but these movements may also be placed into three groups by location:

(a) Most movements are bilateral. The arms, legs, shoulders, neck, chest wall, trunk and all four extremities have been described in some cases, with one or more of these muscle groups predominating in each individual case. Results of electroencephalographic studies suggest that these muscle movements are a manifestation of disinhibition of cortical activity; cortical electroencephalograms, taken during periods when these muscle movements were observed, have failed to reveal seizure activity.

(b) Other movements are described as either unilateral or having a predominance of activity of one side over the other. These movements sometimes resemble a localized response to some stimuli, such as venous pain on injection, in the lightly anesthetized patient (averting movements). Any muscle group or groups may be involved, but a predominance of movement of the arm in which the intravenous infusion is started is frequently noted.

(c) Still other movements probably represent a mixture of the first two types. Skeletal muscle movements appear to be more frequent in patients who also manifest venous pain on injection.

OTHER ADVERSE OBSERVATIONS

Respiratory System: Hyperventilation, hypoventilation, apnea of short duration (5 to 90 seconds with spontaneous recovery), laryngospasm, hiccup and snoring suggestive of partial upper airway obstruction have been observed in some patients. These conditions were managed by conventional countermeasures.

Circulatory System: Hypertension, hypotension, tachycardia, bradycardia and other arrhythmias have occasionally been observed during induction and maintenance of anesthesia. One case of severe hypotension and tachycardia, judged to be anaphylactoid in character, has been reported.

Gastrointestinal System: Postoperative nausea and/or vomiting following induction of anesthesia with etomidate is probably no more frequent than the general incidence. When etomidate was used for both induction and maintenance of anesthesia in short procedures such as dilation and curettage, or when insufficient analgesia was provided, the incidence of postoperative nausea and/or vomiting was higher than that noted in control patients who received thiopental.

OVERDOSAGE:

Overdosage may occur from too rapid or repeated injections. Too rapid injection may be followed by a fall in blood pressure. No adverse cardiovascular or respiratory effects attributable to etomidate overdose have been reported.

In the event of suspected or apparent overdosage, the drug should be discontinued, a patent airway established (intubate, if necessary) or maintained and oxygen administered with assisted ventilation, if necessary.

The LD_{50} of etomidate administered intravenously to rats is 20.4 mg/kg.

DOSAGE AND ADMINISTRATION:

Etomidate injection is intended for administration only by the intravenous route (see CLINICAL PHARMACOLOGY.) The dose for induction of anesthesia in adult patients and in children above the age of ten (10) years will vary between 0.2 and 0.6 mg/kg of body weight, and it must be individualized in each case. The usual dose for induction in these patients 0.3 mg/kg, injected over a period of 30 to 60 seconds. There are inadequate data to make dosage recommendations for induction of anesthesia in patients below the age of ten (10) years; therefore, such use is not recommended.

Smaller increments of intravenous etomidate may be administered to adult patients during short operative procedures to supplement subpotent anesthetic agents, such as nitrous oxide. The dosage employed under these circumstances, although usually smaller than the original induction dose, must be individualized. There are insufficient data to support this use of etomidate for longer adult procedures or for any procedures in children; therefore, such use is not recommended. The use of intravenous fentanyl and other neuroactive drugs employed during the conduct of anesthesia may alter the etomidate dosage requirements. Consult the prescribing information for all other such drugs before using.

Premedication: Etomidate injection is compatible with commonly administered pre-anesthetic medications, which may be employed as indicated. See also CLINICAL PHARMACOLOGY, ADVERSE REACTIONS, and dosage recommendations for maintenance of anesthesia.

Etomidate hypnosis does not significantly alter the usual dosage requirements of neuromuscular blocking agents employed for endotracheal intubation or other purposes shortly after induction of anesthesia.

Parenteral drug products should be inspected visually for particulate matter and discoloration prior to administration, whenever solution and container permit.

To prevent needle-stick injuries, needles should not be recapped, purposely bent, or broken by hand.

Exposure of pharmaceutical products to heat should be minimized. Avoid excessive heat. Protect from freezing. It is recommended that the product be stored at room temperature (25° C); however, brief exposure up to 40° C does not adversely affect the product.

HOW SUPPLIED - RATED THERAPEUTICALLY EQUIVALENT:

Injection, Solution - Intravenous - 2 mg/ml

10 ml	**$23.42**	**AMIDATE, Abbott**	**00074-8062-01**
20 ml	**$26.81**	**AMIDATE, Abbott**	**00074-8061-01**
20 ml	**$27.12**	**AMIDATE, Abbott**	**00074-8060-19**
20 ml	**$28.50**	**AMIDATE, Abbott**	**00074-8060-29**

ETOPOSIDE *(001236)*

CATEGORIES: Antineoplastics; Cancer; Lung Cancer; Oncologic Drugs; Testicular Carcinoma; Tumors; Pregnancy Category D; Sales > $100 Million; FDA Approved 1983 Nov; Patent Expiration 1993 Nov

BRAND NAMES: *Aside*; *Etopos* (Mexico); *Etoposide* (Australia); *Etosid*; *Lastet*; *Medsaposide* (Mexico); *Miantor*; *Peltasol*; *Serozide* (Mexico); **Vepesid**; *Vepeside* (France); *VP-TEC* (Mexico)
(International brand names outside U.S. in italics)

FORMULARIES: Aetna; BC-BS; Medi-Cal; WHO

COST OF THERAPY: $1,741.30 (Lung Cancer; Capsule; 50 mg; 0.143/day; 365 days)

PRIMARY ICD9: 162.9 (Malignant Neoplasm of Bronchus and Lung, Unspecified)

WARNING:
Etoposide should be administered under the supervision of a qualified physician experienced in the use of cancer chemotherapeutic agents. Severe myelosuppression with resulting infection or bleeding may occur.

DESCRIPTION:

Etoposide (also commonly known as VP-16) is a semisynthetic derivative of podophyllotoxin used in the treatment of certain neoplastic diseases. It is 4'-demethylepipodophyllotoxin 9-[4,6-0-(R)-ethylidene-β- D-glucopyranoside]. It is very soluble in methanol and chloroform, slightly soluble in ethanol, and sparingly soluble in water and ether. It is made more miscible with water by means of organic solvents. It has a molecular weight of 588.58 and a molecular formula of $C_{29}H_{32}O_{13}$.

VePesid may be administered either intravenously or orally. VePesid for Injection is available in 100 mg (5 ml), 150 mg (7.5 ml), 500 mg (25 ml), or 1 gram (50 ml), sterile, multiple dose vials.

Toposar is available for intravenous use as a 20 mg/ml solution in 100 mg (5 ml), 200 mg (10 ml) and 500 mg (25 ml) sterile, multiple dose vials.

The pH of the clear yellow solution is 3 to 4. Each ml contains 20 mg etoposide, 2 mg citric acid, 30 mg benzyl alcohol, 80 mg (modified-VePesid) polysorbate 80/tween 80, 650 mg polyethylene glycol 300, and 30.5% (v/v) alcohol. Vial headspace contains nitrogen (VePesid).

VePesid is also available as 50 mg pink capsules. Each liquid filled, soft gelatin capsule contains 50 mg of etoposide in a vehicle consisting of citric acid, glycerin, purified water, and polyethylene glycol 400. The soft gelatin capsules contain gelatin, glycerin, sorbitol, purified water, and parabens (ethyl and propyl) with the following dye system: iron oxide (red) and titanium dioxide; the capsules are printed with edible ink.

CLINICAL PHARMACOLOGY:

Etoposide has been shown to cause metaphase arrest in chick fibroblasts. Its main effect, however, appears to be at the G_2 portion of the cell cycle in mammalian cells. Two different dose-dependent responses are seen. At high concentrations (10 mcg/ml or more), lysis of cells entering mitosis is observed. At low concentrations (0.3 to 10 mcg/ml), cells are inhibited from entering prophase. It does not interfere with microtubular assembly. The predominant macromolecular effect of etoposide appears to be DNA synthesis inhibition.

CLINICAL PHARMACOLOGY: *(cont'd)*

PHARMACOKINETICS

On intravenous administration, the disposition of etoposide is best described as a biphasic process with a distribution half-life of about 1.5 hours and terminal elimination half-life ranging from 4 to 11 hours. Total body clearance values range from 33 to 48 ml/min or 16 to 36 ml/min/m^2 and, like the terminal elimination half-life, are independent of dose over a range 100-600 mg/m^2. Over the same dose range, the areas under the plasma concentration vs time curves (AUC) and the maximum plasma concentration (C_{max}) values increase linearly with dose. Etoposide does not accumulate in the plasma following daily administration of 100 mg/m^2 for 4 to 5 days.

The mean volumes of distribution at steady state fall in the range of 18 to 29 liters or 7 to 17 l/m^2. Etoposide enters the CSF poorly. Although it is detectable in CSF and intracerebral tumors, the concentrations are lower than in extracerebral tumors and in plasma. Etoposide concentrations are higher in normal lung than in lung metastases and are similar in primary tumors and normal tissues of the myometrium. *In vitro,* etoposide is highly protein bound (97%) to human plasma proteins. An inverse relationship between plasma albumin levels and etoposide renal clearance is found in children. In a study determining the effect of other therapeutic agents on the *in vitro* binding of carbon-14 labeled etoposide to human serum proteins, only phenylbutazone, sodium salicylate and aspirin displaced protein-bound etoposide at concentrations achieved *in vivo.*[1]

Etoposide binding ratio correlates directly with serum albumin in patients with cancer and in normal volunteers. The unbound fraction of etoposide significantly correlated with bilirubin in a population of cancer patients.[2,3]

After intravenous administration of ^{3}H-etoposide (70 to 290 mg/m^2), mean recoveries of radioactivity in the urine range from 42% to 67%, and fecal recoveries range from 0% to 16% of the dose. Less than 50% of an intravenous dose is excreted in the urine as etoposide with mean recoveries of 8% to 35% within 24 hours.

In children, approximately 55% of the dose is excreted in the urine as etoposide in 24 hours. The mean renal clearance of etoposide is 7 to 10 ml/min/m^2 or about 35% of the total body clearance over a dose range of 80 to 600 mg/m^2. Etoposide, therefore, is cleared by both renal and nonrenal processes, i.e., metabolism and biliary excretion. The effect of renal disease on plasma etoposide clearance is not known.

Biliary excretion appears to be a minor route of etoposide elimination. Only 6% or less of an intravenous dose is recovered in the bile as etoposide. Metabolism accounts for most of the nonrenal clearance of etoposide. The major urinary metabolite of etoposide in adults and children is the hydroxy acid [4'-demethylepipodophyllic acid-9-(4,6-0- (R)-ethylidene-β-D-glucopyranoside)], formed by opening of the lactone ring. It is also present in human plasma, presumably as the transisomer. Glucuronide and/or sulfate conjugates of etoposide are excreted in human urine and represent 5% to 22% of the dose.

After either intravenous infusion or oral capsule administration, the C_{max} and AUC values exhibit marked intrasubject and intersubject variability. This results in variability in the estimates of the absolute oral bioavailability of etoposide oral capsules.

Cmax and AUC values for orally administered etoposide capsules consistently fall in the same range as the C_{max} and AUC values for an intravenous dose of one-half the size of the oral dose. The overall mean value of oral capsule bioavailability is approximately 50% (range 25-75%). The bioavailability of etoposide capsules appears to be linear up to a dose of at least 250 mg/m^2.

There is no evidence of a first-pass effect for etoposide. For example, no correlation exists between the absolute oral bioavailability of etoposide capsules and nonrenal clearance. No evidence exists for any other differences in etoposide metabolism and excretion after administration of oral capsules as compared to intravenous infusion.

In adults, the total body clearance of etoposide is correlated with creatinine clearance, serum albumin concentration, and nonrenal clearance. In children, elevated serum SGPT levels are associated with reduced drug total body clearance. Prior use of cisplatin may also result in a decrease of etoposide total body clearance in children.

INDICATIONS AND USAGE:

Etoposide is indicated in the management of the following neoplasms:

Refractory Testicular Tumors: Etoposide injection in combination therapy with other approved chemotherapeutic agents in patients with refractory testicular tumors who have already received appropriate surgical, chemotherapeutic, and radiotherapeutic therapy.

Adequate data on the use of VePesid Capsules in the treatment of testicular cancer are not available.

Small Cell Lung Cancer: Etoposide injection and/or capsules in combination with other approved chemotherapeutic agents as first line treatment in patients with small cell lung cancer.

CONTRAINDICATIONS:

Etoposide is contraindicated in patients who have demonstrated a previous hypersensitivity to etoposide or any component of the formulation.

WARNINGS:

Patients being treated with etoposide must be frequently observed for myelosuppression both during and after therapy. Dose-limiting bone marrow suppression is the most significant toxicity associated with etoposide therapy. Therefore, the following studies should be obtained at the start of therapy and prior to each subsequent dose of etoposide: platelet count, hemoglobin, white blood cell count and differential. The occurrence of a platelet count below 50,000/mm^3 or an absolute neutrophil count below 500/mm^3 is an indication to withhold further therapy until the blood counts have sufficiently recovered.

Physicians should be aware of the possible occurrence of an anaphylactic reaction manifested by chills, fever, tachycardia, bronchospasm, dyspnea, and hypotension.

Higher rates of anaphylactic-like reactions have been reported in children who received infusions at concentrations higher than those recommended. The role that concentration of infusion (or rate of infusion) plays in the development of anaphylactic-like reactions is uncertain (VePesid). (See ADVERSE REACTIONS.) Treatment is symptomatic. The infusion should be terminated immediately, followed by the administration of pressor agents, corticosteroids, antihistamines, or volume expanders at the discretion of the physician.

For parenteral administration, etoposide should be given only by slow intravenous infusion (usually over a 30- to 60-minute period) since hypotension has been reported as a possible side effect of rapid intravenous injection.

Pregnancy Category D: Etoposide can cause fetal harm when administered to a pregnant woman. Etoposide has been shown to be teratogenic in mice and rats. There are no adequate and well-controlled studies in pregnant women. If this drug is used during pregnancy, or if the patient becomes pregnant while receiving this drug, the patient should be apprised of the potential hazard to the fetus. Women of childbearing potential should be advised to avoid becoming pregnant.

Etoposide is teratogenic and embryocidal in rats and mice at doses of 1% to 3% of the recommended clinical dose based on body surface area.

WARNINGS: *(cont'd)*

In a teratology study in SPF rats, etoposide was administered intravenously at doses of 0.13, 0.4, 1.2, and 3.6 mg/kg/day on days 6 to 15 of gestation. Etoposide caused dose-related maternal toxicity, embryotoxicity, and teratogenicity at dose levels of 0.4 mg/kg/day and higher. Embryonic resorptions were 90% and 100% at the two highest dosages. At 0.4 and 1.2 mg/kg, fetal weights were decreased and fetal abnormalities including decreased weight, major skeletal abnormalities, exencephaly, encephalocele, and anophthalmia occurred. Even at the lowest dose tested, 0.13 mg/kg, a significant increase in retarded ossification was observed.

Etoposide administered as a single intraperitoneal injection in Swiss-Albino mice at dosages of 1, 1.5, and 2 mg/kg on days 6, 7, or 8 of gestation caused dose-related embryotoxicity, cranial abnormalities, and major skeletal malformations.

PRECAUTIONS:

General: In all instances where the use of etoposide is considered for chemotherapy, the physician must evaluate the need and usefulness of the drug against the risk of adverse reactions. Most such adverse reactions are reversible if detected early. If severe reactions occur, the drug should be reduced in dosage or discontinued and appropriate corrective measures should be taken according to the clinical judgment of the physician. Reinstitution of etoposide therapy should be carried out with caution, and with adequate consideration of the further need for the drug and alertness as to possible recurrence of toxicity.

Laboratory Tests: Periodic complete blood counts should be done during the course of etoposide treatment. They should be performed prior to therapy and at appropriate intervals during and after therapy. At least one determination should be done prior to each dose of etoposide.

Carcinogenesis, Mutagenesis, and Impairment of Fertility: Carcinogenicity tests with etoposide have not been conducted in laboratory animals. Etoposide should be considered a potential carcinogen in humans. The occurrence of acute leukemia with or without a preleukemic phase has been reported rarely in patients treated with etoposide in association with other antineoplastic agents.

The mutagenic and genotoxic potential of etoposide has been established in mammalian cells. Etoposide caused aberrations in chromosome number and structure in embryonic murine cells and human hematopoietic cells; gene mutations in Chinese hamster ovary cells; and DNA damage by strand breakage and DNA-protein cross-links in mouse leukemia cells. Etoposide also caused a dose-related increase in sister chromatid exchanges in Chinese hamster ovary cells.

Treatment of Swiss-Albino mice with 1.5 mg/kg IP of etoposide on day 7 of gestation increased the incidence of intrauterine death and fetal malformations as well as significantly decreased the average fetal body weight. Maternal weight gain was not affected.

Treatment of pregnant SPF rats with 1.2 mg/kg/day IV of etoposide for 10 days led to a prenatal mortality of 92%, and 50% of the implanting fetuses were abnormal.

Pregnancy Category D: (See WARNINGS.)

Nursing Mothers: It is not known whether this drug is excreted in human milk. Because many drugs are excreted in human milk and because of the potential for serious adverse reactions in nursing infants from etoposide, a decision should be made whether to discontinue nursing or to discontinue the drug, taking into account the importance of the drug to the mother.

Pediatric Use: Safety and effectiveness in children have not been established.

Etoposide injection contains polysorbate 80. In premature infants, a life-threatening syndrome consisting of liver and renal failure, pulmonary deterioration, thrombocytopenia, and ascites has been associated with an injectable vitamin E product containing polysorbate 80. Anaphylactic reactions have been reported in children (see WARNINGS, VePesid).

ADVERSE REACTIONS:

The following data on adverse reactions are based on both oral and intravenous administration of etoposide as a single agent, using several different dose schedules for treatment of a wide variety of malignancies.

Hematologic Toxicity: Myelosuppression is dose related and dose limiting, with granulocyte nadirs occurring 7 to 14 days after drug administration and platelet nadirs occurring 9 to 16 days after drug administration. Bone marrow recovery is usually complete by day 20, and no cumulative toxicity has been reported. Fever and infection have also been reported in patients with neutropenia - VePesid.

The occurrence of acute leukemia with or without a preleukemic phase has been reported rarely in patients treated with etoposide in association with other antineoplastic agents. (See WARNINGS, VePesid.)

Gastrointestinal Toxicity: Nausea and vomiting are the major gastrointestinal toxicities. The severity of such nausea and vomiting is generally mild to moderate with treatment discontinuation required in 1% of patients. Nausea and vomiting can usually be controlled with standard antiemetic therapy. Gastrointestinal toxicities are slightly more frequent after oral administration than after intravenous infusion.

Hypotension: Transient hypotension following rapid intravenous administration has been reported in 1% to 2% of patients. It has not been associated with cardiac toxicity or electrocardiographic changes. No delayed hypotension has been noted. To prevent this rare occurrence, it is recommended that etoposide be administered by slow intravenous infusion over a 30- to 60-minute period. If hypotension occurs, it usually responds to cessation of the infusion and administration of fluids or other supportive therapy as appropriate. When restarting the infusion, a slower administration rate should be used.

Allergic Reactions: Anaphylactic-like reactions characterized by chills, fever, tachycardia, bronchospasm, dyspnea, and hypotension have been reported to occur in 0.7% to 2% of patients receiving intravenous etoposide and in less than 1% of the patients treated with the oral capsules. These reactions have usually responded promptly to the cessation of the infusion and administration of pressor agents, corticosteroids, antihistamines, or volume expanders as appropriate; however, the reactions can be fatal. Hypertension and/or flushing have also been reported. Blood pressure usually normalizes within a few hours after cessation of the infusion. Anaphylactic-like reactions have occurred during the initial infusion of etoposide.

Facial/tongue swelling, coughing, diaphoresis, cyanosis, tightness in throat, laryngospasm, back pain, and/or loss of consciousness have sometimes occurred in association with the above reactions. In addition, an apparent hypersensitivity-associated apnea has been reported rarely.

Rash, urticaria, and/or pruritus have infrequently been reported at recommended doses. At investigational doses, a generalized pruritic erythematous maculopapular rash, consistent with perivasculitis, has been reported.

Alopecia: Reversible alopecia, sometimes progressing to total baldness were observed in up to 66% of patients.

Other Toxicities: The following adverse reactions have been infrequently reported: aftertaste, fever, pigmentation, abdominal pain, constipation, dysphagia, transient cortical blindness, and optic neuritis - VePesid, and a single report of radiation recall dermatitis.

ADVERSE REACTIONS: *(cont'd)*

Hepatic toxicity, generally in patients receiving higher doses of the drug than those recommended, has been reported with etoposide. Metabolic acidosis has also been reported in patients receiving these higher doses.

The incidences of adverse reactions in the table (TABLE 1) that follows are derived from multiple databases from studies in 2,081 patients when etoposide was used either orally or by injection as a single agent.

TABLE 1

Adverse Drug Effect	Percent Range of Reported Incidence
Hematologic toxicity	
Leukopenia (less than 1,000 WBC/mm^3)	3-17
Leukopenia (less than 4,000 WBC/mm^3)	60-91
Thrombocytopenia (less than 50,000 platelets/mm^3)	1-20
Thrombocytopenia (less than 100,000 platelets/mm^3	22-41
Anemia	0-33
Gastrointestinal toxicity	
Nausea and vomiting	31-43
Abdominal pain	0-2
Anorexia	10-13
Diarrhea	1-13
Stomatitis	1-6
Hepatic	0-3
Alopecia	8-66
Peripheral neurotoxicity	1-2
Hypotension	1-2
Allergic reaction	1-2

OVERDOSAGE:

No proven antidotes have been established for etoposide overdosage.

DOSAGE AND ADMINISTRATION:

Note: Plastic devices made of acrylic or ABS (a polymer composed of acrylonitrile, butadiene, and styrene) have been reported to crack and leak when used with undiluted etoposide injection.

Etoposide injection: The usual dose of etoposide in testicular cancer in combination with other approved chemotherapeutic agents ranges from 50 to 100 mg/m^2/day on days 1 through 5 to 100 mg/m^2/day on days 1, 3, and 5.

In small cell lung cancer, the etoposide dose in combination with other approved chemotherapeutic drugs ranges from 35 mg/m^2/day for 4 days to 50 mg/m^2/day for 5 days.

Chemotherapy courses are repeated at 3- to 4-week intervals after adequate recovery from any toxicity.

VePesid Capsules: In small cell lung cancer, the recommended dose of VePesid Capsules is two times the IV dose rounded to the nearest 50 mg.

The dosage, by either route, should be modified to take into account the myelosuppressive effects of other drugs in the combination or the effects of prior x-ray therapy or chemotherapy which may have compromised bone marrow reserve.

Administration Precautions: As with other potentially toxic compounds, caution should be exercised in handling and preparing the solution of etoposide. Skin reactions associated with accidental exposure to etoposide may occur. The use of gloves is recommended. If etoposide solution contacts the skin or mucosa, immediately wash the skin or mucosa thoroughly with soap and water.

Preparation for Intravenous Administration: Etoposide must be diluted prior to use with either 5% Dextrose Injection, USP, or 0.9% Sodium Chloride Injection, USP, to give a final concentration of 0.2 to 0.4 mg/ml. If solutions are prepared at concentrations above 0.4 mg/ml, precipitation may occur. Hypotension following rapid intravenous administration has been reported, hence, it is recommended that the etoposide solution be administered over a 30- to 60-minute period. A longer duration of administration may be used if the volume of fluid to be infused is a concern. **Etoposide should not be given by rapid intravenous injection.**

Parenteral drug products should be inspected visually for particulate matter and discoloration (see DESCRIPTION section) prior to administration whenever solution and container permit.

Stability: Unopened vials of etoposide are stable for 24 months at room temperature (25°C). Vials diluted as recommended to a concentration of 0.2 to 0.4 mg/ml are stable for 96 and 24 hours, respectively, at room temperature (25°C) under normal room fluorescent lights in both glass and plastic containers.

VePesid (etoposide) Capsules must be stored under refrigeration 2°-8°C (36°-46°F). The capsules are stable for 24 months under such refrigeration conditions.

Procedures for proper handling and disposal: of anticancer drugs should be considered. Several guidelines on this subject have been published[4-10]. There is no general agreement that all of the procedures recommended in the guidelines are necessary or appropriate.

REFERENCES:

1. Gaver RC, Deeb G.: The Effect of Other Drugs on the *in vitro* Binding of 14C-Etoposide to Human Serum Proteins. Proc Am Assoc Cancer Res 1989; 30:A2132. **2.** Stewart CF, Pieper JA, Arbuck SG, Evans WE.: Altered Protein Binding of Etoposide in Patients with Cancer. Clin Pharmacol Ther 1989; 45:49-55. **3.** Stewart CF, Arbuck SG, Fleming RA, Evans WE.: Prospective Evaluation of a Model for Predicting Etoposide Plasma Protein Binding in Cancer Patients. Proc Am Assoc Cancer Res 1989; 30:A958 **4.** Recommendations for the Safe Handling of Parenteral Antineoplastic Drugs. NIH Publication No. 83-2621. For sale by the Superintendent of Documents, US Government Printing Office, Washington, DC 20402. **5.** AMA Council Report. Guidelines for Handling Parenteral Antineoplastics. JAMA 1985; 253 (11):1590-1592. **6.** National Study Commission on Cytotoxic Exposure - Recommendations for Handling Cytotoxic Agents. Available from Louis P. Jeffrey, ScD, Chairman, National Study Commission on Cytotoxic Exposure, Massachusetts College of Pharmacy and Allied Health Sciences, 179 Longwood Avenue, Boston, Massachusetts 02115. **7.** Clinical Oncological Society of Australia. Guidelines and Recommendations for Safe Handling of Antineoplastic Agents. Med J Australia 1983; 1:426-428. **8.** Jones RB, et al: Safe Handling of Chemotherapeutic Agents: A Report from the Mount Sinai Medical Center. CA-A Cancer Journal for Clinicians 1983; (Sept/Oct)258-263. **9.** American Society of Hospital Pharmacists Technical Assistance Bulletin on Handling Cytotoxic and Hazardous Drugs. Am J Hosp Pharm 1990; 47:1033-1049. **10.** OSHA Work-Practice Guidelines for Personnel Dealing with Cytotoxic (Antineoplastic) Drugs. Am J Hosp Pharm 1986; 43:1193-1204.

HOW SUPPLIED:

VePesid (etoposide) is supplied in vials for injection and 50 mg pink capsules with "Bristol 3091" printed in black blisterpacks of 20 individually labeled blisters, each containing one capsule.

Storage: Capsules are to be stored under refrigeration 2°-8°C (36°-46°F).

DO NOT FREEZE.

Dispense in child-resistant containers.

For information on package sizes available, refer to the current price schedule.

HOW SUPPLIED - RATED THERAPEUTICALLY EQUIVALENT:

Injection, Solution - Intravenous - 20 mg/ml

5 ml	$126.19	Etoposide, Gensia Labs	00703-5643-01
5 ml	**$131.05**	**VEPESID, Mead Johnson**	**00015-3095-30**
5 ml	$136.49	TOPOSAR, Pharmacia & Upjohn	00013-7336-91
10 ml	**$196.58**	**VEPESID, Mead Johnson**	**00015-3084-20**
10 ml	$272.98	TOPOSAR, Pharmacia & Upjohn	00013-7346-94
25 ml	$580.49	Etoposide, Gensia Labs	00703-5646-01
25 ml	**$638.87**	**VEPESID, Mead Johnson**	**00015-3061-20**
25 ml	$665.38	TOPOSAR, Pharmacia & Upjohn	00013-7356-88
50 ml	$1207.33	Etoposide, Gensia Labs	00703-5668-01
50 ml	**$1244.98**	**VEPESID, Mead Johnson**	**00015-3062-20**

Injection, Solution - Intravenous - 100 mg/vial

1's	**$131.05**	**VEPESID 100, Mead Johnson**	**00015-3095-20**

HOW SUPPLIED - NOT RATED EQUIVALENT:

Capsule, Elastic - Oral - 50 mg

20's	**$667.23**	**VEPESID, Mead Johnson**	**00015-3091-45**

ETRETINATE *(001237)*

CATEGORIES: Dermatologicals; Psoriasis; Skin/Mucous Membrane Agents; Skin Infections; Pregnancy Category X; FDA Approved 1986 Sep

BRAND NAMES: **Tegison**; *Tigason* (Germany)
(International brand names outside U.S. in italics)

FORMULARIES: Aetna; BC-BS

WARNING:
Contraindication: Etretinate must not be used by females who are pregnant, who intend to become pregnant, or who are unreliable or may not use reliable contraception while undergoing treatment. The period of time during which pregnancy must be avoided after treatment is concluded has not been determined. Tegison blood levels of 0.5 to 12 ng/ml have been reported in 5 of 47 patients in the range of 2.1 to 2.9 years after treatment was concluded. The length of time necessary to wait after discontinuation of treatment to assure that no drug will be detectable in the blood has not been determined. The significance of undetectable blood levels relative to the risk of teratogenicity is unknown.

Major human fetal abnormalities related to Etretinate administration have been reported, including meningomyelocele, meningoencephalocele, multiple synostoses, facial dysmorphia, syndactylies, absence of terminal phalanges, malformations of hip, ankle and forearm, low set ears, high palate, decreased cranial volume, and alterations of the skull and cervical vertebrae on x-ray.

Women of childbearing potential must not be given Etretinate until pregnancy is excluded. It is strongly recommended that a pregnancy test be performed within two weeks prior to initiating Etretinate therapy. Etretinate therapy should start on the second or third day of the next normal menstrual period. An effective form of contraception must be used for at least one month before Etretinate therapy, during therapy and following discontinuation of Etretinate therapy for an indefinite period of time.

Females should be fully counseled on the serious risks to the fetus should they become pregnant while undergoing treatment or after discontinuation of therapy. If pregnancy does occur, the physician and patient should discuss the desirability of continuing the pregnancy.

DESCRIPTION:

Etretinate, a retinoid, is available in 10-mg and 25-mg gelatin capsules for oral administration. Each capsule also contains corn starch, lactose and talc. Gelatin capsule shells contain parabens (methyl and propyl) and potassium sorbate, with the following dye systems: 10 mg: iron oxide (yellow, black and red), FD&C Blue No. 2 and titanium dioxide: 25 mg: iron oxide (yellow, black, and red) and titanium dioxide.

Chemically, etretinate is ethyl (*all-E*)-9-(4 - methoxy-2,3,6-trimethylphenyl)-3,7-dimethyl-2,4,6,8- nonatetraenoate and is related to both retinoic acid and retinol (vitamin A). It is a greenish-yellow to yellow powder with a calculated molecular weight of 354.5.

CLINICAL PHARMACOLOGY:

The mechanism of action of Etretinate is unknown.

CLINICAL

Improvement in psoriatic patients occurs in association with a decrease in scale, erythema and thickness of lesions, as well as histological evidence of normalization of epidermal differentiation, decreased stratum corneum thickness and decreased inflammation in the epidermis and dermis.

PHARMACOKINETICS

The pharmacokinetic profile of etretinate is predictable and is linear following single and multiple doses. Etretinate is extensively metabolized following oral dosing, with significant first-pass metabolism to the acid form, which also has the all-*trans* structure and is pharmacologically active. Subsequent metabolism results in the 13-*cis* acid form, chain-shortened breakdown products and conjugates that are ultimately excreted in the bile and urine.

After a 6-month course of therapy with doses ranging from 25 mg once daily to 25 mg four times daily, Cmax values ranged from 102 to 389 ng/ml and occurred at Tmax values of 2 to 6 hours. In one study the apparent terminal half-life after six months of therapy was approximately 120 days. In another study of 47 patients treated chronically with etretinate, 5 had detectable serum drug levels (in the range of 0.5 to 12 ng/ml) 2.1 to 2.9 years after therapy was discontinued. The long half-life appears to be due to storage of etretinate in adipose tissue.

Etretinate is more than 99% bound to plasma proteins, predominantly lipoproteins, whereas its active metabolite, the all-*trans* acid form, is predominantly bound to albumin. Concentrations of etretinate in blister fluid after six weeks of dosing were approximately one-tenth of those observed in plasma. Concentrations of etretinate and its all-*trans* acid metabolite in epidermal specimens obtained after 1 to 36 months of therapy were a function of location; subcutis>>serum> epidermis>dermis. Similarly, liver concentrations of etretinate in patients receiving therapy for six months were generally higher than concomitant plasma concentrations and tended to be higher in livers with a higher degree of fatty infiltration.

CLINICAL PHARMACOLOGY: *(cont'd)*

Studies in normal volunteers indicated that, when compared with the fasting state, the absorption of etretinate was increased by whole milk or a high-lipid diet.

INDICATIONS AND USAGE:

Etretinate is indicated for the treatment of severe recalcitrant psoriasis, including the erythrodermic and generalized pustular types. Because of significant adverse effects associated with its use, Etretinate should be prescribed only by physicians knowledgeable in the systemic use of retinoids and reserved for patients with severe recalcitrant psoriasis who are unresponsive to or intolerant of standard therapies: topical tar plus UVB light; psoralens plus UVA light; systemic corticosteroids; and methotrexate.

The use of Etretinate resulted in clinical improvement in the majority of patients treated. Complete clearing of the disease was observed after 4 to 9 months of therapy in 13% of all patients treated for severe psoriasis. This included complete clearing in 16% of patients with erythrodermic psoriasis and 37% of patients with generalized pustular psoriasis.

After discontinuation of Etretinate the majority of patients experience some degree of relapse by the end of 2 months. After relapse, subsequent 4- to 9-month courses of Etretinate therapy resulted in approximately the same clinical response as experienced during the initial course of therapy.

CONTRAINDICATIONS:

Pregnancy Category X See BOXED WARNING.

WARNINGS:

Pseudotumor Cerebri: Etretinate and other retinoids have been associated with cases of pseudotumor cerebri (benign intracranial hypertension). Early signs and symptoms of pseudotumor cerebri include papilledema, headache, nausea and vomiting, and visual disturbances. Patients with these symptoms should be examined for papilledema and, if present, they should discontinue Etretinate immediately and be referred for neurologic diagnosis and care.

Hepatotoxicity: Of the 652 patients treated in U.S. clinical trials, ten had clinical or histologic hepatitis considered possibly or probably related to Etretinate treatment. Liver function tests returned to normal in eight of these patients after Etretinate was discontinued; one patient had histologic changes resembling chronic active hepatitis six months off therapy, and one patient had no follow-up available. There have been four reports of hepatitis-related deaths worldwide; two of these patients had received etretinate for a month or less before presenting with hepatic symptoms. Elevations of AST (SGOT), ALT (SGPT) or LDH have occurred in 18%, 23% and 15%, respectively, of individuals treated with Etretinate. Cases with pathology findings of hepatic fibrosis, necrosis and/or cirrhosis which may be related to Etretinate therapy have been reported. If hepatotoxicity is suspected during treatment with Etretinate, the drug should be discontinued and the etiology further investigated.

Ophthalmic Effects: Corneal erosion, abrasion, irregularity and punctate staining have occurred in patients treated with Etretinate, although these effects were absent or improved after therapy was stopped in those patients who had follow-up examinations. Corneal opacities have occurred in patients receiving isotretinoin; they had either completely resolved or were resolving at follow-up six to seven weeks after discontinuation of the drug. Other ophthalmic effects that have occurred in Etretinate patients include decreased visual acuity and blurring of vision, minimal posterior subcapsular cataract, iritis, blot retinal hemorrhage, scotoma and photophobia. A number of cases of decreased night vision have occurred during Etretinate therapy. Because the onset in some patients was sudden, patients should be advised of this potential problem and warned to be cautious when driving or operating any vehicle at night. Any Etretinate patient experiencing visual difficulties should discontinue the drug and have an ophthalmological examination.

Hyperostosis: There is a very high likelihood of the development of hyperostosis with Etretinate therapy. In one clinical trial, 45 patients with a mean age of 40 years were retrospectively evaluated for evidence of hyperostosis. They had received etretinate at a mean dose of 0.8 mg/kg for a mean duration of 33 months at the time of x-ray. Eleven patients had psoriasis, while 34 patients had a disorder of keratinization. Of these, 38 patients who continued to receive etretinate at an average dose of 0.8 mg/kg/day for an average duration of 60 months, 32 (84%) had radiographic evidence of extraspinal tendon and ligament calcification. The most common sites of involvement were the ankles (76%), pelvis (53%) and knees (42%); spinal changes were uncommon. Involvement tended to be bilateral and multifocal. There were no bone or joint symptoms at the sites of radiographic abnormalities in 47% of the affected patients.

Lipids: Blood lipid determinations should be performed before Etretinate is administered and then at intervals of one or two weeks until the lipid response to Etretinate is established; this usually occurs within four to eight weeks.

Approximately 45% of patients receiving Etretinate during clinical trials experienced an elevation of plasma triglycerides. Approximately 37% developed a decrease in high density lipoproteins and about 16% showed an increase in cholesterol levels. These effects on triglycerides, HDL and cholesterol were reversible after cessation of Etretinate therapy.

Patients with an increased tendency to develop hypertriglyceridemia include those with diabetes mellitus, obesity, increased alcohol intake or a familial history of these conditions.

Hypertriglyceridemia, hypercholesterolemia and lowered HDL may increase a patient's cardiovascular risk status. In addition, elevation of serum triglycerides in excess of 800 mg/dl has been associated with acute pancreatitis. Therefore, every attempt should be made to control significant elevations of triglycerides or cholesterol or significant decreases in HDL. Some patients have been able to reverse triglyceride and cholesterol elevations or HDL decrease by reduction in weight or restriction of dietary fat and alcohol while continuing Etretinate therapy.

Cardiovascular Effects: During clinical trials of 652 patients, 21 significant cardiovascular adverse incidents were reported, all in patients who had a strong history of cardiovascular risk. These incidents were not considered related to Etretinate therapy except for two cases of myocardial infarction: one which was considered possibly related to Etretinate therapy and one for which a relationship was not specified.

Animal Studies: In general, the signs of etretinate toxicity in rats, mice and dogs are dose-related with respect to incidence, onset and severity. In rodents, the most striking manifestations of this toxicity are bone fractures; no evidence of fractures was observed in a one-year dog study. Other dose-related changes in some animals treated with etretinate in subchronic or chronic toxicity studies include alopecia, erythema, reductions in body weight and food consumption, stiffness, altered gait, hematologic changes, elevations in serum alkaline phosphatase and testicular atrophy with microscopic evidence of reduced spermatogenesis.

PRECAUTIONS:

Information for the Patient: Women of childbearing potential should be advised that they must not be pregnant when Etretinate therapy is initiated, and that they should use an effective form of contraception for one month prior to Etretinate therapy, while taking Etretinate and after Etretinate has been discontinued. Etretinate has been found in the blood of some patients two to three years after the drug was discontinued. See BOXED WARNING.

Because of the relationship of Etretinate to vitamin A, patients should be advised against taking vitamin A supplements to avoid possible additive toxic effects.

Patients should be advised that transient exacerbation of psoriasis is commonly seen during the initial period of therapy.

Patients should be informed that they may experience decreased tolerance to contact lenses during and after therapy.

LABORATORY TESTS

See WARNINGS section. In clinical studies, the incidence of hypertriglyceridemia was one patient in two, that of hypercholesterolemia one patient in six, and that of decreased HDL one patient in three during Etretinate therapy. Pretreatment and follow-up blood lipids should be obtained under fasting conditions. If alcohol has been consumed, at least 36 hours should elapse before these determinations are made. It is recommended that these tests be performed at weekly or biweekly intervals until the lipid response to Etretinate is established.

Elevations of AST (SGOT), ALT (SGPT) or LDH have occurred in 18%, 23% and 15%, respectively, of individuals treated with Etretinate. It is recommended that these tests be performed prior to initiation of Etretinate therapy, at one to two week intervals for the first one to two months of therapy and thereafter at intervals of one to three months, depending on the response to Etretinate administration.

CARCINOGENESIS, MUTAGENESIS, AND IMPAIRMENT OF FERTILITY

Carcinogenesis: In a two-year study, male or female Sprague-Dawley rats given etretinate by dietary admixture at doses up to 3 mg/kg/day (two times the maximum recommended human therapeutic dose) had no increase in tumor incidence.

In an 80-week study, Crl:CD-1 (ICR) BR mice were given etretinate by dietary admixture at doses of 1 to 5 mg/kg/day. An increased incidence of blood vessel tumors (hemangiomas and hemangiosarcomas in several different tissue sites) was noted in the high-dose male group (4 to 5 mg/kg/day) but not in the female group.

Mutagenesis: Etretinate was evaluated by the Ames test in a host-mediated assay, in the micronucleus test, and in a "treat and plate" test using the diploid yeast strain *S. cerevisiae* D7. Except for a weakly positive response in the Ames test using the tester strain TA 100, there was no evidence of genotoxicity. No differences in the rate of sister chromatid exchange (SCE) were noted in lymphocytes of patients before and after four weeks of treatment with therapeutic doses of etretinate.

Impairment of Fertility: In a study of fertility and general reproductive performance in rats, no etretinate-related effects were observed at doses up to 2.5 mg/kg/day. At a dose of 5 mg/kg/day (approximately three times the maximum recommended human therapeutic dose) the readiness of the treated animals to copulate was reduced but the pregnancy rate was unaffected. The number of viable young at birth and their postnatal weight gain and survival were adversely affected at the high dose. The pregnancy rate of the untreated first generation animals and postnatal weight gain of the untreated second generation animals were also reduced.

No adverse effects on sperm production were noted in 12 psoriatic patients given 75 mg/day of etretinate for one month and 50 mg/day for an additional two months. However, testicular atrophy was noted in subchronic and chronic rat studies and in a chronic dog study, in some cases at doses approaching those recommended for use in humans. Decreased sperm counts were reported in a 13-week dog study at doses as low as 3 mg/kg/day (approximately twice the maximum recommended human dose). Spermatogenic arrest also was reported with chronic administration of the all-*trans*metabolite to dogs.

PREGNANCY CATEGORY X

See BOXED WARNING.

The following limited preliminary data must not be read or understood to diminish the serious risk of teratogenicity set forth in the Boxed Pregnancy Warning.

Thirty women worldwide have been reported as having taken 1 or more doses of Etretinate during pregnancy. In 29 cases in which information was available, there were a total of ten congenital abnormalities. The occurrence of congenital abnormalities was four of 20 among delivered infants, 2 of 2 among spontaneously aborted fetuses, and 4 of 7 among induced abortions.

A further 38 women are reported to have become pregnant within 24 months after discontinuing Etretinate therapy. Because congenital abnormalities have been reported in these pregnancies, it cannot be stated that there is a "safe" time to become pregnant after Etretinate therapy. In 37 cases in which information was available, there were a total of 3 congenital abnormalities. The occurrence of congenital abnormalities was 2 of 29 among delivered infants, 0 of 1 among spontaneously aborted fetuses, and 1 of 5 among induced abortions. Two stillbirths with no apparent congenital abnormalities were attributed to other causes.

Nonteratogenic Effects: No adverse effects on various parameters of late gestation and lactation were observed in rats at doses of etretinate up to 4 mg/kg/day (approximately three times the maximum human recommended dose). At doses of 8 mg/kg/day (approximately five times the maximum human recommended dose) of etretinate, the rate of stillbirths was increased and neonatal weight gain and survival rate were markedly reduced.

NURSING MOTHERS

Studies have shown that etretinate is excreted in the milk of lactating rats; however, it is not known whether this drug is excreted in human milk. Because of the potential for adverse effects, nursing mothers should not receive Etretinate.

PEDIATRIC USE

No clinical studies have been conducted in the U.S. using Etretinate in children. Ossification of interosseous ligaments and tendons of the extremities has been reported. Two children showed x-ray changes suggestive of premature epiphyseal closure during treatment with Etretinate. Skeletal hyperostosis has also been reported after treatment with isotretinoin. It is not known if any of these effects occur more commonly in children, but concern should be greater because of the growth process. Pretreatment x-rays for bone age including x-rays of the knees, followed by yearly monitoring, are advised. In addition, pain or limitation of motion should be evaluated with appropriate radiological examination. Because of the lack of data on the use of etretinate in children and the possibility of their being more sensitive to effects of the drug, this product should be used only when all alternative therapies have been exhausted.

DRUG INTERACTIONS:

Little information is available on drug interactions with Etretinate; however, concomitant consumption of milk increases the absorption of etretinate. See CLINICAL PHARMACOLOGY, Pharmacokinetics and DOSAGE AND ADMINISTRATION.

ADVERSE REACTIONS:

Clinical: Hepatitis was observed in about 1.5% of patients treated with Etretinate in clinical trials. Pathology findings of hepatic fibrosis, necrosis and/or cirrhosis have been reported. See WARNINGS.

Etretinate has been associated with pseudotumor cerebri. See WARNINGS.

Hypervitaminosis A produces a wide spectrum of signs and symptoms of primarily the mucocutaneous, musculoskeletal, hepatic and central nervous systems. Nearly all of the clinical adverse events reported to date with Etretinate administration resemble those of the hypervitaminosis A syndrome. Table 1 lists the adverse events frequently reported during clinical trials in which 652 patients were treated either for psoriasis (591 patients) or a disorder of keratinization (61 patients). Table 2 lists less frequently reported adverse events in these same patients. However, the number of patients evaluated for each adverse event was not 652 in every case.

TABLE 1 Adverse Events Frequently Reported During Clinical Studies Percent Of Patient Reporting

Body System > 75%	50-75%	25-50%	10-25%
Mucocutaneous			
Dry nose	Excessive thirst	Nosebleed	Cheilitis
Chapped Lips	Sore mouth		
Dermatologic			
Loss of hair	Dry skin	Bruising	Nail Disorder
Palm/sole/fingertip peeling	Itching	Sunburn	Skin peeling
Red scaly face	Skin fragility		
Musculoskeletal			
Hypertosis*	Bone/joint pain	Muscle cramps	
Central Nervous	Fatigue	Headache	Fever
Special Senses	Irritation of eyes Eyelid abnormalities	Eyeball pain - Conjunctiva	Abnormalities of: - cornea - lens - retina Conjunctivitis Decrease in visual acuity Double vision
Gastrointestinal		Abdominal pain	Nausea Changes in appetite

* In a retrospective study of 45 patients, 38 of whom received long-term etretinate therapy, 32 (84%) has radiographic evidence of hyperostosis. See WARNINGS.

Laboratory: Etretinate therapy induces change in serum lipids in a significant number of treated patients. Approximately 45% of patients experienced elevation in serum triglycerides, 37% a decrease in high density lipoproteins and 16% an increase in cholesterol levels.

Approximately 46% of patients had elevations of triglycerides above 250 mg/dl, 54% had decreases of HDL below 36 mg%, and 19% had elevations of cholesterol above 300 mg%. One case of eruptive xanthomas associated with triglyceride levels greater than 1000 mg% has been reported.

Elevations of AST (SGOT), ALT (SGPT) or LDH were experienced by 18%, 23% and 15%, respectively, of individuals treated with Etretinate. In most of the patients, the elevations were slight to moderate and became normal either during therapy or after cessation of treatment. See WARNINGS section.

Table 3 lists the laboratory abnormalities reported during clinical trials. Data for patients who received intermittent courses of therapy for periods up to five years are included. Any instance of two consecutive values outside the range of normal, or an abnormal value with no follow-up during therapy, was considered to be possibly related to Etretinate.

OVERDOSAGE:

There has been no experience with acute overdosage in humans.

The acute oral and intraperitoneal toxicities (LD_{50}) of etretinate capsules in mice and rats were greater than 4000 mg/kg. The acute oral toxicity (LD_{50}) of etretinate substance in 4% solution was 2300 mg/kg in mice and 1300 mg/kg in rats.

DOSAGE AND ADMINISTRATION:

There is intersubject variation in the absorption and the rate of metabolism of Etretinate. Individualization of dosage is required to achieve the maximal therapeutic response with a tolerable degree of side effects. Therapy with Etretinate should generally be initiated at a dosage of 0.75 to 1 mg/kg of body weight/day taken in divided doses. A maximum dose of 1.5 mg/kg/day should not be exceeded. Erythrodermic psoriasis may respond to lower initial doses of 0.25 mg/kg/day increased by 0.25 mg/kg/day each week until optimal initial response is attained.

Maintenance doses of 0.5 to 0.75 mg/kg/day may be initiated after initial response, generally after 8 to 16 weeks of therapy. In general, therapy should be terminated in patients whose lesions have sufficiently resolved. Relapses may be treated as outlined for initial therapy.

Etretinate should be administered with food.

HOW SUPPLIED:

Brown and green capsules, 10 mg, imprinted TEGISON 10 ROCHE.

Brown and caramel capsules, 25 mg, imprinted TEGISON 10 ROCHE.

Storage: Store at 50 to 86°F (15 to 30°C). Protect from light.

HOW SUPPLIED - EQUIVALENTS NOT AVAILABLE:

Capsule, Gelatin - Oral - 10 mg

30's $59.66 TEGISON, Roche 00004-0177-57

Capsule, Gelatin - Oral - 25 mg

30's $93.30 TEGISON, Roche 00004-0179-57

TABLE 2 Less Frequent Adverse Events Reported During Clinical Studies Some Of Which May Bear No Relationship To Therapy) Percent Of Patients Reporting

Body System 1-10%	<1%
Mucocutaneous	
Dry eyes	Decreased mucous secretion
Mucous membrane abnormalities	Rhinorrhea
Dry mouth	
Gingival bleeding/inflammation	
Dermatologic	
Hair abnormalities	Abnormal skin odor
Bullous eruption	Granulation tissue
Cold/clammy skin	Healing impairment
Onycholysis	Herpes simplex
Paronychia	Hirsutism
Pyogenic granuloma	Increased pore size
Changes in perspiration	Sensory skin changes
	Skin atrophy
	Skin fissures
	Skin infection
	Urticaria
Musculoskeletal	
Myalgia	Gout
	Hyperkinesia
	Hypertonia
Central Nervous System	
Dizziness	Abnormal thinking
Lethargy	Amnesia
Changes in sensation	Anxiety
Pain	Depression
Rigors	Pseudotumor cerebri
	Emotional liability
	Faint feeling
	Flu-like symptoms
Special Senses	
Abnormal lacrimation	Changes in equilibrium
Abnormal vision	Ear drainage
Abnormalities of:	Ear infection
-Extraocular musculature	Hearing change
-Ocular tension	Night vision decrease
-Pupil	Photophobia
-Vitreous	Visual change
Earache	Scotoma
Gastrointestinal	
Hepatitis	Constipation
	Diarrhea
	Melena
	Flatulence
	Weight loss
	Oral ulcers
	Taste perversion
	Tooth caries
Cardiovascular	
Cardiovascular thrombotic or obstructive events	Atrial fibrillation
	Chest pain
Edema	Coagulation disorder
	Phlebitis
	Postural hypotension
	Syncope
Respiratory	
Dyspnea	Coughing
	Increased sputum
	Dysphonia
	Pharyngitis
Renal	
	Kidney stones
Urogenital	
	Abnormal menses
	Atrophic vaginitis
	Dysuria
	Polyuria
	Urinary retention
Other	
Malignant neoplasm	

FACTOR IX (HUMAN) *(001245)*

CATEGORIES: Blood Components/Substitutes; Blood Formation/Coagulation; Coagulants and Anticoagulants; Hemophilia; Hemostatics; Orphan Drugs; Pregnancy Category C; FDA Pre 1938 Drugs

BRAND NAMES: Alphanine; Bebulin Vh Immuno; Konyne 80; **Mononine**; Profilnine; Proplex T

FORMULARIES: WHO

DESCRIPTION:

Coagulation Factor IX (Human) Mononine, is a sterile, stable, lyophilized concentrate of Factor IX prepared from pooled human plasma and is intended for use in therapy of Factory IX deficiency, known as Hemophilia B or Christmas disease. Coagulation Factor IX (Human), Mononine is purified of extraneous plasma-derived proteins, including Factors II, VII and X, by use of immunoaffinity chromatography. A murine monoclonal antibody to Factor IX is used as an affinity ligand to isolate Factor IX from source material. Factor IX is then dissociated from the monoclonal antibody, recovered, purified further, formulated and provided as a sterile, lyophilized powder. The immunoaffinity protocol utilized results in a highly pure Factor IX preparation. It shows predominantly a single component by SDS polyacrylamide electrophoretic evaluation and has a specific activity of not less than 150 Factor IX units per mg total protein.

This concentrate has been processed by monoclonal antibody immunoaffinity chromatography during its manufacture which has been shown to be capable of reducing the risk of viral transmission. Additionally, a chemical treatment protocol and an ultrafiltration step used in its manufacture have also been shown to be capable of significant viral reductions. However, no procedure has been shown to be totally effective in removing viral infectivity from coagulation factor concentrates (see CLINICAL PHARMACOLOGY and WARNINGS).

Mononine is a highly purified preparation of Factor IX. When stored as directed, it will maintain its labeled potency for the period indicated on the container and package labels.

DESCRIPTION: *(cont'd)*

TABLE 3 Laboratory Abnormalities Reported During Clinical Studies Percent Of Patients Reporting

Body System 25-50%	10-25%	1-10%
Hematologic		
Increased:	Decreased:	Decreased:
-MCHC (60%)	-Hemoglobin/HCT	-Platelets
-MCH	-RBC	-MCH
-Reticulocytes	-MCV	-MCHC
-PTT	Increased platelets	-PTT
-ESR	Increased or decreased:	Increased:
		-Hemoglobin (HCT)
	-WBC and components	-RBC
	-Prothrombin time	
Urinary		
	WBC in urine	Proteinuria
		Glycosuria
		Microscopic hematuria
		Casts in urine
		Acetonuria
		Hemoglobinuria
Hepatic		
Increased triglycerides	Increased	Increased bilirubin
	-AST (SGOT)	Increased or decreased:
	-ALT (SGPT)	
	-Alkaline phosphatase	-Total protein
		-Albumin
	-GGTP	
	-Globulin	
	-Cholesterol	
Renal		
		Increased:
		-BUN
		-Creatinine
Electrolytes		
Increased or decreased potassium	Increased or decreased:	
	-Venous CO_2	
	-Sodium	
	-Chloride	
Miscellaneous		
Increased or decreased:	Increased or decreased FBS	Increased CPK
-Calcium		
-Phosphorus		

Each vial contains the labeled amount of Factor IX activity expressed in International Units (I.U.). One I.U. represents the activity of Factor IX and non-detectable levels of Factors II, VII and X (<0.0025 units per Factor IX unit using standard coagulation assays). It also contains histidine (approx. 10nM.), sodium chloride (approx. 0.066M) and mannitol (approximately 3%). Hydrochloric acid and/or sodium hydroxide may have been used to adjust pH. Mononine also contains trace amounts (≤50 ng mouse protein/100 Factor IX activity units) of the murine monoclonal antibody used in its purification(see CLINICAL PHARMACOLOGY.)

Mononine is to administered only intravenously.

CLINICAL PHARMACOLOGY:

Hemophilia B, or Christmas Disease, is an X-linked recessively inherited disorder of blood coagulation characterized by insufficient or abnormal synthesis of the clotting protein Factor IX. Factor IX is a vitamin K- dependent coagulation factor which is synthesized in the liver. Factor IX is activated by Factor XIa in the intrinsic coagulation pathway. Activated Factor IX (IXa) in combination with Factor VIII:C, activates Factor X and Factor Xa, resulting ultimately in the conversion of prothrombin to thrombin and the formation of a fibrin clot. The infusion of exogenous Factor IX to replace the deficiency present in Hemophilia B temporarily restores hemostasis. Depending upon the patient's level of biologically active Factor IX, clinical symptoms range from moderate skin bruising or excessive hemorrhage after trauma or surgery to spontaneous hemorrhage into joints, muscles or internal organs including the brain. Severe or recurring hemorrhages can produce death, organ dysfunction or orthopedic deformity.

Infusion of Factor IX Complex concentrates which contain varying but significant amounts of the other liver-dependent blood coagulation proteins, Factors II, VII and X, into patients with Hemophilia B results in Factor X recoveries ranging from approximately 0.57-1.1 IU/dL rise per IU/Kg body weight infused with plasma half-lives for Factor X ranging from approximately 23 hours to 31 hours.[1,2] Infusion of Coagulation Factor IX (Human), Mononine, into ten patients with severe or moderate Hemophilia B has shown a mean recovery of 0.67 IU/dL rise per IU/Kg body weight infused and a mean half-life of 22.6 hours.[7] After six months of experience with repeated infusions performed on the nine patients who remained in the study, it was shown that the half-life and recovery was maintained at a level comparable to that found with the initial infusion. The six-month data showed a mean recovery of 0.68 IU/dL rise in per IU/Kg body weight infused and a mean half-life of 25.3 hours.[7] The data show no statistically significant differences between the initial and six-month values.

The manufacturing procedure for Coagulation Factor IX (human), Mononine, includes multiple processing steps which have been designed to reduce the risk of viral transmission. Validation studies of the monoclonal antibody (MAb) immunoaffinity chromatography/chemical treatment steps and an ultrafiltration step used in the production of Mononine document the viral reduction capacity of the processes employed. These studies were conducted using the Human Immunodeficiency Virus (HIV) and four model viruses representing a broad range of viral characteristics, i.e., Sindbis, Vaccina, Vesicular Stomatitis (VSV) and Murine Encephalomyocarditis (EMC), a non-lipid encapsulated model virus. The results of these validation studies (see TABLE 1) document an HIV viral reduction capacity of ≥11.56 log_{10} and a viral reduction capacity 10.24 log_{10} for Sindbis, 11.64 log_{10} for EMC, ≥14.23 log_{10} for VSV, and ≥10.90 log_{10} for Vaccina.

The viral safety of Coagulation Factor IX (Human), Mononine, is being studied in clinical trials of two cohorts of hemophilia B patients previously unexposed to blood or blood products. One cohort of patients includes those with moderate to severe Factor IX deficiency requiring chronic replacement therapy and the second cohort of patients includes those with a mild deficiency requiring Factor IX replacement for surgical procedures. These patients are being followed for serum ALT levels as well as for a range of viral serologies. Available serum ALT data, representing 22 patients, 13 of whom were followed for 6-15 months and 9 of whom were followed for less than 6 months, and available serology results, representing 19 patients, have continued to show no evidence of transmission of hepatitis or HIV. Although these studies are ongoing, these preliminary results show no evidence of viral transmission resulting from the infusion of Mononine (see WARNINGS.)

CLINICAL PHARMACOLOGY: *(cont'd)*

TABLE 1 Monoclonal Antibody Purified, Clinical Pharmacology Summary of Virus Reduction Studies (Log $_{10}$Reduction)

Processing Step	HIV	Sindbis	EMC	VSV	Vaccina
MAb Chromatography	*	2.76	3.89	≥7.18**	≥3.60
Sodium Thiocyanate Chemical Treatment	≥4.16	0	0	**	0
Ultrafiltration	≥7.4	7.48	7.75	7.05	≥7.30
Total Log_{10} Reduction	≥11.56	10.24	11.64	≥14.23	≥10.90

* MAb Chromatography not studied
** Results are for combined MAb chromatography/sodium thiocyanate step.

Coagulation Factor IX (Human), Mononine, contains trace amounts of the murine monoclonal antibody used in its purification (≤50 ng mouse protein per 100 Factor IX activity units). Using another Murine monoclonal antibody purified concentrate, Antihemophilic Factor (Human) Monoclate, Factor VIII:C, Heat Treated, also containing trace amounts of murine protein (≤50 ng per 100 AHF activity units), a number of patients seronegative for Anti-HIV-1 were monitored to determine whether they would develop antibody to mouse protein or experience adverse reactions as a result of repeated exposure. Pre-study serum measurements of 27 patients for human anti-mouse lgG showed that, prior to treatment, 6 of them had either detectable antibody to mouse proteins or cross- reactive proteins. These patients continued to demonstrate similar or lower antibody levels during the study. of the remaining 21 patients, 6 were shown to have low antibody levels on one or more occasions. In no case was observance of low antibody level associated with an anamnestic response or with any clinical adverse reaction. Patients were observed for time periods ranging from 2 to 30 months.

In similar clinical studies with Mononine, a cohort of nine Anti-HIV seropositive hemophilia B patients were administered Mononine for periods of 15-months. No appreciable increases in levels of lgG, lgM or lgE Human Anti-Mouse Antibodies (HAMA) were observed when compared to pre-study levels.

In clinical studies of Coagulation Factor IX (Human), Mononine, patients were monitored for evidence of disseminated intravascular coagulation. In six patients evaluated after infusion, fibrinogen levels and platelet counts were unchanged, and fibrin degradation products did not appear.[7]

In further clinical evaluations of Coagulation Factor IX (Human), Mononine, in a crossover study with a Factor IX Complex concentrate, Mononine was not associated with the formation of prothrombin activation fragment (F_{1+2}) whereas the Factor IX Complex was.[7,8]Prothrombin activation fragment (F_{1+2}) is indicative of activation of prothrombin.

INDICATIONS AND USAGE:

Coagulation Factor IX (Human), Mononine, is indicated for the prevention and control of bleeding in Factor IX deficiency, also known as Hemophilia B or Christmas disease.

Mononine is not indicated in the treatment or prophylaxis of Hemophilia A patients with inhibitors to Factor VIII.

Coagulation Factor IX (Human) Mononine, contains non-detectable levels of Factors II, VII and X (<0.0025 units per factor IX unit using standard coagulation assays) and is, therefore, not indicated for replacement therapy of these clotting factors.

Mononine is also not indicated in the treatment or reversal of coumarin-induced anticoagulation or in a hemorrhagic state caused by hepatitis- induced lack of production of liver dependent coagulation factors.

CONTRAINDICATIONS:

Known hypersensitivity to mouse protein is a contraindication to Coagulation Factor IX (Human), Mononine.

WARNINGS:

This product is prepared from pooled human plasma which may contain the causative agents of hepatitis and other viral diseases. Prescribed manufacturing procedures utilized at the plasma collection centers, plasma testing laboratories, and the fractionation facilities are designed to reduce the risk of transmitting viral infection. However the risk of viral infectivity from this product cannot be totally eliminated. Accordingly, the benefits and risks of treatment with this concentrate should be carefully assessed prior to use.

Individuals who receive infusions of blood or plasma products may develop signs and/or symptoms of some viral infections, particularly nonA, nonB hepatitis.

Since the use of Factor IX Complex concentrates has historically been associated with the development of thromboembolic complications, the use of Factor IX-containing products may be potentially hazardous in patients with signs of fibrinolysis and in patients with disseminated intravascular coagulation (DIC).

PRECAUTIONS:

The administration of Factor IX Complex concentrates, containing Factors II, VII, IX and X, has been associated with the development of thromboembolic complications. Although Coagulation Factor IX (Human), Mononine, contains highly purified Factor IX, the potential risk of thrombosis or disseminated intravascular coagulation observed with the use of other products containing Factor IX should be recognized. Patients given Mononine should be observed closely for signs or symptoms of intravascular coagulation or thrombosis. Because of the potential risk of thromboembolic complications, caution should be exercised when administering this concentrate to patients with liver disease, to patients post-operatively, to neonates, or to patients at risk of thromboembolic phenomena or disseminated intravascular coagulation[3,4] In each of these situations, the potential benefit of treatment with Mononine should be weighed against risk of these complications.

Coagulation Factor IX (Human), Mononine, should be administered intravenously at a rate that will permit observation of the patient for any immediate reaction. Rates of infusion of up to 225 units per minute have been regularly tolerated with no adverse reactions. If any reaction takes place that is thought to be related to the administration of Mononine, the rate of infusion should be decreased or the infusion stopped, as dictated by the response of the patient.

During the course of treatment, determination of daily Factor IX levels is advised to guide the dose to be administered and the frequency of repeated infusions. Individual patients may vary in the response to Mononine, achieving different levels of *in vivo* recovery and demonstrating different half-lives.

The use of high doses of Factor IX Complex concentrates has been reported to be associated with instances of myocardial infarction, disseminated intravascular coagulation, venous thrombosis and pulmonary embolism. Generally a Factor IX level of 25% to 50% is considered adequate for hemostasis, including major hemorrhages and surgery. Attempting to maintain Factor IX levels of >75% to 100% during treatment is not recommended. To

PRECAUTIONS: *(cont'd)*

achieve Factor IX levels that will remain above 25% between once a day administrations, each daily dose should attempt to raise the level to 50-60%. (See DOSAGE AND ADMINISTRATION.)

No data are available regarding the use of amino caproic acid following an initial infusion of Mononine for the prevention or treatment of oral bleeding following trauma or dental procedures such as extractions.

Formation of Antibodies to Mouse Protein: Although no hypersensitivity reactions have been observed, because Mononine contains trace amounts of mouse protein (≤50 ng per 100 Factor IX activity units), the possibility exists that patients treated with Mononine may develop hypersensitivity to the mouse protein.

INFORMATION FOR THE PATIENT

Patients should be informed of the early signs of hypersensitivity reactions including hives, generalized urticaria, tightness of the chest, wheezing, hypotension, and anaphylaxis, and should be advised to discontinue use of the concentrate and contact their physician if these symptoms occur.

PREGNANCY CATEGORY C

Animal reproduction studies have not been conducted with Coagulation Factor IX (Human), Mononine. It is also not known whether Mononine can cause fetal harm when administered to a pregnant woman or can affect reproduction Capacity. Mononine should be given to a pregnant woman only if clearly needed.

ADVERSE REACTIONS:

As with the administration of any product intravenously, the following reactions may be observed following administration: headache, fever, chills, flushing, nausea, vomiting, tingling, lethargy, hives, stinging or burning at the infusion site or other manifestations of allergic reactions.

There is a potential risk of thromboembolic following the administration of Mononine. (See WARNINGS and PRECAUTIONS).

The patient should be monitored closely during the infusion of Mononine to observe for the development of any reaction. If any reaction takes place that is thought to be related to the administration of Mononine, the rate of infusion should be decreased or the infusion stopped, as dictated by the response of the patient.

DOSAGE AND ADMINISTRATION:

Coagulation Factor IX (Human), Mononine, is intended for intravenous administration only. It should be reconstituted with the volume of Sterile Water for Injection, USP supplied with the lot, and administered within three hours of reconstitution. After administration, any unused solution and the administration equipment should be discarded.

As a general rule, 1 unit of Factor IX activity per Kg can be expected to increase the circulating level of Factor IX by 1% of normal. the following formula provides a guide to dosage calculations:

Number of IX I.U. Required = Body Weight (in Kg) x desired Factor IX increase (%normal) x 1.0 unit/Kg

The amount of Coagulation Factor IX (Human), Mononine, to be infused, as well as the frequency of infusions, will vary with each patient and with the clinical situation.[5,6]

As a general rule, the level of Factor X required for treatment of different conditions is as follows (TABLE 2):

TABLE 2 Monoclonal Antibody Purified, DOSAGE AND ADMINISTRATION

	Minor Spontaneous Hemorrhage, Prophylaxis	Major Trauma or Surgery
Desired Levels of Factor IX for Hemostasis	15-25%	25-50%
Initial loading dose to achieve desired level	up to 20-30 units/kg	up to 75 units/kg
Frequency of dosing depending on $T_{1/2}$ and	once, repeated in 24 hours if necessary	every 18-30 hours, depending on measured Factor IX levels
Duration of treatment	once, repeated if necessary	up to ten days, depending upon nature of insult

Recovery of the loading dose varies from patient to patient. Doses administered should be titrated to the patient's response.

In the presence of an inhibitor to Factor IX, higher doses of Mononine might be necessary to overcome the inhibitor (see PRECAUTIONS.) No data on the treatment of patients with inhibitors to Factor IX with Mononine are available.

For information on the rate of administration, see Rate of Administration, below.

RECONSTITUTION

1. Warm both the diluent and Coagulation Factor IX (Human), Mononine, in unopened vials to room temperature (not above 37°C (98°F)).

2. Remove the caps from both vials to expose the central portions of the rubber stoppers.

3. Treat the surface of the rubber stoppers with antiseptic solution and allow them to dry.

4. Using aseptic technique, insert one end of the double-end needle into the rubber stopper of the diluent vial. Invert the diluent vial and insert the other end of the double-end needle into the rubber stopper of the Mononine vial. Direct the diluent, which will be drawn in by vacuum, over the entire surface of the Mononine cake. (In order to assure transfer of all the diluent, adjust the position of the tip of the needle in the diluent vial to the inside edge of the diluent stopper.) Rotate the vial to ensure complete wetting of the cake during the transfer process.

5. Remove the diluent vial to release the vacuum, then remove the double-end needlefrom the Mononine vial.

6. Gently swirl the vial until the powder is dissolved and the solution is ready for administration. The concentrate routinely and easily reconstitutes within one minute. To assure sterility, Mononine should be administered within three hours of reconstitution.

7. Product should be filtered prior to use as described under Administration. Parenteral drug preparations should be inspected visually for particulate matter and discoloration prior to administration, whenever solution and container permit.

ADMINISTRATION INTRAVENOUS INJECTION

Plastic disposable syringes are recommended with Coagulation Factor IX (Human) Mononine, solution. The ground glass surface of all-glass syringes tend to stick with solutions of this type. Please note, this concentrate is supplied with a SELF-VENTING filter spike.

1. Using aseptic technique, attach the vented filter spike to a sterile disposable syringe. **CAUTION:** The use of other, non-vented filter needles or spikes without the proper procedure may result in an air lock and prevent the complete transfer of the concentrate. **CAUTION:** DO NOT INJECT AIR INTO THE MONONINE VIAL. The self-venting

DOSAGE AND ADMINISTRATION: *(cont'd)*

feature of the vented filter spike precludes the need to inject air in order to facilitate withdrawal of the reconstituted solution. The injection of air could cause partial product loss through the vent filter.

2. Insert the vented filter spike into the stopper of the Mononine vial, invert the vial, and position the filter spike so that the orifice is at the inside edge of the stopper.

3. Withdraw the reconstituted solution into the syringe.

4. Discard the filter spike. Perform venipuncture using the enclosed winged needle with microbore tubing. Attach the syringe to the luer end of the tubing.

CAUTION: Use of other winged needles without microbore tubing, although compatible with the concentrate, will result in a larger retention of solution within the winged infusion set.

RATE OF ADMINISTRATION

The rate of administration should be determined by the response and comfort to the patient; intravenous dosage administration rates of up to 225 units/minute have been regularly tolerated without incident. When reconstituted as directed, i.e, to approximately 100 units/ml, Mononine should be administered at a rate of approximately 2.0 per minute.

STORAGE

When stored at refrigerator temperature, 2° to 8°C (36° to 46°F), Coagulation Factor IX (Human), Mononine, is stable for the period indicated by the expiration date on its label. Within this period, Mononine may be stored at room temperature not to exceed 30°C (86°F), for up to one month.

Avoid freezing which may damage container from the diluent.

REFERENCES:

1. Zauber NP, Levin J: Factor IX levels in patients with hemophilia B (Christmas disease) following transfusion with concentrates of Factor IX or fresh frozen plasma (FFP). *Medicine* (Baltimore) 56(3): 213-24, 1977. **2.** Smith KJ, Thompson AR: Labeled Factor IX Kinetics in Patients with Hemophilia-B. *Blood* 58(3): 625-629, 1981. **3.** Aledort LM: Factor IX and Thrombosis. *Scand J. Haematology*Suppl. 30:40, 1977. **4.** Cederbaum Al, Blatt PM, Roberts HR: Intravascular coagulation with use of human prothrombin complex concentrates. *Ann Intern Med.*84:683-687, 1976. **5.** Kasper CK, Dietrich SL: Comprehensive Management of Hemophilia.*Clin. Haematol.*14(2): 489-512, 1985. **6.** Johnson AJ, Aronson DL, Williams WJ: Preparation and clinical use of plasma and plasma fractions. Chap. 167 in *Hematology* 3rd Edition, Williams WJ, Beutler E, Erslev AJ, Lichtman MA (Eds.), McGraw Hill Book Co., New York: pp 1563-1583, 1983. **7.** Kim HC, McMillan CW, White GC, Bergman GE, Horton MW, Saidi P: Purified Factor IX Using Monoclonal Immunoaffinity Technique: Clinical Trials in Hemophilia B and Comparison to Prothrombin Complex Concentrates. *Blood* 79, No.3: pp 568-575, 1992. **8.** Kim HC, Matts L, Eisele J, Czachur M, Saidi P: Monoclonal Antibody Purified Factor IX—Comparative Thrombogenecity to Prothrombin Complex Concentrate. Seminars in Hematology, Vol.28, No. 3, Suppl. 6, July, 1991, pp. 15-20.

HOW SUPPLIED - EQUIVALENTS NOT AVAILABLE:

Injection, Solution - Intravenous - 250 unit

1's	**$1.10**	**MONONINE, Centeon**	**00053-7668-01**

Injection, Solution - Intravenous - 500 unit

1's	$0.35	Konyne 80, Bayer Pharm	00192-0626-20
1's	$0.35	PROFILNINE, HEAT-TREAT/WET-METH, Alpha Therapeutic	49669-3700-01
1's	**$1.10**	**MONONINE, Centeon**	**00053-7668-02**

Injection, Solution - Intravenous - 1000 unit

1's	$0.35	Konyne 80, Bayer Pharm	00192-0626-50
1's	$0.35	PROFILNINE, HEAT-TREAT/WET-METH, Alpha Therapeutic	49669-3700-02
1's	$1.00	Alphanine, Sd Heat Treat/Solv, Alpha Therapeutic	49669-3800-01
1's	**$1.10**	**MONONINE, Centeon**	**00053-7668-04**
1's	$1.40	ALPHANINE, HEAT-TREAT/SOLV SUSP, Alpha Therapeutic	49669-3900-02

Injection, Solution - Intravenous - 1200 unit

1's	$0.25	PROPLEX T, Baxter Hyland	00944-0581-01
1's	$0.55	BEBULIN VH IMMUNO, Immuno-US	54129-0244-02

FAMCICLOVIR *(003213)*

CATEGORIES: Anti-Infectives; Antimicrobials; Antivirals; Fever Blisters; Herpes Zoster; Infections; Lesions; Varicella; Varicella Zoster; Viral Agents; FDA Class 1S ("Standard Review"); Sales > $100 Million; FDA Approved 1994 Jun

BRAND NAMES: Famvir

FORMULARIES: Medi-Cal; PCS

COST OF THERAPY: $129.15 (Herpes Zoster; Tablet; 500 mg; 3/day; 7 days)

DESCRIPTION:

Famvir contains famciclovir, an orally administered prodrug of the antiviral agent penciclovir. Chemically, famciclovir is known as 2-[2- (2-amino-9*H*-purin-9-yl)ethyl]-1,3-propanediol diacetate. Its molecular formula is $C_{14}H_{19}N_5O_4$; its molecular weight is 321.3. It is a synthetic acyclic guanine derivative.

Famciclovir is a white to pale yellow solid. It is freely soluble in acetone and methanol, and sparingly soluble in ethanol and isopropanol. At 25°C famciclovir is freely soluble (>25% w/v) in water initially, but rapidly precipitates as the sparingly soluble (2-3% w/v) monohydrate. Famciclovir is not hygroscopic below 85% relative humidity. Partition coefficients are: octanol/water (pH 4.8) P=1.09 and octanol/phosphate buffer (pH 7.4) P=2.08.

Tablets for Oral Administration: Each white oval, film-coated tablet contains 500 mg of famciclovir. Inactive ingredients consist of hydroxypropyl cellulose, hydroxypropyl methylcellulose, lactose, magnesium stearate, polyethylene glycols, sodium starch glycolate and titanium dioxide.

CLINICAL PHARMACOLOGY:

Microbiology Mechanism of Antiviral Activity: Famciclovir undergoes rapid biotransformation to the active antiviral compound penciclovir, which has inhibitory activity against herpes simplex virus type 1 (HSV-1) and 2 (HSV-2) and varicella zoster virus (VZV). In HSV-1-, HSV-2- and VZV-infected cells, viral thymidine kinase phosphorylates penciclovir to a monophosphate from which, in turn, is converted to penciclovir triphosphate by cellular kinases. *In vitro* studies demonstrate that penciclovir triphosphate inhibits HSV-2 polymerase competitively with deoxyguanosine triphosphate. Consequently, herpes viral DNA synthesis and, therefore, replication are selectively inhibited.

In uninfected cells, penciclovir does not affect DNA synthesis at concentrations ≥20 times those achieved in clinical usage, because it is phosphorylated only in virus-infected cells. Penciclovir triphosphate has an intracellular half-life of 10 hours in HSV-1-, 20 hours in HSV-2- and 7 hours in VZV-infected cells. The long intracellular half-life of penciclovir triphosphate may ensure prolonged antiviral activity in virus-infected cells.

CLINICAL PHARMACOLOGY: *(cont'd)*

Antiviral Activity *In Vitro* and *In Vivo*: In cell culture studies, penciclovir has antiviral activity against the following herpesviruses (listed in decreasing order of potency): HSV-1, HSV-2, and VZV. However, the degree of inhibition is dependent upon a number of variables, including the assay method, the host cell, virus type and multiplicity of infection MOI). See TABLE 1.

TABLE 1

Method of Assay	Virus Type	Cell Type	IC_{50}	IC_{50} (mcg/ml)
Plaque Reduction	VZV (c.i.)	MRC-5	5.0 ± 3.0	
	VZV (c.i.)	Hs68	0.9 ± 0.4	
	HSV-1 (c.i.)	MRC-5	0.2 - 0.6	
	HSV-1 (c.i.)	WISH	0.04 - 0.5	
	HSV-2 (c.i.)	MRC-5	0.9 - 2.1	
	HSV-2 (c.i.)	WISH	0.1 - 0.8	
Virus Yield	HSV-1 (c.i.)	MRC-5		0.4 - 0.5
Reduction	HSV-2 (c.i.)	MRC-5		0.6 - 0.7
DNA Synthesis	VZV (Ellen)	MRC-5	0.1	
Inhibition	HSV-1 (SC16)	MRC-5	0.04	
	HSV-2 (MS)	MRC-5	0.05	

(c.i.) = clinical isolates

Short-term treatment of HSV-1 or HSV-2-infected MRC-5 cells with 1 mcg/ml penciclovir reduced viral DNA by 76% and 52%, respectively. Studies of VZV-infected MRC-5 cells exposed to pulse-treatment with penciclovir for 8 hours on days, 0, 1, 2, and 3 produced an IC_{50} of 5 mcg/ml.

As there is no appropriate animal model that mimics VZV infection in humans, the antiviral activity of penciclovir has not been evaluated in animal infected with VZV. However, penciclovir has been shown to have inhibitory activity against HSV-1 and HSV-2 infections in mice and guinea pigs. The level of antiviral activity depends on a number of factors, including the route of infection, route of administration of penciclovir, and time between virus infection and treatment with penciclovir.

The clinical significance of inhibitory activity of penciclovir against HSV-1 and HSV-2 in *in vitro* animal studies is unknown at this time.

PHARMACOKINETICS

Absorption and Bioavailability: Famciclovir is the diacetyl 6-deoxy analog of the active antiviral compound penciclovir. Following oral administration, little or no famciclovir is detected in plasma or urine.

The absolute bioavailability of famciclovir is 77 ± 8% as determined following the administration of a 500 mg famciclovir oral dose and a 400 mg penciclovir intravenous dose to 12 healthy male subjects.

Following single oral-dose administration of 500 mg famciclovir to 124 healthy male volunteers across 10 studies the mean ±SD area under the plasma concentration-time profile (AUC) was 8.6 ± 1.9 mcg°hr/ml. The maximum concentration (C_{max}) was 3.3 ± 0.8 mcg/ml and the time to C_{max} (T_{max}) was 0.9 ± 0.5 hours.

Following single oral-dose administration of 500 mg famciclovir to seven patients with herpes zoster, the mean ±SD AUC, C_{max}, and T_{max} were 12.1 ± 1.7 mcg°hr/ml, 4.0 ± 0.7 mcg/ml, and 0.7 ± 0.2 hours, respectively. The AUC of penciclovir was approximately 35% greater in patients with herpes zoster as compared to healthy volunteers. Some of this difference may be due to differences in renal function between the two groups.

There is no accumulation of penciclovir after the administration of 500 mg famciclovir t.i.d. for 7 days. Penciclovir concentrations increased in proportion to dose over a famciclovir dose range of 125 mg to 750 mg administered as a single dose.

Penciclovir C_{max} decreased approximately 50% and T_{max} was delayed by 1.5 hours when a capsule formulation of famciclovir was administered with food (nutritional content was approximately 910 Kcal and 26% fat). There was no effect on the extent of availability (AUC) of penciclovir. There was an 18% decrease in C_{max} and a delay in T_{max} of about 1 hour when famciclovir was given 2 hours after a meal as compared to its administration 2 hours before a meal. Because there was no effect on the extent of systemic availability of penciclovir, it appears that Famciclovir can be taken without regard to meals.

Distribution: After a 1-hour intravenous infusion of penciclovir at doses of 5 mg/kg to 20 mg/kg, the volume of distribution (Vd_{β}) of penciclovir in 18 and 12 healthy male volunteers who received a dose of 5 mg/kg and 400 mg, respectively, was 83.1 ± 7.7 l (1.13 ± 0.11 l/kg) and 125 ± 21.3 l (1.55 ± 0.28 l/kg). Vd_{ss} was 72.6 ± 11.5 l (0.98 ± 0.13 l/kg- and 85.3 ± 10.8 l (1.08 ± 0.17 l/kg).

Penciclovir is <20% bound to plasma proteins over the concentration range of 0.1 to 20 mcg/ml. The blood plasma ratio of penciclovir is approximately 1.

Metabolism: Following oral administration, famciclovir is deacetylated and oxidized to form penciclovir. Metabolites that are inactive include 6-deoxy penciclovir, monoacetylated penciclovir, and 6- deoxy monoacetylated penciclovir (each<0.5% of the dose). Little or no famciclovir is detected in plasma or urine.

An *in vitro* study using human liver microsomes demonstrated that cytochrome P450 does not play an important role in famciclovir metabolism. The conversion of 6-deoxy penciclovir to penciclovir is catalyzed by aldehyde oxidase.

Elimination: Approximately 94% of administered radioactivity was recovered in urine over 24 hours (83% of the dose was excreted in the first 6 hours)after the administration of 5 mg/kg radiolabeled penciclovir as a 1-hour infusion to three healthy male volunteers. Penciclovir accounted for 91% of the radioactivity excreted in the urine.

Following the oral administration of a single 500-mg dose of radiolabeled famciclovir to three healthy male volunteers, 73% and 27% of administered radioactivity were recovered in urine and feces over 72 hours, respectively. Penciclovir accounted for 82% and 6-deoxy penciclovir accounted for 7% of the radioactivity excreted in the urine. Approximately 60% of the administered radiolabeled dose was collected in urine in the first 6 hours.

After intravenous administration of penciclovir in 48 healthy male volunteers, mean ±SD total plasma clearance of penciclovir was 36.6 ± 6.3 l/hr (0.48 ± 0.09 l/hr/kg). Penciclovir renal clearance accounted for 74.5 ± 8.8% of total plasma clearance.

Renal clearance of penciclovir following the oral administration of a single 500 mg dose of famciclovir to 109 healthy male volunteers was 27.7 ± 7.6 l/hr.

Plasma elimination half-life of penciclovir was 2.0 ± 0.3 hours after intravenous administration of penciclovir to 48 healthy male volunteers and 2.3 ± 0.4 hours after oral administration of 500 mg famciclovir to 124 healthy male volunteers. The half-life in seven patients with herpes zoster was 3.1 ± 1.1 hours.

SPECIAL POPULATIONS

Renal Insufficiency: Apparent plasma clearance, renal clearance, and the plasma-elimination rate constant of penciclovir decreased linearly with reduction in renal function. After the administration of a single 500 mg famciclovir oral dose (n=27) to healthy volunteers and to volunteers with varying degrees of renal insufficiency CLCR ranged from 6.4 to 138.8 ml/min.), the following results were obtained (TABLE 2):

CLINICAL PHARMACOLOGY: *(cont'd)*

TABLE 2

Parameter mean ± SD	CL_{CR}*≥60 (ml/min.)	CL_{CR}40-59 (ml/min.)	CL_{CR}20-39 (ml/min.)	CL_{CR}<20 (ml/min.)
Cl_{CR}(ml/min)	88.1 ± 20.6	49.3 ± 5.9	26.5 ± 5.3	12.7 ± 5.9
CL_{β}(l/hr)	30.1 ± 10.6	13.0 ± 1.3**	4.2 ± 0.9	1.6 ± 1.0
CL/F***(l/hr)	66.9 ± 27.5	27.3 ± 2.8	12.8 ± 1.3	5.8 ± 2.8
Half-life(hr)	2.3 ± 0.5	3.4 ± 0.7	6.2 ± 1.6	13.4 ± 10.2
n	15	5	4	3

* CL_{CR} is measured creatinine clearance
** n=4
*** CL/F consists of bioavailability factor and famciclovir to penciclovir conversion factor.

A dosage adjustment is recommended for patients with renal insufficiency (see DOSAGE AND ADMINISTRATION.)

Hepatic Insufficiency: Well-compensated chronic liver disease (chronic hepatitis [n=6], chronic ethanol abuse [n=8], or primary biliary cirrhosis [n=1]) had no effect on the extent of availability (AUC) of penciclovir following a single dose of 500 mg famciclovir. However, there was a 44% decrease in penciclovir mean maximum plasma concentration and the time to maximum plasma concentration was increased by 0.75 hours in patients with hepatic insufficiency compared to normal volunteers. No dosage adjustment is recommended for patients with well- compensated hepatic impairment. The pharmacokinetics of penciclovir have not been evaluated in patients with severe uncompensated hepatic impairment.

Elderly Subjects: Based on cross-study comparisons, mean penciclovir AUC was 40% larger and penciclovir renal clearance was 22% lower after the oral administration of famciclovir in elderly volunteers (n=18, age 65 to 79 years) compared to younger volunteers. Some of this difference may be due to differences in renal function between the two groups.

Gender: The pharmacokinetics of penciclovir was evaluated in 18 healthy male and 18 healthy female volunteers after single-dose oral administration of 500 mg famciclovir. AUC of penciclovir was 9.3 ± 1.9 mcg°hr/ml and 11.1 ± 2.1 mcg°hr/ml in males and females, respectively. Penciclovir renal clearance was 28.5 ± 8.9 l/hr and 21.8 ± 4.3 l/hr, respectively. These differences attributed to differences in renal function between the two groups. No famciclovir dosage adjustment based on gender is recommended.

Pediatric Patients: The pharmacokinetics of famciclovir or penciclovir have not been evaluated in patients <18 years of age.

Race: The pharmacokinetics of famciclovir or penciclovir with respect to race have not been evaluated.

CLINICAL STUDIES:

PLACEBO-CONTROLLED TRIAL

Herpes Zoster: Famciclovir was studied in a placebo-controlled, double-blind trial of 419 otherwise healthy patients with uncomplicated herpes zoster who were treated with Famciclovir 500 mg t.i.d. (n=138). Famciclovir 750 mg t.i.d. (n=135) or placebo (n=146). Treatment was begun within 72 hours of initial lesion appearance and therapy was continued for 7 days.

Dermatology and Virology: The times to full crusting, loss of vesicles, loss of ulcers, and loss of crusts were shorter for Famciclovir 500 mg-treated patients than for placebo-treated patients in the overall study population. The median time to full crusting in Famciclovir 500 mg- treated patients was 5 days compared to 7 days in placebo-treated patients. No additional efficacy was demonstrated with the higher dose of famciclovir (750 mg t.i.d.) when compared to Famciclovir 500 mg t.i.d. In the total population, 65.2% of patients had a positive viral culture at some time during their acute infection. Patients treated with Famciclovir 500 mg had a shorter median duration of viral shedding (time to positive viral culture) than did placebo-treated patients (1 day and 2 days, respectively).

Acute Pain and Postherpetic Neuralgia: There were no overall differences in the duration of acute pain (*i.e.,* pain before rash healing) between Famciclovir and placebo-treated groups. In addition, there was no difference in the incidence of postherpetic neuralgia (*i.e.,* pain after rash healing) between the treatment groups. In the 186 patients (44.4% of total study population) who did develop postherpetic neuralgia, the median duration of postherpetic neuralgia was shorter in patients treated with Famciclovir 500 mg than in those treated with placebo (63 days and 119 days, respectively).

ACTIVE-CONTROL TRIAL

A second double-blind controlled trial in 545 otherwise healthy patients with uncomplicated herpes zoster treated within 72 hours of initial lesion appearance compared Famciclovir 250 mg t.i.d. (n=134), Famciclovir 500 mg t.i.d. (n=134), Famciclovir 750 mg t.i.d. (n=138), and acyclovir 800 mg 5 times per day (n=139) for 7 days. In this study, patients treated with Famciclovir at each dose and acyclovir had comparable times to full lesion crusting and times to loss of acute pain. There were no statistically significant differences in the time to loss of postherpetic neuralgia between Famciclovir and acyclovir-treated groups.

GENITAL HERPES INFECTIONS

Recurrent Episodes: In two placebo-controlled trials, 626 otherwise healthy patients with a recurrence of genital herpes were treated with famciclovir 125 mg b.i.d. (n=160), famciclovir 250 mg b.i.d. (n=169), famciclovir 500 mg b.i.d. (n=154) or placebo (n=143) for 5 days. Treatment was initiated within 6 hours of either symptom onset or lesion appearance. In the two studies combined, the median time to healing in famciclovir 125 mg-treated patients was 4 days compared to 5 days in placebo-treated patients and the median time to cessation of viral shedding was 1.8 vs. 3.4 days in famciclovir 125 mg and placebo recipients, respectively. The median time to loss of all symptoms was 3.2 days in famciclovir 125 mg-treated patients vs. 3.8 days in placebo-treated patients. When used to treat acute recurrent genital herpes, no additional efficacy was demonstrated with higher doses of famciclovir (250 mg b.i.d. or 500 mg b.i.d.) when compared to famciclovir 125 mg b.i.d.

INDICATIONS AND USAGE:

Herpes Zoster: Famciclovir is indicated for the management of acute herpes zoster (shingles).

Genital Herpes: Famciclovir is indicated for the treatment of recurrent episodes of genital herpes.

CONTRAINDICATIONS:

Famciclovir is contraindicated in patients with known hypersensitivity to the product.

PRECAUTIONS:

GENERAL

The efficacy of Famciclovir has not been studied in ophthalmic zoster, disseminated zoster, or in immunocompromised patients.

Dosage adjustment is recommended when administering Famciclovir to patients with creatinine clearance values <60 ml/min. See DOSAGE AND ADMINISTRATION. There is no information from clinical trials about the safety of administering Famciclovir to patients with renal dysfunction.

PRECAUTIONS: *(cont'd)*

CARCINOGENESIS, MUTAGENESIS, AND IMPAIRMENT OF FERTILITY

Famciclovir was administered orally unless otherwise stated.

Carcinogenesis: Two-year dietary carcinogenicity studies on famciclovir were conducted in rats and mice. The high dose tested in rats and mice was lowered after 7 to 8 months of drug administration to ensure long-term survival (female rats and male/female mice from 750 to 600 mg/kg/day; male rats from 300 to 240 mg/kg/day). A significant increase in the incidence of mammary adenocarcinoma was seen in female rats receiving 600 mg/kg/day (1.5 times the human systemic exposure at the recommended oral dose of 500 mg t.i.d. based on area under the plasma concentration curve comparisons [24 hr AUC] for penciclovir). Marginal increases in the incidence of subcutaneous tissue fibrosarcomas or squamous cell carcinomas of the skin were seen in females rats (dosed at 600 mg/kg/day) and male mice (dosed at 600 mg/kg/day; 0.4x the human systemic exposure, based on 24 hr AUC of penciclovir), respectively. No increase in tumor incidence were reported for male rats treated at doses up to 240 mg/kg/day (0.9x the human AUC), or in female mice at doses up to 600 mg/kg/day (0.4x human AUC).

Mutagenesis: Famciclovir and penciclovir (the active metabolite of famciclovir) were tested for genotoxic potential in a battery of *in vitro* and *in vivo* assays. Famciclovir and penciclovir were negative in *in vitro* tests for gene mutation in bacteria (*S. typhimurium* and *E. coli*) and unscheduled DNA synthesis in mammalian HeLa 83 cells (at doses up to 10,000 and 5000 mcg/plate, respectively). Famciclovir was also negative in the L5178Y mouse lymphoma assay (5000 mcg/ml), the *in vivo* mouse micronucleus test (4800 mg/kg), and rat dominant lethal study (5000 mg/kg). Famciclovir induced increases in polyploidy in human lymphocytes *in vitro* in the absence of chromosomal damage (1200 mcg/ml). Penciclovir was positive in the L5178Y mouse lymphoma assay for gene mutation/chromosomal aberrations, with and without metabolic activation (100 mcg/ml). In human lymphocytes, penciclovir caused chromosomal aberrations in the absence of metabolic activation (250 mcg/ml). Penciclovir caused an increased incidence of micronuclei in mouse bone marrow *in vivo* when administered intravenously at doses highly toxic to bone marrow (500 mg/kg), but not when administered orally.

Impairment of Fertility: Testicular toxicity was observed in rats, mice, and dogs following repeated administration of famciclovir or penciclovir. Testicular changes included atrophy of the seminiferous tubules, reduction in sperm count, and/or increased incidence of sperm with abnormal morphology or reduced motility. The degree of toxicity to male reproduction was related to dose and duration of exposure. In male rats, decreased fertility was observed after 10 weeks of dosing at 500 mg/kg/day (1.9x the human AUC). The no observable effect level for sperm and testicular toxicity in rats following chronic administration (26 weeks) was 50 mg/kg/day (0.2x the human systemic exposure based on AUC comparisons). Testicular toxicity was observed following chronic administration to mice (104 weeks) and dogs (26 weeks) at doses of 600 mg/kg/day (0.4x the human AUC) and 150 mg/kg/day (1.7x the human AUC), respectively.

Famciclovir had no effect on general reproductive performance or fertility in female rats at doses up to 1000 mg/kg/day (3.6x the human AUC).

PREGNANCY CATEGORY B

Teratogenic Effects: Famciclovir was tested for effects on embryo-fetal development in rats and rabbits at oral doses up to 1000 mg/kg/day (approximately 3.6x and 1.8x the human systemic exposure to penciclovir based on AUC comparisons for the rat and the rabbit, respectively) and intravenous doses of 360 mg/kg/day in rats (2x the human dose based on body surface area [BSA] comparisons) or 120 mg/kg/day in rabbits (1.5x the human dose [BSA]). No adverse effects were observed on embryo-fetal development. Similarly, no adverse effects were observed following intravenous administration of penciclovir to rats (80mg/kg/day, 0.4x the human dose [BSA]) or rabbits (60 mg/kg/day, 0.7x the human dose [BSA]).

There are, however, no adequate and well-controlled studies in pregnant women. Because animal reproduction studies are not always predictive of human response, famciclovir should be used during pregnancy only if the benefit to the patient clearly exceeds the potential risk to the fetus.

NURSING MOTHERS

Following oral administration of famciclovir to lactating rats, penciclovir was excreted in breast milk at concentrations higher than those seen in the plasma. It is not known whether it is excreted in human milk. Because of the potential for tumorigenicity shown for famciclovir in rats, a decision should be made whether to discontinue nursing or to discontinue the drug, taking into account the importance of the drug to the mother.

PEDIATRIC USE

Safety and efficacy in children under the age of 18 years have not been established.

GERIATRIC USE

Of 816 patients with herpes zoster in clinical studies who were treated with Famciclovir, 248 (30.4%) were ≥65 years of age and 103 (13%) were ≥75 years of age. No overall differences were observed in the incidence or types of adverse events between younger and older patients.

DRUG INTERACTIONS:

Cimetidine: Penciclovir AUC and urinary recovery increased 18 ± 12% (mean ± SD) and 12 ± 16%, respectively, in 12 healthy volunteers following the administration of a single 500 mg famciclovir dose after pre-treatment with cimetidine 400 mg b.i.d. for 7 days. The magnitude of this effect is considered to be of no clinical importance.

Allopurinol: The pharmacokinetics of penciclovir were not altered following a single oral dose of 500 mg famciclovir in 12 healthy volunteers after pre-treatment with allopurinol 300 mg once daily for 7 days.

Theophylline: Penciclovir AUC and C_{max} increased 22 ± 9% and 26 ± 27%, respectively, following a single oral dose of 500 mg famciclovir in 12 healthy volunteers who were pre-treated with theophylline 300 mg b.i.d. for 7 days. Renal clearance of penciclovir decreased by 12 ± 14% (n=10). The magnitude of this effect is considered to be of clinical importance.

Digoxin: After single-dose administration of digoxin and famciclovir in 12 healthy male volunteers, the $C_{max}$of digoxin 19 ± 18% as compared to digoxin administered alone. There was no change in digoxin AUC 0-t where t ranged from 10 to 72 hours.

No clinically significant alterations in penciclovir pharmacokinetics were observed following single-dose administration of 500 mg famciclovir after pre-treatment with multiple doses of cimetidine, allopurinol, or theophylline (See DRUG INTERACTIONS).

Concurrent use with probenecid or other drugs significantly eliminated by active renal tubular secretion mat result in increased plasma concentrations of penciclovir.

The conversions of 6-deoxy penciclovir to penciclovir is catalyzed by aldehyde oxidase. Interactions with other drugs metabolized by this enzyme could potentially occur.

ADVERSE REACTIONS:

HERPES ZOSTER

In four clinical studies involving 816 Famciclovir-treated patients with herpes zoster (Famciclovir, 250 mg t.i.d. to 750 mg t.i.d.), the most frequent adverse events associated with Famciclovir were headache, nausea, fatigue, which occurred in similar frequencies in placebo-treated patients. TABLE 3 lists adverse events occurring on-therapy with an incidence of ≥2%

ADVERSE REACTIONS: *(cont'd)*

per treatment group in the placebo-controlled Famciclovir trial 008. The frequency and types of reported adverse events in trial 008 were representative of the safety experience in the active- controlled herpes zoster Famciclovir trials (007 and 094).

RECURRENT GENITAL HERPES

In three placebo-controlled clinical trials involving 528 famciclovir-treated patients with genital herpes (famciclovir, 125 mg b.i.d. to 500 mg t.i.d.), the most frequent adverse events associated with famciclovir were headache and nausea. Table 3 lists adverse events occurring on-therapy in famciclovir clinical trials with an incidence ≥ 2% per treatment group.

TABLE 3 Adverse Events Reported by ≥2% of Treatment Group in Patients in One Herpes Zoster and Three Placebo-Controlled Recurrent Genital Herpes Famciclovir Trials*

	Incidence			
	Herpes Zoster		Genital Herpes	
Event	Famciclovir (n=273) %	Placebo (n=146) %	Famciclovir (n=640) %	Placebo (n=225) %
Nervous System				
Headache	22.7	17.8	23.6	16.4
Dizziness	3.3	4.1	5.5	4.9
Insomnia	1.5	1.4	2.5	2.2
Somnolence	2.6	2.7	1.6	0.4
Paresthesia	2.6	0.0	1.3	0.0
Gastrointestinal				
Nausea	12.5	11.6	10.0	8.0
Diarrhea	7.7	4.8	4.5	7.6
Abdominal Pain	1.1	3.4	3.9	5.8
Dyspepsia	1.1	1.4	3.4	2.2
Flatulence	1.5	0.7	1.9	2.2
Constipation	4.4	4.8	1.4	0.9
Vomiting	4.8	3.4	1.3	0.9
Anorexia	2.6	4.1	1.1	0.9
Body As A Whole				
Fatigue	4.4	3.4	6.3	4.4
Pain	2.6	2.7	2.0	1.8
Injury	2.6	0.0	0.8	1.3
Fever	3.3	4.1	0.8	0.4
Rigors	1.5	2.7	0.5	0.4
Respiratory				
URI	0.7	0.7	3.3	2.7
Pharyngitis	2.6	4.8	2.7	2.2
Sinusitis	2.6	1.4	1.3	1.3
Musculoskeletal				
Back Pain	1.5	2.7	1.9	2.2
Arthralgia	1.5	2.1	1.3	0.0
Zoster/Genital Herpes-Related Signs/Symptoms /Complications	2.9	3.4	1.7	2.2
Skin And Appendages				
Pruritus	3.7	2.7	0.9	0.0

* Patients may have entered into more than one clinical trial.

OVERDOSAGE:

No acute overdosage has been reported. Appropriate symptomatic and supportive therapy should be given.

It is not known if hemodialysis removes penciclovir from the blood. However, hemodialysis does enhance the elimination of acyclovir, a related nucleoside analog.

DOSAGE AND ADMINISTRATION:

HERPES ZOSTER

The recommended dosage is 500 mg every 8 hours for 7 days. Therapy should be initiated promptly as soon as herpes zoster is diagnosed. In clinical trials, the effect of Famciclovir on rash resolution was more pronounced in patients age 50 years and older. Treatment was begun within 72 hours of rash onset in these studies and was more useful if started within 48 hours. The efficacy of Famciclovir initiated more than 72 hours after rash onset has not been studied.

GENITAL HERPES

For Recurrent Episodes: The recommended dosage is 125 mg b.i.d. for 5 days. Initiate therapy at the first sign or symptom if medical management of a genital herpes recurrence is indicated. The efficacy of famciclovir has not been established when treatment is initiated more than 6 hours after onset of symptoms or lesions.

In patients with reduced renal function, dosage reduction is recommended in TABLE 4.

TABLE 4

Normal Dosage Regimen	Creatinine Clearance (mL/min.)	Adjusted Dosage Regimen	
		Dose (mg)	Dosing Interval
Herpes Zoster			
500 mg every 8 hours	≥60	500	every 8 hours
	40-59	500	every 12 hours
	20-39	500	every 24 hours
	<20	250	every 48 hours
Recurrent Genital Herpes			
125 mg every 12 hours	≥40	125	every 12 hours
	20-39	125	every 24 hours
	<20	125	every 48 hours

Hemodialysis Patients: The recommended dose of famciclovir is 250 mg (herpes zoster) or 125 mg (genital herpes) administered following each dialysis treatment.

ADMINISTRATION WITH FOOD

When famciclovir was administered with food, penciclovir C_{max} decreased approximately 50%. Because the systemic availability of penciclovir (AUC) was not altered, it appears that Famciclovir may be taken without regard to meals.

HOW SUPPLIED:

Famvir is supplied as 500 mg white, oval, film-coated tablets debossed with FAMVIR on one side and 500 on the other, in bottles of 30 and in Single Unit Packages (blister packs) of 50 (intended for institutional use only).

Store at controlled room temperature (15° to 30°C; 59° to 86°F).

HOW SUPPLIED - EQUIVALENTS NOT AVAILABLE:

Tablet, Coated - Oral - 500 mg

30's	$184.50	FAMVIR, SKB Pharms	00007-4117-13
50's	$340.07	FAMVIR, SKB Pharms	00007-4117-19

FAMOTIDINE *(001246)*

CATEGORIES: Acid/Peptic Disorders; Adenoma; Antiulcer Drugs; Duodenal Ulcer; Endocrine Adenomas; Esophagitis; GERD; Gastric Ulcer; Gastrointestinal Drugs; Histamine H2 Receptor Antagonists; Hypersecretory Conditions; Reflux; Ulcer; Zollinger-Ellison Syndrome; Pregnancy Category B; Sales > $500 Million; FDA Approved 1986 Oct; Patent Expiration 2000 Aug; Top 200 Drugs

BRAND NAMES: *Amfamox* (Australia); *Antodine*; *Apo-Famotidine*; *Bestidine*; *Brolin*; *Cepal*; *Durater* (Mexico); *Evatin*; *Facid*; *Fadin*; *Fadine*; *Fagastine*; *Famocid*; *Famodar*; *Famodil*; *Famodine*; *Famodyn*; *Famonit*; *Famopsin*; *Famos*; *Famosan*; *Famotal*; *Famotep*; *Famotin*; *Famovane*; *Famowal*; *Famox*; *Famoxal* (Mexico); *Fanox*; *Farmotex* (Mexico); *Fenox*; *Ferotine*; *Ganor* (Germany); *Gaster* (Japan); *Gastridin*; *Gastrion*; *Gastro*; *Gastrodomina*; *Hacip*; *H2 Bloc*; *Logos*; *Mosul*; *Motiax*; *Panalba*; **Pepcid**; *Pepcid AC*; *Pepcidin*; *Pepcidin Rapitab*; *Pepcidina*; *Pepcidine* (Australia, Mexico); *Pepdine* (France); *Pepdul* (Germany); *Pepfamin*; *Peptan*; *Peptidin*; *Peptifam*; *Pepzan*; *Quamatel*; *Restadin*; *Sedanium-R*; *Sigafam* (Mexico); *Supertidine*; *Tamin*; *Topcid*; *Ulceran*; *Ulcofam*; *Ulfam*; *Ulfinol*; *Ulgarine*; *Weimok*; *Whitidin*

(International brand names outside U.S. in italics)

FORMULARIES: BC-BS; Medi-Cal

COST OF THERAPY: $83.37 (Duodenal Ulcer; Tablet; 40 mg; 1/day; 28 days)

DESCRIPTION:

The active ingredient in Pepcid (Famotidine), is a histamine H_2- receptor antagonist. Famotidine is *N'*-(aminosulfonyl)-3-(((2- ((di-aminomethylene) amino)-4-thiazolyl) methyl) thio)propanimidamide. The empirical formula of famotidine is $C_8H_{15}N_7O_2S_3$ and its molecular weight is 337.43.

Famotidine is a white to pale yellow crystalline compound that is freely soluble in glacial acetic acid, slightly soluble in methanol, very slightly soluble in water, and practically insoluble in ethanol.

Famotidine is supplied in four dosage forms: Pepcid tablets, Pepcid for Oral Suspension, Pepcid Injection and Pepcid Injection Premixed.

Each tablet for oral administration contains either 20 mg or 40 mg of famotidine and the following inactive ingredients: hydroxypropyl cellulose, hydroxypropyl methylcellulose, iron oxides, magnesium stearate, microcrystalline cellulose, starch, talc, titanium dioxide.

Each 5 ml of the oral suspension when prepared as directed contains 40 mg of famotidine and the following inactive ingredients: citric acid, flavors, microcrystalline cellulose and carboxymethylcellulose sodium, sucrose and xanthan gum. Added as preservatives are sodium benzoate 0.1%, sodium methylparaben 0.1%, and sodium propylparaben 0.02%.

Each ml of the solution for intravenous injection contains 10 mg of famotidine and the following inactive ingredients: L-aspartic acid 4 mg, mannitol 20 mg, and Water for Injection q.s. 1 ml. The multidose injection also contains benzyl alcohol 0.9% added as preservative.

CLINICAL PHARMACOLOGY:

GI EFFECTS

Famotidine is a competitive inhibitor of histamine H_2-receptors. The primary clinically important pharmacologic activity of famotidine is inhibition of gastric secretion. Both the acid concentration and volume of gastric secretion are suppressed by famotidine, while changes in pepsin secretion are proportional to volume output.

In normal volunteers and hypersecretors, famotidine inhibited basal and nocturnal gastric secretion, as well as secretion stimulated by food and pentagastrin. After oral administration, the onset of the antisecretory effect occurred within one hour; the maximum effect was dose-dependent, occurring within one to three hours. Duration of inhibition of secretion by doses of 20 and 40 mg was 10 to 12 hours.

After intravenous administration, the maximum effect was achieved within 30 minutes. Single intravenous doses of 10 and 20 mg inhibited nocturnal secretion for a period of 10 to 12 hours. The 20 mg dose was associated with the longest duration of action in most subjects.

Single evening oral doses of 20 and 40 mg inhibited basal and nocturnal acid secretion in all subjects; mean nocturnal gastric acid secretion was inhibited by 86% and 94%, respectively, for a period of at least 10 hours. The same doses given in the morning suppressed food-stimulated acid secretion in all subjects. The mean suppression was 76% and 84% respectively 3 to 5 hours after administration, and 25% and 30% respectively 8 to 10 hours after administration. In some subjects who received the 20 mg dose, however, the antisecretory effect was dissipated within 6-8 hours. There was no cumulative effect with repeated doses. The nocturnal intragastric pH was raised by evening doses of 20 and 40 mg of famotidine to mean values of 5.0 and 6.4, respectively. When famotidine was given after breakfast, the basal daytime interdigestive pH at 3 and 8 hours after 20 or 40 mg of famotidine was raised to about 5.

Famotidine had little or no effect on fasting or postprandial serum gastrin levels. Gastric emptying and exocrine pancreatic function were not affected by famotidine.

OTHER EFFECTS

Systemic effects of famotidine in the CNS, cardiovascular, respiratory or endocrine systems were not noted in clinical pharmacology studies. Also, no antiandrogenic effects were noted. (See ADVERSE REACTIONS.) Serum hormone levels, including prolactin, cortisol, thyroxine (T_4), and testosterone, were not altered after treatment with famotidine.

PHARMACOKINETICS

Famotidine is incompletely absorbed. The bioavailability of oral doses is 40-45%. Famotidine tablets and famotidine oral suspension are bioequivalent. Bioavailability may be slightly increased by food, or slightly decreased by antacids; however, these effects are of no clinical consequence. Famotidine undergoes minimal first-pass metabolism. After oral doses, peak plasma levels occur in 1-3 hours. Plasma levels after multiple doses are similar to those after single doses. Fifteen to 20% of famotidine in plasma is protein bound. Famotidine has an elimination half-life of 2.5-3.5 hours. Famotidine is eliminated by renal (65-70%) and metabolic (30-35%) routes. Renal clearance is 250-450 ml/min, indicating some tubular excretion. Twenty-five to 30% of an oral dose and 65-70% of an intravenous dose are recovered in the urine as unchanged compound. The only metabolite identified in man is the S-oxide.

CLINICAL PHARMACOLOGY: *(cont'd)*

There is a close relationship between creatinine clearance values and the elimination half-life of famotidine. In patients with severe renal insufficiency, i.e. creatinine clearance less than 10 ml/min, famotidine elimination half-life may exceed 20 hours and adjustment of dose or dosing intervals may be necessary (see PRECAUTIONS, DOSAGE AND ADMINISTRATION).)

In elderly patients, there are no clinically significant age-related changes in the pharmacokinetics of famotidine.

CLINICAL STUDIES:

Duodenal Ulcer: In a U.S. multicenter, double-blind study in outpatients with endoscopically confirmed duodenal ulcer, orally administered famotidine was compared to placebo. As shown in TABLE 1, 70% of patients treated with famotidine 40 mg h.s. were healed by week 4.

TABLE 1 Outpatients with Endoscopically Confirmed Healed Duodenal Ulcers

	Pepcid 40 mg h.s. (N = 89)	Pepcid 20 mg b.i.d. (N = 84)	Placebo h.s. (N = 97)
Week 2	*32%	*38%	17%
Week 4	*70%	*67%	31%

* Statistically significantly different than placebo (p<0.001)

Patients not healed by week 4 were continued in the study. By week 8, 83% of patients treated with famotidine had healed versus 45% of patients treated with placebo. The incidence of ulcer healing with famotidine was significantly higher than with placebo at each time point based on proportion of endoscopically confirmed healed ulcers.

In this study, time to relief of daytime and nocturnal pain was significantly shorter for patients receiving famotidine than for patients receiving placebo; patients receiving famotidine also took less antacid than the patients receiving placebo.

TREATMENT OF DUODENAL ULCERS

Long-Term Maintenance: Famotidine, 20 mg p.o.h.s. was compared to placebo h.s. as maintenance therapy in two double-blind, multicenter studies of patients with endoscopically confirmed healed duodenal ulcers. In the U.S. study the observed ulcer incidence within 12 months in patients treated with placebo was 2.4 times greater than in the patients treated with famotidine. The 89 patients treated with famotidine had a cumulative observed ulcer incidence of 23.4% compared to an observed ulcer incidence of 56.6% in the 89 patients receiving placebo (p<0.01). These results were confirmed in an international study where the cumulative observed ulcer incidence within 12 months in the 307 patients treated with famotidine was 35.7%, compared to an incidence of 75.5% in the 325 patients treated with placebo (p<0.01).

GASTRIC ULCER

In both a U.S. and an international multicenter, double-blind study in patients with endoscopically confirmed active benign gastric ulcer, orally administered famotidine, 40 mg h.s., was compared to placebo h.s. Antacids were permitted during the studies, but consumption was not significantly different between the famotidine and placebo groups. As shown in TABLE 2, the incidence of ulcer healing (dropouts counted as unhealed) with famotidine was statistically significantly better than placebo at weeks 6 and 8 in the U.S. study, and at weeks 4, 6 and 8 in the international study, based on the number of ulcers that healed, confirmed by endoscopy.

TABLE 2 Patients with Endoscopically Confirmed Healed Gastric Ulcers

	U.S. Study		International Study	
	Pepcid 40 mg h.s. (N = 74)	Placebo h.s. (N = 75)	Pepcid 40 mg h.s. (N = 149)	Placebo h.s. (N = 145)
Week 4	45%	39%	**47%	31%
Week 6	**66%	44%	**65%	46%
Week 8	*78%	64%	**80%	54%

*, ** Statistically significantly better than placebo (p ≤0.05, p ≤0.01 respectively)

Time to complete relief of daytime and nighttime pain was statistically significantly shorter for patients receiving famotidine than for patients receiving placebo; however, in neither study was there a statistically significant difference in the proportion of patients whose pain was relieved by the end of the study (week 8).

GASTROESOPHAGEAL REFLUX DISEASE (GERD)

Famotidine was compared to placebo in a U.S. study that enrolled patients with symptoms of GERD and without endoscopic evidence of erosion or ulceration of the esophagus. Famotidine 20 mg b.i.d. was statistically significantly superior to 40 mg h.s. and to placebo in providing a successful symptomatic outcome, defined as moderate or excellent improvement of symptoms (TABLE 3).

TABLE 3 % Successful Symptomatic Outcome

	Pepcid 20 mg b.i.d. (N = 154)	Pepcid 40 mg h.s. (N = 149)	Placebo (N = 73)
week 6	82**	69	62

** p ≤0.01 vs Placebo

By two weeks of treatment, symptomatic success was observed in a greater percentage of patients taking famotidine 20 mg b.i.d. compared to placebo (p ≤0.01).

Symptomatic improvement and healing of endoscopically verified erosion and ulceration were studied in two additional trials. Healing was defined as complete resolution of all erosions or ulcerations visible with endoscopy. The U.S. study comparing famotidine 40 mg b.i.d. to placebo and famotidine 20 mg b.i.d., showed a significantly greater percentage of healing for famotidine 40 mg b.i.d. at weeks 6 and 12 (TABLE 4).

TABLE 4 % Endoscopic Healing-U.S. Study

	Pepcid 40 mg b.i.d. (N = 127)	Pepcid 20 mg b.i.d. (N = 125)	Placebo (N = 66)
Week 6	48**,++	32	18
Week 12	69**,+	54**	29

** p ≤0.01 vs Placebo
+ p ≤0.05 vs Pepcid 20 mg b.i.d.
++ p ≤0.01 vs Pepcid 20 mg b.i.d.

CLINICAL STUDIES: *(cont'd)*

As compared to placebo, patients who received famotidine had faster relief of daytime and nighttime heartburn and a greater percentage of patients experienced complete relief of nighttime heartburn. These differences were statistically significant.

In the international study, when famotidine 40 mg b.i.d., was compared to ranitidine 150 mg b.i.d., a statistically significantly greater percentage of healing was observed with famotidine 40 mg b.i.d. at week 12 (TABLE 5). There was, however, no significant difference among treatments in symptom relief.

TABLE 5 % Endoscopic Healing-International Study

	Pepcid 40 mg b.i.d. (N = 175)	Pepcid 20 mg b.i.d. (N = 93)	Ranitidine 150 mg b.i.d. (N = 172)
Week 6	48	52	42
Week 12	71*	68	60

* p ≤0.05 vs Ranitidine 150 mg b.i.d.

PATHOLOGICAL HYPERSECRETORY CONDITIONS

(*e.g.* Zollinger-Ellison Syndrome, Multiple Endocrine Adenomas)

In studies of patients with pathological hypersecretory conditions such as Zollinger-Ellison Syndrome with or without multiple endocrine adenomas, famotidine significantly inhibited gastric acid secretion and controlled associated symptoms. Doses from 20 to 160 mg q 6 h maintained basal acid secretion below 10 mEq/hr; initial doses were titrated to the individual patient need and subsequent adjustments were necessary with time in some patients. Famotidine was well tolerated at these high dose levels for prolonged periods (greater than 12 months) in eight patients, and there were no cases reported of gynecomastia, increased prolactin levels, or impotence which were considered to be due to the drug.

INDICATIONS AND USAGE:

Famotidine is indicated in:

1. Short term treatment of active duodenal ulcer. Most patients heal within 4 weeks; there is rarely reason to use famotidine at full dosage for longer than 6 to 8 weeks. Studies have not assessed the safety of famotidine in uncomplicated active duodenal ulcer for periods of more than eight weeks.

2. Maintenance therapy for duodenal ulcer patients at reduced dosage after healing of an active ulcer. Controlled studies have not extended beyond one year.

3. Short term treatment of active benign gastric ulcer. Most patients heal within 6 weeks. Studies have not assessed the safety or efficacy of famotidine in uncomplicated active benign gastric ulcer for periods of more than 8 weeks.

4. Short term treatment of gastroesophageal reflux disease (GERD). Famotidine is indicated for short term treatment of patients with symptoms of GERD (see CLINICAL STUDIES). Famotidine is also indicated for the short term treatment of esophagitis due to GERD including erosive or ulcerative disease diagnosed by endoscopy (see CLINICAL STUDIES.)

5. Treatment of pathological hypersecretory conditions (*e.g.,* Zollinger-Ellison Syndrome, multiple endocrine adenomas).

Famotidine injection premixed or famotidine injection is indicated in some hospitalized patients with pathological hypersecretory conditions or intractable ulcers, or as an alternative to the oral dosage forms for short-term use in patients who are unable to take oral medication for the above conditions.

CONTRAINDICATIONS:

Hypersensitivity to any component of these products.

PRECAUTIONS:

GENERAL

Symptomatic response to therapy with famotidine does not preclude the presence of gastric malignancy.

Patients with Severe Renal Insufficiency: Longer intervals between doses or lower doses may need to be used in patients with severe renal insufficiency (creatinine clearance <10 ml/min) to adjust for the longer elimination half-life of famotidine. (See CLINICAL PHARMACOLOGY and DOSAGE AND ADMINISTRATION.) However, currently, no drug-related toxicity has been found with high plasma concentrations of famotidine.

INFORMATION FOR THE PATIENT

The patient should be instructed to shake the oral suspension vigorously for 5-10 seconds prior to each use. Unused constituted oral suspension should be discarded after 30 days.

CARCINOGENESIS, MUTAGENESIS,IMPAIRMENT OF FERTILITY

In a 106 week study in rats and a 92 week study in mice given oral doses of up to 2000 mg/kg/day (approximately 2500 times the recommended human dose for active duodenal ulcer), there was no evidence of carcinogenic potential for famotidine.

Famotidine was negative in the microbial mutagen test (Ames test) using *Salmonella typhimurium* and *Escherichia coli* with or without rat liver enzyme activation at concentrations up to 10,000 mcg/plate. In *in vivo* studies in mice, with a micronucleus test and a chromosomal aberration test, no evidence of a mutagenic effect was observed.

In studies with rats given oral doses of up to 2000 mg/kg/day or intravenous doses of up to 200 mg/kg/day fertility and reproductive performance were not affected.

PREGNANCY CATEGORY B

Reproductive studies have been performed in rats and rabbits at oral doses of up to 2000 and 500 mg/kg/day respectively and in both species at IV doses of up to 200 mg/kg/day, and have revealed no significant evidence of impaired fertility or harm to the fetus due to famotidine. While no direct fetotoxic effects have been observed, sporadic abortions occurring only in mothers displaying marked decreased food intake were seen in some rabbits at oral doses of 200 mg/kg/day (250 times the usual human dose) or higher. There are, however, no adequate or well-controlled studies in pregnant women. Because animal reproductive studies are not always predictive of human response, this drug should be used during pregnancy only if clearly needed.

NURSING MOTHERS

Studies performed in lactating rats have shown that famotidine is secreted into breast milk. Transient growth depression was observed in young rats suckling from mothers treated with maternotoxic doses of at least 600 times the usual human dose. It is not known whether this drug is secreted into human milk. Because many drugs are secreted into human milk and because of the potential for serious adverse reactions in nursing infants from famotidine, a decision should be made whether to discontinue nursing or discontinue the drug, taking into account the importance of the drug to the mother.

PEDIATRIC USE

Safety and effectiveness in children have not been established.

PRECAUTIONS: *(cont'd)*

GERIATRIC USE

No dosage adjustment is required based on age (see CLINICAL PHARMACOLOGY, Pharmacokinetics). Dosage adjustment in the case of severe renal impairment may be necessary.

DRUG INTERACTIONS:

No drug interactions have been identified. Studies with famotidine in man, in animal models, and *in vitro* have shown no significant interference with the disposition of compounds metabolized by the hepatic microsomal enzymes, e.g., cytochrome P450 system. Compounds tested in man include warfarin, theophylline, phenytoin, diazepam, aminopyrine and antipyrine. Indocyanine green as an index of hepatic drug extraction has been tested and no significant effects have been found.

ADVERSE REACTIONS:

The adverse reactions listed below have been reported during domestic and international clinical trials in approximately 2500 patient. In those controlled clinical trials in which famotidine tablets were compared to placebo, the incidence of adverse experiences in the group which received famotidine tablets, 40 mg at bedtime, was similar to that in placebo group.

The following adverse reactions have been reported to occur in more than 1% of patients on therapy with famotidine in controlled clinical trials, and may be causally related to the drug: headache (4.7%), dizziness (1.3%), constipation (1.2%) and diarrhea (1.7%).

The following other adverse reactions have been reported infrequently in clinical trials or since the drug was marketed. The relationship to therapy with famotidine has been unclear in many cases. Within each category the adverse reactions are listed in order of decreasing severity:

Body as a Whole: Fever, asthenia, fatigue

Cardiovascular: arrhythmia, AV block, palpitation

Gastrointestinal: Cholestatic jaundice, liver enzyme abnormalities, vomiting, nausea, abdominal discomfort, anorexia, dry mouth

Hematologic: Rare cases of agranulocytosis, pancytopenia, leukopenia, thrombocytopenia

Hypersensitivity: Anaphylaxis, angioedema, orbital or facial edema, urticaria, rash, conjunctival injection

Musculoskeletal: Musculoskeletal pain including muscle cramps, arthralgia

Nervous System/Psychiatric: Grand mal seizure; psychic disturbances, which were reversible in cases for which follow-up was obtained, including hallucinations, confusion, agitation, depression, anxiety, decreased libido; paresthesia; insomnia; somnolence

Respiratory: Bronchospasm

Skin: Toxic epidermal necrolysis (very rare), alopecia, acne, pruritus, dry skin, flushing

Special Senses: Tinnitus, taste disorder

Other: Rare cases of impotence and rare cases of gynecomastia have been reported; however, in controlled clinical trials, the incidence was not greater than that seen with placebo.

The adverse reactions reported for famotidine tablets may also occur with famotidine oral suspension, famotidine injection premixed or famotidine injection. In addition, transient irritation at the injection site has been observed with famotidine injection.

OVERDOSAGE:

There is no experience to date with deliberate overdosage. Dose of up to 640 mg/day have been given to patients with pathological hypersecretory conditions with no serious adverse effects. In the event of overdosage, treatment should be symptomatic and supportive. Unabsorbed material should be removed from the gastrointestinal tract, the patient should be monitored, and supportive therapy should be employed.

The oral LD_{50} of famotidine in male and female rats and mice was greater than 3000 mg/kg and the minimum lethal acute oral dose in dogs exceeded 2000 mg/kg. Famotidine did not produce overt effects at high oral doses in mice, rats, cats and dogs, but induced significant anorexia and growth depression in rabbits starting with 200 mg/kg/day orally. The intravenous LD_{50} of famotidine for mice and rats ranged from 254-563 mg/kg and the minimum lethal single IV dose in dogs was approximately 300 mg/kg. Signs of acute intoxication in IV treated dogs were emesis, restlessness, pallor of mucous membranes or redness of mouth and ears, hypotension, tachycardia and collapse.

DOSAGE AND ADMINISTRATION:

DUODENAL ULCER

Acute Therapy: The recommended adult oral dosage for active duodenal ulcer is 40 mg once a day at bedtime. Most patients heal within 4 weeks; there is rarely reason to use famotidine at full dosage for longer than 6 to 8 weeks. A regimen of 20 mg twice daily is also effective.

Maintenance Therapy: The recommended oral dose is 20 mg once a day at bedtime.

BENIGN GASTRIC ULCER

Acute Therapy: The recommended adult oral dosage for active benign gastric ulcer is 40 mg once a day at bedtime.

GASTROESOPHAGEAL REFLUX DISEASE (GERD)

The recommended oral dosage for treatment of patients with symptoms of GERD is 20 mg twice daily for up to 6 weeks. The recommended oral dosage for the treatment of patients with esophagitis including erosions and ulcerations and accompanying symptoms due to GERD is 20 or 40 mg b.i.d. for up to 12 weeks (see CLINICAL STUDIES.)

PATHOLOGICAL HYPERSECRETORY CONDITIONS

(*e.g.,*Zollinger-Ellison Syndrome, Multiple Endocrine Adenomas)

The dosage of famotidine in patients with pathological hypersecretory conditions varies with the individual patient. The recommended adult oral starting dose for pathological hypersecretory conditions is 20 mg q 6 h. In some patients, a higher starting dose may be required. Doses should be adjusted to individual patient needs and should continue as long as clinically indicated. Doses up to 160 mg q 6 h have been administered to some patients with severe Zollinger-Ellison Syndrome.

ORAL SUSPENSION

Famotidine oral suspension may be substituted for famotidine tablets in any of the above indications. Each five ml contains 40 mg of famotidine after constitution of the powder with 46 ml of Purified Water as directed.

DIRECTIONS FOR PREPARING FAMOTIDINE ORAL SUSPENSION

Prepare suspension at time of dispensing. Slowly add 46 ml of Purified Water. Shake vigorously for 5-10 seconds immediately after adding the water and immediately before use.

STABILITY OF FAMOTIDINE ORAL SUSPENSION

Unused constituted oral suspension should be discarded after 30 days.

INTRAVENOUS ADMINISTRATION

In some hospitalized patients with pathological hypersecretory conditions or intractable ulcers, or in patients who are unable to take oral medication, famotidine I.V. may be administered.

DOSAGE AND ADMINISTRATION: *(cont'd)*

The recommended dosage for famotidine injection premixed is 20 mg every 12 hours, administered as an infusion over a 15-30 minute period.

The recommended dosage for famotidine injection is 20 mg every 12 hours.

The doses and regimen for parenteral administration in patients with GERD have not been established.

DOSAGE ADJUSTMENTS FOR PATIENTS WITH SEVERE RENAL INSUFFICIENCY

In patients with severe renal insufficiency, i.e., with a creatinine clearance less than 10 ml/min, the elimination half-life of famotidine may exceed 20 hours, reaching approximately 24 hours in anuric patients. Although no relationship of adverse effects to high plasma levels has been established, to avoid excess accumulation of the drug, the dose of famotidine injection premixed or famotidine injection may be reduced to 20 mg h.s. or the dosing interval may be prolonged to 36-48 hours as indicated by the patient's clinical response.

PREPARATION OF FAMOTIDINE INJECTION PREMIXED

Pepcid Injection Premixed, supplied in Galaxy containers (PL 2501 Plastic) is a 50 ml iso-osmotic solution premixed with 0.9% sodium chloride for administration as an infusion over a 15-30 minute period.*This premixed solution is for intravenous use only using sterile equipment*

DIRECTIONS FOR USE OF GALAXY CONTAINERS

Check the container for minute leaks prior to use by squeezing the bag firmly. If leaks are found, discard solution as sterility may be impaired. Do not add supplementary medication. Do not use unless solution is clear and seal is intact.

CAUTION: Do not use plastic containers in series connections. Such use could result in air embolism due to residual air being drawn from the primary container before administration of the fluid from the secondary container is complete.

Preparation for administration:

1. Suspend container from eyelet support.

2. Remove plastic protector from outlet port at bottom of container.

3. Attach administration set. Refer to complete directions accompanying set.

PREPARATION OF FAMOTIDINE INJECTION INTRAVENOUS SOLUTIONS

Dilute 2 ml of Pepcid I.V. (solution containing 10 mg/ml) with 0.9% Sodium Chloride Injection or other compatible intravenous solution to a total volume of either 5 ml or 10 ml and inject over a period of not less than 2 minutes.

PREPARATION OF FAMOTIDINE INJECTION FOR INTRAVENOUS INFUSION SOLUTIONS

Famotidine injection may also be administered as an infusion, 2 ml diluted with 100 ml of 5% dextrose or other compatible solution, and infused over a 15-30 minute period.

Parenteral drug products should be inspected visually for particulate matter and discoloration prior to administration whenever solution and container permit.

CONCOMITANT USE OF ANTACIDS

Antacids maybe given concomitantly if needed.

STABILITY OF FAMOTIDINE INJECTION PREMIXED

Pepcid Injection Premixed, as supplied premixed in 0.9% sodium chloride in Galaxy containers (PL 2501 Plastic), is stable through the labeled expiration date when stored under the recommended conditions. (See HOW SUPPLIED, Storage.)

STABILITY OF FAMOTIDINE INJECTION

Famotidine injection is stable for 48 hours at room temperature when added to or diluted with most commonly used intravenous solutions, e.g. Water for Injection, 0.9% Sodium Chloride Injection, 5% and 10% Dextrose Injection, Lactated Ringer's Injection, or Sodium Bicarbonate Injection, 5%.

PATIENT INFORMATION:

Famotidine is used to treat stomach and duodenal (upper small intestine) ulcers; hypersecretory (increased acid secretion) conditions; heartburn and gastroesophageal reflux disease (stomach contents bubbling into the esophagus causing pain). Notify your physician if you are pregnant or nursing. Famotidine may be taken with or without food. Shake the oral suspension vigorously for 5-10 seconds before taking. Unused oral suspension should be discarded after 30 days. Notify your physician if you develop black, tarry stools or coffee-ground vomit.

HOW SUPPLIED:

No. 3535-Pepcid Tablets, 20 mg, are beige colored, U-shaped, film- coated tablets coded MSD 963.

No. 3536-Pepcid Tablets, 40 mg, are light brownish-orange, U-shaped, film-coated tablets coded MSD 964.

No. 3538-Pepcid for Oral Suspension is a white to off-white powder containing 400 mg of famotidine for constitution. When constituted as directed, Pepcid for Oral Suspension is a smooth, mobile, off-white, homogeneous suspension with a cherry-banana-mint flavor, containing 40 mg of famotidine per 5 ml.

STORAGE

Avoid storage of Pepcid tablets at temperatures above 40°C (104°F).

Avoid storage of the powder for oral suspension at temperatures above 40°C (104°F). After constitution store the suspension below 30°C (86°F). Do not freeze. Discard unused suspension after 30 days.

FOR INTRAVENOUS USE ONLY

No. 3537-Pepcid (famotidine) Injection Premixed 20 mg per 50 ml is a clear, non-preserved, sterile solution premixed in a vehicle made iso- osmotic with Sodium Chloride.

50 ml single dose Galaxy containers (PL 2501 Plastic).

No. 3539-Pepcid Injection 10 mg per 1 ml, is a non-preserved, clear, colorless solution.

No. 3541-Pepcid Injection 10 mg per 1 ml, is a clear, colorless solution.

STORAGE

Store Pepcid Injection Premixed in Galaxy containers (PL 2501 Plastic) at room temperature (25°C, 77°F). Exposure of the premixed product to excessive heat should be avoided. Brief exposure to temperatures up to 35°C (95°F) does not adversely affect the product.

Store Pepcid Injection at 2-8°C (36-46°F). If solution freezes, bring to room temperature; allow sufficient time to solubilize all the components.

HOW SUPPLIED - EQUIVALENTS NOT AVAILABLE:

Granule, Reconstitution - Oral - 40 mg/5ml

400 mg x 24	$81.83	PEPCID, Merck	00006-3538-92

Injection, Solution - Intravenous - 10 mg/ml

2 ml x 10	$35.99	PEPCID IV, Merck	00006-3539-04
4 ml	$7.19	PEPCID IV, Merck	00006-3541-14

Injection, Solution - Intravenous - 20 mg/50ml

50 ml	$152.56	PEPCID, Merck	00006-3537-50

HOW SUPPLIED - EQUIVALENTS NOT AVAILABLE: *(cont'd)*

Tablet, Plain Coated - Oral - 20 mg

30's	$46.22	PEPCID, Merck	00006-0963-31
100's	$154.13	PEPCID, Merck	00006-0963-58
100's	$156.85	PEPCID, Merck	00006-0963-28
750's	$1153.13	PEPCID, Merck	00006-0963-62
1000's	$1541.37	PEPCID, Merck	00006-0963-82
1080's	$1664.77	PEPCID, 90 X 12, Merck	00006-0963-94
2160's	$3329.55	PEPCID, 180 X 12, Merck	00006-0963-98
10000's	$14361.25	PEPCID, Merck	00006-0963-87

Tablet, Plain Coated - Oral - 40 mg

30's	$89.33	PEPCID, Merck	00006-0964-31
100's	$297.78	PEPCID, Merck	00006-0964-58
100's	$303.14	PEPCID, Merck	00006-0964-28
750's	$2231.25	PEPCID, Merck	00006-0964-62
1000's	$2977.83	PEPCID, Merck	00006-0964-82
1080's	$3216.16	PEPCID, 90 X 12, Merck	00006-0964-94
10000's	$27745.00	PEPCID, Merck	00006-0964-87

FELBAMATE *(003077)*

CATEGORIES: Anticonvulsants; Antiepileptics; Central Nervous System Agents; Convulsions; Epilepsy; Epilepticus; Lennox-Gastaut Syndrome; Orphan Drugs; Seizures; Tonic-Clonic Seizures; Pregnancy Category C; FDA Class 1P ("Priority Review"); FDA Approved 1993 Jul

BRAND NAMES: Felbamyl; **Felbatol**; Taloxa

FORMULARIES: Medi-Cal; PCS

COST OF THERAPY: $1,165.95 (Epilepsy; Tablet; 600 mg; 4/day; 365 days)

PRIMARY ICD9: 345.90 (Epilepsy, Unspecified, Without Mention of Intractable)

WARNING:

1. APLASTIC ANEMIA: THE USE OF FELBAMATE IS ASSOCIATED WITH A MARKED INCREASE IN THE INCIDENCE OF APLASTIC ANEMIA, ACCORDINGLY, FELBAMATE SHOULD ONLY BE USED IN PATIENTS WHOSE EPILEPSY IS SO SEVERE THAT THE RISK OF APLASTIC ANEMIA IS DEEMED ACCEPTABLE IN LIGHT OF THE BENEFITS CONFERRED BY ITS USE (SEEINDICATIONS AND USAGE). ORDINARILY, A PATIENT SHOULD NOT BE PLACED ON AND/OR CONTINUED ON FELBATOL WITHOUT CONSIDERATION OF APPROPRIATE EXPERT HEMATOLOGIC CONSULTATION.

AMONG FELBAMATE TREATED PATIENTS, APLASTIC ANEMIA (PANCYTOPENIA IN THE PRESENCE OF A BONE MARROW LARGELY DEPLETED OF HEMATOPOIETIC PRECURSORS) OCCURS AT AN INCIDENCE THAT MAY BE MORE THAN A 100 FOLD GREATER THAN THAT SEEN IN THE UNTREATED POPULATION (*I.E.*,2 TO 5 PER MILLION PERSONS PER YEAR). THE RISK OF DEATH IN PATIENTS WITH APLASTIC ANEMIA GENERALLY VARIES AS A FUNCTION OF ITS SEVERITY AND ETIOLOGY; CURRENT ESTIMATES OF THE OVERALL CASE FATALITY RATE ARE IN THE RANGE OF 20 TO 30%, BUT RATES AS HIGH AS 70% HAVE BEEN REPORTED IN THE PAST.

THERE ARE TOO FEW FELBAMATE ASSOCIATED CASES, AND TOO LITTLE KNOWN ABOUT THEM TO PROVIDE A RELIABLE ESTIMATE OF THE SYNDROME'S INCIDENCE OR ITS CASE FATALITY RATE OR TO IDENTIFY THE FACTORS, IF ANY, THAT MIGHT CONCEIVABLY BE USED TO PREDICT WHO IS AT GREATER OR LESSER RISK.

IN MANAGING PATIENTS ON FELBAMATE, IT SHOULD BE BORNE IN MIND THAT THE CLINICAL MANIFESTATION OF APLASTIC ANEMIA MAY NOT BE SEEN UNTIL AFTER A PATIENT HAS BEEN ON FELBAMATE FOR SEVERAL MONTHS (*E.G.*, ONSET OF APLASTIC ANEMIA AMONG FELBAMATE EXPOSED PATIENTS FOR WHOM DATA ARE AVAILABLE HAS RANGED FROM 5 TO 30 WEEKS). HOWEVER, THE INJURY TO BONE MARROW STEM CELLS THAT IS HELD TO BE ULTIMATELY RESPONSIBLE FOR THE ANEMIA MAY OCCUR WEEKS TO MONTHS EARLIER. ACCORDINGLY, PATIENTS WHO ARE DISCONTINUED FROM FELBAMATE REMAIN AT RISK FOR DEVELOPING ANEMIA FOR A VARIABLE, AND UNKNOWN, PERIOD AFTERWARDS.

IT IS NOT KNOWN WHETHER OR NOT THE RISK OF DEVELOPING APLASTIC ANEMIA CHANGES WITH DURATION OF EXPOSURE CONSEQUENTLY, IT IS NOT SAFE TO ASSUME THAT A PATIENT WHO HAS BEEN ON FELBAMATE WITHOUT SIGNS OF HEMATOLOGIC ABNORMALITY FOR LONG PERIODS OF TIME IS WITHOUT RISK.

IT IS NOT KNOWN WHETHER OR NOT THE DOSE OF FELBATOL AFFECTS THE INCIDENCE OF APLASTIC ANEMIA.

IT IS NOT KNOWN WHETHER OR NOT CONCOMITANT USE OF ANTIEPILEPTIC DRUGS AND/OR OTHER DRUGS AFFECTS THE INCIDENCE OF APLASTIC ANEMIA.

APLASTIC ANEMIA TYPICALLY DEVELOPS WITHOUT PREMONITORY CLINICAL OR LABORATORY SIGNS, THE FULL BLOWN SYNDROME PRESENTING WITH SIGNS OF INFECTION, BLEEDING, OR ANEMIA. ACCORDINGLY, ROUTINE BLOOD TESTING CANNOT BE RELIABLY USED TO REDUCE THE INCIDENCE OF APLASTIC ANEMIA, BUT, IT WILL, IN SOME CASES, ALLOW THE DETECTION OF THE HEMATOLOGIC CHANGES BEFORE THE SYNDROME DECLARES ITSELF CLINICALLY. FELBATOL SHOULD BE DISCONTINUED IF ANY EVIDENCE OF BONE MARROW DEPRESSION OCCURS.

2. HEPATIC FAILURE: HEPATIC FAILURE RESULTING IN FATALITIES HAS BEEN REPORTED WITH A MARKED INCREASE IN THE FREQUENCY IN PATIENTS RECEIVING FELBAMATE. ACCORDINGLY, FELBATOL SHOULD ONLY BE USED IN PATIENTS WHOSE EPILEPSY IS SO SEVERE THAT THE RISK OF LIVER FAILURE IS OUTWEIGHED BY THE POTENTIAL BENEFITS OF SEIZURE CONTROL.

ALTHOUGH FULL INFORMATION IS NOT YET AVAILABLE, THE NUMBER OF CASES REPORTED GREATLY EXCEEDS THE NUMBER THAT IS EXPECTED BASED ON THE ANNUAL INCIDENCE OF ACUTE LIVER FAILURE IN THE UNITED STATES (I.E., ABOUT 2,000 CASES PER YEAR).

THERE ARE TOO FEW FELBAMATE ASSOCIATED CASES OF HEPATIC FAILURE AND TOO LITTLE KNOWN ABOUT THEM TO PROVIDE EITHER A RELIABLE ESTIMATE OF ITS INCIDENCE OR TO IDENTIFY THE FACTORS, IF ANY, THAT MIGHT BE USED TO PREDICT WHICH PATIENT IS AT GREATER OR LESSER RISK.

IT IS NOT KNOWN WHETHER OR NOT THE RISK OF DEVELOPING HEPATIC FAILURE CHANGES WITH DURATION OF EXPOSURE.

IT IS NOT KNOWN WHETHER OR NOT THE DOSAGE OF FELBATOL AFFECTS THE INCIDENCE OF HEPATIC FAILURE.

IT IS NOT KNOWN WHETHER CONCOMITANT USE OF OTHER ANTIEPILEPTIC DRUGS AND/OR OTHER DRUGS AFFECT THE INCIDENCE OF HEPATIC FAILURE.

FELBATOL SHOULD NOT BE PRESCRIBED FOR ANYONE WITH A HISTORY OF HEPATIC DYSFUNCTION.

PATIENTS PRESCRIBED FELBAMATE SHOULD HAVE LIVER FUNCTION TESTS (AST, ALT, BILIRUBIN) PERFORMED BEFORE INITIATING FELBATOL AND AT 1- TO 2-WEEK INTERVALS WHILE TREATMENT CONTINUES. A PATIENT WHO DEVELOPS ABNORMAL LIVER FUNCTION TESTS SHOULD BE IMMEDIATELY WITHDRAWN FROM FELBAMATE TREATMENT.

DESCRIPTION:

Before prescribing felbamate, the physician should be thoroughly familiar with the details of this prescribing information.

FELBAMATE SHOULD NOT BE USED BY PATIENTS UNTIL THERE HAS BEEN A COMPLETE DISCUSSION OF THE RISKS AND THE PATIENT, PARENT, OR GUARDIAN HAS PROVIDED WRITTEN INFORMED CONSENT. (SEE PATIENT PACKAGE INSERT/CONSENT SECTION.)

Felbatol (felbamate) is an antiepileptic available as 400 mg and 600 mg tablets and as a 600 mg/5 ml suspension for oral administration. Its chemical name is 2-phenyl-1,3-propanediol dicarbamate.

Felbamate is a white to off-white crystalline powder with a characteristic odor. It is very slightly soluble in water, slightly soluble in ethanol, sparingly soluble in methanol, and freely soluble in dimethyl sulfoxide. The molecular weight is 238.24; felbamate's molecular formula is $C_{11}H_{14}N_2O_4$.

The inactive ingredients for Felbatol (felbamate) tablets 400 mg and 600 mg are starch, microcrystalline cellulose, croscarmellose sodium, lactose, magnesium stearate, FD&C Yellow No. 6, D&C Yellow No. 10, and FD&C Red No. 40 (600 mg tablets only). The inactive ingredients for felbamate suspension 600 mg/5 ml are sorbitol, glycerin, microcrystalline cellulose, carboxymethylcellulose sodium, simethicone, polysorbate 80, methylparaben, saccharin sodium, propylparaben, FD&C Yellow No. 6, FD&C Red No. 40, flavorings, and purified water.

CLINICAL PHARMACOLOGY:

MECHANISM OF ACTION

The mechanism by which felbamate exerts its anticonvulsant activity is unknown, but in animal test systems designed to detect anticonvulsant activity, felbamate has properties in common with other marketed anticonvulsants. Felbamate is effective in mice and rats in the maximal electroshock test, the subcutaneous pentylenetetrazol seizure test, and the subcutaneous picrotoxin seizure test. Felbamate also exhibits anticonvulsant activity against seizures induced by intracerebroventricular administration of glutamate in rats and N-methyl-D,L-aspartic acid in mice. Protection against maximal electroshock- induced seizures suggests that felbamate may reduce seizure spread, an effect possibly predictive of efficacy in generalized tonic-clonic or partial seizures. Protection against pentylenetetrazol-induced seizures suggests that felbamate may increase seizure threshold, an effect considered to be predictive of potential efficacy in absence seizures.

Receptor-binding studies *in vitro* indicate that felbamate has weak inhibitory effects on GABA-receptor binding, benzodiazepine receptor binding, and is devoid of activity at the MK-801 receptor binding site of the NMDA receptor-ionophore complex. However, felbamate does interact as an antagonist at the strychnine-insensitive glycine recognition site of the NMDA receptor-ionophore complex. Felbamate is not effective in protecting chick embryo retina tissue against the neurotoxic effects of the excitatory amino acid agonists NMDA, kainate, or quisqualate *in vitro*.

The monocarbamate, p-hydroxy, and 2-hydroxy metabolites were inactive in the maximal electroshock-induced seizure test in mice. The monocarbamate and p-hydroxy metabolites had only weak (0.2 to 0.6) activity compared with felbamate in the subcutaneous pentylenetetrazol seizure test. These metabolites did not contribute significantly to the anticonvulsant action of felbamate.

PHARMACOKINETICS

The numbers in the pharmacokinetic section are mean $\pm$ standard deviation.

Felbamate is well-absorbed after oral administration. Over 90% of the radioactivity after a dose of 100 mg ^{14}C felbamate was found in the urine. Absolute bioavailability (oral vs. parenteral) has not been measured. The tablet and suspension were each shown to be bioequivalent to the capsule used in clinical trials, and pharmacokinetic parameters of the tablet and suspension are similar. There was no effect of food on absorption of the tablet; the effect of food on absorption of the suspension has not been evaluated.

Following oral administration, felbamate is the predominant plasma species (about 90% of plasma radioactivity). About 40-50% of absorbed dose appears unchanged in urine, and an additional 40% is present as unidentified metabolites and conjugates. About 15% is present as parahydroxyfelbamate, 2-hydroxyfelbamate, and felbamate monocarbamate, none of which have significant anticonvulsant activity.

Binding of felbamate to human plasma protein was independent of felbamate concentrations between 10 and 310 micrograms/ml. Binding ranged from 22% to 25%, mostly to albumin, and was dependent on the albumin concentration.

Felbamate is excreted with a terminal half-life of 20-23 hours, which is unaltered after multiple doses. Clearance after a single 1200 mg dose is 26 ± 3 ml/hr/kg, and after multiple daily doses of 3600 mg is 30 ± 8 ml/hr/kg. The apparent volume of distribution was 756 ± 82 ml/kg after a 1200 mg dose. Felbamate C_{max} and AUC are proportionate to dose after single and multiple doses over a range of 100-800 mg single doses and 1200-3600 mg daily doses. C_{min} (trough) blood levels are also dose proportional. Multiple daily doses of 1200, 2400, and

CLINICAL PHARMACOLOGY: *(cont'd)*

3600 mg gave C_{min} values of 30 ± 5, 55 ± 8, and 83 ± 21 micrograms/ml (N=10 patients). Felbamate gave dose proportional steady-state peak plasma concentrations in children age 4-12 over a range of 15, 30, and 45 mg/kg/day with peak concentrations of 17, 32, and 49 micrograms/ml.

The effects of race and gender on felbamate pharmacokinetics have not been systematically evaluated, but plasma concentrations in males (n=5) and females (N=4) given felbamate have been similar. The effects of felbamate kinetics on renal and hepatic functional impairment have not been evaluated.

PHARMACODYNAMICS

Typical Physiologic Responses:

1. Cardiovascular: In adults, there is no effect of felbamate on blood pressure. Small but statistically significant mean increases in heart rate were seen during adjunctive therapy and monotherapy; however, these mean increases of up to 5 bpm were not clinically significant. In children, no clinically relevant changes in blood pressure or heart rate were seen during adjunctive therapy or monotherapy with felbamate.

2. Other Physiologic Effects: The only other change in vital signs was a mean decrease of approximately 1 respiration per minute in respiratory rate during adjunctive therapy in children. In adults, statistically significant mean reductions in body weight were observed during felbamate monotherapy and adjunctive therapy. In children, there were mean decreases in body weight during adjunctive therapy and monotherapy; however, these mean changes were not statistically significant. These mean reductions in adults and children were approximately 5% of the mean weights at baseline.

CLINICAL STUDIES:

The results of controlled clinical trials established the efficacy of felbamate as monotherapy and adjunctive therapy in adults with partial-onset seizures with or without secondary generalization and in partial and generalized seizures associated with Lennox-Gastaut syndrome in children.

Felbatol Monotherapy Trials in Adults: Felbamate (3600 mg/day given QID) and low-dose valproate (15 mg/kg/day) were compared as monotherapy during a 112-day treatment period in a multicenter and a single-center double-blind efficacy trial. Both trials were conducted according to an identical study design. During a 56-day baseline period, all patients had at least four partial-onset seizures per 28 days and were receiving one antiepileptic drug at a therapeutic level, the most common being carbamazepine. In the multicenter trial, baseline seizure frequencies were 12.4 per 28 days in the felbamate group and 21.3 per 28 days in the low-dose valproate group. In the single-center trial, baseline seizure frequencies were 18.1 per 28 days in the Felbamate group and 15.9 per 28 days in the low-dose valproate group. Patients were converted to monotherapy with Felbamate or low-dose valproic acid during the first 28 days of the 112-day treatment period. Study endpoints were completion of 112 study days or fulfilling an escape criterion. Criteria for escape relative to baseline were: (1) twofold increase in monthly seizure frequency, (2) twofold increase in highest 2-day seizure frequency, (3) single generalized tonic-clonic seizure (GTC) if none occurred during baseline, or (4) significant prolongation of GTCs. The primary efficacy variable was the number of patients in each treatment group who met escape criteria.

In the multicenter trial, the percentage of patients who met escape criteria was 40% (18/45) in the Felbamate group and 78% (39/50) in the low-dose valproate group. In the single-center trial, the percentage of patients who met escape criteria was 14% (3/21) in the Felbatol group and 90% (19/21) in the low-dose valproate group. In both trials, the difference in the percentage of patients meeting escape criteria was statistically significant (P<.001) in favor of Felbamate. These two studies by design were intended to demonstrate the effectiveness of Felbamate monotherapy. The studies were not designed or intended to demonstrate comparative efficacy of the two drugs. For example, valproate was not used at the maximally effective dose.

Felbatol Adjunctive Therapy Trials in Adults: A double-blind, placebo-controlled crossover trial consisted of two 10-week outpatient treatment periods. Patients with refractory partial-onset seizures who were receiving phenytoin and carbamazepine at therapeutic levels were administered felbamate as add-on therapy at a starting dosage of 1400 mg/day in three divided doses, which was increased to 2600 mg/day in three divided doses. Among the 56 patients who completed the study, the baseline seizure frequency was 20 per month. Patients treated with Felbamate had fewer seizures than patients treated with placebo for each treatment sequence. There was a 23% (P=.018) difference in percentage seizure frequency reduction in favor of Felbatol.

Felbamate 3600 mg/day given QID and placebo were compared in a 28-day double-blind add-on trial in patients who had their standard antiepileptic drugs reduced while undergoing evaluations for surgery of intractable epilepsy. All patients had confirmed partial-onset seizures with or without generalization, seizure frequency during surgical evaluation not exceeding an average of four partial seizures per day or more than one generalized seizure per day, and a minimum average of one partial or generalized tonic-clonic seizure per day for the last 3 days of the surgical evaluation. The primary efficacy variable was time to fourth seizure after randomization to treatment with Felbatol or placebo. Thirteen (46%) of 28 patients in the Felbamate group versus 29 (88%) of 33 patients in the placebo group experienced a fourth seizure. The median times to fourth seizure were greater than 28 days in the Felbamate group and 5 days in the placebo group. The difference between Felbamate and placebo in time to fourth seizure was statistically significant (P=.002) in favor of Felbamate.

Felbamate Adjunctive Therapy Trial in Children with Lennox-Gastaut Syndrome: In a 70-day double-blind, placebo-controlled add-on trial in the Lennox-Gastaut syndrome, Felbamate 45 mg/kg/day given QID was superior to placebo in controlling the multiple seizure types associated with this condition. Patients had at least 90 atonic and/or atypical absence seizures per month while receiving therapeutic dosages of one or two other antiepileptic drugs. Patients had a past history of using an average of eight antiepileptic drugs. The most commonly used antiepileptic drug during the baseline period was valproic acid. The frequency of all types of seizures during the baseline period was 1617 per month in the Felbamate group and 716 per month in the placebo group. Statistically significant differences in the effect on seizure frequency favored Felbamate over placebo for total seizures (26% reduction vs 5% increase, P<.001), atonic seizures (44% reduction vs 7% reduction, P=.002), and generalized tonic-clonic seizures (40% reduction vs 12% increase, P=.017). Parent/guardian global evaluations based on impressions of quality of life with respect to alertness, verbal responsiveness, general well-being, and seizure control significantly (P<.001) favored Felbamate over placebo.

When efficacy was analyzed by gender in four well-controlled trials of felbamate as adjunctive and monotherapy for partial-onset seizures and Lennox-Gastaut syndrome, a similar response was seen in 122 males and 142 females.

INDICATIONS AND USAGE:

Felbamate is not indicated as a first line antiepileptic treatment (see WARNINGS). Felbamate is recommended for use only in those patients who respond inadequately to alternative treatments and whose epilepsy is so severe that a substantial risk of aplastic anemia and/or liver failure is deemed acceptable in light of the benefits conferred by its use.

INDICATIONS AND USAGE: *(cont'd)*

If these criteria are met and the patient has been fully advised of the risk and has provided written, informed consent, Felbamate can be considered for either monotherapy or adjunctive therapy in the treatment of partial seizures, with and without generalization, in adults with epilepsy and as adjunctive therapy in the treatment of partial and generalized seizures associated with Lennox-Gastaut syndrome in children.

CONTRAINDICATIONS:

Felbamate is contraindicated in patients with known hypersensitivity to Felbamate, its ingredients, or known sensitivity to other carbamates. It should not be used in patients with a history of any blood dyscrasia or hepatic dysfunction.

WARNINGS:

See BOXED WARNING regarding aplastic anemia and hepatic failure.

Antiepileptic drugs should not be suddenly discontinued because of the possibility of increasing seizure frequency.

PRECAUTIONS:

INFORMATION FOR THE PATIENT

Patients should be informed that the use of Felbamate is associated with aplastic anemia and hepatic failure, potentially fatal conditions acutely or over a long term.

The physician should obtain written, informed consent prior to initiation of Felbamate therapy (see PATIENT PACKAGE INSERT) Consent.

APLASTIC ANEMIA

in the general population is relatively rare. The absolute risk for the individual patient is not known with any degree of reliability, but patients on Felbamate may be at more than a 100 fold greater risk for developing the syndrome than the general population.

The long term outlook for patients with aplastic anemia is variable. Although many patients are apparently cured, others require repeated transfusions and other treatments for relapses, and some, although surviving for years, ultimately develop serious complications that sometimes prove fatal (*e.g.,* leukemia).

At present there is no way to predict who is likely to get aplastic anemia, nor is there a documented effective means to monitor the patient so as to avoid and/or reduce the risk. Patients with a history of any blood dyscrasia should not receive Felbamate.

Patients should be advised to be alert for signs of infection, bleeding, easy bruising, or signs of anemia (fatigue, weakness, lassitude, etc.) and should be advised to report to the physician immediately if any such signs or symptoms appear.

HEPATIC FAILURE

Hepatic failure in the general population is relatively rare. The absolute risk for an individual patient is not known with any degree of reliability but patients on Felbamate are at a greater risk for developing hepatic failure than the general population.

At present, there is no way to predict who is likely to develop hepatic failure, however, patients with a history of hepatic dysfunction should not be started on Felbamate.

Patients should be advised to follow their physician's directives for liver function testing both before starting felbamate and at frequent intervals while taking Felbamate.

LABORATORY TESTS

Full hematologic evaluations should be performed before Felbamate therapy, frequently during therapy, and for a significant period of time after discontinuation of Felbamate therapy. While it might appear prudent to perform frequent CBCs in patients continuing on Felbamate, there is no evidence that such monitoring will allow early detection of marrow suppression before aplastic anemia occurs. (See BOXED WARNING.) Complete pretreatment blood counts, including platelets and reticulocytes should be obtained as a baseline. If any hematologic abnormalities are detected during the course of treatment, immediate consultation with a hematologist is advised. Felbamate should be discontinued if any evidence of bone marrow depression occurs.

Liver Function Testing: (AST, ALT, bilirubin) should be done before Felbamate is started and at 1- to 2-week intervals while the patient is taking Felbamate. If any liver abnormalities are detected during the course of treatment, Felbamate should be discontinued immediately. See PATIENT PACKAGE INSERT, Consent.

DRUG/LABORATORY TEST INTERACTIONS

There are no known interactions of Felbamate with commonly used laboratory tests.

CARCINOGENESIS, MUTAGENESIS, AND IMPAIRMENT OF FERTILITY

Carcinogenicity studies were conducted in mice and rats. Mice received felbamate as a feed admixture for 92 weeks at doses of 300, 600, and 1200 mg/kg and rats were also dosed by feed admixture for 104 weeks at doses of 30, 100, and 300 (males) or 10, 30, and 100 (females) mg/kg. The maximum doses in these studies produced steady-state plasma concentrations that were equal to or less than the steady-state plasma concentrations in epileptic patients receiving 3600 mg/day. There was a statistically significant increase in hepatic cell adenomas in high-dose male and female mice and in high-dose female rats. Hepatic hypertrophy was significantly increased in a dose-related manner in mice, primarily males, but also in females. Hepatic hypertrophy was not found in female rats. The relationship between the occurrence of benign hepatocellular adenomas and the finding of liver hypertrophy resulting from liver enzyme induction has not been examined. There was a statistically significant increase in benign interstitial cell tumors of the testes in high-dose male rats receiving felbamate. The relevance of these findings to humans is unknown.

As a result of the synthesis process, felbamate could contain small amounts of two known animal carcinogens, the genotoxic compound ethyl carbamate (urethane) and the non-genotoxic compound methyl carbamate. It is theoretically possible that a 50 kg patient receiving 3600 mg of felbamate could be exposed to up to 0.72 micrograms of urethane and 1800 micrograms of methyl carbamate. These daily doses are approximately 1/35,000 (urethane) and 1/5,500 (methyl carbamate) on a mg/kg basis, and 1/10,000 (urethane) and 1/1,600 (methyl carbamate) on a mg/m^2 basis, of the dose levels shown to be carcinogenic in rodents. Any presence of these two compounds in felbamate used in the lifetime carcinogenicity studies was inadequate to cause tumors.

Microbial and mammalian cell assays revealed no evidence of mutagenesis in the Ames *Salmonella* microsome plate test, CHO/HGPRT mammalian cell forward gene mutation assay, sister chromatid exchange assay in CHO cells, and bone marrow cytogenetics assay.

Reproduction and fertility studies in rats showed no effects on male or female fertility at oral doses of up to 13.9 times the human total daily dose of 3600 mg on a mg/kg basis, or up to 3 times the human total daily dose on a mg/m^2 basis.

PREGNANCY CATEGORY C

The incidence of malformations was not increased compared to control in offspring of rats or rabbits given doses up to 13.9 times (rat) and 4.2 times (rabbit) the human daily dose on a mg/kg basis, or 3 times (rat) and less than 2 times (rabbit) the human daily dose on a mg/m^2 basis. However, in rats, there was a decrease in pup weight and an increase in pup deaths during lactation. The cause for these deaths is not known. The no effect dose for rat pup mortality was 6.9 times the human dose on a mg/kg basis or 1.5 times the human dose on a mg/m^2 basis.

PRECAUTIONS: *(cont'd)*

Placental transfer of felbamate occurs in rat pups. There are, however, no studies in pregnant women. Because animal reproduction studies are not always predictive of human response, this drug should be used during pregnancy only if clearly needed.

LABOR AND DELIVERY

The effect of felbamate on labor and delivery in humans is unknown.

NURSING MOTHERS

Felbamate has been detected in human milk. The effect on the nursing infant is unknown (see Pregnancy).

PEDIATRIC USE

The safety and effectiveness of Felbamate in children other than those with Lennox-Gastaut syndrome has not been established.

GERIATRIC USE

No systemic studies in geriatric patients have been conducted. Clinical studies of Felbamate did not include sufficient numbers of patients aged 65 and over to determine whether they respond differently from younger patients. Other reported clinical experience has not identified differences in responses between the elderly and younger patients. In general, dosage selection for an elderly patient should be cautious, usually starting at the low end of the dosing range, reflecting the greater frequency of decreased hepatic, renal, or cardiac function, and of concomitant disease or other drug therapy.

DRUG INTERACTIONS:

The drug interaction data described in this section were obtained from controlled clinical trials and studies involving otherwise health adults with epilepsy.

Used in Conjunction with Other Antiepileptic Drugs (See DOSAGE AND ADMINISTRATION): The addition of Felbamate to antiepileptic drugs (AEDs) affects the steady-state plasma concentrations of AEDs.The net effect of these interactions is summarized in TABLE 1.

TABLE 1 Felbamate, Drug Interactions

AED Coadministered	AED Concentration	Felbatol Concentration
Phenytoin	↑	↓
Valproate	↑	↔**
Carbamazepine (CBZ)	↓	↓
*CBZ epoxide	↑	

* Not administered, but an active metabolite of carbamazepine.
** No significant effect.

SPECIAL EFFECTS OF FELBAMATE ON OTHER ANTIEPILEPTIC DRUGS

Phenytoin: Felbamate causes an increase in steady-state phenytoin plasma concentrations. In 10 otherwise healthy subjects with epilepsy ingesting phenytoin, the steady-state trough (C_{min}) phenytoin plasma concentration was 17 ± 5 micrograms/ml. The steady-state C_{min} increased to 21 ± 5 micrograms/ml when 1200 mg/day of felbamate was coadministered. Increasing the felbamate dose to 1800 mg/day in six of these subjects increased the steady-state phenytoin C_{min} to 25 ± 7 micrograms/ml. In order to maintain phenytoin levels, limit adverse experiences, and achieve the felbamate dose of 3600 mg/day, a phenytoin dose reduction of approximately 40% was necessary for eight of these 10 subjects.

In a controlled clinical trial, a 20% reduction of the phenytoin dose at the initiation of Felbamate therapy resulted in phenytoin levels comparable to those prior to Felbamate administration.

Carbamazepine: Felbamate causes a decrease in the steady-state carbamazepine plasma concentration and an increase in the steady- state carbamazepine epoxide plasma concentration. In nine otherwise healthy subjects with epilepsy ingesting carbamazepine, the steady-state trough (Cmin) carbamazepine concentration was 8 ± 2 micrograms/ml. The carbamazepine steady-state Cmin decreased 31% to 5 ± 1 micrograms/ml when felbamate (3000 mg/day, divided into three doses) was coadministered. Carbamazepine epoxide steady-state Cmin concentrations increased 57% from 1.0 ± 0.3 to 1.6 ± 0.4 micrograms/ml with the addition of felbamate.

In clinical trials, similar changes in carbamazepine and carbamazepine epoxide were seen.

Valproate: Felbamate causes an increase in steady-state valproate concentrations. In four subjects with epilepsy ingesting valproate, the steady-state trough (C_{min}) valproate plasma concentration was 63 ± 16 micrograms/ml. The steady-state C_{min} increased to 78 ± 14 micrograms/ml when 1200 mg/day of felbamate was coadministered. Increasing the felbamate dose to 2400 mg/day increased the steady-state valproate C_{min} to 96 ± 25 micrograms/ml. Corresponding values for free valproate C_{min} concentrations were 7 ± 3, 9 ± 4, and 11 ± 6 micrograms/ml for 0, 1200, and 2400 mg/day Felbamate, respectively. The ratios of the AUCs of unbound valproate to the AUCs of the total valproate were 11.1%, 13.0%, and 11.5%, with coadministration of 0, 1200, and 2400 mg/day of Felbamate, respectively. This indicates that the protein binding of valproate did not change appreciably with increasing doses of Felbamate.

EFFECTS OF OTHER ANTIEPILEPTIC DRUGS ON FELBAMATE

Phenytoin: Phenytoin causes an approximate doubling of the clearance of felbamate at steady state and, therefore, the addition of phenytoin causes an approximate 45% decrease in the steady- state trough concentrations of Felbamate as compared to the same dose of Felbamate given as monotherapy.

Carbamazepine: Carbamazepine causes an approximate 50% increase in the clearance of Felbamate at steady state and, therefore, the addition of carbamazepine results in an approximate 40% decrease in the steady-state trough concentrations of Felbamate as compared to the same dose of Felbamate given as monotherapy.

Valproate: Available data suggest that there is no significant effect of valproate on the clearance of Felbamate at steady state. Therefore, the addition of valproate is not expected to cause a clinically important effect on felbamate plasma concentrations.

EFFECTS OF ANTACIDS ON FELBAMATE

The rate and extent of absorption of a 2400 mg dose of Felbamate as monotherapy given as tablets was not affected when coadministered with antacids.

ADVERSE REACTIONS:

The most common adverse reactions seen in association with felbamate in adults during monotherapy are anorexia, vomiting, insomnia, nausea, and headache. The most common adverse reactions seen in association with Felbamate in adults during adjunctive therapy are anorexia, vomiting, insomnia, nausea, dizziness, somnolence, and headache.

The most common adverse reactions seen in association with Felbamate in children during adjunctive therapy are anorexia, vomiting, insomnia, headache, and somnolence.

The dropout rate because of adverse experiences or intercurrent illnesses among adult felbamate patients was 12 percent (120/977). The dropout rate because of adverse experiences or intercurrent illnesses among pediatric felbamate patients was six percent (23/357). In adults, the body systems associated with causing these withdrawals in order of frequency were: digestive (4.3%), psychological (2.2%), whole body (1.7%), neurological (1.5%), and dermatological (1.5%). In children, the body systems associated with causing these withdrawals in order of frequency were: digestive (1.7%), neurological (1.4%), dermatological (1.4%), psychological (1.1%), and whole body (1.0%). In adults, specific events with an incidence of 1% or greater associated with causing these withdrawals, in order of frequency were: anorexia (1.6%), nausea (1.4%), rash (1.2%), and weight decrease (1.1%). In children, specific events with an incidence of 1% or greater associated with causing these withdrawals, in order of frequency was rash (1.1%).

Incidence in Clinical Trials: The prescriber should be aware that the figures cited in TABLE 2 cannot be used to predict the incidence of side effects in the course of usual medical practice where patient characteristics and other factors differ from those which prevailed in the clinical trials. Similarly, the cited frequencies cannot be compared with figures obtained from other clinical investigations involving different investigators, treatments, and uses including the use of felbamate as adjunctive therapy where the incidence of adverse events may be higher due to drug interactions. The cited figures, however, do provide the prescribing physician with some basis for estimating the relative contribution of drug and nondrug factors to the side effect incidence rate in the population studied.

Incidence in Controlled Clinical Trials-Monotherapy Studies in Adults: TABLE 2 enumerates adverse events that occurred at an incidence of 2% or more among 58 adult patients who received Felbamate monotherapy at dosages of 3600 mg/day in double-blind controlled trials. Reported adverse events were classified using standard WHO-based dictionary terminology.

TABLE 2 Felbamate, Adverse Reactions
Adults Treatment-Emergent Adverse Event Incidence in Controlled Monotherapy Trials

Body System/Event	Felbatol* (N=58) %	Low-Dose Valproate** (N=50) %
Body as a Whole		
Fatigue	6.9	4.0
Weight Decrease	3.4	0
Face Edema	3.4	0
Central Nervous System		
Insomnia	8.6	4.0
Headache	6.9	18.0
Anxiety	5.2	2.0
Dermatological		
Acne	3.4	0
Rash	3.4	0
Digestive		
Dyspepsia	8.6	2.0
Vomiting	8.6	2.0
Constipation	6.9	2.0
Diarrhea	5.2	0
SGPT Increased	5.2	2.0
Metabolic/Nutritional		
Hypophosphatemia	3.4	0
Respiratory		
Upper Respiratory Tract Infection	8.6	4.0
Rhinitis	6.9	0
Special Senses		
Diplopia	3.4	4.0
Otitis Media	3.4	0
Urogenital		
Intramenstrual Bleeding	3.4	0
Urinary Tract Infection	3.4	2.0

* 3600 mg/day
** 15 mg/kg/day

Incidence in Controlled Add-On Clinical Studies in Adults: TABLE 3 enumerates adverse events that occurred at an incidence of 2% or more among 114 adult patients who received Felbamate adjunctive therapy in add-on controlled trials at dosages up to 3600 mg/day. Reported adverse events were classified using standard WHO-based dictionary terminology.

Many adverse experiences that occurred during adjunctive therapy may be a result of drug interactions. Adverse experiences during adjunctive therapy typically resolved with conversion to monotherapy, or with adjustment of the dosage of other antiepileptic drugs.

Incidence in a Controlled Add-On Trial in Children with Lennox-Gastaut Syndrome: TABLE 4 enumerates adverse events that occurred more than once among 31 pediatric patients who received Felbamate up to 45 mg/kg/day or a maximum of 3600 mg/day. Reported adverse events were classified using standard WHO-based dictionary terminology.

Other Events Observed in Association with the Administration of Felbamate: In the paragraphs that follow, the adverse clinical events, other than those in the preceding tables, that occurred in a total of 977 adults and 357 children exposed to felbamate and that are reasonably associated with its use are presented. They are listed in order of decreasing frequency. Because the reports cite events observed in open-label and uncontrolled studies, the role of Felbamate in their causation cannot be reliably determined.

Events are classified within body system categories and enumerated in order of decreasing frequency using the following definitions: frequent adverse events are defined as those occurring on one or more occasions in at least 1/100 patients; infrequent adverse events are those occurring in 1/100-1/1000 patients; and rare events are those occurring in fewer than 1/1000 patients.

Event frequencies are calculated as the number of patients reporting an event divided by the total number of patients (N=1334) exposed to Felbamate.

Body as a Whole: *Frequent:* Weight increase, asthenia, malaise, influenza-like symptoms; *Rare:* anaphylactoid reaction, chest pain substernal.

Cardiovascular: *Frequent:* Palpitation, tachycardia; *Rare:* supraventricular tachycardia.

Central Nervous System: *Frequent:* Agitation, psychological disturbance, aggressive reaction; *Infrequent:* hallucination, euphoria, suicide attempt, migraine.

Digestive: *Frequent:* SGOT increased;*Infrequent:* esophagitis, appetite increased; *Rare:* GGT elevated.

Hematologic: *Infrequent:* Lymphadenopathy, leukopenia, leukocytosis, thrombocytopenia, granulocytopenia;*Rare:* antinuclear factor test positive, qualitative platelet disorder, agranulocytosis.

Metabolic/Nutritional: *Infrequent:* Hypokalemia, hyponatremia, LDH increased, alkaline phosphatase increased, hypophosphatemia; *Rare:* creatinine phosphokinase increased.

Musculoskeletal: *Infrequent:* Dystonia.

Dermatological: *Frequent:* Pruritus;*Infrequent:* urticaria, bullous eruption; *Rare:* buccal mucous membrane swelling, Stevens-Johnson Syndrome.

Special Senses: *Rare:* Photosensitivity allergic reaction.

ADVERSE REACTIONS: *(cont'd)*

TABLE 3 Felbamate, Adverse Reactions
Adults Treatment-Emergent Adverse Event Incidence in Controlled Add-On Trials

Body System/Event	Felbatol (N=114) %	Placebo (N=43) %
Body as a Whole		
Fatigue	16.8	7.0
Fever	2.6	4.7
Chest Pain	2.6	0
Central Nervous System		
Headache	36.8	9.3
Somnolence	19.3	7.0
Dizziness	18.4	14.0
Insomnia	17.5	7.0
Nervousness	7.0	2.3
Tremor	6.1	2.3
Anxiety	5.3	4.7
Gait Abnormal	5.3	0
Depression	5.3	0
Paresthesia	3.5	2.3
Ataxia	3.5	0
Mouth Dry	2.6	0
Stupor	2.6	0
Dermatological		
Rash	3.5	4.7
Digestive		
Nausea	34.2	2.3
Anorexia	19.3	2.3
Vomiting	16.7	4.7
Dyspepsia	12.3	7.0
Constipation	11.4	2.3
Diarrhea	5.3	2.3
Abdominal Pain	5.3	0
SGPT Increased	3.5	0
Musculoskeletal		
Myalgia	2.6	0
Respiratory		
Upper Respiratory Tract Infection	5.3	7.0
Sinusitis	3.5	0
Pharyngitis	2.6	0
Special Senses		
Diplopia	6.1	0
Taste Perversion	6.1	0
Vision Abnormal	5.3	2.3

TABLE 4 Felbamate, Adverse Reactions
Children Treatment-Emergent Adverse Event Incidence in a Controlled Add-On Lennox-Gastaut Trial

Body System/Event	Felbatol (N=31) %	Placebo (N=27) %
Body as a Whole		
Fever	22.6	11.1
Fatigue	9.7	3.7
Weight Decrease	6.5	0
Pain	6.5	0
Central Nervous System		
Somnolence	48.4	11.1
Insomnia	16.1	14.8
Nervousness	16.1	18.5
Gait Abnormal	9.7	0
Headache	6.5	18.5
Thinking Abnormal	6.5	3.7
Ataxia	6.5	3.7
Urinary Incontinence	6.5	7.4
Emotional Lability	6.5	0
Miosis	6.5	0
Dermatological		
Rash	9.7	7.4
Digestive		
Anorexia	54.8	14.8
Vomiting	38.7	14.8
Constipation	12.9	0
Hiccup	9.7	3.7
Nausea	6.5	0
Dyspepsia	6.5	3.7
Hematologic		
Purpura	12.9	7.4
Leukopenia	6.5	0
Respiratory		
Upper Respiratory Tract Infection	45.2	25.9
Pharyngitis	9.7	3.7
Coughing	6.5	0
Special Senses		
Otitis Media	9.7	0

Postmarketing Adverse Event Reports: Voluntary reports of adverse events in patients taking Felbamate (usually in conjunction with other drugs) have been received since market introduction and may have no causal relationship with the drug(s). These include the following by body system:

Body as a Whole: neoplasm, sepsis, placental disorder, L.E. syndrome, SIDS, sudden death, fetal death, edema, hypothermia, rigors, microcephaly.

Cardiovascular: atrial fibrillation, atrial arrhythmia, cardiac arrest, torsade de pointes, cardiac failure, hypotension, hypertension, flushing, thrombophlebitis, ischemic necrosis, gangrene, peripheral ischemia.

Central & Peripheral Nervous System: delusion, paralysis, mononeuritis, cerebrovascular disorder, cerebral edema, coma, manic reaction, encephalopathy, paranoid reaction, nystagmus, choreoathetosis, extrapyramidal disorder, confusion, psychosis, status epilepticus, dyskinesia, dysarthria, respiratory depression.

Dermatological: abnormal body odor, sweating, lichen planus, livedo reticularis, alopecia, toxic epidermal necrolysis.

Digestive: (Refer to WARNINGS) hepatitis, hepatic failure, G.I. hemorrhage, hyperammonemia, pancreatitis, hematemesis, gastritis, esophagitis, rectal hemorrhage, flatulence, gingival bleeding, acquired megacolon, ileus, intestinal obstruction, enteritis, ulcerative stomatitis, glossitis, dysphagia, jaundice.

ADVERSE REACTIONS: *(cont'd)*

Hematologic: (Refer to WARNINGS) increased and decreased prothrombin time, anemia, hypochromic anemia, aplastic anemia, pancytopenia, hemolytic uremic syndrome.

Metabolic/Nutritional: hypernatremia, hypoglycemia, SIADH, hypomagnesemia, dehydration.

Musculoskeletal: arthralgia, muscle weakness, involuntary muscle contraction, rhabdomyolysis.

Respiratory: dyspnea, pneumonia, pneumonitis, hypoxia, epistaxis, pleural effusion, respiratory insufficiency, pulmonary hemorrhage.

Special Senses: hemianopsia, decreased hearing, conjunctivitis.

Urogenital: genital malformation, menstrual disorder, acute renal failure, hepatorenal syndrome, hematuria, urinary retention, nephrosis, vaginal hemorrhage.

DRUG ABUSE AND DEPENDENCE:

Abuse: Abuse potential was not evaluated in human studies.

Dependence: Rats administered felbamate orally at doses 8.3 times the recommended human dose 6 days each week for 5 consecutive weeks demonstrated no signs of physical dependence as measured by weight loss following drug withdrawal on day 7 of each week.

OVERDOSAGE:

Four subjects inadvertently received felbamate as adjunctive therapy in dosages ranging from 5400 to 7200 mg/day for durations between 6 and 51 days. One subject who received 5400 mg/day as monotherapy for 1 week reported no adverse experiences. Another subject attempted suicide by ingesting 12,000 mg of Felbamate in a 12-hour period. The only adverse experiences reported were mild gastric distress and resting heart rate of 100 bpm. No serious adverse reactions have been reported.

General supportive measures should be employed if overdosage occurs. It is not known if felbamate is dialyzable.

DOSAGE AND ADMINISTRATION:

Felbamate has been studied as monotherapy and adjunctive therapy in adults and as adjunctive therapy in children with seizures associated with Lennox-Gastaut syndrome. As Felbamate is added to or substituted for existing AEDs, it is strongly recommended to reduce the dosage of those AEDs in the range of 20-33% to minimize side effects (see DRUG INTERACTIONS).

Adults (14 years of age and over): The majority of patients received 3600 mg/day in clinical trials evaluating its use as both monotherapy and adjunctive therapy.

Monotherapy (Initial Therapy): Felbamate has not been systematically evaluated as initial monotherapy. Initiate Felbamate at 1200 mg/day in divided doses three or four times daily. The prescriber is advised to titrate previously untreated patients under close clinical supervision, increasing the dosage in 600-mg increments every 2 weeks to 2400 mg/day based on clinical response and thereafter to 3600 mg/day if clinically indicated.

Conversion to Monotherapy: Initiate Felbamate at 1200 mg/day in divided doses three or four times daily. Reduce the dosage of concomitant AEDs by one-third at initiation of Felbamate therapy. At week 2, increase the Felbamate dosage to 2400 mg/day while reducing the dosage of other AEDs up to an additional one-third of their original dosage. At week 3, increase the Felbamate dosage up to 3600 mg/day and continue to reduce the dosage of other AEDs as clinically indicated.

Adjunctive Therapy: Felbamate should be added at 1200 mg/day in divided doses three to four times daily while reducing present AEDs by 20% in order to control plasma concentrations of concurrent phenytoin, valproic acid, and carbamazepine and its metabolites. Further reductions of the concomitant AEDs dosage may be necessary to minimize side effects due to drug interactions. Increase the dosage of Felbamate by 1200 mg/day increments at weekly intervals to 3600 mg/day. Most side effects seen during Felbamate adjunctive therapy resolve as the dosage of concomitant AEDs is decreased (TABLE 5).

TABLE 5 Felbamate, Dosage Table (Adults)

	WEEK 1	WEEK 2	WEEK 3
Dosage reduction of concomitant AEDs	REDUCE original dose by 20-33%*	REDUCE original dose by up to an additional 1/3*	REDUCE as clinically indicated
Felbatol Dosage	1200 mg/day Initial dose	2400 mg/day Therapeutic dosage range	3600 mg/day Therapeutic dosage range

* See *Adjunctive*and *Conversion to Monotherapy*sections.

While the above Felbamate conversion guidelines may result in a Felbamate 3600 mg/day dose within 3 weeks, in some patients titration to a 3600 mg/day Felbamate dose has been achieved in as little as 3 days with appropriate adjustment of other AEDs.

CHILDREN WITH LENNOX-GASTAUT SYNDROME (AGES 2-14 YEARS)

Adjunctive Therapy: Felbamate should be added at 15 mg/kg/day in divided doses three or four times daily while reducing present AEDs by 20% in order to control plasma levels of concurrent phenytoin, valproic acid, and carbamazepine and its metabolites. Further reductions of the concomitant AED dosage may be necessary to minimize side effects due to drug interactions. Increase the dosage of Felbamate by 15 mg/kg/day increments at weekly intervals to 45 mg/kg/day. Most side effects seen during Felbamate adjunctive therapy resolve as the dosage of concomitant AEDs is decreased.

PATIENT PACKAGE INSERT:

PATIENT INFORMATION CONSENT

FELBAMATE SHOULD NOT BE USED BY PATIENTS UNTIL THERE HAS BEEN A COMPLETE DISCUSSION OF THE RISKS AND WRITTEN INFORMED CONSENT HAS BEEN OBTAINED.

IMPORTANT INFORMATION AND WARNING

Felbamate, taken by itself or with other prescription and/or non-prescription drugs, can result in severe, potentially fatal blood abnormality ("aplastic anemia") and/or severe, potentially fatal liver damage.

SUPPLY OF PATIENT INFORMATION/CONSENT FORMS

A supply of "Patient Information/Consent" forms is available free of charge from your local Wallace representative, or may be obtained by calling 609-655-6147. Permission to use the Patient Information/Consent by photocopy reproduction is also hereby granted by Carter-Wallace, Inc.

Note to Physician: It is strongly recommended that you retain a signed copy of the informed consent with the patient's medical records.

HOW SUPPLIED:

Felbamate Tablets, 400 mg, are yellow, scored, capsule-shaped tablets, debossed "0430" on one side and "WALLACE" on the other.

HOW SUPPLIED: *(cont'd)*

Felbamate Tablets, 600 mg, are peach-colored, scored, capsule- shaped tablets, debossed "0431" on one side and "WALLACE" on the other.

Felbamate Oral Suspension, 600 mg/5 ml, is peach-colored.

Shake suspension well before using.

Store at controlled room temperature 15°-30°C (59°-86°F). Dispense in tight container.

HOW SUPPLIED - EQUIVALENTS NOT AVAILABLE:

Suspension - Oral - 600 mg/5ml

240 ml	$85.67	FELBATOL, Wallace Labs	00037-0442-67
960 ml	$330.34	FELBATOL, Wallace Labs	00037-0442-17

Tablet, Uncoated - Oral - 400 mg

100's	$69.70	FELBATOL, Wallace Labs	00037-0430-01
100's	$69.70	FELBATOL, Wallace Labs	00037-0430-11

Tablet, Uncoated - Oral - 600 mg

100's	$79.86	FELBATOL, Wallace Labs	00037-0431-01
100's	$79.86	FELBATOL, Wallace Labs	00037-0431-11

FELODIPINE *(003059)*

CATEGORIES: Antihypertensives; Calcium Channel Blockers; Cardiovascular Drugs; Hypertension; Pregnancy Category C; FDA Class 1C ("Little or No Therapeutic Advantage"); FDA Approved 1991 Jul

BRAND NAMES: *AGON SR* (Australia); *Felogard*; *Hydac*; *Modip* (Germany); *Munobal* (Germany, Mexico); *Munobal Retard* (Germany); *Penedil*; **Plendil**; *Plendil Depottab*; *Plendil ER* (Australia); *Plendil Retard*; *Renedil* (Canada); *Splendil ER* *(International brand names outside U.S. in italics)*

FORMULARIES: BC-BS; Medi-Cal; PCS

COST OF THERAPY: $311.63 (Hypertension; Tablet; 5 mg; 1/day; 365 days) vs. Potential Cost of $24,027.04 (Coronary Bypass)

PRIMARY ICD9: 401.1 (Essential Hypertension, Benign)

DESCRIPTION:

Plendil (Felodipine) is a calcium antagonist (calcium channel blocker). Felodipine is a dihydropyridine derivative that is chemically described as ± ethyl methyl 4-(2,3 -dichlorophenyl)-1,4-dihydro-2,6-dimethyl-3,5-pyridinedicarboxylate. Its empirical formula is $C_{18}H_{19}Cl_2NO_4$.

Felodipine is a slightly yellowish, crystalline powder with a molecular weight of 384.26. It is insoluble in water and is freely soluble in dichloromethane and ethanol. Felodipine is a racemic mixture.

Felodipine tablets provide extended release of felodipine. They are available as tablets containing 2.5 mg, 5 mg or 10 mg of felodipine for oral administration. In addition to the active ingredient felodipine, the tablets contain the following inactive ingredients: Felodipine 2.5 mg — hydroxypropyl cellulose, lactose, FD&C Blue 2, sodium stearyl fumarate, titanium dioxide, yellow iron oxide and other ingredients. Felodipine 5 mg and 10 mg — cellulose, red and yellow oxide, lactose, polyethylene glycol, sodium stearyl fumarate, titanium dioxide and other ingredients.

CLINICAL PHARMACOLOGY:

MECHANISM OF ACTION

Felodipine is a member of the dihydropyridine class of calcium channel antagonists (calcium channel blockers). It reversibly competes with nitrendipine and/or other calcium channel blockers for dihydropyridine binding sites, blocks voltage-dependent Ca++ currents in vascular smooth muscle and cultured rabbit atrial cells and blocks potassium-induced contracture of the rat portal vein.

In vitro studies show that the effects of felodipine on contractile processes are selective, with greater effects on vascular smooth muscle than cardiac muscle. Negative inotropic effects can be detected *in vitro*, but such effects have not been seen in intact animals.

The effect of felodipine on blood pressure is principally a consequence of a dose-related decrease of peripheral vascular resistance in man, with a modest reflex increase in heart rate (see Cardiovascular Effects). With the exception of a mild diuretic effect seen in several animal species and man, the effects of felodipine are accounted for by its effects on peripheral vascular resistance.

PHARMACOKINETICS AND METABOLISM

Following oral administration, felodipine is almost completely absorbed and undergoes extensive first-pass metabolism. The systemic bioavailability of Felodipine is approximately 20 percent. Mean peak concentrations following the administration of Felodipine are reached in 2.5 to 5 hours. Both peak plasma concentration and the area under the plasma concentration time curve (AUC) increase linearly with doses up to 20 mg. Felodipine is greater than 99 percent bound to plasma proteins.

Following intravenous administration, the plasma concentration of felodipine declined triexponentially with mean disposition half-lives of 4.8 minutes, 1.5 hours and 9.1 hours. The mean contributions of the three individual phases to the overall AUC were 15, 40 and 45 percent, respectively, in the order of increasing $t_{1/2}$.

Following oral administration of the immediate-release formulation, the plasma level of felodipine also declined polyexponentially with a mean terminal $t_{1/2}$ of 11 to 16 hours. The mean peak and trough steady-state plasma concentrations achieved after 10 mg of the immediate-release formulation given once a day to normal volunteers, were 20 and 0.5 nmol/l, respectively. The trough plasma concentration of felodipine in most individuals was substantially below the concentration needed to effect a half-maximal decline in blood pressure (EC_{50}) [4-6 nmol/l for felodipine], thus precluding once a day dosing with the immediate-release formulation.

Following administration of a 10-mg dose of Felodipine, the extended-release formulation, to young, healthy volunteers, mean peak and trough steady-state plasma concentrations of felodipine were 7 and 2 nmol/l, respectively. Corresponding values in hypertensive patients (mean age 64) after a 20-mg dose of Felodipine were 23 and 7 nmol/l. Since the EC_{50} for felodipine is 4 to 6 nmol/l, a 5 to 10-mg dose of Felodipine in some patients, and a 20-mg dose in others, would be expected to provide an antihypertensive effect that persists for 24 hours (see Cardiovascular Effects and DOSAGE AND ADMINISTRATION.

The systemic plasma clearance of felodipine in young healthy subjects is about 0.8 l/min and the apparent volume of distribution is about 10 l/kg.

CLINICAL PHARMACOLOGY: *(cont'd)*

Following an oral or intravenous dose of ^{14}C-labeled felodipine in man, about 70 percent of the dose of radioactivity was recovered in urine and 10 percent in the feces. A negligible amount of intact felodipine is recovered in the urine and feces (<0.5%). Six metabolites, which account for 23 percent of the oral dose, have been identified; none has significant vasodilating activity.

Following administration of Felodipine to hypertensive patients, mean peak plasma concentrations at steady state are about 20 percent higher than after a single dose. Blood pressure response is correlated with plasma concentrations of felodipine.

The bioavailability of Felodipine is not influenced by the presence of food in the gastrointestinal tract. In a study of six patients, the bioavailability of felodipine was increased more than two-fold when taken with doubly concentrated grapefruit juice, compared to when taken with water or orange juice. A similar finding has been seen with some other dihydropyridine calcium antagonists, but to a lesser extent than that seen with felodipine.

Age Effects: Plasma concentrations of felodipine, after a single dose and at steady state, increase with age. Mean clearance of felodipine in elderly hypertensives (mean age 74) was only 45 percent of that of young volunteers (mean age 26). At steady state mean AUC for young patients was 39 percent of that for the elderly. Data for intermediate age ranges suggest that the AUCs fall between the extremes of the young and the elderly.

Hepatic Dysfunction: In patients with hepatic disease, the clearance of felodipine was reduced to about 60 percent of that seen in normal young volunteers.

Renal impairment does not alter the plasma concentration profile of felodipine; although higher concentrations of the metabolites are present in the plasma due to decreased urinary excretion, these are inactive.

Animal studies have demonstrated that felodipine crosses the blood-brain barrier and the placenta.

Cardiovascular Effects Following administration of Felodipine, a reduction in blood pressure generally occurs within two to five hours. During chronic administration, substantial blood pressure control lasts for 24 hours, with trough reductions in diastolic blood pressure approximately 40-50 percent of peak reductions. The antihypertensive effect is dose-dependent and correlates with the plasma concentration of felodipine.

A reflex increase in heart rate frequently occurs during the first week of therapy; this increase attenuates over time. Heart rate increases of 5-10 beats per minute may be seen during chronic dosing. The increase is inhibited by beta-blocking agents.

The P-R interval of the ECG is not affected by felodipine when administered alone or in combination with a beta-blocking agent. Felodipine alone or in combination with a beta-blocking agent has been shown, in clinical and electrophysiologic studies, to have no significant effect on cardiac conduction (P-R, P-Q and H-V intervals).

In clinical trials in hypertensive patients without clinical evidence of left ventricular dysfunction, no symptoms suggestive of a negative inotropic effect were noted; however none would be expected in this population (see PRECAUTIONS.)

Renal/Endocrine Effects: Renal vascular resistance is decreased by felodipine while glomerular filtration rate remains unchanged. Mild diuresis, natriuresis and kaliuresis have been observed during the first week of therapy. No significant effects on serum electrolytes were observed during short- and long-term therapy.

In clinical trials in patients with hypertension increases in plasma noradrenaline levels have been observed.

CLINICAL STUDIES:

Felodipine produces dose-related decreases in systolic and diastolic blood pressure as demonstrated in six placebo-controlled, dose response studies using either immediate-release or extended-release dosage forms. These studies enrolled over 800 patients on active treatment, at total daily doses ranging from 2.5 to 20 mg. In those studies felodipine was administered either as monotherapy or was added to beta blockers. The results of the two studies with Felodipine given once daily as monotherapy are shown in the table (TABLE 1) below:

TABLE 1 Mean Reductions In Blood Pressure (mmHg)* Systolic/Diastolic

Dose	N	Mean Peak Response	Mean Trough Response	Trough/Peak Ratios (%s)
Study 1 (8 weeks)				
2.5 mg	68	9.4/4.7	2.7/2.5	29/53
5 mg	69	9.5/6.3	2.4/3.7	25/59
10 mg	67	18.0/10.8	10.0/6.0	56/56
Study 2 (4 weeks)				
10 mg	50	5.3/7.2	1.5/3.2	33/40**
20 mg	50	11.3/10.2	4.5/3.2	43/34**

* Placebo response subtracted
** Different number of patients available for peak and trough measurements

INDICATIONS AND USAGE:

Felodipine is indicated for the treatment of hypertension. Felodipine may be used alone or concomitantly with other antihypertensive agents.

CONTRAINDICATIONS:

Felodipine is contraindicated in patients who are hypersensitive to this product.

PRECAUTIONS:

GENERAL

Hypotension: Felodipine, like other calcium antagonists, may occasionally precipitate significant hypotension and rarely syncope. It may lead to reflex tachycardia which in susceptible individuals may precipitate angina pectoris. (See ADVERSE REACTIONS.)

Heart Failure: Although acute hemodynamic studies in a small number of patients with NYHA Class II or III heart failure treated with felodipine have not demonstrated negative inotropic effects, safety in patients with heart failure has not been established. Caution therefore should be exercised when using Felodipine in patients with heart failure or compromised ventricular function, particularly in combination with a beta blocker.

Elderly Patients or Patients with Impaired Liver Function: Patients over 65 years of age or patients with impaired liver function may have elevated plasma concentrations of felodipine and may respond to lower doses of Felodipine, therefore a starting dose of 2.5 mg once a day is recommended. These patients should have their blood pressure monitored closely during dosage adjustment of Felodipine. (See CLINICAL PHARMACOLOGYand DOSAGE AND ADMINISTRATION.)

Peripheral Edema: Peripheral edema, generally mild and not associated with generalized fluid retention, was the most common adverse event in the clinical trials. The incidence of peripheral edema was both dose- and age-dependent. Frequency of peripheral edema ranged

PRECAUTIONS: *(cont'd)*

from about 10 percent in patients under 50 years of age taking 5 mg daily to about 30 percent in those over 60 years of age taking 20 mg daily. This adverse effect generally occurs within 2-3 weeks of the initiation of treatment.

INFORMATION FOR THE PATIENT

Patients should be instructed to take Felodipine whole and not to crush or chew the tablets. They should be told that mild gingival hyperplasia (gum swelling) has been reported. Good dental hygiene decreases its incidence and severity.

NOTE: As with many other drugs, certain advice to patients being treated with Felodipine is warranted. This information is intended to aid in the safe and effective use of this medication. It is not a disclosure of all possible adverse or intended effects.

CARCINOGENESIS, MUTAGENESIS, AND IMPAIRMENT OF FERTILITY

In a two-year carcinogenicity study in rats fed felodipine at doses of 7.7, 23.1 or 69.3 mg/kg/day (up to 28 times* the maximum recommended human dose on a mg/m^2 basis), a dose-related increase in the incidence of benign interstitial cell tumors of the testes (Leydig cell tumors) was observed in treated male rats. These tumors were not observed in a similar study in mice at doses up to 138.6 mg/kg/day (28 times* the maximum recommended human dose on a mg/m^2 basis). Felodipine, at the doses employed in the two-year rat study, has been shown to lower testicular testosterone and to produce a corresponding increase in serum luteinizing hormone in rats. The Leydig cell tumor development is possibly secondary to these hormonal effects which have not been observed in man.

In this same rat study a dose-related increase in the incidence of focal squamous cell hyperplasia compared to control was observed in the esophageal groove of male and female rats in all dose groups. No other drug-related esophageal or gastric pathology was observed in the rats or with chronic administration in mice and dogs. The latter species, like man, has no anatomical structure comparable to the esophageal groove.

Felodipine was not carcinogenic when fed to mice at doses of up to 138.6 mg/kg/day (28 times* the maximum recommended human dose on a mg/m^2 basis) for periods of up to 80 weeks in males and 99 weeks in females.

Felodipine did not display any mutagenic activity *in vitro* in the Ames microbial mutagenicity test or in the mouse lymphoma forward mutation assay. No clastogenic potential was seen *in vivo* in the mouse micronucleus test at oral doses up to 2500 mg/kg (506 times* the maximum recommended human dose on a mg/m^2 basis) or *in vitro* in a human lymphocyte chromosome aberration assay.

A fertility study in which male and female rats were administered doses of 3.8, 9.6 or 26.9 mg/kg/day showed no significant effect of felodipine on reproductive performance.

PREGNANCY CATEGORY C

Teratogenic Effects: Studies in pregnant rabbits administered doses of felodipine 0.46, 1.2, 2.3 and 4.6 mg/kg/day (from 0.4 to 4 times* the maximum recommended human dose on a mg/m^{2}basis) showed digital anomalies consisting of reduction in size and degree of ossification of the terminal phalanges in the fetuses. The frequency and severity of the changes appeared dose-related and were noted even at the lowest dose. These changes have been shown to occur with other members of the dihydropyridine class and are possibly a result of compromised uterine blood flow. Similar fetal anomalies were not observed in rats given felodipine.

In a teratology study in cynomolgus monkeys no reduction in the size of the terminal phalanges was observed but an abnormal position of the distal phalanges was noted in about 40 percent of the fetuses.

Nonteratogenic Effects: A prolongation of parturition with difficult labor and an increased frequency of fetal and early postnatal deaths were observed in rats administered doses of 9.6 mg/kg/day (4 times* the maximum human dose on a mg/m^2 basis) and above.

Significant enlargement of the mammary glands in excess of the normal enlargement for pregnant rabbits was found with doses greater than or equal to 1.2 mg/kg/day (equal to the maximum human dose on a mg/m^2 basis). This effect occurred only in pregnant rabbits and regressed during lactation. Similar changes in the mammary glands were not observed in rats or monkeys.

There are no adequate and well-controlled studies in pregnant women. If felodipine is used during pregnancy, or if the patient becomes pregnant while taking this drug, she should be apprised of the potential hazard to the fetus, possible digital anomalies of the infant, and the potential effects of felodipine on labor and delivery, and on the mammary glands of pregnant females.

*Based on patient weight of 50 kg

NURSING MOTHERS

It is not known whether this drug is secreted in human milk and because of the potential for serious adverse reactions from felodipine in the infant, a decision should be made whether to discontinue nursing or to discontinue the drug, taking into account the importance of the drug to the mother.

PEDIATRIC USE

Safety and effectiveness in children have not been established.

DRUG INTERACTIONS:

Beta-Blocking Agents: A pharmacokinetic study of felodipine in conjunction with metoprolol demonstrated no significant effects on the pharmacokinetics of felodipine. The AUC and $C_{max}$of metoprolol, however, were increased approximately 31 and 38 percent, respectively. In controlled clinical trials, however, beta blockers including metoprolol were concurrently administered with felodipine and were well tolerated.

Cimetidine: In healthy subjects pharmacokinetic studies showed an approximately 50 percent increase in the area under the plasma concentration time curve (AUC) as well as the C_{max} of felodipine when given concomitantly with cimetidine. It is anticipated that a clinically significant interaction may occur in some hypertensive patients. Therefore, it is recommended that low doses of Felodipine be used when given concomitantly with cimetidine.

Digoxin: When given concomitantly with Felodipine the pharmacokinetics of digoxin in patients with heart failure were not significantly altered.

Anticonvulsants: In a pharmacokinetic study, maximum plasma concentrations of felodipine were considerably lower in epileptic patients on long-term anticonvulsant therapy (*e.g.,* phenytoin, carbamazepine, or phenobarbital) than in healthy volunteers. In such patients, the mean area under the felodipine plasma concentration-time curve was also reduced to approximately six percent of that observed in healthy volunteers. Since a clinically significant interaction may be anticipated, alternative antihypertensive therapy should be considered in these patients.

Other Concomitant Therapy: In healthy subjects there were no clinically significant interactions when felodipine was given concomitantly with indomethacin or spironolactone.

Interaction with Food: See CLINICAL PHARMACOLOGY, Pharmacokinetics and Metabolism.

ADVERSE REACTIONS:

In controlled studies in the United States and overseas approximately 3000 patients were treated with felodipine as either the extended-release or the immediate-release formulation.

The most common clinical adverse events reported with Felodipine administered as monotherapy at the recommended dosage range of 2.5 mg to 10 mg once a day were peripheral edema and headache. Peripheral edema was generally mild, but it was age- and dose-related and resulted in discontinuation of therapy in about 3 percent of the enrolled patients. Discontinuation of therapy due to any clinical adverse event occurred in about 6 percent of the patients receiving Felodipine, principally for peripheral edema, headache, or flushing.

Adverse events that occurred with an incidence of 1.5 percent or greater at any of the recommended doses of 2.5 mg to 10 mg once a day (Felodipine, N=861; Placebo, N=334), without regard to causality, are compared to placebo and are listed by dose in TABLE 2. These events are reported from controlled clinical trials with patients who were randomized to a fixed dose of Felodipine or titrated from an initial dose of 2.5 mg or 5 mg once a day. A dose of 20 mg once a day has been evaluated in some clinical studies. Although the antihypertensive effect of Felodipine is increased at 20 mg once a day, there is a disproportionate increase in adverse events, especially those associated with vasodilatory effects(see DOSAGE AND ADMINISTRATION.)

TABLE 2 Percent of Patients with Adverse Events in Controlled Trials* of Felodipine (N=861) as Monotherapy without Regard to Causality (Incidence of discontinuations shown in parentheses)

Body System Adverse Events	Placebo N=334	2.5 mg N=255	5 mg N=581	10 mg N=408
Body As A Whole				
Peripheral Edema	3.3 (0.0)	2.0 (0.0)	8.8 (2.2)	17.4 (2.5)
Asthenia	3.3 (0.0)	3.9 (0.0)	3.3 (0.0)	2.2 (0.0)
Warm Sensation	0.0 (0.0)	0.0 (0.0)	0.9 (0.2)	1.5 (0.0)
Cardiovascular				
Palpitation	2.4 (0.0)	0.4 (0.0)	1.4 (0.3)	2.5 (0.5)
Digestive				
Nausea	1.5 (0.9)	1.2 (0.0)	1.7 (0.3)	1.0 (0.7)
Dyspepsia	1.2 (0.0)	3.9 (0.0)	0.7 (0.0)	0.5 (0.0)
Constipation	0.9 (0.0)	1.2 (0.0)	0.3 (0.0)	1.5 (0.2)
Nervous				
Headache	10.2 (0.9)	10.6 (0.4)	11.0 (1.7)	14.7 (2.0)
Dizziness	2.7 (0.3)	2.7 (0.0)	3.6 (0.5)	3.7 (0.5)
Paresthesia	1.5 (0.3)	1.6 (0.0)	1.2 (0.0)	1.2 (0.2)
Respiratory				
Upper Respiratory Infection	1.8 (0.0)	3.9 (0.0)	1.9 (0.0)	0.7 (0.0)
Cough	0.3 (0.0)	0.8 (0.0)	1.2 (0.0)	1.7 (0.0)
Rhinorrhea	0.0 (0.0)	1.6 (0.0)	0.2 (0.0)	0.2 (0.0)
Sneezing	0.0 (0.0)	1.6 (0.0)	0.0 (0.0)	0.0 (0.0)
Skin				
Rash	0.9 (0.0)	2.0 (0.0)	0.2 (0.0)	0.2 (0.0)
Flushing	0.9 (0.3)	3.9 (0.0)	5.3 (0.7)	6.9 (1.2)

* Patients in titration studies may have been exposed to more than one dose level of Plendil.

Adverse events that occurred in 0.5 up to 1.5 percent of patients who received Felodipine in all controlled clinical trials at the recommended dosage range of 2.5 mg to 10 mg once a day and serious adverse events that occurred at a lower rate or events reported during marketing experience (those lower rate events are in italics) are listed below. These events are listed in order of decreasing severity within each category and the relationship of these events to administration of Felodipine is uncertain:

Body as a Whole: Chest pain, facial edema, flu-like illness;

Cardiovascular: Myocardial infarction, hypotension, syncope, angina pectoris, arrhythmia, tachycardia, premature beats;

Digestive: Abdominal pain, diarrhea, vomiting, dry mouth, flatulence, acid regurgitation;

Hematologic: Anemia;

Metabolic: ALT (SGPT) increased;

Musculoskeletal: Arthralgia, back pain, leg pain, foot pain, muscle cramps, myalgia, arm pain, knee pain, hip pain;

Nervous/Psychiatric: Insomnia, depression, anxiety disorders, irritability, nervousness, somnolence, decreased libido;

Respiratory: Dyspnea, pharyngitis, bronchitis, influenza, sinusitis, epistaxis, respiratory infection;

Skin: Contusion, erythema, urticaria;

Special Senses: Visual disturbances;

Urogenital: Impotence, urinary frequency, urinary urgency, dysuria, polyuria.

Gingival Hyperplasia: Gingival hyperplasia, usually mild, occurred in <0.5 percent of patients in controlled studies. This condition may be avoided or may regress with improved dental hygiene. See PRECAUTIONS, Information for Patients.

CLINICAL LABORATORY TEST FINDINGS

Serum Electrolytes: No significant effects on serum electrolytes were observed during short- and long-term therapy (see CLINICAL PHARMACOLOGY, Renal/Endocrine Effects).

Serum Glucose: No significant effects on fasting serum glucose were observed in patients treated with Felodipine in the U.S. controlled study.

Liver Enzymes: One of two episodes of elevated serum transaminases decreased once drug was discontinued in clinical studies; no follow-up was available for the other patient.

OVERDOSAGE:

Oral doses of 240 mg/kg and 264 mg/kg in male and female mice, respectively and 2390 mg/kg and 2250 mg/kg in male and female rats, respectively, caused significant lethality.

In a suicide attempt, one patient took 150 mg felodipine together with 15 tablets each of atenolol and spironolactone and 20 tablets of nitrazepam. The patient's blood pressure and heart rate were normal on admission to hospital; he subsequently recovered without significant sequelae.

Overdosage might be expected to cause excessive peripheral vasodilation with marked hypotension and possibly bradycardia.

If severe hypotension occurs, symptomatic treatment should be instituted. The patient should be placed supine with the legs elevated. The administration of intravenous fluids may be useful to treat hypotension due to overdosage with calcium antagonists. In case of accompanying bradycardia, atropine (0.5-1 mg) should be administered intravenously. Sympathomimetic drugs may also be given if the physician feels they are warranted.

It has not been established whether felodipine can be removed from the circulation by hemodialysis.

DOSAGE AND ADMINISTRATION:

The recommended starting dose is 5 mg once a day. Depending on the patient's response the dosage can be decreased to 2.5 mg or increased to 10 mg once a day. These adjustments should occur generally at intervals of not less than two weeks. The recommended dosage range is 2.5-10 mg once daily. In clinical trials, doses above 10 mg daily showed an increased blood pressure response but a large increase in the rate of peripheral edema and other vasodilatory adverse events (see ADVERSE REACTIONS.) Modification of the recommended dosage is usually not required in patients with renal impairment.

Felodipine should be swallowed whole and not crushed or chewed.

USE IN THE ELDERLY OR PATIENTS WITH IMPAIRED LIVER FUNCTION

Patients over 65 years of age or patients with impaired liver function may develop higher plasma concentrations of felodipine, therefore a starting dose of 2.5 mg once a day is recommended. Dosage may be adjusted as described above. See PRECAUTIONS.

HOW SUPPLIED:

No. 3584 -Felodipine, 2.5 mg, are sage green, round convex tablets, with code 450 on one side and Plendil on the other.

No. 3585 -Felodipine, 5 mg, are light red-brown, round convex tablets, with code 451 on one side and Plendil on the other.

No. 3586 -Felodipine, 10 mg, are red-brown, round convex tablets, with code 452 on one side and Plendil on the other.

Storage: Store below 30°C (86°F). Keep container tightly closed. Protect from light.

HOW SUPPLIED - EQUIVALENTS NOT AVAILABLE:

Tablet, Uncoated, Sustained Action - Oral - 2.5 mg

30's	$25.62	PLENDIL, Astra Merck	61113-0450-31
100's	$85.38	PLENDIL, Astra Merck	61113-0450-58
100's	$89.65	PLENDIL, Astra Merck	61113-0450-28

Tablet, Uncoated, Sustained Action - Oral - 5 mg

30's	$25.62	PLENDIL, Astra Merck	61113-0451-31
100's	$85.38	PLENDIL, Astra Merck	61113-0451-58
100's	$89.65	PLENDIL, Astra Merck	61113-0451-28

Tablet, Uncoated, Sustained Action - Oral - 10 mg

30's	$46.01	PLENDIL, Astra Merck	61113-0452-31
100's	$153.42	PLENDIL, Astra Merck	61113-0452-58
100's	$161.09	PLENDIL, Astra Merck	61113-0452-28

FENFLURAMINE HYDROCHLORIDE *(001252)*

CATEGORIES: Amphetamines; Anorexients/CNS Stimulants; Appetite Suppressants; Central Nervous System Agents; Obesity; Psychostimulants; Respiratory/Cerebral Stimulant; Weight Loss; Pregnancy Category C; DEA Class CIV; FDA Approval Pre 1982; Top 200 Drugs

BRAND NAMES: *Adipomin*; *Deobesan*; *Dexfenfluramine*; *Dietoff*; *Dima-Fen*; *Fenbesy*; *Fendurin*; *Fentrate Retard*; *Flabolin*; *Grazilan*; *Grazilan Extentabs*; *Kataline*; *Miniphage*; *Miniphage Retard*; *Oban 20*; *Obegon*; *Pesos*; *Ponderal* (France, Canada); *Ponderal Retard* (France); *Ponderamin*; *Ponderax* (Germany, England); *Ponderax Pacaps* (Australia); *Ponderax Retard* (Germany); *Ponderax-60*; *Ponderex*; **Pondimin**; *Poneral*; *Ponflural*; *Slimerax*; *Wate Down*
(International brand names outside U.S. in italics)

DESCRIPTION:

Pondimin (fenfluramine hydrochloride) is an anorectic drug for oral administration. Immediate release tablets containing 20 mg fenfluramine hydrochloride are orange, scored, compressed tablets engraved AHR and 6447.

Inactive Ingredients: Corn Starch, FD&C Yellow 6, Magnesium Stearate, Microcrystalline Cellulose, Silicon Dioxide, Sodium Lauryl Sulfate.

Fenfluramine HCl has the following chemical name: N-ethyl-α-methyl-3-(trifluoromethyl) benzeneethanamine hydrochloride.

CLINICAL PHARMACOLOGY:

Fenfluramine is a sympathomimetic amine, the pharmacologic activity of which differs somewhat from that of the prototype drugs of this class used in obesity, the amphetamines, in appearing to produce more central nervous system depression than stimulation.

The mechanism of action of Fenfluramine HCl is unclear but may be related to brain levels (or turnover rates) of serotonin or to increased glucose utilization. The antiappetite effects of Fenfluramine HCl are suppressed by serotonin-blocking drugs and by drugs that lower brain levels of the amine. Furthermore, decreased serotonin levels produced by selective brain lesions suppress the action of Fenfluramine HCl.

In a study of 20 normal males, fenfluramine increased glucose utilization, resulting in decreased blood glucose levels. Experimental work in animals suggested that increased glucose utilization activated the satiety center and decreased the activity of the feeding center. Perhaps by this mechanism Fenfluramine HCl inhibits appetite. The relationship between glucose utilization and serotonin has not been clarified.

Fenfluramine is well-absorbed from the gastrointestinal tract, and a maximal anorectic effect is generally seen after 2 to 4 hours. In man, fenfluramine is de-ethylated to norfenfluramine which is subsequently oxidized to m-trifluoromethyl benzoic acid and excreted as the glycine conjugate, m-trifluoromethylhippuric acid. Other compounds found in the urine include unchanged fenfluramine and norfenfluramine.

The rate of excretion of fenfluramine is pH dependent, with much smaller amounts appearing in an alkaline than in an acid urine.

The half-life of fenfluramine is said to be about 20 hours, compared with 5 hours for amphetamines; however, if urinary excretion is rapid and the pH maintained in the acidic range (below pH 5), half-life can be reduced to 11 hours. Fenfluramine and norfenfluramine reach steady state concentrations in plasma within 3 to 4 days following chronic dosage.

The greatest weight loss is seen in those patients who maintain the highest levels of Fenfluramine HCl. A 2-to-3-kg weight loss over 6 weeks is associated with a plasma level of 0.1 mcg/ml (or 10 mcg/100 ml).

Fenfluramine is widely distributed in almost all body tissues. It is soluble in lipids and crosses the blood-brain barrier. Fenfluramine crosses the placenta readily in monkeys.

INDICATIONS AND USAGE:

Fenfluramine HCl is indicated in the management of exogenous obesity as a short-term (a few weeks) adjunct in a regimen of weight reduction based on caloric restriction.

INDICATIONS AND USAGE: *(cont'd)*

Drugs of this class used in obesity are commonly known as "anorectics" or "anorexigenics." It has not been established, however, that the action of such drugs in treating obesity is primarily one of appetite suppression. Other central nervous system actions or metabolic effects may be involved.

Adult obese subjects instructed in dietary management and treated with "anorectic" drugs, lose more weight on the average than those treated with placebo and diet, as determined in relatively short-term trials.

The average magnitude of increased weight loss of drug-treated patients over placebo-treated is only a fraction of a pound a week. The rate of weight loss is greatest in the first weeks of therapy for both drug and placebo subjects and tends to decrease in succeeding weeks. The possible origins of the increased weight loss due to the various drug effects are not established. The average amount of weight loss associated with the use of an "anorectic" drug varies from trial to trial, and the increased weight loss appears to be related in part to variables other than the drug prescribed such as the physician-investigator, the population treated and the diet prescribed. Studies do not permit conclusions as to the relative importance of the drug and non-drug factors on weight loss.

The natural history of obesity is measured in years, whereas the studies cited are restricted to a few weeks duration; thus, the total impact of drug-induced weight loss over that of diet alone must be considered clinically limited.

CONTRAINDICATIONS:

Fenfluramine is contraindicated in patients with glaucoma or with hypersensitivity to fenfluramine or other sympathomimetic amines. Do not administer fenfluramine during or within 14 days following the administration of monoamine oxidase inhibitors, since hypertensive crises may result. Patients with a history of drug abuse should not receive this drug.

Do not administer fenfluramine to patients with alcoholism since psychiatric symptoms (paranoia, depression, psychosis) have been reported in a few such patients who had been administered this drug.

Fenfluramine should also generally be avoided in patients with psychotic illness. There have been reports of schizophrenic patients who have become agitated, delusional, and assaultive.

A fatal cardiac arrest has been reported shortly after the induction of anesthesia in a patient who had been taking fenfluramine prior to surgery. Fenfluramine may have a catecholamine-depleting effect when administered for prolonged periods of time; therefore, potent anesthetic agents should be administered with caution to patients taking fenfluramine. If general anesthesia cannot be avoided, full cardiac monitoring and facilities for instant resuscitative measures are a minimum necessity.

WARNINGS:

When tolerance to the "anorectic" effect develops, the maximum recommended dose should not be exceeded in an attempt to increase the effect; rather, the drug should be discontinued.

PRECAUTIONS:

GENERAL

Fenfluramine differs in its pharmacological profile from other "anorectic" drugs with which the prescribing practitioner may be familiar. Correspondingly, there are possible adverse effects not associated with other "anorectics"; such effects include those of diarrhea, sedation, and depression. The possibility of these effects should be weighed against the possible advantage of decreased central nervous system stimulation and/or abuse potential.

There have been four cases of pulmonary hypertension reported in association with fenfluramine use. Two cases were apparently reversible after discontinuation of fenfluramine, but evidence of pulmonary hypertension recurred in one of these patients upon rechallenge with fenfluramine. A third patient was initially improved with nifedipine treatment, but was noted to have increased pulmonary arterial pressure again at a four month follow up visit. Finally, an irreversible and fatal case of pulmonary hypertension has been reported in a patient who had seven 1-month courses of fenfluramine in the twelve years prior to death. Patients taking fenfluramine should be advised to report immediately any deterioration in exercise tolerance.

Use only with caution in hypertension, with monitoring of blood pressure, since evidence is insufficient to rule out a possible adverse effect on blood pressure in some hypertensive patients. The drug is not recommended in severely hypertensive patients. The drug is not recommended for patients with symptomatic cardiovascular disease including arrhythmias.

Caution should be exercised in prescribing fenfluramine for patients with a history of mental depression. Further depression of mood may become evident while the patient is on fenfluramine or following withdrawal of fenfluramine. Symptoms of depression occurring immediately following abrupt withdrawal can be readily controlled by reinstituting Fenfluramine HCl, followed by a gradual tapering off of the daily dose.

INFORMATION FOR THE PATIENT

Fenfluramine may impair the ability of the patient to engage in potentially hazardous activities such as operating machinery or driving a motor vehicle (see ADVERSE REACTIONS); the patient should be cautioned accordingly. Patient should also be advised to avoid alcoholic beverages while taking Fenfluramine HCl.

CARCINOGENESIS, MUTAGENESIS, AND IMPAIRMENT OF FERTILITY

No carcinogenic studies or mutagenic studies have been undertaken with this drug.

PREGNANCY CATEGORY C

Fenfluramine HCl was shown to produce a questionable embryotoxic effect in rats and a reduced conception rate when given in a dose of 20 times the human dose. However, additional reproduction studies in rats, rabbits, mice, and monkeys at doses up to, respectively, 5 times, 20 times, 1 time, and 5 times the human dose yielded negative results.

There are no adequate and well-controlled studies in pregnant women. Fenfluramine HCl should be used during pregnancy only if the potential benefit justifies the potential risk to the fetus.

LABOR AND DELIVERY

The effect of fenfluramine during labor or delivery on the mother and the fetus is unknown. The effect on later growth, development, and functional maturation of the child is unknown.

NURSING MOTHERS

It is not known whether this drug is excreted in human milk. Because many drugs are excreted in human milk, caution should be exercised when fenfluramine is administered to a nursing mother.

PEDIATRIC USE

Safety and effectiveness in children below the age of 12 years has not been established.

DRUG INTERACTIONS:

Fenfluramine may increase slightly the effect of antihypertensive drugs, e.g., guanethidine, methyldopa, reserpine.

Other CNS depressant drugs should be used with caution in patients taking fenfluramine, since the effects may be additive.

ADVERSE REACTIONS:

The most common adverse reactions of fenfluramine are drowsiness, diarrhea, and dry mouth. Less frequent adverse reactions reported in association with fenfluramine are:

Central nervous system: Dizziness; confusion; incoordination; headache; elevated mood; depression; anxiety, nervousness, or tension; insomnia; weakness or fatigue; increased or decreased libido; agitation, dysarthria.

Gastrointestinal: Constipation; abdominal pain; nausea.

Autonomic: Sweating; chills; blurred vision.

Genitourinary: Dysuria; urinary frequency.

Cardiovascular: Palpitation; hypotension; hypertension; fainting; pulmonary hypertension.

Skin: Rash; urticaria; burning sensation.

Miscellaneous: Eye irritation; myalgia; fever; chest pain; bad taste.

DRUG ABUSE AND DEPENDENCE:

Fenfluramine hydrochloride is a controlled substance in Schedule IV. Fenfluramine is related chemically to the amphetamines, although it differs somewhat pharmacologically. The amphetamines and related stimulant drugs have been extensively abused and can produce tolerance and severe psychological dependence, as well as other adverse organic and mental changes. In this regard, there has been a report of abuse of fenfluramine by subjects with a history of abuse of other drugs. Abuse of 80 to 400 milligrams of the drug has been reported to be associated with euphoria, derealization, and perceptual changes. Fenfluramine did not produce signs of dependence in animals and appears to produce sedation more often than CNS stimulation at therapeutic doses. Its abuse potential appears qualitatively different from that of amphetamines. The possibility that fenfluramine may induce dependence should be kept in mind when evaluating the desirability of including the drug in the weight reduction programs of individual patients.

OVERDOSAGE:

SIGNS AND SYMPTOMS

Only limited data have been reported concerning clinical effects and management of overdosage of fenfluramine.

Agitation and drowsiness, confusion, flushing, tremor (or shivering), fever, sweating, abdominal pain, hyperventilation, and dilated non-reactive pupils seem frequent in fenfluramine overdosage. Reflexes may be either exaggerated or depressed and some patients may have rotary nystagmus. Tachycardia may be present, but blood pressure may be normal or only slightly elevated. Convulsions, coma, and ventricular extrasystoles, culminating in ventricular fibrillation, and cardiac arrest, may occur at higher dosages.

HUMAN TOXICITY

Less than 5 mg/kg are toxic to humans. Five-ten mg/kg may produce coma and convulsions. Reported single overdoses have ranged from 300 to 2000 mg; the lowest reported fatal dose was a few hundred mg in a small child, and the highest reported nonfatal dose was 1800 mg in an adult. Most deaths were apparently due to respiratory failure and cardiac arrest.

Toxic effects will appear within 30 to 60 minutes and may progress rapidly to potentially fatal complications in 90 to 240 minutes. Symptoms may persist for extended periods depending upon the dose ingested.

MANAGEMENT

After overdosage, only a small percentage of the drug is excreted in the urine. Forced acid diuresis has been recommended only in extreme cases in which the patient survives the early hours of intoxication but fails to show decisive improvement from other measures. Hemodialysis and peritoneal dialysis are of theoretical advantage but have not been used clinically.

Reportedly the treatment of fenfluramine intoxication should include:

Gastric Lavage: (but not drug-induced emesis because the patient may become unconscious at a very early stage.)In the event that gastric lavage is not feasible due to trismus, consult an anesthesiologist for endotracheal intubation after administration of muscle relaxants; only then gastric evacuation should be tried. Administration of activated charcoal after emesis or lavage may reduce absorption of drug.

Monitoring of Vital Functions: If necessary, mechanical respiration, defibrillation, or "cardioversion" should be instituted.

Drug Therapy: Diazepam or phenobarbital for convulsions or muscular hyperactivity. In the presence of extreme tachycardia: propranolol; in the presence of ventricular extrasystoles: lidocaine; in the presence of hyperpyrexia: chlorpromazine.

Since fenfluramine has been shown to have a slight lowering effect on blood sugar in some patients, the theoretical possibility of hypoglycemia should be borne in mind although this effect has not been reported in cases of clinical overdosage.

DOSAGE AND ADMINISTRATION:

The usual dose is one 20 mg tablet three times daily before meals. Depending on the degree of effectiveness and side effects, the dosage may be increased at weekly intervals by one tablet (20 mg) daily until a maximum dosage of two tablets three times daily is attained. Total dosage of fenfluramine should not exceed 120 mg per day.

Store at controlled room temperature, between 15°C and 30°C (59°F and 86°F).

Dispense in well-closed container.

PATIENT INFORMATION:

Fenfluramine is used as part of a diet plan to reduce appetite. Inform your physician if you are pregnant or nursing. Do not take this medication with a monoamine oxidase inhibitor. This medication may cause dizziness, drowsiness, or blurred vision; use caution while driving or operating hazardous machinery. Do not take any other sedating drugs or drink alcohol while taking fenfluramine. This medication may be habit forming. Withdrawal symptoms may occur after you stop taking it. Inform your physician immediately if you develop shortness of breath, breathing difficulty, chest pain, or swelling in feet and lower extremities. May cause nausea, vomiting or constipation; notify your physician if these occur. This medication should be taken on an empty stomach, one hour before meals.

HOW SUPPLIED:

Pondimin is available in 20 mg orange, scored, compressed tablets monogrammed AHR and 6447, in bottles of 100 and 500.

HOW SUPPLIED - EQUIVALENTS NOT AVAILABLE:

Tablet, Uncoated - Oral - 20 mg

100's	**$33.33**	**PONDIMIN, AH Robins**	**00031-6447-63**
500's	**$158.94**	**PONDIMIN, AH Robins**	**00031-6447-70**

FENOPROFEN CALCIUM *(001253)*

CATEGORIES: Analgesics; Anti-Inflammatory Agents; Antianxiety Drugs; Antiarthritics; Antipyretics; Arthritis; Central Nervous System Agents; NSAIDS; Nonsteroidal Anti-Inflammatory; Osteoarthritis; Pain; Migraine*; Vertigo/Motion Sickness/Vomiting*; FDA Approval Pre 1982
* Indication not approved by the FDA

BRAND NAMES: *Fenoprex*; *Fenoprofen*; *Fenopron* (England, Japan); *Fepron*; *Feprona* (Germany); **Nalfon**; *Nalgesic* (France); *Progesic* (England)
(International brand names outside U.S. in italics)

FORMULARIES: Aetna; FHP; Medi-Cal

COST OF THERAPY: $369.56 (Arthritis; Capsule; 300 mg; 3/day; 365 days) vs. Potential Cost of $7,982.49 (Hip Replacement)

PRIMARY ICD9: 715.99 (Osteoarthritis, Unspecified, Multiple Sites)

DESCRIPTION:

Fenoprofen Calcium, USP is a nonsteroidal, anti-inflammatory, antiarthritic drug. Fenoprofen Calcium Pulvules contain fenoprofen calcium as the dihydrate in an amount equivalent to 200 mg (0.826 mmol) or 300 mg (1.24 mmol) of fenoprofen. The Pulvules also contain cellulose, gelatin, iron oxides, silicone, titanium dioxide, and other inactive ingredients. The 300-mg Pulvules also contain D & C Yellow No. 10 and F D & C Yellow No. 6.

Fenoprofen Calcium Tablets contain fenoprofen calcium as the dihydrate in an amount equivalent to 600 mg (2.48 mmol) of fenoprofen. The tablets also contain amberlite, benzyl alcohol, calcium phosphate, corn starch, D & C Yellow No. 10, F D & C Yellow No. 6, hydroxypropyl methylcellulose, magnesium stearate, polyethylene glycol, stearic acid, titanium dioxide, and other inactive ingredients.

Chemically, Fenoprofen Calcium is an arylacetic acid derivative.

Benzeneacetic acid, α-methyl-3-phenoxy-, calcium salt dihydrate (±)-

Fenoprofen Calcium is a white crystalline powder that has the empirical formula $C_{30}H_{26}CaO_6 \cdot 2H_2O$ representing a molecular weight of 558.64. At 25°C, it dissolves to a 15 mg/ml solution in alcohol (95%). It is slightly soluble in water and insoluble in benzene.

The *p*Ka of Fenoprofen Calcium is 4.5 at 25°C.

CLINICAL PHARMACOLOGY:

Fenoprofen Calcium is a nonsteroidal, anti-inflammatory, antiarthritic drug that also possesses analgesic and antipyretic activities. Its exact mode of action is unknown, but it is thought that prostaglandin synthetase inhibition is involved. Fenoprofen Calcium has been shown to inhibit prostaglandin synthetase isolated from bovine seminal vesicles. Reproduction studies in rats have shown Fenoprofen Calcium to be associated with prolonged labor and difficult parturition when given during late pregnancy. Evidence suggests that this may be due to decreased uterine contractility resulting from the inhibition of prostaglandin synthesis. Its action is not mediated through the adrenal gland.

Fenoprofen shows anti-inflammatory effects in rodents by inhibiting the development of redness and edema in acute inflammatory conditions and by reducing soft-tissue swelling and bone damage associated with chronic inflammation. It exhibits analgesic activity in rodents by inhibiting the writhing response caused by the introduction of an irritant into the peritoneal cavities of mice and by elevating pain thresholds that are related to pressure in edematous hindpaws of rats. In rats made febrile by the subcutaneous administration of brewer's yeast, fenoprofen produces antipyretic action. These effects are characteristic of nonsteroidal, anti-inflammatory, antipyretic, analgesic drugs.

The results in humans confirmed the anti-inflammatory and analgesic actions found in animals. The emergence and degree of erythremic response were measured in adult male volunteers exposed to ultraviolet irradiation. The effects of Fenoprofen Calcium, aspirin, and indomethacin were each compared with those of a placebo. All 3 drugs demonstrated antierythemic activity.

In patients with rheumatoid arthritis, the anti-inflammatory action of Fenoprofen Calcium has been evidenced by relief of pain, increase in grip strength, and reductions in joint swelling, duration of morning stiffness, and disease activity (as assessed by both the investigator and the patient). The anti-inflammatory action of Fenoprofen Calcium has also been evidenced by increased mobility (*i.e.,* a decrease in the number of joints having limited motion).

The use of Fenoprofen Calcium in combination with gold salts or corticosteroids has been studied in patients with rheumatoid arthritis. The studies, however, were inadequate in demonstrating whether further improvement is obtained by adding Fenoprofen Calcium to maintenance therapy with gold salts or steroids. Whether or not Fenoprofen Calcium used in conjunction with partially effective doses of a corticosteroid has a "steroid-sparing" effect is unknown.

In patients with osteoarthritis, the anti-inflammatory and analgesic effects of Fenoprofen Calcium have been demonstrated by reduction in tenderness as a response to pressure and reductions in night pain, stiffness, swelling, and overall disease activity (as assessed by both the patient and the investigator). These effects have also been demonstrated by relief of pain with motion and at rest and increased range of motion in involved joints.

In patients with rheumatoid arthritis and osteoarthritis, clinical studies have shown Fenoprofen Calcium to be comparable to aspirin in controlling the aforementioned measures of disease activity, but mild gastrointestinal reactions (nausea, dyspepsia) and tinnitus occurred less frequently in patients treated with Fenoprofen Calcium than in aspirin-treated patients. It is not known whether Fenoprofen Calcium causes less peptic ulceration than does aspirin.

In patients with pain, the analgesic action of Fenoprofen Calcium has produced a reduction in pain intensity, an increase in pain relief, improvement in total analgesia scores, and a sustained analgesic effect.

Under fasting conditions, Fenoprofen Calcium is rapidly absorbed, and peak plasma levels of 50 mcg/ml are achieved within 2 hours after oral administration of 600-mg doses. Good dose proportionality was observed between 200-mg and 600-mg doses in fasting male volunteers. The plasma half-life is approximately 3 hours. About 90% of a single oral dose is eliminated within 24 hours as fenoprofen glucuronide and 4'- hydroxyfenoprofen glucuronide, the major urinary metabolites of fenoprofen. Fenoprofen is highly bound (99%) to albumin.

The concomitant administration of antacid (containing both aluminum and magnesium hydroxide) does not interfere with absorption of Fenoprofen Calcium.

There is less suppression of collagen-induced platelet aggregation with single doses of Fenoprofen Calcium than there is with aspirin.

INDICATIONS AND USAGE:

Fenoprofen Calcium is indicated for relief of the signs and symptoms of rheumatoid arthritis and osteoarthritis. It is recommended for the treatment of acute flare-ups and exacerbations and for the long-term management of these diseases.

INDICATIONS AND USAGE: *(cont'd)*

Fenoprofen Calcium is also indicated for the relief of mild to moderate pain.

CONTRAINDICATIONS:

Fenoprofen Calcium is contraindicated in patients who have shown hypersensitivity to it.

The drug should not be administered to patients with a history of significantly impaired renal function.

Fenoprofen Calcium should not be given to patients in whom aspirin and other nonsteroidal anti-inflammatory drugs induce the symptoms of asthma, rhinitis, or urticaria, because cross-sensitivity to these drugs occurs in a high proportion of such patients.

WARNINGS:

Risk of GI Ulceration, Bleeding and Perforation with NSAID Therapy: Serious gastrointestinal toxicity such as bleeding, ulceration, and perforation, can occur at any time, with or without warning symptoms, in patients treated chronically with NSAID therapy. Although minor upper gastrointestinal problems, such as dyspepsia, are common, usually developing early in therapy, physicians should remain alert for ulceration and bleeding in patients treated chronically with NSAIDs, even in the absence of previous GI tract symptoms. In patients observed in clinical trials of several months to 2 years duration, symptomatic upper GI ulcers, gross bleeding or perforation appear to occur in approximately 1% of patients treated for 3 to 6 months, and in about 2% to 4% of patients treated for 1 year. Physicians should inform patients about the signs and/or symptoms of serious GI toxicity and what steps to take if they occur.

Studies to date have not identified any subset of patients not at risk of developing peptic ulceration and bleeding. Except for a prior history of serious GI events and other risk factors known to be associated with peptic ulcer disease, such as alcoholism, smoking, etc., no risk factors (*e.g.,* age, sex) have been associated with increased risk. Elderly or debilitated patients seem to tolerate ulceration or bleeding less well than other individuals and most spontaneous reports of fatal GI events are in this population. Studies to date are inconclusive concerning the relative risk of various NSAIDs in causing such reactions. High doses of any NSAID probably carry a greater risk of these reactions, although controlled clinical trials showing this do not exist in most cases. In considering the use of relatively large doses (within the recommended dosage range), sufficient benefit should be anticipated to offset the potential increased risk of GI toxicity.

Since Fenoprofen Calcium has been marketed, there have been reports of genitourinary tract problems in patients taking it. The most frequently reported problems have been episodes of dysuria, cystitis, hematuria, interstitial nephritis, and nephrotic syndrome. This syndrome may be preceded by the appearance of fever, rash, arthralgia, oliguria, and azotemia and may progress to anuria. There may also be substantial proteinuria, and, on renal biopsy, electron microscopy has shown foot process fusion and T-lymphocyte infiltration in the renal interstitium. Early recognition of the syndrome and withdrawal of the drug have been followed by rapid recovery. Administration of steroids and the use of dialysis have also been included in the treatment. Because a syndrome with some of these characteristics has also been reported with other nonsteroidal anti-inflammatory drugs, it is recommended that patients who have had these reactions with other such drugs not be treated with Fenoprofen Calcium. In patients with possibly compromised renal function, periodic renal function examinations should be done.

PRECAUTIONS:

GENERAL

Renal Effects: There have been reports of acute interstitial nephritis and nephrotic syndrome (see CONTRAINDICATIONS and WARNINGS).

A second form of renal toxicity has been seen in patients with prerenal conditions leading to a reduction in renal blood flow or blood volume, in which renal prostaglandins play a supportive role in the maintenance of renal perfusion. In these patients, administration of an NSAID may cause a dose-dependent reduction in prostaglandin formation and may precipitate overt renal decompensation at any time. Patients at greatest risk for this reaction are those with impaired renal function, heart failure, liver dysfunction, those taking diuretics, and the elderly. Discontinuation of NSAID therapy is typically followed by recovery to the pretreatment state.

Since Fenoprofen Calcium is primarily eliminated by the kidneys, patients with possibly compromised renal function (such as the elderly) should be monitored periodically, especially during long-term therapy. For such patients, it may be anticipated that a lower daily dosage will avoid excessive drug accumulation.

Miscellaneous: Peripheral edema has been observed in some patients taking Fenoprofen Calcium; therefore, Fenoprofen Calcium should be used with caution in patients with compromised cardiac function or hypertension. The possibility of renal involvement should be considered.

Studies to date have not shown changes in the eyes attributable to the administration of Fenoprofen Calcium. However, adverse ocular effects have been observed with other anti-inflammatory drugs. Eye examinations, therefore, should be performed if visual disturbances occur in patients taking Fenoprofen Calcium.

Caution should be exercised by patients whose activities require alertness if they experience CNS side effects while taking Fenoprofen Calcium.

Since the safety of Fenoprofen Calcium has not been established in patients with impaired hearing, these patients should have periodic tests of auditory function during prolonged therapy with Fenoprofen Calcium.

INFORMATION FOR THE PATIENT

Fenoprofen Calcium, like other drugs of its class, is not free of side effects. The side effects of these drugs can cause discomfort and, rarely, there are more serious side effects, such as gastrointestinal bleeding, which may result in hospitalization and even fatal outcomes.

NSAIDs (Nonsteroidal Anti-Inflammatory Drugs) are often essential agents in the management of arthritis and have a major role in the treatment of pain, but they also may be commonly employed for conditions which are less serious.

Physicians may wish to discuss with their patients the potential risks(see WARNINGS, PRECAUTIONS, and ADVERSE REACTIONS) and likely benefits of NSAID treatment, particularly when the drugs are used for less serious conditions where treatment without NSAIDs may represent an acceptable alternative to both the patient and physician.

LABORATORY TESTS

In chronic studies in rats, high doses of Fenoprofen Calcium caused elevation of serum transaminase and hepatocellular hypertrophy. In clinical trials, some patients developed elevation of serum transaminase, LDH, and alkaline phosphatase that persisted for some months and usually, but not always, declined despite continuation of the drug. The significance of this is unknown. It is recommended, therefore, that Fenoprofen Calcium be discontinued if any significant liver abnormality occurs.

As with other nonsteroidal anti-inflammatory drugs, borderline elevations in 1 or more liver tests may occur in up to 15% of patients. These abnormalities may progress, may remain essentially unchanged, or may be transient with continued therapy. The SGPT (ALT) test is probably the most sensitive indicator of liver dysfunction. Meaningful (*i.e.,* 3 times the upper

PRECAUTIONS: *(cont'd)*

limit of normal) elevations of SGPT or SGOT (AST) occurred in controlled clinical trials in less than 1% of patients. A patient with symptoms and/or signs suggesting liver dysfunction, or in whom an abnormal liver test has occurred, should be evaluated for evidence of the development of more severe hepatic reactions while using Fenoprofen Calcium.

Severe hepatic reactions, including jaundice and cases of fatal hepatitis, have been reported with Fenoprofen Calcium, as with other nonsteroidal anti-inflammatory drugs. As a result, during long-term therapy, liver function tests should be monitored periodically. Although such reactions are rare, if liver tests continue to be abnormal or worsen, if clinical signs and symptoms consistent with liver disease develop, or if systemic manifestations occur (*e.g.,* eosinophilia and rash), Fenoprofen Calcium should be discontinued. If this drug is to be used in the presence of impaired liver function, it must be done under strict observation.

Patients with initial low hemoglobin values who are receiving long-term therapy with Fenoprofen Calcium should have a hemoglobin determination made at reasonable intervals.

Fenoprofen Calcium decreases platelet aggregation and may prolong bleeding time. Patients who may be adversely affected by prolongation of the bleeding time should be carefully observed when Fenoprofen Calcium is administered.

Because serious GI tract ulceration and bleeding can occur without warning symptoms, physicians should follow chronically treated patients for the signs and symptoms of ulceration and bleeding and should inform them of the importance of this follow-up (see WARNINGS, Risk of GI Ulcerations, Bleeding and Perforation with NSAID Therapy.)

LABORATORY TEST INTERACTIONS

Amerlex-M kit assay values of total and free triiodothyronine in patients receiving Fenoprofen Calcium have been reported as falsely elevated on the basis of a chemical cross-reaction that directly interferes with the assay. Thyroid-stimulating hormone, total thyroxine, and thyrotropin-releasing hormone response are not affected.

USAGE IN PREGNANCY

Safe use of Fenoprofen Calcium during pregnancy and lactation has not been established; therefore, administration to pregnant patients and nursing mothers is not recommended. Reproduction studies have been performed in rats and rabbits. When fenoprofen was given to rats during pregnancy and continued until the time of labor, parturition was prolonged. Similar results have been found with other nonsteroidal anti-inflammatory drugs that inhibit prostaglandin synthetase.

USAGE IN CHILDREN

Fenoprofen Calcium is not recommended for use in children because documented clinical experience has been insufficient to establish safety and a suitable dosage regimen in the pediatric age group.

DRUG INTERACTIONS:

The coadministration of aspirin decreases the biologic half-life of fenoprofen because of an increase in metabolic clearance that results in a greater amount of hydroxylated fenoprofen in the urine. Although the mechanism of interaction between fenoprofen and aspirin is not totally known, enzyme induction and displacement of fenoprofen from plasma albumin binding sites are possibilities. Because Fenoprofen Calcium has not been shown to produce any additional effect beyond that obtained with aspirin alone and because aspirin increases the rate of excretion of Fenoprofen Calcium, the concomitant use of Fenoprofen Calcium and salicylates is not recommended.

Chronic administration of phenobarbital, a known enzyme inducer, may be associated with a decrease in the plasma half-life of fenoprofen. When phenobarbital is added to or withdrawn from treatment, dosage adjustment of Fenoprofen Calcium may be required.

In vitro studies have shown that fenoprofen, because of its affinity for albumin, may displace from their binding sites other drugs that are also albumin bound, and this may lead to drug interaction. Theoretically, fenoprofen could likewise be displaced. Patients receiving hydantoin, sulfonamides, or sulfonylureas should be observed for increased activity of these drugs and, therefore, signs of toxicity from these drugs. In patients receiving coumarin-type anticoagulants, the addition of Fenoprofen Calcium to therapy could prolong the prothrombin time. Patients receiving both drugs should be under careful observation. Patients treated with Fenoprofen Calcium may be resistant to the effects of loop diuretics.

In patients receiving Fenoprofen Calcium and a steroid concomitantly, any reduction in steroid dosage should be gradual in order to avoid the possible complications of sudden steroid withdrawal.

ADVERSE REACTIONS:

During clinical studies for rheumatoid arthritis, osteoarthritis, or mild to moderate pain and studies of pharmacokinetics, complaints were compiled from a checklist of potential adverse reactions, and the following data emerged. These encompass observations in 6,786 patients, including 188 observed for at least 52 weeks. For comparison, data are also presented from complaints received from the 266 patients who received placebo in these same trials. During short-term studies for analgesia, the incidence of adverse reactions was markedly lower than that seen in longer-term studies.

INCIDENCE GREATER THAN 1% - PROBABLE CAUSAL RELATIONSHIP

Digestive System: During clinical trials with Fenoprofen Calcium, the most common adverse reactions were gastrointestinal in nature and occurred in 20.8% of patients receiving Fenoprofen Calcium as compared to 16.9% of patients receiving placebo. In descending order of frequency, these reactions included dyspepsia (10.3%, Fenoprofen Calcium, vs 2.3%, placebo), nausea (7.7% vs 7.1%), constipation (7% vs 1.5%), vomiting (2.6% vs 1.9%), abdominal pain (2% vs 1.1%), and diarrhea (1.8% vs 4.1%).

The drug was discontinued because of adverse gastrointestinal reactions in less than 2% of patients during premarketing studies.

Nervous System: The most frequent adverse neurologic reactions were headache (8.7% treated vs 7.5% placebo) and somnolence (8.5% vs 6.4%). Dizziness (6.5% vs 5.6%), tremor (2.2% vs 0.4%), and confusion (1.4% vs none) were noted less frequently.

Fenoprofen Calcium was discontinued in less than 0.5% of patients because of these side effects during premarketing studies.

Skin and Appendages: Increased sweating (4.6% vs 0.4%), pruritus (4.2% vs 0.8%), and rash (3.7% vs 0.4%) were reported.

Fenoprofen Calcium was discontinued in about 1% of patients because of an adverse effect related to the skin during premarketing studies.

Special Senses: Tinnitus (4.5% vs 0.4%), blurred vision (2.2% vs none), and decreased hearing (1.6% vs none) were reported.

Fenoprofen Calcium was discontinued in less than 0.5% of patients because of adverse effects related to the special senses during premarketing studies.

Cardiovascular: Palpitations (2.5% vs 0.4%).

Fenoprofen Calcium was discontinued in about 0.5% of patients because of adverse cardiovascular reactions during premarketing studies.

ADVERSE REACTIONS: *(cont'd)*

Miscellaneous: Nervousness (5.7% vs 1.5%), asthenia (5.4% vs 0.4%), peripheral edema (5.0% vs 0.4%), dyspnea (2.8% vs none), fatigue (1.7% vs 1.5%), upper respiratory infection (1.5% vs 5.6%), and nasopharyngitis (1.2% vs none).

INCIDENCE LESS THAN 1% - PROBABLE CAUSAL RELATIONSHIP

The following adverse reactions, occurring in less than 1% of patients, were reported in controlled clinical trials and voluntary reports made since Fenoprofen Calcium was initially marketed. The probability of a causal relationship exists between Fenoprofen Calcium and these adverse reactions:

Digestive System: Gastritis, peptic ulcer with/without perforation, gastrointestinal hemorrhage, anorexia, flatulence, dry mouth, and blood in the stool. Increases in alkaline phosphatase, LDH, and SGOT, jaundice, and cholestatic hepatitis were observed (see PRECAUTIONS.)

Genitourinary Tract: Dysuria, cystitis, hematuria, oliguria, azotemia, anuria, interstitial nephritis, nephrosis, and papillary necrosis (see WARNINGS.)

Hypersensitivity: Angioedema (angioneurotic edema).

Hematologic: Purpura, bruising, hemorrhage, thrombocytopenia, hemolytic anemia, aplastic anemia, agranulocytosis, and pancytopenia.

Miscellaneous: Anaphylaxis, urticaria, malaise, insomnia, and tachycardia.

INCIDENCE LESS THAN 1% - CAUSAL RELATIONSHIP UNKNOWN

Other reactions reported either in clinical trials or spontaneously, occurred in circumstances in which a causal relationship could not be established. However, with these rarely reported reactions, the possibility of such a relationship cannot be excluded. Therefore, these observations are listed to alert the physician.

Skin and Appendages: Exfoliative dermatitis, toxic epidermal necrolysis, Stevens-Johnson syndrome, and alopecia.

Digestive System: Aphthous ulcerations of the buccal mucosa, metallic taste, and pancreatitis.

Cardiovascular: Atrial fibrillation, pulmonary edema, electrocardiographic changes, and supraventricular tachycardia.

Nervous System: Depression, disorientation, seizures, and trigeminal neuralgia.

Special Senses: Burning tongue, diplopia, and optic neuritis.

Miscellaneous: Personality change, lymphadenopathy, mastodynia, and fever.

OVERDOSAGE:

SIGNS AND SYMPTOMS

Symptoms of overdose appear within several hours and generally involve the gastrointestinal and central nervous systems. They include dyspepsia, nausea, vomiting, abdominal pain, dizziness, headache, ataxia, tinnitus, tremor, drowsiness, and confusion. Hyperpyrexia, tachycardia, hypotension, and acute renal failure may occur rarely following overdose. Respiratory depression and metabolic acidosis have also been reported following overdose with certain NSAIDs.

TREATMENT

To obtain up-to-date information about the treatment of overdose, a good resource is your certified Regional Poison Control Center. Telephone numbers of certified poison control centers are listed in *Physicians GenRx*. In managing overdosage, consider the possibility of multiple drug overdoses, interaction among drugs, and unusual kinetics in your patient.

Protect the patient's airway and support ventilation and perfusion. Meticulously monitor and maintain, within acceptable limits, the patient's vital signs, blood gases, serum electrolytes, etc. Absorption of drugs from the gastrointestinal tract may be decreased by giving activated charcoal, which, in many cases, is more effective than emesis or lavage; consider charcoal instead of or in addition to gastric emptying. Repeated doses of charcoal over time may hasten elimination of some drugs that have been absorbed. Safeguard the patient's airway when employing gastric emptying or charcoal.

Alkalinization of the urine, forced diuresis, peritoneal dialysis, hemodialysis, and charcoal hemoperfusion do not enhance systemic drug elimination.

DOSAGE AND ADMINISTRATION:

Analgesia: For the treatment of mild to moderate pain, the recommended dosage is 200 mg every 4 to 6 hours, as needed.

Rheumatoid Arthritis and Osteoarthritis: The suggested dosage is 300 to 600 mg, 3 or 4 times a day. The dose should be tailored to the needs of the patient and may be increased or decreased depending on the severity of the symptoms. Dosage adjustments may be made after initiation of drug therapy or during exacerbations of the disease. Total daily dosage should not exceed 3,200 mg.

If gastrointestinal complaints occur, Fenoprofen Calcium may be administered with meals or with milk. Although the total amount absorbed is not affected, peak blood levels are delayed and diminished.

Patients with rheumatoid arthritis generally seem to require larger doses of Fenoprofen Calcium than do those with osteoarthritis. The smallest dose that yields acceptable control should be employed.

Although improvement may be seen in a few days in many patients, an additional 2 to 3 weeks may be required to gauge the full benefits of therapy.

Store at controlled room temperature, 59° to 86°F (15° to 30°C).

HOW SUPPLIED - RATED THERAPEUTICALLY EQUIVALENT:

Capsule, Gelatin - Oral - 200 mg

100's	$23.60	Fenoprofen, Watson Labs	52544-0367-01
100's	$27.42	Fenoprofen, H.C.F.A. F F P	99999-1253-01
100's	$27.70	Fenoprofen Calcium, Elkins Sinn	00641-4504-86
100's	$30.15	Fenoprofen, United Res	00677-1306-01
100's	$30.95	Fenoprofen, Harber Pharm	51432-0818-03
100's	**$48.42**	**NALFON, Dista**	**00777-0876-02**

Capsule, Gelatin - Oral - 300 mg

100's	$33.75	Fenoprofen, Schein Pharm (US)	00364-2315-01
100's	$34.50	Fenoprofen, United Res	00677-1307-01
100's	$34.88	Fenoprofen, Geneva Pharms	00781-2862-01
100's	$35.95	Fenoprofen, Harber Pharm	51432-0820-03
100's	**$38.76**	**NALFON, Dista**	**00777-0877-02**
500's	**$272.12**	**NALFON, Dista**	**00777-0877-03**

Tablet, Uncoated - Oral - 600 mg

100's	$18.98	Fenoprofen, H.C.F.A. F F P	99999-1253-02
100's	$19.20	Fenoprofen, United Res	00677-1308-01
100's	$37.80	Fenoprofen, Watson Labs	52544-0366-01
100's	$39.25	Fenoprofen, Raway	00686-0477-20
100's	$40.16	Fenoprofen, Bristol Myers Squibb	00003-0955-02
100's	$44.45	Fenoprofen Calcium, Elkins Sinn	00641-4012-86
100's	$44.80	Fenoprofen, Qualitest Pharms	00603-3578-21
100's	$44.85	Fenoprofen, Rugby	00536-3813-01

HOW SUPPLIED - RATED THERAPEUTICALLY EQUIVALENT: *(cont'd)*

100's	$45.00	Fenoprofen 600, Zenith Labs	00172-4141-60
100's	$45.00	Fenoprofen, Goldline Labs	00182-1902-01
100's	$45.00	Fenoprofen, Mutual Pharm	53489-0287-01
100's	$45.65	Fenoprofen, Purepac Pharm	00228-2317-10
100's	$45.77	Fenoprofen, Lederle Pharm	00005-3559-43
100's	$45.95	Fenoprofen, Geneva Pharms	00781-1863-01
100's	$46.20	Fenoprofen, Schein Pharm (US)	00364-2316-01
100's	$46.70	NAPROFEN, Major Pharms	00904-3786-60
100's	$46.70	Fenoprofen Calcium, Martec Pharms	52555-0473-01
100's	$47.80	Fenoprofen Calcium, Aligen Independ	00405-4424-01
100's	$48.10	Fenoprofen, Mylan	00378-0471-01
100's	$49.75	Fenoprofen, Harber Pharm	51432-0822-03
100's	$62.80	Fenoprofen, Goldline Labs	00182-1902-89
100's	$63.64	Fenoprofen, Vangard Labs	00615-3507-13
500's	$94.90	Fenoprofen, H.C.F.A. F F P	99999-1253-03
500's	$96.00	Fenoprofen Tablets 600 Mg, Mutual Pharm	53489-0287-05
500's	$172.80	Fenoprofen, Elkins Sinn	00641-4012-88
500's	$183.60	Fenoprofen, Watson Labs	52544-0366-05
500's	$198.53	Fenoprofen, Qualitest Pharms	00603-3578-28
500's	$219.25	Fenoprofen, Purepac Pharm	00228-2317-50
500's	$220.80	Fenoprofen 600, Zenith Labs	00172-4141-70
500's	$220.80	Fenoprofen, Goldline Labs	00182-1902-05
500's	$220.88	Fenoprofen, Geneva Pharms	00781-1863-05
500's	$221.70	Fenoprofen, Rugby	00536-3813-05
500's	$221.97	Fenoprofen Calcium, Aligen Independ	00405-4424-02
500's	$222.34	Fenoprofen, Lederle Pharm	00005-3559-31
500's	$226.80	NAPROFEN, Major Pharms	00904-3786-40
500's	$229.75	Fenoprofen, Mylan	00378-0471-05
500's	$248.75	Fenoprofen, Harber Pharm	51432-0822-05
1000's	$189.80	Fenoprofen, H.C.F.A. F F P	99999-1253-04
1000's	$438.50	Fenoprofen, Purepac Pharm	00228-2317-96

FENTANYL *(003010)*

CATEGORIES: Anesthesia; Antipyretics; Central Nervous System Agents; Opiate Agonists (Controlled); Pain; Sedatives; Pregnancy Category C; DEA Class CII; FDA Class 2B ("Modest Therapeutic Advantage"); FDA Approved 1990 Aug

BRAND NAMES: **Duragesic**; *Durogesic* (Mexico); *Fentanest* (Mexico)
(International brand names outside U.S. in italics)

FORMULARIES: Aetna; BC-BS; Medi-Cal; PCS

WARNING:
BECAUSE SERIOUS OR LIFE-THREATENING HYPOVENTILATION COULD OCCUR, DURAGESIC IS CONTRAINDICATED in the management of acute or post-operative pain, including use in out-patient surgeries
In the management of mild or intermittent pain responsive to PRN or non-opioid therapy
In doses exceeding 25 mcg/hour at the initiation of opioid therapy
(See CONTRAINDICATIONS for further information).
DURAGESIC SHOULD NOT BE ADMINISTERED TO CHILDREN UNDER 12 YEARS OF AGE OR PATIENTS UNDER 18 YEARS OF AGE WHO WEIGH LESS THAN 50 KG (110 LBS) EXCEPT IN AN AUTHORIZED INVESTIGATIONAL RESEARCH SETTING. (SEEPediatric Use.)
Duragesic is indicated for chronic pain (such as that of malignancy) that:
cannot be managed by lesser means such as acetaminophen-opioid combinations, non-steroidal analgesics, or PRN dosing with short- acting opioids and
requires continuous opioid administration.
The 50, 75, and 100 mcg/hour dosages should ONLY be used in patients who are already on and are tolerant to opioid therapy.

DESCRIPTION:

Warning: May be habit forming.

Duragesic is a transdermal system providing continuous systemic delivery of fentanyl, a potent opioid analgesic, for 72 hours. The chemical name is N-phenyl- N -(1-2-phenylethyl-4-piperidyl) propanamide.

The molecular weight of fentanyl base is 336.5, and the empirical formula is $C_{22}H_{28}N_2O$. The n-octanol:water partition coefficient is 860:1. The pKa is 8.4.

System Components and Structure: The amount of fentanyl released from each system per hour is proportional to the surface area (25 mcg/h per 10 cm^2). The composition per unit area of all system sizes is identical. Each system also contains 0.1 ml of alcohol USP per 10 cm^2 (TABLE 1):

TABLE 1

Dose* (mcg/h)	Size (cm^2)	Fentanyl Content (mg)
25	10	2.5
50**	20	5
75**	30	7.5
100**	40	10

* Nominal delivery rate per hour
** FOR USE ONLY IN OPIOID TOLERANT PATIENTS

Duragesic is a rectangular transparent unit comprising a protective liner and four functional layers. Proceeding from the outer surface toward the surface adhering to skin, these layers are:

(1) a backing layer of polyester film;

(2) a drug reservoir of fentanyl and alcohol USP gelled with hydroxyethyl cellulose;

(3) an ethylene-vinyl acetate copolymer membrane that controls the rate of fentanyl delivery to the skin surface; and

(4) a fentanyl containing silicone adhesive.

Before use, a protective liner covering the adhesive layer is removed and discarded.

The active component of the system is fentanyl. The remaining components are pharmacologically inactive. Less than 0.2 ml of alcohol is also released from the system during use.

DESCRIPTION: *(cont'd)*

Do not cut or damage Duragesic. If the Duragesic system is cut or damaged, controlled drug delivery will not be possible.

CLINICAL PHARMACOLOGY:

PHARMACOLOGY

Fentanyl is an opioid analgesic. Fentanyl interacts predominately with the opioid μ-receptor. These μ-binding sites are discretely distributed in the human brain, spinal cord, and other tissues.

In clinical settings, fentanyl exerts its principal pharmacologic effects on the central nervous system. Its primary actions of therapeutic value are analgesia and sedation. Fentanyl may increase the patient's tolerance for pain and decrease the perception of suffering, although the presence of the pain itself may still be recognized.

In addition to analgesia, alterations in mood, euphoria and dysphoria, and drowsiness commonly occur. Fentanyl depresses the respiratory centers, depresses the cough reflex, and constricts the pupils. Analgesic blood levels of fentanyl may cause nausea and vomiting directly by stimulating the chemoreceptor trigger zone, but nausea and vomiting are significantly more common in ambulatory than in recumbent patients, as is postural syncope.

Opioids increase the tone and decrease the propulsive contractions of the smooth muscle of the gastrointestinal tract. The resultant prolongation in gastrointestinal transit time may be responsible for the constipating effect of fentanyl. Because opioids may increase biliary tract pressure, some patients with biliary colic may experience worsening rather than relief of pain.

While opioids generally increase the tone of urinary tract smooth muscle, the net effect tends to be variable, in some cases producing urinary urgency, in others, difficulty in urination.

At therapeutic dosages, fentanyl usually does not exert major effects on the cardiovascular system. However, some patients may exhibit orthostatic hypotension and fainting.

Histamine assays and skin wheal testing in man indicate that clinically significant histamine release rarely occurs with fentanyl administration. Assays in man show no clinically significant histamine release in dosages up to 50 mcg/kg.

PHARMACOKINETICS

(See TABLE 2.) Duragesic releases fentanyl from the reservoir at a nearly constant amount per unit time. The concentration gradient existing between the saturated solution of drug in the reservoir and the lower concentration in the skin drives drug release. Fentanyl moves in the direction of the lower concentration at a rate determined by the copolymer release membrane and the diffusion of fentanyl through the skin layers. While the actual rate of fentanyl delivery to the skin varies over the 72 hour application period, each system is labeled with a nominal flux which represents the average amount of drug delivered to the systemic circulation per hour across average skin.

While there is variation in dose delivered among patients, the nominal flux of the systems (25, 50, 75, and 100 mcg of fentanyl per hour) are sufficiently accurate as to allow individual titration of dosage for a given patient. The small amount of alcohol which has been incorporated into the system enhances the rate of drug flux through the rate-limiting copolymer membrane and increases the permeability of the skin to fentanyl.

Following initial Duragesic application, the skin under the system absorbs fentanyl, and a depot of fentanyl concentrates in the upper skin layers. Fentanyl then becomes available to the systemic circulation. Serum fentanyl concentrations increase gradually following initial Duragesic application, generally leveling off between 12 and 24 hours and remaining relatively constant, with some fluctuation, for the remainder of the 72 hour application period. Peak serum levels of fentanyl generally occurred between 24 and 72 hours after a single application. Serum fentanyl concentrations achieved are proportional to the Duragesic delivery rate. With continuous use, serum fentanyl concentrations continue to rise for the first few system applications. After several sequential 72-hour applications, patients reach and maintain a steady state serum concentration that is determined by individual variation in skin permeability and body clearance of fentanyl (see TABLE 2).

After system removal, serum fentanyl concentrations decline gradually, falling about 50% in approximately 17 (range 13-22) hours. Continued absorption of fentanyl from the skin accounts for a slower disappearance of the drug from the serum than is seen after an IV infusion, where the apparent half-life ranges from 3-12 hours (TABLE 2):

TABLE 2 Range Of Pharmacokinetic Parameters Of Fentanyl In Patients

	Clearance Concen. (L/h) Range (70 kg)	Volume of Dist. V_{ss} (L/kg) Range	Half Life $t_{1/2}$(h) Range	Maximal Concen. C_{max} (ng/ml) Range	Time to Maximal (h) Range
IV Fentanyl Surgical Patients	27 - 75	3 - 8	3 - 12		
Hepatically Renally Impaired Patients	30 - 78				
Duragesic 25 mcg/h			*	0.3 - 1.2	26 - 78
Duragesic 50 mcg/h			*	0.6 - 1.8+	24 - 72+
Duragesic 75 mcg/h			*	1.1 - 2.6	24 - 48
Duragesic 100 mcg kg/h			*	1.9 - 3.8	25 - 72

+ Estimated
* After system removal there is continued systemic absorption from residual fentanyl in the skin so that serum concentrations fall 50%, on average, in 17 hours.

Fentanyl plasma protein binding capacity decreases with increasing ionization of the drug. Alterations in pH may affect its distribution between plasma and the central nervous system. Fentanyl accumulates in the skeletal muscle and fat and is released slowly into the blood.

The average volume of distribution for fentanyl is 6 L/kg (range 3-8, N=8). The average clearance in patients undergoing various surgical procedures is 46 L/h (range 27-75, N=8). The kinetics of fentanyl in geriatric patients has not been well studied, but in geriatric patients the clearance of IV fentanyl may be reduced and the terminal half-life greatly prolonged (see PRECAUTIONS).

Fentanyl is metabolized primarily in the liver. In humans, the drug appears to be metabolized primarily by N-dealkylation to norfentanyl and other inactive metabolites that do not contribute materially to the observed activity of the drug. Within 72 hours of IV fentanyl administration, approximately 75% of the dose is excreted in urine, mostly as metabolites with less than 10% representing unchanged drug. Approximately 9% of the dose is recovered in the feces, primarily as metabolites. Mean values for unbound fractions of fentanyl in plasma are estimated to be between 13 and 21%.

CLINICAL PHARMACOLOGY: *(cont'd)*

Skin does not appear to metabolize fentanyl delivered transdermally. This was determined in a human keratinocyte cell assay and in clinical studies in which 92% of the dose delivered from the system was accounted for as unchanged fentanyl that appeared in the systemic circulation.

PHARMACODYNAMICS ANALGESIA

Duragesic is a strong opioid analgesic. In controlled clinical trials in non-opioid tolerant patients, 60 mg/day IM morphine was considered to provide analgesia approximately equivalent to Duragesic 100 mcg/h in an acute pain model.

Minimum effective analgesic serum concentrations of fentanyl in opioid naive patients range from 0.2 to 1.2 ng/ml; side effects increase in frequency at serum levels above 2 ng/ml. Both the minimum effective concentration and the concentration at which toxicity occurs rise with increasing tolerance. The rate of development of tolerance varies widely among individuals.

Ventilatory Effects: At equivalent analgesic serum concentrations, fentanyl and morphine produce a similar degree of hypoventilation. A small number of patients have experienced clinically significant hypoventilation with Duragesic. Hypoventilation was manifest by respiratory rates of less than 8 breaths/minute or a pCO_2 greater than 55 mm Hg. In clinical trials of 357 postoperative (acute pain) treated with Duragesic, 13 patients experienced hypoventilation. As a consequence, 10 of these 13 patients received naloxone, two patients had their dose reduced and one patient required no treatment beyond verbal stimulation. Of the 13 events, seven were associated with Duragesic 100 mcg/h and six were associated with Duragesic 75 mcg/h. In these studies the incidence of hypoventilation was higher in nontolerant women (10) than in men (3) and in patients weighing less than 63 kg (9 of 13). Although patients with impaired respiration were not common in the trials, they had higher rates of hypoventilation.

While most patients using Duragesic chronically develop tolerance to fentanyl induced hypoventilation, episodes of slowed respirations may occur at any time during therapy; medical intervention generally was not required in these instances.

Hypoventilation can occur throughout the therapeutic range of fentanyl serum concentrations. However, the risk of hypoventilation increases at serum fentanyl concentrations greater than 2 ng/ml in non opioid-tolerant patients, especially for patients who have an underlying pulmonary condition or who receive usual doses of opioids or other CNS drugs associated with hypoventilation in addition to Duragesic. The use of Duragesic should be monitored by clinical evaluation. As with other drug level measurements, serum fentanyl concentrations may be useful clinically, although they do not reflect patient sensitivity to fentanyl and should not be used by physicians as a sole indicator of effectiveness or toxicity.

See BOXED WARNING, CONTRAINDICATIONS, WARNINGS, PRECAUTIONS, ADVERSE REACTIONS and OVERDOSAGE for additional information on hypoventilation.

Cardiovascular Effects: Intravenous fentanyl may infrequently produce bradycardia. The incidence of bradycardia in clinical trials with Duragesic was less than 1%.

CNS Effects: In opioid naive patients, central nervous system effects increase when serum fentanyl concentrations are greater than 3 ng/ml.

CLINICAL STUDIES:

Duragesic was studied in patients with acute and chronic pain (postoperative and cancer pain models).

The analgesic efficacy of Duragesic was demonstrated in an acute pain model with surgical procedures expected to produce various intensities of pain (*e.g.*, hysterectomy, major orthopedic surgery). Clinical use and safety was evaluated in patients experiencing chronic pain due to malignancy. Based on the results of these trials, Duragesic was determined to be effective in both populations, but safe only for use in patients with chronic back pain. Because of the risk of hypoventilation (4% incidence) in postoperative patients with acute pain, Duragesic should not be used for postoperative analgesia (see BOXED WARNING and CONTRAINDICATIONS).

Duragesic as therapy for pain due to cancer has been studied in 153 patients. In this patient population, Duragesic has been administered in doses of 25 mcg/h to 600 mcg/h. Individual patients have used Duragesic continuously for up to 866 days. At one month after initiation of Duragesic therapy, patients generally reported lower pain intensity scores as compared to a prestudy analgesic regimen of oral morphine.

INDICATIONS AND USAGE:

Duragesic is indicated in the management of chronic pain in patients who require continuous opioid analgesia for pain that cannot be managed by lesser means such as acetaminophen-opioid combinations, non-steroidal analgesics, or PRN dosing with short-acting opioids.

Duragesic should not be used in the management of acute or postoperative pain because serious or life-threatening hypoventilation could result. (See BOXED WARNING and CONTRAINDICATIONS.)

In patients with chronic pain, it is possible to individually titrate the dose of the transdermal system to minimize the risk of adverse effects while providing analgesia. In properly selected patients, Duragesic is a safe and effective alternative to other opioid regimens (see DOSAGE AND ADMINISTRATION).

CONTRAINDICATIONS:

Because serious or life-threatening hypoventilation could occur, Duragesic is contraindicated:

In the management of acute or post-operative pain, including use in out-patient surgeries because there is no opportunity for proper dose titration (See CLINICAL PHARMACOLOGY and DOSAGE AND ADMINISTRATION).

In the management of mild or intermittent pain that can otherwise be managed by lesser means such as acetaminophen-opioid combinations, non-steroidal analgesics, or PRN dosing with short-acting opioids,

In doses exceeding 25 mcg/hour at the initiation of opioid therapy because of the need to individualize dosing by titrating to the desired analgesic effect.

Duragesic is also contraindicated in patients with known hypersensitivity to fentanyl or adhesives.

WARNINGS:

DURAGESIC SHOULD NOT BE ADMINISTERED TO CHILDREN UNDER 12 YEARS OF AGE OR PATIENTS UNDER 18 YEARS OF AGE WHO WEIGH LESS THAN 50 KG (110 LBS) EXCEPT IN AN AUTHORIZED INVESTIGATIONAL RESEARCH SETTING. (SEEPediatric Use.)

PATIENTS WHO HAVE EXPERIENCED ADVERSE EVENTS SHOULD BE MONITORED FOR AT LEAST 12 HOURS AFTER DURAGESIC REMOVAL SINCE SERUM FENTANYL CONCENTRATIONS DECLINE GRADUALLY AND REACH AN APPROXIMATE 50% REDUCTION IN SERUM CONCENTRATIONS 17 HOURS AFTER SYSTEM REMOVAL.

DURAGESIC SHOULD BE PRESCRIBED ONLY BY PERSONS KNOWLEDGEABLE IN THE CONTINUOUS ADMINISTRATION OF POTENT OPIOIDS, IN THE MANAGEMENT OF PATIENTS RECEIVING POTENT OPIOIDS FOR TREATMENT OF PAIN,

WARNINGS: *(cont'd)*

AND IN THE DETECTION AND MANAGEMENT OF HYPOVENTILATION INCLUDING THE USE OF OPIOID THE CONCOMITANT USE OF OTHER CENTRAL NERVOUS SYSTEM DEPRESSANTS, INCLUDING OTHER OPIOIDS, SEDATIVES OR HYPNOTICS, GENERAL ANESTHETICS, PHENOTHIAZINES, TRANQUILIZERS, SKELETAL MUSCLE RELAXANTS, SEDATING ANTIHISTAMINES, AND ALCOHOL BEVERAGES MAY PRODUCE ADDITIVE DEPRESSANT EFFECTS. HYPOVENTILATION, HYPOTENSION AND PROFOUND SEDATION OR COMA MAY OCCUR. WHEN SUCH COMBINED THERAPY IS CONTEMPLATED, THE DOSE OF ONE OR BOTH AGENTS SHOULD BE REDUCED AT LEAST BY 50%.

ALL PATIENTS SHOULD BE ADVISED TO AVOID EXPOSING THE DURAGESIC APPLICATION SITE TO DIRECT EXTERNAL HEAT SOURCES, SUCH AS HEATING PADS OR ELECTRIC BLANKETS, HEAT LAMPS, SAUNAS, HOT TUBS, AND HEATED WATER BEDS, ETC. WHILE WEARING THE SYSTEM. THERE IS A POTENTIAL FOR TEMPERATURE- DEPENDENT INCREASES IN FENTANYL RELEASE FROM THE SYSTEM. (See PRECAUTIONS, PATIENTS WITH FEVER, EXTERNAL HEAT.)

PRECAUTIONS:

GENERAL

Duragesic doses greater than 25 mcg/h are too high for initiation of therapy in non opioid-tolerant patients and should not be used to begin Duragesic therapy in these patients. (See BOXED WARNING.)

Duragesic may impair mental and/or physical ability required for the performance of potentially hazardous tasks (*e.g.*, driving, operating machinery). Patients who have been given Duragesic should not drive or operate dangerous machinery unless they are tolerant to the side effects of the drug.

Patients should be instructed to keep both used and unused systems out of the reach of children. Used systems should be folded so that the adhesive side of the system adheres to itself and flushed down the toilet immediately upon removal. Patients should be advised to dispose of any system remaining from a prescription as soon as they are no longer needed. Unused systems should be removed from their pouch and flushed down the toilet.

Hypoventilation (Respiratory Depression): Hypoventilation may occur at any time during the use of Duragesic.

Because significant amounts of fentanyl are absorbed from the skin for 17 hours or more after the system is removed, hypoventilation may persist beyond the removal of Duragesic. Consequently, patients with hypoventilation should be carefully observed for degree of sedation and their respiratory rate monitored until respiration has stabilized.

The use of concomitant CNS active drugs requires special patient care and observation. See WARNINGS.

Chronic Pulmonary Disease: Because potent opioids can cause hypoventilation, Duragesic (fentanyl transdermal system) should be administered with caution to patients with preexisting medical conditions predisposing them to hypoventilation. In such patients, normal analgesic doses of opioids may further decrease respiratory drive to the point of respiratory failure.

Head Injuries and Increased Intracranial Pressure: Duragesic should not be used in patients who may be particularly susceptible to the intracranial effects of CO_2 retention such as those with evidence of increased intracranial pressure, impaired consciousness, or coma. Opioids may obscure the clinical course of patients with head injury. Duragesic should be used with caution in patients with brain tumors.

Cardiac Disease: Intravenous fentanyl may produce bradycardia. Fentanyl should be administered with caution to patients with bradyarrhythmias.

Hepatic or Renal Disease: At the present time insufficient information exists to make recommendations regarding the use of Duragesic in patients with impaired renal or hepatic function. If the drug is used in these patients, it should be used with caution because of the hepatic metabolism and renal excretion of fentanyl.

Patients with Fever/External Heat: Based on a pharmacokinetic model, serum fentanyl concentrations could theoretically increase by approximately one third for patients with a body temperature of 40°C (102°F) due to temperature-dependent increases in fentanyl release from the system and increased skin permeability. Therefore, patients wearing Duragesic systems who develop fever should be monitored for opioid side effects and the Duragesic dose should be adjusted if necessary.

ALL PATIENTS SHOULD BE ADVISED TO AVOID EXPOSING THE DURAGESIC APPLICATION SITE TO DIRECT EXTERNAL HEAT SOURCES, SUCH AS HEATING PADS OR ELECTRICAL BLANKETS, HEAT LAMPS, SAUNAS, HOT TUBS AND HEATED WATER BEDS, ETC. WHILE WEARING THE SYSTEM. THERE IS A POTENTIAL FOR TEMPERATURE- DEPENDENT INCREASES IN FENTANYL RELEASE FROM THE SYSTEM.

Central Nervous System Depressants: When patients are receiving Duragesic, the dose of additional opioids or other CNS depressant drugs including benzodiazepines) should be reduced at least by 50%. With the concomitant use of CNS depressants, hypotension may occur.

Drug or Alcohol Dependence: Use of fentanyl in combination with alcoholic beverages and/or other CNS depressants can result in increased risk to the patient. Fentanyl should be used with caution in individuals who have a history of drug or alcohol abuse, especially if they are outside a medically controlled environment.

Ambulatory Patients: Strong opioid analgesics impair the mental or physical abilities required for the performance of potentially dangerous tasks such as driving a car or operating machinery. Patients who have been given fentanyl should not drive or operate dangerous machinery unless they are tolerant to the effects of the drug.

CARCINOGENESIS, MUTAGENESIS, AND IMPAIRMENT OF FERTILITY

Because long-term animal studies have not been conducted, the potential carcinogenic effects of fentanyl are unknown. There was no evidence of mutagenicity in the Ames Salmonella mutagenicity assay, the primary rat hepatocyte unscheduled DNA synthesis assay, the BALB/c-3T3 transformation test, and the human lymphocyte and CHO chromosomal aberration *in vitro* assays.

In the mouse lymphoma assay, fentanyl concentrations 2000 times greater than those seen with chronic fentanyl use were only mutagenic in the presence of metabolic activation.

PREGNANCY CATEGORY C

Fentanyl has been shown to impair fertility and to have an embryocidal effect in rats when given in intravenous doses 0.3 times the human dose for a period of 12 days. No evidence of teratogenic effects has been observed after administration of fentanyl to rats. There are no adequate and well-controlled studies in pregnant women. Fentanyl should be used during pregnancy only if the potential benefit justifies the potential risk to the fetus.

LABOR AND DELIVERY

Fentanyl is not recommended for analgesia during labor and delivery.

NURSING MOTHERS

Fentanyl is excreted in human milk; therefore fentanyl is not recommended for use in nursing women because of the possibility of effects in their infants.

PRECAUTIONS: *(cont'd)*

PEDIATRIC USE

The safety and efficacy of fentanyl in children has not been established. (See BOXED WARNING and CONTRAINDICATIONS.)

FENTANTL SHOULD NOT BE ADMINISTERED TO CHILDREN UNDER 12 YEARS OF AGE OR PATIENTS UNDER 18 YEARS OF AGE WHO WEIGH LESS THAN 50 KG (110 LBS) EXCEPT IN AN AUTHORIZED INVESTIGATIONAL RESEARCH SETTING.

GERIATRIC USE

Information from a pilot study of the pharmacokinetics of IV fentanyl in geriatric patients indicates that the clearance of fentanyl may be greatly decreased in the population above the age of 60. The relevance of these findings to transdermal fentanyl is unknown at this time.

Since elderly, cachectic, or debilitated patients may have altered pharmacokinetics due to poor fat stores, muscle wasting, or altered clearance, they should not be started on fentanyl doses higher than 25 mcg/h unless they are already taking more than 135 mg of oral morphine a day or an equivalent dose of another opioid (see DOSAGE AND ADMINISTRATION).

INFORMATION FOR THE PATIENT

Instructions for the application, removal, and disposal of fentanyl are provided in each carton.

Disposal of Fentanyl: Fentanyl should be kept out of the reach of children. Fentanyl systems should be folded so that the adhesive side of the system adheres to itself, then the system should be flushed down the toilet immediately upon removal. Patients should dispose of any systems remaining from a prescription as soon as they are no longer needed. Unused systems should be removed from their pouch and flushed down the toilet.

If the gel from the drug reservoir accidentally contacts the skin, the area should be washed with clear water.

ADVERSE REACTIONS:

In post-marketing experience, deaths from hypoventilation due to inappropriate use of fentanyl have been reported. (See BOXED WARNING and CONTRAINDICATIONS.)

Post-marketing Clinical Trial Experience: The safety of fentanyl has been evaluated in 357 postoperative patients and 153 cancer patients for a total of 510 patients. Patients with acute pain used fentanyl for 1 to 3 days. The duration of fentanyl use varied in cancer patients; 56% of patients used fentanyl for over 30 days, 28% continued treatment for more than 4 months, and 10% used fentanyl for more than 1 year.

Hypoventilation was the most serious adverse reaction observed in 13 (4%) postoperative patients and in 3 (2%) of the cancer patients. Hypotension and hypertension were observed in 11 (3%) and 4 (1%) of the opioid-naive patients.

Various adverse events were reported; a causal relationship to fentanyl was not always determined. The frequencies presented here reflect the actual frequency of each adverse effect in patients who received fentanyl. There has been no attempt to correct for a placebo effect, concomitant use of other opioids, or to subtract the frequencies reported by placebo-treated patients in controlled trials.

The following adverse reactions were reported in 153 cancer patients at a frequency of 1% or greater; similar reactions were seen in the 357 postoperative patients studied.

Body as a Whole: abdominal pain*, headache*

Cardiovascular: arrhythmia, chest pain

Digestive: nausea**, vomiting**, constipation**, dry mouth**, anorexia*, diarrhea*, dyspepsia*, flatulence

Nervous: somnolence**, confusion**, asthenia**, dizziness*, nervousness*, hallucinations*, anxiety*, depression*, euphoria*, tremor, abnormal coordination, speech disorder, abnormal thinking, abnormal gait, abnormal dreams, agitation, paresthesia, amnesia, syncope, paranoid reaction

Respiratory: dyspnea*, hypoventilation*, hemoptysis, pharyngitis, hiccups

Skin and Appendages: sweating**, pruritus*, rash, application site reaction - erythema, papules, itching, edema

Urogenital: urinary retention*

* Reactions occurring in 3% - 10% of fentanyl patients

** Reactions occurring in 10% or more of fentanyl patients

The following adverse effects have been reported in less than 1% of the 510 postoperative and cancer patients studied; the association between these events and fentanyl administration is unknown. This information is listed to serve as alerting information for the physician.

Digestive: abdominal distention

Nervous: aphasia, hypertonia, vertigo, stupor, hypotonia, depersonalization, hostility

Respiratory: stertorous breathing, asthma, respiratory disorder

Skin and Appendages, General: exfoliative dermatitis, pustules

Special Senses: amblyopia

Urogenital: bladder pain, oliguria, urinary frequency

DRUG ABUSE AND DEPENDENCE:

Fentanyl is a Schedule II controlled substance and can produce drug dependence similar to that produced by morphine. Fentanyl therefore has the potential for abuse. Tolerance, physical and psychological dependence may develop upon repeated administration of opioids. Iatrogenic addiction following opioid administration is relatively rare. Physicians should not let concerns of physical dependence deter them from using adequate amounts of opioids in the management of severe pain when such use is indicated.

OVERDOSAGE:

CLINICAL PRESENTATION

The manifestations of fentanyl overdosage are an extension of its pharmacologic actions with the most serious significant effect being hypoventilation.

TREATMENT

For the management of hypoventilation immediate countermeasures include removing the fentanyl system and physically or verbally stimulating the patient. These actions can be followed by administration of a specific narcotic antagonist such as naloxone. The duration of hypoventilation following an overdose may be longer than the effects of the narcotic antagonist's action (the half-life of naloxone ranges from 30 to 81 minutes). The interval between IV antagonist doses should be carefully chosen because of the possibility of re-narcotization after system removal; repeated administration of naloxone may be necessary. Reversal of the narcotic effect may result in acute onset of pain and the release of catecholamines.

OVERDOSAGE: *(cont'd)*

If the clinical situation warrants, ensure a patent airway is established and maintained, administer oxygen and assist or control respiration as indicated and use an oropharyngeal airway or endotracheal tube if necessary. Adequate body temperature and fluid intake should be maintained.

If severe or persistent hypotension occurs, the possibility of hypovolemia should be considered and managed with appropriate parenteral fluid therapy.

DOSAGE AND ADMINISTRATION:

With all opioids, the safety of patients using the products is dependent on health care practitioners prescribing them in strict conformity with their approved labeling with respect to patient selection, dosing, and proper conditions for use.

As with all opioids, dosage should be individualized. The most important factor to be considered in determining the appropriate dose is the extent of preexisting opioid tolerance. (See BOXED WARNING and CONTRAINDICATIONS.) Initial doses should be reduced in elderly or debilitated patients (see PRECAUTIONS.)

Fentanyl should be applied to non-irritated and non-irradiated skin on a flat surface such as chest, back, flank or upper arm. Hair at the application site should be clipped (not shaved) prior to system application. If the site of fentanyl application must be cleansed prior to application of the system, do so with clear water. Do not use soaps, oils, lotions, alcohol, or any other agents that might irritate the skin or alter its characteristics. Allow the skin to dry completely prior to system application.

Fentanyl should be applied immediately upon removal from the sealed package. Do not alter the system, e.g., cut, in any way prior to application.

The transdermal system should be pressed firmly in place with the palm of the hand for 30 seconds, making sure the contact is complete, especially around the edges.

Each fentanyl may be worn continuously for 72 hours. If analgesia for more than 72 hours is required, a new system should be applied to a different skin site after removal of the previous transdermal system.

Fentanyl should be kept out of the reach of children. Used systems should be folded so that the adhesive side of the system adheres to itself, then the system should be flushed down the toilet immediately upon removal. Patients should dispose of any systems remaining from a prescription as soon as they are no longer needed. Unused systems should be removed from their pouch and flushed down the toilet.

Dose Selection: DOSES MUST BE INDIVIDUALIZED BASED UPON THE STATUS OF EACH PATIENT AND SHOULD BE ASSESSED AT REGULAR INTERVALS AFTER FENTANYL APPLICATION. REDUCED DOSES OF FENTANYL ARE SUGGESTED FOR THE ELDERLY AND OTHER GROUPS DISCUSSED IN PRECAUTIONS.

FENTANYL DOSES GREATER THAM 25 MCG/H SHOULD NOT BE USED FOR INITIATION OF FENTANYL THERAPY IN NON-OPIOID TOLERANT PATIENTS.

In selecting an initial fentanyl dose, attention should be given to 1) the daily dose, potency, and characteristics of the opioid the patient has been taking previously (*e.g.,* whether it is a pure agonist or mixed agonist-antagonist), 2) the reliability of the relative potency estimates used to calculate the fentanyl dose needed (potency estimates may vary with the route of administration), 3) the degree of opioid tolerance, if any, and 4) the general condition and medical status of the patient. Each patient should be maintained at the lowest dose providing acceptable pain control.

Initial Fentanyl Dose Selection: There has been no systematic evaluation of fentanyl as an initial opioid analgesic in the management of chronic pain, since most patients in the clinical trials were converted to fentanyl from other narcotics. Therefore, unless the patient has preexisting opioid tolerance, the lowest fentanyl dose, 25 mcg/h, should be used as the initial dose.

To convert patients from oral or parenteral opioids to fentanyl use the following methodology:

1. Calculate the previous 24-hour analgesic requirement.

2. Convert this amount to the equianalgesic oral morphine dose using TABLE 3.

3. TABLE 4 displays the range of 24-hour oral and IM morphine doses that are approximately equivalent to each fentanyl dose. Use this table to find the calculated 24-hour morphine dose and the corresponding fentanyl dose. Initiate fentanyl treatment using the recommended dose and titrate patients upwards (no more frequently than every 3 days after the initial dose or than every 6 days thereafter) until analgesic efficacy is attained. For delivery rates in excess of 100 mcg/h, multiple systems may be used.

TABLE 3 Equianalgesic Potency Conversion

Name	Equianalgesic Dose (mg) IM[a]	PO
morphine	10	60 (30)[b]
Hydromorphone (Dilaudid)	1.5	7.5
methadone (Dolophine)	10	20
oxycodone (Percocet)	15	30
levorphanol (Levo-Dromoran)	2	4
oxymorphone (Numorphan)	1	10 (PR)
heroin	5	60
meperidine (Demerol)	75	—
codeine	130	200

[a]Based on single-dose studies in which an intramuscular dose of each drug listed was compared with morphine to establish the relative potency. Oral doses are those recommended when changing from parenteral to an oral route.
[b]The conversion ratio of 10 mg parenteral morphine = 30 mg oral morphine is based on clinical experience in patients with chronic pain.
Note: All IM and PO doses in this chart are considered equivalent to 10 mg of IM morphine in analgesic effect. IM denotes intramuscular, PO Oral, and PR rectal.

Note: In clinical trials these ranges of daily oral morphine doses were used as a basis for conversion to fentanyl.

Although controlled studies are not available, in clinical practice it is customary to consider the doses of opioid given IM, IV or subcutaneously to be equivalent. There may be some differences in pharmacokinetic parameters such as C_{max} and T_{max}.

The majority of patients are adequately maintained with fentanyl administered every 72 hours. A small number of patients may not achieve adequate analgesia using this dosing interval and may require systems to be applied every 48 hours rather than every 72 hours. An increase in the fentanyl dose should be evaluated before changing dosing intervals in order to maintain patients on a 72-hour regimen.

DOSAGE AND ADMINISTRATION: *(cont'd)*

TABLE 4 Fentanyl Dose Prescription Based Upon Daily Oral Morphine Dose

Oral 24-hour Morphine (mg/day)	Duragesic Dose (mcg/hr)
45-134	25
135-224	50
225-314	75
315-404	100
405-494	125
495-584	150
585-674	175
675-764	200
765-854	225
855-944	250
945-1034	275
1035-1124	300

Because of the increase in serum fentanyl concentration over the first 24 hours following initial system application, the initial evaluation of the maximum analgesic effect of fentanyl cannot be made before 24 hours of wearing. The initial fentanyl dosage may be increased after 3 days (see Dose Titration.)

During the initial application of fentanyl, patients should use short-acting analgesics for the first 24 hours as needed until analgesic efficacy with fentanyl is attained. Thereafter, some patients still may require periodic supplemental doses of other short-acting analgesics for 'breakthrough' pain.

Dose Titration: The conversion ratio from oral morphine to fentanyl is conservative, and 50% of patients are likely to require a dose increase after initial application of fentanyl. The initial fentanyl dosage may be increased after 3 days, based on the daily dose of supplemental analgesics required by the patient in the second or third day of the initial application.

Physicians are advised that it may take up to 6 days after increasing the dose of fentanyl for the patient to reach equilibrium on the new dose. Therefore, patients should wear a higher dose through two applications before any further increase in dosage is made on the basis of the average daily use of a supplemental analgesic.

Appropriate dosage increments should be based on the daily dose of supplementary opioids, using the ratio of 90 mg/24 hours of oral morphine to a 25 mcg/h increase in fentanyl dose.

Discontinuation of Fentanyl: To convert patients to another opioid, remove fentanyl and titrate the dose of the new analgesic until adequate analgesia has been attained. Upon system removal, 17 hours or more are required for a 50% decrease in serum fentanyl concentrations. For patients requiring discontinuation of opioids, a gradual downward titration is recommended since it is not known at what dose level the opioid may be discontinued without producing the signs and symptoms of abrupt withdrawal.

REFERENCES:

a Foley, K.M. (1985) The treatment of cancer pain. NEJM 313(2):84-95. **b** Ashburn and Lipman (1993) Management of pain in the cancer patient. Anesth Analg 76: 402-416.

PATIENT PACKAGE INSERT:

PLEASE READ THIS SECTION CAREFULLY BEFORE YOU USE FENTANYL.

This leaflet gives a summary of information about fentanyl and will provide you with specific information about how to use fentanyl. If you have any questions or want more information, be sure to discuss your question with your doctor or other health professional. You could ask them for a copy of the information on this product written for health professionals if you wish.

What is Duragesic? Duragesic is a thin, adhesive, rectangular patch that is worn on your skin. Duragesic delivers a strong pain- relieving medicine called "fentanyl" through the skin and into the bloodstream. It should only be used to relieve severe pain that will last more than a few days (chronic pain). It should only be used when other less strong medicines have not been effective and when pain needs to be controlled around the clock.

Fentanyl is NOT INTENDED FOR USE if you have pain that will go away in a few days, such as pain from surgery, medical or dental procedures, or short-lasting painful conditions.

What are the imortant side effects and precautions? Before using fentanyl, you and your household members need to be aware of some important information about using this drug. You should discuss with your doctor the most important side effects of this drug prior to your using it. **ALWAYS FEEL FREE TO CONTACT YOUR DOCTOR WITH ANY QUESTIONS OR CONCERNS YOU MAY HAVE ABOUT FENTANYL AND ANY SUSPECTED SIDE EFFECTS.**

SOME OF THE IMPORTANT THINGS TO HELP YOU USE THIS MEDICATION PROPERLY INCLUDE:

(1) One important side effect is slow, shallow, and/or difficulty in breathing, which can occur if the dose of fentanyl is too high. You and your household members should discuss with your doctor what signs and symptoms to look for and what to do if these develop. if you are uncertain what to do, call your doctor or get other emergency medical help.

(2) Do not take other medications (prescription or over-the-counter) while wearing fentanyl unless specifically told to do so by your doctor. Be especially careful about drugs that can make you sleepy.

(3) Do not drink alcohol while wearing the patch. Also do not drive a vehicle or operate dangerous machinery unless specifically told that you may do so by your doctor.

(4) Direct sources of heat may increase the amount of medication you receive through the skin from the patch. Do not use electric blankets, heating pads, sun lamps, heated water beds, or other sources of direct heat on a patch. Avoid sun bathing, long hot baths, or other sources of heat to the body.

(5) If you develop a fever greater than 102° F, contact your doctor because the increased fever could cause you to receive more medication than you should from the patch.

(6) Do not wear more than one patch at a time unless specifically told to do so by your doctor.

D(7) o not use this patch if you are nursing an infant unless specifically told to do so by your doctor. The medication can get into human milk and can cause serious problems for the infant.

(8) Fentanyl should not be used by children less than 12 years old or patients less than 18 years old who weigh less than 110 pounds, unless your doctor has enrolled the patient in an authorized research program.

(9) Be sure to dispose of used and unused patches so they cannot be touched by any other people or pets.

PATIENT PACKAGE INSERT: *(cont'd)*

How and Where to Apply Duragesic: In the hospital, your doctor or another qualified medical person will apply Duragesic for you. At home, you or a member of your family may apply Duragesic to your skin.

Step 1: Each Duragesic is sealed in its own protective pouch. Until you are ready to use Duragesic, do not remove it from the pouch. When you are ready to put on Duragesic, tear open the pouch and remove the Duragesic system.

Step 2: A stiff, protective liner covers the sticky side of the Duragesic - the side that will be put on your skin. With the oversized, stiff, clear liner facing you, pull the liner from the Duragesic system (try to touch the sticky side as little as possible). Throw away the liner.

Step 3 Immediately after you have taken Duragesic from the pouch, apply the sticky side the Duragesic to a non-hairy, dry area of your chest, back, flank or upper arm. If area you select has body hair, clip (do not shave) the hair close to the skin with scissors. Do not put Duragesic on skin that is excessively oily, burned, broken out, cut, irritated or damaged in any way. If you need to clean the skin where the system will be applied, use only clear water. Do not use soaps, oils, lotions, alcohol or other products that might irritate the skin under the system. Make sure that the skin is completely dry. **Press the Duragesic firmly on your skin with the palm of your hand for about 30 seconds.** Make sure it sticks well to your skin, especially around the edges of the system.

Step 4 Wash your hands when you have finished applying Duragesic.

Step 5 After wearing Duragesic for three days, remove it (see PATIENT PACKAGE INSERT, Disposing of Duragesic.) Then choose a *different* place on your skin to apply a new Duragesic and repeat Steps 1 to 4, in order.

When to Apply Duragesic: If you need continued pain control, wear Duragesic continuously for three days (approximately 72 hours), or as directed by your doctor and then remove the system and replace it as directed by your doctor. Do not apply the new Duragesic to the same place where you removed the last Duragesic.

Your doctor may increase your fentanyl dose if your pain is not adequately controlled. IF YOU CONTINUE TO HAVE PAIN CALL YOUR DOCTOR.

Water and Duragesic: You can bathe, swim or shower while you are wearing the Duragesic. If the system does fall off, put a new Duragesic on your skin. Before putting on a new Duragesic, make sure the new skin area you have selected is dry.

Disposing of the Duragesic: Before putting on a new Duragesic, remove the system you have wearing. Fold the used Duragesic in half so that the sticky side sticks to itself. Flush the used Duragesic down the toilet immediately. Even used Duragesic patches contain enough fentanyl to poison infants, children, pets and adults who have not been prescribed fentanyl.

Throw away any Duragesic systems that are left over from your prescription as soon as they are no longer needed. Remove the leftover systems from their protective pouch and remove the protective liner. Fold the systems in half and flush the system down the system down the toilet. Do not flush the pouch or the protective liner.

Safety and Handling: Fentanyl is supplied in sealed systems which will keep the gel from getting on your hands or body. If the gel from the drug reservoir accidentally contacts the skin, the area should be washed with large amounts of water. Do not use soap, alcohol, or other solvents to remove the gel because they may increase the drug's ability to go through the skin.

Do not cut or damage the Duragesic. Do not use the Duragesic system if it is damaged in any way. The Duragesic will not work properly or may not be safe to use if it is cut or damaged. Too much drug may be released too quickly into your body if the system is damaged.

Storage Instructions: Keep the Duragesic in its protective pouch until you are already to use it.

KEEP DURAGESIC OUT OF THE REACH OF CHILDREN AND PETS.

Do not store the Duragesic above 77° F (25° C). Remember, the inside of your car can reach temperatures much higher than this in the summer.

HOW SUPPLIED:

Fentanyl is supplied in cartons containing 5 individually packaged systems. See TABLE 5 for information regarding individual systems.

TABLE 5

Duragesic Dose (mcg/h)	System Size (cm^2)	Fentanyl Content (mg)
DURAGESIC-25	10	2.5
DURAGESIC-50*	20	5
DURAGESIC-75*	30	7.5
DURAGESIC-100*	40	10

* FOR USE ONLY IN OPIOID TOLERANT PATIENTS

Safety and Handling: Fentanyl is supplied in sealed transdermal systems which pose little risk of exposure to health care workers. If the gel from the drug reservoir accidentally contacts the skin, the area should be washed with copious amounts of water. Do not use soap, alcohol, or other solvents to remove the gel because they may enhance the drug's ability to penetrate the skin. Do not cut or damage fentanyl. If the fentanyl system is cut or damaged, controlled drug delivery will not be possible.

Do not store above 77°F (25°C). Apply immediately after removal from individually sealed package. Do not use if the seal is broken. **For transdermal use only.**

HOW SUPPLIED - EQUIVALENTS NOT AVAILABLE:

Film, Continuous Release - Percutaneous - 25 mcg/hr
5's $49.97 DURAGESIC, Janssen Phar 50458-0033-05

Film, Continuous Release - Percutaneous - 50 mcg/hr
5's $74.92 DURAGESIC, Janssen Phar 50458-0034-05

Film, Continuous Release - Percutaneous - 75 mcg/hr
5's $114.42 DURAGESIC, Janssen Phar 50458-0035-05

Film, Continuous Release - Percutaneous - 100 mcg/hr
5's $142.56 DURAGESIC, Janssen Phar 50458-0036-05

FENTANYL CITRATE *(001254)*

CATEGORIES: Analgesics; Anesthesia; Antipyretics; Central Nervous System Agents; Narcotic Analgesics; Narcotics, Synthetics & Combinations; Opiate Agonists (Controlled); Pain; Pregnancy Category C; DEA Class CII; FDA Approval Pre 1982

BRAND NAMES: *Beatryl*; *Fentanest* (Mexico); Fentanyl Oralet; *Leptanal*; Oralet; **Sublimaze**

(International brand names outside U.S. in italics)

FORMULARIES: BC-BS

WARNING:
LOZENGE: ORAL FENTANYL CONTAINS THE POTENT NARCOTIC FENTANYL CITRATE IN A FORMULATION WHICH:
CARRIES A RISK OF HYPOVENTILATION WITH ITS USE WHICH MAY RESULT IN DEATH IF NOT MONITORED BY TRAINED PERSONNEL SUPPORTED BY APPROPRIATE, IMMEDIATELY AVAILABLE EQUIPMENT.
SHOULD ONLY BE USED AS AN ANESTHETIC PREMEDICATION OR FOR INDUCING CONSCIOUS SEDATION PRIOR TO A DIAGNOSTIC OR THERAPEUTIC PROCEDURE IN A MONITORED ANESTHESIA CARE SETTING.
SHOULD ONLY BE ADMINISTERED IN HOSPITAL SETTINGS SUCH AS THE OPERATING ROOM, EMERGENCY DEPARTMENT, ICU OR OTHER MONITORED ANESTHESIA CARE SETTINGS IN HOSPITALS WHERE THERE IS IMMEDIATE ACCESS TO LIFE SUPPORT EQUIPMENT, OXYGEN, FACILITIES FOR ENDOTRACHEAL INTUBATION, INTRAVENOUS FLUIDS, AND OPIOID ANTAGONISTS.
CAN ONLY BE USED SAFELY IN PATIENTS BEING MONITORED BY BOTH (1) DIRECT VISUAL OBSERVATION BY A HEALTH PROFESSIONAL WHOSE SOLE RESPONSIBILITY IS OBSERVATION OF THE PATIENT AND (2) SOME MEANS OF MEASURING RESPIRATORY FUNCTION SUCH AS PULSE OXIMETRY UNTIL THEY ARE COMPLETELY RECOVERED.
SHOULD ONLY BE ADMINISTERED BY PERSONS SPECIFICALLY TRAINED IN THE USE OF ANESTHETIC DRUGS AND CARDIAC RESUSCITATION OF PATIENTS IN THE AGE GROUP BEING TREATED. SUCH TRAINING MUST INCLUDE THE ESTABLISHMENT AND MAINTENANCE OF A PATENT AIRWAY AND ASSISTED VENTILATION.
SHOULD ONLY BE USED BY HEALTH CARE PRACTITIONERS CREDENTIALED TO USE THE PRODUCT BY THE DIRECTOR OF ANESTHESIA OF THE INSTITUTION IN WHICH THE PRODUCT WILL BE USED.
IS CONTRAINDICATED FOR USE AT ANY OTHER SETTING OUTSIDE A HOSPITAL.
ORAL FENTANYL IS CONTRAINDICATED:
IN CHILDREN WHO WEIGH LESS THAN 15 KILOGRAMS (33 POUNDS).
FOR THE TREATMENT OF ACUTE OR CHRONIC PAIN BECAUSE THE SAFETY OF THIS PRODUCT FOR USE IN THESE INDICATIONS HAS NOT BEEN ESTABLISHED.
IN DOSES ABOVE 15 MCG/KG IN CHILDREN, AND IN DOSES ABOVE 5 MCG/KG IN ADULTS, BECAUSE OF THE EXCESSIVE FREQUENCY OF SIGNIFICANT HYPOVENTILATION AT HIGHER DOSES, THE MAXIMUM DOSE ANY CHILD OR ADULT SHOULD RECEIVE IS 400 MCG, REGARDLESS OF WEIGHT.

DESCRIPTION:

INJECTION

Fentanyl citrate injection is a potent narcotic analgesic. Each milliliter contains fentanyl citrate equivalent to 50 µg of fentanyl base, adjusted to pH 4.0 - 7.5 with sodium hydroxide. Fentanyl citrate is chemically identified as N-(1-phenethyl-4 - piperidyl)propionanilide citrate (1:1) with a molecular weight of 528.61. The empirical formula is $C_{22}H_{28}N_2O{\cdot}C_6H_8O_7$.

Fentanyl citrate is a sterile, non-pyogenic, preservative free aqueous solution for intravenous or intramuscular injection.

Fentanyl Oralet (oral transmucosal fentanyl citrate) is a solid formulation of fentanyl citrate, a potent narcotic analgesic, intended for oral transmucosal administration. It consists of a lozenge on a plastic holder and is consumed by sucking the dosage form.

Fentanyl citrate, USP is N-(1-Phenethyl-4-piperidyl) propionanilide citrate (1:1). Fentanyl is a highly lipophilic compound (octanol-water partition coefficient at pH 7.4 is 816:1) that is freely soluble in organic solvents and sparingly soluble in water (1:40). The molecular weight of the free base is 336.5 (the citrate is 528.6). The pKa of the tertiary nitrogens are 7.3 and 8.4.

Fentanyl Oralet is available in three doses of fentanyl citrate equivalent to 200, 300 or 400 µg of fentanyl base that may be identified by the text on both the outer wrapper and the handle label. Each Fentanyl Oralet is designed for use by a single patient at a single setting. Unconsumed portions of the dose are to be destroyed (see DOSAGE AND ADMINISTRATION, Safety And Handling).

Inactive Ingredients: Each solid dosage form contains sucrose, liquid glucose, raspberry flavor, carmine, and FD&C Blue No. 2 lake dispersion molded into a lozenge on a radiopaque plastic handle that is fracture resistant under normal conditions when used as directed.

CLINICAL PHARMACOLOGY:

INJECTION

Fentanyl citrate is a narcotic analgesic. A dose of 100 µg (0.1 mg) (2 ml) is approximately equivalent in analgesic activity to 10 mg of morphine or 75 mg of meperidine. The principal actions of therapeutic value are analgesia and sedation. Alterations in respiratory rate and alveolar ventilation, associated with narcotic analgesics, may last longer than the analgesic effect. As the dose of narcotic is increased, the decrease in pulmonary exchange becomes greater. Large doses may produce apnea. Fentanyl appears to have less emetic activity than either morphine or meperidine. Histamine assays and skin wheal testing in man indicate that clinically significant histamine release rarely occurs with fentanyl. Recent assays in man show no clinically significant histamine release in dosages up to 50 µg/kg (0.05 mg/kg) (1 ml/kg). Fentanyl preserves cardiac stability and blunts stress-related hormonal changes at higher doses.

Pharmacokinetics

The pharmacokinetics of fentanyl can be described as a three-compartment model, with a distribution time of 1.7 minutes, redistribution of 13 minutes and a terminal elimination half-life of 219 minutes. The volume of distribution for fentanyl is 4 L/kg.

Fentanyl plasma protein binding capacity increases with increasing ionization of the drug. Alterations in pH may affect its distribution between plasma and the central nervous system. It accumulates in skeletal muscle and fat and is released slowly into the blood. Fentanyl, which is primarily transformed in the liver, demonstrates a high first pass clearance and

CLINICAL PHARMACOLOGY: *(cont'd)*

releases approximately 75% of an intravenous dose in urine, mostly as metabolites with less than 10% representing the unchanged drug. Approximately 9% of the dose is recovered in the feces, primarily as metabolites.

The onset of action of fentanyl is almost immediate when the drug is given intravenously; however, the maximal analgesic and respiratory depressant effect may not be noted for several minutes. The usual duration of action of the analgesic effect is 30 to 60 minutes after a single intravenous dose of up to 100 µg (0.1 mg) (2 ml). Following intramuscular administration, the onset of action is from seven to eight minutes, and the duration of action is one to two hours. As with longer acting narcotic analgesics, the duration of the respiratory depressant effect of fentanyl may be longer than the analgesic effect. The following observations have been reported concerning altered respiratory response to CO_2 stimulation following administration of fentanyl citrate to man:

1. DIMINISHED SENSITIVITY TO CO_2 STIMULATION MAY PERSIST LONGER THAN DEPRESSION OF RESPIRATORY RATE. (Altered sensitivity to CO_2 stimulation has been demonstrated for up to four hours following a single dose of 600 µg (0.6 mg) (12 ml) fentanyl to healthy volunteers.) Fentanyl frequently slows the respiratory rate, duration and degree of respiratory depression being dose related.

2. The peak respiratory depressant effect of a single intravenous dose of fentanyl citrate is noted 5 to 15 minutes following injection. See also WARNINGS and PRECAUTIONS concerning respiratory depression.

LOZENGE

Pharmacology: Fentanyl, an opioid analgesic, acts primarily through interaction with opioid µ-receptors located in the brain, spinal cord and smooth muscle. The primary site of therapeutic action for fentanyl is the central nervous system. The most clinically useful pharmacologic effects resulting from the interaction of fentanyl with µ-receptors in the brain are sedation and analgesia.

In addition to these primary effects, opioid effects include hypoventilation, pruritus, dizziness, nausea, diaphoresis, flushing, euphoria, and confusion or difficulty in concentrating. Doses of fentanyl that provide clinically useful therapeutic effects may also cause nausea, vomiting, bradycardia, and postural hypotension.

Fentanyl is a known respiratory depressant and also depresses the cough reflex as a result of its CNS activity. Fentanyl given rapidly in large doses may also interfere with respiration by causing muscle rigidity which may effect the muscles of respiration.

As with other µ agonist opioids, fentanyl increases smooth muscle tone in the gastrointestinal and genitourinary systems. This effect can result in constipation and/or urinary retention, effects that are more common with increasing dose or chronic use.

Pharmacodynamics: The primary effects of fentanyl that are of clinical value are sedation (reduced activity and reduced apprehension) and analgesia (reduced pain). While the onset of action of fentanyl is within 1 to 2 minutes when the drug is given IV, the onset of effects begins 5 to 15 minutes from the start of administration when the drug is delivered as oral fentanyl. Maximum effects are typically noted 20 to 30 minutes from the start of administration. Complete consumption of the oral fentanylunit usually occurs in 10 to 20 minutes.

The analgesic and anesthetic effects of fentanyl are related to the blood level of the drug, if proper allowance is made for the delay into and out of the CNS (a process with a 3 to 5 minute half-life). Fentanyl provides effects ranging from analgesia at blood levels of 1 to 2 ng/ml, all the way to profound respiratory depression and surgical anesthesia at levels of 10 to 20 ng/ml. Fentanyl redistributes into muscle and fat like most other highly lipophilic drugs, and the duration of the effects of fentanyl depends on the route of administration, the duration of administration and the total cumulative dose. Initially, the effects of small single doses are short-lived because the drug is rapidly redistributed into peripheral tissues. With large or repeated doses these tissues begin to accumulate fentanyl. Eventually, the duration of fentanyl effects becomes dependent on clearance of the drug from these tissue reservoirs by metabolic elimination, a slower process than redistribution (see Pharmacokinetics).

In clinical studies of oral fentanyl, both the beneficial effect of the medication and the adverse effect of opioid-induced hypoventilation were related to the dose of fentanyl administered.

In both children and adults, respiratory rate and oxygen saturation typically decrease as fentanyl concentration increases. Typically, peak respiratory depressant effects (decrease in respiratory rate) are seen 15 to 30 minutes from the start of oral fentanyl administration, but such effects may persist for several hours.

The following observations have been reported concerning altered respiratory response after fentanyl administration:

1. Diminished Sensitivity to Carbon Dioxide May Persist Longer Than Slowed Respiration Altered sensitivity to carbon dioxide stimulation has been demonstrated for up to four hours following a single IV dose of 600 µg (0.6 mg) fentanyl to healthy volunteers and up to eight hours after 5 mg of transmucosal fentanyl in healthy adult volunteers.

2. Prolonged Effects On Respiration Are Possible The peak respiratory depressant effects of a oral fentanyl dose (10 to 20 µg/kg) occur 15 to 30 minutes following initiation of administration, but respiratory effects may persist for several hours, especially when oral fentanyl is given in conjunction with other anesthetic agents.

3. Serious Respiratory Depression Can Occur, Even With Proper Doses, Invulnerable Individuals As with other potent anesthetic agents, fentanyl has been associated with cases of serious respiratory depression in individuals with respiratory disorders, cases of excessive or improper dosage, in individuals with unsuspected abnormalities of absorption or metabolism of the drug, and in rare cases where no specific etiology can be identified. **Oral fentanyl should be administered only in specifically monitored settings and by persons specifically trained in the use of anesthetics and the management of the respiratory effects of potent opioids, including establishment and maintenance of a patent airway and assisted ventilation** (see also BOXED WARNING and PRECAUTIONS).

Note: Many of the dosing regimens in this section of the package insert reflect early dosing studies to help characterize the pharmacokinetic properties of this dosage form of fentanyl. They are included here for information on the pharmacokinetic characterization of this product and NOT AS GUIDES TO CLINICAL DOSING. FOR INFORMATION ON APPROPRIATE DOSING AND USE OF THIS PRODUCT, PLEASE SEE DOSAGE AND ADMINISTRATION.

The absorption pharmacokinetics of fentanyl from the Oralet dosage form are a combination of the initial rapid absorption of swallowed fentanyl from the GI tract. Both the blood fentanyl profile and the bioavailability of fentanyl will vary depending on the fraction of the dose that is absorbed through the oral mucosa and the fraction swallowed.

Normally, approximately 25% of the total dose is rapidly absorbed from the buccal mucosa and becomes systemically available. The remaining 75% is swallowed with the saliva and then is slowly absorbed from the GI tract. About 1/3 of this amount (25% of the total dose) escapes hepatic first-pass elimination and becomes systemically available. Therefore, the generally observed 50% bioavailability of oral fentanyl is divided equally between rapid transmucosal and slower GI absorption. Chewed or swallowed fentanyl contributes little to the peak concentration, but is responsible for the prolonged "tail" on the blood level profile as it is slowly absorbed.

CLINICAL PHARMACOLOGY: *(cont'd)*

Dose proportionality among the three available strengths of oral fentanyl (200, 300, and 400 µg) has not been demonstrated. As portrayed in TABLE 1, there is a wide variability in the range of pharmacokinetic parameters of this dosing form of fentanyl, especially in C_{max}, T_{max}, and t1/2. Because of the absorption characteristics of this product in this dosage form, there is a sustained plasma level of the drug. THOSE WHO ADMINISTER THIS PRODUCT MUST BE COGNIZANT OF THE CLINICAL IMPLICATIONS OF THIS PHARMACOKINETIC CHARACTERISTIC AND CONTINUE TO MONITOR AND OBSERVE THE PATIENT UNTIL HE/SHE IS FULLY RECOVERED.

In healthy male volunteers given 15 µg/kg, the mean C_{max} after oral fentanyl is 2.7 ng/ml (see TABLE 1). The median time of maximum plasma concentration (T_{max}) with oral fentanyl is 23 minutes. Absolute bioavailability, as determined by area under the concentration- time curve, of 15 µg/kg of oral fentanyl in 12 healthy male volunteers was 50% compared to intravenous fentanyl. The mean volume of distribution at steady state (V_{ss}) was 4 L/kg and the total plasma clearance of fentanyl was 0.5 L/hr/kg (range 0.3 to 0.7 L/hr/kg).

TABLE 1 Oral Fentanyl Pharmacokinetic Parameters in Adults Receiving 15 µg/kg

Parameter	Unit	N=12
C_{max} (ng/ml)	Mean	2.7
	Absolute Range	1.4 to 4.6
T_{max} (minutes)	Median	23
	Absolute Range	19 to 30
Bioavailability (percent)	Mean	50
	Absolute Range	36 to 71
t1/2 (hours)	Median	6.6
	Absolute Range	5 to 15

In clinical studies in children, a single dose of 10 to 20 (mean 16.50 µg/kg oral fentanyl resulted in a mean peak plasma fentanyl level (C_{max}) of 2 ng/ml that occurred about 20 minutes from the start of administration. In these studies, the C_{max} increased with increasing dose, while the T_{max} increased (slower absorption) with longer consumption times (time to consume the dosage form). In general, the pharmacokinetic profile of oral fentanyl was similar in adults and children.

The plasma protein binding of fentanyl is 80 to 85%. The main binding protein is alpha-1-acid glycoprotein, but both albumin and lipoproteins contribute to some extent. The free fraction of fentanyl increases with acidosis. Following an IV dose, fentanyl is rapidly redistributed from the blood to lung tissue and skeletal muscle and then more slowly to deeper fat compartments. It is then slowly released into the blood from the tissues during its metabolic elimination. Large single doses or many repeated doses can result in the accumulation of a large body burden of fentanyl that may take many hours to clear.

Fentanyl is primarily (more than 90%) eliminated by biotransformation to N-dealkylated and hydroxylated inactive metabolites. Less than 7% of the dose is excreted unchanged in the urine, and only about 1% is excreted unchanged in the feces. The metabolites are mainly excreted in the urine, while fecal excretion is less important.

Special Populations: The absorption, distribution, and metabolism of fentanyl have been shown to be relatively constant over the age range intended for oral fentanyl, although elderly patients have been shown to be approximately twice as sensitive to the same blood level of the drug as younger patients.

Although fentanyl kinetics are known to be altered in both hepatic and renal disease due to alterations in metabolic clearance and plasma proteins, individualized doses of fentanyl have been used successfully in anesthesia in both kinds of disorders. This is because the duration of effect for the initial dose of fentanyl is determined by redistribution of the drug, such that diminished metabolic clearance will only become significant with repeat dosing or with excessively large single doses. For these reasons, reduced doses titrated to clinical effect are recommended in the elderly, and in patients with severe hepatic and/or renal disease.

CLINICAL STUDIES:

Anesthetic Premedication: The efficacy of oral fentanyl was investigated in five randomized, placebo-controlled, clinical trials as premedication for various pediatric surgical procedures (cardiovascular, orthopedic, urological, and general surgery). Single oral fentanyl doses of 5 to 20 µg/kg (18 to 30 patients per treatment group) were compared to placebo in patients 2 to 18 years old. Patients receiving oral fentanyl were significantly more sedated than patients receiving placebo. Median time to peak sedative effect was 30 minutes. Generally, intraoperative and postoperative analgesics were less frequently required in the oral fentanyl group.

The efficacy of oral fentanyl was also compared to an oral solution of meperidine 1.5 mg/kg, diazepam 0.2 mg/kg, and atropine 0.02 mg/kg (MDA solution) as premedication in pediatric patients undergoing cardiovascular surgery. In a study with 20 patients per treatment group, oral fentanyl 20 to 25 µg/kg was compared to MDA solution. In that study, a high incidence of nausea and vomiting suggested that **20 to 25 µg/kg was an excessive oral fentanyl dose.** A second study in patients with a oral fentanyl dose of 15 to 20 µg/kg found that oral fentanyl was similar in efficacy to MDA solution without the excessive vomiting seen in the first study.

The efficacy of oral fentanyl with and without droperidol was also compared to placebo in pediatric general surgery patients. Oral fentanyl with and without droperidol was also compared to placebo in pediatric general surgery patients. Oral fentanyl was administered in doses of 15 to 20 µg/kg with and without droperidol 50 µg/kg versus placebo (also with and without droperidol). Use of oral fentanyl was associated with improved induction and a reduced use of post operative opioids. Droperidol reduced the incidence of nausea and vomiting associated with oral fentanyl, but the combination of droperidol and oral fentanyl resulted in a significantly delayed awakening (the combination of droperidol and oral fentanyl doubled the awakening time after surgery from that of oral fentanyl alone) (see DRUG INTERACTIONS).

Despite the provision of gentle, non-pharmacologic reassurance to all patients, in placebo-controlled studies of a total of 496 children, 42% of patients administered placebo Oralet remained apprehensive 30 minutes following administration of the placebo. Doses of 5 to 10 µg/kg of oral fentanyl reduced the number of apprehensive patients at 30 minutes post drug administration from 42% in the placebo group to about 7% in the oral fentanyl group. Larger doses provided no apparent gain in efficacy, but substantially increased the frequency of adverse events.

About 10 to 20% of the patients who were studied pre-operatively had symptoms of apprehension that were so severe as to unequivocally need premedication. In those cases, oral fentanyl, in doses of 5 to 15 µg/kg produced a dose-related reduction in apprehension that was sufficient to allow a calm, manageable induction of anesthesia within 20 to 30 minutes. Doses above 5 µg/kg (10 and 15 µg/kg) were more effective in managing the already apprehensive patient but were associated with a dose-dependent increase in pruritus, vomiting and hypoventilation.

Conscious Sedation In a Monitored Anesthesia Care Setting: Conscious sedation in a monitored anesthesia care setting in the hospital is commonly required in a patient needing to undergo a painful diagnostic or therapeutic procedure. Oral fentanyl has been evaluated for such monitored anesthesia care outside the operating room environment in two open trials.

CLINICAL STUDIES: *(cont'd)*

Eight (8) adult and 34 pediatric patients have been administered oral fentanyl 10 to 20 μg/kg as a premedicant in the emergency room. Patients who were administered 10 to 15 μg/kg had increased levels of sedation similar to patients administered 15 to 20 μg/kg. However, the lower dose range to 10 to 15 μg/kg was associated with a lower risk od adverse effects. Onset of analgesia occurred at approximately 6 to 8 minutes following oral fentanyl.

In a double-blind, placebo-controlled trial, oral fentanyl 15 to 20 μg/kg was administered to 31 pediatric oncology patients prior to undergoing a painful diagnostic or therapeutic procedure. Some of these children had previous opioid experience. Of the patients who received oral fentanyl, 68% became more sedate over 30 minutes compared to 26% of patients who received placebo. Median time to peak effect in these patients was 20 minutes.

Because of the risk of hypoventilation, the lowest effective dose of oral fentanyl should be used, and it should be administered only in monitored settings and by persons specifically trained in the use of anesthetics and the management of the respiratory effects of potent opioids, including the establishment and maintenance of a patent airway and assisted ventilation.

INDICATIONS AND USAGE:

INJECTION

Fentanyl Citrate Injection is indicated:

for analgesic action of short duration during the anesthetic periods, premedication, induction and maintenance, and in the immediate postoperative period (recovery room) as the need arises.

for use as a narcotic analgesic supplement in general or regional anesthesia.

for administration with a neuroleptic such as droperidol injection as an anesthetic premedication, for the induction of anesthesia and as an adjunct in the maintenance of general and regional anesthesia.

for use as an anesthetic agent with oxygen in selected high risk patients, such as those undergoing open heart surgery or certain complicated neurological or orthopedic procedures.

LOZENGE

Oral fentanyl is only indicated for use in a hospital setting (1) as an anesthetic premedication in the operating room setting or (2) to induce conscious sedation prior to a diagnostic or therapeutic procedure in other monitored anesthesia care settings in the hospital. Appropriate monitored anesthesia care settings are described immediately below in the BOXED WARNING section. Doses must be chosen that minimize the risk of hypoventilation (see DOSAGE AND ADMINISTRATION and WARNINGS).

Caution: Before Administering This Product, Please Note The Following Instructions On The Proper Use Of This Product

Oral fentanyl should only be administered in hospital settings such as the operating room, emergency department, ICU, or other monitored anesthesia care settings in hospitals where there is immediate access to life support equipment, including oxygen, facilities for endotracheal intubation, intravenous fluids, and opioid antagonists.

Oral fentanyl must be given only to patients being monitored by both (1) direct visual observation by a health professional whose sole responsibility is observation of the patient and also by (2) some means of measuring respiratory function such as pulse oximetry until they are completely recovered.

Oral fentanyl should only be administered by persons specifically trained in the use of anesthetic drugs and the management of the respiratory effects of potent opioids, including respiratory and cardiac resuscitation of patients in the age group being treated. Such training must include the establishment and maintenance of a patent airway and assisted ventilation. This product should only be used by health care practitioners credentialed to use the product by the director of anesthesia of the institution in which the product will be used. (See also BOXED WARNING, CLINICAL PHARMACOLOGY, and PRECAUTIONS.

CONTRAINDICATIONS:

INJECTION

Fentanyl citrate injection is contraindicated in patients with known intolerance to the drug.

LOZENGE

Oral Fentanyl is Contraindicated:

In children who weigh less than 15 kilograms (33 pounds).

For the use at home or in any other setting outside a hospital.

For the treatment of acute or chronic pain because the safety of this product for use in these indications has not been established.

In dosages above 15 μg/kg in children, and in doses above 5 μg/kg in adults. Because of the excessive frequency of significant hypoventilation at higher doses, the maximum amount any child or adult should receive is 400 μg, regardless of weight..

In patients with known intolerance or hypersensitivity to any of its components or the drug fentanyl.

WARNINGS:

INJECTION

FENTANYL CITRATE SHOULD BE ADMINISTERED ONLY BY PERSONS SPECIFICALLY TRAINED IN THE USE OF INTRAVENOUS ANESTHETICS AND MANAGEMENT OF THE RESPIRATORY EFFECTS OF POTENT OPIOIDS.

An Opiod Antagonist, Resuscitative and Intubation Equipment and Oxygen Should be Readily Available

See also discussion of narcotic antagonists in PRECAUTIONS and OVERDOSAGE.

If fentanyl is administered with a tranquilizer such as droperidol, the user should become familiar with the special properties of each drug, particularly the widely differing durations of action. In addition, when such a combination is used, fluids and other countermeasures to manage hypotension should be available.

As with other potent narcotics, the respiratory depressant effect of fentanyl may persist longer than the measured analgesic effect. The total dose of all narcotic analgesics administered should be considered by the practitioner before ordering narcotic analgesics during recovery from anesthesia. It is recommended that narcotics, when required, should be used in reduced doses initially, as low as 1/4 to 1/3 those usually recommended.

Fentanyl may cause muscle rigidity, particularly involving the muscles of respiration. In addition, skeletal muscle movements of various groups in the extremities, neck and external eye have been reported during induction of anesthesia with fentanyl; these reported movements have, on rare occasions, been strong enough to pose patient management problems. This effect is related to the dose and speed of injection and its incidence can be reduced by: 1) administration of up to 1/4 of the full paralyzing dose of a non-depolarizing neuromuscular blocking agent just prior to administration of fentanyl citrate; 2) administration of a full paralyzing dose of a neuromuscular blocking agent following loss of eyelash reflex when fentanyl is used in anesthetic doses titrated by slow intravenous infusion; or, 3) simultaneous

WARNINGS: *(cont'd)*

administration of fentanyl citrate and a full paralyzing dose of neuromuscular blocking agent when fentanyl citrate is used in rapidly administered anesthetic dosages. The neuromuscular blocking agent used should be compatible with the patient's cardiovascular status.

Adequate facilities should be available for postoperative monitoring and ventilation of patients administered anesthetic doses of fentanyl. Where moderate or high doses are used (above 10 μg/kg), there must be adequate facilities for postoperative observation, and ventilation if necessary, of patients who have received fentanyl. It is essential that these facilities be fully equipped to handle all degrees of respiratory depression.

Fentanyl may also produce other signs and symptoms characteristic of narcotic analgesics including euphoria, miosis, bradycardia and bronchoconstriction.

Severe and unpredictable potentiation by MAO inhibitors has been reported for other narcotic analgesics. Although this has not been reported for fentanyl, there are insufficient data to establish that this does not occur with fentanyl. Therefore, when fentanyl is administered to patients who have received MAO inhibitors within 14 days, appropriate monitoring and ready availability of vasodilators and beta-blockers for the treatment of hypertension is indicated.

Head Injuries and Increased Intracranial Pressure: Fentanyl should be used with caution in patients who may be particularly susceptible to respiratory depression, such as comatose patients who may have a head injury or brain tumor. In addition, fentanyl may obscure the clinical course of patients with head injury.

Use in Pediatric Premedication: Pediatric premedication, even in critical care areas of a hospital, is not free of risk to the child. Use of potent narcotics, such as fentanyl, is associated with a risk of hypoventilation ranging in severity from mild bradycardia to apnea. This risk cannot be totally eliminated even by proper choice of dose or skillful patient selection. Adverse consequences of hypoventilation, however, can be markedly reduced by appropriate clinical practices. Hypoventilation during monitored anesthetic care is an adverse event that should have no associated morbidity or mortality, provided it is immediately recognized and appropriately managed by stimulation, oxygen, and/or prompt ventilatory support according to severity.

In settings where the practitioner is unable to detect and manage hypoventilation, morbidity due to all forms of pediatric premedication is relatively frequent (10 to 50 human cases per thousand). In anesthetic practice, morbidity due to hypoventilation is rare, occurring approximately once in every 5,000 to 10,000 cases. For this reason, the greatest risk associated with premedication occurs in single-operator settings where qualified personnel are not continually monitoring the patient. Such settings are dental offices without monitored anesthesia care, surgical settings without an anesthetist, single-operator endoscopy suites and radiological settings where access to the patient is restricted by the equipment.

Given these risks, oral fentanyl should only be administered as detailed in the BOXED WARNING, INDICATIONS AND USAGE, and DOSAGE AND ADMINISTRATION sections of this monograph.

See also discussion of narcotic antagonists in PRECAUTIONS and OVERDOSAGE.

Head Injuries and Increased Intracranial Pressure: Oral fentanyl, as with other opioids, should be used with caution in patients who may be particularly susceptible to respiratory depression, such as patients who may have had a head injury or brain tumor. As with all opioids, oral fentanyl may obscure the clinical course of a patient with a head injury and should be used only if clinically indicated.

Use With Other Potent Narcotics: As with other potent narcotics, the respiratory depressant effect of fentanyl may persist longer than the analgesic effect. The total dose all narcotic analgesics administered, including oral fentanyl, should be considered before ordering narcotic analgesic during recovery from anesthesia. For patients who have received oral fentanyl within 6 to 12 hours, it is recommended that, if other narcotic are required, they should be used at starting doses 1/4 to 1/3 those usually recommended.

Other Warnings: Cases of self-administration of fentanyl by health care professionals, including fatalities, have been reported with all fentanyl products. The handling of oral fentanyl should be managed to minimize the risk of diversion, including restriction of access to the appropriate clinical setting and accounting procedures as required by the law.

If fentanyl is administered with a sedative, the user must be familiar with the special properties of combinations of opioids and other CNS depressants, particularly the extended duration of action. Hypotension has also been reported with the concomitant use of fentanyl and droperidol. If it occurs, the possibility of hypovolemia should also be considered and managed with appropriate parenteral fluid therapy.

Fentanyl may cause muscle rigidity, particularly involving the muscles of respiration. Muscle rigidity after IV use is related to the dose and speed of injection. Although muscle rigidity interfering with respiration has not been seen following use of oral fentanyl, the possibility of it happening should be kept in mind. If it occurs, it should be managed by the use of assisted or controlled respiration, by an opioid antagonist, and as a final alternative, by a neuromuscular blocking agent.

Oral fentanyl is not recommended for use in patients who have received MAO inhibitors within 14 days, because severe and unpredictable potentiation by MAO inhibitors has been reported with narcotic analgesics.

PRECAUTIONS:

INJECTION

General: The initial dose of fentanyl citrate should be appropriately reduced in elderly and debilitated patients. The effect of the initial dose should be considered in determining incremental doses.

Nitrous oxide has been reported to produce cardiovascular depression when given with higher doses of fentanyl.

When a tranquilizer such as droperidol is used with fentanyl, pulmonary arterial pressure may be decreased. This fact should be considered by those who conduct diagnostic and surgical procedures where interpretation of pulmonary arterial pressure measurements might determine final management of the patient. When high dose or anesthetic dosages of fentanyl are employed, even relatively small dosages of diazepam may cause cardiovascular depression.

When fentanyl is used with a tranquilizer such as droperidol, hypotension can occur. If it occurs, the possibility of hypovolemia should also be considered and managed with appropriate parenteral fluid therapy. Repositioning the patient to improve venous return to the heart should be considered when operative conditions permit. Care should be exercised in moving and positioning of patients because of the possibility of orthostatic hypotension. If volume expansion with fluids plus other countermeasures do not correct hypotension, the administration of pressor agents other than epinephrine should be considered. Because of the alpha-adrenergic blocking action of droperidol, epinephrine may paradoxically decrease the blood pressure in patients treated with droperidol.

When droperidol is used with fentanyl and the EEG is used for postoperative monitoring, it may be found that the EEG pattern returns to normal slowly.

Vital signs should be monitored routinely.

PRECAUTIONS: *(cont'd)*

Respiratory depression caused by opioid analgesics can be reversed by opioid antagonists such as naloxone. Because the duration of respiratory depression produced by fentanyl may last longer than the duration of the opioid antagonist action, appropriate surveillance should be maintained. As with all potent opioids, profound analgesia is accompanied by respiratory depression and diminished sensitivity to CO_2stimulation which may persist into or recur in the postoperative period. Intraoperative hyperventilation may further alter postoperative response to CO_2. Appropriate postoperative monitoring should be employed to ensure that adequate spontaneous breathing is established and maintained in the absence of stimulation prior to discharging the patient from the recovery area.

Impaired Respiration: Fentanyl should be used with caution in patients with chronic obstructive pulmonary disease, patients with decreased respiratory reserve, and others with potentially compromised respiration. In such patients, narcotics may additionally decrease respiratory drive and increase airway resistance. During anesthesia, this can be managed by assisted or controlled respiration.

Pediatric Use: The safety and efficacy of fentanyl citrate in children under two years of age has not been established.

Rare cases of unexplained clinically significant methemoglobinemia have been reported in premature neonates undergoing emergency anesthesia and surgery which included combined use of fentanyl, pancuronium and atropine. A direct cause and effect relationship between the combined use of these drugs and the reported cases of methemoglobinemia has not been established.

LOZENGE

General: The initial dose of oral fentanyl should be appropriately individualized by assessing the clinical status of the patient in regard to the desired clinical effect(s). The effect(s) of the initial dose should be considered in subsequent administration of any additional CNS depressive agents.

Use in Anesthesia: Nitrous oxide has been reported to produce cardiovascular depression when given with higher doses of IV fentanyl.

Cardiovascular Effects: As with other opioids, orthostatic hypotension is possible (see Use In Ambulatory Surgery).

Use in Children Below 15 Kilograms Weight: USE OF THIS PRODUCT IN CHILDREN LESS THAN 15 KILOGRAMS WEIGHT IS CONTRAINDICATED AS AN APPROPRIATE DOSE CANNOT BE ADMINISTERED WITH THE PRESENT PRESENTATIONS OF THIS PRODUCT. Safety and effectiveness of oral fentanyl in children who weigh less than 15 kilograms have not been established (see DOSAGE AND ADMINISTRATION).

In addition, safety and effectiveness of this product in children less than 2 years of age have not been established.

Use in Elderly Patients: If oral fentanyl is to be used in patients over age 65, the dose should be reduced to 2.5 to 5 µg/kg. Although studies of oral fentanyl in the elderly have not been conducted, elderly patients have been shown to be twice as sensitive as the younger population to the effects of forms of fentanyl. Caution is indicated, because, like all potent opioids, oral fentanyl has the ability to depress respiration and reduce ventilatory drive to a clinically significant extent.

INJECTION AND LOZENGE

General: Certain forms of conduction anesthesia, such as spinal anesthesia and some peridural anesthetics, can alter respiration by blocking intercostal nerves. Through other mechanisms (see CLINICAL PHARMACOLOGY) fentanyl can also alter respiration. Therefore, when fentanyl is used to supplement these forms of anesthesia, the anesthetist should be familiar with the physiological alterations involved, and be prepared to manage them in the patients selected for these forms of anesthesia.

Elevated blood pressure, with and without pre-existing hypertension, has been reported following administration of fentanyl citrate combined with droperidol. This might be due to unexplained alterations in sympathetic activity following large doses; however, it is also frequently attributed to anesthetic and surgical stimulation during light anesthesia.

Impaired Hepatic or Renal Function: Fentanyl citrate should be administered with caution to patients with liver and kidney dysfunction because of the importance of these organs in the metabolism and excretion of drugs.

Cardiovascular Effects: Fentanyl may produce bradycardia, which may be treated with atropine. Fentanyl should be used with caution in patients with cardiac bradyarrhythmias.

Carcinogenesis, Mutagenesis, and Impairment of Fertility: No carcinogenicity or mutagenicity studies have been conducted with fentanyl citrate. Reproduction studies in rats revealed a significant decrease in the pregnancy rate of all experimental groups. This decrease was most pronounced in the high dosed group (1.25 mg/kg—12.5X human dose) in which one of twenty animals became pregnant.

Pregnancy Category C: Fentanyl citrate has been shown to impair fertility and to have an embryocidal effect in rats when given in doses 0.3 times the upper human dose for a period of 12 days. No evidence of teratogenic effects have been observed after administration of fentanyl citrate to rats. There are no adequate and well-controlled studies in pregnant women. Fentanyl should be used during pregnancy only if the potential benefit justifies the potential risk to the fetus.

Labor and Delivery: There are insufficient data to support the use of fentanyl in labor and delivery. Therefore, such use is not recommended.

Nursing Mothers: It is not known whether this drug is excreted in human milk. Because many drugs are excreted in human milk, caution should be exercised when fentanyl citrate is administered to a nursing woman.

DRUG INTERACTIONS:

INJECTION AND LOZENGE

Other CNS depressant drugs (*e.g.,* barbiturates, tranquilizers, narcotics and general anesthetics) will have additive or potentiating effects with fentanyl. When patients have received such drugs, the dose of fentanyl required will be less than usual. Following the administration of fentanyl citrate, the dose of other CNS depressant drugs should be reduced.

LOZENGE

For Use With Other Potent Narcotics, Please See WARNINGS Section. Oral fentanyl is not recommended for use in patients who have received MAO inhibitors within 14 days, because severe and unpredictable potentiation by MAO inhibitors has been reported with narcotic analgesics.

The particular enzyme(s) responsible for fentanyl biotransformation has (have) not been identified even though the major metabolites are well known. Because swallowed fentanyl is known to undergo extensive hepatic first-pass metabolism, oral fentanyl has the potential to have an increased bioavailability in the presence of an inhibitor of drug metabolism (*e.g.,* a food component or another drug). Caution should therefore be exercised in such cases.

The combination of droperidol and oral fentanyl results in a significantly delayed awakening (the combination of droperidol and oral fentanyl doubled the awakening time after surgery from that of oral fentanyl alone).

DRUG INTERACTIONS: *(cont'd)*

Nitrous oxide has been reported to produce cardiovascular depression when given with higher doses of IV fentanyl.

ADVERSE REACTIONS:

INJECTION

As with other narcotic analgesics, the most common serious adverse reactions reported to occur with fentanyl are respiratory depression, apnea, rigidity and bradycardia: if these remain untreated, respiratory arrest, circulatory depression or cardiac arrest could occur. Other adverse reactions that have been reported are hypertension, hypotension, dizziness, blurred vision, nausea, emesis, laryngospasm and diaphoresis.

It has been reported that secondary rebound respiratory depression may occasionally occur postoperatively. Patients should be monitored for this possibility and appropriate countermeasures taken as necessary.

When a tranquilizer such as droperidol is used with fentanyl citrate, the following adverse reactions can occur: chills and/or shivering, restlessness and postoperative hallucinatory episodes (sometimes associated with transient periods of mental depression); extrapyramidal symptoms (dystonia, akathisia and oculogyric crisis) have been observed up to 24 hours postoperatively. When they occur, extrapyramidal symptoms can usually be controlled with anti-parkinson agents. Postoperative drowsiness is also frequently reported following the use of droperidol.

LOZENGE

The safety of oral fentanyl has been formally evaluated across a broad range of doses in a total of 825 patients in clinical trials. THE PRIMARY ADVERSE EVENT OF CONCERN IS OPIOID-INDUCED HYPOVENTILATION, THE SEVERITY OF WHICH IS RELATED TO THE PATIENT'S AGE, PHYSICAL CONDITION, THE DOSE EMPLOYED, AND THE CLINICAL SETTING.

Ventilatory response to oral fentanyl was examined over doses ranging from 5 to 25 µg/kg in both clinical and pharmacokinetic studies. Hypoventilation, usually defined as either desaturation (85 to 90%) or by clinical observation, was the most common potentially serious adverse event and occurred during the first 30 minutes following administration in 6% of patients (14% of adults and 5% of children) participating in clinical trials investigating premedication.

Desaturation and/or hypoventilation was generally dose-related, occurring in 0 to 7% of children across the dose range of 5 to 20 µg/kg and 25 to 42& of adults across the dose range of 5 to 15 µg/kg.

The hypoventilation observed in clinical studies was usually mild, owing in part to prompt response by the monitoring physician, usually responding to gentle stimulation or administration of oxygen. Cases of serious hypoventilation (delayed onset of respirations, and apnea) were observed but were uncommon under the conditions of the clinical trials (8 of 825 cases). All cases of apnea involved doses greater than 15 µg/kg and readily responded to a single dose of naloxone.

Doses above 15 µg/kg are contraindicated regardless of age, and doses above 5 µg/kg (400 µg maximum regardless of weight) are contraindicated in adults, because of this excessive frequency of significant hypoventilation at higher doses.

Besides hypoventilation, other dose-related adverse events occurring in the first 30 minutes following administration in premedication studies included flushing in adults and pruritus in children. Pruritus occurred in over half of the cases studied, and was manifested by the children touching their face and/or complaining of mild itching. Urticaria or generalized pruritus was uncommon.

Common Adverse Events (>1% probably causally related): The following adverse events were reported at a frequency of 1% or more in 189 patients who received oral fentanyl as premedication in anesthesia or in monitored anesthetic care settings at the recommended doses. No adjustment has been made for the rate at which events were observed in placebo treated patients, for causality, or for severity. It should be noted that the reported adverse events include the intraoperative and postoperative period for patients undergoing surgery.

Body as a Whole: headache

Cardiovascular: bradycardia, flushing*, hypertension, pallor, ventricular extrasystole

Digestive: nausea (17%), vomiting (34%),

Nervous: apathy, dizziness (15%), euphoria*, paresthesia

Respiratory: hypoventilation (11%)

Skin: pruritus (56%), rash

Special Senses: vision abnormality

(%) = adverse reaction above 10%;

(*) = adverse reactions 3-9%; all others 1-3%

Uncommon Adverse Events Related to Oral Fentanyl (<1% probably causally related): The following adverse events occurred in less than 1% of patients who received oral fentanyl in the recommended doses, or were only observed in patients who were studied outside the recommended dosage range and indication (N=636).

Body as a Whole: asthenia, hypertonia, spasm

Digestive: anorexia, dyspepsia, dysphagia, gastrointestinal disorder

Musculoskeletal: myasthenia

Nervous: agitation, anxiety, confusion, dry mouth, emotional lability, miosis, somnolence, speech disorder, stupor, urinary retention, vertigo

Respiratory: airway obstruction, apnea, exacerbation of asthma

Skin: urticaria

Special Senses: accommodation abnormality

Uncommon Adverse Events (<1% Relationship Unknown): The following adverse events were uncommon, usually occurred during or after surgery, and their relationship to oral fentanyl is unknown. They are provided as alerting information for the physician.

Body as a Whole: abdominal pain, anaphylactoid reaction, back pain, chest pain, chills, fever

Cardiovascular: bigeminy, tachycardia, ventricular fibrillation

Metabolism and Nutrition: dehydration, hypoglycemia

Musculoskeletal: myalgia

Nervous: abnormal dreams, dystonia, hostility, hypertension, hysteria, nystagmus, twitch

Respiratory: dyspnea, hiccup, increase cough, laryngismus, pharyngitis, rhinitis, voice alteration

Special Senses: ear disorder, lacrimation disorder, photo phobia, perverse taste

DRUG ABUSE AND DEPENDENCE:

INJECTION

Fentanyl citrate injection is a Schedule II controlled drug substance that can produce drug dependence of the morphine type and, therefore, has the potential for being abused.

DRUG ABUSE AND DEPENDENCE: *(cont'd)*

LOZENGE

Fentanyl (the active ingredient in oral fentanyl) is a controlled substance listed in Schedule II by the Drug Enforcement Administration. Fentanyl can produce drug dependence of the morphine type and therefore, has the potential for being abused. The handling of oral fentanyl should be managed to minimize the risk of diversion, including restriction of access and accounting procedures as appropriate to the clinical setting and as required by law.

OVERDOSAGE:

INJECTION

Manifestations: The manifestations of fentanyl overdosage are an extension of its pharmacologic actions (see CLINICAL PHARMACOLOGY) as with other opioid analgesics. The intravenous $LD_{50}$of fentanyl is 3 mg/kg in rats, 1 mg/kg in cats, 14 mg/kg in dogs and 0.03 mg/kg in monkeys.

Treatment: In the presence of hypoventilation or apnea, oxygen should be administered and respiration should be assisted or controlled as indicated. A patent airway must be maintained; an oropharyngeal airway or endotracheal tube might be indicated. If depressed respiration is associated with muscular rigidity, an intravenous neuromuscular blocking agent might be required to facilitate assisted or controlled respiration. The patient should be carefully observed for 24 hours; body warmth and adequate fluid intake should be maintained. If hypotension occurs and is severe or persists, the possibility of hypovolemia should be considered and managed with appropriate parenteral fluid therapy. A specific narcotic antagonist such as nalorphine or naloxone should be available for use as indicated to manage respiratory depression. This does not preclude the use of more immediate countermeasures. The duration of respiratory depression following overdosage of fentanyl may be longer than the duration of narcotic antagonist action. Consult the package insert of the individual narcotic antagonists for details about use.

LOZENGES

Manifestations: The manifestations of oral fentanyl overdosage are expected to be similar to IV fentanyl and are an extension of its pharmacologic actions (see CLINICAL PHARMACOLOGY).

Treatment: Management of severe oral fentanyl overdose includes: securing a patent airway, assisting or controlling ventilation, establishing intravenous access, use of naloxone or other opioid antagonists, and GI decontamination with lavage and/or activated charcoal once the patient's airway is secure. In the presence of hypoventilation or apnea, oxygen should be administered and respiration should be assisted or controlled as indicated. Fentanyl may cause muscle rigidity, particularly involving the muscles of respiration. Although muscle rigidity interfering with respiration has not been seen following the use of oral fentanyl, this is always possible with fentanyl and other opioids. If it occurs, it should be managed by the use of assisted or controlled respiration, by an opioid antagonist, and as a final alternative, by a neuromuscular blocking agent.

The patient should be carefully observed and appropriately managed until his or her condition is well controlled. The duration of respiratory depression following overdosage of fentanyl may be longer than the duration of narcotic antagonist action. Consult the package insert of the individual narcotic antagonists for details about such use.

Dialysis is not likely to be effective because of the large volume of distribution and high lipid solubility of fentanyl.

DOSAGE AND ADMINISTRATION:

INJECTION

50 µg = 0.05 mg = 1 ml

Dosage should be individualized. Some of the factors to be considered in determining the dose are age, body weight, physical status, underlying pathological condition, use of other drugs, type of anesthesia to be used and the surgical procedure involved. Dosage should be reduced in elderly or debilitated patients (see PRECAUTIONS).

Vital signs should be monitored routinely.

I. Premedication: Premedication (to be appropriately modified in the elderly, debilitated and those who have received other depressant drugs) 50 to 100 µg (0.05 to 0.1 mg) (1 to 2 ml) may be administered intramuscularly 30 to 60 minutes prior to surgery.

II. Adjunct to General Anesthesia: See Dosage Range Chart

III. Adjunct to Regional Anesthesia: 50 to 100 µg (0.05 to 0.1 mg) (1 to 2 ml) may be administered intramuscularly or slowly intravenously, over one to two minutes, when additional analgesia is required.

IV. Postoperatively (recovery room): 50 to 100 µg (0.05 to 0.1 mg) (1 to 2 ml) may be administered intramuscularly for the control of pain, tachypnea and emergence delirium. The dose may be repeated in one to two hours as needed.

V. Usage in Children: For induction and maintenance in children 2 to 12 years of age, a reduced dose as low as 2 to 3 µg/kg is recommended.

DOSAGE RANGE CHART

Total Dosage (Expressed as Fentanyl Base)

Low Dose: 2 µg/kg (0.002 mg/kg) (0.04 ml/kg). Fentanyl in small doses is most useful for minor, but painful, surgical procedures. In addition to the analgesia during surgery, fentanyl may also provide some pain relief in the immediate postoperative period.

Moderate Dose: 2 to 20 µg/kg (0.002 to 0.02 mg/kg) (0.04 to 0.4 ml/kg). Where surgery becomes more major, a larger dose is required. With this dose, in addition to adequate analgesia, one would expect to see some abolition of the stress response. However, respiratory depression will be such that artificial ventilation during anesthesia is necessary, and careful observation of ventilation postoperatively is essential.

High Dose: 20 to 50 µg/kg (0.02 to 0.05 mg/kg) (0.4 to 1 ml/kg). During open heart surgery and certain more complicated neurosurgical and orthopedic procedures where surgery is more prolonged, and in the opinion of the anesthesiologist, the stress response to surgery would be detrimental to the well being of the patient, dosages of 20 to 50 µg/kg (0.02 to 0.05 mg/kg) (0.4 to 1 ml/kg) of fentanyl with nitrous oxide oxygen have been shown to attenuate the stress response as defined by increased levels of circulating growth hormone, catecholamine, ADH and prolactin. When dosages in this range have been used during surgery, postoperative ventilation and observation are essential due to extended post-operative respiratory depression. The main objective of this technique would be to produce "stress free" anesthesia.

DOSAGE RANGE CHART

Maintenance Dose

Low Dose: 2 µg/kg (0.002 mg/kg) (0.04 ml/kg). Additional dosages of fentanyl are infrequently needed in these minor procedures.

Moderate Dose: 2-20 µg/kg (0.002 to 0.02 mg/kg) (0.04 to 0.4 ml/kg). 25 to 100 µg (0.025 to 0.1 mg) (0.5 to 2 ml) may be administered intravenously or intramuscularly when movement and/or changes in vital signs indicate surgical stress or lightening of analgesia.

DOSAGE AND ADMINISTRATION: *(cont'd)*

High Dose: 20 to 50 µg/kg (0.02 to 0.05 mg/kg) (0.4 to 1 ml/kg). Maintenance dosage (ranging from 25 µg (0.025 mg) (0.5 ml) to one half the initial loading dose) will be dictated by the changes in vital signs which indicate stress and lightening of analgesia. However, the additional dosage selected must be individualized especially if the anticipated remaining operative time is short.

AS A GENERAL ANESTHETIC

When attenuation of the responses to surgical stress is especially important, doses of 50 to 100 µg/kg (0.05 to 0.1 mg/kg) (1 to 2 ml/kg) may be administered with oxygen and a muscle relaxant. This technique has been reported to provide anesthesia without the use of additional anesthetic agents. In certain cases, doses up to 150 µg/kg (0.15 mg/kg) (3 ml/kg) may be necessary to produce this anesthetic effect. It has been used for open heart surgery and certain other major surgical procedures in patients for whom protection of the myocardium from excess oxygen demand is particularly indicated, and for certain complicated neurological and orthopedic procedures.

As noted above, it is essential that qualified personnel and adequate facilities be available for the management of respiratory depression.

See WARNINGS and PRECAUTIONSfor use of fentanyl with other CNS depressants, and in patients with altered response.

Parenteral drug products should be inspected visually for particulate matter and discoloration prior to administration, whenever solution and container permit.

PROTECT FROM LIGHT. STORE AT ROOM TEMPERATURE 15°C-30°C (59°F-86°F).

LOZENGE

WARNING: BEFORE PRESCRIBING THIS PRODUCT, PLEASE NOT THE FOLLOWING INSTRUCTIONS ON THE PROPER USE OF THIS PRODUCT:

Oral fentanyl should only be administered in hospital settings such as the operating room, emergency department, ICU, or other monitored anesthesia care settings in hospitals where there is immediate access to life support, equipment, including oxygen, facilities for endotracheal intubation, intravenous fluids, and opioid antagonists. Oral fentanyl must be given only to patients being monitored by both (1) direct visual observation by a health professional whose sole responsibility is observation of the patient and also by (2) some means of measuring respiratory function such as pulse oximetry until they are completely recovered.

Oral fentanyl should only be administered by persons specifically trained in the use of anesthetic drugs and the management of the respiratory effects of potent opioids, including respiratory and cardiac resuscitation of patients in the age group being treated. Such training must include the establishment and maintenance of a patent airway and assisted ventilation.

Oral fentanyl should only be used by health care practitioners credentialed to use the product by the director of anesthesia of the institution in which the product will be used.

See also BOXED WARNING, CLINICAL PHARMACOLOGY, INDICATIONS AND USAGE, and PRECAUTIONS.

DOSES SHOULD BE INDIVIDUALIZED BASED UPON THE STATUS OF EACH PATIENT, THE CLINICAL ENVIRONMENT, AND THE DESIRED THERAPEUTIC EFFECT. DOSAGE SHOULD BE REDUCED IN ELDERLY, DEBILITATED OR OTHER VULNERABLE PATIENTS (SEE PRECAUTIONS).

Some of the factors to be considered in determining an individualized dose are age, body weight, physical status, general condition and medical status, underlying pathological condition, use of other drugs, type of anesthesia, and the type and length of the procedure.

Oral fentanyl doses of 5 µg/kg provide effects similar to the usual doses of fentanyl given IM (0.75-1.25 µg/kg). Larger doses have not been shown to increase efficacy. As with all opioids, the dosage should be reduced in vulnerable patients (see PRECAUTIONS). The magnitude of the expected effect will vary from mild with doses of 5 µg/kg to marked with doses of 15 µg/kg. Adults should not receive doses larger than 5 µg/kg (400 µg), and most children not apprehensive at onset may be managed with the same 5 µg/kg dose. Children apprehensive at onset, and some younger children may need doses of 5 to 15 µg/kg, with an attendant increased risk of hypoventilation.

I: Normal Children: Because of the excessive frequency of significant hypoventilation at higher doses, doses above 15 µg/kg (maximum dose 400 µg) are contraindicated in children.

Selection of dosage strength based on patient weight with a dose range of 5 to 15 µg/kg is recommended. Premedication of children below 40 kg may require doses of 10 to 15 µg/kg (TABLE 2).

TABLE 2

Patient Weight Kilograms (kilos)	5 to 10 µg/kg	10 to 15 µg/kg
<15 kilograms	contraindicated	contraindicated
15 kilos	not available	200 µg
20 kilos	200 µg	200 or 300 µg
25 kilos	200 µg	300 µg
30 kilos	300 µg	300 or 400 µg
35 kilos	300 µg	400 µg
40 kilos and over	400 µg	Use 400 µg (seeSection II Normal Adults)

II. Normal Adults: Because of the excessive frequency of significant hypoventilation at higher doses, doses above 5 µg/kg (maximum dose 400 µg) are contraindicated in adults.

III. Vulnerable Patients: Selection of a lower dose should be considered for vulnerable patients, for example: patients with head injury, cardiovascular or pulmonary disease, hepatic disease, or liver dysfunction. If signs of excessive opioid effects appear before the unit is consumed, the dosage unit should be removed from the patient's mouth immediately.

IV. Elderly Patients: If oral fentanyl is to used in patients over age 65, the dose should be reduced to 2.5 to 5 µg/kg. Although studies of oral fentanyl in the elderly has not been conducted, elderly patients have been shown to be twice as sensitive to the effects of other forms of fentanyl as the younger population. Like all potent opioid analgesics, oral fentanyl has the ability to depress respiration and reduce ventilatory drive to a clearly significant extent.

Administration of Oral Fentanyl: The foil overwrap should be removed just prior to administration. After the plastic overcap is removed, the patient should be instructed to place the oral fentanyl unit in his/her mouth and to suck (not chew) it. Chewed or swallowed fentanyl contributes little to the peak concentration, but is responsible for a prolonged "tail" on the blood level profile as it is slowly absorbed.

The oral fentanyl unit should be removed, using the handle, after it is consumed or if the patient has achieved an adequate effect and/or shows signs of respiratory depression. Place any remaining portion of the oral fentanyl unit in the plastic overcap and dispose of the unit appropriately as for Schedule II drugs.

Administration of the oral fentanyl unit should begin 20 to 40 minutes prior to the anticipated need of desired effect. Patients typically take 10 to 20 minutes for complete consumption. Peak effect occurs approximately 20 to 30 minutes after the start of oral

DOSAGE AND ADMINISTRATION: *(cont'd)*

fentanyl administration. In the event that hypoventilation or some other adverse event occurs before the dosage unit is consumed, the unit should be removed from the patient's mouth immediately.

The patient should be attended at all times by a health care professional skilled in airway management and resuscitative measures. Oral fentanyl should be administered only in monitored settings and by persons specifically trained in the use of anesthetics and the management of respiratory effects of potent opioids, including maintenance of a patent airway and assisted ventilation. Some means for measuring respiratory function is recommended, such as pulse oximetry (see BOXED WARNING).

SAFETY AND HANDLING

Oral fentanyl is supplied in individually sealed dosage forms that pose no known risk to health care providers having incidental dermal contact. Accidental dermal exposure to oral fentanyl should be treated by rinsing the affected area with cool water.

Oral fentanyl should be protected from freezing and moisture. Do not store above 30°C (86°F). Store in the protective foil pouch until dispensing. Do not use if the foil pouch has been opened.

Cases of self-administration of fentanyl by health care professionals, including fatalities, have been reported with all fentanyl products. The handling of oral fentanyl should be managed to minimize the risk of diversion, including restriction of access to the appropriate clinical use setting and accounting procedures as required by law.

DISPOSAL OF FENTANYL ORALET

The disposal of Schedule II controlled substances must be consistent with State and Federal Regulations. In general, the following procedure is recommended.

Remove the drug matrix from the handle by grasping it with tissue paper and separate the drug matrix from the handle using a twisting motion. Then flush the drug down the toilet. If any drug matrix remains on the handle, it may be removed by placing the handle under warm running tap water until the remaining portion of the drug matrix is dissolved. The drug-free handle should be disposed of according to institutional protocol. During the disposal process, avoid contact of the drug matrix with the skin, eyes, or mucous membranes. Wash hands thoroughly when complete.

HOW SUPPLIED:

LOZENGE

Fentanyl Oralet (oral transmucosal fentanyl citrate) is supplied in three dosage strengths. Each unit is individually wrapped in protective foil. Each dosage unit has a characteristic red raspberry coated lozenge, but the different doses can be distinguished via color highlighted labels as follows: 200 μg fentanyl base (Yellow), 300 μg fentanyl base (Green), 400 μg fentanyl base (Blue).**Note: Colors are a secondary aid in product identification. Please be sure to confirm the printed dosage before dispensing.**

Store in protective foil pouch at controlled room temperature 15- 30°C (59-86°F) until dispensing.

(Injection: Janssen, 9/92 7614106; Lozenge: Abbott 6/94, 93-3246-20)

HOW SUPPLIED - RATED THERAPEUTICALLY EQUIVALENT:

Injection, Solution - Intramuscular; - 0.05 mg/ml

2 ml	$3.81	Fentanyl Citrate, Abbott	00074-9093-32
2 ml	$7.66	Fentanyl Citrate, Abbott	00074-9094-22
2 ml	$23.14	FENTANYL CITRATE, Abbott	00074-9095-12
2 ml x 10	$9.35	Fentanyl Citrate, Sanofi Winthrop	00024-0682-02
2 ml x 10	$20.63	Fentanyl Citrate, Elkins Sinn	00641-1116-33
5 ml	$7.02	Fentanyl Citrate, Abbott	00074-9093-35
5 ml	$14.00	Fentanyl Citrate, Abbott	00074-9094-25
5 ml x 10	$16.07	Fentanyl Citrate, Sanofi Winthrop	00024-0682-05
5 ml x 10	$37.81	Fentanyl Citrate, Elkins Sinn	00641-1117-33
10 ml	$13.44	Fentanyl Citrate, Abbott	00074-9093-36
10 ml	$13.44	Fentanyl Citrate, Abbott	00074-9094-28
10 ml	$159.72	FENTANYL CITRATE 50 MCG/ML, Abbott	00074-9096-01
10 ml x 5	$35.50	Fentanyl Citrate, Elkins Sinn	00641-1118-34
10 ml x 10	$19.43	FENTANYL CITRATE 50 MCG/ML, Abbott	00074-9096-10
20 ml	$26.36	Fentanyl Citrate, Abbott	00074-9093-38
20 ml	$26.36	Fentanyl Citrate, Abbott	00074-9094-31
20 ml x 5	$69.88	Fentanyl Citrate, Elkins Sinn	00641-1119-34
20 ml x 10	$38.81	FENTANYL CITRATE 50 MCG/ML, Abbott	00074-9096-20
20 ml x 10	$319.44	Fentanyl Citrate, Abbott	00074-9096-02
30 ml	$20.00	FENTANYL CITRATE, Elkins Sinn	00641-2402-41
50 ml	$25.00	FENTANYL CITRATE, Elkins Sinn	00641-2403-41
50 ml	$65.91	Fentanyl Citrate, Abbott	00074-9094-61

HOW SUPPLIED - NOT RATED EQUIVALENT:

Lozenge - Topical; Oral - 200 mcg

1's	$27.99	FENTANYL ORALET, Abbott	00074-2444-05

Lozenge - Topical; Oral - 300 mcg

1's	$27.99	FENTANYL ORALET, Abbott	00074-2445-05

Lozenge - Topical; Oral - 400 mcg

1's	$27.99	FENTANYL ORALET, Abbott	00074-2446-05

Powder

1 gm	$1227.50	Fentanyl Citrate, Mallinckrodt	00406-0662-52

FERRIC SUBSULFATE *(001259)*

CATEGORIES: Pharmaceutical Adjuvants; FDA Pre 1938 Drugs

Prescribing information not available at time of publication.

HOW SUPPLIED - EQUIVALENTS NOT AVAILABLE:

Solution

480 ml	$18.95	Ferric Subsulfate, Millgood	53118-0313-10
500 ml	$16.96	Ferric Subsulfate, Mallinckrodt	00406-5548-03

FERROUS GLUCONATE *(001273)*

CATEGORIES: Antianemia Drugs; Blood Formation/Coagulation; Deficiency Anemias; Homeostatic & Nutrient; Hyperlipidemia; Iron Preparations; FDA Pre 1938 Drugs

BRAND NAMES: *Anemicon; Apo-Ferrous Gluconate* (Canada); *Duroferon; Ercofer; Eryfer; Fefol; Femas; Fenarol; Feospan; Feovit; Fergon; Fergon Elixir; Ferinsol; Feritard; Fermate; Ferral; Ferramat; Ferranina; Ferraton; Ferro 15; Ferro 23; Ferro-Agepha; Ferroblan; Ferrocontin; Ferroglukonat* (Germany); *Ferrokapsul; Ferromax; Ferromikron; Ferrone; Ferronicum; Ferrous Gluconate Sussex; Ferrum; Fersaday; Fersamal; Fertinic* (Canada); *Ferumat; Fesofor; Fespan; Folic; Forcil; Foscofer; Fumafer; Galfer; Glucoferron; Gluferricon; Losferron; Moliron; Novoferrogluc* (Canada); *Novofumar; Orafer; Palafer; Plancaps; Plesmet; Plexafer; Sulfato (International brand names outside U.S. in italics)*

FORMULARIES: Aetna

Prescribing information not available at time of publication.

HOW SUPPLIED - EQUIVALENTS NOT AVAILABLE:

Elixir - Oral

480 ml	$10.20	Ferrous Gluconate, Liquipharm	54198-0143-16

FERROUS SULFATE CACODYLATE *(001277)*

CATEGORIES: Antianemia Drugs; Blood Formation/Coagulation; Iron Preparations; Multivitamins; Vitamins

BRAND NAMES: Octron

Prescribing information not available at time of publication.

HOW SUPPLIED - EQUIVALENTS NOT AVAILABLE:

Injection, Solution - Intravenous - 32.5 mg/ml

2 ml x 10	$32.00	OCTRON, AJ Bart	49326-0183-02
10 ml	$37.00	OCTRON, AJ Bart	49326-0202-10

FERROUS SULFATE; FOLIC ACID; VITAMIN C *(001282)*

CATEGORIES: Antianemia Drugs; Blood Formation/Coagulation; Deficiency Anemias; Iron Preparations; FDA Pre 1938 Drugs

BRAND NAMES: Polytinic

FORMULARIES: Aetna; BC-BS

Prescribing information not available at time of publication.

HOW SUPPLIED - EQUIVALENTS NOT AVAILABLE:

Tablet, Plain Coated - Oral - 304 mg/1 mg/300

100's	$13.82	POLYTINIC, Pharmics	00813-0043-01

FERROUS SULFATE; LIVER EXTRACT; VITAMIN B COMPLEX *(001283)*

CATEGORIES: Antianemia Drugs; Blood Formation/Coagulation; Deficiency Anemias; Liver/Stomach Preparations; FDA Pre 1938 Drugs

BRAND NAMES: Ferlivit; Ferro-Cyte; Primaplex; Thiahep

Prescribing information not available at time of publication.

HOW SUPPLIED - EQUIVALENTS NOT AVAILABLE:

Injection, Solution - Intramuscular - 20 mg/225 mg/50

30 ml	$5.20	THIAHEP, Lannett	00527-0117-58

FERROUS SULFATE; VITAMIN B COMPLEX *(001290)*

CATEGORIES: Anabolic Steroids; Blood Formation/Coagulation; Deficiency Anemias; Homeostatic & Nutrient; Hormones; Multivitamins; Multivitamins W/Minerals; Vitamins; FDA Pre 1938 Drugs

BRAND NAMES: Fero-Vita; Ferro-B; Senilezol; Siderol; Tega-Atric; Vitamed-Im

Prescribing information not available at time of publication.

HOW SUPPLIED - EQUIVALENTS NOT AVAILABLE:

Elixir - Oral - 15 %/5 mg/5 mg/

480 ml	$14.00	SENILEZOL, Edwards Pharms	00485-0038-01

Injection, Solution - Intramuscular - 1.25 mg/15 mcg/

30 ml	$3.60	VITAMED-IM, Med Tek Pharms	52349-0116-30

FEXOFENADINE HYDROCHLORIDE *(003294)*

CATEGORIES: Allergies; Antihistamines; Non-Sedating Antihistamines; Respiratory & Allergy Medications; Rhinitis; Pregnancy Category C; FDA Approved 1996 Jul

BRAND NAMES: **Allegra**

PRIMARY ICD9: 477.9 (Allergic Rhinitis, Cause Unspecified)

DESCRIPTION:

Fexofenadine HCl, the active ingredient of Allegra is a histamine H_1-receptor antagonist with the chemical name (±)-4-[1-hydroxy-4-[4(hydroxydiphenylmethyl)-1—piperidinyl]—butyl]-α,α—dimethyl benzeneacetic acid hydrochloride. The molecular weight is 538.13 and the empirical formula is $C_{32}H_{39}NO_4$·HCl. Fexofenadine HCl is a white to off-white crystalline powder. It is freely soluble in methanol and ethanol, slightly soluble in chloroform and water, and insoluble in hexane. Fexofenadine HCl is a racemate and exists as a zwitterion in aqueous media at a physiological pH.

Fexofenadine HCl is formulated as capsules for oral administration. Each capsule contains 60 mg fexofenadine HCl and the following excipients: croscarmellose sodium, gelatin, lactose, microcrystalline cellulose, and pregelatinized starch. The printed capsule shell is made from gelatin, iron oxide, silicon dioxide, sodium lauryl sulfate, titanium dioxide, and other ingredients.

CLINICAL PHARMACOLOGY:

MECHANISM OF ACTION

Fexofenadine, a metabolite of terfenadine, is an antihistamine with selective peripheral H_1-receptor antagonist activity. Fexofenadine inhibited antigen-induced bronchospasm in sensitized guinea pigs and histamine release from peritoneal mast cells in rats. In laboratory animals, no anticholinergic or alpha$_1$-adrenergic-receptor blocking effects were observed. Moreover, no sedative or other central nervous system effects were observed. Radiolabeled tissue distribution studies in rats indicated that fexofenadine does not cross the blood-brain barrier.

PHARMACOKINETICS

Fexofenadine HCl was rapidly absorbed following oral administration of a single dose of two 60 mg capsules to healthy male volunteers with a mean time to maximum plasma concentration occurring at 2.6 hours postdose. After administration of a single 60 mg dose as an oral solution to healthy subjects, the mean plasma concentration was 209 ng/ml. Mean steady-state peak plasma concentrations of 286 ng/ml were observed when healthy volunteers were administered multiple doses of fexofenadine HCl (60 mg oral solution every 12 hours for 10 doses). Fexofenadine pharmacokinetics were linear for oral doses up to 120 mg twice daily. Although the absolute bioavailability of fexofenadine HCl capsules is unknown, the capsules are bioequivalent to an oral solution. The mean elimination half-life of fexofenadine was 14.4 hours following administration of 60 mg, twice daily, to steady-state in normal volunteers.

Human mass balance studies documented a recovery of approximately 80% and 11% of the [^{14}C] fexofenadine HCl dose in the feces and urine, respectively. Approximately 5% of the total dose was metabolized. Because the absolute bioavailability of fexofenadine HCl has not been established, it is unknown if the fecal component represents unabsorbed drug or the result of biliary excretion. The pharmacokinetics of fexofenadine HCl in seasonal allergic rhinitis patients were similar to those in healthy subjects. Peak fexofenadine plasma concentrations were similar between adolescent (12-16 years of age) and adult patients.

Fexofenadine is 60% to 70% bound to plasma proteins, primarily albumin and α_1-acid glycoprotein.

SPECIAL POPULATIONS

Special population pharmacokinetics (for age and renal hepatic impairment), obtained after a single dose of 80 mg fexofenadine HCl, were compared to those from normal subjects in a separate study of similar design. While subject weights were relatively uniform between studies, these special population patients were substantially older than the healthy, young volunteers. Thus, an age effect may be confounding the pharmacokinetic differences observed in some of the special populations.

Effect of Age: In older subjects ($\geq$65 years old), peak plasma levels of fexofenadine were 99% greater than those observed in normal volunteers (<65 years old). Mean elimination half-lives were similar to those observed in normal volunteers.

Renally Impaired: In patients with mild (creatinine clearance 41-80 ml/min) to severe (creatinine clearance 11-40 ml/min) renal impairment, peak plasma levels of fexofenadine were 87% and 111% greater, respectively, and mean elimination half-lives were 59% and 72% longer, respectively, than observed in normal volunteers. Peak plasma levels in patients on dialysis (creatinine clearance $\leq$10 ml/min) were 82% greater and half-life was 31% longer than observed in normal volunteers. Based on increases in bioavailability and half-life, a dose of 60 mg once daily is recommended as the starting dose in patients with decreased renal function (see DOSAGE AND ADMINISTRATION.)

Hepatically Impaired: The pharmacokinetics of fexofenadine HCl in patients with hepatic disease did not differ substantially from that observed in healthy subjects.

Effect of Gender: Across several trials, no clinically significant gender-related differences were observed in the pharmacokinetics of fexofenadine.

PHARMACODYNAMICS

Wheal and Flare: Human histamine skin wheal and flare studies following single and twice daily doses of 20 mg and 40 mg fexofenadine HCl demonstrated that the drug exhibits an antihistamine effect by 1 hour, achieves maximum effect at 2-3 hours, and an effect is still seen at 12 hours. There was no evidence of tolerance to these effects after 28 days of dosing.

Effects on QTc: In dogs, (10 mg/kg/day, orally for 5 days) and rabbits (10 mg/kg, intravenously over one hour) fexofenadine did not prolong QTc at plasma concentrations that were at least 28 and 63 times, respectively, the therapeutic plasma concentrations in man (based on a 60 mg twice daily fexofenadine HCl dose). No effect was observed on calcium channel current, delayed K^+ channel current, or action potential duration in guinea pig myocytes, Na^+ current in rat neonatal myocytes, or on the delayed rectifier K^+channel cloned from human heart at concentrations up to 1×10^5 M of fexofenadine. This concentration was at least 32 times the therapeutic plasma concentration in man (based on a 60 mg, twice daily fexofenadine HCl dose). No statistically significant increase in mean QTc interval compared to placebo was observed in 714 seasonal allergic rhinitis patients given fexofenadine HCl capsules in doses of 60 mg to 240 mg twice daily for two weeks or in 40 healthy volunteers given fexofenadine HCl as an oral solution at doses up to 400 mg twice daily for 6 days.

CLINICAL STUDIES:

In three, 2-week, multi-center, randomized, double-blind, placebo-controlled trials in patients 12-68 years of age with seasonal allergic rhinitis (n=1634), fexofenadine HCl 60 mg twice daily significantly reduced total symptom scores (the sum of the individual scores for sneezing, rhinorrhea, itchy nose/palate/throat, itchy/watery/red eyes) compared to placebo. Statistically significant reductions in symptom scores were observed following the first 60 mg dose, with the effect maintained throughout the 12 hour interval. In general, there was no additional reduction in total symptom scores with higher doses of fexofenadine up to 240 mg twice daily. Although the number of subjects in some of the subgroups was small, there were no significant differences in the effect of fexofenadine HCl across subgroups of patients defined by gender, age, and race. Onset of action for reduction in total symptom scores, excluding nasal congestion, was observed at 60 minutes compared to placebo following a single 60 mg fexofenadine HCl dose administered to patients with seasonal allergic rhinitis who were exposed to ragweed pollen in an environmental exposure unit.

INDICATIONS AND USAGE:

Fexofenadine HCl is indicated for the relief of symptoms associated with seasonal allergic rhinitis in adults and children 12 years of age and older. Symptoms treated effectively include sneezing, rhinorrhea, itchy nose/palate/throat, itchy/watery/red eyes.

CONTRAINDICATIONS:

Fexofenadine HCl is contraindicated in patients with known hypersensitivity to any of its ingredients.

PRECAUTIONS:

CARCINOGENESIS, MUTAGENESIS, AND IMPAIRMENT OF FERTILITY

The carcinogenic potential and reproductive toxicity of fexofenadine HCl were assessed using terfenadine studies with adequate fexofenadine exposure (based on plasma area-under-the-curve [AUC] values). No evidence of carcinogenicity was observed when mice and rats were

PRECAUTIONS: *(cont'd)*

given daily oral doses of 50 and 150 mg/kg of terfenadine for 18 and 24 months, respectively; these doses resulted in plasma AUC values of fexofenadine that were up to four times the human therapeutic value (based on a 60 mg twice-daily fexofenadine HCl dose).

In *in vitro* Bacterial Reverse Mutation, CHO/HGPRT Forward Mutation, and Rat Lymphocyte Chromosomal Aberration assays) and *in vivo* (Mouse Bone Marrow Micronucleus assay) tests, fexofenadine HCl revealed no evidence of mutagenicity.

In rat fertility studies, dose-related reductions in implants and increases in postimplantation losses were observed at oral doses equal to or greater than 150 mg/kg of terfenadine, these doses produced plasma AUC values or fexofenadine that were equal to or greater than three times the human therapeutic value (based on a 60 mg twice-daily fexofenadine HCl dose).

PREGNANCY CATEGORY C

Teratogenic Effects: There was no evidence of teratogenicity in rats or rabbits at oral terfenadine doses up to 300 mg/kg; these doses produced fexofenadine plasma AUC values that were up to 4 and 37 times the human therapeutic value (based on a 60 mg twice-daily fexofenadine HCl dose), respectively.

There are no adequate and well-controlled studies in pregnant women. Fexofenadine HCl should be used during pregnancy only if the potential benefit justifies the potential risk to the fetus.

Nonteratogenic Effects: Dose-related decreases in pup weight gain and survival were observed in rats exposed to oral doses equal to and greater than 150 mg/kg of terfenadine; at these doses the plasma AUC values of fexofenadine were equal to or greater than 3 times the human therapeutic values (based on a 60 mg twice-daily fexofenadine HCl dose).

NURSING MOTHERS

There are no adequate and well-controlled studies in women during lactation. Because many drugs are excreted in human milk, caution should be exercised when fexofenadine HCl is administered to a nursing woman.

PEDIATRIC USE

Safety and effectiveness of fexofenadine in pediatric patients under the age of 12 years have not been established. Across well-controlled clinical trials in patients with seasonal allergic rhinitis, a total of 205 patients between the ages of 12 and 16 years received doses ranging from 20 mg to 240 mg twice daily for up to two weeks. Adverse events were similar in this group compared to patients above the age of 16 years.

GERIATRIC USE

In placebo-controlled trials, 42 patients, age 60 to 68 years, received doses of 20 mg to 240 mg of fexofenadine twice daily for up to two weeks. Adverse events were similar in this group to patients under age 60 years.

DRUG INTERACTIONS:

In two separate studies, fexofenadine HCl 120 mg twice daily (twice the recommended dose) was co-administered with erythromycin 500 mg every 8 hours or ketoconazole 400 mg once daily under steady-state conditions to normal, healthy volunteers (n=24, each study). No differences in adverse events or QTc interval were observed when subjects were administered fexofenadine HCl alone or in combination with erythromycin or ketoconazole. The findings of these studies are summarized in TABLE 1.

TABLE 1 Effects on Steady-State Fexofenadine Pharmacokinetics After 7 Days of Co-Administration with Fexofenadine HCl 120 mg Every 12 Hours (twice recommended dose) in Normal Human Volunteers (n=24)

Concomitant Drug	C_{max} SS(Peak Plasma Concentration)	AUC_{SS}(0-12*h*) (Extent of Systemic Exposure)
Erythromycin (500 mg every 8 hours)	+82%	+109%
Ketoconazole (400 mg once daily)	+135%	+164%

The mechanisms of these interactions are unknown, and the potential for interaction with other azole antifungal or macrolide agents has not been studied. These changes in plasma levels were within the range of plasma levels achieved in adequate and well-controlled clinical trials. Fexofenadine had no effect on the pharmacokinetics of erythromycin or ketoconazole.

ADVERSE REACTIONS:

In placebo controlled clinical trials, which included 2461 patients receiving fexofenadine HCl at doses of 20 mg to 240 mg twice daily, adverse events were similar in fexofenadine HCl and placebo-treated patients. The incidence of adverse events, including drowsiness, was not dose related and was similar across subgroups defined by age, gender, and race. The percent of patients who withdrew prematurely because of adverse events was 2.2% with fexofenadine HCl vs 3.3% with placebo. All adverse events that were reported by greater than 1% of patients who received the recommended daily dose of fexofenadine HCl (60 mg twice-daily), and that were more common with fexofenadine than placebo, are listed in TABLE 2.

TABLE 2 Adverse Experiences Reported In Placebo-Controlled Seasonal Allergic Rhinitis Clinical Trials at Rates of Greater Than 1%

Adverse Experience	Fexofenadine 60 mg Twice Daily (n=679)	Placebo (n=671)
Viral Infection (cold, flu)	2.5%	1.5%
Nausea	1.6%	1.5%
Dysmenorrhea	1.5%	0.3%
Drowsiness	1.3%	0.9%
Dyspepsia	1.3%	0.6%
Fatigue	1.3%	0.9%

Adverse events occurring in greater than 1% of fexofenadine HCl-treated patients (60 mg twice daily), but that were more common in the placebo-treated group, include headache and throat irritation.

The frequency and magnitude of laboratory abnormalities were similar in fexofenadine HCl and placebo-treated patients.

OVERDOSAGE:

Information regarding acute overdosage is limited to experience from clinical trials conducted during the development of fexofenadine HCl. Single doses of fexofenadine HCl up to 800 mg (6 normal volunteers at this dose level), and doses up to 690 mg twice daily for one month (3 normal volunteers at this dose level), were administered without the development of clinically significant adverse events.

In the event of overdose, consider standard measures to remove any unabsorbed drug. Symptomatic and supportive treatment is recommended.

Hemodialysis did not effectively remove fexofenadine from blood (up to 1.7% removed) following terfenadine administration.

OVERDOSAGE: *(cont'd)*

No deaths occurred at oral doses of fexofenadine HCl up to 5000 mg/kg in mice (170 times the maximum recommended human daily oral dose based on mg/m²) and up to 5000 mg/kg in rats (330 times the maximum recommended human daily oral dose based on mg/m²). Additionally, no clinical signs of toxicity or gross pathological findings were observed. In dogs, no evidence of toxicity was observed at oral doses up to 2000 mg/kg (450 times the maximum recommended human daily oral dose based on mg/m²).

DOSAGE AND ADMINISTRATION:

The recommended dose of fexofenadine is 60 mg twice daily for adults and children 12 years of age and older.

A dose of 60 mg once daily is recommended as the starting dose in patients with decreased renal function (see CLINICAL PHARMACOLOGY.)

PATIENT INFORMATION:

This medication is used for the treatment of allergies.

Inform your doctor if you have kidney disease.

Fexofenadine HCl may cause cold and flu symptoms, nausea, menstrual discomfort, drowsiness, stomach upset, and/or tiredness.

HOW SUPPLIED:

Allegra (fexofenadine HCl) capsules have a white opaque cap and a pink opaque body. The capsules are imprinted in black ink, with "60 mg" on the cap, and "1102" on the body.

Storage: Store fexofenadine HCl capsules at controlled room temperature 20°-25°C (68°-77°F). Foil-backed blister packs should be protected from excessive moisture.

HOW SUPPLIED - EQUIVALENTS NOT AVAILABLE:

Capsule - Oral - 60 mg

100's	$85.94	ALLEGRA, Hoechst Marion Roussel	00088-1102-47
100's	$85.94	ALLEGRA, Hoechst Marion Roussel	00088-1102-49
500's	$429.72	ALLEGRA, Hoechst Marion Roussel	00088-1102-55

FILGRASTIM *(003046)*

CATEGORIES: Anemia; Aplastic Anemia; Biological Response Modifiers; Bone Marrow Transplantation; Cancer; Hematopoietic Agents; Leukemia; Myelodysplastic Syndrome; Neutropenia, Chemotherapy; Neutropenia, Chronic; Orphan Drugs; AIDS Related Complex*; Pregnancy Category C; Recombinant DNA Origin; Sales > $500 Million; FDA Approved 1991 Feb

* Indication not approved by the FDA

BRAND NAMES: G-CSF; Granulocyte Colony Stimulating Factor; *Grasin*; **Neupogen**; *Neupogen 30*; *Neupogen 48*

(International brand names outside U.S. in italics)

FORMULARIES: Aetna

COST OF THERAPY: $2,132.20 (Lung Cancer; Injection; 300 mcg/ml; 1/day; 14 days)

PRIMARY ICD9: 162.9 (Malignant Neoplasm of Bronchus and Lung, Unspecified)

DESCRIPTION:

Filgrastim is a human granulocyte colony stimulating factor (G-CSF), produced by recombinant DNA technology.[1] Neupogen is the Amgen Inc. trademark for Filgrastim, which has been selected as the name for recombinant methionyl human granulocyte colony stimulating factor (r-metHuG-CSF).

Neupogen is a 175 amino acid protein manufactured by recombinant DNA technology.[1] Neupogen is produced by *Escherichia coli* (*E. coli*) bacteria into which has been inserted the human granulocyte colony stimulating factor gene. Neupogen has a molecular weight of 18,800 daltons. The protein has an amino acid sequence that is identical to the natural sequence predicted from human DNA sequence analysis, except for the addition of an N-terminal methionine necessary for expression in *E. coli*. Because Neupogen is produced in *E. coli*, the product is non-glycosylated and thus differs from G-CSF isolated from a human cell.

Neupogen is a sterile, clear, colorless, preservative-free liquid for parenteral administration. Each single-use vial of Neupogen contains 300 mcg/ml of Filgrastim at a specific activity of $1.0 \pm 0.6 \times 10^8$U/mg, (as measured by a cell mitogenesis assay). The product is formulated in a 10 mM sodium acetate buffer at pH 4.0, containing 5% mannitol, and 0.004% Tween® 80. The quantitative composition (per ml) of Neupogen is:

Filgrastim: 300 mcg
Acetate: 0.59 mg
Mannitol: 50.0 mg
Tween® 80: 0.004 %
Sodium: 0.035 mg
Water for injection:
USP q.s. ad: 1.0 ml

CLINICAL PHARMACOLOGY:

Colony Stimulating Factors: Colony stimulating factors are glycoproteins which act on hematopoietic cells by binding to specific cell surface receptors and stimulating proliferation, differentiation commitment, and some end-cell functional activation.

Endogenous G-CSF is a lineage specific colony stimulating factor which is produced by monocytes, fibroblasts and endothelial cells. G-CSF regulates the production of neutrophils within the bone marrow and affects neutrophil progenitor proliferation,[2,3] differentiation[2,4] and selected end cell functional activation (including enhanced phagocytic ability,[5] priming of the cellular metabolism associated with respiratory burst,[6] antibody dependent killing,[7] and the increased expression of some functions associated with cell surface antigens.[8] G-CSF is not species specific and has been shown to have minimal direct *in vivo* or*in vitro* effects on the production of hematopoietic cell types other than the neutrophil lineage.

Pre-Clinical Experience: Filgrastim was administered to monkeys, dogs, hamsters, rats, and mice as part of a comprehensive pre-clinical toxicology program which included both single-dose acute, repeated-dose subacute, subchronic, and chronic studies. Single-dose administration of filgrastim by the oral, intravenous, subcutaneous, or intraperitoneal routes resulted in no significant toxicity in mice, rats, hamsters, or monkeys. Although no deaths were observed in mice, rats, or monkeys at dose levels up to 3,450 mcg/kg and in hamsters using single doses up to approximately 860 mcg/kg, deaths were observed in a subchronic (13 week) study in monkeys. In this study, evidence of neurological symptoms was seen in monkeys treated with doses of filgrastim greater than 1,150 mcg/kg/day for up to 18 days. Deaths were seen in 5 of the 8 treated animals and were associated with 15- to 28-fold increases in peripheral leukocyte counts, and neutrophil-infiltrated hemorrhagic foci were seen in both the cerebrum and cerebellum. In contrast, no monkeys died following 13 weeks of daily intravenous administration of filgrastim at a dose level of 115 mcg/kg. In an ensuing 52 week study, one 115 mcg/kg dose female monkey died after 18 weeks of daily IV administration of filgrastim. Death was attributed to cardiopulmonary insufficiency.

In subacute, repeated-dose studies, changes observed were attributable to the expected pharmacological actions of filgrastim (*i.e.,* dose-dependent increases in white cell counts, increased circulating segmented neutrophils, and increased myeloid: erythroid ratio in bone marrow). In all species, histopathologic examination of the liver and spleen revealed evidence of ongoing extramedullary granulopoiesis; increased spleen weights were seen in all species and appeared to be dose-related. A dose-dependent increase in serum alkaline phosphatase was observed in rats, and may reflect increased activity of osteoblasts and osteoclasts. Changes in serum chemistry values were reversible following discontinuation of treatment.

In rats treated at doses of 1,150 mcg/kg/day for four weeks (5 of 32 animals) and for 13 weeks at doses of 100 mcg/kg/day (4 of 32 animals) and 500 mcg/kg/day (6 of 32 animals) articular swelling of the hind legs was observed. Some degree of hind leg dysfunction was also observed; however, symptoms reversed following cessation of dosing. In rats, osteoclasis and osteoanagenesis were found in the femur, humerus, coccyx, and hind legs (where they were accompanied by synovitis) after intravenous treatment for four weeks (115 to 1150 mcg/kg/day), and in the sternum after intravenous treatment for 13 weeks (115 to 575 mcg/kg/day). These effects reversed to normal within 4 to 5 weeks following cessation of treatment.

In the 52-week chronic, repeated-dose studies performed in rats (intraperitoneal injection up to 57.5 mcg/kg/day), and cynomolgus monkeys (intravenous injection of up to 115 mcg/kg/day), changes observed were similar to those noted in the subacute studies. Expected pharmacological actions of filgrastim included dose-dependent increases in white cell counts, increased circulating segmented neutrophils and alkaline phosphate levels, and increased myeloid: erythroid ratios in the bone marrow. Decreases in platelet counts were also noted in primates. In no animals tested were hemorrhagic complications observed. Rats displayed dose-related swelling of the hind limb, accompanied by some degree of hind limb dysfunction; osteopathy was noted microscopically. Enlarged spleens (both species) and livers (monkeys), reflective of ongoing extramedullary granulopoiesis, as well as myeloid hyperplasia of the bone marrow, were observed in a dose-dependent manner.

Pharmacologic Effects of Filgrastim: In Phase 1 studies involving 96 patients with various non-myeloid malignancies, filgrastim administration resulted in a dose-dependent increase in circulating neutrophil counts over the dose range of 1-70 mcg/kg/day.[9-11] This increase in neutrophil counts was observed whether filgrastim was administered intravenously (1-70 mcg/kg twice daily),[9] subcutaneously (1-3 mcg/kg/daily),[11] or by continuous subcutaneous infusion (3-11 mcg/kg/day).[10] With discontinuation of filgrastim therapy, neutrophil counts returned to baseline, in most cases within four days. Isolated neutrophils displayed normal phagocytic (measured by zymosan- stimulated chemoluminescence) and chemotactic [measured by migration under agarose using N-formyl-methionyl -leucyl-phenylamine (fMLP) as the chemotaxin] activity *in vitro.*

The absolute monocyte count was reported to increase in a dose-dependent manner in most patients receiving filgrastim, however, the percentage of monocytes in the differential count remained within the normal range. In all studies to date, absolute counts of both eosinophils and basophils did not change and were within the normal range following administration of filgrastim. Increases in lymphocyte counts following filgrastim administration have been reported in some normal subjects and cancer patients.

White blood cell differentials obtained during clinical trials have demonstrated a shift towards earlier granulocyte progenitor cells (left shift) including the appearance of promyelocytes and myeloblasts, usually during neutrophil recovery following the chemotherapy-induced nadir. In addition, Dohle bodies, increased granulocyte granulation, as well as hypersegmented neutrophils have been observed. Such changes were transient, and were not associated with clinical sequelae nor were they necessarily associated with infection.

Pharmacokinetics: Absorption and clearance of filgrastim follows first-order pharmacokinetic modeling without apparent concentration dependence. A positive linear correlation occurred between the parenteral dose and both the serum concentration and area under the concentration-time curves. Continuous intravenous infusion of 20 mcg/kg of filgrastim over 24 hours resulted in mean and median serum concentrations of approximately 48 and 56 ng/ml, respectively. Subcutaneous administration of 3.45 mcg/kg and 11.5 mcg/kg resulted in maximum serum concentrations of 4 and 49 ng/ml, respectively, within 2 to 8 hours. The volume of distribution averaged 150 ml/kg in both normal subjects and cancer patients. The elimination half-life, in both normal subjects and cancer patients, was approximately 3.5 hours. Clearance rates of filgrastim were approximately 0.5-0.7 ml/min/kg. Single parenteral doses or daily intravenous doses over a 14 day period, resulted in comparable half-lives. The half-lives were similar for intravenous administration (231 minutes, following doses of 34.5 mcg/kg) and for subcutaneous administration (210 minutes, following filgrastim doses of 3.45 mcg/kg). Continuous 24-hour intravenous infusions at 20 mcg/kg over an 11 to 20 day period produced steady state serum concentrations of filgrastim with no evidence of drug accumulation over the time period investigated.

CLINICAL STUDIES:

Cancer Patients Receiving Myelosuppressive Chemotherapy: Filgrastim has been shown to be safe and effective in accelerating the recovery of neutrophil counts following a variety of chemotherapy regimens. In a Phase 3 clinical trial in small cell lung cancer, patients received subcutaneous administration of filgrastim (4 to 8 mcg/kg/day, days 4-17) or placebo. In this study, the benefits of filgrastim therapy were shown to be prevention of infection as manifested by febrile neutropenia, decreased hospitalization, and decreased intravenous antibiotic usage. No difference in survival or disease progression was demonstrated.

In the Phase 3, randomized, double-blind, placebo-controlled trial conducted in patients with small cell lung cancer, patients were randomized to receive filgrastim (n = 99) or placebo (n = 111) starting on day 4, after receiving standard dose chemotherapy with cyclophosphamide, doxorubicin, and etoposide. A total of 210 patients were evaluated for efficacy and 207 evaluated for safety. Treatment with filgrastim resulted in a clinically and statistically significant reduction in the incidence of infection, as manifested by febrile neutropenia; the incidence of at least one infection over all cycles of chemotherapy was 76% (84/111) for placebo-treated patients, versus 40% (40/99) for filgrastim-treated patients ($p < 0.001$). The following secondary analyses were also performed. The requirements for in-patient hospitalization and antibiotic use were also significantly decreased during the first cycle of chemotherapy; incidence of hospitalization was 69% (77/111) for placebo- treated patients in cycle one, versus 52% (51/99) for filgrastim-treated patients ($p = 0.032$). The incidence of intravenous antibiotic usage was 60% (67/111) for placebo-treated patients in cycle one, versus 38% (38/99) for filgrastim-treated patients ($p = 0.003$). The incidence, severity, and duration of severe neutropenia (ANC < 500/mm³) following chemotherapy were all significantly reduced. The incidence of severe neutropenia in cycle one was 84% (83/99) for patients receiving filgrastim versus 96% (106/110) for patients receiving placebo ($p = 0.004$). Over all cycles, patients randomized to filgrastim had a 57% (286/500 cycles) rate of severe neutropenia versus 77% (416/543 cycles) for patients randomized to placebo. The median duration of severe neutropenia in cycle one was reduced from 6 days (range 0 to 10 days) for patients receiving placebo to 2 days (range 0 to 9 days) for patients receiving filgrastim ($p < 0.001$).

CLINICAL STUDIES: *(cont'd)*

The mean duration of neutropenia in cycle one was 5.64 ± 2.27 for patients receiving placebo versus 2.44 ± 1.90 for patients receiving filgrastim. Over all cycles, the median duration of neutropenia was 3 days for patients randomized to placebo versus 1 day for patients randomized to filgrastim. The median severity of neutropenia (as measured by ANC nadir) was 72/mm^3 (range 0/mm^3 - 7912/mm^3) in cycle one for patients receiving filgrastim versus 38/mm^3 (range 0/mm^3 - 9520/mm^3) for patients receiving placebo (p = 0.012). The mean severity of neutropenia in cycle one was 496/mm^3 ± 1382/mm^3 for patients receiving filgrastim versus 204/mm^3 ± 953/mm^{3}for patients receiving placebo. Over all cycles, the ANC nadir for patients randomized to filgrastim was 403/mm^3, versus 161/mm^3 for patients randomized to placebo. Administration of filgrastim resulted in an earlier ANC nadir following chemotherapy than was experienced by patients receiving placebo (day 10 versus day 12). Neupogen was well tolerated when given subcutaneously daily at doses of 4 to 8 mcg/kg for up to 14 consecutive days following each cycle of chemotherapy (see ADVERSE REACTIONS).

Several other Phase 1/2 studies, which did not directly measure the incidence of infection, but which did measure increases in neutrophils, support the efficacy of Neupogen. The regimens are presented to provide some background on the clinical experience with Neupogen. No claim regarding the safety or efficacy of the chemotherapy regimens is made. The effects of Neupogen on tumor growth or on the anti-tumor activity of the chemotherapy were not assessed. The doses of Neupogen used in these studies are considerably greater than those found to be effective in the Phase 3 study described above. Such phase 1/2 studies are summarized in TABLE 1.

TABLE 1

Type of Malignancy	Regimen	Chemotherapy Dose	No. of Pts. & Trial Phase		Filgrastim Daily Dose
Small Cell Lung Cancer	Cyclophos-phamide	1 g/m^2/day	210	3	4-8 mcg/kg
	Doxorubicin	50 mg/m^2/day			SC
		120 mg/m^2/day x3			
		q 21 days			
Small Cell Lung Cancer[11]	Ifosfamide	5 g/m^2/day	12	1/2	5.75-46 mcg/kg IV
	Doxorubicin	50 mg/m^2/day			days 4-17
	Etoposide	120 mg/m^2/day x3			
	Mesna	8 g/m^2/day			
		q 21 days			
Urothelial Cancer[12]	Methotrexate	30 mg/m^2/day x2	40	1/2	3.45-69 mcg/kg IV
	Vinblastine	3 mg/m^2/day x2			
	Doxorubicin	30 mg/m^2/day			days 4-11
	Cisplatin	70 mg/m^2/day			
		q 28 days			
Various Non- Myeloid Malignancies[13]	Cyclophos-phamide	2.5 g/m^2/day x2	18	1/2	23-69
	Etoposide	500 mg/m^2/day x3			mcg/kg[b] IV
	Cisplatin	50 mg/m^2/day x3			days 8-28
		q 28 days			
Breast/ Ovarian Cancer[14]	Doxorubicin (c)	75 mg/m^2	21	2	11.5 mcg/kg
		100 mg/m^2			days 2-9 IV
		125 mg/m^2			5.75 mcg/kg
		150 mg/m^2			days 10-12 IV
		q 14 days			
Neuroblastoma	Cyclophos-phamide	150 mg/m^2 x7	12	2	5.45-17.25
	Doxorubicin	35 mg/m^2			mcg/kg SC
	Cisplatin	90 mg/m^2			days 6-19
		q 28 days (cycles 1,3,5)[d]			

[a]Neupogen doses were those that accelerated neutrophil production. Doses which provided no additional acceleration beyond that achieved at the next lower dose are not reported.
[b]Lowest dose(s) tested in the study.
[c]Patients received doxorubicin at either 75, 100, 125 or 150 mg/m^2
[d]Cycles 2,6 = cyclophosphamide 150 mg/m^2 × 7 and etoposide 280 mg/m^2 × 3.
Cycle 4 = cisplatin 90 mg/m^2× 1 and etoposide 280 mg/m^2 × 3.

Cancer Patients Receiving Bone Marrow Transplant: In two separate randomized, controlled trials, patients with Hodgkin's and non-Hodgkin's lymphoma were treated with myeloablative chemotherapy and autologous bone marrow transplantation (ABMT). In one study (n = 54), filgrastim was administered at doses of 10 or 30 mcg/kg/day; a third treatment group in this study received no filgrastim. A statistically significant reduction in the median number of days of severe neutropenia (ANC <500/mm^3) occurred in the filgrastim -treated group versus the control group [23 days in the control group, 11 days in the 10 mcg/kg/day group, and 14 days in the 30 mcg/kg/day group, (11 days in combined treatment groups, p = 0.004)]. In the second study (n = 44, 43 patients evaluable), filgrastim was administered at doses of 10 or 20 mcg/kg/day; a third treatment group in this study received no filgrastim. A statistically significant reduction in the median number of days of severe neutropenia occurred in the filgrastim-treated group versus he control group (21.5 days in the control group and 10 days in both treatment groups, p <0.001). The number of days of febrile neutropenia was also reduced significantly in this study [13.5 days in the control group, 5 days in the 10 mcg/kg/day group, and 5.5 days in the 20 mcg/kg/day group, (5 days in the combined treatment groups, p <0.0001)]. Reductions in the number of days of hospitalization and antibiotic use were also seen, although these reductions were not statistically significant. There were no effects on red blood cell or platelet levels.

In a randomized, placebo-controlled trial, 70 patients with myeloid and non-myeloid malignancies were treated with myeloablative therapy and allogeneic bone marrow transplant followed by 300 mcg/m^2/day of a Filgrastim product. A statistically significant reduction in the median number of days of severe neutropenia occurred in the treated group versus the control group (19 days in the control group and 15 days in the treatment group, p <0.001) and time to recovery of ANC to ≥500/mm^3 (21 days in the control group and 16 days in the treatment group, p <0.001).

CLINICAL STUDIES: *(cont'd)*

In three non-randomized studies (n = 119), patients received ABMT and treatment with filgrastim. One study (n = 45) involved patients with breast cancer and malignant melanoma. A second study (n = 39) involved patients with Hodgkin's disease. The third study (n = 35) involved patients with non-Hodgkin's lymphoma, acute lymphoblastic leukemia (ALL), and germ cell tumor. In these studies, the recovery of the ANC to ≥500/mm^{3}ranged from a median of 11.5 to 13 days.

None of the conditioning regimens used in the ABMT studies included radiation therapy.

While these studies were not designed to compare survival, this information was collected and evaluated. The overall survival and disease progression of patients receiving filgrastim in these studies were similar to those observed in the respective control groups and to historical data.

PBPC Collection And Therapy In Cancer Patients: All patients in the Amgen-sponsored trials received a similar mobilization/collection regimen: filgrastim was administered for 6–7 days, with an apheresis procedure on days 5, 6 and 7 (except for a limited number of patients receiving apheresis on days 4, 6 and 8). In a non-Amgen-sponsored study, patients underwent mobilization to a target number of mononuclear cells (MNC), with apheresis starting on day 5. There are no data on the mobilization of PBPCs after days 4–5 that are not confounded by leukapheresis.

Mobilization: Mobilization of PBPC was studied in 50 heavily pre-treated patients (median number of prior chemotherapy cycles=9.5) with non-Hodgkin's lymphoma (NHL), Hodgkin's disease (HD), or acute lymphoblastic leukemia (ALL) [Amgen study 1]. CFU-GM was used as the marker for engraftable PBPC. The median CFU-GM level on each day of mobilization was determined from the data available, (CFU-GM assays were not obtained on all patients on each day of mobilization). These data are presented below.

The data from Amgen study 1 were supported by data from Amgen study 2 in which 22 pre-treated breast cancer patients (median number of prior cycles=3) were studied. Both the CFU-GM and CD34+ cells reached a maximum on day 5 at > 10–fold over baseline and then remained elevated with leukapheresis.

TABLE 2A Peripheral Blood Progenitor Cell Levels by Mobilization Day

Day	Overall Study #1 CFU-GM/ml # Samples	Median (25%, 75%)	Study #2 CFU-GM/ml # Samples	Median (25%, 75%)
Day 1	11	18 (13-62)	20	42 (15-151)
Day 2	7	22 (3-61)	n/a	n/a
Day 3	10	138 (39-364)	n/a	n/a
Day 4	18	365 (158-864)	18	576 (108-1819)
Day 5	36	781 (391-1608)	21	960 (72-1677)
Day 6	46	505 (199-1397)	22	756 (70-3486)
Day 7	37	333 (111-938)	22	597 (118-2009)
Day 8	15	383 (94-815)	12	51 (10-746)

n/a =not available

TABLE 2B Peripheral Blood Progenitor Cell Levels by Mobilization Day

Day	Study #2 # Samples	CD34$^+$ (x 10^4/ml) Median (25%, 75%)
Day 1	20	0.13 (0.02-0.66)
Day 2	n/a	n/a
Day 3	n/a	n/a
Day 4	17	2.11 (0.58-3.93)
Day 5	22	3.16 (1.08-6.11)
Day 6	22	2.67 (1.09-4.40)
Day 7	21	2.64 (0.78-4.22)
Day 8	12	1.61 (0.38-4.31)

n/a =not available

In three studies of patients with prior exposure to chemotherapy, the median CFU-GM yield in the leukapheresis product ranged from 20.9 to 32.7 x 10^4/kg body weight (n=105). In two of these studies where CD34$^+$ yields in the leukapheresis product were also determined, the median CD34$^+$ yields were 3.11 and 2.80 x 10^6/kg respectively (n=56). In an additional study of 18 chemotherapy-nave patients, the median CFU-GM yield was 123.4 x 10^4/kg.

Engraftment: Engraftment following filgrastim-mobilized PBPC is summarized for 101 patients in Table 4. In all studies a Cox regression model showed that the total number of CFU-GM and/or CD34$^+$ cells collected was a significant predictor of time to platelet recovery.

In a randomized unblinded study of patients with HD or NHL undergoing myeloablative chemotherapy (Amgen study 3), 27 patients received filgrastim-mobilized PBPC followed by filgrastim and 31 patients received ABMT followed by filgrastim. Patients randomized to the filgrastim-mobilized PBPC group compared to the ABMT group had significantly fewer days of platelet transfusions (median 6 vs. 10 days), a significantly shorter time to a sustained platelet count >20,000/mm^3 (median 16 vs. 23 days), a significantly shorter time to recovery of a sustained ANC ≥ 500/mm^3 (median 11 vs. 14 days), significantly fewer days of red blood cell transfusions (median 2 vs. 3 days) and a significantly shorter duration of post-transplant hospitalization.

TABLE 4

	Amgen-Sponsored Study 1 (N=13)	Amgen-Sponsored Study 2 (N=22)	Amgen-Sponsored Study 3 (N=27)	Non-Amgen-Sponsored Study (N=39)
Median PBPC/kg Collected:				
MNC	9.5 x 10^8	9.5 x 10^8	8.1 x 10^8	10.3 x 10^8
CD34$^+$	n/a	3.1 x 10^6	2.8 x 10^6	6.2 x 10^6
CFU-GM	63.9 x 10^4	25.3 x 10^4	32.6 x 10^4	n/a
Days to ANC ≥ 500/mm^3:				
Median	9	10	11	10
Range	8-10	8-15	9-38	7-40
Days to Plt. ≥ 20,000/mm^3:				
Median	10	12.5	16	15.5
Range	7-16	10-30	8-52	7-63

n/a =not available

Three of the 101 patients (3%) did not achieve the criteria for engraftment as defined by platelets ≥ 20,000/mm^3 by day 28. In clinical trials of filgrastim for the mobilization of PBPC, filgrastim was administered to patients at 5–24 mcg/kg/day after reinfusion of the collected cells until a sustainable ANC (≥500/mm^3) was reached. The rate of engraftment of these cells in the absence of filgrastim post-transplantation has not been studied.

CLINICAL STUDIES: *(cont'd)*

Patients with Severe Chronic Neutropenia: Severe chronic neutropenia (idiopathic, cyclic, and congenital) is characterized by a selective decrease in the number of circulating neutrophils and an enhanced susceptibility to bacterial infections.

The daily administration of filgrastim has been shown to be safe and effective in causing a sustained increase in the neutrophil count and a decrease in infectious morbidity in children and adults with the clinical syndrome of SCN[15]. In the Phase 3 trial, summarized in TABLE 5, daily treatment with filgrastim resulted in significant beneficial changes in the incidence and duration of infection, fever, antibiotic use, and propharyngeal ulcers. In this trial, 120 patients with a median age of 12 years (range 1 to 76 years) were treated.

TABLE 5 Overall Significant Changes in Clinical Endpoints; Median Incidence [a] (events) or Duration (days) per 28-day period

	Control Patients[b]	Neupogen-treated Patients	p-value
Incidence of Infection	0.50	0.20	< 0.001
Incindence of Fever	0.25	0.20	< 0.001
Duration of Fever	0.63	0.20	0.005
Incidence of Oropharyngeal Ulcers	0.26	0.00	< 0.001
Incidence of Antibiotic Use	0.49	0.20	< 0.001

[a]Incidence values were calculated for each patient, and are defined as the total number of events experienced divided by the number of 28-day periods of exposure (on-study). median incidence values were then reported for each patient group.
[b]Control patients were observed for a 4-month period.

The incidence for each of these five clinical parameters was lower in the filgrastim arm compared to the control arm for cohorts in each of the three major diagnostic categories. All three diagnostic groups showed favorable trends in favor of treatment. An analysis of variance showed no significant interaction between treatment and diagnosis, suggesting that efficacy did not differ substantially reduced neutropenia in all patient groups, in patients with cyclic neutropenia, cycling persisted but the period of neutropenia was shortened to one day.

As a result of the lower incidence and duration of infections, there was also a lower number of episodes of hospitalization [28 hospitalizations in 62 patients in the treated group versus 44 hospitalizations in 60 patients in the control group over a 4 month period (p = 0.0034)]. Patients treated with filgrastim also reported a lower number of episodes of diarrhea, nausea, fatigue, and sore throat.

In the Phase 3 trial, untreated patients had a median ANC of 210/mm^3 (range 0 - 1,550/mm^3). Filgrastim therapy was adjusted to maintain the median ANC between 1,500 and 10,000/mm^3. Overall, the response to filgrastim was observed in 1 to 2 weeks. The median ANC after five months of filgrastim therapy for all patients was 7,460/mm^3 (range 30 to 30,880/mm^3). Filgrastim dosing requirements were generally higher for patients with congenital neutropenia (2.3-40 mcg/kg/day) than for patients with idiopathic (0.6- 11.5 mcg/kg/day) or cyclic (0.5-6 mcg/kg/day) neutropenia.

INDICATIONS AND USAGE:

Cancer Patients Receiving Myelosuppressive Chemotherapy: Filgrastim is indicated to decrease the incidence of infection, as manifested by febrile neutropenia, in patients with non-myeloid malignancies receiving myelosuppressive anti-cancer drugs associated with a significant incidence of severe neutropenia with fever (see CLINICAL STUDIES). A complete blood count and platelet count should be obtained prior to chemotherapy, and twice per week (see PRECAUTIONS, Laboratory Monitoring) during filgrastim therapy to avoid leukocytosis and to monitor the neutrophil count. In Phase 3 clinical studies, filgrastim therapy was discontinued when the absolute neutrophil count (ANC) was ≥ 10,000/cubic mm after the expected chemotherapy-induced nadir.

Cancer Patients Receiving Bone Marrow Transplant (BMT): Filgrastim is indicated to reduce the duration of neutropenia and neutropenia-related clinical sequelae (*e.g.*, febrile neutropenia, in patients with non-myeloid malignancies undergoing myeloablative chemotherapy followed by marrow transplantation (see CLINICAL STUDIES). It is recommended that complete blood counts and platelet counts be obtained at a minimum of three times per week (see PRECAUTIONS, Laboratory Monitoring) following marrow infusion to monitor the recovery of marrow reconstitution.

Patients Undergoing Peripheral Blood Progenitor Cell (PBPC) Collection: Filgrastim is indicated for the mobilization of hematopoietic progenitor cells into the peripheral blood for collection by leukapheresis. Mobilization allows for the collection of increased numbers of progenitor cells capable of engraftment compared with collection by leukapheresis without mobilization or bone marrow harvest. After myeloablative chemotherapy, the transplantation of an increased number of progenitor cells can lead to more rapid engraftment, which may result in a decreased need for supportive care (see CLINICAL STUDIES).

Patients with Severe Chronic Neutropenia (SCN): Filgrastim is indicated for chronic administration to reduce the incidence and duration of sequelae of neutropenia (*e.g.*, fever, infections, oropharyngeal ulcers) in symptomatic patients with congenital neutropenia, cyclic neutropenia, or idiopathic neutropenia (see CLINICAL STUDIES). It is essential that serial complete blood cell counts with differential and platelet counts, and an evaluation of bone marrow morphology and karyotype be performed prior to initiation of filgrastim therapy. The use of filgrastim prior to confirmation of SCN may impair diagnostic efforts and may thus impair or delay evaluation and treatment of an underlying condition, other than SCN, causing the neutropenia.

CONTRAINDICATIONS:

Filgrastim is contraindicated in patients with known hypersensitivity to *E. coli* derived proteins, filgrastim, or any component of the product.

WARNINGS:

Allergic-type reactions occurring on initial or subsequent treatment have been reported in < 1 in 4,000 patients treated with filgrastim. These have generally been characterized by systemic symptoms involving at least two body systems, most often skin (rash, urticaria, facial edema), respiratory (wheezing, dyspnea), and cardiovascular (hypotension, tachycardia). Some reactions occurred on initial exposure. Reactions tended to occur within the first 30 minutes after administration and appeared to occur more frequently in patients receiving filgrastim intravenously. Rapid resolution of symptoms occurred in most cases after administration of antihistamines, steroids, bronchodilators, and/or epinephrine. Symptoms recurred in more than half the patients who were rechallenged.

Patients with Severe Chronic Neutropenia: The safety and efficacy of filgrastim in the treatment of neutropenia due to other hematopoietic disorders (*e.g.*, myelodysplastic disorders or myeloid leukopenia) have not been established. Care should be taken to confirm the diagnosis of SCN, before initiating filgrastim therapy.

While 9 of 325 patients developed myelodysplasia or myeloid leukemia while receiving filgrastim during clinical trials, acute myeloid leukemia (AML) or abnormal cytogenetics have been reported to occur in the natural history of severe chronic neutropenia without cytokine

WARNINGS: *(cont'd)*

therapy.[16] Abnormal cytogenetics have been associated with the eventual development of myeloid leukemia. The effect of filgrastim on the development of abnormal cytogenetics and the effect of continued filgrastim administration in patients with abnormal cytogenetics are unknown. If a patient with SCN develops abnormal cytogenetics, the risks and benefits of continuing filgrastim should be carefully considered (see ADVERSE REACTIONS).

PRECAUTIONS:

GENERAL

Simultaneous Use with Chemotherapy and Radiation Therapy The safety and efficacy of filgrastim given simultaneously with cytotoxic chemotherapy have not been established. Because of the potential sensitivity of rapidly dividing myeloid cells to cytotoxic chemotherapy, do not use filgrastim in the period 24 hours before to 24 hours after the administration of cytotoxic chemotherapy (see DOSAGE AND ADMINISTRATION).

The efficacy of filgrastim has not been evaluated in patients receiving chemotherapy associated with delayed myelosuppression (*e.g.*, nitrosoureas) or with mitomycin C or with myelosuppressive doses of antimetabolites such as 5-fluorouracil or cytosine arabinoside.

The safety and efficacy of filgrastim have not been evaluated in patients receiving concurrent radiation therapy. Simultaneous use of filgrastim with chemotherapy and radiation therapy should be avoided.

Growth Factor Potential: Filgrastim is a growth factor that primarily stimulates neutrophils. However, the possibility that filgrastim can act as a growth factor for any tumor type, particularly myeloid malignancies, cannot be excluded. Therefore, because of the possibility of tumor growth, precaution should be exercised in using this drug in any malignancy with myeloid characteristics.

When filgrastim is used to mobilize PBPC, tumor cells may be released from the marrow and subsequently collected in the leukapheresis product. The effect of reinfusion of tumor cells has not been well-studied, and the limited data available are inconclusive.

Leukocytosis: Cancer Patients Receiving Myelosuppressive Chemotherapy: White blood cell counts of 100,000/mm^{3}or greater were observed in approximately 2% of patients receiving Filgrastim at doses above 5 mcg/kg/day. There were no reports of adverse events associated with this degree of leukocytosis. In order to avoid the potential complications of excessive leukocytosis, a complete blood count (CBC) is recommended twice per week during filgrastim therapy (see PRECAUTIONS, Laboratory Monitoring).

Premature Discontinuation of Filgrastim Therapy: Cancer Patients Receiving Myelosuppressive Chemotherapy: A transient increase in neutrophil counts is typically seen 1 to 2 days after initiation of filgrastim therapy. However, for a sustained therapeutic response, filgrastim therapy should be continued following chemotherapy until the post nadir ANC reaches 10,000/mm^3. Therefore, the premature discontinuation of filgrastim therapy, prior to the time of recovery from the expected neutrophil nadir, is generally not recommended (see DOSAGE AND ADMINISTRATION.)

Other: In studies of filgrastim administration following chemotherapy, most reported side effects were consistent with those usually seen as a result of cytotoxic chemotherapy (see ADVERSE REACTIONS.) Because of the potential of receiving higher doses of chemotherapy (*i.e.*, full doses on the prescribed schedule), the patient may be at greater risk of thrombocytopenia, anemia, and non-hematologic consequences of increased chemotherapy doses (please refer to the prescribing information of the specific chemotherapy agents used). Regular monitoring of the hematocrit and platelet count is recommended. Furthermore, care should be exercised in the administration of filgrastim in conjunction with other drugs known to lower the platelet count. In septic patients receiving filgrastim, the physician should be alert to the theoretical possibility of adult respiratory distress syndrome, due to the possible influx of neutrophils at the site of inflammation.

There have been rare reports (<1 in 7,000 patients) of cutaneous vasculitis in patients treated with filgrastim. In most cases, the severity of cutaneous vasculitis was moderate or severe. Most of the reports involved patients with severe chronic neutropenia receiving long-term filgrastim im therapy. Symptoms of vasculitis generally developed simultaneously with an increase in the ANC and abated when the ANC decreased. Many patients were able to continue filgrastim at a reduced dose.

INFORMATION FOR THE PATIENT

In those situations in which the physician determine that the patient can safely and effectively self-administer filgrastim, the patient should be instructed as to the proper dosage and administration. Patients should be referred to the "Information for Patients" labeling included with the Package Insert in each dispensing carton of filgrastim. This patient information, however, is not intended to be a disclosure of all known or possible effects. If home use is prescribed, patients should be thoroughly instructed in the importance of proper disposal and cautioned against the reuse of needles, syringes, or drug product. A puncture-resistant container for the disposal of used syringes and needles should be available to the patient. The full container should be disposed of according to the directions provided by the physician.

LABORATORY MONITORING

Cancer Patients Receiving Myelosuppressive Chemotherapy: A CBC and platelet count should be obtained prior to chemotherapy, and at regular intervals (twice per week) during filgrastim therapy. Following cytotoxic chemotherapy, the neutrophil nadir occurred earlier during cycles when filgrastim was administered, and white blood cell differentials demonstrated a left shift, including the appearance of promyelocytes and myeloblasts. In addition, the duration of severe neutropenia was reduced, and was followed by an accelerated recovery in the neutrophil counts. Therefore, regular monitoring of white blood cell counts, particularly at the time of the recovery from the post chemotherapy nadir, is recommended in order to avoid excessive leukocytosis.

Cancer Patients Receiving Bone Marrow Transplant: Frequent complete blood counts and platelet counts are recommended (at least three times per week) following marrow transplantation.

Patients with Severe Chronic Neutropenia: During the initial four weeks of filgrastim therapy and during the two weeks following any dose adjustment, a CBC with differential and platelet count should be performed twice weekly. Once a patient is clinically stable, a CBC with differential and platelet count should be performed monthly.

In clinical trials, the following laboratory results were observed.

Cyclic fluctuations in the neutrophil counts were frequently observed in patients with congenital or idiopathic neutropenia after initiation of filgrastim therapy.

Platelet counts were generally at the upper limits of normal prior to filgrastim therapy, platelet counts decreased but usually remained within normal limits (see ADVERSE REACTIONS.)

Early myeloid forms were noted in peripheral blood in most patients, including the appearance of metamyelocytes and myelocytes. Promyelocytes and myeloblasts were noted in some patients.

Relative increases were occasionally noted in the number of circulating eosinophils and basophils. No consistent increases were observed with filgrastim therapy.

PRECAUTIONS: *(cont'd)*

As in other trials, increases were observed in serum uric acid, lactic dehydrogenase, and serum alkaline phosphatase.

Carcinogenesis, Mutagenesis, and Impairment of Fertility: The carcinogenic potential of filgrastim has not been studied. Filgrastim failed to induce bacterial gene mutations in either the presence or absence of a drug metabolizing enzyme system. Filgrastim had no observed effect on the fertility of male or female rats, or on gestation doses up to 500 mcg/kg.

Pregnancy Category C: Filgrastim has been shown to have adverse effects in pregnant rabbits when given in doses 2 to 10 times the human dose. There are no adequate and well-controlled studies in pregnant women. Filgrastim should be used during pregnancy only if the potential benefit justifies the potential risk to the fetus.

In rabbits, increased abortion and embryolethality were observed in animals treated with filgrastim at 80 mcg/kg/day. Filgrastim administered to pregnant rabbits at doses of 80 mcg/kg/day during the period of organogenesis was associated with increased fetal resorption, genitourinary bleeding, developmental abnormalities, and decreased body weight, live births, and food consumption. External abnormalities were not observed in the fetuses of dams treated at 80 mcg/kg/day. Reproductive studies in pregnant rats have shown that filgrastim was not associated with lethal, teratogenic, or behavioral effects on fetuses when administered by daily intravenous injection during the period of organogenesis at dose levels up to 575 mcg/kg/day.

In Segment III studies in rats, offspring of dams treated at >20 mcg/kg/day exhibited a delay in external differentiation (detachment of auricles and descent of testes) and slight growth retardation, possibly due to lower body weight of females during rearing and nursing. Offspring of dams treated at 100 mcg/kg/day exhibited decreased body weights at birth, and a slightly reduced four day survival rate.

Nursing Mothers: It is not known whether filgrastim is excreted in human milk. Because many drugs are excreted in human milk, caution should be exercised if filgrastim is administered to a nursing woman.

Pediatric Use: Serious long-term risks associated with daily administration of filgrastim have not been identified in pediatric patients (ages 4 months to 17 years) with SCN. Limited data from patients who were followed in the Phase 3 study for 1.5 years did not suggest alterations in growth and development, sexual maturation, or endocrine function.

The safety and efficacy in neonates and patients with auto-immune neutropenia of infancy have not been established.

In the cancer setting, 12 pediatric patients with neuroblastoma have received up to six cycles of cyclophosphamide, cisplatin, doxorubicin, and etoposide chemotherapy concurrently with filgrastim; in this population, filgrastim was well tolerated. There was one report of palpable splenomegaly associated with filgrastim therapy, however, the only consistently reported adverse event was musculoskeletal pain, which is no different from the experience in the adult population.

DRUG INTERACTIONS:

Drug interactions between filgrastim and other drugs have not been fully evaluated. Drugs which may potentiate the release of neutrophils, such as lithium, should be used with caution.

ADVERSE REACTIONS:

Cancer Patients Receiving Myelosuppressive Chemotherapy: In clinical trials including over 350 patients receiving filgrastim following non-myeloablative cytotoxic chemotherapy, most adverse experiences were the sequelae of the underlying malignancy or cytotoxic chemotherapy. In all Phase 2 and 3 trials, medullary bone pain, reported in 24% of patients, was the only consistently observed adverse reaction attributed to filgrastim therapy. This bone pain was generally reported to be of mild-to-moderate severity, and could be controlled in most patients with non-narcotic analgesics; infrequently, bone pain was severe enough to require narcotic analgesics. Bone pain was reported more frequently in patients treated with higher doses (20-100 mcg/kg/day) administered intravenously, and less frequently in patients treated with lower subcutaneous doses of filgrastim (3-10 mcg/kg/day).

In the randomized, double-blind, placebo-controlled trial of filgrastim therapy following combination chemotherapy in patients (n = 207) with small cell lung cancer, the following adverse events were reported during blinded cycles of study medication (placebo or filgrastim at 4 to 8 mcg/kg/day). Events are reported as exposure adjusted since patients remained on double-blind filgrastim a median of three cycles versus once cycle for placebo. (Table 6)

TABLE 6

Event	% of Blinded Cycles with Events: Filgrastim N = 384 patient cycles	% of Blinded Cycles with Events: Placebo N = 257 patient cycles
Nausea/Vomiting	57	64
Skeletal Pain	22	11
Alopecia	18	27
Diarrhea	14	23
Neutropenic Fever	13	35
Mucositis	12	20
Fever	12	11
Fatigue	11	16
Anorexia	9	11
Dyspnea	9	11
Headache	7	9
Cough	6	8
Skin Rash	6	9
Chest Pain	5	6
Generalized Weakness	4	7
Sore Throat	4	9
Stomatitis	5	10
Constipation	5	10
Pain (unspecified)	2	7

In this study, there were no serious, life-threatening, or fatal adverse reactions attributed to filgrastim therapy. Specifically, there were no reports of flu-like symptoms, pleuritis, pericarditis, or other major systemic reactions to filgrastim.

Spontaneously reversible elevations in uric acid, lactate dehydrogenase, and alkaline phosphatase occurred in 27% to 58% of 98 patients receiving blinded filgrastim therapy following cytotoxic chemotherapy; increases were generally mild to moderate. Transient decreases in blood pressure (<90/60 mmHg), which did not require clinical treatment, were reported in 7 of 176 patients in Phase 3 clinical studies following administration of filgrastim. Cardiac events (myocardial infarctions, arrhythmias) have been reported in 11 of 375 cancer patients receiving filgrastim in clinical studies; the relationship to filgrastim therapy is unknown. No evidence of interaction of filgrastim with other drugs was observed in the course of clinical trials (see PRECAUTIONS, Simultaneous Use With Chemotherapy and Radiation Therapy.)

There has been no evidence for the development of antibodies or of a blunted or diminished response to filgrastim in treated patients, including those receiving filgrastim daily for almost two years.

ADVERSE REACTIONS: *(cont'd)*

Cancer Patients Receiving Bone Marrow Transplant: In clinical trials, the reported adverse effects were those typically seen in patients receiving intensive chemotherapy followed by bone marrow transplantation. The most common events reported in both the control and treatment groups included stomatitis and nausea and vomiting, generally of mild-to-moderate severity and were considered unrelated to filgrastim. In the randomized studies of BMT involving 167 patients who received study drug, the following events occurred more frequently in patients treated with filgrastim than in controls: nausea (10% vs.4%), vomiting (7% vs. 3%), hypertension (4% vs. 0%), rash (12% vs. 10%), and peritonitis (2% vs. 0%). None of these events were reported by the Investigator to be related to filgrastim. One event of erythema nodosum was reported moderate in severity and possibly related to filgrastim.

Generally, adverse events observed in non-randomized studies were similar to those seen in randomized studies, occurred in a minority of patients, and were of mild to moderate severity. In one study (n = 45), three serious adverse events reported by the Investigator were considered possibly related to filgrastim. These included two events of renal insufficiency and one event of capillary leak syndrome. The relationship of these events to filgrastim remains unclear since they occurred in patients with culture-proven sepsis who were receiving potentially nephrotoxic antibiotic and/or antifungal therapy.

Cancer Patients Undergoing Filgrastim-mobilized PBPC Collection: In clinical trials, 126 patients received filgrastim for PBPC mobilization. In this setting, filgrastim was generally well tolerated. Adverse events related to filgrastim consisted primarily of mild-to-moderate musculoskeletal symptoms, reported in 44% of patients. These symptoms were predominantly events of medullary bone pain (33%). Headache was reported related to filgrastim in 7% of patients. Transient increases in alkaline phosphatase related to filgrastim were reported in 21% of the patients who had serum chemistries measured; most were mild-to-moderate.

All patients had increases in neutrophil counts during mobilization, consistent with the biological effects of trigrastim. Two patients had a white blood cell count >100,000 mm^3. No sequelae were associated with any grade of leukocytosis.

Sixty-five percent of patients had mild-to-moderate anemia and 97% of patients had decreases in platelet counts; five patients (out of 126) had decreased platelet counts to <50,000/mm^3. Anemia and thrombocytopenia have been reported to be related to leukapheresis; however, the possibility that filgrastim mobilization may contribute to anemia or thrombocytopenia has not been ruled out.

Patients with Severe Chronic Neutropenia: Mild to moderate bone pain was reported in approximately 33% of patients in clinical trials. This symptom was readily controlled with non-narcotic analgesics. Generalized musculoskeletal pain was also noted in higher frequency in patients treated with filgrastim. Palpable splenomegaly was observed in approximately 30% of patients. Abdominal or flank pain was seen infrequently and thrombocytopenia (< 50,000/mm^3) was noted in 12% of patients with palpable spleens. Fewer than 3% of all patients underwent splenectomy, and most of these had a pre-study history of splenomegaly. Fewer than 6% of patients had thrombocytopenia (< 50,000/mm^3) during filgrastim therapy, most of whom had a preexisting history of thrombocytopenia. In most cases, thrombocytopenia was managed by filgrastim dose reduction or interruption. An additional 5% of patients had platelet counts between 50,000 to 100,000/mm^3. There were no associated serious hemorrhagic sequelae in these patients. Epistaxis was noted in 15% of patients treated with filgrastim, but was associated with thrombocytopenia in 2% if patients. Anemia was reported in approximately 10% of patients, but in most cases appeared to be related to frequent diagnostic phlebotomy, chronic illness or concomitant medications. In clinical trials, myelodysplasia or myeloid leukemia was reported to have developed during filgrastim threrapy in approximately 3% of patients (9 of 3250 — see WARNINGS, Patients with Severe Chronic Neutropenia). Twelve patients from a subset of 102 who had normal cytogenetic evaluations at baseline were subsequently found to have abnormalities, including monosomy 7, on routine repeat evaluation conducted after 18 to 52 months of filgrastim therapy. It is unknown whether the development of these findings is related to chronic daily filgrastim administration or reflects the natural history of SCN. Other adverse events infrequently observed and possibly related to filgrastim therapy were: injection site reaction, rash, hepatomegaly, arthralgia, osteoporosis, cutaneous vasculitis, hematuria/proteinuria, alopecia, and exacerbation of some preexisting skin disorders (*e.g.*, psoriasis).

OVERDOSAGE:

In cancer patients receiving filgrastim as an adjunct to myelosuppressive chemotherapy, it is recommended, to avoid the potential risks of excessive leukocytosis, that filgrastim therapy be discontinued if the ANC surpasses 10,000/mm^3 after the chemotherapy-induced ANC nadir has occurred. Doses of filgrastim that increase the ANC beyond 10,000/mm^3may not result in any additional clinical benefit.

The maximum tolerated dose of filgrastim has not been determined. Efficacy was demonstrated at doses of 4-8 mcg/kg/day in the Phase 3 study of non- myeloablative chemotherapy. Patients in the BMT studies received up to 138 mcg/kg/day without toxic effects, although there was a flattening of the dose response curve above daily doses of greater than 10 mcg/kg/day.

In filgrastim clinical trials of cancer patients receiving myelosuppressive chemotherapy, white blood cell counts > 100,000/mm^3have been reported in less than 5% of patients, but were not associated with any reported adverse clinical effects.

In cancer patients receiving myelosuppressive chemotherapy, discontinuation of filgrastim therapy usually results in a 50% decrease in circulating neutrophils within 1 to 2 days, with a return to pretreatment levels in 1 to 7 days.

DOSAGE AND ADMINISTRATION:

Cancer Patients Receiving Myelosuppressive Chemotherapy: The recommended starting dose of filgrastim is 5 mcg/kg/day, administered as a single daily injection by subcutaneous bolus injection, by short intravenous infusion (15-30 minutes), or by continuous subcutaneous or continuous intravenous infusion. A CBC platelet count should be obtained before instituting filgrastim therapy, and monitored twice weekly during therapy. Doses may be increased in increments of 5 mcg/kg for each chemotherapy cycle, according to the duration and severity of the ANC nadir.

Filgrastim should be administered no earlier than 24 hours after the administration of cytotoxic chemotherapy. Filgrastim should not be administered in the period 24 hours before the administration of chemotherapy (see PRECAUTIONS.) Filgrastim should be administered daily for up to two weeks, until the ANC has reached 10,000/mm^3following the expected chemotherapy-induced neutrophil nadir. The duration of filgrastim therapy needed to attenuate chemotherapy-induced neutropenia may be dependent on the myelosuppressive potential of the chemotherapy regimen employed. Filgrastim therapy should be discontinued if the ANC surpasses 10,000/mm^3 after the expected chemotherapy-induced neutrophil nadir (see PRECAUTIONS.) In Phase 3 trials, efficacy was observed at doses of 4 to 8 mcg/kg/day.

Cancer Patients Receiving Bone Marrow Transplant: The recommended dose of filgrastim following BMT is 10 mcg/kg/day given as an IV infusion of 4 or 24 hours, or as a continuous 24-hour subcutaneous infusion. For patients receiving bone marrow transplant, the first dose of filgrastim should be administered at least 24 hours after cytotoxic chemotherapy and at least 24 hours after bone marrow infusion.

DOSAGE AND ADMINISTRATION: *(cont'd)*

During the period of neutrophil recovery, the daily dose of filgrastim should be titrated against the neutrophil response as follows (TABLE 7):

TABLE 7

Absolute Neutrophil Count	Neupogen dose adjustment
When ANC > 1,000/mm^3 for 3 consecutive days	Reduce to 5 mcg/kg/day (*see below)
then: If ANC remains > 1,000/mm^3 for 3 more consecutive days	Discontinue Neupogen
then: If ANC decreases to < 1,000/mm^3	Resume at 5 mcg/kg/day

* If ANC decreases to <1,000/mm^{3}at any time during the 5 mcg/kg/day administration, Neupogen should be increased to 10 mcg/kg/day, and the above steps should then be followed.

PBPC Collection and Therapy in Cancer Patients: The recommended dose of filgrastim for the mobilization of PBPC is 10 mcg/kg/day subcutaneously, either as a bolus or a continuous infusion. It is recommended that filgrastim be given for at least 4 days before the first leukapheresis procedure and continued until the last leukapheresis. Although the optimal duration of filgrastim administration and leukapheresis schedule have not been established, administration of filgrastim for 6 to 7 days with leukaphereses on days 5, 6 and 7 was found to be safe and effective (See CLINICAL STUDIES, Response to Filgrastim, PBPC Collection and Therapy in Cancer Patients for schedules used in clinical trials). Neutrophil counts should be monitored after 4 days of filgrastim, and filgrastim dose-modification should be considered for those patients who develop a white blood cell count > 100,000/mm^3.

In all clinical trials of filgrastim for the mobilization of PBPC, filgrastim was also administered after reinfusion of the collected cells (see CLINICAL STUDIES.)

Patients with Severe Chronic Neutropenia: Filgrastim should be administered to those patients in whom a diagnosis of congenital, cyclic, or idiopathic neutropenia has been definitively confirmed. Other diseases associated with neutropenia should be ruled out.

Starting Dose:

Congenital Neutropenia: The recommended daily starting dose is 6 mcg/kg BID subcutaneously every day.

Idiopathic or Cyclic Neutropenia: The recommended daily starting dose is 5 mcg/kg as a single injection subcutaneously every day.

Dose Adjustments: Chronic daily administration is required to maintain clinical benefit. ANC should not be used as the sole indication of efficacy. The dose should be individually adjusted based on the patients' clinical course as well as ANC. In the Phase 3 study, the target ANC was 1,500/mm^3. However, patients may experience clinical benefit with ANC's below this target range. The dose should be reduced if the ANC is persistently greater than 10,000/mm^3.

Dilution: If required, filgrastim may be diluted in 5% dextrose. Filgrastim diluted to concentrations between 5 and 15 mcg/ml should be protected from adsorption to plastic materials by addition of Albumin (Human) to a final concentration of 2 mg/ml. When diluted in 5% dextrose plus Albumin (Human), filgrastim is compatible with glass bottles, PVC and polyolefin IV bags, and polypropylene syringes.

Dilution of filgrastim to a final concentration of less than 5 mcg/ml is not recommended at any time. **Do not dilute with saline at any time; product may precipitate.**

Storage: Filgrastim should be stored in the refrigerator at 2°-8° C (36-46°F). Do not freeze. Avoid shaking. Prior to injection, filgrastim may be allowed to reach room temperature for a maximum of 24 hours. Any vial left at room temperature for greater than 24 hours should be discarded. Parenteral drug products should be inspected visually for particulate matter and discoloration prior to administration, whenever solution and container permit, if particulates or discoloration are observed, the container should not be used.

REFERENCES:

1. Zsebo KM, Cohen AM, Murdock DC, Boone TC, Inque H, Chazin VR, Hines D, and Souza LM. Recombinant human granulocyte colony-stimulating factor: Molecular and biological characterization. Immunobiol.172:175-184 (1986). **2.** Welte K, Bonilla MA, Gillio AP, et al. Recombinant human G-CSF: Effects on hematopoiesis in normal and cyclophosphamide treated primates. J. Exp. Med. 165:941-948 (1987). **3.** Duhrsen U, Villefal JL, Boyd J, et al. Effects of recombinant human granulocyte colony-stimulating factor on hematopoietic progenitor cells in cancer patients. Blood 72:2074-2081 (1988). **4.** Souza LM, Boone TC, Gabrilove J, et al. Recombinant human granulocyte colony-stimulating factor: Effects on normal and leukemic myeloid cells. Science 232:61-65 (1986). **5.** Weisbart RH, Kacena A, Schuh A, Golde DW. GM-CSF induces human neutrophil IgA-mediated phagocytosis by an IgA Fc receptor activation mechanism. Nature332:647-648 (1988). **6.** Kitagawa S, Yuo A, Souza LM, Saito M, Miura Y, Takaku F. Recombinant human granulocyte colony-stimulating factor enhances superoxide release in human granulocyte stimulated by chemotactic peptide. Biochem. Biophys. Res. Commun. 144:1143 (1987). **7.** Glaspy JA, Baldwin GC, Robertson PA, et al. Therapy for neutropenia in hairy cell leukemia with recombinant human granulocyte colony-stimulating factor. Ann. Int. Med. 109:789-795 (1988). **8.** Yuo A, Kitagawa S, Ohsaka A, et al. Recombinant human granulocyte colony-stimulating factor as an activator of human granulocytes: Potentiation of responses triggered by receptor-mediated agonists and stimulation of C3bi receptor expression and adherance.Blood74:2144-2149 (1989). **9.** Gabrilove JL, Jakubowski A, Fain K, et al. Phase I study of granulocyte colony-stimulating factor in patients with transitional cell carcinoma of the urothelium. J. Clin. Invest. 82:1454-1461 (1988). **10.** Morstyn G, Souza L, Keech J, et al. Effect of granulocyte colony-stimulating factor on neutropenia induced by cytotoxic chemotherapy. Lancet March 26:667-672 (1988). **11.** Bronchud MH, Scarffe JH, Thatcher N, et al. Phase I/II study of recombinant human granulocyte colony-stimulating factor in patients receiving intensive chemotherapy for small cell lung cancer.Br. J. Cancer 56:809-813 (1987). **12.** Gabrilove JL, Jakubowski A, Scher H, et al. Effect of granulocyte colony-stimulating factor on neutropenia and associated morbidity due to chemotherapy for transitional cell carcinoma of the urothelium. N. Engl. J. Med.318:1414-1422 (1988). **13.** Neidhart J, Mangalik A, Kohler W, et al. Granulocyte colony-stimulating factor stimulates recovery of granulocytes in patients receiving dose-intensive chemotherapy without bone-marrow transplantation. J. Clin. Oncol. 7:1685-1691 (1989). **14.** Bronchud MH, Howell A, Crowther D, et al. The use of granulocyte colony-stimulating factor to increase the intensity of treatment with doxorubicin in patients with advanced breast and ovarian cancer. Br. J. Cancer 60:121-128 (1989). **15.** Dale DC, Bonilla MA, Davis MW, et al. A randomized controlled phase III trial of recombinant human granulocyte colony-stimulating factor (Filgrastim) for treatment of severe chronic neutropenia. Blood 81:2496-2502 (1993). **16.** Schroeder TM, Kurth R. Spontaneous chromosomal breakage and high incidence of leukemia in inherited disease.Blood 37:96-112 (1971).

HOW SUPPLIED:

Neupogen : Use only one dose per vial; do not reenter the vial. Discard unused portions. Do not save unused drug for later administration.

Single-dose, preservative-free vials containing 300 mcg (1 ml) of Filgrastim (300 mcg/ml).

Single-dose, preservative-free vials containing 480 ml (1.6 ml) of Filgrastim (300 mcg/ml).**Neupogen should be stored at 2°-8° C (36°-46°s F). Do not freeze. Avoid shaking.**

HOW SUPPLIED - EQUIVALENTS NOT AVAILABLE:

Injection, Solution - Intravenous; Su - 300 mcg/ml

1 ml x 10	**$1523.00**	**NEUPOGEN, Amgen**	**55513-0347-10**
1.6 ml x 10	**$2425.00**	**NEUPOGEN, Amgen**	**55513-0348-10**

FINASTERIDE *(003078)*

CATEGORIES: Alpha Reductase Inhibitors; Benign Prostatic Hyperplasia; Prostate Enlargement; Hair Growth Stimulants*; Pregnancy Category X; FDA Class 1P ("Priority Review"); Sales > $100 Million; FDA Approved 1992 Jun
* Indication not approved by the FDA

BRAND NAMES: *Pro-Cure*; **Proscar**; *Proscar 5*
(International brand names outside U.S. in italics)

FORMULARIES: PCS

COST OF THERAPY: $713.42 (BPH; Tablet; 5 mg; 1/day; 365 days) vs. Potential Cost of $3,826.06 (Transurethral Prostatectomy)

PRIMARY ICD9: 600 ((Benign Prostatic Hypertrophy).)

DESCRIPTION:

Finasteride, a synthetic 4-azasteroid compound, is a specific inhibitor of steroid 5α-reductase, an intracellular enzyme that converts testosterone into the potent androgen 5α-dihydrotestosterone (DHT).

Finasteride is 4-azaandrost-1-ene-17-carboxamide,*N*-(1,1-dimethylethyl)-3-oxo-,(5α,17β)-. The empirical formula of finasteride is $C_{23}H_{36}N_2O_2$ and its molecular weight is 372.55.

Finasteride is a white crystalline powder with a melting point near 250°C. It is freely soluble in chloroform and in lower alcohol solvents, but is practically insoluble in water.

Finasteride tablets for oral administration are film-coated tablets that contain 5 mg of finasteride and the following inactive ingredients: docusate sodium, FD&C Blue 2 aluminum lake, hydrous lactose, hydroxypropyl cellulose LF, hydroxypropylmethyl cellulose, magnesium stearate, microcrystalline cellulose, pregelatinized starch, purified water, sodium starch glycolate, talc, titanium dioxide and yellow iron oxide.

CLINICAL PHARMACOLOGY:

Progressive enlargement of the prostate gland is often associated with urinary symptoms and a decrease in urine flow, although a precise correlation between increased gland size and symptoms has not been demonstrated. Benign prostatic hyperplasia (BPH) produces symptoms in the majority of men over the age of 50 and its prevalence increases with age.

The development of the prostate gland is dependent on the potent androgen, 5α-dihydrotestosterone (DHT). The enzyme 5α-reductase metabolizes testosterone to DHT in the prostate gland, liver and skin. DHT induces androgenic effects by binding to androgen receptors in the cell nuclei of these organs.

Finasteride is a competitive and specific inhibitor of 5α-reductase. This has been demonstrated both *in vivo* and *in vitro.* Finasteride has no affinity for the androgen receptor. In man, the 5α-reduced steroid metabolites in blood and urine are decreased after administration of finasteride.

In man, a single 5-mg oral dose of finasteride produces a rapid reduction in serum DHT con centration, with the maximum effect observed 8 hours after the first dose. The suppression of DHT is maintained throughout the 24-hour dosing interval and with continued treatment. Daily dosing of finasteride at 5 mg/day for up to 24 months has been shown to reduce the serum DHT concentration by approximately 70%. The median circulating level of testosterone increased by 10% but remained within the physiologic range.

Adult males with genetically inherited 5α-reductase deficiency also have decreased levels of DHT. Except for the associated urogenital defects present at birth, no other clinical abnormalities related to 5α-reductase deficiency have been observed in these individuals. These individuals have a small prostate gland throughout life and do not develop BPH.

In patients with BPH treated with finasteride (1-100 mg/day) for 7-10 days prior to prostatectomy, an approximate 80% lower DHT content was measured in prostatic tissue removed at surgery, compared to placebo; testosterone tissue concentration was increased up to 10 times over pretreatment levels, relative to placebo. Intraprostatic content of prostate-specific antigen (PSA) was also decreased.

In healthy male volunteers treated with Proscar for 14 days, discontinuation of therapy resulted in a return of DHT levels to pretreatment levels in approximately 2 weeks.

In patients with BPH, finasteride had no effect no circulating levels of cortisol, estradiol, prolactin, thyroid-stimulating hormone, or thyroxine. Nor did it affect the plasma lipid profile (*i.e.,* total cholesterol, low density lipoproteins, high density lipoproteins and triglycerides) of 56 patients receiving finasteride for 12 weeks. The effects of long-term administration of finasteride on the plasma lipid profile are unknown. Increases of about 10% were observed in luteinizing hormone (LH), follicle-stimulating hormone (FSH) and testosterone levels in patients receiving finasteride, but levels remained within the normal range. In healthy volunteers, treatment with finasteride did not alter the response of LH and FSH to gonadotropin-releasing hormone, indicating that the hypothalamic-pituitary -testicular axis was not affected.

PHARMACOKINETICS

Following an oral dose of ^{14}C-finasteride in man, a mean of 39% (range, 32-46%) of the dose was excreted in the urine in the form of metabolites; 57% (range, 51-64%) was excreted in the feces. The major compound isolated from urine was the monocarboxylic acid metabolite; virtually no unchanged drug was recovered. The t-butyl side chain monohydroxylated metabolite has been isolated from plasma. These metabolites possess no more than 20% of the 5α-reductase inhibitory activity of finasteride.

In a study in 15 healthy male subjects, the mean bioavailability of a 5-mg finasteride tablet was 63% (range, 34-108%), based on the ratio of AUC relative to a 5-mg intravenous dose infused over 60 minutes. Maximum finasteride plasma concentration averaged 37 ng/ml (range, 27-49 ng/ml) and was reached 1 to 2 hours postdose. The mean plasma half-life of elimination was 6 hours (range, 3-16 hours). Following the intravenous infusion, mean plasma clearance was 165 ml/min (range, 70-279 ml/min) and mean steady-state volume of distribution was 76 liters (range, 44-96 liters). In a separate study, the bioavailability of finasteride was not affected by food.

Approximately 90% of circulating finasteride is bound to plasma proteins. Finasteride has been found to cross the blood-brain barrier.

There is a slow accumulation phase for finasteride after multiple dosing. After dosing with 5 mg/day of finasteride for 17 days, plasma concentrations of finasteride were 47% and 54% higher than after the first dose in men 45-60 years old (n=12) and ≥ 70 years old (n=12), respectively. Mean trough concentrations after 17 days of dosing were 6.2 ng/ml (range, 2.4-9.8 ng/ml) and 8.1 ng/ml (range, 1.8-19.7 ng/ml), respectively in the two age groups. Although steady state was not reached in this study, mean trough plasma concentration in another study in patients with BPH (mean age, 65 years) receiving 5 mg/day was 9.4 ng/ml (range, 7.1-13.3 ng/ml; n = 22) after over a year of dosing.

The elimination rate of finasteride is decreased in the elderly, but no dosage adjustment is necessary. The mean terminal half-life of finasteride in subjects ≥ 70 years of age was approximately 8 hours (range, 6-15 hours) compared to 6 hours (range, 4-12 hours) in subjects 45-60 years of age. As a result, mean AUC (0-24 hr) after 17 days of dosing was 15% higher in subjects ≥ 70 years of age (p=0.02).

CLINICAL PHARMACOLOGY: *(cont'd)*

No dosage adjustment is necessary in patients with renal insufficiency. In patients with chronic renal impairment, with creatinine clearances ranging from 9.0 to 55 ml/min, area under the curve, maximum plasma concentration, half-life, and protein binding after a single dose of ^{14}C-finasteride were similar to values obtained in healthy volunteers. Urinary excretion of metabolites was decreased in patients with renal impairment. This decrease was associated with an increase in fecal excretion of metabolites. Plasma concentrations of metabolites were significantly higher in patients with renal impairment (based on a 60% increase in total radioactivity AUC). However, finasteride has been well tolerated in BPH patients with normal renal function receiving up to 80 mg/day for 12 weeks where exposure of these patients to metabolites would presumably be much greater.

In 16 subjects receiving finasteride 5 mg/day, finasteride concentrations in semen ranged from undetectable (<1 ng/ml) to 21 ng/ml. Based on a 5 ml ejaculate volume, the amount of finasteride in ejaculate was estimated to be less than 1/50 of the dose of finasteride (5 micrograms) that had no effect on circulating DHT levels in adults.

CLINICAL STUDIES:

TWELVE-MONTH CONTROLLED CLINICAL TRIALS

In a North American and in an international multicenter, double-blind, placebo-controlled, 12-month study in patients with BPH treated with finasteride 5 mg/day, statistically significant regression of the enlarged prostate gland was noted at the first evaluation at 3 months and was maintained during the studies (TABLE 1). In both studies, the maximum urinary flow rates showed statistically significant increases from baseline in patients treated with finasteride from week 2 throughout the 12-month studies. Compared to placebo, statistically significant increases in maximum urinary flow rates were maintained in the North American study from month 4 through 12 in patients treated with finasteride. The maximum urinary flow rates in the international study were statistically significantly greater than placebo at months 7, 8, 11 and 12 (TABLE 2).

TABLE 1

Median % Change in Prostate Volume† from Baseline

	North American Study		International Study	
	Proscar 5 mg (n=297)[a]	Placebo (n=300)[a]	Proscar 5 mg (n=246)[a]	Placebo (n=255)[a]
Baseline volume (cc)	52.1	50	45.5	41.5
	%	%	%	%
Month 3	-12.1***	-2.4	-19.1***	-6.0
Month 6	-17.4***	-2.8	-21.9***	-5.5
Month 12	-19.2***	-3.0	-24.0***	-6.1

† Prostate volume was measured by magnetic resonance imaging (N.Am.) and ultrasound (Int'l). (Prostate volume was not measured at month 9.)
[a] Enrolled at baseline
*** p<0.0001 vs placebo

TABLE 2

Mean Increases in Maximum Urinary Flow Rate (ml/sec)† from Baseline

	North American Study		International Study	
	Proscar 5 mg (n=297)	Placebo (n=300)	Proscar 5 mg (n=246)	Placebo (n=255)
Baseline flow rate (ml/sec)	9.6	9.6	9.2	8.6
Week 2	0.5*	-0.2	0.6	0.2
Month 1	0.5	0.2	0.7	0.3
Month 2	0.9*	0.3	1.1	0.6
Month 3	0.8	0.3	0.8	0.2
Month 4	1.0*	0.4	1.0	0.6
Month 5	1.0**	0.2	0.9	0.8
Month 6	0.8*	0.1	1.1	0.7
Month 7	1.2**	0.4	1.3*	0.4
Month 8	1.4***	0.3	1.3*	0.5
Month 9	1.3**	0.3	1.2	0.4
Month 10	1.5***	0.5	1.3	0.7
Month 11	1.4***	0.3	1.5**	0.4
Month 12	1.6***	0.2	1.3*	0.4

† Maximum urinary flow rates (voided volumes ≥ 150 ml) were measured with a non-invasive urinary flow meter.
* p<0.05 vs placebo, respectively
** p<0.01 vs placebo, respectively
*** p<0.001 vs placebo, respectively

Symptomatic improvement was also evaluated in these multicenter studies. Obstructive and total symptom scores were calculated based on patient responses to a validated questionnaire. The obstructive symptoms evaluated were hesitancy, feeling of incomplete bladder emptying, interruption of urinary stream, impairment of size and force of urinary stream and terminal urinary dribbling. The total symptom score also included straining to start urinary flow, dysuria, frequency of clothes wetting and urgency to urinate. On a scale of 0 (absence of all symptoms) to 36 (worst response for all symptoms), the mean baseline total symptom scores for the North American and international studies were 10.1 and 10.6, respectively.

The mean total symptom scores of patients in the North American and international studies decreased from baseline starting at week 2 of treatment with either finasteride or placebo; from week 2 the scores of the patients treated with finasteride were numerically lower than those of placebo and remained so throughout the 12-month study. These scores became statistically significantly lower than placebo (p<0.05) starting at month 7 in the international study and at month 10 in the North American study. Similar results were observed with the obstructive symptom scores.

Blinded global assessments of overall urinary function and symptoms were performed. Greater improvement in patients treated with finasteride as compared to placebo was demonstrated by both the investigator's assessment (N.Am. and Int'l, p ≤ 0.01) and the patient's own assessment (N.Am., p ≤ 0.01; Int'l, p ≤ 0.1).

In both of these 12-month studies, patients treated with finasteride 5 mg had progressively decreasing prostate volumes, increasing maximum urinary flow rates and improvement of symptoms associated with BPH, suggesting an arrest in the disease process. Controlled clinical data beyond 12 months are not available.

LONG-TERM OPEN EXTENSIONS

In long-term uncontrolled extensions of these studies in approximately 300 patients receiving finasteride 5 mg/day for 24 months, prostate volume was reduced by a median of 25.5% (base line, 52.2 cc), maximum flow rate increased by a mean of 2.2 ml/sec (baseline, 11.3 ml/sec) and the total symptom score improved by a mean of 3.4 points (baseline, 9.6 points).

In addition, regression of the enlarged prostate gland and a decrease in PSA levels were maintained in approximately 50 patients who were treated with finasteride for 36 months.

INDICATIONS AND USAGE:

Finasteride is indicated for the treatment of symptomatic benign prostatic hyperplasia (BPH). Although there is a rapid regression of the enlarged prostate gland in most treated patients, less than 50% of patients experience an increase in urinary flow and improvement in symptoms of BPH when treated with finasteride for 12 months.(See CLINICAL PHARMACOLOGY.)

The long-term effects of finasteride on the incidence of surgery, acute urinary obstruction or other complications of BPH are yet to be determined.

A minimum of 6 months treatment may be necessary to determine whether an individual will respond to finasteride. It is not possible to identify prospectively those patients who will respond.

Prior to initiating therapy with finasteride, appropriate evaluation should be performed to identify other conditions, such as infection, prostate cancer, stricture disease, hypotonic bladder or other neurogenic disorders, that might mimic BPH.

CONTRAINDICATIONS:

Finasteride is contraindicated in the following:

Hypersensitivity to any component of this medication.

Pregnancy. Finasteride is contraindicated in women who are or may become pregnant. Because of the ability of 5α-reductase inhibitors to inhibit the conversion of testosterone to DHT, finasteride may cause abnormalities of the external genitalia of a male fetus of a pregnant woman who receives finasteride. If this drug is used during pregnancy, or if pregnancy occurs while taking this drug, the pregnant woman should be apprised of the potential hazard to the male fetus.

(See also WARNINGS, Exposure of Women - Risk to Male Fetus, and PRECAUTIONS, Information for the Patient and Pregnancy.)

In female rats, low doses of finasteride administered during pregnancy have produced abnormalities of th external genitalia in male offspring.

WARNINGS:

Finasteride is not indicated for use in children (see PRECAUTIONS, Pediatric Use) or women (see also CLINICAL PHARMACOLOGY, Pharmacokinetics;WARNINGS, Exposure of Women - Risk to Male Fetus; and PRECAUTIONS, Information for the Patient and Pregnancy).

EXPOSURE OF WOMEN - RISK TO MALE FETUS

It is not known whether the amount of finasteride that could potentially be absorbed by a pregnant woman through either direct contact with crushed finasteride tablets or from the semen of a patient taking finasteride can adversely affect a developing male fetus (see CLINICAL PHARMACOLOGY, Pharmacokinetics; CONTRAINDICATIONS; and PRECAUTIONS, Information for the Patient and Pregnancy). Therefore, because of the potential risk to a male fetus, a woman who is pregnant or who may become pregnant should not handle crushed finasteride tablets; in addition, when the patient's sexual partner is or may become pregnant, the patient should either avoid exposure of his partner to semen or he should discontinue finasteride.

PRECAUTIONS:

GENERAL

Digital rectal examinations, as well as other evaluations for prostate cancer, should be performed on patients with BPH prior to initiating therapy with finasteride and periodically thereafter. Although currently not indicated for this purpose, serum PSA is being increasingly used as one of the components of the screening process to detect prostate cancer.[1] Generally, a baseline PSA >10 ng/ml (Hybritech) prompts further evaluation and consideration of biopsy; for PSA levels between 4 and 10 ng/ml, further evaluation is generally considered advisable. The physician should be aware that a baseline PSA <4 ng/ml does not exclude the diagnosis of prostate cancer.

Finasteride causes a decrease in serum PSA levels in patients with BPH even in the presence of prostate cancer (see Drug/Laboratory Test Interactions). This reduction of PSA levels should be considered when evaluating PSA laboratory data and does not suggest a beneficial effect of finasteride on prostate cancer. In controlled clinical trials finasteride did not appear to alter the rate of prostate cancer detection.

Any sustained increases in PSA levels while on finasteride should be carefully evaluated, including consideration of non-compliance to therapy with finasteride (see Drug/Laboratory Test Interactions).

Since not all patients demonstrate a response to finasteride, patients with a large residual urinary volume and/or severely diminished urinary flow should be carefully monitored for obstructive uropathy. These patients may not be candidates for this therapy.

Caution should be used in the administration of finasteride in those patients with liver function abnormalities, as finasteride is metabolized extensively in the liver.

INFORMATION FOR THE PATIENT

Crushed finasteride tablets should not be handled by a woman who is pregnant or who may become pregnant because of the potential for absorption of finasteride and the subsequent potential risk to the male fetus. Similarly, when the patient's sexual partner is or may become pregnant, the patient should either avoid exposure of his partner to semen or he should discontinue finasteride (see CLINICAL PHARMACOLOGY, Pharmacokinetics; WARNINGS, Exposure of Women - Risk to Male Fetus; and PRECAUTIONS, Pregnancy).

Physicians should inform patients that the volume of ejaculate may be decreased in some patients during treatment with finasteride. This decrease does not appear to interfere with normal sexual function. However, impotence and decreased libido may occur in patients treated with finasteride (see ADVERSE REACTIONS, Twelve, Month Controlled Clinical Trials.

Physicians should instruct their patients to read the patient package insert before starting therapy with finasteride and to reread it each time the prescription is renewed so that they are aware of current information for patients regarding finasteride.

DRUG/LABORATORY TEST INTERACTIONS

When PSA laboratory determinations are evaluated, consideration should be given to the fact that PSA levels are decreased in patients treated with finasteride. In controlled clinical trials in patients with BPH treated with finasteride, PSA levels decreased from baseline by a median of 41% (95% confidence interval of the median: 38-45%) at month 6 and by a median of 48% (95% confidence interval of the median: 45-52%) at month 12.

CARCINOGENESIS, MUTAGENESIS, AND IMPAIRMENT OF FERTILITY

No evidence of a tumorigenic effect was observed in a 24-month study in Sprague-Dawley rats receiving doses of finasteride up to 160 mg/kg/day in males and 320 mg/kg/day in females. These doses produced respective systemic exposure in rats of 111 and 274 times those observed in man receiving the recommended human dose of 5 mg/day. All exposure calculations were based on calculated AUC(0-24hr) for animals and mean AUC(0-24hr) for man (0.4 mcg* hr/ml).

PRECAUTIONS: *(cont'd)*

In a 19-month carcinogenicity study in CD-1 mice, a statistically significant ($p \leq 0.05$) increase in the incidence of testicular Leydig cell adenomas was observed at a dose of 250 mg/kg/day (228 times the human exposure). In mice at a dose of 25 mg/kg/day (23 times the human exposure, estimated) and in rats at a dose of ≥ 40 mg/kg/day (39 times the human exposure) an increase in the incidence of Leydig cell hyperplasia was observed. A positive correlation between the proliferative changes in the Leydig cells and an increase in serum LH levels (2-3 fold above control) has been demonstrated in both rodent species treated with high doses of finasteride. No drug-related Leydig cell changes were seen in either rats or dogs treated with finasteride for 1 year at doses of 20 mg/kg/day and 45 mg/kg/day (30 and 350 times, respectively, the human exposure) or in mice treated for 19 months at a dose of 2.5 mg/kg/day (2.3 times the human exposure, estimated).

No evidence of mutagenicity was observed in an *in vitro* bacterial mutagenesis, assay, a mammalian cell mutagenesis assay, or in an *in vitro* alkaline elution assay. In an *in vitro* chromosome aberration assay, when Chinese hamster ovary cells were treated with high concentrations (450-550 µmol) of finasteride, there was a slight increase in chromosome aberrations. These concentrations correspond to 4000-5000 times the peak plasma levels in man given a total dose of 5 mg. Further, the concentrations (450-550 µmol) used in *in vitro* studies are not achievable in a biological system. In an *in vivo* chromosome aberration assay in mice, no treatment-related increase in chromosome aberration was observed with finasteride at the maximum tolerated dose of 250 mg/kg/day (228 times the human exposure) as determined in the carcinogenicity studies.

In sexually mature male rabbits treated with finasteride at 80 mg/kg/day (543 times the human exposure) for up to 12 weeks, no effect on fertility, sperm count, or ejaculate volume was seen. In sexually mature male rats treated with 80 mg/kg/day of finasteride (61 times the human exposure), there were no significant effects on fertility after 6 or 12 weeks of treatment; however, when treatment was continued for up to 24 or 30 weeks, there was an apparent decrease in fertility, fecundity and an associated significant decrease in the weights of the seminal vesicles and prostate. All these effects were reversible within 6 weeks of discontinuation of treatment. No drug-related effect on testes or on mating performance has been seen in rats or rabbits. This decrease in fertility in finasteride-treated rats is secondary to its effect on accessory sex organs (prostate and seminal vesicles) resulting in failure to form a seminal plug. The seminal plug is essential for normal fertility in rats and is not relevant in man.

PREGNANCY CATEGORY X

(See CONTRAINDICATIONS.) Finasteride is not indicated for use in women.

Administration of finasteride to pregnant rats at doses ranging from 100 mcg/kg/day to 100 mg/kg/day (1-1000 times the recommended human dose) resulted in dose-dependent development of hypospadias in 3.6 to 100% of male offspring. Pregnant rats produced male offspring with decreased prostatic and seminal vesicular weights, delayed preputial separation and transient nipple development when given finasteride at ≥30 mcg/kg/day (≥3/10 of the recommended human dose) and decreased anogenital distance when given finasteride at ≥3 mcg/kg/day (≥3/100 of the recommended human dose). The critical period during which these effects can be induced in male rats has been defined to be days 16-17 of gestation. The changes described above are expected pharmacological effects of drugs belonging to the class of 5α-reductase inhibitors and are similar to those reported in male infants with a genetic deficiency of 5α-reductase. No abnormalities were observed in female offspring exposed to any dose of finasteride *in utero*.

No developmental abnormalities have been observed in first filial generation (F_1) male or female offspring resulting from mating finasteride-treated male rats (80 mg/kg/day; 61 times the human exposure) with untreated females. Administration of finasteride at 3 mg/kg/day (30 times the recommended human dose) during the late gestation and lactation period resulted in slightly decreased fertility in F_1 male offspring. No effects were seen in female offspring. No evidence of malformations has been observed in rabbit fetuses exposed to finasteride *in utero* from days 6-18 of gestation at doses up to 100 mg/kg/day (1000 times the recommended human dose). However, effects on male genitalia would not be expected since the rabbits were not exposed during the critical period of genital system development.

NURSING MOTHERS

Finasteride is not indicated for use in women.

It is know whether finasteride is excreted in human milk.

PEDIATRIC USE

Finasteride is not indicated for use in children.

Safety and effectiveness in children have not been established.

DRUG INTERACTIONS:

Antipyrine: Antipyrine is used as a model for drugs that are metabolized by the same isoenzymatic cytochrome P450 system. In 12 subjects receiving finasteride 10 mg/day for 28 days, Proscar had no effect on the pharmacokinetic parameters of antipyrine or its metabolites.

Propranolol: In 19 normal volunteers receiving finasteride 5 mg/day for 10 days. Finasteride did not affect the beta-adrenergic blocking activity or plasma concentration of propranolol enantiomers after a single dose of propranolol.

Digoxin: In 17 normal volunteers receiving finasteride 5 mg/day for 10 days, concomitant administration of multiple doses of finasteride and a single dose of digoxin resulted in no effect on plasma concentrations of digoxin and its immunoreactive metabolites.

Theophylline: In 12 normal volunteers receiving finasteride 5 mg/day for 8 days, finasteride significantly increased theophylline clearance by 7% and decreased its half-life by 10% after intravenous administration of aminophylline. These changes were not clinically significant.

Warfarin: In 12 patients chronically treated with warfarin, the prothrombin times and plasma concentrations of warfarin enantiomers were not altered after treatment with finasteride 5 mg/day for 14 days.

Other Concomitant Therapy: Although specific interaction studies were not performed, finasteride was concomitantly used in clinical studies with α-blockers, angiotensin-converting enzyme (ACE) inhibitors, analgesics, anti-convulsants, beta-adrenergic blocking agents, diuretics, calcium channel blockers, cardiac nitrates, HMG-CoA reductase inhibitors, nonsteroidal anti-inflammatory drugs (NSAIDs), benzodiazepines, H_2 antagonists and quinolone antiinfectives without evidence of clinically significant adverse interactions.

ADVERSE REACTIONS:

Finasteride is generally well tolerated; adverse reactions usually have been mild and transient.

TWELVE-MONTH CONTROLLED CLINICAL TRIALS

In North American and international clinical trials, 543 patients were treated with 5 mg of finasteride for 12 months. Seven of these patients (1.3%) were discontinued due to adverse experiences that were considered to be possibly, probably or definitely drug-related; only 1 of these patients (0.2%) discontinued therapy with finasteride because of a sexual adverse experience.

ADVERSE REACTIONS: *(cont'd)*

The following clinical reactions were reported as possibly, probably or definitely drug-related in ≥1% patients treated for 12 months with 5 mg/day of finasteride or placebo, respectively: impotence (3.7%, 1.1%), decreased libido (3.3%, 1.6%), decreased volume of ejaculate (2.8%, 0.9%).

The adverse experience profile for an additional 547 patients treated with 1 mg/day of finasteride of 12 months was similar to that observed in patients treated for 12 months with 5 mg/day of finasteride.

LONG-TERM OPEN EXTENSIONS

The adverse experience profile for approximately 300 patients who were maintained on finasteride 5 mg/day for 24 months was similar to that observed in the controlled studies. In addition, a similar treated with finasteride 5 mg/day for 36 months.

OVERDOSAGE:

Patients have received single doses of finasteride up to 400 mg and multiple doses of finasteride up to 80 mg/day for three months without adverse effects. Until further experience is obtained, no specific treatment for an overdose with finasteride can be recommended.

Significant lethality was observed in male and female mice at single oral doses of 1500 mg/m² (500 mg/kg) and in female and male rats at single oral doses of 2360 mg/m² (400 mg/kg) and 5900 mg/m² (1000 mg/kg), respectively.

DOSAGE AND ADMINISTRATION:

The recommended dose is 5 mg once a day.

Although early improvement may be seen, at least 6 to 12 months of therapy with finasteride may be necessary in some patients to assess whether a beneficial response has been achieved. Periodic follow-up evaluations should be performed to determine whether a clinical response has occurred.

Finasteride may be administered with or without meals.

No dosage adjustment is necessary for patients with renal impairment or for the elderly (see CLINICAL PHARMACOLOGY, Pharmacokinetics).

REFERENCES:

1 Catalona, W.J.; Smith, D.S.; Ratliff, T.I.; Dodds, K.M.; Coplen, M.D.; Yuan, J.J.J.; Petros, J.A.; Andriole, G.L.; Measurement of prostate-specific antigen in serum as a screening test for prostate cancer, N. Eng. J. Med. 324(17): 1156-1161, April 25, 1991.

HOW SUPPLIED:

Storage and Handling: Store at room temperatures below 30°C (86°F). Protect from light and keep container tightly closed.

If the film coating of Proscar has been broken (*e.g.,* crushed), the tablets should not be handled by a woman who is pregnant or who may become pregnant because of the potential for absorption of finasteride and the subsequent potential risk to a male fetus (see CLINICAL PHARMACOLOGY, Pharmacokinetics; WARNINGS, Exposure of Women - Risk to Male Fetus; and PRECAUTIONS, Information for the Patient, and Pregnancy).

(Merck, 9/92, 7735801, 78598/180992)

HOW SUPPLIED - EQUIVALENTS NOT AVAILABLE:

Tablet, Plain Coated - Oral - 5 mg

30's	$58.64	PROSCAR, Merck	00006-0072-31
100's	$195.46	PROSCAR, Merck	00006-0072-28
100's	$195.46	PROSCAR, Merck	00006-0072-58

FLAVOXATE HYDROCHLORIDE *(001297)*

CATEGORIES: Antispasmodics; Dysuria; Genitourinary Muscle Relaxant; Muscle Relaxants; Relaxants/Stimulants, Urinary Tract; Smooth Muscle Relaxants; Urethrocystitis; Urethrotrigonitis; Urinary Tract Infections; FDA Approval Pre 1982

BRAND NAMES: *Baduson*; *Bladderon* (Japan); *Flavogen*; *Fucotin*; *Genurin*; *Harnin* (Japan); *Patricin* (Japan); *Spagerin*; *Spasuret* (Germany); *Spasuri*; *Tonlin*; *Uclean*; *Urispadol*; **Urispas**; *Urispas (200 mg)* (Canada); *Uronid*; *Uroxate*; *Yungken*
(International brand names outside U.S. in italics)

FORMULARIES: Aetna

DESCRIPTION:

Urispas (brand of flavoxate HCl) tablets contain flavoxate hydrochloride, a synthetic urinary tract spasmolytic.

Chemically, flavoxate hydrochloride is 2-piperidinoethyl 3-methyl-4-oxo-2-phenyl-4H-1-benzopyran-8-carboxylate hydrochloride. The empirical formula of flavoxate hydrochloride is: $C_{24}H_{25}NO_4 \cdot HCl$. The molecular weight is 427.94.

Urispas is supplied in tablets for oral administration. Each round, white, film-coated Urispas tablet is debossed URISPAS SKF and contains flavoxate hydrochloride, 100 mg. Inactive ingredients consist of calcium phosphate, castor oil, cellulose acetate phthalate, magnesium stearate, polyethylene glycol, starch and talc.

CLINICAL PHARMACOLOGY:

Flavoxate hydrochloride counteracts smooth muscle spasm of the urinary tract and exerts its effect directly on the muscle.

In a single study of 11 normal male subjects, the time to onset of action was 55 minutes. The peak effect was observed at 112 minutes. 57% of the flavoxate HCl was excreted in the urine within 24 hours.

INDICATIONS AND USAGE:

Flavoxate HCl is indicated for symptomatic relief of dysuria, urgency, nocturia, suprapubic pain, frequency and incontinence as may occur in cystitis, prostatitis, urethritis, urethrocystitis/urethrotrigonitis. Flavoxate HCl is not indicated for definitive treatment, but is compatible with drugs for the treatment of urinary tract infections.

CONTRAINDICATIONS:

Flavoxate HCl is contraindicated in patients who have any of the following obstructive conditions: pyloric or duodenal obstruction, obstructive intestinal lesions or ileus, achalasia, gastrointestinal hemorrhage, and obstructive uropathies of the lower urinary tract.

WARNINGS:

Flavoxate HCl should be given cautiously in patients with suspected glaucoma.

PRECAUTIONS:

INFORMATION FOR THE PATIENT

Patients should be informed that if drowsiness and blurred vision occur they should not operate a motor vehicle or machinery or participate in activities where alertness is required.

CARCINOGENESIS, MUTAGENESIS, AND IMPAIRMENT OF FERTILITY

Mutagenicity studies and long-term studies in animals to determine the carcinogenic potential of Urispas (flavoxate HCl) have not been performed.

PREGNANCY, TERATOGENIC EFFECTS, PREGNANCY CATEGORY B

Reproduction studies have been performed in rats and rabbits at doses up to 34 times the human dose and revealed no evidence of impaired fertility or harm to the fetus due to flavoxate HCl. There are, however, no well-controlled studies in pregnant women. Because animal reproduction studies are not always predictive of human response, this drug should be used during pregnancy only if clearly needed.

NURSING MOTHERS

It is not known whether this drug is excreted in human milk. Because many drugs are excreted in human milk, caution should be exercised when Urispas is administered to a nursing woman.

PEDIATRIC USE

Safety and effectiveness in children below the age of 12 years have not been established.

ADVERSE REACTIONS:

The following adverse reactions have been observed, but there are not enough data to support an estimate of their frequency.

Gastrointestinal: Nausea, vomiting, dry mouth.

CNS: Vertigo, headache, mental confusion, especially in the elderly, drowsiness, nervousness.

Hematologic: Leukopenia (1 case which was reversible upon discontinuation of the drug).

Cardiovascular: Tachycardia and palpitation.

Allergic: Urticaria and other dermatoses, eosinophilia and hyperpyrexia.

Ophthalmic: Increased ocular tension, blurred vision, disturbance in eye accommodation.

Renal: Dysuria.

OVERDOSAGE:

The oral LD_{50} for flavoxate HCl in rats in 4273 mg/kg. The oral LD_{50} for flavoxate HCl in mice in 1837 mg/kg.

It is not known whether flavoxate HCl is dialyzable.

DOSAGE AND ADMINISTRATION:

Adults and children over 12 years of age: One or two 100 mg tablets 3 or 4 times a day. With improvement of symptoms, the dose may be reduced. This drug cannot be recommended for infants and children under 12 years of age because safety and efficacy have not been demonstrated in this age group.

HOW SUPPLIED:

Urispas (flavoxate HCl) tablets, 100 mg, in bottles of 100 and in Single Unit Packages of 100 (intended for institutional use only).

HOW SUPPLIED - EQUIVALENTS NOT AVAILABLE:

Tablet, Plain Coated - Oral - 100 mg

100's	$75.20	URISPAS, SKB Pharms	00007-5290-20
100's	$77.55	URISPAS, SKB Pharms	00007-5290-21

FLECAINIDE ACETATE *(001299)*

CATEGORIES: Antiarrhythmic Agents; Arrhythmia; Atrial Fibrillation; Cardiovascular Drugs; Heart Disease; Heart Flutter; Tachycardia; Pregnancy Category C; FDA Approved 1985 Oct; Patent Expiration 1992 Aug

BRAND NAMES: *Almarytm*; *Apocard*; *Corflene*; *Flecaine* (France); *Tabco*; **Tambocor** *(International brand names outside U.S. in italics)*

FORMULARIES: Aetna; BC-BS

COST OF THERAPY: $490.56 (Arrhythmia; Tablet; 50 mg; 2/day; 365 days) vs. Potential Cost of $3,462.83 (Arrhythmia)

DESCRIPTION:

Tambocor (flecainide acetate) is an antiarrhythmic drug available in tablets of 50, 100, or 150 mg for oral administration.

Flecainide acetate is benzamide, N-(2-piperidinyl-methyl)-2, 5-bis(2,2,2-trifluoroethoxy)-monoacetate.

Flecainide acetate is a white crystalline substance with a pK_a of 9.3. It has an aqueous solubility of 48.4 mg/ml at 37°C.

Tambocor tablets also contain: croscarmellose sodium, hydrogenated vegetable oil, magnesium stearate, microcrystalline cellulose and starch.

CLINICAL PHARMACOLOGY:

Flecainide Acetate has local anesthetic activity and belongs to the membrane stabilizing (Class 1) group of antiarrhythmic agents; it has electrophysiologic effects characteristic of the IC class of antiarrhythmics.

Electrophysiology: In humans, Flecainide Acetate produces a dose-related decrease in intracardiac conduction in all parts of the heart with the greatest effect on the His-Purkinje system (H-V conduction). Effects upon atrioventricular (AV) nodal conduction time and intra-atrial conduction times, although present, are less pronounced than those on ventricular conduction velocity. Significant effects on refractory periods were observed only in the ventricle. Sinus node recovery times (corrected) following pacing and spontaneous cycle lengths are somewhat increased. This latter effect may become significant in patients with sinus node dysfunction. (See WARNINGS.)

Flecainide Acetate causes a dose-related and plasma-level related decrease in single and multiple PVCs and can suppress recurrence of ventricular tachycardia. In limited studies of patients with a history of ventricular tachycardia, Flecainide Acetate has been successful 30-40% of the time in fully suppressing the inducibility of arrhythmias by programmed electrical stimulation. Based on PVC suppression, it appears that plasma levels of 0.2 to 1.0 mcg/ml may be needed to obtain the maximal therapeutic effect. It is more difficult to assess the dose needed to suppress serious arrhythmias, but trough plasma levels in patients successfully treated for recurrent ventricular tachycardia were between 0.2 and 1.0 mcg/ml. Plasma levels above 0.7-1.0 mcg/ml are associated with a higher rate of cardiac adverse experiences such as

CLINICAL PHARMACOLOGY: *(cont'd)*

conduction defects or bradycardia. The relation of plasma levels to proarrhythmic events is not established, but dose reduction in clinical trials of patients with ventricular tachycardia appears to have led to a reduced frequency and severity of such events.

Hemodynamics: Flecainide Acetate does not usually alter heart rate, although bradycardia and tachycardia have been reported occasionally.

In animals and isolated myocardium, a negative inotropic effect of flecainide has been demonstrated. Decreases in ejection fraction, consistent with a negative inotropic effect, have been observed after single administration of 200 to 250 mg of the drug in man; both increases and decreases in ejection fraction have been encountered during multidose therapy in patients at usual therapeutic doses. (See WARNINGS.)

Metabolism in Humans: Following oral administration, the absorption of Flecainide Acetate is nearly complete. Peak plasma levels are attained at about three hours in most individuals (range, 1 to 6 hours). Flecainide does not undergo any consequential presystemic biotransformation (first-pass effect). Food or antacid do not affect absorption.

The apparent plasma half-life averages about 20 hours and is quite variable (range, 12 to 27 hours) after multiple oral doses in patients with premature ventricular contractions (PVCs). With multiple dosing, plasma levels increase because of its long half-life with steady-state levels approached in 3 to 5 days; once at steady-state, no additional (or unexpected) accumulation of drug in plasma occurs during chronic therapy. Over the usual therapeutic range, data suggest that plasma levels in an individual are approximately proportional to dose, deviating upwards from linearity only slightly (about 10 to 15% per 100 mg on average).

In healthy subjects, about 30% of a single oral dose (range, 10 to 50%) is excreted in urine as unchanged drug. The two major urinary metabolites are meta-O-dealkylated flecainide (active, but about one-fifth as potent) and the meta-O-dealkylated lactam of flecainide (non-active metabolite). These two metabolites (primarily conjugated) account for most of the remaining portion of the dose. Several minor metabolites (3% of the dose or less) are also found in urine; only 5% of an oral dose is excreted in feces. In patients, free (unconjugated) plasma levels of the two major metabolites are very low (less than 0.05 mcg/ml).

When urinary pH is very alkaline (8 or higher), as may occur in rare conditions (*e.g.,* renal tubular acidosis, strict vegetarian diet), flecainide elimination from plasma is much slower.

The elimination of flecainide from the body depends on renal function (*i.e.,* 10 to 50% appears in urine as unchanged drug). With increasing renal impairment, the extent of unchanged drug excretion in urine is reduced and the plasma half-life of flecainide is prolonged. Since flecainide is also extensively metabolized, there is no simple relationship between creatinine clearance and the rate of flecainide elimination from plasma. (See DOSAGE AND ADMINISTRATION.)

In patients with NYHA class III congestive heart failure (CHF), the rate of flecainide elimination from plasma (mean half-life, 19 hours) is moderately slower than for healthy subjects (mean half-life, 14 hours), but similar to the rate for patients with PVCs without CHF. The extent of excretion of unchanged drug in urine is also similar. (See DOSAGE AND ADMINISTRATION.)

From age 20 to 80, plasma levels are only slightly higher with advancing age; flecainide elimination from plasma is somewhat slower in elderly subjects than in younger subjects. Patients up to age 80+ have been safely treated with usual dosages.

The extent of flecainide binding to human plasma proteins is about 40% and is independent of plasma drug level over the range of 0.015 to about 3.4 mcg/ml. Thus, clinically significant drug interactions based on protein binding effects would not be expected.

Hemodialysis removes only about 1% of an oral dose as unchanged flecainide.

Small increases in plasma digoxin levels are seen during coadministration of Flecainide Acetate with digoxin. Small increases in both flecainide and propranolol plasma levels are seen during coadministration of these two drugs. (See DRUG INTERACTIONS.)

CLINICAL STUDIES:

In two randomized, crossover, placebo-controlled clinical trials of 16 weeks double-blind duration, 79% of patients with paroxysmal supraventricular tachycardia (PSVT) receiving flecainide were attack free, whereas 15% of patients receiving placebo remained attack free. The median time-before-recurrence of PSVT in patients receiving placebo was 11 to 12 days, whereas over 85% of patients receiving flecainide had no recurrence at 60 days.

In two randomized, crossover, placebo-controlled clinical trials of 16 weeks double-blind duration, 31% of patients with paroxysmal atrial fibrillation/flutter (PAF) receiving flecainide were attack free, whereas 8% receiving placebo remained attack free. The median time-before-recurrence of PAF in patients receiving placebo was about 2 to 3 days, whereas for those receiving flecainide the median time-before-recurrence was 15 days.

INDICATIONS AND USAGE:

In patients without structural heart disease, Flecainide Acetate is indicated for the prevention of:

Paroxysmal supraventricular tachycardias (PSVT), including atrioventricular nodal reentrant tachycardia, atrioventricular reentrant tachycardia and other supraventricular tachycardias of unspecified mechanism associated with disabling symptoms

Paroxysmal atrial fibrillation/flutter (PAF) associated with disabling symptoms

Flecainide Acetate is also indicated for the prevention of:

Documented ventricular arrhythmias, such as sustained ventricular tachycardia (sustained VT), that in the judgment of the physician, are life-threatening.

Use of Flecainide Acetate for the treatment of sustained VT, like other antiarrhythmics, should be initiated in the hospital. The use of Flecainide Acetate is not recommended in patients with less severe ventricular arrhythmias even if the patients are symptomatic.

Because of the proarrhythmic effects of Flecainide Acetate, its use should be reserved for patients in whom, in the opinion of the physician, the benefits of treatment outweigh the risks.

Flecainide Acetate should not be used in patients with recent myocardial infarction. (See box in WARNINGS.)

Use of Flecainide Acetate in chronic atrial fibrillation has not been adequately studied and is not recommended. (See box in WARNINGS.)

As is the case for other antiarrhythmic agents, there is no evidence from controlled trials that the use of Flecainide Acetate favorably affects survival or the incidence of sudden death.

CONTRAINDICATIONS:

Flecainide Acetate is contraindicated in patients with preexisting second- or third-degree AV block, or with right bundle branch block when associated with a left hemiblock (bifascicular block), unless a pacemaker is present to sustain the cardiac rhythm should complete heart block occur. Flecainide Acetate is also contraindicated in the presence of cardiogenic shock or known hypersensitivity to the drug.

WARNINGS:

Mortality: Flecainide Acetate was included in the National Heart Lung and Blood Institute's Cardiac Arrhythmia Suppression Trial (CAST), a long-term, multicenter, randomized, double-blind study in patients with asymptomatic non-life-threatening ventricular arrhythmias who had a myocardial infarction more than six days, but less than two years previously. An excessive mortality or non-fatal cardiac arrest rate was seen in patients treated with Flecainide Acetate compared with that seen in a carefully matched placebo-treated group. This rate was 16/315 (5.1%) for Flecainide Acetate and 7/309 (2.3%) for its matched placebo. The average duration of treatment with Tambocor in this study was 10 months.

Ventricular Proarrhythmic Effects in Patients with Atrial Fibrillation/Flutter. A review of the world literature revealed reports of 568 patients treated with oral Flecainide Acetate for paroxysmal atrial fibrillation/flutter (PAF). Ventricular tachycardia was experienced in 0.4% (2/568) of these patients. Of 19 patients in the literature with chronic atrial fibrillation (CAF), 10.5% (2) experienced VT or VF. FLECAINIDE IS NOT RECOMMENDED FOR USE IN PATIENTS WITH CHRONIC ATRIAL FIBRILLATION. Case reports of ventricular proarrhythmic effects in patients treated with Flecainide Acetate for atrial fibrillation/flutter have included increased PVCs, VT, ventricular fibrillation (VF), and death.

As with other Class I agents, patients treated with Flecainide Acetate for atrial flutter have been reported with 1:1 atrioventricular conduction due to slowing the atrial rate. A paradoxical increase in the ventricular rate also may occur in patients with atrial fibrillation who receive Flecainide Acetate. Concomitant negative chronotropic therapy such as digoxin or beta-blockers may lower the risk of this complication.

The applicability of the CAST results to other populations (*e.g.,* those without recent infarction) is uncertain, but at present it is prudent to consider the risks of Class IC agents, coupled with the lack of any evidence of improved survival, generally unacceptable in patients whose ventricular arrhythmias are not life-threatening, even if the patients are experiencing unpleasant, but not life-threatening, symptoms or signs.

Proarrhythmic Effects: Flecainide Acetate, like other antiarrhythmic agents, can cause new or worsened supraventricular or ventricular arrhythmias. Ventricular proarrhythmic effects range from an increase in frequency of PVCs to the development of more severe ventricular tachycardia, e.g. tachycardia that is more sustained or more resistant to conversion to sinus rhythm, with potentially fatal consequences. In studies of ventricular arrhythmia patients treated with Flecainide Acetate, three-fourths of proarrhythmic events were new or worsened ventricular tachyarrhythmias, the remainder being increased frequency of PVCs or new supraventricular arrhythmias. In patients treated with flecainide for sustained ventricular tachycardia, 80% (51/64) of proarrhythmic events occurred within 14 days of the onset of therapy. In studies of 225 patients with supraventricular arrhythmia (108 with paroxysmal supraventricular tachycardia and 117 with paroxysmal atrial fibrillation), there were 9 (4%) proarrhythmic events, 8 of them in patients with paroxysmal atrial fibrillation. Of the 9, 7 (including the one in a PSVT patient) were exacerbations of supraventricular arrhythmias (longer duration, more rapid rate, harder to reverse) while 2 were ventricular arrhythmias, including one fatal case of VT/VF and one wide complex VT (the patient showed inducible VT, however, after withdrawal of flecainide), both in patients with paroxysmal atrial fibrillation and known coronary artery disease.

It is uncertain if Flecainide Acetate's risk of proarrhythmia is exaggerated in patients with chronic atrial fibrillation (CAF), high ventricular rate, and/or exercise. Wide complex tachycardia and ventricular fibrillation have been reported in two of 12 CAF patients undergoing maximal exercise tolerance testing.

In patients with complex ventricular arrhythmias, it is often difficult to distinguish a spontaneous variation in the patient's underlying rhythm disorder from drug-induced worsening, so that the following occurrence rates must be considered approximations. Their frequency appears to be related to dose and to the underlying cardiac disease.

Among patients treated for sustained VT (who frequently also had CHF, a low ejection fraction, a history of myocardial infarction and/or an episode of cardiac arrest), the incidence of proarrhythmic events was 13% when dosage was initiated at 200 mg/day with slow upward titration, and did not exceed 300 mg/day in most patients. In early studies in patients with sustained VT utilizing a higher initial dose (400 mg/day) the incidence of proarrhythmic events was 26%; moreover, in about 10% of the patients treated proarrhythmic events resulted in death, despite prompt medical attention. With lower initial doses, the incidence of proarrhythmic events resulting in death decreased to 0.5% of these patients. Accordingly, it is extremely important to follow the recommended dosage schedule. (See DOSAGE AND ADMINISTRATION.)

The relatively high frequency of proarrhythmic events in patients with sustained VT and serious underlying heart disease, and the need for careful titration and monitoring, requires that therapy of patients with sustained VT be started in the hospital. (See DOSAGE AND ADMINISTRATION.)

Heart Failure: Flecainide Acetate has a negative inotropic effect and may cause or worsen CHF, particularly in patients with cardiomyopathy, preexisting severe heart failure (NYHA functional class III or IV) or low ejection fractions (less than 30%). In patients with supraventricular arrhythmias new or worsened CHF developed in 0.4% (1/225) of patients. In patients with sustained ventricular tachycardia, during a mean duration of 7.9 months of Flecainide Acetate therapy, 6.3% (20/317) developed new CHF. In patients with sustained ventricular tachycardia and a history of CHF, during a mean duration of 5.4 months of Flecainide Acetate therapy, 25.7% (78/304) developed worsened CHF. Exacerbation of preexisting CHF occurred more commonly in studies which included patients with class III or IV failure than in studies which excluded such patients. Flecainide Acetate should be used cautiously in patients who are known to have a history of CHF or myocardial dysfunction. The initial dosage in such patients should be no more than 100 mg bid (see DOSAGE AND ADMINISTRATION) and patients should be monitored carefully. Close attention must be given to maintenance of cardiac function, including optimization of digitalis, diuretic, or other therapy. In cases where CHF has developed or worsened during treatment with Flecainide Acetate, the time of onset has ranged from a few hours to several months after starting therapy. Some patients who develop evidence of reduced myocardial function while on Flecainide Acetate can continue on Flecainide Acetate with adjustment of digitalis or diuretics, others may require dosage reduction or discontinuation of Flecainide Acetate. When feasible, it is recommended that plasma flecainide levels be monitored. Attempts should be made to keep trough plasma levels below 0.7 to 1.0 mcg/ml.

Effects on Cardiac Conduction: Flecainide Acetate slows cardiac conduction in most patients to produce dose-related increases in PR, QRS, and QT intervals. PR interval increases on average about 25% (0.04 seconds) and as much as 118% in some patients. Approximately one-third of patients may develop new first-degree AV heart block (PR interval ≥0.20 seconds). The QRS complex increases on average about 25% (0.02 seconds) and as much as

WARNINGS: *(cont'd)*

150% in some patients. Many patients develop QRS complexes with a duration of 0.12 seconds or more. In one study, 4% of patients developed new bundle branch block while on Flecainide Acetate. The degree of lengthening of PR and QRS intervals does not predict either efficacy or the development of cardiac adverse effects. In clinical trials, it was unusual for PR intervals to increase to 0.30 seconds or more, or for QRS intervals to increase to 0.18 seconds or more. Thus, caution should be used when such intervals occur, and dose reductions may be considered. The QT interval widens about 8%, but most of this widening (about 60% to 90%) is due to widening of the QRS duration. The JT interval (QT minus QRS) only widens about 4% on the average. Significant JT prolongation occurs in less than 2% of patients. There have been rare cases of Torsade de Pointes-type arrhythmia associated with Flecainide Acetate therapy.

Clinically significant conduction changes have been observed at these rates: sinus node dysfunction such as sinus pause, sinus arrest and symptomatic bradycardia (1.2%), second-degree AV block (0.5%) and third-degree AV block (0.4%). An attempt should be made to manage the patient on the lowest effective dose in an effort to minimize these effects. (See DOSAGE AND ADMINISTRATION.) If second- or third-degree AV block, or right bundle branch block associated with a left hemiblock occur, Flecainide Acetate therapy should be discontinued unless a temporary or implanted ventricular pacemaker is in place to ensure an adequate ventricular rate.

Sick Sinus Syndrome (Bradycardia-Tachycardia Syndrome): Flecainide Acetate should be used only with extreme caution in patients with sick sinus syndrome because it may cause sinus bradycardia, sinus pause, or sinus arrest.

Effects on Pacemaker Thresholds: Flecainide Acetate is known to increase endocardial pacing thresholds and may suppress ventricular escape rhythms. These effects are reversible if flecainide is discontinued. It should be used with caution in patients with permanent pacemakers or temporary pacing electrodes and should not be administered to patients with existing poor thresholds or nonprogrammable pacemakers unless suitable pacing rescue is available.

The pacing threshold in patients with pacemakers should be determined prior to instituting therapy with Flecainide Acetate, again after one week of administration and at regular intervals thereafter. Generally threshold changes are within the range of multiprogrammable pacemakers and, when these occur, a doubling of either voltage or pulse width is usually sufficient to regain capture.

Electrolyte Disturbances: Hypokalemia or hyperkalemia may alter the effects of Class I antiarrhythmic drugs. Preexisting hypokalemia or hyperkalemia should be corrected before administration of Flecainide Acetate.

PRECAUTIONS:

CARCINOGENESIS, MUTAGENESIS, AND IMPAIRMENT OF FERTILITY

Long-term studies with flecainide in rats and mice at doses up to 60 mg/kg/day have not revealed any compound-related carcinogenic effects. Mutagenicity studies (Ames test, mouse lymphoma and *in vivo* cytogenetics) did not reveal any mutagenic effects. A rat reproduction study at doses up to 50 mg/kg/day (seven times the usual human dose) did not reveal any adverse effect on male or female fertility.

PREGNANCY CATEGORY C

Flecainide has been shown to have teratogenic effects (club paws, sternebrae and vertebrae abnormalities, pale hearts with contracted ventricular septum) and an embryotoxic effect (increased resorptions) in one breed of rabbit (New Zealand White) when given doses of 30 and 35 mg/kg/day but not in another breed of rabbit (Dutch Belted) when given doses up to 30 mg/kg/day. No teratogenic effects were observed in rats and mice given doses up to 50 and 80 mg/kg/day, respectively; however, delayed sternebral and vertebral ossification was observed at the high dose in rats. Because there are no adequate and well-controlled studies in pregnant women, Flecainide Acetate should be used during pregnancy only if the potential benefit justifies the potential risk to the fetus.

LABOR AND DELIVERY

It is not known whether the use of Flecainide Acetate during labor or delivery has immediate or delayed adverse effects on the mother or fetus, affects the duration of labor or delivery, or increases the possibility of forceps delivery or other obstetrical intervention.

NURSING MOTHERS

Results from a multiple dose study conducted in mothers soon after delivery indicates that flecainide is excreted in human breast milk in concentrations as high as 4 times (with average levels about 2.5 times) corresponding plasma levels; assuming a maternal plasma level at the top of the therapeutic range (1 mcg/ml), the calculated daily dose to a nursing infant (assuming about 700 ml breast milk over 24 hours) would be less than 3 mg.

PEDIATRIC USE

The safety and effectiveness of Flecainide Acetate in children less than 18 years of age have not been established.

HEPATIC IMPAIRMENT

Since flecainide elimination from plasma can be markedly slower in patients with significant hepatic impairment, Flecainide Acetate should not be used in such patients unless the potential benefits clearly outweigh the risks. If used, frequent and early plasma level monitoring is required to guide dosage (see Plasma Level Monitoring); dosage increases should be made very cautiously when plasma levels have plateaued (after more than four days).

DRUG INTERACTIONS:

Flecainide Acetate has been administered to patients receiving digitalis preparations or beta-adrenergic blocking agents without adverse effects. During administration of multiple oral doses of Flecainide Acetate to healthy subjects stabilized on a maintenance dose of digoxin, a 13% - 19% increase in plasma digoxin levels occurred at six hours postdose. In a study involving healthy subjects receiving Flecainide Acetate and propranolol concurrently, plasma flecainide levels were increased about 20% and propranolol levels were increased about 30% compared to control values. In this formal interaction study, Flecainide Acetate and propranolol were each found to have negative inotropic effects; when the drugs were administered together, the effects were additive. The effects of concomitant administration of Flecainide Acetate and propranolol on the PR interval were less than additive. In Flecainide Acetate clinical trials, patients who were receiving beta blockers concurrently did not experience an increased incidence of side effects. Nevertheless, the possibility of additive negative inotropic effects of beta blockers and flecainide should be recognized.

Flecainide is not extensively bound to plasma proteins. In vitro studies with several drugs which may be administered concomitantly showed that the extent of flecainide binding to human plasma proteins is either unchanged or only slightly less. Consequently, interactions with other drugs which are highly protein bound (*e.g.,* anticoagulants) would not be expected. Flecainide Acetate has been used in a large number of patients receiving diuretics without apparent interaction. Limited data in patients receiving known enzyme inducers (phenytoin, phenobarbital, carbamazepine) indicate only a 30% increase in the rate of flecainide elimination. In healthy subjects receiving cimetidine (1 gm daily) for one week, plasma flecainide levels increased by about 30% and half-life increased by about 10%.

DRUG INTERACTIONS: *(cont'd)*

When amiodarone is added to flecainide therapy, plasma flecainide levels may increase two-fold or more in some patients, if flecainide dosage is not reduced. (See DOSAGE AND ADMINISTRATION.)

There has been little experience with the coadministration of Flecainide Acetate and either disopyramide or verapamil. Because both of these drugs have negative inotropic properties and the effects of coadministration with Flecainide Acetate are unknown, neither disopyramidenor verapamil should be administered concurrently with Flecainide Acetate unless, in the judgment of the physician, the benefits of this combination outweigh the risks. There has been too little experience with the coadministration of Flecainide Acetate with nifedipine or diltiazem to recommend concomitant use.

ADVERSE REACTIONS:

In post-myocardial infarction patients with asymptomatic PVCs and non-sustained ventricular tachycardia, Flecainide Acetate therapy was found to be associated with a 5.1% rate of death and non-fatal cardiac arrest, compared with a 2.3% rate in a matched placebo group. (See WARNINGS.)

Adverse effects reported for Flecainide Acetate, described in detail in the WARNINGS section, were new or worsened arrhythmias which occurred in 1% of 108 patients with PSVT and in 7% of 117 patients with PAF; and new or exacerbated ventricular arrhythmias which occurred in 7% of 1330 patients with PVCs, nonsustained or sustained VT. In patients treated with flecainide for sustained VT, 80% (51/64) of proarrhythmic events occurred within 14 days of the onset of therapy. 198 patients withsustained VT experienced a 13% incidence of new or exacerbated ventricular arrhythmias when dosage was initiated at 200 mg/day with slow upward titration, and did not exceed 300 mg/day in most patients. In some patients, Flecainide Acetate treatment has been associated with episodes of unresuscitatable VT or ventricular fibrillation (cardiac arrest). (See WARNINGS.)New or worsened CHF occurred in 6.3% of 1046 patients with PVCs, non-sustained or sustained VT. Of 297 patients with sustained VT, 9.1% experienced new or worsened CHF. New or worsened CHF was reported in 0.4% of 225 patients with supraventricular arrhythmias. There have also been instances of second- (0.5%) or third-degree (0.4%) AV block. Patients have developed sinus bradycardia, sinus pause, or sinus arrest, about 1.2% altogether (see WARNINGS.) The frequency of most of these serious adverse events probably increases with higher trough plasma levels, especially when these trough levels exceed 1.0 mcg/ml.

There have been rare reports of isolated elevations of serum alkaline phosphatase and isolated elevations of serum transaminase levels. These elevations have been asymptomatic and no cause and effect relationship with Flecainide Acetate has been established. In foreign postmarketing surveillance studies, there have been rare reports of hepatic dysfunction including reports of cholestasis and hepatic failure, and extremely rare reports of blood dyscrasias. Although no cause and effect relationship has been established, it is advisable to discontinue Flecainide Acetate in patients who develop unexplained jaundice or signs of hepatic dysfunction or blood dyscrasias in order to eliminate Flecainide Acetate as the possible causative agent.

Incidence figures for other adverse effects in patients with ventricular arrhythmias are based on a multicenter efficacy study, utilizing starting doses of 200 mg/day with gradual upward titration to 400 mg/day. Patients were treated for an average of 4.7 months, with some receiving up to 22 months of therapy. In this trial, 5.4% of patients discontinued due to noncardiac adverse effects (TABLE 1).

TABLE 1 Flecainide Acetate, Adverse Reactions
Most Common Non-Cardiac Adverse Effects in Ventricular Arrhythmia Patients Treated with Tambocor in the Multicenter Study

Adverse Effect	Incidence In All 429 Patients at Any Dose	Incidence By Dose: During 200 mg/Day (N=426)	Upward 300 mg/Day (N=293)	Titration 400 mg/Day (N=100)
Dizziness*	18.9%	11.0%	10.6%	13.0%
Visual Disturbance†	15.9%	5.4%	12.3%	18.0%
Dyspnea	10.3%	5.2%	7.5%	4.0%
Headache	9.6%	4.5%	6.1%	9.0%
Nausea	8.9%	4.9%	4.8%	6.0%
Fatigue	7.7%	4.5%	4.4%	3.0%
Palpitation	6.1%	3.5%	2.4%	7.0%
Chest Pain	5.4%	3.1%	3.8%	1.0%
Asthenia	4.9%	2.6%	2.0%	4.0%
Tremor	4.7%	2.4%	3.4%	2.0%
Constipation	4.4%	2.8%	2.1%	1.0%
Edema	3.5%	1.9%	1.4%	2.0%
Abdominal Pain	3.3%	1.9%	2.4%	1.0%

* Dizziness includes reports of dizziness, lightheadedness, faintness, unsteadiness, near syncope, etc.
† Visual disturbance includes reports of blurred vision, difficulty in focusing, spots before eyes, etc.

The following additional adverse experiences, possibly related to Flecainide Acetate therapy and occurring in 1% to less than 3% of patients, have been reported in acute and chronic studies:

Body as a Whole: malaise, fever;

Cardiovascular: tachycardia, sinus pause or arrest;

Gastrointestinal: vomiting, diarrhea, dyspepsia, anorexia;

Skin: rash;

Visual: diplopia;

Nervous System: hypoesthesia, paresthesia, paresis, ataxia, flushing, increased sweating, vertigo, syncope, somnolence, tinnitus;

Psychiatric: anxiety, insomnia, depression.

The following additional adverse experiences, possibly related to Tambocor, have been reported in less than 1% of patients:

Body as a Whole: swollen lips, tongue and mouth; arthralgia, bronchospasm, myalgia;

Cardiovascular: angina pectoris, second-degree and third-degree AV block, bradycardia, hypertension, hypotension

Gastrointestinal: flatulence;

Urinary System: polyuria, urinary retention;

Hematologic: leukopenia, thrombocytopenia

Skin: urticaria, exfoliative dermatitis, pruritus, alopecia

Visual: eye pain or irritation, photophobia, nystagmus

Nervous System: twitching, weakness, change in taste, dry mouth, convulsions, impotence, speech disorder, stupor, neuropathy

Psychiatric: amnesia, confusion, decreased libido, depersonalization, euphoria, morbid dreams, apathy.

ADVERSE REACTIONS: *(cont'd)*

For patients with supraventricular arrhythmias, the most commonly reported noncardiac adverse experiences remain consistent with those known for patients treated with Flecainide Acetate for ventricular arrhythmias. Dizziness is possibly more frequent in PAF patients.

OVERDOSAGE:

No specific antidote has been identified for the treatment of Flecainide Acetate overdosage. Overdoses ranging up to 8000 mg have been survived, with pek plasma flecainide concentrations as high as 5 3 mcg/ml. untoward effects in these cases included nausea and vomiting, convulsions, hypotension, bradycardia, syncope, extreme widening of the QRS complex, widening of the QT interval, widening of the PR interval, ventricular tachycardia. AV nodal block, asystole, bundle branch block, cardiac failure, and cardiac arrest. The spectrum of events observed in fatal cases was much the same as that seen in the non=fatal cases. Death has resulted following ingestion of as little as 1000 mg; concomitant overdose of other drugs and or alcohol in many instances undoubtedly contributed to the fatal outcome. Treatment of overdosage should be supportive and may include the following: removal of unabsorbed drug from the gastrointestinal tract, administration of inotropic agents or cardiac stimulants such as dopamine, dobutamine or isoproterenol; mechanically assisted respiration; circulatory assists such as intra-aortic balloon pumping; and transvenous pacing in the event of conduction block. Because of the long plasma half-life of flecainide (12 to 27 hours in patients receiving usual doses), and the possibility of markedly non-linear elimination kinetics at very high doses, these supportive treatments may need to be continued for extended periods of time.

Hemodialysis is not an effective means of removing flecainide from the body. Since flecainide elimination is much slower when urine is very alkaline (pH 8 or higher), theoretically, acidification of urine to promote drug excretion may be beneficial in overdose cases with very alkaline urine. There is no evidence that acidification from normal urinary pH increases excretion.

DOSAGE AND ADMINISTRATION:

For patients with sustained VT, no matter what their cardiac status, Flecainide Acetate, like other antiarrhythmics, should be initiated in-hospital with rhythm monitoring.

Flecainide has a long half-life (12 to 27 hours in patients). Steady-state plasma levels, in patients with normal renal and hepatic function, may not be achieved until the patient has received 3 to 5 days of therapy at a given dose. Therefore, increases in dosage should be made no more frequently than once every four days, since during the first 2 to 3 days of therapy the optimal effect of a given dose may not be achieved.

For patients with PSVT and patients with PAF the recommended starting dose is 50 mg every 12 hours. Flecainide Acetate doses may be increased in increments of 50 mg bid every four days until efficacy is achieved. For PAF patients, a substantial increase in efficacy without a substantial increase in discontinuations for adverse experiences may be achieved by increasing the Flecainide Acetate dose from 50 to 100 mg bid. The maximum recommended dose for patients with paroxysmal supraventricular arrhythmias is 300 mg/day.

For sustained VT the recommended starting dose is 100 mg every 12 hours. This dose may be increased in increments of 50 mg bid every four days until efficacy is achieved. Most patients with sustained VT do not require more than 150 mg every 12 hours (300 mg/day), and the maximum dose recommended is 400 mg/day.

In patients with sustained VT, use of higher initial doses and more rapid dosage adjustments have resulted in an increased incidence of proarrhythmic events and CHF, particularly during the first few days of dosing (see WARNINGS.) Therefore, a loading dose is not recommended.

Intravenous lidocaine has been used occasionally with Flecainide Acetate while awaiting the therapeutic effect of Flecainide Acetate. No adverse drug interactions were apparent. However, no formal studies have been performed to demonstrate the usefulness of this regimen.

An occasional patient not adequately controlled by (or intolerant to) a dose given at 12-hour intervals may be dosed at eight-hour intervals.

Once adequate control of the arrhythmia has been achieved, it may be possible in some patients to reduce the dose as necessary to minimize side effects or effects on conduction. In such patients, efficacy at the lower dose should be evaluated.

Tambocor should be used cautiously in patients with a history of CHF or myocardial dysfunction (see WARNINGS.)

In patients with severe renal impairment (creatinine clearance of 35 ml/min/1.73 square meters or less), the initial dosage should be 100 mg once daily (or 50 mg bid); when used in such patients, frequent plasma level monitoring is required to guide dosage adjustments (see Plasma Level Monitoring.) In patients with less severe renal disease, the initial dosage should be 100 mg every 12 hours; plasma level monitoring may also be useful in these patients during dosage adjustment. In both groups of patients, dosage increases should be made very cautiously when plasma levels have plateaued (after more than four days), observing the patient closely for signs of adverse cardiac effects or other toxicity. It should be borne in mind that in these patients it may take longer than four days before a new steady-state plasma level is reached following a dosage change.

Based on theoretical considerations, rather than experimental data, the following suggestion is made: when transferring patients from another antiarrhythmic drug to Flecainide Acetate allow at least two to four plasma half-lives to elapse for the drug being discontinued before starting Flecainide Acetate at the usual dosage. In patients where withdrawal of a previous anti-arrhythmic agent is likely to produce life-threatening arrhythmias, the physician should consider hospitalizing the patient.

When flecainide is given in the presence of amiodarone, reduce the usual flecainide dose by 50% and monitor the patient closely for adverse effects. Plasma level monitoring is strongly recommended to guide dosage with such combination therapy (see Plasma Level Monitoring.)

Plasma Level Monitoring: The large majority of patients successfully treated with Flecainide Acetate were found to have trough plasma levels between 0.2 and 1.0 mcg/ml. The probability of adverse experiences, especially cardiac, may increase with higher trough plasma levels, especially when these exceed 1.0 mcg/ml. Periodic monitoring of trough plasma levels may be useful in patient management. Plasma level monitoring is required in patients with severe renal failure or severe hepatic disease, since elimination of flecainide from plasma may be markedly slower. Monitoring of plasma levels is strongly recommended in patients on concurrent amiodarone therapy and may also be helpful in patients with CHF and in patients with moderate renal disease.

HOW SUPPLIED:

All tablets are embossed with 3M on one side and TR 50, TR 100, or TR 150 on the other side.

Tambocor is available as 50 mg per white, round tablet; 100 mg per white, round, scored tablet; 150 mg per white, oval, scored tablet

Store at controlled room temperature 15-30°C (59-86°F) in a tight, light-resistant container.

HOW SUPPLIED - EQUIVALENTS NOT AVAILABLE:

Tablet, Uncoated - Oral - 50 mg
100's $67.20 TAMBOCOR, 3M Pharms 00089-0305-10
Tablet, Uncoated - Oral - 100 mg
100's $122.04 TAMBOCOR, 3M Pharms 00089-0307-10
Tablet, Uncoated - Oral - 150 mg
100's $167.94 TAMBOCOR, 3M Pharms 00089-0314-10

FLEROXACIN *(003203)*

CATEGORIES: Anti-Infectives; Antibacterials; Antibiotics; Fluoroquinolones; Gonorrhea; Infections; Quinolones; Urinary Tract Infections; FDA Unapproved

BRAND NAMES: **Megalone**; *Quinodis* (Germany); *Roquinol*
(International brand names outside U.S. in italics)

Prescribing information not available at time of publication.

FLOSEQUINAN *(003147)*

CATEGORIES: Cardiovascular Drugs; Congestive Heart Failure; Fluoroquinolones; Heart Failure; Vasodilating Agents; Pregnancy Category C; FDA Class 1S ("Standard Review"); FDA Approved 1992 Dec

BRAND NAMES: **Manoplax**

DESCRIPTION:

.Manoplax being withdrawn by Boots.

HOW SUPPLIED - EQUIVALENTS NOT AVAILABLE:

Tablet, Uncoated - Oral - 50 mg
30's $75.00 MANOPLAX, Knoll Pharms 00048-0900-30
Tablet, Uncoated - Oral - 75 mg
30's $75.00 MANOPLAX, Knoll Pharms 00048-0901-30
Tablet, Uncoated - Oral - 100 mg
60's $150.00 MANOPLAX, Knoll Pharms 00048-0902-60

FLOXURIDINE *(001300)*

CATEGORIES: Antimetabolites; Antineoplastics; Cancer; Oncologic Drugs; Pregnancy Category D; FDA Approval Pre 1982

BRAND NAMES: **FUDR**; *Tedofuryl*
(International brand names outside U.S. in italics)

FORMULARIES: BC-BS; Medi-Cal

> WARNING:
> FOR INTRA-ARTERIAL INFUSION ONLY.
> It is recommended that Floxuridine be given only by or under the supervision of a qualified physician who is experienced in cancer chemotherapy and intra-arterial drug therapy and is well versed in the use of potent antimetabolites.
> Because of the possibility of severe toxic reactions, all patients should be hospitalized for initiation of the first course of therapy.

DESCRIPTION:

Floxuridine, an antineoplastic antimetabolite, is available as a sterile, nonpyrogenic, lyophilized powder for reconstitution. Each vial contains 500 mg of floxuridine which is to be reconstituted with 5 ml of sterile water for injection. An appropriate amount of reconstituted solution is then diluted with a parenteral solution for intra-arterial infusion (see DOSAGE AND ADMINISTRATION).

Floxuridine is a fluorinated pyrimidine. Chemically, floxuridine is 2'-deoxy-5 - fluorouridine with an empirical formula of $C_9H_{11}FN_2O_5$. It is a white to off-white odorless solid which is freely soluble in water.

The 2% aqueous solution has a pH of between 4.0 and 5.5. The molecular weight of floxuridine is 246.19.

CLINICAL PHARMACOLOGY:

When Floxuridine is given by rapid intraarterial injection it is apparently rapidly catabolized to 5-fluorouracil. Thus, rapid injection of Floxuridine produces the same toxic and antimetabolic effects as does 5-fluorouracil. The primary effect is to interfere with the synthesis of deoxyribonucleic acid (DNA) and to a lesser extent inhibit the formation of ribonucleic acid (RNA). However, when Floxuridine is given by continuous intra-arterial infusion its direct anabolism to Floxuridine-monophosphate is enhanced, thus increasing the inhibition of DNA.

Floxuridine is metabolized in the liver. The drug is excreted intact and as urea, fluorouracil, α-fluoro-β-ureidopropionic acid, dihydrofluorouracil, α-fluoro-β -guanidopropionic acid and α-fluoro-β-alanine in the urine; it is also expired as respiratory carbon dioxide. Pharmacokinetic data on intra-arterial infusion of Floxuridine are not available.

INDICATIONS AND USAGE:

Floxuridine is effective in the palliative management of gastrointestinal adenocarcinoma metastatic to the liver, when given by continuous regional intra-arterial infusion in carefully selected patients who are considered incurable by surgery or other means. Patients with known disease extending beyond an area capable of infusion via a single artery should, except in unusual circumstances, be considered for systemic therapy with other chemotherapeutic agents.

CONTRAINDICATIONS:

Floxuridine therapy is contraindicated for patients in a poor nutritional state, those with depressed bone marrow function or those with potentially serious infections.

WARNINGS:

BECAUSE OF THE POSSIBILITY OF SEVERE TOXIC REACTIONS, ALL PATIENTS SHOULD BE HOSPITALIZED FOR THE FIRST COURSE OF THERAPY.

WARNINGS: *(cont'd)*

Floxuridine should be used with extreme caution in poor risk patients with impaired hepatic or renal function or a history of high-dose pelvic irradiation or previous use of alkylating agents. The drug is not intended as an adjuvant to surgery.

Floxuridine may cause fetal harm when administered to a pregnant woman. It has been shown to be teratogenic in the chick embryo, mouse (at doses of 2.5 to 100 mg/kg) and rat (at doses of 75 to 150 mg/kg). Malformations included cleft palates; skeletal defects; and deformed appendages, paws and tails. The dosages which were teratogenic in animals are 4.2 to 125 times the recommended human therapeutic dose.

There are no adequate and well-controlled studies with Floxuridine in pregnant women. If this drug is used during pregnancy or if the patient becomes pregnant while taking (receiving) this drug, the patient should be apprised of the potential hazard to the fetus. Women of childbearing potential should be advised to avoid becoming pregnant.

Combination Therapy: Any form of therapy which adds to the stress of the patient, interferes with nutrition or depresses bone marrow function will increase the toxicity of Floxuridine.

PRECAUTIONS:

GENERAL

Sterile Floxuridine is a highly toxic drug with a narrow margin of safety. Therefore, patients should be carefully supervised since therapeutic response is unlikely to occur without some evidence of toxicity. Severe hematological toxicity, gastrointestinal hemorrhage and even death may result from the use of Floxuridine despite meticulous selection of patients and careful adjustment of dosage. Although severe toxicity is more likely in poor risk patients, fatalities may be encountered occasionally even in patients in relatively good condition.

Therapy is to be discontinued promptly whenever one of the following signs of toxicity appears:

Myocardial ischemia
Stomatitis or esophagopharyngitis, at the first visible sign
Leukopenia (WBC under 3500) or a rapidly falling white blood count
Vomiting, intractable
Diarrhea, frequent bowel movements or watery stools
Gastrointestinal ulceration and bleeding
Thrombocytopenia (platelets under 100,000)
Hemorrhage from any site

INFORMATION FOR THE PATIENT

Patients should be informed of expected toxic effects, particularly oral manifestations. Patients should be alerted to the possibility of alopecia as a result of therapy and should be informed that it is usually a transient effect.

LABORATORY TESTS

Careful monitoring of the white blood count and platelet count is recommended.

CARCINOGENESIS, MUTAGENESIS, AND IMPAIRMENT OF FERTILITY

Carcinogenesis: Long-term studies in animals to evaluate the carcinogenic potential of floxuridine have not been conducted. On the basis of the available data, no evaluation can be made of the carcinogenic risk of Floxuridine to humans.

Mutagenesis: Oncogenic transformation of fibroblasts from mouse embryo has been induced *in vitro* by Floxuridine, but the relationship between oncogenicity and mutagenicity is not clear. Floxuridine has also been shown to be mutagenic in human leukocytes *in vitro* and in the *Drosophila* test system. In addition, 5-fluorouracil, to which floxuridine is catabolized when given by intra-arterial injection, has been shown to be mutagenic in *in vitro* tests.

Impairment of Fertility: The effects of floxuridine on fertility and general reproductive performance have not been studied in animals. However, because floxuridine is catabolized to 5-fluorouracil, it should be noted that 5-fluorouracil has been shown to induce chromosomal aberrations and changes in chromosome organization of spermatogonia in rats at doses of 125 or 250 mg/kg, administered intraperitoneally.

Spermatogonial differentiation was also inhibited by fluorouracil, resulting in transient infertility. In female rats, fluorouracil, administered intraperitoneally at doses of 25 or 50 mg/kg during the preovulatory phase of oogenesis, significantly reduced the incidence of fertile matings, delayed the development of pre- and postimplantation embryos, increased the incidence of preimplantation lethality and induced chromosomal anomalies in these embryos. Compounds such as Floxuridine, which interfere with DNA, RNA and protein synthesis, might be expected to have adverse effects on gametogenesis.

PREGNANCY CATEGORY D

Teratogenic Effects: See WARNINGS section. Floxuridine has been shown to be teratogenic in the chick embryo, mouse (at doses of 2.5 to 100 mg/kg) and rat (at doses of 75 to 150 mg/kg). Malformations included cleft palates, skeletal defects and deformed appendages, paws and tails. The dosages which were teratogenic in animals are 4.2 to 125 times the recommended human therapeutic dose.

There are not adequate and well-controlled studies with Floxuridine in pregnant women. While there is no evidence of teratogenicity in humans due to, it should be kept in mind that other drugs which inhibit DNA synthesis (*e.g.,* methotrexate and aminopterin) have been reported to be teratogenic in humans. FUDR should be used during pregnancy only if the potential benefit justifies the potential risk to the fetus.

Nonteratogenic Effects: Floxuridine has not been studied in animals for its effects on peri- and postnatal development. However, compounds which inhibit DNA, RNA and protein synthesis might be expected to have adverse effects on peri- and postnatal development.

NURSING MOTHERS

It is not known whether Floxuridine is excreted in human milk. Because Floxuridine inhibits DNA and RNA synthesis, mothers should not nurse while receiving this drug.

PEDIATRIC USE

Safety and effectiveness in children have not been established.

DRUG INTERACTIONS:

See WARNINGS section.

ADVERSE REACTIONS:

Adverse reactions to the arterial infusion of Floxuridine are generally related to the procedural complications of regional arterial infusion.

The more common adverse reactions to the drug are nausea, vomiting, diarrhea, enteritis, stomatitis and localized erythema. The more common laboratory abnormalities are anemia, leukopenia, thrombocytopenia and elevations of alkaline phosphatase, serum transaminase, serum bilirubin and lactic dehydrogenase.

Other adverse reactions are:

Gastrointestinal: Duodenal ulcer, duodenitis, gastritis, bleeding, gastroenteritis, glossitis, pharyngitis, anorexia, cramps, abdominal pain; possible intra- and extrahepatic biliary sclerosis, as well as acalculous cholecystitis.

ADVERSE REACTIONS: *(cont'd)*

Dermatologic: Alopecia, dermatitis, nonspecific skin toxicity, rash.

Cardiovascular: Myocardial ischemia.

Miscellaneous Clinical Reactions: Fever, lethargy, malaise, weakness.

Laboratory Abnormalities: BSP, prothrombin, total proteins, sedimentation rate and thrombopenia.

Procedural Complications of Regional Arterial Infusion: Arterial aneurysm; arterial ischemia; arterial thrombosis; embolism; fibromyositis; thrombophlebitis; hepatic necrosis; abscesses; infection at catheter site; bleeding at catheter site; catheter blocked, displaced or leaking.

The following adverse reactions have not been reported with Floxuridine but have been noted following the administration of 5-fluorouracil. While the possibility of these occurring following Floxuridine therapy is remote because of its regional administration, one should be alert for these reactions following the administration of Floxuridine because of the pharmacological similarity of these two drugs: pancytopenia, agranulocytosis, myocardial ischemia, angina, anaphylaxis, generalized allergic reactions, acute cerebellar syndrome, nystagmus, headache, dry skin, fissuring, photosensitivity, pruritic maculopapular rash, increased pigmentation of the skin, vein pigmentation, lacrimal duct stenosis, visual changes, lacrimation, photophobia, disorientation, confusion, euphoria, epistaxis and nail changes, including loss of nails.

OVERDOSAGE:

The possibility of overdosage with Floxuridine is unlikely in view of the mode of administration. Nevertheless, the anticipated manifestations would be nausea, vomiting, diarrhea, gastrointestinal ulceration and bleeding, bone marrow depression (including thrombocytopenia, leukopenia and agranulocytosis). No specific antidotal therapy exists. Patients who have been exposed to an overdosage of Floxuridine should be monitored hematologically for at least four weeks. Should abnormalities appear, appropriate therapy should be utilized.

The acute intravenous toxicity of floxuridine is detailed in TABLE 1.

TABLE 1

Species	LD_{50} (mg/kg ± S.E.)
Mouse	880 ± 51
Rat	670 ± 73
Rabbit	94 ± 19.6
Dog	157 ± 46

DOSAGE AND ADMINISTRATION:

Each vial must be reconstituted with 5 ml of sterile water for injection to yield a solution containing approximately 100 mg of floxuridine/ml. The calculated daily dose(s) of the drug is then diluted with 5% dextrose or 0.9% sodium chloride injection to a volume appropriate for the infusion apparatus to be used. The administration of FUDR is best achieved with the use of an appropriate pump to overcome pressure in large arteries and to ensure a uniform rate of infusion.

Parenteral drug products should be inspected visually for particulate matter and discoloration prior to administration whenever solution and container permit.

The recommended therapeutic dosage schedule of Floxuridine by continuous arterial infusion is 0.1 to 0.6 mg/kg/day. The higher dosage ranges (0.4 to 0.6 mg) are usually employed for hepatic artery infusion because the liver metabolizes the drug, thus reducing the potential for systemic toxicity. Therapy can be given until adverse reactions appear. (See PRECAUTIONS.) When these side effects have subsided, therapy may be resumed. The patient should be maintained on therapy as long as response to Floxuridine continues.

Procedures for proper handling and disposal of anticancer drugs should be considered. Several guidelines on this subject have been published.[1-6] There is no general agreement that all of the procedures recommended in the guidelines are necessary or appropriate.

The sterile powder should be stored at 59° to 86°F (15° to 30°C). Reconstituted vials should be stored under refrigeration (36° to 46°F, 2° to 8°C) for not more than two weeks.

REFERENCES:

1. Recommendations for the safe handling of parenteral antineoplastic drugs. Washington, DC, U.S. Government Printing Office (NIH Publication No. 83-2621). **2.** AMA Council Report. Guidelines for handling parenteral antineoplastics. *JAMA 253:*1590-1592, Mar 15, 1985. **3.** National Study Commission on Cytotoxic Exposure: Recommendations for handling cytotoxic agents. Available from Louis P. Jeffrey, ScD, Director of Pharmacy Services, Rhode Island Hospital, 593 Eddy Street, Providence, Rhode Island 02902. **4.** Clinical Oncological Society of Australia: Guidelines and recommendations for safe handling of antineoplastic agents. *Med J Aust 1:* 426-428, Apr 30, 1983. **5.** Jones RB, Frank R, Mass T: Safe handling of chemotherapeutic agents: a report from the Mount Sinai Medical Center. *CA 33:*258-263, Sept-Oct 1983. **6.** ASHP technical assistance bulletin on handling cytotoxic drugs in hospitals. *Am J Hosp Pharm 42:*131-137, Jan 1985.

HOW SUPPLIED - EQUIVALENTS NOT AVAILABLE:

Injection, Lyphl-Soln - Intra-Arterial - 500 mg/vial

5 ml $125.40 FUDR, Roche 00004-1935-08

FLUCONAZOLE *(001301)*

CATEGORIES: Anti-Infectives; Antibiotics; Antifungals; Bone Marrow Transplantation; Candidiasis; Fungal Agents; Infections; Meningitis; Peritonitis; Pneumonia; Triazoles; Urinary Tract Infections; Vaginal Preparations; AIDS Related Complex*; Pregnancy Category C; FDA Class 1A ("Important Therapeutic Advantage"); Sales > $500 Million; FDA Approved 1990 Jan; Top 200 Drugs

* Indication not approved by the FDA

BRAND NAMES: *Alflucoz*; *Biozolene*; **Diflucan**; *Flucazol*; *Flukezol* (Mexico); *Fluzone*; *Forcan*; *Fungata* (Germany); *Oxifugol* (Mexico); *Syscan*; *Triflucan* (France); *Zonal* (Mexico)

(International brand names outside U.S. in italics)

FORMULARIES: Aetna; BC-BS; Humana; Kaiser; Medco; Medi-Cal; PCS; PruCare; United

COST OF THERAPY: $86.84 (Candidiasis; Tablet; 100 mg; 1/day; 15 days)

DESCRIPTION:

Diflucan (fluconazole), the first of a new subclass of synthetic triazole antifungal agents, is available as tablets for oral administration, as a powder for oral suspension and as a sterile solution for intravenous use in glass and in Viaflex Plus plastic containers.

Fluconazole is designated chemically as 2,4-difluoro-α,α¹-bis(1H-1,2,4-triazol-1-ylmethyl) benzyl alcohol with an empirical formula of $C_{13}H_{12}F_2N_6O$ and molecular weight 306.3.

Fluconazole is a white crystalline solid which is slightly soluble in water and saline.

DESCRIPTION: *(cont'd)*

Diflucan tablets contain 50, 100, or 200 mg of fluconazole and the following inactive ingredients: microcrystalline cellulose, dibasic calcium phosphate anhydrous, povidone, croscarmellose sodium, FD&C Red No. 40 aluminum lake dye, and magnesium stearate.

Diflucan for oral suspension contains 350 mg or 1400 mg of fluconazole and the following inactive ingredients: sucrose, sodium citrate dihydrate, citric acid anhydrous, sodium benzoate, titanium dioxide, colloidal silicon dioxide, xanthan gum and natural orange flavor. After reconstitution with 24 ml of distilled water or Purified Water (USP), each ml of reconstituted suspension contains 10 mg or 40 mg of fluconazole.

Diflucan injection is an iso-osmotic, sterile, nonpyrogenic solution of fluconazole in a sodium chloride or dextrose diluent. Each ml contains 2 mg of fluconazole and 9 mg of sodium chloride or 56 mg of dextrose, hydrous. The pH ranges from 4.0 to 8.0 in the sodium chloride diluent and from 3.5 to 6.5 in the dextrose diluent. Injection volumes of 100 ml and 200 ml are packaged in glass and in Viaflex Plus plastic containers.

The Viaflex Plus plastic container is fabricated from a specially formulated polyvinyl chloride (PL 146 Plastic) (Viaflex and PL 146 are registered trademarks of Baxter International, Inc.). The amount of water that can permeate from inside the container into the overwrap is insufficient to affect the solution significantly. Solutions in contact with the plastic container can leach out certain of its chemical components in very small amounts within the expiration period, e.g., di-2-ethylhexylphthalate (DEHP), up to 5 parts per million. However, the suitability of the plastic has been confirmed in tests in animals according to USP biological tests for plastic containers as well as by tissue culture toxicity studies.

CLINICAL PHARMACOLOGY:

Mode of Action: Fluconazole is a highly selective inhibitor of fungal cytochrome P-450 sterol C-14 alpha-demethylation. Mammalian cell demethylation is much less sensitive to fluconazole inhibition. The subsequent loss of normal sterols correlates with the accumulation of 14 alpha-methyl sterols in fungi and may be responsible for the fungistatic activity of fluconazole.

Pharmacokinetics and Metabolism: The pharmacokinetic properties of fluconazole are similar following administration by the intravenous or oral routes. In normal volunteers, the bioavailability of orally administered fluconazole is over 90% compared with intravenous administration. Bioequivalence was established between the 100 mg tablet and both suspension strengths when administered as a single 200 mg dose.

Peak plasma concentrations (C_{max}) in fasted normal volunteers occur between 1 and 2 hours with a terminal plasma elimination half-life of approximately 30 hours (range 20-50 hours) after oral administration.

In fasted normal volunteers, administration of a single oral 400 mg dose of fluconazole leads to a mean C_{max} of 6.72 mcg/ml (range: 4.12 to 8.08 mcg/ml) and after single oral doses of 50-400 mg, fluconazole plasma concentrations and AUC (area under the plasma concentration-time curve) are dose proportional.

Administration of a single oral 150 mg tablet of fluconazole to ten lactating women resulted in a mean C_{max} of 2.61 mcg/ml (range: 1.57 to 3.65 mcg/ml).

Steady-state concentrations are reached within 5-10 days following oral doses of 50-400 mg given once daily. Administration of a loading dose (on day 1) of twice the usual daily dose results in plasma concentrations close to steady-state by the second day. The apparent volume of distribution of fluconazole approximates that of total body water. Plasma protein binding is low (11-12%). Following either single- or multiple-oral doses for up to 14 days, fluconazole penetrates into all body fluids studied (see TABLE 1). In normal volunteers, saliva concentrations of fluconazole were equal to or slightly greater than plasma concentrations regardless of dose, route, or duration of dosing. In patients with bronchiectasis, sputum concentrations of fluconazole following a single 150 mg oral dose were equal to plasma concentrations at both 4 and 24 hours post dose. In patients with fungal meningitis, fluconazole concentrations in the CSF are approximately 80% of the corresponding plasma concentrations.

A single oral 150 mg dose of fluconazole administered to 27 patients penetrated into vaginal tissue, resulting in tissue:plasma ratios ranging from 0.94 to 1.14 over the first 48 hours following dosing.

A single oral 150 mg dose of fluconazole administered to 14 patients penetrated into vaginal fluid, resulting in fluid:plasma ratios ranging from 0.36 to 0.71 over the first 72 hours following dosing (TABLE 1).

TABLE 1

Tissue or Fluid	Ratio of FluconazoleTissue (Fluid)/Plasma Concentration*
Cerebrospinal fluid†	.5-.9
Saliva	1
Sputum	1
Blister fluid	1
Urine	10
Normal skin	10
Nails	1
Blister skin	2
Vaginal tissue	1
Vaginal fluid	0.4-0.7

* Relative to concurrent concentrations in plasma in subjects with normal renal function.

† Independent of degree of meningeal inflammation.

In normal volunteers, fluconazole is cleared primarily by renal excretion, with approximately 80% of the administered dose appearing in the urine as unchanged drug. About 11% of the dose is excreted in the urine as metabolites.

The pharmacokinetics of fluconazole are markedly affected by reduction in renal function. There is an inverse relationship between the elimination half-life and creatinine clearance. The dose of fluconazole may need to be reduced in patients with impaired renal function (See DOSAGE AND ADMINISTRATION). A 3-hour hemodialysis session decreases plasma concentrations by approximately 50%.

In normal volunteers, fluconazole administration (doses ranging from 200 mg to 400 mg once daily for up to 14 days) was associated with small and inconsistent effects on testosterone concentrations, endogenous corticosteroid concentrations, and the ACTH-stimulated cortisol response.

Pharmacokinetics in Children: In children, the following pharmacokinetic data [MEAN (% cv)] have been reported (TABLE 2A and TABLE 2B).

Clearance corrected for body weight was not affected by age in these studies. Mean body clearance in adults is reported to be 0.23 (17%) ml/min/kg.

In premature newborns (gestational age 26 to 29 weeks), the mean (% cv) clearance within 36 hours of birth was 0.180 (35%, N=7) ml/min/kg, which increased with time to a mean of 0.218 (31%, N=9) ml/min/kg six days later and 0.333 (56%, N=4) ml/min/kg 12 days later. Similarly, the half- life was 73.6 hours, which decreased with time to a mean of 53.2 hours six days later and 46.6 hours 12 days later.

CLINICAL PHARMACOLOGY: *(cont'd)*

TABLE 2A

Age Studied	Dose (mg/kg)	Clearance (ml/min/kg)
9 Months-13 Years	Single-Oral 2 mg/kg	0.40 (38%) N=14
9 Months-13 Years	Single-Oral 8 mg/kg	0.51 (60%) N=15
5-15 years	Multiple IV 2 mg/kg	0.49 (40%) N=4
5-15 years	Multiple IV 4 mg/kg	0.59 (64%) N=5
5-15 years	Multiple IV 8 mg/kg	0.66 (31%) N=5

TABLE 2B

Half-life (Hours)	C_{max} (mcg/ml)	Vdss (l/kg)
25.0	2.9 (22%) N=16	—
19.5	9.8 (20%) N=15	—
17.4	5.5 (25%) N=5	0.722 (36%) N=4
15.2	11.4 (44%) N=6	0.729 (33%) N=5
17.6	14.1 (22%) N=8	1.069 (37%) N=7

MICROBIOLOGY

Fluconazole exhibits *in vitro* activity against *Cryptococcus neoformans* and *Candida* spp. Fungistatic activity has also been demonstrated in normal and immunocompromised animal models for systemic and intracranial fungal infections due to *Cryptococcus neoformans* and for systemic infections due to *Candida albicans*.

In common with other azole antifungal agents, most fungi show a higher apparent sensitivity to fluconazole *in vivo* than *in vitro*. Fluconazole administered orally and/or intravenously was active in a variety of animal models of fungal infection using standard laboratory strains of fungi. Activity has been demonstrated against fungal infections caused by *Aspergillus flavus* and *Aspergillus fumigatus* in normal mice. Fluconazole has also been shown to be active in animal models of endemic mycoses, including one model of *Blastomyces dermatitidis* pulmonary infections in normal mice; one model of *Coccidioides immitis* intracranial infections in normal mice; and several models of *Histoplasma capsulatum* pulmonary infection in normal and immunosuppressed mice. The clinical significance of results obtained in these studies is unknown.

Concurrent administration of fluconazole and amphotericin B in infected normal and immunosuppressed mice showed the following results: a small additive antifungal effect in systemic infection with *C. albicans*, no interaction in intracranial infection with *Cr. neoformans*, and antagonism of the two drugs in systemic infection with *Asp. fumigatus*. The clinical significance of results obtained in these studies is unknown.

There have been reports of cases of superinfection with Candida species other than *C. albicans*, which are often inherently not susceptible to Diflucan (*e.g., Candida krusei*). Such cases may require alternative antifungal therapy.

CLINICAL STUDIES:

Cryptococcal Meningitis: In a multicenter study comparing fluconazole (200 mg/day) to amphotericin B (0.3 mg/kg/day) for treatment of cryptococcal meningitis in patients with AIDS, a multivariate analysis revealed three pretreatment factors that predicted death during the course of therapy: abnormal mental status, cerebrospinal fluid cryptococcal antigen titer greater than 1:1024, and cerebrospinal fluid white blood cell count of less than 20 cells/mm^3. Mortality among high risk patients was 33% and 40% for amphotericin B and Diflucan patients, respectively (p=0.58), with overall deaths 14% (9 of 63 subjects) and 18% (24 of 131 subjects) for the 2 arms of the study (p=0.48). Optimal doses and regimens for patients with acute cryptococcal meningitis and at high risk for treatment failure remain to be determined. (Saag, *et al*, N Engl J Med 1992;326:83-9)

Vaginal Candidiasis: Two adequate and well-controlled studies were conducted in the U.S. using the 150 mg tablet. In both, the results of the fluconazole regimen were comparable to the control regimen (clotrimazole or miconazole intravaginally for 7 days) both clinically and statistically at the one month post-treatment evaluation.

The therapeutic cure rate, defined as a complete resolution of signs and symptoms of vaginal candidiasis (clinical cure), along with a negative KOH examination and negative culture for *Candida* (microbiologic eradication), was 55% in both the fluconazole group and the vaginal products group (TABLE 3A and TABLE 3B).

TABLE 3A

Fluconazole PO 150 mg tablet	
Enrolled	448
Evaluable at Late Follow-up	347 (77%)
Clinical cure	239/347 (69%)
Mycologic erad.	213/347 (61%)
Therapeutic cure	190/347 (55%)

TABLE 3B

Vaginal Product qhs x 7 days	
Enrolled	422
Evaluable at Late Follow-up	327 (77%)
Clinical cure	235/327 (72%)
Mycologic erad.	196/327 (60%)
Therapeutic cure	179/327 (55%)

Approximately three-fourths of the enrolled patients had acute vaginitis (<4 episodes/12 months) and achieved 80% clinical cure, 67% mycologic eradication and 59% therapeutic cure when treated with a 150 mg fluconazole tablet administered orally. These rates were comparable to control products. The remaining one-fourth of enrolled patients had recurrent vaginitis (≥4 episodes/12 months) and achieved 57% clinical cure, 47% mycologic eradication and 40% therapeutic cure. The numbers are too small to make meaningful clinical or statistical comparisons with vaginal products in the treatment of patients with recurrent vaginitis.

Substantially more gastrointestinal events were reported in the fluconazole group compared to the vaginal product group. Most of the events were mild to moderate. Because fluconazole was given as a single dose, no discontinuations occurred (TABLE 4).

CLINICAL STUDIES: *(cont'd)*

TABLE 4

Parameter	Fluconazole PO	Vaginal Products
Evaluable patients	448	422
With any adverse event	141 (31%)	112 (27%)
Nervous System	90 (20%)	69 (16%)
Gastrointestinal	73 (16%)	18 (4%)
With drug-related event	117 (26%)	67 (16%)
Nervous System	61 (14%)	29 (7%)
Headache	58 (13%)	28 (7%)
With drug-related event (cont.)		
Gastrointestinal	68 (15%)	13 (3%)
Abdominal pain	25 (6%)	7 (2%)
Nausea	30 (7%)	3 (1%)
Diarrhea	12 (3%)	2 (<1%)
Application site event	0 (0%)	19 (5%)
Taste Perversion	6 (1%)	0 (0%)

PEDIATRIC

Oropharyngeal candidiasis: An open-label, comparative study of the efficacy and safety if fluconazole (2-3 mg/kg/day) and oral nystatin (400,000 I.U. 4 times daily) in immunocompromised children with oropharyngeal candidiasis was conducted. Clinical and mycological response rates were higher in the children treated with fluconazole.

Clinical cure at the end of treatment was reported for 86% of fluconazole treated patients compared to 46% of nystatin treated patients. Mycologically, 76% of fluconazole treated patients had the infecting organism eradicated compared to 11% for nystatin treated patients (TABLE 5).

TABLE 5

	Fluconazole	Nystatin
Enrolled	96	90
Clinical Cure	76/88 (86%)	36/78 (46%)
Mycological eradication*	55/72 (76%)	6/54 (11%)

* Subjects without follow-up cultures for any reason were considered nonevaluable for mycological response.

The proportion of patients with clinical relapse 2 weeks after the end of treatment was 14% for subjects receiving fluconazole and 16% for subjects receiving nystatin. At 4 weeks after the end of treatment the percentages of patients with clinical relapse were 22% for Diflucan and 23% for nystatin.

INDICATIONS AND USAGE:

Fluconazole is indicated for the treatment of:

1. Vaginal Candidiasis (vaginal yeast infections due to *Candida*).

2. Oropharyngeal and esophageal candidiasis. In open noncomparative studies of relatively small numbers of patients, fluconazole was also effective for the treatment of Candida urinary tract infections, peritonitis, and systemic Candida infections including candidemia, disseminated candidiasis, and pneumonia.

3. Cryptococcal meningitis. Before prescribing fluconazole for AIDS patients with cryptococcal meningitis, please see CLINICAL STUDIES section. Studies comparing fluconazole to amphotericin B in non-HIV infected patients have not been conducted.

Prophylaxis: Fluconazole is also indicated to decrease the incidence of candidiasis in patients undergoing bone marrow transplantation who receive cytotoxic chemotherapy and/or radiation therapy.

Specimens for fungal culture and other relevant laboratory studies (serology, histopathology) should be obtained prior to therapy to isolate and identify causative organisms. Therapy may be instituted before the results of the cultures and other laboratory studies are known; however, once these results become available, anti-infective therapy should be adjusted accordingly.

CONTRAINDICATIONS:

Fluconazole is contraindicated in patients who have shown hypersensitivity to fluconazole or to any of its excipients. There is no information regarding cross hypersensitivity between fluconazole and other azole antifungal agents. Caution should be used in prescribing fluconazole to patients with hypersensitivity to other azoles.

WARNINGS:

(1) Hepatic injury: Fluconazole has been associated with rare cases of serious hepatic toxicity, including fatalities primarily in patients with serious underlying medical conditions. In cases of fluconazole associated hepatotoxicity, no obvious relationship to total daily dose, duration of therapy, sex or age of the patient has been observed. Fluconazole hepatotoxicity has usually, but not always, been reversible on discontinuation of therapy. Patients who develop abnormal liver function tests during fluconazole therapy should be monitored for the development of more severe hepatic injury. Fluconazole should be discontinued if clinical signs and symptoms consistent with liver disease develop that may be attributable to fluconazole.

(2) Anaphylaxis: In rare cases, anaphylaxis has been reported.

(3) Dermatologic: Patients have rarely developed exfoliative skin disorders during treatment with fluconazole. In patients with serious underlying diseases (predominantly AIDS and malignancy), these have rarely resulted in a fatal outcome. Patients who develop rashes during treatment with fluconazole should be monitored closely and the drug discontinued if lesions progress.

PRECAUTIONS:

GENERAL

Single Dose: The convenience and efficacy of the single dose oral tablet of fluconazole regimen for the treatment of vaginal yeast infections should be weighed against the acceptability of a higher incidence of drug related adverse events with fluconazole (26%) versus intravaginal agents (16%) in U.S. comparative clinical studies. (See ADVERSE REACTIONS and CLINICAL STUDIES.)

CARCINOGENESIS, MUTAGENESIS, AND IMPAIRMENT OF FERTILITY

Fluconazole showed no evidence of carcinogenic potential in mice and rats treated orally for 24 months at doses of 2.5, 5 or 10 mg/kg/day (approximately 2-7x the recommended human dose). Male rats treated with 5 and 10 mg/kg/day had an increased incidence of hepatocellular adenomas.

PRECAUTIONS: *(cont'd)*

Fluconazole, with or without metabolic activation, was negative in tests for mutagenicity in 4 strains of *S. typhimurium*, and in the mouse lymphoma L5178Y system. Cytogenetic studies *in vivo* (murine bone marrow cells, following oral administration of fluconazole) and *in vitro* (human lymphocytes exposed to fluconazole at 1000 mcg/ml) showed no evidence of chromosomal mutations.

Fluconazole did not affect the fertility of male or female rats treated orally with daily doses of 5, 10 or 20 mg/kg or with parenteral doses of 5, 25 or 75 mg/kg, although the onset of parturition was slightly delayed at 20 mg/kg p.o. In an intravenous perinatal study in rats at 5, 20 and 40 mg, dystocia and prolongation of parturition were observed in a few dams at 20 mg/kg (approximately 5-15x the recommended human dose) and 40 mg/kg, but not at 5 mg/kg. The disturbances in parturition were reflected by a slight increase in the number of still-born pups and decrease of neonatal survival at these dose levels. The effects on parturition in rats are consistent with the species specific estrogen-lowering property produced by high doses of fluconazole. Such a hormone change has not been observed in women treated with fluconazole. (See CLINICAL PHARMACOLOGY.)

PREGNANCY, TERATOGENIC EFFECTS, PREGNANCY CATEGORY C

Fluconazole was administered orally to pregnant rabbits during organogenesis in two studies, at 5, 10 and 20 mg/kg and at 5, 25, and 75 mg/kg, respectively. Maternal weight gain was impaired at all dose levels, and abortions occurred at 75 mg/kg (approximately 20-60x the recommended human dose); no adverse fetal effects were detected. In several studies in which pregnant rats were treated orally with fluconazole during organogenesis, maternal weight gain was impaired and placental weights were increased at 25 mg/kg. There were no fetal effects at 5 or 10 mg/kg; increases in fetal anatomical variants (supernumerary ribs, renal pelvis dilation) and delays in ossification were observed at 25 and 50 mg/kg and higher doses. At doses ranging from 80 mg/kg (approximately 20-60x the recommended human dose) to 320 mg/kg embryolethality in rats was increased and fetal abnormalities included wavy ribs, cleft palate and abnormal cranio-facial ossification. These effects are consistent with the inhibition of estrogen synthesis in rats and may be a result of known effects of lowered estrogen on pregnancy, organogenesis and parturition.

There are no adequate and well controlled studies in pregnant women. Fluconazole should be used in pregnancy only if the potential benefit justifies the possible risk to the fetus.

NURSING MOTHERS

Fluconazole is secreted in human milk at concentrations similar to plasma. Therefore, the use of fluconazole in nursing mothers is not recommended.

PEDIATRIC USE

An open-label, randomized, controlled trial has shown Diflucan to be effective in the treatment of oropharyngeal candidiasis in children 6 months to 13 years of age. (See CLINICAL STUDIES.)

The use of fluconazole in children with cryptococcal meningitis, Candida esophagitis, or systemic Candida infections is supported by the efficacy shown for these indications in adults and by the results from several small noncomparative pediatric clinical studies. In addition, pharmacokinetic studies in children (see CLINICAL PHARMACOLOGY), have established a dose proportionality between children and adults. (See DOSAGE AND ADMINISTRATION.)

In a noncomparative study of children with serious systemic fungal infections, most of which were candidemia, the effectiveness of fluconazole was similar to that reported for the treatment of candidemia in adults. Of 17 subjects with culture-confirmed candidemia, 11 of 14 (79%) with baseline symptoms (3 were asymptomatic) had a clinical cure: 13/15 (87%) of evaluable patients had a mycologic cure at the end of treatment but two of these patients relapsed at 10 and 18 days, respectively, following cessation of therapy.

The efficacy of fluconazole for the suppression of cryptococcal meningitis was successful in 4 of 5 children treated in a compassionate-use study of fluconazole for the treatment of life-threatening or serious mycosis. There is no information regarding the efficacy of fluconazole for primary treatment of cryptococcal meningitis in children.

The safety profile of fluconazole in children has been studied in 577 children ages 1 day to 17 years who received doses ranging from 1 to 15 mg/kg/day for 1 to 1,616 days. (See ADVERSE REACTIONS.)

Efficacy of fluconazole has not been established in infants less than 6 months of age. (See CLINICAL PHARMACOLOGY.) A small number of patients (29) ranging in age from 1 day to 6 months have been treated safely with fluconazole.

DRUG INTERACTIONS:

See General.

Clinically or potentially significant drug interactions between fluconazole and the following agents/classes have been observed. These are described in greater detail below:

Oral Hypoglycemics: Clinically significant hypoglycemia may be precipitated by the use of fluconazole with oral hypoglycemic agents: one fatality has been reported from hypoglycemia in association with combined fluconazole and glyburide use. Fluconazole reduces the metabolism of tolbutamide, glyburide, and glipizide and increases the plasma concentration of these agents. When fluconazole is used concomitantly with these or other sulfonylurea oral hypoglycemic agents, blood glucose concentrations should be carefully monitored and the dose of the sulfonylurea should be adjusted as necessary.

Coumarin-Type Anticoagulants: Prothrombin time may be increased in patients receiving concomitant fluconazole and coumarin-type anticoagulants. Careful monitoring of prothrombin time in patients receiving fluconazole and coumarin-type anticoagulants is recommended.

Phenytoin: Fluconazole increases the plasma concentrations of phenytoin. Careful monitoring of phenytoin concentrations in patients receiving fluconazole and phenytoin is recommended.

Cyclosporine: Fluconazole may significantly increase cyclosporine levels in renal transplant patients with or without renal impairment. Careful monitoring of cyclosporine concentrations and serum creatinine is recommended in patients receiving fluconazole and cyclosporine.

Rifampin: Rifampin enhances the metabolism of concurrently administered fluconazole. Depending on clinical circumstances, consideration should be given to increasing the dose of fluconazole when it is administered with rifampin.

Theophylline: Fluconazole increases the serum concentrations of theophylline. Careful monitoring of serum theophylline concentrations in patients receiving fluconazole and theophylline is recommended.

Terfenadine: Because of the occurrence of serious cardiac dysrhythmias in patients receiving other azole antifungals in conjunction with terfenadine, an interaction study has been performed (See DRUG INTERACTIONS), and failed to demonstrate a clinically significant drug interaction. Although these events have not been observed in patients receiving fluconazole, the co-administration of fluconazole and terfenadine should be carefully monitored.

Fluconazole tablets coadministered with ethinyl estradiol- and levonorgestrel -containing oral contraceptives produced an overall mean increase in ethinyl estradiol and levonorgestrel levels; however, in some patients there were decreases up to 47% and 33% of ethinyl estradiol and levonorgestrel levels (See DRUG INTERACTIONS.) The data presently available indicate that the decreases in some individual ethinyl estradiol and levonorgestrel AUC values

DRUG INTERACTIONS: *(cont'd)*

with fluconazole treatment are likely the result of random variation. While there is evidence that fluconazole can inhibit the metabolism of ethinyl estradiol and levonorgestrel, there is no evidence that fluconazole is a net inducer of ethinyl estradiol or levonorgestrel metabolism. The clinical significance of these effects is presently unknown.

Physicians should be aware that interaction studies with medications other than those listed in CLINICAL PHARMACOLOGY have not been conducted, but such interactions may occur.

DRUG INTERACTION STUDIES

Oral Contraceptives: Oral contraceptives were administered as a single dose both before and after the oral administration of fluconazole 50 mg once daily for 10 days in 10 healthy women. There was no significant difference in ethinyl estradiol or levonorgestrel AUC after the administration of 50 mg of fluconazole. The mean increase in ethinyl estradiol AUC was 6% (range: -47 to 108%) and levonorgestrel AUC increased 17% (range: -33 to 141%).

Twenty-five normal females received daily doses of both 200 mg of fluconazole tablets or placebo for two, ten-day periods. The treatment cycles were one month apart with all subjects receiving fluconazole during one cycle and placebo during the other. The order of study treatment was random. Single doses of an oral contraceptive tablet containing levonorgestrel and ethinyl estradiol were administered on the final treatment day (day 10) of both cycles. Following administration of 200 mg of fluconazole, the mean percentage increase of AUC for levonorgestrel compared to placebo was 25% (range: -12 to 82%) and the mean percentage increase for ethinyl estradiol compared to placebo was 38% (range: -11 to 101%). Both of these increases were statistically significantly different from placebo.

Cimetidine: Fluconazole 100 mg was administered as a single oral dose alone and two hours after a single dose of cimetidine 400 mg to six healthy male volunteers. After the administration of cimetidine, there was a significant decrease in fluconazole AUC and C_{max}. There was a mean ± SD decrease in fluconazole AUC of 13% ± 11% (range: -3.4 to -31%) and C_{max} decreased 19% ± 14% (range: -5 to -40%). However, the administration of cimetidine 600 mg to 900 mg intravenously over a four hour period (from one hour before to 3 hours after a single oral dose of fluconazole 200 mg) did not affect the bioavailability or pharmacokinetics of fluconazole in 24 healthy male volunteers.

Antacid: Administration of Maalox (20 ml) to 14 normal male volunteers immediately prior to a single dose of fluconazole 100 mg had no effect on the absorption or elimination of fluconazole.

Hydrochlorothiazide: Concomitant oral administration of 100 mg Diflucan and 50 mg hydrochlorothiazide for 10 days in 13 normal volunteers resulted in a significant increase in fluconazole AUC and C_{max} compared to Diflucan given alone. There was a mean ± SD increase in fluconazole AUC and C_{max} 45% ± 31% (range: 19 to 114%) and 43% ± 31% (range: 19 to 122%), respectively. These changes are attributable to a mean ± SD reduction in renal clearance of 30% ± 12% (range: -10 to -50%).

Rifampin: Administration of a single oral 200 mg dose of fluconazole after 15 days of rifampin administration as 600 mg daily in eight healthy male volunteers resulted in a significant decrease in fluconazole AUC and a significant increase in apparent oral clearance of fluconazole. There was a mean ± SD reduction in fluconazole AUC of 23% ± 9% (range: - 13 to -42%). Apparent oral clearance of fluconazole increased 32% ± 17% (range: 16 to 72%). Fluconazole half-life decreased from 33.4 ± 4.4 hours to 26.8 ± 3.9 hours. (See PRECAUTIONS.)

Warfarin: There was a significant increase in prothrombin time response (area under the prothrombin time-time curve) following a single dose of warfarin (15 mg) administered to 13 normal male volunteers following oral fluconazole 200 mg administered daily for 14 days as compared to the administration of warfarin alone. There was a mean ± SD increase in the prothrombin time response (area under the prothrombin time-time curve) of 7% ± 4% (range: -2 to 13%). (See PRECAUTIONS.)Mean is based on data from 12 subjects as one of 13 subjects experienced a 2-fold increase in his prothrombin time response.

Phenytoin: Phenytoin AUC was determined after 4 days of phenytoin dosing (200 mg daily, orally for 3 days followed by 250 mg intravenously for one dose) both with and without the administration of fluconazole (oral fluconazole 200 mg daily for 16 days) in 10 normal male volunteers. There was a significant increase in phenytoin AUC. The mean ± SD increase in phenytoin AUC was 88% ± 68% (range: 16 to 247%). The absolute magnitude of this interaction is unknown because of the intrinsically nonlinear disposition of phenytoin. (See PRECAUTIONS.)

Cyclosporine: Cyclosporine AUC and C_{max} were determined before and after the administration of fluconazole 200 mg daily for 14 days in eight renal transplant patients who had been on cyclosporine therapy for at least 6 months and on a stable cyclosporine dose for at least 6 weeks. There was a significant increase in cyclosporine AUC, C_{max}, C_{min} (24 hour concentration), and a significant reduction in apparent oral clearance following the administration of fluconazole. The mean ± SD increase in AUC was 92% ± 43% (range: 18 to 147%). The C_{max} increased 60% ± 48% (range: -5 to 133%). The C_{min} increased 157% ± 96% (range: 33 to 360%). The apparent oral clearance decreased 45% ± 15% (range: -15 to -60%). (See PRECAUTIONS.)

Zidovudine: Plasma zidovudine concentrations were determined on two occasions (before and following fluconazole 200 mg daily for 15 days) in 13 volunteers with AIDS or ARC who were on a stable zidovudine dose for at least two weeks. There was a significant increase in zidovudine AUC following the administration of fluconazole. The mean ± SD increase in AUC was 20% ± 32% (range: -27 to 104%). The metabolite, GZDV to parent drug ratio significantly decreased after the administration of fluconazole, from 7.6 ± 3.6 to 5.7 ± 2.2.

Theophylline: The pharmacokinetics of theophylline were determined from a single intravenous dose of aminophylline (6 mg/kg) before and after the oral administration of fluconazole 200 mg daily for 14 days in 16 normal male volunteers. There were significant increases in theophylline AUC, C_{max}, and half-life with a corresponding decrease in clearance. The mean ± SD theophylline AUC increased 21% ± 16% (range: -5 to 48%). The C_{max} increased 13% ± 17% (range: -13 to 40%). Theophylline clearance decreased 16% ± 11% (range: -32 to 5%). The half-life of theophylline increased from 6.6 ± 1.7 hours to 7.9 ± 1.5 hours.

Terfenadine: Six healthy volunteers received terfenadine 60 mg bid for 15 days. Fluconazole 200 mg was administered daily from days 9 through 15. Fluconazole did not affect terfenadine plasma concentrations. Terfenadine acid metabolite AUC increased 36% ± 36% (range: 7 to 102%) from day 8 to 15 with the concomitant administration of fluconazole. There was no change in cardiac repolarization as a measure by Holter QTc intervals.

Oral Hypoglycemics: The effects of fluconazole on the pharmacokinetics of the sulfonylurea oral hypoglycemic agents tolbutamide, glipizide, and glyburide were evaluated in three placebo- controlled studies in normal volunteers. All subjects received the sulfonylurea alone as a single dose and again as a single dose following the administration of fluconazole 100 mg daily for 7 days. In these three studies 22/46 (47.8%) of fluconazole treated patients and 9/22 (40.1%) of placebo treated patients experienced symptoms consistent with hypoglycemia. (See PRECAUTIONS.)

Tolbutamide: In 13 normal male volunteers, there was significant increase in tolbutamide (500 mg single dose) AUC and C_{max} following the administration of fluconazole. There was a mean ± SD increase in tolbutamide AUC of 26% ± 9% (range: 12 to 39%). Tolbutamide C_{max} increased 11% ± 9% (range: -6 to 27%). (See PRECAUTIONS.)

DRUG INTERACTIONS: *(cont'd)*

Glipizide: The AUC and C_{max} of glipizide (2.5 mg single dose) were significantly increased following the administration of fluconazole in 13 normal male volunteers. There was mean ± SD increase in AUC of 49% ± 13% (range: 27 to 73%) and an increase in C_{max} of 19% ± 23% (range: -11 to 79%). (See PRECAUTIONS.)

Glyburide: The AUC and C_{max} of glyburide (5 mg single dose) were significantly increased following the administration of fluconazole in 20 normal male volunteers. There was a mean ± SD increase in AUC of 44% ± 29% (range: -13 to 115%) and C_{max} increased 19% ± 19% (range: -23 to 62%). Five subjects required oral glucose following the ingestion of glyburide after 7 days of fluconazole administration. (See PRECAUTIONS.)

ADVERSE REACTIONS:

In Patients Receiving a Single Dose for Vaginal Candidiasis: During comparative clinical studies conducted in the United States, 448 patients with vaginal candidiasis were treated with Diflucan, 150 mg single dose. The overall incidence of side effects possibly related to Diflucan was 26%. In 422 patients receiving active comparative agents, the incidence was 16%. The most common treatment-related adverse events reported in the patients who received 150 mg single dose fluconazole for vaginitis were headache (13%), nausea (7%), and abdominal pain (6%). Other side effects reported with an incidence equal to or greater than 1% included diarrhea (3%), dyspepsia (1%), dizziness (1%), and taste perversion (1%). Most of the reported side effects were mild to moderate in severity. Rarely, angioedema and anaphylactic reaction have been reported in marketing experience.

In Patients Receiving Multiple Doses for Other Infections: Sixteen percent of over 4000 patients treated with fluconazole in clinical trials of 7 days or more experienced adverse events. Treatment was discontinued in 1.5% of patients due to adverse clinical events and in 1.3% of patients due to laboratory test abnormalities.

Clinical adverse events were reported more frequently in HIV infected patients (21%) than in non-HIV infected patients (13%); however, the patterns in HIV infected and non-HIV infected patients were similar. The proportions of patients discontinuing therapy due to clinical adverse events were similar in the two groups (1.5%).

The following treatment-related clinical adverse events occurred at an incidence of 1% or greater in 4048 patients receiving Diflucan for 7 or more days in clinical trials: nausea 3.7%, headache 1.9%, skin rash 1.8%, vomiting 1.7%, abdominal pain 1.7%, and diarrhea 1.5%.

The following adverse events have occurred under conditions where a casual association is probable:

Hepatobiliary: In combined clinical trials and marketing experience, there have been rare cases of serious hepatic reactions during treatment with fluconazole. (See WARNINGS.) The spectrum of these hepatic reactions has ranged from mild transient elevations in transaminases to clinical hepatitis, cholestasis and fulminant hepatic failure, including fatalities. Instances of fatal hepatic reactions were noted to occur primarily in patients with serious underlying medical conditions (predominantly AIDS or malignancy) and often while taking multiple concomitant medications. Transient hepatic reactions, including hepatitis and jaundice, have occurred among patients with no other identifiable risk factors. In each of these cases, liver function returned to baseline on discontinuation of fluconazole.

In two comparative trials evaluating the efficacy of fluconazole for the suppression of relapse of cryptococcal meningitis, a statistically significant increase was observed in median AST (SGOT) levels from a baseline value of 30 IU/l to 41 IU/l in one trial and 34 IU/l to 66 IU/l in the other. The overall rate of serum transaminase elevations of more than 8 times the upper limit of normal was approximately 1% in fluconazole-treated patients in clinical trials. These elevations occurred in patients with severe underlying disease, predominantly AIDS or malignancies, most of whom were receiving multiple concomitant medications, including many known to be hepatotoxic. The incidence of abnormally elevated serum transaminases was greater in patients taking fluconazole concomitantly with one or more of the following medications: rifampin, phenytoin, isoniazid, valproic acid, or oral sulfonylurea hypoglycemic agents.

Immunological: In rare cases, anaphylaxis has been reported.

The following adverse events have occurred under conditions where a casual association is uncertain:

Central Nervous System: seizures.

Dermatologic: Exfoliative skin disorders including Stevens-Johnson Syndrome and toxic epidermal necroivsis (See WARNINGS, alopecia).

Hematopoietic and Lymphatic: leukopenia, thrombocytopenia.

Metabolic: hypercholesterolemia, hypertriglyceridemia, hypokalemia.

Adverse Reactions in Children: In phase 2/3 clinical trials conducted in the United States and in Europe, 577 pediatric patients, ages 1 day to 17 years were treated with fluconazole at doses up to 15 mg/kg/day for up to 1,616 days. Thirteen percent of children experienced treatment related adverse events. The most commonly reported events were vomiting (5%), abdominal pain (3%), nausea (2%), and diarrhea (2%). Treatment was discontinued inn 2.3% of patients due to adverse clinical events and in 1.4% of patients due to laboratory test abnormalities. The majority of treatment-related laboratory abnormalities were elevations of transaminases or alkaline phosphatase (TABLE 6).

TABLE 6 Percentage of Patients With Treatment-Related Side Effects

	Fluconazole (N=577)	Comparative Agents (N=451)
With any side effect	13.0	9.3
Vomiting	5.4	5.1
Abdominal pain	2.8	1.6
Nausea	2.3	1.6
Diarrhea	2.1	2.2

OVERDOSAGE:

There has been one reported case of overdosage with fluconazole. A 42-year-old patient infected with human immunodeficiency virus developed hallucinations and exhibited paranoid behavior after reportedly ingesting 8200 mg of fluconazole. The patient was admitted to the hospital, and his condition resolved within 48 hours.

In the event of overdose, symptomatic treatment (with supportive measures and gastric lavage if clinically indicated) should be instituted.

Fluconazole is largely excreted in urine. A three hour hemodialysis session decreases plasma levels by approximately 50%.

In mice and rats receiving very high doses of fluconazole, clinical effects in both species included decreased motility and respiration, ptosis, lacrimation, salivation, urinary incontinence, loss of righting reflex and cyanosis; death was sometimes preceded by clonic convulsions.

DOSAGE AND ADMINISTRATION:

DOSAGE AND ADMINISTRATION IN ADULTS

Single Dose: *Vaginal candidiasis:* The recommended dosage of fluconazole for vaginal candidiasis is 150 mg as a single oral dose.

Multiple Dose: SINCE ORAL ABSORPTION IS RAPID AND ALMOST COMPLETE, THE DAILY DOSE OF FLUCONAZOLE IS THE SAME FOR ORAL (TABLETS AND SUSPENSION) AND INTRAVENOUS ADMINISTRATION. In general, a leading dose of twice the daily dose is recommended on the first day of therapy to result in plasma concentrations close to steady-state by the second day of therapy.

The daily dose of fluconazole for the treatment of infections other than vaginal candidiasis should be based on the infecting organism and the patient's response to therapy. Treatment should be continued until clinical parameters or laboratory tests indicate that active fungal infection has subsided. An inadequate period of treatment may lead to recurrence of active infection. Patients with AIDS and cryptococcal meningitis or recurrent oropharyngeal candidiasis usually require maintenance therapy to prevent relapse.

Oropharyngeal Candidiasis: The recommended dosage of fluconazole for oropharyngeal candidiasis is 200 mg on the first day, followed by 100 mg once daily. Clinical evidence of oropharyngeal candidiasis generally resolves within several days, but treatment should be continued for at least 2 weeks to decrease the likelihood of relapse.

Esophageal Candidiasis: The recommended dosage of fluconazole for esophageal candidiasis is 200 mg on the first day, followed by 100 mg once daily. Doses up to 400 mg/day may be used, based on medical judgment of the patient's response to therapy. Patients with esophageal candidiasis should be treated for a minimum of three weeks and for at least two weeks following resolution of symptoms.

Systemic Candida Infections: For systemic Candida infections including candidemia, disseminated candidiasis, and pneumonia, optimal therapeutic dosage and duration of therapy have not been established. In open, noncomparative studies of small numbers of patients, doses of up to 400 mg daily have been used.

Urinary Tract Infection and Peritonitis: For the treatment of Candida urinary tract infections and peritonitis, daily doses of 50-200 mg have been used in open, noncomparative studies of small numbers of patients.

Cryptococcal Meningitis: The recommended dosage for treatment of acute cryptococcal meningitis is 400 mg on the first day, followed by 200 mg once daily. A dosage of 400 mg once daily may be used, based on medical judgment of the patient's response to therapy. The recommended duration of treatment for initial therapy of cryptococcal meningitis is 10-12 weeks after the cerebrospinal fluid becomes culture negative. The recommended dosage of fluconazole for suppression of relapse of cryptococcal meningitis in patients with AIDS is 200 mg once daily.

Prophylaxis in Patients Undergoing Bone Marrow Transplantation: The recommended fluconazole daily dosage for the prevention of candidiasis of patients undergoing bone marrow transplantation is 400 mg once daily. Patients who are anticipated to have severe granulocytopenia (less than 500 neutrophils per cu mm) should start fluconazole prophylaxis several days before the anticipated onset of neutropenia, and continue for 7 days after the neutrophil count rises above 1000 cells per cu mm.

DOSAGE AND ADMINISTRATION IN CHILDREN

The following dose equivalency scheme should generally provide equivalent exposure in pediatric and adult patients (TABLE 7).

TABLE 7

Pediatric Patients	Adults
3 mg/kg	100 mg
6 mg/kg	200 mg
12* mg/kg	400 mg

* Some older children may have clearances similar to that of adults. Absolute doses exceeding 600 mg/day are not recommended.

Experience with fluconazole in neonates is limited to pharmacokinetic studies in premature newborns. (See CLINICAL PHARMACOLOGY.) Based on the prolonged half-life seen in premature newborns (gestational age 26 to 29 weeks), these children, in the first two weeks of life, should receive the same dosage (mg/kg) as in older children, but administered every 72 hours. After the first two weeks, these children should be dosed once daily. No information regarding fluconazole pharmacokinetics in full-term newborns is available.

Oropharyngeal Candidiasis: The recommended dosage of fluconazole for oropharyngeal candidiasis in children is 6 mg/kg on the first day, followed by 3 mg/kg once daily. Treatment should be administered for at least 2 weeks to decrease the likelihood of relapse.

Esophageal Candidiasis: For the treatment of esophageal candidiasis, the recommended dosage of fluconazole in children is 6 mg/kg on the first day, followed by 3 mg/kg once daily. Doses up to 12 mg/kg/day may be used based on medical judgment of the patient's response to therapy. Patients with esophageal candidiasis should be treated for a minimum of three weeks for at least 2 weeks following the resolution of symptoms.

Systemic Candida Infections: For the treatment of candidemia and disseminated Candida infections, daily doses of 6-12 mg/kg/day have been used in an open, noncomparative study of a small number of children.

Cryptococcal Meningitis: For the treatment of acute cryptococcal meningitis, the recommended dosage is 12 mg/kg on the first day, followed by 6 mg/kg once daily. A dosage of 12 mg/kg once daily may be used, based on medical judgment of the patient's response to therapy. The recommended duration of treatment for initial therapy of cryptococcal meningitis is 10-12 weeks after the cerebrospinal fluid becomes culture negative. For suppression of relapse of cryptococcal meningitis in children with AIDS, the recommended dose of fluconazole is 6 mg/kg once daily.

Dosage In Patients With Impaired Renal Function: Fluconazole is cleared primarily by renal excretion as unchanged drug. There is no need to adjust single dose therapy for vaginal candidiasis because of impaired renal function. In patients with impaired renal function who will receive multiple doses of fluconazole, an initial loading dose of 50 to 400 mg should be given. After the loading dose, the daily dose (according to indication) should be based on TABLE 8.

TABLE 8

Creatinine Clearance (ml/min)	Percent of Recommended Dose
>50	100%
11-50	50%
Patients receiving regular hemodialysis	One recommended dose after each dialysis

These are suggested dose adjustments based on pharmacokinetics following administration of multiple doses. Further adjustment may be needed depending upon clinical condition.

DOSAGE AND ADMINISTRATION: *(cont'd)*

When serum creatinine is the only measure of renal function available, the formula found in TABLE 9 (based on sex, weight, and age of the patient) should be used to estimate the creatinine clearance

TABLE 9

Males: [Weight (kg) × (140–Age)] ÷ [72 × Serum Creatnine (mg/100ml]
Females: 0.85 × the above value

Although the pharmacokinetics of fluconazole has not been studied in children with renal insufficiency, dosage reduction in children with renal insufficiency should parallel that recommended for adults. The formula found in TABLE 10 may be used to estimate creatinine clearance in children:

TABLE 10

$$\frac{K \times \text{Linear Length or Height (cm)}}{\text{Serum Creatnine (mg/100 ml)}}$$

K = 0.55 for children older than 1 year and 0.45 for infants.

ADMINISTRATION

Fluconazole may be administered either orally or by intravenous infusion. Diflucan injection has been used safely for up to fourteen days of intravenous therapy. The intravenous infusion of fluconazole should be administered at a maximum rate of approximately 200 mg/hour, given as a continuous infusion.

Fluconazole injections in glass and Viaflex Plus plastic containers are intended only for intravenous administration using sterile equipment.

Parenteral drug products should be inspected visually for particulate matter and discoloration prior to administration whenever solution and container permit.

Do not use if the solution is cloudy or precipitated or if the seal is not intact.

Directions for Mixing the Oral Suspension Prepare a suspension at time of dispensing as follows: tap bottle until all the powder flows freely. To reconstitute, add 24 ml of distilled water or Purified Water (USP) to fluconazole bottle and shake vigorously to suspend powder. Each bottle will deliver 35 ml of suspension. The concentrations of the reconstituted suspensions are as found in TABLE 11.

TABLE 11

Fluconazole Content per Bottle	Concentration of Reconstituted Suspension
350 mg	10 mg/ml
1400 mg	40 mg/ml

Note: Shake oral suspension well before using. Store reconstituted suspension between 86°F (30°C) and 41°F (5°C) and discard unused portion after 2 weeks. Protect from freezing.

Directions for IV Use of Fluconazole in Viaflex Plus Plastic Containers Do not remove unit from overwrap until ready for use. The overwrap is a moisture barrier. The inner bag maintains the sterility of the product.

CAUTION: Do not use plastic containers in series connections. Such use could result in air embolism due to residual air being drawn from the primary container before administration of the fluid from the secondary container is completed.

To Open: Tear overwrap down side at slit and remove solution container. Some opacity of the plastic due to moisture absorption during the sterilization process may be observed. This is normal and does not affect the solution quality or safety. The opacity will diminish gradually. After removing overwrap, check for minute leaks by squeezing inner bag firmly. If leaks are found, discard solution as sterility may be impaired.

DO NOT ADD SUPPLEMENTARY MEDICATION.

PREPARATION FOR ADMINISTRATION

1. Suspend container from eyelet support.
2. Remove plastic protector from outlet port at bottom of container.
3. Attach administration set. Refer to complete directions accompanying set.

PATIENT INFORMATION:

Fluconazole is used to treat fungus infections. Notify your physician if you are pregnant or nursing. This medication may be taken with or without food. Take at regular intervals and complete the entire course of therapy. Notify your physician if you develop severe abdominal pain, yellowing of the skin or eyes, rash, dark urine, or pale stools.

HOW SUPPLIED:

Diflucan Tablets: Pink trapezoidal tablets containing 50, 100 or 200 mg of fluconazole are packaged in bottles or unit dose blisters. The 150 mg fluconazole tablets are pink and oval shaped, packaged in a single dose unit blister. *Storage:* Store tablets below 86°F (30°C).

Diflucan for Oral Suspension: Diflucan for oral suspension is supplied as an orange-flavored powder to provide 35 ml per bottle. *Storage:* Store dry powder below 86°F (30°C). Store reconstituted suspension between 86°F (30°C) and 41°F (5°C) and discard unused portion after 2 weeks. Protect from freezing.

Diflucan Injections: Diflucan injections for intravenous infusion administration are formulated as sterile iso-osmotic solutions containing 2 mg/ml of fluconazole. They are supplied in glass bottles or in Viaflex Plus plastic containers containing volumes of 100 ml or 200 ml affording doses of 200 mg and 400 mg of fluconazole, respectively. *Storage:* Store between 86°F (30°C) and 41°F (5°C). Protect from freezing.Diflucan injections in Viaflex Plus plastic containers are available in both sodium chloride and dextrose diluents. *Storage:* Store between 77°F (25°C) and 41°F (5°C). Brief exposure up to 104°F (40°C) does not adversely affect the product. Protect from freezing.

HOW SUPPLIED - EQUIVALENTS NOT AVAILABLE:

Injection, Solution - Intravenous - 2 mg/ml

100 ml	$410.53	DIFLUCAN, Roerig	00049-3371-26
100 ml	$410.53	DIFLUCAN, Roerig	00049-3435-26
100 ml x 6	$410.53	DIFLUCAN IN DEXTROSE, Roerig	00049-3437-26
200 ml	$600.00	DIFLUCAN, Roerig	00049-3372-26
200 ml	$600.00	DIFLUCAN, Roerig	00049-3436-26
200 ml x 6	$600.00	DIFLUCAN IN DEXTROSE, Roerig	00049-3438-26

Powder - Oral - 50 mg/5ml

60 ml	$23.68	DIFLUCAN, Roerig	00049-3440-19

Powder - Oral - 200 mg/5ml

60 ml	$86.00	DIFLUCAN, Roerig	00049-3450-19

Tablet, Plain Coated - Oral - 50 mg

30's	$110.53	DIFLUCAN, Roerig	00049-3410-30

HOW SUPPLIED - EQUIVALENTS NOT AVAILABLE: *(cont'd)*

Tablet, Plain Coated - Oral - 100 mg

30's	$173.68	DIFLUCAN, Roerig	00049-3420-30
100's	$578.95	DIFLUCAN, Roerig	00049-3420-41

Tablet, Plain Coated - Oral - 150 mg

12's	$107.37	DIFLUCAN, Roerig	00049-3500-79

Tablet, Plain Coated - Oral - 200 mg

30's	$284.21	DIFLUCAN, Roerig	00049-3430-30
100's	$947.37	DIFLUCAN, Roerig	00049-3430-41

FLUCYTOSINE *(001302)*

CATEGORIES: Anti-Infectives; Antibiotics; Antifungals; Antimicrobials; Endocarditis; Fungal Agents; Infections; Meningitis; Pulmonary Infections; Septicemia; Urinary Tract Infections; Pregnancy Category C; FDA Approval Pre 1982

BRAND NAMES: *Alcobon* (England); **Ancobon**; *Ancotil* (France, Germany, Canada, Japan)
(International brand names outside U.S. in italics)

FORMULARIES: Aetna; Medi-Cal; WHO

Use with extreme caution in patients with impaired renal function. Close monitoring of hematologic, renal and hepatic status of all patients is essential. These instructions should be thoroughly reviewed before administration of Ancobon.

DESCRIPTION:

Flucytosine, an antifungal agent, is available as 250-mg and 500-mg capsules for oral administration. Each capsule also contains corn starch, lactose and talc. Ancobon gelatin capsule shells contain parabens (butyl, methyl, propyl) and sodium propionate, with the following dye systems: 250-mg capsules—black iron oxide, FD&C Blue No. 1, FD&C Yellow No. 6, D&C Yellow No. 10 and titanium dioxide; 500-mg capsules—black iron oxide and titanium dioxide. Chemically, flucytosine is 5-fluorocytosine, a fluorinated pyrimidine which is related to fluorouracil and floxuridine. It is a white to off-white crystalline powder with a molecular weight of 129.09.

CLINICAL PHARMACOLOGY:

Flucytosine is rapidly and virtually completely absorbed following oral administration. Bioavailability estimated by comparing the area under the curve of serum concentrations after oral and intravenous administration showed 78% to 89% absorption of the oral dose. Peak blood concentrations of 30 to 40 mcg/ml were reached within two hours of administration of a 2-gm oral dose to normal subjects. The mean blood concentrations were approximately 70 to 80 mcg/ml one to two hours after a dose in patients with normal renal function who received a six-week regimen of flucytosine (150 mg/kg/day given in divided doses every 6 hours) in combination with amphotericin B. The half-life in the majority of normal subjects ranged between 2.4 and 4.8 hours. Flucytosine is excreted via the kidneys by means of glomerular filtration without significant tubular reabsorption. More than 90% of the total radioactivity after oral administration was recovered in the urine as intact drug. Approximately 1% of the dose is present in the urine as the α-fluoro-β-ureido-propionic acid metabolite. A small portion of the dose is excreted in the feces.

The half-life of flucytosine is prolonged in patients with renal insufficiency; the average half-life in nephrectomized or anuric patients was 85 hours (range: 29.9 to 250 hours). A linear correlation was found between the elimination rate constant of flucytosine and creatinine clearance.

In vitro studies have shown that 2.9% to 4% of flucytosine is protein-bound over the range of therapeutic concentrations found in the blood. Flucytosine readily penetrates the blood-brain barrier, achieving clinically significant concentrations in cerebrospinal fluid. Studies in pregnant rats have shown that flucytosine injected intraperitoneally crosses the placental barrier (see PRECAUTIONS).

MICROBIOLOGY

Flucytosine has *in vitro* and *in vivo* activity against Candida and Cryptococcus. Although the exact mode of action is unknown, it has been proposed that flucytosine acts directly on fungal organisms by competitive inhibition of purine and pyrimidine uptake and indirectly by intracellular metabolism to 5-fluorouracil. Flucytosine enters the fungal cell via cytosine permease; thus, flucytosine is metabolized to 5-fluorouracil within fungal organisms. The 5-fluorouracil is extensively incorporated into fungal RNA and inhibits synthesis of both DNA and RNA. The result is unbalanced growth and death of the fungal organism. Antifungal synergism between Ancobon and polyene antibiotics, particularly amphotericin B, has been reported.

Flucytosine has *in vitro* and *in vivo* activity against Candida and Cryptococcus. The exact mode of action against these fungi is not known. Ancobon is not metabolized significantly when given orally to man.

SUSCEPTIBILITY

Cryptococcus: Most strains initially isolated from clinical material have shown flucytosine minimal inhibitory concentrations (MIC's) ranging from.46 to 7.8 mcg/ml. Any isolate with an MIC greater than 12.5 mcg/ml is considered resistant. *In vitro* resistance has developed in originally susceptible strains during therapy. It is recommended that clinical cultures for susceptibility testing be taken initially and at weekly intervals during therapy. The initial culture should be reserved as a reference in susceptibility testing of subsequent isolates.

Candida: As high as 40 to 50 percent of the pretreatment clinical isolates of Candida have been reported to be resistant to flucytosine. It is recommended that susceptibility studies be performed as early as possible and be repeated during therapy. An MIC value greater than 100 mcg/ml is considered resistant.

Interference with *in vitro* activity of flucytosine occurs in complex or semisynthetic media. In order to rely upon the recommended *in vitro* interpretations of susceptibility, it is essential that the broth medium and the testing procedure used be that described by Shadomy.[1]

INDICATIONS AND USAGE:

Ancobon is indicated only in the treatment of serious infections caused by susceptible strains of Candida and/or Cryptococcus.

Candida: Septicemia, endocarditis and urinary system infections have been effectively treated with flucytosine. Limited trials in pulmonary infections justify the use of flucytosine.

Cryptococcus: Meningitis and pulmonary infections have been treated effectively. Studies in septicemias and urinary tract infections are limited, but good responses have been reported.

CONTRAINDICATIONS:

Ancobon should not be used in patients with a known hypersensitivity to the drug.

WARNINGS:

Ancobon must be given with extreme caution to patients with impaired renal function. Since Ancobon is excreted primarily by the kidneys, renal impairment may lead to accumulation of the drug. Ancobon blood concentrations should be monitored to determine the adequacy of renal excretion in such patients.[1] Dosage adjustments should be made in patients with renal insufficiency to prevent progressive accumulation of active drug.

Ancobon must be given with extreme caution to patients with bone marrow depression. Patients may be more prone to depression of bone marrow function if they: 1) have a hematologic disease, 2) are being treated with radiation or drugs which depress bone marrow, or 3) have a history of treatment with such drugs or radiation. Frequent monitoring of hepatic function and of the hematopoietic system is indicated during therapy.

PRECAUTIONS:

General: Before therapy with Ancobon is instituted, electrolytes (because of hypokalemia) and the hematologic and renal status of the patient should be determined (see WARNINGS). Close monitoring of the patient during therapy is essential.

Laboratory tests: Since renal impairment can cause progressive accumulation of the drug, blood concentrations and kidney function should be monitored during therapy. Hematologic status (leucocyte and thrombocyte count) and liver function (alkaline phosphatase, SGOT and SGPT) should be determined at frequent intervals during treatment as indicated.

Drug/laboratory test interactions: Measurement of serum creatinine levels should be determined by the Jaffe method, since Ancobon does not interfere with the determination of creatinine values by this method, as it does when the dry-slide enzymatic method with the Kodak Ektachem analyzer is used.

Carcinogenesis, mutagenesis, impairment of fertility: Ancobon has not undergone adequate animal testing to evaluate carcinogenic potential. The mutagenic potential of Ancobon was evaluated in Ames-type studies with five different mutants of *S. typhimurium* and no mutagenicity was detected in the presence or absence of activating enzymes. Ancobon was nonmutagenic in three different repair assay systems.

There have been no adequate trials in animals on the effects of Ancobon on fertility or reproductive performance. The fertility and reproductive performance of the offspring (F_1 generation) of mice treated with 100, 200 or 400 mg/kg/day of flucytosine on days 7 to 13 of gestation was studied; the *in utero* treatment had no adverse effect on the fertility or reproductive performance of the offspring.

Pregnancy, Teratogenic Effects, Pregnancy Category C: Ancobon has been shown to be teratogenic in the rat and mouse at doses of 40 mg/kg/day (*i.e.,* 0.27 times the maximum recommended human dose). There are no adequate and well-controlled studies in pregnant women. Ancobon should be used during pregnancy only if the potential benefit justifies the potential risk to the fetus.

The teratogenicity of Ancobon is apparently species-related. Although there is confirmation of rat teratogenicity in the published literature, three studies in the mouse and studies in the rabbit and monkey have failed to reveal a teratogenic liability.

Nursing Mothers: It is not known whether this drug is excreted in human milk. Because many drugs are excreted in human milk and because of the potential for serious adverse reactions in nursing infants from Ancobon, a decision should be made whether to discontinue nursing or to discontinue the drug, taking into account the importance of the drug to the mother.

Pediatric Use: Safety and effectiveness in children have not been established.

DRUG INTERACTIONS:

Cytosine arabinoside, a cytostatic agent, has been reported to inactivate the antifungal activity of Ancobon by competitive inhibition. Drugs which impair glomerular filtration may prolong the biological half-life of flucytosine. Antifungal synergism between Ancobon and polyene antibiotics, particularly amphotericin B, has been reported.

ADVERSE REACTIONS:

The adverse reactions which have occurred during treatment with Ancobon are grouped according to organ system affected.

Cardiovascular: Cardiac arrest.

Respiratory: Respiratory arrest, chest pain, dyspnea.

Dermatologic: Rash, pruritus, urticaria, photosensitivity.

Gastrointestinal: Nausea, emesis, abdominal pain, diarrhea, anorexia, dry mouth, duodenal ulcer, gastrointestinal hemorrhage, hepatic dysfunction, jaundice, ulcerative colitis, bilirubin elevation.

Genitourinary: Azotemia, creatinine and BUN elevation, crystalluria, renal failure.

Hematologic: Anemia, agranulocytosis, aplastic anemia, eosinophilia, leukopenia, pancytopenia, thrombocytopenia.

Neurologic: Ataxia, hearing loss, headache, paresthesia, parkinsonism, peripheral neuropathy, pyrexia, vertigo, sedation.

Psychiatric: Confusion, hallucinations, psychosis.

Miscellaneous: Fatigue, hypoglycemia, hypokalemia, weakness.

OVERDOSAGE:

There is no experience with intentional overdosage. It is reasonable to expect that overdosage may produce pronounced manifestations of the known clinical adverse reactions. Prolonged serum concentrations in excess of 100 mcg/ml may be associated with an increased incidence of toxicity, especially gastrointestinal (diarrhea, nausea, vomiting), hematologic (leukopenia, thrombocytopenia) and hepatic (hepatitis).

In the management of overdosage, prompt gastric lavage or the use of an emetic is recommended. Adequate fluid intake should be maintained, by the intravenous route if necessary, since Ancobon is excreted unchanged via the renal tract. The hematologic parameters should be monitored frequently; liver and kidney function should be carefully monitored. Should any abnormalities appear in any of these parameters, appropriate therapeutic measures should be instituted. Since hemodialysis has been shown to rapidly reduce serum concentrations in anuric patients, this method may be considered in the management of overdosage.

DOSAGE AND ADMINISTRATION:

The usual dosage of Ancobon is 50 to 150 mg/kg/day administered in divided doses at 6-hour intervals. Nausea or vomiting may be reduced or avoided if the capsules are given a few at a time over a 15-minute period. If the BUN or the serum creatinine is elevated, or if there are other signs of renal impairment, the initial dose should be at the lower level (see WARNINGS).

REFERENCES:

1. Shadomy S: *Appl Microbiol 17*:871-877, June 1969.

HOW SUPPLIED - EQUIVALENTS NOT AVAILABLE:

Capsule, Gelatin - Oral - 250 mg

100's $104.39 ANCOBON, Roche 00004-0077-01

Capsule, Gelatin - Oral - 500 mg

100's $200.92 ANCOBON, Roche 00004-0079-01

FLUDARABINE PHOSPHATE *(003047)*

CATEGORIES: Antineoplastics; Cancer; Leukemia; Orphan Drugs; Pregnancy Category D; FDA Class 1A ("Important Therapeutic Advantage"); FDA Approved 1991 Apr

BRAND NAMES: **Fludara**

FORMULARIES: Medi-Cal

WARNING:
Fludarabine Phosphate FOR INJECTION should be administered under the supervision of a qualified physician experienced in the use of antineoplastic therapy. Fludarabine Phosphate for injection can severely suppress bone marrow function. When used at high doses in dose-ranging studies in patients with acute leukemia, Fludarabine Phosphate for injection was associated with severe neurologic effects, including blindness, coma, and death. This severe central nervous system toxicity occurred in 36% of patients treated with doses approximately four times greater (96 mg/square meter/day for 5-7 days) than the recommended dose. Similar severe central nervous system toxicity has been rarely (</= 0.2%) reported in patients treated at doses in the range of the dose recommended for chronic lymphocytic leukemia.
Instances of life-threatening and sometimes fatal autoimmune hemolytic anemia have been reported to occur after one or more cycles of treatment with Fludarabine Phosphate for injection. Patients undergoing treatment with Fludarabine Phosphate for injection should be evaluated and closely monitored for hemolysis.
In a clinical investigation using Fludarabine Phosphate for injection in combination with pentostatin (deoxycoformycin) for the treatment of refractory chronic lymphocytic leukemia (CLL), there was an unacceptably high incidence of fatal pulmonary toxicity. Therefore, the use of Fludarabine Phosphate for injection in combination with pentostatin is not recommended.

DESCRIPTION:

For Injection; For Intravenous Use Only: Fludarabine Phosphate For Injection Contains Fludarabine Phosphatebine Phosphate, A Fluorinated Nucleotide Analog Of The Antiviral Agent Vidarabine, 9-β-D- Arabinofuranosyladenine (Ara-A) That Is Relatively Resistant To Deamination By Adenosine Deaminase. Each Vial Of Sterile Lyophilized Solid Cake Contains 50 Mg Of The Active Ingredient Fludarabine Phosphatebine Phosphate, 50 Mg Of Mannitol, And Sodium Hydroxide To Adjust Ph To 7.7. The Ph Range For The Final Product Is 7.2-8.2. Reconstitution With 2 Ml Of Sterile Water For Injection Usp Results In A Solution Containing 25 Mg/Ml Of Fludarabine Phosphate Intended For Intravenous Administration.

The chemical name for fludarabine phosphate is 9H-Purin-6-amine, 2-fluoro-9-(5-O-phosphono-β-d-arabinofuranosyl).

The molecular formula of fludarabine phosphate is:
$C_{10}H_{13}FN_5O_7P$ (MW 365.2).

CLINICAL PHARMACOLOGY:

Fludarabine phosphate is rapidly dephosphorylated to 2-fluoro-ara-A and then phosphorylated intracellularly by deoxycytidine kinase to the active triphosphate, 2-fluoro-ara-ATP. This metabolite appears to act by inhibiting DNA polymerase alpha, ribonucleotide reductase and DNA primase, thus inhibiting DNA synthesis. The mechanism of action of the antimetabolite is not completely characterized and may be multi- faceted.

CLINICAL STUDIES:

Phase 1 studies in humans have demonstrated that fludarabine phosphate is rapidly converted to the active metabolite, 2-fluoro-ara-A, within minutes after intravenous infusion. Consequently, clinical pharmacology studies have focused on 2-fluoro-ara-A pharmacokinetics. In a study with 4 patients treated with 25 mg/m^2/day for 5 days, the half-life of 2-fluoro-ara-A was approximately 10 hours. The mean total plasma clearance was 8.9 l/hr/m^2 and the mean volume of distribution was 98 l/m^2. Approximately 23% of the dose was excreted in the urine as unchanged 2-fluoro-ara-A. The mean C_{max} after the Day 1 dose was 0.57 mcg/ml and after the Day 5 dose was 0.54 mcg/ml. No information is available on pharmacokinetic parameters, other than C_{max}, following the Day 5 dose of 25 mg/m^2. Total body clearance of 2-fluoro-ara-A has been shown to be inversely correlated with serum creatinine, suggesting renal elimination of the compound.

A correlation was noted between the degree of absolute granulocyte count nadir and increased area under the concentration x time curve (AUC).

Two single-arm open-label studies of Fludarabine Phosphate for injection have been conducted in patients with CLL refractory to at least one prior standard alkylating-agent containing regimen. In a study conducted by M.D. Anderson Cancer Center (MDAH), 48 patients were treated with a dose of 22-40 mg/m^2 daily for 5 days every 28 days. Another study conducted by the Southwest Oncology Group (SWOG) involved 31 patients treated with a dose of 15-25 mg/m^2 daily for 5 days every 28 days. The overall objective response rates were 48% and 32% in the MDAH and SWOG studies, respectively. The complete response rate in both studies was 13%; the partial response rate was 35% in the MDAH study and 19% in the SWOG study. These response rates were obtained using standardized response criteria developed by the National Cancer Institute CLL Working Group were achieved in heavily pre-treated patients. The ability of Fludarabine Phosphate for injection to induce a significant rate of response in refractory patients suggests minimal cross- resistance with commonly used anti-CLL agents.

The median time to response in the MDAH and SWOG studies was 7 weeks (range of 1 to 68 weeks) and 21 weeks (range of 1 to 53 weeks) respectively. The median duration of disease control was 91 weeks (MDAH) and 65 weeks (SWOG). The median survival of all refractor CLL patients treated with Fludarabine Phosphate for injection was 43 weeks and 52 weeks in the MDAH and SWOG studies, respectively.

CLINICAL STUDIES: *(cont'd)*

Rai stage improved to Stage II or better in 7 of 12 MDAH responders (58%) and in 5 of 7 SWOG responders (71%) who were Stage III or IV at baseline. In the combined studies, mean hemoglobin concentration improved from 9.0 g/dl at baseline to 11.8 g/dl at the time of response in a subgroup of anemic patients. Similarly, average platelet count improved from 63,500/mm^3 to 103,3000/mm^3 at the time of response in a subgroup of patients who were thrombocytopenic at baseline.

INDICATIONS AND USAGE:

Fludarabine Phosphate for injection is indicated for the treatment of patients with B- cell chronic lymphocytic leukemia (CLL) who have not responded to or whose disease has progressed during treatment with at least one standard alkylating-agent containing regimen. The safety and effectiveness of Fludarabine Phosphate for injection in previously untreated or non-refractory patients with CLL have not been established.

CONTRAINDICATIONS:

Fludarabine Phosphate for injection is contraindicated in those patients who are hypersensitive to this drug or its components.

WARNINGS:

See BOXED WARNING.

There are clear dose dependent toxic effect seen with Fludarabine Phosphate for Injection. Dose levels approximately 4 times greater (96 mg/m^2/day for 5 to 7 days) than that recommended for CLL (25 mg/m^2 /day for 5 days) were associated with a syndrome characterized by delayed blindness, coma and death. Symptoms appeared from 21 to 60 days following the last dose. Thirteen of 36 patients (36%) who received Fludarabine Phosphate for injection at high doses (96 mg/m^2/day for 5 to 7 days) developed this severe neurotoxicity. This syndrome has been reported rarely in patients treated with doses in the range of the recommended CLL dose of 25 mgm^2/day for 5 days every 28 days. The effect of chronic administration of Fludarabine Phosphate for injection on the central nervous system is unknown, however, patients have received the recommended dose for up to 15 courses of therapy.

Severe bone marrow suppression, notably anemia, thrombocytopenia and neutropenia, has been reported in patients treated with Fludarabine Phosphate for injection. In a Phase I study in solid tumor patients, the median time to nadir counts was 13 days (range, 3-25 days) for granulocytes and 16 days (range,,2-32) for platelets. Most patients had hematologic impairment at baseline either as a result of disease or as a result of prior myelosuppressive therapy. Cumulative myelosuppression may be seen. While chemotherapy-induced myelosuppression is often reversible, administration of Fludarabine Phosphate for injection requires careful hematologic monitoring.

Instances of life-threatening and sometimes fatal autoimmune hemolytic anemia have been reported to occur after one or more cycles of treatment with Fludarabine Phosphate for injection in patients with or without a previous history of autoimmune hemolytic anemia or a positive Coombs test and who may or may not be in remission for their disease. Steroids may or may not be effective in controlling these hemolytic episodes. The majority of patients rechallenged with Fludarabine Phosphate for injection developed a recurrence in the hemolytic process. The mechanism(s) which predispose patients to the development of this complication has not been identified. Patients undergoing treatment with Fludarabine Phosphate for injection should be evaluated and closely monitored for hemolysis.

In a clinical investigation using Fludarabine Phosphate for injection in combination with pentostatin (deoxycoformycin) for the treatment of refractory chronic lymphocytic leukemia (CLL), there was an unacceptably high incidence of fatal pulmonary toxicity. Therefore, the use of Fludarabine Phosphate for injection in combination with pentostatin is not recommended.

Of the 133 CLL patients in the two trials, there were 29 fatalities during study. Approximately 50% of the fatalities were due to infection and 25% due to progressive disease.

Pregnancy Category D: Fludarabine Phosphate for Injection may cause fetal harm when administered to a pregnant woman. Fludarabine Phosphatebine phosphate was teratogenic in rats and in rabbits. Fludarabine Phosphatebine phosphate was administered intravenously at doses of 0, 1, 10 or 30 mg/kg/day to pregnant rats on days 6 to 15 of gestation. At 10 and 30 mg/kg/day in rats, there was an increased incidence of various skeletal malformations. Fludarabine Phosphatebine phosphate was administered intravenously at doses of 0,1,5 or 8 mg/kg/day to pregnant rabbits on days 6 to 15 of gestation. Dose-related teratogenic effects manifested by external deformities and skeletal malformations were observed in the rabbits at 5 and 8 mg/kg/day. Drug related deaths or toxic effects on maternal and fetal weights were not observed. There are no adequate and well-controlled studies in pregnant women.

If Fludarabine Phosphate for injection is used during pregnancy, or if the patient becomes pregnant while taking this drug, the patient should be apprised of the potential hazard to the fetus. Women of childbearing potential should be advised to avoid becoming pregnant.

PRECAUTIONS:

General: Fludarabine Phosphate for injection is a potent antineoplastic agent with potentially significant toxic side effects. Patients undergoing therapy should be closely observed for signs of hematologic and hematologic and nonhematologic toxicity. Periodic assessment of peripheral blood counts is recommended to detect the development of anemia, neutropenia and thrombocytopenia.

Tumor lysis syndrome associated with Fludarabine Phosphate for injection treatment has been reported in CLL patients with large tumor burdens. Since Fludarabine Phosphate for injection can induce a response as early as the first week of treatment, precautions should be taken in those patients at risk of developing this complication.

There are adequate data on dosing of patients with renal insufficiency. Fludarabine Phosphate for injection must be administered cautiously in patients with renal insufficiency. The total body clearance of 2-fluoro-ara-A has been shown to be inversely correlated with serum creatinine, suggesting renal elimination of the compound.

Laboratory Tests: During treatment,the patient's hematologic profile (particularly neutrophils and platelets) should be monitored regularly to determine the degree of hematopoietic suppression.

Carcinogenesis: No animal carcinogenicity studies with Fludarabine Phosphate for injection have been conducted.

Mutagenesis: Fludarabine Phosphatebine phosphate has been shown to be non- mutagenic to several strains of Salmonella typhimurium, including TA-98, TA-100, TA-1535 and TA-1537. In addition, Fludarabine Phosphatebine phosphate was non- mutagenic to Chinese hamster ovary (CHO) cells at the hypoxanthine-guanine-phosphoribosyltransferase (HGPRT) locus under both activated and non-activated metabolic conditions. Chromosomal aberrations were observed in an *in vitro* assay using CHO cells under metabolically activated conditions. In addition, Fludarabine Phosphatebine phosphate was determined to cause increased sister chromatid exchanges using an*in vitro* sister chromatid exchange (SCE) assay under both metabolically activated and non-activated conditions.

PRECAUTIONS: *(cont'd)*

Impairment of Fertility: Studies in mice, rats and dogs have demonstrated dose-related adverse effects on the male reproductive system. Observations consisted of a decrease in mean testicular weights in mice and rats with a trend toward decreased testicular weights in dogs and degeneration and necrosis of spermatogenic epithelium of the testes in mice, rats, and dogs. The possible adverse effects of fertility in humans have not been adequately evaluated.

Pregnancy Category D: See WARNINGS.

Nursing Mothers: It is not known whether this drug is excreted in human milk. Because many drugs are excreted in human milk and because of the potential for serious adverse reactions in nursing infants from Fludarabine Phosphate for injection, a decision should be made to discontinue nursing or discontinue the drug, taking into account the importance of the drug for the mother.

Pediatric Use: The safety and effectiveness of Fludarabine Phosphate for injection in children have not been established.

DRUG INTERACTIONS:

The use of this drug in combination with pentostatin is not recommended due to the risk of severe pulmonary toxicity (See WARNINGS).

ADVERSE REACTIONS:

The most common adverse events include myelosuppression (neutropenia, thrombocytopenia and anemia), fever and chills, infection, and nausea and vomiting. Other commonly reported events include malaise, fatigue,anorexia, and weakness. Serious opportunistic infections have occurred in CLL patients treated with Fludarabine Phosphate for injection. The most frequently reported adverse events and those reactions which are more clearly related to the drug are arranged below according to body system.

Hematopoietic Systems: Hematologic events (neutropenia, thrombocytopenia, and anemia) were reported in the majority of CLL patients treated with Fludarabine Phosphate for injection. During Fludarabine Phosphate for injection treatment of 133 patients with CLL, the absolute neutrophil count decreased to less than 500/mm^3 in 59% of patients, hemoglobin decreased from pretreatment values by at least 2 grams percent in 60%, and platelet count decreased from pretreatment values by at least 50% in 55%. Myelosuppression may be severe and cumulative. Bone marrow fibrosis occurred in one CLL patient treated with Fludarabine Phosphate for injection.

Life-threatening and sometimes fatal autoimmune hemolytic anemia have been reported to occur in patients receiving Fludarabine Phosphate for Injection (see WARNINGS). The majority of patients rechallenged with Fludarabine Phosphate for injection developed a recurrence in the hemolytic process.

Metabolic: Tumor lysis syndrome has been reported in CLL patients treated with Fludarabine Phosphate for injection. This complication may include hyperuricemia, hyperphosphatemia, hypocalcemia, metabolic acidosis, hyperkalemia, hematuria, urate crystalluria, and renal failure. The onset of this syndrome may be heralded by flank pain and hematuria.

Nervous System: See WARNINGS. Objective weakness, agitation, confusion, visual disturbances, and coma have occurred in CLL patients treated with Fludarabine Phosphate for injection at the recommended dose. Peripheral neuropathy has been observed in patients treated with Fludarabine Phosphate for injection and one case of wrist-drop was reported.

Pulmonary System: Pneumonia, a frequent manifestation of infection in CLL patients, occurred in 16%, and 22% of those treated with Fludarabine Phosphate for injection in the MDAH and SWOG studies, respectively. Pulmonary hypersensitivity reactions to Fludarabine Phosphate for injection characterized by dyspnea, cough and interstitial pulmonary infiltrate have been observed.

Gastrointestinal System: Gastrointestinal disturbances such as nausea and vomiting, anorexia, diarrhea, stomatitis and gastrointestinal bleeding have been reported in patients treated with Fludarabine Phosphate for injection.

Cardiovascular: Edema has been frequently reported. One patient developed a pericardial effusion possibly related to treatment with Fludarabine Phosphate for injection. No other severe cardiovascular events were considered to be drug related.

Genitourinary System: Rare cases of hemorrhagic cystitis have been reported in patients treated with Fludarabine Phosphate for injection.

Skin: Skin toxicity, consisting primarily of skin rashes, has been reported in patients treated with Fludarabine Phosphate for injection.

Data in TABLE 1 are derived from the 133 patients with CLL who received Fludarabine Phosphate for injection in the MDAH and SWOG studies.

More than 3000 patients received Fludarabine Phosphate for injection in studies of other leukemias, lymphomas, and other solid tumors. The spectrum of adverse effects reported in these studies was consistent with the data presented in TABLE 1.

OVERDOSAGE:

High doses of Fludarabine Phosphate for injection (see WARNINGS) have been associated with an irreversible central nervous system toxicity characterized by delayed blindness, coma and death. High doses are also associated with severe thrombocytopenia and neutropenia due to bone marrow suppression. There is no known specific antidote for Fludarabine Phosphate for injection overdosage. Treatment consists of drug discontinuation and supportive therapy.

DOSAGE AND ADMINISTRATION:

Usual Dose: The recommended dose of Fludarabine Phosphate for injection is 25 mg/m^2 administered intravenously over a period of approximately 30 minutes daily for five consecutive days. Each 5 day course of treatment should commence every 28 days. Dosage maybe decreased or delayed based on evidence on evidence of hematologic or nonhematologic toxicity. Physicians should consider delaying or discontinuing the drug if neurotoxicity occurs.

A number of clinical settings may predispose to increased toxicity from Fludarabine Phosphate for injection. These include advanced age, renal insufficiency, and bone marrow impairment. Such patients should be monitored closely for excessive toxicity and the dose modified accordingly.

The optimal duration of treatment has not been clearly established. It is recommended that three additional cycles of Fludarabine Phosphate for injection be administered following the achievement of a maximal response and then the drug should be discontinued.

PREPARATION OF SOLUTIONS

Fludarabine Phosphate for injection should be prepared for parenteral use by aseptically adding Sterile Water for Injection USP. When reconstituted with 2 ml of Sterile Water for Injection, USP, the solid cake should fully dissolve in 15 seconds or less; each ml of the resulting solution will contain 25 mg of Fludarabine Phosphatebine phosphate, 25 mg of mannitol, and sodium hydroxide to adjust the pH to 7.7. The pH range for the final product is 7.2-8.2. In clinical studies, the product has been diluted to 100 cc or 125 cc of 5% Dextrose Injection USP or 0.9% Sodium Chloride USP.

DOSAGE AND ADMINISTRATION: *(cont'd)*

TABLE 1 Fludarabine Phosphate, Adverse Reactions
PERCENT OF CLL PATIENTS REPORTING NON-HEMATOLOGIC ADVERSE EVENTS

ADVERSE EVENTS	MDAH (N=101)	SWOG (N=32)
ANY ADVERSE EVENT	88%	91%
Body As A Whole	72	84
Fever	60	69
Chills	11	19
Fatigue	10	38
Infection	33	44
Pain	20	22
Malaise	8	6
Diaphoresis	1	13
Alopecia	0	3
Anaphylaxis	1	0
Hemorrhage	1	0
Hyperglycemia	1	6
Dehydration	1	0
Neurological	21	69
Weakness	9	65
Paresthesia	4	12
Headache	3	0
Visual Disturbance	3	15
Hearing Loss	2	6
Sleep Disorder	1	3
Depression	1	0
Cerebellar Syndrome	1	0
Impaired Mentation	1	0
Pulmonary	35	69
Cough	10	44
Pneumonia	16	22
Dyspnea	9	22
Sinusitis	5	0
Pharyngitis	0	9
Upper Respiratory Infection	2	16
Allergic Pneumonitis	0	6
Epistaxis	1	0
Hemoptysis	1	6
Bronchitis	1	0
Hypoxia	1	0
Gastrointestinal	46	63
Nausea/Vomiting	36	31
Diarrhea	15	13
Anorexia	7	34
Stomatitis	9	0
GI Bleeding	3	13
Esophagitis	3	0
Mucositis	2	0
Liver Failure	1	0
Abnormal Liver Function Test	1	3
Cholelithiasis	0	3
Constipation	1	3
Dysphagia	1	0
Cutaneous	17	18
Rash	15	15
Pruritus	1	3
Seborrhea	1	0
Genitourinary	12	22
Dysuria	4	3
Urinary Infection	2	15
Hematuria	2	3
Renal Failure	1	0
Abnormal Liver Function Test	1	0
Proteinuria	1	0
Hesitancy	0	3
Cardiovascular	12	38
Edema	8	19
Angina	0	6
Congestive Heart Failure	0	3
Arrhythmia	0	3
Supraventricular Tachycardia	0	3
Myocardial Infarction	0	3
Deep Venous Thrombosis	1	3
Phlebitis	1	3
Transient Ischemic Attack	1	0
Aneurysm	1	0
Cerebrovascular Accident	0	3
Musculoskeletal	7	16
Myalgia	4	16
Osteoporosis	2	0
Arthralgia	1	0
Tumor Lysis Syndrome	1	0

Reconstituted Fludarabine Phosphate for injection contains no antimicrobial preservative and thus should be used within 8 hours of reconstitution. Care must be taken to assure the sterility of prepared solutions. Parenteral drug products should be inspected visually for particulate matter and discoloration prior to administration.

HANDLING AND DISPOSAL

Procedures for handling and disposal should be considered. Consideration should be given to handling and disposal according to guidelines issued for cytotoxic drugs. Several guidelines on this subject have been published. There is no general agreement that all of the procedures recommended in the guidelines are necessary or appropriate.

Caution should be exercised in the handling and preparation of Fludarabine Phosphate for injection solution. The use of latex gloves and safety glasses is recommended to avoid exposure in case of breakage of the vial or other accidental spillage. If the solution contacts the skin or mucous membranes, wash thoroughly with soap and water; rinse eyes thoroughly with plain water. Avoid exposure by inhalation or by direct contact of the skin or mucous membranes.

Storage: Store under refrigeration, between 2°-8°C (36°-46°F).

HOW SUPPLIED - EQUIVALENTS NOT AVAILABLE:

Injection, Solution - Intravenous - 50 mg

1's	$179.52	FLUDARA, Berlex Labs	50419-0511-06

FLUDEOXYGLUCOSE, F-18 *(003217)*

CATEGORIES: Diagnostic Agents; Epilepsy; PET Scanning; FDA Class 1P ("Priority Review"); FDA Approved 1994 Aug

Prescribing information not available at time of publication.

FLUDROCORTISONE ACETATE *(001303)*

CATEGORIES: Addison's Disease; Adrenal Corticosteroids; Adrenocortical Insufficiency; Adrenogenital Syndrome; Hormones; Steroids; Pregnancy Category C; FDA Approval Pre 1982

BRAND NAMES: *Astonin; Astonin H* (Germany); **Florinef**
(International brand names outside U.S. in italics)

FORMULARIES: Aetna; BC-BS; Medi-Cal; PCS; WHO

DESCRIPTION:

Fludrocortisone Acetate Tablets USP contain fludrocortisone acetate, a synthetic adrenocortical steroid possessing very potent mineralocorticoid properties and high glucocorticoid activity; it is used only for its mineralocorticoid effects. The chemical name for fludrocortisone acetate is 9-fluoro-11β,17,21-trihydroxypregn-4-ene-3,20-dione 21-acetate.

$C_{23}H_{31}FO_6$

Molecular Weight: 422.49 (CAS 514-36-3)

Fludrocortisone Acetate is available for oral administration as scored tablets providing 0.1 mg fludrocortisone acetate per tablet. Inactive ingredients: calcium phosphate, color additive (D&C Red No. 27), corn starch, lactose, magnesium stearate, sodium benzoate, and talc.

CLINICAL PHARMACOLOGY:

Corticosteroids are thought to act, at least in part, by controlling the rate of synthesis of proteins. Although there are a number of instances in which the synthesis of specific proteins is known to be induced by corticosteroids, the links between the initial actions of the hormones and final metabolic effects have not been completely elucidated.

The physiologic action of fludrocortisone acetate is similar to that of hydrocortisone. However, the effects of fludrocortisone acetate, particularly on electrolyte balance, but also on carbohydrate metabolism, are considerably heightened and prolonged. Mineralocorticoids act on the distal tubules of the kidney to enhance the reabsorption of sodium ions from the tubular fluid into the plasma; they increase the urinary excretion of both potassium and hydrogen ions. The consequence of these three primary effects together with similar actions on cation transport in other tissues appear to account for the entire spectrum of physiological activities that are characteristic of mineralocorticoids. In small oral doses, fludrocortisone acetate produces marked sodium retention and increased urinary potassium excretion. It also causes a rise in blood pressure, apparently because of these effects on electrolyte levels.

In larger doses, fludrocortisone acetate inhibits endogenous adrenal cortical secretion, thymic activity, and pituitary corticotropin excretion; promotes the deposition of liver glycogen; and, unless protein intake is adequate, induces negative nitrogen balance.

The approximate plasma half-life of fludrocortisone (fluorohydrocortisone) is 3.5 hours or more and the biological half-life is 18 to 36 hours.

INDICATIONS AND USAGE:

Fludrocortisone Acetate is indicated as partial replacement therapy for primary and secondary adrenocortical insufficiency in Addison's disease and for the treatment of salt-losing adrenogenital syndrome.

CONTRAINDICATIONS:

Corticosteroids are contraindicated in patients with systemic fungal infections and in those with a history of possible or known hypersensitivity to these agents.

WARNINGS:

BECAUSE OF ITS MARKED EFFECT ON SODIUM RETENTION, THE USE OF FLUDROCORTISONE ACETATE IN THE TREATMENT OF CONDITIONS OTHER THAN THOSE INDICATED HEREIN IS NOT ADVISED.

Corticosteroids may mask some signs of infection, and new infections may appear during their use. There may be decreased resistance and inability to localize infection when corticosteroids are used. If an infection occurs during fludrocortisone acetate therapy, it should be promptly controlled by suitable antimicrobial therapy.

Prolonged use of corticosteroids may produce posterior subcapsular cataracts, glaucoma with possible damage to the optic nerves, and may enhance the establishment of secondary ocular infections due to fungi or viruses.

Average and large doses of hydrocortisone or cortisone can cause elevation of blood pressure, salt and water retention, and increased excretion of potassium. These effects are less likely to occur with the synthetic derivatives except when used in large doses. However, since fludrocortisone acetate is a potent mineralocorticoid, both the dosage and salt intake should be carefully monitored in order to avoid the development of hypertension, edema, or weight gain. **Periodic checking of serum electrolyte levels is advisable during prolonged therapy; dietary salt restriction and potassium supplementation may be necessary.** All corticosteroids increase calcium excretion.

Patients should not be vaccinated against smallpox while on corticosteroid therapy. Other immunization procedures should not be undertaken in patients who are on corticosteroids, especially on high dose, because of possible hazards of neurological complications and a lack of antibody response.

The use of Fludrocortisone Acetate Tablets in active tuberculosis should be restricted to those cases of fulminating or disseminated tuberculosis in which the corticosteroid is used for the management of the disease in conjunction with an appropriate antituberculous regimen. If corticosteroids are indicated in patients with latent tuberculosis or tuberculin reactivity, close observation is necessary since reactivation of the disease may occur. During prolonged corticosteroid therapy these patients should receive chemoprophylaxis.

Children who are on immunosuppressant drugs are more susceptible to infections than healthy children. Chicken pox and measles, for example, can have a more serious or even fatal course in children on immunosuppressant corticosteroids. In such children, or in adults who have not had these diseases, particular care should be taken to avoid exposure. If exposed, therapy with varicella zoster immune globulin (VZIG) or pooled intravenous immunoglobulin (IVIG), as appropriate, may be indicated. If chicken pox develops, treatment with antiviral agents may be considered.

PRECAUTIONS:

GENERAL

Adverse reactions to corticosteroids may be produced by too rapid withdrawal or by continued use of large doses.

To avoid drug-induced adrenal insufficiency, supportive dosage may be required in times of stress (such as trauma, surgery, or severe illness) both during treatment with fludrocortisone acetate and for a year afterwards.

There is an enhanced corticosteroid effect in patients with hypothyroidism and in those with cirrhosis.

Corticosteroids should be used cautiously in patients with ocular herpes simplex because of possible corneal perforation.

The lowest possible dose of corticosteroid should be used to control the condition being treated. A gradual reduction in dosage should be made when possible.

Psychic derangements may appear when corticosteroids are used. These may range from euphoria, insomnia, mood swings, personality changes, and severe depression to frank psychotic manifestations. Existing emotional instability or psychotic tendencies may also be aggravated by corticosteroids.

Aspirin should be used cautiously in conjunction with corticosteroids in patients with hypoprothrombinemia.

Corticosteroids should be used with caution in patients with nonspecific ulcerative colitis if there is a probability of impending perforation, abscess or other pyrogenic infection. Corticosteroids should also be used cautiously in patients with diverticulitis, fresh intestinal anastomoses, active or latent peptic ulcer, renal insufficiency, hypertension, osteoporosis, and myasthenia gravis.

INFORMATION FOR THE PATIENT

The physician should advise the patient to report any medical history of heart disease, high blood pressure, or kidney or liver disease and to report current use of any medicines to determine if these medicines might interact adversely with fludrocortisone acetate (see DRUG INTERACTIONS).

Patients who are on immunosuppressant doses of corticosteroids should be warned to avoid exposure to chicken pox or measles, and, if exposed, to obtain medical advice.

The patient's understanding of his steroid-dependent status and increased dosage requirement under widely variable conditions of stress is vital. Advise the patient to carry medical identification indicating his dependence on steroid medication and, if necessary, instruct him to carry an adequate supply of medication for use in emergencies.

Stress to the patient the importance of regular follow-up visits to check his progress and the need to promptly notify the physician of dizziness, severe or continuing headaches, swelling of feet or lower legs, or unusual weight gain.

Advise the patient to use the medicine only as directed, to take a missed dose as soon as possible, unless it is almost time for the next dose, and not to double the next dose.

Inform the patient to keep this medication and all drugs out of the reach of children.

LABORATORY TESTS

Patients should be monitored regularly for blood pressure determinations and serum electrolyte determinations (see WARNINGS).

DRUG/LABORATORY TEST INTERACTIONS

Corticosteroids may affect the nitrobluetetrazolium test for bacterial infection and produce false-negative results.

CARCINOGENESIS, MUTAGENESIS, AND IMPAIRMENT OF FERTILITY

Adequate studies have not been performed in animals to determine whether fludrocortisone acetate has carcinogenic or mutagenic activity or whether it affects fertility in males or females.

PREGNANCY CATEGORY C

Adequate animal reproduction studies have not been conducted with fludrocortisone acetate. However, many corticosteroids have been shown to be teratogenic in laboratory animals at low doses. Teratogenicity of these agents in man has not been demonstrated. It is not known whether fludrocortisone acetate can cause fetal harm when administered to a pregnant woman or can affect reproduction capacity. Fludrocortisone acetate should be given to a pregnant woman only if clearly needed.

Nonteratogenic Effects: Infants born of mothers who have received substantial doses of fludrocortisone acetate during pregnancy should be carefully observed for signs of hypoadrenalism.

Maternal treatment with corticosteroids should be carefully documented in the infant's medical records to assist in follow up.

NURSING MOTHERS

Corticosteroids are found in the breast milk of lactating women receiving systemic therapy with these agents. Caution should be exercised when fludrocortisone acetate is administered to a nursing woman.

PEDIATRIC USE

Safety and effectiveness in children have not been established.

Growth and development of infants and children on prolonged corticosteroid therapy should be carefully observed.

DRUG INTERACTIONS:

When administered concurrently, the following drugs may interact with adrenal corticosteroids.

Amphotericin B or Potassium-Depleting Diuretics: (Benzothiadiazines and related drugs, ethacrynic acid and furosemide) - enhanced hypokalemia. Check serum potassium levels at frequent intervals; use potassium supplements if necessary (see WARNINGS).

Digitalis Glycosides: Enhanced possibility of arrhythmias of digitalis toxicity associated with hypokalemia. Monitor serum potassium levels; use potassium supplements if necessary.

Oral Anticoagulants: Decreased prothrombin time response. Monitor prothrombin levels and adjust anticoagulant dosage accordingly.

Antidiabetic Drugs: (Oral agents and insulin)—diminished antidiabetic effect. Monitor for symptoms of hyperglycemia; adjust dosage of antidiabetic drug upward if necessary.

Aspirin: Increased ulcerogenic effect; decreased pharmacologic effect of aspirin. Rarely salicylate toxicity may occur in patients who discontinue steroids after concurrent high-dose aspirin therapy. Monitor salicylate levels or the therapeutic effect for which aspirin is given; adjust salicylate dosage accordingly if effect is altered (see PRECAUTIONS, General).

Barbiturates, Phenytoin, Or Rifampin: Increased metabolic clearance of fludrocortisone acetate because of the induction of hepatic enzymes. Observe the patient for possible diminished effect of steroid and increase the steroid dosage accordingly.

Anabolic Steroids (Particularly C-17 alkylated androgens such as oxymetholone, methandrostenolone, norethandrolone, and similar compounds)—enhanced tendency toward edema. Use caution when giving these drugs together, especially in patients with hepatic or cardiac disease.

DRUG INTERACTIONS: *(cont'd)*

Vaccines: Neurological complications and lack of antibody response (see WARNINGS).

Estrogen: increased levels of corticosteroid-binding globulin, thereby increasing the bound (inactive) fraction; this effect is at least balanced by decreased metabolism of corticosteroids. When estrogen therapy is initiated, a reduction in corticosteroid dosage may be required, and increased amounts may be required when estrogen is terminated.

ADVERSE REACTIONS:

Most adverse reactions are caused by the drug's mineralocorticoid activity (retention of sodium and water) and include hypertension, edema, cardiac enlargement, congestive heart failure, potassium loss, and hypokalemic alkalosis.

When fludrocortisone is used in the small dosages recommended, the glucocorticoid side effects often seen with cortisone and its derivatives are not usually a problem; however the following untoward effects should be kept in mind, particularly when fludrocortisone is used over a prolonged period of time or in conjunction with cortisone or a similar glucocorticoid.

Musculoskeletal: Muscle weakness, steroid myopathy, loss of muscle mass, osteoporosis, vertebral compression fractures, aseptic necrosis of femoral and humeral heads, pathologic fracture of long bones, and spontaneous fractures.

Gastrointestinal: Peptic ulcer with possible perforation and hemorrhage, pancreatitis, abdominal distention, and ulcerative esophagitis.

Dermatologic: Impaired wound healing, thin fragile skin, bruising, petechiae and ecchymoses, facial erythema, increased sweating, subcutaneous fat atrophy, purpura, striae, hyperpigmentation of the skin and nails, hirsutism, acneiform eruptions, and hives and/or allergic skin rash; reactions to skin tests may be suppressed.

Neurological: Convulsions, increased intracranial pressure with papilledema (pseudotumor cerebri) usually after treatment, vertigo, headache, and severe mental disturbances.

Endocrine: Menstrual irregularities; development of the cushingoid state; suppression of growth in children; secondary adrenocortical and pituitary unresponsiveness, particularly in times of stress (*e.g.,* trauma, surgery, or illness); decreased carbohydrate tolerance; manifestations of latent diabetes mellitus; and increased requirements for insulin or oral hypoglycemic agents in diabetics.

Ophthalmic: Posterior subcapsular cataracts, increased intraocular pressure, glaucoma, and exophthalmos.

Metabolic: Hyperglycemia, glycosuria, and negative nitrogen balance due to protein catabolism.

Other adverse reactions that may occur following the administration of a corticosteroid are necrotizing angitis, thrombophlebitis, aggravation or masking of infections, insomnia, syncopal episodes, and anaphylactoid reactions.

OVERDOSAGE:

Development of hypertension, edema, hypokalemia, excessive increase in weight, and increase in heart size are signs of overdosage of fludrocortisone acetate. When these are noted, administration of the drug should be discontinued, after which the symptoms will usually subside within several days; subsequent treatment with fludrocortisone acetate should be with a reduced dose. Muscular weakness may develop due to excessive potassium loss and can be treated by administering a potassium supplement. Regular monitoring of blood pressure and serum electrolytes can help to prevent overdosage (see WARNINGS).

DOSAGE AND ADMINISTRATION:

Dosage depends on the severity of the disease and the response of the patient. Patients should be continually monitored for signs that indicate dosage adjustment is necessary, such as remissions or exacerbations of the disease and stress (surgery, infection, trauma) (see WARNINGS and PRECAUTIONS, General).

ADDISON'S DISEASE: In Addison's disease, the combination of Fludrocortisone Acetate tablets with a glucocorticoid such as hydrocortisone or cortisone provides substitution therapy approximating normal adrenal activity with minimal risks of unwanted effects.

The usual dose is 0.1 mg of Fludrocortisone Acetate daily, although dosage ranging from 0.1 mg three times a week to 0.2 mg. daily has been employed. In the event transient hypertension develops as a consequence of therapy, the dose should be reduced to 0.05 mg. daily. Fludrocortisone Acetate is preferably administered in conjunction with cortisone (10 mg. to 37.5 mg. daily in divided doses) or hydrocortisone (10 mg. to 30 mg. daily in divided doses).

Salt-Losing Adrenogenital Syndrome: The recommended dosage for treating the salt-losing adrenogenital syndrome is 0.1 mg. to 0.2 mg. of Fludrocortisone Acetate daily.

Storage: Store at room temperature; avoid excessive heat.

HOW SUPPLIED - EQUIVALENTS NOT AVAILABLE:

Tablet, Uncoated - Oral - 0.1 mg

100's	**$44.86**	**FLORINEF ACETATE, Bristol Myers Squibb**	**00003-0429-50**

FLUMAZENIL *(003104)*

CATEGORIES: Antagonists and Antidotes; Benzodiazepine Antagonists; Pregnancy Category C; FDA Class 1B ("Modest Therapeutic Advantage"); FDA Approved 1991 Dec

BRAND NAMES: *Anexate* (Australia, England, France, Germany); *Lanexat* (Mexico); **Mazicon**; Romazicon
(International brand names outside U.S. in italics)

DESCRIPTION:

Romazicon (flumazenil) is a benzodiazepine receptor antagonist. Chemically, flumazenil is ethyl 8-fluoro-5,6-dihydro- 5-methyl-6-oxo-4H-imidazo[1,5-a](1,4) benzodiazepine-3-carboxylate. Flumazenil has an imidazobenzodiazepine structure and a calculated molecular weight of 303.3.

Flumazenil is a white to off-white crystalline compound with an octanol:buffer partition coefficient of 14 to 1 at pH 7.4. It is insoluble in water but slightly soluble in acidic aqueous solutions. Flumazenil is available as a sterile parenteral dosage form for intravenous administration. Each ml contains 0.1 mg of flumazenil compounded with 1.8 mg of methylparaben, 0.2 mg of propylparaben, 0.9% sodium chloride, 0.01% edetate disodium, and 0.01% acetic acid; the pH is adjusted to approximately 4 with hydrochloric acid and/or, if necessary, sodium hydroxide.

CLINICAL PHARMACOLOGY:

Flumazenil, an imidazobenzodiazepine derivative, antagonizes the actions of benzodiazepines on the central nervous system. Flumazenil competitively inhibits the activity at the benzodiazepine recognition site on the GABA/benzodiazepine receptor complex. Flumazenil is a weak partial agonist in some animal models of activity, but has little or no agonist activity in man.

CLINICAL PHARMACOLOGY: *(cont'd)*

Flumazenil does not antagonize the central nervous system effects of drugs affecting GABA-ergic neurons by means other than the benzodiazepine receptor (including ethanol, barbiturates, or general anesthetics) and does not reverse the effects of opioids.

PHARMACODYNAMICS

Intravenous Flumazenil has been shown to antagonize sedation, impairment of recall and psychomotor impairment produced by benzodiazepines in healthy human volunteers.

The duration and degree of reversal of benzodiazepine effects are related to the dose and plasma concentrations of flumazenil.

Generally, doses of approximately 0.1 to 0.2 mg (corresponding to peak plasma levels of 3 to 6 ng/ml) produce partial antagonism, whereas higher doses of 0.4 to 1.0 mg (peak plasma levels of 12 to 28 ng/ml) usually produce complete antagonism in patients who have received the usual sedating doses of benzodiazepines. The onset of reversal is usually evident within 1 to 2 minutes after the injection is completed. Eighty percent response will be reached within 3 minutes, with the peak effect occurring at 6 to 10 minutes. The duration and degree of reversal are related to the plasma concentration of the sedating benzodiazepine as well as the dose of Flumazenil given.

In healthy volunteers, Flumazenil did not alter intraocular pressure when given alone and reversed the decrease in intraocular pressure seen after administration of midazolam.

PHARMACOKINETICS

After IV administration, plasma concentrations of flumazenil follow a two compartment open pharmacokinetic model with an initial distribution half-life of 7 to 15 minutes and a terminal half-life of 41 to 79 minutes. Peak concentrations of flumazenil are proportional to dose, with an apparent initial volume of distribution of 0.5 L/kg. After redistribution the apparent volume of distribution (V_{ss}) ranges from 0.77 to 1.60 L/kg. Protein binding is approximately 50% and the drug shows no preferential partitioning into red blood cells.

Flumazenil is a highly extracted drug. Clearance of flumazenil occurs primarily by hepatic metabolism and is dependent on hepatic blood flow. In pharmacokinetic studies of normal volunteers, total clearance ranges from 0.7 to 1.3 L/hr/kg, with less than 1% of the administered dose eliminated unchanged in the urine. The major metabolites of flumazenil identified in urine are the de-ethylated free acid and its glucuronide conjugate. In preclinical studies there was no evidence of pharmacologic activity exhibited by the de-ethylated free acid. Elimination of radiolabeled drug is essentially complete within 72 hours, with 90% to 95% of the radioactivity appearing in urine and 5% to 10% in the feces.

Pharmacokinetic Parameters Following a 5-minute infusion of a total of 1 mg of Flumazenil Mean (Coefficient of variation, Range) (TABLE 1).

TABLE 1

C_{max} (ng/ml)	24 (38%, 11-43)
AUC (ng * hr/ml)	15 (22%, 10-22)
V_{ss} (L/kg)	1 (24%, 0.8-1.6)
Cl (L/hr/kg)	1 (20%, 0.7-1.4)
Half-life (min)	54 (21%, 41-79)

The pharmacokinetics of flumazenil are not significantly affected by gender, age, renal failure (creatinine clearance <10 ml/min), or hemodialysis beginning 1 hour after drug administration. Mean total clearance is decreased to 40% to 60% of normal in patients with moderate liver dysfunction and to 25% of normal in patients with severe liver dysfunction compared with age-matched healthy subjects. This results in a prolongation of the half-life from 0.8 hours in healthy subjects to 1.3 hours in patients with moderate hepatic impairment and 2.4 hours in severely impaired patients. Ingestion of food during an intravenous infusion of the drug results in a 50% increase in clearance, most likely due to the increased hepatic blood flow that accompanies a meal. The pharmacokinetic profile of flumazenil is unaltered in the presence of benzodiazepine agonists and the kinetic profiles of those benzodiazepines are unaltered by flumazenil.

INDIVIDUALIZATION OF DOSAGES

General Principles: The serious adverse effects of Flumazenil are related to the reversal of benzodiazepine effects. Using more than the minimally effective dose of Flumazenil is tolerated by most patients but may complicate the management of patients who are physically dependent on benzodiazepines or patients who are depending on benzodiazepines for therapeutic effect (such as suppression of seizures in cyclic antidepressant overdose).

In high-risk patients, it is important to administer the smallest amount of Flumazenil that is effective. The 1-minute wait between individual doses in the dose-titration recommended for general clinical populations may be too short for high risk patients. This is because it takes 6 to 10 minutes for any single dose of flumazenil to reach full effects. Practitioners should slow the rate of administration of Flumazenil administered to high risk patients as recommended below.

Anesthesia And Conscious Sedation: Flumazenil is well tolerated at the recommended doses in individuals who have no tolerance to (or dependence on) benzodiazepines. The recommended dosages and titration rates in anesthesia and conscious sedation (0.2 to 1 mg given at 0.2 mg/min) are well tolerated in patients receiving the drug for reversal of a single benzodiazepine exposure in most clinical settings (see ADVERSE REACTIONS). The major risk will be resedation because the duration of effect of a long-acting (or large dose of a short-acting) benzodiazepine may exceed that of Flumazenil. Resedation may be treated by giving a repeat dose at no less than 20-minute intervals. For repeat treatment, no more than 1 mg (at 0.2 mg/min doses) should be given at any one time and no more than 3 mg should be given in any one hour.

Overdose Patients: The risk of confusion, agitation, emotional lability and perceptual distortion with the doses recommended in patients with benzodiazepine overdose (3 to 5 mg administered as 0.5 mg/min) may be greater than that expected with lower doses and slower administration. The recommended doses represent a compromise between a desirable slow awakening and the need for prompt response and a persistent effect in the overdose situation. If circumstances permit, the physician may elect to use the 0.2 mg/minute titration rate to slowly awaken the patient over 5 to 10 minutes, which may help to reduce signs and symptoms on emergence.

Flumazenil has no effect in cases where benzodiazepines are not responsible for sedation. Once doses of 3 to 5 mg have been reached without clinical response, additional Flumazenil is likely to have no effect.

Patients Tolerant To Benzodiazepines: Flumazenil may cause benzodiazepine withdrawal symptoms in individuals who have been taking benzodiazepines long enough to have some degree of tolerance. Patients who had been taking benzodiazepines prior to entry into the Flumazenil trials who were given flumazenil in doses over 1 mg experienced withdrawal-like events 2 to 5 times more frequently than patients who received less than 1 mg.

In patients who may have tolerance to benzodiazepines, as indicated by clinical history or by the need for larger than usual doses of benzodiazepine, slower titration rates of 0.1 mg/min and lower total doses may help reduce the frequency of emergent confusion and agitation. In such cases special care must be taken to monitor the patients for resedation because of the lower doses of Flumazenil used.

CLINICAL PHARMACOLOGY: *(cont'd)*

Patients Physically Dependent On Benzodiazepines: Flumazenil is known to precipitate withdrawal seizures in patients who are physically dependent on benzodiazepines, even if such dependence was established in a relatively few days of high dose sedation in Intensive Care Unit environments. The risk of either seizures or resedation in such cases is high and patients have experienced seizures before regaining consciousness. Flumazenil should be used in such settings with extreme caution, since the use of flumazenil in this situation has not been studied and no information as to dose and rate of titration is available. Flumazenil should be used in such patients only if the potential benefits of using the drug outweigh the risks of precipitated seizures. Physicians are directed to the scientific literature for the most current information in this area.

CLINICAL STUDIES:

Flumazenil has been administered to reverse the effects of benzodiazepines in conscious sedation, general anesthesia, and the management of suspected benzodiazepine overdose.

Conscious Sedation: Flumazenil was studied in four trials in 970 patients who received an average of 30 mg diazepam or 10 mg midazolam for sedation (with or without a narcotic) in conjunction with both inpatient and outpatient diagnostic or surgical procedures. Flumazenil was effective in reversing the sedating and psychomotor effects of the benzodiazepine, however, amnesia was less completely and less consistently reversed. In these studies, Flumazenil was administered as an initial dose of 0.4 mg IV (two doses of 0.2 mg) with additional 0.2 mg doses as needed to achieve complete awakening, up to a maximum total dose of 1 mg.

Seventy-eight percent of patients receiving flumazenil responded by becoming completely alert. Of those patients, approximately half responded to doses of 0.4 to 0.6 mg, while the other half responded to doses of 0.8 to 1 mg. Adverse effects were infrequent in patients who received 1 mg of Flumazenil or less, although injection site pain, agitation and anxiety did occur. Reversal of sedation was not associated with any increase in the frequency of inadequate analgesia or increase in narcotic demand in these studies. While most patients remained alert throughout the 3 hour post-procedure observation period, resedation was observed to occur in 3% to 9% of the patients, and was most common in patients who had received high doses of benzodiazepine. (See PRECAUTIONS.)

General Anesthesia: Flumazenil was studied in four trials in 644 patients who received midazolam as an induction and/or maintenance agent in both balanced and inhalational anesthesia. Midazolam was generally administered in doses ranging from 5 to 80 mg, alone and/or in conjunction with muscle relaxants, nitrous oxide, regional or local anesthetics, narcotics and/or inhalational anesthetics. Flumazenil was given as an initial dose of 0.2 mg IV, with additional 0.2 mg doses as needed to reach a complete response, up to a maximum total dose of 1 mg. These doses were effective in reversing sedation and restoring psychomotor function, but did not completely restore memory as tested by picture recall. Flumazenil was not as effective in the reversal of sedation in patients who had received multiple anesthetic agents in addition to benzodiazepines.

Eighty-one percent of patients sedated with midazolam responded to flumazenil by becoming completely alert or just slightly drowsy. Of those patients, 36% responded to doses of 0.4 to 0.6 mg, while 64% responded to doses of 0.8 to 1 mg.

Resedation in patients who responded to Flumazenil occurred in 10% to 15% of patients studied and was more common with larger doses of midazolam (>20 mg), long procedures (>60 minutes) and use of neuromuscular blocking agents. (See PRECAUTIONS.)

Management Of Suspected Benzodiazepine Overdose: Flumazenil was studied in two trials in 497 patients who were presumed to have taken an overdose of a benzodiazepine, either alone or in combination with a variety of other agents. In these trials, 299 patients were proven to have taken a benzodiazepine as part of the overdose, and 80% of the 148 who received Flumazenil responded by an improvement in level of consciousness. Of the patients who responded to flumazenil, 75% responded to a total dose of 1 to 3 mg.

Reversal of sedation was associated with an increased frequency of symptoms of CNS excitation. Of the patients treated with flumazenil, 1% to 3% were treated for agitation or anxiety. Serious side effects were uncommon, but six seizures were observed in 446 patients treated with flumazenil in these studies. Four of these 6 patients had ingested a large dose of cyclic antidepressants, which increased the risk of seizures. (See WARNINGS.)

INDICATIONS AND USAGE:

Flumazenil is indicated for the complete or partial reversal of the sedative effects of benzodiazepines in cases where general anesthesia has been induced and/or maintained with benzodiazepines, where sedation has been produced with benzodiazepines for diagnostic and therapeutic procedures, and for the management of benzodiazepine overdose.

CONTRAINDICATIONS:

Flumazenil is contraindicated:

In patients with a known hypersensitivity to flumazenil or to benzodiazepines.

In patients who have been given a benzodiazepine for control of a potentially life-threatening condition (*e.g.,* control of intracranial pressure or status epilepticus).

In patients who are showing signs of serious cyclic antidepressant overdose. (See WARNINGS.)

WARNINGS:

THE USE OF Flumazenil HAS BEEN ASSOCIATED WITH THE OCCURRENCE OF SEIZURES.
THESE ARE MOST FREQUENT IN PATIENTS WHO HAVE BEEN ON BENZODIAZEPINES FOR LONG-TERM SEDATION OR IN OVERDOSE CASES WHERE PATIENTS ARE SHOWING SIGNS OF SERIOUS CYCLIC ANTIDEPRESSANT OVERDOSE.
PRACTITIONERS SHOULD INDIVIDUALIZE THE DOSAGE OF Flumazenil AND BE PREPARED TO MANAGE SEIZURES.

Risk of Seizures: The reversal of benzodiazepine effects may be associated with the onset of seizures in certain high-risk populations. Possible risk factors for seizures include: concurrent major sedative-hypnotic drug withdrawal, recent therapy with repeated doses of parenteral benzodiazepines, myoclonic jerking or seizure activity prior to flumazenil administration in overdose cases, or concurrent cyclic anti-depressant poisoning.

Flumazenil is not recommended in cases of serious cyclic antidepressant poisoning, as manifested by motor abnormalities (twitching, rigidity, focal seizure), dysrhythmia (wide QRS, ventricular dysrhythmia, heart block), anticholinergic signs (mydriasis, dry mucosa, hypo-peristalsis), and cardiovascular collapse at presentation. In such cases Flumazenil should be withheld and the patient should be allowed to remain sedated (with ventilatory and circulatory support as needed) until the signs of antidepressant toxicity have subsided. Treatment with Flumazenil has no known benefit to the seriously ill mixed-overdose patient other than reversing sedation and should not be used in cases where seizures (from any cause) are likely.

WARNINGS: *(cont'd)*

Most convulsions associated with flumazenil administration require treatment and have been successfully managed with benzodiazepines, phenytoin or barbiturates. Because of the presence of flumazenil, higher than usual doses of benzodiazepines may be required.

Hypoventilation: Patients who have received Flumazenil for the reversal of benzodiazepine effects (after conscious sedation or general anesthesia) should be monitored for resedation, respiratory depression, or other residual benzodiazepine effects for an appropriate period (up to 120 minutes) based on the dose and duration of effect of the benzodiazepine employed.

This is because Flumazenil has not been established as an effective treatment for hypoventilation due to benzodiazepine administration. In healthy male volunteers, Flumazenil is capable of reversing benzodiazepine induced depression of the ventilatory responses to hypercapnia and hypoxia after a benzodiazepine alone. However, such depression may recur because the ventilatory effects of typical doses of Flumazenil (1 mg or less) may wear off before the effects of many benzodiazepines. The effects of Flumazenil on ventilatory response following sedation with a benzodiazepine in combination with an opioid are inconsistent and have not been adequately studied. The availability of flumazenil does not diminish the need for prompt detection of hypoventilation and the ability to effectively intervene by establishing an airway and assisting ventilation.

Overdose cases should always be monitored for resedation until the patients are stable and resedation is unlikely.

PRECAUTIONS:

Return Of Sedation: Flumazenil may be expected to improve the alertness of patients recovering from a procedure involving sedation or anesthesia with benzodiazepines, but should not be substituted for an adequate period of post-procedure monitoring. The availability of Flumazenil does not reduce the risks associated with the use of large doses of benzodiazepines for sedation.

Patients should be monitored for resedation, respiratory depression (See WARNINGS), or other persistent or recurrent agonist effects for an adequate period of time after administration of Flumazenil.

Resedation is least likely in cases where Flumazenil is administered to reverse a low dose of a short-acting benzodiazepine (<10 mg midazolam). It is most likely in cases where a large single or cumulative dose of a benzodiazepine has been given in the course of a long procedure along with neuromuscular blocking agents and multiple anesthetic agents.

Profound resedation was observed in 1% to 3% of patients in the clinical studies. In clinical situations where resedation must be prevented, physicians may wish to repeat the initial dose (up to 1 mg of Flumazenil given at 0.2 mg/min) at 30 minutes and possibly again at 60 minutes. This dosage schedule, although not studied in clinical trials, was effective in preventing resedation in a pharmacologic study in normal volunteers.

Use In The ICU: Flumazenil should be used with caution in the Intensive Care Unit because of the increased risk of unrecognized benzodiazepine dependence in such settings. Flumazenil may produce convulsions in patients physically dependent on benzodiazepines. See WARNINGS and CLINICAL PHARMACOLOGY,Individualization Of Dosage.

Administration of Flumazenil to diagnose benzodiazepine-induced sedation in the Intensive Care Unit is not recommended due to the risk of adverse events as described above. In addition, the prognostic significance of a patient's failure to respond to flumazenil in cases confounded by metabolic disorder, traumatic injury, drugs other than benzodiazepines, or any other reasons not associated with benzodiazepine receptor occupancy is not known.

Use In Overdose: Flumazenil is intended as an adjunct to, not as a substitute for proper management of airway, assisted breathing, circulatory access and support, internal decontamination by lavage and charcoal, and adequate clinical evaluation.

Necessary measures should be instituted to secure airway, ventilation and intravenous access prior to administering flumazenil. Upon arousal patients may attempt to withdraw endotracheal tubes and/or intravenous lines as the result of confusion and agitation following awakening.

Head Injury: Flumazenil should be used with caution in patients with head injury as it may be capable of precipitating convulsions or altering cerebral blood flow in patients receiving benzodiazepines. It should be used only by practitioners prepared to manage such complications should they occur.

Use With Neuromuscular Blocking Agents: Flumazenil should not be used until the effects of neuromuscular blockade have been fully reversed.

Use In Psychiatric Patients: Flumazenil has been reported to provoke panic attacks in patients with a history of panic disorder.

Pain On Injection: To minimize the likelihood of pain or inflammation at the injection site, Flumazenil should be administered through a freely flowing intravenous infusion into a large vein. Local irritation may occur following extravasation into perivascular tissues.

Use In Respiratory Disease: The primary treatment of patients with serious lung disease who experience serious respiratory depression due to benzodiazepines should be appropriate ventilatory support (See PRECAUTIONS) rather than the administration of Flumazenil. Flumazenil is capable of partially reversing benzodiazepine-induced alterations in ventilatory drive in healthy volunteers, but has not been shown to be clinically effective.

Use In Cardiovascular Disease: Flumazenil did not increase the work of the heart when used to reverse benzodiazepines in cardiac patients when given at a rate of 0.1 mg/min in total doses of less than 0.5 mg in studies reported in the clinical literature. Flumazenil alone had no significant effects on cardiovascular parameters when administered to patients with stable ischemic heart disease.

Use In Liver Disease: The clearance of Flumazenil is reduced to 40% to 60% of normal in patients with mild to moderate hepatic disease and to 25% of normal in patients with severe hepatic dysfunction see CLINICAL PHARMACOLOGY, Pharmacokinetics. While the dose of flumazenil used for initial reversal of benzodiazepine effects is not affected, repeat doses of the drug in liver disease should be reduced in size or frequency.

Use In Drug And Alcohol Dependent Patients: Flumazenil should be used with caution in patients with alcoholism and other drug dependencies due to the increased frequency of benzodiazepine tolerance and dependence observed in these patient populations.

Flumazenil is not recommended either as a treatment for benzodiazepine dependence or for the management of protracted benzodiazepine abstinence syndromes, as such use has not been studied.

The administration of flumazenil can precipitate benzodiazepine withdrawal in animals and man. This has been seen in healthy volunteers treated with therapeutic doses of oral lorazepam for up to 2 weeks who exhibited effects such as hot flushes, agitation and tremor when treated with cumulative doses of up to 3 mg doses of flumazenil.

Similar adverse experiences suggestive of flumazenil precipitation of benzodiazepine withdrawal have occurred in some patients in clinical trials. Such patients had a short-lived syndrome characterized by dizziness, mild confusion, emotional lability, agitation (with signs and symptoms of anxiety), and mild sensory distortions. This response was dose-related, most common at doses above 1 mg, rarely required treatment other than reassurance and was usually short lived. When required (5 to 10 cases), these patients were successfully treated with usual doses of a barbiturate, a benzodiazepine, or other sedative drug.

PRECAUTIONS: *(cont'd)*

Practitioners should assume that flumazenil administration may trigger dose-dependent withdrawal syndromes in patients with established physical dependence on benzodiazepines and may complicate the management of withdrawal syndrome for alcohol, barbiturates and cross-tolerant sedatives.

Use In Ambulatory Patients: The effects of Flumazenil may wear off before a long-acting benzodiazepine is completely cleared from the body. In general, if a patient shows no signs of sedation within 2 hours after a 1 mg dose of flumazenil, serious resedation at a later time is unlikely. An adequate period of observation must be provided for any patient in whom either long-acting benzodiazepines (such as diazepam) or large doses of short-acting benzodiazepines (such as >10 mg of midazolam) have been used. See CLINICAL PHARMACOLOGY, Individualization Of Dosage.

Because of the increased risk of adverse reactions in patients who have been taking benzodiazepines on a regular basis, it is particularly important that physicians query carefully about benzodiazepine, alcohol and sedative use as part of the history prior to any procedure in which the use of Flumazenil is planned. See PRECAUTIONS, Drug And Alcohol Dependent Patients.

INFORMATION FOR THE PATIENT

Flumazenil does not consistently reverse amnesia. Patients cannot be expected to remember information told to them in the post-procedure period and instructions given to patients should be reinforced in writing or given to a responsible family member. Physicians are advised to discuss with their patients, both before surgery and at discharge, that although the patient may feel alert at the time of discharge, the effects of the benzodiazepine may recur. As a result, the patient should be instructed, preferably in writing, that their memory and judgement may be impaired and specifically advised:

1. Not to engage in any activities requiring complete alertness, and not to operate hazardous machinery or a motor vehicle until at least 18 to 24 hours after discharge, and it is certain no residual sedative effects of the benzodiazepine remain.

2. Not to take any alcohol or non-prescription drugs for 18 to 24 hours after flumazenil administration or if the effects of the benzodiazepine persist.

LABORATORY TESTS

No specific laboratory tests are recommended to follow the patient's response or to identify possible adverse reactions.

DRUG/LABORATORY TEST INTERACTIONS

The possible interaction of flumazenil with commonly used laboratory tests has not been evaluated.

CARCINOGENESIS, MUTAGENESIS, AND IMPAIRMENT OF FERTILITY

Carcinogenesis: No studies in animals to evaluate the carcinogenic potential of flumazenil have been conducted.

Mutagenesis: No evidence for mutagenicity was noted in the Ames test using five different tester strains. Assays for mutagenic potential in *S. cerevisiae* D7 and in Chinese hamster cells were considered to be negative as were blastogenesis assays *in vitro* in peripheral human lymphocytes and *in vivo* in a mouse micronucleus assay. Flumazenil caused a slight increase in unscheduled DNA synthesis in rat hepatocyte culture at concentrations which were also cytotoxic; no increase in DNA repair was observed in male mouse germ cells in an *in vivo* DNA repair assay.

Impairment of Fertility: A reproduction study in male and female rats did not show any impairment of fertility at oral dosages of 125 mg/kg/day. From the available data on the area under the curve (AUC) in animals and man the dose represented 120 x the human exposure from a maximum recommended intravenous dose of 5 mg.

PREGNANCY CATEGORY C:

There are no adequate and well-controlled studies of the use of flumazenil in pregnant women. Flumazenil should be used during pregnancy only if the potential benefit justifies the potential risk to the fetus.

Teratogenic Effects: Flumazenil has been studied for teratogenicity in rats and rabbits following oral treatments of up to 150 mg/kg/day. The treatments during the major organogenesis were on days 6 to 15 of gestation in the rat and days 6 to 18 of gestation in the rabbit. No teratogenic effects were observed in rats or rabbits at 150 mg/kg; the dose, based on the available data on the area under the plasma concentration-time curve (AUC) represented 120 x to 600 x the human exposure from a maximum recommended intravenous dose of 5 mg in humans. In rabbits, embryocidal effects (as evidenced by increased pre-implantation and post-implantation losses) were observed at 50 mg/kg or 200 x the human exposure from a maximum recommended intravenous dose of 5 mg. The no-effect dose of 15 mg/kg in rabbits represents 60 x the human exposure.

Nonteratogenic Effects: An animal reproduction study was conducted in rats at oral dosages of 5, 25 and 125 mg/kg/day of flumazenil. Pup survival was decreased during the lactating period, pup liver weight at weaning was increased for the high-dose group (125 mg/kg/day) and incisor eruption and ear opening in the offspring were delayed; the delay in ear opening was associated with a delay in the appearance of the auditory startle response. No treatment-related adverse effects were noted for the other dose groups. Based on the available data from AUC, the effect level (125 mg/kg), represents 120 x the human exposure from 5 mg, the maximum recommended intravenous dose in humans. The no-effect level represents 24 x the human exposure from an intravenous dose of 5 mg.

LABOR AND DELIVERY

The use of Flumazenil to reverse the effects of benzodiazepines used during labor and delivery is not recommended because the effects of the drug in the newborn are unknown.

NURSING MOTHERS

Caution should be exercised when deciding to administer Flumazenil to a nursing woman because it is not known whether flumazenil is excreted in human milk.

PEDIATRIC USE

Flumazenil is not recommended for use in children (either for the reversal of sedation, the management of overdose or the resuscitation of the newborn), as no clinical studies have been performed to determine the risks, benefits and dosages to be used.

GERIATRIC USE

The pharmacokinetics of flumazenil have been studied in the elderly and are not significantly different from younger patients. Several studies of Flumazenil in patients over the age of 65 and one study in patients over the age of 80 suggest that while the doses of benzodiazepine used to induce sedation should be reduced, ordinary doses of Flumazenil may be used for reversal.

DRUG INTERACTIONS:

Interaction with central nervous system depressants other than benzodiazepines has not been specifically studied; however, no deleterious interactions were seen when Flumazenil was administered after narcotics, inhalational anesthetics, muscle relaxants and muscle relaxant antagonists administered in conjunction with sedation or anesthesia.

DRUG INTERACTIONS: *(cont'd)*

Particular caution is necessary when using Flumazenil in cases of mixed drug overdosage since the toxic effects (such as convulsions and cardiac dysrhythmias) of other drugs taken in overdose (especially cyclic antidepressants) may emerge with the reversal of the benzodiazepine effect by flumazenil. (See WARNINGS.)

The pharmacokinetics of benzodiazepines are unaltered in the presence of flumazenil.

ADVERSE REACTIONS:

SERIOUS ADVERSE REACTIONS

Deaths have occurred in patients who received Flumazenil in a variety of clinical settings. The majority of deaths occurred in patients with serious underlying disease or in patients who had ingested large amounts of non-benzodiazepine drugs, (usually cyclic antidepressants) as part of an overdose.

Serious adverse events have occurred in all clinical settings, and convulsions are the most common serious adverse event-reported. Flumazenil administration has been associated with the onset of convulsions in patients who are relying on benzodiazepine effects to control seizures, are physically dependent on benzodiazepines, or who have ingested large doses of other drugs. (See WARNINGS.)

Two of the 446 patients who received Flumazenil in controlled clinical trials for the management of a benzodiazepine overdosage had cardiac dysrhythmias (1 ventricular tachycardia, 1 junctional tachycardia).

ADVERSE EVENTS IN CLINICAL STUDIES

The following adverse reactions were considered to be related to Flumazenil administration (both alone and for the reversal of benzodiazepine effects) and were reported in studies involving 1875 individuals who received flumazenil in controlled trials. Adverse events most frequently associated with flumazenil alone were limited to dizziness, injection site pain, increased sweating, headache and abnormal or blurred vision (3% to 9%).

Body As A Whole: Fatigue (asthenia, malaise), Headache, Injection Site Pain*, Injection Site Reaction (thrombophlebitis, skin abnormality, rash)

Cardiovascular System: Cutaneous vasodilation (sweating, flushing, hot flushes)

Digestive System: Nausea and Vomiting (11%)

Nervous System: Agitation (anxiety, nervousness, dry mouth, tremor, palpitations, insomnia, dyspnea, hyperventilation)*, Dizziness (vertigo, ataxia) (10%), Emotional lability (crying abnormal, depersonalization, euphoria, increased tears, depression, dysphoria, paranoia).

Special Senses: Abnormal Vision (visual field defect, diplopia), Paresthesia (sensation abnormal, hypoesthesia)

(All adverse reactions occurred in 1% to 3% of cases unless otherwise marked.)

*indicates reaction in 3% to 9% of cases.

Observed percentage reported if greater than 9%.

The following adverse events were observed infrequently (less than 1%) in the clinical studies, but were judged as probably related to Flumazenil administration and/or reversal of benzodiazepine effects:

Nervous System: Confusion (difficulty concentrating, delirium), Convulsions (See WARNINGS), Somnolence (stupor).

Special Senses: Abnormal Hearing (transient hearing impairment, hyperacusis, tinnitus).

The following adverse events occurred with frequencies less than 1% in the clinical trials. Their relationship to Flumazenil administration is unknown, but they are included as alerting information for the physician.

Body As A Whole: Rigors, shivering.

Cardiovascular: Arrhythmia (atrial, nodal, ventricular extrasystoles), bradycardia, tachycardia, hypertension, chest pain.

Digestive System: Hiccup.

Nervous System: Speech disorder (dysphoria, thick tongue).

Not included in this list is operative site pain that occurred with the same frequency in patients receiving placebo as in patients receiving flumazenil for reversal of sedation following a surgical procedure.

DRUG ABUSE AND DEPENDENCE:

Flumazenil acts as a benzodiazepine antagonist, blocks the effects of benzodiazepines in animals and man, antagonizes benzodiazepine reinforcement in animal models, produces dysphoria in normal subjects, and has had no reported abuse in foreign marketing.

Although Flumazenil has a benzodiazepine-like structure it does not act as a benzodiazepine agonist in man and is not a controlled substance.

OVERDOSAGE:

Large intravenous doses of Flumazenil, when administered to healthy normal volunteers in the absence of a benzodiazepine agonist, produced no serious adverse reactions, severe signs or symptoms, or clinically significant laboratory test abnormalities. In clinical studies, most adverse reactions to flumazenil were an extension of the pharmacologic effects of the drug in reversing benzodiazepine effects.

Reversal with an excessively high dose of Flumazenil may produce anxiety, agitation, increased muscle tone, hyperesthesia and possibly convulsions. Convulsions have been treated with barbiturates, benzodiazepines and phenytoin, generally with prompt resolution of the seizures. (See WARNINGS.)

DOSAGE AND ADMINISTRATION:

Flumazenil is recommended for intravenous use only. It is compatible with 5% dextrose in water, lactated Ringer's and normal saline solutions. If Flumazenil is drawn into a syringe or mixed with any of these solutions, it should be discarded after 24 hours. For optimum sterility, Flumazenil should remain in the vial until just before use. As with all parenteral drug products, Flumazenil should be inspected visually for particulate matter and discoloration prior to administration, whenever solution and container permit.

To minimize the likelihood of pain at the injection site, Flumazenil should be administered through a freely running intravenous infusion into a large vein.

Reversal Of Conscious Sedation Or In General Anesthesia: For the reversal of the sedative effects of benzodiazepines administered for conscious sedation or general anesthesia, the recommended initial dose of Flumazenil is 0.2 mg (2 ml) administered intravenously over 15 seconds. If the desired level of consciousness is not obtained after waiting an additional 45 seconds, a further dose of 0.2 mg (2 ml) can be injected and repeated at 60-second intervals where necessary (up to a maximum of 4 additional times) to a maximum total dose of 1 mg (10 ml). The dose should be individualized based on the patient's response, with most patients responding to doses of 0.6 to 1 mg. See CLINICAL PHARMACOLOGY, Individualization Of Dosage.

In the event of resedation, repeated doses may be administered at 20 minute intervals as needed. For repeat treatment, no more than 1 mg (given as 0.2 mg/min) should be administered at any one time, and no more than 3 mg should be given in any one hour.

DOSAGE AND ADMINISTRATION: *(cont'd)*

It is recommended that Flumazenil be administered as the series of small injections described (not as a single bolus injection) to allow the practitioner to control the reversal of sedation to the approximate endpoint desired and to minimize the possibility of adverse effects. SeeCLINICAL PHARMACOLOGY, Individualization Of Dosage.

Management Of Suspected Benzodiazepine Overdose: For initial management of a known or suspected benzodiazepine overdose, the recommended initial dose of Flumazenil is 0.2 mg (2 ml) administered intravenously over 30 seconds. If the desired level of consciousness is not obtained after waiting 30 seconds, a further dose of 0.3 mg (3 ml) can be administered over another 30 seconds. Further doses of 0.5 mg (5 ml) can be administered over 30 seconds at 1-minute intervals up to a cumulative dose of 3 mg.

Do not rush the administration of Flumazenil. Patients should have a secure airway and intravenous access before administration of the drug and be awakened gradually. (See PRECAUTIONS.)

Most patients with benzodiazepine overdose will respond to a cumulative dose of 1 to 3 mg of Flumazenil, and doses beyond 3 mg do not reliably produce additional effects. On rare occasions, patients with a partial response at 3 mg may require additional titration up to a total dose of 5 mg (administered slowly in the same manner).

If a patient has not responded 5 minutes after receiving a cumulative dose of 5 mg Flumazenil, the major cause of sedation is likely not to be due to benzodiazepines, and additional Flumazenil is likely to have no effect.

In the event of resedation, repeated doses may be given at 20-minute intervals if needed. For repeat treatment, no more than 1 mg (given as 0.5 mg/min) should be given at any one time and no more than 3 mg should be given in any one hour.

Safety And Handling: Flumazenil is supplied in sealed dosage forms and poses no known risk to the health care provider. Routine care should be taken to avoid aerosol generation when preparing syringes for injection, and spilled medication should be rinsed from the skin with cool water.

Store at 59° to 86°F (15° to 30°C).

HOW SUPPLIED - EQUIVALENTS NOT AVAILABLE:

Injection, Solution - Intravenous - 0.1 mg/ml

5 ml x 10	$292.66	ROMAZICON, Roche	00004-6911-06
10 ml x 10	$465.60	ROMAZICON, Roche	00004-6912-06

FLUNISOLIDE *(001305)*

CATEGORIES: Adrenal Corticosteroids; Airway Obstruction; Allergies; Anti-Inflammatory Agents; Asthma; EENT Drugs; Eye, Ear, Nose, & Throat Preparations; Hormones; Nasal Congestion; Respiratory & Allergy Medications; Rhinitis; Steroids; Topical; Pregnancy Category C; FDA Approval Pre 1982

BRAND NAMES: Aerobid; Aerobid-M; *Bronalide* (Canada); *Bronilide* (France); *Flunase*; *Gibiflu*; *Inhacort* (Germany); *Locasyn*; *Lokilan*; *Lokilan Nasal*; *Lunibron-A*; *Lunis*; **Nasalide**; Nasarel; *Rhinalar* (Canada); *Rhinalar Nasal Mist*; *Rhinalar Nasal Spray*; *Sanergal*; *Synaclyn* (Japan); *Syntaris* (Germany, England); *Syntaris Nasal Spray*
(International brand names outside U.S. in italics)

FORMULARIES: Aetna; BC-BS; CIGNA; FHP; Humana; Kaiser; Medco; Medi-Cal; PruCare; United

COST OF THERAPY: $564.18 (Asthma; Aerosol; 250 mcg; 0.2/day; 365 days)

PRIMARY ICD9: 493.90 (Asthma, Unspecified, Without Mention of Status Asthmaticus)

DESCRIPTION:

NASAL SOLUTION

Flunisolide nasal solution is intended for administration as a spray to the nasal mucosa. Flunisolide, the active component of Flunisolide nasal solution, is an anti-inflammatory steroid with the chemical name: 6α-fluoro-11β, 16α, 17, 21-tetrahydroxypregna-1,4-diene-3,20- dione cyclic 16,17-acetal with acetone (USAN).

Flunisolide is a white to creamy white crystalline powder with a molecular weight of 434.49. It is insoluble in acetone, sparingly soluble in chloroform, slightly soluble in methanol, and practically insoluble in water. It has a melting point of about 245°C.

Each 25 ml spray bottle contains flunisolide 6.25 mg (0.25 mg/ml) in a solution of propylene glycol, polyethylene glycol 3350, citric acid, sodium citrate, butylated hydroxyanisole, edetate disodium, benzalkonium chloride, and purified water, with NaOH and/or HCl added to adjust the pH to approximately 5.3. It contains no fluorocarbons.

After priming the delivery system for Flunisolide, each actuation of the unit delivers a metered droplet spray containing approximately 25 mcg of flunisolide. The size of the droplets produced by the unit is in excess of 8 microns to facilitate deposition on the nasal mucosa. The contents of one nasal spray bottle deliver at least 200 sprays.

ORAL INHALER

Flunisolide, the active component of Aerobid Inhaler System, is an anti-inflammatory steroid having the chemical name 6α-fluoro-11β, 16α, 17, 21-tetrahydroxypregna-1, 4-diene-3, 20-dione cyclic-16, 17- acetal with acetone.

Flunisolide is a white to creamy white crystalline powder with a molecular weight of 434.49. It is insoluble in acetone, sparingly soluble in chloroform, slightly soluble in methanol, and practically insoluble in water. It has a melting point of about 245°C.

Aerobid (flunisolide) inhaler is delivered in a metered dose aerosol system containing a microcrystalline suspension of flunisolide as the hemihydrate in propellants (trichloromonofluoromethane, dichlorodifluoromethane and dichlorotetrafluoroethane) with sorbitan trioleate as a dispersing agent, (and Menthol as a flavoring agent in Aerobid-M). Each activation delivers approximately 250 mcg of Flunisolide to the patient. One Aerobid Inhaler System is designed to deliver at least 100 metered inhalations.

CLINICAL PHARMACOLOGY:

NASAL SOLUTION

Flunisolide has demonstrated potent glucocorticoid and weak mineralocorticoid activity in classical animal test systems. As a glucocorticoid it is several hundred times more potent than the cortisol standard. Clinical studies with flunisolide have shown therapeutic activity on nasal mucous membranes with minimal evidence of systemic activity at the recommended doses.

A study in approximately 100 patients which compared the recommended dose of flunisolide nasal solution with an oral dose providing equivalent systemic amounts of flunisolide has shown that the clinical effectiveness of Flunisolide, when used topically as recommended, is due to its direct local effect and not to an indirect effect through systemic absorption.

CLINICAL PHARMACOLOGY: *(cont'd)*

Following administration to flunisolide to man, approximately half of the administered dose is recovered in the urine and half in the stool; 65-70% of the dose recovered in urine is the primary metabolite, which has undergone loss of the 6α fluorine and addition of a 6β hydroxy group. Flunisolide is well absorbed but is rapidly converted by the liver to the much less active primary metabolite and to glucuronate and/or sulfate conjugates. Because of first-pass liver metabolism, only 20% of the flunisolide reaches the systemic circulation when it is given orally whereas 50% of the flunisolide administered intranasally reaches the systemic circulation unmetabolized. The plasma half-life of flunisolide is 1-2 hours.

The effects of flunisolide on hypothalamic-pituitary-adrenal (HPA) axis function has been studied in volunteers. Flunisolide was administered intranasally as a spray in total doses over 7 times the recommended dose (2200 mcg equivalent to 88 sprays/days) in 2 subjects for 4 days, about 3 times the recommended dose (800 mcg, equivalent to 32 sprays/day) in 4 subjects for 10 days. Early morning plasma cortisol concentrations and 24-hour urinary 17-ketogenic steroids were measured daily. There was evidence of decreased endogenous cortisol production at all three doses.

In controlled studies, Flunisolide was found to be effective in reducing symptoms of stuffy nose, runny nose and sneezing in most patients. These controlled clinical studies have been conducted in 488 adult patients at doses ranging from 8 to 16 sprays (200-400 mcg) per day and 127 children at doses ranging from 6 to 8 sprays (150-200 mcg) per day for periods as long as 3 months. In 170 patients who had cortisol levels evaluated at baseline and after 3 months or more of flunisolide treatment, there was no unequivocal flunisolide-related depression of plasma cortisol levels.

The mechanisms responsible for the anti-inflammatory action of corticosteroids and for the activity of the aerosolized drug on the nasal mucosa are unknown.

ORAL INHALER

Flunisolide has demonstrated marked anti-inflammatory and anti-allergic activity in classical test systems. It is a corticosteroid that is several hundred times more potent in animal anti-inflammatory assays than the cortisol standard. The molar dose of each activation of flunisolide in this preparation is approximately 2.5 to 7 times that of comparable inhaled corticosteroid products marketed for the same indication. The dose of flunisolide delivered per activation in this preparation is 10 times that per activation of flunisolide nasal solution. Clinical studies have shown therapeutic activity on bronchial mucosa with minimal evidence of systemic activity at recommended doses.

After oral inhalation of 1 mg flunisolide, total systemic availability was 40%. The flunisolide that is swallowed is rapidly and extensively converted to the 6β-OH metabolite and to water-soluble conjugates during the first pass through the liver. This offers a metabolic explanation for the low systemic activity of oral flunisolide itself since the metabolite has low corticosteroid potency (on the order of the cortisol standard). The inhaled flunisolide absorbed through the bronchial tree is converted to the metabolites. Repeated inhalation of 2.0 mg of flunisolide per day (the maximum recommended dose) of 14 days did not show accumulation of the drug in plasma. The plasma half-life of flunisolide is approximately 1.8 hours.

The following observations relevant to systemic absorption were made in clinical studies. In one uncontrolled study a statistically significant decrease in responsiveness to metyrapone was noted in 15 adult steroid- independent patients treated with 2.0 mg of flunisolide per day (the maximum recommended dose) for 3 months. A small but statistically significant drop in eosinophils from 11.5% to 7.4% of total circulating leukocytes was noted in another study in children who were not taking oral corticosteroids simultaneously. A 5% incidence of menstrual disturbances was reported during open studies, in which there were no control groups for comparison.

Aerosol administration of flunisolide 2.0 mg twice daily for one week to 6 healthy male subjects revealed neither suppression of adrenal function as measured by early morning cortisol levels nor impairment of HPA axis function as determined by insulin hypoglycemia tests.

Controlled clinical studies have included over 500 patients with asthma, among them 150 children age 6 and over. More than 120 patients have been treated in open trials for two years or more. No significant adrenal suppression attributed to flunisolide was seen in these studies.

Significant decreases of systemic steroid dosages have been possible in flunisolide-treated patients. Asthma patients have had further symptomatic improvement with flunisolide treatment even while reducing concomitant medication.

INDICATIONS AND USAGE:

NASAL SOLUTION

Flunisolide is indicated for the topical treatment of the symptoms of seasonal or perennial or perennial rhinitis when effectiveness of or tolerance to conventional treatment is unsatisfactory.

Clinical studies have shown that improvement is based on a local effect rather than systemic absorption, and is usually apparent within a few days starting Flunisolide. However, symptomatic relief may not occur in some patients for as long as two weeks. Although systemic effects are minimal at recommended doses, Flunisolide should not be continued beyond 3 weeks in the absence of significant symptomatic improvement.

Flunisolide should not be used in the presence of untreated localized infection involving nasal mucosa.

ORAL INHALER

Flunisolide Inhaler is indicated only for patients who require chronic treatment with corticosteroids for control of the symptoms of bronchial asthma. Such patients would include those already receiving systemic corticosteroids, and selected patients who are inadequately controlled on a non-steroid regimen and in whom steroid therapy has been withheld because of concern over potential adverse effects.

As with any topically applied medication, flunisolide is absorbed through the mucous membrane and is systemically available. For these reasons, Flunisolide Inhaler should be used with caution for initial therapy and the recommended dosage not be exceeded. When the drug is used chronically at 2 mg/day, patients should be monitored periodically for effects on the hypothalamic-pituitary-adrenal axis.

Flunisolide Inhaler in NOT indicated for:

1. For relief of asthma that can be controlled by bronchial dilators and other non-steroid medications.

2. In patients who require systemic corticosteroid treatment infrequently.

3. In the treatment of non-asthmatic bronchitis.

There is insufficient information is available to warrant use in children under the age of 6.

CONTRAINDICATIONS:

NASAL SOLUTION

Hypersensitivity to any of the ingredients.

ORAL INHALER

Flunisolide Inhaler is contraindicated in the primary treatment of status asthmaticus or other acute episodes of asthma where intensive measures are required.

CONTRAINDICATIONS: *(cont'd)*

Hypersensitivity to any of the ingredients of this preparation contraindicates its use.

WARNINGS:

NASAL SOLUTION

The replacement of a systemic corticosteroid with a topical corticoid can be accompanied by signs of adrenal insufficiency, and in addition some patients may experience symptoms of withdrawal *e.g.,* joint and/or muscular pain, lassitude and depression. Patients previously treated for prolonged periods with systemic corticosteroids and transferred to flunisolide should be carefully monitored to avoid acute adrenal insufficiency in response to stress.

When transferred to Flunisolide, careful attention must be given to patients previously treated for prolonged periods with systemic corticosteroids. This is particularly important in those patients who have associated asthma or other clinical conditions, where too rapid a decrease in systemic corticosteroids may cause a severe exacerbation of their symptoms.

The use of Flunisolide with alternate-day prednisone systemic treatment could increase the likelihood of HPA suppression compared to a therapeutic dose of either one alone. Therefore, Flunisolide treatment should be used with caution in patients already on alternate-day prednisone regimens for any disease.

ORAL INHALER

WARNINGS:
Oral Inhaler: Particular care is needed in patients who are transferred from systemically active corticosteroids to Aerobid Inhaler because deaths due to renal insufficiency have occurred in asthmatic patients during and after transfer from systemic corticosteroids to aerosol corticosteroids. After withdrawal from systemic corticosteroids, a number of months are required for recovery of hypothalamic-pituitary-adrenal (HPA) function. During this period of HPA suppression, patients may exhibit signs and symptoms of adrenal insufficiency when exposed to trauma, surgery, or infections, particularly gastroenteritis. Although Aerobid Inhaler may provide control of asthmatic symptoms during these episodes, it does NOT provide the systemic steroid that is necessary for coping with emergencies.
During periods of stress or a severe asthmatic attack, patients who have been withdrawn from systemic corticosteroids should be instructed to resume systemic steroids (in larger doses) immediately and to contact their physicians for further instruction. These patients should also be instructed to carry a warning card indicating that they may need supplementary systemic steroids during periods of stress or a severe asthma attack. To assess the risk of adrenal insufficiency in emergency situations, routine tests of adrenal cortical function, including measurement of early morning cortisol levels, should be performed periodically in all patients. An early morning resting cortisol level may be accepted as normal if it falls at or near the normal mean level.

Localized infections with *Candida albicans* or *Aspergillus niger* have occurred in the mouth and pharynx and occasionally in the larynx. Positive cultures for oral *Candida* may be present in up to 34% of patients. Although the frequency of clinically apparent infection is considerably lower, these infections may require treatment with appropriate antifungal therapy or discontinuance of treatment with Aerobid (flunisolide) Inhaler.

Aerobid (flunisolide) Inhaler is not to be regarded as a bronchodilator and is not indicated for rapid relief of bronchospasm.

Patients should be instructed to contact their physician immediately when episodes of asthma that are not responsive to bronchodilators occur during the course of treatment. During such episodes, patients may require therapy with systemic corticosteroids.

There is no evidence that control of asthma can be achieved by administration of the drug in amounts greater than the recommended doses, which appear to be the therapeutic equivalent of approximately 10 mg/day of oral prednisone. Theoretically, the use of inhaled corticosteroids with alternate day prednisone systemic treatment should be accompanied by more HPA suppression than a therapeutically equivalent regimen of either alone.

Transfer of patients from systemic steroid therapy to Aerobid Inhaler may unmask allergic conditions previously suppressed by the systemic steroid therapy, *e.g.,* rhinitis, conjunctivitis, eczema.

Children who are on immunosuppressant drugs are more susceptible to infections than healthy children. Chicken pox and measles for example, can have a more serious or even fatal course in children on immunosuppressant corticosteroids. In such children, or in adults who have not had these diseases, particular care should be taken to avoid exposure. If exposed, therapy with varicella zoster immune globulin (VZIG) or pooled intravenous immunoglobulin (IVIG), as appropriate, may be indicated. If chicken pox develops, treatment with antiviral agents maybe considered.

PRECAUTIONS:

NASAL SOLUTION

General: In clinical studies with flunisolide administered intranasally, the development of localized infections of the nose and pharynx with *Candida albicans* has occurred only rarely. When such an infection develops it may require treatment with appropriate local therapy or discontinuance of treatment with flunisolide.

Flunisolide is absorbed into the circulation. Use of excessive doses of Flunisolide may suppress hypothalamic-pituitary-adrenal function.

Flunisolide should be used with caution, if at all in patients with active quiescent tuberculosis infections of the respiratory tract or in treated fungal, bacterial or systemic viral infections or ocular herpes simplex.

Because of the inhibitory effect of corticosteroids on wound healing, in patients who have experienced recent nasal septal ulcers, recurrent epistaxis, nasal surgery or trauma, a nasal corticosteroid should be used with caution until healing has occurred.

Although systemic effects have been minimal with recommended doses, this potential increases with excessive dosages. Therefore, larger than recommended doses should be avoided.

Information for the Patient: Patients should use Flunisolide at regular intervals since its effectiveness depends on its regular use. The patient should take the medication as directed. It is not acutely effective and the prescribed dosage should not be increased. Instead, nasal vasoconstrictors or oral antihistamines may be needed until the effects of Flunisolide are fully manifested. One or two weeks may pass before full relief is obtained. The patient should contact the physician if symptoms do not improve, or if the condition worsens, or if sneezing or nasal irritation occurs.

For the proper use of this unit and to attain maximum improvement, the patient should read and follow the accompanying Patient Instructions carefully. (Contact the manufacturer for this information).

PRECAUTIONS: *(cont'd)*

Carcinogenesis, Mutagenesis, and Impairment of Fertility: Long-term studies were conducted in mice and rats using oral administration to evaluate the carcinogenic potential of the drug. There was an increase in the incidence of pulmonary adenomas in mice, but not in rats.

Female rats receiving the highest oral dose had an increased incidence of mammary adenocarcinoma compared to control rats. An increased incidence of this tumor type has been reported for other corticosteroids.

Impairment of Fertility: Female rats receiving high doses of flunisolide (200 mcg/kg/day) showed some evidence of impaired fertility. Reproductive performance in low (8 mcg/kg/day) and mid-dose (40 mcg/kg/day) groups was comparable to controls.

Pregnancy, Teratogenic Effects, Pregnancy Category C: As with other corticosteroids, flunisolide has been shown to be teratogenic in rabbits and rats at doses of 40 and 200 mcg/kg/day respectively. It was also fetotoxic in these animal reproductive studies. There are no adequate and well-controlled studies in pregnant women. Flunisolide should be used during pregnancy only if the potential benefit justifies the potential risk to the fetus.

Nursing Mothers: It not known whether this drug is excreted in human milk. Because other corticosteroids are excreted in human milk, caution should be exercised when flunisolide is administered to nursing women.

ORAL INHALER

General: Because of the relatively high molar dose of flunisolide per activation in this preparation, and because of the evidence suggesting higher levels of systemic absorption with flunisolide than with other comparable inhaled corticosteroids (see CLINICAL PHARMACOLOGY), patients treated with Aerobid (flunisolide) should be observed carefully for any evidence of systemic corticosteroid effect, including suppression of bone growth in children. Particular care should be taken in observing patients post-operatively or during periods of stress for evidence of a decrease in adrenal function. During withdrawal from oral steroids, some patients may experience symptoms of systemically active steroids withdrawal, e.g., joint and/or muscular pain, lassitude and depression, despite maintenance of even improvement of respiratory function (see DOSAGE AND ADMINISTRATION for details).

In responsive patients, flunisolide may permit control of asthmatic symptoms without suppression of HPA function. Since flunisolide is absorbed into the circulation and can be systemically active, the beneficial effects of Aerobid Inhaler in minimizing or preventing HPA dysfunction may be expected only when recommended dosages are not exceeded.

The long-term effects of the drug in human subjects are still unknown. In particular, the local effects of the agent on developmental or immunologic processes in the mouth, pharynx, trachea, and lung are unknown. There is also no information about the possible long-term systemic effects of the agent.

The potential effects of the drug on acute, recurrent, or chorionic pulmonary infections, including active or quiescent tuberculosis, are not known. Similarly, the potential effects of long-term administration of the drug on lung or other tissues are unknown.

Pulmonary infiltrates with eosinophilia may occur in patients on Aerobid Inhaler therapy. Although it is possible that in some patients this state may become manifest because of systemic steroid withdrawal when inhalational steroids are administered, a causative role for the drug and/or its vehicle cannot be ruled out

INFORMATION FOR THE PATIENT

There is no evidence that better control of asthma can be achieved by the administration of Aerobid Inhaler in amounts greater than the recommended doses; higher doses may induce adrenal suppression.

Since the relief from Aerobid Inhaler depends on its regular use and on proper inhalation technique, patients must be instructed to take inhalations at regular intervals. They should also be instructed in the correct method of use (see PATIENT PACKAGE INSERT).

Patients receiving bronchodilators by inhalation should be advised to use the bronchodilator before Aerobid Inhaler in order to enhance penetration of flunisolide into the bronchial tree. After use of an aerosol bronchodilator, several minutes should elapse before using Aerobid Inhaler.

Patients whose systemic corticosteroids have been reduced or withdrawn should be instructed to carry a warning card indicating that they may need supplemental systemic steroids during periods of stress or a severe asthmatic attack that is not responsive to bronchodilators.

Patients who are on immunosuppressant doses of corticosteroids should be warned to avoid exposure to chicken pox or measles and, if exposed, to obtain medical advice.

An illustrated leaflet of patient instructions for proper use accompanies each Aerobid Inhaler System.

CONTENTS UNDER PRESSURE

Do not puncture. Do not use or store near heat or open flame. Exposure to temperatures above 120°F (49°C) may cause container to explode. Never throw container into fire or incinerator. Keep out of reach of children.

Carcinogenesis, Mutagenesis, and Impairment of Fertility: Please refer to the appropriate subheading above under Nasal Solution.

Nursing Mothers: Please refer to the appropriate subheading above under Nasal Solution

ADVERSE REACTIONS:

NASAL SOLUTION

Adverse reactions reported in controlled clinical trials and long-term open studies in 595 patients treated with Flunisolide are described below. Of these patients, 409 were treated for 3 months or longer, 323 for 6 months or longer, 259 for 1 year or longer, and 91 for 2 years or longer.

In general, side effects elicited in the clinical studies have been primarily associated with the nasal mucous membranes. The most frequent complaints were those of mild transient nasal burning and stinging, which were reported in approximately 45% of the patients treated with Flunisolide in placebo-controlled and long-term studies. These complaints do not usually interfere with treatment; in only 3% of patients was it necessary to decrease dosage or stop treatment because of these symptoms. Approximately the same incidence of mild transient nasal burning and stinging was reported in patients on placebo as was reported in patients treated with Flunisolide in controlled studies, implying that these complaints may be related to the vehicle or the delivery system.

The incidence of complaints of nasal burning and stinging decreased with increasing duration of treatment.

Other side effects reported at frequency of 5% or less were: nasal congestion, sneezing, epistaxis and/or bloody mucus, nasal irritation, watery eyes, sore throat, nausea and/or vomiting, headache and loss of sense of smell and taste. As is the case with other nasally inhaled corticosteroids, nasal septal perforations have been observed in rare instances.

Systemic corticosteroid side effects were not reported during the controlled clinical trials. If recommended doses are exceeded or if individuals are particularly sensitive, symptoms of hypercorticism, i.e., Cushing's syndrome, could occur.

ADVERSE REACTIONS: *(cont'd)*

ORAL INHALER

Adverse events reported in controlled clinical trials and long-term open studies in 514 patients treated with Aerobid (flunisolide) are described below. Of those patients, 463 were treated for 3 months or longer, 407 for 6 months or longer, 287 for 1 year or longer, and 122 for 2 years or longer.

Musculoskeletal reactions were reported in 35% of steroid-dependent patients in whom the dose of oral steroid was being tapered. This is a well-known effect of steroid withdrawal.

INCIDENCE 10% OR GREATER

Gastrointestinal: diarrhea (10%), nausea and/or vomiting (25%), upset stomach (10%)

General: flu (10%)

Mouth and Throat: sore throat (20%)

Nervous system: headache (25%)

Respiratory: cold symptoms (15%), nasal congestion (15%), upper respiratory infection (25%).

Special Senses: unpleasant tastes (10%)

INCIDENCE 3-9%

Cardiovascular: palpitations

Gastrointestinal: abdominal pain, heartburn

General: chest pain, decreased appetite, edema, fever

Mouth and Throat: *Candida*Infection

Nervous System: dizziness, irritability, nervousness, shakiness

Reproductive: menstrual disturbances

Respiratory: chest congestion, cough*, hoarseness, rhinitis, runny nose, sinus congestion, sinus drainage, sinus infection, sinusitis, sneezing, sputum, wheezing*

Skin: eczema, itching (pruritus), rash

Special Senses: ear infection, loss of smell or taste

INCIDENCE 1-3%

General: chills, increased appetite and weight gain, malaise, peripheral edema, sweating, weakness.

Cardiovascular: hypertension, tachycardia

Gastrointestinal: Constipation, dyspepsia, gas

Hemic/Lymph: capillary fragility, enlarged lymph nodes

Mouth and Throat: dry throat, glossitis, mouth irritation, pharyngitis, phlegm, throat irritation

Nervous System: anxiety, depression, faintness, fatigue, hyperactivity, hypoactivity, insomnia, moodiness, numbness, vertigo

Respiratory: bronchitis, chest tightness*, dyspnea, epistaxis, head stuffiness, laryngitis, nasal irritation, pleurisy, pneumonia, sinus discomfort

Skin: acne, hives, or urticaria

Special Senses: blurred vision, earache, eye discomfort, eye infection

Incidence less than 1%, judged by investigators as possibly or probably drug related: abdominal fullness, shortness of breath.

* The incidences as shown of cough, wheezing, and chest tightness were judged by investigators to be possibly or probably drug-related. In placebo-controlled trials, the *overall* incidences of these adverse events (regardless of investigators' judgement of drug relationship) were similar for drug and placebo-treated groups. They may be related to the vehicle or delivery system.

OVERDOSAGE:

NASAL SOLUTION

IV flunisolide in animals at doses up to 4 mg/kg showed no effect. One spray bottle contains 6.25 mg of Flunisolide; therefore acute overdosage is unlikely.

DOSAGE AND ADMINISTRATION:

NASAL SOLUTION

The therapeutic effects of corticosteroids, unlike those of decongestants, are not immediate. This should be explained to the patient in advance in order to ensure cooperation and continuation of treatment with the prescribed dosage regimen. Full therapeutic benefit requires regular use, and is usually evident within a few days. However, a longer period of therapy may be required may be required for some patients to achieve maximum benefit (up to 3 weeks). If no improvement is evidence by that time, flunisolide should not be continued.

Patients with blocked nasal passages should be encouraged to use a decongestant just before Flunisolide administration to ensure adequate penetration of the spray. Patients should also be advised to clear nasal passages of secretions prior to use.

Adults: The recommended starting dose of Flunisolide is 2 sprays (50 mcg) in each nostril 2 times a day (total dose 200 mcg/day). If needed, this dose may be increased to 2 sprays in each nostril 3 times a day (total dose 300 mcg/day).

Children: 6-14 years: The recommended starting dose of Flunisolide is one spray (25 mcg) in each nostril 3 times a day or two sprays (50 mcg) in each nostril 2 times a day (total dose 150-200 mcg/day). Flunisolide is not recommended for use for children less than 6 years of age as safety and efficacy studies, including possible adverse effects on growth, have not been conducted.

Maximum total daily doses should not exceed 8 sprays in each nostril for adults (total dose 400 mcg/day) and 4 sprays in each nostril for children under 14 years of age (total dose 200 mcg/day). Since there is no evidence that exceeding the maximum recommended dosage is more effective and increased systemic absorption would occur, higher doses should be avoided.

After the desired clinical effect is obtained, the maintenance dose should be reduced to the smallest amount necessary to control the symptoms. Approximately 15% of the patients with perennial rhinitis may be maintained on as little as 1 spray in each nostril per day.

Store at controlled room temperature, 15°-30°C (59°-86°F).

ORAL INHALER

The flunisolide Inhaler System is for oral inhalation only.

Adults: The recommended starting dose is 2 inhalations twice daily morning and evening for a total daily dose of 1 mg. The maximum daily dose should not exceed 4 inhalations twice a day for a total daily dose of 2 mg. When the drug is used chronically at 2 mg/day, patients should be monitored periodically for effects on the hypothalamic- pituitary-adrenal axis.

Children: For children 6-15 years of age, two inhalations may be administered twice daily for a total daily dose of 1 mg. Higher doses have not been studied. Insufficient information is available to warrant use in children under age 6. With chronic use, children should be monitored for growth as well as for effects on the HPA axis.

DOSAGE AND ADMINISTRATION: *(cont'd)*

Rinsing the mouth after inhalation is advised. Patients receiving bronchodilators by inhalation should be advised to use the bronchodilator before Aerobid (flunisolide) Inhaler in order to enhance penetration of flunisolide into bronchial tree. After use of an aerosol bronchodilator, several minutes should elapse before use of the Aerobid Inhaler to reduce the potential toxicity from the inhaled fluorocarbon propellants in the two aerosols.

Different considerations must be given to the following groups of patients in order to obtain the full therapeutic benefit of Aerobid (flunisolide) Inhaler.

Patients not receiving systemic steroids: The use of Aerobid Inhaler is straightforward in patients who are inadequately controlled with non-steroid medications but in whom systemic steroid therapy has been withheld because of concern over potential adverse reactions. In patients who respond to the drug, an improvement in pulmonary function is usually apparent within one to four weeks after the start of treatment.

Patients receiving systemic steroids: In those patients dependent on systemic steroids, transfer to Aerobid (flunisolide) and subsequent management may be more difficult because recovery from impaired adrenal function is usually slow. Such suppression has been known to last for up to 12 months. Clinical studies, however, have demonstrated that Aerobid may be effective in the management of these asthmatic patients and may permit replacement or significant reduction in the dosage of systemic corticosteroids.

Inhaled corticosteroids generally are not recommended for chronic use with alternate day prednisone regimens (see WARNINGS).

The patient's asthma should be reasonably stable before treatment with Aerobid (flunisolide) Inhaler is started. Initially, the aerosol should be used concurrently with patient's usual maintenance dose of systemic steroid. After approximately one week, gradual withdrawal of the systemic steroid is started by reducing the daily or alternate daily dose. The next reduction is made after an interval of one or two weeks, depending on the response of the patient. Generally, these decrements should not exceed 2.5 mg of prednisone or its equivalent. A slow rate of withdrawal cannot be overemphasized. During withdrawal, some patients may experience symptoms of systemically active steroid withdrawal, *e.g.,* joint and/or muscular pain, lassitude and depression, despite maintenance or even improvement of respiratory function. Such patients should be encouraged to continue with the Inhaler but should be watched carefully for objective signs of adrenal insufficiency, such as hypotension, and weight loss. If evidence of adrenal insufficiency occurs, the systemic steroid dose should be boosted temporarily and thereafter further withdrawal should continue more slowly. *During periods of stress or severe asthma attack, transfer patients will require supplementary treatment with systemic steroids.* Exacerbations of asthma that occur during the course of treatment with Aerobid (flunisolide) Inhaler should be treated with a short course of systemic steroid that is gradually tapered as these symptoms subside. There is no evidence that control of asthma can be achieved by administration of the drug in amounts greater than the recommended doses.

PATIENT PACKAGE INSERT:

ORAL INHALER

Directions For Use: Before using your new Aerobid Inhaler System, it is important that you read over the following simple instructions and familiarize yourself with the inhaler and its metal cartridge.

As your doctor has probably told you, the Aerobid Inhaler System must be used for a few days before it begins working, and then should be used regularly to help reduce the frequency and severity of your asthma attacks. It is not a bronchodilator and will not provide relief during an actual asthmatic attack but can cut down the number of bad attacks if used regularly every day.

(For graphic illustrations, please refer to the original, manufacturer's package insert.)

1. Before the first use, place the Aerobid metal cartridge inside the plastic container as shown.

2. Shake the inhaler system before each inhalation.

3. Before each use, remove dustcap and inspect mouthpiece for foreign objects.

4. Replace dustcap after each use.

5. Breathe out as completely as possible.

6. Hold the inhaler system upright and put plastic mouthpiece in your mouth as shown, being sure to close your lips tightly around the mouthpiece.

7. Breathe in deeply and steadily through your mouth. At the same time firmly press down on the metal cartridge with your index finger.

8. Hold your breath as long as you can.

9. While holding your breath, stop pressing on the cartridge and remove the mouthpiece from your mouth.

10. If your doctor has prescribed two or more inhalations at each use, wait a minute to allow pressure to build up again in the metal canister, then repeat steps two through nine (2-9). Be sure to shake the inhaler system *again* before each inhalation.

11. After the prescribed number of inhalations, rinse out your mouth thoroughly with water.

12. Clean the inhaler system every few days. To do so, remove the metal cartridge, then rinse the plastic inhaler and cap with briskly running warm water. Dry thoroughly. Replace the cartridge and cap.

Note: If your mouth becomes sore or develops a rash, be sure to mention this to your physician, but do not stop using your inhaler system unless he tells you.

Warning: The contents of the metal cartridge are under pressure. Do not puncture. Do not use or store near heat or open flame. Exposure to temperature above 120°F (49°C) may cause cartridge to explode. Never throw cartridge into fire or incinerator. Use by children should always be supervised by an adult.

(Nasal Solution, Syntex Labs, 7/88)

(Oral Inhaler, Forest Pharm (3M), 3/92)

HOW SUPPLIED - EQUIVALENTS NOT AVAILABLE:

Aerosol - Inhalation - 250 mcg

7 gm	$54.10	AEROBID-M, Forest Pharms	00456-0670-99
7 gm	$54.10	AEROBID, Forest Pharms	00456-0672-99

Aerosol, Spray - Nasal - 0.025 %

25 ml	$34.80	NASAREL, Roche	00004-1708-09

Solution - Nasal - 0.25 mg/ml

25 ml	**$27.59**	**NASALIDE, Syntex Labs**	**00033-2906-40**

FLUOCINOLONE ACETONIDE *(001306)*

CATEGORIES: Adrenal Corticosteroids; Anti-Inflammatory Agents; Dermatologicals; Dermatoses; Hormones; Inflammation; Ocular Infections; Ophthalmics; Pruritus; Skin/Mucous Membrane Agents; Steroids; Topical; FDA Approval Pre 1982

BRAND NAMES: *Alfabios*; *Alvadermo-Fuerte*; *Alvadermo Fuerte*; *Aplosyn*; Bio-Syn; *Cinolon*; *Clofeet* (Japan); *Colurene*; *Cortalar*; *Cortoderm*; *Cremisona* (Mexico); Derma-Smoothe Fs; *Dermacril-IFSA*; *Dermalar*; *Dermoran* (Japan); *Esacinone*; *Fluciderm*; *Flucort* (Japan); *Flulone*; *Flumort*; *Flunolone-V*; Fluocet; *Fluocinil*; *Fluoderm* (Canada); *Fluolar* (Canada); Fluonid; Flurosyn; *Flusonlen*; *Fluzon* (Japan); *Fusalar* (Mexico); *Gelidina*; *Jellin* (Germany); Lidex; *Luci*; *Patroncort*; *Radiocin*; *Supralan*; **Synalar**; *Synalar 25*; Synalar-Hp; Synemol; *Ultraderm*
(International brand names outside U.S. in italics)

FORMULARIES: Aetna; BC-BS; FHP; Medi-Cal

DESCRIPTION:

Synemol cream, Fluocinolone Acetonide-HP cream, and Fluocinolone Acetonide (fluocinolone acetonide) creams, ointment and solution are intended for topical administration. The active component is the corticosteroid fluocinolone acetonide, which has the chemical name: pregna-1, 4-diene-3,20-dione,6,9-difluoro-11,21-dihydroxy-16,17-((1-methylethylidene)bis (oxy))-,(6α,11β,16α)-.

Synemol cream contains fluocinolone acetonide 0.25 mg/g in a water-washable aqueous emollient base of cetyl alcohol, citric acid, mineral oil, polysorbate 60, propylene glycol, sorbitan monostearate, stearyl alcohol and water (purified).

Fluocinolone Acetonide-HP cream contains fluocinolone acetonide 2 mg/g in a water- washable aqueous base of cetyl alcohol, citric acid, methylparaben and propylparaben (preservatives), mineral oil, polysorbate 60, propylene glycol, sorbitan monostearate, stearyl alcohol and water (purified).

Fluocinolone Acetonide creams contain fluocinolone acetonide 0.25 mg/g or 0.1 mg/g in a water-washable aqueous base of butylated hydroxytoluene, cetyl alcohol, citric acid, edetate disodium, methylparaben and propylparaben (preservatives), mineral oil, polyoxyl 20 cetostearyl ether, propylene glycol, simethicone, stearyl alcohol, water (purified) and white wax.

Fluocinolone Acetonide ointment contains fluocinolone acetonide 0.25 mg/g in a white petroleum USP vehicle.

Fluocinolone Acetonide solution contains fluocinolone acetonide 0.1 mg/ml in a water washable base of citric acid and propylene glycol.

CLINICAL PHARMACOLOGY:

Topical corticosteroids share anti-inflammatory, anti-pruritic and vasoconstrictive actions.

The mechanism of anti-inflammatory activity of the topical corticosteroids is unclear. Various laboratory methods, including vasoconstrictor assay, are used to compare and predict potencies and/or clinical efficacies of the topical corticosteroids. There is some evidence to suggest that a recognizable correlation exists between vasoconstrictor potency and therapeutic efficacy in man.

PHARMACOKINETICS

The extent of percutaneous absorption of topical corticosteroids is determined by many factors including the vehicle, the integrity of the epidermal barrier, and the use of occlusive dressings.

Topical corticosteroids can be absorbed from normal intact skin. Inflammation and/or other disease processes in the skin increase percutaneous absorption. Occlusive dressings substantially increase the percutaneous absorption of topical corticosteroids. Thus, occlusive dressings may be a valuable therapeutic adjunct for treatment of resistant dermatoses. (See DOSAGE AND ADMINISTRATION.)

Once absorbed through the skin, topical corticosteroids are handled through pharmacokinetic pathways similar to systemically administered corticosteroids. Corticosteroids are bound to plasma proteins in varying degrees. Corticosteroids are metabolized primarily in the liver and are then excreted by the kidneys. Some of the topical corticosteroids and their metabolites are also excreted into the bile.

INDICATIONS AND USAGE:

Fluocinolone acetonide creams, ointment, and solution are indicated for the relief of the inflammatory and pruritic manifestations of corticosteroid-responsive dermatoses.

CONTRAINDICATIONS:

Topical corticosteroids are contraindicated in those patients with a history of hypersensitivity to any of the components of the preparation.

PRECAUTIONS:

GENERAL

Systemic absorption of topical corticosteroids has produced reversible hypothalamic-pituitary-adrenal (HPA) axis suppression, manifestations of Cushing's syndrome, hyperglycemia, and glucosuria in some patients.

Conditions which augment systemic absorption include the application of the more potent steroids, use over large surface areas, prolonged use, and the addition of occlusive dressings.

Therefore, patients receiving a large dose of a potent topical corticosteroid applied to large surface area or under an occlusive dressing should be evaluated periodically for evidence of HPA axis suppression by using the urinary free cortisol and ACTH stimulation tests. If HPA axis suppression is noted, an attempt should be made to withdraw the drug, to reduce the frequency of application, or to substitute a less potent steroid.

Recovery of HPA axis function is generally prompt and complete upon discontinuation of the drug. Infrequently, signs and symptoms of steroid withdrawal may occur, requiring supplemental systemic corticosteroids.

Children may absorb proportionately larger amounts of topical corticosteroids and thus be more susceptible to systemic toxicity. (See PRECAUTIONS, Pediatric Use.) If irritation develops, topical corticosteroids should be discontinued and appropriate therapy instituted.

In the presence of dermatological infections, the use of an appropriate antifungal or antibacterial agent should be instituted. If factorable response does not occur promptly, the corticosteroid should be discontinued until the infection has been adequately controlled.

Fluocinolone Acetonide-HP (fluocinolone acetonide) cream should not be used for prolonged periods and the quantity per day should not exceed 2 g of formulated material.

INFORMATION FOR THE PATIENT

Patients using topical corticosteroids should receive the following information and instructions:

1. This medication is to be used as directed by the physician. It is for external use only. Avoid contact with the eyes.

2. Patients should be advised not to use this medication for any disorder other than for which it was prescribed.

3. The treated skin area should not be bandaged or otherwise covered or wrapped as to be occlusive unless directed by the physician.

PRECAUTIONS: *(cont'd)*

4. Patients should report any signs of local adverse reactions especially under occlusive dressing.

5. Parents of pediatric patients should be advised not to use tight-fitting diapers or plastic pants on a child being treated in the diaper area, as these garments may constitute occlusive dressings.

LABORATORY TESTS

The following tests may be helpful in evaluating the HPA axis suppression:

Urinary free cortisol test

ACTH stimulation test

CARCINOGENESIS,MUTAGENESIS, AND IMPAIRMENT OF FERTILITY

Long-term animal studies have not been performed to evaluate the carcinogenic potential or the effect on fertility of topical corticosteroids.

Studies to determine mutagenicity with prednisolone and hydrocortisone have revealed negative results.

PREGNANCY CATEGORY C

Corticosteroids are generally teratogenic in laboratory animals when administered systemically at relatively low dosage levels. The more potent corticosteroids have been shown to be teratogenic after dermal application in laboratory animals. There are no adequate and well-controlled studies in pregnant women on teratogenic effects from topically applied corticosteroids. Therefore, topical corticosteroids should be used during pregnancy only if the potential benefit justifies the potential risk to the fetus. Drugs of this class should not be used extensively on pregnant patients, in large amounts, or for prolonged periods of time.

NURSING MOTHERS

It is not known whether topical administration of corticosteroids could result in sufficient systemic absorption to produce detectable quantities in breast milk. Systemically administered corticosteroids are secreted into breast milk in quantities *not* likely to have a deleterious effect on the infant. Nevertheless, caution should be exercised when topical corticosteroids are administered to a nursing woman.

PEDIATRIC USE

Pediatric patients may demonstrate greater susceptibility to topical corticosteroid-induced HPA axis suppression and Cushing's syndrome than mature patients because of a large skin surface area to body weight ratio.

Hypothalamic-pituitary-adrenal (HPA) axis suppression, Cushing's syndrome, and intracranial hypertension have been reported in children receiving topical corticosteroids. Manifestations of adrenal suppression in children include linear growth retardation, delayed weight gain, low plasma cortisol levels, and absence of response to ACTH stimulation.

Manifestations of intracranial hypertension include bulging fontanelles, headaches, and bilateral papilledema.

Administration of topical corticosteroids to children should be limited to the least amount compatible with an effective therapeutic regime. Chronic corticosteroid therapy may interfere with the growth and development of children.

ADVERSE REACTIONS:

The following local adverse reactions are reported infrequently with topical corticosteroids, but may occur more frequently with the use of occlusive dressings.

These reactions are listed in an approximate decreasing order of occurrence:

Burning; itching; irritation; dryness; folliculitis; hypertrichosis; acneiform eruptions; hypopigmentation; perioral dermatitis; allergic contact dermatitis; maceration of the skin; secondary infection; skin atrophy; striae; miliaria.

OVERDOSAGE:

Topically applied corticosteroids can be absorbed in sufficient amounts to produce systemic effects (See PRECAUTIONS.)

DOSAGE AND ADMINISTRATION:

CREAMS ONLY

Synemol, Fluocinolone Acetonide-HP, and fluocinolone acetonide creams are generally applied to the affected area as a thin film from two to four times daily depending on the severity of the condition. In hairy sites, the hair should be parted to allow direct contact with the lesion.

Occlusive dressings may be used for the management of psoriasis or recalcitrant conditions. Some plastic films may be flammable and due care should be exercised in their use. Similarly, caution should be employed when such films are used on children or left in their proximity, to avoid the possibility of accidental suffocation.

If an infection develops, the use of occlusive dressings should be discontinued and appropriate antimicrobial therapy instituted.

Storage: *Fluocinolone Acetonide:* Store tubes at room temperature; avoid freezing and excessive heat, above 40°C (104°F). Store jars at controlled room temperature, 15-30° (59- 86°F). *Synemol and Fluocinolone Acetonide-HP:* Store tubes at room temperature. Avoid excessive heat, above 40°C (104°F).

OINTMENT ONLY

Fluocinolone acetonide ointment is generally applied to the affected area as a film from two to four times daily depending on the severity of the condition.

Occlusive dressings may be used for the management of psoriasis or recalcitrant conditions. Some plastic films may be flammable and due care should be exercised in their use. Similarly, caution should be employed when such films are used on children or left in their proximity, to avoid the possibility of accidental suffocation.

If an infection develops, the use of occlusive dressings should be discontinued and appropriate antimicrobial therapy instituted.

Storage: Store at room temperature. Avoid excessive heat, above 40°C (104°F).

SOLUTION ONLY

Fluocinolone acetonide topical solution 0.01% is generally applied to the affected area as a thin film two to four times daily depending on the severity of the condition. In hairy sites, the hair should be parted to allow direct contact with the lesion.

Occlusive dressings may be used for the management of psoriasis or recalcitrant conditions.

If an infection develops, the use of occlusive dressings should be discontinued and appropriate antimicrobial therapy instituted.

Storage: Store at room temperature. Avoid freezing.

(Synemol Cream: Syntex, 4/91)(Synalar-HP Cream: Syntex, 4/91)(Synalar Creams: Syntex, 4/91)(Synalar Ointment: Syntex, 4/91)(Synalar Solution: Syntex, 4/91)

HOW SUPPLIED - RATED THERAPEUTICALLY EQUIVALENT:

Cream - Topical - 0.01 %

15 gm	$1.26	Fluocinolone, United Res	00677-0713-40
15 gm	$1.26	Fluocinolone, GW Labs	00713-0223-15
15 gm	$1.26	Fluocinolone, H.C.F.A. F F P	99999-1306-01
15 gm	$1.34	Fluocinolone Acetonide, Clay Park Labs	45802-0067-35
15 gm	$1.50	Fluocinolone, Thames Pharma	49158-0142-20
15 gm	$1.50	Fluocinolone Acetonide, Harber Pharm	51432-0720-10
15 gm	$1.60	Fluocinolone, HL Moore Drug Exch	00839-6346-47
15 gm	$1.66	Fluocinolone, Qualitest Pharms	00603-7747-74
15 gm	$1.95	Fluocinolone Acetonide, Consolidated Midland	00223-4297-15
15 gm	$1.95	FLUROSYN, Rugby	00536-4431-20
15 gm	$2.04	Fluocinolone, Fougera	00168-0058-15
15 gm	$2.10	Fluocinolone Acetonide, Major Pharms	00904-2660-36
30 gm	$2.52	Fluocinolone, H.C.F.A. F F P	99999-1306-02
60 gm	$2.47	Fluocinolone, H.C.F.A. F F P	99999-1306-03
60 gm	$2.85	Fluocinolone Acetonide, Clay Park Labs	45802-0067-37
60 gm	$3.20	Fluocinolone, Thames Pharma	49158-0142-24
60 gm	$3.20	Fluocinolone Acetonide, Harber Pharm	51432-0720-17
60 gm	$3.36	Fluocinolone, HL Moore Drug Exch	00839-6346-50
60 gm	$3.74	Fluocinolone, Qualitest Pharms	00603-7747-88
60 gm	$4.06	FLUROSYN, Rugby	00536-4431-25
60 gm	$4.10	Fluocinolone Acetonide, Major Pharms	00904-2660-02
60 gm	$4.20	Fluocinolone, Fougera	00168-0058-60
60 gm	$4.20	Fluocinolone, Goldline Labs	00182-1149-52
60 gm	$4.25	Fluocinolone Acetonide, Consolidated Midland	00223-4297-60
60 gm	$5.04	Fluocinolone, United Res	00677-0713-43
60 gm	$5.04	Fluocinolone, GW Labs	00713-0223-60
60 gm	**$19.72**	**SYNALAR, Syntex Labs**	**00033-2502-17**
425 gm	$11.88	Fluocinolone Acetonide, Clay Park Labs	45802-0067-38
425 gm	$35.70	Fluocinolone, H.C.F.A. F F P	99999-1306-04

Cream - Topical - 0.025 %

15 gm	$1.57	Fluocinolone, United Res	00677-0712-40
15 gm	$1.57	Fluocinolone, GW Labs	00713-0222-15
15 gm	$1.57	Fluocinolone, H.C.F.A. F F P	99999-1306-05
15 gm	$1.67	Fluocinolone, HL Moore Drug Exch	00839-6347-47
15 gm	$1.79	Fluocinolone Acetonide, Clay Park Labs	45802-0068-35
15 gm	$1.80	Fluocinolone, Thames Pharma	49158-0143-20
15 gm	$1.80	Fluocinolone Acetonide, Harber Pharm	51432-0721-10
15 gm	$2.25	FLUOCINOLNE ACETONIDE, IDE-Interstate	00814-3190-93
15 gm	$2.35	Fluocinolone Acetonide, Major Pharms	00904-2659-36
15 gm	$2.44	FLUROSYN, Rugby	00536-4401-20
15 gm	$2.50	Fluocinolone Acetonide, Consolidated Midland	00223-4296-15
15 gm	$2.70	Fluocinolone, Goldline Labs	00182-1150-51
15 gm	$2.90	Fluocinolone, Qualitest Pharms	00603-7748-74
15 gm	$3.05	Fluocinolone, Fougera	00168-0060-15
15 gm	$9.50	FLUONID, Allergan	00023-0873-15
15 gm	**$14.27**	**SYNALAR, Syntex Labs**	**00033-2501-13**
15 gm	$14.88	SYNEMOL, Syntex Labs	00033-2509-13
30 gm	$3.15	Fluocinolone, H.C.F.A. F F P	99999-1306-06
60 gm	$3.67	Fluocinolone, H.C.F.A. F F P	99999-1306-07
60 gm	$3.67	Fluocinolone, H.C.F.A. F F P	99999-1306-08
60 gm	$3.81	Fluocinolone, HL Moore Drug Exch	00839-6347-50
60 gm	$4.20	Fluocinolone, Thames Pharma	49158-0143-24
60 gm	$4.20	Fluocinolone Acetonide, Harber Pharm	51432-0721-17
60 gm	$4.32	Fluocinolone Acetonide, Clay Park Labs	45802-0068-37
60 gm	$4.41	Fluocinolone, Qualitest Pharms	00603-7748-88
60 gm	$4.75	Fluocinolone, Goldline Labs	00182-1150-52
60 gm	$6.30	Fluocinolone, United Res	00677-0712-43
60 gm	$6.30	Fluocinolone, GW Labs	00713-0222-60
60 gm	$6.58	Fluocinolone Acetonide, Major Pharms	00904-2659-02
60 gm	$7.20	Fluocinolone, Fougera	00168-0060-60
60 gm	$7.25	Fluocinolone Acetonide, Consolidated Midland	00223-4296-60
60 gm	$7.81	FLUROSYN, Rugby	00536-4401-25
60 gm	$12.30	Fluocinolone, Goldline Labs	00182-5015-52
60 gm	$18.81	FLUONID, Allergan	00023-0873-60
60 gm	**$33.54**	**SYNALAR, Syntex Labs**	**00033-2501-17**
425 gm	$24.94	FLUROSYN, Rugby	00536-4401-98
425 gm	$25.38	Fluocinolone Acetonide, Clay Park Labs	45802-0068-38
425 gm	$27.50	Fluocinolone, HL Moore Drug Exch	00839-6347-99
425 gm	$27.50	Fluocinolone, Thames Pharma	49158-0143-23
425 gm	$44.62	Fluocinolone, H.C.F.A. F F P	99999-1306-09

Ointment - Topical - 0.025 %

15 gm	$2.86	Fluocinolone 0.25, GW Labs	00713-0224-15
15 gm	$2.86	Fluocinolone, H.C.F.A. F F P	99999-1306-10
15 gm	$3.88	Fluocinolone, Fougera	00168-0064-15
15 gm	$4.00	Fluocinolone, Major Pharms	00904-2580-36
15 gm	$4.15	FLUROSYN, Rugby	00536-4462-20
15 gm	$4.95	Fluocinolone Acetonide, Consolidated Midland	00223-4290-15
15 gm	**$14.27**	**SYNALAR, Syntex Labs**	**00033-2504-13**
30 gm	$4.08	Fluocinolone, H.C.F.A. F F P	99999-1306-11
30 gm	$10.75	Fluocinolone Acetonide, Consolidated Midland	00223-4290-60
60 gm	$5.80	Fluocinolone, H.C.F.A. F F P	99999-1306-12
60 gm	$9.08	Fluocinolone, Fougera	00168-0064-60
60 gm	$9.44	Fluocinolone, HL Moore Drug Exch	00839-7615-50
60 gm	$9.95	FLUROSYN, Rugby	00536-4462-25
60 gm	$9.95	Fluocinolone, Major Pharms	00904-2580-02
60 gm	$11.46	Fluocinolone 0.25, GW Labs	00713-0224-60

Solution - Topical - 0.01 %

20 ml	$3.52	Fluocinolone, H.C.F.A. F F P	99999-1306-13
20 ml	$4.17	Fluocinolone Acetonide, HL Moore Drug Exch	00839-6660-97
20 ml	$4.45	Fluocinolone Topical, Goldline Labs	00182-1564-65
20 ml	$4.45	Fluocinolone, Qualitest Pharms	00603-1231-43
20 ml	$4.79	Fluocinolone, Rugby	00536-0720-73
20 ml	$4.97	Fluocinolone, Schein Pharm (US)	00364-7343-55
20 ml	$5.00	Fluocinolone Acetonide, Consolidated Midland	00223-6180-20
20 ml	$14.50	FLUONID, Allergan	00023-0878-20
20 ml	**$17.88**	**SYNALAR, Syntex Labs**	**00033-2506-44**
60 ml	$5.62	Fluocinolone, H.C.F.A. F F P	99999-1306-14
60 ml	$7.30	Fluocinolone Topical, Thames Pharma	49158-0209-32
60 ml	$8.64	Fluocinolone, Qualitest Pharms	00603-1231-49
60 ml	$9.00	Fluocinolone, Schein Pharm (US)	00364-7343-58
60 ml	$9.30	Fluocinolone Acetonide, IDE-Interstate	00814-3195-74
60 ml	$9.30	Fluocinolone, HL Moore Drug Exch	00839-6660-64
60 ml	$9.99	Fluocinolone, Fougera	00168-0059-60
60 ml	$10.57	Fluocinolone, Rugby	00536-0720-61
60 ml	$10.57	Fluocinolone, United Res	00677-0790-25
60 ml	$10.60	Fluocinolone Acetonide, Major Pharms	00904-2661-03
60 ml	$10.80	Fluocinolone Topical, Goldline Labs	00182-1564-68
60 ml	$11.50	Fluocinolone Acetonide, Consolidated Midland	00223-6180-60
60 ml	$33.02	FLUONID, Allergan	00023-0878-60
60 ml	**$35.40**	**SYNALAR, Syntex Labs**	**00033-2506-46**

HOW SUPPLIED - NOT RATED EQUIVALENT:

Cream - Topical - 0.2 %

12 gm	$27.32	SYNALAR-HP, Syntex Labs	00033-2503-12

Shampoo - Topical - 0.01 %

4 oz	$12.35	FS SHAMPOO, Hill Dermac	28105-0249-04

Solution - Topical - 0.01 %

120 ml	$17.00	DERMA SMOOTHE/FS 0.01% TOPICAL OIL, Hill Dermac	28105-0149-04

FLUOCINONIDE *(001310)*

CATEGORIES: Adrenal Corticosteroids; Anti-Inflammatory Agents; Dermatologicals; Dermatoses; Hormones; Skin/Mucous Membrane Agents; Steroids; Topical; Pruritus*; FDA Approval Pre 1982
*** Indication not approved by the FDA**

BRAND NAMES: *Adidas*; *Bestasone* (Japan); *Biscosal* (Japan); *Cusigel*; Dermacin; *Flu-21*; *Flubiol* (Japan); Fluex; Fluocin; Fluonex; *Garia*; *Gelisyn* (Mexico); *Klariderm*; *Lamagram*; Licon; *Lidemol* (Canada); **Lidex**; Lidex-E; *Lyderm* (Canada); *Metosyn* (England); *Novoter*; *Rawracid* (Japan); *Supracort*; *Tohsino* (Japan); *Topsym* (Germany, Japan); *Topsym F*; *Topsymin*; *Topsyn* (Canada); *Topsyne* (France); Vasoderm
(International brand names outside U.S. in italics)

FORMULARIES: BC-BS; FHP; PCS

DESCRIPTION:

Fluocinonide creams, ointment, gel, and topical solution are intended for topical administration. The active component is the corticosteroid fluocinonide, which is the 21-acetate ester of fluocinolone acetonide, has the chemical name pregna-1,4- diene -3,20-dione,21-(acetyloxy)-6,9- difluoro-11-hydroxy -16,17-((1- methylethylidene) bis(oxy))-,(6α,11β,16α)-.

CREAMS

Fluocinonide cream contains fluocinonide 0.5 mg/g in FAPG cream, a specially formulated cream base consisting of citric acid, 1,2,6-hexanetriol, polyethylene glycol 8000, propylene glycol and stearyl alcohol. This white cream vehicle is greaseless, non-staining, anhydrous and completely water miscible. The base provides emollient and hydrophilic properties.

In this formulation, the active ingredient is totally in solution.

Fluocinonide-E cream contains fluocinonide 0.5 mg/g in a water- washable aqueous emollient base of cetyl alcohol, citric acid, mineral oil, polysorbate 60, propylene glycol, sorbitan monostearate, stearyl alcohol and water (purified).

OINTMENT

Fluocinonide ointment contains fluocinonide 0.5 mg/g in a specially formulated ointment base consisting of glyceryl monostearate, white petrolatum, propylene carbonate, propylene glycol and white wax. It provides the occlusive and emollient effects desirable in an ointment.

In this formulation, the active ingredient is totally in solution.

GEL

Fluocinonide gel contains fluocinonide 0.5 mg/g in a specially formulated gel base consisting of carbomer 940, edetate disodium, propyl gallate, propylene glycol, sodium hydroxide and/or hydrochloric acid (to adjust the pH) and water (purified). This clear, colorless, thixotropic vehicle is greaseless, non-staining and completely water miscible.

In this formulation, the active ingredient is totally in solution.

SOLUTION

Fluocinonide topical solution contains fluocinonide 0.5 mg/ml in a solution of alcohol (35%), citric acid, diisopropyl adipate, and propylene glycol. In this formulation, the active ingredient is totally in solution.

CLINICAL PHARMACOLOGY:

Topical corticosteroids share anti-inflammatory, anti-pruritic and vasoconstrictive actions.

The mechanism of anti-inflammatory activity of the topical steroids is unclear. Various laboratory methods, including vasoconstrictor assays, are used to compare and predict potencies and/or clinical efficacies of the topical corticosteroids. There is some evidence to suggest that a recognizable correlation exists between vasoconstrictor potency and therapeutic efficacy in man.

PHARMACOKINETICS

The extent of percutaneous absorption of topical corticosteroids is determined by many factors including the vehicle, the integrity of the epidermal barrier, and the use of occlusive dressings.

Topical corticosteroids can be absorbed from normal intact skin. Inflammation and/or other disease processes in the skin increase the percutaneous absorption of topical corticosteroids. Thus, occlusive dressings may be a valuable therapeutic adjunct for treatment of resistant dermatoses. (See DOSAGE AND ADMINISTRATION.)

Once absorbed through the skin, topical corticosteroids are handled through pharmacokinetic pathways similar to systemically administered corticosteroids. Corticosteroids are bound to plasma proteins in varying degrees. Corticosteroids are metabolized primarily in the liver and are then excreted by the kidneys. Some of the topical corticosteroids and their metabolites are also excreted into the bile.

INDICATIONS AND USAGE:

Fluocinonide creams, ointment, gel, and topical solution are indicated for the relief of the inflammatory and pruritic manifestations of corticosteroid-responsive dermatoses.

CONTRAINDICATIONS:

Topical corticosteroids are contraindicated in those patients with a history of hypersensitivity to any of the components of the preparation.

PRECAUTIONS:

GENERAL

Systemic absorption of topical corticosteroids has produced reversible hypothalamic-pituitary-adrenal (HPA) axis suppression, manifestations of Cushing's syndrome, hyperglycemia, and glucosuria in some patients.

Conditions which augment systemic absorption include the application of the more potent steroids, use over large areas, prolonged use, and the addition of occlusive dressings.

Therefore, patients receiving a large dose of a potent topical steroid applied to a large surface area or under an occlusive dressing should be evaluated periodically for evidence of HPA axis suppression by using the urinary free cortisol and ACTH stimulation tests. If HPA axis suppression is noted, an attempt should be made to withdraw the drug, to reduce the frequency of application, or to substitute a less potent steroid.

PRECAUTIONS: *(cont'd)*

Recovery of HPA axis function is generally prompt and complete upon discontinuation of the drug. Infrequently, signs and symptoms of steroid withdrawal may occur, requiring supplemental systemic corticosteroids.

Children may absorb proportionally larger amounts of topical corticosteroids and thus be more susceptible to systemic toxicity. (See PRECAUTIONS, Pediatric Use.) If irritation develops, topical corticosteroids should be discontinued and appropriate therapy instituted.

As with any topical corticosteroid product, prolonged use may produce atrophy of the skin and subcutaneous tissues. When used on intertriginous or flexor areas, or on the face, this may occur even with short-term use.

In the presence of dermatological infections, the use of an appropriate antifungal or antibacterial agent should be instituted. If a favorable response does not occur promptly, the corticosteroid should be discontinued until the infection has been adequately controlled.

Topical Solution Only: This preparation is not for ophthalmic use. Severe irritation is possible if fluocinonide solution hits the eye. If that should occur, immediate flushing of the eye with a large volume of water is recommended.

If irritation develops, topical corticosteroids should be discontinued and appropriate therapy instituted.

INFORMATION FOR THE PATIENT

Patients using corticosteroids should receive the following information and instructions:

1. This medication is to be used as directed by the physician. It is for external use only. Avoid contact with the eyes.

2. Patients should be advised not to use this medication for any disorder other than that for which it was prescribed.

3. The treated skin area should not be bandaged or otherwise covered or wrapped as to be occlusive unless directed by the physician.

4. Patients should report any signs of local adverse reactions especially under occlusive dressing.

5. Parents of pediatric patients should be advised not to use tight- fitting diapers or plastic pants on a child being treated in the diaper area, as these garments may constitute occlusive dressings.

LABORATORY TESTS

The following tests may be helpful in evaluating the HPA axis suppression:

Urinary free cortisol test

ACTH stimulation test

CARCINOGENESIS, MUTAGENESIS, AND IMPAIRMENT OF FERTILITY

Long-term animal studies have not been performed to evaluate the carcinogenic potential or the effect on fertility of topical corticosteroids.

Studies to determine mutagenicity with prednisolone and hydrocortisone have revealed negative results.

PREGNANCY CATEGORY C

Corticosteroids are generally teratogenic in laboratory animals when administered systemically at relatively low dosage levels. The more potent corticosteroids have been shown to be teratogenic after dermal application in laboratory animals. There are no adequate and well-controlled studies in pregnant women on teratogenic effects from topically applied corticosteroids. Therefore, topical corticosteroids should be used during pregnancy only if the potential benefit justifies the potential risk to the fetus. Drugs of this class should not be used extensively on pregnant patients, in large amounts, or for prolonged periods of time.

NURSING MOTHERS

It is not known whether topical administration of corticosteroids could result in sufficient systemic absorption to produce detectable quantities in breast milk. Systemically administered corticosteroids are administered into breast milk in quantities *not* likely to have a deleterious effect on the infant. Nevertheless, caution should be exercised when topical corticosteroids are administered to a nursing woman.

PEDIATRIC USE

Pediatric patients may demonstrate greater susceptibility to topical corticosteroid-induced HPA axis suppression and Cushing's syndrome than mature patients because of a larger skin surface to body weight ratio.

Hypothalamic-pituitary-adrenal (HPA) axis suppression, Cushing's Syndrome, and intracranial hypertension have been reported in children receiving topical corticosteroids. Manifestations of adrenal suppression include linear growth retardation, delayed weight gain, low plasma cortisol levels, and absence of response to ACTH stimulation. Manifestations of intracranial hypertension include bulging fontanelles, headaches, and bilateral papilledema.

Administration of topical corticosteroids to children should be limited to the least amount compatible with an effective therapeutic regimen. Chronic corticosteroid therapy may interfere with the growth and development of children.

ADVERSE REACTIONS:

The following local adverse reactions are reported frequently with topical corticosteroids, but may occur more frequently with the use of occlusive dressings. These reactions are listed in an approximate decreasing order of occurrence:

Burning; Itching; Irritation; Dryness; Folliculitis; Hypertrichosis; Acneiform eruptions; Hypopigmentation; Perioral dermatitis; Allergic contact dermatitis; Maceration of the skin; Secondary infection; Skin atrophy; Striae; Miliaria

OVERDOSAGE:

Topically applied corticosteroids can be absorbed in sufficient amounts to produce systemic effects. (See PRECAUTIONS.)

DOSAGE AND ADMINISTRATION:

Fluocinonide creams, ointment, gel, and solution are generally applied to the affected area as a thin film from two to four times daily depending on the severity of the condition.

Occlusive dressings may be used for the management of psoriasis or recalcitrant conditions.

If an infection develops, the use of occlusive dressings should be discontinued and appropriate antimicrobial therapy instituted.

STORAGE

Creams And Solution: Store at room temperature. Avoid excessive heat, above 40°C (104°F).

Ointment: Store at room temperature. Avoid temperature above 30°C (86°F).

Gel: Store at controlled room temperature, 15°- 30°C (59°-86°F).

(Lidex Cream: Syntex, 4/91, 02-2511-14-02)(Lidex-E Cream: Syntex, 4/91, 02-2513-14-01)(Ointment: Syntex, 4/91, 02-2514-14-01)(Gel: Syntex, 4/91, 02-2507-14-01)(Solution: Syntex, 4/91, 02-2517-44-04)

HOW SUPPLIED - RATED THERAPEUTICALLY EQUIVALENT:

Cream - Topical - 0.05 %

15 gm	$3.52	Fluocinonide, United Res	00677-0735-40
15 gm	$3.52	Fluocinonide, H.C.F.A. F F P	99999-1310-01
15 gm	$4.80	Fluocinonide, Thames Pharma	49158-0212-20
15 gm	$4.86	Fluocinonide, Clay Park Labs	45802-0017-35
15 gm	$5.93	Fluocinonide, IDE-Interstate	00814-3200-93
15 gm	$6.24	Fluocinonide Cream 0.05% (Taro), NMC Labs	23317-0390-15
15 gm	$6.60	Fluocinonide, HL Moore Drug Exch	00839-7698-47
15 gm	$7.30	LICON, Major Pharms	00904-0770-36
15 gm	$7.32	Fluocinonide, Qualitest Pharms	00603-7759-74
15 gm	$7.90	Fluocinonide, HL Moore Drug Exch	00839-7013-47
15 gm	$8.25	Fluocinonide, Hamilton Pharma	60322-0511-13
15 gm	$8.50	Fluocinonide, Rugby	00536-4350-20
15 gm	$8.55	Fluocinonide, Teva	00093-0262-15
15 gm	$8.55	Fluocinonide, Geneva Pharms	00781-7008-27
15 gm	$8.60	Fluocinonide, Schein Pharm (US)	00364-0857-72
15 gm	$8.64	Fluocinonide, Fougera	00168-0139-15
15 gm	$8.85	Fluocinonide, Goldline Labs	00182-1731-51
15 gm	$9.50	Fluocinonide, Taro Pharms (US)	51672-1253-01
15 gm	$9.50	Fluocinonide-E, Taro Pharms (US)	51672-1254-01
15 gm	$10.45	Fluocinonide, Major Pharms	00904-0773-36
15 gm	$11.95	Fluocinonide-E, HL Moore Drug Exch	00839-0758-47
15 gm	$11.95	Fluocinonide, HL Moore Drug Exch	00839-7758-47
15 gm	$12.35	Fluocinonide-E, Qualitest Pharms	00603-7763-74
15 gm	$12.35	Fluocinonide-E, Hamilton Pharma	60322-0513-13
15 gm	$12.50	Fluocinonide-E, Teva	00093-0263-15
15 gm	**$17.98**	**LIDEX, Syntex Labs**	**00033-2511-13**
15 gm	**$17.98**	**LIDEX-E, Syntex Labs**	**00033-2513-13**
30 gm	$5.47	Fluocinonide, H.C.F.A. F F P	99999-1310-02
30 gm	$7.05	Fluocinonide, United Res	00677-1404-45
30 gm	$7.30	Fluocinonide, Thames Pharma	49158-0212-68
30 gm	$8.10	Fluocinonide, Clay Park Labs	45802-0017-11
30 gm	$8.58	Fluocinonide Cream 0.05% (Taro), NMC Labs	23317-0390-30
30 gm	$9.68	Fluocinonide, Qualitest Pharms	00603-7759-78
30 gm	$10.15	LICON, Major Pharms	00904-0770-31
30 gm	$10.25	Fluocinonide, HL Moore Drug Exch	00839-7013-49
30 gm	$10.25	Fluocinonide, HL Moore Drug Exch	00839-7698-49
30 gm	$11.30	FLUEX, Ocusoft	54799-0801-30
30 gm	$12.00	Dermacin, Pedinol Pharma	00884-5793-01
30 gm	$12.25	Fluocinonide, Rugby	00536-4350-28
30 gm	$12.29	Fluocinonide, Fougera	00168-0139-30
30 gm	$12.40	Fluocinonide, Teva	00093-0262-30
30 gm	$12.40	Fluocinonide, Goldline Labs	00182-1731-56
30 gm	$12.45	Fluocinonide, Schein Pharm (US)	00364-0857-56
30 gm	$12.45	Fluocinonide, Geneva Pharms	00781-7008-03
30 gm	$14.16	Fluocinonide, Taro Pharms (US)	51672-1253-02
30 gm	$14.16	Fluocinonide-E, Taro Pharms (US)	51672-1254-02
30 gm	$15.75	Fluocinonide, Major Pharms	00904-0773-31
30 gm	$16.60	Fluocinonide-E, Goldline Labs	00182-5051-56
30 gm	$17.48	Fluocinonide-E, HL Moore Drug Exch	00839-0758-49
30 gm	$17.48	Fluocinonide, HL Moore Drug Exch	00839-7758-49
30 gm	$17.50	Fluocinonide-E, Teva	00093-0263-30
30 gm	**$24.92**	**LIDEX, Syntex Labs**	**00033-2511-14**
30 gm	**$24.92**	**LIDEX-E, Syntex Labs**	**00033-2513-14**
60 gm	$9.75	Fluocinonide, H.C.F.A. F F P	99999-1310-03
60 gm	$9.75	Fluocinonide, H.C.F.A. F F P	99999-1310-04
60 gm	$12.40	Fluocinonide, Thames Pharma	49158-0212-24
60 gm	$12.96	Fluocinonide, Clay Park Labs	45802-0017-37
60 gm	$13.37	Fluocinonide, HL Moore Drug Exch	00839-7698-50
60 gm	$13.88	Fluocinonide, IDE-Interstate	00814-3200-91
60 gm	$14.10	Fluocinonide, United Res	00677-0735-43
60 gm	$14.10	Fluocinonide, United Res	00677-1404-43
60 gm	$14.60	Fluocinonide Cream 0.05% (Taro), NMC Labs	23317-0390-60
60 gm	$16.05	Fluocinonide, HL Moore Drug Exch	00839-7013-50
60 gm	$16.26	Fluocinonide, Qualitest Pharms	00603-7759-88
60 gm	$16.35	Fluocinonide, Geneva Pharms	00781-7008-35
60 gm	$16.50	LICON, Major Pharms	00904-0770-02
60 gm	$19.00	Fluocinonide, Hamilton Pharma	60322-0511-17
60 gm	$20.50	Fluocinonide, Fougera	00168-0139-60
60 gm	$20.80	Fluocinonide, Teva	00093-0262-92
60 gm	$20.83	Fluocinonide, Schein Pharm (US)	00364-0857-58
60 gm	$20.85	Fluocinonide, Goldline Labs	00182-1731-52
60 gm	$22.60	Fluocinonide, Taro Pharms (US)	51672-1253-03
60 gm	$22.60	Fluocinonide-E, Taro Pharms (US)	51672-1254-03
60 gm	$24.50	Fluocinonide, Rugby	00536-4350-25
60 gm	$25.68	Fluocinonide, Geneva Pharms	00781-7103-35
60 gm	$25.91	Fluocinonide-E, HL Moore Drug Exch	00839-7589-50
60 gm	$27.75	Fluocinonide-E, Goldline Labs	00182-5051-52
60 gm	$27.75	Fluocinonide-E, Qualitest Pharms	00603-7763-88
60 gm	$28.00	Fluocinonide, Rugby	00536-0781-25
60 gm	$28.35	Fluocinonide Cream 0.05% (Taro), Major Pharms	00904-0773-02
60 gm	$28.65	Fluocinonide-E, Hamilton Pharma	60322-0513-17
60 gm	$28.70	Fluocinonide, Teva	00093-0263-92
60 gm	$40.10	Fluocinonide, HL Moore Drug Exch	00839-7731-50
60 gm	**$41.78**	**LIDEX, Syntex Labs**	**00033-2511-17**
60 gm	**$41.78**	**LIDEX-E, Syntex Labs**	**00033-2513-17**
120 gm	$21.99	Fluocinonide, HL Moore Drug Exch	00839-7698-53
120 gm	$23.55	Fluocinonide, H.C.F.A. F F P	99999-1310-05
120 gm	$24.60	Fluocinonide, Thames Pharma	49158-0212-25
120 gm	$25.25	Fluocinonide, Harber Pharm	51432-0719-18
120 gm	$26.95	Fluocinonide, Major Pharms	00904-0770-22
120 gm	$28.08	Fluocinonide, Clay Park Labs	45802-0017-13
120 gm	$30.33	Fluocinonide, Taro Pharms (US)	51672-1253-04
120 gm	$35.05	Fluocinonide, Goldline Labs	00182-1731-57
120 gm	**$70.24**	**LIDEX, Syntex Labs**	**00033-2511-22**

Gel - Topical - 0.05 %

15 gm	$8.96	Fluocinonide, H.C.F.A. F F P	99999-1310-06
15 gm	$12.00	Fluocinonide, Fougera	00168-0135-15
15 gm	**$17.98**	**LIDEX GEL 0.05%, Syntex Labs**	**00033-2507-13**
30 gm	$17.93	Fluocinonide, H.C.F.A. F F P	99999-1310-07
30 gm	**$24.92**	**LIDEX GEL 0.05%, Syntex Labs**	**00033-2507-14**
60 gm	$25.68	Fluocinonide Topical Gel, Geneva Pharms	00781-7101-35
60 gm	$26.95	Fluocinonide, Harber Pharm	51432-0577-17
60 gm	$30.68	Fluocinonide Gel, Teva	00093-0265-92
60 gm	$35.86	Fluocinonide, H.C.F.A. F F P	99999-1310-08
60 gm	$39.60	Fluocinonide, Fougera	00168-0135-60
60 gm	$41.46	Fluocinonide, HL Moore Drug Exch	00839-7590-50
60 gm	**$41.78**	**LIDEX GEL 0.05%, Syntex Labs**	**00033-2507-17**
120 gm	$71.73	Fluocinonide, H.C.F.A. F F P	99999-1310-09

Ointment - Topical - 0.05 %

15 gm	$14.50	Fluocinonide, Harber Pharm	51432-0753-10
15 gm	$15.25	Fluocinonide, Goldline Labs	00182-5075-51

HOW SUPPLIED - RATED THERAPEUTICALLY EQUIVALENT: *(cont'd)*

15 gm	$15.25	Fluocinonide, Major Pharms	00904-7677-36
15 gm	$15.90	Fluocinonide, Teva	00093-0264-15
15 gm	$15.95	Fluocinonide, Qualitest Pharms	00603-7761-74
15 gm	$17.22	Fluocinonide, H.C.F.A. F F P	99999-1310-10
15 gm	$17.54	Fluocinonide, HL Moore Drug Exch	00839-7731-47
15 gm	$17.95	Fluocinonide, Rugby	00536-7501-20
15 gm	**$17.98**	**LIDEX, Syntex Labs**	**00033-2514-13**
30 gm	$19.50	Fluocinonide, Harber Pharm	51432-0753-11
30 gm	$21.75	Fluocinonide, Rugby	00536-7501-28
30 gm	$21.80	Fluocinonide, Qualitest Pharms	00603-7761-78
30 gm	$21.85	Fluocinonide, Goldline Labs	00182-5075-56
30 gm	$21.85	Fluocinonide, Major Pharms	00904-7677-31
30 gm	$21.90	Fluocinonide, Teva	00093-0264-30
30 gm	$24.42	Fluocinonide, HL Moore Drug Exch	00839-7731-49
30 gm	**$24.92**	**LIDEX, Syntex Labs**	**00033-2514-14**
30 gm	$25.27	Fluocinonide, H.C.F.A. F F P	99999-1310-11
60 gm	$34.35	Fluocinonide, Qualitest Pharms	00603-7761-88
60 gm	$34.50	Fluocinonide, Harber Pharm	51432-0753-17
60 gm	$35.25	Fluocinonide, Rugby	00536-7501-25
60 gm	$35.35	Fluocinonide, Teva	00093-0264-92
60 gm	$35.90	Fluocinonide, Goldline Labs	00182-5075-52
60 gm	$35.90	Fluocinonide, Major Pharms	00904-7677-02
60 gm	$40.08	Fluocinonide, H.C.F.A. F F P	99999-1310-12
60 gm	**$41.78**	**LIDEX, Syntex Labs**	**00033-2514-17**
120 gm	**$70.24**	**LIDEX, Syntex Labs**	**00033-2514-22**
120 gm	$137.76	Fluocinonide, H.C.F.A. F F P	99999-1310-13

Solution - Topical - 0.05 %

20 ml	$5.47	Fluocinonide, H.C.F.A. F F P	99999-1310-14
20 ml	**$20.45**	**LIDEX, Syntex Labs**	**00033-2517-44**
60 ml	$16.42	Fluocinonide, H.C.F.A. F F P	99999-1310-15
60 ml	$17.50	Fluocinonide, Copley Pharm	38245-0623-12
60 ml	$18.75	Fluocinonide Topical, Thames Pharma	49158-0316-48
60 ml	$20.48	Fluocinonide, Qualitest Pharms	00603-1230-49
60 ml	$20.81	Fluocinonide, Rugby	00536-0780-61
60 ml	$21.59	Fluocinonide, HL Moore Drug Exch	00839-7583-64
60 ml	$23.58	Fluocinonide Topical, Geneva Pharms	00781-6308-61
60 ml	$23.80	Fluocinonide, Teva	00093-0266-39
60 ml	$23.85	Fluocinonide, Hamilton Pharma	60322-0517-46
60 ml	$23.90	Fluocinonide, NMC Labs	23317-0393-60
60 ml	$24.00	Fluocinonide, Fougera	00168-0134-60
60 ml	$24.00	Fluocinonide Topical, Goldline Labs	00182-5050-68
60 ml	$24.00	Fluocinonide Topical, Schein Pharm (US)	00364-2412-58
60 ml	$25.45	Fluocinonide, Major Pharms	00904-0769-03
60 ml	**$40.50**	**LIDEX, Syntex Labs**	**00033-2517-46**

FLUOROMETHOLONE *(001317)*

CATEGORIES: Anti-Inflammatory Agents; Conjunctivitis; Corneal Inflammation; Corneal Injury; EENT Drugs; Eye, Ear, Nose, & Throat Preparations; Ocular Infections; Ophthalmic Corticosteroids; Ophthalmics; Uveitis; Pregnancy Category C; FDA Approved 1982 Jul

BRAND NAMES: *Cortilet*; *Cortisdin*; *Delmeson*; *Efemoline*; *Efflumidex*; Eflone; *F.M.L.*; *Flarex*; Floromet; *Fluaton*; *Flucon*; *Flumetol-Ofteno*; *Flumex*; Fluor-Op; FML; *Liquifilm*; *Regresin*
(International brand names outside U.S. in italics)

FORMULARIES: Aetna; BC-BS; Medi-Cal

DESCRIPTION:

Fluorometholone ophthalmic suspension is a topical anti-inflammatory agent for ophthalmic use.

Chemical Name: Fluorometholone: 9-Fluor-11β, 17-dihydroxy-6- α-methylpregna-1, 4-diene-3, 20-dione.

Contains: Fluorometholone - 0.1% (or 0.25%, for the 0.25% strength)

with Liquifilm (polyvinyl alcohol) 1.4%; benzalkonium chloride 0.004% (0.005% for the 0.25% strength); edetate disodium; sodium chloride, monobasic; sodium phosphate, monobasic; sodium phosphate, dibasic; polysorbate 80; sodium hydroxide to adjust the pH; and purified water.

CLINICAL PHARMACOLOGY:

Corticosteroids inhibit the inflammatory response to a variety of inciting agents and probably delay or slow healing. They inhibit the edema, fibrin deposition, capillary dilation, leukocyte migration, capillary proliferation, fibroblast proliferation, deposition of collagen, and scar formation associated with inflammation.

There is no generally accepted explanation for the mechanism of action of ocular corticosteroids. However, corticosteroids are thought to act by the induction of phospholipase A_2 inhibitory proteins, collectively called lipocortins. It is postulated that these proteins control the biosynthesis of potent mediators of inflammation such as prostaglandins and leukotrienes by inhibiting the release of their common precursor arachidonic acid. Arachidonic acid is released from membrane phospholipids by phospholipase A_2.

0.1% OPHTHALMIC SUSPENSION

Corticosteroids are capable of producing a rise in intraocular pressure. In clinical studies on patients's eyes treated with dexamethasone and Fluorometholone 0.1% suspensions, fluorometholone demonstrated a lower propensity to increase intraocular pressure than did dexamethasone.

0.25% OPHTHALMIC SUSPENSION

Corticosteroids are capable of producing a rise in intraocular pressure. In clinical studies of documented steroid-responders, fluorometholone demonstrated a significantly longer average time to produce a rise in intraocular pressure than dexamethasone phosphate; however, in a small percentage of individuals a significant rise in intraocular pressure occurred within one week. The ultimate magnitude of the rise was equivalent for both drugs.

INDICATIONS AND USAGE:

Fluorometholone ophthalmic suspension is indicated for the treatment of corticosteroid-responsive inflammation of the palpebral and bulbar conjunctiva, cornea and anterior segment of the globe.

CONTRAINDICATIONS:

Fluorometholone ophthalmic suspension is contraindicated in most viral diseases of the cornea and conjunctiva, including epithelial herpes simplex keratitis (dendritic keratitis), vaccina, and varicella, and also in mycobacterial infection of the eye and fungal diseases of

CONTRAINDICATIONS: *(cont'd)*

ocular structures. Fluorometholone ophthalmic suspension is also contraindicated in patients in individuals with known or suspected hypersensitivity to any of the ingredients of this preparation and to other corticosteroids.

WARNINGS:

Prolonged use of corticosteroids may result in glaucoma with damage to the optic nerve, defects in visual acuity and fields of vision, and in posterior subcapsular cataract formation. Prolonged may also suppress the host immune response and thus increase the hazard of secondary ocular infections.

Various ocular diseases and long-term use of topical corticosteroids have been known to cause corneal and scleral thinning. Use of topical corticosteroids in the presence of thin corneal or scleral tissue may lead to perforation.

Acute purulent untreated infections of the eye may be masked or activity enhanced by the presence of corticosteroid medication.

If this product is used for 10 days or longer, intraocular pressure should be routinely monitored even though it may be difficult in children and uncooperative patients. Steroids should be used with caution in the presence of glaucoma. Intraocular pressure should be checked frequently.

The use of steroids after cataract surgery may delay healing and increase the incidence of bleb formation.

Use of ocular steroids may prolong the course and may exacerbate the severity of many viral infections of the eye (including herpes simplex). Employment of a corticosteroid medication in the treatment of patients with a history of herpes simplex requires great caution; frequent slit lamp microscopy is recommended.

Corticosteroids are not effective in mustard gas keratitis and Sjogren's keratoconjunctivitis,

PRECAUTIONS:

GENERAL

The initial prescription and renewal of the medication order beyond 20 milliliters of Fluorometholone ophthalmic suspension should be made by a physician only after examination of the patient with the aid of magnification, such as lamp biomicroscopy and, where appropriate, fluorescein staining. If signs and symptoms fail to improve after two days, the patient should be re-evaluated.

As fungal infections of the cornea are particularly prone to develop coincidentally wit long-term local corticosteroid applications, fungal invasion should be suspected in any persistent corneal ulceration where a corticosteroid has been used or is in use. Fungal cultures should be taken when appropriate.

If this product is used for 10 days or longer, intraocular pressure should be monitored (see WARNINGS.)

INFORMATION FOR THE PATIENT

If inflammation or pain persists longer than 48 hours or becomes aggravated, the patient should be advised to discontinue the use of the medication and consult a physician.

This product is sterile when packaged. To prevent contamination, care should be taken to avoid touching the bottle tip to eyelids or to any other surface. The use of this bottle by more than one person may spread infection. Keep bottle tightly closed when not in use Keep out of reach of children.

CARCINOGENESIS, MUTAGENESIS, AND IMPAIRMENT OF FERTILITY

No studies have been conducted in animals or in humans to evaluate the possibility of these effects with fluorometholone.

PREGNANCY, TERATOGENIC EFFECTS, PREGNANCY CATEGORY C

Fluorometholone has been shown to be embryocidal and teratogenic in rabbits when administered at low multiples of the human ocular dose. Fluorometholone was applied ocularly to rabbits daily on days 6-18 of gestation, and dose-related fetal loss and fetal abnormalities including cleft palate, deformed rib cage, anomalous limbs and neural abnormalities such as encephalocele, craniorachischisis, and spina bifida were observed. There are no adequate and well-controlled studies of fluorometholone in pregnant women, and it is not known whether fluorometholone can cause fetal harm when administered to a pregnant woman. Fluorometholone should be used during pregnancy only if the potential benefit justifies the potential risk to the fetus.

NURSING MOTHERS

It is not known whether topical ophthalmic administration of corticosteroids could result in sufficient systemic absorption to produce detectable quantities in human milk and could suppress growth, interfere with endogenous corticosteroid production, or cause other untoward effects. Because of the potential for serious adverse reactions in nursing infants from fluorometholone, a decision should be made whether to discontinue nursing or to discontinue the drug, taking into account the importance of the drug to the mother.

PEDIATRIC USE

Safety and effectiveness in children below the age of two years have not been established.

ADVERSE REACTIONS:

Adverse reactions include, in decreasing order of frequency, elevation of intraocular pressure (IOP) with possible development of glaucoma and infrequent optic nerve damage, posterior subcapsular cataract formation, and delayed wound healing.

Although systemic effects are extremely uncommon, there have been rare occurrences of systemic hypercorticoidism after the use of topical steroids.

Corticosteroids-containing preparations have also been reported to cause uveitis and perforation of the globe. Keratitis, conjunctivitis, corneal ulcers, mydriasis, conjunctival hyperemia, loss of accommodation and ptosis have occasionally been reported following local use of corticosteroids.

The development of secondary ocular infection (bacterial, fungal, and viral) has occurred. Fungal and viral infections of the cornea are particularly prone to develop coincidentally with long-term application of steroids. The possibility of fungal invasions should be considered in any persistent corneal ulceration where steroid treatment has been used(see WARNINGS.)

DOSAGE AND ADMINISTRATION:

0.1% OPHTHALMIC SUSPENSION

Instill one drop into the conjunctival sac two to four times daily. During the initial 24 to 48 hours, the dosage may be increased to one application every four hours. Care should be taken not to discontinue therapy prematurely.

If signs and symptoms fail to improve after two days, the patient should be re-evaluated (see PRECAUTIONS.)

The dosing of Fluorometholone ophthalmic suspension (0.1%) may be reduced, but care should be taken not to discontinue therapy prematurely. In chronic conditions, withdrawal of treatment should be carried out by gradually decreasing the frequency of applications.

DOSAGE AND ADMINISTRATION: *(cont'd)*

0.25% OPHTHALMIC SUSPENSION

Instill one drop into the conjunctival sac two to four times daily. Care should be taken not to discontinue therapy prematurely.

If signs and symptoms fail to improve after two days, the patient should be re-evaluated (see PRECAUTIONS.)

The dosing of Fluorometholone ophthalmic suspension (0.25%) may be reduced, but care should be taken not to discontinue therapy prematurely. In chronic conditions, withdrawal of treatment should be carried out by gradually decreasing the frequency of applications.

Note: Store at or below 25°C (77°F), protect from freezing. **Shake well before using.**

(Allergan, 0.1%: 70198 31-6T, 0.25%:70199 31-6T)

HOW SUPPLIED - RATED THERAPEUTICALLY EQUIVALENT:

Solution - Ophthalmic - 0.1 %

5 ml	$9.38	Fluorometholone, H.C.F.A. F F P	99999-1317-01

Suspension - Ophthalmic - 0.1 %

1 ml	$1.88	Fluorometholone, H.C.F.A. F F P	99999-1317-02
1 ml	$4.69	FML, OPHTHALMIC, Allergan-Amer	11980-0211-01
5 ml	$9.38	Fluorometholone, H.C.F.A. F F P	99999-1317-03
5 ml	$9.78	FLUOR-OP, OPHTHALMIC, Ciba Vision	00058-2358-05
5 ml	$14.94	FML, OPHTHALMIC, Allergan-Amer	11980-0211-05
10 ml	$15.66	FLUOR-OP, OPHTHALMIC, Ciba Vision	00058-2358-10
10 ml	$18.75	Fluorometholone, H.C.F.A. F F P	99999-1317-04
10 ml	$22.94	FML, OPHTHALMIC, Allergan-Amer	11980-0211-10
15 ml	$19.50	FLUOR-OP, OPHTHALMIC, Ciba Vision	00058-2358-15
15 ml	$28.13	Fluorometholone, H.C.F.A. F F P	99999-1317-05
15 ml	$32.07	FML, OPHTHALMIC, Allergan-Amer	11980-0211-15

HOW SUPPLIED - NOT RATED EQUIVALENT:

Ointment - Ophthalmic; Top - 0.1 %

3.5 gm	$18.01	FML S.O.P., Allergan	00023-0316-04

Powder - Ophthalmic - 0.1 %

5 ml	$12.06	Eflone, Ciba Vision	58768-0107-05
10 ml	$18.60	Eflone, Ciba Vision	58768-0107-10

Solution - Ophthalmic - 0.1 %

5 ml	$12.50	Floromet, Cooper Vision Pharm	59426-0336-05

Suspension - Ophthalmic - 0.25 %

2 ml	$5.40	FML FORTE, STERILE OPHTHALMIC, Allergan-Amer	11980-0228-02
5 ml	$12.89	FML FORTE, STERILE OPHTHALMIC, Allergan-Amer	11980-0228-05
10 ml	$22.03	FML FORTE, STERILE OPHTHALMIC, Allergan-Amer	11980-0228-10
15 ml	$30.91	FML FORTE, STERILE OPHTHALMIC, Allergan-Amer	11980-0228-15

FLUOROMETHOLONE ACETATE *(003177)*

CATEGORIES: Anti-Inflammatory Agents; Antibacterials; Antibiotics; Conjunctivitis; Corneal Inflammation; Corneal Injury; EENT Drugs; Eye, Ear, Nose, & Throat Preparations; Ocular Infections; Ophthalmic Corticosteroids; Ophthalmics; Uveitis; FDA Approved 1982 Jul

BRAND NAMES: *Efflumidex* (Germany); **Flarex**; *Fluaton*; *Flucon* (Australia, France); *Flumetholon*; *Flumetol Ofteno* (Mexico); *Flumex*; *Flurexol*; *Flurolón*; *Flurop*; *F.M.L.*; *FML* (England, Canada); *FML Forte* (Canada); *FML Liquifilm* (Australia); *Fumelon*; *Isopto Flucon*
(International brand names outside U.S. in italics)

DESCRIPTION:

Fluorometholone acetate is a corticosteroid prepared as a sterile topical ophthalmic suspension. The active ingredient, fluorometholone acetate, is a white to creamy white powder with an empirical formula of $C_{24}H_{31}FO_5$ and a molecular weight of 418.5. Its chemical name is 9-fluoro-11β, 17-dihydroxy-6α-methylpregna-1,4-diene-3, 20-dione 17-acetate.

Each ml Contains: *Active:* fluorometholone acetate 1 mg (0.1%). *Preservative:* benzalkonium chloride 0.01%. *Inactive:* sodium chloride, monobasic sodium phosphate, edetate disodium, hydroxyethyl cellulose, tyloxapol, hydrochloric acid and/or sodium hydroxide (to adjust pH), and purified water.

CLINICAL PHARMACOLOGY:

Corticosteroids suppress the inflammatory response to inciting agents of mechanical, chemical, or immunological nature. No generally accepted explanation of this steroid property has been advanced. Clinical studies demonstrate that Fluorometholone Acetate is significantly more efficacious than Fluorometholone for the treatment of external ocular inflammation.[1] Corticosteroids cause a rise in intraocular pressure in susceptible individuals. In a small study, fluorometholone acetate ophthalmic suspension demonstrated a significantly longer average time to produce a rise in intraocular pressure than did dexamethasone phosphate; however, the ultimate magnitude of the rise was equivalent for both drugs and in a small percentage of individuals a significant rise in intraocular pressure occurred within three days.[2]

INDICATIONS AND USAGE:

Fluorometholone acetate ophthalmic suspension is indicated for use in the treatment of steroid responsive inflammatory conditions of the palpebral and bulbar conjunctiva, cornea, and anterior segment of the eye.

CONTRAINDICATIONS:

Contraindicated in acute superficial herpes simplex keratitis, vaccinia, varicella, and most other viral diseases of cornea and conjunctiva; tuberculosis; fungal diseases; acute purulent untreated infections which, like other diseases caused by microorganisms, may be masked or enhanced by the presence of the steroid; and in those persons who have known hypersensitivity to any component of this preparation.

WARNINGS:

Not for injection. Use in the treatment of herpes simplex infection requires great caution. prolonged use may result in glaucoma, damage to the optic nerve, defects in visual acuity and visual field, cataract formation and/or may aid in the establishment of secondary ocular infections from pathogens due to suppression of host response. Acute purulent infections of the eye may be masked or exacerbated by presence of steroid medication. In those diseases causing thinning of the cornea or sclera, perforation has been known to occur with chronic use of topical steroids. It is advisable that the intraocular pressure be checked frequently.

PRECAUTIONS:

General: Fungal infections of the cornea are particularly prone to develop coincidentally with long-term local steroid application. Fungus invasion must be considered in any persistent corneal ulceration where a steroid has been used or is in use.

Carcinogenesis, Mutagenesis, and Impairment of Fertility: No studies have been conducted in animals or in humans to evaluate the possibility of these effects with fluorometholone.

Pregnancy Category C: Fluorometholone has been shown to be embryocidal and teratogenic in rabbits when administered at low multiples of the human ocular dose. Fluorometholone was applied ocularly to rabbits daily on days 6-18 of gestation, and dose-related fetal loss and fetal abnormalities including cleft palate, deformed rib cage, anomalous limbs and neural abnormalities, such as encephalocele, craniorachischisis, and spina bifida were observed. There are no adequate and well controlled studies of fluorometholone in pregnant women, and it is not known whether fluorometholone can cause fetal harm when administered to a pregnant woman. Fluorometholone should be used during pregnancy only if the potential benefit justifies the potential risk to the fetus.

Nursing Mothers: It is not known whether topical administration of corticosteroids could result in sufficient systemic absorption to produce detectable quantities in human milk. Systemically-administered corticosteroids appear in human milk and could suppress growth, interfere with endogenous corticosteroid production, or cause other untoward effects. Because of the potential for serious adverse reactions in nursing infants from fluorometholone, a decision should be made whether to discontinue nursing or to discontinue the drug.

Pediatric Use: Safety and effectiveness in children have not been established.

ADVERSE REACTIONS:

Glaucoma with optic nerve damage, visual acuity and field defects, cataract formation, secondary ocular infection and following suppression of host response, and perforation of the globe may occur.

DOSAGE AND ADMINISTRATION:

One to two drugs instilled into the conjunctival sac(s) four times daily. During the initial 24 to 48 hours the dosage may be safely increased to two drops every two hours. If no improvement after two weeks, consult physician. Care should be taken not to discontinue therapy prematurely.

HOW SUPPLIED:

5 ml and 10 ml in plastic DROP-TAINER dispensers.

Storage: Store upright between 36° and 80° F. **Shake Well Before Using.**

HOW SUPPLIED - EQUIVALENTS NOT AVAILABLE:

Solution - Ophthalmic - 0.1 %

2.5 ml	$4.38	FLAREX, Alcon	00065-0096-25
5 ml	$15.00	FLAREX, Alcon	00065-0096-05
10 ml	$22.81	FLAREX, Alcon	00065-0096-10

FLUOROMETHOLONE; SULFACETAMIDE SODIUM *(003035)*

CATEGORIES: Adrenal Corticosteroids; Conjunctivitis; Corneal Injury; EENT Drugs; Eye, Ear, Nose, & Throat Preparations; Inflammation; Inflammatory Conditions; Ocular Infections; Ophthalmic Corticosteroids; Ophthalmics; Steroids; Uveitis; Pregnancy Category C; FDA Approved 1989 Sep

BRAND NAMES: FML-S

FORMULARIES: BC-BS

DESCRIPTION:

This drug is abbreviated here as: "Fluorometholone-S". Fluorometholone-S polyvinyl alcohol sterile ophthalmic suspension is a topical anti-inflammatory/anti-infective combination product for ophthalmic use.

Chemical Names: *Fluorometholone:* 9-Fluoro-11 beta, 17-dihydroxy-6 alpha-methylpregna-1,4-diene-3,20-dione. *Sulfacetamide sodium:* N-Sulfanilylacetamide monosodium salt monohydrate.

FML-S Contains: fluorometholone: 0.1%; sulfacetamide sodium: 10%; with: polyvinyl alcohol 1.4%; benzalkonium chloride 0.006%; edetate disodium; polysorbate 80; povidone; sodium chloride; sodium phosphate; dibasic; sodium phosphate, monobasic; sodium thiosulfate; hydrochloric acid and/or sodium hydroxide to adjust the pH; and purified water.

CLINICAL PHARMACOLOGY:

Corticosteroids suppress the inflammatory response to a variety of agents and they probably delay or slow healing. Corticosteroids and their derivatives are capable of producing a rise in intraocular pressure. Since corticosteroids may inhibit the body's defense mechanism against infection, a concomitant antimicrobial drug may be used when this inhibition is considered to be clinically significant in a particular case.

In clinical studies of documented steroid-responders, fluorometholone demonstrated a significantly longer average time to produce a rise in intraocular pressure than dexamethasone phosphate; however, in a small percentage of individuals, a significant rise in intraocular pressure occurred within one week. The ultimate magnitude of the rise was equivalent for both drugs.

The anti-infective component in Fluorometholone-S is included to provide action against specific organisms susceptible to it. Sulfacetamide sodium is active *in vitro* against susceptible strains of the following microorganisms: *Escherichia coli, Staphylococcus Aureus, Streptococcus Pneumoniae, Streptococcus* (viridans group),*Haemophilus Influenzae, Klebsiella* species, and *Enterobacter* species. Some strains of these bacteria may be resistant to sulfacetamide or resistant strains may emerge *in vivo*..

When a decision to administer both a corticosteroid and an antimicrobial is made, the administration of such drugs in combination has the advantage of greater patient compliance and convenience, with the added assurance that the appropriate dosage of both drugs is administered. When both types of drugs are in the same formulation, compatibility of ingredients is assured and the correct volume of drug is delivered and retained.

The relative potency of corticosteroid formulations depends on the molecular structure, concentration, and release from the vehicle.

INDICATIONS AND USAGE:

Fluorometholone-S is indicated for steroid-responsive inflammatory ocular conditions for which a corticosteroid is indicated and where superficial bacterial ocular infection or a risk of bacterial ocular infection exists.

INDICATIONS AND USAGE: *(cont'd)*

Ocular steroids are indicated in inflammatory conditions of the palpebral and bulbar conjunctiva, cornea, and anterior segment of the globe, where the inherent risk of steroid use in certain infective conjunctivitises is accepted to obtain a diminution in edema and inflammation. They are also indicated in chronic anterior uveitis and corneal injury from chemical, radiation or thermal burns or penetration of foreign bodies.

The use of a combination drug with an anti-infective component is indicated where the risk of superficial ocular infection is high or where there is an expectation that potentially dangerous numbers of bacteria will be present in the eye.

The anti-infective drug in this product, sulfacetamide, is active against the following common bacterial eye pathogens: *Escherichia coli, Staphylococcus Aureus, Streptococcus Pneumoniae, Streptococcus* (viridans group),*Haemophilus Influenzae, Klebsiella* species, and *Enterobacter* species.

This product does not provide adequate coverage against *Neisseria* species and *Serratia Marcescens.* A significant percentage of staphylococcal isolates are completely resistant to sulfa drugs.

CONTRAINDICATIONS:

Epithelial herpes simplex keratitis (dendritic keratitis) and vaccinia. Fungal diseases of the ocular structures. Hypersensitivity to any component of the medication.

WARNINGS:

Not For Injection Into The Eye.

Prolonged use of steroids may result in glaucoma, with damage to the optic nerve, defects in visual acuity and fields of vision, and in posterior subcapsular cataract formation. If used for longer than 10 days, intraocular pressure should be routinely monitored even though it may be difficult in children and uncooperative patients.

Prolonged use of steroids may suppress the host immune response in ocular tissues and thus increase the hazard of secondary ocular infections. Various ocular diseases and long-term use of topical corticosteroids have been known to cause corneal and scleral thinning. Use of topical corticosteroids in the presence of thin corneal or scleral tissue may lead to perforation. In acute purulent conditions of the eye, corticosteroids may mask infection or enhance existing infection.

Use of ocular steroids may prolong the course and may exacerbate the severity of many viral infections of the eye. Employment of a corticosteroid medication in the treatment of patients with a history of herpes simplex requires great caution.

Fatalities have occurred, although rarely, due to severe reactions to sulfonamides including Stevens-Johnson syndrome, toxic epidermal necrolysis, fulminant hepatic necrosis, agranulocytosis, aplastic anemia, and other blood dyscrasias. Sensitizations may recur when a sulfonamide is readministered, irrespective of the route of administration. If signs of hypersensitivity or other serious reactions occur, discontinue use of this preparation. (See ADVERSE REACTIONS.)

Cross-sensitivity among corticosteroids has been demonstrated.

A significant percentage of staphylococcal isolates are completely resistant to sulfa drugs.

PRECAUTIONS:

General: The initial prescription and renewal of the medication order beyond 20 milliliters should be made only by a physician after evaluation of the patient's intraocular pressure, examination of the patient with the aid of magnification, such as slit lamp biomicroscopy and, where appropriate, fluorescein staining.

Carcinogenesis, Mutagenesis, and Impairment of Fertility: No studies have been conducted in animals or in humans to evaluate the possibility of these effects with fluorometholone or sulfacetamide.

Pregnancy Category C: Animal studies have not been conducted with Fluorometholone-S polyvinyl alcohol ophthalmic suspension. Fluorometholone has been shown to be embryocidal and teratogenic in rabbits when administered at low multiples of the human dose. Fluorometholone was applied ocularly to rabbits daily on days 6-18 of gestation, and dose-related fetal loss and fetal abnormalities including cleft palate, deformed rib cage, anomalous limbs and neural abnormalities such as encephalocele, craniorrhachischisis, and spina bifida were observed. Kernicterus may be precipitated in infants by sulfonamides being given systemically during the third trimester of pregnancy. There are no adequate and well-controlled studies of Fluorometholone-S polyvinyl alcohol ophthalmic suspension in pregnant women, and it is not known whether Fluorometholone-S can cause fetal harm when administered to a pregnant woman. Fluorometholone-S polyvinyl alcohol ophthalmic suspension should be used during pregnancy only if the potential benefit justifies the potential risk to the fetus.

Nursing Mothers: It is not known whether topical administration of corticosteroids could result in sufficient systemic absorption to produce detectable quantities in breast milk. Systemically administered corticosteroids appear in breast milk and could suppress growth, interfere with endogenous corticosteroid production, or cause other untoward effects. Systemically administered sulfonamides are capable of producing kernicterus in infants of lactating women. Because of the potential for serious adverse reactions in nursing infants from Fluorometholone-S, a decision should be made whether to discontinue nursing or to discontinue the medication.

Pediatric Use: Safety and effectiveness in children have not been established.

DRUG INTERACTIONS:

Sulfacetamide preparations are incompatible with silver preparations.

ADVERSE REACTIONS:

Adverse reactions have occurred with corticosteroid/anti-infective combination drugs which can be attributed to the corticosteroid component, the anti-infective component, or the combination. Exact incidence figures are not available, since no denominator of treated patients is available.

Reactions occurring most often from the presence of the anti-infective ingredient are allergic sensitizations. Fatalities have occurred, although rarely, due to severe reactions to sulfonamides including Stevens-Johnson syndrome, toxic epidermal necrolysis, fulminant hepatic necrosis, agranulocytosis, aplastic anemia, and other blood dyscrasias (see WARNINGS). Sulfacetamide sodium may cause local irritation.

The reactions due to the corticosteroid component in decreasing order of frequency are; elevation of intraocular pressure (IOP) with possible development of glaucoma, and infrequent optic nerve damage; posterior subcapsular cataract formation; and delayed wound healing.

Secondary Infection: The development of secondary infection has occurred after use of combinations containing corticosteroids and antimicrobials. Fungal infections of the cornea are particularly prone to develop coincidentally with long-term applications of corticosteroids. When signs of chronic ocular inflammation persist following prolonged corticosteroid dosing, the possibility of fungal infections of the cornea should be considered.

DOSAGE AND ADMINISTRATION:

One drop of Fluorometholone-S should be instilled into the conjunctival sac four times daily. Care should be taken not to discontinue therapy prematurely.

Not more than 20 milliliters should be prescribed initially, and the prescription should not be refilled without further evaluation as outlined in PRECAUTIONS.

Note: Store at controlled room temperature, 15°-30°C (59°-86°F). Protect from freezing and light.

Shake Well Before Using. Do not use suspension if it is dark brown.

HOW SUPPLIED - EQUIVALENTS NOT AVAILABLE:

Suspension - Ophthalmic - 0.1 %/10 %

5 ml	$14.35	FML-S STERILE OPHTHALMIC, Allergan-Amer	11980-0422-05
10 ml	$19.34	FML-S STERILE OPHTHALMIC, Allergan-Amer	11980-0422-10

FLUOROURACIL *(001319)*

CATEGORIES: Actinic Keratosis; Antimetabolites; Antineoplastics; Breast Carcinoma; Colon Carcinoma; Dermatologicals; Keratolytic Agents; Keratoses; Lesions; Mucous Membrane Agents; Oncologic Drugs; Rectal Carcinoma; Skin Cancer; Skin/Mucous Membrane Agents; Stomach Carcinoma; Topical; Pregnancy Category D; FDA Approval Pre 1982

BRAND NAMES: Adrucil; Efudex; *Efudix* (Australia, England, France, Germany, Mexico, Japan); *Efurix*; Fluoroplex; *Fluoroplex Topical Solution*
(International brand names outside U.S. in italics)

FORMULARIES: BC-BS; Medi-Cal; WHO

> **WARNING:**
> It is recommended that Fluorouracil be given only by or under the supervision of a qualified physician who is experienced in cancer chemotherapy and who is well versed in the use of potent antimetabolites.
> Because of the possibility of severe toxic reactions, it is recommended that patients be hospitalized at least during the initial course of therapy.

DESCRIPTION:

INJECTION

Fluorouracil Injection, an antineoplastic antimetabolite, is a sterile, nonpyrogenic injectable solution for intravenous administration. Each 10-ml contains 500 mg Fluorouracil; pH is adjusted to approximately 9.2 with sodium hydroxide.

Chemically, Fluorouracil, a fluorinated pyrimidine, is 5-fluoro-2,4 (1*H*,3*H*)-pyrimidinedione. It is a white to practically white crystalline powder which is sparingly soluble in water. The molecular weight of Fluorouracil is 130.08.

TOPICAL SOLUTIONS AND CREAMS

Fluorouracil topical solutions and cream are chemotherapeutic agents for the treatment of solar keratoses and superficial basal cell carcinomas. They contain the fluorinated pyrmidine 5-fluorouracil, antineoplastic antimetabolite. Fluorouracil solution consists of 2% or 5% Fluorouracil on a weight/weight basis, compounded with propylene glycol, tris (hydroxymethyl), aminomethane, hydroxypropyl cellulose, parabens (methyl and propyl) and disodium edetate.

Fluorouracil cream contains 5% Fluorouracil in a vanishing cream base consisting of white petrolatum, stearyl alcohol, propylene glycol, polysorbate 60 and parabens (methyl and propyl).

CLINICAL PHARMACOLOGY:

ALL FORMS

There is evidence that the metabolism of Fluorouracil in the anabolic pathway blocks the methylation reaction of deoxyuridylic acid to thymidylic acid. In this manner, Fluorouracil interferes with the synthesis of deoxyribonucleic acid (DNA) and to a lesser extent inhibits the formation of ribonucleic acid (RNA). Since DNA and RNA are essential for cell division and growth, the effect of Fluorouracil may be to create a thymine deficiency which provokes unbalanced growth and death of the cell. The effects of DNA and RNA deprivation are most marked on those cells which grow more rapidly and which take up Fluorouracil at a more rapid rate.

Following intravenous injection, Fluorouracil distributes into tumors, intestinal mucosa, bone marrow, liver and other tissues throughout the body. In spite of its limited lipid solubility, Fluorouracil diffuses readily across the blood-brain barrier and distributes into cerebrospinal fluid and brain tissue.

Seven to twenty percent of the parent drug is excreted unchanged in the urine in six hours; of this over 90% is excreted in the first hour. The remaining percentage of the administered dose is metabolized, primarily in the liver. The catabolic metabolism of Fluorouracil results in degradation products (*e.g.*, CO_2, urea and α-fluoro-β-alanine) which are inactive. The inactive metabolites are excreted in the urine over the next 3 to 4 hours. When Fluorouracil is labeled in the six carbon position, thus preventing the ^{14}C metabolism to CO_2, approximately 90% of the total radioactivity is excreted in the urine. When Fluorouracil is labeled in the two carbon position approximately 90% of the total radioactivity is excreted in expired CO_2. Ninety percent of the dose is accounted for during the first 24 hours following intravenous administration.

Following intravenous administration of Fluorouracil, the mean half-life of elimination from plasma is approximately 16 minutes, with a range of 8 to 20 minutes, and is dose dependent. No intact drug can be detected in the plasma three hours after an intravenous injection.

Additional Information For Topicals: Studies in man with topical application of ^{14}C-labeled Fluorouracil demonstrated insignificant absorption as measured by ^{14}C content of plasma, urine, and respiratory CO_2.

INDICATIONS AND USAGE:

INJECTION

Fluorouracil is effective in the palliative management of carcinoma of the colon, rectum, breast, stomach and pancreas.

TOPICAL SOLUTIONS AND CREAMS

Fluorouracil is recommended for the topical treatment of multiple actinic or solar keratoses. In the 5% strength it is also useful in the treatment of superficial basal cell carcinomas, when conventional methods are impractical, such as with multiple lesions or difficult treatment sites. The diagnosis should be established prior to treatment, since this new method has not been proven effective in other types of basal cell carcinomas. With isolated, easily accessible lesions, conventional techniques are preferred since success with such lesions is almost 100%

INDICATIONS AND USAGE: *(cont'd)*

with these methods. The success rate with Fluorouracil topicals is approximately 93%. This 93% success rate is based on 113 lesions in 54 patients. Twenty-five lesions treated with the solution produced one failure and 88 lesions treated with the cream produced 7 failures.

CONTRAINDICATIONS:

INJECTION

Fluorouracil therapy is contraindicated for patients in a poor nutritional state, those with depressed bone marrow function, those with potentially serious infections or those with a known hypersensitivity to Fluorouracil.

TOPICAL SOLUTIONS AND CREAMS

Contraindicated in patients with known hypersensitivity to any of its components.

WARNINGS:

INJECTION

THE DAILY DOSE OF FLUOROURACIL IS NOT TO EXCEED 800 MG. IT IS RECOMMENDED THAT PATIENTS BE HOSPITALIZED DURING THEIR FIRST COURSE OF TREATMENT.

Fluorouracil should be used with extreme caution in poor risk patients with a history of high-dose pelvic irradiation or previous use of alkylating agents, those who have a widespread involvement of bone marrow by metastatic tumors or those with impaired hepatic or renal function.

Use in Pregnancy: Pregnancy, Teratogenic Effects, Pregnancy Category D. See Pregnancy, Teratogenic Effects, Pregnancy Category D.

Combination Therapy: Any form of therapy which adds to the stress of the patient, interferes with nutrition or depresses bone marrow function will increase the toxicity of Fluorouracil.

TOPICAL SOLUTIONS AND CREAMS

If an occlusive dressing is used, there may be an increase in the incidence of inflammatory reactions in the adjacent normal skin. A porous gauze dressing may be applied for cosmetic reasons without an increase in reaction.

Prolonged exposure to ultraviolet rays should be avoided while under treatment with Fluorouracil because the intensity of the reaction may be increased.

Use in Pregnancy: Safety for use in pregnancy has not been established.

PRECAUTIONS:

INJECTION

General

Fluorouracil is a highly toxic drug with a narrow margin of safety. Therefore, patients should be carefully supervised, since therapeutic response is unlikely to occur without some evidence of toxicity. Severe hematological toxicity, gastrointestinal hemorrhage and even death may result from the use of Fluorouracil despite meticulous selection of patients and careful adjustment of dosage. Although severe toxicity is more likely in poor risk patients, fatalities may be encountered occasionally even in patients in relatively good condition.

Therapy is to be discontinued promptly whenever one of the following signs of toxicity appears:

Stomatitis or esophagopharyngitis, at the first visible sign.

Leukopenia (WBC under 3500) or a rapidly falling white blood count.

Vomiting, intractable.

Diarrhea, frequent bowel movements or watery stools.

Gastrointestinal ulceration and bleeding.

Thrombocytopenia (platelets under 100,000).

Hemorrhage from any site.

The administration of 5-fluorouracil has been associated with the occurrence of palmar-plantar erythrodysesthesia syndrome, also known as hand-foot syndrome. This syndrome has been characterized as a tingling sensation of hands and feet which may progress over the next few days to pain when holding objects or walking. The palms and soles become symmetrically swollen and erythematous with tenderness of the distal phalanges, possibly accompanied by desquamation. Interruption of therapy is followed by gradual resolution over 5 to 7 days. Although pyridoxine has been reported to ameliorate the palmar-plantar erythrodysesthesia syndrome, its safety and effectiveness have not been established.

Information for the Patient

Patients should be informed of expected toxic effects, particularly oral manifestations. Patients should be alerted to the possibility of alopecia as a result of therapy and should be informed that it is usually a transient effect.

Laboratory Tests

White blood counts with differential are recommended before each dose.

Pregnancy, Teratogenic Effects, Pregnancy Category D

Fluorouracil may cause fetal harm when administered to a pregnant woman. Fluorouracil has been shown to be teratogenic in laboratory animals. Fluorouracil exhibited maximum teratogenicity when given to mice as single intraperitoneal injections of 10 to 40 mg/kg on day 10 or 12 of gestation. Similarly, intraperitoneal doses of 12 to 37 mg/kg given to rats between days 9 and 12 of gestation and intramuscular doses of 3 to 9 mg given to hamsters between days 8 and 11 of gestation were teratogenic. Malformations included cleft palates, skeletal defects and deformed appendages, paws and tails. The dosages which were teratogenic in animals are 1 to 3 times the maximum recommended human therapeutic dose. In monkeys, divided doses of 40 mg/kg given between days 20 and 24 of gestation were not teratogenic.

There are no adequate and well-controlled studies with Fluorouracil in pregnant women. While there is no evidence of teratogenicity in humans due to Fluorouracil, it should be kept in mind that other drugs which inhibit DNA synthesis (*e.g.*, methotrexate and aminopterin) have been reported to be teratogenic in humans. Women of childbearing potential should be advised to avoid becoming pregnant. If the drug is used during pregnancy, or if the patient becomes pregnant while taking the drug, the patient should be told of the potential hazard to the fetus. Fluorouracil should be used during pregnancy only if the potential benefit justifies the potential risk to the fetus.

Carcinogenesis, Mutagenesis, and Impairment of Fertility

Carcinogenesis: Long-term studies in animals to evaluate the carcinogenic potential of Fluorouracil have not been conducted. However, there was no evidence of carcinogenicity in small groups of rats given Fluorouracil orally at doses of 0.01, 0.3, 1 or 3 mg per rat 5 days per week for 52 weeks, followed by a six-month observation period. Also, in other studies, 33 mg/kg of Fluorouracil was administered intravenously to male rats once a week for 52 weeks followed by observation for the remainder of their lifetimes with no evidence of carcinogenicity. Female mice were given 1 mg of Fluorouracil intravenously once a week for 16 weeks with no effect on the incidence of lung adenomas. On the basis of the available data, no evaluation can be made of the carcinogenic risk of Fluorouracil to humans.

PRECAUTIONS: *(cont'd)*

Mutagenesis: Oncogenic transformation of fibroblasts from mouse embryo has been induced *in vitro* by Fluorouracil, but the relationship between oncogenicity and mutagenicity is not clear. Fluorouracil has been shown to be mutagenic to several strains of *Salmonella typhimurium*, including TA 1535, TA 1537 and TA 1538, and to*Saccharomyces cerevisiae*, although no evidence of mutagenicity was found with *Salmonella typhimurium* strains TA 92, TA 98 and TA 100. In addition, a positive effect was observed in the micronucleus test on bone marrow cells of the mouse, and Fluorouracil at very high concentrations produced chromosomal breaks in hamster fibroblasts *in vitro*.

Impairment of Fertility: Fluorouracil has not been adequately studied in animals to permit an evaluation of its effects on fertility and general reproductive performance. However, doses of 125 or 250 mg/kg, administered intraperitoneally, have been shown to induce chromosomal aberrations and changes in chromosomal organization of spermatogonia in rats. Spermatogonial differentiation was also inhibited by Fluorouracil, resulting in transient infertility. However, in studies with a strain of mouse which is sensitive to the induction of sperm head abnormalities after exposure to a range of chemical mutagens and carcinogens, Fluorouracil did not produce any abnormalities at oral doses of up to 80 mg/kg/day. In female rats, Fluorouracil, administered intraperitoneally at weekly doses of 25 or 50 mg/kg for three weeks during the pre-ovulatory phase of oogenesis, significantly reduced the incidence of fertile matings, delayed the development of pre- and post-implantation embryos, increased the incidence of pre-implantation lethality and induced chromosomal anomalies in these embryos. In a limited study in rabbits, a single 25 mg/kg dose of Fluorouracil or 5 daily doses of 5 mg/kg had no effect on ovulation, appeared not to affect implantation and had only a limited effect in producing zygote destruction. Compounds such as Fluorouracil, which interfere with DNA, RNA and protein synthesis, might be expected to have adverse effects on gametogenesis.

Pregnancy, Nonteratogenic Effects: Fluorouracil has not been studied in animals for its effects on peri- and postnatal development. However, Fluorouracil has been shown to cross the placenta and enter into fetal circulation in the rat. Administration of Fluorouracil has resulted in increased resorptions and embryolethality in rats. In monkeys, maternal doses higher than 40 mg/kg resulted in abortion of all embryos exposed to Fluorouracil. Compounds which inhibit DNA, RNA and protein synthesis might be expected to have adverse effects on peri- and postnatal development.

Nursing Mothers

It is known whether Fluorouracil is excreted in human milk. Because Fluorouracil inhibits DNA, RNA and protein synthesis, mothers should not nurse while receiving this drug.

Pediatric Use

Safety and effectiveness in children have not been established.

TOPICAL SOLUTIONS AND CREAMS

If Fluorouracil is applied with the fingers, the hands should be washed immediately afterward. Fluorouracil should be applied with care near the eyes, nose, and mouth. Solar keratoses which do no not respond should be biopsied to confirm the diagnosis. Patients should be forewarned that the reaction in the treated areas may be unsightly during therapy, and, in some cases, for several weeks following the cessation of therapy.

Follow-up biopsies should be performed as indicated in the management of superficial basal cell carcinoma.

DRUG INTERACTIONS:

Leucovorin calcium may enhance the toxicity of Fluorouracil.

Also see WARNINGS section.

ADVERSE REACTIONS:

INJECTION

Stomatitis and esophagopharyngitis (which may lead to sloughing and ulceration), diarrhea, anorexia, nausea and emesis are commonly seen during therapy.

Leukopenia usually follows every course of adequate therapy with Fluorouracil. The lowest white blood cell counts are commonly observed between the 9th and 14th days after the first course of treatment, although uncommonly the maximal depression may be delayed for as long as 20 days. By the 30th day the count has usually returned to the normal range.

Alopecia and dermatitis may be seen in a substantial number of cases. The dermatitis most often seen is a pruritic maculopapular rash usually appearing on the extremities and less frequently on the trunk. It is generally reversible and usually responsive to symptomatic treatment.

Other Adverse Reactions Are:

Hematologic: pancytopenia, thrombocytopenia, agranulocytosis, anemia.

Cardiovascular: myocardial ischemia, angina.

Gastrointestinal: gastrointestinal ulceration and bleeding.

Allergic reactions: anaphylaxis and generalized allergic reactions.

Neurologic: acute cerebellar syndrome (which may persist following discontinuance of treatment), nystagmus, headache.

Dermatologic: dry skin; fissuring; photosensitivity, as manifested by erythema or increased pigmentation of the skin; vein pigmentation; palmar-plantar erythrodysesthesia syndrome, as manifested by tingling of the hands and feet followed by pain, erythema and swelling.

Ophthalmic: lacrimal duct stenosis, visual changes, lacrimation, photophobia.

Psychiatric: disorientation, confusion, euphoria.

Miscellaneous: thrombophlebitis, epistaxis, nail changes (including loss of nails).

TOPICAL SOLUTIONS AND CREAMS

The most frequently encountered local reactions are pain, pruritus, hyperpigmentation and burning at the site of the application. Other local reactions include allergic contact dermatitis, scarring, soreness, tenderness, suppuration, scaling, and swelling.

Also reported are alopecia, insomnia, stomatitis, irritability. medicinal taste, photosensitivity, lacrimation, telangiectasia and urticaria, although a causal relationship is remote.

Laboratory abnormalities reported are leukocytosis, thrombocytopenia, toxic granulation and eosinophilia.

OVERDOSAGE:

The possibility of overdosage with Fluorouracil is unlikely in view of the mode of administration. Nevertheless, the anticipated manifestations would be nausea, vomiting, diarrhea, gastrointestinal ulceration and bleeding, bone marrow depression (including thrombocytopenia, leukopenia and agranulocytosis). No specific antidotal therapy exists. Patients who have been exposed to an overdose of Fluorouracil should be monitored hematologically for at least four weeks. Should abnormalities appear, appropriate therapy should be utilized.

The acute intravenous toxicity of Fluorouracil is as seen in TABLE 1.

TABLE 1

Species	LD_{50} (mg/kg ± S.E.)
Mouse	340 ± 17
Rat	165 ± 26
Rabbit	27 ± 5.1
Dog	31.5 ± 3.8

DOSAGE AND ADMINISTRATION:

INJECTION

General Instructions: Fluorouracil Injection should be administered only intravenously, using care to avoid extravasation. No dilution is required.

All dosages are based on the patient's actual weight. However, the estimated lean body mass (dry weight) is used if the patient is obese or if there has been a spurious weight gain due to edema, ascites or other forms of abnormal fluid retention.

It is recommended that prior to treatment each patient be carefully evaluated in order to estimate as accurately as possible the optimum initial dosage of Fluorouracil.

Dosage: Twelve mg/kg are given intravenously once daily for four successive days. The daily dose should not exceed 800 mg.

If no toxicity is observed: 6 mg/kg are given on the 6th, 8th, 10th and 12th days *unless toxicity occurs.* No therapy is given on the 5th, 7th, 9th or 11th days. *Therapy is to be discontinued at the end of the 12th day, even if no toxicity has become apparent.* (See WARNINGS and PRECAUTIONS.)

Poor risk patients or those who are not in an adequate nutritional state (see CONTRAINDICATIONS and WARNINGS) should receive 6 mg/kg/day for three days. *If no toxicity is observed*, 3 mg/kg may be given on the 5th, 7th and 9th days *unless toxicity occurs.* No therapy is given on the 4th, 6th or 8th days. The daily dose should not exceed 400 mg.

A sequence of injections on either schedule constitutes a "course of therapy".

Maintenance Therapy: In instances where toxicity has not been a problem, it is recommended that therapy be continued using either of the following schedules:

1. Repeat dosage of first course every 30 days after the last day of the previous course of treatment.

2. When toxic signs resulting from the initial course of therapy have subsided, administer a maintenance dosage of 10 to 15 mg/kg/week as a single dose. Do not exceed 1 g per week.

The patient's reaction to the previous course of therapy should be taken into account in determining the amount of the drug to be used, and the dosage should be adjusted accordingly. Some patients have received from 9 to 45 courses of treatment during periods which ranged from 12 to 60 months.

Procedures for proper handling and disposal of anticancer drugs should be considered. Several guidelines on this subject have been published[1-6]. There is no general agreement that all of the procedures recommended in the guidelines are necessary or appropriate.

Note: Parenteral drug products should be inspected visually for particulate matter and discoloration prior to administration, whenever solution and container permit. Although the Fluorouracil solution may discolor slightly during storage, the potency and safety are not adversely affected. If a precipitate occurs due to exposure to low temperatures, resolubilize by heating to 140°F and shaking vigorously; allow to cool to body temperature before using.

Store at room temperature (59° to 86°F; 15° to 30°C). Protect from light.

TOPICAL SOLUTIONS AND CREAMS

When Fluorouracil is applied to a lesion, a response occurs with the following sequence: erythema, usually followed by vesiculation, erosion, ulceration, necrosis and epithelization.

Actinic Or Solar Keratosis: Apply cream or solution twice daily in an amount sufficient to cover the lesions. Medication should be continued until the inflammatory response reaches the erosion, necrosis and the ulceration stage, at which time use of the drug should be terminated. The usual duration of therapy is from two to four weeks. Complete healing of the lesions may not be evident for one to two months following cessation of Fluorouracil therapy.

Superficial Basal Cell Carcinomas: Only the 5% strength is recommended. Apply cream or solution twice daily in an amount sufficient to cover the lesions. Treatment should be continued for at least three to six weeks. Therapy may be required for as long as 10 to 12 weeks before the lesions are obliterated. As in any neoplastic condition, the patient should be followed for a reasonable period of time to determine if a cure has been obtained.

REFERENCES:

1. Recommendations for the safe handling of parenteral antineoplastic drugs. Washington, DC, U.S. Government Printing Office (NIH Publication No. 83-2621). **2.** AMA Council Report. Guidelines for handling parenteral antineoplastics. *JAMA 253:* 1590-1592, Mar 15, 1985. **3.** National Study Commission on Cytotoxic Exposure: Recommendations for handling cytotoxic agents. Available from Louis P. Jeffrey, ScD, Director of Pharmacy Services, Rhode Island Hospital, 593 Eddy Street, Providence, Rhode Island 02902. **4.** Clinical Oncological Society of Australia: Guidelines and recommendations for safe handling of antineoplastic agents. *Med J Aust 1:* 426-428, Apr 30, 1983. **5.** Jones RB, Frank R, Mass T: Safe handling of chemotherapeutic agents: a report from the Mount Sinai Medical Center. *CA 33:* 258-263, Sept-Oct 1983. **6.** ASHP technical assistance bulletin on handling cytotoxic drugs in hospitals. *Am J Hosp Pharm 42:* 131-137, Jan 1985.

HOW SUPPLIED - RATED THERAPEUTICALLY EQUIVALENT:

Injection, Solution - Intravenous - 50 mg/ml

10 ml	$37.50	Fluorouracil, Solopak Labs	39769-0012-10
10 ml x 10	$1.54	ADRUCIL, Pharmacia & Upjohn	00013-1036-91
10 ml x 10	$14.79	Fluorouracil, Roche	00004-1977-01
10 ml x 25	$40.50	Fluorouracil, Harber Pharm	51432-0470-10
20 ml x 10	$31.25	Fluorouracil, Harber Pharm	51432-0409-10
50 ml x 5	$7.69	ADRUCIL, Pharmacia & Upjohn	00013-1046-94
100 ml	$15.38	ADRUCIL, Pharmacia & Upjohn	00013-1056-94
100 ml	$250.00	Fluorouracil, Solopak Labs	39769-0012-90

HOW SUPPLIED - NOT RATED EQUIVALENT:

Cream - Topical - 1 %

30 gm	$32.89	FLUOROPLEX, Allergan	00023-0812-30

Cream - Topical - 5 %

25 gm	$35.82	EFUDEX, Roche	00004-1506-03

Solution - Topical - 1 %

30 ml	$32.89	FLUOROPLEX, Allergan	00023-0810-30

Solution - Topical - 2 %

10 ml	$22.30	EFUDEX, Roche	00004-1704-06

Solution - Topical - 5 %

10 ml	$31.61	EFUDEX, Roche	00004-1705-06

FLUOXETINE HYDROCHLORIDE *(001320)*

CATEGORIES: Antidepressants; Attention Deficit Disorders*; Bulimia; Central Nervous System Agents; Depression; Depressive Disorder; Fatigue; Obesity*; Obsessive-Compulsive Disorder; Panic Disorder*; Psychotherapeutic Agents; Selective Serotonin Reuptake Inhibitors; Weight Loss*; Pregnancy Category B; Sales > $1 Billion; FDA Approved 1987 Dec; Patent Expiration 2001 Dec; Top 200 Drugs
* Indication not approved by the FDA

BRAND NAMES: *Adofen*; *Deproxin*; *Fluctin* (Germany); *Fluctine*; *Fludac*; *Flufran*; *Flunil*; *Fluoxac* (Mexico); *Fluoxeren*; *Fluoxil*; *Fluoxeron*; *Flutine*; *Fluxil*; *Fontex*; Lovan; *Margrilan*; *Oxetine*; *Prodep*; **Prozac**; *Prozac 20* (Mexico); *Rowexetina*
(International brand names outside U.S. in italics)

FORMULARIES: Aetna; BC-BS; Kaiser; Medco; Medi-Cal; PCS; United

COST OF THERAPY: $202.08 (Depression; Capsule; 20 mg; 1/day; 90 days)

PRIMARY ICD9: 311 (Depressive Disorder, Not Elsewhere Classified)

DESCRIPTION:

Fluoxetine hydrochloride is an antidepressant for oral administration; it is chemically unrelated to tricyclic, tetracyclic, or other available antidepressant agents. It is designated (±)-N-methyl-3-phenyl-3-[(α,α,α-trifluoro-*p*-tolyl)-oxy]propylamine hydrochloride and has the empirical formula of $C_{17}H_{18}F_3NO{\cdot}HCl$. Its molecular weight is 345.79.

Fluoxetine hydrochloride is a white to off-white crystalline solid with a solubility of 14 mg/ml in water.

Each Pulvule contains fluoxetine hydrochloride equivalent to 10 mg (32.3 μmol) or 20 mg (64.7 μmol) of fluoxetine. The Pulvules also contain F D & C Blue No. 1, gelatin, iron oxide, silicone, starch, titanium dioxide, and other inactive ingredients.

The oral solution contains fluoxetine hydrochloride equivalent to 20 mg/5 ml (64.7 μmol) of fluoxetine. It also contains alcohol 0.23%, benzoic acid, flavoring agent, glycerin, purified water, and sucrose.

CLINICAL PHARMACOLOGY:

PHARMACODYNAMICS

The antidepressant, antiobsessive-compulsive, and antibulimic actions of fluoxetine are presumed to be linked to its inhibition of CNS neuronal uptake of serotonin. Studies at clinically relevant doses in man have demonstrated that fluoxetine blocks the uptake of serotonin into human platelets. Studies in animals also suggest that fluoxetine is a much more potent uptake inhibitor of serotonin than of norepinephrine.

Antagonism of muscarinic, histaminergic, and α_1-adrenergic receptors has been hypothesized to be associated with various anticholinergic, sedative, and cardiovascular effects of classical tricyclic antidepressant drugs. Fluoxetine binds to these and other membrane receptors from brain tissue much less potently *in vitro* than do the tricyclic drugs.

ABSORPTION, ELIMINATIONMETABOLISM,

Systemic Bioavailability: In man, following a single oral 40 mg dose, peak plasma concentrations of fluoxetine from 15 to 55 ng/ml are observed after 6 to 8 hours.

The Pulvule and oral solution dosage forms of fluoxetine are bioequivalent. Food does not appear to affect the systemic bioavailability of fluoxetine, although it may delay its absorption inconsequentially. Thus, fluoxetine may be administered with or without food.

Protein Binding: Over the concentration range from 200 to 1000 ng/ml, approximately 94.5% of fluoxetine is bound *in vitro* to human serum proteins, including albumin and α_1-glycoprotein. The interaction between fluoxetine and other highly protein-bound drugs has not been fully evaluated, but may be important (see PRECAUTIONS).

Enantiomers: Fluoxetine is a racemic mixture (50/50) of *R*-fluoxetine and *S*-fluoxetine enantiomers. In animal models, both enantiomers are specific and potent serotonin uptake inhibitors with essentially equivalent pharmacologic activity. The *S*-fluoxetine enantiomer is eliminated more slowly and is the predominant enantiomer present in plasma at steady state.

Metabolism: Fluoxetine is extensively metabolized in the liver to norfluoxetine and a number of other, unidentified metabolites. The only identified active metabolite, norfluoxetine, is formed by demethylation of fluoxetine. In animal models, *S*-norfluoxetine is a potent and selective inhibitor of serotonin uptake and has activity essentially equivalent to *R*- or *S*-fluoxetine. *R*-norfluoxetine is significantly less potent than the parent drug in the inhibition of serotonin uptake. The primary route of elimination appears to be hepatic metabolism to inactive metabolites excreted by the kidney.

Clinical Issues Related to Metabolism/Elimination: The complexity of the metabolism of fluoxetine has several consequences that may potentially affect fluoxetine's clinical use.

Variability in Metabolism: A subset (about 7%) of the population has reduced activity of the drug metabolizing enzyme cytochrome P450IID6. Such individuals are referred to as "poor metabolizers" of drugs such as debrisoquin, dextromethorphan, and the tricyclic antidepressants. In a study involving labeled and unlabeled enantiomers administered as a racemate, these individuals metabolized *S*-fluoxetine at a slower rate and thus achieved higher concentrations of *S*-fluoxetine. Consequently, concentrations of *S*-norfluoxetine at steady state were lower. The metabolism of *R*-fluoxetine in these poor metabolizers appears normal. When compared with normal metabolizers, the total sum at steady state of the plasma concentrations of the 4 active enantiomers was not significantly greater among poor metabolizers. Thus, the net pharmacodynamic activities were essentially the same. Alternative, nonsaturable pathways (non-IID6) also contribute to the metabolism of fluoxetine. This explains how fluoxetine achieves a steady-state concentration rather than increasing without limit.

Because fluoxetine's metabolism, like that of a number of other compounds including tricyclic and other selective serotonin antidepressants, involves the P450IID6 system, concomitant therapy with drugs also metabolized by this enzyme system (such as the tricyclic antidepressants) may lead to drug interactions (see DRUG INTERACTIONS).

Accumulation and Slow Elimination: The relatively slow elimination of fluoxetine (elimination half-life of 1 to 3 days after acute administration and 4 to 6 days after chronic administration) and its active metabolite, norfluoxetine (elimination half-life of 4 to 16 days after acute and chronic administration), leads to significant accumulation of these active species in chronic use and delayed attainment of steady state, even when a fixed dose is used. After 30 days of dosing at 40 mg/day, plasma concentrations of fluoxetine in the range of 91 to 302 ng/ml and norfluoxetine in the range of 72 to 258 ng/ml have been observed. Plasma concentrations of fluoxetine were higher than those predicted by single-dose studies, because fluoxetine's metabolism is not proportional to dose. Norfluoxetine, however, appears to have linear pharmacokinetics. Its mean terminal half-life after a single dose was 8.6 days and after multiple dosing was 9.3 days. Steady state levels after prolonged dosing are similar to levels seen at 4-5 weeks.

The long elimination half-lives of fluoxetine and norfluoxetine assure that, even when dosing is stopped, active drug substance will persist in the body for weeks (primarily depending on individual patient characteristics, previous dosing regimen, and length of previous therapy at discontinuation). This is of potential consequence when drug discontinuation is required or when drugs are prescribed that might interact with fluoxetine and norfluoxetine following the discontinuation of fluoxetine.

Liver Disease: As might be predicted from its primary site of metabolism, liver impairment can affect the elimination of fluoxetine. The elimination half-life of fluoxetine was prolonged in a study of cirrhotic patients, with a mean of 7.6 days compared to the range of 2 to 3 days seen in subjects without liver disease; norfluoxetine elimination was also delayed, with a mean duration of 12 days for cirrhotic patients compared to the range of 7 to 9 days in normal subjects. This suggests that the use of fluoxetine in patients with liver disease must be approached with caution. If fluoxetine is administered to patients with liver disease, a lower or less frequent dose should be used (see PRECAUTIONS and DOSAGE AND ADMINISTRATION).

Renal Disease: In single dose studies, the pharmacokinetics of fluoxetine and norfluoxetine were similar among subjects with all levels of impaired renal function including anephric patients on chronic hemodialysis. However, with chronic administration, additional accumulation of fluoxetine or its metabolites (possibly including some not yet identified) may occur in patients with severely impaired renal function and use of a lower or less frequent dose is advised (see PRECAUTIONS).

Age: The disposition of single doses of fluoxetine in healthy elderly subjects (greater than 65 years of age) did not differ significantly from that in younger normal subjects. However, given the long half-life and nonlinear disposition of the drug, a single-dose study is not adequate to rule out the possibility of altered pharmacokinetics in the elderly, particularly if they have systemic illness or are receiving multiple drugs for concomitant diseases. The effects of age upon the metabolism of fluoxetine have been investigated in 260 elderly but otherwise healthy depressed patients (≥60 years of age) who received 20 mg fluoxetine for 6 weeks. Combined fluoxetine plus norfluoxetine plasma concentrations were 209.3 ± 85.7 ng/ml at the end of 6 weeks. No unusual age-associated pattern of adverse events was observed in those elderly patients.

CLINICAL STUDIES:

DEPRESSION

The efficacy of fluoxetine HCl for the treatment of patients with depression (≥18 years of age) has been studied in 5- and 6-week placebo-controlled trials. Fluoxetine HCl was shown to be significantly more effective than placebo as measured by the Hamilton Depression Rating Scale (HAM-D). Fluoxetine HCl was also significantly more effective than placebo on the HAM-D subscores for depressed mood, sleep disturbance, and the anxiety subfactor.

Two 6-week controlled studies comparing fluoxetine HCl, 20 mg, and placebo have shown fluoxetine HCl, 20 mg daily, to be effective in the treatment of elderly patients (≥60 years of age) with depression. In these studies, fluoxetine HCl produced a significantly higher rate of response and remission as defined respectively by a 50% decrease in the HAM-D score and a total endpoint HAM-D score of ≤7. Fluoxetine HCl was well tolerated and the rate of treatment discontinuations due to adverse events did not differ between fluoxetine HCl (12%) and placebo (9%).

OBSESSIVE COMPULSIVE DISORDER

The effectiveness of fluoxetine HCl for the treatment for obsessive compulsive disorder (OCD) was demonstrated in two 13-week, multicenter, parallel group studies (Studies 1 and 2) of adult outpatients who received fixed fluoxetine HCl doses of 20, 40, or 60 mg/day (on a once a day schedule, in the morning) or placebo. Patients in both studies had moderate to severe OCD (DSM-III-R), with mean baseline ratings on the Yale-Brown Obsessive Compulsive Scale (YBOCS, total score) ranging from 22 to 26. In Study 1, patients receiving fluoxetine HCl experienced mean reductions of approximately 4 to 6 units on the YBOCS total score, compared to a 1-unit reduction for placebo patients. In Study 2, patients receiving fluoxetine HCl experienced mean reductions of approximately 4 to 9 units on the YBOCS total score, compared to a 1-unit reduction for placebo patients. While there was no indication of a dose response relationship for effectiveness in Study 1, a dose response relationship was observed in Study 2, with numerically better responses in the 2 higher dose groups. TABLE 1 provides the outcome classification by treatment group on the Clinical Global Impression (CGI) improvement scale for studies 1 and 2 combined.

TABLE 1 Outcome Classification (%) on CGI Improvement Scale for Completers in Pool of Two OCD Studies

Outcome Classification	Placebo	Fluoxetine Hydrochloride 20 mg	40 mg	60 mg
Worse	8%	0%	0%	0%
No Change	64%	41%	33%	29%
Minimally Improved	17%	23%	28%	24%
Much Improved	8%	28%	27%	28%
Very Much Improved	3%	8%	12%	19%

Exploratory analyses for age and gender effects on outcome did not suggest any differential responsiveness on the basis of age or sex.

BULIMIA NERVOSA

The effectiveness of fluoxetine HCl for the treatment of bulimia was demonsrated in two 8-week and one 16-week, multicenter, parallel group studies of adult outpatients meeting DSM-III-R criteria for bulimia. Patients in the 8-week studies received either 20 mg/day or 60 mg/day of fluoxetine HCl or placebo in the morning. Patients in the 16-week study received a fixed fluoxetine HCl dose of 60 mg/day (once a day) or placebo. Patients in these 3 studies had moderate to severe bulimia with median binge-eating and vomiting frequencies ranging from 7 to 10 per week and 5 to 9 per week, respectively. In these 3 studies, fluoxetine HCl, 60 mg, but not 20 mg, was statistically significantly superior to placebo in reducing the number of binge-eating and vomiting episodes per week. The statistically significantly superior effect of 60 mg vs. placebo was present as early as week 1 and persisted throughout each study. The fluoxetine HCl related reduction in bulimic episodes appeared to be independent of baseline depression as assessed by the Hamilton Depression Rating Scale. In each of these 3 studies, the treatment effect, as measured by differences between fluoxetine HCl, 60 mg, and placebo on median reduction from baseline in frequency of bulimic behaviors at endpoint, ranged from 1 to 2 episodes per week for binge-eating and 2 to 4 episodes per week for vomiting. The size of the effect was related to baseline frequency, with greater reductions seen in patients with higher baseline frequencies. Although, some patients achieved freedom from binge-eating and purging as a result of treatment, for the majority, the benefit was a partial reduction in the frequency of binge-eating and purging.

INDICATIONS AND USAGE:

DEPRESSION

Fluoxetine HCl is indicated for the treatment of depression. The efficacy of fluoxetine HCl was established in 5- and 6-week trials with depressed outpatients (≥18 years of age) whose diagnoses corresponded most closely to the DSM-III category of major depressive disorder (see CLINICAL STUDIES).

INDICATIONS AND USAGE: *(cont'd)*

A major depressive episode implies a prominent and relatively persistent depressed or dysphoric mood that usually interferes with daily functioning (nearly every day for at least 2 weeks); it should include at least 4 of the following 8 symptoms: change in appetite, change in sleep, psychomotor agitation or retardation, loss of interest in usual activities or decrease in sexual drive, increased fatigue, feelings of guilt or worthlessness, slowed thinking or impaired concentration, and a suicide attempt or suicidal ideation.

The antidepressant action of fluoxetine HCl in hospitalized depressed patients has not been adequately studied.

The effectiveness of fluoxetine HCl in long-term use, that is, for more than 5 to 6 weeks, has not been systematically evaluated in controlled trials. Therefore, the physician who elects to use fluoxetine HCl for extended periods should periodically reevaluate the long-term usefulness of the drug for the individual patient.

OBSESSIVE-COMPULSIVE DISORDER

Fluoxetine HCl is indicated for the treatment of obsessions and compulsions in patients with obsessive-compulsive disorder (OCD), as defined in the DSM-III-R (*i.e.,* the obsessions or compulsions caused marked distress) are time-consuming, or significantly interfere with social or occupational functioning.

The efficacy of fluoxetine HCl was established in 13-week trials with obsessive-compulsive outpatients whose diagnoses corresponded most closely to the DSM-III-R category of obsessive-compulsive disorder (see CLINICAL STUDIES).

Obsessive-compulsive disorder is characterized by recurrent and persistent ideas, thoughts, impulses, or images (obsessions) that are ego-dystonic and/or repetitive, purposeful, and intentional behaviors (compulsions) that are recognized by the person as excessive or unreasonable.

The effectiveness of fluoxetine HCl in long-term use (*i.e.,* for more than 13 weeks) has not been systematically evaluated in placebo-controlled trials. Therefore, the physician who elects to use fluoxetine HCl for extended periods should periodically reevaluate the long-term usefulness of the drug for the individual patient (see DOSAGE AND ADMINISTRATION).

BULIMIA NERVOSA

Fluoxetine HCl is indicated for the treatment of binge-eating and vomiting behaviors in patients with moderate to severe bulimia nervosa.

The efficacy of fluoxetine HCl was established in 8 to 16 week trials for adult outpatients with moderate to severe bulimia nervosa (*i.e.,* at least 3 bulimic episodes per week for 6 months) (see CLINICAL STUDIES).

The effectiveness of fluoxetine HCl in long-term use (*i.e.,* for more than 16 weeks) has not been systemically evaluated in placebo-controlled trials. Therefore, the physician who elects to use fluoxetine HCl for extended periods should periodically reevaluate the long-term usefulness of the drug for the individual patient (see DOSAGE AND ADMINISTRATION).

CONTRAINDICATIONS:

Fluoxetine HCl is contraindicated in patients known to be hypersensitive to it.

Monoamine Oxidase Inhibitors: There have been reports of serious, sometimes fatal, reactions (including hyperthermia, rigidity, myoclonus, autonomic instability with possible rapid fluctuations of vital signs, and mental status changes that include extreme agitation progressing to delirium and coma) in patients receiving fluoxetine in combination with a monoamine oxidase inhibitor (MAOI), and in patients who have recently discontinued fluoxetine and are then started on an MAOI. Some cases presented with features resembling neuroleptic malignant syndrome. Therefore, fluoxetine HCl should not be used in combination with an MAOI, or within 14 days of discontinuing therapy with an MAOI. Since fluoxetine and its major metabolite have very long elimination half-lives, at least 5 weeks perhaps longer, especially if fluoxetine has been prescribed chronically and/or at higher doses (see CLINICAL PHARMACOLOGY, Accumulation and Slow Elimination) should be allowed after stopping fluoxetine HCl before starting an MAOI.

WARNINGS:

Rash and Possibly Allergic Events: In U.S. fluoxetine clinical trials, 7% of 10782 patients developed various types of rashes and/or urticaria. Among these cases of rash and/or urticaria reported in premarketing clinical trials, almost a third were withdrawn from treatment because of the rash and/or systemic signs or symptoms associated with the rash. Clinical findings reported in association with rash include fever, leukocytosis, arthralgias, edema, carpal tunnel syndrome, respiratory distress, lymphadenopathy, proteinuria, and mild transaminase elevation. Most patients improved promptly with discontinuation of fluoxetine and/or adjunctive treatment with antihistamines or steroids, and all patients experiencing these events were reported to recover completely.

In premarketing clinical trials, 2 patients are known to have developed a serious cutaneous systemic illness. In neither patient was there an unequivocal diagnosis, but 1 was considered to have a leukocytoclastic vasculitis, and the other, a severe desquamating syndrome that was considered variously to be a vasculitis or erythema multiforme. Other patients have had systemic syndromes suggestive of serum sickness.

Since the introduction of fluoxetine HCl, systemic events, possibly related to vasculitis, have developed in patients with rash. Although these events are rare, they may be serious, involving the lung, kidney, or liver. Death has been reported to occur in association with these systemic events.

Anaphylactoid events, including bronchospasm, angioedema, and urticaria alone and in combination, have been reported.

Pulmonary events, including inflammatory processes of varying histopathology and/or fibrosis, have been reported rarely. These events have occurred with dyspnea as the only preceding symptom.

Whether these systemic events and rash have a common underlying cause or are due to different etiologies or pathogenic processes is not known. Furthermore, a specific underlying immunologic basis for these events has not been identified. Upon the appearance of rash or of other possibly allergic phenomena for which an alternative etiology cannot be identified, fluoxetine HCl should be discontinued.

PRECAUTIONS:

GENERAL

Anxiety and Insomnia: In U.S. placebo-controlled clinical trials for depression, 12% to 16% of patients treated with fluoxetine HCl and 7% to 9% of patients treated with placebo reported anxiety, nervousness, or insomnia.

In U.S. placebo-controlled clinical trials for obsessive-compulsive disorder, insomnia was reported in 30% of patients treated with fluoxetine HCl and in 28% of patients treated with placebo. Anxiety was reported in 14% of patients treated with fluoxetine HCl and in 7% of patients treated with placebo.

In U.S. placebo-controlled clinical trials for bulimia nervosa, insomnia was reported in 33% of patients treated with fluoxetine, 60 mg, and 13% of patients treated with placebo. Anxiety and nervousness were reported respectively in 15% and 11% of patients treated with fluoxetine HCl, 60 mg, and in 9% and 5% of patients treated with placebo.

PRECAUTIONS: *(cont'd)*

Among the most common adverse events associated with discontinuation in U.S. placebo-controlled fluoxetine clinical trials were anxiety (≤2%), insomnia (≤2%), and nervousness (≤1%) (see TABLE 4).

Altered Appetite and Weight: Significant weight loss, especially in underweight depressed or bulimic patients may be an undesirable result of treatment with fluoxetine HCl.

In U.S. placebo-controlled clinical trials for depression, 11% of patients treated with fluoxetine HCl and 2% of patients treated with placebo reported anorexia (decreased appetite). Weight loss was reported in 1.4% of patients treated with fluoxetine HCl and in 0.5% of patients treated with placebo. However, only rarely have patients discontinued treatment with fluoxetine HCl because of anorexia or weight loss.

In U.S. placebo-controlled clinical trials for OCD, 17% of patients treated with fluoxetine HCl and 10% of patients treated with placebo reported anorexia (decreased appetite). One patient discontinued treatment with fluoxetine HCl because of anorexia.

In U.S. placebo-controlled clinical trials for bulimia nervosa, 8% of patients treated with fluoxetine HCl, 60 mg, and 4% of patients treated with placebo reported anorexia (decreased appetite). Patients treated with fluoxetine HCl, 60 mg, on average lost 0.45 kg compared with a gain of 0.16 kg by patients treated with placebo in the 16-week doublble-blind trial. Weight change should be monitored during therapy.

Activation of Mania/Hypomania: In U.S. placebo-controlled clinical trials for depression, mania/hypomania was reported in 0.1% of patients treated with fluoxetine HCl and 0.1% of patients treated with placebo. Activation of mania/hypomania has also been reported in a small proportion of patients with Major Affective Disorder treated with other marketed antidepressants.

In U.S. placebo-controlled clinical trials for OCD, mania/hypomania was reported in 0.8% of patients treated with fluoxetine HCl and no patients treated with placebo. No patients reported mania/hypomania in U.S. placebo-controlled clinical trials for bulimia. In all U.S. fluoxetine HCl clinical trials, 0.7% of 10782 patients reported mania/hypomania.

Seizures: In U.S. placebo-controlled clinical trials for depression, convulsions (or events described as possibly having been seizures) were reported in 0.1% of patients treated with fluoxetine HCl and 0.2% of patients treated with placebo. No patients reported convulsions in U.S. placebo-controlled clinical trials for either OCD or bulimia. In all U.S. fluoxetine HCl clinical trials, 0.2% of 10782 patients reported convulsions. The percentage appears to be similar to that associated with other marketed antidepressants. Fluoxetine HCl should be introduced with care in patients with a history of seizures.

Suicide: The possibility of a suicide attempt is inherent in depression and may persist until significant remission occurs. Close supervision of high risk patients should accompany initial drug therapy. Prescriptions for fluoxetine HCl should be written for the smallest quantity of capsules consistent with good patient management, in order to reduce the risk of overdose.

Because of well-established comorbidity between both OCD and depression and bulimia and depression, the same precautions observed when treating patients with depression should be observed when treating patients with OCD or bulimia.

The Long Elimination Half-Lives of Fluoxetine and Its Metabolites: Because of the long elimination half-lives of the parent drug and its major active metabolite, changes in dose will not be fully reflected in plasma for several weeks, affecting both strategies for titration to final dose and withdrawal from treatment (see CLINICAL PHARMACOLOGY and DOSAGE AND ADMINISTRATION).

Use in Patients With Concomitant Illness: Clinical experience with fluoxetine HCl in patients with concomitant systemic illness is limited. Caution is advisable in using fluoxetine HCl in patients with diseases or conditions that could affect metabolism or hemodynamic responses.

Fluoxetine has not been evaluated or used to any appreciable extent in patients with a recent history of myocardial infarction or unstable heart disease. Patients with these diagnoses were systematically excluded from clinical studies during the product's premarket testing. However, the electrocardiograms of 312 patients who received fluoxetine HCl in double-blind trials were retrospectively evaluated; no conduction abnormalities that resulted in heart block were observed. The mean heart rate was reduced by approximately 3 beats/min.

In subjects with cirrhosis of the liver, the clearances of fluoxetine and its active metabolite, norfluoxetine, were decreased, thus increasing the elimination half-lives of these substances. A lower or less frequent dose should be used in patients with cirrhosis.

Since fluoxetine is extensively metabolized, excretion of unchanged drug in urine is a minor route of elimination. However, until adequate numbers of patients with severe renal impairment have been evaluated during chronic treatment with fluoxetine, it should be used with caution in such patients.

In patients with diabetes, fluoxetine HCl may alter glycemic control. Hypoglycemia has occurred during therapy with fluoxetine HCl, and hyperglycemia has developed following discontinuation of the drug. As is true with many other types of medication when taken concurrently by patients with diabetes, insulin and/or oral hypoglycemic dosage may need to be adjusted when therapy with fluoxetine HCl is instituted or discontinued.

Interference With Cognitive and Motor Performance: Any psychoactive drug may impair judgment, thinking, or motor skills, and patients should be cautioned about operating hazardous machinery, including automobiles, until they are reasonably certain that the drug treatment does not affect them adversely.

INFORMATION FOR THE PATIENT

Physicians are advised to discuss the following issues with patients for whom they prescribe fluoxetine HCl:

Because fluoxetine HCl may impair judgment, thinking, or motor skills, patients should be advised to avoid driving a car or operating hazardous machinery until they are reasonably certain that their performance is not affected.

Patients should be advised to inform their physician if they are taking or plan to take any prescription or over-the-counter drugs, or alcohol.

Patients should be advised to notify their physician if they become pregnant or intend to become pregnant during therapy.

Patients should be advised to notify their physician if they are breast feeding an infant.

Patients should be advised to notify their physician if they develop a rash or hives.

LABORATORY TESTS

There are no specific laboratory tests recommended.

CARCINOGENESIS, MUTAGENESIS, AND IMPAIRMENT OF FERTILITY

There is no evidence of carcinogenicity, mutagenicity, or impairment of fertility with fluoxetine HCl.

The dietary administration of fluoxetine to rats and mice for 2 years at levels equivalent to approximately 7.5 and 9.0 times the maximum human dose (80 mg) respectively produced no evidence of carcinogenicity.

Fluoxetine and norfluoxetine have been shown to have no genotoxic effects based on the following assays: bacterial mutation assay, DNA repair assay in cultured rat hepatocytes, mouse lymphoma assay, and *in vivo* sister chromatid exchange assay in Chinese hamster bone marrow cells.

PRECAUTIONS: *(cont'd)*

Two fertility studies conducted in rats at doses of approximately 5 and 9 times the maximum human dose (80 mg) indicated that fluoxetine had no adverse effects on fertility. A slight decrease in neonatal survival was noted, but this was probably associated with depressed maternal food consumption and suppressed weight gain.

PREGNANCY, TERATOGENIC EFFECTS, PREGNANCY CATEGORY B

Reproduction studies have been performed in rats and rabbits at doses 9 and 11 times the maximum daily human dose (80 mg) respectively and have revealed no evidence of harm to the fetus due to fluoxetine HCl. There are, however, no adequate and well-controlled studies in pregnant women. Because animal reproduction studies are not always predictive of human response, this drug should be used during pregnancy only if clearly needed.

LABOR AND DELIVERY

The effect of fluoxetine HCl on labor and delivery in humans is unknown.

NURSING MOTHERS

Because fluoxetine HCl is excreted in human milk, nursing while on fluoxetine HCl is not recommended. In 1 breast milk sample, the concentration of fluoxetine plus norfluoxetine was 70.4 ng/ml. The concentration in the mother's plasma was 295.0 ng/ml. No adverse effects on the infant were reported. In another case, an infant nursed by a mother on fluoxetine HCl developed crying, sleep disturbance, vomiting, and watery stools. The infant's plasma drug levels were 340 ng/ml of fluoxetine and 208 ng/ml of norfluoxetine on the second day of feeding.

PEDIATRIC USE

Safety and effectiveness in children have not been established.

GERIATRIC USE

Evaluation of patients over the age of 60 who received fluoxetine HCl 20 mg daily revealed no unusual pattern of adverse events relative to the clinical experience in younger patients. However, these data are insufficient to rule out possible age-related differences during chronic use, particularly in elderly patients who have concomitant systemic illnesses or who are receiving concomitant drugs (see CLINICAL PHARMACOLOGY, Age).

HYPONATREMIA

Several cases of hyponatremia (some with serum sodium lower than 110 mmol/l) have been reported. The hyponatremia appeared to be reversible when fluoxetine HCl was discontinued. Although these cases were complex with varying possible etiologies, some were possibly due to the syndrome of inappropriate antidiuretic hormone secretion (SIADH). The majority of these occurrences have been in older patients and in patients taking diuretics or who were otherwise volume depleted. In a placebo-controlled, double-blind trial, 10 of 313 fluoxetine patients and 6 of 320 placebo recipients had a lowering of serum sodium below the reference range; this difference was not statistically significant. The lowest observed concentration was 129 mmol/l. The observed decreases were not clinically significant.

PLATELET FUNCTION

There have been rare reports of altered platelet function and/or abnormal results from laboratory studies in patients taking fluoxetine. While there have been reports of abnormal bleeding in several patients taking fluoxetine, it is unclear whether fluoxetine had a causative role.

DRUG INTERACTIONS:

As with all drugs, the potential for interaction by a variety of mechanisms (*e.g.*, pharmacodynamic, pharmacokinetic drug inhibition or enhancement, etc.) is a possibility (see CLINICAL PHARMACOLOGY, Accumulation and Slow Elimination).

DRUGS METABOLIZED BY P450IID6

Approximately 7% of the normal population has a genetic defect that leads to reduced levels of activity of the cytochrome P450 isoenzyme P450IID6. Such individuals have been referred to as "poor metabolizers" of drugs such as debrisoquin, dextromethorphan, and tricyclic antidepressants. Many drugs, such as most antidepressants, including fluoxetine and other selective uptake inhibitors of serotonin, are metabolized by this isoenzyme; thus, both the pharmacokinetic properties and relative proportion of metabolites are altered in poor metabolizers. However, for fluoxetine and its metabolite the sum of the plasma concentrations of the 4 active enantiomers is comparable between poor and extensive metabolizers (see CLINICAL PHARMACOLOGY, Variability in Metabolism).

Fluoxetine, like other agents that are metabolized by P450IID6, inhibits the activity of this isoenzyme, and thus may make normal metabolizers resemble "poor metabolizers." Therapy with medications that are predominantly metabolized by the P450IID6 system and that have a relatively narrow therapeutic index (see list), should be initiated at the low end of the dose range if a patient is receiving fluoxetine concurrently or has taken it in the previous 5 weeks. Thus, his/her dosing requirements resemble those of "poor metabolizers." If fluoxetine is added to the treatment regimen of a patient already receiving a drug metabolized by P450IID6, the need for decreased dose of the original medication should be considered. Drugs with a narrow therapeutic index represent the greatest concern:

flecainide

vinblastine

tricyclic antidepressants

DRUGS METABOLIZED BY CYTOCHROME P450IIIA4

In an *in vivo* interaction study involving co-administration of fluoxetine with single doses of terfenadine (a cytochrome P450IIIA4 substrate), no increase in plasma terfenadine concentrations occurred with concomitant fluoxetine. In addition, *in vitro* studies have shown ketoconazole, a potent inhibitor of P450IIIA4 activity, to be at least 100 times more potent than fluoxetine or norfluoxetine as an inhibitor of the metabolism of several substrates for this enzyme, including astemizole, cisapride, and midazolam. These data indicate the fluoxetine's extent of inhibition of cytochrome P450IIIA4 activity is not likely to be of clinical significance.

CNS ACTIVE DRUGS

The risk of using fluoxetine HCl in combination with other CNS active drugs has not been systematically evaluated. Nonetheless, caution is advised if the concomitant administration of fluoxetine HCl and such drugs is required. In evaluating individual cases, consideration should be given to using lower initial doses of the concomitantly administered drugs, using conservative titration schedules, and monitoring of clinical status (see CLINICAL PHARMACOLOGY, Accumulation and Slow Elimination).

Anticonvulsants: Patients on stable doses of phenytoin and carbamazepine have developed elevated plasma anticonvulsant concentrations and clinical anticonvulsant toxicity following initiation of concomitant fluoxetine treatment.

Antipsychotics: Some clinical data suggests a possible pharmacodynamic and/or pharmacokinetic interaction between serotonin specific reuptake inhibitors (SSRIs) and antipsychotics. Elevation of blood levels of haloperidol and clozapine has been observed in patients receiving concomitant fluoxetine. A single case report has suggested possible additive effects of pimozide and fluoxentine leading to bradycardia.

DRUG INTERACTIONS: *(cont'd)*

Benzodiazepines: The half-life of concurrently administered diazepam may be prolonged in some patients (see CLINICAL PHARMACOLOGY, Accumulation and Slow Elimination). Coadministration of alprazolam and fluoxetine has resulted in increased alprazolam plasma concentrations and in further psychomotor performance due to increased alprazolam levels.

Lithium: There have been reports of both increased and decreased lithium levels when lithium was used concomitantly with fluoxetine. Cases of lithium toxicity and increased serotonergic effects have been reported. Lithium levels should be monitored when these drugs are administered concomitantly.

Tryptophan: Five patients receiving fluoxetine HCl in combination with tryptophan experienced adverse reactions, including agitation, restlessness, and gastrointestinal distress.

Monoamine Oxidase Inhibitors: See CONTRAINDICATIONS.

Other Antidepressants: In two studies, previously stable plasma levels of imipramine and desipramine have increased greater than 2 to 10-fold when fluoxetine has been administered in combination. This influence may persist for three weeks or longer after fluoxetine is discontinued. Thus, the dose of tricyclic antidepressant (TCA) may need to be reduced and plasma TCA concentrations may need to be monitored temporarily when fluoxetine is coadministered or has been recently discontinued (see CLINICAL PHARMACOLOGY, Accumulation and Slow Elimination).

POTENTIAL EFFECTS OF COADMINISTRATION OF DRUGS TIGHTLY BOUND TO PLASMA PROTEINS

Because fluoxetine is tightly bound to plasma protein, the administration of fluoxetine to a patient taking another drug that is tightly bound to protein (*e.g.*, Coumadin, digitoxin) may cause a shift in plasma concentrations potentially resulting in an adverse effect. Conversely, adverse effects may result from displacement of protein bound fluoxetine by other tightly bound drugs (see CLINICAL PHARMACOLOGY, Accumulation and Slow Elimination).

Warfarin: Altered anti-coagulant effects, including increased bleeding, have been reported when fluoxetine is co-administered with warfarin. Patients receiving warfarin therapy should receive careful coagulation monitoring when fluoxetine is initiated or stopped.

Electroconvulsive Therapy: There are no clinical studies establishing the benefit of the combined use of ECT and fluoxetine. There have been rare reports of prolonged seizures in patients on fluoxetine receiving ECT treatment.

ADVERSE REACTIONS:

Multiple doses of fluoxetine HCl had been administered to 10782 patients with various diagnoses in U.S. clinical trials as of May 8, 1995. Adverse events were recorded by clinical investigators using descriptive terminology of their own choosing. Consequently, it is not possible to provide a meaningful estimate of the proportion of individuals experiencing adverse events without first grouping similar types of events into a limited (*i.e.*, reduced) number of standardized event categories.

In TABLE 3 and TABLE 4 the COSTART Dictionary terminology has been used to classify reported adverse events. The stated frequencies represent the proportion of individuals who experienced, at least once, a treatment-emergent adverse event of the type listed. An event was considered treatment-emergent if it occurred for the first time or worsened while receiving therapy following baseline evaluation. It is important to emphasize that event reported during therapy were not necessarily caused by it.

The prescriber should be aware that the figures in the tables and tabulations cannot be used to predict the incidence of side effects in the course of usual medical practice where patient characteristics and other factors differ from those that prevailed in the clinical trials. Similarly, the cited frequencies cannot be compared with figures obtained from other clinical investigations involving different treatments, uses, and investigators. The cited figures, however, do provide the prescribing physician with some basis for estimating the relative contribution of drug and nondrug factors to the side effect incidence rate in the population studied.

INCIDENCE IN U.S. PLACEBO-CONTROLLED CLINICAL TRIALS (EXCLUDING DATA FROM EXTENSIONS OF TRIALS)

TABLE 2A, TABLE 2B, and TABLE 2C enumerate the most common treatment-emergent adverse events associated with the use of fluoxetine HCl (incidence of at least 5% for fluoxetine and depression, OCD, and bulimia in U.S. controlled clinical trials. TABLE 3 enumerates treatment-emergent adverse events that occurred in 2% or more patients treated with fluoxetine HCl and with incidence greater than placebo who participated in U.S. controlled clinical trials comparing fluoxetine HCl with placebo in the treatment of depression, OCD, or bulimia. TABLE 3 provides combined data for the pool of studies that are provided separately by indication in TABLE 2A, TABLE 2B, and TABLE 2C.

ASSOCIATED WITH DISCONTINUATION IN U.S. PLACEBO-CONTROLLED CLINICAL TRIALS (EXCLUDING DATA FROM EXTENSIONS OF TRIALS)

TABLE 4 lists the adverse events associated with discontinuation of fluoxetine HCl treatment (incidence at least twice that for placebo and at least 1% for fluoxetine HCl in clinical trials) in depression, OCD, and bulimia.

Other Events Observed During Premarketing Evaluation of Fluoxetine HCl: Following is a list of all treatment-emergent adverse events reported at anytime by individuals taking fluoxetine in U.S. clinical trials (10782 patients) except (1) those listed in the body or footnotes of TABLE 2A, TABLE 2B, TABLE 2C or TABLE 3 or elsewhere in labeling; (2) those for which the COSTART terms were uninformative or misleading; (3) those events for which a causal relationship to fluoxetine HCl use was considered remote; and (4) events occurring in only 1 patient treated with fluoxetine HCl and which did not have a substantial probability of being acutely life-threatening.

Events are further classified within body system categories using the following definitions: frequent adverse events are defined as those occurring on 1 or more occasions in at least 1/100 patients; infrequent adverse events are those occurring in 1/100 to 1/1,000 patients; rare events are those occurring in less than 1/1,000 patients.

Body as a Whole: *Frequent:* chills; *Infrequent:* chills and fever, face edema, intentional overdose, malaise, pelvic pain, suicide attempt; *Rare:* abdomen acute syndrome, hypothermia, intentional injury, neuroleptic malignant syndrome, photosensitivity.

Cardiovascular System: *Frequent:* hemorrhage, hypertension; *Infrequent:* angina pectoris, arrhythmia, congestive heart failure, hemorrhage, hypotension, migraine, myocardial infarct, postural hypotension, syncope, and tachycardia, vascular headache; *Rare:* atrial fibrillation, bradycardia, cerebral embolism, cerebral ischemia, cerebrovascular accident, extrasystoles, heart arrest, heart block, pallor, peripheral vascular disorder, phlebitis, shock, thrombophlebitis, thrombosis, vasospasm, ventricular arrhythmia, ventricular extrasystoles, ventricular fibrillation.

Digestive System: *Frequent:* increased appetite, nausea and vomiting; *Infrequent:* aphthous stomatitis, cholelithiasis, colitis, dysphagia, eructation, esophagitis, gastritis, gastroenteritis, glossitis, gum hemorrhage, hyperchlorhydria, increased salivation, liver function tests abnormal, melena, mouth ulceration, nausea/vomiting/diarrhea, stomach ulcer, stomatitis, thirst; *Rare:* biliary pain, bloody diarrhea, cholecystitis, duodenal ulcer, enteritis, esophageal ulcer, fecal incontinence, gastrointestinal hemorrhage, hematemesis, hemorrhage of colon, hepatitis, intestinal obstruction, liver fatty deposit, pancreatitis, peptic ulcer, rectal hemorrhage, salivary gland enlargement, stomach ulcer hemorrhage, tongue edema.

ADVERSE REACTIONS: *(cont'd)*

TABLE 2A Most Common Treatment-Emergent Adverse Events: Incidence In U.S. Placebo-Controlled Clinical Trials

	Percentage of Patients Reporting Event Depression	
Body System/Adverse Event	**Fluoxetine HCl (N=1,728)**	**Placebo (N=975)**
Body as a Whole		
Asthenia	9	5
Flu syndrome	3	4
Cardiovascular System		
Vasodilation	3	2
Digestive System		
Nausea	21	9
Anorexia	11	2
Dry mouth	10	7
Dyspepsia	7	5
Nervous System		
Insomnia	16	9
Anxiety	12	7
Nervousness	14	9
Somnolence	13	6
Tremor	10	3
Libido decreased	3	—
Abnormal dreams	1	1
Respiratory System		
Pharyngitis	3	3
Sinusitis	1	4
Yawn	—	—
Skin and Appendages		
Sweating	8	3
Rash	4	3
Urogenital		
Impotence*	2	—
Abnormal ejaculation*	—	—

* Denominator used was males only (N=690 fluoxetine HCl depression; N=410 placebo depression; N=116 fluoxetine HCl OCD; N=43 placebo OCD; N=14 fluoxetine HCl bulimia; N=1 placebo bulimia).
— Incidence less than 1%.

TABLE 2B Most Common Treatment-Emergent Adverse Events: Incidence In U.S. Placebo-Controlled Clinical Trials

	Percentage of Patients Reporting Event OCD	
Body System/Adverse Event	**Fluoxetine HCl (N=266)**	**Placebo (N=89)**
Body as a Whole		
Asthenia	15	11
Flu syndrome	10	7
Cardiovascular System		
Vasodilation	5	—
Digestive System		
Nausea	26	13
Anorexia	17	10
Dry mouth	12	3
Dyspepsia	10	4
Nervous System		
Insomnia	28	22
Anxiety	14	7
Nervousness	14	15
Somnolence	17	7
Tremor	9	1
Libido decreased	11	2
Abnormal dreams	5	2
Respiratory System		
Pharyngitis	11	9
Sinusitis	5	2
Yawn	7	—
Skin and Appendages		
Sweating	7	—
Rash	6	3
Urogenital		
Impotence*	—	—
Abnormal ejaculation*	7	—

* Denominator used was males only (N=690 fluoxetine HCl depression; N=410 placebo depression; N=116 fluoxetine HCl OCD; N=43 placebo OCD; N=14 fluoxetine HCl bulimia; N=1 placebo bulimia).
— Incidence less than 1%.

Endocrine System: *Infrequent:* hypothyroidism;*Rare:* diabetic acidosis, diabetes mellitus.

Hemic and Lymphatic System: *Infrequent:* anemia and lymphadenopathy; *Rare:* blood dyscrasia, hypochromic anemia, leukopenia, lymphedema, lymphocytosis, petechia, purpura, thrombocythemia, thrombocytopenia.

Metabolic and Nutritional: *Frequent:* weight gain; *Infrequent:* dehydration, generalized edema, gout, hypocholesteremia, hyperlipemia, hypokalemia, peripheral edema; *Rare:* alcohol intolerance, alkaline phosphatase increased, BUN increased, creatine phosphokinase increased, hyperkalemia, hyperuricemia, hypocalcemia, iron deficiency anemia, SGPT increased.

Musculoskeletal System: *Infrequent:* arthritis, bone pain, bursitis, leg cramps, tenosynovitis; *Rare:*arthrosis, chondrodystrophy, myasthenia, myopathy, myositis, osteomyelitis, osteoporosis, rheumatoid arthritis.

Nervous System: *Frequent:* agitation, amnesia, confusion, emotional lability, sleep disorder; *Infrequent:* abnormal gait, acute brain syndrome, akathisia, apathy, ataxia, buccoglossal syndrome, CNS depression, CNS stimulation, depersonalization, euphoria, hallucinations, hostility, hyperkinesia, hypertonia, hypesthesia, incoordination, libido increased, myoclonus, neuralgia, neuropathy, neurosis, paranoid reaction, personality disordert, psychosis, and vertigo; *Rare:* abnormal electroencephalogram, antisocial reaction, circumoral paresthesia, coma, delusions, dysarthria, dystonia, extrapyramidal syndrome, foot drop, hyperesthesia, neuritis, paralysis, reflexes decreased, reflexes increased, stupor.

Respiratory System: *Infrequent:* asthma, epistaxis, hiccup, hyperventilation; *Rare:* apnea, atelectasis, cough decreased, emphysema, hemoptysis, hypoventilation, hypoxia, larynx edema, lung edema, pneumothorax, stridor.

Skin and Appendages: *Infrequent:* acne, alopecia, contact dermatitis, eczema, maculopapular rash, skin discoloration, skin ulcer, vesiculobullous rash; *Rare:* furunculosis, herpes zoster, hirsutism, petecial rash, psoriasis, purpuric rash, pustular rash, seborrhea.

ADVERSE REACTIONS: *(cont'd)*

TABLE 2C Most Common Treatment-Emergent Adverse Events: Incidence In U.S. Placebo-Controlled Clinical Trials

	Percentage of Patients Reporting Event Bulimia	
Body System/Adverse Event	**Fluoxetine HCl (N=450)**	**Placebo (N=267)**
Body as a Whole		
Asthenia	21	9
Flu syndrome	8	3
Cardiovascular System		
Vasodilation	2	1
Digestive System		
Nausea	29	11
Anorexia	8	4
Dry mouth	9	6
Dyspepsia	10	6
Nervous System		
Insomnia	33	13
Anxiety	15	9
Nervousness	11	5
Somnolence	13	5
Tremor	13	1
Libido decreased	5	1
Abnormal dreams	5	3
Respiratory System		
Pharyngitis	10	5
Sinusitis	6	4
Yawn	11	—
Skin and Appendages		
Sweating	8	3
Rash	4	4
Urogenital		
Impotence*	7	—
Abnormal ejaculation*	7	—

* Denominator used was males only (N=690 fluoxetine HCl depression; N=410 placebo depression; N=116 fluoxetine HCl OCD; N=43 placebo OCD; N=14 fluoxetine HCl bulimia; N=1 placebo bulimia).
— Incidence less than 1%.

TABLE 3 Treatment-Emergent Adverse Events: Incidence In U.S. Depression, OCD, and Bulimia Placebo-Controlled Clinical Trials

	Percentage of Patients Reporting Event Depression, OCD, and Bulimia	
Body System/Adverse Event*	**Fluoxetine HCl (N=2444)**	**Placebo (N=1331)**
Body as a Whole		
Headache	21	20
Asthenia	12	6
Flu syndrome	5	4
Fever	2	1
Cardiovascular System		
Vasodilation	3	1
Palpitation	2	1
Digestive System		
Nausea	23	10
Diarrhea	12	8
Anorexia	11	3
Dry mouth	10	7
Dyspepsia	8	5
Flatulence	3	2
Vomiting	3	2
Metabolic and Nutritional Disorders		
Weight loss	2	1
Nervous System		
Insomnia	20	11
Anxiety	13	8
Nervousness	13	9
Somnolence	13	6
Tremor	10	3
Libido decreased	4	—
Respiratory System		
Pharyngitis	5	4
Yawn	3	—
Skin and Appendages		
Sweating	8	3
Rash	4	3
Pruritus	3	2
Special Senses		
Abnormal vision	3	1

* Included are events reported by at least 2% of patients taking fluoxetine HCl, except the following events, which had an incidence on placebo ≥fluoxetine HCl (depression, OCD, and bulimia combined): abnormal pain, abnormal dreams, accidental injury, back pain, chest pain, constipation, cough increased, depression (includes suicidal thoughts), dysmenorrhea, gastrointestinal disorder, infection, myalgia, pain, paresthesia, rhinitis, sinusitus, thinking abnormal.
— Incidence less than 1%.

TABLE 4 Most Common Adverse Events Associated with Discontinuation in U.S. Depression, OCD, and Bulimia Placebo-controlled Clinical Trials

Depression, OCD, and bulima combined	Depression	OCD	Bulimia
—	—	Anxiety (2%)	—
Insomnia (1%)	Insomnia (1%)	—	Insomnia (2%)
—	Nausea (1%)	—	—
Nervousness (1%)	Nervousness (1%)	—	—
—	—	Rash (3%)	—

Special Senses: *Frequent:* ear pain, taste perversion, tinnitus; *Infrequent:* conjunctivitis, dry eyes, mydriasis, photophobia; *Rare:*blepharitis, deafness, diplopia, exophthalmos, eye hemorrhage, glaucoma, hyperacusis, iritis, parosmia, scleritis, strabismus, taste loss, visual field defect.

Urogenital System: *Frequent:* urinary frequency; *Infrequent:*abortion*, albuminuria, amenorrhea*, anorgasmia*, breast enlargement, breast pain, cystitis, dysuria, female lactation*, fibrocystic breast*, hematuria, leukorrhea*, menorrhagia*, metrorrhagia*, nocturia, polyuria,

ADVERSE REACTIONS: *(cont'd)*

urinary incontinence, urinary retention, urinary urgency, vaginal hemorrhage*; *Rare:* breast engorgement, glycosuria, hypomenorrhea*, kidney pain, oliguria, priapism*, uterine hemorrhage*, uterine fibroids enlarged*.

†Personality disorder is the COSTART term for designating non-aggresive objectionable behavior.

*Adjusted for gender.

Postintroduction Reports: Voluntary reports of adverse events temporally associated with fluoxetine HCl that have been received since market introduction, and that may have no causal relationship with the drug include the following: aplastic anemia, atrial fibrillation, cerebral vascular accident, cholestatic jaundice, confusion, dyskinesia (including, for example, a case of buccal-lingual-masticatory syndrome with involuntary tongue protrusion reported to develop in a 77-year-old female after 5 weeks of fluoxetine therapy and which completely resolved over the next few months following drug discontinuation), eosinophilic pneumonia, epidermal necrolysis, exfoliative dermatitis, gynecomastia, heart arrest, hepatic failure/necrosis, hyperprolactinemia, immune-related hemolytic anemia, kidney failure, misuse/abuse, movement disorders developing in patients with risk factors including drugs associated with such events and worsening or preexisting movement disorders, neuroleptic malignant syndrome-like events, pancreatitis, pancytopenia, priapism, pulmonary embolism, QT prolongation, Steven-Johnson syndrome, sudden unexpected death, suicidal ideation, thrombocytopenia, thrombocytopenic purpura, vaginal bleeding after drug withdrawal, and violent behaviors.

DRUG ABUSE AND DEPENDENCE:

Controlled Substance Class: Fluoxetine HCl is not a controlled substance.

Physical and Psychological Dependence: Fluoxetine HCl has not been systematically studied, in animals or humans, for its potential for abuse, tolerance, or physical dependence. While the premarketing clinical experience with fluoxetine HCl did not reveal any tendency for a withdrawal syndrome or any drug seeking behavior, these observations were not systematic and it is not possible to predict on the basis of this limited experience the extent to which a CNS active drug will be misused, diverted, and/or abused once marketed. Consequently, physicians should carefully evaluate patients for history of drug abuse and follow such patients closely, observing them for signs of misuse or abuse of fluoxetine HCl (*e.g.*, development of tolerance, incrementation of dose, drug-seeking behavior).

OVERDOSAGE:

HUMAN EXPERIENCE

As of December 1987, there were 2 deaths among approximately 38 reports of acute overdose with fluoxetine, either alone or in combination with other drugs and/or alcohol. One death involved a combined overdose with approximately 1,800 mg of fluoxetine and an undetermined amount of maprotiline. Plasma concentrations of fluoxetine and maprotiline were 4.57 mg/L and 4.18 mg/L, respectively. A second death involved 3 drugs yielding plasma concentrations as follows: fluoxetine, 1.93 mg/L; norfluoxetine, 1.10 mg/L; codeine, 1.80 mg/L; temazepam, 3.80 mg/L.

One other patient who reportedly took 3,000 mg of fluoxetine experienced 2 grand mal seizures that remitted spontaneously without specific anticonvulsant treatment (see Management of Overdose). The actual amount of drug absorbed may have been less due to vomiting.

Nausea and vomiting were prominent in overdoses involving higher fluoxetine doses. Other prominent symptoms of overdose included agitation, restlessness, hypomania, and other signs of CNS excitation. Except for the 2 deaths noted above, all other overdose cases recovered without residua.

Since introduction, reports of death attributed to overdosage of fluoxetine alone have been extremely rare.

ANIMAL EXPERIENCE

Studies in animals do not provide precise or necessarily valid information about the treatment of human overdose. However, animal experiments can provide useful insights into possible treatment strategies.

The oral median lethal dose in rats and mice was found to be 452 and 248 mg/kg respectively. Acute high oral doses produced hyperirritability and convulsions in several animal species.

Among 6 dogs purposely overdosed with oral fluoxetine, 5 experienced grand mal seizures. Seizures stopped immediately upon the bolus intravenous administration of a standard veterinary dose of diazepam. In this short term study, the lowest plasma concentration at which a seizure occurred was only twice the maximum plasma concentration seen in humans taking 80 mg/day, chronically.

In a separate single-dose study, the ECG of dogs given high doses did not reveal prolongation of the PR, QRS, or QT intervals. Tachycardia and an increase in blood pressure were observed. Consequently, the value of the ECG in predicting cardiac toxicity is unknown. Nonetheless, the ECG should ordinarily be monitored in cases of human overdose (see Management of Overdose).

MANAGEMENT OF OVERDOSE

Establish and maintain an airway; ensure adequate oxygenation and ventilation. Activated charcoal, which may be used with sorbitol, may be as or more effective than emesis or lavage, and should be considered in treating overdose.

Cardiac and vital signs monitoring is recommended, along with general symptomatic and supportive measures. Based on experience in animals, which may be relevant to humans, fluoxetine-induced seizures that fail to remit spontaneously may respond to diazepam.

There are no specific antidotes for fluoxetine HCl.

Due to the large volume of distribution of fluoxetine HCl, forced diuresis, dialysis, hemoperfusion, and exchange transfusion are unlikely to be of benefit.

In managing overdosage, consider the possibility of multiple drug involvement. A specific caution involves patients taking or recently having taken fluoxetine who might ingest by accident or intent, excessive quantities of a tricyclic antidepressant. In such a case, accumulation of the parent tricyclic and an active metabolite may increase the possibility of clinically significant sequelae and extend the time needed for close medical observation (see DRUG INTERACTIONS, Other Antidepressants).

The physician should consider contacting a poison control center on the treatment of any overdose.

DOSAGE AND ADMINISTRATION:

DEPRESSION

Initial Treatment: In controlled trials used to support the efficacy of fluoxetine, patients were administered morning doses ranging from 20 mg to 80 mg/day. Studies comparing fluoxetine 20, 40, and 60 mg/day to placebo indicate that 20 mg/day is sufficient to obtain a satisfactory antidepressant response in most cases. Consequently, a dose of 20 mg/day, administered in the morning, is recommended as the initial dose.

DOSAGE AND ADMINISTRATION: *(cont'd)*

A dose increase may be considered after several weeks if no clinical improvement is observed. Doses above 20 mg/day may be administered on a once a day (morning) or twice a day schedule (*i.e.*, morning and noon) and should not exceed a maximum dose of 80 mg/day.

As with other antidepressants, the full antidepressant effect may be delayed until 4 weeks of treatment or longer.

As with many other medications, a lower or less frequent dosage should be used in patients with renal and/or hepatic impairment. A lower or less frequent dosage should also be considered for patients, such as the elderly (see PRECAUTIONS, Usage in the Elderly), with concurrent disease or on multiple medications.

Maintenance/Continuation/Extended Treatment: There is no body of evidence available to answer the question of how long the patient treated with fluoxetine should remain on it. It is generally agreed among expert psychopharmacologists (circa 1987) that acute episodes of depression require several months or longer of sustained pharmacologic therapy. Whether the dose of antidepressant needed to induce remission is identical to the dose needed to maintain and/or sustain euthymia is unknown.

OBSESSIVE-COMPULSIVE DISORDER:

Initial Treatment: In the controlled clinical trials of fluoxetine supporting its effectiveness in the treatment of obsessive-compulsive disorder, patients were administered fixed daily doses of 20, 40, or 60 mg of fluoxetine or placebo (see CLINICAL STUDIES). In one of these studies, no dose response relationship for effectiveness was demonstrated. Consequently, a dose of 20 mg/day, administered in the morning, is recommended as the initial dose. Since there was a suggestion of a possible dose response relationship for effectiveness in the second study, a dose increase may be considered after several weeks if insufficient clinical improvement is observed. The full therapeutic effect may be delayed until 5 weeks of treatment or longer.

Doses above 20 mg/day may be administered on a once a day (*i.e.*, morning) or twice a day schedule (*i.e.*, morning and noon). A dose range of 20 to 60 mg/day is recommended, however, doses of up to 80 mg/day have been well tolerated in open studies of OCD. The maximum fluoxetine dose should not exceed 80 mg/day.

As with the use of fluoxetine HCl in depression, a lower or less frequent dosage should be used in patients with renal and/or hepatic impairment. A lower or less frequent dosage should also be considered for patients, such as the elderly (see PRECAUTIONS, Usage in the Elderly), with concurrent disease or on multiple medications.

Maintenance/Continuation Treatment: While there are no systematic studies that answer the question of how long to continue fluoxetine HCl, OCD is a chronic condition and it is reasonable to consider continuation for a responding patient. Although the efficacy of fluoxetine HCl after 13 weeks has not been documented in controlled trials, patients have been continued in therapy under double-blind conditions for up to an additional 6 months without loss of benefit. However, dosage adjustments should be made to maintain the patient on the lowest effective dosage, and patients should be periodically reassessed to determine the need for treatment.

BULIMIA NERVOSA

Initial Treatment: In the controlled clinical trials of fluoxetine supporting its effectiveness in the treatment of bulimia nervosa, patients were administered fixed daily fluoxetine doses of 20 or 60 mg, or placebo (see CLINICAL STUDIES). Only the 60 mg dose was statistically significantly superior to placebo in reducing the frequency of binge-eating and vomiting. Consequently, the recommended dose is 60 mg/day, administered in the morning. For some patients it may be advisable to titrate up to this target dose over several days. Fluoxetine doses above 60 mg/day have not been systematically studied in patients with bulimia.

As with the use of fluoxetine HCl in depression and OCD, a lower or less frequent dosage should be used in patients with renal and/or hepatic impairment. A lower or less frequent dosage should also be considered for patients, such as the elderly (see PRECAUTIONS, Geriatric Use), with concurrent disease or on multiple medications.

Maintenance/Continuation Treatment: While there are no systemic studies that answer the question of how long to continue fluoxetine HCl, bulimia is a chronic condition and it is reasonable to consider continuation for a responding patient. Although the efficacy of fluoxetine HCl after 16 weeks has not been documented in controlled trials, some patients have been continued in therapy under double-blind conditions for up to an additional 6 months without loss of benefit. However, patients should be periodically reassessed to determine the need for continued treatment.

Switching Patients to a Tricyclic Antidepressant (TCA): Dosage of a TCA may need to be reduced, and plasma TCA concentrations may need to be monitored temporarily when fluoxetine is coadministered or has been recently discontinued (see DRUG INTERACTIONS).

Switching Patients To or From a Monoamine Oxidase Inhibitor: At least 14 days should elapse between discontinuation of an MAOI and initiation of therapy with fluoxetine HCl. In addition, at least 5 weeks, perhaps longer, should be allowed after stopping fluoxetine HCl before starting an MAOI (see CONTRAINDICATIONS).

ANIMAL PHARMACOLOGY:

Animal Toxicology: Phospholipids are increased in some tissues of mice, rats, and dogs given fluoxetine chronically. This effect is reversible after cessation of fluoxetine treatment. Phospholipid accumulation in animals has been observed with many cationic amphiphilic drugs, including fenfluramine, imipramine, and ranitidine. The significance of this effect in humans is unknown.

PATIENT INFORMATION:

Fluoxetine is used for the treatment of depression, obsesive-compulsive disorder, and bulimia.

Notify your physician if you are pregnant or breast-feeding.

Do not take any other drugs, including over-the-counter medicines and alcohol, without consulting your physician.

Fluoxetine may cause dizziness or drowsiness, use caution while driving or operating hazardous machinery.

May cause rash or hive, notify your physician if these occur.

May cause anxiety, nervousness, drowsiness, dizziness, lightheadedness, insomnia, fatigue, or weakness, tremor, and sweating, stomache complaints, including anorexia, nausea, and diarrhea.

May be taken with or without food.

HOW SUPPLIED:

Store at controlled room temperature, 59° to 86°F (15° to 30°C).

HOW SUPPLIED - EQUIVALENTS NOT AVAILABLE:

Capsule, Gelatin - Oral - 10 mg

100's	$218.91	PROZAC, Dista	00777-3104-02
620's	$1373.04	PROZAC, Dista	00777-3104-82

HOW SUPPLIED - EQUIVALENTS NOT AVAILABLE: *(cont'd)*

Capsule, Gelatin - Oral - 20 mg

30's	$67.37	PROZAC, Dista	00777-3105-30
100's	$224.54	PROZAC, Dista	00777-3105-02
100's	$228.92	PROZAC, Dista	00777-3105-33
620's	$1407.95	PROZAC, Dista	00777-3105-82

Solution - Oral - 20 mg/5ml

5 ml x 50	$339.60	PROZAC, Xactdose	50962-0500-05
120 ml	$99.71	PROZAC, Dista	00777-5120-58

FLUOXYMESTERONE *(001321)*

CATEGORIES: Anabolic Steroids; Androgens; Antineoplastics; Breast Carcinoma; Cancer; Cryptorchidism; Delayed Puberty; Hormones; Hypogonadism; Oncologic Drugs; Tumors; Pregnancy Category X; DEA Class CIII; FDA Approval Pre 1982

BRAND NAMES: *Alomon*; Android-F; *Fluoron*; *Fuloan*; **Halotestin**; Hysterone; Ora-Testryl; *Oratestin*; *Stenox* (Mexico); *Vewon*
(International brand names outside U.S. in italics)

FORMULARIES: BC-BS; Medi-Cal

DESCRIPTION:

Halotestin Tablets contain fluoxymesterone, an androgenic hormone.

Fluoxymesterone is a white or nearly white, odorless, crystalline powder, melting at or about 240°C, with some decomposition. It is practically insoluble in water, sparingly soluble in alcohol, and slightly soluble in chloroform.

The chemical name for fluoxymesterone is androst-4-en-3-one, 9-fluoro-11,17-dihydroxy-17-methyl-, (11β,17β)-. The molecular formula is $C_{20}H_{29}FO_3$ and the molecular weight is 336.45.

Each Halotestin tablet, for oral administration, contains 2 mg, 5 mg or 10 mg fluoxymesterone. Inactive ingredients: calcium stearate, corn starch, FD&C yellow no. 5, lactose, sorbic acid, sucrose, tragacanth. In addition, the **2 mg** tablet contains FD&C yellow no. 6 and the**5 mg** and **10 mg** contain FD&C blue no. 2.

CLINICAL PHARMACOLOGY:

Endogenous androgens are responsible for normal growth and development of the male sex organs and for maintenance of secondary sex characteristics. These effects include growth and maturation of the prostate, seminal vesicles, penis, and scrotum; development of male hair distribution, such as beard, pubic, chest, and axillary hair; laryngeal enlargement, vocal cord thickening, and alterations in body musculature and fat distribution. Drugs in this class also cause retention of nitrogen, sodium, potassium, and phosphorus, and decreased urinary excretion of calcium. Androgens have been reported to increase protein anabolism and decrease protein catabolism. Nitrogen balance is improved only when there is sufficient intake of calories and protein.

Androgens are responsible for the growth spurt of adolescence and for eventual termination of linear growth, brought about by fusion of the epiphyseal growth centers. In children, exogenous androgens accelerate linear growth rates, but may cause disproportionate advancement in bone maturation. Use over long periods may result in fusion of the epiphyseal growth centers and termination of the growth process. Androgens have been reported to stimulate production of red blood cells by enhancing production of erythropoietic stimulation factor.

During exogenous administration of androgens, endogenous testosterone release is inhibited through feedback inhibition of pituitary luteinizing hormone (LH). At large doses of exogenous androgens, spermatogenesis may also be suppressed through feedback inhibition of pituitary follicle stimulating hormone (FSH).

Inactivation of testosterone occurs primarily in the liver.

The half-life of fluoxymesterone after oral administration is approximately 9.2 hours.

INDICATIONS AND USAGE:

In the Male: Fluoxymesterone tablets are indicated for:

1. Replacement therapy in conditions associated with symptoms of deficiency or absence of endogenous testosterone.

a. Primary hypogonadism (congenital or acquired)-testicular failure due to cryptorchidism, bilateral torsion, orchitis, vanishing testis syndrome; or orchidectomy.

b. Hypogonadotropic hypogonadism (congenital or acquired)-idiopathic gonadotropin or LHRH deficiency, or pituitary-hypothalamic injury from tumors, trauma, or radiation.

2. Delayed puberty, provided it has been definitely established as such, and is not just a familial trait.

In the Female: Fluoxymesterone Tablets are indicated for palliation of androgen-responsive recurrent mammary cancer in women who are more than one year but less than five years postmenopausal, or who have been proven to have a hormone-dependent tumor as shown by previous beneficial response to castration.

CONTRAINDICATIONS:

1. Known hypersensitivity to the drug
2. Males with carcinoma of the breast
3. Males with known or suspected carcinoma of the prostate gland
4. Women known or suspected to be pregnant
5. Patients with serious cardiac, hepatic or renal disease

WARNINGS:

Hypercalcemia may occur in immobilized patients and in patients with breast cancer. If this occurs, the drug should be discontinued.

Prolonged use of high doses of androgens (principally the 17-α alkyl-androgens) has been associated with development of hepatic adenomas, hepatocellular carcinoma, and peliosis hepatis-all potentially life-threatening complications.

Cholestatic hepatitis and jaundice may occur with 17-α-alkyl-androgens. Should this occur, the drug should be discontinued. This is reversible with discontinuation of the drug.

Geriatric patients treated with androgens may be at an increased risk of developing prostatic hypertrophy and prostatic carcinoma although conclusive evidence to support this concept is lacking.

Edema, with or without congestive heart failure, may be a serious complication in patients with pre-existing cardiac, renal or hepatic disease.

Gynecomastia may develop and occasionally persists in patients being treated for hypogonadism.

WARNINGS: *(cont'd)*

Androgen therapy should be used cautiously in males with delayed puberty. Androgens can accelerate bone maturation without producing compensatory gain in linear growth. The effect on bone maturation should be monitored by assessing bone age of the wrist and hand every six months.

This drug has not been shown to be safe and effective for the enhancement of athletic performance. Because of the potential risk of serious adverse health effects, this drug should not be used for such purpose.

PRECAUTIONS:

GENERAL

Women should be observed for signs of virilization which is usual following androgen use at high doses. Discontinuation of drug therapy at the time of evidence of mild virilism is necessary to prevent irreversible virilization. A decision may be made by the patient and the physician that some virilization will be tolerated during treatment for breast carcinoma.

Patients with benign prostatic hypertrophy may develop acute urethral obstruction. Priapism or excessive sexual stimulation may develop. Oligospermia may occur after prolonged administration or excessive dosage. If any of these effects appear, the androgen should be stopped and if restarted, a lower dosage should be utilized.

This product contains FD&C Yellow no. 5 (tartrazine) which may cause allergic-type reactions (including bronchial asthma) in certain susceptible individuals. Although the overall incidence of FD&C Yellow no. 5 (tartrazine) sensitivity in the general population is low, it is frequently seen in patients who also have aspirin hypersensitivity.

INFORMATION FOR THE PATIENT

Patients should be instructed to report any of the following: nausea, vomiting, changes in skin color, and ankle swelling. Males should be instructed to report too frequent or persistent erections of the penis and females any hoarseness, acne, changes in menstrual periods or increase in facial hair.

LABORATORY TESTS

Women with disseminated breast carcinoma should have frequent determination of urine and serum calcium levels during the course of androgen therapy (See WARNINGS).

Because of the hepatotoxicity associated with the use of 17-alpha-alkylated androgens, liver function tests should be obtained periodically.

Periodic (every six months) X-ray examinations of bone age should be made during treatment of prepubertal males to determine the rate of bone maturation and the effects of androgen therapy on the epiphyseal centers.

Hemoglobin and hematocrit levels (to detect polycythemia) should be checked periodically in patients receiving long-term androgen administration.

Serum cholesterol may increase during androgen therapy.

DRUG/LABORATORY TEST INTERACTIONS

Androgens may decrease levels of thyroxine-binding globulin, resulting in decreased total T_4 serum levels and increased resin uptake of T_3 and T_4. Free thyroid hormone levels remain unchanged, however, and there is no clinical evidence of thyroid dysfunction.

CARCINOGENESIS, MUTAGENESIS, AND IMPAIRMENT OF FERTILITY

Animal data: Testosterone has been tested by subcutaneous injection and implantation in mice and rats. The implant induced cervical-uterine tumors in mice, which metastasized in some cases. There is suggestive evidence that injection of testosterone into some strains of female mice increases their susceptibility to hepatoma. Testosterone is also known to increase the number of tumors and decrease the degree of differentiation of chemically-induced carcinomas of the liver in rats.

Human data: There are rare reports of hepatocellular carcinoma in patients receiving long-term therapy with androgens in high doses. Withdrawal of the drugs did not lead to regression of the tumors in all cases.

Geriatric patients treated with androgens may be at an increased risk of developing prostatic hypertrophy and prostatic carcinoma although conclusive evidence to support this concept is lacking.

This compound has not been tested for mutagenic potential. However, as noted above, carcinogenic effects have been attributed to treatment with androgenic hormones. The potential carcinogenic effects likely occur through a hormonal mechanism rather than by a direct chemical interaction mechanism.

Impairment of fertility was not tested directly in animal species. However, as noted below under Adverse Reactions, oligospermia in males and amenorrhea in females are potential adverse effects of treatment with Fluoxymeterone Tablets. Therefore, impairment of fertility is a possible outcome of treatment with Fluoxymeterone (fluoxymesterone).

PREGNANCY, TERATOGENIC EFFECTS, PREGNANCY CATEGORY X

See CONTRAINDICATIONS.

NURSING MOTHERS

Fluoxymeterone is not recommended for use in nursing mothers.

PEDIATRIC USE

Androgen therapy should be used very cautiously in children and only by specialists aware of the adverse effects on bone maturation. Skeletal maturation must be monitored every six months by an X-ray of the hand and wrist (See WARNINGS).

DRUG INTERACTIONS:

Androgens may increase sensitivity to oral anticoagulants. Dosage of the anticoagulant may require reduction in order to maintain satisfactory therapeutic hypoprothrombinemia.

Concurrent administration of oxyphenbutazone and androgens may result in elevated serum levels of oxyphenbutazone.

In diabetic patients, the metabolic effects of androgens may decrease blood glucose and, therefore, insulin requirements.

ADVERSE REACTIONS:

ENDOCRINE AND UROGENITAL

Female: The most common side effects of androgen therapy are amenorrhea and other menstrual irregularities; inhibition of gonadotropin secretion; and virilization, including deepening of the voice and clitoral enlargement. The latter usually is not reversible after androgens are discontinued. When administered to a pregnant woman, androgens can cause virilization of external genitalia of the female fetus.

Male: Gynecomastia, and excessive frequency and duration of penile erections. Oligospermia may occur at high dosage.

SKIN AND APPENDAGES

Hirsutism, male pattern of baldness, seborrhea, and acne.

FLUID AND ELECTROLYTE DISTURBANCES

Retention of sodium, chloride, water, potassium, calcium, and inorganic phosphates.

ADVERSE REACTIONS: *(cont'd)*

GASTROINTESTINAL

Nausea, cholestatic jaundice, alterations in liver function tests, rarely hepatocellular neoplasms and peliosis hepatis (see WARNINGS).

HEMATOLOGIC

Suppression of clotting factors II, V, VII, and X, bleeding in patients on concomitant anticoagulant therapy, and polycythemia.

NERVOUS SYSTEM

Increased or decreased libido, headache, anxiety, depression, and generalized paresthesia.

ALLERGIC

Hypersensitivity, including skin manifestations and anaphylactoid reactions.

DRUG ABUSE AND DEPENDENCE:

Controlled Substance Class: Fluoxymesterone is a controlled substance under the Anabolic Steroids Control Act, and Fluoxymesterone Tablets has been assigned to Schedule III.

OVERDOSAGE:

There have been no reports of acute overdosage with the androgens.

DOSAGE AND ADMINISTRATION:

The dosage will vary depending upon the individual, the condition being treated, and its severity. The total daily oral dose may be administered singly or in divided (three or four) doses.

Male Hypogonadism: For complete replacement in the hypogonadal male, a daily dose of 5 to 20 mg will suffice in the majority of patients. It is usually preferable to begin treatment with full therapeutic doses which are later adjusted to individual requirements. Priapism is indicative of excessive dosage and is indication for temporary withdrawal of the drug.

Delayed Puberty: Dosage should be carefully titrated utilizing a low dose, appropriate skeletal monitoring, and by limiting the duration of therapy to four to six months.

Inoperable Carcinoma of the Breast in the Female: The recommended total daily dose for palliative therapy in advanced inoperable carcinoma of the breast is 10 to 40 mg. Because of its short action, fluoxymesterone should be administered to patients in divided, rather than single, daily doses to ensure more stable blood levels. In general, it appears necessary to continue therapy for at least one month for a satisfactory subjective response, and for two to three months for an objective response.

Store at controlled room temperature 15-30°C (59-86°F)

HOW SUPPLIED - EQUIVALENTS NOT AVAILABLE:

Tablet, Uncoated - Oral - 2 mg

100's	**$44.82**	**HALOTESTIN, Pharmacia & Upjohn**	**00009-0014-01**

Tablet, Uncoated - Oral - 5 mg

100's	**$109.96**	**HALOTESTIN, Pharmacia & Upjohn**	**00009-0019-06**

Tablet, Uncoated - Oral - 10 mg

30's	**$50.29**	**HALOTESTIN, Pharmacia & Upjohn**	**00009-0036-03**
100's	$82.38	Fluoxymesterone, United Res	00677-0934-01
100's	$89.75	Fluoxymesterone, Rosemont	00832-0086-00
100's	$93.48	Fluoxymesterone, Qualitest Pharms	00603-3645-21
100's	$95.95	HYSTERONE, Major Pharms	00904-1218-60
100's	$111.00	Fluoxymesterone, IDE-Interstate	00814-3240-14
100's	$143.44	Fluoxymesterone, Rugby	00536-3826-01
100's	**$163.52**	**HALOTESTIN, Pharmacia & Upjohn**	**00009-0036-04**

FLUPHENAZINE DECANOATE *(001322)*

CATEGORIES: Antipsychotics/Antimanics; Central Nervous System Agents; Neuroleptics; Phenothiazine Tranquilizers; Psychotherapeutic Agents; Psychotic Disorders; Tranquilizers; FDA Approval Pre 1982

BRAND NAMES: *Anatensol*; *Anatensol Decanoato*; *Dapotum d*; *Dapotum D*; *Dapatum D25* (Germany); *Dapotum Depot*; *Deca*; *Decafen*; *Flucan*; *Fludecate*; *Fludecate Multidose*; Fluphenazine; *Modecate* (Australia, England, France); *Moditen*; *Moditen Depot*; *Phenazine*; *Prolixin-D*; **Prolixin Decanoate**; *Siqualone*; *Sydepres* *(International brand names outside U.S. in italics)*

FORMULARIES: Aetna; WHO

DESCRIPTION:

Fluphenazine Decanoate is the decanoate ester of a trifluoromethyl phenothiazine derivative. It is a highly potent behavior modifier with a markedly extended duration of effect. Fluphenazine Decanoate is available for intramuscular or subcutaneous administration, providing 25 mg fluphenazine decanoate per ml in a sesame oil vehicle with 1.2% (w/v) benzyl alcohol as a preservative. At the time of manufacture, the air in the vials is replaced by nitrogen.

CLINICAL PHARMACOLOGY:

The basic effects of fluphenazine decanoate appear to be no different from those of fluphenazine HCl, with the exception of duration of action. The esterification of fluphenazine markedly prolongs the drug's duration of effect without unduly attenuating the its beneficial action.

Fluphenazine Decanoate has activity at all levels of the central nervous system as well as on multiple organ systems. The mechanism whereby its therapeutic action is exerted is unknown.

Fluphenazine differs from other phenothiazine derivatives in several respects: it is more potent on a milligram basis, it has less potentiating effect on central nervous system depressants and anesthetics than do some of the phenothiazines to produce hypotension (nevertheless, appropriate cautions should be observed — see PRECAUTIONS and ADVERSE REACTIONS).

INDICATIONS AND USAGE:

Fluphenazine Decanoate Injection is a long-acting parenteral antipsychotic drug intended for use in the management of patients requiring prolonged parenteral neuroleptic therapy (*e.g.,* chronic schizophrenics).

Fluphenazine Decanoate has not been shown effective in the management of behavioral complications in patients with mental retardation.

CONTRAINDICATIONS:

Phenothiazines are contraindicated in patients with suspected or established or established subcortical brain damage.

Phenothiazine compounds should not be used in patients receiving large doses of hypnotics.

CONTRAINDICATIONS: *(cont'd)*

Fluphenazine Decanoate Injection is contraindicated in comatose or severely depressed states.

The presence of blood dyscrasia or liver damage precludes the use of fluphenazine decanoate.

Fluphenazine decanoate is not intended for use in children under 12 years of age.

Fluphenazine Decanoate is contraindicated in patients who have shown hypersensitivity to fluphenazine; cross-sensitivity to phenothiazine derivatives may occur.

WARNINGS:

TARDIVE DYSKINESIA

Tardive dyskinesia, a syndrome consisting of potentially irreversible, involuntary, dyskinetic movements may develop in patients treated with neuroleptic (antipsychotic) drugs. Although the prevalence of the syndrome appears to be highest among the elderly, especially elderly women, it is impossible to rely upon prevalence estimates to predict, at the inception of neuroleptic treatment, which patients are likely to develop the syndrome. Whether neuroleptic drug products differ in their potential to cause tardive dyskinesia is unknown.

Both the risk of developing the syndrome and the likelihood that it will become irreversible are believed to increase as the duration of treatment and the total cumulative dose of neuroleptic drugs administered to the patient increase. However, the syndrome can develop, although much less commonly, after relatively brief treatment periods at low doses.

There is no known treatment for established cases of tardive dyskinesia, although the syndrome may remit, partially or completely, if neuroleptic treatment is withdrawn. Neuroleptic treatment, itself, however, may suppress (or partially suppress) the signs and symptoms of the syndrome and thereby may possibly mask the underlying disease process. The effect that symptomatic suppression has upon the long-term course of the syndrome is unknown.

Given these considerations, neuroleptics should be prescribed in a manner that is most likely to minimize the occurrence of tardive dyskinesia. Chronic neuroleptic treatment should generally be reserved for patients who suffer from a chronic illness that, 1) is known to respond to neuroleptic drugs, and, 2) for whom alternative, equally effective, but potentially less harmful treatments are *not* available or appropriate. In patients who do require chronic treatment, the smallest dose and the shortest duration of treatment producing a satisfactory clinical response should be sought. The need for continued treatment should be reassessed periodically.

If signs and symptoms of tardive dyskinesia appear in a patient on neuroleptics, drug discontinuation should be considered. However, some patients may require treatment despite the presence of the syndrome. (For further information about the description of tardive dyskinesia and its clinical detention, please refer to the sections on PRECAUTIONS,Information for Patients and ADVERSE REACTIONS,Tardive Dyskinesia.)

NEUROLEPTIC MALIGNANT SYNDROME (NMS)

A potentially fatal symptom complex sometimes referred to as Neuroleptic Malignant Syndrome (NMS) has been reported in association with antipsychotic drugs. Clinical manifestations of NMS are hyperpyrexia, muscle rigidity, altered mental status and evidence of autonomic instability (irregular pulse or blood pressure, tachycardia, diaphoresis, and cardiac dysrhythmias).

The diagnostic evaluation of patients with this syndrome is complicated. In arriving at a diagnosis, it is important to identify cases where the clinical presentation includes both serious mental illness (*e.g.,* pneumonia, systemic infection, etc.) and untreated or inadequately treated extrapyramidal signs and symptoms (EPS). Other important considerations in the differential diagnosis include anticholinergic toxicity, heat stroke, drug fever and primary central nervous system (CNS) pathology.

The management of NMS should include 1) immediate discontinuation of antipsychotic drugs and other drugs not essential to concurrent therapy, 2) intensive symptomatic treatment and medical monitoring, and 3) treatment of any concomitant serious medical problems for which specific treatments are available. There is no general agreement about specific pharmacological treatment regimens for uncomplicated NMS.

If a patient requires antipsychotic drug treatment after recovery from NMS, the potential reintroduction of drug therapy should be carefully considered. The patient should be carefully monitored, since recurrences of NMS have been reported.

The use of this drug may impair the mental and physical abilities required for driving a car or operating heavy machinery.

Physicians should be alert to the possibility that severe reactions may which require immediate medical attention.

Potentiation of the effects of alcohol may occur with use of this drug.

Since there is no adequate experience in children who have received this drug, safety and efficacy in children have not been established.

USAGE IN PREGNANCY

The safety for the use of the drug during pregnancy has not been established; therefore, the possible hazards should be weighed against the potential benefits when administering this drug to pregnant patients.

PRECAUTIONS:

GENERAL

Because of the possibility of cross-sensitivity, fluphenazine decanoate should be used cautiously in patients who have developed cholestatic jaundice, dermatoses, or other allergic reactions to phenothiazine derivatives.

Psychotic patients on large doses of a phenothiazine drug who are undergoing surgery should be watched carefully for possible hypotensive phenomena. Moreover, it should be remembered that reduced amounts of anesthetics or central nervous system depressants may be necessary.

The effects of atropine may be potentiated in some patients receiving fluphenazine because of added anticholinergic effects.

Fluphenazine decanoate should be used cautiously in patients exposed to extreme heat or phosphorus insecticides.

The preparation should be used with caution in patients with a history of convulsive disorders, since grand mal convulsions have been know to occur.

Use with caution in patients with special medical disorders such as mitral insufficiency or other cardiovascular diseases and pheochromocytoma.

The possibility of liver damage, pigmentary retinopathy, lenticular and corneal deposits, and development of irreversible dyskinesia should be remembered when patients are on prolonged therapy.

Outside state hospitals or psychiatric institutions, fluphenazine decanoate should be administered under the direction of a physician experienced in the clinical use of psychotropic drugs, particularly phenothiazine derivatives. Furthermore, facilities should be available for periodic checking of hepatic function, renal function, and the blood picture. Renal function of patients on long-term therapy should be monitored; If BUN (blood urea nitrogen) becomes abnormal, treatment should be discontinued.

As with any phenothiazine, the physician should be alert to the possible development of "silent pneumonias" in patients under treatment with fluphenazine decanoate.

PRECAUTIONS: *(cont'd)*

Neuroleptic drugs elevate prolactin levels; the elevation persists during chronic administration. Tissue culture experiments indicate that approximately one-third of human breast cancers are prolactin dependent*in vitro*, a factor of potential importance if the prescription of these drugs is contemplated in a patient with previously detected breast cancer. Although disturbances such as galactorrhea, amenorrhea, gynecomastia, and impotence have been reported, the clinical significance of elevated serum prolactin levels is unknown for most patients. An increase in mammary neoplasms has been found in rodents after chronic administration of neuroleptic drugs. Neither clinical studies nor epidemiologic studies conducted to date, however, have shown an association between chronic administration of these drugs and mammary tumorigenesis; the available evidence is considered too limited to be conclusive at this time.

INFORMATION FOR THE PATIENT

Given the likelihood that a substantial proportion of patients exposed chronically to neuroleptics will develop tardive dyskinesia, it is advised that patients in whom chronic use is contemplated to be given, if possible, full information about this risk. The decision to inform patients and/or their guardians must obviously take into account the clinical circumstances and the competency of the patient to understand the information provided.

ADVERSE REACTIONS:

Central Nervous System: The side effects most frequently reported with phenothiazine compounds are extrapyramidal symptoms including pseudoparkinsonism, dystonia, dyskinesia, akathisia, oculogyric crises, opisthotonos, and hyperreflexia. Muscle rigidity sometimes accompanied by hyperthermia has been reported following use of fluphenazine decanoate. Most often these extrapyramidal symptoms are reversible; however, they may be persistent (see below). The frequency of such reactions is related in part to chemical structure: one can expect a higher incidence with fluphenazine decanoate than with less potent piperazine derivatives or with straight-chain phenothiazines such as chlorpromazine. With any given phenothiazine derivative, the incidence and severity of such reactions depend more on individual patient sensitivity than on other factors, but dosage level and patient age are also determinants.

Extrapyramidal reactions may be alarming, and the patient should be forewarned and reassured. These reactions can usually be controlled by administration of antiparkinsonism drugs such as Benztropine Mesylate or intravenous Caffeine and Sodium Benzoate Injection, and by subsequent reduction in dosage.

Tardive Dyskinesia: See WARNINGS. The syndrome is characterized by involuntary choreoathetoid movements which variously involve the tongue, face, mouth, lips, or jaw (*e.g.*, protrusion of the tongue, puffing of cheeks, puckering of mouth, chewing movements), trunk and extremities. The severity of the syndrome and the degree of impairment produced may vary widely.

The syndrome may become clinically recognizable either during treatment, upon dosage reduction, or upon withdrawal of treatment. Early detection of tardive dyskinesia is important. To increase the likelihood of detecting the syndrome at the earliest possible time, the dosage of neuroleptic drug should be reduced periodically (if clinically possible) and the patient observed for signs of the disorder. This maneuver is critical, since neuroleptic drugs may mask the signs of the syndrome.

Other CNS Effects: Occurrence of neuroleptic malignant syndrome (NMS) have been reported in patients on neuroleptic therapy (see WARNINGS, Neuroleptic Malignant Syndrome) ; leukocytosis, elevated CPK, liver function abnormalities, and acute renal failure may also occur with NMS.

Drowsiness or lethargy, if they occur, may necessitate a reduction in dosage; the induction of a catatonic-like state has been known to occur with dosages of fluphenazine far in excess of the recommended amounts. As with other phenothiazine compounds, reactivation or aggravation of psychotic processes may be encountered.

Phenothiazine derivatives have been known to cause, in some patients, restlessness, excitement, or bizarre dreams.

Autonomic Nervous System: Hypertension and fluctuations in blood pressure have been reported with fluphenazine.

Hypotension has rarely presented a problem with fluphenazine. However, patients with pheochromocytoma, cerebral vascular or renal insufficiency, or a severe cardiac reserve deficiency such as mitral insufficiency appear to be particularly prone to hypotensive reactions with phenothiazine compounds, and should therefore be observed closely when the drug is administered. If severe hypotension should occur, supportive measures including the use of intravenous vasopressor drugs should be instituted immediately. Levarterenol Bitartrate Injection is the most suitable drug for this purpose; *epinephrine should not be used* since phenothiazine derivatives have been found to reverse its action, resulting in a further lowering of blood pressure.

Autonomic reactions including nausea and loss of appetite, salivation, polyuria, perspiration, dry mouth, headache, and constipation may occur. Autonomic effects can usually be controlled by reducing or temporarily discontinuing dosage.

In some patients, phenothiazine derivatives have caused blurred vision, glaucoma, bladder paralysis, fecal impaction, paralytic ileus, tachycardia, or nasal congestion.

Metabolic and Endocrine: Weight change, peripheral edema, abnormal lactation, gynecomastia, menstrual irregularities, false results on pregnancy tests, impotency in men and increased libido in women have all been known to occur in some patients on phenothiazine therapy.

Allergic Reactions: Skin disorders such as itching, erythema, urticaria, seborrhea, photosensitivity, eczema and even exfoliative dermatitis have been reported with phenothiazine derivatives. The possibility of anaphylactoid reactions occurring in some patients should be borne in mind.

Hematologic: Routine blood counts are advisable during therapy since blood dyscrasias including leukopenia, agranulocytosis, thrombocytopenic or nonthrombocytopenic purpura, eosinophilia, and pancytopenia have been observed with phenothiazine derivatives. Furthermore, if any soreness of the mouth, gums, or throat, or any symptoms of upper respiratory infection occur and confirmatory leukocyte count indicates cellular depression, therapy should be discontinued and other appropriate measures instituted immediately.

Hepatic: Liver damage as manifested by cholestatic jaundice may be encountered, particularly during the first months of therapy; treatment should be discontinued if this occurs. An increase in cephalin flocculation, sometimes accompanied by alterations in other liver function tests, has been reported in patients receiving the enanthate ester of fluphenazine (a closely related compound) who have had no clinical evidence of liver damage.

Other: Sudden, unexpected and unexplained deaths have been reported in hospitalized psychotic patients receiving phenothiazines. Previous brain damage or seizures may be predisposing factors; high doses should be avoided in known seizure patients. Several patients have shown sudden flare-ups of psychotic behavior patterns shortly before death. Autopsy findings have usually revealed acute fulminating pneumonia or pneumonitis, aspiration of gastric contents, or intramyocardial lesions.

Although this is not a general feature of fluphenazine, potentiation of central nervous system depressants (opiates, analgesics, antihistamines, barbiturates, alcohol) may occur.

ADVERSE REACTIONS: *(cont'd)*

The following adverse reactions have also occurred with phenothiazine derivatives: systemic lupus erythematosus-like syndrome, hypotension severe enough to cause fatal cardiac arrest, altered electrocardiographic and electroencephalographic tracings, altered cerebrospinal fluid proteins, cerebral edema, asthma, laryngeal edema, angioneurotic edema; with long-term use—skin pigmentation, and lenticular and corneal opacities.

Injections of fluphenazine decanoate are extremely well tolerated, local tissue reactions occurring only rarely.

DOSAGE AND ADMINISTRATION:

Parenteral drug products should be inspected visually for particulate matter and discoloration prior to administration, whenever solution and container permit.

Fluphenazine Decanoate Injection may be given intramuscularly or subcutaneously. A dry syringe and needle of at least 21 gauge should be used. Use of a wet needle or syringe may cause the solution to become cloudy.

To begin therapy with Fluphenazine Decanoate the following regimens are suggested:

For most patients: a dose of 12.5 to 25 mg (0.5 to 1 ml) may be given to initiate therapy. The onset of action generally appears between 24 and 72 hours after injection and the effects of the drug on psychotic symptoms becomes significant within 48 to 96 hours. Subsequent injections and the dosage interval are determined in accordance with the patient's response. When administered as maintenance therapy, a single injection may be effective in controlling schizophrenic symptoms up to four weeks or longer. The response to a single dose has been found to last as long as six weeks in a few patients on maintenance therapy.

It may be advisable that patients who have no history of taking phenothiazines should be treated initially with a shorter-acting form of fluphenazine before administering the decanoate to determine the patient's response to fluphenazine and to establish appropriate dosage. For psychotic patients who have been stabilized on a fixed daily dosage of Fluphenazine HCl Tablets USP, Fluphenazine HCl Elixir USP), or Fluphenazine HCL Oral Solution, conversion of therapy from these short-acting oral forms to the long-acting injectable Fluphenazine Decanoate may be indicated.

Appropriate dosage of Fluphenazine Decanoate Injection should be individualized for each patient and responses carefully monitored. No precise formula can be given to convert to use of Fluphenazine Decanoate; however, a controlled multicenter study,* in patients receiving oral doses from 5 to 60 mg fluphenazine HCl daily, showed that 20 mg fluphenazine HCl daily was equivalent to 25 mg (1 ml) Fluphenazine Decanoate every three weeks. This represents an approximate conversion ratio of 0.5 ml (12.5 mg) of decanoate every three weeks for every 10 mg of fluphenazine HCl daily.

Once conversion to Fluphenazine Decanoate is made, careful clinical monitoring of the patient and appropriate dosage adjustment should be made at the time of each injection.

Severely Agitated Patients: may be treated initially with a rapid- acting phenothiazine compound such as Fluphenazine HCl Injection USP. When acute symptoms have subsided, 25 mg (1 ml) of Fluphenazine Decanoate may be administered; subsequent dosage is adjusted as necessary.

"Poor risk" Patients: (those with known hypersensitivity to phenothiazines, or with disorders that predispose to undue reactions): Therapy may be initiated cautiously with oral or parenteral fluphenazine HCl. When the pharmacologic effects and an appropriate dosage are apparent, an equivalent dose of Fluphenazine Decanoate may be administered. Subsequent dosage adjustments are made in accordance with the response of the patient.

The optimal amount of the drug and the frequency of administration must be determined for each patient, since dosage requirements have been found to vary with clinical circumstances as well as with individual response to the drug.

Dosage should not exceed 100 mg. If doses greater than 50 mg are deemed necessary, the next dose and succeeding doses should be increased cautiously in increments of 12.5 mg.

Storage Store at room temperature; avoid freezing and excessive heat. Protect from light.

REFERENCES:

* The initiation of Long-Term Pharmacotherapy in Schizophrenia: Dosage and Side Effect Comparisons Between Oral and Depot Fluphenazine; N.R. Schooler; Pharmakopsych. 9:159-169, 1976.(Princeton, J4-474)

HOW SUPPLIED - RATED THERAPEUTICALLY EQUIVALENT:

Injection, Solution - Intramuscular; - 25 mg/ml

1 ml	$13.15	Fluphenazine Decanoate, Pasadena	00418-2720-01
1 ml x 500	**$23.28**	**PROLIXIN DECANOATE, Bristol Myers Squibb**	**00003-0569-02**
5 ml	$20.99	Fluphenazine Decanoate, Balan	00304-2130-55
5 ml	$62.00	Fluphenazine Decanoate, Pasadena	00418-2720-10
5 ml	$66.00	Fluphenazine Decanoate, Fujisawa USA	00469-2720-20
5 ml	$67.44	Fluphenazine Decanoate, Insource	58441-1126-05
5 ml	**$103.75**	**PROLIXIN DECANOATE, Bristol Myers Squibb**	**00003-0569-15**

FLUPHENAZINE ENANTHATE *(001323)*

CATEGORIES: Antipsychotics/Antimanics; Central Nervous System Agents; Neuroleptics; Otic Preparations; Otologic; Phenothiazine Tranquilizers; Psychotherapeutic Agents; Psychotic Disorders; Tranquilizers; Vertigo/Motion Sickness/Vomiting; FDA Approval Pre 1982

BRAND NAMES: *Flunanthate*; *Moditen depot*; **Prolixin Enanthate**
(International brand names outside U.S. in italics)

DESCRIPTION:

Prolixin Enanthate (Fluphenazine Enanthate Injection) is an esterified trifluoromethyl phenothiazine derivative chemically designated as 2-(4-(3-(2-(Trifluoromethyl) phenothiazin-10-yl) propyl)-1-piperazinyl)ethyl heptanoate. It is a highly potent behavior modifier with a markedly extended duration of effect. Prolixin Enanthate is available for intramuscular or subcutaneous, providing 25 mg fluphenazine enanthate per ml in a sesame oil vehicle with 1.5% (w/v) benzyl alcohol as a preservative. At the time of manufacture, the air in the vials is replaced by nitrogen.

CLINICAL PHARMACOLOGY:

The basic effects of fluphenazine enanthate appear to be no different from those of fluphenazine HCl, with the exception of duration of action. The esterification of fluphenazine markedly prolongs the drug's duration of effect without unduly attenuating its beneficial action. The onset of action generally appears between 24 to 72 hours after injection, and the effects of the drug on psychotic symptoms become significant within 48 to 96 hours. Amelioration of symptoms then continues for one to three weeks or longer, with an average duration of effect of about two weeks.

Prolixin has activity at all levels of the central nervous system as well as on multiple organ systems. The mechanism whereby its therapeutic action is exerted is unknown.

CLINICAL PHARMACOLOGY: *(cont'd)*

Fluphenazine differs from other phenothiazine derivatives in several respects: it is more potent on a milligram basis, it has less potentiating effect on central nervous system depressants and anesthetics than do some of the phenothiazines and appears to be less sedating, and it is less likely than some of the older phenothiazines to produce hypotension (nevertheless, appropriate cautions should be observed—see sections on PRECAUTIONS and ADVERSE REACTIONS.).

INDICATIONS AND USAGE:

Prolixin Enanthate is a long-acting parenteral antipsychotic drug intended for use in the management of patients requiring prolonged parenteral neuroleptic therapy (*e.g.,* chronic schizophrenics).

Prolixin Enanthate (Fluphenazine Enanthate Injection) has not been shown effective in the management of behavioral complications in patients with mental retardation.

CONTRAINDICATIONS:

Phenothiazines are contraindicated in patients with suspected or established subcortical brain damage.

Phenothiazine compounds should not be used in patients receiving large doses of hypnotics.

Prolixin Enanthate is contraindicated in comatose or severely depressed states.

The presence of blood dyscrasia or liver damage precludes the use fluphenazine enanthate.

Fluphenazine enanthate is not intended for use in children under 12 years of age.

Prolixin Enanthate is contraindicated in patients who have shown hypersensitivity to fluphenazine; cross-sensitivity to phenothiazine derivatives may occur.

WARNINGS:

TARDIVE DYSKINESIA

Tardive dyskinesia, a syndrome consisting of potentially irreversible, involuntary, dyskinetic movements may develop in patients treated with neuroleptic (antipsychotic) drugs. Although the prevalence of the syndrome appears to be highest among the elderly, especially elderly women, it is impossible to rely upon prevalence estimates to predict, at the inception of neuroleptic treatment, which patients are likely to develop the syndrome. Whether neuroleptic drug products differ in their potential to cause tardive dyskinesia is unknown.

Both the risk of developing the syndrome and the likelihood that it will become irreversible are believed to increase as the duration of treatment and the total cumulative dose of neuroleptic drugs administered to the patient increase. however, the syndrome can develop, although much less commonly, after relatively brief treatment periods at low doses.

There is no known treatment for established cases of tardive dyskinesia, although the syndrome may remit, partially or completely, if neuroleptic treatment is withdrawn. Neuroleptic treatment, itself, however, may suppress (or partially suppress) the signs and symptoms of the syndrome and thereby may possibly mask the underlying disease process. The effect that symptomatic suppression has upon the long-term course of the syndrome is unknown.

Given these considerations, neuroleptics should be prescribed in a manner that is most likely to minimize the occurrence of tardive dyskinesia. Chronic neuroleptic treatment should generally be reserved for patients who suffer from a chronic illness that, 1) is known to respond to neuroleptic drugs, and, 2) for whom alternative, equally effective, but potentially less harmful treatments are *not* available or appropriate. In patients who do require chronic treatment, the smallest dose and the shortest duration of treatment producing a satisfactory clinical response should be sought. The need for continued treatment should be reassessed periodically.

If signs and symptoms of tardive dyskinesia appear in a patient on neuroleptics, drug discontinuation should be considered. However, some patients may require treatment despite the presence of the syndrome.

(For further information about the description of tardive dyskinesia and its clinical detection, please refer to the sections PRECAUTIONS, Information for Patients and ADVERSE REACTIONS, Tardive Dyskinesia.)

NEUROLEPTIC MALIGNANT SYNDROME (NMS)

A potentially fatal symptom complex sometimes referred to as Neuroleptic Malignant Syndrome (NMS) has been reported in association with antipsychotic drugs. Clinical manifestations of NMS are hyperpyrexia, muscle rigidity, altered mental status and evidence of autonomic instability (irregular pulse or blood pressure, tachycardia, diaphoresis, and cardiac dysrhythmias).

The diagnostic evaluation of patients with this syndrome is complicated. In arriving at a diagnosis, it is important to identify cases where the clinical presentation includes both serious mental illness (*e.g.,* pneumonia, systemic infection, etc.) Other important considerations in the differential diagnosis include central anticholinergic toxicity, heat stroke, drug fever and primary central nervous system (CNS) pathology.

The management of NMS should include 1) immediate discontinuation of antipsychotic drugs and other drugs not essential to concurrent therapy, 2) intensive symptomatic treatment and medical monitoring, and 3) treatment of any concomitant serious medical problems for which specific treatments are available. There is no general agreement about specific pharmacological treatment regimens for uncomplicated NMS.

If a patient requires antipsychotic drug treatment after recovery from NMS, the potential reintroduction of drug therapy should be carefully considered. The patient should be carefully monitored, since recurrences of NMS have been reported.

The use of this drug may impair the mental and physical abilities required for driving a car or operating heavy machinery.

Physicians should be alert to the possibility that severe adverse reactions may occur which require immediate medical attention.

Potentiation of the effects of alcohol may occur with the use of this drug.

Since there is no adequate experience in children who have received this drug, safety and efficacy in children have not been established.

USAGE IN PREGNANCY

The safety for the use of this drug during pregnancy has not been established; therefore, the possible hazards should be weighed against the potential benefits when administering the drug to pregnant patients.

PRECAUTIONS:

GENERAL

Because of the possibility of cross-sensitivity, fluphenazine enanthate should be used cautiously in patients who have developed cholestatic jaundice, dermatoses, or other allergic reactions phenothiazine derivatives.

Psychotic patients on large doses of phenothiazine drug who are undergoing surgery should be watched carefully for possible hypotensive phenomena. Moreover, it should be remembered that reduced amounts of anesthetics or central nervous system depressants may be necessary.

PRECAUTIONS: *(cont'd)*

The effects of atropine may be potentiated in some patients receiving fluphenazine because of added anticholinergic effects.

Fluphenazine enanthate should be used cautiously in patients exposed to extreme heat or phosphorus insecticides.

The preparation should be used with caution in patients with a history of convulsive disorders, since grand mal convulsions have been known to occur.

Use with caution in patients with special medical disorders such as mitral insufficiency or other cardiovascular diseases and pheochromocytoma.

The possibility of liver damage, pigmentary retinopathy, lenticular and corneal deposits, and development of irreversible dyskinesia should be remembered when patients are on prolonged therapy.

Outside state hospitals or other psychiatric institutions, fluphenazine enanthate should be administered under the direction of a physician experienced in the clinical use of psychotropic drugs, particularly phenothiazine derivatives. Furthermore, facilities should be available for periodic checking of hepatic function, renal function, and the blood picture. Renal function of patients on long-term therapy should be monitored; if BUN (blood urea nitrogen) becomes abnormal, treatment should be discontinued.

As with any phenothiazine, the physician should be alert to the possible development of "silent pneumonias" in patients under treatment with fluphenazine enanthate.

Neuroleptics drugs elevate prolactin levels; the elevation persists during chronic administration. Tissue culture experiments indicate that approximately one-third of human breast cancers are prolactin dependent *in vitro,* a factor of potential importance if the prescription of these drugs is contemplated in a patient with a previously detected breast cancer. Although disturbances such as galactorrhea, amenorrhea, gynecomastia, and impotence have been reported, the clinical significance of elevated serum prolactin levels is unknown for most patients. An increase in mammary neoplasms has been found in rodents after chronic administration of neuroleptic drugs. Neither clinical studies nor epidemiologic studies conducted to date, however, have shown an association between chronic administration of these drugs and mammary tumorigenesis; the available evidence is considered too limited to be conclusive at this time.

INFORMATION FOR THE PATIENT

Given the likelihood that some patients exposed chronically to neuroleptics will develop tardive dyskinesia, it is advised that all patients in whom chronic use is contemplated be given, if possible, full information about this risk. The decision to inform patients and/or their guardians must obviously take into account the clinical circumstances and the competency of the patient to understand the information provided.

ADVERSE REACTIONS:

Central Nervous System: The side effects most frequently reported with phenothiazine compounds are extrapyramidal symptoms including pseudoparkinsonism, dystonia, dyskinesia, akathisia, oculogyric crises, opisthotonos, and hyperreflexia. Most often these extrapyramidal symptoms are reversible; however, they may be persistent see below. The frequency of such reactions is related in part to chemical structure: one can expect a higher incidence with fluphenazine enanthate than with less potent piperazine derivatives or with straight-chain phenothiazines such as chlorpromazine. With any given phenothiazine derivative, the incidence and severity of such reactions depend more on individual patient sensitivity than on other factors, but dosage level and patient age are also determinants.

Extrapyramidal reactions may be alarming, and the patient should be forewarned and reassured. These reactions can usually be controlled by administration of antiparkinsonian drugs such as Benztropine Mesylate or intravenous Caffeine and Sodium Benzoate Injection, and by subsequent reduction in dosage.

Tardive Dyskinesia: See WARNINGS. The syndrome is characterized by involuntary choreoathetoid movements which variously involve the tongue, face, mouth, lips, or jaw (*e.g.,* protrusion of the tongue, puffing of the cheeks, puckering of the mouth, chewing movements), trunk and extremities. The severity of the syndrome and the degree of impairment produced vary widely.

The syndrome may become clinically recognizable either during treatment, upon dosage reduction, or upon withdrawal of treatment. Early detection of tardive dyskinesia is important. To increase the likelihood of detecting the syndrome at the earliest possible time, the dosage of neuroleptic drug should be reduced periodically (if clinically possible) and the patient observed for signs of the disorder. This maneuver is critical, since neuroleptic drugs may mask the signs of the syndrome.

Other CNS Effects: Occurrences of neuroleptic malignant syndrome (NMS) have been reported in patients on neuroleptic therapy (see WARNINGS, Neuroleptic Malignant Syndrome); leukocytosis, elevated CPK, liver function abnormalities, and acute renal failure may also occur with NMS.

Drowsiness or lethargy, if they occur, may necessitate a reduction in dosage; the induction of a catatonic-like state has been known to occur with dosages of fluphenazine far in excess of the recommended amounts. As with other phenothiazine compounds, reactivation or aggravation of psychotic processes may be encountered.

Phenothiazine derivatives have been known to cause, in some patients, restlessness, excitement, or bizarre dreams.

Autonomic Nervous System: Hypertension and fluctuations in blood pressure have been reported with fluphenazine enanthate.

Hypotension has rarely presented a problem with fluphenazine. However, patients with pheochromocytoma, cerebral vascular or renal insufficiency, or a severe cardiac reserve deficiency such as mitral insufficiency appear to be a particularly prone to hypotensive reactions with phenothiazine compounds, and should therefore be observed closely when the drug is administered. If severe hypotension should occur, supportive measures including the use of intravenous vasopressor drugs should be instituted immediately. Levarterenol Bitartrate Injection is the most suitable drug for this purpose; *epinephrine should not be used* since phenothiazine derivatives have been found to reverse its action, resulting in a further lowering of blood pressure.

Autonomic reactions including nausea and loss of appetite, salivation, polyuria, perspiration, dry mouth, headache, and constipation may occur. Autonomic effects can usually be controlled by reducing or temporarily discontinuing dosage.

In some patients, phenothiazine derivatives have caused blurred vision, glaucoma, bladder paralysis, fecal impaction, paralytic ileus, tachycardia, or nasal congestion.

Metabolic and Endocrine: Weight change, peripheral edema, abnormal lactation, gynecomastia, menstrual irregularities, false results on pregnancy tests, impotency in men and increased libido in women have all been known to occur in some patients on phenothiazine therapy.

Allergic Reactions: Skin disorders such as itching, erythema, urticaria, seborrhea, photosensitivity, eczema and even exfoliative dermatitis have been reported with phenothiazine derivatives. The possibility of anaphylactoid reactions occurring in some patients should be borne in mind.

ADVERSE REACTIONS: *(cont'd)*

Hematologic: Routine blood counts are advisable during therapy since blood dyscrasias including leukopenia, agranulocytosis, thrombocytopenic or nonthrombocytopenic purpura, eosinophilia, and pancytopenia have been observed with phenothiazine derivatives. Furthermore, if any soreness of the mouth, gums, or throat, or any symptoms of upper respiratory infection occur and confirmatory leukocyte count indicates cellular depression, therapy should be discontinued and other appropriate measures instituted immediately.

Hepatic: Liver damage as manifested by cholestatic jaundice may be encountered, particularly during the first months of therapy; treatment should be discontinued if this occurs. An increase in cephalin flocculation, sometimes accompanied by alterations in other liver function tests, has been reported in patients receiving the fluphenazine enanthate who have had no evidence of liver damage.

Others: Sudden, unexpected and unexplained deaths have been reported in hospitalized psychotic patients receiving phenothiazines. Previous brain damage or seizures may be predisposing factors; high doses should be avoided in known seizure patients. Several patients have shown sudden flare-ups of psychotic behavior patterns shortly before death. Autopsy findings have usually revealed acute fulminating pneumonia or pneumonitis, aspiration of gastric contents, or intramyocardial lesions.

Although this is not a general feature of fluphenazine, potentiation of central nervous system depressants (opiates, analgesics, antihistamines, barbiturates, alcohol) may occur.

The following adverse reactions have also occurred with phenothiazine derivatives: systemic lupus erythematosus-like syndrome, hypotension severe enough to cause fatal cardiac arrest, altered electrocardiographic and electroencephalographic tracings, altered cerebrospinal fluid proteins, cerebral edema, asthma, laryngeal edema, and angioneurotic edema; with long-term use—skin pigmentation, and lenticular and corneal opacities.

Injections of fluphenazine enanthate are extremely well tolerated, local tissue reactions occurring only rarely.

DOSAGE AND ADMINISTRATION:

Prolixin Enanthate (Fluphenazine Enanthate Injection USP) may be given intramuscularly or subcutaneously. A dry syringe and needle of at least 21 gauge should be used. Use of a wet needle or syringe may cause the solution to become cloudy.

To begin therapy with Prolixin Enanthate the following regimens are suggested:

Most patients: For *most patients* a dose of 25 mg (1 ml) every two weeks should prove to be adequate, and therapy may be started on that basis. Subsequent adjustments in the amount and the dosage interval may be made, if necessary, in accordance with the patient's response.

It may be advisable that patients who have no history of taking phenothiazines should be treated initially with a shorter-acting form of fluphenazine before administering the enanthate to determine the patient's response to fluphenazine and to establish appropriate dosage. Since the dosage comparability of the shorter-acting forms of fluphenazine to the longer-acting enanthate is not known, special caution should be exercised when switching from the shorter-acting forms to the enanthate.

Severely agitated patients may be treated initially with a rapid-acting phenothiazine compound such as Prolixin Injection (Fluphenazine HCl Injection USP—see package insert accompanying that product for complete information). When acute symptoms have subsided, 25 mg (1 ml) of Prolixin Enanthate may be administered; subsequent dosage is adjusted as necessary.

'Poor risk' patients (those with known hypersensitivity to phenothiazines, or with disorders that predispose to undue reactions): Therapy may be initiated cautiously with oral or parenteral fluphenazine HCl. (See package inserts accompanying these products for complete information.) When the pharmacologic effects and an appropriate dosage are apparent, an equivalent dose of Prolixin Enanthate may be administered. Subsequent dosage adjustments are made in accordance with the response of the patient.

The optimal amount of the drug and the frequency of administration must be determined for each patient, since dosage requirements have been found to vary with clinical circumstances as well as with individual response to the drug. Although in a large series of patients the optimal dose was usually 25 mg every two weeks, the amount required ranged from 12.5 to 100 mg (0.5 to 4 ml). The interval between doses ranged from one to three weeks in most instances. The response to a single dose was found to last as long as six weeks in a few patients on maintenance therapy.

Dosage should not exceed 100 mg. If doses greater than 50 mg are deemed necessary, the next dose and succeeding doses should be increased cautiously in increments of 12.5 mg.

HOW SUPPLIED:

Prolixin Enanthate (Fluphenazine Enanthate Injection USP) is available in vials providing 25 mg fluphenazine enanthate per ml.

Storage: Store at room temperature; avoid freezing and excessive heat. Protect from light.

HOW SUPPLIED - EQUIVALENTS NOT AVAILABLE:

Injection, Solution - Subcutaneous - 25 mg/ml

5 ml $110.53 PROLIXIN ENANTHATE, Bristol Myers Squibb 00003-0824-05

FLUPHENAZINE HYDROCHLORIDE *(001324)*

CATEGORIES: Antipsychotics/Antimanics; Central Nervous System Agents; Neuroleptics; Phenothiazine Tranquilizers; Psychotherapeutic Agents; Psychotic Disorders; Schizophrenia; Tranquilizers; Vertigo/Motion Sickness/Vomiting; FDA Approval Pre 1982

BRAND NAMES: *Anatensol* (Australia); *Apo-Fluphenazine*; *Cenilene*; *Dapotum* (Germany); *Flunazine*; Fluphenazine Hcl; *Fluzine*; *Fluzine-P*; *Funazine*; *Lyogen* (Germany); *Lyogen Depot* (Germany); *Lyogen Retard*; *Moditen* (England, France, Canada); *Omca* (Germany); *Pacinol*; *Pacinol Prolong*; Permitil; *Potensone*; **Prolixin**; *Sediten*; *Selecten*; *Siqualone*
(International brand names outside U.S. in italics)

FORMULARIES: Medi-Cal; PCS

COST OF THERAPY: $81.86 (Schizophrenia; Tablet; 1 mg; 1/day; 365 days) vs. Potential Cost of $3,628.44 (Psychoses)

DESCRIPTION:

TABLETS AND ELIXIR

Fluphenazine Hydrochloride is a trifluoroethyl phenothiazine derivative intended for the management of schizophrenia.

Fluphenazine HCl tablets contain 1, 2.5, 5, and 10 mg Fluphenazine HCl per tablet. Inactive ingredients: acacia, carnauba wax for 1 and 2.5 only, castor oil; Aluminum Lakes of the following colorants: (D&C Red No. 27 for 1 and 10 mg only; D&C Yellow No. 10 for 5 and 10 mg only; FD&C Blue No.1 for 5 and 10 mg only; FD&C Blue No.2 for 2.5 mg only; FD&C Yellow No. 5 (tartrazine) for 2.5, 5 an 10 mg only; FC&C Yellow No. 6 for 1 mg only); corn starch; ethylcellulose; gelatin; lactose; magnesium carbonate; magnesium stearate; pharmaceutical glaze; polyethylene glycol for 1 and 2.5 mg only; povidone for 1,2.5, and 10 mg only; precipitated calcium carbonate; sodium benzoate; sucrose; synthetic iron oxide; talc; titanium dioxide; white wax for 1 and 2.5 mg only; and other ingredients.

Fluphenazine HCl elixir contains 0.5 mg fluphenazine hydrochloride per ml. Inactive ingredients: alcohol (14%(v/v)) colorant (FD&C Yellow No.6), flavors, glycerin, polysorbate 40, purified water, sodium benzoate, and sucrose.

INJECTION

Fluphenazine HCl Injection is available in multiple dose vials providing 2.5 mg fluphenazine HCl per ml. The preparation also includes sodium chloride for isotonicity, sodium hydroxide or hydrochloric acid to adjust the pH to 4.8-5.2, and 0.1% methylparaben and 0.01% propylparaben as preservatives. At the time of manufacture, the air in the vials is replaced by nitrogen.

CLINICAL PHARMACOLOGY:

Fluphenazine HCl has activity at all levels of the central nervous system as well as on multiple organ systems. The mechanism whereby its therapeutic action is extended action exerted is unknown.

INDICATIONS AND USAGE:

Fluphenazine HCl is indicated in the management of manifestations of psychotic disorders.

Fluphenazine HCl has not been shown effective in the management of behavioral complications in patients with mental retardation.

CONTRAINDICATIONS:

Phenothiazines are contraindicated in patients with suspected or established subcortical brain damage, in patients receiving large doses of hypnotics, & in comatose or severely depressed states. The presence of blood dyscrasia or liver damage precludes the use of fluphenazine HCl. This drug is contraindicated in patients who have shown hypersensitivity to fluphenazine; cross-sensitivity to phenothiazine derivatives may occur.

WARNINGS:

TARDIVE DYSKINESIA

Tardive Dyskinesia a syndrome consisting of potentially irreversible, involuntary, dyskinetic movements may develop in patients treated with neuroleptic (antipsychotic) drugs. Although the prevalence of the syndrome appears to be highest among the elderly, especially elderly women, it is impossible to rely upon prevalence estimates to predict, at the inception of neuroleptic treatment, which patients are likely to develop the syndrome. Whether neuroleptic drug products differ in their potential to cause tardive dyskinesia is unknown.

Both the risk of developing the syndrome and the likelihood that it will become irreversible are believed to increase as the duration of treatment and the total cumulative dose of neuroleptic drugs administered to the patient increase. However, the syndrome can develop, although much less commonly, after relatively brief treatment periods at low doses.

There is no known treatment for established cases of tardive dyskinesia, although the syndrome may remit, partially or completely, if neuroleptic treatment is withdrawn. Neuroleptic treatment, itself, however, amy suppress (or partially suppress) the signs and symptoms of the syndrome and thereby may possibly mask the underlying disease process. The effect that symptomatic suppression has upon the long-term course of the syndrome is unknown.

Given these considerations, neuroleptics should be prescribed in a manner that is most likely to minimize the occupance of tardive dyskinesia. Chronic neuroleptic treatment should generally be reserved for patients who suffer from a chronic illness that 1) ia known to respond to neuroleptic drugs, and, 2) for whom alternative, equally effective, but potentially less harmful treatments are *not* available or appropriate. In patients who do require chronic treatment, the smallest dose and the shortest duration of treatment of treatment producing a satisfactory clinical response should be sought. The need for continued treatment should be reassessed periodically.

If signs and symptoms of tardive dyskinesia appear in a patient on neuroleptics, drug discontinuation should be considered. However, some patients may require treatment despite the presence of the syndrome.

(For further information about the description of tardive dyskinesia and its clinical detection, please refer to the sections on PRECAUTIONS, Information for Patients, and ADVERSE REACTIONS, Tardive Dyskinesia).

NEUROLEPTIC MALIGNANT SYNDROME (NMS)

A potentially fatal symptom complex sometimes referred to as Neuroleptic Malignant Syndrome (NMS) has been reported in association with antipsychotic drugs. Clinical manifestations of NMS are hyperpyrexia, muscle rigidity, altered mental status and evidence of automatic instability (irregular pulse or blood pressure, tachycardia, diaphoresis, and cardiac dysrhythmias).

The diagnostic evaluation of patients with this syndrome is complicated. In arriving at a diagnosis, it is important to identify cases where the clinical presentation includes both serious medical illness (*e.g.,* pneumonia, systemic infection, etc.) and untreated or inadequately treated extrapyramidal signs and symptoms. Other important considerations in the differential diagnosis include central anticholinergic toxicity, heat stroke, drug fever and primary central nervous system pathology.

The management of NMS should include: 1) immediate discontinuation of antipsychotic and other drugs not essential to concurrent therapy; 2) intensive symptomatic treatment and medical monitoring; and 3) treatment of any concomitant serious medical problems for which specific treatments are available. There is no general agreement about specific pharmacologic treatment regimens for uncomplicated NMS.

If a patient requires antipsychotic drug treatment after recovery from NMS, the potential reintroduction of drug therapy should be carefully considered. The patient should be carefully monitored, since recurrences of NMS have been reported.

The use of this drug may impair the mental and physical abilities for driving or operating heavy machinery.

Potentiation of the effects of alcohol may occur with the use of this drug.

Since there is no adequate experience in children who have received this drug, safety and efficacy in children have not been established.

USAGE IN PREGNANCY

The safety for the use of this drug during pregnancy has not been established; therefore, the possible hazards should be weighed against the potential benefits when administering this drug to pregnant patients.

PRECAUTIONS:

GENERAL

Because of the possibility of cross-sensitivity, fluphenazine HCl should be used cautiously in patients who have developed cholestatic jaundice, dermatoses, or other allergic reactions to phenothiazine derivatives.

Fluphenazine HCl tablets 2.5, 5. and 10 mg contain FD&C Yellow No.5 (tartrazine) which may cause allergic-type reactions (including bronchial asthma) in certain susceptible individuals. Although the overall incidence of FD&C yellow No.5 (tartrazine) sensitivity in the general population is low, it is frequently seen in patients who also have aspirin hypersensitivity.

Psychotic patients on large doses of a phenothiazine drug who are undergoing surgery should be watched carefully for possible hypotensive phenomena. Moreover, it should be remembered that reduced amounts of anesthetics or central nervous system depressants may be necessary.

The effects of atropine may be potentiated in some patients receiving fluphenazine HCl because of added anticholinergic effects.

Fluphenazine HCl should be used cautiously in patients exposed to extreme heat or phosphorus insecticides; in patients with a history of convulsive disorders, since grand mal convulsions have been known to occur; and in patients with a special medical disorders, such as mitral insufficiency or other cardiovascular diseases and pheochromocytoma.

The possibility of liver damage, pigmentary retinopathy, lenticular and corneal deposits, and development of irreversible dyskinesia should be remembered when patients are on prolonged therapy.

Neuroleptic drugs elevate prolactin levels; the elevation persists during chronic administration. Tissue culture experiments indicate that approximately one-third of human breast cancers are prolactin dependent *in vitro*, a factor of potential importance if the prescription of these drugs is contemplated in a patient with previously detectable breast cancer. Although disturbances such as galactorrhea, amenorrhea, gynecomastia, and impotence have been reported, the clinical significance of elevated serum prolactin levels is unknown for most patients. An increase in mammary neoplasms have been found in rodents after chronic administration of neuroleptic drugs. Neither clinical studies nor epidemiologic studies conducted to date, however, have shown an association between chronic administration of these drugs and mammary tumorigenesis; the available evidence is considered too limited to be conclusive at this time.

INFORMATION FOR THE PATIENT

Given the likelihood that some patients exposed chronically to neuroleptics will develop tardive dyskinesia, it is advised that all patients in whom chronic use is contemplated be given, if possible, full information about this risk. The decision to inform patients and/or their guardians must obviously take into account the clinical circumstances and the competency of the patient to understand the information provided.

ABRUPT WITHDRAWAL

In general, phenothiazines do not produce psychic dependence; however, gastritis, nausea and vomiting, dizziness, and tremulousness have been reported following abrupt cessation of high dose therapy. Reports suggest that these symptoms can be reduced if concomitant antiparkinsonian agents are continued for several weeks after the phenothiazine is withdrawn.

Facilities should be available for periodic checking of the hepatic function, renal function and the blood picture. Renal function of the patient on long-term therapy should be monitored; if BUN (blood urea nitrogen) becomes abnormal, treatment should be discontinued.

As with any phenothiazines, the physicians should be alert to the possible development of "silent pneumonias" in patients under treatment with fluphenazine HCl.

ADVERSE REACTIONS:

CENTRAL NERVOUS SYSTEM

The side effects most frequently reported with phenothiazine compounds are extrapyramidal symptoms, including pseudoparkinsonism, dystonia, dyskinesia, akathisia, oculogyric crises, opisthotonos, and hyperreflexia. Most often these extrapyramidal symptoms are reversible; however, they may be persistent see below. With any given phenothiazine derivative, the incidence and severity of such reactions depend more on the individual patient sensitivity than on other factors, but dosage level and patient age are also determinants.

Extrapyramidal reactions may be alarming, and the patient should be forewarned and reassured. These reactions can usually be controlled by administration of antiparkinsonian drugs such as benztropine mesylate or IV caffeine and sodium benzoate injection, and by subsequent reduction in dosage.

TARDIVE DYSKINESIA

See WARNINGS. The syndrome is characterized by involuntary choreoathetoid movements which variously involve the tongue, face, mouth, lips, or jaw (*e.g.,* protrusion of the tongue, puffing of cheeks, puckering of the mouth, chewing movements), trunk and extremities. The severity of the syndrome and the degree of impairment produced vary widely.

The syndrome may become clinically recognizable either during treatment, upon dosage reduction, or upon withdrawal of treatment. Early detection of tardive dyskinesia is important. To increase the likelihood of detecting the syndrome at the earliest possible time, the dosage of neuroleptic drug should be reduced periodically (if clinically possible) and the patient observed for signs of the disorder. This maneuver is critical, since neuroleptic drugs may mask the signs of the syndrome.

OTHER CNS EFFECTS

Occurrences of neuroleptic malignant syndrome (NMS) have been reported in patients on neuroleptic therapy (see WARNINGS, Neuroleptic Malignant Syndrome.) Leukocytosis, elevated CPK, liver function abnormalities, and acute renal failure may also occur with NMS.

Drowsiness or lethargy, if they occur, may necessitate a reduction in dosage; the induction of a catatonic-like state has been known to occur with dosages of fluphenazine far in excess of the compounds, reactivation or aggravation of psychotic processes may be encountered.

Phenothiazine derivatives have been known to cause, in some patients, restlessness, excitement, or bizarre dreams.

Automatic Nervous System: Hypertension and fluctuation in blood pressure have been reported with fluphenazine HCl.

Hypotension has rarely presented a problem with fluphenazine HCl. However, patients with pheochromocytoma, cerebral vascular or renal insufficiency, or a severe cardiac reserve deficiency (such as mitral insufficiency) appear to be particularly prone to hypotensive reactions with phenothiazine compounds, and should therefore be observed closely when the drug is administered. If severe hypotension should occur, supportive measures including the use of IV vasopressor drugs should be instituted immediately. Levarterenol Bitartrate Injection is the most suitable drug for this purpose; *epinephrine should not be used* since phenothiazine derivatives have been found to reverse its action, resulting in a further lowering of blood pressure.

Autonomic reactions including nausea and loss of appetite, salivation, polyuria, perspiration, dry mouth, headache, and constipation may occur. Autonomic effects can usually be controlled by reducing or temporarily discontinuing dosage.

ADVERSE REACTIONS: *(cont'd)*

In some patients, phenothiazine derivatives have caused blurred vision, glaucoma, bladder paralysis, fecal impaction, paralytic ileus, tachycardia, or nasal congestion.

METABOLIC AND ENDOCRINE

Weight change, peripheral edema, abnormal lactation, gynecomastia, menstrual irregularities, false results on pregnancy tests, impotency in men and increased libido in women have all been known to occur in some patients on phenothiazine therapy.

ALLERGIC REACTIONS

Skin disorders such as itching, erythema, urticaria, seborrhea, photosensitivity, eczema and even exfoliative dermatitis have been reported with phenothiazine derivatives. The possibility of anaphylactoid reactions occurring in some patients should be borne in mind.

HEMATOLOGIC

Routine blood counts are advisable during therapy since blood dyscrasias including leukopenia, agranulocytosis, thrombocytopenic or nonthrombocytopenic purpura, eosinophilia, and pancytopenia have been observed with phenothiazine derivatives. Furthermore, if any soreness of the mouth, gums, or throat, or any symptoms of upper respiratory infection occur and confirmatory leukocyte indicates cellular depression, therapy should be discontinued and other appropriate measures instituted immediately.

HEPATIC

Liver damage as manifested by cholestatic jaundice may be encountered, particularly during the first months of therapy; treatment should be discontinued if this occurs. An increase in cephalin flocculation, sometimes accompanied by alterations in other liver function tests, has been reported in patients receiving fluphenazine HCl who have had no clinical evidence of liver damage.

OTHERS

Sudden, unexpected and unexplained deaths have been reported in hospitalized psychotic patients receiving phenothiazines. Previous brain damage or seizures may be predisposing factors; high doses should be avoided in known seizure patients. Several patients have shown sudden flare-ups of psychotic behavior patterns shortly before death. Autopsy findings have usually revealed acute fulminating pneumonia or pneumonitis, aspiration of gastric contents, or intramyocardial lesions.

Although this is not a general feature of fluphenazine HCl, potentiation of central nervous system depressants (opiates, analgesics, antihistamines, barbiturates, alcohol) may occur.

The following adverse reactions have also occurred with phenothiazine derivatives: systemic lupus erythematosus-like syndrome, hypotension severe enough to cause fatal cardiac arrest, altered electrocardiographic and electroencephalographic tracings, altered cerebrospinal fluid proteins, cerebral edema, asthma, laryngeal edema, and angioneurotic edema; with long-term use- skin pigmentation, and lenticular and corneal opacities.

DOSAGE AND ADMINISTRATION:

TABLETS AND ELIXIR

Fluphenazine HCl elixir should be inspected prior to use. Upon standing a slight wispy precipitate or globular material may develop due to the flavoring oils separating from the solution (potency is not affected). Gentle shaking redisperses the oils and the solution becomes clear. Solutions that do not clarify should not be used.

Depending on the severity and duration of symptoms, total dosage for*adult* psychotic patients may range initially from 2.5 to 10.0 mg and should be divided and given at six-to eight-hour intervals.

The smallest amount that will produce the desired results must be carefully determined for each individual, since optimal dosage levels of the potent drug vary from patient to patient. In general, the oral dose has been found to be approximately two to three times the parenteral dose of fluphenazine HCl. Treatment is best instituted with a *low initial dosage*, which may be increased, if necessary, until the desired clinical effects are achieved. Therapeutic effect is often achieved with doses under 20 mg daily. Patients remaining severely distributed or inadequately controlled may require upward titration of dosage. Daily doses up to 40 mg may be necessary; controlled clinical studies have not been performed to demonstrate safety of prolonged administration of such doses.

When symptoms are controlled, dosage can generally be reduced gradually to daily maintenance doses of 1.0 or 5.0 mg, often given as a single daily dose. Continued treatment is needed to achieve maximum therapeutic benefits; further adjustments in dosage may be necessary during the course of therapy to meet the patient's requirements.

For psychotic patients who have been stabilized on a fixed daily dosage or orally administered fluphenazine HCl dosage forms, conversion to the long-acting injectable Fluphenazine Decanoate may be indicated (see package insert for Fluphenazine Decanoate Injection for conversion information).

For *geriatric* patients, the suggested starting dose is 1.0 to 2.5 mg daily, adjusted according to the response of the patient.

Fluphenazine HCl Injection, USP is useful when psychotic patients are unable or unwilling to take oral therapy.

STORAGE

Store tablets and elixir at room temperature. Protect from light. Keep tightly closed.

Tablets: Avoid excessive heat.

Elixir : Avoid freezing.

INJECTION

The average well-tolerated starting dose for adult psychotic patients is 1.25 mg (0.5 ml) intramuscularly. Depending on the severity and duration of symptoms, initial total daily dosage may range from 2.5 to 10.0 mg and should be divided and given at six- to eight-hour intervals.

The smallest amount that will produce the desired results must be carefully determined for each individual, since optimal dosage levels of this potent drug very from patient to patient. In general, the parenteral dose for fluphenazine has been found to be approximately 1/3 to 1/2 the oral dose. Treatment may be instituted with a *low initial dosage*, which may be increased, if necessary, until the desired clinical effects are achieved. Dosages exceeding 10.0 mg daily should be used with caution.

When symptoms are controlled, oral maintenance therapy can generally be instituted, often with single daily doses. Continued treatment, by the oral route if possible, is needed to achieve maximum therapeutic benefits; further adjustments in dosage may be necessary during the course of therapy to meet the patient's requirements.

STORAGE

Solutions should be protected from exposure to light. Parenteral solutions may vary in color from essentially colorless to light amber. If a solution has become any darker than light amber or is discolored in any other way it should not be used.

Store at room temperature; avoid freezing.

(Tablets and Elixir: Apothecon, 10/93, P2237-02)

(Injection: Apothecon, 7/87, J4-479A)

HOW SUPPLIED - RATED THERAPEUTICALLY EQUIVALENT:

Concentrate - Oral - 5 mg/ml

1 ml x 100	$163.95	PERMITIL, Xactdose	50962-0379-01
120 ml	$74.16	PERMITIL, Schering	00085-0296-05
120 ml	$91.15	Fluphenazine Hcl, Copley Pharm	38245-0630-14
120 ml	**$113.71**	**PROLIXIN, Bristol Myers Squibb**	**00003-0801-10**
120 ml	$136.72	Fluphenazine Hcl, H.C.F.A. F F P	99999-1324-01

Elixir - Oral - 2.5 mg/5ml

60 ml	$15.90	Fluphenazine Elixir USP, 0.5 mg/mL, Copley Pharm	38245-0686-12
60 ml	**$18.08**	**PROLIXIN, Bristol Myers Squibb**	**00003-0820-30**
473 ml	$126.80	Fluphenazine, Copley Pharm	38245-0686-07
480 ml	**$144.11**	**PROLIXIN, Bristol Myers Squibb**	**00003-0820-50**

Injection, Solution - Intramuscular - 2.5 mg/ml

10 ml	$26.50	Fluphenazine Hcl, Pasadena	00418-2720-20
10 ml	$30.25	Fluphenazine Hcl, Fujisawa USA	00469-2810-30
10 ml	**$59.20**	**PROLIXIN, Bristol Myers Squibb**	**00003-0586-30**

Tablet, Plain Coated - Oral - 1 mg

50's	$11.21	Fluphenazine HCl, H.C.F.A. F F P	99999-1324-02
50's	$26.10	Fluphenazine HCl, Geneva Pharms	00781-1436-50
100's	$22.43	Fluphenazine HCl, H.C.F.A. F F P	99999-1324-03
100's	$23.63	Fluphenazine Hcl, United Res	00677-1217-01
100's	$34.44	Fluphenazine Hcl, Vangard Labs	00615-3573-13
100's	$42.80	Fluphenazine Hcl, Qualitest Pharms	00603-3666-21
100's	$45.00	Fluphenazine Hcl, Goldline Labs	00182-1365-01
100's	$45.90	Fluphenazine Hcl, Par Pharm	49884-0061-01
100's	$46.08	Fluphenazine HCl, Schein Pharm (US)	00364-2265-01
100's	$47.95	Fluphenazine Hcl, Parmed Pharms	00349-8983-01
100's	$48.18	Fluphenazine Hcl, HL Moore Drug Exch	00839-6440-06
100's	$48.31	Fluphenazine Hcl, Aligen Independ	00405-4439-01
100's	$49.75	Fluphenazine HCl, Geneva Pharms	00781-1436-01
100's	$51.95	Fluphenazine Hcl, Mylan	00378-6004-01
100's	$62.99	Fluphenazine HCl, Geneva Pharms	00781-1436-13
100's	$63.00	Fluphenazine Hydrochloride, Goldline Labs	00182-1365-89
100's	$65.24	Fluphenazine HCl, Rugby	00536-3805-01
100's	$74.43	Fluphenazine Hcl, Major Pharms	00904-3673-61
100's	**$83.03**	**PROLIXIN, Bristol Myers Squibb**	**00003-0863-50**
100's	**$91.50**	**PROLIXIN, Bristol Myers Squibb**	**00003-0863-55**
100's UD	$47.05	PHENAZIDE, Major Pharms	00904-3673-60
500's	$112.15	Fluphenazine HCl, H.C.F.A. F F P	99999-1324-04
500's	$172.45	Fluphenazine Hcl 1, Harber Pharm	51432-0813-05
500's	$229.50	Fluphenazine Hcl, Par Pharm	49884-0061-05
500's	$233.79	Fluphenazine HCl, Geneva Pharms	00781-1436-05
500's	$235.95	Fluphenazine Hcl, Mylan	00378-6004-05
500's	**$392.83**	**PROLIXIN, Bristol Myers Squibb**	**00003-0863-70**
1000's	$224.30	Fluphenazine HCl, H.C.F.A. F F P	99999-1324-05

Tablet, Plain Coated - Oral - 2.5 mg

50's	$16.69	Fluphenazine HCl, H.C.F.A. F F P	99999-1324-06
50's	$40.57	Fluphenazine HCl, Geneva Pharms	00781-1437-50
100's	$33.38	Fluphenazine HCl, H.C.F.A. F F P	99999-1324-07
100's	$34.73	Fluphenazine Hcl, United Res	00677-1218-01
100's	$48.95	Fluphenazine HCl 2.5, Harber Pharm	51432-0814-03
100's	$60.80	Fluphenazine Hcl, Qualitest Pharms	00603-3667-21
100's	$64.00	Fluphenazine Hcl, Goldline Labs	00182-1366-01
100's	$64.98	Fluphenazine Hcl, Par Pharm	49884-0062-01
100's	$66.54	Fluphenazine HCl, Schein Pharm (US)	00364-2266-01
100's	$67.25	PHENAZIDE, Major Pharms	00904-3674-60
100's	$68.24	Fluphenazine Hcl, HL Moore Drug Exch	00839-6441-06
100's	$68.95	Fluphenazine HCl, Parmed Pharms	00349-8981-01
100's	$75.42	Fluphenazine HCl, Aligen Independ	00405-4440-01
100's	$75.75	Fluphenazine HCl, Geneva Pharms	00781-1437-01
100's	$78.95	Fluphenazine Hcl, Mylan	00378-6009-01
100's	$90.99	Fluphenazine HCl, Geneva Pharms	00781-1437-13
100's	$91.00	Fluphenazine Hydrochloride, Goldline Labs	00182-1366-89
100's	$92.51	Fluphenazine HCl, Rugby	00536-3806-01
100's	**$113.21**	**PROLIXIN, Bristol Myers Squibb**	**00003-0864-50**
100's	**$124.45**	**PROLIXIN, Bristol Myers Squibb**	**00003-0864-52**
500's	$166.90	Fluphenazine HCl, H.C.F.A. F F P	99999-1324-08
500's	$198.45	Fluphenazine HCl, Major Pharms	00904-3674-40
500's	$244.75	Fluphenazine HCl 2.5, Harber Pharm	51432-0814-05
500's	$324.90	Fluphenazine Hcl, Par Pharm	49884-0062-05
500's	$330.74	Fluphenazine HCl, Geneva Pharms	00781-1437-05
500's	$331.95	Fluphenazine Hcl, Mylan	00378-6009-05
500's	**$534.11**	**PROLIXIN, Bristol Myers Squibb**	**00003-0864-70**
1000's	$333.80	Fluphenazine HCl, H.C.F.A. F F P	99999-1324-09

Tablet, Plain Coated - Oral - 5 mg

50's	$20.81	Fluphenazine HCl, H.C.F.A. F F P	99999-1324-10
50's	$47.17	Fluphenazine HCl, Geneva Pharms	00781-1438-50
100's	$41.63	Fluphenazine HCl, H.C.F.A. F F P	99999-1324-11
100's	$42.75	Fluphenazine Hcl, United Res	00677-1219-01
100's	$57.79	Fluphenazine Hcl, Vangard Labs	00615-1501-13
100's	$78.74	Fluphenazine Hcl, Qualitest Pharms	00603-3668-21
100's	$83.00	08903, Goldline Labs	00182-1367-01
100's	$83.75	Fluphenazine Hcl 5, Par Pharm	49884-0076-01
100's	$83.88	Fluphenazine HCl, Aligen Independ	00405-4441-01
100's	$84.25	PHENAZIDE, Major Pharms	00904-3675-60
100's	$84.42	Fluphenazine HCl, Schein Pharm (US)	00364-2267-01
100's	$87.95	Fluphenazine HCl, Parmed Pharms	00349-8982-01
100's	$87.95	Fluphenazine Hcl, HL Moore Drug Exch	00839-6442-06
100's	$89.95	Fluphenazine HCl, Geneva Pharms	00781-1438-01
100's	$91.95	Fluphenazine Hcl, Mylan	00378-6074-01
100's	$123.50	Fluphenazine Hcl, Rugby	00536-3807-01
100's	$134.99	Fluphenazine HCl, Geneva Pharms	00781-1438-13
100's	$135.00	08903, Goldline Labs	00182-1367-89
100's	$136.49	Fluphenazine Hcl, Major Pharms	00904-3675-61
100's	**$151.88**	**PROLIXIN, Bristol Myers Squibb**	**00003-0877-50**
100's	**$167.38**	**PROLIXIN, Bristol Myers Squibb**	**00003-0877-52**
500's	$208.15	Fluphenazine HCl, H.C.F.A. F F P	99999-1324-12
500's	$300.55	PHENAZIDE, Major Pharms	00904-3675-40
500's	$313.95	Fluphenazine HCl 5, Harber Pharm	51432-0815-05
500's	$323.70	Fluphenazine Hcl, HL Moore Drug Exch	00839-6442-12
500's	$373.95	Fluphenazine HCl, Qualitest Pharms	00603-3668-28
500's	$418.75	Fluphenazine Hcl 5, Par Pharm	49884-0076-05
500's	$423.70	Fluphenazine HCl, Geneva Pharms	00781-1438-05
500's	$423.95	Fluphenazine Hcl, Mylan	00378-6074-05
500's	**$703.89**	**PROLIXIN, Bristol Myers Squibb**	**00003-0877-70**
1000's	$416.30	Fluphenazine HCl, H.C.F.A. F F P	99999-1324-13

Tablet, Plain Coated - Oral - 10 mg

50's	$25.12	Fluphenazine HCl, H.C.F.A. F F P	99999-1324-14
50's	$60.24	Fluphenazine HCl Usp, Geneva Pharms	00781-1439-50
100's	$50.25	Fluphenazine HCl, H.C.F.A. F F P	99999-1324-15
100's	$52.88	Fluphenazine Hcl, United Res	00677-1220-01

HOW SUPPLIED - RATED THERAPEUTICALLY EQUIVALENT: *(cont'd)*

100's	$70.19	Fluphenazine HCl, Vangard Labs	00615-3574-13
100's	$81.85	Fluphenazine HCl, Harber Pharm	51432-0816-03
100's	$102.36	Fluphenazine Hcl, Qualitest Pharms	00603-3669-21
100's	$108.00	Fluphenazine Hcl, Goldline Labs	00182-1368-01
100's	$109.05	Fluphenazine HCl 10, Aligen Independ	00405-4442-01
100's	$109.05	Fluphenazine Hcl, Par Pharm	49884-0064-01
100's	$110.81	Fluphenazine HCl 10, Schein Pharm (US)	00364-2268-01
100's	$111.40	PHENAZIDE, Major Pharms	00904-3676-60
100's	$114.48	Fluphenazine Hcl, HL Moore Drug Exch	00839-7452-06
100's	$114.75	Fluphenazine HCl Usp, Geneva Pharms	00781-1439-01
100's	$117.95	Fluphenazine Hcl, Mylan	00378-6097-01
100's	$128.50	Fluphenazine HCl, Rugby	00536-3808-01
100's	$170.30	Fluphenazine Hydrochloride, Goldline Labs	00182-1368-89
100's	$170.30	Fluphenazine HCl Usp, Geneva Pharms	00781-1439-13
100's	**$190.08**	**PROLIXIN, Bristol Myers Squibb**	**00003-0956-50**
100's	**$209.55**	**PROLIXIN, Bristol Myers Squibb**	**00003-0956-52**
500's	$251.25	Fluphenazine HCl, H.C.F.A. F F P	99999-1324-16
500's	$339.45	PHENAZIDE, Major Pharms	00904-3676-40
500's	$409.25	Fluphenazine, Harber Pharm	51432-0816-05
500's	$485.90	Fluphenazine HCl, Qualitest Pharms	00603-3669-28
500's	$545.25	Fluphenazine HCl, Geneva Pharms	00781-1439-05
500's	$545.25	Fluphenazine Hcl, Par Pharm	49884-0064-05
500's	$546.95	Fluphenazine Hcl, Mylan	00378-6097-05
500's	**$915.00**	**PROLIXIN, Bristol Myers Squibb**	**00003-0956-70**
1000's	$502.50	Fluphenazine HCl, H.C.F.A. F F P	99999-1324-17

HOW SUPPLIED - NOT RATED EQUIVALENT:

Tablet, Plain Coated - Oral - 2.5 mg

100's	$103.75	PERMITIL, Schering	00085-0442-04

Tablet, Plain Coated - Oral - 5 mg

100's	$138.50	PERMITIL, Schering	00085-0550-04

Tablet, Plain Coated - Oral - 10 mg

100's	$110.15	Fluphenazine Hcl, Parmed Pharms	00349-8979-01
1000's	$1643.41	PERMITIL, Schering	00085-0316-05

FLUPIRTINE MALEATE *(003079)*

CATEGORIES: Analgesics; Pain; Pain, Episiotomy; FDA Unapproved

Prescribing information not available at time of publication.

FLURANDRENOLIDE *(001325)*

CATEGORIES: Adrenal Corticosteroids; Anti-Inflammatory Agents; Dermatologicals; Dermatoses; Skin/Mucous Membrane Agents; Steroids; Topical; Pregnancy Category C; FDA Approval Pre 1982

BRAND NAMES: **Cordran**; Cordran Tape Patch; *Drenison* (Canada); *Drenison 1 4* (Canada); *Haelan*; *Sermaka* (Germany)
(International brand names outside U.S. in italics)

FORMULARIES: Medi-Cal

DESCRIPTION:

(Please note this monograph contains information for Cordran Ointment and SP Cream, Lotion, and Tape).

All Forms: Flurandrenolide, USP is a potent corticosteroid intended for topical use. It occurs as white to off-white, fluffy, crystalline powder and is odorless. Flurandrenolide is practically insoluble in water and in ether. One g dissolves in 72 ml of alcohol and in 10 ml of chloroform. The molecular weight of Flurandrenolide is 436.52.

The chemical name of flurandrenolide is pregn-4-ene-3,20-dione, 6-fluro-11,21-dihydroxy-16,17-[(1-methylethylidene)bis (oxy)]-, (6α-11β, 16α)-; its empirical formula is $C_{24}H_{33}FO_6$.

Ointment and SP Cream: Each g of Flurandrenolide Cream, USP contains 0.5 mg (1.145 µmol; 0.05%) or 0.25 mg (0.57 µmol; 0.025%) flurandrenolide in an emulsified base composed of cetyl alcohol, citric acid, mineral oil, polyoxyl 40 stearate, propylene glycol, sodium citrate, stearic acid, and purified water.

Lotion: Each ml of Lotion contains 0.5 mg (1.145 µmol) (0.05%) flurandrenolide in an oil-in-water emulsion base composed of glycerin, cetyl alcohol, stearic acid, glyceryl monostearate, mineral oil, polyoxyl 40 stearate, menthol, benzyl alcohol, and purified water.

Tape: Flurandrenolide Tape, USP is a transparent, inconspicuous plastic surgical tape, impervious to moisture.

Each square centimeter contains 4 mcg (0.00916 µmol) flurandrenolide uniformly distributed in the adhesive layer. The tape is made of a thin, matte-finish poly-ethylene film that is slightly elastic and highly flexible.

The adhesive is a synthetic copolymer of acrylate ester and acrylic acid that is free from substances of plant origin. The pressure-sensitive adhesive surface is covered with a protective paper liner to permit handling and trimming before application.

CLINICAL PHARMACOLOGY:

Flurandrenolide is primarily effective because of its anti-inflammatory, antipruritic, and vasoconstrictive actions.

The mechanism of the anti-inflammatory effect of topical corticosteroids is not completely understood. Various laboratory methods, including vasoconstrictor assays, are used to compare and predict potencies and/or clinical efficacies of the topical corticosteroids. There is some evidence to suggest that a recognizable correlation exists between vasoconstrictor potency and therapeutic efficacy in man. Corticosteroids with anti-inflammatory activity may stabilize cellular and lysosomal membranes. There is also the suggestion that the effect on the membranes of lysosomes prevents the release of proteolytic enzymes and, thus, plays a part in reducing inflammation.

Evaporation of water from the lotion vehicle produces a cooling effect which is often desirable in the treatment of acutely inflamed or weeping lesions.

Tape: The tape serves as both a vehicle and an occlusive dressing. Retention of insensible perspiration by the tape results in hydration of the stratum corneum and improved diffusion of the medication. The skin is protected from scratching, rubbing, desiccation, and chemical irritation. The tape acts as mechanical splint to fissured skin. Since it prevents removal of the medication by washing or the rubbing action of clothing, the tape formulation provides a sustained action.

CLINICAL PHARMACOLOGY: *(cont'd)*

PHARMACOKINETICS

The extent of percutaneous absorption of topical corticosteroids is determined by many factors, including the vehicle, the integrity of the epidermal barrier, and the use of occlusive dressings.

Topical corticosteroids can be absorbed from normal intact skin. Inflammation and/or other disease processes in the skin increase percutaneous absorption. Occlusive dressings substantially increase the percutaneous absorption of topical corticosteroids. Thus, occlusive dressings may be a valuable therapeutic adjunct for treatment of resistant dermatoses. (see DOSAGE AND ADMINISTRATION).

Once absorbed through the skin, topical corticosteroids are handled through pharmacokinetic pathways similar to those of systemically administered corticosteroids. Corticosteroids are bound to plasma proteins in varying degrees. Corticosteroids are metabolized primarily in the liver and then excreted in the kidneys. Some of the topical corticosteroids and their metabolites are also excreted into the bile.

INDICATIONS AND USAGE:

Flurandrenolide is indicated for the relief of the inflammatory and pruritic manifestations of corticosteroid-responsive dermatoses, (particularly dry, scale localized lesions -Tape only).

CONTRAINDICATIONS:

Topical corticosteroids are contraindicated in patients with a history of hypersensitivity to any of the components of these preparations.

Tape: Use of Flurandrenolide Tape is not recommended for lesions exuding serum or in intertriginous areas.

PRECAUTIONS:

General: Systemic absorption of topical corticosteroids has produced reversible hypothalamic-pituitary-adrenal (HPA) axis suppression, manifestations of Cushing's syndrome, hyperglycemia, and glucosuria in some patients.

Conditions that augment systemic absorption include application of the more potent steroids, use over large surface areas, prolonged use, and the addition of occlusive dressings.

Therefore, patients receiving a large dose of a potent topical steroid applied to a large surface area or under an occlusive dressing should be evaluated periodically for evidence of HPA axis suppression by using urinary-free cortisol and ACTH stimulation tests. If HPA axis suppression is noted, an attempt should be made to withdraw the drug, to reduce the frequency of application, or to substitute a less potent steroid.

Recovery of HPA axis function is generally prompt and complete on discontinuation of the drug. Infrequently, signs and symptoms of steroid withdrawal may occur, so that supplemental systemic corticosteroids are required.

Children may absorb proportionately larger amounts of topical corticosteroids and thus be more susceptible to systemic toxicity (see Pediatric Use).

If irritation develops, topical corticosteroids should be discontinued and appropriate therapy instituted.

In the presence of dermatologic infections, the use of an appropriate antifungal or antibacterial agent should be instituted. If a favorable response does not occur promptly, Flurandrenolide should be discontinued until the infection has been adequately controlled.

Information for the Patient: Patients using topical corticosteroids should receive the following information and instructions:

1. This medication is to be used as directed by the physician. It is for external us only. Avoid contact with the eyes.

2. Patients should be advised not to use this medication for any disorder other than that for which it was prescribed.

3. The treated skin area should not be bandaged or otherwise covered or wrapped in order to be occlusive unless the patient is directed to do so by the physician.

4. Patients should report any signs of local adverse reactions, especially under occlusive dressing.

5. Parents of pediatric patients should be advised not to use tight-fitting diapers or plastic pants on a child being treated in the diaper area, because these garments may constitute occlusive dressings.

Laboratory Tests: The following tests may be helpful in evaluating the HPA axis suppression:

Urinary-free cortisol test

ACTH stimulation test

Carcinogenesis, Mutagenesis, and Impairment of Fertility: Long-term animal studies have not been performed to evaluate the carcinogenic potential or the effect on fertility of topical corticosteroids.

Studies to determine mutagenicity with prednisolone and hydrocortisone have revealed negative results.

Pregnancy Category C: Corticosteroids are generally teratogenic in laboratory animals when administered systemically at relatively low dosage levels. The more potent corticosteroids have been shown to be teratogenic after dermal application in laboratory animals. There are no adequate and well-controlled studies in pregnant women on teratogenic effects from topically applied corticosteroids. Therefore, topical corticosteroids should be used during pregnancy only if the potential benefit justifies the potential risk to the fetus. Drugs of this class should not be used extensively on pregnant patients or in large amounts or for prolonged periods of time.

Nursing Mothers: It is not known whether topical administration of corticosteroids could result in sufficient systemic absorption to produce detectable quantities in breast milk. Systemically administered corticosteroids are secreted into breast milk in quantities *not* likely to have a deleterious effect on the infant. Nevertheless, caution should be exercised when topical corticosteroids are administered to a nursing woman.

Pediatric Use: Pediatric patients may demonstrate greater susceptibility to topical-corticosteroid-induced HPA axis suppression and Cushing's syndrome than do mature patients because of a larger skin surface area to body weight ratio.

Hypothalamic-pituitary-adrenal (HPA) axis suppression, Cushing's syndrome, and intracranial hypertension have been reported in children receiving topical corticosteroids. Manifestations of adrenal suppression in children include linear growth retardation, delayed weight gain, low plasma-cortisol levels, and absence of response to ACTH stimulation. Manifestations of intracranial hypertension include bulging fontanelles, headaches, and bilateral papilledema.

Administration of topical corticosteroids to children should be limited to the least amount compatible with an effective therapeutic regimen. Chronic corticosteroid therapy may interfere with the growth and development of children.

ADVERSE REACTIONS:

The following local adverse reactions are reported infrequently with topical corticosteroids but may occur more frequently with the use of occlusive dressings. These reactions are listed in an approximate decreasing order of occurrence:

Burning
Itching
Irritation
Dryness
Folliculitis
Hypertrichosis
Acneform eruptions
Hypopigmentation
Perioral dermatitis
Allergic contact dermatitis
Maceration of the skin
Secondary infection
Skin atrophy
Striae
Miliaria

OVERDOSAGE:

Topically applied corticosteroids can be absorbed in sufficient amounts to produce systemic effects (see PRECAUTIONS).

DOSAGE AND ADMINISTRATION:

SP Cream, Ointment, and Lotion: Topical corticosteroids are generally applied to the affected area as a thin film from 1 to 4 times daily, depending on the severity of the condition.

A small quantity of Flurandrenolide SP Cream or Lotion should be rubbed gently into the affected area 2 or 3 times daily.

Occlusive dressings may be used for the management of psoriasis or recalcitrant conditions.

If an infection develops, the use of occlusive dressings should be discontinued and appropriate antimicrobial therapy instituted.

Use with Occlusive Dressings: The technique of occlusive dressings (for management of psoriasis and other persistent dermatoses) is as follows:

1. Remove as much as possible of the superficial scaling before applying Flurandrenolide SP Cream, Ointment or Lotion. Soaking in a bath will help soften the scales and permit easier removal by brushing, picking, or rubbing.

2. Rub the lotion thoroughly into the affected areas.

3. Cover with an occlusive plastic film, such as polyethylene, Saran Wrap, or Handi-Wrap. (Added moisture may be provided by placing a slightly dampened cloth or gauze over the lesion before the plastic film is applied.)

4. Seal the edges to adjacent normal skin with tape or hold in place by a gauze wrapping.

5. For convenience, the patient may remove the dressing during the day. The dressing should then be reapplied each night.

6. For daytime therapy, the condition may be treated by rubbing Flurandrenolide SP Cream, Ointment or Lotion sparingly into the affected areas.

7. In more resistant cases, leaving the dressing in place for 3 to 4 days at a time may result in a better response.

8. Thin polyethylene gloves are suitable for treatment of the hands and fingers; plastic garment bags may be utilized for treating lesions on the trunk or buttocks. A tight shower cap is useful in treating lesions on the scalp.

OCCLUSIVE DRESSINGS HAVE THE FOLLOWING ADVANTAGES

1. Percutaneous penetration of the corticosteroid is enhanced.

2. Medication is concentrated on the areas of skin where it is most needed.

3. This method of administration frequently is more effective in very resistant dermatoses than is the conventional application of Flurandrenolide.

Precautions to Be Observed in Therapy with Occlusive Dressings: Treatment should be continued for at least a few days after clearing of the lesions. If it is stopped too soon, a relapse may occur. Reinstitution of treatment frequently will cause remission.

Because of the increased hazard of secondary infection from resistant strains of staphylococci among hospitalized patients, it is suggested that the use of occlusive plastic films for corticosteroid therapy in such cases be restricted.

Generally, occlusive dressings should not be used on weeping, or exudative, lesions.

When large areas of the body are covered, thermal homeostasis may be impaired. If elevation of body temperature occurs, use of the occlusive dressing should be discontinued.

Rarely, a patient may develop miliaria, folliculitis, or a sensitivity to either the particular dressing material or a combination of Flurandrenolide and the occlusive dressing. If miliaria or folliculitis occurs, use of the occlusive dressing should be discontinued. Treatment by inunction with Flurandrenolide may be continued. If the sensitivity is caused by the particular material of the dressing, substitution of a different material may be tried.

Warnings: Some plastic films are readily flammable. Patients should be cautioned against the use of any such material.

When plastic films are used on infants and children, the persons caring for the patients must be reminded of the danger of suffocation if the plastic material accidentally covers the face.

Tape: Occlusive dressings may be used for the management of psoriasis or recalcitrant conditions.

If an infection develops, the use of Flurandrenolide Tape and other occlusive dressings should be discontinued and appropriate antimicrobial therapy instituted.

Replacement of the tape every 12 hours produces the lowest incidence of adverse reactions, but it may be left in place for 24 hours it is well tolerated and adheres satisfactorily. When necessary, the tape may be used at night only and removed during the day.

If ends of the tape loosen prematurely, they may be trimmed off and replaced with fresh tape.

The directions given below are included on a separate package insert for the patient to follow unless otherwise instructed by the physician.

APPLICATION OF FLURANDRENOLIDE TAPE

DOSAGE AND ADMINISTRATION: *(cont'd)*

Important: Skin should be **Clean and Dry before tape is applied. Tape should always be cut, never torn.**

Directions For Use:

1. Prepare skin as directed by your physician or as follows: Gently clean the area to be covered to remove scales, crusts, dried exudates, and any previously used ointments or creams. A germicidal soap or cleanser should be used to prevent the development of odor under the tape. Shave or clip the hair in the treatment area to allow food contact with the skin and comfortable removal. If shower or tub bath is to be taken, it should be completed before the tape is applied. The skin should be dry before application of the tape.

2. Remove tape from package and cut a piece slightly larger than area to be covered. Round off corners.

3. Pull white paper from transparent tape. Be careful that tape does not stick to itself.

4. Apply tape, keeping skin smooth; press tape into place.

Replacement of Tape: Unless instructed otherwise by your physician, replace tape after 12 hours. Cleanse skin and allow it to dry for 1 hour before applying new tape.

If Irritation Or Infection Develops, Remove Tape And Consult Physician.

(SP Cream and Ointment, Oclassen Pharmaceuticals, Inc., 9/92, PA 7560 UCP)

(Lotion, Oclassen Pharmaceuticals, Inc., 9/92, PA 5080 UCP)

(Tape, Oclassen Pharmaceuticals, Inc., 1/95, PA 2032 UCP)

HOW SUPPLIED - RATED THERAPEUTICALLY EQUIVALENT:

Lotion - Topical - 0.05 %

15 ml	$12.35	CORDRAN, Oclassen Pharms	55515-0052-15
60 ml	$32.45	CORDRAN, Oclassen Pharms	55515-0052-60

Tape, Medicated - Topical - 4 mcg/sq cm

12's	$13.56	CORDRAN TAPE, Oclassen Pharms	55515-0014-12
24' x 3'	$13.56	CORDRAN, Oclassen Pharms	55515-0014-24
80' x 3'	$29.13	CORDRAN, Oclassen Pharms	55515-0014-80

HOW SUPPLIED - NOT RATED EQUIVALENT:

Cream - Topical - 0.025 %

30 gm	$14.07	CORDRAN SP, Oclassen Pharms	55515-0034-30
60 gm	$19.88	CORDRAN SP, Oclassen Pharms	55515-0034-60

Cream - Topical - 0.05 %

15 gm	$12.70	CORDRAN SP, Oclassen Pharms	55515-0035-15
30 gm	$17.96	CORDRAN SP, Oclassen Pharms	55515-0035-30
60 gm	$33.37	CORDRAN SP, Oclassen Pharms	55515-0035-60
225 gm	$86.45	CORDRAN SP, Dista	00777-6035-88

Ointment - Topical - 0.025 %

30 gm	$14.07	CORDRAN, Oclassen Pharms	55515-0024-30
60 gm	$19.88	CORDRAN, Oclassen Pharms	55515-0024-60
225 gm	$49.36	CORDRAN, Dista	00777-1824-88

Ointment - Topical - 0.05 %

15 gm	$12.70	CORDRAN, Oclassen Pharms	55515-0026-15
30 gm	$17.96	CORDRAN, Oclassen Pharms	55515-0026-30
60 gm	$33.37	CORDRAN, Oclassen Pharms	55515-0026-60

FLURANDRENOLIDE; NEOMYCIN SULFATE

(001326)

CATEGORIES: Anti-Infectives; Antibiotics; Dermatologicals; Dermatoses; Infections; Skin/Mucous Membrane Agents; Steroids; FDA Approval Pre 1982

BRAND NAMES: **Cordran-N**; *Drenison con neomicina*; *Drenison-N*; *Drenison-neomicina*; *Sermaka N* (Germany)
(International brand names outside U.S. in italics)

FORMULARIES: Aetna

DESCRIPTION:

Cordran (Flurandrenolide, USP) is a potent corticosteroid intended for topical use. The chemical formula of Cordran is 6α-fluoro-16α-hydroxyhydrocortisone 16,17-acetonide.

Each g of Cordran-N (flurandrenolide with neomycin sulfate) cream contains 0.5 mg (0.05%) flurandrenolide and 5 mg neomycin sulfate (equivalent to 3.5 mg neomycin base) in a base composed of stearic acid, cetyl alcohol, mineral oil, polyoxyl 40 stearate, ethylparaben, glycerin, and purified water.

Each g of Cordran-N ointment contains 0.5 mg (0.05%) flurandrenolide and 5 mg neomycin sulfate (equivalent to 3.5 mg neomycin base) in a base composed of white wax, cetyl alcohol, sorbitan sesquioleate, and white petrolatum.

CLINICAL PHARMACOLOGY:

Cordran is primarily effective because of its anti-inflammatory, antipruritic, and vasoconstrictive actions.

The addition of neomycin broadens the usefulness of Cordran so that dermatoses complicated by actual skin infections may be treated more effectively and with safety.

INDICATIONS AND USAGE:

On the basis of a review of this drug by the National Academy of Sciences-National Research Council and/or other information, FDA has classified the following indications as "possibly" effective.
For relief of the inflammatory manifestations of corticosteroid-responsive dermatoses complicated by bacterial infections.
Final classification of the less-than-effective indications requires further investigation.

CONTRAINDICATIONS:

Topical corticosteroids are contraindicated in patients with a history of hypersensitivity to any of the components of these preparations.

WARNINGS:

Because of the potential hazard of nephrotoxicity and ototoxicity, prolonged use of large amounts of this product should be avoided in the treatment of skin infections following extensive burns, trophic ulceration, and other conditions in which absorption of neomycin is possible.

PRECAUTIONS:

If irritation develops, the product should be discontinued and appropriate therapy instituted.

Patients with superficial fungus or yeast infections should be treated with additional appropriate methods and observed frequently.

Prolonged use of neomycin preparations may result in the overgrowth of nonsusceptible organisms. If this occurs, appropriate measures should be taken.

There are articles in the current medical literature that indicate an increase in the prevalence of persons who are sensitive to neomycin.

If extensive areas are treated or if the occlusive technique is used, there will be increased systemic absorption of the corticosteroid, and suitable precautions should be taken, particularly in children and infants.

Although topical corticosteroids have not been reported to have an adverse effect on human pregnancy, the safety of their use on pregnant women has not been absolutely established. In laboratory animals, increases in incidence of fetal abnormalities have been associated with exposure of gestating females to topical corticosteroids, in some cases at rather low dosage levels. Therefore, drugs of this class should not be used extensively, in large amounts, or for prolonged periods of time on pregnant patients.

These products are not for ophthalmic use.

ADVERSE REACTIONS:

The following local adverse reactions (TABLE 1) have been reported with topical corticosteroid formulations:

TABLE 1

Acneform eruptions	Hypertrichosi
Allergic contact dermatitis	Hypopigmentation
Burning	Irritation
Dryness	Itching
Folliculitis	Perioral dermatitis
The following may occur more frequently with occlusive dressings:	
Maceration of the skin	Skin atrophy
Miliaria	Striae
Secondary infection	

Topical neomycin has been reported to cause allergic contact dermatitis, ototoxicity, and nephrotoxicity.

DOSAGE AND ADMINISTRATION:

For moist lesions, a small quantity of the cream should be rubbed gently into the affected areas 2 or 3 times a day. For dry, scaly lesions, the ointment is applied as a thin film to affected areas 2 or 3 times daily.

USE WITH OCCLUSIVE DRESSINGS

The technique of occlusive dressings (for management of psoriasis and other persistent dermatoses complicated by bacterial infection) is as follows:

1. Remove as much as possible of the superficial scaling before applying Cordran-N cream or ointment. Soaking in a bath will help soften the scales and permit easier removal by brushing, picking, or rubbing.

2. Rub Cordran-N thoroughly into the affected areas.

3. Cover with an occlusive plastic film, such as polyethylene, Saran Wrap, or Handi-Wrap. When Cordran-N cream is used, added moisture may be provided by placing a slightly dampened cloth or gauze over the lesion before the plastic film is applied.

4. Seal the edges to adjacent normal skin with tape or hold in place by a gauze wrapping.

5. For convenience, the patient may remove the dressing during the day. The dressing should then be reapplied each night.

6. For daytime therapy, the condition may be treated by rubbing Cordran-N cream or ointment sparingly into the affected areas.

7. In more resistant cases, leaving the dressing in place for 3 to 4 days at a time may result in a better response.

8. Thin polyethylene gloves are suitable for treatment of the hands and fingers; plastic garment bags may be utilized for treating lesions on the trunk or buttocks. A tight shower cap is useful in treating lesions on the scalp.

Occlusive Dressings Have the Following Advantages-

1. Percutaneous penetration of the corticosteroid is enhanced.

2. Medication is concentrated on the areas of skin where it is most needed.

3. This method of administration frequently is more effective in very resistant dermatoses than is the conventional application of Cordran-N.

*Precautions to Be Observed in Therapy with Occlusive Dressings-*Treatment should be continued for at least a few days after clearing of the lesions. If it is stopped too soon, a relapse may occur. Reinstitution of treatment frequently will cause remission.

Because of the increased hazard of secondary infection from resistant strains of staphylococci among hospitalized patients, it is suggested that the use of occlusive plastic films for corticosteroid therapy in such cases be restricted.

Generally, occlusive dressings should not be used on weeping, or exudative, lesions.

When large areas of the body are covered, thermal homeostasis may be impaired. If elevation of body temperature occurs, use of the occlusive dressing should be discontinued.

Rarely, a patient may develop miliaria, folliculitis, or a sensitivity, to either the particular dressing material or the combination of Cordran-N and the occlusive dressing. If miliaria or folliculitis occurs, use of the occlusive dressing should be discontinued. Treatment by inunction with Cordran-N may be continued. If the sensitivity is caused by the particular material of the dressing, substitution of a different material may be tried.

*Warnings-*Some plastic films are readily flammable. Patients should be cautioned against the use of any such material.

When plastic films are used on infants and children, the persons caring for the patients must be reminded of the danger of suffocation if the plastic material accidentally covers the face.

HOW SUPPLIED - EQUIVALENTS NOT AVAILABLE:

Ointment - Topical - 0.5 mg/5 mg

15 gm	$10.93	CORDRAN-N, Dista	00777-1827-47
15 gm	$12.43	CORDRAN-N, Dista	00777-1884-47
30 gm	$15.59	CORDRAN-N, Dista	00777-1827-67

HOW SUPPLIED - EQUIVALENTS NOT AVAILABLE: *(cont'd)*

30's	**$17.74**	**CORDRAN-N, Dista**	**00777-1884-67**
60 gm	**$28.75**	**CORDRAN-N, Dista**	**00777-1827-97**
60 gm	**$32.72**	**CORDRAN-N, Dista**	**00777-1884-97**

FLURAZEPAM HYDROCHLORIDE *(001327)*

CATEGORIES: Anxiolytics, Sedatives, Hypnotic; Benzodiazepines; Central Nervous System Agents; Hypnotics; Insomnia; Sedatives; Sedatives/Hypnotics; DEA Class CIV; FDA Approval Pre 1982

BRAND NAMES: *Apo-Flurazepam* (Canada); *Benozil* (Japan); *Dalmadorm* (Germany); **Dalmane**; *Dalmate* (Japan); *Dormodor*; *Felison*; *Fluleep*; *Flunox*; *Fluzepam*; *Fordrim*; *Insumin* (Japan); *Irdal*; *Midorm*; *Midorm AR*; *Natam*; *Nergart* (Japan); *Nindral*; *Niotal*; *Novoflupam* (Canada); *Paxane*; *Remdue*; *Somlan*; *Staurodorm* (Germany); *Valdorm*
(International brand names outside U.S. in italics)

FORMULARIES: Aetna; BC-BS; Foundation; Medi-Cal

COST OF THERAPY: $0.47 (Insomnia; Capsule; 30 mg; 1/day; 7 days) vs. Potential Cost of $3,628.44 (Psychoses)

DESCRIPTION:

Flurazepam hydrochloride is available as capsules containing 15 mg or 30 mg flurazepam HCl. Each 15-mg capsule also contains corn starch, lactose, magnesium stearate and talc; gelatin capsule shells may contain methyl and propyl parabens and potassium sorbate, with the following dye systems: FD&C Red No. 3, FD&C Yellow No. 6 and D&C Yellow No. 10. Each 30-mg capsule also contains corn starch, lactose and magnesium stearate; gelatin capsule shells may contain methyl and propyl parabens and potassium sorbate, with the following dye systems: FD&C Blue No. 1, FD&C Yellow No. 6, D&C Yellow No. 10 and either FD&C Red No. 3 or FD&C Red No. 40.

Flurazepam HCl is chemically 7-chloro-1-(2-(diethylamino)ethyl)-5-(*o*-fluorophenyl)-1,3-dihydro-*2H*-1,4-benzodiazepin-2-one dihydrochloride. It is a pale yellow, crystalline compound, freely soluble in U.S.P. alcohol and very soluble in water. It has a molecular weight of 460.826.

CLINICAL PHARMACOLOGY:

Flurazepam HCl is rapidly absorbed from the G.I. tract. Flurazepam is rapidly metabolized and is excreted primarily in the urine. Following a single oral dose, peak flurazepam plasma concentrations ranging from 0.5 to 4.0 ng/ml occur at 30 to 60 minutes post-dosing. The harmonic mean apparent half-life of flurazepam is 2.3 hours. The blood level profile of flurazepam and its major metabolites was determined in man following the oral administration of 30 mg daily for 2 weeks. The N_1-hydroxyethyl-flurazepam was measurable only during the early hours after a 30-mg dose and was not detectable after 24 hours. The major metabolite in blood was N_1-desalkyl-flurazepam, which reached steady-state (plateau) levels after 7 to 10 days of dosing, at levels approximately five-to sixfold greater than the 24-hour levels observed on Day 1. The half-life of elimination of N_1-desalkyl-flurazepam ranged from 47 to 100 hours. The major urinary metabolite is conjugated N_1-hydroxyethyl-flurazepam which accounts for 22% to 55% of the dose. Less than 1% of the dose is excreted in the urine as N_1-desalkyl-flurazepam.

This pharmacokinetic profile may be responsible for the clinical observation that flurazepam is increasingly effective on the second or third night of consecutive use and that for one or two nights after the drug is discontinued both sleep latency and total wake time may still be decreased.

INDICATIONS AND USAGE:

Flurazepam HCl is a hypnotic agent useful for the treatment of insomnia characterized by difficulty in falling asleep, frequent nocturnal awakenings, and/or early morning awakening. Flurazepam hydrochloride can be used effectively in patients with recurring insomnia or poor sleeping habits, and in acute or chronic medical situations requiring restful sleep. Sleep laboratory studies have objectively determined that flurazepam hydrochloride is effective for at least 28 consecutive nights of drug administration. Since insomnia is often transient and intermittent, short-term use is usually sufficient. Prolonged use of hypnotics is usually not indicated and should only be undertaken concomitantly with appropriate evaluation of the patient.

CONTRAINDICATIONS:

Flurazepam hydrochloride is contraindicated in patients with known hypersensitivity to the drug.

Usage in Pregnancy: Benzodiazepines may cause fetal damage when administered during pregnancy. An increased risk of congenital malformations associated with the use of diazepam and chlordiazepoxide during the first trimester of pregnancy has been suggested in several studies.

Flurazepam HCl is contraindicated in pregnant women. Symptoms of neonatal depression have been reported; a neonate whose mother received 30 mg of flurazepam HCl nightly for insomnia during the 10 days prior to delivery appeared hypotonic and inactive during the first four days of life. Serum levels of N_1-desalkyl-flurazepam in the infant indicated transplacental circulation and implicate this long-acting metabolite in this case. If there is a likelihood of the patient becoming pregnant while receiving flurazepam, she should be warned of the potential risks to the fetus. Patients should be instructed to discontinue the drug prior to becoming pregnant. The possibility that a woman of child-bearing potential may be pregnant at the time of institution of therapy should be considered.

WARNINGS:

Patients should also be cautioned about engaging in hazardous occupations requiring complete mental alertness such as operating machinery or driving a motor vehicle after ingesting the drug, including potential impairment of the performance of such activities which may occur the day following ingestion of flurazepam HCl.

USAGE IN CHILDREN

Clinical investigations of flurazepam hydrochloride have not been carried out in children. Therefore, the drug is not currently recommended for use in persons under 15 years of age.

Withdrawal symptoms of the barbiturate type have occurred after the discontinuation of benzodiazepines. (See DRUG ABUSE AND DEPENDENCE.)

PRECAUTIONS:

Since the risk of the development of oversedation, dizziness, confusion and/or ataxia increases substantially with larger doses in elderly and debilitated patients, it is recommended that in such patients the dosage be limited to 15 mg. If flurazepam hydrochloride is to be combined with other drugs having known hypnotic properties or CNS-depressant effects, due consideration should be given to potential additive effects.

PRECAUTIONS: *(cont'd)*

The usual precautions are indicated for severely depressed patients or those in whom there is any evidence of latent depression; particularly the recognition that suicidal tendencies may be present and protective measures may be necessary.

The usual precautions should be observed in patients with impaired renal or hepatic function and chronic pulmonary insufficiency.

Information for the Patient: To assure the safe and effective use of benzodiazepines, patients should be informed that since benzodiazepines may produce psychological and physical dependence, it is advisable that they consult with their physician before either increasing the dose or abruptly discontinuing this drug.

DRUG INTERACTIONS:

Patients receiving flurazepam HCl should be cautioned about possible combined effects with alcohol and other CNS depressants. Also, caution patients that an additive effect may occur if alcoholic beverages are consumed during the day following the use of flurazepam hydrochloride for nighttime sedation. The potential for this interaction continues for several days following discontinuance of flurazepam, until serum levels of psychoactive metabolites have declined.

ADVERSE REACTIONS:

Dizziness, drowsiness, light-headedness, staggering, ataxia and falling have occurred, particularly in elderly or debilitated persons. Severe sedation, lethargy, disorientation and coma, probably indicative of drug intolerance or overdosage, have been reported.

Also reported were headache, heartburn, upset stomach, nausea, vomiting, diarrhea, constipation, gastrointestinal pain, nervousness, talkativeness, apprehension, irritability, weakness, palpitations, chest pains, body and joint pains and genitourinary complaints. There have also been rare occurrences of leukopenia, granulocytopenia, sweating, flushes, difficulty in focusing, blurred vision, burning eyes, faintness, hypotension, shortness of breath, pruritus, skin rash, dry mouth, bitter taste, excessive salivation, anorexia, euphoria, depression, slurred speech, confusion, restlessness, hallucinations, and elevated SGOT, SGPT, total and direct bilirubins, and alkaline phosphatase. Paradoxical reactions, *e.g.*, excitement, stimulation and hyperactivity, have also been reported in rare instances.

DRUG ABUSE AND DEPENDENCE:

Withdrawal symptoms, similar in character to those noted with barbiturates and alcohol (convulsions, tremor, abdominal and muscle cramps, vomiting and sweating), have occurred following abrupt discontinuance of benzodiazepines. The more severe withdrawal symptoms have usually been limited to those patients who had received excessive doses over an extended period of time. Generally milder withdrawal symptoms (*e.g.*, dysphoria and insomnia) have been reported following abrupt discontinuance of benzodiazepines taken continuously at therapeutic levels for several months. Consequently, after extended therapy, abrupt discontinuation should generally be avoided and a gradual dosage tapering schedule followed. Addiction-prone individuals (such as drug addicts or alcoholics) should be under careful surveillance when receiving flurazepam or other psychotropic agents because of the predisposition of such patients to habituation and dependence.

OVERDOSAGE:

Manifestations of flurazepam hydrochloride overdosage include somnolence, confusion and coma. Respiration, pulse and blood pressure should be monitored as in all cases of drug overdosage. General supportive measures should be employed, along with immediate gastric lavage. Intravenous fluids should be administered and an adequate airway maintained. Hypotension and CNS depression may be combated by judicious use of appropriate therapeutic agents. The value of dialysis has not been determined. If excitation occurs in patients following flurazepam hydrochloride overdosage, barbiturates should not be used. As with the management of intentional overdosage with any drug, it should be borne in mind that multiple agents may have been ingested.

Flumazenil, a specific benzodiazepine-receptor antagonist, is indicated for the complete or partial reversal of the sedative effects of benzodiazepines and may be useful in situations when an overdose with a benzodiazepine is known or suspected. Prior to the administration of flumazenil, necessary measures should be instituted to secure airway, ventilation and intravenous access. Flumazenil is intended as an adjunct to, not as a substitute for, proper management of benzodiazepine overdose. Patients treated with flumazenil should be monitored for resedation, respiratory depression and other residual benzodiazepine effects for an appropriate period after treatment. **The prescriber should be aware of a risk of seizure in association with flumazenil treatment, particularly in long-term benzodiazepine users and in cyclic, antidepressant overdose.** The complete flumazenil package insert, including CONTRAINDICATIONS, WARNINGS, and PRECAUTIONS, should be consulted prior to use.

DOSAGE AND ADMINISTRATION:

Dosage should be individualized for maximal beneficial effects. The usual adult dosage is 30 mg before retiring. In some patients, 15 mg may suffice. In elderly and/or debilitated patients, 15 mg is usually sufficient for a therapeutic response and it is therefore recommended that therapy be initiated with this dosage.

HOW SUPPLIED - RATED THERAPEUTICALLY EQUIVALENT:

Capsule, Gelatin - Oral - 15 mg

50's	$2.62	Flurazepam HCl, H.C.F.A. F F P	99999-1327-01
100's	$5.25	Flurazepam Hcl, United Res	00677-1065-01
100's	$5.25	Flurazepam HCl, H.C.F.A. F F P	99999-1327-02
100's	$15.00	Flurazepam HCl, West Ward Pharm	00143-3367-01
100's	$19.91	Flurazepam Hcl, Qualitest Pharms	00603-3691-21
100's	$21.50	Flurazepam, Schein Pharm (US)	00364-0801-01
100's	$21.50	Flurazepam, Major Pharms	00904-2800-60
100's	$21.65	Flurazepam HCl, Geneva Pharms	00781-2806-01
100's	$22.00	Flurazepam Hcl, Halsey Drug	00879-0534-01
100's	$22.05	Flurazepam HCl, Rugby	00536-3795-01
100's	$22.10	Flurazepam Hcl, Goldline Labs	00182-1817-01
100's	$22.10	Flurazepam Hcl, Purepac Pharm	00228-2021-10
100's	$22.10	Flurazepam Hcl, Aligen Independ	00405-0085-01
100's	$22.10	Flurazepam Hcl, Par Pharm	49884-0193-01
100's	$22.80	Flurazepam Hcl, HL Moore Drug Exch	00839-7154-06
100's	$23.63	Flurazepam HCl 15, Warner Chilcott	00047-0988-24
100's	$23.95	Flurazepam Hcl, Mylan	00378-4415-01
100's	$26.17	Flurazepam Hcl, Vangard Labs	00615-0460-13
100's	$26.17	Flurazepam Hcl, Vangard Labs	00615-0460-47
100's	$29.85	Flurazepam Hcl, Medirex	57480-0510-01
100's	$32.00	Flurazepam HCl, West Ward Pharm	00143-3367-25
100's	$34.46	Flurazepam, Major Pharms	00904-2800-61
100's	$38.88	Flurazepam Hcl, Voluntary Hosp	53258-0612-01
100's	$39.45	Flurazepam Hcl, Voluntary Hosp	53258-0612-13
100's	**$47.50**	**DALMANE, Roche Prod**	**00140-0065-50**
100's	**$49.70**	**DALMANE, Roche Prod**	**00140-0065-49**
100's	**$50.20**	**DALMANE, Roche Prod**	**00140-0065-03**
100's	**$54.26**	**DALMANE, Roche Prod**	**00140-0065-01**

HOW SUPPLIED - RATED THERAPEUTICALLY EQUIVALENT: *(cont'd)*

500's	$26.25	Flurazepam HCl, H.C.F.A. F F P	99999-1327-03
500's	$75.00	Flurazepam HCl, West Ward Pharm	00143-3367-05
500's	$90.58	Flurazepam, Schein Pharm (US)	00364-0801-05
500's	$96.51	Flurazepam Hcl, HL Moore Drug Exch	00839-7154-12
500's	$96.95	Flurazepam, Major Pharms	00904-2800-40
500's	$97.75	Flurazepam HCl, Geneva Pharms	00781-2806-05
500's	$98.63	Flurazepam Hcl, Goldline Labs	00182-1817-05
500's	$98.63	Flurazepam Hcl, Purepac Pharm	00228-2021-50
500's	$103.82	Flurazepam Hcl, Aligen Independ	00405-0085-02
500's	$104.35	Flurazepam Hcl, Par Pharm	49884-0193-05
500's	$105.22	Flurazepam Hcl, Halsey Drug	00879-0534-05
500's	$105.25	Flurazepam HCl, Rugby	00536-3795-05
500's	$111.50	Flurazepam Hcl, Mylan	00378-4415-05
500's	**$270.09**	**DALMANE, Roche Prod**	**00140-0065-14**
600's	$193.00	Flurazepam Hcl, Medirex	57480-0510-06

Capsule, Gelatin - Oral - 30 mg

50's	$3.37	Flurazepam HCl, H.C.F.A. F F P	99999-1327-04
100's	$6.75	Flurazepam Hcl, United Res	00677-1066-01
100's	$6.75	Flurazepam HCl, H.C.F.A. F F P	99999-1327-05
100's	$15.00	Flurazepam HCl, West Ward Pharm	00143-3370-01
100's	$21.86	Flurazepam Hcl, Qualitest Pharms	00603-3692-21
100's	$23.85	Flurazepam, Major Pharms	00904-2801-60
100's	$23.86	Flurazepam Hcl, Lederle Pharm	00005-3058-23
100's	$24.00	Flurazepam HCl, Geneva Pharms	00781-2807-01
100's	$24.55	Flurazepam Hcl, Goldline Labs	00182-1818-01
100's	$24.55	Flurazepam Hcl, Purepac Pharm	00228-2022-10
100's	$24.55	Flurazepam Hcl, Aligen Independ	00405-0086-01
100's	$24.65	Flurazepam Hcl, Par Pharm	49884-0194-01
100's	$24.68	Flurazepam Hcl, Schein Pharm (US)	00364-0802-01
100's	$25.10	Flurazepam Hcl, HL Moore Drug Exch	00839-7155-06
100's	$26.70	Flurazepam HCl, Warner Chilcott	00047-0989-24
100's	$26.70	Flurazepam Hcl, Mylan	00378-4430-01
100's	$26.70	Flurazepam HCl, Rugby	00536-3796-01
100's	$29.92	Flurazepam Hcl, Vangard Labs	00615-0461-13
100's	$29.92	Flurazepam Hcl, Vangard Labs	00615-0461-47
100's	$31.81	Flurazepam Hcl, Medirex	57480-0511-01
100's	$34.00	Flurazepam HCl, West Ward Pharm	00143-3370-25
100's	$34.87	Flurazepam, Major Pharms	00904-2801-61
100's	$41.40	Flurazepam Hcl, Voluntary Hosp	53258-0613-01
100's	$43.17	Flurazepam Hcl, Voluntary Hosp	53258-0613-13
100's	**$51.46**	**DALMANE, Roche Prod**	**00140-0066-50**
100's	**$53.90**	**DALMANE, Roche Prod**	**00140-0066-49**
100's	**$54.40**	**DALMANE, Roche Prod**	**00140-0066-03**
100's	**$59.02**	**DALMANE, Roche Prod**	**00140-0066-01**
500's	$33.75	Flurazepam HCl, H.C.F.A. F F P	99999-1327-06
500's	$85.00	Flurazepam HCl, West Ward Pharm	00143-3370-05
500's	$103.94	Flurazepam Hcl, HL Moore Drug Exch	00839-7155-12
500's	$106.80	Flurazepam Hcl, Qualitest Pharms	00603-3692-28
500's	$110.50	Flurazepam, Major Pharms	00904-2801-40
500's	$113.59	Flurazepam Hcl, Goldline Labs	00182-1818-05
500's	$113.59	Flurazepam Hcl, Purepac Pharm	00228-2022-50
500's	$116.35	Flurazepam HCl, Geneva Pharms	00781-2807-05
500's	$116.35	Flurazepam Hcl, Par Pharm	49884-0194-05
500's	$119.57	Flurazepam Hcl, Aligen Independ	00405-0086-02
500's	$127.95	Flurazepam Hcl, Mylan	00378-4430-05
500's	$127.95	Flurazepam HCl, Rugby	00536-3796-05
500's	**$293.96**	**DALMANE, Roche Prod**	**00140-0066-14**
600's	$214.00	Flurazepam Hcl, Medirex	57480-0511-06

FLURBIPROFEN *(001328)*

CATEGORIES: Analgesics; Anti-Inflammatory Agents; Antiarthritics; Antipyretics; Arthritis; Central Nervous System Agents; Cystoid Macular Edema; NSAIDS; Nonsteroidal Anti-Inflammatory; Osteoarthritis; Pain; Headache*; Migraine*; Pregnancy Category B; Sales > $100 Million; FDA Approved 1988 Oct; Patent Expiration 1993 Feb

* Indication not approved by the FDA

BRAND NAMES: **Ansaid**; *Apo-Flurbiprofen* (Canada); *Arflur, Cebutid* (France); *Florphen*; *Flupen*; *Flurofen*; *Flurozin*; *Froben* (England, Germany, Canada, Japan); *Froben SR* (Canada); *Lapole* (Japan)
(International brand names outside U.S. in italics)

FORMULARIES: Aetna; BC-BS; Medi-Cal

COST OF THERAPY: $414.49 (Arthritis; Tablet; 100 mg; 2/day; 365 days)

PRIMARY ICD9: 715.99 (Osteoarthritis, Unspecified, Multiple Sites)

DESCRIPTION:

Flurbiprofen is a nonsteroidal anti-inflammatory agent. Flurbiprofen is a phenylalkanoic acid derivative designated chemically as (1,1'-biphenyl)-4-acetic acid, 2-fluoro-alpha-methyl-, (±)-. The empirical formula is $C_{15}H_{13}FO_2$, with a molecular weight of 244.26. Flurbiprofen is a white or slightly yellow crystalline powder. It is slightly soluble in water at pH 7.0 and readily soluble in most polar solvents.

Flurbiprofen is available as 50 mg and 100 mg tablets for oral administration. Inactive ingredients for both strengths are carnauba wax, colloidal silicon dioxide, croscarmellose sodium, hydroxypropyl methylcellulose, lactose, magnesium stearate, microcrystalline cellulose, propylene glycol, and titanium dioxide. In addition, the 100 mg tablet contains FD&C blue No. 2.

CLINICAL PHARMACOLOGY:

Flurbiprofen is a nonsteroidal anti-inflammatory agent which has shown anti-inflammatory, analgesic, and antipyretic properties in pharmacologic studies. As with other such drugs, its mode of action is not known. However, it is a potent prostaglandin synthesis inhibitor, and this property may be involved in its anti-inflammatory effect.

Flurbiprofen is well absorbed after oral administration, reaching peak blood levels in approximately 1.5 hours (range 0.5 to 4 hours). Administration with food alters the rate of absorption but does not affect the extent of drug availability. The elimination half-life is 5.7 hours with 90% of the half-life values from 3 to 9 hours. Individual half-life values ranged from 2.8 to 12 hours. There is no evidence of drug accumulation and flurbiprofen does not induce enzymes that alter its metabolism. Excretion of flurbiprofen is 88% to 98% complete 24 hours after the last dose.

Flurbiprofen is extensively metabolized and excreted primarily in the urine, about 20% as free and conjugated drug and about 50% as hydroxylated metabolites. About 90% of the flurbiprofen in urine is present as conjugates. The major metabolite, 4'-hydroxy-flurbiprofen, has been detected in human plasma, but in animal models of inflammation this metabolite showed little anti-inflammatory activity. Flurbiprofen is more than 99% bound to human serum proteins.

CLINICAL PHARMACOLOGY: *(cont'd)*

The average maximum serum concentration of flurbiprofen, following a 100 mg oral dose of Flurbiprofen in normal volunteers (n=184), was 15.2 mcg/ml, with 90% of the values between 10 and 22 mcg/ml. In geriatric subjects (n=7) between the ages of 58 and 77 years, 100 mg Flurbiprofen resulted in an average peak drug level of 18.0 mcg/ml and an average elimination half-life of 6.5 hours (range 3-10 hours). In geriatric rheumatoid arthritis patients (n=13) between the ages of 65 and 83 years receiving 100 mg Flurbiprofen, the average maximum blood level was 12.7 mcg/ml and the average elimination half-life was 5.6 hours (range 4-10 hours).

In a study assessing flurbiprofen pharmacokinetics in end stage renal disease (ESRD), mean urinary recovery of a 100 mg dose was 73% in 48 hours for 9 normal subjects and 17% in 96 hours for 8 ESRD patients undergoing continuous ambulatory peritoneal dialysis. Plasma concentrations of flurbiprofen were about 40% lower in the ESRD patients; the elimination half-life of flurbiprofen was unchanged. Elimination of the 4'-hydroxy-flurbiprofen metabolite was markedly reduced in the ESRD patients. The pharmacokinetics of flurbiprofen in patients with decreased renal function but not ESRD have not been determined.

The pharmacokinetics of flurbiprofen in patients with hepatic disease have not been determined.

The efficacy of flurbiprofen has been demonstrated in patients with rheumatoid arthritis and osteoarthritis. Using standard assessments of therapeutic response, Flurbiprofen (200-300 mg/day) demonstrated effectiveness comparable to aspirin (2000-4000 mg/day), ibuprofen (2400-3200 mg/day), and indomethacin (75-150 mg/day).

In patients with rheumatoid arthritis, Flurbiprofen may be used in combination with gold salts or corticosteroids.

INDICATIONS AND USAGE:

Flurbiprofen is indicated for the acute or long-term treatment of the signs and symptoms of rheumatoid arthritis and osteoarthritis.

CONTRAINDICATIONS:

Flurbiprofen is contraindicated in patients who have previously demonstrated hypersensitivity to it. Flurbiprofen should not be given to patients in whom Flurbiprofen, aspirin, or other nonsteroidal anti-inflammatory drugs induce asthma, urticaria, or other allergic-type reactions. Flurbiprofen should not be given to patients with the aspirin triad. The triad typically occurs in asthmatic patients who experience rhinitis with or without nasal polyps or who exhibit severe, potentially fatal bronchospasm after taking aspirin or other nonsteroidal anti-inflammatory drugs. Fatal asthmatic and anaphylactoid reactions have been reported in such patients.

WARNINGS:

RISK OF GASTROINTESTINAL (GI) ULCERATIONS, BLEEDING AND PERFORATION WITH NONSTEROIDAL ANTI-INFLAMMATORY THERAPY

Serious gastrointestinal toxicity, such as bleeding, ulceration, and perforation, can occur at any time, with or without warning symptoms, in patients treated chronically with nonsteroidal anti-inflammatory drugs. Although minor upper GI problems, such as dyspepsia, are common, usually developing early in therapy, physicians should remain alert for ulceration and bleeding in patients treated chronically with nonsteroidal anti-inflammatory drugs, even in the absence of previous GI tract symptoms. In patients observed in clinical trials of such agents for several months to two years, symptomatic upper GI ulcers, gross bleeding, or perforation appear to occur in approximately 1% of patients treated for 3-6 months, and in about 2-4% of patients treated for one year. Physicians should inform patients about the signs and/or symptoms of serious GI toxicity and what steps to take if they occur.

Studies to date have not identified any subset of patients not at risk of developing peptic ulceration and bleeding. Except for a prior history of serious GI events and other risk factors known to be associated with peptic ulcer disease, such as alcoholism, smoking, etc., no risk factors (*e.g.,* age, sex) have been associated with increased risk. Elderly or debilitated patients seem to tolerate ulceration or bleeding less well than other individuals and most spontaneous reports of fatal GI events are in this population. Studies to date are inconclusive concerning the relative risk of various nonsteroidal anti-inflammatory agents in causing such reactions. High doses of any such agent probably carry a greater risk of these reactions, although controlled clinical trials showing this do not exist in most cases. In considering the use of relatively large doses (within the recommended dosage range), sufficient benefit should be anticipated to offset the potential increased risk of GI toxicity.

Because serious GI tract ulceration and bleeding can occur without warning symptoms, physicians should follow chronically treated patients for the signs and symptoms of ulceration and bleeding and should inform the patients of the importance of this follow-up.

PRECAUTIONS:

GENERAL

Impaired Renal or Hepatic Function: As with other nonsteroidal anti-inflammatory drugs, flurbiprofen should be used with caution in patients with impaired renal or hepatic function, or a history of kidney or liver disease. Studies to assess the pharmacokinetics of Flurbiprofen in patients with decreased liver function have not been done.

Renal Effects: Toxicology studies in rats have shown renal papillary necrosis at dosage levels equivalent on a mg/kg basis to those used clinically in humans. Similar findings were seen in monkeys given high doses (50-100 mg/kg, or approximately 20-40 times the human therapeutic dose) for 90 days.

In Upjohn clinical studies, kidney function tests were done at least monthly in patients taking flurbiprofen. In these studies, renal effects of flurbiprofen were similar to those seen with other nonsteroidal anti-inflammatory drugs.

A second form of renal toxicity has been seen in patients with prerenal conditions leading to a reduction in renal blood flow or blood volume, where the renal prostaglandins have a supportive role in the maintenance of renal perfusion. In these patients administration of a nonsteroidal anti-inflammatory drug may cause a dose-dependent reduction in prostaglandin formation, which may precipitate overt renal decompensation. Patients at greatest risk of this reaction are those with impaired renal function, heart failure, liver dysfunction, those taking diuretics, and the elderly. Discontinuation of nonsteroidal anti-inflammatory drug therapy is typically followed by recovery to the pretreatment state. Those patients at high risk who chronically take flurbiprofen should have renal function monitored if they have signs or symptoms that may be consistent with mild azotemia, such as malaise, fatigue, loss of appetite, etc. Occasional patients may develop some elevation of serum creatinine and BUN levels without signs or symptoms.

The elimination half-life of flurbiprofen was unchanged in patients with end stage renal disease (ESRD). Flurbiprofen metabolites are primarily eliminated by the kidneys and elimination of 4'-hydroxy-flurbiprofen was markedly reduced in ESRD patients. Therefore,

PRECAUTIONS: *(cont'd)*

patients with significantly impaired renal function may require a reduction of dosage to avoid accumulation of flurbiprofen metabolites and should be monitored. (See also CLINICAL PHARMACOLOGY).

Liver Tests: As with other nonsteroidal anti-inflammatory drugs, borderline elevations of one or more liver tests may occur in up to 15% of patients. These abnormalities may progress, may remain essentially unchanged, or may disappear with continued therapy. The ALT (SGPT) test is probably the most sensitive indicator of liver injury. Meaningful (3 times the upper limit of normal) elevations of ALT or AST (SGOT) have been reported in controlled clinical trials in less than 1% of patients. A patient with symptoms and/or signs suggesting liver dysfunction, or in whom an abnormal liver test has occurred, should be evaluated for evidence of the development of a more severe hepatic reaction while on therapy with flurbiprofen.

Anemia: Anemia is commonly observed in rheumatoid arthritis and is sometimes aggravated by nonsteroidal anti-inflammatory drugs, which may produce fluid retention or minor gastrointestinal blood loss in some patients. Therefore, patients who have initial hemoglobin values of 10 g/dl or less, and who are to receive long-term therapy, should have hemoglobin values determined periodically.

Fluid Retention and Edema: Fluid retention and edema have been reported; therefore, flurbiprofen should be used with caution in patients with cardiac decompensation, hypertension, or similar conditions.

Vision Changes: Blurred and/or diminished vision has been reported with the use of Flurbiprofen and other nonsteroidal anti-inflammatory drugs. Patients experiencing eye complaints should have ophthalmologic examinations.

Effect on Platelets and Coagulation: Flurbiprofen inhibits collagen-induced platelet aggregation. Prolongation of bleeding time by flurbiprofen has been demonstrated in humans after single and multiple oral doses. Patients who may be adversely affected by prolonged bleeding time should be carefully observed when Flurbiprofen is administered.

INFORMATION FOR THE PATIENT

Flurbiprofen, like other drugs of its class, is not free of side effects. The side effects of these drugs can cause discomfort and, rarely, there are more serious side effects, such as gastrointestinal bleeding, which may result in hospitalization and even fatal outcomes. Nonsteroidal anti-inflammatory drugs are often essential agents in the management of arthritis, but they also may be commonly employed for conditions which are less serious. Physicians may wish to discuss with their patients the potential risks (see WARNINGS, PRECAUTIONS, and ADVERSE REACTIONS) and likely benefits of nonsteroidal anti-inflammatory drug treatment, particularly when the drugs are used for less serious conditions where treatment without such agents may represent an acceptable alternative to both the patient and the physician.

Pre-existing Asthma: About 10% of patients with asthma may have aspirin-sensitive asthma. The use of aspirin in patients with aspirin-sensitive asthma has been associated with severe bronchospasm which can be fatal. Since cross-reactivity, including bronchospasm, between aspirin and other nonsteroidal anti-inflammatory drugs has been reported in such aspirin-sensitive patients. Flurbiprofen tablets should not be administered to patients with this form of aspirin sensitivity and should be used with caution in all patients with pre-existing asthma.

CARCINOGENESIS, MUTAGENESIS, AND IMPAIRMENT OF FERTILITY

An 80-week study in mice at doses of 2, 5, and 12 mg/kg/day and a 2-year study in rats at doses of 0.5, 2, and 4 mg/kg/day did not show evidence of carcinogenicity at maximum tolerated doses of flurbiprofen.

Flurbiprofen did not impair the fertility of male or female rats treated orally at 2.25 mg/kg/day for 65 days and 16 days, respectively, before mating.

PREGNANCY CATEGORY B

In teratology studies flurbiprofen, given to mice in doses up to 12 mg/kg/day, to rats in doses up to 25 mg/kg/day, and to rabbits in doses up to 7.5 mg/kg/day, showed no teratogenic effects.

Because there are no adequate and well-controlled studies in pregnant women, and animal teratology studies do not always predict human response, Ansaid is not recommended for use in pregnancy.

LABOR AND DELIVERY

Ansaid's effects on labor and delivery in women are not known. As with other drugs known to inhibit prostaglandin synthesis, an increased incidence of dystocia and delayed parturition occurred in rats treated throughout pregnancy. Because of the known effects of prostaglandin-inhibiting drugs on the fetal cardiovascular system (closure of the ductus arteriosus), use of Ansaid during late pregnancy is not recommended.

NURSING MOTHERS

Concentrations of flurbiprofen in breast milk and plasma of nursing mothers suggested that a nursing infant could receive approximately 0.10 mg flurbiprofen per day in the established milk of a woman taking 200 mg/day. Because of possible adverse effects of prostaglandin-inhibiting drugs on neonates, Flurbiprofen is not recommended for use in nursing mothers.

PEDIATRIC USE

Safety and effectiveness in children have not been established.

DRUG INTERACTIONS:

Antacids: Administration of flurbiprofen to volunteers under fasting conditions, or with antacid suspension, yielded similar serum flurbiprofen-time profiles in young subjects (n=12). In geriatric subjects (n=7) there was a reduction in the rate but not the extent of flurbiprofen absorption.

Anticoagulants: Flurbiprofen, like other nonsteroidal anti-inflammatory drugs, has been shown to affect bleeding parameters in patients receiving anticoagulants, and serious clinical bleeding has been reported. The physician should be cautious when administering Flurbiprofen to patients taking anticoagulants.

Aspirin: Concurrent administration of aspirin and flurbiprofen resulted in 50% lower serum flurbiprofen concentrations. This effect of aspirin (which also lowers serum concentrations of other nonsteroidal anti-inflammatory drugs given with it) has been demonstrated in patients with rheumatoid arthritis (n=15) as well as normal volunteers (n=16). Concurrent use of Flurbiprofen and aspirin is therefore not recommended.

Beta-adrenergic Blocking Agents: The effect of flurbiprofen on blood pressure response to propranolol and atenolol was evaluated in men with mild uncomplicated hypertension (n=10). Flurbiprofen pretreatment attenuated the hypotensive effect of a single dose of propranolol but not atenolol. Flurbiprofen did not appear to affect the beta-blocker-mediated reduction in heart rate. Flurbiprofen did not affect the pharmacokinetic profile of either drug, and the mechanism underlying the interference with propranolol's hypotensive effect is unknown. Patients taking both flurbiprofen and a beta-blocker should be monitored to ensure that a satisfactory hypotensive effect is achieved.

Cimetidine, Ranitidine: In normal volunteers (n=9), pretreatment with cimetidine or ranitidine did not affect flurbiprofen pharmacokinetics, except that a small (13%) but statistically significant increase in the area under the serum concentration curve of flurbiprofen resulted with cimetidine.

DRUG INTERACTIONS: *(cont'd)*

Digoxin: Studies of concomitant administration of flurbiprofen and digoxin to healthy men (n=14) did not show a change in the steady state serum levels of either drug.

Diuretics: Studies in normal volunteers have shown that flurbiprofen, like other nonsteroidal anti-inflammatory drugs, can interfere with the effects of furosemide. Although results have varied from study to study, effects have been shown on furosemide-stimulated diuresis, natriuresis, and kaliuresis. Other nonsteroidal anti-inflammatory drugs that inhibit prostaglandin synthesis have been shown to interfere with thiazide diuretics in some studies, and with potassium-sparing diuretics. Patients receiving Flurbiprofen and furosemide or other diuretics should be observed closely to determine if the desired effect is obtained.

Oral Hypoglycemic Agents: In one study, flurbiprofen was given to adult diabetics who were already receiving glyburide (n=4), metformin (n=2), chlorpropamide with phenformin (n=3), or glyburide with phenformin (n=6). Although there was a slight reduction in blood sugar concentrations during concomitant administration of flurbiprofen and hypoglycemic agents, there were no signs or symptoms of hypoglycemia.

ADVERSE REACTIONS:

Adverse reaction information was derived from patients who received flurbiprofen in blinded-controlled and open-label clinical trials, and from worldwide marketing experience and from publications. In the description below, rates of the more common events (greater than 1%) and many of the less common events (less than 1%) represent clinical study results. For rarer events that were derived principally from worldwide marketing experience and the literature (printed in italics), accurate rate estimates are generally impossible.

Of the 4123 patients in premarketing studies, 2954 were treated for at least 1 month, 1448 for at least 3 months, 948 for at least 6 months, 356 for at least 1 year, and 100 for at least 2 years. Of the 4123 patients, 9.4% dropped out of the studies because of an adverse drug reaction, principally involving the gastrointestinal tract (5.8%) central nervous system and special senses (1.4%), skin (0.6%) and genitourinary tract (0.5%).

INCIDENCE GREATER THAN 1%

An asterisk after a reaction identifies reactions which occurred in 3-9% of patients treated with flurbiprofen. Reactions occurring in 1-3% of the patients are unmarked.

Gastrointestinal: Dyspepsia*, diarrhea*, abdominal pain*, nausea*, constipation, GI bleeding, flatulence, elevated liver enzymes, and vomiting

Central Nervous System: Headache*, nervousness, and other manifestations of CNS "stimulation" (*e.g.*, anxiety, insomnia, reflexes increased, and tremor), and symptoms associated with CNS "inhibition" (*e.g.*, amnesia, asthenia, somnolence, malaise, and depression)

Respiratory: Rhinitis

Dermatological: Rash

Special Senses: Dizziness, tinnitus, and changes in vision

Genitourinary: Signs and symptoms suggesting urinary tract infection*

Body as a Whole: Edema*

Metabolic/Nutritional: Body weight changes

INCIDENCE LESS THAN 1% (CAUSAL RELATIONSHIP PROBABLE)

The reactions listed in this category occurred in <1% of patients in the clinical trials or were reported during postmarketing experience from other countries. Adverse reactions reported only in worldwide postmarketing experience or the literature (which presumably indicates that they are rarer) are italicized.

Gastrointestinal: Peptic ulcer disease (see also WARNINGS, Risk of Gastrointestinal (GI) Ulcerations, Bleeding and Perforation with Nonsteroidal Anti-inflammatory Therapy), gastritis, bloody diarrhea, stomatitis, esophageal disease, hematemesis, and hepatitis; *cholestatic and non-cholestatic jaundice*

Central Nervous System: Ataxia, cerebrovascular ischemia, confusion, paresthesia, and twitching

Hematologic: Decrease in hemoglobin and hematocrit, iron deficiency anemia, *hemolytic anemia* and *aplastic anemia*; leukopenia; eosinophilia; ecchymosis *and thrombocytopenia.* (See also PRECAUTIONS, Effect On Platelets and Coagulation)

Respiratory: Asthma and epistaxis

Dermatological: Angioedema, urticaria, eczema, and pruritus; *photosensitivity, toxic epidermal necrolysis,* and *exfoliative dermatitis*

Special Senses: Conjunctivitis and parosmia

Genitourinary: Hematuria and renal failure; *interstitial nephritis*

Body as a Whole: Chills and fever; *anaphylactic reaction*

Metabolic/Nutritional: Hyperuricemia

Cardiovascular: Heart failure, hypertension, vascular diseases and vasodilation

INCIDENCE LESS THAN 1% (CAUSAL RELATIONSHIP UNKNOWN)

The following reactions have been reported in patients taking flurbiprofen under circumstances that do not permit a clear attribution of the reaction to flurbiprofen. These reactions are being included as alerting information for physicians. Adverse reactions reported only in worldwide postmarketing experience or the literature (which presumably indicates that they are rarer) are italicized.

Gastrointestinal: Periodontal abscess, appetite changes, cholecystitis, dry mouth, colitis, exacerbation of inflammatory bowel disease, and small intestine inflammation with loss of blood and protein

Central Nervous System: Convulsion, meningitis, hypertonia, cerebrovascular accident, emotional lability, and subarachnoid hemorrhage

Hematologic: Lymphadenopathy

Respiratory: Bronchitis, laryngitis, dyspnea, pulmonary embolism, pulmonary infarct, and hyperventilation

Dermatological: Alopecia, nail disorder, herpes simplex, zoster, dry skin, and sweating

Special Senses: Ear disease, corneal opacity, glaucoma, retrobulbar neuritis, changes in taste, and transient hearing loss; *retinal hemorrhage*

Genitourinary: Menstrual disturbances, vaginal and uterine hemorrhage, vulvovaginitis, and prostate disease

Metabolic/Nutritional: Hyperkalemia

Cardiovascular: Arrhythmias, angina pectoris, and myocardial infarction

Musculoskeletal: Myasthenia

DRUG ABUSE AND DEPENDENCE:

No drug abuse or drug dependence has been observed with flurbiprofen.

OVERDOSAGE:

Information on overdosage is available for 13 children and 12 adults. Nine of the 13 children were less than 6 years old. Drowsiness occurred after doses of 150 to 800 mg in 3 of these young children (with dilated pupils in 1), and in a 2-year-old who also had semiconsciousness, pinpoint pupils, diminished tone, and elevated liver enzymes. Other children who ingested doses of 200 mg to 2.5 g showed no symptoms.

Among the adults, a 70-year-old man with a history of chronic obstructive airway disease died. Toxicological analysis showed acute flurbiprofen overdose and a blood ethanol concentration of 100 mg/dl. In the other cases, symptoms were as follows: coma and respiratory depression after 3-6 g; drowsiness, nausea and epigastric pain after 2.5-5 g; epigastric pain and dizziness after 3 g; headache and nausea after ≤ 2 g; agitation after 1.5 g; and drowsiness after 1.0 g. One patient, who took 200-400 mg flurbiprofen and 2.4 g fenoprofen, had disorientation and diplopia. Three adults had no symptoms after 3-5 g flurbiprofen.

Treatment of an overdose: the stomach should be emptied by vomiting or lavage, though little drug will likely be recovered if more than an hour has elapsed since ingestion. Supportive treatment should be instituted as necessary. Some patients have been given supplemental oral or intravenous fluids and required no other treatment.

In mice, the flurbiprofen LD_{50} was 750 mg/kg when administered orally and 200 mg/kg when administered intraperitoneally. The primary signs of toxicity were prostration, ataxia, loss of righting reflex, labored respiration, twitches, convulsions, CNS depression, and splayed hind limbs. In rats, the flurbiprofen LD_{50} was 160 mg/kg when administered orally and 400 mg/kg when administered intraperitoneally. The primary signs of toxicity were tremors, convulsions, labored respiration, and prostration. These were observed mostly in the intraperitoneal studies.

DOSAGE AND ADMINISTRATION:

Flurbiprofen is administered orally.

Rheumatoid arthritis and osteoarthritis: Recommended starting dose is 200 to 300 mg total daily dose administered BID, TID, or QID. (Most experience in rheumatoid arthritis has been with TID or QID dosage.) The largest recommended single dose in a multiple-dose daily regimen is 100 mg. The dose should be tailored to each patient according to the severity of the symptoms and the response to therapy.

Although a few patients have received higher doses, doses above 300 mg per day are not recommended until more clinical experience with flurbiprofen is obtained.

Store at controlled room temperature 15-30°C (59-86°F).

HOW SUPPLIED - RATED THERAPEUTICALLY EQUIVALENT:

Tablet - Oral - 50 mg

100's	$66.27	Flurbiprofen, H.C.F.A. F F P	99999-1328-01

Tablet - Oral - 100 mg

100's	$56.78	Flurbiprofen, H.C.F.A. F F P	99999-1328-02

Tablet, Coated - Oral - 50 mg

100's	$68.02	Flurbiprofen, Novopharm (US)	55953-0573-40
100's	$68.02	Flurbiprofen, Warrick Pharms	59930-1771-01
100's	$68.15	Flurbiprofen, Greenstone	59762-3723-01
100's	$71.34	FLURBIPROFEN, Aligen Independ	00405-4443-01
100's	$71.90	Flurbiprofen, Zenith Labs	00172-4361-60
100's	$72.00	Flurbiprofen, Geneva Pharms	00781-1031-01
100's	$73.97	Flurbiprofen, Novopharm (US)	55953-0573-41
100's	$75.03	Flurbiprofen, Mylan	00378-0076-01
100's	**$80.09**	**ANSAID, Pharmacia & Upjohn**	**00009-0170-07**
100's	**$85.96**	**ANSAID, Pharmacia & Upjohn**	**00009-0170-08**
500's	$334.27	Flurbiprofen, Novopharm (US)	55953-0573-70
500's	$349.20	Flurbiprofen, Zenith Labs	00172-4361-70
500's	**$388.44**	**ANSAID, Pharmacia & Upjohn**	**00009-0170-09**
1000's	$601.68	Flurbiprofen, Novopharm (US)	55953-0573-80
1000's	$687.90	Flurbiprofen, Zenith Labs	00172-4361-80

Tablet, Coated - Oral - 100 mg

100's	$74.99	Flurbiprofen, United Res	00677-1568-01
100's	$106.25	Flurbiprofen, Major Pharms	00904-5019-60
100's	$106.38	Flurbiprofen, Greenstone	59762-3724-01
100's	$106.95	Flurbiprofen, Qualitest Pharms	00603-3700-21
100's	$107.58	Flurbiprofen, Novopharm (US)	55953-0577-40
100's	$107.58	Flurbiprofen, Warrick Pharms	59930-1772-01
100's	$108.25	Flurbiprofen, Teva	00093-0711-01
100's	$111.25	Flurbiprofen, Rugby	00536-3789-01
100's	$111.98	FLURBIPROFEN, Aligen Independ	00405-4444-01
100's	$112.25	Flurbiprofen, Zenith Labs	00172-4362-60
100's	$112.50	Flurbiprofen, Schein Pharm (US)	00364-2647-01
100's	$112.50	Flurbiprofen, Geneva Pharms	00781-1033-01
100's	$112.62	Flurbiprofen, Novopharm (US)	55953-0577-41
100's	$117.11	Flurbiprofen, Mylan	00378-0093-01
100's	$122.49	Flurbiprofen, Geneva Pharms	00781-1033-13
100's	$123.10	FLURBIPROFEN, Vangard Labs	00615-3575-13
100's	**$125.00**	**ANSAID, Pharmacia & Upjohn**	**00009-0305-03**
100's	**$130.85**	**ANSAID, Pharmacia & Upjohn**	**00009-0305-06**
500's	$515.35	Flurbiprofen, Major Pharms	00904-5019-40
500's	$517.46	Flurbiprofen, Greenstone	59762-3724-03
500's	$518.85	Flurbiprofen, Qualitest Pharms	00603-3700-28
500's	$519.50	Flurbiprofen, Teva	00093-0711-05
500's	$521.76	Flurbiprofen, Novopharm (US)	55953-0577-70
500's	$521.76	Flurbiprofen, Warrick Pharms	59930-1772-02
500's	$539.60	Flurbiprofen, Rugby	00536-3789-05
500's	$544.60	Flurbiprofen, Zenith Labs	00172-4362-70
500's	$545.20	Flurbiprofen, Schein Pharm (US)	00364-2647-05
500's	$545.20	Flurbiprofen, Geneva Pharms	00781-1033-05
500's	$568.00	Flurbiprofen, Mylan	00378-0093-05
500's	**$606.30**	**ANSAID, Pharmacia & Upjohn**	**00009-0305-05**
1000's	$939.17	Flurbiprofen, Novopharm (US)	55953-0577-80
1000's	$1072.85	Flurbiprofen, Zenith Labs	00172-4362-80
2000's	**$2350.14**	**ANSAID, Pharmacia & Upjohn**	**00009-0305-30**

FLURBIPROFEN SODIUM *(001329)*

CATEGORIES: Anti-Inflammatory Agents; EENT Drugs; Eye, Ear, Nose, & Throat Preparations; Miosis; Ophthalmics; Surgical Aid, Ophthalmic; Pregnancy Category C; FDA Approved 1986 Dec

BRAND NAMES: *Froben*; **Ocufen**; *Ocufen A*; *Ocuflur* (Germany)
(International brand names outside U.S. in italics)

DESCRIPTION:

Flurbiprofen Sodium 0.03% Liquifilm sterile ophthalmic solution is a topical nonsteroidal anti-inflammatory product for ophthalmic use.

DESCRIPTION: *(cont'd)*

Chemical Name: Sodium (±)-2-fluoro-α-methyl-4-biphenyl-acetate dihydrate.

Contains: Flurbiprofen sodium: 0.03%; with Liquifilm (polyvinyl alcohol) 1.4%; thimerosal 0.005%; edetate disodium; potassium chloride; sodium chloride; sodium citrate; citric acid; hydrochloric acid and/or sodium hydroxide to adjust the pH; and purified water.

CLINICAL PHARMACOLOGY:

Flurbiprofen Sodium is one of a series of phenylalkanoic acids that have shown analgesic, antipyretic, and anti-inflammatory activity in animal inflammatory diseases. Its mechanism of action is believed to be through inhibition of the cyclo-oxygenase enzyme that is essential in the biosynthesis of prostaglandins.

Prostaglandins have been shown in many animal models to be mediators of certain kinds of intraocular inflammation. In studies performed on animal eyes, prostaglandins have been shown to produce disruption of the blood- aqueous humor barrier, vasodilation, increased vascular permeability, leukocytosis, and increased intraocular pressure.

Prostaglandins also appear to play a role in the miotic response produces during ocular surgery by constricting the iris sphincter independently of cholinergic mechanisms. In clinical studies, Flurbiprofen Sodium has been shown to inhibit the miosis induced during the course of cataract surgery.

Results from clinical studies indicate that flurbiprofen sodium has no significant effect upon intraocular pressure.

INDICATIONS AND USAGE:

Flurbiprofen Sodium is indicated for the inhibition of intraoperative miosis.

CONTRAINDICATIONS:

Flurbiprofen Sodium is contraindicated in individuals who are hypersensitive to any components of the medication.

WARNINGS:

With nonsteroidal anti-inflammatory drugs, there exists the potential for increased bleeding due to interference with thrombocyte aggregation. There have been reports that Flurbiprofen Sodium may cause increased bleeding of ocular tissue (including hyphemas) in conjunction with ocular surgery.

There exists the potential for cross-sensitivity to acetylsalicylic acid and other non-steroidal anti-inflammatory drugs. Therefore, caution should be used when treating individuals who have previously exhibited sensitivities to these drugs.

PRECAUTIONS:

GENERAL

Wound healing may be delayed with the use of Flurbiprofen Sodium.

It is recommended that flurbiprofen sodium 0.03% Liquifilm sterile ophthalmic solution be used with caution in surgical patients with known bleeding tendencies or who are receiving other medications which may prolong bleeding time.

CARCINOGENESIS, MUTAGENESIS, AND IMPAIRMENT OF FERTILITY

Long-term studies with mice and/or rats have shown no evidence of carcinogenicity or impairment of fertility with flurbiprofen.

Long-term mutagenicity studies in animals have not been performed.

PREGNANCY CATEGORY C

Flurbiprofen has been shown to be embryocidal, delay parturition, prolong gestation, reduce weight, and/or slightly retard growth of fetuses when given to rats in daily oral doses of 0.4 mg/kg (approximately 185 times the human daily topical dose) and above. There are no adequate and well-controlled studies in pregnant women. Flurbiprofen Sodium should only be used during pregnancy only if the potential benefit justifies the potential risk to the fetus.

NURSING MOTHERS

It is not known whether this drug is excreted in human milk. Because many drugs are excreted in human milk and because of the potential for serious adverse in nursing infants from flurbiprofen sodium, a decision should be made whether to discontinue the drug, taking into account the importance of the drug to the mother.

PEDIATRIC USE

Safety and effectiveness in children have not been established.

DRUG INTERACTIONS:

Interaction of Flurbiprofen Sodium with other ophthalmic medications has not been fully investigated.

Although clinical studies with acetylcholine choline and animal studies with acetylcholine choline or carbachol revealed no interference and there is no known pharmacological basis for an interaction, there have been reports that acetylcholine choline or carbachol have been ineffective when used in patients treated with Flurbiprofen Sodium.

ADVERSE REACTIONS:

The most frequent adverse reactions reported with the use of Flurbiprofen Sodium are transient burning and stinging upon instillation and other minor symptoms of ocular irritation.

Increased bleeding tendency of ocular tissues in conjunction with ocular surgery has also been reported.

OVERDOSAGE:

Overdosage will not ordinarily cause acute problems. If accidentally ingested, drink fluids to dilute.

DOSAGE AND ADMINISTRATION:

A total of four (4) drops of Flurbiprofen Sodium should be administered by instilling 1 drop approximately every 1/2 hour beginning 2 hours before surgery.

Note: Store at room temperature.

HOW SUPPLIED - RATED THERAPEUTICALLY EQUIVALENT:

Solution - Ophthalmic - 0.03 %

2.5 ml	**$14.49**	**OCUFEN 0.03%, Allergan-Amer**	**11980-0801-03**

FLUTAMIDE *(001330)*

CATEGORIES: Androgen Inhibitors; Antineoplastics; Cancer; Oncologic Drugs; Oral Androgen Blockers; Prostatic Carcinoma; Pregnancy Category D; FDA Class 1A ("Important Therapeutic Advantage"); Sales > $100 Million; FDA Approved 1989 Jan; Patent Expiration 2001 Dec

BRAND NAMES: *Drogenil* (England); *Euflex* (Canada); **Eulexin**; *Eulexine* (France); *Flucinom*; *Flucinome*; *Flugerel*; *Fluken* (Mexico); *Flulem* (Mexico); *Fugerel* (Germany); *Plutamid*; *Prostamid*
(International brand names outside U.S. in italics)

FORMULARIES: Aetna; BC-BS; Medi-Cal

COST OF THERAPY: $3,603.42 (Prostatic Carcinoma; Capsule; 125 mg; 6/day; 365 days)

DESCRIPTION:

Flutamide capsules contain flutamide, an acetanilid, nonsteroidal, orally active antiandrogen having the chemical name, 2-methyl-*N*- [4-nitro-3-(trifluoromethyl)phenyl] propanamide.

Each capsule contains 125 mg flutamide. The compound is a buff to yellow powder with a molecular weight of 276.2.

The inactive ingredients for flutamide capsules include: corn starch, lactose, magnesium stearate, povidone, and sodium lauryl sulfate. Gelatin capsule shells may contain methylparaben, propylparaben, butylparaben and the following dye systems: FD&C Blue 1, FD&C Yellow 6 and either FD&C Red 3 or FD&C Red 40 plus D&C Yellow 10, with titanium dioxide and other inactive ingredients.

CLINICAL PHARMACOLOGY:

General: In animal studies, flutamide demonstrates potent antiandrogenic effects. It exerts its antiandrogenic action by inhibiting androgen uptake and/or by inhibiting nuclear binding of androgen in target tissues or both. Prostatic carcinoma is known to be androgen-sensitive and responds to treatment that counteracts the effect of androgen and/or removes the source of androgen, *e.g.,* castration.

Pharmacokinetics: Analysis of plasma, urine, and feces following a single oral 200 mg dose of tritium-labeled flutamide to human volunteers showed that the drug is rapidly and completely absorbed. It is excreted mainly in the urine with only 4.2% of the dose excreted in the feces over 72 hours. The composition of plasma radioactivity showed that flutamide is rapidly and extensively metabolized, with flutamide comprising only 2.5% of plasma radioactivity 1 hour after administration. At least six metabolites have been identified in plasma. The major plasma metabolite is a biologically active alpha-hydroxylated derivative which accounts for 23% of the plasma tritium 1 hour after drug administration.

The major urinary metabolite is 2-amino-5-nitro-4- (trifluoromethyl)phenol.

Following a single 250 mg oral dose to normal adult volunteers, low plasma levels of varying amounts of flutamide were detected. The biologically active alpha-hydroxylated metabolite reaches maximum plasma levels in about 2 hours, indicating that it is rapidly formed from flutamide. The plasma half-life for this metabolite is about 6 hours.

Following multiple oral dosing of 250 mg three times daily in normal geriatric volunteers, flutamide and its active metabolite approached steady-state plasma levels (based on pharmacokinetic simulations) after the fourth flutamide dose. The half-life of the active metabolite in geriatric volunteers after a single flutamide dose is about 8 hours and at steady-state is 9.6 hours.

Flutamide, *in vivo*, at steady-state plasma concentrations of 24 to 78 ng/ml is 94% to 96% bound to plasma proteins. The active metabolite of flutamide, *in vivo*, at steady-state plasma concentrations of 1556 to 2284 ng/ml, is 92% to 94% bound to plasma proteins.

In male rats neither flutamide nor any of its metabolites is preferentially accumulated in any tissue except the prostate after an oral 5 mg/kg dose of ^{14}C-flutamide. Total drug levels were highest 6 hours after drug administration in all tissues. Levels declined at roughly similar rates to low levels at 18 hours. The major metabolite was present at higher concentrations than flutamide in all tissues studied.

Elevations of plasma testosterone and estradiol levels have been noted following flutamide administration.

CLINICAL STUDIES:

Flutamide has been demonstrated to interfere with testosterone at the cellular level. This can complement medical castration achieved with leuprolide, which suppresses testicular androgen production by inhibiting luteinizing hormone secretion.

To study the effects of combination therapy, 617 patients (311 leuprolide + flutamide, 306 leuprolide + placebo) with previously untreated advanced prostatic carcinoma were enrolled in a large multicentered, controlled clinical trial.

Three and one-half years after the study was initiated, median survival had been reached. The median actuarial survival time was 34.9 months for patients treated with leuprolide and flutamide versus 27.9 months for patients treated with leuprolide alone. This 7-month increment represents a 25% improvement in overall survival time with the flutamide therapy. Analysis of progression-free survival showed a 2.6 month improvement in patients who received leuprolide plus flutamide, a 19% increment over leuprolide and placebo.

INDICATIONS AND USAGE:

Flutamide capsules are indicated for use in combination with LHRH agonists (such as leuprolide acetate) for the treatment of metastatic prostatic carcinoma (stage D_2). To achieve the benefit of the adjunctive therapy with Flutamide, treatment must be started simultaneously using both drugs.

CONTRAINDICATIONS:

Flutamide capsules are contraindicated in patients who are hypersensitive to flutamide or any component of this preparation.

WARNINGS:

Gynecomastia occurred in 9% of patients receiving flutamide together with medical castration.

Flutamide may cause fetal harm when administered to a pregnant woman. There was decreased 24-hour survival in the offspring of rats treated with flutamide at doses of 30, 100, or 200 mg/kg/day (approximately 3, 9, and 19 times the human dose) during pregnancy. A slight increase in minor variations in the development of the sternebrae and vertebrae was seen in fetuses of rats at the two higher doses. Feminization of the males also occurred at the two higher dose levels. There was a decreased survival rate in the offspring of rabbits receiving the highest dose (15 mg/kg/day; equal to 1.4 times the human dose).

Hepatic Injury: Since transaminase abnormalities, cholestatic jaundice, hepatic necrosis, and hepatic encephalopathy have been reported with the use of flutamide, periodic liver function tests should be considered. (See ADVERSE REACTIONS.) Appropriate laboratory testing should be done at the first symptom/sign of liver dysfunction (*e.g.,* pruritus, dark urine, persistent anorexia, jaundice, right upper quadrant tenderness or unexplained "flu-like" symptoms). If the patient has jaundice or laboratory evidence of liver injury, in the absence of biopsy-confirmed liver metastases, Flutamide therapy should be discontinued or the dosage reduced. The hepatic injury is usually reversible after discontinuation of therapy, and in some patients, after dosage reduction. However, there have been reports of death following severe hepatic injury associated with use of flutamide.

PRECAUTIONS:

Information for the Patient: Patients should be informed that flutamide capsules and the drug used for medical castration should be administered concomitantly, and that they should not interrupt their dosing or stop taking these medications without consulting their physician.

Laboratory Tests: See WARNINGS, Hepatic Injury.

Carcinogenesis, Mutagenesis, and Impairment of Fertility: Daily administration of flutamide to rats for 52 weeks at doses of 30, 90, or 180 mg/kg/day (approximately 3, 8, or 17 times the human dose), produced testicular interstitial cell adenomas at all doses.

In a 24-month carcinogenicity study conducted in male rats, daily administration of flutamide at doses of 10, 30 and 50 mg/kg/day (*i.e.,* up to approximately 5 times the human dose) was associated with an increased number of testicular interstitial cell adenomas at all doses tested and with dose-related increases in mammary gland adenomas and/or carcinomas.

Flutamide did not demonstrate DNA modifying activity in the Ames *Salmonella*/microsome Mutagenesis Assay. Dominant lethal tests in rats were negative.

Reduced sperm counts were observed during a 6-week study of flutamide monotherapy in normal human volunteers.

Flutamide did not affect estrous cycles or interfere with the mating behavior of male and female rats when the drug was administered at 25 and 75 mg/kg/day prior to mating. Males treated with 150 mg/kg/day (30 times the minimum effective antiandrogenic dose) failed to mate; mating behavior returned to normal after dosing was stopped. Conception rates were decreased in all dosing groups. Suppression of spermatogenesis was observed in rats dosed for 52 weeks at approximately 3, 8, or 17 times the human dose and in dogs dosed for 78 weeks at 1.4, 2.3, and 3.7 times the human dose.

Pregnancy Category D: See WARNINGS.

DRUG INTERACTIONS:

Interactions between flutamide capsules and leuprolide have not occurred. Increases in prothrombin time have been noted in patients receiving long-term warfarin therapy after flutamide was initiated. Therefore close monitoring of prothrombin time is recommended and adjustment of the anticoagulant dose may be necessary when flutamide capsules are administered concomitantly with warfarin.

ADVERSE REACTIONS:

The following adverse experiences were reported during a multicenter clinical trial comparing flutamide + LHRH agonist versus placebo + LHRH agonist.

The most frequently reported (greater than 5%) adverse experiences during treatment with flutamide capsules in combination with an LHRH agonist are listed in TABLE 1. For comparison, adverse experiences seen with an LHRH agonist and placebo are also listed in TABLE 1.

TABLE 1 Flutamide, Adverse Reactions

	(n = 294) Flutamide + LHRH agonist % All	(n = 285) Placebo + LHRH agonist % All
Hot Flashes	61	57
Loss of Libido	36	31
Impotence	33	29
Diarrhea	12	4
Nausea/Vomiting	11	10
Gynecomastia	9	11
Other	7	9
Other GI	6	4

As shown in TABLE 1, for both treatment groups, the most frequently occurring adverse experiences (hot flashes, impotence, loss of libido) were those known to be associated with low serum androgen levels and known to occur with LHRH agonists alone.

The only notable difference was the higher incidence of diarrhea in the flutamide + LHRH agonist group (12%), which was severe in 5% as opposed to the placebo + LHRH agonist (4%), which was severe in less than 1%.

In addition, the following adverse reactions were reported during treatment with flutamide + LHRH agonist. No causal relatedness of these reactions to drug treatment has been made, and some of the adverse experiences reported are those that commonly occur in elderly patients.

Cardiovascular System: hypertension in 1% of patients.

Central Nervous System: CNS (drowsiness/ confusion/ depression /anxiety/nervousness) reactions occurred in 1% of patients.

Gastrointestinal System: anorexia 4%, and other GI disorders occurred in 6% of patients.

Hematopoietic System: anemia occurred in 6%, leukopenia in 3%, and thrombocytopenia in 1% of patients.

Liver and Biliary System: hepatitis and jaundice in less than 1% of patients.

Skin: irritation at the injection site and rash occurred in 3% of patients.

Other: edema occurred in 4%, genitourinary and neuromuscular symptoms in 2%, and pulmonary symptoms in less than 1% of patients.

In addition, the following spontaneous adverse experiences have been reported during the marketing of flutamide: hemolytic anemia, macrocytic anemia, methemoglobinemia, photosensitivity reactions (including erythema, ulceration, bullous eruptions, and epidermal necrolysis) and urine discoloration. The urine was noted to change to an amber or yellow-green appearance which can be attributed to the flutamide and/or its metabolites. Also reported were cholestatic jaundice, hepatic encephalopathy, and hepatic necrosis. The hepatic conditions were usually reversible after discontinuing therapy; however, there have been reports of death following severe hepatic injury associated with use of flutamide.

Two reports of malignant breast neoplasms occurring in male patients being dosed with flutamidehave been reported. One involved a pre-existing nodule which was first detected 3-4 months before initiation of flutamidemonotherapy. After excision, this nodule was diagnosed as a poorly differentiated ductal carcinoma. The other report involved gynecomastia and a breast nodule noted 2 and 6 months, respectively, after initiation of flutamidemonotherapy. The nodule was excised and diagnosed as a moderately differentiated invasive ductal tumor.

Abnormal Laboratory Test Values: Laboratory abnormalities including elevated SGOT, SGPT, bilirubin values, SGGT, BUN, and serum creatinine have been reported.

OVERDOSAGE:

In animal studies with flutamide alone, signs of overdose included hypoactivity, piloerection, slow respiration, ataxia, and/or lacrimation, anorexia, tranquilization, emesis, and methemoglobinemia.

OVERDOSAGE: *(cont'd)*

Clinical trials have been conducted with flutamide in doses up to 1500 mg per day for periods up to 36 weeks with no serious adverse effects reported. Those adverse reactions reported included gynecomastia, breast tenderness, and some increases in SGOT. The single dose of flutamide ordinarily associated with symptoms of overdose or considered to be life-threatening has not been established.

Since flutamide is highly protein bound, dialysis may not be of any use as treatment for overdose. As in the management of overdosage with any drug, it should be borne in mind that multiple agents may have been taken. If vomiting does not occur spontaneously, it should be induced if the patient is alert. General supportive care, including frequent monitoring of the vital signs and close observation of the patient, is indicated.

DOSAGE AND ADMINISTRATION:

The recommended dosage is two capsules three times a day at 8-hour intervals for a total daily dose of 750 mg.

Store between 2° and 30°C (36° and 86°F).

Protect the Unit Dose packages from excessive moisture.

HOW SUPPLIED:

Eulexin Capsules, 125 mg, are available as opaque, two-toned brown capsules, imprinted with "Schering 525".

HOW SUPPLIED - EQUIVALENTS NOT AVAILABLE:

Capsule, Gelatin - Oral - 125 mg

100's	$164.54	EULEXIN, Schering	00085-0525-03
180's	$279.38	EULEXIN, Schering	00085-0525-06
500's	$776.20	EULEXIN, Schering	00085-0525-05

FLUTICASONE PROPIONATE *(003011)*

CATEGORIES: Adrenal Corticosteroids; Allergies; Anti-Inflammatory Agents; Dermatoses; Eye, Ear, Nose, & Throat Preparations; Rhinitis; Skin/Mucous Membrane Agents; Steroids; Dermatitis*; Eczema*; Pregnancy Category C; FDA Class 1C ("Little or No Therapeutic Advantage"); FDA Approved 1990 Dec; Top 200 Drugs
* Indication not approved by the FDA

BRAND NAMES: **Cutivate**; *Flixonase* (England); *Flixonase Nasal Spray*; *Flixotide* (England); *Flixotide Disk*; *Flixotide Disks*; *Flixotide Inhaler*, Flonase; Flonase Aq; Flovent; *Flutide* (Germany); *Flutivate* (Germany)
(International brand names outside U.S. in italics)

FORMULARIES: BC-BS; Medi-Cal

COST OF THERAPY: $534.03 (Rhinitis; Aerosol; 0.05 %; 0.53 gm/day; 365 days)

DESCRIPTION:

Cream and Ointment: Fluticasone Propionate Cream (0.05%) and Fluticasone Propionate Ointment (0.005%) each contain fluticasone propionate [(6α,11β,16α,17α)-6,9,-difluoro-11-hydroxy-16-methyl-3-oxo-17-(1-oxopropoxy)androsta-1,4-diene-17-carbothioic acid, S-fluoromethyl ester], a synthetic fluorinated corticosteroid, for topical dermatologic use. The topical corticosteroids constitute a class of primarily synthetic steroids used as anti-inflammatory and antipruritic agents.

Chemically, fluticasone propionate is $C_{25}H_{31}F_3O_5S$.

Fluticasone propionate has a molecular weight of 500.6. It is a white to off-white powder and is insoluble in water.

Cream: Each gram of Fluticasone Propionate Cream, 0.05% contains fluticasone propionate 0.5 mg in a base of propylene glycol, mineral oil, cetostearyl alcohol, Ceteth-20, isopropyl myristate, dibasic sodium phosphate, citric acid, purified water, and imidurea as preservative.

Ointment: Each gram of Fluticasone Propionate Ointment, 0.005% contains fluticasone propionate 0.05 mg in a base of propylene glycol, sorbitan sesquioleate, microcrystalline wax, and liquid paraffin.

Nasal Spray: Fluticasone propionate, the active ingredient of Flonase Nasal Spray is a glucocorticoid with the chemical name of S-fluoromethyl 6α,9α-difluoro-11β-hydroxy-16α-methyl-3-oxo-17α-propionyloxyandrosta -1, 4-diene-17β-carbothioate.

Fluticasone propionate is a white to off-white powder with a molecular weight of 500.6. It is practically insoluble in water, freely soluble in dimethyl sulfoxide and dimethylformamide, and slightly soluble in methanol and 95% ethanol.

Fluticasone propionate nasal spray (0.05% w/w) is an aqueous suspension of microfine fluticasone propionate for topical administration to the nasal mucosa by means of a metering, atomizing spray pump. Fluticasone propionate nasal spray also contains microcrystalline cellulose and carboxymethylcellulose sodium, dextrose, 0.02% w/w benzalkonium chloride, polysorbate 80, and 0.25% w/w phenylethyl alcohol.

After initial priming (three to four actuations), each 100-mg spray delivered by the nasal adapter contains 50 mcg of fluticasone propinate. Each 16-g bottle of fluticasone propionate nasal spray will provide at least 120 metered sprays. Each 9-g bottle will provide at least 60 metered sprays.

CLINICAL PHARMACOLOGY:

Cream and Ointment: Like other topical corticosteroids, fluticasone propionate has anti-inflammatory, antipruritic, and vasoconstrictive properties. The mechanism of the anti-inflammatory activity of the topical steroids, in general, is unclear. However, corticosteroids are thought to act by the induction of phospholipase A_2 inhibitory proteins, collectively called lipocortins. It is postulated that these proteins control the biosynthesis of potent mediators of inflammation such as prostaglandins and leukotrienes by inhibiting the release of their common precursor, arachidonic acid, which is released from membrane phospholipids by phospholipase A_2.

Nasal Spray: Fluticasone propionate is a synthetic, trifluorinated glucocorticoid with anti-inflammatory activity. *In vitro* dose response studies on a cloned human glucocorticoid receptor system involving binding and gene expression afforded 50% responses at 1.25 and 0.17 nM concentrations, respectively. Fluticasone propionate was three-to five-fold more potent than dexamethasone in these assays. Data from the McKenzie vasoconstrictor assay in man also support its potent glucocorticoid activity.

In preclinical studies, fluticasone propionate revealed progesteronelike activity similar to the natural hormone. However, the clinical significance of these findings in relation to the low plasma levels (see Pharmacokinetics) is not known.

The precise mechanism through which glucocorticoids affect allergic rhinitis symptoms is not known. Glucocorticoids have been shown to have a wide range of effects on multiple cell types (*e.g.*, mast cells, eosinophils, neutrophils, macrophages, and lymphocytes) and mediators (*e.g.*, histamine, eicosanoids, leukotrienes, and cytokines) involved in inflammation. In seven

CLINICAL PHARMACOLOGY: *(cont'd)*

trials, fluticasone propionate nasal spray has decreased nasal mucosal eosinophils in 66% (35% for placebo) of patients and basophils in 39% (28% for placebo) of patients. The direct relationship of these findings to long-term symptom relief is not known.

Fluticasone propionate nasal spray, like other glucocorticoids, is an agent that does not have an immediate effect on allergic symptoms. A decrease in nasal symptoms has been noted in some patients 12 hours after initial treatment with fluticasone propionate nasal spray. Maximum benefit may not be reached for several days.

Similarly, when glucocorticoids are discontinued, symptoms may not return for several days.

PHARMACOKINETICS

Cream and Ointment

The extent of percutaneous absorption of topical corticosteroids is determined by many factors, including the vehicle and the integrity of the epidermal barrier. Occlusive dressing with hydrocortisone for up to 24 hours has not been demonstrated to increase penetration; however, occlusion of hydrocortisone for 96 hours markedly enhances penetration. Topical corticosteroids can be absorbed from normal intact skin, while inflammation and/or other disease processes in the skin increase percutaneous absorption.

Studies performed with Fluticasone Propionate Cream 0.05% and Fluticasone Propionate Ointment 0.005% indicate that these are in the medium range of potency as compared with other topical corticosteroids.

Nasal Spray

Absorption: The activity of fluticasone propionate nasal spray is due to the parent drug, fluticasone propionate. Indirect calculations indicate that fluticasone propionate delivered by the intranasal route has absolute bioavailability averaging less than 2%. After intranasal treatment of patients with allergic rhinitis for 3 weeks, fluticasone propionate plasma concentrations were above the level of detection (50 pg/ml) only when recommended doses were exceeded and then only in occasional samples at low plasma levels. Due to the low bioavailability by the intranasal route, the majority of the pharmacokinetic data was obtained via other routes of administration. Studies using oral dosing of radiolabeled drug have demonstrated that fluticasone propionate is highly extracted from plasma and absorption is low. Oral bioavailability is negligible, and the majority of the circulating radioactivity is due to an inactive metabolite.

Distribution: Following intravenous administration, the distribution of fluticasone propionate follows a three-compartment open model with an apparent volume of distribution of approximately 3.7 l/kg. The percentage of fluticasone propionate bound to human plasma proteins averaged 91% with no obvious concentration relationship. Fluticasone propionate is weakly and reversibly bound to erythrocytes and freely equilibrates between erythrocytes and plasma. Fluticasone propionate is not significantly bound to human transcortin.

Metabolism

The total blood clearance of fluticasone propionate approximates that of liver blood flow, with renal clearance accounting for less than 1% of total. The only circulating metabolite detected in man is the 17β-carboxylic acid derivative of fluticasone propionate. This metabolite detected *in vitro* using cultured human hepatoma cells have not been detected in man.

Excretion

Following intravenous dosing, fluticasone propionate had an elimination half-life of approximately 3 hours. Less than 5% of a radiolabeled oral dose was excreted in the urine as metabolites, with the remainder excreted in the feces as parent drug and metabolites.

Special Populations

Fluticasone propionate was not studied in any special populations, and no gender-specific pharmacokinetic data have been obtained.

PHARMACODYNAMICS

In a trial to evaluate the potential systemic and topical effects of fluticasone propionate nasal spray on allergic rhinitis symptoms, the benefits of comparable drug blood levels produced by fluticasone propionate nasal spray and oral fluticasone propionate were compared. The doses used were 200 mcg of fluticasone propionate nasal spray, the nasal spray vehicle (plus oral placebo), and 5 and 10 mg of oral fluticasone propionate (plus nasal spray vehicle) per day for 14 days. Plasma levels were undetectable in the majority of patients after intranasal dosing, but present at low levels in the majority after oral dosing. Fluticasone propionate nasal spray was significantly more effective in reducing symptoms of allergic rhinitis than either the oral fluticasone propionate or the nasal vehicle. This trial demonstrated that the therapeutic effect of fluticasone propionate nasal spray can be attributed to the topical effects of fluticasone propionate.

In another trial, the potential systemic effects of fluticasone propionate nasal spray on the hypothalamic-pituitary-adrenal (HPA) axis were also studied in allergic patients. Fluticasone propionate nasal spray given as 200 mcg once daily or 400 mcg twice daily was compared with placebo or oral prednisone 7.5 or 15 mg given in the morning. Fluticasone propionate nasal spray at either dose for 4 weeks did not affect the adrenal response to 6-hour cosyntropin stimulation, while both doses of oral prednisone significantly reduced the response to cosyntropin.

CLINICAL STUDIES:

A total of 11 pivotal, randomized, double-blind, parallel, multicenter, vehicle-controlled clinical trials were conducted in adults and adolescents (children over 12 years of age) with seasonal of perennial allergic rhinitis. The trials included 2,633 adults (1,439 men and 1,194 women) with mean age of 37 (range, 18 to 79). A total of 440 adolescents (405 boys and 35 girls), mean age of 14 (range, 12 to 17), were also studied. The overall racial distribution was 88% white, 4% black, and 8% other. These trials evaluated the total nasal symptoms scores (TNSS) that included rhinorrhea, nasal obstruction, sneezing, and nasal itching in known allergic patients who were treated for 2 to 24 weeks. Subjects treated with fluticasone propionate nasal spray noted relief of these symptoms and exhibited significant decreases in TNSS. Nasal mucosal basophils and eosinophils were also reduced at the end of treatment; however, the clinical significance of this decrease is not known.

There were no significant differences between fluticasone propionate regimens whether administered as a single daily dose of 200 mcg (two 50- mcg sprays in each nostril) or as 100 mcg (one 50-mcg spray in each nostril) twice daily in six clinical trials. A clear dose response could not be identified in clinical trials. In one trial, 200 mcg per day was slightly more effective than 50 mcg per day during the first few days of treatment, thereafter, no difference was seen. Doses higher than 200 mcg per day were not more effective.

Individualization of Dosage: Patients may be started on 200-mcg once-a-day regimen (two 50-mcg sprays in each nostril once a day). An alternative 200-mcg per day dosage regimen can be given as 100 mcg twice daily (one 50-mcg spray in each nostril twice a day). Individual patients will experience a variable time to onset and different degree of symptom relief. A decrease in nasal symptoms may occur as soon as 12 hours after treatment onset. Maximum effect may take several days. Patients who have responded may be able to maintain (after 4 to 7 days) on 100 mcg per day (one spray in each nostril be maintained once daily. Most adolescents (12 years of age and older) should be started with 100 mcg (one spray in each nostril). Treatment with 200 mcg (two sprays in each nostril once daily or one spray in each nostril twice daily) should be reserved for adolescents not adequately responding to 100 mcg daily or as a starting dosage for adolescents with more severe symptoms. In the latter case,

CLINICAL STUDIES: *(cont'd)*

depending upon the patient's response, dosage may be decreased to 100 mcg (one spray in each nostril) daily. Maximum total daily doses should not exceed two sprays in each nostril (total dose, 200 mcg per day). There is no evidence that exceeding the recommended dose is more effective.

INDICATIONS AND USAGE:

Cream and Ointment: Fluticasone Propionate is a medium potency corticosteroid indicated for the relief of the inflammatory and pruritic manifestations of corticosteroid-responsive dermatoses.

Nasal Spray: Fluticasone propionate nasal spray is indicated for the management of seasonal and perennial allergic rhinitis in adults and adolescents 12 years of age and older.

It is not indicated for the treatment of nonallergic rhinitis since efficacy has not been adequately demonstrated in patients with this condition.

Children: It is not recommended for treatment of children below the age of 12 years with either seasonal rhinitis or allergic or nonallergic perennial rhinitis. Safety and effectiveness of fluticasone propionate nasal spray in children below 12 years of age have not been adequately established.

CONTRAINDICATIONS:

Cream and Ointment: Fluticasone propionate cream, 0.05% and ointment, 0.005% are contraindicated in those patients with a history of hypersensitivity to any of the components of the preparation.

Nasal Spray: Fluticasone propionate nasal spray is contradicted in patients with a hypersensitivity to any of its ingredients.

WARNINGS:

Nasal Spray: The replacement of a systemic glucocorticoid with a topical glucocorticoid can be accompanied by signs of adrenal insufficiency, and in addition some patients may experience symptoms of withdrawal, e.g., joint and/or muscular pain, lassitude, and depression. Patients previously treated for prolonged periods with systemic glucocorticoids and transferred to topical glucocorticoids should be carefully monitored for acute adrenal insufficiency in response to stress. In those patients who have asthma or other clinical conditions requiring long-term systemic glucocorticoid treatment, too rapid a decrease in systemic glucocorticoids may cause a severe exacerbation of their symptoms.

The use of fluticasone propionate nasal spray with alternate-day systemic prednisone could increase the likelihood of HPA suppression compared with a therapeutic dose of either one alone. Therefore, fluticasone propionate nasal spray should be used with caution in patients already receiving alternate-day prednisone treatment for any disease. In addition, the concomitant use of fluticasone propionate nasal spray with other inhaled glucocorticoids could increase the risk of signs or symptoms of hypercorticism and/or suppression of the HPA axis.

Patients who are on immunosuppressant drugs are more susceptible to infections than healthy individuals. Chickenpox and measles, for example, can have a more serious or even fatal course in patients on immunosuppressant doses of corticosteroids. In such patients who have not had these diseases, particular care should be taken to avoid exposure. How the dose, route, and duration of corticosteroid administration affects the risk of developing a disseminated infection is not known. The contribution of the underlying disease and/or prior corticosteroid treatment to the risk is also not known. If exposed to chickenpox, prophylaxis will varicella zoster immune globulin (VZIG) may be indicated. If exposed to measles, prophylaxis with pooled intramuscular immunoglobulin (IG) may be indicated. (See the respective package inserts for complete VZIG and IG prescribing information.) If chickenpox develops, treatment with antiviral agents may be considered.

PRECAUTIONS:

GENERAL

Cream and Ointment: Systemic absorption of topical corticosteroids can produce reversible hypothalamic-pituitary-adrenal (HPA) axis suppression with the potential for glucocorticosteroid insufficiency after withdrawal from treatment. Manifestations of Cushing's syndrome, hyperglycemia, and glucosuria can also be produced in some patients by systemic absorption of topical corticosteroids while on therapy.

Patients receiving a large dose of a potent topical steroid applied to a large surface area or under an occlusive dressing should be evaluated periodically for evidence of HPA axis suppression. This may be done by using the ACTH stimulation, a.m. plasma cortisol, and urinary free cortisol tests.

If HPA axis suppression is noted, an attempt should be made to withdraw the drug, to reduce the frequency of application, or to substitute a less potent steroid. Recovery of HPA axis function is generally prompt and complete upon discontinuation of topical corticosteroids. Infrequently, signs and symptoms of glucocorticosteroid insufficiency may occur that require supplemental systemic corticosteroids. For information on systemic supplementation, see prescribing information for those products.

Children may be more susceptible to systemic toxicity from equivalent doses due to their larger skin surface to body mass ratios (see PRECAUTIONS, Pediatric Use).

If irritation develops, fluticasone propionate cream, 0.05% and ointment, 0.005% should be discontinued and appropriate therapy instituted. Allergic contact dermatitis with corticosteroids is usually diagnosed by observing *failure to heal* rather than noting a clinical exacerbation as with most topical products not containing corticosteroids. Such an observation should be corroborated with appropriate diagnostic patch testing.

If concomitant skin infections are present or develop, an appropriate antifungal or antibacterial agent should be used. If a favorable response does not occur promptly, use of fluticasone propionate cream, 0.05% and ointment, 0.005% should be discontinued until the infection has been adequately controlled.

Fluticasone propionate cream, 0.05% and ointment, 0.005% should not be used in the treatment of rosacea and perioral dermatitis.

Cream: Fluticasone propionate cream, 0.05% produced HPA axis suppression with 7 days when used at a dose of 30 g per day in diseased patients. In a study of the effects of fluticasone propionate cream, 0.05% on the HPA axis, a total of 30 g per day was used in two applications daily for 7 days to six patients with psoriasis or atopic dermatitis involving at least 30% of the body surface. One patient developed evidence of adrenal suppression after 6 days of treatment with a below normal plasma cortisol level that returned to low normal levels the following day. Another patient developed a 60% decrease (although never below normal) in the plasma cortisol level from pretreatment values after 2 days of treatment. This suppression persisted at this level for 48 hours before recovering by day 6 of treatment. The results of this study indicate that fluticasone propionate cream, 0.05% may be able to suppress the HPA axis within a few days with a dose of 30 mg per day.

Ointment: Fluticasone propionate ointment, 0.05% (a concentration 10 times that of fluticasone propionate ointment, 0.005%) did not suppress plasma cortisol in any of 30 g per day six patients but did moderately suppress 24-hour urinary free cortisol levels in two of six patients when used at a dose of 30 g per day for a week in patients with psoriasis or eczema. In a second study, fluticasone propionate ointment, 0.05% caused a minimal depression of a.m. plasma cortisol levels in 3 of 12 normal volunteers when applied at doses of 50 g per day for 21 days. Morning plasma levels returned to normal levels within the first week upon discontinuation of fluticasone propionate. In this study there was no corresponding decrease in 24-hour urinary free cortisol levels.

Nasal Spray: Rarely, immediate hypersensitivity reactions or contact dermatitis may occur after the intranasal administration of fluticasone propionate. Rare instances of wheezing, nasal septum perforation, cataracts, glaucoma and increased intraocular pressure have been reported following the intranasal application of glucocorticoids.

Use of excessive doses of glucocorticoids may lead to signs or symptoms of hypercorticism, suppression of HPA function, and/or suppression of growth in children or teenagers. Knemometry studies in asthmatic children on orally inhaled glucocorticoids showed inhibitory effects on short-term growth rate. The relationship between short-term changes in lower leg growth and long-term effects on growth is unclear at this time. Physicians should closely follow the growth of adolescents taking glucocorticosteroids, by any route, and weigh the benefit of glucocorticoid therapy against the possibility of growth suppression if an adolescents growth appears slowed.

Although systemic effects have been minimal with recommended doses of fluticasone propionate nasal spray, potential risk increases with larger doses. Therefore, larger than recommended doses of fluticasone propionate nasal spray should be avoided.

When used at larger doses, systemic glucocorticoid effects such as hypercorticism and adrenal suppression may appear. If such changes occur, the dosage of fluticasone propionate nasal spray should be discontinued slowly consistent with accepted procedures for discontinuing oral glucocorticoid therapy.

In clinical studies with fluticasone propionate administered intranasally, the development of localized infections of the nose and pharynx with *Candida albicans* has occurred only rarely. When such an infection develops, it may require treatment with appropriate local therapy and discontinuation of treatment with fluticasone propionate nasal spray. Patients using fluticasone propionate nasal spray over several months or longer should be examined periodically for evidence of *Candida* infection or other signs of adverse effects on the nasal mucosa.

Fluticasone propionate nasal spray should be used with caution, if at all, in patients with active or quiescent tuberculous infections; untreated fungal, bacterial, or systemic viral infections; or ocular herpes simplex.

Because of the inhibitory effect of glucocorticoids on wound healing, patients who have experienced recent nasal septal ulcers, nasal surgery, or nasal trauma should not use a nasal glucocorticoid until healing has occurred.

INFORMATION FOR THE PATIENT

Cream and Ointment: Patients using topical corticosteroids should receive the following information and instructions:

1. This medication is to be used as directed by the physician. It is for external use only. Avoid contact with the eyes.

2. This medication should not be used for any disorder other than that for which it was prescribed.

3. The treated skin area should not be bandaged or otherwise covered or wrapped so as to be occlusive unless directed by the physician.

4. Patients should report to their physician any signs of local adverse reactions.

Nasal Spray: Patients being treated with fluticasone propionate nasal spray should receive the following information and instructions. This information is intended to aid them in the safe and effective use of this medication. It is not a disclosure of all possible adverse or intended effects.

Patients should be warned to avoid exposure to chickenpox or measles and, if exposed, to consult their physician without delay.

Patients should use fluticasone propionate nasal spray at regular intervals as directed since its effectiveness depends on its regular use. A decrease in nasal symptoms may occur as soon as 12 hours after starting therapy with fluticasone propionate nasal spray. Results in several clinical trials indicate statistically significant improvement within the first day or two of treatment; however, the full benefit of fluticasone propionate nasal spray may not be achieved until treatment has been administered for several days. The patient should not increase the prescribed dosage but should contact the physician if symptoms do not improve or if the condition worsens. For the proper use of the nasal spray and to attain maximum improvement, the patient should read and follow carefully the accompanying patient's instructions.

LABORATORY TESTS

Cream and Ointment: The following tests may be helpful in evaluating patients for HPA axis suppression:

ACTH stimulation test

A.M. plasma cortisol test

Urinary free cortisol test

CARCINOGENESIS, MUTAGENESIS, AND IMPAIRMENT OF FERTILITY

Cream and Ointment: Long-term animal studies have not been performed to evaluate the carcinogenic potential of fluticasone propionate.

Fluticasone propionate was not mutagenic in the standard Ames test, *E. coli* fluctuation test, *S. cerevisiae* gene conversion test, or Chinese Hamster ovarian cell assay. It was not clastogenic in mouse micronucleus or cultured human lymphocyte tests.

In a fertility and general reproductive performance study in rats, fluticasone propionate administered subcutaneously to females at up to 50 mcg/kg per day and to males at up to 100 mcg/kg per day (later reduced to 50 mcg/kg per day) had no effect upon mating performance or fertility. In Fluticasone Propionate Cream, 0.05%, these doses are approximately 15 and 30 times, and in Fluticasone Propionate Ointment, 0.05%, these doses are approximately 150 and 300 times, respectively, the human systemic exposure following use of the recommended human topical dose, assuming human percutaneous absorption of approximately 3% and the use in a 70-kg person of 15 g per day.

Nasal Spray: Fluticasone propionate demonstrated no tumorigenic potential in studies of oral doses up to 1.0 mg/kg (3 mg/m^2 as calculated on a surface area basis) for 78 weeks in the mouse or inhalation of up to 57 mcg/kg (336 mcg/m^2) for 104 weeks in the rat.

Fluticasone propionate did not induce gene mutation in prokaryotic or eukaryotic cells *in vitro*. No significant clastogenic effect was seen in cultured human peripheral lymphocytes *in vitro* or in the mouse micronucleus test when administered at high doses by the oral or subcutaneous routes. Furthermore, the compound did not delay erythroblast division in bone marrow.

No evidence of impairment of fertility was observed in reproductive studies conducted in rats dosed subcutaneously with doses up to 50 mcg/kg (295 mcg/m^2) in males and females. However, prostate weight was significantly reduced in rats.

PREGNANCY, TERATOGENIC EFFECTS, PREGNANCY CATEGORY C

Cream and Ointment: Corticosteroids have been shown to be teratogenic in laboratory animals when administered systemically at relatively low dosage levels. The more potent corticosteroids have been shown to be teratogenic after dermal application in laboratory

PRECAUTIONS: *(cont'd)*

animals. Teratology studies in the mouse demonstrated fluticasone propionate to be teratogenic (cleft palate) when administered subcutaneously in doses of 45 mcg/kg per day and 150 mcg/kg per day. This dose is approximately 14 and 45 times, respectively, the human topical dose of fluticasone propionate cream, 0.05% and ointment, 0.005%. There are no adequate and well-controlled studies in pregnant women. Fluticasone propionate cream, 0.05% and ointment, 0.005% should be used during pregnancy only if the potential benefit justifies the potential risk to the fetus.

Nasal Spray: Subcutaneous studies in the mouse and rat and 45 and 100 mcg/kg, respectively (135 and 590 mcg/m^2, respectively, as calculated on a surface area basis), revealed fetal toxicity characteristic of potent glucocorticoid compounds, including embryonic growth retardation, omphalocele cleft palate, and retarded cranial ossification.

In the rabbit, fetal weight reduction and cleft palate were observed following subcutaneous doses of 4 mcg/kg (48 mcg/m^2).

However, following oral administration of up to 300 mcg/kg (3.6 mg/m^2) of fluticasone propionate to the rabbit, there were no maternal effects nor increased incidence of external, visceral, or skeletal fetal defects. No fluticasone propionate was detected in the plasma in this study, consistent with the established low bioavailability following oral administration (see CLINICAL PHARMACOLOGY).

Less than 0.008% of the dose crosses the placenta following oral administration to rats (100 mcg/kg, 590 mcg/m^2) or rabbits (300 mcg/kg, 3.6 mg/m^2).

There are no adequate and well-controlled studies in pregnant women. Fluticasone propionate should be used during pregnancy only if the potential benefit justifies the potential risk to the fetus. Experience with oral glucocorticoids since their introduction in pharmacologic, as opposed to physiologic, doses suggests that rodents are more prone to teratogenic effects from glucocorticoids than humans. In addition, because there is a natural increase in glucocorticoid production during pregnancy, most women will require a lower exogenous glucocorticoid dose and many will not need glucocorticoid treatment during pregnancy.

NURSING MOTHERS

Cream and Ointment: Systemically administered corticosteroids appear in human milk and could suppress growth, interfere with endogenous corticosteroid production, or cause other untoward effects. It is not known whether topical administration of corticosteroids could result in sufficient systemic absorption to produce detectable quantities in human milk. Because many drugs are excreted in human milk, caution should be exercised when fluticasone propionate cream, 0.05% or ointment, 0.005% is administered to a nursing woman.

Nasal Spray: It is not known whether fluticasone propionate is excreted in human breast milk. Subcutaneous administration of titrated drug to lactating rats (10 mcg/kg, 59 mcg/m^2) resulted in measurable radioactivity in both plasma and milk. Because other glucocorticoids are excreted in human milk, caution should be exercised when fluticasone propionate nasal spray is administered to a nursing woman.

PEDIATRIC USE

Cream and Ointment: Safety and effectiveness in children and infants have not been established. Because of a higher ratio of skin surface area to body mass, children are at a greater risk than adults of HPA axis suppression when they are treated with topical corticosteroids. They are therefore also at greater risk of glucocorticosteroid insufficiency after withdrawal of treatment and of Cushing's syndrome while on treatment. Adverse effects including striae have been reported with inappropriate use of topical corticosteroids in infants and children (see PRECAUTIONS).

HPA axis suppression, Cushing's syndrome, and intracranial hypertension have been reported in children receiving topical corticosteroids. Manifestations of adrenal suppression in children include linear growth retardation, delayed weight gain, low plasma cortisol levels, and absence of response to ACTH stimulation. Manifestations of intracranial hypertension include bulging fontanelles, headaches, and bilateral papilledema.

Nasal Spray: The safety and effectiveness of fluticasone propionate nasal spray in children below 12 years of age have not been established. Oral glucocorticoids have been shown to cause growth suppression in children and teenagers with extended use. If a child or teenager on any glucocorticoid appears to have growth suppression, the possibility that they are particularly sensitive to this effect of glucocorticoids should be considered (see PRECAUTIONS).

Geriatric Use: A limited number of patients above 60 years of age (n=132) have been treated with fluticasone propionate nasal spray in US and non-US clinical trials. While the number of patients is too small to permit separate analysis of efficacy and safety, the adverse reactions reported in this population were similar to those reported by younger patients.

ADVERSE REACTIONS:

Cream and Ointment: In controlled clinical trials, the total incidence of adverse reactions associated with the use of fluticasone propionate cream, 0.05% and ointment, 0.005% was approximately 4%.

The following additional local adverse reactions have been reported infrequently with other topical corticosteroids, and they may occur more frequently with the use of occlusive dressings, especially with higher potency corticosteroids. These reactions are listed in an approximately decreasing order of occurrence: irritation, folliculitis, acneiform eruptions, hypopigmentation, perioral dermatitis, allergic contact dermatitis, secondary infection, skin atrophy, striae, and miliaria. Also, there are reports of the development of pustular psoriasis from chronic plaque psoriasis following reduction or discontinuation of potent topical corticosteroid products.

Cream: The adverse reactions were mild, usually self-limiting, and consisted primarily of pruritus, dryness, numbness of fingers, and burning. These events occurred in 2.9%, 1.2%, 1.0%, and 0.6% of patients, respectively.

Ointment: The adverse reactions were mild, usually self-limiting, and consisted primarily of pruritus, burning, hypertrichosis, increased erythema, hives, irritation, and lightheadedness. Each of these events occurred individually in less than 1% of patients.

Nasal Spray: In controlled US studies, 2,427 patients received treatment with intranasal fluticasone propionate. In general, adverse reactions in clinical studies have been primarily associated with irritation of the nasal mucous membranes, and the adverse reactions were reported with approximately the same frequency by patients treated with vehicle itself. The complaints did not usually interfere with treatment. Less than 2% of patients in clinical trials discontinued because of adverse events; this rate was similar for vehicle and active comparators.

Systemic glucocorticoid side effects were not reported during controlled clinical studies up to 6 months' duration with fluticasone propionate nasal spray. If recommended doses are exceeded, however, or if individuals are particularly sensitive or if in conjunction with systemically administered glucocorticoids, symptoms or hypercorticism, e.g., Cushing's syndrome, could occur.

The following incidence of common adverse reactions is based upon seven controlled clinical trials in which 536 patients (57 girls and 108 boys aged 4 to 11 years, 137 female and 234 male adolescents and adults) were treated with fluticasone propionate nasal spray 200 mcg

ADVERSE REACTIONS: *(cont'd)*

once daily over 2 to 4 weeks and two controlled clinical trials in which 246 patients (119 female and 127 adolescents and adults) were treated with fluticasone propionate nasal spray 200 mcg once daily over 6 months.

INCIDENCE GREATER THAN 1% (CAUSAL RELATIONSHIP POSSIBLE)

Respiratory: Epistaxis, nasal burning (incidence 3% to 6%); blood in nasal mucus, pharyngitis, nasal irritation (incidence 1% to 3%).

Neurological: Headache (incidence 1% to 3%).

INCIDENCE LESS THAN 1% (CAUSAL RELATIONSHIP POSSIBLE)

Respiratory: Sneezing, runny nose, nasal dryness, sinusitis, nasal congestion, bronchitis, nasal ulcer, nasal septum excoriation.

Neurological: Dizziness.

Special Senses: Eye disorder, unpleasant taste.

Digestive: Nausea and vomiting, xerostomia.

Skin and Appendages: Urticaria.

OVERDOSAGE:

Cream and Ointment: Topically applied fluticasone propionate cream, 0.05% or ointment, 0.005% can be absorbed in sufficient amounts to produce systemic effects (see PRECAUTIONS).

Nasal Spray: There are no data available on the effects of acute or chronic overdosage with fluticasone propionate nasal spray. Intranasal administration of 2 mg (10 times the recommended dose) of fluticasone propionate twice daily for 7 days to healthy human volunteers was well tolerated. Single oral doses up to 16 mg have been studied in human volunteers with no acute toxic effects reported. Repeat oral doses up to 80 mg daily for 10 days in volunteers and repeat oral doses up to 10 mg daily for 14 days in patients were well tolerated. Adverse reactions were of mild or moderate severity, and incidences were similar in active and placebo treatment groups. Acute overdosage with this dosage form is unlikely since one bottle of fluticasone propionate nasal spray contains approximately 8 mg of fluticasone propionate. Chronic overdosage may result in signs/symptoms of hypercorticism (see PRECAUTIONS).

DOSAGE AND ADMINISTRATION:

Cream and Ointment: Apply a thin film of Fluticasone Propionate Cream, 0.05% or Ointment, 0.005% to the affected skin areas twice daily. Rub in gently.

Nasal Spray: Patients should use fluticasone propionate nasal spray at regular intervals as directed since its effectiveness depends on its regular use.

Adults and Adolescents 12 Years of Age and Older: The recommended starting dosage in **adults** is two sprays (50 mcg of fluticasone propionate each) in each nostril once a day (total daily dose, 200 mcg). The same dosage divided into 100 mcg given twice a day (*e.g.,* 8 am and 8 p.m.) is also effective. After the first few days, patients may be able to reduce their dosage to 100 mcg (one spray in each nostril) once daily for maintenance therapy.

Most **adolescents** should be started with 100 mcg (one spray in each nostril). Adolescents not adequately responding to 100 mcg or adolescents with more severe symptoms may use 200 mcg (two sprays in each nostril). Depending upon the patient's response, dosage may be decreased to 100 mcg (one spray in each nostril) daily.

The maximum total daily dosage should not exceed two sprays in each nostril (22 mcg per day). (See Individualization Of Dosage and CLINICAL PHARMACOLOGY.)

Fluticasone propionate nasal spray is not recommended for children under 12 years of age or for patients with nonallergic rhinitis.

Directions for Use: Illustrated patient's instructions for proper use accompany each package of fluticasone propionate nasal spray.

PATIENT INFORMATION:

Fluticasone propionate is a corticosteroid used to decrease inflammation and irritation. It is available as a nasal spray to treat allergies and as a cream or ointment to relieve itchy irritation skin. Creams and ointments should be applied only to the affected area. Keep the medicine away from the eyes. Do not cover the affected skin with a tight bandage or covering. Wash hands after applying so there is no risk of contact with the eyes or mouth. When using the nasal spray, proper technique for administering the medication is important. Please read the information pamphlet you were provide. Within a few days the nasal spray may help with symptoms of allergies. If there is no improvement within a week, contact your physician. The nasal spray should not be discontinued abruptly. This medication should be used regularly and not in an attempt to relieve an immediate situation.

HOW SUPPLIED:

CREAM

Cutivate Cream, 0.05% is supplied in 15g, 30g, and 60g tubes.

Storage: Store between 2° and 30°C (36° and 86°F).

OINTMENT

Cutivate Ointment, 0.005% is supplied in 15g, 30g, and 60g tubes.

Storage: Store between 2° and 30°C (36° and 86°F).

NASAL SPRAY

Fluticasone Propionate Nasal Spray, 0.05% w/w is supplied in a 16g amber glass bottle providing 120 actuations and in a 9g amber glass bottle providing 60 actuations. Each actuation delivers 100 mg of the suspension, which contains 50 mcg of fluticasone propionate. Each bottle is fitted with a metering atomizing pump, nasal adapter, and dust cover in a box of one with patient's instructions for use.

Storage: Store between 4° and 30°C (39° and 86°F).

HOW SUPPLIED - EQUIVALENTS NOT AVAILABLE:

Aerosol, Spray - Nasal - 0.05 %

9 gm	$33.12	FLONASE AQ, Glaxo Wellcome	00173-0472-00
16 gm	$44.17	FLONASE AQ, Glaxo Wellcome	00173-0453-01

Cream - Topical - 0.05 %

15 gm	**$13.52**	**CUTIVATE, Glaxo Wellcome**	**00173-0430-00**
30 gm	**$20.83**	**CUTIVATE, Glaxo Wellcome**	**00173-0430-01**
60 gm	**$31.68**	**CUTIVATE, Glaxo Wellcome**	**00173-0430-02**

Ointment - Topical - 0.005 %

15 gm	**$13.52**	**CUTIVATE, Glaxo Wellcome**	**00173-0431-00**
30 gm	**$20.83**	**CUTIVATE, Glaxo Wellcome**	**00173-0431-01**
60 gm	**$31.68**	**CUTIVATE, Glaxo Wellcome**	**00173-0431-02**

FLUVASTATIN SODIUM *(003193)*

CATEGORIES: Antilipemic Agents; Atherosclerosis; Cardiovascular Drugs; Cholesterol; HMG-COA Reductase Inhibitors; Heart Disease; Hypercholesterolemia; Hyperlipidemia; Hyperlipoproteinemia; Hypolipidemics; Vascular Disease; Pregnancy Category X; FDA Class 1S ("Standard Review"); Sales > $100 Million; FDA Approved 1993 Dec; Top 200 Drugs

BRAND NAMES: *Cranoc* (Germany); **Lescol**; *Locol* (Germany)
(International brand names outside U.S. in italics)

FORMULARIES: Medi-Cal; PCS

COST OF THERAPY: $419.38 (Hypercholesterolemia; Capsule; 20 mg; 1/day; 365 days)

DESCRIPTION:

Fluvastatin sodium is a water soluble cholesterol lowering agent which acts through the inhibition of 3-hydroxy-3-methylglutaryl- coenzyme A (HMG-CoA) reductase.

Fluvastatin sodium is [*R**, *S**- (*E*)]-(±)-7-[3-(4- fluorophenyl)-1-(1-methylethyl)-1*H*-indol-2-yl]-3,5-dihydroxy-6- heptenoic acid, monosodium salt.

This molecular entity is the first entirely synthetic HMG-CoA reductase inhibitor, and is in part structurally distinct from the fungal derivatives of this therapeutic class.

Fluvastatin sodium is a white to pale yellow, hygroscopic powder soluble in water, ethanol and methanol. Fluvastatin sodium is supplied as capsules containing fluvastatin sodium, equivalent to 20 mg or 40 mg of fluvastatin, for oral administration.

Active Ingredient: fluvastatin sodium

Inactive Ingredients: gelatin, magnesium stearate, microcrystalline cellulose, pregelatinized starch, red iron oxide, sodium lauryl sulfate, talc, titanium dioxide, yellow iron oxide, and other ingredients.

May Also Include: benzyl alcohol, black iron oxide, butylparaben, carboxymethylcellulose sodium, edetate calcium disodium, methylparaben, propylparaben, silicon dioxide and sodium propionate.

CLINICAL PHARMACOLOGY:

A variety of clinical studies have demonstrated that elevated levels of total cholesterol (Total-C), low density lipoprotein cholesterol (LDL-C), and apolipoprotein B (a membrane transport complex for LDL-C) promote human atherosclerosis. Similarly, decreased levels of HDL-cholesterol (HDL-C) and its transport complex, apolipoprotein A, are associated with the development of atherosclerosis. Epidemiologic investigations have established that cardiovascular morbidity and mortality vary directly with the level of Total-C and LDL-C and inversely with the level of HDL- C. The Lipid Research Clinics Coronary Primary Prevention Trial (LRC- CPPT) was a multicenter, randomized, double-blind study involving 3,806 asymptomatic middle-aged men in the United States with Type II hyperlipoproteinemia treated with diet and cholestyramine. Results of this trial demonstrated that a statistically significant reduction of 19% in the incidence of definite myocardial infarction and/or coronary heart disease death was associated with an 8% decrease in blood cholesterol and 11% decrease in LDL-C levels. In other multicenter clinical trials, those pharmacologic and/or nonpharmacologic interventions that simultaneously lowered LDL-C and increased HDL-C also have reduced the rate of cardiovascular events (both fatal and nonfatal myocardial infarctions).

In patients with hypercholesterolemia,treatment with fluvastatin sodium reduced Total-C, LDL-C, and apolipoprotein B. Lescol (fluvastatin sodium) also moderately reduced triglycerides (TG) while producing an increase in HDL-C of variable magnitude. The agent had no consistent effect on either Lp(a) or fibrinogen. The effect of fluvastatin sodium- induced changes in lipoprotein levels on the evolution of atherosclerosis has not been established.

MECHANISM OF ACTION

Fluvastatin sodium is a competitive inhibitor of HMG-CoA reductase, which is responsible for the conversion of 3-hydroxy-3-methyl- glutaryl-coenzyme A (HMG-CoA) to mevalonate, a precursor of sterols, including cholesterol. The inhibition of cholesterol biosynthesis reduces the cholesterol in hepatic cells, which stimulates the synthesis of LDL receptors and thereby increases the uptake of LDL particles. The end result of these biochemical processes is a reduction of the plasma cholesterol concentration.

PHARMACOKINETICS AND METABOLISM

Fluvastatin sodium is administered orally in the active form. Fluvastatin is absorbed rapidly and completely (98%) following oral administration to fasted volunteers. In a fed state, even up to 4 hours post prandial, the drug is also completely absorbed, but at a reduced rate ($C_{max}$is reduced by 40%-70%). The action of HMGR inhibitors occurs within the liver. The absolute systemic bioavailability for this drug class is low. The absolute bioavailability of fluvastatin following a 10 mg oral dose was 24% (range 9%-50%). At doses above 20 mg, fluvastatin exhibits nonlinear kinetics, at least in the fasting state, resulting in dose normalized AUC values 20%-40% higher than expected for the 40 mg dose. The volume of distribution (VD_{SS}) for the drug is calculated to be 34.4 liters. More than 98% of the circulating drug is bound to plasma proteins, and this binding is unaffected by drug concentration.

Biotransformation pathways for fluvastatin include: a) hydroxylation of the indole ring at the 5- and 6-positions; b) N-dealkylation; and c) beta-oxidation. The major circulating blood components are fluvastatin and the pharmacologically inactive N-desisopropyl-propionic acid metabolite. The hydroxylated metabolites have pharmacological activity but do not circulate systemically. Both enantiomers of fluvastatin are metabolized in a similar manner resulting in only minor differences in systemic exposure.

Following administration of ^{3}H-fluvastatin sodium to healthy volunteers, excretion of radioactivity was about 5% in the urine and 90% in the feces, with the parent, fluvastatin, accounting for less than 2% of the total radioactivity excreted. The plasma clearance for fluvastatin in man is calculated to be 39.2 ± 4.4 liters per hour. Steady-state plasma concentrations show no evidence of fluvastatin accumulation following administration of 40 mg daily; however, after 6 days of dosing with 40 mg ^{3}H-fluvastatin sodium solution, total radioactivity - which includes parent compound and pharmacologically inactive metabolites - accumulated by a factor of 2 based on C_{min}values. Following oral administration of 20 mg of fluvastatin sodium, the beta elimination half-life for fluvastatin is 1.2 hours (range of 0.53-3.1 hours).

The bioavailability of fluvastatin sodium 20 mg capsules is equivalent to a solution of fluvastatin sodium except that the time to peak under fasted conditions is about 0.7 hours following administration of the capsule compared to about 0.4 hours for the solution. Following ingestion of a single 20 mg fluvastatin sodium capsule under fasted conditions, measurable plasma concentrations of fluvastatin appear systemically within 10 minutes after dosing and reach a peak of 147 ± 86 ng/ml at 0.66 ± 0.3 hours. fluvastatin sodium, like the other HMGR inhibitors, has variable systemic bioavailability. The coefficient of variation (based on the inter-subject variability) was 47%-57% for AUC, and 58%-69% for C_{max}.

CLINICAL PHARMACOLOGY: *(cont'd)*

Results from an overnight pharmacokinetic evaluation following steady-state administration of fluvastatin sodium with the evening meal or 4 hours after the evening meal for 15 weeks showed that administration of fluvastatin sodium with the evening meal results in a two-fold decrease in $C_{max}$and more than a two-fold increase in T_{max} as compared to patients receiving the drug 4 hours after the evening meal. No significant difference in AUC was observed between the 2 treatment groups, and there were no differences in the lipid-lowering effects of fluvastatin sodium administered with the evening meal or 4 hours after the evening meal.

The effects of gender and age on the pharmacokinetics of fluvastatin sodium were evaluated in 4 patient subgroups; young and elderly males and females. All patients were administered 20 mg fluvastatin daily, at least 2 hours after the evening meal, for 21 days. Results from an overnight pharmacokinetic evaluation indicate that for the general patient population plasma concentrations of fluvastatin do not vary either as a function of age or gender. Due to their generally small body weight, young female patients show higher fluvastatin plasma concentrations after administration of 1-40 mg of fluvastatin compared to young males.

Since fluvastatin is eliminated primarily via the biliary route and is subject to significant presystemic metabolism, the potential exists for drug accumulation in patients with hepatic insufficiency. In a single- dose study the kinetics of fluvastatin sodium in subjects with cirrhosis (n=11) and in healthy age- and sex-matched subjects (n=11) were compared. The mean AUC and C_{max} parameters were about 2.5 times higher in the subjects with hepatic insufficiency. There was a 28% decrease in plasma clearance and a 31% smaller volume of distribution. No apparent difference was observed in the plasma elimination half-lives for the 2 groups. Caution should be exercised when fluvastatin sodium is administered to patients with a history of liver disease or heavy alcohol ingestion (see WARNINGS).

CLINICAL STUDIES:

Fluvastatin sodium has been studied in 4 controlled Phase 3 trials. These studies involved 1605 North American patients with Type IIa or IIb hyperlipoproteinemia. Lescol (fluvastatin sodium) was administered to 946 patients in these trials of 24-54 weeks duration. In the largest single randomized study with Lescol (fluvastatin sodium) (n=292), treatment at a dose of 20 mg QPM resulted in a highly significant decrease in LDL-C of 22.2% after 9 weeks of study. In the largest single study (n=210) of patients randomized to 40 mg daily and limited to FH patients, a mean LDL-C reduction of 24.0% was observed. Reductions in Apo B were also seen as a result of treatment with fluvastatin sodium. Small but statistically significant increases in HDL-C and corresponding decreases in TG were also noted. No consistent effect on Lp(a) was found.

INDICATIONS AND USAGE:

Fluvastatin sodium is indicated as an adjunct to diet in the treatment of elevated total cholesterol (total-C) and LDL-C levels in patients with primary hypercholesterolemia (Type IIa and IIb) whose response to dietary restriction of saturated fat and cholesterol and other nonpharmacological measures has not been adequate.

Therapy with lipid-altering agents should be considered only after secondary causes for hyperlipidemia such as poorly controlled diabetes mellitus, hypothyroidism, nephrotic syndrome, dysproteinemias, obstructive liver disease, other medication, or alcoholism, have been excluded. Prior to initiation of fluvastatin sodium, a lipid profile should be performed to measure Total-C, HDL-C and TG. For patients with TG <400 mg/dl (<4.5 mmol/L), LDL-C can be estimated using the following equation:

LDL-C = Total-C - HDL-C - 1/5 TG

For TG levels >400 mg/dl (>4.5 mmol/L), this equation is less accurate and LDL-C concentrations should be determined by ultracentrifugation. In many hypertriglyceridemic patients LDL-C may be low or normal despite elevated Total-C. In such cases, fluvastatin sodium is not indicated.

Lipid determinations should be performed at intervals of no less than 4 weeks and dosage adjusted according to the patient's response to therapy.

The Natural Cholesterol Education Program (NCEP) Treatment Guidelines are summarized below:

TABLE 1 Fluvastatin Sodium, INDICATIONS AND USAGE

Definite Atherosclerotic Disease	LDL-Cholesterol Two or More Other Risk Factors**	mg/dL (mmol/L) Initiation Level	Goal
NO	NO	≥190 (≥4.9)	<160 (<4.1)
NO	YES	≥160 (≥4.1)	<130 (<3.4)
YES	YES or NO	≥130 (≥3.4)	<100 (<2.6)

* Coronary heart disease or peripheral vascular disease (including symptomatic carotid artery disease).
** Other risk factors for coronary heart disease (CHD) include: age (males: ≥45 years; females: ≥55 years or premature menopause without estrogen replacement therapy); family history of premature CHD; current cigarette smoking; hypertension; confirmed HDL-C <35 mg/dL (<0.91 mmol/L); and diabetes mellitus.
Subtract one risk factor if HDL is ≥60 mg/dL (≥1.6 mmol/L).

Since the goal of treatment is to lower LDL-C, the NCEP recommends that the LDL-C levels be used to initiate and assess treatment response. Only if LDL-C levels are not available, should the Total-C be used to monitor therapy.

TABLE 2 Classification of Hyperlipoproteinemias

Type	Lipoproteins Elevated	Lipid Elevations Major	Minor
I (rare)	Chylomicrons	TG	↑ → C
IIa	LDL	C	-
IIb	LDL, VLDL	C	TG
III (rare)	IDL	C/TG	-
IV	VLDL	TG	↑ → C
V (rare)	Chylomicrons, VLDL	TG	↑ → C

C = cholesterol
TG = triglycerides
LDL = low density lipoprotein
VLDL = very low density lipoprotein
IDL = intermediate density lipoprotein

Fluvastatin sodium has not been studied in conditions where the major abnormality is elevation of chylomicrons, VLDL, or IDL (*i.e.*, hypolipoproteinemia Types I, III, IV, or V).

INDICATIONS AND USAGE: *(cont'd)*

The effect of fluvastatin sodium-induced changes in lipoprotein levels on cardiovascular morbidity or mortality has not been established.

CONTRAINDICATIONS:

Hypersensitivity to any component of this medication. Fluvastatin sodium is contraindicated in patients with active liver disease or unexplained, persistent elevations in serum transaminases (see WARNINGS).

USE IN PREGNANCY

Atherosclerosis is a chronic process and discontinuation of lipid- lowering drugs during pregnancy should have little impact on the outcome of long-term therapy of primary hypercholesterolemia. Cholesterol and other products of cholesterol biosynthesis are essential components for fetal development (including synthesis of steroids and cell membranes). Since HMG-CoA reductase inhibitors decrease cholesterol synthesis and possibly the synthesis of other biologically active substances derived from cholesterol, they may cause fetal harm when administered to pregnant women. Therefore, HMG-CoA reductase inhibitors are contraindicated during pregnancy and in nursing mothers. **Fluvastatin sodium should be administered to women of childbearing age only when such patients are highly unlikely to conceive and have been informed of the potential hazards.** If the patient becomes pregnant while taking this class of drug, therapy should be discontinues and the patient apprised of the potential hazard to the fetus.

WARNINGS:

LIVER ENZYMES

Biochemical abnormalities of liver function have been associated with HMG-CoA reductase inhibitors and other lipid-lowering agents. A small number of patients treated with fluvastatin sodium in United States controlled trials (N=17, 1.1%) developed persistent elevations of transaminase levels to more than 3 times the upper limit of normal. Ten of these patients (0.7%) were discontinued from therapy. Most of these (10/17) abnormalities occurred within the first 6 weeks of treatment and resolved rapidly to pretreatment values. In a long-term open-label extension study, 5 of 824 (0.6%) patients exposed to fluvastatin sodium at a dose of 40 mg developed persistent transaminase elevations. Only 2 of these patients were discontinued from the study. The majority of these abnormal biochemical findings were asymptomatic.

It is recommended that liver function tests be performed before the initiation of treatment, at 6 and 12 weeks after initiation of therapy or elevation in persistent, and periodically thereafter (*e.g.*, semiannually).

Liver enzyme changes generally occur in the first 3 months of treatment with fluvastatin sodium. Patients who develop increased transaminase levels should be monitored with a second liver function evaluation to confirm the finding and be followed thereafter with frequent liver function tests until the abnormality(ies) return to normal. Should an increase in AST or ALT of three times the upper limit of normal or greater persist, withdrawal of fluvastatin sodium therapy is recommended.

Active liver disease or unexplained transaminase elevations are contraindications to the use of fluvastatin sodium (see CONTRAINDICATIONS.) Caution should be exercised when fluvastatin sodium is administered to patients with a history of liver disease or heavy alcohol ingestion (see CLINICAL PHARMACOLOGY, Pharmacokinetics and Metabolism). Such patients should be closely monitored.

Skeletal Muscle: Rhabdomyolysis with renal dysfunction secondary to myoglobinuria has been reported with other drugs in this class.To this date, this has not occurred with fluvastatin sodium. Myopathy, defined as muscle aching or muscle weakness in conjunction with increases in creatine phosphokinase (CPK) values to greater than 10 times the upper limit of normal, has been reported in 1 fluvastatin sodium patient to date and was related to physical exertion. An additional case was reported in a patient receiving placebo.

Myopathy should be considered in any patients with diffuse myalgias, muscle tenderness or weakness, and/or marked elevation of CPK. Patients should be advised to report promptly unexplained muscle pain, tenderness or weakness, particularly if accompanied by malaise or fever. Fluvastatin sodium therapy should be discontinued if markedly elevated CPK levels occur or myopathy is diagnosed or suspected. Fluvastatin sodium therapy should also be temporarily withheld in any patient experiencing an acute or serious condition predisposing to the development of renal failure secondary to rhabdomyolysis, e.g., sepsis; hypotension, major surgery; trauma; severe metabolic, endocrine, or electrolyte disorders; or uncontrolled epilepsy.

The risk of myopathy during treatment with another HMG-CoA reductase inhibitor was found to be increased if therapy with either cyclosporine, gemfibrozil, erythromycin, or niacin is administered concurrently. Myopathy was not observed in a clinical trial in 74 patients involving patients who were treated with fluvastatin sodium together with niacin.

Uncomplicated myalgia has been observed infrequently in patients treated with fluvastatin sodium at rates indistinguishable from placebo.

The use of fibrates alone may occasionally be associated with myopathy. The combined use of HMG-CoA inhibitors and fibrates should generally be avoided.

PRECAUTIONS:

GENERAL

Before instituting therapy with fluvastatin sodium, an attempt should be made to control hypercholesterolemia with appropriate diet, exercise, and weight reduction in obese patients, and to treat other underlying medical problems (see INDICATIONS AND USAGE).

The HMG-CoA reductase inhibitors may cause elevation of creatine phosphokinase and transaminase levels (see WARNINGS and ADVERSE REACTIONS). This should be considered in the differential diagnosis of chest pain in a patient on therapy with fluvastatin sodium.

HOMOZYGOUS FAMILIAL HYPERCHOLESTEROLEMIA

HMG-CoA reductase inhibitors are reported to be less effective in patients with rare homozygous familial hypercholesterolemia, possibly because these patients have few functional LDL receptors.

INFORMATION FOR THE PATIENT

Patients should be advised to report promptly unexplained muscle pain, tenderness or weakness, particularly if accompanied by malaise or fever.

CNS TOXICITY

CNS effects, as evidenced by decreased activity, ataxia. loss of righting reflex, and ptosis were seen in the following animal studies: the 18-month mouse carcinogenicity study at 50 mg/kg/day, the 6-month dog study at 36 mg/kg/day, the 6-month hamster study at 40 mg/kg/day, and in acute, high-dose studies in rats and hamsters (50 mg/kg),rabbits (300 mg/kg) and mice (1500 mg/kg). CNS toxicity in the acute high-dose studies was characterized (in mice) by conspicuous vacuolation in the ventral white columns of the spinal cord at a dose of 5000 mg/kg and (in rat) by edema with separation of myelinated fibers of the ventral spinal tracts and sciatic nerve at a dose of 1500 mg/kg. CNS toxicity, characterized by periaxonal vacuolization, was observed in the medulla of dogs that after treatment for 5 weeks with 48 mg/kg/day; this finding was not observed in the remaining dogs when the dose level was lowered to 36 mg/kg/day. CNS vascular lesions, characterized by perivascular hemorrhages,

PRECAUTIONS: *(cont'd)*

edema, and mononuclear cell infiltration of perivascular spaces, have been observed in dogs treated with other members of this class. No CNS lesions have been observed after chronic treatment for up to 2 years with fluvastatin in the mouse (at doses up to 350 mg/kg/day), rat (up to 24 mg/kg/day), or dog (up to 16 mg/kg/day).

CARCINOGENESIS, MUTAGENESIS, AND IMPAIRMENT OF FERTILITY

A 2-year study was performed in rats at dose levels of 6, 9, and 18-24 (escalated after 1 year) mg/kg/day. These treatment levels represented plasma drug levels of approximately 9, 13, and 26-35 times the mean human plasma drug concentration after a 40 mg oral dose. A low incidence of forestomach squamous papillomas and 1 carcinoma of the forestomach at the 24 mg/kg/day dose level was considered to reflect the prolonged hyperplasia induced by direct contact exposure to fluvastatin sodium rather than to a systemic effect of the drug. In addition, an increased incidence of thyroid follicular cell neoplasm in male rats with fluvastatin sodium appears to be consistent with species specific findings from other HMG-CoA reductase inhibitors. In contrast to other HMG-CoA reductase inhibitors, no hepatic adenomas or carcinomas were observed.

The carcinogenicity study conducted in mice at dose levels of 0.3, 15 and 30 mg/kg/day revealed, as in rats, a statistically significant increase in forestomach squamous cell papillomas in males and females at 30 mg/kg/day and in females at 15 mg/kg/day. These treatment levels represented plasma drug levels of approximately 0.05, 2, and 7 times the mean human plasma drug concentration after a 40 mg oral dose.

No evidence of mutagenicity was observed *in vitro*, with or without rat liver metabolic activation, in the following studies: microbial mutagen tests using mutant strains of *Salmonella typhimurium* or *Escherichia coli*, malignant transformation assay in BALB/3T3 cells; unscheduled DNA synthesis in rat primary hepatocytes; chromosomal aberrations in V79 Chinese Hamster cells; HGPRT V79 Chinese Hamster cells. In addition, there was no evidence of mutagenicity *in vivo* in either a rat or mouse micronucleus test.

In a study in rats at dose levels for females of 0.6, 2 and 6 mg/kg/day and for males at 2, 10 and 20 mg/kg/day fluvastatin sodium had no adverse effects on the fertility or reproductive performance at any of the dose levels studied. A study in which female rats were dosed during the third trimester at 12 and 14 mg/kg/day resulted in maternal mortality at or near term and postpartum. In addition, fetal and neonatal lethality were apparent. No effects on the dam or fetus occurred at the low dose level of 2 mg/kg/day. A second study at levels of 2, 6, 12 and 24 mg/kg/day confirmed the findings in the first study. A modified Segment III study was performed at dose levels of 12 or 24 mg/kg/day with or without the presence of concurrent supplementation with mevalonic acid, a product of HMG-CoA reductase which is essential for cholesterol biosynthesis. The concurrent administration of mevalonic acid completely prevented the maternal and neonatal mortality. Therefore, the maternal and neonatal lethality observed with fluvastatin sodium reflect its exaggerated pharmacologic effect during pregnancy.

PREGNANCY CATEGORY X

See CONTRAINDICATIONS.

Fluvastatin sodium was not teratogenic in rats at doses up to 36 mg/kg daily or in rabbits at doses of up to 10 mg/kg/day. There are no data in pregnant women.

NURSING MOTHERS

Based on preclinical data, drug is present in breast milk in a 2:1 ratio (milk:plasma). Because of the potential for serious adverse reactions in nursing infants, nursing women should not take fluvastatin sodium (see CONTRAINDICATIONS.)

PEDIATRIC USE

Safety and effectiveness in individuals less than 18 years old have not been established. Treatment in patients less than 18 years of age is not recommended at this time.

GERIATRIC USE

The effect of age on the pharmacokinetics of fluvastatin sodium was evaluated. Results indicate that for the general patient population plasma concentrations of fluvastatin sodium do not vary either as a function of age or gender. (See CLINICAL PHARMACOLOGY, Pharmacokinetics and Metabolism.) Elderly patients (≥65 years of age) demonstrated a greater treatment response in respect to LDL-C, Total-C and LDL/HDL ratio than patients <65 years of age.

DRUG INTERACTIONS:

IMMUNOSUPPRESSIVE DRUGS, GEMFIBROZIL, NIACIN (NICOTINIC ACID), ERYTHROMYCIN

See WARNINGS, Skeletal Muscle.

Antipyrine: Administration of fluvastatin sodium does not influence the metabolism and excretion of antipyrine, either by induction or inhibition. Antipyrine is a model for drugs metabolized by the microsomal hepatic enzyme system; therefore, interactions with other drugs metabolized by this mechanism are not expected.

Niacin/Propranolol: Concomitant administration of fluvastatin sodium with niacin or propranolol has no effect on the bioavailability of fluvastatin sodium.

Cholestyramine: Administration of fluvastatin sodium concomitantly with, or up to 4 hours after cholestyramine, results in fluvastatin decreases of more than 50% for AUC and 50%-80% for C^{max}. However, administration of fluvastatin sodium 4 hours after cholestyramine resulted in a clinically significant additive effect compared with that achieved with either component drug.

Digoxin: In a crossover study involving 18 patients chronically receiving digoxin, a single 40 mg dose of fluvastatin had no effect on digoxin AUC, but had an 11% increase in digoxin $C^{max}$and small increase in digoxin urinary clearance. Patients taking digoxin should be monitored appropriately when fluvastatin therapy is initiated.

Cimetidine/Ranitidine/Omeprazole: Concomitant administration of fluvastatin sodium with cimetidine, ranitidine and omeprazole results in a significant increase in the fluvastatin C^{max} (43%, 70% and 50%, respectively) and AUC (24%-33%), with an 18%-23% decrease in plasma clearance.

Rifampicin: Administration of fluvastatin sodium to subjects pretreated with rifampicin results in significant reduction in C^{max} (59%) and AUC (51%), with a large increase (95%) in plasma clearance.

Warfarin: *In vitro* protein binding studies demonstrated no interaction at therapeutic concentrations.

Other Concomitant Therapy: Although specific interaction studies were not performed, in clinical studies, fluvastatin sodium was used concomitantly with angiotensin-converting enzyme (ACE) inhibitors, beta blockers, calcium-channel blockers, diuretics and nonsteroidal antiinflammatory drugs (NSAIDs) without evidence of clinically significant adverse interactions.

ENDOCRINE FUNCTION

HMG-CoA reductase inhibitors interfere with cholesterol synthesis and lower circulating cholesterol levels and, as such, might theoretically blunt adrenal or gonadal steroid hormone production.

DRUG INTERACTIONS: *(cont'd)*

Fluvastatin exhibited no effect upon non-stimulated cortisol levels and demonstrated no effect upon thyroid metabolism as assessed by TSH. Small declines in total testosterone have been noted in treated groups, but no commensurate elevation in LH occurred, suggesting that the observation was not due to a direct effect upon testosterone production. No effect upon FSH in males was noted. Due to the limited number of premenopausal females studied to date, no conclusions regarding the effect of fluvastatin upon female sex hormones may be made.

Two investigational clinical studies in patients receiving fluvastatin at doses up to 80 mg daily (twice the recommended dose) for periods of 24-28 weeks demonstrated no effect of treatment upon the adrenal response to ACTH stimulation. Although the mean total testosterone response was significantly reduced ($p<0.05$) relative to baseline in the 80 mg group, it was not significant in comparison to the changes noted in groups receiving either 40 mg of fluvastatin or placebo.

Patients treated with fluvastatin sodium who develop clinical evidence of endocrine dysfunction should be evaluated appropriately. Caution should be exercised if an HMG-CoA reductase inhibitor or other agent used to lower cholesterol levels is administered to patients receiving other drugs (e.g. ketoconazole, spironolactone, or cimetidine) that may decrease the levels of endogenous steroid hormones.

ADVERSE REACTIONS:

In the controlled clinical studies and their open extensions, fluvastatin sodium was discontinued in 1.0% of 1881 patients due to adverse experiences (mean exposure approximately 14 months ranging in duration from 1->24 months). This results in an exposure adjusted rate of 0.9% per patient-year in fluvastatin patients compared to an incidence of 1.3% in placebo patients. Fluvastatin sodium has been studied in more than 2200 patients. Adverse reactions have usually been mild and similar in incidence to placebo.

Adverse experiences occurring with a frequency >2% regardless of causality include the following:

TABLE 3 Fluvastatin Sodium, Adverse Reactions

Adverse Event	Lescol (fluvastatin sodium) (%) (N=620)	Placebo (%) (N=411)
Integumentary		
Rash	2.7	3.6
Musculoskeletal		
Back Pain	6.1	8.5
Arthropathy	4.0	3.2
Exercise-Related Muscle Pain	3.4	2.4
Respiratory		
Upper Respiratory Tract Infection	11.6	15.3
Pharyngitis	4.5	4.9
Rhinitis	4.5	6.1
Sinusitis	2.7	1.5
Coughing	2.6	3.2
Bronchitis	2.3	1.2
Gastrointestinal		
Dyspepsia	8.1	4.9
Diarrhea	6.0	5.6
Abdominal Pain	5.5	4.1
Nausea	3.2	2.4
Constipation	2.6	4.9
Flatulence	2.6	4.1
Misc. Tooth Disorder	2.1	1.9
Central Nervous System		
Dizziness	2.6	2.9
Psychiatric Disorders		
Insomnia	2.6	1.7
Miscellaneous		
Headache	8.7	8.8
Influenza-Like Symptoms	5.3	5.4
Accidental Trauma	5.3	5.1
Fatigue	3.5	3.4
Allergy	2.6	3.6

The following effects have been reported with drugs in this class. Not all the effects listed below have necessarily been associated with fluvastatin sodium therapy.

Skeletal: myopathy, rhabdomyolysis, arthralgias.

Neurological: dysfunction of certain cranial nerves (including alteration of taste, impairment of extra-ocular movement, facial paresis), tremor, vertigo, memory loss, paresthesia, peripheral neuropathy, peripheral nerve palsy, anxiety, insomnia, depression.

Hypersensitivity Reactions: An apparent hypersensitivity syndrome has been reported rarely which has included one or more of the following features: anaphylaxis, angioedema, lupus erythematosus-like syndrome, polymyalgia rheumatica, vasculitis, purpura, thrombocytopenia, leukopenia, hemolytic anemia, positive ANA, ESR increase, eosinophilia, arthritis, arthralgia, urticaria, asthenia, photosensitivity, fever, chills, flushing, malaise, dyspnea, toxic epidermal necrolysis, erythema multiforme, including Stevens-Johnson syndrome.

Gastrointestinal: pancreatitis, hepatis, including chronic active hepatitis, cholestatic jaundice, fatty change in liver, and, rarely, cirrhosis, fulminant hepatic necrosis, and hepatoma; anorexia, vomiting.

Skin: alopecia, pruritus. A variety of skin changes (*e.g.,* nodules, discoloration, dryness of skin/mucous membranes, changes to hair/nails) have been reported.

Reproductive: gynecomastia, loss of libido, erectile dysfunction.

Eye: progression of cataracts (lens opacities), ophthalmoplegia.

Laboratory Abnormalities: elevated transaminases, alkaline phosphatase, and bilirubin; thyroid function abnormalities.

CONCOMITANT THERAPY

Fluvastatin sodium has been administered concurrently with cholestyramine and nicotinic acid. No adverse reactions unique to the combination or in addition to those previously reported for this class of drugs alone have been reported. Myopathy and rhabdomyolysis (with or without acute renal failure) have been reported when another HMG-CoA reductase inhibitor was used in combination with immunosuppressive drugs, gemfibrozil, erythromycin, or lipid-lowering doses of nicotinic acid. Concomitant therapy with HMG-CoA reductase inhibitors and these agents is generally not recommended (see WARNINGS, Skeletal Muscle.)

OVERDOSAGE:

The approximate oral LD_{50} is greater than 2 g/kg in mice and greater than 0.7 g/kg in rats.

The maximum single oral dose received by healthy volunteers was 60 mg. No clinically significant adverse experiences were seen at this dose. There has been a single report of 2 children, one 2 years old and the other 3 years of age, either of whom may have possibly ingested fluvastatin sodium. The maximum amount of fluvastatin sodium that could have been ingested was 80 mg (4 x 20 mg capsules). Vomiting was induced by ipecac in both children and no capsules were noted in their emesis. Neither child experienced any adverse symptoms and both recovered from the incident without problems.

No specific information on the treatment of overdosage can be recommended. Should an accidental overdose occur, treat symptomatically and institute supportive measures as required. The dialyzability of fluvastatin sodium and of its metabolites in humans is not known at present.

DOSAGE AND ADMINISTRATION:

The patient should be placed on a standard cholesterol-lowering diet before receiving fluvastatin sodium and should continue on this diet during treatment with fluvastatin sodium. (See NCEP Treatment Guidelines for details on dietary therapy.)

The recommended starting dose for the majority of patients is 20 mg once daily at bedtime. The recommended dosing range is 20-40 mg/day as a single dose in the evening. Splitting the 40 mg QPM dose into a BID regimen provides a modest improvement in LDL-C response. Fluvastatin sodium may be taken without regard to meals, since there are no apparent differences in the lipid-lowering effects of fluvastatin sodium administered with the evening meal or 4 hours after the evening meal. Since the maximal reductions in LDL-C of a given dose are seen within 4 weeks, periodic lipid determinations should be performed during this time with dosage adjusted according to the patient's response to therapy and established treatment guidelines. The therapeutic effect of fluvastatin sodium is maintained with prolonged administration.

CONCOMITANT THERAPY

Lipid-lowering effects on total cholesterol and LDL cholesterol are additive when fluvastatin sodium is combined with a bile-acid binding resin or niacin. When administering a bile-acid resin (*e.g.,* cholestyramine) and fluvastatin sodium, fluvastatin sodium should be administered at bedtime, at least 2 hours following the resin to avoid a significant interaction due to drug binding to resin. (See also ADVERSE REACTIONS, Concomitant Therapy).

DOSAGE IN PATIENTS WITH RENAL INSUFFICIENCY

Since fluvastatin sodium is cleared hepatically with less than 5% of the administered dose excreted into the urine, dose adjustments for mild to moderate renal impairment are not necessary. Caution should be exercised with severe impairment.

PATIENT INFORMATION:

Fluvastatin sodium is used to treat high cholesterol. This drug is called an HMG Co-A reductase inhibitor because it inhibits an enzyme in your body that makes cholesterol. It is important to continue with dietary modification and exercise programs. This drug should not be taken by those with liver disease. It should not be taken by pregnant or nursing women. If pregnancy results while taking this medication, it may be necessary to discontinue the medication temporarily. Please consult your physician. Because this drug works in the liver, you will be asked to have your liver function assessed periodically. If you experience any muscle pain, tenderness, weakness, or fever please inform your physician. This drug also has several drug interactions, please inform your physician or pharmacist of all medications, prescription and over-the-counter, you are taking.

HOW SUPPLIED:

20 mg capsules: Brown and light brown imprinted twice with "S" (surrounded by a triangle) and "20" on one half and "LESCOL" and the Lescol© (fluvastatin sodium) logo twice on the other half of the capsule.

40 mg capsules: Brown and gold imprinted twice with "S" (surrounded by a triangle) and "40" on one half and "LESCOL" and the Lescol© (fluvastatin sodium) logo twice on the other half of the capsule.

Store and Dispense: Below 86°F (30°C) in a tight container. Protect from light.

(Sandoz, 12/93, 30153901))

HOW SUPPLIED - EQUIVALENTS NOT AVAILABLE:

Capsule, Gelatin - Oral - 20 mg

30's	$34.50	LESCOL, Novartis	00078-0176-15
100's	$114.90	LESCOL, Novartis	00078-0176-05

Capsule, Gelatin - Oral - 40 mg

30's	$38.58	LESCOL, Novartis	00078-0234-15
100's	$128.46	LESCOL, Novartis	00078-0234-05

FLUVOXAMINE MALEATE *(003080)*

CATEGORIES: Antidepressants; Central Nervous System Agents; Obsessive-Compulsive Disorder; Psychotherapeutic Agents; Selective Serotonin Reuptake Inhibitors; Depression*; Pregnancy Category C; FDA Class 1S ("Standard Review"); FDA Approved 1994 Dec

* Indication not approved by the FDA

BRAND NAMES: *Dumirox*; *Dumyrox*; *Faverin* (England); *Favoxil*; *Fevarin* (Germany); Floxyfral; **Luvox**; *Maveral*

(International brand names outside U.S. in italics)

FORMULARIES: Medi-Cal

COST OF THERAPY: $139.06 (Obsessive-Compulsive Disorder; Tablet; 50 mg; 1/day; 70 days)

PRIMARY ICD9: 300.3 (Obsessive-Compusive Disorders)

DESCRIPTION:

Fluvoxamine maleate is a selective serotonin (5-HT) reuptake inhibitor (SSRI) belonging to a new chemical series, the 2-aminoethyl oxime ethers of aralkylketones. It is chemically unrelated to other SSRIs and clomipramine. It is chemically designated as 5-methoxy-4'-(trifluoromethyl)valerophenone-(E)-O-(2-aminoethyl)oxime maleate (1:1) and has the empirical formula $C_{15}H_{21}O_2N_2F_3{\cdot}C_4H_4O_4$. Its molecular weight is 434.4.

Fluvoxamine maleate is a white or off white, odorless, crystalline powder which is sparingly soluble in water, freely soluble in ethanol and chloroform and practically insoluble in diethyl ether.

DESCRIPTION: *(cont'd)*

Luvox (fluvoxamine maleate) tablets are available in 50 mg and 100 mg strengths for oral administration. In addition to the active ingredient, fluvoxamine maleate, each tablet contains the following inactive ingredients: carnauba wax, hydroxypropyl methylcellulose, mannitol, polyethylene glycol, polysorbate 80, pregelatinized starch, silicon dioxide, sodium stearyl fumarate, starch, synthetic iron oxides, and titanium dioxide.

CLINICAL PHARMACOLOGY:

PHARMACODYNAMICS

The mechanism of action of fluvoxamine maleate in Obsessive Compulsive Disorder is presumed to be linked to its specific serotonin reuptake inhibition in brain neurons. In preclinical studies, it was found that fluvoxamine inhibited neuronal uptake of serotonin.

In *in vitro* studies fluvoxamine maleate had no significant affinity for histaminergic, alpha or beta adrenergic, muscarinic, or dopaminergic receptors. Antagonism of some of these receptors is thought to be associated with various sedative, cardiovascular, anticholinergic, and extrapyramidal effects of some psychotic drugs.

PHARMACOKINETICS

Bioavailability: The absolute bioavailability of fluvoxamine maleate is 53%. Oral bioavailability is not significantly affected by food.

In a dose proportionality study involving fluvoxamine maleate at 100, 200 and 300 mg/day for 10 consecutive days in 30 normal volunteers, steady state was achieved after about a week of dosing. Maximum plasma concentrations at steady state occurred within 3-8 hours of dosing and reached concentrations averaging 88, 283 and 546 ng/ml, respectively. Thus, fluvoxamine had nonlinear pharmacokinetics over this dose range, i.e., higher doses of fluvoxamine maleate produced disproportionately higher concentrations than predicted from the lower dose.

Distribution/Protein Binding: The mean apparent volume of distribution for fluvoxamine is approximately 25 l/kg, suggesting extensive tissue distribution.

Approximately 80% of fluvoxamine is bound to plasma protein, mostly albumin, over a concentration range of 20 to 2000 ng/ml.

Metabolism: Fluvoxamine maleate is extensively metabolized by the liver; the main metabolic routes are oxidative demethylation and deamination. Nine metabolites were identified following a 5 mg radiolabelled dose of fluvoxamine maleate, constituting approximately 85% of the urinary excretion products of fluvoxamine. The main human metabolite was fluvoxamine acid which, together with its N- acetylated analog, accounted for about 60% of the urinary excretion products. A third metabolite, fluvoxethanol, formed by oxidative deamination, accounted for about 10%. Fluvoxamine acid and fluvoxethanol were tested in an *in vitro* assay of serotonin and norepinephrine reuptake inhibition in rats; they were inactive except for a weak effect of the former metabolite on inhibition of serotonin uptake (1-2 orders of magnitude less potent than the parent compound). Approximately 2% of fluvoxamine was excreted in urine unchanged. (See DRUG INTERACTIONS)

Elimination: Following a ^{14}C-labelled oral dose of fluvoxamine maleate (5 mg), an average of 94% of drug-related products was recovered in the urine within 71 hours.

The mean plasma half-life of fluvoxamine at steady state after multiple oral doses of 100 mg/day in healthy, young volunteers was 15.6 hours.

Elderly Subjects: In a study of fluvoxamine maleate at 50 and 100 mg comparing elderly (aged 66-73) and young subjects (aged 19-35), mean maximum plasma concentrations in the elderly were 40% higher. The multiple dose elimination half-life of fluvoxamine was 17.4 and 25.9 hours in the elderly compared to 13.6 and 15.6 hours in the young subjects at steady state for 50 and 100 mg doses, respectively.

In elderly patients, the clearance of fluvoxamine was reduced by about 50% and, therefore, fluvoxamine maleate should be slowly titrated during initiation of therapy.

Hepatic and Renal Disease: A cross study comparison (healthy subjects vs. patients with hepatic dysfunction) suggested a 30% decrease in fluvoxamine clearance in association with hepatic dysfunction. The mean minimum plasma concentrations in renally impaired patients (creatinine clearance of 5 to 45 ml/min) after 4 and 6 weeks of treatment (50 mg bid, N=13) were comparable to each other, suggesting no accumulation of fluvoxamine in these patients. See PRECAUTIONS, Use in Patients with Concomitant Illness,

CLINICAL STUDIES:

The effectiveness of fluvoxamine maleate for the treatment of Obsessive Compulsive Disorder (OCD) was demonstrated in two 10-week multicenter, parallel group studies of adult outpatients. Patients in these trials were titrated to a total daily fluvoxamine maleate dose of 150 mg/day over the first two weeks of the trial, following which the dose was adjusted within a range of 100-300 mg/day (on a bid schedule), on the basis of response and tolerance. Patients in these studies had moderate to severe OCD (DSM-III-R), with mean baseline ratings on the Yale-Brown Obsessive Compulsive Scale (Y-BOCS), total score of 23. Patients receiving fluvoxamine maleate experienced mean reductions of approximately 4 to 5 units on the Y-BOCS total score, compared to a 2 unit reduction for placebo patients.

TABLE 1 provides the outcome classification by treatment group on the Global Improvement item of the Clinical Global Impressions (CGI) scale for both studies combined.

TABLE 1 Outcome Classification (%) on CGI-Global Improvemnet Item for Completers in Pool of Two OCD Studies

Outcome Classification	Fluvoxamine (N = 120)	Placebo (N = 134)
Worse	4%	6%
No Change	31%	51%
Minimally Improved	22%	32%
Much Improved	30%	10%
Very Much Improved	13%	2%

Exploratory analyses for age and gender effects on outcomes did not suggest any differential responsiveness on the basis of age or sex.

INDICATIONS AND USAGE:

Fluvoxamine maleate are indicated for the treatment of obsessions and compulsions in patients with Obsessive Compulsive Disorder (OCD), as defined in the DSM-III-R. The obsessions or compulsions cause marked distress, are time-consuming, or significantly interfere with social or occupational functioning.

The efficacy of fluvoxamine maleate was established in two 10-week trials with obsessive compulsive outpatients with the diagnosis of Obsessive Compulsive Disorder as defined in DSM-III-R. (See CLINICAL STUDIES.)

Obsessive Compulsive Disorder is characterized by recurrent and persistent ideas, thoughts, impulses or images (obsessions) that are ego- dystonic and/or repetitive, purposeful, and intentional behaviors (compulsions) that are recognized by the person as excessive or unreasonable.

INDICATIONS AND USAGE: *(cont'd)*

The effectiveness of fluvoxamine maleate for long-term use, i.e., for more than 10 weeks, has not been systematically evaluated in placebo-controlled trials. Therefore, the physician who elects to use fluvoxamine maleate for extended periods should periodically re-evaluate the long-term usefulness of the drug for the individual patient. (See DOSAGE AND ADMINISTRATION.)

CONTRAINDICATIONS:

Co-administration of terfenadine, astemizole, or cisapride with fluvoxamine maleate is contraindicated (see WARNINGS and PRECAUTIONS).

Fluvoxamine maleate are contraindicated in patients with a history of hypersensitivity to fluvoxamine maleate.

WARNINGS:

POTENTIAL FOR INTERACTION WITH MONOAMINE OXIDASE INHIBITORS

In patients receiving another serotonin reuptake inhibitor drug in combination with monoamine oxidase inhibitors (MAOI), there have been reports of serious, sometimes fatal, reactions including hyperthermia, rigidity, myoclonus, autonomic instability with possible rapid fluctuations of vital signs, and mental status changes that include extreme agitation progressing to delirium and coma. These reactions have also been reported in patients who have discontinued that drug and have been started on a MAOI. Some cases presented with features resembling neuroleptic malignant syndrome. Therefore, it is recommended that fluvoxamine maleate not be used in combination with a MAOI, or within 14 days of discontinuing treatment with a MAOI. After stopping fluvoxamine maleate, at least 2 weeks should be allowed before starting a MAOI.

OTHER POTENTIALLY IMPORTANT DRUG INTERACTIONS

See DRUG INTERACTIONS

Benzodiazepines: Benzodiazepines metabolized by hepatic oxidation (*e.g.*, alprazolam, midazolam, triazolam, etc.) should be used with caution because the clearance of these drugs is likely to be reduced by fluvoxamine. The clearance of benzodiazepines metabolized by glucuronidation (*e.g.*, lorazepam, oxazepam, temazepam) is unlikely to be affected by fluvoxamine.

Alprazolam: When fluvoxamine maleate (100 mg qd) and alprazolam (1 mg qid) were co-administered to steady state, plasma concentrations and other pharmacokinetic parameters (AUC, C_{max}, $T_{1/2}$) of alprazolam were approximately twice those observed when alprazolam was administered alone; oral clearance was reduced by about 50%. The elevated plasma alprazolam concentrations resulted in decreased psychomotor performance and memory. This interaction, which has not been investigated using higher doses of fluvoxamine, may be more pronounced if a 300 mg daily dose is co-administered, particularly since fluvoxamine exhibits non-linear pharmacokinetics over the dosage range 100-300 mg. If alprazolam is co-administered with fluvoxamine maleate, the initial alprazolam dosage should be at least halved and titration to the lowest effective dose is recommended. No dosage adjustment is required for fluvoxamine maleate.

Diazepam: The co-administration of fluvoxamine maleate and diazepam is generally not advisable. Because fluvoxamine reduces the clearance of both diazepam and its active metabolite, N-desmethyldiazepam, there is a strong likelihood of substantial accumulation of both species during chronic co-administration.

Evidence supporting the conclusion that is inadvisable to co-administer fluvoxamine and diazepam is derived from a study in which healthy volunteers taking 150 mg/day of fluvoxamine were administered a single oral dose of 10 mg of diazepam. In these subjects (n=8), the clearance of diazepam was reduced 65% and that of N-desmethyldiazepam to a level that was too low to measure over the course of the 2 week long study.

It is likely that this experience significantly underestimates the degree of accumulation that might occur with repeated diazepam administration. Moreover, as noted with alprazolam, the effect of fluvoxamine may even be more pronounced when it is administered at higher doses. Accordingly, diazepam and fluvoxamine should not ordinarily be co-administered.

POTENTIAL TERFENADINE, ASTEMIZOLE, AND CISAPRIDE INTERACTIONS

Terfenadine, astemizole, and cisapride are all metabolized by the cytochrome P450IIIA4 isozyme, and it has been demonstrated that ketoconazole, a potent inhibitor of IIIA4, blocks the metabolism of these drugs, resulting in increased plasma concentrations of parent drug. Increased plasma concentrations of terfenadine, astemizole, and cisapride cause QT prolongation and have been associated with torsades de pointes- type ventricular tachycardia, sometimes fatal. As noted below, a substantial pharmacokinetic interaction has been observed for fluvoxamine in combination with alprazolam, a drug that is known to be metabolized by the IIIA4 isozyme. Although it has not been definitively demonstrated that fluvoxamine is a potent IIIA4 inhibitor, it is likely to be, given the substantial interaction of fluvoxamine with alprazolam. Consequently, it is recommended that fluvoxamine not be used in combination with either terfenadine, astemizole, or cisapride (see CONTRAINDICATIONS and PRECAUTIONS).

Theophylline: The effect of steady-state fluvoxamine (50 mg bid) on the pharmacokinetics of a single dose of theophylline (375 mg as 442 mg aminophylline) was evaluated in 12 healthy non-smoking, male volunteers. The clearance of theophylline was decreased approximately 3-fold. Therefore, if theophylline is co-administered with fluvoxamine maleate, its dose should be reduced to one third of the usual daily maintenance dose and plasma concentrations of theophylline should be monitored. No dosage adjustment is required for fluvoxamine maleate.

Warfarin: When fluvoxamine maleate (50 mg tid) was administered concomitantly with warfarin for two weeks, warfarin plasma concentrations increased by 98% and prothrombin times were prolonged. Thus patients receiving oral anticoagulants and fluvoxamine maleate should have their prothrombin time monitored and their anticoagulant dose adjusted accordingly. No dosage adjustment is required for fluvoxamine maleate.

PRECAUTIONS:

GENERAL

Activation of Mania/Hypomania: During premarketing studies involving primarily depressed patients, hypomania or mania occurred in approximately 1% of patients treated with fluvoxamine. Activation of mania/hypomania has also been reported in a small proportion of patients with major affective disorder who were treated with other marketed antidepressants. As with all antidepressants, fluvoxamine maleate should be used cautiously in patients with a history of mania.

Seizures: During premarketing studies, seizures were reported in 0.2% of fluvoxamine-treated patients. Fluvoxamine maleate should be used cautiously in patients with a history of seizures. It should be discontinued in any patient who develops seizures.

Suicide: The possibility of a suicide attempt is inherent in patients with depressive symptoms, whether these occur in primary depression or in association with another primary disorder such as OCD. Close supervision of high risk patients should accompany initial drug therapy. Prescriptions for fluvoxamine maleate should be written for the smallest quantity of tablets consistent with good patient management in order to reduce the risk of overdose.

PRECAUTIONS: *(cont'd)*

Use in Patients with Concomitant Illness: Closely monitored clinical experience with fluvoxamine maleate in patients with concomitant systemic illness is limited. Caution is advised in administering fluvoxamine maleate to patients who diseases or conditions that could affect hemodynamic responses or metabolism.

Fluvoxamine maleate have not been evaluated or used to any appreciable extent in patients with a recent history of myocardial infarction or unstable heart disease. Patients with these diagnoses were systematically excluded from many clinical studies during the product's premarketing testing. Evaluation of the electrocardiograms for patients with depression or OCD who participated in premarketing studies revealed no differences between fluvoxamine and placebo in the emergence of clinically important ECG changes.

In patients with liver dysfunction, fluvoxamine clearance was decreased by approximately 30%. Fluvoxamine maleate should be slowly titrated in patients with liver dysfunction during the initiation of treatment.

INFORMATION FOR THE PATIENT

Physicians are advised to discuss the following issues with patients for whom they prescribe fluvoxamine maleate:

Interference with Cognitive or Motor Performance: Since any psychoactive drug may impair judgement, thinking, or motor skills, patients should be cautioned about operating hazardous machinery, including automobiles, until they are certain that fluvoxamine maleate therapy does not adversely affect their ability to engage in such activities.

Pregnancy: Patients should be advised to notify their physicians if they become pregnant or intend to become pregnant during therapy with fluvoxamine maleate.

Nursing: Patients receiving fluvoxamine maleate should be advised to notify their physicians if they are breast feeding an infant.(See PRECAUTIONS, Nursing Mothers)

Concomitant Medication: Patients should be advised to notify their physicians if they are taking, or plan to take, any prescription or over-the-counter drugs, since there is a potential for clinically important interactions with fluvoxamine maleate.

Alcohol: As with other psychotropic medications, patients should be advised to avoid alcohol while taking fluvoxamine maleate.

Allergic Reactions: Patients should be advised to notify their physicians if they develop a rash, hives, or a related allergic phenomenon during therapy with fluvoxamine maleate.

LABORATORY TESTS

There are no specific laboratory tests recommended.

CARCINOGENESIS, MUTAGENESIS, AND IMPAIRMENT OF FERTILITY

Carcinogenesis: There is no evidence of carcinogenicity, mutagenicity or impairment of fertility with fluvoxamine maleate.

There was no evidence of carcinogenicity in rats treated orally with fluvoxamine maleate for 30 months or hamsters treated orally with fluvoxamine maleate for 20 (females) or 26 (males) months. The daily doses in the high dose groups in these studies were increased over the course of the study from a minimum of 160 mg/kg to a maximum of 240 mg/kg in rats, and from a minimum of 135 mg/kg to a maximum of 240 mg/kg in hamsters. The maximum dose of 240 mg/kg is approximately 6 times the maximum human daily dose on a mg/m^2 basis.

Mutagenesis: No evidence of mutagenic potential was observed in a mouse micronucleus test, an *in vitro* chromosome aberration test, or the Ames microbial mutagen test with or without metabolic activation.

Impairment of Fertility: In fertility studies of male and female rats, up to 80 mg/kg/day orally of fluvoxamine maleate (approximately 2 times the maximum human daily dose on a mg/m^{2}basis) had no effect on mating performance, duration of gestation, or pregnancy rate.

Pregnancy, Teratogenic Effects, Pregnancy Category C: In teratology studies in rats and rabbits, daily oral doses of fluvoxamine maleate of up to 80 and 40 mg/kg, respectively (approximately 2 times the maximum human daily dose on a mg/m^2 basis) caused no fetal malformations. However, in other reproduction studies in which pregnant rats were dosed through weaning there was (1) an increase in pup mortality at birth (seen at 80 mg/kg and above but not at 20 mg/kg), and (2) decreases in postnatal pup weights (seen at 160 but not at 80 mg/kg) and survival (seen at all doses; lowest dose tested = 5 mg/kg). (Doses of 5, 20, 80, and 160 mg/kg are approximately 0.1, 0.5, 2, and 4 times the maximum human daily dose on a mg/m^2 basis.) While the results of a cross-fostering study implied that at least some of these results likely occurred secondarily to maternal toxicity, the role of a direct drug effect on the fetuses or pups could not be ruled out. There are no adequate and well-controlled studies in pregnant women. Fluvoxamine maleate should be used during pregnancy only if the potential benefit justifies the potential risk to the fetus.

Labor and Delivery: The effect of fluvoxamine on labor and delivery in humans in unknown.

Nursing Mothers: As for many other drugs, fluvoxamine is secreted in human breast milk. The decision of whether to discontinue nursing or to discontinue the drug should take into account the potential for serious adverse effects from exposure to fluvoxamine in the nursing infant as well as the potential benefits of fluvoxamine maleate therapy to the mother.

Pediatric Use: Safety and effectiveness of fluvoxamine maleate in individuals below 18 years of age have not been established.

Geriatric Use: Approximately 230 patients participating in controlled premarketing studies with fluvoxamine maleate were 65 years of age or over. No overall differences in safety were observed between these patients and younger patients. Other reported clinical experience has not identified differences in response between the elderly and younger patients. However, the clearance of fluvoxamine is decreased by about 50% in elderly compared to younger patients (see Pharmacokinetics under CLINICAL PHARMACOLOGY, and greater sensitivity of some older individuals also cannot be ruled out. Consequently, fluvoxamine maleate should be slowly titrated during initiation of therapy.

DRUG INTERACTIONS:

Potential Interactions with Drugs that Inhibit or are Metabolized by Cytochrome P450 Isozymes: Multiple hepatic cytochrome P450 (CYP450) enzymes are involved in the oxidative biotransformation of a large number of structurally different drugs and endogenous compounds. The available knowledge concerning the relationship of fluvoxamine and the CYP450 enzyme system has been obtained mostly from pharmacokinetic interaction studies conducted in healthy volunteers, but some preliminary *in vitro* data are also available. Based on a finding of substantial interactions of fluvoxamine with certain of these drugs (seeWARNINGS for details) and limited *in vitro* data for the IIIA4 isozyme, it appears that fluvoxamine inhibits the following isozymes that are known to be involved in the metabolism of the listed drugs found in TABLE 2.

TABLE 2

IA2	IIC9	IIIA4
Warfarin	Warfarin	Alprazolam
Theophylline		
Propranolol		

DRUG INTERACTIONS: *(cont'd)*

In vitro data suggest that fluvoxamine is a relatively weak inhibitor of the IID6 isozyme.

None of the drugs studied for drug interactions significantly affected the pharmacokinetics of fluvoxamine. However, the metabolism of fluvoxamine has not been fully characterized and the effects of potent inhibitors of IID6, such as quinidine, or of IIIA4 such as ketoconazole, on fluvoxamine metabolism have not been studied.

A clinically significant fluvoxamine interaction is possible with drugs having a narrow therapeutic ratio such as terfenadine, astemizole, or cisapride, warfarin, theophylline, certain benzodiazepines and phenytoin. If fluvoxamine maleate are to be administered together with a drug that is eliminated via oxidative metabolism and has a narrow therapeutic window, plasma levels and/or pharmacodynamic effects of the latter drug should be monitored closely, at least until steady-state conditions are reached (See CONTRAINDICATIONS and WARNINGS).

CNS ACTIVE DRUGS

Monoamine Oxidase Inhibitors: See WARNINGS

Alprazolam: See WARNINGS.

Diazepam: See WARNINGS.

Lorazepam: A study of multiple doses of fluvoxamine maleate (50 mg 2 × daily) in healthy male volunteers (N=12) and a single dose of lorazepam (4 mg single dose) indicated no significant pharmacokinetic interaction. On average, both lorazepam alone and lorazepam with fluvoxamine produced substantial decrements in cognitive functioning; however, the co-administration of fluvoxamine and lorazepam did not produce larger mean decrements compared to lorazepam alone.

Lithium: As with other serotonergic drugs, lithium may enhance the serotonergic effects of fluvoxamine and, therefore, the combination should be used with caution. Seizures have been reported with the co-administration of fluvoxamine maleate and lithium.

Tryptophan: Tryptophan may enhance the serotonergic effects of fluvoxamine, and the combination should, therefore, be used with caution. Severe vomiting has been reported with the co-administration of fluvoxamine maleate and tryptophan.

Clozapine: Elevated serum levels of clozapine have been reported in patients taking fluvoxamine maleate and clozapine. Since clozapine related seizures and orthostatic hypotension appear to be dose related, the risk of these adverse events may be higher when fluvoxamine and clozapine are co-administered. Patients should be closely monitored when fluvoxamine maleate and clozapine are used concurrently.

Alcohol: Studies involving single 40 g doses of ethanol (oral administration in one study and intravenous in the other) and multiple dosing with fluvoxamine maleate (50 mg bid) revealed no effect of either drug on the pharmacokinetics or pharmacodynamics of the other.

Tricyclic Antidepressants (TCAs): Significantly increased plasma TCA levels have been reported with the co-administration of fluvoxamine maleate and amitriptyline, clomipramine or imipramine. Caution is indicated with the co-administration of fluvoxamine maleate and TCAs.

Carbamazepine: Elevated carbamazepine levels and symptoms of toxicity have been reported with the co-administration of fluvoxamine maleate and carbamazepine.

Methadone: Significantly increased methadone (plasma level:dose) ratios have been reported when fluvoxamine maleate was administered to patients receiving maintenance methadone treatment, with symptoms of opioid intoxication in one patient. Opioid withdrawal symptoms were reported following fluvoxamine maleate discontinuation in another patient.

OTHER DRUGS

Theophylline: See WARNINGS

Propranolol and Other Beta-Blockers: Co-administration of fluvoxamine maleate 100 mg per day and propranolol 160 mg per day in normal volunteers resulted in a mean five-fold increase (range 2 to 17) in minimum propranolol plasma concentrations. In this study, there was a slight potentiation of the propranolol-induced reduction in heart rate and reduction in the exercise diastolic pressure.

One case of bradycardia and hypotension and a second case of orthostatic hypotension have been reported with the co-administration of fluvoxamine and metoprolol.

If propranolol or metoprolol is co-administered with fluvoxamine maleate, a reduction in the initial beta-blocker dose and more cautious dose titration is recommended. No dosage adjustment is required for fluvoxamine maleate.

Co-administration of fluvoxamine maleate 100 mg per day with atenolol 100 mg per day (N=6) did not affect the plasma concentrations of atenolol. Unlike propranolol and metoprolol which undergo hepatic metabolism, atenolol is eliminated primarily by renal excretion.

Warfarin: See WARNINGS

Digoxin: Administration of fluvoxamine maleate 100 mg daily for 18 days (N=8) did not significantly affect the pharmacokinetics of a 1.25 mg single intravenous dose of digoxin.

Diltiazem: Bradycardia has been reported with the co-administration of fluvoxamine maleate and diltiazem.

Effects of Smoking on Fluvoxamine Metabolism: Smokers had a 25% increase in the metabolism of fluvoxamine compared to nonsmokers.

Electroconvulsive Therapy (ECT): There are no clinical studies establishing the benefits or risks of combined use of ECT and fluvoxamine maleate.

ADVERSE REACTIONS:

Associated with Discontinuation of Treatment: Of the 1087 OCD and depressed patients treated with fluvoxamine maleate in controlled clinical trials conducted in North America, 22% discontinued treatment due to an adverse event. The most common events (≥ 1%) associated with discontinuation and considered to be drug related (*i.e.,* those events associated with dropout at a rate at least twice that of placebo) included those listed in TABLE 3.

INCIDENCE IN CONTROLLED TRIALS

Commonly Observed Adverse Events in Controlled Clinical Trials: Fluvoxamine maleate have been studied in controlled trials of OCD (N=320) and depression (N=1350). In general, adverse event rates were similar in the two data sets. The most commonly observed adverse events associated with the use of fluvoxamine maleate and likely to be drug-related (incidence of 5% or greater and at least twice that for placebo) derived from TABLE 4 were: *somnolence, insomnia, nervousness, tremor, nausea, dyspepsia, anorexia, vomiting, abnormal ejaculation, asthenia, and sweating.*In a pool of two studies involving only patients with OCD, the following additional events were identified using the above rule: *dry mouth, decreased libido, urinary frequency, anorgasmia, rhinitis and taste perversion.*

Adverse Events Occurring at an Incidence of 1%: TABLE 4 enumerates adverse events that occurred at a frequency of 1% or more, and were more frequent than in the placebo group, among patients treated with fluvoxamine maleate in two short-term placebo controlled OCD trials (10 week) and depression trials (6 week) in which patients were dosed in a range of generally 100 to 300 mg/day. This table shows the percentage of patients in each group who had at least one occurrence of an event at some time during their treatment. Reported adverse events were classified using a standard COSTART-based Dictionary terminology.

ADVERSE REACTIONS: *(cont'd)*

TABLE 3 Adverse Events Associated with Discontinuation of Treatment in OCD and Depression Populations

BODY SYSTEM/ ADVERSE EVENT	PERCENTAGE OF PATIENTS FLUVOXAMINE	PLACEBO
BODY AS A WHOLE		
Headache	3%	1%
Asthenia	2%	< 1%
Abdominal Pain	1%	0%
DIGESTIVE		
Nausea	9%	1%
Diarrhea	1%	< 1%
Vomiting	2%	< 1%
Anorexia	1%	< 1%
Dyspepsia	1%	< 1%
NERVOUS SYSTEM		
Insomnia	4%	1%
Somnolence	4%	< 1%
Nervousness	2%	< 1%
Agitation	2%	< 1%
Dizziness	2%	< 1%
Anxiety	1%	< 1%
Dry Mouth	1%	< 1%

The prescriber should be aware that these figures cannot be used to predict the incidence of side effects in the course of usual medical practice where patient characteristics and other factors may differ from those that prevailed in the clinical trials. Similarly, the cited frequencies cannot be compared with figures obtained from other clinical investigations involving different treatments, uses, and investigators. The cited figures, however, do provide the prescribing physician with some basis for estimating the relative contribution of drug and non-drug factors to the side-effect incidence rate in the population studied.

Adverse Events in OCD Placebo Controlled Studies Which are Markedly Different (defined as at least a two-fold difference) in rate from the Pooled Event Rates in OCD and Depression Placebo Controlled Studies: The events in OCD studies with a two-fold decrease in rate compared to event rates in OCD and depression studies were dysphagia and amblyopia (mostly blurred vision). Additionally, there was an approximate 25% decrease in nausea.

The events in OCD studies with a two-fold increase in rate compared to event rates in OCD and depression studies were: *asthenia, abnormal ejaculation (mostly delayed ejaculation), anxiety, infection, rhinitis, anorgasmia (in males), depression, libido decreased, pharyngitis, agitation, impotence, myoclonus/twitch, thirst, weight loss, leg cramps, myalgia and urinary retention.* These events are listed in order of decreasing rates in the OCD trials.

Vital Sign Changes: Comparisons of fluvoxamine maleate and placebo groups in separate pools of short-term OCD and depression trials on (1) median change from baseline on various vital signs variables and on (2) incidence of patients meeting criteria for potentially important changes from baseline on various vital signs variables revealed no important differences between fluvoxamine maleate and placebo.

Laboratory Changes: Comparisons of fluvoxamine maleate and placebo groups in separate pools of short-term OCD and depression trials on (1) median change from baseline on various serum chemistry, hematology, and urinalysis variables and on (2) incidence of patients meeting criteria for potentially important changes from baseline on various serum chemistry, hematology, and urinalysis variables revealed no important differences between fluvoxamine maleate and placebo.

ECG Changes: Comparisons of fluvoxamine maleate and placebo groups in separate pools of short-term OCD and depression trials on (1) mean change from baseline on various ECG variables and on (2) incidence of patients meeting criteria for potentially important changes from baseline on various ECG variables revealed no important differences between fluvoxamine maleate and placebo (TABLE 4).

Other Events Observed During the Premarketing Evaluation of Fluvoxamine Maleate: During premarketing clinical trials conducted in North America and Europe, multiple doses of fluvoxamine maleate were administered for a combined total of 2737 patient exposures in patients suffering OCD or Major Depressive Disorder. Untoward events associated with this exposure were recorded by clinical investigators using descriptive terminology of their own choosing. Consequently, it is not possible to provide a meaningful estimate of the proportion of individuals experiencing adverse events without first grouping similar types of untoward events into a limited (*i.e.,* reduced) number of standard event categories.

In the tabulations which follow, a standard COSTART-based Dictionary terminology has been used to classify reported adverse events. If the COSTART term for an event was so general as to be uninformative, it was replaced with a more informative term. The frequencies presented, therefore, represent the proportion of the 2737 patient exposures to multiple doses of fluvoxamine maleate who experienced an event of the type cited on at least one occasion while receiving fluvoxamine maleate. All reported events are included in the list below, with the following exceptions: 1) those events already listed in TABLE 4, which tabulates incidence rates of common adverse experiences in placebo-controlled OCD and depression clinical trials, are excluded; 2) those events for which a drug cause was considered remote (*i.e.,* neoplasia, gastrointestinal carcinoma, herpes simplex, herpes zoster, application site reaction, and unintended pregnancy) are omitted; and 3) events which were reported in only one patient and judged to not be potentially serious are not included. It is important to emphasize that, although the events reported did occur during treatment with fluvoxamine maleate, a casual relationship to fluvoxamine maleate has not been established.

Events are further classified within body system categories and enumerated in order of decreasing frequency using the following definitions: frequent adverse events are defined as those occurring on one or more occasions in at least 1/100 patients; infrequent adverse events are those occurring between 1/100 and 1/1000 patients; and rare adverse events are those occurring in less than 1/1000 patients.

Body as a Whole: *Frequent:* accidental injury, malaise; *Infrequent:* allergic reaction, neck pain, neck rigidity, overdose, photosensitivity reaction, suicide attempt; *Rare:* cyst, pelvic pain, sudden death.

Cardiovascular System: *Frequent:* hypertension, hypotension, syncope, tachycardia;*Infrequent:* angina pectoris, bradycardia, cardiomyopathy, cardiovascular disease, cold extremities, conduction delay, heart failure, myocardial infarction, pallor, pulse irregular, ST segment changes; *Rare:* AV block, cerebrovascular accident, coronary artery disease, embolus, pericarditis, phlebitis, pulmonary infarction, supraventricular extrasystoles.

Digestive System: *Frequent:* elevated liver transaminases;*Infrequent:* colitis, eructation, esophagitis, gastritis, gastroenteritis, gastrointestinal hemorrhage, gastrointestinal ulcer, gingivitis, glossitis, hemorrhoids, melena, rectal hemorrhage, stomatitis; *Rare:* biliary pain, cholecystitis, cholelithiasis, fecal incontinence, hematemesis, intestinal obstruction, jaundice.

Endocrine System: *Infrequent:* hypothyroidism;*Rare:* goiter

Hemic and Lymphatic Systems: *Infrequent:* anemia, ecchymosis, leukocytosis, lymphadenopathy, thrombocytopenia;*Rare:* leukopenia, purpura.

ADVERSE REACTIONS: *(cont'd)*

TABLE 4 Treatment-Emergent Adverse Event Icidence Rates by Body System in OCD and Depression Populations Combined [1]

BODY SYSTEM/ ADVERSE EVENT	Percentage of Patients Reporting Event FLUVOXAMINE N = 892	PLACEBO N = 778
BODY AS WHOLE		
Headache	22	20
Asthenia	14	6
Flu Syndrome	3	2
Chills	2	1
CARDIOVASCULAR		
Palpitations	3	2
DIGESTIVE SYSTEM		
Nausea	40	14
Diarrhea	11	7
Constipation	10	8
Dyspepsia	10	5
Anorexia	6	2
Vomiting	5	2
Flatulence	4	3
Tooth Disorder[2]	3	1
Dysphagia	2	1
NERVOUS SYSTEM		
Somnolence	22	8
Insomnia	21	10
Dry Mouth	14	10
Nervousness	12	5
Dizziness	11	6
Tremor	5	1
Anxiety	5	3
Vasodilatation[3]	3	1
Hypertonia	2	1
Agitation	2	1
Decreased Libido	2	1
Depression	2	1
CNS Stimulation	2	1
RESPIRATORY SYSTEM		
Upper Respiratory Infection	9	5
Dyspnea	2	1
Yawn	2	0
SKIN		
Sweating	7	3
SPECIAL SENSES		
Taste Perversion	3	1
Amblyopia[4]	3	2
UROGENITAL		
Abnormal Ejaculation[5,6]	8	1
Urinary Frequency	3	2
Impotence[6]	2	1
Anorgasmia	2	0
Urinary Retention	1	0

1 Events for which fluvoxamine maleate incidence was equal to or less than placebo are not listed in the table above, but include the following: abdominal pain, abnormal dreams, appetite increase, back pain, chest pain, confusion, dysmenorrhea, fever, infection, leg cramps, migraine, myalgia, pain, paresthesia, pharyngitis, postural hypotension, pruritus, rash, rhinitis, thirst and tinnitus.
2 Includes "toothache," "tooth extraction and abscess," and "caries."
3 Mostly feeling warm, hot, or flushed.
4 Mostly "blurred vision."
5 Mostly "delayed ejaculation."
6 Incidence based on number of male patients.

Metabolic and Nutritional Systems: *Frequent:* edema, weight gain, weight loss; *Infrequent:* dehydration, hypercholesterolemia; *Rare:* diabetes mellitus, hyperglycemia, hyperlipidemia, hypoglycemia, hypokalemia, lactate dehydrogenase increased.

Musculoskeletal System: *Infrequent:* arthralgia, arthritis, bursitis, generalized muscle spasm, myasthenia, tendinous contracture, tenosynovitis; *Rare:* arthrosis, myopathy, pathological fracture.

Nervous System: *Frequent:* amnesia, apathy, hyperkinesia, hypokinesia, manic reaction, myoclonus, psychotic reaction;*Infrequent:* agoraphobia, akathisia, ataxia, CNS depression, convulsion, delirium, delusion, depersonalization, drug dependence, dyskinesia, dystonia, emotional lability, euphoria, extrapyramidal syndrome, gait unsteady, hallucinations, hemiplegia, hostility, hypersomnia, hypochondriasis, hypotonia, hysteria, incoordination, increased salivation, increased libido, neuralgia, paralysis, paranoid reaction, phobia, psychosis, sleep disorder, stupor, twitching, vertigo;*Rare:* akinesia, coma, fibrillations, mutism, obsessions, reflexes decreased, slurred speech, tardive dyskinesia, torticollis, trismus, withdrawal syndrome.

Respiratory System: *Frequent:* cough increased, sinusitis; *Infrequent:* asthma, bronchitis, epistaxis, hoarseness, hyperventilation; *Rare:* apnea, congestion of upper airway, hemoptysis, hiccups, laryngismus, obstructive pulmonary disease, pneumonia.

Skin: *Infrequent:* acne, alopecia, dry skin, eczema, exfoliative dermatitis, furunculosis, seborrhea, skin discoloration, urticaria.

Special Senses: *Infrequent:* accommodation abnormal, conjunctivitis, deafness, diplopia, dry eyes, ear pain, eye pain, mydriasis, otitis media, parosmia, photophobia, taste loss, visual field defect; *Rare:* corneal ulcer, retinal detachment.

Urogenital System: *Infrequent:* anuria, breast pain, cystitis, delayed menstruation[1], dysuria, female lactation[1], hematuria, menopause[1], menorrhagia[1], metrorrhagia[1], nocturia, polyuria, premenstrual syndrome[1], urinary incontinence, urinary tract infection, urinary urgency, urination impaired, vaginal hemorrhage[1], vaginitis[1]; *Rare:* kidney calculus, hematospermia[2], oliguria.

[1] Based on the number of females.

[2] Based on the number of males.

Non-US Postmarketing Reports: Voluntary reports of adverse events in patients taking fluvoxamine maleate that have been received since market introduction and are of unknown casual relationship to fluvoxamine maleate use include: toxic epidermal necrolysis, Stevens-Johnson syndrome, Henoch- Schoenlein purpura, bullous eruption, priapism, agranulocytosis, neuropathy, aplastic anemia, anaphylactic reaction, hyponatremia, acute renal failure, and severe akinesia with fever when fluvoxamine was co- administered with antipsychotic medication.

DRUG ABUSE AND DEPENDENCE:

Controlled Substance Class: Fluvoxamine maleate tablets are not controlled substances.

Physical and Psychological Dependence: The potential for abuse, tolerance and physical dependence with fluvoxamine maleate has been studied in a nonhuman primate model. No evidence of dependency phenomena was found. The discontinuation effects of fluvoxamine

DRUG ABUSE AND DEPENDENCE: *(cont'd)*

maleate were not systematically evaluated in controlled clinical trials. fluvoxamine maleate were not systematically studied in clinical trials for potential for abuse, but there was no indication of drug-seeking behavior in clinical trials. It should be noted, however, that patients at risk for drug dependency were systematically excluded from investigational studies of fluvoxamine maleate. Generally, it is not possible to predict on the basis of preclinical or premarketing clinical experience the extent to which a CNS active drug will be misused, diverted, and/or abused once marketed. Consequently, physicians should carefully evaluate patients for a history of drug abuse and follow such patients closely, observing them for signs of fluvoxamine maleate misuse or abuse (*i.e.,* development of tolerance, incrementation of dose, drug-seeking behavior).

OVERDOSAGE:

Human Experience: Worldwide exposure to fluvoxamine maleate includes over 37,000 patients treated in clinical trials and an estimated exposure of 4,500,000 patients treated during foreign marketing experience (circa 1992). Of the 354 cases of deliberate or accidental overdose involving fluvoxamine maleate reported from this population, there were 19 deaths. Of the 19 deaths, 2 were in patients taking fluvoxamine maleate alone and the remaining 17 were in patients taking fluvoxamine maleate along with other drugs. In the remaining 335 patients, 309 had complete recovery after gastric lavage or symptomatic treatment. One patient had persistent mydriasis after the event, and a second patient had a bowel infarction requiring a hemicolectomy. In the remaining 24 patients the outcome was unknown. The highest reported overdose of fluvoxamine maleate involved a non-lethal ingestion of 10,000 mg (equivalent of 1-3 months' dosage). The patient fully recovered with no sequelae.

Commonly observed adverse events associated with fluvoxamine maleate overdose included drowsiness, vomiting, diarrhea, and dizziness. Other notable signs and symptoms seen with fluvoxamine maleate overdose (single or mixed drugs) included coma, tachycardia, bradycardia, hypotension, ECG abnormalities, liver function abnormalities, convulsions, and symptoms such as aspiration pneumonitis, respiratory difficulties or hypokalemia that may occur secondary to loss of consciousness or vomiting.

MANAGEMENT OF OVERDOSE

1. An unobstructed airway should be established with maintenance of respiration as required. Vital signs and ECG should be monitored.

2. Administration of activated charcoal may be as effective as emesis or lavage and should be considered in treating overdose. Since absorption with overdose may be delayed, measures to minimize absorption may be necessary for up to 24 hours post-ingestion.

3. Maintain close observation as clinically indicated.

4. There are no specific antidotes for fluvoxamine maleate.

5. In managing overdosage, consider the possibility of multiple drug involvement. The physician should consider contacting a poison control center for additional information on the treatment of any overdosage.

6. Dialysis is not believed to be beneficial.

DOSAGE AND ADMINISTRATION:

The recommended starting dose for fluvoxamine maleate is 50 mg, administered as a single daily dose at bedtime. In the controlled clinical trials establishing the effectiveness of fluvoxamine maleate in OCD, patients were titrated within a dose range of 100 to 300 mg/day. Consequently, the dose should be increased in 50 mg increments every 4 to 7 days, as tolerated, until maximum therapeutic benefit is achieved, not exceed 300 mg per day. It is advisable that a total daily dose of more than 100 mg should be given in two divided doses. If the doses are not equal, the larger dose should be given at bedtime.

Dosage for Elderly or Hepatically Impaired Patients: Elderly patients and those with hepatic impairment have been observed to have a decreased clearance of fluvoxamine maleate. Consequently, it may be appropriate to modify the initial dose and the subsequent dose titration for these patient groups.

Maintenance/Continuation Extended Treatment: Although the efficacy of fluvoxamine maleate beyond 10 weeks of dosing for OCD has not been documented in controlled trials, OCD is a chronic condition, and it is reasonable to consider continuation for a responding patient. Dosage adjustments should be made to maintain the patient on the lowest effective dosage, and patients should be periodically reassessed to determine the need for continued treatment.

HOW SUPPLIED:

50 mg Tablets: scored, yellow, elliptical, film-coated (debossed "Solvay" and "4205" on one side and scored on the other)

100 mg Tablets: scored, beige, elliptical, film-coated (debossed "Solvay" and "4210" on one side and scored on the other)

Fluvoxamine maleate should be protected from high humidity and stored at controlled room temperature, 15°-30° C (59°- 86° F).

Dispense in tight containers.

HOW SUPPLIED - EQUIVALENTS NOT AVAILABLE:

Tablet, Uncoated - Oral - 50 mg

100's	**$198.67**	**LUVOX, Solvay Pharms**	**00032-4205-01**
100's	**$198.67**	**LUVOX, Solvay Pharms**	**00032-4205-11**

Tablet, Uncoated - Oral - 100 mg

100's	**$204.37**	**LUVOX, Solvay Pharms**	**00032-4210-01**
100's	**$204.37**	**LUVOX, Solvay Pharms**	**00032-4210-11**

FOLIC ACID *(001331)*

CATEGORIES: Anemia; Blood Formation/Coagulation; Central Nervous System Agents; Deficiency Anemias; Homeostatic & Nutrient; Pharmaceutical Adjuvants; Pregnancy; Vitamin B Complex; Vitamins; Spina Bifida*; FDA Approval Pre 1982
* Indication not approved by the FDA

BRAND NAMES: *Acfol*; *Acido*; *Acido Folico*; *Apo-Folic* (Canada); *Filicine*; *Folacin*; *Folasic*; *Foliamin*; *Folic Acid DHA*; *Folic Acid Sussex*; Folicet; *Folicid*; *Folico*; *Folina*; *Folinsyre*; *Folitab* (Mexico); *Folivit*; *Folsan* (Germany); **Folvite**; *Lexpec* (England); *Megafol*; *Nifolin*; *Novofolacid* (Canada); Renal Multivit Form Forte Zinc
(International brand names outside U.S. in italics)

FORMULARIES: BC-BS; FHP; Medi-Cal; WHO; PCS

DESCRIPTION:

Folic Acid, N-(p(((2-Amino-4-hydroxy-6-pteridinyl)-methyl)Amino)benzoyl) glutamic acid, is a complex organic compound present in liver, yeast and other substances, and which may be prepared synthetically.

Tablets: 1 mg folic acid

DESCRIPTION: *(cont'd)*

Parenteral: Each ml of folic acid-Solution contains sodium folate equivalent to 5 mg of FOLIC ACID.

Inactive ingredients: Sequestrene Sodium 0.2% and Water for Injection q.s. 100%. Sodium Hydroxide to approx. pH 9.

Preservative: Benzyl Alcohol 1.5%

CLINICAL PHARMACOLOGY:

In man, an exogenous source of folate is required for nucleoprotein synthesis and the maintenance of normal erythropoiesis. Folic acid, whether given by mouth or parenterally, stimulates specifically the production of red blood cells, white blood cells, and platelets in persons suffering from certain megaloblastic anemias.

INDICATIONS AND USAGE:

Folic acid is effective in the treatment of megaloblastic anemias due to a deficiency of folic acid as may be seen in tropical or non-tropical sprue, in anemias of nutritional origin, pregnancy, infancy, or childhood.

WARNINGS:

Folic acid alone is improper therapy in the treatment of pernicious anemia and other megaloblastic anemias where Vitamin B12 is deficient.

PRECAUTIONS:

Folic acid in doses above 0.1 mg daily may obscure pernicious anemia in that hematologic remission can occur while neurological manifestations remain progressive.

ADVERSE REACTIONS:

Allergic sensitization has been reported following both oral and parenteral administration of folic acid.

DOSAGE AND ADMINISTRATION:

Oral Administration: Folic acid is well absorbed and may be administered orally with satisfactory results except in severe instances of intestinal malabsorption.

Parenteral Administration: Intramuscular, intravenous, and subcutaneous routes may be used if the disease is exceptionally severe, or if gastrointestinal absorption may be, or is known to be, impaired.

Usual Therapeutic Dosage: Adults and children regardless of age-up to 1.0 mg daily. Resistant cases may require larger doses.

Maintenance Level: When clinical symptoms have subsided and the blood picture has become normal, a maintenance level should be used, i.e., 0.1 mg for infants and up to 0.3 mg for children under four years of age, 0.4 mg for adults and children four or more years of age, and 0.8 mg for pregnant and lactating women, per day, but never less than 0.1 mg per day. Patients should be kept under close supervision and adjustment of the maintenance level made if relapse appears imminent.

In the presence of alcoholism, hemolytic anemia, anticonvulsant therapy, or chronic infection, the maintenance level may need to be increased.

HOW SUPPLIED - RATED THERAPEUTICALLY EQUIVALENT:

Injection, Solution - Intramuscular; - 5 mg/ml

10 ml	$11.85	Folic Acid, Fujisawa USA	00469-1840-30
10 ml	$12.50	Folic Acid, Bedford Labs	55390-0410-10
10 ml	**$14.33**	**FOLVITE, Lederle Parenterals**	**00205-4154-34**

Tablet, Uncoated - Oral - 1 mg

30's	$1.85	Folic Acid, Major Pharms	00904-0625-46
100's	$.89	Folic Acid, H.C.F.A. F F P	99999-1331-01
100's	$0.98	Folic Acid, Lannett	00527-1098-01
100's	$2.30	Folic Acid, Paddock Labs	00574-0060-01
100's	$2.40	Folic Acid, Rugby	00536-3843-01
100's	$2.70	Folic Acid, Voluntary Hosp	53258-0128-01
100's	$2.75	Folic Acid, Consolidated Midland	00223-1002-01
100's	$2.80	Folic Acid, Major Pharms	00904-0625-60
100's	$2.86	Folic Acid, Schein Pharm (US)	00364-0137-01
100's	$3.00	Folic Acid, West Ward Pharm	00143-1248-01
100's	$4.75	Folic Acid, Paddock Labs	00574-0060-11
100's	$5.31	Folic Acid, Voluntary Hosp	53258-0128-13
100's	$5.40	Folic Acid, Raway	00686-0041-20
100's	$5.89	Folic Acid, Major Pharms	00904-0625-61
100's	$7.85	Folic Acid 1, Vangard Labs	00615-0664-13
100's	$8.13	Folic Acid, Medirex	57480-0327-01
100's	$8.37	Folic Acid, HL Moore Drug Exch	00839-5066-06
100's	$8.50	Folic Acid, West Ward Pharm	00143-1248-25
100's	$11.60	Folic Acid, Schein Pharm (US)	00364-0137-90
100's	$15.65	Folic Acid, Goldline Labs	00182-0507-89
600's	$66.40	Folic Acid, Medirex	57480-0327-06
1000's	$5.20	Folic Acid, Lannett	00527-1098-10
1000's	$8.00	Folic Acid, C O Truxton	00463-6096-10
1000's	$8.90	Folic Acid, West Ward Pharm	00143-1248-10
1000's	$8.90	Folic Acid, H.C.F.A. F F P	99999-1331-02
1000's	$9.75	Folic Acid, Consolidated Midland	00223-1001-02
1000's	$10.80	Folic Acid, Qualitest Pharms	00603-3714-32
1000's	$12.10	BLUE CROSS FOLIC ACID, Halsey Drug	00879-0081-10
1000's	$12.90	Folic Acid, Major Pharms	00904-0625-80
1000's	$13.17	Folic Acid, Aligen Independ	00405-4447-03
1000's	$13.17	Folic Acid, United Res	00677-0449-10
1000's	$13.35	Folic Acid, Goldline Labs	00182-0507-10
1000's	$14.08	Folic Acid, Schein Pharm (US)	00364-0137-02
1000's	$20.19	Folic Acid, Rugby	00536-3845-10
1000's	$21.26	Folic Acid, HL Moore Drug Exch	00839-5066-16

HOW SUPPLIED - NOT RATED EQUIVALENT:

Injection, Solution - Intravenous - 10 mg/ml

10 ml	$3.10	Folic Acid, Americal Pharm	54945-0572-52
10 ml	$17.85	Folic Acid, Merit Pharms	30727-0389-70

Powder

10 gm	$12.46	Folic Acid, Millgood	53118-0519-10
25 gm	$24.50	Folic Acid, Millgood	53118-0519-25
100 gm	$84.00	Folic Acid, Millgood	53118-0519-01

FOLIC ACID; MULTIVITAMINS; POLY-FERROUS SULFATE *(001334)*

CATEGORIES: Antianemia Drugs; Blood Formation/Coagulation; Deficiency Anemias; Homeostatic & Nutrient; Iron Preparations; Polysaccharide-Iron Complex; Vitamins; FDA Pre 1938 Drugs

FORMULARIES: PCS

Prescribing information not available at time of publication.

HOW SUPPLIED - EQUIVALENTS NOT AVAILABLE:

Tablet, Coated - Oral - 312 mg/3 mcg/40

100's	$20.40	NU-IRON-V, Mayrand Pharms	00259-0331-01

FORMALDEHYDE *(001337)*

CATEGORIES: Anti-Infectives; Antifungals; Dermatologicals; Drying Agents; Hyperhidrosis; Local Infections; Mucous Membrane Agents; Skin/Mucous Membrane Agents; Warts; FDA Pre 1938 Drugs

BRAND NAMES: Forma-Ray; Formalin; Formalyde-10; Lazer Formalyde; **Lazerformalyde**; Scrip Super Dri

Prescribing information not available at time of publication.

HOW SUPPLIED - EQUIVALENTS NOT AVAILABLE:

Aerosol, Spray - Topical

60 ml	$5.75	FORMALYDE-10, Pedinol Pharma	00884-4789-02

Solution - 10 %

90 ml	**$6.75**	**LAZERFORMALYDE, Pedinol Pharma**	**00884-3986-03**

FOSCARNET SODIUM *(003061)*

CATEGORIES: AIDS Related Complex; Anti-Infectives; Antimicrobials; Antivirals; Cytomegalovirus Infections; Herpes Simplex; HIV Infection; Immunodeficiency; Immunodeficiency Syndrome; Infections; Ocular Infections; Retinitis; Viral Agents; Pregnancy Category C; FDA Class 1A ("Important Therapeutic Advantage"); FDA Approved 1991 Sep; Patent Expiration 1997 Jul

BRAND NAMES: **Foscavir**; *Foscovir*
(International brand names outside U.S. in italics)

FORMULARIES: Medi-Cal

COST OF THERAPY: $26,632.22 (AIDS Retinitis; Solution - Intravenous; 24 mg/ml; 250/day; 365 days)

> WARNING:
> RENAL IMPAIRMENT IS THE MAJOR TOXICITY OF FOSCARNET SODIUM, AND OCCURS TO SOME DEGREE IN MOST PATIENTS. CONSEQUENTLY, CONTINUAL ASSESSMENT OF A PATIENT'S RISK AND FREQUENT MONITORING OF SERUM CREATININE WITH DOSE ADJUSTMENT FOR CHANGES IN RENAL FUNCTION ARE IMPERATIVE.
> FOSCARNET SODIUM HAS BEEN SHOWN TO CAUSE ALTERATIONS IN PLASMA MINERALS AND ELECTROLYTES THAT HAVE LED TO SEIZURES. THEREFORE, PATIENTS MUST BE MONITORED FREQUENTLY FOR SUCH CHANGES AND THEIR POTENTIAL SEQUELAE.
> FOSCARNET SODIUM IS INDICATED FOR USE ONLY IN THE TREATMENT OF CMV RETINITIS AND MUCOCUTANEOUS ACYCLOVIR-RESISTANT HSV INFECTIONS IN IMMUNOCOMPROMISED PATIENTS. (SEE INDICATIONS AND USAGE.)

DESCRIPTION:

The chemical name of foscarnet sodium is phosphonoformic acid, trisodium salt. Foscarnet sodium is a white, crystalline powder containing 6 equivalents of water of hydration with an empirical formula of $Na_3CO_5P \cdot 6\ H_2O$ and a molecular weight of 300.1.

Foscarnet sodium has the potential to chelate divalent metal ions, such as calcium and magnesium, to form stable coordination compounds. Foscarnet sodium injection is a sterile, isotonic aqueous solution for intravenous administration only. The solution is clear and colorless. Each milliliter of Foscavir contains 24 mg of foscarnet sodium hexahydrate in Water for Injection, USP. Hydrochloric acid and/or sodium hydroxide may have been added to adjust the pH of the solution to 7.4. Foscavir Injection contains no preservatives.

CLINICAL PHARMACOLOGY:

MICROBIOLOGY

Mechanism of Action: Foscarnet sodium is an organic analogue of inorganic pyrophosphate that inhibits replication of all known herpesviruses *in vitro* including cytomegalovirus (CMV), herpes simplex virus types 1 and 2 (HSV-1, HSV-2), human herpesvirus 6 (HHV-6), Epstein-Barr virus (EBV), and varicella-zoster virus (VZV).

Foscarnet sodium exerts its antiviral activity by a selective inhibition at the pyrophosphate binding site on virus-specific DNA polymerases and reverse transcriptases at concentrations that do not affect cellular DNA polymerases. Foscarnet sodium does not require activation (phosphorylation) by thymidine kinase or other kinases, and therefore is active *in vitro* against HSV TK deficient mutants and CMV UL97 mutants. Thus, HSV strains resistant to acyclovir or CMV strains resistant to ganciclovir may be sensitive to foscarnet sodium. However, acyclovir or ganciclovir resistant mutants with alterations in the viral DNA polymerase may be resistant to foscarnet sodium and may not respond to therapy with foscarnet sodium.

Antiviral Activity: The quantitative relationship between the *in vitro* susceptibility of human cytomegalovirus (CMV) or mucocutaneous herpes simplex virus 1 and 2 (HSV-1 and HSV-2) to foscarnet sodium and clinical response to therapy has not been clearly established in man and virus sensitivity testing has not been standardized. Sensitivity test results, expressed as the concentration of drug required to inhibit by 50% the growth of virus in cell culture (IC_{50}), vary greatly depending on the assay method used, cell type employed and the laboratory performing the test. A number of sensitive viruses and their IC_{50} values are listed in TABLE 1.

TABLE 1
Foscarnet Inhibition of virus multiplication in cell culture

Virus	IC_{50} (µM)
CMV	50-800*
HSV-1, HSV-2	10-130
VZV	48-90
EBV	< 500**
HHV-6	< 67***
Ganciclovir resistant CMV	190
HSV-TK minus mutant	67
HSV-DNA polymerase mutants	5-443

* Mean = 269 µM
** 97% of viral antigen synthesis inhibited at 500 µM
*** IC_{100} = 67 µM

Clinical isolates of CMV taken from patients show different sensitivities to foscarnet sodium *in vitro*. Statistically significant decreases in positive CMV cultures from blood and urine have been demonstrated in two studies (FOS-03 and ACTG-015/915) of patients treated with foscarnet sodium. Although median time to progression of CMV retinitis was increased in patients treated with the drug, reductions in positive blood or urine cultures have not been shown to correlate with clinical efficacy in individual patients.

Table 2 Blood And Urine Culture Results From Cmv Retinitis Patients*

Blood	+CMV	-CMV
Baseline	27	34
End of Induction**	1	60
Urine	+CMV	-CMV
Baseline	52	6
End of Induction**	21	37

* A combined total of 77 patients were treated with Foscavir in two clinical trials (FOS-03 and ACTG-015/915). Not all patients had blood or urine cultures done and some patients had results from both cultures.
** (60 mg/kg Foscavir TID for 2-3 weeks).

Drug Resistance: Strains of both HSV and CMV that are resistant to foscarnet sodium can be readily selected *in vitro* by passage of wild type virus in the presence of increasing concentrations of the drug. All foscarnet sodium resistant mutants are known to be generated through mutation in the viral DNA polymerase gene. If no clinical response to foscarnet sodium is observed, viral isolates should be tested for sensitivity to foscarnet as naturally resistant mutants may emerge under selective pressure both *in vitro* and *in vivo*. The latent state of any of the human herpesviruses is not known to be sensitive to foscarnet sodium and viral reactivation of CMV occurs after foscarnet sodium therapy is terminated. In patients treated with foscarnet sodium for mucocutaneous acyclovir-resistant HSV infections, reactivation may be with HSV sensitive to acyclovir. Therefore, in the case of a relapse, sensitivity testing of the viral isolate is advised.

PHARMACOKINETICS

Protein Binding: *In vitro* studies have shown that 14-17% of foscarnet is bound to plasma protein at plasma drug concentrations of 1-1000 µM.

Plasma Concentrations: The pharmacokinetics of foscarnet sodium infusions have been determined when administered as an intermittent infusion during induction therapy in AIDS patients with CMV retinitis. Observed plasma foscarnet concentrations in two studies (FOS-01 and ACTG-015 respectively) are summarized in TABLE 3.

TABLE 3

Mean ± SD Dose mg/kg * (Infusion Time)	Day of Sampling	Mean Plasma Concentration (µM) C_{MAX}** [range]	C_{MIN}*** [range]
FOS-01			
57 ± 6 78 [<33-139] (1 hour)	Q8h	1	573 [213-1305]
47 ± 12 Q8h (1 hour)	14 or 15	579 [246-922]	110 [<33-148]
ACTG-015			
55 ± 6 Q8h (2 hours)	3	445 [306-720]	88 [<33-162])
57 ± 7 Q8h (2 hours)	14 or 15	517 [348-789]	105 [43-205]

* Planned dose = 60 mg/kg Q8h in both studies.
** Observed Maximum Concentration:**FOS-01:**Day 1 (N=14): Observed 0.9-2.0 hr after start of infusion. Day 14/15 (N=10): Observed 0.8-1.3 hr after start of infusion.**ACTG-015:**Day 3 (N=12): Observed 1.8-2.4 hr after start of infusion. Day 14/15 (N=12): Observed 1.7-2.6 hr after start of infusion.
*** Observed Minimum Concentration:**FOS-01:**Day 1 (N=13): Observed 4-8 hr after start of infusion. (Mean represents 5/13 observations, 8/13 <33 µM) Day 14/15 (N=10): Observed 6.3-8 hr after start of infusion. (Mean represents 9/10 observations, 1/10 <33 µM)**ACTG-015:** Day 3 (N=12): Observed 7.8-8.1 hr after start of infusion. (Mean represents 9/12 observations, 3/12 <33 µM) Day 14/15 (N=12): Observed 6.4-8.7 hr after start of infusion. (Mean represents 12/12 observations)

Clearance: Mean (± SD) plasma clearances were 130 ± 44 and 178 ± 48 ml/min in two studies in which foscarnet sodium was given by intermittent infusion (ACTG-015 and FOS-01 respectively), and 152 ± 59 and 214 ± 25 ml/min/1.73 m^2in two studies using continuous infusion. Approximately 80-90% of IV foscarnet sodium is excreted unchanged in the urine of patients with normal renal function. Urinary excretion data suggest that both tubular secretion and glomerular filtration account for urinary elimination of foscarnet. In one study, plasma clearance was less than creatinine clearance, suggesting that foscarnet sodium may also undergo tubular reabsorption. In three studies, decreases in plasma clearance of foscarnet sodium were proportional to decreases in creatinine clearance.

Half-life: Two studies (FOS-01 and ACTG-015) in patients with initially normal renal function who were treated with intermittent infusions of foscarnet sodium showed average drug plasma half-lives of about three hours determined on days 1 or 3 of therapy. This may be an underestimate of the effective half-life of foscarnet sodium due to the limited duration of the observation period. The plasma half-life of foscarnet sodium increases with the severity of renal impairment. Half-lives of 2-8 hours have been reported in patients having estimated or measured 24-hour creatinine clearances of 44-90 ml/min. Careful monitoring of renal function and dose adjustment in patients on foscarnet sodium is imperative (see WARNINGSand DOSAGE AND ADMINISTRATION).

CLINICAL PHARMACOLOGY: *(cont'd)*

Following the continuous infusion of foscarnet sodium for 72 hours in six HIV + patients, plasma half-lives of 0.45 ± 0.32 and 3.3 ± 1.3 hours were determined. A terminal half-life (lambda 3) of 18 ± 2.8 hours was estimated from the urinary excretion of foscarnet over 48 hours after stopping the infusion. When foscarnet sodium was administered as a continuous infusion to 13 patients with HIV infection for 8 to 21 days, plasma half-lives of 1.4 ± 0.6 and 6.8 ± 5.0 hours were determined. A terminal half-life of 87.5 ± 41.8 hours was estimated from the urinary excretion of foscarnet over six days after the last infusion; however, the renal function of these patients at the time of discontinuing the foscarnet sodium infusion was not known.

Measurements of urinary excretion are required to detect the longer terminal half-life assumed to represent release of foscarnet from bone. In animal studies (mice), 40% of an intravenous dose of foscarnet sodium is deposited in bone in young animals and 7% in adults. Postmortem data on several patients in European clinical trials provide evidence that foscarnet does accumulate in bone in humans; however, the extent to which this occurs has not been determined.

Volume of Distribution: Mean volumes of distribution at steady state range from 0.3-0.6 l/kg.

Cerebrospinal Fluid: Variable penetration of foscarnet sodium into cerebrospinal fluid has been observed. Intermittent infusion of 50 mg/kg of foscarnet sodium every 8 hours for 28 days in 9 patients produced foscarnet CSF levels 3 hours after the end of the infusion of 150-260 μM or 39-103% of plasma levels. In another 4 patients, the CSF concentrations of foscarnet were 35-69% of the plasma drug level after a dose of 230 mg/kg/day by continuous infusion for 2-13 days; however, the CSF:plasma ratio was only 13% in one patient while receiving a continuous infusion of foscarnet sodium at a rate of 274 mg/kg/day. Disease-related defects in the blood-brain barrier may be responsible for the variations seen.

Pharmacodynamics: A pharmacodynamic analysis of patient data form one U.S. clinical trial (FOS-01) revealed a relationship between cumulative exposure to foscarnet (product of plasma foscarnet concentration *x* time) and changes in renal function (serum creatinine) during induction. All patients had their doses adjusted according to the recommended foscarnet sodium dosing nomogram. Seventeen of 24 patients (72%) showed evidence of renal impairment (>20% suppression from baseline estimated creatinine clearance) during induction. This occurred in 3 patients on days 5-6, in 11 patients on days 7-14 and in 3 patients after day 14. Eleven patients had at least 40% suppression from baseline estimated creatinine clearance and six patients had more than 50% suppression, demonstrating that patients vary in their degree of sensitivity to foscarnet sodium-induced renal impairment. No specific factors were identified that predicted patients at higher risk. No relationship was found between a patient's initial creatinine clearance or initial drug clearance and renal impairment. Thus initial renal function may not be predictive of a patient's potential for renal impairment induced by foscarnet sodium.

CLINICAL STUDIES:

CMV RETINITIS

Controlled clinical trials of foscarnet sodium have been conducted in the treatment of CMV retinitis. In most studies, treatment was begun with an induction dosage regimen of 60 mg/kg every 8 hours for the first 2-3 weeks, followed by a once-daily maintenance regimen at doses ranging from 60-120 mg/kg.

A prospective, randomized, masked, controlled clinical trial (FOS-03) was conducted in 24 patients with AIDS and CMV retinitis. All diagnoses and determinations of retinitis progression were made from retinal photographs by ophthalmologists who were masked to the patient's treatment assignment. Patients received induction treatment of foscarnet sodium, 60 mg/kg every 8 hours for 3 weeks, followed by maintenance treatment with 90 mg/kg/day until retinitis progression (appearance of a new lesion or advancement of the border of a posterior lesion greater than 750 microns in diameter). The 13 patients randomized to treatment with foscarnet sodium had a significant delay in progression of CMV retinitis compared to untreated controls. Median times to retinitis progression from study entry were 93 days (range 21- >364) and 22 days (range 7-42), respectively, p<0.001.

In another prospective clinical trial of CMV retinitis in patients with AIDS (ACTG-915), 33 patients were treated with two to three weeks of foscarnet sodium induction (60 mg/kg TID) and then randomized to two maintenance dose groups, 90 mg/kg/day and 120 mg/kg/day. Median times from study entry to retinitis progression were 96 (range 14- >176) days and 140 (range 16- >233) days, respectively (FDA analysis). This difference was not statistically significant. The same criteria for retinitis progression were used as described above for FOS-03.

Mucocutaneous Acyclovir-Resistant HSV Infections: A prospective, comparative trial was conducted in 25 AIDS patients with mucocutaneous, acyclovir-resistant HSV infections. Fourteen patients were randomized to either foscarnet sodium (N=8) at a dose of 40 mg/kg TID or vidarabine (N=6) at a dose of 15 mg/kg per day; eleven patients received foscarnet sodium without being randomized. Lesions in the eight patients randomized to foscarnet sodium healed after 11 to 25 days; seven of the 11 patients non-randomly treated with foscarnet sodium healed their lesions in 10 to 30 days. Vidarabine was discontinued because of intolerance in four patients and poor therapeutic response in two patients. Five of these patients were subsequently treated with foscarnet sodium and two healed their lesions in 15 and 24 days. In a second prospective, randomized trial, forty AIDS patients and three bone marrow transplant recipients with mucocutaneous, acyclovir-resistant HSV infections were randomized to receive foscarnet sodium at a dose of either 40 mg/kg BID or 40 mg/kg TID. Fifteen of the 43 patients had healing of their lesions in 11 to 72 days with no difference in response between the two treatment groups.

INDICATIONS AND USAGE:

CMV Retinitis: Foscarnet sodium is indicated for the treatment of CMV retinitis in patients with acquired immunodeficiency syndrome (AIDS). SAFETY AND EFFICACY OF FOSCARNET SODIUM HAVE NOT BEEN ESTABLISHED FOR TREATMENT OF OTHER CMV INFECTIONS (*E.G.,* PNEUMONITIS, GASTROENTERITIS); CONGENITAL OR NEONATAL CMV DISEASE; OR NON-IMMUNOCOMPROMISED INDIVIDUALS.

The diagnosis of CMV retinitis should be made by indirect ophthalmoscopy. Other conditions in the differential diagnosis of CMV retinitis include candidiasis, toxoplasmosis, and other diseases producing a similar retinal pattern, any of which may produce a retinal appearance similar to CMV. For this reason it is essential that the diagnosis of CMV retinitis be established by an ophthalmologist familiar with the retinal presentation of these conditions. The diagnosis of CMV retinitis may be supported by culture of CMV from urine, blood, throat, or other sites, but a negative CMV culture does not rule out CMV retinitis.

Mucocutaneous Acyclovir-Resistant HSV Infections: Foscarnet sodium is indicated for the treatment of acyclovir-resistant mucocutaneous HSV infections in immunocompromised patients. SAFETY AND EFFICACY OF FOSCARNET SODIUM HAVE NOT BEEN ESTABLISHED FOR TREATMENT OF OTHER HSV INFECTIONS (*e.g.,* RETINITIS, ENCEPHALITIS); CONGENITAL OR NEONATAL HSV DISEASE; OR HSV IN NON-IMMUNOCOMPROMISED INDIVIDUALS.

CONTRAINDICATIONS:

Foscarnet sodium is contraindicated in patients with clinically significant hypersensitivity to foscarnet sodium.

WARNINGS:

RENAL IMPAIRMENT

THE MAJOR TOXICITY OF FOSCARNET SODIUM IS RENAL IMPAIRMENT, WHICH OCCURS TO SOME DEGREE IN MOST PATIENTS. Approximately 33% of 189 patients with AIDS and CMV retinitis who received intravenous foscarnet sodium in clinical studies developed significant impairment of renal function, manifested by a rise in serum creatinine concentration to 2.0 mg/dl or greater. Foscarnet sodium must therefore be used with caution in all patients, especially those with a history of impairment of renal function. Patients vary in their sensitivity to nephrotoxicity induced by foscarnet sodium and initial function may not be predictive of the potential for drug induced renal impairment (see CLINICAL PHARMACOLOGY, Pharmacodynamics). Foscarnet sodium has not been studied in patients with baseline serum creatinine levels greater than 2.8 mg/dl or measured 24-hour creatinine clearances <50 ml/min.

Analysis of data in one clinical trial (FOS-01) demonstrated renal impairment is most likely to become clinically evident, as assessed by increasing serum creatinine, during the second week of induction therapy at 60 mg/kg TID (see CLINICAL PHARMACOLOGY, Pharmacodynamics). Renal impairment, however, may occur at any time in any patient during foscarnet sodium treatment and renal function should therefore be monitored especially carefully (see PATIENT MONITORING).

Elevations in serum creatinine are usually, but not uniformly, reversible following discontinuation or dose adjustment of foscarnet sodium. In the U.S. studies, recovery of renal function after foscarnet sodium-induced impairment usually occurred within one week if drug discontinuation. However, of 35 patients in the U.S. controlled clinical studies who experienced grade II renal impairment (serum creatinine 2-3 times the upper limit of normal), two died with renal failure within four weeks of stopping foscarnet sodium, and three others died with renal insufficiency still present less than four weeks after drug cessation.

BECAUSE OF FOSCARNET SODIUM'S POTENTIAL TO CAUSE RENAL IMPAIRMENT, DOSE ADJUSTMENT FOR DECREASED BASELINE RENAL FUNCTION AND ANY CHANGE IN RENAL FUNCTION DURING TREATMENT IS NECESSARY. In addition, it may be beneficial for adequate hydration to be established (*e.g.,* by inducing diuresis) prior to and during foscarnet sodium administration.

MINERAL AND ELECTROLYTE IMBALANCES

Foscarnet sodium has been associated with changes in serum electrolytes including hypocalcemia (15%), hypophosphatemia (8%) and hyperphosphatemia (6%), hypomagnesemia (15%), and hypokalemia (16%). Administration of foscarnet sodium has been shown to be associated with a transient, dose-related decrease in ionized serum calcium, which may not be reflected in total serum calcium. This effect most likely is related to foscarnet's chelation of divalent metal ions such as calcium. Therefore, patients should be advised to report symptoms of low ionized calcium such as perioral tingling, numbness in the extremities and paresthesias. Physicians should be prepared to treat these as well as severe manifestations of electrolyte abnormalities such as tetany and seizures. The rate of foscarnet sodium infusion may affect the transient decrease in ionized calcium. Slowing the rate may decrease or prevent symptoms.

Transient changes in calcium or other electrolytes (including magnesium, potassium or phosphate) may also contribute to a patient's risk for cardiac disturbances and seizures (see WARNINGS, Neurotoxicity and Seizures). Therefore, particular caution is advised in patients with altered calcium or other electrolyte levels before treatment, especially those with neurologic or cardiac abnormalities and those receiving other drugs known to influence minerals and electrolytes (see DOSAGE AND ADMINISTRATION, Patient Monitoring and DRUG INTERACTIONS).

NEUROTOXICITY AND SEIZURES

Foscarnet sodium treatment has been associated with seizures in 18/189 (10%) of AIDS patients in five controlled studies. Three patients were not taking foscarnet sodium at the time of seizure. In most cases (15/18), the patients had an active CNS condition (*e.g.,* toxoplasmosis, HIV encephalopathy) or a history of CNS diseases. The rate of seizures did not increase with duration of treatment. Three cases were associated with overdoses of foscarnet sodium (see OVERDOSAGE.)

A logistic regression analysis was performed comparing the 18 patients in these five studies who had seizures with the 161 who did not. Statistically significant (p<0.05) risk factors associated with seizures were low baseline absolute neutrophil count (ANC), impaired baseline renal function, and low total serum calcium. Several cases of seizures were associated with death. However, occurrence of seizures did not always necessitate discontinuation of foscarnet sodium; ten of fifteen patients with seizures that occurred while receiving the drug continued or resumed foscarnet sodium following treatment of their underlying disease, electrolyte disturbances, and/or dose decreases. If factors predisposing a patient to seizures are present, electrolytes, including calcium and magnesium, must be monitored especially carefully (see DOSAGE AND ADMINISTRATION, Patient Monitoring).

PRECAUTIONS:

General: In controlled clinical studies with foscarnet sodium, the maximum single dose administered was 120 mg/kg by intravenous infusion over 2 hours. It is likely that larger doses, or more rapid infusions, would result in increased toxicity. Care must be taken to infuse solutions containing foscarnet sodium only into veins with adequate blood flow to permit rapid dilution and distribution, and avoid local irritation (see DOSAGE AND ADMINISTRATION). Local irritation and ulcerations of penile epithelium have been reported in male patients receiving foscarnet sodium, possibly related to the presence of drug in urine. One case of vulvovaginal ulcerations in a female receiving foscarnet sodium has been reported. Adequate hydration with close attention to personal hygiene may minimize the occurrence of such events.

Hemopoietic System: Anemia has been reported in 33% of patients receiving foscarnet sodium in controlled studies. This anemia was usually manageable with transfusions and required discontinuation of foscarnet sodium in less than 1% (1/189) of patients in the studies. Granulocytopenia has been reported in 17% of patients receiving foscarnet sodium in controlled studies; however, only 1% (2/189) were terminated from these studies because of neutropenia.

INFORMATION FOR THE PATIENT

CMV Retinitis: Patients should be advised that foscarnet sodium is not a cure for CMV retinitis, and that they may continue to experience progression of retinitis during or following treatment. They should be advised to have regular ophthalmologic examinations.

Mucocutaneous Acyclovir-Resistant HSV Infections: Patients should be advised that foscarnet sodium is not a cure for HSV infections. While complete healing may occur, relapse occurs in most patients. Because relapse may be due to acyclovir-sensitive HSV, sensitivity testing of the viral isolate is advised. In addition, repeated treatment with foscarnet sodium has led to the development of resistance associated with poorer response. In the case of poor therapeutic response, sensitivity testing of the viral isolate also is advised.

PRECAUTIONS: *(cont'd)*

General: Patients should be informed that the major toxicities of foscarnet are renal impairment, electrolyte disturbances, and seizures, and that dose modifications and possibly discontinuation may be required. The importance of close monitoring while on therapy must be emphasized. Patients should be advised of the importance of perioral tingling, numbness in the extremities or paresthesias during or after infusion as possible symptoms of electrolyte abnormalities. Should such symptoms occur, the infusion of foscarnet sodium should be stopped, appropriate laboratory samples for assessment of electrolyte concentrations obtained, and a physician consulted before resuming treatment. The rate of infusion must be no more than 1 mg/kg/minute. The potential for renal impairment may be minimized by accompanying foscarnet sodium administration with hydration adequate to establish and maintain a diuresis during dosing.

Carcinogenesis, Mutagenesis, and Impairment of Fertility: Carcinogenicity studies were conducted in rats and mice at oral doses of 500 mg/kg/day and 250 mg/kg/day. Oral bioavailability in unfasted rodents is <20%. No evidence of oncogenicity was reported at plasma drug levels equal to 1/3 and 1/5, respectively, of those in humans (at the maximum recommended human daily dose) as measured by the area-under-the-time/concentration curve (AUC).

Foscarnet sodium showed genotoxic effects in the BALB/3T3 *in vitro* transformation assay at concentrations greater than 0.5 mcg/ml and an increased frequency of chromosome aberrations in the sister chromatid exchange assay at 1000 mcg/ml. A high dose of foscarnet (350 mg/kg) caused an increase in micronucleated polychromatic erythrocytes *in vivo* in mice at doses that produced exposures (Area Under Curve) comparable to that anticipated clinically.

Pregnancy, Teratogenic Effects, Pregnancy Category C: Foscarnet sodium did not adversely affect fertility and general reproductive performance in rats. The results of peri- and post-natal studies in rats were also negative. However, these studies used exposures that are inadequate to define the potential for impairment of fertility at human drug exposure levels.

Daily subcutaneous doses up to 75 mg/kg administered to female rats prior to and during mating, during gestation, and 21 days post-partum caused a slight increase (<5%) in the number of skeletal anomalies compared with the control group. Daily subcutaneous doses up to 75 mg/kg administered to rabbits and 150 mg/kg administered to rats during gestation caused an increase in the frequency of skeletal anomalies/variations. On the basis of estimated drug exposure (as measured by AUC), the 150 mg/kg dose in rats and 75 mg/kg dose in rabbits were approximately one-eighth (rat) and one-third (rabbit) the estimated maximal daily human exposure. These studies are inadequate to define the potential teratogenicity at levels to which women will be exposed.

There are no adequate and well controlled studies in pregnant women. Because animal reproductive studies are not always predictive of human response, foscarnet sodium should be used during pregnancy only if clearly needed.

Nursing Mothers: It is not known whether foscarnet sodium is excreted in human milk; however, in lactating rats administered 75 mg/kg, foscarnet sodium was excreted in maternal milk at concentrations three times higher than peak maternal blood concentrations. Because many drugs are excreted in human milk, caution should be exercised if foscarnet sodium is administered to a nursing woman.

Pediatric Use: The safety and effectiveness of foscarnet sodium in children have not been studied. Foscarnet sodium is deposited in teeth and bone and deposition is greater in young and growing animals. Foscarnet sodium has been demonstrated to adversely affect development of tooth enamel in mice and rats. The effects of this deposition on skeletal development have not been studied. Since deposition in human bone also occurs, it is likely that it does so to a greater degree in developing bone in children. Administration to children should be undertaken only after careful evaluation and only if the potential benefits for treatment outweigh the risks.

Geriatric Use: No studies of the efficacy or safety of foscarnet sodium in persons over age 65 have been conducted. Since these individuals frequently have reduced glomerular filtration, particular attention should be paid to assessing renal function before and during foscarnet sodium administration (see DOSAGE AND ADMINISTRATION).

DRUG INTERACTIONS:

Coadministration of foscarnet sodium with other drugs could theoretically alter its antiviral activity, toxicity or pharmacokinetics.

A possible drug interaction of foscarnet sodium and intravenous pentamidine has been described. Concomitant treatment of four patients in the United Kingdom with foscarnet sodium and intravenous pentamidine may have caused hypocalcemia; one patient died with severe hypocalcemia. Toxicity associated with concomitant use of aerosolized pentamidine has not been reported.

The elimination of foscarnet may be impaired by drugs that inhibit renal tubular secretion; however, no studies have been conducted to determine whether this occurs. Nonetheless, because of foscarnet's tendency to cause renal impairment, the use of foscarnet sodium should be avoided in combination with potentially nephrotoxic drugs such as aminoglycosides, amphotericin B and intravenous pentamidine (see DRUG INTERACTIONS) unless the potential benefits outweigh the risks to the patient.

Since foscarnet sodium decreases serum levels of ionized calcium, concurrent treatment with other drugs known to influence serum calcium levels should be used with particular caution.

Foscarnet sodium was used concomitantly with zidovudine in approximately one-third of patients in the U.S. studies. Although the combination was generally well tolerated, additive effects on anemia may have occurred. In one study of 24 patients (FOS-03), anemia was reported as an adverse event in 60% (3/5) of patients receiving foscarnet sodium only, 88% (7/8) of patients receiving both zidovudine and foscarnet sodium, 29% (2/7) of patients receiving only zidovudine and 25% (1/4) of patients receiving neither drug. However, no evidence of increased myelosuppression was seen with foscarnet sodium in combination with zidovudine.

ADVERSE REACTIONS:

In five controlled U.S. clinical trials in which 189 patients with AIDS and CMV retinitis were treated with foscarnet sodium, the most frequently reported events were the following: fever 65% (123/189), nausea 47% (88/189), anemia 33% (63/189), diarrhea 30% (57/189), abnormal renal function including acute renal failure, decreased creatinine clearance and increased serum creatinine 27% (51/189), vomiting 26% (50/189), headache 26% (49/189), and seizure 10% (18/189) (see WARNINGS and PRECAUTIONS). These incidence figures were calculated without reference to drug relationship or severity.

From the same controlled studies, adverse events categorized by investigator as "severe" were death (14%), abnormal renal function (14%), marrow suppression (10%), anemia (9%), and seizures (7%). Although death was specifically attributed to foscarnet sodium in only one case, other complications of foscarnet (*i.e.,* renal impairment, electrolyte abnormalities, and seizures) may have contributed to patient deaths (see WARNINGS and PRECAUTIONS).

From the five U.S. controlled clinical trials of foscarnet sodium, the following list of adverse events has been compiled regardless of causal relationship to foscarnet sodium. Evaluation of these reports was difficult because of the diverse manifestations of the underlying disease and because most patients received numerous concomitant medications.

Incidence 5% or Greater

ADVERSE REACTIONS: *(cont'd)*

Body as a Whole: fever, fatigue, rigors, asthenia, malaise, pain, infection, sepsis, death

Central and Peripheral Nervous System: headache, paresthesia, dizziness, involuntary muscle contractions, hypoesthesia, neuropathy, seizures including grand mal seizures (see WARNINGS.)

Gastrointestinal System: anorexia, nausea, diarrhea, vomiting, abdominal pain

Hematologic: anemia, granulocytopenia, leukopenia (see PRECAUTIONS.)

Metabolic and Nutritional: mineral and electrolyte imbalances (see WARNINGS.) including hypokalemia, hypocalcemia, hypomagnesemia, hypophosphatemia, hyperphosphatemia

Psychiatric: depression, confusion, anxiety

Respiratory System: coughing, dyspnea

Skin and Appendages: rash, increased sweating

Urinary: alterations in renal function including increased serum creatinine, decreased creatinine clearance, and abnormal renal function (see WARNINGS)

Special Senses: vision abnormalities

Incidence between 1% and 5%

Application Site: injection site pain, injection site inflammation

Body as a Whole: back pain, chest pain, edema, influenza-like symptoms, bacterial infections, moniliasis, fungal infections, abscess

Cardiovascular: hypertension, palpitations, ECG abnormalities including sinus tachycardia, first degree AV block and non-specific ST-T segment changes, hypotension, flushing, cerebrovascular disorder (see WARNINGS)

Central and Peripheral Nervous System: tremor, ataxia, dementia, stupor, generalized spasms, sensory disturbances, meningitis, aphasia, abnormal coordination, leg cramps, EEG abnormalities (see WARNINGS)

Gastrointestinal: constipation, dysphagia, dyspepsia, rectal hemorrhage, dry mouth, melena, flatulence, ulcerative stomatitis, pancreatitis

Hematologic: thrombocytopenia, platelet abnormalities, thrombosis, white blood cell abnormalities, lymphadenopathy

Liver and Biliary: abnormal A-G ratio, abnormal hepatic function, increased SGPT, increased SGOT

Metabolic and Nutritional: hyponatremia, decreased weight, increased alkaline phosphatase, increased LDH, increased BUN, acidosis, cachexia, thirst, hypercalcemia (see WARNINGS)

Musculo-Skeletal: arthralgia, myalgia

Neoplasms: lymphoma-like disorder, sarcoma

Psychiatric: insomnia, somnolence, nervousness, amnesia, agitation, aggressive reaction, hallucination

Respiratory System: pneumonia, sinusitis, pharyngitis, rhinitis, respiratory disorders, respiratory insufficiency, pulmonary infiltration, stridor, pneumothorax, hemoptysis, bronchospasm

Skin and Appendages: pruritus, skin ulceration, seborrhea, erythematous rash, maculo-papular rash, skin discoloration

Special Senses: taste perversions, eye abnormalities, eye pain, conjunctivitis

Urinary System: albuminuria, dysuria, polyuria, urethral disorder, urinary retention, urinary tract infections, acute renal failure, nocturia, facial edema

Incidence less than 1%

Body as a Whole: hypothermia, leg edema, peripheral edema, syncope, ascites, substernal chest pain, abnormal crying, malignant hyperpyrexia, herpes simplex, viral infection, toxoplasmosis

Cardiovascular: cardiomyopathy, cardiac failure, cardiac arrest, bradycardia, extrasystole, arrhythmias, atrial arrhythmias, atrial fibrillation, phlebitis, superficial thrombophlebitis of the arm, mesenteric vein thrombophlebitis

Central and Peripheral Nervous System: vertigo, coma, encephalopathy, abnormal gait, hyperesthesia, hypertonia, visual field defects, dyskinesia, extrapyramidal disorders, hemiparesis, hyperkinesia, vocal cord paralysis, paralysis, paraplegia, speech disorders, tetany, hyporeflexia, neuralgia, neuritis, peripheral neuropathy, hyperreflexia, cerebral edema, nystagmus

Endocrine: antidiuretic hormone disorders, decreased gonadotropins, gynecomastia

Gastrointestinal System: enteritis, enterocolitis, glossitis, proctitis, stomatitis, tenesmus, increased amylase, pseudomembranous colitis, gastroenteritis, oral leukoplakia, oral hemorrhage, rectal disorders, colitis, duodenal ulcer, hematemesis, paralytic ileus, esophageal ulceration, ulcerative proctitis, tongue ulceration

Hematologic: pulmonary embolism, coagulation disorders, decreased coagulation factors, epistaxis, decreased prothrombin, hypochromic anemia, pancytopenia, hemolysis, leukocytosis, cervical lymphadenopathy, lymphopenia

Special Senses: deafness, earache, tinnitus, otitis

Liver and Biliary System: cholecystitis, cholelithiasis, hepatitis, cholestatic hepatitis, hepatosplenomegaly, jaundice

Metabolic and Nutritional: dehydration, glycosuria, increased creatine phosphokinase, diabetes mellitus, abnormal glucose tolerance, hypervolemia, hypochloremia, periorbital edema, hypoproteinemia

Musculo-Skeletal System: arthrosis, synovitis, torticollis

Neoplasms: malignant lymphoma, skin hypertrophy

Psychiatric: impaired concentration, emotional lability, psychosis, suicide attempt, delirium, personality disorders, sleep disorders

Reproductive: perineal pain in women, penile inflammation

Respiratory System: bronchitis, laryngitis, respiratory depression, abnormal chest x-ray, pleural effusion, lobar pneumonia, pulmonary hemorrhage, pneumonitis

Skin and Appendages: acne, alopecia, dermatitis, anal pruritus, genital pruritus, aggravated psoriasis, psoriaform rash, skin disorders, dry skin, urticaria, verruca

Urinary System: hematuria, glomerulonephritis, micturition disorders, micturition frequency, toxic nephropathy, nephrosis, urinary incontinence, renal tubular disorders, pyelonephritis, urethral irritation, uremia

Special Senses: diplopia, blindness, retinal detachment, mydriasis, photophobia

The types and incidences of adverse events reported worldwide in post-marketing surveillance for foscarnet sodium have not been different from or greater in frequency than those observed in U.S. clinical trials. Rare events that have appeared in post-marketing surveillance include: ventricular arrhythmia, prolongation of QT interval, nephrogenic diabetes insipidus, and muscular weakness.

OVERDOSAGE:

In controlled clinical trials performed in the United States, overdosage with foscarnet sodium was reported in 10 out of 189 patients. All 10 patients experienced adverse events and all except one made a complete recovery. One patient died after receiving a total daily dose of 12.5 g for three days instead of the intended 10.9 g. The patient suffered a grand mal seizure

OVERDOSAGE: *(cont'd)*

and became comatose. Three days later the patient expired with the cause of death listed as respiratory/cardiac arrest. The other nine patients received doses ranging from 1.14 times to 8 times their recommended doses with an average of 4 times their recommended doses. Overall, three patients had seizures, three patients had renal function impairment, four patients had paresthesia either in limbs or periorally, and five patients had documented electrolyte disturbances primarily involving calcium and phosphate.

The pattern of adverse events associated with overdose in post-marketing surveillance is consistent with the symptoms previously observed during foscarnet therapy.

There is no specific antidote for foscarnet sodium overdose. Hemodialysis and hydration may be of benefit in reducing drug plasma levels in patients who receive an overdosage of foscarnet sodium, but the effectiveness of these interventions has not been evaluated. The patient should be observed for signs and symptoms of renal impairment and electrolyte imbalance. Medical treatment should be instituted if clinically warranted.

DOSAGE AND ADMINISTRATION:

CAUTION: DO NOT ADMINISTER FOSCARNET SODIUM BY RAPID OR BOLUS INTRAVENOUS INJECTION. THE TOXICITY OF FOSCARNET SODIUM MAY BE INCREASED AS A RESULT OF EXCESSIVE PLASMA LEVELS. CARE SHOULD BE TAKEN TO AVOID UNINTENTIONAL OVERDOSE BY CAREFULLY CONTROLLING THE RATE OF INFUSION. THEREFORE, AN INFUSION PUMP MUST BE USED. IN SPITE OF THE USE OF AN INFUSION PUMP, OVERDOSES HAVE OCCURRED.

ADMINISTRATION

Foscarnet sodium is administered by controlled intravenous infusion, either by using a central venous line by using a peripheral vein. The standard 24 mg/ml solution may be used without dilution when using a central venous catheter for infusion. When a peripheral vein catheter is used, the 24 mg/ml solution **must**be diluted to 12 mg/ml with 5% dextrose in water or with a normal saline solution prior to administration to avoid local irritation of peripheral veins. Since the dose of foscarnet sodium is calculated on the basis of body weight, it may be desirable to remove and discard any unneeded quantity from the bottle before starting with the infusion to avoid overdosage. Dilutions and/or removals of excess quantities should be accomplished under aseptic conditions. Solutions thus prepared should be used within 24 hours of first entry into a sealed bottle.

Other drugs and supplements can be administered to a patient receiving foscarnet sodium. However, care must be taken to ensure that foscarnet sodium is only administered with normal saline or 5% dextrose solution and that no other drug or supplement is administered concurrently via the same catheter. Foscarnet has been reported to be chemically incompatible with 30% dextrose, amphotericin B, and solutions containing calcium such as Ringer's lactate and TPN. Physical incompatibility with other IV drugs has also been reported including acyclovir sodium, ganciclovir, trimetrexate glucuronate, pentamidine isethionate, vancomycin, trimethoprim/sulfamethoxazole, diazepam, midazolam, digoxin, phenytoin, leucovorin, and prochlorperazine. Because of foscarnet's chelating properties, a precipitate can potentially occur when divalent cations are administered concurrently in the same catheter.

Parenteral drug products must be inspected visually for particulate matter and discoloration prior to administration whenever the solution and container permit. Solutions that are discolored or contain particulate matter should not be used.

Accidental Exposure: Accidental skin and eye contact with foscarnet sodium solution may cause local irritation and burning sensation. If accidental contact occurs, the exposed area should be flushed with water.

DOSAGE

THE RECOMMENDED DOSAGE, FREQUENCY, OR INFUSION RATES SHOULD NOT BE EXCEEDED. ALL DOSES MUST BE INDIVIDUALIZED FOR PATIENTS' RENAL FUNCTION.

Induction Treatment

The recommended initial dose of foscarnet sodium for patients with normal renal function is 60 mg/kg (minimum one hour infusion) every eight hours for CMV retinitis patients over 2-3 weeks depending on clinical response, and 40 mg/kg (minimum one hour infusion) either every 8 or 12 hours for acyclovir-resistant HSV patients for 2-3 weeks or until healed.

An infusion pump must be used to control the rate of infusion. Adequate hydration is recommended to establish a diuresis, both prior to and during treatment to minimize renal toxicity (see WARNINGS), provided there are no clinical contraindications.

Maintenance Treatment: Following induction treatment the recommended maintenance dose of foscarnet sodium is 90 mg/kg/day to 120 mg/kg/day (individualized for renal function) given as an intravenous infusion over 2 hours. Because the superiority of the 120 mg/kg/day has not been established in controlled trials, and given the likely relationship of higher plasma foscarnet levels to toxicity, it is recommended that most patients be started on maintenance treatment with a dose of 90 mg/kg/day. Escalation to 120 mg/kg/day may be considered should early reinduction be required because of retinitis progression. Some patients who show excellent tolerance to foscarnet sodium may benefit from initiation of maintenance treatment at 120 mg/kg/day earlier in their treatment. An infusion pump must be used to control the rate of infusion with all doses. Again, hydration to establish diuresis both prior to and during treatment is recommended to minimize renal toxicity, provided there are no clinical contraindications (see WARNINGS).

Patients who experience progression of retinitis while receiving foscarnet sodium maintenance therapy may be retreated with the induction and maintenance regimens given above.

Use in Patients with Abnormal Renal Function: Foscarnet sodium should be used with caution in patients with abnormal renal function because reduced plasma clearance of foscarnet will result in elevated plasma levels (see CLINICAL PHARMACOLOGY). In addition, foscarnet sodium has the potential to further impair renal function (see WARNINGS). Foscarnet sodium has not been specifically studied in patients with creatinine clearances <50 ml/min or serum creatinines >2.8 mg/dl. Renal function must be monitored carefully at baseline and during induction and maintenance therapy with appropriate dose adjustments for foscarnet sodium as outlined below (see DOSAGE AND ADMINISTRATION, Dose Adjustment and Patient Monitoring). During foscarnet sodium therapy if creatinine clearance falls below the limits of the dosing nomograms (0.4 ml/min/kg), foscarnet sodium should be discontinued and the patient monitored daily until resolution of renal impairment is ensured.

Dose Adjustment

Foscarnet sodium dosing must be individualized according to the patient's renal function status. Refer to TABLE 5 for recommended doses and adjust the dose as indicated.

To use this dosing guide, actual 24-hour creatinine clearance (ml/min) must be divided by body weight (kg), or the estimated creatinine clearance in ml/min/kg can be calculated from serum creatinine (mg/dl) using the formula (modified Cockcroft and Gault equation) found in TABLE 4.

TABLE 4

For males: [140 - age] ÷ [serum creatinine × 72]
For females: Above value × 0.85

DOSAGE AND ADMINISTRATION: *(cont'd)*

TABLE 5 Foscarnet Sodium Dosing Guide Induction

CrCl (ml/min/kg)	HSV Equivalent to 40 mg/kg Q12h	HSV Equivalent to 40 mg/kg Q8h	CMV Equivalent to 60 mg/kg Q8h
≥1.6	40	40	60
1.5	38	38	57
1.4	36	35	53
1.3	34	33	49
1.2	32	31	46
1.1	31	28	42
1.0	30	26	39
0.9	28	24	35
0.8	26	21	32
0.7	24	19	28
0.6	23	17	25
0.5	21	14	21
0.4	19	12	18
MAINTENANCE:			
CrCl (ml/min/kg)		**Equivalent to 90 mg/kg Q24h**	**CMV Equivalent to 120 mg/kg Q24h**
≥1.4		90	120
1.2-1.4		78	104
1.0-1.2		75	100
0.8-1.0		71	94
0.6-0.8		63	84
0.4-0.6		57	76

Patient Monitoring

The majority of patients will experience some decrease in renal function due to foscarnet sodium administration. Therefore it is recommended that creatinine clearance, either measured or estimated using the modified Cockcroft and Gault equation based on serum creatinine, be determined at baseline, 2-3 times per week during induction therapy and at least once every one to two weeks during maintenance therapy, with foscarnet sodium dose adjusted accordingly (see DOSAGE AND ADMINISTRATION, Dose Adjustment). More frequent monitoring may be required for some patients. It is also recommended that a 24-hour creatinine clearance be determined at baseline and periodically thereafter to ensure correct dosing (assuming verification of an adequate collection using creatinine index). Foscarnet sodium should be discontinued if creatinine clearance drops below 0.4 ml/min/kg.

Due to foscarnet sodium's propensity to chelate divalent metal ions and alter levels of serum electrolytes, patients must be monitored closely for such changes. It is recommended that a schedule similar to that recommended for serum creatinine see DOSAGE AND ADMINISTRATION, Dose Adjustment be used to monitor serum calcium, magnesium, potassium and phosphorus. Particular caution is advised in patients with decreased total serum calcium or other electrolyte levels before treatment, as well as in patients with neurologic or cardiac abnormalities, and in patients receiving other drugs known to influence serum calcium levels. Any clinically significant metabolic changes should be corrected. Also, patients who experience mild (*e.g.,* perioral numbness or paresthesias) or severe (*e.g.,* seizures) symptoms of electrolyte abnormalities should have serum electrolyte and mineral levels assessed as close in time to the event as possible.

Careful monitoring and appropriate management of electrolytes, calcium, magnesium and creatinine are of particular importance in patients with conditions that may predispose them to seizures (see WARNINGS).

HOW SUPPLIED:

Foscavir Injection, 24 mg/ml for intravenous infusion, is supplied in glass bottles.

Foscarnet sodium injection should be stored at controlled room temperature 15°-30°C (59°-86°F), and should be protected from excessive heat (above 40°C) and from freezing. Foscarnet sodium injection should be used only if the bottle and seal are intact, a vacuum is present, and the solution is clear and colorless.

HOW SUPPLIED - EQUIVALENTS NOT AVAILABLE:

Solution - Intravenous - 24 mg/ml

250 ml	$73.28	FOSCAVIR, Astra USA	00186-1905-01
500 ml	$145.93	FOSCAVIR, Astra USA	00186-1906-01

FOSINOPRIL SODIUM *(003052)*

CATEGORIES: ACE Inhibitors; Angiotensin Converting Enzyme Inhibitors; Antihypertensives; Cardiovascular Drugs; Heart Failure; Hypertension; Pregnancy Category D; FDA Class 1C ("Little or No Therapeutic Advantage"); FDA Approved 1991 May; Top 200 Drugs; Top 200 Drugs

BRAND NAMES: *Acenor-M*; *Dynacil* (Germany); *Fosinorm* (Germany); *Fozitec* (France); **Monopril**; *Staril* (England); *Vasopril*
(International brand names outside U.S. in italics)

FORMULARIES: PCS

COST OF THERAPY: $266.37 (Hypertension; Tablet; 10 mg; 1/day; 365 days) vs. Potential Cost of $24,027.04 (Coronary Bypass)

PRIMARY ICD9: 401.1 (Essential Hypertension, Benign)

WARNING:
Use In Pregnancy: When used in pregnancy during the second and third trimesters, ACE inhibitors can cause injury and even death to the developing fetus When pregnancy is detected, fosinopril sodium should be discontinued as soon as possible. See WARNINGS, Fetal/Neonatal Morbidity and Mortality.

DESCRIPTION:

Fosinopril sodium is the sodium salt of fosinopril, the ester prodrug of an angiotensin converting enzyme (ACE) inhibitor, fosinoprilat. It contains a phosphinate group capable of specific binding to the active site of angiotensin converting enzyme. Fosinopril sodium is designated chemically as: L-proline, 4-cyclohexyl-1-[[[2-methyl-1-(1-oxopropoxy) propoxyl](4-phenyl-butyl) phosphinyl]acetyl]-,sodium salt, *trans-*.

Fosinopril sodium is a white to off-white crystalline powder. It is soluble in water (100 mg/ml), methanol, and ethanol and slightly soluble in hexane.

DESCRIPTION: *(cont'd)*

Its empiric formula is $C_{30}H_{45}NNaO_7P$, and its molecular weight is 585.65.

Monopril is available for oral administration as 10 mg and 20 mg tablets. Inactive ingredients include: lactose, microcrystalline cellulose, crospovidone, povidone, and sodium stearyl fumarate.

CLINICAL PHARMACOLOGY:

MECHANISM OF ACTION

In animals and humans, fosinopril sodium is hydrolyzed by esterases to the pharmacologically active form, fosinoprilat, a specific competitive inhibitor of angiotensin converting enzyme (ACE).

ACE is a peptidyl dipeptidase that catalyzes the conversion of angiotensin I to the vasoconstrictor substance, angiotensin II. Angiotensin II also stimulates aldosterone secretion by the adrenal cortex. Inhibition of ACE results in decreased plasma angiotensin II, which leads to decreased vasopressor activity and to decreased aldosterone secretion. The latter decrease may result in a small increase of serum potassium.

In 647 hypertensive patients treated with fosinopril alone for an average of 29 weeks, mean increases in serum potassium of 0.1 mEq/L were observed. Similar increases were observed among all patients treated with fosinopril, including those receiving concomitant diuretic therapy. Removal of angiotensin II negative feedback on renin secretion leads to increased plasma renin activity.

ACE is identical to kininase, an enzyme that degrades bradykinin. Whether increased levels of bradykinin, a potent vasopressor peptide, play a role in the therapeutic effects of fosinopril sodium remains to be elucidated.

While the mechanism through which fosinopril sodium lowers blood pressure is believed to be primarily suppression of the renin-angiotensin-aldosterone system, fosinopril sodium has an antihypertensive effect even inpatients with low-renin hypertension. Although fosinopril sodium was antihypertensive in all races studied, black hypertensive patients(usually a low-renin hypertensive population) had a smaller average response to ACE inhibitor monotherapy than non-black patients.

PHARMACOKINETICS AND METABOLISM

Following oral administration, fosinopril (the prodrug) is absorbed slowly. The absolute absorption of fosinopril averaged 36% of an oral dose. The primary site of absorption is the proximal small intestine (duodenum/jejunum). While the rate of absorption may be slowed by the presence of food in the gastrointestinal tract, the extent of absorption of fosinopril is essentially unaffected.

Fosinoprilat is highly protein-bound ($\geq$ 95%), has a relatively small volume of distribution, and has negligible binding to cellular components in blood. After single and multiple oral doses, plasma levels, areas under plasma concentration-time curves (AUCs) and peak concentrations (C_{max}) are directly proportional to the dose of fosinopril. Times to peak concentrations are independent of dose and are achieved in approximately 3 hours.

After an oral dose of radiolabeled fosinopril, 75% of radioactivity in plasma was present as active fosinoprilat, 20-30% as a glucuronide conjugate of fosinoprilat, and 1-5% as a *p*-hydroxy metabolite of fosinoprilat. Since fosinoprilat is not biotransformed after intravenous administration, fosinopril, not fosinoprilat, appears to be the precursor for the glucuronide and *p*-hydroxy metabolites. In rats, the*p*- hydroxy metabolite of fosinoprilat is as potent an inhibitor of ACE as fosinoprilat; the glucuronide conjugate is devoid of ACE inhibitor activity.

After intravenous administration, fosinoprilat was eliminated approximately equally by the liver and kidney. After oral administration of radiolabeled fosinopril, approximately half of the absorbed dose is excreted and the urine and the remainder is excreted in the feces. In two studies involving healthy subjects, the mean body clearance of intravenous fosinoprilat was between 26 and 39 ml/min.

In healthy subjects, the terminal elimination half-life (t1/2) of an intravenous dose of radiolabeled fosinoprilat is approximately 12 hours. In hypertensive patients with normal renal and hepatic function, who received repeated doses of fosinopril, the effective t1/2 for accumulation of fosinoprilat averaged 11.5 hours.

In patients with renal insufficiency: (creatinine clearance < 80 ml/min/1.73 m^2), the total body clearance of fosinoprilat is approximately one-half of that in patients with normal renal function, while absorption, bioavailability, and protein-binding are not appreciably altered. The clearance of fosinoprilat does not differ appreciably with the degree of renal insufficiency,because the diminished renal elimination is offset by increased hepatobiliary elimination. A modest increase in plasma AUC levels (less than two times that in normals) was observed in patients with various degrees of renal insufficiency, including end-stage renal failure (creatinine clearance < 10 ml/min/ 1.73 m^2). (See DOSAGE AND ADMINISTRATION.)

Fosinopril is not well dialyzed. Clearance of fosinoprilat by hemodialysis and peritoneal dialysis averages 2% and 7%, respectively, of urea clearances.

In patients with hepatic insufficiency (alcoholic or biliary cirrhosis): , the extent of hydrolysis of fosinopril is not appreciably reduced, although the rate of hydrolysis may be slowed;the apparent total body clearance of fosinoprilat is approximately one-half of that in patients with normal hepatic function.

In elderly (male) subjects: (65-74 years old) with clinically normal renal and hepatic function, there appear to be no significant differences in pharmacokinetic parameters for fosinoprilat compared to those of younger subjects (20-35 years old).

Fosinoprilat was found to cross the placenta of pregnant animals.

Studies in animals indicate that fosinopril and fosinoprilat do not cross the blood-brain barrier.

PHARMACODYNAMICS AND CLINICAL EFFECTS

Serum ACE activity was inhibited $\geq$ 90% at 2 to 12 hours after single doses of 10 to 40 mg of fosinopril. At 24 hours, serum ACE activity remained suppressed by 85%, 93%, and 93% in the 10, 20 and 40 mg dose groups, respectively.

Administration of fosinopril sodium to patients with mild to moderate hypertension results in a reduction of both supine and standing blood pressure to about the same extent with no compensatory tachycardia. Symptomatic postural hypotension is infrequent,although in can occur in patients who are salt-and/or volume-depleted (see WARNINGS.) Use of fosinopril sodium in combination with thiazide diuretics gives a blood pressure-lowering effect greater than that seen with either agent alone.

Following oral administration of single doses of 10-40 mg, fosinopril sodium lowered blood pressure within one hour, with peak reductions achieved 2-6 hours after dosing. The antihypertensive effect of a single dose persisted for 24 hours. Following four weeks of monotherapy in placebo-controlled trials in patients with mild to moderate hypertension, once daily doses of 20-80 mg lowered supine or seated systolic and diastolic blood pressures at 24 hours after dosing by an average of 8-9/6-7 mmHg more than placebo. The trough effect was about 50-60% of the peak diastolic response and about 80% of the peak systolic response.

CLINICAL PHARMACOLOGY: *(cont'd)*

In most trials, the antihypertensive effect of fosinopril sodium increased during the first several weeks of repeated measurements. The antihypertensive effect of fosinopril sodium has been shown to continue during long-term therapy for at least 2 years. Abrupt withdrawal of fosinopril sodium has not resulted in a rapid increase in blood pressure.

Limited experience in controlled and uncontrolled trials combining fosinopril with a calcium channel blocker or a loop diuretic has indicated no unusual drug-drug interactions. Other ACE inhibitors have had less than additive effects with beta-adrenergic blockers, presumably because both drugs lower blood pressure by inhibiting parts of the renin-angiotensin system.

ACE inhibitors are generally less effective in blacks than in non-blacks. The effectiveness of fosinopril sodium was not influenced by age, sex, or weight.

In hemodynamic studies in hypertensive patients after three months of therapy, responses (changes in BP, heart rate, cardiac index,and PVR) to various stimuli (*e.g.,* isometric exercise, 45° head-up tilt, and mental challenge) were unchanged compared to baseline, suggesting that fosinopril sodium does not affect the activity of the sympathetic nervous system. Reduction in systemic blood pressure appears to have been mediated by a decrease in peripheral vascular resistance without reflex cardiac effects. Similarly, renal, splanchnic, cerebral, and skeletal muscle blood flow were unchanged compared to baseline, as was glomerular filtration rate.

INDICATIONS AND USAGE:

Fosinopril sodium is indicated for the treatment of hypertension. It may be used alone or in combination with thiazide diuretics.

In using fosinopril sodium, consideration should be given to the fact that another angiotensin converting enzyme inhibitor, captopril, has caused agranulocytosis, particularly in patients with renal impairment or collagen-vascular disease. Available data are insufficient to show that fosinopril sodium does not have a similar risk (see WARNINGS.)

CONTRAINDICATIONS:

Fosinopril sodium is contraindicated in patients who are hypersensitive to this product or to any other angiotensin converting enzyme inhibitor (*e.g.,* a patient who has experienced angioedema with any other ACE inhibitor therapy).

WARNINGS:

ANAPHYLACTOID AND POSSIBLY RELATED REACTIONS

Presumably because angiotensin-converting enzyme inhibitors affect the metabolism of eicosanoids and polypeptides, including endogenous bradykinin, patients receiving ACE inhibitors (including fosinopril sodium) may be subject to a variety of adverse reactions, none of them serious.

Angioedema: Angioedema involving the extremities, face, lips, mucous membranes,tongue, glottis, or larynx has been reported in patients treated with ACE inhibitors. If angioedema involves the tongue, glottis,or larynx, airway obstruction may occur and be fatal. If laryngeal stridor or angioedema of the face, lips, mucous membranes, tongue, glottis or extremities occurs, treatment with fosinopril sodium should be discontinued and appropriate therapy instituted immediately. **Where there is involvement of the tongue, glottis, or larynx, likely to cause airway obstruction, appropriate therapy, e.g., subcutaneous epinephrine solution 1:1000 (0.3 ml to 0.5 ml) should be promptly administered** (see PRECAUTIONS, Information For Patients and ADVERSE REACTIONS.

Anaphylactoid reactions during desensitization: Two patients undergoing desensitizing treatment with hymenoptera venom while receiving ACE inhibitors sustained life-threatening anaphylactoid reactions. In the same patients, these reactions were avoided when ACE inhibitors were temporarily withheld, but they reappeared upon inadvertent rechallenge.

Anaphylactoid reactions during membrane exposure: Anaphylactoid reactions have been reported in patients dialyzed with high-flux membranes and treated concomitantly with an ACE inhibitor. Anaphylactoid reactions have also been reported in patients undergoing low-density lipoprotein apheresis with dextran sulfate absorption (a procedure dependent upon devices not approved in the United States).

HYPOTENSION

Fosinopril sodium can cause symptomatic hypotension. Like other ACE inhibitors, fosinopril has been only rarely associated with hypotension in uncomplicated hypertensive patients. Symptomatic hypotension is most likely to occur in patients who have been volume- and/or salt-depleted as a result of prolonged diuretic therapy, dietary salt restriction, dialysis, diarrhea, or vomiting. Volume and/or salt depletion should be corrected before initiating therapy with fosinopril sodium.

In patients with congestive heart failure, with or without associated renal insufficiency, ACE inhibitor therapy may cause excessive hypotension, which may be associated with oliguria or azotemia and, rarely, with acute renal failure and death. In such patients, fosinopril sodium therapy should be started under close medical supervision; they should be followed closely for the first 2 weeks of treatment and whenever the dose of fosinopril or diuretic is increased.

If hypotension occurs, the patient should be placed in a supine position, and, if necessary, treated with intravenous infusion of physiological saline. Fosinopril sodium treatment usually can be continued following restoration of blood pressure and volume.

NEUTROPENIA/AGRANULOCYTOSIS

Another angiotensin converting enzyme inhibitor, captopril, has been shown to cause agranulocytosis and bone marrow depression, rarely in uncomplicated patients, but more frequently in patients with renal impairment, especially if they also have a collagen-vascular disease such as systemic lupus erythematosus or scleroderma. Available data from clinical trials of fosinopril are insufficient to show that fosinopril does not cause agranulocytosis at similar rates. Monitoring of white blood cell counts should be considered on patients with collagen vascular-disease, especially if the disease is associated with impaired renal function.

FETAL/NEONATAL MORBIDITY AND MORTALITY

ACE inhibitors can cause fetal and neonatal morbidity and mortality when administered to pregnant women. Several dozen cases have been reported in the world literature. When pregnancy is detected, ACE inhibitors should be discontinued as soon as possible.

The use of ACE inhibitors during the second and third trimesters of pregnancy has been associated with fetal and neonatal injury, including hypotension, neonatal skull hypoplasia, anuria, reversible or irreversible renal failure, and death. Oligohydramnios has also been reported, presumably resulting from decreased fetal renal function,; oligohydramnios in this setting has been associated with fetal limb contractures, craniofacial malformation, and hypoplastic lung development. Prematurity, intrauterine growth retardation, and patent ductus arteriosus have also been reported, although it is not clear whether these occurrences were due to the ACE-inhibitor exposure.

These adverse effects do not appear to have resulted from intrauterine ACE-inhibitor exposure that has been limited to the first trimester. Mothers whose embryos and fetuses are exposed to ACE inhibitors only during the first trimester should be so informed. Nonetheless, when patients become pregnant, physicians should make every effort to discontinue the use of fosinopril as soon as possible.

WARNINGS: *(cont'd)*

When ACE inhibitors have been used during the second and third trimesters of pregnancy there have been reports of neonatal hypotension, renal failure, skull hypoplasia, and death. Oligohydramnios has also been reported, presumably resulting from decreased fetal renal function; oligohydramnios has been associated with fetal limb contractures, craniofacial malformations,hypoplastic lung development, and intrauterine growth retardation. Prematurity and patent ductus arteriosus have been reported,although it is not clear whether these occurrences were due to the ACE inhibitor exposure or to the mother's underlying disease.

Rarely (probably less often than once in every thousand pregnancies), no alternative to ACE inhibitors will be found. In these rare cases, the mothers should be apprised of the potential hazards to their fetuses, and serial ultrasound examinations should be performed to assess the intramniotic environment.

If oligohydramnios is observed, fosinopril should be discontinued unless it is considered life-saving for the mother. Contraction stress testing (CST), a non-stress test (NST), or biophysical profiling (BPP) may be appropriate, depending upon the week of pregnancy. Patients and physicians should be aware, however, that oligohydramnios may not appear until after the fetus has sustained irreversible injury.

Infants with histories of *in utero* exposure to ACE inhibitors should be closely observed for hypotension, oliguria, and hyperkalemia. If oliguria occurs, attention should be directed toward support of blood pressure and renal perfusion. Exchange transfusion or dialysis may be required as a means of reversing hypotension and/or substituting for disordered renal function. Fosinopril is poorly dialyzed from the circulation of adults by hemodialysis and peritoneal dialysis. There is no experience with ant procedure for removing fosinopril from the neonatal circulation.

When fosinopril was given to pregnant rats at doses about 80 to 250 times (on a mg/kg basis) the maximum recommended human dose, three similar orofacial malformations and one fetus with *situs inversus* were observed among the off spring. No teratogenic effects of fosinopril were seen in studies in pregnant rabbits at doses up to 25 times (on a mg/kg basis) the maximum recommended human dose.

HEPATIC FAILURE

Rarely, ACE inhibitors have been associated with a syndrome that starts with cholestatic jaundice and progresses to fulminant hepatic necrosis and (sometimes) death. The mechanism of this syndrome is not understood. Patients receiving ACE inhibitors who develop jaundice or marked elevations of hepatic enzymes should discontinue the ACE inhibitor and receive appropriate medical follow-up.

PRECAUTIONS:

GENERAL

Impaired Renal Function: As a consequence of inhibiting the renin-angiotensin-aldosterone system, changes in renal function may be anticipated in susceptible individuals. In patients with severe congestive heart failure whose renal function may depend on the activity of the renin-angiotensin-aldosterone system, treatment with angiotensin converting enzyme inhibitors, including fosinopril sodium,may be associated with oliguria and/or progressive azotemia and (rarely) with acute renal failure and/or death.

In hypertensive patients with renal artery stenosis in a solitary kidney or bilateral renal artery stenosis, increases in blood urea nitrogen and serum creatinine may occur. Experience with another angiotensin converting enzyme inhibitor suggests that these increases are usually reversible upon discontinuation of ACE inhibitor and/or diuretic therapy. In such patients, renal function should be monitored during the first few weeks f therapy. Some hypertensive patients with no apparent pre-existing renal vascular disease have developed increases in blood urea nitrogen and serum creatinine, usually minor and transient, especially when fosinopril sodium has been given concomitantly with a diuretic. This is more likely to occur in patients with pre-existing renal impairment. Dosage reduction of fosinopril sodium and/or discontinuation of the diuretic may be required.

Evaluation of the hypertensive patient should always include assessment of renal function (see DOSAGE AND ADMINISTRATION.)

Impaired renal function decreases total clearance of fosinoprilat and approximately doubles AUC. In general, however, no adjustment of dosing is needed (See CLINICAL PHARMACOLOGY.)

Hyperkalemia: In clinical trials, hyperkalemia (serum potassium greater that 10% above the upper limit of normal) has occurred in approximately 2.6% of hypertensive patients receiving fosinopril sodium. In most cases, these were isolates values which resolved despite continued therapy. In clinical trials, 0.1% of patients (two patients) were discontinued from therapy due to an elevated serum potassium. Risk factors for the development of hyperkalemia include renal insufficiency, diabetes mellitus, and concomitant use of potassium-sparing diuretics, potassium supplements, and/or potassium-containing salt substitutes, which should be used cautiously, if at all, with fosinopril sodium (see DRUG INTERACTIONS.)

Cough: Presumable due to the inhibition of the degradation of endogenous bradykinin, persistent nonproductive cough has been reported with all ACE inhibitors, always resolving after discontinuation of therapy. ACE inhibitor-induced cough should be considered in the differential diagnosis of cough.

Impaired Liver Function: Since fosinopril is primarily metabolized by hepatic and gut wall esterases to its active moiety, fosinoprilat, patients with impaired liver function could develop elevated plasma levels of unchanged fosinopril. In a study in patients with alcoholic or biliary cirrhosis, the extent of hydrolysis was unaffected, although the rate was slowed. In these patients, the apparent total body clearance of fosinoprilat was decreased and the plasma AUC approximately doubled.

Surgery/Anesthesia: In patients undergoing surgery or during anesthesia with agents that produce hypotension, fosinopril will block the angiotensin II formation that could otherwise occur secondary to compensatory renin release. Hypotension that occurs as a result of this mechanism can by corrected by volume expansion.

HEMODIALYSIS

Recent clinical observations have shown an association of hypersensitivity-like (anaphylactoid) reactions during hemodialysis with high-flux dialysis membranes (*e.g.,* AN69) in patients receiving ACE inhibitors as medication. In these patients, consideration should be given to using a different type of dialysis membrane or a different class of medication. See WARNINGS, Anaphylactoid reactions during membrane exposure.

INFORMATION FOR THE PATIENT

Angioedema: Angioedema, including laryngeal edema, can occur with treatment with ACE inhibitor, especially following the first dose.Patients should be advised to immediately report to their physician any signs or symptoms suggesting angioedema (*e.g.,* swelling of face, eyes, lips, tongue, larynx, mucous membranes, and extremities; difficulty in swallowing or breathing; hoarseness) and to discontinue therapy. See WARNINGS, Angioedema and ADVERSE REACTIONS

Symptomatic Hypotension: Patients should be cautioned that lightheadedness can occur, especially during the first days of therapy, and it should be reported to a physician. Patients should be told that if syncope occurs, fosinopril sodium should be discontinued until the physician has been consulted.

PRECAUTIONS: *(cont'd)*

All patients should be cautioned that inadequate fluid intake or excessive perspiration, diarrhea, or vomiting can lead to an excessive fall in blood pressure, with the same consequences of lightheadedness and possible syncope.

Hyperkalemia: Patients should be told not to use potassium supplements or salt substitutes containing potassium without consulting the physician.

Neutropenia: Patients should be told to promptly report any indication of infection (*e.g.,* sore throat, fever), which could be a sign of neutropenia.

Pregnancy: Female patients of childbearing age should be told about the consequences of second- and third-trimester exposure to ACE inhibitors, and they should also be told that these consequences do not appear to have resulted from intrauterine ACE-inhibitor exposure that has been limited to the first trimester. These patients should be asked to report pregnancies to their physicians as soon as possible.

DRUG/LABORATORY TEST INTERACTION

Fosinopril may cause a false low measurement of serum digoxin levels with the Digi-Tab RIA Kit for Digoxin. Other kits, such as the Coat-A-Count RIA Kit, may be used.

CARCINOGENESIS, MUTAGENESIS, AND IMPAIRMENT OF FERTILITY

No evidence of a carcinogenic effect was found when fosinopril was given in the diet to mice and rats for up to 24 months at doses up to 400 mg/kg/day. On a body weight basis, the highest dose in mice and rats is about 250 times the maximum human dose of 80 mg,assuming a 50 kg subject. On a body surface area basis, in mice, this dose is 20 times the maximum human dose; in rats, this dose is 40 times the maximum human dose. Male rats given the highest dose level had a slightly higher incidence of mesentery/omentum lipomas.

Neither fosinopril nor the active fosinoprilat was mutagenic in the Ames microbial mutagen test, the mouse lymphoma forward mutation assay, or a mitotic gene conversion assay. Fosinopril was also not genotoxic in a mouse micronucleus test *in vivo* and a mouse bone marrow cytogenic assay *in vivo.*

In the Chinese hamster ovary cell cytogenic assay, fosinopril increased the frequency of chromosomal aberrations when tested without metabolic activation at a concentration that was toxic to the cells. However, there was no increase in chromosomal aberrations at lower drug concentration without metabolic activation or at any concentration with metabolic activation.

There were no adverse reproductive effects in male and female rats treated with 15 or 60 mg/kg/daily. On a body weight basis, the high dose of 60 mg/kg is about 38 times the maximum recommended human dose. On a body surface area basis, this dose is 6 times the maximum recommended human dose. There was no effect on pairing time prior to mating in rats until a daily dose of 240 mg/kg, atoxic dose, was given; at this dose, a slight increase in pairing time was observed. On a body weight basis, this dose is 150 times the maximum recommended human dose. On a body surface area basis,this dose is 24 times the maximum recommended human dose.

PREGNANCY CATEGORIES C (FIRST TRIMESTER) AND D (SECOND AND THIRD TRIMESTERS)

See WARNINGS, Fetal/Neonatal Morbidity and Mortality.

NURSING MOTHERS

Ingestion of 20 mg daily for three days resulted in detectable levels of fosinoprilat in breast milk. Fosinopril sodium should not be administered to nursing mothers.

GERIATRIC USE

Of the total number of patients who received fosinopril in US clinical studies of fosinopril sodium, 13% were 65 and older whole 1.3% were 75 and older. No overall differences in effectiveness or safety were observed between these patients and younger patients, and other reported clinical experience has not identified differences in response between the elderly and younger patients, but greater sensitivity of some older individuals cannot be ruled out.

In a pharmacokinetic study comparing elderly (65-74 years old) and non-elderly (20-35 years old) healthy volunteers, there were no differences between the groups in peak fosinoprilat levels or area under the plasma concentration time curve (AUC).

PEDIATRIC USE

Safety and effectiveness in children have not been established.

DRUG INTERACTIONS:

With diuretics: Patients on diuretic, especially those with intravascular volume depletion, may occasionally experience an excessive reduction of blood pressure after initiation of therapy with fosinopril sodium. The possibility of hypotensive effects can be minimized by either discontinuing the diuretic or increasing salt intake prior to initiation of treatment with fosinopril sodium. If this is not possible, the starting dose should be reduced and the patient should be observed closely for several hours following an initial dose and until blood pressure has stabilized(see DOSAGE AND ADMINISTRATION.)

With potassium supplements and potassium-sparing diuretics: Fosinopril sodium can attenuate potassium loss caused by thiazide diuretics. Potassium-sparing diuretics (spironolactone, amiloride,triamterene, and others) or potassium supplements can increase the risk of hyperkalemia. Therefore, if concomitant use of such agents is indicated, they should be given with caution, and the patient's serum potassium should be monitored frequently.

With lithium: Increased serum lithium levels and symptoms of lithium toxicity have been reported in patients receiving ACE inhibitors during therapy with lithium. These drugs should be coadministered with caution, and frequent monitoring of serum lithium levels is recommended. If a diuretic is also used, the risk of lithium toxicity may be increased.

With antacids: In a clinical pharmacology study, coadministration of an antacid (aluminum hydroxide, magnesium hydroxide, and simethicone) with fosinopril reduced serum levels and urinary excretion of fosinoprilat as compared with fosinopril administered alone, suggesting that antacids may impair absorption of fosinopril. Therefore, if concomitant administration of these agents is indicated, dosing should be separated by 2 hours.

Other: Neither fosinopril sodium nor its metabolites have been found interact with food. In separate single or multiple dose pharmacokinetic interaction studies with chlorthalidone,nifedipine, propanolol, hydrochlorothiazide, cimetidine,metoclopramide, propantheline, digoxin, and warfarin, the bioavailability of fosinoprilat was not altered by coadministration of fosinopril with any one of these drugs. In a study with concomitant administration of aspirin and fosinopril sodium, the bioavailability of unbound fosinoprilat was not altered.

In a pharmacokinetic interaction study with warfarin, bioavailability parameters, the degree of protein binding, and the anticoagulant effect (measured by prothrombin time) of warfarin were not significantly changed.

ADVERSE REACTIONS:

Fosinopril sodium has been evaluated for safety in more than 1500 individuals in hypertension trials, including approximately 450 patients treated for a year or more. Generally adverse events were mild and transient, and their frequency was not prominently related to dose within the recommended daily dosage range.

ADVERSE REACTIONS: *(cont'd)*

In placebo-controlled clinical trials (688 fosinopril-treated patients), the usual duration of therapy was two to three months. Discontinuations due to any clinical or laboratory adverse event were 4.1 and 1.1 percent in fosinopril-treated and placebo-treated patients, respectively. The most frequent reasons (0.4 to 0.9%) were headache, elevated transaminases, fatigue, cough (see PRECAUTIONS, general, cough, diarrhea, and nausea and vomiting).

During clinical trial with any fosinopril regimen, the incidence of adverse events in the elderly (≥ 65 years old) was similar to that seen in younger patients.

Clinical adverse events probably or possibly related or of uncertain relationship to therapy, occurring in at least 1% of patients treated with fosinopril sodium alone in placebo-controlled clinical trials are shown in the table below.

TABLE 1 Clinical Adverse Events In Placebo-Controlled Trials

	Fosinopril Sodium (N = 688) Incidence (Discontinuation)	Placebo (N = 184) Incidence (Discontinuation)
Headache	3.2 (0.9)	3.3
Cough	2.2 (0.4)	0.0
Dizziness	1.6	0.0
Diarrhea	1.5 (0.4)	1.6
Fatigue	1.5 (0.6)	1.6
Nausea/Vomiting	1.2 (0.4)	0.5
Sexual Dysfunction	1.0 (0.1)	1.1 (0.5)

Other clinical events probably or possibly related, or of uncertain relationship to therapy occurring 0.2 to 1.0% of patients (except as noted) treated with fosinopril sodium in controlled or uncontrolled clinical trials (N = 1479) and less frequent, clinically significant events include (listed by body system):

General: Chest pain, edema, weakness, excessive sweating.

Cardiovascular: Angina/myocardial infarction, cerebrovascular accident, hypertensive crisis, rhythm disturbances, palpitations,hypotension, syncope, flushing, claudication. Orthostatic hypotension occurred in 4.1% of patients treated with fosinopril monotherapy. Hypotension or orthostatic hypotension was a cause for discontinuation of therapy in 0.1% patients.

Dermatologic: Urticaria, rash, photosensitivity, pruritus.

Endocrine/Metabolic: Gout, decreased libido.

Gastrointestinal: Pancreatitis, hepatitis, dysphagia, abdominal distention, abdominal pain, flatulence, constipation, heartburn,appetite/weight change, dry mouth.

Hematologic: Lymphadenopathy.

Immunologic: Angioedema. (See WARNINGS, Angioedema.)

Musculoskeletal: Arthralgia, musculoskeletal pain, myalgia/muscle cramp.

Nervous/Psychiatric: Memory disturbance, tremor, confusion, mood change, paresthesia, sleep disturbance, drowsiness, vertigo.

Respiratory: Bronchospasm, pharyngitis, sinusitis/rhinitis, laryngitis/hoarseness, epistaxis. A symptom-complex of cough,bronchospasm, and eosinophilia has been observed in two patients treated with fosinopril.

Special Senses: Tinnitus, vision disturbance, taste disturbance, eye irritation.

Urogenital: Renal insufficiency, urinary frequency.

FETAL NEONATAL MORBIDITY AND MORTALITY

See WARNINGS: Fetal Neonatal Morbidity and Mortality

POTENTIAL ADVERSE EFFECTS REPORTED WITH ACE INHIBITORS

Body as a whole: Anaphylactoid reactions (see WARNINGS: Anaphylactoid and possible related reactions and PRECAUTIONS: Hemodialysis).

Other medically important adverse effects reported with ACE inhibitors include: Cardiac arrest; eosinophilic pneumonitis; neutropenia/agranulocytosis, pancytopenia, anemia (including hemolytic and aplastic), thrombocytopenia; acute renal failure;hepatic failure, jaundice (hepatocellular or cholestatic);symptomatic hyponatremia; bullous pemphigus, exfoliative dermatitis; a syndrome which may include: arthralgia/arthritis, vasculitis, serositis, myalgia, fever rash or other dermatologic manifestations, a positive ANA, leukocytosis, eosinophilia, or an elevated ESR.

LABORATORY TEST ABNORMALITIES

Serum Electrolytes: Hyperkalemia, (see PRECAUTIONS); hyponatremia, (see DRUG INTERACTIONS, with diuretics).

BUN/Serum Creatinine: Elevations, usually transient and minor, of BUN or serum creatinine have been observed. In placebo-controlled clinical trials, there were no significant differences in the number of patients experiencing increases in serum creatinine(outside the normal range or 1.33 times the pre-treatment value)between fosinopril and placebo treatment groups. Rapid reduction of longstanding or markedly elevated blood pressure by any antihypertensive therapy can result in decreases in the glomerular filtration rate and, in turn, lead to increases in BUN or serum creatinine. See PRECAUTIONS, General.

Hematology: In controlled trials, a mean *hemoglobin* decrease of 0.1g/dL was observed in fosinopril-treated patients. In individual patients decreases in hemoglobin or hematocrit were usually transient, small, and not associated with symptoms. No patient was discontinued from therapy due to the development of anemia.

Other: Neutropenia (see WARNINGS), leukopenia and eosinophilia.

Liver Function Tests: Elevations of transaminases, LDH, alkaline phosphatase and serum bilirubin have been reported. Fosinopril therapy was discontinued because of serum transaminase elevations in 0.7% of patients. In the majority of cases, the abnormalities were either present at baseline or were associated with other etiologic factors. In those cases which were possibly related to fosinopril therapy, the elevations were generally mild and transient and resolved after discontinuation of therapy.

OVERDOSAGE:

Oral doses of fosinopril at 2600 mg/kg in rats were associated with significant lethality. Human overdoses of fosinopril have not been reported, but the most common manifestation of human fosinopril overdosage is likely to be hypotension.

Laboratory determinations of serum levels of fosinoprilat and its metabolites are not widely available, and such determinations, have in any event, no established role in the management of fosinopril overdose. No data are available to suggest the physiological maneuvers (*e.g.,* maneuvers to change the pH of the urine) that might accelerate elimination of fosinopril and its metabolites. Fosinoprilat is poorly removed from the body by both hemodialysis and peritoneal dialysis.

Angiotensin II could presumably serve as a specific antagonist-antidote in the setting of fosinopril overdose, but angiotensin II is essentially unavailable outside of scattered research facilities. Because the hypotensive effect of fosinopril is achieved through vasodilation and effective hypovolemia, it is reasonable to treat fosinopril overdose by infusion of normal saline solution.

DOSAGE AND ADMINISTRATION:

The recommended initial dose of fosinopril sodium is 10 mg once a day, both as monotherapy and when the drug is added to a diuretic. Dosage should then be adjusted according to blood pressure response at peak (2-6 hours) and trough (about 24 hours after dosing) blood levels. The usual dosage range needed to maintain a response at trough is 20-40 mg but some patients appear to have a further response to 80 mg. In some patients treated with once daily dosing, the antihypertensive effect may diminish toward the end of the dosing interval. If trough response is inadequate, dividing the daily dose should be considered. If blood pressure is not adequately controlled with fosinopril sodium alone, a diuretic may be added.

Concomitant administration of fosinopril sodium with potassium supplements,potassium salt substitutes, or potassium-sparring diuretics can lead to increases of serum potassium (see PRECAUTIONS.)

In patients who are currently being treated with a diuretic,symptomatic hypotension occasionally can occur following the initial dose of fosinopril sodium. To reduce the likelihood of hypotension,the diuretic should, if possible, be discontinued two to three days prior to beginning therapy with fosinopril sodium (see WARNINGS.) Then, if blood pressure is not controlled with fosinopril sodium alone, diuretic therapy should be resumed. If diuretic therapy can not be discontinued, an initial dose of 10 mg of fosinopril sodium should be used with careful medical supervision for several hours and until blood pressure has stabilized. See WARNINGS; PRECAUTIONS, Information for Patients and DRUG INTERACTIONS.

Since concomitant administration of fosinopril sodium with potassium supplements, or potassium-containing salt substitutes or potassium-sparing diuretics may lead to increases in serum potassium, they should be used with caution.

For hypertensive Patients With Renal Impairment: In patients with impaired renal function, the total body clearance of fosinoprilat is approximately 50% slower than in patients with normal renal function. Since hepatobiliary elimination partially compensates for diminished renal elimination, the total body clearance of fosinoprilat does not differ appreciably with any degree of renal insufficiency (creatinine clearances < 80 ml/min/1.73 m^2), including end-stage renal failure (creatinine clearance < 80 ml/min/1.73 m^2. This relative constancy of body clearance of active fosinoprilat,resulting from the dual route of elimination, permits use of the usual dose in patients with any degree of renal impairment. See WARNINGS: Anaphylactoid reactions during membrane exposure and PRECAUTIONS: Hemodialysis

PATIENT INFORMATION:

Fosinopril sodium is known as an ACE-inhibitor. It used in the treatment of high blood pressure, alone or with other medications. This medication should not be used during pregnancy and should be discontinued when pregnancy is determined. A nonproductive, persistent cough has been reported with the use of ACE inhibitors. The cough normally disappears when the medication is discontinued. A rare condition called angioedema can occur with ACE inhibitors, especially following the first dose. If you experience swelling of the face, eyes, lips, or tongue, difficulty in breathing) do not take additional medication and contact your physician immediately. Dizziness and lightheadedness can result when the mediation is first started. If this persists longer than one week, contact your physician. Signs of infections (sore throat or fever) should be reported to your physician as well to assure these are not drug related. Your blood pressure should be checked regularly to assure adequate control.

HOW SUPPLIED:

10 mg tablets: White to off-white, biconvex flat-end diamond shaped, compressed tablets with unilog number **158** and **MJ** on one side and **m**on the other.

20 mg tablets: White to off-white, oval shaped, compressed tablets with unilog number **609** and **MJ** on one side and **m**on the other.

Storage Store between 15°C (59°F) and 30°C (86°F). Avoid prolonged exposure to temperatures above 30°C (86°F).Keep bottles tightly closed (protect from moisture).

HOW SUPPLIED - EQUIVALENTS NOT AVAILABLE:

Tablet, Uncoated - Oral - 10 mg

30's	$21.89	MONOPRIL, Bristol Myers Squibb	00087-0158-22
90's	$65.68	MONOPRIL, Bristol Myers Squibb	00087-0158-46
100's	$72.98	MONOPRIL, Bristol Myers Squibb	00087-0158-45
100's	$72.98	MONOPRIL, Bristol Myers Squibb	00087-0158-50
1000's	$729.85	MONOPRIL, Bristol Myers Squibb	00087-0158-85

Tablet, Uncoated - Oral - 20 mg

30's	$21.89	MONOPRIL, Bristol Myers Squibb	00087-0609-41
90's	$65.68	MONOPRIL, Bristol Myers Squibb	00087-0609-42
100's	$78.11	MONOPRIL, Bristol Myers Squibb	00087-0609-45
1000's	$729.85	MONOPRIL, Bristol Myers Squibb	00087-0609-85

FOSINOPRIL SODIUM; HYDROCHLOROTHIAZIDE *(003245)*

CATEGORIES: ACE Inhibitors; Angiotensin Converting Enzyme Inhibitors; Antihypertensives; Cardiovascular Drugs; Diuretics; Hypertension; Thiazides; Pregnancy Category D; FDA Class 4S ("Standard Review"); FDA Approved 1994 Nov

BRAND NAMES: **Monopril-HCT**

Prescribing information not available at time of publication.

FOSPHENYTOIN SODIUM *(003298)*

CATEGORIES: Anticonvulsants; Antiepileptics; Central Nervous System Agents; Convulsions; Epilepsy; Hydantoin Anticonvulsants; Neuromuscular; Seizures; Pregnancy Category D; FDA Approved 1996 Aug

BRAND NAMES: **Cerebyx**

DESCRIPTION:

Fosphenytoin is a prodrug intended for parenteral administration; its active metabolite is phenytoin. Each Cerebyx vial contains 75 mg/ml fosphenytoin sodium (here-after referred to as fosphenytoin) **equivalent to 50 mg/ml phenytoin sodium** after administration.

Cerebyx is supplied in vials as a ready-mixed solution in Water for Injection, USP, and Tromethamine, USP (TRIS), buffer adjusted to pH 8.6 to 9.0 with either Hydrochloric Acid, NF, or Sodium Hydroxide, NF.

Fosphenytoin is a clear, colorless to pale yellow sterile solution. The chemical name of fosphenytoin is 5,5-diphenyl-3-[(phosphonooxy)methyl]-2,4-imidazolidine-dione disodium salt. The molecular weight of fosphenytoin is 406.24.

DESCRIPTION: *(cont'd)*

IMPORTANT NOTE: Throughout its product labeling, the amount and concentration of fosphenytoin is expressed in terms of phenytoin sodium equivalents (PE). Fosphenytoin's weight is expressed as phenytoin sodium equivalents to avoid the need to perform molecular weight-based adjustments when converting between fosphenytoin and phenytoin sodium doses. Fosphenytoin should always be prescribed and dispensed in phenytoin sodium equivalent units (PE) (see DOSAGE AND ADMINISTRATION).

CLINICAL PHARMACOLOGY:

INTRODUCTION

Following parenteral administration of fosphenytoin, it is converted to the anticonvulsant phenytoin. For every mmol of fosphenytoin administered, one mmol of phenytoin is produced. The pharmacological and toxicological effects of fosphenytoin include those of phenytoin. However, the hydrolysis of fosphenytoin to phenytoin yields two metabolites, phosphate and formaldehyde. Formaldehyde is subsequently converted to formate, which is in turn metabolized via a folate dependent mechanism. Although phosphate and formaldehyde (formate) have potentially important biological effect, these effects typically occur at concentrations considerably in excess of those obtained when fosphenytoin is administered under conditions of use recommended in this labeling.

MECHANISM OF ACTION

Fosphenytoin is a prodrug of phenytoin and accordingly, its anticonvulsant effects are attributable to phenytoin.

After IV administration to mice, fosphenytoin blocked the tonic phase of maximal electroshock seizures at doses equivalent to those effective for phenytoin. In addition to its ability to suppress maximal electroshock seizures in rats and mice, phenytoin exhibits anticonvulsant activity against kindled seizures in rats, audiogenic seizures in mice, and seizures produced by electrical stimulation of the brainstem in rats. The cellular mechanisms of phenytoin thought to be responsible for its anticonvulsant actions include modulation of voltage-dependent sodium channels of neurons, inhibition of calcium flux across neuronal membranes, modulation of voltage-dependent calcium channels of neurons, and enhancement of the sodium-potassium ATPase activity of neurons and glial cells. The modulation of sodium channels may be a primary anticonvulsant mechanism because this property is shared with several other anticonvulsants in addition to phenytoin.

PHARMACOKINETICS AND DRUG METABOLISM

Fosphenytoin

Absorption/Bioavailability

Intravenous: When fosphenytoin is administered by IV infusion, maximum plasma fosphenytoin concentrations are achieved at the end of the infusion. Fosphenytoin has a half-life of approximately 15 minutes.

Intramuscular: Fosphenytoin is completely bioavailable following IM administration of fosphenytoin. Peak concentrations occur at approximately 30 minutes postdose. Plasma fosphenytoin concentrations following IM administration are lower but more sustained than those following IV administration due to the time required for absorption of fosphenytoin from the injection site.

Distribution: Fosphenytoin is extensively bound (95% to 99%) to human plasma proteins, primarily albumin. Binding to plasma proteins is saturable with the result that the percent bound decreases as total fosphenytoin concentrations increase. Fosphenytoin displaces phenytoin from protein binding sites. The volume of distribution of fosphenytoin increases with fosphenytoin dose and rate, and ranges from 4.3 to 10.8 liters.

Metabolism and Elimination: The conversion half-life of fosphenytoin to phenytoin is approximately 15 minutes. The mechanism of fosphenytoin conversion has not been determined, but photophatases probably play a major role. Fosphenytoin is not excreted in urine. Each mmol of fosphenytoin is metabolized to 1 mmol of phenytoin, phosphate, and formate (see CLINICAL PHARMACOLOGY, Introduction and PRECAUTIONS, Phosphate Load for Renally Impaired Patients).

Phenytoin (After Fosphenytoin Administration)

In general, IM administration of fosphenytoin generates systemic phenytoin concentrations that are similar enough to oral phenytoin sodium to allow essentially interchangeable use.

The pharmacokinetics of fosphenytoin following IV administration of fosphenytoin, however, are complex, and when used in an emergency setting (*e.g.,* status epilepticus), differences in rate of availability of phenytoin could be critical. Studies have therefore empirically determined an infusion rate for fosphenytoin that gives a rate and extent of phenytoin systemic availability similar to that of a 50 mg/min phenytoin sodium infusion.

A dose of 15 to 20 mg PE/kg of fosphenytoin infused at 100 to 150 mg PE/min yields plasma free phenytoin concentrations over time that approximate those achieved when an equivalent dose of phenytoin sodium (*e.g.,* parenteral Dilantin) is administered at 50 mg/min (see DOSAGE AND ADMINISTRATION and WARNINGS).

Following administration of single IV fosphenytoin doses of 400 to 1200 mg PE, mean maximum total phenytoin concentrations increase in proportion to dose, but do not change appreciably with changes in infusion rate. In contrast, mean maximum unbound protein concentrations increase with both dose and rate.

Absorption/Bioavailability: Fosphenytoin is completely converted to phenytoin following IV administration, with a half-life of approximately 15 minutes. Fosphenytoin is also completely converted to phenytoin following IM administration and plasma total phenytoin concentrations peak in approximately 3 hours.

Distribution: Phenytoin is highly bound to plasma proteins, primarily albumin, although to a lesser extent than fosphenytoin. In the absence of fosphenytoin, approximately 12% of total plasma phenytoin is unbound over the clinically relevant concentration range. However, fosphenytoin displaces phenytoin from plasma protein binding sites. This increases the fraction of phenytoin unbound (up to 30% unbound) during the period required for conversion of fosphenytoin to phenytoin (approximately 0.5 to 1 hour postinfusion).

Metabolism and Elimination: Phenytoin derived from administration of fosphenytoin is extensively metabolised in the liver and excreted in urine primarily as 5-(p-hydroxyphenyl)-5-phenylhydantoin and its glucuronide; little unchanged phenytoin (1%-5% of the fosphenytoin dose) is recovered in urine. Phenytoin hepatic metabolism is satuable, and following administration of single IV fosphenytoin doses of 400 to 1200 mg PE, total and unbound phenytoin AUC values increase disproportionately with dose. Mean total phenytoin half-life values (12.0 to 28.9 hr) following fosphenytoin administration at these doses are similar to those after equal doses of parenteral phenytoin sodium and tend to be greater at higher plasma phenytoin concentrations.

SPECIAL POPULATIONS

Patients with Renal or Hepatic Disease: Due to an increased fraction of unbound phenytoin in patients with renal or hepatic disease, or in those with hypoalbuminemia, the interpretation of total phenytoin plasma concentrations should be made with caution (see DOSAGE AND ADMINISTRATION). Unbound phenytoin concentration may be more useful in these patient populations. After IV administration of fosphenytoin to patients with renal and/or hepatic disease, or in those with hypoalbuminemia, fosphenytoin clearance to phenytoin may be increased without similar increase in phenytoin clearance. This has the potential to increase the frequency and severity of adverse events (see PRECAUTIONS).

CLINICAL PHARMACOLOGY: *(cont'd)*

Age: The effect of age was evaluated in patients 5 to 98 years of age. Patient age had no significant impact on fosphenytoin pharmacokinetics. Phenytoin clearance tends to decrease with increasing age (20% less in patients over 70 years of age relative to that in patients 20-30 years of age). Phenytoin dosing requirements are highly variable and must be individualized (see DOSAGE AND ADMINISTRATION).

Gender and Race: Gender and race have no significant impact on fosphenytoin or phenytoin pharmacokinetics.

Pediatrics: Only limited pharmacokinetic data are available in children (N=8; age 5 to 10 years). In these patients with status epilepticus who received loading doses of fosphenytoin, the plasma fosphenytoin, total phenytoin, and unbound phenytoin concentration-time profiles did not signal any major differences from those in adult patients with status epilepticus receiving comparable doses.

CLINICAL STUDIES:

Infusion tolerance was evaluated in clinical studies. One double-blind study assessed infusion-site tolerance of equivalent loading dose (15–20 mg PE/kg) of fosphenytoin infused at 150 mg PE/min or phenytoin infused 50 mg/min. The study demonstrated better local tolerance (pain and burning at the infusion site), fewer disruptions of the infusion, and a shorter infusion period for fosphenytoin-treated patients (TABLE 1).

TABLE 1 Infusion Tolerance of Equivalent Loading Doses of IV Fosphenytoin and IV Phenytoin

	IV Fosphenytoin N=90	IV Phenytoin N=22
Local Intolerance	9%[a]	90%
Infusion Disrupted	21%	67%
Average Infusion Time	13 min	44 min

a Percent of Patients

Fosphenytoin-treated patients, however, experienced more systemic sensory disturbances (see PRECAUTIONS, Sensory Disturbances).

Infusion disruptions in fosphenytoin-treated patients were primarily due to systemic burning, pruritus, and/or paresthesia while those in phenytoin-treated patients were primarily due to pain and burning at the infusion site (see TABLE 1).

In a double-blind study investigating temporary substitution of fosphenytoin for oral phenytoin, IM fosphenytoin was as well-tolerated as IM placebo. IM fosphenytoin resulted in a slight increase in transient, mild to moderate local itching (23% of patients vs 11% of IM placebo-treated patients at any time during the study). This study also demonstrated that equimolar doses of IM fosphenytoin may be substituted for oral phenytoin sodium with no dosage adjustments needed when initiating IM or returning to oral therapy. In contrast, switching between IM and oral phenytoin requires dosage adjustments because of slow and erratic phenytoin absorption from muscle.

INDICATIONS AND USAGE:

Fosphenytoin is indicated for short-term parenteral administration when other means of phenytoin administration are unavailable, inappropriate or deemed less advantageous. The safety and effectiveness of fosphenytoin in this use has not been systemically evaluated for more than 5 days.

Fosphenytoin can be used for the control of generalized convulsive status epilepticus and prevention and treatment of seizures occurring during neuosurgery. It can also be substituted, short-term, for oral phenytoin.

CONTRAINDICATIONS:

Fosphenytoin is contraindicated in patients who have demonstrated hypersensitivity to fosphenytoin or its ingredients, or to phenytoin or other hydantoins.

Because of the effect of parenteral phenytoin on ventricular automaticity, fosphenytoin is contraindicated in patients with sinus bradycardia, sino-atrial block and third degree A-V block, and Adams-Stokes syndrome.

WARNINGS:

DOSES OF FOSPHENYTOIN ARE EXPRESSED AS THEIR PHENYTOIN SODIUM EQUIVALENTS IN THIS LABELING (PE=Phenytoin Sodium Equivalent).

DO NOT, THEREFORE, MAKE ANY ADJUSTMENT IN THE RECOMMENDED DOSES WHEN SUBSTITUTING FOSPHENYTOIN FOR PHENYTOIN SODIUM OR VICE VERSA.

The following warnings are based on experience with fosphenytoin or phenytoin.

STATUS EPILEPTICUS DOSING REGIMEN

Do not administer fosphenytoin at a rate greater than 150 mg PE/min.

The dose of IV fosphenytoin (15 to 20 mg PE/kg) that is used to treat status epilepticus is administered at a maximum rate of 150 mg PE/min. The typical fosphenytoin infusion administered to a 50 kg patient would take between 5 and 7 minutes. Note that the delivery of an identical molar dose of phenytoin using parenteral Dilantin or generic phenytoin sodium injection cannot be accomplished in less than 15 to 20 minutes because of the untoward cardiovascular effects that accompany the direct intravenous administration of phenytoin at rates greater than 50 mg/min.

If rapid phenytoin loading is a primary goal, IV administration of fosphenytoin is preferred because the time to achieve therapeutic plasma phenytoin concentrations is greater following IM than that following IV administration (see DOSAGE AND ADMINISTRATION).

WITHDRAWL PRECIPITATED SEIZURE, STATUS EPILEPTICUS

Antiepileptic drugs should not be abruptly discontinued because of the possibility of increased seizure frequency, including status epilepticus. When, in the judgement of the clinician, the need for dosage reduction, discontinuation, or substitution of alternative antiepileptic medication arises, this should be done gradually. However, in the event of an allergic or hypersensitivity reaction, rapid substitution of alternative therapy may be necessary. In this case, alternative therapy should be an antiepileptic drug not belonging to the hydantoin chemical class.

CARDIOVASCULAR DEPRESSION

Hypotension may occur, especially after IV administration at high doses and high rates of administration. Following administration of phenytoin, severe cardiovascular reactions and fatalities have been reported with atrial and ventricular conduction depression and ventricular fibrillation. Severe complications are most commonly encountered in elderly or gravely ill patients. Therefore, careful cardiac monitoring is needed when administering IV loading doses of fosphenytoin. Reduction in rate of administration or discontinuation of dosing may be needed.

Fosphenytoin should be used with caution in patients with hypotension and severe myocardial insufficiency.

WARNINGS: *(cont'd)*

RASH

Fosphenytoin should be discontinued if a skin rash appears. If the rash is exfoliative purpuric, or bullous, or if lupus erythematosus, Stevens-Johnson syndrome or toxic epidermal necrolysis is suspected, use of this drug should not be resumed and alternative therapy should be considered. If the rash is of a milder type (measles-like or scarlatiniform), therapy may be resumed after the rash has completely disappeared. If the rash recurs upon reinstitution of therapy, further fosphenytoin or phenytoin administration is contraindicated.

HEPATIC INJURY

Cases of acute hepatotoxicity, including infrequent cases of acute hepatic failure, have been reported with phenytoin. These incidents have been associated with a hypersensitivity syndrome characterized by fever, skin eruptions, and lymphadenopathy, and usually occur within the first 2 months of treatment. Other common manifestations include jaundice, hepatomegaly, elevated serum transaminase levels, leukocytosis, and eosinophilia. The clinical course of acute phenytoin hepatotoxicity ranges from prompt recovery to fatal outcomes. In these patients with acute hepatotoxicity, fosphenytoin should be immediately discontinued and not readministered.

HEMOPOIETIC SYSTEM

Hemopoietic complications, some fatal, have occasionally been reported in association with administration of phenytoin. These have included thrombocytopenia, leukopenia, granulocytopenia, agranulocytosis, and pancytopenia with or without bone marrow suppression.

There have been a number of reports that have suggested a relationship between phenytoin and the development of lymphadenopathy (local or generalized), including benign lymph node hyperplasia, pseudolymphoma, lymphoma, and Hodgkin's disease. Although a cause and effect relationship has not been established, the occurrence of lymphadenopathy indicates the need to differentiate such a condition from other types of lymph node pathology. Lymph node involvement may occur with or without symptoms and signs resembling serum sickness *e.g.,* fever, rash and liver involvement. In all cases of lymphadenopathy, follow-up observation for an extended period is indicated and every effort should be made to achieve seizure control using alternative antiepileptic drugs.

ALCOHOL USE

Acute alcohol intake may increase plasma phenytoin concentrations while chronic alcohol use may decrease plasma concentrations.

USAGE IN PREGNANCY

Clinical

A. Risks to Mother: An increase in seizure frequency may occur during pregnancy because of altered phenytoin pharmacokinetics. Periodic measurement of plasma phenytoin concentrations may be valuable in the management of pregnant women as a guide to appropriate adjustment of dosage (see PRECAUTIONS, Laboratory Tests). However, postpartum restoration of the original dosage will probably be indicated.

B. Risks to the Fetus: If this drug is used during pregnancy, or if the patient becomes pregnant while taking the drug, the patient should be apprised of the potential harm to the fetus.

Prenatal exposure to phenytoin may increase the risks for congenital malformations and other adverse developmental outcomes. Increased frequencies of major malformations (such as orofacial clefts and cardiac defects), minor anomalies (dysmorphic facial features, nail and digit hypoplasia), growth abnormalities (including microcephaly), and mental deficiency have been reported among children born to epileptic women who took phenytoin alone or in combination with other antiepileptic drugs during pregnancy. There have also been several reported cases of malignancies, including neuroblastoma, in children whose mothers received phenytoin during pregnancy. The overall incidence of malformations for children of epileptic women treated with antiepileptic drugs (phenytoin and/or others) during pregnancy is about 10%, or two-to three-fold that in the general population. However, the relative contributions of antiepileptic drugs and other factors associated with epilepsy to this increased risk are uncertain and in most cases it has not been possible to attribute specific developmental abnormalities to particular antiepileptic drugs.

Patients should consult with their physicians to weigh the risks and benefits of phenytoin during pregnancy.

C. Postpartum Period: A potentially life-threatening bleeding disorder related to decreased levels of vitamin K-dependent clotting factors may occur in newborns exposed to phenytoin *in utero*. This drug-induced condition can be prevented with vitamin K administration to the mother before delivery and to the neonate after birth.

Preclinical: Increased frequencies of malformations (brain, cardiovascular, digit, and skeletal anomalies), death, growth retardation, and functional impairment (chromodacryorrhea, hyperactivity, circling) were observed among the offspring of rats receiving fosphenytoin during pregnancy. Most of the adverse reflects on embryo-fetal development occurred at doses of 33 mg PE/kg or higher (approximately 30% of the maximum human loading dose or higher on a mg/m^2 basis), which produced peak maternal plasma phenytoin concentrations of approximately 20 mcg/ml or greater. Maternal toxicity was often associated with these doses and plasma concentrations, however, there is no evidence to suggest that the developmental effects were secondary to the maternal effects. The single occurrence of a rare brain malformation at a non-maternotoxic dose of 17 mg PE/kg (approximately 10% of the maximum human loading dose on a mg/m^{2}basis) was also considered drug-induced. The developmental effects of fosphenytoin in rats were similar to those which have been reported following administration of phenytoin to pregnant rats.

No effects on embryo-fetal development were observed when rabbits were given up to 33 mg PE/kg of fosphenytoin (approximately 50% of the maximum human loading dose on a mg/m^2 basis) during pregnancy. Increased resorption and malformation rates have been reported following administration of phenytoin doses of 75 mg/kg or higher (approximately 120% of the maximum human loading dose or higher on a mg/m^2 basis) to pregnant rabbits.

PRECAUTIONS:

GENERAL: (FOSPHENYTOIN SPECIFIC)

Sensory Disturbances

Severe burning, itching, and/or paresthesia were reported by 7 of 16 normal volunteers administered IV fosphenytoin at a dose of 1200 mg PE at the maximum rate of administration (150 mg PE/min). The severe sensory disturbance lasted from 3 to 50 minutes in 6 of these subjects and for 14 hours in the seventh subject. In some cases, milder sensory disturbances persisted for as long as 24 hours. The location of the discomfort varied among subjects with the groin mentioned most frequently as an area of discomfort. In a separate cohort of 16 normal volunteers (taken from 2 other studies) who were administered IV fosphenytoin at a dose of 1200 mg PE at the maximum rate of administration (150 mg PE/min), none experienced severe disturbances, but most experienced mild to moderate itching or tingling.

Patients administered fosphenytoin at doses of 20 mg PE kg at 150 mg PE/min are expected to experience discomfort of some degree. The occurrence and intensity of the discomfort can be lessened by slowing or temporarily stopping the infusion.

PRECAUTIONS: *(cont'd)*

The effect of continuing infusion unaltered in the presence of these sensations is unknown. No permanent sequelae have been reported thus far. The pharmacologic basis for these positive sensory phenomena is unknown, but other phosphate ester drugs, which deliver smaller phosphate loads, have been associated with burning, itching, and/or tingling predominantly in the groin area.

Phosphate Load

The phosphate load provided by fosphenytoin (0.0037 mmol phosphate/mg PE fosphenytoin) should be considered when treating patients who require phosphate restriction, such as those with severe renal impairment.

IV Loading in Renal and/or Hepatic Disease or in Those With Hypoalbuminemia

After IV administration to patients with renal and/or hepatic disease or in those with hypoalbuminemia, fosphenytoin clearance to phenytoin may be increased without a similar increase in phenytoin clearance. This has the potential to increase the frequency and severity of adverse events see CLINICAL PHARMACOLOGY, Special Populations and DOSAGE AND ADMINISTRATION, Dosing in Special Populations.

GENERAL: (PHENYTOIN ASSOCIATED)

Fosphenytoin is *not* indicated for the treatment of *absence seizures.*

A small percentage of individuals who have been treated with phenytoin have been shown to metabolize the drug slowly. *Slow metabolism* may be due to limited enzyme availability and lack of induction; it appears to be genetically determined.

Phenytoin and other hydantoins are contraindicated in patients who have experienced phenytoin hypersensitivity. Additionally, caution should be exercised if using structurally similar (*e.g.* barbiturates, succinimides, oxazolidinediones, and other related compounds) in these same patients.

Phenytoin has been infrequently associated with the exacerbation of *porphyria*. Caution should be exercised when fosphenytoin is used in patients with this disease.

Hyperplycemia, resulting from phenytoin's inhibitory effect on insulin release has been reported. Phenytoin may also raise the serum glucose concentrations in diabetic patients. Plasma concentrations of phenytoin sustained above the optimal range may produce confusional states referred to as "delirium," "psychosis," or "encephalopathy," or rarely, irreversible cerebellar dysfunction. Accordingly, at the first sign of *acute toxicity,* determination of plasma phenytoin concentrations is recommended (see PRECAUTIONS, Laboratory Tests). Fosphenytoin dose reduction is indicated if phenytoin concentrations are excessive; if symptoms persist, administration of fosphenytoin should be discontinued.

The liver is the primary site of biotransformation of phenytoin; patients with impaired liver function, elderly patients, or those who are gravely ill may show early signs of toxicity.

Phenytoin and other hydantoins are not indicated for seizures due to hypoglycemic or other metabolic causes. Appropriate diagnostic procedures should be performed as indicated.

Phenytoin has the potential to lower serum folate levels.

LABORATORY TESTS

Phenytoin doses are usually selected to attain therapeutic plasma total phenytoin concentrations of 10 to 20 mcg/ml, (unbound phenytoin concentrations of 1 to 2 mcg/ml). Following fosphenytoin administration, it is recommended that phenytoin concentrations not be monitored until conversion to phenytoin is essentially complete. This occurs within approximately 2 hours after the end of IV infusion and 4 hours after IM injection.

Prior to complete conversion commonly used immunoanalytical techniques such as TDx/TDx/FLx (fluorescence polarization) and Emit 2000 (enzyme multiplied), may significantly overestimate plasma phenytoin concentrations because of cross-reactivity with fosphenytoin. The error is dependent on plasma phenytoin and fosphenytoin concentration (influenced by fosphenytoin dose, route and rate of administration, and time of sampling relative to dosing), and analytical method. Chromatographic assay methods accurately quantitate phenytoin concentrations in biological fluids in the presence of fosphenytoin. Prior to complete conversion, blood samples for phenytoin monitoring should be collected in tubes containing EDTA as an anticoagulant to minimize *ex vivo* conversion of fosphenytoin to phenytoin. However, even with specific assay methods, phenytoin concentrations measured before conversion of fosphenytoin is complete will not reflect phenytoin concentrations ultimately achieved.

DRUG/LABORATORY TEST INTERACTIONS

Phenytoin may decrease serum concentrations of T_4. It may also produce artifactually low results in dexamethasone or metyrapone tests. Phenytoin may also cause increased serum concentrations of glucose, alkaline phosphatase, and gamma glutamyl transpeptidase (GGT).

Care should be taken when using immunoanalytical methods to measure plasma phenytoin concentrations following fosphenytoin administration (see Laboratory Testls).

CARCINOGENESIS, MUTAGENESIS, AND IMPAIRMENT OF FERTILITY

The carcinogenic potential of fosphenytoin has not been studied. Assessment of the carcinogenic potential of phenytoin in mice and rats is ongoing.

Structural chromosome aberration frequency in cultured V79 Chinese hamster lung cells was increased by exposure to fosphenytoin in the presence of metabolic activation. No evidence of mutagenicity was observed in bacteria (Ames test) or Chinese hamster lung cells *in vitro*, and no evidence for clastogenic activity was observed in an *in vivo* mouse bone marrow micronucleus test.

No effects on fertility were noted in rats of either sex given fosphenytoin. Maternal toxicity and altered estrous cycles, delayed mating, prolonged gestation length, and developmental toxicity were observed following administration of fosphenytoin during mating, gestation, and lactation at doses of 50 mg PE kg or higher (approximately 40% of the maximum human loading dose or higher on a mg/m^2 basis).

Pregnancy Category D: See WARNINGS.

Nursing Mothers: It is not known whether fosphenytoin is excreted in human milk.

Following administration of phenytoin sodium, phenytoin appears to be excreted in low concentrations in human milk. Therefore, breast-feeding is not recommended for women receiving fosphenytoin.

Pediatric Use: The safety of fosphenytoin in pediatric patients has not been established.

Geriatric Use: No systematic studies in geriatric patients have been conducted. Phenytoin clearance tends to decrease with increasing age (see CLINICAL PHARMACOLOGY, Special Populations).

DRUG INTERACTIONS:

No drugs are known to interfere with the conversion of fosphenytoin to phenytoin. Conversion could be affected by alterations in the level of phosphatase activity, but given the abundance and wide distribution of phosphatases in the body it is unlikely that drugs would affect this activity enough to affect conversion of fosphenytoin to phenytoin. Drugs highly bound to albumin could increase the unbound fraction of fosphenytoin. Although, it is unknown whether this could result in clinically significant effects, caution is advised when administering fosphenytoin with other drugs that significantly bind to serum albumin.

The pharmacokinetics and protein binding of fosphenytoin, phenytoin, and diazepam were not altered when diazepam and fosphenytoin were concurrently administered in single submaximal doses.

DRUG INTERACTIONS: *(cont'd)*

The most significant drug interactions following administration of fosphenytoin are expected to occur with drugs that interact with phenytoin. Phenytoin is extensively bound to serum plasma proteins and is prone to competitive displacement. Phenytoin is metabolized by hepatic cytochrome P450 enzymes and is particularly susceptible to inhibitory drug interactions because it is subject to saturable metabolism. Inhibition of metabolism may produce significant increases in circulating phenytoin concentrations and enhance the risk of drug toxicity. Phenytoin is a potent inducer of hepatic drug-metabolizing enzymes.

The most commonly occurring drug interactions are listed below:

Drugs that may increase plasma phenytoin concentrations include: acute alcohol intake, amiodarone, chloramphenicol, chlordiazepoxide, cimetidine, diazepam, dicumarol, disulfiram, estrogens, ethosuximide, fluoxetine, H_2-antagonists, halothane, isoniazid, methylphenidate, phenothiazines, phenylbutazone, salicylates, succinimides, sulfonamides, tolbutamide, trazodone.

Drugs that may decrease plasma phenytoin concentrations include: carbamazepine, chronic alcohol abuse, reserpine.

Drugs that may either increase or decrease plasma phenytoin concentrations include: phenobarbital, valproic acid, and sodium valproate. Similarly, the effects of phenytoin on phenobarbital, valproic acid and sodium plasma valproate concentrations are unpredictable.

Although not a true drug interaction, tricyclic antidepressants may precipitate seizures in susceptible patients and fosphenytoin dosage may need to be adjusted.

Drugs whose efficacy is impaired by phenytoin include: anticoagulants, corticosteroids, coumarin, digitoxin, doxycycline, estrogens, furosemide, oral contraceptives, rifampin, quinidine, theophylline, vitamin D.

Monitoring of plasma phenytoin concentrations may be helpful when possible drug interactions are suspected (see Laboratory Tests).

ADVERSE REACTIONS:

The more important adverse clinical events caused by the IV use of fosphenytoin or phenytoin are cardiovascular collapse and/or central nervous system depression. Hypotension can occur when either drug is administered rapidly by the IV route. The rate of administration is very important; for fosphenytoin, it should not exceed 150 mg PE/min.

The adverse clinical events most commonly observed with the use of fosphenytoin in clinical trials were nystagmus, dizziness, pruritus, paresthesia, headache, somnolence, and ataxia. With two exceptions, these events are commonly associated with the administration of IV phenytoin. Paresthesia and pruritus, however, were seen much more often following fosphenytoin administration and occurred more often with IV fosphenytoin administration than with IM fosphenytoin administration. These events were dose and rate related; most alert patients (41 of 64; 64%) administered doses of ≥15 mg PE/kg at 150 mg PE/min experienced discomfort of some degree. These sensations, generally described as itching, burning or tingling, were usually not at the infusion site. The location of the discomfort varied with the groin mentioned most frequently as a site of involvement. The paresthesia and pruritus were transient events that occurred within several minutes of the start of infusion and generally resolved within 10 minutes after completion of fosphenytoin infusion. Some patients experienced symptoms for hours. These events did not increase in severity with repeated administration. Concurrent adverse events or clinical laboratory change suggesting an allergic process were not seen (see PRECAUTIONS, Sensory Disturbances).

Approximately 2% of the 859 individuals who received fosphenytoin in premarketing clinical trials discontinued treatment because of an adverse event. The adverse events most commonly associated with withdrawal were pruritus (0.5%), hypotension (0.3%), and bradycardia (0.2%).

Dose and Rate Dependency of Adverse Events Following IV Fosphenytoin: The incidence of adverse events tended to increase as both dose and infusion rate increased. In particular, at doses of ≥15 mg PE/kg and rates ≥150 mg PE/min, transient pruritus, tinnitus, nystagmus, somnolence, and ataxia occurred 2 to 3 times more often than at lower doses or rates.

INCIDENCE IN CONTROLLED CLINICAL TRIALS

All adverse events were recorded during the trials by the clinical investigators using terminology of their own choosing. Similar types of events were grouped into standardized categories using modified COSTART dictionary terminology. These categories are used in the tables and listings with the frequencies representing the proportion of individuals exposed to fosphenytoin or comparative therapy.

The prescriber should be aware that these figures cannot be used to predict the frequency of adverse events in the course of usual medical practice where patient characteristics and other factors may differ from those prevailing during clinical studies. Similarly, the cited frequencies cannot be directly compared with figures obtained from other clinical investigations involving different treatments uses or investigators. An inspection of these frequencies, however, does provide the prescribing physician with one basis to estimate the relative contribution of drug and nondrug factors to the adverse event incidences in the population studied.

Incidence in Controlled Clinical Trials - IV Administration To Patients With Epilepsy or Neurosurgical Patients: TABLE 2 lists treatment-emergent adverse events that occurred in at least 2% of patients treated with IV fosphenytoin at the maximum dose and rate in a randomized, double blind, controlled clinical trial where the rates for phenytoin and fosphenytoin administration would have resulted in equivalent systemic exposure to phenytoin.

Incidence In Controlled Trials - IM Administration to Patients With Epilepsy: TABLE 3 lists treatment-emergent adverse events that occurred in at least 2% of fosphenytoin-treated patients in a double-blind, randomized, controlled clinical trial of adult epilepsy patients receiving either IM fosphenytoin substituted for oral phenytoin sodium or continuing oral phenytoin sodium. Both treatments were administered for 5 days.

ADVERSE EVENTS DURING ALL CLINICAL TRIALS

Fosphenytoin has been administered to 859 individuals during all clinical trials. All adverse events seen at least twice are listed in the following except those already included in previous tables and listings. Events are further classified within body system categories and enumerated in order of increasing frequency using the following definitions: frequent adverse events are defined as those occurring in greater than 1/100 individuals infrequent adverse events are those occurring in 1/100 to 1/1000 individuals.

Body As a Whole: *Frequent:* fever, injection-site reaction, infection, chills, face edema, injection pain; *Infrequent:* sepsis, injection-site inflammation, injection-site edema, injection-site hemorrhage, flu syndrome, malaise, generalized edema, shock, photosensitivity reaction, cachexia, cryptococcosis

Cardiovascular: *Frequent:* hypertension *Infrequent:* cardiac arrest, migraine, syncope cerebral hemorrhage, palpitation, sinus bradycardia, atrial flutter, bundle branch block, cardiomegaly, cerebral infarct, postural hypotension, pulmonary embolus, QT interval prolongation, thrombophlebitis, ventricular extrasystoles, congestive heart failure.

Digestive: *Frequent:* constipation *Infrequent:* dyspepsia, diarrhea, anorexia, gastrointestinal hemorrhage, increased salivation, liver function tests abnormal, tenesmus, tongue edema, dysphagia, flatulence, gastritis, ileus.

ADVERSE REACTIONS: *(cont'd)*

TABLE 2 Treatment-Emergent Adverse Event Incidence Following IV Administration at the Maximum Dose and Rate to Patients With Epilepsy or Neurosurgical Patients (Events in at Least 2% of Fosphenytoin-Treated Patients)

Body System / Adverse Event	IV Fosphenytoin N=90	IV Phenytoin N=22
Body as a Whole		
Pelvic Pain	4.4	0.0
Asthenia	2.2	0.0
Back Pain	2.2	0.0
Headache	2.2	4.5
Cardiovascular		
Hypotension	7.7	9.1
Vasodilatation	5.6	4.5
Tachycardia	2.2	0.0
Digestive		
Nausea	8.9	13.6
Tongue Disorder	4.4	0.0
Dry Mouth	4.4	4.5
Vomiting	2.2	9.1
Nervous		
Nystagmus	44.4	59.1
Dizziness	31.1	27.3
Somnolence	21.0	27.3
Ataxia	11.1	18.2
Stupor	7.7	4.5
Incoordination	4.4	4.5
Paresthesia	4.4	0.0
Extrapyramidal Syndrome	4.4	0.0
Tremor	3.3	9.1
Agitation	3.3	0.0
Hypesthesia	2.2	9.1
Dysarthria	2.2	0.0
Vertigo	2.2	0.0
Brain Edema	2.2	4.5
Skin and Appendages		
Pruritus	48.9	4.5
Special Senses		
Tinnitus	8.9	9.1
Diplopia	3.3	0.0
Taste Perversion	3.3	0.0
Amblyopia	2.2	9.1
Deafness	2.2	0.0

TABLE 3 Treatment-Emergent Adverse Event Incidence Following Substitution of IM Fosphenytoin for Oral Phenytoin Sodium in Patients With Epilepsy (Events in at Least 2% of Fosphenytoin -Treated Patients)

Body System / Adverse Event	IV Fosphenytoin N=179	Oral Phenytoin Sodium N=61
Body as a Whole		
Headache	8.9	4.9
Asthenia	3.9	3.3
Accidental Injury	3.4	6.6
Digestive		
Nausea	4.5	0.0
Vomiting	2.8	0.0
Hematologic and Lymphatic		
Ecchymosis	7.3	4.9
Nervous		
Nystagmus	15.1	8.2
Tremor	9.5	13.1
Ataxia	8.4	8.2
Incoordination	7.8	4.9
Somnolence	6.7	9.8
Dizziness	5.0	3.3
Paresthesia	3.9	3.3
Reflexes Decreased	2.8	4.9
Skin and Appendages		
Pruritus	2.8	0.0

Endocrine: *Infrequent:* diabetes insipidus.

Hematologic and Lymphatic: *Infrequent:* thrombocytopenia, anemia, leukocytosis, cyanosis, hypochromic anemia, leukopenia, lymphadenopathy, petechia.

Metabolic and Nutritional: *Frequent:* hypokalemia; *Infrequent:* hyperglycemia, hypophosphatemia, alkalosis, acidosis, dehydration, hyperkalemia, ketosis.

Musculoskeletal: *Frequent:* myasthenia; *Infrequent:* myopathy, leg cramps, arthralgia, myalgia.

Nervous: *Frequent:* reflexes increased, speech disorder, dysarthria, intracranial hypertension, thinking abnormal, nervousness, hypesthesia; *Infrequent:* confusion, twitching, Babinski sign positive, circumoral paresthesia, hemiplegia, hypotonia, convulsion, extrapyramidal syndrome, insomnia, meningitis, depersonalization, CNS depression, depression, hypokinesia, hyperkinesia, brain edema, paralysis, psychosis, aphasia, emotional lability, coma, hyperesthesia, myoclonus, personality disorder, acute brain syndrome, encephalitis, subdural hematoma, encephalopathy, hostility, akathisia, amnesia, neurosis.

Respiratory: *Frequent:* pneumonia; *Infrequent:* pharyngitis, sinusitis, hyperventilation, rhinitis, apnea, aspiration pneumonia, asthma, dyspnea, atelectasis, cough increased, sputum increased, epistaxis, hypoxia, pneumothorax, hemoptysis, bronchitis.

Skin and Appendages: *Frequent:* rash; *Infrequent:* maculopapular rash, urticaria, sweating, skin discoloration, contact dermatitis, pustular rash, skin nodule.

Special Senses: *Frequent:* taste perversion; *Infrequent:* deafness, visual field defect, eye pain, conjunctivitis, photophobia, hyperacusis, mydriasis, parosmia, ear pain, taste loss.

Urogenital: *Infrequent:* urinary retention, oliguria, dysuria, vaginitis, albuminuria, genital edema, kidney failure, polyuria, urethral pain, urinary incontinence, vaginal moniliasis.

OVERDOSAGE:

There is no experience with fosphenytoin overdosage in humans. The median lethal dose of fosphenytoin given intravenously in mice and rats was 156 mg PE/kg and approximately 250 mg PE/kg, or about 0.6 and 2 times, respectively, the maximum human loading dose on a mg/m^2 basis. Signs of acute toxicity in animals included ataxia, labored breathing, ptosis, and hypoactivity.

Because fosphenytoin is a prodrug of phenytoin the following information may be helpful. Initial symptoms of acute phenytoin toxicity are nystagmus, ataxia, and dysarthria. Other signs include tremor, hyperreflexia, lethargy, slurred speech, nausea, vomiting, coma, and hypotension. Depression of respiratory and circulatory systems leads to death. There are

OVERDOSAGE: *(cont'd)*

marked variations among individuals with respect to plasma phenytoin concentrations where toxicity occurs. Lateral gaze nystagmus usually appears at 20 mcg/ml, ataxia at 30 mcg/ml, and dysarthria and lethargy appear when the plasma concentration is over 40 mcg/ml. However, phenytoin concentrations as high as 50 mcg/ml have been reported without evidence of toxicity. As much as 25 times the therapeutic phenytoin dose has been taken, resulting in plasma phenytoin concentrations over 100 mcg/ml, with complete recovery.

Treatment is nonspecific since there is no known antidote to fosphenytoin or phenytoin overdosage. The adequacy of the respiratory and circulatory systems should be carefully observed, and appropriate supportive measures employed. Hemodialysis can be considered since phenytoin is not completely bound to plasma proteins. Total exchange transfusion has been used in the treatment of severe intoxication in children. In acute overdosage the possibility of other CNS depressants, including alcohol, should be borne in mind.

Formate and phosphate are metabolites of fosphenytoin and therefore may contribute to signs of toxicity following overdosage. Signs of formate toxicity are similar to those of methanol toxicity and are associated with severe anion-gap metabolic acidosis. Large amounts of phosphate, delivered rapidly, could potentially cause hypocalcemia with paresthesia, muscle spasms, and seizures. Ionized free calcium levels can be measured and, if low, used to guide treatment.

DOSAGE AND ADMINISTRATION:

The dose, concentration in dosing solutions, and infusion rate of IV fosphenytoin is expressed as phenytoin sodium equivalents (PE) to avoid the need to perform molecular weight-based adjustments when converting between fosphenytoin and phenytoin sodium doses. Fosphenytoin should always be prescribed and dispensed in phenytoin sodium equivalent units (PE). Fosphenytoin has important differences in administration from those for parenteral phenytoin sodium.

Products with particulate matter or discoloration should not be used. Prior to IV infusion, dilute fosphenytoin in 5% dextrose or 0.9% saline solution for injection to a concentration ranging from 1.5 to 25 mg PE/ml.

STATUS EPILEPTICUS

The loading dose of fosphenytoin is 15 to 20 mg PE/kg administered at 100 to 150 mg PE/min.

Because of the risk of hypotension, fosphenytoin should be administered no faster than 150 mg PE/min. Continuous monitoring of the electrocardiogram, blood pressure, and respiratory function is essential and the patient should be observed throughout the period where maximal serum phenytoin concentrations occur, approximately 10 to 20 minutes after the end of fosphenytoin infusions.

Because the full antiepileptic effect of phenytoin whether given as fosphenytoin or parenteral phenytoin, is not immediate, other measures, including concomitant administration of an IV benzodiazepine, will usually be necessary for the control of status epilepticus.

The loading dose should be followed by maintenance doses of fosphenytoin, or phenytoin either orally or parenterally.

If administration of fosphenytoin does not terminate seizures, the use of other anticonvulsants and other appropriate measures should be considered.

IM fosphenytoin should not be used in the treatment of status epilepticus because therapeutic phenytoin concentrations may not be reached as quickly as with IV administration. If IV access is impossible, loading doses of fosphenytoin have been given by the IM route for other indications.

NONEMERGENT LOADING AND MAINTENANCE DOSING

The loading dose of fosphenytoin is 10 - 20 mg PE/kg given IV or IM. The rate of administration for IV fosphenytoin should be no greater than 150 mg PE/min. Continuous monitoring of the electrocardiogram, blood pressure, and respiratory function is essential and the patient should be observed throughout the period where maximal serum phenytoin concentrations occur, approximately 10 to 20 minutes after the end of fosphenytoin infusions.

The initial daily maintenance dose of fosphenytoin is 4 - 6 mg PE/kg/day.

IM OR IV SUBSTITUTION FOR ORAL PHENYTOIN THERAPY

Fosphenytoin can be substituted for oral phenytoin sodium therapy at the same total daily dose.

Phenytoin sodium capsules are approximately 90% bioavailable by the oral route. Phenytoin, supplied as fosphenytoin, is 100% bioavailable by both the IM and IV routes. For this reason, plasma phenytoin concentrations may increase modestly when IM or IV fosphenytoin is substituted for oral phenytoin sodium therapy.

The rate of administration for IV fosphenytoin should be no greater than 150 mg PE/min.

In controlled trials, IM fosphenytoin was administered as a single daily dose utilizing either 1 or 2 injection sites. Some patients may require more frequent dosing.

DOSING IN SPECIAL POPULATIONS

Patients with Renal or Hepatic Disease: Due to an increased fraction of unbound phenytoin in patients with renal or hepatic disease, or in those with hypoalbuminemia, the interpretation of total phenytoin plasma concentrations should be made with caution (see CLINICAL PHARMACOLOGY, Special Populations). Unbound phenytoin concentrations may be more useful in these patient populations. After IV fosphenytoin administration to patients with renal and/or hepatic disease, or in those with hypoalbuminemia, fosphenytoin clearance to phenytoin may be increased without a similar increase in phenytoin clearance. This has the potential to increase the frequency and severity of adverse events (see PRECAUTIONS).

Elderly Patients: Age does not have a significant impact on the pharmacokinetics of fosphenytoin following fosphenytoin administration. Phenytoin clearance is decreased slightly in elderly patients and lower or less frequent dosing may be required.

Pediatric: The safety of fosphenytoin in pediatric patients has not been established.

HOW SUPPLIED:

Cerebyx Injection is supplied as follows: Each 10 ml vial contains fosphenytoin sodium 750 mg equivalent to 500 mg of phenytoin sodium. Each 2 ml vial contains fosphenytoin sodium 150 mg equivalent to 100 mg of phenytoin sodium. Both sizes of vials contain Tromethamine, USP (TRIS), Hydrochloric Acid, NF, or Sodium Hydroxide, NF, and Water for Injection, USP.

Fosphenytoin should always be prescribed in phenytoin sodium equivalent units (PE) (see DOSAGE AND ADMINISTRATION).

Storage: Store under refrigeration at 2°C to 8°C (36°F to 46°F). The product should not be stored at room temperature for more than 48 hours. Vials that develop particulate matter should not be used.

HOW SUPPLIED - EQUIVALENTS NOT AVAILABLE:

Injection - Intravenous - 75 mg/ml

25 x 2 ml	$450.00	CEREBYX, Parke-Davis	00071-4007-05

FRUCTOSE *(001339)*

CATEGORIES: Caloric Agents; Electrolytic, Caloric-Water Balance; Pharmaceutical Adjuvants; FDA Pre 1938 Drugs

Prescribing information not available at time of publication.

HOW SUPPLIED - EQUIVALENTS NOT AVAILABLE:

Injection, Solution - Intravenous - 10 %

1000 ml	$18.25	10% FRUCTOSE INJ., Abbott	00074-1537-05
1000 ml x 6	$13.76	10% FRUCTOSE, McGaw	00264-1160-00

Powder

454 gm	$10.55	Fructose, Millgood	53118-0520-10

FURAZOLIDONE *(001341)*

CATEGORIES: Anti-Infectives; Antibacterials; Antidiarrhea Agents; Antiprotozoals; Diarrhea; Enteritis; Gastrointestinal Drugs; Parasiticidal; FDA Approval Pre 1982

BRAND NAMES: *Furion*; *Furoxona* (Mexico); **Furoxone**
(International brand names outside U.S. in italics)

FORMULARIES: Medi-Cal

DESCRIPTION:

Furazolidone is one of the synthetic antimicrobial nitrofurans.

Inactive Ingredients: Furoxone tablets contain calcium pyrophosphate, FD&C Blue #2, magnesium stearate, starch, and sucrose. Furoxone liquid contains carboxy-methylcellulose sodium, flavors, glycerin, magnesium aluminum silicate, methylparaben, propylparaben, purified water, and saccharin sodium.

CLINICAL PHARMACOLOGY:

Furazolidone has a broad antibacterial spectrum covering the majority of gastrointestinal tract pathogens including *E. coli*, staphylococci, *Salmonella, Shigella, Proteus, Aerobacter aerogenes, Vibrio cholerae*[9,10,11] and *Giardia lamblia.*[5,6] Its bactericidal activity is based upon its interference with several bacterial enzyme systems; this antimicrobial action minimizes the development of resistent organisms. It neither significantly alters the normal bowel flora nor results in fungal overgrowth. The brown color found in the urine with adequate dosage is of no clinical significance.

INDICATIONS AND USAGE:

Indicated in the specific and symptomatic treatment of bacterial or protozoal diarrhea and enteritis caused by susceptible organisms. Furazolidone products are well tolerated, have a very low incidence of adverse reactions.

CONTRAINDICATIONS:

1. To obviate an antabuse-like reaction which may occur in some patients, the ingestion of alcohol should be avoided during or within four days after furazolidone therapy (see ADVERSE REACTIONS.)

2. IN GENERAL, MAOI DRUGS, TYRAMINE-CONTAINING FOODS AND INDIRECTLY-ACTING SYMPATHOMIMETIC AMINES ARE CONTRAINDICATED OR SHOULD BE USED WITH CAUTION IN PATIENTS RECEIVING FURAZOLIDONE (SEE PRECAUTIONS.)

3. INFANTS UNDER 1 MONTHS SHOULD NOT RECEIVE FURAZOLIDONE (SEE ADVERSE REACTIONS AND DOSAGE FOR CHILDREN).[4] THE FURAZOLIDONE CONCENTRATION IN THE BREAST MILK OF LACTATING WOMEN HAS NOT BEEN DETERMINED, THEREFORE THE SAFETY IN THIS CIRCUMSTANCE HAS NOT BEEN ESTABLISHED.

4. Prior sensitivity to furazolidone is a contraindication.

WARNINGS:

See CONTRAINDICATIONS.

Use in Pregnancy: The safety of furazolidone during the childbearing age has not been established; as with any potent antibacterial, furazolidone must be administered with caution during the childbearing age. However, animal breeding studies have revealed no evidence of teratogenicity following the administration of furazolidone for long periods of time and at doses far in excess of those recommended for the human. There have been no clinical reports regarding this possible adverse effect on the fetus or the newborn infant.

PRECAUTIONS:

Monoamine Oxidase Inhibition:[7]Effective inhibition of monoamine oxidase by furazolidone has been demonstrated experimentally in man by the enhancement of tyramine and amphetamine sensitivity and by directly measured monoamine oxidase inhibition.

A period of five days of furazolidone administration in the recommended doses in these patients was required to give an enhancement of the tyramine and amphetamine sensitivities by two to threefold. Administration of furazolidone in the recommended dose of 400 mg/day for a period of five days should not subject the adult patient to an undue hazard of hypertensive crisis due to monoamine oxidase inhibition. Hypertensive crises have never been reported even after the peroral administration of larger doses and/or for longer periods of time. Controlled studies reveal no signs or symptoms of hypertensive crisis even after the peroral administration of furazolidone in doses of 400 mg/day in excess of 48 consecutive months.[8]

If administered in doses larger than recommended or in excess of five days, the indications must be weighed against the possible hazards of hypertensive crisis related to the accumulation of monoamine oxidase inhibition. If indications are sufficient, the patients should be informed of drugs and foods which predispose of hypertensive crises:

A. Other known MAOI drugs; however, when indicated they should be prescribed with caution and at a reduced dosage.

B. Tyramine-containing foods such as broad beans, yeast extracts, strong unpasteurized cheeses, beer, wine, pickled herring, chicken livers, and fermented products are contraindicated.

C. Indirectly-acting sympathomimetic amines such as those found in nasal decongestants (phenylephrine, ephedrine) and anorectics (amphetamines) are contraindicated.

D. Likewise, sedatives, antihistamines, tranquilizers, and narcotics should be used in reduced dosages and with caution. Orthostatic hypotension and hypoglycemia may occur.

CARCINOGENESIS, MUTAGENESIS, AND IMPAIRMENT OF FERTILITY

Furazolidone has shown evidence of tumorigenic activity in several studies involving chronic, high-dose oral administration to rodents. Promotion of the development of mammary neoplasia has been demonstrated in rats of two strains. Prominent among the finding in mice

PRECAUTIONS: *(cont'd)*

was that furazolidone caused significant increases in malignant lung tumors. The relevance of these animal findings, particularly relationship to short-term therapy in humans, is not established.

ADVERSE REACTIONS:

A few hypersensitivity reactions of furazolidone have been reported including a fall in blood pressure, urticaria, fever, arthralgia, and a vesicular morbilliform rash. These reactions subsided following withdrawal of the drug.

Nausea, emesis, headache, or malaise occur occasionally and may be minimized or eliminated by reduction in dosage or withdrawal of the drug.

Rarely, individuals receiving furazolidone have exhibited an antabuse-like reaction to alcohol characterized by flushing, slight temperature elevation, dyspnea, and in some instances, a sense of constriction within the chest. All symptomatology disappeared within 24 hours with no lasting ill effects. During nine years of clinical use and approximately 3.5 million courses of therapy (in the U.S.A alone) in the published literature and documented case reports 43 cases have been reported—of which 14 were produced under experimental conditions with planned doses of the compound in excess of those recommended.

Three of these experienced a fall in blood pressure necessitating active therapy. Indications are that levarterenol may be used to combat such hypotensive episodes since human studies shown that this drug is not potentiated in patients treated with furazolidone. (Indirectly acting pressor agents should be avoided.) The ingestion of alcohol in any form should be avoided during furazolidone therapy and for four days thereafter to prevent this reaction.

Furazolidone may cause mild reversible intravascular hemolysis in certain ethnic groups, of Mediterranean and Near-Eastern origin, and Negroes.[1,3] This is due to an intrinsic defect of red blood cell metabolism in a small percentage of these ethnic groups, making them unusually susceptible to hemolysis by numerous compounds.[2] It is necessary to observe such patients closely while receiving furazolidone and to discontinue its use if there is any indication of hemolysis.

Should not be administered to infants under 1 month of age because of the possibility of producing a hemolytic anemia due to immature enzyme systems (glutathione instability) in the early neonatal period.[4]

Colitis, proctitis, anal pruritus, staphylococcic enteritis, renal or hepatic toxicity have not been a significant problem with furazolidone.

DOSAGE AND ADMINISTRATION:

Furoxone tablets, 100 mg each, are green and scored to facilitate adjustment of dosage.

Average Adult Dosage: One 100-mg tablet four times daily.

Average Dosage for Children: Those 5 years of age or older should receive 25 to 50 mg (1/4 to 1/2 tablet) four times daily. The tablet dosage may be crushed and given in a spoonful of corn syrup.

Furoxone liquid composition: each 15 ml tablespoonful contains Furoxone 50 mg per 15 ml (3.33 mg per ml) in a light-yellow aqueous vehicle. Suitable flavoring, suspending and preservative agents complete the formulation. (See Inactive Ingredients.) It is stable in storage. Prior to administering Furoxone Liquid shake the bottle vigorously. It should be dispensed in amber bottles.

Average Adult Dosage: Two tablespoonfuls four times daily.

AVERAGE DOSAGE FOR CHILDREN

5 years or older: 1/2 to 1 tablespoonful four times daily (7.5-15.0 ml)

1 to 4 years old: 1 to 1 1/2 teaspoonfuls four times daily (5.0-7.5 ml)

1 month to 1 year: 1/2 to 1 teaspoonful four times daily (2.5-5.0 ml)

This dosage is based on an average dose of 5 mg of Furoxone per Kg (2.3 mg per lb) of body weight given in four equally divided doses during 24 hours. The maximal dose of 8.8 mg of Furoxone per Kg (4 mg per lb) of body weight per 24 hours should probably not be exceeded because of the possibility of producing nausea or emesis. If these are severe, the dosage should be reduced.

The average case of diarrhea treated with Furoxone will respond within 2 to 5 days of therapy. Occasional patients may require a longer term of therapy. If satisfactory clinical response is not obtained within 7 days it indicates that the pathogen is refractory to Furoxone and the drug should be discontinued. Adjunctive therapy with other antibacterial agents or bismuth salts is not contraindicated. (N.B. Refer to WARNINGS.)

In order to administer furazolidone in doses larger than recommended or in excess of five days the indications must be weighed against the possible hazards of hypertensive crisis related to the accumulation of monoamine oxidase inhibition. If indications are sufficient, the patient should be informed of drugs and foods which predispose to hypertensive crises. (See PRECAUTIONS.)

REFERENCES:

(1) Kellermeyer, R.S., Tarlov, A.R., Schrier, S.L., and Alving, A.S. J. Lab. Clin. Med. 52:827-828 (Nov) 1958. **(2)** Tarlov et al. Arch. Int. med. 109:209-234, 1962. **(3)** Kellermeyer et al. J.A.M.A. 180: No. 5, 388-394, 1962. **(4)** Zinkham, Pediatrics 23:18-32, 1959; Gross & Hurwitz, Pediatrics 22:453, 1958. **(5)** Fallas Vargas, M. Un Nuevo Tratamiento para la Giardiasis (A New Treatment for Giardiasis). Rev. Med. Costa Rica 19:269-284 (July) 1962. **(6)** Webster, B.H. Furazolidone in the Treatment of Giardiasis. Amer. J. Dig. Diseases 5:618-622 (July) 1960. **(7)** Oates, J.A., Pettinger, W.A. Inhibition of Monoamine Oxidase by Furazolidone in Man. Data on file: Office of the Medical Director, Norwich Eaton Pharmaceuticals, Inc. Available upon request. **(8)** Kirsner, Joseph B., M.D., Ph.D. Data on file: Office of the Medical Director, Norwich Eaton Pharmaceuticals, Inc. Available upon request. **(9)** Neogy, K.N., et al. Furazolidone in Cholera, Journ. Indian Med. Assoc. 48:137, 1967. **(10)** Chaudhuri, R.N. et al. Furazolidone in Cholera. Lancet 2:909 (Oct 30) 1965. **(11)** Curlin, G. Comparison of Antibiotic Regimens in Cholera. Abstracts of papers, Epidemiological Intelligence Service Conference, Atlanta, Ga., April 11-14, 1967, p. 11.Furoxone (Furazolidone) Sensi-Discs for laboratory determination of bacterial sensitivity are available from BBL, division of BioQuest.

HOW SUPPLIED - EQUIVALENTS NOT AVAILABLE:

Liquid - Oral - 50 mg/15 ml

60 ml	**$14.48**	**FUROXONE, Roberts Labs**	**54092-0430-60**
473 ml	**$84.80**	**FUROXONE, Roberts Labs**	**54092-0430-16**

Tablet, Coated - Oral - 100 mg

20's	**$48.17**	**FUROXONE, Roberts Labs**	**54092-0130-20**
100's	**$232.61**	**FUROXONE, Roberts Labs**	**54092-0130-01**

FUROSEMIDE *(001342)*

CATEGORIES: Antihypertensives; Cirrhosis; Congestive Heart Failure; Diuresis; Diuretics; Edema; Electrolytic, Caloric-Water Balance; Heart Failure; Hypertension; Loop Diuretics; Nephrotic Syndrome; Pulmonary Edema; Renal Drugs; Vertigo/Motion Sickness/Vomiting; Pregnancy Category C; Sales > $100 Million; FDA Approval Pre 1982; Top 200 Drugs

BRAND NAMES: *Aldic*; *Aluzine*; *Anfuramaide*; *Apo-Frusemide*; *Apo-Furosemide* (Canada); *Aquarid*; *Aquamide*; *Aquasin*; *Arasemide* (Japan); *Bioretic*; *Cetasix*; Detue; *Dirine*; *Discoid* (Germany); *Disemide*; *Diural*; *Diuresal*; *Diurema*; *Diurin*; *Diurolasa*; *Diusil*; *Dranex*; *Dryptal* (England); *Durafurid* (Germany); *Edenol* (Mexico); *Errolon*; *Eutensin* (Japan); *Fluidrol*; *Franyl* (Japan); *Frumex*; *Furmid*; *Frusedan*; *Frusema*; *Frusemid*; *Frusemide*; *Frusetic*; *Frusid* (England); *Frusix*; *Furantril*; *Furanturil*; *Furetic*; *Furex*; *Furix*; *Frumide*; *Furo-Basan*; Furocot; *Furodiurol*; *Furomen*; *Furomex*; Furomide M.D.; *Furo-Puren* (Germany); *Furorese* (Germany); *Furosan*; *Furoside* (Canada); *Furosix*; *Furoter*; *Furovite*; *Fusid* (Germany); *Golan*; *Hissuflux*; *Hydrex*; *Hydro*; *Impugan*; *Kofuzon*; *Kutrix* (Japan); *Lasemid*; *Lasiletten*; *Lasilix* (France); **Lasix**; *Lasix Retard*; *Laxur*; *Liside*; Lo-Aqua; Luramide; *Marsemide*; Myrosemide; *Naclex*; *Nadis*; *Nelsix*; *Nephron*; *Nildema*; *Novosemide* (Canada); *Odemase*; *Odemex*; *Oedemex*; *Promedes* (Japan); *Promide*; *Radisemide*; *Radonna*; *Rasitol*; *Retep*; Ro-Semide; Rose-40; *Rosis*; *Salinex*; *Salurid*; *Seguril*; *Sigasalur* (Germany); *Trofurit*; *Uremide* (Australia); *Urenil* (Japan); *Uresix*; *Urex* (Australia, Japan); *Urex-M* (Australia); *Urian*; *Uridon*; *Uritol* (Canada); *Yidoli*
(International brand names outside U.S. in italics)

FORMULARIES: Aetna; BC-BS; CIGNA; DoD; FHP; Humana; Kaiser; Medco; Medi-Cal; PCS; PruCare; United; WHO

COST OF THERAPY: $15.91 (Hypertension; Tablet; 40 mg; 2/day; 365 days) vs. Potential Cost of $24,027.04 (Coronary Bypass)

PRIMARY ICD9: 401.1 (Essential Hypertension, Benign)

Furosemide is a potent diuretic which, if given in excessive amounts, can lead to a profound diuresis with water and electrolyte depletion. Therefore, careful medical supervision is required and dose and dose schedule must be adjusted to the individual patient's needs. (See DOSAGE AND ADMINISTRATION.)

DESCRIPTION:

Tablets: Furosemide is a diuretic which is an anthranilic acid derivative. Furosemide for oral administration contains furosemide as the active ingredient and the following inactive ingredients: lactose USP, magnesium stearate NF, starch NF, and talc USP.

Chemically, it is 4-chloro-N-furfuryl-5-sulfamoylanthranilic acid. Furosemide is available as white tablets for oral administration in dosage strengths of 20, 40 and 80 mg.

Furosemide is a white, off-white to slightly yellow odorless crystalline powder. It is practically insoluble in water, sparingly soluble in alcohol, freely soluble in dilute alkali solutions and insoluble in dilute acids.

The CAS Registry Number is 54-31-9.

Injection: Furosemide Injection is composed of 4-chloro-N-furfuryl-5- sulfamoylanthranilic acid, sodium chloride for isotonicity and sodium hydroxide to adjust pH.

Furosemide Injection 10 mg/ml is a sterile, non-pyrogenic solution in ampules, disposable syringes and single dose vials for intravenous and intramuscular injection.

Oral Solution: Furosemide Oral Solution contains furosemide as the active ingredient and the following inactive ingredients: alcohol USP 11.5%, D&C yellow #10, FD&C yellow #6 as color additives, flavors, glycerin USP, parabens NF, purified water USP, sorbitol NF; sodium hydroxide NF added to adjust pH. Furosemide Oral Solution 10 mg/ml is an orange flavored liquid for oral administration.

CLINICAL PHARMACOLOGY:

Investigations into the mode of action of furosemide have utilized micropuncture studies in rats, stop flow experiments in dogs and various clearance studies in both humans and experimental animals. It has been demonstrated that furosemide inhibits primarily the absorption of sodium and chloride not only in the proximal and distal tubules but also in the loop of Henle. The high degree of efficacy is largely due to this unique site of action. The action on the distal tubule is independent of any inhibitory effect on carbonic anhydrase and aldosterone.

Recent evidence suggests that furosemide glucuronide is the only or at least the major biotransformation product of furosemide in man. Furosemide is extensively bound to plasma proteins, mainly to albumin. Plasma concentrations ranging from 1 to 400 mcg/ml are 91 to 99% bound in healthy individuals. The unbound fraction averages 2.3 to 4.1% at therapeutic concentrations.

The onset of diuresis following oral administration is within 1 hour. The peak effect occurs within the first or second hour. The duration of diuretic effect is 6 to 8 hours.

The onset of diuresis following intravenous administration is within 5 minutes and somewhat later after intramuscular administration. The peak effect occurs within the first half hour. The duration of diuretic effect is approximately 2 hours.

In fasted normal men, the mean bioavailability of furosemide from furosemide Tablets and furosemide Oral Solution is 64% and 60%, respectively, of that from an intravenous injection of the drug. Although furosemide is more rapidly absorbed from the oral solution (50 minutes) than from the tablet (87 minutes), peak plasma levels and area under the plasma concentration-time curves do not differ significantly. Peak plasma concentrations increase with increasing dose but times-to-peak do not differ among doses. The terminal half-life of furosemide is approximately 2 hours.

Significantly more furosemide is excreted in urine following the IV injection than after the tablet or oral solution. There are no significant differences between the two oral formulations in the amount of unchanged drug excreted in urine.

INDICATIONS AND USAGE:

Parenteral therapy should be reserved for patients unable to take oral medication or for patients in emergency clinical situations.

TABLETS, INJECTION, AND ORAL SOLUTION

Edema: Furosemide is indicated in adults, infants, and children for the treatment of edema associated with congestive heart failure, cirrhosis of the liver, and renal disease, including the nephrotic syndrome. Furosemide is particularly useful when an agent with greater diuretic potential is desired.

TABLETS AND ORAL SOLUTION

Hypertension: Oral furosemide may be used in adults for the treatment of hypertension alone or in combination with other antihypertensive agents. Hypertensive patients who cannot be adequately controlled with thiazides will probably also not be adequately controlled with furosemide alone.

INJECTION

Furosemide is indicated as adjunctive therapy in acute pulmonary edema. The intravenous administration of furosemide is indicated when a rapid onset of diuresis is desired, e.g., in acute pulmonary edema.

If gastrointestinal absorption is impaired or oral medication is not practical for any reason, furosemide is indicated by the intravenous or intramuscular route. Parenteral use should be replaced with oral furosemide as soon as practical.

CONTRAINDICATIONS:

Furosemide is contraindicated in patients with anuria and in patients with a history of hypersensitivity to furosemide.

WARNINGS:

TABLETS, INJECTION, AND ORAL SOLUTION

In patients with hepatic cirrhosis and ascites, furosemide therapy is best initiated in the hospital. In hepatic coma and in states of electrolyte depletion, therapy should not be instituted until the basic condition is improved. Sudden alterations of fluid and electrolyte balance in patients with cirrhosis may precipitate hepatic coma; therefore, strict observation is necessary during the period of diuresis. Supplemental potassium chloride and, if required, an aldosterone antagonist are helpful in preventing hypokalemia and metabolic alkalosis.

If increasing azotemia and oliguria occur during treatment of severe progressive renal disease, furosemide should be discontinued.

Cases of tinnitus and reversible or irreversible hearing impairment have been reported. Usually, reports indicate that furosemide ototoxicity is associated with rapid injection, severe renal impairment, doses exceeding several times the usual recommended dose, or concomitant therapy with aminoglycoside antibiotics, ethacrynic acid, or other ototoxic drugs. If the physician elects to use high dose parenteral therapy, controlled intravenous infusion is advisable (for adults, an infusion rate not exceeding 4 mg furosemide per minute has been used).

INJECTION

Pediatric Use: In premature neonates with respiratory distress syndrome, diuretic treatment with furosemide in the first few weeks of life may increase the risk of persistent patent ductus arteriosus (PDA), possibly through a prostaglandin-E-mediated process.

Hearing loss in neonates has been associated with the use of furosemide injection (see WARNINGS).

PRECAUTIONS:

TABLETS, INJECTION, AND ORAL SOLUTION

General: Excessive diuresis may cause dehydration and blood volume reduction with circulatory collapse and possibly vascular thrombosis and embolism, particularly in elderly patients. As with any effective diuretic, electrolyte depletion may occur during furosemide therapy, especially in patients receiving higher doses and a restricted salt intake. Hypokalemia may develop with furosemide, especially with brisk diuresis, inadequate oral electrolyte intake, when cirrhosis is present, or during concomitant use of corticosteroids or ACTH. Digitalis therapy may exaggerate metabolic effects of hypokalemia, especially myocardial effects.

All patients receiving furosemide therapy should be observed for these signs or symptoms of fluid or electrolyte imbalance (hyponatremia, hypochloremic alkalosis, hypokalemia, hypomagnesemia or hypocalcemia): dryness of mouth, thirst, weakness, lethargy, drowsiness, restlessness, muscle pains or cramps, muscular fatigue, hypotension, oliguria, tachycardia, arrhythmia, or gastrointestinal disturbances such as nausea and vomiting. Increases in blood glucose and alterations in glucose tolerance tests (with abnormalities of the fasting and 2-hour postprandial sugar) have been observed, and rarely precipitation of diabetes mellitus has been reported.

Asymptomatic hyperuricemia can occur and gout may rarely be precipitated.

ORAL SOLUTION

The sorbitol present in the vehicle may cause diarrhea (especially in children) when higher doses of furosemide Oral Solution are given.

TABLETS, INJECTION, AND ORAL SOLUTION

Patients allergic to sulfonamides may also be allergic to furosemide. The possibility exists of exacerbation or activation of systemic lupus erythematosus.

As with many other drugs, patients should be observed regularly for the possible occurrence of blood dyscrasias, liver or kidney damage, or other idiosyncratic reactions.

Information for the Patient: Patients receiving furosemide should be advised that they may experience symptoms from excessive fluid and/or electrolyte losses. The postural hypotension that sometimes occurs can usually be managed by getting up slowly. Potassium supplements and/or dietary measures may be needed to control or avoid hypokalemia.

Patients with diabetes mellitus should be told that furosemide may increase blood glucose levels and thereby affect urine glucose tests. The skin of some patients may be more sensitive to the effects of sunlight while taking furosemide.

Hypertensive patients should avoid medications that may increase blood pressure, including over-the-counter products for appetite suppression and cold symptoms.

Laboratory Tests: Serum electrolytes (particularly potassium), CO_2, creatinine and BUN should be determined frequently during the first few months of furosemide therapy and periodically thereafter. Serum and urine electrolyte determinations are particularly important when the patient is vomiting profusely or receiving parenteral fluids. Abnormalities should be corrected or the drug temporarily withdrawn. Other medications may also influence serum electrolytes.

Reversible elevations of BUN may occur and are associated with dehydration, which should be avoided, particularly in patients with renal insufficiency.

Urine and blood glucose should be checked periodically in diabetics receiving furosemide, even in those suspected of latent diabetes.

Furosemide may lower serum levels of calcium (rarely cases of tetany have been reported) and magnesium. Accordingly, serum levels of these electrolytes should be determined periodically.

Carcinogenesis, Mutagenesis, and Impairment of Fertility: Furosemide was tested for carcinogenicity by oral administration in one strain of mice and one strain of rats. A small but significantly increased incidence of mammary gland carcinomas occurred in female mice at a dose 17.5 times the maximum human dose of 600 mg. There were marginal increases in uncommon tumors in male rats at a dose of 15 mg/kg (slightly greater than the maximum human dose) but not at 30 mg/kg.

Furosemide was devoid of mutagenic activity in various strains of *Salmonella typhimurium* when tested in the presence or absence of an *in vitro* metabolic activation system, and questionably positive for gene mutation in mouse lymphoma cells in the presence of rat liver S9 at the highest dose tested. Furosemide did not induce sister chromatid exchange in human cells *in vitro*, but other studies on chromosomal aberrations in human cells *in vitro* gave conflicting results. In Chinese hamster cells it induced chromosomal damage but was questionably positive for sister chromatid exchange. Studies

PRECAUTIONS: *(cont'd)*

on the induction by furosemide of chromosomal aberrations in mice were inconclusive. The urine of rats treated with this drug did not induce gene conversion in *Saccharomyces cerevisiae*.

Furosemide produced no impairment of fertility in male or female rats, at 100 mg/kg/day (the maximum effective diuretic dose in the rat and 8 times the maximal human dose of 600 mg/day).

Pregnancy Category C: Furosemide has been shown to cause unexplained maternal deaths and abortions in rabbits at 2, 4 and 8 times the maximal recommended human dose. There are no adequate and well-controlled studies in pregnant women. Furosemide should be used during pregnancy only if the potential benefit justifies the potential risk to the fetus.

The effects of furosemide on embryonic and fetal development and on pregnant dams were studied in mice, rats and rabbits.

Furosemide caused unexplained maternal deaths and abortions in the rabbit at the lowest dose of 25 mg/kg (2 times the maximal recommended human dose of 600 mg/day). In another study, a dose of 50 mg/kg (4 times the maximal recommended human dose of 600 mg/day) also caused maternal deaths and abortions when administered to rabbits between days 12 and 17 of gestation. In a third study, none of the pregnant rabbits survived a dose of 100 mg/kg. Data from the above studies indicate fetal lethality that can precede maternal deaths.

The results of the mouse study and one of the three rabbit studies also showed an increased incidence and severity of hydronephrosis (distention of the renal pelvis and in some cases of the ureters) in fetuses derived from the treated dams as compared with the incidence in fetuses from the control group.

Nursing Mothers: Because it appears in breast milk, caution should be exercised when furosemide is administered to a nursing mother.

INJECTION

Pediatric Use: Renal calcifications (from barely visible on x-ray to staghorn) have occurred in some severely premature infants treated with intravenous furosemide for edema due to patent ductus arteriosus and hyaline membrane disease. The concurrent use of chlorothiazide has been reported to decrease hypercalciuria and dissolve some calculi.

DRUG INTERACTIONS:

Furosemide may increase the ototoxic potential of aminoglycoside antibiotics, especially in the presence of impaired renal function. Except in life-threatening situations, avoid this combination.

Furosemide should not be used concomitantly with ethacrynic acid because of the possibility of ototoxicity. Patients receiving high doses of salicylates concomitantly with furosemide, as in rheumatic disease, may experience salicylate toxicity at lower doses because of competitive renal excretory sites.

Furosemide has a tendency to antagonize the skeletal muscle relaxing effect of tubocurarine and may potentiate the action of succinylcholine.

Lithium generally should not be given with diuretics because they reduce lithium's renal clearance and add a high risk of lithium toxicity.

Furosemide may add to or potentiate the therapeutic effect of other antihypertensive drugs. Potentiation occurs with ganglionic or peripheral adrenergic blocking drugs.

Furosemide may decrease arterial responsiveness to norepinephrine. However, norepinephrine may still be used effectively.

TABLETS

Simultaneous administration of sucralfate and furosemide tablets may reduce the natriuretic and antihypertensive effects of furosemide. Patients receiving both drugs should be observed closely to determine if the desired diuretic and/or antihypertensive effect of furosemide is achieved. The intake of furosemide and sucralfate should be separated by at least two hours.

TABLETS, INJECTION, AND ORAL SOLUTION

One study in six subjects demonstrated that the combination of furosemide and acetylsalicylic acid temporarily reduced creatinine clearance in patients with chronic renal insufficiency. There are case reports of patients who developed increased BUN, serum creatinine and serum potassium levels, and weight gain when furosemide was used in conjunction with NSAIDs.

Literature reports indicate that coadministration of indomethacin may reduce the natriuretic and antihypertensive effects of furosemide in some patients by inhibiting prostaglandin synthesis. Indomethacin may also affect plasma renin levels, aldosterone excretion, and renin profile evaluation. Patients receiving both indomethacin and furosemide should be observed closely to determine if the desired diuretic and/or antihypertensive effect of furosemide is achieved.

ADVERSE REACTIONS:

Adverse reactions are categorized below by organ system and listed by decreasing severity:

Gastrointestinal System Reactions

1. Pancreatitis
2. Jaundice (intrahepatic cholestatic juandice)
3. Anorexia
4. Oral and gastric irritation
5. Cramping
6. Diarrhea
7. Constipation
8. Nausea
9. Vomiting

Systemic Hypersensitivity Reactions

1. Systemic vasculitis
2. Interstitial nephritis
3. Necrotizing angiitis

Central Nervous System Reactions

1. Tinnitus and hearing loss
2. Paresthesias
3. Vertigo
4. Dizziness
5. Headache
6. Blurred vision
7. Xanthopsia

ADVERSE REACTIONS: *(cont'd)*

Hematologic Reactions

1. Aplastic anemia (rare)
2. Thrombocytopenia
3. Agranulocytosis (rare)
4. Hemolytic anemia
5. Leukopenia
6. Anemia

Dermatologic-Hypersensitivity Reactions

1. exfoliative dermatitis
2. erythema multiforme
3. purpura
4. photosensitivity
5. urticaria
6. rash
7. pruritus

Cardiovascular Reaction: Orthostatic hypotension may occur and be aggravated by alcohol, barbiturates or narcotics.

Other Reactions

1. hyperglycemia
2. glycosuria
3. hyperuricemia
4. muscle spasm
5. weaknesses
6. restlessness
7. urinary bladder spasm
8. thrombophlebitis
9. transient injection site pain following intramuscular injection
10. fever

Whenever adverse reactions are moderate or severe, furosemide dosage should be reduced or therapy withdrawn.

OVERDOSAGE:

The principal signs and symptoms of overdose with furosemide are dehydration, blood volume reduction, hypotension, electrolyte imbalance, hypokalemia and hypochloremic alkalosis, and are extensions of its diuretic action.

The acute toxicity of furosemide has been determined in mice, rats and dogs. In all three, the oral LD_{50} exceeded 1000 mg/kg body weight while the intravenous LD_{50} ranged from 300 to 680 mg/kg. The acute intragastric toxicity in neonatal rats is 7 to 10 times that of adult rats.

The concentration of furosemide in biological fluids associated with toxicity or death is not known.

Treatment of overdosage is supportive and consists of replacement of excessive fluid and electrolyte losses. Serum electrolytes, carbon dioxide level and blood pressure should be determined frequently. Adequate drainage must be assured in patients with urinary bladder outlet obstruction (such as prostatic hypertrophy).

Hemodialysis does not accelerate furosemide elimination.

DOSAGE AND ADMINISTRATION:

TABLETS AND ORAL SOLUTION

Edema: Therapy should be individualized according to patient response to gain maximal therapeutic response and to determine the minimal dose needed to maintain that response.

Adults: The usual initial dose of furosemide is 20 to 80 mg given as a single dose. Ordinarily a prompt diuresis ensues. If needed, the same dose can be administered 6 to 8 hours later or the dose may be increased. The dose may be raised by 20 or 40 mg and given not sooner than 6 to 8 hours after the previous dose until the desired diuretic effect has been obtained. This individually determined single dose should then be given once or twice daily (*e.g.,* at 8 am and 2 pm). The dose of furosemide may be carefully titrated up to 600 mg/day in patients with clinically severe edematous states.

Edema may be most efficiently and safely mobilized by giving furosemide on 2 to 4 consecutive days each week.

When doses exceeding 80 mg/day are given for prolonged periods, careful clinical observation and laboratory monitoring are particularly advisable. (See PRECAUTIONS, Laboratory Tests.)

Infants and Children: The usual initial dose of oral furosemide in infants and children is 2 mg/kg body weight, given as a single dose. If the diuretic response is not satisfactory after the initial dose, dosage may be increased by 1 or 2 mg/kg no sooner than 6 to 8 hours after the previous dose. Doses greater than 6 mg/kg body weight are not recommended. For maintenance therapy in infants and children, the dose should be adjusted to the minimum effective level. For ease of administration, and to allow maximum flexibility in dosing, the use of furosemide oral solution is suggested.

Hypertension: Therapy should be individualized according to the patient's response to gain maximal therapeutic response and to determine the minimal dose needed to maintain the therapeutic response.

Adults: The usual initial dose of furosemide for hypertension is 80 mg, usually divided into 40 mg twice a day. Dosage should then be adjusted according to response. If response is not satisfactory, add other antihypertensive agents.

Changes in blood pressure must be carefully monitored when furosemide is used with other antihypertensive drugs, especially during initial therapy. To prevent excessive drop in blood pressure, the dosage of other agents should be reduced by at least 50 percent when furosemide is added to the regimen. As the blood pressure falls under the potentiating effect of furosemide, a further reduction in dosage or even discontinuation of other antihypertensive drugs may be necessary.

TABLETS

Note: Dispense in well-closed, light-resistant containers. Exposure to light might cause a slight discoloration. Discolored tablets should not be dispensed.

ORAL SOLUTION

Note: Store at controlled room temperature (59 to 86° F). Dispense in light-resistant containers. Discard opened bottle after 60 days.

INJECTION

Adults: Parenteral therapy with furosemide Injection should be used only in patients unable to take oral medication or in emergency situations and should be replaced with oral therapy as soon as practical.

DOSAGE AND ADMINISTRATION: *(cont'd)*

Edema: The usual initial dose of furosemide is 20 to 40 mg given as a single dose, injected intramuscularly or intravenously. The intravenous dose should be given slowly (1 to 2 minutes). Ordinarily a prompt diuresis ensues. If needed, another dose may be administered in the same manner 2 hours later or the dose may be increased. The dose may be raised by 20 mg and given not sooner than 2 hours after the previous dose until the desired diuretic effect has been obtained. This individually determined single dose should then be given once or twice daily.

Therapy should be individualized according to patient response to gain maximal therapeutic response to determine the minimal dose needed to maintain that response. Close medical supervision is necessary.

If the physician elects to use high dose parenteral therapy, add the furosemide to either Sodium Chloride Injection USP, Lactated Ringer's Injection USP, or Dextrose (5%) Injection USP after pH has been adjusted to above 5.5, and administer as a controlled intravenous infusion at a rate not greater than 4 mg/min. Furosemide Injection is a buffered alkaline solution with a pH of about 9 and the drug may precipitate at pH values below 7. Care must be taken to ensure that the pH of the prepared infusion solution is in the weakly alkaline to neutral range. Acid solutions, including other parenteral medications (*e.g.,* labetalol, ciprofloxacin, amrinone, and milrinone) must not be administered concurrently in the same infusion because they may cause precipitation of the furosemide. In addition, furosemide injection should not be added to a running intravenous line containing any of these acidic products.

Acute Pulmonary Edema: The usual initial dose of furosemide is 40 mg injected slowly intravenously (over 1 to 2 minutes). If a satisfactory response does not occur within 1 hour, the dose may be increased to 80 mg injected slowly intravenously (over 1 to 2 minutes).

If necessary, additional therapy (*e.g.,* digitalis, oxygen) may be administered concomitantly.

Infants and Children: Parenteral therapy should be used only in patients unable to take oral medication or in emergency situations and should be replaced with oral therapy as soon as practical.

The usual initial dose of furosemide Injection (intravenously or intramuscularly) in infants and children is 1 mg/kg body weight and should be given slowly under close medical supervision. If the diuretic response to the initial dose is not satisfactory, dosage may be increased by 1 mg/kg not sooner than 2 hours after the previous dose, until the desired diuretic effect has been obtained. Doses greater than 6 mg/kg body weight are not recommended.

Furosemide Injection should be inspected visually for particulate matter and discoloration before administration. Do not use if solution is discolored.

To insure patient safety, this needle should be handled with care and should be destroyed and discarded if damaged in any manner. If cannula is bent, no attempt should be made to straighten.

To prevent needle-stick injuries, needles should not be recapped, purposely bent, or broken by hand.

Store at controlled room temperature (59 to 86° F).

Do not use if solution is discolored.

Protect syringes from light. Do not remove syringe from individual package until time of use.

PATIENT INFORMATION:

Furosemide is a diuretic (water pill) used to treat fluid retention and high blood pressure. Do not take this medication if you are allergic to sulfa medicine. Notify your physician if you are pregnant or nursing. Notify your physician if you have diabetes mellitus. Blood glucose levels may be increased in patients with diabetes mellitus. Take this medication early in the day. Furosemide may be taken with or without food. Take with food or milk if stomach upset occurs. Notify your physician if you develop weakness, cramps, or nausea. Dizziness or lightheadedness may occur with therapy; avoid sudden changes in posture. Furosemide may cause increased sensitivity to sunlight. Use sunscreens and wear protective clothing until degree of sensitivity is determined.

HOW SUPPLIED - RATED THERAPEUTICALLY EQUIVALENT:

Injection, Solution - Intramuscular; - 10 mg/ml

2 ml	$1.50	Furosemide, Rugby	00536-4662-67
2 ml	$2.03	Furosemide, Abbott	00074-6101-02
2 ml	$2.46	Furosemide, Abbott	00074-6102-02
2 ml	$3.56	Furosemide Inj. 20, Abbott	00074-6054-02
2 ml	$28.13	Furosemide, Fujisawa USA	00469-7500-10
2 ml x 5	**$5.50**	**LASIX, AMPULS, Hoechst Marion Roussel**	**00039-0061-15**
2 ml x 5	**$8.30**	**LASIX, PREFILLED SYRINGES, Hoechst Marion Roussel**	**00039-0062-08**
2 ml x 10	$7.12	Furosemide, Sanofi Winthrop	00024-0611-03
2 ml x 10	$11.06	FUROSEMIDE, Sanofi Winthrop	00024-0611-13
2 ml x 25	$8.77	Furosemide, Pasadena	00418-0361-02
2 ml x 25	$13.18	Furosemide, Elkins Sinn	00641-1425-35
2 ml x 25	$19.76	Furosemide, Elkins Sinn	00641-0382-25
2 ml x 25	$22.19	Furosemide, Am Regent	00517-5702-25
2 ml x 25	$27.25	Furosemide, Consolidated Midland	00223-7700-02
2 ml x 25	**$33.75**	**LASIX, Hoechst Marion Roussel**	**00039-0162-25**
2 ml x 25	$34.38	Furosemide 1%, Astra USA	00186-1114-13
2 ml x 50	$35.59	Furosemide, Sanofi Winthrop	00024-0611-50
2 ml x 50	**$51.50**	**LASIX, AMPULS, Hoechst Marion Roussel**	**00039-0061-05**
4 ml	$3.92	Furosemide, Abbott	00074-6101-04
4 ml	$4.20	Furosemide, Abbott	00074-6102-04
4 ml	$4.86	Furosemide, Abbott	00074-6055-14
4 ml	$34.38	Furosemide, Fujisawa USA	00469-7500-70
4 ml x 5	**$9.25**	**LASIX, PREFILLED SYRINGES, Hoechst Marion Roussel**	**00039-0061-45**
4 ml x 5	**$11.00**	**LASIX, PREFILLED SYRINGES, Hoechst Marion Roussel**	**00039-0064-08**
4 ml x 10	$26.25	Furosemide 1%, Astra USA	00186-0635-01
4 ml x 25	$19.76	Furosemide, Elkins Sinn	00641-1426-35
4 ml x 25	$29.65	Furosemide, Elkins Sinn	00641-2311-25
4 ml x 25	$35.94	Furosemide, Am Regent	00517-5704-25
4 ml x 25	$37.50	Furosemide, Consolidated Midland	00223-7704-04
4 ml x 25	**$45.00**	**LASIX, AMPULS, Hoechst Marion Roussel**	**00039-0061-65**
4 ml x 25	**$51.50**	**LASIX, Hoechst Marion Roussel**	**00039-0163-25**

HOW SUPPLIED - RATED THERAPEUTICALLY EQUIVALENT:
(cont'd)

4 ml x 25	$57.75	Furosemide 1%, Astra USA	00186-1115-13
8 ml	$7.03	Furosemide, Abbott	00074-6056-17
8 ml x 25	$108.29	Furosemide 1%, Astra USA	00186-1116-12
10 ml	$2.36	Furosemide, HL Moore Drug Exch	00839-6677-30
10 ml	$4.69	Furosemide, Rugby	00536-4662-70
10 ml	$4.94	Furosemide, Rugby	00536-4663-70
10 ml	$5.05	Furosemide, Major Pharms	00904-1485-10
10 ml	$8.11	Furosemide, Intl Medication	00548-1431-00
10 ml	$9.49	Furosemide, Abbott	00074-6102-10
10 ml	$9.94	Furosemide, Abbott	00074-6101-10
10 ml	$11.32	Furosemide, Abbott	00074-6102-11
10 ml	$12.31	Furosemide, Abbott	00074-6056-18
10 ml	$78.13	Furosemide, Fujisawa USA	00469-7500-30
10 ml x 5	**$26.15**	**LASIX, AMPULS, Hoechst Marion Roussel**	**00039-0061-08**
10 ml x 5	**$27.50**	**LASIX, Hoechst Marion Roussel**	**00039-0065-08**
10 ml x 10	$68.88	Furosemide 1%, Astra USA	00186-0636-01
10 ml x 25	$57.19	Furosemide, Am Regent	00517-5710-25
10 ml x 25	$72.49	Furosemide, Elkins Sinn	00641-2312-25
10 ml x 25	$105.00	Furosemide 1%, Astra USA	00186-1117-12
10 ml x 25	$125.00	Furosemide, Consolidated Midland	00223-7707-10
10 ml x 25	**$126.50**	**LASIX, AMPULS, Hoechst Marion Roussel**	**00039-0061-25**
10 ml x 25	**$132.00**	**LASIX, Hoechst Marion Roussel**	**00039-0164-25**

Solution - Oral - 10 mg/ml

60 ml	$6.60	Furosemide, HL Moore Drug Exch	00839-7431-64
60 ml	$8.88	Furosemide, Qualitest Pharms	00603-1250-52
60 ml	$9.05	Furosemide, Aligen Independ	00405-2832-56
60 ml	$9.10	Furosemide, Roxane	00054-3294-46
60 ml	$9.46	Furosemide, Morton Grove	60432-0613-60
60 ml	$9.75	Furosemide, Major Pharms	00904-1477-03
60 ml	$9.82	Furosemide, United Res	00677-1423-25
60 ml	$9.87	Furosemide, Rugby	00536-0709-96
60 ml	$10.00	Furosemide, Goldline Labs	00182-6053-68
60 ml	$10.00	Furosemide, Geneva Pharms	00781-6302-02
60 ml	**$11.10**	**LASIX, BOTTLE W/DROPPER, Hoechst Marion Roussel**	**00039-0063-06**
120 ml	$12.60	Furosemide, Major Pharms	00904-1477-20
120 ml	$12.90	Furosemide, Goldline Labs	00182-6053-37
120 ml	$12.98	Furosemide, Morton Grove	60432-0613-04
120 ml	$17.67	Furosemide, Roxane	00054-3294-50
120 ml	**$18.40**	**LASIX, BOTTLE W/DROPPER, Hoechst Marion Roussel**	**00039-0063-40**

Tablet, Uncoated - Oral - 20 mg

30's	$.63	Furosemide, H.C.F.A. F F P	99999-1342-05
30's	$1.85	Furosemide, Major Pharms	00904-1580-46
90's	$1.89	Furosemide, H.C.F.A. F F P	99999-1342-01
90's	$2.80	Furosemide, Major Pharms	00904-1580-89
100's	$2.10	Furosemide, H.C.F.A. F F P	99999-1342-02
100's	$3.08	Furosemide, IDE-Interstate	00814-3300-14
100's	$3.60	Furosemide, Voluntary Hosp	53258-0129-01
100's	$3.90	LURAMIDE, Major Pharms	00904-1480-60
100's	$3.90	Furosemide, Major Pharms	00904-1580-60
100's	$3.95	Furosemide, Watson Labs	52544-0300-01
100's	$3.95	Furosemide, Watson Labs	52544-0311-01
100's	$4.00	Furosemide, Raway	00686-0072-20
100's	$4.15	Furosemide, United Res	00677-0662-01
100's	$4.25	Furosemide, HL Moore Drug Exch	00839-6345-06
100's	$4.29	Furosemide, PRL Enterpr	53633-0259-11
100's	$4.98	Furosemide, Aligen Independ	00405-4452-01
100's	$5.10	Furosemide, Geneva Pharms	50752-0286-05
100's	$5.20	Furosemide, Qualitest Pharms	00603-3736-21
100's	$5.25	Furosemide, Roxane	00054-4297-25
100's	$5.25	Furosemide, Zenith Labs	00172-2908-60
100's	$5.25	Furosemide, Goldline Labs	00182-1170-01
100's	$5.25	Furosemide, Geneva Pharms	00781-1818-01
100's	$6.00	Furosemide, Schein Pharm (US)	00364-0568-01
100's	$6.05	Furosemide, Rugby	00536-3840-01
100's	$6.06	Furosemide, HL Moore Drug Exch	00839-7782-06
100's	$6.39	LURAMIDE, Major Pharms	00904-1480-61
100's	$6.87	Furosemide, Voluntary Hosp	53258-0129-13
100's	$7.05	Furosemide, Bristol Myers Squibb	00003-0359-50
100's	$7.57	Furosemide, Roxane	00054-8297-25
100's	$8.75	Furosemide, Schein Pharm (US)	00364-0568-90
100's	$8.88	Furosemide, Lederle Pharm	00005-3708-60
100's	$9.20	Furosemide, Medirex	57480-0328-01
100's	$11.24	Furosemide, TIE Pharm	55496-2201-09
100's	$11.36	Furosemide, Lederle Pharm	00005-3708-23
100's	$11.50	Furosemide, Mylan	00378-0208-01
100's	$11.95	Furosemide, Goldline Labs	00182-1170-89
100's	$12.78	Furosemide, Major Pharms	00904-1580-61
100's	$12.90	Furosemide, Vangard Labs	00615-1569-13
100's	**$15.75**	**LASIX, Hoechst Marion Roussel**	**00039-0067-10**
100's	**$16.65**	**LASIX, Hoechst Marion Roussel**	**00039-0067-11**
500's	$9.90	Furosemide, Geneva Pharms	00781-1818-05
500's	$10.50	Furosemide, H.C.F.A. F F P	99999-1342-03
500's	$18.75	Furosemide Tablets 20 Mg, Watson Labs	52544-0300-05
500's	$18.75	Furosemide, Watson Labs	52544-0311-05
500's	$19.50	Furosemide, Zenith Labs	00172-2908-70
500's	$26.64	Furosemide, Lederle Pharm	00005-3708-31
500's	$27.50	Furosemide, Rugby	00536-3840-05
500's	**$74.40**	**LASIX, Hoechst Marion Roussel**	**00039-0067-50**
600's	$65.00	Furosemide, Medirex	57480-0328-06
750's	$90.00	Furosemide, Glasgow Pharm	60809-0133-55
750's	$90.00	Furosemide, Glasgow Pharm	60809-0133-72
1000's	$17.55	Furosemide, IDE-Interstate	00814-3300-30
1000's	$18.50	Furosemide, Mova Pharms	55370-0514-09
1000's	$19.90	LURAMIDE, Major Pharms	00904-1480-80
1000's	$19.90	Furosemide, Major Pharms	00904-1580-80
1000's	$21.00	Furosemide, H.C.F.A. F F P	99999-1342-04
1000's	$25.50	Furosemide, United Res	00677-0662-10
1000's	$25.65	Furosemide, HL Moore Drug Exch	00839-6345-16
1000's	$25.95	Furosemide, Qualitest Pharms	00603-3736-32
1000's	$31.96	Furosemide, Geneva Pharms	00781-1818-10
1000's	$34.95	Furosemide, Watson Labs	52544-0300-10
1000's	$34.95	Furosemide, Watson Labs	52544-0311-10
1000's	$36.05	Furosemide, Roxane	00054-4297-31
1000's	$36.05	Furosemide, Zenith Labs	00172-2908-80
1000's	$36.05	Furosemide, Goldline Labs	00182-1170-10
1000's	$38.03	Furosemide, Aligen Independ	00405-4452-03
1000's	$41.90	Furosemide, Schein Pharm (US)	00364-0568-02
1000's	$48.25	Furosemide, Geneva Pharms	50752-0286-09
1000's	$52.95	Furosemide, Parmed Pharms	00349-8486-10

HOW SUPPLIED - RATED THERAPEUTICALLY EQUIVALENT:
(cont'd)

1000's	$53.73	Furosemide, HL Moore Drug Exch	00839-7782-16
1000's	$53.75	Furosemide, Mylan	00378-0208-10
1000's	$53.75	Furosemide, Rugby	00536-3840-10
1000's	$63.57	Furosemide, Bristol Myers Squibb	00003-0359-75
1000's	**$141.35**	**LASIX, Hoechst Marion Roussel**	**00039-0067-70**

Tablet, Uncoated - Oral - 40 mg

30's	$.76	Furosemide, H.C.F.A. F F P	99999-1342-06
30's	$1.90	Furosemide, Major Pharms	00904-1481-46
90's	$2.28	Furosemide, H.C.F.A. F F P	99999-1342-07
90's	$2.95	Furosemide, Major Pharms	00904-1481-89
100's	$2.18	Furosemide, Talbert Phcy	44514-0376-88
100's	$2.54	Furosemide, H.C.F.A. F F P	99999-1342-08
100's	$3.50	Furosemide, Mova Pharms	55370-0515-07
100's	$3.68	Furosemide, IDE-Interstate	00814-3301-14
100's	$3.75	Furosemide, Voluntary Hosp	53258-0220-01
100's	$4.75	Furosemide, Raway	00686-0073-20
100's	$4.85	Furosemide, Major Pharms	00904-1481-60
100's	$5.00	Furosemide, Watson Labs	52544-0301-01
100's	$5.05	Furosemide, United Res	00677-0659-01
100's	$5.32	Furosemide, Aligen Independ	00405-4453-01
100's	$5.54	Furosemide, Roxane	00054-4299-25
100's	$5.66	Furosemide, HL Moore Drug Exch	00839-6323-06
100's	$5.85	Furosemide, Geneva Pharms	50752-0287-05
100's	$5.98	Furosemide, Zenith Labs	00172-2907-60
100's	$5.98	Furosemide, Goldline Labs	00182-1161-01
100's	$6.20	Furosemide, Schein Pharm (US)	00364-0514-01
100's	$6.28	Furosemide, HL Moore Drug Exch	00839-7783-06
100's	$6.93	Furosemide, Rugby	00536-3841-01
100's	$6.93	Furosemide, Geneva Pharms	00781-1966-01
100's	$7.20	Furosemide, Voluntary Hosp	53258-0220-13
100's	$7.86	Furosemide, Roxane	00054-8299-25
100's	$9.91	Furosemide, Bristol Myers Squibb	00003-0360-50
100's	$11.39	Furosemide, Medirex	57480-0329-01
100's	$12.30	Furosemide, Lederle Pharm	00005-3709-60
100's	$13.56	Furosemide, Lederle Pharm	00005-3709-23
100's	$13.75	Furosemide, Mylan	00378-0216-01
100's	$14.76	Furosemide, TIE Pharm	55496-2202-09
100's	$15.75	Furosemide 40, H & H Labs	46703-0040-10
100's	$16.35	Furosemide, Goldline Labs	00182-1161-89
100's	$18.20	Furosemide, Vangard Labs	00615-0446-13
100's	$18.46	Furosemide, Major Pharms	00904-1481-61
100's	**$22.10**	**LASIX, Hoechst Marion Roussel**	**00039-0060-13**
100's	**$23.00**	**LASIX, Hoechst Marion Roussel**	**00039-0060-11**
100's	$59.70	Furosemide, Mylan	00378-0216-10
500's	$12.50	Furosemide, Geneva Pharms	00781-1966-05
500's	$12.70	Furosemide, H.C.F.A. F F P	99999-1342-10
500's	$23.75	Furosemide Tablets 40 Mg, Watson Labs	52544-0301-05
500's	$23.90	Furosemide, Zenith Labs	00172-2907-70
500's	$30.45	Furosemide, Rugby	00536-3841-05
500's	**$104.75**	**LASIX, Hoechst Marion Roussel**	**00039-0060-50**
600's	$91.60	Furosemide, Medirex	57480-0329-06
750's	$120.00	Furosemide, Glasgow Pharm	60809-0134-55
750's	$120.00	Furosemide, Glasgow Pharm	60809-0134-72
1000's	$2.50	Furosemide 40, H & H Labs	46703-0040-01
1000's	$15.00	Detue, Macnary	55982-0011-01
1000's	$20.48	Furosemide, IDE-Interstate	00814-3301-30
1000's	$21.55	Furosemide, Mova Pharms	55370-0515-09
1000's	$22.00	FUROCOT, C O Truxton	00463-6283-10
1000's	$23.75	Furosemide, Major Pharms	00904-1481-80
1000's	$25.40	Furosemide, H.C.F.A. F F P	99999-1342-09
1000's	$41.90	Furosemide, Roxane	00054-4299-31
1000's	$43.14	Furosemide, United Res	00677-0659-10
1000's	$43.19	Furosemide, HL Moore Drug Exch	00839-6323-16
1000's	$44.95	Furosemide, Zenith Labs	00172-2907-80
1000's	$44.95	Furosemide, Goldline Labs	00182-1161-10
1000's	$44.95	Furosemide, Watson Labs	52544-0301-10
1000's	$44.98	Furosemide, Aligen Independ	00405-4453-03
1000's	$45.00	Furosemide, Schein Pharm (US)	00364-0514-02
1000's	$45.95	Furosemide, Qualitest Pharms	00603-3737-32
1000's	$46.95	Furosemide, Parmed Pharms	00349-2337-10
1000's	$47.55	Furosemide, Geneva Pharms	50752-0287-09
1000's	$53.11	Furosemide, Geneva Pharms	00781-1966-10
1000's	$59.46	Furosemide, Lederle Pharm	00005-3709-34
1000's	$59.67	Furosemide, HL Moore Drug Exch	00839-7783-16
1000's	$59.70	Furosemide, Rugby	00536-3841-10
1000's	$89.46	Furosemide, Bristol Myers Squibb	00003-0360-75
1000's	$89.95	Rose-40, Quality Res Pharms	52765-1351-00
1000's	**$199.00**	**LASIX, Hoechst Marion Roussel**	**00039-0060-70**

Tablet, Uncoated - Oral - 80 mg

50's	$2.81	Furosemide, H.C.F.A. F F P	99999-1342-11
50's	$8.85	Furosemide, Voluntary Hosp	53258-0131-04
50's	**$17.95**	**LASIX, Hoechst Marion Roussel**	**00039-0066-05**
100's	$5.63	Furosemide, United Res	00677-0976-01
100's	$5.63	Furosemide, H.C.F.A. F F P	99999-1342-12
100's	$6.25	Furosemide Tablets 80 Mg, H & H Labs	46703-0077-01
100's	$8.25	Furosemide, IDE-Interstate	00814-3303-14
100's	$11.75	Furosemide, Major Pharms	00904-1482-60
100's	$12.20	Furosemide, Qualitest Pharms	00603-3738-21
100's	$12.49	Furosemide, Roxane	00054-4301-25
100's	$13.05	Furosemide, Geneva Pharms	50752-0288-05
100's	$13.07	Furosemide, HL Moore Drug Exch	00839-6777-06
100's	$14.70	Furosemide, Voluntary Hosp	53258-0131-13
100's	$15.63	Furosemide, Geneva Pharms	00781-1446-01
100's	$16.23	Furosemide, Roxane	00054-8301-25
100's	$17.04	Furosemide, Lederle Pharm	00005-3100-60
100's	$19.60	Furosemide, Schein Pharm (US)	00364-0700-01
100's	$19.63	Furosemide, Medirex	57480-0330-01
100's	$19.95	Furosemide, Watson Labs	52544-0302-01
100's	$19.98	Furosemide, Aligen Independ	00405-4454-01
100's	$20.69	Furosemide, Lederle Pharm	00005-3100-23
100's	$20.75	Furosemide, Parmed Pharms	00349-8353-01
100's	$20.99	Furosemide, Schein Pharm (US)	00364-0700-90
100's	$22.30	Furosemide, Goldline Labs	00182-1736-89
100's	$22.72	Furosemide, Vangard Labs	00615-1571-13
100's	$23.44	Furosemide, Geneva Pharms	00781-1446-13
100's	$24.50	Furosemide, Goldline Labs	00182-1736-01
100's	$24.95	Furosemide, Mylan	00378-0232-01
100's	$24.95	Furosemide, Rugby	00536-3835-01
100's	$29.75	Furosemide, Major Pharms	00904-1482-61
100's	**$36.55**	**LASIX, Hoechst Marion Roussel**	**00039-0066-11**
500's	$28.15	Furosemide, H.C.F.A. F F P	99999-1342-13

HOW SUPPLIED - RATED THERAPEUTICALLY EQUIVALENT: *(cont'd)*

500's	$54.70	Furosemide, Qualitest Pharms	00603-3738-28
500's	$54.95	FUROSEMIDE 80, Major Pharms	00904-1482-40
500's	$56.16	Furosemide, HL Moore Drug Exch	00839-6777-12
500's	$60.45	Furosemide, Parmed Pharms	00349-8353-05
500's	$62.48	Furosemide, Roxane	00054-4301-29
500's	$63.00	Furosemide, Schein Pharm (US)	00364-0700-05
500's	$65.13	Furosemide, Lederle Pharm	00005-3100-31
500's	$65.40	Furosemide, Geneva Pharms	50752-0288-08
500's	$65.63	Furosemide, Geneva Pharms	00781-1446-05
500's	$94.75	Furosemide, Goldline Labs	00182-1736-05
500's	$94.75	Furosemide, Watson Labs	52544-0302-05
500's	$94.80	Furosemide, Aligen Independ	00405-4454-02
500's	$118.50	Furosemide, Rugby	00536-3835-05
500's	$118.95	Furosemide, Mylan	00378-0232-05
500's	**$169.30**	**LASIX, Hoechst Marion Roussel**	**00039-0066-50**
600's	$133.40	Furosemide, Medirex	57480-0330-06
750's	$165.00	Furosemide, Glasgow Pharm	60809-0160-55
750's	$165.00	Furosemide, Glasgow Pharm	60809-0160-72

HOW SUPPLIED - NOT RATED EQUIVALENT:

Injection, Solution - Intramuscular; - 10 mg/ml

4 ml x 10	$8.19	Furosemide, Sanofi Winthrop	00024-0609-40
4 ml x 10	$12.81	FUROSEMIDE, Sanofi Winthrop	00024-0609-23
4 ml x 25	$20.46	Furosemide, Sanofi Winthrop	00024-0609-25

Solution - Oral - 40 mg/5ml

5 ml x 40	$47.50	Furosemide, Roxane	00054-8298-16
10 ml x 40	$68.11	Furosemide, Roxane	00054-8300-16
500 ml	$29.04	Furosemide, Roxane	00054-3298-63

GABAPENTIN *(003175)*

CATEGORIES: Anticonvulsants; Antiepileptics; Central Nervous System Agents; Convulsions; Epilepsy; Epilepticus; Neuromuscular; Orphan Drugs; Seizures; Tonic-Clonic Seizures; Amyotrophic Lateral Sclerosis*; FDA Class 1P ("Priority Review"); FDA Approved 1993 Dec

* Indication not approved by the FDA

BRAND NAMES: **Neurontin**

FORMULARIES: Medi-Cal; PCS

COST OF THERAPY: $1,034.77 (Epilepsy; Capsule; 300 mg; 3/day; 365 days)

PRIMARY ICD9: 345.90 (Epilepsy, Unspecified, Without Mention of Intractable)

DESCRIPTION:

Neurontin (gabapentin capsules) is supplied as imprinted hard shell capsules containing 100 mg, 300 mg, and 400 mg of gabapentin. The inactive ingredients are lactose, corn starch, and talc. The 100-mg capsule shell contains gelatin and titanium dioxide. The 300-mg capsule shell contains gelatin, titanium oxide, and yellow iron oxide. The 400-mg capsule shell contains gelatin, red iron oxide, titanium dioxide, and yellow iron oxide. The imprinting ink contains FD&C Blue No. 2 and titanium dioxide.

Gabapentin is described as 1-(aminomethyl)cyclohexanacetic acid with an empirical formula of $C_9H_{17}NO_2$ and a molecular weight of 171.24.

Gabapentin is a white to off-white crystalline solid. It is freely soluble in water and both basic and acidic aqueous solutions.

CLINICAL PHARMACOLOGY:

MECHANISM OF ACTION

The mechanism by which gabapentin exerts its anticonvulsant action is unknown, but in animal test systems designed to detect anticonvulsant activity, gabapentin prevents seizures as do other marketed anticonvulsants. Gabapentin exhibits anti-seizure activity in mice and rats in both the maximal electroshock and pentylenetetrazol seizure models and other preclinical models (*e.g.,* strains with genetic epilepsy, etc.). The relevance of these models to human epilepsy is not known.

Gabapentin is structurally related to the neurotransmitter GABA (gamma-aminobutyric acid) but it does not interact with GABA receptors, it is not converted metabolically into GABA or a GABA agonist, and it is not an inhibitor of GABA uptake or degradation. Gabapentin was tested in radioligand binding assays at concentrations up to 100 mcM and did not exhibit affinity for a number of other common receptor sites, including benzodiazepine, glutamate, N-methyl-D-aspartate (NMDA), quisqualate, kainate, strychnine-insensitive or strychnine-sensitive glycine, alpha 1, alpha 2, or beta adrenergic, adenosine A1 or A2, cholinergic muscarinic or nicotinic, dopamine D1 or D2, histamine H1, serotonin S1 or S2, opiate mu, delta or kappa, voltage-sensitive calcium channel sites labeled with nitrendipine or diltiazem, or at voltage-sensitive sodium channel sites with batrachotoxinin A 20-alpha-benzoate.

Several test systems ordinarily used to assess activity at the NMDA receptor have been examined. Results are contradictory. Accordingly, no general statement about the effects, if any, of gabapentin at the NMDA receptor can be made.

In vitro studies with radiolabeled gabapentin have revealed a gabapentin binding site in areas of rat brain including neocortex and hippocampus. The identity and function of this binding site remain to be elucidated.

PHARMACOKINETICS AND DRUG METABOLISM

All pharmacological actions following gabapentin administration are due to the activity of the parent compound; gabapentin is not appreciably metabolized in humans.

Oral Bioavailability: Gabapentin bioavailability is not dose proportional; i.e., as dose is increased, bioavailability decreases. A 400 mg dose, for example is about 25% less bioavailable than 100 mg dose. Over the recommended dose range of 300 to 600 mg T.I.D., however, the differences in bioavailability is about 60 percent. Food has no effect on the rate and extent of absorption of gabapentin.

Distribution: Gabapentin circulates largely unbound (<3%) to plasma protein. The apparent volume of distribution of gabapentin after 150 mg intravenous administration is 58 ± 6 L (Mean $\pm$SD). In patients with epilepsy, steady-state predose (Cmin) concentrations of gabapentin in cerebrospinal fluid were approximately 20% of the corresponding plasma concentrations.

Elimination: Gabapentin is eliminated from the systemic circulation by renal excretion as unchanged drug. Gabapentin is not appreciably metabolized in humans.

CLINICAL PHARMACOLOGY: *(cont'd)*

Gabapentin elimination half-life is 5 to 7 hours and is unaltered by dose or following multiple dosing. Gabapentin elimination rate constant, plasma clearance, and renal clearance are directly proportional to creatinine clearance (see Special Populations). In elderly patients, and in patients with impaired renal function, gabapentin plasma clearance is reduced. Gabapentin can be removed from plasma by hemodialysis.

Dosage adjustment in patients with compromised renal function or undergoing hemodialysis is recommended (see DOSAGE AND ADMINISTRATION, TABLE 2).

SPECIAL POPULATIONS

Patients With Renal Insufficiency: Subjects (N=60) with renal insufficiency (mean creatinine clearance ranging from 13-114 ml/min) were administered single 400 mg oral doses of gabapentin. The mean gabapentin half-life ranged from about 6.5 hours (patients with creatinine clearance >60 ml/min) to 52 hours (creatinine clearance <30 ml/min) and gabapentin renal clearance from about 90 ml/min (>60 ml/min group) to about 10 ml/min (<30 ml/min). Mean plasma clearance (CL/F) decreased from approximately 190 ml/min to 20 ml/min.

Dosage adjustment in patients with compromised renal function is necessary (see DOSAGE AND ADMINISTRATION).

Hemodialysis: In a study in anuric subjects (n=11), the apparent elimination half-life of gabapentin on non-dialysis days was about 132 hours; dialysis three times a week (4 hours duration) lowered the apparent half-life of gabapentin by about 60%, from 132 hours to 51 hours. Hemodialysis thus has a significant effect on gabapentin elimination in anuric subjects.

Dosage adjustment in patients undergoing hemodialysis is necessary (see DOSAGE AND ADMINISTRATION).

Hepatic Disease: Because gabapentin is not metabolized, no study was performed in patients with hepatic impairment.

Age: The effect of age was studied in subjects 20-80 years of age. Apparent oral clearance (CL/F) of gabapentin decreased as age increased, from about 225 ml/min in those under 30 years of age to about 125 ml/min in those over 70 years of age. Renal clearance (CLr) and CLr adjusted for body surface area also declined with age; however, the decline in the renal clearance of gabapentin with age can largely be explained by the decline in renal function. reduction of gabapentin dose may be required in patients who have age related compromised renal function. (See PRECAUTIONS, Geriatric Use, and DOSAGE AND ADMINISTRATION.)

Pediatric: No pharmacokinetic data are available in children below the age of 18 years.

Gender: Although no formal study has been conducted to compare the pharmacokinetics of gabapentin in men and women, it appears that the pharmacokinetic parameters for males and females are similar and there are no significant gender differences.

Race: Pharmacokinetic differences due to race have not been studied. Because gabapentin is primarily renally excreted and there are no important racial differences in creatinine clearance, pharmacokinetic differences due to race are not expected.

CLINICAL STUDIES:

The effectiveness of gabapentin as adjunctive therapy (added to other antiepileptic drugs) was established in three multicenter placebo- controlled, double-blind, parallel-group clinical trials in 705 adults with refractory partial seizures. The patients enrolled had a history of at least 4 partial seizures per month in spite of receiving one or more antiepileptic drugs at therapeutic levels and were observed on their established antiepileptic drug regimen during a 12-week baseline period. In patients continuing to have at least 2 (or 4 in some studies) seizures per month, gabapentin or placebo was then added on to the existing therapy during a 12-week treatment period.

Effectiveness was assessed primarily on the basis of the percent of patients with a 50% or greater reduction in seizure frequency from baseline to treatment (the "responder rate") and a derived measure called response ratio, a measure os change defined as (T - B)/(T + B), where B is the patient's baseline seizure frequency and T is the patient's seizure frequency during treatment. Response ratio is distributed within the range -1 to +1. A zero value indicates no change while complete elimination of seizures would give a value of -1; increased seizure rates would give positive values. A response ratio of -0.33 corresponds to a 50% reduction in seizure frequency. The results given below are for all partial seizures in the intent-to-treat (all patients who recieved any doses of treatment) population in each study, unless otherwise indicated.

One study compared gabapentin 1200 mg/day TID with placebo. Responder rate was 23% (14/61) in the gabapentin group and 9% (6/66) in the placebo group; the difference between groups was statistically significant. Response ratio was also better in the gabapentin group (-0.199) than in the placebo group (-0.044), a difference that also achieved statistical significance.

A second study compared primarily 1200 mg/day T.I.D. Gabapentin (N = 101) with placebo (N = 98). Additional smaller gabapentin dosage groups (600 mg/day, N = 53; 1800 mg/day, N = 54) were also studied for information regarding dose response. Responder rate was higher in the gabapentin 1200 mg/day group (16%) than in the placebo group (8%), but the difference was not statistically significant. The responder rate at 600 mg (17%) was also not significantly higher than in the placebo, but the responder rate in the 1800 mg group (26%) was statistically significantly superior to the placebo rate. Response ratio was better in the gabapentin 1200 mg/day group (-0.103) than in the placebo group (-0.022); but this difference was also not statistically significant (p = 0.224). A better response was seen in the gabapentin 600 mg/day group (-0.105) and 1800 mg/day group (- 0.222) than in the 1200 mg/day group, with the 1800 mg/day group achieving statistical significance compared to the placebo group.

A third study compared gabapentin 900 mg/day T.I.D. (N = 111) and placebo (N = 109). An additional gabapentin 1200 mg/day dosage group (N = 52) provided dose-response data. A statistically significant difference in responder rate was seen in the gabapentin 900 mg/day group (22%) compared to that in the placebo group (10%). Response ratio was also statistically significantly superior in the gabapentin 900 mg/day group (-0.119) compared to that in the placebo group (-0.027), as was response ratio in 1200 mg/day gabapentin (-0.184) compared to placebo.

Analyses were also performed in each study to examine the effect of gabapentin on preventing secondarily generalized tonic-clonic seizures. Patients who experienced a secondarily generalized tonic-clonic seizure in either the baseline or in the treatment period in all three placebo controlled studies were included in these analyses. There were several response ratio comparisons that showed a statistically significant advantage for gabapentin compared to placebo and favorable trends for almost all comparisons.

Analysis of responder rate using combined data from all three studies and all doses (N = 162, gabapentin; N = 89, placebo) also showed a significant advantage for gabapentin over placebo in reducing the frequency of secondarily generalized tonic-clonic seizures.

In two of the three controlled studies, more than one dose of gabapentin was used. Within each study the results did not show a consistently increased response to dose. However, looking across studies, a trend toward increasing efficacy with increasing dose is evident.

CLINICAL STUDIES: *(cont'd)*

Although no formal analysis by gender has been performed, estimates of response (Response Ratio) derived from clinical trials (398 men, 307 women) indicate no important gender differences exist. There was no consistent pattern indicating that age had any effect on the response to gabapentin. There were insufficient numbers of patients of races other than Caucasian to permit a comparison of efficacy among racial groups.

INDICATIONS AND USAGE:

Gabapentin is indicated as adjunctive therapy in the treatment of partial seizures with and without secondary generalization in adults with epilepsy.

CONTRAINDICATIONS:

Gabapentin is contraindicated in patients who have demonstrated hypersensitivity to the drug or its ingredients.

WARNINGS:

WITHDRAWAL PRECIPITATED SEIZURE, STATUS EPILEPTICUS

Antiepileptic drugs should not be abruptly discontinued because of the possibility of increasing seizure frequency.

In the placebo-controlled studies, the incidence of status epilepticus in patients receiving gabapentin was 0.6% (5 of 543) versus 0.5% in patients receiving placebo (2 of 378). Among the 2074 patients treated with gabapentin across all studies (controlled and uncontrolled) 31 (1.5%) had status epilepticus. Of these, 14 patients had no prior history of status epilepticus either before treatment or while on other medications. Because adequate historical data are not available, it is impossible to say whether or not treatment with gabapentin is associated with a higher or lower rate of status epilepticus than would be expected to occur in a similar population not treated with gabapentin.

TUMORIGENIC POTENTIAL

In standard preclinical *in-vivo* lifetime carcinogenicity studies, an unexpectedly high incidence of pancreatic acinar adenocarcinomas was identified in male, but not female, rats. (See PRECAUTIONS, Carcinogenesis, Mutagenesis, and Impairment of Fertility.) The clinical significance of this finding is unknown. Clinical experience during gabapentin's pre-marketing development provides no direct means to assess its potential for inducing tumors in humans.

In clinical studies comprising 2085 patient-years of exposure, new tumors were reported in 10 patients (2 breast, 3 brain, 2 lung, 1 adrenal, 1 non-Hodgkin's lymphoma, 1 endometrial carcinoma *in situ*), and pre-existing tumors worsened in 11 patients (9 brain, 1 breast, 1 prostate) during or up to 2 years following discontinuation of gabapentin. Without knowledge of the background incidence and recurrence in a similar population not treated with gabapentin, it is impossible to know whether the incidence seen in this cohort is or is not affected by treatment.

SUDDEN AND UNEXPLAINED DEATHS

During the course of premarketing development of gabapentin, 8 sudden and unexplained deaths were recorded among a cohort of 2203 patients treated (2103 patient-years of exposure).

Some of these could represent seizure-related deaths in which the seizure was not observed, e.g., at night. This represents an incidence of 0.0038 deaths per patient-year. Although this rate exceeds that expected in a healthy population matched for age and sex, it is within the range of estimates for the incidence of sudden unexplained deaths in patients with epilepsy not receiving gabapentin (ranging from 0.0005 for the general population of epileptics, to 0.003 for a clinical trial population similar to that in the gabapentin program, to 0.005 for patients with refractory epilepsy).

Consequently, whether these figures are reassuring or raise further concern depends on comparability of the populations reported upon to the gabapentin cohort and the accuracy of the estimates provided.

PRECAUTIONS:

INFORMATION FOR THE PATIENT

Patients should be instructed to take gabapentin only as prescribed.

Patients should be advised that gabapentin may cause dizziness, somnolence and other symptoms and signs of CNS depression. Accordingly, they should be advised neither to drive a car nor to operate other complex machinery until they have gained sufficient experience on gabapentin to gauge whether or not it affects their mental and/or motor performance adversely.

LABORATORY TESTS

Clinical trials do not indicate that routine monitoring of clinical laboratory parameters is necessary for the safe use of gabapentin. The value of monitoring gabapentin blood concentrations has not been established. Gabapentin may be used in combination with other antiepileptic drugs without concern for alteration of the blood concentrations of gabapentin or of other antiepileptic drugs.

DRUG/LABORATORY TESTS INTERACTIONS

Because false positive readings were reported with the Ames N-Multistix SG dipstick test for urinary protein when gabapentin was added to other antiepileptic drugs, the more specific sulfosalicylic acid precipitation procedure is recommended to determine the presence of urine protein.

CARCINOGENESIS, MUTAGENESIS, AND IMPAIRMENT OF FERTILITY

Gabapentin was given in the diet to mice at 200, 600, and 2000 mg/kg/day and to rats at 250, 1000, and 2000 mg/kg/day for 2 years. A statistically significant increase in the incidence of pancreatic acinar cell adenomas and carcinomas was found in male rats receiving the high dose; the no- effect dose for the occurrence of carcinomas was 1000 mg/kg/day. Peak plasma concentrations of gabapentin in rats receiving the high dose of 2000 mg/kg were 10 times higher than plasma concentrations in humans receiving 3600 mg per day and in rats receiving 1000 mg/kg/day peak plasma concentrations were 6.5 times higher than in humans receiving 3600 mg/day. The pancreatic acinar cell carcinomas did not affect survival, did not metastasize and were not locally invasive. Studies to attempt to define a mechanism by which this relatively rare tumor type is occurring are in progress. The relevance of this finding to carcinogenic risk in humans is unclear.

Gabapentin did not demonstrate mutagenic or genotoxic potential in three*in vitro* and two *in vivo* assays. It was negative in the Ames test and the *in vitro* HGPRT forward mutation assay in Chinese hamster lung cells; it did not produce significant increases in chromosomal aberrations in the *in vitro* Chinese hamster lung cell assay; it was negative in the *in vivo* chromosomal aberration assay and in the *in vivo* micronucleus test in Chinese hamster bone marrow.

No adverse effects on fertility or reproduction were observed in rats at doses up to 2000 mg/kg (approximately 7 times the maximum recommended human dose on a mg/m^2 basis).

PREGNANCY

Pregnancy Category C: Gabapentin has been shown to be fetotoxic in rodents, causing delayed ossification of several bones in the skull, vertebrae, forelimbs and hindlimbs. These effects occurred when pregnant mice received oral doses of 1000 or 3000 mg/kg/day during the period of organogenesis, or approximately 1 to 4 times the maximum dose of 3600 mg/day given to epileptic patients on a mg/m^2 basis. The no effect level was 500 mg/kg/day or approximately 1/2 of the human dose on a mg/m^{2}basis.

When rats were dosed prior to and during mating, and throughout gestation, pups from all dose groups (500, 1000 and 2000 mg/kg/day) were affected. These doses are equivalent to less than approximately 1 to 5 times the maximum human dose on a mg/m^2 basis. There was an increased incidence of hydroureter and/or hydronephrosis in rats in a study of fertility and general reproductive performance at 2000 mg/kg/day with no effect at 1000 mg/kg/day, in a teratology study at 1500 mg/kg/day with no effect at 300 mg/kg/day, and in a perinatal and postnatal study at all doses studied (500, 1000 and 2000 mg/kg/day). The doses at which the effects occurred are approximately 1 to 5 times the maximum human dose of 3600 mg/day on a mg/m^{2}basis; the no effect doses were approximately 3 times (Fertility and General Reproductive Performance study) and approximately equal to (Teratogenicity study) the maximum human dose on a mg/m^2 basis. Other than hydroureter and hydronephrosis, the etiologies of which are unclear, the incidence of malformations was not increased compared to controls in offspring of mice, rats, or rabbits given doses up to 50 times (mice), 30 times (rats), and 25 times (rabbits) the human daily dose on a mg/kg basis, or 4 times (mice), 5 times (rat), or 8 times (rabbit) the human daily dose on a mg/m^2 basis.

In a teratology study in rabbits, an increased incidence of postimplantation fetal loss occurred in dams exposed to 60, 300 and 1500 mg/kg/day, or less than approximately 1/4 to 8 times the maximum human dose on a mg/m^2 basis. There are no adequate and well controlled studies in pregnant women. Because animal reproduction studies are not always predictive of human response, this drug should be used during pregnancy only if the potential benefit justifies the potential risk to the fetus.

USE IN NURSING MOTHERS

It is not known if gabapentin is excreted in human milk and the effect on the nursing infant is unknown. However, because many drugs are excreted in human milk, gabapentin should be used in women who are nursing only if the benefits clearly outweigh the risks.

PEDIATRIC USE

Safety and effectiveness in children below the age of 12 years have not been established.

GERIATRIC USE

No systematic studies in geriatric patients have been conducted. Adverse clinical events reported among 59 gabapentin exposed patients over age 65 did not differ in kind from those reported for younger individuals. The small number of older individuals evaluated, however, limits the strength of any conclusions reached about the influence, if any, of age on the kind and incidence of adverse events or laboratory abnormality associated with the use of gabapentin.

Because gabapentin is eliminated primarily by renal excretion, the dose of gabapentin should be adjusted as noted in **DOSAGE AND ADMINISTRATION**, (TABLE 2) for elderly patients with compromised renal function. Creatinine clearance is difficult to measure in outpatients and serum creatinine may be reduced in the elderly because of decreased muscle mass. Creatinine clearance (C_{Cr}) can be reasonably well estimated using the equation of Cockcroft and Gault:

for females C_{Cr}=(0.85)(140-age)(wt)/(72)(S_{Cr})

for males C_{Cr}=(140-age)(wt)/(72)(S_{Cr})

where age is in years, wt is in kilograms and $S_{Cr}$is serum creatinine in mg/dl.

DRUG INTERACTIONS:

Gabapentin is not appreciably metabolized nor does it interfere with the metabolism of commonly co-administered anti-epileptic drugs.

The drug interaction data described in this section were obtained from studies involving healthy adults and patients with epilepsy.

Phenytoin: In a single and multiple dose study of gabapentin (400 mg T.I.D.) in epileptic patients (N = 8) maintained on phenytoin monotherapy for at least 2 months, gabapentin had no effect on gabapentin had no effect on the steady-state trough plasma concentrations of phenytoin and phenytoin had no effect on gabapentin pharmacokinetics.

Carbamazepine: Steady-state trough plasma carbamazepine and carbamazepine 10, 11 epoxide concentrations were not affected by concomitant gabapentin (400 mg T.I.D.; N = 12) administration. Likewise, gabapentin pharmacokinetics were unaltered by carbamazepine administration.

Valproic Acid: The mean steady state trough serum valproic acid concentrations prior to and during concomitant gabapentin administration (400 mg T.I.D.; N = 17) were not different and neither were gabapentin pharmacokinetic parameters affected by valproic acid.

Phenobarbital: Estimates of steady-state pharmacokinetic parameters for phenobarbital or gabapentin (300 mg T.I.D.; N = 12) are identical whether the drugs are administered alone or together.

Cimetidine: In the presence of cimetidine at 300 mg Q.I.D. (N = 12) the mean apparent oral clearance of gabapentin fell by 14% and creatinine clearance fell by 10%. Thus cimetidine appeared to alter the renal excretion of both gabapentin and creatinine, and endogenous marker of renal function. This small decrease in excretion of gabapentin by cimetidine is not expected to be of clinical importance. The effect of gabapentin on cimetidine was not evaluated.

Oral Contraceptive: Based on AUC and half-life, multiple-dose pharmacokinetic profiles of norethindrone and ethinyl estradiol following administration of tablets containing 2.5 mg of norethindrone acetate and 50 mcg of ethinyl estradiol were similar with and without coadministration of gabapentin (400 mg TID; N = 13). The Cmax of norethindrone was 13% higher when coadministered with gabapentin; this interaction is not expected to be of clinical importance.

Antacid (Maalox): Maalox reduced the bioavailability of gabapentin (N = 16) by about 20%. This decrease in bioavailability was about 5% when gabapentin was administered 2 hours after Maalox. It is recommended that gabapentin be taken at least 2 hours following Maalox administration.

Effect of Probenecid: Probenecid is a blocker of renal tubular secretion. Gabapentin pharmacokinetic parameters without and with probenecid were comparable. This indicates that gabapentin does not undergo renal tubular secretion by the pathway that is blocked by probenecid.

ADVERSE REACTIONS:

The most commonly observed adverse events associated with the use of gabapentin in combination with other antiepileptic drugs, not seen at an equivalent frequency among placebo-treated patients, were somnolence, dizziness, ataxia, fatigue and nystagmus.

Approximately 7% of the 2074 individuals who received gabapentin in premarketing clinical trials discontinued treatment because of an adverse event. The adverse events most commonly associated with withdrawal were somnolence (1.2%), ataxia (0.8%), fatigue (0.6%), nausea and/or vomiting (0.6%), and dizziness (0.6%).

ADVERSE REACTIONS: *(cont'd)*

INCIDENCE IN CONTROLLED CLINICAL TRIALS

TABLE 1 lists treatment-emergent signs and symptoms that occurred in at least 1% of gabapentin-treated patients with epilepsy participating in placebo-controlled trials and were numerically more common in the gabapentin group. In these studies, either gabapentin or placebo was added to the patient's current antiepileptic drug therapy. Adverse events were usually mild to moderate in intensity.

The prescriber should be aware that these figures, obtained when gabapentin was added to concurrent antiepileptic drug therapy, cannot be used to predict the frequency of adverse events in the course of usual medical practice where patient characteristics and other factors may differ from those prevailing during clinical studies. Similarly, the cited frequencies cannot be directly compared with figures obtained from other clinical investigations involving different treatments, uses, or investigations. An inspection of these frequencies, however, does provide the prescribing physician with one basis to estimate the relative contribution of drug and non-drug factors to the adverse event incidences in the population studied.

TABLE 1 Treatment-Emergent Adverse Event Incidence in Controlled Add-On Trials (Events in at least 1% of Gabapentin patients and numerically more frequent than in the placebo group)

Body System/ Adverse Event	Gabapentin[a] N = 543 %	Placebo[a] N = 378 %
Body As A Whole		
Fatigue	11.0	5.0
Weight Increase	2.9	1.6
Back Pain	1.8	0.5
Peripheral Edema	1.7	0.5
Cardiovascular		
Vasodilation	1.1	0.3
Digestive System		
Dyspepsia	2.2	0.5
Mouth or Throat Dry	1.7	0.5
Constipation	1.5	0.8
Dental Abnormalities	1.5	0.3
Increased Appetite	1.1	0.8
Hematologic and Lymphatic Systems		
Leukopenia	1.1	0.5
Musculoskeletal System		
Myalgia	2.0	1.9
Fracture	1.1	0.8
Somnolence	19.3	8.7
Dizziness	17.1	6.9
Ataxia	12.5	5.6
Nystagmus	8.3	4.0
Tremor	6.8	3.2
Nervousness	2.4	1.9
Dysarthria	2.4	0.5
Amnesia	2.2	0.0
Depression	1.8	1.1
Thinking Abnormal	1.7	1.3
Twitching	1.3	0.5
Coordination Abnormal	1.1	0.3
Respiratory System		
Rhinitis	4.1	3.7
Pharyngitis	2.8	1.6
Coughing	1.8	1.3
Skin and Appendages		
Abrasion	1.3	0.0
Pruritus	1.3	0.5
Urogenital System		
Impotence	1.5	1.1
Special Senses		
Diplopia	5.9	1.9
Amblyopia[b]	4.2	1.1
Laboratory Deviations		
WBC Decreased	1.1	0.5

[a]Plus background antiepileptic drug therapy
[b]Amblyopia was often described as blurred vision

Other events in more than 1% of patients but equally or more frequent in the placebo group included: headache, viral infection, fever, nausea and/or vomiting, abdominal pain, diarrhea, convulsions, confusion, insomnia, emotional liability, rash, acne.

Among the treatment-emergent adverse events occurring at an incidence of at least 10% of gabapentin-treated patients, somnolence and ataxia appeared to exhibit a positive dose-response relationship.

The overall incidence of adverse events and the types of adverse events seen were similar among men and women treated with gabapentin. The incidence of adverse events increased slightly with increasing age in patients treated with either gabapentin or placebo. Because only 3% of patients (28/921) in placebo-controlled studies were identified as nonwhite (black or other), there are insufficient data to support a statement regarding the distribution of adverse events by race.

OTHER ADVERSE EVENTS OBSERVED DURING ALL CLINICAL TRIALS

Gabapentin has been administered to 2074 individuals during all clinical trials, only some of which were placebo-controlled. During these trials, all adverse events were recorded by the clinical investigators using terminology of their own choosing. To provide a meaningful estimate of the proportion of individuals having adverse events, similar types of events were grouped into a smaller number of standardized categories using modified COSTART dictionary terminology. These categories are used in the listing below. The frequencies presented represent the proportion of the 2074 individuals exposed to gabapentin who experienced an event of the type cited on at least one occasion while receiving gabapentin. All reported events are included except those already listed in the previous table, those too general to be informative, and those not reasonably associated with the use of the drug.

Events are further classified within body system categories and enumerated in order of decreasing frequency using the following definitions: frequent adverse events are defined as those occurring in 1/100 to 1/1000 patients; rare events are those occurring in fewer than 1/1000 patients.

Body As A Whole: *Frequent:* asthenia, malaise, face edema;*Infrequent:* allergy, generalized edema, weight decrease, chill;*Rare:* strange feelings, lassitude, alcohol intolerance, hangover effect.

Cardiovascular System: *Frequent:* hypertension;*Infrequent:* hypotension, angina pectoris, peripheral vascular disorder, palpitation, tachycardia, migraine, murmur; *Rare:* atrial fibrillation, heart failure, thrombophlebitis, deep thrombophlebitis, myocardial infarction, cerebrovascular accident, pulmonary thrombosis, ventricular extrasystoles, bradycardia, premature atrial contraction, pericardial rub, heart block, pulmonary embolus, hyperlipidemia, hypercholesterolemia, pericardial effusion, pericarditis.

ADVERSE REACTIONS: *(cont'd)*

Digestive System: *Frequent:* anorexia, flatulence, gingivitis;*Infrequent:*glossitis, gum hemorrhage, thirst, stomatitis, increased salivation, gastroenteritis, hemorrhoids, bloody stools, fecal incontinence, hepatomegaly; *Rare:* dysphagia, eructation, pancreatitis, peptic ulcer, colitis, blisters in mouth, tooth discolor, perleche, salivary gland enlarged, lip hemorrhage, esophagitis, hiatal hernia, hematemesis, proctitis, irritable bowel syndrome, rectal hemorrhage, esophageal spasm.

Endocrine System: *Rare:* hyperthyroid, hypothyroid, goiter, hypoestrogen, ovarian failure, epididymitis, swollen testicle, cushingoid appearance.

Hematologic and Lymphatic System: *Frequent:* purpura most often described as bruises resulting from physical trauma; *Infrequent:* anemia, thrombocytopenia, lymphadenopathy; *Rare:* WBC count increased, lymphocytosis, non-Hodgkin's lymphoma, bleeding time increased.

Musculoskeletal System: *Frequent:* arthralgia; *Infrequent:* tendinitis, arthritis, joint stiffness, joint swelling, positive Romberg test; *Rare:* costochondritis, osteoporosis, bursitis, contracture.

Nervous System: *Frequent:* vertigo, hyperkinesia, paresthesia, decreased or absent reflexes, increased reflexes, anxiety, hostility;*Infrequent:*CNS tumors, syncope, dreaming abnormal, aphasia, hypesthesia, intracranial hemorrhage, hypotonia, dysesthesia, paresis, dystonia, hemiplegia, facial paralysis, stupor, cerebellar dysfunction, positive Babinski sign, decreased position sense, subdural hematoma, apathy, hallucination, decrease or loss of libido, agitation, paranoia, depersonalization, euphoria, feeling high, doped-up sensation, suicidal, psychosis; *Rare:* choreoathetosis, orofacial dyskinesia, encephalopathy, nerve palsy, personality disorder, increased libido, subdued temperament, apraxia, fine motor control disorder, meningismus, local myoclonus, hyperesthesia, hypokinesia, mania, neurosis, hysteria, antisocial reaction, suicide gesture.

Respiratory System: *Frequent:* pneumonia; *Infrequent:* epistaxis, dyspnea, apnea; *Rare:* mucositis, aspiration pneumonia, hyperventilation, hiccup, laryngitis, nasal obstruction, snoring, bronchospasm, hypoventilation, lung edema.

Dermatological: *Infrequent:* alopecia, eczema, dry skin, increased sweating, urticaria, hirsutism, seborrhea, cyst, herpes simplex;*Rare:* herpes zoster, skin discolor, skin papules, photosensitive reaction, leg ulcer, scalp seborrhea, psoriasis, desquamation, maceration, skin nodules, subcutaneous nodule, melanosis, skin necrosis, local swelling.

Urogenital System: *Infrequent:* hematuria, dysuria, urination frequency, cystitis, urinary retention, urinary incontinence, vaginal hemorrhage, amenorrhea, dysmenorrhea, menorrhagia, breast cancer, unable to climax, ejaculation abnormal; *Rare:* kidney pain, leukorrhea, pruritus genital, renal stone, acute renal failure, anuria, glycosuria, nephrosis, nocturia, pyuria, urination urgency, vaginal pain, breast pain, testicle pain.

Special Senses: *Frequent:* abnormal vision; *Infrequent:* cataract, conjunctivitis, eyes dry, eye pain, visual field defect, photophobia, bilateral or unilateral ptosis, eye hemorrhage, hordeolum, hearing loss, earache, tinnitus, inner ear infection, otitis, taste loss, unusual taste, eye twitching, ear fullness; *Rare:* eye itching, abnormal accommodation, perforated ear drum, sensitivity to noise, eye focusing problem, watery eyes, retinopathy, glaucoma, iritis, corneal disorders, lacrimal dysfunction, degenerative eye changes, blindness, retinal degeneration, miosis, chorioretinitis, strabismus, eustachian tube dysfunction, labyrinthitis, otitis externa, odd smell.

DRUG ABUSE AND DEPENDENCE:

The abuse and dependence potential of gabapentin has not been evaluated in human studies.

OVERDOSAGE:

A lethal dose of gabapentin was not identified in mice and rats receiving single oral doses as high as 8000 mg/kg. Signs of acute toxicity in animals included ataxia, labored breathing, ptosis, sedation, hypoactivity, or excitation.

Acute oral overdoses of gabapentin up to 49 grams have been reported. In these cases, double vision, slurred speech, drowsiness, lethargy and diarrhea were observed. All patients recovered with supportive care.

Gabapentin can be removed by hemodialysis. Although hemodialysis has not been performed in the few overdose cases reported, it may be indicated by the patient's clinical state or in patients with significant renal impairment.

DOSAGE AND ADMINISTRATION:

Gabapentin is recommended for add-on therapy in patients over 12 years of age. Evidence bearing on its safety and effectiveness in children is not available.

Gabapentin is given orally with or without food.

The effective dose of gabapentin is 900 to 1800 mg/day and given in divided doses (three times a day) using 300- or 400-mg capsules. Titration to an effective dose can take place rapidly, over a few days, giving 300 mg on Day 1, 300 mg twice a day on Day 2, and 300 mg three times a day on Day 3. To minimize potential side effects, especially somnolence, dizziness, fatigue, and ataxia, the first dose on Day 1 may be administered at bedtime. If necessary, the dose may be increased using 300- or 400-mg capsules three times a day up to 1800 mg/day. Dosages up to 2400 mg/day have been well-tolerated in long-term clinical studies. Doses of 3600 mg/day have also been administered to a small number of patients for a relatively short duration, and have been well tolerated. The maximum time between doses in the T.I.D. schedule should not exceed 12 hours.

It is not necessary to monitor gabapentin plasma concentrations to optimize gabapentin therapy. Further, because there are no significant pharmacokinetic interactions among gabapentin and other commonly used anti-epileptic drugs, the addition of gabapentin does not alter the plasma levels of these drugs appreciably.

If gabapentin is discontinued and/or an alternate anticonvulsant medication is added to the therapy, this should be done gradually over a minimum of 1 week.

Dosage adjustment in patients with compromised renal function or undergoing hemodialysis is recommended as follows (TABLE 2):

TABLE 2 Gabapentin Dosage Based on Renal Function

Renal Function/Creatinine Clearance (ml/min)	Total Daily Dose (mg/day)	Dose Regimen (mg)
>60	1200	400 TID
30 - 60	600	300 BID
15 - 30	300	300 QD
<15	150	300 QOD[a]
Hemodialysis	-	200- 300[b]

[a]Every other day
[b]Loading dose of 300 to 400 mg in patients who have never received Neurontin, then 200 to 300 mg Neurontin following each 4 hours of hemodialysis

HOW SUPPLIED:

Neurontin (gabapentin capsules) are supplied as follows:

100-mg capsules — White hard gelatin capsules printed with "PD" on one side and "Neurontin/100 mg" on the other

300-mg capsules — Yellow hard gelatin capsules printed with "PD" on one side and "Neurontin/300 mg" on the other

400-mg capsules — Orange hard gelatin capsules printed with "PD" on one side and "Neurontin/400 mg" on the other

STORAGE

Store at controlled room temperature 15°-30°C (59°-86°F).

Caution — Federal law prohibits dispensing without prescription.

HOW SUPPLIED - EQUIVALENTS NOT AVAILABLE:

Capsule, Gelatin - Oral - 100 mg

50's	$24.00	NEURONTIN, Parke-Davis	00071-0803-40
100's	$37.80	NEURONTIN, Parke-Davis	00071-0803-24

Capsule, Gelatin - Oral - 300 mg

50's	$54.00	NEURONTIN, Parke-Davis	00071-0805-40
100's	$94.50	NEURONTIN, Parke-Davis	00071-0805-24

Capsule, Gelatin - Oral - 400 mg

50's	$60.00	NEURONTIN, Parke-Davis	00071-0806-40
100's	$113.40	NEURONTIN, Parke-Davis	00071-0806-24

GADOTERIDOL *(003141)*

CATEGORIES: Cancer; Diagnostic Agents; Intracranial Lesions; Magnetic Resonance Imaging; Roentgenography; Pregnancy Category C; FDA Class 1S ("Standard Review"); FDA Approved 1992 Nov

BRAND NAMES: **Prohance**

DESCRIPTION:

Prohance (Gadoteridol Injection) is a nonionic contrast medium for magnetic resonance imaging (MRI), available as a 0.5M sterile clear colorless to slightly yellow aqueous solution in vials for IV injection. Gadoteridol is the gadolinium complex of 10-(2, hydroxypropyl)-1,4,7,10- tetraazacyclodode-cane-1,4,7, triacetic acid with a molecular weight of 558.7 and an empirical formula of $C_{17}H_{29}N_4O_7Gd$.

Each ml of Prohance contains 279.3 mg gadoteridol, 0.23 mg calteridol calcium, 1.21 mg tromethamine and water for injection. Prohance contains no antimicrobial preservative.

Gadoteridol has a pH of 6.5 to 8.0. Pertinent physiochemical data are noted in TABLE 1.

TABLE 1

PARAMETER	
Osmolality (mOsmol/kg water) - at 37°C	630
Viscosity	
- (cP) at 20°C	2.0
- at 37°C	1.3
Specific Gravity - at 25°C	1.140

Gadoteridol has an osmolality 2.2 times that of plasma (285 mOsmol/kg water) and is hypertonic under conditions of use.

CLINICAL PHARMACOLOGY:

The pharmacokinetics of IV administered gadoteridol in normal subjects conforms to a two-compartment open model with mean distribution and elimination half-lives (reported as mean ± SD) of about 0.20 ± 0.04 hours and 1.57 ± 0.08 hours, respectively.

Gadoteridol is eliminated in the urine with 94.4 ± 4.8% (mean ± SD) of the dose excreted within 24 hours post-injection. It is unknown if biotransformation or decomposition of Gadoteridol occur *in vivo.*

The renal and plasma clearance rates (1.41 ± 0.33 ml/min/kg and 1.50 ± 0.35 ml/min/kg, respectively) of Gadoteridol are essentially identical, indicating no alteration in elimination kinetics on passage through the kidneys and that the drug is essentially cleared through the kidney. The volume of distribution (204 ± 58 ml/kg) is equal to that of extracellular water, and clearance is similar to that of glomerular filtration.

It is unknown if protein binding of gadoteridol occurs *in vivo.*

Gadoteridol is a paramagnetic agent and, as such, develops a magnetic moment when placed in a magnetic field. The relatively large magnetic moment produced by the paramagnetic agent, results in a relatively large local magnetic field, which can enhance the relaxation rates of water protons in the vicinity of the paramagnetic agent.

In magnetic resonance imaging (MRI), visualization or normal and pathologic brain tissue depends in part on variations in the radiofrequency signal intensity that occur with 1) differences in proton density; 2) differences of the spin-lattice or longitudinal relaxation times (T1); and 3) differences in the spin-spin or transverse relaxation time (T2). When placed in a magnetic field, Gadoteridol decreases T1 relaxation times in the target tissues. At recommended doses, the effect is observed with greatest sensitivity in the T1-weighted sequences.

Gadoteridol does not cross the intact blood-brain barrier and, therefore, does not accumulate in normal blood-brain barrier and, therefore, does not accumulate in normal brain lesions that have a normal blood-brain barrier, *e.g.,* cysts, mature post-operative scars, etc. However, disruption of the blood-brain barrier or abnormal vascularity allows accumulation of Gadoteridol in lesions such as neoplasms, abscesses, and subacute infarcts. The pharmacokinetics of gadoteridol in various lesions is not known.

INDICATIONS AND USAGE:

Using magnetic resonance imaging (MRI), Prohance (Gadoteridol Injection) provides contrast enhancement of the brain, spine and surrounding tissues resulting in improved visualization (compared with unenhanced MRI) of lesions with abnormal vascularity or those thought to cause a disruption of the normal blood-brain barrier. Prohance (Gadoteridol Injection) has been shown to facilitate visualization of central nervous system lesions including but not limited to tumors.

CONTRAINDICATIONS:

None known.

WARNINGS:

Deoxygenated sickle erythrocytes have been shown to *in vitro* studies to align perpendicular to a magnetic field which may result in vaso-occlusive complications *in vivo.* The enhancement of magnetic moment by gadoteridol may possibly potentiate sickle erythrocyte alignment. Gadoteridol in patients with sickle cell anemia and other hemoglobinopathies has not been studied.

Patients with other hemolytic anemias have not been adequately evaluated following administration of Prohance to exclude the possibility of increased hemodialysis.

Patients with history of allergy or drug reaction should be observed for several hours after drug administration.

PRECAUTIONS:

GENERAL

Diagnostic procedures that involve the use of contrast agents should be carried out under direction of a physician with the prerequisite training and a thorough knowledge of the procedure to be performed. In a patient with a history of grand mal seizure, the possibility to induce such a seizure by gadoteridol is unknown.

Since Gadoteridol is cleared from the body by glomerular filtration, caution should be exercised in patients with severely impaired renal function. An alternate route of excretion frequently observed in patients with severe renal impairment receiving iodinated contrast media, is the hepato-biliary enteric pathway, although this has not yet been demonstrated with gadoteridol. However, caution should be exercised in patients with either renal or hepatic impairment.

The possibility of a reaction, including serious anaphylaxis or cardiovascular reactions or other idiosyncratic reactions should be considered, especially in those patients with a history of a known clinical hypersensitivity.

When gadoteridol Iinjection is to be injected using nondisposable equipment, scrupulous care should be taken to prevent residual contamination with traces of cleansing agents. After Prohance is drawn into a syringe, the solution should be used immediately.

Repeat Procedures: Data for repeated examination are not available. If in the clinical judgement of the physician, repeat examinations are required, a suitable interval of time between administrations should be observed to allow for normal clearance of the drug from the body.

INFORMATION FOR THE PATIENT

Patients scheduled to receive gadoteridol should be instructed to:

1. Inform their physicians if they are pregnant or are breastfeeding.

2. Inform the physician if they have anemia or diseases that affect the red blood cells.

3. Inform the physician if they have had a history of renal or hepatic disease, seizure, asthma, or allergic respiratory diseases.

CARCINOGENESIS, MUTAGENESIS, AND IMPAIRMENT OF FERTILITY

No animal studies have been performed to evaluate the carcinogenic potential of Gadoteridol or potential effects on fertility.

Gadoteridol did not demonstrate genotoxic activity in bacterial reverse mutation assays using *Salmonella typhimurium* and *Escherichia coli,* in a mouse lymphoma forward mutation assay, in an *in vitro* cytogenetic assay measuring chromosomal aberration frequencies in Chinese hamster ovary cells, nor in an *in vivo* mouse micronucleus assay at IV doses as high as 5.0 mmol/kg.

PREGNANCY CATEGORY C

Gadoteridol administered to rats at 10 mmol/kg/day (33 times the maximum recommended human dose of 0.3 mmol/kg) for 12 days during gestation double the incidence of postimplantation loss. This may have been related to maternal toxicity.

When rats were administered 6.0 or 1.0 mmol/kg/day for 12 days, an increase in spontaneous locomotor activity was observed in the offspring.

Prohance increased the incidence of spontaneous abortion and early delivery in rabbits administered 6 mmol/kg day (20 times the maximum recommended human dose) for 13 days during gestation. This may have been related to maternal toxicity.

There are no adequate and well-controlled studies in pregnant women. Prohance (Gadoteridol Injection) should be used during pregnancy only if the potential benefit justifies the potential risk to the fetus.

NURSING MOTHERS

It is not known whether this drug is excreted in human milk. Because many drugs are excreted in human milk, caution should be exercised when gadoteridol is administered to a nursing woman.

PEDIATRIC USE

Safety and effectiveness of gadoteridol in children have not yet been established.

ADVERSE REACTIONS:

The most commonly noted adverse experiences were nausea and taste perversion with an incidence of 1.4%. These events were mild to moderate in severity:

The following additional events occurred in fewer than 1% of the patients:

Body as a Whole: Facial Edema; Neck Rigidity; Pain at Injection Site; Chest Pain; Headache; Fever; Itching Watery Eyes; Abdominal Cramps; Tingling Sensation in Throat; Flushed Feeling.

Cardiovascular: Prolonged P-R Interval; Hypotension; Elevated Heart Rate; A-V Nodal Rhythm.

Digestive: Edema-tongue; Gingivitis; Dry Mouth; Loose Bowel; Vomiting; Itching Tongue.

Nervous System: Anxiety; Dizziness; Paresthesia; Mental Status Decline; Loss of Coordination in Arm; Staring Episode; Syncope.

Respiratory System: Dyspnea; Rhinitis; Cough.

Skin and Appendages: Pruritus; Rash, Rash Macular Papular; Urticaria; Hives Tingling Sensation of Extremity and Digits.

Special Senses: Tinnitus.

OVERDOSAGE:

The minimum single lethal dose of gadoteridol in mice was found to be between 7 and 10 mmol/kg (23 to 33 times the human dose of 0.3 mmol/kg). Overt clinical signs noted prior to death included ataxia, convulsions, collapse, bloody exudate from nares and decreased activity. Prohance (Gadoteridol Injection) was not lethal to rats at single doses up to 10 mmol/kg.

DOSAGE AND ADMINISTRATION:

The recommended dose of gadoteridol is 0.1 mmol/kg (0.2 ml/kg) administered as a rapid IV infusion or bolus. However, in patients suspected of having cerebral metastases or other poorly enhancing lesions, in the presence of negative scans, after 0.1 mmol/kg injection, at the clinician's discretion, a second dose of 0.2 mmol/kg (0.4 ml/kg) can be administered up to 30 minutes after the first dose for further evaluation. Any unused potion must be discarded.

To ensure complete injection of the contrast medium, the injection should be followed by a 5 ml normal saline flush. The imaging procedure should be completed within 1 hour of the first injection of gadoteridol.

Parenteral products should be inspected visually for particulate matter and discoloration prior to administration. Do not use the solution if it is discolored or particulate matter is present.

STORAGE

Gadoteridol should be stored at controlled room temperature room temperature, between 15 and 30°C (59 - 86°F) and protected from light. Do not freeze. Should freezing occur in the vial, gadoteridol should be brought to room temperature before use. If allowed to stand at room temperature for a minimum of 60 minutes, gadoteridol should return to a clear, colorless to slightly yellow solution. Before use, examine this product to assure that all solids are redissolved and that the container and closure have not been damaged. Should solids persist, discard vial.

For How Supplied Information, Contact Bristol Myer (NDA# 020131)

GALLAMINE TRIETHIODIDE *(003226)*

CATEGORIES: Analeptics; Anesthesia; Autonomic Drugs; Muscle Relaxants; Neuromuscular Blocking Agents; Skeletal Muscle Relaxants; FDA Approval Pre 1982

BRAND NAMES: **Flaxedil**; *Garosan*; *Miowas G*; *Myraxan*
(International brand names outside U.S. in italics)

Prescribing information not available at time of publication.

GALLIUM NITRATE *(003030)*

CATEGORIES: Antineoplastics; Cancer; Hypercalcemia; Orphan Drugs; Pregnancy Category C; FDA Class 1B ("Modest Therapeutic Advantage"); FDA Approved 1991 Jan

BRAND NAMES: **Ganite**

WARNING:
Concurrent use of gallium nitrate with other potentially nephrotoxic drugs (*e.g.,* aminoglycosides, amphotericin B) may increase the risk for developing severe renal insufficiency in patients with cancer-related hypercalcemia. If use of a potentially nephrotoxic drug is indicated during gallium nitrate therapy, gallium nitrate administration should be discontinued and it is recommended that hydration be continued for several days after administration of the potentially nephrotoxic drug. Serum creatinine and urine output should be closely monitored during and subsequent to this period. Gallium nitrate therapy should be discontinued if the serum creatinine level exceeds 2.5 mg/Dl.

DESCRIPTION:

Gallium nitrate injection is a clear, colorless, odorless, sterile solution of gallium nitrate, a hydrated nitrate salt of the group IIIa element gallium. Gallium nitrate is formed by the reaction of elemental gallium with nitric acid, followed by crystallization of the drug from the solution. The stable, nonahydrate, (Ga(NO3)3. 9(H20) is a white, slightly hygroscopic, crystalline powder of molecular weight 417.87, that is readily soluble in water.

Each ml of gallium nitrate injection contains gallium nitrate 25 mg (on an anhydrous basis) and sodium citrate dihydrate 28.75 mg. The solution may contain sodium hydroxide for pH adjustment to 6.0 - 7.0.

CLINICAL PHARMACOLOGY:

MECHANISM OF ACTION

Gallium Nitrate exerts a hypocalcemic effect by inhibiting calcium resorption from bone, possibly by reducing increased bone turnover. Although *in vitro* and animal studies have been performed to investigate the mechanism of action of gallium nitrate, the precise mechanism for inhibiting calcium resorption has not been determined. No cytotoxic effects were observed on bone cells in drug-treated animals.

PHARMACOKINETICS

Gallium nitrate was infused at a daily dose of 200 mg/square meter for 5 (n=2) or 7(n=10) consecutive days to 12 cancer patients. In most patients apparent steady-state is achieved by 24 to 48 hours. The range of average steady-state plasma levels of gallium observed among 7 fully evaluable patients was between 1134 and 2399 ng/ml. The average plasma clearance of gallium (n=7) following daily infusion of gallium nitrate at a dose of 200 mg/square meter for 5 or 7 days was 0.15 L/hr/kg (range: 0.12 to 0.20 L/hr/kg). In one patient who received daily infusion doses of 100, 150, and 200 mg/square meter the apparent steady-state levels of gallium did not increase proportionally with an increase in dose. Gallium nitrate is not metabolized either by the liver or the kidney and appears to be significantly excreted via the kidney. Urinary excretion data for a dose of 200 mg/square meter has not been determined.

CANCER-RELATED HYPERCALCEMIA

Hypercalcemia is a common problem in hospitalized patients with malignancy. It may affect 10 - 20 % of patients with cancer. Different types of malignancy seem to vary in their propensity to cause hypercalcemia. A higher incidence of hypercalcemia has been observed in patients with non-small-cell lung cancer, breast cancer, multiple myeloma, kidney cancer, and cancer of head and neck. Hypercalcemia of malignancy seems to result from an imbalance between the net resorption of bone and urinary excretion of calcium. Patients with extensive osteolytic bone metastases frequently develop hypercalcemia; this type of hypercalcemia is common with primary breast cancer. Some of these patients have been reported to have increased renal tubular calcium resorption. Breast cancer cells have been reported to produce several potential bone-resorbing factors which stimulate the local osteoclast activity. Humoral hypercalcemia is common with the solid tumors of the lung, head and neck, kidney, and ovaries. Systemic factors (*e.g.,* PTH-rP) produced either by the tumor or host cells have been implicated for the altered calcium fluxes between the extracellular fluid, the kidney and the skeleton. About 30% of patients with myeloma develop hypercalcemia associated with extensive osteolytic lesions and impaired glomerular filtration. Myeloma cells have been reported to produce local factors that stimulate adjacent osteoclasts.

CLINICAL PHARMACOLOGY: *(cont'd)*

Hypercalcemia may produce a spectrum of signs and symptoms including: anorexia, lethargy, fatigue, nausea, vomiting, constipation, dehydration, renal insufficiency, impaired mental status, coma and cardiac arrest. A rapid rise in serum calcium may cause more severe symptoms for a given level of hypercalcemia. Since calcium is bound to serum proteins, which may fluctuate in concentration as a response to changes in blood volume, changes in total serum calcium (especially during rehydration) may not accurately reflect changes in the concentration of free-ionized calcium. In the absence of a direct measurement of free-ionized calcium, measurement of the serum albumin concentration and correction of the total serum calcium concentration may help in assessing the severity of hypercalcemia. The patient's acid-base status should also be taken into consideration while assessing the degree of hypercalcemia. Mild or asymptomatic hypercalcemia may be treated with conservative measures (*i.e.,* saline hydration, with or without diuretics). The patient's cardiovascular status should be taken into consideration in the use of saline. In patients who have an underlying cancer type that may be sensitive to corticosteroids (*e.g.,* hematologic cancers), the use or addition of corticosteroid therapy may be indicated.

HYPOCALCEMIC ACTIVITY

A randomized double-blind clinical study comparing Gallium Nitrate with calcitonin was conducted in patients with a serum calcium concentration (corrected for albumin) ≥ 12.0 mg/dL following 2 days of hydration. Gallium Nitrate was given as a continuous intravenous infusion at a dose of 200 mg/m²/day for 5 days and calcitonin was given intramuscularly at a dose of 8 I.U./kg every 6 hours for 5 days. Elevated serum calcium (corrected for albumin) was normalized in 75% (18 of 24) of the patients receiving Gallium Nitrate and in 27% (7 of 26) of the patients receiving calcitonin (p = 0.0016). The time-course of effect on serum calcium (corrected for albumin) is summarized in the following table.

TABLE 1
CHANGE IN CORRECTED SERUM CALCIUM BY TIME FROM INITIATION OF TREATMENT

Time Period (1) (hours)	Mean Change in Serum Calcium (mg/dL) (2)	
	Gallium Nitrate	Calcitonin
24	- 0.4	- 1.6*
48	- 0.9	- 1.4
72	- 1.5	- 1.1
96	- 2.9*	- 1.1
120	- 3.3*	- 1.3

(1) Time after initiation of therapy in hours.
(2) Change from baseline in serum calcium (corrected for albumin)
* Comparison between treatment groups (p < 0.01)

The median duration of normocalcemia/hypocalcemia was 7.5 days for patients treated with Gallium Nitrate and 1 day for patients treated with calcitonin. A total of 92% patients treated with Gallium Nitrate had a decrease in serum calcium (corrected for albumin) ≥ 2.0 mg/dl as compared to 54% of the patients treated with calcitonin (p = 0.004).

An open-label, non-randomized study was conducted to examine a range of doses and dosing schedules of Gallium Nitrate for control of cancer-related hypercalcemia. The principal dosing regimens were 100 and 200 mg/square meter/day, administered as continuous intravenous infusions for 5 days. Gallium Nitrate, at a dose of 200 mg/square meter/day for 5 days was found to normalize elevated serum calcium levels (corrected for albumin) in 83% of patients as compared to 50% of patients receiving a dose of 100 mg/m²/day for 5 days. A decrease in serum calcium (corrected for albumin) ≥ mg/dL was observed in 83% and 94% of patients treated with Gallium Nitrate at dosages of 100 and 200 mg/square meter/day for 5 days, respectively. There were no significant differences in the proportion of patients responding to Gallium Nitrate when considering wither the presence or absence of bone metastasis, or whether the tumor histology was epidermoid or nonepidermoid.

INDICATIONS AND USAGE:

Gallium Nitrate is indicated for the treatment of clearly symptomatic cancer-related hypercalcemia that has not responded to adequate hydration. In general, patients with a serum calcium (corrected for albumin) < 12 mg/dL would not be expected to be symptomatic. Mild or asymptomatic hypercalcemia may be treated with conservative measures (*i.e.,* saline hydration, with or without diuretics). In the treatment of cancer-related hypercalcemia, it is important first to establish adequate hydration, preferably with intravenous saline, in order to increase the renal excretion of calcium and correct dehydration caused by hypercalcemia.

CONTRAINDICATIONS:

Gallium Nitrate should not be administered to patients with severe renal impairment (serum creatinine > 2.5 mg/dL).

WARNINGS:

(See BOXED WARNING.) The hypercalcemic state in cancer patients of commonly associated with impaired renal function. Abnormalities in renal function (elevated BUN and/or serum creatinine) have been observed in clinical trials with Gallium Nitrate. IT IS STRONGLY RECOMMENDED THAT SERUM CREATININE BE MONITORED DURING GALLIUM NITRATE THERAPY. Since patients with cancer-related hypercalcemia are frequently dehydrated, it is important that such patients be adequately hydrated with and/or intravenous fluids (preferably saline) and that a satisfactory urine output (a urine output of 2 L/day is recommended) be established before therapy with Gallium Nitrate is started. Adequate hydration should be maintained throughout the treatment period, with careful attention to avoid over hydration in patients with compromised cardiovascular status. Diuretic therapy should not be employed prior to correction of hypovolemia. Gallium Nitrate therapy should be discontinued if the serum creatinine level exceeds 2.5 mg/dL.

The use of Gallium Nitrate in patients with marked renal insufficiency (serum creatinine > 2.5 mg/dL) has not been systematically examined. If therapy is undertaken in patients with moderately impaired renal function (serum creatinine 2.0 to 2.5 mg/dL), frequent monitoring of the patient's renal status is recommended. Treatment should be discontinued if the serum creatinine level exceeds 2.5 mg/dL.

PRECAUTIONS:

GENERAL

Asymptomatic of mild to moderate hypocalcemia (6.5 - 8.0 mg/dL, corrected for serum albumin) occurred in approximately 38% of patients treated with Gallium Nitrate in the controlled clinical trial. One patient exhibited a positive Chvostek's sign. If hypocalcemia occurs, Gallium Nitrate therapy should be stopped and short-term calcium therapy may be necessary.

LABORATORY TESTS

Renal function (serum creatinine and BUN) and serum calcium must be closely monitored during Gallium Nitrate therapy. In addition to baseline assessment, the suggested frequency of calcium and phosphorus determinations is daily and twice weekly, respectively. Gallium Nitrate should be discontinued if the serum creatinine exceeds 2.5 mg/dL.

PRECAUTIONS: *(cont'd)*

CARCINOGENESIS, MUTAGENESIS, AND IMPAIRMENT OF FERTILITY

Long-term studies in animals have not been performed to evaluate the carcinogenic potential of gallium nitrate. Gallium nitrate is not mutagenic in standard tests (*i.e.,* Ames test and chromosomal aberration studies on human lymphocytes).

USAGE IN PREGNANCY

Pregnancy Category C. Animal reproduction studies have not been conducted with gallium nitrate. It is also not known whether gallium nitrate can cause fetal harm when administered to a pregnant woman or can affect reproductive capacity. Gallium Nitrate should be administered to a pregnant woman only if clearly needed.

NURSING MOTHERS

It is not known whether gallium nitrate is excreted in human milk. Because if the potential for serious adverse reactions in nursing infants from gallium nitrate, a decision should be made whether to discontinue nursing or discontinue the drug, taking into account the importance of the drug to the mother.

PEDIATRIC USE

The safety and effectiveness of Gallium Nitrate in children have not been established.

DRUG INTERACTIONS:

Combined use of Gallium Nitrate with other potentially nephrotoxic drugs (*e.g.,* amino glycosides, amphotericin B) may increase the risk for developing renal insufficiency in patients with cancer-related hypercalcemia (see BOXED WARNING).

The concomitant use of highly nephrotoxic drugs in combination with Gallium Nitrate may increase the risk for development of renal insufficiency. Available information does not indicate any adverse interaction with diuretics such as furosemide.

ADVERSE REACTIONS:

KIDNEY

Adverse renal effects, as demonstrated by rising BUN and creatinine, have been reported in about 12.5% of patients treated with Gallium Nitrate. In a controlled clinical trial of patients with cancer-related hypercalcemia, two patients receiving Gallium Nitrate and one patient receiving calcitonin developed acute renal failure. Due to the serious nature of the patient's underlying conditions, the relationship of these events to the drug was unclear. Gallium Nitrate should not be administered to patients with serum creatinine > 2.5 mg/dl (see CONTRAINDICATIONS and WARNINGS).

METABOLIC

Hypercalcemia may occur after Gallium Nitrate treatment (see PRECAUTIONS).

Transient hypophosphatemia of mild-to-moderate degree may occur in up to 79% of hypercalcemic patients following treatment with Gallium Nitrate. In a controlled clinical trial, 33% of patients had at least 1 serum phosphorus value < 1.5 mg/dl. Patients who develop hypophosphatemia may require oral phosphorus therapy.

Decreased serum bicarbonate, possibly secondary to mild respiratory diagnosis was reported in 40 - 50% of cancer patients treated with Gallium Nitrate. The cause for this effect is not clear. This effect has been asymptomatic and has not required specific treatment.

HEMATOLOGIC

The use of very high doses of gallium nitrate (up to 1400 mg/square meter) in treating patients for advanced cancer has been associated with anemia, and several patients have received red blood cell transfusions. Due to the serious nature of the underlying illness, it is uncertain that the anemia was caused by gallium nitrate.

BLOOD PRESSURE

A decrease in mean systolic and diastolic blood pressure was observed several days after treatment with gallium nitrate in a controlled clinical trial. The decrease in blood pressure was asymptomatic and did not require specific treatment.

VISUAL AND AUDITORY

In cancer chemotherapy trials, a small proportion (< 1%) of patients treated with multiple high doses of gallium nitrate combined with other investigational anticancer drugs, have developed acute optic neuritis. While these patients were critically ill and had received multiple drugs, a reaction to high- dose gallium nitrate is possible. Most patients had full visual recovery; however, at least one case of persistent visual impairment has been reported. One patient with cancer-related hypercalcemia was reported to develop decreased hearing following gallium nitrate administration. Due to the patient's underlying condition and concurrent therapies, the relationship of this event to gallium nitrate administration is unclear. Tinnitus and partial loss of auditory acuity have been reported rarely (< 1%) in patients who received high-dose gallium nitrate as anticancer treatment.

MISCELLANEOUS

Other clinical events reported in association with gallium nitrate treatment for cancer as well as cancer-related hypercalcemia include: nausea and/or vomiting, tachycardia, lethargy, confusion, diarrhea, constipation, lower extremity edema, hypothermia, fever, dyspnea, rales and rhonchi, anemia, leukopenia, paresthesia, skin rash, pleural effusion, and pulmonary infiltrates. Due to the serious nature of the underlying condition of these patients, the relationship of these events to therapy with gallium nitrate is unknown.

OVERDOSAGE:

Rapid intravenous infusions of gallium nitrate or use of doses higher than recommended (200 mg/m^2) may cause nausea and vomiting and a substantially increased risk of renal insufficiency. In the event of overdosage, further drug administration should be discontinued, serum calcium should be monitored, and the patient should receive vigorous intravenous hydration, with or without diuretics, for 2 - 3 days. During this time period, renal function and urinary output should be carefully monitored so that fluid intake and output are balanced.

DOSAGE AND ADMINISTRATION:

The usual recommended dose of Gallium Nitrate is 200 mg per square meter of body surface area (200 mg/square meter) daily for 5 consecutive days. In patients with mild hypercalcemia and few symptoms, a lower dosage of 100/mg/square meter/day for 5 days may be considered. If serum calcium levels are lowered are lowered into their normal range in less than 5 days, treatment may be discontinued early. The daily dose must be administered as an intravenous infusion over 24 hours. The daily dose should be diluted, preferably in 1,000 ml of 0.9% Sodium Chloride Injection, USP, or in 5% Dextrose Injection, USP, for administration as an intravenous infusion over 24 hours. Adequate hydration must be maintained throughout the treatment period, with careful attention to avoid over hydration in patients with compromised cardiovascular status. Controlled studies have not been undertaken to evaluate the safety and effectiveness of retreatment with gallium nitrate.

When Gallium Nitrate is added to either 0.9% Sodium Chloride Injection, USP, or 5% Dextrose Injection, USP, is stable for at least 48 hours at room temperature (15-30°C) and for seven (7) days if stored under refrigeration (2-8°C). Parenteral drug products should be inspected visually for particulate matter and discoloration prior to administration whenever solution and container permit.

Store at controlled room temperature 15-30°C (59-86°F).

DOSAGE AND ADMINISTRATION: *(cont'd)*

Contains no preservative. Discard unused portion.

HOW SUPPLIED - EQUIVALENTS NOT AVAILABLE:

Injection, Solution - Intravenous - 25 mg/ml

20 ml x 10 $1155.00 GANITE, Solopak Labs 39769-0342-20

GANCICLOVIR SODIUM *(001343)*

CATEGORIES: AIDS Related Complex; Anti-Infectives; Antimicrobials; Antivirals; Cytomegalovirus Infections; HIV Infection; Infections; Orphan Drugs; Retinitis; Pregnancy Category C; FDA Approved 1989 Jun

BRAND NAMES: *Cymevan* (France); *Cymeven* (Germany); *Cymevene* (Australia, Asia, Europe, Mexico); **Cytovene**

(International brand names outside U.S. in italics)

FORMULARIES: Medi-Cal; PCS

COST OF THERAPY: $12,702.00 (AIDS Retinitis; Injection; 500 mg/vial; 1/day; 365 days)

WARNING:
THE CLINICAL TOXICITY OF GANCICLOVIR SODIUM AND GANCICLOVIR SODIUM IV INCLUDES GRANULOCYTOPENIA, ANEMIA, AND THROMBOCYTOPENIA. IN ANIMAL STUDIES GANCICLOVIR WAS CARCINOGENIC, TERATOGENIC, AND CAUSED ASPERMATOGENESIS.
GANCICLOVIR SODIUM-IV IS INDICATED FOR USE ONLY IN THE TREATMENT OF CYTOMEGALOVIRUS (CMV) RETINITIS IN IMMUNOCOMPROMISED PATIENTS AND FOR THE PREVENTION OF CMV DISEASE IN TRANSPLANT PATIENTS AT RISK FOR CMV DISEASE (SEE INDICATIONS AND USAGE.)
BECAUSE GANCICLOVIR SODIUM CAPSULES ARE ASSOCIATED WITH A RISK OF MORE RAPID RATE OF CMV RETINITIS PROGRESSION, THEY SHOULD BE USED ONLY IN THOSE PATIENTS FOR WHOM THIS RISK IS BALANCED BY THE BENEFIT ASSOCIATED WITH AVOIDING DAILY INTRAVENOUS INFUSIONS.

DESCRIPTION:

Ganciclovir is a synthetic guanine derivative active against cytomegalovirus (CMV). Cytovene-IV and Cytovene are the brand names for ganciclovir sodium for injection and ganciclovir capsules, respectively.

Cytovene-IV is available as sterile lyophilized powder in strength of 500 mg per vial for intravenous administration only. Each vial of Cytovene-IV contains the equivalent of 500 mg ganciclovir as the sodium salt (46 mg sodium). Reconstitution with 10 ml of Sterile Water for Injection, USP, yields a solution with pH 11 and a ganciclovir concentration of approximately 50 mg/ml. Further dilution in an appropriate intravenous solution must be performed before infusion (see DOSAGE AND ADMINISTRATION.)

Cytovene is available as 250 mg capsules. Each capsule contains 250 mg ganciclovir and inactive ingredients croscarmellose sodium, magnesium stearate, and povidone. The hard gelatin shell consists of gelatin, titanium dioxide, yellow iron oxide, and FD&C Blue #2.

Ganciclovir is a white to off-white crystalline powder with a molecular formula of $C_9H_{13}N_5O_4$ and a molecular weight of 255.23. The chemical name for ganciclovir is 9-[[2-hydroxy-1-(hydroxymethyl)-ethoxy]methyl]guanine. Ganciclovir is a polar hydrophilic compound with a solubility of 2.6 mg/ml in water at 25°C and an n-octanol/water partition coefficient of 0.022. The pK_as for ganciclovir are 2.2 and 9.4.

Ganciclovir, when formulated as monosodium salt in the IV dosage form, is a white to off-white lyophilized powder with a molecular formula of $C_9H_{12}N_5NaO_4$, and molecular weight of 277.22. The chemical name for ganciclovir sodium is 9-[[2-hydroxy-1- (hydroxymethyl)-ethoxy]methyl]guanine, monosodium salt. The lyophilized powder has an aqueous solubility of greater than 50 mg/ml at 25°C. At physiological pH, ganciclovir sodium exists as the un-ionized form with a solubility of approximately 6 mg/ml at 37°C.

All doses in this insert are specified in terms of ganciclovir.

CLINICAL PHARMACOLOGY:

VIROLOGY

Mechanism of Action: Ganciclovir is an acyclic nucleoside analogue of 2'-deoxyguanosine that inhibits replication of herpes viruses both *in vitro* and *in vivo.* Sensitive human viruses include cytomegalovirus (CMV), herpes simplex virus-1 and -2, herpesvirus type 6, Epstein-Barr virus, varicella zoster virus, and hepatitis B virus.[1-4] Clinical studies have been limited to assessment of efficacy in patients with CMV infection.

Ganciclovir must be converted to the corresponding triphosphate in order to exert its antiviral activity. In herpes simplex virus-infected cells, the initial conversion to the monophosphate is catalyzed by a viral thymidine kinase.[5] In contrast, in CMV-infected cells a protein kinase homologue, encoded by the CMV gene UL97, may be responsible for the initial phosphorylation of ganciclovir.[6,7] Cellular kinases, in CMV-infected cells, subsequently phosphorylate ganciclovir monophosphate to the diphosphate and active triphosphate moieties.[8,9]It has been shown that the levels of ganciclovir- triphosphate are as much as 100-fold greater in CMV-infected cells than in uninfected cells, indicating a preferential phosphorylation of ganciclovir in virus-infected cells.[9]

Ganciclovir triphosphate, once formed, appears quite stable and persists for days in the CMV-infected cell.[9] The antiviral activity of ganciclovir-triphosphate is believed to be the result of inhibition of viral DNA synthesis by two known modes: (1) competitive inhibition of viral DNA polymerases; (2) direct incorporation into viral DNA, resulting in eventual termination of viral DNA elongation. The cellular DNA polymerase alpha is also inhibited, but at a higher concentration than required for inhibition of viral DNA polymerase.

Antiviral Activity: The median concentration of ganciclovir which effectively inhibits the replication of either laboratory strains or clinical isolates of CMV (ED_{50}) has ranged from 0.02 to 3.48 mcg/ml. The relationship of *in vitro* sensitivity of CMV to ganciclovir and clinical response has not been established. Ganciclovir inhibits mammalian cell proliferation *in vitro* at higher concentrations: IC_{50}values range from 30 to 725 mcg/ml[4,10] with the exception of bone marrow-derived colony- forming cells which are more sensitive with IC_{50} values ranging from 0.028 to 0.7 mcg/ml.[4,11]

CLINICAL PHARMACOLOGY: *(cont'd)*

CLINICAL ANTIVIRAL EFFECT OF GANCICLOVIR SODIUM IV AND GANCICLOVIR SODIUM CAPSULES

Ganciclovir Sodium IV: Of 314 immunocompromised patients enrolled in an open label study of the treatment of life- or sight-threatening CMV disease with ganciclovir sodium IV solution, 121 patients were identified who had a positive culture for CMV within 7 days prior to treatment and had sequential viral cultures after treatment with ganciclovir sodium IV.[12] Post-treatment virologic response was defined as conversion to culture negativity, or a greater than 100-fold decrease in CMV infectious units, as shown in TABLE 1.

TABLE 1 Virologic Response

Culture Source	No. Patients Cultured	No. (%) Patients Responding	Median Days to Response
Urine	107	93 (87)	8
Blood	41	34 (83)	8
Throat	21	19 (90)	7
Semen	6	6 (100)	15

The antiviral activity of ganciclovir sodium IV solution was demonstrated in two separate placebo-controlled studies for the prevention of CMV disease in transplant recipients. One hundred and forty-nine heart allograft recipients who were either CMV seropositive or had received seropositive heart allografts were randomized to treatment with ganciclovir sodium IV solution (5 mg/kg BID for 14 days followed by 6 mg/kg QD for 5 days/week for an additional 14 days) or placebo.[13] Seventy-two CMV culture- positive allogeneic bone marrow[14] transplant recipients were randomized to treatment with ganciclovir sodium IV solution (5 mg/kg BID for 7 days followed by 5 mg/kg QD) or placebo until day 100 post- transplant.[12] Ganciclovir sodium IV suppressed CMV shedding in heart allograft and bone marrow allograft recipients. The antiviral effect of ganciclovir sodium IV solution in these patients is summarized in TABLE 2.

TABLE 2 Patients With Positive CMV Cultures

Time	Heart Allograft: Ganciclovir Sodium-IV	Heart Allograft: Placebo	Bone Marrow Allograft: Ganciclovir Sodium-IV	Bone Marrow Allograft: Placebo
Pre- Treatment	1/67 (2%)	5/64 (8%)	37/37 (100%)	35/35 (100%)
Week 2	2/75 (3%)	11/67 (16%)	2/31 (6%)	19/28 (68%)
Week 4	3/66 (5%)	28/66 (43%)	0/24 (0%)	16/20 (80%)

Ganciclovir Sodium Capsules: The antiviral activity of ganciclovir sodium capsules was confirmed in two randomized, controlled trials comparing ganciclovir sodium IV solution with ganciclovir sodium capsules for the maintenance treatment of CMV retinitis in patients with AIDS. Serial cultures of urine were obtained, and cultures of semen, biopsy specimens, blood, and other sources also were obtained when available. Only a small proportion of patients remained culture-positive during maintenance therapy with either ganciclovir sodium IV solution or ganciclovir sodium capsules. There were no statistically significant differences in the rates of positive cultures between the treatment groups. The antiviral effect of ganciclovir sodium capsules in the patients in the two studies is summarized in TABLE 3.

TABLE 3 Patients With Positive CMV Cultures In Two Controlled Clinical Studies with Ganciclovir Sodium

	Patients With Newly Diagnosed CMV Retinitis*: IV Solution	Patients With Newly Diagnosed CMV Retinitis*: Capsules	Patients With Stable, Previously Treated CMV Retinitis†: IV Solution	Patients With Stable, Previously Treated CMV Retinitis†: Capsules‡
At Start of Maintenance	5/37 (13.5%)	9/27 (24.3)	2/66 (3.0%)	5/137 (3.6%)
Anytime During Maintenance	3/48 (6.3%)	4/44 (9.1%)	1/45 (2.2%)	7/99 (7.1%)

* Study ISM 1653. 3 weeks of treatment with IV ganciclovir before start og maintenance.
† Study ICM 1774. 4weeks to 4 months treatment with IV ganciclovir
‡ Data from 6 times daily and 3 times daily regimens pooled

Viral Resistance: The current working definition of CMV resistance to ganciclovir is IC_{50}>2.9 mcg/ml (11.4 µm) or IC_{90} >7.4 mcg/ml (29 µm). CMV resistance to ganciclovir in individuals with AIDS and CMV retinitis who have not previously been treated with ganciclovir does occur but appears to be infrequent. Viral resistance has been observed in patients receiving prolonged treatment with ganciclovir sodium IV.[15-19] However, due to the limited number of viral isolates tested, it is difficult to estimate the overall frequency of reduced sensitivity in patients receiving ganciclovir. Nonetheless, the possibility of viral resistance should be considered in patients who show poor clinical response or experience persistent viral excretion during therapy. The principal mechanism of resistance to ganciclovir in CMV is the decreased ability to form the active triphosphate moiety; resistant viruses have been described which contain mutations in the UL97 gene of CMV which controls phosphorylation of ganciclovir.[6, 7, 20- 24] Mutations in the viral DNA polymerase have also been reported to confer viral resistance to ganciclovir.[23,24]

In two randomized controlled trials, the incidence of reduced sensitivity appeared to be no more common during treatment with ganciclovir sodium capsules than during treatment with ganciclovir sodium IV solution.

Pharmacokinetics: BECAUSE THE MAJOR ELIMINATION PATHWAY FOR GANCICLOVIR IS RENAL, DOSAGE MUST BE REDUCED ACCORDING TO CREATININE CLEARANCE. FOR DOSING INSTRUCTIONS IN PATIENTS WITH RENAL IMPAIRMENT, REFER TO THE SECTION ON DOSAGE AND ADMINISTRATION.

Absorption: The absolute bioavailability of oral ganciclovir under fasting conditions was approximately 5% (n=6) and following food was 6-9% (n=32). When ganciclovir was administered orally with food at a total daily dose of 3 g/day (500 mg q3h, 6 times daily and 1000 mg TID), the steady-state absorption as measured by area under the serum concentration vs. time curve (AUC) over 24 hours and maximum serum concentrations (C_{max}) were similar following both regimens with an AUC_{0-24} of 15.9 ± 4.2 (mean ± SD) and 15.4 ± 4.3 mcg·hr/ml and C_{max} of 1.02 ± 0.24 and 1.18 ± 0.36 mcg/ml, respectively (n=16).

At the end of a one-hour intravenous infusion of 5 mg/kg ganciclovir, total AUC ranged between 22.1 ± 3.2 (n=16) and 26.8 ± 6.1 mcg·hr/ml (n=16) and C_{max} ranged between 8.27 ± 1.02 (n=16) and 9.0 ± 1.4 mcg/ml (n=16).

Food Effects: When ganciclovir sodium capsules were given with a meal containing 602 calories and 46.5% fat at a dose of 1000 mg every 8 hours to 20 HIV-positive subjects, the steady-state AUC increased by 22 ± 22% (range: -6% to 68%) and there was a significant prolongation of time to peak serum concentrations (T_{max}) from 1.8 ± 0.8 to 3.0 ± 0.6 hours and a higher C_{max}(0.85 ± 0.25 vs. 0.96 ± 0.27 mcg/ml) (n=20).

Distribution: The steady-state volume of distribution of ganciclovir after intravenous administration was 0.74 ± 0.15 l/kg (n=98). For ganciclovir sodium capsules, no correlation was observed between AUC and reciprocal weight (range of 55-128 kg); oral dosing according to weight is not required. Cerebrospinal fluid concentrations obtained 0.25 and 5.67 hours post-dose in 3 patients who received 2.5 mg/kg ganciclovir intravenously q8h or q12h ranged from 0.31 to 0.68 mcg/ml[25] representing 24 to 70% of the respective plasma concentrations. Binding to plasma proteins was 1-2% over ganciclovir concentrations of 0.5 and 51 mcg/ml.

Metabolism: Following oral administration of a single 1000 mg dose of ^{14}C-labelled ganciclovir, 86 ± 3% of the administered dose was recovered in the feces and 5 ± 1% was recovered in the urine (n = 4). No metabolite accounted for more than 1 to 2% of the radioactivity recovered in urine or feces.

Elimination: When administered intravenously, ganciclovir exhibits linear pharmacokinetics over the range of 1.6 to 5.0 mg/kg and when administered orally, it exhibits linear kinetics up to a total daily dose of 4 g/day. Renal excretion of unchanged drug by glomerular filtration and active tubular secretion is the major route of elimination of ganciclovir. In patients with normal renal function, 91.3 ± 5.0% (n=4) of intravenously administered ganciclovir was recovered unmetabolized in the urine. Systemic clearance of intravenously administered ganciclovir was 3.52 ± 0.80 ml/min/kg (n=98) while renal clearance was 3.20 ± 0.80 ml/min/kg (n=47), accounting for 91 ± 11% of the systemic clearance (n=47). After oral administration of ganciclovir, steady-state is achieved within 24 hours. Renal clearance following oral administration was 3.1 ± 1.2 ml/min/kg (n=22). Half- life was 3.5 ± 0.9 hours (n=98) following IV administration and 4.8 ± 0.9 (n=39) following oral administration.

SPECIAL POPULATIONS

Renal Impairment: The pharmacokinetics following intravenous administration of ganciclovir sodium IV solution were evaluated in 10 immunocompromised patients with renal impairment who received doses ranging from 1.25 to 5 mg/kg (TABLE 4).

TABLE 4

CrCl (ml/min)	n	Dose	Clearance (ml/min) Mean ± SD	Half-life (hours) Mean ± SD
50-79	4	3.2 - 5 mg/kg	128 ± 63	4.6 ± 1.4
25-49	3	3 - 5 mg/kg	57 ± 8	4.4 ± 0.4
<25	3	1.25 - 5 mg/kg	30 ± 13	10.7 ± 5.7

The pharmacokinetics following oral administration of ganciclovir sodium capsules were evaluated in 8 solid organ transplant recipients; dose was modified according to estimated creatinine clearance (TABLE 5):

TABLE 5

CrCl (ml/min)	n	Dose	AUC_{0-24}[a] (mcg·hr/ml) Mean ± SD	Half-life (hours)
50-69	4	1000 mg q8h	49.1 ± 12.2	NC[b]
25-49	1	1000 mg QD	27.4	18.2
10-24	1	500 mg QD	10.7	15.7
<10	2	500 mg TIW[b]	25.6 ± 5.9	NC[c]

[a] Estimated or actual
[b] Three times weekly, after hemodialysis
[c] Not Calculated since half-life exceeded sampling interval

Hemodialysis reduces plasma concentrations of ganciclovir by about 50% after both intravenous and oral administration.

Race and Gender: The effects of race and gender were studied in subjects receiving a dose regimen of 1000 mg every 8 hours. Although the numbers of blacks (16%) and Hispanics (20%) were small, there appeared to be a trend towards a lower steady-state C_{max} and AUC_{0-8} in these subpopulations as compared to Caucasians. No definitive conclusions regarding gender differences could be made because of the small number of females (12%); however, no differences between males and females were observed.

Pediatrics: Ganciclovir pharmacokinetics were studied in 27 neonates, aged 2 to 49 days. At an intravenous dose of 4 mg/kg (n=14) or 6 mg/kg (n=13), the pharmacokinetic parameters were, respectively, C_{max} of 5.5 ± 1.6 and 7.0 ± 1.6 mcg/ml, systemic clearance of 3.14 ± 1.75 and 3.56 ± 1.27 ml/min/kg, and $t_{1/2}$ of 2.4 hours (harmonic mean) for both.[26]

Elderly: No studies have been conducted in adults older than 65 years of age.

CLINICAL STUDIES:

CMV Retinitis: The diagnosis of CMV retinitis should be made by indirect ophthalmoscopy. Other conditions in the differential diagnosis of CMV retinitis include candidiasis, toxoplasmosis, histoplasmosis, retinal scars, and cotton wool spots, any of which may produce a retinal appearance similar to CMV. For this reason it is essential that the diagnosis of CMV be established by an ophthalmologist familiar with the retinal presentation of these conditions. The diagnosis of CMV retinitis may be supported by culture of CMV from urine, blood, throat, or other sites, but a negative CMV culture does not rule out CMV retinitis.

Studies with Ganciclovir Sodium IV: In a retrospective, non- randomized, single-center analysis of 41 patients with AIDS and CMV retinitis diagnosed by ophthalmologic examination between August 1983 and April 1988, treatment with ganciclovir sodium IV solution resulted in a significant delay in mean (median) time to first retinitis progression compared to untreated controls [105 (71) days from diagnosis versus 35 (29) days from diagnosis].[27] Patients in this series received induction treatment of ganciclovir sodium IV 5 mg/kg BID for 14 to 21 days followed by maintenance treatment with either 5 mg/kg once daily, 7 days per week or 6 mg/kg once daily, 5 days per week (see DOSAGE AND ADMINISTRATION).

In a controlled, randomized, study (ICM 1697), conducted between February 1989 and December 1990, immediate treatment with ganciclovir sodium IV was compared to delayed treatment in 42 patients with AIDS and peripheral CMV retinitis; 35 of 42 patients (13 in the immediate-treatment group and 22 in the delayed-treatment group) were included in the analysis of time to retinitis progression. Based on masked assessment of fundus photographs, the mean [95% CI] and median [95% CI] times to progression of retinitis were 66 days and 50 days [40, 84], respectively, in the immediate- treatment group compared to 19 days and 13.5 days [8, 18], respectively, in the delayed-treatment group (TABLE 6).

ICM 1653: In this randomized, open label, parallel group trial, conducted between March 1991 and November 1992, patients with AIDS and newly diagnosed CMV retinitis received a 3-week induction course of ganciclovir sodium IV solution, 5 mg/kg BID for 14 days followed by 5 mg/kg once daily for 1 additional week. Following the 21-day intravenous induction course, patients with stable CMV retinitis were randomized to receive 20 weeks of maintenance treatment with either ganciclovir sodium IV solution, 5 mg/kg once daily, or ganciclovir sodium capsules, 500 mg 6 times daily (3000 mg/day). The study showed that the mean [95% CI] and median [95% CI] times to progression of CMV retinitis, as assessed by masked reading of fundus photographs, were 57 days [44, 70] and 29 days [28, 43],

CLINICAL STUDIES: *(cont'd)*

TABLE 6 Studies comparing Ganciclovir Sodium Capsules to Ganciclovir Sodium IV Solution: Demography of Populations in Studies ICM 1653, ICM 1774 and AVI 034

		ICM 1653 (n=121)	ICM 1774 (n=225)	AVI 034 (n=159)
Median age (years)		38	37	39
Range		24-62	22-56	23-62
Sex	Males	116 (96%)	222 (99%)	148 (93%)
	Females	5 (4%)	3 (1%)	1 (1%)
Ethnicity	Asian	3 (3%)	5 (2%)	7 (4%)
	Black	11 (9%)	9 (4%)	3 (2%)
	Caucasian	98 (81%)	186 (83%)	140 (88%)
	Other	9 (7%)	25 (11%)	8 (5%)
Median CD4 Count		9.5	7.0	10.0
Range		0 - 141	0 - 80	0 - 320
Mean (S.D.) Observation Time (days)		107.9 (43.0)	97.6 (42.5)	80.9 (47.0)

respectively, for patients on oral therapy compared to 62 days [50, 73] and 49 days [29, 61], respectively, for patients on intravenous therapy. The difference [95% CI] in the mean time to progression between the oral and intravenous therapies (oral - IV) was -5 days [-22, 12].

ICM 1774: In this three-arm, randomized, open label, parallel group trial, conducted between June 1991 and August 1993, patients with AIDS and stable CMV retinitis following from 4 weeks to 4 months of treatment with ganciclovir sodium IV solution were randomized to receive maintenance treatment with ganciclovir sodium IV solution, 5 mg/kg once daily, ganciclovir sodium capsules, 500 mg 6 times daily, or ganciclovir sodium capsules, 1000 mg TID for 20 weeks. The study showed that the mean [95% CI] and median [95% CI] times to progression of CMV retinitis, as assessed by masked reading of fundus photographs, were 54 days [48, 60] and 42 days [31, 54], respectively, for patients on oral therapy compared to 66 days [56, 76] and 54 days [41, 69], respectively, for patients on intravenous therapy. The difference [95% CI] in the mean time to progression between the oral and intravenous therapies (oral - IV) was -12 days [-24, 0].

AVI 034: In this randomized, open-label, parallel group trial, conducted between June 1991 and February 1993, patients with AIDS and newly diagnosed (81%) or previously treated (19%) CMV retinitis who had tolerated 10 to 21 days of induction treatment with ganciclovir sodium IV, 5 mg/kg twice daily, were randomized to receive 20 weeks of maintenance treatment with either ganciclovir sodium capsules, 500 mg 6 times daily or ganciclovir sodium IV solution, 5 mg/kg/day. The study showed that the mean [95% CI] and median [95% CI] times to progression of CMV retinitis, as assessed by masked reading of fundus photographs, were 51 days [44, 57] and 41 days [31, 45], respectively, for patients on oral therapy compared to 62 days [52, 72] and 60 days [42, 83], respectively, for patients on intravenous therapy. The difference [95% CI] in the mean time to progression between the oral and intravenous therapies (oral - IV) was -11 days [-24, 1].

Other CMV retinitis outcomes as assessed by masked reading of fundus photographs in the three studies, and visual acuity data, are presented in TABLE 7A, 7B, 7C, and 7D. Because of low event rates among these endpoints, these studies are underpowered to rule out significant differences in these endpoints.

TABLE 7A Other Ophthalmologic Endpoints Assessed Using Fundus Photographs During Maintenance Treatment of CMV Retinitis With Ganciclovir Sodium Capsules, 3 g/day, versus Ganciclovir Sodium IV Solution, 5 mg/kg/day, in Three Controlled Clinical Trials

	Study ICM 1653		Study ICM 1774	
	IV n=57	Oral n=58	IV n=63	Oral n=136*
Subjects Developing Bilateral Retinitis‡	3/34 (9%)	9/42 (21%)	7/52 (13%)	17/89 (19%)
95% Confidence Interval	[0%, 18%]	[9%, 34%]	[4%, 22%]	[11%, 27%]
Oral-IV Difference	13%		6%	
95% Confidence Interval	[-3%, +28%]		[-7%, +18%]	
Subjects with Progression into Zone 1‡	3/52 (6%)	6/56 (11%)	7/59 (12%)	20/127 (16%)
95% Confidence Interval	[0%, 12%]	[3%, 18%]	[4%, 20%]	[9%, 22%]
Oral-IV Difference	5%		4%	
95% Confidence Interval	[-5%, +15%]		[-7%, +14%]	

* Data from 6 times daily and 3 times daily dosage regimens pooled.
‡ The rates of development of bilateral CMV retinitis and of progression into Zone 1 in studies 1774 and 034 may be underestimated when assessed by photography because photographic assessment was discontinued at the time of funduscopically-determined progression, which may have occurred earlier.

TABLE 7B Other Ophthalmologic Endpoints Assessed Using Fundus Photographs During Maintenance Treatment of CMV Retinitis With Ganciclovir Sodium Capsules, 3 g/day, versus Ganciclovir Sodium IV Solution, 5 mg/kg/day, in Three Controlled Clinical Trials

	Study ACI 034	
	IV n=37	Oral n=104
Subjects Developing Bilateral Retinitis‡	6/31 (19%)	7/70 (10%)
95% Confidence Interval	[5%, 33%]	[3%, 17%]
Oral-IV Difference	-9%	
95% Confidence Interval	[-25%, +6%]	
Subjects with Progression into Zone 1‡	1/33 (3%)	1/86 (1%)
95% Confidence Interval	[0%, 9%]	[0%, 3%]
Oral-IV Difference	-2%	
95% Confidence Interval	[-8%, +4%]	

‡ The rates of development of bilateral CMV retinitis and of progression into Zone 1 in studies 1774 and 034 may be underestimated when assessed by photography because photographic assessment was discontinued at the time of funduscopically-determined progression, which may have occurred earlier.

PREVENTION OF CMV DISEASE IN TRANSPLANT RECIPIENTS

Ganciclovir sodium IV solution was evaluated in three randomized, controlled trials of prevention of CMV disease in organ transplant recipients.

ICM 1496: In a randomized, double-blind, placebo-controlled study of 149 heart transplant recipients[15] at risk for CMV infection (CMV seropositive, or a seronegative recipient of an organ from a CMV seropositive donor), there was a statistically significant reduction in the overall incidence of CMV disease in patients treated with ganciclovir sodium- IV. Immediately post-transplant, patients received ganciclovir sodium IV solution 5 mg/kg BID for 14 days followed by 6 mg/kg QD for 5 days/week for an additional 14 days. Twelve of the 76 (16%) patients treated with ganciclovir sodium IV versus 31 of the 73 (43%) placebo-treated patients developed CMV disease during the 120-day post-transplant observation period. No significant differences in hematologic toxicities were seen between the two treatment groups (TABLE 8).

TABLE 7C Other Ophthalmologic Endpoints Assessed Using Fundus Photographs During Maintenance Treatment of CMV Retinitis With Ganciclovir Sodium Capsules, 3 g/day, versus Ganciclovir Sodium IV Solution, 5 mg/kg/day, in Three Controlled Clinical Trials

	Study ICM 1653		Study ICM 1774	
	IV n=57	Oral n=58	IV n=63	Oral n=136*
Subjects with Deterioration of Visual Acuity	14/57 (25%)	12/60 (20%)	11/69 (16%)	28/150 (19%)
95% Confidence Interval	[13%, 36%]	[10%, 30%]	[7%, 25%]	[12%, 25%]
Oral-IV Difference	-5%		-3%	
95% Confidence Interval	[-20%, +11%]		[-8%, +13%]	

* Data from 6 times daily and 3 times daily dosage regimens pooled.

TABLE 7D Other Ophthalmologic Endpoints Assessed Using Fundus Photographs During Maintenance Treatment of CMV Retinitis With Ganciclovir Sodium Capsules, 3 g/day, versus Ganciclovir Sodium IV Solution, 5 mg/kg/day, in Three Controlled Clinical Trials

	Study ACI 034	
	IV n=37	Oral n=104
Subjects with Deterioration of Visual Acuity	5/44 (11%)	18/110 (16%)
95% Confidence Interval	[2%, 21%]	[9%, 23%]
Oral-IV Difference	-5%	
95% Confidence Interval	[-7%, +17%]	

ICM 1689: In a randomized, double-blind, placebo-controlled study of 72 bone marrow transplant recipients[16] with asymptomatic CMV infection (CMV positive culture of urine, throat, or blood) there was a statistically significant reduction in the incidence of CMV disease in patients treated with ganciclovir sodium IV solution following successful hematopoietic engraftment. Patients with virologic evidence of CMV infection received ganciclovir sodium IV 5 mg/kg BID for 7 days followed by 5 mg/kg QD through day 100 post-transplant. One of the 37 (3%) patients treated with ganciclovir sodium IV versus 15 of the 35 (43%) placebo-treated patients developed CMV disease during the study. At 6 months post-transplant, there continued to be a statistically significant reduction in the incidence of CMV disease in patients treated with ganciclovir sodium IV. Six of 37 (16%) patients treated with ganciclovir sodium IV versus 15 of the 35 (43%) placebo-treated patients developed disease through 6 months post- transplant. The overall rate of survival was statistically significantly higher in the group treated with ganciclovir sodium IV, both at day 100 and day 180 post-transplant. Although the differences in hematologic toxicities were not statistically significant, the incidence of neutropenia was higher in the group treated with ganciclovir sodium IV solution (TABLE 8).

ICM 1570: A second, randomized, unblinded, study evaluated 40 allogeneic bone marrow transplant recipients at risk for CMV disease.[28] Patients underwent bronchoscopy and bronchoalveolar lavage (BAL) on day 35 post-transplant. Patients with histologic, immunologic, or virologic evidence of CMV infection in the lung were then randomized to observation or treatment with ganciclovir sodium IV solution (5 mg/kg BID for 14 days followed by 5 mg/kg QD 5 days/week until day 120). Four of 20 (20%) patients treated with ganciclovir sodium IV and 14 of 20 (70%) control patients developed interstitial pneumonia. The incidence of CMV disease was significantly lower in the group treated with ganciclovir sodium IV solution, consistent with the results observed in ICM 1689.

INDICATIONS AND USAGE:

Ganciclovir sodium IV is indicated for the treatment of CMV retinitis in immunocompromised patients, including patients with acquired immunodeficiency syndrome (AIDS). Ganciclovir sodium IV is also indicated for the prevention of CMV disease in transplant recipients at risk for CMV disease (see CLINICAL STUDIES.)

Ganciclovir sodium capsules are indicated as an alternative to the intravenous formulation for maintenance treatment of CMV retinitis in immunocompromised patients, including patients with AIDS, in whom retinitis is stable following appropriate induction therapy and for whom the risk of more rapid progression is balanced by the benefit associated with avoiding daily IV infusions (see CLINICAL STUDIES.)

SAFETY AND EFFICACY OF GANCICLOVIR SODIUM IV AND GANCICLOVIR SODIUM HAVE NOT BEEN ESTABLISHED FOR CONGENITAL OR NEONATAL CMV DISEASE; NOR FOR THE TREATMENT OF ESTABLISHED CMV DISEASE OTHER THAN RETINITIS; NOR FOR USE IN NON- IMMUNOCOMPROMISED INDIVIDUALS. THE SAFETY AND EFFICACY OF GANCICLOVIR SODIUM CAPSULES HAVE NOT BEEN ESTABLISHED FOR TREATING ANY MANIFESTATION OF CMV DISEASE OTHER THAN MAINTENANCE TREATMENT OF CMV RETINITIS.

CONTRAINDICATIONS:

Ganciclovir sodium IV and ganciclovir sodium are contraindicated in patients with hypersensitivity to ganciclovir or acyclovir.

WARNINGS:

Hematologic: Ganciclovir sodium IV and ganciclovir sodium should not be administered if the absolute neutrophil count is less than 500 cells/μl or the platelet count is less than 25,000 cells/μl. Granulocytopenia (neutropenia), anemia and thrombocytopenia have been observed in patients treated with ganciclovir sodium IV and ganciclovir sodium. The frequency and severity of these events vary widely in different patient populations (see ADVERSE REACTIONS.)

Ganciclovir sodium IV and ganciclovir sodium should, therefore, be used with caution in patients with pre-existing cytopenias, or with a history of cytopenic reactions to other drugs, chemicals, or irradiation. Granulocytopenia usually occurs during the first or second week of treatment, but may occur at any time during treatment. Cell counts usually begin to recover within 3 to 7 days of discontinuing drug. Colony-stimulating factors have been shown to increase neutrophil and white blood cell counts in patients receiving ganciclovir sodium IV solution for treatment of CMV retinitis.[29-30]

Impairment of Fertility: Animal data indicate that administration of ganciclovir causes inhibition of spermatogenesis and subsequent infertility. These effects were reversible at lower doses and irreversible at higher doses (see Carcinogenesis, Mutagenesis, and Impairment of Fertility). Although data in humans have not been obtained regarding this effect, it is considered probable that ganciclovir at the recommended doses causes temporary or permanent inhibition of spermatogenesis. Animal data also indicate that suppression of fertility in females may occur.

WARNINGS: *(cont'd)*

Teratogenesis: Because of the mutagenic and teratogenic potential of ganciclovir, women of childbearing potential should be advised to use effective contraception during treatment. Similarly, men should be advised to practice barrier contraception during and for at least 90 days following treatment with ganciclovir sodium IV or ganciclovir sodium (see Pregnancy, Category C.)

PRECAUTIONS:

General: In clinical studies with ganciclovir sodium IV, the maximum single dose administered was 6 mg/kg by intravenous infusion over 1 hour. Larger doses have resulted in increased toxicity. It is likely that more rapid infusions would result in increased toxicity (see OVERDOSAGE.) Administration of ganciclovir sodium IV solution should be accompanied by adequate hydration.

Initially, reconstituted solutions of ganciclovir sodium IV have a high pH (pH 11). Despite further dilution in intravenous fluids, phlebitis and/or pain may occur at the site of intravenous infusion. Care must be taken to infuse solutions containing ganciclovir sodium IV only into veins with adequate blood flow to permit rapid dilution and distribution (see DOSAGE AND ADMINISTRATION.)

Since ganciclovir is excreted by the kidneys, normal clearance depends on adequate renal function. IF RENAL FUNCTION IS IMPAIRED, DOSAGE ADJUSTMENTS ARE REQUIRED. Such adjustments should be based on measured or estimated creatinine clearance values. (see DOSAGE AND ADMINISTRATION).

Information for the Patient: All patients should be informed that the major toxicities of ganciclovir are granulocytopenia (neutropenia), anemia, and thrombocytopenia and that dose modifications may be required, including discontinuation. The importance of close monitoring of blood counts while on therapy should be emphasized.

Patients should be instructed to take ganciclovir sodium capsules with food to maximize bioavailability.

Patients should be advised that ganciclovir has caused decreased sperm production in animals and may cause infertility in humans. Women of childbearing potential should be advised that ganciclovir causes birth defects in animals and should not be used during pregnancy. Women of childbearing potential should be advised to use effective contraception during treatment with ganciclovir sodium IV or ganciclovir sodium. Similarly, men should be advised to practice barrier contraception during and for at least 90 days following treatment with ganciclovir sodium IV or ganciclovir sodium.

Patients should be advised that ganciclovir causes tumors in animals. Although there is no information from human studies, ganciclovir should be considered a potential carcinogen.

Patients With AIDS and CMV Retinitis: Ganciclovir is not a cure for CMV retinitis, and immunocompromised patients may continue to experience progression of retinitis during or following treatment. Patients should be advised to have ophthalmologic followup examinations at a minimum of every 4 to 6 weeks while being treated with ganciclovir sodium IV or ganciclovir sodium. Some patients will require more frequent followup. Patients with AIDS may be receiving zidovudine (Retrovir). Patients should be counseled that treatment with both ganciclovir and zidovudine simultaneously may not be tolerated by some patients and may result in severe granulocytopenia (neutropenia). Patients with AIDS may be receiving didanosine (Videx). Patients should be counseled that concomitant treatment with both ganciclovir and didanosine can cause didanosine levels to be significantly increased.

Transplant Recipients: Transplant recipients should be counseled regarding the high frequency of impaired renal function in transplant recipients with received ganciclovir sodium IV solution in controlled clinical trials, particularly in patients receiving concomitant administration of nephrotoxic agents such as cyclosporine and amphotericin B. Although the specific mechanism of this toxicity, which in most cases was reversible, has not been determined, the higher rate of renal impairment in patients receiving ganciclovir sodium IV solution compared with those who received placebo in the same trials may indicate that ganciclovir sodium IV played a significant role.

Laboratory Tests: Due to the frequency of neutropenia, anemia and thrombocytopenia in patients receiving ganciclovir sodium IV and ganciclovir sodium (see ADVERSE REACTIONS), it is recommended that complete blood counts and platelet counts be performed frequently, especially in patients in whom ganciclovir or other nucleoside analogues have previously resulted in leukopenia, or in whom neutrophil counts are less than 1,000 cells/µl at the beginning of treatment. Because dosing with ganciclovir sodium IV and ganciclovir sodium must be modified in patients with renal impairment, and because of the incidence of increased serum creatinine levels that have been observed in transplant recipients treated with ganciclovir sodium IV solution, patients should have serum creatinine or creatinine clearance values followed carefully.

Carcinogenesis, Mutagenesis, and Impairment of Fertility: Ganciclovir was carcinogenic in the mouse at oral doses of 20 and 1000 mg/kg/day (approximately 0.1x and 1.4x, respectively, the mean drug exposure in humans following the recommended intravenous dose of 5 mg/kg, based on area under the plasma concentration curve (AUC) comparisons). At the dose of 1000 mg/kg/day there was a significant increase in the incidence of tumors of the preputial gland in males, forestomach (nonglandular mucosa) in males and females, and reproductive tissues (ovaries, uterus, mammary gland, clitoral gland, and vagina) and liver in females. At the dose of 20 mg/kg/day, a slightly increased incidence of tumors was noted in the preputial and harderian glands in males, forestomach in males and females, and liver in females. No carcinogenic effect was observed in mice administered ganciclovir at 1 mg/kg/day (estimated as 0.01x the human dose based on AUC comparison). Except for histiocytic sarcoma of the liver, ganciclovir induced tumors were generally of epithelial or vascular origin. Although the preputial and clitoral glands, forestomach, and harderian glands of mice do not have human counterparts, ganciclovir should be considered a potential carcinogen in humans.

Ganciclovir increased mutations in mouse lymphoma cells and DNA damage in human lymphocytes *in vitro* at concentrations between 50-500 and 250-2000 mcg/ml, respectively. In the mouse micronucleus assay, ganciclovir was clastogenic at doses of 150 and 500 mg/kg (IV) (2.8-10x human exposure based on AUC) but not 50 mg/kg (exposure approximately comparable to the human based on AUC). Ganciclovir was not mutagenic in the Ames Salmonella assay at concentrations of 500-5000 mcg/ml.

Impairment of Fertility*: Ganciclovir caused decreased mating behavior, decreased fertility, and an increased incidence of embryolethality in female mice following intravenous doses of 90 mg/kg/day (approximately 1.7x the mean drug exposure in humans following the dose of 5 mg/kg, based on AUC comparisons). Ganciclovir caused decreased fertility in male mice and hypospermatogenesis in mice and dogs following daily oral or intravenous administration of doses ranging from 0.2-10 mg/kg. Systemic drug exposure (AUC) at the lowest dose showing toxicity in each species ranged from 0.03-0.1x the AUC of the recommended human intravenous dose.

Pregnancy, Teratogenic Effects, Pregnancy Category C*: Ganciclovir has been shown to be embryotoxic in rabbits and mice following intravenous administration and teratogenic in rabbits. Fetal resorptions were present in at least 85% of rabbits and mice administered 60 mg/kg/day and 108 mg/kg/day (2x the human exposure based on AUC comparisons), respectively. Effects observed in rabbits included: fetal growth retardation, embryolethality,

PRECAUTIONS: *(cont'd)*

teratogenicity, and/or maternal toxicity. Teratogenic changes included cleft palate, anophthalmia/microphthalmia, aplastic organs (kidney and pancreas), hydrocephaly, and brachygnathia. In mice, effects observed were maternal/fetal toxicity and embryolethality.

Daily intravenous doses of 90 mg/kg administered to female mice prior to mating, during gestation, and during lactation caused hypoplasia of the testes and seminal vesicles in the month-old male offspring, as well as pathologic changes in the nonglandular region of the stomach (see Carcinogenesis, Mutagenesis, and Impairment of Fertility.) The drug exposure in mice as estimated by the AUC was approximately 1.7x the human AUC.

Ganciclovir may be teratogenic or embryotoxic at dose levels recommended for human use. There are no adequate and well-controlled studies in pregnant women. Ganciclovir sodium IV or ganciclovir sodium should be used during pregnancy only if the potential benefits justify the potential risk to the fetus.

* All dose comparisons presented in the Carcinogenesis, Mutagenesis, Impairment of Fertility, and Pregnancy subsections are based on the human AUC following administration of a single 5 mg/kg intravenous infusion of ganciclovir sodium IV as used during the maintenance phase of treatment. Compared with the single 5 mg/kg intravenous infusion, human exposure is doubled during the intravenous induction phase (5 mg/kg BID) and approximately halved during maintenance treatment with ganciclovir sodium capsules (1000 mg TID). The cross-species dose comparisons should be divided by two for intravenous induction treatment with ganciclovir sodium IV and multiplied by two for ganciclovir sodium capsules.

Nursing Mothers: It is not known whether ganciclovir is excreted in human milk. However, many drugs are excreted in human milk and, because carcinogenic and teratogenic effects occurred in animals treated with ganciclovir, the possibility of serious adverse reactions from ganciclovir in nursing infants is considered likely (see Pregnancy, Category C.) Mothers should be instructed to discontinue nursing if they are receiving ganciclovir sodium IV or ganciclovir sodium. The minimum interval before nursing can safely be resumed after the last dose of ganciclovir sodium IV or ganciclovir sodium is unknown.

Pediatric Use: SAFETY AND EFFICACY OF GANCICLOVIR SODIUM IV AND GANCICLOVIR SODIUM IN CHILDREN HAVE NOT BEEN ESTABLISHED. THE USE OF GANCICLOVIR SODIUM IV OR GANCICLOVIR SODIUM IN CHILDREN WARRANTS EXTREME CAUTION DUE TO THE PROBABILITY OF LONG-TERM CARCINOGENICITY AND REPRODUCTIVE TOXICITY. ADMINISTRATION TO CHILDREN SHOULD BE UNDERTAKEN ONLY AFTER CAREFUL EVALUATION AND ONLY IF THE POTENTIAL BENEFITS OF TREATMENT OUTWEIGH THE RISKS.

The spectrum of adverse events reported in 120 immunocompromised pediatric clinical trial participants with serious CMV infections receiving ganciclovir sodium IV solution were similar to those reported in adults. Granulocytopenia (17%) and thrombocytopenia (10%) were the most common adverse events reported.

Sixteen children (8 months to 15 years of age) with life- or sight-threatening CMV infections were evaluated in an open-label ganciclovir sodium IV solution pharmacokinetics study. Adverse events reported for more than one child were as follows: hypokalemia (4/16, 25%), abnormal kidney function (3/16, 19%), sepsis (3/16, 19%), thrombocytopenia (3/16, 19%), leukopenia (2/16, 13%), coagulation disorder (2/16, 13%), hypertension (2/16, 13%), pneumonia (2/16, 13%), and immune system disorder (2/16, 13%).

There has been very limited clinical experience using ganciclovir sodium IV for the treatment of CMV retinitis in patients under the age of 12 years. Two children (ages 9 and 5 years) showed improvement or stabilization of retinitis for 23 and 9 months, respectively. These children received induction treatment with 2.5 mg/kg TID followed by maintenance therapy with 6 to 6.5 mg/kg once per day, 5 to 7 days per week. When retinitis progressed during once-daily maintenance therapy, both children were treated with the 5 mg/kg BID regimen. Two other children (ages 2.5 and 4 years) who received similar induction regimens showed only partial or no response to treatment. Another child, a 6-year old with T-cell dysfunction, showed stabilization of retinitis for 3 months while receiving continuous infusions of ganciclovir sodium IV at doses of 2-5 mg/kg/24 hours. Continuous infusion treatment was discontinued due to granulocytopenia.

Eleven of the 72 patients in the placebo-controlled trial in bone marrow transplant recipients were children, ranging from 3 to 10 years of age (5 treated with ganciclovir sodium IV solution and 6 with placebo). Five of the pediatric patients treated with ganciclovir sodium IV received 5 mg/kg intravenously BID for up to 7 days; 4 patients went on to receive 5 mg/kg QD up to day 100 post-transplant. Results were similar to those observed in adult transplant recipients treated with ganciclovir sodium IV solution. Two of the 6 placebo-treated pediatric patients developed CMV pneumonia, versus none of the 5 patients treated with ganciclovir sodium IV. The spectrum of adverse events in the pediatric group was similar to that observed in the adult patients.

Ganciclovir sodium capsules have not been studied in children under age 13.

Use in Patients with Renal Impairment: Ganciclovir sodium IV and ganciclovir sodium should be used with caution in patients with impaired renal function because the half-life and plasma/serum concentrations of ganciclovir will be increased due to reduced renal clearance (see DOSAGE AND ADMINISTRATIONand ADVERSE REACTIONS, Renal Toxicity.)

Hemodialysis has been shown to reduce plasma levels of ganciclovir by approximately 50%.

Use in Elderly Patients: The pharmacokinetic profiles of ganciclovir sodium IV and ganciclovir sodium in elderly patients have not been established. Since elderly individuals frequently have a reduced glomerular filtration rate, particular attention should be paid to assessing renal function before and during administration of ganciclovir sodium IV or ganciclovir sodium (see DOSAGE AND ADMINISTRATION.)

DRUG INTERACTIONS:

Didanosine: At an oral dose of 1000 mg of ganciclovir sodium every 8 hours and didanosine, 200 mg every 12 hours, the steady-state didanosine $AUC_{0\text{-}12}$ increased 111 ± 114% (range: 10% to 493%) when didanosine was administered either 2 hours prior to or concurrent with administration of ganciclovir sodium (n=12 patients, 23 observations). A decrease in steady-state ganciclovir AUC of 21 ± 17% (range: -44% to 5%) was observed when didanosine was administered 2 hours prior to administration of ganciclovir sodium, but ganciclovir AUC was not affected by the presence of didanosine when the two drugs were administered simultaneously (n=12). There were no significant changes in renal clearance for either drug.

Zidovudine: At an oral dose of 1000 mg of ganciclovir sodium every 8 hours, mean steady-state ganciclovir $AUC_{0\text{-}8}$decreased 17 ± 25% (range: -52% to 23%) in the presence of zidovudine, 100 mg every 4 hours (n=12). Steady-state zidovudine $AUC_{0\text{-}4}$increased 19 ± 27% (range: 11% to 74%) in the presence of ganciclovir.

Since both zidovudine and ganciclovir have the potential to cause neutropenia and anemia, some patients may not tolerate concomitant therapy with these drugs at full dosage.

Probenecid: At an oral dose of 1000 mg of ganciclovir sodium every 8 hours (n=10), ganciclovir $AUC_{0\text{-}8}$ increased 53 ± 91% (range: -14% to 299%) in the presence of probenecid, 500 mg every 6 hours. Renal clearance of ganciclovir decreased 22 ± 20% (range: -54% to -4%), which is consistent with an interaction involving competition for renal tubular secretion.

Imipenem-cilastatin: Generalized seizures have been reported in patients who received ganciclovir and imipenem-cilastatin. These drugs should not be used concomitantly unless the potential benefits outweighs the risks.

DRUG INTERACTIONS: *(cont'd)*

Other Medications: It is possible that drugs that inhibit replication of rapidly dividing cell populations such as bone marrow, spermatogonia, and germinal layers of skin and gastrointestinal mucosa may have additive toxicity when administered concomitantly with ganciclovir. Therefore, drugs such as dapsone, pentamidine, flucytosine, vincristine, vinblastine, adriamycin, amphotericin B, trimethoprim/sulfamethoxazole combinations or other nucleoside analogues, should be considered for concomitant use with ganciclovir only if the potential benefits are judged to outweigh the risks.

No formal drug interaction studies of ganciclovir sodium IV solution or ganciclovir sodium and drugs commonly used in transplant recipients have been conducted. Increases in serum creatinine were observed in patients treated with ganciclovir sodium IV plus either cyclosporine or amphotericin B, drugs with known potential for nephrotoxicity (see ADVERSE REACTIONS.)

ADVERSE REACTIONS:

Adverse events that occurred during clinical trials of ganciclovir sodium IV solution and ganciclovir sodium capsules are summarized below, according to the participating study subject population.

Subjects with AIDS: Three controlled, randomized, phase-3 trials comparing ganciclovir sodium IV solution and ganciclovir sodium capsules for maintenance treatment of CMV retinitis have been completed. During these trials, ganciclovir sodium IV or ganciclovir sodium was prematurely discontinued because of adverse events, new or worsening intercurrent illnesses, or laboratory abnormalities in 9% of the subjects. Laboratory data and adverse events reported during the conduct of these controlled trials are summarized below.

Laboratory Data: Minimum ANC, Hemoglobin, Platelet Counts, and Maximum Serum Creatinine Values During Treatment with ganciclovir sodium or ganciclovir sodium IV in Three Controlled Clinical Trials* (TABLE 8)

TABLE 8

	% of subjects Capsules† 3000 mg/day (n=320)	% of subjects Intravenous Solution‡ (n=175)
Neutropenia ANC/µl		
<500	18	25
500 to <750	17	14
50 to <1000	19	26
Total ANC ≤1000	54	66
Anemia Hemoglobin g/dl		
<6.5	2	5
6.5 to <8.0	10	16
8.0 to <9.5	25	26
Total Hgt <9.5	36	46

* Data from Study 1653, Study ICM 1774, and Study AVI 034 pooled.
† Mean time on therapy = 91 days, including allowed reinduction treatment periods
‡ Mean time on therapy = 103 days, including allowed reinduction treatment periods (see discussion of clinical trials under INDICATIONS AND USAGEsection).

Overall, subjects treated with ganciclovir sodium IV solution experienced lower minimum ANC's and hemoglobin levels, consistent with more neutropenia and anemia, compared with those who received ganciclovir sodium capsules (p=0.024 for neutropenia; p=0.027 for anemia).

For the majority of subjects, maximum serum creatinine levels were less than 1.5 mg/dl and no difference was noted between ganciclovir sodium IV solution and ganciclovir sodium capsules for the occurrence of renal impairment. Serum creatinine elevations ≥ 2.5 mg/dl occurred in < 2% of all subjects and no significant differences were noted in the time from the start of maintenance to the occurrence of elevations in serum creatinine values.

Adverse Events: The following table (TABLE 9) shows selected adverse events reported in 5% or more of the subjects in three controlled clinical trials during treatment with either ganciclovir sodium IV solution (5 mg/kg/day) or ganciclovir sodium capsules (3000 mg/day).

TABLE 9 Selected Adverse Events Reported ≥ 5% of Subjects in Three Randomized Phase 3 Studies Comparing Ganciclovir Sodium Capsules to Ganciclovir Sodium IV Solution Maintenance Treatment

Body System	Adverse Event	Capsules (n=326)	IV (n=179)
Body as a Whole	Fever	38%	48%
	Abdominal Pain	17%	19%
	Infection	9%	13%
	Chills	7%	10%
	Sepsis	4%	15%
Digestive System	Diarrhea	41%	44%
	Nausea	26%	25%
	Anorexia	15%	14%
	Vomiting	13%	13%
	Flatulence	6%	3%
Hemic and Lymphatic System	Leukopenia	29%	41%
	Anemia	19%	25%
	Thrombocytopenia	6%	6%
Respiratory System	Pneumonia	6%	8%
Nervous System	Neuropathy	8%	9%
	Paresthesia	6%	10%
Other	Rash	15%	10%
	Sweating	11%	12%
	Pruritus	6%	5%
	Vitreous Disorder	6%	4%
Catheter Related[1]	Total Catheter Events	6%	22%
	Catheter Infection	4%	9%
	Catheter Sepsis	1%	8%

[1]Some of these events also appear under other body systems.

Retinal Detachment: Retinal detachment has been observed in subjects with CMV retinitis both before and after initiation of therapy with ganciclovir. Its relationship to therapy with ganciclovir is unknown. Retinal detachment occurred in 11% of patients treated with ganciclovir sodium IV solution and in 8% of patients treated with ganciclovir sodium capsules. Patients with CMV retinitis should have frequent ophthalmologic evaluations to monitor the status of their retinitis and to detect any other retinal pathology.

Transplant Recipients: There have been three controlled clinical trials of ganciclovir sodium IV solution for the prevention of CMV disease in transplant recipients.[15,16,35] Laboratory data and adverse events reported during these trials are summarized below.

Laboratory Data: The following table (TABLE 10A and B) shows the frequency of granulocytopenia (neutropenia) and thrombocytopenia observed:

ADVERSE REACTIONS: *(cont'd)*

TABLE 10A Controlled Trials - Transplant Recipients

	Heart Allograft* Ganciclovir Sodium-IV (n=76)	Heart Allograft* Placebo (n=73)
Neutropenia		
Minimum ANC < 500/µl	4%	3%
Minimum ANC 500-1000/µl	3%	8%
TOTAL ANC ≤1000/µl	7%	11%
Thrombocytopenia		
Platelet count < 25,000/µl	3%	1%
Platelet count 25,000-50,000/µl	5%	3%
TOTAL Platelet 50,000/µl	8%	4%

* Study ICM 1496. Mean duration of treatment = 28 days
† Study ICM 1570 and ICM 1689. Mean duration of treatment = 45 days (see discussion of clinical trials under INDICATIONS AND USAGE section.)

TABLE 10B Controlled Trials - Transplant Recipients

Bone Marrow Allograft†	Ganciclovir Sodium-IV (n=57)	Control (n=55)
Neutropenia		
Minimum ANC < 500/µl	12%	6%
Minimum ANC 500-1000/µl	29%	17%
TOTAL ANC ≤1000/µl	41%	23%
Thrombocytopenia		
Platelet count < 25,000/µl	32%	28%
Platelet count 25,000-50,000/µl	25%	37%
TOTAL Platelet 50,000/µl	57%	65%

* Study ICM 1496. Mean duration of treatment = 28 days
† Study ICM 1570 and ICM 1689. Mean duration of treatment = 45 days (see CLINICAL STUDIES.)

The following table (TABLE 11A and B) shows the frequency of elevated serum creatinine values in these controlled clinical trials.

TABLE 11A Controlled Trials - Transplant Recipients

Maximum Serum Creatinine Levels	Heart Allograft ICM 1496 Ganciclovir Sodium-IV (n=76)	Heart Allograft ICM 1496 Placebo (n=73)
Serum Creatinine ≥ 2.5 mg/dl	18%	4%
Serum Creatinine ≥ 1.5 - <2.5 mg/dl	58%	69%

TABLE 11B

	Bone Marrow Allograft			
	ICM 1570		ICM 1689	
Maximum Serum Creatinine Levels	Ganciclovir Sodium-IV (n=20)	Control (n=20)	Ganciclovir Sodium-IV (n=37)	Placebo (n=35)
Serum Creatinine ≥ 2.5 mg/dl	20%	0%	0%	0%
Serum Creatinine ≥ 1.5 - <2.5 mg/dl	50%	35%	43%	44%

In a placebo-controlled clinical trial conducted in heart allograft recipients (ICM 1496), more patients receiving ganciclovir sodium IV solution had elevation of serum creatinine to values exceeding 2.5 mg/dl than patients receiving placebo (18% vs. 4%, respectively). These increases in serum creatinine, up to 5.5 mg/dl in one patient, were transient and occurred primarily during the first week of treatment with ganciclovir sodium IV solution. In a randomized, open-label study of ganciclovir sodium IV solution in bone marrow allograft recipients (ICM 1570), more patients treated with ganciclovir sodium IV solution experienced serum creatinine values exceeding 1.5 mg/dl than patients who were not treated (70% vs. 35%, respectively). These elevations in serum creatinine, up to 3.2 mg/dl in one patient, were transient and occurred intermittently throughout the 3-month study. Most patients in these studies also received cyclosporine. In a second study in bone marrow transplant patients that was placebo-controlled (ICM 1689), no differences in elevations of serum creatinine were seen between the patients receiving ganciclovir sodium IV solution and those receiving placebo. The mechanism of impairment of renal function is not known. However, careful monitoring of renal function during therapy with ganciclovir sodium IV solution is essential, especially for those patients receiving concomitant agents that may cause nephrotoxicity.

General: Other adverse events that were thought to be "probably" or "possibly" related to ganciclovir sodium IV solution or ganciclovir sodium capsules in clinical studies in either subjects with AIDS or transplant recipients are listed below. These events all occurred with a frequency of 1% or less unless otherwise noted.

Body as a Whole: abdomen enlarged, abscess, asthenia (6%), back pain, cellulitis, chest pain, chills and fever, drug level increased (ganciclovir), edema, face edema, headache (4%), injection site abscess, injection site edema, injection site hemorrhage, injection site inflammation (2%), injection site pain, injection site phlebitis, laboratory test abnormality, malaise, pain (2%), photosensitivity reaction, neck pain, neck rigidity.

Digestive System: abnormal liver function test (2%), constipation, dyspepsia (2%), dysphagia, eructation, fecal incontinence, hemorrhage, hepatitis, melena, mouth ulceration, nausea and vomiting (2%), tongue disorder.

Hemic and Lymphatic System: eosinophilia, hypochromic anemia, marrow depression, pancytopenia.

Respiratory System: cough increased, dyspnea.

Nervous System: abnormal dreams, abnormal gait, agitation, amnesia, anxiety, ataxia, coma, confusion, depression, dizziness, dry mouth, euphoria, hypertonia, hypesthesia, insomnia, libido decreased, manic reaction, nervousness, psychosis, seizures, somnolence, thinking abnormal, tremor, trismus. (Overall, probably or possibly related neurologic system events occurred in approximately 5% of patients).

ADVERSE REACTIONS: *(cont'd)*

Skin and Appendages: acne, alopecia, dry skin, fixed eruption, herpes simplex, maculopapular rash, skin discoloration, urticaria, vesiculobullous rash.

Special Senses: abnormal vision, amblyopia, blindness, conjunctivitis, deafness, eye pain, glaucoma, retinitis, photophobia, taste perversion, tinnitus.

Metabolic and Nutritional Disorders: alkaline phosphatase increased, creatinine increased, creatine phosphokinase increased, hypokalemia, lactic dehydrogenase increased, pancreatitis, SGOT increased, SGPT increased.

Cardiovascular System: arrhythmia, deep thrombophlebitis, hypertension, hypotension, migraine, phlebitis (2%), vasodilation.

Urogenital System: breast pain, creatinine clearance decreased, hematuria, increased blood urea nitrogen (BUN), kidney failure, kidney function abnormal, urinary frequency, urinary tract infection.

Laboratory Abnormalities: decreased blood sugar.

Musculoskeletal System: myalgia, myasthenia.

The following adverse events reported in patients receiving ganciclovir may be potentially fatal: pancreatitis, sepsis, and multiple organ failure.

Adverse Events Reported in Post-Market Surveillance of Ganciclovir Sodium- IV Solution: The following are adverse events reported since the marketing introduction of ganciclovir sodium IV, and which are not listed under adverse events above. These events may also occur as part of the underlying disease process. There is insufficient data from the post- marketing reports to establish a relationship to ganciclovir use or to estimate incidence.

Reported on two or more occasions: acidosis, anaphylactic reaction, cardiac arrest, cataracts, cholestasis, cholangitis, congenital anomaly, encephalopathy, hyponatremia, impotence, infertility, intracranial hypertension, leukemia, lymphoma, myocardial infarction, pericarditis, Stevens-Johnson syndrome, stroke, transverse myelitis, unexplained death.

Reported once: Allograft rejection, arthritis, asthma, bleeding disorder, cachexia, corneal erosion, cyanosis, diplopia, dry eyes, dysesthesia, ear infection, elevated triglyceride levels, endocarditis, exfoliative dermatitis, exacerbation of psoriasis, facial palsy, gangrene, gingival hypertrophy, Guillain-Barre syndrome, hemolytic-uremic syndrome, hypernatremia, hypomagnesemia, icterus, inappropriate serum ADH, increased sweating, irritability, loss of memory, loss of sense of smell, multiple organ failure, myelopathy, myocarditis, nephritis, ophthalmoplegia, parathyroid disorder, Parkinsonism-like reaction, pneumothorax, peripheral ischemia, perforated intestine, pneumonia, proteinuria, pseudotumor cerebri, pulmonary fibrosis, pulmonary embolism, respiratory distress syndrome, rhabdomyolysis, sperm production abnormal, testicular hypotrophy, thyroid disorder, Wolff-Parkinson-White syndrome.

OVERDOSAGE:

Ganciclovir Sodium IV Solution: Overdosage with ganciclovir sodium IV solution has been reported in seventeen patients (13 adults and 4 children under 2 years of age). Five patients experienced no adverse events following overdosage at the following doses: 7 doses of 11 mg/kg over a 3-day period (adult), single dose of 3500 mg (adult), single dose of 500 mg (72.5 mg/kg) followed by 48 hours of peritoneal dialysis (4 month-old), single dose of approximately 60 mg/kg followed by exchange transfusion (18 month-old), 2 doses of 500 mg instead of 31 mg (21 month-old).

Irreversible pancytopenia developed in one adult with AIDS and CMV colitis after receiving 3000 mg of ganciclovir sodium IV solution on each of two consecutive days. He experienced worsening GI symptoms and acute renal failure which required short-term dialysis. Pancytopenia developed and persisted until his death from a malignancy several months later. Other adverse events reported following overdosage included: persistent bone marrow suppression (one adult with neutropenia and thrombocytopenia after a single dose of 6000 mg), reversible neutropenia or granulocytopenia (four adults, overdoses ranging from 8 mg/kg daily for 4 days to a single dose of 25 mg/kg), hepatitis (one adult receiving 10 mg/kg daily, and one 2 kg infant after a single 40 mg dose), renal toxicity (one adult with transient worsening of hematuria after a single 500 mg dose, and one adult with elevated creatinine (5.2 mg/dl) after a single 5000-7000 mg dose), and seizure (one adult with known seizure disorder after 3 days of 9 mg/kg). In addition, one adult received 0.4 ml (instead of 0.1 ml) ganciclovir sodium IV solution by intravitreal injection, and experienced temporary loss of vision and central retinal artery occlusion secondary to increased intraocular pressure related to the injected fluid volume.

Ganciclovir Sodium Capsules: There have been no reports of overdosage with ganciclovir sodium capsules. Doses as high as 6000 mg/day, given either as 1000 mg 6 times daily or as 2000 mg TID, did not result in overt toxicity other than transient neutropenia. Daily doses of more than 6000 mg have not been studied.

Since ganciclovir is dialyzable, dialysis may be useful in reducing serum concentrations. Adequate hydration should be maintained. The use of hematopoietic growth factors should be considered.

DOSAGE AND ADMINISTRATION:

CAUTION — DO NOT ADMINISTER GANCICLOVIR SODIUM IV SOLUTION BY RAPID OR BOLUS INTRAVENOUS INJECTION. THE TOXICITY OF GANCICLOVIR SODIUM-IV MAY BE INCREASED AS A RESULT OF EXCESSIVE PLASMA LEVELS.

CAUTION — INTRAMUSCULAR OR SUBCUTANEOUS INJECTION OF RECONSTITUTED GANCICLOVIR SODIUM-IV SOLUTION MAY RESULT IN SEVERE TISSUE IRRITATION DUE TO HIGH pH (11).

Dosage: THE RECOMMENDED DOSE FOR GANCICLOVIR SODIUM-IV SOLUTION AND GANCICLOVIR SODIUM CAPSULES SHOULD NOT BE EXCEEDED. THE RECOMMENDED INFUSION RATE FOR GANCICLOVIR SODIUM-IV SOLUTION SHOULD NOT BE EXCEEDED.

FOR TREATMENT OF CMV RETINITIS IN PATIENTS WITH NORMAL RENAL FUNCTION

Induction Treatment: The recommended initial dose for patients with normal renal function is 5 mg/kg (given intravenously at a constant rate over 1 hour) every 12 hours for 14 to 21 days. Ganciclovir sodium capsules should not be used for induction treatment.

Maintenance Treatment: *Ganciclovir sodium IV Solution:* Following induction treatment, the recommended maintenance dose of ganciclovir sodium IV solution is 5 mg/kg given as a constant-rate intravenous infusion over 1 hour once daily, 7 days per week, or 6 mg/kg once daily, 5 days per week. *Ganciclovir Sodium Capsules:* Following induction treatment, the recommended maintenance dose of ganciclovir sodium capsules is 1000 mg TID with food. Alternatively, the dosing regimen of 500 mg 6 times daily every three hours with food, during waking hours, may be used.

For patients who experience progression of CMV retinitis while receiving maintenance treatment with either formulation of ganciclovir, reinduction treatment is recommended.

FOR THE PREVENTION OF CMV DISEASE IN TRANSPLANT RECIPIENTS

The recommended initial dose of ganciclovir sodium IV solution for patients with normal renal function is 5 mg/kg (given intravenously at a constant rate over 1 hour) every 12 hours for 7 to 14 days, followed by 5 mg/kg once daily 7 days per week, or 6 mg/kg once daily 5 days per week.

DOSAGE AND ADMINISTRATION: *(cont'd)*

The duration of treatment with ganciclovir sodium IV solution in transplant recipients is dependent upon the duration and degree of immunosuppression. In controlled clinical trials in bone marrow allograft recipients, treatment was continued until day 100 to 120 post-transplantation. CMV disease occurred in several patients who discontinued treatment with ganciclovir sodium IV solution prematurely. In heart allograft recipients, the onset of newly diagnosed CMV disease occurred after treatment with ganciclovir sodium IV was stopped at day 28 post-transplant, suggesting that continued dosing may be necessary to prevent late occurrence of CMV disease in this patient population (see INDICATIONS AND USAGE.)

RENAL IMPAIRMENT

Ganciclovir Sodium IV Solution: For patients with impairment of renal function, refer to the table (TABLE 12) below for recommended doses of ganciclovir sodium IV solution and adjust the dosing interval as indicated.

TABLE 12

Creatinine Clearance* (ml/min)	Ganciclovir Sodium-IV Induction Dose (mg/kg)	Dosing Interval (hours)	Ganciclovir Sodium-IV Maintenance Dose (mg/kg)	Dosing Interval (hours)
≥70	5.0	12	5.0	24
50 to 69	2.5	12	2.5	24
25 to 49	2.5	24	1.25	24
10 to 24	1.25	24	0.625	24
<10	1.25	3 times per week, following hemodialysis	0.625	3 times per week, following hemodialysis

* Creatinine clearance can be related to serum creatinine by the formulae given below.

Dosing for patients undergoing hemodialysis should not exceed 1.25 mg/kg three times per week, following each hemodialysis session. Ganciclovir sodium IV should be given shortly after completion of the hemodialysis session, since hemodialysis has been shown to reduce plasma levels by approximately 50%.

Ganciclovir Sodium Capsules: In patients with renal impairment, the dose of ganciclovir sodium capsules should be modified as shown below (TABLE 13).

TABLE 13

Creatinine Clearance* ml/min	Ganciclovir Sodium Capsule Doses
≥70	1000 mg TID or 500 mg q3h, 6x/day
50 to 69	1500 mg QD or 500 mg TID
25 to 49	1000 mg QD or 500 mg BID
10 to 24	500 mg QD
<10	500 mg three times per week, following hemodialysis

* Creatinine clearance can be related to serum creatinine by the following formulae:
Creatinine clearance for males = [(140 - age [yrs]) (body wt [kg])] ÷ [(72) (serum creatinine [mg/dl])]
Creatinine clearance for females = 0.85 × male value

Patient Monitoring: Due to the frequency of granulocytopenia and thrombocytopenia in patients receiving ganciclovir (see ADVERSE REACTIONS), it is recommended that neutrophil counts and platelet counts be performed frequently, especially in patients in whom ganciclovir or other nucleoside analogues have previously resulted in leukopenia, or in whom neutrophil counts are less than 1000 cells/µl at the beginning of treatment. Because dosing with ganciclovir sodium- IV or ganciclovir sodium must be modified in patients with renal impairment, and because of the incidence of increased serum creatinine levels that have been observed in transplant recipients treated with ganciclovir sodium IV solution, patients should have serum creatinine or creatinine clearance values followed carefully.

Reduction of Dose: Dose reductions are required for patients with renal impairment (see Renal Impairment) and for those with neutropenia and/or thrombocytopenia (see ADVERSE REACTIONS.)

The most frequently observed adverse event following treatment with ganciclovir is leukopenia/neutropenia (see ADVERSE REACTIONS.) Therefore, frequent white blood cell counts should be performed. Severe neutropenia (ANC less than 500/µl) or severe thrombocytopenia (platelets less than 25,000/µl) require a dose interruption until evidence of marrow recovery is observed (ANC > 750/µl).

Method of Preparation of Ganciclovir Sodium IV Solution: Each 10 ml clear glass vial contains ganciclovir sodium equivalent to 500 mg of the free base form of ganciclovir sodium and 46 mg of sodium. The contents of the vial should be prepared for administration in the following manner:

1. Reconstituted Solution:

a. Reconstitute lyophilized ganciclovir sodium IV by injecting 10 ml of Sterile Water for Injection, USP, into the vial. DO NOT USE BACTERIOSTATIC WATER FOR INJECTION CONTAINING PARABENS. IT IS INCOMPATIBLE WITH GANCICLOVIR SODIUM IV AND MAY CAUSE PRECIPITATION.

b. Shake the vial to dissolve the drug.

c. Visually inspect the reconstituted solution for particulate matter and discoloration prior to proceeding with infusion solution. Discard the vial if particulate matter or discoloration is observed.

d. Reconstituted solution in the vial is stable at room temperature for 12 hours. It should not be refrigerated.

2. Infusion Solution: Based on the patient weight, the appropriate volume of the reconstituted solution (ganciclovir concentration 50 mg/ml) should be removed from the vial and added to an acceptable infusion fluid (typically 100 ml) for delivery over the course of one hour. Infusion concentrations greater than 10 mg/ml are not recommended. The following infusion fluids have been determined to be chemically and physically compatible with ganciclovir sodium IV solution: 0.9% Sodium Chloride, 5% Dextrose, Ringer's Injection, and Lactated Ringer's Injection, USP.

Note: Because nonbacteriostatic infusion fluid must be used with ganciclovir sodium IV solution, the infusion solution must be used within 24 hours of dilution to reduce the risk of bacterial contamination. The infusion solution should be refrigerated. Freezing is not recommended.

Handling and Disposal: Caution should be exercised in the handling and preparation of solutions of ganciclovir sodium IV and in the handling of ganciclovir sodium capsules. Solutions of ganciclovir sodium IV are alkaline (pH 11). Avoid direct contact with the skin or mucous membranes of the powder contained in ganciclovir sodium capsules or ganciclovir sodium IV solutions. If such contact occurs, wash thoroughly with soap and water; rinse eyes thoroughly with plain water.

Ganciclovir sodium capsules should not be opened or crushed.

DOSAGE AND ADMINISTRATION: *(cont'd)*

Because ganciclovir shares some of the properties of antitumor agents (*i.e.*, carcinogenicity and mutagenicity), consideration should be given to handling and disposal according to guidelines issued for antineoplastic drugs. Several guidelines on this subject have been published.[31-36]

There is no general agreement that all of the procedures recommended in the guidelines are necessary or appropriate.

REFERENCES:

1. Agut H, Huraux J-M, Collandre H, Montagnier L. Susceptibility of human herpesvirus 6 to acyclovir and ganciclovir. Lancet. 1989; 2:626. Letter. **2.** Russler SK, Tapper MA, Carrigan DR. Susceptibility of human herpesvirus 6 to acyclovir and ganciclovir. Lancet. 1989; 2:382. Letter. **3.** Locarnini S, Guo K, Lucas R, Gust I. Inhibition of HBV DNA replication by ganciclovir in patients with AIDS. Lancet. 1989; 2:1225-1226. Letter. **4.** Faulds D, Heel RC. Ganciclovir: a review of its antiviral activity, pharmacokinetic properties and therapeutic efficacy in cytomegalovirus infections. Drugs. 1990; 39:597-638. **5.** Field AK, Biron KK. The End of Innocence Revisited: Resistance of Herpes-viruses to Antiviral Drugs. Clin Microbiology Rev. 1994; 7:1-13. **6.** Littler E, Stuart AD, Chee MS. Human cytomegalovirus UL97 open reading frame encodes a protein that phosphorylates the antiviral nucleoside analogue ganciclovir. Nature. 1992; 358:160-162. **7.** Sullivan V, Talarico CL, Stanat SC, Davis M, Coen DM, Biron KK. A protein kinase homologue controls phosphorylation of ganciclovir in human cytomegalovirus-infected cells. [Published erratum appears in Nature 1992; 359:85] Nature. 1992; 358:162-164. **8.** Smee DF. Interaction of 9-(1,3,-dihydroxy-2-propoxymethyl) guanine with cytosol and mitochondrial deoxyguanosine kinases: possible role in anti-cytomegalovirus activity. Mol Cell Biochem. 1985; 69:75-81. **9.** Biron KK, Stanat SC, Sorrell JB, Fyfe JA, Keller PM, Lambe CU, Nelson DJ. Metabolic activation of the nucleoside analog 9-([2-hydroxy-1-(hydroxymethyl)ethoxy]methyl)guanine in human diploid fibroblasts infected with human cytomegalovirus. Proc Natl Acad Sci (USA). 1985; 82:2473-2777. **10.** Freitas VR, Smee DF, Chernow M, Boehme R, Matthews TR. Activity of 9-(1,3-dihydroxy-2-propoxymethyl)guanine compared with that of acyclovir against human, monkey, and rodent cytomegaloviruses. Anti-microb Agents Chemother. 1985; 28:240-245. **11.** Sommadossi J-P, Carlisle R. Toxicity of 3'-azido-3'- deoxythymidine and 9-(1,3-dihydroxy-2-propoxymethyl) guanine for normal human hematopoietic progenitor cells *in vitro*. Antimicrob Agents Chemother. 1987; 31:452-454. **12.** Buhles WC, Mastre BJ, Tinker AJ, Strand V, Koretz SH, the Syntex Collaborative Ganciclovir Treatment Study Group. Ganciclovir treatment of life- or sight-threatening cytomegalovirus infection: experience in 314 immunocompromised patients. Rev Infect Dis. 1988; 10:495-506. **13.** Merigan TC, Renlund DG, Keay S, et al. A controlled trial of ganciclovir to prevent cytomegalovirus disease after heart transplantation. New Engl J Med. 1992; 326:1182-1186. **14.** Goodrich JM, Mori M, Gleaves CA, et al. Early treatment with ganciclovir to prevent cytomegalovirus disease after allogeneic bone marrow transplantation. New Engl J Med. 1991; 325:1601-1607. **15.** Erice A, Chou S, Biron KK, Stanat SC, Balfour HH Jr, Jordan MC. Progressive disease due to ganciclovir-resistant cytomegalovirus in immunocompromised patients. New Eng J Med. 1989; 320:289-293. **16.** Drew WL, Miner RC, Busch DF, et al. Prevalence of resistance in patients receiving ganciclovir for serious cytomegalovirus infection. J Infect Dis. 1991; 163:716-719. **17.** Jacobson MA, Drew WL, Feinberg J, O'Donnell JJ, Whitmore PV, Miner RD, Parenti D. Foscarnet therapy for ganciclovir-resistant cytomegalovirus retinitis in patients with AIDS. J Infect Dis. 1991; 163:1348-1351. **18.** Pepin J-M, Simon F, Dussault A, Collin G, Dazza M-C, Brun- Vezinet F. Rapid determination of human cytomegalovirus susceptibility to ganciclovir directly from clinical specimen primocultures. J Clin Microbiol. 1992; 30:2917-2920. **19.** Tseng LF. Rapid and simple antiviral sensitivity testing of cytomegalovirus (CMV). In: Abstract Book of the 92nd General Meeting of the American Society for Microbiology; May 26 - 30, 1992; New Orleans, LA. Abstract. **20.** Biron KK, Fyfe JA, Stanat SC, Leslie LK, Sorrell JB, Lambe CU, Coen DM. A human cytomegalovirus mutant resistant to the nucleoside analog 9-([2-hydroxy- 1-(hydroxymethyl)ethoxy]methyl)guanine (BW B759U) induces reduced levels of BW B759U triphosphate. Proc Natl Acad Sci (USA). 1986; 83:8769-8773. **21.** Stanat SC, Reardon JE, Erice A, Jordan MC, Drew WL, Biron KK. Ganciclovir-resistant cytomegalovirus clinical isolates: mode of resistance to ganciclovir. Antimicrob Agents Chemother. 1991; 35:2191- 2197. **22.** Lurain NS, Spafford LE, Thompson KD. Mutation in the UL97 open reading frame of human cytomegalovirus strains resistant to ganciclovir. J. Virol. 1994; 68:4427-4431. **23.** Sullivan V, Biron KK, Talarico C, Stanat SC, Davis M, Pozzi L, Coen DM. A point mutation in the human cytomegalovirus DNA polymerase gene confers resistance to ganciclovir and phosphonylmethoxyalkyl derivatives. Antimicrob Agents Chemother. 1993: 37:19-25. **24.** Lurain NS, Thompson KD, Holmes EW, Sullivan Read G. Point mutations in the DNA polymerase gene of human cytomegalovirus strains resistant to ganciclovir. J Virol. 1992; 66:7146- 7152. **25.** Fletcher C, Sawchuk R, Chinnock B, deMiranda P, Balfour HH Jr. Human pharmacokinetics of the antiviral drug DHPG. Clin Pharmacol Ther. 1986; 40:281-286. **26.** Trang JM, Kidd L, Gruber W, Storch G, Demmler G, Jacobs R, Dankner W, Starr S, Pass R, Stagno S, Alford C, Soong S-J, Whitley RJ, Sommadossi J-P. Linear single-dose pharmacokinetics of ganciclovir in newborns with congenital cytomegalovirus infections. Clin Pharmacol Ther. 1993; 53:15-21. **27.** Jabs DA, Enger C, Bartlett JG. Cytomegalovirus retinitis and acquired immunodeficiency syndrome. Arch Ophthalmol. 1989; 170:75-80. **28.** Schmidt GM, Horak DA, Niland JC, Duncan SR, Forman SJ, Zaia JA, The City of Hope-Stanford-Syntex CMV Study Group. A randomized, controlled trial of prophylactic ganciclovir for cytomegalovirus pulmonary infection in recipients of allogeneic bone marrow transplants. New Engl J Med. 1991; 15:1005-1011. **29.** Hardy WD. Combined ganciclovir and recombinant human granulocyte-macrophage colony- stimulating factor in the treatment of cytomegalovirus retinitis in AIDS patients. J Acquir Immune Defic Syndr. 1991; 4:S22-S28. **30.** Jacobson MA, Stanley HD, Heartd SE. Ganciclovir with recombinant methionyl human granulocyte-stimulating factor for treatment of cytomegalovirus disease in AIDS patients. AIDS. 1992; 6:515-517. **31.** Recommendations for the Safe Handling of Cytotoxic Drugs. Washington, DC: Superintendent of Documents; 1992. US Government Printing Office publication NIH 92-2621. **32.** Council on Scientific Affairs: Guidelines for Handling Parenteral Antineoplastics. JAMA. 1985; 253:1590-1592. **33.** Recommendations for Handling Cytotoxic Agents, September 1987. National Study Commission of Cytotoxic Exposure. Available from: Louis P. Jeffrey, Sc. D., President Emeritus, Massachusetts College of Pharmacy and Allied Health Sciences, Boston, MA. **34.** Guidelines and recommendations for safe handling of antineoplastic agents. Med J Aust. 1983; (April 30):426-428. **35.** Jones RB, Frank R, Mass T. Safe handling of chemotherapeutic agents: a report from the Mount Sinai Medical Center, CA. Cancer J Clin. 1983; 33:258-263. **36.** American Society of Hospital Pharmacists technical assistance bulletin on handling cytotoxic and hazardous drugs. Am J Hosp Pharm. 1990; 47:1033-1049.

HOW SUPPLIED:

Cytovene-IV (ganciclovir sodium for injection) is supplied in 10 ml sterile vials, each containing ganciclovir sodium equivalent to 500 mg of ganciclovir, in cartons of 25.

Store vials at temperatures below 40°C (104°F).

Cytovene (ganciclovir capsules) 250 mg are two-pieced, size #1, opaque green hard gelatin capsules with the Syntex logo and "CY250" imprinted on the cap in dark blue ink and with two blue lines partially encircling the capsule body. Each capsule contains 250 mg of ganciclovir as a white to off-white powder. Cytovene capsules are supplied as follows: Bottles of 180 capsules

Store at controlled room temperature, 15° -30°C (59° - 86°F).

HOW SUPPLIED - EQUIVALENTS NOT AVAILABLE:

Capsule, Gelatin - Oral - 250 mg

180's $702.00 CYTOVENE, Syntex Labs 00033-2913-50

Injection, Lyphl-Soln - Intravenous - 500 mg/vial

25's $870.00 CYTOVENE 500, 10ML VIALS, Syntex Labs 00033-2903-48

GEMCITABINE HYDROCHLORIDE *(003266)*

CATEGORIES: Antineoplastics; Chemotherapy; Oncologic Drugs; Pancreatic Cancer; FDA Approved 1996 May

BRAND NAMES: **Gemzar**

DESCRIPTION:

Gemcitabine hydrochloride is a nucleoside analogue that exhibits antitumor activity. Gemcitabine HCl is 2'-deoxy-2',2'-difluorocytidine monohydrochloride (β-isomer). The empirical formula for gemcitabine HCl is $C_9H_{11}F_2N_3O_4 \cdot HCl$. It has a molecular weight of 299.66.

Gemcitabine HCl is a white to off-white solid. It is soluble in water, slightly soluble in methanol, and practically insoluble in ethanol and polar organic solvents.

The clinical formulation is supplied in a sterile form for intravenous use only. Vials of Gemzar contain either 200 mg or 1 g of gemcitabine HCl (expressed as free base) formulated with mannitol (200 mg or 1 g, respectively) and sodium acetate (12.5 mg or 62.5 mg, respectively) as a sterile lyophilized powder. Hydrochloric acid and/or sodium hydroxide may have been added for pH adjustment.

CLINICAL PHARMACOLOGY:

Gemcitabine exhibits cell phase specificity, primarily killing cells undergoing DNA synthesis (S-phase) and also blocking the progression of cells through the G1/S-phase boundary. Gemcitabine is metabolized intracellularly by nucleoside kinases to the active diphosphate (dFdCDP) and triphosphate (dFdCTP) nucleosides. The cytotoxic effect of gemcitabine is attributed to a combination of two actions of the diphosphate and the triphosphate nucleosides, which leads to inhibition of DNA synthesis. First, gemcitabine diphosphate inhibits ribonucleotide reductase, which is responsible for catalyzing the reactions that generate the deoxynucleoside triphosphates for DNA synthesis. Inhibition of this enzyme by the diphosphate nucleoside causes a reduction in the concentrations of deoxynucleotides, including dCTP. Second, gemcitabine triphosphate competes with dCTP for incorporation into DNA. The reduction in the intracellular concentration of dCTP (by the action of the diphosphate) enhances the incorporation of gemcitabine triphosphate into DNA (self-potentiation). After the gemcitabine nucleotide is incorporated into DNA, only one additional nucleotide is added to the growing DNA strands. After this addition, there is inhibition of further DNA synthesis. DNA polymerase epsilon is unable to remove the gemcitabine nucleotide and repair the growing DNA strands (masked chain termination). In CEM T lymphoblastoid cells, gemcitabine induces internucleosomal DNA fragmentation, one of the characteristics of programmed cell death.

HUMAN PHARMACOKINETICS

Gemcitabine disposition was studied in five patients who received a single 1000 mg/m²/30 minute infusion of radiolabeled drug. Within one (1) week, 92% to 98% of the dose was recovered, almost entirely in the urine. Gemcitabine (<10%) and the inactive uracil metabolite, 2'-deoxy-2',2'-difluorouridine (dFdU), accounted for 99% of the excreted dose. The metabolite dFdU is also found in plasma. Gemcitabine plasma protein binding is negligible.

The pharmacokinetics of gemcitabine were examined in 353 patients, about 2/3 men, with various solid tumors. Pharmacokinetic parameters were derived using data from patients treated for varying durations of therapy given weekly with periodic rest weeks and using both short infusions (<70 minutes) and long infusions (70 to 285 minutes). The total gemcitabine dose varied from 500 to 3600 mg/m².

Gemcitabine pharmacokinetics are linear and are described by a 2-compartment model. Population pharmacokinetic analyses of combined single and multiple dose studies showed that the volume of distribution of gemcitabine was significantly influenced by duration of infusion and gender. Clearance was affected by age and gender. Differences in either clearance or volume of distribution based on patient characteristics or the duration of infusion result in changes in half-life and plasma concentrations. Table 1 shows plasma clearance and half-life of gemcitabine following short infusions for typical patients by age and gender.

TABLE 1 Gemcitabine Clearance and Half-Life for the "Typical" Patient

Age	Clearance Men (L/hr/m²)	Clearance Women (L/hr/m²)	Half-Life[a] Men (min)	Half-Life[a] Women (min)
29	92.2	69.4	42	49
45	75.7	57.0	48	57
65	55.1	41.5	61	73
79	40.7	30.7	79	94

[a]Half-life for patients receiving a short infusion (<70 min)

Gemcitabine half-life for short infusions ranged from 32 to 94 minutes, and the value for long infusions varied from 245 to 638 minutes, depending on age and gender, reflecting a greatly increased volume of distribution with longer infusions. The lower clearance in women and the elderly results in higher concentrations of gemcitabine for any given dose.

The volume of distribution was increased with infusion length. Volume of distribution of gemcitabine was 50 L/m² following infusions lasting <70 minutes, indicating that gemcitabine, after short infusions, is not extensively distributed into tissues. For long infusions, the volume of distribution rose to 370 L/m², reflecting slow equilibration of gemcitabine within the tissue compartment.

The maximum plasma concentrations of dFdU (inactive metabolite) were achieved up to 30 minutes after discontinuation of the infusions and the metabolite is excreted in urine without undergoing further biotransformation. The metabolite did not accumulate with weekly dosing, but its elimination is dependent on renal excretion, and could accumulate with decreased renal function.

The effects of significant renal or hepatic insufficiency on the disposition of gemcitabine have not been assessed.

The active metabolite, gemcitabine triphosphate, can be extracted from peripheral blood mononuclear cells. The half-life of the terminal phase for gemcitabine triphosphate from mononuclear cells ranges from 1.7 to 19.4 hours.

CLINICAL STUDIES:

Data from two clinical trials evaluated the use of gemcitabine in patients with locally advanced or metastatic pancreatic cancer. The first trial compared gemcitabine to 5-Fluorouracil (5-FU) in patients who had received no prior chemotherapy. A second trial studied the use of gemcitabine in pancreatic cancer patients previously treated with 5-FU or a 5-FU-containing regimen. In both studies, the first cycle of gemcitabine was administered intravenously at a dose of 1000 mg/m² over 30 minutes once weekly for up to 7 weeks (or until toxicity necessitated holding a dose) followed by a week of rest from treatment with gemcitabine. Subsequent cycles consisted of injections once weekly for 3 consecutive weeks out of every 4 weeks.

The primary efficacy parameter in these studies was "clinical benefit response," which is a measure of clinical improvement based on analgesic consumption, pain intensity, performance status and weight change. Definitions for improvement in these variables were formulated prospectively during the design of the two trials. A patient was considered a clinical benefit responder if either:

i) the patient showed a ≥ 50% reduction in pain intensity (Memorial Pain Assessment Card) or analgesic consumption, or a twenty point or greater improvement in performance status (Karnofsky Performance Scale) for a period of at least four consecutive weeks, without showing any sustained worsening in any of the other parameters. Sustained worsening was defined as four consecutive weeks with either any increase in pain intensity or analgesic consumption or a 20 point decrease in performance status occurring during the first 12 weeks of therapy. Or:

ii) the patient was stable on all of the aforementioned parameters, and showed a marked, sustained weight gain (≥ 7% increase maintained for ≥ 4 weeks) not due to fluid accumulation.

The first study was a multicenter (17 sites in US and Canada), prospective, single-blinded, two-arm, randomized, comparison of gemcitabine and 5-FU in patients with locally advanced or metastatic pancreatic cancer who had received no prior treatment with chemotherapy. 5-FU was administered intravenously at a weekly dose of 600 mg/m² for 30 minutes. The

CLINICAL STUDIES: *(cont'd)*

results from this randomized trial are shown in Table 2. Patients treated with gemcitabine had statistically significant increases in clinical benefit response, survival, and time to progressive disease compared to 5-FU. The Kaplan-Meier curve for survival is shown in Figure 1 of the manufacturer's original drug package insert. No confirmed objective tumor responses were observed with either treatment.

TABLE 2 Gemcitabine Versus 5–FU in Pancreatic Cancer

	Gemcitabine	5-FU	
NUMBER OF PATIENTS	63	63	
Male	34	34	
Female	29	29	
MEDIAN AGE	62 years	61 years	
Range	37 to 79	36 to 77	
Stage IV disease	71.4%	76.2%	
Baseline KPS[a] ≤ 70	69.8%	68.3%	
Clinical benefit response	22.2% (N[c]=14)	4.8% (N=3)	p=0.004
SURVIVAL			p=0.0009
Median	5.7 months	4.2 months	
6-month probability[b]	(N=30) 46%	(N=19) 29%	
9-month probability[b]	(N=14) 24%	(N=4) 5%	
1-year probability[b]	(N=9) 18%	(N=2) 2%	
Range	0.2 to 18.6 months	0.4 to 15.1+ months	
95% C.I. of the median	4.7 to 6.9 months	3.1 to 5.1 months	
TIME TO PROGRESSIVE DISEASE			p=0.0013
Median	2.1 months	0.9 months	
Range	0.1+ to 9.4 months	0.1 to 12.0+ months	
95% C.I. of the median	1.9 to 3.4 months	0.9 to 1.1 months	

[a]Karnofsky Performance Status
[b]Kaplan-Meier estimates
[c]N=number of patients
+ No progression at last visit; remains alive
The p-value for clinical benefit response was calculated using the 2-sided test for difference in binomial proportions. All other p-values were calculated using the Log Rank test for difference in overall time to an event.

Clinical benefit response was achieved by 14 patients treated with gemcitabine and 3 patients treated with 5-FU. One patient on the gemcitabine arm showed improvement in all three primary parameters (pain intensity, analgesic consumption, and performance status). Eleven patients on the gemcitabine arm and two patients on the 5-FU arm showed improvement in analgesic consumption and/or pain intensity with stable performance status. Two patients on the gemcitabine arm showed improvement in analgesic consumption or pain intensity with improvement in performance status. One patient on the 5-FU arm was stable with regard to pain intensity and analgesic consumption with improvement in performance status. No patient on either arm achieved a clinical benefit response based on weight gain.

The second trial was a multicenter (17 US and Canadian centers), open-label study of gemcitabine in 63 patients with advanced pancreatic cancer previously treated with 5-FU or a 5-FU-containing regimen. The study showed a clinical benefit response rate of 27% and median survival of 3.9 months.

When gemcitabine was administered more frequently than once weekly or with infusions longer than 60 minutes, increased toxicity was observed. Results of a Phase 1 study of gemcitabine to assess the maximum tolerated dose (MTD) on a daily x 5 schedule showed that patients developed significant hypotension and severe flu-like symptoms that were intolerable at doses above 10 mg/m^2. The incidence and severity of these events were dose-related. Other Phase 1 studies using a twice-weekly schedule reached MTDs of only 65 mg/m^2 (30-minute infusion) and 150 mg/m^2(5-minute bolus). The dose-limiting toxicities were thrombocytopenia and flu-like symptoms, particularly asthenia. In a Phase 1 study to assess the maximum tolerated infusion time, clinically significant toxicity, defined as myelosuppression, was seen with weekly doses of 300 mg/m^2 at or above a 270-minute infusion time. The half-life of gemcitabine is influenced by the length of the infusion (see CLINICAL PHARMACOLOGY) and the toxicity appears to be increased if gemcitabine is administered more frequently than once weekly or with infusions longer than 60 minutes (see WARNINGS).

In a single trial where gemcitabine at a dose of 1000 mg/m^2 was administered for up to six (6) consecutive weeks concurrently with therapeutic thoracic radiation to patients with NSCLC, significant toxicity in the form of severe, and potentially life-threatening, esophagitis and pneumonitis was observed, particularly in patients receiving large volumes of radiotherapy. The optimum regimen for safe administration of gemcitabine with therapeutic doses of radiation has not yet been determined (see PRECAUTIONS).

INDICATIONS AND USAGE:

Therapeutic Indication: Gemzar is indicated as first-line treatment for patients with locally advanced (nonresectable Stage II or Stage III) or metastatic (Stage IV) adenocarcinoma of the pancreas. Gemcitabine is indicated for patients previously treated with 5-FU.

CONTRAINDICATIONS:

Gemzar is contraindicated in those patients with a known hypersensitivity to the drug (see ADVERSE REACTIONS, Allergic).

WARNINGS:

Caution: Prolongation of the infusion time beyond 60 minutes and more frequent than weekly dosing have been shown to increase toxicity (see CLINICAL STUDIES).

Gemcitabine can suppress bone marrow function as manifested by leukopenia, thrombocytopenia and anemia (see ADVERSE REACTIONS), and myelosuppression is usually the dose-limiting toxicity. Patients should be monitored for myelosuppression during therapy. See DOSAGE AND ADMINISTRATION for recommended dose adjustments.

Hemolytic-Uremic Syndrome (HUS) has been reported rarely with the use of gemcitabine. (see ADVERSE REACTIONS, Renal).

Pregnancy Category D: Gemcitabine can cause fetal harm when administered to a pregnant woman. Gemcitabine is embryotoxic causing fetal malformations (cleft palate, incomplete ossification) at doses of 1.5 mg/kg/day in mice (about 1/200 the recommended human dose on a mg/m^2 basis). Gemcitabine is fetotoxic causing fetal malformations (fused pulmonary artery, absence of gall bladder) at doses of 0.1 mg/kg/day in rabbits (about 1/600 the recommended human dose on a mg/m^2 basis). Embryotoxicity was characterized by decreased fetal viability, reduced live litter sizes, and developmental delays. There are no studies of gemcitabine in pregnant women. If gemcitabine is used during pregnancy, or if the patient becomes pregnant while taking gemcitabine, the patient should be apprised of the potential hazard to the fetus.

PRECAUTIONS:

GENERAL

Patients receiving therapy with gemcitabine should be monitored closely by a physician experienced in the use of cancer chemotherapeutic agents. Most adverse events are reversible and do not need to result in discontinuation, although doses may need to be withheld or reduced. There was a greater tendency in women, especially older women, not to proceed to the next cycle.

LABORATORY TESTS

Patients receiving gemcitabine should be monitored prior to each dose with a complete blood count (CBC), including differential and platelet count. Suspension or modification of therapy should be considered when marrow suppression is detected (see DOSAGE AND ADMINISTRATION).

Laboratory evaluation of renal and hepatic function should be performed prior to initiation of therapy and periodically thereafter.

CARCINOGENESIS, MUTAGENESIS, IMPAIRMENT OF FERTILITY

Long-term animal studies to evaluate the carcinogenic potential of gemcitabine have not been conducted. Gemcitabine induced forward mutations *in vitro*in a mouse lymphoma (L5178Y) assay and was clastogenic in an *in vivo* mouse micronucleus assay. Gemcitabine was negative when tested using the Ames, *in vivo* sister chromatic exchange, and *in vitro* chromosomal aberration assays, and did not cause unscheduled DNA synthesis *in vitro*. Gemcitabine I.P. doses of 0.5 mg/kg/day (about 1/700 the human dose on a mg/m^{2}basis) in male mice had an effect on fertility with moderate to severe hypospermatogenesis, decreased fertility, and decreased implantations. In female mice, fertility was not affected but, maternal toxicities were observed at 1.5 mg/kg/day I.V. (about 1/200 the human dose on a mg/m^2 basis) and fetotoxicity or embryolethality was observed at 0.25 mg/kg/day I.V. (about 1/1300 the human dose on a mg/m^2 basis).

PREGNANCY

Category D. See WARNINGS.

NURSING MOTHERS

It is not known whether gemcitabine or its metabolites are excreted in human milk. Because many drugs are excreted in human milk and because of the potential for serious adverse reactions from gemcitabine in nursing infants, the mother should be warned and a decision should be made whether to discontinue nursing or to discontinue the drug, taking into account the importance of the drug to the mother and the potential risk to the infant.

ELDERLY PATIENTS

Gemzar clearance is affected by age (see CLINICAL PHARMACOLOGY). There is no evidence, however, that unusual dose adjustments, (*i.e.*, other than those already recommended in the DOSAGE AND ADMINISTRATION section) are necessary in patients over 65, and, in general adverse reaction rates were similar in patients above and below 65. Grade 3/4 thrombocytopenia was more common in the elderly.

GENDER

Gemzar clearance is affected by gender (see CLINICAL PHARMACOLOGY). There is no evidence, however, that unusual dose adjustments (*i.e.*, other than those already recommended in the DOSAGE AND ADMINISTRATION section) are necessary in women. In general, adverse reaction rates were similar in men and women but women, especially older women were more likely not to proceed to a subsequent cycle and to experience grade 3/4 neutropenia and thrombocytopeni.

PEDIATRIC PATIENTS

Gemzar has not been studied in pediatric patients. Safety and effectiveness in pediatric patients have not been established.

PATIENTS WITH RENAL OR HEPATIC IMPAIRMENT

Gemcitabine should be used with caution in patients with preexisting renal impairment or hepatic insufficiency. Gemcitabine has not been studied in patients with significant renal or hepatic impairment.

COMBINATION THERAPY

Safe and effective regimens for the administration of gemcitabine with therapeutic doses of radiation have not yet been determined (See CLINICAL STUDIES).

DRUG INTERACTIONS:

No confirmed interactions have been reported with the use of gemcitabine. No specific drug interaction studies have been conducted.

ADVERSE REACTIONS:

Myelosuppression is the principal dose-limiting factor with gemcitabine therapy. Dosage adjustments for hematologic toxicity are frequently needed and are described in the DOSAGE AND ADMINISTRATION section.

Data in Table 3 are based on 22 clinical studies (N = 979) of gemcitabine administered as a single agent, using starting doses in the range of 800 to 1250 mg/m^2 administered weekly as a 30-minute infusion for treatment of a wide variety of malignancies. Data are also shown for the subset of patients with pancreatic cancer treated in 5 clinical studies. The frequency of all grades and severe (WHO Grade 3 or 4) adverse events were generally similar for the overall safety database and the subset of patients with pancreatic cancer. Adverse reactions reported in the overall database resulted in discontinuation of gemcitabine therapy in about 10% of patients. In the comparative trial, the discontinuation rate for adverse reactions was 14.3% for the gemcitabine arm and 4.8% for the 5-FU arm. All WHO-graded laboratory events are listed in Tables 3A and 3B regardless of causality. Nonlaboratory adverse events listed in Tables 3A and 3B or discussed below were those reported, regardless of causality, for at least 10% of all patients, except the categories of Extravasation, Allergic, and Cardiovascular and certain specific events under the Renal, Pulmonary, and Infection categories. Table 4 presents the data from the comparative trial of gemcitabine and 5-FU for the same adverse events as Table 3A and 3B regardless of incidence.

Hematologic: Myelosuppression is the dose-limiting toxicity with gemcitabine, but <1% of patients discontinued therapy for either anemia, leukopenia, or thrombocytopenia. Red blood cell transfusions were required by 19% of patients. The incidence of sepsis was less than 1 %. Petechiae or mild blood loss (hemorrhage), from any cause, were reported in 16% of patients; less than 1% of patients required platelet transfusions. Patients should be monitored for myelosuppression during gemcitabine therapy and dosage modified or suspended according to the degree of hematologic toxicity (see DOSAGE AND ADMINISTRATION).

Gastrointestinal: Nausea and vomiting were commonly reported (69%) but were usually mild to moderate. Severe nausea and vomiting (WHO grade 3/4) occurred in <15% of patients. Diarrhea was reported by 19% of patients, and stomatitis by 11% of patients.

Hepatic: Gemcitabine HCl was associated with transient elevations of serum transaminases in approximately two-thirds of patients, but there was no evidence of increasing hepatic toxicity with either longer duration of exposure to gemcitabine HCl or with greater total cumulative dose.

Renal: Mild proteinuria and hematuria were commonly reported. Clinical findings consistent with the hemolytic uremic syndrome (HUS) were reported in 6 of 2429 patients (0.25%) receiving gemcitabine in clinical trials. Four patients developed HUS on gemcitabine therapy,

ADVERSE REACTIONS: *(cont'd)*

two immediately posttherapy. Renal failure may not be reversible even with discontinuation of therapy and dialysis may be required.

TABLE 3A Selected WHO-Graded Adverse Events in Patients Receiving Gemcitabine

	WHO Grades (% incidence)			Discontinuations (LT (%)[c]
	All Patients[a] All Grades	Grade 3	Grade 4	All Patients
LABORATORY[d]				
HEMATOLOGIC				
Anemia	68	7	1	<1
Leukopenia	62	9	<1	<1
Neutropenia	63	19	6	-
Thrombocytopenia	24	4	1	<1
HEPATIC				<1
ALT	68	8	2	
AST	67	6	2	
Alkaline Phosphatase	55	7	2	
Bilirubin	13	2	<1	
RENAL				<1
Proteinuria	45	<1	0	
Hematuria	35	<1	0	
BUN	16	0	0	
Creatinine	8	<1	0	
NONLABORATORY[e]				
Nausea and Vomiting	69	13	1	<1
Pain	48	9	<1	<1
Fever	41	2	0	<1
Rash	30	<1	0	<1
Dyspnea	23	3	<1	<1
Constipation	23	1	<1	0
Diarrhea	19	1	0	0
Hemorrhage	17	<1	<1	<1
Infection	16	1	<1	<1
Alopecia	15	<1	0	0
Stomatitis	11	<1	0	<1
Somnolence	11	<1	<1	<1
Parasthesias	10	<1	0	0

Grade based on criteria from the World Health Organization (WHO)
[a]N=699-974; all patients with data
[b]N=161-241; all pancreatic cancer patients with data
[c]N=979
[d]Regardless of causality
[e]Table includes nonlaboratory data with incidence for all patients ≥10%. For approximately 60% of the patients, nonlaboratory events were graded only if assessed to be possibly drug-related.

TABLE 3B Selected WHO-Graded Adverse Events in Patients Receiving Gemcitabine

	WHO Grades (% incidence) Pancreatic Cancer Patients[b]			Discontinuations (%)[c]
	All Grades	Grade 3	Grade 4	All Patients
LABORATORY[d]				
HEMATOLOGIC				
Anemia	73	8	2	<1
Leukopenia	64	8	1	<1
Neutropenia	61	17	7	-
Thrombocytopenia	36	7	<1	<1
HEPATIC				<1
ALT	72	10	1	
AST	78	12	5	
Alkaline Phosphatase	77	16	4	
Bilirubin	26	6	2	
RENAL				<1
Proteinuria	32	<1	0	
Hematuria	23	0	0	
BUN	15	0	0	
Creatinine	6	0	0	
NONLABORATORY[e]				
Nausea and Vomiting	71	10	2	<1
Pain	42	6	<1	<1
Fever	38	2	0	<1
Rash	28	<1	0	<1
Dyspnea	10	0	<1	<1
Constipation	31	3	<1	0
Diarrhea	30	3	0	0
Hemorrhage	4	2	<1	<1
Infection	10	2	<1	<1
Alopecia	16	0	0	0
Stomatitis	10	<1	0	<1
Somnolence	11	2	<1	<1
Paresthesias	10	<1	0	0

Grade based on criteria from the World Health Organization (WHO)
[a]N=699-974; all patients with data
[b]N=161-241; all pancreatic cancer patients with data
[c]N=979
[d]Regardless of causality
[e]Table includes nonlaboratory data with incidence for all patients ≥10%. For approximately 60% of the patients, nonlaboratory events were graded only if assessed to be possibly drug-related.

Fever: The overall incidence of fever was 41%. This is in contrast to the incidence of infection (16%) and indicates that gemcitabine may cause fever in the absence of clinical infection. Fever was frequently associated with other flu-like symptoms and was usually mild and clinically manageable.

Rash: Rash was reported in 30% of patients. The rash was typically a macular or finely granular maculopapular pruritic eruption of mild to moderate severity involving the trunk and extremities. Pruritus was reported for 13% of patients.

Pulmonary: Dyspnea was reported in 23% of patients, severe dyspnea in 3%. Dyspnea may be due to underlying disease such as lung cancer (40% of study population) or pulmonary manifestations of other malignancies. Dyspnea was occasionally accompanied by bronchospasm (<2% of patients.) Rare reports of parenchymal lung toxicity consistent with drug induced pneumonitis have been associated with the use of gemcitabine.

ADVERSE REACTIONS: *(cont'd)*

Edema: Edema (13%), peripheral edema (20%) and generalized edema (<1%) were reported. Less than 1% of patients discontinued due to edema.

Flu-like Symptoms: 'Flu syndrome' was reported for 19% of patients. Individual symptoms of fever, asthenia, anorexia, headache, cough, chills, and myalgia were commonly reported. Fever and asthenia were also reported frequently as isolated symptoms. Insomnia, rhinitis, sweating, and malaise were reported infrequently. Less than 1% of patients discontinued due to flu-like symptoms.

TABLE 4A Selected WHO-Graded Adverse Events from Comparative Trial of Gemcitabine and 5–FU

	WHO Grades (% incidence) Gemcitabine[a]		
	All Grades	Grade 3	Grade 4
LABORATORY[c]			
HEMATOLOGIC			
Anemia	65	7	3
Leukopenia	71	10	0
Neutropenia	62	19	7
Thrombocytopenia	47	10	0
HEPATIC			
ALT	72	8	2
AST	72	10	2
Alkaline Phosphatase	71	16	0
Bilirubin	16	2	2
RENAL			
Proteinuria	10	0	0
Hematuria	13	0	0
BUN	8	0	0
Creatinine	2	0	0
NONLABORATORY[d]			
Nausea and Vomiting	64	10	3
Pain	10	2	0
Fever	30	0	0
Rash	24	0	0
Dyspnea	6	0	0
Constipation	10	3	0
Diarrhea	24	2	0
Hemorrhage	0	0	0
Infection	8	0	0
Alopecia	18	0	0
Stomatitis	14	0	0
Somnolence	5	2	0
Paresthesias	2	0	0

Grade based on criteria from the World Health Organization (WHO)
[a]N=58-63; all gemcitabine HCl patients with data
[b]N=61-63; all 5-FU patients with data
[c]Regardless of causality
[d]Nonlaboratory events were graded only if assessed to be possibly drug-related.

TABLE 4B Selected WHO-Graded Adverse Events from Comparative Trial of Gemcitabine and 5–FU

	WHO Grades (% incidence) 5-FU[b]		
	All Grades	Grade 3	Grade 4
LABORATORY[c]			
HEMATOLOGIC			
Anemia	45	0	0
Leukopenia	15	2	0
Neutropenia	18	2	3
Thrombocytopenia	15	2	0
HEPATIC			
ALT	38	0	0
AST	52	2	0
Alkaline Phosphatase	64	10	3
Bilirubin	25	6	3
RENAL			
Proteinuria	2	0	0
Hematuria	0	0	0
BUN	10	0	0
Creatinine	0	0	0
NONLABORATORY[d]			
Nausea and Vomiting	58	5	0
Pain	7	0	0
Fever	16	0	0
Rash	13	0	0
Dyspnea	3	0	0
Constipation	11	2	0
Diarrhea	31	5	0
Hemorrhage	2	0	0
Infection	3	2	0
Alopecia	16	0	0
Stomatitis	15	0	0
Somnolence	7	2	0
Paresthesias	2	0	0

Grade based on criteria from the World Health Organization (WHO)
[a]N=58-63; all gemcitabine HCl patients with data
[b]N=61-63; all 5-FU patients with data
[c]Regardless of causality
[d]Nonlaboratory events were graded only if assessed to be possibly drug-related.

Infection: Infections were reported for 16% of patients. Sepsis was rarely reported (<1%).

Alopecia: Hair loss, usually minimal, was reported by 15% of patients.

Neurotoxicity: There was a 10% incidence of mild paresthesias and a <1% rate of severe paresthesias.

Extravasation: Injection-site related events were reported for 4% of patients. There were no reports of injection site necrosis. Gemcitabine is not a vesicant.

Allergic: Bronchospasm was reported for less than 2% of patients. Anaphylactoid reaction has been reported rarely. Gemcitabine should not be administered to patients with a known hypersensitivity to this drug (see CONTRAINDICATIONS).

ADVERSE REACTIONS: *(cont'd)*

Cardiovascular: Two percent of patients discontinued therapy with gemcitabine due to cardiovascular events such as myocardial infarction, cerebrovascular accident, arrhythmia, and hypertension. Many of these patients had a prior history of cardiovascular disease.

OVERDOSAGE:

There is no known antidote for overdoses of gemcitabine. Myelosuppression, paresthesias and severe rash were the principal toxicities seen when a single dose as high as 5700 mg/m^{2}was administered by IV infusion over 30 minutes every 2 weeks to several patients in a Phase 1 study. In the event of suspected overdose, the patient should be monitored with appropriate blood counts and should receive supportive therapy, as necessary.

DOSAGE AND ADMINISTRATION:

Gemcitabine is for intravenous use only.

ADULTS

Gemcitabine should be administered by intravenous infusion at a dose of 1000 mg/m^{2}over 30 minutes once weekly for up to 7 weeks (or until toxicity necessitates reducing or holding a dose), followed by a week of rest from treatment. Subsequent cycles should consist of infusions once weekly for 3 consecutive weeks out of every 4 weeks. Dosage adjustment is based upon the degree of hematologic toxicity experienced by the patient (see WARNINGS). Clearance in women and the elderly is reduced and women were somewhat less able to progress to subsequent cycles (see **HUMAN PHARMACOKINETICS** and PRECAUTIONS).

Patients receiving gemcitabine should be monitored prior to each dose with a complete blood count (CBC), including differential and platelet count. If marrow suppression is detected, therapy should be modified or suspended according to the guidelines in Table 5.

TABLE 5 Dosage Reduction Guidelines

Absolute granulocyte count (x 10^6/L)		Platelet count (x 10^6/L)	% of full dose
≥1,000	and	≥100,000	100
500-999	or	50,000-99,000	75
<500	or	<50,000	hold

Laboratory evaluation of renal and hepatic function, including transaminases and serum creatinine, should be performed prior to initiation of therapy and periodically thereafter. Gemcitabine should be administered with caution in patients with evidence of significant renal or hepatic impairment. Patients who complete an entire 7 week initial cycle of gemcitabine therapy or a subsequent 3 week cycle at a dose of 1000 mg/m^2 may have the dose for subsequent cycles increased by 25% (to 1250 mg/m^2), provided that the absolute granulocyte count (AGC) and platelet nadirs exceed 1500 x 10^6/L and 100,000 x 10^6/L, respectively, and if nonhematologic toxicity has not been greater than WHO Grade 1. If patients tolerate the subsequent course of gemcitabine at a dose of 1250 mg/m^2, the dose for the next cycle can be increased to 1500 mg/m^2, provided again that the AGC and platelet nadirs exceed 1500 x 10^6/L and 100,000 x 10^6/L, respectively, and again, if nonhematologic toxicity has not been greater than WHO Grade 1.

Gemcitabine may be administered on an outpatient basis.

INSTRUCTIONS FOR USE/HANDLING

The recommended diluent for reconstitution of gemcitabine is 0.9% Sodium Chloride Injection without preservatives. Due to solubility considerations, the maximum concentration for gemcitabine upon reconstitution is 40 mg/mL. Reconstitution at concentrations greater than 40 mg/mL may result in incomplete dissolution, and should be avoided.

To reconstitute, add 5 mL of 0.9% Sodium Chloride Injection to the 200 mg vial or 25 mL of 0.9% Sodium Chloride Injection to the 1 g vial. Shake to dissolve. These dilutions each yield a gemcitabine concentration of 40 mg/mL. The appropriate amount of drug may be administered as prepared or further diluted with 0.9% Sodium Chloride Injection to concentrations as low as 0.1 mg/mL.

Reconstituted gemcitabine is a clear, colorless to light straw-colored solution. After reconstitution with 0.9% Sodium Chloride Injection, the pH of the resulting solution lies in the range of 2.7 to 3.3. The solution should be inspected visually for particulate matter and discoloration, prior to administration, whenever solution or container permit. If particulate matter or discoloration is found, do not administer.

When prepared as directed, gemcitabine solutions are stable for 24 hours at controlled room temperature 20° to 25°C (68° to 77°F). Discard unused portion. Solutions of reconstituted gemcitabine should not be refrigerated, as crystallization may occur.

The compatibility of gemcitabine with other drugs has not been studied. No incompatibilities have been observed with infusion bottles or polyvinyl chloride bags and administration sets.

Unopened vials of gemcitabine are stable until the expiration date indicated on the package when stored at controlled room temperature 20° to 25°C (68° to 77°F).

Caution should be exercised in handling and preparing gemcitabine solutions. The use of gloves is recommended. If gemcitabine solution contacts the skin or mucosa, immediately wash the skin thoroughly with soap and water or rinse the mucosa with copious amounts of water. Although acute dermal irritation has not been observed in animal studies, two of three rabbits exhibited drug-related systemic toxicities (death, hypoactivity, nasal discharge, shallow breathing) due to dermal absorption.

Procedures for proper handling and disposal of anti-cancer drugs should be considered. Several guidelines on this subject have been published.[1-7]There is no general agreement that all of the procedures recommended in the guidelines are necessary or appropriate.

REFERENCES:

1. Recommendations for the safe handling of parenteral antineoplastic drugs. NIH publication No. 83-2621. US Government Printing Office, Washington, DC 20402. **2.** Council on Scientific Affairs: Guidelines for handling parenteral antineoplastics. JAMA 1985;253:1590. **3.** National Study Commission on Cytotoxic Exposure—Recommendations for handling cytotoxic agents, 1987. Available from Louis P Jeffrey, ScD, Director of Pharmacy Services, Rhode Island Hospital, 593 Eddy Street, Providence, Rhode Island 02902. **4.** Clinical Oncological Society of Australia: Guidelines and recommendations for safe handling of antineoplastic agents. Med J Aust 1983;1:426. **5.** Jones RB, et al. Safe handling of chemotherapeutic agents: A report from the Mount Sinai Medical Center. CA 1983;33(Sept/Oct): 258. **6.** American Society of Hospital Pharmacists: Technical assistance bulletin on handling cytotoxic drugs in hospitals. Am J Hosp Pharm 1990;47:1033. **7.** Yodaiken RE, Bennet D, OSHA work-practice guidelines for personnel dealing with cytotoxic (antineoplastic) drugs. Am J Hosp Pharm 1988;43:1193-1204.

HOW SUPPLIED:

Vials: 200 mg white, lyophilized powder in a 10 mL size sterile single use vial (No. 7501). 1 g white, lyophilized powder in a 50 mL size sterile single use vial (No. 7502).

Storage: Store at controlled room temperature (20° to 25°C) (68° to 77°F). The USP has defined controlled room temperature as "A temperature maintained thermostatically that encompasses the usual and customary working environment of 20° to 25°C (68° to 77°F); that

HOW SUPPLIED: *(cont'd)*

results in a mean kinetic temperature calculated to be not more than 25°C; and that allows for excursions between 15° and 30°C (59° and 86°F) that are experienced in pharmacies, hospitals, and warehouses."

HOW SUPPLIED - EQUIVALENTS NOT AVAILABLE:

Injectable - Intravenous - 1 g

1 g x 1 $318.29 GEMZAR, Lilly 00002-7502-01

Injectable - Intravenous - 200 mg

200 mg x 1 $63.66 GEMZAR, Lilly 00002-7501-01

GEMFIBROZIL *(001351)*

CATEGORIES: Antilipemic Agents; Cardiovascular Drugs; Cholesterol; Coronary Artery Disease; Fibrates; Heart Disease; Hypercholesterolemia; Hyperlipidemia; Hyperlipoproteinemia; Hypertriglyceridemia; Hypolipidemics; Pancreatitis; Pregnancy Category B; Sales > $500 Million; FDA Approval Pre 1982; Patent Expiration 1993 Jan; Top 200 Drugs

BRAND NAMES: *Apo-Gemfibrozil*; *Bolutol*; *Clearol*; *Decrelip*; *Elmogan*; *Fetinor*; *Fibrocit*; *Gelidin*; *Gemd*; *Gemfibril*; *Gemlipid*; *Gemnpid*; *Gempar*; *Gem-S*; *Gevilon* (Germany); *Gevilon Uno* (Germany); *Gozid*; *Hidil*; *Ipolipid*; *Jezil* (Australia); *Lanaterom*; *Lifibron*; *Lipigem*; *Lipira*; *Lipizyl*; *Lipur* (France); **Lopid**; *Low-Lip*; *Normolip*; *Polyxit*; *Progemzal*; *Regulip*; *Scantipid*; *Tripid*; *Zilop*
(International brand names outside U.S. in italics)

FORMULARIES: Aetna; BC-BS; CIGNA; FHP; Humana; Kaiser; Medco; Medi-Cal; PCS; PruCare; United

COST OF THERAPY: $547.50 (Hyperlipidemia; Tablet; 600 mg; 2/day; 365 days)

DESCRIPTION:

Lopid is a lipid regulating agent. It is available as tablets for oral administration. Each tablet contains 600 mg gemfibrozil. Each also contains calcium stearate, NF; candelilla wax FCC; microcrystalline cellulose, NF; hydroxypropyl cellulose, NF; hydroxypropyl methylcellulose, USP; methylparaben, NF; Opaspray white; polyethylene glycol, NF; polysorbate 80, NF; propylparaben, NF; colloidal silicon dioxide, NF; pregelatinized starch, NF. The chemical name is 5- (2,5-dimethylphenoxy)-2,2-dimethylpentanoic acid.

The empirical formula is $C_{15}H_{22}O_3$ and the molecular weight is 250.35; the solubility in water and acid is 0.0019% and in dilute base it is greater than 1%. The melting point is 58°-61°C. Gemfibrozil is a white solid which is stable under ordinary conditions.

CLINICAL PHARMACOLOGY:

Gemfibrozil is a lipid regulating agent which decreases serum triglycerides and very low density lipoprotein (VLDL) cholesterol, and increases high density lipoprotein (HDL) cholesterol. While modest decreases in total and low density lipoprotein (LDL) cholesterol may be observed with gemfibrozil therapy, treatment of patients with elevated triglycerides due to Type IV hyperlipoproteinemia often results in a rise in LDL-cholesterol. LDL-cholesterol levels in Type IIb patients with elevations of both serum LDL-cholesterol and triglycerides are, in general, minimally affected by gemfibrozil treatment; however, gemfibrozil usually raises HDL-cholesterol significantly in this group. Gemfibrozil increases levels of high density lipoprotein (HDL) subfractions $HDL_2$and HDL_3, as well as apolipoproteins AI and AII. Epidemiological studies have shown that both low HDL-cholesterol and high LDL-cholesterol are independent risk factors for coronary heart disease.

In the primary prevention component of the Helsinki Heart Study (refs. 1,2), in which 4081 male patients between the ages of 40 and 55 were studied in a randomized, double-blind, placebo-controlled fashion, gemfibrozil therapy was associated with significant reductions in total plasma triglycerides and a significant increase in high density lipoprotein cholesterol. Moderate reductions in total plasma cholesterol and low density lipoprotein cholesterol were observed for the gemfibrozil treatment group as a whole, but the lipid response was heterogeneous, especially among different Fredrickson types. The study involved subjects with serum non-HDL-cholesterol of over 200 mg/dl and no previous history of coronary heart disease. Over the 5-year study period, the gemfibrozil group experienced a 1.4% absolute (34% relative) reduction in the rate of serious coronary events (sudden cardiac deaths plus fatal and nonfatal myocardial infarctions) compared to placebo, p = 0.04 (see TABLE 1A and TABLE B). There was a 37% relative reduction in the rate of nonfatal myocardial infarction compared to placebo, equivalent to a treatment-related difference of 13.1 events per thousand persons. Deaths from any cause during the double-blind portion of the study totaled 44 (2.2%) in the gemfibrozil randomization group and 43 (2.1%) in the placebo group.

TABLE 1A Reduction in CHD Rates (events per 1000 patients) by Baseline Lipids [1] in the Helsinki Heart Study, Years 0-5 [2]

	All Patients			LDL-C > 175; HDL-C > 46.4		
	P	G	Dif3	P	G	Dif
Incidence of Events	41	27	14	32	29	3

1 lipid values in mg/dl at baseline
2 P = placebo group; G = gemfibrozil group
3 difference in rates between placebo and gemfibrozil groups

TABLE 1B

	LDL-C > 175; TG> 177			LDL-C > 175; TG>200; HDL-C < 35		
	P	G	Dif	P	G	Dif
Incidence of Events[4]	71	44	27	149	64	85

4 fatal and nonfatal myocardial infarctions plus sudden cardiac deaths (events per 1000 patients over 5 years)

Among Fredrickson types, during the 5-year double-blind portion of the primary prevention component of the Helsinki Heart Study, the greatest reduction in the incidence of serious coronary events occurred in Type IIb patients who had elevations of both LDL-cholesterol and total plasma triglycerides. This subgroup of Type IIb gemfibrozil group patients had a lower mean HDL-cholesterol level at baseline than the Type IIa subgroup that had elevations

CLINICAL PHARMACOLOGY: *(cont'd)*

of LDL-cholesterol and normal plasma triglycerides. The mean increase in HDL-cholesterol among the Type IIb patients in this study was 12.6% compared to placebo. The mean change in LDL-cholesterol among Type IIb patients was - 4.1% with gemfibrozil compared to a rise of 3.9% in the placebo subgroup. The Type IIb subjects in the Helsinki Heart Study had 26 fewer coronary events per thousand persons over 5 years in the gemfibrozil group compared to placebo. The difference in coronary events was substantially greater between gemfibrozil and placebo for that subgroup of patients with the triad of LDL-cholesterol > 175 mg/dl (>4.5 mmol), triglycerides >200 mg/dl (>2.2 mmol), and HDL-cholesterol <35 mg/dl (<0.90 mmol) (see TABLE 1A and TABLE 1B).

Further information is available from a 3.5 year (8.5 year cumulative) follow-up of all subjects who had participated in the Helsinki Heart Study. At the completion of the Helsinki Heart Study, subjects could choose to start, stop, or continue to receive gemfibrozil; without knowledge of their own lipid values or double-blind treatment, 60% of patients originally randomized to placebo began therapy with gemfibrozil and 60% of patients originally randomized to gemfibrozil continued medication. After approximately 6.5 years following randomization, all patients were informed of their original treatment group and lipid values during the 5 years of the double-blind treatment. After further elective changes in gemfibrozil treatment status, 61% of patients in the group originally randomized to gemfibrozil were taking drug; in the group originally randomized to placebo, 65% were taking gemfibrozil.

The event rate per 1000 occurring during the open-label follow-up period is detailed in TABLE 2.

TABLE 2 Cardiac Events and All-Cause Mortality (events per 1000 patients) Occurring during the 3.5 Year Open-Label Follow-up to the Helsinki Heart Study[1]

Group:	PDrop N = 215	PN N = 494	PG N = 1283	GDrop N = 221	GN N = 574	GG N = 1207
Cardiac Events	38.8	22.9	22.5	37.2	28.3	25.4
All-Cause Mortality	41.9	22.3	15.6	72.3	19.2	24.9

[1]The six open-label groups are designated first by the original randomization (P = placebo, G = gemfibrozil) and then by the drug taken in the follow-up period (N = Attend clinic but took no drug, G= gemfibrozil, Drop = No attendance at clinic during open-label).

Cumulative mortality through 8.5 years showed a 20% relative excess of deaths in the group originally randomized to gemfibrozil versus the originally randomized placebo group and a 20% relative decrease in cardiac events in the group originally randomized to gemfibrozil versus the originally randomized placebo group (see TABLE 3.) This analysis of the originally randomized "intent-to-treat" population neglects the possible complicating effects of treatment switching during the open-label phase. Adjustment of hazard ratios taking into account open-label treatment status from years 6.5 to 8.5 could change the reported hazard ratios for mortality toward unity.

TABLE 3 Cardiac Events, Cardiac Deaths, Non-Cardiac Deaths and All-Cause Mortality in the Helsinki Heart Study, Years 0-8.5.[1]

Event	Gemfibrozil at Study Start	Placebo at Study Start	Gemfibrozil:Placebo Hazard Ratio[2]	CI Hazard Ratio[3]
Cardiac Events[4]	110	131	0.80	0.62-1.03
Cardiac Deaths	36	38	0.98	0.63-1.54
Non-Cardiac Deaths	65	45	1.40	0.95-2.05
All-Cause Mortality	101	83	1.20	0.90-1.61

[1]Intention-to-Treat Analysis of originally randomized patients neglecting the open-label treatment switches and exposure to study conditions.
[2]Hazard ratio for risk of event in the group originally randomized to gemfibrozil compared to the group originally randomized to placebo neglecting open-label treatment switch and exposure to study condition.
[3]95% confidence intervals of gemfibrozil:placebo group hazard ratio.
[4]Fatal and non-fatal myocardial infarctions plus sudden cardiac deaths over the 8.5 year period.

It is not clear to what extent the findings of the primary prevention component of the Helsinki Heart Study can be extrapolated to other segments of the dyslipidemic population not studied (such as women, younger or older males, or those with lipid abnormalities limited solely to HDL-cholesterol) or to other lipid-altering drugs.

The secondary prevention component of the Helsinki Heart Study was conducted over 5 years in parallel and at the same centers in Finland in 628 middle-aged males excluded from the primary prevention component of the Helsinki Heart Study because of a history of angina, myocardial infarction or unexplained ECG changes. The primary efficacy endpoint of the study was cardiac events (the sum of fatal and non-fatal myocardial infarctions and sudden cardiac deaths). The hazard ratio (gemfibrozil:placebo) for cardiac events was 1.47 (95% confidence limits 0.88-2.48, p=0.14). Of the 35 patients in the gemfibrozil group who experienced cardiac events, 12 patients suffered events after discontinuation from the study. Of the 24 patients in the placebo group with cardiac events, 4 patients suffered events after discontinuation from the study. There were 17 cardiac deaths in the gemfibrozil group and 8 in the placebo group (hazard ratio 2.18; 95% confidence limits 0.94-5.05, p=0.06). Ten of these deaths in the gemfibrozil group and 3 in the placebo group occurred after discontinuation from therapy. In this study of patients with known or suspected coronary heart disease, no benefit from gemfibrozil treatment was observed in reducing cardiac events or cardiac deaths. Thus, gemfibrozil has shown benefit only in selected dyslipidemic patients *without* suspected or established coronary heart disease. Even in patients with coronary heart disease and the triad of elevated LDL-cholesterol, elevated triglycerides, plus low HDL- cholesterol, the possible effect of gemfibrozil on coronary events has not been adequately studied.

No efficacy in the patients with established coronary heart disease was observed during the Coronary Drug Project with the chemically and pharmacologically related drug, clofibrate. The Coronary Drug Project was a 6-year randomized, double-blind study involving 1000 clofibrate, 1000 nicotinic acid, and 3000 placebo patients with known coronary heart disease. A clinically and statistically significant reduction in myocardial infarctions was seen in the concurrent nicotinic acid group compared to placebo; no reduction was seen with clofibrate.

The mechanism of action of gemfibrozil has not been definitely established. In man, gemfibrozil has been shown to inhibit peripheral lipolysis and to decrease the hepatic extraction of free fatty acids, thus reducing hepatic triglyceride production. Gemfibrozil inhibits synthesis and increases clearance of VLDL carrier apolipoprotein B, leading to a decrease in VLDL production.

Animal studies suggest that gemfibrozil may, in addition to elevating HDL-cholesterol, reduce incorporation of long-chain fatty acids into newly formed triglycerides, accelerate turnover and removal of cholesterol from the liver, and increase excretion of cholesterol in the feces. Gemfibrozil is well absorbed from the gastrointestinal tract after oral administration. Peak

CLINICAL PHARMACOLOGY: *(cont'd)*

plasma levels occur in 1 to 2 hours with a plasma half-life of 1.5 hours following multiple doses. Plasma levels appear proportional to dose and do not demonstrate accumulation across time following multiple doses.

Gemfibrozil mainly undergoes oxidation of a ring methyl group to successively form a hydroxymethyl and a carboxyl metabolite. Approximately seventy percent of the administered human dose is excreted in the urine, mostly as the glucuronide conjugate, with less than 2% excreted as unchanged gemfibrozil. Six percent of the dose is accounted for in the feces.

INDICATIONS AND USAGE:

Gemfibrozil is indicated as adjunctive therapy to diet for:

1. Treatment of adult patients with very high elevations of serum triglyceride levels (Types IV and V hyperlipidemia) who present a risk of pancreatitis and who do not respond adequately to a determined dietary effort to control them. Patients who present such risk typically have serum triglycerides over 2000 mg/dl and have elevations of VLDL- cholesterol as well as fasting chylomicrons (Type V hyperlipidemia). Subjects who consistently have total serum or plasma triglycerides below 1000 mg/dl are unlikely to present a risk of pancreatitis. Gemfibrozil therapy may be considered for those subjects with triglyceride elevations between 1000 and 2000 mg/dl who have a history of pancreatitis or of recurrent abdominal pain typical of pancreatitis. It is recognized that some Type IV patients with triglycerides under 1000 mg/dl may, through dietary or alcoholic indiscretion, convert to a Type V pattern with massive triglyceride elevations accompanying fasting chylomicronemia, but the influence of gemfibrozil therapy on the risk of pancreatitis in such situations has not been adequately studied. Drug therapy is not indicated for patients with Type I hyperlipoproteinemia, who have elevations of chylomicrons and plasma triglycerides, but who have normal levels of very low density lipoprotein (VLDL). Inspection of plasma refrigerated for 14 hours is helpful in distinguishing Types I, IV, and V hyperlipoproteinemia (ref. 3).

2. Reducing the risk of developing coronary heart disease **only** in Type IIb patients without history of or symptoms of existing coronary heart disease who have had an inadequate response to weight loss, dietary therapy, exercise, and other pharmacologic agents (such as bile acid sequestrants and nicotinic acid, known to reduce LDL- and raise HDL- cholesterol) **and** who have the following triad of lipid abnormalities: low HDL-cholesterol levels in addition to elevated LDL- cholesterol) and elevated triglycerides (see WARNINGS,PRECAUTIONS, and CLINICAL PHARMACOLOGY.) The National Cholesterol Education Program has defined a serum HDL-cholesterol value that is consistently below 35 mg/dl as constituting an independent risk factor for coronary heart disease (ref. 4). Patients with significantly elevated triglycerides should be closely observed when treated with gemfibrozil. In some patients with high triglyceride levels, treatment with gemfibrozil is associated with a significant increase in LDL- cholesterol. BECAUSE OF POTENTIAL TOXICITY SUCH AS MALIGNANCY, GALLBLADDER DISEASE, ABDOMINAL PAIN LEADING TO APPENDECTOMY AND OTHER ABDOMINAL SURGERIES, AN INCREASED INCIDENCE IN NONCORONARY MORTALITY, AND THE 44% RELATIVE INCREASE DURING THE TRIAL PERIOD IN AGE-ADJUSTED ALL- CAUSE MORTALITY SEEN WITH THE CHEMICALLY AND PHARMACOLOGICALLY RELATED DRUG, CLOFIBRATE, THE POTENTIAL BENEFIT OF GEMFIBROZIL IN TREATING TYPE IIA PATIENTS WITH ELEVATIONS OF LDL-CHOLESTEROL ONLY IS NOT LIKELY TO OUTWEIGH THE RISKS. GEMFIBROZIL IS ALSO NOT INDICATED FOR THE TREATMENT OF PATIENTS WITH LOW HDL-CHOLESTEROL AS THEIR ONLY LIPID ABNORMALITY.

In a subgroup analysis of patients in the Helsinki Heart Study with above-median HDL-cholesterol values at baseline (greater than 46.4 mg/dl), the incidence of serious coronary events was similar for gemfibrozil and placebo subgroups (see TABLE 1A and TABLE 1B).

The initial treatment for dyslipidemia is dietary therapy specific for the type of lipoprotein abnormality. Excess body weight and excess alcohol intake may be important factors in hypertriglyceridemia and should be managed prior to any drug therapy. Physical exercise can be an important ancillary measure, and has been associated with rises in HDL- cholesterol. Diseases contributory to hyperlipidemia such as hypothyroidism or diabetes mellitus should be looked for and adequately treated. Estrogen therapy is sometimes associated with massive rises in plasma triglycerides, especially in subjects with familial hypertriglyceridemia. In such cases, discontinuation of estrogen therapy may obviate the need for specific drug therapy of hypertriglyceridemia. The use of drugs should be considered only when reasonable attempts have been made to obtain satisfactory results with nondrug methods. If the decision is made to use drugs, the patient should be instructed that this does not reduce the importance of adhering to diet.

CONTRAINDICATIONS:

1. Hepatic or severe renal dysfunction, including primary biliary cirrhosis.

2. Preexisting gallbladder disease (see WARNINGS).

3. Hypersensitivity to gemfibrozil.

WARNINGS:

1. Because of chemical, pharmacological, and clinical similarities between gemfibrozil and clofibrate, the adverse findings with clofibrate in two large clinical studies may also apply to gemfibrozil. In the first of those studies, the Coronary Drug Project, 1000 subjects with previous myocardial infarction were treated for 5 years with clofibrate. There was no difference in mortality between the clofibrate-treated subjects and 3000 placebo-treated subjects, but twice as many clofibrate-treated subjects developed cholelithiasis and cholecystitis requiring surgery. In the other study, conducted by the World Health Organization (WHO), 5000 subjects without known coronary heart disease were treated with clofibrate for 5 years and followed one year beyond. There was a statistically significant, 44%, higher age-adjusted total mortality in the clofibrate-treated than in a comparable placebo-treated control group during the trial period. The excess mortality was due to a 33% increase in non-cardiovascular causes, including malignancy, post-cholecystectomy complications, and pancreatitis. The higher risk of clofibrate-treated subjects for gallbladder disease was confirmed.

Because of the more limited size of the Helsinki Heart Study, the observed difference in mortality from any cause between the gemfibrozil and placebo group is not statistically significantly different from the 29% excess mortality reported in the clofibrate group in the separate WHO study at the 9 year follow-up (see CLINICAL PHARMACOLOGY.) Noncoronary heart disease related mortality showed an excess in the group originally randomized to gemfibrozil primarily due to cancer deaths observed during the open-label extension.

During the 5 year primary prevention component of the Helsinki Heart Study mortality from any cause was 44 (2.2%) in the gemfibrozil group and 43 (2.1%) in the placebo group; including the 3.5 year follow-up period since the trial was completed, cumulative mortality from any cause was 101 (4.9%) in the gemfibrozil group and 83 (4.1%) in the group originally randomized to placebo (hazard ratio 1.20 in favor of placebo). Because of the more limited size of the Helsinki Heart Study, the observed difference in mortality from any cause between the gemfibrozil and placebo groups at year-5 or at year-8.5 is not statistically significantly different from the 29% excess mortality reported in the clofibrate group in the separate WHO

WARNINGS: *(cont'd)*

study at the 9 year follow-up. Noncoronary heart disease related mortality showed an excess in the group originally randomized to gemfibrozil at the 8.5 year follow-up (65 gemfibrozil versus 45 placebo noncoronary deaths).

The incidence of cancer (excluding basal cell carcinoma) discovered during the trial and in the 3.5 years after the trial was completed was 51 (2.5%) in both originally randomized groups. In addition, there were 16 basal cell carcinomas in the group originally randomized to gemfibrozil and 9 in the group randomized to placebo (p = 0.22). There were 30 (1.5%) deaths attributed to cancer in the group originally randomized to gemfibrozil and 18 (0.9%) in the group originally randomized to placebo (p = 0.11). Adverse outcomes, including coronary events, were higher in gemfibrozil patients in a corresponding study in men with a history of known or suspected coronary heart disease in the secondary prevention component of the Helsinki Heart Study. (See CLINICAL PHARMACOLOGY.)

2. A gallstone prevalence substudy of 450 Helsinki Heart Study participants showed a trend toward a greater prevalence of gallstones during the study within the gemfibrozil treatment group (7.5% vs 4.9% for the placebo group, a 55% excess for the gemfibrozil group). A trend toward a greater incidence of gallbladder surgery was observed for the gemfibrozil group (17 vs 11 subjects, a 54% excess). This result did not differ statistically from the increased incidence of cholecystectomy observed in the WHO study in the group treated with clofibrate. Both clofibrate and gemfibrozil may increase cholesterol excretion into the bile leading to cholelithiasis. If cholelithiasis is suspected, gallbladder studies are indicated. gemfibrozil therapy should be discontinued if gallstones are found.

3. Since a reduction of mortality from coronary heart disease has not been demonstrated and because liver and interstitial cell testicular tumors were increased in rats, gemfibrozil should be administered only to those patients described in INDICATIONS AND USAGE. If a significant serum lipid response is not obtained, gemfibrozil should be discontinued.

4. Concomitant Anticoagulants: Caution should be exercised when anticoagulants are given in conjunction with gemfibrozil. The dosage of the anticoagulant should be reduced to maintain the prothrombin time at the desired level to prevent bleeding complications. Frequent prothrombin determinations are advisable until it has been definitely determined that the prothrombin level has stabilized.

5. Concomitant therapy with gemfibrozil and lovastatin has been associated with rhabdomyolysis, markedly elevated creatine kinase (CK) levels and myoglobinuria, leading in a high proportion of cases to acute renal failure. IN VIRTUALLY ALL PATIENTS WHO HAVE HAD AN UNSATISFACTORY LIPID RESPONSE TO EITHER DRUG ALONE, ANY POTENTIAL LIPID BENEFIT OF COMBINED THERAPY WITH LOVASTATIN AND GEMFIBROZIL DOES NOT OUTWEIGH THE RISKS OF SEVERE MYOPATHY, RHABDOMYOLYSIS, AND ACUTE RENAL FAILURE (SEE DRUG INTERACTIONS). The use of fibrates alone, including gemfibrozil, may occasionally be associated with myositis. Patients receiving gemfibrozil and complaining of muscle pain, tenderness, or weakness should have prompt medical evaluation for myositis, including serum creatine kinase level determination. If myositis is suspected or diagnosed, gemfibrozil therapy should be withdrawn.

6. Cataracts: Subcapsular bilateral cataracts occurred in 10% and unilateral in 6.3% of male rats treated with gemfibrozil at 10 times the human dose.

PRECAUTIONS:

Initial Therapy: Laboratory studies should be done to ascertain that the lipid levels are consistently abnormal. Before instituting gemfibrozil therapy, every attempt should be made to control serum lipids with appropriate diet, exercise, weight loss in obese patients, and control of any medical problems such as diabetes mellitus and hypothyroidism that are contributing to the lipid abnormalities.

Continued Therapy: Periodic determination of serum lipids should be obtained, and the drug withdrawn if lipid response is inadequate after 3 months of therapy.

Carcinogenesis, Mutagenesis, and Impairment of Fertility: Long- term studies have been conducted in rats at 0.2 and 2 times the human dose (based on surface area, mg/meter^2). Based on two-week toxicokinetic studies; exposure (AUC) of the dose groups was estimated to be 0.2 and 1.3 times the human exposure. The incidence of benign liver nodules and liver carcinomas was significantly increased in high dose male rats. The incidence of liver carcinomas increased also in low dose males, but this increase was not statistically significant (p = 0.1). Male rats had a dose-related and statistically significant increase of benign Leydig cell tumors. The higher dose female rats had a significant increase in the combined incidence of benign and malignant liver neoplasms.

Long-term studies have been conducted in mice at 0.1 and 1 times the human dose (based on surface area). Based on two-week toxicokinetic studies, exposure (AUC) of the two dose groups was estimated to be 0.1 and 0.7 times the human exposure. There were no statistically significant differences from controls in the incidence of liver tumors, but the doses tested were lower than those shown to be carcinogenic with other fibrates.

Electron microscopy studies have demonstrated a florid hepatic peroxisome proliferation following gemfibrozil administration to the male rat. An adequate study to test for peroxisome proliferation has not been done in humans but changes in peroxisome morphology have been observed. Peroxisome proliferation has been shown to occur in humans with either of two other drugs of the fibrate class when liver biopsies were compared before and after treatment in the same individual.

Administration of approximately 0.6 and 2 times the human dose (based on surface area) to male rats for 10 weeks resulted in a dose-related decrease of fertility. Subsequent studies demonstrated that this effect was reversed after a drug-free period of about eight weeks, and it was not transmitted to the offspring.

Pregnancy Category C: Gemfibrozil has been shown to produce adverse effects in rats and rabbits at doses between 0.5 and 3 times the human dose (based on surface area) but no developmental toxicity or teratogenicity among offspring of either species. There are no adequate and well-controlled studies in pregnant women. Gemfibrozil should be used during pregnancy only if the potential benefit justifies the potential risk to the fetus.

Administration of gemfibrozil to female rats at 0.6 and 2 times the human dose (based on surface area) before and throughout gestation caused a dose- related decrease in conception rate and, at the high dose, an increase in stillborns and a slight reduction in pup weight during lactation. There were also dose-related increased skeletal variations. Anophthalmia occurred, but rarely.

Administration of 0.6 and 2 times the human dose (based on surface area) of gemfibrozil to female rats from gestation day 15 through weaning caused dose-related decreases in birth weight and suppressions of pup growth during lactation.

Administration of 1 and 3 times the human dose (based on surface area) of gemfibrozil to female rabbits during organogenesis caused a dose-related decrease in litter size and, at the high dose, an increased incidence of parietal bone variations.

Nursing Mothers: It is not known whether this drug is excreted in human milk. Because many drugs are excreted in human milk and because of the potential for tumorigenicity shown for gemfibrozil in animal studies, a decision should be made whether to discontinue nursing or to discontinue the drug, taking into account the importance of the drug to the mother.

PRECAUTIONS: *(cont'd)*

Hematologic Changes: Mild hemoglobin, hematocrit and white blood cell decreases have been observed in occasional patients following initiation of gemfibrozil therapy. However, these levels stabilize during long- term administration. Rarely, severe anemia, leukopenia, thrombocytopenia, and bone marrow hypoplasia have been reported. Therefore, periodic blood counts are recommended during the first 12 months of gemfibrozil administration.

Liver Function: Abnormal liver function tests have been observed occasionally during gemfibrozil administration, including elevations of AST (SGOT), ALT (SGPT), LDH, bilirubin, and alkaline phosphatase. These are usually reversible when gemfibrozil is discontinued. Therefore periodic liver function studies are recommended and gemfibrozil therapy should be terminated if abnormalities persist.

Kidney Function: There have been reports of worsening renal insufficiency upon the addition of gemfibrozil therapy in individuals with baseline plasma creatinine >2.0 mg/dl. In such patients, the use of alternative therapy should be considered against the risks and benefits of a lower dose of gemfibrozil.

Use in Children: Safety and efficacy in children and adolescents have not been established.

DRUG INTERACTIONS:

HMG-CoA reductase inhibitors: Rhabdomyolysis has occurred with combined gemfibrozil and lovastatin therapy. It may be seen as early as 3 weeks after initiation of combined therapy or after several months. In most subjects who have had an unsatisfactory lipid response to either drug alone, the possible benefit of combined therapy with lovastatin (or other HMG-CoA reductase inhibitors) and gemfibrozil does not outweigh the risks of severe myopathy, rhabdomyolysis, and acute renal failure. There is no assurance that periodic monitoring of creatine kinase will prevent the occurrence of severe myopathy and kidney damage.

Anticoagulants: CAUTION SHOULD BE EXERCISED WHEN ANTICOAGULANTS ARE GIVEN IN CONJUNCTION WITH GEMFIBROZIL. THE DOSAGE OF THE ANTICOAGULANT SHOULD BE REDUCED TO MAINTAIN THE PROTHROMBIN TIME AT THE DESIRED LEVEL TO PREVENT BLEEDING COMPLICATIONS. FREQUENT PROTHROMBIN DETERMINATIONS ARE ADVISABLE UNTIL IT HAS BEEN DEFINITELY DETERMINED THAT THE PROTHROMBIN LEVEL HAS STABILIZED.

ADVERSE REACTIONS:

In the double-blind controlled phase of the primary prevention component of the Helsinki Heart Study, 2046 patients received gemfibrozil for up to 5 years. In that study, the following adverse reactions were statistically more frequent in subjects in the gemfibrozil group (TABLE 4):

TABLE 4

	Gemfibrozil (N = 2046)	Placebo (N = 2035)
	Frequency in percent of subjects	
Gastrointestinal reactions	34.2	23.8
Dyspepsia	19.6	11.9
Abdominal pain	9.8	5.6
Acute appendicitis (histologically confirmed in most cases where data were available)	1.2	0.6
Atrial fibrillation	0.7	0.1
Adverse events reported by more than 1% subjects, but without a significant difference between groups:		
Diarrhea	7.2	6.5
Fatigue	3.8	3.5
Nausea/Vomiting	2.5	2.1
Eczema	1.9	1.2
Rash	1.7	1.3
Vertigo	1.5	1.3
Constipation	1.4	1.3
Headache	1.2	1.1

Gallbladder surgery was performed in 0.9% of gemfibrozil and 0.5% of placebo subjects in the primary prevention component, a 64% excess, which is not statistically different from the excess of gallbladder surgery observed in the clofibrate compared to the placebo group of the WHO study. Gallbladder surgery was also performed more frequently in the gemfibrozil group compared to placebo (1.9% vs 0.3%, p=0.07) in the secondary prevention component. A statistically significant increase in appendectomy in the gemfibrozil group was seen also in the secondary prevention component (6 on gemfibrozil vs 0 on placebo, p=0.014).

Nervous system and special senses adverse reactions were more common in the gemfibrozil group. These included hypesthesia, paresthesias, and taste perversion. Other adverse reactions that were more common among gemfibrozil treatment group subjects but where a causal relationship was not established include cataracts, peripheral vascular disease, and intracerebral hemorrhage.

From other studies it seems probable that gemfibrozil is causally related to the occurrence of MUSCULOSKELETAL SYMPTOMS (see WARNINGS), and to ABNORMAL LIVER FUNCTION TESTS and HEMATOLOGIC CHANGES (see PRECAUTIONS).

Reports of viral and bacterial infections (common cold, cough, urinary tract infections) were more common in gemfibrozil treated patients in other controlled clinical trials of 805 patients. Additional adverse reactions that have been reported for gemfibrozil are listed below by system (TABLE 5). These are categorized according to whether a causal relationship to treatment with gemfibrozil is probable or not established:

OVERDOSAGE:

While there has been no reported case of overdosage, symptomatic supportive measures should be taken should it occur.

DOSAGE AND ADMINISTRATION:

The recommended dose for adults is 1200 mg administered in two divided doses 30 minutes before the morning and evening meal.

REFERENCES:

1. Frick MH, Elo O, Haapa K, et al: Helsinki Heart Study: Primary prevention trial with gemfibrozil in middle-aged men with dyslipidemia. *N Engl J Med* 1987; 317:1237-1245. **2.** Manninen V, Elo O, Frick MH, et al: Lipid alterations and decline in the incidence of coronary heart disease in the Helsinki Heart Study. *JAMA* 1988; 260: 641-651. **3.** Nikkila EA: Familial lipoprotein lipase deficiency and related disorders of chylomicron metabolism. In Stanbury JB et al. (eds.):*The Metabolic Basis of Inherited Disease,* 5th ed., McGraw-Hill, 1983, Chap. 30, pp. 622-642. **4.** Report of the National Cholesterol Education Program Expert Panel on Detection, Evaluation, and Treatment of High Blood Cholesterol. *Arch Int Med* 1988;148:36-69.

REFERENCES: *(cont'd)*

TABLE 5

	PROBABLE	CAUSAL RELATIONSHIP NOT ESTABLISHED
General		Weight loss
Cardiac		extrasystoles
Gastrointestinal	cholestatic jaundice	pancreatitis hepatoma colitis
Central Nervous System	dizziness somnolence paresthesia peripheral neuritis decreased libido depression headache	confusion convulsions syncope
Eye	blurred vision	retinal edema
Genitourinary	impotence	decreased male fertility dysfunction
Musculoskeletal	myopathy myasthenia myalgia painful extremities arthralgia synovitis rhabdomyolysis (seeWARNINGS and DRUG INTERACTIONS)	
Clinical Laboratory	increased creatine phosphokinase increased bilirubin increased liver transaminases (AST (SGOT), ALT (SGPT) increased alkaline phophatase	positive antinuclear antibody
Hematopoietic	anemia leukopenia bone marrow hypoplasia eosinophilia	thrombocytopenia
Immunologic	angioedema laryngeal edema urticaria	anaphylaxis Lupus-like syndrome vasculitis
Integumentary	exfoliative dermatitis rash dermatitis pruritus	alopecia

PATIENT INFORMATION:

Gemfibrozil is used to lower high triglyceride and cholesterol levels. Notify your physician if you are pregnant or nursing. Gemfibrozil should be taken 30 minutes before the morning and evening meals. This medication may cause dizziness or blurred vision; use caution while driving or operating hazardous machinery. Gemfibrozil may cause an increase in blood sugar. If you have diabetes mellitus, carefully monitor blood sugar levels. Notify your physician if you develop severe stomach pain, muscle pain or weakness, or unexplained fever.

HOW SUPPLIED:

Lopid (Tablet 737), white, elliptical, film-coated, scored tablets, each containing 600 mg gemfibrozil.

Storage: Store below 30°C (86°F).

HOW SUPPLIED - RATED THERAPEUTICALLY EQUIVALENT:

Tablet, Plain Coated - Oral - 600 mg

30's	$5.40	Gemfibrozil, H.C.F.A. F F P	99999-1351-01
50's	$9.00	Gemfibrozil, H.C.F.A. F F P	99999-1351-03
60's	$10.80	Gemfibrozil, H.C.F.A. F F P	99999-1351-02
60's	$13.98	Gemfibrozil, United Res	00677-1473-06
60's	$13.98	Gemfibrozil, Geneva Pharms	00781-1056-60
60's	$51.00	Gemfibrozil, Sidmak Labs	50111-0857-04
60's	$52.50	Gemfibrozil, Rugby	00536-5668-08
60's	$53.50	Gemfibrozil, Aligen Independ	00405-4456-31
60's	$54.05	Gemfibrozil, Purepac Pharm	00228-2552-06
60's	$54.92	Gemfibrozil, Qualitest Pharms	00603-3750-20
60's	$54.95	Gemfibrozil, Harber Pharm	51432-0787-02
60's	$55.65	Gemfibrozil, West Point Pharma	59591-0017-68
60's	$55.89	Gemfibrozil, Watson Labs	52544-0454-60
60's	$56.50	Gemfibrozil, Martec Pharms	52555-0634-60
60's	$56.60	Gemfibrozil, Lederle Pharm	00005-3160-32
60's	$56.63	Gemfibrozil, HL Moore Drug Exch	00839-7787-05
60's	$57.10	Gemfibrozil, Geneva Pharms	50752-0310-80
60's	$57.20	Gemfibrozil, Major Pharms	00904-7732-52
60's	$59.10	Gemfibrozil, Teva	00093-0670-06
60's	$59.10	Gemfibrozil, Goldline Labs	00182-1956-26
60's	$59.55	Gemfibrozil, Warner Chilcott	00047-0084-20
60's	$64.75	Gemfibrozil, Mylan	00378-0517-91
60's	$64.75	Gemfibrozil, Rugby	00536-3854-08
60's	**$71.99**	**LOPID, Parke-Davis**	**00071-0737-20**
100's	$75.00	Gemfibrozil, Raway	00686-0787-20
100's	$89.50	Gemfibrozil, Purepac Pharm	00228-2552-10
100's	$96.91	Gemfibrozil, Vangard Labs	00615-3559-13
100's	$115.50	Gemfibrozil, Goldline Labs	00182-1956-89
100's	**$137.94**	**LOPID, Parke-Davis**	**00071-0737-40**
500's	$90.00	Gemfibrozil, H.C.F.A. F F P	99999-1351-04
500's	$116.50	Gemfibrozil, Geneva Pharms	00781-1056-05
500's	$418.00	Gemfibrozil, Sidmak Labs	50111-0857-02
500's	$447.35	Gemfibrozil, Purepac Pharm	00228-2552-50
500's	$456.90	Gemfibrozil, Qualitest Pharms	00603-3750-28
500's	$457.90	Gemfibrozil, Harber Pharm	51432-0787-05
500's	$459.00	Gemfibrozil, Rugby	00536-5668-05
500's	$465.65	Gemfibrozil, Watson Labs	52544-0454-05
500's	$465.70	Gemfibrozil, Martec Pharms	52555-0634-05
500's	$466.50	Gemfibrozil, Geneva Pharms	50752-0310-08
500's	$469.10	Gemfibrozil, Major Pharms	00904-7732-40
500's	$471.14	Gemfibrozil, Lederle Pharm	00005-3160-31
500's	$471.14	Gemfibrozil, HL Moore Drug Exch	00839-7787-12
500's	$492.45	Gemfibrozil, Teva	00093-0670-05
500's	$492.50	Gemfibrozil, Goldline Labs	00182-1956-05
500's	$493.00	Gemfibrozil, Schein Pharm (US)	00364-2566-05

HOW SUPPLIED - RATED THERAPEUTICALLY EQUIVALENT: *(cont'd)*

500's	$493.50	Gemfibrozil, Warner Chilcott	00047-0084-30
500's	$493.75	Gemfibrozil, Mylan	00378-0517-05
500's	$493.75	Gemfibrozil, Rugby	00536-3854-05
500's	**$599.87**	**LOPID, Parke-Davis**	**00071-0737-30**
750's	$739.72	Gemfibrozil, Glasgow Pharm	60809-0122-55
750's	$739.72	Gemfibrozil, Glasgow Pharm	60809-0122-72

GENTAMICIN SULFATE *(001352)*

CATEGORIES: Aminoglycosides; Anti-Infectives; Antibacterials; Antibiotics; Anti-hypertensives; Antimicrobials; Antitussives/Expectorants/Mucolytics; Bacterial Sepsis; Blepharoconjunctivitis; Bone Infections; Burns; Central Nervous System Agents; Conjunctivitis; Corneal Ulcer; Dacryocystitis; Dermatologicals; EENT Drugs; Endocarditis; Eye, Ear, Nose, & Throat Preparations; Joint Infections; Keratitis; Keratoconjunctivitis; Meningitis; Ocular Blepharitis; Ocular Infections; Ophthalmics; Pneumonia; Respiratory & Allergy Medications; Respiratory Tract Infections; Septicemia; Skin/Mucous Membrane Agents; Skin Infections; Topical; Urinary Tract Infections; FDA Approval Pre 1982

BRAND NAMES: *Alcomicin* (Canada); Apogen; *Biogaracin*; *Biogenta*; *Biogenta Oftalmica*; Bristagen; *Cidomycin* (Australia, England, Canada); *Danigen*; *Dermogen*; *Diakarmon*; Ed-Mycin; *Fermentmycin*; G-Mycin; G-Myticin; *Garalen* (Mexico); *Garamicin*; *Garamicina* (Mexico); *Garamicina Cream*; *Garamicina Crema* (Mexico); *Garamicina Oftalmica* (Mexico); **Garamycin**; *Garalone*; *Garasone*; *Garbilocin*; Garramycin Topical; *Gencin*; *Genemicin* (Mexico); Genoptic; *Genrex* (Mexico); *Gensumycin*; *Gentabiotic*; Gentacidin; *Gentacin* (Japan); *Gentacyl*; Gentafair; Gentak; *Gental*; *Gentalline* (France); *Gentalol* (Japan); *Gentalyn*; *Gentalyn Oftalmico-Otico*; Gentamar; *Gentamax*; *Gentamen*; *Gentamerck*; *Gentamil Ofteno*; *Gentamin*; *Gentamina*; *Gentamytrex* (Germany); *Gentamytrex Ophthiole*; *Gentarad*; *Gentarex*; Gentasol; *Gentasporin*; *Gentatrim*; *Genticin* (England); *Genticol*; *Genticyn*; *Gentiderm*; *Gentotal*; Gentrasul; *Geomycine*; *Gevramycin*; *Grammicin*; *Gramosol*; *Hexamycin*; I-Gent; *Ifigencin*; Infa-Gen; Isotonic Gentamicin; Jenamicin; *Jintamycin*; *Lacromycin*; *Lisagent*; *Lisarin*; *Lugacin*; *Lyramycin*; *Megental*; *Miramycin*; *Nichogencin*; Ocu-Mycin; *Oftalmogenta*; *Ophtagram* (Germany); *Optigen*; *Optimycin*; *Ottogenta*; *Pyogenta*; Qualamycin; *Refobacin* (Germany); *Rocy Gen*; *Rovixida*; *Sedanazin* (Japan); *Servigenta*; Spectro-Genta; Storz-G; *Sulmycin* (Germany); U-Gencin; *Versigen*; *Yectamicina* (Mexico)

(International brand names outside U.S. in italics)

FORMULARIES: Aetna; BC-BS; DoD; FHP; Medi-Cal; PCS; WHO

WARNING:

PARENTERAL Patients treated with aminoglycosides should be under close clinical observation because of the potential toxicity associated with their use.

As with other aminoglycosides, gentamicin sulfate pediatric injectable is potentially nephrotoxic. The risk of nephrotoxicity is greater in patients with impaired renal function and in those who receive high dosage or prolonged therapy.

Neurotoxicity manifested by ototoxicity, both vestibular and auditory, can occur in patients treated with gentamicin sulfate pediatric injectable, primarily in those with pre-existing renal damage and in patients with normal renal function treated with higher doses and/or for longer periods than recommended.

Aminoglycoside induced ototoxicity is usually irreversible. Other manifestations of neurotoxicity may include numbness, skin tingling, muscle twitching, and convulsions.

Renal and eighth cranial nerve functions should be closely monitored, especially in patients with known or suspected reduced renal function at onset of therapy, and also in those whose renal function is initially normal but who develop signs of renal dysfunction during therapy. Urine should be examined for decreased specific gravity, increased excretion of protein, and the presence of cells or casts. Blood urea nitrogen, serum creatinine, or creatinine clearance should be determined periodically. When feasible, it is recommended that serial audiograms be obtained in patients old enough to be tested, particularly high-risk patients.

Evidence of ototoxicity (dizziness, vertigo, tinnitus, roaring in the ears, or hearing loss) or nephrotoxicity requires dosage adjustment or discontinuance of the drug. As with the other aminoglycosides, on rare occasions changes in renal and eighth cranial nerve function may not become manifest until soon after completion of therapy.

Serum concentrations of aminoglycosides should be monitored when feasible to assure adequate levels and to avoid potentially toxic levels. When monitoring gentamicin peak concentrations, dosage should be adjusted so that prolonged levels above 12 mcg/ml are avoided. When monitoring gentamicin through concentrations, dosage should be adjusted so that levels above 2 mcg/ml are avoided.

Excessive peak and/or through serum concentrations of aminoglycosides may increase the risk of renal and eighth cranial nerve toxicity. In the event of overdose or toxic reactions, hemodialysis may aid in the removal of gentamicin from the blood, especially if renal function is, or becomes, compromised. The rate of removal of gentamicin is considerably less by peritoneal dialysis than by hemodialysis. In the newborn infant, exchange transfusions may also be considered.

Concurrent and/or sequential systemic or topical use of other potentially neurotoxic and/or nephrotoxic drugs, such as cisplatin, cephaloridine, kanamycin, amikacin, neomycin, polymyxin B, colistin, paromomycin, streptomycin, tobramycin, vancomycin, and viomycin, should be avoided. Another factor which may increase patient risk of toxicity is dehydration. The concurrent use of gentamicin with potent diuretics, such as ethacrynic acid or furosemide, should be avoided, since certain diuretics by themselves may cause ototoxicity. In addition, when administered intravenously, diuretics may enhance aminoglycoside toxicity by altering the antibiotic concentration in serum and tissue.

WARNING:
GENTAMICIN INTRATHECAL INJECTION is intended as adjunctive therapy in patients with central nervous system infections.
Since patients considered for treatment with gentamicin intrathecal injection will usually be receiving concomitant treatment with IM or IV gentamicin sulfate, all warnings and precautions for this or other concomitantly administered agents must be observed. Moreover, when the drug is administered by more than one route, additive effects must be considered (see gentamicin sulfate injectable or gentamicin sulfate pediatric injectable product information). Laboratory studies in animals have shown that gentamicin sulfate, when administered directly into the central nervous system, has caused neurologic disturbances, including adverse effects on the eighth cranial nerve.
The risk of direct administration of a potentially neurotoxic drug into the cerebrospinal fluid spaces of the central nervous system must be weighed against the potential benefit to be derived from this route of administration.

DESCRIPTION:

PARENTERAL

Gentamicin sulfate, USP, a water-soluble antibiotic of the aminoglycoside group, is derived from *Micromonospora purpurea*, an actinomycete. Gentamicin sulfate pediatric injectable is a sterile, aqueous solution for parenteral administration. Each ml contains gentamicin sulfate, USP equivalent to 10 mg gentamicin base; 1.3 mg methylparaben and 0.2 mg propylparaben as preservatives; 3.2 mg sodium bisulfite and 0.1 mg edetate disodium.

INTRATHECAL

Gentamicin sulfate, USP, a water-soluble antibiotic of the aminoglycoside group, is derived from *Micromonospora purpurea*, an actinomycete. Gentamicin sulfate pediatric injectable is a sterile, aqueous solution for parenteral administration. Each ml contains gentamicin sulfate, USP equivalent to 2.0 mg gentamicin base and 8.5 mg sodium chloride.

OPHTHALMIC SOLUTION/OINTMENT

Gentamicin sulfate is a water-soluble antibiotic of the aminoglycoside group.

Gentamicin sulfate ophthalmic solution is a sterile, aqueous solution buffered to approximately pH 7 for ophthalmic use. Each ml contains gentamicin sulfate USP (equivalent to 3.0 mg gentamicin), disodium phosphate, monosodium phosphate, sodium chloride, and benzalkonium chloride (0.1 mg) as a preservative.

Gentamicin sulfate ophthalmic ointment is a sterile ointment, each gram containing gentamicin sulfate, USP (equivalent to 3.0 mg gentamicin) in a base of white petrolatum, with methylparaben (0.5 mg) and propylparaben (0.1 mg) as preservatives.

Gentamicin is obtained from cultures of *Micromonospora purpurea*. It is a mixture of the sulfate salts of gentamicin C_1, C_2, and C_{1A}. All three components appear to have similar antimicrobial activities. Gentamicin sulfate occurs as a white powder and is soluble in water and insoluble in alcohol.

CLINICAL PHARMACOLOGY:

PARENTERAL

After intramuscular administration of gentamicin sulfate pediatric injectable, peak serum concentrations usually occur between 30 and 60 minutes and serum levels are measurable for 6 to 12 hours. In infants, a single dose of 2.5 mg/kg usually provides a peak serum level in the range of 3 to 5 mcg/ml. When gentamicin is administered by intravenous infusion over a 2-hours period, the serum concentrations are similar to those obtained by intramuscular administration. Age markedly affects the peak concentrations: in one report, a 1 mg/kg dose produced mean peak concentrations: in one report, a 1 mg/kg dose produced mean peak concentrations of 1.58, 2.03 and 2.81 mcg/ml in patients 6 months to 5 years old, 5 to 10 years old, and over 10 years old, respectively.

In infants 1 week to 6 months of age, the half-life is 3 to 3 1/2 hours. In full-term and large premature infants less than 1 week old, the approximate serum half-life of gentamicin is 5 1/2 hours. In small premature infants, the half-life is inversely related to birth weight. In premature infants weighing less than 150 grams, the half-life is 11 1/2 hours; in those weighing 1500 to 2000 grams, the half-life is 8 hours; in those weighing over 2000 grams, the half-life is approximately 5 hours. While some variation is to be expected due to a number of variables such as age, body temperature, surface area, and physiologic differences, the individual patients given the same dose tends to have similar levels in repeated determinations.

Gentamicin, like all aminoglycosides, may accumulate in the serum and tissues of patients treated with higher doses and/or for prolonged periods, particularly in the presence of impaired or immature renal function. In patients with immature or impaired renal function, gentamicin is cleared from the body more slowly than in patients with normal renal function. The more severe the impairment, the slower the clearance. (Dosage must be adjusted.)

Since gentamicin is distributed in extracellular fluid, peak serum concentrations may be lower than usual in patients who have a large volume of this fluid. Serum concentrations of gentamicin in febrile patients may be lower than those in afebrile patients given the same dose. When body temperature returns to normal, serum concentrations of the drug may rise. Febrile and anemic states may be associated with a shorter than usual serum half-life. (Dosage adjustment is usually not necessary.) In severely burned patients, the half-life may be significantly decreased and resulting serum concentrations may be lower than anticipated from the mg/kg dose.

Protein-binding studies have indicated that the degree of gentamicin binding is low; depending upon the methods used for testing, this may be between 0 and 30%.

In neonates less than 3 days old, approximately 10% of the administered dose is excreted in 12 hours; in infants 5 to 40 days old, approximately 40% is excreted over the same period. Excretion of gentamicin correlates with postnatal age and creatinine clearance. Thus, with increasing postnatal age and concomitant increase in renal maturity, gentamicin is excreted more rapidly. Little, if any, metabolic transformation occurs; the drug is excreted principally by glomerular filtration. After several days of treatment, the amount of gentamicin excreted in the urine approaches, but does not equal, the daily dose administered. As with other aminoglycosides, a small amount of the gentamicin dose may be retained in the tissues, especially in the kidneys. Minute quantities of aminoglycosides have been detected in the urine of some patients weeks after drug administration was discontinued. Renal clearance of gentamicin is similar to that of endogenous creatinine.

In patients with marked impairment of renal function, there is a decrease in the concentration of aminoglycosides in urine and in their penetration into defective renal parenchyma. This decreased drug excretion, together with the potential nephrotoxicity of aminoglycosides, should be considered when treating such patients who have urinary tract infections.

Probenecid dose not affect renal tubular transport of gentamicin.

CLINICAL PHARMACOLOGY: *(cont'd)*

The endogenous creatinine clearance rate and the serum creatinine level have a high correlation with the half-life of gentamicin in serum. Results of these tests may serve as guides for adjusting dosage in patients with renal impairment (see DOSAGE AND ADMINISTRATION.)

Following parenteral administration, gentamicin can be detected in serum, lymph, tissues, sputum, and in pleural, synovial, and peritoneal fluids. Concentrations in renal cortex sometimes may be eight times higher than the usual serum levels. Concentrations in bile, in general, have been low and have suggested minimal biliary excretion. Gentamicin crosses the peritoneal as well as the placental membranes. Since aminoglycosides diffuse poorly into the subarachnoid space after parenteral administration, concentrations of gentamicin in cerebrospinal fluid are often low and dependent upon dose, rate of penetration and degree of meningeal inflammation. There is minimal penetration of gentamicin into ocular tissues following intramuscular or intravenous administration.

MICROBIOLOGY

Parenteral and Intrathecal

In vitro tests have demonstrated that gentamicin is a bactericidal antibiotic which acts by inhibiting normal protein synthesis in susceptible microorganisms. It is active against a wide variety of pathogenic bacteria including *Escherichia coli, Proteus* species (indole-positive and indole-negative),*Pseudomonas aeruginosa*, species of the*Klebsiella-Enterobacter-Serratia* group, *Citrobacter* species, and *Staphylococcus* species (including penicillin- and methicillin-resistant strains). Gentamicin is also active *in vitro* against species of *Salmonella* and *Shigella*. The following bacteria are usually resistant to aminoglycosides:*Streptococcus pneumoniae*, most species of streptococci, particularly group D and anaerobic organisms, such as*Bacteroides* species or *Clostridium* species.

In vitro studies have shown that an aminoglycoside combined with an antibiotic that interferes with cell wall synthesis may act synergistically against some group D streptococcal strains. The combination of gentamicin and penicillin G has a synergistic bactericidal effect against virtually all strains of *Streptococcus faecalis* and its varieties (*S. faecalis var. liquefaciens, S. faecalis var. zymogens*), *S. faecium* and *S. durans*. An enhanced killing effect against many of these strains has also been shown *in vitro* with combinations of gentamicin and ampicillin, carbenicillin, nafcillin, or oxacillin, the combined effect of gentamicin and carbenicillin is synergistic for many strains of*Pseudomonas aeruginosa*. *In vitro* synergism against other gram-negative organisms has been shown with combinations of gentamicin and cephalosporins.

Gentamicin may be active against clinical isolates of bacteria resistant to other aminoglycosides. Bacteria resistant to one aminoglycoside may be resistant to one or more other aminoglycosides. Bacterial resistance to gentamicin is generally developed slowly.

Ophthalmic Solution/Ointment

Gentamicin sulfate is active *in vitro* against many strains of the following microorganisms:

Staphylococcus aureus, Staphylococcus epidermidis, Streptococcus pyogenes, Streptococcus pneumoniae, Enterobacter aerogenes, Escherichia coli, Haemophilus influenzae, Klebsiella pneumoniae, Neisseria gonorrhoeae, Pseudomonas aeruginosa and *Serratia marcescens*.

SUSCEPTIBILITY TESTING

If the disc method of susceptibility testing used is that described by Bauer *et al* (*Am J Clin Path* 45: 493, 1966; *Federal Register* 37:20525-20529, 1972), a disc containing 10 mcg of gentamicin should give a zone of inhibition of 15 mm or more to indicate susceptibility of the infecting organism. A zone of 12 mm or less indicates that the infecting organism is likely to be resistant. Zones greater than 12 mm and less than 15 mm indicate intermediate susceptibility. In certain conditions it may be desirable to do additional susceptibility testing by the tube or agar dilution method; gentamicin substance is available for this purpose.

INDICATIONS AND USAGE:

PARENTERAL

Gentamicin sulfate pediatric injectable is indicated in the treatment of serious infections caused by susceptible strains of the following microorganisms; *Pseudomonas aeruginosa, Proteus* species (indole-positive and indole-negative), *Escherichia coli, Klebsiella-Enterobacter-Serratia* species, *Citrobacter* species, and *Staphylococcus* species (coagulase-positive and coagulase-negative).

Clinical studies have shown gentamicin sulfate pediatric injectable to be effective in bacterial neonatal sepsis; bacterial septicemia; and serious bacterial infections of the central nervous system (meningitis), urinary tract, respiratory tract, gastrointestinal tract (including peritonitis), skin, bone and soft tissue (including burns).

Aminoglycosides, including gentamicin, are not indicated in uncomplicated initial episodes or urinary tract infections unless the causative organisms are susceptible to these antibiotics and are not susceptible to antibiotics having less potential for toxicity.

Specimens for bacterial culture should be obtained to isolate and identify causative organisms and to determine their susceptibility to gentamicin.

Gentamicin sulfate may be considered as initial therapy in suspected or confirmed gram-negative infections, and therapy may be instituted before obtaining results of susceptibility testing. The decision to continue therapy with this drug should be based on the results of susceptibility tests, the severity of the infection, and the important additional concepts contained in the BOXED WARNING above. If the causative organisms are resistant to gentamicin, other appropriate therapy should be instituted.

In serious infections when the causative organisms are unknown, gentamicin sulfate may be administered as initial therapy in conjunction with a penicillin-type or cephalosporin-type drug before obtaining results of susceptibility testing. If anaerobic organisms are suspected as etiologic agents, consideration should be given to using other suitable antimicrobial therapy in conjunction with gentamicin. Following identification of the organism and its susceptibility, appropriate antibiotic therapy should then be continued.

Gentamicin sulfate has been used effectively in combination with carbenicillin for the treatment of life-threatening infections caused by*Pseudomonas aeruginosa*. It has also been found effective when used in conjunction with a penicillin-type drug for the treatment of endocarditis caused by group D streptococci.

Gentamicin sulfate pediatric injectable has also been shown to be effective in the treatment of serious staphylococcal infections. While not the antibiotic of first choice, gentamicin sulfate pediatric injectable may be considered when penicillins or other less potentially toxic drugs are contraindicated and bacterial susceptibility tests and clinical judgment indicate its use. It may also be considered in mixed infections caused by susceptible strains of staphylococci and gram-negative organisms.

In the neonate with suspected bacterial sepsis or staphylococcal pneumonia, a penicillin-type drug is also usually indicated as concomitant therapy with gentamicin.

(For the Indications for the intrathecal form, please see the BOXED WARNING at the beginning of this monograph).

INDICATIONS AND USAGE: *(cont'd)*

OPHTHALMIC SOLUTION/OINTMENT

Gentamycin sterile ophthalmic solution and ointment are indicated in the topical treatment of ocular bacterial infections, including conjunctivitis, keratitis, keratoconjunctivitis, corneal ulcers, blepharitis, blepharoconjunctivitis, acute meibomianitis, and dacryocystitis caused by susceptible strains of the following microorganisms:

Staphylococcus aureus, Staphylococcus epidermidis, Streptococcus pyogenes, Streptococcus pneumoniae, Enterobacter aerogenes, Escherichia coli, Haemophilus influenzae, Klebsiella pneumoniae, Neisseria gonorrhoeae, Pseudomonas aeruginosa and *Serratia marcescens.*

CONTRAINDICATIONS:

PARENTERAL

Hypersensitivity to gentamicin is a contraindication to its use. A history of hypersensitivity or serious toxic reactions to other aminoglycosides may contraindicate use of gentamicin because of the known cross-sensitivity of patients to drugs in this class.

OPHTHALMIC SOLUTION/OINTMENT

Gentamicin ophthalmic solution and ointment are contraindicated in patients with known hypersensitivity to any of the components.

WARNINGS:

PARENTERAL

(See BOXED WARNING.) Aminoglycosides can cause fetal harm when administered to a pregnant woman. Aminoglycoside antibiotics cross the placenta, and there have been several reports of total irreversible bilateral congenital deafness in children whose mothers received streptomycin during pregnancy. Serious side effects to mother, fetus, or newborn have not been reported in the treatment of pregnant women with other aminoglycosides. Animal reproduction studies conducted on rats and rabbits did not reveal evidence of impaired fertility or harm to the fetus due to gentamicin sulfate.

It is not known whether gentamicin sulfate can cause fetal harm when administered to a pregnant woman or can affect reproduction capacity. If gentamicin is used during pregnancy of if the patient becomes pregnant while taking gentamicin, she should be apprised of the potential hazard to the fetus.

Gentamicin sulfate pediatric injectable contains sodium bisulfite, a sulfite that may cause allergic-type reactions including anaphylactic symptoms and life-threatening or less severe asthmatic episodes in certain susceptible people. The overall prevalence of sulfite sensitivity in the general population is unknown and probably low. Sulfite sensitivity is seen more frequently in asthmatic than in nonasthmatic people.

OPHTHALMIC SOLUTION/OINTMENT

NOT FOR INJECTION INTO THE EYE. Gentamicin sulfate ophthalmic solution and ointment are not for injection. They should never be injected subconjunctivally, nor should they be directly introduced into the anterior chamber of the eye.

PRECAUTIONS:

PARENTERAL

Neurotoxic and nephrotoxic antibiotics may be absorbed in significant quantities from body surfaces after local irrigation or application. The potential toxic effect of antibiotics administered in this fashion should be considered.

Increased nephrotoxicity has been reported following concomitant administration of aminoglycoside antibiotics and cephalosporins.

Neuromuscular blockade and respiratory paralysis have been reported in the cat receiving high doses (40 mg/kg) of gentamicin. The possibility of these phenomena occurring in man should be considered if aminoglycosides are administered by any route to patients receiving anesthetics, or to patients receiving neuromuscular blocking agents, such as succinylcholine, tubocurarine, or decamethonium, or in patients receiving massive transfusions of citrate-anticoagulated blood. If neuromuscular blockade occurs, calcium salts may reverse it.

Aminoglycosides should be used with caution in patients with neuromuscular disorders, such as myasthenia gravis, since these drugs may aggravate muscle weakness because of their potential curare-like effects on the neuromuscular junction. During or following gentamicin therapy, paresthesias, tetany, positive Chvostek and Trousseau signs, and mental confusion have been described in patients with hypomagnesemia, hypocalcemia, and hypokalemia. When this has occurred in infants, tetany and muscle weakness has been described. Both adults and infants required appropriate corrective electrolyte therapy.

A Fanconi-like syndrome, with aminoaciduria and metabolic acidosis, has been reported in some adults and infants being given gentamicin injection.

Cross-allergenicity among aminoglycosides has been demonstrated. Patients should be well hydrated during treatment.

Treatment with gentamicin may result in overgrowth of nonsusceptible organisms. If this occurs, appropriate therapy is indicated.

See BOXED WARNING regarding concurrent use of potent diuretics and regarding concurrent and/or sequential use of other neurotoxic and/or nephrotoxic antibiotics and for other essential information.

Usage in Pregnancy: Safety for use in pregnancy has not been established.

OPHTHALMIC SOLUTION/OINTMENT

General

Prolonged use of topical antibiotics may give rise to overgrowth of nonsusceptible organisms including fungi. Bacterial resistance to gentamicin may also develop. If purulent discharge, inflammation or pain becomes aggravated, the patient should discontinue use of medication and consult a physician.

If irritation or hypersensitivity to any component of the drug develops, the patient should discontinue use of this preparation, and appropriate therapy should be instituted.

Ophthalmic ointments may retard corneal healing.

Information for the Patient

To avoid contamination, do not touch tip of container to the eye, eyelid, or any surface.

Carcinogenesis, Mutagenesis, and Impairment of Fertility

There are no published carcinogenicity or impairment of fertility studies on gentamicin. Aminoglycoside antibiotics have been found to be non-mutagenic.

Pregnancy Category C

Gentamicin has been shown to depress body weights, kidney weights, and median glomerular counts in newborn rats when administered systemically to pregnant rats in daily doses approximately 500 times the maximum recommended ophthalmic human dose. There are no adequate and well- controlled-studies in pregnant women. Gentamicin should be used during pregnancy only if the potential benefit justifies the potential risk to the fetus.

DRUG INTERACTIONS:

Although the *in vitro* mixing of gentamicin and carbenicillin results in a rapid and significant inactivation of gentamicin, this interaction has not been demonstrated in patients with normal renal function who received both drugs by different routes of administration. A reduction in gentamicin serum half-life has been reported in patients with severe renal impairment receiving carbenicillin concomitantly with gentamicin.

ADVERSE REACTIONS:

PARENTERAL

Nephrotoxicity: Adverse renal effects, as demonstrated by the presence of casts, cells, or protein in the urine or by rising BUN, NPN, serum creatinine or oliguria, have been reported. They occur more frequently in patients treated for longer periods or with larger dosages than recommended.

Neurotoxicity: Serious adverse effects on both vestibular and auditory branches of the eighth cranial nerve have been reported, primarily in patients with renal impairment (especially if dialysis is required) and in patients on high doses and/or prolonged therapy. Symptoms include dizziness, vertigo, tinnitus, roaring in the ears and hearing loss, which, as with the other aminoglycosides, may be irreversible. Hearing loss is usually manifested initially by diminution of high-tone acuity. Other factors which may increase the risk of toxicity include excessive dosage, dehydration and previous exposure to other ototoxic drugs.

Peripheral neuropathy or encephalopathy, including numbness, skin tingling, muscle twitching, convulsions, and a myasthenia gravis-like syndrome, have been reported.

Note: The risk of toxic reactions is low in neonates, infants, and children with normal renal function who do not receive gentamicin sulfate pediatric injectable at higher doses or for longer periods of time than recommended.

Other reported adverse reactions possibly related to gentamicin include: respiratory depression, lethargy, confusion, depression, visual disturbances, decreased appetite, weight loss, and hypotension and hypertension; rash, itching, urticaria, generalized burning, laryngeal edema, anaphylactoid reactions, fever, and headache; nausea, vomiting, increased salivation, and stomatitis; purpura, pseudotumor cerebri, acute organic brain syndrome, pulmonary fibrosis, joint pain, transient hepatomegaly, and splenomegaly.

Laboratory abnormalities possibly related to gentamicin include: increased levels of serum transaminase (SGOT, SGPT), serum LDH and bilirubin; decreased serum calcium, magnesium, sodium and potassium; anemia, leukopenia, granulocytopenia, transient agranulocytosis, eosinophilia, increased and decreased reticulocyte counts, and thrombocytopenia.

While clinical laboratory test abnormalities may be isolated findings, they may also be associated with clinically related signs and symptoms. For example, tetany and muscle weakness may be associated with hypomagnesemia, hypocalcemia, and hypokalemia.

While local tolerance of gentamicin sulfate pediatric injectable is generally excellent, there has been an occasional report of pain at the injection site. Subcutaneous atrophy or fat necrosis suggesting local irritation has been reported rarely.

OPHTHALMIC SOLUTION/OINTMENT

Bacterial and fungal corneal ulcers have developed during treatment with gentamicin ophthalmic preparations.

The most frequently reported adverse reactions are ocular burning and irritation upon drug instillation, non-specific conjunctivitis, conjunctival epithelial defects, and conjunctival hyperemia.

Other adverse reactions which have occurred rarely are allergic reactors, thrombocytopenic purpura, and hallucinations.

OVERDOSAGE:

PARENTERAL

In the event of overdose or toxic reactions, hemodialysis may aid in the removal of gentamicin from the blood, and is especially important if renal function is, or becomes, compromised. The rate of removal of gentamicin is considerably less by peritoneal dialysis than it is by hemodialysis. In the newborn infant, exchange transfusions may also be considered.

DOSAGE AND ADMINISTRATION:

PARENTERAL

Gentamicin sulfate pediatric injectable may be given intramuscularly or intravenously. The patient's pretreatment body weight should be obtained for calculation of correct dosage. The dosage of aminoglycosides in obese patients should be based on an estimate of the lean body mass. It is desirable to limit the duration of treatment with aminoglycosides to short term.

DOSAGE FOR PATIENTS WITH NORMAL RENAL FUNCTION

Children: 6 to 7.5 mg/kg/day. (2.0 to 2.5 mg/kg administered every 8 hours.)

Infants and Neonates: 7.5 mg/kg/day. (2.5 mg/kg administered every 8 hours.)

Premature or Full-Term Neonates One Week of Age or Less: 5 mg/kg/day. (2.5 mg/kg administered every 12 hours.)

It is desirable to measure periodically both peak and trough serum concentrations of gentamicin when feasible during therapy to assure adequate but not excessive drug levels. For example, the peak concentration (at 30 to 60 minutes after intramuscular injection) is expected to be in the range of 3 to 5 mcg/ml. When monitoring peak concentrations after intramuscular or intravenous administration, dosage should be adjusted so that prolonged levels above 12 mcg/ml are avoided. When monitoring trough concentrations (just prior to the next dose), dosage should be adjusted so that levels above 2 mcg/ml are avoided. Determination of the adequacy of a serum level for a particular patient must take into consideration the susceptibility of the causative organism, the severity of the infection, and the status of the patient's host-defense mechanisms.

In patients with extensive burns, altered pharmacokinetics may result in reduced serum concentrations of aminoglycosides. In such patients treated with gentamicin, measurement of serum concentrations is recommended as a basis for dosage adjustment.

The usual duration of treatment is 7 to 10 days. In difficult and complicated infections, a longer course of therapy may be necessary. In such cases monitoring of renal, auditory, and vestibular functions is recommended, since toxicity is more apt to occur with treatment extended for more than 10 days. Dosage should be reduced if clinically indicated.

FOR INTRAVENOUS ADMINISTRATION

The intravenous administration of gentamicin may be particularly useful for treating patients with bacterial septicemia or those in shock. It may also be the preferred route of administration for some patients with congestive heart failure, hematologic disorders, severe burns, or those with reduced muscle mass.

For intermittent intravenous administration, a single dose of gentamicin sulfate pediatric injectable may be diluted in sterile isotonic saline solution or in a sterile solution of dextrose 5% in water. The solution may be infused over a period of one-half to two hours.

The recommended dosage for intravenous and intramuscular administration is identical.

DOSAGE AND ADMINISTRATION: *(cont'd)*

Gentamicin sulfate pediatric injectable should not be physically premixed with other drugs, but should be administered separately in accordance with the recommended route of administration and dosage schedule.

DOSAGE FOR PATIENTS WITH IMPAIRED RENAL FUNCTION

Dosage must be adjusted in patients with impaired renal function to assure therapeutically adequate, but not excessive, blood levels. Whenever possible, serum concentrations of gentamicin should be monitored. One method of dosage adjustment is to increase the interval between administration of the usual doses. Since the serum creatinine concentration has a high correlation with the serum half-life of gentamicin, this laboratory test may provide guidance for adjustment of the interval between doses. In adults, the interval between doses (in hours) may be approximated by multiplying the serum creatinine level (mg/100 ml) by 8. For example, a patient weighing 60 kg with a serum creatinine level of 0.2 mg/100 ml could be given 60 mg (1 mg/kg) every 16 hours (2 x 8). These guidelines may be considered when treating infants and children with serious renal impairment.

In patients with serious systemic infections and renal impairment, it may be desirable to administer the antibiotic more frequently but in reduced dosage. In such patients, serum concentrations of gentamicin should be measured so that adequate but not excessive levels result. A peak and trough concentration measured intermittently during therapy will provide optimal guidance for adjusting dosage. After the usual initial dose, a rough guide for determining reduced dosage at 8-hour intervals is to divide the normally recommended dose by the serum creatinine level (TABLE 1). For example, after an initial dose of 20 mg (2.0 mg/kg), a child weighing 10 kg with a serum creatinine level of 2.0 mg/100 ml could be given 10 mg every 8 hours (20 divided by 2). It should be noted that the status of renal function may be changing over the course of the infectious process. It is important to recognize that deteriorating renal function may require a greater reduction in dosage than that specified in the above guidelines for patients with stable renal impairment (TABLE 1):

TABLE 1
(Dosage at Eight-Hour Intervals After the Usual Initial Dose)

Serum Creatinine (mg %)	Approximate Creatinine Clearance Rate (ml/min/1.73M^2)	Percent of Usual Doses Shown Above
≤<1.0	>100	100
1.1-1.3	70-100	80
1.4-1.6	55-70	65
1.7-1.9	45-55	55
2.0-2.2	40-45	50
2.3-2.5	35-40	40
2.6-3.0	30-35	35
3.1-3.5	25-30	30
3.6-4.0	20-25	25
1.4-5.1	15-20	20
5.2-6.6	10-15	15
6.7-8.0	<10	10

In patients with renal failure undergoing hemodialysis, the amount of gentamicin removed from the blood may vary depending upon several factors including the dialysis method used. An 8-hour hemodialysis may reduce serum concentrations of gentamicin by approximately 50%. In children the recommended dose at the end of each dialysis period is 2.0 to 2.5 mg/kg depending upon the severity of infection.

The above dosage schedules are not intended as rigid recommendations but are provided as guides to dosage when the measurement of gentamicin serum levels is not feasible.

A variety of methods are available to measure gentamicin concentrations in body fluids; these include microbiologic, enzymatic and radioimmunoassay techniques.

INTRATHECAL

Gentamicin intrathecal injection is intended for administration directly into the cerebrospinal fluid spaces of the central nervous system.

The dosage will vary depending upon factors, such as age and weight of the patient, site of injection, degree of obstruction to cerebrospinal fluid estimated to be present. In general, the recommended dose for infants 3 months of age and older and children is 1 to 2 mg once a day. for adults, 4 to 8 mg may be administered once a day.

Administration of gentamicin intrathecal injection should be continued as long as sensitive organisms are demonstrated in the cerebrospinal fluid. Since the intralumbar or intraventricular dose is administered immediately after specimens are taken for laboratory study, treatment should usually be continued for at least one day after negative results have been obtained from CSF cultures and/or strained smears.

The suggested method for administering gentamicin intrathecal injection into the lumbar area is as follows: the desired quantity of gentamicin Intrathecal Injection is drawn up carefully from the ampul into a 5- or 10- ml sterile syringe. After the lumbar puncture is performed and a specimen of the spinal fluid is removed for laboratory tests, the syringe containing gentamicin is inserted into the hub of the spinal needle. A quantity of cerebrospinal fluid (appr. 10% of the estimated total CSF volume) is allowed to flow into the syringe and mix with the gentamicin Intrathecal Injection. The resultant solution is then injected over a period of 3 to 5 minutes with the bevel of the needle directed upward.

If the cerebrospinal fluid is grossly purulent, or if it is unobtainable, gentamicin intrathecal injection may be diluted with sterile normal saline before injection.

Gentamicin intrathecal injection may also be administered directly into the subdural space or directly into the ventricles, including administration by use of an implanted reservoir.

NOTE: This preparation does not contain any preservative. Once opened, contents should be used immediately and unused portions should be discarded.

OPHTHALMIC SOLUTION

Instill one or two drops into the affected eye every four hours. In severe infections, dosage may to as much as two drops once every hour.

OPHTHALMIC OINTMENT

Apply a small amount (about 1/2 inch) to the affected eye two to three times a day.

STORAGE

Store (parental and ophthalmic forms) between 2 and 30°C (36 and 86°F).

Store (intrathecal) below 30°C (86°F).

(Sterile Ophthalmic Solution and Ointment: Schering, 4/92, 132272)

HOW SUPPLIED - RATED THERAPEUTICALLY EQUIVALENT:

Cream - Topical - 0.1 %

15 gm	$2.02	Gentamicin, United Res	00677-0709-40
15 gm	$2.02	Gentamicin, H.C.F.A. F F P	99999-1352-02
15 gm	$2.40	Gentamicin, Thames Pharma	49158-0162-20
15 gm	$2.59	Gentamicin, Clay Park Labs	45802-0056-35
15 gm	$2.90	Gentamicin, Qualitest Pharms	00603-7769-74
15 gm	$3.10	Gentamicin, Schein Pharm (US)	00364-7305-72
15 gm	$3.10	Gentamicin, Geneva Pharms	00781-7310-27

HOW SUPPLIED - RATED THERAPEUTICALLY EQUIVALENT: *(cont'd)*

15 gm	$3.10	Gentamicin Sulfate, Major Pharms	00904-2663-36
15 gm	$3.12	Gentamicin, Rugby	00536-4480-20
15 gm	$3.15	Gentamicin, Goldline Labs	00182-1403-51
15 gm	$3.23	Gentamicin, HL Moore Drug Exch	00839-6492-47
15 gm	$3.25	Gentamicin Sulfate, Consolidated Midland	00223-4304-15
15 gm	$3.60	Gentamicin, Fougera	00168-0071-15
15 gm	$3.60	Gentamicin, Rugby	00536-4470-20
15 gm	$3.75	G-MYTICIN, Pedinol Pharma	00884-3684-15
15 gm	**$17.40**	**GARAMYCIN, Schering**	**00085-0008-05**
30 gm	$4.00	Gentamicin, Clay Park Labs	45802-0056-11
30 gm	$4.75	Gentamicin, Schein Pharm (US)	00364-7305-56
30 gm	$6.19	Gentamicin, Rugby	00536-4480-28
30 gm	$7.20	Gentamicin, Rugby	00536-4470-28
454 gm	$86.40	Gentamicin, Clay Park Labs	45802-0056-05

Injection, Solution - Intramuscular; - 2 mg/ml

2 ml x 25	**$67.46**	**GARAMYCIN INTRATHECAL, Schering**	**00085-0337-03**

Injection, Solution - Intramuscular; - 10 mg/ml

2 ml	$1.75	Gentamicin Sulfate, Consolidated Midland	00223-7715-02
2 ml	$29.38	Gentamicin, Fujisawa USA	00469-1730-10
2 ml	$32.81	Gentamicin, Solopak Labs	39769-0001-02
2 ml x 10	**$22.49**	**GARAMYCIN PEDIATRIC INJ, Schering**	**00085-0013-06**
2 ml x 25	$15.00	Gentamicin, Voluntary Hosp	53258-5130-02
2 ml x 25	$17.71	Gentamicin, Elkins Sinn	00641-0394-25
2 ml x 25	$26.40	Gentamicin, Gensia Labs	00703-9642-04
2 ml x 25	$29.38	PEDIATRIC GENTAMICIN, Fujisawa USA	00469-5130-25
2 ml x 25	$37.50	Gentamicin Sulfate, Consolidated Midland	00223-7714-02
6 ml	$5.59	Gentamicin, Abbott	00074-3400-01
8 ml	$5.97	Gentamicin, Abbott	00074-3401-01
10 ml	$6.42	Gentamicin, Abbott	00074-3402-01

Injection, Solution - Intramuscular; - 40 mg/ml

1.5 ml	**$3.61**	**GARAMYCIN, Schering**	**00085-0069-05**
2 ml	$1.26	Gentamicin Sulfate, Insource	58441-0125-02
2 ml	$1.74	Gentamicin, HL Moore Drug Exch	00839-6503-23
2 ml	$2.13	Gentamicin, Abbott	00074-1207-03
2 ml	$2.25	Gentamicin Sulfate, Consolidated Midland	00223-7719-02
2 ml	$3.00	Gentamicin, Goldline Labs	00182-1424-61
2 ml	$3.00	G MYCIN, Bolan Pharm	44437-0559-02
2 ml	$3.10	Gentamicin, Steris Labs	00402-0559-02
2 ml	**$4.02**	**GARAMYCIN, Schering**	**00085-0069-06**
2 ml	$4.95	Gentamicin, Rugby	00536-4690-67
2 ml	$46.88	Gentamicin, Fujisawa USA	00469-1000-10
2 ml	$51.56	Gentamicin, Solopak Labs	39769-0014-02
2 ml x 25	$12.00	Gentamicin, Voluntary Hosp	53258-1000-01
2 ml x 25	$26.04	Gentamicin, Elkins Sinn	00641-0395-25
2 ml x 25	$26.70	Gentamicin, Gensia Labs	00703-9652-04
2 ml x 25	$50.00	Gentamicin Sulfate, Consolidated Midland	00223-7721-02
2 ml x 25	$81.38	Gentamicin, Schein Pharm (US)	00364-6739-48
2 ml x 25	**$109.16**	**GARAMYCIN, Schering**	**00085-0069-04**
15 gm	$3.00	Gentamicin Sulfate, IDE-Interstate	00814-3446-93
20 ml	$3.93	Gentamicin Sulfate, Insource	58441-0125-20
20 ml	$7.74	Gentamicin Sulfate, Major Pharms	00904-0799-55
20 ml	$8.25	Gentamicin Sulfate, Consolidated Midland	00223-7717-20
20 ml	$9.35	Gentamicin, Goldline Labs	00182-1424-65
20 ml	$10.21	Gentamicin, Steris Labs	00402-0559-20
20 ml	$11.25	Gentamicin Sulfate, Rugby	00536-4690-73
20 ml	$11.87	Gentamicin, Schein Pharm (US)	00364-6739-55
20 ml	$109.38	Gentamicin, Fujisawa USA	00469-1000-40
20 ml	$387.50	Gentamicin, Solopak Labs	39769-0014-20
20 ml x 5	**$152.52**	**GARAMYCIN, Schering**	**00085-0069-08**
20 ml x 10	$104.12	Gentamicin, Elkins Sinn	00641-2331-43
20 ml x 25	$97.50	Gentamicin, Pasadena	00418-0011-20
20 ml x 25	$127.80	Gentamicin, Gensia Labs	00703-9665-04
25 x 2 ml	$45.50	Gentamicin, Pasadena	00418-0010-20
50 ml	$87.50	Gentamicin, Fujisawa USA	00469-1000-60

Injection, Solution - Intravenous - 0.6 mg/ml

100 ml plastic	$10.03	Gentamicin, McGaw	00264-5806-32

Injection, Solution - Intravenous - 0.8 mg/ml

100 ml	$8.21	Gentamicin In 0.9% Sodium, Abbott	00074-1395-11
100 ml	$10.51	Gentamicin, Abbott	00074-7884-23
100 ml plastic	$10.06	Gentamicin, McGaw	00264-5808-32
100 ml x 24	$132.00	Gentamicin Inj 80, Elkins Sinn	00641-7130-99

Injection, Solution - Intravenous - 0.9 mg/ml

100 ml	$11.12	Gentamicin, Abbott	00074-7886-23

Injection, Solution - Intravenous - 1 mg/ml

100 ml	$7.03	Gentamicin In 0.9% Sodium, Abbott	00074-1399-11
100 ml	$11.42	Gentamicin, Abbott	00074-7889-23
100 ml plastic	$8.83	Gentamicin, McGaw	00264-5810-32
100 ml x 24	$144.00	Gentamicin, Elkins Sinn	00641-7140-99

Injection, Solution - Intravenous - 1.2 mg/ml

50 ml	$7.21	Gentamicin In 0.9% Sodium, Abbott	00074-1390-01
50 ml	$9.84	Gentamicin, Abbott	00074-7879-13
50 ml plastic b	$9.52	Gentamicin, McGaw	00264-5812-38
50 ml x 24	$120.00	Gentamicin Inj 60, Elkins Sinn	00641-7100-99

Injection, Solution - Intravenous - 1.4 mg/ml

50 ml	$10.43	Gentamicin, Abbott	00074-7881-13

Injection, Solution - Intravenous - 1.6 mg/ml

50 ml plastic b	$10.06	GENTAMICN, McGaw	00264-5816-38
50 ml x 24	$132.00	Gentamicin Inj 160, Elkins Sinn	00641-7120-99

Injection, Solution - Intravenous - 40 mg/50ml

50 ml	$8.90	Isotonic Gentamicin, Baxter Hlthcare	00338-0503-41
100 ml	$9.91	Isotonic Gentamicin, Baxter Hlthcare	00338-0503-48

Injection, Solution - Intravenous - 60 mg/50ml

50 ml	$9.29	Isotonic Gentamicin, Baxter Hlthcare	00338-0507-41
100 ml	$11.00	Isotonic Gentamicin, Baxter Hlthcare	00338-0507-48

Injection, Solution - Intravenous - 60 mg/100 ml

100 ml	$9.19	Gentamicin In Ns, Abbott	00074-7880-23
100's	$9.29	Isotonic Gentamicin, Baxter Hlthcare	00338-0501-48

Injection, Solution - Intravenous - 80 mg/50ml

50 ml	$9.91	Isotonic Gentamicin, Baxter Hlthcare	00338-0509-41
50 ml	$10.51	Gentamicin In Ns, Abbott	00074-7883-13

Injection, Solution - Intravenous - 100 mg/50ml

50 ml	$10.66	Gentamicin In Ns, Abbott	00074-7888-13
50 ml	$10.78	Isotonic Gentamicin, Baxter Hlthcare	00338-0511-41

HOW SUPPLIED - RATED THERAPEUTICALLY EQUIVALENT: *(cont'd)*

Injection, Solution - Intravenous - 100 mg/100ml

60 ml x 5	$16.07	Gentamicin, Fujisawa USA	00469-1983-00
80 ml x 5	$19.63	Gentamicin, Fujisawa USA	00469-1993-00
100 ml	$10.78	Isotonic Gentamicin, Baxter Hlthcare	00338-0505-48
100 ml x 5	$23.80	Gentamicin, Fujisawa USA	00469-2013-00

Ointment - Ophthalmic - 3 mg/gm

3.5 gm	$3.85	INFA-GEN, Infinity Pharm	58154-0575-55
3.5 gm	$5.50	Gentamicin, United Res	00677-1401-18
3.5 gm	$5.70	Gentamicin, Rugby	00536-4490-91
3.5 gm	$5.95	Spectro Genta, Spectrum Scitfc	53268-0575-55
3.5 gm	$9.00	GENTAK, Akorn	17478-0284-35
3.5 gm	$11.22	Gentamicin Sulfate, Ciba Vision	00058-0151-05
3.5 gm	$13.51	GENOPTIC S.O.P., Allergan	00023-0320-04
3.5 gm	**$15.75**	**GARAMYCIN OPHTHALMIC, Schering**	**00085-0151-05**

Ointment - Ophthalmic; Top - 0.3 %

3.5 gm	$13.50	Gentamicin, H.C.F.A. F F P	99999-1352-05

Ointment - Topical - 0.1 %

15 gm	$2.03	Gentamicin, H.C.F.A. F F P	99999-1352-06
30 gm	$4.22	Gentamicin, H.C.F.A. F F P	99999-1352-07

Ointment - Topical - 1 mg/gm

15 g	$3.50	Gentamicin, Schein Pharm (US)	00364-7338-72
15 gm	$2.02	Gentamicin, United Res	00677-0710-40
15 gm	$2.40	Gentamicin, Thames Pharma	49158-0191-20
15 gm	$2.59	Gentamicin, Clay Park Labs	45802-0046-35
15 gm	$2.90	Gentamicin, Qualitest Pharms	00603-7770-74
15 gm	$3.00	Gentamicin, IDE-Interstate	00814-3447-93
15 gm	$3.1	Gentamicin, Geneva Pharms	00781-7320-27
15 gm	$3.10	Gentamicin Sulfate, Major Pharms	00904-2664-36
15 gm	$3.23	Gentamicin, HL Moore Drug Exch	00839-6599-47
15 gm	$3.25	Gentamicin Sulfate, Consolidated Midland	00223-4306-15
15 gm	$3.60	Gentamicin, Fougera	00168-0078-15
15 gm	$3.75	Gentamicin, Goldline Labs	00182-1474-51
15 gm	$3.75	G-MYTICIN, Pedinol Pharma	00884-3784-15
15 gm	**$17.40**	**GARAMYCIN, Schering**	**00085-0343-05**
30 g	$4.75	Gentamicin, Schein Pharm (US)	00364-7338-56
30 gm	$4.00	Gentamicin, Clay Park Labs	45802-0046-11
30 gm	$4.50	Gentamicin Sulfate, Goldline Labs	00182-1474-56
30 gm	$8.00	ED-MYCIN, Edwards Pharms	00485-0060-30
454 gm	$70.00	Gentamicin, Thames Pharma	49158-0191-16
454 gm	$86.40	Gentamicin, Clay Park Labs	45802-0046-05

Solution - Ophthalmic - 0.3 %

5 ml	$2.52	Gentamicin, H.C.F.A. F F P	99999-1352-10
15 ml	$6.23	Gentamicin, H.C.F.A. F F P	99999-1352-11

Solution - Ophthalmic - 3 mg/ml

1 ml	$2.96	GENOPTIC STERILE OPHTHALMIC, Allergan-Amer	11980-0117-01
5 ml	$3.15	Gentamicin, United Res	00677-0901-20
5 ml	$4.70	Gentamicin, Goldline Labs	00182-1695-62
5 ml	$4.78	Gentamicin Sulfate Ophthalmic, IDE-Interstate	00814-3448-38
5 ml	$5.40	GENTAFAIR, Qualitest Pharms	00603-7158-37
5 ml	$5.52	Gentamicin Ophthalmic, HL Moore Drug Exch	00839-6745-25
5 ml	$5.60	Gentamicin Sulfate, Major Pharms	00904-1907-05
5 ml	$5.89	Gentamicin Opthalmic, Parmed Pharms	00349-8579-75
5 ml	$6.10	Gentamicin Ophthalmic, Geneva Pharms	00781-7110-75
5 ml	$6.12	Gentamicin, Steris Labs	00402-0749-05
5 ml	$6.14	Gentamicin, Aligen Independ	00405-6060-05
5 ml	$6.35	GENTASOL, Ocusoft	54799-0510-05
5 ml	$6.77	Gentamicin Sulfate, Fougera	00168-0248-03
5 ml	$7.10	Gentamicin Ophthalmic, Schein Pharm (US)	00364-7388-53
5 ml	$7.62	GENTACIDIN OPHTHALMIC, Ciba Vision	00058-2365-05
5 ml	$8.10	GENTAK, Akorn	17478-0283-10
5 ml	$8.75	Gentamicin Ophthalmic, Rugby	00536-0925-65
5 ml	$13.43	GENOPTIC STERILE OPHTHALMIC, Allergan-Amer	11980-0117-05
5 ml	**$15.75**	**GARAMYCIN OPHTHALMIC, Schering**	**00085-0899-05**
15 ml	$7.13	Gentamicin Sulfate Ophthalmic, IDE-Interstate	00814-3448-42
15 ml	$7.35	Gentamicin Ophthalmic, Rugby	00536-0925-72
15 ml	$7.52	Gentamicin, Aligen Independ	00405-6060-15
15 ml	$7.60	Gentamicin, Steris Labs	00402-0749-15
15 ml	$8.95	Gentamicin Ophthalmic, Schein Pharm (US)	00364-7388-72
15 ml	$8.95	Gentamicin Ophthalmic, Geneva Pharms	00781-7110-85
15 ml	$10.35	GENTAK, Akorn	17478-0283-12

HOW SUPPLIED - NOT RATED EQUIVALENT:

Injection, Solution - Intravenous - 0.6 mg/ml

100 ml x 24	$120.00	Gentamicin Inj 60, Elkins Sinn	00641-7110-99

Ointment - Ophthalmic - 3 mg/gm

3.5 gm	$5.50	Gentamicin Ophth, Harber Pharm	51432-0863-35

Powder

100 gm	$221.50	Gentamicin, Paddock Labs	00574-0419-01
1000 gm	$1830.00	Gentamicin, Paddock Labs	00574-0419-00

Solution - Ophthalmic - 3 mg/ml

5 ml	$3.05	Gentamicin Sulfate, Raway	00686-6580-60
5 ml	$3.63	INFA-GEN, Infinity Pharm	58154-0580-60
5 ml	$4.75	Qualamycin, Quality Res Pharms	52765-0749-05
5 ml	$4.95	Gentamicin Sulfate Ophthalmic, Harber Pharm	51432-0509-05
5 ml	$5.95	SPECTRO GENTA, Spectrum Scitfc	53268-0580-10
15 ml	$3.40	Gentamicin Sulfate, Raway	00686-6580-64
15 ml	$5.75	Gentamicin Sulfate, Harber Pharm	51432-0509-15

GENTAMICIN SULFATE; PREDNISOLONE ACETATE *(001353)*

CATEGORIES: Anti-Infectives; Antibiotics; Burns; Conjunctivitis; Corneal Inflammation; Corneal Injury; EENT Drugs; Edema; Eye, Ear, Nose, & Throat Preparations; Hemophilus; Inflammatory Conditions; Ocular Infections; Ophthalmics; Steroids; Uveitis; FDA Approved 1988 Jun

BRAND NAMES: **Pred-G**; *Pred G*
(International brand names outside U.S. in italics)

FORMULARIES: Aetna; BC-BS

DESCRIPTION:

Pred-G liquifilm sterile ophthalmic suspension and Pred-G S.O.P. sterile ophthalmic ointment are topical anti-inflammatory/anti-infective combination products for ophthalmic use.

Chemical Names: Prednisolone acetate: 11β, 17,21-Trihydroxypregna-1,4-diene-3,20-dione 21-acetate.

Gentamicin sulfate is the sulfate salt of gentamicin C_1, gentamicin C_2, and gentamicin C_{1A}which are produced by the growth of **Micromonospora purpura**.

Liquifilm Sterile Ophthalmic Suspension Contains: Prednisolone acetate (microfine suspension) - 1.0% Gentamicin sulfate - equivalent to 0.3% gentamicin base with: liquifilm (polyvinyl alcohol) 1.4%; benzalkonium chloride 0.005%; edetate disodium; hydroxypropyl methylcellulose; polysorbate 80; sodium citrate, dihydrate; sodium chloride; sodium hydroxide and/or hydrochloric acid to adjust the pH; and purified water.

Sterile Ophthalmic Ointment Contains: Prednisolone acetate 0.6% gentamicin sulfate - equivalent to 0.3 gentamicin base with: chlorobutanol (chloral derivative) 0.5%; white petroleum; mineral oil; petrolatum (and) lanolin alcohol; and purified water.

CLINICAL PHARMACOLOGY:

Corticosteroids suppress the inflammatory response to a variety of agents and they probably delay or slow healing. Since corticosteroids may inhibit the body's defense mechanism against infection, a concomitant antimicrobial drug may be used when this inhibition is considered to be clinically significant in a particular case.

The anti-infective component in gentamicin sulfate-prednisolone acetate is included to provide action against specific organisms susceptible to it. Gentamicin sulfate is active *in vitro* against susceptible strains of the following microorganisms: *Staphylococcus aureus, Streptococcus pyones, Streptococcus pneumoniae, Enterobacter aerogenes, Escherichia coli, Haemophilus influenzae, Klebsiella pneumoniae, Neisseria gonorrhoeae, Pseudomonas aeruginosa,* and *Serratia marcescens.*

When a decision to administer both a corticosteroid and an antimicrobial is made, the administration of such drugs in combination has the advantage of greater patient compliance and conveniences, with the added assurance that the appropriate dosage of both drugs is administered. When both types of drugs are in the same formulation, compatibility of ingredients is assured and the correct volume of drug is delivered and retained.

The relative potency of corticosteroids depends on the molecular structure, concentration, and release from the vehicle.

INDICATIONS AND USAGE:

gentamicin sulfate-prednisolone acetate suspension and ointment are indicated for steroid-responsive inflammatory ocular conditions for which a corticosteroid is indicated and where superficial bacterial ocular infection or a risk of bacterial ocular infection exists.

Ocular steroids are indicated in inflammatory conditions of the palpebral and bulbar conjunctiva, cornea, and anterior segment of the globe where the inherent risk of steroid use in certain infective conjunctivitises is accepted to obtain a diminution in edema and inflammation. They are also indicated in chronic anterior uveitis and corneal injury from chemical, radiation, or thermal burns or penetration of foreign bodies.

The use of a combination drug with an anti-infective component is indicated where the risk of superficial ocular infection is high or where there is an expectation that potentially dangerous numbers of bacteria will be present in the eye.

The particular anti-infective drug in this product is active against the following common bacterial eye pathogens: *Staphylococcus aureus,Streptococcus pyogenes, Streptococcus pneumoniae;Enterobacter aerogens, Escherichia coli, Haemophilus influenzae; Klebsiella pneumoniae, Neisseria gonorrhoeae, Pseudomonas aeruginosa,* and *Serratia marcescens.*

CONTRAINDICATIONS:

Liquifilm Sterile Ophthalmic Suspension: gentamicin sulfate-prednisolone acetate suspension is contraindicated in most viral diseases of the cornea and conjunctiva including epithelial herpes simplex keratitis (dendritic keratitis), vaccinia, and varicella, and also in mycobacterial infection of the eye and fungal diseases of the ocular structures. Gentamicin sulfate-prednisolone acetate suspension is also contraindicated in individuals with known or suspected hypersensitivity to any ingredients of this preparation or to other corticosteroids.

Sterile Ophthalmic Ointment: Epithelial herpes simplex keratitis (dendritic keratitis), vaccinia, varicella and many other viral diseases of the cornea and conjunctiva. Mycobacterial infection of the eye. Fungal diseases of the ocular structures. Hypersensitivity to a component of the mediation. (Hypersensitivity to the antibiotic component occurs at a higher rate than for other components.)

Gentamicin sulfate-prednisolone acetate S.O.P. is always contraindicated after uncomplicated removal of a corneal foreign body.

WARNINGS:

Liquifilm Sterile Ophthalmic Suspension: Prolonged use of corticosteroids may result in glaucoma with damage to the optic nerve, defects in visual acuity and fields of vision, and in posterior subcapsular cataract formation.

Prolonged use of corticosteroids may suppress the host response and thus increase the hazard of secondary ocular infections.

Various ocular diseases and long-term use of topical corticosteroids have been known to cause corneal and scleral thinning. Use of topical corticosteroids in the presence of thin corneal or scleral tissue may lead to perforation.

Acute purulent infections of the eye may be masked or enhanced by the prescience of corticosteroid medication.

If this product is used for 10 days or longer, intraocular pressure should be routinely monitored even though it may be difficult in children and uncooperative patients. Steroids should be used with caution in the presence of glaucoma. Intraocular pressure should be checked frequently.

The use of steroids after cataract surgery may delay healing and increase the incidence of bleb formation.

Use of ocular steroids may prolong the course and may exacerbate the severity of many viral infections of the eye (including herpes simplex). Employment of a corticosteroid medication in the treatment of patients with a history of herpes simplex requires great caution; frequent slit lamp microscopy is recommended.

Gentamicin sulfate-prednisolone acetate liquifilm sterile ophthalmic suspension is not for injection. It should never be injected subconjunctivally, nor should it be directly introduced into the anterior chamber of the eye.

Sterile Ophthalmic Ointment: Prolonged use may result in glaucoma, with damage to the optic nerve, defects in visual acuity and fields of vision, and in posterior subcapsular cataract formation. Prolonged use may suppress the host immune response and thus increase the hazard of secondary ocular infections. In those diseases causing thinning of the cornea or sclera, perforations have been known to occur with the use of topical steroids. In acute

WARNINGS: *(cont'd)*

purulent conditions of the eye, steroids may mask infection or enhance existing infection. If these products are used for 10 days or longer, intraocular pressure should be routinely monitored even though it may be difficult in children and uncooperative patients.

Employment of a steroid medication in the treatment of patients with a history of herpes simplex requires great caution. Gentamicin sulfate-prednisolone acetate is contraindicated in patients with active herpes simplex keratitis.

PRECAUTIONS:

General: Ocular irritation and punctuate keratitis have been associated with the use of gentamicin sulfate-prednisolone acetate. The initial prescription and renewal of the medication order beyond 20 milliliters should be made by a physician only after examination of the patient's intraocular pressure, examination of the patient with the aid of magnification such as slit lamp biomicroscopy and, where appropriate, fluorescein staining.

As fungal infections of the cornea are particularly prone to develop coincidentally with long-term local corticosteroid applications, fungal invasion should be suspected in any persistent corneal ulceration where a corticosteroid has been used or is in use.

Fungal cultures should be taken when appropriate.

Carcinogenesis, Mutagenesis, and Impairment of Fertility: There are no published carcinogenicity or impairment of fertility studies on gentamicin. Aminoglycoside antibiotics have been found to be non- mutagenic.

There are no published mutagenicity or impairment of fertility studies on prednisolone. Prednisolone has been reported to be non-carcinogenic.

Pregnancy Category C: Gentamicin has been shown to depress body weight, kidney weight and median glomerular counts in newborn rats when administered systemically to pregnant rats in daily doses approximately 500 times the maximum recommended ophthalmic human dose. There are no adequate and well-controlled studies in pregnant women. Gentamicin should be used during pregnancy only if the potential benefit justifies the potential risk to the fetus.

Prednisolone has been shown to be teratogenic in mice when given in doses 1-10 times the human ocular dose. Dexamethasone, hydrocortisone and prednisolone were applied to both eyes of pregnant mice five times per day on days 10 through 13 of gestation. A significant increase in the incidence of cleft palate was observed in the fetuses of the treated mice. There are no adequate well-controlled studies in pregnant women. Gentamicin sulfate-prednisolone acetate suspension should be used during pregnancy only if the potential benefit justifies the potential risk to the fetus.

Nursing Mothers: It is not known whether topical codministration of corticosteroids could result in sufficient systemic absorption to produce detectable quantities in human milk. Systemically administered corticosteroids appear in human milk and could suppress growth, interfere with endogenous corticosteroid production, or cause other untoward effects. Because of the potential for serious adverse reactions in nursing infants from gentamicin sulfate-prednisolone acetate suspension, a decision should be made whether to discontinue the nursing while the drug is being administered or to discontinue the medication.

Pediatric Use: Safety and effectiveness in children have not been established.

Information for the Patient: (Gentamicin sulfate-prednisolone acetate liquifilm sterile ophthalmic suspension only) If inflammation or pain persists longer than 48 hours or becomes aggravated, the patient should be advised to discontinue use of the medication and consult a physician.

This product is sterile when packaged. To prevent contamination, care should be taken to avoid touching the bottle tip to eyelids or to any other surface. The use of this bottle by more than one person may spread infection. Protect from freezing and from heat of 40°C (104° F) and above. Keep out of reach of children. Shake well before using.

ADVERSE REACTIONS:

Adverse reactions have occurred with steroid/anti-infective combination drugs which can be attributed to the steroid component, the anti- infective component, or the combination. Exact incidence figures are not available since no denominator of treated patients is available.

Reactions occurring most often from the presence of the anti-infective ingredient are allergic sensitizations. The reactions due to the steroid component in decreasing order of frequency are: elevation of intraocular pressure (IOP) with possible development of glaucoma, and infrequent optic nerve damage; posterior subcapsular cataract formation; and delayed wound healing.

Burning, stinging and other symptoms of irritation have been reported with gentamicin sulfate-prednisolone acetate. Superficial punctate keratitis has been reported occasionally with onset occurring typically after several days of use.

Secondary Infection: The development of secondary infection has occurred after use of combinations containing steroids and antimicrobials. Fungal infections of the cornea are particularly prone to develop coincidentally with long-term applications of steroid. The possibility of fungal invasion must be considered in any persistent corneal ulceration where steroid treatment has been used. (See WARNINGS)

Secondary bacterial ocular infection following suppression of host responses also occurs.

DOSAGE AND ADMINISTRATION:

Liquifilm Sterile Opthalmic Suspension: Instill one drop into the conjunctival sac two to four times daily. During the initial 24 to 48 hours, the dosing frequency may be increased, if necessary. Care should be taken not to discontinue therapy prematurely.

Not more than 20 milliliters should be prescribed initially, and the prescription should not be refilled without further evaluation as outlined in PRECAUTIONS above.

Sterile Ophthalmic Ointment: A small amount (1/2 inch ribbon) of ointment should be applied in the conjunctival sac one to three times daily. Care should be taken not to discontinue therapy prematurely.

Not more than 8 grams should be prescribed initially and the prescription should not be refilled without further evaluation as outlined in PRECAUTIONS above.

HOW SUPPLIED:

Liquifilm Sterile Opthalmic Suspension: Gentamicin sulfate-prednisolone acetate liquifilm sterile ophthalmic suspension is supplied in plastic dropper bottles.

Note: Store at room temperature. Avoid excessive heat, 40°C (104°F) and above. Protect from freezing. **Shake well before using.**

Sterile Opthalmic Suspension: Gentamicin sulfate-prednisolone acetate S.O.P. sterile opthalmic ointment is supplied in ophthalmic ointment tubes.

Note: Store at controlled room temperature between 15° - 30°C (59°-86°F).

(Pred-G Liquifilm, Allergan, Inc., 3/94)

(Pred-G S.O.P., Allergan, Inc., 12/89)

HOW SUPPLIED - EQUIVALENTS NOT AVAILABLE:

Ointment - Ophthalmic - 0.3 %/0.6 %

3.5 g	$17.77	PRED-G SOP STERILE OPHTHALMIC, Allergan	00023-0066-04

Solution - Ophthalmic - 1 %

2 ml	**$6.69**	**PRED-G, Allergan**	**00023-0106-02**
5 ml	**$18.29**	**PRED-G, Allergan**	**00023-0106-05**
10 ml	**$33.11**	**PRED-G, Allergan**	**00023-0106-10**

GLATIRAMER ACETATE *(003332)*

CATEGORIES: Autonomic Drugs; Biologicals; Immuno Response Modifier; Multiple Sclerosis; Relapsing-Remitting Multiple Sclerosis; Pregnancy Category B; FDA Approved 1997 Feb

BRAND NAMES: **Copaxone**

PRIMARY ICD9: 340 (Multiple Sclerosis)

DESCRIPTION:

Copaxone is a steril lyophilized material containing 20 mg of glatiramer acetate and 40 mg of mannitol. Glatiramer acetate is the acetate salts of synthetic polypeptides, containing four naturally occurring amino acids: L-glutamic acid, L-alanine, L-tyrosine and L-lysine with an average molar fraction of 0.141, 0.095 and 0.338, respectively. The average molecular weight of glatiramer acetate is 4700-11,000 daltons. Copaxone is a white to off-white lyophilized powder supplied in single-use vials for subcutaneous administration after reconstitution with diluent supplied (Sterile Water for Injection).

CLINICAL PHARMACOLOGY:

MECHANISM OF ACTION

The mechanism(s) by which glatiramer acetate exerts its effects in patients with Multiple Sclerosis (MS) is (are) unknown.

Glatiramer acetate is thought to act, however, by modifying immune processes that are currently held to be responsible for the pathogensis of MS. This view of glatiramer acetate derive from knowledge that reduces the incidence and severity of experimental allergic encephalomyelitise (EAE) - a condition induced in several animal species through immunization against CNS derived material containing myelin and often used as an experimental animal model of MS.

Because glatiramer acetate can modify immune function, concerns exist about its potential to alter naturally occurring immune responses. Results of a limited battery of tests designed to evaluate the risk produced no finding of concern; nevertheless, there is no logical way to absolutely exclude this possibility (see PRECAUTIONS).

PHARMACOKINETICS

Pharmacokinetics studies in humans have not been performed. It is assumed, however, based in part on the results of animal studies, that a substantial fraction of subcutaneous injection of glatiramer acetate is hydrolyzed locally. Some fraction of injection material is presumed to enter the lymphatic circulation, enabling it to reach regionaly lymph nodes, and some may enter the systemic circulation intact.

CLINICAL STUDIES:

Evidence supporting the effectiveness of glatiramer acetate in decreasing the frequency of relapses in patients with Relapsing-Remitting Multiple Sclerosis (RR MS) derives from two placebo controlled trials, both of which used a glatiramer acetate dose of 20 mg/day. (No other dose has been studied in placebo controlled trials of Relapsing-Remitting Multiple Sclerosis.)

One trial was performed at a single center. It enrolled 50 patients (glatiramer acetate, 25; placebo, 25) who were randomized to receive daily doses of glatiramer acetate, 20 mg subcutaneously, or placebo. Patients were diagnosed with RR MS by standard criteria, and had at least 2 exacerbations during the 2 years immediately preceding enrollment. Patients were ambulatory, as evidenced by a score of no more than 6 on the Kurtzke Expanded Disability Scale Score (EDSS), a standard scale ranging from 0-Normal to 10-Death due to MS. A score of 6 is defined as one at which a patient is still ambulatory with assistance; a score of 7 means the patient must use a wheelchair.

Patients were seen every 3 months for 2 years, as well as within several days of a presumed exacerbation. In order for an exacerbation to be confirmed, a blinded neurologist had to document objective neurologic signs, as well as document the existence of other criteria (*e.g.,* the persistence of the lesion for at least 48 hours).

The protocol specified primary outcome measure was the proportion of patients in each treatment group who remained exacerbation free for the 2 years of the trial, but two other important outcomes were also specified as endpoints: the frequency of attacks during the trial, and the change in number of attacks compared to the rate of attacks in the previous 2 years.

TABLE 1 presents the results of analyses of the three outcomes described above, as well as several protocol specified secondary measures. These analyses are based on the intent-to-treat population (*i.e.,* all patients who received at least 1 dose of treatment and who had at least 1 on-treatment assessment):

TABLE 1

Outcome	Glatiramer Acetate (N=25)	Placebo (N=25)	P-Value
% Relapse Free	14/25 (56%)	7/25 (28%)	0.085
Mean Relapse Frequency	0.6/2 years	2.4/2 years	0.005
Change in Relapse Rate	3.2	1.6	0.025
Mean Time to First Relapse (days)	>700	150	0.03
% of Patients Progression Free*	20/25 (80%)	13/25 (52%)	0.07

* Progression defined as an increase of at least 1 point on the EDSS that persists for at least 3 consecutive months.

The second trial was multicenter trial of design similiar to the first study, and was performed in 11 U.S. centers. A total of 251 patients (glatiramer acetate 125; placebo, 126) were enrolled. The primary outcome measure was the Mean 2 Year Relapse Rate. TABLE 2 presents the results of the analysis of this outcome for the intent-to-treat population, as well as other secondary measures:

In both sudies glatiramer acetate exhibited a clear beneficial effect on relapse rate, and it is on this basis that glatiramer acetate is considered effective.

TABLE 2

Outcome	Glatiramer Acetate	Placebo	P-Value
Mean Relapse Rate	1.19/2 years	1.68/2 years	0.055
% Relapse Free	42/125 (34%)	34/126 (27%)	0.25
Mean Time to First Relapse (days)	287	198	0.23
% of Patients Progression Free	98/125 (78%)	95/126 (75%)	0.48
Mean Change in EDSS	-0.05	+0.21	0.023

INDICATIONS AND USAGE:

Glatiramer acetate is indicated for reduction of the frequency of relapses in patients with Relapsing-Remitting Multiple Scelerosis.

CONTRAINDICATIONS:

Glatiramer acetate is contraindicated in patients with known hypersensitivity to glatiramer acetate or mannitol.

WARNINGS:

The only recommended route to administration of glatiramer acetate injection is by the subcutaneous route. Glatiramer acetate should not be administered by the intravenous route.

PRECAUTIONS:

GENERAL

Patients should be instructed in self-injection techniques to assure the safe administration of glatiramer acetate. (see Information for the Patient and the glatiramer acetate PATIENT PACKAGE INSERT). Based on current data, no special caution is required for patients operating an automobile or using complex machinery.

CONSIDERATIONS INVOLVING THE USE OF A PRODUCT CAPABLE OF MODIFYING IMMUNE RESPONSE

Because glatiramer acetate can modify immune response, consideration must be given to the possiblity that it could interfere with useful immune function. For example, treatment with glatiramer acetate might in theory interfere with the recognition of foreign antigens in a way that would undermine the body's defenses against infections and tumor surveillance. There is no evidence that it does so, but there has as yet been no systematic evaluation of this risk.

Because glatiramer acetate is an antigenic material it is possible that its use may lead to the induction of host responses that are untoward. Although there is no evidence that this occurs in humans, systematic surveillance for these effects has not been undertaken. Studies in both the rat and monkey, however, have suggested that immune complexes are deposited in the renal glomeruli. Furthermore, in a controlled trial of 125 patients with Relapsing-Remitting Multiple Sclerosis (RR MS) given glatiramer acetate, 20 mg subcutaneously every day for 2 years, serum IgG levels reached approximately 3 times baseline values of 80% of patients within 3 to 6 months of initiation of treatment. These values returned to about 50% greater than baseline during the remainder of treatment.

Although glatiramer acetate is intended to minimize the autoimmune response to myelin, there is the possibility that continued alteration of cellular immunity due to chronic treatment with glatiramer acetate might result in untoward effects.

INFORMATION FOR THE PATIENT

To assure safe and effective use of glatiramer acetate, the following information and instructions should be given to the patients.

1. Inform your physician if you are pregnant, if you are planning to have a child, or it you become pregnant while taking this medication.

2. Inform your physician if you are nursing.

3. Do not change the dose or dosing schedule without consulting your physician.

4. Do not stop taking the drug without consulting your physician.

Patients should be instructed in the use of aseptic techniques when administering glatiramer acetate. Appropriate instructions for reconstitution of glatiramer acetate and self-injection should be given, including a careful review of the glatiramer acetate PATIENT PACKAGE INSERT. The first injection should be performed under the supervision of an appropriately qualified health care professional. Patient understanding and use of aseptic self-injection techniques and procedures should be periodically reevaluated. Patients should be cautioned against the re-use of needles or syringes and instructed in safe disposal procedures. A puncture-resistant container for disposal of used needles and syringes should be used by the patient. Patients should be instructed on the safe disposal of full containers.

Awareness of Adverse Reactions: Patients should be advised about the common adverse events associated with the use of glatiramer acetate (see ADVERSE REACTIONS).

LABORATORY TESTS

Data collected during premarketing development do not suggest the necessity for routine laboratory monitoring.

DRUG/LABORATORY TEST INTERACTIONS

None known.

CARCINOGENESIS, MUTAGENESIS, AND IMPAIRMENT OF FERTILITY

Results of tests to assess the carcinogenic potential of glatiramer acetate in mice and rats are unavailable; these studies are in progress.

Glatiramer acetate was not mutagenic in four strains of *Salmonella typhimurium* and two strains of *Escherichia coli* (Ames test) or in the *in vitro* mouse lymphoma assay in L5178Y cells. Glatiramer acetate was clastogenic in two separate *in vitro* chromosomal aberation assays in cultured human lymphocytes; it was not clastogenic in an *in vitro* mouse bone marrow micronucleus assay.

In a multi-generation reproduction and fertility study in rats, glatiramer acetate at subcutaneous doses up to 36 mg/kg (18 times the recommended human daily dose of 20 mg on a mg/m^2 basis) had no adverse effects on reproductive parameters.

PREGNANCY CATEGORY B

Teratogenic Effects: No adverse effects on embryofetal development occurred in reproduction studies in rats and rabbits receiving subcutaneous doses up to 37.5 mg/kg of glatiramer acetate during the period of organogenesis (18 and 36 times the human dose of 20 mg on a mg/m^2 basis, respectively). In a prenatal and postnatal study, in which rats received subcutaneous glatiramer acetate at doses up to 36 mg/kg for day 15 of pregnancy throughout lactation, no significant effects on delivery or on offspring growth and development were observed. There are, however, no adequate and well-controlled studies in pregnant women. Because animal reproduction studies are not always predictive of human response, glatiramer acetate should be used during pregnancy only if clearly needed.

Non-Teratogenic Effects: In a prenatal and postnatal study, in which rats received subcutaneous glatiramer acetate at doses up to 36 mg/kg from day 15 of pregnancy throughout lactation, no significant effects on delivery or on offspring growth and development were observed.

PRECAUTIONS: *(cont'd)*

LABOR AND DELIVERY

In a prenatal and postnatal study, in which rats received subcutaneous glatiramer acetate at doses up to 36 mg/kg from day 15 of pregnancy throughout lactation, no significant effects on delivery or on offspring growth and development were observed. The relevance of these findings to humans is unknown.

NURSING MOTHERS

It is not known whether glatiramer acetate is excreted in human milk. Because many drugs are excreted in human milk, caution should be exercised when glatiramer acetate is administered to a nursing woman.

PEDIATRIC USE

The safety and effectiveness of glatiramer acetate have not been established in individuals below 18 years of age.

GERIATRIC USE

Glatiramer acetate has not been studied specifically in elderly patients.

IMPAIRED RENAL FUNCTION

The pharmacokinetics of glatiramer acetate in patients with impaired renal function has not been determined.

DRUG INTERACTIONS:

Interactions between glatiramer acetate and other drugs have not been fully evaluated. Results from existing clinical trials do not suggest any significant interactions of glatiramer acetate with therapies commonly used in MS patients. This includes the concurrent use of corticosteroids for up to 28 days. Glatiramer acetate has not been formally evaluated in combination with Interferon beta. However, 10 patients who switched from therapy with Interferon beta to glatiramer acetate have not reported any serious and unexpected adverse events thought to be related to treatment.

ADVERSE REACTIONS:

Approximately 850 patients with MS and 50 healthy volunteers have received at least one dose for glatiramer acetate. In controlled clinical trials the most commonly observed adverse experiences associated with the use of glatiramer acetate and not seen at an equivalent frequency among placebo treated patients were: injection site reactions, vasodilation, chest pain, asthenia, infection, pain, nausea, arthralgia, anxiety, and hypertonia.

Approximately 8% of the 893 subjects receiving glatiramer acetate discontinued treatment due to an adverse event. The adverse events most commonly associated with discontinuation were: injection site reaction (6.5%), vasodilation, unintended pregnancy, depression, dyspnea, urticaria, tachycardia, dizziness, and tremor.

IMMEDIATE POST-INJECTION REACTION

Approximately 10% of patients with Multiple Sclerosis exposed to glatiramer acetate in premarketing studies experienced a constellation of symptoms immediately after injection that could include flushing, chest pain, palpitations, anxiety, dyspnea, constriction of the throat, and urticaria. The symptoms were invariably transient and self-limited and did not require specific treatment. In general, these symptoms have their onset several months after the initiation of treatment, although they may occur earlier in the course of treatment, and a given patient may experience one or several episodes of these symptoms. Whether or not this constellation of symptoms actually represents a specific syndrome is uncertain.

Whether these episodes are mediated by an immunologic or non-immunologic mechanism, or whether several similar episodes seen in a given patient have identical mechanisms is unknown.

CHEST PAIN

Approximately 26% of glatiramer acetate patients in the multicenter controlled trial (compared to 10% of placebo patients) experienced at least one episode of what was described as transient chest pain. While some of these episodes occurred in the context of Immediate Post-Injection Reaction, many did not. The temporal relationship of the chest pain to an injection of glatiramer acetate was not always known, although the pain was transient (usually lasting only a few minutes), often unassociated with other symptoms, and appeared to have no important clinical sequelae. EKG monitoring was not performed during any of these episodes. Some patients experienced more than one such episode, and episodes usually began at least 1 month after the initiation of treatment. The pathogenesis of this symptom is unknown.

INCIDENCE IN CONTROLLED CLINICAL STUDIES

The following table lists treatment emergent signs and symptoms that occurred in at least 2% of patients with MS treated with glatiramer acetate in placebo controlled trials and that were numerically more common in the patients treated with glatiramer acetate than in placebo-treated patients. These trials include the two controlled trials in Relapsing-Remitting Multiple Sclerosis patients and a controlled trial in patients with Chronic Progressive Multiple Sclerosis. Adverse events were usually mild in intensity.

The prescriber should be aware that these figures cannot be used to predict the frequency of adverse experiences in the course of usual medical practice where patient characteristics and other factors may differ from those prevailing during clinical studies. Similarly, the cited frequencies cannot be directly compared with figures obtained from other clinical investigations involving different treatments, uses, or investigators. An inspection of these frequencies, however, does provide the prescriber with one basis to estimate relative contribution of drug and non-drug factors to the adverse event incidences in the population studied.

Other events which occurred in at least 2% of patients but were present at equal or greater rates in the placebo group included:

Body as a whole: Headache, injection site ecchymosis, accidental injury, abdominal pain, allergic rhinitis, neck rigidity, and malaise.

Digestive System: Dyspepsia, constipation, dysphagia, fecal incontinence, flatulence, nausea and vomiting, gastritis, gingivitis, periodontal abscess, and dry mouth.

Musculoskeletal: Myasthenia and myalgia.

Nervous System: Dizziness, hypesthesia, paresthesia, insomnia, depression, dysesthesia, incoordination, somnolence, abnormal gait, amnesia, emotional liability, Lhermitte's sign, abnormal thinking, twitching, euphoria, and sleep disorder.

Respiratory System: Pharyngitis, sinusitis, increased cough and laryngitis.

Skin and Appendages: Acne, alopecia, and nail disorder.

Special Senses: Abnormal vision, diplopia, amblyopia, eye pain, conjunctivitis, tinnitus, taste perversion, and deafness.

Urogenital System: Urinary tract infection, urinary frequency, urinary incontinence, urinary retention, dysuria, metrorrhagia, breast pain, and vaginitis.

Data on adverse events occurring in the controlled clinical trials were analyzed to evaluate differences based on sex. No clinically significant differences were identified. Ninety-two percent of patients in these clinical trials were caucasian. This is representative of the population of patients with Multiple Sclerosis. In addition, the vast majority of patients

ADVERSE REACTIONS: *(cont'd)*

TABLE 3 Controlled Trials in Patients with Multiple Sclerosis: Incidence of Glatiramer Acetate Adverse Experience ≥2% and More Frequent than Placebo

Preferred Term	Glatiramer Acetate (N=201) N	%	Placebo (N=206) N	%
Body as Whole				
Asthenia	83	41	78	38
Back Pain	33	16	30	15
Bacterial Infection	11	5	9	4
Chest Pain	43	21	22	11
Chills	8	4	2	1
Cyst	5	2	1	0
Face Edema	12	6	2	1
Fever	17	8	15	7
Flu Syndrome	38	19	35	17
Infection	101	50	99	48
Injection Site Erythema	132	66	40	19
Injection Site Hemorrhage	11	5	6	3
Injection Site Induration	26	13	1	0
Injection Site Inflammation	98	49	22	11
Injection Site Mass	54	27	21	10
Injection Site Pain	147	73	78	38
Injection Site Pruritus	80	40	12	6
Injection Site Urticaria	10	5	0	0
Injection Site Welt	22	11	5	2
Neck Pain	16	8	9	4
Pain	56	28	52	25
Cardiovascular System				
Migraine	10	5	5	2
Palpitations	35	17	16	8
Syncope	10	5	5	2
Tachycardia	11	5	8	4
Vasodilation	55	27	21	10
Digestive System				
Anorexia	17	8	15	7
Diarrhea	25	12	23	11
Gastroenteritis	6	3	2	1
Gastroitestinal Disorder	10	5	8	4
Nausea	44	22	34	17
Vomiting	13	6	8	4
Hemic and Lymphatic System				
Ecchymosis	16	8	13	6
Lymphadenopathy	25	12	12	6
Metabolic and Nutritional				
Edema	5	3	1	0
Peripheral Edema	14	7	8	4
Weight Gain	7	3	0	0
Musculoskeletal System				
Arthralgia	49	24	39	19
Nervous System				
Agitation	8	4	4	2
Anxiety	46	23	40	19
Confusion	5	2	1	0
Foot Drop	6	3	4	2
Hypertonia	44	22	37	18
Nervousness	4	2	2	1
Nystagmus	5	2	2	1
Speech Disorder	5	2	3	1
Tremor	14	7	7	3
Vertigo	12	6	11	5
Respiratory System				
Bronchitis	18	9	12	6
Dyspnea	38	19	15	7
Laryngismus	10	5	7	3
Rhinitis	29	14	27	13
Skin and Appendages				
Erythema	8	4	4	2
Herpes Simplex	8	4	6	3
Pruritus	36	18	26	13
Rash	37	18	30	15
Skin Nodule	4	2	1	0
Sweating	31	15	21	10
Urticaria	9	4	5	2
Special Senses				
Ear Pain	15	7	12	6
Eye Disorder	8	4	1	0
Urogenital System				
Dysmenorrhea	12	6	10	5
Urinary Urgency	20	10	17	8
Vaginal Moniliasis	16	8	9	4

treated with glatiramer acetate were between the ages of 18 and 45. Consequently, inadequate data are available to perform an analysis of the incidence of adverse events related to clinically relevant age subgroups.

Laboratory analyses were performed on all patients participating in the clinical program for glatiramer acetate. Clinically significant laboratory values for hematology, chemistry, and urinalysis were similar for both glatiramer acetate and placebo groups in blinded clinical trials. No patient receiving glatiramer acetate withdrew from any trial due to abnormal laboratory findings.

OTHER ADVERSE EXPERIENCE OBSERVED DURING ALL CLINICAL TRIALS

Other Adverse Events: Glatiramer acetate has been administered to approximately 900 individuals during all clinical trials, only some of which were placebo-controlled. During these trials, all adverse events were recorded by the clinical investigators using terminology of their own choosing. To provide a meaningful estimate of the proportion of individuals having adverse events, similar types of events were grouped into a smaller number of standardized categories using COSTART II dictionary terminology. The frequencies presented represent the proportion of the 860 individuals exposed to glatiramer acetate who had data available for this determination. All reported events that occurred at least twice and potentially important events occurring once, are included except those already listed in the previous table, those too general to be informative, trival events, and those not reasonably related to the drug.

Events are further classified within body system categories and enumerated in order of decreasing frequency using the following definitions: Frequent adverse events are defined as those occurring in at least 1/100 patients; infrequent adverse events are those occurring in 1/100 to 1/1000 patients.

ADVERSE REACTIONS: *(cont'd)*

Body as a Whole: *Frequent:* Injection site edema, injection site atrophy, abscess; *Infrequent:* Injection site hematoma, injection site fibrosis, moon face, cellulitis, generalized edema, hernia, injection site abscess, serum sickness, suicide attempt, injection site hypertrophy, injection site melanosis, lipoma and photosensitivity reaction.

Cardiovascular: *Frequent:*Hypertension; *Infrequent:*Hypotension, midsystolic click, systolic murmur, atrial fibrillation, bradycardia, fourth heart sound, postural hypotension, and varicose veins.

Digestive: *Infrequent:*Dry mouth, stomatitis, burning sensation on tongue, cholecystis, colitis, esophageal ulcer, esophagitis, gastrointestinal carcinoma, gum hemorrhage, hepatomegaly, increased appetite, melena, mouth ulceration, pancreas disorder, pancreatitis, rectal hemorrhage, tenesmus, tongue discoloration, and duodenal ulcer.

Endocrine: *Infrequent:*Goiter, hyperthyroidism, and hypothyroidism.

Gastrointestinal: *Frequent:*Bowel urgency, oral moniliasis, salivary gland enlargement, tooth carries, and ulcerative stomatitis.

Hemic and Lymphatic: *Infrequent:*Leukopenia, anemia, cyanosis, eosinophilia, hematemesis, lymphedema, pancytopenia, and splenomegaly.

Metabolic and Nutritional: *Infrequent:*Weight loss, alcohol intolerance, Cushing's syndrome, gout, abnormal healing, and xanthoma.

Musculoskeletal: *Infrequent:* Arthritis, muscle atrophy, bone pain, bursitis, kidney pain, muscle disorder, myopathy, osteomyelitis, tendon pain, and tenosynovitis.

Nervous: *Frequent:*Abnormal dreams, emotional lability, and stupor; *Infrequent:*Ataxia, circumoral paresthesia, depersonalization, hallucinations, hostility, hypokinesia, coma, concentration disorder, facial paralysis, decreased libido, manic reaction, memory impairment, myoclonus, paranoid reaction, paraplegia, psychotic depression, and transient stupor.

Respiratory: *Frequent:* Hyperventilation; *Infrequent:*Asthma, pneumonia, epistaxis, hypoventilation, and voice alteration.

Skin and Appendages: *Frequent:* Eczema, herpes zoster, pustular rash, skin atrophy, and warts; *Infrequent:*Dry skin, skin hypertrophy, dermatitis, furunculosis, psoriasis, angioedema, contact dermatitis, erythema nodosum, fungal dermatitis, maculopapular rash, pigmentation, benign skin neoplasm, skin carcinoma, skin striae, and vesiculobullous rash.

Special Senses: *Infrequent:*Dry eyes, otitis externa, ptosis, cataract, corneal ulcer, mydriasis, optic neuritis, photophobia, and taste loss.

Urogenital: *Frequent:*Amenorrhea, hematuria, impotence, menorrhagia, suspicious papanicolaou smear, and vaginal hemorrhage; *Infrequent:*Vaginitis, flank pain (kidney), abortion, breast engorgement, breast enlargement, carcinoma *in situ* cervix, fibocystic breast, kidney calculus, nocturia, ovarian cyst, priapism, pyelonephritis, abnormal sexual function, and urethritis.

DRUG ABUSE AND DEPENDENCE:

No evidence or experience suggests that abuse or dependence occurs with glatiramer acetate therapy; however the risk of dependence has not been systematically evaluated.

DOSAGE AND ADMINISTRATION:

The recommended dose of glatiramer acetate for the treatment of Relapsing-Remitting MS is 20 mg/day injected subcutaneously.

INSTRUCTIONS FOR USE

To reconstitute lyophilized glatiramer acetate for injection, use sterile syringe and needle to transfer the diluent supplied, Sterile Water for Injection, into the glatiramer acetate vial. Gently swirl the vial of glatiramer acetate and let stand at room temperature until solid material is completely dissolved. Inspect the reconstituted product visually and discard or return the product to the pharmacist before use if it contains particulate matter.

Soon after reconstitution, withdraw the solution into a sterile syringe fitted with a new 27 gauge needle and inject the solution subcutaneously. Sites for self-injection include arm, abdomen, hips, and thighs. A vial is suitable for single use only; unused portions should be discarded. (See PATIENT PACKAGE INSERT for self-injection procedure.)

STABILITY

The reconstituted product contains no preservative; it should be used immediately. Before reconstitution with diluent, store at -20° C to -10° C (freeze).

PATIENT PACKAGE INSERT:

To reconstitute lyophilized glatiramer acetate (glatiramer acetate for injection, formerly known as copolymer-1) use a sterile syringe and needle to transfer the diluent (Sterile Water for Injection) supplied into the glatiramer acetate vial.

1. Extract the diluent from the clear glass vial into the syringe.

2. Inject the diluent from the syringe into the amber glass vial containing the sterile lyophilized material.

3. Swirl the vial gently and allow it to stand at room temperature until the solid material is completely dissolved (this process takes about 5 minutes).

SELF-INJECTION PROCEDURE

Your physician has prescribed glatiramer acetate a drug that has been shown to be effective in treating Relapsing-Remitting Multiple Sclerosis. Although it is not a cure, patients treated with glatiramer acetate experience fewer relapses.

Glatiramer acetate is not recommended for use in pregnancy. Therefore, inform your physician if you are pregnant, if you are planning to have a child, or if you become pregnant while you are taking this medication.

Inform your physician if you are nursing.

Do not change the dose or dosing schedule without consulting your physician.

Do not stop taking the drug without consulting your physician.

The most commonly observed adverse reactions associated with the use of glatiramer acetate are redness, pain, inflammation, itching, or a lump at the of injection. These reactions are usually mild and most often do not require professional treatment.

Some patients have reported a transient, self-limited reaction immediately after injecting glatiramer acetate. This reaction is characterized by flushing or chest tightness with heart palpitations, anxiety, and difficulty in breathing. In clinical trials these symptoms occurred rarely, generally appeared within minutes of an injection, lasted approximately 15 minutes, and resolved without further problems.

After you inject glatiramer acetate, if you notice hives (an itchy, blotchy swelling of the skin) or severe pain at the injection site, call your physician immediately.

Your Copaxone prescription includes two types of vials: brown vials containing glatiramer acetate and clear vials of sterile water. Separate the vials.

Store the vials of glatiramer acetate in the freezer immediately after bringing them home.

Store the vials labeled "Sterile Water for Injection" (diluent) at room temperature.

Keep out of the reach of children.

PATIENT PACKAGE INSERT: *(cont'd)*

INSTRUCTIONS FOR INJECTING GLATIRAMER ACETATE

The following instructions will help you through three basic steps – gathering the materials, adding sterile water (diluent) to the dry glatiramer acetate, and finally injecting yourself.

Gathering the Materials

1) First, assemble the items you will need on a clean cloth or towel in a well-lighted area:

One brown vial of glatiramer acetate

One clear vial of diluent

One 3 cc* syringe with 25 gauge, 5/8" needle (used for adding diluent to the glatiramer acetate)

One 1 cc syringe with 27 gauge, 1/2" needle (used for the actual injection into your body)

A few alcohol wipes

A dry cotton ball

***Please Note:** One cubic meter centimeter (cc) represents the same amount as one milliliter (ml). In this labeling, we always refer to measured volume as "cc" but you will also find volume presented as "ml" in other articles and brochures.

2) To prevent infection, wash and dry your hands. Do not touch your hair or skin afterwards.

3) Remove one 3 cc syringe from its protective wrapper by peeling back the paper label.

4) Make sure the needle is tightly in place by slightly twisting the plastic cover over the needle. Do not touch the needle itself, and do not remove the plastic cover yet.

5) Place the syringe on the clean surface.

6) Remove the plastic cover from the brown glatiramer acetate vial, and use the alcohol wipe to clean the rubber top. Do not touch the rubber top after it is cleaned.

7) Next, remove the plastic cover from the diluent vial, and clean the rubber top with a fresh alcohol wipe. Do not touch the rubber top after it is cleaned.

8) Let both rubber tops dry a few seconds.

Important:

Don't touch the top of the vial or the needle in order to keep things sterile.

Use only the sterile water provided when reconstituting glatiramer acetate.

Questions? Contact your physician or nurse before reconstituting and injecting glatiramer acetate. You may also contact your nurse counselor if you have enrolled in the Shared Solutions program by calling 1-800-887-8100.

Reconstituting Glatiramer Acetate

1) Take the larger syringe (3 cc) in one hand and pull the cover straight off the needle with the other hand. Never touch the needle.

2) Pull the plunger back to draw 1.1 cc of air into the syringe.

Read the Syringe

Syringes often have two scales for measuring volume printed on the barrel. Use the scale labeled "cc" or "ml." Do not use the scale labeled "M."

3) Insert the needle through the rubber top of the sterile water vial and push the plunger all the way in.

4) Then turn the vial upside down, make sure the needle tip is below the level of liquid, and pull the plunger back to withdraw 1.1 cc of diluent into the syringe.

5) Pull the syringe out of the vial, and place the vial on the clean surface.

Are You Left Handed? If you are left-handed, do what comes naturally. You will probably find it most comfortable to hold the syringe in your left hand, and hold the vial between thumb and forefinger of your right hand.

6) With the glatiramer acetate vial still on the table, insert the needle through the rubber top and slowly inject the diluent into the vial. The best way is to point the needle toward the inside wall of the vial, instead of injecting the diluent directly onto the cake of drug.

7) Remove the needle and syringe from the glatiramer acetate vial.

8) Replace the plastic needle cover and dispose of the needle and syringe in a safe, hard-walled container, according to your physician's instructions.

9) Gently swirl the vial until all the medication dissolves and the solution looks clear. Do not shake the vial. Inspect it for particles. Do not use it if any are present.

10) Let the vial sit and warm up for about 5 minutes.

Preparing the Injection Syringe

1) Take the smaller syringe (1.0 cc) from its package and twist the plastic needle cover slightly to make sure the needle is tightly in place. Remove the cover from the needle without touching the needle.

2) Pull the plunger back to the 1.0 cc mark.

3) Insert the needle into the rubber top of the reconstituted glatiramer acetate vial and push the plunger all the way in to inject the air.

4) Then slowly withdraw the solution into the syringe to the 1.0 cc mark. Make sure the needle tip is below the level of the solution.

5) With the vial and syringe still upside down, and the needle still in the vial, check the syringe for air bubbles.

6) Tap the side of the syringe to make the air bubbles float to the top of the syringe.

7) Inject the air back into the vial. Now you will probably need to draw a little more solution into the syringe to bring the level back to the 1.0 cc mark.

8) Make sure your dose is correct by checking that the position of the plunger is at the 1.0 cc mark.

9) Then remove the needle from the vial, put the plastic cover back into the needle, and place it on a clean surface.

Giving Yourself the Injection

Before you begin the procedure to self-inject the glatiramer acetate dose, note these important points:

Decide where you will inject yourself. There are seven injection sites on your body, and you should not use any site more than once each week. (Marking a calendar will help you keep track of the sites you have used each day.)

Be consistent. Give yourself the injection at the same time each day. Choose a time when you feel strongest.

Have a friend or relative with you. You may have had a friend attend the injection training session as your assistant. Especially when you fist start giving yourself injections, your assistant should be with you.

Injection Sites

1) Clean the injection site with a fresh alcohol wipe, and let it dry.

2) Pick up the 1.0 cc syringe you already filled with glatiramer acetate as you would a pencil, using the hand you write with. Remove the plastic cover from the needle.

3) Then pinch about a 2-inch fold of skin between thumb and index finger.

PATIENT PACKAGE INSERT: *(cont'd)*

4) Insert the needle into the 2-inch fold of skin. It may help to steady your hand by resting the heel of your hand against your body.

5) When the needle is all the way in, release the fold of skin.

6) Inject the medication by holding the syringe steady while pushing down on the plunger. The injection should take just a few seconds.

How Do I Reach The Upper Back Portions Of My Arms: For these two injection sites, it is not possible to pinch 2 inches of skin with one hand and inject yourself with the other hand. Ask your nurse for instruction on how to use these sites.

7) Pull the needle straight out.

8) Press a dry cotton ball on the injection site for a few seconds, but do not massage it.

9) Put the plastic cover back on the needle.

10) Dispose of both needles, both syringes, and the used vials in a safe, hard-walled container, according to your physician's instructions and the laws of your state.

If you experience dizziness, skin eruptions with irritation, sweating, chest pain, difficulty breathing, or other uncomfortable changes in your general health, call your physician immediately.

If symptoms become severe, call 911 or the appropriate emergency phone number in your area. Make no more injections until the physician tells you to begin again. Be sure to inform your physician about any side effects.

Proper Use Of Needles And Syringes: Needles, syringes, and vials should be used for only one injection. Place all used syringes, needles, and vials in a hard-walled plastic container, such as a liquid laundry detergent container. Keep the cover of this container tight and out of reach of children. When the container is full, check with your physician or nurse about proper disposal, as laws vary from state to state.

Storage: Store the vials of sterile lyophilized material for subcutaneous injection in a freezer (-20° C to -10° C/-4° F to 14° F). The vials of diluent may be stored at room temperature.

HOW SUPPLIED:

Copaxone is supplied as a sterile lyophilized material containing 20 mg of glatiramer acetate and 40 mg mannitol, USP. The drug is packaged in a USP Type I amber glass, single use 2 ml vial. A separate vial, containing 1 ml of diluent (Sterile Water for Injection) is included for each vial of drug. Store glatiramer acetate in a freezer (-20° C to -10° C/4° F to 14° F). The diluent may be stored at room temperature. Glatiramer acetate is available in packs of 32 amber vials of sterile lyophilized material for subcutaneous injection.

Shelf-Life: The shelf-life of glatiramer acetate as packaged for sale is 18 months when stored in a freezer (-20° C to -10° C). This product contains no preservatives and should be used immediately after reconstitution or discarded. Protect glatiramer acetate from light.

GLIMEPIRIDE *(003279)*

CATEGORIES: Antidiabetic Agents; Blood Glucose Regulators; Diabetes; Diabetes Mellitus; Hormones; Hyperglycemia; Sulfonylureas; FDA Class 1S ("Standard Review"); FDA Approved 1995 Nov

BRAND NAMES: **Amaryl**

DESCRIPTION:

Glimepiride tablets are an oral blood-glucose-lowering drug of the sulfonylurea class. Glimepiride is a white to yellowish-white, crystalline, odorless to practically odorless powder formulated into tablets of 1-mg, 2-mg, and 4-mg strengths for oral administration. Glimepiride tablets contain the active ingredient glimepiride and the following inactive ingredients: lactose (hydrous), sodium starch glycolate, povidone, microcrystalline cellulose, and magnesium stearate.

Amaryl 1-mg tablets contain Ferric Oxide Red, Amaryl 2-mg tablets contain Ferric Oxide Yellow and FD&C Blue #2 Aluminum Lake, and Amaryl 4-mg tablets contain FD&C Blue #2 Aluminum Lake.

Chemically, glimepiride is identified as 1-[[p-[2-(3-ethyl-4-methyl-2-oxo-3-pyrroline-1-carboxamido) ethyl]phenyl]sulfonyl]-3-(trans-4-methylcyclohexyl)urea.

Molecular Formula: $C_{24}H_{34}N_4O_5S$

Molecular Weight: 490.62

Glimepiride is practically insoluble in water.

CLINICAL PHARMACOLOGY:

MECHANISM OF ACTION

The primary mechanism of action of glimepiride in lowering blood glucose appears to be dependent on stimulating the release of insulin from functioning pancreatic beta cells. In addition, extrapancreatic effects may also play a role in the activity of sulfonylureas such as glimepiride. This is supported by both preclinical and clinical studies demonstrating that glimepiride administration can lead to increased sensitivity of peripheral tissues to insulin. These findings are consistent with the results of a long term, randomized, placebo-controlled trial in which glimepiride therapy improved postprandial insulin/C-peptide responses and overall glycemic control without producing clinically meaningful increases in fasting insulin/C-peptide levels. However, as with other sulfonylureas, the mechanism by which glimepiride lowers blood glucose during long-term administration has not been clearly established.

PHARMACODYNAMICS

A mild glucose-lowering effect first appeared following single oral doses as low as 0.5-0.6 mg in healthy subjects. The time required to reach the maximum effect (*i.e.,* minimum blood glucose level [T_{min}]) was about 2 to 3 hours. In noninsulin-dependent (Type II) diabetes mellitus (NIDDM) patients, both fasting and 2-hour postprandial glucose levels were significantly lower with glimepiride (1, 2, 4, and 8 mg once daily) than with placebo after 14 days of oral dosing. The glucose-lowering effect in all active treatment groups was maintained over 24 hours.

In larger dose-ranging studies, blood glucose and HbA1c were found to respond in a dose-dependent manner over the range of 1 to 4 mg/day of glimepiride. Some patients, particularly those with higher fasting plasma glucose (FPG) levels, may benefit from doses of glimepiride up to 8 mg once daily. No difference in response was found when glimepiride was administered once or twice daily.

In two 14-week, placebo-controlled studies in 720 subjects, the average net reduction in HbA1c for glimepiride patients treated with 8 mg once daily was 2.0% in absolute units compared with placebo-treated patients. In a long-term, randomized, placebo-controlled study of NIDDM patients unresponsive to dietary management, glimepiride therapy improved postprandial insulin/C-peptide responses, and 75% of patients achieved and maintained control of blood glucose and HbA1c. Efficacy results were not affected by age, gender, weight, or race.

CLINICAL PHARMACOLOGY: *(cont'd)*

In long-term extension trials with previously-treated patients, no meaningful deterioration in mean fasting blood glucose (FBG) or HbA1c levels was seen after 2 1/2 years of glimepiride therapy.

Combination therapy with glimepiride and insulin (70% NPH/30% regular) was compared to placebo/insulin in secondary failure patients whose body weight was > 130% of their ideal body weight. Initially, 5-10 units of insulin were administered with the main evening meal and titrated upward weekly to achieve predefined FPG values. Both groups in this double-blind study achieved similar reductions in FPG levels but the glimepiride/insulin therapy group used approximately 38% less insulin.

Glimepiride therapy is effective in controlling blood glucose without deleterious changes in the plasma lipoprotein profiles of patients treated for NIDDM.

PHARMACOKINETICS

Absorption: After oral administration, glimepiride is completely (100%) absorbed from the GI tract. Studies with single oral doses in normal subjects and with multiple oral doses in patients with NIDDM have shown significant absorption of glimepiride within 1 hour after administration and peak drug levels (C_{max}) at 2 to 3 hours. When glimepiride was given with meals, the mean T_{max} (time to reach C_{max}) was slightly increased (12%) and the mean C_{max} and AUC (area under the curve) were slightly decreased (8% and 9%, respectively).

Distribution: After intravenous (IV) dosing in normal subjects, the volume of distribution (Vd) was 8.8 L (113 mL/kg), and the total body clearance (CL) was 47.8 mL/min. Protein binding was greater than 99.5%.

Metabolism: Glimepiride is completely metabolized by oxidative biotransformation after either an IV or oral dose. The major metabolites are the cyclohexyl hydroxy methyl derivative (M1) and the carboxyl derivative (M2). Cytochrome P450 II C9 has been shown to be involved in the biotransformation of glimepiride to M1. M1 is further metabolized to M2 by one or several cytosolic enzymes. M1, but not M2, possesses about 1/3 of the pharmacological activity as compared to its parent in an animal model; however, whether the glucose-lowering effect of M1 is clinically meaningful is not clear.

Excretion: When ^{14}C-glimepiride was given orally, approximately 60% of the total radioactivity was recovered in the urine in 7 days and M1 (predominant) and M2 accounted for 80-90% of that recovered in the urine. Approximately 40% of the total radioactivity was recovered in the feces and M1 and M2 (predominant) accounted for about 70% of that recovered in feces. No parent drug was recovered from urine or feces. After IV dosing in patients, no significant biliary excretion of glimepiride or its M1 metabolite has been observed.

Pharmacokinetic Parameters: The pharmacokinetic parameters of glimepiride obtained from a single-dose, crossover, dose-proportionality (1, 2, 4, and 8 mg) study in normal subjects and from a single- and multiple-dose, parallel, dose-proportionality (4 and 8 mg) study in patients with NIDDM are summarized in TABLE 1.

TABLE 1

	Volunteers	Patients with NIDDM	
	Single Dose Mean ± SD	Single Dose (Day 1) Mean ± SD	Multiple Dose (Day 10) Mean ± SD
C_{max}(ng/mL)			
1 mg	103 ± 34 (12)	—	—
2 mg	177 ± 44 (12)	—	—
4 mg	308 ± 69 (12)	352 ± 222 (12)	309 ± 134 (12)
8 mg	557 ± 152 (12)	591 ± 232 (14)	578 ± 265 (11)
T_{max}(h)	2.4 ± 0.8 (48)	2.5 ± 1.2 (26)	2.8 ± 2.2 (23)
CL/f(mL/min)	52.1 ± 16.0 (48)	48.5 ± 29.3 (26)	52.7 ± 40.3 (23)
Vd/f(L)	21.8 ± 13.9 (48)	19.8 ± 12.7 (26)	37.1 ± 18.2 (23)
T 1/2 (h)	5.3 ± 4.1 (48)	5.0 ± 2.5 (26)	9.2 ± 3.6 (23)

() No. of subjects
CL/f Total body clearance after oral dosing
Vd/f Volume of distribution calculated after oral dosing

These data indicate that glimepiride did not accumulate in serum, and the pharmacokinetics of glimepiride were not different in healthy volunteers and in NIDDM patients. Oral clearance of glimepiride did not change over the 1-8 mg dose range, indicating linear pharmacokinetics.

Variability: In normal healthy volunteers, the intra-individual variabilities of C_{max}, AUC, and CL/f for glimepiride were 23%, 17%, and 15%, respectively, and the inter-individual variabilities were 25%, 29%, and 24%, respectively.

SPECIAL POPULATIONS

Geriatric: Comparison of glimepiride pharmacokinetics in NIDDM patients ≥ 65 years and those > 65 years was performed in a study using a dosing regimen of 6 mg daily. There were no significant differences in glimepiride pharmacokinetics between the two age groups. The mean AUC at steady state for the older patients was about 13% lower than that for the younger patients; the mean weight-adjusted clearance for the older patients was about 11% higher than that for the younger patients.

Pediatric: No studies were performed in pediatric patients.

Gender: There were no differences between males and females in the pharmcokinetics of glimepiride when adjustment was made for differences in body weight.

Race: No pharmacokinetic studies to assess the effects of race have been performed, but in placebo-controlled studies of glimepiride in patients with NIDDM, the antihyperglycemic effect was comparable in whites (n=536), blacks (n=63), and Hispanics (n=63).

Renal Insufficiency: A single-dose, open-label study was conducted in 15 patients with renal impairment. Glimepiride (3m) was administered to 3 groups of patients with different levels of mean creatinine clearance (CLcr); (Group I, CLcr=77.7 mL/min, n=5), (Group II, CLcr=27.7 mL/min, n=3), and (Group III, CLcr=9.4 mL/min, n=7). Glimepiride was found to be well tolerated in all 3 groups. The results showed that glimepiride serum levels decreased as renal function decreased. However, M1 and M2 serum levels (mean AUC values) increased 2.3 and 8.6 times from Group I to Group III. The apparent terminal half-life ($T_{1/2}$) for glimepiride did not change, while the half-lives for M1 and M2 increased as renal function decreased. Mean urinary excretion of M1 plus M2 as percent of dose, however, decreased (44.4%, 21.9%, and 9.3% for Groups I to III).

A multiple-dose titration study was also conducted in 16 NIDDM patients with renal impairment using doses ranging from 1-8 mg daily for 3 months. The results were consistent with those observed after single doses. All patients with a CLcr less than 22 mL/min had adequate control of their glucose levels with a dosage regimen of only 1 mg daily. The result from this study suggested that a starting dose of 1 mg glimepiride may be given to NIDDM patients with kidney disease, and the dose may be titrated based on fasting blood glucose levels.

Hepatic Insufficiency: No studies were performed in patients with hepatic insufficiency.

Other Populations: There were no important differences in glimepiride metabolism in subjects identified as phenotypically different drug-metabolizers by their metabolism of sparteine.

CLINICAL PHARMACOLOGY: *(cont'd)*

The pharmacokinetics of glimepiride in morbidly obese patients were similar to those in the normal weight group, except for a lower C_{max} and AUC. However, since neither C_{max} nor AUC values were normalized for body surface area, the lower values of C_{max} and AUC for the obese patients were likely the result of their excess weight and not due to a difference in the kinetics of glimepiride.

CLINICAL STUDIES:

Human Ophthalmology Data: Ophthalmic examinations were carried out in over 500 subjects during long-term studies using the methodology of Taylor and West and Laties et al. No significant differences were seen between glimepiride and glyburide in the number of subjects with clinically important changes in visual acuity, intra-ocular tension, or in any of the five lens-related variables examined.

Ophthalmic examinations were carried out during long-term studies using the method of Chylack et al. No significant or clinically meaningful differences were seen between glimepiride and glipizide with respect to cataract progression by subjective LOCS II grading and objective image analysis systems, visual acuity, intra-ocular pressure, and general ophthalmic examination.

INDICATIONS AND USAGE:

Glimepiride is indicated as an adjunct to diet and exercise to lower the blood glucose in patients with noninsulin-dependent (Type II) diabetes mellitus (NIDDM) whose hyperglycemia cannot be controlled by diet and exercise alone.

Glimepiride is also indicated for use in combination with insulin to lower blood glucose in patients whose hyperglycemia cannot be controlled by diet and exercise in conjunction with an oral hypoglycemic agent. Combined use of glimepiride and insulin may increase the potential for hypoglycemia.

In initiating treatment for noninsulin-dependent diabetes, diet and exercise should be emphasized as the primary form of treatment. Caloric restriction, weight loss, and exercise are essential in the obese diabetic patient. Proper dietary management and exercise alone may be effective in controlling the blood glucose and symptoms of hyperglycemia. In addition to regular physical activity, cardiovascular risk factors should be identified and corrective measures taken where possible.

If this treatment program fails to reduce symptoms and/or blood glucose, the use of an oral sulfonylurea or insulin should be considered. Use of glimepiride must be viewed by both the physician and patient as a treatment in addition to diet and exercise and not as substitute for diet and exercise or as a convenient mechanism for avoiding dietary restraint. Furthermore, loss of blood glucose control on diet and exercise alone may be transient, thus requiring only short-term administration of glimepiride.

During maintenance programs, glimepiride monotherapy should be discontinued if satisfactory lowering of blood glucose is no longer achieved. Judgements should be based on regular clinical and laboratory evaluations. Secondary failures to glimepiride monotherapy can be treated with glimepiride-insulin combination therapy.

In considering the use of glimepiride in asymptomatic patients, it should be recognized that blood glucose control in NIDDM has not definitely been established to be effective in preventing the long-term cardiovascular and neural complications of diabetes. However, the Diabetes Control and Complications Trial (DCCT) demonstrated that control of HbA1c and glucose was associated with a decrease in retinopathy, neuropathy, and nephropathy for insulin-dependent diabetic (IDDM) patients.

CONTRAINDICATIONS:

Glimepiride is contraindicated in patients with:

1. Known hypersensitivity to the drug.
2. Diabetic ketoacidosis, with or without come. This condition should be treated with insulin.

WARNINGS:

SPECIAL WARNING ON INCREASED RISK OF CARDIOVASCULAR MORTALITY

The administration of oral hypoglycemic drugs has been reported to be associated with increased cardiovascular mortality as compared to treatment with diet alone or diet plus insulin. This warning is based on the study conducted by the University Group Diabetes Program (UGDP), a long-term, prospective clinical trial designed to evaluate the effectiveness of glucose-lowering drugs in preventing or delaying vascular complications in patients with non-insulin-dependent diabetes. The study involved 823 patients who were randomly assigned to one of four treatment groups (Diabetes, 19 supp. 2: 747-830, 1970).

UGDP reported that patients treated for 5 to 8 years with diet plus a fixed dose of tolbutamide (1.5 grams per day) had a rate of cardiovascular mortality approximately 2-1/2 times that of patients treated with diet alone. A significant increase in total mortality was not observed, but the use of tolbutamide was discontinued based on the increase in cardiovascular mortality, thus limiting the opportunity for the study to show an increase in overall mortality. Despite controversy regarding the interpretation of these results, the finding of the UGDP study provide an adequate basis for this warning. The patient should be informed of the potential risks and advantages of glimepiride tablets and of alternative modes of therapy.

Although only one drug in the sulfonylurea class (tolbutamide) was included in this study, it is prudent from a safety standpoint to consider that this warning may also apply to other oral hypoglycemic drugs in this class, in view of their close similarities in mode of action and chemical structure.

PRECAUTIONS:

GENERAL

Hypoglycemia: All sulfonylurea drugs are capable of producing severe hypoglycemia. Proper patient selection, dosage, and instructions are important to avoid hypoglycemic episodes. Patients with impaired renal function may be more sensitive to the glucose-lowering effect of glimepiride. A starting dose of 1 mg once daily followed by appropriate dose titration is recommended in those patients. Debilitated or malnourished patients, and those with adrenal, pituitary, or hepatic insufficiency are particularly susceptive to the hypoglycemic action of glucose-lowering drugs. Hypoglycemia may be difficult to recognize in the elderly and in people who are taking beta-adrenergic blocking drugs or other sympatholytic agents. Hypoglycemia is more likely to occur when caloric intake is deficient, after severe or prolonged exercise, when alcohol is ingested, or when more than one glucose-lowering drug is used.

Loss Of Control Of Blood Glucose: When a patient stabilized on any diabetic regimen is exposed to stress such as fever, trauma, infection, or surgery, a loss of control may occur. At such times, it may be necessary to add insulin in combination with glimepiride or even use insulin monotherapy. The effectiveness of any oral hypoglycemic drug, including glimepiride, in lowering blood glucose to a desired level decreases in many patients over a period of time, which may be due to progression of the severity of the diabetes or to diminished responsiveness to the drug. This phenomenon is known as secondary failure, to distinguish it from primary failure in which the drug is ineffective in an individual patient when first given.

PRECAUTIONS: *(cont'd)*

Should secondary failure occur with glimepiride monotherapy, glimepiride-insulin combination therapy may be instituted. Combined use of glimepiride and insulin may increase the potential for hypoglycemia.

LABORATORY TESTS

Fasting blood glucose should be monitored periodically to determine therapeutic response. Glycosylated hemoglobin should also be monitored, usually every 3 to 6 months, to more precisely assess long-term glycemic control.

CARCINOGENESIS, MUTAGENESIS, AND IMPAIRMENT OF FERTILITY

Studies in rats at doses of up to 5000 ppm in complete feed (approximately 340 times the maximum recommended human dose, based on surface area) for 30 months showed no evidence of carcinogenesis. In mice, administration of glimepiride for 24 months resulted in an increase in benign pancreatic adenoma formation which was dose related and is thought to be the result of chronic pancreatic stimulation. The no-effect dose for adenoma formation in mice in this study was 320 ppm in complete feed, or 46-54 mg/kg body weight/day. This is about 35 times the maximum human recommended dose of 8 mg once daily based on surface area.

Glimepiride was non-mutagenic in a battery of *in vitro* and *in vivo* mutagenicity studies (Ames test, somatic cell mutation, chromosomal aberration, unscheduled DNA synthesis, mouse micronucleus test). There was no effect of glimepiride on male mouse fertility in animals exposed up to 2500 mg/kg body weight (> 1,700 times the maximum recommended human dose based on surface area). Glimepiride had no effect on the fertility of male and female rats administered up to 4000 mg/kg body weight (approximately 4,000 times the maximum recommended human dose based on surface area).

PREGNANCY, TERATOGENIC EFFECTS, PREGNANCY CATEGORY C

Glimepiride did not produce teratogenic effects in rats exposed orally up to 4000 mg/kg body weight (approximately 4,000 times the maximum recommended human dose based on surface area) or in rabbits exposed up to 32 mg/kg body weight (approximately 60 times the maximum recommended human dose based on surface area). Glimepiride has been shown to be associated with intrauterine fetal death in rats when given in doses as low as 50 times the human dose based on surface area and in rabbits when given in doses as low as 0.1 times the human dose based on surface area. This fetotoxicity, observed only at dose inducing maternal hypoglycemia, has been similarly noted with other sulfonylureas, and is believed to be directly related to the pharmacologic (hypoglycemic) action of glimepiride.

There are no adequate and well-controlled studies in pregnant women. On the basis of results from animal studies, glimepiride should not be used during pregnancy. Because recent information suggests that abnormal blood glucose levels during pregnancy are associated with a higher incidence of congenital abnormalities, many experts recommend that insulin be used during pregnancy to maintain glucose levels as close to normal as possible.

Nonteratogenic Effects: In some studies in rats, offspring of dams exposed to high levels of glimepiride during pregnancy and lactation developed skeletal deformities consisting of shortening, thickening, and bending of the humerus during the postnatal period. Significant concentrations of glimepiride were observed in the serum and breast milk of the dams as well as in the serum of the pups. These skeletal deformations were determined to be the result of nursing from mothers exposed to glimepiride.

Prolonged severe hypoglycemia (4 to 10 days) has been reported in neonates born to mothers who were receiving a sulfonylurea drug at the time of delivery. This has been reported more frequently with the use of agents with prolonged half-lives. Patients who are planning a pregnancy should consult their physician, and it is recommended that they change over to insulin for the entire course of pregnancy and lactation.

NURSING MOTHERS

In rat reproduction studies, significant concentrations of glimpiride were observed in the serum and breast milk of the dams, as well as in the serum of the pups. Although it is not known whether glimepiride is excreted in human milk, other sulfonylureas are excreted in human milk. Because the potential for hypoglycemia in nursing infants may exist, and because of the effects on nursing animals, glimepiride should be discontinued in nursing mothers. If glimepiride is discontinued, and if diet and exercise alone are in adequate for controlling blood glucose, insulin therapy should be considered. (See Pregnancy, Teratogenic Effects, Pregnancy Category C.)

PEDIATRIC USE

Safety and effectiveness in pediatric patients have not been established.

DRUG INTERACTIONS:

The hypoglycemic action of sulfonylureas may be potentiated by certain drugs, including nonsteroidal anti-inflammatory drugs and other drugs that are highly protein bound, such as salicylates, sulfonamides, chloramphenicol, coumarins, probenecid, monamine oxidase inhibitors, and beta adrenergic blocking agents. When these drugs are administered to a patient receiving glimepiride the patient should be observed closely for hypoglycemia. When these drugs are withdrawn from a patient receiving glimepiride, the patient should be observed closely for loss of glycemic control.

Certain drugs tend to produce hyperglycemia and may lead to loss of control. These drugs include the thiazides and other diurectics, corticosteroids, phenothiazines, thyroid products, estrogens, oral contraceptives, phenytoin, nicotinic acid, sympathomimetics, and isoniazid. When these drugs are administered to a patient receiving glimepiride the patient should be closely observed for loss of control. When these drugs are withdrawn from a patient receiving glimepiride, the patient should be observed closely for hypoglycemia.

Coadministration of aspirin (1 g tid) and glimepiride led to a 34% decrease in the mean glimepiride AUC and, therefore, a 34% increase in the mean CL/f. The mean C_{max} had a decrease of 4%. Blood glucose and serum C-peptide concentrations were unaffected and no hypoglycemic symptoms were reported. Pooled data from clinical trials showed no evidence of clinically significant adverse interactions with uncontrolled concurrent administration of aspirin and other salicylates. Coadministration of either cimetidine (800 mg once daily) or ranitidine (150 mg bid) with a single 4-mg oral dose of glimepiride did not significantly alter the absorption and disposition of glimepiride, and no differences were seen in hypoglycemic symptomatology. Pooled data from clinical trials showed no evidence of clinically significant adverse interactions with uncontrolled concurrent administration of H2-receptor antagonists.

Concomitant administration of propranolol (40 mg tid) and glimepiride significantly increased C_{max}, AUC, and $T_{1/2}$ of glimepiride by 23%, 22%, and 15%, respectively, and it decreased CL/f by 18%. The recovery of M1 and M2 from urine, however, did not change. The pharmacodynamic responses to glimepiride were nearly identical in normal subjects receiving propranolol and placebo. Pooled data from clinical trials in patients with NIDDM showed no evidence of clinically significant adverse interactions with uncontrolled concurrent administration of beta-blockers. However, if beta blockers are used, caution should be exercised and patients should be warned about the potential for hypoglycemia.

Concomitant administration of glimepiride (4 mg once daily) did not alter the pharmacokinetic characteristics of R- and S-warfarin enantiomers following administration of a single dose (25 mg) of racemic warfarin to healthy subjects. No changes were observed in warfarin plasma protein binding. Glimepiride treatment did result in a slight, but statistically significant, decrease in the pharmacodynamic response to warfarin. The reductions in mean area

DRUG INTERACTIONS: *(cont'd)*

under the prothrombin time (PT) curve and maximum PT values during glimepiride treatment were very small (3.3% and 9.9%, respectively) and are unlikely to be clinically important.

The responses of serum glucose, insulin, C-peptide, and plasma glucagon to 2 mg glimepiride were unaffected by coadministration of ramipril (an ACE inhibitor) 5 mg once daily in normal subjects. No hypoglycemic symptoms were reported. Pooled data from clinical trials in patients with NIDDM showed no evidence of clinically significant adverse interactions with uncontrolled concurrent administration of ACE inhibitors.

A potential interaction between oral miconazole and oral hypoglycemic agents leading to severe hypoglycemia has been reported. Whether this interaction also occurs with the intravenous, topical, or vaginal preparations of miconazole is not known. Potential interactions of glimepiride with other drugs metabolized by cytochrome P450 II C9 also include phenytoin, diclofenac, ibuprofen, naproxen, and mefenamic acid.

Although no specific interaction studies were performed, pooled data from clinical trials showed no evidence of clinically significant adverse interactions with uncontrolled concurrent administration of calcium-channel blockers, estrogens, fibrates, NSAIDS, HMG CoA reductase inhibitors, sulfonamides, or thyroid hormone.

ADVERSE REACTIONS:

The incidence of hypoglycemia with glimepiride, as documented by blood glucose values >60 mg/dL, ranged from 0.9-1.7% in two large, well-controlled, 1-year studies. (See WARNINGS and PRECAUTIONS.)

Glimepiride has been evaluated for safety in 2,013 patients in US controlled trials, and in 1,551 patients in foreign controlled trials. More than 1,650 of these patients were treated for at least 1 year.

Adverse events, other than hypoglycemia, considered to be possibly or probably related to study drug that occurred in US placebo-controlled trials in more than 1% of patients treated with glimepiride are shown in TABLE 2.

TABLE 2 Adverse Events Occurring in ≥ 1% Glimepiride patients

	Glimepiride		Placebo	
	No.	%	No.	%
Total Treated	746	100	294	100
Dizziness	13	1.7	1	0.3
Asthenia	12	1.6	3	1.0
Headache	11	1.5	4	1.4
Nausea	8	1.1	0	0.0

Gastrointestinal Reactions: Vomiting, gastrointestinal pain, and diarrhea have been reported, but the incidence in placebo-controlled trials was less than 1%. Isolated transaminase elevations have been reported. Cholestatic jaundice has been reported to occur rarely with sulfonylureas.

Dermatologic Reactions: Allergic skin reactions, e.g., pruritus, erythema, urticaria, and morbilliform or maculopapular eruptions, occur in less than 1% of treated patients. These may be transient and may disappear despite continued use of glimepiride; if skin reactions persist, the drug should be discontinued. Porphyria cutanea tarda and photosensitivity reactions have been reported with sulfonylureas.

Hematologic Reactions: Leukopenia, agranulocytosis, thrombocytopenia, hemolytic anemia, aplastic anemia, and pancytopenia have been reported with sulfonylureas.

Metabolic Reactions: Hepatic porphyria reactions and disulfiram-like reactions have been reported with sulfonylureas; however, no cases have yet been reported with glimepiride. Cases of hyponatremia have been reported with glimepiride and all other sulfonylureas, most often in patients who are on other medications or have medical conditions known to cause hyponatremia or increase release of antidiuretic hormone. The syndrome of inappropriate antidiuretic hormone (SIADH) secretion has been reported with certain other sulfonylureas, and it has been suggested that these sulfonylureas may augment the peripheral (anti-diuretic) action of ADH and/or increase release of ADH.

Other Reactions: Changes in accommodation and/or blurred vision may occur with the use of glimepiride. This is thought to be due to changes in blood glucose, and may be more pronounced when treatment is initiated. This condition is also seen in untreated diabetic patients, and may actually be reduced by treatment. In placebo-controlled trials of glimepiride, the incidence of blurred vision was placebo, 0.7%, and glimepiride, 0.4%.

OVERDOSAGE:

Overdosage of sulfonylureas, including glimepiride, can produce hypoglycemia. Mild hypoglycemic symptoms without loss of consciousness or neurologic findings should be treated aggressively with oral glucose and adjustments in drug dosage and/or meal patterns. Close monitoring should continue until the physician is assured that the patient is out of danger. Severe hypoglycemic reactions with coma, seizure, or other neurological impairment occur infrequently, but constitute medical emergencies requiring immediate hospitalization. If hypoglycemic coma is diagnosed or suspected, the patient should be given a rapid intravenous injection of concentrated (50%) glucose solution. This should be followed by a continuous infusion of a more dilute (10%) glucose solution at a rate that will maintain the blood glucose at a level above 100 mg/dL. Patients should be closely monitored for a minimum of 24 to 48 hours, because hypoglycemia may recur after apparent clinical recovery.

DOSAGE AND ADMINISTRATION:

There is no fixed dosage regimen for the management of diabetes mellitus with glimepiride or any other hypoglycemic agent. The patient's fasting blood glucose and HbA1c must be measured periodically to determine the minimum effective dose for the patient; to detect primary failure, i.e., inadequate lowering of blood glucose at the maximum recommended dose of medication; and to detect secondary failure, i.e., loss of adequate blood glucose lowering response after an initial period of effectiveness. Glycosylated hemoglobin levels should be performed to monitor the patient's response to therapy.

Short-term administration of glimepiride may be sufficient during periods of transient loss of control in patients usually controlled well on diet and exercise.

USUAL STARTING DOSE

The usual starting dose of glimepiride as initial therapy is 1-2 mg once daily, administered with breakfast or the first main meal. Those patients who may be more sensitive to hypoglycemic drugs should be started at 1mg once daily, and should be titrated carefully. (See PRECAUTIONS Section for patients at increased risk.)

No exact dosage relationship exists between glimepiride and the other oral hypoglycemic agents. The maximum starting dose of glimepiride should be no more than 2 mg.

Failure to follow an appropriate dosage regimen may precipitate hypoglycemia. Patients who do not adhere to their prescribed dietary and drug regimen are more prone to exhibit unsatisfactory response to therapy.

DOSAGE AND ADMINISTRATION: *(cont'd)*

USUAL MAINTENANCE DOSE

The usual maintenance dose is 1 to 4 mg once daily. The maximum recommended dose is 8 mg once daily. After reaching a dose of 2 mg, dosage increases should be made in increments of no more than 2 mg at 1-2 week intervals based upon the patient's blood glucose response. Long-term efficacy should be monitored by measurement of HbA1c levels, for example, every 3 to 6 months.

GLIMEPIRIDE-INSULIN COMBINATION THERAPY

Combination therapy with glimepiride and insulin may be used in secondary failure patients. The fasting glucose level for instituting combination therapy is in the range of > 150 mg/dL in plasma or serum depending on the patient. The recommended glimepiride dose is 8 mg once daily administered with the first main meal. After starting with lowdose insulin, upward adjustments of insulin can be done approximately weekly as guided by frequent measurements of fasting blood glucose. Once stable, combination-therapy patients should monitor their capillary blood glucose on an ongoing basis, preferably daily. Periodic adjustments of insulin may also be necessary during maintenance as guided by glucose and HbA1c levels.

SPECIFIC PATIENT POPULATIONS

Glimepiride is not recommended for use in pregnancy, nursing mothers, or children. In elderly, debilitated, or malnourished patients, or in patients with renal or hepatic insufficiency, the initial dosing, dose increments, and maintenance dosage should be conservative to avoid hypoglycemic reactions (See CLINICAL PHARMACOLOGY, Special Populations and PRECAUTIONS, General)

PATIENTS RECEIVING OTHER ORAL HYPOGLYCEMIC AGENTS

As with other sulfonylurea hypoglycemic agents, no transition period is necessary when transferring patients to glimepiride. Patients should be observed carefully (1-2 weeks) for hypoglycemia when being transferred from longer half-life sulfonylureas (*e.g.*, chlorpropamide) to glimepiride due to potential overlapping of drug effect.

ANIMAL PHARMACOLOGY:

Animal Toxicology: Reduced serum glucose values and degranulation of the pancreatic beta cells were observed in beagle dogs exposed to 320 mg glimepiride/kg/day for 12 months (approximately 1,000 times the recommended human dose based on surface area). No evidence of tumor formation was observed in any organ. One female and one male dog developed bilateral subscapsular cataracts. Non-GLP studies indicated that glimepiride was unlikely to exacerbate cataract formation. Evaluation of the co-cataractogenic potential of glimepiride in several diabetic and cataract rat models was negative and there was no adverse effect of glimepiride on bovine ocular lens metabolism in organ culture.

PATIENT INFORMATION:

Glimepiride is used with diet and exercise to lower blood sugur (glucose) in diabetics. Do not use if you are pregnant or nursing. Inform your doctor if you are taking any other medications. Take once daily with breakfast or the first main meal. Glimepiride is not a substitute for a good diet, regular exercise and regular urine or blood glucose testing. May cause decreased blood sugar, dizziness, weakness, headache or nausea. Inform your doctor or pharmacist if these effects occur.

HOW SUPPLIED:

Store between 59 and 86°F (15 to 30°C). Dispense in well-closed containers with safety closures.

HOW SUPPLIED - EQUIVALENTS NOT AVAILABLE:

Tablet - Oral - 1 mg

100's	$21.59	AMARYL, Hoechst Marion Roussel	00039-0221-10
100's UD	$21.59	AMARYL, Hoechst Marion Roussel	00039-0221-11

Tablet - Oral - 2 mg

100's	$31.44	AMARYL, Hoechst Marion Roussel	00039-0222-10
100's UD	$31.44	AMARYL, Hoechst Marion Roussel	00039-0222-11

Tablet - Oral - 4 mg

100's	$56.79	AMARYL, Hoechst Marion Roussel	00039-0223-10
100's UD	$56.79	AMARYL, Hoechst Marion Roussel	00039-0223-11

GLIPIZIDE *(001357)*

CATEGORIES: Antidiabetic Agents; Blood Glucose Regulators; Diabetes; Diabetes Mellitus; Hormones; Hyperglycemia; Sulfonylureas; Weight Loss; Pregnancy Category C; Sales > $100 Million; FDA Approved 1984 May; Patent Expiration 1994 May; Top 200 Drugs

BRAND NAMES: *Digrin*; *Dipazide*; *Glibenese* (England, France, Germany); *Glibetin*; *Glican*; *Glidiab*; *Glipid*; *Glucolip*; *Gluco-Rite*; **Glucotrol**; Glucotrol Xl; *Glucozide*; *Glupizide*; *Glyco*; *Glyde*; *Glynase*; *Melizide* (Australia); *Mindiab*; *Minidab*; *Minidiab* (Australia, France); *Minodiab* (England, Mexico); *Napizide*; *Sucrazide*
(International brand names outside U.S. in italics)

FORMULARIES: BC-BS; Medi-Cal; PCS

COST OF THERAPY: $23.83 (Diabetes; Tablet; 5 mg; 1/day; 365 days)

DESCRIPTION:

IMMEDIATE AND EXTENDED RELEASE TABLETS

Glucotrol (glipizide) is an oral blood-glucose-lowering drug of the sulfonylurea class.

The chemical abstracts name of glipizide is 1-cyclohexyl-3-([p-(2-(5-methylpyrazinecarboxamido)ethyl]phenyl]-sulfonyl) urea. The molecular formula is $C_{21}H_{27}N_5O_4S$; the molecular weight is 445.55.

Glipizide is a whitish, odorless powder with a pKa of 5.9. It is insoluble in water and alcohols, but soluble in 0.1 *N*NaOH; it is freely soluble in dimethylformamide. Glucotrol tablets for oral use are available in 5 and 10 mg strengths.

Inert ingredients are: colloidal silicon dioxide; lactose; microcrystalline cellulose; starch; stearic acid.

EXTENDED RELEASE TABLET

Glucotrol XL Extended Release Tablet is similar in appearance to a conventional tablet. It consists, however, of an osmotically active drug core surrounded by a semipermeable membrane. The core itself is divided into two layers : an "active" layer containing the drug, and a "push" layer containing pharmacologically insert (but osmotically active) components. The membrane surrounding the tablet is permeable to water but not to drug or osmotic excipients. As water from the gastrointestinal tract enters the tablet pressure increases in the osmotic layer and "pushes" against the drug layer, resulting in the release of through a small laser-drilled orifice in the membrane on the drug side of the tablet.

DESCRIPTION: *(cont'd)*

The Glucotrol XL Extended Release Tablet is designed to provide a controlled rate of delivery of glipizide. into the gastrointestinal lumen which is independent of pH or gastrointestinal motility. The function of the Glucotrol XL Extended Release Tablet depends upon the existence of an osmotic gradient between the contents of the bi-layer core and fluid in the GI tract. Drug delivery is essentially constant as long as the osmotic gradient remains constant, and then gradually falls to zero. The bio logically inert components of the tablet remain intact during drug GI transit and are eliminated in the feces as an insoluble shell.

CLINICAL PHARMACOLOGY:

Mechanism of Action: The primary mode of action of glipzide in experimental animals appears to be the stimulation of insulin secretion from the beta cells of pancreatic islet tissue and is thus dependent on functioning beta cells in the pancreatic islets. In humans glipzide appears to lower the blood glucose acutely by stimulating the release of insulin from the pancreas, an effect dependent upon functioning beta cells in the pancreatic islets. The mechanism by which glipzide lowers blood glucose during long-term administration has not been clearly established. In man, stimulation of insulin secretion by glipizide in response to a meal is undoubtedly of major importance. Fasting insulin levels are not elevated even on long-term glipzide administration, but the postprandial insulin response continues to be enhanced after at least 6 months of treatment. The insulinotropic response to a meal occurs within 30 minutes after an oral dose of glipzide in diabetic patients, but elevated insulin levels do not persist beyond the time of the meal challenge. Extrapancreatic effects may play a part in the mechanism of action of oral sulfonylurea hypoglycemic drugs.

Blood sugar control persists in some patients for up to 24 hours after a single dose of glipzide, even though plasma levels have declined to a small fraction of peak levels by that time (see Pharmacokinetics).

Some patients fail to respond initially, or gradually lose their responsiveness to sulfonylurea drugs, including glipzide. Alternatively, glipzide may be effective in some patients who have not responded or have ceased to respond to other sulfonylureas.

PHARMACOKINETICS

Gastrointestinal absorption of glipzide in man is uniform, rapid, and essentially complete. Peak plasma concentrations occur 1-3 hours after a single oral dose. The half-life of elimination ranges from 2-4 hours in normal subjects, whether given intravenously or orally. The metabolic and excretory patterns are similar with the two routes of administration, indicating that first-pass metabolism is not significant. glipzide does not accumulate in plasma on repeated oral administration. Total absorption and disposition of an oral dose was unaffected by food in normal volunteers, but absorption was delayed by about 40 minutes. Thus glipzide was more effective when administered about 30 minutes before, rather than with, a test meal in diabetic patients. Protein binding was studied in serum from volunteers who received either oral or intravenous glipzide and found to be 98-99% one hour after either route of administration. The apparent volume of distribution of glipzide after intravenous administration was 11 liters, indicative of localization within the extracellular fluid compartment. In mice no glipzide or metabolites were detectable autoradiographically in the brain or spinal cord of males or females, nor in the fetuses of pregnant females. In another study, however, very small amounts of radioactivity were detected in the fetuses of rats given labelled drug.

The metabolism of glipzide is extensive and occurs mainly in the liver. The primary metabolites are inactive hydroxylation products and polar conjugates and are excreted mainly in the urine. Less than 10% unchanged glipzide is found in the urine.

EXTENDED RELEASE TABLETS

Mechanism of Action: Glipizide appears to lower blood glucose acutely by stimulating the release of insulin from the pancreas, an effect dependent upon functioning beta cells in the pancreatic islets. Extrapancreatic effects also may play a part in the mechanism of action of oral sulfonylurea hypoglycemic drugs. Two extrapancreatic effects shown to be important in the action of glipizide are an increase in insulin sensitivity and a decrease in hepatic glucose production. However, the mechanism by which glipizide lowers blood glucose during long-term administration has not been clearly established. Stimulation of insulin secretion by glipizide in response to a meal is of major importance. The insulinotropic response to a meal is enhanced with glipizide extended-release administration in diabetic patients. The postprandial insulin and C-peptide responses continue to be enhanced after at least 6 months of treatment. In 2 randomized, double blind, dose-response studies comprising a total of 347 patients, there was no significant increase in fasting insulin in all glipizide extended-release-treated patients combined compared to placebo, although minor elevations were observed at some doses. There was no increase in fasting insulin over the long-term.

Some patients fail to respond initially, or gradually lose their responsiveness to sulfonylurea drugs, including glipizide. Alternatively, glipizide may be effective in some patients who have not responded or have ceased to respond to other sulfonylurea.

EFFECTS ON BLOOD GLUCOSE

The effectiveness of glipizide extended-release tablets in NIDDM at doses from 5-60 mg once daily has been evaluated in 4 therapeutic clinical trials each with long-term open extensions involving a total 598 patients. Once daily administration of 5, 10, and 20 mg produced statistically significant reductions from placebo in hemoglobin A_1c, fasting plasma glucose and postprandial glucose in mild to severe NIDDM patients. In a pooled analysis of the patients treated with 5 mg and 20 mg, the relationship between dose and glipizide extended-release's effect of reducing hemoglobin A_1c was not established. However, in the case of fasting plasma glucose patients treated with 20 mg had a statistically significant reduction of fasting plasma glucose compared to the 5 mg-treated group.

The reductions in hemoglobin A_1c and fasting plasma glucose were similar in younger and older patients. Efficacy of glipizide extended-release was not affected by gender, race, or weight (as assessed by body mass index). In long term extension trials, efficacy of glipizide extended-release was maintained in 81% of patients for up to 12 months.

In an open, two-way crossover study 132 patients were randomly assigned to either glipizide extended-release or glipizide for 8 weeks and then crossed over to the other drug for an additional 8 weeks. Glipizide extended-release administration resulted in significantly lower fasting plasma glucose levels and equivalent hemoglobin A_1c levels, as compared to glipizide.

Pharmacokinetics and Metabolism: Glipizide is rapidly and completely absorbed following oral administration in an immediate release dosage form. The absolute bioavailability of glipizide was 100% after single doses in patients with NIDDM. Beginning 2 to 3 hours after administration of glipizide extended-release tablets, plasma drug concentrations gradually rise reaching maximum concentrations within 6 to 12 hours after dosing. With subsequent once daily dosing of glipizide extended-release tablets, effective plasma glipizide concentrations are maintained throughout the 24 hour dosing interval with less peak to through fluctuation than that observed with twice daily dosing of immediate release glipizide. The mean relative bioavailability of glipizide in 21 males with NIDDM after administration of 20 mg glipizide extended-release tablets, compared to immediate release glipzide (10 mg given twice daily), was 90% at steady state. Steady state plasma concentrations were achieved by at least the fifth day of dosing with glipizide extended-release tablets in 21 male with NIDDM and patients younger than 65 years. Approximately 1 to 2 days longer were required to reach steady state in 24 elderly (≥65 years) males and females with NIDDM. No accumulation of drug was observed in patients with NIDDM during chronic dosing with glipizide extended-re-

CLINICAL PHARMACOLOGY: *(cont'd)*

lease tablets. Administration of glipzide extended-release with food has no effect on the 2 to 3 hour lag time in drug absorption. In a single dose, food effect study in 21 healthy males subjects, the administration of glipizide extended-release immediately before a high fat breakfast resulted in a 40% increase in the glipizide mean C_{max} value, which was significant, but the effect on the AUC was not significant. There was no change in glucose response between the fed and fasting state. Markedly reduced GI retention times of the glipzide extended-release tablets over prolonged periods (*e.g.,* short bowel syndrome) may influence the pharmacokinetic profile of the drug and potentially result in lower plasma concentrations.In a multiple dose study in 26 males with NIDDM, the pharmacokinetics of glipizide were linear over the dose range of 5 to 60 mg of glipizide extended-release in that the plasma drug concentrations increased proportionately with dose. In a single dose study in 24 healthy subjects, four 5 mg, two 10 mg, and one 20 mg glipizide extended-release tablets were bioequivalent.

Glipizide is eliminated primarily by hepatic biotransformation: less than 10% of a dose is excreted as unchanged drug in urine and feces; approximately 90% of a dose is excreted as biotransformation products in urine (80%) and feces (10%). The major metabolites of glipizide are products of aromatic hydroxylation and have no hypoglycemic activity. A minor metabolite which accounts for less than 2% of a dose, an acetylaminoethyl benzine derivatives, is reported to have 1/10 to 1/3 as much hypoglycemic activity as the parent compound. The mean total body clearance of glipizide was approximately 3 liters per hour after single intravenous doses in patients with NIDDM. The mean apparent volume of distribution was approximately 10 liters. Glipizide is 98-99% bound to serum proteins, primarily to albumin. The mean terminal elimination half-life of glipizide ranged from 2 to 5 hours after single or multiple doses in patients with NIDDM. There were no significant differences in the pharmacokinetics of glipizide after single dose administration to older diabetic subjects compared to younger healthy subjects. There is only limited information regarding the effects of renal impairment on the disposition of glipizide and no information regarding the effects of hepatic disease. However, since glipizide is highly protein bound and hepatic biotransformation is the predominant route of elimination the pharmacokinetics and/or pharmacodynamics of glipizide may be altered in patients with renal or hepatic impairment.

In mice no glipizide or metabolites were detectable autoradiographically in the brain or spinal cord of males or females, nor in the fetuses of pregnant females. In another study, however, very small amounts of radioactivity were detected in the fetuses of rats given labeled drug.

IMMEDIATE AND EXTENDED RELEASE TABLETS

Other Effects: It has been shown that glipzide therapy was effective in controlling blood sugar without deleterious changes in the plasma lipoprotein profiles of patients treated for NIDDM.

In a placebo-controlled, crossover study in normal volunteers, glipzide had no anti-diuretic activity, and, in fact, led to a slight increase in free water clearance.

INDICATIONS AND USAGE:

IMMEDIATE AND EXTENDED RELEASE TABLETS

Glipzide is indicated as an adjunct to diet for the control of hyperglycemia and its associated symptomatology in patients with non- insulin-dependent diabetes mellitus (NIDDM; type II), formerly known as maturity-onset diabetes, after an adequate trial of dietary therapy has proved unsatisfactory.

In initiating treatment for non-insulin-dependent diabetes, diet should be emphasized as the primary form of treatment. Caloric restriction and weight loss are essential in the obese diabetic patient. Proper dietary management alone may be effective in controlling the blood glucose and symptoms of hyperglycemia. The importance of regular physical activity should also be stressed, and cardiovascular risk factors should be identified, and corrective measures taken where possible.

If this treatment program fails to reduce symptoms and/or blood glucose, the use of an oral sulfonylurea or insulin should be considered. Use of glipzide must be viewed by both the physician and patient as a treatment in addition to diet, and not as a substitute for diet or as a convenient mechanism for avoiding dietary restraint. Furthermore, loss of blood glucose control on diet alone also may be transient, thus requiring only short-term administration of glipzide.

During maintenance programs, glipzide should be discontinued if satisfactory lowering of blood glucose is no longer achieved. Judgments should be based on regular clinical and laboratory evaluations.

In considering the use of glipzide in asymptomatic patients, it should be recognized that controlling the blood glucose in non-insulin-dependent diabetes has not been definitely established to be effective in preventing the long-term cardiovascular or neural complications of diabetes.

EXTENDED RELEASE TABLET

Glipzide extended-release is indicated when diet alone has been unsuccessful in correcting hyperglycemia, but even after the introduction of the drug in the patients regimen, dietary measures should continue to be considered as important. I 12 week, well-controlled studies there was a maximal average net reduction in hemoglobin A_{1C} of 1.7% in absolute units between placebo-treated and glipzide extended-release-treated patients.

In insulin-dependent diabetes mellitus controlling blood glucose has been effective in slowing the progression of diabetic retinopathy, nephropathy, and neuropathy.

CONTRAINDICATIONS:

IMMEDIATE AND EXTENDED RELEASE TABLETS

Glipzide is contraindicated in patients with:

1. Known hypersensitivity to the drug.

2. Diabetic ketoacidosis, with or without coma. This condition should be treated with insulin.

WARNINGS:

IMMEDIATE AND EXTENDED RELEASE TABLETS

SPECIAL WARNING ON INCREASED RISK OF CARDIOVASCULAR MORTALITY:

The administration of oral hypoglycemic drugs has been reported to be associated with increased cardiovascular mortality as compared to treatment with diet alone or diet plus insulin. This warning is based on the study conducted by the University Group Diabetes Program (UGDP), a long-term prospective clinical trial designed to evaluate the effectiveness of glucose-lowering drugs in preventing or delaying vascular complications in patients with non-insulin-dependent diabetes. The study involved 823 patients who were randomly assigned to one of four treatment groups (*Diabetes*, 19, supp. 2: 747-830, 1970).

UGDP reported that patients treated for 5 to 8 years with diet plus a fixed dose of tolbutamide (1.5 grams per day) had a rate of cardiovascular mortality approximately 21/2 times that of patients treated with diet alone. A significant increase in total mortality was not observed, but the use of tolbutamide was discontinued based on the increase in cardiovascular mortality, thus limiting the opportunity for the study to show an increase in overall mortality. Despite controversy regarding the interpretation of these results, the findings of the UGDP study provide an adequate basis for this warning. The patient should be informed of the potential risks and advantages of glipzide and of alternative modes of therapy.

WARNINGS: *(cont'd)*

Although only one drug in the sulfonylurea class (tolbutamide) was included in this study, it is prudent from a safety standpoint to consider that this warning may also apply to other oral hypoglycemic drugs in this class, in view of their close similarities in mode of action and chemical structure.

As with any other non-deformable material, caution should be used when administering glipzide extended-release tablets in patients with preexisting severe gastrointestinal narrowing (pathologic or iatrogenic). There have been rare reports of obstructive symptoms in patients with known structures in association with the ingestion of another drug in this non-deformable sustained release formulation.

PRECAUTIONS:

GENERAL

Renal and Hepatic Disease: The metabolism and excretion of glipzide may be slowed in patients with impaired renal and/or hepatic function. If hypoglycemia should occur in such patients, it may be prolonged and appropriate management should be instituted.

Hypoglycemia: All sulfonylurea drugs are capable of producing severe hypoglycemia. Proper patient selection, dosage, and instructions are important to avoid hypoglycemic episodes. Renal or hepatic insufficiency may cause elevated blood levels of glipzide and the latter may also diminish gluconeogenic capacity, both of which increase the risk of serious hypoglycemic reactions. Elderly, debilitated or malnourished patients, and those with adrenal or pituitary insufficiency are particularly susceptible to the hypoglycemic action of glucose-lowering drugs. Hypoglycemia may be difficult to recognize in the elderly, and in people who are taking beta-adrenergic blocking drugs. Hypoglycemia is more likely to occur when caloric intake is deficient, after severe or prolonged exercise, when alcohol is ingested, or when more than one glucose-lowering drug is used.

Loss of Control of Blood Glucose: When a patient stabilized on any diabetic regimen is exposed to stress such as fever, trauma, infection, or surgery, a loss of control may occur. At such times, it may be necessary to discontinue glipzide and administer insulin.

The effectiveness of any oral hypoglycemic drug, including glipzide, in lowering blood glucose to a desired level decreases in many patients over a period of time, which may be due to progression of the severity of the diabetes or to diminished responsiveness to the drug. This phenomenon is known as secondary failure, to distinguish it from primary failure in which the drug is ineffective in an individual patient when first given.

Laboratory Tests: Blood and urine glucose should be monitored periodically. Measurement of glycosylated hemoglobin may be useful.

Carcinogenesis, Mutagenesis, and Impairment of Fertility: A twenty month study in rats and an eighteen month study in mice at doses up to 75 times the maximum human dose revealed no evidence of drug-related carcinogenicity. Bacterial and *in vivo* mutagenicity tests were uniformly negative. Studies in rats of both sexes at doses up to 75 times the human dose showed no effects on fertility.

Pregnancy Category C: Glipizide was found to be mildly fetotoxic in rat reproductive studies at all dose levels (5-50 mg/kg). This fetotoxicity has been similarly noted with other sulfonylureas, such as tolbutamide and tolazamide. The effect is perinatal and believed to be directly related to the pharmacologic (hypoglycemic) action of glipzide. In studies in rats and rabbits no teratogenic effects were found. There are no adequate and well controlled studies in pregnant women. glipzide should be used during pregnancy only if the potential benefit justifies the potential risk to the fetus.

Because recent information suggests that abnormal blood glucose levels during pregnancy are associated with a higher incidence of congenital abnormalities, many experts recommend that insulin be used during pregnancy to maintain blood glucose levels as close to normal as possible.

NONTERATOGENIC EFFECTS

Prolonged severe hypoglycemia (4 to 10 days) has been reported in neonates born to mothers who were receiving a sulfonylurea drug at the time of delivery. This has been reported more frequently with the use of agents with prolonged half-lives. If glipzide is used during pregnancy, it should be discontinued at least one month before the expected delivery date.

NURSING MOTHERS

Although it is not known whether glipzide is excreted in human milk, some sulfonylurea drugs are known to be excreted in human milk. Because the potential for hypoglycemia in nursing infants may exist, a decision should be made whether to discontinue nursing or to discontinue the drug, taking into account the importance of the drug to the mother. If the drug is discontinued and if diet alone is inadequate for controlling blood glucose, insulin therapy should be considered.

Pediatric Use: Safety and effectiveness in children have not been established.

IMMEDIATE RELEASE TABLETS

Information for Patients: Patients should be informed of the potential risks and advantages of glipzide and of alternative modes of therapy. They should also be informed about the importance of adhering to dietary instructions, of a regular exercise program, and of regular testing of urine and/or blood glucose.

The risks of hypoglycemia, its symptoms and treatment, and conditions that predispose to its development should be explained to patients and responsible family members. Primary and secondary failure should also be explained.

EXTENDED RELEASE TABLETS

GI Disease: Markedly reduced GI retention times of the glipzide extended-release tablets may influence the pharmacokinetic profile and hence the clinical efficacy of the drug.

Adequate adjustment of dose and adherence to diet should be assessed before classifying a patient as a secondary failure.

Information for the Patient: Patients should be informed that glipzide extended-release tablets should be swallowed whole. Patients should not chew, divide or crush tablets. Patients should not be concerned if they occasionally notice in their something that looks like a tablet. In the glipzide extended-release tablet, the medication is contained within a shell that has been specially designed to slowly release the drug so the body can absorb it. When this process is completed, the empty tablet is eliminated from the body.

Patients should be informed of the potential risks and advantages of glipzide extended-release and of alternative modes of therapy. They should also be informed about the importance of adhering to dietary instructions,of a regular exercise program, and of regular testing of urine and/or blood glucose.

The risk of hypoglycemia, its symptoms and treatment, and conditions that predispose to its development should be explained to patients and responsible family members. Primary and secondary failure also should be explained.

Geriatric Use: Of the total number of patients in clinical studies of glipzide extended-release 33 percent were 65 and over. No overall differences in effectiveness or safety were observed between these patients and younger patients, but greater sensitivity of some individuals cannot be ruled out. Approximately 1-2 days longer were required to reach steady state in the elderly. (See CLINICAL PHARMACOLOGY and DOSAGE AND ADMINISTRATION).

DRUG INTERACTIONS:

IMMEDIATE AND EXTENDED RELEASE TABLETS

The hypoglycemic action of sulfonylureas may be potentiated by certain drugs including nonsteroidal anti-inflammatory agents and other drugs that are highly protein bound, salicylates, sulfonamides, chloramphenicol, probenecid, coumarins, monoamine oxidase inhibitors, and beta adrenergic blocking agents. When such drugs are administered to a patient receiving glipzide, the patient should be observed closely for hypoglycemia. When such drugs are withdrawn from a patient receiving glipzide, the patient should be observed closely for loss of control. *In vitro* binding studies with human serum proteins indicate that glipzide binds differently than tolbutamide and does not interact with salicylate or dicumarol. However, caution must be exercised in extrapolating these findings to the clinical situation and in the use of glipzide with these drugs.

Certain drugs tend to produce hyperglycemia and may lead to loss of control. These drugs include the thiazides and other diuretics, corticosteroids, phenothiazines, thyroid products, estrogens, oral contraceptives, phenytoin, nicotinic acid, sympathomimetics, calcium channel blocking drugs, and isoniazid. When such drugs are administered to a patient receiving glipzide, the patient should be closely observed for loss of control. When such drugs are withdrawn from a patient receiving glipzide, the patient should be observed closely for hypoglycemia.

A potential interaction between oral miconazole and oral hypoglycemic agents leading to severe hypoglycemia has been reported. Whether this interaction also occurs with the intravenous, topical, or vaginal preparations of miconazole is not known.

The effect of concomitant administration of fluconazole and glipzide has been demonstrated in a placebo-controlled crossover study in normal volunteers. All subjects received glipzide alone and following treatment with 100 mg of fluconazole as a single daily oral dose for 7 days. The mean percentage increase in the glipzide AUC after fluconazole administration was 56.9% (range: 35 to 81).

ADVERSE REACTIONS:

IMMEDIATE RELEASE TABLETS

In U.S. and foreign controlled studies, the frequency of serious adverse reactions reported was very low. Of 702 patients, 11.8% reported adverse reactions and in only 1.5% was glipzide discontinued.

Hypoglycemia: See PRECAUTIONSand OVERDOSAGE.

Gastrointestinal: Gastrointestinal disturbances are the most common reactions. Gastrointestinal complaints were reported with the following approximate incidence: nausea and diarrhea, one in seventy; constipation and gastralgia, one in one hundred. They appear to be dose-related and may disappear on division or reduction of dosage. Cholestatic jaundice may occur rarely with sulfonylureas: glipzide should be discontinued if this occurs.

Dermatologic: Allergic skin reactions including erythema, morbilliform or maculopapular eruptions, urticaria, pruritus, and eczema have been reported in about one in seventy patients. These may be transient and may disappear despite continued use of glipzide; if skin reactions persist, the drug should be discontinued. Porphyria cutanea tarda and photosensitivity reactions have been reported with sulfonylureas.

Miscellaneous: Dizziness, drowsiness, and headache have each been reported in about one in fifty patients treated with glipzide. They are usually transient and seldom require discontinuance of therapy.

In U.S. controlled studies the frequency of serious adverse experiences reported was very low and causal relationship has not been established. The 580 patients from 31 to 87 years of age who recieved glipzide extended-release tablets in doses from 5 mg to 60 mg in both controlled and open trials were included in the evaluation of adverse experiences. All adverse experiences reported were tabulated independently of their possible causal relation to medication.

Hypoglycemia: See PRECAUTIONS and OVERDOSAGEsections.

Only 3.4% of patients receiving glipzide extended-release tablets had hypoglycemia documented by/ a blood glucose measurement <60 mg/dl and or symptoms believed to be associated with hypoglycemia. In a comparative efficacy study of glipzide extended-release and glipzide, hypoglycemia occurred rarely with an incidence of less than 1% with both drugs.

In double-blind, placebo-controlled studies the adverse experiences reported with an incidence of 3% or more in glipzide extended-release-treated patients include:

TABLE 1

	Glucotrol XL (N=278)	Placebo % (N=69)
Adverse effect		
Asthenia	10.1	13.0
Headache	8.6	8.7
Dizziness	6.8	5.8
Nervousness	3.6	2.9
Tremor	3.6	0.0
Diarrhea	5.4	0.0
Flatulence	3.2	1.4

The following adverse experiences occurred with an incidence of less than 3% in glipzide extended-release-treated patients:

Body as a Whole: pain

Nervous System: insomnia, paresthesia, anxiety, depression and hypesthesia

Gastrointestinal: nausea, dyspepsia, constipation and vomiting

Metabolic: hypoglycemia

Musculoskeletal: arthralgia, leg cramps and myalgia

Cardiovascular: syncope

Skin: sweating and pruritus

Respiratory: rhinitis

Special Senses: blurred vision

Urogenital: polyuria

Other adverse experiences occurred with an incidence of less than 1% in glipzide extended-release-treated patients:

Body as a Whole: chills

Nervous System: hypertonia, confusion, vertigo, somnolence, gait abnormality and decreases libido

Gastrointestinal: anorexia and trace blood in stool

Metabolic: thirst and edema

Cardiovascular: arrhythmia, migraine, flushing and hypertension

Skin: rash and urticaria

Respiratory: pharyngitis and dyspnea

Special Senses: pain in the eye, conjunctivitis and retinal hemorrhage

ADVERSE REACTIONS: *(cont'd)*

Urogenital: dysuria

Although these adverse experiences occurred in patients treated with glipzide extended-release, a causal relationship to the medication has not been established in all cases.

There have been rare reports of gastrointestinal irritation and gastrointestinal bleeding with use of another drug in this non-deformable sustained release formulation, although causal relationships to the drug is uncertain.

IMMEDIATE AND EXTENDED RELEASE TABLETS

The following are adverse experiences reported with immediate release glipzide and other sulfonylureas, but have not been observed with glipzide extended-release:

Hematologic: Leukopenia, agranulocytosis, thrombocytopenia, hemolytic anemia, aplastic anemia, and pancytopenia have been reported with sulfonylureas.

Metabolic: Hepatic porphyria and disulfiram-like reactions have been reported with sulfonylureas. In the mouse, glipzide pretreatment did not cause an accumulation of acetaldehyde after ethanol administration. Clinical experience to date has shown that glipzide has an extremely low incidence of disulfiram-like alcohol reactions.

Endocrine Reactions: Cases of hyponatremia and the syndrome of inappropriate antidiuretic hormone (SIADH) secretion have been reported with this and other sulfonylureas.

Laboratory Tests: The pattern of laboratory test abnormalities observed with glipzide was similar to that for other sulfonylureas. Occasional mild to moderate elevations of SGOT, LDH, alkaline phosphatase, BUN and creatinine were noted. One case of jaundice was reported. The relationship of these abnormalities to glipzide is uncertain, and they have rarely been associated with clinical symptoms.

OVERDOSAGE:

There is no well documented experience with glipzide overdosage. The acute oral toxicity was extremely low in all species tested (LD_{50} greater than 4 g/kg).

Overdosage of sulfonylureas including glipzide can produce hypoglycemia. Mild hypoglycemic symptoms without loss of consciousness or neurologic findings should be treated aggressively with oral glucose and adjustments in drug dosage and/or meal patterns. Close monitoring should continue until the physician is assured that the patient is out of danger. Severe hypoglycemic reactions with coma, seizure, or other neurological impairment occur infrequently, but constitute medical emergencies requiring immediate hospitalization. If hypoglycemic coma is diagnosed or suspected, the patient should be given a rapid intravenous injection of concentrated (50%) glucose solution. This should be followed by a continuous infusion of a more dilute (10%) glucose solution at a rate that will maintain the blood glucose at a level above 100 mg/dl. Patients should be closely monitored for a minimum of 24 to 48 hours since hypoglycemia may recur after apparent clinical recovery. Clearance of glipzide from plasma would be prolonged in persons with liver disease. Because of the extensive protein binding of glipzide, dialysis is unlikely to be of benefit.

EXTENDED RELEASE TABLETS

There have been no known suicide attempts associated with purposeful overdosing with glipzide extended-release.

DOSAGE AND ADMINISTRATION:

IMMEDIATE AND EXTENDED RELEASE TABLETS

There is no fixed dosage regimen for the management of diabetes mellitus with glipzide or any other hypoglycemic agent. In addition to the usual monitoring of urinary glucose, the patient's blood glucose must also be monitored periodically to determine the minimum effective dose for the patient; to detect primary failure, i.e., inadequate lowering of blood glucose at the maximum recommended dose of medication; and to detect secondary failure, i.e., loss of an adequate blood-glucose-lowering response after an initial period of effectiveness. Glycosylated hemoglobin levels may also be of value in monitoring the patient's response to therapy.

Short-term administration of glipzide may be sufficient during periods of transient loss of control in patients usually controlled well on diet.

Patients Receiving Insulin: As with other sulfonylurea-class hypoglycemics, many stable non-insulin-dependent diabetic patients receiving insulin may be safely placed on glipzide. When transferring patients from insulin to glipzide, the following general guidelines should be considered:

For patients whose daily insulin requirement is 20 units or less, insulin may be discontinued and glipzide therapy may begin at usual dosages. Several days should elapse between glipzide titration steps.

For patients whose daily insulin requirement is greater than 20 units, the insulin dose should be reduced by 50% and glipzide therapy may begin at usual dosages. Subsequent reductions in insulin dosage should depend on individual patient response. Several days should elapse between glipzide titration steps.

During the insulin withdrawal period, the patient should test urine samples for sugar and ketone bodies at least three times daily. Patients should be instructed to contact the prescriber immediately if these tests are abnormal. In some cases, especially when patient has been receiving greater than 40 units of insulin daily, it may be advisable to consider hospitalization during the transition period.

PATIENTS RECEIVING OTHER ORAL HYPOGLYCEMIC AGENTS

As with other sulfonylurea-class hypoglycemics, no transition period is necessary when transferring patients to glipzide. Patients should be observed carefully (1-2 weeks) for hypoglycemia when being transferred from longer half-life sulfonylureas (*e.g.,* chlorpropamide) to glipzide due to potential over-lapping of drug effect.

EXTENDED RELEASE TABLETS

Recommended Dosing: The recommended stating dose of glipzide extended-release is 5 mg per day, given with breakfast. The recommended dose for geriatric patients is also 5 mg per day.

Dosage adjustment should be based on laboratory measures of glycemic control. While fasting blood glucose levels generally reach steady state following initiation of change in glipzide dosage, a single fasting glucose determination may not accurately reflect the response to therapy. In most cases, hemoglobin A_1c level measured at three month intervals is the preferred means of monitoring response to therapy.

Hemoglobin A_1c should be measured as glipzide extended-release therapy is initiated at the 5 mg dose and repeated approximately three months later, if the result of this test suggests that glycemic control over the preceding three months was inadequate, the glipzide extended-release dose may be increased to 10 mg. Subsequent dosage adjustments should be made on the basis of hemoglobin A_1c levels measured at three month intervals. If no improvement is seen after three months of therapy with a higher dose, the previous dose should be resumed. Decisions which utilize fasting blood glucose to adjust glipzide extended-release therapy should be based on at least two or more similar, consecutive values obtained seven days or more after the previous dose adjustment.

DOSAGE AND ADMINISTRATION: *(cont'd)*

Most patients will be controlled with 5 mg or 10 mg taken once daily. However, some patients may require up to the maximum recommended daily dose of 20 mg. While the glycemic control of selected patients may improve with doses which exceed 10 mg, clinical studies conducted to date have not demonstrated an additional group average reduction of hemoglobin A_1c beyond what was achieved with the 10 mg dose.

Based on the results of a randomized crossover study patients receiving immediate release glipizide may be switched safely to glipzide extended-release tablets once-a-day at the nearest equivalent total daily dose. Patients receiving immediate release glipzide also may be titrated to the appropriate dose of glipzide extended-release starting with 5 mg once daily. The decision to switch to the nearest equivalent dose ir to titrate should be based on clinical judgement.

In elderly patients, debilitated or malnourished patients, and patients with impaired renal or hepatic function, the initial and maintenance dosing should be conservative to avoid hypoglycemic reactions (see PRECAUTIONS.)

IMMEDIATE RELEASE TABLETS

In general, glipzide should be given approximately 30 minutes before a meal to achieve the greatest reduction in postprandial hyperglycemia.

INITIAL DOSE

The recommended starting dose is 5 mg, given before breakfast. Geriatric patients or those with liver disease may be started on 2.5 mg.

TITRATION

Dosage adjustments should ordinarily be in increments of 2.5-5 mg, as determined by blood glucose response. At least several days should elapse between titration steps. If response to a single dose is not satisfactory, dividing that dose may prove effective. The maximum recommended once daily dose is 15 mg. Doses above 15 mg should ordinarily be divided and given before meals of adequate caloric content. The maximum recommended total daily dose is 40 mg.

MAINTENANCE

Some patients may be effectively controlled on a once-a-day regimen, while others show better response with divided dosing. Total daily doses above 15 mg should ordinarily be divided. Total daily doses above 30 mg have been safely given on a b.i.d. basis to long-term patients.

In elderly patients, debilitated or malnourished patients, and patients with impaired renal or hepatic function, the initial and maintenance dosing should be conservative to avoid hypoglycemic reactions (see PRECAUTIONS).

IMMEDIATE RELEASE TABLETS

Patients Receiving Other Oral Hypoglycemic Agents: As with other sulfonylurea-class hypoglycemics, no transition period is necessary when transferring patients to glipzide. Patients should be observed carefully (1-2 weeks) for hypoglycemia when being transferred from longer half-life sulfonylureas (*e.g.*, chlorpropamide) to glipzide due to potential overlapping of drug effect.

PATIENT INFORMATION:

Glipizide is a sulfonylurea used in patients with diabetes mellitus to lower blood sugar. Notify your physician if you are pregnant or nursing. Do not change the dose or stop taking glipizide without talking with your physician. Immediate-release glipizide tablets should be taken on an empty stomach, 30 minutes before a meal. Extended-release glipizide tablets may be taken with food. Do not break, crush, or chew extended-release glipizide tablets. Patients taking extended release glipizide tablets may notice something that looks like a tablet in their stool. This is the leftover tablet after the medicine has been absorbed and is normal. Avoid drinking alcohol while taking this medication. Alcohol may cause flushing, weakness, dizziness, a tingling sensation and headache. Avoid taking aspirin with this medication. Notify your physician if you develop unexplained fever, sore throat, yellowing of the skin or eyes, dark urine, or skin rash. Notify your physician if you develop fatigue, nausea, confusion, agitation, excessive hunger, profuse sweating, numbness or tingling of lips, tongue or extremities (may indicate low blood sugar), or if you develop excessive thirst or urination, or glucose or ketones in the urine or blood (may indicate high blood sugar).

HOW SUPPLIED:

IMMEDIATE RELEASE TABLETS

Glucotrol tablets are white, dye-free, scored, diamond-shaped, and imprinted as follows:

5 mg-Pfizer 411

10 mg-Pfizer 412.

Recommended Storage: Store below 86°F (30°C).

EXTENDED RELEASE TABLETS

Glucotrol XL Extended Release Tablets are supplied as 5 mg and 10 mg round, biconvex tablets and imprinted with black ink with color coating.

The tablets should be protected from moisture and humidity and stored at controlled room temperature, 59° to 86°F (15° to 30°C).

HOW SUPPLIED - RATED THERAPEUTICALLY EQUIVALENT:

Tablet - Oral - 5 mg

100's	$6.53	Glipizide, H.C.F.A. F F P	99999-1357-01

Tablet - Oral - 10 mg

100's	$11.63	Glipizide, H.C.F.A. F F P	99999-1357-02

Tablet, Uncoated - Oral - 5 mg

100's	$18.23	Glipizide, United Res	00677-1544-01
100's	$27.30	Glipizide, Circa	71114-0221-01
100's	$28.97	Glipizide, Watson Labs	52544-0460-01
100's	$30.25	Glipizide, Schein Pharm (US)	00364-2604-01
100's	$30.35	Glipizide, Qualitest Pharms	00603-3755-21
100's	$30.62	Glipizide, Endo Labs	60951-0711-70
100's	$30.65	Glipizide, Major Pharms	00904-7924-60
100's	$30.67	Glipizide, Goldline Labs	00182-1994-01
100's	$30.67	Glipizide, Aligen Independ	00405-5380-01
100's	**$30.89**	**GLUCOTROL, Roerig**	**00049-4110-66**
100's	$31.09	Glipizide, Par Pharm	49884-0451-01
100's	$31.85	Glipizide, Geneva Pharms	00781-1452-01
100's	$31.85	Glipizide, HL Moore Drug Exch	00839-7939-06
100's	$31.90	Glipizide, Warner Chilcott	00047-0463-24
100's	$31.90	Glipizide, Rugby	00536-5702-01
100's	**$32.44**	**GLUCOTROL, Roerig**	**00049-4110-41**
100's	$34.60	Glipizide, Geneva Pharms	00781-1452-13
100's	**$35.45**	**GLUCOTROL, Roerig Pfizer**	**00662-4110-66**
100's	$36.50	Glipizide, Mylan	00378-1105-01
100's	**$37.23**	**GLUCOTROL, Roerig Pfizer**	**00662-4110-41**
500's	$129.68	Glipizide, Circa	71114-0221-05
500's	$137.63	Glipizide, Watson Labs	52544-0460-05
500's	$144.00	Glipizide, Schein Pharm (US)	00364-2604-05

HOW SUPPLIED - RATED THERAPEUTICALLY EQUIVALENT: *(cont'd)*

500's	$144.05	Glipizide, Qualitest Pharms	00603-3755-28
500's	$145.70	Glipizide, Major Pharms	00904-7924-40
500's	$145.73	Glipizide, Goldline Labs	00182-1994-05
500's	$145.73	Glipizide, Aligen Independ	00405-5380-02
500's	$146.05	Glipizide, Par Pharm	49884-0451-05
500's	**$146.77**	**GLUCOTROL, Roerig**	**00049-4110-73**
500's	$151.29	Glipizide, HL Moore Drug Exch	00839-7939-12
500's	$151.55	Glipizide, Endo Labs	60951-0711-85
500's	$151.75	Glipizide, Warner Chilcott	00047-0463-30
500's	$151.85	Glipizide, Rugby	00536-5702-05
500's	$156.85	Glipizide, Mylan	00378-1105-05
500's	**$168.39**	**GLUCOTROL, Roerig Pfizer**	**00662-4110-73**
1000's	$259.36	Glipizide, Circa	71114-0221-00
1000's	$261.50	Glipizide, Watson Labs	52544-0460-10
1000's	$275.85	Glipizide, Major Pharms	00904-7924-80
1000's	$288.32	Glipizide, Geneva Pharms	00781-1452-10

Tablet, Uncoated - Oral - 10 mg

10 mg x 500	**$269.41**	**GLUCOTROL, Roerig**	**00049-4120-73**
100's	$33.53	Glipizide, United Res	00677-1545-01
100's	$50.12	Glipizide, Circa	71114-0222-01
100's	$53.18	Glipizide, Watson Labs	52544-0461-01
100's	$55.50	Glipizide, Schein Pharm (US)	00364-2605-01
100's	$55.70	Glipizide, Qualitest Pharms	00603-3756-21
100's	$56.22	Glipizide, Endo Labs	60951-0714-70
100's	$56.30	Glipizide, Major Pharms	00904-7925-60
100's	$56.31	Glipizide, Goldline Labs	00182-1995-01
100's	$56.31	Glipizide, Aligen Independ	00405-5381-01
100's	**$56.72**	**GLUCOTROL, Roerig**	**00049-4120-66**
100's	$57.09	Glipizide, Par Pharm	49884-0452-01
100's	$58.47	Glipizide, HL Moore Drug Exch	00839-7940-06
100's	$58.50	Glipizide, Geneva Pharms	00781-1453-01
100's	$58.53	Glipizide, Warner Chilcott	00047-0464-24
100's	$58.54	Glipizide, Rugby	00536-5703-01
100's	**$59.56**	**GLUCOTROL, Roerig**	**00049-4120-41**
100's	$60.50	Glipizide, Geneva Pharms	00781-1453-13
100's	$63.95	Glipizide, Mylan	00378-1110-01
100's	**$65.08**	**GLUCOTROL, Roerig Pfizer**	**00662-4120-66**
100's	**$68.33**	**GLUCOTROL, Roerig Pfizer**	**00662-4120-41**
500's	$238.07	Glipizide, Circa	71114-0222-05
500's	$252.61	Glipizide, Watson Labs	52544-0461-05
500's	$253.35	Glipizide, Major Pharms	00904-7925-40
500's	$264.50	Glipizide, Schein Pharm (US)	00364-2605-05
500's	$264.50	Glipizide, Qualitest Pharms	00603-3756-28
500's	$264.52	Glipizide, Goldline Labs	00182-1995-05
500's	$264.52	Glipizide, Aligen Independ	00405-5381-02
500's	$268.19	Glipizide, Par Pharm	49884-0452-05
500's	$277.75	Glipizide, HL Moore Drug Exch	00839-7940-12
500's	$278.21	Glipizide, Endo Labs	60951-0714-85
500's	$278.25	Glipizide, Warner Chilcott	00047-0464-30
500's	$280.58	Glipizide, Rugby	00536-5703-05
500's	$288.50	Glipizide, Mylan	00378-1110-05
500's	**$309.11**	**GLUCOTROL, Roerig Pfizer**	**00662-4120-73**
1000's	$476.14	Glipizide, Circa	71114-0222-00
1000's	$479.96	Glipizide, Watson Labs	52544-0461-10
1000's	$506.70	Glipizide, Major Pharms	00904-7925-80
1000's	$528.67	Glipizide, Geneva Pharms	00781-1453-10

HOW SUPPLIED - NOT RATED EQUIVALENT:

Tablet, Coated, Sustained Action - Oral - 5 mg

100's	**$26.73**	**GLUCOTROL XL, Roerig**	**00049-1550-66**
500's	**$133.68**	**GLUCOTROL XL, Roerig**	**00049-1550-73**

Tablet, Coated, Sustained Action - Oral - 10 mg

100's	**$52.90**	**GLUCOTROL XL, Roerig**	**00049-1560-66**
500's	**$264.47**	**GLUCOTROL XL, Roerig**	**00049-1560-73**

GLUCAGON HYDROCHLORIDE *(001358)*

CATEGORIES: Antagonists and Antidotes; Antidiabetic Agents; Antidotes; Blood Glucose Regulators; Diabetes; Diagnostic Agents; Hormones; Hyperglycemia; Hypoglycemia; Shock; Pregnancy Category B; FDA Approval Pre 1982

FORMULARIES: BC-BS; Medi-Cal

DESCRIPTION:

Glucagon is extracted from beef and pork pancreas.

Chemically unrelated to insulin, glucagon is a single-chain polypeptide containing 29 amino acid residues and having a molecular weight of 3,483.

The empirical formula is $C_{153}H_{225}N_{43}O_{49}S$.

Crystalline glucagon is a white powder containing less than 0.05% zinc. It is relatively insoluble in water but is soluble at a pH of less than 3 or more than 9.5. Glucagon is stable in lyophilized form at room temperatures.

Glucagon for Injection contains glucagon as the hydrochloride. The 1-mg vials contain 1 mg (1 unit) of glucagon and 49 mg of lactose. The 10-mg vial contains 10 mg (10 units) of glucagon and 133 mg lactose. One USP unit of is equivalent to 1 International Unit of glucagon and also to about 1 mg of glucagon.[1] The diluent contains glycerin, 1.6%, with 0.2% phenol as a preservative. Sodium hydroxide and/or hydrochloric acid may have been added during manufacture to adjust the pH.

CLINICAL PHARMACOLOGY:

Glucagon causes an increase in blood glucose concentration and is used in the treatment of hypoglycemia. It is effective in small doses, and no evidence of toxicity has been reported with its use. Glucagon acts only on liver glycogen, converting it to glucose.

Parenteral administration of glucagon produces relaxation of the smooth muscle of the stomach, duodenum, small bowel, and colon.

The half-life of glucagon in plasma is approximately 3 to 6 minutes, which is similar to that of insulin.

INDICATIONS AND USAGE:

For the treatment of hypoglycemia: Glucagon is useful in counteracting severe hypoglycemic reactions.

The patient with type I diabetes does not have as great a response in blood glucose levels as does the stable type II diabetes patient. Therefore, supplementary carbohydrate should be given as soon as possible, especially to the child or adolescent patient.

INDICATIONS AND USAGE: *(cont'd)*

For use as a diagnostic aid: Glucagon is indicated as a diagnostic aid in the radiologic examination of the stomach, duodenum, small bowel, and colon when a hypotonic state would be advantageous.

Glucagon is as effective for this examination as are the anticholinergic drugs, but it has fewer side effects. When glucagon is administered concomitantly with an anticholinergic agent, the response is not significantly greater than when either drug is used alone. However, the addition of the anticholinergic agent results in increased side effects.

CONTRAINDICATIONS:

Glucagon is contraindicated in patients with known hypersensitivity to it or in patients with pheochromocytoma.

WARNINGS:

Glucagon should be administered cautiously to patients with a history suggestive of insulinoma and/or pheochromocytoma. In patients with insulinoma, intravenous administration of glucagon will produce an initial increase in blood glucose; however, because of glucagon's insulin-releasing effect, it may cause the insulinoma to release its insulin and subsequently cause hypoglycemia. A patient developing symptoms of hypoglycemia after a dose of glucagon should be given glucose orally, intravenously, or by gavage, whichever is more appropriate.

Exogenous glucagon also stimulates the release of catecholamines. In the presence of pheochromocytoma, glucagon can cause the tumor to release catecholamines, which results in a sudden and marked increase in blood pressure. If a patient suddenly develops a marked increase in blood pressure, 5 to 10 mg of phentolamine mesylate may be administered intravenously in an attempt to control the blood pressure.

Generalized allergic reactions, including urticaria, respiratory distress, and hypotension, have been reported in patients who received glucagon injection.

PRECAUTIONS:

General: Glucagon is helpful in hypoglycemia only if liver glycogen is available. Because glucagon is of little or no help in states of starvation, adrenal insufficiency, or chronic hypoglycemia, glucose should be considered for the treatment of hypoglycemia.

Laboratory Tests: Blood glucose determinations may be obtained to follow the patient in hypoglycemic shock until he or she is asymptomatic.

Carcinogenesis, Mutagenesis, and Impairment of Fertility: Because glucagon is usually given in a single dose and has a very short half-life (3 to 6 minutes), no studies have been done regarding carcinogenesis.

Reproduction studies have been performed in rats at doses up to 2 mg/kg b.i.d. (up to 120 times the human dose) and have revealed no evidence of impaired fertility.

Usage in Pregnancy: Pregnancy Category B: Reproduction studies have been performed in rats at doses up to 2 mg/kg b.i.d., (up to 120 times the human dose), and have revealed no evidence of harm to the fetus due to glucagon. There are, however, no adequate and well-controlled studies in pregnant women. Because animal reproduction studies are not always predictive of human response, this drug should be used during pregnancy only if clearly needed.

Nursing Mothers: It is not known whether this drug is excreted in human milk. Because many drugs are excreted in human milk, caution should be exercised when glucagon is administered to a nursing woman. If the drug is excreted in human milk during its short half-life, it will be handled like any other polypeptide, i.e. it will be hydrolyzed and absorbed. Glucagon is not active when taken orally because it is destroyed in the gastrointestinal tract before it can be absorbed.

ADVERSE REACTIONS:

Glucagon is relatively free of adverse reactions except for occasional nausea and vomiting, which may also occur with hypoglycemia. Generalized allergic reactions have been reported (see WARNINGS.)

OVERDOSAGE:

Signs and Symptoms: No cases of human overdosage of glucagon have been reported. Glucagon is generally well tolerated. If overdosage occurred, it would not be expected to cause consequential toxicity, but would be expected to be associated with nausea, vomiting, gastric hypotonicity, and diarrhea.

Intravenous administration of glucagon has been shown to have a positive inotropic and chronotropic effect. A transient increment in both blood pressure and pulse rate may occur following the administration of glucagon. Patients taking β-blockers might be expected to have a greater increment in both pulse and blood pressure. This increase will be transient because of glucagon's short half-life. The increase in blood pressure and pulse rate may require therapy in patients with pheochromocytoma, insulinomas, or coronary artery disease.

When glucagon was given in large doses to cardiac patients, investigators reported a positive inotropic effect. These investigators administered glucagon in doses of 5 to 166 hours. Total doses ranged from 25 to 996 mg, and a 21-month-old child received approximately 8.25 mg in 165 hours. Side effects included nausea, vomiting, and decreasing serum potassium concentration. Serum potassium could be maintained within normal limits with supplemental potassium.

The intravenous median lethal dose for glucagon in mice is approximately 300 mg/kg. Because glucagon is a polypeptide, it would be rapidly destroyed in the gastrointestinal tract if it were to be accidentally ingested.

Treatment: To obtain up-to-date information about the treatment of overdose, a good resource is your certified Regional Poison Control Center. Telephone numbers of certified poison control centers are listed in *Physicians GenRx*.In managing overdosage, consider the possibility of multiple drug overdoses, interaction among drugs, and unusual drug kinetics in your patient.

In view of the extremely short half-life of glucagon and its prompt destruction and excretion, the treatment of overdosage is symptomatic, primarily for nausea, vomiting, and possible hypokalemia.

If the patient develops a dramatic increase in blood pressure, 5 to 10 mg of phentolamine has been shown to be effective in lowering blood pressure for the short time that control would be needed.

Forced diuresis, peritoneal dialysis, hemodialysis, or charcoal hemoperfusion have not been established as beneficial for an overdose of glucagon; it is extremely unlikely that one of these procedures would ever be indicated.

DOSAGE AND ADMINISTRATION:

For the treatment of hypoglycemia: The diluent is provided for use only in the preparation of glucagon for *intermittent*parenteral injection and for no other use.

If glucagon is to be given at doses higher than 2 mg, it should be reconstituted with Sterile Water for Injection instead of the supplied diluting solution supplied and used immediately.

DOSAGE AND ADMINISTRATION: *(cont'd)*

Directions for Use of Glucagon

1. Dissolve the lyophilized glucagon in the accompanying solvent.
2. Glucagon should not be used at concentrations greater than 1 mg (1 unit/ml).
3. Glucagon solutions should not be used unless they are clear and of a water-like consistency.
4. For adults and for children weighing more than 20 kg, give 1 mg (1 unit) by subcutaneous, intramuscular, or intravenous injection.
5. For children weighing less than 20 kg, give 0.5 mg (0.5 unit) or a dose equivalent to 20-30 mcg/kg.[2,3,4,5,6]
6. The patient will usually awaken within 15 minutes. If the response is delayed, there is no contraindication to the administration of 1 or 2 additional doses of glucagon; however, in view of the deleterious effects of cerebral hypoglycemia and depending on the duration and depth of coma, the use of parenteral glucose *must* be considered by the physician.
7. Intravenous glucose *must* be given if the patient fails to respond to glucagon.
8. When the patient responds, give supplemental carbohydrate to restore the liver glycogen and prevent secondary hypoglycemia.

Instructions to the Family: Instructions describing the method of using, this preparation are included in the literature that accompanies the patient's package. It is advisable for the patient and family members to become familiar with the technique of preparing Glucagon for Injection, before and emergency arises. Patients are instructed to use 1 mg (1 unit) for adults and, if recommended by a doctor, 1/2 the adult dose (0.5 mg) [0.5 unit] for children weighing less than 44 lb (20 kg).

General Management of Hypoglycemia: The following are helpful measures in the prevention of hypoglycemic reactions due to insulin:

1. Reasonable uniformity from day to day with regard to diet, insulin, and exercise.
2. Careful adjustment of the insulin program so that the type (or types) of insulin, dose, and time (or times) of administration are suited to the individual patient.
3. Frequent testing of the blood or urine for glucose so that a change in insulin requirements can be foreseen.
4. Routine carrying of sugar, candy, or other readily absorbable carbohydrate by the patient so that it may be taken at the first warning of an oncoming reaction.

If the patient is unaware of the symptoms of hypoglycemia, he/she may lapse into insulin shock; therefore, the physician should instruct the patient in this regard when feasible.

It is important that the patient be aroused as quickly as possible, because prolonged hypoglycemic reactions may result in cortical damage. Glucagon or intravenous glucose will awaken the patient sufficiently so that oral carbohydrates may be taken.

CAUTION-Although glucagon may be used for the treatment of hypoglycemia during an emergency, the physician must still be notified when hypoglycemic reactions occur so that the treatment regimen may be adjusted if necessary.

For use as a diagnostic aid: Dissolve the lyophilized glucagon in the accompanying diluting solution.

Glucagon should not be used at concentrations greater than 1 mg (1 unit/ml).

The following doses may be administered for relaxation of the stomach, duodenum, and small bowel, depending on the time of onset of action and the duration of effect required for the examination. Since the stomach is less sensitive to the effect of glucagon, 0.5 mg (0.5 units) IV or 2 units mg (2 units) IM are recommended. (TABLE 1)

TABLE 1

Dose	Route of Administration	Time of Onset of Action	Approximate Duration of Effect
0.25-0.5 mg	IV	1 minute	9-17 minutes
1 mg	IM	8-10 minutes	12-27 minutes
2 mg*	IV	1 minute	22-25 minutes
2 mg*	IM	4-7 minutes	21-32 minutes

* Administration of 2-mg (2 units) doses produces a higher incidence of nausea and vomiting than do lower doses.

For examination of the colon, it is recommended that a 2-mg (2 units) dose be administered intramuscularly approximately 10 minutes prior to initiation of the procedure.

Relaxation of the colon and reduction of discomfort to the patient will allow the radiologist to perform a more satisfactory examination.

STABILITY AND STORAGE

Before Reconstitution: Vials of Glucagon as well as the Diluting Solution for Glucagon for Injection, USP, may be stored at controlled room temperature, 59° to 86°F (15° to 30°C).

After Reconstitution: Glucagon in 1-ml vials or Hyporets should be used immediately. Glucagon reconstituted with the Diluting Solution for Glucagon for Injection in multiple dose vials may be stored at 41°F (5°C) for up to 48 hours if necessary. Glucagon reconstituted with Diluting Solution for Glucagon for Injection should be used immediately.

REFERENCES:

1. *Drug Information for the Health Care Professional.* 11th ed. Rockville, Maryland: The United States Pharmacopeial Convention, Inc; 1991; IA:1380. **2.** Gibbs et al: Use of Glucagon to terminate insulin reactions in diabetic children. *Nebr Med J* 1958;43:56-57. **3.** Cornblath M, et al: Studies of carbohydrate metabolism in the newborn: Effect of glucagon on concentration of sugar in capillary blood of newborn infant. *Pediatrics*1958;21:885-892. **4.** Carson MJ Koch R, Clinical studies with glucagon in children. *J Pediatr*1955;47:167-170. **5.** Shipp JC, et al: Treatment of insulin hypoglycemia in diabetic campers. *Diabetes* 1964;13:645-648. **6.** Amos J, Wranne L: Hypoglycemia in childhood diabetes II: Effect of subcutaneous or intramuscular injection of different doses of glucagon. *Acta Pediatr Scand* 1988;77:548-553.

PATIENT PACKAGE INSERT:

INFORMATION FOR THE USER

BECOME FAMILIAR WITH THE FOLLOWING INSTRUCTIONS BEFORE AN EMERGENCY ARISES. DO NOT USE GLUCAGON FOR INJECTION AFTER DATE STAMPED ON THE BOTTLE LABEL. IF YOU HAVE QUESTIONS CONCERNING THE USE OF THIS PRODUCT, CONSULT A DOCTOR.

IMPORTANT

Act quickly. Prolonged unconsciousness may be harmful.

Turn patient on his/her side to prevent patient from choking.

Do not prepare Glucagon for Injection until you are ready to use it.

Indications for Use: Use glucagon to treat insulin coma or insulin reaction resulting from severe hypoglycemia (low blood sugar). Symptoms of severe hypoglycemia include disorientation, unconsciousness, and seizures or convulsions. Administer glucagon if (1) the patient is unconscious, (2) the patient is unable to eat sugar or a sugar-sweetened product, or (3) repeated administration of sugar or a sugar-sweetened product does not improve the patient's

PATIENT PACKAGE INSERT: *(cont'd)*

condition. Milder cases of hypoglycemia should be treated promptly by eating sugar or a sugar- sweetened product. (See Information On Hypoglycemia for more information on the symptoms of hypoglycemia.)

DIRECTIONS FOR USE TO PREPARE GLUCAGON INJECTION

1. Remove the flip-off seals on bottle Nos. 1 and 2.

2. Wipe the rubber stoppers on both bottles with alcohol swab.

3. Use a sterile U-100 (1-ml) insulin syringe and needle. Remove the needle protector from the syringe.

4. Draw the plunger of the syringe back to the 50-unit mark on a U-100 syringe. The syringe now contains 1/2 ml of air.

5. Pick up the white-labeled, brown bottle (No. 1) containing the diluting solution. Pierce the center of the stopper with the needle attached to the syringe containing 1/2 ml of air.

6. Turn the bottle upside down and slowly inject air from the syringe into the bottle. It will now be possible to remove the diluting solution more easily.

7. Keep the tip of the needle in the diluting solution and withdraw all of the solution into the syringe.

8. Remove syringe from bottle No. 1 and insert same needle into the clear bottle with green-striped label (No. 2) containing the glucagon. Inject all the diluting solution from the syringe into bottle No. 2

9. Remove the syringe. Shake bottle gently until glucagon dissolves and the solution becomes clear. GLUCAGON SHOULD NOT BE USED UNLESS THE SOLUTION IS CLEAR AND OF A WATER-LIKE CONSISTENCY. Inject Glucagon immediately after mixing.

To Inject Glucagon: Using Same Technique as for Injecting Insulin

10. Using the same syringe, withdraw all of the solution (100-unit mark on syringe) from bottle. The usual adult dose is 1 mg (1 unit). For children weighing less than 44 lbs (20 kg) give 1/2 adult dose (0.5mg). For children, withdraw 1/2 of the solution from the bottle (50-unit mark on syringe).

11. Cleanse injection site on buttock, arm, or thigh with alcohol swab.

12. Insert the needle into the loose tissue under the cleansed injection site, and inject all of the glucagon solution. THERE IS NO DANGER OF OVERDOSE. Apply light pressure at the injection site, and withdraw the needle. Press an alcohol swab against the injection site.

13. Turn the patient on his/her side. When an unconscious person awakens, he/she may vomit. Turning the patient on his/her side will prevent him/her from choking.

14. FEED THE PATIENT AS SOON AS HE/SHE AWAKENS AND IS ABLE TO SWALLOW. Give the patient a fast-acting source of sugar (such as a regular soft drink or orange juice) and a long-acting source of sugar (such as crackers and cheese or a meat sandwich). If the patient does not awaken within 15 minutes, give another dose of glucagon and INFORM A DOCTOR IMMEDIATELY.

WARNING: THE PATIENT MAY BE IN A COMA FROM SEVERE HYPERGLYCEMIA (HIGH BLOOD GLUCOSE) RATHER THAN HYPOGLYCEMIA. IN SUCH A CASE, THE PATIENT WILL **NOT** RESPOND TO GLUCAGON AND REQUIRES IMMEDIATE MEDICAL ATTENTION.

15. Even if the glucagon revives the patient, his/her doctor should be promptly notified. A doctor should be notified whenever severe hypoglycemic reactions occur.

Information on Hypoglycemia: Early symptoms of hypoglycemia (low blood glucose include: sweating, drowsiness, dizziness, sleep disturbances, palpitation, anxiety, tremor, blurred vision, hunger, slurred speech, restlessness, depressive mood, tingling in the hands, feet, lips, or tongue, irritability, lightheadedness, abnormal behavior, unsteady movement, inability to concentrate, personality changes, headache.

If not treated, the patient may progress to severe hypoglycemia that can include: disorientation, seizures, unconsciousness, death.

The occurrence of early symptoms calls for prompt and, if necessary, repeated administration of some for of carbohydrate. Patients should always carry a quick source of sugar, such as candy mints or glucose tablets. The prompt treatment of mild hypoglycemic symptoms can prevent severe hypoglycemic reactions. If improvement does not occur or if administration of carbohydrate is impossible, glucagon should be given at a medical facility. Glucagon, a naturally occurring substance produced by the pancreas, is helpful because it enables the patient to produce his/her own blood glucose to correct the hypoglycemic state.

*Hyporet (disposable syringe, Lilly)

HOW SUPPLIED - EQUIVALENTS NOT AVAILABLE:

Injection, Dry-Soln - Intramuscular; - 10 mg/10ml

10 ml x 1	$270.06	Glucagon, Lilly	00002-1451-01

Injection, Solution - Intramuscular; - 1 mg/vial

1 mg x 10	$36.28	Glucagon Emergency Kit, Lilly	00002-8030-01
1 ml x 1	$28.42	Glucagon, Lilly	00002-1450-01

GLUCOSE *(001360)*

CATEGORIES: EENT Drugs; Eye, Ear, Nose, & Throat Preparations; Ophthalmics; FDA Pre 1938 Drugs

FORMULARIES: WHO

Prescribing information not available at time of publication.

GLUCOSE; LIDOCAINE *(001362)*

CATEGORIES: Anesthesia; Antiarrhythmic Agents; Local Anesthetics; Renal Drugs; FDA Pre 1938 Drugs

BRAND NAMES: Xylocaine HCl For Spinal; Xylocaine W/Glucose

Prescribing information not available at time of publication.

HOW SUPPLIED - RATED THERAPEUTICALLY EQUIVALENT:

Injection, Solution - Intraspinal; In - 75 mg/50 mg

2 ml x 10	$87.64	XYLOCAINE 5%, WITH GLUCOSE 7.5%, Astra USA	00186-0225-03

GLUTETHIMIDE *(001366)*

CATEGORIES: Anxiolytics, Sedatives, Hypnotic; Central Nervous System Agents; Hypnotics; Insomnia; Sedatives/Hypnotics; Pregnancy Category C; DEA Class CII; DEA Class CIII; FDA Approval Pre 1982

BRAND NAMES: **Doriden**; Doriglute; Dorimide; *Orimeten*
(International brand names outside U.S. in italics)

COST OF THERAPY: $0.73 (Insomnia; Tablet; 500 mg; 1/day; 7 days)

DESCRIPTION:

Glutethimide, an oral hypnotic, is a piperidinedione derivative that occurs as a white, crystalline powder and is practically insoluble in water, soluble in alcohol. Its chemical name is 2-ethyl-2-phenylglutarimide.

The tablets also contain corn starch, magnesium aluminum silicate, methylcellulose, colloidal silica, and stearic acid.

CLINICAL PHARMACOLOGY:

Glutethimide is erratically absorbed from the gastrointestinal tract. Following single oral doses of 500 mg, wide variations in absorption of the drug were observed, and the peak plasma concentration occurred from one to six hours after administration. The average plasma half-life is 10-12 hours. Glutethimide is a racemate; both isomers are hydroxylated; the d-isomer on the piperidinedione ring and the l-isomer the phenyl substituent. Both hydroxylates are conjugated with glucuronic acid; the glucuronides pass into the enterohepatic circulation, and thence are excreted in the urine.

Less than 2% of a usual dose is excreted in the urine unchanged. About 50% of the drug is bound to plasma proteins.

Glutethimide exhibits pronounced anticholinergic activity, which is manifested by mydriasis, inhibition of salivary secretions, and decreased intestinal motility.

INDICATIONS AND USAGE:

Glutethimide has been shown to be effective as a hypnotic for three to seven days. It is not indicated for chronic administration. Should insomnia persist, a drug-free interval of one or more weeks should elapse before retreatment is considered. Attempts should be made to find alternative nondrug therapy in chronic insomnia.

CONTRAINDICATIONS:

Glutethimide is contraindicated in patients with known hypersensitivity to the drug. It is also contraindicated in patients with porphyria.

WARNINGS:

The concomitant use of alcohol or other CNS depressants may produce additive CNS depressant effects.

PRECAUTIONS:

Information for the Patient: The patient should be warned about the possible additive effects when glutethimide is taken concomitantly with other central nervous system depressants such as alcohol.

The patient on glutethimide must be warned against driving a car or operating dangerous machinery while on the drug, since glutethimide may impair the ability to perform hazardous activities requiring mental alertness or physical coordination.

Carcinogenesis: No carcinogenicity studies in animals have been performed.

PREGNANCY, TERATOGENIC EFFECTS, PREGNANCY CATEGORY C

Animal reproduction studies have not been conducted with glutethimide. It is also not known whether glutethimide can cause fetal harm when administered to a pregnant woman or can affect reproduction capacity. Glutethimide should be given to a pregnant woman only if clearly needed.

Nursing Mothers: Because of the potential for serious adverse reactions in nursing infants from glutethimide, a decision should be made whether to discontinue nursing or to discontinue the drug, taking into account the importance of the drug to the mother.

Pediatric Use: Glutethimide is not recommended for use in children, because its safety and effectiveness in the pediatric age group have not been established by clinical trials.

DRUG INTERACTIONS:

Glutethimide induces hepatic microsomal enzymes resulting in increased metabolism of coumarin anticoagulants and decreased anticoagulant response.

ADVERSE REACTIONS:

In clinical studies in more than 796 patients, 8.6% exhibited skin rash, 2.7% reported nausea, 1.1% hangover, and 1% reported drowsiness. The following reactions occurred in less than 1% of the patient population: vertigo, headache, depression, dizziness, ataxia, confusion, edema, indigestion, lightheadedness, nocturnal diaphoresis, vomiting, dry mouth, euphoria, impaired memory, slurred speech, and tinnitus. Paradoxical excitation, blurred vision, acute hypersensitivity, porphyria, and blood dyscrasia such as thrombocytopenic purpura, aplastic anemia, and leukopenia are rare.

In cases in which a generalized skin rash occurs, the medication should be withdrawn. This rash usually clears spontaneously within a few days after drug withdrawal.

DRUG ABUSE AND DEPENDENCE:

Controlled Substance: This drug is controlled in Schedule III.

Dependence: Both physical and psychological dependence have occurred; therefore patients should be carefully evaluated before prescribing glutethimide. Ordinarily, an amount adequate for one week is sufficient. The patient should be reevaluated before represcribing, after an interval of one or more weeks. Withdrawal symptoms include nausea, abdominal discomfort, tremors, convulsions, and delirium. Newborn infants of mothers dependent on glutethimide may also exhibit withdrawal symptoms. In the presence of dependence, dosage, should be reduced gradually.

OVERDOSAGE:

Acute Overdosage: The single acute lethal dose of glutethimide in humans ranges from 10 g to 20 g. Although the majority of fatalities have resulted from single doses in this range, patients have died from single doses as low as 5 g and have recovered from single doses as high as 35 g. A single oral dose of 5 g usually produces severe intoxication. A plasma level of 3 mg/100 ml is indicative of severe poisoning, but the level may be higher if the patient is tolerant to the drug.

OVERDOSAGE: *(cont'd)*

However, the level may also be lower because of sequestration of the drug in body fat depots and in the gastrointestinal tract. A lower level does not preclude the possibility of severe poisoning; therefore, the extent of intoxication may not be accurately reflected by single glutethimide plasma level determinations. Serial determinations are mandatory for proper patient evaluation.

Ingestion of acutely excessive dosage of glutethimide can give rise to a life-threatening situation. The effects of glutethimide are exaggerated by concomitant ingestion of other hypnotics or sedatives such as alcohol, barbiturates, etc., and suicidal effects commonly involve multiple drugs of the sedative-hypnotic-tranquilizer types.

Signs and Symptoms: The principal signs and symptoms caused by glutethimide intoxication vary in severity in ratio to the ingested dosage, in general, and are indistinguishable from those caused by barbiturate intoxication. The degree of CNS depression often fluctuates, possibly due to irregular absorption of the drug and/or accumulation of an active toxic metabolite, 4-hydroxy-2-ethyl-2-phenyl-glutarimide (4-HG). They are: CNS depression, including coma (Profound And Prolonged in Severe Intoxication); hypothermia, which may be followed by fever even without apparent infection; depressed or lost deep tendon reflexes; depression or absence of corneal and pupillary reflexes; dilation of pupils; depressed or absent response to painful stimuli; inadequate ventilation (even with relatively normal respiratory rate), sometimes with cyanosis; sudden apnea, especially with manipulation such as gastric lavage or endotracheal intubation; diminished or absent peristalsis. Severe hypotension unresponsive to volume expansion, tonic muscular spasms, twitching and convulsions may occur.

Treatment: As with all forms of acute intoxication, the sooner adequate treatment is instituted, the better the prognosis. Early and vigorous cardiopulmonary supportive measures should be employed and should include:

1. Maintenance of a patent airway with assisted ventilation if necessary.

2. Monitoring of vital signs and level of consciousness.

3. Continuous electrocardiogram to detect arrhythmias.

4. Maintenance of blood pressure with plasma volume expanders and, if absolutely essential, pressor drugs.

Blood for glutethimide levels and other chemical determinations should be obtained as well as arterial blood for blood gas determinations.

Vomiting should be induced if the patient is fully conscious. Gastric lavage should be done in all cases regardless of elapsed time since drug ingestion, with due caution to prevent aspiration of gastric contents or respiratory arrest during manipulation, including prior insertion of a cuffed endotracheal tube or employment of tracheostomy. Lavage with a 1:1 mixture of castor oil and water is capable of removing larger amounts of glutethimide from the stomach than with aqueous lavage. Fifty ml of castor oil should be left in the stomach as a cathartic.

Intestinal lavage is used to remove unabsorbed glutethimide from the intestines (100-250 ml of 20-40% sorbitol or mannitol). If emesis or gastric lavage cannot be effected in the fully conscious patient, delay absorption of glutethimide by giving one pint of water, milk or fruit juice; flour or cornstarch suspension, or activated charcoal in water. Follow up as soon as possible with production of emesis or gastric lavage.

Adequate respiratory gas exchange must be maintained and may require tracheostomy and mechanical assistance. If coma is prolonged, urine output must be monitored and maintained while preventing overhydration which might contribute to pulmonary or cerebral edema.

In severe intoxication, in addition to intensive supportive measures and symptomatic care, consideration should be given to dialysis or hemoperfusion in the following circumstances: Grade III or Grade IV coma, but the level of coma per se is not a mandatory indication for the procedure. Hemodialysis may also be required when renal shutdown or impaired renal function are manifest and in life-threatening overdose situations complicated by (a) pulmonary edema, (b) heart failure, (c) circulatory collapse, (d) significant liver disease, (e) major metabolic disturbance, (f) uremia. While aqueous hemodialysis is less effective for glutethimide than for readily water-soluble compounds that are not bound by proteins or sequestered in body fat depots, glutethimide blood levels may decline more rapidly with hemodialysis and the duration of coma may be shortened; efficacy of the procedure, however, is largely controversial. As long as significant amounts of glutethimide remain in fat deposits or as an unabsorbed bolus in the intestinal tract, the fall in serum level accelerated by hemodialysis may be followed by increased absorption into the bloodstream on termination of dialysis and may require further dialysis.

Recent clinical data indicate that use of pure food-grade soybean oil as the dialysate enhances removal of glutethimide and some other lipid-soluble substances by means of hemodialysis. Peritoneal dialysis, while able to remove some glutethimide, apparently is of minimal value.

Hemoperfusion appears to be a promising technique for eliminating glutethimide from the body. Charcoal hemoperfusion utilizing acrylic hydrogel microencapsulation of activated charcoal has been reported to be simpler and more effective than hemodialysis.

Similarly, a microcapsule artificial kidney has been developed utilizing activated charcoal granules encapsulated with cellulose nitrate and albumin. Resin hemoperfusion utilizing a column containing Amerberlite XAD-2 has demonstrated exceptionally high clearance capabilities in glutethimide intoxication and has been reported to be clinically superior to hemodialysis in patients with profound life-threatening coma and potentially lethal blood concentrations of intoxicant drugs.

Drug extraction techniques should be continued for at least two hours after the patient regains consciousness. Glutethimide is highly lipid soluble and therefore, rapidly accumulated in lipoid tissue. As the drug is removed from the bloodstream by any technique, it is gradually released from fat storage depots back into the bloodstream. Even after substantial quantities of the drug have been extracted, this blood-level rebound can cause coma to persist or recur.

As in the case of any prolonged coma, appropriate antibiotic therapy is indicated if pulmonary or other infection intervenes.

Chronic Overdosage: Signs and symptoms of chronic glutethimide intoxication (and for all drugs producing barbiturate-alcohol type of dependence in chronic overdosage) include impairment of memory and ability to concentrate, impaired gait, ataxia, tremors, hyporeflexia, and slurring of speech. Abrupt discontinuance of glutethimide after prolonged overdosage will in most cases cause withdrawal reactions ranging from nervousness and anxiety to grand mal seizures, and may include abdominal cramping, chills, numbness of extremities, and dysphagia.

Treatment: Chronic glutethimide intoxication may be treated by gradual, stepwise reduction of dosage over a period of days or weeks. Watch patient carefully. If withdrawal reactions occur, they can be controlled by readministration of glutethimide, or substitution of pentobarbital, and subsequent gradual withdrawal.

DOSAGE AND ADMINISTRATION:

For use as a hypnotic, dosage should be individualized. The usual adult dosage is 0.25 to 0.5 g at bedtime. For elderly or debilitated patients, the initial daily dosage should not exceed 0.5 g at bedtime, in order to avoid oversedation.

HOW SUPPLIED - RATED THERAPEUTICALLY EQUIVALENT:

Tablet, Uncoated - Oral - 500 mg

100's	$10.50	Glutethimide, Rugby	00536-3870-01
100's	$12.00	Glutethimide, MD Pharm	43567-0529-07
100's	$16.95	Glutethimide, Halsey Drug	00879-0550-01
500's	$61.95	Glutethimide, Halsey Drug	00879-0550-05
1000's	$79.38	Glutethimide, Rugby	00536-3870-10
1000's	$110.00	Glutethimide, MD Pharm	43567-0529-12
1000's	$111.95	Glutethimide, Halsey Drug	00879-0550-10

GLYBURIDE *(001368)*

CATEGORIES: Antidiabetic Agents; Blood Glucose Regulators; Diabetes; Diabetes Mellitus; Hormones; Hyperglycemia; Sulfonylureas; Pregnancy Category C; Sales > $100 Million; FDA Approved 1984 May; Patent Expiration 1994 May; Top 200 Drugs

BRAND NAMES: *Antibet*; *Apo-Glibenclamide*; *Azuglucon*; *Bastiverit*; *Benclamin*; *Betanase*; *Betanese 5*; *Calabren* (England); *Cytagon*; *D.B.T.*; *Daonil* (Australia, Asia, England, France); *Debtan*; *Diaben*; Diabeta; *Dibelet*; *Euglucan* (France); *Euglucon* (Australia, Asia, England, Germany); *GBN*; *GBN 5*; *Gilbesyn*; *Gilemal*; *Glamide*; *Gliban*; *Gliben*; *Glibenil* (Mexico); *Glibesyn*; *Glibetic*; *Glibil*; *Gliboral*; *Glidiabet*; *Glimel* (Australia); *Glimide*; *Glisulin*; *Glitisol*; *Gluben*; *Glucal* (Mexico); *Glucobene*; *Glucohexal*; *Glucolon*; *Glucomid*; *Glucoven*; *Glukovital*; *Glyben*; *Glycomin*; Glynase; *Glynor*; *Hemi-Daonil* (France); *Libanil*; *Med-Glionil*; *Melix*; **Micronase**; *Miglucan* (France); *Norboral* (Mexico); *Orabetic*; *Pira*; *Prodiabet*; *Renabetic*; *Semi-Daonil* (Australia); *Semi-Euglucon* (Australia); *Sugril*; *Yuglucon*
(International brand names outside U.S. in italics)

FORMULARIES: Aetna; BC-BS; CIGNA; FHP; Humana; Kaiser; Medco; Medi-Cal; PCS; PruCare; United

COST OF THERAPY: $107.85 (Diabetes; Tablet; 2.5 mg; 1/day; 365 days)

DESCRIPTION:

Micronase Tablets: Contain glyburide, which is an oral blood-glucose-lowering drug of the sulfonylurea class. Glyburide is a white, crystalline compound, formulated as Micronase tablets of 1.25, 2.5, and 5 mg strength for oral administration. Inactive ingredients: colloidal silicon dioxide, dibasic calcium phosphate, magnesium stearate, microcrystalline cellulose, sodium alginate, talc. In addition, the **2.5 mg** contains aluminum oxide and FD&C Red No. 40 and the **5 mg** contains aluminum oxide and FD&C Blue No. 1. The chemical name for glyburide is 1-[[p-[2-(5-chloro-o-anisamido)-ethyl]phenyl]-sulfonyl]-3-cyclohexylurea and the molecular weight is 493.99.

Glynase Prestab Tablets: Contain micronized (smaller particle size) glyburide, which is an oral blood-glucose-lowering drug of sulfonylurea class. Glyburide is a white, crystalline compound formulated as Glynase Prestab tablets of 1.5 and 3 mg strengths for oral administration. Inactive ingredients: colloidal silicon dioxide, corn starch, lactose, magnesium stearate. In addition the **3 mg** strength contains aluminum oxide and FD&C Blue No. 1.

Diabeta: (Glyburide) is an oral blood-glucose-lowering drug of the sulfonylurea class. It is a white, crystalline compound, formulated as tablets of 1.25 mg, 2.5 mg. and 5 mg strengths for oral administration. Diabeta tablets contain the active ingredient glyburide and the following inactive ingredients: dibasic calcium phosphate USP, magnesium stearate NF, microcrystalline cellulose NF, sodium alginate NF, talc USP. Diabeta 2.5 mg tablets also contain FD&C Red #40. Diabeta 5 mg tablets also contain D&C Yellow #10 Aluminum Lake, and FD&C Blue #1.

The chemical name for glyburide is 1-((p-(2-(5-chloro-o-anisamido)-ethyl)phenyl)-sulfonyl)-3-cyclohexylurea and the molecular weight is 493.99. The aqueous solubility of Diabeta increases with pH as a result of salt formation.

CAS Number: 10238-21-8.

CLINICAL PHARMACOLOGY:

MECHANISM OF ACTION

Glyburide appears to lower the blood glucose acutely by stimulating the release of insulin from the pancreas, an effect dependent upon functioning beta cells in the pancreatic islets. The mechanism by which glyburide lowers blood glucose during long-term administration has not been clearly established. With chronic administration in Type II diabetic patients, the blood glucose lowering effect persists despite a gradual decline in the insulin secretory response to the drug. Extrapancreatic effects may be involved in the mechanism of action of oral sulfonylurea hypoglycemic drugs.

Some patients who are initially responsive to oral hypoglycemic drugs, including glyburide, may become unresponsive or poorly responsive over time. Alternatively, glyburide tablets may be effective in some patients who have become unresponsive to one or more other sulfonylurea drugs.

In addition to its blood glucose lowering actions, glyburide produces a mild diuresis by enhancement of renal free water clearance. Disulfiram-like reactions have very rarely been reported in patients treated with glyburide tablets.

PHARMACOKINETICS

Single dose studies with glyburide tablets in normal subjects demonstrate significant absorption of glyburide within one hour, peak drug levels at about four hours, and low but detectable levels at twenty-four hours. Mean serum levels of glyburide, as reflected by areas under the serum concentration-time curve, increase in proportion to corresponding increases in dose. Multiple dose studies with glyburide in diabetic patients demonstrate drug level concentration-time curves similar to single dose studies, indicating no buildup of drug in tissue depots. The decrease of glyburide in the serum of normal healthy individuals is biphasic; the terminal half-life is about 10 hours. In single dose studies in fasting normal subjects, the degree and duration of blood glucose lowering is proportional to the dose administered and to the area under the drug level concentration-time curve. The blood glucose lowering effect persists for 24 hours following single morning doses in nonfasting diabetic patients. Under conditions of repeated administration in diabetic patients, however, there is no reliable correlation between blood drug levels and fasting blood glucose levels. A one year study of diabetic patients treated with glyburide showed no reliable correlation between administered dose and serum drug level.

The major metabolite of glyburide is the 4-transhydroxy derivative. A second metabolite, the 3-cishydroxy derivative, also occurs. These metabolites probably contribute no significant hypoglycemic action in humans since they are only weakly active (1/400th and 1/40th as active, respectively, as glyburide) in rabbits.

Glyburide is excreted as metabolites in the bile and urine, approximately 50% by each route. This dual excretory pathway is qualitatively different from that of other sulfonylureas, which are excreted primarily in the urine.

CLINICAL PHARMACOLOGY: *(cont'd)*

Sulfonylurea drugs are extensively bound to serum proteins. Displacement from protein binding sites by other drugs may lead to enhanced hypoglycemic action. *In vitro,* the protein binding exhibited by glyburide is predominantly non-ionic, whereas that of other sulfonylureas (chlorpropamide, tolbutamide, tolazamide) is predominantly ionic. Acidic drugs such as phenylbutazone, warfarin, and salicylates displace the ionic-binding sulfonylureas from serum proteins to a far greater extent than the non-ionic binding glyburide. It has not been shown that this difference in protein binding will result in fewer drug-drug interactions with glyburide tablets in clinical use.

INDICATIONS AND USAGE:

Glyburide tablets are indicated as an adjunct to diet to lower the blood glucose in patients with non-insulin-dependent diabetes mellitus (type II) whose hyperglycemia cannot be satisfactorily controlled by diet alone.

In initiating treatment for non-insulin-dependent diabetes, diet should be emphasized as the primary form of treatment. Caloric restriction and weight loss are essential in the obese diabetic patient. Proper dietary management alone may be effective in controlling the blood glucose and symptoms of hyperglycemia. The importance of regular physical activity should also be stressed, and cardiovascular risk factors should be identified and corrective measures taken where possible. If this treatment program fails to reduce symptoms and/or blood glucose, the use of an oral sulfonylurea or insulin should be considered. Use of glyburide must be viewed by both the physician and patient as a treatment in addition to diet and not as a substitution or as a convenient mechanism for avoiding dietary restraint. Furthermore, loss of blood glucose control on diet alone may be transient, thus requiring only short-term administration of glyburide.

During maintenance programs, glyburide should be discontinued if satisfactory lowering of blood glucose is no longer achieved. Judgment should be based on regular clinical and laboratory evaluations.

In considering the use of glyburide in asymptomatic patients, it should be recognized that controlling blood glucose in non-insulin-dependent diabetes has not been definitely established to be effective in preventing the long-term cardiovascular or neural complications of diabetes.

CONTRAINDICATIONS:

Glyburide tablets are contraindicated in patients with:

1. Known hypersensitivity or allergy to the drug.
2. Diabetic ketoacidosis, with or without coma. This condition should be treated with insulin.
3. Type I diabetes mellitus, as sole therapy.

WARNINGS:

SPECIAL WARNING ON INCREASED RISK OF CARDIOVASCULAR MORTALITY

The administration of oral hypoglycemic drugs has been reported to be associated with increased cardiovascular mortality as compared to treatment with diet alone or diet plus insulin. This warning is based on the study conducted by the University Group Diabetes Program (UGDP), a long-term prospective clinical trial designed to evaluate the effectiveness of glucose-lowering drugs in preventing or delaying vascular complications in patients with non-insulin-dependent diabetes. The study involved 823 patients who were randomly assigned to one of four treatment groups (*Diabetes*, 19 (Suppl. 2):747-830, 1970).

UGDP reported that patients treated for 5 to 8 years with diet plus a fixed dose of tolbutamide (1.5 grams per day) had a rate of cardiovascular mortality approximately 2 1/2 times that of patients treated with diet alone. A significant increase in total mortality was not observed, but the use of tolbutamide was discontinued based on the increase in cardiovascular mortality, thus limiting the opportunity for the study to show an increase in overall mortality. Despite controversy regarding the interpretation of these results, the findings of the UGDP study provide an adequate basis for this warning. The patient should be informed of the potential risks and advantages of glyburide and of alternative modes of therapy.

Although only one drug in the sulfonylurea class (tolbutamide) was included in this study, it is prudent from a safety standpoint to consider that this warning may also apply to other oral hypoglycemic drugs in this class, in view of their close similarities in mode of action and chemical structure.

PRECAUTIONS:

Bioavailability studies have demonstrated that Glynase PresTab tablets 3 mg provide serum glyburide concentrations that are not bioequivalent to those from glyburide tablets 5 mg. Therefore, patients should be re-titrated when transferred from glyburide or Diabeta or other oral hypoglycemic agents.

GENERAL

Hypoglycemia: All sulfonylureas are capable of producing severe hypoglycemia. Proper patient selection and dosage and instructions are important to avoid hypoglycemic episodes. Renal or hepatic insufficiency may cause elevated drug levels of glyburide and the latter may also diminish gluconeogenic capacity, both of which increase the risk of serious hypoglycemic reactions. Elderly, debilitated or malnourished patients, and those with adrenal or pituitary insufficiency, are particularly susceptible to the hypoglycemic action of glucose-lowering drugs. Hypoglycemia may be difficult to recognize in the elderly and in people who are taking beta-adrenergic blocking drugs. Hypoglycemia is more likely to occur when caloric intake is deficient, after severe or prolonged exercise, when alcohol is ingested, or when more than one glucose lowering drug is used.

Loss of Control of Blood Glucose: When a patient stabilized on any diabetic regimen is exposed to stress such as fever, trauma, infection or surgery, a loss of control may occur. At such times it may be necessary to discontinue glyburide and administer insulin.

The effectiveness of any hypoglycemic drug, including glyburide, in lowering blood glucose to a desired level decreases in many patients over a period of time which may be due to progression of the severity of diabetes or to diminished responsiveness to the drug. This phenomenon is known as secondary failure, to distinguish it from primary failure in which the drug is ineffective in an individual patient when glyburide is first given. Adequate adjustment of dose and adherence to diet should be assessed before classifying a patient as a secondary failure.

INFORMATION FOR THE PATIENT

Patients should be informed of the potential risks and advantages of glyburide and of alternative modes of therapy. They also should be informed about the importance of adherence to dietary instructions, of a regular exercise program, and of regular testing of urine and/or blood glucose.

The risks of hypoglycemia, its symptoms and treatment, and conditions that predispose to its development should be explained to patients and responsible family members. Primary and secondary failure also should be explained.

PRECAUTIONS: *(cont'd)*

LABORATORY TESTS

Therapeutic response to glyburide tablets should be monitored by frequent urine glucose tests and periodic blood glucose tests. Measurement of glycosylated hemoglobin levels may be helpful in some patients.

CARCINOGENESIS, MUTAGENESIS, AND IMPAIRMENT OF FERTILITY

Studies in rats at doses up to 300 mg/kg/day for 18 months showed no carcinogenic effects. Glyburide is nonmutagenic when studied in the Salmonella microsome test (Ames test) and in the DNA damage/alkaline elution assay. No drug related effects were noted in any of the criteria evaluated in the two year oncogenicity study of glyburide in mice.

PREGNANCY

Teratogenic Effects: Pregnancy Category C: Glyburide has been shown to effect the maturation of the long bones (humerous and femur) in rat pups when given in doses 6250 times the maximum recommended human dose. These effects, which were seen during organogenesis, are a shortening of the bones with effects to various structures of the long bones, especially the humerous and femur.

Reproduction studies have been performed in rats and rabbits at doses up to 500 times the human dose and have revealed no evidence of impaired fertility or harm to the fetus due to glyburide. There are, however, no adequate and well controlled studies in pregnant women. Because animal reproduction studies are not always predictive of human response, this drug should be used during pregnancy only if clearly needed.

Because recent information suggests that abnormal blood glucose levels during pregnancy are associated with a higher incidence of congenital abnormalities, many experts recommend that insulin be used during pregnancy to maintain blood glucose as close to normal as possible.

Nonteratogenic Effects: Prolonged severe hypoglycemia (4 to 10 days) has been reported in neonates born to mothers who were receiving a sulfonylurea drug at the time of delivery. This has been reported more frequently with the use of agents with prolonged halflives. If glyburide is used during pregnancy, it should be discontinued at least two weeks before the expected delivery date.

NURSING MOTHERS

Although it is not known whether glyburide is excreted in human milk, some sulfonylurea drugs are known to be excreted in human milk. Because the potential for hypoglycemia in nursing infants may exist, a decision should be made whether to discontinue nursing or to discontinue the drug, taking into account the importance of the drug to the mother. If the drug is discontinued, and if diet alone is inadequate for controlling blood glucose, insulin therapy should be considered.

PEDIATRIC USE

Safety and effectiveness in children have not been established.

DRUG INTERACTIONS:

The hypoglycemic action of sulfonylureas may be potentiated by certain drugs including nonsteroidal anti-inflammatory agents and other drugs that are highly protein bound, salicylates, sulfonamides, chloramphenicol, probenecid, coumarins, monoamine oxidase inhibitors, and beta adrenergic blocking agents. When such drugs are administered to a patient receiving glyburide, the patient should be observed closely for hypoglycemia. When such drugs are withdrawn from a patient receiving glyburide, the patient should be observed closely for loss of control.

Possible interactions betweenglyburide and coumarin derivatives have been reported that may either potentiate or weaken the effects of coumarin derivatives. The mechanism of these interactions is not known.

Certain drugs tend to produce hyperglycemia and may lead to loss of control. These drugs include the thiazides and other diuretics, corticosteroids, phenothiazines, thyroid products, estrogens, oral contraceptives, phenytoin, nicotinic acid, sympathomimetics, calcium channel blocking drugs, and isoniazid. When such drugs are administered to a patient receiving glyburide, the patient should be closely observed for loss of control. When such drugs are withdrawn from a patient receiving glyburide, the patient should be observed closely for hypoglycemia.

A possible interaction between glyburide and ciprofloxacin, a fluoroquinolone antibiotic, has been reported, resulting in a potentiation of the hypoglycemic action of glyburide. The mechanism for this interaction is not known.

A potential interaction between oral miconazole and oral hypoglycemic agents leading to severe hypoglycemia has been reported. Whether this interaction also occurs with the intravenous, topical or vaginal preparations of miconazole is not known.

ADVERSE REACTIONS:

Hypoglycemia: See PRECAUTIONS and OVERDOSAGE Sections.

Gastrointestinal Reactions: Cholestatic jaundice and hepatitis may occur rarely; glyburide tablets should be discontinued if this occurs.

Liver function abnormalities, including isolated transaminase elevations, have been reported.

Gastrointestinal disturbances, *e.g.,* nausea, epigastric fullness, and heartburn are the most common reactions, having occurred in 1.8% of treated patients during clinical trials. They tend to be dose related and may disappear when dosage is reduced.

Dermatologic Reactions: Allergic skin reactions, *e.g.,* pruritus, erythema, urticaria, and morbilliform or maculopapular eruptions occurred in 1.5% of treated patients during clinical trials. These may be transient and may disappear despite continued use of glyburide; if skin reactions persist, the drug should be discontinued.

Porphyria cutanea tarda and photosensitivity reactions have been reported with sulfonylureas.

Hematologic Reactions: Leukopenia, agranulocytosis, thrombocytopenia, hemolytic anemia, aplastic anemia, and pancytopenia have been reported with sulfonylureas.

Metabolic Reactions: Hepatic porphyria and disulfiram-like reactions have been reported with sulfonylureas; however, hepatic porphyria has not been reported with glyburide and disulfiram-like reactions have been reported very rarely.

Cases of hyponatremia have been reported with glyburide and all other sulfonylureas, most often in patients who are on other medications or have medical conditions known to cause hyponatremia or increase release of antidiuretic hormone. The syndrome of inappropriate antidiuretic hormone (SIADH) secretion has been reported with certain other sulfonylureas, and it has been suggested that these sulfonylureas may augment the peripheral (antidiuretic) action of ADH and/or increase release of ADH.

Other Reactions: Changes in accommodation and/or blurred vision have been reported with glyburide and other sulfonylureas. These are thought to be related to fluctuation in glucose levels.

In addition to dermatologic reactions, allergic reactions such as angioedema, arthralgia, myalgia and vasculitis have been reported.

OVERDOSAGE:

Overdosage of sulfonylureas, including glyburide tablets, can produce hypoglycemia. Mild hypoglycemic symptoms, without loss of consciousness or neurological findings, should be treated aggressively with oral glucose and adjustments in drug dosage and/or meal patterns. Close monitoring should continue until the physician is assured that the patient is out of danger. Severe hypoglycemic reactions with coma, seizure, or other neurological impairment occur infrequently, but constitute medical emergencies requiring immediate hospitalization. If hypoglycemic coma is diagnosed or suspected, the patient should be given a rapid intravenous injection of concentrated (50%) glucose solution. This should be followed by a continuous infusion of a more dilute (10%) glucose solution at a rate which will maintain the blood glucose at a level above 100 mg/dl. Patients should be closely monitored for a minimum of 24 to 48 hours, since hypoglycemia may recur after apparent clinical recovery.

DOSAGE AND ADMINISTRATION:

There is no fixed dosage regimen for the management of diabetes mellitus with glyburide tablets or any other hypoglycemic agent. In addition to the usual monitoring of urinary glucose, the patient's fasting blood glucose must also be monitored periodically to determine the minimum effective dose for the patient; to detect primary failure, *i.e.,* inadequate lowering of blood glucose at the maximum recommended dose of medication; and to detect secondary failure, *i.e.,* loss of adequate blood glucose lowering response after an initial period of effectiveness. Glycosylated hemoglobin levels may also be of value in monitoring the patient's response to therapy.

Short-term administration of glyburide may be sufficient during periods of transient loss of control in patients usually controlled well on diet.

USUAL STARTING DOSE

The usual starting dose of glyburide/Diabeta tablets is 2.5 to 5 mg daily (Glynase tablets: 1.5 to 3 mg daily), administered with breakfast or the first main meal. Those patients who may be more sensitive to hypoglycemic drugs should be started at 1.25 mg daily. (See PRECAUTIONS for patients at increased risk.)Failure to follow an appropriate dosage regimen may precipitate hypoglycemia. Patients who do not adhere to their prescribed dietary and drug regimen are more prone to exhibit unsatisfactory response to therapy.

Bioavailability studies have demonstrated that Glynase PresTab tablets 3 mg are not bioequivalent to Diabeta tablets 5 mg. Therefore, these products are not substitutable and patients should be retitrated if transferred.

TRANSFER FROM OTHER HYPOGLYCEMIC THERAPY PATIENTS RECEIVING OTHER ORAL ANTIDIABETIC THERAPY

Micronase/Diabeta: Transfer of patients from other oral antidiabetic regimens to Micronase should be done conservatively and the initial daily dose should be 2.5 to 5 mg. When transferring patients from oral hypoglycemic agents other than chlorpropamide to Micronase/ Diabeta, no transition period and no initial or priming dose are necessary. When transferring patients from chlorpropamide, particular care should be exercised during the first two weeks because the prolonged retention of chlorpropamide in the body and subsequent overlapping drug effects may provoke hypoglycemia.

Glynase: Patients should be re-titrated when transferring from Micronase or other oral hypoglycemic agents. The initial daily dose should be 1.5 to 3 mg. When transferring patients from oral hypoglycemic agents other than chlorpropamide to Glynase Prestab, no transition period and no initial or priming dose are necessary. When transferring patients from chlorpropamide, particular care should be exercised during the first two weeks because the prolonged retention of chlorpropamide in the body and subsequent overlapping drug effects may provoke hypoglycemia.

Patients Receiving Insulin: Some Type II diabetic patients being treated with insulin may respond satisfactorily to glyburide. If the insulin dose is less than 20 units daily, substitution of Micronase/Diabeta tablets 2.5 to 5 mg (Glynase tablets 1.5 to 3 mg) as a single daily dose may be tried. If the insulin dose is between 20 and 40 units daily, the patient may be placed directly on Micronase/Diabeta tablets 5 mg (Glynase tablets 3 mg) daily as a single dose. If the insulin dose is more than 40 units daily, a transition period is required for conversion to Micronase/Diabeta/Glynase. In these patients insulin dosage is decreased by 50% and Micronase/Diabeta tablets 5 mg (Glynase tablets 3 mg) daily is started. Please refer to Titration to Maintenance Dose for further explanation.

TITRATION TO MAINTENANCE DOSE

Micronase/Diabeta: The usual maintenance dose is in the range of 1.25 to 20 mg daily, which may be given as a single dose or in divided doses (See Dosage Interval). Dosage increases should be made in increments of no more than 2.5 mg at weekly intervals based upon the patient's blood glucose response.

No exact dosage relationship exists between Micronase/Diabeta and the other oral hypoglycemic agents. Although patients may be transferred from the maximum dose of other sulfonylureas, the maximum starting dose of 5 mg of Micronase/Diabeta tablets should be observed. A maintenance dose of 5 mg of Micronase/Diabeta tablets provides approximately the same degree of blood glucose control as 250 to 375 mg chlorpropamide, 250 to 375 mg tolazamide, 500 to 750 mg acetohexamide, or 1000 to 1500 mg tolbutamide.

When transferring patients receiving more than 40 units of insulin daily, they may be started on a daily dose of Micronase/Diabeta tablets 5 mg concomitantly with a 50% reduction in insulin dose. Progressive withdrawal of insulin and increase of Micronase/Diabeta in increments of 1.25 to 2.5 mg every 2 to 10 days is then carried out. During this conversion period when both insulin and Micronase/Diabeta are being used, hypoglycemia may rarely occur. During insulin withdrawal, patients should test their urine for glucose and acetone at least three times daily and report results to their physician. Self-testing of urinary glucose is a less desirable alternative. The appearance of persistent acetonuria with glycosuria indicates that the patient is a Type I diabetic who requires insulin therapy.

Glynase: The usual maintenance dose is in the range of 0.75 to 12 mg daily, which may be given as a single dose or in divided doses (See Dosage Interval). Dosage increases should be made in increments of no more than 1.5 mg at weekly intervals based upon the patient's blood glucose response.

No exact dosage relationship exists between Glynase Prestab and the other oral hypoglycemic agents including Micronase/Diabeta or Diabeta. Although patients may be transferred from the maximum dose of other sulfonylureas, the maximum starting dose of 3 mg of Glynase tablets should be observed. A maintenance dose of 3 mg of Glynase tablets provides approximately the same degree of blood glucose control as 250 to 375 mg chlorpropamide, 250 to 375 mg tolazamide, 5 mg of glyburide (non-micronized tablets), 500 to 750 mg acetohexamide, or 1000 to 1500 mg tolbutamide.

When transferring patients receiving more than 40 units of insulin daily, they may be started on a daily dose of Glynase tablets 3 mg concomitantly with a 50% reduction in insulin dose. Progressive withdrawal of insulin and increase of Glynase tablets in increments of 0.75 to 1.5 mg every 2 to 10 days is then carried out. During this conversion period when both insulin and Glynase tablets are being used, hypoglycemia may rarely occur. During insulin withdrawal, patients should test their urine for glucose and acetone at least three times daily and report results to their physician. The appearance of persistent acetonuria with glycosuria indicates that the patient is a type I diabetic who requires insulin therapy.

DOSAGE AND ADMINISTRATION: *(cont'd)*

MAXIMUM DOSE

Micronase/Diabeta: Daily doses of more than 20 mg are not recommended.

Glynase: Daily doses of more than 12 mg are not recommended.

DOSAGE INTERVAL

Micronase/Diabeta: Once-a-day therapy is usually satisfactory, based upon usual meal patterns and a 10 hour half-life. Some patients, particularly those receiving more than 10 mg daily, may have a more satisfactory response with twice-a-day dosage.

Glynase: Once-a-day therapy is usually satisfactory. Some patients, particularly those receiving more than 6 mg daily, may have a more satisfactory response with twice-a-day dosage.

SPECIFIC PATIENT POPULATIONS

Micronase and Glynase are not recommended for use in pregnancy or for use in children.

In elderly patients, debilitated or malnourished patients, and patients with impaired renal or hepatic function, the initial and maintenance dosing should be conservative to avoid hypoglycemic reactions. (See PRECAUTIONS).

PATIENT INFORMATION:

Glyburide is a sulfonylurea used in patients with diabetes mellitus to lower blood sugar. Notify your physician if you are pregnant or nursing. Do not change the dose or stop taking glyburide without talking with your physician. This medication should be taken on an empty stomach, 30 minutes before a meal. May be taken with food if nausea or stomach upset occurs. Avoid drinking alcohol while taking this medication. Alcohol may cause flushing, weakness, dizziness, a tingling sensation and headache. Avoid taking aspirin with this medication. Notify your physician if you develop unexplained fever, sore throat, yellowing of the skin or eyes, dark urine, or skin rash. Notify your physician if you develop fatigue, nausea, confusion, agitation, excessive hunger, profuse sweating, numbness or tingling of lips, tongue or extremities (may indicate low blood sugar), or if you develop excessive thirst or urination, or glucose or ketones in the urine or blood (may indicate high blood sugar).

HOW SUPPLIED:

Micronase tablets are supplied as follows:

Micronase Tablets 1.25 mg (White, Round, Scored)

Micronase Tablets 2.5 mg (Dark Pink, Round, Scored)

Micronase Tablets 5 mg (Blue, Round, Scored)

Store at controlled room temperature 15°-30°C (59°-86°F).

Dispense in well-closed containers with safety closures.

HOW SUPPLIED - RATED THERAPEUTICALLY EQUIVALENT:

Tablet, Uncoated - Oral - 1.25 mg

100's	$18.32	Glyburide, Major Pharms	00904-5075-60
100's	$18.32	Glyburide, Greenstone	59762-3725-01
100's	**$21.52**	**MICRONASE, Pharmacia & Upjohn**	**00009-0131-01**

Tablet, Uncoated - Oral - 1.5 mg

100's	$23.97	Glyburide Micronized, Copley Pharm	38245-0725-10

Tablet, Uncoated - Oral - 2.5 mg

30's	**$10.80**	**MICRONASE, Pharmacia & Upjohn**	**00009-0141-06**
100's	$29.55	Glyburide, Goldline Labs	00182-1220-01
100's	$30.53	Glyburide, Major Pharms	00904-5076-60
100's	$30.53	Glyburide, Greenstone	59762-3726-03
100's	$30.54	Glyburide, United Res	00677-1580-01
100's	$30.60	Glyburide, Novopharm (US)	55953-0343-40
100's	$31.05	Glyburide, Geneva Pharms	00781-1456-01
100's	$31.55	Glyburide, Geneva Pharms	00781-1456-13
100's	$31.95	Glyburide, Rugby	00536-5751-01
100's	$32.14	GLYBURIDE, Aligen Independ	00405-5375-01
100's	**$35.87**	**MICRONASE, Pharmacia & Upjohn**	**00009-0141-01**
100's	**$35.87**	**MICRONASE, Pharmacia & Upjohn**	**00009-0141-02**
500's	$123.50	Glyburide, Goldline Labs	00182-1220-05
500's	$131.45	Glyburide, Novopharm (US)	55953-0343-70
1000's	$226.10	Glyburide, Novopharm (US)	55953-0343-80
1000's	$255.90	Glyburide, Goldline Labs	00182-1220-10

Tablet, Uncoated - Oral - 3 mg

100's	$40.32	Glyburide Micronized, Copley Pharm	38245-0381-10
500's	$189.15	Glyburide Micronized, Copley Pharm	38245-0381-50
1000's	$372.19	Glyburide Micronized, Copley Pharm	38245-0381-20

Tablet, Uncoated - Oral - 5 mg

30's	**$18.16**	**MICRONASE, Pharmacia & Upjohn**	**00009-0171-11**
60's	**$36.37**	**MICRONASE, Pharmacia & Upjohn**	**00009-0171-12**
100's	$51.17	Glyburide, Rugby	00536-5643-01
100's	$51.58	Glyburide, Major Pharms	00904-5077-60
100's	$51.58	Glyburide, Greenstone	59762-3727-04
100's	$52.50	Glyburide, United Res	00677-1581-01
100's	$52.95	Glyburide, Rugby	00536-5752-01
100's	$53.00	Glyburide, Novopharm (US)	55953-0344-40
100's	$53.05	Glyburide, Geneva Pharms	00781-1457-01
100's	$53.44	Glyburide, Geneva Pharms	00781-1457-13
100's	$54.30	GLYBURIDE, Aligen Independ	00405-5376-01
100's	**$60.62**	**MICRONASE, Pharmacia & Upjohn**	**00009-0171-03**
100's	**$60.62**	**MICRONASE, Pharmacia & Upjohn**	**00009-0171-05**
500's	$213.48	Glyburide, Rugby	00536-5643-05
500's	$226.60	Glyburide, Rugby	00536-5752-05
500's	$226.60	Glyburide, Major Pharms	00904-5077-40
500's	$226.60	Glyburide, Greenstone	59762-3727-06
500's	$226.75	Glyburide, United Res	00677-1581-05
500's	$228.00	Glyburide, Novopharm (US)	55953-0344-70
500's	$228.05	Glyburide, Geneva Pharms	00781-1457-05
500's	**$266.29**	**MICRONASE, Pharmacia & Upjohn**	**00009-0171-06**
1000's	$435.00	Glyburide, Major Pharms	00904-5077-80
1000's	$438.57	Glyburide, Greenstone	59762-3727-07
1000's	$440.00	Glyburide, Novopharm (US)	55953-0344-80
1000's	$440.05	Glyburide, Geneva Pharms	00781-1457-10
1000's	$461.65	GLYBURIDE, Aligen Independ	00405-5376-03
1000's	**$515.36**	**MICRONASE, Pharmacia & Upjohn**	**00009-0171-07**

HOW SUPPLIED - NOT RATED EQUIVALENT:

Tablet, Uncoated - Oral - 1.25 mg

50's	$7.20	Glyburide, Goldline Labs	00182-1219-19
50's	$7.47	Glyburide, Copley Pharm	38245-0477-49
50's	$8.30	DIABETA, Hoechst Marion Roussel	00039-0053-05
100's	$18.35	Glyburide, Novopharm (US)	55953-0342-40
100's	$18.40	Glyburide, Geneva Pharms	00781-1455-01
100's	$19.28	GLYBURIDE, Aligen Independ	00405-5374-01
500's	$78.90	Glyburide, Novopharm (US)	55953-0342-70

HOW SUPPLIED - NOT RATED EQUIVALENT: *(cont'd)*

Tablet, Uncoated - Oral - 1.5 mg

100's	$32.50	GLYNASE, Pharmacia & Upjohn	00009-0341-01
100's	$32.50	GLYNASE, Pharmacia & Upjohn	00009-0341-02

Tablet, Uncoated - Oral - 2.5 mg

100's	$30.15	Glyburide, Rugby	00536-5642-01
100's	$30.53	Glyburide, Copley Pharm	38245-0433-10
100's	$30.53	Glyburide, Copley Pharm	38245-0433-55
100's	$31.00	Glyburide, Schein Pharm (US)	00364-2577-01
100's	$32.10	DIABETA, Hoechst Marion Roussel	00039-0051-10
100's	$32.10	DIABETA, Hoechst Marion Roussel	00039-0051-11
500's	$123.50	Glyburide, Schein Pharm (US)	00364-2577-05
500's	$123.50	Glyburide, Copley Pharm	38245-0433-50
500's	$137.10	DIABETA, Hoechst Marion Roussel	00039-0051-50
1000's	$260.40	Glyburide, Copley Pharm	38245-0433-20

Tablet, Uncoated - Oral - 3 mg

100's	$54.93	GLYNASE, Pharmacia & Upjohn	00009-0352-01
100's	$54.93	GLYNASE, Pharmacia & Upjohn	00009-0352-02
500's	$240.87	GLYNASE, Pharmacia & Upjohn	00009-0352-03
1000's	$465.72	GLYNASE, Pharmacia & Upjohn	00009-0352-04

Tablet, Uncoated - Oral - 5 mg

100's	$50.99	Glyburide, Goldline Labs	00182-1221-01
100's	$50.99	Glyburide, Schein Pharm (US)	00364-2578-01
100's	$53.01	Glyburide, Copley Pharm	38245-0364-10
100's	$53.01	Glyburide, Copley Pharm	38245-0364-55
100's	$58.90	DIABETA, Hoechst Marion Roussel	00039-0052-10
100's	$58.90	DIABETA, Hoechst Marion Roussel	00039-0052-11
500's	$218.00	Glyburide, Goldline Labs	00182-1221-05
500's	$218.00	Glyburide, Schein Pharm (US)	00364-2578-05
500's	$226.60	Glyburide, Copley Pharm	38245-0364-50
500's	$246.70	DIABETA, Hoechst Marion Roussel	00039-0052-50
1000's	$423.00	Glyburide, Goldline Labs	00182-1221-10
1000's	$438.57	Glyburide, Copley Pharm	38245-0364-20
1000's	$441.30	DIABETA, Hoechst Marion Roussel	00039-0052-70

Tablet, Uncoated - Oral - 6 mg

100's	$82.40	GLYNASE, Pharmacia & Upjohn	00009-3449-01
500's	$361.31	GLYNASE, Pharmacia & Upjohn	00009-3449-03

GLYCERIN *(001370)*

CATEGORIES: Antiglaucomatous Agents; Corneal Inflammation; EENT Drugs; Edema; Emollients; Eye, Ear, Nose, & Throat Preparations; Glaucoma; Hyperosmotic Agents; Keratitis; Ocular Hypertension; Ophthalmics; Skin/Mucous Membrane Agents; Pregnancy Category C; FDA Pre 1938 Drugs

BRAND NAMES: Ophthalgan; **Osmoglyn**

DESCRIPTION:

Glycerin is 1,2,3-propanetriol: CH_2OH-$CHOH$-CH_2OH.

It is a clear, colorless, viscous liquid. Ophthalgan is a sterile glycerin ophthalmic solution.

CLINICAL PHARMACOLOGY:

Glycerin ophthalmic solution is used only for topical application to the cornea. By virtue of its osmotic action, it promptly reduces edema and causes clearing of corneal haze. The action of glycerin is transient, and it is, therefore, used primarily for diagnostic purposes.

INDICATIONS AND USAGE:

Glycerin is indicated to clear an edematous cornea in order to facilitate ophthalmoscopic and gonioscopic examination especially in acute glaucoma, bullous keratitis, Fuchs's endothelial dystrophy, and so forth. In gonioscopy of an edematous cornea, additional glycerin may be used as the lubricant. A local anesthetic should be instilled shortly before use of glycerin.

CONTRAINDICATIONS:

Hypersensitivity to the active or inactive ingredients.

PRECAUTIONS:

Because glycerin is an irritant and may cause pain, a local anesthetic should be instilled shortly before its use.

Carcinogenesis, Mutagenesis, and Impairment of Fertility: No long-term studies in animals or humans have been conducted.

Pregnancy Category C: Animal reproduction studies have not been conducted with glycerin. It is also not known whether glycerin can cause fetal harm when administered to a pregnant woman or can affect reproduction capacity. Glycerin should be given to a pregnant woman only if clearly needed.

Nursing Mothers: It is not known whether this drug is excreted in human milk. Because many drugs are excreted in human milk, caution should be exercised when glycerin is administered to a nursing woman.

Pediatric Use: Safety and effectiveness in children have not been established.

ADVERSE REACTIONS:

Some pain and/or irritation may occur upon instillation.

DOSAGE AND ADMINISTRATION:

One or two drops prior to examination. In gonioscopy of an edematous cornea, additional glycerin may be used as the lubricant.

DISCARD THIS PRODUCT SIX MONTHS AFTER DROPPER IS FIRST PLACED IN THE DRUG SOLUTION.

(Glycerin contains not more than 1.0% water. Chlorobutanol (chloral derivative) 0.55% is incorporated as preservative. The pH of this solution may differ from that specified in the U.S.P.)

HOW SUPPLIED - EQUIVALENTS NOT AVAILABLE:

Solution - Ophthalmic - 99.5 %

7.5 ml	$22.29	OPHTHALGAN, Ayerst	00046-1013-07

Solution - Oral - 50 %

220 ml	**$262.47**	**OSMOGLYN, Alcon**	**00065-0035-08**

GLYCINE *(001375)*

CATEGORIES: Electrolytic, Caloric-Water Balance; Irrigating Solutions; Pharmaceutical Aids; Surgical Aids; FDA Approval Pre 1982

BRAND NAMES: Aminoacetic Acid

DESCRIPTION:

NONELECTROLYTE IRRIGATING FLUID FOR TRANSURETHRAL SURGICAL PROCEDURES.

For Urologic Irrigation Only; Not For Injection By Usual Parenteral Routes

Flexible Irrigation Container; Semi-rigid Irrigation Container

1.5% Glycine Irrigation, USP is a sterile, nonpyrogenic, hypotonic, aqueous solution of glycine intended only for urologic irrigation during transurethral surgical procedures.

Each 100 ml contains 1.5 g of glycine in water for injection. The solution is nonelectrolytic, hypotonic and has an osmolarity of 200 mOsmol/liter (calc.); pH 6.0 (4.5 to 6.5).

The solution contains no bacteriostat, antimicrobial agent or added buffer and is intended only for use as a single-dose irrigation. When smaller volumes are required, the unused portion should be discarded.

1.5% Glycine Irrigation is a urologic nonelectrolyte irrigant.

Glycine, USP is chemically designated aminoacetic acid ($C_2H_5NO_2$), a white crystalline powder freely soluble in water. It has the following structural formula: NH_2CH_2COOH

Water for Injection, USP is chemically designated H_2O.

The flexible plastic container is fabricated from a specially formulated polyvinylchloride. Water can permeate from inside the container into the overwrap but not in amounts sufficient to affect the solution significantly. Solutions inside the plastic container also can leach out certain of its chemical components in very small amounts before the expiration period is attained. However, the safety of the plastic has been confirmed by tests in animals according to USP biological standards for plastic containers.

The semi-rigid container is fabricated from a specially formulated polyolefin. It is a copolymer of ethylene and propylene. The safety of the plastic has been confirmed by tests in animals according to USP biological standards for plastic containers. The container requires no vapor barrier to maintain the proper drug concentration.

CLINICAL PHARMACOLOGY:

Glycine is an amino acid and a nonelectrolyte. A solution of glycine in water is therefore nonconductive and suitable for urologic irrigation during electrosurgical procedures. A 1.5% concentration of glycine in water (200 mOsmol/liter calc.) is sufficient to minimize the risk of intravascular hemolysis which can occur from absorption of plain water through open prostatic veins during transurethral resection (TUR). It is hypotonic in relation to the extracellular fluid (280 mOsmol/liter). Any solution absorbed intravascularly during transurethral prostatic or bladder surgery, although variable in amount depending primarily on the extent of surgery, will be excreted by the kidney. Studies have shown that the absorption of glycine does not cause significant hemolysis (increase of free hemoglobin) or release significant amounts of free ammonia in the blood. Glycine is rapidly degraded in the liver by glycine oxidase.

Water is an essential constituent of all body tissues and accounts for approximately 70% of total body weight. Average normal adult daily requirement ranges from two to three liters (1.0 to 1.5 liters each for insensible water loss by perspiration and urine production).

Water balance is maintained by various regulatory mechanisms. Water distribution depends primarily on the concentration of electrolytes in the body compartments and sodium (Na+) plays a major role in maintaining physiologic equilibrium.

INDICATIONS AND USAGE:

1.5% Glycine Irrigation, USP is indicated for use as irrigating fluid during transurethral prostatic resection and other transurethral surgical procedures.

CONTRAINDICATIONS:

NOT FOR INJECTION BY USUAL PARENTERAL ROUTES.

Do not use in patients with anuria.

WARNINGS:

FOR UROLOGIC IRRIGATION ONLY.

Solutions for urologic irrigation must be used with caution in patients with severe cardiopulmonary or renal dysfunction. Irrigating fluids used during transurethral prostatectomy have been demonstrated to enter the systemic circulation in relatively large volumes. Thus, glycine irrigating solution must be regarded as a systemic drug. Absorption of large amounts of fluids containing glycine may significantly alter cardiopulmonary and renal dynamics.

Do not heat container over 66°C (150°F).

PRECAUTIONS:

Cardiovascular status, especially of the patient with cardiac disease, should be carefully observed before and during transurethral resection of the prostate when using glycine irrigating solution, because the quantity of fluid absorbed into the systemic circulation by opened prostatic veins may produce significant expansion of the extracellular fluid and lead to fulminating congestive heart failure. Shift of sodium free intracellular fluid into the extracellular compartment following systemic absorption of solution may lower serum sodium concentration and aggravate pre-existing hyponatremia.

Care should be exercised if impaired liver function is known or suspected. Under such conditions, ammonia resulting from metabolism of glycine may accumulate in the blood.

Aseptic technique is essential with the use of sterile solutions for irrigation. The administration set should be attached promptly. Unused portions should be discarded and a fresh container of appropriate size used for the start-up of each cycle or repeat procedure.

Do not administer unless solution is clear, seal is intact and container is undamaged. Discard unused portion.

DRUG INTERACTIONS:

Additives may be incompatible. Consult with pharmacist, if available. When introducing additives, use aseptic technique, mix thoroughly and do not store.

Parenteral drug products should be inspected visually for particulate matter and discoloration prior to administration, whenever solution container permits. See PRECAUTIONS.

ADVERSE REACTIONS:

Adverse reactions may result from intravascular absorption of glycine. Large intravenous doses of glycine are known to cause salivation, nausea and lightheadedness. Other consequences of absorption of urologic irrigating solutions include fluid and electrolyte disturbances such as acidosis, electrolyte loss, marked diuresis, urinary retention, edema, dryness of mouth, thirst, dehydration, coma from hyponatremia, secondary hyponatremia due to fluid

ADVERSE REACTIONS: *(cont'd)*

overload, and hyperammonemia with resultant coma and/or encephalopathy; cardiovascular disorders such as hypotension, tachycardia, angina-like pains; pulmonary disorders such as pulmonary congestion; and other general reactions such as blurred vision, convulsions, nausea, vomiting, rhinitis, chills, vertigo, backache, transient blindness and urticaria. Allergic reactions from glycine are unknown or exceedingly rare.

Should any adverse reaction occur, discontinue the irrigant, evaluate the patient, institute appropriate therapeutic countermeasures and save the remainder of the fluid for examination if deemed necessary.

OVERDOSAGE:

In the event of overhydration or solute overload, re-evaluate the patient and institute appropriate corrective measures. See WARNINGS, PRECAUTIONS and ADVERSE REACTIONS.

DOSAGE AND ADMINISTRATION:

1.5% Glycine Irrigation, USP should be administered only by transurethral instillation with appropriate urologic instrumentation. A disposable irrigation set should be used. The total volume of solution used for irrigation is solely at the discretion of the surgeon.

Height of container(s) above the operating table in excess of 60 cm (approx. 2 ft.) has been reported to increase intravascular absorption of the irrigating fluid.

Exposure of pharmaceutical products to heat should be minimized. Avoid excessive heat. Protect from freezing. It is recommended that the product be stored at room temperature (25°C); however, brief exposure up to 40°C does not adversely affect the product.

HOW SUPPLIED - RATED THERAPEUTICALLY EQUIVALENT:

Solution - Irrigation - 15 mg/ml

1500 ml	$24.00	1.5% GLYCINE, Abbott	00074-6142-06
2000 ml x 6	$21.04	AMINOACETIC ACID, McGaw	00264-2302-50
3000 ml	$15.51	Glycine Urologic, Baxter Hlthcare	00338-0289-47
3000 ml	$21.33	Glycine, Abbott	00074-7974-08
4000 ml x 4	$25.68	AMINOACETIC ACID, McGaw	00264-2302-70
5000 ml	$25.05	Glycine Urologic, Baxter Hlthcare	00338-0289-49

GLYCOPYRROLATE *(001377)*

CATEGORIES: Anesthesia; Anticholinergic Agents; Antimuscarinics/Antispasmodics; Antispasmodics & Anticholinergics; Autonomic Drugs; Central Nervous System Agents; Gastrointestinal Drugs; Parasympatholytics; Peptic Ulcer; Sedatives/Hypnotics; FDA Approval Pre 1982

BRAND NAMES: *Gastrodyn Inj; Glycopyrrolate Inj;* Robinul; *Robinul Forte* (Canada); *Robinul Inj.* (Australia, England, Germany); *Sroton* (Japan); *Strodin (International brand names outside U.S. in italics)*

FORMULARIES: Medi-Cal

DESCRIPTION:

Glycopyrrolate is a quaternary ammonium compound with the following chemical name: 3-((cyclopentylhydroxyphenylacetyl)oxy)-1, 1-dimethylpyrrolidinium bromide.

TABLETS

Glycopyrrolate and glycopyrrolate extra strength tablets contain the synthetic anticholinergic, glycopyrrolate.

Robinul: Tablets are scored, compressed white tablets engraved AHR. *Each tablet contains:* Glycopyrrolate, USP 1 mg

Robinul Forte: Tablets are scored, compressed white tablets engraved AHR. *Each tablet contains:* Glycopyrrolate, USP 2 mg

Inactive Ingredients: Dibasic calcium phosphate, lactose, magnesium stearate, povidone, sodium starch glycolate.

INJECTION

Glycopyrrolate is a synthetic anticholinergic agent. Each 1 ml contains:

Glycopyrrolate, USP 0.2 mg

Water for Injection, USP q.s.

Benzyl Alcohol, NF 0.9%

(preservative)

pH adjusted, when necessary, with hydrochloric acid and/or sodium hydroxide.

For intramuscular or intravenous administration.

Unlike atropine, glycopyrrolate is completely ionized at physiological pH values.

Glycopyrrolate injectable is a clear, colorless, sterile liquid; pH 2.0- 3.0.

CLINICAL PHARMACOLOGY:

Glycopyrrolate, like other anticholinergic (antimuscarinic) agents, inhibits the action of acetylcholine on structures innervated by postganglionic cholinergic nerves and on smooth muscles that respond to acetylcholine but lack cholinergic innervation. These peripheral cholinergic receptors are present in the autonomic effector cells of smooth muscle, cardiac muscle, the sino-atrial node, the atrioventricular node, exocrine glands, and, to a limited degree, in the autonomic ganglia. Thus, it diminishes the volume and free acidity of gastric secretions and controls excessive pharyngeal, tracheal, and bronchial secretions.

Glycopyrrolate antagonizes muscarinic symptoms (*e.g.,* bronchorrhea, bronchospasm, bradycardia, and intestinal hypermotility) induced by cholinergic drugs such as the anticholinesterases.

The highly polar quaternary ammonium group of glycopyrrolate limits its passage across lipid membranes, such as the blood-brain barrier, in contrast to atropine sulfate and scopolamine hydrobromide, which are non-polar tertiary amines which penetrate lipid barriers easily.

Injection: Peak effects occur approximately 30 to 45 minutes after intramuscular administration. The vagal blocking effects persist for 2 to 3 hours and the antisialagogue effects persist up to 7 hours, periods longer than for atropine. With intravenous injection, the onset of action is generally evident within one minute.

INDICATIONS AND USAGE:

TABLETS

For use as adjunctive therapy in the treatment of peptic ulcer.

INJECTION

In Anesthesia: Glycopyrrolate injectable is indicated for use as a preoperative antimuscarinic to reduce salivary, tracheobronchial, and pharyngeal secretions; to reduce the volume and free acidity of gastric secretions; and, to block cardiac vagal inhibitory reflexes during induction of anesthesia and intubation. When indicated, glycopyrrolate injectable may be used intraoperatively to counteract drug-induced or vagal traction reflexes with the associated arrhythmias. Glycopyrrolate protects against the peripheral muscarinic effects (*e.g.,* bradycardia and excessive secretions) of cholinergic agents such as neostigmine and pyridostigmine given to reverse the neuromuscular blockade due to nondepolarizing muscle relaxants.

In Peptic Ulcer: For use in adults as adjunctive therapy for the treatment of peptic ulcer when rapid anticholinergic effect is desired or when oral medication is not tolerated.

CONTRAINDICATIONS:

Glaucoma; obstructive uropathy (for example, bladder neck obstruction due to prostatic hypertrophy); obstructive disease of the gastrointestinal tract (as in achalasia, pyloroduodenal stenosis, etc.); paralytic ileus; intestinal atony of the elderly or debilitated patient; unstable cardiovascular status in acute hemorrhage; severe ulcerative colitis; toxic megacolon complicating ulcerative colitis; myasthenia gravis.

Glycopyrrolate tablets are contraindicated in those patients with a hypersensitivity to glycopyrrolate.

Injection: Due to its benzyl alcohol content, glycopyrrolate injectable should not be used in newborns (children less than 1 month of age).

WARNINGS:

In the presence of a high environmental temperature, heat prostration (fever and heat stroke due to decreased sweating) can occur with use of glycopyrrolate.

Diarrhea may be an early symptom of incomplete intestinal obstruction, especially in patients with ileostomy or colostomy. In this instance treatment with this drug would be inappropriate and possibly harmful.

Glycopyrrolate may produce drowsiness or blurred vision. In this event, the patient should be warned not to engage in activities requiring mental alertness such as operating a motor vehicle or other machinery, or performing hazardous work while taking this drug.

Tablets: Theoretically, with overdosage, a curare-like action may occur, i.e., neuromuscular blockade leading to muscular weakness and possible paralysis.

Injection: This drug should be used with great caution, if at all, in patients with glaucoma or asthma.

PRECAUTIONS:

TABLETS

Use Glycopyrrolate with caution in the elderly and in all patients with:

Autonomic neuropathy.

Hepatic or renal disease.

Ulcerative colitis-large doses may suppress intestinal motility to the point of producing a paralytic ileus and for this reason may precipitate or aggravate "toxic megacolon," a serious complication of the disease.

Hyperthyroidism, coronary heart disease, congestive heart failure,cardiac tachyarrhythmias, tachycardia, hypertension and prostatic hypertrophy.

Hiatal hernia associated with reflux esophagitis, since anticholinergic drugs may aggravate this condition.

Pregnancy: The safety of this drug during pregnancy has not been established. The use of any drug during pregnancy requires that the potential benefits of the drug be weighed against possible hazards to mother and child. Reproduction studies in rats revealed no teratogenic effects from glycopyrrolate; however, the potent anticholinergic action of this agent resulted in diminished rates of conception and of survival at weaning, in a dose-related manner. Other studies in dogs suggest that this may be due to diminished seminal secretion which is evident at high doses of glycopyrrolate. Information on possible adverse effects in the pregnant female is limited to uncontrolled data derived from marketing experience. Such experience has revealed no reports of teratogenic or other fetus- damaging potential. No controlled studies to establish the safety of the drug in pregnancy have been performed.

Nursing Mothers: It is not known whether this drug is excreted in human milk. As a general rule, nursing should not be undertaken while a patient is on a drug since many drugs are excreted in human milk.

Pediatric Use: Since there is no adequate experience in children who have received this drug, safety and efficacy in children have not been established.

INJECTION

General: Investigate any tachycardia before giving glycopyrrolate since an increase in the heart rate may occur.

Use with caution in patients with: coronary artery disease; congestive heart failure; cardiac arrhythmias; hypertension; hyperthyroidism.

In managing ulcer patients, use glycopyrrolate with caution in the elderly and in all patients with autonomic neuropathy, hepatic or renal disease, ulcerative colitis or hiatal hernia, since anticholinergic drugs may aggravate these conditions.

With overdosage, a curare-like action may occur.

Carcinogenesis, Mutagenesis, and Impairment of Fertility: Long-term studies in animals have not been performed to evaluate carcinogenic potential. In the teratology studies, diminished rates of conception and of survival at weaning were observed in rats, in a dose-related manner. Studies in dogs suggest that this may be due to diminished seminal secretion which is evident at high doses of glycopyrrolate.

Pregnancy Category B: Reproduction studies have been performed in rats and rabbits up to 1000 times the human dose and have revealed no teratogenic effects from glycopyrrolate. There are, however, no adequate and well-controlled studies in pregnant women. Because animal reproduction studies are not always predictive of human response, this drug should be used during pregnancy only if clearly needed.

Nursing Mothers: It is not known whether this drug is excreted in human milk. Because many drugs are excreted in human milk, caution should be exercised when glycopyrrolate is administered to a nursing woman.

Pediatric Use: Safety and effectiveness in children below the age of 12 years have not been established for the management of peptic ulcer.

DRUG INTERACTIONS:

TABLETS: There are no known drug interactions.

Injection: The intravenous administration of any anticholinergic in the presence of cyclopropane anesthesia can result in ventricular arrhythmias; therefore, caution should be observed if glycopyrrolate injectable is used during cyclopropane anesthesia. If the drug is given in small incremental doses of 0.1 mg or less, the likelihood of producing ventricular arrhythmias is reduced.

ADVERSE REACTIONS:

Anticholinergics produce certain effects, most of which are extensions of their fundamental pharmacological actions. Adverse reactions to anticholinergics in general may include xerostomia; decreased sweating; urinary hesitancy and retention; blurred vision; tachycardia; palpitations; dilatation of the pupil; cycloplegia; increased ocular tension; loss of taste; headaches; nervousness; mental confusion; drowsiness; weakness; dizziness; insomnia; nausea; vomiting; constipation; bloated feeling; impotence; suppression of lactation; severe allergic reaction or drug idiosyncrasies including anaphylaxis, urticaria and other dermal manifestations.

Glycopyrrolate is chemically a quaternary ammonium compound; hence, its passage across lipid membranes, such as the blood-brain barrier, is limited in contrast to atropine sulfate and scopolamine hydrobromide. For this reason the occurrence of CNS related side effects is lower, in comparison to their incidence following administration of anticholinergics which are chemically tertiary amines that can cross this barrier readily.

OVERDOSAGE:

TABLETS

The symptoms of overdosage of glycopyrrolate are peripheral in nature rather than central.

1. To Guard Against Further Absorption Of The Drug: Use gastric lavage, cathartics and/or enemas.

2. To Combat Peripheral Anticholinergic Effects (Residual Mydriasis Dry Mouth, Etc.): Utilize a quaternary ammonium anticholinesterase such as neostigmine methylsulfate.

3. To Combat Hypotension: Use pressor amines (nor-epinephrine metaraminol) IV; and supportive care.

4. To Combat Respiratory Depression: Administer oxygen; utilize a respiratory stimulant such as dopram IV; artificial respiration

INJECTION

To combat peripheral anticholinergic effects, a quaternary ammonium anticholinergic effects, a quaternary ammonium anticholinergic such as neostigmine methylsulfate (which does not cross the blood-brain barrier) may be given intravenously in increments of 0.25 mg in adults. This dosage may be repeated every five to ten minutes until anticholinergic overactivity id reversed or up to a maximum od 2.5 mg. Proportionately smaller doses should be used in children. Indication for repetitive doses of neostigmine should be based on close monitoring of the decrease in heart rate and the return of bowel sounds.

In the unlikely event that CNS symptoms (excitement, restlessness, convulsions, psychotic behavior) occur, physostigmine (which does not cross the blood-brain barrier) should be used. Physostigmine (0.5 to 2 mg should be slowly administered intervenously and repeated as necessary up to a total of 5 mg in adults. Proportionately smaller doses should be used in children.

Fever should be treated symptomatically. In the event of a curare-like effect on respiratory muscles, artificial respiration should be instituted and maintained until effective respiratory action returns.

DOSAGE AND ADMINISTRATION:

TABLETS

The dosage of glycopyrrolate or glycopyrrolate extra strength should be adjusted to the needs of the individual patient to assure symptomatic control with a minimum of adverse reactions. The presently recommended maximum daily dosage of glycopyrrolate is 8 mg.

Glycopyrrolate: *1 mg Tablets:* The recommended initial dosage of glycopyrrolate for adults is one tablet three times daily (in the morning, early afternoon, and at bedtime). Some patients may require two tablets at bedtime to assure overnight control of symptoms. For maintenance, a dosage of one tablet twice a day is frequently adequate.

Glycopyrrolate Extra Strength: *2 mg Tablets:* The recommended dosage of glycopyrrolate extra strength for adults is one tablet two or three times daily at equally spaced intervals.

Glycopyrrolate tablets are not recommended for use in children under the age of 12 years.

INJECTION

Glycopyrrolate injectable may be administered intramuscularly, or intravenously, without dilution, in the following indications:

Adults

Preanesthetic Medication: The recommended dose of glycopyrrolate injectable is 0.002 mg (0.01 ml) per pound of body weight by intramuscular injection, given 30 to 60 minutes prior to the anticipated time of induction of anesthesia or at the time the preanesthetic narcotic and/or sedative are administered.

Intraoperative Medication: Glycopyrrolate injectable may be used during surgery to counteract drug induced or vagal taction reflexes with the associated arrhythmias (*e.g.,* bradycardia). It should be administered intravenously as single doses of 0.1 mg (0.5 ml) and repeated, as needed, at intervals of 2-3 minutes. The usual attempts should be made to determine the etiology of the arrhythmia, and the surgical or anesthetic manipulations necessary to correct parasympathetic imbalance should be performed.

Reversal of Neuromuscular Blockade: The recommended dose of glycopyrrolate injectable is 0.2 mg (1.0 ml) for each 1.0 mg of neostigmine or 5.0 mg of pyridostigmine. In order to minimize the appearance of cardiac side effects, the drugs may be administered simultaneously by intravenous injection and may be mixed in the same syringe.

Peptic Ulcer: The usual recommended dose of glycopyrrolate injectable is 0.1 mg (0.5 ml) administered at 4-hour intervals. 3 or 4 times daily intravenously or intramuscularly. Where more profound effect is required, 0.2 mg (1.0 ml) may be given. Some patients may be given. Some patients may need only a single dose, and frequency of administration should be dictated by patient response up to a maximum of four times daily.

Children

(Read CONTRAINDICATIONS.)

Preanesthetic Medication: The recommended dose of glycopyrrolate injectable in children 1 month to 12 years of age is 0.002 mg (0.01 ml) per pound of body weight intramuscularly, given 30 to 60 minutes prior to the anticipated time of induction of anesthesia or at the time the preanesthetic narcotic and/or sedative are administered.

Children 1 month to 2 years of age may require up to 0.004 mg (0.02 ml) per pound of body weight.

Intraoperative Medication: Because of the long duration of action of glycopyrrolate if used as preanesthetic medication, additional glycopyrrolate injectable for anticholinergic effect intraoperatively is rarely needed; in the event it is required the recommended pediatric dose 0.002 mg (0.01 ml) per pound of body weight intravenously, not to exceed 0.1 mg (0.5 ml) in a single dose which may be repeated, as needed, at intervals of 2-3 minutes. The usual attempts should be made to determine the etiology of the arrhythmia, and the surgical or anesthetic manipulations necessary to correct parasympathetic imbalance should be performed.

DOSAGE AND ADMINISTRATION: *(cont'd)*

Reversal of Neuromuscular Blockade: The recommended pediatric dose of glycopyrrolate injectable is 0.2 mg (1.0 ml) for each 1.0 mg of neostigmine or 5.0 mg of pyridostigmine. In order to minimize the appearance of cardiac side effects, the drugs may be administered simultaneously by intravenous injection and may be mixed in the same syringe.

Glycopyrrolate injectable is not recommended for peptic ulcer in children under 12 years of age. (See PRECAUTIONS.)

Note: Parenteral drug products should be inspected visually for particulate matter and discoloration prior to administration whenever solution and container permit.

Admixture Compatibilities: Glycopyrrolate injectable is compatible for mixing and injection with the following injectable dosage forms: 5% and 10% glucose in water or saline; atropine sulfate, USP; physostigmine salicylate; diphenhydramine HCl; codeine phosphate, USP; benzquinamide HCl; hydromorphone HCl, USP; droperidol; droperidol and fentabyl citrate; propiomazine HCl; levorphanol tartrate); lidocaine, USP; meperidine and promethazine HCls; meperidine HCl, USP; pyridostigmine bromide; morphine sulfate, USP; alphaprodine HCl; nalbuphine HCl; oxymorphone HCl; opium alkaloids HCls; procaine HCl, USP; promethazine HCl, USP; neostigmine methylsulfate, USP; scopolamine HBr, USP; promazine HCl; butorphanol tartrate; fentanyl citrate; pentazocine lactate; tri-methobenzamide HCl; triflupromazine HCl; hydroxyzine HCl. Glycopyrrolate injectable may be administered via the tubing of a running infusion of physiological saline or lactated Ringer's solution.

Since the stability of glycopyrrolate is questionable above a pH of 6.0 do *not* combine glycopyrrolate injectable in the same syringe with methohexital Na; chloramphenicol Na succinate; dimenhydrinate; pentobarbital Na; thiopental Na; secobarbital Na; sodium bicarbonate; or diazepam. A gas will evolve or precipitate may form. Mixing with dexamethazone Na phosphate or a buffered solution of lactated Ringer's solution will result in a pH higher than 6.0. Mixing chlorpromazine HCl, USP, or prochlorperazine with other agents in a syringe is not recommended by the manufacturer, although the mixture with glycopyrrolate is physically compatible.

Store at controlled room temperature between 15°C and 30°C (59°F and 86°F).

HOW SUPPLIED - RATED THERAPEUTICALLY EQUIVALENT:

Injection, Solution - Intramuscular; - 0.2 mg/ml

1 ml x 5	$3.04	ROBINUL, AH Robins	00031-7890-87
1 ml x 25	$14.69	ROBINUL, AH Robins	00031-7890-11
1 ml x 25	$15.00	Glycopyrrolate, Gensia Labs	00703-2601-04
1 ml x 25	$17.65	Glycopyrrolate, Schein Pharm (US)	00364-3013-46
1 ml x 25	$22.19	Glycopyrrolate, Am Regent	00517-4601-25
2 ml x 25	$21.00	Glycopyrrolate, Gensia Labs	00703-2612-04
2 ml x 25	$26.66	ROBINUL, AH Robins	00031-7890-95
2 ml x 25	$35.94	Glycopyrrolate, Am Regent	00517-4602-25
5 ml	$2.74	Glycopyrrolate 0.2, Abbott	00074-1098-01
5 ml	$2.86	ROBINUL, AH Robins	00031-7890-93
5 ml	$3.30	Glycopyrrolate, Schein Pharm (US)	00364-3013-53
5 ml x 25	$23.25	Glycopyrrolate, Voluntary Hosp	53258-3400-02
5 ml x 25	$48.00	Glycopyrrolate, Gensia Labs	00703-2623-04
5 ml x 25	$78.44	Glycopyrrolate, Am Regent	00517-4605-25
20 ml	$1.35	Glycopyrrolate, Voluntary Hosp	53258-3400-04
20 ml	$2.88	Glycopyrrolate, Gensia Labs	00703-2635-01
20 ml	$4.59	ROBINUL, AH Robins	00031-7890-83
20 ml x 25	$155.94	Glycopyrrolate, Am Regent	00517-4620-25

Tablet, Uncoated - Oral - 1 mg

100's	$18.41	ROBINUL, AH Robins	00031-7824-63

Tablet, Uncoated - Oral - 2 mg

100's	$29.34	ROBINUL FORTE, AH Robins	00031-7840-63

GOLD SODIUM THIOMALATE *(001379)*

CATEGORIES: Antiarthritics; Arthritis; Gold; Pain; Pregnancy Category C; FDA Pre 1938 Drugs

BRAND NAMES: Aurolate; *Aurothio*; *Miocrin*; **Myochrysine**; *Myocrisin* (Australia, England); *Myocrisine*; *Shiosol* (Japan); *Tauredon* (Germany)
(International brand names outside U.S. in italics)

> **WARNING:**
> Physicians planning to use gold sodium thiomalate should thoroughly familiarize themselves with its toxicity and its benefits. The possibility of toxic reactions should always be explained to the patient before starting therapy. Patients should be warned to report promptly any symptoms suggesting toxicity. Before each injection of gold sodium thiomalate the physician should review the results of laboratory work, and see the patient to determine the presence or absence of adverse reactions since some of these can be severe or even fatal.

DESCRIPTION:

Gold sodium thiomalate is a sterile aqueous solution of gold sodium thiomalate. It contains 0.5 percent benzyl alcohol added as a preservative. The pH of the product is 5.8-6.5.

Gold sodium thiomalate is a mixture of the mono- and di-sodium salts of gold thiomalic acid.

The molecular weight for $C_4H_3AuNa_2O_4S$ (the disodium salt) is 390.07 and for $C_4H_4AuNaO_4S$ (the mono-sodium salt) is 368.09.

Gold sodium thiomalate is supplied as a solution for intramuscular injection containing 25 mg or 50 mg of gold sodium thiomalate per ml.

CLINICAL PHARMACOLOGY:

The mode of action of gold sodium thiomalate is unknown. The predominant action appears to be a suppressive effect on the synovitis of active rheumatoid disease.

INDICATIONS AND USAGE:

Gold sodium thiomalate is indicated in the treatment of selected cases of active rheumatoid arthritis—both adult and juvenile type. The greatest benefit occurs in the early active stage. In late stages of the illness when cartilage and bone damage have occurred, gold can only check the progression of rheumatoid arthritis and prevent further structural damage to joints. It cannot repair damage caused by previously active disease.

Gold sodium thiomalate should be used only as *one part* of a complete program of therapy; alone it is not a complete treatment.

CONTRAINDICATIONS:

Hypersensitivity to any component of this product.

Severe toxicity resulting from previous exposure to gold or other heavy metals.

Severe debilitation.

Systemic lupus erythematosus.

WARNINGS:

Before treatment is started, the patient's hemoglobin, erythrocyte, white blood cell, differential and platelet counts should be determined, and urinalysis should be done to serve as basic reference. Urine should be analyzed for protein and sediment changes prior to each injection. Complete blood counts including platelet estimation should be made before every second injection throughout treatment. The occurrence of purpura or ecchymoses at any time always requires a platelet count.

Danger signals of possible gold toxicity include: rapid reduction of hemoglobin, leukopenia below 4000 WBC/mm^3, eosinophilia above 5 percent, platelet decrease below 100,000/mm^3, albuminuria, hematuria, pruritus, skin eruption, stomatitis, or persistent diarrhea. No additional injections of gold sodium thiomalate should be given unless further studies show these abnormalities to be caused by conditions other than gold toxicity.

PRECAUTIONS:

GENERAL

Gold salts should not be used concomitantly with penicillamine.

The safety of coadministration with cytotoxic drugs has not been established.

Caution is indicated in the use of gold sodium thiomalatein patients with the following:

1. a history of blood dyscrasias such as granulocytopenia or anemia caused by drug sensitivity,

2. allergy or hypersensitivity to medications,

3. skin rash,

4. previous kidney or liver disease,

5. marked hypertension,

6. compromised cerebral or cardiovascular circulation.

Diabetes mellitus or congestive heart failure should be under control before gold therapy is instituted.

CARCINOGENICITY

Renal adenomas have been reported in long-term toxicity studies of rats receiving gold sodium thiomalate at high dose levels (2 mg/kg weekly for 45 weeks, followed by 6 mg/kg daily for 47 weeks), approximately 2 to 42 times the usual human dose. These adenomas are histologically similar to those produced in rats by chronic administration of experimental gold compounds and other heavy metals, such as lead. No reports have been received of renal adenomas in man in association with the use of gold sodium thiomalate.

PREGNANCY CATEGORY C

Gold sodium thiomalate has been shown to be teratogenic during the organogenetic period in rats and rabbits when given in doses, respectively, of 140 and 175 times the usual human dose. Hydrocephaly and microphthalmia were the malformations observed in rats when gold sodium thiomalate was administered subcutaneously at a dose of 25 mg/kg day from 6 through day 15 of gestation. In rabbits, limb malformations and gastroschisis were the malformations observed when gold sodium thiomalate was administered subcutaneously at doses of 20-45 mg/kg/day from day 6 through day 18 of gestation.

There are no adequate and well-controlled studies in pregnant women. Gold sodium thiomalate should be used during pregnancy only if the potential benefit to the mother justifies the potential risk to the fetus.

NURSING MOTHERS

The presence of gold has been demonstrated in the milk of lactating mothers. In addition, gold has been found in the serum and red blood cells of a nursing infant. In view of the above findings and because of the potential for serious adverse reactions in nursing infants from gold sodium thiomalate, a decision should be made whether to discontinue nursing or to discontinue the drug, taking into account the importance of the drug to the mother. The slow excretion and persistence of gold in the mother, even after therapy is discontinued, must also be kept in mind.

ADVERSE REACTIONS:

A variety of adverse reactions may develop during the initial phase (weekly injections) of therapy or during maintenance treatment. Adverse reactions are observed most frequently when the cumulative dose of gold sodium thiomalate administered is between 400 and 800 mg. Very uncommonly, complications occur days to months after cessation of treatment.

Cutaneous Reactions: Dermatitis is the most common reaction. *Any eruption, especially if pruritic, that develops during treatment with* gold sodium thiomalate *should be considered a reaction to gold until proven otherwise.* Pruritus often exists before dermatitis becomes apparent, and therefore should be considered a warning signal of impending cutaneous reaction. The most serious form of cutaneous reaction is generalized exfoliative dermatitis which may lead to alopecia and shedding of nails. Gold dermatitis may be aggravated by exposure to sunlight or an actinic rash may develop.

Mucous Membrane Reactions: Stomatitis is the second most common adverse reaction. Shallow ulcers on the buccal membranes, on the borders of the tongue, and on the palate or in the pharynx may occur as the only adverse reaction, or along with dermatitis. Sometimes diffuse glossitis or gingivitis develops. A metallic taste may precede these oral mucous membrane reactions and should be considered a warning signal.

Conjunctivitis is a rare reaction.

Renal Reactions: Gold may be toxic to the kidney and produce a nephrotic syndrome or glomerulitis with hematuria. These renal reactions are usually relatively mild and subside completely if recognized early and treatment is discontinued. They may become severe and chronic if treatment is continued after onset of the reaction. Therefore, it is important to perform a *urinalysis before every injection,* and to discontinue treatment promptly if proteinuria or hematuria develops.

Hematologic Reactions: Blood dyscrasia due to gold toxicity is rare, but because of the potential serious consequences it must be constantly watched for and recognized early by frequent blood examinations done throughout treatment. Granulocytopenia; thrombocytopenia, with or without purpura; hypoplastic and aplastic anemia; and eosinophilia have all been reported. These hematologic disorders may occur separately or in combinations.

Nitritoid and Allergic Reactions: Reactions of the "nitritoid type" which may resemble anaphylactoid effects have been reported. Flushing, fainting, dizziness and sweating are most frequently reported. Other symptoms that may occur include: nausea, vomiting, malaise, headache, and weakness.

ADVERSE REACTIONS: *(cont'd)*

More severe, but less common effects include: anaphylactic shock, syncope, bradycardia, thickening of the tongue, difficulty in swallowing and breathing, and angioneurotic edema. These effects may occur almost immediately after injection or as late as 10 minutes following injection. They may occur at any time during the course of therapy and if observed, treatment with gold sodium thiomalate should be discontinued.

Miscellaneous Reactions: Gastrointestinal reactions have been reported, including nausea, vomiting, anorexia abdominal cramps and diarrhea. Ulcerative enterocolitis, which can be severe or even fatal, has been reported rarely.

There have been rare reports of reactions involving the eye such as iritis, corneal ulcers, and gold deposits in ocular tissues. Peripheral and central nervous system complications have been reported rarely. Peripheral neuropathy, with or without fasciculations, sensorimotor effects (including Guillain-Barre syndrome) and elevated spinal fluid protein have been reported. Central nervous system complications have included confusion, hallucinations and seizures. Usually these signs and symptoms cleared upon discontinuation of gold therapy.

Hepatitis, jaundice, with or without cholestasis, gold bronchitis, pulmonary injury manifested by interstitial pneumonitis and fibrosis, partial or complete hair loss and fever have also been reported.

Sometimes arthralgia occurs for a day or two after an injection of gold sodium thiomalate; this reaction usually subsides after the first few injections.

MANAGEMENT OF ADVERSE REACTIONS

Treatment with gold sodium thiomalate should be discontinued, immediately when toxic reactions occur. Minor complications such as localized dermatitis, mild stomatitis, or slight proteinuria generally require no other therapy and resolve spontaneously with suspension of gold sodium thiomalate. Moderately severe skin and mucous membrane reactions often benefit from topical corticosteroids, oral antihistaminics, and soothing or anesthetic lotions.

If stomatitis or dermatitis becomes severe or more generalized, systemic corticosteroids (generally, prednisone 10 to 40 mg daily in divided doses) may provide symptomatic relief.

For serious renal, hematologic, pulmonary, and enterocolitic complications, high doses of systemic corticosteroids (prednisone 40 to 100 mg daily in divided doses) are recommended. The optimum duration of corticosteroid treatment varies with the response of the individual patient. Therapy may be required for many months when adverse effects are unusually severe or progressive.

In patients whose complications do not improve with high-dose corticosteroid treatment, or who develop significant steroid-related adverse reactions, a chelating agent may be given to enhance gold excretion. Dimercaprol (BAL) has been used successfully, but patients must be monitored carefully as numerous untoward reactions may attend its use. Corticosteroids and a chelating agent may be used concomitantly.

Gold sodium thiomalate *should not be reinstituted after severe or idiosyncratic reactions.*

Gold sodium thiomalate may be readministered following resolution of mild reactions, using a reduced dosage schedule. If an initial test dose of 5 mg gold sodium thiomalate is well-tolerated, progressively larger doses (5 to 10 mg increments) may be given at weekly to monthly intervals until a dose of 25 to 50 mg is reached.

DOSAGE AND ADMINISTRATION:

Gold sodium thiomalate should be administered only by intramuscular injection, preferably intragluteally. It should be given with the patient lying down. He should remain recumbent for approximately 10 minutes after the injection.

Therapeutic effects from gold sodium thiomalate occur slowly. Early improvement, often limited to a reduction in morning stiffness, may begin after six to eight weeks of treatment, but beneficial effects may not be observed until after months of therapy.

Parenteral drug products should be inspected visually for particulate matter and discoloration prior to administration. Do not use if material has darkened. Color should not exceed pale yellow.

For the adult of average size the following dosage schedule is suggested:

Weekly Injections:

1st Injection: 10 mg

2nd Injection: 25 mg

3rd and subsequent injections, 25 to 50 mg until there is toxicity or major clinical improvement, or, in the absence of either of these, the cumulative dose of gold sodium thiomalate reaches one gram.

Gold sodium thiomalate is continued until the cumulative dose reaches one gram unless toxicity or major clinical improvement occurs. If significant clinical improvement occurs before a cumulative dose of one gram has been administered, the dose may be decreased or the interval between injections increased as with maintenance therapy. Maintenance doses of 25 to 50 mg every other week for two to 20 weeks are recommended. If the clinical course remains stable, injections of 25 to 50 mg may be given every third and subsequently every fourth week indefinitely. Some patients may require maintenance treatment at intervals of one to three weeks. Should the arthritis exacerbate during maintenance therapy, weekly injections may be resumed temporarily until disease activity is suppressed.

Should a patient fail to improve during initial therapy (cumulative dose of one gram), several options are available:

1. the patient may be considered to be unresponsive and gold sodium thiomalate is discontinued

2. the same dose (25 to 50 mg) of gold sodium thiomalate may be continued for approximately ten additional weeks

3. the dose of gold sodium thiomalate may be increased by increments of 10 mg every one to four weeks, not to exceed 100 mg in a single injection.

If significant clinical improvement occurs using option 2 or 3, the maintenance schedule described above should be initiated. If there is no significant improvement or if toxicity occurs, therapy with gold sodium thiomalate should be stopped. The higher the individual dose of gold sodium thiomalate, the greater the risk of gold toxicity. Selection of one of these options for chrysotherapy should be based upon a number of factors including the physician's experience with gold salt therapy, the course of the patient's condition, the choice of alternative treatments, and the availability of the patient for the close supervision required.

JUVENILE RHEUMATOID ARTHRITIS

The pediatric dose of gold sodium thiomalate is proportional to the adult dose on a weight basis. After the initial test dose of 10 mg, the recommended dose for children is one mg per kilogram body weight, not to exceed 50 mg for a single in injection. Otherwise, the guidelines given above for administration to adults also apply to children.

Concomitant Drug Therapy: Gold salts should not be used concomitantly with penicillamine. The safety of coadministration with cytotoxic drugs has not been established. Other measures, such as salicylates, other non-steroidal anti-inflammatory drugs, or systemic corticosteroids, may be continued when gold sodium thiomalate is initiated. After improvement commences, analgesic and anti-inflammatory drugs may be discontinued slowly as symptoms permit.

DOSAGE AND ADMINISTRATION: *(cont'd)*

Storage: Protect from light. Store container in carton until contents have been used.

HOW SUPPLIED - EQUIVALENTS NOT AVAILABLE:

Injection, Solution - Intramuscular - 25 mg/ml

1 ml x 6	**$43.41**	**MYOCHRYSINE, Merck**	**00006-7764-64**

Injection, Solution - Intramuscular - 50 mg/ml

1 ml	$16.75	Gold Sodium Thiomalate, Yorpharm	61147-8006-00
1 ml x 6	$55.04	Aurolate, Pasadena	00418-4450-01
1 ml x 6	**$66.35**	**MYOCHRYSINE, Merck**	**00006-7762-64**
10 ml	$82.97	Gold Sodium Thiomalate, Insource	58441-1124-01
10 ml	$82.97	Gold Sodium Thiomalate, King Pharms	60793-0109-10
10 ml	$85.75	Aurolate, Pasadena	00418-4450-10
10 ml	**$103.59**	**MYOCHRYSINE, Merck**	**00006-7762-10**
10 ml	$156.86	Gold Sodium Thiomalate, Yorpharm	61147-8006-03

GONADORELIN ACETATE *(003027)*

CATEGORIES: Amenorrhea; Central Nervous System Agents; Gonadotropins; Hormones; Hypogonadism; Infertility; Orphan Drugs; Pituitary; Pregnancy Category B; FDA Approved 1989 Oct

BRAND NAMES: *Cryptocur*; *Fertiral* (England); *H.R.F.*; *H.R.F. Inj.*; *Kryptocur* (Germany); *Luforan*; *Lutrelef*; **Lutrepulse**; *Relefact*; *Relefact LH-RH* (Germany); *Relisorm-L* (Mexico); *Stimu-LH* (France); *Wyeth-Ayerst HRF*; *Zyklomat*
(International brand names outside U.S. in italics)

FORMULARIES: Aetna

DESCRIPTION:

Lutrepulse (gonadorelin acetate) for Injection is used for the induction of ovulation in women with primary hypothalamic amenorrhea. Gonadorelin acetate is a synthetic decapeptide that is identical in amino acid sequence to endogenous gonadotropin-releasing hormone (GnRH) synthesized in the human hypothalamus and in various neurons terminating in the hypothalamus. The molecular formula of gonadorelin acetate is:

$C_{55}H_{75}N_{17}O_{13} \cdot xC_2H_4O_2 \cdot yH_2O$

Its molecular weight is 1182.3 + x60 +y18, where$x$ and y represent a non-stoichiometric ratio of acetate and water associated with the peptide, and $x$ranges from 1-2 and y ranges from 2-3. The amino acid sequence of GnRH is:

5-oxoPro-His-Trp-Ser-Tyr-Gly-Leu-Arg-Pro-Gly-NH_2

Lutrepulse for Injection is a sterile, lyophilized powder intended for intravenous pulsatile injection after reconstitution. It is white and very soluble in water. Vials are available containing 0.8 mg or 3.2 mg gonadorelin acetate (expressed as the diacetate) and 10.0 mg mannitol as a carrier. After reconstituting with 8 ml of diluent (sterile 0.9% Sodium Chloride Solution and hydrochloric acid to adjust the pH) for lutrepulse for injection, the concentration of gonadorelin acetate is 5 mcg per 50 µl in each vial containing 0.8 mg lyophilized hormone, and 20 mcg per 50 µl in each vial containing 3.2 mg lyophilized hormone. Lutrepulse (gonadorelin acetate) for injection is intended for use with the lutrepulse for injection kits and/or its individual components as listed below. The volumes and concentrations are specific for use with the lutrepulse pump for appropriate dosing.

CLINICAL PHARMACOLOGY:

Under physiologic conditions, gonadotropin-releasing hormone (GnRH) is released by the hypothalamus in a pulsatile fashion. The primary effect of GnRH is the synthesis and release of luteinizing hormone (LH) in the anterior pituitary gland. GnRH also stimulates the synthesis and release of follicle stimulating hormone (FSH), but this effect is less pronounced. LH and FSH subsequently stimulate the gonads to produce steroids which are instrumental in regulating reproductive hormonal status. Unlike human menopausal gonadotropin (hMG) which supplies pituitary hormones, pulsatile administration of gonadorelin acetate injection replaces defective hypothalamic secretion of GnRH. The pulsatile administration of gonadorelin acetate injection approximates the natural hormonal secretory pattern, causing pulsatile release of pituitary gonadotropins. Accordingly, gonadorelin acetate injection is useful in treating conditions of infertility caused by defective GnRH stimulation from the hypothalamus (see INDICATIONS AND USAGE). The following information summarizes clinical efficacy of gonadorelin acetate administered by pulsatile intravenous injection to patients with primary hypothalamic amenorrhea.

44 patients with primary hypothalamic amenorrhea (HA)

93% (41/44) patients ovulatory with gonadorelin acetate therapy

62% (24/39)* patients pregnant

100% (7/7) of those failing past attempts at ovulation induction by other methods were ovulatory on gonadorelin acetate.

* Five patients did not desire pregnancy.

Following intravenous injection of GnRH into normal subjects and/or hypogonadotropic patients, plasma GnRH concentrations rapidly decline with initial and terminal half-lives of 2-10 min. and 10-40 min., respectively. In these studies, high clearance values (500-1500 l/day) and low volumes of distribution (10-15 l) were calculated. The pharmacokinetics of GnRH in normal subjects and in hypogonadotropic patients were similar. GnRH was rapidly metabolized to various biologically inactive peptide fragments which are readily excreted in urine. Renal failure, but not hepatic disease, prolonged the half-life and reduced the clearance of GnRH.

INDICATIONS AND USAGE:

Gonadorelin acetate injection is indicated in the treatment of primary hypothalamic amenorrhea.

Differential Diagnosis: Proper diagnosis is critical for successful treatment with gonadorelin acetate injection. It must be established that hypothalamic amenorrhea or hypogonadism is, in fact, due to a deficiency in quantity or pulsing of endogenous GnRH. The diagnosis of hypothalamic amenorrhea or hypogonadism is based on the exclusion of other causes of the dysfunction, since there is currently no practical technique to directly assess hypothalamic function. Prior to initiation of therapy with gonadorelin acetate injection, the physician should rule out disorders of general health, reproductive organs, anterior pituitary, and central nervous system, other than abnormalities of GnRH secretion.

CONTRAINDICATIONS:

Gonadorelin acetate injection is contraindicated in women with any condition that could be exacerbated by pregnancy. For example, pituitary prolactinoma should be considered one such condition. Additionally, any history of sensitivity to gonadorelin acetate, gonadorelin hydrochloride or any component of gonadorelin acetate injection is a contraindication.

Patients who have ovarian cysts or causes of anovulation other than those of hypothalamic origin should not receive gonadorelin acetate injection.

CONTRAINDICATIONS: *(cont'd)*

Gonadorelin acetate injection is intended to initiate events including the production of reproductive hormones (*e.g.*, estrogens and progestins). Therefore, any condition that may be worsened by reproductive hormones, such as a hormonally-dependent tumor, is a contraindication to the use of gonadorelin acetate injection.

WARNINGS:

Therapy with gonadorelin acetate injection should be conducted by physicians familiar with pulsatile GnRH delivery and the clinical ramifications of ovulation induction. While there have been few cases of hyperstimulation (<1%) this possibility must be considered. If hyperstimulation should occur, therapy should be discontinued and spontaneous resolution can be expected. The preservation of the endogenous feedback mechanisms makes severe hyperstimulation (with ascites and pleural effusion) rare. However, the physician should be aware of the possibility and be alert for any evidence of ascites, pleural effusion, hemoconcentration, rupture of a cyst, fluid or electrolyte imbalance, or sepsis.

Multiple pregnancy is a possibility that can be minimized by careful attention to the recommended doses and ultrasonographic monitoring of the ovarian response to therapy. Following a baseline pelvic ultrasound, follow-up studies should be conducted at a minimum on day 7 and day 14 of therapy.

Serious hypersensitivity reactions (anaphylaxis) have been reported following gonadotropin-releasing hormone administration, including gonadorelin acetate. Clinical manifestations may include: cardiovascular collapse, hypotension, tachycardia, loss of consciousness, angioedema, bronchospasm, dyspnea, urticaria, flushing and pruritus. If any allergic reaction occurs, therapy with gonadorelin should be discontinued. Serious acute hypersensitivity reactions may require emergency medical treatment.

As with any intravenous medication, scrupulous attention to asepsis is important. The infusion area must be monitored as with all indwelling parenteral approaches. The catheter and IV site should be monitored and changed at appropriate intervals for the type of intravenous catheter utilized for the delivery of therapy.

PRECAUTIONS:

General: Ovarian hyperstimulation has been reported. This may be related to pulse dosage or concomitant use of other ovulation stimulators. Hyperstimulation may be a greater risk in patients where spontaneous variations in endogenous GnRH secretion occur. Multiple follicle development, multiple pregnancy, and spontaneous termination of pregnancy have been reported. Multiple pregnancy can be minimized by appropriate monitoring of follicle formation; nonetheless, the patient and her partner should be advised on the frequency (12%) and potential risks of multiple pregnancy before starting treatment.

Ovarian hyperstimulation, a syndrome of sudden ovarian enlargement, ascites with or without pain, and/or pleural effusion, is rare with pulsatile GnRH therapy. Among 268 patients participating in clinical trials, once case of moderate hyperstimulation has been reported, but this cycle included the concomitant use of clomiphene citrate.

Antibody formation (IgE and IgG) has been reported following administration of gonadorelin. The safety and efficacy implication of antibody development are uncertain (see WARNINGS).

Gonadorelin acetate injection should be administered only with the Lutrepulse Pump. The patient should be provided with detailed oral and written instructions regarding infusion pump usage and potential sepsis in order to minimize the frequency of infusion pump malfunction and inflammation, infection, mild phlebitis, or hematoma at the catheter site.

Information for the Patient: The patient should be advised to discontinue the drug and seek medical attention at the first sign of skin rash, urticaria, rapid heart beat, difficulty in swallowing and breathing, or any swelling which may suggest angioedema (see WARNINGS and ADVERSE REACTIONS).

Laboratory Tests: Following a diagnosis of primary hypothalamic amenorrhea, initiation of gonadorelin acetate injection therapy may be monitored by the following:

1. Ovarian ultrasound - baseline, therapy day 7, therapy day 14.

2. Mild-luteal phase serum progesterone.

3. Clinical observation of infusion site at each visit as needed.

4. Physical examination including pelvic at regularly scheduled visits.

Drug/Laboratory Test Interactions: None are known.

Carcinogenesis, Mutagenesis, and Impairment of Fertility: Since GnRH is a natural substance normally present in humans, long-term studies in animals have not been performed to evaluate carcinogenic potential. Mutagenicity testing was not done.

Pregnancy Category B: Reproduction studies (teratology and embryo-toxicity) performed in rats and rabbits have not revealed any evidence of harm to the fetus due to gonadorelin acetate. There was no evidence of teratogenicity when gonadorelin acetate was administered intravenously up to 120 mcg/kg/day (>70 times the recommended human dose of 5 mcg per pulse) in rats and rabbits.

Studies in pregnant women have shown that gonadorelin acetate does not increase the risk abnormalities when administered during the first trimester of pregnancy. It appears that the possibility of fetal harm is remote, if the drug is used during pregnancy. In clinical studies, 47 pregnant patients have used gonadorelin acetate during the first trimester of pregnancy (51 pregnancies) and the drug had no apparent adverse effect on the course of pregnancy. Available follow-up reports on infants born to these women reveal no adverse effects or complications that were attributable to gonadorelin acetate. Nevertheless, because the studies in humans cannot rule out the possibility of harm, gonadorelin acetate should be used during pregnancy only for maintenance of the corpus luteum in ovulation induction cycles.

Nursing Mothers: It is not known whether this drug is excreted in human milk. There is no indication for use of gonadorelin acetate injection in a nursing woman.

Pediatric Use: Safety and effectiveness in children under the age of 18 have not been established.

DRUG INTERACTIONS:

None are known. Gonadorelin acetate injection should not be used concomitantly with other ovulation stimulators.

ADVERSE REACTIONS:

Adverse reactions have been reported in approximately 10% of treatment regimens. Ten of 268 patients interrupted therapy because of an adverse reaction but subsequently resumed treatment. One other subject did not resume treatment.

In clinical studies involving 268 women, one case of moderate ovarian hyperstimulation has been reported. This cycle included concomitant use of clomiphene citrate. This low incidence of hyperstimulation appears to be due to the preservation of normal feedback mechanisms of the pituitary-ovarian axis.

Despite the preservation of feedback mechanisms, some incidents of multiple follicle development, multiple pregnancy, and spontaneous termination of pregnancy have been reported.

ADVERSE REACTIONS: *(cont'd)*

Multiple pregnancy can be minimized by appropriate monitoring of follicle formation; nonetheless, the patient and her partner should be advised of the frequency and potential hazards of multiple pregnancy before starting treatment. In clinical studies involving 142 pregnancies, delivery information was available on 89 pregnancies. Eleven of these gonadorelin acetate injection-induced pregnancies (12%) were multiple (10 sets of twins, 1 set of triplets).

The following adverse reactions have occurred at the injection site: urticaria, pruritus, inflammation, infection, mild phlebitis, or hematoma at the catheter site. Additionally, infusion set malfunction and interruption of infusion may occur; this has no known adverse effect other than interruption of therapy. Acute generalized (anaphylaxis, angioedema, urticaria, etc.) hypersensitivity reactions have been reported (see WARNINGS and PRECAUTIONS).

Anaphylaxis (bronchospasm, tachycardia, flushing, urticaria, induration at injection site) has also been reported with the related polypeptide hormone gonadorelin hydrochloride (Factrel), Wyeth-Ayerst.

OVERDOSAGE:

Continuous, non-pulsatile exposure to gonadorelin acetate could temporarily reduce pituitary responsiveness. If the pump should malfunction and deliver the entire contents of the 3.2 mg system, no harmful effects would be expected. Bolus doses as high as 3000 mcg of gonadorelin hydrochloride have not been harmful. Pituitary hyperstimulation and multiple follicle development can be minimized by adhering to recommended doses, and appropriate monitoring of follicle formation (see PRECAUTIONS).

Administration of 640 mcg/kg in monkeys as a single intravenous bolus resulted in no compound-related effects in clinical observations or gross morphologic evaluations.

DOSAGE AND ADMINISTRATION:

Dosage: Dosages between 1 and 20 mcg have been successfully used in clinical studies. The recommended dose in primary hypothalamic amenorrhea is 5 mcg every 90 minutes. This is delivered by lutrepulse pump using the 0.8 mg solution at 50 µl per pulse (see physician pump manual.) Sixty-eight percent of the 5 mcg every 90 minutes regimens induced ovulation in patients with primary hypothalamic amenorrhea.

The lutrepulse pump is capable of delivering 2.5, 5, 10, or 20 mcg of gonadorelin acetate every 90 minutes. Some women may require a reduction in the recommended dose of 5 mcg should laboratory testing and patient monitoring indicate an inappropriate response. While most primary hypothalamic amenorrhea patients will ovulate during the first cycle of 5 mcg therapy, some may be refractory to this dose. The recommended treatment interval is 21 days. It may be necessary to raise the dose cautiously, and in stepwise fashion if there is no response after three treatment intervals. All dose changes should be carefully monitored for inappropriate response.

The following table can be used to calculate the dose per pulse when individualizing treatment (TABLE 1):

TABLE 1

VIAL	DILUENT	VOLUME/PULSE	DOSE/PULSE
0.8 mg	8 ml	25 µl	2.5 mcg
0.8 mg	8 ml	50 µl	5 mcg
3.2 mg	8 ml	25 µl	10 mcg
3.2 mg	8 ml	50 µl	20 mcg

The response to gonadorelin acetate injection usually occurs within two to three weeks after therapy initiation. When ovulation occurs with the lutrepulse pump in place, therapy should be continued for another two weeks to maintain the corpus luteum. A comparison of gonadorelin acetate injection to hCG or hCG + gonadorelin acetate injection for corpus luteum maintenance revealed the following information (TABLE 2):

TABLE 2

hCG	
Delivered = 43 ÷ 63 = 68%	
Aborted = 20 ÷ 63 = 32%	
lutrepulse for injection	
Delivered = 19 ÷ 26 = 73%	
Aborted = 7 ÷ 26 = 27%	
hCG + lutrepulse for injection	
Delivered = 19 ÷ 25 = 76%	
Aborted = 6 ÷ 25 = 24%	

Gonadorelin acetate injection alone was able to maintain the corpus luteum during pregnancy.

Administration: Gonadorelin acetate injection is to be reconstituted aseptically with 8 ml of diluent for gonadorelin acetate injection. *The drug product should be reconstituted immediately prior to use and transferred to the plastic reservoir.* First withdraw the required volume of the saline diluent and inject it gently onto the lyophile (drug product) cake. The product is then gently rolled for a few seconds to produce a solution which should be clear, colorless, and free of particulate matter. Parenteral drug products should be inspected visually for particular matter and discoloration prior to administration, whenever solution and container permit. If particulate matter or discoloration are present, the solution should not be used. A presterilized reservoir (bag) with the infusion catheter set supplied with the gonadorelin acetate injection is filled with the reconstituted solution, and administered intravenously using the Lutrepulse Pump. The pump should be set to deliver 25 or 50 µl of solution, based upon the dose selected, over a pulse period of one minute and at a pulse frequency of 90 minutes. The solution will supply 90 minute pulsatile doses for approximately 7 or 14 consecutive days, depending upon the vial size and dose used.

HOW SUPPLIED:

Lutrepulse (gonadorelin acetate) for Injection is supplied in drug product alone, kits and Lutrepulse Pump component packages.

Each Lutrepulse for Injection drug product contains one 10 ml vial of 0.8 mg or 3.2 mg Lutrepulse for Injection as a lyophilized, sterile powder and one 10 ml vial of Lutrepulse for Injection Diluent. These should be stored at controlled room temperature (15°-30°C, 50°-86°F).

The following components are included in each lutrepulse for injection kit:

Sterile catheter tubing	Sterile syringe needle
Sterile reservoir catheter with double-female luer adaptor	Alcohol swabs (four supplied)
	Elastic belt
Sterile IV cannula units (four supplied)	9-V battery
Sterile 10 ml syringe	

Physician package insert, physician pump manual, and patient instructions

HOW SUPPLIED: *(cont'd)*

The lutrepulse pump kit contains the following components:

Lutrepulse pump	Physician pump manual
9-V batteries (two supplied)	Physician package insert
3-V lithium battery	Warranty card

HOW SUPPLIED - EQUIVALENTS NOT AVAILABLE:

Injection, Solution - Intravenous - 0.8 mg
1's $144.94 LUTREPULSE, Ferring Labs 55566-7208-00

Injection, Solution - Intravenous - 3.2 mg
1's $437.44 LUTREPULSE, Ferring Labs 55566-7232-00

Kit - Intravenous - 0.8 mg
1's $282.44 LUTREPULSE, Ferring Labs 55566-7208-05

Kit - Intravenous - 3.2 mg
1's $574.44 LUTREPULSE, Ferring Labs 55566-7232-05

GONADOTROPIN, CHORIONIC *(001381)*

CATEGORIES: Anterior Pituitary/Hypothalmic Function; Cryptorchidism; Gonadotropins; Hormones; Hypogonadism; Infertility; Pregnancy; Pregnancy Category X; FDA Approval Pre 1982

BRAND NAMES: A.P.L.; *APL* (Canada); Chorex; Chorigon; *Choriomon*; Chorionic Gonadotropin; Choron 10; Corgonject-5; *Corion*; Follutein; Glukor Revised; *Gonadotrophine Chorionique "Endo"* (France); *Gonadotrophon L.H.*; *Gonadotrophon LH*; *Gonadotropyl C* (Mexico); Gonatrin-L; Gonic; *IVF-C*; *Pregnesin* (Germany); Pregnyl; *Primogonyl* (Germany); Profasi; *Profasi HP* (Canada); *Pubergen*; Tega-Gonad

(International brand names outside U.S. in italics)

FORMULARIES: Aetna; BC-BS

DESCRIPTION:

Human chorionic gonadotropin (HCG), a polypeptide hormone produced by the human placenta, is composed of an alpha and a beta sub-unit. The alpha sub-unit is essentially identical to the alpha sub-units of the human pituitary gonadotropins, luteinizing hormone (LH) and follicle-stimulating hormone (FSH), as well as to the alpha sub-unit of human thyroid-stimulating hormone (TSH). The beta subunits of these hormones differ in amino acid sequence.

Chorionic Gonadotropin is a water soluble glycoprotein derived from human pregnancy urine. The sterile lyophilized powder is stable. When reconstituted the solution should be refrigerated and used within 30 days.

Each vial, when reconstituted with provided diluent (Bacteriostatic Water for Injection, USP), will contain:

A. Chorionic Gonadotropin **2,000, 5,000, 10,000 or 20,000** USP Units, Mannitol 100 mg, Dibasic Sodium Phosphate 16 mg, Monobasic Sodium Phosphate 4 mg, with Benzyl Alcohol 0.9% as preservative, in Water for Injection. Sodium Hydroxide and/or Hydrochloric Acid may have been used to adjust pH of the diluent; or;

B. Chorionic Gonadotropin **15,000** USP Units, Mannitol 300 mg, Dibasic Sodium Phosphate 48 mg, Monobasic Sodium Phosphate 12 mg, with Benzyl Alcohol 0.9% as preservative, in Water for Injection. Sodium Hydroxide and/or Hydrochloric Acid may have been used to adjust pH of the diluent.

CLINICAL PHARMACOLOGY:

The action of HCG is virtually identical to that of pituitary LH, although HCG appears to have a small degree of FSH activity as well. It stimulates production of gonadal steroid hormones by stimulating the interstitial cells (Leydig cells) of the testis to produce androgens and the corpus luteum of the ovary to produce progesterone. Androgen stimulation in the male leads to the development of secondary sex characteristics and may stimulate testicular descent when no anatomical impediment to descent is present. This descent is usually reversible when HCG is discontinued. During the normal menstrual cycle LH participates with FSH in the development and maturation of the normal ovarian follicle, and the mid-cycle LH surge triggers ovulation. HCG can substitute for LH in this function.

During a normal pregnancy, HCG secreted by the placenta maintains the corpus luteum after LH secretion decreases, supporting continued secretion of estrogen and progesterone and preventing menstruation. HCG HAS NO KNOWN EFFECT ON FAT MOBILIZATION, APPETITE OR SENSE OF HUNGER, OR BODY FAT DISTRIBUTION.

INDICATIONS AND USAGE:

HCG HAS NOT BEEN DEMONSTRATED TO BE EFFECTIVE ADJUNCTIVE THERAPY IN THE TREATMENT OF OBESITY. THERE IS NO SUBSTANTIAL EVIDENCE THAT IT INCREASES WEIGHT LOSS BEYOND THAT RESULTING FROM CALORIC RESTRICTION, THAT IT CAUSES A MORE ATTRACTIVE OR "NORMAL" DISTRIBUTION OF FAT OR THAT IT DECREASES THE HUNGER AND DISCOMFORT ASSOCIATED WITH CALORIE-RESTRICTED DIETS.

1. Prepubertal cryptorchidism not due to anatomical obstruction. In general HCG is thought to induce testicular descent in situations when descent would have occurred at puberty. HCG thus may help predict whether or not orchiopexy will be needed in the future. Although in some cases descent following HCG administration is permanent, in most cases, the response is temporary. Therapy is usually instituted between the ages of 4 and 9.

2. Selected cases of hypogonadotropic hypogonadism (hypogonadism secondary to a pituitary deficiency) in males.

3. Induction of ovulation and pregnancy in the anovulatory, infertile woman in whom the cause of anovulation is secondary and not due to primary ovarian failure, and who has been appropriately pre-treated with human menotropins.

CONTRAINDICATIONS:

Precocious puberty, prostatic carcinoma or other androgen-dependent neoplasm, prior allergic reaction to HCG.

WARNINGS:

HCG should be used in conjunction with human menopausal gonadotropins only by physicians experienced with infertility problems who are familiar with the criteria for patient selection, contraindications, warnings, precautions and adverse reactions described in the package insert for menotropins. The principal serious adverse reactions during this use are: (1) Ovarian hyperstimulation, a syndrome of sudden ovarian enlargement, ascites with or without pain and/or pleural effusion, (2) Rupture of ovarian cysts with resultant hemoperitoneum, (3) Multiple births, and (4) Arterial thromboembolism.

PRECAUTIONS:

GENERAL

1. Induction of androgen secretion by HCG may induce precocious puberty in patients treated for cryptorchidism. Therapy should be discontinued if signs of precocious puberty occur.

2. Since androgens may cause fluid retention, HCG should be used with caution in patients with cardiac or renal disease, epilepsy, migraine, or asthma.

Pregnancy Category C: Animal reproduction studies have not been conducted with HCG. It is also not known whether HCG can cause fetal harm when administered to a pregnant woman or can affect reproduction capacity. HCG should be given to a pregnant woman only if clearly needed.

ADVERSE REACTIONS:

Headache, irritability, restlessness, depression, fatigue, edema, precocious puberty, gynecomastia, pain at the site of injection. Hypersensitivity reactions both localized and systemic in nature, including erythema, uticaria, rash, angioedema, dyspnea and shortness of breath, have been reported. The relationship of these allergic-like events to the polypeptide hormone or the diluent containing benzyl alcohol is not clear.

DOSAGE AND ADMINISTRATION:

Intramuscular Use Only: The dosage regimen employed in any particular case will depend upon the indication for use, the age and weight of the patient and the physician's preference. The following regimens have been advocated by various authorities.

Prepubertal cryptorchidism not due to anatomical obstruction

1. 4,000 USP Units three times weekly for three weeks.
2. 5,000 USP Units every second day for four injections.
3. 15 injections of 500 to 1,000 USP Units over a period of six weeks.
4. 500 USP Units three times weekly for four to six weeks. If this course of treatment is not successful, another is begun one month later, giving 1,000 USP Units per injection.

Selected cases of hypogonadotropic hypogonadism in males

1. 500 to 1,000 USP Units three times a week for three weeks, followed by the same dose twice a week for three weeks.
2. 4,000 USP Units three times weekly for six to nine months, following which the dosage may be reduced to 2,000 USP Units three times weekly for an additional three months.

Induction of ovulation and pregnancy in the anovulatory, infertile woman in whom the cause of anovulation is secondary and not due to primary ovarian failure and who has been appropriately pre-treated with human menotropins (See prescribing information for menotropins for dosage and administration for that drug product).

5,000 to 10,000 USP Units one day following the last dose of menotropins (A dosage of 10,000 USP Units is recommended in the labeling for menotropins).

Parenteral drug products should be inspected visually for particulate matter and discoloration prior to administration, whenever the solution and container permit.

Store dry product at controlled room temperature 15 - 30°C (59 - 86 F). AFTER RECONSTITUTION REFRIGERATE THE PRODUCT AT 2 - 8°C (36 - 46°F) AND USE WITHIN 30 DAYS.

(Steris Labs, June 1992, 695101250402*B1)

HOW SUPPLIED - RATED THERAPEUTICALLY EQUIVALENT:

Injection, Lyphl-Soln - Intramuscular - 5,000 unit/vial

1's	$21.27	PROFASI, Serono Labs	44087-8005-03
10 ml	$13.95	Chorionic Gonadotropin, Steris Labs	00402-0125-10
10 ml	$16.40	Chorionic Gonadotropin, Pasadena	00418-5811-42
10 ml	$105.00	Chorionic Gonadotropin, Fujisawa USA	00469-1511-30
10 ml	$105.00	Chorionic Gonadotropin, Fujisawa USA	00469-1512-30
10 ml w/sterile	**$86.69**	**A.P.L., Ayerst**	**00046-0970-10**

Injection, Lyphl-Soln - Intramuscular - 10,000 unit/via

1's	$22.50	Chorionic Gonadotropin, Consolidated Midland	00223-7770-10
1's	$34.41	PREGNYL, Organon	00052-0315-10
1's	$41.20	PROFASI, Serono Labs	44087-8010-03
10 ml	$15.79	Chorionic Gonadotropin, McGuff	49072-0127-10
10 ml	$18.13	Chorionic Gonadotropin, Fujisawa USA	00469-1501-30
10 ml	$19.29	Chrionic Gonadotropin, HL Moore Drug Exch	00839-5564-30
10 ml	$23.00	CHORON, Forest Pharms	00456-1013-10
10 ml	$23.13	Chorionic Gonadotropin With Diluent, Rugby	00536-0500-70
10 ml	$23.13	Chorionic Gonadotropin With Diluent, Rugby	00536-5130-70
10 ml	$23.65	Chorionic Gonadotropin, Major Pharms	00904-1189-10
10 ml	$24.35	Chorionic Gonadotropin, Pasadena	00418-5821-42
10 ml	$24.94	Chorionic Gonadotropin With Diluent, Schein Pharm (US)	00364-6584-54
10 ml	$24.94	Chorionic Gonadotropin, Schein Pharm (US)	00364-6706-54
10 ml	$24.94	Chorionic Gonadotropin, Steris Labs	00402-0126-10
10 ml	$24.94	Chorionic Gonadotropin, Steris Labs	00402-0126-11
10 ml	$33.07	CHOREX-10, Hyrex Pharms	00314-0618-70
10 ml	$36.20	Chorionic Gonadotropin, Goldline Labs	00182-0805-63
10 ml	$36.20	Chorionic Gonadotropin, Goldline Labs	00182-1165-63
10 ml	$96.81	FOLLUTEIN, Bristol Myers Squibb	00003-0419-40
10 ml	$220.00	Chorionic Gonadotropin, Fujisawa USA	00469-1502-30
10 ml w/sterile	**$162.06**	**A.P.L., Ayerst**	**00046-0971-10**

Injection, Lyphl-Soln - Intramuscular - 20,000 unit/via

1's	$30.00	Chorionic Gonadotropin, Consolidated Midland	00223-7775-10
10 ml	**$329.90**	**A.P.L., Ayerst**	**00046-0972-10**
10 ml	$350.00	Chorionic Gonadotropin, Fujisawa USA	00469-1532-30

HOW SUPPLIED - NOT RATED EQUIVALENT:

Injection, Lyphl-Soln - Intramuscular - 5,000 unit/vial

1's	$19.47	Chorionic Gonadotropin, Eveready Drugs	57548-0125-10

Injection, Lyphl-Soln - Intramuscular - 10,000 unit/via

10 ml	$20.00	Chorionic Gonadotropin, Bolan Pharm	44437-0126-22
10 ml	$24.50	EVEREADY-HCG 1000, Eveready Drugs	57548-0126-10

GOSERELIN ACETATE *(001382)*

CATEGORIES: Antineoplastics; Cancer; Endometriosis; Gonadotropins; Hormones; Lh-Rh Analog; Prostatic Carcinoma; Breast Carcinoma*; Testicular Carcinoma*; Pregnancy Category X; FDA Class 1C ("Little or No Therapeutic Advantage"); Sales > $100 Million; FDA Approved 1989 Dec; Patent Expiration 1997 Jul

* Indication not approved by the FDA

BRAND NAMES: *Prozoladex* (Mexico); **Zoladex**; *Zoladex Depot*; *Zoladex Implant* (Europe); *Zoladex Inj.*

(International brand names outside U.S. in italics)

FORMULARIES: Medi-Cal

DESCRIPTION:

Goserelin acetate implant contains a potent synthetic decapeptide analogue of luteinizing hormone-releasing hormone (LHRH), also known as a gonadotropin releasing hormone (GnRH) agonist analogue. Goserelin acetate is chemically described as an acetate salt of [D- Ser(Bu^t)^6, Azgly^{10}]LHRH. Its chemical structure is pyro-Glu-His-Trp-Ser-Tyr-D-Ser(Bu^t)-Leu-Arg-Pro-Azgly-NH_2 acetate [$C_{59}H_{84}N_{18}O_{14}\cdot(C_2H_4O_2)_x$ where x = 1 to 2.4].

Goserelin acetate is an off-white powder with a molecular weight of 1269 Daltons (free base). It is freely soluble in glacial acetic acid. It is soluble in water, 0.1 M hydrochloric acid, 0.1 M sodium hydroxide, dimethylformamide and dimethyl sulfoxide. Goserelin acetate is practically insoluble in acetone, chloroform and ether.

Zoladex is supplied as a sterile, biodegradable product containing goserelin acetate equivalent to 3.6 mg (or 10.8 mg) of goserelin. Zoladex is designed for subcutaneous injection with continuous release over a 28-day (or 12-week) period. Goserelin acetate is dispersed in a matrix of D,L-lactic and glycolic acids copolymer (13.3-14.3 mg/dose) or (12.82–14.76 mg/dose) containing less than 2.5% (2%) acetic acid and up to 12% (10%) goserelin-related substances and presented as a sterile, white to cream colored 1-mm (1.5 mm) diameter cylinder, preloaded in a special single use syringe with a 16 gauge (14 gauge) needle and overwrapped in a sealed, light- and moisture-proof, aluminum foil laminate pouch containing a desiccant capsule.

Studies of the D,L-lactic and glycolic acids copolymer have indicated that it is completely biodegradable and has no demonstrable antigenic potential.

CLINICAL PHARMACOLOGY:

MECHANISM OF ACTION

Goserelin acetate is a synthetic decapeptide analogue of LHRH. Goserelin acetate acts as a potent inhibitor of pituitary gonadotropin secretion when administered in the biodegradable formulation.

Following initial administration in males, goserelin acetate causes an initial increase in serum luteinizing hormone (LH) and follicle stimulating hormone (FSH) levels with subsequent increases in serum levels of testosterone. Chronic administration of goserelin acetate leads to sustained suppression of pituitary gonadotropins, and serum levels of testosterone consequently fall into the range normally seen in surgically castrated men approximately 21 days after initiation of therapy. This leads to accessory sex organ regression.

In animal and in *in vitro* studies, administration of goserelin resulted in the regression or inhibition of growth of the hormonally sensitive dimethylbenzanthracene (DMBA)-induced rat mammary tumor and Dunning R3327 prostate tumor.

In clinical trials using goserelin 3.6 mg with follow-up of more than 2 years, suppression of serum testosterone to castrate levels has been maintained for the duration of therapy.

In females (3.6 mg only), a similar down-regulation of the pituitary gland by chronic exposure to goserelin acetate leads to suppression of gonadotropin secretion, a decrease in serum estradiol to levels consistent with the postmenopausal state, and would be expected to lead to a reduction of ovarian size and function, reduction in the size of the uterus and mammary gland, as well as a regression of sex hormone-responsive tumors, if present. Serum estradiol is suppressed to levels similar to those observed in postmenopausal women within 3 weeks following initial administration; however, after supression was attained, isolated elevations of estradiol were seen in 10% of the patients enrolled in clinical trials. Serum LH and FSH are suppressed to follicular phase levels within 4 weeks after initial administration of the drug and are usually maintained in that range with continued use of goserelin acetate. In 5% or less of women treated with goserelin, FSH and LH levels may not be suppressed to follicular phase levels on day 28 post treatment with use of a single 3.6 mg depot injection. In certain individuals, suppression of any of these hormones to such levels may not be achieved with goserelin. Estradiol, LH and FSH levels return to pretreatment values within 12 weeks following the last implant administration in all but rare cases.

3.6 MG IMPLANT

Pharmacokinetics: The pharamcokinetics of goserelin have been determined in both male and female healthy volunteers and patients. In these studies, goserelin was administered as a single 250 mcg (aqueous solution) dose and as a single or multiple 3.6 mg depot dose by subcutaneous route. The absorption of radiolabeled drug was rapid, and the peak blood radioactivity levels occurred between 0.5 and 1.0 hour after dosing. The pharamcokinetic parameter estimates of goserelin after administration of 3.6 mg depot for 2 months in males and females are presented in TABLE 1.

TABLE 1 Pharmacokinetic Parameters of 3.6 mg Implant

Parameters (Units)	Males (n=7)	Females (n=9)
Peak Plasma Concentration (ng/ml)	2.84 ± 1.81	1.46 ± 0.82
Time to Peak Concentration (days)	12-15	8-22
Area Under the Curve (0-28 days)(ng.h/ml)	27.8 ± 15.3	18.5 ± 10.3
Systemic Clearance (ml/min)	110.5 ± 47.5	163.9 ± 71.0
*Apparent Volume of Distribution (L)	44.1 ± 13.6	20.3 ± 4.1
*Elimination Half-life (h)	4.2 ± 1.1	2.3 ± 0.6

* The apparent volume of distribution and the elimination half-life were determined after subcutaneous administration of 250 mcg aqueous solution of goserelin.

Pharmacokinetic data were obtained using a nonspecific RIA method.

Goserelin is released from the depot at a much slower rate initially for the first 8 days, and then there is more rapid and continuous release for the remainder of the 28–day dosing period. Despite the change in the releasing rate of goserelin, administration of goserelin every 28 days resulted in testosterone levels that were suppressed to and maintained in the range normally seen in surgically castrated men.

When goserelin 3.6 mg depot was used for treating male and female patients with normal renal and hepatic function, there was no significant evidence of drug accumulation. However, in clinical trials the minimum serum levels of a few patients were increased. These levels can be attributed to interpatient variation.

Distribution: The apparent volumes of distribution determined after subcutaneous administration of 250 mcg aqueous solution of goserelin were 44.1 and 20.3 liters for males and females, respectively. The plasma protein binding of goserelin obtained from one sample was found to be 27.3%.

Metabolism: Metabolism of goserelin, by hydrolysis of the C-terminal amino acids, is the major clearance mechanism. The major circulating component in serum appeared to be 1-7 fragment, and the major component presented in urine of one healthy male volunteer was 5-10 fragment. The metabolism of goserelin in humans yields a similar but narrow profile of metabolites to that found in other species. All metabolites found in humans have also been found in toxicology species.

CLINICAL PHARMACOLOGY: *(cont'd)*

Excretion: Clearance of goserelin following subcutaneous administration of the solution formulation of goserelin is very rapid and occurs via a combination of hepatic metabolism and urinary excretion. More than 90% of a subcutaneous, radiolabeled solution formulation dose of goserelin is excreted in urine. Approximately 20% of the dose in urine is accounted for by unchanged goserelin. The total body clearance of goserelin (administered subcutaneously as 3.6 mg depot) was significantly ($p<0.05$) greater (163.9 versus 110.5 ml/min) in females compared to males.

Special Populations: In clinical trials with the solution formulation of goserelin, male patients with impaired renal function (creatinine clearance <20 ml/min) had a total body clearance and serum elimination half-life of 31.5 ml/min and 12.1 hours, respectively, compared to 133 ml/min and 4.2 hours for subjects with normal renal function (creatinine clearance >70 ml/min). In females, the effects of reduced goserelin clearance due to impaired renal function on drug efficacy and toxicity are unknown. The total body clearances and serum elimination half-lives were similar between normal and hepatic impaired patients receiving 250 mcg solution formulation of goserelin. Pharmacokinetic studies using the aqueous formulation of goserelin in patients with renal and hepatic impairment do not indicate a need for dose adjustment with the use of the depot formulation.

10.8 MG IMPLANT

Pharmacokinetics: The pharmacokinetics of goserelin have been determined in healthy male volunteers and prostate cancer patients using an RIA method, which has been shown to be specific for goserelin in the presence of its metabolites.

The profiles for serum goserelin concentrations in prostate cancer patients administered three 3.6 mg depots followed by one 10.8 are primarily dependent upon the rate of drug release from the depots. For the 3.6 mg depot, mean concentrations gradually rise to reach a peak of about 3 ng/ml at around 15 days after administration and then decline to approximately 0.5 ng/ml by the end of the treatment period. For the 10.8 mg depot, mean concentrations increase to reach a peak of about 8 ng/ml within the first 24 hours and then decline rapidly up to Day 4. Thereafter, mean concentrations remain relatively stable in the range of about 0.3 to 1 ng/ml up to the end of the treatment period.

Absorption: The absorption of radiolabelled drug was rapid following administration as a single 250 mcg (aqueous solution) dose to volunteers by the subcutaneous route. The pharmacokinetics of goserelin following administration of goserelin acetate 10.8 mg depot to patients with prostate cancer are determined by the release of drug from the depot; representative data are summarized in TABLE 2.

Release of goserelin from the depot was relatively rapid shortly after administration resulting in peak concentration being observed 2 hours after dosing. Sustained release of goserelin produced a reasonably stable systemic exposure from Day 4 until the end of the 12-week dosing interval. This overall profile resulted in testosterone levels that were suppressed to and maintained within the range normally observed in surgically castrated men (0-1.73 nmol/L or 0-50 ng/dl), over the dosing interval in approximately 91% (145/160) of patients studied. In 6 of 15 patients that escaped from castrate range, serum testosterone levels were maintained below 2.0 nmol/L (58 ng/dl) and in only one of the 15 patients did the depot completely fail to maintain serum testosterone levels to within the recognized castrate range over a 336-day period (4 depot injections). In the 8 additional patients, a transient escape was followed 14 days later by a level within the castrate range. There is no clinically significant accumulation of goserelin following administration of four depots administered at 12-week intervals.

Distribution: The plasma protein-binding of goserelin is low (<30%).

Metabolism/Elimination: Clearance of goserelin following subcutaneous administration of the solution formulation of goserelin is very rapid and occurs via a combination of hepatic metabolism and urinary excretion. The metabolism of goserelin in humans yields a similar but narrow profile of metabolites to that found in other species. All the human metabolites have also been found in the toxicology species. The major component in serum was the 1-7 fragment formed by hydrolysis of the C-terminal amino acid.

Excretion: More than 90% of a subcutaneous radiolabelled solution formulation dose of goserelin is excreted in urine. Approximately 20% of the dose recovered in urine is accounted for by unchanged goserelin.

Special Populations

Renal Insufficiency: In clinical trials with the solution formulation of goserelin, subjects with impaired renal function (creatinine clearance less than 20 ml/min) had a serum elimination half-life of 12.1 hours compared to 4.2 hours for subjects with normal renal function (creatinine clearance greater than 70 ml/min). However, there was no evidence for any accumulation of goserelin on multiple dosing of the goserelin acetate 10.8 mg depot to subjects with impaired renal function. There was no evidence for any increase in incidence of adverse events in renally impaired patients administered the 10.8 mg depot. These data indicate that there is no need for any dosage adjustment when administering goserelin 10.8 mg to subjects with impaired renal function.

Hepatic Insufficiency: The clearance and half-life of goserelin administered as an aqueous solution are not affected by hepatic impairment. These data indicate that there is no need for any dosage adjustment when administering goserelin acetate 10.8 mg to subjects with impaired hepatic function.

Geriatric: There is no need for any dosage adjustment when administering goserelin acetate 10.8 mg to geriatric patients.

Body Weight: A decline of approximately 1 to 2.5% in the AUC after administration of a 10.8 mg depot was observed with a kilogram increase in body weight. In obese patients who have not responded clinically, testosterone levels should be monitored closely.

TABLE 2 Goserelin Pharmacokinetic Parameters for the 10.8 mg Depot

Parameter	n	Mean	SE	95% CI Lower	95% CI Upper
Systemic clearance (ml/min)	41	121	6.6	108	134
C_{max} (ng/ml)	41	8.85	0.44	7.96	9.74
T_{max} (h)	41	1.80	0.05	1.70	1.92
C_{min} (ng/ml)	44	0.37	0.03	0.30	0.43
Elimination Half-life (h)*	7	4.16	0.40	3.12	5.20

* determined after subcutaneous administration of 250 mcg aqueous soltion of goserelin.
SE =standard error of the mean
95% CI =95% confidence interval

CLINICAL STUDIES:

Endometriosis: In controlled clinical studies using the 3.6 mg formulation every 28 days for 6 months, goserelin was shown to be as effective as danazol therapy in relieving clinical symptoms (dysmenorrhea, dyspareunia and pelvic pain) and signs (pelvic tenderness, pelvic induration) of endometriosis and decreasing the size of endometrial lesions as determined by laparoscopy. In one study comparing goserelin with danazol (800 mg/day), 63% of goserelin-treated patients and 42% of danazol-treated patients had a greater than or equal to 50% reduction in the extent of endometrial lesions. In the second study comparing goserelin with danazol (600 mg/day), 62% of goserelin-treated and 51% of danazol-treated patients had a greater than or equal to 50% reduction in the extent of endometrial lesions. The clinical significance of a decrease in endometriotic lesions is not known at this time; and in addition, laparoscopic staging of endometriosis does not necessarily correlate with severity of symptoms.

In these two studies, goserelin led to amenorrhea in 92% and 80%, respectively, of all treated women within 8 weeks after initial administration. Menses usually resumed within 8 weeks following completion of therapy.

Within 4 weeks following initial administration, clinical symptoms were significantly reduced, and at the end of treatment were, on average, reduced by approximately 84%.

During the first two months of goserelin use, some women experience vaginal bleeding of variable duration and intensity. In all likelihood, this bleeding represents estrogen withdrawal bleeding, and is expected to stop spontaneously.

There is insufficient evidence to determine whether pregnancy rates are enhanced or adversely affected by the use of goserelin.

Breast Cancer: The Southwest Oncology Group conducted a prospective, randomized clinical trial (SWOG-8692 [INT-0075]) in premenopausal women with advanced estrogen receptor positive or progesterone receptor positive breast cancer which compared goserelin with oophorectomy. On the basis of interim data from 124 women, the best objective response (CR+PR) for the goserelin group is 22% versus 12% for the oophorectomy group. The median time to treatment failure is 6.7 months for patients treated with goserelin and 5.5 months for patients treated with oophorectomy. The median survival time for the goserelin arm is 33.2 months and for the oophorectomy arm is 33.6 months.

Subjective responses based on measures of pain control and performance status were observed with both treatments; 48% of the women in the goserelin treatment group and 50% in the oophorectomy group had subjective responses. In the clinical trial (SWOG-8692 [INT 0075]), the mean post treatment estradiol level was reported as 17.8 pg/ml. (The mean estradiol level in postmenopausal women as reported in the literature as 13 pg/ml.) During the conduct of the clinical trial, women whose estradiol levels were not reduced to the postmenopausal range received two goserelin depots, thus, increasing the dose of goserelin from 3.6 mg to 7.2 mg.

Findings were similar in uncontrolled clinical trials involving patients with hormone receptor positive and negative breast cancer. Premenopausal women with estrogen receptor (ER) status of positive, negative, or unknown participated in the uncontrolled (Phase II and Trial 2302) clinical trials. Objective tumor responses were seen regardless of ER status, see TABLE 3

TABLE 3 Objective Response By ER Status

ER status	CR + PR/Total No. (%) Phase II (n=228)	Trial 2302 (n=159)
Positive	43/119 (36)	31/86 (36)
Negative	6/33 (18)	3/26 (10)
Unknown	20/76 (26)	18/44 (41)

Prostate Cancer: In two controlled clinical trials, 160 patients with prostate cancer were randomized to receive either one 3.6 mg goserelin acetate implant every four weeks or a single 10.8 mg goserelin acetate implant every 12–weeks. Mean serum testosterone suppression was similar between the two arms. PSA falls at three months were 94% in patients who received the 10.8 mg implant and 92.5% in the patients that received three 3.6 mg implants.

Periodic monitoring of the serum testosterone should be considered if the anticipated clinical or biochemical response to treatment has not been achieved. A clinical outcome similar to that produced with the use of the 3.6 mg implant administered every 28 days is predicted with goserelin 10.8 mg implant administered every 12 weeks (84 days). Total testosterone was measured by the DPC Coat-a-Count radioimmunoassay method which, as defined by the manufacturers, is highly specific and accurate. Acceptable variability of approximately 20% at low testosterone levels has been demonstrated in the clinical studies performed with the goserelin 10.8 mg depot.

INDICATIONS AND USAGE:

Prostatic Carcinoma: Goserelin acetate is indicated in the palliative treatment of advanced carcinoma of the prostate. Goserelin offers an alternative treatment of prostatic cancer when orchiectomy or estrogen administration are either not indicated or unacceptable to the patient.

In controlled studies of patients with advanced prostatic cancer comparing goserelin 3.6 mg to orchiectomy, the long-term endocrine responses and objective responses were similar between the two treatment arms. Additionally, duration of survival was similar between the two treatment arms in a major comparative trial.

In controlled studies of patients with advanced prostatic cancer comparing goserelin acetate 10.8 mg implant produced pharmacodynamically similar effect in terms of supression of serum testosterone to that achieved with goserelin 3.6 mg implant. Clinical outcome similar to that produced with the use of the goserelin acetate 3.6 mg implant administered every 28 days is predicted with the goserelin acetate 10.8 mg implant administered every 12 weeks.

Endometriosis: Goserelin is indicated for the management of endometriosis; including pain relief and reduction of endometriotic lesions for the duration of therapy. Experience with goserelin for the management of endometriosis has been limited to women 18 years of age and older treated for 6 months.

Advanced Breast Cancer: Goserelin is indicated for use in the palliative treatment of advanced breast cancer in pre- and perimenopausal women.

The estrogen and progesterone receptor values may help to predict whether goserelin therapy is likely to be beneficial. (See CLINICAL PHARMACOLOGY.)

CONTRAINDICATIONS:

A report of anaphylactic reaction to synthetic GnRH (Factrel) has been reported in medical literature. Goserelin is contraindicated in those patients who have a known hypersensitivity to LHRH, LHRH agonist analogues or any of the components in goserelin acetate.

Goserelin acetate 10.8 mg implant is not indicated in women as the data are insufficient to support reliable suppression of serum estradiol. (See INDICATIONS AND USAGE for female patients requiring treatment with goserelin.)

Goserelin is contraindicated in women being treated for endometriosis who are or may become pregnant while receiving the drug. In studies in rats and rabbits, goserelin increased preimplantation loss, resorptions, and abortions (see PRECAUTIONS, Pregnancy). In rats and dogs, goserelin suppressed ovarian function, decreased ovarian weight and size, and led to atropic changes in secondary sex organs. Further evidence suggests that fertility was reduced in female rats that became pregnant after goserelin was stopped. These effects are an expected consequence of the hormonal alterations produced by goserelin in humans. If a patient becomes pregnant during treatment, the drug must be discontinued and the patient must be apprised of the potential risk for loss of the pregnancy due to possible hormonal imbalance as a result of the expected pharmacologic action of goserelin treatment. In animal

CONTRAINDICATIONS: *(cont'd)*

studies, there was no evidence that goserelin possessed the potential to cause teratogenicity in rabbits; however, in rats the incidence of umbilical hernia was significantly increased with treatment. (See PRECAUTIONS, Pregnancy, Teratogenic Effects)

Goserelin can cause fetal harm when administered to a pregnant woman. Effects on reproductive function, as a result of antigonadotrophic properties of the drug, are expected to occur on chronic administration.

Effective nonhormonal contraception must be used by all premenopausal women during goserelin therapy and for 12 weeks following discontinuation of therapy. There are no adequate and well-controlled studies in pregnant women using goserelin. If this drug is used during pregnancy, or the patient being treated for endometriosis becomes pregnant while taking this drug, the patient should be apprised of the potential hazard to the fetus or potential risk for loss of the pregnancy. Women of childbearing potential should be advised to avoid becoming pregnant.

For a description of findings in animal reproductive toxicity studies, (see WARNINGS).

Goserelin is contraindicated in women who are breast feeding (see PRECAUTIONS, Nursing Mothers).

WARNINGS:

Before starting treatment with goserelin, pregnancy must be excluded. Safe use of goserelin in pregnancy has not been established. Goserelin can cause fetal harm when administered to a pregnant woman. Goserelin has been found to cross the placenta following subcutaneous administration of 50 and 1000 mcg/kg in rats and rabbits, respectively. Studies in both rats and rabbits at doses equal to or greater than 2 and 20 mcg/kg/day, respectively (about 1/10 and 2 times the daily maximum recommended dose, respectively, on a mg/m^2 basis), administered during the period of organogenesis, have confirmed that goserelin will increase pregnancy loss, and is embryotoxic/fetotoxic (characterized by increased preimplantation loss, increased resorption and an increase in umbilical hernia in rats at a dose of $\geq$10 mcg/kg/day [about 1/2 the recommended human dose on a mg/m^2 basis]; effects were dose-related. In additional reproduction studies in rats, goserelin was found to decrease fetus and pup survival.

There are no adequate and well-controlled studies in pregnant women using goserelin. Women of childbearing potential should be advised to avoid becoming pregnant.

When used every 28 days, goserelin usually inhibits ovulation and stops menstruation. Contraception is not ensured, however, by taking goserelin. During treatment, pregnancy must be avoided by the use of nonhormonal methods of contraception. If goserelin is used during pregnancy in a patient with advanced breast cancer or the patient becomes pregnant while receiving this drug, the patient must be apprised of the potential risk for loss of the pregnancy due to possible hormonal imbalance as a result of the expected pharmacologic action of goserelin treatment.

Following the last goserelin injection, nonhormonal methods of contraception must be continued until the return of menses or for at least 12 weeks. (See CONTRAINDICATIONS.)

Prostate and Breast Cancer: Initially, goserelin, like other LHRH agonists, causes transient increases in serum levels of testosterone in men with prostate cancer, and estrogen in women with breast cancer. Transient worsening of symptoms, or the occurrence of additional signs and symptoms of prostate or breast cancer, may occasionally develop during the first few weeks of goserelin treatment. A small number of patients may experience a temporary increase in bone pain, which can be managed symptomatically. As with other LHRH agonists, isolated cases of ureteral obstruction and spinal cord compression have been observed in patients with prostate cancer. If spinal cord compression or renal impairment develops, standard treatment of these complications should be instituted. For extreme cases in prostate cancer patients, an immediate orchiectomy should be considered.

As with other LHRH agonists or hormonal therapies (antiestrogens, estrogens, etc.), hypercalcemia has been reported in some prostate and breast cancer patients with bone metastases after starting treatment with goserelin. If hypercalcemia does occur, appropriate treatment measures should be initiated.

PRECAUTIONS:

GENERAL

Hypersensitivity, antibody formation and anaphylactic reactions have been reported with LHRH agonist analogues.

Of 115 women worldwide treated with goserelin and tested for development of binding to goserelin following treatment with goserelin, one patient showed low-titer binding to goserelin. On further testing of this patient's plasma obtained following treatment, her goserelin binding component was found not to be precipitated with rabbit antihuman immunoglobulin polyvalent sera. These findings suggest the possibility of antibody formation.

INFORMATION FOR THE PATIENT

Males: The use of goserelin in patients at particular risk of developing ureteral obstruction or spinal cord compression should be considered carefully and the patients monitored closely during the first month of therapy. Patients with ureteral obstruction or spinal cord compression should have appropriate treatment prior to initiation of goserelin therapy.

Females: Patients must be made aware of the following information

1. Since menstruation should stop with effective doses of goserelin the patient should notify her physician if regular menstruation persists. Patients missing one or more successive doses of goserelin may experience breakthrough menstrual bleeding.

2. Goserelin should not be prescribed if the patient is pregnant, breast feeding, lactating, has nondiagnosed abnormal vaginal bleeding, or is allergic to any of the components of goserelin.

3. Use of goserelin in pregnancy is contraindicated in women being treated for endometriosis. Therefore, a nonhormonal method of contraception should be used during treatment. Patients should be advised that if they miss one or more successive doses of goserelin, breakthrough menstrual bleeding or ovulation may occur with the potential for conception. If a patient becomes pregnant during treatment for endometriosis, goserelin treatment should be discontinued and the patient should be advised of the possible risks to the pregnancy and fetus. (See CONTRAINDICATIONS.) For patients being treated for advanced breast cancer (see WARNINGS).

4. Those adverse events occurring most frequently in clinical studies with goserelin are associated with hypoestrogenism; of these the most frequently reported are hot flashes (flushes), headaches, vaginal dryness, emotional lability, change in libido, depression, sweating and change in breast size.

5. As with other LHRH agonist analogues, treatment with goserelin induces a hypoestrogenic state which results in a loss of bone mineral density (BMD) over the course of treatment, some of which may not be reversible. In patients with a history of prior treatment that may have resulted in bone mineral density loss and/or in patients with major risk factors for decreased bone mineral density such as chronic alcohol abuse and/or tobacco abuse, significant family history of osteoporosis, or chronic use of drugs that can reduce bone density such as anticonvulsants or corticosteroids, goserelin therapy may pose an additional risk. In these patients the risks and benefits must be weighed carefully before therapy with goserelin is instituted.

6. Currently, there are no clinical data on the effects of retreatment or treatment of benign gynecological conditions with goserelin for periods in excess of 6 months.

7. As with other hormonal interventions that disrupt the pituitary-gonadal axis, some patients may have delayed return to menses. The rare patient, however, may experience persistent amenorrhea.

DRUG/LABORATORY TEST INTERACTIONS

Administration of goserelin in therapeutic doses results in suppression of the pituitary-gonadal system. Because of this suppression, diagnostic tests of pituitary-gonadotropic and gonadal functions conducted during treatment and until the resumption of menses may show results which are misleading. Normal function is usually restored within 12 weeks after treatment is discontinued.

CARCINOGENESIS, MUTAGENESIS, AND IMPAIRMENT OF FERTILITY

The subcutaneous implant of goserelin in male and female rats once every 4 weeks for 1 year and recovery for 23 weeks at doses of about 80 and 150 mcg/kg (males) and 50 and 100 mcg/kg (females) daily (about 3 to 9 times the recommended human dose on a mg/m^2 basis) resulted in an incresed incidence of pituitary adenomas. An increased incidence of pituitary adenomas was also observed following subcutaneous implant of goserelin in rats at similar dose levels for a period of 72 weeks in males and 101 weeks in females. The relevance of the rat pituitary adenomas to humans has not been established. Subcutaneous implants of goserelin every 3 weeks for 2 years delivered to mice at doses of up to 2400 mcg/kg/day (about 70 times the recommended human dose on a mg/m^2 basis) resulted in an increased incidence of histiocytic sarcoma of the vertebral column and femur.

Mutagenicity tests using bacterial and mammalian systems for point mutations and cytogenetic effects have provided no evidence for mutagenic potential.

Administration of goserelin led to changes that were consistent with gonadal suppression in both male and female rats as a result of its endocrine action. In male rats administered 500-1000 mcg/kg/day (about 30-60 times the recommended human dose on a mg/m^2 basis), a decrease in weight and atrophic histological changes were observed in the testes, epididymis, seminal vesicle, and prostate gland with complete suppression of spermatogenesis. In female rats administered 50-1000 mcg/kg/day (about 3-60 times the recommended human dose on a mg/m^2 basis), suppression of ovarian function led to decreased size and weight of ovaries and secondary sex organs; follicular development was arrested at the antral stage and the corpora lutea were reduced in size and number. Except for the testes, almost complete histologic reversal of these effects in males and females was observed several weeks after dosing was stopped; however, fertility and general reproductive performance were reduced in those that became pregnant after goserelin was discontinued. Fertile matings occurred within 2 weeks after cessation of dosing, even though total recovery of reproductive function may not have occurred before mating took place; and, the ovulation rate, the corresponding implantation rate, and number of live fetuses were reduced.

Based on histological examination, drug effects on reproductive organs were reversible in male and female dogs administered 107-214 mcg/kg/day (about 20-40 times the recommended human dose on a mg/m^2 basis) when drug treatment was stopped after continuous administration for 1 year.

PREGNANCY: TERATOGENIC EFFECTS: PREGNANCY CATEGORY X

(See CONTRAINDICATIONS.) Goselerin 10.8 mg is not indicated in women as the data are insufficient to support reliable suppression of serum estradiol. Studies in both rats and rabbits at doses of 2, 10, 20 and 50 mcg/kg/day and 20, 250, and 1,000 mcg/kg/day, respectively (up to 1/10 to 3 times and 2 to 100 times the maximum recommended human dose, respectively, on a mg/m^2 basis) administered during the period of organogenesis, have confirmed that goserelin will increase pregnancy loss in a dose-related manner. While there was no evidence that goserelin possessed the potential to cause teratogenicity in rabbits, in rats the incidence of umbilical hernia was significantly increased at doses greater than 10 mcg/kg/day (about 1/2 the recommended dose on a mg/m^2 basis).

Nursing Mothers: Goserelin has been shown to be excreted in the milk of lactating rats. It is not known if this drug is excreted in human milk. Because many drugs are excreted in human milk and because of the potential for serious adverse reactions from goserelin in nursing infants, mothers receiving goserelin should discontinue nursing prior to taking the drug. (See CONTRAINDICATIONS.)

Pediatric Use: The safety and efficacy of goserelin in pediatric patients have not been established.

DRUG INTERACTIONS:

No formal drug interaction studies with other drugs have been conducted with goserelin. No confirmed interactions have been reported between goserelin and other drugs.

ADVERSE REACTIONS:

General: Rarely, hypersensitivity reactions (including urticaria and anaphylaxis) have been reported in patients receiving goserelin.

MALES

As with other endocrine therapies, hypercalcemia (increased calcium) has rarely been reported in cancer patients with bone metastases following initiation of treatment with goserelin or other LHRH agonists.

Goserelin has been found to be generally well tolerated in clinical trials. Adverse reactions reported in these trials were rarely severe enough to result in the patients' withdrawal from goserelin treatment. As seen with other hormonal therapies, the most commonly observed adverse events during goserelin therapy were due to the expected physiological effects from decreased testosterone levels. These included hot flashes, sexual dysfunction and decreased erections.

Initially, goserelin, like other LHRH agonists, causes transient increases in serum levels of testosterone. A small percentage of patients experienced a temporary worsening of signs and symptoms (see WARNINGS), usually manifested by an increase in cancer-related pain which was managed symptomatically. Isolated cases of exacerbation of disease symptoms, either ureteral obstruction or spinal cord compression, occurred at similar rates in controlled clinical trials with both goserelin and orchiectomy. The relationship of these events to therapy is uncertain.

In the controlled clinical trails of goserelin versus orchiectomy, the following events were reported as adverse reactions in greater than 5% of the patients.

The following additional adverse reactions were reported in greater than 1% but less than 5% of the patients treated with goserelin:

Cardiovascular: arrhythmia, cerebrovascular accident, hypertension, myocardial infarction, peripheral vascular disorder, chest pain;

Central Nervous System: anxiety, depression, headache;

Gastrointestinal: constipation, diarrhea, ulcer, vomiting;

Hematologic: anemia;

ADVERSE REACTIONS: *(cont'd)*

TABLE 4 Treatment Received

Adverse Event	Goserelin (n=242) %	Orchiectomy (n=254) %
Hot Flashes	62	53
Sexual Dysfunction	21	15
Decreased Erections	18	16
Lower Urinary Tract Symptoms	13	8
Lethargy	8	4
Pain (worsened in the first 30 days)	8	3
Edema	7	8
Upper Respiratory Infection	7	2
Rash	6	1
Sweating	6	4
Anorexia	5	2
Chronic Obstructive Pulmonary Disease	5	3
Congestive Heart Failure	5	1
Dizziness	5	4
Insomnia	5	1
Nausea	5	2
Complications of Surgery	0	18†

† Complications related to surgery were reported in 18% of the orchiectomy patients, while only 3% of goserelin patients reported adverse reactions at the injection site. The surgical complications included scrotal infection (5.9%), groin pain (4.7%), wound seepage (3.1%), scrotal hematoma (2.8%), incisional discomfort (1.6%), and skin necrosis (1.2%).

Metabolic/ Nutritional: gout, hyperglycemia, weight increase;

Miscellaneous: chills, fever;

Urogenital: renal insufficiency, urinary tract obstruction, urinary tract infection, breast swelling and tenderness.

FEMALES

As would be expected with a drug that results in hypoestrogenism, the most frequently reported adverse reactions were those related to this effect.

Endometriosis: In controlled clinical trials comparing goserelin every 28 days and danazol daily for the treatment of endometriosis, the events in TABLE 5 were reported at a frequency of 5% or greater.

TABLE 5 Treatment Received

Adverse Event	Goserelin (n=411) %	Danazol (n=207) %
Hot Flushes	96	67
Vaginitis	75	43
Headache	75	63
Emotional Lability	60	56
Libido Decreased	61	44
Sweating	45	30
Depression	54	48
Acne	42	55
Breast Atrophy	33	42
Seborrhea	26	52
Peripheral Edema	21	34
Breast Enlargement	18	15
Pelvic Symptoms	18	23
Pain	17	16
Dyspareunia	14	5
Libido Increased	12	19
Infection	13	11
Asthenia	11	13
Nausea	8	14
Hirsutism	7	15
Insomnia	11	4
Breast Pain	7	4
Abdominal Pain	7	7
Back Pain	7	13
Flu Syndrome	5	5
Dizziness	6	4
Application Site Reaction	6	-
Voice Alterations	3	8
Pharyngitis	5	2
Hair Disorders	4	11
Myalgia	3	11
Nervousness	3	5
Weight Gain	3	23
Leg Cramps	2	6
Increased Appetite	2	5
Pruritus	2	6
Hypertonia	1	10

The following adverse events not already listed above were reported at a frequency of 1% or greater, regardless of causality, in goserelin-treated women from all clinical trials:

Whole Body: allergic reaction, chest pain, fever, malaise;

Cardiovascular: hemorrhage, hypertension, migraine, palpitations, tachycardia;

Digestive: anorexia, constipation, diarrhea, dry mouth, dyspepsia, flatulence;

Hematologic: ecchymosis;

Metabolic and Nutritional: edema;

Musculoskeletal: arthralgia, joint disorder;

CNS: anxiety, paresthesia, somnolence, thinking abnormal;

Respiratory: bronchitis, cough increased, epistaxis, rhinitis, sinusitis;

Skin: alopecia, dry skin, rash, skin discoloration;

Special Senses: amblyopia, dry eyes;

Urogenital: dysmenorrhea, urinary frequency, urinary tract infection, vaginal hemorrhage.

Changes in Bone Mineral Density: After 6 months of goserelin treatment, 109 female patients treated with goserelin showed an average 4.3% decrease of vertebral trabecular bone mineral density (BMD) as compared to pretreatment values. BMD was measured by dual-photon absorptiometry or dual energy x-ray absorptiometry. Sixty-six of these patients were assessed for BMD loss 6 months after the completion (posttherapy) of the 6-month therapy period. Data from these patients showed an average 2.4% BMD loss compared to pretreatment values. Twenty-eight of the 109 patients were assessed for BMD at 12 months posttherapy. Data from these patients showed an average decrease of 2.5% in BMD compared to pretreatment values. These data suggest a possibility of partial reversibility.

ADVERSE REACTIONS: *(cont'd)*

CHANGES IN LABORATORY VALUES DURING TREATMENT

Plasma Enzymes: Elevation of liver enzymes (AST, ALT) have been reported in female patients exposed to goserelin 3.6 mg (representing less than 1% of all patients). There was no other evidence of abnormal liver function. Causality between these changes and goserelin have not been established.

Lipids: In a controlled trial, goserelin 3.6 mg therapy resulted in a minor, but statistically significant effect on serum lipids. In patients treated for endometriosis at 6 months following initiation of therapy, danazol treatment resulted in a mean increase in LDL cholesterol of 33.3 mg/dl and a decrease in HDL cholesterol of 21.3 mg/dl compared to increases of 21.3 and 2.7 mg/dl in LDL cholesterol and HDL cholesterol, respectively, for goserelin-treated patients. Triglycerides increased by 8.0 mg/dl in goserelin-treated patients compared to a decrease of 8.9 mg/dl in danazol-treated patients.

In patients treated for endometriosis, goserelin increased total cholesterol and LDL cholesterol during 6 months of treatment. However, goserelin therapy resulted in HDL cholesterol levels which were significantly higher relative to danazol therapy. At the end of 6 months of treatment, HDL cholesterol fractions (HDL_2 and HDL_3) were decreased by 13.5 and 7.7 mg/dl, respectively, for danazol-treated patients compared to treatment increases of 1.9 and 0.8 mg/dl, respectively, for goserelin treated patients.

Breast Cancer: The adverse event profile for women with advanced breast cancer treated with goserelin is consistent with the profile described above for women treated with goserelin for endometriosis. In a controlled clinical trial (SWOG-8692) comparing goserelin with oophorectomy in premenopausal and perimenopausal women with advanced breast cancer, the following events were reported at a frequency of 5% or greater in either treatment group regardless of causality.

TABLE 6 Treatment Received

Adverse Event	Goserelin (n=57) %	Oophorectomy (n=55) %
Hot Flashes	70	47
Tumor Flare	23	4
Nausea	11	7
Edema	5	0
Malaise/Fatigue/Lethargy	5	2
Vomiting	4	7

In the Phase II clinical trial program in 333 pre- and perimenopausal women with advanced breast cancer, hot flashes were reported in 75.9% of patients and decreased libido was noted in 47.7% of patients. These two adverse events reflect the pharmacological actions of goserelin.

Injection site reactions were reported in less than 1% of patients.

OVERDOSAGE:

The pharmacologic properties of goserelin and its mode of administration make accidental or intentional overdosage unlikely. There is no experience of overdosage from clinical trials. Animal studies indicate that no increased pharmacologic effect occurred at higher doses or more frequent administration. Subcutaneous doses of the drug as high as 1 mg/kg/day in rats and dogs did not produce any nonendocrine related sequelae; this dose is greater than 400 times that proposed for human use. If overdosage occurs, it should be managed symptomatically.

DOSAGE AND ADMINISTRATION:

Goserelin, at a dosage of 3.6 mg, should be administered subcutaneously every 28 days into the upper abdominal wall using an aseptic technique under the supervision of a physician.

Goserelin, at a dosage of 10.8 mg, should be administered subcutaneously every 12 weeks into the upper abdominal wall using an aseptic technique under the supervision of a physician.

While a delay of a few days is permissible, every effort should be made to adhere to the 28-day or 12 week schedule.

For the management of advanced prostate cancer, goserelin is intended for long-term administration unless clinically inappropriate.

For the management of endometriosis, the recommended duration of administration is 6 months.

Currently, there are no clinical data on the effect of treatment of benign gynecological conditions with goserelin for periods in excess of 6 months.

Retreatment cannot be recommended for the management of endometriosis since safety data for retreatment are not available. If the symptoms of endometriosis recur after a course of therapy, and further treatment with goserelin is contemplated, consideration should be given to monitoring bone mineral density.

No dosage adjustment in necessary for patients with renal or hepatic impairment.

Administration Technique: The proper method of administration of goserelin is described in the instructions that follow.

1. The package should be inspected for damage prior to opening. If the package is damaged, the syringe should not be used. Do not remove the sterile syringe from the package until immediately before use. Examine the syringe for damage, and check that goserelin is visible in the translucent chamber.

2. Clean an area of skin of the upper abdominal wall with an alcohol swab. (A local anesthetic may be used in the normal fashion at the option of the administrator or patient.)

3. Grasp red (blue for 10.8 mg) plastic safety clip tab, pull out and away from needle, and discard immediately. Then remove needle cover.

4. Using an aseptic technique, stretch or pinch the patient's skin with one hand, and grip the syringe barrel. Insert the hypodermic needle into the subcutaneous tissue. *Note:*The goserelin syringe cannot be used for aspiration. If the hypodermic needle penetrates a large vessel, blood will be seen instantly in the syringe chamber. If a vessel is penetrated, withdraw the needle and inject with a new syringe elsewhere.

5. Change the direction of the needle so it parallels the abdominal wall. Push the needle in until the barrel hub touches the patient's skin. Withdraw the needle one centimeter to create a space to discharge goserelin. Fully depress the plunger to discharge goserelin.

6. Withdraw the needle. Then bandage the site. Confirm discharge of goserelin by ensuring tip of the plunger is visible within the tip of the needle. Dispose of the used needle and syringe in a safe manner. *Note:*In the unlikely event of the need to surgically remove goserelin, it may be localized by ultrasound.

HOW SUPPLIED:

Zoladex is supplied as a sterile and totally biodegradable D,L-lactic and glycolic acids copolymer (13.3-14.3 mg/dose) impregnated with goserelin acetate equivalent to 3.6 mg or 10.8 mg of goserelin in a disposable syringe device fitted with a 16 gauge or 14 gauge hypodermic needle. The unit is sterile and comes in a sealed, light and moisture proof, aluminum foil laminate pouch containing a desiccant capsule.

Storage: Store at room temperature (do not exceed 25°C).

HOW SUPPLIED - EQUIVALENTS NOT AVAILABLE:

Implant, Continuous Release - Subcutaneous - 3.6 mg

1's	**$383.65**	**ZOLADEX, Zeneca Pharms**	**00310-0960-36**

Implant, Continuous Release - Subcutaneous - 10.8 mg

1's	**$1208.49**	**ZOLADEX, Zeneca Pharms**	**00310-0961-30**

GRAMICID; NEOMYCIN; NYSTATIN; TRIAMCINOLONE *(001383)*

CATEGORIES: Anti-Infectives; Antibacterials; Antibiotics; Antifungals; Candidiasis; DESI Drugs; Dermatitis; Dermatologicals; Fungal Agents; Hormones; Pruritus; Skin/Mucous Membrane Agents; Steroids; Topical; Pregnancy Category C; FDA Pre 1938 Drugs

BRAND NAMES: Myco-Aricin; Myco-Bal; Myco-Par; Myco-Tac; Myco-Triacet; Myconel; Myocidin; **Mytrex**; Tri-Statin

Prescribing information not available at time of publication.

HOW SUPPLIED - EQUIVALENTS NOT AVAILABLE:

Cream - Topical - 0.03 %/0.3 %/10

454 gm	$55.94	TRI-STATIN, Rugby	00536-4850-98

Ointment - Topical - 0.25 mg/100000

15 gm	$2.50	TRI-STATIN, Rugby	00536-4870-20
30 gm	$4.06	TRI-STATIN, Rugby	00536-4870-28

GRAMICIDIN; NEOMYCIN SULFATE; POLYMYXIN B SULFATE *(001385)*

CATEGORIES: Anti-Infectives; Antibacterials; Antibiotics; Antihypertensives; Burns; Diuretics; EENT Drugs; Eye, Ear, Nose, & Throat Preparations; Ocular Infections; Ophthalmics; Renal Drugs; Topical; Vascular Disorders, Cerebral/Peripheral; FDA Approval Pre 1982

BRAND NAMES: Ak-Spore; Alba-3; Bio-Triple; Infa-3; Neocidin; Neocin-Pg; Neomycin Polymyxin Gramicidin; Neopolygram; **Neosporin**; Neotricin; Ocu-Spor-G; Ocusporin; Ocutricin; P. N. Ophthalmic; *Polixin-Ofteno*; *Polixin Ofteno*; Spectro-Sporin; Storz P-N-G; *Sulned*; Tri-Ophthalmic; Tri-Thalmic; Tribiotic; Triple Antibiotic
(International brand names outside U.S. in italics)

FORMULARIES: Aetna; BC-BS; DoD

DESCRIPTION:

Neosporin Ophthalmic Solution (polymyxin B sulfate-neomycin sulfate-gramicidin) is a sterile antimicrobial solution for ophthalmic use. Each ml contains: polymyxin B sulfate 10,000 units, neomycin sulfate equivalent to 1.75 mg neomycin base and gramicidin 0.025 mg. The vehicle contains alcohol 0.5%, thimerosal 0.001% (added as a preservative) and the inactive ingredients propylene glycol, polyoxyethylene polyoxypropylene compound, sodium chloride and water for injection.

Polymyxin B sulfate is the sulfate salt of polymyxin B_1 and B_2 which are produced by the growth of *Bacillus polymyxa* (Prazmowski) Migula (Fam. Bacillaceae). It has a potency of not less than 6,000 polymyxin B units per mg, calculated on an anhydrous basis.

Neomycin sulfate is the sulfate salt of neomycin B and C, which are produced by the growth of *Streptomyces fradiae* Waksman (Fam. Streptomycetaceae). It has a potency equivalent of not less than 600 mcg of neomycin standard per mg, calculated on an anhydrous basis.

Gramicidin (also called Gramicidin D) is a mixture of three pairs of antibacterial substances (Gramicidin A, B and C) produced by the growth of *Bacillus brevis* Dubos (Fam. Bacillaceae). It has a potency of not less than 900 mcg of standard gramicidin per mg.

CLINICAL PHARMACOLOGY:

A wide range of antibacterial action is provided by the overlapping spectra of polymyxin B sulfate, neomycin and gramicidin. The spectrum of action encompasses most bacterial pathogens capable of causing external infections of the eye and its adnexa.

Polymyxin B is bactericidal for a variety of gram-negative organisms. It increases the permeability of the bacterial cell membrane by interacting with the phospholipid components of the membrane.

Neomycin is bactericidal for many gram-positive and gram-negative organisms. It i+an aminoglycoside antibiotic which inhibits protein synthesis by binding with ribosomal RNA and causing misreading of the bacterial genetic code.

Gramicidin is bactericidal for a variety of gram-positive organisms. It increases the permeability of the bacterial cell membrane to inorganic cations by forming a network of channels through the normal lipid bilayer of the membrane.

When used topically, polymyxin B, neomycin and gramicidin are rarely irritating, and absorption from the intact skin or mucous membrane is insignificant. The incidence of skin sensitization to this combination has been shown to be low on normal skin.[1,2] Since these antibiotics are seldom used systemically, the patient is spared sensitization to those antibiotics which might later be required systemically.

Microbiology: Polymyxin B sulfate, neomycin sulfate and gramicidin together are considered active against the following microorganisms: *Staphylococcus aureus,* streptococci, including*Streptococcus pneumoniae, Escherichia coli, Haemophilus influenzae, Klebsiella-Enterobacter* species, *Neisseria* species and *Pseudomonas aeruginosa.* The product does not provide adequate coverage against *Serratia marcescens.*

INDICATIONS AND USAGE:

Neosporin Ophthalmic Solution is indicated in the short-term treatment of superficial external ocular infections caused by organisms susceptible to one or more of the antibiotics contained therein.

CONTRAINDICATIONS:

This product is contraindicated in those individuals who have shown hypersensitivity to any of its components.

WARNINGS:

The manifestations of sensitization to neomycin are usually itching, reddening and edema of the conjunctiva and eyelid. It may be manifest simply as a failure to heal. During long-term use of neomycin-containing products, periodic examination for such signs is advisable, and the patient should be told to discontinue the product if they are observed. These symptoms subside quickly on withdrawing the medication. Neomycin-containing applications should be avoided for the patient thereafter.

PRECAUTIONS:

General: As with other antibiotic preparations, prolonged use may result in overgrowth of nonsusceptible organisms including fungi. Appropriate measures should be taken if this occurs.

Allergic cross-reactions may occur which could prevent the use of any or all of the following antibiotics for the treatment of future infections: kanamycin, paromomycin, streptomycin, and possibly gentamicin.

Information for the Patient: If redness, irritation, swelling or pain persists or increases, discontinue use and contact your physician.

Avoid contaminating the applicator tip with material from the eye, fingers, or other source. This caution is necessary if the sterility of the drops is to be preserved.

ADVERSE REACTIONS:

Neomycin Sulfate may cause cutaneous and conjunctival sensitization. A precise incidence of hypersensitivity reactions (primarily skin rash) due to topical neomycin is not known.

DOSAGE AND ADMINISTRATION:

The suggested dosage is one or two drops in the affected eye two to four times daily, or more frequently as required, for 7 to 10 days. In acute infections, initiate therapy with one or two drops every 15 to 30 minutes, reducing the frequency of instillation gradually as the infection is controlled.

Store at 15°-25°C (59°-77°F) and protect from light.

REFERENCES:

1. Leyden JJ, and Kligman AM. Contact Dermatitis to Neomycin Sulfate. JAMA *242* (12): 1276-1278, 1979. **2.** Prystowsky SD, Allen AM, Smith RW, Nonomura JH, Odom RB and Akers WA. Allergic Contact Hypersensitivity to Nickel, Neomycin, Ethylenediamine, and Benzocaine. Arch Dermatol *115*: 959-962, 1979.

HOW SUPPLIED - RATED THERAPEUTICALLY EQUIVALENT:

Solution - Ophthalmic - 0.025 mg/1.75 m

10 ml	$3.11	Infa-3 Ophthalmic Solution, Infinity Pharm	58154-0790-62
10 ml	$4.52	OCUSPORIN, HL Moore Drug Exch	00839-6662-90
10 ml	$4.60	TRIPLE ANTIBIOTIC, Parmed Pharms	00349-8328-70
10 ml	$5.02	OCUTRICIN, United Res	00677-0906-21
10 ml	$5.25	Triple Antibiotic, Harber Pharm	51432-0387-10
10 ml	$6.35	NEOCIDIN, Ocusoft	54799-0511-05
10 ml	$7.20	TRIBIOTIC, IDE-Interstate	00814-8012-40
10 ml	$7.50	TRI-BIOTIC, Quality Res Pharms	52765-0747-10
10 ml	$8.30	Neomycin/Polymyxin/Gramicidin, Steris Labs	00402-0747-10
10 ml	$8.55	Neomycin/Polymixin/Gramicidin, Aligen Independ	00405-6110-10
10 ml	$8.55	P.N. OPHTHALMIC, Geneva Pharms	00781-7250-70
10 ml	$9.56	Neomycin/Polymyxin/Gramicidin, Rugby	00536-1890-70
10 ml	$11.48	AK-SPORE, Akorn	17478-0790-11
10 ml	**$17.75**	**NEOSPORIN, Glaxo Wellcome**	**00173-0728-69**
10 ml	$18.30	ALBA-3, Alba Pharma	10023-0186-10

Solution/Drops - Ophthalmic - 0.025 mg/ml/1.7

10 ml	$5.02	Gramicidin; Neomycin Sulfate; Polymyxin, H.C.F.A. F F P	99999-1385-01

HOW SUPPLIED - NOT RATED EQUIVALENT:

Solution - Ophthalmic - 0.025 mg/1.75 m

2 ml	$3.75	Neomycin/Polymyxin/Gramicidin, Consolidated Midland	00223-6755-02
2 ml	$6.35	Neocin-Pg, Ocusoft	54799-0511-02
10 ml	$2.40	Ocutricin, Raway	00686-6790-62
10 ml	$3.80	Neopolygram, Logen Pharm	00820-0107-24
10 ml	$5.95	SPECTRO SPORIN, Spectrum Scitfc	53268-0790-62
15 ml	$4.50	Neomycin/Polymyxin/Gramicidin, Consolidated Midland	00223-6755-15

GRANISETRON HYDROCHLORIDE *(003157)*

CATEGORIES: Antiemetics; Autonomic Drugs; Cancer; Central Nervous System Agents; Chemotherapy; 5-HT3 Receptor Antagonist; Gastrointestinal Drugs; Nausea; Nausea and Vomiting; Serotonin Antagonists; Sympatholytic Agents; Vomiting; FDA Class 1S ("Standard Review"); Sales > $100 Million; FDA Approved 1993 Dec

BRAND NAMES: *Kevatril* (Germany); **Kytril**
(International brand names outside U.S. in italics)

FORMULARIES: Aetna; BC-BS; Harvard; Medi-Cal

COST OF THERAPY: $166.00 (Nausea; Injection; 1 mg/ml; 1/day; 1 days)

DESCRIPTION:

Kytril (granisetron hydrochloride) is an antinauseant and antiemetic agent. Chemically it is *endo*-N-(9-methyl-9-azabicyclo[3.3.1]non-3-yl)-1-methyl-1H-indazole-3-carboxamide hydrochloride with a molecular weight of 348.9 (312.4 free base). Its empirical formula is $C_{18}H_{24}N_4O{\cdot}HCl$.

Granisetron hydrochloride is a white to off-white solid that is readily soluble in water and normal saline at 20°C. Granisetron HCl injection is a clear, colorless, sterile, nonpyrogenic, aqueous solution for intravenous administration.

Each 1 ml of preservative-free aqueous solution contains 1.12 mg granisetron hydrochloride equivalent to granisetron, 1.0 mg and sodium chloride, 9.0 mg. The solution's pH ranges from 4.7 to 7.3.

Tablets for Oral Administration: Each white, triangular, biconvex, film-coated Kytril Tablet contains 1.12 mg granisetron hydrochloride equivalent to granisetron, 1 mg. Inactive ingredients are: hydroxypropyl methylcellulose, lactose, magnesium stearate, microcrystalline cellulose, polyethylene glycol, polysorbate 80, sodium starch glycolate and titanium dioxide.

CLINICAL PHARMACOLOGY: *(cont'd)*

Granisetron is a selective 5-hydroxytryptamine$_3$(5-HT_3) receptor antagonist with little or no affinity for other serotonin receptors, including 5-HT_1; 5-HT_{1A}; 5-$HT_{1B/C}$; 5- HT_2; for alpha$_1$-, alpha$_2$-, or beta- adrenoreceptors; for dopamine-D_2; or for histamine-H_1; benzodiazepine; picrotoxin, or opioid receptors.

Serotonin receptors of the 5-HT_3 type are located peripherally on vagal nerve terminals and centrally in the chemoreceptor trigger zone of the area postrema. During chemotherapy that induces vomiting, mucosal enterochromaffin cells release serotonin, which stimulates 5-HT_3 receptors. This evokes vagal afferent discharge, inducing vomiting. Animal studies demonstrate that, in binding to 5-HT_3 receptors, granisetron blocks serotonin stimulation and subsequent vomiting after emetogenic stimuli such as cisplatin. In the ferret animal model, a single granisetron injection prevented vomiting due to high-dose cisplatin or arrested vomiting within 5 to 30 seconds.

In most human studies, granisetron has had little effect on blood pressure, heart rate or ECG. No evidence of an effect on plasma prolactin or aldosterone concentrations has been found in other studies.

Following single and multiple oral doses, granisetron HCl slowed colonic transit in normal volunteers. However, granisetron HCl had no effect on oro-cecal transit time in normal volunteers when given as a single intravenous (IV) infusion of 50 mcg/kg or 200 mcg/kg.

PHARMACOKINETICS

Injection

In adult cancer patients undergoing chemotherapy and in volunteers, infusion of a single 40 mcg/kg dose of granisetron HCl injection produced the following mean pharmacokinetic data (TABLE 1):

TABLE 1 Pharmacokinetic Parameters in Adult Cancer Patients Undergoing Chemotherapy and in Volunteers, Following a Single Intravenous 40 mcg/kg Dose of Granisetron HCl Injection

	Peak Plasma Concentration (ng/ml)	Terminal Phase Plasma Half-Life (h)	Total Clearance (l/h/kg)	Volume of Distribution (l/kg)
Cancer Patients				
Mean	63.8*	8.95*	0.38*	3.07*
Range	18.0 to 176	0.90 to 31.1	0.14 to 1.54	0.85 to 10.4
Volunteers				
21 to 42 years				
Mean	64.3†	4.91†	0.79†	3.04†
Range	11.2 to 182	0.88 to 15.2	0.20 to 2.56	1.68 to 6.13
65 to 81 years				
Mean	57.0†	7.69†	0.44†	3.97†
Range	14.6 to 153	2.65 to 17.7	0.17 to 1.06	1.75 to 7.01

* 5-minute infusion
† 3-minute infusion

There was high inter and intrasubject variability noted in these studies. No difference in mean AUC was found between males and females, although males had a higher C_{max} generally.

Granisetron metabolism involves N-demethylation and aromatic ring oxidation followed by conjugation. Animal studies suggest that some of the metabolites may also have 5-HT_3 receptor antagonist activity.

Clearance is predominantly by hepatic metabolism. In normal volunteers, approximately 12% of the administered dose is eliminated unchanged in the urine in 48 hours. The remainder of the dose is excreted as metabolites, 49% in the urine and 34% in the feces.

In vitro liver microsomal studies show that granisetron's major route of metabolism is inhibited by ketoconazole, suggestive of metabolism mediated by the cytochrome P-450 3A subfamily.

Plasma protein binding is approximately 65% and granisetron distributes freely between plasma and red blood cells.

Tablets

In healthy volunteers and adult cancer patients undergoing chemotherapy, administration of oral granisetron HCl produced the following mean pharmacokinetic data (TABLES 2A and 2B):

TABLE 2A Pharmacokinetic Parameters (Median [range]) Following Granisetron Hydrochloride

	Peak Plasma Concentration (ng/ml)	Terminal Phase Plasma Half-Life (h)
Cancer Patients 1.0 mg b.i.d., 7 days (n=27)	5.99 [0.63 to 30.9]	N.D.*
Volunteers single 1.0 mg dose (n=39)	3.63 [0.27 to 9.14]	6.23 [0.96 to 19.9]

* Not determined after oral administration; following a single intravenous dose of 40 mcg/kg, terminal phase half-life was determined to be 8.95 hours.
N.D. Not determined

TABLE 2B Pharmacokinetic Parameters (Median [range]) Following Granisetron Hydrochloride

	Volume of Distribution (l/kg)	Total Clearance (l/h/kg)
Cancer Patients 1.0 mg b.i.d., 7 days (n=27)	N.D.*	0.52 [0.09 to 7.37]
Volunteers single 1.0 mg dose (n=39)	3.94 [1.89 to 39.4]	0.41 [0.11 to 24.6]

* Not determined after oral administration; following a single intravenous dose of 40 mcg/kg, terminal phase half-life was determined to be 8.95 hours.
N.D. Not determine

The effects of gender on the pharmacokinetics of oral granisetron HCl have not been studied. However, after intravenous infusion of granisetron HCl, no difference in mean AUC was found between males and females, although males had a higher C_{max} generally.

CLINICAL PHARMACOLOGY: *(cont'd)*

When oral granisetron HCl was administered with food, AUC was decreased by 5% and C_{max} increased by 30% in non-fasted healthy volunteers who received a single dose of 10 mg.

Granisetron metabolism involves N-demethylation and aromatic ring oxidation followed by conjugation. Animal studies suggest that some of the metabolites may also have 5-HT_3 receptor antagonist activity.

Clearance is predominantly by hepatic metabolism. In normal volunteers, approximately 11% of the orally administered dose is eliminated unchanged in the urine in 48 hours. The remainder of the dose is excreted as metabolites, 48% in the urine and 38% in the feces.

In vitro liver microsomal studies show that granisetron's major route of metabolism is inhibited by ketoconazole, suggestive of metabolism mediated by the cytochrome P-450 3A subfamily.

Plasma protein binding is approximately 65% and granisetron distributes freely between plasma and red blood cells.

In the elderly and in patients with renal failure or hepatic impairment, the pharmacokinetics of granisetron was determined following administration of intravenous granisetron HCl:

Elderly: The ranges of the pharmacokinetic parameters in elderly volunteers (mean age 71 years), given a single 40 mcg/kg intravenous dose of granisetron HCl injection, were generally similar to those in younger healthy volunteers; mean values were lower for clearance and longer for half-life in the elderly.

Renal Failure Patients: Total clearance of granisetron was not affected in patients with severe renal failure who received a single 40 mcg/kg intravenous dose of granisetron HCl injection.

Hepatically Impaired Patients: A pharmacokinetic study with intravenous granisetron HCl in patients with hepatic impairment due to neoplastic liver involvement showed that total clearance was approximately halved compared to patients without hepatic impairment. Given the wide variability in pharmacokinetic parameters noted in patients and the good tolerance of doses well above the recommended 1.0 mg b.i.d. dose, dosage adjustment in patients with possible hepatic functional impairment is not necessary.

Pediatrics: The pharmacokinetics of granisetron has not been adequately studied in children.

CLINICAL STUDIES:

INJECTION

Granisetron HCl injection has been shown to prevent nausea and vomiting associated with single-day and repeat cycle cancer chemotherapy.

SINGLE-DAY CHEMOTHERAPY

Cisplatin-Based Chemotherapy: In a double-blind, placebo-controlled study in 28 cancer patients, granisetron HCl injection, administered as a single intravenous infusion of 40 mcg/kg, was significantly more effective than placebo in preventing nausea and vomiting induced by cisplatin chemotherapy. See TABLE 3

TABLE 3 Prevention of Chemotherapy-Induced Nausea and Vomiting—Single-Day Cisplatin Therapy [1]

	Kytril Injection	Placebo	P-Value
Number of Patients	14	14	
Response Over 24 Hours			
Complete Response[2]	93%	7%	<0.001
No Vomiting	93%	14%	<0.001
No More Than Mild Nausea	93%	7%	<0.001

1 Cisplatin administration began within 10 minutes of Kytril Injection infusion and continued for 1.5 to 3.0 hours. Mean cisplatin dose was 86 mg/m^2 in the Kytril Injection group and 80 mg/m^2 in the placebo group.
2 No vomiting and no moderate or severe nausea.

Granisetron HCl injection was also evaluated in a randomized dose response study of cancer patients receiving cisplatin ≥75 mg/m^2. Additional chemotherapeutic agents included: anthracyclines, carboplatin, cytostatic antibiotics, folic acid derivatives, methylhydrazine, nitrogen mustard analogs, podophyllotoxin derivatives, pyrimidine analogs and vinca alkaloids. Granisetron HCl injection doses of 10 and 40 mcg/kg were superior to 2 mcg/kg in preventing cisplatin-induced nausea and vomiting, but 40 mcg/kg was not significantly superior to 10 mcg/kg. See TABLE 4

TABLE 4 Prevention of Chemotherapy-Induced Nausea and Vomiting—Single-Day High-Dose Cisplatin Therapy [1]

	Kytril Injection (mcg/kg) 2	10	40	P-Value (vs. 2 mcg/kg) 10	40
Number of Patients	52	52	53		
Response Over 24 Hours					
Complete Response[2]	31%	62%	68%	<0.002	<0.001
No Vomiting	38%	65%	74%	<0.001	<0.001
No More Than Mild Nausea	58%	75%	79%	NS	0.007

1 Cisplatin administration began within 10 minutes of Kytril Injection infusion and continued for 2.6 hours (mean). Mean cisplatin doses were 96 to 99 mg/m^2.
2 No vomiting and no moderate or severe nausea.

Granisetron HCl injection was also evaluated in a double-blind, randomized dose response study of 353 patients stratified for high (≥80 to 120 mg/m^2) or low (50 to 79 mg/m^2) cisplatin dose. Response rates of patients for both cisplatin strata are given in TABLE 5.

For both the low and high cisplatin strata, the 10, 20 and 40 mcg/kg doses were more effective than the 5 mcg/kg dose in preventing nausea and vomiting within 24 hours of chemotherapy administration. The 10 mcg/kg was at least as effective as the higher doses.

Moderately Emetogenic Chemotherapy: Granisetron HCl injection, 40 mcg/kg, was compared with the combination of chlorpromazine (50 to 200 mg/24 hours) and dexamethasone (12 mg) in patients treated with moderately emetogenic chemotherapy, including primarily carboplatin >300 mg/m^2, cisplatin 20 to 50 mg/m^2 and cyclophosphamide >600 mg/m^2. Granisetron HCl injection was superior to the chlorpromazine regimen in preventing nausea and vomiting. See TABLE 6.

In other studies of moderately emetogenic chemotherapy, no significant difference in efficacy was found between granisetron HCl doses of 40 mcg/kg and 160 mcg/kg doses.

Repeat-Cycle Chemotherapy: In an uncontrolled trial, 512 cancer patients received granisetron HCl injection, 40 mcg/kg, prophylactically, for two cycles of chemotherapy, 224 patients received it for at least four cycles and 108 patients received it for at least six cycles. Granisetron HCl injection efficacy remained relatively constant over the first six repeat cycles, with complete response rates (no vomiting and no moderate or severe nausea in 24 hours) of 60% to 69%. No patients were studied for more than 15 cycles.

CLINICAL STUDIES: *(cont'd)*

TABLE 5 Prevention of Chemotherapy-Induced Nausea and Vomiting—Single-Day High-Dose and Low-Dose Cisplatin Therapy [1]

	Kytril Injection (mcg/kg) 5	10	20	40	P-Value (vs. 5 mcg/kg) 10	20	40
High-Dose Cisplatin							
Number of Patients	40	49	48	47			
Response Over 24 Hours							
Complete Response[2]	18%	41%	40%	47%	0.018	0.025	0.004
No Vomiting	28%	47%	44%	53%	NS	NS	0.016
No Nausea	15%	35%	38%	43%	0.036	0.019	0.005
Low-Dose Cisplatin							
Number of Patients	42	41	40	46			
Response Over 24 Hours							
Complete Response[2]	29%	56%	58%	41%	0.012	0.009	NS
No Vomiting	36%	63%	65%	43%	0.012	0.008	NS
No Nausea	29%	56%	38%	33%	0.012	NS	NS

1 Cisplatin administration began within 10 minutes of Kytril Injection infusion and continued for 2 hours (mean). Mean cisplatin doses were 64 and 98 mg/m^2 for low and high strata.
2 No vomiting and no use of rescue antiemetic.

TABLE 6 Prevention of Chemotherapy-Induced Nausea and Vomiting—Single-Day Moderately Emetogenic Chemotherapy

	Kytril Injection	Chlorpromazine [1]	P-Value
Number of Patients	133	133	
Response Over 24 Hours			
Complete Response[2]	68%	47%	<0.001
No Vomiting	73%	53%	<0.001
No More Than Mild Nausea	77%	59%	<0.001

1 Patients also received dexamethasone, 12 mg.
2 No vomiting and no moderate or severe nausea.

Pediatric: A randomized double-blind study evaluated the 24-hour response of 80 pediatric cancer patients (age 2 to 16 years) to granisetron HCl injection 10, 20 or 40 mcg/kg. Patients were treated with cisplatin ≥60 mg/m^2, cytarabine ≥3 g/m^2, cyclophosphamide ≥1 g/m^2 or nitrogen mustard ≥6 mg/m^2. See TABLE 7

TABLE 7 Prevention of Chemotherapy-Induced Nausea and Vomiting in Pediatric Patients

	Kytril Injection Dose (mcg/kg) 10	20	40
Number of Patients	29	26	25
Median Number of Vomiting Episodes	2	3	1
Complete Response Over 24 Hours[1]	21%	31%	32%

1 No vomiting and no moderate or severe nausea.

A second pediatric study compared granisetron HCl injection 20 mcg/kg to chlorpromazine plus dexamethasone in 88 patients treated with ifosfamide ≥3 g/m^2/day for two or three days. Granisetron HCl injection was administered on each day of ifosfamide treatment. At 24 hours, 22% of granisetron HCl injection patients achieved complete response (no vomiting and no moderate or severe nausea in 24 hours) compared with 10% on the chlorpromazine regimen. The median number of vomiting episodes with granisetron HCl injection was 1.5; with chlorpromazine it was 7.0.

TABLETS

Oral granisetron HCl prevents nausea and vomiting associated with emetogenic cancer therapy as shown by 24-hour efficacy data from three double-blind studies. The first trial compared oral granisetron HCl doses of 0.25 to 2.0 mg b.i.d. in 930 cancer patients receiving, principally, cyclophosphamide, carboplatin and cisplatin (20 mg/m^2 to 50 mg/m^2). Efficacy was based on: complete response (*i.e.,* no vomiting, no moderate or severe nausea, no rescue medication), no vomiting and no nausea. TABLE 8 summarizes the results of this study.

TABLE 8 Prevention of Nausea and Vomiting 24 Hours Post-Chemotherapy [1]

Efficacy Measures	Percentage of Patients Oral Kytril Dose: 0.25 mg b.i.d. (n=229) %	0.5 mg b.i.d. (n=235) %	1.0 mg b.i.d. (n=233) %	2.0 mg b.i.d. (n=233) %
Complete Response[2]	61	70*	81*†	72*
No Vomiting	66	77*	88*	79*
No Nausea	48	57	63*	54

1 Chemotherapy included oral and injectable cyclophosphamide, carboplatin, cisplatin (20 mg/m^2 to 50 mg/m^2), dacarbazine, doxorubicin, epirubicin.
2 No vomiting, no moderate or severe nausea, no rescue medication.
* Statistically significant (*P*<0.01) vs. 0.25 mg b.i.d.
† Statistically significant (*P*<0.01) vs. 0.5 mg b.i.d.

A second double-blind, randomized trial compared oral granisetron HCl 1.0 mg b.i.d. with prochlorperazine sustained release capsules 10.0 mg b.i.d., in 230 cancer patients receiving moderately emetogenic chemotherapeutic agents. Oral granisetron HCl was significantly better than prochlorperazine in preventing nausea and vomiting (see TABLE 9.)

A third double-blind trial compared oral granisetron HCl 1.0 mg b.i.d., relative to placebo (historical control), in 119 cancer patients receiving high-dose cisplatin (mean dose 80 mg/m^2). At 24 hours, oral granisetron HCl 1.0 mg b.i.d. was significantly (*P*<0.001) superior to placebo (historical control) in all efficacy parameters: complete response (52%), no vomiting (56%) and no nausea (45%). The placebo rates were 7%, 14% and 7%, respectively, for the three efficacy parameters.

No controlled study comparing granisetron injection with the oral formulation to prevent chemotherapy-induced nausea and vomiting has been performed.

TABLE 9 Prevention of Nausea and Vomiting 24 Hours Post-Chemotherapy [1] Percentage of Patients Antiemetic Regimen

Efficacy Measures	Kytril 1.0 mg b.i.d. (n = 119) %	Prochlorperazine 10.0 mg b.i.d. (n = 111) %
Complete Response[2]	74*	41
No Vomiting	82*	48
No Nausea	58*	35

1 Chemotherapy included injectable cyclophosphamide, carboplatin, cisplatin (20 mg/m^2 to 50 mg/m^2), dacarbazine, doxorubicin, epirubicin.
2 No vomiting, no moderate or severe nausea, no rescue medication.
* Statistically significant (*P*<0.001) vs. prochlorperazine.

INDICATIONS AND USAGE:

Granisetron HCl is indicated for the prevention of nausea and vomiting associated with initial and repeat courses of emetogenic cancer therapy, including high-dose cisplatin.

CONTRAINDICATIONS:

Granisetron HCl is contraindicated in patients with known hypersensitivity to the drug or any of its components.

PRECAUTIONS:

CARCINOGENESIS, MUTAGENESIS, AND IMPAIRMENT OF FERTILITY

Injection

In a 24-month carcinogenicity study, rats were treated orally with granisetron 1, 5 or 50 mg/kg/day (6, 30 or 300 mg/m^2/day). The 50 mg/kg/day dose was reduced to 25 mg/kg/day (150 mg/m^2/day) during week 59 due to toxicity. For a 50 kg person of average height (1.46 m^2 body surface area), these doses represent 16, 81 and 405 times the recommended clinical dose (0.37 mg/m^2, IV) on a body surface area basis. There was a statistically significant increase in the incidence of hepatocellular carcinomas and adenomas in males treated with 5 mg/kg/day (30 mg/m^2/day, 81 times the recommended human dose based on body surface area) and above, and in females treated with 25 mg/kg/day (150 mg/m^2/day, 405 times the recommended human dose based on body surface area). No increase in liver tumors was observed at a dose of 1 mg/kg/day (6 mg/m^2/day, 16 times the recommended human dose based on body surface area) in males and 5 mg/kg/day (30 mg/m^2/day, 81 times the recommended human dose based on body surface area) in females. In a 12-month oral toxicity study, treatment with granisetron 100 mg/kg/day (600 mg/m^2/day, 1622 times the recommended human dose based on body surface area) produced hepatocellular adenomas in male and female rats while no such tumors were found in the control rats. A 24-month mouse carcinogenicity study of granisetron did not show a statistically significant increase in tumor incidence, but the study was not conclusive.

Because of the tumor findings in rat studies, granisetron HCl injection should be prescribed only at the dose and for the indication recommended (see INDICATIONS AND USAGE, and DOSAGE AND ADMINISTRATION).

Granisetron was not mutagenic in *in vitro* Ames test and mouse lymphoma cell forward mutation assay, and *in vivo* mouse micronucleus test and *in vitro* and *ex vivo* rat hepatocyte UDS assays. It, however, produced a significant increase in UDS in HeLa cells *in vitro* and a significant increased incidence of cells with polyploidy in an *in vitro* human lymphocyte chromosomal aberration test.

Granisetron at subcutaneous doses up to 6 mg/kg/day (36 mg/m^2/day, 97 times the recommended human dose based on body surface area) was found to have no effect on fertility and reproductive performance of male and female rats.

Tablets

In a 24-month carcinogenicity study, rats were treated orally with granisetron 1, 5 or 50 mg/kg/day (6, 30 or 300 mg/m^2/day). The 50 mg/kg/day dose was reduced to 25 mg/kg/day (150 mg/m^2/day) during week 59 due to toxicity. For a 50 kg person of average height (1.46 m^2 body surface area), these doses represent 4, 20 and 101 times the recommended clinical dose (1.48 mg/m^2, oral) on a body surface area basis. There was a statistically significant increase in the incidence of hepatocellular carcinomas and adenomas in males treated with 5 mg/kg/day (30 mg/m^2/day, 20 times the recommended human dose based on body surface area) and above, and in females treated with 25 mg/kg/day (150 mg/m^2/day, 101 times the recommended human dose based on body surface area). No increase in liver tumors was observed at a dose of 1 mg/kg/day (6 mg/m^2/day, 4 times the recommended human dose based on body surface area) in males and 5 mg/kg/day (30 mg/m^2/day, 20 times the recommended human dose based on body surface area) in females. In a 12-month oral toxicity study, treatment with granisetron 100 mg/kg/day (600 mg/m^2/day, 405 times the recommended human dose based on body surface area) produced hepatocellular adenomas in male and female rats while no such tumors were found in the control rats. A 24-month mouse carcinogenicity study of granisetron did not show a statistically significant increase in tumor incidence, but the study was not conclusive.

Because of the tumor findings in rat studies, granisetron hydrochloride tablets should be prescribed only at the dose and for the indication recommended (see INDICATIONS AND USAGE, and DOSAGE AND ADMINISTRATION).

Granisetron was not mutagenic in *in vitro* Ames test and mouse lymphoma cell forward mutation assay, and *in vivo* mouse micronucleus test and *in vitro* and *ex vivo* rat hepatocyte UDS assays. It, however, produced a significant increase in UDS in HeLa cells *in vitro* and a significant increased incidence of cells with polyploidy in an *in vitro* human lymphocyte chromosomal aberration test.

Granisetron at oral doses up to 100 mg/kg/day (600 mg/m^2/day, 405 times the recommended human dose based on body surface area) was found to have no effect on fertility and reproductive performance of male and female rats.

PREGNANCY, TERATOGENIC EFFECTS, PREGNANCY CATEGORY B

Injection

Reproduction studies have been performed in pregnant rats at intravenous doses up to 9 mg/kg/day (54 mg/m^2/day, 146 times the recommended human dose based on body surface area) and pregnant rabbits at intravenous doses up to 3 mg/kg/day (35.4 mg/m^2/day, 96 times the recommended human dose based on body surface area) and have revealed no evidence of impaired fertility or harm to the fetus due to granisetron. There are, however, no adequate and well-controlled studies in pregnant women. Because animal reproduction studies are not always predictive of human response, this drug should be used during pregnancy only if clearly needed.

Tablets

Reproduction studies have been performed in pregnant rats at oral doses up to 125 mg/kg/day (750 mg/m^2/day, 507 times the recommended human dose based on body surface area) and pregnant rabbits at oral doses up to 32 mg/kg/day (378 mg/m^2/day, 255 times the recommended human dose based on body surface area) and have revealed no evidence of impaired fertility or harm to the fetus due to granisetron. There are, however, no adequate

PRECAUTIONS: *(cont'd)*

and well-controlled studies in pregnant women. Because animal reproduction studies are not always predictive of human response, this drug should be used during pregnancy only if clearly needed.

NURSING MOTHERS

It is not known whether granisetron is excreted in human milk. Because many drugs are excreted in human milk, caution should be exercised when granisetron HCl is administered to a nursing woman.

PEDIATRIC USE

Injection: See DOSAGE AND ADMINISTRATION for use in children 2 to 16 years of age. Safety and effectiveness in children under 2 years of age have not been established.

Tablets: Safety and effectiveness in children have not been established.

GERIATRIC USE

Injection: During clinical trials, 713 patients 65 years of age or older received granisetron HCl injection. Effectiveness and safety were similar in patients of various ages.

Tablets: During clinical trials, 325 patients 65 years of age or older received oral granisetron HCl; 298 were 65 to 74 years of age and 27 were 75 years of age or older. Efficacy and safety were maintained with increasing age.

DRUG INTERACTIONS:

Granisetron does not induce or inhibit the cytochrome P-450 drug-metabolizing enzyme system. There have been no definitive drug-drug interaction studies to examine pharmacokinetic or pharmacodynamic interaction with other drugs but, in humans, granisetron HCl injection has been safely administered with drugs representing benzodiazepines, neuroleptics and anti-ulcer medications commonly prescribed with antiemetic treatments. Granisetron HCl injection also does not appear to interact with emetogenic cancer chemotherapies. Because granisetron is metabolized by hepatic cytochrome P-450 drug-metabolizing enzymes, inducers or inhibitors of these enzymes may change the clearance and, hence, the half-life of granisetron.

ADVERSE REACTIONS:

INJECTION

TABLE 10 gives the comparative frequencies of the five most commonly reported adverse events (≥3%) in patients receiving granisetron HCl injection, in single-day chemotherapy trials. These patients received chemotherapy, primarily cisplatin, and intravenous fluids during the 24-hour period following granisetron HCl injection administration. Events were generally recorded over seven days post-granisetron HCl injection administration. In the absence of a placebo group, there is uncertainty as to how many of these events should be attributed to granisetron HCl, except for headache, which was clearly more frequent than in comparison groups.

TABLE 10 Principal Adverse Events in Clinical Trials—Single-Day Chemotherapy

	Number of Patients with Event	
	Kytril Injection 40 mcg/kg (n=1,268)	Comparator[1] (n=422)
Headache	14%	6%
Asthenia	5%	6%
Somnolence	4%	15%
Diarrhea	4%	6%
Constipation	3%	3%

1 Metoclopramide/dexamethasone and phenothiazines/ dexamethasone.

In over 3,000 patients receiving granisetron HCl injection (2 to 160 mcg/kg) in single-day and multiple-day clinical trials with emetogenic cancer therapies, adverse events, other than those in TABLE 10, were observed; attribution of many of these events to granisetron HCl is uncertain:

Hepatic: In comparative trials, mainly with cisplatin regimens, elevations of AST and ALT (>2 times the upper limit of normal) following administration of granisetron HCl injection occurred in 2.8% and 3.3% of patients, respectively. These frequencies were not significantly different from those seen with comparators (AST: 2.1%; ALT: 2.4%).

Cardiovascular: Hypertension (2%); hypotension, arrhythmias such as sinus bradycardia, atrial fibrillation, varying degrees of A-V block, ventricular ectopy including non-sustained tachycardia, and ECG abnormalities have been observed rarely.

Central Nervous System: Agitation, anxiety, CNS stimulation and insomnia were seen in less than 2% of patients. Extrapyramidal syndrome occurred rarely and only in the presence of other drugs associated with this syndrome.

Hypersensitivity: Rare cases of anaphylactoid reactions, other allergic reactions and skin rashes have been reported.

Other: Taste disorder (2%), fever (3%). In multiple-day comparative studies, fever occurred more frequently with granisetron HCl injection (8.6%) than with comparative drugs (3.4%, $P<0.014$), which usually included dexamethasone.

TABLETS

Over 2,600 patients have received oral granisetron HCl in clinical trials with emetogenic cancer therapies consisting primarily of cyclophosphamide or cisplatin regimens.

In patients receiving oral granisetron HCl 1 mg b.i.d. for 1, 7 or 14 days, the following table (TABLE 11) lists adverse experiences reported in more than 5% of the patients with comparator and placebo incidences.

TABLE 11 Principal Adverse Events in Clinical Trials

	Oral Kytril[1] 1 mg b.i.d. (n=978)	Comparator[2] (n=599)	Placebo (n=185)
Headache[3]	21%	13%	12%
Constipation	18%	16%	9%
Asthenia	14%	10%	4%
Diarrhea	8%	10%	4%
Abdominal pain	6%	6%	3%

1 Adverse events were recorded for 7 days when oral Kytril was given on a single day and for up to 28 days when oral Kytril was administered for 7 or 14 days.
2 Metoclopramide/dexamethasone; phenothiazines/dexamethasone; dexamethasone alone; prochlorperazine.
3 Usually mild to moderate in severity.

Gastrointestinal: In single-day dosing studies in which adverse events were collected for 7 days, nausea (15%) and vomiting (9%) were recorded as adverse events after the 24-hour efficacy assessment period.

ADVERSE REACTIONS: *(cont'd)*

Hepatic: In comparative trials, elevation of AST and ALT (>2 times the upper limit of normal) following the administration of oral granisetron HCl occurred in 5% and 6% of patients, respectively. These frequencies were not significantly different from those seen with comparators (AST: 2%; ALT: 9%).

Cardiovascular: Hypertension (1%); hypotension, angina pectoris, atrial fibrillation and syncope have been observed rarely.

Central Nervous System: Dizziness (3%), insomnia (3%), anxiety (2%), somnolence (1%). One case compatible with but not diagnostic of extrapyramidal symptoms has been reported in a patient treated with oral granisetron HCl.

Hypersensitivity: Rare cases of hypersensitivity reactions, sometimes severe (*e.g.,* anaphylaxis, shortness of breath, hypotension, urticaria) have been reported.

Other: Fever (5%). Events often associated with chemotherapy also have been reported: leukopenia (11%), decreased appetite (5%), anemia (4%), alopecia (3%), thrombocytopenia (3%).

Over 5,000 patients have received injectable granisetron HCl in clinical trials.

TABLE 12 gives the comparative frequencies of the five commonly reported adverse events (≥3%) in patients receiving granisetron HCl injection, 40 mcg/kg, in single-day chemotherapy trials. These patients received chemotherapy, primarily cisplatin, and intravenous fluids during the 24-hour period following granisetron HCl injection administration.

TABLE 12 Principal Adverse Events in Clinical Trials—Single-Day Chemotherapy

	Number of Patients with Event	
	Kytril Injection[1] 40 mcg/kg (n=1,268)	Comparator[2] (n=422)
Headache	14%	6%
Asthenia	5%	6%
Somnolence	4%	15%
Diarrhea	4%	6%
Constipation	3%	3%

1 Adverse events were generally recorded over 7 days post-Kytril Injection administration.
2 Metoclopramide/ dexamethasone and phenothiazines/ dexamethasone.

In the absence of a placebo group, there is uncertainty as to how many of these events should be attributed to granisetron HCl, except for headache, which was clearly more frequent than in comparison groups.

OVERDOSAGE:

There is no specific treatment for granisetron hydrochloride overdosage. In case of overdosage, symptomatic treatment should be given. Overdosage of up to 38.5 mg of granisetron hydrochloride injection has been reported without symptoms or only the occurrence of a slight headache.

DOSAGE AND ADMINISTRATION:

INJECTION

The recommended dosage for granisetron HCl injection is 10 mcg/kg infused intravenously over 5 minutes, beginning within 30 minutes before initiation of chemotherapy, and only on the day(s) chemotherapy is given.

Pediatric Use: The recommended dose in children 2 to 16 years of age is 10 mcg/kg (see CLINICAL STUDIES). Children under 2 years of age have not been studied.

Use in the Elderly, Renal Failure Patients or Hepatically Impaired Patients: No dosage adjustment is recommended. (See CLINICAL PHARMACOLOGY, Pharmacokinetics.)

Infusion Preparation: Granisetron HCl injection should be diluted in 0.9% Sodium Chloride or 5% Dextrose to a total volume of 20 to 50 ml.

Stability: Intravenous infusion of granisetron HCl injection should be prepared at the time of administration. However, granisetron HCl injection has been shown to be stable for at least 24 hours when diluted in 0.9% sodium chloride or 5% Dextrose and stored at room temperature under normal lighting conditions.

As a general precaution, granisetron HCl injection should not be mixed in solution with other drugs. Parenteral drug products should be inspected visually for particulate matter and discoloration before administration whenever solution and container permit.

TABLETS

The recommended adult dosage of oral granisetron HCl is 1 mg twice daily. The first 1 mg tablet is given up to 1 hour before chemotherapy, and the second tablet, 12 hours after the first, only on the day(s) chemotherapy is given. Continued treatment, while not on chemotherapy, has not been found to be useful.

Use in the Elderly, Renal Failure Patients or Hepatically Impaired Patients: No dosage adjustment is recommended. (See CLINICAL PHARMACOLOGY, Pharmacokinetics.)

Pediatric Use: Data on oral granisetron HCl are not available.

HOW SUPPLIED:

Injection: Kytril (granisetron hydrochloride) Injection, 1 mg/ml (free base), is supplied in 1 ml Single-Use Vials.

Store vials at 30°C (86°F) or below. Do not freeze. Protect from light.

Tablets: White, triangular, biconvex, film-coated tablets debossed K1 on one face.

Store between 15° and 30°C (59° and 86°F). Protect from light.

HOW SUPPLIED - EQUIVALENTS NOT AVAILABLE:

Injection, Solution - Intravenous - 1 mg/ml

1 ml	$166.00	KYTRIL, Beecham	00029-4149-01

Tablet, Uncoated - Oral - 1 mg

2's	$78.75	KYTRIL, Beecham	00029-4151-39
20's	$787.50	KYTRIL, Beecham	00029-4151-05

GRISEOFULVIN, MICROCRYSTALLINE *(001388)*

CATEGORIES: Anti-Infectives; Antibiotics; Antifungals; Antimicrobials; Dermatologicals; Fungal Agents; Infections; Onychomycosis; Skin Infections; Tinea Barbae; Tinea Capitis; Tinea Corporis; Tinea Cruris; Tinea Pedis; Tinea Unguium; FDA Approval Pre 1982

BRAND NAMES: *Brofulin*; *Fulcin*; *Fulcin 500*; Fulvicin U F; *Fungin*; *Grifulin*; Grifulvin V; **Grisactin**; *Grisefuline* (France); *Griseofulvin* (England); *Griseofulvin Prafa*; *Griseofulvina*; *Griseofulvine*; *Grisflavin*; *Grisfulvin*; *Grisfulvin V*; *Grisovin*

(Australia); *Grisovin-FP* (Canada, Mexico); *Grisuvin*; *Grivin*; *Krisovin*; *Likuden M* (Germany); *Microfulvin*; *Microfulvin-500*; *Microgris*; *Mycostop*; *Rasovin*; *Taidin* *(International brand names outside U.S. in italics)*

FORMULARIES: Aetna; BC-BS; FHP; Medi-Cal; WHO

DESCRIPTION:

Griseofulvin Tablets contain microsize crystals of griseofulvin, an antibiotic derived from a species of *Penicillium*.

Each griseofulvin tablet contains 250 or 500 mg of microsized griseofulvin.

The inactive ingredients for Griseofulvin Tablets, 250 or 500 mg, include: magnesium stearate, pluronic F-68 (poloxamer 188), potato starch, and silica.

CLINICAL PHARMACOLOGY:

Microbiology: Griseofulvin is fungistatic with an *in vitro* activity against various species of *Microsporum, Epidermophyton,* and *Trichophyton*. It has no effect on bacteria or on other genera of fungi.

Human Pharmacology: Griseofulvin absorption from the gastrointestinal tract varies considerably among individuals mainly because of insolubility of the drug in aqueous media of the upper G.I. tract. The peak serum level found in fasting adults given 0.5 g occurs at about four hours and ranges between 0.5 to 1.5 mcg/ml. The serum level may be increased by giving the drug with a meal with a high fat content.

Griseofulvin is deposited in the keratin precursor cells and has a greater affinity for diseased tissue. The drug is tightly bound to the new keratin which becomes highly resistant to fungal invasions.

INDICATIONS AND USAGE:

Tablets are indicated for the treatment of ringworm infections of the skin, hair, and nails, namely: tinea corporis, tinea pedis, tinea cruris, tinea barbae, tinea capitis, tinea unguium (onychomycosis) when caused by one or more of the following genera of fungi: Tr*ichophyton rubrum, Trichophyton tonsurans, Trichophyton mentagrophytes, Trichophyton interdigitale, Trichophyton verrucosum, Trichophyton megninii, Trichophyton gallinae, Trichophyton crateriforme, Trichophyton sulphureum, Trichophyton schoenleinii, Microsporum audouini, Microsporum canis, Microsporum gypseum and Epidermophyton floccosum.*

Note: Prior to therapy, the type of fungi responsible for the infection should be identified.

The use of the drug is not justified in minor or trivial infections which will respond to topical agents alone.

Griseofulvin is not effective in the following: bacterial infections, candidiasis (moniliasis), histoplasmosis, actinomycosis, sporotrichosis, chromoblastomycosis, coccidioidomycosis, North American blastomycosis, cryptococcosis (torulosis), tinea versicolor, and nocardiosis.

CONTRAINDICATIONS:

This drug is contraindicated in patients with porphyria, hepatocellular failure, and in individuals with a history of hypersensitivity to griseofulvin.

Rare cases of conjoined twins have been reported in patients taking griseofulvin during the first trimester of pregnancy. Griseofulvin should not be prescribed to patients or women contemplating pregnancy.

WARNINGS:

Prophylactic Usage: Safety and efficacy of griseofulvin for prophylaxis of fungal infections have not been established.

Since griseofulvin has demonstrated harmful effects *in vitro* on the genotype in bacteria, plants, and fungi, males should wait at least six months after completing griseofulvin therapy before fathering a child. Females should avoid risk of pregnancy while receiving griseofulvin therapy.

Animal Toxicology: Chronic feeding of griseofulvin, at levels ranging from 0.5-2.5% of the diet, resulted in the development of liver tumors in several strains of mice, particularly in males. Smaller particle sizes result in an enhanced effect. Lower oral dosage levels have not been tested. Subcutaneous administration of relatively small doses of griseofulvin once a week during the first three weeks of life has also been reported to induce hepatomata in mice. Thyroid tumors, mostly adenomas but some carcinomas, have been reported in male rats receiving griseofulvin at levels of 2.0%, 1.0%, and 0.2% of the diet, and in female rats receiving the two higher dose levels. Although studies in other animal species have not yielded evidence of tumorigenicity, these studies were not of adequate design to form a basis for conclusions in this regard.

In subacute toxicity studies, orally administered griseofulvin produced hepatocellular necrosis in mice, but this has not been seen in other species. Disturbances in porphyrin metabolism have been reported in griseofulvin-treated laboratory animals. Griseofulvin has been reported to have a colchicine-like effect in mitosis and cocarcinogenicity with methylcholanthrene in cutaneous tumor induction in laboratory animals.

Griseofulvin interferes with chromosomal distribution during cell division, causing aneuploidy in plant and mammalian cells. These effects have been demonstrated *in vitro* at concentrations that may be achieved in the serum with the recommended therapeutic dose.

Usage in Pregnancy: Griseofulvin should not be prescribed to pregnant patients or to women contemplating pregnancy (see CONTRAINDICATIONS.)

Animal Reproduction Studies: It has been reported in the literature that griseofulvin was found to be embryotoxic and teratogenic on oral administration to pregnant rats. Pups with abnormalities have been reported in the litters of a few bitches treated with griseofulvin.

Suppression of spermatogenesis has been reported to occur in rats, but investigation in man failed to confirm this.

PRECAUTIONS:

Patients on prolonged therapy with any potent medication should be under close observation. Periodic monitoring of organ system functions, including renal, hepatic, and hematopoietic, should be done.

Since griseofulvin is derived from species of *Penicillium*, the possibility of cross-sensitivity with penicillin exists; however, known penicillin-sensitive patients have been treated without difficulty.

Since a photosensitivity reaction is occasionally associated with griseofulvin therapy, patients should be warned to avoid exposure to intense natural or artificial sunlight.

Lupus erythematosus or lupus-like syndromes, or exacerbation of existing lupus, have been reported in patients receiving griseofulvin.

DRUG INTERACTIONS:

Griseofulvin decreases the activity of warfarin-type anticoagulants so that patients receiving these drugs concomitantly may require dosage adjustment of the anticoagulant during and after griseofulvin therapy.

DRUG INTERACTIONS: *(cont'd)*

Barbiturates usually depress griseofulvin activity and concomitant administration may require a dosage adjustment of the antifungal agent.

The effects of alcohol may be potentiated by griseofulvin, producing such effects as tachycardia and flush.

Griseofulvin may potentiate an increase in hepatic enzymes that metabolize estrogens at an increased rate, including the estrogen component of oral contraceptives, thereby causing possible decreased contraceptive effects and menstrual irregularities.

ADVERSE REACTIONS:

When adverse reactions occur, they are most commonly of the hypersensitivity type, such as skin rashes and urticaria; and rarely, angioneurotic edema and epidermal necrolysis (Lyell's syndrome), and may necessitate withdrawal of therapy and appropriate countermeasures. Paresthesias of the hands and feet have been reported rarely after extended therapy. Other side effects reported occasionally are oral thrush, nausea, vomiting, epigastric distress, diarrhea, headache, fatigue, dizziness, insomnia, mental confusion, and impairment of performance of routine activities.

Proteinuria nephrosis, leukopenia, hepatic toxicity, GI bleeding and menstrual irregularities have been reported rarely. Administration of the drug should be discontinued if granulocytopenia occurs.

When rare, serious reactions occur with griseofulvin, they are usually associated with high dosages, long periods of therapy, or both.

DOSAGE AND ADMINISTRATION:

Accurate diagnosis of the infecting organism is essential. Identification should be made either by direct microscopic examination of a mounting of infected tissue in a solution of potassium hydroxide or by culture on an appropriate medium.

Medication must be continued until the infecting organism is completely eradicated as indicated by appropriate clinical or laboratory examination. Representative treatment periods are for tinea capitis, 4 to 6 weeks; tinea corporis, 2 to 4 weeks; tinea pedis, 4 to 8 weeks; tinea unguium — depending on rate of growth — fingernails, at least 4 months; toenails, at least 6 months.

General measures in regard to hygiene should be observed to control sources of infection or reinfection. Concomitant use of appropriate topical agents is usually required, particularly in treatment of tinea pedis. In some in some forms of athlete's foot, yeasts and bacteria may be involved as well as fungi. Griseofulvin will not eradicate the bacterial or monilial infection.

Adults: Daily administration of 500 mg (as a single dose or in divided amounts) will give a satisfactory response in most patients with tinea corporis, tinea cruris, and tinea capitis.

For those fungus infections more difficult to eradicate, such as tinea pedis and tinea unguium, a daily dosage of 1.0 g is recommended.

Children: Approximately 5 mg per pound of body weight per day is an effective dose for most children. On this basis the following dosage schedule for children is suggested.

Children weighing 30 to 50 pounds — 125 mg to 250 mg daily.

Children weighing over 50 pounds — 250 mg to 500 mg daily.

Clinical experience with griseofulvin in children with tinea capitis indicates that a single daily dose is effective. Clinical relapse will occur if the medication is not continued until the infecting organism is eradicated.

Store between 2° and 30°C (36° and 86°F).

HOW SUPPLIED - RATED THERAPEUTICALLY EQUIVALENT:

Tablet, Uncoated - Oral - 250 mg

60's	$45.02	FULVICIN-U/F, Schering	00085-0948-03
100's	$32.50	Grivate, Fujisawa Pharm (US)	57317-0660-10
100's	$68.52	GRIFULVIN V, Ortho Pharm	00062-0211-60
250's	$177.66	FULVICIN-U/F, Schering	00085-0948-06

Tablet, Uncoated - Oral - 500 mg

60's	$71.92	FULVICIN-U/F, Schering	00085-0496-03
60's	**$77.25**	**GRISACTIN 500, Ayerst**	**00046-0444-60**
100's	$51.25	Grivate, Fujisawa Pharm (US)	57317-0661-10
100's	$106.32	GRIFULVIN V, Ortho Pharm	00062-0214-60
250's	$283.67	FULVICIN-U/F, Schering	00085-0496-06
500's	$461.22	GRIFULVIN V, Ortho Pharm	00062-0214-70

HOW SUPPLIED - NOT RATED EQUIVALENT:

Capsule, Gelatin - Oral - 125 mg

100's	**$27.98**	**GRISACTIN 125, Ayerst**	**00046-0442-81**

Capsule, Gelatin - Oral - 250 mg

100's	**$73.11**	**GRISACTIN 250, Ayerst**	**00046-0443-81**
500's	**$342.09**	**GRISACTIN 250, Ayerst**	**00046-0443-85**

Suspension - Oral - 125 mg/5ml

120 ml	$22.32	GRIFULVIN V, Ortho Pharm	00062-0206-04

GRISEOFULVIN, ULTRAMICROCRYSTALLINE

(001389)

CATEGORIES: Anti-Infectives; Antibiotics; Antifungals; Antimicrobials; Dermatologicals; Fungal Agents; Infections; Skin Infections; Tinea Barbae; Tinea Capitis; Tinea Corporis; Tinea Cruris; Tinea Pedis; Tinea Unguium; FDA Approval Pre 1982

BRAND NAMES: Fulvicin P G; *Fulvina*; *Fulvina P G* (Mexico); **Gris-Peg**; Grisactin Ultra; *Griseofort*; Griseofulvin Ultramicrosize; *Griseostatin* (Australia); *Polygris* (Germany); *Polygris-OD*; *Sporostatin*; *Sporostatin P G*; *Sporostatin U F*; Ultramicrosize Griseofulvin
(International brand names outside U.S. in italics)

FORMULARIES: Aetna; BC-BS; DoD; FHP; Medi-Cal; PCS

DESCRIPTION:

Griseofulvin tablets contain ultramicrosize crystals of griseofulvin, an antibiotic derived from a species of *Penicillium*. Griseofulvin crystals are partly dissolved in polyethylene glycol 6000 and partly dispersed throughout the tablet matrix.

Each griseofulvin tablet contains 125 mg, 165 mg, 250 mg, or 330 mg griseofulvin ultramicrosize.

The inactive ingredients for griseofulvin tablets, 125 mg or 250 mg, include: corn starch, lactose, magnesium stearate, PEG, and sodium lauryl sulfate.

CLINICAL PHARMACOLOGY:

Microbiology: Griseofulvin is fungistatic with *in vitro* activity against various species of *Microsporum, Epidermophyton,* and *Trichophyton.* It has no effect on bacteria or on the other genera of fungi.

Human Pharmacology: Following oral administration, griseofulvin is deposited in the keratin precursor cells and has a greater affinity for diseased tissue. The drug is tightly bound to the new keratin which becomes highly resistant to fungal invasions.

The efficiency of gastrointestinal absorption of ultramicrocrystalline griseofulvin is approximately one and one-half times that of the conventional microsize griseofulvin. This factor permits the oral intake of two-thirds as much ultramicrocrystalline griseofulvin as the microsize form. However, there is currently no evidence that this lower dose confers any significant clinical difference with regard to safety and/or efficacy.

INDICATIONS AND USAGE:

Griseofulvin tablets are indicated for the treatment of ringworm infections of the skin, hair, nails, namely: tinea corporis, tinea pedis, tinea cruris, tinea barbae, tinea capitis, tinea unguium (onychomycosis) when caused by one or more of the following genera of fungi: *trichophyton rubrum, trichophyton tonsurans, trichophyton mentagrophytes, trichophyton interdigitale, trichophyton verrucosum, trichophyton megninii, trichophyton gallinae, trichophyton craterifome, trichophyton sulphureum, trichophyton schoenleinii, microsporum audouini, microsporum canis, microsporum gypseum, and epidermophyton floccosum.*

Note: Prior to therapy, the type of fungi responsible for the infection should be identified.

The use of this drug is not justified in minor or trivial infections which will respond to topical agents alone.

Griseofulvin is not effective in the following: bacterial infections, candidiasis (moniliasis), histoplasmosis, actinomycosis, sporotrichosis, chromoblastomycosis, coccidioidomycosis, North American blastomycosis, cryptococcosis, (torulosis), tinea versicolor, and nocardiosis.

CONTRAINDICATIONS:

This drug is contraindicated in patients with porphyria, hepatocellular failure, and in individuals with a history of hypersensitivity to griseofulvin.

Rare cases of conjoined twins have been reported in patients taking griseofulvin during the first trimester of pregnancy. Griseofulvin should not be prescribed to pregnant patients or women contemplating pregnancy.

WARNINGS:

Prophylactic Usage: Safety and efficacy of griseofulvin for prophylaxis of fungal infections has not been established.

Animal Toxicology: Chronic feeding of griseofulvin, at levels ranging from 0.5-2.5% of the diet, resulted in the development of liver tumors in several strains of mice, particularly in males. Smaller particle sizes result in an enhanced effect. Lower oral dosage levels have not been tested. Subcutaneous administration of relatively small doses of griseofulvin, once a week during the first three weeks of life has also been reported to induce hepatomata in mice. Thyroid tumors, mostly adenomas but some carcinomas, have been reported in male rats receiving griseofulvin at levels of 2.0%, 1.0%, and 0.2% of the diet, and in female rats receiving the two higher dose levels. Although studies in other animal species have not yielded evidence of tumorigenicity, these studies were not of adequate design to form a basis for conclusions in this regard.

In subacute toxicity studies, orally administered griseofulvin produced hepatocellular necrosis in mice, but this has not been seen in other species. Disturbances in porphyrin metabolism have been reported in griseofulvin-treated laboratory animals. Griseofulvin has been reported to have a colchicine-like effect on mitosis and cocarcinogenicity with methylcholanthrene in cutaneous tumor induction in laboratory animals.

Usage in Pregnancy: The safety of this drug during pregnancy has not been established.

Animal Reproduction Studies: It has been reported in the literature that griseofulvin was found to be embryotoxic and teratogenic on oral administration to pregnant rats. Pups with abnormalities have been reported in the litters of a few bitches treated with griseofulvin. Additional animal reproduction studies are in progress.

Suppression of spermatogenesis has been reported to occur in rats, but investigation in man failed to confirm this.

PRECAUTIONS:

Patients on prolonged therapy with any potent medication should be under close observation. Periodic monitoring of organ system function, including renal, hepatic, and hematopoietic, should be done.

Since griseofulvin is derived from species of *Penicillium*, the possibility of cross-sensitivity with penicillin exists; however, known penicillin sensitive patients have been treated without difficulty.

Since a photosensitivity reaction is occasionally associated with griseofulvin therapy, patients should be warned to avoid exposure to intense natural or artificial sunlight.

Lupus erythematosus, lupus-like syndromes, or exacerbation of existing lupus erythematosus have been reported in patients receiving griseofulvin.

DRUG INTERACTIONS:

Griseofulvin decreases the activity of warfarin-type anticoagulants so that patients receiving these drugs concomitantly may require dosage adjustment of the anticoagulant during and after griseofulvin therapy.

Barbiturates usually depress griseofulvin activity and concomitant administration may require a dosage adjustment of the antifungal agent.

The effect of alcohol may be potentiated by griseofulvin, producing such effects as tachycardia and flush.

Griseofulvin may potentiate an increase in hepatic enzymes that metabolize estrogens at an increased rate, including the estrogen components of oral contraceptive effects and menstrual irregularities.

ADVERSE REACTIONS:

When adverse reactions occur, they are most commonly of the hypersensitivity type such as skin rashes, urticaria, and rarely, angioneurotic edema, and may necessitate withdrawal of therapy and appropriate countermeasures. Paresthesias of the hands and feet have been reported rarely after extended therapy. Other side effects reported occasionally are oral thrush, nausea, vomiting, epigastric distress, diarrhea, headache, fatigue, dizziness, insomnia, mental confusion, and impairment of performance of routine activities.

Proteinuria and leukopenia have been reported rarely. Administration of the drug should be discontinued if granulocytopenia occurs.

When rare, serious reactions occur with griseofulvin, they are usually associated with high dosages, long periods of therapy, or both.

DOSAGE AND ADMINISTRATION:

Accurate diagnosis of the infecting organism is essential. Identification should be made either by direct microscopic examination of a mounting of infected tissue in a solution of potassium hydroxide or by culture on an appropriate medium.

Medication must be continued until the infecting organism is completely eradicated as indicated by appropriate clinical or laboratory examination. Representative treatment periods are - *tinea capitis,* 4 to 6 weeks; *tinea corporis,* 2 to 4 weeks;*tinea pedis,* 4 to 8 weeks; *tinea unguium* - depending on rate of growth - fingernails, at least 4 months; toenails, at least 6 months.

General measures in regard to hygiene should be observed to control sources of infection or reinfection. Concomitant use of appropriate topical agents is usually required, particularly in treatment of *tinea pedis.* In some forms of athlete's foot, yeasts and bacteria may be involved as well as fungi. Griseofulvin will not eradicate the bacterial or monilial infection.

Adults: Daily administration of 330 mg (as a single dose or in divided doses) will give a satisfactory response in most patients with tinea corporis, tinea cruris, and tinea capitis. For those fungal infections more difficult to eradicate such as tinea pedis and tinea unguium, a divided dose of 660 mg is recommended.

Children: Approximately 3.3 mg per pound of body weight per day of ultramicrosize griseofulvin is an effective dose for most children. On this basis, the following dosage schedules are suggested:

Children weighing 35 to 50 pounds: 82.5 mg to 165 mg daily. Children weighing over 50 pounds: 165 mg to 330 mg daily.

Children 2 years of age and younger: dosage has not been established.

Clinical experience with griseofulvin in children with tinea capitis indicates that a single daily dose is effective. Clinical relapse will occur if the medication is not continued until the infecting organism is eradicated.

Store between 2 and 30°C (36 and 86°F).

HOW SUPPLIED - RATED THERAPEUTICALLY EQUIVALENT:

Tablet - Oral - 125 mg

100's	$38.93	Griseofulvin, Ultramicrocrystalline, H.C.F.A. F F P	99999-1389-01

Tablet - Oral - 165 mg

100's	$67.50	Griseofulvin, Ultramicrocrystalline, H.C.F.A. F F P	99999-1389-02

Tablet - Oral - 250 mg

100's	$74.93	Griseofulvin, Ultramicrocrystalline, H.C.F.A. F F P	99999-1389-03

Tablet - Oral - 330 mg

100's	$67.43	Griseofulvin, Ultramicrocrystalline, H.C.F.A. F F P	99999-1389-04

Tablet, Uncoated - Oral - 125 mg

100's	$33.11	Griseofulvin, Warrick Pharms	59930-1620-01
100's	$34.10	Griseofulvin Ultramicrosize, Martec Pharms	52555-0583-01
100's	$36.05	GRISACTIN ULTRA, Ayerst	00046-0434-81
100's	**$43.91**	**GRIS-PEG, Allergan**	**00023-0763-04**
100's	$44.00	FULVICIN P/G, Schering	00085-0228-03
500's	**$171.44**	**GRIS-PEG, Allergan**	**00023-0763-99**

Tablet, Uncoated - Oral - 165 mg

100's	$53.15	Ultra Griseofulvin, Sidmak Labs	50111-0415-01
100's	$63.51	FULVICIN P/G, Schering	00085-0654-03

Tablet, Uncoated - Oral - 250 mg

100's	$64.96	Griseofulvin, Warrick Pharms	59930-1621-01
100's	$66.95	Griseofulvin Ultramicrosize, Martec Pharms	52555-0584-01
100's	$68.21	Griseofulvin, HL Moore Drug Exch	00839-7965-06
100's	$69.20	Griseofulvin Ultramicrosize, Goldline Labs	00182-1490-01
100's	$73.28	Griseofulvin Ultramicrosize, Rugby	00536-5552-01
100's	**$76.58**	**GRIS-PEG, Allergan**	**00023-0773-04**
100's	$86.32	FULVICIN P/G, Schering	00085-0507-03
100's	$87.59	GRISACTIN ULTRA, Ayerst	00046-0435-81
500's	**$340.65**	**GRIS-PEG, Allergan**	**00023-0773-50**

Tablet, Uncoated - Oral - 330 mg

100's	$81.75	Griseofulvin, United Res	00677-1412-01
100's	$82.47	Griseofulvin, Warrick Pharms	59930-1624-01
100's	$82.48	Griseofulvin Ultramicrosize, Qualitest Pharms	00603-3771-21
100's	$84.50	Ultra Griseofulvin, Sidmak Labs	50111-0416-01
100's	$84.95	Griseofulvin Ultramicrosize, Martec Pharms	52555-0585-01
100's	$87.85	Griseofulvin Ultramicrosize, Goldline Labs	00182-1500-01
100's	$93.05	Griseofulvin Ultramicrosize, Rugby	00536-5551-01
100's	$109.60	FULVICIN P/G 330, Schering	00085-0352-03
100's	$120.14	GRISACTIN ULTRA, Ayerst	00046-0437-81

HOW SUPPLIED - NOT RATED EQUIVALENT:

Tablet, Uncoated - Oral - 330 mg

100's	$86.59	Griseofulvin, HL Moore Drug Exch	00839-7947-06

GUAIFENESIN *(001391)*

CATEGORIES: Antitussives/Expectorants/Mucolytics; Asthma; Bronchitis; Congestion; Cough Preparations; Decongestants; Expectorants; Mucolytic Agents; Pharyngitis; Respiratory & Allergy Medications; Respiratory Tract Infections; Sinusitis; Pregnancy Category C; FDA Pre 1938 Drugs

BRAND NAMES: Allfen-M; *Balminil Expectorant* (Canada); *Breacol*; *Codimal*; *Dextricyl*; *Ecolate*; *Expectorin Cough*; Fenex La; Fenesin; *Flemonex*; G-600; Guaibid L.A.; **Humibid L.A.**; Hydro-Spec; Liquidid; Muco-Fen-La; Mucobid-L.A.; Nortussin; Numobid; Organidin Nr; *Pantussin*; *Pecbyal*; Pneumomist; *Polibronquiol*; Prolex; Q-Mibid-La; *Resyl S*; *Robitussin* (England, Canada); *Suprekof*; *Tintus*; Touro Ex; Tussin

(International brand names outside U.S. in italics)

FORMULARIES: Aetna

COST OF THERAPY: $93.44 (Asthma; Tablet; 600 mg; 2/day; 365 days)

PRIMARY ICD9: 493.90 (Asthma, Unspecified, Without Mention of Status Asthmaticus)

DESCRIPTION:

Each Humibid L.A. light green scored, sustained-release tablet provides 600 mg guaifenesin. Inactive ingredients: Dicalcium Phosphate, Methocel, Magnesium Stearate, Silicon Dioxide, Stearic Acid, FD&C Blue #1 Lake, D&C Yellow #10 Lake. Chemically, guaifenesin is 3-(2-methoxyphenoxy)-1, 2-propanediol.

CLINICAL PHARMACOLOGY:

Guaifenesin is an expectorant which increases respiratory tract fluid secretions & helps to loosen phlegm and bronchial secretions. By reducing the viscosity of secretions, guaifenesin increases the efficiency of the cough reflex and of ciliary action in removing accumulated secretions from the trachea and bronchi. Guaifenesin is readily absorbed from the gastrointestinal tract and is rapidly metabolized and excreted in the urine. Guaifenesin has a plasma half-life of one hour. The major urinary metabolite is B-(2-methoxyphenoxy) lactic acid.

INDICATIONS AND USAGE:

Guaifenesin tablets are indicated for the temporary relief of coughs associated with respiratory tract infections and related conditions such as sinusitis, pharyngitis, bronchitis, and asthma, when these conditions are complicated by tenacious mucus and/or mucus plugs and congestion. The drug is effective in productive as well as non-productive cough, but is of particular value in dry, non-productive cough which tends to injure the mucous membrane of the air passages.

CONTRAINDICATIONS:

This drug is contraindicated in patients with hypersensitivity to guaifenesin.

PRECAUTIONS:

General: Before prescribing medication to suppress or modify cough, it is important to ascertain that the underlying cause of cough is identified, that modification of cough does not increase the risk of clinical or physiological complications, and that appropriate therapy for the primary disease is instituted.

Drug/Laboratory Test Interactions: Guaifenesin may increase renal clearance for urate and thereby lower serum uric acid levels. Guaifenesin may produce an increase in urinary 5-hydroxy-indoleacetic acid and may therefore interfere with the interpretation of this test for the diagnosis of carcinoid syndrome. It may also falsely elevate the VMA test for catechols. Administration of this drug should be discontinued 48 hours prior to the collection of urine specimens for such tests.

Carcinogenesis, Mutagenesis, and Impairment of Fertility: No data are available on the long-term potential for carcinogenesis, mutagenesis, or impairment of fertility in animals or humans.

Pregnancy Category C: Animal reproduction studies have not been conducted with guaifenesin. It is also not known whether guaifenesin can cause fetal harm when administered to a pregnant woman or can affect reproduction capacity. Guaifenesin should be given to a pregnant woman only if clearly needed.

Nursing Mothers: It is not known whether guaifenesin is excreted in human milk. Because many drugs are excreted in human milk, caution should be exercised when guaifenesin is administered to a nursing woman and a decision should be made whether to discontinue nursing or to discontinue the drug, taking into account the importance of the drug to the mother.

ADVERSE REACTIONS:

No serious side effects from guaifenesin have been reported.

OVERDOSAGE:

Overdosage to with Guaifenesin is unlikely to produce toxic effects since its toxicity is low. Guaifenesin, when administered by stomach tube to test animals in doses up to 5 grams/kg, produced no signs of toxicity. In severe cases of overdosage, treatment should be aimed at reducing further absorption of the drug. Gastric emptying (Syrup of Ipecac) and/or lavage is recommended as soon as possible after ingestion.

DOSAGE AND ADMINISTRATION:

Adults and children over 12 years of age: One or two tablets every 12 hours not to exceed 4 tablets (2400 mg) in 24 hours.

Children 6 to 12 years: One tablet every 12 hours not to exceed 2 tablets (1200 mg) in 24 hours.

Children 2 to 6 years: $\frac{1}{2}$ tablet every 12 hours not to exceed 1 tablet (600 mg) in 24 hours.

Store at controlled room temperature between 15° and 30°C (59° and 86°F). Dispense in tight containers.

HOW SUPPLIED - EQUIVALENTS NOT AVAILABLE:

Capsule, Sprinkle - Oral - 300 mg

100's	$43.55	HUMIBID, Medeva Pharms	53014-0018-10

Liquid - Oral - 100 mg/5ml

480 ml	$13.00	Guaifenesin, Morton Grove	60432-0079-16
480 ml	$36.95	Ganidin Nr, Cypress Pharm	60258-0256-16
480 ml	$57.98	Iofen-Nf, Superior	00144-0636-16
480 ml	$72.48	ORGANIDIN NR, Wallace Labs	00037-4214-10

Tablet, Coated, Sustained Action - Oral - 600 mg

100's	$22.50	Guaibid La, Vintage Pharms	00254-5312-28
100's	$22.50	Q-MIBID-LA, Qualitest Pharms	00603-5543-21
100's	$23.40	Guaifenesin La, United Res	00677-1475-01
100's	$23.40	Guaifenesin Long Acting, United Res	00677-1475-02
100's	$23.60	Guaifenex La, Ethex	58177-0205-04
100's	$23.95	Guaifenesin La, Major Pharms	00904-7759-60
100's	$24.00	Respa-Gf, Respa Pharms	60575-0786-19
100's	$24.15	Guaifenesin 600, Alphagen Labs	59743-0018-01
100's	$24.92	Fenex La, Tmk Pharm	59582-0001-01
100's	$25.00	Guaifenesin Er 600, Trinity Technologies	61355-0501-10
100's	$25.20	Pneumomist, ECR Pharms	00095-0600-01
100's	$25.98	Guaifenesin, HL Moore Drug Exch	00839-7655-06
100's	$25.99	Touro Ex, Dartmouth Pharms	58869-0321-01
100's	$26.00	Guaifenesin, Duramed Pharms	51285-0417-02
100's	$26.20	Guaifenesin, Aligen Independ	00405-4457-01
100's	$26.25	Muco-Fen-La, Wakefield Pharms	59310-0102-10
100's	$26.55	Guaifenesin, Goldline Labs	00182-1188-01
100's	$27.00	Liquidid, Ion	11808-0300-01
100's	$28.43	Guaifenesin La, Rugby	00536-4447-01
100's	$30.26	Fenesin, Dura	51479-0009-01
100's	$31.50	Allfen-M, Am Pharms	58605-0509-01
100's	$50.48	HUMABID L.A., Medeva Pharms	53014-0012-10
100's	$80.00	NUMOBID, Teral Labs	51234-0151-90
250's	$53.40	Guaibid La, Vintage Pharms	00254-5312-33
250's	$53.40	Q-Bid La, Qualitest Pharms	00603-5543-24
250's	$53.95	MUCOBID-L.A., Econolab	55053-0040-02
250's	$54.90	Guaifenesin-Sr, Alphagen Labs	59743-0018-25
250's	$55.45	Guaifenesin La, Major Pharms	00904-7759-70
250's	$56.79	Guaifenesin, Aligen Independ	00405-4457-04
250's	$64.95	Guaifenesin, Trinity Technologies	61355-0501-25
500's	$99.50	Guaifenesin-Sr, Alphagen Labs	59743-0018-05

HOW SUPPLIED - EQUIVALENTS NOT AVAILABLE: *(cont'd)*

500's	$101.20	Guaibid La, Vintage Pharms	00254-5312-35
500's	$101.20	Q-Bid La, Qualitest Pharms	00603-5543-28
500's	$112.10	Guaifenex La, Ethex	58177-0205-08
500's	$123.50	Guaifenesin, Duramed Pharms	51285-0417-04
500's	$128.25	Liquibid, Ion	11808-0300-05
500's	$129.29	Guaifenesin Er 600, Trinity Technologies	61355-0501-50
500's	$135.04	Guaifenesin La, Rugby	00536-4447-05
500's	$247.29	HUMABID L.A., Medeva Pharms	53014-0012-50
600's	$163.06	Fenesin, Dura	51479-0009-06
1000's	$215.26	Guaifenesin, Aligen Independ	00405-4457-03

Tablet, Uncoated - Oral - 200 mg

100's	$10.94	Guaifenesin, HL Moore Drug Exch	00839-7977-06
100's	$15.70	Guaifenesin, Goldline Labs	00182-2614-01
100's	$19.95	Organ-I Nr, Qualitest Pharms	00603-4885-21
100's	$21.00	GUAIFENESIN, United Res	00677-1554-01
100's	$23.95	IODROL NR, Econolab	55053-0270-01
100's	$24.92	Gg 200 Nr, Alphagen Labs	59743-0019-01
100's	$26.26	GUAIFENESIN, Aligen Independ	00405-4455-01
100's	$27.19	ORGANIDIN NR, Wallace Labs	00037-4312-01
500's	$108.00	IODROL NR, Econolab	55053-0270-05

GUAIFENESIN; HYDROCODONE BITARTRATE *(001395)*

CATEGORIES: Antipyretics; Antitussives; Antitussives/Expectorants/Mucolytics; Central Nervous System Agents; Common Cold; Cough Preparations; Decongestants; Opiate Agonists (Controlled); Respiratory & Allergy Medications; Pregnancy Category C; DEA Class CIII; FDA Pre 1938 Drugs

BRAND NAMES: Atuss Ex; Bertuss; Cleartuss Dh; Co-Tuss V; Co-Tussin; Codiclear Dh; Codotuss; Cotuss-V; Entuss; Fentuss; Hycosin; **Hycotuss;** Hydrocodone W/Guaifenesin; Hydrotuss; Kwelcof; Pneumotussin Hc; Prolex Dh; Propatuss; Protuss; Vi-Q-Tuss; Vicoclear Dh; Vicodin Tuss; Vitussin

DESCRIPTION:

Vicodin Tuss Expectorant Syrup contains hydrocodone (dihydrocodeinone) bitartrate, semi-synthetic centrally-acting narcotic antitussive and guaifenesin, an expectorant for oral administration.

Each teaspoonful (5 ml) contains:

Hydrocodone bitartrate USP 5 mg

WARNING: May be habit forming

Guaifenesin USP 100 mg

Vicodin Tuss Expectorant Syrup also contains: glycerin, L-menthol, methylparaben, propylparaben, propylene glycol, sodium saccharin, sorbitol solution, artificial flavoring, and purified water.

CLINICAL PHARMACOLOGY:

Clinical trials have proven hydrocodone bitartrate to be an effective antitussive agent which is pharmacologically 2 to 8 times as potent as codeine. At equi-effective doses, its sedative action is greater than codeine. The precise mechanism of action of hydrocodone and other opiates is not known, however, hydrocodone is believed to act by directly depressing the cough center. In excessive doses hydrocodone, like other opium derivatives, can depress respiration. The effects of hydrocodone in therapeutic doses on the cardiovascular system is insignificant. The constipation effects of hydrocodone are much weaker than that of morphine and no stronger than that of codeine. Hydrocodone can produce miosis, euphoria, physical and psychological dependence. At therapeutic antitussive doses, it does exert analgesic effects. Following a 10 mg oral dose of hydrocodone administered to five male human subjects the mean peak concentration was 23.6 ± 5.2 ng/ml. Maximum serum levels were achieved at 1.3 ± 0.3 hours and half-life was determined to be 3.8 ± 0.3 hours. Hydrocodone exhibits a complex pattern of metabolism including O-demethylation, N-demethylation and 6-keto reduction to the corresponding 6-α- and c-β-hydroxymetabolites.

The exact mechanism of action is not established but guaifenesin is believed to act by stimulating receptors in the gastric mucosa that initiates a reflex secretion of respiratory tract fluid, thereby increasing the volume and decreasing the viscosity of bronchial secretions. Studies with guaifenesin indicate that it is rapidly absorbed from the gastrointestinal tract and has a half-life of one hour.

INDICATIONS AND USAGE:

Guaifenesin-hydrocodone bitartrate is indicated for the symptomatic relief of irritating non-productive cough associated with upper and lower respiratory tract congestion.

CONTRAINDICATIONS:

Guaifenesin-hydrocodone bitartrate is contraindicated in patients hypersensitive to hydrocodone or guaifenesin. Patients known to be hypersensitive to other opioids may exhibit cross sensitivity to guaifenesin-hydrocodone bitartrate. Hydrocodone is contraindicated in the presence of an intracranial lesion associated with increased intracranial pressure; and whenever ventilatory function is depressed.

WARNINGS:

May be habit forming. Hydrocodone can produce drug dependence of the morphine type and therefore has the potential for being abused. Psychic dependence, physical dependence and tolerance may develop upon repeated administration of guaifenesin-hydrocodone bitartrate and it should be prescribed and administered with the same degree of caution appropriate to the use of other narcotic drugs (see DRUG ABUSE AND DEPENDENCE).

Respiratory Depression: Guaifenesin-hydrocodone bitartrate produces dose-related respiratory depression by directly acting on the brain stem respiratory centers. If respiratory depression occurs, it may be antagonized by the use of naloxone and other supportive measures when indicated.

Head Injury and Increased Intracranial Pressure: The respiratory depressant properties of narcotics and their capacity to elevate cerebrospinal fluid pressure may be markedly exaggerated in the presence of head injury, other intracranial lesions or a pre-existing increase in intracranial pressure. Furthermore, narcotics produce adverse reactions which may obscure the clinical course of patients with head injuries.

Acute Abdominal Conditions: The administration of guaifenesin-hydrocodone bitartrate or other opioids may obscure the diagnosis or clinical course of patients with acute abdominal conditions.

PRECAUTIONS:

Before prescribing medication to suppress or modify cough, it is important to ascertain that the underlying cause of cough is identified, that modification of cough does not increase the risk of clinical or physiologic complications, and that appropriate therapy for the primary disease is provided.

Usage in Ambulatory Patients: Hydrocodone, like all narcotics, may impair the mental and/or physical abilities required for the performance of potentially hazardous tasks such as driving a car or operating machinery, and patients should be warned accordingly.

Laboratory Interactions: The metabolite of guaifenesin has been found to produce an apparent increase in urinary 5-hydroxyindoleacetic acid, and guaifenesin therefore may interfere with the interpretation of this test for the diagnosis of carcinoid syndrome. Guaifenesin administration should be discontinued 24 hours prior to the collection of urine specimens for the determination of 5-hydroxyindoleacetic acid.

Carcinogenesis, Mutagenesis, and Impairment of Fertility: Carcinogenicity, mutagenicity and reproduction studies have not been conducted with guaifenesin-hydrocodone bitartrate.

Usage in Pregnancy: Pregnancy Category C. Animal reproduction studies have not been conducted with guaifenesin-hydrocodone bitartrate.

It is also not known whether guaifenesin-hydrocodone bitartrate can cause fetal harm when administered to a pregnant woman or can effect reproductive capacity. Guaifenesin-hydrocodone bitartrate should be given to a pregnant woman only if clearly needed.

Nonteratogenic Effects: Babies born to mothers who have been taking opioids regularly prior to delivery will be physically dependent. The withdrawal signs include irritability and excessive crying, tremors, hyperactive reflexes, increased respiratory rate, increased stools, sneezing, yawning, vomiting and fever. The intensity of the syndrome does not always correlate with the duration of maternal opioid use or dose. There is no consensus on the best method of managing withdrawal. Chlorpromazine 0.7-1.0 mg/kg q 6 h, phenobarbital 2 mg/kg q 6 h, and paregoric 2-4 drops/kg q 4 h, have been used to treat withdrawal symptoms in infants. The duration of therapy is 4 to 28 days, with the dosages decreased as tolerated.

Nursing Mothers: It is not known whether this drug is excreted in human milk. Because many drugs are excreted in human milk and because of the potential for serious adverse reactions in nursing infants from guaifenesin-hydrocodone bitartrate, a decision should be made whether to discontinue the drug, taking into account the importance of the drug to the mother.

DRUG INTERACTIONS:

Patients receiving other narcotic analgesics, general anesthetics, phenothiazines, other tranquilizers, sedative hypnotics or other CNS depressants (including alcohol) concomitantly with hydrocodone may exhibit an additive CNS depression. When such combined therapy is contemplated, the dose of one or both agents should be reduced (see WARNINGS).

ADVERSE REACTIONS:

Respiratory System: Hydrocodone produces dose-related respiratory depression by acting directly on brain stem respiratory centers.

Cardiovascular System: Hypertension, postural hypotension and palpitations.

Genitourinary System: Ureteral spasm, spasm of vesical sphincters and urinary retention have been reported with opiates.

Central Nervous System: Sedation, drowsiness, mental clouding, lethargy, impairment of mental and physical performance, anxiety, fear, dysphoria, dizziness, psychic dependence, mood changes and blurred vision.

Gastrointestinal System: Nausea and vomiting occur more frequently in ambulatory than in recumbent patients.

DRUG ABUSE AND DEPENDENCE:

Special care should be exercised in prescribing hydrocodone for emotionally unstable patients and for those with a history of drug misuse. Such patients should be closely supervised when long-term therapy is contemplated.

Guaifenesin-hydrocodone bitartrate is a Schedule III narcotic. Psychic dependence, physical dependence and tolerance may develop upon repeated administration of narcotics; therefore, guaifenesin-hydrocodone bitartrate should always be prescribed and administered with caution. Physical dependence is the condition in which continued administration of the drug is required to prevent the appearance of a withdrawal syndrome.

Patients physically dependent on opioids will develop an abstinence syndrome upon abrupt discontinuation of the opioid or following the administration of a narcotic antagonist. The character and severity of the withdrawal symptoms are related to the degree of physical dependence. Manifestations of opioid withdrawal are similar to but milder than that of morphine and include lacrimation, rhinorrhea, yawning, sweating, restlessness, dilated pupils, anorexia, goose-flesh, irritability and tremor. In more severe forms, nausea, vomiting, intestinal spasm and diarrhea, increased heart rate and blood pressure, chills, and pains in bones and muscles of the back and extremities may occur. Peak effects will usually be apparent at 48 to 72 hours.

Treatment of withdrawal is usually managed by providing sufficient quantities of an opioid to suppress **severe** withdrawal symptoms and then gradually reducing the dose of opioid over a period of several days.

OVERDOSAGE:

Signs and Symptoms: Serious overdosage with guaifenesin-hydrocodone bitartrate is characterized by respiratory depression (a decrease in respiratory rate and/or tidal volume, Cheyne-Stokes respiration, cyanosis), extreme somnolence progressing to stupor or coma, skeletal muscle flaccidity, cold and clammy skin, and sometimes bradycardia and hypotension. In severe overdosage apnea, circulatory collapse, cardiac arrest, and death may occur.

Treatment: Primary attention should be given to the reestablishment of adequate respiratory exchange through provision of a patent airway and the institution of assisted or controlled ventilation. The narcotic antagonist naloxone hydrochloride is a specific antidote for respiratory depression which may result from overdosage or unusual sensitivity to narcotics including hydrocodone. Therefore, an appropriate dose of naloxone should be administered, preferably by the intravenous route, simultaneously with efforts at respiratory resuscitation. For further information, see full prescribing information for naloxone hydrochloride. An antagonist should not be administered in the absence of clinically significant respiratory depression. Oxygen, intravenous fluids, vasopressors and other supportive measures should be employed as indicated. Gastric emptying may be useful in removing unabsorbed drug. Activated charcoal may be of benefit.

DOSAGE AND ADMINISTRATION:

Usual Adult Dose: One teaspoonful (5 ml) after meals and at bedtime, not less than 4 hours apart (not to exceed 6 teaspoonfuls in a 24 hour period). Treatment should be initiated with one teaspoonful and subsequent doses, up to a maximum single dose of 3 teaspoonfuls, adjusted if required.

DOSAGE AND ADMINISTRATION: *(cont'd)*

USUAL CHILDREN'S DOSE

Over 12 Years: Initial dose 1 teaspoonful; maximum single dose, 2 teaspoonfuls.

6 to 12 Years: Initial dose 1/2 teaspoonful; maximum single dose, 1 teaspoonful.

Store at controlled room temperature 59°-86°F (15°-30°C).

HOW SUPPLIED - EQUIVALENTS NOT AVAILABLE:

Syrup - Oral - 100 mg/5 mg

120 ml	$7.06	HYCOCLEAR TUSS, Ethex	58177-0881-03
120 ml	$11.45	Protuss, Horizon Pharm	59630-0100-04
120 ml	$121.40	CODICLEAR DH SYRUP, Schwarz Pharma (US)	00131-5134-64
473 ml	$26.88	Co-Tussin, Am Generics	58634-0032-01
473 ml	$28.95	Cleartuss Dh, Econolab	55053-0770-16
473 ml	$31.25	Atuss Ex, Atley Pharms	59702-0005-16
480 ml	$20.95	COTATE DH, Major Pharms	00904-1235-16
480 ml	$21.21	Hydrocodone W/Guaifenesin, HL Moore Drug Exch	00839-7855-69
480 ml	$23.52	HYCOCLEAR TUSS, Ethex	58177-0881-07
480 ml	$24.95	Vi-Q-Tuss, Qualitest Pharms	00603-1853-58
480 ml	$30.00	Pneumotussin HC, ECR Pharms	00095-0065-16
480 ml	$30.20	Hydrocodone W/Guaifenesin, Goldline Labs	00182-0159-40
480 ml	$30.20	Codotuss, Major Pharms	00904-7888-16
480 ml	$31.37	Co-Tuss V, Rugby	00536-2704-85
480 ml	$32.00	Cotuss-V, Alphagen Labs	59743-0020-16
480 ml	$32.28	Vitussin, Cypress Pharm	60258-0730-16
480 ml	$33.50	PROPATUSS, H N Norton Co.	50732-0878-16
480 ml	$33.60	VICODIN TUSS, Knoll Labs	00044-0730-16
480 ml	$33.98	Hydrocodone W/Guaifenesin, Aligen Independ	00405-0095-16
480 ml	$35.30	CODICLEAR DH SYRUP, Schwarz Pharma (US)	00131-5134-70
480 ml	$37.00	Hydrocodone W/Guaifenesin, Schein Pharm (US)	00364-2517-16
480 ml	$38.25	HYDROTUSS EXPECTORANT, Rugby	00536-2660-85
480 ml	$39.50	Protuss, Horizon Pharm	59630-0100-16
480 ml	$39.95	Hycosin, Alpharma	00472-0077-16
480 ml	$44.40	KWELCOF, Ascher	00225-0420-45
480 ml	$45.75	Hydrocodone W/Guaifenesin, Goldline Labs	00182-0158-40
480 ml	**$53.40**	**HYCOTUSS, Dupont Pharma**	**00056-0235-16**

Tablet, Uncoated, Sustained Action - Oral - 300 mg/20 mg

100's	$17.71	CHEMDAL, H N Norton Co.	50732-0754-01
500's	$69.87	CHEMDAL, H N Norton Co.	50732-0754-05

GUAIFENESIN; HYDROCODONE BITARTRATE; PHENIRAMINE MALEATE; PHENYLPROPANOLAMINE HYDROCHLORIDE *(001396)*

CATEGORIES: Allergies; Antitussives; Antitussives/Expectorants/Mucolytics; Common Cold; Congestion; Cough Preparations; Decongestants; Expectorants; Hay Fever; Influenza; Lacrimation; Pruritus; Respiratory & Allergy Medications; Rhinitis; Sympathomimetic Agents; Pregnancy Category C; DEA Class CIII; FDA Pre 1938 Drugs

BRAND NAMES: Triaminic Dh; **Triaminic Expectorant Dh**

Prescribing information not available at time of publication.

HOW SUPPLIED - EQUIVALENTS NOT AVAILABLE:

Syrup - Oral

120 ml	$7.19	S-T FORTE, Scot Tussin	00372-0004-04
240 ml	$12.35	S-T FORTE, Scot Tussin	00372-0004-08
240 ml	$12.35	S-T FORTE SUGAR FREE, Scot Tussin	00372-0005-08
480 ml	$24.70	S-T FORTE SUGAR FREE, Scot Tussin	00372-0005-16
480 ml	$25.27	S-T FORTE, Scot Tussin	00372-0004-16
480 ml	**$39.01**	**TRIAMINIC EXPECTORANT DH, Novartis**	**00043-0521-16**
840 ml	$176.80	S-T FORTE SUGAR FREE, Scot Tussin	00372-0005-28
840 ml	$180.81	S-T FORTE, Scot Tussin	00372-0004-28

GUAIFENESIN; HYDROCODONE BITARTRATE; PSEUDOEPHEDRINE HYDROCHLORIDE *(001397)*

CATEGORIES: Antitussives; Antitussives/Expectorants/Mucolytics; Bronchitis; Common Cold; Cough Preparations; Expectorants; Nasal Congestion; Respiratory & Allergy Medications; Sinusitis; DEA Class CIII; FDA Pre 1938 Drugs

BRAND NAMES: Cophene-S; Cophene-Xp; Deconamine Cx; Detussin; Duratuss HD; Entuss-D; Hydro-Coff; Hyphed; Hytussin; Kg-Tuss Hd; Med-Hist; Pancof Xp; Poly-Tussin Xp; Protuss-D; Spantuss Hd; Src Expectorant; Tussadur-Hd; Tussafin; Tussend; Tussgen; Vanacon; Vanex

DESCRIPTION:

Hydrocodone Bitartrate: 2.5 mg (WARNING: May be habit forming)

Pseudoephedrine Hydrochloride: 30 mg

Guaifenesin: 100 mg

Alcohol: 5%

Also contains citric acid anhydrous, glucose liquid, methylparaben, propylene glycol, propylparaben, purified water, saccharin sodium, sorbitol solution, sucrose, FD&C Red #40, natural and artificial flavoring.

Hydrocodone bitartrate is an antitussive. The chemical name is: 4,5α-epoxy-3-methoxy-17-methylmorphian-6-one tartrate (1:1) hydrate (2:5). M.W. 494.50.

$C_{18}H_{21}NO_3 \cdot C_4H_6O_6 \cdot 2\ 1/2\ H_2O$

Pseudoephedrine hydrochloride is a nasal decongestant. The chemical name is: [S-(R*,R*)]-α-[1-(methylamino)ethyl] benzenemethanol hydrochloride. M.W. 201.70.

Guaifenesin is an expectorant. The chemical name is: 3-(O- (methoxyphenoxy)-1,2 propanediol. M.W. 198.22.

CLINICAL PHARMACOLOGY:

Hydrocodone is a semisynthetic narcotic analgesic and antitussive with multiple actions qualitatively similar to those of codeine. Most of these involve the central nervous system and smooth muscle. Hydrocodone suppresses the cough reflex by depressing the medullary

CLINICAL PHARMACOLOGY: *(cont'd)*

cough center. The precise mechanism of action of hydrocodone and other opiates is not known, although it is believed to relate to the existence of opiate receptors in the central nervous system.

Pseudoephedrine hydrochloride is an orally effective nasal decongestant that acts on alpha-adrenergic receptors in the mucosa of the respiratory tract producing vasoconstriction. Pseudoephedrine shrinks swollen nasal mucous membranes, reduces tissue hyperemia, edema and nasal congestion and increases nasal airway patency. Drainage of sinus secretions is increased and obstructed Eustachian ostia may be opened. Pseudoephedrine produces little if any rebound congestion.

Guaifenesin is an expectorant which enhances the flow of respiratory tract secretions. The enhanced flow of less viscid secretions lubricates irritated respiratory tract membranes, promotes cilliary action and facilitates the removal of inspissated mucus. As a result, sinus and bronchial drainage is improved and nonproductive coughs become more productive and less frequent.

INDICATIONS AND USAGE:

For exhausting, nonproductive cough accompanying respiratory tract congestion associated with the common cold, sinusitis and bronchitis.

CONTRAINDICATIONS:

This combination elixir is contraindicated in patients with severe hypertension, severe coronary artery disease, and in patients on MAO inhibitor therapy.

Hypersensitivity: Contraindicated in patients with hypersensitivity or idiosyncrasy to sympathomimetic amines, phenanthrene derivatives, or to any other formula ingredients.

Nursing Mothers: Contraindicated because of the higher than usual risk for infants for sympathomimetic amines.

WARNINGS:

Hydrocodone should be prescribed and administered with the same degree of caution as all oral medications containing a narcotic analgesic. Extreme caution should be exercised in the use of hydrocodone in patients with severe respiratory impairment or patients with impaired respiratory drive.

If sympathomimetic amines are used in patients with hypertension, diabetes mellitus, ischemic heart disease, hyperthyroidism, increased intraocular pressure or prostatic hypertrophy, judicious caution should be exercised (see CONTRAINDICATIONS.)

Use in Elderly: The elderly (60 years and older) are more likely to have adverse reactions to sympathomimetics. Overdosage of sympathomimetics in this age group may cause hallucinations, convulsions, CNS depression and death.

PRECAUTIONS:

General: Caution should be exercised if used in patients with diabetes, hypertension, cardiovascular diseases, hyperreactivity to ephedrine, or decreased respiratory drive (see CONTRAINDICATIONS.)

Information for the Patient: Hydrocodone may produce drowsiness. Persons who perform hazardous tasks requiring mental alertness or physical coordination should be cautioned accordingly. Concomitant use of hydrocodone with tranquilizers, alcohol or other depressants may produce additive depressant effects. Do not exceed the prescribed dosage.

Laboratory Test Interactions: Guaifenesin interferes with the colorimetric determination of 5-hydroxyindoleacetic acid (5-HIAA) and Vanillylmandelic acid (VMA).

Pregnancy Category C: Animal reproduction studies have not been conducted with pseudoephedrine, guaifenesin, or hydrocodone. It is also not known whether pseudoephedrine, guaifenesin or hydrocodone can cause fetal harm when administered to a pregnant woman or can affect reproduction capacity. Pseudoephedrine, guaifenesin or hydrocodone may be given to a pregnant woman only if clearly needed.

Nursing Mothers: Because of the potential for serious adverse reactions in nursing infants from sympathomimetic amines, pseudoephedrine is contraindicated in nursing mothers.

DRUG INTERACTIONS:

Hydrocodone may potentiate the effects of other narcotics, general anesthetics, tranquilizers, sedatives and hypnotics, tricyclic antidepressants, MAO inhibitors, alcohol, and other CNS depressants. Beta-adrenergic blockers and MAO inhibitors potentiate the sympathomimetic effects of pseudoephedrine. Sympathomimetics may reduce the antihypertensive effects of methyldopa, mecamylamine, reserpine and veratrum alkaloids.

ADVERSE REACTIONS:

Gastrointestinal upset, nausea, drowsiness and constipation. A slight elevation in serum transaminase levels has been noted.

Individuals hyperreactive to pseudoephedrine may display ephedrine-like reactions such as tachycardia, palpitations, headache, dizziness or nausea. Sympathomimetic drugs have been associated with certain untoward reactions including fear, anxiety, tenseness, restlessness, tremor, weakness, pallor, respiratory difficulty, dysuria, insomnia, hallucinations, convulsions, CNS depression, arrhythmias, and cardiovascular collapse with hypotension. Patient idiosyncrasy to adrenergic agents may be manifested by insomnia, dizziness, weakness, tremor or arrhythmias.

DRUG ABUSE AND DEPENDENCE:

Controlled Substance: Hydrocodone in this combination elixir is controlled by the Drug Enforcement Administration. This combination elixir is a Schedule III controlled substance.

Abuse: Hydrocodone is a narcotic drug related to codeine with similar abuse potential.

Dependence: Hydrocodone can produce drug dependence of the morphine type. Psychic dependence, physical dependence and tolerance may develop if dosage recommendations are greatly exceeded over a prolonged period of time.

OVERDOSAGE:

Acute overdosage with this combination elixir may produce variable clinical signs as hydrocodone produces CNS depression and cardiovascular depression while pseudoephedrine produces CNS stimulation and variable cardiovascular effects. Hydrocodone is likely to be responsible for most of the severe reactions from overdosage. Pressor amines should be used with great caution when taking pseudoephedrine. Patients with signs of stimulation should be treated conservatively and depressant medications should be avoided if possible because of potential drug interaction with hydrocodone.

DOSAGE AND ADMINISTRATION:

This combination expectorant is administered orally. The usual doses are: *Adults:* 2 teaspoonfuls (10 ml) every 4-6 hours. *Children: 6-12 years of age:* 1 teaspoonful (5 ml) every 4-6 hours. May be given four times a day as needed. May be taken with meals.

HOW SUPPLIED:

Storage: Store at controlled room temperature, 15°–30°C (59°–86°F). Dispense in a tight, light-resistant container as described in USP.

HOW SUPPLIED - EQUIVALENTS NOT AVAILABLE:

Liquid - Oral - 200 mg/5 mg/60

120 ml	$11.45	PROTUSS-D, Horizon Pharm	59630-0105-04
473 ml	$18.00	Cophene-S, Dunhall Pharms	00217-0411-11
473 ml	$25.95	Spantuss Hd, Econolab	55053-0780-16
473 ml	$32.75	Vanacon, GM Pharms	58809-0929-01
480 ml	$12.90	DETUSSIN, Qualitest Pharms	00603-1131-58
480 ml	$14.95	Detussin, Consolidated Midland	00223-6133-01
480 ml	$15.40	DETUSSIN, Major Pharms	00904-0965-16
480 ml	$16.59	DETUSSIN EXPECTORANT, Alpharma	00472-0957-16
480 ml	$17.65	TUSSGEN EXPECTORANT, Goldline Labs	00182-1164-40
480 ml	$24.50	Tussadur-Hd, Alphagen Labs	59743-0056-16
480 ml	$25.00	SRC EXPECTORANT, Edwards Pharms	00485-0042-16
480 ml	$26.45	Kg-Tuss Hd, King Pharms	60793-0025-16
480 ml	$30.13	POLY-TUSSIN XP, Poly Pharms	50991-0925-16
480 ml	$31.45	MED-HIST, Med Tek Pharms	52349-0450-16
480 ml	$35.56	VANEX EXPECTORANT, Abana Pharms	12463-0123-16
480 ml	$37.39	DURATUSS HD, UCB Pharma	50474-0610-16
480 ml	$37.94	TUSSEND, Monarch	61570-0005-16
480 ml	$39.50	PROTUSS-D, Horizon Pharm	59630-0105-16
480 ml	$41.00	DECONAMINE CX, Bradley Pharms	00482-0186-16
3840 ml	$63.55	TUSSAFIN, Rugby	00536-0540-90
3840 ml	$99.49	Detussin, Consolidated Midland	00223-6133-02
3840 ml	$272.18	Duratuss Hd, UCB Pharma	50474-0610-28

Tablet, Uncoated - Oral

100's	$41.00	DECONAMINE CX, Bradley Pharms	00482-0182-10

GUAIFENESIN; HYDROCODONE; PHENYLEPHRINE HYDROCHLORIDE *(001393)*

CATEGORIES: Antitussives; Antitussives/Expectorants/Mucolytics; Cough Preparations; Expectorants; Respiratory & Allergy Medications; DEA Class CIII; FDA Pre 1938 Drugs

BRAND NAMES: **Donatussin Dc**

Prescribing information not available at time of publication.

HOW SUPPLIED - EQUIVALENTS NOT AVAILABLE:

Syrup - Oral - 50 mg/2.5 mg/7.

120 ml	**$8.57**	**DONATUSSIN DC SYRUP, Laser**	**00277-0171-34**
480 ml	**$31.18**	**DONATUSSIN DC SYRUP, Laser**	**00277-0171-41**

GUAIFENESIN; HYDROMORPHONE *(001398)*

CATEGORIES: Antitussives; Antitussives/Expectorants/Mucolytics; Cough Preparations; Respiratory & Allergy Medications; Pregnancy Category C; DEA Class CII; FDA Pre 1938 Drugs

BRAND NAMES: **Dilaudid**

FORMULARIES: Aetna

Prescribing information not available at time of publication.

HOW SUPPLIED - EQUIVALENTS NOT AVAILABLE:

Syrup - Oral - 100 mg/1 mg

480 ml	**$33.90**	**DILAUDID, Knoll Labs**	**00044-1080-01**

GUAIFENESIN; OXTRIPHYLLINE *(001401)*

CATEGORIES: Antiasthmatics/Bronchodilators; Asthma; Bronchitis; Bronchospasm; Emphysema; Pulmonary Emphysema; Respiratory & Allergy Medications; Respiratory Muscle Relaxant; Smooth Muscle Relaxants; FDA Pre 1938 Drugs

BRAND NAMES: Brondecon; Brondelate; *Choledyl*; *Choledyl Expectorant* (Canada); *Euspirax Comp.*; Oxyfenesin; Theocon
(International brand names outside U.S. in italics)

COST OF THERAPY: $521.80 (Asthma; Tablet; 100 mg/200 mg; 4/day; 365 days) vs. Potential Cost of $3,576.99 (Bronchitis & Asthma)

PRIMARY ICD9: 493.90 (Asthma, Unspecified, Without Mention of Status Asthmaticus)

DESCRIPTION:

Each tablet contains 200 mg oxtriphylline, USP and 100 mg guaifenesin, USP. Also contains acacia, NF; colloidal silicon dioxide, NF; corn starch, NF; ethylcellulose, NF; FD&C red No. 40; FD&C yellow No. 6; hydrogenated vegetable oil, NF; lactose, NF; magnesium stearate, NF; methylcellulose, USP; pregelatinized starch, NF; saccharin sodium, USP; sucrose, NF.

NOTE: 100 mg oxtriphylline is equivalent to 64 mg anhydrous theophylline.

CLINICAL PHARMACOLOGY:

Oxtriphylline w/ guaifenesin, a bronchodilator and expectorant, helps to relieve symptoms of bronchospasm as well as obstruction caused by viscid mucus in the bronchioles. Oxtriphylline, the choline salt of theophylline, is a xanthine bronchodilating agent. Compared to aminophylline, oxtriphylline is less irritating to the gastric mucosa, better absorbed from the gastrointestinal tract, more stable and more soluble. The expectorant component of oxtriphylline w/ guaifenesin is guaifenesin which tends to increase the secretion and decrease the viscosity of fluids of the respiratory tract. These physiologic fluids help to lubricate the inflamed mucous membranes of the bronchi and also help the patient to expel viscid mucus, thus making cough more productive.

INDICATIONS AND USAGE:

Oxtriphylline w/ guaifenesin is an adjunct in the management of bronchitis, bronchial asthma, asthmatic bronchitis, pulmonary emphysema, and similar chronic obstructive lung disease. It is indicated when both relaxation of bronchospasm and expectorant action are desirable.

PRECAUTIONS:

Concurrent use of other xanthine preparations may lead to adverse reactions, particularly CNS stimulation in children.

ADVERSE REACTIONS:

Gastric distress and, occasionally, palpitation and CNS stimulation have been reported.

DOSAGE AND ADMINISTRATION:

Tablets - over 12 years of age: one tablet, 4 times a day.

Above recommendations are averages. Dosage should be individualized.

Store between 15-30°C (59-86°F).

HOW SUPPLIED - EQUIVALENTS NOT AVAILABLE:

Elixir - Oral - 50 mg/100 mg

120 ml	$5.90	THEOCON, H N Norton Co.	50732-0896-04
480 ml	$16.00	Brondelate, Consolidated Midland	00223-6434-01
480 ml	$16.20	BRONDELATE, Harber Pharm	51432-0540-20
480 ml	$17.00	THEOCON, H N Norton Co.	50732-0896-16
480 ml	$17.01	BRONDELATE, Alpharma	00472-0709-16
480 ml	$37.96	BRONDECON, Parke-Davis	00071-2201-23
3840 ml	$76.99	THEOCON, H N Norton Co.	50732-0896-28
3840 ml	$89.47	Brondelate, Consolidated Midland	00223-6434-02

Tablet, Plain Coated - Oral - 100 mg/200 mg

100's	$35.74	BRONDECON, Parke-Davis	00071-0200-24

GUAIFENESIN; PHENYLEPHRINE HYDROCHLORIDE *(001402)*

CATEGORIES: Allergies; Antihistamines; Antitussives/Expectorants/Mucolytics; Autonomic Drugs; Common Cold; Cough Preparations; Decongestants; Expectorants; Respiratory & Allergy Medications; Sympathomimetic Agents; Pregnancy Category C; FDA Pre 1938 Drugs

BRAND NAMES: Chemdal; **Deconsal**; Endal; Guiaphen; Liquibid-D; Numonyl; Numonyl Pediatric; Pneumax; Quindal; Sinupan

FORMULARIES: Aetna

DESCRIPTION:

Each Deconsal Sprinkle Capsule provides 10 mg phenylephrine hydrochloride and 300 mg guaifenesin in a sustained-release formulation intended for oral administration. The microencapsulated contents of a capsule may be sprinkled on a small amount of soft food immediately prior to ingestion, making the product ideal for pediatric patients and other patients unable to swallow capsules or tablets. Capsules are oversized facilitate opening but may also be swallowed whole.

Phenylephrine hydrochloride is an orally effective nasal decongestant. Chemically, it is (R)-3-hydroxy-α-[(methyl-amino) methyl]benzenemethanol hydrochloride. The chemical formula is $C_9H_{13}NO_2 \cdot HCl$ and the molecular weight is 203.67.

Guaifenesin is an expectorant. Chemically, it is 3-(2-methoxyphenoxy)-1,2-propanediol and it has a chemical formula of $C_{10}H_{14}O_4$ and a molecular weight of 198.22.

CLINICAL PHARMACOLOGY:

Phenylephrine hydrochloride effects its vasoconstrictor activity by releasing noradrenaline from sympathetic nerve endings, and from direct stimulation of α-adrenoreceptors in blood vessels in the nasal mucosa helps relieve nasal congestion. In therapeutic doses the drug causes little, if any, central nervous system stimulation.

Guaifenesin is an expectorant which increases respiratory tract fluid secretions and helps to loosen phlegm and bronchial secretions. By reducing the viscosity of secretions, guaifenesin increases the efficiency of the mucociliary mechanism in removing accumulated secretions from the upper and lower airway. Guaifenesin is readily absorbed from the gastrointestinal tract and is rapidly metabolized and excreted in the urine. Guaifenesin has a plasma half-life of one hour. The major urinary metabolite is β-(2-methoxyphenoxy) lactic acid.

INDICATIONS AND USAGE:

Guaifenesin-phenylephrine HCl sprinkle capsules are indicated for the temporary relief of nasal congestion and cough associated with respiratory tract infections and related conditions such as sinusitis, pharyngitis, bronchitis, and asthma, when these conditions are complicated by tenacious mucus and/or mucus plugs and congestion. The product is effective as well as non-productive cough, but is of particular value in dry, non-productive cough which tends to injure the mucous membrane of the air passages. Guaifenesin-phenylephrine HCl sprinkle capsules are particularly suitable for use in pediatric patients and other patients unable to swallow tablets or capsules.

CONTRAINDICATIONS:

This product is contraindicated in patients with hypersensitivity to guaifenesin, or with hypersensitivity or idiosyncrasy to sympathomimetic amines which may be manifested by insomnia, dizziness, weakness, tremor or arrhythmias.

Patients known to be hypersensitive to other sympathomimetic amines may exhibit cross sensitivity with phenylephrine. Phenylephrine is contraindicated in patients with severe hypertension, severe coronary artery disease and patients on monoamine oxidase inhibitor (MAOI) therapy and for 14 days after stopping MAOI therapy. (See DRUG INTERACTIONS.)

WARNINGS:

Sympathomimetic amines should be used with caution in patients with hypertension, ischemic heart disease, diabetes, mellitus, increased intraocular pressure, hyperthyroidism, or prostatic hypertrophy. Sympathomimetics may produce central nervous system stimulation with convulsions or cardiovascular collapse with accompanying hypotension. **Do not exceed recommended dosage.**

Hypertensive crises can occur with concurrent use of phenylephrine and MAOI, and for 14 days after stopping MAOI therapy, indomethacin or with beta-blockers and methyldopa. If hypertensive crisis occurs, these drugs should be discontinued immediately and therapy to lower blood pressure should be instituted. Fever should be managed by means of external cooling.

PRECAUTIONS:

General: Use with caution in patients with diabetes, hypertension, cardiovascular disease and intolerance to ephedrine.

PRECAUTIONS: *(cont'd)*

Before prescribing medication to suppress or modify cough, it is important to ascertain that the underlying cause of cough is identified, that modification of cough does not increase the risk of clinical or physiologic complications, and that appropriate therapy for the primary disease is instituted.

Information for the Patient: Capsules may be swallowed whole or the entire contents sprinkled on a small amount of soft food (jam, etc.) immediately prior to ingestion. Capsule contents should not be subdivided. Capsule contents should not be crushed or chewed. Patients should be instructed to check with physician if symptoms do not improve within 5 days or if fever is present.

Pediatric Use: This product is not recommended for use in pediatric patients under 2 years of age.

Use In Elderly: The elderly (60 years and older) are more likely to experience adverse reactions to sympathomimetics. Overdosage of sympathomimetics in this age group may cause hallucinations, convulsions, CNS depression, and death.

Drug/Laboratory Test Interactions: Guaifenesin may increase renal clearance for urate and thereby lower serum uric acid levels. Guaifenesin may produce an increase in urinary 5-hydroxy-in-doleacetic acid and may therefore interfere with the interpretation of this test for the diagnosis of carcinoid syndrome. It may also falsely elevate the VMA test for catechols. Administration of this drug should be discontinued 48 hours prior to the collection of urine specimens for such tests.

Carcinogenesis, Mutagenesis, and Impairment of Fertility: No data are available on the long-term potential of the components of this product for carcinogenesis, mutagenesis, or impairment of fertility in animals or humans.

Pregnancy Category C: Animal reproduction studies have not been conducted with guaifenesin-phenylephrine HCl sprinkle capsules. It is also not known whether guaifenesin-phenylephrine HCl sprinkle capsules can cause fetal harm when administered to a pregnant woman or can affect reproduction capacity. Guaifenesin-phenylephrine HCl sprinkle capsules should be given to a pregnant women only if clearly needed.

Nursing Mothers: Use of this product by nursing mothers is not recommended because of the higher than usual risk for pediatric patients from sympathomimetic amines.

DRUG INTERACTIONS:

Do not prescribe this product for use in patients that are now taking a prescription MAOI (certain drugs for depression, psychiatric or emotional conditions, or Parkinson's disease), or for 14 days after stopping the MAOI drug therapy. Beta-adrenergic blockers and MAOI may potentiate the pressor effect of phenylephrine (see WARNINGS). Concurrent use of digitalis glycosides may increase the possibility of cardiac arrhythmias. Sympathomimetics may reduce the hypotensive effects of guanethidine, mecamylamine, methyldopa, reserpine and veratrum alkaloids. Concurrent use of tricyclic antidepressants may antagonize the effect of phenylephrine.

ADVERSE REACTIONS:

Hyper-reactive individuals may display ephedrine-like reactions such as tachycardia, palpitations, headache, dizziness, or nausea. Sympathomimetics have been associated with certain untoward reactions including fear, anxiety, nervousness, restlessness, tremor, weakness, pallor, respiratory difficulty, dysuria, insomnia, hallucinations, convulsions, CNS depression, arrhythmias, and cardiovascular collapse with hypotension. No serious side effects have been reported with the use of guaifenesin.

OVERDOSAGE:

Since guaifenesin-phenylephrine HCl sprinkle capsules contain two pharmacologically different compounds, treatment of overdosage should be based upon the symptomatology of the patient as it relates to the individual ingredients. Treatment of acute overdosage should be based upon the symptomatology of the patient as it relates to the individual ingredients. Treatment of acute overdosage would probably be based upon treating the patient for phenylephrine toxicity which may manifest itself as excessive CNS stimulation resulting in excitement, tremor, restlessness, and insomnia. Other effects may include tachycardia, hypertension, pallor, mydriasis, hyperglycemia and urinary retention. may cause tachypnea or hyperpnea, hallucinations, convulsions or delirium, but in some individuals there may be CNS depression with somnolence, stupor or respiratory depression. Arrhythmias (including ventricular fibrillation) may lead to hypotension and circulatory collapse. Severe hypokalemia can occur, probably due to a compartmental shift rather than a depletion of potassium. Overdosage with guaifenesin is unlikely to produce toxic effects since its toxicity is much lower than that of phenylephrine. In severe case of overdose, it is recommended to monitor the patient in an intensive care setting.

The LD_{50} of phenylephrine (single oral dose) has been reported to be 120 mg/kg in the mouse and 350 mg/kg in the rat. The toxic and lethal concentrations in human biologic fluids are not known. Guaifenesin, when administered by stomach tube to test animals in doses up to 5 grams/kg, produced no signs of toxicity.

Since the action of sustained-release products may continue for as long as 12 hours, treatment of overdosage should be directed toward reducing further absorption and supporting the patient for at least that length of time. Gastric emptying (Syrup of Ipecac) and/or lavage is recommended as soon as possible after ingestion, even if the patient has vomited spontaneously. Either isotonic or half-isotonic saline may used for lavage. Administration of an activated charcoal slurry is beneficial after lavage and/or emesis if less than 4 hours have passed since ingestion. Saline cathartics, such as Milk of Magnesia, are useful for hastening the evacuation of unreleased medication.

Adrenergic receptor blocking agents are antidotes to phenylephrine. In practice, the most useful is the beta-blocker propranolol which is indicated when there are signs of cardiac toxicity. Theoretically, phenylephrine is dialyzable but procedures have not been clinically established.

DOSAGE AND ADMINISTRATION:

Adults and Adolescents Over 12 Years of Age: Two to three capsules every 12 hours not to exceed 6 capsules in 24 hours.

Children 6 to 12 Years: One or two capsules every 12 hours not to exceed 4 capsules in 24 hours.

Children 2 to 6 yYears: One capsule every 12 hours not to exceed 2 capsules in 24 hours. Capsules may be swallowed whole or the entire contents sprinkled on a small amount of soft food immediately prior to ingestion. **Subdividing the contents of a capsule is not recommended.**

HOW SUPPLIED:

White beads in a blue and clear capsule imprinted with "Adams/019". Store at controlled room temperature between 15° C and 30° C (59° F and 86° F).

HOW SUPPLIED - EQUIVALENTS NOT AVAILABLE:

Capsule, Gelatin - Oral - 200 mg/40 mg

100's	$60.90	SINUPAN, Ion	11808-0140-01

HOW SUPPLIED - EQUIVALENTS NOT AVAILABLE: *(cont'd)*

Capsule, Sprinkle - Oral - 300 mg/10 mg

100's	**$49.46**	**DECONSAL, Medeva Pharms**	**53014-0019-10**

Liquid - Oral - 250 mg/10 mg

120 ml	$14.50	NUMONYL, Teral Labs	51234-0158-04
120 ml	$14.50	NUMONYL, Teral Labs	51234-0170-04

Solution - Oral - 50 mg/2 mg

30 ml	$14.40	NUMONYL PEDIATRIC, Teral Labs	51234-0159-70
30 ml	$14.40	NUMONYL PEDIATRIC, Teral Labs	51234-0169-77

Tablet, Coated, Sustained Action - Oral - 300 mg/20 mg

	$16.45	EFASIN, Major Pharms	00904-3540-60
	$60.55	EFASIN, Major Pharms	00904-3540-40
100's	$15.85	Phenylephrine/Guaifenesin, Goldline Labs	00182-1206-01
100's	$17.40	GUIAPHEN, Rugby	00536-4393-01
100's	$17.88	Quindal, Qualitest Pharms	00603-5571-21
100's	$31.56	ENDAL, UAD Labs	00785-2204-01
100's	**$99.00**	**DECONSAL, Medeva Pharms**	**53014-0015-10**

Tablet, Coated, Sustained Action - Oral - 600 mg/15 mg

100's	$100.00	NUMONYL SR, Teral Labs	51234-0152-90

Tablet, Coated, Sustained Action - Oral - 600 mg/40 mg

100's	$37.83	LIQUIBID-D, Ion	11808-0141-01

GUAIFENESIN; PHENYLEPHRINE HYDROCHLORIDE; PHENYLPROPANOLAMINE HYDROCHLORIDE *(001403)*

CATEGORIES: Antitussives/Expectorants/Mucolytics; Autonomic Drugs; Bronchitis; Common Cold; Congestion; Cough Preparations; DESI Drugs; Decongestants; Expectorants; Mucolytic Agents; Nasal Congestion; Pharyngitis; Respiratory & Allergy Medications; Sinusitis; Sympathomimetic Agents; Pregnancy Category C; FDA Pre 1938 Drugs

BRAND NAMES: Altex; Ami-Tex; Banex; Coldloc; Conex; Contuss; Crantex; Cyntex; Decon-E; Despec; Despec-Sf; Dura-Gest; Duratex; Endix; Enomine; **Entex**; Epicap; Episol; Equi-Tex; Fentex; Gentex; Guaifenex; Guiafen-La; Guiatex; Harber-Tex; Miraphen; Mytex; P-Tex; Phentex; Phenylfenesin; Profen; Quentex; Quintex; Rymed; Sil-Tex; Tri-Tex; Trintex; Ulr

FORMULARIES: Aetna

DESCRIPTION:

Entex Capsules: Each orange and white capsule for oral administration contains

phenylephrine hydrochloride... 5 mg

phenylpropanolamine hydrochloride... 45 mg

guaifenesin... 200 mg

Inactive Ingredients: Each capsule contains D&C Red No. 28, D&C Yellow No. 10, edible black ink, FD&C Red No. 40, gelatin, silica gel, starch, titanium dioxide, FD&C Yellow #6, and zinc stearate.

Liquid: Each 5ml (one teaspoonful) for oral administration contains

phenylephrine hydrochloride... 5 mg

phenylpropanolamine hydrochloride... 20 mg

guaifenesin... 100 mg

alcohol... 5%

Inactive Ingredients: The liquid form contains citric acid, FD&C Yellow No. 6, flavoring, glycerin, purified water, saccharin sodium, sodium benzoate, sodium chloride, sorbitol solution, and sucrose.

This product contains ingredients of the following therapeutic classes: decongestant and expectorant.

Phenylephrine hydrochloride is a decongestant having the chemical name, 3-hydroxy-α-[(methylamino)methyl] benzenemethanol hydrochloride.

Phenylpropanolamine hydrochloride is a decongestant having the chemical name, benzenemethanol, α-(1-aminoethyl)-,hydrochloride(R*, S*),(±).

Guaifenesin is an expectorant having the chemical name, 1,2-propanediol,3-(2-methoxyphenoxy).

CLINICAL PHARMACOLOGY:

Phenylephrine hydrochloride and phenylpropanolamine hydrochloride are α-adrenergic receptor agonists (sympathomimetics) which produce vasoconstriction by stimulating α-receptors within the mucosa of the respiratory tract. Clinically, phenylephrine and phenylpropanolamine shrink swollen mucous membranes, reduce tissue hyperemia, edema, and nasal congestion, and increase nasal airway patency. Guaifenesin promotes lower respiratory tract drainage by thinning bronchial secretions, lubricates irritated respiratory tract membranes through increased mucous flow, and facilitates removal of viscous, inspissated mucus. As a result of these drugs, sinus and bronchial drainage is improved, and dry, nonproductive coughs become more productive and less frequent.

INDICATIONS AND USAGE:

This drug is indicated for the symptomatic relief of sinusitis,bronchitis, pharyngitis, and coryza when these conditions are associated with nasal congestion and viscous mucus in the lower respiratory tract.

CONTRAINDICATIONS:

This drug is contraindicated in individuals with known hypersensitivity to sympathomimetics, severe hypertension, or in patients receiving monoamine oxidase inhibitors.

WARNINGS:

Sympathomimetic amines should be used with caution in patients with hypertension, diabetes mellitus, heart disease, peripheral vascular disease, increased intraocular pressure, hyperthyroidism, or prostatic hypertrophy.

PRECAUTIONS:

Drug/Laboratory Test Interactions: Guaifenesin has been reported to interfere with clinical laboratory determinations of urinary 5-hydroxyindoleacetic acid (5-HIAA) and urinary vanillylmandelic acid (VMA).

PRECAUTIONS: *(cont'd)*

Pregnancy: Pregnancy Category C. Animal reproduction studies have not been conducted with this drug. It is also not known whether this drug can cause fetal harm when administered to a pregnant woman or can affect reproduction capacity. This drug should be given to a pregnant woman only if clearly needed.

Nursing Mothers: It is not known whether the drugs in this product are excreted in human milk. Because many drugs are excreted in human milk and because of the potential for serious adverse reactions in nursing infants, a decision should be made whether to discontinue nursing or to discontinue the product, taking into account the importance of the drug to the mother.

PEDIATRIC USE: *Capsules:* Safety and effectiveness of this drug in capsule format in children below the age of 12 have not been established.*Liquid:* Safety and effectiveness of this drug in liquid format in children below the age of 2 have not been established.

DRUG INTERACTIONS:

This drug should not be used in patients taking monoamine oxidase inhibitors or other sympathomimetics.

ADVERSE REACTIONS:

Possible adverse reactions include nervousness, insomnia, restlessness, headache, nausea, or gastric irritation. These reactions seldom, if ever, require discontinuation of therapy. Urinary retention may occur in patients with prostatic hypertrophy.

OVERDOSAGE:

The treatment of overdosage should provide symptomatic and supportive care. If the amount ingested is considered dangerous or excessive, induce vomiting with ipecac syrup unless the patient is convulsing, comatose, or has lost the gag reflex, in which case perform gastric lavage using a large-bore tube. If indicated, follow with activated charcoal and a saline cathartic.

DOSAGE AND ADMINISTRATION:

Capsules: *Adults and Children 12 Years of Age and Older:* one capsule four times daily (every 6 hours) with food or fluid. This drug in capsule format is not recommended for children under 12 years of age.

LIQUID

All dosages should be administered four times daily (every 6 hours).

Children

2 to under 4 years... ½ teaspoonful (2.5 ml)

4 to under 6 years... 1 teaspoonful (5 ml)

6 to under 12 years... 1 ½ teaspoonfuls (7.5 ml)

Adults and Children 12 Years of Age and Older: 2 teaspoonfuls (10 ml)

Store below 86°F (30°C). DO NOT REFRIGERATE LIQUID FORM.

HOW SUPPLIED - EQUIVALENTS NOT AVAILABLE:

Capsule, Gelatin - Oral - 200 mg/5 mg/45

100's	$7.65	QUINTEX, Qualitest Pharms	00603-5665-21
100's	$8.69	GUIATEX, Rugby	00536-4459-01
100's	$9.50	ULR, Geneva Pharms	00781-2510-01
100's	$11.70	ENOMINE, Major Pharms	00904-3263-60
100's	$17.04	Duratex, Duramed Pharms	51285-0293-02
100's	$19.25	Phenylfenesin, Goldline Labs	00182-1998-01
100's	$19.25	BANEX, H N Norton Co.	50732-0789-01
100's	$20.45	Guaifenesin/Pe/Phenylprop, HL Moore Drug Exch	00839-7201-06
100's	**$43.85**	**ENTEX, Procter Gamble Pharm**	**00149-0412-01**
100's	$53.30	DESPEC, Intl Ethical	11584-1028-01
500's	$96.25	BANEX, H N Norton Co.	50732-0789-05
500's	**$203.10**	**ENTEX, Procter Gamble Pharm**	**00149-0412-05**

Liquid - Oral - 100 mg/20

120 ml	$6.95	Conex, Llorens Pharm	54859-0511-04
120 ml	$7.00	Decon-E, Norega Labs	51724-0014-04
120 ml	$8.30	DESPEC, Intl Ethical	11584-1030-04
120 ml	$9.15	DESPEC-SF, Intl Ethical	11584-0453-04
240 ml	$8.00	Mytex, Morton Grove	60432-0051-08
473 ml	$19.29	Cyntex, Cypress Pharm	60258-0320-16
480 ml	$11.00	PHENYLFENESIN LIQUID, Goldline Labs	00182-6100-40
480 ml	$13.75	Equi-Tex, Equipharm	57779-0112-09
480 ml	$14.00	PHENTEX, Hi Tech Pharma	50383-0111-16
480 ml	$14.25	ULR LIQUID, Geneva Pharms	00781-6702-16
480 ml	$14.28	BANEX LIQUID, H N Norton Co.	50732-0833-16
480 ml	$14.61	CRANTEX, HL Moore Drug Exch	00839-7562-69
480 ml	$14.80	Guaifenesin/Phenyleph/P-Prop, United Res	00677-1354-33
480 ml	$15.40	Mytex, Morton Grove	60432-0051-16
480 ml	$15.76	Altex, Aligen Independ	00405-2138-16
480 ml	$15.90	ENTAC, Alpharma	00472-0650-16
480 ml	$16.37	GUIATEX, Rugby	00536-2395-85
480 ml	$16.45	ENOMINE, Major Pharms	00904-3262-16
480 ml	$17.00	RYMED, Edwards Pharms	00485-0044-16
480 ml	$17.38	CONTUSS LIQUID, Parmed Pharms	00349-8508-16
480 ml	$17.91	QUINTEX, Qualitest Pharms	00603-1634-58
480 ml	$18.76	Sil-Tex, Silarx Pharms	54838-0503-80
480 ml	$21.56	SYRUP #7, Mikart	46672-0608-16
480 ml	$21.79	P-TEX, Poly Pharms	50991-0916-01
480 ml	$21.79	P-Tex, Poly Pharms	50991-0916-16
480 ml	$22.77	Guaifenex, Ethex	58177-0882-07
480 ml	$28.80	COLDLOC, Flemming Pharms	60976-0125-16
480 ml	**$33.02**	**ENTEX, Procter Gamble Pharm**	**00149-0414-16**

Tablet, Coated - Oral - 400 mg/75 mg

100's	$19.95	RYMED-TR, Edwards Pharms	00485-0045-01
100's	$30.96	PROFEN LA, Primus	55762-0125-02

Tablet, Coated - Oral - 600 mg/120 mg

100's	$39.98	QUINTEX PSE, Qualitest Pharms	00603-5668-21

GUAIFENESIN; PHENYLPROPANOLAMINE HYDROCHLORIDE *(001404)*

CATEGORIES: Antitussives/Expectorants/Mucolytics; Autonomic Drugs; Bronchitis; Common Cold; Congestion; Cough Preparations; Decongestants; Expectorants; Influenza; Mucolytic Agents; Nasal Congestion; Pharyngitis; Respiratory & Allergy Medications; Sinusitis; Sympathomimetic Agents; Sales > $100 Million; FDA Pre 1938 Drugs; Top 200 Drugs

BRAND NAMES: Ami-Tex La; Banex-La; Bestex La; Biotuss La; Contuss-Xt; Despec; Dura-Vent; Endix La; Enomine La; Entex; **Entex LA**; Ephenesin; Ephensin-La; Epibid; Exgest La; Exo-D-La; Gentex-La; Guaioax; Guaipax; Guiatex-La; Harber-Tex; Histacon-X; Lantex-La; Medex-La; Miraphen La; Nolex La; Partuss-La; Phenylfenesin; Profen Ii; Rotex-La; Sinuvent; Stamoist La; Tega D & E; Trintex; Ulr; Vanex-La

FORMULARIES: Aetna; FHP; PCS

DESCRIPTION:

Entex LA is an orange, scored, long-acting tablet for oral administration and contains

phenylpropanolamine hydrochloride... 75 mg

guaifenesin... 400 mg

in a special base to provide a prolonged therapeutic effect.

This product contains ingredients of the following therapeutic classes: decongestant and expectorant.

Phenylpropanolamine hydrochloride is a decongestant having the chemical name, benzenemethanol, α-(1-aminoethyl)-, hydrochloride (R*, S*), (±).

Guaifenesin is an expectorant having the chemical name, 1,2-propanediol, 3-(2-methoxyphenoxy)-.

Entex LA Inactive Ingredients: Each tablet contains carbomer 934 P, compressible sugar, docusate sodium, FD&C Yellow No. 6 Aluminum Lake, hydroxypropyl cellulose, hydroxypropyl methylcellulose, polyethylene glycol, silicon dioxide, stearic acid, titanium dioxide, and zinc stearate.

CLINICAL PHARMACOLOGY:

Phenylpropanolamine hydrochloride is an α-adrenergic receptor agonist (sympathomimetic) which produces vasoconstriction by stimulating α-receptors within the mucosa of the respiratory tract. Clinically, phenylpropanolamine shrinks swollen mucous membranes, reduces tissue hyperemia, edema, and nasal congestion, and increases nasal airway patency. Guaifenesin promotes lower respiratory tract drainage by thinning bronchial secretions, lubricates irritated respiratory tract membranes through increased mucous flow, and facilitates removal of viscous, inspissated mucus. As a result of these drugs, sinus and bronchial drainage is improved, and dry, nonproductive coughs become more productive and less frequent.

INDICATIONS AND USAGE:

Phenylpropanolamine HCl w/guaifenesin long acting tablets are indicated for the symptomatic relief of sinusitis, bronchitis, pharyngitis, and coryza when these conditions are associated with nasal congestion and viscous mucus in the lower respiratory tract.

CONTRAINDICATIONS:

Phenylpropanolamine HCl w/guaifenesin long acting tablets are contraindicated in individuals with known hypersensitivity to sympathomimetics, severe hypertension, or in patients receiving monoamine oxidase inhibitors.

WARNINGS:

Sympathomimetic amines should be used with caution in patients with hypertension, diabetes mellitus, heart disease, peripheral vascular disease, increased intraocular pressure, hyperthyroidism, or prostatic hypertrophy.

PRECAUTIONS:

Information for the Patient: Do not crush or chew phenylpropanolamine HCl w/ guaifenesin long acting tablets prior to swallowing.

Drug/Laboratory Test Interactions: Guaifenesin has been reported to interfere with clinical laboratory determinations of urinary 5-hydroxyindole-acetic acid (5-HIAA) and urinary vanillylmandelic acid (VMA).

Pregnancy: Pregnancy Category C. Animal reproduction studies have not been conducted with phenylpropanolamine HCl w/guaifenesin long acting tablets. It is also not known whether phenylpropanolamine HCl w/guaifenesin long acting tablets, can cause fetal harm when administered to a pregnant woman or can affect reproduction capacity. Phenylpropanolamine HCl w/guaifenesin long acting tablets, should be given to a pregnant woman only if clearly needed.

Nursing Mothers: It is not known whether the drugs in phenylpropanolamine HCl w/ guaifenesin long acting tablets, are excreted in human milk. Because many drugs are excreted in human milk and because of the potential for serious adverse reactions in nursing infants, a decision should be made whether to discontinue nursing or to discontinue the product, taking into account the importance of the drug to the mother.

Pediatric Use: Safety and effectiveness of phenylpropanolamine HCl w/guaifenesin long acting tablets, in children below the age of 6 have not been established.

DRUG INTERACTIONS:

Phenylpropanolamine HCl w/guaifenesin long acting tablets should not be used in patients taking monoamine oxidase inhibitors or other sympathomimetics.

ADVERSE REACTIONS:

Possible adverse reactions include nervousness, insomnia, restlessness, headache, nausea, or gastric irritation. These reactions seldom, if ever, require discontinuation of therapy. Urinary retention may occur in patients with prostatic hypertrophy.

OVERDOSAGE:

The treatment of overdosage should provide symptomatic and supportive care. If the amount ingested is considered dangerous or excessive, induce vomiting with ipecac syrup unless the patient is convulsing, comatose, or has lost the gag reflex, in which case perform gastric lavage using a large-bore tube. If indicated, follow with activated charcoal and a saline cathartic. Since the effects of phenylpropanolamine HCl w/guaifenesin long acting tablet may last up to 12 hours, treatment should be continued for at least that length of time.

DOSAGE AND ADMINISTRATION:

Adults and children 12 years of age and older: one tablet twice daily (every 12 hours).

Children 6 to under 12 years: one-half (1/2) tablet twice daily (every 12 hours). Phenylpropanolamine HCl w/guaifenesin long acting tablets are not recommended for children under 6 years of age.

Tablets may be broken in half for ease of administration without affecting release of medication but should not be crushed or chewed prior to swallowing.

PATIENT INFORMATION:

Guaifenesin with phenylpropanolamine is used for the symptomatic relief of a respiratory condition characterized by a stuffy nose, mucous in the respiratory tract, and dry, nonproductive cough caused by colds, flu, or hay fever. Inform your physician if you are pregnant or nursing. Inform your physician or pharmacist if you have high blood pressure, diabetes, glaucoma, heart disease, or an overactive thyroid. Do not take diet pills while taking this medication. Do not take this medication with a monoamine oxidase inhibitor. This medication may be taken with or without food. Drink a glass of water with each dose. Guaifenesin with phenylpropanolamine may cause trouble sleeping; take your last dose of the day several hours before bedtime. Notify your physician if you develop trouble breathing or a fast, pounding or irregular heart beat. Notify your physician if your cough lasts for more than one week.

HOW SUPPLIED - EQUIVALENTS NOT AVAILABLE:

Tablet, Coated, Sustained Action - Oral - 400 mg/75 mg

14's	$2.35	ENOMINE LA, Major Pharms	00904-3264-54
20's	$2.80	ENOMINE LA, Major Pharms	00904-3264-95
30's	$2.30	Guaifenesin/Phenylprop, Talbert Phcy	44514-0348-18
60's	$4.60	Guaifenesin/Phenylprop, Talbert Phcy	44514-0348-36
100's	$4.95	GUAIPAX, Eon Labs Mfg	00185-0745-01
100's	$7.45	PARTUSS LA, Parmed Pharms	00349-8483-01
100's	$7.75	ENOMINE LA, Major Pharms	00904-3264-60
100's	$8.20	Guaifenesin/Phenylprop, Qualitest Pharms	00603-5214-21
100's	$8.25	Phenylpropanolamine Hcl & Guaifen, Duramed Pharms	51285-0295-02
100's	$8.31	Guaitex La, Vintage Pharms	00254-5052-28
100's	$8.34	Guaitex La, Vintage Pharms	00254-5051-28
100's	$8.93	Phenylpropanolamine/Guaifenesin, United Res	00677-1026-01
100's	$8.95	PHENYLFENESIN LA, Goldline Labs	00182-1798-01
100's	$8.95	Guaifenesin/Phenylprop, Qualitest Pharms	00603-5215-21
100's	$9.00	Guaifenesin Phenylpropanolamine La, Interpharm	53746-0096-01
100's	$9.08	Phenylpropanolamine/Guaifenesin, Sidmak Labs	50111-0385-01
100's	$9.08	Phenylpropanolamine/Guaifenesin, Sidmak Labs	50111-0522-01
100's	$9.10	Guaifenesin W/Phenylpropanoline HCl, Schein Pharm (US)	00364-2138-01
100's	$9.11	Guaifenesin/Phenylprop, HL Moore Drug Exch	00839-7884-06
100's	$9.30	GUIATEX LA, Rugby	00536-3871-01
100's	$9.35	Phenylpropanolamine/Guaifenesin, Martec Pharms	52555-0385-01
100's	$9.42	PARTUSS-LA, Parmed Pharms	00349-8931-01
100's	$9.56	Phenylpropanolamine/Guaifenesin, Aligen Independ	00405-4740-01
100's	$11.00	ULR-LA, Geneva Pharms	00781-1503-01
100's	$11.00	BANEX-LA, H N Norton Co.	50732-0788-01
100's	$19.65	LANTEX-LA, Bolan Pharm	44437-0111-01
100's	$23.75	STAMOIST LA, Huckaby Pharma	58407-0374-01
100's	$33.60	Phenesin L.A., Bergmar Pharm	58173-0003-01
100's	$35.95	CONEX LA, Llorens Pharm	54859-0102-10
100's	$36.70	EXGEST LA, Carnrick	00086-0063-10
100's	$73.92	ENTEX LA, Procter Gamble Pharm	00149-0436-01
500's	$24.50	GUAIPAX, Eon Labs Mfg	00185-0745-05
500's	$31.85	Enomine La, Major Pharms	00904-3264-40
500's	$37.50	PHENYLFENESIN LA, Goldline Labs	00182-1798-05
500's	$38.00	Guaifenesin/Phenylprop, HL Moore Drug Exch	00839-7884-12
500's	$38.30	Guaifenesin/Phenylprop, Qualitest Pharms	00603-5214-28
500's	$38.36	Phenylpropanolamine Hcl & Guaifen, Duramed Pharms	51285-0295-04
500's	$38.75	Guaitex La, Vintage Pharms	00254-5052-35
500's	$38.80	Guaitex La, Vintage Pharms	00254-5051-35
500's	$40.80	Guaifenesin/Phenylprop, Qualitest Pharms	00603-5215-28
500's	$41.00	Guaifenesin/Phenylprop, United Res	00677-1026-05
500's	$42.00	Guaifenesin W/Phenylpropanoline HCl, Schein Pharm (US)	00364-2138-05
500's	$42.20	Phenylpropanolamine/Guaifenesin, Sidmak Labs	50111-0385-02
500's	$42.20	Phenylpropanolamine/Guaifenesin, Sidmak Labs	50111-0522-02
500's	$44.42	Guaifenesin/Phenylprop, Aligen Independ	00405-4740-02
500's	$44.90	PARTUSS-LA, Parmed Pharms	00349-8931-05
500's	$44.94	PARTUSS LA, Parmed Pharms	00349-8483-05
500's	$52.00	ULR-LA, Geneva Pharms	00781-1503-05
500's	$52.00	BANEX-LA, H N Norton Co.	50732-0788-05
500's	$59.30	Phenylpropanolamine/Guaifenesin, Martec Pharms	52555-0385-05
500's	$59.85	Guaifenesin/Phenylprop, Interpharm	53746-0096-05
500's	$156.50	EXGEST LA, Carnrick	00086-0063-50
500's	$358.48	ENTEX LA, Procter Gamble Pharm	00149-0436-05
1000's	$47.50	GUAIPAX, Eon Labs Mfg	00185-0745-10
1000's	$66.60	Guaifenesin/Phenylprop, Major Pharms	00904-3264-80
1000's	$85.95	GUIATEX LA, Rugby	00536-3871-10

Tablet, Coated, Sustained Action - Oral - 600 mg/37.5 mg

100's	$37.14	PROFEN II, Wakefield Pharms	59310-0107-10

Tablet, Coated, Sustained Action - Oral - 600 mg/75 mg

50's	$34.80	Coldloc-La, Flemming Pharms	60976-0675-05
100's	$39.70	PROFEN LA, Wakefield Pharms	59310-0104-10
100's	$42.45	Guaivent, Qualitest Pharms	00603-3778-21
100's	$42.95	G-Vent, Pharmacist Choice	54979-0165-01
100's	$49.95	Guaivent, Pecos	59879-0108-01
100's	$50.00	Sinuvent, WE Pharm	59196-0001-01
100's	$50.33	Guaifenex Ppa 75, Ethex	58177-0204-04
100's	$52.45	Guaivent, HL Moore Drug Exch	00839-8018-06
100's	$59.45	Guiavent, Rugby	00536-5635-01
100's	$62.40	Coldloc-La, Flemming Pharms	60976-0675-10
100's	$63.44	DESPEC-SR, Intl Ethical	11584-0441-01
600's	$260.00	Sinuvent, WE Pharm	59196-0001-06

Tablet, Uncoated, Sustained Action - Oral - 200 mg/75 mg

100's	$9.11	Phenylpropanolamine & Guaifenesin La, HL Moore Drug Exch	00839-7130-06
500's	$35.03	Phenylpropanolamine & Guaifenesin La, HL Moore Drug Exch	00839-7130-12

GUAIFENESIN; PSEUDOEPHEDRINE HYDROCHLORIDE *(001405)*

CATEGORIES: Allergies; Antihistamines; Antitussives/Expectorants/Mucolytics; Autonomic Drugs; Common Cold; Congestion; Cough Preparations; Decongestants; Expectorants; Hay Fever; Mucolytic Agents; Nasal Congestion; Respiratory & Allergy Medications; Sympathomimetic Agents; Pregnancy Category C; FDA Pre 1938 Drugs

BRAND NAMES: Altex Pse; Anatuss La; Congess Jr; Congess Jr.; Congess Sr; Congess Sr.; Conpec L.A.; Decongestant Ii; **Deconsal**; Deconsal Ii; Demibid Ii; Duogest; Entex Pse; Eudal Sr; Eudal-Sr; Ex-Span; Fenex-Pse; G-Phed; G-Phed-Pd;

G-Tuss; Gp 500; Guai-Sudo; Guaibid D; Guaifed; Guaifed-Pd; Guaifen Pse; Guaifen-P; Guaifen-P-Pd; Guaifenesin W/Pseudoephedrine; Guaifenesin/Pseudoephedrine; Guaimax-D; Guaitab; Guiadrine Ii; Guiadrine Pse; Guiafed; Guiafenesin/Pseudoephedrine; Guiatex Ii; Guiatex Pse; Histalet X; Iotex Pse; K-Gest, S.A.; Maxifed; Maxifed-G; Medent; Nalex; Nasabid; Nasatab La; Pan-Mist La; Profed; Pseudo G/Psi; Pseudo-G/Psi; Pseudocot-G; Pseudofen; Pseudofen-Pd; Quintex Pse; Respaire-120; Respaire-120 Sr; Respaire-60; Respaire-60 Sr; Respinol La; Respinol-G; Ru-Tuss De; Rymed; Sinufed; Sinumist-Sr; Stamoist E; Suda-X; Sudex; Syn-Rx; T-Moist; Touro La; Tuss-La; V-Dec-M; Zaptec Pse; Zephrex; Zephrex La; Zephrex-La

FORMULARIES: Aetna

DESCRIPTION:

Please note the brand names, Deconsal II Tablets and Deconsal L.A. Tablets have been used in this monograph where noted to avoid confusion.

Deconsal II: Each scored, dark blue Deconsal II Tablet provides 60 mg pseudoephedrine hydrochloride and 600 mg guaifenesin in a sustained-release formulation intended for oral administration. Inactive ingredients: Stearic acid, dibasic calcium phosphate, FD&C Blue #1 Lake, sodium lauryl sulfate, ethylcellulose, magnesium stearate.

Deconsal L.A.: Each scored, light blue Deconsal L.A. Tablet provides 120 mg pseudoephedrine hydrochloride and 400 mg guaifenesin in a sustained-release formulation intended for oral administration.

Pseudoephedrine hydrochloride is a nasal decongestant. Chemically, it is [S-(R*,R*)]-α-[1-(methylamino)ethyl]-, benzenemethanol hydrochloride and has the following formula: $C_{10}H_{15}NO°HCl$ and a molecular weight of 201.70.

Guaifenesin is an expectorant. Chemically it is, 3-(2-methoxyphenoxy)-1,2 propanediol and has the following chemical formula: $C_{10}H_{14}O_4$ and a molecular weight of 198.22.

CLINICAL PHARMACOLOGY:

Pseudoephedrine hydrochloride is an orally indirect acting sympathomimetic amine and exerts a decongestant action on the nasal mucosa. It does this by vasoconstriction which results in reduction of tissue hyperemia, edema, nasal congestion, and an increase in nasal airway patency. The vasoconstriction action of pseudoephedrine is similar to that of ephedrine. In the usual dose it has minimal vasopressor effects. Pseudoephedrine is rapidly and almost completely absorbed from the gastrointestinal tract. It has a plasma half-life of 6 to 8 hours. Alkaline urine is associated with slower elimination of the drug. The drug is distributed to body tissues and fluids, including the central nervous system (CNS). Approximately 50% to 75% of the administered dose is excreted unchanged in the urine; the remainder is apparently metabolized in the liver to inactive compounds by N-demethylation, parahydroxylation and oxidative deamination.

Guaifenesin is an expectorant which increases respiratory tract fluid secretions and helps loosen phlegm and bronchial secretions. By reducing the viscosity of secretions, guaifenesin increases the efficiency of the mucociliary mechanism in removing accumulated secretions from the upper and lower airway. Guaifenesin is readily absorbed from the gastrointestinal tract and is rapidly metabolized and excreted in the urine. Guaifenesin has a plasma half-life of one hour. The major urinary metabolite is β-(2-methoxyphenoxy) lactic acid.

INDICATIONS AND USAGE:

Pseudoephedrine HCl w/ guaifenesin tablets are indicated for the temporary relief of nasal congestion and cough associated with respiratory tract infections and related conditions such as sinusitis, pharyngitis, bronchitis, and asthma, when these conditions are complicated by tenacious mucus and/or mucus plugs and congestion. The product is effective in productive as well as non-productive cough which tends to injure the mucus membrane of the air passages.

CONTRAINDICATIONS:

Pseudoephedrine HCl w/ guaifenesin tablets are contraindicated in patients with hypersensitivity to guaifenesin, or with hypersensitivity or idiosyncrasy to sympathomimetic amines which may be manifested by insomnia, dizziness, weakness and tremor or arrhythmias.

Sympathomimetic amines are contraindicated in patients with severe hypertension, severe coronary artery disease and patients on monoamine oxidase inhibitor (MAOI) therapy and for 14 days after stopping MAOI therapy. (See DRUG INTERACTIONS.)

WARNINGS:

Sympathomimetic amines should be used with caution in patients with hypertension, ischemic heart disease, diabetes mellitus, increased intraocular pressure, hyperthyroidism, or prostatic hypertrophy. Sympathomimetics may produce central nervous system stimulation with convulsions or cardiovascular collapse with accompanying hypotension.

Do not exceed recommended dosage.

Hypertensive crises can occur with concurrent use of pseudoephedrine or phenylephrine and MAOI, and for 14 days after stopping MAOI therapy, indomethacin, or with beta-blockers and methyldopa. If a hypertensive crisis occurs, these drugs should be discontinued immediately and therapy to lower blood pressure should be instituted. Fever should be managed by means of external cooling.

PRECAUTIONS:

General: Use with caution in patients with diabetes, hypertension, cardiovascular disease and intolerance to ephedrine.

Before prescribing medication to suppress or modify cough, it is important too ascertain that the underlying cause of cough is identified, that modification of cough does not increase the risk of clinical or physiologic complications, and that appropriate therapy for the primary disease is instituted.

Information for the Patient: Patients should be instructed to check with physician if symptoms do not improve within 5 days or fever is present.

Pediatric Use: This product is not recommended for use in pediatric patients under 2 years of age.

Use in Elderly: The elderly (60 years and older) are more likely to experience adverse reactions to sympathomimetics. Overdosage of sympathomimetics in this age group may cause hallucinations, convulsions, CNS depression, and death.

Drug/Laboratory Interactions: Guaifenesin may increase renal clearance for urate and thereby lower serum uric acid levels. Guaifenesin may produce an increase in urinary 5-hydroxyindoleacetic acid and may therefore interfere with the interpretation of this test for the diagnosis of carcinoid syndrome. It may also falsely elevate the VMA test for catechols. Administration of this drug should be discontinued 48 hours prior to the collection of urine specimens for such tests.

Carcinogenesis, Mutagenesis, and Impairment of Fertility: No data are available on the long-term potential of the components of this product for carcinogenesis, mutagenesis, or impairment of fertility in animals or or humans.

PRECAUTIONS: *(cont'd)*

Pregnancy Category C: Animal reproduction studies have not been conducted with pseudoephedrine HCl w/ guaifenesin tablets. It is also not known whether pseudoephedrine HCl w/ guaifenesin tablets can cause fetal harm when administered to a pregnant woman or can affect reproduction capacity. Pseudoephedrine HCl w/ guaifenesin should be given to a pregnant woman only if clearly needed.

Nursing Mothers: Pseudoephedrine is excreted in breast milk. Use of this product by nursing mothers is not recommended because of the higher than usual risk for infants from sympathomimetic amines.

DRUG INTERACTIONS:

Do not prescribe this product for use in patients that are now taking a prescription MAOI (certain drugs for depression, psychiatric or emotional conditions, or Parkinson's disease), or for 14 days after stopping the MAOI drug therapy. Beta-adrenergic blockers and MAOI may potentiate the pressor effect of pseudoephedrine. (see WARNINGS.) Concurrent use of digitalis glycosides may increase the possibility of cardiac arrhythmias. Sympathomimetics may reduce the hypotensive effects of guanethidine, mecamylamine, methyldopa, reserpine and veratrum alkaloids. Concurrent use of tricyclic antidepressants may antagonize the effects of pseudoephedrine.

ADVERSE REACTIONS:

Hyper-reactive individuals may display ephedrine-like reactions such as tachycardia, palpitations, headache, dizziness, or nausea. Sympathomimetics have been associated with certain untoward reactions including fear, anxiety, nervousness, restlessness, tremor, weakness, pallor, respiratory difficulty, dysuria, insomnia, hallucinations, convulsions, CNS depression, arrhythmias, and cardiovascular collapse with hypotension. No serious side effects have been reported with the use of guaifenesin.

OVERDOSAGE:

Since pseudoephedrine HCl w/ guaifenesin tablets contain two pharmacologically different compounds, treatment of overdosage should be based upon the symptomatology of the patient as it relates to the individual ingredients. Treatment of acute overdosage would probably be based upon treating the patient for pseudoephedrine toxicity which may manifest itself as excessive CNS stimulation resulting the excitement tremor, restlessness, and insomnia. Other effects may include tachycardia, hypertension, pallor, mydriasis, hyperglycemia and urinary retention. Severe overdosage may cause tachypnea or hyperpnea, hallucinations, convulsions or delirium, but in some individuals there may be CNS depression. Arrhythmias (including ventricular fibrillation) may lead to hypotension and circulatory collapse. Severe hypokalemia can occur, probably due to a compartmental shift rather than a depletion of potassium. No organ damage or significant metabolic derangement is associated with pseudoephedrine overdosage. Overdosage with guaifenesin is unlikely to produce toxic effects since its toxicity is much lower than that of pseudoephedrine. In severe cases of overdose, it is recommended to monitor the patient in an intensive care setting.

The LD_{50} of pseudoephedrine (single oral dose) has been reported to be 726 mg/kg in the mouse, 2206 mg/kg in the rat and 1177 mg/kg in the rabbit. The toxic and lethal concentrations in human biologic fluids are not known. Urinary excretion increases with acidification and decreases with alkalization of the urine. There are few published reports of toxicity due to pseudoephedrine and no case of fatal overdosage has been reported. Guaifenesin, when administered by stomach tube to test animals in doses up to 5 grams/kg, produced no signs of toxicity.

Since the action of sustained release products may continue for as long as 12 hours, treatment of overdosage should be directed toward reducing further absorption and supporting the patient for at least that length of time. Gastric emptying (Syrup of Ipecac) and/or lavage is recommended as soon as possible after ingestion, even if the patient has vomited spontaneously. Either isotonic or half-isotonic saline may be used for lavage. Administration of an activated charcoal slurry is beneficial after lavage and/or emesis if less than 4 hours have passed since ingestion. Saline cathartics, such as Milk of Magnesia, are useful for hastening the evacuation of unreleased medication.

Adrenergic receptor blocking agents are antidotes to pseudoephedrine. In practice, the most useful is the beta-blocker propranolol which is indicated where there are signs of cardiac toxicity. Theoretically, pseudoephedrine is dialyzable but procedures have not been clinically established.

DOSAGE AND ADMINISTRATION:

Adults and adolescents over 12 years of age: One or two tablets every 12 hours not to exceed 4 tablets in 24 hours.

Children 6 to under 12 years: 1 tablet every 12 hours not to exceed 2 tablets in 24 hours.

Children 2 to 6 years: 1/2 tablet every 12 hours not to exceed 1 tablet in 24 hours.

Store at controlled room temperature between 15° C and 30° C (59°F and 86°F). Dispense in tight, light- resistant containers.

HOW SUPPLIED - RATED THERAPEUTICALLY EQUIVALENT:

Capsule - Oral - 250/120 mg

100's	$30.50	Guaifenesin; Pseudoephedrine Hcl, Duramed Pharms	51285-0855-02

Capsule - Oral - 300/60 mg

100's	$28.25	Guaifenesin; Pseudoephedrine Hcl, Duramed Pharms	51285-0856-02

Capsule, Gelatin, Sustained Action - Oral - 250 mg/120 mg

100's	$56.80	Guaivent, Ethex	58177-0016-04

Capsule, Gelatin, Sustained Action - Oral - 300 mg/60 mg

100's	$45.28	Guaivent-Pd, Ethex	58177-0015-04

HOW SUPPLIED - NOT RATED EQUIVALENT:

Capsule, Gelatin - Oral - 250 mg/30 mg

100's	$18.00	RYMED, Edwards Pharms	00485-0043-01

Capsule, Gelatin, Sustained Action - Oral - 125 mg/60 mg

100's	$25.00	CONGESS JR., Fleming	00256-0174-01
1000's	$163.00	CONGESS JR., Fleming	00256-0174-02

Capsule, Gelatin, Sustained Action - Oral - 200 mg/60 mg

100's	$33.88	RESPAIRE-60 SR, Laser	00277-0174-01

Capsule, Gelatin, Sustained Action - Oral - 250 mg/120 mg

100's	$27.00	CONGESS SR, Fleming	00256-0173-01
100's	$28.20	Pseudofen, Rugby	00536-5626-01
100's	$29.76	Guaifen-P, Qualitest Pharms	00603-3776-21
100's	$35.03	Guaifenesin W/Pseudoephedrine, HL Moore Drug Exch	00839-7925-06
100's	$39.00	G-Phed, Alphagen Labs	59743-0002-01
100's	$39.99	RESPAIRE-SR 120, Laser	00277-0169-01
100's	$45.00	Guaifenesin W/Pseudoephedrine, United Res	00677-1503-01
100's	$56.80	G-Fed, Pecos	59879-0508-01

HOW SUPPLIED - NOT RATED EQUIVALENT: *(cont'd)*

100's	$58.42	Guaibid D, Econolab	55053-0860-01
100's	$61.50	Guaifenesin W/Pseudoephedrine, Aligen Independ	00405-4466-01
100's	$78.28	GUAIFED, Muro Pharm	00451-4002-50
500's	$371.71	GUAIFED, Muro Pharm	00451-4002-60
1000's	$186.50	CONGESS SR, Fleming	00256-0173-02

Capsule, Gelatin, Sustained Action - Oral - 300 mg/60 mg

100's	$25.50	Pseudofen-Pd, Rugby	00536-5627-01
100's	$27.82	Guaifen-P-Pd, Qualitest Pharms	00603-3777-21
100's	$30.80	Guaifenesin W/Pseudoephedrine, HL Moore Drug Exch	00839-7924-06
100's	$35.00	G-Phed-Pd, Alphagen Labs	59743-0003-01
100's	$36.00	Guaifenesin W/Pseudoephedrine, United Res	00677-1502-01
100's	$45.25	G-Fed Ped, Pecos	59879-0509-01
100's	$46.49	Guaibid D, Econolab	55053-0870-01
100's	$48.94	Guaifenesin W/Pseudoephedrine, Aligen Independ	00405-4465-01
100's	$62.40	GUAIFED PD, Muro Pharm	00451-4003-50
500's	$295.75	GUAIFED PD, Muro Pharm	00451-4003-60

Syrup - Oral

480 ml	$9.31	GUIAFED, Rugby	00536-0890-85

Tablet, Coated, Sustained Action - Oral - 400 mg/120 mg

100's	$34.50	Nasatab La, ECR Pharms	00095-0225-01
100's	$35.16	SUDA-X, H N Norton Co.	50732-0117-01
100's	$42.36	EUDAL-S.R., UAD Labs	00785-6301-01
100's	$54.00	ANATUSS LA, Mayrand Pharms	00259-0379-01

Tablet, Coated, Sustained Action - Oral - 500 mg/60 mg

100's	$24.67	Sudal, Atley Pharms	59702-0060-01
100's	$27.50	Venbid, Venture Pharm	59785-0102-10
100's	$38.95	Maxifed-G, Am Pharms	58605-0506-01

Tablet, Coated, Sustained Action - Oral - 500 mg/120 mg

100's	$21.70	GP-500, Marnel Pharceut	00682-0500-01
100's	$24.78	TUSS-LA, Hyrex Pharms	00314-8050-01
100's	$28.75	Stamoist E, Huckaby Pharma	58407-0375-01
100's	$43.62	Touro La, Dartmouth Pharms	58869-0536-01
100's	$100.00	CONPEC L A, Teral Labs	51234-0129-90

Tablet, Coated, Sustained Action - Oral - 600 mg/60 mg

56's	$31.20	SYN-RX, Medeva Pharms	53014-0308-14
100's	$25.00	Profed, Am Pharms	58605-0510-01
100's	$30.62	Guaifenex Pse, Ethex	58177-0214-04
100's	$32.50	Guiadrine Ii, Pharmacist Choice	54979-0149-01
100's	$32.50	Demibid Ii, Econolab	55053-0140-01
100's	$34.21	Guaifenesin W/Pseudoephedrine, Aligen Independ	00405-4467-01
100's	$34.45	Guiatex Ii, Rugby	00536-5590-01
100's	$35.85	Guaifenesin W/Pseudoephedrine, United Res	00677-1487-01
100's	$35.95	D-Feda Ii, WE Pharm	59196-0005-01
100's	$37.30	Defen-La, Horizon Pharm	59630-0110-10
100's	$38.00	Respa-1St, Respa Pharms	60575-0108-19
100's	$38.80	Guaifenesin W/Pseudoephedrine, Goldline Labs	00182-1037-01
100's	$38.90	Decongestant Ii, Qualitest Pharms	00603-3116-21
100's	$38.90	Desal-Ii, Alphagen Labs	59743-0050-01
100's	$39.95	Decongestant Ii, Pecos	59879-0116-01
100's	$42.60	Guaifenesin W/Pseudoephedrine, Trinity Technologies	61355-0201-10
100's	$42.65	Guiadrine II, HL Moore Drug Exch	00839-7898-06
100's	**$62.01**	**DECONSAL II, Medeva Pharms**	**53014-0017-10**
500's	**$303.81**	**DECONSAL II, Medeva Pharms**	**53014-0017-50**

Tablet, Coated, Sustained Action - Oral - 600 mg/120 mg

100's	$24.50	Sudal, Atley Pharms	59702-0600-01
100's	$33.00	Maxifed, Am Pharms	58605-0505-01
100's	$34.80	Duraphen, Qualitest Pharms	00603-3507-21
100's	$39.95	Guiafenesin/Pseudoephedrine, Harber Pharm	51432-0647-03
100's	$39.95	Guaifed-Pse, Pecos	59879-0112-01
100's	$39.98	Fenex-Pse, Tmk Pharm	59582-0003-01
100's	$42.00	Guaifenesin/Pseudoephedrine, Duramed Pharms	51285-0401-02
100's	$42.95	G-Tuss, Pharmacist Choice	54979-0162-01
100's	$45.00	Guaipax Pse, Eon Labs Mfg	00185-0784-01
100's	$45.16	Altex Pse, Aligen Independ	00405-4040-01
100's	$45.44	Guaifen Pse, Vintage Pharms	00254-6211-28
100's	$45.85	Guaifenesin W/Pseudoephedrine, Goldline Labs	00182-1740-01
100's	$47.50	Guaimax-D, Schwarz Pharma (US)	00131-2055-37
100's	$47.75	Guiadrine Pse, Pharmacist Choice	54979-0142-01
100's	$49.90	Guaifenesin with Pseudoephedrine, United Res	00677-1476-01
100's	$49.94	Pseudo & Guafenesin, HL Moore Drug Exch	00839-7754-06
100's	$51.50	Guaifenex Pse, Ethex	58177-0208-04
100's	$52.54	ZEPHREX LA, Bock Pharma	00563-2627-01
100's	$52.90	Guaifenesin W/Pseudoephedrine, Trinity Technologies	61355-0202-10
100's	$53.30	Guiatex Pse, Rugby	00536-5535-01
100's	$54.94	Guai-Sudo, MD Pharm	43567-0451-07
100's	$56.05	Altex-Pse, Alphagen Labs	59743-0059-01
100's	$56.56	DURATUSS, UCB Pharma	50474-0612-01
100's	$56.70	Pseudo G/Psi, Major Pharms	00904-7689-60
100's	$56.70	Pseudo-G/Psi, Major Pharms	00904-7861-60
100's	$56.86	Zaptec Pse, Am Generics	58634-0033-01
100's	$61.90	RU-TUSS DE, Knoll Pharms	00048-0090-01
100's	$73.92	ENTEX PSE, Procter Gamble Pharm	00149-0427-02
250's	$106.90	Guaipax Pse, Eon Labs Mfg	00185-0784-52
250's	$113.40	Pseudo G/Psi, Major Pharms	00904-7689-70
250's	$113.40	Pseudo-G/Psi, Major Pharms	00904-7861-70
500's	$152.67	Guaifenesin W/Pseudoephedrine, HL Moore Drug Exch	00839-7754-12
500's	$179.88	Guaifen-Pse, Vintage Pharms	00254-6211-35
500's	$179.88	Guaifen-Pse, Qualitest Pharms	00603-5668-28
500's	$191.00	Guiadrine Pse, Pharmacist Choice	54979-0142-05
500's	$193.00	Altex-Pse, Alphagen Labs	59743-0059-05
500's	$208.75	Guaifenesin/Pseudoephedrine, Duramed Pharms	51285-0401-04
500's	$213.75	Guaipax Pse, Eon Labs Mfg	00185-0784-05
500's	$235.40	Guaifenesin W/Pseudoephedrine, Trinity Technologies	61355-0202-50

Tablet, Uncoated - Oral - 100 mg/60 mg

100's	$8.50	PSEUDOCOT G LAYTAB, C O Truxton	00463-7014-01

Tablet, Uncoated - Oral - 400 mg/60 mg

100's	$29.21	GUAITAB, Muro Pharm	00451-4600-50
100's	$46.56	ZEPHREX, Bock Pharma	00563-2624-01

GUAIFENESIN; PSEUDOEPHEDRINE; THEOPHYLLINE *(001406)*

CATEGORIES: Antiasthmatics/Bronchodilators; Antitussives/Expectorants/Mucolytics; Expectorants; Respiratory & Allergy Medications; Respiratory Muscle Relaxant; Smooth Muscle Relaxants; FDA Pre 1938 Drugs

BRAND NAMES: Broncomar; Hycoff-A Nn

Prescribing information not available at time of publication.

HOW SUPPLIED - EQUIVALENTS NOT AVAILABLE:

Liquid - Oral - 15 mg/100 mg/45

pint only	$16.00	HYCOFF-A NN, Saron	00834-6046-73

Tablet, Uncoated - Oral - 100 mg/30 mg/10

100's	$18.79	BRONCOMAR, Marlop Pharms	12939-0112-02
1000's	$168.60	BRONCOMAR, Marlop Pharms	12939-0112-90

GUAIFENESIN; THEOPHYLLINE *(001407)*

CATEGORIES: Airway Obstruction; Antiasthmatics/Bronchodilators; Antitussives/Expectorants/Mucolytics; Asthma; Bronchial Dilators; Bronchitis; Bronchospasm; Chronic Bronchitis; Decongestants; Emphysema; Respiratory & Allergy Medications; Respiratory Muscle Relaxant; Smooth Muscle Relaxants; Xanthine Derivatives; Pregnancy Category C; FDA Pre 1938 Drugs

BRAND NAMES: *Amilex*; Asbron-G; *Asianbron*; Bronchial; *Bronchil*; *Broncophylin*; *Broncophylline*; *Dilabron*; Ed-Bron G; **Elixophyllin-Gg**; *Equibran*; Equibron G; Glyceryl-T; Glynazan; Lanophyllin-Gg; *Polyphed*; *Pulmatropine Con Teofilina*; Q-B; Quelan; Quiatex; *Quibran*; Quibron; Slo-Phyllin Gg; Solu-Phyllin Gg; Synophylate-Gg; Theo-G; Theocolate; Theolate; Uni-Bronchial
(International brand names outside U.S. in italics)

FORMULARIES: Aetna

COST OF THERAPY: $46.86 (Asthma; Capsule; 90 mg/150 mg; 3/day; 365 days)

PRIMARY ICD9: 493.90 (Asthma, Unspecified, Without Mention of Status Asthmaticus)

DESCRIPTION:

Each theophylline w/guaifenesin gelatin capsule or tablespoonful (15 ml) of liquid contains 100 mg of theophylline (anhydrous) and 100 mg of guaifenesin, as an oral bronchodilator-expectorant.

Theophylline (1 *H*-Purine-2,6-dione, 3,7-dihydro-1,3-dimethyl-), a xanthine compound, is a white, odorless, crystalline powder, having a bitter taste.

Guaifenesin (1,2-Propanediol, 3-(2-methoxyphenoxy)-), a guaiacol compound, is a white to slightly yellow crystalline powder with a bitter, aromatic taste.

Theophylline w/guaifenesin inactive ingredients: black iron oxide, dimethylpolysiloxane, FD&C Blue No. 1, gelatin, glycerin, lecithin, methylparaben, pharmaceutical glaze, polyethylene glycol, propylparaben, sorbitol, titanium dioxide.

Elixophyllin Elixir Inactive Ingredients: Citric acid, flavors, glycerin, methylparaben, propylene glycol, sodium benzoate, saccharin sodium, sorbitol, sucrose, purified water.

CLINICAL PHARMACOLOGY:

Theophylline: Theophylline directly relaxes the smooth muscle of the bronchial airways and pulmonary blood vessels, thus acting mainly as a bronchodilator, pulmonary vasodilator and smooth muscle relaxant. The drug also possesses other actions typical of the xanthine derivatives: coronary vasodilator, diuretic, cardiac stimulant, cerebral stimulant, and skeletal muscle stimulant. The actions of theophylline may be mediated through inhibition of phosphodiesterase and a resultant increase in intracellular cyclic AMP which could mediate smooth muscle relaxation. At concentrations higher than attained *in vivo,* theophylline also inhibits the release of histamine by mast cells.

In vitro, theophylline has been shown to react synergistically with beta agonists that increase intracellular cyclic AMP through the stimulation of adenyl cyclase (isoproterenol), but synergism has not been demonstrated in patient studies and more data are needed to determine if theophylline and beta agonists have clinically important additive effects *in vivo.*

Apparently, no development of tolerance occurs with chronic use of theophylline. The half-life is shortened with cigarette smoking. The half-life is prolonged in alcoholism, reduced hepatic or renal function, congestive heart failure, and in patients receiving antibiotics such as TAO (troleandomycin), erythromycin and clindamycin. High fever for prolonged periods may decrease theophylline elimination (TABLE 1).

TABLE 1 Theophylline Elimination Characteristics

	Theophylline Clearance Rates (mean ± S.D.)	Half-life Average (mean ± S.D.)
Children (over 1 year of age)	1.45 ± .58 ml/kg/min	3.7 ± 1.1 hours
Adult nonsmokers with uncomplicated asthma	.65 ± .19 ml/kg/min	8.7 ± 2.2 hours

Newborn infants have extremely slow clearances and half-lives exceeding 24 hours which approach those seen for older children after about 3-6 months.

Older adults with chronic obstructive pulmonary disease, any patients with cor pulmonale or other causes of heart failure, and patients with liver pathology may have much lower clearances with half-lives that may exceed 24 hours.

The half-life of theophylline in smokers (1 to 2 packs/day) averaged 4 to 5 hours among various studies, much shorter than the half-life in nonsmokers, who averaged about 7 to 9 hours. The increase in theophylline clearance caused by smoking is probably the result of induction of drug-metabolizing enzymes that do not readily normalize after cessation of smoking. It appears that between 3 months and 2 years may be necessary for normalization of the effect of smoking on theophylline pharmacokinetics.

Guaifenesin: Guaifenesin increases respiratory tract secretions, possibly by stimulating the Goblet cells.

Guaifenesin appears to be well absorbed, but its pharmacokinetics have not been thoroughly studied.

INDICATIONS AND USAGE:

For relief and/or prevention of symptoms of asthma and reversible bronchospasm associated with chronic bronchitis and emphysema.

CONTRAINDICATIONS:

Theophylline w/guaifenesin is contraindicated in individuals who have shown hypersensitivity to any of the components of this product or to xanthine derivatives.

WARNINGS:

Status asthmaticus is a medical emergency. Optimal therapy frequently requires additional medication including corticosteroids when the patient is not rapidly responsive to bronchodilators. Excessive theophylline doses may be associated with toxicity. Therefore, monitoring of serum theophylline levels is recommended to ensure maximal benefit without excessive risk. Incidence of toxicity increases at levels greater than 20 mcg/ml. Morphine, curare, and stilbamidine should be used with caution in patients with airflow obstruction since they stimulate histamine release and can induce asthmatic attacks. They may also suppress respiration leading to respiratory failure. Alternative drugs should be chosen whenever possible.

There is an excellent correlation between high blood levels of theophylline resulting from conventional doses and associated clinical manifestations of toxicity in (1) patients with lowered body plasma clearances (due to transient cardiac decompensation), (2) patients with liver dysfunction or chronic obstructive pulmonary disease, and (3) patients who are older than 55 years of age, particularly males. There are often no early signs of less serious theophylline toxicity such as nausea and restlessness, which may appear in up to 50 percent of patients prior to onset of convulsions. Ventricular arrhythmias or seizures may be the first signs of toxicity.

Many patients who have higher theophylline serum levels exhibit tachycardia.

Theophylline products may cause or worsen arrhythmias and any significant change in rate and/or rhythm warrants monitoring and further investigation.

Decreased clearance of theophylline may be associated with either influenza immunization or active influenza, and with other viral infections.

It is important to consider reduction of dosage and measurement of serum theophylline levels in the above individuals.

PRECAUTIONS:

GENERAL

Theophylline: Mean half-life in smokers is shorter than nonsmokers; therefore, smokers may require larger doses of theophylline. Theophylline should not be administered concurrently with other xanthine medications. Use with caution in patients with severe cardiac disease, severe hypoxemia, hypertension, hyperthyroidism, acute myocardial injury, cor pulmonale, congestive heart failure, liver disease, and in the elderly (especially males) and in neonates. Great caution should especially be used in giving theophylline to patients in congestive heart failure. Such patients have shown markedly prolonged theophylline blood level curves with theophylline persisting in serum for long periods following discontinuation of the drug.

Use theophylline cautiously in patients with a history of peptic ulcer. Theophylline may occasionally act as a local irritant to G.I. tract although gastrointestinal symptoms are more commonly central and associated with serum concentrations over 20 mcg/ml.

Xanthines can potentiate hypokalemia resulting from $beta_2$ agonist therapy, steroids, diuretics, other xanthines and hypoxia. Particular caution is advised in severe asthma. It is recommended that serum potassium levels be monitored in such situations.

DRUG/LABORATORY TEST INTERACTIONS

Theophylline may increase uric acid levels and urinary catecholamines. Metabolites of guaifenesin may contribute to increased urinary 5-hydroxy-indoleacetic acid readings, when determined with nitrosonaphthol reagent.

CARCINOGENESIS, MUTAGENESIS, AND IMPAIRMENT OF FERTILITY

Long-term animal studies have not been performed to evaluate the carcinogenic potential, mutagenic potential, or the effect on fertility by xanthine compounds.

USAGE IN PREGNANCY: PREGNANCY CATEGORY C

Teratogenic Effects: Reproduction studies performed in mice and rats at oral doses from 7 to 17 times the human dose (maximum human dose for adults assumed to be 13 mg/kg/day) have indicated that theophylline may cause malformations, but these effects only occurred at or near doses that were toxic to the maternal animals. There are no adequate and well-controlled studies in pregnant women. It is not known whether theophylline can cause fetal harm when administered to a pregnant woman or can affect reproduction capacity. Theophylline w/guaifenesin should be used during pregnancy only if the potential benefit justifies the potential risk to the fetus.

Nonteratogenic Effects: Theophylline may be excreted in the milk and cause irritability in the nursing infant. Therefore, caution should be exercised when theophylline w/guaifenesin is administered to a nursing mother.

NURSING MOTHERS

Theophylline is distributed into breast milk and may cause irritability or other signs of toxicity in nursing infants. Because of the potential for serious adverse reactions in nursing infants from theophylline, a decision should be made whether to discontinue nursing or to discontinue the drug, taking into account the importance of the drug to the mother.

PEDIATRIC USE

Sufficient numbers of infants under the age of 1 year have not been studied in clinical trials to support use in this age group; however, there is evidence recorded that the use of dosage recommendations for older infants and young children (16 mg/kg/24 hours) may result in the development of toxic serum levels. Such findings very probably reflect differences in the metabolic handling of the drug related to absent or undeveloped enzyme systems. Consequently, prescribers of the drug for this age group should carefully consider the associated benefits and risks. If used, the maintenance dose must be conservative and in accord with the following guidelines:

INITIAL MAINTENANCE DOSAGE OF THEOPHYLLINE ANHYDROUS

Premature Infants: Up to 24 days postnatal age-1.0 mg/kg every 12 hours.

Beyond 24 Days Postnatal Age: 1.5 mg/kg every 12 hours.

Infants 6 to 52 Weeks: ((0.2 × age in weeks) + 5.0) × kg body wt=24 hours dose in mg.

Up to 26 Weeks: divide into dosing intervals every 8 hours.

From 26-52 Weeks: divide into dosing intervals every 6 hours.Final dosage should be guided by serum concentration after a steady state (no further accumulation of drug) has been achieved.

DRUG INTERACTIONS:

Drug-Drug: Toxic synergism with ephedrine has been documented and may occur with some other sympathomimetic bronchodilators. In addition, the following drug interactions have been demonstrated (TABLE 2):

TABLE 2

Drug	Effect
Theophylline with:	
Allopurinol (high dose)	Increased serum theophylline levels
Cimetidine	Increased serum theophylline levels
Ciprofloxacin	Increased serum theophylline levels
Erythromycin, Troleandomycin	Increased serum theophylline levels
Lithium carbonate	Increased renal excretion of lithium
Oral contraceptives	Increased serum theophylline levels
Propranolol	Increased serum theophylline levels
Phenytoin	Decreased theophylline and phenytoin serum levels
Rifampin	Decreased serum theophylline levels

ADVERSE REACTIONS:

The frequency of adverse reactions is related to serum theophylline levels and is usually not a problem at levels below 20 mcg/ml. The most consistent adverse reactions are usually due to overdosage and, while all have not been reported with theophylline w/guaifenesin, the following reactions may be considered when theophylline is administered.

Central Nervous System: clonic and tonic generalized convulsions, muscle twitching, reflex hyperexcitability, headaches, insomnia, restlessness, and irritability.

Cardiovascular: circulatory failure, life-threatening ventricular arrhythmias, hypotension, extrasystoles, tachycardia, palpitation, and flushing.

Gastrointestinal: hematemesis, vomiting, diarrhea, epigastric pain, and nausea.

Renal: increased excretion of renal tubular cells and red blood cells, albuminuria, and potentiation of diuresis.

Respiratory: tachypnea.

Other: hyperglycemia and inappropriate ADH syndrome.

OVERDOSAGE:

Symptoms: Nervousness, agitation, headache, insomnia, vomiting, tachycardia, extrasystoles, hyperreflexia, fasciculations and clonic and tonic convulsions. Children may be particularly prone to restlessness and hyperactivity that can proceed to convulsions.

Management:

A. If potential oral overdose is established and seizure has not occurred:

1) Induce vomiting.

2) Administer a cathartic (this is particularly important if extended-release preparations have been taken).

3) Administer activated charcoal.

4) Monitor vital signs, maintain blood pressure and provide adequate hydration.

5) Monitor serum potassium.

B. If patient is having a seizure:

1) Establish an airway.

2) Administer oxygen.

3) Treat the seizure with intravenous diazepam, 0.1 to 0.3 mg/kg, up to 10 mg.

4) Monitor vital signs, maintain blood pressure and provide adequate hydration.

C. Postseizure Coma:

1) Maintain airway and oxygenation.

2) If a result of oral medication, follow above recommendations to prevent absorption of drug, but intubation and lavage will have to be performed instead of inducing emesis, and the cathartic and charcoal will need to be introduced via a large-bore gastric lavage tube.

3) Continue to provide full supportive care and adequate hydration while waiting for drug to be metabolized. In general, the drug is metabolized sufficiently rapidly enough so as to not warrant consideration of dialysis.

D. Animal studies suggest that phenobarbital may decrease theophylline toxicity. There are as yet, however, insufficient data to recommend pretreatment of an overdosage with phenobarbital.

GENERAL

The oral LD_{50} of theophylline in mice is 350 mg/kg. The oral LD_{50} of guaifenesin in mice is 1725 mg/kg. In humans, adverse reactions often occur when serum theophylline levels exceed 20 mcg/ml. Information on physiological variables which influence excretion of theophylline can be found under the heading CLINICAL PHARMACOLOGY.

DOSAGE AND ADMINISTRATION:

Therapeutic serum levels associated with optimal likelihood for benefit and minimal risk of toxicity are considered to be between 10 mcg/ml and 20 mcg/ml. Levels above 20 mcg/ml may produce toxic effects. There is great variation from patient to patient in dosage needed in order to achieve a therapeutic blood level because of variable rates of elimination. Because of this wide variation from patient to patient, and the relatively narrow therapeutic blood level range, dosage must be individualized and monitoring of serum theophylline levels is highly recommended.

Dosage should be calculated on the basis of lean (ideal) body weight where mg/kg doses are stated. Theophylline does not distribute into fatty tissue.

Giving theophylline with food may prevent the rare case of stomach irritation, and although absorption may be slower, it is still complete.

When rapidly absorbed products such as solutions and soft gelatin capsules with rapid dissolution are used, dosing to maintain "around the clock" blood levels generally requires administration every 6 hours to obtain the greatest efficacy for clinical use in children; dosing intervals up to 8 hours may be satisfactory for adults because of their slower elimination. Children and adults requiring higher-than-average doses may benefit from products with slower absorption which may allow longer dosing intervals and/or less fluctuation in serum concentration over a dosing interval during chronic therapy.

ACUTE SYMPTOMS OF ASTHMA REQUIRING RAPID THEOPHYLLINIZATION

Note: Due to their slower rate of absorption, extended-release theophylline products are not designed for use in conditions requiring rapid theophyllinization.

I. Not currently receiving theophylline products.

II. Those currently receiving theophylline products: Determine, where possible, the time, amount, route of administration and form of the patient's last dose.

The loading dose for theophylline will be based on the principle that each 0.5 mg/kg of theophylline administered as a loading dose will result in a 1 mcg/ml increase in serum theophylline concentration. Ideally, then, the loading dose should be deferred if a serum theophylline concentration can be rapidly obtained. If this is not possible, the clinician must exercise his judgment in selecting a dose based on the potential for benefit and risk. When there is sufficient respiratory distress to warrant a small risk, 2.5 mg/kg of theophylline is

DOSAGE AND ADMINISTRATION: *(cont'd)*

likely to increase the serum concentration when administered as a loading dose in rapidly absorbed form by only about 5 mcg/ml. If the patient is not already experiencing theophylline toxicity, this is unlikely to result in dangerous adverse effects.

Subsequent to the modified decision regarding loading dose in this group of patients, the subsequent maintenance dosage recommendations are the same as those described above (TABLE 3).

TABLE 3

Group	Oral Loading Dose (theophylline)	Maintenance Dose for Next 12 Hours (theophylline)	Maintenance Dose Beyond 12 Hours (theophylline)
1. Children age 1 to under 9 years	5 mg/kg	4 mg/kg q4hrs	4 mg/kg q6hrs
2. Children age 9 to under 16 years; and smokers	5 mg/kg	3 mg/kg q4hrs	3 mg/kg q6hrs
3. Otherwise healthy non-smoking adults	5 mg/kg	3 mg/kg q6hrs	3 mg/kg q8hrs
4. Older patients and patients with cor pulmonale	5 mg/kg	2 mg/kg q6hrs	2 mg/kg q8hrs
5. Patients with congestive heart failure, liver failure	5 mg/kg	2 mg/kg q8hrs	1-2 mg/kg q12hrs

COMMENTS

To achieve optimal therapeutic theophylline dosage, it is recommended to monitor serum theophylline concentration. However, it is not always possible or practical to obtain a serum theophylline level.

Patients should be closely monitored for signs of toxicity. The present data suggest that the above dosage recommendations will achieve therapeutic serum concentrations with minimal risk of toxicity for most patients. However, some risk of toxic serum concentrations is still present. Adverse reactions to theophylline often occur when serum theophylline levels exceed 20 mcg/ml.

CHRONIC ASTHMA

Theophyllinization is a treatment of first choice for the management of chronic asthma (to prevent symptoms and maintain patent airways). Slow clinical titration is generally preferred to ensure acceptance and safety of the medication.

Initial Dose: 16 mg/kg/day or 400 mg/day (whichever is lower) in 3 to 4 divided doses at 6- to 8-hour intervals for the Syrup and Capsules.

Increased Dose: The above dosage may be increased in approximately 25 percent increments at 2- to 3-day intervals so long as no intolerance is observed, until the maximum indicated below is reached.

Maximum Dose Without Measurement of Serum Concentration: Not to exceed the following: **(WARNING: DO NOT ATTEMPT TO MAINTAIN ANY DOSE THAT IS NOT TOLERATED.)** (See TABLE 4.)

TABLE 4

Age 1-under 9 years	24 mg/kg/day
Age 9-under 12 years	20 mg/kg/day
Age 12-under 16 years	18 mg/kg/day
Age 16 years or older (WHICHEVER IS LESS)	13 mg/kg/day or 900 mg/day

Note: Use ideal body weight for obese patients.

MEASUREMENT OF SERUM THEOPHYLLINE CONCENTRATION DURING CHRONIC THERAPY

If the above maximum doses are to be maintained or exceeded, serum theophylline measurement is recommended. This should be obtained at the approximate time of peak absorption during chronic therapy for the product used (1 to 2 hours for liquids, soft gelatin capsules, and plain uncoated tablets that undergo rapid dissolution, 3 to 5 hours for extended-release preparations). It is important that the patient will have missed *no* doses during the previous 48 hours and that dosing intervals will have been reasonably typical with no added doses during that period of time. **DOSAGE ADJUSTMENT BASED ON SERUM THEOPHYLLINE MEASUREMENTS WHEN THESE INSTRUCTIONS HAVE NOT BEEN FOLLOWED MAY RESULT IN RECOMMENDATIONS THAT PRESENT RISK OF TOXICITY TO THE PATIENT.**

Final Dosage Adjustment: Caution should be exercised for younger children who cannot complain of minor side effects. Older adults, those with cor pulmonale, congestive heart failure, and/or liver disease may have unusually low dosage requirements and thus may experience toxicity at the maximal dosage recommended above.

It is important that no patient be maintained on any dosage that he is not tolerating. In instructing patients to increase dosage according to the schedule above, they should be instructed not to take a subsequent dose if apparent side effects occur and to resume therapy at a lower dose once adverse effects have disappeared.

KEEP THIS AND ALL MEDICATION OUT OF THE REACH OF CHILDREN.

HOW SUPPLIED - EQUIVALENTS NOT AVAILABLE:

Capsule, Elastic - Oral - 90 mg/150 mg

100's	$4.28	GLYCERYL-T, Rugby	00536-3868-01
100's	$4.44	BRONCHIAL CAPS, HL Moore Drug Exch	00839-6697-06
100's	$4.80	BRONCHIAL, Geneva Pharms	00781-2890-01
100's	$9.02	Q-B CAPS, Major Pharms	00904-2282-61
100's	$37.38	SLO-PHYLLIN GG, Rhone-Poulenc Rorer	00075-0358-00
100's	$41.05	QUIBRON, Roberts Labs	54092-0067-01
100's	$53.32	QUIBRON, Roberts Labs	54092-0067-52
250's	$10.60	Q-B CAPS, Major Pharms	00904-2282-70
1000's	$32.25	GLYCERYL-T, Rugby	00536-3868-10
1000's	$37.20	Q-B CAPS, Major Pharms	00904-2282-80
1000's	$358.87	QUIBRON, Bristol Myers Squibb	00087-0516-02
1000's	$389.37	QUIBRON, Roberts Labs	54092-0067-10

Capsule, Elastic - Oral - 180 mg/300 mg

100's	$65.65	QUIBRON-300, Roberts Labs	54092-0068-01

Elixir - Oral - 90 mg/150 mg

480 ml	$4.66	Theolate, HL Moore Drug Exch	00839-6348-69
480 ml	$4.80	THEOLATE, Harber Pharm	51432-0676-20
480 ml	$4.90	GLYCERYL-T-LIQUID, Rugby	00536-0760-85
480 ml	$4.91	THEOPHYLLINE & GUAIFENESIN, Schein Pharm (US)	00364-7264-16
480 ml	$4.94	Q-B, Major Pharms	00904-0070-16

HOW SUPPLIED - EQUIVALENTS NOT AVAILABLE: *(cont'd)*

480 ml	$5.04	THEOLATE, Alpharma	00472-1540-16
480 ml	$5.50	Theolate, Consolidated Midland	00223-6622-01
480 ml	$25.06	QUIBRON, Bristol Myers Squibb	00087-0510-03
480 ml	$40.17	SLO-PHYLLIN GG, Rhone-Poulenc Rorer	00075-0357-16
3840 ml	$24.04	GLYCERYL-T-LIQUID, Rugby	00536-0760-90
3840 ml	$27.26	THEOLATE, Harber Pharm	51432-0676-21
3840 ml	$28.99	Theolate, Consolidated Midland	00223-6622-02
3840 ml	$170.27	QUIBRON, Bristol Myers Squibb	00087-0510-01

Elixir - Oral - 100 mg/137 mg

480 ml	$37.50	EQUIBRON G, Equipharm	57779-0115-09

Liquid - Oral - 100 mg/100 mg

240 ml	$38.15	ELIXOPHYLLIN GG, Berlex Labs	50419-0136-08
240 ml	$48.69	ELIXOPHYLLIN GG, Forest Pharms	00456-0648-08
480 ml	$60.31	ELIXOPHYLLIN GG, Berlex Labs	50419-0136-16
480 ml	$93.56	ELIXOPHYLLIN GG, Forest Pharms	00456-0648-16

Liquid - Oral - 100 mg/150 mg

473 ml	$28.00	ED-BRON G, Edwards Pharms	00485-0059-16

GUANABENZ ACETATE *(001408)*

CATEGORIES: Alpha Adrenoreceptor Agonists; Antihypertensives; Cardiovascular Drugs; Hypertension; Pregnancy Category C; FDA Approved 1982 Sep

BRAND NAMES: *Rexitene*; *Wytens* (Japan); **Wytensin**
(International brand names outside U.S. in italics)

FORMULARIES: BC-BS; Medi-Cal

COST OF THERAPY: $369.59 (Hypertension; Tablet; 4 mg; 2/day; 365 days)

PRIMARY ICD9: 401.1 (Assential Hypertension, Benign)

DESCRIPTION:

Wytensin (guanabenz acetate), an antihypertensive agent for oral administration, is an aminoguanidine derivative, 2,6-dichlorobenzylideneamino-guanidine monoacetate.

It is an odorless, white to off-white, crystalline substance, sparingly soluble in water and soluble in alcohol, with a molecular weight of 291.14. Each tablet of Wytensin is equivalent to 4 mg or 8 mg of free guanabenz base. The inactive ingredients present are cellulose, iron oxide, lactose, and magnesium stearate. The 8 mg dosage strength also contains FD&C Blue 2.

Wytensin is available as 4 mg or 8 mg tablets for oral administration.

CLINICAL PHARMACOLOGY:

Guanabenz acetate is an orally active central alpha-2 adrenergic agonist. Its antihypertensive action appears to be mediated via stimulation of central alpha adrenergic receptors, resulting in a decrease of sympathetic outflow from the brain at the bulbar level to the peripheral circulatory system.

PHARMACOKINETICS

In human studies, about 75% of an orally administered dose of guanabenz acetate is absorbed and metabolized with less than 1% of unchanged drug recovered from the urine. Peak plasma concentrations of unchanged drug occur between two and five hours after a single oral dose. The average half-life for guanabenz acetate is about 6 hours. The site or sites of metabolism of guanabenz acetate have not been determined. The effect of meals on the absorption of guanabenz acetate has not been studied.

PHARMACODYNAMICS

The onset of the antihypertensive action of guanabenz acetate begins within 60 minutes after a single oral dose and reaches a peak effect within two to four hours. The effect of an acute single dose is reduced appreciably six to eight hours after administration, and blood pressure approaches baseline values within 12 hours of administration.

The acute antihypertensive effect of guanabenz acetate occurs without major changes in peripheral resistance, but its chronic effect appears to be a decrease in peripheral resistance. A decrease in blood pressure is seen in both the supine and standing positions without alterations of normal postural mechanisms, so that postural hypotension has not been observed. Guanabenz decreases pulse rate by about 5 beats per minute. Cardiac output and left ventricular ejection fraction are unchanged during long-term therapy.

In clinical trials, guanabenz, given orally to hypertensive patients, effectively controlled blood pressure without any significant effect on glomerular filtration rate, renal blood flow, body fluid volume or body weight. Guanabenz given parenterally to dogs has produced a natriuresis. Similarly, hypertensive subjects, 24 hours after salt loading, have shown a decrease in blood pressure and a natriuresis (5% to 240% increase in sodium excretion) following a single oral dose of guanabenz. After seven consecutive days of administration and effective blood-pressure control, no significant change on glomerular filtration rate, renal blood flow, or body weight was observed. However, in clinical trials of six to thirty months duration, hypertensive patients with effective blood-pressure control by guanabenz lost one to four pounds of body weight. The mechanism of this weight loss has not been established. Tolerance to the antihypertensive effect of guanabenz has not been observed.

During long-term administration of guanabenz, there is a small decrease in serum cholesterol and total triglycerides without any change in the high density lipoprotein fraction. Plasma norepinephrine, serum dopamine beta-hydroxylase, and plasma renin activity are decreased during chronic administration of guanabenz. No changes in serum electrolytes, uric acid, blood urea nitrogen, calcium, or glucose have been observed.

Guanabenz and hydrochlorothiazide have been shown to have at least partially additive effects in patients not responding adequately to either drug alone.

INDICATIONS AND USAGE:

Guanabenz acetate is indicated in the treatment of hypertension. It may be employed alone or in combination with a thiazide diuretic.

CONTRAINDICATIONS:

Guanabenz acetate is contraindicated in patients with a known sensitivity to the drug.

PRECAUTIONS:

1. Sedation: Guanabenz causes sedation or drowsiness in a large fraction of patients. When guanabenz is used with centrally active depressants, such as phenothiazines, barbiturates, and benzodiazepines, the potential for additive sedative effects should be considered.

2. Patients with Vascular Insufficiency: Guanabenz, like other antihypertensive agents, should be used with caution in patients with severe coronary insufficiency, recent myocardial infarction, cerebrovascular disease, or severe hepatic or renal failure.

PRECAUTIONS: *(cont'd)*

3. Rebound: Sudden cessation of therapy with central alpha agonists like guanabenz may rarely result in "overshoot" hypertension and more commonly produces an increase in serum catecholamines and subjective symptomatology.

4. Patients with Hepatic Impairment: The disposition of orally administered guanabenz is altered in patients with alcohol-induced liver disease. Mean plasma concentrations of guanabenz were higher in these patients than in healthy subjects. The clinical significance of this finding is unknown. However, careful monitoring of blood pressure is suggested when guanabenz is administered to patients with hypertension and coexisting chronic hepatic dysfunction.

5. Patients with Renal Impairment: The disposition of orally administered guanabenz is altered modestly in patients with renal impairment. Guanabenz's half-life is prolonged and clearance decreased, more so in patients on hemodialysis. The clinical significance of these findings is unknown. Careful monitoring of blood pressure during guanabenz dose titration is suggested in patients with coexisting hypertension and renal impairment.

INFORMATION FOR THE PATIENT

Patients who receive guanabenz should be advised to exercise caution when operating dangerous machinery or driving motor vehicles until it is determined that they do not become drowsy or dizzy from the medication. Patients should be warned that their tolerance for alcohol and other CNS depressants may be diminished. Patients should be advised not to discontinue therapy abruptly.

LABORATORY TESTS

In clinical trials, no clinically significant laboratory-test abnormalities were identified during either acute or chronic therapy with guanabenz. Tests carried out included CBC, urinalysis, electrolytes, SGOT, bilirubin, alkaline phosphatase, uric acid, BUN, creatinine, glucose, calcium, phosphorus, total protein, and Coombs' test. During long-term administration of guanabenz, there was a small decrease in serum cholesterol and total triglycerides without any change in the high-density lipoprotein fraction. In rare instances an occasional nonprogressive increase in liver enzymes has been observed. However, no clinical evidence of hepatic disease has been found.

DRUG/LABORATORY TEST INTERACTIONS

No laboratory-test abnormalities were identified with the use of guanabenz.

CARCINOGENESIS, MUTAGENESIS, AND IMPAIRMENT OF FERTILITY

No evidence of carcinogenic potential emerged in rats during a two-year oral study with guanabenz at doses up to 9.5 mg/kg/day, i.e., about 10 times the maximum recommended human dose. In the Salmonella microsome mutagenicity (Ames) test system, guanabenz at 200 to 500 mcg per plate or at 30 to 50 mcg/ml in suspension gave dose-related increases in the number of mutants in one (TA 1537) of five *Salmonella typhimurium* strains with or without inclusion of rat liver microsomes. No mutagenic activity was seen at doses up to those which inhibit growth in the eukaryotic microorganism, *Schizosaccharomyces pombe*, or in Chinese hamster ovary cells at doses up to those which were lethal to the cells in culture. In another eukaryotic system, *Saccharomyces cerevisiae*, guanabenz produced no activity in an assay measuring induction of repairable DNA damage. Reproductive studies showed a decreased pregnancy rate in rats administered high oral doses (9.6 mg/kg) of guanabenz, suggesting an impairment of fertility. The fertility of treated males (9.6 mg/kg) may also have been affected, as suggested by the decreased pregnancy rate of their mates, even though the females received Guanabenz only during the last third of pregnancy.

PREGNANCY CATEGORY C

GUANABENZ MAY HAVE ADVERSE EFFECTS ON THE FETUS WHEN ADMINISTERED TO PREGNANT WOMEN. A teratology study in mice has indicated a possible increase in skeletal abnormalities when guanabenz is given orally at doses of 3 to 6 times the maximum recommended human dose of 1.0 mg/kg. These abnormalities, principally costal and vertebral, were not noted in similar studies in rats and rabbits. However, increased fetal loss has been observed after oral guanabenz administration to pregnant rats (14 mg/kg) and rabbits (20 mg/kg). Reproductive studies of guanabenz in rats have shown slightly decreased live-birth indices, decreased fetal survival rate, and decreased pup body weight at oral doses of 6.4 and 9.6 mg/kg. There are no adequate, well controlled studies in pregnant women. Guanabenz should be used during pregnancy only if the potential benefit justifies the potential risk to the fetus.

NURSING MOTHERS

Because no information is available on the excretion of guanabenz in human milk, it should not be administered to nursing mothers.

PEDIATRIC USE

The safety and effectiveness of guanabenz acetate in children less than 12 years of age have not been demonstrated. Therefore, its use in this age group cannot be recommended at this time.

DRUG INTERACTIONS:

Guanabenz acetate has not been demonstrated to cause any drug interactions when administered with other drugs, such as digitalis, diuretics, analgesics, anxiolytics, and antiinflammatory or antiinfective agents, in clinical trials. However, the potential for increased sedation when guanabenz acetate is administered concomitantly with CNS-depressant drugs should be noted.

ADVERSE REACTIONS:

The incidence of adverse effects has been ascertained from controlled clinical studies conducted in the United States and is based on data from 859 patients who received guanabenz acetate for up to 3 years. There is some evidence that the side effects are dose-related.

The following table (TABLE 1) shows the incidence of adverse effects, occurring in at least 5% of patients in a study comparing guanabenz acetate to placebo, at a starting dose of 8 mg b.i.d.

TABLE 1

Adverse Effect	Placebo (%) n=102	Wytensin (%) n=109
Dry mouth	7	28
Drowsiness or sedation	12	39
Dizziness	7	17
Weakness	7	10
Headache	6	5

In other controlled clinical trials at the starting dose of 16 mg/day in 476 patients, the incidence of dry mouth was slightly higher (38%) and that of dizziness was slightly lower (12%), but the incidence of the most frequent adverse effects was similar to the placebo-controlled trial. Although these side effects were not serious, they led to discontinuation of treatment about 15% of the time. In more recent studies using an initial dose of 8 mg/day in 274 patients, the incidence of drowsiness or sedation was lower, about 20%.

Other adverse effects were reported during clinical trials with guanabenz acetate but are not clearly distinguishable from placebo effects and occurred with a frequency of 3% or less:

ADVERSE REACTIONS: *(cont'd)*

Cardiovascular: chest pain, edema, arrhythmias, palpitations.

Gastrointestinal: nausea, epigastric pain, diarrhea, vomiting, constipation, abdominal discomfort.

Central Nervous System: anxiety, ataxia, depression, sleep disturbances.

ENT Disorders: nasal congestion.

Eye Disorders: blurring of vision.

Musculoskeletal: aches in extremities, muscle aches.

Respiratory: dyspnea.

Dermatologic: rash, pruritus.

Urogenital: urinary frequency, disturbances of sexual function (decreased libido, impotence).

Other: gynecomastia, taste disorders.

In very rare instances atrioventricular dysfunction, up to and including complete AV block, has been caused by guanabenz acetate.

DRUG ABUSE AND DEPENDENCE:

No reported dependence or abuse has been associated with the administration of guanabenz acetate.

OVERDOSAGE:

Accidental ingestion of guanabenz acetate caused hypotension, somnolence, lethargy, irritability, miosis, and bradycardia in two children aged one and three years. Gastric lavage and administration of pressor substances, fluids, and oral activated charcoal resulted in complete and uneventful recovery within 12 hours in both patients.

Since experience with accidental overdosage is limited, the suggested treatment is mainly supportive while the drug is being eliminated from the body and until the patient is no longer symptomatic. Vital signs and fluid balance should be carefully monitored. An adequate airway should be maintained and, if indicated, assisted respiration instituted. There are no data available on the dialyzability of guanabenz acetate.

DOSAGE AND ADMINISTRATION:

Dosage with guanabenz acetate should be individualized. A starting dose of 4 mg twice a day is recommended, whether guanabenz acetate is used alone or with a thiazide diuretic. Dosage may be increased in increments of 4 to 8 mg per day every one to two weeks, depending on the patients's response. The maximum dose studied to date has been 32 mg twice daily, but doses as high as this are rarely needed.

Keep tightly closed.Protect from light.

HOW SUPPLIED - RATED THERAPEUTICALLY EQUIVALENT:

Tablet - Oral - 4 mg

100's	$50.63	Guanabenz Acetate, H.C.F.A. F F P	99999-1408-01

Tablet - Oral - 8 mg

100's	$75.75	Guanabenz Acetate, H.C.F.A. F F P	99999-1408-02

Tablet, Uncoated - Oral - 4 mg

100's	$53.17	Guanabenz Acetate, Watson Labs	52544-0451-01
100's	$53.20	Guanabenz Acetate, Qualitest Pharms	00603-3779-21
100's	$54.75	Guanabenz Acetate, Martec Pharms	52555-0555-01
100's	$59.33	Guanabenz Acetate, HL Moore Drug Exch	00839-7932-06
100's	$61.92	Guanabenz Acetate, Zenith Labs	00172-4226-60
100's	$61.92	Guanabenz Acetate, Goldline Labs	00182-1951-01
100's	$66.20	Guanabenz Acetate, Copley Pharm	38245-0717-10
100's	**$73.61**	**WYTENSIN, Wyeth Labs**	**00008-0073-01**
500's	$321.00	Guanabenz Acetate, Copley Pharm	38245-0717-50
500's	**$357.30**	**WYTENSIN, Wyeth Labs**	**00008-0073-04**

Tablet, Uncoated - Oral - 8 mg

100's	$79.80	Guanabenz Acetate, Qualitest Pharms	00603-3780-21
100's	$79.82	Guanabenz Acetate, Watson Labs	52544-0452-01
100's	$82.25	Guanabenz Acetate, Martec Pharms	52555-0556-01
100's	$89.10	Guanabenz Acetate, HL Moore Drug Exch	00839-7933-06
100's	$91.27	Guanabenz Acetate, Zenith Labs	00172-4227-60
100's	$91.27	Guanabenz Acetate, Goldline Labs	00182-1952-01
100's	$99.40	Guanabenz Acetate, Warner Chilcott	00047-0561-24
100's	$99.40	Guanabenz Acetate, Copley Pharm	38245-0711-10
100's	**$110.51**	**WYTENSIN, Wyeth Labs**	**00008-0074-01**

GUANADREL SULFATE *(001409)*

CATEGORIES: Antihypertensives; Cardiovascular Drugs; Hypertension; Pregnancy Category B; FDA Approved 1982 Dec

BRAND NAMES: **Hylorel**

FORMULARIES: BC-BS

COST OF THERAPY: $546.55 (Hypertension; Tablet; 10 mg; 2/day; 365 days) vs. Potential Cost of $24,027.04 (Coronary Bypass)

PRIMARY ICD9: 401.1 (Essential Hypertension, Benign)

DESCRIPTION:

Hylorel Tablets for oral administration contain guanadrel sulfate, an antihypertensive agent belonging to the class of adrenergic neuron blocking drugs. Guanadrel sulfate is (1,4-Dioxaspiro[4.5] dec-2-ylmethyl) guanidine sulfate with a molecular weight of 524.63. The empirical formula is $(C_{10}H_{19}N_3O_2)_2 \cdot H_2SO_4$. It is a white to off-white crystalline powder, which melts with decomposition at about 235° C. It is soluble in water to the extent of 76 mg/ml.

Hylorel Tablets are available in two strengths: 10 mg and 25 mg. Inactive ingredients: colloidal silicon dioxide, corn starch, lactose monohydrate, magnesium stearate, microcrystalline cellulose and talc. The 10 mg tablet also contains FD&C Yellow No. 6.

CLINICAL PHARMACOLOGY:

Guanadrel sulfate is an orally effective antihypertensive agent that lowers both systolic and diastolic arterial blood pressures. Guanadrel sulfate inhibits sympathetic vasoconstriction by inhibiting norepinephrine release from neuronal storage sites in response to stimulation of the nerve and also causes depletion of norepinephrine from the nerve ending. This results in relaxation of vascular smooth muscle which decreases total peripheral resistance, and decreases venous return, both of which reduce the ability to maintain blood pressure in the upright position. The result is a hypotensive effect that is greater in the standing than in the supine position by about 10 mmHg systolic and 3.5 mmHg diastolic, on the average. Heart

CLINICAL PHARMACOLOGY: *(cont'd)*

rate is also decreased usually by about 5 beats/minute. Fluid retention occurs during treatment with guanadrel, particularly when it is not accompanied by a diuretic. The drug does not inhibit parasympathetic nerve function nor does it enter the central nervous system.

Guanadrel sulfate is rapidly absorbed after oral administration. Plasma concentrations generally peak 1 1/2 to 2 hours after ingestion. The half-life is about 10 hours, but individual variability is great. Approximately 85% of the drug is eliminated in the urine. Urinary excretion is approximately 85% complete within 24 hours after administration; about 40% of the dose is excreted as unchanged drug. The disposition of guanadrel sulfate is significantly altered in patients with impaired renal function. A study in such patients has shown that as renal function (measured as creatinine clearance) declines, apparent total body clearance, renal and apparent nonrenal clearances decrease, and the terminal elimination half-life is prolonged. Dosage adjustments may be necessary, especially in patients with creatinine clearances of less than 60 ml/min (see DOSAGE AND ADMINISTRATION.)

Guanadrel sulfate begins to decrease blood pressure within two hours and produces maximal decreases in four to six hours. No significant change in cardiac output accompanies the blood pressure decline in normal individuals.

Because drugs of the adrenergic neuron blocking class are transported into the neuron by the "norepinephrine pump", drugs that compete for the pump may block their effects. Tricyclic antidepressants have been shown to block the norepinephrine-depleting effect of guanadrel sulfate in rats and monkeys, and the blood pressure lowering effect of guanadrel sulfate in monkeys. Similar effects have been seen with guanethidine and inhibition of the antihypertensive effects of guanadrel sulfate by tricyclic antidepressants in humans should be presumed.

Therefore caution is recommended if guanadrel sulfate and a tricyclic antidepressant are used concomitantly. Should patients be on both a tricyclic antidepressant and guanadrel sulfate, caution is advised upon discontinuation of the tricyclic antidepressant, especially if discontinued abruptly, as an enhanced effect of guanadrel sulfate may occur.

Chlorpromazine seems to have a similar effect on guanethidine and may affect guanadrel as well. Indirectly acting adrenergic amines are transported into the neuron by the "norepinephrine pump" and may interfere with uptake or may displace blocking agents. Ephedrine rapidly reverses the effects of guanadrel but other agents have not been studied.

Agents of the guanethidine class cause increased sensitivity to circulating norepinephrine, probably by preventing uptake of norepinephrine by adrenergic neurons, the usual mechanism for terminating norepinephrine effects. Agents of this class are thus dangerous in the presence of excess norepinephrine, e.g., in the presence of a pheochromocytoma.

In controlled clinical studies comparing guanadrel to guanethidine and methyldopa, involving about 2000 patients exposed to guanadrel, patients with initial supine blood pressures averaging 160-170/105-110 mmHg had decreases in blood pressure of 20-25/15-20 mmHg in the standing position. The decreases in supine blood pressure were less than the decreases in standing blood pressure by 6-10/2-7 mmHg in different studies. Guanethidine and guanadrel were very similar in effectiveness while methyldopa had a larger effect on supine systolic pressure. Side effects of guanadrel and guanethidine were generally similar in type (see ADVERSE REACTIONS) while methyldopa had more central nervous system effects (depression, drowsiness) but fewer orthostatic effects and less diarrhea.

INDICATIONS AND USAGE:

Hylorel Tablets are indicated for the treatment of hypertension in patients not responding adequately to a thiazide type diuretic. Hylorel should be added to a diuretic regimen for optimum blood pressure control.

CONTRAINDICATIONS:

Hylorel Tablets are contraindicated in known or suspected pheochromocytoma.

Hylorel should not be used concurrently with, or within one week of, monoamine oxidase inhibitors.

Hylorel should not be used in patients hypersensitive to the drug.

Hylorel should not be used in patients with frank congestive heart failure.

WARNINGS:

a. Orthostatic Hypotension: Orthostatic hypotension and its consequences (dizziness and weakness) are frequent in people treated with Hylorel Tablets. Rarely, fainting upon standing or exercise is seen. Careful instructions to the patient can minimize these symptoms, as can recognition by the physician that the supine blood pressure does not constitute an adequate assessment of the effects of this drug. Patients with known regional vascular disease (cerebral, coronary) are at particular risk from marked orthostatic hypotension and Hylorel should be avoided in them unless drugs with lesser degrees of orthostatic hypotension are ineffective or unacceptable. In such patients hypotensive episodes should be avoided, even if this requires accepting a poorer degree of blood pressure control.

Instructions to patients: Patients should be advised about the risk of orthostatic hypotension and told to sit or lie down immediately at the onset of dizziness or weakness so that they can prevent loss of consciousness. They should be told that postural hypotension is worst in the morning and upon arising, and may be exaggerated by alcohol, fever, hot weather, prolonged standing, or exercise.

Surgery: To reduce the possibility of vascular collapse during anesthesia, guanadrel should be discontinued 48-72 hours before elective surgery. If emergency surgery is required, the anesthesiologist should be made aware that the patient has been taking Hylorel and that preanesthetic and anesthetic agents should be administered cautiously in reduced dosage. If vasopressors are needed they must be used cautiously, as guanadrel can enhance the pressor response to such agents and increase their arrhythmogenicity.

c. Asthmatic patients: Special care is needed in patients with bronchial asthma, as their condition may be aggravated by catecholamine depletion and sympathomimetic amines may interfere with the hypotensive effect of guanadrel.

PRECAUTIONS:

General: Salt and water retention may occur with the use of Hylorel Tablets. In clinical studies major problems did not arise because of concomitant diuretic use. Patients with heart failure have not been studied on Hylorel, but guanadrel could interfere with the adrenergic mechanisms that maintain compensation.

In patients with a history of peptic ulcer, which could be aggravated by a relative increase in parasympathetic tone, Hylorel should be used cautiously.

In patients with compromised renal function, decreases in renal and nonrenal clearances and an increase in the elimination half-life of guanadrel sulfate have been found. This could possibly lead to an increased incidence of side effects if standard doses are used in these patients. Titration of dose based on the blood pressure response is necessary because of marked interpatient variability (see DOSAGE AND ADMINISTRATION.)

A transient increase in blood pressure has been observed in some patients.

Information for the Patient: See WARNINGS section.

PRECAUTIONS: *(cont'd)*

Carcinogenesis, Mutagenesis, and Impairment of Fertility: No evidence of carcinogenic potential appeared in a 2-year mouse study of guanadrel sulfate. In a 2-year rat study, an increased number of benign testicular interstitial cell tumors was observed at dosages of 100 mg/kg/day and 400 mg/kg/day. These are common spontaneous tumors in aged rats and their significance to therapy with Hylorel in man is unknown. Salmonella testing (Ames test) showed no evidence of mutagenic activity.

A reproduction study was performed in male and female rats at dosages of 0, 10, 30, and 100 mg/kg/day. Suppressed libido and reduced fertility were noted at 100 mg/kg/day (12 times the maximum human dose in a 50 kg subject) and libido was suppressed to a lesser extent at 30 mg/kg/day.

Pregnancy Category B: Teratology studies performed in rats and rabbits at doses up to 12 times the maximum recommended human dose (in a 50 kg subject) revealed no significant harm to the fetus due to guanadrel sulfate. There are, however, no adequate and well-controlled studies in pregnant women. Because animal reproduction studies are not always predictive, Hylorel should be used in pregnant women only when the potential benefit outweighs the potential risk to mother and infant.

Nursing Mothers: Whether guanadrel sulfate is excreted in human milk is not known, but because many drugs are excreted in human milk and because of the potential for serious adverse reactions in nursing infants from guanadrel, a decision should be made whether to discontinue nursing or discontinue the drug, taking into account the importance of the drug to the mother.

Pediatric Use: Safety and effectiveness in children have not been established.

DRUG INTERACTIONS:

As discussed in CLINICAL PHARMACOLOGY, tricyclic antidepressants and indirect-acting sympathomimetics such as ephedrine or phenylpropanolamine, and possibly phenothiazines, can reverse the effects of neuronal blocking agents. IN VIEW OF THE PRESENCE OF SYMPATHOMIMETIC AMINES IN MANY NON-PRESCRIPTION DRUGS FOR THE TREATMENT OF COLDS, ALLERGY, OR ASTHMA, PATIENTS GIVEN GUANADREL SHOULD BE SPECIFICALLY WARNED NOT TO USE SUCH PREPARATIONS WITHOUT THEIR PHYSICIAN'S ADVICE.

Guanadrel enhances the activity of direct-acting sympathomimetics, like norepinephrine, by blocking neuronal uptake.

Drugs that affect the adrenergic response by the same or other mechanisms would be expected to potentiate the effects of guanadrel, causing excessive postural hypotension and bradycardia. These include alpha- or beta-adrenergic blocking agents and reserpine. There is no clinical experience with the combination of Hylorel with alpha-adrenergic blocking agents or reserpine.

When Hylorel was added to the treatment regimen in hypertensive patients inadequately controlled with a diuretic and propranolol, no significant adverse effects, including bradycardia, were reported in the 26 patients treated concomitantly with the three drugs.

The use of Hylorel with vasodilators has not been adequately studied and is not generally recommended because concomitant use may increase the potential for symptomatic orthostatic hypotension.

ADVERSE REACTIONS:

The adverse reaction data for guanadrel is derived principally from comparative long-term (6 months to 3 years) studies with methyldopa and guanethidine in which side effects were assessed through use of periodic questionnaires, a method that tends to give high adverse reaction rates. In the tables that follow, some of the adverse effects reported may not be drug-related, but in the absence of a placebo-treated group, these cannot be readily distinguished. Comparative results with two well-known drugs, methyldopa and guanethidine should aid in interpretation of these adverse reaction rates.

TABLE 1 displays the frequency of side effects which are believed to be related to sympathetic blocking agents: orthostatic faintness, increased bowel movements and ejaculation disturbances for peripherally acting drugs such as guanadrel and drowsiness for centrally acting drugs such as methyldopa. The frequencies observed were generally higher during the first 8 weeks of therapy. Week O frequencies, which were recorded just prior to administration of the antihypertensive drugs while the patients were receiving diuretics, serve as a reference point. Frequency while on therapy are shown for the first 8 weeks and for weeks 9 to 52.

TABLE 1 Frequency Of Side Effects
Percent of Clinic Visits in Which Side Effect was Reported

Week	Guanadrel Pre-Drug 0	1-8	9-52
Number of clinic visits analyzed	470	3003	4260
Side Effect			
Morning orthostatic faintness	6.6	9.4	6.8
Orthostatic faintness during the day	7.5	10.8	8.5
Other faintness	7.8	4.8	4.5
Increased bowel movements	4.9	7.9	6.1
Drowsiness	15.3	14.4	8.7
Fatigue	25.7	26.6	23.7
Ejaculation disturbance	7.0	17.5	12.0

Week	Methyldopa Pre-Drug 0	1-8	9-52
Number of clinic visits analyzed	266	1610	2216
Side Effect			
Morning orthostatic faintness	6.8	8.1	7.4
Orthostatic faintness during the day	7.5	8.0	7.8
Other faintness	6.2	3.7	3.8
Increased bowel movements	4.9	5.9	3.8
Drowsiness	13.2	21.2	18.6
Fatigue	32.9	22.6	27.6
Ejaculation disturbance	10.3	13.4	11.5

The frequency of side effects over time may be reduced by the discontinuation of drugs in patients who experience intolerable side effects. Reasons for discontinuation of therapy with guanadrel are shown in TABLE 2.

The following paragraph shows the incidence of reactions often associated with adrenergic neuron blockers as the percent of patients who reported the event at least once over the treatment periods of 6 months to 3 years. For such long-term studies these incidence rates of

ADVERSE REACTIONS: *(cont'd)*

Week	Guanethidine Pre-Drug 0	1-8	9-52
Number of clinic visits analyzed	215	1421	2009
Side Effect			
Morning orthostatic faintness	4.6	10.7	7.9
Orthostatic faintness during the day	5.6	8.9	6.3
Other faintness	5.9	2.7	2.0
Increased bowel movements	3.7	7.9	9.4
Drowsiness	10.2	10.3	6.4
Fatigue	21.4	20.5	17.5
Ejaculation disturbance	6.9	16.6	18.2

TABLE 2 Percent Of Patients Who Discontinued

	Guanadrel	Methyldopa	Guanethidine
Orthostatic faintness	0.6	0.7	6.0*
Syncope	0.4	0.3	2.0
Other faintness	1.2	0.0	0.0
Increased bowel movements	0.8	0.7	1.4
Drowsiness	0.0	1.9*	0.0
Fatigue	0.2	2.6*	0.0
Ejaculation disturbances	0.4	0.0	0.0

* significantly greater than Hylorel, p<0.003

side effects, which are found often in untreated patients, tend to be high and accumulate with time. The incidence rates for two well-known comparison drugs, methyldopa and guanethidine should aid in interpreting the high rates. It can be seen that the serious consequences of the orthostatic effect of guanadrel, such as syncope, were very uncommon.

1544 guanadrel, 743 methyldopa and 330 guanethidine patients were evaluated in comparison studies. The observed incidence rates of major drug related side effects for guanadrel, methyldopa and guanethidine, respectively, are as follows: orthostatic faintness: 49%, 41%, 48%; other faintness: 47%, 46%, 45%; increased bowel movements: 31%, 28%, 36%; ejaculation disturbances: 18%, 21%, 22%; impotence: 5.1%, 12.2%, 7.2%; syncope: 0.4%, 0.3%, 2%; urine retention: 0.2%, 0%, 0%.

Apart from these adverse effects, many others were reported. Relationship to therapy is less clear, although some (such as peripheral edema with all three drugs, depression with methyldopa) are in part drug related. All adverse effects reported in at least 1% of guanadrel patients are listed in TABLE 3.

TABLE 3

Drug No. pts. treated Event	Guanadrel 1544 %	Methyldopa 743 %	Guanethidine 330 %
Cardiovascular-Respiratory			
Chest Pain	27.9	37.4	27.3
Coughing	26.9	36.2	21.5
Palpitations	29.5	35.0	24.5
Shortness of breath at rest	18.3	22.3	17.0
Shortness of breath on exertion	45.9	53.2	48.8
Central Nervous System-Special Senses			
Confusion	14.8	22.6	10.9
Depression	1.9	3.9	1.8
Drowsiness	44.6	64.1	28.5
Headache	58.1	69.0	49.7
Paresthesias	25.1	35.1	16.4
Psychological problems	3.8	4.8	3.9
Sleep disorders	2.1	2.3	2.7
Visual disturbances	29.2	35.3	26.1
Gastrointestinal			
Abdominal distress or pain	1.7	1.9	1.5
Anorexia	18.7	23.0	17.6
Constipation	21.0	29.1	20.3
Dry mouth, dry throat	1.7	4.0	0.6
Gas pain	32.0	39.7	29.4
Glossitis	8.4	10.8	4.8
Indigestion	23.7	30.8	18.5
Nausea and/or vomiting	3.9	4.8	3.6
Genitourinary			
Hematuria	2.3	4.2	2.1
Nocturia	48.4	52.4	41.5
Peripheral edema	28.6	37.4	22.7
Urination urgency or frequency	33.6	39.8	27.6
Miscellaneous			
Excessive weight gain	44.3	53.7	42.4
Excessive weight loss	42.2	51.1	41.5
Fatigue	63.6	76.2	57.0
Musculoskeletal			
Aching limbs	42.9	51.7	33.9
Backache or neckache	1.5	1.1	1.8
Joint pain or inflammation	1.7	2.0	2.4
Leg cramps during the day	21.1	26.0	20.0
Leg cramps during the night	25.6	32.6	21.2

OVERDOSAGE:

Overdosage usually produces marked dizziness and blurred vision related to postural hypotension and may progress to syncope on standing. The patient should lie down until these symptoms subside.

If excessive hypotension occurs and persists despite conservative treatment, intensive therapy may be needed to support vital functions. A vasoconstrictor such as phenylephrine will ameliorate the effect of Hylorel Tablets, but great care must be used because patients may be hypersensitive to such agents.

DOSAGE AND ADMINISTRATION:

As with other sympathetic suppressant drugs, the dose response to Hylorel Tablets varies widely and must be adjusted for each patient until the therapeutic goal is achieved. With long-term therapy, some tolerance may occur and the dosage may have to be increased.

DOSAGE AND ADMINISTRATION: *(cont'd)*

Because Hylorel has a substantial orthostatic effect, monitoring both supine and standing pressures is essential, especially while dosage is being adjusted.

Hylorel should be administered in divided doses. The usual starting dosage for treating hypertension is 10 mg per day, which can be given as 5 mg b.i.d. by breaking the 10 mg tablet. The dosage should be adjusted weekly or monthly until blood pressure is controlled. Most patients will require daily dosage in the range of 20 to 75 mg usually in twice daily doses. For larger doses 3 or 4 times daily dosing may be needed. A dosage of more than 400 mg/day is rarely required.

Dosage should be adjusted for patients with impaired renal function (see CLINICAL PHARMACOLOGY and PRECAUTIONS). As a general guideline, it is recommended that initial therapy with Hylorel in patients with creatinine clearances of 30 to 60 ml/min be reduced to 5 mg every 24 hours. In patients with creatinine clearances less than 30 ml/min, the dosing interval should be increased to 48 hours. The time to achieve steady state will be increased. Dosage increases should be made cautiously at intervals not less than 7 days in patients with moderate renal insufficiency and not less than 14 days in patients with severe renal insufficiency. These recommendations are based upon human pharmacokinetic data and not clinical experience.

HOW SUPPLIED:

Hylorel Tablets are available as follows:

10 mg, scored elliptical tablets (light orange)

25 mg, scored elliptical tablets (white)

Store at controlled room temperature 15°-30° C (59°-86° F). Keep out of the reach of children.

(Fisons Pharmaceuticals, 4/94, RF253, 814 438 104, 691015)

HOW SUPPLIED - EQUIVALENTS NOT AVAILABLE:

Tablet, Uncoated - Oral - 10 mg

100's $74.87 HYLOREL, Medeva Pharms 53014-0787-71

Tablet, Uncoated - Oral - 25 mg

100's $108.36 HYLOREL, Fisons 00585-0788-71

GUANETHIDINE MONOSULFATE *(001410)*

CATEGORIES: Amyloidosis; Antihypertensives; Cardiovascular Drugs; Hypertension; Pyelonephritis; Renal Function; Renal Drugs; Stenosis; Vasodilating Agents; Pregnancy Category C; FDA Approval Pre 1982

BRAND NAMES: *Antipres*; *Apo-Guanethidine* (Canada); *Declindin*; Ingadine; **Ismelin**; *Ismeline*; *Normalin*; *Sanotensin*
(International brand names outside U.S. in italics)

FORMULARIES: Aetna; BC-BS; Medi-Cal

COST OF THERAPY: $181.29 (Hypertension; Tablet; 10 mg; 1/day; 365 days)

PRIMARY ICD9: 401.1 (Essential Hypertension, Benign)

DESCRIPTION:

Ismelin, guanethidine monosulfate USP, is an antihypertensive, available as tablets of 10 mg and 25 mg for oral administration. Each 10-mg and 25-mg tablet contains guanethidine monosulfate USP equivalent to 10 mg and 25 mg of guanethidine sulfate USP. Its chemical name is (2-(hexahydro-1(*2H*)-azocinyl)ethyl)guanidine sulfate 1:1.

Guanethidine monosulfate USP is a white to off-white crystalline powder with a molecular weight of 296.38. It is very soluble in water, sparingly soluble in alcohol, and practically insoluble in chloroform.

Ismelin Inactive Ingredients: Calcium stearate, colloidal silicon dioxide, D&C Yellow No. 10 (10-mg tablets), lactose, starch, stearic acid, and sucrose.

CLINICAL PHARMACOLOGY:

Guanethidine monosulfate acts at the sympathetic neuroeffector junction by inhibiting or interfering with the release and/or distribution of the chemical mediator (presumably the catecholamine norepinephrine), rather than acting at the effector cell by inhibiting the association of the transmitter with its receptors. In contrast to ganglionic blocking agents, guanethidine monosulfate suppresses equally the responses mediated by alpha-and beta-adrenergic receptors but does not produce parasympathetic blockade. Since sympathetic blockade results in modest decreases in peripheral resistance and cardiac output, guanethidine monosulfate lowers blood pressure in the supine position. It further reduces blood pressure by decreasing the degree of vasoconstriction that normally results from reflex sympathetic nervous activity upon assumption of the upright posture, thus reducing venous return and cardiac output more. The inhibition of sympathetic venoconstrictive mechanisms results in venous pooling of blood. Therefore, the effect of guanethidine monosulfate is especially pronounced when the patient is standing. Both the systolic and diastolic pressures are reduced.

Other actions at the sympathetic nerve terminal include depletion of norepinephrine. Once it gains access to the neuron, guanethidine monosulfate accumulates within the intraneuronal storage vesicles and causes depletion of norepinephrine stores within the nerve terminal. Prolonged oral administration of guanethidine monosulfate produces a denervation sensitivity of the neuroeffector junction, probably resulting from the chronic reduction in norepinephrine released by the sympathetic nerve endings. Systemic responses to catecholamines released from the adrenal medulla are not prevented and may even be augmented as a result of this denervation sensitivity. A paradoxical hypertensive crisis may occur if guanethidine monosulfate is given to patients with pheochromocytoma or if norepinephrine is given to a patient receiving the drug.

Due to its poor lipid solubility, guanethidine monosulfate does not readily cross the blood-brain barrier. In contrast to most neural blocking agents, guanethidine monosulfate does not appear to suppress plasma renin activity in many patients.

PHARMACOKINETICS

The pharmacokinetics of guanethidine monosulfate are complex. The amount of drug in plasma and in urine is linearly related to dose, although large differences occur between individuals because of variation in absorption and metabolism. Adrenergic blockade occurs with a minimum concentration in plasma of 8 ng/ml; this concentration is achieved in different individuals with dosages of 10-50 mg/day at steady state. Guanethidine monosulfate is eliminated slowly because of extensive tissue binding. After chronic oral administration, the initial phase of elimination with a half-life of 1.5 days is followed by a second phase of elimination with a half-life of 4-8 days. The renal clearance of guanethidine monosulfate is 56 ml/min. Guanethidine monosulfate is converted by the liver to three metabolites, which are excreted in the urine. The metabolites are pharmacologically less active than guanethidine monosulfate.

INDICATIONS AND USAGE:

Guanethidine monosulfate is indicated for the treatment of moderate and severe hypertension, either alone or as an adjunct, and for the treatment of renal hypertension, including that secondary to pyelonephritis, renal amyloidosis, and renal artery stenosis.

CONTRAINDICATIONS:

Known or suspected pheochromocytoma; hypersensitivity; frank congestive heart failure not due to hypertension; use of monoamine oxidase (MAO) inhibitors.

WARNINGS:

Guanethidine monosulfate is a potent drug and its use can lead to disturbing and serious clinical problems. Before prescribing, physicians should familiarize themselves with the details of its use and warn patients not to deviate from instructions.

Orthostatic hypotension can occur frequently, and patients should be properly instructed about this potential hazard. Fainting spells may occur unless the patient is forewarned to sit or lie down with the onset of dizziness or weakness. Postural hypotension is most marked in the morning and is accentuated by hot weather, alcohol, or exercise. Dizziness or weakness may be particularly bothersome during the initial period of dosage adjustment and with postural changes, such as arising the morning. The potential occurrence of these symptoms may require alteration of previous daily activity. The patient should be cautioned to avoid sudden or prolonged standing or exercise while taking the drug.

Inhibition of ejaculation has been reported in animals (see PRECAUTIONS, Carcinogenesis, Mutagenesis, and Impairment of Fertility) as well as in men given guanethidine monosulfate. This effect, which result from the sympathetic blockade caused by the drug's action, is reversible after guanethidine monosulfate has been discontinued for several weeks. The drug does not cause parasympathetic blockade, and erectile potency is usually retained during administration of guanethidine monosulfate. The possible occurrence of inhibition of ejaculation should be kept in mind when considering the use of guanethidine in men or reproductive age.

If possible, therapy should be withdrawn 2 weeks prior to surgery to reduce the possibility of vascular collapse and cardiac arrest during anesthesia. If emergency surgery is indicated, preanesthetic and anesthetic agents should be administered cautiously in reduced dosage. Oxygen, atropine, vasopressors, and adequate solutions for volume replacement should be ready for immediate use to counteract vascular collapse in the surgical patient. Vasopressors should be used only with extreme caution, since guanethidine monosulfate augments responsiveness to exogenously administered norepinephrine and vasopressors; specially; blood pressure may rise and cardiac arrhythmias may be produced.

PRECAUTIONS:

GENERAL

Dosage requirements may be reduced in the presence of fever.

Special care should be exercised when treating patients with a history of bronchial asthma; asthmatic patients are more apt to be hypersensitive to catecholamine depletion, and their condition may be aggravated.

The effects of guanethidine monosulfate are cumulative over long periods; initial doses should be small and increased gradually in small increments.

Guanethidine monosulfate should be used very cautiously in hypertensive patients with: renal disease and nitrogen retention or rising BUN levels, since decreased blood pressure may further compromise renal function; coronary insufficiency or recent myocardial infarction; and cerebrovascular disease, especially with encephalopathy.

Guanethidine monosulfate should not be given to patients with severe cardiac failure except with extreme caution, since guanethidine monosulfate may interfere with the compensatory role of the adrenergic system in producing circulatory adjustment in patients with congestive heart failure.

Patients with incipient cardiac decompensation should be watched for weight gain or edema, which may be averted by the concomitant administration of a thiazide.

Guanethidine monosulfate should be used cautiously in patients with a history of peptic ulcer or other chronic disorders that may be aggravated by a relative increase in parasympathetic tone.

INFORMATION FOR THE PATIENT

The patient should be advised to take guanethidine monosulfate exactly as directed. If the patient misses a dose, he or she should be told to take only the next scheduled dose (without doubling it).

The patient should be advised to avoid sudden or prolonged standing or exercise and to arise slowly, especially in the morning, to reduce the orthostatic hypotensive effects of dizziness, lightheadedness, or fainting.

The patient should be cautioned about ingesting alcohol, since it aggravates the orthostatic hypotensive effects of guanethidine monosulfate.

Male patients should be advised that guanethidine may interfere with ejaculation.

CARCINOGENESIS, MUTAGENESIS, AND IMPAIRMENT OF FERTILITY

Long-term carcinogenicity studies in animals have not been conducted with guanethidine monosulfate.

While inhibition of sperm passage and accumulation of sperm debris have been reported in rats and rabbits after several weeks of administration of guanethidine monosulfate, 5 or 10 mg/kg per day, subcutaneously or intraperitoneally, recovery of ejaculatory function and fertility has been demonstrated in rats given guanethidine monosulfate intramuscularly, 25 mg/kg per day, for 8 weeks. Inhibition of ejaculation has also been reported in men (see WARNINGSand ADVERSE REACTIONS). This effect, which is attributable to the sympathetic blockade caused by the drug, is reversible several weeks after discontinuance of the drug.

PREGNANCY CATEGORY C

Animal reproduction studies have not been conducted with guanethidine monosulfate. It is also not known whether guanethidine monosulfate can cause fetal harm when administered to a pregnant woman or can affect reproduction capacity. Guanethidine monosulfate should be given to a pregnant woman only if clearly needed.

NURSING MOTHERS

Guanethidine monosulfate is excreted in breast milk in very small quantity. Caution should be exercised when guanethidine monosulfate is administered to a nursing woman.

PEDIATRIC USE

Safety and effectiveness in children have not been established.

DRUG INTERACTIONS:

Concurrent use of guanethidine monosulfate and rauwolfia derivatives may cause excessive postural hypotension, bradycardia, and mental depression.

Both digitalis and guanethidine monosulfate slow the heart rate.

Thiazide diuretics enhance the antihypertensive action of guanethidine monosulfate (see DOSAGE AND ADMINISTRATION).

Amphetamine-like compounds, stimulants (*e.g.,* ephedrine, methylphenidate), tricyclic antidepressants (*e.g.,* amitriptyline, imipramine, desipramine) and other psychopharmacologic agents (*e.g.,* phenothiazines and related compounds), as well as oral contraceptives, may reduce the hypotensive effect of guanethidine monosulfate.

MAO inhibitors should be discontinued for at least 1 week before starting therapy with guanethidine monosulfate.

ADVERSE REACTIONS:

The following adverse reactions have been observed, but there are not enough data to support an estimate of their frequency. Consequently the reactions are categorized by organ system and are listed in decreasing order of severity and not frequency.

Digestive : Diarrhea, which may be severe at times and necessitate discontinuance of medication; vomiting; nausea; increased bowel movements; dry mouth; parotid tenderness.

Cardiovascular: Chest pains (angina); bradycardia; a tendency toward fluid retention and edema with occasional development of congestive heart failure.

Respiratory: Dyspnea; asthma in susceptible individuals; nasal congestion.

Neurologic: Syncope resulting from either postural or exertional hypotension; dizziness; blurred vision; muscle tremor; ptosis of the lids; mental depression; chest paresthesias; weakness; lassitude; fatigue.

Muscular: Myalgia.

Genitourinary: Rise in BUN; urinary incontinence; inhibition of ejaculation; nocturia.

Metabolic: Weight gain.

Skin and Appendages: Dermatitis; scalp hair loss.

Although a causal relationship has not been established, a few instances of blood dyscrasias (anemia, thrombocytopenia, and leukopenia) and of priapism or impotence have been reported.

OVERDOSAGE:

Acute Toxicity: No deaths due to acute poisoning have been reported.

Oral LD_{50} in rats: 1262 mg/kg.

Signs and Symptoms: Postural hypotension (with dizziness, blurred vision, and possibly syncope when standing), shock, and bradycardia are most likely to occur; diarrhea (possibly severe), nausea, and vomiting may also occur. Unconsciousness is unlikely if adequate blood pressure and cerebral perfusion can be maintained by placing the patient in the supine position and by administering other treatment as required.

Treatment: There is no specific antidote.

Treatment should consist of gastric lavage. An activated charcoal slurry should be instilled and laxatives given, if conditions permit.

In sinus bradycardia, atropine should be administered.

In previously normotensive patients, treatment has consisted essentially of restoring blood pressure and heart rate to normal by keeping the patient in the supine position. Normal homeostatic control usually returns gradually over a 72-hour period in these patients.

In previously hypertensive patients, particularly those with impaired cardiac reserve or other cardiovascular-renal disease, intensive treatment may be required to support vital functions and to control cardiac irregularities that might be present. The supine position must be maintained; if vasopressors are required, they must be used with extreme caution, since guanethidine monosulfate may increase responsiveness, causing a rise in blood pressure and development of cardiac arrhythmias.

Diarrhea, if severe or persistent, should be treated with anticholinergic agents to reduce intestinal hypermotility; hydration and electrolyte balance should be maintained.

Since guanethidine monosulfate is excreted slowly, cardiovascular and renal function should be monitored for a few days.

DOSAGE AND ADMINISTRATION:

Better control may be obtained, especially in the initial phases of treatment, if the patient can have his blood pressure recorded regularly at home.

AMBULATORY PATIENTS

Initial doses should be small (10 mg) and increased gradually, depending upon the patient's response. Guanethidine monosulfate has a long duration of action; therefore, dosage increases should not be made more often than every 5-7 days, unless the patient is hospitalized.

Blood pressure should be measured in the supine position, after standing for 10 minutes, and immediately after exercise if feasible. Dosage may be increased only if there has been no decrease in the standing blood pressure from previous levels. The average daily dose is 25-50 mg; only one dose a day is usually required (**TABLE 1**).

TABLE 1 Dosage Chart for Ambulatory Patients

Visits (Intervals of 5 - 7 Days)	Daily Dose
Visit 1 (Patient may be started on 10-mg tablets)	10 mg
Visit 2	20 mg
Visit 3 (Patient may be changed to 25-mg tablets whenever convenient)	30 mg (three 10-mg tablets) or 37.5 mg (one and one-half 25-mg tablets)
Visit 4	50 mg
Visit 5 and subsequent	Dosage may be increased by 12.5 mg or 25 mg if necessary.

The dosage should be reduced in any of the following situations: (1) normal supine pressure; (2) excessive orthostatic fall in pressure; (3) severe diarrhea.

HOSPITALIZED PATIENTS

Initial oral dose is 25-50 mg, increased by 25 mg or 50 mg daily or every other day, as indicated. This higher dosage is possible because hospitalized patients can be watched carefully. Unless absolutely impossible, the standing blood pressure should be measured regularly. Patients should not be discharged from the hospital until the effect of the drug on the standing blood pressure is known. Patients should be told about the possibility of orthostatic hypotension and warned not to get out of bed without help during the period of dosage adjustment.

DOSAGE AND ADMINISTRATION: *(cont'd)*

COMBINATION THERAPY

Guanethidine monosulfate may be added gradually to thiazides and/or hydralazine. Thiazide diuretics enhance the effectiveness of guanethidine monosulfate and may reduce the incidence of edema. When thiazide diuretics are added to the regimen in patients taking guanethidine monosulfate, it is usually necessary to reduce the dosage of guanethidine monosulfate. After control is established, the dosage of all drugs should be reduced to the lowest effective level.

Note: When guanethidine monosulfate is replacing MAO inhibitors, at least 1 week should elapse before commencing treatment with guanethidine monosulfate (see CONTRAINDICATIONS). If ganglionic blockers have not been discontinued before guanethidine monosulfate is started, they should be gradually withdrawn to prevent a spiking blood pressure response during the transfer period.

Do not store above 86° F (30° C). *Dispense in tight container (USP).*

HOW SUPPLIED - EQUIVALENTS NOT AVAILABLE:

Tablet, Uncoated - Oral - 10 mg

100's $49.67 ISMELIN, Novartis 00083-0049-30

Tablet, Uncoated - Oral - 25 mg

100's $81.17 ISMELIN, Novartis 00083-0103-30

GUANETHIDINE MONOSULFATE; HYDROCHLOROTHIAZIDE *(001411)*

CATEGORIES: Antihypertensives; Cardiovascular Drugs; Diuretics; Hypertension; Renal Drugs; Vasodilating Agents; Pregnancy Category B; FDA Approval Pre 1982

BRAND NAMES: **Esimil**; *Ismelin-Esidrix* (Canada)
(International brand names outside U.S. in italics)

FORMULARIES: Aetna

WARNING:
This fixed-combination drug is not indicated for initial therapy of hypertension. Hypertension requires therapy titrated to the individual patient. If the fixed combination represents the dosage so determined, its use may be more convenient in patient management. The treatment of hypertension is not static but be must be reevaluated as conditions in each patient warrant.

DESCRIPTION:

Esimil is an antihypertensive-diuretic combination, available as tablets for oral administration. Each tablet contains Ismelin (guanethidine monosulfate USP), 10 mg, and Esidrix (hydrochlorothiazide USP), 25 mg.

FOR COMPLETE PRESCRIBING INFORMATION REFER TO THE INDIVIDUAL DRUG MONOGRAPHS (GUANETHIDINE MONOSULFATE, HYDROCHLOROTHIAZIDE).

INDICATIONS AND USAGE:

Guanethidine monosulfate HCTZ is indicated for the treatment of hypertension.

DOSAGE AND ADMINISTRATION:

Dosage should be determined by individual titration.

The usual dosage is two tablets daily. Depending upon the degree of hypertension, the patient should be started on the lowest possible dose (usually one tablet daily) and the dose gradually increased at weekly intervals until the desired response is obtained. Blood pressure should be recorded with the patient in the supine position and again after 10 minutes of standing. Dosage should be increased only if standing blood pressure has not been reduced to desired levels. Dosage adjustment should be made at not less than weekly intervals; maximal dosage should not exceed four tablets daily. If additional effect is desirable, guanethidine tablets may be supplemented individually.

Before starting therapy with guanethidine monosulfate HCTZ, at least 1 week should elapse after MAO inhibitors or ganglionic blockers are discontinued.

When guanethidine monosulfate HCTZ is to be substituted for other antihypertensive agents, the change should be made gradually. In general, dosage of the agent to be discontinued should be halved, and guanethidine monosulfate HCTZ should be started at one tablet daily. This schedule should be followed for at least 1 week; then, dosage of the previous therapy may be halved again and the dosage of guanethidine monosulfate HCTZ increased to two tablets daily. At the next weekly interval, the previously used drugs can generally be discontinued. The dosage of guanethidine monosulfate HCTZ should be titrated at weekly intervals, as mentioned above.

Patients receiving more than 75 mg of guanethidine alone may do well on a smaller dose if also given hydrochlorothiazide. Because of the ratio of the combination, these patients are probably not candidates for guanethidine monosulfate HCTZ.

Do not store above 86°F (30°C).

HOW SUPPLIED - EQUIVALENTS NOT AVAILABLE:

Tablet, Uncoated - Oral - 10 mg/25 mg

100's $66.46 ESIMIL, Novartis 00083-0047-30

GUANFACINE HYDROCHLORIDE *(001412)*

CATEGORIES: Alpha Adrenoreceptor Agonists; Antihypertensives; Cardiovascular Drugs; Hypertension; Pregnancy Category B; FDA Approved 1986 Oct

BRAND NAMES: *Entulic*; *Estulic* (France, Germany, Japan); **Tenex**
(International brand names outside U.S. in italics)

FORMULARIES: BC-BS; Medi-Cal

COST OF THERAPY: $87.52 (Hypertension; Tablet; 1 mg; 1/day; 365 days)

PRIMARY ICD9: 401.1 (Essential Hypertension, Benign)

DESCRIPTION:

Guanfacine HCl is a centrally acting antihypertensive with α_2-adrenoceptor agonist properties in tablet form for oral administration.

DESCRIPTION: *(cont'd)*

The chemical name of guanfacine HCl is N-amidino-2- (2,6-dichlorophenyl) acetamide hydrochloride and its molecular weight is 282.56.

Guanfacine hydrochloride is a white to off-white powder; sparingly soluble in water and alcohol and slightly soluble in acetone. The tablets contain the following inactive ingredients:

Tenex 1 mg: FD&C Red 40 aluminum lake, Lactose, Microcrystalline cellulose, Povidone, Stearic Acid.

Tenex 2 mg: D&C Yellow 10 aluminum lake, Lactose, Microcrystalline cellulose, Povidone, Stearic Acid.

CLINICAL PHARMACOLOGY:

Guanfacine HCl is an orally active antihypertensive agent whose principal mechanism of action appears to be stimulation of central α_2-adrenergic receptors. By stimulating these receptors, guanfacine reduces sympathetic nerve impulses from the vasomotor center to the heart and blood vessels. This results in a decrease in peripheral vascular resistance and a reduction in heart rate.

Controlled clinical trials in patients with mild to moderate hypertension who were receiving a thiazide-type diuretic have defined the dose- response relationship for blood pressure response and adverse reactions of guanfacine given at bedtime and have shown that the blood pressure response to guanfacine can persist for 24 hours after a single dose. In the dose-response study, patients were randomized to placebo or to doses of 0.5, 1, 2, and 3 mg of guanfacine, each given at bedtime. The observed mean changes from baseline, tabulated in TABLE 1, indicate the similarity of response for placebo and the 0.5 mg dose. Doses of 1, 2, and 3 mg resulted in decreased blood pressure in the sitting position with no real differences among the three doses. In the standing position there was some increase in response with dose.

TABLE 1 Mean Decrease in Seated and Standing Blood Pressure (BP) by Guanfacine Dosage Group

Vital Sign	n =	Placebo 63	0.5 mg 63	1 mg 64	2 mg 58	3 mg 59
Change in Systolic (seated)	BP	-5	-5	-14	-12	-16
Change in Diastolic (seated)	BP	-7	-6	-13	-13	-13
Change in Systolic (standing)	BP	-3	-5	-11	-9	-15
Change in Diastolic (standing)	BP	-5	-4	-9	-10	-12

While most of the effectiveness of guanfacine was present at 1 mg, adverse reactions at this dose were not clearly distinguishable from those associated with placebo. Adverse reactions were clearly present at 2 and 3 mg (see ADVERSE REACTIONS.)

In a placebo-controlled study of guanfacine HCl a significant decrease in blood pressure was maintained for a full 24 hours after dosing. While there was no significant difference between the 12 and 24 hour blood pressure readings, the fall in blood pressure at 24 hours was numerically smaller, suggesting possible escape of blood pressure in some patients and the need for individualization of therapy.

In a double-blind, randomized trial, either guanfacine or clonidine was given at recommended doses with 25 mg chlorthalidone for 24 weeks and then abruptly discontinued. Results showed equal degrees of blood pressure reduction with the two drugs and there was no tendency for blood pressures to increase despite maintenance of the same daily dose of the two drugs. Signs and symptoms of rebound phenomena were infrequent upon discontinuation of either drug. Abrupt withdrawal of clonidine produced a rapid return of diastolic and especially, systolic blood pressure to approximately pre-treatment levels, with occasional values significantly greater than baseline, whereas guanfacine withdrawal produced a more gradual increase to pre-treatment levels, but also with occasional values significantly greater than baseline.

Pharmacodynamics: Hemodynamic studies in man showed that the decrease in blood pressure observed after single-dose or long-term oral treatment with guanfacine was accompanied by a significant decrease in peripheral resistance and a slight reduction in heart rate (5 beats/min). Cardiac output under conditions of rest or exercise was not altered by guanfacine.

Guanfacine HCl lowered elevated plasma renin activity and plasma catecholamine levels in hypertensive patients, but this does not correlate with individual blood-pressure responses.

Growth hormone secretion was stimulated with single oral doses of 2 and 4 mg of guanfacine. Long-term use of guanfacine HCl had no effect on growth hormone levels.

Guanfacine had no effect on plasma aldosterone. A slight but insignificant decrease in plasma volume occurred after one month of guanfacine therapy. There were no changes in mean body weight or electrolytes.

Pharmacokinetics: Relative to an intravenous dose of 3 mg, the absolute oral bioavailability of guanfacine is about 80%. Peak plasma concentrations occur from 1 to 4 hours with an average of 2.6 hours after single oral doses or at steady state.

The area under the concentration-time curve (AUC) increases linearly with the dose.

In individuals with normal renal function, the average elimination half-life is approximately 17 hr (range 10-30 hr). Younger patients tend to have shorter elimination half-lives (13-14 hr) while older patients tend to have half-lives at the upper end of the range. Steady state blood levels were attained within 4 days in most subjects.

In individuals with normal renal function, guanfacine and its metabolites are excreted primarily in the urine. Approximately 50% (40-75%) of the dose is eliminated in the urine as unchanged drug; the remainder is eliminated mostly as conjugates of metabolites produced by oxidative metabolism of the aromatic ring.

The guanfacine-to-creatinine clearance ratio is greater than 1.0, which would suggest that tubular secretion of drug occurs.

The drug is approximately 70% bound to plasma proteins, independent of drug concentration.

The whole body volume of distribution is high (a mean of 6.3 L/kg), which suggests a high distribution of drug to the tissues.

The clearance of guanfacine in patients with varying degrees of renal insufficiency is reduced, but plasma levels of drug are only slightly increased compared to patients with normal renal function. When prescribing for patients with renal impairment, the low end of the dosing range should be used. Patients on dialysis also can be given usual doses of guanfacine hydrochloride as the drug is poorly dialyzed.

INDICATIONS AND USAGE:

Guanfacine HCl is indicated in the management of hypertension. Since dosing information (see DOSAGE AND ADMINISTRATION) has been established in the presence of a thiazide-type diuretic; guanfacine HCl should, therefore, be used in patients who are already receiving a thiazide-type diuretic.

CONTRAINDICATIONS:

Guanfacine HCl is contraindicated in patients with known hypersensitivity to guanfacine hydrochloride.

PRECAUTIONS:

GENERAL

Like other antihypertensive agents, guanfacine HCl should be used with caution in patients with severe coronary insufficiency, recent myocardial infarction, cerebrovascular disease or chronic renal or hepatic failure.

Sedation: Guanfacine HCl, like other orally active central alpha-2 adrenergic agonists, causes sedation or drowsiness, especially when beginning therapy. These symptoms are dose-related (see ADVERSE REACTIONS.) When guanfacine HCl is used with other centrally active depressants (such as phenothiazines, barbiturates, or benzodiazepines), the potential for additive sedative effects should be considered.

Rebound: Abrupt cessation of therapy with orally active central alpha-2 adrenergic agonists may be associated with increases (from depressed on-therapy levels) in plasma and urinary catecholamines, symptoms of "nervousness and anxiety" and, less commonly, increases in blood pressure to levels significantly greater than those prior to therapy.

INFORMATION FOR THE PATIENT

Patients who receive guanfacine HCl should be advised to exercise caution when operating dangerous machinery or driving motor vehicles until it is determined that they do not become drowsy or dizzy from the medication. Patients should be warned that their tolerance for alcohol and other CNS depressants may be diminished. Patients should be advised not to discontinue therapy abruptly.

LABORATORY TESTS

In clinical trials, no clinically relevant laboratory test abnormalities were identified as causally related to drug during short-term treatment with guanfacine HCl.

DRUG/LABORATORY TEST INTERACTIONS

No laboratory test abnormalities related to the use of guanfacine HCl have been identified.

CARCINOGENESIS, MUTAGENESIS, AND IMPAIRMENT OF FERTILITY

No carcinogenic effect was observed in studies of 78 weeks in mice at doses more than 150 times the maximum recommended human dose and 102 weeks in rats at doses more than 100 times the maximum recommended human dose. In a variety of test models guanfacine was not mutagenic.

No adverse effects were observed in fertility studies in male and female rats.

PREGNANCY CATEGORY B

Administration of guanfacine to rats at 70 times the maximum recommended human dose and rabbits at 20 times the maximum recommended human dose resulted in no evidence of impaired fertility or harm to the fetus. Higher doses (100 and 200 times the maximum recommended human dose in rabbits and rats respectively) were associated with reduced fetal survival and maternal toxicity. Rat experiments have shown that guanfacine crosses the placenta.

There are, however, no adequate and well-controlled studies in pregnant women. Because animal reproduction studies are not always predictive of human response, this drug should be used during pregnancy only if clearly needed.

LABOR AND DELIVERY

Guanfacine HCl is not recommended in the treatment of acute hypertension associated with toxemia of pregnancy. There is no information available on the effects of guanfacine on the course of labor and delivery.

NURSING MOTHERS

It is not known whether guanfacine HCl is excreted in human milk. Because many drugs are excreted in human milk, caution should be exercised when guanfacine HCl is administered to a nursing woman. Experiments with rats have shown that guanfacine is excreted in the milk.

PEDIATRIC USE

Safety and effectiveness in children under 12 years of age have not been demonstrated. Therefore, the use of guanfacine HCl in this age group is not recommended.

DRUG INTERACTIONS:

The potential for increased sedation when guanfacine HCl is given with other CNS- depressant drugs should be appreciated.

The administration of guanfacine concomitantly with a known microsomal enzyme inducer (phenobarbital or phenytoin) to two patients with renal impairment reportedly resulted in significant reductions in elimination half-life and plasma concentration. In such cases, therefore, more frequent dosing may be required to achieve or maintain the desired hypotensive response. Further, if guanfacine is to be discontinued in such patients, careful tapering of the dosage may be necessary in order to avoid rebound phenomena (see Rebound.)

Anticoagulants: Ten patients who were stabilized on oral anticoagulants were given guanfacine, 1-2 mg/day, for 4 weeks. No changes were observed in the degree of anticoagulation.

In several well-controlled studies, guanfacine was administered together with diuretics with no drug interactions reported. In the long-term safety studies, guanfacine HCl was given concomitantly with many drugs without evidence of any interactions. The principal drugs given (number of patients in parentheses) were: cardiac glycosides (115), sedatives and hypnotics (103), coronary vasodilators (52), oral hypoglycemics (45), cough and cold preparations (45), NSAIDs (38), anti-hyperlipidemics (29), antigout drugs (24), oral contraceptives (18), bronchodilators (13), insulin (10), and beta blockers (10).

ADVERSE REACTIONS:

Adverse reactions noted with guanfacine HCl are similar to those of other drugs of the central α-2 adrenoreceptor agonist class: dry mouth, sedation (somnolence), weakness (asthenia), dizziness, constipation, and impotence. While the reactions are common, most are mild and tend to disappear on continued dosing.

Skin rash with exfoliation has been reported in a few cases; although clear cause and effect relationships to guanfacine HCl could not be established, should a rash occur, guanfacine HCl should be discontinued and the patient monitored appropriately.

In a 12-week placebo-controlled, dose-response study the frequency of the most commonly observed adverse reactions showed a clear dose relationship from 0.5 to 3 mg, as follows (TABLE 2):

There were 41 premature terminations because of adverse reactions in this study. The percent of patients who terminated and the dose at which they terminated were as follows (TABLE 3):

Reasons for dropouts among patients who received guanfacine were: somnolence, headache, weakness, dry mouth, dizziness, impotence, insomnia, constipation, syncope, urinary incontinence, conjunctivitis, paresthesia, and dermatitis. In a second placebo-controlled study in which the dose should be adjusted upward to 3 mg per day in 1-mg increments at 3-week intervals, i.e., a setting more similar to ordinary clinical use, the most commonly recorded reactions were: dry mouth 47%, constipation 16%, fatigue 12%, somnolence 10%, asthenia 6%, dizziness 6%, headache 4%, and insomnia 4%.

ADVERSE REACTIONS: *(cont'd)*

TABLE 2

Adverse Reaction	Placebo	Assigned Treatment Group 0.5 mg	1.0 mg	2.0 mg	3.0 mg
n =	73	72	72	72	72
Dry Mouth	5 (7%)	4 (5%)	6 (8%)	8 (11%)	20 (28%)
Somnolence	1 (1%)	3 (4%)	0 (0%)	1 (1%)	10 (14%)
Asthenia	0 (0%)	2 (3%)	0 (0%)	2 (2%)	7 (10%)
Dizziness	2 (2%)	1 (1%)	3 (4%)	6 (8%)	3 (4%)
Headache	3 (4%)	4 (3%)	3 (4%)	1 (1%)	2 (2%)
Impotence	1 (1%)	1 (0%)	0 (0%)	1 (1%)	3 (4%)
Constipation	0 (0%)	0 (0%)	0 (0%)	1 (1%)	1 (1%)
Fatigue	3 (3%)	2 (3%)	2 (3%)	5 (6%)	3 (4%)

TABLE 3

Dose:	Placebo	0.5 mg	1 mg	2 mg	3 mg
Terminated:	6.9%	4.2%	3.2%	6.9%	8.3%

Reasons for dropouts among patients who received guanfacine were: somnolence, dry mouth, dizziness, impotence, constipation, confusion, depression, and palpitations.

In the clonidine/guanfacine comparison described in Clinical Pharmacology, the most common adverse reactions noted were (TABLE 4):

TABLE 4

	Guanfacine (n=279)	Clonidine (n=278)
Dry mouth	30%	37%
Somnolence	21%	35%
Dizziness	11%	8%
Constipation	10%	5%
Fatigue	9%	8%
Headache	4%	4%
Insomnia	4%	3%

Adverse reactions occurring in 3% or less of patients in the three controlled trials were:

Cardiovascular: bradycardia, palpitations, substernal pain

Gastrointestinal: abdominal pain, diarrhea, dyspepsia, dysphagia, nausea

CNS: amnesia, confusion, depression, insomnia, libido decrease

ENT disorders: rhinitis, taste perversion, tinnitus

Eye disorders: conjunctivitis, iritis, vision disturbance

Musculoskeletal: leg cramps, hypokinesia

Respiratory: dyspnea

Dermatologic: dermatitis, pruritus, purpura, sweating

Urogenital: testicular disorder, urinary incontinence

Other: malaise, paresthesia, paresis

Adverse reaction reports tend to decrease over time. In an open-label trial of one year's duration, 580 hypertensive subjects were given guanfacine, titrated to achieve goal blood pressure, alone (51%), with diuretic (38%), with beta blocker (3%), with diuretic plus beta blocker (6%), or with diuretic plus vasodilator (2%). The mean daily dose of guanfacine reached was 4.7 mg (TABLE 5):

TABLE 5

Adverse Reaction	Incidence of adverse reactions at any time during the study	Incidence of adverse at end of one year
N	580	580
Dry mouth	60%	15%
Drowsiness	33%	6%
Dizziness	15%	1%
Constipation	14%	3%
Weakness	5%	1%
Headache	4%	0.2%
Insomnia	5%	0%

There were 52 (8.9%) dropouts due to adverse effects in this 1-year trial. The causes were: dry mouth (n = 20), weakness (n = 12), constipation (n = 7), somnolence (n = 3), nausea (n = 3), orthostatic hypotension (n = 2), insomnia (n = 1), rash (n = 1), nightmares (n = 1), headache (n = 1), and depression (n = 1).

Postmarketing Experience: An open-label postmarketing study involving 21,718 patients was conducted to assess the safety of guanfacine HCl 1 mg/day given at bedtime for 28 days. Guanfacine HCl was administered with or without other antihypertensive agents. Adverse events reported in the postmarketing study at an incidence greater than 1% included dry mouth, dizziness, somnolence, fatigue, headache and nausea. The most commonly reported adverse events in this study were the same as those observed in controlled clinical trials.

Less frequent, possibly guanfacine HCl-related events observed in the postmarketing study and/or reported spontaneously include:

Body As A Whole: asthenia, chest pain, edema, malaise, tremor

Cardiovascular: bradycardia, palpitations, syncope, tachycardia

Central Nervous System: paresthesias, vertigo

Eye Disorders: blurred vision

Gastrointestinal System: abdominal pain, constipation, diarrhea, dyspepsia

Liver And Biliary System: abnormal liver function tests

Musculo-Skeletal System: arthralgia, leg cramps, leg pain, myalgia

Psychiatric: agitation, anxiety, confusion, depression, insomnia, nervousness

Reproductive System, Male: impotence

Respiratory System: dyspnea

Skin And Appendages: alopecia, dermatitis, exfoliative pruritus, rash, dermatitis,

Special Senses: alterations in taste

Urinary System: nocturia, urinary frequency

Rare, serious disorders with no definitive cause and effect relationship to guanfacine HCl have been reported spontaneously and/or in the postmarketing study. These events include acute renal failure, cardiac fibrillation, cerebrovascular accident, congestive heart failure, heart block, and myocardial infarction.

DRUG ABUSE AND DEPENDENCE:

No reported abuse or dependence has been associated with the administration of guanfacine HCl.

OVERDOSAGE:

Signs and Symptoms: Drowsiness, lethargy, bradycardia and hypotension have been observed following overdose with guanfacine.

A 25-year-old female intentionally ingested 60 mg. She presented with severe drowsiness and bradycardia of 45 beats/minute. Gastric lavage was performed and an infusion of isoproterenol (0.8 mg in 12 hours) was administered. She recovered quickly and without sequelae.

A 28-year-old female who ingested 30-40 mg developed only lethargy, was treated with activated charcoal and a cathartic, was monitored for 24 hours, and was discharged in good health.

A 2-year-old male weighing 12 kg, who ingested up to 4 mg of guanfacine, developed lethargy. Gastric lavage (followed by activated charcoal and sorbitol slurry via NG tube) removed some tablet fragments within 2 hours after ingestion, and vital signs were normal. During 24-hour observation in ICU, systolic pressure was 58 and heart rate 70 at 16 hours post- ingestion. No intervention was required, and child was discharged fully recovered the next day.

Treatment: Gastric lavage and infusion of isoproterenol, as appropriate.

Guanfacine is not dialyzable in clinically significant amounts (2.4%).

DOSAGE AND ADMINISTRATION:

The recommended dose of guanfacine HCl is 1 mg daily given at bedtime to minimize somnolence. Patients should already be receiving a thiazide type diuretic.

If after 3 to 4 weeks of therapy, 1 mg does not give a satisfactory result, doses of 2 and then subsequently 3 mg may be given, although most of the effect of guanfacine HCl is seen at 1 mg (see CLINICAL PHARMACOLOGY.) Some patients may show a rise in pressure toward the end of the dosing interval; in this event a divided dose may be utilized.

Higher daily doses (rarely up to 40 mg/day, in divided doses) have been used, but adverse reactions increase significantly with doses above 3 mg/day and there is no evidence of increased efficacy. No studies have established an appropriate dose or dosing interval when guanfacine HCl is given as the sole antihypertensive agent.

The frequency of rebound hypertension is low, but rebound can occur. When rebound occurs, it does so after 2-4 days, which is delayed compared with clonidine hydrochloride. This is consistent with the longer half-life of guanfacine. In most cases, after abrupt withdrawal of guanfacine, blood pressure returns to pretreatment levels slowly (within 2-4 days) without ill effects.

Store at controlled room temperature, between 15 and 30°C (59 and 86°F).

HOW SUPPLIED - RATED THERAPEUTICALLY EQUIVALENT:

Tablet - Oral - 1.0 mg

100's	$81.08	Guanfacine, Mylan	00378-1160-01

Tablet - Oral - 2.0 mg

100's	$111.15	Guanfacine, Mylan	00378-1190-01

Tablet, Uncoated - Oral - 1 mg

100's	$70.58	Guanfacine HCl, Watson Labs	52544-0444-01
100's	**$87.11**	**TENEX, AH Robins**	**00031-8901-63**
100's	**$93.90**	**TENEX, AH Robins**	**00031-8901-64**
500's	**$413.44**	**TENEX, AH Robins**	**00031-8901-70**

Tablet, Uncoated - Oral - 2 mg

100's	$96.77	Guanfacine HCl, Watson Labs	52544-0453-01
100's	**$119.43**	**TENEX 2, AH Robins**	**00031-8903-63**

GUANIDINE HYDROCHLORIDE *(001413)*

CATEGORIES: Autonomic Drugs; Cancer; Eaton-Lambert Syndrome; Parasympathomimetic Agents; Myasthenia Gravis*; FDA Approval Pre 1982

* Indication not approved by the FDA

DESCRIPTION:

Chemically, guanidine (aminomethanamidine) hydrochloride is a crystalline powder, freely soluble in water and alcohol. The aqueous solution is neutral.

Each tablet contains 125 mg of guanidine hydrochloride with no color additive in the base.

CLINICAL PHARMACOLOGY:

Guanidine apparently acts by enhancing the release of acetylcholine following a nerve impulse. It also appears to slow the rates of depolarization and repolarization of muscle cell membranes.

INDICATIONS AND USAGE:

Guanidine is indicated for the reduction of the symptoms of muscle weakness and easy fatigability associated with the myasthenic syndrome of Eaton-Lambert. It is not indicated for treating myasthenia gravis. The Eaton-Lambert syndrome is ordinarily differentiated from myasthenia gravis by the usual association of the syndrome with a small cell carcinoma of the lung, but myography may be necessary to make the diagnosis.

CONTRAINDICATIONS:

Guanidine is contraindicated in individuals with a history of intolerance or allergy to this drug.

WARNINGS:

Fatal bone-marrow suppression, apparently dose related, can occur with guanidine.

Safe use of guanidine hydrochloride in pregnancy has not been established. Therefore, the benefits of therapy must be weighed against the potential hazards. Because guanidine is excreted in milk, patients on this drug should discontinue breast feeding.

Since there is inadequate experience in children who have received this drug, safety and efficacy in children have not been established.

PRECAUTIONS:

Baseline blood studies should be followed by frequent red and white blood cell and differential counts. The drug should be discontinued upon appearance of bone-marrow suppression. Concurrent therapy with other drugs that may cause bone-marrow suppression should be avoided.

Renal function may be affected in some patients receiving guanidine. Patients should therefore have regular urine examinations and serum creatinine determinations while taking this drug.

PRECAUTIONS: *(cont'd)*

Physicians should be given adequate precautions pertaining to the gastrointestinal side effects and the possibility of induced behavior disorders.

Treatment should not be continued longer than necessary.

ADVERSE REACTIONS:

Anemia, leukopenia, and thrombocytopenia resulting from bone-marrow depression attributable to guanidine have been reported. Other adverse reactions that have been observed are:

General: sore throat, rash, fever.

Neurologic: paresthesia of lips, face, hands, feet; cold sensations in hands and feet; nervousness, lightheadedness, jitteriness, increased irritability; tremor, trembling sensation; ataxia; emotional lability; psychotic state; confusion; mood changes and hallucinations.

Gastrointestinal: dry mouth; gastric irritation; anorexia, nausea; diarrhea; abdominal cramping. Gastrointestinal side effects may preclude the use of guanidine as a desired form of therapy.

Dermatologic: rash, flushing or pink complexion; folliculitis; petechiae, purpura, ecchymoses; sweating; skin eruptions; dryness and scaling of the skin.

Renal: elevation of blood creatinine; uremia; chronic interstitial nephritis and renal tubular necrosis.

Hepatic: abnormal liver function tests.

Cardiac: palpitation, tachycardia, atrial fibrillation, hypotension.

OVERDOSAGE:

Mild gastrointestinal disorders, such as anorexia, increased peristalsis, or diarrhea are early warnings that tolerance is being exceeded. These symptoms may be relieved by atropine, but nevertheless note should be taken of these symptoms, and dosage reductions considered. Slight numbness or tingling of the lips and fingertips shortly after taking a dose of guanidine has been reported. This per se is not an indication to discontinue the treatment and/or reduce dosage.

Severe guanidine intoxication is characterized by nervous hyperirritability, fibrillary tremors and convulsive contractions of muscle, salivation, vomiting, diarrhea, hypoglycemia, and circulatory disturbances. Administration of intravenous calcium gluconate may control the neuromuscular and convulsive symptoms and provide some relief of other toxic manifestations.

Atropine is more effective than calcium in relieving the G.I. symptoms, circulatory disturbances, and changes in blood sugar.

DOSAGE AND ADMINISTRATION:

Initial dosage is usually between 10 and 15 mg/kg (5 to 7 mg/pound) of body weight per day in 3 or 4 divided doses. This dosage may be gradually increased to a total daily dosage of 35 mg/kg (16 mg/pound) of body weight per day or up to the development of side effects. As individual tolerance is highly variable, the dosage must be carefully titrated. Once a tolerable dose has been established it should be continued. Occasionally removal of the primary neoplastic lesion may result in an improvement of symptoms, permitting the discontinuance of guanidine.

Store between 15° and 30°C (59° and 86°F)

HOW SUPPLIED - EQUIVALENTS NOT AVAILABLE:

Tablet, Uncoated - Oral - 125 mg

100's	$18.34	GUANIDINE HCL, Schering	00085-0492-01

HAEMOPHILUS B CONJUGATE VACCINE *(001414)*

CATEGORIES: Biologicals; Immunologic; Influenza; Serums, Toxoids and Vaccines; Toxoids; Vaccines; Pregnancy Category C; FDA Approved 1988 Dec

BRAND NAMES: ActHIB; HibTITER; **PedvaxHIB**; ProHIBIT

DESCRIPTION:

PEDVAXHIB

PedvaxHIB (Haemophilus b Conjugate Vaccine (Meningococcal Protein Conjugate)) is a highly purified capsular polysaccharide (polyribosylribitol phosphate or PRP) of *Haemophilus influenzae* type b (Haemophilus b, Ross strain) that is covalently bound to an outer membrane protein complex (OMPC) of the B11 strain of *Neisseria meningitidis* serogroup B. The covalent bonding of the PRP to the OMPC which is necessary for enhanced immunogenicity of the PRP is confirmed by analysis of the conjugate's components by chemical treatment which yields a unique amino acid. This PRP-OMPC conjugate vaccine is a lyophilized preparation containing lactose as a stabilizer.

PedvaxHIB, when reconstituted as directed, is a sterile suspension for intramuscular use formulated to contain: 15 mcg of Haemophilus b PRP, 250 mcg of *Neisseria meningitidis* OMPC, 225 mcg of aluminum as aluminum hydroxide, thimerosal (a mercury derivative) at 1:20,000 as a preservative, and 2.0 mg of lactose, in 0.9% sodium chloride.

HIBTITER

HibTITER Haemophilus b Conjugate Vaccine (Diphtheria CRM_{197} Protein Conjugate) is a sterile solution of a conjugate of oligosaccharides of the capsular antigen of *Haemophilus influenzae* type b (Haemophilus b) and diphtheria CRM_{197}protein (CRM_{197}) dissolved in 0.9% sodium chloride. The oligosaccharides are derived from highly purified capsular polysaccharide, polyribosylribitol phosphate, isolated from Haemophilus b strain Eagan grown in a chemically defined medium (a mixture of mineral salts, amino acids, and cofactors). The oligosaccharides are purified and sized by diafiltrations through a series of ultrafiltration membranes, and coupled by reductive amination directly to highly purified CRM_{197}.[1,2] CRM_{197} is a nontoxic variant of diphtheria toxin isolated from cultures of *Corynebacterium diphtheriae* C7 (β197) grown in a casamino acids and yeast extract- based medium that is ultrafiltered before use. CRM_{197} is purified through ultrafiltration, ammonium sulfate precipitation and ion-exchange chromatography to high purity. The conjugate is purified to remove unreacted protein, oligosaccharides, and reagents; sterilized by filtration; and filled into vials. HibTITER is intended for intramuscular use.

The vaccine is a clear, colorless solution. Each single dose of 0.5 ml is formulated to contain 10 mcg of purified Haemophilus b saccharide and approximately 25 mcg of CRM_{197} protein. Multidose vials contain thimerosal (mercurial derivative) 1:10,000 as a preservative.

CLINICAL PHARMACOLOGY:

PEDVAXHIB

Haemophilus influenzae type b (Haemophilus b) is the most frequent cause of bacterial meningitis and a leading cause of serious, systemic bacterial disease in young children worldwide.[1,2,3,4]

CLINICAL PHARMACOLOGY: *(cont'd)*

Haemophilus b disease occurs primarily in children under 5 years of age and in the United States prior to the initiation of a vaccine program was estimated to account for nearly 20,000 cases of invasive infections annually, approximately 12,000 of which are meningitis. The mortality rate from Haemophilus b meningitis is about 5%. In addition, up to 35% of survivors develop neurologic sequelae including seizures, deafness, and mental retardation.[5,6] Other invasive diseases caused by this bacterium include cellulitis, epiglottitis, sepsis, pneumonia, septic arthritis, osteomyelitis and pericarditis.

It has been estimated that 17% of all cases of Haemophilus b disease occur in infants less than 6 months of age.[7] The peak incidence of Haemophilus b meningitis occurs between 6 to 11 months of age. Forty- seven percent of all cases occur by one year of age with the remaining 53% of cases occurring over the next four years.[2,20]

Among children under 5 years of age, the risk of invasive Haemophilus b disease is further increased in certain populations including the following:

Daycare attendees[8,9]

Lower socio-economic groups[10]

Blacks[11] (especially those who lack the Km(1) immunoglobulin allotype)[12]

Caucasians who lack the G2m(n or 23) immunoglobulin allotype[13]

Native Americans[14,15,16]

Household contacts of cases[17]

Individuals with asplenia, sickle cell disease, or antibody deficiency syndromes[18,19]

An important virulence factor of the Haemophilus b bacterium is its polysaccharide capsule (PRP). Antibody to PRP (anti-PRP) has been shown to correlate with protection against Haemophilus b disease.[3,21] While the anti-PRP level associated with protection using conjugated vaccines has not yet been determined, the level of anti-PRP associated with protection in studies using bacterial polysaccharide immune globulin or nonconjugated PRP vaccines ranged from ≥0.15 to ≥1.0 mcg/ml.[22,23,24,25,26,27,28]

Nonconjugated PRP vaccines are capable of stimulating B-lymphocytes to produce antibody without the help of T-lymphocytes (T-independent). The responses to many other antigens are augmented by helper T-lymphocytes (T-dependent). PedvaxHIB is a PRP-conjugate vaccine in which the PRP is covalently bound to the OMPC carrier[29] producing an antigen which is postulated to convert the T-independent antigen (PRP alone) into a T-dependent antigen resulting in both an enhanced antibody response and immunologic memory.

CLINICAL EVALUATION OF PEDVAXHIB

The protective efficacy, safety, and antibody responses to PedvaxHIB were evaluated in 3,486 Native American (Navajo) infants who completed the primary two-dose regimen in a randomized, double-blind, placebo-controlled study (The Protective Efficacy Study). This population has a much higher incidence of Haemophilus b disease than the United States population as a whole and also has a lower antibody response to Haemophilus b conjugate vaccines, including PedvaxHIB.[14,15,16,30,34]

Each infant in this study received two doses of either placebo or PedvaxHIB with the first dose administered at a mean of 8 weeks of age and the second administered approximately two months later; DTP and OPV were administered concomitantly. Antibody levels were measured in a subset of each group (TABLE 1).

TABLE 1 Antibody Responses in Navajo Infants

Vaccine No. of Subjects	Time	% Subjects with >0.15 (mcg/ml)	% Subjects with >1.0 (mcg/ml)	Anti-PRP GMT (mcg/ml)
Haemophilus b Conjugate Vaccine				
416	Pre-Vaccination	44	10	0.16
416	Dose 1	88	52	0.95
416	Dose 2	91	60	1.43
Placebo*				
461†	Pre-Vaccination	44	9	0.16
461	Dose 1	21	2	0.09
461	Dose 2	14	1	0.08
Haemophilus b Conjugate Vaccine				
27‡	Prebooster	70	33	0.51
27	Postbooster§	100	89	8.39

* Post vaccination values obtained approximately 1-3 months after each dose.
† The Protective Efficacy Study.
‡ Immunogenicity Trial.[34]
§ Booster given at 12 months of age; post vaccination values obtained 1 month after administration of booster dose.

In this study, 22 cases of invasive Haemophilus b disease occurred in the placebo group (8 cases after the first dose and 14 cases after the second dose) and only 1 case in the vaccine group (none after the first dose and 1 after the second dose). Following the recommended two-dose regimen, the protective efficacy of PedvaxHIB was calculated to be 93% with a 95% confidence interval of 57%-98% (p = 0.001, two-tailed). In the two months between the first and second doses, the difference in number of cases of disease between placebo and vaccine recipients (8 vs 0 cases, respectively) was statistically significant (p = 0.008, two-tailed); however, a primary two-dose regimen is required for infants 2-14 months of age. A subset of 1,368 infants from this study was followed to 15 months of age with no additional cases of invasive Haemophilus b disease occurring after the primary two-dose regimen of PedvaxHIB (see DOSAGE AND ADMINISTRATION, including Booster Dose.)

Since protective efficacy with PedvaxHIB was demonstrated in such a high risk population, it would be expected to be predictive of efficacy in other populations.

The safety and immunogenicity of PedvaxHIB were evaluated in infants and children in other clinical studies that were conducted in various locations throughout the United States. PedvaxHIB was highly immunogenic in all age groups studied.[31,32]

Antibody responses from these clinical studies (excluding Native Americans) are shown in TABLE 2.[34] These data were derived by evaluating the sera in one laboratory using a radioimmunoassay which correlated with both the Finnish National Public Health Institute assay[33] and that recommended by the Center for Biologics Evaluation and Research of the FDA (TABLE 1, TABLE 2).

Since the magnitude of initial antibody response is lower among younger infants, a booster dose is required in infants who complete the primary two-dose regimen before 12 months of age (see TABLE 1 and DOSAGE AND ADMINISTRATION).

Antibodies to the OMPC of *N. meningitidis* (see DESCRIPTION) have been demonstrated in vaccinee sera but the clinical relevance of these antibodies has not been established.[34]

In a multicenter study of immunogenicity and safety in different subpopulations in the United States, antibody responses to PedvaxHIB were evaluated in infants initially vaccinated between the ages of 2 and 3 months (TABLE 3).

PedvaxHIB induced antibody levels greater than 1.0 mcg/ml in children who were poor responders to nonconjugated PRP vaccines. In a study involving such a subpopulation[34, 35] 34 children ranging in age from 27 to 61 months who developed invasive Haemophilus b disease despite previous vaccination with nonconjugated PRP vaccines were randomly assigned to 2 groups. One group (n = 14) was immunized with PedvaxHIB and the other group (n = 20) with a nonconjugated PRP vaccine at a mean interval of approximately 12 months after recovery from disease. All 14 children immunized with PedvaxHIB but only 6 of 20 children re-immunized with a nonconjugated PRP vaccine achieved an antibody level of > 1.0 mcg/ml. The 14 children who had not responded to revaccination with the nonconjugated PRP vaccine were then immunized with a single dose of PedvaxHIB; following this vaccination, all achieved antibody levels of > 1.0 mcg/ml.

CLINICAL PHARMACOLOGY: *(cont'd)*

TABLE 2 Antibody Responses* to PedvaxHIB in Other Clinical Studies

Age (Months)	Time	No of Subjects	% Subjects Responding with >0.15 mcg/ml	% Subjects Responding with >1.0 mcg/ml	Post Vaccination Anti-PRP (mcg/ml)
2-3	Dose 1**	113	97	81	2.48
	Dose 2***	113	98	88	4.60
4-14	Dose 1**	252	98	75	2.53
	Dose 2***	252	100	92	6.04
15-1	Single Dose***	59	100	83	3.11
18-2	Single	59	98	97	7.43
24-71	Dose***	52	98	92	10.55

* Only subjects with prevaccination anti-PRP ≤0.15 mcg/ml are include in this table (excluding Native Americans).
** Two months post vaccination.
*** One month post vaccination.

TABLE 3 Antibody Responses* After Two Doses of PedvaxHIB Among Infants Initially Vaccinated at 2-3

Months of Age By Racial/Ethnic Group

Racial/Ethnic Groups	No. of Subjects	% With Anti-PRP >0.15 mcg/ml	% With Anti-PRP >1.0 mcg/ml	GMT (mcg/ml)
Native American†	44	95	68	2.24
Caucasian	155	99	85	4.00
Hispanic	16	100	94	4.60
Black	18	100	94	8.57

† Apache and Navajo
* One month after the second dose

In addition, PedvaxHIB has been studied in children at high risk of Haemophilus b disease because of genetically-related deficiencies (Blacks who were Km (1) allotype negative and Caucasians who were G2m (23) allotype negative) and are considered hyporesponsive to nonconjugated PRP vaccines on this basis.[36] The hyporesponsive children had anti-PRP responses comparable to those of allotype positive children of similar age range when vaccinated with PedvaxHIB. All children achieved anti-PRP levels of > 1.0 mcg/ml.

HIBTITER

For several decades, *Haemophilus influenzae* type b (Haemophilus b) was the most common cause of invasive bacterial disease, including meningitis, in young children in the United States. Although nonencapsulated *H. influenzae* are common and six capsular polysaccharide types are known, strains with the type b capsule cause most of the invasive Haemophilus diseases.[3]

Haemophilus b diseases occurred primarily in children under 5 years of age prior to immunization with *Haemophilus influenzae* type b vaccines. In the US, the cumulative risk of developing invasive Haemophilus b disease during the first 5 years of life was estimated to be about 1 in 200. Approximately 60% of cases were meningitis. Cellulitis, epiglottitis, pericarditis, pneumonia, sepsis, or septic arthritis made up the remaining 40%. An estimated 12,000 cases of Haemophilus b meningitis occurred annually prior to the routine use of conjugate vaccines in toddlers.[3,4] The mortality rate can be 5%, and neurologic sequelae have been observed in up to 38% of survivors.[5]

The incidence of invasive Haemophilus b disease peaks between 6 months and 1 year of age, and approximately 55% of disease occurs between 6 and 18 months of age.[3] Interpersonal transmission of Haemophilus b occurs and risk of invasive disease is increased in children younger than 4 years of age who are exposed in the household to a primary case of disease. Clusters of cases in children in day care have been reported and recent studies suggest that the rate of secondary cases may also be increased among children exposed to a primary case in the day-care setting.[3,6]

The incidence of invasive Haemophilus b disease is increased in certain children, such as those who are native Americans, black, or from lower socioeconomic status, and those with medical conditions such as asplenia, sickle cell disease, malignancies associated with immunosuppression, and antibody deficiency syndromes.[3,4,6]

The protective activity of antibody to Haemophilus b polysaccharide was demonstrated by passive antibody studies in animals and in children with agammaglobulinemia or with Haemophilus b disease[7] and confirmed with the efficacy study of Haemophilus b polysaccharide (HbPs) vaccine.[8] Data from passive antibody studies indicate that a preexisting titer of antibody to HbPs of 0.15 mcg/ml correlates with protection.[9] Data from a Finnish field trial in children 18 to 71 months of age indicate that a titer of > 1.0 mcg/ml 3 weeks after vaccination is associated with long-term protection.[10]

Linkage of Haemophilus b saccharides to a protein such as CRM^{197} converts the saccharide (Hbo) to a T-dependent (HbOC) antigen, and results in an enhanced antibody response to the saccharide in young infants that primes for an anamnestic response and is predominantly of the IgG class.[11] Laboratory evidence indicates that the native state of the CRM_{197} protein and the use of oligosaccharides in the formulation of HibTITER enhances its immunogenicity.[12-14] Haemophilus b conjugate vaccines with other carrier proteins will be recognized differently by the immune system.

Prior to licensure, the immunogenicity of HibTITER was evaluated in US infants and children.[14] Infants 1 to 6 months of age at first immunization received three doses at approximately 2-month intervals.[15]

Children 7 to 11 and 12 to 14 months of age received 2 doses at the same interval.[14] Children 15 to 23 months of age received a single dose.[16] HibTITER was highly immunogenic in all age groups studied, with 97% to 100% of 1,232 infants attaining titers of ≥ 1 mcg/ml and 92% to 100% for bactericidal activity.[14-16]

Long-term persistence of the antibody response was observed. More than 80% of 235 infants who received three doses of vaccine had an anti-HbPs antibody level ≥ 1 mcg/ml at 2 years of age.[17]

CLINICAL PHARMACOLOGY: *(cont'd)*

The vaccine generated an immune response characteristic of a protein antigen. IgG anti-HbPs antibodies of IgG_1 subclass predominated and the immune system was primed for a booster response to HibTITER. There is some evidence suggesting natural increases in antibody levels over time after vaccination, most probably the result of contact with Haemophilus type b organisms of cross-reactive antigens.[17] These studies were carried out at a time when significant levels of Haemophilus b disease were still present in the community.

Antibody generated by HibTITER has been found to have high avidity, a measure of the functional affinity of antibody to bind to antigen. High-avidity antibody is more potent than low-avidity antibody in serum bactericidal assays.[18] The contribution to clinical protection is unknown.

Immunogenicity of HibTITER was evaluated in 26 children 22 months to 5 years of age who had not responded to earlier vaccination with Haemophilus b polysaccharide vaccine. One dose of HibTITER was immunogenic in all 26 children and generated titers of ≥ 1 mcg/ml in 25 of the 26 infants.[19] HibTITER has been found to be immunogenic in children with sickle cell disease, a condition which may cause increased susceptibility to Haemophilus b disease.[20] HibTITER has also been shown to be immunogenic in native American infants, such as the group of 50 studied in Alaska who received three doses at 2, 4, and 6 months of age.[19] Antibody levels achieved were comparable to those seen in healthy US infants who received their first dose at 1 to 2 months of age and subsequent doses at 4 to 6 months of age.[14,15,19]

Postlicensure surveillance of immunogenicity was conducted during the distribution of the first 30 million doses of HibTITER and during the time period over which Haemophilus b disease in children has been decreasing significantly in areas of extensive vaccine usage.[19,21-28]

After three doses, titers ranged from 2.37 to 8.45 mcg/ml with 67% to 94% attaining ≥ 1 mcg/ml.[19,23,24]

Persistence of antibody was examined in several cohorts of subjects that received either a selected commercial lot or that were part of the initial efficacy trial in northern California. Geometric mean titers for these cohorts were between 0.51 and 1.96 just prior to boosting at 15 to 18 months. These lots not only induced persistent antibody but also provided effective priming for a booster dose with commercial lots, with postboosting titers greater than 1.0 mcg/ml in 80% to 97% of subjects.[19]

HibTITER (HbOC) was shown to be effective in a large-scale controlled clinical trial in a multiethnic population in northern California carried out between February 1988 and June 1990.[29,30] There was no (O) vaccine failures in infants who received three doses of HibTITER and 12 cases of Haemophilus b disease (6 cases of meningitis) in the control group. The estimate of efficacy is 100% (*P*=.0002) with 95% Confidence Intervals of 68% to 100%. Through the end of 1991, with an additional 49,000 person-years of follow-up, there were still no cases of Haemophilus b disease in fully vaccinated infants less than 2 years of age.[21-22] One case of disease has been reported in a 3 1/2 -year- old child who did not receive a booster dose as recommended.

A comparative clinical trial was performed in Finland where approximately 53,000 infants received HibTITER at 4 and 6 months of age and a booster dose at 14 months in a trial conducted from January 1988 through December 1990. Only two children developed Haemophilus b disease after receiving the two-dose primary immunization schedule. One child became ill at 15 months of age and the other at 18 months of age; neither child received the scheduled booster at 14 months of age. No vaccine failure has been reported in children who received the two-dose primary series and the booster dose at 14 months of age. Based on more than 32,000 person-years of follow-up time, the estimate of efficacy is about 95% when compared to historical control groups followed between 1985 and 1988.[19] Historical controls were used since all infants received one of two Haemophilus b conjugate vaccines during the period of the trial.

Evidence of efficacy postlicensure includes significant reduction in Haemophilus b disease tat are closely associated with increases in the net doses of Haemophilus b Conjugate Vaccine distributed in the US.[19, 21-28]

In the northern California Kaiser Permanente there has been a 94% decrease in Haemophilus disease incidence in 1991 for children younger than 18 months of age, compared to 1984-1988, when HibTITER was not available for this age group.[21,22] Furthermore, active surveillance by the Centers for Disease Control and Prevention (CDC) has shown a 71% decrease in Haemophilus b disease in children less than 15 months old, between 1989 and 1991, which corresponds temporally and geographically with increases in net doses of Haemophilus b conjugate vaccine distributed in the US.[25] AS with all vaccines, this conjugate vaccine cannot be expected to be 100% effective. There have been rare reports to the Vaccine Adverse Event Reporting System (VAERS) of Haemophilus b disease following full primary immunization.

INDICATIONS AND USAGE:

PEDVAXHIB

PedvaxHIB is indicated for routine immunization against invasive disease caused by *Haemophilus influenzae* type b in infants and children 2 to 71 months of age.

PedvaxHIB will not protect against disease caused by *Haemophilus influenzae* other than type b or against other microorganisms that cause invasive disease such as meningitis or sepsis.

Revaccination

Infants completing the primary two-dose regimen before 12 months of age should receive a booster dose (see DOSAGE AND ADMINISTRATION.)

Use with Other Vaccines

Studies have been conducted in which PedvaxHIB has been administered concomitantly with the primary vaccination series of DTP and OPV, or concomitantly with M-M-R* II (Measles, Mumps, and Rubella Virus Vaccine Live,) (using separate sites and syringes) or with a booster dose of OPV plus DTP (using separate sites and syringes for PedvaxHIB and DTP). No impairment of immune response to individual tested vaccine antigens was demonstrated. The type, frequency and severity of adverse experiences observed in these studies with PedvaxHIB were similar to those seen when the other vaccines were given alone.

PedvaxHIB IS NOT RECOMMENDED FOR USE IN INFANTS YOUNGER THAN 2 MONTHS OF AGE.

HIBTITER

HibTITER Haemophilus b Conjugate Vaccine (Diphtheria CRM_{197}Protein Conjugate) is indicated for the immunization of children 2 months to 71 months of age against invasive diseases caused by *H. influenzae* type b.

As with any vaccine, HibTITER may not protect 100% of individuals receiving the vaccine.

HibTITER may be administered simultaneously but at different sites from other routine pediatric vaccines, e.g., Diphtheria and Tetanus Toxoids and Pertussis Vaccine Adsorbed (DTP), Oral Poliovirus Vaccine (OPV), and Measles-Mumps-Rubella Vaccine (MMR).[31,32]

CONTRAINDICATIONS:

PedvaxHIB: Hypersensitivity to any component of the vaccine or the diluent.

HibTITER: Hypersensitivity to any component of the vaccine, including diphtheria toxoid, or thimerosal in the multidose presentation, is a contraindication to use of HibTITER.

WARNINGS:

PEDVAXHIB

USE ONLY THE ALUMINUM HYDROXIDE DILUENT SUPPLIED.

If PedvaxHIB is used in persons with malignancies or those receiving immunosuppressive therapy or who are otherwise immunocompromised, the expected immune response may not be obtained.

HIBTITER

HibTITER WILL NOT PROTECT AGAINST *H. INFLUENZAE* OTHER THAN TYPE b STRAINS, NOR WILL HibTITER PROTECT AGAINST OTHER MICROORGANISMS THAT CAUSE MENINGITIS OR SEPTIC DISEASE.

AS WITH ANY INTRAMUSCULAR INJECTION, HibTITER SHOULD BE GIVEN WITH CAUTION TO INFANTS OR CHILDREN WITH THROMBOCYTOPENIA OR ANY COAGULATION DISORDER THAT WOULD CONTRAINDICATE INTRAMUSCULAR INJECTION (SEE DRUG INTERACTIONS).

ANTIGENURIA HAS BEEN DETECTED FOLLOWING RECEIPT OF HAEMOPHILUS b CONJUGATE VACCINE[33] AND THEREFORE ANTIGEN DETECTION IN URINE MAY NOT HAVE DIAGNOSTIC VALUE IN SUSPECTED HAEMOPHILUS b DISEASE WITHIN 2 WEEKS OF IMMUNIZATION.

PRECAUTIONS:

GENERAL

PedvaxHIB

As for any vaccine, adequate treatment provisions, including epinephrine, should be available for immediate use should an anaphylactoid reaction occur.

As with other vaccines, PedvaxHIB may not induce protective antibody levels immediately following vaccination.

As with any vaccine, vaccination with PedvaxHIB may not result in a protective antibody response in all individuals given the vaccine.

As reported with Haemophilus b Polysaccharide Vaccine[37] and another Haemophilus b Conjugate Vaccine[38], cases of Haemophilus b disease may occur in the week after vaccination, prior to the onset of the protective effects of the vaccines.

There is insufficient evidence that PedvaxHIB given immediately after exposure to natural *Haemophilus influenzae* type b will prevent illness.

Any acute infection or febrile illness is reason for delaying use of PedvaxHIB except when in the opinion of the physician, withholding the vaccine entails a greater risk.

HibTITER

1. CARE IS TO BE TAKEN BY THE HEALTH CARE PROVIDER FOR SAFE AND EFFECTIVE USE OF THIS PRODUCT.

2. PRIOR TO ADMINISTRATION OF ANY DOSE OF HibTITER, THE PATIENT OR GUARDIAN SHOULD BE ASKED ABOUT THE PERSONAL HISTORY, FAMILY HISTORY, AND RECENT HEALTH STATUS OF THE VACCINE RECIPIENT. THE HEALTH CARE PROVIDER SHOULD ASCERTAIN PREVIOUS IMMUNIZATION HISTORY, CURRENT HEALTH STATUS, AND OCCURRENCE OF ANY SYMPTOMS AND/OR SIGNS OF AN ADVERSE EVENT AFTER PREVIOUS IMMUNIZATION IN THE CHILD TO BE IMMUNIZED, IN ORDER TO DETERMINE THE EXISTENCE OF ANY CONTRAINDICATIONS TO IMMUNIZATION WITH HibTITER AND TO ALLOW AN ASSESSMENT OF BENEFITS AND RISKS.

3. BEFORE THE INJECTION OF ANY BIOLOGICAL, THE HEALTH CARE PROVIDER SHOULD TAKE ALL PRECAUTIONS KNOWN FOR THE PREVENTION OF ALLERGIC OR ANY OTHER SIDE REACTIONS. This should include: a review of the patient's history regarding possible sensitivity; the ready availability of epinephrine 1:1000 and other appropriate agents used for control of immediate allergic reactions; and a knowledge of the recent literature pertaining to use of the biological concerned, including the nature of side effects and adverse reactions that may follow its use.

4. Children with impaired immune responsiveness, whether due to the use of immunosuppressive therapy (including irradiation, corticosteroids, antimetabolites, alkylating agents, and cytotoxic agents), a genetic defect, human immunodeficiency virus (HIV) infection, or other causes, may have reduced antibody response to active immunization procedures.[34,35] Deferral of administration of vaccine may be considered in individuals receiving immunosuppressive therapy.[34] Other groups should receive this vaccine according to the usual recommended schedule.[34-36] (See DRUG INTERACTIONS.)

5. This product is not contraindicated based on the presence of human immunodeficiency virus infection.[37]

6. Any acute infection or febrile illness is reason for delaying use of HibTITER except when in the opinion of the physician, withholding the vaccine entails a greater risk. A minor afebrile illness, such as mild upper respiratory infection, is not usually reason to defer immunization.

7. As reported with Haemophilus b polysaccharide vaccine, cases of Haemophilus b disease may occur prior to the onset of the protective effects of the vaccine.[3,38]

8. The vaccine should not be injected intradermally since the safety and immunogenicity of this route have not been evaluated. The vaccine should be given intramuscularly.

9. A separate sterile syringe and needle or a sterile disposable unit should be used for each individual patient to prevent transmission of infectious agents from one person to another. Needles should be disposed of properly and should not be recapped.

10. Special care should be taken to prevent injection into a blood vessel.

The US Department of Health and Human Services has established a new Vaccine Adverse Event Reporting System (VAERS) to accept all reports of suspected adverse events after the administration of any vaccine, including but not limited to the reporting of events required by the National Childhood Vaccine Injury Act of 1986.[39] The VAERS toll- free number for VAERS forms and information is 800-822-7967.

ALTHOUGH SOME ANTIBODY RESPONSE TO DIPHTHERIA TOXIN OCCURS, IMMUNIZATION WITH HiBTITER DOES NOT SUBSTITUTE FOR ROUTINE DIPHTHERIA IMMUNIZATION.

INFORMATION FOR THE PATIENT

HibTITER: PRIOR TO ADMINISTRATION OF HibTITER, HEALTH CARE PERSONNEL SHOULD INFORM THE PATIENT, GUARDIAN, OR OTHER RESPONSIBLE ADULT, OF THE RECOMMENDED IMMUNIZATION SCHEDULE FOR PROTECTION AGAINST HAEMOPHILUS b DISEASE AND THE BENEFITS AND RISKS TO THE CHILD RECEIVING THIS VACCINE. GUIDANCE SHOULD BE PROVIDED ON MEASURES TO BE TAKEN SHOULD ADVERSE EVENTS OCCUR, SUCH AS, ANTIPYRETIC MEASURES FOR ELEVATED TEMPERATURES AND THE NEED TO REPORT ADVERSE EVENTS TO THE HEALTH CARE PROVIDER. Parents should be provided with vaccine information pamphlets at the time of each vaccination, as stated in the National Childhood Vaccine Injury Act.[39]

PATIENTS, PARENTS, OR GUARDIANS SHOULD BE INSTRUCTED TO REPORT ANY SERIOUS ADVERSE REACTIONS TO THEIR HEALTH CARE PROVIDER.

PRECAUTIONS: *(cont'd)*

LABORATORY TEST INTERACTIONS

PedvaxHIB Sensitive tests (*e.g.* Latex Agglutination Kits) may detect PRP derived from the vaccine in urine of some vaccinees for up to seven days following vaccination with PedvaxHIB[39]; in clinical studies with PedvaxHIB, such children demonstrated normal immune response to the vaccine.

CARCINOGENESIS, MUTAGENESIS, AND IMPAIRMENT OF FERTILITY:

PedvaxHIB and HibTITER have not been evaluated for carcinogenic, mutagenic potential, or impairment of fertility.

PREGNANCY CATEGORY C

Animal reproduction studies have not been conducted with PedvaxHIB or HibTITER. It is also not known whether PedvaxHIB or HibTITER can cause fetal harm when administered to a pregnant woman or can affect reproduction capability. PedvaxHIB or HibTITER is not recommended for use in a pregnant woman.

PEDIATRIC USE

HibTITER: The safety and effectiveness of HibTITER in children below the age of 6 weeks have not been established.

DRUG INTERACTIONS:

No impairment of the antibody response to the individual antigens was demonstrated when HibTITER was given at the same time but at separate sites as DTP plus OPV to children 2 to 20 months of age or MMR to children 15 ± 1 month of age.[19,40]

As with other intramuscular injections, HibTITER should be given with caution to children on anticoagulant therapy.

ADVERSE REACTIONS:

PEDVAXHIB

In early clinical studies involving the administration of 8,086 doses of PedvaxHIB alone to 5,027 healthy infants and children 2 months to 71 months of age, PedvaxHIB was generally well tolerated. No serious adverse reactions were reported.

During a two-day period following vaccination with PedvaxHIB in a subset of these infants and children, the most frequently reported adverse reactions, excluding those shown in TABLE 4, in decreasing order of frequency included irritability, sleepiness, respiratory infection/symptoms and ear infection/otitis media. Urticaria was reported in two children. Thrombocytopenia was seen in one child. A cause and effect relationship between these side effects and the vaccination has not been established.

Selected objective observations reported by parents over a 48-hours period in infants and children 2 to 71 months of age following primary vaccination with PedvaxHIB alone are summarized in TABLE 3.

In The Protective Efficacy Study (see CLINICAL PHARMACOLOGY) 4459 healthy Navajo infants 6 to 12 weeks of age received PedvaxHIB or placebo. Most of these infants received DTP/OPV concomitantly. No differences were seen in the type and frequency of serious health problems expected in this Navajo population or in serious adverse experiences reported among those who received PedvaxHIB and those who received placebo, and none was reported to be related to PedvaxHIB. Only one serious reaction (tracheitis) was reported as possibly related to PedvaxHIB and only one (diarrhea) as possibly related to placebo. Seizures occurred infrequently in both groups (9 occurred in vaccine recipients, 8 of whom also received DTP; 8 occurred in placebo recipients, 7 of whom also received DTP) and were not reported to be related to PedvaxHIB. The frequencies of fever and local reactions occurring in a subset of these infants during a 48-hour period following each dose were similar to those seen in early clinical studies (TABLE 4).

TABLE 4 Fever or Local Reactions in Subjects 2 to 71 Months of Age Vaccinated with PedvaxHIB Alone Other Clinical Studies

Age (Months)	Reaction	Number of Subjects Evaluated	Dose 1		
			6hr	24	48
2-14*	Fever >38.3°C (101°F)	532	2.4	3.8	1.9
	Rectal Erythema >2.5cm diameter	1026	0.2	1.0	0.4
	Swelling/ Induration >2.5cm diameter	1026	0.6	1.5	1.6
15-71**	Fever >38.3°C (101°F)				
	Rectal Erythema >2.5cm diameter	572	0.0	0.3	0.2
	Swelling/ Induration >2.5cm diameter	572	0.9	2.1	1.4

* Additional complaints reported following vaccination with the first and second dose of PedvaxHIB, respectively, in the indicated number of subjects were: nausea, vomiting and/or diarrhea (101, 41), cryingfor more than one-half hour (43, 15), rash (16, 17), and unusual high-pitched crying (4, 4).

** Additional complaints reported following vaccination with 1 dose of PedvaxHIB in the indicated number of subjects were: nausea, vomiting and/or diarrhea (44), crying for more than one-half hour (19), rash (12), and unusual high-pitched crying (0).

TABLE 4A Fever or Local Reactions in Subjects 2 to 71 Months of Age Vaccinated with PedvaxHIB Alone Other Clinical Studies

Age (Months)	Reaction	Number of Subjects Evaluated	Dose 2		
			6hr	24	48
2-14*	Fever >38.3°C (101°F)	329	3.0	4.3	3.6
	Rectal Erythema >2.5cm diameter	585	0.9	1.2	0.7
	Swelling/ Induration >2.5cm diameter	585	0.9	2.8	3.7

As with any vaccine, there is the possibility that broad use of PedvaxHIB could reveal adverse reactions not observed in clinical trials.

POTENTIAL ADVERSE REACTIONS

The use of Haemophilus b Polysaccharide Vaccines and another Haemophilus b Conjugate Vaccine has been associated with the following additional adverse effects: early onset Haemophilus b disease and Guillain-Barre syndrome. A cause and effect relationship between these side effects and the vaccination was not established.[37,38,40,41,42]

HIBTITER

Adverse reactions with HibTITER have been evaluated in 401 infants who were vaccinated initially at 1 to 6 months of age and were given 1,118 doses independent of DTP vaccine. Observations were made during the day of vaccination and days 1 and 2 postvaccination. A temperature > 38.3°C was recorded at least once during the observation period following 2% of the vaccinations. Local erythema, warmth, or swelling (≥ 2 cm) was observed following 3.3% of vaccinations. The incidence of temperature > 38.3°C was greater during the first postvaccination day than during the day of vaccination or the second postvaccination day. The incidence of local erythema, warmth, or swelling was similar during the day of vaccination and the first postvaccination day; it was lower during the second postvaccination day. All side effects have been infrequent, mild, and transient with no serious sequelae (TABLE 5A, TABLE 5B, and TABLE 5C). No difference in the rates of these complaints was reported after dose 1, 2, or 3.

TABLE 5A Number of Subjects (Percent) Manifesting Side Effects Associated with HibTITER Administered Independently from DTP* (Infants Vaccinated Initially at 1-6 Months of Age)

Symptoms	Same Day As Vacc.	Dose 1 n = 401 +1 Day	+2 Days
Temp > 38.3°C	0 -	2 <1%	2 <1%
Redness ≥ 2 cm	1 <1%	0 -	0 -
Warmth ≥ 2 cm	1 <1%	1 <1%	0 -
Swelling ≥ 2 cm	5 1.2%	1 <1%	0 -

* DTP and HibTITER given 2 weeks apart with DTP having been given first.

TABLE 5B Number of Subjects (Percent) Manifesting Side Effects Associated with HibTITER Administered Independently from DTP* (Infants Vaccinated Initially at 1-6 Months of Age)

Symptoms	Same Day As Vacc.	Dose 2 n = 383 +1 Day	+2 Days
Temp > 38.3°C	2 <1%	3 <1%	2 <1%
Redness ≥ 2 cm	1 <1%	6 1.6%	0 -
Warmth ≥ 2 cm	2 <1%	1 <1%	0 -
Swelling ≥ 2 cm	2 <1%	2 <1%	0 -

* DTP and HibTITER given 2 weeks apart with DTP having been given first.

TABLE 5C Number of Subjects (Percent) Manifesting Side Effects Associated with HibTITER Administered Independently from DTP* (Infants Vaccinated Initially at 1-6 Months of Age)

Symptoms	Same Day As Vacc.	Dose 3 n = 334 +1 Day	+2 Days
Temp > 38.3°C	2 <1%	6 1.8%	5 1.5%
Redness ≥ 2 cm	5 1.5%	4 1.2%	0 -
Warmth ≥ 2 cm	1 <1%	6 1.8%	0 -
Swelling ≥ 2 cm	1 <1%	0 -	0 -

* DTP and HibTITER given 2 weeks apart with DTP having been given first.

The following complaints were also observed after 1,118 vaccinations with HibTITER: irritability (133), sleepiness (91), prolonged crying [≥ 4 hours] (38), appetite loss (23), vomiting (9), diarrhea (2), and rash (1).

Additional safety data with HibTITER are available from the efficacy studies in young infants.[29] There were 79,483 doses given to 30,844 infants at approximately 2, 4, and 6 months of age in California, usually at the same time as DTP (but at a separate injection site) and OPV; approximately 100,000 doses have been given to 53,000 infants at 4 and 6 months in Finland at the same time as a combined DTP and inactivated polio (IPV) vaccine (but at a separate injection site). The rate and type of reactions associated with the vaccinations were no different from those seen when DTP or DTP-IPV was administered alone. These included fever, local reactions, rash, and one hyporesponsive episode with a single seizure. The safety of HibTITER was also evaluated in the California study by direct phone questioning of the parents or guardians of 6,887 vaccine recipients. The incidence and type of side effects reported within 24 hours of vaccination were similar to those cited in TABLE 5. In addition, analysis of emergency (ER) visits within 30 days and hospitalization within 60 days after receipt of 23,800 doses of HibTITER showed no increase in the rates of any type of ER visit or hospitalization.

TABLE 6 details the side effects associated with a single vaccination of HibTITER given (without DTP) to infants of 15 to 23 months of age.

Similar results have been observed in the analysis of 2,285 subjects of 18 to 60 months of age, vaccinated as part of a post-marketing safety study of HibTITER.[19] These data were collected by telephone survey 24 to 48 hours postvaccination. Additional observations included irritability, restless sleep, and GI symptoms (diarrhea, vomiting, and loss of appetite) in the group that received HibTITER alone. A cause and effect relationship between these observations and the vaccinations has not been established (TABLE 6).

DOSAGE AND ADMINISTRATION:

PEDVAXHIB

2 to 14 Months of Age: FOR INTRAMUSCULAR ADMINISTRATION. DO NOT INJECT INTRAVENOUSLY. Infants 2 to 14 months of age should receive a 0.5 ml dose of vaccine ideally beginning at 2 months of age followed by a 0.5 ml dose 2 months later (or as soon as possible thereafter). When the primary two-dose regimen is completed before 12 months of age, a booster dose is required (see Booster Dose as well as TABLE 4).

15 Months of Age and Older: Children 15 months of age and older previously unvaccinated against Haemophilus b disease should receive a single 0.5 ml dose of vaccine.

DOSAGE AND ADMINISTRATION: *(cont'd)*

TABLE 6 Selected Adverse Reactions* in Children of 15-23 Months of Age Following Vaccination with HibTITER

Adverse Reaction	No. of Subjects	Reaction Within 24 hrs	% Postvaccination At 48 hrs
Fever > 38.3°C	354	1.4	0.6
Erythema	354	2.0	-
Swelling	354	1.7	-
Tenderness	354	3.7	0.3

* The following complaints were reported after vaccination of these 354 children in the indicated number of children: diarrhea (9), vomiting (5), prolonged crying [> 4 hours] (4), and rashes (2). Rash, hives (urticaria), erythema multiforme, convulsions,[41] vomiting/diarrhea,[41] and Guillain-Barre syndrome[42] have been observed following the administration of Haemophilus b polysaccharide and Haemophilus b conjugate vaccines. However, a cause and effect relationship among any of these events and the vaccination has not been established.

BOOSTER DOSE

In infants completing the primary two-dose regimen before 12 months of age, a booster dose (0.5 ml) should be administered at 12 to 15 months of age but not earlier than 2 months after the second dose. DATA ARE NOT AVAILABLE REGARDING THE INTERCHANGEABILITY OF OTHER HAEMOPHILUS b CONJUGATE VACCINES AND PedvaxHIB.

Vaccination regimens by age group are outlined in TABLE 7.

TABLE 7

Age (Months) at First Dose	Primary	Age (Months) at Booster Dose
2 - 10	2 doses, 2 mo. apart	12 - 15
11 - 14	2 doses, 2 mo. apart	—
15 - 71	1 dose	—

TO RECONSTITUTE, USE ONLY THE ALUMINUM HYDROXIDE DILUENT SUPPLIED.

First, agitate the diluent vial, then, using sterile technique, withdraw the entire volume of aluminum hydroxide diluent into the syringe to be used for reconstitution. Inject all the aluminum hydroxide diluent in the syringe into the vial of lyophilized vaccine, and agitate to mix thoroughly.

Withdraw the entire contents into the syringe and inject the total volume of reconstituted vaccine (0.5 ml) intramuscularly, preferably into the anterolateral thigh or the outer aspect of the upper arm.

It is recommended that the vaccine be used as soon as possible after reconstitution. Store reconstituted vaccine in the vaccine vial at 2°-8°C (36°-46°F) and discard if not used within 24 hours. Agitate prior to injection.

Parenteral drug products should be inspected visually for extraneous particulate matter and discoloration prior to administration whenever solution and container permit. Aluminum hydroxide diluent and PedvaxHIB when reconstituted are slightly opaque white suspensions.

Special care should be taken to ensure that the injection does not enter a blood vessel.

It is important to use a separate sterile syringe and needle for each patient to prevent transmission of hepatitis B or other infectious agents from one person to another.

HibTITER is for intramuscular use only: Any parenteral drug product should be inspected visually for extraneous particulate matter and/or discoloration prior to administration whenever solution and container permit. If these conditions exist, HibTITER should not be administered.

Before injection, the skin over the site to be injected should be cleansed with a suitable germicide. After insertion of the needle, aspirate to help avoid inadvertent injection into a blood vessel.

The vaccine should be injected intramuscularly, preferably into the midlateral muscles of the thigh or deltoid, with care to avoid major peripheral nerve trunks.

HibTITER is indicated for children 2 months to 71 months of age for the prevention of invasive Haemophilus b disease. For infants 2 to 6 months of age, the immunizing dose is three separate injections of 0.5 ml given at approximately 2 months apart. Children from 12 through 14 months of age who have not been vaccinated previously receive one injection. All vaccinated children receive a single booster dose at 15 months of age or older, but not less than 2 months after the previous dose. Previously unvaccinated children 15 to 71 months of age receive a single injection of HibTITER.[31,32] Preterm infants should be vaccinated with HibTITER according to their chronological birth [31] (TABLE 8).

TABLE 8 Recommended Immunization Schedule

Age at First Immunization (Mo)	No. of Doses	Booster
2 - 6	3	Yes
7 - 11	2	Yes
12 - 14	1	Yes
15 and over	1	No

Interruption of the recommended schedules with a delay between doses does not interfere with the final immunity achieved nor does it necessitate starting the series over again, regardless of the length of time elapsed between doses.[31, 32]

NO DATA ARE AVAILABLE TO SUPPORT THE INTERCHANGEABILITY OF HibTITER OR OTHER HAEMOPHILUS b CONJUGATE VACCINES WITH ONE ANOTHER FOR THE PRIMARY IMMUNIZATION SERIES. THEREFORE, IT IS RECOMMENDED THAT THE SAME CONJUGATE VACCINE BE USED THROUGHOUT EACH IMMUNIZATION SCHEDULE, CONSISTENT WITH THE DATA SUPPORTING APPROVAL AND LICENSURE OF THE VACCINE.

Each dose of 0.5 ml is formulated to contain 10 mcg of purified Haemophilus b saccharide and approximately 25 mcg of CRM_{197} protein.

REFERENCES:

PedvaxHIB 1. Cochi, S. L., et al: Immunization of U.S. children with *Haemophilus influenzae* type b polysaccharide vaccine: A cost-effectiveness model of strategy assessment. JAMA 253: 521-529, 1985. **2.** Schlech, W. F., III, et al: Bacterial meningitis in the United States, 1978 through 1981. The National Bacterial Meningitis Surveillance Study. JAMA 253: 1749-1754, 1985. **3.** Peltola, H., et al: Prevention of *Haemophilus influenzae* type b bacteremic infections with the capsular polysaccharide vaccine. N Engl J Med 310: 1561-1566, 1984. **4.** Cadoz, M., et al: Etude epidemiologique des cas de meningitis purulentes hospitalises a Dakar pendant la decemie 1970-1979. Bull WHO 59: 575-584, 1981. **5.** Sell, S. H., et al: Long-term Sequelae of *Haemophilus influenzae* meningitis. Pediatr 49: 206-217, 1972. **6.** Taylor, H. G., et al: Intellectual, neuropsychological and achievement outcomes in children six to eight years after recovery from *Haemophilus influenzae* meningitis. Pediatr 74: 198-205, 1984. 7. Hay, J. W., et al: Cost-benefit analysis of two strategies for prevention of *Haemophilus influenzae* type b infection. Pediatr 80(3): 319-329, 1987. **8.** Redmond, S. R., et al: *Haemophilus influenzae* type b disease: an epidemiologic study with special reference to daycare centers. JAMA 252: 2581-2584, 1984. **9.** Istre, G. R., et

REFERENCES: *(cont'd)*

al: Risk factors for primary invasive *Haemophilus influenzae* disease: increased risk from daycare attendance and school age household members. J Pediatr 106: 190-195, 1985. **10.** Fraser, D. W., et al: Risk factors in bacterial meningitis: Charleston County, South Carolina. J Infect Dis 127: 271-277, 1973. **11.** Tarr, P. I., et al: Demographic factors in the epidemiology of Haemophilus influenzae meningitis in young children. J Pediatr 92: 884-888, 1978. **12.** Granoff, D. M., et al: Response to immunization with *Haemophilus influenzae* type b polysaccharide-pertussis vaccine and risk of Haemophilus meningitis in children with Km(1) immunoglobulin allotype. J Clin Invest 74: 1708-1714, 1984. **13.** Ambrosino, D. M., et al: Correlation between G2m(n) immunoglobulin allotype and human antibody response and susceptibility to polysaccharide encapsulated bacteria. J Clin Invest 75: 1935-1942, 1985. **14.** Coulehan, J.L., et al: Epidemiology of *Haemophilus influenzae* type b disease among Navajo Indians. Pub Health Rep 99: 404-409, 1984. **15.** Losonsky, G. A., et al: *Haemophilus influenzae* disease in the White Mountain Apaches: molecular epidemiology of a high risk population. Pediatr Infect Dis J 3: 539-547, 1985. **16.** Ward, J. I., et al: *Haemophilus influenzae*disease in Alaskan Eskimos: characteristics of a population with an unusual incidence of disease. Lancet 1: 1281-1285, 1981. **17.** Ward, J. I., et al: *Haemophilus influenzae* meningitis: a national study of secondary spread in household contacts. N Engl J Med 301: 122-126, 1979. **18.** Ward, J., et al: *Haemophilus influenzae* bacteremia in children with sickle cell disease. J Pediatr 88: 261-263, 1976. **19.** Bartlett, A. V., et al: Unusual presentations of *Haemophilus influenzae* infections in immunocompromised patients. J Pediatr 102: 55-58, 1983. **20.** Recommendations of the Immunization Practices Advisory Committee. Polysaccharide vaccine for prevention of *Haemophilus influenzae* type b disease. MMWR 34(15): 201-205, 1985. **21.** Santosham, M., et al: Prevention of *Haemophilus influenzae* type b infections in high-risk infants treated with bacterial polysaccharide immune globulin. N Engl J Med 317: 923-929, 1987. **22.** Siber, G. R., et al: Preparation of human hyperimmune globulin to *Haemophilus influenzae* b, *Streptococcus pneumoniae,* and *Neisseriameningitidis.*Infect Immun 45: 248-254, 1984. **23.** Smith, D. H., et al: Responses of children immunized with the capsular polysaccharide of *Haemophilus influenzae* type b. Pediatr 52: 637-645, 1973. **24.** Robbins, J. B., et al: Quantitative measurement of "natural" and immunization-induced *Haemophilus influenzae* type b capsular polysaccharide antibodies. Pediatr Res 7: 103-110, 1973. **25.** Kaythy, H., et al: The protective level of serum antibodies to the capsular polysaccharide of *Haemophilus influenzae* type b. J Infect Dis 147: 1100, 1983. **26.** Peltola, H., et al: *Haemophilus influenzae* type b capsular polysaccharide vaccine in children: a double-blind field study of 100,000 vaccinees 3 months to 5 years of age in Finland. Pediatr 60: 730-737, 1977. **27.** Ward, J. I., et al: *Haemophilus influenzae* type b vaccines: Lessons For the Future. Pediatr 81: 886-893, 1988. **28.** Daum, R. S., et al: *Haemophilus influenzae* type b vaccines: Lessons From the Past. Pediatr 81: 893-897, 1988. **29.** Marburg, S., et al: Bimolecular chemistry of macromolecules: Synthesis of bacterial polysaccharide conjugates with *Neisseria meningitidis*membrane protein. J Am Chem Soc 108: 5282-5287, 1986. **30.** Letson, G. W., et al: Comparison of active and combined passive/active immunization of Navajo children against *Haemophilus influenzae* type b. Pediatr Infect Dis J 7(111): 747-752, 1988. **31.** Einhorn, M. S., et al: Immunogenicity in infants of *Haemophilus influenzae* type b polysaccharide in a conjugate vaccine with *Neisseria meningitidis* outer-membrane protein. Lancet 2: 299-302, 1986. **32.** Ahonkhai, V. I., et al: *Haemophilus influenzae* Type b Conjugate Vaccine (Meningococcal Protein Conjugate) (PedvaxHIB TM): Clinical Evaluation. Pediatr 85(4): 676-681, 1990. **33.** Ward, J. I., et al: Variable quantitation of *Haemophilus influenzae* type b anticapsular antibody by radioantigen-binding assay. J Clin Microbiol 26: 72-78, 1988. **34.** Data on file at Merck Sharp & Dohme Research Laboratories. **35.** Granoff, D. M., et al: Immunogenicity of*Haemophilus influenzae* type b polysaccharide—outer membrane protein conjugate vaccine in patients who acquired *Haemophilus*disease despite previous vaccination with type b polysaccharide vaccine. J. Pediatr 114(6): 925-933, June, 1989. **36.** Lenoir, A. A., et al: Response to *Haemophilus influenzae* type b (*H influenzae* type b) polysaccharide *N. meningitidis* outer membrane protein (PS-OMP) conjugate vaccine in relation to Km(1) and G2m(23) allotypes. Twenty-sixth Interscience Conference on Antimicrobial Agents and Chemotherapy (Abstract #216) 133, 1986. **37.** Mortimer, E. A.; Efficacy of Haemophilus b polysaccharide vaccine An enigma. JAMA 260: 1454, 1988. **38.** Meekison, W., et al: Post-marketing surveillance of adverse effects following ProHIBiT vaccine—British Columbia Canada Diseases Weekly Report 15-28: 143-145, 1989. **39.** Sood, S. K., et al: *Haemophilus influenzae* type b (Hib) antigen and antibody kinetics in the week following immunization with Hib capsular polysaccharide-*N. meningitidis* outer membrane protein conjugate (PRP-OMP). Pediatr Res 25: 1130, 1989. **40.** Milstein, J. B., et al: Adverse reactions reported following receipt of *Haemophilus influenzae* type b vaccine: An analysis after one year of marketing. Pediatr 80: 270, 1987. **41.** Black, S., et al: b-CAPSA 1*Haemophilus influenzae* type b capsular polysaccharide vaccine safety: Pediatr 79: 321-325, 1987. **42.** D'Cruz, O. F., et al: Acute inflammatory demyelinating poly radiculoneuropathy (Guillain-Barre syndrome) after immunization with *Haemophilus influenzae* type b conjugate vaccine. J Pediatr 115: 743-746, 1989. **HibTITER 1.** United States Patent Number 4,902,506 by Anderson PW, Eby RJ filed May 5, 1986 issued February 20, 1990. **2.** Seid RC Jr, Boykins RA, Liu DF, et al. Chemical evidence for covalent linkage of a semi-synthetic glycoconjugate vaccine for *Haemophilusinfluenzae* type b disease. *Glycoconjugate J.* 1989;6:489-498. **3.** Wenger JD, Ward JL, Broome CV. Prevention of*Haemophilus influenzae* type b disease: vaccines and passive prophylaxis. In: Remington JS, Swartz MS, eds. *Current Clinical Topics in Infectious Diseases.* New York, NY:McGraw-Hill Inc;1989;10:306-339. **4.** Recommendations of the Immunization Practices Advisory Committee (ACIP) — polysaccharide vaccine for prevention of *Haemophilus influenzae* type b disease.*MMWR.* 1985;34:201-205. **5.** Sell SH. Long term sequelae of bacterial meningitis in children. *Pediatr Infect Dis J.*1983;2:90-93. **6.** Broome CV. Epidemiology of *Haemophilus influenzae* type b infections in the United States. *Pediatr Infect Dis J.* 1987;6:779-782. **7.** Alexander HE. The productive or curative element in type b *Haemophilus influenzae* rabbit serum.*Yale J Biol Med.* 1944;16:425-434. **8.** Peltola H, Kayhty H, Sivonen A. *Haemophilus influenzae* type b capsular polysaccharide vaccine in children: a double-blinded field study of 100,000 vaccinees 3 months to 5 years of age in Finland. *Pediatrics.*1977;60:730-737. **9.** Robbins JB, Parke JC Jr, Schneerson R. Quantitative measurement of "natural" and immunization-induced *Haemophilus influenzae* type b capsular polysaccharide antibodies. *Pediatr Res.* 1973;7:103-110. **10.** Kayhty H, Peltola H, Karanko V, et al. The protective level of serum antibodies to the capsular polysaccharide of *Haemophilus influenzae* type b. *J Infect Dis.* 1983;147:1100. **11.** Weinberg GA, Granoff DM. Polysaccharide-protein conjugate vaccines for the prevention of*Haemophilus influenzae* type b disease. *J Pediatr.*1988;113:621-631. **12.** Makela O, Peterfy F, Outshoom IG, et al. Immunogenic properties of a (1-6) dextran, its protein conjugates, and conjugates of its breakdown products in mice. *Scand J Immunol.*1984;19:541-550. **13.** Anderson P, Pichichero ME, Insel RA. Immunogens consisting of oligosaccharides from *Haemophilus influenzae* type b coupled to diphtheria toxoid or the toxin protein CRM_{197}.*J Clin Invest.* 1985;76:52-59. **14.** Madore DV, Phipps DC, Eby R, et al. Immune response of young children vaccinated with *Haemophilus influenzae* type b conjugate vaccines. In: Cruse JM, Lewis RE, eds. *Contributions to Microbiology and Immunology: Conjugate Vaccines.*New York, NY: Karger Medical and Scientific Publishers; 1989;10:125-150. **15.** Madore DV, Phipps DC, Eby R, et al. Safety and immunologic response to *Haemophilus influenzae* type b oligosaccharide-CRM_{197} conjugate vaccine in 1- to 6-month- old infants. *Pediatrics.* 1990;85:331-337. **16.** Madore DV, Johnson CL, Phipps DC, et al. Safety and immunogenicity of*Haemophilus influenzae* type b oligosaccharide-CRM_{197}conjugate vaccine in infants aged 15-23 months. Pediatrics. 1990;86:527- 534. **17.** Rothstein EP, Madore DV, Long S. Antibody persistence four years after primary immunization of infants and toddlers with*Haemophilus influenzae* type b CRM_{197}conjugate vaccine.*J Pediatrics.*1991;119:655-657. **18.** Schlesinger Y, Granoff DM. Avidity and bactericidal activity of antibodies elicited by different *Haemophilus influenzae* type b conjugate vaccines.*JAMA.*1992;267:1489-1494. **19.** Unpublished data available from Praxis Biologics, Inc. **20.** Gigliotti F, Feldman S, Wang WC, et al. Immunization of young infants with sickle cell disease with a*Haemophilus influenzae* type b saccharide-diphtheria CRM_{197}protein conjugate vaccine. *J Pediatr.*1989;114:1006-1010. **21.** Black SB, Shinefield HR, The Kaiser Permanente Pediatric Vaccine Study Group. Immunization with oligosaccharide conjugate *Haemophilus influenzae* type b (HbOC) vaccine on a large health maintenance organization population: extended follow-up and impact on *Haemophilus influenzae* disease epidemiology. *Pediatr Infect Dis J.* 1992;11:610-613. **22.** Black SB, Shinefield HR, Fireman B, et al. Safety, immunogenicity, and efficacy in infancy of oligosaccharide conjugate *Haemophilus influenzae* type b vaccine in a United States Population: possible implications for optimal use. *J Infect Dis.* 1992;165 (suppl 1):S139-S143. **23.** Granoff DM, Anderson EL, Osterholm MT, et al. Differences in the immunogenicity of three *Haemophilus influenzae* type b conjugate vaccines in infants. *J Pediatr.*1992;121:187-194. **24.** Decker MD, Edwards KM, Bradley R, et al. Comparative trial in infants of four conjugate *Haemophilus influenzae* type b vaccines. *J. Pediatr.* 1992;120:184-189. **25.** Adams WG, Deaver KA, Cochi SL, et al. Decline of childhood *Haemophilusinfluenzae* type b (Hib) disease in the Hib vaccine era.*JAMA.*1993;269:221-226. **26.** Murphy TV, White KE, Pastor P, et al. Declining incidence of *Haemophilus influenzae* type b disease since introduction of vaccination. *JAMA.* 1993;269:246- 248. **27.** Broadhurst LE, Erickson RL, Kelley PW. Decreases in invasive *Haemophilus influenzae* diseases in US Army children, 1984 through 1991. *JAMA.*1993;269:227-231. **28.** Shapiro ED. Infections caused by *Haemophilus influenzae* type b: the beginning of the end? *JAMA.* 1993;269:264-266. **29.** Black SB, Shinefield HR, Lampert D, et al. Safety and immunogenicity of oligosaccharide conjugate *Haemophilus influenzae* type b (HbOC) vaccine in infancy. *Pediatr Infect Dis J.* 1991;10:92-96. **30.** Black SB, Shinefield HR, Fireman B, et al. Efficacy in infancy of oligosaccharide conjugate *Haemophilus influenzae* type b (HbOC) vaccine in a United States Population of 61,080 children.*Pediatr Infect Dis J.* 1991;10:97-104. **31.** Recommendations of the AAP: *Haemophilus influenzae* type b conjugate vaccines: recommendations for immunization of infants and children 2 months of age and older: update. *Pediatrics.* 1991;88:169-172. **32.** Recommendations of the ACIP: Haemophilus b conjugate vaccines for prevention of *Haemophilus influenzae* type b disease among infants and children two months of age and older. *MMWR.* 1991;40:1-7. **33.** Jones RG, Bass JW, Weisse ME, et al. Antigenuria after immunization with *Haemophilus influenzae*oligosaccharide CRM_{197}conjugate (HbOC) vaccine. *Pediatr Infect Dis J.*1991;10:557-559. **34.** American Academy of Pediatrics: Report of the Committee on Infectious Diseases. 22nd ed. Elk Grove Village, Ill: American Academy of Pediatrics; 1991. **35.** Recommendations of the ACIP — immunization of children infected with human T-lymphotrophic virus type III/lymphadenopathy-associated virus. *MMWR.*1986;35(38):595-606. **36.** Immunization of children infected with human immunodeficiency virus - supplementary ACIP statement.*MMWR.* 1988;37(12):181-183. **37.** General Recommendations on Immunization — recommendations of the Immunization Practices Advisory Committee (ACIP). *MMWR.* 1989;38(13):221. **38.** Spinola SM, Sheaffer Cl, Philbrick KB, et al. Antigenuria after *Haemophilus influenzae* type b polysaccharide immunization: a prospective study.*J Pediatrics.* 1986;109:835-837. **39.** CDC. Vaccine Adverse Event Reporting System — United States. *MMWR.* 1990;39:730-733. **40.** Paradiso PR. Combined childhood immunizations. *JAMA.*1992;268:1685. **41.** Milstein JB, Gross TP, Kuritsky JN. Adverse reactions reported following receipt of *Haemophilus influenzae* type b vaccine: an analysis after one year of marketing.*Pediatrics.* 1987;80:270-274. **42.** D'Cruz DF, Shapiro ED, Spiegelman KN, et al. Acute inflammatory demyelinating polyradiculoneuropathy (Guillain-Barre syndrome) after immunization with*Haemophilus influenzae* type b conjugate vaccine. *J Pediatr.*1989;115:743-746.

HOW SUPPLIED:

Before reconstitution, store at 2°-8°C (36°-46°F).

Store reconstituted vaccine in the vaccine vial at 2°-8°C (36°-46°F) and discard if not used within 24 hours.

DO NOT FREEZE the aluminum hydroxide diluent or the reconstituted vaccine.

(PedvaxHIB: Merck, 1/92, 7611805)

HOW SUPPLIED: *(cont'd)*

(HibTITER: Lederle, 8/93, 32450-93)

HOW SUPPLIED - EQUIVALENTS NOT AVAILABLE:

Injection, Solution - Intramuscular

.5 ml x 5	$99.38	PROHIBIT, Connaught Labs	49281-0541-01
0.5 ml	$16.00	HIBTITER, Lederle-Praxis	53124-0201-01
0.5 ml x 4	$90.68	Hibtiter 35 M, Lederle-Praxis	53124-0104-41
1 ml	$20.00	PEDVAXHIB, Merck	00006-4792-00
1 ml x 5	$100.00	PEDVAXHIB, Merck	00006-4797-00
5 ml	$204.56	HIBTITER, Lederle-Praxis	53124-0201-10
5's	$87.13	PROHIBIT, Connaught Labs	49281-0541-05
10's	$174.25	PROHIBIT, Connaught Labs	49281-0541-10

HAEMOPHILUS B; TETANUS TOXOID *(001415)*

CATEGORIES: Biologicals; Immunologic; Serums, Toxoids and Vaccines; Toxoids; Vaccines; FDA Pre 1938 Drugs

BRAND NAMES: Acthib; OmniHib

DESCRIPTION:

OmniHIB, Haemophilus b Conjugate Vaccine (Tetanus Toxoid Conjugate), produced by Pasteur Merieux Serums & Vaccins, S.A., for intramuscular use, is a sterile, lyophilized powder which is reconstituted at the time of use with saline diluent (0.4% Sodium Chloride). The vaccine consists of the Haemophilus b polysaccharide, a high molecular weight polymer prepared from the *Haemophilus influenzae* type b strain 1482 grown in a semi-synthetic medium, covalently bound to tetanus toxoid.[1] The lyophilized powder and saline diluent contain no preservatives. Each single dose of 0.5 ml is formulated to contain 10 mcg of purified capsular polysaccharide, 24 mcg of tetanus toxoid and 8.5% of sucrose. The tetanus toxoid is prepared by extraction, ammonium sulfate purification, and formalin inactivation of the toxin from cultures of *Clostridium tetani* (Harvard strain) grown in a modified Mueller and Miller medium.[2] The toxoid is filter sterilized prior to the conjugation process. Potency of OmniHIB is specified on each lot by limits on the content of PRP polysaccharide and protein in each dose and the proportion of polysaccharide and protein in the vaccine which is characterized as high molecular weight conjugate. The reconstituted vaccine is clear and colorless.

CLINICAL PHARMACOLOGY:

H influenzae type b was the leading cause of invasive bacterial disease among children in the Unites States prior to licensing of*Haemophilus* b conjugate vaccines. Based on its active surveillance areas, the Centers for Disease Control and Prevention (CDC) now estimate that *H influenzae* type b disease in children under the age of 5 years has been reduced by 95%.[3] Before effective vaccines were introduced, it was estimated that one in 200 children developed invasive *H influenzae* type b disease by the age of 5 years. In children less than 5 years of age, the mortality rate for invasive Hib disease ranged between 3% and 6%.[3] In more than 60% of these children, meningitis was the clinical syndrome and permanent sequelae ranging from mild hearing loss to mental retardation affecting 20% to 30% of all survivors.[3] Ninety-five percent of the cases of invasive *H influenzae* disease among children <5 years of age were caused by organisms with the type b polysaccharide capsule. Approximately two-thirds of all cases of invasive *H influenzae* type b disease affected infants and children <15 months of age, a group for which a vaccine was not available until late 1990.[4,5]

Incidence rates of invasive *H influenzae* type b disease have been shown to be increased in certain high-risk groups, such as native Americans (both American Indians and Eskimos), blacks, individuals of lower socioeconomic status, and patients with asplenia, sickle cell disease, Hodgkin's disease, and antibody deficiency syndromes.[5,6]Studies also have suggested that the risk of acquiring primary invasive*H influenzae* type b disease for children under 5 years of age appears to be greater for those who attend day-care facilities.[7,8,9,10]

The potential for person to person transmission of the organism among susceptible individuals has been recognized. Studies of secondary spread of disease in household contacts of index patients have shown a substantially increased risk among exposed household contacts under 4 years of age.[11] Adults can be colonized with *H influenzae* type b from children infected with the organism.[12]

The response to OmniHIB is typical of a T-dependent immune response to antigen. The predominant isotype of anti-capsular polysaccharide (polyribosyl-ribitol-phosphate or PRP) antibody induced by OmniHIB is IgG.[13] A substantial booster response has been demonstrated in children 12 months of age or older who previously received two or three doses. Bactericidal activity against *H influenzae* type b is demonstrated in serum after immunization and statistically correlates with the anti-PRP antibody response induced by OmniHIB.[14]

Antibody to *H influenzae* capsular polysaccharide (anti-PRP) titers of >1.0 mcg/ml following vaccination with unconjugated PRP vaccine correlated with long-term protection against invasive *H influenzae* type b disease in children older than 24 months of age.[15] Although the relevance of this threshold to clinical protection after immunization with conjugate vaccines is not known, particularly in light of the induced, immunologic memory, this level continues to be considered as indicative of long-term protection.[4] The immunogenicity and safety of OmniHIB has been demonstrated in the United States and worldwide, OmniHIB induced, on average anti-PRP levels $\geq$1.0 mcg/ml in 90% of infants after the primary series and in more than 98% of infants after a booster dose.[14]

Two clinical trials supported by the National Institutes of Health (NIH) have compared the anti-PRP antibody responses to three Haemophilus b conjugate vaccines in a racially mixed population of children. These studies were done in Tennessee[16] (TABLE 1) and in Minnesota, Missouri and Texas[17] (TABLE 2) in infants immunized with OmniHIB and other Haemophilus b conjugate vaccines at 2, 4 and 6 months of age. All Haemophilus b conjugate vaccines were administered concomitantly with Poliovirus Vaccine Live Oral and DTP vaccines at separate sites.

N/A Not applicable in this comparison trial although third dose data have been published.[16,17]

Native American populations have high rates of *H influenzae* type b disease and have been observed to have low immune responses to Haemophilus b conjugate vaccines. Following three doses of OmniHIB at six weeks, four and six months of age, 75% of Native Americans in Alaska showed an anti-PRP antibody titer of $\geq$1.0 mcg/ml.[18]

In three U.S. trials in 12- to 15-month-old children and one trial in 17- to 24-month-old children who had not previously received Haemophilus b conjugate vaccination, a single dose of OmniHIB produced an anti-PRP antibody response comparable to those seen after three doses were administered in infants (TABLE 3).[18]

These trials demonstrated that OmniHIB consistently conferred an anti-PRP antibody response previously shown to correlate with protection, when administered either as a regimen of three doses at least four to eight weeks apart in infants 2 to 6 months of age or as single dose in children 12 months of age and older.[18]

CLINICAL PHARMACOLOGY: *(cont'd)*

TABLE 1 Anti-PRP Antibody Responses in 2-Month-Old infants NIH Trial in Tennessee

Vaccine Immunization	N* Immunization	Geometric Mean Titer (GMT) (mcg/ml) Pre-Immunization % $\geq$1.0 mcg/ml	Post Second	Post Third	Post Third Immunization
PRP-T† (OmniHIB)	65	0.10	0.30	3.64	83%
PRP-OMPπ (PedvaxHIB)	64	0.11	0.84	N/A	50%**
HbOC‡ (HibTITER)	61	0.07	0.13	3.08	75%

* N = Number of Children
† Haemophilus b Conjugate Vaccine (Tetanus Toxoid Conjugate)
π Haemophilus b Conjugate Vaccine (Meningococcal Protein Conjugate)
** Serconversion after the recommended 2-dose primary immunization series is shown.
‡ Haemophilus b Conjugate Vaccine (Diphtheria CRM_{197}Protein Conjugate)

TABLE 2 Anti-PRP Antibody Responses in 2-Month-Old Infants NIH Trial in Minnesota, Missouri And Texas

Vaccine Immunization	N * Immunization	Geometric Mean Titer (GMT) (mcg/ml) Pre-Immunization % $\geq$1.0 mcg/ml	Post Second	Post Third	Post Third(S) Immunization (S)
PRP-T† (OmniHIB)	142	0.25	1.25	6.37	97%
PRP-OMPπ (PedvaxHIB)	149	0.18	4.00	N/A	85%**
HbOC‡ (HibTITER)	167	0.17	0.45	6.31	90%

* N = Number of Children
(S) *(S)* Sera were obtained after the third dose from 86 and 110 infants, in PRP-T and HbOC vaccine groups, respectively.
† Haemophilus b Conjugate Vaccine (Tetanus Toxoid Conjugate)
π Haemophilus b Conjugate Vaccine (Meningococcal Protein Conjugate)
** Serconversion after the recommended 2-dose primary immunization series is shown.
‡ Haemophilus b Conjugate Vaccine (Diphtheria CRM_{197}Protein Conjugate)

TABLE 3 Anti-PRP Antibody Responses in 12- to 24-Month-Old Children Immunized With A Single Dose of OmniHIB

Age Group	N	Responding With GMT (mcg/ml) Pre	Post	% Subjects $\geq$1.0 mcg/ml Pre	Post
12 to 15 months	256	0.06	5.12	1.6	90.2
17 to 24 months	81	0.10	4.4	3.7	81.5

OmniHIB has been found to be immunogenic in children with sickle cell anemia, a condition which may cause increased susceptibility to Haemophilus b disease. Two doses of OmniHIB given at two month intervals induced anti-PRP antibody titers of > 1.0 mcg/ml in 89% of these children with a mean age of 11 months. This is comparable to anti-PRP antibody levels demonstrated in normal children of similar age following two doses of OmniHIB.[19]

Although OmniHIB produces an antibody response to tetanus toxoid, data do not exist to substantiate the correlation of this response with protection against tetanus. IMMUNIZATION WITH OmniHIB ALONE DOES NOT SUBSTITUTE FOR ROUTINE TETANUS IMMUNIZATION.

INDICATIONS AND USAGE:

OmniHIB is indicated for the active immunization of infants and children 2 months through 5 years of age for the prevention of invasive disease caused by *H influenzae* type b.

Antibody levels associated with protection may not be achieved earlier than two weeks following the last recommended dose.

CONTRAINDICATIONS:

As with any vaccine, vaccination with OmniHIB may not protect 100% of susceptible individuals: OmniHIB IS CONTRAINDICATED IN CHILDREN WITH A HISTORY OF HYPERSENSITIVITY TO ANY COMPONENT OF THIS VACCINE, INCLUDING TETANUS TOXOID.

WARNINGS:

If OmniHIB is administered to immunosuppressed persons or persons receiving immunosuppressive therapy, the expected antibody response may not be obtained. This includes patients with asymptomatic or symptomatic HIV-infection,[20] severe combined immunodeficiency, hypogammaglobulinemia, or agammaglobulinemia; altered immune states due to diseases such as leukemia, lymphoma, or generalized malignancy; or an immune system compromised by treatment with corticosteroids, alkylating drugs, antimetabolites or radiation.[21]

IMMUNIZATION WITH OmniHIB ALONE DOES NOT SUBSTITUTE FOR ROUTINE TETANUS IMMUNIZATION.

PRECAUTIONS:

General: EPINEPHRINE INJECTION (1:1000) MUST BE IMMEDIATELY AVAILABLE SHOULD AN ANAPHYLACTIC OR OTHER ALLERGIC REACTION OCCUR DUE TO ANY COMPONENT OF THE VACCINE.

Prior to an injection of any vaccine, all known precautions should be taken to prevent adverse reactions. This includes a review of the patient's history with respect to possible hypersensitivity to this vaccine or similar vaccines.

The health-care provider should ask the parent or guardian about the recent health status of the infant or child to be immunized including the infant's or child's previous immunization history prior to administration of OmniHIB.

PRECAUTIONS: *(cont'd)*

Any acute infection or febrile illness is reason for delaying use of OmniHIB except when in the opinion of the physician, withholding the vaccine entails a greater risk.

As reported with Haemophilus b polysaccharide vaccines,[22] cases of *H influenzae* type b disease may occur subsequent to vaccination and prior to the onset of protective effects of the vaccine.[18] (See INDICATIONS AND USAGE)

Antigenuria has been detected in some instances following receipt of OmniHIB; therefore, urine antigen detection may not have definitive diagnostic value in suspected *H influenzae* type b disease within one week of immunization.[23]

Special care should be taken to ensure that OmniHIB is not injected into a blood vessel.

Administration of OmniHIB is not contraindicated in individuals with an HIV infection.[21]

A separate, sterile syringe and needle or a sterile disposable unit should be used for each patient to prevent transmission of hepatitis or other infectious agents from person to person. Needles should not be recapped and should be properly disposed.

Information for the Patient: The health-care provider should inform the patient or guardian of the benefits and risks of the vaccine.

The physician should inform the parent or guardian about the significant adverse reactions that have been temporally associated with OmniHIB administration. The parent or guardian should be instructed to report any serious adverse reactions to the health-care provider.

As part of the child's immunization record, the date, lot number and manufacturer of the vaccine administered should be recorded.[24,25,26]

The U.S. Department of Health and Human Services has established a new vaccine Adverse Event Reporting System (VAERS) to accept all reports of suspected adverse events after the administration of any vaccine, including but not limited to the reporting of events required by the National Childhood Vaccine Injury Act of 1986.[24] The toll-free number for VAERS forms and information is 1-800-822-7967.

The National Vaccine Injury Compensation Program, established by the National Childhood Vaccine Injury Act of 1986, requires physicians and other health-care providers who administer vaccines to maintain permanent vaccination records and to report occurrences of certain adverse events to the U.S. Department of Health and Human Services. Reportable events include those listed in the Act for each vaccine and events specified in the package insert as contraindications to further doses of the vaccine.[25,26]

The health-care provider should inform the parent or guardian of the importance of completing the immunization series.

The health-care provider should provide the Vaccine Information Materials (VIMs) which are required to be given with each immunization.

Carcinogenesis, Mutagenesis, and Impairment of Fertility: OmniHIB has not been evaluated for its carcinogenic, mutagenic potential or impairment of fertility.

Pregnancy Category C: Animal reproduction studies have not been conducted with OmniHIB. It is also not known whether OmniHIB can cause fetal harm when administered to a pregnant woman or can affect reproduction capacity. OmniHIB is NOT recommended for use in a pregnant woman.

Pediatric Use: *SAFETY AND EFFECTIVENESS OF OmniHIB IN INFANTS BELOW THE AGE OF SIX WEEKS HAVE NOT BEEN ESTABLISHED.* (See DOSAGE AND ADMINISTRATION.)

DRUG INTERACTIONS:

There are no known interactions of OmniHIB with drugs or food.

In clinical trials, OmniHIB was routinely administered, at separate sites, concomitantly with one or more of the following vaccines: DTP vaccine, Poliovirus Vaccine Live Oral, Measles, Mumps and Rubella vaccine (MMR), Hepatitis B vaccine and occasionally Inactivated Polio Vaccine (IPV). No significant impairment of the antibody response to any antigen was observed in three clinical trials when Connaught Laboratories, Inc. (CLI) DTP vaccine was given concurrently with OmniHIB at separate sites.[18] Interference with the antibody response to the pertussis component has been suggested with DTP vaccine unlicensed in the U.S.[27] No impairment of the antibody response to the individual antigens was demonstrated when OmniHIB was given at the same time, at separate sites, with Inactivated Polio Vaccine (IPV) or Measles, Mumps and Rubella Vaccine (MMR).[18] In addition, more than 47,000 infants in Finland have received a third dose of OmniHIB concomitantly with MMR vaccine.[18]

ADVERSE REACTIONS:

More than 7,000 infants and young children (≤2 years of age) have received at least one dose of OmniHIB during U.S. clinical trials. Of these, 1,064 subjects 12 to 24 months of age who received OmniHIB alone reported no serious or life threatening adverse reactions.

Summarized in (TABLE 4) are adverse reactions temporally associated with OmniHIB immunization in 188 subjects 12 to 15 months of age.[18]

TABLE 4 Percentage of 12- to 15-Month-Old Children Presenting With Local or Systemic Reactions Within The First 24 Hours of Immunization With OmniHIB (N=188)

Reactions	Dose 1*	Dose 2*
Local		
Pain	9.0%	6.4%
Erythema (1 to 5 cm)	24.0%	18.6%
Induration	9.6%	9.0%
Systemic		
Fever (>100.6°F)	7.4%	6.4%
Irritability	30.9%	28.2%
Lethargy	18.6%	17.0%
Anorexia	9.0%	8.5%
Rhinorrhea	24.5%	21.3%
Diarrhea	5.8%	8.5%
Vomiting	4.3%	3.7%
Cough	9.6%	4.3%

* DTP was not administered concomitantly with OmniHIB.

When OmniHIB was administered to infants at 2, 4, and 6 months of age concomitantly, at separate sites, with CLI DTP vaccine, the systemic adverse experience profile was not different from that seen when CLI DTP vaccine was administered alone.[18] *Refer to product insert for CLI whole-cell DTP.*

Adverse reactions from a U.S. multicenter trial in 2-, 4- and 6-month-old infants are summarized in TABLE 5 A and B. Systemic adverse reactions listed in TABLE 5 A and B are more prominent than those in TABLE 4 because infants also received concomitant immunization with DTP.[14,18]

In general, the rates of minor systemic reactions after OmniHIB and DTP immunization were comparable to those usually reported after DTP vaccine alone.[28,29,30,31]

Adverse reactions associated with OmniHIB generally subsided after 24 hours and usually do not persist beyond 48 hours after immunization.

ADVERSE REACTIONS: *(cont'd)*

TABLE 5A percentage of Infants Presenting With Local or Systemic Reactions At 6, 24, And 48 Hours of Immunization With OmniHIB Administered Simultaneously, At Separate Sites, With CLI DTP Vaccine

Reaction	2 Months (n=365)			Age At Immunization 4 Months (n=364)		
	6 Hrs.	24 Hrs.	48 Hrs.	6 Hrs.	24 Hrs.	48 Hrs.
Local (S)						
Tenderness	46.3%	11.5%	2.2%	23.4%	7.4%	1.1%
Erythema	14.3%	4.1%	0.3%	8.8%	5.8%	0.6%
Induration	22.5%	6.3%	1.9%	12.4%	4.7%	0.8%
Systemic*						
Fever >100.8°F†	20.1%	1.3%	0.6%	14.6%	6.6%	1.4%
Irritability	72.6%	21.9%	12.6%	48.4%	25.0%	13.2%
Drowsiness	57.5%	29.9%	10.4%	44.2%	18.1%	7.4%
Anorexia	15.3%	5.8%	4.9%	8.0%	5.0%	3.0%
Diarrhea	4.4%	6.6%	5.2%	5.0%	4.7%	4.7%
Vomiting	2.7%	4.1%	2.7%	2.5%	3.3%	2.8%
Persistent Crying	Percentage of infants within 72 hours after immunization was 1.6% after dose one, 0.6% after dose two, and 0.3% after dose three.					

* The adverse reaction profile is defined by the concomitant use of CLI DTP vaccine.
† The number of individuals observed at each time point for fever varied from 357 to 363.
***(S)* Local reactions were evaluated at the OmniHIB injection site.**

Table 5B Percentage Of Infants Presenting With Local Or Systemic Reactions At 6, 24, And 48 Hours Of Immunization With OmniHIB Administered Simultaneously, At Separate Sites, With Cli Dtp Vaccine

Reaction	Age At Immunization 6 Months		(n=365)
	6 Hrs.	24 Hrs.	48 Hrs.
Local (S)			
Tenderness	19.2%	6.0%	1.1%
Erythema	11.5%	6.9%	1.6%
Induration	9.6%	3.8%	1.1%
Systemic*			
Fever >100.8°F†	15.7%	8.8%	0.8%
Irritability	44.1%	25.2%	10.1%
Drowsiness	32.6%	13.4%	2.5%
Anorexia	5.5%	4.9%	2.2%
Diarrhea	4.7%	6.3%	3.6%
Vomiting	2.2%	2.7%	1.9%
Persistent Crying	Percentage of infants within 72 hours after immunization was 1.6% after dose one, 0.6% after dose two, and 0.3% after dose three.		

* The adverse reaction profile is defined by the concomitant use of CLI DTP vaccine.
† The number of individuals observed at each time point for fever varied from 357 to 363.
***(S)* Local reactions were evaluated at the OmniHIB injection site.**

In a randomized, double-blind U.S. clinical trial, OmniHIB was given concomitantly with DTP to more than 5,000 infants and hepatitis B vaccine was given with DTP to a similar number. In this large study, deaths due to sudden infant death syndrome (SIDS) and other causes were observed but were not different in the two groups. In the first 48 hours following immunization, two definite and three possible seizures were observed after OmniHIB and DTP in comparison with none after hepatitis B vaccine and DTP.[18] This rate of seizures following OmniHIB and DTP was not greater than previously reported in infants receiving DTP alone. Other adverse reactions reported with administration of other Haemophilus b conjugate vaccines include urticaria, seizures, hives, renal failure and Guillain-Barre syndrome (GBS).[18,32] A cause and effect relationship among any of these events and the vaccination has not been established.

When OmniHIB was given with DTP and inactivated poliovirus vaccine to more than 100,000 Finnish infants, the rate and extent of serious adverse reactions were not different from those seen when other Haemophilus b conjugate vaccines were evaluated in Finland (*i.e.*, HibTITER, ProHIBiT).[18]

Reporting of Adverse Events: Reporting by the parent or guardian of all adverse events occurring after vaccination administration should be encouraged. Adverse events following immunization with vaccine should be reported by the health-care provider to the U.S. Department of Health and Human Services (DHHS) Vaccine Adverse Event Reporting System (VAERS). Reporting forms and information about reporting requirements or completion of the form can be obtained from VAERS through a toll-free number 1-800-822-7967.[24,25,26]

Health-care providers also should report these events to the Director of Medical Affairs, Connaught Laboratories, Inc., Route 611, P.O. Box 187, Swiftwater, PA 18370 or call 1-800-822-2463.

DOSAGE AND ADMINISTRATION:

Parenteral drug products should be inspected visually for particulate matter and/or discoloration prior to administration, whenever solution and container permit. If these conditions exist, the vaccine should not be administered.

Reconstitution with Supplied Diluent: Prior to reconstitution, cleanse the vaccine vial rubber barrier with a suitable germicide and inject the entire volume of diluent contained in the syringe into the vial of lyophilized vaccine. Thorough agitation is advised to ensure complete rehydration. The entire volume of reconstituted vaccine is then drawn back into a new syringe before injection of one 0.5 ml dose. The vaccine will appear clear and colorless.

Reconstitution instructions for diluent supplied:

Administer OmniHIB intramuscularly after reconstitution with diluent supplied. (In the event of coagulation disorders, OmniHIB may be given subcutaneously in the mid-lateral aspect of the thigh.[14]) **Vaccine should be used immediately after reconstitution.**

1. Insert syringe needle through the rubber barrier into the OmniHIB vial and inject 0.6 ml of diluent supplied.

2. Agitate vial thoroughly to ensure complete reconstitution.

3. After reconstitution, discard syringe and withdraw total volume of reconstituted vaccine in a new syringe and administer 0.5 ml intramuscularly (or subcutaneously if coagulation disorders exist).

Each 0.5 ml dose is formulated to contain 10 mcg of purified capsular polysaccharide conjugated to 24 mcg of inactivated tetanus toxoid and 8.5% of sucrose.

DOSAGE AND ADMINISTRATION: *(cont'd)*

Before injection, the skin over the site to be injected should be cleansed with a suitable germicide. After insertion of the needle, aspirate to ensure that the needle has not entered a blood vessel.

DO NOT INJECT INTRAVENOUSLY.

Each dose of OmniHIB is administered intramuscularly in the outer aspect of the vastus lateralis (mid-thigh) or deltoid. The vaccine should not be injected into the gluteal area or areas where there may be a nerve trunk. During the course of primary immunizations, injections should not be made more than once at the same site.

OmniHIB is indicated for infants and children 2 months through 5 years of age for intramuscular administration in accordance with the schedule indicated in (TABLE 6).[14,16]

Infants between 2 and 6 months of age should receive three 0.5 ml doses at eight week intervals, followed by a booster dose at 15 to 18 months of age. Infants 7 to 11 months of age who have not been previously immunized should receive two 0.5 ml doses at eight week intervals, followed by a booster dose at 15 to 18 months of age; children 12 to 14 months of age who have not been previously immunized should receive one 0.5 ml dose, followed by a booster dose at 15 to 18 months of age; and children 15 to 60 months of age who have not been previously immunized should receive a single 0.5 ml dose.

TABLE 6

Age At First Dose	Primary Series	Booster
2 to 6 months	3 Doses, 8 weeks apart	1 Dose, 15 to 18 months
7 to 11 months	2 Doses, 8 weeks apart	1 Dose, 15 to 18 months
12 to 14 months	1 Dose	1 Dose, 15 to 18 months*
15 to 60 months	1 Dose	None

* Administer vaccine not earlier than 2 months after the previous dose.

Preterm infants should be vaccinated according to their chronological age from birth.[33]

Interruption of the recommended schedule with a delay between doses should not interfere with the final immunity achieved with OmniHIB. There is no need to start the series over again, regardless of the time elapsed between doses.

No data are available to support the interchangeability of OmniHIB and ActHIB with other Haemophilus b conjugate vaccines. Therefore, it is recommended that the same conjugate vaccine be used throughout each immunization schedule, consistent with the data supporting approval and licensure of the vaccine. Since OmniHIB and ActHIB are the same vaccine these may be used interchangeably.

REFERENCES:

1. Chu CY, et al. Further studies on the immunogenicity of*Haemophilus influenzae* type b and pneumococcal type 6A polysaccharide-protein conjugate. Infect Immun 40: 245-246, 1983 **2.** Mueller JH, et al. Production of diphtheria toxin of high potency (100 Lf) on a reproductive medium. J Immunol 40: 21-32, 1941 **3.** Adams WG, et al. Decline of Childhood *Haemophilus influenzae* Type b (Hib) Disease in the Hib Vaccine Era. JAMA 269: 221-226, 1993 **4.** Recommendations of the Immunization Practices Advisory Committee (ACIP). Haemophilus b Conjugate Vaccines for prevention of *Haemophilus influenzae* type b disease among infants and children two months of age and older. MMWR 40: No. RR-1, 1991 **5.** Broome CV. Epidemiology of *Haemophilus influenzae* type b infections in the United States. Pediatr Infect Dis J 6: 779-782, 1987 **6.** ACIP. Polysaccharide vaccine for prevention of *Haemophilus influenzae* type b disease. MMWR 34: 201-205, 1985 **7.** Istre GR, et al. Risk factors for primary invasive *Haemophilus influenzae* disease: Increased risk from day care attendance and school-aged household members. J Pediatr 106: 190-195, 1985 **8.** Redmond SR, et al. *Haemophilus influenzae* type b disease. An epidemiologic study with special reference to day-care centers. JAMA 252: 2581-2584, 1984 **9.** Murphy TV, et al. County-wide surveillance of invasive Haemophilus infections: Risk of associated cases in Child Care Programs (CCPs). Twenty-third Interscience Conference on Antimicrobial Agents and Chemotherapy (Abstract #788) 229, 1983 **10.** Fleming D, et al. *Haemophilus influenzae* b (Hib) disease-secondary spread in day care. Twenty-fourth Interscience Conference on Antimicrobial Agents and Chemotherapy (Abstract #967) 261, 1984 **11.** CDC. Prevention of secondary cases of *Haemophilus influenzae* type b disease. MMWR 31: 672-680, 1982 **12.** Michaels RH, et al. Pharyngeal colonization with *Haemophilus influenzae* type b: A longitudinal study of families with a child with meningitis or epiglottis due to *H. influenzae* type b. J Infect Dis 136: 222-227, 1977 **13.** Holmes SJ, et al. Immunogenicity of four *Haemophilus influenzae* type b conjugate vaccines in 17- to 19-month-old children. J Pediatr 118: 364- 371, 1991 **14.** Data on file, Pasteur Merieux Serums & Vaccins, S.A. **15.** Peltola H, et al. Prevention of *Haemophilus influenzae* type b bacteremic infections with the capsular polysaccharide vaccine. N Engl J Med 310: 1561-1566, 1984 **16.** Decker MD, et al. Comparative trial in infants of four conjugate*Haemophilus influenzae* type b vaccines. J Pediatr 120: 184-189, 1992 **17.** Granoff DM, et al. Differences in the immunogenicity of three *Haemophilus influenzae* type b conjugate vaccines in infants. J Pediatr 121: 187-194, 1992 **18.** Data on file, Connaught Laboratories, Inc. **19.** Kaplan SL, et al. Immunogenicity of*Haemophilus influenzae* type b polysaccharide-tetanus protein conjugate vaccine in children with sickle hemoglobinopathy or malignancies, and after systemic *Haemophilus influenzae* type b infection. J Pediatr Vol 120: 360-370, 1992 **20.** Steinhoff MC, et al. Antibody responses to *Haemophilus influenzae* type b vaccines in men with human immunodeficiency virus infection. N Engl J Med 325(26): 1837-1842, 1991 **21.** ACIP. General recommendations on immunization. MMWR 38: 205-227, 1989 **22.** FDA Workshop on Haemophilus b Polysaccharide Vaccine-A Preliminary Report. MMWR 36: 529- 531, 1987 **23.** Rothstein EP, et al. Comparison of antigenuria after immunization with three *Haemophilus influenzae* type b conjugate vaccines. Pediatr Infect Dis J 10: 311-314, 1991 **24.** Vaccine Adverse Event Reporting System-United States. MMWR 39: 730-733, 1990 **25.** CDC. National Childhood Vaccine Injury Act: Requirements for permanent vaccination records and for reporting of selected events after vaccination. MMWR 37: 197-200, 1988 **26.** National Childhood Vaccine Injury Act of 1986 (Amended 1987) **27.** Clemens JD, et al. Impact of *Haemophilus influenzae* Type b Polysaccharide-Tetanus Protein Conjugate Vaccine on responses to concurrently administered Diphtheria-Tetanus-Pertussis Vaccine. JAMA 267: 673-678, 1992 **28.** Cody CL, et al. Nature and rates of adverse reactions associated with DTP and DT immunizations in infants and children. Pediatr 68: 650-660, 1981 **29.** Barkin RM, et al. Diphtheria-tetanus-pertussis vaccine: reactogenicity of commercial products. Pediatr 63: 256-260, 1979 **30.** Baraff LJ, et al. DTP-associated reactions: an analysis by injection site, manufacturer, prior reactions and dose. Pediatr 73: 31- 39, 1984 **31.** Long SS, et al. Longitudinal study of adverse reactions following diphtheria-tetanus-pertussis vaccine in infancy. Pediatr 85: 294-302, 1990 **32.** D'Cruz OF, et al. Acute inflammatory demyelinating polyradiculoneuropathy (Guillain-Barre Syndrome) after immunization with *Haemophilus influenzae* type b conjugate vaccine. J Pediatr 115: 743-746, 1989 **33.** Report of the Committee on Infectious Diseases. American Academy of Pediatrics. Twenty- second Edition, 1991

HOW SUPPLIED:

Vial, 1 Dose, lyophilized vaccine (5 x 1 Dose vials per package), packaged with prefilled 0.6 ml Syringe containing diluent (5 x 0.6 ml syringes per package)-Product No. 0007-4408-05.

Administer vaccine immediately after reconstitution.

Store lyophilized vaccine and prefilled syringe containing diluent between 2°-8°C (35°- 46°F). DO NOT FREEZE.

HOW SUPPLIED - EQUIVALENTS NOT AVAILABLE:

Injection, Solution - Intramuscular

10's	$315.54	ACTHIB, Connaught Labs	49281-0549-10

Kit - Intravenous

5's	$89.05	OMNIHIB, SKB Pharms	00007-4408-05

HALCINONIDE *(001417)*

CATEGORIES: Anti-Inflammatory Agents; Dermatologicals; Dermatoses; Skin/Mucous Membrane Agents; Steroids; Topical; Pregnancy Category C; FDA Approval Pre 1982; Patent Expiration 1992 Jul

BRAND NAMES: *Adcortin* (Japan); *Alcinon*; *Alcinon-BC*; *Ascochrom*; *Cortilate*; *Dermalog*; *Dermalog Simple Al* (Mexico); *Halciderm* (England); *Halciderm Crema Al*; *Halcimat* (Germany); *Halocort*; **Halog**; Halog-E; *Volog*
(International brand names outside U.S. in italics)

DESCRIPTION:

The topical corticosteroids constitute a class primarily synthetic steroids used an anti-inflammatory and antipruritic agents. The steroids in this class include halcinonide. Halcinonide is designated chemically as 21-Chloro-9-fluoro-11β, 16α, 17-trihydroxypregn-4-ene-3,20- dione cyclic 16,17-acetal with acetone.

The molecular formula is $C_{24}H_{32}ClFO_{51}$, with a molecular weight of 454.96.

Cream: Each gram of 0.025% Halog Cream (Halcinonide Cream) contains 0.25 mg halcinonide in a specially formulated cream base consisting of glyceryl monostearate NF XII, cetyl esters wax, polysorbate 60, propylene glycol, dimethicone 350, and purified water.

Each gram of 0.1% Halog Cream (Halcinonide Cream) contains 1 mg halcinonide in a specially formulated cream base consisting of glyceryl monostearate NF XII, cetyl alcohol, isopropyl palmitate, dimethicone 350, polysorbate 60, titanium dioxide, propylene glycol, and purified water.

Ointment: Each gram of 1.0% Halog Ointment (Halcinonide Ointment) contains 1 mg halcinonide in plasticized hydrocarbon gel), a polyethylene and mineral oil base with polyethylene glycol 400, polyethylene glycol 6000, distearate, polyethylene glycol 300, polyethylene glycol 1450, and butylated hydroxytoluene as an antioxidant.

Solution: Each ml of 0.1% Halog Solution (Halcinonide Topical Solution) contains 1 mg Halcinonide with edetate disodium, polyethylene glycol 300, purified water, and butylated hydroxytoluene as an antioxidant.

CLINICAL PHARMACOLOGY:

Topical corticosteroids share anti-inflammatory, antipruritic and vasoconstrictive actions.

The mechanism of anti-inflammatory activity of the topical corticosteroids is unclear. Various laboratory methods, including vasoconstrictor assays, are used to compare and predict potencies and/or clinical efficacious of the topical corticosteroids. There is some evidence to suggest that a recognizable correlation exists between vasoconstrictor potency and therapeutic efficacy in man.

Pharmacokinetics: The extent of percutaneous absorption of topical corticosteroids is determined by many factors including the vehicle, the integrity of the epidermal barrier, and the use of occlusive dressings.

Topical corticosteroids can be absorbed from normal intact skin. Inflammation and/or other disease processes in the skin increase percutaneous absorption. Occlusive dressings substantially increase the percutaneous absorption of topical corticosteroids. Thus, occlusive dressings may be a valuable therapeutic adjunct for treatment of resistant dermatoses (see DOSAGE AND ADMINISTRATION).

Once absorbed through the skin, topical corticosteroids are handled through pharmacokinetic pathways similar to systemically administered corticosteroids. Corticosteroids are bound to plasma proteins in varying degrees. Corticosteroids are metabolized primarily in the liver and are then excreted by the kidneys. Some of the topical corticosteroids and their metabolites are also excreted into the bile.

INDICATIONS AND USAGE:

Halcinonide is indicated for the relief of the inflammatory and pruritic manifestations of corticosteroid-responsive dermatoses.

CONTRAINDICATIONS:

Topical corticosteroids are contraindicated in those patients with a history of hypersensitivity to any of the components of the preparations.

PRECAUTIONS:

GENERAL

Systemic absorption of topical corticosteroids has produced reversible hypothalamic-pituitary-adrenal (HPA) axis suppression, manifestations of Cushing's syndrome, hyperglycemia, and glucosuria in some patients.

Conditions which augment systemic absorption include the application of the more potent steroids, use over large surface areas, prolonged use, and the addition of occlusive dressings.

Therefore, patients receiving a large dose of any potent topical steroid applied to a large surface area or under an occlusive dressing should be evaluated periodically for evidence of HPA axis suppression by using the urinary free cortisol and ACTH stimulation tests, and for impairment of thermal homeostasis. If HPA axis suppression or elevation of the body temperature occurs, an attempt should be made ot withdraw the drug, to reduce the frequency of application, substitute a less potent steroid, or use a sequential approach when utilizing the occlusive technique.

Recovery of HPA axis function and thermal homeostasis are generally prompt and complete upon discontinuation of the drug. Infrequently, signs and symptoms of steroid withdrawal may occur, requiring supplemental systemic corticosteroids. Occasionally, a patient may develop a sensitivity reaction to a particular occlusive dressing material or adhesive and a substitute material may be necessary.

Children may absorb proportionally larger amounts of topical corticosteroids and thus be more susceptible to systemic toxicity (see PRECAUTIONS, Pediatric Use).

If irritation develops, topical corticosteroids should be discontinued and appropriate therapy instituted.

In the presence of dermatological infections, the use of an appropriate antifungal or antibacterial agent should be instituted. If a favorable response does not occur promptly, the corticosteroid should be discontinued until the infection has been adequately controlled.

These preparations are not for ophthalmic use.

INFORMATION FOR THE PATIENT

Patients using topical corticosteroids should receive the following information and instructions:

1. This medication is to be used as directed by the physician. It is for dermatologic use only. Avoid contact with the eyes.

2. Patients should be advised not to use this medication for any disorder other than for which it was prescribed.

3. The treated skin area should not be bandaged or otherwise covered or wrapped as to be occlusive unless directed by the physician.

4. Patients should report any signs of local adverse reactions especially under occlusive dressing.

5. Parents of pediatric should be advised not to use tight-fitting diapers or plastic pants on a child being treated in the diaper area, as these garments may constitute occlusive dressings.

LABORATORY TESTS

A urinary free cortisol test and ACTH stimulation test may be helpful in evaluating HPA axis suppression.

CARCINOGENESIS, MUTAGENESIS, AND IMPAIRMENT OF FERTILITY

Long-term animal studies have not been performed ot evaluate the carcinogenic potential or the effect on fertility of topical corticosteroids.

PRECAUTIONS: *(cont'd)*

Studies to determine mutagenicity with prednisolone and hydrocortisone showed negative results.

PREGNANCY, TERATOGENIC EFFECTS, PREGNANCY CATEGORY C

Corticosteroids are generally teratogenic in laboratory animals when administered systemically at relatively low dosage levels. The more potent corticosteroids have been shown to be teratogenic after dermal application in laboratory animals. There are no adequate and well-controlled studies in pregnant women on teratogenic effects from topically applied corticosteroids. Therefore, topical corticosteroids should be used during pregnancy only if the potential benefit just potential risk to the fetus. Drugs of this class should not be used extensively on pregnant patients, in large amounts, of for prolonged periods of time.

NURSING MOTHERS

It is not known whether topical administration of corticosteroids could result insufficient systemic absorption to produce detectable quantities in breast milk. Systemically administered corticosteroids are secreted into breast milk in quantities not likely to have a deleterious effect on the infant. Nevertheless, caution should be exercised when topical corticosteroids are administered to a nursing woman.

PEDIATRIC USE

Pediatric patients may demonstrate greater susceptibility to topical corticosteroid-induced HPA axis suppression and Cushing's syndrome than mature patients because of a larger skin surface area to body weight ratio.

HPA axis suppression, Cushing's syndrome, and intracranial hypertension have been reported in children receiving topical corticosteroids. Manifestations of adrenal suppression in children include linear growth retardation, delayed weight gain, low plasma cortisol levels, and absence of response to ACTH stimulation. Manifestations of intracranial hypertension include bulging fontanelles, headaches, and bilateral papilledema.

Administration of topical corticosteroids to children should be limited to the least amount compatible with an effective therapeutic regimen. Chronic corticosteroid therapy may interfere with the growth and development of children.

ADVERSE REACTIONS:

The following local adverse reactions are reported in frequently with topical corticosteroids, but may occur more frequently with the use of occlusive dressings (reactions are listed in an approximate decreasing order of occurrence): burning, itching, irritation, dryness, folliculitis, hypertrichosis, acneiform eruptions, hypopigmentation, perioral dermatitis, allergic contact dermatitis maceration of the skin, secondary infection, skin atrophy, striae, and miliaria.

OVERDOSAGE:

Topically applied corticosteroids can be absorbed in sufficient amounts to produce systemic effects (see PRECAUTIONS, General).

DOSAGE AND ADMINISTRATION:

CREAM

Apply the 0.025% or the 0.1% halcinonide cream to the affected area two to three times daily. Rub in gently.

OCCLUSIVE DRESSING TECHNIQUE

Occlusive dressings may be used for the management of psoriasis or other recalcitrant conditions. Gently run a small amount of cream into the lesion until it disappears. Reapply the preparation leaving a thin coating on the lesion, cover with a pliable nonporous film, a seal the edges. If needed, additional moisture may be provided by covering the lesion with a dampened clean cotton cloth before the nonporous film is applied or by briefly wetting the affected area with water immediately prior to applying the medication. The frequency of changing dressings is best determined on an individual basis. It may be convenient to apply halcinonide cream under an occlusive dressing in the evening and to remove the dressing in the morning (*i.e.,* 12-hour occlusion). When utilizing the 12- hour occlusion regimen, additional cream should be applied, without occlusion, during day. Reapplication is essential at each dressing change.

If an infection develops, the use of occlusive dressings should be discontinued and appropriate antimicrobial therapy instituted.

OINTMENT

Apply a thin film of 0.1% halcinonide ointment to the affected area two to three times daily.

OCCLUSIVE DRESSING TECHNIQUE

Occlusive dressings may be used for the management of psoriasis or other recalcitrant conditions. Apply a thin film the to the lesion, cover with a pliable nonporous film, and seal the edges. If needed, additional moisture may be provided by covering the lesion with a dampened clean cotton cloth before the nonporous film is applied or by briefly wetting the affected area with water immediately prior to applying the medication. The frequency of changing dressings is best determined on an individual basis. It may be convenient to apply halcinonide ointment under an occlusive dressing in the evening and to remove the dressing in the morning (*i.e.,* 12-hour occlusion). When utilizing the 12-hour occlusion regimen, additional cream should be applied, without occlusion, during day. Reapplication is essential at each dressing change.

If an infection develops, the use of occlusive dressings should be discontinued and appropriate antimicrobial therapy instituted.

SOLUTION

Apply halcinonide solution to the affected area two to three times daily.

See above for Occlusive Dressing Techniques (under Ointment).

Store (all forms) at room temperature; avoid excessive heat (104° F).

HOW SUPPLIED - EQUIVALENTS NOT AVAILABLE:

Cream - Topical - 0.1 %

15 gm	$17.84	HALOG-E 0.1 %, Bristol Myers Squibb	00003-1494-14
15 gm	$18.64	HALOG 0.1 %, Bristol Myers Squibb	00003-1482-15
30 gm	$29.95	HALOG 0.1 %, Bristol Myers Squibb	00003-1482-20
30 gm	$29.95	HALOG-E 0.1 %, Bristol Myers Squibb	00003-1494-21
60 gm	$50.95	HALOG 0.1 %, Bristol Myers Squibb	00003-1482-30
60 gm	$50.95	HALOG-E 0.1 %, Bristol Myers Squibb	00003-1494-31
240 gm	$162.06	HALOG, Bristol Myers Squibb	00003-1482-40

Ointment - Topical - 0.1 %

15 gm	$18.64	HALOG, Bristol Myers Squibb	00003-0248-15
30 gm	$29.95	HALOG, Bristol Myers Squibb	00003-0248-20
60 gm	$50.95	HALOG, Bristol Myers Squibb	00003-0248-30
240 gm	$162.06	HALOG, Bristol Myers Squibb	00003-0248-40

Solution - Topical - 0.1 %

20 ml	$22.08	HALOG 0.1%, Bristol Myers Squibb	00003-0249-15
60 ml	$49.45	HALOG 0.1%, Bristol Myers Squibb	00003-0249-20

HALOBETASOL PROPIONATE *(003012)*

CATEGORIES: Adrenal Corticosteroids; Anti-Inflammatory Agents; Dermatoses; Skin/Mucous Membrane Agents; Steroids; Topical; Dermatitis*; Eczema*; Pregnancy Category C; FDA Class 1C ("Little or No Therapeutic Advantage"); FDA Approved 1990 Dec

* Indication not approved by the FDA

BRAND NAMES: **Ultravate**

DESCRIPTION:

Ultravate (halobetasol propionate) Cream and Ointment contains the active compound halobetasol propionate, a synthetic corticosteroid for topical dermatological use.

Chemically, halobetasol propionate is 21-chloro-6α,9-difluoro- 11β,17-dihydroxy-16β-methylpregna-1,4-diene-3-20-dione, 17- propionate, with the empirical formula $C_{25}H_{31}ClF_2O_5$, and a molecular weight of 485.

Halobetasol propionate is a white crystalline powder insoluble in water.

Ultravate cream contains halobetasol propionate 0.5 mg/g in a cream base of cetyl alcohol, glycerin, isopropyl isostearate, isopropyl palmitate, steareth-21, diazolidinyl urea, methylchloroisothiazolinone (and) methylisothiazolinone and water.

Ultravate ointment contains halobetasol propionate 0.5 mg/g in a base of aluminum stearate, beeswax, pentaerythritol cocoate, petroleum, propylene glycol, sorbitan sesquioleate and stearyl citrate.

CLINICAL PHARMACOLOGY:

Like other topical corticosteroids, halobetasol propionate has anti-inflammatory, anti-pruritic and vasoconstrictive actions. The mechanism of the anti-inflammatory activity of the topical corticosteroids, in general, is unclear. However, corticosteroids are thought to act by the induction of phospholipase A_2 inhibitory proteins, collectively called lipocortins. It is postulated that these proteins control the biosynthesis of potent mediators of inflammation such as prostaglandins and leukotrienes by inhibiting the release of their common precursor arachidonic acid. arachidonic acid is released from membrane phospholipids by phospholipase A_2.

Pharmacokinetics: The extent of percutaneous absorption of topical corticosteroids is determined by many factors, including the vehicle and the integrity of the epidermal barrier. Occlusive dressings with hydrocortisone for up to 24 hours have not been demonstrated to increase penetration, however, occlusion of hydrocortisone for 96 hours markedly enhances penetration. Topical corticosteroids can be absorbed from normal intact skin while inflammation and/or other disease processes in the skin may increase percutaneous absorption.

Human and animal studies indicate that approximately 2% of the applied dose of halobetasol propionate enters the circulation within 96 hours following topical administration of the cream (3% for the ointment).

Studies performed the halobetasol propionate ointment indicate that it is in the super-high range of potency as compared with other topical corticosteroids. In one of three studies conducted with halobetasol propionate cream, its potency was comparable to halobetasol propionate ointment. However, in two other studies, halobetasol propionate cream did not appear to be as potent as halobetasol propionate ointment.

INDICATIONS AND USAGE:

Halobetasol propionate cream/ointment is a high to super-high potency corticosteroid (See CLINICAL PHARMACOLOGY) indicated for the relief of the inflammatory and pruritic manifestations of corticosteroid- responsive dermatoses. Treatment beyond two consecutive weeks is not recommended, and the total dosage should not exceed 50 g/week because of the potential for the drug to suppress the hypothalamic-pituitary-adrenal (HPA) axis.

CONTRAINDICATIONS:

Halobetasol propionate cream/ointment is contraindicated in those patients with a history of hypersensitivity to any of the components of the preparation.

PRECAUTIONS:

GENERAL

Systemic absorption of topical corticosteroids can produce reversible hypothalamic-pituitary-adrenal (HPA) axis suppression with the potential for glucocorticosteroid insufficiency after withdrawal of treatment. Manifestations of Cushing's syndrome, hyperglycemia, and glucosuria can also be produced in some patients by systemic absorption of topical corticosteroids while on treatment.

Patients receiving a large dose of a higher potency topical steroid applied to a large surface area or under an occlusive dressing should be evaluated periodically for evidence of HPA axis suppression. This may be done by using the ACTH stimulation, A.M. plasma cortisol, and urinary free-cortisol tests. Patients receiving super-potent corticosteroids should not be treated for more than 2 weeks at a time and only small areas should be treated at any one time due to the increased risk of HPA suppression.

Halobetasol propionate ointment produced HPA axis suppression when used in divided doses at 7 grams per day for one week in patients with psoriasis. These effects were reversible upon discontinuation of treatment.

If HPA axis suppression is noted, an attempt should be made to withdraw the drug, to reduce the frequency of application, or to substitute a less potent corticosteroid. Recovery of PHA axis function is generally prompt and complete upon discontinuation of topical corticosteroids. Infrequently, signs and symptoms of glucocorticosteroid insufficiency may occur, requiring supplemental systemic corticosteroids. For information on systemic supplementation, see prescribing information for those products.

Children may be more susceptible to systemic toxicity from equivalent doses due to their larger skin surface to body mass ratios (see PRECAUTIONS, Pediatric Use).

If irritation develops, halobetasol propionate cream/ointment should be discontinued and appropriate therapy instituted. Allergic contact dermatitis with corticosteroids is usually diagnosed by observing failure to heal rather than noting a clinical exacerbation as with most topical products not containing corticosteroids. Such an observation should be corroborated with appropriate diagnostic patch testing.

If concomitant skin infections are present or develop, an appropriate antifungal or antibacterial agent should be used. If a favorable response does not occur promptly, use of halobetasol propionate cream/ointment should be discontinued until the infection has been adequately controlled.

Halobetasol propionate cream/ointment should not be used in the treatment of rosacea or perioral dermatitis, and it should not be used on the face, groin, or axillae.

INFORMATION FOR THE PATIENT

Patients using topical corticosteroids should receive the following information and instructions:

1. The medication is to be used as directed by the physician. It is for external use only. Avoid contact with the eyes.

PRECAUTIONS: *(cont'd)*

2. The medication should not be used for any disorder other than that for which it was prescribed.
3. The treated skin area should not be bandaged or otherwise covered or wrapped so as to be occlusive unless directed by the physician.
4. Patients should report to their physician any signs of local adverse reactions.

LABORATORY TESTS

The following tests may be helpful in evaluating patients for HPA axis suppression: ACTH-stimulation test, A.M. plasma-cortisol test; Urinary free-cortisol test.

CARCINOGENESIS, MUTAGENESIS AND IMPAIRMENT OF FERTILITY

Long-term animal studies have not been performed to evaluate the carcinogenic potential of halobetasol propionate.

Studies in the rat following oral administration at dose levels up to 50 mcg/kg/day indicated no impairment of fertility or general reproductive performance.

Positive mutagenicity effects were observed in two genotoxicity assays. halobetasol propionate was positive in a Chinese hamster micronucleus test, and in a mouse lymphoma gene mutation assay *in vitro*.

In other genotoxicity testing halobetasol propionate was not found to be genotoxic in the Ames/Salmonella assay, in the sister chromatid exchange test in somatic cells of the Chinese hamster, in chromosome aberration studies of germinal and somatic cells of rodents, and in a mammalian spot test to determine point mutations.

PREGNANCY, TERATOGENIC EFFECTS, PREGNANCY CATEGORY C

Corticosteroids have been shown to be teratogenic in laboratory animals when administered systemically at relatively low dosage levels. Some corticosteroids have been shown to be teratogenic after dermal application to laboratory animals.

Halobetasol propionate has been shown to be teratogenic in SPF rats and chinchilla-type rabbits when given systemically during gestation at doses of 0.04 to 0.1 mg/kg in rats and 0.01 mg/kg in rabbits. These doses are approximately 13, 33 and 3 times, respectively, the human topical dose of halobetasol propionate cream/ointment. Halobetasol propionate was embryotoxic in rabbits but not in rats.

Cleft palate was observed in both rats and rabbits. Omphalocele was seen in rats, but not in rabbits.

There are no adequate and well-controlled studies of the teratogenic potential of halobetasol propionate in pregnant women. Therefore, halobetasol propionate cream/ointment should be used during pregnancy only if the potential benefit justifies the potential risk to the fetus.

NURSING MOTHERS

Systemically administered corticosteroids appear in human milk and could suppress growth, interfere with endogenous corticosteroid production, or cause other untoward effects. It is not known whether topical administration of corticosteroids could result in sufficient systemic absorption to produce detectable quantities in human milk. Because many drugs are excreted in human milk, caution should be exercised when halobetasol propionate cream/ointment is administered to a nursing woman.

PEDIATRIC USE

Safety and effectiveness of halobetasol propionate cream/ointment in children have not been established. Because of a higher ratio of skin surface area to body mass, children are at a greater risk than adults of HPA-axis suppression when they are treated with topical corticosteroids. They are therefore also at greater risk of glucocorticosteroid insufficiency after withdrawal of treatment and of Cushing's syndrome while on treatment. Adverse effects including striae have been reported with inappropriate use of topical corticosteroids in infants and children. (See PRECAUTIONS.)

HPA axis suppression, Cushing's syndrome, and intracranial hypertension have been reported in children receiving topical corticosteroids. Manifestations of adrenal suppression in children include linear growth retardation, delayed weight gain, low plasma cortisol levels, and absence of response to ACTH stimulation. Manifestations of intracranial hypertension include bulging fontanelles, headaches, and bilateral papilledema.

ADVERSE REACTIONS:

In controlled clinical trials, the most frequent adverse events reported for halobetasol propionate cream included stinging, burning or itching in 4.4% (2.4% for the ointment) of the patients. Less frequently reported adverse reactions were dry skin, erythema, skin atrophy, leukoderma, vesicles and rash.

The following additional local adverse reactions are reported infrequently with topical corticosteroids, but may occur more frequently with high potency corticosteroids, such as halobetasol propionate cream/ointment. These reactions are listed in an approximate decreasing order of occurrence: folliculitis, hypertrichosis, acneiform eruptions, hypopigmentation, perioral dermatitis, allergic contact dermatitis, secondary infection, striae, and miliaria.

OVERDOSAGE:

Topically applied halobetasol propionate cream/ointment can be absorbed in sufficient amount to produce systemic effects (see PRECAUTIONS.)

DOSAGE AND ADMINISTRATION:

Apply a thin layer of halobetasol propionate cream/ointment to the affected skin once or twice daily, as directed by your physician, and rub in gently and completely.

Halobetasol propionate cream/ointment is a high potency topical corticosteroid; therefore, treatment should be limited to two weeks, and amounts greater then 50 g/wk should not be used. Halobetasol propionate cream should not be used with occlusive dressings.

Store between 15 and 30°C (59 and 86°F).

HOW SUPPLIED - EQUIVALENTS NOT AVAILABLE:

Cream - Topical - 0.05 %

15 gm	$20.90	ULTRAVATE, Westwood Squibb	00072-1400-15
50 gm	$51.19	ULTRAVATE, Westwood Squibb	00072-1400-50

Ointment - Topical - 0.05 %

15 gm	$20.90	ULTRAVATE, Westwood Squibb	00072-1450-15
50 gm	$51.19	ULTRAVATE, Westwood Squibb	00072-1450-50

HALOFANTRINE HYDROCHLORIDE *(003128)*

CATEGORIES: Anti-Infectives; Antibiotics; Antimalarial Agents; Malaria; Orphan Drugs; FDA Class 1P ("Priority Review"); FDA Approved 1992 Jul

BRAND NAMES: **Halfan**

DESCRIPTION:

Release being delayed by SmithKline Beecham.

HALOPERIDOL *(001418)*

CATEGORIES: Antipsychotics/Antimanics; Behavior Problems; Butyrophenones; Central Nervous System Agents; Neuroleptics; Neuromuscular; Psychotherapeutic Agents; Psychotic Disorders; Sedatives/Hypnotics; Skeletal Muscle Hyperactivity; Tics; Tourette Syndrome; Tranquilizers; Schizophrenia*; Vertigo/Motion Sickness/ Vomiting*; FDA Approval Pre 1982
* Indication not approved by the FDA

BRAND NAMES: *Alased*; *Aloperidin*; *Apo-Haloperidol* (Canada); *Avant*; *Binison*; *Brotopon* (Japan); *Cereen*; *Depidol*; *Dozic* (England); *Duraperidol* (Germany); *Einalon*; *Einalon S* (Japan); *Eukystol*; **Haldol**; *Halidol*; *Halojust* (Japan); *Halomed*; *Halo-P*; *Haloper* (Germany); *Haloperil* (Mexico); Haloperidol Lactate; *Haloperin*; *Halopidol*; *Halopol*; *Halosten* (Japan); *Haricon*; *Inin*; *Linton* (Japan); *Mixidol* (Japan); *Novoperidol* (Canada); *Pacedol*; *Peluces* (Japan); *Pericate*; *Perida*; *Peridol* (Canada); *Peridor*; *Selezyme* (Japan); *Seranace* (England); *Seranase*; *Serenace* (Australia, Asia); *Serenase*; *Serenelfi*; *Sigaperidol* (Germany); *Trancodol-5*; *Trancodol-10*
(International brand names outside U.S. in italics)

FORMULARIES: Aetna; BC-BS; CIGNA; FHP; Humana; Kaiser; Medco; Medi-Cal; PCS; PruCare; United; WHO

DESCRIPTION:

Haloperidol is the first of the butyrophenone series of major tranquilizers. The chemical designation is 4-[4-(p-chlorophenyl)-4-hydroxy-piperidino]-4'-fluorobutyrophenone.

Haloperidol dosage forms include: tablets (1/2, 1, 2, 5*, 10* and 20 mg); a concentrate with 2 mg per ml haloperidol (as the lactate); and a sterile parenteral form for intramuscular injection. The injection provides 5 mg haloperidol (as the lactate) with 1.8 mg methylparaben and 0.2 mg propylparaben per ml, and lactic acid for pH adjustment between 3.0 - 3.6.

Inactive ingredients: tablets - calcium phosphate, calcium stearate, corn starch and flavor-1 mg contains FD&C Yellow No. 10 and FD&C Red No. 40; 2 mg contains D&C Red No. 33 and FD&C Blue No. 2; 5 mg contains FD&C Blue No. 1 and FD&C Yellow No. 10 and D&C Red No. 30; 10 mg contains FD&C Blue No. 1 and FD&C Yellow No. 5*; and 20 mg contains FD&C Red No. 40; concentrate - lactic acid and methylparaben.

CLINICAL PHARMACOLOGY:

The precise mechanism of action has not been clearly established.

INDICATIONS AND USAGE:

Haloperidol is indicated for use in the management of manifestations of psychotic disorders.

Haloperidol is indicated for the control of tics and vocal utterances of Tourette's Disorder in children and adults.

Haloperidol is effective for the treatment of severe behavior problems in children of combative, explosive hyperexcitability (which cannot be accounted for by immediate provocation).

Haloperidol is also effective in the short-term treatment of hyperactive children who show excessive motor activity with accompanying conduct disorders consisting of some or all of the following symptoms: impulsivity, difficulty sustaining attention, aggressivity, mood lability and poor frustration tolerance. Haloperidol should be reserved for these two groups of children only after failure to respond to psychotherapy or medications other than antipsychotics.

CONTRAINDICATIONS:

Haloperidol is contraindicated in severe toxic central nervous system depression or comatose states from any cause and in individuals who are hypersensitive to this drug or have Parkinson's disease.

WARNINGS:

Tardive Dyskinesia: A syndrome consisting of potentially irreversible, involuntary, dyskinetic movements may develop in patients treated with antipsychotic drugs. Although the prevalence of the syndrome appears to be highest among the elderly, especially elderly women, it is impossible to rely upon prevalence estimates to predict, at the inception of antipsychotic treatment, which patients are likely to develop the syndrome. Whether antipsychotic drug products differ in their potential to cause tardive dyskinesia is unknown.

Both the risk of developing tardive dyskinesia and the likelihood that it will become irreversible are believed to increase as the duration of treatment and the cumulative dose of antipsychotic drugs administered to the patient increase. However, the syndrome can develop, although much less commonly, after relatively brief treatment periods at low doses.

There is no known treatment for established cases of tardive dyskinesia, although the syndrome may remit, partially or completely, if antipsychotic treatment is withdrawn. Antipsychotic treatment, itself, however, may suppress (or partially suppress) the signs and symptoms of the syndrome and thereby may possible mask the underlying process. The effect that symptomatic suppression has upon the long-term course of the syndrome is unknown.

Given these considerations, antipsychotic drugs should be prescribed in a manner that is most likely to minimize the occurrence of tardive dyskinesia. Chronic antipsychotic treatment should generally be reserved for patients who suffer from a chronic illness that, 1) is known to respond to antipsychotic drugs, and 2) for whom alternative, equally effective, but potentially less harmful treatments are **not** available or appropriate. In patients who do require chronic treatment, the smallest dose and the shortest duration of treatment producing a satisfactory clinical response should be sought. The need for continued treatment should be reassessed periodically.

If signs and symptoms of tardive dyskinesia appear in a patient on antipsychotics, drug discontinuation should be considered. However, some patients may require treatment despite the presence of the syndrome.

(For further information about the description of tardive dyskinesia and its clinical detection, please refer to ADVERSE REACTIONS.)

Neuroleptic Malignant Syndrome (NMS): A potentially fatal symptom complex sometimes referred to as Neuroleptic Malignant Syndrome (NMS) has been reported in association with antipsychotic drugs. Clinical manifestations of NMS are hyperpyrexia, muscle rigidity, altered mental status (including catatonic signs) and evidence of autonomic instability (irregular pulse or blood pressure, tachycardia, diaphoresis, and cardiac dysrhythmias). Additional signs may include elevated creatine phosphokinase, myoglobinuria (rhabdomyolysis) and acute renal failure.

The diagnostic evaluation of patients with this syndrome is complicated. In arriving at a diagnosis, it is important to identify cases where the clinical presentation includes both serious medical illness (*e.g.,* pneumonia, systemic infection, etc.) and untreated or inadequately treated extrapyramidal signs and symptoms (EPS). Other important considerations in the differential diagnosis include central anticholinergic toxicity, heat stroke, drug fever and primary central nervous system (CNS) pathology.

WARNINGS: *(cont'd)*

The management of NMS should include 1) immediate discontinuation of antipsychotic drugs and other drugs not essential to concurrent therapy, 2) intensive symptomatic treatment and medical monitoring, and 3) treatment of any concomitant serious medical problems for which specific treatments are available. There is no general agreement about specific pharmacological treatment regimens for uncomplicated NMS.

If a patient requires antipsychotic drug treatment after recovery from NMS, the potential reintroduction of drug therapy should be carefully considered. The patient should be carefully monitored, since recurrences of NMS have been reported.

Hyperpyrexia and heat stroke, not associated with the above symptom complex, have also been reported with haloperidol.

Usage in Pregnancy: Rodents given 2 to 20 times the usual maximum human dose of haloperidol by oral or parenteral routes showed an increase in incidence of resorption, reduced fertility, delayed delivery and pup mortality. No teratogenic effect has been reported in rats, rabbits or dogs at dosages within this range, but cleft palate has been observed in mice given 15 times the usual maximum human dose. Cleft palate in mice appears to be a non-specific response to stress or nutritional imbalance as well as to a variety of drugs, and there is no evidence to relate this phenomenon to predictable human risk for most of these agents.

There are no well controlled studies with haloperidol in pregnant women. There are reports, however, of cases of limb malformations observed following maternal use of haloperidol along with other drugs which have suspected teratogenic potential during the first trimester of pregnancy. Causal relationships were not established in these cases. Since such experience does not exclude the possibility of fetal damage due to haloperidol, this drug should be used during pregnancy or in women likely to become pregnant only if the benefit clearly justifies a potential risk to the fetus. Infants should not be nursed during drug treatment.

General: A number of cases of bronchopneumonia, some fatal, have followed the use of antipsychotic drugs, including haloperidol. It has been postulated that lethargy and decreased sensation of thirst due to central inhibition may lead to dehydration, hemoconcentration and reduced pulmonary ventilation. Therefore, if the above signs and symptoms appear, especially in the elderly, the physician should institute remedial therapy promptly.

Although not reported with haloperidol, decreased serum cholesterol and/or cutaneous and ocular changes have been reported in patients receiving chemically-related drugs.

Haloperidol may impair the mental and/or physical abilities required for the performance of hazardous tasks such as operating machinery or driving a motor vehicle. The ambulatory patient should be warned accordingly.

The use of alcohol with this drug should be avoided due to possible additive effects and hypotension.

PRECAUTIONS:

Haloperidol should be administered cautiously to patients:

with severe cardiovascular disorders, because of the possibility of transient hypotension and/or precipitation of anginal pain. Should hypotension occur and a vasopressor be required, epinephrine should not be used since haloperidol may block its vasopressor activity and paradoxical further lowering of the blood pressure may occur. Instead, metaraminol, phenylephrine or norepinephrine should be used.

receiving anticonvulsant medications, with a history of seizures, or with EEG abnormalities, because haloperidol may lower the convulsive threshold. If indicated, adequate anticonvulsant therapy should be concomitantly maintained.

with known allergies, or with a history of allergic reactions to drugs.

receiving anticoagulants, since an isolated instance of interference occurred with the effects of one anticoagulant (phenindione).

If concomitant antiparkinson medication is required, it may have to be continued after haloperidol is discontinued because of the difference in excretion rates. If both are discontinued simultaneously, extrapyramidal symptoms may occur. The physician should keep in mind the possible increase in intraocular pressure when anticholinergic drugs, including antiparkinson agents, are administered concomitantly with haloperidol.

As with other antipsychotic agents, it should be noted that haloperidol may be capable of potentiating CNS depressants such as anesthetics, opiates, and alcohol.

When haloperidol is used to control mania in cyclic disorders, there may be a rapid mood swing to depression.

Severe neurotoxicity (rigidity, inability to walk or talk) may occur in patients with thyrotoxicosis who are also receiving antipsychotic medication, including haloperidol.

No mutagenic potential of haloperidol was found in the Ames Salmonella microsomal activation assay. Negative or inconsistent positive findings have been obtained in *in vitro* and *in vivo* studies of effects of haloperidol on chromosome structure and number. The available cytogenetic evidence is considered too inconsistent to be conclusive at this time.

Carcinogenicity studies using oral haloperidol were conducted in Wistar rats (dosed at up to 5 mg/kg daily for 24 months) and in Albino Swiss mice (dosed at up to 5 mg/kg daily for 18 months). In the rat study survival was less than optimal in all dose groups, reducing the number of rats at risk for developing tumors. However, although a relatively greater number of rats survived to the end of the study in high dose male and female groups, these animals did not have a greater incidence of tumors than control animals. Therefore, although not optimal, this study does suggest the absence of a haloperidol related increase in the incidence of neoplasia in rats at doses up to 20 times the usual daily human dose for chronic or resistant patients.

In female mice at 5 and 20 times the highest initial daily dose for chronic or resistant patients, there was a statistically significant increase in mammary gland neoplasia and total tumor incidence; at 20 times the same daily dose there was a statistically significant increase in pituitary gland neoplasia. In male mice, no statistically significant differences in incidences of total tumors or specific tumor types were noted.

Antipsychotic drugs elevate prolactin levels; the elevation persists during chronic administration. Tissue culture experiments indicate that approximately one-third of human breast cancers are prolactin dependent*in vitro,* a factor of potential importance if the prescription of these drugs is contemplated in a patient with a previously detected breast cancer. Although disturbances such as galactorrhea, amenorrhea, gynecomastia, and impotence have been reported, the clinical significance of elevated serum prolactin levels is unknown for most patients. An increase in mammary neoplasms has been found in rodents after chronic administration of antipsychotic drugs. Neither clinical studies nor epidemiologic studies conducted to date, however, have shown an association between chronic administration of these drugs and mammary tumorigenesis; the available evidence is considered too limited to be conclusive this time.

DRUG INTERACTIONS:

Combined Use of Haloperidol and Lithium: An encephalopathic syndrome (characterized by weakness, lethargy, fever, tremulousness and confusion, extrapyramidal symptoms, leukocytosis, elevated serum enzymes, BUN, and FBS) followed by irreversible brain damage has occurred in a few patients treated with lithium plus haloperidol. A causal relationship between these events and the concomitant administration of lithium and haloperidol has not been established; however, patients receiving such combined therapy should be monitored closely for early evidence of neurological toxicity and treatment discontinued promptly if such signs appear.

ADVERSE REACTIONS:

CNS EFFECTS

Extrapyramidal Symptoms (EPS): EPS during the administration of haloperidol have been reported frequently, often during the first few days of treatment. EPS can be categorized generally as Parkinson-like symptoms, akathisia, or dystonia (including opisthotonos and oculogyric crisis). While all can occur at relatively low doses, they occur more frequently and with greater severity at higher doses. The symptoms may be controlled with dose reductions or administration of antiparkinson drugs such as benztropine mesylate USP or trihexyphenidyl hydrochloride USP. It should be noted that persistent EPS have been reported; the drug may have to be discontinued in such cases.

Withdrawal Emergent Neurological Signs: Generally, patients receiving short term therapy experience no problems with abrupt discontinuation of antipsychotic drugs. However, some patients on maintenance treatment experience transient dyskinetic signs after abrupt withdrawal. In certain of these cases the dyskinetic movements are indistinguishable from the syndrome described below under "Tardive Dyskinesia" except for duration. It is not known whether gradual withdrawal of antipsychotic drugs reduce the rate of occurrence of withdrawal emergent neurological signs but until further evidence becomes available, it seems reasonable to gradually withdraw use of haloperidol.

Tardive Dyskinesia: As with all antipsychotic agents haloperidol has been associated with persistent dyskinesias. Tardive dyskinesia, a syndrome consisting of potentially irreversible, involuntary, dyskinetic movements, may appear in some patients on long-term therapy or may occur after drug therapy has been discontinued. The risk appears to be greater in elderly patients on high-dose therapy, especially females. The symptoms are persistent and in some patients appear irreversible. The syndrome is characterized by rhythmical involuntary movements of tongue, face, mouth or jaw (*e.g.,* protrusion of tongue, puffing of cheeks, puckering of mouth, chewing movements). Sometimes these may be accompanied by involuntary movements of extremities and the trunk.

There is no known effective treatment for tardive dyskinesia; antiparkinson agents usually do not alleviate the symptoms of this syndrome. It is suggested that all antipsychotic agents be discontinued if these symptoms appear. Should it be necessary to reinstitute treatment, or increase the dosage of the agents, or switch to a different antipsychotic agent, this syndrome may be masked.

It has been reported that fine vermicular movement of the tongue may an early sign of tardive dyskinesia and if the medication is stopped at that time the full syndrome may not develop.

Tardive Dystonia: Tardive dystonia, not associated with the above syndrome, has also been reported. Tardive dystonia is characterized by delayed onset of choreic or dystonic movements, is often persistent, and has the potential of becoming irreversible.

Other CNS Effects: Insomnia, restlessness, anxiety, euphoria, agitation, drowsiness, depression, lethargy, headache, confusion, vertigo, grand mal seizures, exacerbation of psychotic symptoms including hallucinations, and catatonic-like behavioral states which may be responsive to drug withdrawal and/or treatment with anticholinergic drugs.

Body as a Whole: Neuroleptic malignant syndrome (NMS), hyperpyrexia and heat stroke have been reported with haloperidol. (See WARNINGS for further information concerning NMS.)

Cardiovascular Effects: Tachycardia, hypotension, hypertension and ECG changes including prolongation of the Q-T interval and ECG pattern changes compatible with the polymorphous configuration of torsades de pointes.

Hematologic Effects: Reports have appeared citing the occurrence of mild and usually transient leukopenia and leukocytosis, minimal decreases in red blood cell counts, anemia, or a tendency toward lymphomonocytosis. Agranulocytosis has rarely been reported to have occurred with the use of haloperidol, and then only in association with other medication.

Liver Effects: Impaired liver function and/or jaundice have been reported.

Dermatologic Reactions: Maculopapular and acneiform skin reactions and isolated cases of photosensitivity and loss of hair.

Endocrine Disorders: Lactation, breast engorgement, mastalgia, menstrual irregularities, gynecomastia, impotence, increased libido, hyperglycemia, hypoglycemia and hyponatremia.

Gastrointestinal Effects: Anorexia, constipation, diarrhea, hypersalivation, dyspepsia, nausea and vomiting.

Autonomic Reactions: Dry mouth, blurred vision, urinary retention, diaphoresis and priapism.

Respiratory Effects: Laryngospasm, bronchospasm and increased depth of respiration.

Special Senses: Cataracts, retinopathy and visual disturbances.

Other: Cases of sudden and unexpected death have been reported in association with the administration of haloperidol. The nature of the evidence makes it impossible to determine definitively what role, if any, haloperidol played in the outcome of the reported cases. The possibility that haloperidol caused death cannot, of course, be excluded, but it is to be kept in mind that sudden and unexpected death may occur in psychotic patients when they go untreated or when they are treated with other antipsychotic drugs.

Postmarketing Events: Hyperammonemia has been reported in a 5 1/2 year old child with citrullinemia, an inherited disorder of ammonia excretion, following treatment with haloperidol.

OVERDOSAGE:

Manifestations: In general, the symptoms of overdosage would be an exaggeration of known pharmacologic effects and adverse reactions, the most prominent of which would be: 1) severe extrapyramidal reactions, 2) hypotension, or 3) sedation. The patient would appear comatose with respiratory depression and hypotension which could be severe enough to produce a shock-like state. The extrapyramidal reaction would be manifest by muscular weakness or rigidity and a generalized or localized tremor as demonstrated by the akinetic or agitans types respectively. With accidental overdosage, hypertension rather than hypotension occurred in a two-year old child. The risk of ECG changes associated with torsades de pointes should be considered. (For further information regarding torsades de pointes, please refer to ADVERSE REACTIONS.)

Treatment: Gastric lavage or induction of emesis should be carried out immediately followed by administration of activated charcoal. Since there is no specific antidote, treatment is primarily supportive. A patent airway must be established by use of an oropharyngeal airway or endotracheal tube or, in prolonged cases of coma, by tracheostomy. Respiratory depression may be counteracted by artificial respiration and mechanical respirators. Hypotension and circulatory collapse may be counteracted by use of intravenous fluids, plasma, or concentrated albumin, and vasopressor agents such as metaraminol, phenylephrine and norepinephrine. Epinephrine should not be used. In case of severe extrapyramidal reactions, antiparkinson medication should be administered. ECG and vital signs should be monitored

OVERDOSAGE: *(cont'd)*

especially for signs of Q-T prolongation or dysrhythmias and monitoring should continue until the ECG is normal. Severe arrhythmias should be treated with appropriate anti-arrhythmic measures.

DOSAGE AND ADMINISTRATION:

There is considerable variation from patient to patient in the amount of medication required for treatment. As with all antipsychotic drugs, dosage should be individualized according to the needs and response of each patient. Dosage adjustments, either upward or downward, should be carried out as rapidly as practicable to achieve optimum therapeutic control.

To determine the initial dosage, consideration should be given to the patient's age, severity of illness, previous response to other antipsychotic drugs, and any concomitant medication or disease state. Children, debilitated or geriatric patients, as well as those with a history of adverse reactions to antipsychotic drugs, may require less haloperidol. The optimal response in such patients is usually obtained with more gradual dosage adjustments and at lower dosage levels, as recommended below.

Clinical experience suggests the following recommendations:

INITIAL ORAL DOSAGE RANGE

Adults: Moderate Symptomatology: 0.5 mg to 2.0 mg b.i.d. or t.i.d.

Severe Symptomatology: 3.0 mg to 5.0 mg b.i.d. or t.i.d.

To achieve prompt control, higher doses may be required in some cases.

Geriatric or Debilitated Patients: 0.5 mg to 2.0 mg b.i.d. or t.i.d.

Chronic or Resistant Patients: 3.0 mg to 5.0 mg b.i.d. or t.i.d.

Patients who remain severely disturbed or inadequately controlled may require dosage adjustment. Daily dosages up to 100 mg may be necessary in some cases to achieve an optimal response. Infrequently, haloperidol has been used in doses above 100 mg for severely resistant patients; however, the limited clinical usage has not demonstrated the safety of prolonged administration of such doses.

Children: The following recommendations apply to children between the ages of 3 and 12 years (weight range 15 to 40 kg). Haloperidol is not intended for children under 3 years old. Therapy should begin at the lowest dose possible (0.5 mg per day). If required, the dose should be increased by an increment of 0.5 mg at 5 to 7 day intervals until the desired therapeutic effect is obtained.

The total dose may be divided, to be given b.i.d. of t.i.d.

Psychotic Disorders: 0.05 mg/kg/day to 0.15 mg/kg/day

Non-Psychotic Behavior Disorders and Tourette's Disorder:

0.05 mg/kg/day to 0.75 mg/kg/day

Severely disturbed psychotic children may require higher doses.

In severely disturbed, non-psychotic children or in hyperactive children with accompanying conduct disorders, who have failed to respond to psychotherapy or medications other than antipsychotics, it should be noted that since these behaviors may be short-lived, short-term administration of haloperidol may suffice. There is no evidence establishing a maximum effective dosage. There is little evidence that behavior improvement is further enhanced in dosages beyond 6 mg per day.

Maintenance Dosage: Upon achieving a satisfactory therapeutic response, dosage should then be gradually reduced to the lowest effective maintenance level.

INTRAMUSCULAR ADMINISTRATION

Adults: Parenteral medication, administered intramuscularly in doses of 2 to 5 mg, is utilized for prompt control of the acutely agitated patient with moderately severe to very severe symptoms. Depending on the response of the patient, subsequent doses may be given, administered as often as every hour, although 4 to 8 hour intervals may be satisfactory.

Controlled trials to establish the safety and effectiveness of intramuscular administration in children have not been conducted.

Parenteral drug products should be inspected visually for particulate matter and discoloration prior to administration, whenever solution and container permit.

Switchover Procedure: The oral form should supplant the injectable as soon as practicable. In the absence of bioavailability studies establishing bioequivalence between these two dosage forms the following guidelines for dosage are suggested. For an initial approximation of the total daily dose required, the parenteral dose administered in the preceding 24 hours may be used. Since this dose is only an initial estimate, it is recommended that careful monitoring of clinical signs and symptoms, including clinical efficacy, sedation, and adverse effects, be carried out periodically for the first several days following the initiation of switchover. In this way, dosage adjustments, either upward or downward, can be quickly accomplished. Depending on the patient's clinical status, the first oral dose should be given within 12-24 hours following the last parenteral dose.

HOW SUPPLIED - RATED THERAPEUTICALLY EQUIVALENT:

Concentrate - Oral - 2 mg/ml

2.5 ml x 100	$100.00	Haloperidol Lactate, Xactdose	50962-0326-03
5 ml x 100	$136.64	Haloperidol, Xactdose	50962-0325-05
10 ml x 100	$245.28	Haloperidol, Xactdose	50962-0325-10
15 ml	$6.95	Haloperidol, Harber Pharm	51432-0001-00
15 ml	$7.75	Haloperidol Lactate, Consolidated Midland	00223-6525-15
15 ml	$7.93	Haloperidol, H.C.F.A. F F P	99999-1418-01
15 ml	$8.44	Haloperidol, Alpharma	00472-0766-99
15 ml	$9.30	Haloperidol Lactate, Silarx Pharms	54838-0501-15
15 ml	$9.45	Haloperidol, Goldline Labs	00182-6059-64
15 ml	$9.50	Haloperidol, Copley Pharm	38245-0604-15
15 ml	$9.60	Haloperidol, Major Pharms	00904-1729-35
15 ml	$9.76	Haloperidol Intensol, Roxane	00054-3350-41
15 ml	$9.88	Haloperidol Concentrate, Geneva Pharms	00781-6205-47
15 ml	$10.35	Haloperidol Concentrate, Schein Pharm (US)	00364-0854-72
15 ml	**$23.03**	**HALDOL, McNeil Lab**	**00045-0250-15**
120 ml	$15.75	Haloperidol, H.C.F.A. F F P	99999-1418-02
120 ml	$28.95	Haloperidol, Harber Pharm	51432-0001-08
120 ml	$31.84	Haloperidol Intensol, Roxane	00054-3350-50
120 ml	$31.85	Haloperidol Lactate, Cypress Pharm	60258-0464-04
120 ml	$32.00	Haloperidol Lactate, Consolidated Midland	00223-6525-04
120 ml	$32.70	Haloperidol, Alpharma	00472-0766-94
120 ml	$32.70	Haloperidol Concentrate, Geneva Pharms	00781-6205-04
120 ml	$32.75	Haloperidol, Qualitest Pharms	00603-1290-54
120 ml	$32.95	Haloperidol, Major Pharms	00904-1729-20
120 ml	$33.00	Haloperidol, Goldline Labs	00182-6059-71
120 ml	$33.50	Haloperidol, Rugby	00536-1011-97
120 ml	$33.50	Haloperidol, Copley Pharm	38245-0604-14
120 ml	$36.12	Haloperidol Lactate, Silarx Pharms	54838-0501-40
120 ml	$37.10	Haloperidol Concentrate, Schein Pharm (US)	00364-0854-77
120 ml	$41.86	Haloperidol, Teva	00093-0553-12
120 ml	**$96.23**	**HALDOL, McNeil Lab**	**00045-0250-04**

HOW SUPPLIED - RATED THERAPEUTICALLY EQUIVALENT: *(cont'd)*

Injection, Solution - Intramuscular - 5 mg/ml

1 ml	$37.50	Haloperidol, Solopak Labs	39769-0088-02
1 ml x 10	**$60.18**	**HALDOL, McNeil Lab**	**00045-0255-01**
1 ml x 10	**$65.21**	**HALDOL, McNeil Lab**	**00045-0255-31**
1 ml x 25	$74.08	Haloperidol Lactate, Fujisawa USA	00469-3620-00
1 ml x 25	$74.69	Haloperidol, Fujisawa USA	00469-2250-00
10 ml	$16.68	Haloperidol Lactate, Voluntary Hosp	53258-2250-03
10 ml	$27.93	Haloperidol, Fujisawa USA	00469-2250-30
10 ml	**$58.67**	**HALDOL, McNeil Lab**	**00045-0255-49**

Tablet, Uncoated - Oral - 0.5 mg

100's	$1.88	Haloperidol, United Res	00677-1115-01
100's	$1.88	Haloperidol, H.C.F.A. F F P	99999-1418-03
100's	$6.75	Haloperidol, Consolidated Midland	00223-1020-01
100's	$10.20	Haloperidol, Raway	00686-2594-13
100's	$11.01	Haloperidol, US Trading	56126-0335-11
100's	$11.50	Haloperidol, Major Pharms	00904-1730-60
100's	$13.10	Haloperidol, Medirex	57480-0376-01
100's	$13.44	Haloperidol, Roxane	00054-8342-25
100's	$13.49	Haloperidol, Purepac Pharm	00228-2289-10
100's	$13.78	Haloperidol, Roxane	00054-4342-25
100's	$14.70	Haloperidol, Schein Pharm (US)	00364-2204-01
100's	$14.95	Haloperidol, Major Pharms	00904-1830-60
100's	$17.65	Haloperidol, Parmed Pharms	00349-8944-01
100's	$17.65	Haloperidol, Mova Pharms	55370-0802-07
100's	$17.68	Haloperidol, Aligen Independ	00405-4459-01
100's	$17.95	Haloperidol, Rugby	00536-3869-01
100's	$18.55	Haloperidol, Qualitest Pharms	00603-3782-21
100's	$18.56	Haloperidol, HL Moore Drug Exch	00839-7346-06
100's	$18.81	Haloperidol, TIE Pharm	55496-3001-09
100's	$18.89	Haloperidol, Par Pharm	49884-0223-01
100's	$18.95	Haloperidol, Goldline Labs	00182-1262-01
100's	$19.75	Haloperidol, Geneva Pharms	00781-1391-01
100's	$19.95	Haloperidol, Mylan	00378-0351-01
100's	$24.35	Haloperidol, Vangard Labs	00615-2594-13
100's	$27.82	Haloperidol, Geneva Pharms	00781-1391-13
100's	$28.47	Haloperidol, Major Pharms	00904-1830-61
100's	**$41.24**	**HALDOL, McNeil Lab**	**00045-0240-60**
500's	$9.40	Haloperidol, H.C.F.A. F F P	99999-1418-04
500's	$43.43	Haloperidol, Rugby	00536-3869-05
500's	$48.90	Haloperidol, Major Pharms	00904-1830-40
500's	$67.45	Haloperidol, Purepac Pharm	00228-2289-50
500's	$94.43	Haloperidol, Par Pharm	49884-0223-05
500's	$94.70	Haloperidol, Goldline Labs	00182-1262-05
600's	$119.20	Haloperidol, Medirex	57480-0376-06
1000's	$18.80	Haloperidol, H.C.F.A. F F P	99999-1418-05
1000's	$42.50	Haloperidol, Consolidated Midland	00223-1020-02
1000's	$82.30	Haloperidol, Major Pharms	00904-1730-80
1000's	$82.30	Haloperidol, Major Pharms	00904-1830-80
1000's	$178.45	Haloperidol, Qualitest Pharms	00603-3782-32
1000's	$179.75	Haloperidol, HL Moore Drug Exch	00839-7346-16
1000's	$183.19	Haloperidol, Par Pharm	49884-0223-10
1000's	$183.26	Haloperidol, Geneva Pharms	00781-1391-10
1000's	$183.95	Haloperidol, Mylan	00378-0351-10
1000's	**$343.17**	**HALDOL, McNeil Lab**	**00045-0240-80**

Tablet, Uncoated - Oral - 1 mg

100's	$2.10	Haloperidol, United Res	00677-1116-01
100's	$2.10	Haloperidol, H.C.F.A. F F P	99999-1418-06
100's	$7.95	Haloperidol, Consolidated Midland	00223-1021-01
100's	$13.95	Haloperidol, Raway	00686-2595-13
100's	$18.08	Haloperidol, US Trading	56126-0336-11
100's	$18.50	Haloperidol, Major Pharms	00904-1731-60
100's	$18.50	Haloperidol, Major Pharms	00904-1831-60
100's	$18.55	Haloperidol, Mova Pharms	55370-0803-07
100's	$19.13	Haloperidol, Roxane	00054-8343-25
100's	$19.25	Haloperidol, Medirex	57480-0377-01
100's	$20.15	Haloperidol, Purepac Pharm	00228-2280-10
100's	$20.22	Haloperidol, Roxane	00054-4343-25
100's	$21.89	Haloperidol, Rugby	00536-3877-01
100's	$23.68	Haloperidol, Aligen Independ	00405-4460-01
100's	$24.69	Haloperidol, Schein Pharm (US)	00364-2205-01
100's	$25.13	Haloperidol, Searle	00014-0841-34
100's	$26.31	Haloperidol, HL Moore Drug Exch	00839-7347-06
100's	$26.78	Haloperidol, TIE Pharm	55496-3002-09
100's	$27.00	Haloperidol, Parmed Pharms	00349-8945-01
100's	$27.25	Haloperidol, Qualitest Pharms	00603-3783-21
100's	$27.49	Haloperidol, Par Pharm	49884-0224-01
100's	$27.95	Haloperidol, Goldline Labs	00182-1263-01
100's	$28.26	Haloperidol, Geneva Pharms	00781-1392-01
100's	$28.95	Haloperidol, Mylan	00378-0257-01
100's	$38.42	Haloperidol, Vangard Labs	00615-2595-13
100's	$38.62	Haloperidol, Major Pharms	00904-1731-61
100's	$39.80	Haloperidol, Geneva Pharms	00781-1392-13
100's	$45.43	Haloperidol, Major Pharms	00904-1831-61
100's	**$61.04**	**HALDOL, McNeil Lab**	**00045-0241-60**
500's	$10.50	Haloperidol, H.C.F.A. F F P	99999-1418-07
500's	$60.83	Haloperidol, Rugby	00536-3877-05
500's	$97.63	Haloperidol, Aligen Independ	00405-4460-02
500's	$100.09	Haloperidol, Par Pharm	49884-0224-05
500's	$100.75	Haloperidol, Purepac Pharm	00228-2280-50
500's	$139.70	Haloperidol, Goldline Labs	00182-1263-05
600's	$169.20	Haloperidol, Medirex	57480-0377-06
1000's	$21.00	Haloperidol, H.C.F.A. F F P	99999-1418-08
1000's	$54.50	Haloperidol, Consolidated Midland	00223-1021-02
1000's	$132.30	Haloperidol, Major Pharms	00904-1831-80
1000's	$190.67	Haloperidol, Roxane	00054-4343-31
1000's	$214.71	Haloperidol, Searle	00014-0841-52
1000's	$236.99	Haloperidol, HL Moore Drug Exch	00839-7347-16
1000's	$250.85	Haloperidol, Qualitest Pharms	00603-3783-32
1000's	$251.19	Haloperidol, Par Pharm	49884-0224-10
1000's	$258.29	Haloperidol, Geneva Pharms	00781-1392-10
1000's	$258.95	Haloperidol, Mylan	00378-0257-10

Tablet, Uncoated - Oral - 2 mg

100's	$2.03	Haloperidol, United Res	00677-1117-01
100's	$2.03	Haloperidol, H.C.F.A. F F P	99999-1418-09
100's	$10.95	Haloperidol, Consolidated Midland	00223-1022-01
100's	$11.25	Haloperidol, US Trading	56126-0337-11
100's	$18.00	Haloperidol, Raway	00686-2596-13
100's	$25.82	Haloperidol, Roxane	00054-8344-25
100's	$26.38	Haloperidol, Medirex	57480-0378-01
100's	$27.37	Haloperidol, Purepac Pharm	00228-2281-10

HOW SUPPLIED - RATED THERAPEUTICALLY EQUIVALENT: *(cont'd)*

100's	$28.08	Haloperidol, Roxane	00054-4344-25
100's	$30.65	Haloperidol, Major Pharms	00904-1832-60
100's	$31.70	Haloperidol, SCS Pharm	00905-0851-31
100's	$31.88	Haloperidol, Schein Pharm (US)	00364-2206-01
100's	$33.20	Haloperidol, Harber Pharm	51432-0594-03
100's	$33.83	Haloperidol, SCS Pharm	00905-0851-34
100's	$36.10	Haloperidol, Mova Pharms	55370-0804-07
100's	$36.15	Haloperidol, TIE Pharm	55496-3003-09
100's	$36.20	Haloperidol, Aligen Independ	00405-4461-01
100's	$36.50	Haloperidol, Rugby	00536-3878-01
100's	$37.00	Haloperidol, Parmed Pharms	00349-8946-01
100's	$37.60	Haloperidol, Qualitest Pharms	00603-3784-21
100's	$37.87	Haloperidol, HL Moore Drug Exch	00839-7348-06
100's	$37.95	Haloperidol, Goldline Labs	00182-1264-01
100's	$38.65	Haloperidol, Par Pharm	49884-0225-01
100's	$38.86	Haloperidol, Geneva Pharms	00781-1393-01
100's	$39.95	Haloperidol, Mylan	00378-0214-01
100's	$47.75	Haloperidol, Vangard Labs	00615-2596-13
100's	$53.80	Haloperidol, Geneva Pharms	00781-1393-13
100's	$56.80	Haloperidol, Major Pharms	00904-1832-61
100's	**$80.82**	**HALDOL, McNeil Lab**	**00045-0242-10**
100's	**$84.19**	**HALDOL, McNeil Lab**	**00045-0242-60**
100's	$223.40	Haloperidol, Medirex	57480-0378-06
500's	$10.15	Haloperidol, H.C.F.A. F F P	99999-1418-10
500's	$62.70	Haloperidol, Rugby	00536-3878-05
500's	$136.85	Haloperidol, Purepac Pharm	00228-2281-50
500's	$190.00	Haloperidol, Aligen Independ	00405-4461-02
500's	$193.15	Haloperidol, Par Pharm	49884-0225-05
1000's	$20.30	Haloperidol, H.C.F.A. F F P	99999-1418-11
1000's	$72.50	Haloperidol, Consolidated Midland	00223-1022-02
1000's	$179.25	Haloperidol, Major Pharms	00904-1832-80
1000's	$267.15	Haloperidol, Roxane	00054-4344-31
1000's	$301.39	Haloperidol, SCS Pharm	00905-0851-52
1000's	$332.00	Haloperidol, Harber Pharm	51432-0594-06
1000's	$365.75	Haloperidol, Qualitest Pharms	00603-3784-32
1000's	$367.61	Haloperidol, HL Moore Drug Exch	00839-7348-16
1000's	$374.68	Haloperidol, Par Pharm	49884-0225-10
1000's	$374.99	Haloperidol, Geneva Pharms	00781-1393-10
1000's	$377.95	Haloperidol, Mylan	00378-0214-10
1000's	**$686.24**	**HALDOL, McNeil Lab**	**00045-0242-80**

Tablet, Uncoated - Oral - 5 mg

100's	$2.93	Haloperidol, United Res	00677-1118-01
100's	$2.93	Haloperidol, H.C.F.A. F F P	99999-1418-12
100's	$16.00	Haloperidol, Consolidated Midland	00223-1023-01
100's	$23.00	Haloperidol, Raway	00686-2597-13
100's	$38.95	Haloperidol, Major Pharms	00904-1833-60
100's	$39.84	Haloperidol, Purepac Pharm	00228-2282-10
100's	$41.23	HALOPRIDOL, Roxane	00054-8345-25
100's	$44.15	Haloperidol, Medirex	57480-0379-01
100's	$45.96	Haloperidol, Roxane	00054-4345-25
100's	$45.97	Haloperidol, Schein Pharm (US)	00364-2207-01
100's	$47.75	Haloperidol, Rugby	00536-3879-01
100's	$51.80	Haloperidol, SCS Pharm	00905-0861-31
100's	$53.93	Haloperidol, SCS Pharm	00905-0861-34
100's	$54.25	Haloperidol, Harber Pharm	51432-0595-03
100's	$57.73	Haloperidol, TIE Pharm	55496-3004-09
100's	$59.00	Haloperidol, Qualitest Pharms	00603-3785-21
100's	$59.02	Haloperidol, Aligen Independ	00405-4462-01
100's	$59.02	Haloperidol, Mova Pharms	55370-0805-07
100's	$59.50	Haloperidol, Parmed Pharms	00349-8947-01
100's	$61.97	Haloperidol, HL Moore Drug Exch	00839-7349-06
100's	$63.15	Haloperidol, Par Pharm	49884-0226-01
100's	$64.85	Haloperidol, Goldline Labs	00182-1265-01
100's	$66.09	Haloperidol, Geneva Pharms	00781-1396-01
100's	$66.95	Haloperidol, Mylan	00378-0327-01
100's	$80.41	Haloperidol, Vangard Labs	00615-2597-13
100's	$86.09	Haloperidol, Geneva Pharms	00781-1396-13
100's	$95.29	Haloperidol, Major Pharms	00904-1833-61
100's	**$129.36**	**HALDOL, McNeil Lab**	**00045-0245-10**
100's	**$137.60**	**HALDOL, McNeil Lab**	**00045-0245-60**
500's	$14.65	Haloperidol, H.C.F.A. F F P	99999-1418-13
500's	$82.28	Haloperidol, Rugby	00536-3879-05
500's	$118.65	Haloperidol, Major Pharms	00904-1833-40
500's	$194.95	Haloperidol, Goldline Labs	00182-1265-05
500's	$199.20	Haloperidol, Purepac Pharm	00228-2282-50
500's	$265.40	Haloperidol, Qualitest Pharms	00603-3785-28
500's	$301.12	Haloperidol, Aligen Independ	00405-4462-02
500's	$315.75	Haloperidol, Par Pharm	49884-0226-05
600's	$353.40	Haloperidol, Medirex	57480-0379-06
1000's	$29.30	Haloperidol, H.C.F.A. F F P	99999-1418-14
1000's	$99.50	Haloperidol, Consolidated Midland	00223-1023-02
1000's	$438.36	Haloperidol, Roxane	00054-4345-31
1000's	$494.46	Haloperidol, SCS Pharm	00905-0861-52
1000's	$542.50	Haloperidol, Harber Pharm	51432-0595-06
1000's	$619.65	Haloperidol, HL Moore Drug Exch	00839-7349-16
1000's	$631.52	Haloperidol, Par Pharm	49884-0226-10
1000's	$633.95	Haloperidol, Mylan	00378-0327-10
1000's	**$1125.87**	**HALDOL, McNeil Lab**	**00045-0245-80**

Tablet, Uncoated - Oral - 10 mg

100's	$4.05	Haloperidol, United Res	00677-1203-01
100's	$4.05	Haloperidol, H.C.F.A. F F P	99999-1418-15
100's	$22.50	Haloperidol, Consolidated Midland	00223-1024-01
100's	$22.82	Haloperidol, Schein Pharm (US)	00364-2236-01
100's	$42.67	Haloperidol, Purepac Pharm	00228-2286-10
100's	$46.40	Haloperidol, Major Pharms	00904-1734-60
100's	$62.55	Haloperidol, Roxane	00054-8346-25
100's	$62.75	Haloperidol, Rugby	00536-3880-01
100's	$64.20	Haloperidol, Parmed Pharms	00349-8948-01
100's	$65.00	Haloperidol, Roxane	00054-4346-25
100's	$65.00	Haloperidol, Mova Pharms	55370-0806-07
100's	$65.63	Haloperidol 10, Aligen Independ	00405-4463-01
100's	$65.70	Haloperidol, Qualitest Pharms	00603-3786-21
100's	$66.71	Haloperidol, Searle	00014-0871-31
100's	$68.24	Haloperidol, HL Moore Drug Exch	00839-7398-06
100's	$68.84	Haloperidol, Searle	00014-0871-34
100's	$69.55	Haloperidol, Goldline Labs	00182-1854-01
100's	$69.55	Haloperidol, Geneva Pharms	00781-1397-01
100's	$69.55	Haloperidol, Par Pharm	49884-0227-01
100's	$98.98	Haloperidol, Geneva Pharms	00781-1397-13
100's	$101.25	Haloperidol, Major Pharms	00904-1834-61
100's	$119.17	Haloperidol, Major Pharms	00904-1734-61

HOW SUPPLIED - RATED THERAPEUTICALLY EQUIVALENT: *(cont'd)*

100's	**$155.94**	**HALDOL, McNeil Lab**	**00045-0246-10**
100's	**$176.53**	**HALDOL, McNeil Lab**	**00045-0246-60**
500's	$20.25	Haloperidol, H.C.F.A. F F P	99999-1418-16
500's	$165.00	Haloperidol, Major Pharms	00904-1734-40
500's	$195.10	Haloperidol, Rugby	00536-3880-05
500's	$202.43	Haloperidol, HL Moore Drug Exch	00839-7398-12
500's	$213.35	Haloperidol, Purepac Pharm	00228-2286-50
500's	$318.65	Haloperidol, Qualitest Pharms	00603-3786-28
500's	$347.75	Haloperidol, Goldline Labs	00182-1854-05
500's	$347.75	Haloperidol, Par Pharm	49884-0227-05
1000's	$40.50	Haloperidol, H.C.F.A. F F P	99999-1418-17
1000's	$175.00	Haloperidol, Consolidated Midland	00223-1024-02
1000's	$202.43	Haloperidol, HL Moore Drug Exch	00839-7398-16
1000's	$639.07	Haloperidol, Searle	00014-0871-52
1000's	$650.00	Haloperidol, Roxane	00054-4346-31
1000's	**$1455.16**	**HALDOL, McNeil Lab**	**00045-0246-80**

Tablet, Uncoated - Oral - 20 mg

100's	$12.00	Haloperidol, H.C.F.A. F F P	99999-1418-18
100's	$45.00	Haloperidol, Schein Pharm (US)	00364-2237-01
100's	$47.00	Haloperidol, Squibb-Mark	57783-6830-01
100's	$55.00	Haloperidol 20, Aligen Independ	00405-4464-01
100's	$63.50	Haloperidol, Major Pharms	00904-1735-60
100's	$63.52	Haloperidol, Purepac Pharm	00228-2287-10
100's	$67.73	Haloperidol, Parmed Pharms	00349-8953-01
100's	$112.49	Haloperidol, Geneva Pharms	00781-1398-01
100's	$112.50	Haloperidol, Roxane	00054-8347-25
100's	$115.57	Haloperidol, Roxane	00054-4347-25
100's	$129.50	Haloperidol, Harber Pharm	51432-0597-03
100's	$130.15	Haloperidol, Searle	00014-0881-34
100's	**$338.66**	**HALDOL, McNeil Lab**	**00045-0248-60**
500's	$60.00	Haloperidol, H.C.F.A. F F P	99999-1418-19
500's	$206.40	Haloperidol, Major Pharms	00904-1735-40
500's	$265.60	Haloperidol, Rugby	00536-3881-05
500's	$317.60	Haloperidol, Purepac Pharm	00228-2287-50

HALOPERIDOL DECANOATE *(001419)*

CATEGORIES: Antipsychotics/Antimanics; Central Nervous System Agents; Neuroleptics; Psychotherapeutic Agents; Psychotic Disorders; Tourette Syndrome; Tranquilizers; Vertigo/Motion Sickness/Vomiting; Pregnancy Category C; FDA Approved 1986 Jan

BRAND NAMES: *Aloperidin*; *Haldol*; *Haldol Decanoas*; *Haldol Decanoas* (France, Mexico); *Haldol Decanoat* (Germany); *Haldol Decanoaat*; **Haldol Decanoate**; *Halidol Decanoas*; *Haridol Decanoate*; *Pericate*; *Serenase*; *Serenase Dekanoat* *(International brand names outside U.S. in italics)*

DESCRIPTION:

Haloperidol decanoate is the decanoate ester of the butyrophenone, haloperidol. It has a markedly extended duration of effect. It is available in sesame oil in sterile form for intramuscular (IM) injection. Haloperidol decanoate, 4-(4-chlorophenyl)-1[4-(4-fluoro-phenyl)-4-oxobutyl]-4 piperidinyl decanoate.

Haloperidol decanoate is almost insoluble in water (0.01 mg/ml), but is soluble in most organic solvents.

Each ml of haloperidol decanoate 50 for IM injection contains 50 mg haloperidol (present as haloperidol decanoate 70.52 mg) in a sesame oil vehicle, with 1.2% (w/v) benzyl alcohol as a preservative.

Each ml of haloperidol decanoate 100 for IM injection contains 100 mg haloperidol (present as haloperidol decanoate 141.04 mg) in a sesame oil vehicle, with 1.2% (w/v) benzyl alcohol as a preservative.

CLINICAL PHARMACOLOGY:

Haloperidol decanoate is the long-acting form of haloperidol. The basic effects of haloperidol decanoate are no different from those of haloperidol with the exception of duration of action. Haloperidol blocks the effects of dopamine and increases its turnover rate; however, the precise mechanism of action is unknown.

Administration of haloperidol decanoate in sesame oil results in slow and sustained release of haloperidol. The plasma concentrations of haloperidol gradually rise, reaching a peak at about 6 days after the injection, and falling thereafter, with an apparent half-life of about 3 weeks. Steady state plasma concentrations are achieved after the third or fourth dose. The relationship between dose of haloperidol decanoate and plasma haloperidol concentration is roughly linear for doses below 450 mg. It should be noted, however, that pharmacokinetics of haloperidol decanoate following intramuscular injections can be quite variable between subjects.

INDICATIONS AND USAGE:

Haloperidol decanoate is a long-acting parenteral antipsychotic drug intended for use in the management of patients requiring prolonged parenteral antipsychotic therapy (*e.g.,* patients with chronic schizophrenia).

CONTRAINDICATIONS:

Since the pharmacologic and clinical actions of haloperidol decanoate is attributed to haloperidol as the active medication, CONTRAINDICATIONS, WARNINGS, and additional information are those of haloperidol, modified only to reflect the prolonged action.

Haloperidol is contraindicated in severe toxic central nervous system depression or comatose states from any cause and in individuals who are hypersensitive to this drug or have Parkinson's disease.

WARNINGS:

Tardive Dyskinesia: A syndrome consisting of potentially, irreversible, involuntary, dyskinetic movements may develop in patients treated with antipsychotic drugs. Although the prevalence of the syndrome appears to be highest among the elderly, especially elderly women, it is impossible to rely upon prevalence estimates to predict, at the inception of antipsychotic treatment, which patients are likely to develop the syndrome. Whether antipsychotic drug products differ in their potential to cause tardive dyskinesia is unknown.

Both the risk of developing tardive dyskinesia and the likelihood that it will become irreversible are believed to increase as the duration of treatment, and the total cumulative dose of antipsychotic drugs administered to the patient increase. However, the syndrome can develop, although much less commonly, after relatively brief treatment periods at low doses.

WARNINGS: *(cont'd)*

There is no known treatment for established cases of tardive dyskinesia, although the syndrome may remit, partially or completely, if antipsychotic treatment is withdrawn. Antipsychotic treatment, itself, however, may suppress (or partially suppress) the signs and symptoms of the syndrome and thereby may possibly mask the underlying process. The effect that symptomatic suppression has upon the long-term course of the syndrome is unknown.

Given these considerations, antipsychotic drugs should be prescribed in a manner that is most likely to minimize the occurrence of tardive dyskinesia. Chronic antipsychotic treatment should generally be reserved for patients who suffer from a chronic illness that 1) is known to respond to antipsychotic drugs, and 2) for whom alternative, equally effective, but potentially less harmful treatments are **not** available or appropriate. In patients who do not require chronic treatment, the smallest dose and the shortest duration of treatment producing a satisfactory clinical response should be sought. The need for continued treatment should be reassessed periodically.

If signs and symptoms of tardive dyskinesia appear in a patient on antipsychotics, drug discontinuation should be considered.

However, some patients may require treatment despite the presence of the syndrome. (For further information about description of tardive dyskinesia and its clinical detection, please refer to ADVERSE REACTIONS.)

Neuroleptic Malignant Syndrome (NMS): A potentially fatal symptom complex sometimes referred to as Neuroleptic Malignant Syndrome (NMS) has been reported in association with antipsychotic drugs. Clinical manifestations of NMS are hyperpyrexia, muscle rigidity, altered mental status (including catatonic signs) and evidence of autonomic instability (irregular pulse or blood pressure, tachycardia, diaphoresis, and cardiac dysrhythmias). Additional signs may include elevated creatine phosphokinase, myoglobinuria (rhabdomyolysis) and acute renal failure.

The diagnostic evaluation of patients with this syndrome is complicated. In arriving at a diagnosis, it is important to identify cases where the clinical presentation includes both serious medical illness (*e.g.,* pneumonia, systemic infection, etc.) and untreated or inadequately treated extrapyramidal signs and symptoms (EPS). Other important consideration in the differential diagnosis include central anticholinergic toxicity, heat stroke, drug fever and primary central nervous system (CNS) pathology.

The management of NMS should include 1) immediate discontinuation of antipsychotic drugs and other drugs not essential to concurrent therapy, 2) intensive symptomatic treatment and medical monitoring, and 3) treatment of any concomitant serious medical problems for which specific treatments are available. there is no general agreement about specific pharmacological treatment regimens for uncomplicated NMS.

If a patient requires antipsychotic drug treatment after recovery from NMS, the potential reintroduction of drug therapy should be carefully considered. The patient should be carefully monitored, since recurrences of NMS have been reported.

Hyperpyrexia and heat stroke, not associated with the above symptom complex, have also been reported with haloperidol.

General: A number of cases of bronchopneumonia, some fatal, have followed the use of antipsychotic drugs, including haloperidol. It has been postponed that lethargy and decreased sensation of thirst due to central inhibition may lead to dehydration, hemoconcentration and reduced pulmonary ventilation. Therefore, if the above signs and symptoms appear, especially in the elderly, the physician should institute remedial therapy promptly.

Although not reported with haloperidol, decreased serum cholesterol and/or cutaneous and ocular changes have been reported in patients receiving chemically-related drugs.

PRECAUTIONS:

Haloperidol decanoate 40 and haloperidol decanoate 100 should be administered cautiously to patients:

with severe cardiovascular disorders, because of the possibility of transient hypotension and/or precipitation of anginal pain.

receiving anticonvulsant medications, with a history of seizures, or with EEG abnormalities, because haloperidol may lower the convulsive threshold. If indicated, adequate anticonvulsant therapy should be concomitantly maintained.

with known allergies, or with a history of allergic reactions to drugs.

receiving anticoagulants, since an isolated instance of interference occurred with the effects of one anticoagulant (phenindione).

Should hypotension occur and a vasopressor be required, epinephrine should not be used since haloperidol may block its vasopressor activity, and paradoxical further lowering of the blood pressure may occur. Instead, metaraminol, phenylephrine or norepinephrine should be used.

If concomitant antiparkinson medication is required, it may have to be continued after haloperidol decanoate is discontinued because of the prolonged action of haloperidol decanoate. If both drugs are discontinued simultaneously, extrapyramidal symptoms may occur. The physician should keep in mind the possible increase in intraocular pressure when anticholinergic drugs, including antiparkinson agents, are administered concomitantly with haloperidol decanoate.

In patients with thyrotoxicosis who are also receiving antipsychotic medication, including haloperidol decanoate, severe neurotoxicity (rigidity, inability to walk or talk) may occur.

When haloperidol is used to control mania in bipolar disorders, there may be a rapid mood swing to depression.

Information for the Patient: Haloperidol decanoate may impair the mental or physical abilities required for the performance of hazardous tasks such as operating machinery or driving a motor vehicle. The ambulatory patient should be warned accordingly.

The use of alcohol with this drug should be avoided due to possible additive effects and hypotension.

Carcinogenesis, Mutagenesis, and Impairment of Fertility: No mutagenic potential of haloperidol decanoate was found in the Ames Salmonella microsomal activation assay. Negative or inconsistent positive findings have been obtained *in vitro* and *in vivo* studies of effects of short-acting haloperidol on chromosome structure and number. The available cytogenic evidence is considered too inconsistent to be conclusive at this time.

Carcinogenicity studies using oral haloperidol were conducted in Wistar rats (dosed at up to 5 mg/kg daily for 24 months) and in Albino Swiss mice (dosed at up to 5 mg/kg daily for 18 months). In the rat study survival was less than optimal in all dose groups, reducing the number of rats at risk for developing tumors. However, although a relatively greater number of rats survived to the end of the study in high dose male and female groups, these animals did not have a greater incidence of tumors than control animals. Therefore, although not optimal, this study does suggest the absence of a haloperidol related increase in the incidence of neoplasia in rats at doses up to 20 times the usual daily human dose for chronic or resistant patients.

PRECAUTIONS: *(cont'd)*

In female mice at 5 and 20 times the highest initial daily dose for chronic or resistant patients, there was a statistically significant increase in mammary gland neoplasia and total tumor incidence; at 20 times the same daily dose there was a statistically significant increase in pituitary gland neoplasia. In male mice, no statistically significant difference in incidences of total tumors or specific tumor types were noted.

Antipsychotic drugs elevate prolactin levels; the elevation persists during chronic administration. Tissue culture experiments indicated that approximately one-third of human breast cancers are prolactin dependent*in vitro*, a factor of potential importance if the prescription of these drugs is contemplated in a patient with a previously detected breast cancer. Although disturbances such as galactorrhea, amenorrhea, gynecomastia, and impotence have been reported, the clinical significance of elevated serum prolactin levels is unknown for most patients.

An increase in mammary neoplasms has been found in rodents after chronic administration of antipsychotic drugs. Neither clinical studies nor epidemiologic studies conducted to date, however, have shown an association between chronic administration of these drugs and mammary tumorigenesis; the available evidence is considered too limited to be conclusive at this time.

Pregnancy Category C: Rodents given up to 3 times the usual maximum human dose of haloperidol decanoate showed an increase in incidence of resorption, fetal mortality, and pup mortality. No fetal abnormalities were observed.

Cleft palate has been observed in mice given oral haloperidol at 15 times the usual maximum human dose. Cleft palate in mice appears to be a non-specific response to stress or nutritional imbalance as well as to a variety of drugs, and there is no evidence to relate this phenomenon to predictable human risk for most of these agents.

There are no adequate and well-controlled studies in pregnant women. There are reports, however, of cases of limb malformations observed following maternal use of haloperidol along with other drugs which have suspected teratogenic potential during the first trimester of pregnancy. Casual relationships were not established with these cases. Since such experience does not exclude the possibility of fetal damage due to haloperidol, haloperidol decanoate should be used during pregnancy or in women likely to become pregnant only if the benefit clearly justifies a potential risk to the fetus.

Nursing Mothers: Since haloperidol is excreted in human breast milk, infants should not be nursed during drug treatment with haloperidol decanoate.

Pediatric Use: Safety and effectiveness of haloperidol decanoate in children have not been established.

DRUG INTERACTIONS:

An encephalopathic syndrome (characterized by weakness, lethargy, fever, tremulousness and confusion, extrapyramidal symptoms leukocytosis, elevated serum enzymes, BUN, and FBS) followed by irreversible brain damage has occurred in a few patients treated with lithium plus haloperidol. A casual relationship between these events and the concomitant administration of lithium and haloperidol has not been established; however, patients receiving such combined therapy should be monitored closely for early evidence of neurological toxicity and treatment discontinued promptly if such signs appear.

As with other antipsychotic agents, it should be noted that haloperidol may be capable of potentiating CNS depressants such as anesthetics, opiates, and alcohol.

ADVERSE REACTIONS:

Adverse reactions following the administration of haloperidol decanoate are those of haloperidol. Since vast experience has accumulated with haloperidol, the adverse reactions are reported for that compound as well as for haloperidol decanoate. As with all injectable medications, local tissue reactions have been reported with haloperidol decanoate.

CNS EFFECTS

Extrapyramidal Symptoms (EPS): EPS during the administration of haloperidol have been reported frequently, often during the first few days of treatment. EPS can be categorized generally as Parkinson-like symptoms, akathisia, or dystonia (including opisthotonos and oculogyric crisis). While all can occur at relatively low doses, they occur more frequently and with greater severity at higher doses. The symptoms may be controlled with dose reductions or administration of antiparkinson drugs such as benztropine mesylate USP or trihexyphenidyl hydrochloride USP. It should be noted that persistent EPS have been reported; the drug may have to be discontinued in such cases.

Withdrawal Emergent Neurological Signs: Generally, patients receiving short term memory therapy experience no problems with abrupt discontinuation of antipsychotic drugs. However, some patients on maintenance treatment experience transient dyskinetic signs after abrupt withdrawal. In certain of these cases the dyskinetic movements are indistinguishable from the syndrome described below under, "Tardive Dyskinesia" except for duration. Although the long acting properties of haloperidol decanoate provide gradual withdrawal, it is not known Whether gradual withdrawal of antipsychotic drugs will reduce the rate of occurrence of withdrawal emergent neurological signs.

Tardive Dyskinesia: As with all antipsychotic agents haloperidol has been associated with persistent dyskinesias. Tardive dyskinesia, a syndrome consisting of potentially irreversible, involuntary, dyskinetic movements, may appear in some patients on long-term therapy with haloperidol decanoate or may occur after drug therapy has been discontinued. The risk appears to be greater in elderly patients on high-dose therapy, especially females. The symptoms are persistent and in some patients appear irreversible. The syndrome is characterized by rhythmical involuntary movements of tongue, face, mouth, or jaw (*e.g.,* protrusion of tongue, puffing of cheeks, puckering of mouth, chewing movements). Sometimes these may be accompanied by involuntary movements of extremities and the trunk.

There is no known effective treatment for tardive dyskinesia; antiparkinson agents usually do not alleviate the symptoms of this syndrome. It is suggested that all antipsychotic agents be discontinued if these symptoms appear. Should it be necessary to reinstitute treatment, or increase the dosage of the agent, or switch to a different antipsychotic agent, this syndrome maybe masked.

It has been reported that since vermicular movement of the tongue may be an early sign of tardive dyskinesia and if the medication is stopped at that time the full syndrome may not develop.

Tardive Dystonia: Tardive dystonia, not associated with the above syndrome, has also been reported. Tardive dystonia is characterized by delayed onset of choreic or dystonic movements is often persistent, and has the potential of becoming irreversible.

Other CNS Effects: Insomnia, restlessness, anxiety, euphoria, agitation, drowsiness, depression, lethargy, headache, confusion, vertigo, grand mal seizures, exacerbation of psychotic symptoms including hallucinations and catatonic-like behavioral states which may be response to drug withdrawal and/or treatment with anticholinergic drugs.

Body as a Whole: Neuroleptic malignant syndrome (NMS), hyperpyrexia and heat stroke have been reported with haloperidol. (See WARNINGS for further information concerning NMS.)

ADVERSE REACTIONS: *(cont'd)*

Cardiovascular Effects: Tachycardia, hypotension, hypertension and ECG changes including prolongation of the Q-T interval and ECG pattern changes compatible with the polymorphous configuration of torsades de pointes.

Hematologic Effects: Reports have appeared citing the occurrence of mild and usually transient leukopenia and leukocytosis, minimal decreases in red blood cell counts, anemia, or a tendency toward lymphomonocytosis. Agranulocytosis has rarely been reported to have occurred with the use of haloperidol, and then only in association with other medication.

Liver Effects: Impaired liver function and/or jaundice have been reported.

Dermatologic Reactions: Maculopapular and acneiform skin reactions isolated cases of photosensitivity and loss of hair.

Endocrine Disorders: Lactation, breast engorgement, mastalgia, menstrual irregularities, gynecomastia, impotence, increased libido, hyperglycemia, hypoglycemia and hyponatremia.

Gastrointestinal Effects: Anorexia, constipation, diarrhea, hypersalivation, dyspepsia, nausea and vomiting.

Autonomic Reactions: Dry mouth, blurred vision, urinary retention, diaphoresis and priapism.

Respiratory Effects : Laryngospasm, bronchospasm and increased depth of respiration.

Special Senses: Cataracts, retinopathy and visual disturbances.

Other: Cases of sudden and unexpected death have been reported in association with the administration of haloperidol. The nature of the evidence makes it impossible to determine definitively what role, if any, haloperidol played in the outcome of the reported cases. The possibility that haloperidol caused death, cannot, of course, be excluded, but it is to be kept in mind that sudden and unexpected death may occur in psychotic patients when they go untreated or when they are treated with other antipsychotic drugs.

Postmarketing Events: Hyperammonemia has been reported in a 5 1/2 year old child with citrullinemia, an inherited disorder of ammonia excretion, following treatment with haloperidol.

OVERDOSAGE:

While overdosage is less likely to occur with a parenteral than with an oral medication, information pertaining to haloperidol is presented, modified only to reflect the extended duration of action of haloperidol decanoate.

Manifestations In general, the symptoms of overdosage would be exaggeration of known pharmacologic effects and adverse reactions, the most prominent of which would be: 1) severe extrapyramidal reactions, 2) hypotension, or 3) sedation. The patient would appear comatose with respiratory depression and hypotension which could be severe enough to produce a shock-like state. The extrapyramidal reactions would be manifested by muscular weakness or rigidity and a generalized or localized tremor, as demonstrated by the akinetic or agitans types, respectively. With accidental overdosage, hypertension rather hypotension occurred in a two-year old child. The risk of ECG changes associated with torsades de pointes should be considered. (For further information regarding torsades de pointes, please refer to ADVERSE REACTIONS.)

Treatment: Since there is no specific antidote, treatment is primarily supportive. A patent airway must be established by use be counteracted by artificial respiration and mechanical respirators. Hypotension and circulatory collapse may be counteracted by use of intravenous fluids, plasma, or concentrated albumin, and vasopressor agents such as metaraminol, phenylephrine and norepinephrine. Epinephrine should not be used. In case of severe extrapyramidal reactions, antiparkinson medication should be administered, and should be continued for several weeks, and then withdrawn gradually as extrapyramidal symptoms may emerge. ECG and vital signs should be monitored especially for signs of Q-T prolongation or dysrhythmias and monitoring should continue until the ECG is normal. Severe arrhythmias should be treated with appropriate anti-arrhythmic measures.

DOSAGE AND ADMINISTRATION:

Haloperidol decanoate should be administered by deep intramuscular injection. A 21 gauge needle is recommended. The maximum volume per injection site should not exceed 3 ml. DO NOT ADMINISTER INTRAVENOUSLY.

Parenteral drug products should be inspected visually for particulate matter and discoloration prior to administration, whenever solution and container permit.

Haloperidol decanoate is intended for use in chronic psychotic patients who require prolonged parenteral antipsychotic therapy. These patients should be previously stabilized on antipsychotic medication before considering a conversion to haloperidol decanoate. Furthermore, it is recommended that patients being considered for haloperidol decanoate therapy have been treated with, and tolerate well, short-acting haloperidol in order to reduce the possibility of an unexpected adverse sensitivity to haloperidol. Close clinical supervision is required during the initial period of dose adjustment in order to minimize the risk of overdosage or reappearance of psychotic symptoms before the next injection. During dose adjustment or episodes of exacerbation of psychotic symptoms, haloperidol decanoate therapy can be supplemented with short-acting forms of haloperidol.

The dose of haloperidol decanoate should be expressed in terms of its haloperidol content. The starting dose of haloperidol decanoate should be based on the patient's age, clinical history, physical condition, and response to previous antipsychotic therapy. The preferred approach to determining the minimum effective dose is to begin with lower initial doses and to adjust the dose upward as needed. For patients previously maintained on low doses of antipsychotics (*e.g.,* up to the equivalent of 10 mg/day oral haloperidol), it is recommended that the initial dose of haloperidol decanoate be 10-15 times the previous daily dose in oral haloperidol equivalents, limited clinical experience suggests that lower initial doses may be adequate.

Initial Therapy: Conversion from oral haloperidol decanoate can be achieved by using an initial dose of haloperidol decanoate that is 10 to 20 times the previous daily dose in oral haloperidol equivalents.

In patients who are elderly, debilitated, or stable on low doses of oral haloperidol (*e.g.,* up to the equivalent of 10 mg/day oral haloperidol), a range of 10 to 15 times the previous daily dose in oral haloperidol equivalents is appropriate for initial conversion.

In patients previously maintained on higher doses of antipsychotics for whom a low dose approach risks recurrence of psychiatric decompensation and in patients whose long term use of haloperidol has resulted in a tolerance to the drug, 20 times the previous daily dose in oral haloperidol equivalents should be considered for initial conversion, with downward titration on succeeding injections.

The initial dose of haloperidol decanoate should not exceed 100 mg regardless of previous antipsychotic dose requirements. If, therefore, conversion requires more than 100 mg of haloperidol decanoate as an initial dose, that dose should be administered in two injections, i.e., a maximum of 100 mg initially followed by the balance in 3 to 7 days.

Maintenance Therapy: The maintenance dosage of haloperidol decanoate must be individualized with titration upward or downward based on therapeutic response. The usual maintenance range is 10 to 15 times the previous daily dose in oral haloperidol equivalents dependent on the clinical response of the patient. (TABLE 1)

DOSAGE AND ADMINISTRATION: *(cont'd)*

TABLE 1

Patients	Monthly 1st Month	Maintenance
Stabilized on low daily doses (up to 10 mg/day) Elderly or Debilitated	10-15 x Daily Oral Dose	10-15 x Previous Oral Dose
High Dose Risk of relapse Tolerent to oral haloperidol	20 x Daily Oral Dose	10-15 x Previous Daily Oral Dose

Close clinical supervision is required during initiation and stabilization of haloperidol decanoate therapy.

Haloperidol decanoate is usually administered monthly or every 4 weeks. However, variation in patient response may dictate a need for adjustment of the dosing interval as well as the dose. (See CLINICAL PHARMACOLOGY.)

Clinical experience with haloperidol decanoate at doses greater than 450 mg per month has been limited.

Store at controlled room temperature (15°-30° C, 59°-86° F). Do not refrigerate or freeze. Protect from light.

HOW SUPPLIED - EQUIVALENTS NOT AVAILABLE:

Injection, Solution - Intramuscular - 50 mg/ml

1 ml x 3	$83.84	HALDOL DECANOATE, McNeil Lab	00045-0253-03
1 ml x 10	$279.44	HALDOL DECANOATE, McNeil Lab	00045-0253-01
5 ml	$139.76	HALDOL DECANOATE, McNeil Lab	00045-0253-46

Injection, Solution - Intramuscular - 100 mg/ml

1 ml ampul x 5	$256.36	HALDOL DECANOATE 100, McNeil Lab	00045-0254-14
5 ml	$256.36	HALDOL DECANOATE 100, McNeil Lab	00045-0254-46

HEPARIN LOCK FLUSH *(001427)*

CATEGORIES: Anticoagulants; Anticoagulants/Thrombolytics; Blood Clotting; Blood Formation/Coagulation; Coagulants and Anticoagulants; Pregnancy Category C; FDA Pre 1938 Drugs

BRAND NAMES: Cvc Heparin Flush Kit; Hep Flush; Hep-Lock; Lok-Pak-N

DESCRIPTION:

Heparin Lock Flush Solution, USP, is a sterile preparation of Heparin Sodium Injection, USP, with sufficient sodium chloride to make it isotonic with blood.

Heparin Sodium Injection, USP, is a mixture of substances having the property of prolonging the clotting time of blood, and is usually obtained from the lungs and intestinal mucosa of domestic animals used for food by man. The potency is determined by biological assay using a USP reference standard based upon units of heparin activity per milligram.

Carpuject Sterile Cartridge-Needle Unit contains a sterile solution of Heparin Lock Flush Solution, USP. Each ml contains either 10 or 100 USP heparin units of heparin sodium derived from porcine intestinal mucosa in Water for Injection, benzyl alcohol 1%, and sufficient sodium chloride to render the solution isotonic. The pH is adjusted with hydrochloric acid or sodium hydroxide.

HEP-PAK Convenience Package contains two cartridges of Sodium Chloride Injection, USP, 0.9%, and one cartridge of Heparin Lock Flush Solution either 10 USP heparin units/ ml or 100 USP heparin units/ml.

HEP-PAK 2 Convenience Package contains one cartridge of Sodium Chloride Injection, USP, 0.9%, and one cartridge of Heparin Lock Flush Solution either 10 USP heparin units/ ml or 100 USP heparin units/ml.

HEP-PAK CVC Convenience Package contains two cartridges of Sodium Chloride Injection, USP, 0.9%, and one cartridge of Heparin Lock Flush Solution either 10 USP heparin units/ ml or 100 USP heparin units/ml, both in a 2 ml fill.

CLINICAL PHARMACOLOGY:

Heparin inhibits reactions that lead to the clotting of blood and the formation of fibrin clots both in vitro and in vivo. Heparin acts at multiple sites in the normal coagulation system. Small amounts of heparin in combination with antithrombin III (heparin cofactor) can inhibit thrombosis by inactivating activated Factor X and inhibiting the conversion of prothrombin to thrombin. Once active thrombosis has developed, larger amounts of heparin can inhibit further coagulation by inactivating thrombin and preventing the conversion of fibrinogen to fibrin. Heparin also prevents the formation of a stable fibrin clot by inhibiting the activation of the fibrin stabilizing factor.

Bleeding time is usually unaffected by heparin. Clotting time is prolonged by full therapeutic doses of heparin; in most cases, it is not measurably affected by low doses of heparin.

Peak plasma levels of heparin are achieved 2 to 4 hours following subcutaneous administration, although there are considerable individual variations. Loglinear plots of heparin plasma concentrations with time for a wide range of dose levels are linear, which suggest the absence of zero order processes. The liver and the reticulo-endothelial system are the site of biotransformation. The biphasic elimination curve, a rapidly declining alpha phase (t1/2 = 10') and after the age of 40, a slower beta phase, indicates uptake in organs. The absence of a relationship between anticoagulant half-life and concentration half-life may reflect factors such as protein binding of heparin.

Heparin does not have fibrinolytic activity; therefore, it will not lyse existing clots.

INDICATIONS AND USAGE:

Heparin lock flush solution, is intended to maintain patency of an indwelling venipuncture device designed for intermittent injection or infusion therapy, or blood sampling. Heparin lock flush solution, may be used following initial placement of the device in the vein, after each injection of a medication, or after withdrawal of blood for laboratory tests.

Heparin lock flush solution, is not to be used for anticoagulant therapy.

CONTRAINDICATIONS:

Severe thrombocytopenia.

Inability to perform suitable blood coagulation tests, e.g., the whole-blood clotting time, partial thromboplastin time, etc, at appropriate intervals (this contraindication refers to full-dose heparin—there is usually no need to monitor coagulation parameters in patients receiving low-dose heparin).

An uncontrollable active bleeding state (see WARNINGS), except when this is due to disseminated intravascular coagulation.

WARNINGS:

Heparin is not intended for intramuscular use.

Hypersensitivity: Patients with documented hypersensitivity to heparin should be given the drug only in clearly life-threatening situations.

Hemorrhage: Hemorrhage can occur at virtually any site in patients receiving heparin. An unexplained fall in hematocrit, fall in blood pressure, or any other unexplained symptom should lead to serious consideration of a hemorrhagic event.

Heparin sodium should be used with extreme caution in disease states in which there is increased danger of hemorrhage. Some of the conditions in which increased danger of hemorrhage exists are:

Cardiovascular: Subacute bacterial endocarditis, severe hypertension.

Surgical: During and immediately following (a) spinal tap or spinal anesthesia or (b) major surgery, especially involving the brain, spinal cord, or eye.

Hematologic: Conditions associated with increased bleeding tendencies, such as hemophilia, thrombocytopenia, and some vascular purpuras.

Gastrointestinal: Ulcerative lesions and continuous tube drainage of the stomach or small intestine.

Other: Menstruation, liver disease with impaired hemostasis.

Coagulation Testing: When heparin sodium is administered in therapeutic amounts, its dosage should be regulated by frequent blood coagulation tests. If the coagulation test is unduly prolonged or if hemorrhage occurs, heparin sodium should be discontinued promptly (see OVERDOSAGE.)

Thrombocytopenia: Thrombocytopenia has been reported to occur in patients receiving heparin with a reported incidence of 0% to 30%. Mild thrombocytopenia (count greater than 100,000/mm^3) may remain stable or reverse even if heparin is continued. However, thrombocytopenia of any degree should be monitored closely. If the count falls below 100,000/mm^3 or if recurrent thrombosis develops (see White Clot Syndrome,PRECAUTIONS), the heparin product should be discontinued. If continued heparin therapy is essential, administration of heparin from a different organ source can be reinstituted with caution.

Miscellaneous: This product contains benzyl alcohol as preservative. Benzyl alcohol has been reported to be associated with a fatal "Gasping Syndrome" in premature infants.

PRECAUTIONS:

GENERAL

White Clot Syndrome: It has been reported that patients on heparin may develop new thrombus formation in association with thrombocytopenia resulting from irreversible aggregation of platelets induced by heparin, the so-called "white clot syndrome." The process may lead to severe thromboembolic complications like skin necrosis, gangrene of the extremities that may lead to amputation, myocardial infarction, pulmonary embolism, stroke, and possibly death. Therefore, heparin administration should be promptly discontinued if a patient develops new thrombosis in association with thrombocytopenia.

Heparin Resistance: Increased resistance to heparin is frequently encountered in fever, thrombosis, thrombophlebitis, infections with thrombosing tendencies, myocardial infarction, cancer, and in postsurgical patients.

Increased Risk in Older Women: A higher incidence of bleeding has been reported in women over 60 years of age.

LABORATORY TESTS

Periodic platelet counts, hematocrits, and tests for occult blood in stool are recommended during the entire course of heparin therapy, regardless of the route of administration (see DOSAGE AND ADMINISTRATION.)

DRUG/LABORATORY TEST INTERACTIONS

Hyperaminotransferasemia: Significant elevations of aminotransferase (SGOT (S-AST) and SGPT (S-ALT)) levels have occurred in a high percentage of patients (and healthy subjects) who have received heparin. Since aminotransferase determinations are important in the differential diagnosis of myocardial infarction, liver disease, and pulmonary emboli, rises that might be caused by drugs (like heparin) should be interpreted with caution.

CARCINOGENESIS, MUTAGENESIS, AND IMPAIRMENT OF FERTILITY

No long-term studies in animals have been performed to evaluate the carcinogenic potential of heparin. Also, no reproduction studies in animals have been performed concerning mutagenesis or impairment of fertility.

PREGNANCY CATEGORY C

Teratogenic Effects: Animal reproduction studies have not been conducted with heparin sodium. It is also not known whether heparin sodium can cause fetal harm when administered to a pregnant woman or can affect reproduction capacity. Heparin sodium should be given to a pregnant woman only if clearly needed.

Nonteratogenic Effects: Heparin does not cross the placental barrier.

Nursing Mothers: Heparin is not excreted in human milk.

Pediatric Use: See DOSAGE AND ADMINISTRATION.

DRUG INTERACTIONS:

Oral Anticoagulants: Heparin sodium may prolong the one-stage prothrombin time. Therefore, when heparin sodium is given with dicumarol or warfarin sodium, a period of at least 5 hours after the last intravenous dose or 24 hours after the last subcutaneous dose should elapse before blood is drawn if a valid prothrombin time is to be obtained.

Platelet Inhibitors: Drugs such as acetylsalicylic acid, dextran, phenylbutazone, ibuprofen, indomethacin, dipyridamole, hydroxychloroquine, and others that interfere with platelet-aggregation reactions (the main hemostatic defense of heparinized patients) may induce bleeding and should be used with caution in patients receiving heparin sodium.

Other Interactions: Digitalis, tetracyclines, nicotine, or antihistamines may partially counteract the anticoagulant action of heparin sodium.

ADVERSE REACTIONS:

HEMORRHAGE

Hemorrhage is the chief complication that may result from heparin therapy(see WARNINGS.) An overly prolonged clotting time or minor bleeding during therapy can usually be controlled by withdrawing the drug (see OVERDOSAGE.) It should be appreciated that gastrointestinal or urinary tract bleeding during anticoagulant therapy may indicate the presence of an underlying occult lesion. Bleeding can occur at any site but certain specific hemorrhagic complications may be difficult to detect:

Adrenal hemorrhage, with resultant acute adrenal insufficiency, has occurred during anticoagulant therapy. Therefore, such treatment should be discontinued in patients who develop signs and symptoms of acute adrenal hemorrhage and insufficiency. Initiation of corrective therapy should not depend on laboratory confirmation of the diagnosis, since any delay in an acute situation may result in the patient's death.

ADVERSE REACTIONS: *(cont'd)*

Ovarian (corpus luteum) hemorrhage developed in a number of women of reproductive age receiving short- or long-term anticoagulant therapy. This complication if unrecognized may be fatal.

Retroperitoneal hemorrhage.

LOCAL IRRITATION

Local irritation, erythema, mild pain, hematoma, or ulceration may follow deep subcutaneous (intrafat) injection or heparin sodium. These complications are much more common after intramuscular use, and such use is not recommended.

HYPERSENSITIVITY

Generalized hypersensitivity reactions have been reported, with chills, fever, and urticaria as the most usual manifestations, and asthma, rhinitis, lacrimation, headache, nausea and vomiting, and anaphylactoid reactions, including shock, occurring more rarely. Itching and burning, especially on the plantar site of the feet may occur.

Thrombocytopenia has been reported to occur in patients receiving heparin with a reported incidence of 0% to 30%. While often mild and of no obvious clinical significance, such thrombocytopenia can be accompanied by severe thromboembolic complications such as skin necrosis, gangrene of the extremities that may lead to amputation, myocardial infarction, pulmonary embolism, stroke, and possibly death. (See WARNINGS, PRECAUTIONS.)

Certain episodes of painful, ischemic, and cyanosed limbs have in the past been attributed to allergic vasospastic reactions. Whether these are in fact identical to the thrombocytopenia-associated complications remains to be determined.

OTHER

Osteoporosis following long-term administration of high doses of heparin, cutaneous necrosis after systemic administration, suppression of aldosterone synthesis, delayed transient alopecia, priapism, and rebound hyperlipemia on discontinuation of heparin sodium have also been reported.

Significant elevations of aminotransferase (SGOT (S-AST) and SGPT (S-ALT)) levels have occurred in a high percentage of patients (and healthy subjects) who have received heparin.

OVERDOSAGE:

Symptoms: Bleeding is the chief sign of heparin overdosage. Nosebleeds, blood in urine, or tarry stools may be noted as the first sign of bleeding. Easy bruising or petechial formations may precede frank bleeding.

Treatment: Neutralization of heparin effect.

When clinical circumstances (bleeding) require reversal of heparinization, protamine sulfate (1% solution) by slow infusion will neutralize heparin sodium. No more than 50 mg should be administered, very slowly, in any 10 minute period. Each mg of protamine sulfate neutralizes approximately 100 USP heparin units. The amount of protamine required decreases over time as heparin is metabolized. Although the metabolism of heparin is complex, it may, for the purpose of choosing a protamine dose, be assumed to have a half-life of about 30 minutes after intravenous injection.

Administration of protamine sulfate can cause severe hypotensive and anaphylactoid reactions. Because fatal reactions often resembling anaphylaxis have been reported, the drug should be given only when resuscitation techniques and treatment of anaphylactoid shock are readily available.

For additional information, the labeling of Protamine Sulfate Injection, USP, products should be consulted.

DOSAGE AND ADMINISTRATION:

HEP-PAK Convenience Package and HEP-PAK CVC Convenience Package should be utilized for "SASH" Procedures (*i.e.,* Sodium Chloride Injection, Administration of medication or the aspiration of a blood sample, Sodium Chloride Injection, Heparin Lock Flush Solution).

HEP-PAK 2 Convenience Package should be utilized whenever a two-step procedure to maintain venous patency is required, using one cartridge of Sodium Chloride Injection, and one cartridge of Heparin Lock Flush Solution. The two-step procedure consists of flushing the set with one cartridge of Sodium Chloride Injection, USP, 0.9% followed by injecting Heparin Lock Flush Solution into the device in sufficient quantity (usually 1 ml) to fill the set. This procedure is used only when the administration of medication or the aspiration of a blood sample is not required.

CLEARING INTERMITTENT INFUSION (HEPARIN LOCK) SETS

To prevent clot formation in a heparin lock set following its proper insertion, dilute heparin solution (heparin lock flush solution) is injected via the injection hub in a quantity sufficient to fill the entire set to the needle tip. This solution should be replaced each time the heparin lock is used. Aspirate before administering any solution via the lock in order to confirm patency and location of needle or catheter tip. If the medication to be administered is incompatible with heparin, the entire heparin lock set should be flushed with sterile water or normal saline before and after the medication is administered; following the second flush, the dilute heparin solution may be reinstilled into the set. The set manufacturer's instructions should be consulted for specifics concerning the heparin lock set in use at a given time.

Note: Since repeated injections of small doses of heparin can alter tests for activated partial thromboplastin time (APTT), a baseline value for APTT should be obtained prior to insertion of a heparin lock set.

Usually this dilute heparin solution will maintain anticoagulation within the device for up to 4 hours.

WITHDRAWAL OF BLOOD SAMPLES

Heparin lock flush solution, may also be used after each withdrawal of blood for laboratory tests. When heparin (or sodium chloride) would interfere with or alter the results of blood tests, the heparin solution should be cleared from the device by aspirating and discarding it before withdrawing the blood sample.

PARENTERAL DRUG PRODUCTS SHOULD BE INSPECTED VISUALLY FOR PARTICULATE MATTER AND DISCOLORATION PRIOR TO ADMINISTRATION, WHENEVER SOLUTION AND CONTAINER PERMIT.

Discard unused portion after initial use.

Keep at room temperature. Do not freeze.

HOW SUPPLIED - RATED THERAPEUTICALLY EQUIVALENT:

Injection, Solution - Intravenous - 10 unit/ml

1 ml	$4.04	Heparin Lock Flush, Abbott	00074-4822-01
1 ml	$13.13	Heparin Lock Flush, Solopak Labs	39769-0018-01
1 ml x 25	$10.23	HEP-LOCK, Elkins Sinn	00641-0392-25
1 ml x 25	$11.63	HEP-LOCK U/P, Elkins Sinn	00641-0414-25
1 ml x 50	$35.94	HEP-LOCK 10 UNT/ML, Elkins Sinn	00641-3260-09
1 ml x 50	$37.49	Heparin Lock Flush 1Ml/2Ml, Sanofi Winthrop	00024-0721-12
1 ml x 50	$53.25	Heparin Lock Flush, Wyeth Labs	00008-0523-50
1 ml x 50	$62.35	Heparin Lock Flush, Sanofi Winthrop	00024-0721-16
1 ml x 120	$181.50	Heparin Lock Flush, Solopak Mdcl	59747-0106-71

HOW SUPPLIED - RATED THERAPEUTICALLY EQUIVALENT: *(cont'd)*

1 ml x 120	$181.50	Heparin Flush, Solopak Mdcl	59747-0106-81
2 ml	$15.00	Heparin Lock Flush, Solopak Labs	39769-0018-02
2 ml x 25	$11.80	HEP-LOCK, Elkins Sinn	00641-0393-25
2 ml x 50	$48.82	Heparin Lock Flush 2Ml/2Ml, Sanofi Winthrop	00024-0721-13
2 ml x 50	$62.35	Heparin Lock Flush, Sanofi Winthrop	00024-0721-17
2.5 ml x 50	$73.24	Heparin Lock Flush, Wyeth Labs	00008-0523-51
3 ml x 25	$27.53	Heparin Lock Flush, Sanofi Winthrop	00024-0721-14
3 ml x 25	$40.15	Heparin Lock Flush, Sanofi Winthrop	00024-0721-32
3 ml x 120	$264.00	Heparin Lock Flush, Solopak Mdcl	59747-0106-73
3 ml x 120	$264.00	Heparin Flush, Solopak Mdcl	59747-0106-83
5 ml	$18.13	Heparin Lock Flush, Solopak Labs	39769-0018-05
5 ml x 25	$32.88	Heparin Lock Flush, Sanofi Winthrop	00024-0721-15
5 ml x 25	$50.09	Heparin Lock Flush, Sanofi Winthrop	00024-0721-34
5 ml x 120	$304.50	Heparin Lock Flush, Solopak Mdcl	59747-0106-75
5 ml x 120	$304.50	Heparin Flush, Solopak Mdcl	59747-0106-85
10 ml	$1.06	Heparin Lock Flush, Abbott	00074-1151-71
10 ml	$1.26	Heparin Lock, Abbott	00074-1151-70
10 ml	$40.31	Heparin Lock Flush, Solopak Labs	39769-0035-10
10 ml	$92.19	HEPFLUSH-10, Fujisawa USA	00469-1700-30
10 ml x 25	$16.85	HEP-LOCK, Elkins Sinn	00641-2438-45
30 ml	$2.46	Heparin Lock Flush, Abbott	00074-1151-73
30 ml	$2.92	Heparin Lock, Abbott	00074-1151-78
30 ml	$47.49	Heparin Lock Flush, Solopak Labs	39769-0035-30
30 ml x 25	$33.00	Heparin Lock Flush, Voluntary Hosp	53258-3030-02
30 ml x 25	$43.03	HEP-LOCK, Elkins Sinn	00641-2442-45

Injection, Solution - Intravenous - 100 unit/ml

1 ml	$13.13	Heparin Lock Flush, Solopak Labs	39769-0011-01
1 ml x 25	$6.50	Heparin Lock Flush, Voluntary Hosp	53258-3101-01
1 ml x 25	$10.23	HEP-LOCK, Elkins Sinn	00641-0389-25
1 ml x 25	$11.63	HEP-LOCK U/P 100 UNT/ML, Elkins Sinn	00641-0411-25
1 ml x 50	$35.94	HEP-LOCK, Elkins Sinn	00641-3262-09
1 ml x 50	$37.49	Heparin Lock Flush 1Ml/2Ml, Sanofi Winthrop	00024-0722-12
1 ml x 50	$53.25	Heparin Lock Flush, Wyeth Labs	00008-0487-50
1 ml x 50	$62.35	Heparin Lock Flush, Sanofi Winthrop	00024-0722-16
1 ml x 120	$181.50	Heparin Lock Flush, Solopak Mdcl	59747-0107-71
1 ml x 120	$181.50	Heparin Flush, Solopak Mdcl	59747-0107-81
2 ml	$15.00	Heparin Lock Flush, Solopak Labs	39769-0011-02
2 ml x 25	$11.80	HEP-LOCK, Elkins Sinn	00641-0387-25
2 ml x 50	$48.82	Heparin Lock Flush 2Ml/2Ml, Sanofi Winthrop	00024-0722-13
2 ml x 50	$62.35	Heparin Lock Flush, Sanofi Winthrop	00024-0722-17
2.5 ml x 50	$56.80	HEP-LOCK 250 UNT/2.5 ML, Elkins Sinn	00641-3263-09
2.5 ml x 50	$73.24	Heparin Lock Flush, Wyeth Labs	00008-0487-51
3 ml x 25	$27.53	Heparin Lock Flush, Sanofi Winthrop	00024-0722-14
3 ml x 25	$40.15	Heparin Lock Flush, Sanofi Winthrop	00024-0722-33
3 ml x 120	$264.00	Heparin Lock Flush, Solopak Mdcl	59747-0107-73
3 ml x 120	$264.00	Heparin Flush, Solopak Mdcl	59747-0107-83
5 ml	$18.13	Heparin Lock Flush, Solopak Labs	39769-0011-05
5 ml x 25	$22.19	Heparin Lock Flush, Fujisawa USA	00469-3105-25
5 ml x 25	$50.09	Heparin Lock Flush, Sanofi Winthrop	00024-0722-35
5 ml x 120	$304.50	Heparin Lock Flush, Solopak Mdcl	59747-0107-75
5 ml x 120	$304.50	Heparin Flush, Solopak Mdcl	59747-0107-85
10 ml	$1.21	Heparin Lock Flush, Abbott	00074-1152-71
10 ml	$1.44	Heparin Lock, Abbott	00074-1152-70
10 ml	$40.31	Heparin Lock Flush, Solopak Labs	39769-0036-10
10 ml x 25	$18.60	Hep-Lock, Elkins Sinn	00641-2436-41
10 ml x 25	$18.60	HEP-LOCK, Elkins Sinn	00641-2436-45
30 ml	$2.79	Heparin Lock Flush, Abbott	00074-1152-73
30 ml	$3.32	Heparin Lock, Abbott	00074-1152-78
30 ml	$47.49	Heparin Lock Flush, Solopak Labs	39769-0036-30
30 ml x 25	$48.84	HEP-LOCK 100 UNITS/ML, Elkins Sinn	00641-2443-45

Injection, Solution - Intravenous - 10000 unit/ml

1 ml x 25	$37.50	Hep-Lock, Consolidated Midland	00223-7861-01
2 ml x 25	$25.00	Hep-Lock, Consolidated Midland	00223-7863-02

Injection, Solution - Misc - 25 unit

2.5 ml x 50	$56.80	HEP-LOCK, Elkins Sinn	00641-3261-09

Kit - Intravenous - 10 unit/ml

200's	$832.50	Lok-Pak-N-1Ml, Solopak Mdcl	59747-0117-71
200's	$1005.00	Lok-Pak-N-3Ml, Solopak Mdcl	59747-0117-73
200's	$1542.50	Lok-Pak-N-5Ml, Solopak Mdcl	59747-0117-75

Kit - Intravenous - 100 unit/ml

200's	$832.50	Lok-Pak-N-1Ml, Solopak Mdcl	59747-0118-71
200's	$1005.00	Lok-Pak-N-3Ml, Solopak Mdcl	59747-0118-73
200's	$1542.50	Lok-Pak-N-5Ml, Solopak Mdcl	59747-0118-75

Package - Intravenous - 10 unit/ml

30's	$88.15	HEP-PAK CVC, Sanofi Winthrop	00024-0725-02
50's	$114.76	HEP-PAK, Sanofi Winthrop	00024-0725-03
200's	$252.28	Hep Flush, Fujisawa USA	00469-0030-15

Package - Intravenous - 100 unit/ml

30's	$88.15	HEP-PAK CVC, Sanofi Winthrop	00024-0736-02
50's	$114.76	HEP-PAK, Sanofi Winthrop	00024-0736-03
200's	$252.28	Hep Flush, Fujisawa USA	00469-0031-25

HOW SUPPLIED - NOT RATED EQUIVALENT:

Injection, Solution - Intravenous - 10 unit/ml

combination pac	$103.98	CVC HEPARIN FLUSH KITS, Wyeth Labs	00008-2528-01
30 unit of use	$81.02	CVC HEPARIN FLUSH KITS, Wyeth Labs	00008-2528-02
50 kit	$103.98	CVC HEPARIN FLUSH KITS, Wyeth Labs	00008-2528-03

Injection, Solution - Intravenous - 100 unit/ml

combination pac	$103.98	CVC HEPARIN FLUSH KITS, Wyeth Labs	00008-2529-01
30 unit of use	$81.02	CVC HEPARIN FLUSH KITS, Wyeth Labs	00008-2529-02
50 kit	$103.98	CVC HEPARIN FLUSH KITS, Wyeth Labs	00008-2529-03

Kit - Intravenous - 10 unit/ml

50's	$160.23	Heparin Flush, Wyeth Labs	00008-2528-52

Kit - Intravenous - 100 unit/ml

30's	$114.77	Heparin Flush, Wyeth Labs	00008-2529-51

Package - Intravenous - 10 unit/ml

50's	$72.78	HEP-PAK 2, Sanofi Winthrop	00024-0741-12

Package - Intravenous - 100 unit/ml

50's	$72.78	HEP-PAK 2, Sanofi Winthrop	00024-0742-12

HEPARIN SODIUM *(001428)*

CATEGORIES: Anticoagulants; Anticoagulants/Thrombolytics; Atrial Fibrillation; Blood Clotting; Blood Formation/Coagulation; Coagulants and Anticoagulants; Coagulopathies; Embolism; Fibrillation; Pulmonary Embolism; Thrombosis; Angina*; Pregnancy Category C; FDA Approval Pre 1982
* Indication not approved by the FDA

BRAND NAMES: *Beparine*; *Helberina* (Mexico); *Hepaflex*; *Hepalean* (Canada); *Heparin* (Germany, England); Heparin Flush; *Heparin Injection*; *Heparin Injection B.P.*; *Heparin Leo* (Canada); Heparin Lok-Pak; *Heparin Novo*; Heparin Porcine; *Heparin Sodium B Braun*; *Heparin Subcutaneous*; *Heparina Leo*; *Heparina*; *Heparine*; *Heparine Choay* (France); *Heparine Novo*; *Inhepar* (Mexico); Liquaemin Sodium; *Liquemin* (Germany); *Liquemine*; *Minihep*; *Monoparin*; *Multiparin*; Sodium Heparin; *Triheparine*; *Thromboliquine*; *Unihep*; *Uniparin*
(International brand names outside U.S. in italics)

FORMULARIES: BC-BS; Medi-Cal; WHO

DESCRIPTION:

Heparin is a heterogenous group of straight-chain anionic mucopolysaccharides, called glycosaminoglycans, having anticoagulant properties. Although others may be present, the main sugars occurring in heparin are: (1) α-L-iduronic acid 2-sulfate, (2) 2-deoxy-2-sulfamino-α-D-glucose 6-sulfate, (3) β-D-glucuronic acid, (4) 2-acetamido-2-deoxy-α-D-glucose, and (5) α-L-iduronic acid. These sugars are present in decreasing amounts, usually in the order: (2)> (1)> (4)> (3)> (5), and are joined by glycosidic linkages, forming polymers of varying sizes. Heparin is strongly acidic because of its content of covalently linked sulfate and carboxylic acid groups. In heparin sodium, the acidic protons of the sulfate units are partially replaced by sodium ions.

Heparin Sodium Injection, USP, is a sterile solution of heparin sodium derived from porcine intestinal mucosa, standardized for anticoagulant activity. It is to be administered by intravenous or deep subcutaneous routes. The potency is determined by a biological assay using a USP reference standard based on units of heparin activity per milligram.

Carpuject Sterile Cartridge-Needle Unit contains a sterile solution of Heparin Sodium Injection, USP. Each ml contains 5,000 USP heparin units of heparin sodium and benzyl alcohol 1% in Water for Injection. The pH is adjusted with hydrochloric acid or sodium hydroxide.

Each half ml of preservative-free Heparin Sodium Injection contains 5,000 USP heparin units of heparin sodium in Water for Injection. The pH is adjusted with hydrochloric acid or sodium hydroxide as required.

CLINICAL PHARMACOLOGY:

Heparin inhibits reactions that lead to the clotting of blood and the formation of fibrin clots both *in vitro* and *in vivo*. Heparin acts at multiple sites in the normal coagulation system. Small amounts of heparin in combination with antithrombin III (heparin cofactor) can inhibit thrombosis by inactivating activated Factor X and inhibiting the conversion of prothrombin to thrombin. Once active thrombosis has developed, larger amounts of heparin can inhibit further coagulation by inactivating thrombin and preventing the conversion of fibrinogen to fibrin. Heparin also prevents the formation of a stable fibrin clot by inhibiting the activation of the fibrin stabilizing factor.

Bleeding time is usually unaffected by heparin. Clotting time is prolonged by full therapeutic doses of heparin; in most cases, it is not measurably affected by low doses of heparin.

Peak plasma levels of heparin are achieved 2 to 4 hours following subcutaneous administration, although there are considerable individual variations. Loglinear plots of heparin plasma concentrations with time for a wide range of dose levels are linear, which suggest the absence of zero order processes. The liver and the reticulo-endothelial system are the site of biotransformation. The biphasic elimination curve, a rapidly declining alpha phase ($t_{1/2}$ = 10') and after the age of 40, a slower beta phase, indicates uptake in organs. The absence of a relationship between anticoagulant half-life and concentration half-life may reflect factors such as protein binding of heparin.

Heparin does not have fibrinolytic activity; therefore, it will not lyse existing clots.

INDICATIONS AND USAGE:

Heparin sodium is indicated for anticoagulant therapy in prophylaxis and treatment of venous thrombosis and its extension; (in a low-dose regimen) for prevention of postoperative deep venous thrombosis and pulmonary embolism in patients undergoing major abdominothoracic surgery or who, for other reasons, are at risk of developing thromboembolic disease (see DOSAGE AND ADMINISTRATION); for prophylaxis and treatment of pulmonary embolism; for atrial fibrillation with embolization; for diagnosis and treatment of acute and chronic consumption coagulopathies (disseminated intravascular coagulation); for prevention of clotting in arterial and heart surgery; for prophylaxis and treatment of peripheral arterial embolism; as an anticoagulant in blood transfusions, extracorporeal circulation and dialysis procedures, and in blood samples for laboratory purposes.

CONTRAINDICATIONS:

Severe thrombocytopenia.

Inability to perform suitable blood coagulation tests, e.g., the whole-blood clotting time, partial thromboplastic time, etc, at appropriate intervals (this contraindication refers to full dose heparin—there is usually no need to monitor coagulation parameters in patients receiving low-dose heparin).

An uncontrollable active bleeding state (see WARNINGS), except when this is due to disseminated intravascular coagulation.

WARNINGS:

Heparin is not intended for intramuscular use.

Hypersensitivity: Patients with documented hypersensitivity to heparin should be given the drug only in clearly life-threatening situations.

Hemorrhage: Hemorrhage can occur at virtually any site in patients receiving heparin. An unexplained fall in hematocrit, fall in blood pressure, or any other unexplained symptom should lead to serious consideration of a hemorrhagic event.

Heparin sodium should be used with extreme caution in disease states in which there is increased danger of hemorrhage. Some of the conditions in which increased danger of hemorrhage exists are:

Cardiovascular: Subacute bacterial endocarditis. Severe hypertension.

Surgical: During and immediately following (a) spinal tap or spinal anesthesia or (b) major surgery, especially involving the brain, spinal cord, or eye.

Hematologic: Conditions associated with increased bleeding tendencies, such as hemophilia, thrombocytopenia, and some vascular purpuras.

WARNINGS: *(cont'd)*

Gastrointestinal: Ulcerative lesions and continuous tube drainage of the stomach or small intestine.

Other: Menstruation, liver disease with impaired hemostasis.

Coagulation Testing: When heparin sodium is administered in therapeutic amounts, its dosage should be regulated by frequent blood coagulation tests. If the coagulation test is unduly prolonged or if hemorrhage occurs, heparin sodium should be discontinued promptly (see OVERDOSAGE).

Thrombocytopenia: Thrombocytopenia has been reported to occur in patients receiving heparin with a reported incidence of 0% to 30%. Mild thrombocytopenia (count greater than 100,000/mm^3) may remain stable or reverse even if heparin is continued. However, thrombocytopenia of any degree should be monitored closely. If the count falls below 100,000/mm^3 or if recurrent thrombosis develops (see PRECAUTIONS, White Clot Syndrome), the heparin product should be discontinued. If continued heparin therapy is essential, administration of heparin from a different organ source can be reinstituted with caution.

Miscellaneous: This product contains benzyl alcohol as preservative. Benzyl alcohol has been reported to be associated with a fatal "Gasping Syndrome" in premature infants.

PRECAUTIONS:

GENERAL

White Clot Syndrome: It has been reported that patients on heparin may develop new thrombus formation in association with thrombocytopenia resulting from irreversible aggregation of platelets induced by heparin, the so-called "white clot syndrome." The process may lead to severe thromboembolic complications like skin necrosis, gangrene of the extremities that may lead to amputation, myocardial infarction, pulmonary embolism, stroke, and possibly death. Therefore, heparin administration should be promptly discontinued if a patient develops new thrombosis in association with thrombocytopenia.

Heparin Resistance: Increased resistance to heparin is frequently encountered in fever, thrombosis, thrombophlebitis, infections with thrombosing tendencies, myocardial infarction, cancer, and in postsurgical patients.

Increased Risk in Older Women: A higher incidence of bleeding has been reported in women over 60 years of age.

LABORATORY TESTS

Periodic platelet counts, hematocrits, and tests for occult blood in stool are recommended during the entire course of heparin therapy, regardless of the route of administration (see DOSAGE AND ADMINISTRATION).

DRUG/LABORATORY TEST INTERACTIONS

Hyperaminotransferasemia: Significant elevations of aminotransferase (SGOT (S-AST) and SGPT (S-ALT) levels have occurred in a high percentage of patients (and healthy subjects) who have received heparin. Since aminotransferase determinations are important in the differential diagnosis of myocardial infarction, liver disease, and pulmonary emboli, rises that might be caused by drugs (like heparin) should be interpreted with caution.

CARCINOGENESIS, MUTAGENESIS, AND IMPAIRMENT OF FERTILITY

No long-term studies in animals have been performed to evaluate the carcinogenic potential of heparin. Also, no reproduction studies in animals have been performed concerning mutagenesis or impairment of fertility.

PREGNANCY CATEGORY C

Teratogenic Effects: Animal reproduction studies have not been conducted with heparin sodium. It is also not known whether heparin sodium can cause fetal harm when administered to a pregnant woman or can affect reproduction capacity. Heparin sodium should be given to a pregnant woman only if clearly needed.

Nonteratogenic Effects: Heparin does not cross the placental barrier.

NURSING MOTHERS

Heparin is not excreted in human milk.

PEDIATRIC USE

See DOSAGE AND ADMINISTRATION.

DRUG INTERACTIONS:

Oral Anticoagulants: Heparin sodium may prolong the one-stage prothrombin time. Therefore, when heparin sodium is given with dicumarol or warfarin sodium, a period of at least 5 hours after the last intravenous dose or 24 hours after the last subcutaneous dose should elapse before blood is drawn if a valid prothrombin time is to be obtained.

Platelet Inhibitors: Drugs such as acetylsalicylic acid, dextran, phenylbutazone, ibuprofen, indomethacin, dipyridamole, hydroxychloroquine, and others that interfere with platelet-aggregation reactions (the main hemostatic defense of heparinized patients) may induce bleeding and should be used with caution in patients receiving heparin sodium.

Other Interactions: Digitalis, tetracyclines, nicotine, or antihistamines may partially counteract the anticoagulant action of heparin sodium.

ADVERSE REACTIONS:

HEMORRHAGE

Hemorrhage is the chief complication that may result from heparin therapy (see WARNINGS). An overly prolonged clotting time or minor bleeding during therapy can usually be controlled by withdrawing the drug (see OVERDOSAGE). It should be appreciated that gastrointestinal or urinary tract bleeding during anticoagulant therapy may indicate the presence of an underlying occult lesion. Bleeding can occur at any site but certain specific hemorrhagic complications may be difficult to detect:

Adrenal hemorrhage, with resultant acute adrenal insufficiency, has occurred during anticoagulant therapy. Therefore, such treatment should be discontinued in patients who develop signs and symptoms of acute adrenal hemorrhage and insufficiency. Initiation of corrective therapy should not depend on laboratory confirmation of the diagnosis, since any delay in an acute situation may result in the patient's death.

Ovarian (corpus luteum) hemorrhage developed in a number of women of reproductive age receiving short- or long-term anticoagulant therapy. This complication if unrecognized may be fatal.

Retroperitoneal hemorrhage.

LOCAL IRRITATION

Local irritation, erythema, mild pain, hematoma, or ulceration may follow deep subcutaneous (intrafat) injection of heparin sodium. These complications are much more common after intramuscular use, and such use is not recommended.

HYPERSENSITIVITY

Generalized hypersensitivity reactions have been reported, with chills, fever, and urticaria as the most usual manifestations, and asthma, rhinitis, lacrimation, headache, nausea and vomiting, and anaphylactoid reactions, including shock, occurring more rarely. Itching and burning, especially on the plantar site of the feet, may occur.

ADVERSE REACTIONS: *(cont'd)*

Thrombocytopenia has been reported to occur in patients receiving heparin with a reported incidence of 0% to 30%. While often mild and of no obvious clinical significance, such thrombocytopenia can be accompanied by severe thromboembolic complications such as skin necrosis, gangrene of the extremities that may lead to amputation, myocardial infarction, pulmonary embolism, stroke, and possibly death. (See WARNINGS, PRECAUTIONS.)

Certain episodes of painful, ischemic, and cyanosed limbs have in the past been attributed to allergic vasospastic reactions. Whether these are in fact identical to the thrombocytopenia-associated complications remains to be determined.

OTHER

Osteoporosis following long-term administration of high doses of heparin, cutaneous necrosis after systemic administration, suppression of aldosterone synthesis, delayed transient alopecia, priapism, and rebound hyperlipemia on discontinuation of heparin sodium have also been reported.

Significant elevations of aminotransferase (SGOT (S-AST) and SGPT (S-ALT)) levels have occurred in a high percentage of patients (and healthy subjects) who have received heparin.

OVERDOSAGE:

Symptoms: Bleeding is the chief sign of heparin overdosage. Nosebleeds, blood in urine, or tarry stools may be noted as the first sign of bleeding. Easy bruising or petechial formations may precede frank bleeding.

Treatment: Neutralization of heparin effect.

When clinical circumstances (bleeding) require reversal of heparinization, protamine sulfate (1% solution) by slow infusion will neutralize heparin sodium. No more than 50 mg should be administered very slowly, in any 10-minute period. Each mg of protamine sulfate neutralizes approximately 100 USP heparin units. The amount of protamine required decreases over time as heparin is metabolized. Although the metabolism of heparin is complex, it may, for the purpose of choosing a protamine dose, be assumed to have a half-life of about 30 minutes after intravenous injection.

Administration of protamine sulfate can cause severe hypotensive and anaphylactoid reactions. Because fatal reactions often resembling anaphylaxis have been reported, the drug should be given only when resuscitation techniques and treatment of anaphylactoid shock are readily available.

For additional information, the labeling of Protamine Sulfate Injection, USP, products should be consulted.

DOSAGE AND ADMINISTRATION:

When heparin is added to an infusion solution for continuous intravenous administration, the container should be inverted at least six times to insure adequate mixing and prevent pooling of the heparin in the solution.

Heparin sodium is not effective by oral administration and should be given by intermittent intravenous injection, intravenous infusion or deep subcutaneous (intrafat, i.e., above the iliac crest or abdominal fat layer) injection. The intramuscular route of administration should be avoided because of the frequent occurrence of hematoma at the injection site.

The dosage of heparin sodium should be adjusted according to the patient's coagulation test results. When heparin is given by continuous intravenous infusion, the coagulation time should be determined approximately every 4 hours in the early stages of treatment. When the drug is administered intermittently by intravenous injection, coagulation tests should be performed before each injection during the early stages of treatment and at appropriate intervals thereafter. Dosage is considered adequate when the activated partial thromboplastin time (APTT) is 1.5 to 2 times normal or when the whole blood clotting time is elevated approximately 2.5 to 3 times the control value. After deep subcutaneous (intrafat) injections, tests for adequacy of dosage are best performed on samples drawn 4 to 6 hours after the injections.

Periodic platelet counts, hematocrits, and tests for occult blood in stool are recommended during the entire course of heparin therapy, regardless of the route of administration.

CONVERTING TO ORAL ANTICOAGULANT

When an oral anticoagulant of the coumarin or similar type is to be begun in patients already receiving heparin sodium, baseline and subsequent tests of prothrombin activity must be determined at a time when heparin activity is too low to affect the prothrombin time. This is about 5 hours after the last IV bolus and 24 hours after the last subcutaneous dose. If continuous IV heparin infusion is used, prothrombin time can usually be measured at any time.

In converting from heparin to an oral anticoagulant, the dose of the oral anticoagulant should be the usual initial amount and thereafter prothrombin time should be determined at the usual intervals. To ensure continuous anticoagulation, it is advisable to continue full heparin therapy for several days after the prothrombin time has reached the therapeutic range. Heparin therapy may then be discontinued without tapering.

THERAPEUTIC ANTICOAGULANT EFFECT WITH FULL-DOSE HEPARIN

Although dosage must be adjusted for the individual patient according to the results of suitable laboratory tests, the following dosage schedules may be used as guidelines (TABLE 1):

TABLE 1

Method Of Administration	Frequency	Recommended Dose*
Deep Subcutaneous (Intrafat injection)	Initial Dose	5,000 units by IV injection, followed by 10,000 to 20,000 units of a concentrated solution, subcutaneously
A different site should be used for each injection to prevent the development of massive hematoma.	Every 8 hrs. or	8,000 to 10,000 units of a concentrated solution
	Every 12 hrs.	15,000 to 20,000 units of a concentrated solution
Intermittent Intravenous Injection	Initial dose	10,000 units, either undiluted or in 50 ml to 100 ml of Sodium Chloride Injection, USP, 0.9%
	Every 4 to 6 hours	5,000 to 10,000 units, either undiluted or in 50 ml to 100 ml of Sodium Chloride Injection USP, 0.9%
Continuous Intravenous Infusion	Initial dose	5,000 units by IV Injection
	Continuous	20,000 to 40,000 units/24 hours in 1,000 ml of Sodium Chloride Injection, USP, 0.9% (or in any compatible solution) for infusion

* Based on 150 lb (68 kg) patient.

PEDIATRIC USE

Follow recommendations of appropriate pediatric reference texts. (See WARNINGS, Miscellaneous.) In general, the following dosage schedule may be used as a guideline:

DOSAGE AND ADMINISTRATION: *(cont'd)*

Initial Dose: 50 units/kg (IV, drip)

Maintenance Dose: 100 units/kg (IV, drip) every four hours, or 20,000 units/M^2/24 hours continuously

SURGERY OF THE HEART AND BLOOD VESSELS

Patients undergoing total body perfusion for open-heart surgery should receive an initial dose of not less than 150 units of heparin sodium per kilogram of body weight. Frequently, a dose of 300 units per kilogram is used for procedures estimated to last less than 60 minutes or 400 units per kilogram for those estimated to last longer than 60 minutes.

LOW-DOSE PROPHYLAXIS OF POSTOPERATIVE THROMBOEMBOLISM

A number of well-controlled clinical trials have demonstrated that low-dose heparin prophylaxis, given just prior to and after surgery, will reduce the incidence of postoperative deep vein thrombosis in the legs (as measured by the 1-125 fibrinogen technique and venography) and of clinical pulmonary embolism. The most widely used dosage has been 5,000 units 2 hours before surgery and 5,000 units every 8 to 12 hours thereafter for 7 days or until the patient is fully ambulatory, whichever is longer. The heparin is given by deep subcutaneous (intrafat, i.e., above the iliac crest or abdominal fat layer, arm, or thigh) injection with a fine (25- to 26-gauge) needle to minimize tissue trauma. A concentrated solution of heparin sodium is recommended. Such prophylaxis should be reserved for patients over the age of 40 who are undergoing major surgery. Patients with bleeding disorders and those having brain or spinal cord surgery, spinal anesthesia, eye surgery, or potentially sanguineous operations should be excluded, as should patients receiving oral anticoagulants or platelet-active drugs (see WARNINGS). The value of such prophylaxis in hip surgery has not been established. The possibility of increased bleeding during surgery or postoperatively should be borne in mind. If such bleeding occurs, discontinuance of heparin and neutralization with protamine sulfate are advisable. If clinical evidence of thromboembolism develops despite low-dose prophylaxis, full therapeutic doses of anticoagulants should be given unless contraindicated. Prior to initiating heparinization the physician should rule out bleeding disorders by appropriate history and laboratory tests, and appropriate coagulation tests should be repeated just prior to surgery. Coagulation tests values should be normal or only slightly elevated at these times.

EXTRACORPOREAL DIALYSIS

Follow equipment manufacturers' operating directions carefully.

BLOOD TRANSFUSION

Addition of 400 to 600 USP units per 100 ml of whole blood is usually employed to prevent coagulation. Usually, 7,500 USP units of heparin sodium are added to 100 ml of Sodium Chloride Injection, USP, 0.9% (or 75,000 USP units per 1,000 ml of Sodium Chloride Injection, USP, 0.9%) and mixed; from this sterile solution, 6 ml to 8 ml are added per 100 ml of whole blood.

LABORATORY SAMPLES

Addition of 70 to 150 units of heparin sodium per 10 ml to 20 ml sample of whole blood is usually employed to prevent coagulation of the sample. Leukocyte counts should be performed on heparinized blood within 2 hours after addition of the heparin. Heparinized blood should not be used for isoagglutinin, complement, or erythrocyte fragility tests or platelet counts.

PARENTERAL DRUG PRODUCTS SHOULD BE INSPECTED VISUALLY FOR PARTICULATE MATTER AND DISCOLORATION PRIOR TO ADMINISTRATION, WHENEVER SOLUTION AND CONTAINER PERMIT.

Discard unused portion after initial use.

Keep at room temperature. Do not freeze.

HOW SUPPLIED - RATED THERAPEUTICALLY EQUIVALENT:

Injection, Solution - Intramuscular; - 40,000 unit/ml

1 ml x 25	$78.00	LIQUAEMIN SODIUM, Organon	00052-0816-25
1 ml x 25	$187.50	Heparin Sodium, Schein Pharm (US)	00364-2364-46
2 ml x 25	$333.38	Heparin Sodium, Schein Pharm (US)	00364-2364-48
5 ml	$16.50	Heparin Sodium, Steris Labs	00402-0519-05
5 ml	$17.41	Heparin Sodium, Schein Pharm (US)	00364-2364-53
5 ml	$22.75	Heparin Sodium, Porcine Mucosa, Pasadena	00418-4461-05

Injection, Solution - Intravenous - 2 unit/ml

500 ml	$6.87	Heparin Sodium/0.9% Sodium Chloride, Baxter Hlthcare	00338-0431-03
500 ml	$14.27	HEPARIN SODIUM IN NS, McGaw	00264-9872-10
1000 ml	$7.32	Heparin Sodium/0.9% Sodium Chloride, Baxter Hlthcare	00338-0433-04

Injection, Solution - Intravenous - 10 unit/ml

1 ml x 25	$16.56	Heparin Lock Flush, Fujisawa USA	00469-5044-01
1 ml x 50	$34.50	Heparin Sodium, Wyeth Labs	00008-0523-01
2.5 ml x 50	$54.49	Heparin Sodium, Wyeth Labs	00008-0523-02
30's	$114.77	Heparin Flush, Wyeth Labs	00008-2528-51
50's	$160.23	Heparin Flush, Wyeth Labs	00008-2528-50
200's	$832.50	Heparin Lok-Pak, Solopak Mdcl	59747-0060-02
200's	$1005.00	Heparin Lok-Pak, Solopak Mdcl	59747-0060-03
200's	$1542.50	Heparin Lok-Pak, Solopak Mdcl	59747-0060-05

Injection, Solution - Intravenous - 40 unit/ml

500 ml	$11.57	HEPARIN SODIUM IN %5 DEXTROSE, Abbott	00074-7760-03
500 ml	$21.94	HEPARIN SODIUM/5% DEXTROSE, McGaw	00264-9567-10

Injection, Solution - Intravenous - 50 unit/ml

100 ml	$11.88	HEPARIN SODIUM IN 5% DEXTROSE, Abbott	00074-7794-23
150 ml	$11.87	HEPARIN SODIUM IN 5% DEXTROSE, Abbott	00074-7794-61
200 ml	$11.87	HEPARIN SODIUM IN 5% DEXTROSE, Abbott	00074-7794-12
250 ml	$11.88	HEPARIN SODIUM IN 5% DEXTROSE, Abbott	00074-7794-62
500 ml	$13.37	HEPARIN SODIUM IN 5% DEXTROSE, Abbott	00074-7761-03
500 ml	$22.02	HEPARIN SODIUM IN DEXTROSE, McGaw	00264-9577-10
500 ml x 10	$20.52	Heparin Sodium, McGaw	00264-5577-10

Injection, Solution - Intravenous - 100 unit/ml

1 ml x 25	$13.75	Heparin Sodium, Consolidated Midland	00223-7865-01
1 ml x 25	$14.69	Heparin Lock Flush, Fujisawa USA	00469-5045-01
1 ml x 50	$34.50	Heparin Sodium In Normal Saline, Wyeth Labs	00008-0487-01
1 ml x 50	$42.64	Heparin Lock Flush, Sanofi Winthrop	00024-0722-26
2 ml x 25	$20.00	Heparin Sodium, Consolidated Midland	00223-7867-02
2 ml x 50	$58.53	Heparin Lock Flush, Sanofi Winthrop	00024-0722-27
2.5 ml x 50	$54.49	Heparin Sodium In Normal Saline, Wyeth Labs	00008-0487-03
50's	$160.23	Heparin Flush, Wyeth Labs	00008-2529-50
50's	$160.23	Heparin Flush, Wyeth Labs	00008-2529-52
100 ml	$9.38	HEPARIN SODIUM IN 5% DEXTROSE, Abbott	00074-7813-23
100 ml	$14.25	HEPARIN SODIUM IN 5% DEXTROSE, Abbott	00074-7793-23
150 ml	$14.25	HEPARIN SODIUM IN 5% DEXTROSE, Abbott	00074-7793-61
200 ml	$11.87	HEPARIN SODIUM IN 5% DEXTROSE, Abbott	00074-7793-12
200's	$832.50	Heparin Lok-Pak, Solopak Mdcl	59747-0037-02
200's	$1005.00	Heparin Lok-Pak, Solopak Mdcl	59747-0037-03
200's	$1542.50	Heparin Lok-Pak, Solopak Mdcl	59747-0037-05

HOW SUPPLIED - RATED THERAPEUTICALLY EQUIVALENT: *(cont'd)*

250 ml	$10.53	HEPARIN SODIUM IN 0.45% NS, Abbott	00074-7650-62
250 ml	$11.21	HEPARIN SODIUM IN 5% DEXTROSE, Abbott	00074-7813-62
250 ml	$11.88	HEPARIN SODIUM IN 5% DEXTROSE, Abbott	00074-7793-62
250 ml	$22.81	Heparin Sodium/5% Dextrose, McGaw	00264-9587-20

Injection, Solution - Intravenous - 1000 unit/ml

1 ml x 10	$7.44	Sodium Heparin, Wyeth Labs	00008-0275-01
1 ml x 10	$11.19	Heparin Sodium, Wyeth Labs	00008-0275-50
1 ml x 25	$11.59	Heparin Sodium, Elkins Sinn	00641-0391-25
1 ml x 25	$20.00	Heparin Sodium, Consolidated Midland	00223-7808-01
1 ml x 25	$24.38	Heparin Sodium, Fujisawa USA	00469-5040-01
1 ml x 50	$15.71	Heparin Sodium, Fujisawa USA	00469-7507-50
2 ml x 25	$92.19	Heparin Sodium, Fujisawa USA	00469-2760-10
5 ml x 25	$74.17	Heparin Sodium, Perservative Free, Marsam	00209-4220-14
5 ml x 25	$90.94	Heparin Sodium, Bristol Myers Squibb	00003-2963-20
10 ml	$3.03	Heparin Sodium, Pharmacia & Upjohn	00009-0268-01
10 ml	$4.50	Heparin Sodium, Consolidated Midland	00223-7843-10
10 ml	$4.75	Heparin Sodium, Consolidated Midland	00223-7810-10
10 ml	$39.06	Heparin Sodium, Solopak Labs	39769-0019-10
10 ml	$64.06	Heparin Sodium, Fujisawa USA	00469-0813-30
10 ml x 1	$2.70	Heparin Sodium, Elkins Sinn	00641-2440-41
10 ml x 25	$23.03	Heparin Sodium, Elkins Sinn	00641-2440-45
10 ml x 25	$25.50	LIQUAEMIN SODIUM, Organon	00052-0811-10
10 ml x 25	$48.25	Heparin Sodium, Organon	00052-0801-10
10 ml x 25	$75.69	Heparin Sodium, Pharmacia & Upjohn	00009-0268-12
25 x 10 ml	$81.25	Heparin Sodium, Beef Lung, Pasadena	00418-5301-10
25's	$82.41	Heparin Sodium, Geneva Pharms	00781-3734-75
30 ml	$1.98	Heparin Sodium, Insource	58441-0110-30
30 ml	$3.75	Heparin, IDE-Interstate	00814-3650-46
30 ml	$8.63	Heparin Sodium, Pharmacia & Upjohn	00009-0268-02
30 ml	$10.64	Heparin Sodium, Rugby	00536-4860-75
30 ml	$12.50	Heparin Sodium, Consolidated Midland	00223-7811-30
30 ml	$12.50	Heparin Sodium, Consolidated Midland	00223-7844-30
30 ml	$68.75	Heparin Sodium, Solopak Labs	39769-0019-30
30 ml	$127.18	Heparin Sodium, Fujisawa USA	00469-0813-50
30 ml x 1	$7.21	Heparin Sodium, Elkins Sinn	00641-2450-41
30 ml x 25	$40.47	Heparin Sodium, Elkins Sinn	00641-2450-45
30 ml x 25	$66.95	LIQUAEMIN SODIUM, Organon	00052-0811-75
30 ml x 25	$81.25	Heparin Sodium, Porcine Mucosa, Pasadena	00418-4301-61
30 ml x 25	$100.00	Heparin Sodium, Beef Lung, Pasadena	00418-5301-61
30 ml x 25	$122.50	Heparin Sodium, Organon	00052-0801-30
500 ml	$9.90	Heparin Sodium, Abbott	00074-7620-03

Injection, Solution - Intravenous - 2500 unit/ml

ml x 10	$13.46	Heparin Sodium, Wyeth Labs	00008-0482-01
5 ml	$3.41	Heparin Sodium, Abbott	00074-2582-02
10 ml	$6.56	Heparin Sodium, Abbott	00074-2584-02

Injection, Solution - Intravenous - 5000 unit/ml

0.5 ml x 10	$16.05	Heparin Sodium, Elkins Sinn	00641-3266-03
1 ml x 10	$10.25	Heparin Sodium, Sanofi Winthrop	00024-0793-02
1 ml x 10	$15.98	Sodium Heparin, Wyeth Labs	00008-0278-02
1 ml x 10	$16.05	Heparin Sodium, Elkins Sinn	00641-3267-03
1 ml x 25	$15.98	Heparin Sodium, Elkins Sinn	00641-0400-25
1 ml x 25	$26.88	Heparin Sodium, Fujisawa USA	00469-1262-15
1 ml x 25	$33.90	Heparin Sodium, Organon	00052-0802-01
1 ml x 50	$51.29	Heparin Sodium, Sanofi Winthrop	00024-0793-12
10 ml	$7.50	Heparin, Schein Pharm (US)	00364-6538-54
10 ml	$7.50	Heparin Sodium, Steris Labs	00402-0418-10
10 ml	$7.50	Heparin Sodium, United Res	00677-0275-21
10 ml	$10.08	Heparin Sodium With Diluent, Rugby	00536-4900-70
10 ml	$14.06	Heparin Sodium, Pharmacia & Upjohn	00009-0291-01
10 ml	$112.19	Heparin Sodium, Fujisawa USA	00469-0923-30
10 ml x 1	$9.63	Heparin Sodium, Elkins Sinn	00641-2460-41
10 ml x 25	$60.23	Heparin Sodium, Elkins Sinn	00641-2460-45
10 ml x 25	$92.40	LIQUAEMIN SODIUM, Organon	00052-0812-10
10 ml x 25	$196.75	Heparin Sodium, Organon	00052-0802-10
30 ml x 25	$215.00	Heparin Sodium, Porcine Mucosa, Pasadena	00418-4451-41
250 ml	$8.84	Heparin Sodium, Abbott	00074-7651-02
250 ml	$19.12	Heparin Sodium In 5%, Abbott	00074-6287-02
500 ml	$9.20	Heparin Sodium & 5% Dextrose, Baxter Hlthcare	00338-0449-03
500 ml	$9.94	Heparin Sodium & 5% Dextrose, Baxter Hlthcare	00338-0450-03
500 ml	$10.53	Heparin Sodium, Abbott	00074-7651-03
500 ml	$22.94	Heparin Sodium In 5%, Abbott	00074-6287-03

Injection, Solution - Intravenous - 10000 unit/ml

0.5 ml x 10	$10.25	Heparin Sodium, Sanofi Winthrop	00024-0733-05
0.5 ml x 50	$51.29	Heparin Sodium, Sanofi Winthrop	00024-0733-15
0.5 ml x 50	$78.05	Sodium Heparin, Wyeth Labs	00008-0277-03
0.5 nk x 10	$15.98	Sodium Heparin, Wyeth Labs	00008-0277-02
1 ml	$4.75	HEPARIN SODIUM, Consolidated Midland	00223-7846-01
1 ml x 10	$17.12	Heparin Sodium, Sanofi Winthrop	00024-0733-02
1 ml x 10	$22.05	Sodium Heparin, Wyeth Labs	00008-0277-01
1 ml x 10	$22.19	Heparin Sodium 10000 Unt/Ml, Elkins Sinn	00641-3268-03
1 ml x 20	$18.35	Heparin Sodium, Sanofi Winthrop	00024-0733-50
1 ml x 20	$26.35	Heparin Sodium, Sanofi Winthrop	00024-0733-59
1 ml x 25	$3.03	Heparin Sodium, Pharmacia & Upjohn	00009-0317-08
1 ml x 25	$21.56	Heparin Sodium, Elkins Sinn	00641-0410-25
1 ml x 25	$26.25	Heparin Sodium, Voluntary Hosp	53258-2152-01
1 ml x 25	$35.00	Heparin Sodium, Consolidated Midland	00223-7828-01
1 ml x 25	$36.88	Heparin Sodium, Fujisawa USA	00469-5042-01
1 ml x 25	$51.60	Heparin Sodium, Organon	00052-0805-01
1 ml x 50	$85.59	Heparin Sodium, Sanofi Winthrop	00024-0733-12
4 ml	$11.28	Heparin Sodium, Pharmacia & Upjohn	00009-0317-02
4 ml x 1	$8.40	Heparin Sodium, Elkins Sinn	00641-2470-41
4 ml x 25	$56.46	Heparin Sodium, Elkins Sinn	00641-2470-45
4 ml x 25	$63.25	LIQUAEMIN SODIUM, Organon	00052-0815-04
4 ml x 25	$90.00	Heparin Sodium, Consolidated Midland	00223-7830-04
4 ml x 25	$168.95	Heparin Sodium, Organon	00052-0805-04
4 ml x 25	$225.00	Heparin Sodium, Voluntary Hosp	53258-0833-07
4 ml x 25	$268.50	Heparin Sodium, Beef Lung, Pasadena	00418-5302-01
4 ml x 25	$282.10	Heparin Sodium, Pharmacia & Upjohn	00009-0317-11
5 ml	$3.74	Heparin Sodium, Balan	00304-1326-55
5 ml	$3.90	Heparin Sodium, Consolidated Midland	00223-7831-05
5 ml	$113.75	Sodium Heparin, Porcine Mucosa, Pasadena	00418-4351-05
5 ml x 1	$24.58	Heparin Sodium 10000 U/Ml, Lilly	00002-7217-01
10 ml	$8.25	Heparin Sodium, Steris Labs	00402-0049-10
10 ml	$11.50	Heparin Sodium, Consolidated Midland	00223-7832-10
10 ml	$11.90	Heparin, Schein Pharm (US)	00364-6539-54
10 ml	$13.20	Heparin Sodium, Porcine Mucosa, Pasadena	00418-4351-41
10 ml	$14.50	Heparin Sodium, Ortega Pharm	00191-2033-21
10 ml	$17.25	Heparin Sodium With Diluent, Rugby	00536-4925-70
25 x 4 ml	$268.50	Heparin Sodium, Beef Lung, Pasadena	00418-5301-01
100 ml	$17.98	Heparin Sodium In 5% Dextrose, Abbott	00074-6286-11

HOW SUPPLIED - RATED THERAPEUTICALLY EQUIVALENT: *(cont'd)*

250 ml	$8.84	Heparin Sodium, Abbott	00074-7650-02
250 ml	$9.94	Heparin Sodium & 5% Dextrose, Baxter Hlthcare	00338-0451-02
250 ml	$22.94	Heparin Sodium In 5% Dextrose, Abbott	00074-6286-02

Injection, Solution - Intravenous - 20000 unit/ml

1 ml	$7.61	Heparin Sodium, Lilly	00002-7218-01
1 ml x 10	$41.30	Sodium Heparin, Wyeth Labs	00008-0276-01
1 ml x 25	$36.00	LIQUAEMIN SODIUM, Organon	00052-0813-25
1 ml x 25	$63.75	Heparin Sodium, Voluntary Hosp	53258-1155-01
1 ml x 25	$65.63	Heparin Sodium, Fujisawa USA	00469-1155-15
1 ml x 25	$93.75	Heparin, Schein Pharm (US)	00364-6540-46
2 ml	$14.38	Heparin Sodium, Lilly	00002-7219-01
2 ml x 25	$60.00	LIQUAEMIN SODIUM, Organon	00052-0813-02
2 ml x 25	$166.65	Heparin, Schein Pharm (US)	00364-6540-48
5 ml	$7.44	LIQUAEMIN SODIUM, Organon	00052-0813-05
5 ml	$11.95	Heparin Sodium, Consolidated Midland	00223-7840-05
5 ml	$12.65	Sodium Heparin, Porcine Mucosa, Pasadena	00418-4341-05
5 ml	$15.83	Heparin Sodium, Steris Labs	00402-0050-05
5 ml	$15.90	Heparin Sodium With Diluent, Rugby	00536-4950-65
5 ml	$16.62	Heparin, Schein Pharm (US)	00364-6540-53
25 x 1 ml	$80.00	Heparin Sodium, Porcine Mucosa, Pasadena	00418-1155-15

HOW SUPPLIED - NOT RATED EQUIVALENT:

Injection, Solution - Intramuscular; - 7,500 unit/ml

1 ml x 10	$18.30	Sodium Heparin, Wyeth Labs	00008-0293-01

Injection, Solution - Intravenous - 2 unit/ml

500 ml x 10	$9.37	Heparin Sodium, McGaw	00264-8872-10
1000 ml	$9.90	HEPARIN SODIUM IN NS, Abbott	00074-7620-59

Injection, Solution - Intravenous - 50 unit/ml

250 ml	$9.71	HEPARIN SODIUM IN 5% DEXTROSE, Abbott	00074-7814-62
250 ml	$9.93	Heparin Sodium In 0.45% Sodium, Abbott	00074-7651-62
500 ml x 10	$6.02	Heparin Sodium, McGaw	00264-8877-10

Injection, Solution - Intravenous - 2000 unit/ml

5 ml	$2.83	Heparin Sodium, Abbott	00074-2581-02
10 ml	$5.05	Heparin Sodium, Abbott	00074-2583-02
10 ml	$22.75	Sodium Heparin, Porcine Mucosa, Pasadena	00418-4341-41

Injection, Solution - Intravenous - 2500 unit/ml

1 ml x 10	$9.53	Heparin Sodium, Sanofi Winthrop	00024-0733-03

Injection, Solution - Intravenous - 5000 unit/ml

1 ml	$1.00	Heparin Sodium, Consolidated Midland	00223-7818-01
10 ml	$17.50	Heparin Sodium, Consolidated Midland	00223-7820-10

Injection, Solution - Intravenous - 7500 unit/ml

1 ml x 10	$12.12	Heparin Sodium, Sanofi Winthrop	00024-0733-04

HEPATITIS A VACCINE *(003158)*

CATEGORIES: Biologicals; Hepatitis A; Immunologic; Jaundice; Serums, Toxoids and Vaccines; Vaccines; Sales > $100 Million; FDA Approved 1995 Feb

BRAND NAMES: Havrix

DESCRIPTION:

Havrix (Hepatitis A Vaccine, Inactivated) is a noninfectious hepatitis A vaccine developed and manufactured by SmithKline Beecham Biologicals. The virus (strain HM175) is propagated in MRC_5 human diploid cells. After removal of the cell culture medium, the cells are lysed to form a suspension, then purified and concentrated by ultrafiltration and gel chromatography. Treatment of this lysate with formalin ensures viral inactivation. Havrix contains a sterile suspension of inactivated virus; viral antigen activity is referenced to a standard using an enzyme linked immunosorbent assay (ELISA), and is therefore expressed in terms of ELISA Units (EL.U.).

Havrix is supplied as a sterile suspension for intramuscular administration. The vaccine is ready for use without reconstitution; it must be shaken before administration to assure a uniform suspension.

Each 1 ml adult dose of vaccine consists of not less than 1440 EL.U. of viral antigen, adsorbed on 0.5 mg of aluminum, as aluminum hydroxide.

Each 0.5 ml pediatric dose of vaccine consists of not less than 360 EL.U. of viral antigen, adsorbed onto 0.25 of aluminum, as aluminum hydroxide.

The vaccine preparations also contain 0.5% (w/v) of 2-phenoxyethanol as a preservative. Other excipients are: amino acid supplement (0.3% w/v) in a phosphate-buffered saline solution and polysorbate 20 (0.05 mg/ml). Residual MRC_5 cellular proteins (not more than 5 mcg/adult dose) and traces of formalin (not more than 0.1 mg/ml) are present.

CLINICAL PHARMACOLOGY:

The hepatitis A virus (HAV) belongs to the picornavirus family. Only one serotype of HAV has been described.[1]

Hepatitis A is highly contagious with the predominant mode of transmission being person-to-person via the fecal-oral route. Infection has been shown to be spread (1) by contaminated water or food; (2) by infected food handlers[2]; (3) after breakdown in usual sanitary conditions or after floods or natural disasters; (4) by ingestion of raw or undercooked shellfish (oysters, clams, mussels) from contaminated waters[3]; (5) during travel to areas of the world with poor hygienic conditions[4,5]; (6) among institutionalized children and adults[6]; (7) in day-care centers where children have not been toilet trained[7]; (8) by parenteral transmission, either blood transfusions or sharing needles with infected people.[1]

The level of economic development influences the prevalence of hepatitis A and the age at which it is most likely to occur. In developing countries with poor hygiene and sanitation, about 90% of children are infected by age 5 years.[1] As conditions improve, the prevalence decreases and the age at which infection occurs increases. Hence it is more likely to occur in adulthood, when disease is generally more severe and more likely to be fatal.[1] In the United States, attack rates for hepatitis A infection are cyclical and vary by population. The rates have increased gradually from 9.2 per 100,000 in 1983 to 14.6 per 100,000 in 1989.[8]

The incubation period for hepatitis A averages 28 days (range: 15 to 50 days).[9] The course of hepatitis A infection is extremely variable, ranging from asymptomatic infection to icteric hepatitis. However, most adults (76% to 97%)[10] become symptomatic. Symptoms range from mild and transient to severe and prolonged and may include fever, nausea, vomiting and diarrhea in the prodromal phase, followed by jaundice in up to 88% of adults, as well as hepatomegaly and biochemical evidence of hepatocellular damage.[10] Recovery is generally complete and followed by protection against HAV infection. However, illness may be prolonged, and relapse of clinical illness and viral shedding have been described.[11]

CLINICAL PHARMACOLOGY: *(cont'd)*

Hepatitis A infection is often asymptomatic in children under 2 years of age, who nonetheless excrete the virus in their stool and thereby serve as a source of infection.[10] In older patients and persons with underlying liver disease[1], it is generally much more severe. This is reflected in mortality rates. While an overall case fatality rate of 0.6% has been reported, a case fatality rate of 2.7% has been reported in patients ≥49 years of age.[1]Indeed, while 67% of cases occur in children, over 70% of deaths occur in those over the age of 49 years.[1]

There is no chronic carrier state. The virus replicates in the liver and is excreted in bile. The highest concentrations of HAV are found in stools of infected persons during the 2-week period immediately before the onset of jaundice and decline after jaundice appears.[12]Children and infants may shed HAV for longer periods than adults, possibly lasting as long as several weeks after the onset of clinical illness.[13] Chronic shedding of HAV in feces has not been demonstrated, but relapses of hepatitis A can occur in as many as 20% of patients[1,14] and fecal shedding of HAV may recur at this time.[11]

The presence of antibodies to HAV (anti-HAV) confers protection against hepatitis A infection. However, the lowest titer needed to confer protection has not been determined.

In a chimpanzee challenge study, the quality of protection afforded by immune globulin (IG) prepared from initially seronegative human volunteers vaccinated with hepatitis A vaccine was comparable to that afforded by commercial IG. In this experiment chimpanzees immunized with either preparation developed passive-active immunity, when challenged with wild-type HAV. No animal in either group developed clinical illness.

In vitro studies in a randomly selected subset of human subjects (n=80) showed anti-HAV induced by hepatitis A vaccine to have functional activity. This was demonstrated by a neutralization assay and a competitive inhibition assay using a panel of monoclonal antibodies known to have neutralizing activity.

Immunogenicity in Adults: In three clinical studies involving over 400 healthy adult volunteers given a single 1440 EL.U. dose of hepatitis A vaccine, specific humoral antibodies against HAV were elicited in more than 96% of subjects when measured 1 month after vaccination. By day 15, 80% to 98% of vaccines had already seroconverted (anti-HAV ≥20 mIU/ml [the lower limit of antibody measurement by current assay]). Geometric mean titers (GMTs) of seroconverters ranged from 264 to 339 mIU/ml at day 15 and increased to a range of 335 to 637 mIU/ml by 1 month following vaccination.[15]

The GMTs obtained following a single dose of hepatitis A vaccine are at least several times higher than that expected following receipt of IG.

In a clinical study using 2.5 to 5 times the standard dose of IG (standard dose = 0.02 to 0.06 ml/kg), the GMT in recipients was 146 mIU/ml at 5 days post-administration, 77 mIU/ml at month 1 and 63 mIU/ml at month 2.[15]

In two clinical trials in which a booster dose of 1440 EL.U. was given 6 months following the initial dose, 100% of vaccines (n=269) were seropositive 1 month after the booster dose, with GMTs ranging from 3318 mIU/ml to 5925 mIU/ml. The titers obtained from this additional dose approximate those observed several years after natural infection.

In a subset of vaccinees (n=89), a single dose of Havrix 1440 EL.U. elicited specific anti-HAV neutralizing antibodies in more than 94% of vaccinees when measured 1 month after vaccination. These neutralizing antibodies persisted until month 6. One hundred percent of vaccinees had neutralizing antibodies when measured 1 month after a booster dose given at month 6.

Immunogenicity in Children: In six clinical studies involving children (n=762) ranging from 1 to 18 years of age, the GMT following two doses of hepatitis A vaccine 360 EL.U. given 1 month apart ranged from 197 to 660 mIU/ml. Ninety-nine percent of subjects seroconverted following two doses. When a booster (third) dose of hepatitis A vaccine 360 EL.U. was administered 6 months following the initial dose, all subjects were seropositive 1 month following the booster dose with GMTs rising to a range of 3388 to 4643 mIU/ml. In one study in which children were followed for an additional 6 months, all subjects remained seropositive. Solicited adverse effects were similar in frequency and nature to those seen following administration of Engerix-B [Hepatitis B Vaccine (Recombinant)]. Also, hepatitis A vaccine has been found to be highly efficacious in a clinical study of children at high risk of HAV infection (see CLINICAL PHARMACOLOGY, Protective Efficacy).

At present, the duration of protection afforded by hepatitis A vaccine has not been established. Therefore it is unknown if the protection provided to immunized children will last until adulthood.

PROTECTIVE EFFICACY

Protective efficacy with hepatitis A vaccine has been demonstrated in a double-blind, randomized controlled study in school children (age 1 to 16 years) in Thailand who were at high risk of HAV infection. A total of 40,119 children were randomized to be vaccinated with either hepatitis A vaccine 360 EL.U. or Engerix-B at 0, 1, 12 months. 19,037 children received a primary course (0, 1 months) of hepatitis A vaccine and 19,120 children received a primary course (0, 1 months) of Engerix-B. 38,157 children entered surveillance at day 138 and were observed for an additional 8 months. Using the protocol-defined endpoint (≥2 days absence from school, ALT level >45 U/ml, and a positive result in the HAVAB-M test), 32 cases of clinical hepatitis A occurred in the control group; in the hepatitis A vaccine group, two cases were identified. These two cases were mild both in terms of biochemical and clinical indices of hepatitis A disease. Thus the calculated efficacy rate for prevention of clinical hepatitis A was 94% (95% confidence intervals 74% to 98%).[16]

In outbreak investigations occurring in the trial, 26 clinical cases of hepatitis A (of total of 34 occurring in the trial) occurred. No cases occurred in hepatitis A vaccine vaccinees.

Using additional virological and serological analyses post hoc, the efficacy of hepatitis A vaccine was confirmed. Up to three additional cases of very mild clinical illness may have occurred in vaccinees. Using available testing, these illnesses could neither be proven nor disproven to have been caused by HAV. By including these as cases, the calculated efficacy rate for prevention of clinical hepatitis A would be 84% (95% confidence intervals 60% to 94%).

INDICATIONS AND USAGE:

Hepatitis A vaccine is indicated for active immunization of person ≥2 years of age against disease caused by hepatitis A virus (HAV).

Hepatitis A vaccine will not prevent hepatitis caused by other agents such as hepatitis B virus, hepatitis C virus, hepatitis E virus or other pathogens known to infect the liver.

Immunization with Hepatitis A vaccine is indicated for those people desiring protection against hepatitis A. Primary immunization should be completed at least 2 weeks prior to expected exposure to HAV. Individuals who are, or will be, at increased risk of infection by HAV include:

Travelers: Persons traveling to area of higher endemicity for hepatitis A. These areas include, but are not limited to, Africa, Asia (except Japan), the Mediterranean basin, Eastern Europe, the Middle East, Central and South America, Mexico, and parts of the Caribbean. Current CDC advisories should be consulted with regard to specific locales.

Military personnel.

People living in, or relocating to, areas of high endemicity.

INDICATIONS AND USAGE: *(cont'd)*

Certain ethnic and geographic populations that experience cyclic hepatitis A epidemics such as: Native peoples of Alaska and the Americas.

Others:

Persons engaging in high-risk sexual activity (such as men having sex with men)

Residents of a community experiencing an outbreak of hepatitis A

Users of illicit injectable drugs

Although the epidemiology of hepatitis A does not permit the identification of other specific populations at high risk of disease, outbreaks of hepatitis A exposure to hepatitis A virus have been described in a variety of populations in which hepatitis A vaccine may be useful:

Certain institutional workers (*e.g.*, caretakers for the developmentally challenged

Employees of child day-care centers

Laboratory workers who handle live hepatitis A virus

Handlers of primate animals that may be harboring HAV

People exposed to hepatitis A: For those requiring both immediate and long-term protection, heptatitis A vaccine may be administered concomitantly with IG.

CONTRAINDICATIONS:

Hepatitis A vaccine is contraindicated in people with known hypersensitivity to any component of the vaccine.

WARNINGS:

There have been rare reports of anaphylaxis/anaphylactoid reactions following commercial use of the vaccine in other countries. Patients experiencing hypersensitivity reactions after a hepatitis A vaccine injection should not receive further Havrix injections. (See CONTRAINDICATIONS.)

Hepatitis A has a relatively long incubation period (15 to 50 days). Hepatitis A vaccine may not prevent hepatitis A infection in individuals who have an unrecognized hepatitis A infection at the time of vaccination. Additionally, it may not prevent infection in individuals who do not achieve protective antibody titers (although the lowest titer needed to confer protection has not been determined).

PRECAUTIONS:

General: As with any parenteral vaccine, epinephrine should be available for use in case of anaphylaxis or anaphylactoid reaction.

As with any vaccine, administration of hepatitis A vaccine should be delayed, if possible, in people with any febrile illness, except when, in the opinion of the physician, withholding vaccine entails the greater risk.

Hepatitis A vaccine should be administered with caution to people with thrombocytopenia or a bleeding disorder since bleeding may occur following an intramuscular administration to these subjects.

As with any vaccine, if administered to immunosuppressed persons or persons receiving immunosuppressive therapy, the expected immune response may not be obtained.[17]

Care is to be taken by the health-care provider for the safe and effective use of hepatitis A vaccine.

Prior to an injection of any vaccine, all known precautions should be taken to prevent adverse reactions. This includes a review of the patient's history with respect to possible hypersensitivity to the vaccine or similar vaccines.

A separate sterile syringe and needle (for single-dose vial) or a sterile disposable unit (prefilled syringe) must be used for each patient to prevent the transmission of infectious agents from person to person. Needles should not be recapped and should be properly disposed. Special care should be taken to ensure that hepatitis A vaccine is not injected into a blood vessel.

Information for the Patient: Patients, parents or guardians should be fully informed of the benefits and risks of immunization with hepatitis A vaccine.

Hepatitis A vaccine is indicated in a variety of situations (see INDICATIONS AND USAGE.) For persons traveling to endemic or epidemic areas, current CDC advisories should be consulted with regard to specific locales.

Travelers should take all necessary precautions to avoid contact with or ingestion of contaminated food or water.

The duration of immunity following a complete schedule of immunization with Havrix has not been established.

Carcinogenesis, Mutagenesis, and Impairment of Fertility: Hepatitis A vaccine has not been evaluated for its carcinogenic potential, mutagenic potential or potential for impairment of fertility.

Pregnancy Category C: Animal reproduction studies have not been conducted with hepatitis A vaccine. It is also not known whether hepatitis A vaccine can cause fetal harm when administered to a pregnant woman or can affect reproduction capacity. Hepatitis A vaccine should be given to a pregnant woman only if clearly needed.

Nursing Mothers: It is not known whether hepatitis A vaccine is excreted in human milk. Because many drugs are excreted in human milk, caution should be exercised when hepatitis A vaccine is administered to a nursing woman.

Pediatric Use: Hepatitis A vaccine is well tolerated and highly immunogenic and effective in children ≥2 years of age. (See CLINICAL PHARMACOLOGYfor immunogenicity and efficacy data. See DOSAGE AND ADMINISTRATIONfor recommended dosage.)

DRUG INTERACTIONS:

Preliminary results suggest that the concomitant administration of a wide variety of other vaccines is unlikely to interfere with the immune response to hepatitis A vaccine.

As with other intramuscular injections, hepatitis A vaccine should be given with caution to individuals on anticoagulant therapy.

When concomitant administration of other vaccines or IG is required, they should be given with different syringes and at different injection sites.

ADVERSE REACTIONS:

During clinical trials involving more than 31,000 individuals receiving doses ranging from 360 EL.U. to 1440 EL.U. and during extensive postmarketing experience in Europe, hepatitis A vaccine has been generally well tolerated. As with all pharmaceuticals, however, it is possible that expanded commercial use of the vaccine could reveal rare adverse events not observed in clinical studies.

The frequency of solicited adverse events tended to decrease with successive doses of hepatitis A vaccine. Most events reported were considered by the subjects as mild and did not last for more than 24 hours.

ADVERSE REACTIONS: *(cont'd)*

Of solicited adverse events in clinical trials, the most frequently reported by volunteers was injection-site soreness (56% of adults and 21% of children); however, less than 0.5% of soreness was reported as severe. Headache was reported by 14% of adults and less than 9% of children. Other solicited and unsolicited events occurring during clinical trials are listed below:

Incidence 1% to 10% of Injections

Local reactions at injection site: induration, redness, swelling.

Body as a whole: fatigue, fever (>37.5°C), malaise.

Gastrointestinal: anorexia, nausea.

Incidence <1% of Injections

Local reaction at injection site: hematoma.

Dermatologic: pruritus, rash, urticaria.

Respiratory: pharyngitis, other upper respiratory tract infections.

Gastrointestinal: abdominal pain, diarrhea, dysgeusia, vomiting.

Musculoskeletal: arthralgia, elevation of creatine phosphokinase, myalgia.

Hematologic: lymphadenopathy.

Central nervous system: hypertonic episode, insomnia, photophobia, vertigo.

ADDTIONAL SAFETY DATA: Safety data were obtained from two additional sources in which large populations were vaccinated. In an outbreak setting in which 4,930 individuals were immunized with a single dose of either 720 EL.U. or 1440 EL.U. of hepatitis A vaccine, the vaccine was well-tolerated and no serious adverse events due to vaccination were reported. Overall, less than 10% of vaccines reported solicited general adverse events following the vaccine. The most common solicited local adverse event was pain at the injection site, reported in 22.3% of subjects at 24 hours and decreasing to 2.4% by 72 hours.

In a field efficacy trial, 19,037 children received the 360 EL.U. dose of hepatitis A vaccine. The most commonly reported adverse events following administration of hepatitis A vaccine were injection-site pain (9.5%) and tenderness (8.1%), which were reported following first doses of hepatitis A vaccine. Other adverse events were infrequent and comparable to the control vaccine Engerix-B. Additionally, no serious adverse events due to the vaccine were reported. The large trial further allowed for analysis of rare adverse events, including hospitalization and death. No significant differences were found between the cohorts.

Postmarketing Reports: Rare voluntary reports of adverse events in people receiving hepatitis A vaccine that have been reported since market introduction of the vaccine include the following:

Local: localized edema.

While no causal relationship has been established, the following rare events have been reported:

Body as a whole: anaphylaxis/anaphylactoid reactions, somnolence.

Cardiovascular: syncope.

Hepatobiliary: jaundice, hepatitis.

Dermatologic: erythema multiforme, hyperhydrosis, angioedema.

Respiratory: dyspnea.

Hematologic: lymphadenopathy.

Central nervous system: convulsions, encephalopathy, dizziness, neuropathy, myelitis, paresthesia, Guillain-Barre syndrome, multiple sclerosis.

Other: congenital abnormality.

Reporting of Adverse Events: The U.S. Department of Health and Human Services has established the Vaccine Adverse Events Reporting System (VAERS) to accept reports of suspected adverse events after the administration of any vaccine, including, but not limited to, the reporting of events required by the National Childhood Vaccine Injury Act of 1986. The toll-free number for VAERS forms and information is 1- 800-822-7967.[18]

DOSAGE AND ADMINISTRATION:

Hepatitis A vaccine should be administered by intramuscular injection. *Do not inject intravenously, intradermally or subcutaneously.* In adults, the injection should be given in the deltoid region. Hepatitis A vaccine should not be administered in the gluteal region; such injections may result in suboptimal response.

Hepatitis A vaccine may be administered concomitantly with IG, although the ultimate antibody titer obtained is likely to be lower than when the vaccine is given alone. Hepatitis A vaccine has been administered simultaneously with Engerix-B without interference with their respective immune responses.

When concomitant administration of other vaccines or IG is required, they should be given with different syringes and at different injection sites.

Preparation for Administration: Shake vial or syringe well before withdrawal and use. Parenteral drug products should be inspected visually for particulate matter or discoloration prior to administration. With thorough agitation, hepatitis A vaccine is an opaque white suspension. Discard if it appears otherwise.

The vaccine should be used as supplied; no dilution or reconstitution is necessary. The full recommended dose of the vaccine should be used. After removal of the appropriate volume from a single-dose vial, any vaccine remaining in the vial should be discarded.

Primary immunization for adults consists of single dose of 1440 EL.U. in 1 ml. Primary immunization for children and adolescents (2 to 18 years of age) may follow either of these two schedules:

TABLE 1

Group	Dose	Schedule
Children and adolescents (2 through 18 years of age)	Primary course: 360 EL.U./0.5 mL	two doses, given 1 month apart (month 0 and month 1)
	Booster: 360 EL.U./0.5 mL	6 to 12 months after primary course
	OR	
	Primary course: 720 EL.U./0.5 mL	one dose (month 0)
	Booster: 720 EL.U./0.5 mL	6 to 12 months after primary course

Individuals should not be alternated between the 360EL.U. and 720 EL.U. doses. Those who receive an intial 360 EL.U. dose should continue on the 360 EL.U. dosing schedule. Likewise, those individuals who receive a single 720 EL.U. primary dose should receive a 720 EL.U. booster dose.

For all age groups, a booster dose is recommended anytime between 6 and 12 months after the initiation of the primary dose in order to ensure the highest antibody titers.

DOSAGE AND ADMINISTRATION: *(cont'd)*

In those with an impaired immune system, adequate anti-HAV response may not be obtained after the primary immunization course. Such patients may therefore require administration of additional doses of vaccine.

Storage: Store between 2° and 8°C (36° and 47°F). Do not freeze; discard if product has been frozen. Do not dilute to administer.

REFERENCES:

1. Hadler SC: Global impact of hepatitis A virus infection changing patterns. In Hollinger FB, Lemon SM, Margolis H (eds):*Viral Hepatitis and Liver Disease.* Baltimore, Williams & Wilkins, 1991, pp. 14-20. **2.** Dienstag JL, Routenberg JA, Purcell RH, et al: Foodhandler-associated outbreak of hepatitis type A. An immune electron microscopic study. *Ann Intern Med.* 1975;83:647. **3.** Mackowiak PA, Caraway CT, Portnoy BL: Oyster-associated hepatitis. Lessons from the Louisiana experience. *Am J Epidemiol.* 1976;103:181. **4.** Woodson RD, Clinton JJ: Hepatitis prophylaxis abroad. Effectiveness of immune serum globulin in protecting Peace Corps volunteers. *JAMA.* 1969;1009:1053. **5.** Krugman S, Giles JP: Viral hepatitis. New light on an old disease. *JAMA.* 1970;212: 1019. **6.** Mosley JW: Hepatitis types B and non-B. Epidemiologic background. *JAMA.* 1975;233:967. **7.** Hadler SC, Erben JJ, Francis DP, et al: Risk factors for hepatitis A in daycare centers. *J Infect Dis.* 1982;145:255. **8.** Shapiro CN, Shaw SE, Mandel EJ, Hadler SC: Epidemiology of hepatitis A in the United States. In Hollinger FB, Lemon SM, Margolis H (eds): *Viral Hepatitis and Liver Disease.* Baltimore, Williams & Wilkins, 1991, pp. 71-76. **9.** Centers for Disease Control: Protection against viral hepatitis: Recommendations of the Immunization Practices Advisory Committee (ACIP). *MMWR.* 1990;39(No. RR-2):1- 26. **10.** Lemon SM: Type A viral hepatitis: new developments in an old disease. *N. Engl J Med.* Oct. 24, 1985;313(17):1059-1067. **11.** Sjogren MH, Tanno H, Fay O, et al: Hepatitis A virus in stool during clinical relapse. *Ann Intern Med.* 1987;106:221-226. **12.** Hollinger FB, Ticehurst J: Hepatitis A Virus. In Hollinger FB, Robinson WS, Purcell RH, et al (eds): *Viral Hepatitis.* New York, Raven Press, 1990, pp. 1-37. **13.** Tassopoulos NC, Papaevangelou GJ, Ticehurst JR, et al: Fecal excretion of Greek strains of hepatitis A virus in patients with hepatitis A and in experimentally infected chimpanzees. *J Infect Dis.* 1986; 154:231-237. **14.** Chiriaco P, Gaudalupi C, Armigliato MK, et al: Polyphasic course of hepatitis type A in children. *J Infect Dis.*1986; 153:378. **15.** Data on file, SmithKline Beecham Pharmaceuticals. **16.** Innis BL, Snitbhan R, Kunasol P, et al: Protection against hepatitis A by an inactivated vaccine. *JAMA,*1994;271(17):1328-1364. **17.** ACIP: Use of vaccines and immune globulins in persons with altered immunocompetence. *MMWR.*1993;42 (No. RR-4). **18.** Centers for Disease Control; Vaccine Adverse Event Reporting System-United States. *MMWR.* 1990;39:730- 733.(SmithKine Beecham Pharmaceuticals, 2/95, HA: L3A)

HOW SUPPLIED - EQUIVALENTS NOT AVAILABLE:

Injection, Solution - Intramuscular - 360 unit/0.5 ml

0.5 ml	**$18.75**	**HAVRIX, SKB Biols**	**58160-0836-01**

Injection, Solution - Intramuscular - 720 unit/0.5 mL

0.5 mL	$28.45	HAVRIX, SKB Biols	58160-0837-01
0.5 mL	$28.45	HAVRIX, SKB Biols	58160-0837-02

Injection, Solution - Intramuscular - 1440 unit/ml

1 ml	**$54.70**	**HAVRIX, SKB Biols**	**58160-0835-01**
1 ml	**$54.70**	**HAVRIX, SKB Biols**	**58160-0835-02**

HEPATITIS B IMMUNE GLOBULIN *(001429)*

CATEGORIES: Antiserum; Biologicals; Hepatitis B; Immunologic; Serums, Toxoids and Vaccines; Vaccines; Pregnancy Category C; FDA Pre 1938 Drugs

BRAND NAMES: H-Big; **Hep-B-Gammagee**; Hyperhep

DESCRIPTION:

Hepatitis B Immune Globulin (Human)) is a sterile solution of human immunoglobulin (10-18% protein) intended for intramuscular injection. The high levels of antibody to hepatitis B surface antigen (anti-HBs) found in the product are derived from a small group of well-monitored individuals who were hyperimmunized with hepatitis B vaccine. The potency is adjusted by the addition of IgG obtained from large pools of normal plasma. Each unit of plasma was found to be nonreactive when tested for hepatitis B surface antigen (HBsAg) by an FDA approved test. The pooled plasma is processed by and/or Armour Pharmaceutical Company using Cohn cold ethanol fractionation procedures. The product is dissolved in 0.3 molar glycine and contains thimerosal (mercury derivative) 1:10,000 added as a preservative. The solution has a pH of 6.8 ± 0.4 adjusted with hydrochloric acid or sodium hydroxide. Each vial of Hep-B-Gammagee contains anti-HBs equivalent to or exceeding the potency of anti-HBs in a U.S. reference Hepatitis B Immune Globulin (Office of Biologics Research and Review FDA).

There is no evidence to suggest that the causative virus of AIDS (HIV) has been transmitted by Hep-B-Gammagee prepared by the Cohn cold ethanol process.[8]

CLINICAL PHARMACOLOGY:

Hepatitis B immune globulin (human) provides passive immunization for individuals exposed to the hepatitis B virus (HBV) as evidenced by a reduction in the attack rate of hepatitis B following its use.[1-3] The administration of the usual recommended dose of hepatitis B immune globulin (human) generally results in a detectable level of circulating antibody to hepatitis B surface antigen (anti-HBs) which persists for approximately 2 months or longer. Peak serum levels of anti-HBs are seen at 3-7 days after intramuscular administration of hepatitis B immunoglobulin. The half-life of this antibody ranges from 17.5-25 days.[4] The possibility of hepatitis B transmission is remote, as it is with other immune globulins prepared by the cold ethanol process.

INDICATIONS AND USAGE:

Hepatitis B immune globulin (human) is indicated for post-exposure prophylaxis[5] following either parenteral exposure, direct mucous membrane contact, sexual exposure[5] or oral ingestion involving HBsAg-positive materials such as blood, plasma or serum. Such exposures might occur by accidental "needle-stick", accidental splash, or a pipetting accident. Hepatitis B immune globulin (human) is also indicated for post-exposure prophylaxis in infants born to hepatitis B-positive (HBsAg-positive) mothers.

CONTRAINDICATIONS:

Hypersensitivity to any component of the product.

WARNINGS:

Persons with isolated immunoglobulin A deficiency have the potential for developing antibodies to immunoglobulin A and could have anaphylactic reactions to subsequent administration of blood products that contain immunoglobulin A.[6] Therefore, as with any immunoglobulin preparation, hepatitis B immune globulin (human) should be given to such persons only if the expected benefits outweigh the potential risks.

In patients who have severe thrombocytopenia or any coagulation disorder that would contraindicate intramuscular injections, hepatitis B immune globulin (human) should be given only if the expected benefits outweigh the potential risks.

PRECAUTIONS:

GENERAL

Hepatitis B immune globulin (human) should be given with caution to patients with a history of prior systemic allergic reactions following the administration of human immune globulin preparations. Hypersensitivity reactions to injections of immunoglobulin occur rarely. The incidence of these reactions may be increased in patients receiving large intramuscular doses or in patients receiving repeated injections of immunoglobulin.[7]

Hepatitis B immune globulin (human) *must not be administered intravenously* because of the potential for serious reactions. Injections should be made intramuscularly. Care should be taken to draw back on the plunger of the syringe before injection in order to be certain that the needle is not in a blood vessel.

Epinephrine should be available for treatment of acute allergic symptoms.

There is no evidence that the causative virus of AIDS (HIV-1) is transmitted by hepatitis B immune globulin (human) which is prepared by the Cohn cold ethanol process.[8]

Some investigational intravenous immunoglobulin products have been linked to transmission of non-A, non-B hepatitis;[15] however, there have been no reports of this in association with hepatitis B immune globulin (human).

PREGNANCY CATEGORY C

Animal reproduction studies have not been conducted with hepatitis B immune globulin (human). It is also not known whether hepatitis B immune globulin (human) can cause fetal harm when administered to a pregnant woman or can affect reproduction capacity. Hepatitis B immune globulin (human) should be given to a pregnant woman only if clearly needed.

NURSING MOTHERS

It is not known whether this drug is excreted in human milk. Because many drugs are excreted in human milk, caution should be exercised when hepatitis B immune globulin (human) is administered to a nursing woman.

DRUG INTERACTIONS:

Antibodies present in immunoglobulin preparations may interfere with the immune response to live virus vaccines such as measles, mumps, and rubella. Therefore, vaccination with live virus vaccines should be deferred until approximately three months after administration of hepatitis B immune globulin (human). It may be necessary to revaccinate persons who received hepatitis B immune globulin (human) shortly after live virus vaccination.

ADVERSE REACTIONS:

Local pain and tenderness at the injection site, urticaria and angioedema may occur. Anaphylactic reactions, although rare, have been reported following the injection of human immunoglobulin preparations.[6] Anaphylaxis is more likely to occur if hepatitis B immune globulin (human) is given intravenously; therefore, hepatitis B immune globulin (human) must be administered *only* intramuscularly. In highly allergic individuals, repeated injections may lead to anaphylactic shock.[9,10]

OVERDOSAGE:

Although no data are available, clinical experience with other immunoglobulin preparations suggests that the only manifestations would be pain and tenderness at the injection site.

DOSAGE AND ADMINISTRATION:

Parenteral drug products should be inspected visually for particulate matter and discoloration prior to administration, whenever solution and container permit. Hepatitis B immune globulin (human) is a clear, very slightly amber, moderately viscous liquid.

Hepatitis B immune globulin (human) is administered *intramuscularly. It must not be injected intravenously.*

It is important to use a separate sterile syringe and needle for each individual patient to prevent transmission of hepatitis B and other infectious agents from one person to another.

KNOWN OR PRESUMED EXPOSURE TO HBSAG

There are no prospective studies directly testing the efficacy of a combination of hepatitis B immune globulin (human) and hepatitis B vaccine or hepatitis B vaccine (Recombinant) in preventing clinical hepatitis B following percutaneous, ocular or mucous membrane exposure to hepatitis B virus. However, since most persons with such exposures (*e.g.,* health-care workers) are candidates for the hepatitis B vaccine and since combined hepatitis B immune globulin (human) plus vaccine is more efficacious than hepatitis B immune globulin (human) alone in perinatal exposures, the following guidelines are recommended for persons who have been exposed to hepatitis B virus such as through (1) percutaneous (needlestick), ocular, mucous membrane exposure to blood known or presumed to contain HBsAg, (2) human bites by known or presumed HBsAg carriers, that penetrate the skin, or (3) following intimate sexual contact with known or presumed HBsAg carriers:

Recommendations For Adults Who Have Not Been Previously Vaccinated Against Hepatitis B: Hepatitis B immune globulin (human) (0.06 ml/kg) should be given intramuscularly as soon as possible after exposure and within 24 hours if possible. Hepatitis B vaccine (see Heptavax, B (Hepatitis B Vaccine or Recombivax HB (Hepatitis B Vaccine (Recombinant)) circular for appropriate dosage recommendations) should be given intramuscularly within 7 days of exposure and second and third doses given one and six months, respectively, after the first dose.

Recommendations For Adults Who Have Been Previously Vaccinated Against Hepatitis B: Prior recipients of a recommended course of hepatitis B vaccine should have their anti-HBs titer checked promptly. For those with known adequate antibody (10 MIU/ml anti-HBs, approximately equal to 10 SRU) nothing is required. Those with inadequate or unknown titers should receive a dose of hepatitis B immune globulin (human) and a dose of hepatitis B vaccine simultaneously at two different sites as soon as possible.

Dosage for Infants Born of HBsAg Positive Mothers: Infants born to HBsAg positive mothers are at high risk of becoming chronic carriers of hepatitis B virus and of developing the chronic sequelae of hepatitis B virus infection. Well-controlled studies have shown that administration of three 0.5 ml doses of hepatitis B immune globulin (human) starting at birth is 75% effective in preventing establishment of the chronic carrier state in these infants during the first year of life.[11] Protection can be transient, whereupon the effectiveness of the hepatitis B immune globulin (human) would decline thereafter. Results from clinical studies indicate that administration of one 0.5 ml dose of hepatitis B immune globulin (human) at birth and the recommended three doses of Heptavax-B (Hepatitis B Vaccine) or Recombivax HB (Hepatitis B Vaccine (Recombinant)) (TABLE 1), were effective in preventing establishment of the chronic carrier state in infants born to HBsAg and HBeAg positive mothers.[3,12,13,14]

Testing for HBsAg and anti-HBs is recommended at 12-15 months of age. If HBsAg is not detectable, and anti-HBs is present, the child has been protected.[5]

The recommended dosage for infants born to HBsAg positive mothers can be found in TABLE 1.

STORAGE

Store at 2-8°C (36-46°F). Do not freeze. Do not use after expiration date.

TABLE 1

	Birth	Within 7 days	1 month	6 months
Hepatitis B Vaccine**		0.5 ml*	0.5 ml	0.5 ml
Hepatitis B Immune Globulin (Human)	0.5 ml	-	-	-

* The first dose of hepatitis B vaccine may be given at birth at the same time as Hepatitis B Immune Globulin (Human); but should be administered in the opposite anterolateral thigh.
** See DOSAGE AND ADMINISTRATIONsection of Hepatitis B Vaccine or Hepatitis B Vaccine (Recombinant).

REFERENCES:

1. Seeff, L. B.; Hoofnagle, J. H.: Immunoprophylaxis of viral hepatitis, Gastroenterology *77:*161-182, 1979. **2.** Seeff. L. B.; Wright, E. C.; Zimmerman, H. J.; et al: Type B hepatitis after needle-stick exposure: Prevention with hepatitis B immune globulin — Final report of the Veterans Administration Cooperative Study, Ann. Int. Med. *88:* 285-293, 1978. **3.** Beasley, R. P.; Lin, C. C.; Wang, K. Y.; Hsieh, F. J.; Hwang, L. Y.; Stevens, C. E.; Sun, T. S.; Szmuness, W.: Hepatitis B immune globulin (HBIG) efficacy in the interruption of perinatal transmission of hepatitis B virus carrier state, Lancet *2* (8243): 388-393, Aug. 22, 1981. **4.** Scheiermann, N.; Kuwert, E. K.: Absorption and Elimination of Hepatitis-B immune globulin after intramuscular application, Dtsch. Med. Wochenschr. *107* (50): 1918-1922, Dec. 17, 1982 (German). **5.** Centers for Disease Control: Recommendations for protection against viral hepatitis. MMWR *34* (22): 313-335, June 7, 1985. **6.** Fudenberg, H. H.: Sensitization to immunoglobulins and hazards of gamma globulin therapy, in Immunoglobulins. Biologic Aspects and Clinical Uses. Edited by Ezio Merler, National Academy of Sciences, Washington, D. C., 1970, pp. 211-220. **7.** Bruhl, H. H.: Adverse reaction to large doses of human immune serum globulin (ISG). Clinical observations, Minn. Med. *60* (9): 673-676, Sept. 1977. **8.** Zuck, T. F.; Preston, M. S.; Tankersley, D. L.; Wells, M. A.; Wittck, A. E.; Epstein, J. E.; Daniel, S., Phelan, M.; and Quinnan, G. V.: N. Eng. J. Med. *314* (22): 1454-1455, May 1986. **9.** Owings, W. J.: Hypersensitivity to gamma globulin. A case report, J. Med. Ass. Alabama *23:* 74, Sept. 1953. **10.** Baybutt, J. E.: Hypersensitivity to immune serum globulin. Report of a case, J. Amer. Med. Ass. *171:*415, Sept. 26, 1959. **11.** Beasley, R. P., Hwang, L.; Stevens, C. E.; Lin, C.; Hsieh, F.; Wang, K.; Sun, T.; Szmuness, W.: Efficacy of Hepatitis B Immune Globulin for Prevention of Perinatal Transmission of the Hepatitis B Virus Carrier State: Final Report of a Randomized Double-Blind, Placebo-Controlled Trial, Hepatology *3:* 135-141, 1983. **12.** Beasley, R. P.; Hwang, L.; Lee, G. C.; Lan, C., Roan, C.; Hwang, F.; Chen, C.: Prevention of Perinatally Transmitted Hepatitis B Virus infections with Hepatitis B Immune Globulin and Hepatitis B Vaccine, Lancet ii: 1099-1102, November 12, 1983. **13.** Stevens, C. E.: Taylor, P. E.; Tong, M. J.; Toy, P. T.; Vyas, G. N.: Hepatitis B Vaccine: an Overview, In Viral Hepatitis and Liver Disease, Vyas, G. N., Deinstag, J. L., Hoofnagle, J. H. (eds); Grune & Stratton Inc., 275-291, 1984. **14.** Stevens, C. E.; Toy, P. T.; Long, M. J.; Taylor P. E.; Vyas, G. N.; Nair, P. V.; Gudavalli, M.; Krugman, S.: Perinatal hepatitis B virus transmission in the United States, JAMA; *253* (12): 1740-1745, 1985. **15.** Lever, A.M.L., et al.: Non-A, Non-B hepatitis occurring in agammaglobulinemic patients after intravenous immunoglobulin, The Lancet: 1062-1064, November 10, 1984.

HOW SUPPLIED - EQUIVALENTS NOT AVAILABLE:

Injection, Solution - Intramuscular

0.5 ml	$43.75	Hyperhep, Bayer Pharm	00192-0616-00
0.5 ml	$56.25	H-BIG, N Am Biologicals	59730-0399-11
1 ml	$56.25	H-BIG, N Am Biologicals	59730-0399-01
1 ml	$93.75	Hyperhep, Bayer Pharm	00192-0616-01

Injection, Solution - Intramuscular - 1 unit/vial

5 ml	**$393.84**	**HEP-B-GAMMAGEE, Merck**	**00006-4692-00**

Injection, Solution - Intramuscular

5 ml	$212.50	H-BIG, N Am Biologicals	59730-0399-05
5 ml	$343.75	Hyperhep, Bayer Pharm	00192-0616-05

HEPATITIS B VACCINE, RECOMBINANT

(001431)

CATEGORIES: Biologicals; Hepatitis B; Immunologic; Serums, Toxoids and Vaccines; Vaccines; Pregnancy Category C; Recombinant DNA Origin; Sales > $500 Million; FDA Approved 1986 Jul

BRAND NAMES: Engerix-B; Recombivax Hb; **Recombivax-HB**

COST OF THERAPY: $85.57 (Vaccination; Injection; 10 mcg/ml; 1/day; 3 days)

DESCRIPTION:

Recombivax B: Hepatitis B Vaccine (Recombinant) is a noninfectious subunit viral vaccine derived from hepatitis B surface antigen (HBsAg) produced in yeast cells. A portion of the hepatitis B virus gene, coding for HBsAg, is cloned into yeast, and the vaccine for hepatitis B is produced from cultures of this recombinant yeast strain according to methods developed in the Merck Sharp & Dohme Research Laboratories.

The antigen is harvested and purified from fermentation cultures of a recombinant strain of the yeast *Saccharomyces cerevisiae* containing the gene for the *adw* subtype of HBsAg. The HBsAg protein is released from the yeast cells by cell disruption and purified by a series of physical and chemical methods. The vaccine contains no detectable yeast DNA but may contain not more than 1% yeast protein. The vaccine produced by the Merck method has been shown to be comparable to the plasma-derived vaccine in terms of animal potency (mouse, monkey, and chimpanzee) and protective efficacy (chimpanzee and human).

The vaccine against hepatitis B, prepared from recombinant yeast cultures, is free of association with human blood or blood products.

Each lot of hepatitis B vaccine is tested for safety, in mice and guinea pigs, and for sterility.

Recombivax HB is a sterile suspension for intramuscular injection. However, for persons at risk of hemorrhage following intramuscular injection, the vaccine may be administered subcutaneously (see DOSAGE AND ADMINISTRATION).

Hepatitis B Vaccine (Recombinant), is supplied in two dosage strengths.

Recombivax HB (Hepatitis B Vaccine (Recombinant)) contains 10 mcg of HBsAg/ml. Each 1 ml dose of Recombivax HB contains 10 mcg of hepatitis B surface antigen adsorbed onto approximately 0.5 mg of aluminum provided as aluminum hydroxide; each 0.5 ml dose contains 5 mcg of hepatitis B surface antigen adsorbed onto approximately 0.25 mg of aluminum provided as aluminum hydroxide; and each 0.25 ml dose contains 2.5 mcg of hepatitis B surface antigen adsorbed onto approximately 0.125 mg of aluminum provided as aluminum hydroxide.

Recombivax HB (Hepatitis B Vaccine (Recombinant)) Dialysis Formulation is a sterile suspension for intramuscular injection. Recombivax HB Dialysis Formulation contains 40 mcg of HBsAg/ml. Each 1 ml dose of Recombivax HB Dialysis Formulation contains 40 mcg of hepatitis B surface antigen adsorbed onto approximately 0.5 mg of aluminum provided as aluminum hydroxide.

Both dosage strengths contain thimerosal (mercury derivative) 1:20,000 added as a preservative and have been treated with formaldehyde prior to adsorption onto aluminum hydroxide. The vaccine is of the *adw* subtype. Recombivax HB is indicated for vaccination of persons at risk of infection from hepatitis B virus including all known subtypes. Recombivax HB Dialysis Formulation is indicated for vaccination of adult predialysis and dialysis patients against infection caused by all known subtypes of hepatitis B virus.

Engerix-B: Hepatitis B Vaccine (Recombinant) is a noninfectious recombinant DNA hepatitis B vaccine developed and manufactured by SmithKline Beecham Biologicals. It contains purified surface antigen of the virus obtained by culturing genetically engineered *Saccharomyces cerevisiae* cells, which carry the surface antigen gene of the hepatitis B virus. The

DESCRIPTION: *(cont'd)*

surface antigen expressed in *Saccharomyces cerevisiae* cells is purified by several physiochemical steps and formulated as a suspension of the antigen absorbed on aluminum hydrochloride. The procedures used to manufacture Engerix-B result in a product that contains no more than 5% yeast protein.

No substances of human origin are used its manufacture.

Engerix-B is supplied as a sterile suspension for IM administration. The vaccine is ready for use without reconstitution; it must be shaken before administration since a fine white deposit with a clear colorless supernatant may form on storage.

Each 1 ml of adult dose of vaccine consists of 20 mcg of hepatitis B surface antigen absorbed on 0.5 mg aluminum as aluminum HCl. Each 0.5 ml pediatric dose of vaccine consists of 10 mcg of hepatitis B surface antigen absorbed on 0.25 mg aluminum as aluminum HCl. Both formulations contain 1:20,000 thimerosal (mercury derivative) as a preservative, sodium chloride (9 mg/ml) and phosphate buffers (disodium phosphate dihydrate, 0.98 mg/ml; sodium dihydrogen phosphate dihydrate, 0.71 mg/ml).

CLINICAL PHARMACOLOGY:

Hepatitis B virus is one of at least three hepatitis viruses that cause a systemic infection, with a major pathology in the liver. The others are hepatitis A virus, and non-A, non-B hepatitis viruses.

Hepatitis B virus is an important cause of viral hepatitis. There is no specific treatment for this disease. The incubation period for hepatitis B is relatively long; six weeks to six months may elapse between exposure and the onset of clinical symptoms. The prognosis following infection with hepatitis B virus is variable and dependent on at least three factors: (1) Age—Infants and younger children usually experience milder initial disease than older persons;[1] (2) Dose of Virus—The higher the dose, the more likely acute icteric hepatitis B will result;[1] and, (3) Severity of associated underlying disease—underlying malignancy or pre-existing hepatic disease predisposes to increased mortality and morbidity.[1]

Persistence of viral infection (the chronic hepatitis B Virus carrier state) occurs in 5-10% of persons following acute hepatitis B, and occurs more frequently after initial anicteric hepatitis B than after initial icteric disease. Consequently, carriers of hepatitis B surface antigen (HBsAg) frequently give no history of having had recognized acute hepatitis. It has been estimated that more than 170 million people in the world today are persistently infected with hepatitis B virus.[1] The Centers for Disease Control (CDC) estimates that there are approximately 0.75 to 1 million chronic carriers of hepatitis B virus in the USA.[2] Chronic carriers represent the largest human reservoir of hepatitis B virus.

The serious complications and sequelae of hepatitis B virus infection include massive hepatic necrosis, cirrhosis of the liver, chronic active hepatitis, and hepatocellular carcinoma. Chronic carriers of HBsAg appear to be at increased risk of developing hepatocellular carcinoma. Although a number of etiologic factors are associated with development of hepatocellular carcinoma, the single most important etiologic factor appears to be active infection with the hepatitis B virus.[2]

There is also evidence that several diseases other than hepatitis have been associated with hepatitis B virus infection through an immunologic mechanism involving antigen-antibody complexes. Such diseases include a syndrome with rash, urticaria, and arthralgia resembling serum sickness; periarteritis nodosa; membranous glomerulonephritis; and infantile papular acrodermatitis.

Although the vehicles for transmission of the virus are often blood and blood products, viral antigen has also been found in tears, saliva, breast milk, urine, semen and vaginal secretions. Hepatitis B virus is capable of surviving for days on environmental surfaces exposed to body fluids containing hepatitis B virus. Infection may occur when hepatitis B virus, transmitted by infected body fluids, is implanted via mucous surfaces or percutaneously introduced through accidental or deliberate breaks in the skin.

Transmission of hepatitis B virus infection is often associated with close interpersonal contact with an infected individual and with crowded living conditions. In such circumstances, transmission by inoculation via routes other than overt percutaneous ones may be quite common.[1]Perinatal transmission of hepatitis B infection from infected mother to child at or shortly after birth, can occur if the mother is a hepatitis B surface antigen (HBsAg) carrier or if the mother has an acute hepatitis B infection in the third trimester. Infection in infancy by the hepatitis B virus usually leads to the chronic carrier state. Among infants born to women whose sera are positive for both the hepatitis B and surface antigen and the e antigen, 85-90% are infected and become chronic carriers.[3,4]Well-controlled studies have shown that administration of three 0.5 ml doses of Hepatitis B Immune Globulin (Human) starting at birth is 75% effective in preventing establishment of the chronic carrier state in these infants during the first year of life.[4] However, the protective effect of Hepatitis B Immune Globulin (Human) is transient.

Hepatitis B is endemic throughout the world and is a serious medical problem in population groups at increased risk. (Refer to INDICATIONS AND USAGE.)

Numerous epidemiological studies have shown that persons who develop anti-HBs following active infection with the hepatitis B virus are protected against the disease on re-exposure to the virus.

CLINICAL STUDIES:

Clinical studies have established that Recombivax HB when injected into the deltoid muscle induced protective levels of antibody in 96% of 1213 healthy adults who received the recommended 3-dose regimen. Antibody responses varied with age; a protective level of antibody was induced in 98% of 787 young adults 20-29 years of age, 94% of 249 adults 30-39 years of age and in 89% of 177 adults ≥40 years of age.[14] Studies with Hepatitis B vaccine derived from plasma have shown that a lower response rate (81%) to vaccine may be obtained if the vaccine is administered as a buttock injection.[5] Seroconversion rates and geometric mean antibody titers were measured 1 to 2 months after the 3rd dose. A protective antibody (anti-HBs) level has been defined as 1) 10 or more sample ratio units (SRU) as determined by radioimmunoassay or 2) a positive result as determined by enzyme immunoassay.[2] Note: 10 SRU is comparable to 10 mIU/ml of antibody.[7]

Recombivax HB is highly immunogenic in younger individuals. In clinical studies, 99% of 94 infants under 1 year of age born of non-carrier mothers, 96% of 48 children 1-10 years of age, and 99% of 112 children and adolescents 11-19 years of age developed a protective level of antibody following the recommended 3-dose regimen of vaccine (see DOSAGE AND ADMINISTRATION).

The protective efficacy of three 5 mcg doses of Recombivax HB has been demonstrated in neonates born of mothers positive for both HBsAg and HBeAg (a core-associated antigenic complex which correlates with high infectivity). In a clinical study of infants who received one dose of Hepatitis B Immune Globulin at birth followed by the recommended three dose regimen of Recombivax HB, chronic infection had not occurred in 96% of 130 infants after nine months of follow up.[13] The estimated efficacy in prevention of chronic hepatitis B infection was 95% as compared to the infection rate in untreated historical controls.[15] Significantly fewer neonates became chronically infected when given one dose of Hepatitis B Immune Globulin at birth followed by the recommended three dose regimen of Recombivax

CLINICAL STUDIES: *(cont'd)*

HB when compared to historical controls who received only a single dose of Hepatitis B Immune Globulin.[4] Testing for HBsAg and anti-HBs is recommended at 12 - 15 months of age. If HBsAg is not detectable, and anti-HBs is present, the child has been protected.

As demonstrated in the above study, Hepatitis B Immune Globulin, when administered simultaneously with Recombivax HB at separate body sites, did not interfere with the induction of protective antibodies against hepatitis B virus elicited by the vaccine.

Predialysis and Dialysis Patients: Predialysis and dialysis adult patients respond less well to hepatitis B vaccines than do healthy individuals. In addition, the responses to these vaccines may be lower if the vaccine is administered as a buttock injection. When 40 mcg of Hepatitis B Vaccine (Recombinant), was administered in the deltoid muscle, 89% of 28 participants developed anti-HBs with 86% achieving levels ≥10 mIU/ml. However, when the same dosage of this vaccine was administered inappropriately either in the buttock or a combination of buttock and deltoid, 62% of 47 participants developed anti-HBs with 55% achieving levels of ≥10 mIU/ml.[14]

The duration of protective effect of Recombivax HB is unknown at present, and the need for booster doses is not yet defined. However, a booster dose or revaccination with Recombivax HB Dialysis Formulation may be considered in predialysis/dialysis patients if the anti-HBs level is less than 10 mIU/ml 1 to 2 months after the 3rd dose.[16]

Reports in the literature describe a more virulent form of hepatitis B associated with superinfections or coinfections by delta virus, an incomplete RNA virus. Delta virus can only infect and cause illness in persons infected with hepatitis B virus since the delta agent requires a coat of HBsAg in order to become infectious. Therefore, persons immune to hepatitis B virus infection should also be immune to delta virus infection.[2]

Interchangeability of Plasma-Derived and Recombinant Hepatitis B Vaccines: Recombinant-derived vaccine is produced in yeast by the hepatitis B virus gene which codes for the hepatitis B surface antigen (HBsAg). Like plasma-derived vaccine, recombinant-derived vaccine is a protein aggregate or particle visible by electron microscopy containing important vaccine antigen epitopes as determined by monoclonal antibody analyses.[8]

Recombinant-derived vaccine has been shown by *in vitro* analyses to induce antibodies (anti-HBs) which are biochemically and immunologically comparable by extent of binding, and both avidity and affinity of binding to virus-derived antigen, to antibodies induced by plasma-derived vaccine. In cross absorption studies, the spectra of antibodies induced in man to plasma-derived or to recombinant hepatitis B vaccines were indistinguishable.[8,9]

The recommended doses of Heptavax-B (Hepatitis B Vaccine) and Recombivax HB have resulted in similar seroconversion rates in healthy persons; the geometric mean titers (GMTs) following Recombivax HB have been lower in some studies and equivalent in others but were many times greater than the minimum level associated with protection (≥10 mIU/ml).[6,10,11,12] A single injection of the recommended dose of Recombivax HB induced significant anamnestic antibody responses in 97% of 31 healthy adults vaccinated 5 to 7 years previously with Heptavax-B (Hepatitis B Vaccine).[6]

There have been no clinical studies in which a three-dose vaccine series was initiated with Heptavax-B (Hepatitis B Vaccine) and completed with Recombivax HB, or vice versa. However, based on the comparability of the plasma-derived and recombinant-derived vaccines in extensive *in vitro* and *in vivo* studies as described above, it is possible to interchange the use of these two vaccines (but see CONTRAINDICATIONS).

Several hepatitis viruses are known to cause a systemic infection resulting in major pathologic changes in the liver (*e.g.,* A,B,C,D,E). The estimated lifetime risk of HBV infection in the U.S varies from almost 100% for the highest-risk groups to approximately 5% for the population as a whole.[1]

Hepatitis B infection can have serious consequences including acute massive hepatic necrosis, chronic active hepatitis and cirrhosis of the liver. Sixty to 80% of neonates and 6 to 10% of adults who are infected in the United States will become hepatitis B carriers.[1] It has been estimated that more than 170 million people in the world today are persistently infected with hepatitis B virus.[2] The Centers for Disease Control (CDC) estimates that there are approximately 0.75 to 1.0 million chronic carriers of hepatitis B virus in the United States.[1] Those patients who become chronic carriers can infect others and are at increased risk of developing primary hepatocellular carcinoma. Among other factors, infection with hepatitis B may be the single most important factor for the development of this carcinoma.[1,3] Considering the serious consequences of infection, immunization should be considered for all persons at potential risk of exposure to the hepatitis B virus.

Mothers infected with hepatitis B virus can infect their infants at, or shortly after, birth if they are carriers of the HBsAg antigen or develop an active infection during the third trimester of pregnancy. Infected infants usually become chronic carriers. Therefore, screening of pregnant women for hepatitis B is recommended.[4,5]

Because a vaccination strategy limited to high-risk individuals has failed to substantially lower the overall incidence of hepatis B infection, both the Immunization Practices Advisory Committee (ACIP) and the Committee on Infectious Diseases of the American Academy of Pediatrics (AAP) have endorsed universal infant immunization as part of a comprehensive strategy for the control of hepatitis B infection.[4,5] These advisory groups further recommend broad-based vaccination of adolescents. The ACIP encourages universal hepatis B vaccination of adolescents in communities where use of illicit injectable drugs, pregnancy among teenagers, and/or sexually transmitted diseases are common.[4] Similarly, the AAP recommends that universal immunization of all adolescents should be implemented when resources permit with emphasis on those individuals in high-risk settings.[5] (See INDICATIONS AND USAGE.)

There is no specific treatment for acute hepatitis B infection. However, those who develop anti-HBs antibodies after active infection are usually protected against subsequent infection.

Antibody titers ≥10 mIU/ml against HBsAg are recognized as conferring protection against hepatitis B[6]. Seroconversion is usually defined as antibody titers ≥1 mIU/ml.

Immunogenicity in Healthy Adults and Adolescents: Clinical trials in healthy adult and adolescent subjects have shown that following a course of three doses of 20 mcg Engerix-Bgiven according to the Immunization Practices Advisory Committee (ACIP) recommended schedule of injections at months 0,1, and 6, the seroprotection (antibody titers ≥10 mIU/ml) rate for all individuals was 79% at month 6 and 96% at month 7; the geometric mean antibody titer (GMT) for seroconverters at month 7 was 2,204 mIU/ml. On an alternate schedule (injections at months 0,1 and 2) designed for certain populations (eg., neonates born of hepatitis B infected mothers, individuals who have or might have been recently exposed to the virus, and certain travelers to high-risk areas — see INDICATIONS AND USAGE), 99% of all individuals were seroprotected at month 3 and remained protected through month 12. On the alternate schedule, an additional dose at 12 months produced a GMT for seroconverters at month 13 of 9,163 mIU/ml.

Immunogenicity in Adolescents: In clinical trials with healthy adolescent subjects 11 through 19 years of age, immunization with 10 mcg using a 0,1,6-month schedule produced a seroprotection rate of 97% at months 8 (N=119) with a GMT of 1,989 mIU/ml (N=118, 95% confidence intervals=1,318-3,020). Immunization with 20 mcg using a 0, 1, 6-month schedule produced a seroprotection rate of 99% at month 8 (N=122) with a GMT of 7,672 mIU/ml (N=122, 95% confidence intervals=5,248-10,965).

CLINICAL STUDIES: *(cont'd)*

Immunogenicity in Neonates: Immunization with 10 mcg at 0,1, and 2 months of age produced a seroprotection rate of 96% in infants by month 4, with a GMT among seroconverters of 210 mIU/ml (N=311); an additional dose at month 12 produced a GMT among seroconverters of 2,941 mIU/ml at month 13 (N=126).

Immunization with 10 mcg at 0,1, and 6 months of age produced seroconversion in 100% of infants by month 7 with a GMT of 713 mIU/ml (N=52), and the seroprotection rate was 97%.

Clinical trials indicate that administration of hepatitis B immune globulin at birth does not alter response to Engerix-B.

Immunogenicity in Children: In clinical trials with 242 children ages 6 months to, and including, 10 years given 10 mcg at months 0,1 and 6, the seroprotection rate was 98% one to two months after the third dose; the GMT of seroconverters was 4,023 mIU/ml.

Immunogenicity in Older Subjects: Among older subjects given 20 mcg at months 0,1, and 6, the seroprotection rate one month after the third dose was 88%. However, as with other hepatitis B vaccines, in adults over 40 years of age, Engerix-B vaccine produced anti-HBs titers that were lower than those in younger adults (GMT among seroconverters one month after the third 20 mcg dose with a 0,1, 6-month schedule; 610 mIU/ml for individuals over 40 years of age, N=50).

Hemodialysis Patients: Hemodialysis patients given hepatitis B vaccines respond with lower titers[7], which remain at protective levels for shorter durations than in normal subjects. In a study in which patients on chronic hemodialysis (mean time on dialysis was 24 months; N=562) received 40 mcg of the plasma derived vaccine at months 0,1, and 6 approximately 50% of patients achieved antibody titers ≥10 mIU/ml[7].

Since a fourth dose of Engerix-B given to healthy adults at month 12 following the 0,1,2 month schedule resulted in a substantial increase in the GMT (see Immunogenicity in Healthy Adults and Adolescents above), a four-dose regimen was studied in hemodialysis patients. In a clinical trial of adults who had been on hemodialysis for a mean of 56 months (N=43), 67% of patients were seroprotected two months after the last dose of 40 mcg of Engerix-B (two x 20 mcg) given on a 0,1,2,6-month schedule; the GMT among seroconverters was 93 mIU/ml.

Protective Efficacy: Protective efficacy withEngerix-B has been demonstrated in a clinical trial in neonates at high risk of hepatitis B infection.[8,9] Fifty-eight neonates born of mothers who were both HBsAg and HBeAG positive, were givenEngerix-B (10 mcg at 0,1, and 2 months) without concomitant hepatitis B immune globulin. Two infants became chronic carriers in the 12 month follow-up period after initial inoculation. Assuming an expected carrier rate of 70%[1], the protective efficacy rate against the chronic carrier state during the first 12 months of life was 95%.

Other Clinical Studies: In one study[10], four of 244 (1.6%) adults (homosexual men) at high risk of contracting hepatitis B virus became infected during the period prior to completion of three doses of Engerix-B (20 mcg at 0,1 and 6 months). No additional patients became infected during the 18 month follow-up period after the completion of the immunization course.

Interchangeability of Other Hepatitis B Vaccines: Recombinant DNA vaccines are produced in yeast by expression of a hepatitis B virus gene sequence that codes for the hepatitis B surface antigen. Like plasma-derived vaccine, the yeast derived vaccines are protein particles visible by electron microscopy and have hepatitis B surface antigen epitopes as determined by monoclonal antibody analyses. Yeast-derived vaccines have been shown by *in vitro* analyses to induce antibodies (anti-HBs) which are immunologically comparable by epitope specificity and binding affinity to antibodies induced by plasma-derived vaccine[11]. In cross absorption studies, no differences were detected in the spectra of the antibodies induced in man to plasma-derived or to yeast-derived hepatitis B vaccines[11].

Additionally, patients immunized approximately three years previously with plasma-derived vaccine and whose antibody titers were <100 mIU/ml (GMT: 35 mIU/ml; range: 9-94) were given a 20 mcg of Engerix-B. All patients, including two who had not responded to the plasma-derived vaccine, showed a response to Engerix-B (GMT: 5,069 mIU/ml; range: 624-15,019). There have been no clinical studies in which a three-day dose vaccine series was initiated with a plasma-derived hepatitis B vaccine and completed with Engerix-B, or vise-versa. However, because the *in vitro* and *in vivo* studies described above indicate the comparability of the antibody produced in response to plasma-derived vaccine and Engerix-B, it should be possible to interchange the use of Engerix-B plasma derived vaccines (but see CONTRAINDICATIONS).

A controlled study (N=48) demonstrated that completion of a course of immunization with one dose of Engerix-B (20 mcg, month 6) following two doses of Recombivax HB* (10 mcg, months 0 and 1) produced a similar GMT (4,077 mIU/ml) to immunization with three doses of Recombivax HB (10 mcg, months 0 and 1) produced a similar GMT (4,077 mIU/ml) to immunization with three doses of Recombivax HB (10 mcg, months 0,1, and 6; 2,654 mIU/ml). Thus, Engerix-B can be used to complete a vaccination initiated with Recombivax HB.

INDICATIONS AND USAGE:

RECOMBIVAX HB

Recombivax HB is indicated for vaccination against infection caused by all known subtypes of hepatitis B virus. **Recombivax HB Dialysis Formulation** is indicated for vaccination of adult predialysis and dialysis patients against infection caused by all known subtypes of hepatitis B virus.

Vaccination with Recombivax HB is recommended in persons of all ages, who are or will be at increased risk of infection with hepatitis B virus.[2] In areas with high prevalence of infection, most of the population are at risk of acquiring hepatitis B infection at a young age. Therefore, vaccination should be targeted to prevent such transmission in areas of low prevalence, vaccination should be limited to those who are in groups identified as being at increased risk of infection, for example:

Health Care Personnel:

Dentists and oral surgeons.

Physicians and surgeons.

Nurses.

Paramedical personnel and custodial staff who may be exposed to the virus via blood or other patient specimens.

Dental hygienists and dental nurses.

Laboratory personnel handling blood, blood products, and other patient specimens.

Dental, medical and nursing students.

Selected Patients and Patient Contacts:

Staff in hemodialysis units and hematology/oncology units.

Patients requiring frequent and/or large volume blood transfusions or clotting factor concentrates (*e.g.,* persons with hemophilia, thalassemia).

Clients (residents) and staff of institutions for the mentally handicapped.

Classroom contacts of deinstitutionalized mentally handicapped persons who have persistent hepatitis B surface antigenemia and who show aggressive behavior.

INDICATIONS AND USAGE: *(cont'd)*

Household and other intimate contacts of persons with persistent hepatitis B surface antigenemia.

Infants Born to HBsAg Positive Mothers whether HBeAg positive or negative (see DOSAGE AND ADMINISTRATION)

Adolescents (see CLINICAL PHARMACOLOGY.)

Sub-populations with a known high incidence of the disease, such as:

Alaskan Eskimos.

Indochinese refugees.

Haitian refugees.

Military Personnel identified as being at increased risk

Morticians and Embalmers

Blood bank and plasma fractionation workers

Persons at increased risk of the disease due to their sexual practices, such as:

Persons who have heterosexual activity with multiple partners.

Persons who repeatedly contract sexually transmitted diseases.

Homosexually active males.

Prostitutes.

Prisoners

Users Of Illicit Injectable Drugs: Neither dosage strength will prevent hepatitis caused by other agents, such as hepatitis A virus, non-A, non-B hepatitis viruses, or other viruses known to infect the liver.

Others: Police and fire department personnel who render first aid or medical assistance, and any others who, through their work or personal life-style, may be exposed to the hepatitis B virus.

Adoptees from countries of high HBV endemicity.

Use with Other Vaccines: The Immunization Practices Advisory Committee states that, in general, simultaneous administration of certain live and inactivated pediatric vaccines has not resulted in impaired antibody responses or increased rates of adverse reactions.[17] Separate sites and syringes should be used for simultaneous administration of injectable vaccines.

Revaccination: See CLINICAL PHARMACOLOGY.

ENGERIX-B

Engerix-B is indicated for immunization against infection caused by all known subtypes of hepatitis B virus. As hepatitis D (caused by the delta virus) does not occur in the absence of hepatitis B infection, it can be expected that hepatitis D will also be prevented by Engerix-B vaccination.

Engerix-B will not prevent hepatitis caused by other agents, such as A,C, and E viruses, or other pathogens known to infect the liver.

Immunization is recommended in persons of all ages, especially those who are, or will be, at increased risk of exposure to hepatitis B virus[1] (please see above list under Recombivax HB)

CONTRAINDICATIONS:

Hypersensitivity to yeast or any component of the vaccine.

WARNINGS:

Patients who develop symptoms suggestive of hypersensitivity after an injection should not receive further injections of the vaccine (see CONTRAINDICATIONS).

Because of the long incubation period for hepatitis B, it is possible for unrecognized infection to be present at the time the vaccine is given. The vaccine may not prevent hepatitis B in such patients.

PRECAUTIONS:

GENERAL

As with any percutaneous vaccine, epinephrine should be available for immediate use should an anaphylactoid reaction occur.

Any serious active infection is reason for delaying use of the vaccine except when in the opinion of the physician, withholding the vaccine entails a greater risk.

Caution and appropriate care should be exercised in administering the vaccine to individuals with severely compromised cardiopulmonary status or to others in whom a febrile or systemic reaction could pose a significant risk.

PREGNANCY CATEGORY C

Animal reproduction studies have not been conducted with the vaccine. It is also not known whether the vaccine can cause fetal harm when administered to a pregnant woman or can affect reproduction capacity. The vaccine should be given to a pregnant woman only if clearly needed.

NURSING MOTHERS

It is not known whether the vaccine is excreted in human milk. Because many drugs are excreted in human milk, cautions should be exercised when the vaccine is administered to a nursing woman.

PEDIATRIC USE

Recombivax HB and Engerix-B has been shown to be usually well-tolerated and highly immunogenic in infants and children of all ages. Newborns also respond well; maternally transferred antibodies do not interfere with the active immune response to the vaccine. See DOSAGE AND ADMINISTRATION for recommended pediatric dosage and for recommended dosage for infants born to HBsAg positive mothers.

The safety and effectiveness of Recombivax HB Dialysis Formulation in children have not been established.

ADVERSE REACTIONS:

RECOMBIVAX HB

Recombivax HB and Recombivax HB Dialysis Formulation are generally well-tolerated. No serious adverse reactions attributable to the vaccine have been reported during the course of clinical trials. No adverse experiences were reported during clinical trials which could be related to changes in the titers of antibodies to yeast. As with any vaccine, there is the possibility that broad use of the vaccine could reveal adverse reactions not observed in clinical trials.

In a group of studies, 3258 doses of Recombivax HB were administered to 1252 healthy adults who were monitored for 5 days after each dose. Injection site and systemic complaints were reported following 17% and 15% of the injections, respectively. The following adverse reactions were reported:

Incidence Equal to or Greater Than 1% of Injections

Local Reaction (Injection Site): Injection site reactions consisting principally of soreness and including pain, tenderness, pruritus, erythema, ecchymosis, swelling, warmth, and nodule formation.

ADVERSE REACTIONS: *(cont'd)*

Body as a Whole: The most frequent systemic complaints include fatigue/weakness; headache, fever (≥100 F); and malaise.

Digestive System: Nausea; and diarrhea

Respiratory System: Pharyngitis; and upper respiratory infection

Incidence Less Than 1% of Injections

Body as a Whole: Sweating; achiness; sensation of warmth; lightheadedness; chills; and flushing

Digestive System: Vomiting; abdominal pain/cramps; dyspepsia; and diminished appetite

Respiratory System: Rhinitis; influenza; and cough

Nervous System: Vertigo/dizziness; and paresthesia

Integumentary System: Pruritus; rash (non-specified); angioedema; and urticaria

Musculoskeletal System: Arthralgia including monoarticular; myalgia; back pain, neck pain; shoulder pain; and neck stiffness

Hemic/Lymphatic System: Lymphadenopathy

Psychiatric/Behavioral: Insomnia/disturbed sleep

Special Senses: Earache

Urogenital System: Dysuria

Cardiovascular System: Hypotension

The following additional adverse reactions have been reported with use of the marketed vaccine. In many instances, the relationship to the vaccine was unclear.

Hypersensitivity: Anaphylaxis and symptoms of immediate hypersensitivity reactions including rash, pruritus, urticaria, edema, angioedema, dyspnea, chest discomfort, bronchial spasm, palpitation, or symptoms consistent with a hypotensive episode have been reported within the first few hours after vaccination. An apparent hypersensitivity syndrome (serum-sickness-like) of delayed onset has been reported days to weeks after vaccination including: arthralgia/arthritis (usually transient), fever, and dermatologic reactions such as urticaria, erythema multiforme, ecchymoses and erythema nodosum (see WARNINGS and PRECAUTIONS).

Digestive System: Elevation of liver enzymes; constipation.

Nervous System: Peripheral neuropathy including Bell's Palsy; muscle weakness; Guillain-Barre syndrome; radiculopathy; herpes zoster; hypesthesia; migraine.

Integumentary System: Stevens-Johnson Syndrome; petechiae.

Hematologic: Increased erythrocyte sedimentation rate.

Psychiatric/Behavioral: Irritability; agitation; somnolence.

Special Senses: Optic neuritis; tinnitus; conjunctivitis.

Cardiovascular System: Syncope; tachycardia

Potential Adverse Effects: In addition, a variety of adverse effects not observed in clinical trials with Recombivax HB, or Recombivax HB Dialysis Formulation have been reported with Heptavax-B (plasma-derived hepatitis B vaccine). Those listed below are to serve as alerting information to physicians:

Nervous System: Neurological disorders such as myelitis including transverse myelitis.

Hematologic: Thrombocytopenia

Special Senses: Visual disturbances

The following adverse reaction has been reported with another Hepatitis B Vaccine (Recombinant) but not with Recombivax HB: keratitis.

ENGERIX-B

Engerix-B (Hepatitis B Vaccine) is generally well tolerated. As with any vaccine, however, it is possible that expanded commercial use of the vaccine could reveal rare adverse reactions.

Ten double-blind studies involving 2,252 subjects showed no significant difference in the frequency or severity of adverse experiences betweenEngerix-B and plasma derived vaccines. In 36 clinical studies, a total of 13, 495 doses of Engerix-B were administered to 5,071 healthy adults and children who were initially seronegative for hepatitis B markers, and healthy neonates. All subjects were monitored for 4 days post-administration. Frequency of adverse experiences tended to decrease with successive doses of Engerix-B. Using a system checklist‡, the most frequently reported adverse reactions were injection site soreness (22%) and fatigue‡ (14%). Other reactions are listed below.

Incidence 1% to 10% of Injections

Local Reactions at injection site: Induration; erythema; swelling.

Body As Whole: Fever (>37.5°C).

Nervous System: Headache‡, dizziness‡

‡Parent or guardian completed forms for children and neonates. Neonatal checklist did not include headache, fatigue, or dizziness.

Incidence < 1% of Injections

Local reactions at injection site: Pain; pruritus; ecchymosis.

Body As A Whole: Sweating; malaise; chills; weakness; flushing, tingling.

Cardiovascular System: Hypotension.

Respiratory System: Influenza-like symptoms; upper respiratory tract illnesses.

Gastrointestinal System: Nausea; anorexia; abdominal pain/ cramps; vomiting; constipation; diarrhea.

Lymphatic System: Lymphadenopathy.

Musculoskeletal System: Pain/stiffness in arm, shoulder or neck; arthralgia; myalgia; back pain.

Skin And Appendages: Rash; urticaria; petechiae; pruritus, erythema.

Nervous System: Somnolence; insomnia; irritability; agitation

Additional adverse experiences have been reported with the commercial use of Engerix-B. Those listed below are to serve as alerting information to physicians.

Hypersensitivity: Anaphylaxis; erythema multiforme including Stevens-Johnson syndrome; angiodema; arthritis.

Cardiovascular system: Tachycardia/palpitations.

Respiratory system: Bronchospasm including asthma-like symptoms.

Gastrointestinal system: Abnormal liver function tests; dyspepsia.

Nervous system: Migraine; syncope; paresis; neuropathy including hypoesthesia; paresthesia, Guillain-Barre syndrome and Bell's palsy, transverse myelitis; optic neuritis, multiple sclerosis.

Hematologic: Thrombocytopenia.

Skin and appendages: Eczema; purpura; herpes zoster; erythema nodosum.

Special Senses: Conjunctivitis; keratitis; visual disturbances; vertigo; tinnitus; earache.

Potential Adverse Experiences: In addition, certain other adverse experiences not observed with Engerix-Bhave been reported with Heptavax-B‡ and/or Recombivax HB. Those listed below are to serve as alerting information to physicians:

ADVERSE REACTIONS: *(cont'd)*

Urogenital System: Dysuria

DOSAGE AND ADMINISTRATION:

RECOMBIVAX HB

Do not inject intravenously or intradermally.

Recombivax HB (Hepatitis B Vaccine (Recombinant)) DIALYSIS FORMULATION (40 mcg/ml) IS INTENDED ONLY FOR ADULT PREDIALYSIS/DIALYSIS PATIENTS

Recombivax HB (Hepatitis B Vaccine (Recombinant)) (10 mcg/ml) IS NOT INTENDED FOR USE IN PREDIALYSIS/DIALYSIS PATIENTS

Recombivax HB and Recombivax HB Dialysis Formulation are for intramuscular injection. The *deltoid muscle* is the preferred site for intramuscular injection in adults. Data suggests that injections given in the buttocks frequently are given into fatty tissue instead of into muscle. Such injections have resulted in a lower seroconversion rate than was expected. The *anterolateral thigh* is the recommended site for intramuscular injection in infants and young children.

For persons at risk of hemorrhage following intramuscular injection, Recombivax HB may be administered subcutaneously. However, when other aluminum-adsorbed vaccines have been administered subcutaneously, an increased incidence of local reactions including subcutaneous nodules has been observed. Therefore, subcutaneous administration should be used only in persons (*e.g.,* hemophiliacs) who are at risk of hemorrhage following intramuscular injections.

The vaccine should be used as supplied; no dilution or reconstitution is necessary. The full recommended dose of the vaccine should be used.

It is important to use a separate sterile syringe and needle for each individual patient to prevent transmission of hepatitis and other infectious agents one person to another.

Shake well before withdrawal and use. Thorough agitation at the time of administration is necessary to maintain suspension of the vaccine.

Parenteral drug products should be inspected visually for particulate matter and discoloration prior to administration. After thorough agitation, the vaccine is a slightly opaque, white suspension.

Recombivax HB: The vaccination regimen consists of 3 doses of vaccine given according to the following schedule:

1st dose: at elected date

2nd dose: 1 month later

3rd dose: 6 months after the first dose

The volume of vaccine to be given on each occasion is as enumerated in TABLE 1.

TABLE 1

Age Group	Initial	1 month	6 months
Birth* 10 years of age	0.25 ml (2.5 mcg)	0.25 ml (2.5 mcg)	0.25 ml (2.5 mcg)
11-19 years of age	0.5 ml (5 mcg)	0.5 ml (5 mcg)	0.5 ml (5 mcg)
≥20 years	1 ml (10 mcg)	1 ml (10 mcg)	1 ml (10 mcg)

* Infants born of HBsAg negative mothers.

For Syringe Use Only: Withdraw the recommended dose from the vial using a sterile needle and syringe free of preservatives, antiseptics and detergents.

Use of a 1 ml hubless syringe, one in which the needle is permanently attached to the syringe, will permit accurate withdrawal of 0.25 ml doses for pediatric use. However, injection must be accomplished with a needle long enough to ensure intramuscular deposition of the vaccine.

Revaccination: Whenever revaccination or administration of a booster dose is appropriate, Recombivax HB may be used (see CLINICAL PHARMACOLOGY).

Dosage For Infants Born of HBsAg Positive Mothers: The recommended regimen for infants born of HBsAg positive mothers is as enumerated in TABLE 2.

TABLE 2

	Birth	Within 7 days	1 month	6 months
Recombivax HB		0.5 ml** (5 mcg)	0.5 ml (5 mcg)	0.5 ml (5 mcg)
Hepatitis B Immune Globulin	0.5 ml		-	-

** The first 0.5 ml dose of Recombivax HB may be given at birth at the same time as Hepatitis B Immune Globulin but should be administered in the opposite anterolateral thigh.

Known or Presumed Exposure to HBsAg: There are no prospective studies directly testing the efficacy of a combination of Hepatitis B Immune Globulin (Human) and Recombivax HB in preventing clinical hepatitis B following percutaneous, ocular or mucous membrane exposure to hepatitis B virus. However, since most persons with such exposures (*e.g.,* health-care workers) are candidates for Recombivax HB and since combined Hepatitis B Immune Globulin (Human) plus vaccine is more efficacious than Hepatitis B Immune Globulin (Human) alone in perinatal exposures, the following guidelines are recommended for persons who have been exposed to hepatitis B virus such as through (1) percutaneous (needlestick), ocular, mucous membrane exposure to blood known or presumed to contain HBsAg, (2) human bites by known or presumed HBsAg carriers, that penetrate the skin, or (3) following intimate sexual contact with known or presumed HBsAg carriers:

Hepatitis B Immune Globulin (Human) (0.06 ml kg) should be given intramuscularly as soon as possible after exposure and within 24 hours if possible. Recombivax HB (see Dosage Recommendation) should be given intramuscularly at a separate site within 7 days of exposure and second and third doses given one and six months, respectively, after the first dose.

Recombivax HB Dialysis Formulation: The recommended vaccination regimen for predialysis/dialysis patients is as enumerated in TABLE 3.

TABLE 3

Group	Formulation	Initial	1 month	6 months
Predialysis and Dialysis Patients	Dialysis 40 mcg/ml	1 ml	1 ml	1 ml

For Syringe Use Only: Withdraw the recommended dose from the vial using a sterile needle and syringe free of preservatives, antiseptics, and detergents.

DOSAGE AND ADMINISTRATION: *(cont'd)*

Revaccination: A booster dose or revaccination with Recombivax HB Dialysis Formulation may be considered in predialysis/dialysis patients if the anti-HBs level is less than 10 mIU/ml 1 to 2 months after the 3rd dose.[16]

Storage: Store vials at 2-8° C (36-46° F). Storage above or below the recommended temperature may reduce potency.

Do not freeze since freezing destroys potency.

ENGERIX-B INJECTION:

Engerix-B should be administered by intramuscular injection. *Do not inject intravenously or intradermally.* In adults, the injection should be given in the deltoid region but it may be preferable to inject in the anterolateral thigh in neonates and infants, who have smaller deltoid muscles.Engerix-B should not be administered in the gluteal region; such injections may result in suboptimal response. The attending physician should determine final selection of the injection site and needle size, depending upon the patient's age and size of the target muscle. A 1-inch 23 gauge needle is sufficient to penetrate the anterolateral thigh in infants younder than 12 months of age. A 5/8 inch 25-gauge needle may be used to administer the vaccine in the deltoid region of toddlers and children up to, and including, 10 years of age. The 1-inch 23-gauge needle is appropriate for use in older children and adults.[13]

Engerix-B may be administered subcutaneously to persons at risk of hemorrhage (*e.g.,* hemophiliacs). However, hepatitis B vaccines administered subcutaneously are known to result in lower GMTs. Additionally, when other aluminum-absorbed vaccines have been administered subcutaneously, an increased incidence of local reactions including subcutaneous nodules has been observed. Therefore, subcutaneous administration should be used only in persons who are at risk of hemorrhage with intramuscular injections.

Preparation for Administration: *Shake well before withdrawal and use.* Parenteral drug products should be inspected visually for particulate matter and discoloration prior to administration. With thorough agitation, Engerix-B is a slightly opaque white suspension. Discard it if it appears otherwise. The vaccine should be used as supplied; no dilution or reconstitution is necessary. The full recommended dose of the vaccine should be used.

Dosing Schedules: The usual immunization regimen (see TABLE 4) consists of 3 doses of vaccine given according to the following schedule: 1st dose: at elected date, 2nd dose: 1 month later, 3rd dose: six months after first dose.

There is an alternate schedule with injections at 0, 1, and 2 months designed for certain populations (*e.g.,* neonates born of hepatitis B infected mothers, others who have or might have been recently exposed to the virus, certain travellers to high-risk areas. See INDICATIONS AND USAGE). On this alternate schedule, an additional dose at 12 months is recommended for infants born of infected mothers and for others for whom prolonged maintenance of protective titers is desired. (see TABLE 4)

TABLE 4

Group	Dose	Schedule*
Infants born of:		
HBsAg-negative mothers	10 mcg/0.5 ml	Usual
HBsAg-positive mothers	10 mcg/0.5 ml	Either
Children:		
0 through 10 years of age	10 mcg/0.5 ml	Either
Adolescents:		
11 through 19 years of age	10 mcg/0.5 ml	Usual
	20 mcg/1.0 ml	Either
Adults (>19 years):	20 mcg/1.0 ml	Either
Adults hemodialysis	40 mcg/2.0 ml**	0, 1, 2, 6 months

* Usual dosing schedule is 0, 1, 6 months alternate dosing scjedule is 0, 1, 2, 12 months. When the alternate scehdule is used for adolescents, the 20 mcg/1.0 ml dose should be used.
** Two X 20 mcg in one or two injections.

For hemodialysis patients, in whom vaccine-induced protection is less complete and may persist only as long as antibody levels remain above 10 mIU/ml, the need for booster doses should be assessed by annual antibody testing. 40 mcg (two x 20 mcg) booster doses with Engerix-B should be given when antibody levels decline below 10 mIU/ml[1]. Data shows individuals given a booster with Engerix-B achieve high antibody titers (see CLINICAL PHARMACOLOGY).

Booster Vaccinations: Whenever administration of a booster is appropriate, the dose of Engerix-B is 10 mcg for children under 10 years of age and under; 20 mcg for other children and adults. Studies have demonstrated a substantial increase in antibody titers after Engerix-B booster vaccination following an initial course with both plasma-and yeast-derived vaccines. (See CLINICAL PHARMACOLOGY.)

See previous section for discussion on a booster vaccination for adult hemodialysis patients.

Known Or Presumed Exposure To Hepatitis B Virus: Unprotected individuals with known or presumed exposure to the hepatitis B virus (*e.g.,* neonates born of infected mothers, others experiencing percutaneous or permucosal exposure) should be given hepatitis B immune globulin (HBIG) in addition to Engerix-B in accordance with ACIP recommendations[1] and with the package insert for HBIG. Engerix-B can be given on either dosing schedule (see above).

Storage: Store between 2 and 8°C (35° to 46°F). *Do not freeze*; discard if product has been frozen. Do not dilute to administer.

REFERENCES:

Recombivax HB 1. Robinson, W.S.: Hepatitis B Virus and the Delta Virus, in "Principles and Practice of Infectious Diseases," G.L. Mandell; R.G.Douglas; J.E. Bennett (eds), vol. 2, New York, John Wiley & Sons,1985, pp. 1002-1029. **2.** Recommendation of the Immunization Practices Advisory Committee (ACIP): Protection against viral hepatitis, MMWR *39* (RR-2): 5-22, Feb. 9, 1990. **3.** Stevens, C.E.; Toy, P.T.; Tong, M.J.; Taylor, P.E.; Vyas, G.N.; Nair, P.V.; Gudavalli, M.; Krugman, S.: Perinatal hepatitis B virus transmission in the United States, JAMA; *253* (12):1740-1745, 1985. **4.** Beasley, R.P.; Hwang, L.; Stevens, C.E.; Lin, C.; Hsieh, F.; Wang, K.; Sun, T.; Szmuness, W.: Efficacy of Hepatitis B Immune Globulin for prevention of Perinatal Transmission of the Hepatitis B Virus Carrier State: Final Report of a Randomized Double-Blind, Placebo-Controlled Trial, Hepatology *3*:135-141, 1983. **5.** Centers for Disease Control: Suboptimal response to hepatitis B vaccine given by injection into the buttock MMWR; *34* (8): 105-113, March 1, 1985. **6.** Davidson, M.; and Krugman S.: Recombinant yeast hepatitis B vaccine compared with plasma-derived vaccine: Immunogenicity and effect of booster dose; J. of Infection, *13* (Sup. A), 31-38, 1986. **7.** Hadler, S.C., et al: Long-term Immunogenicity and Efficacy of Hepatitis B Vaccine in Homosexual Men, NEJM *315* (4): 209-214 (1986). **8.** Emini, E.A.; Ellis, R.W.; Miller, W.J.; McAleer, W.J.; Scolnick, E.M. and Gerety, R.J.: Production and immunological analysis of recombinant hepatitis B vaccine, J. of Infection, *13* (Sup. A): 3-9,1986. **9.** Brown, S.E.; Stanley, C.; Howard, C.R.; Zuckerman, A.J.; Steward, M.W., Antibody responses to recombinant and plasma derived hepatitis B vaccines, Brit. Med. J., *292:*159-161, 1986. **10.** Yamamoto, S.; Kuroki, T.; Kurai, K.; Iino, S.: Comparison of results for Phase I studies with recombinant and plasma-derived hepatitis B vaccines, and controlled study comparing intramuscular and subcutaneous injections of recombinant hepatitis B vaccine, J. of Infection,*13* (Sup. A) 53-60, 1986 **11.** Jilg, W.; Schmidt, M.; Zoulek, G.; Lorbeer, B.; Wilske, B.; Deinhardt, F.: Clinical evaluation of a recombinant hepatitis B vaccine, Lancet 1174-1175, Nov. 24, 1984. **12.** Schalm, S. W.; Heytink, R. A.; Kruining, H.; Bakker-Bendik, M.:Immunogenicity of recombinant yeast hepatitis-B vaccine, Neth. J. Med.*29:* 28 1986. **13.** Stevens, C.E., Taylor, P.E., Tong, M.J.*et al.:* Prevention of perinatal hepatitis B virus infection with hepatitis B immunoglobulin and hepatitis B vaccine. *IN:*Zuckerman, A.J. (ed), *Viral Hepatitis and Liver Diseases* Alan R. Liss, 1988, pp. 982-983. **14.** Data on file at Merck Sharp & Dohme Research Laboratories. **15.** Stevens, C.E.; Taylor, P.E.; Tong, M.J., et al.: Yeast-Recombinant. Hepatitis B Vaccine, Efficacy with hepatitis B immune globulin in prevention of perinatal hepatitis B virus transmission, JAMA 257(19):2612-2616, 1987. **16.** Recommendations of the Immunization Practices Advisory Committee (ACIP): Update on Hepatitis B Prevention, MMWR 36(23): 353-366, June 29, 1987. **Engerix-B 1.** Centers for Disease Control: Protection against viral hepatitis: recommendations of the Immunization Practices Advisory Committee (ACIP). *MMWR.* 39(No. RR-2)

REFERENCES: *(cont'd)*

1990. **2.** Robinson, W.S.: Hepatitis B virus and the delta virus. In Mandell, G.L, Douglas, R.G., Bennett, J.E. (eds): *Principles and practice of infectious diseases,* vol. 3, New York, John Wiley & Sons, 1990, pp. 1204-1231. **3.** Beasley, R.P., et. al.: Efficacy of hepatitis B immune globulin for prevention of perinatal transmission of hepatitis B virus carrier state: final report of a randomized double-blind, placebo-controlled trial. *Hepatology* 3: 135-141, 1983. **4.** Centers for Disease Control: Hepatits B virus: a comprehensive strategy for eliminating transmission in the United States through universal childhood vaccination: recommendations of the Immunization Practices Advisory Committee (ACIP). *MMWR.*40 (No. RR-13):1-25, 1991. **5.** Committee on Infectious Diseases: Universal hepatitis B immunization.*Pediatrics.*89(4):795-800, 1992. **6.** Ambrosch F.: Persistanc of vaccine-induced antibodies to hepatitis B surface antigen-the need for booster vaccination in adult subjects. *Postgrad. Med. J.*63(Suppl. 2):129-135, 1987. **7.** Stevens, C.E. et al:Hepatitis B vaccine in patients receiving hemodialysis. *N. Engl. J. Med.* 311:496-501 **8.** Andre, F.E. and Safary, A., Clinical experience with a yeast-derived hepatits B vaccine. In Zuckerman, A.J. (ed): *Viral hepatitis and liver disease*, Alan R. Liss, Inc., 1988,pp. 1025-1030. **9.** Poovorawan, Y., et al.: Protective efficacy of a recombinant DNA hepatitis B vaccine in neonates of HBe antigen-positive mothers. *JAMA.* 261(22):3278-3281, June 9, 1989. **10.** Goilav, C., et al.: Immunization of homosexual men with a recombinant DNA vaccine against hepatitis B: immunogenicity and protection. In Zuckerman, A.J. (ed): *Viral hepatitis and liver disease,*Alan R. Liss, Inc., 1988, pp. 1057-1058. **11.** Hauser, P., et al.: Immunological properties of recombinant HBsAg produced in yeast. *Postgrad. Med. J.* 63 (Suppl. 2):83-91, 1987. **12.** Centers for Disease COntrol: Recommendations of the Immunization Practices Advisory Committee (ACIP): General Recommendations on Immunization, *MMWR.* 38(13): April 7, 1989. **13.** Centers for Disease Control and Prevention: General Recommendations on Immunization: Recommendations of the Advisory Committee on Immunization Practices (ACIP).*MMWR.*1994.;43(RR-1):6.

HOW SUPPLIED - EQUIVALENTS NOT AVAILABLE:

Injection, Susp - Intramuscular - 5 mcg/ml

0.5 ml	$22.50	RECOMBIVAX HB, Merck	00006-4799-00
0.5 ml x 10	$212.88	RECOMBIVAX HB, Merck	00006-4874-00
3 ml	$121.25	RECOMBIVAX HB, Merck	00006-4761-00
3 ml x 10	$1141.50	RECOMBIVAX HB, Merck	00006-4875-00

Injection, Susp - Intramuscular - 10 mcg/ml

0.5 ml	$28.84	RECOMBIVAX-HB, Merck	00006-4769-00
0.5 ml x 10	$285.25	RECOMBIVAX HB, Merck	00006-4876-00
1 ml	$47.92	RECOMBIVAX HB, Merck	00006-4775-00
1 ml x 10	$474.09	RECOMBIVAX HB, Merck	00006-4872-00
3 ml	$143.82	RECOMBIVAX-HB, Merck	00006-4773-00
3 ml x 10	$1422.70	RECOMBIVAX HB, Merck	00006-4873-00

Injection, Susp - Intramuscular - 10 mcg/5ml

0.5 ml x 1	$23.45	ENGERIX-B, SKB Biols	58160-0859-01

Injection, Susp - Intramuscular - 20 mcg/ml

0.5 ml x 5	$117.25	ENGERIX-B, SKB Biols	58160-0859-05
0.5 ml x 5	$117.25	ENGERIX-B, SKB Biols	58160-0859-06
1 ml x 5	$271.75	ENGERIX-B, SKB Biols	58160-0861-05
20 mcg/ml x 1	$54.35	ENGERIX-B, SKB Biols	58160-0860-01
20 mcg/ml x 10	$522.75	ENGERIX-B, SKB Biols	58160-0860-11
20 mcg/ml x 25	$1359.10	ENGERIX-B, SKB Biols	58160-0860-16

Injection, Susp - Intramuscular - 40 mcg/ml

1 ml x 1425	$134.33	RECOMBIVAX HB, Merck	00006-4776-00

HEXACHLOROPHENE *(001436)*

CATEGORIES: Anti-Infectives; Antibacterials; Antiseptics/Disinfectants; Dermatologicals; Detergents; Local Infections; Skin/Mucous Membrane Agents; Pregnancy Category C; FDA Approval Pre 1982

BRAND NAMES: Dial; E-Z Scrub; *Fisohex*; Gamophen; Germa-Medica; Hexa-Germ; Hexascrub; Phiso-Scrub; **Phisohex**; Pre-Op; Septisol; *Ster-Zac*; Turgex *(International brand names outside U.S. in italics)*

FORMULARIES: Aetna; BC-BS

DESCRIPTION:

Hexachlorophene detergent cleanser, is an antibacterial sudsing emulsion for topical administration. Hexachlorophene contains a colloidal dispersion of hexachlorophene 3% (w/w) in a stable emulsion consisting of entsufon sodium, petrolatum, lanolin cholesterols, methylcellulose, polyethylene glycol, polyethylene glycol monostearate, lauryl myristyl diethanolamide, sodium benzoate, and water. pH is adjusted with hydrochloric acid. Entsufon sodium is a synthetic detergent.

Chemically, hexachlorophene is Phenol, 2,2'-methylenebis(3,4,6-trichloro-).

CLINICAL PHARMACOLOGY:

Hexachlorophene is a bacteriostatic cleansing agent. It cleanses the skin thoroughly and has bacteriostatic action against staphylococci and other gram-positive bacteria. Cumulative antibacterial action develops with repeated use. Cleansing with alcohol or soaps containing alcohol removes the antibacterial residue.

Detectable blood levels of hexachlorophene following absorption through intact skin have been found in subjects who regularly scrubbed with hexachlorophene emulsion 3%. (See WARNINGS for additional information.)

Hexachlorophene has the same slight acidity as normal skin (pH value 5.0 to 6.0).

INDICATIONS AND USAGE:

Hexachlorophene is indicated for use as a surgical scrub and a bacteriostatic skin cleanser. It may also be used to control an outbreak of gram-positive infection where other infection control procedures have been unsuccessful. Use only as long as necessary for infection control.

CONTRAINDICATIONS:

Hexachlorophene should not be used on burned or denuded skin.

It should not be used as an occlusive dressing, wet pack, or lotion.

It should not be used routinely for prophylactic total body bathing.

It should not be used as a vaginal pack or tampon, or on any mucous membranes.

Hexachlorophene should not be used on persons with sensitivity to any of its components. It should not be used on persons who have demonstrated primary light sensitivity to halogenated phenol derivatives because of the possibility of cross-sensitivity to hexachlorophene.

WARNINGS:

RINSE THOROUGHLY AFTER EACH USE.

Patients should be closely monitored and use should be immediately discontinued at the first sign of any of the symptoms described below.

Rapid absorption of hexachlorophene may occur with resultant toxic blood levels when preparations containing hexachlorophene are applied to skin lesions such as ichthyosis congenita, the dermatitis of Letterer-Siwe's syndrome, or other generalized dermatological conditions. Application to burns has also produced neurotoxicity and death.

HEXACHLOROPHENE SHOULD BE DISCONTINUED PROMPTLY IF SIGNS OR SYMPTOMS OF CEREBRAL IRRITABILITY OCCUR.

WARNINGS: *(cont'd)*

Infants, especially premature infants or those with dermatoses, are particularly susceptible to hexachlorophene absorption. Systemic toxicity may be manifested by signs of stimulation (irritation) of the central nervous system, sometimes with convulsions.

Infants have developed dermatitis, irritability, generalized clonic muscular contractions and decerebrate rigidity following application of a 6 percent hexachlorophene powder. Examination of brainstems of those infants revealed vacuolization like that which can be produced in newborn experimental animals following repeated topical application of 3 percent hexachlorophene. Moreover, a study of histologic sections of premature infants who died of unrelated causes has shown a positive correlation between hexachlorophene baths and lesions in white matter of brains.

PRECAUTIONS:

GENERAL

Avoid accidental contact of hexachlorophene with the eyes.

If contact occurs, promptly rinse thoroughly with water. To assist in the detection of ocular irritation, applications to the head and periorbital skin areas should be performed only in responsive patients with unanesthetized eyes.

RINSE THOROUGHLY AFTER USE, especially from sensitive areas such as the scrotum and perineum.

Hexachlorophene is intended for external use only. If swallowed, hexachlorophene is harmful, especially to infants and children.**Hexachlorophene should not be poured into measuring cups, medicine bottles, or similar containers since it may be mistaken for baby formula or other medications.**

CARCINOGENESIS, MUTAGENESIS, AND IMPAIRMENT OF FERTILITY

Carcinogenicity Studies In Animals: Hexachlorophene was tested in one experiment in rats by oral administration; it had no carcinogenic effect.

Hexachlorophene was not mutagenic in *Salmonella typhimurium* and was negative in a dominant lethal assay in male mice. Cytogenetic tests with cultured human lymphocytes were also negative.

Human Data: No case reports or epidemiological studies were available.

Impairment of Fertility: Topical exposure of neonatal rats to 3% hexachlorophene solution caused reduced fertility in 7-month-old males, due to inability to ejaculate.

Embryotoxicity and Teratogenicity: Placental transfer of hexachlorophene has been demonstrated in rats.

Hexachlorophene is embryotoxic and produces some teratogenic effects.

PREGNANCY CATEGORY C

There are no adequate and well-controlled studies in pregnant women. Hexachlorophene should be used during pregnancy only if the potential benefit justifies potential risk to the fetus.

Hexachlorophene has been shown to be teratogenic and embryotoxic in rats when given by mouth or instilled into the vagina in large doses.

Administration of 500 mg/kg diet or 20 to 30 mg/kg bw/day by gavage to rats caused some malformations (angulated ribs, cleft palate, micro- and anophthalmia) and reduction in litter size.

Placental transfer and excretion in milk of hexachlorophene has been demonstrated in rats.

In another study, doses of up to 50 mg/kg diet failed to produce any effects in 3 generations of rats. Hexachlorophene did not interfere with reproduction in hamsters.

NURSING MOTHERS

It is not known whether this drug is excreted in human milk. Because many drugs are excreted in human milk and because of the potential for serious adverse reactions in nursing infants from hexachlorophene, a decision should be made whether to discontinue nursing or to discontinue the drug taking into account the importance of the drug to the mother.

PEDIATRIC USE

Hexachlorophene should not be used routinely for bathing infants. See WARNINGS. For premature infants: see WARNINGS.

ADVERSE REACTIONS:

Adverse reactions to hexachlorophene may include dermatitis and photosensitivity. Sensitivity to hexachlorophene is rare; however, persons who have developed photoallergy to similar compounds also may become sensitive to hexachlorophene.

In persons with highly sensitive skin the use of hexachlorophene may at times produce a reaction characterized by redness and/or mild scaling or dryness, especially when it is combined with such mechanical factors as excessive rubbing or exposure to heat or cold.

OVERDOSAGE:

The accidental ingestion of hexachlorophene in amounts from 1 oz to 4 oz has caused anorexia, vomiting, abdominal cramps, diarrhea, dehydration, convulsions, hypotension, and shock, and in several reported instances, fatalities.

If patients are seen early, the stomach should be evacuated by emesis or gastric lavage. Olive oil or vegetable oil (60 ml or 2 fl oz) may then be given to delay absorption of hexachlorophene, followed by a saline cathartic to hasten removal. Treatment is symptomatic and supportive; intravenous fluids (5 percent dextrose in physiologic saline solution) may be given for dehydration. Any other electrolyte derangement should be corrected. If marked hypotension occurs, vasopressor therapy is indicated. Use of opiates may be considered if gastrointestinal symptoms (cramping, diarrhea) are severe. Scheduled medical or surgical procedures should be postponed until the patient's condition has been evaluated and stabilized.

DOSAGE AND ADMINISTRATION:

SURGICAL HAND SCRUB

1. Wet hands and forearms with water. Apply approximately 5 ml of hexachlorophene over the hands and rub into a copious lather by adding small amounts of water. Spread suds over hands and forearms and scrub well with a wet brush for 3 minutes. Pay particular attention to the nails and interdigital spaces. A separate nail cleaner may be used. *Rinse thoroughly* under running water.

2. Apply 5 ml of hexachlorophene to hands again and scrub as above for another 3 minutes. *Rinse thoroughly* with running water and dry.

3. For repeat surgical scrubs during the day, scrub thoroughly with the same amount of hexachlorophene for 3 minutes only. *Rinse thoroughly* with water and dry.

BACTERIOSTATIC CLEANSING

Wet hands with water. Dispense approximately 5 ml of hexachlorophene into the palm, work up a lather with water and apply to area to be cleansed.

Rinse thoroughly after each washing.

Infant Care: Hexachlorophene should not be used routinely for bathing infants. See WARNINGS.

Premature Infants: See WARNINGS.

DOSAGE AND ADMINISTRATION: *(cont'd)*

Use of baby skin products containing alcohol may decrease the antibacterial action of Hexachlorophene.

ANIMAL PHARMACOLOGY:

Toxicity: The oral LD_{50} of hexachlorophene in male rats is 66 mg/kg bw, in females 56 mg/kg bw, and in weaning rats 120 mg/kg bw.

In suckling rats (10 days old), it is 9 mg/kg bw.

HOW SUPPLIED - EQUIVALENTS NOT AVAILABLE:

Liquid - Topical - 3 %

8 ml x 50	$30.28	PHISOHEX, Sanofi Winthrop	00024-1535-05
148 ml	$12.51	PHISOHEX, Sanofi Winthrop	00024-1535-02
148 ml x 48	$435.97	PHISOHEX, Sanofi Winthrop	00024-1535-48
473 ml x 24	$420.82	PHISOHEX, Sanofi Winthrop	00024-1535-24
480 ml	$24.13	PHISOHEX, Sanofi Winthrop	00024-1535-06
3840 ml	$119.50	PHISOHEX, Sanofi Winthrop	00024-1535-08
3840 ml x 4	$346.37	PHISOHEX, Sanofi Winthrop	00024-1535-04

HISTRELIN ACETATE *(003105)*

CATEGORIES: Adrenal Hyperplasia; Hormones; Luteinizing Hormone Agonist; Precocious Puberty; FDA Class 1A ("Important Therapeutic Advantage"); FDA Approved 1991 Dec

BRAND NAMES: **Supprelin**

DESCRIPTION:

Supprelin (histrelin acetate) Injection contains a synthetic nonapeptide agonist of the naturally occurring gonadotropin releasing hormone (GnRH or LHRH). The analog possesses a greater potency than the natural sequence hormone. The amino acid sequence and chemical name of histrelin acetate is:

5-oxo-L-prolyl-L-histidyl-L-tryptophyl-L-seryl- L-tyrosyl-N-benzyl -D-histidyl-L-leucyl-L-arginyl-N-ethyl-L-prolinamide acetate (salt)

($C_{66}H_{86}N_{18}O_{12}$.(1.7-2.8 moles) CH_3COOH. (0.6-7.0 moles) H_2O).

The molecular weight of the peptide base is 1323.52.

Supprelin Injection is a sterile, aqueous solution for subcutaneous administration available in single-use vials of 0.6 ml. It contains histrelin equivalent to either 200 mcg/ml, 500 mcg/ml, or 1000 mcg/ml peptide base with 0.9% sodium chloride and 10% mannitol. The pH of the 200 mcg/ml solution is 4.5 - 6.5 and the pH of the 500 mcg/ml and 1000 mcg/ml solutions is 4.5 - 6.0. All solutions are unbuffered, hypertonic and contain no preservative.

CLINICAL PHARMACOLOGY:

Supprelin Injection, a GnRH agonist, is a potent inhibitor of gonadotropin secretion when administered daily in therapeutic doses. Both animal and human studies indicate that following an initial stimulatory phase, chronic, subcutaneous administration of histrelin acetate desensitizes responsiveness of the pituitary gonadotropin which, in turn, causes a reduction in ovarian and testicular steroidogenesis.

Although animal studies have shown that acute administration of Supprelin (histrelin acetate) injection results in stimulation of the reproductive system, chronic Supprelin Injection administration in the rat delays sexual development, inhibits estrous cyclicity and pregnancy, reduces reproductive organ weight and inhibits ovarian and testicular steroidogenesis in a reversible fashion. In the rabbit, chronic administration of Supprelin Injection resulted in decreased reproductive organ weights.

In human studies, chronic administration of Supprelin Injection controls the secretion of pituitary gonadotropins resulting in decreased sex steroid levels and in the regression of secondary sexual characteristics in children with precocious puberty. In girls, menses cease, serum estradiol levels are decreased to prepubertal levels, linear growth velocities decrease, skeletal maturation is slowed and adult height predictions increase. In boys, testicular steroidogenesis is inhibited and testicular volume is reduced.

Continuous Supprelin Injection administration to patients with central precocious puberty can be monitored by standard GnRH testing and by serial determinations of sex steroid levels. The decreases in LH, FSH, and sex steroid levels are evident within three months of the initiation of therapy. These effects have been demonstrated in the 10 female patients who were studied for periods up to eighteen months. The metabolism, distribution, and excretion of Supprelin Injection in humans have not been determined.

INDICATIONS AND USAGE:

Supprelin Injection is indicated for the control of the biochemical and clinical manifestations of central precocious puberty.

Selection of Patients

1. Only patients with centrally mediated precocious puberty (either idiopathic or neurogenic and occurring before age 8 years in girls or 9.5 years in boys) should receive Supprelin Injection treatment.

2. Before treatment with Supprelin (histrelin acetate) Injection is instituted, a thorough physical and endocrinologic evaluation should be performed. This should include:

a. Height and weight as baseline for serial monitoring.

b. Hand and wrist x-ray for bone age determination, to document advanced skeletal age and as baseline for serially monitoring predicted height.

c. Total sex steroid level (estradiol or testosterone).

d. Adrenal steroid level, to exclude congenital adrenal hyperplasia.

e. Beta-Human Chorionic Gonadotropin level, to rule out a chorionic gonadotropin-secreting tumor.

f. GnRH stimulation test, to demonstrate activation of the Hypothalamic-Pituitary-Gonadal (HPG) axis.

g. Pelvic/adrenal/testicular ultrasound, to rule out a steroid-secreting tumor and to document gonadal size for serial monitoring.

h. Computerized tomography of the head, to rule out previously undiagnosed intracranial tumor.

3. Patients must be able to maintain compliance with a *daily* regimen of injections.

CONTRAINDICATIONS:

Supprelin Injection should not be administered to patients known to be hypersensitive to any of its components.

Supprelin Injection is contraindicated in women who are or may become pregnant while receiving the drug and in nursing mothers. There was increased fetal size and mortality in rats and increased fetal mortality in rabbits but not in mice after Supprelin Injection administration. Other responses to Supprelin Injection included dystocia, a greater incidence of unilateral hydroureter, and incomplete ossification in rat fetuses in all treated groups. When administered to rabbits on days 6-18 of pregnancy at doses of 20 to 80 mcg/kg/day (2 to 8 times the human dose), Supprelin Injection produced early termination of pregnancy and increased fetal death. In rats administered Supprelin Injection on days 7-20 of pregnancy at doses of 1 to 15 mcg/kg/day (0.1 to 1.5 times the human dose) there was an increase in fetal resorptions. In mice treated on days 6-15 of pregnancy at 10 to 100 times the human dose, Supprelin Injection had no adverse effects. The effects on fetal mortality are expected consequences of the alterations in hormonal levels brought about by the drug. If this drug is inadvertently used during pregnancy or in the rare event that a patient becomes pregnant while taking this drug, she should be apprised of the potential hazard to the fetus.

It is not known if this drug is excreted in human milk, but because many drugs are excreted in human milk and because of the potential for serious adverse reactions in nursing infants from Supprelin Injection, the drug should not be given to nursing mothers.

WARNINGS:

Non-compliance with drug regimen or inadequate dosing may result in inadequate control of the pubertal process. The consequences of poor control include the return of pubertal signs such as menses, breast development, and testicular growth. The long-term consequences of inadequate control of gonadal steroid secretion are unknown, but may include a further compromise of adult stature.

Serious hypersensitivity reactions (angioedema, urticaria) have been reported following Supprelin (histrelin acetate) Injection administration. Clinical manifestations may include: cardiovascular collapse, hypotension, tachycardia, loss of consciousness, angioedema, bronchospasm, dyspnea, urticaria, flushing and pruritus. If any allergic reaction occurs, therapy with Supprelin Injection should be discontinued. Serious acute hypersensitivity reactions may require emergency medical treatment.

PRECAUTIONS:

General: Studies in rats and monkeys have indicated that all of the known biochemical and antifertility effects of Supprelin Injection are reversible. Because animal studies are not always predictive of human response, and because children who have received Supprelin Injection have not been followed sufficiently long to ensure reactivation of the HPG axis following long-term therapy, this drug should be used only when the benefits to the patient outweigh the potential risks. In addition, the patient (and/or guardian) should be advised that hypogonadism may result if the HPG axis fails to reactivate after the drug is discontinued.

Information for the Patient: Prior to Supprelin Injection therapy, patients and their families should be informed of the importance of complying with the schedule of single, *daily* Injections, given at approximately the same time each day. If injections are not given daily, the pubertal process may be reactivated. Supprelin Injection contains no preservative. Patients should be informed that vials are to be used once and any unused solution is to be discarded. Medication should be allowed to reach room temperature before injecting. Daily injections should be rotated through different body sites (upper arms, thighs, abdomen).

Patients should be made aware of the required monitoring of their condition and of the potential risks of therapy. Within the first month of therapy, girls being treated with Supprelin (histrelin acetate) Injection may experience a light menstrual flow. This menstrual flow is common and likely is related to the lower estrogen levels brought about by treatment, and the withdrawal of estrogen support from the endometrium.

Irritation, redness, or swelling at the injection sites may occur. If these reactions are severe, or do not go away, the patient's doctor should be notified.

The patients and their families should be advised to discontinue the drug and seek medical attention at the first sign of skin rash, urticaria, rapid heartbeat, difficulty in swallowing and breathing, or any swelling which may suggest angioedema (See WARNINGS and ADVERSE REACTIONS.)

Clinical Evaluations/Laboratory Tests: An initial pelvic ultrasound should be performed to exclude other conditions before treating with Supprelin Injection. The patient should be monitored carefully after 3 months and every 6 to 12 months thereafter by serial clinical evaluations, repeated height measurements, bone age determinations (yearly), and serial GnRH testing to document that gonadotropin responsiveness of the pituitary remains prepubertal while on therapy. During the initial agonistic phase of treatment, the patient may demonstrate transient increases in breast tissue, moodiness, vaginal secretions, or testicular volume. After this initial agonistic phase (usually one to three weeks), control of the biochemical and physical manifestations of puberty should remain as long as chronic therapy is in effect. Treatment should be discontinued when the onset of puberty is desired. Following the discontinuation of Supprelin Injection treatment, the onset of normal puberty should be documented. In addition, patients should be monitored to assess menstrual cyclicity, reproductive function, and ultimate adult height.

Carcinogenesis, Mutagenesis, and Impairment of Fertility: Carcinogenicity studies were conducted in rats for 2 years at doses of 5, 25, or 150 mcg/kg/day (up to 15 times the human dose) and in mice for 18 months at doses of 20, 200 or 2000 mcg/kg/day (up to 200 times the human dose). As seen with other GnRH agonists, Supprelin (histrelin acetate) Injection administration was associated with an increase in tumors of hormonally responsive tissues. There was a significant increase in pituitary adenomas in rats. There was an increase in pancreatic islet-cell adenomas in treated female rats and a non-dose-related increase in testicular Leydig-cell tumors (highest incidence in the low-dose group). In mice, there was a significant increase in mammary-gland adenocarcinomas in all treated females. In addition, there were increases in stomach papillomas in male rats given high doses, and an increase in histiocytic sarcomas in female mice at the highest dose.

Mutagenicity studies have not been performed. Fertility studies have been conducted in rats and monkeys given subcutaneous daily doses of Supprelin Injection up to 180 mcg/kg for 6 months and full reversibility of fertility suppression was demonstrated. The development and reproductive performance of offspring from parents treated with Supprelin Injection has not been investigated.

Pregnancy, Teratogenic Effects, Pregnancy Category X: See CONTRAINDICATIONS.

Nursing Mothers: See CONTRAINDICATIONS section.

Pediatric Use: Safety and effectiveness in children below the age of two years have not been established.

ADVERSE REACTIONS:

At least one adverse experience was reported for 139 of the 183 (76%) children in clinical studies of central precocious puberty. Three of the 183 children (2%) stopped therapy due to a hypersensitivity reaction.

Adverse experiences considered related or probably related to drug therapy included (TABLE 1):

Other adverse experiences considered possibly related to drug therapy and reported in at least 1% of patients are as follows:

Cardiovascular: (1-3%) - palpitations, tachycardia, epistaxis, hypertension, migraine headache, pallor.

ADVERSE REACTIONS: *(cont'd)*

TABLE 1	
Skin reactions at the medication site (redness, swelling, and itching)	45%
Vaginal bleeding (usually only one episode within 1 to 3 weeks of starting therapy lasting several days)	22%
Urticaria	4%
Purpura	2%
Convulsions (increased frequency)	2%
Visual disturbances	2%
Hot flashes/flushes	2%
Edema (other than at medication site)	2%
Mood changes	2%
Erythema (other than at medication site)	1%
Conduct disorder	1%

Endocrine: (6%) - leukorrhea; (1%) - goiter, hyperlipidemia, anemia, breast edema, breast pain, breast discharge, glycosuria

Gastrointestinal: (3-10%)-gastrointestinal pain, abdominal pain, nausea, vomiting, diarrhea; (1-3%) - GI cramps, GI distress, constipation, decreased appetite, and increased thirst

Miscellaneous: (14%) - pyrexia; (6%) - extremity pain; (1-3%) - fatigue, chills, malaise, neck or chest or trunk pain, viral infection

Musculoskeletal: (4%) - arthralgia; (1%) - pain, hypotonia

Nervous System: (22%) - headache; (1-3%) - somnolence, lethargy, dizziness, impaired consciousness, syncope, tremor, hyperkinesia, nervousness, anxiety, depression

Respiratory: (3-10%) - cough, pharyngitis; (1-3%) - hyperventilation, upper respiratory infection

Skin: (7%) - rash; (1-3%) - pruritus, dyschromia, keratoderma, alopecia, sweating

Special Senses: (1-3%) - abnormal pupillary function, otalgia, hearing loss, polyopia, photophobia

Urogenital: (1-3%)-irritation or odor or pruritus or infections of the female genitalia, polyuria, dysuria, urinary frequency, incontinence, hematuria, nocturia

Acute generalized (angioedema, urticaria) hypersensitivity reactions have been reported (See: Warnings and Precautions).

Other patients

Supprelin (histrelin acetate) Injection has been studied in other patients for various indications (N = 196). Adverse experiences occurring in 2% or more of the study population are:

Cardiovascular: (35%) - vasodilation; (3%) - edema, migraine headache, hypertension

Endocrine: (12%) - vaginal dryness; (3-10%) -metrorrhagia, breast pain, breast edema; (2-3%) - leukorrhea, breast discharge, decreased breast size, tenderness of female genitalia

Gastrointestinal: (3-10%) - nausea, GI pain, flatulence, decreased appetite, dyspepsia; (2-3%) - vomiting, constipation, diarrhea, GI cramps, gastritis

Miscellaneous: (12%) - abdominal pain; (3-10%) - pain in trunk, body, or extremities, fatigue, pyrexia, weight gain, chest pain, viral infection; (2-3%) - chills, malaise, head/face pain, neck pain, purpura

Musculoskeletal: (3-10%) - arthralgia, joint stiffness, muscle cramp; (2-3%) - muscle stiffness, myalgia

Nervous System: (22%) - headache; (3-10%) - mood changes, nervousness, dizziness, depression, libido changes, insomnia, anxiety; (2-3%) - paresthesia, cognitive changes, syncope

Respiratory: (3-10%) - upper respiratory infection, pharyngitis, respiratory congestion; (2-3%) - cough, asthma, breathing disorder, rhinorrhea, bronchitis, sinusitis

Skin: (12%) - skin reaction at the medication site: (3-10%) - acne, rash, sweating; (2-3%) - keratoderma, pruritus, pain

Special Senses: (6%) - visual disturbances; (2-3%) - ear congestion, otalgia

Urogenital: (3-10%) - pain of female genitalia, vaginitis, dysmenorrhea; (2-3%)-dyspareunia, dysuria, hypertrophy of female genitalia, pruritus of external female genitalia

Urticaria, which was reported by less than 2% of the population, may be clinically significant.

DRUG ABUSE AND DEPENDENCE:

No instances of drug abuse or dependence have been reported.

OVERDOSAGE:

Supprelin (histrelin acetate) Injection of up to 200 mcg/kg (rats, rabbits), or 2000 mcg/kg (mice) resulted in no systemic toxicity. This represents 20 to 200 times the maximal recommended human dose of 10 mcg/kg/day.

DOSAGE AND ADMINISTRATION:

The dose of Supprelin Injection that is recommended for the treatment of central precocious puberty is 10 mcg/kg of body weight administered as a single, daily subcutaneous injection. If prepubertal levels of sex steroids and/or a prepubertal gonadotropin response to GnRH testing are not achieved within the first 3 months of treatment, the patient should be reevaluated. Doses greater than 10 mcg/kg/day have not been evaluated in clinical trials. The injection site should be varied daily.

NOTE: Parenteral drug products should be inspected visually for discoloration and particulate matter before use. Supprelin Injection contains no preservative. Vials are to be used once. Any unused solution is to be discarded.

Store refrigerated at 2-8°C (36-46°F) and protect from light. Remove vial from packaging only at time of use. Allow vial to reach room temperature before injecting contents. Discard unused portion of the vial after administration.

HOW SUPPLIED - EQUIVALENTS NOT AVAILABLE:

Injection, Solution - Subcutaneous - 200 mcg/ml

0.6 ml x 30 $413.66 SUPPRELIN, Roberts Labs 54092-0637-75

Injection, Solution - Subcutaneous - 500 mcg/ml

0.6 ml x 30 $413.66 SUPPRELIN, Roberts Labs 54092-0638-75

Injection, Solution - Subcutaneous - 1000 mcg/ml

0.6 ml x 30 $413.66 SUPPRELIN, Roberts Labs 54092-0639-75

HOMATROPINE HYDROBROMIDE *(001442)*

CATEGORIES: Anticholinergic Agents; Antimuscarinics/Antispasmodics; Autonomic Drugs; Corneal Ulcer; Cycloplegics/Mydriatics; EENT Drugs; Eye, Ear, Nose, & Throat Preparations; Inflammatory Conditions; Lens Opacities; Mydriasis; Mydriatics; Mydriatics & Cycloplegics; Ophthalmics; Refraction; Conjunctivitis*; Pregnancy Category C; FDA Pre 1938 Drugs
* Indication not approved by the FDA

BRAND NAMES: Ak-Homatropine; *Allergan-Homatropine*; *Bell Homatropine Eye*; *Hom ofteno al*; *Hom Ofteno Al 2%* (Mexico); *Homatro*; *Homatrocil*; *Homatropin*; *Homatropin DAK*; *Homatropin Dispersa*; *Homatropin-POS* (Germany); *Homatropina*; *Homatropine*; *Homatropine Eye*; I-Homatrine; *Isopto-Homatropine*; **Isopto Homatropine**; *Minims-Homatropine*; *Minims Homatropine* (Canada); *Minims Homatropine HBr*; *Minims Homatropine Hydrobromide* (England); *Mydryn Eye*; *Omatropina Lux*; Spectro-Homatropine
(International brand names outside U.S. in italics)

FORMULARIES: Aetna; FHP; Medi-Cal

DESCRIPTION:

Homatropine hydrobromide ophthalmic solution is a sterile solution for ophthalmic administration in drop form, having the following composition:

Plastic squeeze bottle

Homatropine Hydrobromide: 20 or 50 mg/ml

(cycloplegic-mydriatic)

in a buffered aqueous solution containing boric acid, potassium chloride, sodium carbonate and purified water, preserved with benzalkonium chloride.

The chemical name is 1αH, 3αH-Tropan-3α-o1 mandelate (ester) hydrobromide.

CLINICAL PHARMACOLOGY:

Homatropine hydrobromide causes wide dilation of the pupil and paralysis of accommodation. Dilation is more rapid than with atropine but cycloplegia is not as pronounced and does not last as long.

INDICATIONS AND USAGE:

Homatropine hydrobromide is indicated for treatment of iritis and iridocyclitis, for relief of ciliary spasm, and also as an aid in refraction. It is frequently employed as a cycloplegic and mydriatic in preoperative and postoperative conditions.

CONTRAINDICATIONS:

Contraindicated in the presence of an anatomically narrow angle or in individuals with primary glaucoma and in individuals hypersensitive to any components of this preparation including the belladonna alkaloid group.

WARNINGS:

In infants and small children, use with extreme caution. Excessive use in children or certain individuals with a history of susceptibility to belladonna alkaloids may produce systemic symptoms of homatropine poisoning (see OVERDOSAGE.)

PRECAUTIONS:

Caution should be exercised when driving with dilated pupils or when engaging in hazardous activities. Parents of children should be cautious not to get the drug into the child's mouth and to wash both the child's and their hands after use of the drug.

If eye pain occurs from use of this medication, the patient should be advised to discontinue use and see prescribing physician immediately as this may indicate undiagnosed glaucoma. Use cautiously in elderly or hypertensive patients.

To avoid excessive systemic absorption, the lacrimal sac should be compressed by digital pressure for one minute after instillation.

Not for internal use. To prevent contaminating the dropper tip and solution, care should be taken not to touch the eyelids or surrounding area with the dropper tip of the bottle.

Carcinogenesis, Mutagenesis, and Impairment of Fertility: There have been no long-term studies using homatropine in animals to evaluate carcinogenic potential.

Pregnancy: Pregnancy Category C. Animal reproduction studies have not been done with homatropine. It is also not known whether homatropine hydrobromide can cause fetal harm when administered to a pregnant woman or can affect reproduction capacity. Homatropine should be given to a pregnant woman only if clearly needed.

Nursing Mothers: Since homatropine is absorbed systematically and since it is detectable in very small amounts in human milk, and because of the potential for serious adverse reactions in nursing infants from homatropine, a decision should be made whether to discontinue nursing or to discontinue the drug, taking into account the importance of the drug to the mother.

Pediatric Use: Homatropine should not be used during the first three months of life due to a possible association between the cycloplegia produced and the development of amblyopia. Safety and effectiveness in children have not been established.

ADVERSE REACTIONS:

Prolonged use may produce local irritation characterized by follicular conjunctivitis, vascular congestion, edema, exudate, and an eczematoid dermatitis. Systemic homatropine toxicity is manifested by flushing and dryness of the skin (a rash may be present in children), dryness of the mouth, anhidrosis, blurred vision, photophobia, loss of neuromuscular coordination (ataxic gait), a rapid and irregular pulse, fever, abdominal and bladder distention, dysarthric quality of speech, and mental aberration (hallucinosis) with recovery frequently followed by retrograde amnesia.

OVERDOSAGE:

When signs and symptoms of homatropine toxicity develop (see ADVERSE REACTIONS), physostigmine should be administered parenterally (for dosage refer to Goodman and Gilman or other pharmacology reference). In infants and children, the body surface must be kept moist.

DOSAGE AND ADMINISTRATION:

Usual dosage is one or two drops of the 2% or 5% solution in the eye(s) two or three times a day, modified at the discretion of the physician.

For refraction: One to two drops of the 2% solution every 10 to 15 minutes for 5 doses or one to two drops of the 5% solution repeated in 15 minutes, modified at the discretion of the physician.

Keep bottle tightly closed when not in use. Store at controlled room temperature 15°-30°C (59°-86°F).

HOW SUPPLIED - EQUIVALENTS NOT AVAILABLE:

Solution - Ophthalmic - 2 %

5 ml	**$11.25**	**ISOPTO HOMATROPINE, Alcon-PR**	**00998-0311-05**
15 ml	**$16.25**	**ISOPTO HOMATROPINE, Alcon-PR**	**00998-0311-15**

Solution - Ophthalmic - 5 %

2 ml x 12	$46.37	Homatropine Hydrobromide, Alcon	00065-0712-12
5 ml	$10.02	Homatropine Hydrobromide Ophthalmic, Ciba Vision	00058-2467-05

HOW SUPPLIED - EQUIVALENTS NOT AVAILABLE: *(cont'd)*

5 ml	$13.13	ISOPTO HOMATROPINE, Alcon-PR	00998-0315-05
15 ml	$17.50	ISOPTO HOMATROPINE, Alcon-PR	00998-0315-15

Solution - Ophthalmic; Top - 5 % 1 ml units

1 ml x 12	$25.80	Homatropine Hydrobromide Ophthalmic, Ciba Vision	00058-0778-12

HOMATROPINE METHYLBROMIDE *(001443)*

CATEGORIES: Anticholinergic Agents; Antimuscarinics/Antispasmodics; Autonomic Drugs; Gastrointestinal Drugs; Peptic Ulcer; Pregnancy Category C; FDA Approval Pre 1982

BRAND NAMES: Equipin; **Homapin**; Lantro

DESCRIPTION:

Homatropine methylbromide tablets contain homatropine methylbromide, an anticholinergic, which occurs as white crystals, or as a white odorless crystalline powder. Homatropine methylbromide melts at about 190°. The drug is very soluble in water, freely soluble in alcohol and practically insoluble in acetone.

The chemical name for homatropine methylbromide is 8- Azoniabicyclo(3.2.1) octane, 3-((hydroxyphenylacetyl)oxy)-8,8-dimethyl-,bromide, endo-.

3 α -Hydroxy-8-methyl-l α H,5 α H-tropanium bromide mandelate and the molecular weight is 370.29.

Each homatropine methylbromide tablet for oral administration, contains 5 mg or 10 mg of homatropine methylbromide. Inactive ingredients: lactose, microcrystalline cellulose and magnesium stearate. The homatropine methylbromide 10 mg tablet also contains FD&C Blue #1 Lake.

CLINICAL PHARMACOLOGY:

Homatropine methylbromide is an anticholinergic agent which possesses most of the pharmacologic actions of that drug class. These include reduction in volume & total acid content of gastric secretion inhibition of gastrointestinal motility, inhibition of salivary excretion, dilation of the pupil and inhibition of accommodation with resulting blurring of vision. Large doses may result in tachycardia.

Pharmacokinetics: Homatropine methylbromide is a quaternary ammonium derivative of scopolamine. As a class, these agents are poorly an unreliably absorbed.[1,2] Total absorption of quaternary ammonium derivatives of the alkaloids is 10-25%. Rate of absorption is not available. Quaternary ammonium salts have limited absorption from intact skin and conjunctival penetration is poor.[1] Little is known of the fate and excretion of most of these agents.[1] Homatropine methylbromide has limited ability to cross the blood-brain barrier.[3,4,5]The drug is excreted primarily in the urine and bile, or as unabsorbed drug in the feces.[2] There is no data on the presence of homatropine in breast milk; traces of atropine have been found after administration of atropine.[1]

INDICATIONS AND USAGE:

Adjunctive therapy for the treatment of peptic ulcer.

HOMATROPINE METHYLBROMIDE HAS NOT BEEN SHOWN TO BE EFFECTIVE IN CONTRIBUTING TO THE HEALING OF PEPTIC ULCER, DECREASING THE RATE OF RECURRENCE OR PREVENTING COMPLICATIONS.

CONTRAINDICATIONS:

Glaucoma; obstructive uropathy (*e.g.,* bladder neck obstruction due to prostatic hypertrophy), obstructive disease of the gastrointestinal tract (*e.g.,* pyloroduodenal stenosis); paralytic ileus; intestinal atony of the elderly or debilitated patient; unstable cardiovascular status in acute hemorrhage; severe ulcerative colitis; toxic megacolon complicating ulcerative colitis; myasthenia gravis.

Homatropine methylbromide is contraindicated in patients who are hypersensitive to it or related drugs.

WARNINGS:

In the presence of high environmental temperature, heat prostration (fever and heat strike due to decreased sweating) can occur with drug use.

Diarrhea may be an early symptom of incomplete intestinal obstruction, especially in patients with ileostomy or colostomy, In this instance treatment with this drug would be in appropriate and possibly harmful.

Homatropine methylbromide may produce drowsiness or blurred vision. The patient should be cautioned regarding activities requiring mental alertness such as operating a motor vehicle or other machinery or performing hazardous work while taking this drug.

With overdosage, a curare-like action may occur, i.e., neuromuscular blockade leading to muscular weakness and possible paralysis.

Homatropine methylbromide should be used in pregnancy, lactation, or in women of childbearing age only when in judgement of the physician, the expected benefits outweigh the potential hazards to the mother and child.

PRECAUTIONS:

General: Use homatropine methylbromide with caution in the elderly and in all patients with: autonomic neuropathy; hepatic or renal disease; or ulcerative colitis—large doses may suppress intestinal mobility to the point of producing a paralytic ileus and for this reason precipitate or aggravate "toxic megacolon," a serious complication of the disease.

The drug should also be used with caution in patients having hyperthyroidism, coronary heart disease, congestive heart failure, tachyarrhythmia, tachycardia, hypertension, or prostatic hypertrophy.

Information for the Patient: See statement under WARNINGS.

Laboratory Tests: Progress of the peptic ulcer under treatment should be followed by upper gastrointestinal contrast radiology or endoscopy to insure healing. Stool tests for occult blood and blood hemoglobin or hemocrit values should be followed to rule out bleeding from the ulcer.

Carcinogenesis, Mutagenesis, and Impairment of Fertility: No long-term studies in animals have been performed to evaluate carcinogenic potential.

Pregnancy, Teratogenic Effects, Pregnancy Category C: Animal reproduction studies have not been conducted with homatropine methylbromide. It is also not known whether homatropine methylbromide can cause fetal harm wen administered to a pregnant woman or can affect reproduction capacity.. Homatropine methylbromide should be given to a pregnant woman only if clearly needed.

Nursing Mothers: It is not known whether this drug is excreted in human milk. Because many drugs are excreted in human milk, caution should be exercised when homatropine methylbromide is administered to a nursing woman.

Anticholinergic drugs may suppress lactation.

PRECAUTIONS: *(cont'd)*

Pediatric Use: Safety and efficacy in children have not been established.

DRUG INTERACTIONS:

Additive anticholinergic effects may result from concomitant use with antipsychotics, tricyclic antidepressants, and other drugs with anticholinergic effects. Concomitant administration with antacids may interfere with the absorption of homatropine methylbromide.

ADVERSE REACTIONS:

The following adverse reactions have been observed, but there are not enough data to support an estimate of frequency.

Cardiovascular: Tachycardia, palpitation.

Allergic: Severe allergic reaction or drug idiosyncrasies including anaphylaxis.

CNS: Headaches, nervousness, mental confusion, drowsiness, dizziness.

Special Senses: Blurred vision, dilatation of the pupil, cystoplegia, increased ocular tension, loss of taste.

Renal: Urinary hesitancy and retention.

Gastrointestinal: Nausea, vomiting, constipation, bloated feeling.

Dermatologic: Decreased sweating, urticaria and other dermal manifestations.

Miscellaneous: Xerostomia, weakness, insomnia, impotence, suppression of lactation.

OVERDOSAGE:

The symptoms of overdosage with homatropine methylbromide progress from intensification of the usual side effects to CNS disturbances (from restlessness and excitement to psychotic behavior), circulatory changes (flushing, fall in blood pressure, circulatory failure), respiratory failure, paralysis, and coma.

Measures to be taken are (1) induction of emesis and (2) injection of physostigmine 0.5 to 2 mg Intravenously, and repeated as necessary up to a total of 5 mg. Fever may be treated symptomatically (alcohol, sponging, ice packs). Excitement of a degree which demands attention may be managed with sodium thiopental 2% solution given slowly intravenously or chloral hydrate (100-200 ml of a 2% solution) by rectal infusion. In the event of progression of the curare-like effect to paralysis of the respiratory muscles, artificial respiration should be instituted and maintained until effective respiratory action returns.

DOSAGE AND ADMINISTRATION:

Usual Adult Dosage: The average dosage of homatropine methylbromide is 5 mg or 10 mg 3 or 4 times daily, one-half hour before meals and at bedtime. Dosage should be adjusted to individual patient's needs.

Patients whose dosage should has been reduced to eliminate or modify side effects often continue to show adequate response both subjectively in relief of symptoms and objectively as measured by antisecretory effects.

The ultimate aim of therapy is to arrive at a dosage which provides maximal clinical effectiveness with a minimum of unpleasant side effects. Many patients report no side effects on a dosage which gives complete relief of symptoms. On the other hand, some patients have reported severe side effects without appreciable sympathetic relief. Such patients must be considered unsuited for this therapy. Usually they have been or will prove to be similarly intolerant to other anticholinergic drugs. If homatropine methylbromide is to be used in a patient who gives a history of such intolerance, it should be started at a low dosage.

Store at controlled room temperature 15-30°C (59-65°F).

REFERENCES:

1. *The Pharmacological Basis of Therapeutics.* Gilman and Goodman, MacMillan Publ. Co., New York, 6th Ed. 1980. **2.** *American Hospital Formulary Service.*American Society of Hospital Pharmacists. Bethesda, Maryland. **3.** Domino, E.F., Corasen, G., Central and Peripheral Effects of Muscarinic Cholinergic Blocking Agents in Man. *Anesthesiology* 28:568-574 (1967) **4.** Mogensen, L. and Orinius, E. Arrhythmic Complications after Parasympathetic Treatment of Bradyarrhythmias in a Coronary Care Unit.*Acts Med. Scan.* 190:495-498 (1971) **5.** Neeld, J.B., Jr., et al; Cardiac Rate and Rhythm Changes with Atropine and Methscopolamine. Clin. *Pharmacol. Ther.*17(3):290-295 (March) 1975.

HOW SUPPLIED - EQUIVALENTS NOT AVAILABLE:

Tablet, Uncoated - Oral - 10 mg

100's	$125.92	HOMAPIN, Mission Pharma	00178-0141-01

HOMATROPINE METHYLBROMIDE; HYDROCODONE BITARTRATE *(001444)*

CATEGORIES: Antitussives; Antitussives/Expectorants/Mucolytics; Cough Preparations; Respiratory & Allergy Medications; Pregnancy Category C; DEA Class CIII; FDA Approved 1983 Mar

BRAND NAMES: Histussin-Hc; **Hycodan**; Hycomar; Hydrocodone Compound; Hydrocone/Mycodone; Hydromet; Hydropane; Hydrotropine; Mycodone; Tussigon

FORMULARIES: Aetna; PCS

DESCRIPTION:

The product contains hydrocodone bitartrate, a semisynthetic centrally acting narcotic antitussive. Homatropine methylbromide is included in a subtherapeutic amount to discourage deliberate overdosage.

Each tablet or teaspoonful (5 ml) contains:

Hydrocodone bitartrate, USP: 5 mg WARNING: May be habit forming.

Homatropine methylbromide, USP: 1.5 mg

Hycodane tablets also contain: calcium phosphate dibasic, colloidal silicon dioxide, lactose, magnesium stearate, starch and stearic acid.

Hycodan syrup: caramel coloring, FD&C Red 40, liquid sugar, methylparaben, propylparaben, sorbitol solution and wild cherry imitation flavor.

The hydrocodone component is 4,5α-epoxy-3-methoxy-17-methylmorphinan-6-one tartrate (1: 1) hydrate (2:5), a fine white crystal or crystalline powder, which is derived from the opium alkaloid, thebaine, has a molecular weight of (494.50).

Hydrocodone Bitartrate: $C_{18}H_{21}NO_3C_4H_6O_6$ 2 1/2H_2O

Homatropine Methylbromide: $C_{17}H_{24}BrNO_3$

Homatropine Methylbromide is 8-Azoniabicyclo [3.2.1.]octane,3- [(hydroxyphenylacetyl)oxy]-8,8-dimethyl-, bromide, endo-; a white crystal or fine white crystalline powder, with a molecular weight of (370.29).

CLINICAL PHARMACOLOGY:

Hydrocodone is a semisynthetic narcotic antitussive and analgesic with multiple actions qualitatively similar to those of codeine. The precise mechanism of action of hydrocodone and other opiates is not known; however, hydrocodone is believed to act directly on the cough center. In excessive doses, hydrocodone, like other opium derivatives, will depress respiration. The effects of hydrocodone in therapeutic doses on the cardiovascular system are insignificant. Hydrocodone can produce miosis, euphoria, physical and physiological dependence.

Following a 10 mg oral dose of hydrocodone administered to five adult male subjects, the mean peak concentration was 23.6 ± 5.2 ng/ml. Maximum serum levels were achieved at 1.3 ± 0.3 hours and the half-life was determined to be 3.8 ± 0.3 hours. Hydrocodone exhibits a complex pattern of metabolism including O-demethylation, N-demethylation and 6-keto reduction to the corresponding 6-α and 6-β-hydroxymetabolites.

INDICATIONS AND USAGE:

Hydrocodone w/homatropine is indicated for the symptomatic relief of cough.

CONTRAINDICATIONS:

Hydrocodone w/homatropine should not be administered to patients who are hypersensitive to hydrocodone or homatropine methylbromide.

WARNINGS:

May be habit forming. Hydrocodone can produce drug dependence of the morphine type and, therefore, has the potential for being abused. Psychic dependence, physical dependence and tolerance may develop upon repeated administration of hydrocodone w/homatropine and it should be prescribed and administered with the same degree of caution appropriate to the use of other narcotic drugs (See DRUG ABUSE AND DEPENDENCE.)

Respiratory Depression: Hydrocodone w/homatropine produces dose-related respiratory depression by directly acting on brain stem respiratory centers. If respiratory depression occurs, it may be antagonized by the use of naloxone hydrochloride and other supportive measures when indicated.

Head Injury And Increased Intracranial Pressure: The respiratory depression properties of narcotics and their capacity to elevate cerebrospinal fluid pressure may be markedly exaggerated in the presence of head injury, other intracranial lesions or a pre-existing increase in intracranial pressure. Furthermore, narcotics produce adverse reactions which may obscure the clinical course of patients with head injuries.

Acute Abdominal Conditions: The administration of hydrocodone w/homatropine or other narcotics may obscure the diagnosis or clinical course of patients with acute abdominal conditions.

Pediatric Use: In young children, as well as adults, the respiratory center is sensitive to the depressant action of narcotic cough suppressants in a dose-dependent manner. Benefit-to-risk ratio should be carefully considered especially in children with respiratory embarrassment (*e.g.,* croup).

PRECAUTIONS:

GENERAL

Before prescribing medication to suppress or modify cough, it is important to ascertain that the underlying cause of cough is identified, that modification of cough does not increase the risk of clinical or physiological complications, and that appropriate therapy for the primary disease is provided.

Special Risk Patients: Hydrocodone w/homatropine should be given with caution to certain patients such as the elderly or debilitated, and those with severe impairment of hepatic or renal functions, hypothyroidism, Addison's disease, prostatic hypertrophy or urethral stricture, asthma, and narrow-angle glaucoma.

INFORMATION FOR THE PATIENT

Hydrocodone may impair the mental and/or physical abilities required for the performance of potentially hazardous tasks such as driving a car or operating machinery. The patient using hydrocodone w/homatropine should be cautioned accordingly.

CARCINOGENESIS, MUTAGENESIS, AND IMPAIRMENT OF FERTILITY

Studies of hydrocodone w/homatropine in animals to evaluate the carcinogenic and mutagenic potential and the effect of fertility have not been conducted.

PREGNANCY CATEGORY C

Teratogenic Effects: Animal reproduction studies have not been conducted with hydrocodone w/homatropine. It is also not known whether hydrocodone w/homatropine can cause fetal harm when administered to a pregnant woman or can affect reproduction capacity. hydrocodone w/homatropine should be given to a pregnant woman only if clearly needed.

Nonteratogenic Effects: Babies born to mothers who have been taking opioids regularly prior to delivery will be physically dependent. The withdrawal signs include irritability and excessive crying, tremors, hyperactive reflexes, increased respiratory rate, increased stools, sneezing, yawning, vomiting, and fever. The intensity of the syndrome does not always correlate with the duration of maternal opioid use or dose.

LABOR AND DELIVERY

As with all narcotics, administration of hydrocodone w/homatropine to the mother shortly before delivery may result in some degree of respiratory depression in the newborn, especially if higher doses are used.

NURSING MOTHERS

It is not known whether this drug is excreted in human milk. Because many drugs are excreted in human milk and because of the potential for serious adverse reactions in nursing infants from hydrocodone w/homatropine, a decision should be made whether to discontinue nursing or to discontinue the drug, taking into account the importance of the drug to the mother.

PEDIATRIC USE

Safety and effectiveness of hydrocodone w/homatropine in children under six have not been established.

DRUG INTERACTIONS:

Patients receiving narcotics, antihistamines, antipsychotics, antianxiety agents or other CNS depressants (including alcohol) concomitantly with hydrocodone w/homatropine, may exhibit an additive CNS depression. When combined therapy is contemplated, the dose of one or both agents should be reduced. The use of MAO inhibitors or tricyclic antidepressants with hydrocodone preparations may increase the effect of either the antidepressant or hydrocodone.

ADVERSE REACTIONS:

Central Nervous System: Sedation, drowsiness, mental clouding, lethargy, impairment of mental and physical performance, anxiety, fear, dysphoria, dizziness, psychic dependence, mood changes.

ADVERSE REACTIONS: *(cont'd)*

Gastrointestinal System: Nausea and vomiting may occur; they are more frequent in ambulatory than in recumbent patients. Prolonged administration of hydrocodone w/homatropine may produce constipation.

Genitourinary System: Ureteral spasm, spasm of vesicle sphincters and urinary retention have been reported with opiates.

Respiratory Depression: Hydrocodone w/homatropine may produce dose-related respiratory depression by acting directly on the brain stem respiratory centers (see OVERDOSAGE.)

Dermatological: Skin rash, pruritus.

DRUG ABUSE AND DEPENDENCE:

Hydrocodone w/homatropine is a schedule III narcotic. Psychic dependence, physical dependence and tolerance may develop upon repeated administration of narcotics; therefore, hydrocodone w/homatropine should be prescribed and administered with caution. However, psychic dependence is unlikely to develop when hydrocodone w/homatropine is used for a short time for the treatment of cough. Physical dependence, the condition in which continued administration of the drug is required to prevent the appearance of a withdrawal syndrome, assumes clinically significant proportions only after several weeks of continued oral narcotic use, although some mild degree of physical dependence may develop after a few days of narcotic therapy.

OVERDOSAGE:

Signs and Symptoms: Serious overdosage with hydrocodone is characterized by respiratory depression (a decrease in respiratory rate and/or tidal volume, Cheyne-Stokes respiration, cyanosis), extreme somnolence progressing to stupor or coma, skeletal muscle flaccidity, cold and clammy skin, and sometimes bradycardia and hypotension. In severe overdosage, apnea, circulatory collapse, cardiac arrest and death may occur. The ingestion of very large amounts of hydrocodone w/homatropine may, in addition, result in acute homatropine intoxication.

Treatment: Primary attention should be given to the reestablishment of adequate respiratory exchange through provision of a patent airway and the institution of assisted or controlled ventilation. The narcotic antagonist naloxone hydrochloride is a specific antidote for respiratory depression which may result from overdosage or unusual sensitivity to narcotics including hydrocodone. Therefore, an appropriate dose of naloxone hydrochloride should be administered, preferably by the intravenous route, simultaneously with efforts at respiratory resuscitation. For further information, see full prescribing information for naloxone hydrochloride. An antagonist should not be administered in the absence of clinically significant respiratory depression. Oxygen, intravenous fluids, vasopressors and other supportive measures should be employed as indicated. Gastric emptying may be useful in removing unabsorbed drug.

DOSAGE AND ADMINISTRATION:

Adults: One (1) tablet or one (1) teaspoonful (5 ml) of the syrup every 4 to 6 hours as needed; do not exceed six (6) tablets or six (6) teaspoonfuls in 24 hours.

Children 6 to 12 years of age: One-half (1/2) tablet or one-half (1/2) teaspoonful (2.5 ml) of the syrup every 4 to 6 hours as needed; do not exceed three (3) tablets or three (3) teaspoonfuls in 24 hours.

Store at controlled room temperature (59°-86°F, 15°-30°C).

HOW SUPPLIED - RATED THERAPEUTICALLY EQUIVALENT:

Syrup - Oral - 1.5 mg/5 mg/5ml

473 ml	$13.13	HYDROMET SYRUP, Alpharma	00472-1030-16
480 ml	$8.93	Hydrocodone & Homatropine Syrup, H.C.F.A. F F P	99999-1444-02
480 ml	$10.71	Hydrocodone Compound, Qualitest Pharms	00603-1296-58
480 ml	$11.50	Hydrocodone Homatropine Syrup, Geneva Pharms	00781-6526-16
480 ml	$12.35	Hydrocodone, Goldline Labs	00182-1155-40
480 ml	$12.50	HYDROMIDE, Major Pharms	00904-0956-16
480 ml	$12.95	HYDROTROPINE, Rugby	00536-0920-85
480 ml	$13.10	Hydrocodone/Homatropine, Aligen Independ	00405-0098-16
480 ml	$13.10	Hydrocodone Compound, Morton Grove	60432-0455-16
480 ml	$13.25	HYDROPANE SYRUP, Halsey Drug	00879-0455-16
480 ml	$13.50	Hydrocodone/Homatropine Methyl, IDE-Interstate	00814-3729-82
480 ml	$14.24	HYDROMET, HL Moore Drug Exch	00839-6555-69
480 ml	**$54.50**	**HYCODAN, Dupont Pharma**	**00056-0234-16**
3785 ml	$91.88	HYDROMET SYRUP, Alpharma	00472-1030-28
3840 ml	$71.42	Hydrocodone & Homatropine Syrup, H.C.F.A. F F P	99999-1444-01
3840 ml	$71.46	HYDROTROPINE, Rugby	00536-0920-90
3840 ml	$91.95	HYDROPANE SYRUP, Halsey Drug	00879-0455-28

Tablet, Uncoated - Oral - 1.5 mg/5 mg

100's	**$46.85**	**HYCODAN, Dupont Pharma**	**00056-0042-70**
500's	**$231.00**	**HYCODAN, Dupont Pharma**	**00056-0042-85**

HOW SUPPLIED - NOT RATED EQUIVALENT:

Syrup - Oral - 1.5 mg/5 mg/5ml

480 ml	$32.15	HISTUSSIN HC, Bock Pharma	00563-0860-16

HOMATROPINE; PAREGORIC; PECTIN *(001445)*

CATEGORIES: Antidiarrhea Agents; Gastrointestinal Drugs; DEA Class CV; FDA Pre 1938 Drugs

BRAND NAMES: Dia-Quel

Prescribing information not available at time of publication.

HYDRALAZINE HYDROCHLORIDE *(001450)*

CATEGORIES: Antihypertensives; Cardiovascular Drugs; Hypertension; Vasodilating Agents; Pregnancy Category C; FDA Approval Pre 1982

BRAND NAMES: *Alphapress* (Australia); *Apdormin* (Japan); *Apo-Hydralazine*; *Apresolin*; *Apresolin Retard*; *Apresolina* (Mexico); **Apresoline**; Apresrex; *Apulon*; *Asozart*; *Deselazin* (Japan); Dralzine; *Hydrapres*; *Hypatol* (Japan); *Hyperphen*; *Hyperex*; *Ipolina*; *Naselin*; *Nepresol*; *Nonpolin* (Japan); *Novo-Hylazin* (Canada); *Resporidin* (Japan); *Slow-Apresoline*; *Solesorin* (Japan); *Solezorin*; *Stable*; *Sulesorin*; *Supres*; *Tetrasoline* (Japan); *Travinon* (Japan); *Zinepress*
(International brand names outside U.S. in italics)

FORMULARIES: Aetna; BC-BS; FHP; Medi-Cal; PCS; WHO

COST OF THERAPY: $27.44 (Hypertension; Tablet; 10 mg; 4/day; 365 days) vs. Potential Cost of $24,027.04 (Coronary Bypass)

PRIMARY ICD9: 401.1 (Essential Hypertension, Benign)

DESCRIPTION:

Hydralazine hydrochloride USP, is an antihypertensive. Its chemical name is 1-hydrazinophthalazine monohydrochloride.

Hydralazine HCl USP is a white to off-white, odorless crystalline powder. It is soluble in water, slightly soluble in alcohol, and very slightly soluble in ether. It melts at about 275°C, with decomposition, and has a molecular weight of 196.64.

Hydralazine HCl is available as 10-,25-,50-, and 100-mg tablets for oral administration.

Inactive Ingredients. Acacia, D&C Yellow No. 10(10-mg tablets), FD&C Blue No.1(25-mg and 50-mg tablets), FD&C Yellow No. 5 and FD&C Yellow No. 6(100-mg tablets), lactose, magnesium stearate, mannitol, polyethylene glycol, sodium starch glycolate, starch, and stearic acid.

Hydralazine HCl is available in 1-ml ampuls for intravenous and intramuscular administration. Each milliliter of the sterile, colorless solution contains hydralazine hydrochloride USP, 20 mg; methylparaben NF, 0.65 mg; propylparaben NF, 0.35 mg; propene glycol USP, 103.6 mg. The pH of the solution is 3.4-4.0.

CLINICAL PHARMACOLOGY:

Although the precise mechanism of action of hydralazine is not fully understood, the major effects are on the cardiovascular system. Hydralazine apparently lowers blood pressure by exerting a peripheral vasodilating effect through a direct relaxation of vascular smooth muscle. Hydralazine, by altering cellular calcium metabolism, interferes with calcium movements within the vascular smooth muscle that are responsible for initiating or maintaining the contractile state.

The peripheral vasodilating effect of hydralazine results in decreased arterial blood pressure (diastolic more than systolic); decreased peripheral vascular resistance; and an increased heart rate, stroke volume, and cardiac output. The preferential dilatation of arterioles, as compared to veins, minimizes postural hypotension and promotes the increase in cardiac output. Hydralazine usually increases renin activity in plasma, presumably as a result of increased secretion of renin by the renal juxtaglomerular cells in response to reflex sympathetic discharge. This increase in renin activity leads to the production of angiotensin II, which then causes stimulation of aldosterone and consequent sodium reabsorption. Hydralazine also maintains or increases renal and cerebral blood flow.

TABLETS

Hydralazine is rapidly absorbed after oral administration, and peak plasma levels are reached at 1-2 hours. Plasma levels of apparent hydralazine decline with a half-life of 3-7 hours. Binding to human plasma protein is 87%. Plasma levels of hydralazine vary widely among individuals. Hydralazine is subject to polymorphic acetylation; slow acetylators generally have higher plasma levels of hydralazine and require lower doses to maintain control of blood pressure. Hydralazine undergoes extensive hepatic metabolism; it is excreted mainly in the form of metabolites in the urine.

INJECTION

The average maximal decrease in blood pressure usually occurs 10-80 minutes after administration of parenteral hydralazine HCl. No other pharmacokinetic data on parenteral hydralazine HCl are available.

INDICATIONS AND USAGE:

Essential hypertension, alone or as an adjunct.

CONTRAINDICATIONS:

Hypersensitivity to hydralazine; coronary artery disease; mitral valvular rheumatic heart disease.

WARNINGS:

In a few patients hydralazine may produce a clinical picture simulating systemic lupus erythematosus including glomerulonephritis. In such patients hydralazine should be discontinued unless the benefit-to-risk determination requires continued antihypertensive therapy with this drug. Symptoms and signs usually regress when the drug is discontinued but residua have been detected many years later. Long-term treatment with steroids may be necessary. (See PRECAUTIONS, Laboratory Tests.)

PRECAUTIONS:

GENERAL

Myocardial stimulation produced by hydralazine HCl can cause anginal attacks and ECG changes of myocardial ischemia. The drug has been implicated in the production of myocardial infarction. It must, therefore, be used with caution in patients with suspected coronary artery disease.

The "hyperdynamic" circulation caused by hydralazine HCl may accentuate specific cardiovascular inadequacies. For example, hydralazine HCl may increase pulmonary artery pressure in patients with mitral valvular disease. The drug may reduce the pressor responses to epinephrine. Postural hypotension may result from hydralazine HCl but is less common than with ganglionic blocking agents. It should be used with caution in patients with cerebral vascular accidents.

In hypertensive patients with normal kidneys who are treated with hydralazine HCl, there is evidence of increased renal blood flow and a maintenance of glomerular filtration rate. In some instances where control values were below normal, improved renal function has been noted after administration of hydralazine HCl. However, as with any antihypertensive agent, hydralazine HCl should be used with caution in patients with advanced renal damage.

Peripheral neuritis, evidenced by paresthesia, numbness, and tingling, has been observed. Published evidence suggests an antipyridoxine effect, and that pyridoxine should be added to the regimen if symptoms develop.

LABORATORY TESTS

Complete blood counts and antinuclear antibody titer determinations are indicated before and periodically during prolonged therapy with hydralazine even though the patient is asymptomatic. These studies are also indicated if the patient develops arthralgia, fever, chest pain, continued malaise, or other unexplained signs or symptoms.

A positive antinuclear antibody titer requires that the physician carefully weigh the implications of the test results against the benefits to be derived from antihypertensive therapy with hydralazine.

Blood dyscrasias, consisting of reduction in hemoglobin and red cell count, leukopenia, agranulocytosis, and purpura, have been reported. If such abnormalities develop, therapy should be discontinued.

CARCINOGENESIS, MUTAGENESIS, AND IMPAIRMENT OF FERTILITY

In a life-time study in Swiss albino mice, there was a statistically significant increase in the incidence of lung tumors (adenomas and adenocarcinomas) of both male and female mice given hydralazine continuously in their drinking water at a dosage of about 250 mg/kg per day (about 80 times the maximum recommended human dose). In a 2-year carcinogenicity study of rats given hydralazine by gavage at dose levels of 15, 30, and 60 mg/kg/day (approximately 5 to 20 times the recommended human daily dosage), microscopic examination of the liver revealed a small, but statistically significant, increase in benign neoplastic nodules in male and female rats from the high-dose group and in female rats from the intermediate-dose group. Benign interstitial cell tumors of the testes were also significantly increased in male rats from the high-dose group. The tumors observed are common in aged rats and a significantly increased incidence was not observed until 18 months of treatment. hydralazine was shown to be mutagenic in bacterial systems (Gene Mutation and DNA Repair) and in one of two rat and one rabbit hepatocyte *in vitro*DNA repair studies. Additional *in vivo* and *in vitro* studies using lymphoma cells, germinal cells, and fibroblasts from mice, bone marrow cells from Chinese hamsters and fibroblasts from human cell lines did not demonstrate any mutagenic potential for hydralazine.

The extent to which these findings indicate a risk to man is uncertain. While long-term clinical observation has not suggested that human cancer is associated with hydralazine use, epidemiologic studies have so far been insufficient to arrive at any conclusions.

PREGNANCY CATEGORY C

Animal studies indicate that hydralazine is teratogenic in mice at 20-30 times the maximum daily human dose of 200-300 mg and possibly in rabbits at 10-15 times the maximum daily human dose, but that it is nonteratogenic in rats. Teratogenic effects observed were cleft palate and malformations of facial and cranial bones.

There are no adequate and well-controlled studies in pregnant women. Although clinical experience does not include any positive evidence of adverse effects on the human fetus, hydralazine should be used during pregnancy only if the expected benefit justifies the potential risk to the fetus.

NURSING MOTHERS

It is not known whether this drug is excreted in human milk. Because many drugs are excreted in human milk, caution should be exercised when hydralazine HCl is administered to a nursing woman.

PEDIATRIC USE

Safety and effectiveness in children have not been established in controlled clinical trails, although there is experience with the use of hydralazine HCl in children.

GENERAL

The hydralazine HCl tablets (100 mg) contain FD&C Yellow No. 5 (tartrazine), which may cause allergic-type reactions (including bronchial asthma) in certain susceptible individuals. Although the overall incidence of FD&C Yellow No. 5 (tartrazine) sensitivity in the general population is low, it is frequently seen in patients who are also hypersensitive to aspirin.

INFORMATION FOR THE PATIENT

Patients should be informed of possible side effects and advised to take the medication regularly and continuously as directed.

PEDIATRIC USE

Tablets: The usual recommended oral starting dosage is 0.75 mg/kg of body weight daily in four divided doses. Dosage may be increased gradually over the next 3-4 weeks to a maximum of 7.5 mg/kg or 200 mg daily.

Injection: The usual recommended parenteral dosage, administered intramuscularly or intravenously, is 1.7-3.5 mg/kg of body weight daily, divided into four to six doses.

DRUG INTERACTIONS:

MAO inhibitors should be used with caution in patients receiving hydralazine.

When other potent parenteral antihypertensive drugs, such as diazoxide, are used in combination with hydralazine, patients should be continuously observed for several hours for any excessive fall in blood pressure. Profound hypotensive episodes may occur when diazoxide injection and hydralazine HCl are used concomitantly.

Drug/Food Interactions with Tablets: Administration of hydralazine with food results in higher plasma levels.

ADVERSE REACTIONS:

Adverse reactions with hydralazine HCl are usually reversible when dosage is reduced. However, in some cases it may be necessary to discontinue the drug.

The following adverse reactions have been observed, but there has not been enough systematic collection of data to support an estimate of their frequency.

Common: Headache, anorexia, vomiting, diarrhea, palpitations, tachycardia, angina pectoris.

Less Frequent

Digestive: constipation, paralytic ileus.

Cardiovascular: hypotension, paradoxical pressor response, edema.

Respiratory: dyspnea.

Neurologic: peripheral neuritis, evidenced by paresthesia, numbness, and tingling; dizziness; tremors; muscle cramps; psychotic reactions characterized by depression, disorientation, or anxiety.

Genitourinary: difficulty in urination.

Hematologic: blood dyscrasias, consisting of reduction in hemoglobin and red cell count, leukopenia, agranulocytosis, purpura; lymphadenopathy; splenomegaly.

Hypersensitive Reactions: rash, urticaria, pruritus, fever, chills, arthralgia, eosinophilia, and, rarely, hepatitis.

Other: nasal congestion, flushing, lacrimation, conjunctivitis.

OVERDOSAGE:

Acute Toxicity: No deaths due to acute poisoning have been reported.

Highest known dose survived : adults, 10 g orally.

Oral LD_{50} in rats: 173 and 187 mg/kg.

Signs and Symptoms: Signs and symptoms of overdosage include hypotension, tachycardia, headache, and generalized skin flushing.

Complications can include myocardial ischemia and subsequent myocardial infarction, cardiac arrhythmia, and profound shock.

Treatment: There is no specific antidote.

Support of the cardiovascular system is of primary importance. Shock should be treated with plasma expanders. If possible, vasopressors should not be not be given, but if a vasopressor is required, care should be taken not to precipitate or aggravate cardiac arrhythmia. Tachycardia responds to beta blockers. Digitalization may be necessary, and renal function should be monitored and supported as required.

No experience has been reported with extracorporeal or peritoneal dialysis.

Tablets Only: The gastric contents should be evacuated, taking adequate precautions against aspiration and for protection of the airway. An activated charcoal slurry may be instilled if conditions permit. These manipulations may have to be omitted or carried out after cardiovascular status has been stabilized, since they might precipitate cardiac arrhythmias or increase the depth of shock.

DOSAGE AND ADMINISTRATION:

TABLETS

Initiate therapy in gradually increasing dosages; adjust according to individual response. Start with 10 mg four times daily for the first 2-4 days, increase to 25 mg four times daily for the balance of the first week. For the second and subsequent weeks, increase dosage to 50 mg four times daily. For maintenance, adjust dosage to the lowest effective levels.

The incidence of toxic reactions, particularly the L.E. cell syndrome, is high in the group of patients receiving large doses of hydralazine HCl.

In a few resistant patients, up to 300 mg of hydralazine HCl daily may be required for a significant antihypertensive effect. In such cases, a lower dosage of hydralazine HCl combined with a thiazide and/or reserpine or a bete blocker may be considered. However, when combining therapy, individual titration is essential to ensure the lowest possible therapeutic dose of each drug.

Do not store above 86°F (30° C).

Dispense in tight, light-resistant container (USP).

INJECTION

When there is urgent need, therapy in the hospitalized patient may be initiated intramuscularly or as a rapid intravenous bolus injection directly into the vein. Parenteral hydralazine HCl should be used only when the drug cannot be given orally. The usual dose is 20-40 mg, repeated as necessary. Certain patients (especially those with marked renal damage) may require a lower dose. Blood pressure should be checked frequently. It may begin to fall within a few minutes after injection, with the average maximal decrease occurring in 10-80 minutes. In cases where there has been increased intracranial pressure, lowering the blood pressure may increase cerebral ischemia. Most patients can be transferred to oral hydralazine HCl within 24-48 hours.

The product should be used immediately after the ampul is opened. It should not be added to infusion solutions. Apresoline hydrochloride parenteral may discolor upon contact with metal; discolored solutions should be discarded.

Parenteral drug products should be inspected visually for particulate matter and discoloration prior to administration, whenever solution and container permit.

Store between 59°-86°F (15°-30°C).

(Tablets: Ciba, 4/92, 666691)

(Injection: Ciba, 4/92, 665803)

HOW SUPPLIED - RATED THERAPEUTICALLY EQUIVALENT:

Injection, Solution - Intramuscular; - 20 mg/ml

1 ml	**$28.39**	**APRESOLINE, Novartis**	**00083-2626-05**
1 ml	$65.63	Hydralazine Hcl, Fujisawa USA	00469-2490-00
1 ml	$147.85	Hydralazine Hcl, Solopak Labs	39769-0021-01

Tablet, Uncoated - Oral - 10 mg

100's	$1.88	Hydralazine HCl, H.C.F.A. F F P	99999-1450-01
100's	$2.50	Hydralazine Hcl, Squibb-Mark	57783-6640-01
100's	$2.63	Hydralazine Hcl, HL Moore Drug Exch	00839-6114-06
100's	$2.65	Hydralazine, United Res	00677-0650-01
100's	$2.65	Hydralazine Hcl, Mutual Pharm	53489-0123-01
100's	$2.75	Hydralazine Hcl, Consolidated Midland	00223-1060-01
100's	$2.75	Hydralazine Hcl, Halsey Drug	00879-0535-01
100's	$3.00	Hydralazine Hcl, Major Pharms	00904-2338-60
100's	$3.08	Hydralazine Hcl, Camall	00147-0255-10
100's	$3.40	Hydralazine Hcl, Qualitest Pharms	00603-3830-21
100's	$3.50	Hydralazine Hcl, Goldline Labs	00182-0905-01
100's	$3.50	Hydralazine Hcl 10, Aligen Independ	00405-4469-01
100's	$3.50	Hydralazine Hcl, Sidmak Labs	50111-0398-01
100's	$3.51	Hydralazine HCl, Schein Pharm (US)	00364-0647-01
100's	$3.57	Hydralazine Hcl, Martec Pharms	52555-0029-01
100's	$3.60	Hydralazine Hcl, Rugby	00536-3890-01
100's	$3.70	Hydralazine Hcl, Par Pharm	49884-0029-01
100's	$4.25	Hydralazine Hcl, Raway	00686-0074-20
100's	$4.58	Hydralazine Hcl, Major Pharms	00904-2338-61
100's	$11.50	Hydralazine Hcl, Goldline Labs	00182-0905-89
100's	$11.84	Hydralazine Hcl, Vangard Labs	00615-0516-13
100's	**$20.60**	**APRESOLINE, Novartis**	**00083-0037-30**
1000's	$9.90	Hydralazine Hcl, Camall	00147-0255-20
1000's	$12.50	Hydralazine Hcl, Major Pharms	00904-2338-80
1000's	$13.75	Hydralazine Hcl, Squibb-Mark	57783-6640-03
1000's	$15.05	Hydralazine Hcl, Sidmak Labs	50111-0398-03
1000's	$15.11	Hydralazine Hcl, HL Moore Drug Exch	00839-6114-16
1000's	$16.50	Hydralazine Hcl, Mutual Pharm	53489-0123-10
1000's	$16.79	Hydralazine, United Res	00677-0650-10
1000's	$16.84	Hydralazine Hcl, Qualitest Pharms	00603-3830-32
1000's	$17.50	Hydralazine Hcl, Consolidated Midland	00223-1060-02
1000's	$17.50	Hydralazine Hcl, Halsey Drug	00879-0535-10
1000's	$17.65	Hydralazine Hcl, Rugby	00536-3890-10
1000's	$18.80	Hydralazine HCl, H.C.F.A. F F P	99999-1450-02
1000's	$33.95	Hydralazine Hcl 10, Aligen Independ	00405-4469-03
1000's	$33.95	Hydralazine Hcl, Par Pharm	49884-0029-10

Tablet, Uncoated - Oral - 25 mg

100's	$1.68	Hydralazine Hcl, Rugby	00536-3917-01
100's	$1.88	Hydralazine HCl, H.C.F.A. F F P	99999-1450-03
100's	$3.18	Hydralazine Hcl, Voluntary Hosp	53258-0176-01
100's	$3.20	Hydralazine Hcl, Halsey Drug	00879-0536-01
100's	$3.25	Hydralazine Hcl, Consolidated Midland	00223-1061-01
100's	$3.30	Hydralazine Hcl, Squibb-Mark	57783-6650-01
100's	$3.50	Hydralazine Hcl, United Res	00677-0447-01
100's	$3.51	Hydralazine Hcl, Qualitest Pharms	00603-3831-21
100's	$3.65	Hydralazine Hcl, HL Moore Drug Exch	00839-1361-06
100's	$3.65	Hydralazine Hcl, Mutual Pharm	53489-0124-01
100's	$3.78	Hydralazine Hcl, US Trading	56126-0027-11
100's	$3.95	Hydralazine Hcl, Major Pharms	00904-2339-60
100's	$4.20	Hydralazine Hcl, Goldline Labs	00182-0554-01
100's	$4.20	Hydralazine Hcl, Sidmak Labs	50111-0327-01
100's	$4.25	Hydralazine HCl, Rugby	00536-3862-01
100's	$4.32	Hydralazine Hcl 25, Aligen Independ	00405-4470-01
100's	$4.34	Hydralazine Hcl, Martec Pharms	52555-0027-01
100's	$4.35	Hydralazine Hcl, Raway	00686-0075-20
100's	$4.79	Hydralazine Hydrochloride, Camall	00147-0256-10
100's	$4.85	Hydralazine HCl, Schein Pharm (US)	00364-0144-01
100's	$4.89	Hydralazine Hcl, Par Pharm	49884-0027-01
100's	$6.21	Hydralazine Hcl, Major Pharms	00904-2339-61
100's	$6.45	Hydralazine Hcl, Voluntary Hosp	53258-0176-13
100's	$14.50	Hydralazine Hcl, Goldline Labs	00182-0554-89
100's	$15.02	Hydralazine Hcl, Vangard Labs	00615-0531-13
100's	**$29.44**	**APRESOLINE, Novartis**	**00083-0039-30**
600's	$110.00	Hydralazine Hcl, Medirex	57480-0332-06
1000's	$16.04	Hydralazine Hcl, Camall	00147-0256-20
1000's	$17.25	Hydralazine Hcl, Sidmak Labs	50111-0327-03

HOW SUPPLIED - RATED THERAPEUTICALLY EQUIVALENT: *(cont'd)*

1000's	$18.80	Hydralazine HCl, H.C.F.A. F F P	99999-1450-04
1000's	$19.00	Hydralazine Hcl, Squibb-Mark	57783-6650-03
1000's	$19.12	Hydralazine Hcl, Halsey Drug	00879-0536-10
1000's	$19.50	Hydralazine Hcl, Consolidated Midland	00223-1061-02
1000's	$20.70	Hydralazine Hcl, Qualitest Pharms	00603-3831-32
1000's	$20.93	Hydralazine HCl, Rugby	00536-3862-10
1000's	$20.95	Hydralazine, Major Pharms	00904-2339-80
1000's	$24.65	Hydralazine Hcl, Goldline Labs	00182-0554-10
1000's	$24.65	Hydralazine Hcl, United Res	00677-0447-10
1000's	$24.65	Hydralazine Hcl, Mutual Pharm	53489-0124-10
1000's	$28.01	Hydralazine Hcl, HL Moore Drug Exch	00839-1361-16
1000's	$33.83	Hydralazine Hcl, Lederle Pharm	00005-3564-34
1000's	$35.10	Hydralazine HCl, Schein Pharm (US)	00364-0144-02
1000's	$41.23	Hydralazine Hcl 25, Aligen Independ	00405-4470-03
1000's	$41.23	Hydralazine Hcl, Par Pharm	49884-0027-10
1000's	$42.05	Hydralazine Hcl, Martec Pharms	52555-0027-10

Tablet, Uncoated - Oral - 50 mg

100's	$2.05	Hydralazine Hcl, Rugby	00536-3911-01
100's	$2.63	Hydralazine HCl, H.C.F.A. F F P	99999-1450-05
100's	$3.40	Hydralazine Hcl, Squibb-Mark	57783-6660-01
100's	$3.50	Hydralazine Hydrochloride, Camall	00147-0257-10
100's	$3.50	Hydralazine Hcl, Consolidated Midland	00223-1062-01
100's	$3.50	Hydralazine Hcl, US Trading	56126-0028-11
100's	$3.67	Hydralazine Hcl, Halsey Drug	00879-0537-01
100's	$3.75	Hydralazine Hcl, United Res	00677-0451-01
100's	$3.78	Hydralazine Hcl, Qualitest Pharms	00603-3832-21
100's	$3.84	Hydralazine Hcl, Voluntary Hosp	53258-0132-01
100's	$4.00	Hydralazine Hcl, Sidmak Labs	50111-0328-01
100's	$4.60	Hydralazine Hcl, Mutual Pharm	53489-0125-01
100's	$4.66	Hydralazine Hcl, Lederle Pharm	00005-3565-62
100's	$4.66	Hydralazine Hcl, HL Moore Drug Exch	00839-1363-06
100's	$4.70	Hydralazine HCl, Rugby	00536-3863-01
100's	$4.75	Hydralazine Hcl, Goldline Labs	00182-0555-01
100's	$4.75	Hydralazine Hcl 50, Aligen Independ	00405-4471-01
100's	$4.85	Hydralazine Hcl, Martec Pharms	52555-0028-01
100's	$5.00	Hydralazine Hcl, Major Pharms	00904-2340-60
100's	$5.10	Hydralazine HCl, Schein Pharm (US)	00364-0145-01
100's	$5.15	Hydralazine Hcl, Raway	00686-0076-20
100's	$5.19	Hydralazine Hcl, Par Pharm	49884-0028-01
100's	$7.45	Hydralazine Hcl, Major Pharms	00904-2340-61
100's	$7.80	Hydralazine Hcl, Voluntary Hosp	53258-0132-13
100's	$17.70	Hydralazine Hcl, Goldline Labs	00182-0555-89
100's	$18.42	Hydralazine Hcl, Vangard Labs	00615-0532-13
100's	**$43.90**	**APRESOLINE, Novartis**	**00083-0073-30**
1000's	$24.50	Hydralazine Hcl, Consolidated Midland	00223-1062-02
1000's	$24.75	Hydralazine Hcl, Sidmak Labs	50111-0328-03
1000's	$25.25	Hydralazine Hcl, Squibb-Mark	57783-6660-03
1000's	$25.46	Hydralazine Hcl, Qualitest Pharms	00603-3832-32
1000's	$26.08	Hydralazine Hcl, Halsey Drug	00879-0537-10
1000's	$26.25	Hydralazine Hcl, Goldline Labs	00182-0555-10
1000's	$26.25	Hydralazine Hcl, Major Pharms	00904-2340-80
1000's	$26.25	Hydralazine Hcl, Major Pharms	00904-3340-80
1000's	$26.30	Hydralazine HCl, H.C.F.A. F F P	99999-1450-06
1000's	$27.32	Hydralazine Hcl, Camall	00147-0257-20
1000's	$27.75	Hydralazine Hcl, United Res	00677-0451-10
1000's	$27.75	Hydralazine Hcl, Mutual Pharm	53489-0125-10
1000's	$33.28	Hydralazine Hcl, HL Moore Drug Exch	00839-1363-16
1000's	$37.25	Hydralazine HCl, Rugby	00536-3863-10
1000's	$39.07	Hydralazine Hcl, Lederle Pharm	00005-3565-34
1000's	$40.00	Hydralazine HCl, Schein Pharm (US)	00364-0145-02
1000's	$46.08	Hydralazine Hcl 50, Aligen Independ	00405-4471-03
1000's	$47.00	Hydralazine Hcl, Martec Pharms	52555-0028-10
1000's	$47.09	Hydralazine Hcl, Par Pharm	49884-0028-10

Tablet, Uncoated - Oral - 100 mg

100's	$4.28	Hydralazine Hcl, United Res	00677-0922-01
100's	$4.28	Hydralazine HCl, H.C.F.A. F F P	99999-1450-07
100's	$5.16	Hydralazine Hcl, Camall	00147-0258-10
100's	$5.51	Hydralazine Hcl, Qualitest Pharms	00603-3833-21
100's	$6.90	Hydralazine Hcl, Major Pharms	00904-2341-60
100's	$7.75	Hydralazine Hcl, Goldline Labs	00182-1553-01
100's	$7.75	Hydralazine Hcl, Sidmak Labs	50111-0397-01
100's	$7.85	Hydralazine Hcl, Martec Pharms	52555-0026-01
100's	$7.95	Hydralazine Hcl, Rugby	00536-3891-01
100's	$8.09	Hydralazine Hcl, HL Moore Drug Exch	00839-6761-06
100's	$8.11	Hydralazine Hcl, Aligen Independ	00405-4472-01
100's	$8.12	Hydralazine HCl, Schein Pharm (US)	00364-0696-01
100's	$8.25	Hydralazine Hcl, Raway	00686-0183-20
100's	$8.29	Hydralazine Hcl, Par Pharm	49884-0121-01
100's	**$61.76**	**APRESOLINE, Novartis**	**00083-0101-30**
1000's	$42.80	Hydralazine Hcl, Sidmak Labs	50111-0397-03
1000's	$42.80	Hydralazine HCl, H.C.F.A. F F P	99999-1450-08
1000's	$48.22	Hydralazine Hcl, Camall	00147-0258-20
1000's	$74.69	Hydralazine Hcl, Par Pharm	49884-0121-10

HYDRALAZINE HYDROCHLORIDE; HYDROCHLOROTHIAZIDE *(001451)*

CATEGORIES: Antihypertensives; Cardiovascular Drugs; Diuretics; Hypertension; Renal Drugs; Sulfonamides; Vasodilating Agents; Pregnancy Category C; FDA Approval Pre 1982

BRAND NAMES: **Apresazide**; Apresodex; Apresoline-Esidrix; HH 25/25; Hy-Zide; Hydra-Zide

FORMULARIES: Medi-Cal

> **WARNING:**
> This fixed combination drug is not indicated for initial therapy of hypertension. Hypertension requires therapy titrated to the individual patient. If the fixed combination represents the dosage so determined, its use may be more convenient in patient management. The treatment of hypertension is not static but must be reevaluated as conditions in each patient warrant.

DESCRIPTION:

Hydralazine hydrochloride and hydrochlorothiazide, is an antihypertensive-diuretic combination available as capsules for oral administration. Hydralazine HCl w/ HCTZ capsules of 25/25 contain 25 mg of hydralazine hydrochloride USP and 25 mg of hydrochlorothiazide USP; capsules of 50/50 contain 50 mg of hydralazine hydrochloride USP and 50 mg of hydrochlorothiazide USP; and capsules of 100/50 contain 100 mg of hydralazine hydrochloride USP and 50 mg of hydrochlorothiazide USP.

FOR COMPLETE PRESCRIBING INFORMATION REFER TO THE INDIVIDUAL DRUG MONOGRAPHS (HYDRALAZINE HYDROCHLORIDE, HYDROCHLOROTHIAZIDE).

INDICATIONS AND USAGE:

Hypertension.

DOSAGE AND ADMINISTRATION:

Dosage should be determined by individual titration (see BOXED WARNING).

The usual dosage is one capsule twice daily, the strength depending upon individual requirement following titration. For maintenance, the dosage should be adjusted to the lowest effective level.

When necessary, other antihypertensive agents such as sympathetic inhibitors may be added gradually in reduced dosages, and the effects should be watched carefully.

Do not store above 86° F.

HOW SUPPLIED - RATED THERAPEUTICALLY EQUIVALENT:

Capsule, Gelatin - Oral - 25 mg/25 mg

100's	$7.88	Hydralazine / Hydrochlorothiazide, United Res	00677-0773-01
100's	$7.88	Hydralazine W/Hctz, H.C.F.A. F F P	99999-1451-01
100's	$13.30	Hydralazine W/Hctz, Qualitest Pharms	00603-3834-21
100's	$13.43	Hydralazine Plus, Rugby	00536-3885-01
100's	$13.45	Hydralazine W/Hctz, Goldline Labs	00182-1509-01
100's	$13.45	H H 25/25 Capsules, Major Pharms	00904-2852-60
100's	$13.45	APROZIDE, Major Pharms	00904-2855-60
100's	$13.72	Hydralazine W/Hctz, Martec Pharms	52555-0143-01
100's	$13.99	Hydralazine W/Hctz, Solvay Pharms	00032-4410-06
100's	$13.99	H H 25/25, Intl Labs	00665-4410-06
100's	$14.11	Hydralazine Hcl/Hydrochlorothiazide, HL Moore Drug Exch	00839-6582-06
100's	$14.29	HYDRA-ZIDE, Par Pharm	49884-0143-01
100's	$15.82	Hydralazine W/Hctz, Aligen Independ	00405-4477-01
100's	**$39.15**	**APRESAZIDE, Novartis**	**00083-0139-30**
500's	$39.40	Hydralazine W/Hctz, H.C.F.A. F F P	99999-1451-02
500's	$65.23	HYDRA-ZIDE, Par Pharm	49884-0143-05
1000's	$78.80	Hydralazine W/Hctz, H.C.F.A. F F P	99999-1451-03
1000's	$102.20	Hydralazine W/Hctz, HL Moore Drug Exch	00839-6582-16

Capsule, Gelatin - Oral - 50 mg/50 mg

100's	$9.15	Hydralazine Hcl, United Res	00677-0774-01
100's	$9.15	Hydralazine W/Hctz, H.C.F.A. F F P	99999-1451-04
100's	$19.90	Hydralazine W/Hctz, Qualitest Pharms	00603-3835-21
100's	$20.15	Hydralazine HCl, Rugby	00536-3886-01
100's	$20.20	HYDRAZIDE 50/50, Goldline Labs	00182-1484-01
100's	$20.20	Hydralazine W/Hctz, Goldline Labs	00182-1510-01
100's	$20.20	H H 50/50 Capsules, Major Pharms	00904-2853-60
100's	$20.20	APROZIDE, Major Pharms	00904-2856-60
100's	$20.66	Hydralazine W/Hctz, Martec Pharms	52555-0144-01
100's	$20.90	Hydralazine W/Hctz, Solvay Pharms	00032-4420-06
100's	$20.90	H H 50/50, Intl Labs	00665-4420-06
100's	$21.25	HYDRA-ZIDE, Par Pharm	49884-0144-01
100's	$21.26	Hydralazine Hcl, HL Moore Drug Exch	00839-6583-06
100's	$21.32	Hydralazine W/Hctz, Aligen Independ	00405-4478-01
100's	**$58.50**	**APRESAZIDE, Novartis**	**00083-0149-30**
500's	$45.75	Hydralazine W/Hctz, H.C.F.A. F F P	99999-1451-05
500's	$61.88	Hydralazine Hcl, Rugby	00536-3886-05
500's	$98.21	HYDRA-ZIDE, Par Pharm	49884-0144-05
1000's	$91.50	Hydralazine W/Hctz, H.C.F.A. F F P	99999-1451-06

Capsule, Gelatin - Oral - 100 mg/50 mg

100's	$19.28	Hydralazine W/Hctz, H.C.F.A. F F P	99999-1451-07
100's	$28.71	Hydralazine W/Hctz, Qualitest Pharms	00603-3836-21
100's	$31.32	HYDRA-ZIDE, Par Pharm	49884-0145-01
100's	**$71.28**	**APRESAZIDE, Novartis**	**00083-0159-30**
500's	$96.40	Hydralazine W/Hctz, H.C.F.A. F F P	99999-1451-08
1000's	$192.80	Hydralazine W/Hctz, H.C.F.A. F F P	99999-1451-09

HYDRALAZINE HYDROCHLORIDE; HYDROCHLOROTHIAZIDE; RESERPINE *(001452)*

CATEGORIES: Antihypertensives; Cardiovascular Drugs; Diuretics; Hypertension; Renal Drugs; Vasodilating Agents; Pregnancy Category C; FDA Approval Pre 1982

BRAND NAMES: Cam-Ap-Es; Diuretic Ap-Es; *Esi-Dri* (Japan); H.H.R.; Hydrap-Es; *Hydrares*; Hydro-Ap-Es; Hydroap-Es; Hydroserpazine; Hydroserpine Plus; Hyserp; Marpres; *Reser*; Sae; Ser-A-Gen; **Ser-Ap-Es**; Seralazide; Serathide; Serpazide; Serpex; Tri-Hydroserpine; Uni-Serp; Unipres
(International brand names outside U.S. in italics)

FORMULARIES: BC-BS; Medi-Cal

> **WARNING:**
> This fixed-combination drug is not indicated for initial therapy of hypertension. Hypertension requires therapy titrated to the individual patient. If the fixed combination represents the dosage so determined, its use may be more convenient in patient management. The treatment of hypertension is not static but must be reevaluated as conditions in each patient warrant.

DESCRIPTION:

Hydralazine HCTZ w/reserpine is an antihypertensive-diuretic combination, available as tablets for oral administration. Each tablet contains Serpasil (reserpine USP), 0.1 mg; Apresoline (hydralazine hydrochloride USP), 25 mg; and Esidrix (hydrochlorothiazide USP), 15 mg.

FOR COMPLETE PRESCRIBING INFORMATION REFER TO THE INDIVIDUAL DRUG MONOGRAPHS (HYDRALAZINE HYDROCHLORIDE, HYDROCHLOROTHIAZIDE, RESERPINE).

INDICATIONS AND USAGE:

Hypertension.

DOSAGE AND ADMINISTRATION:

Dosage should be determined by individual titration.

Dosage regimens that exceed 0.25 mg of reserpine per day are not recommended.

Do not store above 86°F (30°C).

HOW SUPPLIED - EQUIVALENTS NOT AVAILABLE:

Tablet, Uncoated - Oral - 25 mg/15 mg/0.1

100's	$3.45	SERPAZIDE, Major Pharms	00904-2335-60
100's	$5.25	SERPAZIDE, Major Pharms	00904-2334-60
100's	$5.73	Hydralazine/HCTZ/Reserpine, Schein Pharm (US)	00364-0361-01
100's	$6.40	UNI SERP, United Res	00677-0415-01
100's	$6.75	TRI-HYDROSERPINE, Rugby	00536-4909-01
100's	$7.15	SER A GEN, Goldline Labs	00182-1820-01
100's	$8.07	Hctz/Reserpine/Hydralazine, Qualitest Pharms	00603-3807-21
100's	$11.44	CAM-AP-ES, Camall	00147-0124-10
100's	$12.01	DIURETIC-APRES, HL Moore Drug Exch	00839-1282-06
100's	**$49.49**	**SER-AP-ES, Novartis**	**00083-0071-30**
1000's	$26.25	SERPAZIDE, Major Pharms	00904-2335-80
1000's	$35.95	SERPAZIDE, Major Pharms	00904-2334-80
1000's	$36.10	UNI SERP, United Res	00677-0415-10
1000's	$37.49	Hydralazine/HCTZ/Reserpine, Schein Pharm (US)	00364-0361-02
1000's	$39.30	TRI-HYDROSERPINE, Rugby	00536-4909-10
1000's	$49.75	Hctz/Reserpine/Hydralazine, Qualitest Pharms	00603-3807-32
1000's	$50.65	SER A GEN, Goldline Labs	00182-1820-10
1000's	$62.00	HYDRAP-ES, Parmed Pharms	00349-2076-10
1000's	$77.94	CAM-AP-ES, Camall	00147-0124-20
1000's	$77.96	DIURETIC-APRES, HL Moore Drug Exch	00839-1282-16
1000's	**$489.84**	**SER-AP-ES, Novartis**	**00083-0071-40**

HYDROCHLORIC ACID *(001455)*

CATEGORIES: Acidifying Agents; Digestants; Electrolytic, Caloric-Water Balance; Gastrointestinal Drugs; FDA Pre 1938 Drugs

Prescribing information not available at time of publication.

HOW SUPPLIED - EQUIVALENTS NOT AVAILABLE:

Injection, Solution - Intravenous - 2 mg/ml

100 ml	$3.10	Hydrochloric Acid, Americal Pharm	54945-0575-45
100 ml	$8.75	Hydrochloric Acid, Merit Pharms	30727-0331-95

HYDROCHLOROTHIAZIDE *(001456)*

CATEGORIES: Antihypertensives; Cardiovascular Drugs; Congestive Heart Failure; Diuretics; Edema; Electrolytic, Caloric-Water Balance; Glomerulonephritis; Heart Failure; Hypertension; Nephrotic Syndrome; Renal Drugs; Renal Failure; Thiazides; Pregnancy Category B; Sales > $100 Million; FDA Approval Pre 1982

BRAND NAMES: *Apo-Hydro* (Canada); Aquazide H; Carozide; *Clothia* (Japan); Diaqua; *Dichlotride* (Australia, Japan); *Dichlozid*; *Diclotride* (Mexico); *Didralin*; *Di-Ertride*; *Disothiazide*; *Diu-Melsin* (Germany); *Diuchlor H* (Canada); *Diurace*; *Diuret-P*; *Diurex*; *Esidrex* (Australia, England, France, Japan); **Esidrix**; *H.C.T.*; *Hidrenox*; *Hidrosaluretil*; *Hydrex*; *Hydrex-semi*; Hydro Par; Hydro-D; Hydro-T; Hydrochlorulan; *Hydrochlorzide*; Hydrocot; Hydrodiuril; Hydromal; Hydrorex; *Hydrosaluric* (England); *Hydrozide*; *Idrodiuvis*; Loqua-50; M-Zide; *Manschitt*; *Maschitt* (Japan); Mictrin; *Natrimax*; *Nefrol*; *Neoflumen*; *Neo-codema* (Canada); *Newtolide* (Japan); *Novohydrazide* (Canada); Oretic; *Pantemon* (Japan); *Servithiazid*; *Tandiur*; *Urirex*; *Urozide* (Canada); Zide
(International brand names outside U.S. in italics)

FORMULARIES: Aetna; BC-BS; CIGNA; DoD; FHP; Foundation; Humana; Kaiser; Medco; Medi-Cal; PCS; PruCare; United; WHO

COST OF THERAPY: $3.68 (Hypertension; Tablet; 50 mg; 1/day; 365 days)

PRIMARY ICD9: 401.1 (Essential Hypertension, Benign)

DESCRIPTION:

Hydrochlorothiazide is a diuretic and antihypertensive. It is the 3,4-dihydro derivative of chlorothiazide. Its chemical name is 6-chloro-3,4-dihydro-2*H*-1,2,4-benzothiadiazine-7-sulfonamide 1,1-dioxide. Its empirical formula is $C_7H_8ClN_3O_4S_2$.

It is a white, or practically white, crystalline powder with a molecular weight of 297.72, which is slightly soluble in water, but freely soluble in sodium hydroxide solution.

Hydrochlorothiazide is supplied as 25 mg, 50 mg and 100 mg tablets for oral use. Each tablet contains the following inactive ingredients: calcium phosphate, FD&C Yellow 6, gelatin, lactose, magnesium stearate, starch and talc.

CLINICAL PHARMACOLOGY:

The mechanism of the antihypertensive effect of thiazides is unknown. Hydrochlorothiazide does not usually affect normal blood pressure.

Hydrochlorothiazide affects the distal renal tubular mechanism of electrolyte reabsorption. At maximal therapeutic dosage all thiazides are approximately equal in their diuretic efficacy.

Hydrochlorothiazide increases excretion of sodium and chloride in approximately equivalent amounts. Natriuresis may be accompanied by some loss of potassium and bicarbonate.

After oral use diuresis begins within 2 hours, peaks in about 4 hours and lasts about 6 to 12 hours.

Pharmacokinetics and Metabolism: Hydrochlorothiazide is not metabolized but is eliminated rapidly by the kidney. When plasma levels have been followed for at least 24 hours, the plasma half-life has been observed to vary between 5.6 and 14.8 hours. At least 61 percent of the oral dose is eliminated unchanged within 24 hours. Hydrochlorothiazide crosses the placental but not the blood-brain barrier and is excreted in breast milk.

INDICATIONS AND USAGE:

Hydrochlorothiazide is indicated as adjunctive therapy in edema associated with congestive heart failure, hepatic cirrhosis, and corticosteroid and estrogen therapy.

Hydrochlorothiazide has also been found useful in edema due to various forms of renal dysfunction such as nephrotic syndrome, acute glomerulonephritis, and chronic renal failure.

INDICATIONS AND USAGE: *(cont'd)*

Hydrochlorothiazide is indicated in the management of hypertension either as the sole therapeutic agent or to enhance the effectiveness of other antihypertensive drugs in the more severe forms of hypertension.

Use in Pregnancy: Routine use of diuretics during normal pregnancy is inappropriate and exposes mother and fetus to unnecessary hazard. Diuretics do not prevent development of toxemia of pregnancy and there is no satisfactory evidence that they are useful in the treatment of toxemia.

Edema during pregnancy may arise from pathologic causes or from the physiologic and mechanical consequences of pregnancy. Thiazides are indicated in pregnancy when edema is due to pathologic causes, just as they are in the absence of pregnancy (see PRECAUTIONS, Pregnancy). Dependent edema in pregnancy, resulting from restriction of venous return by the gravid uterus, is properly treated through elevation of the lower extremities and use of support stockings. Use of diuretics to lower intravascular volume in this instance is illogical and unnecessary. During normal pregnancy there is hypervolemia which is not harmful to the fetus or the mother in the absence of cardiovascular disease. However, it may be associated with edema, rarely generalized edema. If such edema causes discomfort, increased recumbency will often provide relief. Rarely this edema may cause extreme discomfort which is not relieved by rest. In these instances, a short course of diuretic therapy may provide relief and be appropriate.

CONTRAINDICATIONS:

Anuria.

Hypersensitivity to this product or to other sulfonamide-derived drugs.

WARNINGS:

Use with caution in severe renal disease. In patients with renal disease, thiazides may precipitate azotemia. Cumulative effects of the drug may develop in patients with impaired renal function.

Thiazides should be used with caution in patients with impaired hepatic function or progressive liver disease, since minor alterations of fluid and electrolyte balance may precipitate hepatic coma.

Thiazides may add to or potentiate the action of other antihypertensive drugs.

Sensitivity reactions may occur in patients with or without a history of allergy or bronchial asthma.

The possibility of exacerbation or activation of systemic lupus erythematosus has been reported.

Lithium generally should not be given with diuretics (see DRUG INTERACTIONS.)

PRECAUTIONS:

GENERAL

All patients receiving diuretic therapy should be observed for evidence of fluid or electrolyte imbalance: namely, hyponatremia, hypochloremic alkalosis, and hypokalemia. Serum and urine electrolyte determinations are particularly important when the patient is vomiting excessively or receiving parenteral fluids. Warning signs or symptoms of fluid and electrolyte imbalance, irrespective of cause, include dryness of mouth, thirst, weakness, lethargy, drowsiness, restlessness, confusion, seizures, muscle pains or cramps, muscular fatigue, hypotension, oliguria, tachycardia, and gastrointestinal disturbance such as nausea or vomiting.

Hypokalemia may develop, especially with brisk diuresis, when severe cirrhosis is present or after prolonged therapy.

Interference with adequate oral electrolyte intake will also contribute to hypokalemia. Hypokalemia may cause cardiac arrhythmia and may also sensitize or exaggerate the response of the heart to the toxic effects of digitalis (*e.g.,* increased ventricular irritability). Hypokalemia may be avoided or treated by use of potassium sparing diuretics or potassium supplements such as foods with a high potassium content.

Although any chloride deficit is generally mild and usually does not require specific treatment except under extraordinary circumstances (as in liver disease or renal disease), chloride replacement may be required in the treatment of metabolic alkalosis.

Dilutional hyponatremia may occur in edematous patients in hot weather; appropriate therapy is water restriction, rather than administration of salt, except in rare instances when the hyponatremia is life threatening. In actual salt depletion, appropriate replacement is the therapy of choice.

Hyperuricemia may occur or acute gout may be precipitated in certain patients receiving thiazides.

In diabetic patients dosage adjustments of insulin or oral hypoglycemic agents may be required. Hyperglycemia may occur with thiazide diuretics. Thus latent diabetes mellitus may become manifest during thiazide therapy.

The antihypertensive effects of the drug may be enhanced in the post-sympathectomy patient.

If progressive renal impairment becomes evident, consider withholding or discontinuing diuretic therapy.

Thiazides have been shown to increase the urinary excretion of magnesium; this may result in hypomagnesemia.

Thiazides may decrease urinary calcium excretion. Thiazides may cause intermittent and slight elevation of serum calcium in the absence of known disorders of calcium metabolism. Marked hypercalcemia may be evidence of hidden hyperparathyroidism. Thiazides should be discontinued before carrying out tests for parathyroid function.

Increases in cholesterol and triglyceride levels may be associated with thiazide diuretic therapy.

LABORATORY TESTS

Periodic determination of serum electrolytes to detect possible electrolyte imbalance should be done at appropriate intervals.

DRUG/LABORATORY TEST INTERACTIONS

Thiazides should be discontinued before carrying out tests for parathyroid function (see PRECAUTIONS, General.)

CARCINOGENESIS, MUTAGENESIS, AND IMPAIRMENT OF FERTILITY

Two-year feeding studies in mice and rats conducted under the auspices of the National Toxicology Program (NTP) uncovered no evidence of a carcinogenic potential of hydrochlorothiazide in female mice (at doses of up to approximately 600 mg/kg/day) or in male and female rats (at doses of up to approximately 100 mg/kg/day). The NTP, however, found equivocal evidence for hepatocarcinogenicity in male mice.

Hydrochlorothiazide was not genotoxic *in vitro* in the Ames mutagenicity assay of *Salmonella typhimurium* strains TA 98, TA 100, TA 1535, TA 1537, and TA 1538 and in the Chinese Hamster Ovary (CHO) test for chromosomal aberrations, or *in vivo* in assays using mouse germinal cell chromosomes, Chinese hamster bone marrow chromosomes, and the *Drosophila* sex-linked recessive lethal trait gene. Positive test results were obtained only in the *in*

PRECAUTIONS: *(cont'd)*

*vitro*CHO Sister Chromatid Exchange (clastogenicity) and in the Mouse Lymphoma Cell (mutagenicity) assays, using concentrations of hydrochlorothiazide from 43 to 1300 mcg/ml, and in the *Aspergillus nidulans* non-disjunction assay at an unspecified concentration.

Hydrochlorothiazide had no adverse effects on the fertility of mice and rats of either sex in studies wherein these species were exposed, via their diet, to doses of up to 100 and 4 mg/kg, respectively, prior to conception and throughout gestation.

PREGNANCY

Teratogenic Effects: Studies in which hydrochlorothiazide was orally administered to pregnant mice and rats during their respective periods of major organogenesis at doses up to 3000 and 1000 mg hydrochlorothiazide/kg, respectively, provided no evidence of harm to the fetus.

There are, however, no adequate and well-controlled studies in pregnant women. Because animal reproduction studies are not always predictive of human response, this drug should be used during pregnancy only if clearly needed.

Nonteratogenic Effects: Thiazides cross the placental barrier and appear in cord blood. There is a risk of fetal or neonatal jaundice, thrombocytopenia, and possibly other adverse reactions that have occurred in adults.

NURSING MOTHERS

Thiazides are excreted in breast milk. Because of the potential for serious adverse reactions in nursing infants, a decision should be made whether to discontinue nursing or to discontinue hydrochlorothiazide, taking into account the importance of the drug to the mother.

PEDIATRIC USE

Safety and effectiveness in pediatric patients have not been established.

DRUG INTERACTIONS:

When given concurrently the following drugs may interact with thiazide diuretics.

Alcohol, barbiturates, or narcotics: potentiation of orthostatic hypotension may occur.

Antidiabetic drugs: (oral agents and insulin) - dosage adjustment of the antidiabetic drug may be required.

Other antihypertensive drugs: additive effect or potentiation.

Cholestyramine and colestipol resins: Absorption of hydrochlorothiazide is impaired in the presence of anionic exchange resins. Single doses of either cholestyramine or colestipol resins bind the hydrochlorothiazide and reduce its absorption from the gastrointestinal tract by up to 85 and 43 percent, respectively.

Corticosteroids, ACTH: intensified electrolyte depletion, particularly hypokalemia.

Pressor amines (*e.g.,* norepinephrine): possible decreased response to pressor amines but not sufficient to preclude their use.

Skeletal muscle relaxants, nondepolarizing (*e.g.,* tubocurarine): possible increased responsiveness to the muscle relaxant.

Lithium: generally should not be given with diuretics. Diuretic agents reduce the renal clearance of lithium and add a high risk of lithium toxicity. Refer to the package insert for lithium preparations before use of such preparations with Hydrochlorothiazide.

Non-steroidal Anti-inflammatory Drugs: In some patients, the administration of a non-steroidal anti-inflammatory agent can reduce the diuretic, natriuretic, and antihypertensive effects of loop, potassium-sparing and thiazide diuretics. Therefore, when Hydrochlorothiazide and non-steroidal anti-inflammatory agents are used concomitantly, the patient should be observed closely to determine if the desired effect of the diuretic is obtained.

ADVERSE REACTIONS:

The following adverse reactions have been reported and, within each category, are listed in order of decreasing severity.

Body as a Whole: Weakness.

Cardiovascular: Hypotension including orthostatic hypotension (may be aggravated by alcohol, barbiturates, narcotics or antihypertensive drugs).

Digestive: Pancreatitis, jaundice (intrahepatic cholestatic jaundice), diarrhea, vomiting, sialadenitis, cramping, constipation, gastric irritation, nausea, anorexia.

Hematologic: Aplastic anemia, agranulocytosis, leukopenia, hemolytic anemia, thrombocytopenia.

Hypersensitivity: Anaphylactic reactions, necrotizing angiitis (vasculitis and cutaneous vasculitis), respiratory distress including pneumonitis and pulmonary edema, photosensitivity, fever, urticaria, rash, purpura.

Metabolic: Electrolyte imbalance (see PRECAUTIONS), hyperglycemia, glycosuria, hyperuricemia.

Musculoskeletal: Muscle spasm.

Nervous System/Psychiatric: Vertigo, paresthesias, dizziness, headache, restlessness.

Renal: Renal failure, renal dysfunction, interstitial nephritis. (See WARNINGS.)

Skin: Erythema multiforme including Stevens-Johnson syndrome, exfoliative dermatitis including toxic epidermal necrolysis, alopecia.

Special Senses: Transient blurred vision, xanthopsia.

Urogenital: Impotence.

Whenever adverse reactions are moderate or severe, thiazide dosage should be reduced or therapy withdrawn.

OVERDOSAGE:

The most common signs and symptoms observed are those caused by electrolyte depletion (hypokalemia, hypochloremia, hyponatremia) and dehydration resulting from excessive diuresis. If digitalis has also been administered, hypokalemia may accentuate cardiac arrhythmias.

In the event of overdosage, symptomatic and supportive measures should be employed. Emesis should be induced or gastric lavage performed. Correct dehydration, electrolyte imbalance, hepatic coma and hypotension by established procedures. If required, give oxygen or artificial respiration for respiratory impairment. The degree to which hydrochlorothiazide is removed by hemodialysis has not been established.

The oral LD_{50} of hydrochlorothiazide is greater than 10 g/kg in the mouse and rat.

DOSAGE AND ADMINISTRATION:

Therapy should be individualized according to patient response. Use the smallest dosage necessary to achieve the required response.

ADULTS

For Edema: The usual adult dosage is 25 to 100 mg daily as a single or divided dose. Many patients with edema respond to intermittent therapy, i.e., administration on alternate days or on three to five days each week. With an intermittent schedule, excessive response and the resulting undesirable electrolyte imbalance are less likely to occur.

DOSAGE AND ADMINISTRATION: *(cont'd)*

For Control of Hypertension: The usual initial dose in adults is 25 mg daily given as a single dose. The dose may be increased to 50 mg daily, given as a single or two divided doses. Doses above 50 mg are often associated with marked reductions in serum potassium (see also PRECAUTIONS).

Patients usually do not require doses in excess of 50 mg of hydrochlorothiazide daily when used concomitantly with other antihypertensive agents.

INFANTS AND CHILDREN

For Diuresis and for Control of Hypertension: The usual pediatric dosage is 0.5 to 1.0 mg of Hydrochlorothiazide per pound of body weight per day in two doses not to exceed 37.5 mg per day. Infants under 6 months of age may require up to 1.5 mg per pound per day in two doses.

On this basis, infants up to 2 years of age may be given 12.5 to 37.5 mg daily in two doses. Children from 2 to 12 years of age may be given 37.5 to 100 mg daily in two doses. Dosage in both age groups should be based on body weight. However, pediatric patients with hypertension only rarely will benefit from doses larger than 50 mg daily.

Storage: Keep container tightly closed. Protect from light, moisture, freezing, -20°C (-4°F) and store at room temperature, 15-30°C (59-86°F).

HOW SUPPLIED - RATED THERAPEUTICALLY EQUIVALENT:

Tablet, Uncoated - Oral - 25 mg

30's	$.50	Hydrochlorothiazide, H.C.F.A. F F P	99999-1456-01
30's	$2.25	Hydrochlorothiazide, Major Pharms	00904-2083-46
90's	$1.51	Hydrochlorothiazide, H.C.F.A. F F P	99999-1456-02
90's	$5.40	Hydrochlorothiazide, Major Pharms	00904-2083-89
100's	$1.68	Hydrochlorothiazide, H.C.F.A. F F P	99999-1456-03
100's	$1.72	Hydrochlorothiazide, Talbert Phcy	44514-0410-88
100's	$1.75	Hydrochlorothiazide, Consolidated Midland	00223-1069-01
100's	$2.40	HYDRO PAR, Parmed Pharms	00349-2070-01
100's	$2.52	Hydrochlorothiazide, Voluntary Hosp	53258-0133-01
100's	$2.75	Hydrochlorothiazide, West Point Pharma	59591-0241-68
100's	$2.75	Hydrochlorothiazide, Endo Labs	60951-0770-70
100's	$2.86	Hydrochlorothiazide, Qualitest Pharms	00603-3858-21
100's	$2.86	Hydrochlorothiazide, United Res	00677-0346-01
100's	$2.88	Hydrochlorothiazide, Schein Pharm (US)	00364-0322-01
100's	$2.95	Hydrochlorothiazide, Major Pharms	00904-2083-60
100's	$3.03	Hydrochlorothiazide, Lederle Pharm	00005-3752-23
100's	$3.45	Hydrochlorothiazide, Geneva Pharms	00781-1480-01
100's	$3.95	Hydrochlorothiazide, Rugby	00536-3922-01
100's	$4.22	Hydrochlorothiazide, Camall	00147-0116-10
100's	$4.36	ORETIC, Abbott	00074-6978-01
100's	$4.44	Hydrochlorothiazide, HL Moore Drug Exch	00839-5135-06
100's	$4.80	Hydrochlorothiazide, Medirex	57480-0334-01
100's	$4.95	Hydrochlorothiazide, Raway	00686-0049-20
100's	$5.11	Hydrochlorothiazide, Major Pharms	00904-2083-61
100's	$5.25	Hydrochlorothiazide, Voluntary Hosp	53258-0133-13
100's	$5.55	ORETIC, Abbott	00074-6978-05
100's	$10.35	Hydrochlorothiazide, Goldline Labs	00182-0556-89
100's	$10.83	Hydrochlorothiazide, Vangard Labs	00615-1561-13
100's	**$12.02**	**ESIDRIX, Novartis**	**00083-0022-30**
100's	$13.48	HYDRODIURIL, Merck	00006-0042-68
600's	$62.40	Hydrochlorothiazide, Medirex	57480-0334-06
1000's	$6.95	Hydrochlorothiazide, Calvin Scott	17224-0510-10
1000's	$8.33	Hydrochlorothiazide, Qualitest Pharms	00603-3858-32
1000's	$8.58	Hydrochlorothiazide, Balan	00304-0139-00
1000's	$9.95	Hydrochlorothiazide, Consolidated Midland	00223-1069-02
1000's	$10.50	Hydrochlorothiazide, Major Pharms	00904-2083-80
1000's	$12.80	Hydrochlorothiazide, West Point Pharma	59591-0241-82
1000's	$12.80	Hydrochlorothiazide, Endo Labs	60951-0770-90
1000's	$13.05	Hydrochlorothiazide, Martec Pharms	52555-0577-10
1000's	$13.55	Hydrochlorothiazide, Camall	00147-0116-20
1000's	$14.24	Hydrochlorothiazide, HL Moore Drug Exch	00839-5135-16
1000's	$15.12	Hydrochlorothiazide, Lederle Pharm	00005-3752-34
1000's	$15.20	Hydrochlorothiazide, United Res	00677-0346-10
1000's	$15.25	Hydrochlorothiazide, Schein Pharm (US)	00364-0322-02
1000's	$15.93	Hydrochlorothiazide, Roxane	00054-4385-31
1000's	$15.95	Hydrochlorothiazide, Zenith Labs	00172-2083-80
1000's	$15.95	Hydrochlorothiazide, Goldline Labs	00182-0556-10
1000's	$16.25	HYDRO PAR, Parmed Pharms	00349-2070-10
1000's	$16.80	Hydrochlorothiazide, H.C.F.A. F F P	99999-1456-04
1000's	$17.21	Hydrochlorothiazide, Purepac Pharm	00228-2221-96
1000's	$17.21	Hydrochlorothiazide, Geneva Pharms	00781-1480-10
1000's	$18.27	ORETIC, Abbott	00074-6978-02
1000's	$19.25	Hydrochlorothiazide, Rugby	00536-3922-10
1000's	$129.66	HYDRODIURIL, Merck	00006-0042-82
5000's	$60.45	Hydrochlorothiazide, Parmed Pharms	00349-2070-51

Tablet, Uncoated - Oral - 50 mg

30's	$.69	Hydrochlorothiazide, H.C.F.A. F F P	99999-1456-05
30's	$1.70	Hydrochlorothiazide, Major Pharms	00904-2089-46
60's	$1.38	Hydrochlorothiazide, H.C.F.A. F F P	99999-1456-06
100's	$1.01	Hydrochlorothiazide, Talbert Phcy	44514-0411-88
100's	$2.31	Hydrochlorothiazide, H.C.F.A. F F P	99999-1456-07
100's	$2.67	Hydrochlorothiazide, Voluntary Hosp	53258-0134-01
100's	$2.75	Hydrochlorothiazide, Consolidated Midland	00223-1070-01
100's	$3.00	Hydrochlorothiazide, Zenith Labs	00172-2089-60
100's	$3.00	Hydrochlorothiazide, Goldline Labs	00182-0557-01
100's	$3.40	Hydrochlorothiazide, Major Pharms	00904-2089-60
100's	$3.50	Hydrochlorothiazide, West Point Pharma	59591-0243-68
100's	$3.50	Hydrochlorothiazide, Endo Labs	60951-0771-70
100's	$3.65	Hydrochlorothiazide, Schein Pharm (US)	00364-0328-01
100's	$3.66	Hydrochlorothiazide, United Res	00677-0347-01
100's	$3.70	Hydrochlorothiazide, Qualitest Pharms	00603-3859-21
100's	$3.71	Hydrochlorothiazide, Lederle Pharm	00005-3753-23
100's	$3.90	HYDRO PAR, Parmed Pharms	00349-2071-01
100's	$3.90	Hydrochlorothiazide, Rugby	00536-3919-01
100's	$3.94	EZIDE, CALCIUM-FREE, Embrex Economed	38130-0020-01
100's	$3.95	Hydrochlorothiazide, Geneva Pharms	00781-1481-01
100's	$4.63	Hydrochlorothiazide, Camall	00147-0108-10
100's	$4.86	Hydrochlorothiazide, HL Moore Drug Exch	00839-5136-06
100's	$5.25	Hydrochlorothiazide, Raway	00686-0111-20
100's	$5.26	Hydrochlorothiazide, Major Pharms	00904-2089-61
100's	$5.37	Hydrochlorothiazide, Voluntary Hosp	53258-0134-13
100's	$6.90	ORETIC, Abbott	00074-6985-01
100's	$6.95	Hydrochlorothiazide, Medirex	57480-0335-01
100's	$8.09	ORETIC, Abbott	00074-6985-06
100's	$9.80	CAROZIDE, Seneca Pharms	47028-0003-01
100's	$12.50	Hydrochlorothiazide, Goldline Labs	00182-0557-89
100's	$13.29	Hydrochlorothiazide, Vangard Labs	00615-1562-13
100's	**$19.05**	**ESIDRIX, Novartis**	**00083-0046-30**
100's	$21.35	HYDRODIURIL, Merck	00006-0105-68
600's	$97.40	Hydrochlorothiazide, Medirex	57480-0335-06

HOW SUPPLIED - RATED THERAPEUTICALLY EQUIVALENT: *(cont'd)*

1000's	$7.95	Hydrochlorothiazide, Calvin Scott	17224-0511-10
1000's	$9.18	HYDROCHLOROYHIAZIDE, Balan	00304-0140-00
1000's	$10.59	Hydrochlorothiazide, Voluntary Hosp	53258-0134-10
1000's	$11.25	Hydrochlorothiazide, Consolidated Midland	00223-1070-02
1000's	$14.05	Hydrochlorothiazide, Qualitest Pharms	00603-3859-32
1000's	$15.87	Hydrochlorothiazide, Camall	00147-0108-20
1000's	$16.50	Hydrochlorothiazide, Major Pharms	00904-2089-80
1000's	$16.59	Hydrochlorothiazide, HL Moore Drug Exch	00839-5136-16
1000's	$17.50	HYDRO PAR, Parmed Pharms	00349-2071-10
1000's	$17.90	Hydrochlorothiazide, Martec Pharms	52555-0578-10
1000's	$18.00	HYDROCOT, C O Truxton	00463-6268-10
1000's	$18.48	Hydrochlorothiazide, Camall	00147-0123-20
1000's	$18.80	Hydrochlorothiazide, West Point Pharma	59591-0243-82
1000's	$18.80	Hydrochlorothiazide, Endo Labs	60951-0771-90
1000's	$21.00	Hydrochlorothiazide, Schein Pharm (US)	00364-0328-02
1000's	$21.08	Hydrochlorothiazide, Lederle Pharm	00005-3753-34
1000's	$23.10	EZIDE, CALCIUM-FREE, Embrex Economed	38130-0020-10
1000's	$23.10	Hydrochlorothiazide, H.C.F.A. F F P	99999-1456-08
1000's	$23.92	Hydrochlorothiazide, United Res	00677-0347-10
1000's	$23.98	Hydrochlorothiazide, Zenith Labs	00172-2089-80
1000's	$23.98	Hydrochlorothiazide, Goldline Labs	00182-0557-10
1000's	$23.98	Hydrochlorothiazide, Purepac Pharm	00228-2222-96
1000's	$24.50	Hydrochlorothiazide, Geneva Pharms	00781-1481-10
1000's	$24.51	ORETIC, Abbott	00074-6985-02
1000's	$25.21	Hydrochlorothiazide, Amer Preferred	53445-0557-00
1000's	$26.35	Hydrochlorothiazide, Rugby	00536-3919-10
1000's	$26.62	Hydrochlorothiazide, Aligen Independ	00405-4490-03
5000's	$38.85	Hydrochlorothiazide, Major Pharms	00904-2089-90
5000's	$48.50	Hydrochlorothiazide, Aligen Independ	00405-4490-07
5000's	$53.35	Hydrochlorothiazide, HL Moore Drug Exch	00839-5136-20
5000's	$54.05	Hydrochlorothiazide, United Res	00677-0347-50
5000's	$67.65	Hydrochlorothiazide, Zenith Labs	00172-2089-85
5000's	$67.65	Hydrochlorothiazide, Goldline Labs	00182-0557-50
5000's	$70.50	Hydrochlorothiazide, Camall	00147-0108-30
5000's	$75.19	Hydrochlorothiazide, Geneva Pharms	00781-1481-51
5000's	$115.50	Hydrochlorothiazide, H.C.F.A. F F P	99999-1456-09
5000's	$125.16	Hydrochlorothiazide, Rugby	00536-3919-50
5000's	$953.05	HYDRODIURIL, Merck	00006-0105-86

Tablet, Uncoated - Oral - 100 mg

100's	$2.75	Hydrochlorothiazide, Consolidated Midland	00223-1068-01
100's	$4.43	Hydrochlorothiazide, United Res	00677-0764-01
100's	$4.80	Hydrochlorothiazide, H.C.F.A. F F P	99999-1456-10
100's	$5.25	HYDRO-T, Major Pharms	00904-2478-60
100's	$5.95	Hydrochlorothiazide, Rugby	00536-3923-01
100's	$5.97	Hydrochlorothiazide, Schein Pharm (US)	00364-0421-01
100's	$6.00	Hydrochlorothiazide, Zenith Labs	00172-2485-60
100's	$6.20	Hydrochlorothiazide, Martec Pharms	52555-0299-01
100's	$6.87	Hydrochlorothiazide, HL Moore Drug Exch	00839-6013-06
1000's	$14.95	Hydrochlorothiazide, Consolidated Midland	00223-1068-02
1000's	$45.00	Hydrochlorothiazide, Zenith Labs	00172-2485-80
1000's	$48.00	Hydrochlorothiazide, H.C.F.A. F F P	99999-1456-11

HOW SUPPLIED - NOT RATED EQUIVALENT:

Solution - Oral - 50 mg/5ml

500 ml	$15.37	Hydrochlorothiazide, Roxane	00054-3383-63

HYDROCHLOROTHIAZIDE; LISINOPRIL

(001458)

CATEGORIES: ACE Inhibitors; Angiotensin Converting Enzyme Inhibitors; Antihypertensives; Cardiovascular Drugs; Diuretics; Hypertension; Renal Drugs; Thiazides; Pregnancy Category C; FDA Approved 1989 Feb

BRAND NAMES: *Carace Plus* (England); *Novazyd*; **Prinzide**; *Vivazid*; Zestoretic *(International brand names outside U.S. in italics)*

FORMULARIES: BC-BS

COST OF THERAPY: $358.35 (Hypertension; Tablet; 12.5 mg/20 mg; 1/day; 365 days) vs. Potential Cost of $24,027.04 (Coronary Bypass)

PRIMARY ICD9: 401.1 (Essential Hypertension, Benign)

DESCRIPTION:

Lisinopril-hydrochlorothiazide combines an angiotensin converting enzyme inhibitor, lisinopril, and a diuretic, hydrochlorothiazide.

FOR COMPLETE PRESCRIBING INFORMATION REFER TO THE INDIVIDUAL DRUG MONOGRAPHS (HYDROCHLOROTHIAZIDE; LISINOPRIL).

INDICATIONS AND USAGE:

Lisinopril-hydrochlorothiazide is indicated for the treatment of hypertension.

These fixed dose combinations are not indicated for initial therapy. Patients already receiving a diuretic when lisinopril is initiated, or given a diuretic and lisinopril simultaneously, can develop symptomatic hypotension. In the initial titration of the individual entities, it is important, if possible, to stop the diuretic for several days before starting lisinopril or, if this is not possible, begin lisinopril at a low initial dose. (See DOSAGE AND ADMINISTRATION.)

In using lisinopril-hydrochlorothiazide, consideration should be given to the fact that an angiotensin converting enzyme inhibitor, captopril, has caused agranulocytosis, particularly in patients with renal impairment or collagen vascular disease, and that available data are insufficient to show that lisinopril does not have a similar risk.

In considering the use of Hydrochlorothiazide Lisinopril, it should be noted that in controlled trials ACE inhibitors have an effect on blood pressure that is less in black patients than in nonblacks. In addition, ACE inhibitors have been associated with a higher rate of angioedema in black than in nonblack patients.

DOSAGE AND ADMINISTRATION:

DOSAGE MUST BE INDIVIDUALIZED. THE FIXED COMBINATIONS ARE NOT FOR INITIAL THERAPY. THEY MAY BE SUBSTITUTED FOR THE TITRATED INDIVIDUAL COMPONENTS. ALTERNATIVELY, PATIENTS WHO HAVE RECEIVED LISINOPRIL MONOTHERAPY 10 MG MAY BE GIVEN LISINOPRIL-HYDROCHLOROTHIAZIDE 10-12.5; PATIENTS WHO HAVE RECEIVED LISINOPRIL MONOTHERAPY 20 OR 40 MG MAY BE GIVEN LISINOPRIL-HYDROCHLOROTHI-

DOSAGE AND ADMINISTRATION: *(cont'd)*

AZIDE 20-12.5 THEN LISINOPRIL-HYDROCHLOROTHIAZIDE 20-25, THUS TITRATING THE HYDROCHLOROTHIAZIDE COMPONENT USING THE COMBINATION.

The usual dose is one or two tablets of lisinopril-hydrochlorothiazide 20-12.5 or lisinopril-hydrochlorothiazide 20-25 once daily. The recommended dose of lisinopril-hydrochlorothiazide 10-12.5 is one tablet once daily. (See INDICATIONS AND USAGE.) Data from clinical trials suggest that the mean group antihypertensive response is similar when lisinopril 10 mg or 20 mg is combined with hydrochlorothiazide 12.5 mg or 25 mg; therefore, patients whose blood pressure is controlled with lisinopril 20 mg plus hydrochlorothiazide 25 mg ordinarily should be given a trial of lisinopril-hydrochlorothiazide 20-12.5 before lisinopril-hydrochlorothiazide 20-25 is used.

Patients usually do not require doses in excess of 50 mg of hydrochlorothiazide daily, particularly when it is combined with other antihypertensive agents.

For lisinopril monotherapy the recommended initial dose in patients not on diuretics is 10 mg of lisinopril once a day. Dosage should be adjusted according to blood pressure response. The usual dosage range of lisinopril is 20 to 40 mg administered in a single daily dose; the maximum recommended dose is 80 mg in a single daily dose. Blood pressure should be measured at the interdosing interval to ensure that there is an adequate antihypertensive response at that time. If blood pressure is not controlled with lisinopril alone, a diuretic may be added. Hydrochlorothiazide 12.5 mg has been shown to provide an additive effect. After addition of the diuretic it may be possible to reduce the dose of lisinopril.

In patients who are currently being treated with a diuretic, symptomatic hypotension occasionally may occur following the initial dose of lisinopril. The diuretic should, if possible, be discontinued for two to three days before beginning therapy with lisinopril to reduce the likelihood od hypotension. If the patient's blood pressure is not controlled with lisinopril alone, diuretic therapy may be resumed.

If the diuretic cannot be discontinued an initial dose of 5 mg of lisinopril should be used under medical supervision for at least two hours and until blood pressure has stabilized for at least an additional hour.

Concomitant administration of lisinopril-hydrochlorothiazide with potassium supplements, potassium salt substitutes, or potassium sparing diuretics may lead to increases of serum potassium.

Dosage Adjustment in Renal Impairment: The usual dose of lisinopril-hydrochlorothiazide is recommended for patients with a creatinine clearance > 30 ml/min (serum creatinine of up to approximately 3 mg/dl).

When concomitant diuretic therapy is required in patients with severe renal impairment, a loop diuretic rather than a thiazide diuretic is preferred for use with lisinopril; therefore, for patients with severe renal dysfunction the lisinopril-hydrochlorothiazide combination tablet is not recommended.

Use in Elderly: In general, blood pressure response and adverse experiences were similar in younger and older patients given lisinopril-hydrochlorothiazide. However, in a multiple dose pharmacokinetic study in elderly versus young patients using the lisinopril/hydrochlorothiazide combination, area under the plasma concentration time curve (AUC) increased approximately 120% for lisinopril and approximately 80% for hydrochlorothiazide in older patients. Therefore, dosage adjustments in elderly patients should be made with particular caution.

Storage: Store at controlled room temperature, 15-30°C (59-86°F). Protect from excessive light and humidity.

Dispense in a well-closed container, if product package is subdivided.

HOW SUPPLIED - RATED THERAPEUTICALLY EQUIVALENT:

Tablet, Uncoated - Oral - 12.5 mg/10 mg

30's	**$27.22**	**PRINZIDE, Merck**	**00006-0145-31**
100's	**$90.72**	**PRINZIDE, Merck**	**00006-0145-58**
100's	$90.72	Zestoretic, Stuart Pharm	00038-0141-10

Tablet, Uncoated - Oral - 12.5 mg/20 mg

30's	**$29.46**	**PRINZIDE 12-5, Merck**	**00006-0140-31**
100's	**$98.18**	**PRINZIDE 12-5, Merck**	**00006-0140-58**
100's	$98.18	ZESTORETIC, Stuart Pharm	00038-0142-10

Tablet, Uncoated - Oral - 25 mg/20 mg

30's	**$29.82**	**PRINZIDE 25, Merck**	**00006-0142-31**
100's	**$99.40**	**PRINZIDE 25, Merck**	**00006-0142-58**
100's	$99.40	ZESTORETIC, Stuart Pharm	00038-0145-10

HYDROCHLOROTHIAZIDE; LOSARTAN POTASSIUM *(003260)*

CATEGORIES: Angiotensin II Inhibitors; Antihypertensives; Cardiovascular Drugs; Hypertension; FDA Class 4S ("Standard Review"); FDA Approved 1995 Apr

BRAND NAMES: **Hyzaar**

DESCRIPTION:

Hyzaar (losartan potassium-hydrochlorothiazide), combines an angiotensin II receptor (type AT_1) antagonist and a diuretic, hydrochlorothiazide.

FOR COMPLETE PRESCRIBING INFORMATION REFER TO THE INDIVIDUAL DRUG MONOGRAPHS (HYDROCHLOROTHIAZIDE; LOSARTAN POTASSIUM).

INDICATIONS AND USAGE:

Losartan potassium-HCTZ is indicated for the treatment of hypertension. This fixed dose combination is not indicated for initial therapy (see DOSAGE AND ADMINISTRATION.)

DOSAGE AND ADMINISTRATION:

The usual starting dose of losartan is 50 mg once daily, with 25 mg recommended for patients with intravascular volume depletion (*e.g.,* patients treated with diuretics), and patients with a history of hepatic impairment. Losartan can be administered once or twice daily at total daily doses of 25 to 100 mg. If the antihypertensive effect measured at trough using once-a-day dosing is inadequate, a twice-a-day regimen at the same total daily dose or an increase in dose may give a more satisfactory response.

Hydrochlorothiazide is effective in doses of 12.5 to 100 mg once daily and can be given at doses of 12.5 to 25 mg as losartan potassium-HCTZ.

To minimize dose-independent side effects, it is usually appropriate to begin combination therapy only after a patient has failed to achieve the desired effect with monotherapy.

The side effects of losartan are generally rare and apparently independent of dose; those of hydrochlorothiazide are a mixture of dose-dependent (primarily hypokalemia) and dose-independent phenomena (*e.g.,* pancreatitis), the former much more common than the latter. Therapy with any combination of losartan and hydrochlorothiazide will be associated with both sets of dose-independent side effects.

DOSAGE AND ADMINISTRATION: *(cont'd)*

Replacement Therapy: The combination may be substituted for the titrated components.

Dose Titration by Clinical Effect: A patient whose blood pressure is not adequately controlled with losartan monotherapy may be switched to losartan potassium-HCTZ (losartan 50 mg/hydrochlorothiazide 12.5 mg) once daily. If blood pressure remains uncontrolled after about 3 weeks of therapy, the dose may be increased to two tablets once daily.

A patient whose blood pressure is inadequately controlled by 25 mg once daily of hydrochlorothiazide, or is controlled but who experiences hypokalemia with this regimen, may be switched to losartan potassium-HCTZ (losartan 50 mg/hydrochlorothiazide 12.5 mg once daily, reducing the dose of hydrochlorothiazide without reducing the overall expected antihypertensive response. The clinical response to losartan potassium-HCTZ should be subsequently evaluated and if blood pressure remains uncontrolled after about 3 weeks of therapy, the dose may be increased to two tablets once daily.

The usual dose of losartan potassium-HCTZ is one tablet once daily. More than two tablets once daily is not recommended. The maximal antihypertensive effect is attained about 3 weeks after initiation of therapy.

Use in Patients with Renal Impairment: The usual regimens of therapy with losartan potassium-HCTZ may be followed as long as the patient's creatinine clearance is > 30 ml/min. In patients with more severe renal impairment, loop diuretics are preferred to thiazides, so losartan potassium-HCTZ is not recommended.

Patients with Hepatic Impairment: Losartan potassium-HCTZ is not recommended for titration in patients with hepatic impairment because the appropriate 25 mg starting dose of losartan cannot be given.

Losartan potassium-HCTZ may be administered with other antihypertensive agents.

Losartan potassium-HCTZ may be administered with or without food.

HOW SUPPLIED:

No. 3502 - Tablets Hyzaar, 50-12.5 are yellow, teardrop shaped film-coated tablets, coded MRK 717 on one side and Hyzaar on the other. Each tablet contains 50 mg of losartan potassium and 12.5 mg of hydrochlorothiazide.

Storage: Store at controlled room temperature, 15-30°C (59-86°F). Keep container tightly closed. Protect from light.

HOW SUPPLIED - EQUIVALENTS NOT AVAILABLE:

Tablet, Uncoated - Oral - 12.5 mg/50 mg

30's	**$33.00**	**HYZAAR, Merck**	**00006-0717-31**
90's	**$99.00**	**HYZAAR, Merck**	**00006-0717-54**
100's	**$110.00**	**HYZAAR, Merck**	**00006-0717-28**
100's	**$110.00**	**HYZAAR, Merck**	**00006-0717-58**

HYDROCHLOROTHIAZIDE; METHYLDOPA

(001459)

CATEGORIES: Antihypertensives; Cardiovascular Drugs; Diuretics; Edema; Hypertension; Renal Drugs; Thiazides; Pregnancy Category C; FDA Approval Pre 1982; Top 200 Drugs

BRAND NAMES: **Aldoril**; *Apo-Methiazide* (Canada); *Dopatens-H*; *Hydromet* (England, Mexico, Japan); Methyldopa Hydrochlorothiazide; *Sembrina Compound*; *Tensifort*

(International brand names outside U.S. in italics)

FORMULARIES: BC-BS; Medi-Cal

> WARNING:
> This fixed combination drug is not indicated for initial therapy of hypertension. Hypertension requires therapy titrated to the individual patient. If the fixed combination represents the dosage so determined, its use may be more convenient in patient management. The treatment of hypertension is not static, but must be reevaluated as conditions in each patient warrant.

DESCRIPTION:

Methyldopa-hydrochlorothiazide (abbreviated here as methyldopa w/HCTZ). combines two antihypertensives: methyldopa and hydrochlorothiazide.

FOR COMPLETE PRESCRIBING INFORMATION REFER TO THE INDIVIDUAL DRUG MONOGRAPHS (HYDROCHLOROTHIAZIDE ; METHYLDOPA).

INDICATIONS AND USAGE:

Hypertension.

DOSAGE AND ADMINISTRATION:

DOSAGE MUST BE INDIVIDUALIZED AS DETERMINED BY TITRATION OF THE INDIVIDUAL COMPONENTS (see BOXED WARNING). Once the patient has been successfully titrated, methyldopa w/HCTZ may be substituted if the previously determined titrated doses are the same as in the combination. The usual starting dosage is one tablet of methyldopa w/HCTZ 15 two or three times a day or one tablet of methyldopa w/HCTZ 25 two times a day. For those patients requiring higher doses, one tablet of methyldopa w/ HCTZ 30 or methyldopa w/HCTZ 50 two times a day may be used.

Patients usually do not require doses of hydrochlorothiazide in excess of 50 mg daily when combined with other antihypertensive agents. The usual daily dosage of methyldopa is 500 mg to 2 g. To minimize the sedation associated with methyldopa, start dosage increases in the evening.

Occasionally tolerance to methyldopa may occur, usually between the second and third month of therapy. Additional separate doses of methyldopa or replacement of methyldopa w/ HCTZ with single entity agents is necessary until the new effective dose ratio is re-established by titration. The maximum recommended daily dose of methyldopa is 3 g and of hydrochlorothiazide is 200 mg.

If methyldopa w/HCTZ does not adequately control blood pressure, additional doses of other agents may be given. When methyldopa w/HCTZ is given with antihypertensives other than thiazides, the initial dosage of methyldopa should be limited to 500 mg daily in divided doses and the dose of these other agents may need to be adjusted to effect a smooth transition.

Since both components of methyldopa w/HCTZ have a relatively short duration of action, withdrawal is followed by return of hypertension usually within 48 hours. This is not complicated by an overshoot of blood pressure.

DOSAGE AND ADMINISTRATION: *(cont'd)*

Since methyldopa is largely excreted by the kidney, patients with impaired renal function may respond to smaller doses. Syncope in older patients may be related to an increased sensitivity and advanced arteriosclerotic vascular disease. This may be avoided by lower dose.

Storage: Keep container tightly closed. Protect from light, moisture, freezing, - 20°C (-4°F) and store at room temperature, 15-30°C (59-86°F).

PATIENT INFORMATION:

Hydrochlorothiazide with methyldopa is used for the treatment of high blood pressure. This medication should be taken even if you feel fine because high blood pressure may not produce physical symptoms. Do not discontinue this medication suddenly without consulting your physician. Inform your physician if you are pregnant or nursing. Inform your physician and pharmacist if you are allergic to sulfites. Do not take this medication with a monoamine oxidase inhibitor. This medication may be taken with or without food. Take with food if stomach upset occurs. This medication may cause dizziness or drowsiness, especially during the first days of therapy; use caution while driving or operating hazardous machinery. Avoid sudden changes in posture. Do not drink alcohol while taking hydrochlorothiazide with methyldopa. Hydrochlorothiazide with methyldopa may cause increased sensitivity to sunlight. Use sunscreens and wear protective clothing until degree of sensitivity is determined. This medication may cause an increase in blood sugar. If you have diabetes mellitus, carefully monitor blood sugar levels. This medication may worsen gout. When urine is exposed to the air after voiding, it may darken. This is normal. Notify your physician if you develop unusual weakness, muscle cramps, unusual bleeding or bruising, yellow eyes or skin, or a rash.

HOW SUPPLIED - RATED THERAPEUTICALLY EQUIVALENT:

Tablet, Plain Coated - Oral - 15 mg/250 mg

100's	$10.43	Methyldopa w/HCTZ, United Res	00677-1051-01
100's	$10.43	Methyldopa w/HCTZ, H.C.F.A. F F P	99999-1459-01
100's	$18.52	Methyldopa w/HCTZ, Watson Labs	52544-0357-01
100's	$20.23	Methyldopa w/HCTZ, Bristol Myers Squibb	00003-0630-50
100's	$21.95	Methyldopa w/HCTZ, Major Pharms	00904-2403-60
100's	$21.95	Methyldopa/Hydrochlorothiazide, Major Pharms	00904-7813-60
100's	$22.70	Methyldopa w/HCTZ, Qualitest Pharms	00603-4543-21
100's	$23.30	Methyldopa w/HCTZ, Lederle Pharm	00005-3852-23
100's	$25.23	Methyldopa w/HCTZ, Schein Pharm (US)	00364-0827-01
100's	$25.80	Methyldopa/Hydrochlorothiazide, West Point Pharma	59591-0179-68
100's	$25.80	Methyldopa/Hydrochlorothiazide, Endo Labs	60951-0778-70
100's	$25.99	Methyldopa/HCTZ, HL Moore Drug Exch	00839-7141-06
100's	$26.00	Methyldopa w/HCTZ, Goldline Labs	00182-1830-01
100's	$26.20	Methyldopa/Hydrochlorothiazide, Rugby	00536-5651-01
100's	$26.39	Methyldopa w/HCTZ, Vangard Labs	00615-3524-13
100's	$26.54	Methyldopa w/HCTZ, Aligen Independ	00405-4658-01
100's	$27.00	Methyldopa/Hydrochlorothiazide, Consolidated Midland	00223-1587-01
100's	$27.50	Methyldopa w/HCTZ, Geneva Pharms	00781-1809-01
100's	$27.80	Methyldopa & Hydrochlorothiazide, Par Pharm	49884-0186-01
100's	$28.07	Methyldopa w/HCTZ, Major Pharms	00904-2403-61
100's	$30.95	Methyldopa w/HCTZ, Mylan	00378-0507-01
100's	**$46.43**	**ALDORIL 15, Merck**	**00006-0423-68**
500's	$52.15	Methyldopa w/HCTZ, H.C.F.A. F F P	99999-1459-02
500's	$87.97	Methyldopa w/HCTZ, Watson Labs	52544-0357-05
500's	$126.10	Methyldopa & Hydrochlorothiazide, Par Pharm	49884-0186-05
1000's	$104.30	Methyldopa w/HCTZ, H.C.F.A. F F P	99999-1459-03
1000's	$170.55	Methyldopa w/HCTZ, Major Pharms	00904-2403-80
1000's	$170.55	Methyldopa/Hydrochlorothiazide, Major Pharms	00904-7813-80
1000's	$172.11	Methyldopa w/HCTZ, HL Moore Drug Exch	00839-7141-16
1000's	$175.94	Methyldopa w/HCTZ, Watson Labs	52544-0357-10
1000's	$200.30	Methyldopa w/HCTZ, Qualitest Pharms	00603-4543-32
1000's	$215.00	Methyldopa/Hydrochlorothiazide, West Point Pharma	59591-0179-82
1000's	$215.00	Methyldopa/Hydrochlorothiazide, Endo Labs	60951-0778-90
1000's	$221.42	Methyldopa w/HCTZ, Lederle Pharm	00005-3852-34
1000's	$252.20	Methyldopa & Hydrochlorothiazide, Par Pharm	49884-0186-10
1000's	**$450.67**	**ALDORIL 15, Merck**	**00006-0423-82**

Tablet, Plain Coated - Oral - 25 mg/250 mg

100's	$10.43	Methyldopa w/HCTZ, United Res	00677-1052-01
100's	$10.43	Methyldopa w/HCTZ, H.C.F.A. F F P	99999-1459-04
100's	$19.42	Methyldopa w/HCTZ, Watson Labs	52544-0358-01
100's	$22.91	Methyldopa w/HCTZ, Bristol Myers Squibb	00003-0645-50
100's	$23.68	Methyldopa w/HCTZ, Qualitest Pharms	00603-4544-21
100's	$24.70	Methyldopa w/HCTZ, Major Pharms	00904-2404-60
100's	$24.70	Methyldopa/Hydrochlorothiazide, Major Pharms	00904-7814-60
100's	$25.79	Methyldopa w/HCTZ, Lederle Pharm	00005-3853-23
100's	$27.50	Methyldopa/Hydrochlorothiazide, Rugby	00536-5652-01
100's	$29.25	Methyldopa/Hydrochlorothiazide, West Point Pharma	59591-0153-68
100's	$29.25	Methyldopa/Hydrochlorothiazide, Endo Labs	60951-0779-70
100's	$29.60	Methyldopa w/HCTZ, Vangard Labs	00615-3525-13
100's	$31.12	Methyldopa w/HCTZ, HL Moore Drug Exch	00839-7142-06
100's	$31.30	Methyldopa/Hydrochlorothiazide, Goldline Labs	00182-1310-01
100's	$31.48	Methyldopa w/HCTZ, Major Pharms	00904-2404-61
100's	$33.19	Methyldopa w/HCTZ, Aligen Independ	00405-4659-01
100's	$33.39	Methyldopa & Hydrochlorothiazide, Par Pharm	49884-0187-01
100's	$33.70	Methyldopa w/HCTZ, Schein Pharm (US)	00364-0828-01
100's	$35.95	Methyldopa w/HCTZ, Mylan	00378-0711-01
100's	**$54.69**	**ALDORIL 25, Merck**	**00006-0456-68**
500's	$52.15	Methyldopa w/HCTZ, H.C.F.A. F F P	99999-1459-05
500's	$92.25	Methyldopa w/HCTZ, Watson Labs	52544-0358-05
500's	$151.80	Methyldopa & Hydrochlorothiazide, Par Pharm	49884-0187-05
1000's	$104.30	Methyldopa w/HCTZ, H.C.F.A. F F P	99999-1459-06
1000's	$180.35	Methyldopa/Hydrochlorothiazide, Major Pharms	00904-7814-80
1000's	$184.49	Methyldopa w/HCTZ, Watson Labs	52544-0358-10
1000's	$208.10	Methyldopa w/HCTZ, Qualitest Pharms	00603-4544-32
1000's	$220.11	Methyldopa w/HCTZ, Schein Pharm (US)	00364-0828-02
1000's	$222.47	Methyldopa w/HCTZ, Bristol Myers Squibb	00003-0645-75
1000's	$243.60	Methyldopa/Hydrochlorothiazide, West Point Pharma	59591-0153-82
1000's	$243.60	Methyldopa/Hydrochlorothiazide, Endo Labs	60951-0779-90
1000's	$244.92	Methyldopa w/HCTZ, Lederle Pharm	00005-3853-34
1000's	$268.10	Methyldopa & Hydrochlorothiazide, HL Moore Drug Exch	00839-7142-16
1000's	$303.61	Methyldopa & Hydrochlorothiazide, Par Pharm	49884-0187-10
1000's	$306.95	Methyldopa w/HCTZ, Mylan	00378-0711-10
1000's	**$531.13**	**ALDORIL 25, Merck**	**00006-0456-82**

Tablet, Plain Coated - Oral - 30 mg/500 mg

100's	$38.44	Methyldopa w/HCTZ, Watson Labs	52544-0359-01
100's	$42.75	Methyldopa/Hydrochlorothiazide, Consolidated Midland	00223-1589-01
100's	$45.43	Methyldopa w/HCTZ, Schein Pharm (US)	00364-2400-01
100's	$48.95	Methyldopa/Hydrochlorothiazide, Harber Pharm	51432-0273-03
100's	$49.00	Methyldopa & Hydrochlorothiazide, Aligen Independ	00405-4660-01
100's	$51.00	Methyldopa & Hydrochlorothiazide, Par Pharm	49884-0188-01

HOW SUPPLIED - RATED THERAPEUTICALLY EQUIVALENT: *(cont'd)*

100's	$57.66	Methyldopa w/HCTZ, H.C.F.A. F F P	99999-1459-07
100's	**$86.96**	**ALDORIL D30, Merck**	**00006-0694-68**
250's	$144.15	Methyldopa w/HCTZ, H.C.F.A. F F P	99999-1459-08
500's	$182.59	Methyldopa w/HCTZ, Watson Labs	52544-0359-05
500's	$197.50	Methyldopa/Hydrochlorothiazide, Consolidated Midland	00223-1589-05
500's	$288.30	Methyldopa w/HCTZ, H.C.F.A. F F P	99999-1459-09

Tablet, Plain Coated - Oral - 50 mg/500 mg

100's	$39.46	Methyldopa w/HCTZ, Watson Labs	52544-0360-01
100's	$48.87	Methyldopa w/HCTZ, Schein Pharm (US)	00364-2401-01
100's	$49.95	Methyldopa/Hydrochlorothiazide, Harber Pharm	51432-0275-03
100's	$51.00	Methyldopa & Hydrochlorothiazide, Aligen Independ	00405-4661-01
100's	$53.55	Methyldopa & Hydrochlorothiazide, Par Pharm	49884-0189-01
100's	$59.19	Methyldopa w/HCTZ, H.C.F.A. F F P	99999-1459-10
100's	**$93.50**	**ALDORIL D50, Merck**	**00006-0935-68**
250's	$147.97	Methyldopa w/HCTZ, H.C.F.A. F F P	99999-1459-11
500's	$187.44	Methyldopa w/HCTZ, Watson Labs	52544-0360-05
500's	$295.95	Methyldopa w/HCTZ, H.C.F.A. F F P	99999-1459-12

HYDROCHLOROTHIAZIDE; METOPROLOL TARTRATE *(001460)*

CATEGORIES: Antihypertensives; Beta Adrenergic Blocking Agents; Beta Blockers; Cardiovascular Drugs; Hypertension; Renal Drugs; Angina*; Myocardial Infarction*; Pregnancy Category C; FDA Approved 1984 Dec

* Indication not approved by the FDA

BRAND NAMES: *Beloc Comp* (Germany); *Betaloc Comp*; *Betazide*; *Co-Betaloc* (England); **Lopressor HCT**; *Seloken Retard Comp.*; *Selokomb*; *Selokomb 200*; *Selokomb Zoc 100*; *Selopresin*; *Selozide*

(International brand names outside U.S. in italics)

FORMULARIES: BC-BS

COST OF THERAPY: $340.61 (Hypertension; Tablet; 25 mg/100 mg; 1/day; 365 days) vs. Potential Cost of $24,027.04 (Coronary Bypass)

PRIMARY ICD9: 401.1 (Essential Hypertension, Benign)

DESCRIPTION:

Lopressor HCT has the antihypertensive effect of Lopressor, metoprolol tartrate, a selective $beta_1$-adrenoreceptor blocking agent, and the antihypertensive and diuretic actions of hydrochlorothiazide. It is available as tablets for oral administration. The 50/25 tablets contain 50 mg of metoprolol tartrate USP and 25 mg of hydrochlorothiazide USP; the 100/25 tablets contain 100 mg of metoprolol tartrate USP and 25 mg of hydrochlorothiazide USP; and the 100/50 tablets contain 100 mg of metoprolol tartrate USP and 50 mg of hydrochlorothiazide USP.

Metoprolol tartrate is (±)-1-isopropylamino-3-(*p*-(2-methoxyethyl)phenoxy)-2-propanol 2:1 *dextro*-tartrate salt.

FOR COMPLETE PRESCRIBING INFORMATION REFER TO THE INDIVIDUAL DRUG MONOGRAPHS (HYDROCHLOROTHIAZIDE; METOPROLOL TARTRATE).

INDICATIONS AND USAGE:

Lopressor HCT is indicated for the management of hypertension.

This fixed-combination drug is not indicated for initial therapy of hypertension. If the fixed combination represents the dose titrated to the individual patient's needs, therapy with the fixed combination may be more convenient than with the separate components.

DOSAGE AND ADMINISTRATION:

Dosage should be determined by individual titration.

Hydrochlorothiazide is usually given at a dosage of 25 to 100 mg per day. The usual initial dosage of Lopressor is 100 mg daily in single or divided doses. Dosage may be increased gradually until optimum blood pressure control is achieved. The effective dosage range is 100 to 450 mg per day. While once-daily dosing is effective and can maintain a reduction in blood pressure throughout the day, lower doses (especially 100 mg) may not maintain a full effect at the end of the 24-hour period, and larger or more frequent daily doses may be required. This can be evaluated by measuring blood pressure near the end of the dosing interval to determine whether satisfactory control is being maintained throughout the day. $Beta_1$ selectivity diminishes as dosage of Lopressor is increased.

The following dosage schedule may be used to administer from 100 to 200 mg of Lopressor per day and from 25 to 50 mg of hydrochlorothiazide per day (TABLE 1) :

TABLE 1

Lopressor HCT	Dosage
Tablets of 50/25	2 tablets per day in single or divided doses
Tablets of 100/25	1 to 2 tablets per day in single or divided doses
Tablets of 100/50	1 tablet per day in single or divided doses

Dosing regimens that exceed 50 mg of hydrochlorothiazide per day are not recommended. When necessary, another antihypertensive agent may be added gradually, beginning with 50% of the usual recommended starting dose to avoid an excessive fall in blood pressure.

Store between 59-86° F (15-30° C). Protect from moisture.

Dispense in tight, light-resistant container (USP).

HOW SUPPLIED - EQUIVALENTS NOT AVAILABLE:

Tablet, Uncoated - Oral - 25 mg/50 mg

100's	$59.72	LOPRESSOR HCTZ, Novartis	00028-0035-01

Tablet, Uncoated - Oral - 25 mg/100 mg

100's	$93.32	LOPRESSOR HCTZ, Novartis	00028-0053-01

Tablet, Uncoated - Oral - 50 mg/100 mg

100's	$98.98	LOPRESSOR HCTZ, Novartis	00028-0073-01

HYDROCHLOROTHIAZIDE; PROPRANOLOL HYDROCHLORIDE *(001461)*

CATEGORIES: Antihypertensives; Beta Adrenergic Blocking Agents; Beta Blockers; Cardiovascular Drugs; Diuretics; Hypertension; Renal Drugs; Pregnancy Category C; FDA Approval Pre 1982

BRAND NAMES: *Artensol H; Ciplar-H;* **Inderide**; Inderide LA
(International brand names outside U.S. in italics)

FORMULARIES: BC-BS

COST OF THERAPY: $44.23 (Hypertension; Tablet; 25 mg/40 mg; 2/day; 365 days) vs. Potential Cost of $24,027.04 (Coronary Bypass)

PRIMARY ICD9: 401.1 (Essential Hypertension, Benign)

DESCRIPTION:

Inderide Tablets for oral administration combine two antihypertensive agents: Propranolol Hydrochloride, a beta-adrenergic blocking agent, and hydrochlorothiazide, a thiazide diuretic-antihypertensive. Inderide 40/25 Tablets contain 40 mg propranolol hydrochloride and 25 mg hydrochlorothiazide; Inderide 80/25 Tablets contain 80 mg propranolol hydrochloride and 25 mg hydrochlorothiazide.

FOR COMPLETE PRESCRIBING INFORMATION REFER TO THE INDIVIDUAL DRUG MONOGRAPHS (HYDROCHLOROTHIAZIDE; PROPRANOLOL HYDROCHLORIDE).

INDICATIONS AND USAGE:

Inderide is indicated in the management of hypertension.

This fixed combination is not indicated for initial therapy of hypertension. Hypertension requires therapy titrated to the individual patient. If the fixed combination represents the dosage so determined, its use may be more convenient in patient management. The treatment of hypertension is not static, but must be reevaluated as conditions in each patient warrant.

DOSAGE AND ADMINISTRATION:

The dosage must be determined by individual titration.

Hydrochlorothiazide can be given at doses of 25 to 100 mg per day when used alone, but in most patients, 50 mg exerts a maximal effect. The initial dose of propranolol is 80 mg daily, and it may be increased gradually until optimal blood pressure control is achieved. The usual effective dose when used alone is 160 to 480 mg per day.

TABLETS

One Inderide Tablet twice daily can be used to administer up to 160 mg of propranolol and 50 mg of hydrochlorothiazide. For doses of propranolol greater than 160 mg the combination products are not appropriate, because their use would lead to an excessive dose of the thiazide component.

When necessary, another antihypertensive agent may be added gradually beginning with 50 percent of the usual recommended starting dose to avoid an excessive fall in blood pressure.

Store at room temperature (approximately 25° C).

Dispense in well-closed, light-resistant containers.

Protect from moisture, freezing, and excessive heat.

LONG ACTING CAPSULES

One Inderide LA Capsule once-a-day can be used to administer up to 160 mg of propranolol and 50 mg of hydrochlorothiazide. For doses of propanolol greater than 160 mg, the combination products are not appropriate because their use would lead to an excessive dose of the thiazide component.

Inderide LA provides propanolol hydrochloride in a sustained-release form and hydrochlorothiazide in conventional formulation, for once-daily administration. If patients are switched from Inderide tablets (or propanolol plus hydrochlorothiazide) to Inderide LA, care should be taken to ensure that the desired therapeutic effect is maintained. Inderide LA should not be considered a mg-for-mg substitute for Inderide or propanolol plus hydrochlorothiazide. Inderide LA has different kinetics and produces lower blood levels. Retitration may be necessary, especially to maintain effectiveness at the end of the 24-hour dosing interval.

When necessary, another antihypertensive agent may be added gradually, beginning with 50% of the usual recommended starting dose, to avoid an excessive fall in blood pressure.

HOW SUPPLIED - RATED THERAPEUTICALLY EQUIVALENT:

Tablet, Uncoated - Oral - 25 mg/40 mg

100's	$6.06	Propranolol w/HCTZ, H.C.F.A. F F P	99999-1461-01
100's	$6.75	Propranolol w/HCTZ, United Res	00677-1106-01
100's	$16.78	Propranolol w/HCTZ, Sidmak Labs	50111-0473-01
100's	$21.04	Propranolol w/HCTZ, Barr	00555-0427-02
100's	$24.90	Propranolol w/HCTZ, Goldline Labs	00182-1833-01
100's	$25.12	Propranolol Hcl W/Hctz, Qualitest Pharms	00603-5503-21
100's	$25.75	Propranolol w/HCTZ, Purepac Pharm	00228-2358-10
100's	$26.50	Propranolol Hcl & Hydrochlorothia, Major Pharms	00904-0434-60
100's	$27.85	Propranolol w/HCTZ, Schein Pharm (US)	00364-0838-01
100's	$30.00	Propranolol Hcl & Hychlorothiad 40, Harber Pharm	51432-0395-03
100's	$31.12	Propranolol w/HCTZ, Geneva Pharms	00781-1431-01
100's	$31.12	Propranolol Hcl & Hctz, HL Moore Drug Exch	00839-7197-06
100's	$31.25	Propranolol Hcl & HCTZ, Mylan	00378-0731-01
100's	$31.25	Propranolol w/HCTZ, Rugby	00536-4402-01
100's	$34.10	Propranolol w/HCTZ, Geneva Pharms	00781-1431-13
100's	$35.58	Propranolol Hcl & HCTZ, Aligen Independ	00405-4894-01
100's	**$75.39**	**INDERIDE, Ayerst**	**00046-0484-99**
100's	**$98.16**	**INDERIDE, Ayerst**	**00046-0484-81**
500's	$30.30	Propranolol w/HCTZ, H.C.F.A. F F P	99999-1461-02
500's	$80.58	Propranolol w/HCTZ, Sidmak Labs	50111-0473-02
500's	$110.45	Propranolol Hcl W/Hctz, Qualitest Pharms	00603-5503-28
500's	$112.38	Propranolol w/HCTZ, Rugby	00536-4402-05
500's	$128.75	Propranolol w/HCTZ, Purepac Pharm	00228-2358-50
1000's	$60.60	Propranolol w/HCTZ, H.C.F.A. F F P	99999-1461-03
1000's	$96.85	Propranolol w/HCTZ, Major Pharms	00904-0434-80
1000's	$173.24	Propranolol/Hydrochlorothiazide, Barr	00555-0427-05
1000's	$220.22	Propranolol Hcl W/Hctz, Aligen Independ	00405-4894-03
1000's	$338.22	Propranolol w/HCTZ, Purepac Pharm	00228-2358-96
1000's	**$942.12**	**INDERIDE, Ayerst**	**00046-0484-91**

Tablet, Uncoated - Oral - 25 mg/80 mg

100's	$9.06	Propranolol w/HCTZ, H.C.F.A. F F P	99999-1461-04
100's	$9.23	Propranolol w/HCTZ, United Res	00677-1107-01
100's	$9.23	Propranolol Hcl & Hctz, HL Moore Drug Exch	00839-7198-06
100's	$23.43	Propranolol w/HCTZ, Sidmak Labs	50111-0474-01
100's	$29.60	Propranolol w/HCTZ, Barr	00555-0428-02
100's	$34.10	Propranolol w/HCTZ, Goldline Labs	00182-1834-01

HOW SUPPLIED - RATED THERAPEUTICALLY EQUIVALENT: *(cont'd)*

100's	$34.44	Propranolol Hcl W/Hctz, Qualitest Pharms	00603-5504-21
100's	$35.99	Propranolol w/HCTZ, Purepac Pharm	00228-2360-10
100's	$37.90	IPRAZIDE, Major Pharms	00904-0438-60
100's	$38.95	Propranolol w/HCTZ, Schein Pharm (US)	00364-0839-01
100's	$38.95	Propranolol Hcl & HCTZ, Mylan	00378-0347-01
100's	$38.95	Propranolol HCL & HCTZ, Aligen Independ	00405-4895-01
100's	$38.95	Propranolol w/HCTZ, Rugby	00536-4403-01
100's	$46.95	Propranolol w/HCTZ, Geneva Pharms	00781-1432-13
100's	**$131.83**	**INDERIDE, Ayerst**	**00046-0488-81**
500's	$45.30	Propranolol w/HCTZ, H.C.F.A. F F P	99999-1461-05
500's	$112.64	Propranolol w/HCTZ, Sidmak Labs	50111-0474-02
1000's	$90.60	Propranolol w/HCTZ, H.C.F.A. F F P	99999-1461-06
1000's	$155.94	Propranolol w/HCTZ, Rugby	00536-4403-05
1000's	$349.43	Propranolol w/HCTZ, Purepac Pharm	00228-2360-96
1000's	$349.43	Propranolol Hcl W/Hctz, Aligen Independ	00405-4895-03

HOW SUPPLIED - NOT RATED EQUIVALENT:

Capsule, Gelatin, Sustained Action - Oral - 50 mg/80 mg

100's	**$140.44**	**INDERIDE LA 80/50, Ayerst**	**00046-0455-81**

Capsule, Gelatin, Sustained Action - Oral - 50 mg/120 mg

100's	**$166.86**	**INDERIDE LA 120/50, Ayerst**	**00046-0457-81**

Capsule, Gelatin, Sustained Action - Oral - 50 mg/160 mg

100's	**$187.09**	**INDERIDE LA 160/50, Ayerst**	**00046-0459-81**

HYDROCHLOROTHIAZIDE; RESERPINE *(001462)*

CATEGORIES: Antihypertensives; Cardiovascular Drugs; Diuretics; Edema; Hypertension; Renal Drugs; Vasodilating Agents; Pregnancy Category C; FDA Approval Pre 1982

BRAND NAMES: *Dichlotride*; *Dichlotride S* (Japan); Hydro-Reserp; Hydroplus-50; Hydropres; Hydrorex; Hydroserp; Hydroserpalan; Hydroserpine; Mallopress; *Medeserpine Co*; **Serpasil-Esidrix**
(International brand names outside U.S. in italics)

FORMULARIES: BC-BS; Medi-Cal

> WARNING:
> This fixed combination drug is not indicated for initial therapy of hypertension. Hypertension requires therapy titrated to the individual patient. If the fixed combination represents the dosage so determined, its use may be more convenient in patient management. The treatment of hypertension is not static but must be reevaluated as conditions in each patient warrant.

DESCRIPTION:

FOR COMPLETE PRESCRIBING INFORMATION REFER TO THE INDIVIDUAL DRUG MONOGRAPHS (HYDROCHLOROTHIAZIDE; RESERPINE).

INDICATIONS AND USAGE:

Hypertension.

DOSAGE AND ADMINISTRATION:

The initial dosage of reserpine w/HCTZ should conform to the dosages of the individual components established during titration.

The usual adult dosage of reserpine w/HCTZ 25mg is 1 or 2 tablets once a day; that of reserpine w/HCTZ 50mg is 1 tablet once a day. Patients usually do not require doses in excess of 50 mg of hydrochlorothiazide daily when combined with other antihypertensive agents. Dosage may require adjustment according to the blood pressure response of the patient. For maintenance, dosage should be adjusted to the lowest requirements of the individual patient. Doses higher than 0.25 daily of reserpine should be used cautiously, because occurrence of serious mental depression and other side effects may increase considerably.

Storage: Keep container tightly closed. Protect from light, moisture, freezing, - 20°C (-4°F) and store at room temperature, 15-30°C (59-86°F).

HOW SUPPLIED - EQUIVALENTS NOT AVAILABLE:

Tablet, Uncoated - Oral - 25 mg/0.125 mg

100's	$3.77	HYDROSERPINE #1, HL Moore Drug Exch	00839-5137-06
100's	$3.95	Reserpine & HCTZ, Aligen Independ	00405-4495-01
100's	$4.03	Reserpine & Hctz, Schein Pharm (US)	00364-0354-01
100's	$4.79	HYDROSERPINE NO.1, Rugby	00536-3915-01
100's	$28.15	HYDROPRES 25, Merck	00006-0053-68
1000's	$27.00	Reserpine & Hctz, Schein Pharm (US)	00364-0354-02

Tablet, Uncoated - Oral - 50 mg/0.125 mg

100's	$4.15	HYDROSINE, Major Pharms	00904-2168-60
100's	$4.16	Reserpine & Hctz, Schein Pharm (US)	00364-0355-01
100's	$5.94	HYDROSERPINE NO.2, Rugby	00536-3916-01
100's	$17.44	HYDROPINE H P 50, Rugby	00536-3884-01
100's	$43.91	HYDROPRES 50, Merck	00006-0127-68
500's	$83.13	HYDROPINE H P 50, Rugby	00536-3884-05
1000's	$22.28	HYDROSERPINE #2, HL Moore Drug Exch	00839-5138-16
1000's	$29.84	Reserpine & Hctz, Schein Pharm (US)	00364-0355-02
1000's	$32.80	HYDROSINE, Major Pharms	00904-2168-80
1000's	$403.96	HYDROPRES 50, Merck	00006-0127-82

HYDROCHLOROTHIAZIDE; SPIRONOLACTONE *(001463)*

CATEGORIES: Antihypertensives; Cardiovascular Drugs; Cirrhosis; Congestive Heart Failure; Diuretics; Edema; Electrolytic, Caloric-Water Balance; Heart Failure; Hypertension; Hypokalemia; Nephrotic Syndrome; Potassium Sparing Diuretics; Renal Drugs; Thiazides; FDA Approval Pre 1982

BRAND NAMES: **Aldactazide**; *Diuren*; Hydrotone; *Slosat*; Spironazide; *Spironothiazid* (Germany); Spirozide
(International brand names outside U.S. in italics)

FORMULARIES: Aetna; Medi-Cal

WARNING:
Spironolactone has been shown to be a tumorigen in chronic toxicity studies in rats (see Spironolactone, WARNINGS). Spironolactone with Hydrochlorothiazide should be used only in those conditions described under "Indications". Unnecessary use of this drug should be avoided.
Fixed-dose combination drugs are not indicated for initial therapy of edema or hypertension. Edema or hypertension requires therapy titrated to the individual patient. If the fixed combination represents the dosage so determined, its use may be more convenient in patient management. The treatment of hypertension and edema is not static, but must be reevaluated as conditions in each patient warrant.

DESCRIPTION:

Each tablet of spironolactone with hydrochlorothiazide contains 25 mg of spironolactone, USP and 25 mg of hydrochlorothiazide, USP Spironolactone is Pregn-4-ene-21-carboxylic acid, 7-(acetylthio)-17-hydroxy-3-oxo-, γ-lactone, (7α, 17α)-.

Hydrochlorothiazide is 2H-1,2,4-Benzothiadiazine-7-sulfonamide, 6-chloro-3,4-dihydro-, 1,1-dioxide.

FOR COMPLETE PRESCRIBING INFORMATION REFER TO THE INDIVIDUAL DRUG MONOGRAPHS (HYDROCHLOROTHIAZIDE ; SPIRONOLACTONE).

INDICATIONS AND USAGE:

Spironolactone has been shown to be a tumorigen in chronic toxicity studies in rats. Spironolactone with Hydrochlorothiazide should be used only in those conditions described below. Unnecessary use of this drug should be avoided.

Spironolactone with Hydrochlorothiazide is indicated for: EDEMATOUS conditions for patients with:

Congestive heart failure: For the management of edema and sodium retention when the patient is only partially responsive to, or is intolerant of, other therapeutic measures. The treatment of diuretic-induced hypokalemia in patients with congestive heart failure when other measures are considered inappropriate. The treatment of patients with congestive heart failure taking digitalis when other therapies are considered inadequate or inappropriate.

Cirrhosis of the liver accompanied by edema and/or ascites: Aldosterone levels may be exceptionally high in this condition. Spironolactone with Hydrochlorothiazide is indicated for maintenance therapy together with bed rest and the restriction of fluid and sodium.

The nephrotic syndrome: For nephrotic patients when treatment of the underlying disease, restriction of fluid and sodium intake, and the use of other diuretics do not provide an adequate response.

Essential hypertension: For patients with essential hypertension in whom other measures are considered inadequate or inappropriate. In hypertensive patients for the treatment of a diuretic-induced hypokalemia when other measures are considered inappropriate.

Usage in Pregnancy: The routine use of diuretics in an otherwise healthy woman is inappropriate, and exposes mother and fetus to unnecessary hazard. Diuretics do not prevent development of toxemia of pregnancy, and there is no satisfactory evidence that they are useful in the treatment of developing toxemia.

Edema during pregnancy may arise from pathologic causes or from the physiologic and mechanical consequences of pregnancy. Spironolactone with Hydrochlorothiazide is indicated in pregnancy when edema is due to pathologic causes just as it is in the absence of pregnancy (however, see WARNINGS, Hydrochlorothiazide and Spironolactone). Dependent edema in pregnancy, resulting from the restriction of venous return by the expanded uterus, is properly treated through elevation of the lower extremities and use of support hose; use of diuretics to lower intravascular volume in this case is unsupported and unnecessary. There is hypervolemia during normal pregnancy which is harmful to neither the fetus nor the mother (in the absence of cardio-vascular disease) but which is associated with edema, including generalized edema, in the majority of pregnant women. If this edema produces discomfort, increased recumbency will often provide relief. In rare instances, this edema may cause extreme discomfort which is not relieved by rest. In these cases, a short course of diuretics may provide relief and may be appropriate.

DOSAGE AND ADMINISTRATION:

Optimal dosage should be established by individual titration of the components.

Edema in adults (congestive heart failure, hepatic cirrhosis of nephrotic syndrome). The usual maintenance dose of Spironolactone with Hydrochlorothiazide is four tablets daily administered in a single dose or in divided doses but may range from one to eight tablets daily depending on the response to the initial titration. In some instances it may be desirable to administer separate tablets of either spironolactone with hydrochlorothiazide in addition to Spironolactone with Hydrochlorothiazide in order to provide optimal individual therapy.

The onset of diuresis with Spironolactone with Hydrochlorothiazide occurs promptly and, due to prolonged effect of the spironolactone component, persists for two to three days after Spironolactone with Hydrochlorothiazide is discontinued.

Edema in children. The usual daily maintenance dose of spironolactone with hydrochlorothiazide should be that which provides 0.75 to 1.5 mg of spironolactone per pound of body weight (1.65 to 3.3 mg/kg).

Essential hypertension. Although the dosage will vary depending on the results of titration of the individual ingredients, many patients will be found to have an optimal response to the amount of hydrochlorothiazide and spironolactone contained in two to four tablets of spironolactone with hydrochlorothiazide per day given in a single dose or in divided doses.

Concurrent potassium supplementation is not recommended when spironolactone with hydrochlorothiazide is used in the long-term management of hypertension or in the treatment of most edematous conditions, since the spironolactone content of spironolactone with hydrochlorothiazide is usually sufficient to minimize loss induced by the hydrochlorothiazide component.

STORE AT 15-30°C (59-86°F), PROTECTED FROM LIGHT.

HOW SUPPLIED - RATED THERAPEUTICALLY EQUIVALENT:

Tablet, Plain Coated - Oral - 25 mg/25 mg

100's	$5.33	Spironolactone w/HCTZ, H.C.F.A. F F P	99999-1463-01
100's	$5.65	Spironolactone & HCTZ, Major Pharms	00904-0344-60
100's	$7.30	Spironolactone W/Hctz, Qualitest Pharms	00603-5767-21
100's	$7.50	Spironolactone w/HCTZ, Goldline Labs	00182-1158-01
100's	$7.50	Spironolactone With Hctz, Mutual Pharm	53489-0144-01
100's	$7.74	Spironolactone, United Res	00677-0624-01

HOW SUPPLIED - RATED THERAPEUTICALLY EQUIVALENT: *(cont'd)*

100's	$7.84	Spironolactone W/Hctz, Caremark	00339-5357-12
100's	$8.00	SPIROZIDE, Rugby	00536-4576-01
100's	$8.03	Spironolactone, HL Moore Drug Exch	00839-6322-06
100's	$8.12	Spironolactone W/Hctz, Voluntary Hosp	53258-0160-13
100's	$8.18	Spironolactone w/HCTZ, Aligen Independ	00405-4946-01
100's	$8.60	Spironolactone w/HCTZ, Parmed Pharms	00349-2306-01
100's	$8.85	Spironolactone W/Hctz, Voluntary Hosp	53258-0160-01
100's	$9.30	Spironolactone w/HCTZ, Geneva Pharms	00781-1149-01
100's	$9.60	Spironolactone & HCTZ, Mylan	00378-0141-01
100's	$9.70	Spironolactone W/Hctz, Amer Preferred	53445-1095-01
100's	$9.87	Spironolactone W/Hctz, US Trading	56126-0305-11
100's	$10.50	Spironolactone W/Hctz, Raway	00686-3887-13
100's	$11.10	Spironolactone & HCTZ, Major Pharms	00904-0344-61
100's	$25.07	Spironolactone w/HCTZ, Geneva Pharms	00781-1149-13
100's	**$41.64**	**ALDACTAZIDE, Searle**	**00025-1011-31**
250's	$11.95	Spironolactone & HCTZ, Major Pharms	00904-0344-70
250's	$13.32	Spironolactone w/HCTZ, H.C.F.A. F F P	99999-1463-02
500's	$24.40	Spironolactone W/Hctz, Major Pharms	00904-0344-40
500's	$26.65	Spironolactone w/HCTZ, H.C.F.A. F F P	99999-1463-03
500's	$31.66	Spironolactone W/Hctz, Qualitest Pharms	00603-5767-28
500's	$32.50	Spironolactone W/Hctz, United Res	00677-0624-05
500's	$32.50	Spironolactone With Hctz, Mutual Pharm	53489-0144-05
500's	$32.60	SPIROZIDE, Rugby	00536-4576-05
500's	$43.95	Spironolactone & HCTZ, Mylan	00378-0141-05
1000's	$33.75	Spirono Hct, H & H Labs	46703-0058-10
1000's	$45.71	Spironolactone W/Hctz, Qualitest Pharms	00603-5767-32
1000's	$53.26	Spironolactone, United Res	00677-0624-10
1000's	$53.30	Spironolactone w/HCTZ, Geneva Pharms	00781-1149-10
1000's	$53.30	Spironolactone w/HCTZ, H.C.F.A. F F P	99999-1463-04
1000's	$64.20	Spironolactone With Hctz, Mutual Pharm	53489-0144-10
1000's	$65.00	HCTZ & Spironolactone, Schein Pharm (US)	00364-0513-02
1000's	$65.50	Spironolactone w/HCTZ, Goldline Labs	00182-1158-10
1000's	$65.50	SPIROZIDE, Rugby	00536-4576-10
1000's	$67.95	Spironolactone w/HCTZ, Parmed Pharms	00349-2306-10
1000's	$72.23	Spironolactone, HL Moore Drug Exch	00839-6322-16
1000's	$73.49	Spironolactone w/HCTZ, Aligen Independ	00405-4946-03
1000's	$95.50	SPIRONOLACTONE 250, Harber Pharm	51432-0430-06
1000's	$179.95	Hydrotone, Quality Res Pharms	52765-1080-00
1000's	**$383.14**	**ALDACTAZIDE, Searle**	**00025-1011-52**
2500's	$133.25	Spironolactone w/HCTZ, H.C.F.A. F F P	99999-1463-05
2500's	**$930.80**	**ALDACTAZIDE, Searle**	**00025-1011-55**

HOW SUPPLIED - NOT RATED EQUIVALENT:

Tablet, Plain Coated - Oral - 50 mg/50 mg

100's	**$73.15**	**ALDACTAZIDE, Searle**	**00025-1021-31**

HYDROCHLOROTHIAZIDE; TIMOLOL MALEATE *(001464)*

CATEGORIES: Antihypertensives; Beta Adrenergic Blocking Agents; Beta Blockers; Cardiovascular Drugs; Diuretics; Hypertension; Renal Drugs; Pregnancy Category C; FDA Approval Pre 1982

BRAND NAMES: **Timolide**

FORMULARIES: Aetna; BC-BS

COST OF THERAPY: $470.92 (Hypertension; Tablet; 25 mg/10 mg; 2/day; 365 days) vs. Potential Cost of $24,027.04 (Coronary Bypass)

PRIMARY ICD9: 401.1 (Essential Hypertension, Benign)

DESCRIPTION:

Timolol Maleate-Hydrochlorothiazide is for the treatment of hypertension. It combines the antihypertensive activity of two agents: a non-selective beta-adrenergic receptor blocking agent (timolol maleate) and a diuretic (hydrochlorothiazide).

FOR COMPLETE PRESCRIBING INFORMATION REFER TO THE INDIVIDUAL DRUG MONOGRAPHS (HYDROCHLOROTHIAZIDE; TIMOLOL MALEATE).

INDICATIONS AND USAGE:

Timolol maleate w/ HCTZ is indicated for the treatment of hypertension.

This fixed combination drug is not indicated for initial therapy of hypertension. If the fixed combination represents the dose titrated to an individual patient's needs, it may be more convenient than the separate components.

DOSAGE AND ADMINISTRATION:

The recommended starting and maintenance dosage is 1 tablet twice a day or 2 tablets once a day. Patients usually do not require doses in excess of 50 mg of hydrochlorothiazide daily when combined with other antihypertensive agents. If the antihypertensive response is not satisfactory, another nondiuretic antihypertensive agent may be added.

Storage: Store in a well-closed container, protected from light.

HOW SUPPLIED - EQUIVALENTS NOT AVAILABLE:

Tablet, Uncoated - Oral - 25 mg/10 mg

100's	**$64.51**	**TIMOLIDE 10-25, Merck**	**00006-0067-68**

HYDROCHLOROTHIAZIDE; TRIAMTERENE *(001465)*

CATEGORIES: Antihypertensives; Cardiovascular Drugs; Diuretics; Edema; Electrolytic, Caloric-Water Balance; Hypertension; Potassium Sparing Diuretics; Renal Drugs; Thiazides; Pregnancy Category C; Sales > $500 Million; FDA Approval Pre 1982; Top 200 Drugs

BRAND NAMES: *Anjal*; *Apo-triazide* (Canada); *Dazid*; *Dinazide*; **Dyazide**; *Dyberzide*; *Dytenzide*; *Dytide H* (Germany); *Esiteren* (Germany); *Hydrene* (Australia); Maxzide; *Renezide*; *Slimin*; *Triamizide*; *Triazide*; *Trizid*; *Turfa* (Germany)
(International brand names outside U.S. in italics)

FORMULARIES: Aetna; BC-BS; CIGNA; FHP; Humana; Kaiser; Medco; Medi-Cal; PruCare; United; PCS

COST OF THERAPY: $19.45 (Hypertension; Tablet; 50 mg/75 mg; 1/day; 365 days) vs. Potential Cost of $24,027.04 (Coronary Bypass)

PRIMARY ICD9: 401.1 (Essential Hypertension, Benign)

DESCRIPTION:

Hydrochlorothiazide is a diuretic/antihypertensive agent and triamterene is an antikaliuretic agent.

FOR COMPLETE PRESCRIBING INFORMATION REFER TO THE INDIVIDUAL DRUG MONOGRAPHS (HYDROCHLOROTHIAZIDE; TRIAMTERENE).

INDICATIONS AND USAGE:

This fixed combination drug is not indicated for the initial therapy of edema or hypertension except in individuals in whom the development of hypokalemia cannot be risked.

Triamterene w/HCTZ is indicated for the treatment of hypertension or edema in patients who develop hypokalemia on hydrochlorothiazide alone.

Triamterene w/HCTZ is also indicated for those patients who require a thiazide diuretic and in whom the development of hypokalemia cannot be risked (*e.g.,* patients on concomitant digitalis preparations, or with a history of cardiac arrhythmias, etc.).

Triamterene w/HCTZ may be used alone or as an adjunct or in combination with other antihypertensive drugs, such as beta-blockers. Since triamterene w/HCTZ may enhance the action(s) of these agents/drugs, dosage adjustments may be necessary.

DOSAGE AND ADMINISTRATION:

CAPSULES

The usual dose of triamterene w/HCTZ is one or two capsules given once daily, with appropriate monitoring of serum potassium and of the clinical effect. (See Triamterene, WARNINGS regarding hyperkalemia.)

Store between 15° and 30°C (59° and 86°F). Protect from light. Dispense in a tight, light-resistant container.

TABLETS

The usual dose of triamterene w/HCTZ-25 mg is one or two tablets daily, given as a single dose, with appropriate monitoring of serum potassium. The usual dose of triamterene w/ HCTZ is one tablet daily, with appropriate monitoring of serum potassium. There is no experience with the use of more than one triamterene w/HCTZ tablet daily or more than two triamterene w/HCTZ-25 mg tablets daily. Clinical experience with the administration of two triamterene w/HCTZ-25 mg tablets daily in divided doses (rather than as a single dose) suggests an increased risk of electrolyte imbalance and renal dysfunction.

Patients receiving 50 mg of hydrochlorothiazide who become hypokalemic may be transferred to triamterene w/HCTZ directly. Patients receiving 25 mg hydrochlorothiazide who become hypokalemic may be transferred to triamterene w/HCTZ-25 mg (37.5 mg triamterene/25 mg hydrochlorothiazide) directly.

In patients requiring hydrochlorothiazide therapy and in whom hypokalemia cannot be risked therapy may be initiated with triamterene w/HCTZ-25 mg. If an optimal blood pressure response is not obtained with triamterene w/HCTZ-25 mg, the dose should be increased to two triamterene w/HCTZ-25 mg tablets daily as a single dose, or one triamterene w/HCTZ tablet daily. If blood pressure still is not controlled, another antihypertensive agent may be added.

Clinical studies have shown that patients taking less bioavailable formulations of triamterene and hydrochlorothiazide in daily doses 25-50 mg hydrochlorothiazide and 50-100 mg triamterene may be safely changed to one triamterene w/HCTZ-25 mg tablet daily. All patients changed from less bioavailable formulations to triamterene w/HCTZ should be monitored clinically and for serum potassium after the transfer.

Store at Controlled Room Temperature 15-30°C (59-86°F).

Protect from Light.

Dispense in a tight, light resistant, child-resistant container.

PATIENT INFORMATION:

Hydrochlorothiazide with triamterene is used for the treatment of fluid accumulation and to lower blood pressure. This medication should be taken even if you feel fine because high blood pressure may not produce physical symptoms. Inform your physician if you are pregnant or nursing. Inform your physician if you have diabetes mellitus. Blood glucose levels may be increased in patients with diabetes mellitus. This medication may worsen gout. Hydrochlorothiazide with triamterene may be taken with or without food and should be taken early in the day. Dizziness or lightheadedness may occur with therapy; avoid sudden changes in posture. Hydrochlorothiazide with triamterene may cause increased sensitivity to sunlight. Use sunscreens and wear protective clothing until degree of sensitivity is determined.

HOW SUPPLIED - RATED THERAPEUTICALLY EQUIVALENT:

Capsule - Oral - 25 mg/ 37.5 mg

100's	$37.53	HCTZ & Triamterene, Mylan	00378-2537-01
1000's	$360.68	HCTZ & Triamterene, Mylan	00378-2537-10

Capsule, Gelatin - Oral - 25 mg/37.5 mg

100's	$37.53	Triamterene W/Hctz, Geneva Pharms	00781-2056-01
1000's	$360.68	Triamterene W/Hctz, Geneva Pharms	00781-2056-10

Capsule, Gelatin - Oral - 25 mg/50 mg

24's	$7.40	Triamterene W/Hctz, Zenith Labs	00172-2950-43
100's	$17.70	Triamterene w/HCTZ, H.C.F.A. F F P	99999-1465-01
100's	$27.95	Triamterene W/Hctz, Zenith Labs	00172-2950-60
100's	$27.95	Triamterene W/Hctz, Geneva Pharms	00781-2540-01
100's	$27.95	Triamterene W/HCTZ, Geneva Pharms	00781-2715-01
100's	$28.00	Triamterene W/Hctz, Goldline Labs	00182-1750-01
100's	$28.00	Triamterene and HCTZ, Sidmak Labs	50111-0850-01
100's	$29.95	Triamterene W/HCTZ, Major Pharms	00904-1936-60
100's	$32.00	Triamterene W/Hctz, Geneva Pharms	00781-2540-13
100's	$32.00	Triamterene W/HCTZ, Geneva Pharms	00781-2715-13
100's	**$36.80**	**DYAZIDE, SKB Pharms**	**00108-3590-22**
100's	**$38.80**	**DYAZIDE, SKB Pharms**	**00108-3590-21**
1000's	$177.00	Triamterene w/HCTZ, H.C.F.A. F F P	99999-1465-02
1000's	$255.70	Triamterene W/HCTZ, Major Pharms	00904-1936-80
1000's	$267.50	Triamterene W/HCTZ, Qualitest Pharms	00603-6181-32
1000's	$268.00	Triamterene W/Hctz, Goldline Labs	00182-1750-10
1000's	$268.00	Triamterene and HCTZ, Sidmak Labs	50111-0850-03
1000's	$269.00	Triamterene W/Hctz, Zenith Labs	00172-2950-80
1000's	$269.00	Triamterene W/Hctz, Geneva Pharms	00781-2540-10
1000's	$269.00	Triamterene W/HCTZ, Geneva Pharms	00781-2715-10
1000's	**$353.20**	**DYAZIDE, SKB Pharms**	**00108-3590-30**

Tablet - Oral - 37.5/25 mg

100's	$37.72	Triamterene, Mylan	00378-1352-01
500's	$160.17	Triamterene, Mylan	00378-1352-05

HOW SUPPLIED - RATED THERAPEUTICALLY EQUIVALENT: *(cont'd)*

Tablet - Oral - 75/50 mg

100's	$40.42	Triamterene, Mylan	00378-1355-01
500's	$206.38	Triamterene, Mylan	00378-1355-05

Tablet, Uncoated - Oral - 25 mg/37.5 mg

100's	$29.90	Triamterene W/Hctz, Qualitest Pharms	00603-6180-21
100's	$30.75	Triamterene w/HCTZ, H.C.F.A. F F P	99999-1465-03
100's	$30.86	Triamterene W/Hctz, Watson Labs	52544-0424-01
100's	$32.48	Triamterene W/Hctz, Aligen Independ	00405-5049-01
100's	$32.67	Triamterene W/Hctz, Rugby	00536-5665-01
100's	$33.04	Triamterene W/Hctz, Caremark	00339-5837-12
100's	$33.50	Triamterene W/Hctz, Geneva Pharms	50752-0300-05
100's	$33.65	Triamterene W/Hctz, Goldline Labs	00182-1903-01
100's	$33.65	Triamterene w/HCTZ, Major Pharms	00904-7873-60
100's	$33.95	Triamterene W/Hctz, Geneva Pharms	00781-1123-01
100's	$33.95	Triamterene W/Hctz, HL Moore Drug Exch	00839-7950-06
100's	$35.00	Triamterene W/Hctz, Harber Pharm	51432-0797-03
100's	$41.26	MAXZIDE, Lederle Pharm	00005-4464-43
100's	$45.79	MAXZIDE, Lederle Pharm	00005-4464-60
500's	$146.59	Triamterene W/Hctz, Watson Labs	52544-0424-05
500's	$153.75	Triamterene w/HCTZ, H.C.F.A. F F P	99999-1465-04
500's	$154.31	Triamterene W/Hctz, Aligen Independ	00405-5049-02
500's	$155.18	Triamterene W/Hctz, Rugby	00536-5665-05
500's	$161.26	Triamterene W/Hctz, Geneva Pharms	00781-1123-05
500's	$164.15	Triamterene W/Hctz, Geneva Pharms	50752-0300-08
500's	$167.95	Triamterene w/HCTZ, Major Pharms	00904-7873-40
500's	$168.00	Triamterene W/Hctz, Goldline Labs	00182-1903-05

Tablet, Uncoated - Oral - 50 mg/75 mg

15's	$2.40	Triamterene w/HCTZ, Major Pharms	00904-1965-48
30's	$1.59	Triamterene w/HCTZ, H.C.F.A. F F P	99999-1465-05
30's	$3.45	Triamterene w/HCTZ, Major Pharms	00904-1965-46
100's	$5.33	Triamterene w/HCTZ, H.C.F.A. F F P	99999-1465-06
100's	$5.78	Triamterene w/HCTZ, United Res	00677-1212-01
100's	$8.93	Triamterene W/Hctz, IDE-Interstate	00814-8011-14
100's	$22.83	Triamterene w/HCTZ, Bristol Myers Squibb	00003-0851-50
100's	$28.46	Triamterene w/HCTZ, Qualitest Pharms	00603-6182-21
100's	$28.50	Triamterene w/HCTZ, Rugby	00536-4956-01
100's	$28.50	Triamterene w/HCTZ, Major Pharms	00904-1965-60
100's	$28.78	Triamterene & Hydrochlorothiazide 75, Barr	00555-0444-02
100's	$28.90	Triamterene w/ HCTZ, Aligen Independ	00405-5048-01
100's	$33.10	Triamterene W/Hctz, Geneva Pharms	50752-0304-05
100's	$35.44	Triamterene W/Hctz, Caremark	00339-5625-12
100's	$36.25	Triamterene w/HCTZ, Medirex	57480-0373-01
100's	$37.42	Triamterene w/HCTZ, Parmed Pharms	00349-8749-01
100's	$37.55	Triamterene & HCTZ, Schein Pharm (US)	00364-2242-01
100's	$38.02	Triamterene w/HCTZ, Vangard Labs	00615-0567-13
100's	$43.10	Triamterene & HCTZ, Schein Pharm (US)	00364-2242-90
100's	$46.77	Triamterene w/HCTZ, Major Pharms	00904-1965-61
100's	$49.98	Triamterene w/HCTZ, Warner Chilcott	00047-0833-24
100's	$49.98	Triamterene w/HCTZ 75, Goldline Labs	00182-1872-01
100's	$49.98	Triamterene w/HCTZ, Par Pharm	49884-0279-01
100's	$49.98	Triamterene w/HCTZ 75, Watson Labs	52544-0348-01
100's	$49.98	Triamterene w/HCTZ, Martec Pharms	52555-0974-01
100's	$50.02	Triamterene W/Hctz, HL Moore Drug Exch	00839-7422-06
100's	$51.00	Triamterene w/HCTZ, Goldline Labs	00182-1872-89
100's	$55.60	Triamterene w/HCTZ, Geneva Pharms	00781-1008-01
100's	$69.05	Triamterene w/HCTZ, Geneva Pharms	00781-1008-13
100's	$83.46	MAXZIDE, Lederle Pharm	00005-4460-43
100's	$89.41	MAXZIDE, Lederle Pharm	00005-4460-60
500's	$26.65	Triamterene w/HCTZ, H.C.F.A. F F P	99999-1465-07
500's	$28.90	Triamterene w/HCTZ, United Res	00677-1212-05
500's	$101.84	Triamterene w/HCTZ, Qualitest Pharms	00603-6182-28
500's	$101.96	Triamterene W/Hctz, Barr	00555-0444-04
500's	$102.20	Triamterene w/HCTZ, Major Pharms	00904-1965-40
500's	$102.22	Triamterene W/ HCTZ, Aligen Independ	00405-5048-02
500's	$109.28	Triamterene w/HCTZ, Bristol Myers Squibb	00003-0851-60
500's	$142.50	Triamterene w/HCTZ, Rugby	00536-4956-05
500's	$162.10	Triamterene W/Hctz, Geneva Pharms	50752-0304-08
500's	$175.10	Triamterene & HCTZ, Schein Pharm (US)	00364-2242-05
500's	$241.95	Triamterene w/HCTZ, Warner Chilcott	00047-0833-30
500's	$241.95	Triamterene w/HCTZ 75, Goldline Labs	00182-1872-05
500's	$241.95	Triamterene/Hydrochlorothiazide, HL Moore Drug Exch	00839-7422-12
500's	$241.95	Triamterene & HCTZ, Par Pharm	49884-0279-05
500's	$241.95	Triamterene w/HCTZ 75, Watson Labs	52544-0348-05
500's	$241.95	Triamterene w/HCTZ, Martec Pharms	52555-0974-05
500's	$264.10	Triamterene w/HCTZ, Geneva Pharms	00781-1008-05
500's	$417.31	MAXZIDE, Lederle Pharm	00005-4460-31
600's	$223.60	Triamterene w/HCTZ, Medirex	57480-0373-06
1000's	$53.30	Triamterene w/HCTZ, H.C.F.A. F F P	99999-1465-08
1000's	$173.40	Triamterene w/HCTZ, Major Pharms	00904-1965-80
1000's	$218.56	Triamterene w/HCTZ, Bristol Myers Squibb	00003-0851-75
1000's	$225.00	Triamterene & HCTZ, Schein Pharm (US)	00364-2242-02
1000's	$277.00	Triamterene W/HCTZ, Rugby	00536-4956-10
1000's	$321.05	Triamterene W/Hctz, Geneva Pharms	50752-0304-09
1000's	$459.71	Triamterene W/HCTZ, Watson Labs	52544-0348-10
1000's	$459.71	Triamterene W/Hctz, Martec Pharms	52555-0974-10

HOW SUPPLIED - NOT RATED EQUIVALENT:

Capsule, Gelatin - Oral - 25 mg/37.5 mg

100's	**$40.10**	**DYAZIDE, SKB Pharms**	**00007-3650-22**
100's	**$42.35**	**DYAZIDE, SKB Pharms**	**00007-3650-21**
1000's	**$385.35**	**DYAZIDE, SKB Pharms**	**00007-3650-30**

Capsule, Gelatin - Oral - 25 mg/50 mg

100's	$27.95	Triamterene W/Hctz, Rugby	00536-4961-01
1000's	$255.70	Triamterene W/Hctz, Major Pharms	00904-5016-80
1000's	$269.00	Triamterene W/Hctz, Rugby	00536-4961-10

Tablet, Uncoated - Oral - 50 mg/75 mg

100's	$6.29	Triamterene w/HCTZ, Balan	00304-1892-01
100's	$8.39	Triamterene w/HCTZ, US Trading	56126-0394-11
500's	$23.99	Triamterene w/HCTZ, Balan	00304-1892-05
500's	$145.90	Triamterene W/HCTZ, Elkins Sinn	00641-4033-88

HYDROCODONE BITARTRATE; PHENYLEPHRINE HYDROCHLORIDE; PHENYLPROPANOLAMINE HYDROCHLORIDE; PYRILAMINE *(001468)*

CATEGORIES: Allergies; Antihistamines; Antitussives; Antitussives/Expectorants/Mucolytics; Common Cold; Congestion; Cough Preparations; DESI Drugs; Decongestants; Hay Fever; Influenza; Lacrimation; Narcotic Analgesics; Otitis Media; Respiratory & Allergy Medications; Rhinitis; Sinus Congestion; DEA Class CIII; DEA Class CV; FDA Pre 1938 Drugs

BRAND NAMES: Ban-Tuss Hc; G-Tuss; Iogreen; Novatuss; Q-Tuss Hc; Qrp Tussin Syrup; Rolatuss W/Hydrocodone; Roni-Tuss Green; Ru-Tuss W/Hydrocodone; Statuss Green; Tri-Phen-Pyrl Hc; Vetuss Hc

Prescribing information not available at time of publication.

HOW SUPPLIED - EQUIVALENTS NOT AVAILABLE:

Liquid - Oral - 10 mg/20 mg/30

480 ml	$14.25	Rolatuss W/Hydrocodone, Major Pharms	00904-1201-16
480 ml	$16.80	Q-Tuss Hc, Qualitest Pharms	00603-1596-58
480 ml	$18.67	BAN-TUSS HC, H N Norton Co.	50732-0607-16
480 ml	$20.00	Tri-Phen-Pyrl Hc, Goldline Labs	00182-0157-40
480 ml	$25.00	STATUSS GREEN, Huckaby Pharma	58407-0372-16
480 ml	$29.50	Vetuss Hc, Cypress Pharm	60258-0767-16
480 ml	$43.20	RU-TUSS WITH HYDROCODONE LIQUID, Knoll Pharms	00048-1007-16
3840 ml	$124.72	BAN-TUSS HC, H N Norton Co.	50732-0607-28

HYDROCODONE BITARTRATE; PHENYLEPHRINE HYDROCHLORIDE; PYRILAMINE MALEATE *(001469)*

CATEGORIES: Allergies; Antihistamines; Antitussives; Antitussives/Expectorants/Mucolytics; Cough Preparations; Decongestants; Hay Fever; Narcotic Analgesics; Respiratory & Allergy Medications; Rhinitis; Pregnancy Category C; DEA Class CIII; FDA Pre 1938 Drugs

BRAND NAMES: **Codimal Dh**; Dicomal-Dh; Hycomal Dh

Prescribing information not available at time of publication.

HOW SUPPLIED - EQUIVALENTS NOT AVAILABLE:

Syrup - Oral - 1.66 mg/5 mg/8.

118 ml	$5.52	Dicomal-Dh, Econolab	55053-0900-04
120 ml	**$84.88**	**CODIMAL DH, Schwarz Pharma (US)**	**00131-5129-64**
473 ml	$17.95	Dicomal-Dh, Econolab	55053-0900-16
480 ml	$18.05	Hycomal Dh, Alphagen Labs	59743-0021-16
480 ml	**$23.86**	**CODIMAL DH, Schwarz Pharma (US)**	**00131-5129-70**
3840 ml	**$160.57**	**CODIMAL DH, Schwarz Pharma (US)**	**00131-5129-72**

HYDROCODONE BITARTRATE; PHENYLPROPANOLAMINE HYDROCHLORIDE *(001470)*

CATEGORIES: Antitussives; Antitussives/Expectorants/Mucolytics; Common Cold; Cough Preparations; Narcotic Analgesics; Nasal Congestion; Respiratory & Allergy Medications; Pregnancy Category C; DEA Class CIII; FDA Approved 1990 Aug

BRAND NAMES: Baycomine; Codamine; **Hycomine**; Hycophen; Hydro-Propanolamine; Hydromine; Hydrophen; Morcomine; Propachem

FORMULARIES: Aetna

DESCRIPTION:

Hydrocodone bitratrate w/phenylpropanolamine HCl contains hydrocodone (dihydrocodeinone) bitartrate, a semisynthetic centrally-acting narcotic antitussive and phenylpropanolamine hydrochloride, a sympathomimetic amine decongestant for oral administration.

The pH of hydrocodone bitartrate syrup and pediatric syrup is 3.2-4.2. The hydrocodone component is (5α)-4,5-epoxy-3-methoxy-17- methylmorphinan-6-one[R-(R*,R*)]-2,3-dihydroxybutanedioate (1:1) hydrate (2:5), a fine white crystal or crystalline powder, which is derived from the opium alkaloid, thebaine, has a molecular weight of (494.50). The phenylpropanolamine component is (±)-(R*,S*)-α-(1-aminoethyl) benzenemethanol hydrochloride and has a molecular weight of (187.67). (TABLE 1):

TABLE 1

	Pediatric Syrup	Adult Syrup
Each Teaspoonful (5 ml) contains		
Hydrocodone Bitartrate, USP	2.5 mg	5 mg
WARNING: May be habit forming		
Phenylpropanolamine HCl, USP	12.5 mg	25 mg

Also hydrocodone bitartrate and phenylpropanolamine HCl, both strengths contain: artificial cherry flavor, glycerin, methylparaben, propylparaben, saccharin, sodium, and sorbitol solution. Hydrocodone bitartrate and phenylpropanolamine HCl Pediatric syrup contains D&C Yellow 10 and FD&C Green 3. Hydrocodone bitartrate w/phenylpropanolamine HCl syrup: FD&C Red 40 and FD&C Yellow 6.

CLINICAL PHARMACOLOGY:

Hydrocodone is a semisynthetic narcotic antitussive and analgesic with multiple actions qualitatively similar to those of codeine. The precise mechanism of action of hydrocodone and other opiates is not known; however, hydrocodone is believed to act directly on the cough center. In excessive doses, hydrocodone, like other opium derivatives, will depress respiration. The effects of hydrocodone in therapeutic doses on the cardiovascular system are insignificant. Hydrocodone can produce miosis, euphoria, physical and physiological dependence.

CLINICAL PHARMACOLOGY: *(cont'd)*

Following a 10 mg oral dose of hydrocodone administered to five adult male subjects, the mean peak concentration was 23.6 ± 5.2 ng/ml. Maximum serum levels were achieved at 1.3 ± 0.3 hours and half-life was determined to be 3.8 ± 0.3 hours. Hydrocodone exhibits a complex pattern of metabolism including O-demethylation, N-demethylation and 6-keto reduction to the corresponding 6-α- and 6-β-hydroxymetabolites. Phenylpropanolamine effects its vasoconstrictor activity by releasing noradrenaline from sympathetic nerve endings, and from direct stimulation of α-adrenoreceptors of blood vessels.

INDICATIONS AND USAGE:

Hydrocodone bitratrate and phenylpropanolamine HCl is indicated for the symptomatic relief of cough and nasal congestion.

CONTRAINDICATIONS:

Hydrocodone bitratrate and phenylpropanolamine HCl is contraindicated in patients hypersensitive to hydrocodone or phenylpropanolamine, and in patients on current MAO inhibitor therapy. Patients known to be hypersensitive to other opioids or sympathomimetic amines may exhibit cross sensitivity to hydrocodone bitratrate and phenylpropanolamine HCl. Phenylpropanolamine is contraindicated in patients with heart disease, hypertension, diabetes or hyperthyroidism. Hydrocodone is contraindicated in the presence of an intracranial lesion associated with increased intracranial pressure; and whenever ventilatory function is depressed.

WARNINGS:

May be habit forming. Hydrocodone can produce drug dependence of the morphine type and, therefore, has the potential for being abused. Psychic dependence, physical dependence and tolerance may develop upon repeated administration of hydrocodone bitratrate and phenylpropanolamine HCl and it should be prescribed and administered with the same degree of caution appropriate to the use of other narcotic drugs (see DRUG ABUSE AND DEPENDENCE.)

Respiratory Depression: Hydrocodone bitratrate and phenylpropanolamine HCl produces dose-related respiratory depression by directly acting on brain stem respiratory centers. If respiratory depression occurs, it may be antagonized by the use of naloxone hydrochloride and other supportive measures when indicated.

Head Injury and Increased Intracranial Pressure: The respiratory depression properties of narcotics and their capacity to elevate cerebrospinal fluid pressure may be markedly exaggerated in the presence of head injury, other intracranial lesions or a preexisting increase in intracranial pressure. Furthermore, narcotics produce adverse reactions which may obscure the clinical course of patients with head injuries.

Acute Abdominal Conditions: The administration of hydrocodone bitratrate and phenylpropanolamine HCl or other narcotics may obscure the diagnosis or clinical course of patients with acute abdominal conditions.

Pediatric Use: In young children, as well as adults, the respiratory center is sensitive to the depressant action of narcotic cough suppressants in a dose-dependent manner. Benefit to risk ratio should be carefully considered especially in children with respiratory embarrassment (*e.g.,* croup).

Phenylpropanolamine: Hypertensive crises can occur with concurrent use of phenylpropanolamine and monoamine oxidase (MAO) inhibitors, indomethacin or with beta-blockers and methyldopa.

If hypertensive crisis occurs, these drugs should be discontinued immediately and therapy to lower blood pressure should be instituted immediately. Fever should be managed by means of external cooling.

PRECAUTIONS:

GENERAL

Before prescribing medication to suppress or modify cough, it is important to ascertain that the underlying case of cough is identified, that modification of cough does not increase the risk of clinical or physiologic complication and that appropriate therapy for the primary disease is provided.

Special Risk Patients: Hydrocodone bitratrate and phenylpropanolamine HCl should be given with caution to certain patients such as the elderly or debilitated, and those with severe impairment of hepatic or renal functions, hypothyroidism, Addison's disease, prostatic hypertrophy or urethral stricture, asthma, narrow-angle glaucoma, and uncontrolled hypertension.

INFORMATION FOR THE PATIENT

Hydrocodone may impair the mental and/or physical abilities required for the performance of potentially hazardous tasks such as driving a car or operating machinery; phenylpropanolamine may produce a rapid pulse, dizziness or palpitations. The patient using hydrocodone bitratrate and phenylpropanolamine HCl should be cautioned accordingly.

CARCINOGENESIS, MUTAGENESIS, AND IMPAIRMENT OF FERTILITY

Carcinogenicity, mutagenicity and reproduction studies have not been conducted with this drug.

PREGNANCY CATEGORY C

Teratogenic Effects: Animal reproduction studies have not been conducted with hydrocodone bitratrate and phenylpropanolamine HCl. It is also not known whether hydrocodone bitratrate and phenylpropanolamine HCl can cause fetal harm when administered to a pregnant woman or can affect reproductive capacity. This drug should be given to a pregnant woman only if clearly needed.

Nonteratogenic Effects: Babies born to mothers who have been taking opioids regularly prior to delivery will be physically dependent. The withdrawal signs include irritability and excessive crying, tremors, hyperactive reflexes, increased respiratory rate, increased stools, sneezing, yawning, vomiting and fever. The intensity of the syndrome does not always correlate with the duration of maternal opioid use or dose.

LABOR AND DELIVERY

As with all narcotics, administration of hydrocodone bitratrate and phenylpropanolamine HCl to the mother shortly before delivery may result in some degree of respiratory depression in the newborn, especially if higher doses are used.

NURSING MOTHERS

It is not known whether this drug is excreted in human milk. Because many drugs are excreted in human milk and because of the potential for serious adverse reactions in nursing infants from hydrocodone bitratrate and phenylpropanolamine HCl, a decision should be made whether to continue nursing or discontinue the drug, taking into account the importance of the drug to the mother.

PEDIATRIC USE

Safety and effectiveness of hydrocodone bitratrate and phenylpropanolamine HCl in children under six have not been established.

DRUG INTERACTIONS:

Patients receiving other narcotic analgesics, general anesthetics, phenothiazines, other tranquilizers, sedative-hypnotics or other CNS depressants (including alcohol) concomitantly with hydrocodone may exhibit an additive CNS depression. When such combined therapy is contemplated, the dose of one or both agents should be reduced. The use of phenylpropanolamine with other sympathomimetic amines and MAO inhibitors may produce an additive elevation of blood pressure (See WARNINGS.)

ADVERSE REACTIONS:

Respiratory System: Hydrocodone produces dose-related respiratory depression by acting directly on brain stem respiratory centers. (see OVERDOSAGE.)

Cardiovascular System: Hypertension, postural hypotension, tachycardia and palpitations.

Genitourinary System: Urethral spasm, spasm of vesical sphincters and urinary retention have been reported with opiates.

Central Nervous System: Sedation, drowsiness, mental clouding, lethargy, impairment of mental and physical performance, anxiety, fear, dysphoria, dizziness, psychic dependance, mood changes and blurred vision.

Gastrointestinal System: Nausea and vomiting occur more frequently in ambulatory than in recumbent patients. Prolonged administration of this drug may produce constipation.

Dermatological: Skin rash, pruritus.

DRUG ABUSE AND DEPENDENCE:

Hydrocodone bitratrate and phenylpropanolamine HCl is a Schedule III narcotic. Psychic dependence, physical dependence, and tolerance may develop upon repeated administration of narcotics; therefore, this drug should be prescribed and administered with caution. However, psychic dependence is unlikely to develop when hydrocodone bitratrate and phenylpropanolamine HCl is used for a short time for the treatment of cough. Physical dependence, the condition in which continued administration of the drug is required to prevent the appearance of a withdrawal syndrome, assumes clinically significant proportions only after several weeks of continued oral narcotic use, although some mild degree of physical dependence may develop after a few days of narcotic therapy.

OVERDOSAGE:

Signs and Symptoms: Serious overdosage with hydrocodone bitratrate and phenylpropanolamine HCl is characterized by respiratory depression (a decrease in respiratory rate and/or tidal volume, Cheyne-Stokes respiration, cyanosis), extreme somnolence progressing to stupor or coma, skeletal muscle flaccidity, cold and clammy skin, and sometimes bradycardia and hypotension. In severe overdosage apnea, circulatory collapse, cardiac arrest, and death may occur.

The signs and symptoms of overdosage of the individual components of this drug may be modified in varying degrees by the presence of other active ingredients. Overdosage with phenylpropanolamine alone may result in tremor, restlessness, increased motor activity, agitation and hallucinations.

Treatment: Primary attention should be given to the reestablishment of adequate respiratory exchange through provision of a patent airway and the institution of assisted or controlled ventilation. The narcotic antagonist naloxone HCl is a specific antidote for respiratory depression which may result from overdosage or unusual sensitivity to narcotics including hydrocodone. Therefore, an appropriate dose of naloxone HCl should be administered preferably by the IV route, simultaneously with efforts at respiratory resuscitation. For further information, see full prescribing information for naloxone HCl. An antagonist should not be administered in the absence of clinically significant respiratory depression. Oxygen, IV fluids, vasopressors, and other supportive measures should be employed as indicated. Gastric emptying may be useful in removing unabsorbed drug.

DOSAGE AND ADMINISTRATION:

Adults: The usual dose for adults is one teaspoonful hydrocodone bitartrate and phenylpropanolamine HCl syrup (hydrocodone bitartrate 5 mg and phenylpropanolamine HCl 25 mg/5 cc) every four hours as needed, not to exceed six teaspoonfuls in a 24–hour period.

Children 6 to 12 years of age: The usual dose for children 6 to 12 years of age is one teaspoonful hydrocodone bitratrate and phenylpropanolamine HCl pediatric syrup (hydrocodone bitartrate 2.5 mg and phenylpropanolamine HCl 12.5 mg/5 cc) every four hours as needed, not to exceed six teaspoonfuls in a 24–hour period.

Store at controlled room temperature (59°-86°F, 15°-30°C).

HOW SUPPLIED - EQUIVALENTS NOT AVAILABLE:

Syrup - Oral - 2.5 mg/12.5 mg

480 ml	$9.13	HYDROPHEN PEDIATRIC, Rugby	00536-0910-85
480 ml	$13.02	CODAMINE PEDIATRIC, Alpharma	00472-0748-16
480 ml	$13.40	CODAMINE PEDIATRIC, Qualitest Drugs	52446-0810-58
480 ml	$15.10	Codamin, Goldline Labs	00182-0069-40
480 ml	**$47.20**	**HYCOMINE PEDIATRIC, Dupont Pharma**	**00056-0247-16**

Syrup - Oral - 5 mg/25 mg

480 ml	$10.44	HYDROPHEN, Rugby	00536-0905-85
480 ml	$12.40	HYPAMINE, Major Pharms	00904-0954-16
480 ml	$13.91	CODAMINE, Alpharma	00472-0749-16
480 ml	$15.00	CODAMINE, Goldline Labs	00182-1153-40
480 ml	$15.44	HYDROCODONE/PHENYLPROPANOLAMINE, Schein Pharm (US)	00364-7255-16
480 ml	**$54.20**	**HYCOMINE, Dupont Pharma**	**00056-0246-16**
3840 ml	$64.93	HYDROPHEN, Rugby	00536-0905-90
3840 ml	$84.33	Codamine, Major Pharms	00904-0954-28

HYDROCODONE; PHENIRAMINE; POTASSIUM CITRATE; PYRILAMINE; VITAMIN C *(001466)*

CATEGORIES: Cough Preparations; Narcotic Analgesics; DEA Class CIII

BRAND NAMES: Citra Forte

Prescribing information not available at time of publication.

HOW SUPPLIED - EQUIVALENTS NOT AVAILABLE:

Syrup - Oral

480 ml	$11.25	CITRA FORTE, Boyle Pharm	00222-0257-16

HYDROCODONE; PHENYLEPHRINE HYDROCHLORIDE *(001471)*

CATEGORIES: Antitussives; Antitussives/Expectorants/Mucolytics; Cough Preparations; Narcotic Analgesics; Respiratory & Allergy Medications; DEA Class CIII; FDA Pre 1938 Drugs

BRAND NAMES: Dicomal Dh; Nalex Dh

Prescribing information not available at time of publication.

HOW SUPPLIED - EQUIVALENTS NOT AVAILABLE:

Syrup - Oral

480 ml	$19.78	Dicomal Dh, HL Moore Drug Exch	00839-7978-69

HYDROCODONE; PSEUDOEPHEDRINE *(001472)*

CATEGORIES: Antiasthmatics/Bronchodilators; Antitussives; Antitussives/Expectorants/Mucolytics; Cough Preparations; DESI Drugs; Narcotic Analgesics; Nasal Congestion; Respiratory & Allergy Medications; DEA Class CIII; DEA Class CV; FDA Pre 1938 Drugs

BRAND NAMES: Detussin; Dihistine Dh; Entuss-D; Hydrophen; Hytussin; Ordrine At; P-V-Tussin; Tussafin; Tussend; Tussgen; Tussogest

Prescribing information not available at time of publication.

HOW SUPPLIED - EQUIVALENTS NOT AVAILABLE:

Capsule, Gelatin, Sustained Action - Oral - 40 mg/75 mg

100's	$16.10	TUSSOGEST, EXTENDED-RELEASE, Major Pharms	00904-0322-60
100's	$48.75	Ordrine At, Eon Labs Mfg	00185-0345-01
500's	$74.25	TUSSOGEST, EXTENDED-RELEASE, Major Pharms	00904-0322-40

Liquid - Oral - 5 mg/60 mg/5ml

480 ml	$9.13	TUSSAFIN, Rugby	00536-0532-85
480 ml	$12.20	DETUSSIN, Qualitest Pharms	00603-1130-58
480 ml	$13.00	DETUSSIN, Major Pharms	00904-0967-16
480 ml	$13.50	Detussin, Consolidated Midland	00223-6134-01
480 ml	$13.65	Detussin, Alpharma	00472-0958-16
480 ml	$14.55	TUSSGEN, Goldline Labs	00182-1163-40
3840 ml	$89.47	Detussin, Consolidated Midland	00223-6134-02

Tablet, Uncoated - Oral

100's	$63.85	P-V-TUSSIN, Solvay Pharms	00032-1091-01

HYDROCORTISONE *(001476)*

CATEGORIES: Adrenal Corticosteroids; Adrenal Hyperplasia; Adrenal Insufficiency; Adrenocortical Insufficiency; Airway Obstruction; Allergic Reactions; Allergies; Anemia; Ankylosing Spondylitis; Anorectal Products; Anterior Pituitary/Hypothalmic Function; Anti-Inflammatory Agents; Antiarthritics; Antiseptics/Disinfectants; Arthritis; Aspiration Pneumonitis; Asthma; Atopic Dermatitis; Bursitis; Cancer; Carditis; Chemotherapy; Chorioretinitis; Choroiditis; Colitis; Conjunctivitis; Corneal Ulcer; Cryptitis; Dermatitis; Dermatitis Herpetiformis; Dermatologicals; Dermatomyositis; Dermatoses; Diuresis; Drug Hypersensitivity; Edema; Enteritis; Epicondylitis; Erythema Multiforme; Erythroblastopenia; Gastrointestinal Drugs; Glucocorticoids; Gouty Arthritis; Herpes; Herpes Zoster; Hormones; Hypercalcemia; Infertility; Inflammation; Iridocyclitis; Keratitis; Leukemia; Lupus Erythematosus; Lymphoma; Meningitis; Mucous Membrane Agents; Mycosis Fungoides; Nephrotic Syndrome; Osteoarthritis; Pain; Pemphigus; Pharmaceutical Adjuvants; Pneumoconiosis; Pneumonitis; Proteinuria; Pruritus; Psoriasis; Purpura; Retinochoroiditis; Rhinitis; Sarcoidosis; Serum Sickness; Skin/Mucous Membrane Agents; Spondylitis; Steroids; Synovitis; Synovitis of Osteoarthritis; Tenosynovitis; Thrombocytopenia; Thrombocytopenic Purpura; Thyroiditis; Topical; Trichinosis; Tuberculosis; Ulcerative Colitis; Uveitis; Pregnancy Category C; FDA Approval Pre 1982

BRAND NAMES: Acticort; Aeroseb-Hc; Ala-Cort; Ala-Scalp; *Algicortis*; Albacort; Allercort; Alphaderm; Anusol-Hc; Balneol-Hc; Beta-Hc; Cetacort; Coracin; *Coreton*; Cort-Dome; *Cortate* (Canada); Cortef; Cortenema; *Cortes*; *Cortesal*; *Corticrem*; Cortril; Cotacort; *Covocort*; *Cremicort-H*; *Cutaderm*; *Daniel Hydrocortisone*; *Dermocortal*; *Derm-Aid*; *Derm-Aid Cream* (Australia); Dermacort; Dermol Hc; *Dioderm* (England); *Eczacort*; *Efcortelan*; *Egocort Cream* (Australia); Eldecort; *Emo-Cort* (Canada); Epicort; *Ficortril* (Germany); *Filocot*; Flexicort; Glycort; H-Cort; Hi-Cor; *Hidroaltesona*; Hidromar; *Hidrotisona*; *Hycor*; Hycort; Hycortole; Hydro-Tex; *Hydrocortemel*; *Hydrocortison* (Germany); *Hydrocortisone* (France); *Hydrocortisone Astier* (France); *Hydrocortisonum*; *Hydrocortistab* (England); *Hydrocortisyl* (England); Hydrocortone; *Hydroderm* (Germany); *Hydrokort*; *Hydrokortison*; *Hydrotopic*; Hymac; *Hysone*; *Hytisone*; Hytone; IVocort; *Kyypakkaus*; Lacticare; *Lacticare HC* (Mexico); Lemoderm; *Lenirit*; Lidex; *Mildison*; *Mildison-Fatty*; *Mildison Lipocream* (England); Nogenic Hc; **Nutracort**; *Otozonbase*; Penecort; Procto-Hc; Proctocort; *Procutan*; Rederm; S-T Cort; *Sanatison* (Germany); *Schericur*; *Schericur 0.25%*; *Skincalm*; Stie-Cort; Synacort; Tega-Cort; Texacort; Topisone; *Unicort* (Canada); *Uniderm*

(International brand names outside U.S. in italics)

FORMULARIES: Aetna; BC-BS; CIGNA; DoD; FHP; Humana; Kaiser; Medco; Medi-Cal; PCS; PruCare; United; WHO

COST OF THERAPY: $29.20 (Asthma; Tablet; 20 mg; 1/day; 365 days)

PRIMARY ICD9: 493.90 (Asthma, Unspecified, Without Mention of Status Asthmaticus)

DESCRIPTION:

ORAL TABLETS

Glucocorticoids are adrenocortical steroids, both naturally occurring and synthetic, which are readily absorbed from the gastrointestinal tract. Hydrocortisone USP is a white to practically white, odorless, crystalline powder with a melting point of about 215°. It is very slightly soluble in water and ether; sparingly soluble in acetone and in alcohol; slightly soluble in chloroform.

The chemical name for hydrocortisone is pregn-4-ene-3, 20-dione, 11,17,21-trihydroxy-,(11β). Its molecular weight is 362.

DESCRIPTION: *(cont'd)*

Hydrocortisone tablets are available for oral administration in three strengths: each tablet contains either 5 mg, 10 mg, or 20 mg of hydrocortisone.

TOPICAL CREAM

The topical corticosteroids constitute a class of primarily synthetic steroids used as anti-inflammatory and antipruritic agents. Hydrocortisone cream, 2.5% is a topical corticosteroid with hydrocortisone 2.5% (active ingredient) in a water-washable cream containing the following inactive ingredients: benzyl alcohol, petrolatum, stearyl alcohol, propylene glycol, isopropyl myristate, polyoxyl 40 stearate, carbomer 934, sodium lauryl sulfate, edetate disodium, sodium hydroxide to adjust the pH and purified water.

CLINICAL PHARMACOLOGY:

ORAL TABLETS

Naturally occurring glucocorticoids (hydrocortisone and cortisone), which also have salt-retaining properties, are used as replacement therapy in adrenocortical deficiency states. Their synthetic analogs are primarily used for their potent anti-inflammatory effects in disorders of many organ systems.

Glucocorticoids cause profound and varied metabolic effects. In addition, they modify the body's immune responses to diverse stimuli.

TOPICAL CREAM

Topical corticosteroids share antiinflammatory, antipruritic and vasoconstrictive actions.

The mechanism of antiinflammatory activity of the topical corticosteroids is unclear. Various laboratory methods, including vasoconstrictor assays, are used to compare and predict potencies and/or clinical efficacies of the topical corticosteroids. There is some evidence to suggest that a recognizable correlation exists between vasoconstrictor potency and therapeutic efficacy

Pharmacokinetics: The extent of percutaneous absorption of topical corticosteroids is determined by many factors including the vehicle, the integrity of the epidermal barrier, and the use of occlusive dressings.

Topical corticosteroids can be absorbed from normal intact skin. Inflammation and/or other disease processes in the skin increase percutaneous absorption. Occlusive dressings substantially increase the percutaneous absorption of topical corticosteroids. Thus, occlusive dressings may be a valuable therapeutic adjunct for treatment of resistant dermatoses (See DOSAGE AND ADMINISTRATION.)

Once absorbed through the skin, topical corticosteroids are handled through pharmacokinetic pathways similar to systemically administered corticosteroids. Corticosteroids are bound to plasma proteins in varying degrees. Corticosteroids are metabolized primarily in the liver and are then excreted by the kidneys. Some of the topical corticosteroids and their metabolites are also excreted into the bile.

INDICATIONS AND USAGE:

ORAL TABLETS

Hydrocortisone tablets are indicated in the following conditions:

1. Endocrine Disorders: Primary or secondary adrenocortical insufficiency (hydrocortisone or cortisone is the first choice; synthetic analogs may used in conjunction with mineralocorticoids where applicable; in infancy mineralocorticoid supplementation is of particular importance). Congenital adrenal hyperplasia, Hypercalcemia associated with cancer, Nonsuppurative thyroiditis.

2. Rheumatic Disorders: As adjunctive therapy for short-term administration (to tide the patient over an acute episode or exacerbation) in: psoriatic arthritis, rheumatoid arthritis, including juvenile rheumatoid arthritis (selected cases may require low-dose maintenance therapy), ankylosing spondylitis, acute and subacute bursitis, acute nonspecific tenosynovitis, acute gouty arthritis, post-traumatic osteoarthritis, synovitis of osteoarthritis, epicondylitis.

3. Collagen Diseases: During an exacerbation or as maintenance therapy in selected cases of: systemic lupus erythematosus, systemic dermatomyositis (polymyositis), acute rheumatic carditis.

4. Dermatologic Diseases: Pemphigus, bullous dermatitis herpetiformis, severe erythema multiforme (Stevens-Johnson syndrome), exfoliative dermatitis, mycosis fungoides, severe psoriasis, severe seborrheic dermatitis.

5. Allergic States: Control of severe or incapacitating allergic conditions intractable to adequate trials of conventional treatment:, seasonal or perennial allergic rhinitis, serum sickness, bronchial asthma, contact dermatitis, atopic dermatitis, drug hypersensitivity reactions.

6. Ophthalmic Diseases: Severe acute and chronic allergic and inflammatory processes involving the eye and its adnexa such as: allergic conjunctivitis, keratitis, allergic corneal marginal ulcers, herpes zoster ophthalmicus, iritis and iridocyclitis, chorioretinitis, anterior segment inflammation, diffuse posterior uveitis and choroiditis, optic neuritis, sympathetic ophthalmia.

7. Respiratory Diseases: Symptomatic sarcoidosis, Loeffler's syndrome not manageable by other means, berylliosis, fulminating or disseminated pulmonary tuberculosis when used concurrently with appropriate antituberculous chemotherapy, Aspiration pneumonitis.

8. Hematologic Disorders: Idiopathic thrombocytopenic purpura in adults, secondary thrombocytopenia in adults, acquired (autoimmune) hemolytic anemia erythroblastopenia (rbc anemia), congenital (erythroid) hypoplastic anemia.

9. Neoplastic Diseases: For palliative management of: leukemias and lymphomas in adults, acute leukemia of childhood.

10. Edematous States: To induce a diuresis or remission of proteinuria in the nephrotic syndrome, without uremia, of the idiopathic type or that due to lupus erythematosus.

11. Gastrointestinal Diseases: To tide that patient over a critical period of the disease in: ulcerative colitis, regional enteritis.

12. Miscellaneous: Tuberculous meningitis with subarachnoid block or impending block when used concurrently with appropriate antituberculous chemotherapy, trichinosis with neurologic or myocardial involvement.

TOPICAL CREAM

Topical corticosteroids are indicated for the relief of the inflammatory and pruritic manifestations of corticosteroid-responsive dermatoses.

CONTRAINDICATIONS:

Oral Tablets: Systemic fungal infections.

Topical Cream: Topical corticosteroids are contraindicated in those patients with a history of hypersensitivity to any of the components of the preparation.

WARNINGS:

In patients on corticosteroid therapy subjected to unusual stress, increased dosage of rapidly acting corticosteroids before, during, and after the stressful situation of indicated.

WARNINGS: *(cont'd)*

Corticosteroids may mask some signs of infection and new infections may appear during their use. There may be decreased resistance and inability to localize infection when corticosteroids are used.

Prolonged use of corticosteroids may produce posterior subcapsular cataracts, glaucoma with possible damage to the optic nerves, and may enhance the establishment of secondary ocular infections due to fungi or viruses.

Usage In Pregnancy: Since adequate human reproduction studies have not been done with corticosteroids, the use of these drugs in pregnancy, nursing mothers or women of childbearing potential requires that the possible benefits of the drug be weighed against the potential hazards to the mother and embryo or fetus. Infants born of mothers who have received substantial doses of corticosteroids during pregnancy should be carefully observed for signs of hypoadrenalism.

Average and large doses of hydrocortisone or cortisone can cause elevation of blood pressure, salt and water retention, and increased excretion of potassium. These effects are less likely to occur with the synthetic derivatives except when used in large doses. Dietary salt restriction and potassium supplementation may be necessary. All corticosteroids increase calcium excretion.

While on corticosteroid therapy patients should not be vaccinated against smallpox. Other immunization procedures should not be undertaken in patients who are on corticosteroids, especially on high dose, because of possible hazards of neurological complications and a lack of antibody response.

The use of Hydrocortisone in active tuberculosis should be restricted to those cases of fulminating or disseminated tuberculosis in which the corticosteroid is used for the management of the disease in conjunction with an appropriate antituberculous regimen.

If corticosteroids are indicated in patients with latent tuberculosis or tuberculin reactivity, close observation in necessary as reactivation of the disease may occur. During prolonged corticosteroid therapy, these patients should receive chemoprophylaxis.

PRECAUTIONS:

ORAL TABLETS

Drug-induced secondary adrenocortical insufficiency may be minimized by gradual reduction of dosage. This type of relative insufficiency may persist for months after discontinuation of therapy; therefore, in any situation of stress occurring during at period; hormone therapy should be reinstituted. Since mineralocorticoid secretion may be impaired, salt and/or a mineralocorticoid should be administered concurrently.

There is an enhanced effect of corticosteroids on patients with hypothyroidism and in those with cirrhosis.

Corticosteroids should be used cautiously in patients with ocular herpes simplex because of possible corneal perforation.

The lowest possible dose of corticosteroid should be used to control the condition under treatment, and when reduction in dosage is possible, the reduction should be gradual.

Psychic derangements may appear when corticosteroids are used, ranging from euphoria, insomnia, mood swings, personality changes, are severe depression, to frank psychotic manifestations. Also, existing emotional instability or psychotic tendencies may be aggravated by corticosteroids.

Aspirin should be used cautiously in conjunction with corticosteroids in hypoprothrombinemia.

Steroids should be used with caution in nonspecific ulcerative colitis, if there is a probability of impending perforation, abscess or other pyogenic infection; diverticulitis; fresh intestinal anastomoses; active or latent peptic ulcer; renal insufficiency; hypertension; osteoporosis; and myasthenia gravis.

Growth and development of infants and children on prolonged corticosteroid therapy should be carefully observed.

TOPICAL CREAM

General: Systemic absorption of topical corticosteroids has produced reversible hypothalamic-pituitary-adrenal (HPA) axis-suppression, manifestations of Cushing's syndrome, hyperglycemia, and glucosuria in some patients.

Conditions which augment systemic absorption include the application of the more potent steroids, use over large surface areas, prolonged used, and the addition of occlusive dressings.

If HPA axis suppression is noted (by using the urinary free cortisol and ACTH stimulation tests) an attempt should be made to withdraw the drug or to reduce the frequency of application.

Recovery of HPA axis suppression is noted (by using the urinary free cortisol and ACTH stimulation tests) an attempt should be made to withdraw the drug or reduce the frequency of application.

Recovery of HPA axis function is generally prompt and complete upon discontinuation of the drug. Infrequently, signs and symptoms of steroid withdrawal may occur, requiring supplemental systemic corticosteroids.

Children may absorb proportionally larger amounts of topical corticosteroids and thus be more susceptible to systemic toxicity (See PRECAUTIONS, Pediatric Use).

If irritation develops, topical corticosteroids should be discontinued and appropriate therapy instituted. In the presence of dermatological infections, the use of an appropriate antifungal or antibacterial agent should be instituted. If a favorable response does not occur promptly, the corticosteroid should be discontinued until the infection had been adequately controlled.

Information for the Patient: Patients using topical corticosteroids should receive the following information and instructions:

1. This medication is to be used as directed by the physician. It is for external use only. Avoid contact with the eyes.

2. Patients should be advised not to use this medication for any disorder other than that for which it had been prescribed.

3. The treated skin area should not be bandaged or otherwise covered or wrapped as to be occlusive unless directed by the physician.

4. Patients should report any signs of local adverse reactions especially under occlusive dressing.

5. Parents of pediatric patients should be advised not to use tight-fitting diapers or plastic pants on a child being treated in the diaper area, as these garments may constitute occlusive dressings.

Laboratory Tests: The urinary free cortisol test and the ACTH stimulation test may be helpful in evaluating the HPA axis suppression.

Carcinogenesis, Mutagenesis, and Impairment of Fertility: Long-term animal studies have not been performed to evaluate the carcinogenic potential or the effect on fertility of topical corticosteroids. Studies to determine mutagenicity with hydrocortisone have revealed negative results.

PRECAUTIONS: *(cont'd)*

Pregnancy Category C: Corticosteroids are generally teratogenic in laboratory animals when administered systemically at relatively low dosage levels. The more potent corticosteroids have been shown to be teratogenic after dermal application in laboratory animals. There are no adequate and well-controlled studies in pregnant women of teratogenic effects from topically applied corticosteroids.

Therefore, topical corticosteroids should be used during pregnancy only if the potential benefit justifies the potential risk to the fetus. Drugs of this class should not be used extensively on pregnant patients, in large amounts, or for prolonged periods of time.

Nursing Mothers: It is not known whether topical administration of corticosteroids could result in sufficient systemic absorption to produce detectable quantities in breast milk. Systemically administered corticosteroids are secreted into breast milk in quantities not likely to have a deleterious effect on the infant. Nevertheless, caution should be exercised when topical corticosteroids are administered to a nursing woman.

Pediatric Use: PEDIATRIC PATIENTS MAY DEMONSTRATE GREATER SUSCEPTIBILITY TO TOPICAL CORTICOSTEROID-INDUCED HPA AXIS SUPPRESSION AND CUSHING'S SYNDROME THAN MATURE PATIENTS BECAUSE OF A LARGER SKIN SURFACE AREA TO BODY WEIGHT RATIO.

Hypothalamic-pituitary-adrenal (HPA) axis suppression, Cushing's syndrome, and intracranial hypertension have been reported in children receiving topical corticosteroids. Manifestations of adrenal suppression in children include linear growth retardation, delayed weight gain, low plasma cortisol levels, and absence of response ACTH stimulation. Manifestations of intracranial hypertension include bulging fontanelles, headaches, and bilateral papilledema.

Administration of topical corticosteroids to children should be limited to the least amount compatible with an effective therapeutic regimen. Chronic corticosteroid therapy may interfere with the growth and development of children.

ADVERSE REACTIONS:

ORAL TABLETS

Fluid and Electrolyte Disturbances: Sodium retention, fluid retention, congestive heart failure in susceptible patients, potassium loss, hypokalemic alkalosis, hypertension

Musculoskeletal: Muscle weakness, steroid myopathy, loss of muscle mass, osteoporosis, vertebral compression fractures, aseptic necrosis of femoral and humeral heads, pathologic fracture of long bones.

Gastrointestinal: Peptic ulcer with possible perforation and hemorrhage, pancreatitis, abdominal distention, ulcerative esophagitis.

Dermatologic: Impaired wound healing, thin fragile skin, petechiae and ecchymoses, facial erythema, increased sweating, may suppress reactions to skin tests.

Neurological: Increased intracranial pressure with papilledema (pseudotumor cerebri) usually after treatment, convulsions, vertigo, headache.

Endocrine: Development of cushingoid state, suppression of growth in children, secondary adrenocortical and pituitary unresponsiveness, particularly in times of stress, as in trauma, surgery or illness, menstrual irregularities, decreased carbohydrate tolerance, manifestations of latent diabetes mellitus, increased requirements for insulin or oral hypoglycemic agents in diabetics.

Ophthalmic: Posterior subcapsular cataracts, increased intraocular pressure, glaucoma, exophthalmos.

Metabolic: Negative nitrogen balance due to protein catabolism.

TOPICAL CREAM

The following adverse reactions are reported infrequently with topical corticosteroids, but may occur more frequently with the use of occlusive dressings. These reactions are listed in an approximate decreasing order of occurrence: burning, itching, irritation, dryness, folliculitis, hypertrichosis, acneiform eruptions, hypopigmentation, perioral dermatitis, allergic contact dermatitis, maceration of the skin, secondary infection, skin atrophy, striae, miliaria.

DOSAGE AND ADMINISTRATION:

ORAL TABLETS

The initial dosage of Hydrocortisone may vary from 20 mg to 240 mg per day depending on the specific disease entity being treated. In situations of less severity lower doses will generally suffice while in selected patients higher initial doses may be required. The initial dosage should be maintained or adjusted until a satisfactory response is noted. If after a reasonable period of time there is a lack of satisfactory clinical response, Hydrocortisone should be discontinued and the patient transferred to other appropriate therapy. **IT SHOULD BE EMPHASIZED THAT DOSAGE REQUIREMENTS ARE VARIABLE AND MUST BE INDIVIDUALIZED ON THE BASIS OF THE DISEASE UNDER TREATMENT AND THE RESPONSE OF THE PATIENT.** After a favorable response is noted, the proper maintenance dosage should be determined by decreasing the initial drug dosage in small decrements at appropriate time intervals until the lowest dosage which will maintain an adequate clinical response is reached. It should be kept in mind that constant monitoring is needed in regard to drug dosage. Included in the situations which may make dosage adjustments necessary are changes in clinical status secondary to remissions or exacerbations in the disease process, the patient's individual drug responsiveness, and the effect of patient exposure to stressful situations not directly related to the disease entity under treatment; in this latter situation it may be necessary to increase the dosage of Hydrocortisone for a period of time consistent with the patient's condition. If after long-term therapy the drug is to be stopped, it is recommended that it be withdrawn gradually, rather than abruptly.

TOPICAL CREAM

2.5% hydrocortisone cream should be applied to the affected area two to four times daily depending on the severity of the condition.

Occlusive dressings may be used for the management of psoriasis or recalcitrant conditions. If an infection develops, the use of occlusive dressings should be discontinued and appropriate antimicrobial therapy instituted.

Store hydrocortisone cream at controlled room temperature 15-30°C (59-86°F). Store away from heat. Protect from freezing.

HOW SUPPLIED - RATED THERAPEUTICALLY EQUIVALENT:

Cream - Rectal - 1 %

30 gm	$14.98	PROCTO-HC, Am Generics	58634-0024-01

Cream - Rectal - 2.5 %

30 gm	$4.65	Hydrocortisone, H.C.F.A. F F P	99999-1476-01
30 gm	$14.15	PROCTOSOL-HC, Am Generics	58634-0025-01

Cream - Rectal; Topical - 2.5 %/1 %

15 gm	$1.59	Hydrocortisone, H.C.F.A. F F P	99999-1476-03
15 gm	$1.80	Hydrocortisone, H.C.F.A. F F P	99999-1476-02
28.35 gm	$3.01	Hydrocortisone, H.C.F.A. F F P	99999-1476-05
28.4 gm	$5.85	Hydrocortisone, H.C.F.A. F F P	99999-1476-04
30 gm	$3.18	Hydrocortisone, H.C.F.A. F F P	99999-1476-08
30 gm	$3.60	Hydrocortisone, H.C.F.A. F F P	99999-1476-07

HOW SUPPLIED - RATED THERAPEUTICALLY EQUIVALENT: *(cont'd)*

30 gm	$6.19	Hydrocortisone, H.C.F.A. F F P	99999-1476-06
60 gm	$12.37	Hydrocortisone, H.C.F.A. F F P	99999-1476-09
90 gm	$10.80	Hydrocortisone, H.C.F.A. F F P	99999-1476-10
454 gm	$93.66	Hydrocortisone, H.C.F.A. F F P	99999-1476-11

Cream - Topical - 0.5 %

1 gm	$0.03	Hydrocortisone, H.C.F.A. F F P	99999-1476-12
2 gm	$0.05	Hydrocortisone, H.C.F.A. F F P	99999-1476-13
15 gm	$1.50	Hydrocortisone, Consolidated Midland	00223-4162-12
15 gm	$1.71	Hydrocortisone, H.C.F.A. F F P	99999-1476-14
22.5 gm	$2.56	Hydrocortisone, H.C.F.A. F F P	99999-1476-15
30 gm	$1.20	Hydrocortisone, H.C.F.A. F F P	99999-1476-16
30 gm	$1.90	Hydrocortisone, Consolidated Midland	00223-4162-30
30 gm	$1.95	Hydrocortisone, Geneva Pharms	00781-7017-24
30 gm	$2.32	Hydrocortisone, Rugby	00536-8310-95
30 gm	$12.31	CORT-DOME, Bayer	00026-1631-81
45 gm	$5.13	Hydrocortisone, H.C.F.A. F F P	99999-1476-17
60 gm	$6.84	Hydrocortisone, H.C.F.A. F F P	99999-1476-18
120 gm	$4.86	Hydrocortisone, H.C.F.A. F F P	99999-1476-19
120 gm	$5.85	Hydrocortisone, Rugby	00536-8310-97
120 gm	$6.50	Hydrocortisone, Consolidated Midland	00223-4162-11
425 gm	$16.45	Hydrocortisone, H.C.F.A. F F P	99999-1476-20
454 gm	$13.30	Hydrocortisone, H.C.F.A. F F P	99999-1476-21
454 gm	$14.17	Hydrocortisone, Rugby	00536-8310-98
480 gm	$18.58	Hydrocortisone, H.C.F.A. F F P	99999-1476-22
15890 gm	$643.54	Hydrocortisone, H.C.F.A. F F P	99999-1476-23

Cream - Topical - 1 %

1 oz	$2.36	Hydrocortisone, NMC Labs	23317-0321-28
5 gm	$1.40	Hydrocortisone, Consolidated Midland	00223-4124-05
15 gm	$1.80	Hydrocortisone, H.C.F.A. F F P	99999-1476-25
15 gm	$2.00	Hydrocortisone, Consolidated Midland	00223-4124-15
20 gm	$1.64	Hydrocortisone, Clay Park Labs	45802-0003-02
20 gm	$1.90	Hydrocortisone, Thames Pharma	49158-0101-07
20 gm	$1.95	Hydrocortisone, Harber Pharm	51432-0724-32
20 gm	$2.15	Hydrocortisone, HL Moore Drug Exch	00839-5207-45
20 gm	$2.25	Hydrocortisone, C O Truxton	00463-8045-20
20 gm	$2.40	Hydrocortisone, Consolidated Midland	00223-4124-20
20 gm	$2.40	Hydrocortisone, H.C.F.A. F F P	99999-1476-26
20 gm	$2.90	Hydrocortisone, Rugby	00536-0501-99
27 gm	$1.74	Hydrocortisone, H.C.F.A. F F P	99999-1476-27
28 gm	$2.06	Hydrocortisone, Clay Park Labs	45802-0278-03
28 gm	$3.36	Hydrocortisone, H.C.F.A. F F P	99999-1476-28
28.35 gm	$3.40	Hydrocortisone, H.C.F.A. F F P	99999-1476-30
28.4 gm	$3.41	Hydrocortisone, H.C.F.A. F F P	99999-1476-29
30 gm	$1.93	Hydrocortisone, H.C.F.A. F F P	99999-1476-24
30 gm	$2.00	HYCORT, Everett Labs	00642-0071-01
30 gm	$2.00	Hydrocortisone, Thames Pharma	49158-0101-08
30 gm	$2.05	Hydrocortisone, Clay Park Labs	45802-0003-03
30 gm	$2.27	Hydrocortisone, Harber Pharm	51432-0724-33
30 gm	$2.30	Hydrocortisone, Qualitest Pharms	00603-7780-78
30 gm	$2.42	Hydrocortisone, HL Moore Drug Exch	00839-5207-49
30 gm	$2.50	Hydrocortisone, Consolidated Midland	00223-4124-30
30 gm	$2.60	Hydrocortisone, Schein Pharm (US)	00364-7087-56
30 gm	$2.85	Hydrocortisone, Rugby	00536-5108-95
30 gm	$2.95	Hydrocortisone, Major Pharms	00904-0749-31
30 gm	$2.97	Hydrocortisone, Rugby	00536-0501-95
30 gm	$3.10	Hydrocortisone, Fougera	00168-0015-31
30 gm	$3.95	NOGENIC HC, Syosset Labs	47854-0660-05
30 gm	$4.69	ALA CORT, Del Ray Lab	00316-0126-01
30 gm	$5.95	HYDROTEX, Syosset Labs	47854-0567-05
30 gm	$7.11	PENECORT, Allergan	00023-0510-30
30 gm	**$7.13**	**NUTRACORT, Galderma**	**00299-5821-30**
30 gm	$8.00	ALBACORT, Alba Pharma	10023-0116-30
30 gm	$15.84	ANUSOL-HC, Parke-Davis	00071-3124-13
30 gm	$20.25	PROCTOCORT, Solvay Pharms	00032-1920-61
30 gm	$29.90	Hydrocortisone, Geneva Pharms	00781-7018-24
45 gm	$5.40	Hydrocortisone, H.C.F.A. F F P	99999-1476-31
60 gm	$7.20	Hydrocortisone, H.C.F.A. F F P	99999-1476-32
90 gm	$8.19	ALA CORT, Del Ray Lab	00316-0126-03
120 gm	$7.13	Hydrocortisone, HL Moore Drug Exch	00839-5207-53
120 gm	$7.20	Hydrocortisone, Rugby	00536-5108-97
120 gm	$7.45	Hydrocortisone, Clay Park Labs	45802-0278-04
120 gm	$7.50	Hydrocortisone, Thames Pharma	49158-0101-12
120 gm	$8.75	Hydrocortisone, Consolidated Midland	00223-4124-11
120 gm	$11.39	Hydrocortisone, Rugby	00536-0501-97
120 gm	$14.40	Hydrocortisone, H.C.F.A. F F P	99999-1476-33
425 gm	$25.50	Hydrocortisone, H.C.F.A. F F P	99999-1476-35
454 gm	$14.95	HYDROTEX, Syosset Labs	47854-0567-13
454 gm	$21.60	Hydrocortisone, Clay Park Labs	45802-0003-05
454 gm	$21.60	Hydrocortisone, Clay Park Labs	45802-0278-05
454 gm	$21.60	Hydrocortisone, Thames Pharma	49158-0101-16
454 gm	$24.35	Hydrocortisone, Major Pharms	00904-0749-27
454 gm	$25.95	DERMACORT, Solvay Pharms	00032-6002-68
454 gm	$27.50	Hydrocortisone, Geneva Pharms	00781-7018-16
454 gm	$27.52	Hydrocortisone, HL Moore Drug Exch	00839-5207-60
454 gm	$27.52	Hydrocortisone, NMC Labs	23317-0321-16
454 gm	$28.95	Hydrocortisone, Fougera	00168-0015-16
454 gm	$32.67	Hydrocortisone, Rugby	00536-0501-98
454 gm	$54.48	Hydrocortisone, H.C.F.A. F F P	99999-1476-34

Cream - Topical - 2.5 %

5 gm	$2.25	Hydrocortisone, Consolidated Midland	00223-4159-05
20 gm	$3.71	Hydrocortisone, HL Moore Drug Exch	00839-6376-45
20 gm	$3.80	Hydrocortisone, Thames Pharma	49158-0200-07
20 gm	$4.00	Hydrocortisone, Harber Pharm	51432-0726-32
20 gm	$4.10	Hydrocortisone, Clay Park Labs	45802-0004-02
20 gm	$4.12	Hydrocortisone, United Res	00677-0718-38
20 gm	$4.12	Hydrocortisone, H.C.F.A. F F P	99999-1476-36
20 gm	$4.65	Hydrocortisone, Major Pharms	00904-0756-29
20 gm	$4.70	Hydrocortisone 2.5%, NMC Labs	23317-0322-20
20 gm	$4.75	Hydrocortisone, Consolidated Midland	00223-4159-20
20 gm	$5.45	Hydrocortisone, Goldline Labs	00182-5005-48
20 gm	$5.49	Hydrocortisone, Geneva Pharms	00781-7011-22
20 gm	$5.88	Hydrocortisone, Rugby	00536-0611-99
28.35 gm	$5.85	Hydrocortisone, H.C.F.A. F F P	99999-1476-39
28.4 gm	$5.86	Hydrocortisone, H.C.F.A. F F P	99999-1476-38
30 gm	$4.65	Hydrocortisone, H.C.F.A. F F P	99999-1476-37
30 gm	$5.25	Hydrocortisone, Schein Pharm (US)	00364-2446-56
30 gm	$5.80	Hydrocortisone, Thames Pharma	49158-0200-08
30 gm	$5.85	Hydrocortisone, Qualitest Pharms	00603-7781-78
30 gm	$5.94	Hydrocortisone, Clay Park Labs	45802-0004-03
30 gm	$6.24	Hydrocortisone, NMC Labs	23317-0322-30
30 gm	$6.75	Hydrocortisone, Major Pharms	00904-0756-31

HOW SUPPLIED - RATED THERAPEUTICALLY EQUIVALENT:
(cont'd)

30 gm	$6.85	Hydrocortisone, Harber Pharm	51432-0726-11
30 gm	$7.02	Hydrocortisone, Clay Park Labs	45802-0287-03
30 gm	$8.10	Hydrocortisone, Geneva Pharms	00781-7011-24
30 gm	$8.22	Hydrocortisone, HL Moore Drug Exch	00839-6376-49
30 gm	$8.38	Hydrocortisone, Fougera	00168-0080-31
30 gm	$10.32	Hydrocortisone, Rugby	00536-0611-95
30 gm	$12.06	PENECORT, Allergan	00023-0550-30
30 gm	$18.27	HYTONE, Dermik Labs	00066-0095-01
30 gm	$21.68	ANUSOL-HC 2.5%, Parke-Davis	00071-3131-13
60 gm	$12.38	Hydrocortisone, H.C.F.A. F F P	99999-1476-40
60 gm	$29.21	HYTONE, Dermik Labs	00066-0095-02
454 gm	$56.70	Hydrocortisone, Thames Pharma	49158-0200-16
454 gm	$58.32	Hydrocortisone, Clay Park Labs	45802-0004-05
454 gm	$68.24	Hydrocortisone 2.5%, NMC Labs	23317-0322-16
454 gm	$85.03	Hydrocortisone, H.C.F.A. F F P	99999-1476-41

Lotion - Topical - 0.5 %

30 ml	$1.19	Hydrocortisone, H.C.F.A. F F P	99999-1476-44
60 ml	$2.38	Hydrocortisone, H.C.F.A. F F P	99999-1476-42
60 ml	$3.75	Hydrocortisone, Consolidated Midland	00223-4163-60
60 ml	$15.62	CETACORT 0.5%, Galderma	00299-3948-02
120 ml	$4.80	Hydrocortisone, H.C.F.A. F F P	99999-1476-43
120 ml	$5.00	COTACORT, C O Truxton	00463-8010-04
120 ml	$6.62	S-T CORT, Scot Tussin	00372-0011-04
120 ml	$7.75	Hydrocortisone, Consolidated Midland	00223-4163-11

Lotion - Topical - 1 %

4 oz	$14.21	HYDRO LOT, Glades Pharms	59366-2707-04
30 ml	$22.65	CORT-DOME, Bayer	00026-1642-81
60 ml	$4.35	Hydrocortisone, H.C.F.A. F F P	99999-1476-46
60 ml	$5.40	Hydrocortisone, Clay Park Labs	45802-0283-46
60 ml	$6.80	GLY-CORT, Heran Pharm	50434-0003-02
60 ml	**$15.50**	**NUTRACORT, Galderma**	**00299-5830-01**
60 ml	$17.81	CETACORT 1%, Galderma	00299-3949-02
75 ml	$5.15	Hydrocortisone, H.C.F.A. F F P	99999-1476-47
118 ml	$8.11	Hydrocortisone, H.C.F.A. F F P	99999-1476-48
120 ml	$6.07	Hydrocortisone, H.C.F.A. F F P	99999-1476-45
120 ml	$7.30	Hydrocortisone, Thames Pharma	49158-0203-12
120 ml	$7.98	Hydrocortisone, Balan	00304-0816-74
120 ml	$8.09	Hydrocortisone, Rugby	00536-5105-97
120 ml	$8.10	Hydrocortisone, Clay Park Labs	45802-0023-06
120 ml	$8.10	Hydrocortisone, Clay Park Labs	45802-0283-06
120 ml	$8.22	Hydrocortisone, HL Moore Drug Exch	00839-6233-53
120 ml	$8.25	Hydrocortisone, Geneva Pharms	00781-7071-04
120 ml	$8.75	Hydrocortisone, Qualitest Pharms	00603-7784-54
120 ml	$9.31	DERMACORT, Solvay Pharms	00032-6008-74
120 ml	$11.18	ALA CORT, Del Ray Lab	00316-0131-04
120 ml	$14.24	Hydrocortisone, Qualitest Pharms	00603-7783-54
120 ml	$15.00	LACTICARE HC, Stiefel Labs	00145-2537-04
120 ml	**$23.12**	**NUTRACORT, Galderma**	**00299-5830-02**

Lotion - Topical - 2.5 %

60 ml	$13.95	Hydrocortisone, Harber Pharm	51432-0479-17
60 ml	$15.69	Hydrocortisone, Qualitest Pharms	00603-7785-52
60 ml	$16.49	Hydrocortisone, Glades Pharms	59366-2708-02
60 ml	$17.25	Hydrocortisone, H.C.F.A. F F P	99999-1476-49
60 ml	$17.39	LACTICARE HC, Stiefel Labs	00145-2538-02
60 ml	**$19.69**	**NUTRACORT, Galderma**	**00299-5825-01**
60 ml	$27.26	HYTONE, Dermik Labs	00066-0098-02
120 ml	**$30.75**	**NUTRACORT, Galderma**	**00299-5825-02**
120 ml	$34.50	Hydrocortisone, H.C.F.A. F F P	99999-1476-50

Ointment - Topical - 1 %

15 gm	$0.77	Hydrocortisone, H.C.F.A. F F P	99999-1476-51
15 gm	$1.95	Hydrocortisone, Consolidated Midland	00223-4161-15
20 gm	$1.73	Hydrocortisone, Clay Park Labs	45802-0013-02
20 gm	$1.90	Hydrocortisone, Thames Pharma	49158-0103-07
20 gm	$2.25	Hydrocortisone, Consolidated Midland	00223-4161-20
20 gm	$2.36	Hydrocortisone, HL Moore Drug Exch	00839-5208-45
20 gm	$2.58	Hydrocortisone, H.C.F.A. F F P	99999-1476-52
20 gm	$2.60	Hydrocortisone, United Res	00677-0722-38
20 gm	$4.00	Hydrocortisone, C O Truxton	00463-8005-20
28.35 gm	$3.66	Hydrocortisone, H.C.F.A. F F P	99999-1476-53
28.4 gm	$3.66	Hydrocortisone, H.C.F.A. F F P	99999-1476-55
30 gm	$1.93	Hydrocortisone, H.C.F.A. F F P	99999-1476-54
30 gm	$2.00	HYCORT, Everett Labs	00642-0073-01
30 gm	$2.00	Hydrocortisone, Thames Pharma	49158-0103-08
30 gm	$2.16	Hydrocortisone, Clay Park Labs	45802-0013-03
30 gm	$2.25	Hydrocortisone, Major Pharms	00904-0751-31
30 gm	$2.27	Hydrocortisone, Harber Pharm	51432-0730-11
30 gm	$2.36	Hydrocortisone 10, NMC Labs	23317-0326-28
30 gm	$2.50	Hydrocortisone, Consolidated Midland	00223-4161-30
30 gm	$2.69	Hydrocortisone, HL Moore Drug Exch	00839-5208-49
30 gm	$2.85	Hydrocortisone, Rugby	00536-5107-95
30 gm	$2.90	Hydrocortisone, Schein Pharm (US)	00364-0785-56
30 gm	$2.97	Hydrocortisone, Rugby	00536-0515-95
30 gm	$3.22	Hydrocortisone, Fougera	00168-0020-31
30 gm	$4.68	HYDROCORTISONE 1% IN ABSORBASE, Carolina Med	46287-0003-01
60 gm	$3.87	Hydrocortisone, H.C.F.A. F F P	99999-1476-56
120 gm	$7.14	Hydrocortisone, HL Moore Drug Exch	00839-5208-53
120 gm	$7.74	Hydrocortisone, H.C.F.A. F F P	99999-1476-57
120 gm	$7.88	Hydrocortisone, Clay Park Labs	45802-0013-04
120 gm	$9.00	HYDROCORTISONE 1% IN ABSORBASE, Carolina Med	46287-0003-04
454 gm	$21.60	Hydrocortisone, Thames Pharma	49158-0103-16
454 gm	$21.72	Hydrocortisone, HL Moore Drug Exch	00839-5208-60
454 gm	$23.27	Hydrocortisone, Rugby	00536-2570-98
454 gm	$23.76	Hydrocortisone, Clay Park Labs	45802-0013-05
454 gm	$27.90	Hydrocortisone 10, NMC Labs	23317-0326-16
454 gm	$29.28	Hydrocortisone, H.C.F.A. F F P	99999-1476-58
454 gm	$29.37	Hydrocortisone, Fougera	00168-0020-16
454 gm	$29.82	HYDROCORTISONE 1% IN ABSORBASE, Carolina Med	46287-0003-16
480 gm	$24.30	Hydrocortisone, Harber Pharm	51432-0730-20
480 gm	$28.80	Hydrocortisone, H.C.F.A. F F P	99999-1476-59

Ointment - Topical - 2.5 %

5 gm	$2.25	Hydrocortisone, Consolidated Midland	00223-4125-05
20 gm	$4.00	Hydrocortisone, Harber Pharm	51432-0732-32
20 gm	$4.32	Hydrocortisone, Clay Park Labs	45802-0014-02
20 gm	$4.75	Hydrocortisone, Consolidated Midland	00223-4159-03
20 gm	$4.93	Hydrocortisone, HL Moore Drug Exch	00839-5209-45
20 gm	$4.95	Hydrocortisone, Consolidated Midland	00223-4125-20

HOW SUPPLIED - RATED THERAPEUTICALLY EQUIVALENT:
(cont'd)

20 gm	$5.01	Hydrocortisone, Schein Pharm (US)	00364-7088-55
20 gm	$5.47	Hydrocortisone, United Res	00677-0724-38
20 gm	$5.47	Hydrocortisone, H.C.F.A. F F P	99999-1476-60
20 gm	$5.88	Hydrocortisone, Rugby	00536-0620-99
20 gm	$5.95	Hydrocortisone, Major Pharms	00904-0757-29
28.4 gm	$7.77	Hydrocortisone, H.C.F.A. F F P	99999-1476-61
30 gm	$8.21	Hydrocortisone, H.C.F.A. F F P	99999-1476-62
30 gm	$8.38	Hydrocortisone, Fougera	00168-0146-30
30 gm	$19.67	HYTONE, Dermik Labs	00066-0085-01
454 gm	$58.32	Hydrocortisone, Clay Park Labs	45802-0014-05
454 gm	$124.30	Hydrocortisone, H.C.F.A. F F P	99999-1476-63

Powder

5 gm	$27.05	Hydrocortisone, Mallinckrodt	00406-8830-03
5 gm	$61.18	Hydrocortisone, Merck	00006-7595-05
10 gm	$28.60	Hydrocortisone, Paddock Labs	00574-0420-10
10 gm	$38.00	Hydrocortisone, Mallinckrodt	00406-8830-05
25 gm	$57.10	Hydrocortisone, Paddock Labs	00574-0420-25
100 gm	$130.00	Hydrocortisone, Millgood	53118-0203-01
100 gm	$218.40	Hydrocortisone, Paddock Labs	00574-0420-01

Solution - Topical - 1 %

30 ml	$8.00	TEXACORT, Genderm Corp	29936-0247-01
30 ml	$8.00	TEXACORT, Genderm	52761-0247-01
30 ml	$8.03	PENECORT, Allergan	00023-0889-30
60 ml	$14.04	PENECORT, Allergan	00023-0889-60

HOW SUPPLIED - NOT RATED EQUIVALENT:

Aerosol - Topical - 0.5 %

58 gm	$17.57	AEROSEB-HC, Allergan	00023-0804-90

Cream - Rectal - 2.5 %

30 gm	$11.95	Proctosol Hc, Major Pharms	00904-7806-31
30 gm	$36.95	PROCTO-HC, Am Generics	58634-0028-01

Cream - Rectal; Topical - 2.5 %/1 %

30 gm	$20.24	PROCTOCREAM-HC, Reed & Carnrick	00021-4640-24

Enema - Rectal - 100 mg/60ml

60 ml	$8.58	CORTENEMA, Solvay Pharms	00032-1904-73
60 ml x 7	$50.00	CORTENEMA, Solvay Pharms	00032-1904-82

Lotion - Topical - 0.25 %

120 ml	$15.62	CETACORT 0.25 %, Galderma	00299-3947-04
120 ml	$16.29	CORT-DOME, Bayer	00026-1622-04

Lotion - Topical - 2 %

30 ml	$6.22	ALA SCALP, Del Ray Lab	00316-0140-01

Solution - Topical - 2.5 %

30 ml	$15.41	TEXACORT, Genderm Corp	29936-0293-01
30 ml	$15.41	TEXACORT, Genderm	52761-0293-01

Tablet, Uncoated - Oral - 5 mg

50's	$5.57	CORTEF, Pharmacia & Upjohn	00009-0012-01

Tablet, Uncoated - Oral - 10 mg

100's	$19.69	CORTEF, Pharmacia & Upjohn	00009-0031-01
100's	$20.09	HYDROCORTONE, Merck	00006-0619-68

Tablet, Uncoated - Oral - 20 mg

100's	$8.00	Hydrocortisone, West Ward Pharm	00143-1254-01
100's	$8.10	Hydrocortisone, United Res	00677-0076-01
100's	$8.25	Hydrocortisone, West Ward Pharm	00143-1254-25
100's	$8.65	Hydrocortisone, Major Pharms	00904-2674-60
100's	$9.25	Hydrocortisone, HL Moore Drug Exch	00839-1365-06
100's	$11.55	Hydrocortisone, Rugby	00536-3913-01
100's	$37.35	CORTEF, Pharmacia & Upjohn	00009-0044-01
100's	$38.35	HYDROCORTONE, Merck	00006-0625-68
100's	$42.50	Hydrocortisone, Consolidated Midland	00223-1063-01
1000's	$400.00	Hydrocortisone, Consolidated Midland	00223-1063-02

HYDROCORTISONE ACETATE *(001477)*

CATEGORIES: Adrenal Corticosteroids; Alopecia; Anti-Inflammatory Agents; Antiarthritics; Arthritis; Bursitis; Colitis; Cryptitis; Dental; Dermatologicals; Dermatoses; Gastrointestinal Drugs; Glucocorticoids; Granuloma Annulare; Hemorrhoids; Hormones; Inflammatory Conditions; Lupus Erythematosus; Mucous Membrane Agents; Osteoarthritis; Pain; Pharmaceutical Adjuvants; Proctitis; Pruritus; Skin/Mucous Membrane Agents; Steroids; Tenosynovitis; Topical; Ulcerative Colitis; FDA Approval Pre 1982

BRAND NAMES: *Allocort*; Anucort-Hc; Anurx Hc; *Anusol + H*; Anusol Hc; *Apocort*; *Calacort*; *Colifoam* (Australia, England, Germany); *Colofoam* (France); *Cordes H* (Germany); *Cortaid*; *Cortaid Cream*; Cort-Dome Suppository; Corta-Plex Hc; *Cortamed* (Canada); *Cortef* (Canada); Cortef Acetate; *Cortef Cream* ; *Cortic Cream*; *Corticreme* (Canada); Cortifoam; *Cortoderm* (Canada); *Cortril*; *Dermacort*; *DHAcort*; *Dicaldox*; *Dilucort*; Dricort; *Ekzemsalbe*; *Enkacort*; *Ficortril* (Germany); Hemorrhoidal Hc; Hemril-Hc; *Hycor Eye Ointment*; *Hyderm* (Canada); Hydrocorten-A; *Hydrocortison* (Germany); *Hydrocortison Berco* (Germany); *Hydrocortison Dispersa*; *Hydrocortison Streuli* (Germany); **Hydrocortone Acetate**; *Hydrokortison*; *Hytisone*; *Lanacort*; *Mylocort*; *Novohydrocort* (Canada); *Nutracort*; Orabase Hca; *Pannocort*; *Proctocort* (France); Proctosol-Hc; Rectasol-Hc; *Rectoparin H* (Germany); *Scherosona F Pomada*; *Sigmacort*; *Siquent Hycor*, *Squibb-HC*; *Steroderm*; *Stopitch*; *Wycort*
(International brand names outside U.S. in italics)

FORMULARIES: BC-BS; FHP; PCS

DESCRIPTION:

The topical corticosteroids constitute a class of primarily synthetic steroids used as anti-inflammatory and anti-pruritic agents.

Topical Cream: Hydrocortisone Acetate Cream, USP 1% is a topical corticosteroid with micronized hydrocortisone acetate 1% (active ingredient) in a buffered, water-washable cream containing the following inactive ingredients: citric acid, USP; glyceryl stearate; imidurea, NF; methylparaben, NF; mineral oil, USP; PEG-100 stearate; polysorbate 60, NF; propylene glycol, USP; propylparaben, NF; purified water, USP; sodium citrate, USP hydrous; sorbitan monostearate, NF; and white petrolatum, USP. Hydrocortisone acetate has the chemical name Pregn-4-ene-3,20-dione, 21-(acetyloxy)-11, 17-dihydroxy-, (11β)-.

DESCRIPTION: *(cont'd)*

Suppository: Each Hydrocortisone Acetate 25 mg suppository contains 25 mg hydrocortisone acetate in a hydrogenated cocoglyceride base. Hydrocortisone acetate is a corticosteroid.

Sterile Suspension: Hydrocortisone Acetate sterile suspension is a sterile suspension of hydrocortisone acetate (pH 5.0 to 7.0) in a suitable aqueous medium. It is supplied in two strengths, one containing 25 mg hydrocortisone acetate per milliliter, the other containing 50 mg per milliliter. Inactive ingredients per ml: sodium chloride, 9 mg; polysorbate 80, 4 mg; sodium carboxymethylcellulose, 5 mg; and Water for Injection, q.s., 1 ml. Benzyl alcohol, 9 mg, added as a preservative.

Oral Paste: Hydrocortisone Acetate oral paste is an adrenocorticoid topical dental paste for application to the oral mucosa. Each gram contains hydrocortisone acetate 5 g (0.5%) in a paste vehicle containing pectin, gelatin, sodium carboxymethylcellulose dispersed in a plasticized hydrocarbon gel composed of 5% polyethylene in mineral oil, flavored with imitation vanilla. Hydrocortisone acetate is also known as cortisol acetate. Structural formula; Pregn-4-ene-3, 20-dione, 21-(acetyloxy)-11, 17 dihydroxy-, (11β)

Rectal Foam: Contains hydrocortisone acetate 10% as the sole active ingredianet in 20 g of a foam containing propylene glycol, emulsifying wax, polyoxyethylene-10-stearyl ether, cetyl alcohol, methylparaben and propylparaben, trolamine, purified water and inert propellants, dichlorodifluoromethane and dichlorotetrafluoroethane.

Each application delivers approximately 900 mg of foam containing 80 mg of hydrocortisone (90 mg of hydrocortisone acetate).

Solubility of hydrocortisone acetate in water: 1 mg/100 ml

CLINICAL PHARMACOLOGY:

Topical corticosteroids share anti-inflammatory, anti-pruritic and vasoconstrictive actions.

TOPICAL CREAM

The mechanism of anti-inflammatory activity of the topical corticosteroids is unclear. Various laboratory methods, including vasoconstrictor assays, are used to compare and predict potencies and/or clinical efficacies of the topical corticosteroids. There is some evidence to suggest that a recognizable correlation exists between vasoconstrictor potency and therapeutic efficacy in man.

Pharmacokinetics: The extent of percutaneous absorption of topical corticosteroids is determined by many factors including the vehicle, the integrity of the epidermal barrier, and the use of occlusive dressings.

Topical corticosteroids can be absorbed from normal intact skin. Inflammation and/or other disease processes in the skin increase percutaneous absorption. Occlusive dressings substantially increase the percutaneous absorption of topical corticosteroids. Thus, occlusive dressings may be a valuable therapeutic adjunct for treatment of resistant dermatoses (see DOSAGE AND ADMINISTRATION.)

Once absorbed through the skin, topical corticosteroids are handled through pharmacokinetic pathways similar to systemically administered corticosteroids. Corticosteroids are bound to plasma proteins in varying degrees. Corticosteroids are metabolized primarily in the liver and are then excreted by the kidneys. Some of the topical corticosteroids and their metabolites are also excreted into the bile.

SUPPOSITORY

In normal subjects, about 26 percent of hydrocortisone acetate is absorbed when the hydrocortisone acetate suppository is applied to the rectum. Absorption of hydrocortisone acetate may vary across abraded or inflamed surfaces.

STERILE SUSPENSION

Hydrocortisone Acetate sterile suspension has a slow onset but long duration of action when compared with more soluble preparations. Because of its insolubility, it is suitable for intra-articular, intralesional, and soft tissue injection where its anti-inflammatory effects are confined mainly to the area in which it has been injected, although it is capable of producing systemic hormonal effects.

Naturally occurring glucocorticoids (hydrocortisone and cortisone), which also have salt-retaining properties, are used as replacement therapy in adrenocortical deficiency states. They are also used for their potent anti-inflammatory effect in disorders of many organ systems.

Glucocorticoids cause profound and varied metabolic effects. In addition, they modify the body's immune responses to diverse stimuli.

ORAL PASTE

The paste acts as an adhesive vehicle for applying the active medication to oral tissues. The protective action of the adhesive vehicle may serve to reduce oral irritation.

The mechanism of anti-inflammatory activity of the topical steroids is unclear. Various laboratory methods, including vasoconstrictor assays, are used to compare and predict potencies and/or clinical efficacies of the topical corticosteroids. There is some evidence to suggest that a recognizable correlation exists between vasoconstrictor potency and therapeutic efficacy in man.

Once absorbed, topical corticosteroids are handled through pharmacokinetic pathways similar to systemically administered corticosteroids. Corticosteroids are bound to plasma proteins in varying degrees. Corticosteroids are metabolized primarily in the liver and are then excreted by the kidneys. Some of the topical corticosteroids and their metabolites are also excreted into the bile.

RECTAL FOAM

Hydrocortisone acetate rectal foam provides effective topical administration of an anti-inflammatory corticosteroid as adjunctive therapy of ulcerative proctitis.

INDICATIONS AND USAGE:

TOPICAL CREAM

Topical corticosteroids are indicated for the relief of the inflammatory and pruritic manifestations of corticosteroid-responsive dermatoses.

SUPPOSITORY

For use in inflamed hemorrhoids, post irradiation (factitial) proctitis, as an adjunct in the treatment of chronic ulcerative colitis, cryptitis, other inflammatory conditions of the anorectum, and pruritus ani.

STERILE SUSPENSION

A. By intra-articular or soft tissue injection: As adjunctive therapy for short-term administration (to tide the patient over an acute episode or exacerbation) in: Synovitis of osteoarthritis, Rheumatoid arthritis, Acute and sub acute bursitis, Acute gouty arthritis, Epicondylitis, Acute nonspecific tenosynovitis, Post-traumatic osteoarthritis

B. By intralesional injection: Keloids, Localized hypertrophic, infiltrated, inflammatory lesions of: lichen planus, psoriatic plaques, granuloma annulare, and lichen simplex chronicus (neurodermatitis), Discoid lupus erythematosus, Necrobiosis lipoidica diabeticorum, Alopecia areata, May also be useful in cystic tumors of an aponeurosis or tendon (ganglia).

ORAL PASTE

Indicated for adjunctive treatment and for temporary relief of symptoms associated with oral inflammatory lesions and ulcerative lesions resulting from trauma.

INDICATIONS AND USAGE: *(cont'd)*

RECTAL FOAM

HCTZ acetate foam is indicated as adjunctive therapy in the topical treatment of ulcerative proctitis of the distal portion of the rectum in patients who cannot retain hydrocortisone or other corticosteroid enemas. Direct observations of methylene blue-containing foam have shown staining about 10 centimeters into the rectum.

CONTRAINDICATIONS:

Topical Cream and Suppository: Topical/suppository corticosteroids are contraindicated in those patients with a history of hypersensitivity to any of the components of the preparation/suppository.

Sterile Suspension: Systemic fungal infections

Hypersensitivity to any component of this product.

Oral Paste: Topical corticosteroids are contraindicated in those patients with a history of hypersensitivity to any of the components of the preparation. Because it contains a corticosteroid, the preparation is contraindicated in the presence of fungal, viral, or bacterial infections of the mouth or throat.

Rectal Foam: Local contraindications to the use of intrarectal steroids include obstruction, abscess, perforation, peritonitis, fresh intestinal anastomoses, extensive fistulas and sinus tracts. Tuberculosis (active, latent or questionably healed), ocular herpes simplex and acute psychosis are usually considered absolute contraindications to the use of corticosteroids. Relative contraindications include active peptic ulcer, acute glomerulonephritis, myasthenia gravis, osteoporosis, diverticulitis, thrombophlebitis, psychic disturbances, pregnancy, diabetes, hyperthyroidism, acute coronary disease, hypertension, limited cardiac reserve, and local and systemic infections, including fungal or exanthematous diseases. Where these conditions exist, the expected benefits from steroid therapy must be weighed against the risks involved in its use. Pregnancy is a relative contraindication to corticosteroids, particularly during third trimester. If corticosteroids must be administered in pregnancy, watch newborn infant closely for signs of hypoadrenalism, and administered appropriate therapy if needed.

WARNINGS:

STERILE SUSPENSION

Because rare instances of anaphylactoid reactions have occurred in patients receiving corticosteroid therapy, appropriate precautionary measures should be taken prior to administration, especially when the patient has a history of allergy to any drug.

In patients on corticosteroid therapy subjected to any unusual stress, increased dosage of rapidly acting corticosteroids before, during, and after the stressful situation is indicated.

Drug-induced secondary adrenocortical insufficiency may result from too rapid withdrawal of corticosteroids and may be minimized by gradual reduction of dosage. This type of relative insufficiency may persist for months after discontinuation of therapy; therefore, in any situation of stress occurring during that period, hormone therapy should be reinstituted. If the patient is receiving steroids already, dosage may have to be increased. Since mineralocorticoid secretion may be impaired, salt and/or a mineralocorticoid should be administered concurrently.

Corticosteroids may mask some signs of infection, and new infections may appear during their use. There may be decreased resistance and inability to localize infection when corticosteroids are used. Moreover, corticosteroids may affect the nitroblue-tetrazolium test for bacterial infection and produce false negative results.

In cerebral malaria, a double-blind trial has shown that the use of corticosteroids is associated with prolongation of coma and a higher incidence of pneumonia and gastrointestinal bleeding.

Corticosteroids may activate latent amebiasis. Therefore, it is recommended that latent or active amebiasis be ruled out before initiating corticosteroid therapy in any patient who has spent time in the tropics or any patient with unexplained diarrhea.

Prolonged use of corticosteroids may produce posterior subcapsular cataracts, glaucoma with possible damage to the optic nerves, and may enhance the establishment of secondary ocular infections due to fungi or viruses.

Usage in Pregnancy: Since adequate human reproduction studies have not been done with corticosteroids, use of these drugs in pregnancy or in women of childbearing potential requires that the anticipated benefits be weighed against the possible hazards to the mother and embryo or fetus. Infants born of mothers who have received substantial doses of corticosteroids during pregnancy should be carefully observed for signs of hypoadrenalism.

Corticosteroids appear in breast milk and could suppress growth, interfere with endogenous corticosteroid production, or cause other unwanted effects. Mothers taking pharmacologic doses of corticosteroids should be advised not to nurse.

Average and large doses of cortisone or hydrocortisone can cause elevation of blood pressure, salt and water retention, and increased excretion of potassium. These effects are less likely to occur with the synthetic derivatives except when used in large doses. Dietary salt restriction and potassium supplementation may be necessary. All corticosteroids increase calcium excretion.

Administration of live virus vaccines, including smallpox, is contraindicated in individuals receiving immunosuppressive doses of corticosteroids. If inactivated viral or bacterial vaccines are administered to individuals receiving immunosuppressive doses of corticosteroids, the expected serum antibody response may not be obtained.

If corticosteroids are indicated in patients with latent tuberculosis or tuberculin reactivity, close observation is necessary as reactivation of the disease may occur. During prolonged corticosteroid therapy, these patients should receive chemoprophylaxis.

Literature reports suggest an apparent association between use of corticosteroids and left ventricular free wall rupture after a recent myocardial infarction; therefore, therapy with corticosteroids should be used with great caution in these patients.

RECTAL FOAM

Do not insert any part of the aerosol container into the anus. Contents of the container are under pressure, but not flammable. Do not burn or puncture the aerosol container. Store at room temperature and not over 120°F. Because HCTZ acetate rectal foam is not expelled, systemic hydrocortisone absorption may be greater from HCTZ acetate rectal foam than from corticosteroid enema formulations. If there is not evidence of clinical or proctologic improvement within two or three weeks after starting HCTZ acetate rectal foam therapy, or if the patient's condition worsens, discontinue the drug. Children who are on immunosuppressant drugs are more susceptible to infections than healthy children. Chickenpox and measles, for example, can have a more serious or even fatal course in children on immunosuppressant corticosteroids. In such children, or in adults who have not had these diseases, particular care should be taken to avoid exposure. if exposed, therapy with varicella zoster immune globulin (VZIG) or pooled intravenous immunoglobulin (IVIG), as appropriate, may be indicated. If chicken pox develops, treatment with antiviral agents may be considered.

PRECAUTIONS:

GENERAL

Topical Cream and Oral Paste: Systemic absorption of topical corticosteroids has produced reversible hypothalamic-pituitary-adrenal (HPA) axis suppression, manifestations of Cushing's syndrome, hyperglycemia, and glucosuria in some patients.

Conditions which augment systemic absorption include the application of the more potent steroids, use over large surface areas, prolonged use, and the addition of occlusive dressings.

Therefore, patients receiving a large dose of a potent topical steroid applied to a large surface area or under an occlusive dressing should be evaluated periodically for evidence of HPA axis suppression by using the urinary free cortisol and ACTH stimulation tests. If HPA axis suppression is noted, an attempt should be made to withdraw the drug, to reduce the frequency of application, or to substitute a less potent steroid.

Recovery of HPA axis function is generally prompt and complete upon discontinuation of the drug. Infrequently, signs and symptoms of steroid withdrawal may occur, requiring supplemental systemic corticosteroids.

Children may absorb proportionally larger amounts of topical corticosteroids and thus be more susceptible to systemic toxicity (see PRECAUTIONS, Pediatric Use.)

If irritation develops, topical corticosteroids should be discontinued and appropriate therapy instituted. In the presence of dermatological infections, the use of an appropriate antifungal or antibacterial agent should be instituted. If a favorable response does not occur promptly, the corticosteroid should be discontinued until the infection has been adequately controlled.

Suppository: Do not use unless adequate proctologic examination is made.

If irritation develops, the product should be discontinued and appropriate therapy instituted.

In the presence of an infection, the use of an appropriate antifungal or antibacterial agent should be instituted. If a favorable response does not occur promptly, the corticosteroid should be discontinued until the infection has been adequately controlled.

No long-term studies in animals have been performed to evaluate the carcinogenic potential of corticosteroid suppositories.

Sterile Suspension: This product, like many other steroid formulations, is sensitive to heat. Therefore, it should not be autoclaved when it is desirable to sterilize the exterior of the vial.

Following prolonged therapy, withdrawal of corticosteroids may result in symptoms of the corticosteroid withdrawal syndrome including fever, myalgia, arthralgia, and malaise. This may occur in patients even without evidence of adrenal insufficiency.

There is an enhanced effect of corticosteroids in patients with hypothyroidism and in those with cirrhosis.

Corticosteroids should be used cautiously in patients with ocular herpes simplex for fear of corneal perforation.

Psychic derangements may appear when corticosteroids are used, ranging from euphoria, insomnia, mood swings, personality changes, and severe depression to frank psychotic manifestations. Also, existing emotional instability or psychotic tendencies may be aggravated by corticosteroids.

Aspirin should be used cautiously in conjunction with corticosteroids in hypothrombinemia.

Steroids should be used with caution in nonspecific ulcerative colitis, if there is a probability of impending perforation, abscess, or other pyogenic infection, also in diverticulitis, fresh intestinal anastomoses, active or latent peptic ulcer, renal insufficiency, hypertension, osteoporosis, and myasthenia gravis. Signs of peritoneal irritation following gastrointestinal perforation in patients receiving large doses of corticosteroids may be minimal or absent. Fat embolism has been reported as a possible complication of hypercortisonism.

When large doses are given, some authorities advise that antacids be administered between meals to prevent peptic ulcer.

Growth and development of infants and children on prolonged corticosteroid therapy should be carefully followed.

Steroids may increase or decrease motility and number of spermatozoa in some patients.

Phenytoin, phenobarbital, ephedrine, and rifampin may enhance the metabolic clearance of corticosteroids resulting in decreased blood levels and lessened physiologic activity, thus requiring adjustment in corticosteroid dosage.

The prothrombin time should be checked frequently in patients who are receiving corticosteroids and coumarin anticoagulants at the same time because of reports that corticosteroids have altered the response to these anticoagulants. Studies have shown that the usual effect produced by adding corticosteroids is inhibition of response to coumarins, although there have been some conflicting reports of potentiation not substantiated by studies.

When corticosteroids are administered concomitantly with potassium-depleting diuretics, patients should be observed closely for development of hypokalemia.

Intra-articular injection of a corticosteroid may produce systemic as well as local effects.

Appropriate examination of any joint fluid present is necessary to exclude a septic process.

A marked increase in pain accompanied by local swelling, further restriction of joint motion, fever, and malaise is suggestive of septic arthritis. If this complication occurs and the diagnosis of sepsis is confirmed, appropriate antimicrobial therapy should be instituted.

Injection of a steroid into an infected site is to be avoided.

Corticosteroids should not be injected into unstable joints.

Patients should be impressed strongly with the importance of not overusing joints in which symptomatic benefit has been obtained as long as the inflammatory process remains active.

Frequent intra-articular injection may result in damage to joint tissues.

Rectal Foam: Steroid therapy should be administered with caution in patients with severe ulcerative disease because these patients are predisposed to perforation of the bowel wall. Where surgery is imminent, it is hazardous to wait more than a few days for satisfactory response to medical treatment. General precautions common to all corticosteroid therapy should be observed during treatment with HCTZ acetate rectal foam. These include gradual withdrawal of therapy to allow for possible adrenal insufficiency and awareness to possible growth suppression in children. Patients should be kept under close observation, for, as with all drugs, rare individuals may react unfavorably under certain conditions. If severe reactions or idiosyncrasies occur, steroids should be discontinued immediately and appropriate measures instituted. Do not employ in immediate or early postoperative period following ileorectostomy.

INFORMATION FOR THE PATIENT

Patients who are on immunosuppressive doses of corticosteroids should be warned to avoid exposure to chicken pox or measles and, if exposed, to obtain medical advice.

Topical Cream and Oral Paste: Patients using topical corticosteroids should receive the following information and instructions:

1. This medication is to be used as directed by the dentist or physician. (The **Topical Cream** is for external use only.) Avoid contact with the eyes.

2. Patients should be advised not to use this medication for any disorder other than for which it has been prescribed.

3. The treated skin area should not be bandaged or otherwise covered or wrapped as to be occlusive unless directed by the physician.

PRECAUTIONS: *(cont'd)*

4. Patients should report any signs of local adverse reactions especially under occlusive dressing.

5. Parents of pediatric patients should be advised not to use tight-fitting diapers or plastic pants on a child being treated in the diaper area, as these garments may constitute occlusive dressings.

LABORATORY TESTS

Topical Cream and Oral Paste: The following tests may be helpful in evaluating the HPA axis suppression:

Urinary free cortisol test

ACTH stimulation test

CARCINOGENESIS, MUTAGENESIS, AND IMPAIRMENT OF FERTILITY

Topical Cream and Oral Paste: Long-term animal studies have not been performed to evaluate the carcinogenic potential or the effect on fertility of topical corticosteroids. Studies to determine mutagenicity with prednisolone and hydrocortisone have revealed negative results.

NURSING MOTHERS

Topical Cream and Oral Paste: It is not known whether topical administration of corticosteroids could result in sufficient systemic absorption to produce detectable quantities in breast milk. Systemically administered corticosteroids are secreted into breast milk in quantities not likely to have a deleterious effect on the infant. Nevertheless, caution should be exercised when topical corticosteroids are administered to a nursing woman.

PEDIATRIC USE

Topical Cream and Oral Paste: PEDIATRIC PATIENTS MAY DEMONSTRATE GREATER SUSCEPTIBILITY TO TOPICAL CORTICOSTEROID-INDUCED HPA AXIS SUPPRESSION AND CUSHING'S SYNDROME THAN MATURE PATIENTS BECAUSE OF A LARGER SKIN SURFACE AREA TO BODY WEIGHT RATIO.

Hypothalamic-pituitary-adrenal (HPA) axis suppression, Cushing's syndrome, and intracranial hypertension have been reported in children receiving topical corticosteroids. Manifestations of adrenal suppression in children include linear growth retardation, delayed weight gain, low plasma cortisol levels, and absence of response to ACTH stimulation. Manifestations of intracranial hypertension include bulging fontanelles, headaches, and bilateral papilledema.

Administration of topical corticosteroids to children should be limited to the least amount compatible with an effective therapeutic regimen. Chronic corticosteroid therapy may interfere with the growth and development of children.

PREGNANCY CATEGORY C

Topical Cream, Suppositories and Oral Paste: Corticosteroids are generally teratogenic in laboratory animals when administered systemically at relatively low dosage levels. The more potent corticosteroids have been shown to be teratogenic after dermal application in laboratory animals. There are no adequate and well-controlled studies in pregnant women on teratogenic effects from topically applied corticosteroids.

Therefore, topical corticosteroids should be used during pregnancy only if the potential benefit justifies the potential risk to the fetus. Drugs of this class should not be used extensively on pregnant patients, in large amounts, or for prolonged periods of time.

NURSING MOTHERS

Topical Cream, Suppositories and Oral Paste: It is not known whether this drug is excreted in human milk, and because many drugs are excreted in human milk and because of the potential for serious adverse reactions in nursing infants from hydrocortisone acetate suppositories, a decision should be made whether to discontinue nursing or to discontinue the drug, taking into account the importance of the drug to the mother.

ADVERSE REACTIONS:

TOPICAL CREAM

The following local adverse reactions are reported infrequently with topical corticosteroids, but may occur more frequently with the use of occlusive dressings. These reactions are listed in an approximate decreasing order of occurrence.

Burning	Perioral dermatitis
Itching	Allergic contact dermatitis
Irritation	Maceration of the skin
Dryness	Secondary infection
Folliculitis	Skin atrophy
Hypertrichosis	Striae
Acneiform eruptions	Miliaria
Hypopigmentation	

SUPPOSITORY

The following local adverse reactions have been reported with corticosteroid suppositories:

Burning	Folliculitis
Itching	Hypopigmentation
Irritation	Allergic Contact Dermatitis
Dryness	Secondary Infection.

STERILE SUSPENSION

Fluid and electrolyte disturbances: Sodium retention, Fluid retention, Congestive heart failure in susceptible patients, Potassium loss, Hypokalemic alkalosis, Hypertension.

Musculoskeletal: Muscle weakness, Steroid myopathy, Loss of muscle mass, Osteoporosis, Vertebral compression fractures, Aseptic necrosis of femoral and humeral heads, Pathologic fracture of long bones, Tendon rupture.

Gastrointestinal: Peptic ulcer with possible subsequent perforation and hemorrhage, Perforation of the small and large bowel, particularly in patients with inflammatory bowel disease, Pancreatitis, Abdominal distension, Ulcerative esophagitis.

Dermatologic: Impaired wound healing, Thin fragile skin, Petechiae and ecchymoses, Erythema, Increased sweating, May suppress reactions to skin tests, Other cutaneous reactions, such as allergic dermatitis, urticaria, angioneurotic edema.

Neurologic: Convulsions, Increased intracranial pressure with papilledema (pseudotumor cerebri) usually after treatment, Vertigo, Headache, Psychic disturbances.

Endocrine: Menstrual irregularities, Development of cushingoid state, Suppression of growth in children, Secondary adrenocortical and pituitary unresponsiveness, particularly in times of stress, as in trauma, surgery or illness, Decreased carbohydrate tolerance, Manifestation of latent diabetes mellitus, Increased requirements for insulin or oral hypoglycemic agents in diabetics, Hirsutism.

Ophthalmic: Posterior subcapsular cataracts, Increased intraocular pressure, Glaucoma, Exophthalmos.

Metabolic: Negative nitrogen balance due to protein catabolism.

Cardiovascular: Myocardial rupture following recent myocardial infarction (see WARNINGS.)

Other: Anaphylactoid or hypersensitivity reactions, Thromboembolism, Weight gain, Increased appetite, Nausea, Malaise.

ADVERSE REACTIONS: *(cont'd)*

The following *additional* adverse reactions are related to injection of corticosteroids: Rare instances of blindness associated with intralesional therapy around the face and head, Hyperpigmentation or hypopigmentation, Subcutaneous and cutaneous atrophy, Sterile abscess, Postinjection flare (following intra-articular use), Charcot-like arthropathy

ORAL PASTE

The following local adverse reactions are reported infrequently with topical corticosteroids. These reactions are listed in an approximate decreasing order of occurrence: Burning, itching, irritation, dryness, hypopigmentation, perioral dermatitis, allergic contact dermatitis, secondary infection, striae, miliaria.

RECTAL FOAM

Corticosteroid therapy may produce side effects which include moon face, fluid retention excessive appetite and weight gain, abnormal fat deposits, mental symptoms, hypertrichosis, acne, ecchymosis, increased sweating, pigmentation, dry scaly skin, thinning scalp hair, thrombophlebitis, decreased resistance to infection, negative nitrogen balance with delayed bone and wound healing, menstrual disorders, neuropathy, peptic ulcer, decreased glucose tolerance, hypopotassemia, adrenal insufficiency, necrotizing angitis, hypertension, pancreatitis and increased intraocular pressure. In children, suppression of growth may occur. Increased intracranial pressure may occur and possibly account for headache, insomnia, and fatigue. Subcapsular cataracts may result from prolonged usage. Long-term use of all corticosteroids results in catabolic effects characterized by negative protein and calcium balance. Osteoporosis, spontaneous fractures and aseptic necrosis of the hip and humerus may occur as part of this catabolic phenomenon. Where hypopotassemia and other symptoms associated with fluid and electrolyte imbalance call for potassium supplementation and salt poor or salt-free diets, these may be instituted and are compatible with diet requirements for ulcerative proctitis.

DRUG ABUSE AND DEPENDENCE:

Suppository: Drug abuse and dependence have not been reported in patients treated with Hydrocortisone Acetate suppositories.

OVERDOSAGE:

Topical Cream and Oral Paste: Topically applied corticosteroids can be absorbed in sufficient amounts to produce systemic effects. (See PRECAUTIONS.)

Suppository: If signs and symptoms of systemic overdosage occur, discontinue use.

Sterile Suspension: Reports of acute toxicity and/or death following overdosage of glucocorticoids are rare. In the event of overdosage, no specific antidosage is available; treatment is supportive and symptomatic.

DOSAGE AND ADMINISTRATION:

TOPICAL CREAM

Topical corticosteroids are generally applied to the affected area as a thin film from two to four times daily depending on the severity of the condition.

Occlusive dressings may be used for the management of psoriasis or recalcitrant conditions. If an infection develops, the use of occlusive dressings should be discontinued and appropriate antimicrobial therapy instituted.

Storage: Store at controlled room temperature 15°-30°C (59°-86°F).

SUPPOSITORY

Usual Dosage: One suppository in the rectum morning and night for two weeks, in nonspecific proctitis. In more severe cases, one suppository three times daily; or two suppositories twice daily. In factitial proctitis, recommended therapy is six to eight weeks or less, according to response.

Storage: Store below 30°C (86°F). Protect from freezing.

STERILE SUSPENSION

For intra-articular, intralesional, and soft tissue injection only. NOT FOR INTRAVENOUS USE.

DOSAGE AND FREQUENCY OF INJECTION ARE VARIABLE AND MUST BE INDIVIDUALIZED ON THE BASIS OF THE DISEASE AND THE RESPONSE OF THE PATIENT.

The initial dose varies from 5 to 75 mg depending on the disease being treated and the size of the area to be injected. Frequency of injection depends on symptomatic response, and usually is once every two or three weeks. Severe conditions may require injection once a week. Frequent intra-articular injection may result in damage to joint tissues. If satisfactory clinical response does not occur after a reasonable period of time, discontinue hydrocortisone acetate sterile suspension and transfer the patient to other therapy.

Patients should be observed closely for signs that might require dosage adjustment, including changes in clinical status resulting from remissions or exacerbations of the disease, and individual responsiveness.

Some of the usual single doses are:

Large Joints (*e.g.,* Knee): 25 mg, occasionally 37.5 mg. Doses over 50 mg not recommended

Small Joints (*e.g.,* Interphalangeal, Temporomandibular): 10 to 25 mg

Bursae: 25 to 37.5 mg

Tendon Sheaths: 5 to 12.5 mg

Soft Tissue Infiltration: 25 to 50 mg, occasionally 75 mg

Ganglia: 12.5 to 25 mg

For rapid onset of action, a soluble adrenocortical hormone preparation, such as Dexamethasone Sodium Phosphate injection or Prednisolone Sodium Phosphate injection, may be given with Hydrocortisone Acetate sterile suspension.

If desired, a local anesthetic may be used, and may be injected before Hydrocortisone Acetate sterile suspension or mixed in a syringe with Hydrocortisone Acetate sterile suspension and given simultaneously.

If used prior to intra-articular injection of the steroid, inject most of the anesthetic into the soft tissues of the surrounding area and instill a small amount into the joint.

If given together, mixing should be done in the injection syringe by drawing the steroid in *first*, then the anesthetic. In this way, the anesthetic will not be introduced inadvertently into the vial of steroid. *The mixture must be used immediately and any unused portion discarded.*

Storage: Sensitive to heat. Do not autoclave. Protect from freezing.

ORAL PASTE

Dab, **do not rub**, on the lesion until the paste adheres. (Rubbing this preparation on lesions may result in a granular, gritty sensation.) After application, a smooth, slippery film develops.

Usual adult dose: Topical, to the oral mucous membrane, 2 or 3 times a day following meals and at bedtime.

Usual pediatric dose: Dosage has not been established.

DOSAGE AND ADMINISTRATION: *(cont'd)*

RECTAL FOAM

Usual dose is one applicatorful once or twice daily for two or three weeks, and every second day thereafter, administered rectally. The patient direction package with the applicator describes how to use the aerosol container and applicator. Satisfactory response usually occurs within five to seven days marked by a decrease in symptoms. Symptomatic improvement in ulcerative proctitis should not be used as the sole criterion for evaluating efficacy. Sigmoidoscopy is also recommended to judge dosage adjustment, duration of therapy and rate of improvement.

Directions for use: 1) Shake foam container vigorously before use. Hold container upright and insert into the opening of the tip of the applicator. **Be sure applicator plunger is drawn all the way out.** Container must be held upright to obtain proper flow of medication. 2) To fill, press down slowly on container cap. When foam reaches fill line in the applicator, it is ready for use. **Caution:** The aerosol container should never be inserted directly into the anus. 3) Remove applicator from container. Allow some foam to remain on the applicator tip. hold applicator by barrel and gently insert tip into the anus. With applicator in place, push plunger in order to expel foam, then withdraw applicator. (Applicator parts should be pulled apart for thorough cleaning with warm water.)

Storage: Store upright at controlled room temperature 15-30°C (59- 86°F).

(Topical Cream: Parke-Davis, 5/89, 3124G011) (Suppository: Parke-Davis, 1/89, 1726G010) (Sterile Suspension: Merck, 3/88, 7348726) (Oral Paste: Colgate, 5/92, LIPI-900) (Rectal Foam: Reed & Carnrick, 12/91)

HOW SUPPLIED - EQUIVALENTS NOT AVAILABLE:

Aerosol, Foam - Rectal - 10 %

20 gm	$47.07	CORTIFOAM, Reed & Carnrick	00021-0695-20

Injection, Susp - Intra-Articular - 25 mg/ml

5 ml	$4.75	Hydrocortisone Acetate, Consolidated Midland	00223-7880-05
10 ml	$1.48	Hydrocortisone Acetate, Lannett	00527-0168-55
10 ml	$4.45	Hydrocortisone Acetate, Major Pharms	00904-0855-10
10 ml	$4.80	Hydrocortisone Acetate, Steris Labs	00402-0051-10
10 ml	$5.00	Hydrocortisone Acetate, Consolidated Midland	00223-7881-10
10 ml	$5.76	Hydrocortisone Acetate, Schein Pharm (US)	00364-6624-54
10 ml	$7.00	Hydrocortisone Acetate, United Res	00677-0278-21
10 ml	$7.87	Hydrocortisone Acetate, HL Moore Drug Exch	00839-5176-30

Injection, Susp - Intra-Articular - 50 mg/ml

5 ml	**$26.96**	**HYDROCORTONE ACETATE, Merck**	**00006-7519-03**
10 ml	$2.48	Hydrocortisone Acetate, Lannett	00527-0201-55
10 ml	$5.05	Hydrocortisone Acetate, Major Pharms	00904-0853-10
10 ml	$5.10	Sterile Hydrocortisone Acetate, United Res	00677-0279-21
10 ml	$5.75	Hydrocortisone Acetate, Consolidated Midland	00223-7891-10
10 ml	$6.00	Hydrocortisone Acetate, C O Truxton	00463-1037-10

Paste - Dental; Topical - 0.5 %

5 gm	$76.94	ORABASE HCA, Colgate Oral	00126-0101-45

Powder

5 gm	$19.17	Hydrocortisone Acetate, Purepac Pharm	00228-2215-52
25 gm	$57.10	Hydrocortisone Acetate, Paddock Labs	00574-0421-25
100 gm	$218.40	Hydrocortisone Acetate, Paddock Labs	00574-0421-01

Suppository - Rectal - 25 mg

12's	$1.55	Rectasol-Hc, Bio Pharm	59741-0310-12
12's	$4.00	Hydrocortisone Acetate, Clay Park Labs	45802-0725-30
12's	$4.14	Hydrocortisone Acetate, NMC Labs	23317-0511-12
12's	$4.65	Anurx Hc, Rose Laboratories	42037-0132-12
12's	$5.75	ANUCORT-HC, GW Labs	00713-0503-12
12's	$5.78	Hemorrhoidal Hc, Vintage Pharms	00254-8400-06
12's	$5.95	ANUCORT-HC, Raway	00686-0503-12
12's	$7.35	Hemorrhoidal Hc, Qualitest Pharms	00603-8127-11
12's	$7.50	Hydrocortisone Acetate, Goldline Labs	00182-7038-11
12's	$8.70	Hydrocortisone Acetate, United Res	00677-1377-12
12's	$8.75	HEMORRHOIDAL HC, Rugby	00536-1406-12
12's	$8.99	Hydrocortisone Acetate, Cypress Pharm	60258-0501-12
12's	$9.85	Hydrocortisone Acetate, Paddock Labs	00574-7090-12
12's	$9.90	HEMORRHOIDAL/HYDROCORTISONE ACETATE, Schein Pharm (US)	00364-2423-12
12's	$9.96	HEMORRHOIDAL HC SUPPOSITORIES 25, Geneva Pharms	00781-7700-32
12's	$10.95	Hemorrhoidal Hc, Consolidated Midland	00223-5555-12
12's	$13.00	Anudil Hc, Llorens Pharm	54859-0601-12
12's	$14.90	Hydrocortisone Acetate, Elge	58298-0150-12
12's	$15.90	Rectasol-Hc, Bio Pharm	59741-0301-12
12's	$18.38	Proctosol-Hc, Am Generics	58634-0036-01
12's	$24.12	ANUSOL-HC SUPPOSITORIES 25, Parke-Davis	00071-1726-07
12's	$37.70	CORT-DOME, Bayer	00026-5005-12
12's UD	$5.93	HEMRIL-HC, Upsher Smith	00245-0111-12
24's	$2.95	Rectasol-Hc, Bio Pharm	59741-0310-24
24's	$4.86	Hydrocortisone Acetate, Clay Park Labs	45802-0725-31
24's	$7.78	Hydrocortisone Acetate, NMC Labs	23317-0511-24
24's	$10.97	Hemorrhoidal Hc, Vintage Pharms	00254-8400-15
24's	$11.25	ANUCORT-HC, GW Labs	00713-0503-24
24's	$12.00	HEMORRHOIDAL HC, Goldline Labs	00182-7038-16
24's	$13.97	Hemorrhoidal Hc, Qualitest Pharms	00603-8127-18
24's	$14.90	HYDROCORTISONE ACETATE, Schein Pharm (US)	00364-2423-24
24's	$14.94	HEMORRHOIDAL HC SUPPOSITORIES 25, Geneva Pharms	00781-7700-40
24's	$25.00	Hydrocortisone Acetate, Elge	58298-0150-24
24's	$26.95	Rectasol-Hc, Bio Pharm	59741-0301-24
24's	$32.19	Proctosol-Hc, Am Generics	58634-0036-02
24's	$42.25	ANUSOL-HC SUPPOSITORIES 25, Parke-Davis	00071-1726-13
50's	$6.15	Rectasol-Hc, Bio Pharm	59741-0310-50
50's	$18.95	Anurx Hc, Rose Laboratories	42037-0132-50
50's	$49.50	Rectasol-Hc, Bio Pharm	59741-0301-50
100's	$12.25	Rectasol-Hc, Bio Pharm	59741-0310-49
100's	$39.95	Rectasol-Hc, Bio Pharm	59741-0301-49
100's	$51.25	ANUCORT-HC, GW Labs	00713-0503-01
100's	$59.24	HEMORRHOIDAL-HC, Rugby	00536-1406-01
100's	$89.50	Hemorrhoidal Hc, Consolidated Midland	00223-5555-01
1000's	$297.54	Hydrocortisone Acetate, Clay Park Labs	45802-0725-14

HYDROCORTISONE ACETATE; NEOMYCIN SULFATE *(001478)*

CATEGORIES: Anti-Infectives; Antibiotics; Dermatologicals; Dermatoses; EENT Drugs; Eye, Ear, Nose, & Throat Preparations; Ocular Infections; Ophthalmics; Otic Hydrocortisones; Skin/Mucous Membrane Agents; Skin Infections; FDA Approval Pre 1982

BRAND NAMES: Ak-Neo-Cort; Cor-Oticin; Eye-Cort; Hydro-Neomycin; Neo-Cort-Dome; **Neo-Cortef**

FORMULARIES: Medi-Cal

DESCRIPTION:

Hydrocortisone with neomycin ointment contains the anti-inflammatory agent hydrocortisone acetate in three concentrations, 0.5%, 1%, and 2.5%, and the broad-spectrum antibiotic neomycin sulfate equivalent to 3.5 mg neomycin. Each gram of ointment also contains methylparaben 0.2 mg and butylparaben 1.8 mg in a bland base composed of white petrolatum, microcrystalline wax, mineral oil and cholesterol.

CLINICAL PHARMACOLOGY:

Topical steroids are primarily effective because of their anti-inflammatory, antipruritic and vasoconstrictive actions.

Hydrocortisone exerts a marked anti-inflammatory effect through its controlling influence on the vascular and connective tissue components. In inhibiting the inflammatory reaction, hydrocortisone does not appear to interfere with antibody formation or with antigen-antibody union.

Applied topically on the skin, hydrocortisone inhibits more markedly than cortisone, similarly employed, the various aspects of inflammation (particularly of the allergic type) including edema, hyperemia, cellular infiltration, and pruritus. In acute allergic dermatitis topical application has been found to be rapidly effective. In many instances objective signs of improvement, subsidence of erythema and edema with symptomatic relief, occur within a few hours of the first application. Following discontinuance of the applications no "rebound" activation of the lesions has been observed. Even in acute exudative lesions the application of hydrocortisone with neomycin ointment is effective. The results are questionable in dermatitic lesions in which there is considerable thickening or scaling of the skin.

Neomycin is an antibacterial substance derived from cultures of the soil organism, Streptomyces fradiae. It exhibits a wider spectrum of antibacterial activity than either bacitracin, streptomycin, or penicillin and is active against a variety of gram-positive and gram-negative organisms including staphylococci, Escherichia coli, and Hemophilius influenzae. It is not active against fungi. Neomycin rarely causes resistant strains of microorganisms to develop; in addition, it is unusually nontoxic for human epithelial cells in tissue culture and is nonirritating topically in therapeutic concentrations.

INDICATIONS AND USAGE:

For the treatment of corticosteroid-responsive dermatoses with secondary infection. It has not been demonstrated that this steroid-antibiotic combination provides greater benefit than the steroid component alone after seven days of treatment.(See WARNINGS.)

CONTRAINDICATIONS:

This preparation is contraindicated in cutaneous tuberculosis, fungus infections and certain virus infections (herpes simplex, vaccinia and varicella) for which an effective antibiotic or chemotherapeutic agent is not available for simultaneous application, and in those patients with a history of hypersensitivity to any of its components.

WARNINGS:

Because of the potential hazard of nephrotoxicity and ototoxicity, prolonged use or use of large amounts of this product should be avoided in the treatment of skin infections following extensive burns, trophic ulceration and other conditions where absorption of neomycin is possible.

Because of the concern of nephrotoxicity associated with neomycin, this combination product should not be used over a wide area or for extended periods of time.

PRECAUTIONS:

This preparation is unusually well tolerated. However, neomycin may occasionally induce sensitivity reactions. If signs of irritation or sensitivity should develop, application should be discontinued.

If extensive areas are treated or if the occlusive technique is used, The possibility exists of increased absorption of the corticoid and suitable precautions should be taken.

The safety of the use of topical steroid preparations during pregnancy has not been fully established. Therefore, they should not be used unnecessarily during pregnancy, on extended areas, in large amounts, or for prolonged periods of time.

This product should not be put in the eyes or, if the ear drum is perforated, in the external ear canal.

NOTE: The prolonged use of antibiotic-containing preparations may result in overgrowth of of nonsusceptible organisms, particularly fungi. If new infections appear during treatment, appropriate therapy should be instituted.

ADVERSE REACTIONS:

When steroid preparations are used for long periods in intertriginous areas or under occlusive dressing, localized atrophy and striae may occur.

Other local adverse reactions associated with topically applied corticoids either with or without occlusive dressings include: burning sensations, itching, irritation, dryness, folliculitis, secondary infection, atrophy of the skin, acneiform eruption and hypopigmentation.

Ototoxicity and nephrotoxicity have been reported following absorption of topically applied neomycin.

According to current medical literature there has been an increase in the prevalence of neomycin hypersensitivity.

DOSAGE AND ADMINISTRATION:

After thorough cleansing of the affected skin, a small amount of the ointment is applied and rubbed gently into the involved areas. Application may be made one to three times daily. In many instances the the amount of the ointment required is small and applications at intervals as long as two or three days may be sufficient. Hydrocortisone with neomycin ointment 2.5% is recommended for beginning treatment of more severe types of dermatoses and the 1% or 0.5% strengths for maintenance therapy. In less severe conditions the 0.5% or 1% concentrations may be employed initially.

HOW SUPPLIED - EQUIVALENTS NOT AVAILABLE:

Ointment - Topical - 10 mg/5 mg

20 gm	$22.31	NEO-CORTEF, Pharmacia & Upjohn	00009-0622-02

HYDROCORTISONE ACETATE; NEOMYCIN SULFATE; POLYMYXIN B SULFATE *(003037)*

CATEGORIES: Adrenal Corticosteroids; Dermatologicals; Dermatoses; Infections; Otic Hydrocortisones; Skin/Mucous Membrane Agents; Skin Infections; Topical; Pregnancy Category C; FDA Approved 1985 Aug

BRAND NAMES: **Cortisporin**; *Cortisporin Otico* (Mexico); *Neosporin-H Ear*, *Oticomycin*; *Otosporin* (Germany, England)
(International brand names outside U.S. in italics)

FORMULARIES: Medi-Cal

DESCRIPTION:

Cortisporin Cream (polymyxin B sulfate-neomycin sulfate- hydrocortisone acetate) is a topical antibacterial cream. Each gram contains: polymyxin B sulfate 10,000 units, neomycin sulfate equivalent to 3.5 mg neomycin base, and hydrocortisone acetate 5 mg (0.5%). The inactive ingredients are liquid petrolatum, white petrolatum, propylene glycol, polyoxyethylene polyoxypropylene compound, emulsifying wax, purified water, and 0.25% methylparaben added as a preservative. Sodium hydroxide or sulfuric acid may be added to adjust pH.

Polymyxin B sulfate is the sulfate salt of polymyxin B_1 and B_2, which are produced by the growth of*Bacillus polymyxa* (Prazmowski) Migula (Fam. Bacillaceae). It has a potency of not less than 6,000 polymyxin B units per mg, calculated on an anhydrous basis.

Neomycin sulfate is the sulfate salt of neomycin B and C, which are produced by the growth of *Streptomyces fradiae* Waksman (Fam. Streptomycetaceae). It has the potency equivalent of not less than 600 mcg of neomycin standard per mg calculated on an anhydrous basis.

Hydrocortisone acetate is the acetate ester of hydrocortisone, an anti-inflammatory hormone. Its chemical name is 21-(acetyloxy)-11β, 17- dihydroxypregn-4-ene-3,20 dione. The base is a smooth vanishing creme with a pH of approximately 5.0

CLINICAL PHARMACOLOGY:

Corticoids suppress the inflammatory response to a variety of agents and they may delay healing. Since corticoids may inhibit the body's defense mechanism against infection, a concomitant antimicrobial drug may be used when this inhibition is considered to be clinically significant in a particular case.

The anti-infective components in the combination are included to provide action against specific organisms susceptible to them. Polymyxin B sulfate and neomycin sulfate together are considered active against the following microorganisms: *Staphylococcus aureus, Escherichia coli, Haemophilus influenzae, Klebsiella-Enterobacter* species,*Neisseria* species, and *Pseudomonas aeruginosa.* This product does not provide adequate coverage against *Serratia marcescens* and streptococci, including *Streptococcus pneumonia.*

The relative potency of corticosteroids depends on the molecular structure, concentration, and release from the vehicle.

The acid pH helps restore normal cutaneous acidity. Owing to its excellent spreading and penetrating properties, the cream facilitates treatment of hairy and intertriginous areas. It may also be of value in selective cases where the lesions are moist.

INDICATIONS AND USAGE:

For the treatment of corticosteroid-responsive dermatoses with secondary infection. It has not been demonstrated that this steroid-antibiotic combination provides greater benefit than the steroid component alone after 7 days of treatment. (see WARNINGS.)

CONTRAINDICATIONS:

Not for use in the eyes or in the external ear canal if the eardrum is perforated. This product is contraindicated in tuberculous, fungal or viral lesions of the skin (herpes simplex, vaccina and varicella). This product is contraindicated in those individuals who have shown hypersensitivity to any of its components.

WARNINGS:

Because of the concern of nephrotoxicity and ototoxicity associated with neomycin, this combination should not be used over a wide area or for extended periods of time.

PRECAUTIONS:

General: As with any antibacterial preparation, prolonged use may result in overgrowth of nonsusceptible organisms, including fungi. Appropriate measures should be taken if this occurs. Use of steroids on infected areas should be supervised with care as anti-inflammatory steroids may encourage spread of infection. If this occurs, steroid therapy should be stopped and appropriate antibacterial drugs used. Generalized dermatological conditions may require systemic therapy.

Signs and symptoms of exogenous hyperadrenocorticism can occur with the use of topical corticosteroids, including adrenal suppression. Systemic absorption of topically applied steroids will be increased if extensive body surface areas are treated or if occlusive dressings are used. Under these circumstances, suitable precautions should be taken when long term use is anticipated.

Information for the Patient: Avoid contaminating the dropper with material from the ear, fingers, or other source. This caution is necessary if the sterility of the drops is to be preserved.

If sensitization or irritation occurs, discontinue use immediately and contact your physician.

Laboratory Tests: Systemic effects of excessive levels of hydrocortisone may include a reduction in the number of circulating eosinophils and a decrease in urinary excretion of 17-hydroxycorticosteroids.

Carcinogenesis, Mutagenesis, and Impairment of Fertility: Long-term studies in animals (rats, rabbits, mice) showed no evidence of carcinogenicity attributable to oral administration of corticosteroids.

Pregnancy: Teratogenic effects: Pregnancy Category C. Corticosteroids have been shown to be teratogenic in rabbits when applied topically at concentrations of 0.5% on days 6 to 18 of gestation and in mice when applied topically at a concentration of 15% on days 10 to 13 of gestation. There are no adequate and well-controlled studies in pregnant women. Corticosteroids should be used during pregnancy only if the potential benefit justifies the potential risk to the fetus.

Nursing Mothers: Hydrocortisone appears in human milk following oral administration of the drug. Since systemic absorption of hydrocortisone may occur when applied topically, caution should be exercised when Cortisporin Otic Suspension is used by a nursing woman.

Pediatric Use: Sufficient percutaneous absorption of hydrocortisone can occur in infants and children during prolonged use to cause cessation of growth as well as other systemic signs and symptoms of hyperadrenocorticism.

ADVERSE REACTIONS:

Neomycin occasionally causes skin sensitization. Ototoxicity and nephrotoxicity have also been reported (See WARNINGS.) Adverse reactions have occurred with topical use of antibiotic combinations including neomycin and polymyxin B. Exact incidence figures are not available since no denominator of treated patients is available. The reaction occurring most often is allergic sensitization. In one clinical study, using a 20% neomycin patch, neomycin-induced allergic skin reactions occurred in two of 2,175 (0.09%) individuals in the general population. In another study, the incidence was found to be approximately 1%.

The following local adverse reactions have been reported with local topical corticosteroids, especially under occlusive dressings: burning, itching, irritation, dryness, folliculitis, hypertrichosis, acneform eruptions, hypopigmentation, perioral dermatitis, maceration of the skin, secondary infection, skin atrophy, striae, and miliaria.

When steroid preparations are used for long periods of time in intertriginous areas or over extensive body areas, with or without occlusive non-permeable dressings, striae may occur; also there exists the possibility of systemic side effects when steroid preparations are used over large areas for a long period of time.

DOSAGE AND ADMINISTRATION:

A small quantity of the cream should be applied 2 to 4 times daily, as required. The cream should, if conditions permit, be gently rubbed into the affected areas.

Store at 15-25°C (59° to 77°F).

REFERENCES:

1 Leyden JJ, Kligman AM. Contact dermatitis to neomycin sulfate. *JAMA* 1979;242(12):1276-1278. 2 Prystowsky SD, Allen AM, Smith RW, et al: Allergic contact hypersensitivity to nickel, neomycin, ethylenediamine, and benzocaine. *Arch Dermatol* 1979;115:959-962.

HOW SUPPLIED - EQUIVALENTS NOT AVAILABLE:

Cream - Topical - 5 mg/10000 unit

7.5 gm $17.38 CORTISPORIN, Glaxo Wellcome 00173-0185-98

HYDROCORTISONE ACETATE; OXYTETRACYCLINE HYDROCHLORIDE

(001479)

CATEGORIES: Adrenal Corticosteroids; Anti-Infectives; Antibacterials; Antibiotics; Burns; Corneal Injury; EENT Drugs; Edema; Eye, Ear, Nose, & Throat Preparations; Inflammation; Inflammatory Conditions; Ocular Infections; Ophthalmics; Steroids; Uveitis; FDA Approval Pre 1982

BRAND NAMES: **Terra-Cortril**; *Terracortril; Terracortril Eye Ear Suspension (International brand names outside U.S. in italics)*

DESCRIPTION:

Terra-Cortril suspension combines the antibiotic, oxytetracycline HCl ($C_{22}H_{24}N_2O_9$.HCl) and the adrenocorticoid, hydrocortisone acetate ($C_{23}H_{32}O_6$). **Each ml of Terra-Cortril contains Terramycin (oxytetracycline HCl) equivalent to 5 mg of oxytetracycline, and 15 mg of Cortril (hydrocortisone acetate) incorporated in mineral oil with aluminum tristearate.**

For Ophthalmic Use Only.

CLINICAL PHARMACOLOGY:

Corticosteroids suppress the inflammatory response to a variety of agents and they probably delay or slow healing. Since corticoids may inhibit the body's defense mechanism against infection, a concomitant antimicrobial drug may be used when this inhibition is considered to be clinically significant in a particular case.

The anti-infective component in the combination is included to provide action against specific organisms susceptible to it.

Oxytetracycline HCl is considered active against the following microorganisms:

Rickettsiae (Rocky Mountain spotted fever, typhus fever and the typhus group, Q fever, rickettsialpox and tick fevers),

Mycoplasma pneumoniae (PPLO, Eaton Agent),

Agents of psittacosis and ornithosis,

Agents of lymphogranuloma venereum and granuloma inguinale,

The spirochetal agent of relapsing fever (*Borrelia recurrentis*).

The following gram-negative microorganisms:

Haemophilus ducreyi (chancroid),

Pasteurella pestis and Pasteurella tularensis,

Bartonella bacilliformis,

Bacteroides species,

Vibrio comma and Vibrio fetus,

Brucella species (in conjunction with streptomycin).

Because many strains of the following groups of microorganisms have been shown to be resistant to tetracyclines, culture and susceptibility testing are recommended.

Oxytetracycline is indicated for treatment of infections caused by the following gram-negative microorganisms, when bacteriologic testing indicates appropriate susceptibility to the drug:

Escherichia coli,

Enterobacter aerogenes (formerly *Aerobacter aerogenes*),

Shigella species,

Mima species and *Herellea* species,

Haemophilus influenzae (respiratory infections),

Klebsiella species (respiratory and urinary infections).

Oxytetracycline is indicated for treatment of infections caused by the following gram-positive microorganisms when bacteriologic testing indicates appropriate susceptibility to the drug:

Streptococcus species:

Up to 44 percent of strains of *Streptococcus pyogenes* and 74 percent of *Streptococcus faecalis* have been found to be resistant to tetracycline drugs. Therefore, tetracyclines should not be used for streptococcal disease unless the organism has been demonstrated to be sensitive.

For upper respiratory infections due to Group A beta-hemolytic streptococci, penicillin is the usual drug of choice, including prophylaxis of rheumatic fever.

Diplococcus pneumoniae,

Staphylococcus aureus, skin and soft tissue infections. Oxytetracycline is not the drug of choice in the treatment of any type of staphylococcal infections.

CLINICAL PHARMACOLOGY: *(cont'd)*

When penicillin is contraindicated, tetracyclines are alternative drugs in the treatment of infections due to:

Neisseria gonorrhoeae,

Treponema pallidum and *Treponema pertenue* (syphilis and yaws),

Listeria monocytogenes,

Clostridium species,

Bacillus anthracis,

Fusobacterium fusiforme (Vincent's infection),

Actinomyces species.

Tetracyclines are indicated in the treatment of trachoma, although the infectious agent is not always eliminated, as judged by immunofluorescence.

Inclusion conjunctivitis may be treated with oral tetracyclines or with a combination of oral and topical agents.

When a decision to administer both a corticoid and an antimicrobial is made, the administration of such drugs in combination has the advantage of greater patient compliance and convenience, with the added assurance that the appropriate dosage of both drugs is administered, plus assured compatibility of ingredients when both types of drug are in the same formulation and, particularly, that the correct volume of drug is delivered and retained.

The relative potency of corticosteroids depends on the molecular structure, concentration, and release from the vehicle.

INDICATIONS AND USAGE:

For steroid-responsive inflammatory ocular conditions for which a corticosteroid is indicated and where bacterial infection or a risk of bacterial ocular infection exists.

Ocular steroids are indicated in inflammatory conditions of the palpebral and bulbar conjunctiva, cornea, and anterior segment of the globe where the inherent risk of steroid use in certain infective conjunctivitides is accepted to obtain a diminution in edema and inflammation. They are also indicated in chronic anterior uveitis and corneal injury from chemical radiation, thermal burns, or penetration of foreign bodies.

The use of a combination drug with an anti-infective component is indicated where the risk of infection is high or where there is an expectation that potentially dangerous numbers of bacteria will be present in the eye.

The particular anti-infective drug in this product is active against the following common bacterial eye pathogens:

Staphylococcus aureus

Streptococci, including *Streptococcus pneumoniae*

Escherichia coli

Neisseria species

The product does not provide adequate coverage against:

Haemophilus influenzae

Klebsiella/Enterobacter species

Pseudomonas aeruginosa

Serratia marcescens

CONTRAINDICATIONS:

Epithelial herpes simplex keratitis (dendritic keratitis), vaccinia, varicella, and many other viral diseases of the cornea and conjunctiva. Mycobacterial infection of the eye. Fungal diseases of ocular structures. Hypersensitivity to a component of the medication. (Hypersensitivity to the antibiotic component occurs at a higher rate than for other components.)

The use of these combinations is always contraindicated after uncomplicated removal of a corneal foreign body.

WARNINGS:

Prolonged use may result in glaucoma, with damage to the optic nerve, defects in visual acuity and fields of vision, and posterior subcapsular cataract formation. Prolonged use may suppress the host response and thus increase the hazard of secondary ocular infections. In those diseases causing thinning of the cornea or sclera, perforations have been known to occur with the use of topical steroids. In acute purulent conditions of the eye, steroids may mask infection or enhance existing infection. If these products are used for 10 days or longer, intraocular pressure should be routinely monitored even though it may be difficult in children and uncooperative patients.

Employment of steroid medication in the treatment of herpes simplex requires great caution.

PRECAUTIONS:

The initial prescription and renewal of the medication order beyond 20 milliliters should be made by a physician only after examination of the patient with the aid of magnification, such as slit lamp biomicroscopy and, where appropriate, fluorescein staining.

The possibility of persistent fungal infections of the cornea should be considered after prolonged steroid dosing.

ADVERSE REACTIONS:

Adverse reactions have occurred with steroid/anti-infective combination drugs which can be attributed to the steroid component, the anti-infective component, or the combination. Exact incidence figures are not available since no denominator of treated patients is available.

Reactions occurring most often from the presence of the anti-infective ingredient are allergic sensitizations. The reactions due to the steroid component in decreasing order of frequency are: elevation of intraocular pressure (IOP) with possible development of glaucoma, and infrequent optic nerve damage; posterior subcapsular cataract formation; and delayed wound healing.

Secondary Infection: The development of secondary infection has occurred after use of combinations containing steroids and antimicrobials. Fungal infections of the cornea are particularly prone to develop coincidentally with long-term applications of steroid. The possibility of fungal invasion must be considered in any persistent corneal ulceration where steroid treatment has been used.

Secondary bacterial ocular infection following suppression of host responses also occurs.

DOSAGE AND ADMINISTRATION:

Instill 1 or 2 drops of Terra-Cortril Ophthalmic Suspension into the affected eye three times daily.

Not more than 20 milliliters should be prescribed initially and the prescription should not be refilled without further evaluation as outlined in PRECAUTIONS above.

HOW SUPPLIED - EQUIVALENTS NOT AVAILABLE:

Suspension - Ophthalmic - 1.5 %

5 ml	$18.43	TERRA-CORTRIL, Roerig	00049-0670-48

HYDROCORTISONE ACETATE; PRAMOXINE HYDROCHLORIDE *(001480)*

CATEGORIES: Anesthesia; Anorectal Products; Anti-Inflammatory Agents; Antipruritics/Local Anesthetics; Dermatologicals; Dermatoses; EENT Drugs; Eye, Ear, Nose, & Throat Preparations; Gastrointestinal Drugs; Glucocorticoids; Hormones; Mucous Membrane Agents; Otic Hydrocortisones; Otic Preparations; Otologic; Pruritus; Skin/Mucous Membrane Agents; Steroids; Topical Anesthetics; Pregnancy Category C; FDA Approval Pre 1982

BRAND NAMES: Analpram-Hc; Cortane; Derma-Sone; Enzone; **Epifoam**; Oticol; Pramosone; *Prasone*; Proctocream-Hc; *Proctofoam* (England, Germany); Proctofoam-Hc; *Proctofoam-HC*; Zone-A
(International brand names outside U.S. in italics)

FORMULARIES: Aetna; BC-BS

DESCRIPTION:

A topical corticosteroid in an aerosol foam containing hydrocortisone acetate 1% and pramoxine hydrochloride 1% in a base containing: propylene glycol, cetyl alcohol, glyceryl stearate, PEG-100 stearate, laureth-23, polyoxyl-40 stearate, methylparaben, propylparaben, trolamine or hydrochloric acid to adjust pH, purified water, propellants (inert): butane and propane.

This drug contains a synthetic steroid used as an anti-inflammatory and anti-pruritic agent, and a local anesthetic. Molecular weight: Hydrocortisone acetate 404.51. Solubility of hydrocortisone acetate in water: 1 mg/100 ml. Chemical name: Pregn-4-ene,3,20-dione, 21-(acetyloxy)-11, 17-dihydroxy-(11β).

CLINICAL PHARMACOLOGY:

Topical corticosteroids share anti-inflammatory, anti-pruritic and vasoconstrictive actions.

The mechanism of anti-inflammatory activity of the topical corticosteroids is unclear. Various laboratory methods, including vasoconstrictor assays, are used to compare and predict potencies and/or clinical efficacies of the topical corticosteroids. There is some evidence to suggest that a recognizable correlation exists between vasoconstrictor potency and therapeutic efficacy in man.

PRAMOXINE HYDROCHLORIDE

A surface or local anesthetic which is not chemically related to the "caine" types of local anesthetics. Its unique chemical structure is likely to minimize the danger of cross-sensitivity reactions in patients allergic to other local anesthetics.

PHARMACOKINETICS

The extent of percutaneous absorption of topical corticosteroids is determined by many factors including the vehicle, the integrity of the epidermal barrier, and the use of occlusive dressings.

Topical corticosteroids can be absorbed from normal intact skin. Inflammation and/or disease processes in the skin increase the percutaneous absorption of topical corticosteroids. Occlusive dressings substantially increase the percutaneous absorption of topical corticosteroids. Thus, occlusive dressings may be a valuable therapeutic adjunct for treatment of resistant dermatoses. (See DOSAGE AND ADMINISTRATION.)

Once absorbed through the skin, topical corticosteroids are handled through pharmacokinetic pathways similar to systemically administered corticosteroids. Corticosteroids are bound to plasma proteins in varying degrees. Corticosteroids are metabolized primarily in the liver and are then excreted by the kidneys. Some of the topical corticosteroids and their metabolites are also excreted into the bile.

INDICATIONS AND USAGE:

Topical corticosteroids are indicated for the relief of the inflammatory and pruritic manifestations of corticosteroid-responsive dermatoses.

CONTRAINDICATIONS:

Topical corticosteroid products are contraindicated in those patients with a history of hypersensitivity to any of the components of the preparation.

WARNINGS:

Not for prolonged use. If redness, pain irritation or swelling persists, discontinue use and consult a physician. Contents of the container are under pressure, but not flammable. Do not burn or puncture the aerosol container. Store at temperatures below 120°F. Keep this and all medicines out of the reach of children.

PRECAUTIONS:

GENERAL

Systemic absorption of topical corticosteroids has produced reversible hypothalamic-pituitary-adrenal (HRA) axis suppression, manifestations of Cushing's syndrome, hyperglycemia and glucosuria in some patients.

Conditions which augment systemic absorption include the application of the more potent steroids, use over large surface areas, prolonged use and the addition of occlusive dressings.

Therefore, patients receiving a large dose of a potent topical steroid applied to a large surface area or under an occlusive dressing should be evaluated periodically for evidence of HPA axis suppression by using the urinary hydrocortisone and ACTH stimulation tests. If HPA axis suppression is noted, an attempt should be made to withdraw the drug, to reduce the frequency of application, or to substitute a less potent steroid.

Recovery of HPA axis function is generally prompt and complete upon discontinuation of the drug. Infrequently, signs and symptoms of steroid withdrawal may occur, requiring supplemental systemic corticosteroids.

In children absorption may result if higher blood levels and thus more susceptibility to systemic toxicity. (See PRECAUTIONS, Pediatric Use.) If irritation develops, topical corticosteroids should be discontinued and appropriate therapy instituted.

In the presence of dermatological infections, the use of an appropriate antifungal or antibacterial agent should be instituted. If a favorable response does not occur promptly, the corticosteroid should be discontinued until the infection has been adequately controlled.

INFORMATION FOR THE PATIENT

Patient using topical corticosteroids should receive the following information and instructions:

PRECAUTIONS: *(cont'd)*

1. This medication is to be used as directed by the physician. It is for external use only. Avoid contact with the eyes.

2. Do not use this medication for any disorder other than for which it has been prescribed.

3. The treated skin area should not be bandaged or otherwise covered or wrapped as to be occlusive unless directed by the physician.

4. Report any signs of local adverse reactions especially under occlusive dressings.

5. Do not use any tight fitting diapers or plastic pants on a child being treated in the diaper area, as these garments may constitute occlusive dressings.

LABORATORY TESTS

The following tests may be helpful in evaluating the HPA axis suppression:

Urinary hydrocortisone test

ACTH stimulation test

CARCINOGENESIS, MUTAGENESIS, AND IMPAIRMENT OF FERTILITY

Long-term animal studies have not been performed to evaluate carcinogenic potential or the effect on fertility of topical corticosteroids.

Studies to determine mutagenicity with prednisolone and hydrocortisone have revealed negative results.

PREGNANCY CATEGORY C

Corticosteroids are generally teratogenic in laboratory animals when administered systemically at relatively low dosage levels. The more potent corticosteroids have been shown to be teratogenic after dermal application in laboratory animals. There are no adequate and well-controlled studies in pregnant women of teratogenic effects from topically applied corticosteroids. Therefore, topical corticosteroids should be used during pregnancy only if the potential benefit justifies the potential risk to the fetus. Drugs of those class should not be used extensively on pregnant patients, in large amounts, or for prolonged periods of time.

NURSING MOTHERS

It is not known whether topical administration of corticosteroids could result in sufficient systemic absorption to produce detectable quantities in breast milk. Systemically administered corticosteroids into breast milk in quantities not likely to have a deleterious effect on the infant. Caution should be exercised when any topical corticosteroids are administered to a nursing woman.

PEDIATRIC USE

Pediatric patients may demonstrate greater susceptibility to topical corticosteroid-induced HPA axis suppression and Cushing's syndrome than mature patients because of a large skin surface area to body weight ratio.

Hypothalamic-pituitary-adrenal (HPA) axis suppression, Cushing's syndrome and intracranial hypertension have been reported in children receiving topical corticosteroids. Manifestations of adrenal suppression in children include liner growth retardation, delayed weight gain, low plasma cortisone levels and absence of response to ACTH stimulation. Manifestations of intracranial hypertension include bulging fontanelles, headaches and bilateral papilledema.

Administration of topical corticosteroids to children should be limited to the least amount compatible with an effective therapeutic regimen. Chronic corticosteroid therapy may interfere with the growth and development of children.

ADVERSE REACTIONS:

The following local adverse reactions are reported infrequently with topical corticosteroids, but may occur more frequently with the use of occlusive dressings. These reactions are listed in an approximate decreasing order of occurrence:

Burring, Itching, Irritation, Dryness, Folliculitis, Hypopigmentation, Perioral dermatitis, Allergic contact dermatitis, Maceration of the skin, Secondary infection, Skin atrophy, Striae, Miliaria.

OVERDOSAGE:

Topically applied corticosteroids can be absorbed in sufficient amounts to produce systemic effects. (See PRECAUTIONS.)

DOSAGE AND ADMINISTRATION:

Apply of affected area 3 or 4 times daily.

Directions for Use

1. Shake foam container vigorously before use.

2. Hold container upright and dispense medication onto a pad by depressing the container cap several times. A small amount of foam is all that is needed on the pad. Apply to affected areas. Alternatively, the foam may be applied directly to affected areas.

3. The container and cap should be disassembled and rinsed with warm water after use.

NOTE: The aerosol container should never be inserted into the vagina or anus.

HOW SUPPLIED - EQUIVALENTS NOT AVAILABLE:

Aerosol, Foam - Rectal - 1 %/1 %

10 gm	$11.49	Pramoxine Hcl W/Hydrocortisone, HL Moore Drug Exch	00839-7535-90
10 gm	$11.51	Pramoxine Hcl W/Hydrocortisone, Qualitest Pharms	00603-1565-72
10 gm	$11.70	Hydrocortisone Acetate/Pramoxine, Copley Pharm	38245-0624-05
10 gm	$15.03	Pramoxine Hc, Rugby	00536-2145-19

Aerosol, Foam - Topical - 1 %/1 %

10 gm	**$11.68**	**EPIFOAM, Reed & Carnrick**	**00021-0740-10**
10 gm	$23.20	PROCTOFOAM HC, Reed & Carnrick	00021-0690-10

Cream - Rectal - 1 %

28.35 gm	$17.95	RECTOCORT-HC, Econolab	55053-0156-30
30 gm	$14.65	ANALPRAM-HC, Ferndale Labs	00496-0778-04

Cream - Rectal; Topical - 0.5 %/1 %

30 gm	$14.14	DIBUCORT, H N Norton Co.	50732-0780-30

Cream - Rectal; Topical - 2.5 %/1 %

30 gm	$21.55	ANALPRAM-HC 2.5%, Ferndale Labs	00496-0800-04

Cream - Topical - 1 %/1 %

15 gm	$15.96	ZONE-A, UAD Labs	00785-5505-04
30 gm	$8.80	PRAMOSONE, Ferndale Labs	00496-0716-04
30 gm	$17.18	PROCTOCREAM-HC, Reed & Carnrick	00021-4620-10
30 gm	$18.24	ENZONE, UAD Labs	00785-5510-04
60 gm	$14.00	PRAMOSONE, Ferndale Labs	00496-0716-03

Cream - Topical - 2.5 %/1 %

30 gm	$17.55	PRAMASONE, Ferndale Labs	00496-0717-04
60 gm	$28.10	PRAMASONE, Ferndale Labs	00496-0717-03

HOW SUPPLIED - EQUIVALENTS NOT AVAILABLE: *(cont'd)*

Lotion - Topical - 1 %/1 %

60 ml	$14.75	PRAMOSONE, Ferndale Labs	00496-0729-06
60 ml	$17.50	ZONE-A, UAD Labs	00785-5500-02
120 ml	$23.50	PRAMOSONE, Ferndale Labs	00496-0729-04
240 ml	$37.60	PRAMOSONE, Ferndale Labs	00496-0729-03

Lotion - Topical - 2.5 %/1 %

60 ml	$21.84	ZONE-A-FORTE, UAD Labs	00785-5502-02
60 ml	$26.10	PRAMOSONE, Ferndale Labs	00496-0726-06
120 ml	$41.75	PRAMOSONE, Ferndale Labs	00496-0726-04

Ointment - Topical - 1 %

30 gm	$10.35	PRAMOSONE, Ferndale Labs	00496-0763-04

Ointment - Topical - 2.5 %

30 gm	$18.90	PRAMOSONE, Ferndale Labs	00496-0777-04

HYDROCORTISONE ACETATE; UREA *(001481)*

CATEGORIES: Anti-Inflammatory Agents; Dermatologicals; Dermatoses; Pruritus; Skin/Mucous Membrane Agents; Steroids; FDA Approval Pre 1982

BRAND NAMES: Alphaderm; Calmurid Hc; Carmol Hc; **Carmol-Hc**; *Handlife*; Lidex; *Sential* (Canada)
(International brand names outside U.S. in italics)

FORMULARIES: BC-BS

DESCRIPTION:

The topical corticosteroids constitute a class of primarily synthetic steroids used as anti-inflammatory and antipruritic agents. Hydrocortisone acetate cream is a member of this class. Hydrocortisone Acetate has the chemical name pregn-4-ene-3,20-dione,21-(acetyloxy)-11, 17-dihydroxy-11β)-. It has a Molecular Weight of 404.50. The Molecular Formula is $C_{23}H_{32}O_6$.

Each gram of the cream contains 10 mg Hydrocortisone Acetate, USP in a water-washable vanishing cream base containing urea (10%), purified water, stearic acid, propylene glycol, isopropyl myristate, isopropyl palmitate, PPG-26 oleate, sodium laureth sulfate, triethanolamine, xanthan gum, sodium bisulfite, cetyl alcohol, edetate disodium, carbomer 940 with hypoallergenic perfume. It is non-occlusive, and contains no mineral oil, petrolatum, lanolin or parabens.

CLINICAL PHARMACOLOGY:

Topical corticosteroids share anti-inflammatory, anti-pruritic and vasoconstrictive actions.

The mechanism of anti-inflammatory activity of the topical corticosteroids is unclear. Various laboratory methods, including vasoconstrictor assays, are used to compare and predict potencies and/or clinical efficacies of the topical corticosteroids. There is some evidence to suggest that a recognizable correlation exists between vasoconstrictor potency and therapeutic efficacy in man.

Pharmacokinetics: The extent of percutaneous absorption of topical corticosteroids is determined by many factors including the vehicle, the integrity of the epidermal barrier, and the use of occlusive dressings.

Topical corticosteroids can be absorbed from normal intact skin. Inflammation and/or other disease processes in the skin increase percutaneous absorption. Occlusive dressings substantially increase the percutaneous absorption of topical corticosteroids. Thus, occlusive dressings may be a valuable therapeutic adjunct for treatment of resistant dermatoses. (See DOSAGE AND ADMINISTRATION.)

Once absorbed through the skin, topical corticosteroids are handled through pharmacokinetic pathways similar to systemically administered corticosteroids. Corticosteroids are bound to plasma proteins in varying degrees. Corticosteroids are metabolized primarily in the liver and are then excreted by the kidneys. Some of the topical corticosteroids and their metabolites are also excreted into the bile.

INDICATIONS AND USAGE:

Hydrocortisone acetate-urea cream is indicated for the relief of the inflammatory and pruritic manifestations of corticosteroid-responsive dermatoses.

CONTRAINDICATIONS:

Topical corticosteroids are contraindicated in those patients with a history of hypersensitivity to any of the components of the preparation.

WARNINGS:

Hydrocortisone acetate-urea contains sodium bisulfite, a sulfite that may cause allergic-type reactions including anaphylactic symptoms and life-threatening or less severe asthmatic episodes in certain susceptible people. The overall prevalence of sulfite sensitivity in the general population is unknown and probably low. Sulfite sensitivity is seen more frequently in asthmatic than in non-asthmatic people.

PRECAUTIONS:

General: Systemic absorption of topical corticosteroids has produced reversible hypothalamic-pituitary-adrenal (HPA) axis suppression, manifestations of Cushing's syndrome, hyperglycemia, and glucosuria in some patients.

Conditions which augment systemic absorption include the application of the more potent steroids, use over large surface areas, prolonged use, and the addition of occlusive dressings.

Therefore, patients receiving a large dose of a potent topical corticosteroid applied to large surface area or under an occlusive dressing, should be evaluated periodically for evidence of HPA axis suppression by using the urinary free cortisol and ACTH stimulation tests. If HPA axis suppression is noted, an attempt should be made to withdraw the drug, to reduce the frequency of application, or to substitute a less potent steroid.

Recovery of HPA axis function is generally prompt and complete upon discontinuation of the drug. Infrequently, signs and symptoms of steroid withdrawal may occur requiring supplemental systemic corticosteroids.

Children may absorb proportionately larger amounts of topical corticosteroids and thus be more susceptible to systemic toxicity. (See PRECAUTIONS, Pediatric Use.)

If irritation develops, topical corticosteroids should be discontinued and appropriate therapy instituted.

In the presence of dermatological infections, the use of an appropriate antifungal or antibacterial agent should be instituted. If a favorable response does not occur promptly, the corticosteroid should be discontinued until the infection has been adequately controlled.

Information for the Patient: Patients using topical corticosteroids should receive the following information and instructions:

PRECAUTIONS: *(cont'd)*

1. This medication is to be used as directed by the physician. It is for external use only. Avoid contact with the eyes.

2. Patients should be advised not to use this medication for any disorder other than for which it was prescribed.

3. The treated skin area should not be bandaged or otherwise covered or wrapped as to be occlusive unless directed by the physician.

4. Patients should report any signs of local adverse reactions especially under occlusive dressing.

5. Parents of pediatric patients should be advised not to use tight-fitting diapers or plastic paints on a child being treated in the diaper area, as these garments may constitute occlusive dressings.

Laboratory Tests: The following tests may be helpful in evaluating the HPA axis suppression:
Urinary free cortisol test
ACTH stimulation test

Carcinogenesis, Mutagenesis, and Impairment of Fertility: Long-term animal studies have not been performed to evaluate the carcinogenic potential or the effect on fertility of topical corticosteroids.

Studies to determine mutagenicity with prednisolone and hydrocortisone have revealed negative results.

Pregnancy Category C: Corticosteroids are generally teratogenic in laboratory animals when administered systemically at relatively low dosage levels. The more potent corticosteroids have been shown to be teratogenic after dermal application in laboratory animals. There are no adequate and well-controlled studies in pregnant women on teratogenic effects from topically applied corticosteroids. Therefore, topical corticosteroids should be used during pregnancy only if the potential benefit justifies the potential risk to the fetus. Drugs of this class should not be used extensively on pregnant patients, in large amounts, or for prolonged periods of time.

Nursing Mothers: It is not known whether topical corticosteroids could result in sufficient systemic absorption to produce detectable quantities in breast milk. Systemically administered corticosteroids are secreted into breast milk in quantities *not* likely to have a deleterious effect on the infant. Nevertheless, caution should be exercised when topical corticosteroids are administered to a nursing woman.

Pediatric Use: *Pediatric patients may demonstrate greater susceptibility to topical corticosteroid-induced HPA axis suppression and Cushing's syndrome than mature patients because of a large skin surface area to body weight ratio.*

Hypothalamic-pituitary-adrenal (HPA) axis suppression, Cushing's syndrome, and intracranial hypertension have been reported in children receiving topical corticosteroids. Manifestations of adrenal suppression in children include linear growth retardation, delayed weight gain, low plasma cortisol levels, and absence of response to ACTH stimulation. Manifestations of intracranial hypertension include bulging fontanelles, headaches, and bilateral papilledema.

Administration of topical corticosteroids to children should be limited to the least amount compatible with an effective therapeutic regimen. Chronic corticosteroid therapy may interfere with the growth and development of children.

ADVERSE REACTIONS:

The following local adverse reactions are reported infrequently with topical corticosteroids, but may occur more frequently with the use of occlusive dressings. These reactions are listed in an approximate decreasing order of occurrence:

Burning, itching, irritation, dryness, folliculitis, hypertrichosis, acneiform eruptions, hypopigmentation, perioral dermatitis, allergic contact dermatitis, maceration of the skin, secondary infection, skin atrophy, striae, miliaria.

OVERDOSAGE:

Topically applied corticosteroids can be absorbed in sufficient amounts to produce systemic effects (See PRECAUTIONS.)

DOSAGE AND ADMINISTRATION:

Hydrocortisone acetate-urea cream is generally applied to the affected areas as a thin film from two to four times daily depending on the severity of the condition.

Occlusive dressings may be used for the management of psoriasis or recalcitrant conditions.

If an infection develops, the use of occlusive dressings should be discontinued an appropriate antimicrobial therapy instituted.

Store at controlled room temperature 15°-30°C (59°-86°F).

Protect from freezing.

Storage: Dispense in tight containers as specified in USP.

(Doak Dermatologics, MG #10769)

HOW SUPPLIED - RATED THERAPEUTICALLY EQUIVALENT:

Cream - Topical - 1 %

30 gm	$11.94	CARMOL HC, Doak Dermatologics	10337-0550-52

HYDROCORTISONE BUTEPRATE *(003333)*

CATEGORIES: Antipruritics/Local Anesthetics; Dermatoses; Inflammation; Topical; Vasoconstrictors; Pregnancy Category C; FDA Approved 1997 Feb

BRAND NAMES: **Pandel**

DESCRIPTION:

Pandel Cream contains hydrocortisone buteprate, a synthetic adrenocorticosteroid, for dermatologic use. The topical corticosteroids constitute a class of primarily synthetic steroids used as anti-inflammatory and anti-pruitic agents.

Hydrocortisone buteprate is a tasteless and odorless white crystalline powder practically insoluble in hexane or water, slightly soluble in ether, and very soluble in dichloromethane, methanol and acetone. Chemically, it is 11β,17,21-trihydroxypregn-4-ene-3,20-dione 17-butyrate 21-propionate.

The molecular formula is $C_{28}H_{40}O_7$. The molecular weight is 488.62.

Each gram of Pandel (hydrocortisone buteprate cream) Cream, 0.1% contains: 1 mg of hydrocortisone buteprate in a cream base of propylene glycol, white petrolatum, light mineral oil, stearyl alcohol, polysorbate 60, sorbitan monostearate, glyceryl monostearate, PEG-20 stearate, glyceryl stearate SE, methylparaben, butylparaben, citric acid anhydrous, sodium citrate anhydrous, and purified water.

CLINICAL PHARMACOLOGY:

Topical corticosteroids share anti-inflammatory, anti-pruritic and vasoconstrictive actions. The mechanism of anti-inflammatory activity of the topical corticosteroids is unclear. However, corticosteroids are thought to act by the induction of phospholipase A_2 inhibitory proteins, collectively called lipocortins. It is postulated that these proteins control the biosynthesis of potent rnediators of inflammation such as prostaglandins and leukotrienes by inhibiting the release of their common precursor arachidonic acid. Arachidonic acid is released from membrane phospholipids by phospholipase A_2.

Pharmacokinetics: The extent of percutaneous absorption of topical corticosteroids is determined by many factors, including the vehicle and the integrity of the epidermal barrier. Use of occlusive dressings with hydrocortisone for up to 24 hours has not been shown to increase penetration; however, occlusion of hydrocortisone for 96 hours does markedly enhance penetration. Topical corticosteroids can be absorbed from normal intact skin. Inflammation and/or other disease processes in the skin increase percutaneous absorption. Studies performed with hydrocortisone buteprate cream, 0.1% indicate that it is in the medium range of potency compared with other topical corticosteroids

INDICATIONS AND USAGE:

Hydrocortisone buteprate cream, 0.1% is a medium potency corticosteroid indicated for the relief of the inflammatory and pruritic manifestations of corticosteroid responsive dermatoses in patients 18 years of age or older.

CONTRAINDICATIONS:

Hydrocortisone buteprate cream, 0.1% is contraindicated in those patients who are hypersensitive to hydrocortisone buteprate or to any of the components of the preparation.

PRECAUTIONS:

General: Systemic absorption of topical corticosteroids can produce reversible hypothalamic-pituitary-adrenal (HPA) axis suppression with the potential for glucocorticosteroid insufficiency after withdrawal of treatment. Manifestations of Cushing's syndrome, hyperglycemia, and glucosuria can also be produced in some patients by systemic absorption of topical corticosteroids while on treatment.

Patients applying a topical steroid to a large surface area or to areas under occluslon should be evaluated periodically for evidence of HPA-axis suppression. This may be done by using the ACTH stimulation, A.M. plasma cortisol, or urinary free cortisol tests.

If HPA axis suppression is noted, an attempt should be made to withdraw the drug, to reduce the frequency of application, or to substitute a less potent steroid. Recovery of HPA axis function is generally prompt and complete upon discontinuation of the drug. Infrequently, signs and symptoms of steroid withdrawal may occur, requiring supplemental systemic corticosteroids. For information on systemic supplementation, see prescribing information for those products.

Pediatric patients may be more susceptible to systemic toxicity from equivalent doses due to their larger skin surface to body mass ratios. (See PRECAUTIONSPediatric Use).

If irritation develops, hydrocortisone buTepratc cream, 0.1% should be discontinued and appropriate therapy instituted. Allergic contact dermatitis with corticosteroids is usually diagnosed by observing a failure to heal rather than noting a clinical exacerbation, as observed with most topical products not containing corticosteroids. If concomitant skin infections are present or develop, an appropriate antifungal or antibacterial agent should be used. If a favorable response does not occur promptly, use of hydrocortisone buteprate cream, 0.1% should be discontinued until the infection has been adequately controlled.

Information for the Patient: Patients using hydrocortisone buteprate cream, 0.1% should receive the following information and instructions:

1. This medication is to be used as directed by the physician. It is for external use only. Avoid contact with the eyes

2. This medication should not be used for any disorder other than that for which it was prescribed.

3. The treated skin area should not be bandaged or otherwise covered or wrapped so as to be occlusive, unless directed by the physician.

4. Patients should report to their physician any signs of local adverse reactions.

5. Parents of pediatric patients should be advised not to use hydrocortisone buteprate cream, 0.1% in the treatment of diaper dermatitis. Hydrocortisone buteprate cream, 0.1% should not be applied in the diaper area as diapers or plastic pants may constitute occlusive dressings (See DOSAGE AND ADMINISTRATION).

6. This medication should not be used on the face, underarms, or groin areas unless directed by the physician.

7. As with other corticosteroids, therapy should be discontinued when control is achieved. If no improvement is seen within two weeks, contact the physician.

Laboratory Tests: The following tests may be helpful in evaluating if HPA axis suppression does occur:

ACTH stimulation test

A.M. plasma cortisol test

Urinary free Gortisol test

Carcinogenesis, Mutagenesis, and Impairment of Fertility: Long-term animal studies have not been performed to evaluate the carcinogenic potential or the effect on fertility of topical corticosteroids. In two mutagenicity experiments using hydrocortisone buteprate, negative responses were observed in the occurrence of micronuclei in the bone marrow of mice and in the Ames reverse mutation test bacterial assay with and without metabolic activation.

Pregnancy:Pregnancy Category C: Corticosteroids have been shown to be teratogenic in laboratory animals when administe~ed systemically at relatl~ely low dosage levels. Some corticosteroids have been shown to be teratogenic after dermal application to laboratory animals.

Hydrocortisone buteprate has not been tested for teratogenicity when applied topically; however, it is absorbed percutaneously, and studies in Wistar rats using the subcutaneous route resulted in teratogenicity at dose levels equal to or greater than 1 mg/kg. This dose is approximately 12 times the human average topical dose of hydrocortisone buteprate cream, 0.1% assuming 3% absorption and an application of 30 g/day on a 70 kg individual. Abnormalities seen included delayed ossification of the caudal vertebrae and other skeletal variations, cleft palate, umbilical hernia, edema. and exencephalia.

In rabbits, hydrocortisone buteprate given by the subeutaneous route was teratogenic at doses equal to or greater than 0.1 mg/kg. This dose is approximately 2 times the human average topical dose of hydrocortisone buteprate cream, 0.1% assuming 3% absorption and an application of 30 g/day on a 70 kg individual. Abnormalities seen included delayed ossification of the caudal vertebrae and other skeletal abnormalities, cleft palate and increased fetal mortality.

PRECAUTIONS: *(cont'd)*

The differences between the doses used in animal studies and the proposed human dose may not fully predict the human outcome. The animals received a bolus subcutaneous dose, whereas humans receive a dermal application, where absorption is lower and highly dependent on various factors (*e.g.,* vehicle, integrity of epidermal barrier, occlusion).

There are no adequate and well-controlled studies of the teratogenic potential of hydrocortisone buteprate in pregnant women. Although human epidemiological studies do not indicate an increased incidence of teratogenicity with the use of topical corticosteroids, hydrocortisone butepaprate cream should be used during pregnancy only if the potential benefit justifies the potential risk to the fetus.

Nursing Mothers: Systemically administered corticosteroids appear in human milk and could suppress growth, interfere with endogenous corticosteroid production, or cause other untoward effects. It is not known whether topical administration of corticosteroids could result in sufficient systemic absorption to produce detectable quantities in human milk. Because many drugs are excreted in human milk, caution should be exercised when hydrocortisone buteprate cream, 0.1% is administered to a nursing woman.

Pediatric Use: Safety and effectiveness in pediatric patients have not been established. Because of a higher ratio of skin surface area to body mass, pediatric patients are at a greater risk than adults of HPA axis suppression and Cushing's syndrome when they are treated with topical corticosteroids. They are therefore also at a greater risk of adrenal insufficiency during and/or after withdrawal of treatment. Adverse effects including striae have been reported with inappropriate use of topical corticosteroids in infants and children.

Hypothalamic-pituitary-adrenal (HPA) axis suppression, Cushing's syndrome, linear growth retardation, delayed weight gain, and intracranial hypertension have been reported in children receiving topical corticosteroids. Manifestations of adrenal suppression in children include low plasrna cortisol levels and an absence of response to ACTH stimulation. Manifestations of intracranial hypertension include bulging fontanelles, headaches, and bilateral papilledema.

ADVERSE REACTIONS:

The most frequent adverse reactions reported for hydrocortisone buteprate cream, 0.1% have included burning in 4, stinging in 2, and moderate paresthesia in 1 out of 226 patients.

The following local adverse reactions as reported with topical corticosteroids, and they may occur more frequently with the use of occlusive dressings. These reactions are listed in an approximate decreasing order of occurrence: burning, itching, irritation, dryness, folliculitis, hypertrichosis, acneiform eruptions, hypopigmentation, perioral dermatitis, allergic contact dermatitis, secondary infections, skin atrophy, striae, miliaria.

OVERDOSAGE:

Topically applied corticosteroids can be absorbed in sufficient amounts to produce systemic effects. (See PRECAUTIONS).

DOSAGE AND ADMINISTRATION:

Apply a thin film of hydrocortisone buteprate cream, 0.1% to the affected area once or twice a day depending on the severity of the condition. Massage gently until the medication disappears.

Occlusive dressings may be used for the management of refractory lesions of psoriasis and other deep-seated dermatoses, such as localized neurodermatitis (lichen simplex chronicus).

As with other corticosteroids, therapy should be discontinued when control is achieved If no improvement is seen within 2 weeks, reassessment of the diagnosis may be necessary. Hydrocortisone buteprate cream, 0.1% should not be used with occlusive dressings unless directed by the physician. Hydrocortisone buteprate cream, 0.1% should not be applied in the diaper area, as diapers or plastic pants may constitute occlusive dressings.

HOW SUPPLIED:

Pandel (hydrocortisone buteprate cream) Cream, O.1%, is a white to off-white opaque cream.

Storage: Store at controlled room temperature 15°- 30°C (S9° - 86°F).

HYDROCORTISONE BUTYRATE *(001482)*

CATEGORIES: Anti-Inflammatory Agents; Dermatologicals; Dermatoses; Pruritus; Skin/Mucous Membrane Agents; Steroids; Dermatitis*; Pregnancy Category C; FDA Approved 1983 Jan

* Indication not approved by the FDA

BRAND NAMES: *Alfason* (Germany); *Hyde*; **Locoid**; *Locoidon*; *Plancol*
(International brand names outside U.S. in italics)

DESCRIPTION:

Locoid cream contains the topical corticosteroid, hydrocortisone butyrate, a non-fluorinated ester of hydrocortisone. It has the chemical name: pregn-4-ene-3,20-dione, 11,21-dihydroxy-17-((1-oxobutyi)oxy)-, (11β)-: the empirical formula: $C_{26}H_{26}O_6$; the molecular weight: 432.54 and the CAS registry number: 13609-67-1.

Each gram of Locoid cream contains 1 mg of hydrocortisone butyrate in a hydrophilic base consisting of cetearyl alcohol, ceteth-20, mineral oil, white petrolatum, citric acid, sodium citrate, methyl paraben (preservative) and purified water.

CLINICAL PHARMACOLOGY:

Topical corticosteroids share anti-inflammatory, anti-pruritic and vasoconstrictive actions.

The mechanism of anti-inflammatory activity of the topical corticosteroids is unclear[1]. Various laboratory methods, including vasoconstrictor assays, are used to compare and predict potencies and/or clinical efficacious of the topical corticosteroids[2,3,4]. There is some evidence to suggest that a recognizable correlation exists between vasoconstrictor potency and therapeutic efficacy in man[3].

PHARMACOKINETICS

The extent of percutaneous absorption of topical corticosteroids is determined by many factors including the vehicle, the integrity of the epidermal barrier, and the use of occlusive dressings[5].

Topical corticosteroids can be absorbed from normal intact skin[5]. Inflammation and/or other disease processes in the skin increase percutaneous absorption[5]. Occlusive dressings substantially increase the percutaneous absorption of topical corticosteroids[5,6].

Thus, occlusive dressings may be a valuable therapeutic adjunct for treatment of resistant dermatoses. (See DOSAGE AND ADMINISTRATION.)

Once absorbed through the skin, topical corticosteroids are handled through pharmacokinetic pathways similar to systemically administered corticosteroids. Corticosteroids are bound to plasma proteins in varying degrees. Corticosteroids are metabolized primarily in the liver and are then excreted by the kidneys. Some of the topical corticosteroids and their metabolites are also excreted into the bile.

INDICATIONS AND USAGE:

Locoid cream 0.1% (hydrocortisone butyrate) is indicated for the relief of the inflammatory and pruritic manifestations of corticosteroid-responsive dermatoses[7,8,9,10,11].

CONTRAINDICATIONS:

Topical corticosteroids are contraindicated in those patients with a history of hypersensitivity to any of the components of the preparation.

PRECAUTIONS:

General: Systemic absorption of topical corticosteroids has produced reversible hypothalamic-pituitary-adrenal (HPA) axis suppression, manifestations of Cushing's syndrome, hyperglycemia, and glucosuria in some patients[12].

Conditions which augment systemic absorption include the application of the more potent steroids, use over large surface areas, prolonged use, and the addition of occlusive dressings[13].

Therefore, patients receiving a large dose of a potent topical steroid applied to a large surface area or under an occlusive dressing should be evaluated periodically for evidence of HPA axis suppression by using the urinary free cortisol and ACTH stimulation tests. If HPA axis suppression is noted, an attempt should be made to withdraw the drug, to reduce the frequency of application, or to substitute a less potent steroid.

Recovery of HPA axis function is generally prompt and complete upon discontinuation of the drug[13,14]. Infrequently, signs and symptoms of steroid withdrawal may occur, requiring supplemental systemic corticosteroids[15,16]. Children may absorb proportionally larger amounts of topical corticosteroids and thus be more susceptible to systemic toxicity [17,18] (See PRECAUTIONS, Pediatric Use.)

If irritation develops, topical corticosteroids should be discontinued and appropriate therapy instituted.

In the presence of dermatological infections, the use of an appropriate antifungal or antibacterial agent should be instituted. If a favorable response does not occur promptly, the corticosteroid should be discontinued until the infection has been adequately controlled.

INFORMATION FOR THE PATIENT

Patients using topical corticosteroids should receive the following information and instructions:

1. This medication is to be used as directed by the physician. It is for external use only. Avoid contact with the eyes.
2. Patients should be advised not to use this medication for any disorder other than for which it was prescribed.
3. The treated skin area should not be bandaged or otherwise covered or wrapped as to be occlusive unless directed by the physician.
4. Patients should report any signs of local adverse reactions especially under occlusive dressing.
5. Parents of pediatric patients should be advised not to use tight-fitting diapers or plastic pants on a child being treated in the diaper area, as these garments may constitute occlusive dressings.

LABORATORY TESTS

The following tests may be helpful in evaluating the HPA axis suppression:

Urinary free cortisol test

ACTH stimulation test

CARCINOGENESIS, MUTAGENESIS, AND IMPAIRMENT OF FERTILITY

Long-term animal studies have not been performed to evaluate the carcinogenic potential or the effect on fertility of topical corticosteroids.

Studies to determine mutagenicity with prednisolone and hydrocortisone have revealed negative results [19,20].

PREGNANCY CATEGORY C

Corticosteroids are generally teratogenic in laboratory animals when administered systemically relatively low dosage levels. The more potent corticosteroids have been shown to be teratogenic after dermal application in laboratory animals. There are no adequate and well-controlled studies in pregnant women on teratogenic effects from topically applied corticosteroids. Therefore, topical corticosteroids should be used during pregnancy only if the potential benefit justifies the potential risk to the fetus. Drugs of this class should not be used extensively on pregnant patients, in large amounts, or for prolonged periods of time.

NURSING MOTHERS

It is not known whether topical administration of corticosteroids could result in sufficient systemic absorption to produce detectable quantities in breast milk. Systemically administered corticosteroids are secreted into breast milk in quantities not likely to have a deleterious effect on the infant[21,22]. Nevertheless, caution should be exercised when topical corticosteroids are administered to a nursing woman.

PEDIATRIC USE

Pediatric patients may demonstrate greater susceptibility to topical corticosteroid-induced HPA axis suppression and Cushing's syndrome than mature patients because of a larger skin surface area to body weight ratio.

Hypothalamic-pituitary-adrenal (HPA) axis suppression, Cushing's syndrome, and intracranial hypertension have been reported in children receiving topical corticosteroids. Manifestations of adrenal suppression in children include linear growth retardation, delayed weight gain, low plasma cortisol levels, and absence of response to ACTH stimulation. Manifestations of intracranial hypertension include bulging fontanelles, headaches, and bilateral papilledema.

Administration of topical corticosteroids to children should be limited to the least amount compatible with an effective therapeutic regimen[23]. Chronic corticosteroid therapy may interfere with the growth and development of children.

ADVERSE REACTIONS:

The following local adverse reactions are reported infrequently with topical corticosteroids, but may occur more frequently with the use of occlusive dressings. These reactions are listed in an approximate decreasing order of occurrence: burning, itching, irritation, dryness, folliculitis, hypertrichosis, acneiform eruptions, hypopigmentation, perioral dermatitis, allergic contact dermatitis, maceration of the skin, secondary infection, skin atrophy, striae, miliaria.

OVERDOSAGE:

Topically applied corticosteroids can be absorbed in sufficient amounts to produce systemic effects (See PRECAUTIONS.)

DOSAGE AND ADMINISTRATION:

Locoid cream 0.1% (hydrocortisone butyrate) should be applied to the affected area as a thin film from two to four times daily depending on the severity of the condition. Occlusive dressings may be used for the management of psoriasis or recalcitrant conditions.

If an infection develops, the use of occlusive dressings should be discontinued and appropriate antimicrobial therapy instituted.

DOSAGE AND ADMINISTRATION: *(cont'd)*

Store between 46 and 77°F (8 and 25°C).

REFERENCES:

1. Maibach, H.I. and R.B. Stoughton. 'Topical corticosteroids'. *Medical Clinics of North America*, 57:1253-1264, 1973. **2.** Engel, J.C., et al., 'Topically active corticosteroids (A quantitative evaluation of McKenzie's skin-blanching test)', *Archives of Dermatology*, 109:863-865, 1974. **3.** Barry, B.W., 'Bioavailability of topical steroids', *Dermatologics*, 152 (Supp. 1): 47-65, 1976. **4.** Barry, B.W. and R. Woodford, 'Vasoconstrictor activities and bioavailabilities of seven proprietary corticosteroid creams assessed using a non-occluded multiple dosage regimen; clinical implications', *British Journal of Dermatology*, 97:555-560, 1977. **5.** Kukita, A.K. Yamada and Y. Takeda, 'Systemic effects and percutaneous absorption of topically applied 0.1% hydrocortisone 17-butyrate'. *Dermatologics*, 152 (Supp. 1): 197-207, 1976. **6.** Feldmann, R.J. and H.I. Maibach, 'Penetration of ^{14}C hydrocortisone through normal skin', *Archives of Dermatology*, 91: 661-666, 1965. **7.** Polano, M.K. et al., 'A clinical trial with hydrocortisone butyrate cream in psoriasis' *British Journal of Dermatology*, 83:93-97, 1970. **8.** Ashurst, P.J., 'Hydrocortisone 17-butyrate, a new synthetic topical corticosteroid', *British Journal of Clinical Practice*, 26:263-266, 1972. **9.** Alexander, S. and C. Lyne. 'A preliminary clinical trial of hydrocortisone 17-butyrate'. *British Journal of Clinical Practice*, 27:177-179, 1973. **10.** Polano, M.K. and P. Kanaar, 'A clinical trial with hydrocortisone butyrate cream in eczema', *British Journal of Dermatology*, 88:83-85, 1973. **11.** Gip, L. 'Hydrocortisone 17-butyrate 0.1% cream and fluocinolone acetonide 0.025% cream: a double-blind comparison in patients suffering from psoriasis of the scalp', *Current Therapeutic Research*, 29:198-201, 1981. **12.** Hendrikse, J.C.M. and A.J. Moolenaar, 'Adrenal and pituitary functions during long-term topical steroid therapy', *Dermatologics*, 144:179-186, 1972. **13.** Munro, D.D., 'The effect of percutaneously absorbed steroids on hypothalamic-pituitary-adrenal function after intensive use in in-patients'. *British Journal of Dermatology*, 94 (Supp. 12): 67-76, 1976. **14.** Hendrikse, J.C.M. and A.J. Moolenaar, 'Adrenal suppression with topical hydrocortisone butyrate', *Dermatologics*, 147:191-197, 1973. **15.** Nathan, A.W. and G.L. Rose, 'Fatal iatrogenic Cushing's syndrome'. *Lancet*, 1:207, 1979. **16.** May, P. et al., 'Cushing syndrome from percutaneous absorption of triamcinolone cream', *Archives of Internal Medicine*, 136:612-613, 1976. **17.** Johns, A.M. and B.D. Bower, 'Wasting of napkin area after repeated use of fluorinated steroid ointment', *British Medical Journal*, 1:347-348, 1970. **18.** Feiwel, M.V.H.T. James, and E.S. Barrett,'Effects of potent topical steroids on plasma-cortisol levels of infants and children with eczema', *Lancet*, 1:485-487, 1969. **19.** Seino, Y. et al., 'Mutagenicity of several classes of antitumor agents to Salmonella typhimurium TA 98, TA 100 and TA 92', *Cancer Research*, 38: 2148-2156, 1978. **20.** Hemmerly, J. and M. Demeree, 'Chemical tests for mutagenicity', *Cancer Research*, 15 (Supp. 3): 69-75, 1955. **21.** Mckenzie, S.A., J.A. Selley, and J.E. Agnew, 'Secretion of prednisolone into 'breast milk', *Archives of Disease in Childhood*, 50:894-896, 1975. **22.** Katz, F.H. and B.R. Duncan, 'Entry of prednisone into human milk', *New England Journal of Medicine*, 293:1154, 1975. **23.** Marten, R.H. et al., 'Study of the effects of hydrocortisone and hydrocortisone 17-butyrate ointments on plasma ACTH levels and Synacthen responses in children with eczema' *Dermatologics*, 160:261-269, 1980.

HOW SUPPLIED - EQUIVALENTS NOT AVAILABLE:

Cream - Topical - 0.1 %

15 gm	**$12.95**	**LOCOID, Ferndale Labs**	**00496-0802-15**
45 gm	**$26.95**	**LOCOID, Ferndale Labs**	**00496-0802-45**

Ointment - Topical - 0.1 %

15 gm	**$12.95**	**LOCOID, Ferndale Labs**	**00496-0803-15**
45 gm	**$26.95**	**LOCOID, Ferndale Labs**	**00496-0803-45**

Solution - Topical - 0.1 %

20 ml	**$18.40**	**LOCOID, Ferndale Labs**	**00496-0804-20**
60 ml	**$36.80**	**LOCOID, Ferndale Labs**	**00496-0804-60**

HYDROCORTISONE CYPIONATE *(001483)*

CATEGORIES: Adrenal Corticosteroids; Adrenal Hyperplasia; Adrenocortical Insufficiency; Anemia; Ankylosing Spondylitis; Arthritis; Aspiration Pneumonitis; Asthma; Atopic Dermatitis; Bursitis; Cancer; Carditis; Chemotherapy; Chorioretinitis; Choroiditis; Colitis; Conjunctivitis; Dermatitis; Dermatitis Herpetiformis; Dermatomyositis; Diuresis; Drug Hypersensitivity; Enteritis; Epicondylitis; Erythema Multiforme; Erythroblastopenia; Gouty Arthritis; Herpes; Herpes Zoster; Hormones; Hypercalcemia; Inflammation; Keratitis; Leukemia; Lupus Erythematosus; Meningitis; Mycosis Fungoides; Nephrotic Syndrome; Neuritis; Osteoarthritis; Pemphigus; Pneumonitis; Proteinuria; Psoriasis; Purpura; Rhinitis; Serum Sickness; Spondylitis; Synovitis; Synovitis of Osteoarthritis; Tenosynovitis; Thrombocytopenia; Thrombocytopenic Purpura; Thyroiditis; Trichinosis; Ulcerative Colitis; Uveitis; FDA Approval Pre 1982

BRAND NAMES: Cortef

COST OF THERAPY: $498.80 (Asthma; Suspension; 10 mg/5ml; 10/day; 365 days)

PRIMARY ICD9: 493.90 (Asthma, Unspecified, Without Mention of Status Asthmaticus)

DESCRIPTION:

Cortef Oral Suspension contains hydrocortisone cypionate which is a glucocorticoid. Glucocorticoids are adrenocortical steroids, both naturally occurring and synthetic, which are readily absorbed from the gastrointestinal tract. Hydrocortisone cypionate is the water-insoluble cypionate ester of hydrocortisone. It is both tasteless and odorless, and by the oral route and in equimolar doses, is equivalent to hydrocortisone free alcohol in biologic activity (rat liver-glycogen assay). Determinations of plasma and urinary 17-hydroxycorticoid levels in man following oral administration indicate that this ester is as efficiently absorbed and metabolized as the free alcohol.

The chemical name for hydrocortisone cypionate is pregn-4-ene-3,20-dione,21-(3-cyclopentyl-1-oxopropoxy)-11,17-dihydroxy-,(11β)- and the molecular weight is 486.65.

Cortef, a preparation for oral use, contains 13.4 mg hydrocortisone cypionate (equivalent to 10 mg hydrocortisone) in each 5 ml. Cortef also contains the following inactive ingredients: benzoic acid, citric acid, FD&C yellow #6 (sunset yellow) as a color additive, flavors, glycerin, methylparaben, propylparaben, sucrose, tragacanth, and purified water. Cortef is stable at room temperature. The pH within the USP specified range of 2.8 to 3.2.

CLINICAL PHARMACOLOGY:

Naturally occurring glucocorticoids (hydrocortisone and cortisone), which also have salt-retaining properties, are used as replacement therapy in adrenocortical deficiency states. Their synthetic analogs are primarily used for their potent anti-inflammatory effects in disorders of many organ systems.

Glucocorticoids cause profound and varied metabolic effects. In addition, they modify the body's immune responses to diverse stimuli.

INDICATIONS AND USAGE:

Hydrocortisone cypionate oral suspension is indicated in the following conditions:

Endocrine Disorders Primary or secondary adrenocortical insufficiency (hydrocortisone or cortisone is the first choice; synthetic analogs may be used in conjunction with mineralocorticoids where applicable; in infancy mineralocorticoid supplementation is of particular importance).

Congenital adrenal hyperplasia

Nonsuppurative thyroiditis

Hypercalcemia associated with cancer

Rheumatic Disorders

Psoriatic arthritis

Rheumatoid arthritis, including juvenile

Acute nonspecific tenosynovitis

Acute gouty arthritis

INDICATIONS AND USAGE: *(cont'd)*

rheumatoid arthritis (selected cases may require low-dose maintenance therapy)	Post-traumatic osteoarthritis
Ankylosing spondylitis	Synovitis of osteoarthritis
Acute and subacute bursitis	Epicondylitis

Collagen Diseases During an exacerbation or as maintenance therapy in selected cases of:

Systemic lupus erythematosus	Acute rheumatic carditis
Systemic dermatomyositis (polymyositis)	

Dermatologic Diseases

Pemphigus	Exfoliative dermatitis
Bullous dermatitis herpetiformis	Mycosis fungoides
Severe erythema multiforme (Stevens-Johnson syndrome)	Severe psoriasis
	Severe seborrheic dermatitis

Allergic States Control of severe or incapacitating allergic conditions intractable to adequate trials of conventional treatment:

Seasonal or perennial allergic rhinitis	Atopic dermatitis
Serum sickness	Contact dermatitis
Bronchial asthma	Drug hypersensitivity reactions

Ophthalmic Diseases Severe acute and chronic allergic and inflammatory processes involving the eye and its adnexa such as:

Allergic corneal marginal ulcers	Allergic conjunctivitis
Herpes zoster ophthalmicus	Keratitis
Anterior segment inflammation	Chorioretinitis
Diffuse posterior uveitis and choroiditis	Optic neuritis
Sympathetic ophthalmia	Iritis and iridocyclitis

Respiratory Diseases

Symptomatic sarcoidosis	Fulminating or disseminated pulmonary tuberculosis when used concurrently with appropriate antituberculous chemotherapy
Loeffler's syndrome not manageable by other means	
Berylliosis	Aspiration pneumonitis.

Hematologic Disorders

Idiopathic thrombocytopenic purpura in adults	Acquired (autoimmune) hemolytic anemia
	Erythroblastopenia (RBC anemia)
Secondary thrombocytopenia in adults	Congenital (erythroid) hypoplastic anemia

Neoplastic Diseases For palliative management of:

Leukemias and lymphomas in adults	Acute leukemia of childhood

Edematous States
To induce a diuresis or remission of proteinuria in the nephrotic syndrome, without uremia, of the idiopathic type or that due to lupus erythematosus.

Gastrointestinal Diseases To tide the patient over a critical period of the disease in:

Ulcerative colitis	Regional enteritis

Miscellaneous
Tuberculous meningitis with subarachnoid block or impending block when used concurrently with appropriate antituberculous chemotherapy
Trichinosis with neurologic or myocardial involvement

CONTRAINDICATIONS:

Systemic fungal infections and known hypersensitivity to components.

WARNINGS:

In patients on corticosteroid therapy subjected to unusual stress, increased dosage of rapidly acting corticosteroids before, during, and after the stressful situation is indicated.

Corticosteroids may mask some signs of infection, and new infections may appear during their use. There may be decreased resistance and inability to localize infection when corticosteroids are used. Prolonged use of corticosteroids may produce posterior subcapsular cataracts, glaucoma with possible damage to the optic nerves, and may enhance the establishment of secondary ocular infections due to fungi or viruses.

Usage in pregnancy: Since adequate human reproduction studies have not been done with corticosteroids, the use of these drugs in pregnancy, nursing mothers or women of childbearing potential requires that the possible benefits of the drug be weighted against the potential hazards to the mother and embryo or fetus. Infants born of mothers who have received substantial doses of corticosteroids during pregnancy should be carefully observed for sings of hypoadrenalism.

Average and large doses of hydrocortisone or cortisone can cause elevation of blood pressure, salt and water retention, and increased excretion of potassium. These effects are less likely to occur with the synthetic derivatives except when used in large doses. Dietary salt restriction and potassium supplementation may be necessary. All corticosteroids increase calcium excretion.

While on corticosteroid therapy patients should not be vaccinated against smallpox. Other immunization procedures should not be undertaken in patients who are on corticosteroids, especially on high dose, because of possible hazards of neurological complications and a lack of antibody response.

The use of hydrocortisone cypionate oral suspension in active tuberculosis should be restricted to those cases of fulminating or disseminated tuberculosis in which the corticosteroid is used for the management of the disease in conjunction with an appropriate antituberculous regimen.

If corticosteroids are indicated in patients with latent tuberculosis or tuberculin reactivity, close observation is necessary as reactivation of the disease may occur. During prolonged corticosteroid therapy, these patients should receive chemoprophylaxis.

Children who are on immunosuppressant drugs are more susceptible to infections than healthy children. Chickenpox and measles, for example, can have a more serious or even fatal course in children on immunosuppressant corticosteroids. In such children, or in adults who have not had these diseases, particular care should be taken to avoid exposure. If exposed, therapy with varicella zoster immune globulin (VZIG) or pooled intravenous immunoglobin (IVIG), as appropriate, may be indicated. If chickenpox develops, treatment with antiviral agents may be considered.

PRECAUTIONS:

GENERAL

Drug-induced secondary adrenocortical insufficiency may be minimized by gradual reduction of dosage. This type of relative insufficiency may persist for months after discontinuation of therapy; therefore, in any situation of stress occurring during that period, hormone therapy should be reinstituted. Since mineralocorticoid secretion may be impaired, salt and/or a mineralocorticoid should be administered concurrently.

There is an enhanced effect of corticosteroids on patients with hypothyroidism and in those with cirrhosis.

Corticosteroids should be used cautiously in patients with ocular herpes simplex because of possible corneal perforation.

The lowest possible doses of corticosteroid should be used to control the condition under treatment, and when reduction in dosage is possible, the reduction should be gradual.

PRECAUTIONS: *(cont'd)*

Psychic derangements may appear when corticosteroids are used, ranging from euphoria, insomnia, mood swings, personality changes, and severe depression, to frank psychotic manifestations. Also, existing emotional instability or psychotic tendencies may be aggravated by corticosteroids.

Aspirin should be used cautiously in conjunction with corticosteroids in hypoprothrombinemia.

Steroids should be used with caution in nonspecific ulcerative colitis, if there is a probability of impending perforation, abscess or other pyogenic infection; diverticulitis; fresh intestinal anastomoses; active or latent peptic ulcer; renal insufficiency; hypertension; osteoporosis; and myasthenia gravis.

Growth and development of infants and children on prolonged corticosteroid therapy should be carefully observed.

INFORMATION FOR THE PATIENT

Patients who are on immunosuppressant doses of corticosteroids should be warned to avoid exposure to chickenpox or measles and, if exposed, to obtain medical advice.

ADVERSE REACTIONS:

Fluid and Electrolyte Disturbances

Sodium retention	Potassium loss
Fluid retention	Hypokalemic alkalosis
Congestive heart failure in susceptible patients	Hypertension

Musculoskeletal

Muscle weakness	Vertebral compression fractures
Steroid myopathy	Aseptic necrosis of femoral and humeral heads
Loss of muscle mass	Pathologic fracture of long bones
Osteoporosis	

Gastrointestinal

Peptic ulcer with possible perforation and hemorrhage	Abdominal distention
	Ulcerative esophagitis
Pancreatitis	

Dermatologic

Impaired wound healing	Facial erythema
Thin fragile skin	Increased sweating
Petechiae and ecchymoses	May suppress reactions to skin tests

Metabolic
Negative nitrogen balance due to protein catabolism

Neurological

Increased intracranial pressure with papilledema (pseudo-tumor cerebri) usually after treatment	Convulsions
	Vertigo
	Headache

Endocrine

Menstrual irregularities	Suppression of growth in children
Development of Cushingoid state	Decreased carbohydrate tolerance
Secondary adrenocortical and pituitary unresponsiveness, particularly in times of stress, as in trauma, surgery or illness	Manifestations of latent diabetes mellitus
	Increased requirements for insulin or oral hypoglycemic agents in diabetics

Ophthalmic

Posterior subcapsular cataracts	Glaucoma
Increased intraocular pressure	Exophthalmos

DOSAGE AND ADMINISTRATION:

The initial dosage of hydrocortisone cypionate oral suspension may vary from 2 to 24 teasoonfuls (10-120 ml) per day depending on the specific disease entity being treated. This provides a daily dosage of 26.8 mg to 321.6 mg of hydrocortisone cypionate, equivalent in activity to 20 to 240 mg of hydrocortisone. In situations of less severity lower doses will generally suffice while in selected patients higher initial doses may be required. The initial dosage should be maintained or adjusted until a satisfactory response is noted. If after a reasonable period of time there is a lack of satisfactory clinical response, hydrocortisone cypionate should be discontinued and the transferred to other appropriate therapy.**IT SHOULD BE EMPHASIZED THAT DOSAGE REQUIREMENTS ARE VARIABLE AND MUST BE INDIVIDUALIZED ON THE BASIS OF THE DISEASE UNDER TREATMENT AND THE RESPONSE OF THE PATIENT.** After a favorable response is noted, the proper maintenance dosage should be determined by decreasing the initial drug dosage in small decrements at appropriate time intervals until the lowest dosage which will maintain an adequate clinical response is reached. It should be kept in mind that constant monitoring is needed in regard to drug dosage. Included in the situations which may make dosage adjustments necessary are changes in clinical status secondary to remissions or exacerbations in the disease process, the patient's individual drug responsiveness, and the effect of patient exposure to stressful situations not directly related to the disease entity under treatment; in this latter situation it may be necessary to increase tp the dosage of hydrocortisone cypionate for a period of time consistent with the patient's condition. If after long-term therapy the drug is to be stopped, it is recommended that it be withdrawn gradually rather than abruptly.

HOW SUPPLIED - EQUIVALENTS NOT AVAILABLE:

Suspension - Oral - 10 mg/5ml

120 ml	$16.40	CORTEF, Pharmacia & Upjohn	00009-0142-01

HYDROCORTISONE SODIUM PHOSPHATE

(001484)

CATEGORIES: Adrenal Corticosteroids; Adrenal Hyperplasia; Adrenal Insufficiency; Adrenocortical Insufficiency; Airway Obstruction; Allergies; Anemia; Ankylosing Spondylitis; Anti-Inflammatory Agents; Arthritis; Asthma; Atopic Dermatitis; Berylliosis; Bursitis; Cancer; Carditis; Chemotherapy; Chorioretinitis; Choroiditis; Colitis; Conjunctivitis; Corneal Ulcer; Dermatitis; Dermatitis Herpetiformis; Dermatomyositis; Diuresis; Drug Hypersensitivity; Enteritis; Epicondylitis; Erythema Multiforme; Glucocorticoids; Gouty Arthritis; Herpes; Herpes Zoster; Hormones; Hypercalcemia; Inflammation; Iridocyclitis; Keratitis; Laryngeal Edema; Leukemia; Lupus Erythematosus; Lymphoma; Meningitis; Mycosis Fungoides; Nephrotic Syndrome; Neuritis; Osteoarthritis; Pemphigus; Pneumoconiosis; Proteinuria; Psoriasis; Purpura; Retinochoroiditis; Rhinitis; Sarcoidosis; Serum Sickness; Shock; Spondylitis; Steroids; Synovitis; Synovitis of Osteoarthritis; Tenosynovitis; Thrombocytopenia; Thyroiditis; Transfusion Reactions; Trichinosis; Tuberculosis; Ulcerative Colitis; Urticaria; Uveitis; FDA Approval Pre 1982

BRAND NAMES: **Hydrocortone Phosphate**

DESCRIPTION:

Hydrocortisone sodium phosphate, a synthetic adrenocortical steroid, is a white to light yellow, odorless or practically odorless powder. It is freely soluble in water and is exceedingly hygroscopic. The molecular weight is 486.41. It is designated chemically as 11β, 17-dihydroxy-21-(phosphonooxy) pregn-4-ene-3,20-dione disodium salt. The empirical formula is $C_{21}H_{29}Na_2O_8P$.

Hydrocortisone sodium phosphate injection is a sterile solution (pH 7.5 to 8.5) sealed under nitrogen, for intravenous, intramuscular, and subcutaneous administration.

Each milliliter contains hydrocortisone sodium phosphate equivalent to 50 mg hydrocortisone. Inactive ingredients per ml; 8 mg creatinine, 10 mg sodium citrate, sodium hydroxide to adjust pH, and Water for Injection, q.s. 1 ml, with 3.2 mg sodium bisulfite, 1.5 mg methylparaben, and 0.2 mg propylparaben added as preservatives.

CLINICAL PHARMACOLOGY:

Hydrocortisone sodium phosphate injection has a rapid onset but short duration of action when compared with less soluble preparations. Because of this, it is suitable for the treatment of acute disorders responsive to adrenocortical steroid therapy.

Naturally occurring glucocorticoids (hydrocortisone and cortisone) which also have salt-retaining properties, are used as replacement therapy in adrenocortical deficiency states. They are also used for their potent anti-inflammatory effects in disorders of many organ systems.

Glucocorticoids cause profound and varied metabolic effects. In addition, they modify the body's immune responses to diverse stimuli.

INDICATIONS AND USAGE:

When oral therapy is not feasible:

Endocrine disorders: Primary or secondary adrenocortical insufficiency (hydrocortisone or cortisone is the drug of choice; synthetic analogs may be used in conjunction with mineralocorticoids where applicable; in infancy, mineralocorticoid supplementation is of particular importance).

Acute adrenocortical insufficiency (hydrocortisone or cortisone is the drug of choice; mineralocorticoid supplementation may be necessary, particularly when synthetic analogs are used).

Preoperatively, and in the event of serious trauma or illness, in patients with known adrenal insufficiency or when adrenocortical reserve is doubtful.

Shock unresponsive to conventional therapy if adrenocortical insufficiency exists or is suspected.

Congenital adrenal hyperplasia

Nonsuppurative thyroiditis

Hypercalcemia associated with cancer

Rheumatic disorders:

Post-traumatic osteoarthritis	Epicondylitis
Synovitis of osteoarthritis	Acute nonspecific tenosynovitis
Rheumatoid arthritis, including juvenile rheumatoid arthritis (selected cases may require low-dose maintenance therapy)	Acute gouty arthritis
	Psoriatic arthritis
	Ankylosing spondylitis
Acute and subacute bursitis	

Collagen diseases: During an exacerbation or as maintenance therapy in selected cases of:

Systemic lupus erythematosus	Systemic dermatomyositis (polymyositis)
Acute rheumatic carditis	

Dermatologic diseases:

Pemphigus	Bullous dermatitis herpetiformis
Severe erythema multiforme (Stevens-Johnson syndrome)	Severe seborrheic dermatitis
	Severe psoriasis
Exfoliative dermatitis	Mycosis fungoides

Allergic States: Control of severe or incapacitating allergic conditions intractable to adequate trials of conventional treatment in:

Bronchial asthma	Drug hypersensitivity reactions
Contact dermatitis	Urticarial transfusion reactions
Atopic dermatitis	Acute noninfectious laryngeal edema
Serum sickness	(epinephrine is the drug of first choice)
Seasonal or perennial allergic rhinitis	

Ophthalmic diseases: Severe acute and chronic allergic and inflammatory processes involving the eye such as:

Herpes zoster ophthalmicus	Sympathetic ophthalmia
Iritis, iridocyclitis	Anterior segment inflammation
Chorioretinitis	Allergic conjunctivitis
Diffuse posterior uveitis and choroiditis	Keratitis
Optic neuritis	Allergic corneal marginal ulcers

Gastrointestinal diseases: To tide the patient over a critical period of the disease in:

Ulcerative colitis (Systemic therapy)	Regional enteritis (Systemic therapy)

Respiratory Diseases

Symptomatic sarcoidosis	appropriate antituberculous chemotherapy.
Berylliosis	Loeffler's syndrome not manageable by other means.
Fulminating or disseminated pulmonary tuberculosis when used concurrently with	Aspiration pneumonitis

Hematologic disorders

Acquired (autoimmune) hemolytic anemia	Secondary thrombocytopenia in adults
Idiopathic thrombocytopenia purpura in adults (IV only; IM administration is contraindicated)	Erythroblastopenia (RBC anemia)
	Congenital (erythroid) hypoplastic anemia

Neoplastic diseases: For palliative management of:

Leukemias and lymphomas in adults	Acute leukemia of childhood

Edematous states: To induce diuresis or remission of proteinuria in the nephrotic syndrome, without uremia, of the idiopathic type, or that due to lupus erythematosus

Miscellaneous: Tuberculous meningitis with subarachnoid block or impending block when used concurrently with appropriate antituberculous chemotherapy, Trichinosis with neurologic or myocardial involvement.

CONTRAINDICATIONS:

Systemic fungal infections (see WARNINGS) regarding amphotericin B

Hypersensitivity to any component of this product, including sulfites(see WARNINGS.)

WARNINGS:

Because rare instances of anaphylactoid reactions have occurred in patients receiving parenteral corticosteroid therapy, appropriate precautionary measures should be taken prior to administration, especially when the patient has a history of allergy to any drug. Anaphylactoid and hypersensitivity reactions have been reported for injection hydrocortisone sodium phosphate (see ADVERSE REACTIONS.)

WARNINGS: *(cont'd)*

Injection Hydrocortone Phosphate contains sodium bisulfite, a sulfite that may cause allergic-type reactions including anaphylactic symptoms and life-threatening or less severe asthmatic episodes in certain susceptible people. The overall prevalence of sulfite sensitivity in the general population is unknown and probably low. Sulfite sensitivity is seen more frequently in asthmatic than in nonasthmatic people.

Corticosteroids may exacerbate systemic fungal infections and therefore should not be used in the presence of such infections unless they are needed to control drug reactions due to amphotericin B. Moreover, there have been cases reported in which concomitant use of amphotericin B and hydrocortisone was followed by cardiac enlargement and congestive failure.

In patients on corticosteroid therapy subjected to any unusual stress, increased dosage of rapidly acting corticosteroids before, during, and after the stressful situation is indicated.

Drug-induced secondary adrenocortical insufficiency may result from too rapid withdrawal of corticosteroids and may be minimized by gradual reduction of dosage. This type of relative insufficiency may persist for months after discontinuation of therapy; therefore, in any situation of stress occurring during that period, hormone therapy should be reinstituted. If the patient is receiving steroids already, dosage may have to be increased. Since mineralocorticoid secretion may be impaired, salt and/or a mineralocorticoid should be administered concurrently.

Corticosteroids may mask some signs of infection, and new infections may appear during their use. There may be decreased resistance and inability to localize infection when corticosteroids are used. Moreover, corticosteroids may affect the nitroblue-tetrazolium test for bacterial infection and produce false negative results.

In cerebral malaria, a double-blind trial has shown that the use of corticosteroids is associated with prolongation of coma and a higher incidence of pneumonia and gastrointestinal bleeding.

Corticosteroids may activate latent amebiasis. Therefore, it is recommended that latent or active amebiasis be ruled out before initiating corticosteroid therapy in any patient who has spent time in the tropics or any patient with diarrhea.

Prolonged use of corticosteroids may produce posterior subcapsular cataracts, glaucoma with possible damage to the optic nerves, and may enhance the establishment of secondary ocular infections due to fungi or viruses.

Usage in pregnancy: Since adequate human reproduction studies have not been done with corticosteroids, use of these drugs in pregnancy or in women of childbearing potential requires that the anticipated benefits be weighed against the possible hazards to the mother and embryo or fetus. Infants born of mothers who have received substantial doses of corticosteroids during pregnancy should be carefully observed for signs of hypoadrenalism.

Corticosteroids appear in breast milk and could suppress growth, interfere with endogenous corticosteroid production, or cause other unwanted effects. Mothers taking pharmacologic doses of corticosteroids should be advised not to nurse.

Average and large doses of cortisone or hydrocortisone can cause elevation of blood pressure, salt and water retention, and increased excretion of potassium. These effects are less likely to occur with the synthetic derivatives except when used in large doses. Dietary salt restriction and potassium supplementation may be necessary. All corticosteroids increase calcium excretion.

Administration of live virus vaccines, including smallpox, is contraindicated in individuals receiving immunosuppressive doses of corticosteroids. If inactivated viral or bacterial vaccines are administered to individuals receiving immunosuppressive doses of steroids, the expected serum antibody response may not be obtained. However, immunization procedures may be undertaken in patients who are receiving corticosteroids as replacement therapy, e.g., for Addison's disease.

Patients who are on drugs which suppress the immune system are more susceptible to infections than healthy individuals. Chickenpox and measles, for example, can have a more serious or even fatal course in non-immune children or adults on corticosteroids. In such children or adults who have not had these diseases, particular care should be taken to avoid exposure. The risk of developing a disseminated infection varies among individuals and can be related to the dose, route and duration of corticosteroid administration as well as to the underlying disease. If exposed to chickenpox, prophylaxis with varicella zoster immune globulin (VZIG) may be indicated. If chickenpox develops, treatment with antiviral agents may be considered. If exposed to measles, prophylaxis with immune globulin (IG) may be indicated. (See the respective package inserts for VZIG and IG for complete prescribing information.)

The use of Hydrocortone Phosphate injection in active tuberculosis should be restricted to those cases of fulminating or disseminated tuberculosis in which the corticosteroid is used for the management of the disease in conjunction with an appropriate anti-tuberculosis regimen.

If corticosteroids are indicated in patients with latent tuberculosis or tuberculin reactivity, close observation is necessary as reactivation of the disease may occur. During prolonged corticosteroid therapy, these patients should receive chemoprophylaxis.

Literature reports suggest an apparent association between use of corticosteroids and left ventricular free wall rupture after a recent myocardial infarction; therefore, therapy with corticosteroids should be used with great caution in these patients.

PRECAUTIONS:

This product, like many other steroid formulations, is sensitive to heat. Therefore, it should not be autoclaved when it is desirable to sterilize the exterior of the vial.

Following prolonged therapy, withdrawal of corticosteroids may result in symptoms of the corticosteroid withdrawal syndrome including fever, myalgia, arthralgia and malaise. This may occur in patients even without evidence of adrenal insufficiency.

There is an enhanced effect of corticosteroids in patients with hypothyroidism and in those with cirrhosis.

Corticosteroids should be used cautiously in patients with ocular herpes simplex for fear of corneal perforation.

The lowest possible dose of corticosteroid should be used to control the condition under treatment, and when reduction in dosage is possible, the reduction must be gradual.

Psychic derangements may appear when corticosteroids are used, ranging from euphoria, insomnia, mood swings, personality changes and severe depression to frank psychotic manifestations. Also, existing emotional instability or psychotic tendencies may be aggravated by corticosteroids.

Aspirin should be used cautiously in conjunction with corticosteroids in hypoprothrombinemia.

Steroids should be used with caution in non-specific ulcerative colitis, if there is a probability of impending perforation, abscess, or other pyogenic infection, also in diverticulitis, fresh intestinal anastomoses, active or latent peptic ulcer, renal insufficiency, hypertension, osteoporosis, and myasthenia gravis. Signs of peritoneal irritation following gastrointestinal perforation in patients receiving large doses of corticosteroids may be minimal or absent. Fat embolism has been reported as a possible complication of hypercortisonism.

PRECAUTIONS: *(cont'd)*

When large doses are given, some authorities advise that antacids be administered between meals to help prevent peptic ulcer.

Growth and development of infants and children on prolonged corticosteroid therapy should be carefully followed.

Steroids may increase or decrease motility and number of spermatozoa in some patients.

Phenytoin, phenobarbital, ephedrine, and rifampin may enhance the metabolic clearance of corticosteroids, resulting in decreased blood levels and lessened physiologic activity, thus requiring adjustment in corticosteroid dosage.

The prothrombin time should be checked frequently in patients who are receiving corticosteroids and coumarin anticoagulants at the same time because of reports that corticosteroids have altered the response to these anticoagulants. Studies have shown that the usual effect produced by adding corticosteroids is inhibition of response to coumarins, although there have been some conflicting reports of potentiation not substantiated by studies.

When corticosteroids are administered concomitantly with potassium-depleting diuretics, patients should be observed closely for development of hypokalemia.

Injection of a steroid into an infected site is to be avoided.

The slower rate of absorption by intramuscular administration should be recognized.

INFORMATION FOR THE PATIENT

Susceptible patients who are on immunosuppressant doses of corticosteroids should be warned to avoid exposure to chickenpox or measles. Patients should also be advised that if they are exposed, medical advice should be sought without delay.

ADVERSE REACTIONS:

Fluid and electrolyte disturbances: Sodium retention; Fluid retention; Congestive heart failure in susceptible patients; Potassium loss; Hypokalemic alkalosis; Hypertension

Musculoskeletal: Muscle weakness; Steroid myopathy; Loss of muscle mass; Osteoporosis; Vertebral compression fractures; Aseptic necrosis of femoral and humeral heads; Pathologic fracture of long bones; Tendon rupture

Gastrointestinal: Peptic ulcer with possible subsequent perforation and hemorrhage; Perforation of the small and large bowel, particularly in patients with inflammatory bowel disease; Pancreatitis; Abdominal distention; Ulcerative esophagitis

Dermatologic: Impaired wound healing; Thin fragile skin; Petechiae and ecchymoses; Erythema; Increased sweating; May suppress reactions to skin tests; Burning or tingling, especially in the perineal area (after IV injection); Other cutaneous reactions, such as allergic dermatitis, urticaria, angioneurotic edema

Neurologic: Convulsions; Increased intracranial pressure with papilledema (pseudotumor cerebri) usually after treatment; Vertigo; Headache; Psychic disturbances

Endocrine: Menstrual irregularities; Development of cushingoid state; Suppression of growth in children; Secondary adrenocortical and pituitary unresponsiveness, particularly in times of stress, as in trauma, surgery, or illness; Decreased carbohydrate tolerance; Manifestations of latent diabetes mellitus; Increased requirements for insulin or oral hypoglycemic agents in diabetics; Hirsutism

Ophthalmic: Posterior subcapsular cataracts; Increased intraocular pressure; Glaucoma; Exophthalmos

Metabolic: Negative nitrogen balance due to protein catabolism

Cardiovascular: Myocardial rupture following recent myocardial infarction (see WARNINGS)

Other: Anaphylactoid or hypersensitivity reactions; Thromboembolism; Weight gain; Increased appetite; Nausea; Malaise

The following *additional* adverse reactions are related to parenteral corticosteroid therapy:

Rare instances of blindness associated with intralesional therapy around the face and head

Hyperpigmentation or hypopigmentation

Subcutaneous and cutaneous atrophy

Sterile abscess

OVERDOSAGE:

Reports of acute toxicity and/or death following overdosage of glucocorticoids are rare. In the event of overdosage, no specific antidote is available; treatment is supportive and symptomatic.

The intraperitoneal LD_{50} of hydrocortisone in female mice was 1740 mg/kg.

DOSAGE AND ADMINISTRATION:

For intravenous, intramuscular, and subcutaneous injection.

Hydrocortisone sodium phosphate injection can be given directly from the vial, or it can be added to Sodium Chloride Injection or Dextrose Injection and administered by intravenous drip.

Benzyl alcohol as a preservative has been associated with toxicity in premature infants. Solutions used for intravenous administration or further dilution of this product should be preservative-free when used in the neonate, especially the premature infant.

When it is mixed with an infusion solution, sterile precautions should be observed. Since infusion solutions generally do not contain preservatives, mixtures should be used within 24 hours.

DOSAGE REQUIREMENTS ARE VARIABLE AND MUST BE INDIVIDUALIZED ON THE BASIS OF THE DISEASE AND THE RESPONSE OF THE PATIENT.

The initial dosage varies from 15 to 240 mg a day depending on the disease being treated. In less severe diseases doses lower than 15 mg may suffice, while in severe diseases doses higher than 240 mg may be required. Usually the parenteral dosage ranges are one-third to one-half the oral dose given every 12 hours. However, in certain overwhelming, acute, life-threatening situations, administration in dosages exceeding the usual dosages may be justified and may be in multiples of the oral dosages.

The initial dosage should be maintained or adjusted until the patient's response is satisfactory. If a satisfactory response does not occur after a reasonable period of time, discontinue Hydrocortone Phosphate injection and transfer the patient to other therapy.

After a favorable initial response, the proper maintenance dosage should be determined by decreasing the initial dosage in small amounts to the lowest dosage that maintains an adequate clinical response.

Patients should be observed closely for signs that might require dosage adjustment, including changes in clinical status resulting from remissions or exacerbations of the disease, individual drug responsiveness, and the effect of stress (*e.g.,* surgery, infection, trauma.) During stress it may be necessary to increase dosage temporarily.

If the drug is to be stopped after more than a few days of treatment, it usually should be withdrawn gradually.

HOW SUPPLIED:

No. 7633 -Injections Hydrocortone Phosphate, 50 mg hydrocortisone equivalent per ml, is a clear, light yellow solution.

Storage: Sensitive to heat. Do not autoclave.

(Merck, 2/93, 7498326)

HOW SUPPLIED - EQUIVALENTS NOT AVAILABLE:

Injection, Solution - Intramuscular; - 50 mg/ml

2 ml	$10.43	HYDROCORTONE PHOSPHATE, Merck	00006-7633-04
10 ml	$50.53	HYDROCORTONE PHOSPHATE, Merck	00006-7633-10

HYDROCORTISONE SODIUM SUCCINATE

(001485)

CATEGORIES: Adrenal Corticosteroids; Adrenal Hyperplasia; Adrenal Insufficiency; Adrenocortical Insufficiency; Airway Obstruction; Allergies; Anemia; Ankylosing Spondylitis; Anti-Inflammatory Agents; Arthritis; Asthma; Atopic Dermatitis; Berylliosis; Bursitis; Cancer; Carditis; Chemotherapy; Chorioretinitis; Choroiditis; Colitis; Conjunctivitis; Corneal Ulcer; Dermatitis; Dermatitis Herpetiformis; Dermatomyositis; Diuresis; Drug Hypersensitivity; Enteritis; Epicondylitis; Erythema Multiforme; Glucocorticoids; Gouty Arthritis; Herpes; Herpes Zoster; Hormones; Hypercalcemia; Inflammation; Iridocyclitis; Keratitis; Laryngeal Edema; Leukemia; Lupus Erythematosus; Lymphoma; Meningitis; Multiple Sclerosis; Mycosis Fungoides; Nephrotic Syndrome; Neuritis; Osteoarthritis; Pemphigus; Pneumoconiosis; Proteinuria; Psoriasis; Purpura; Retinochoroiditis; Rhinitis; Sarcoidosis; Serum Sickness; Shock; Spondylitis; Steroids; Synovitis; Synovitis of Osteoarthritis; Tenosynovitis; Thrombocytopenia; Thyroiditis; Transfusion Reactions; Trichinosis; Tuberculosis; Ulcerative Colitis; Urticaria; Uveitis; FDA Approval Pre 1982

BRAND NAMES: A-Hydrocort; *Efcortelan Soluble*; *Flebocortid* (Mexico); *Hycortil*; *Hydro-Adreson Aquosum*; *Hydro Adreson Aquosum*; *Hydrocort*; *Hydrocortison* (Germany); *Hydrocortisone Roussel* (France); *Hydrocortisone Upjohn* (France); *Hydroson Organon*; *Hydrotopic*; *Nordicort*; *Nositrol* (Mexico); *Radicortin*; *Silacort*; **Solu-Cortef**; *Solu Cortef* (Asia, England, Canada)

(International brand names outside U.S. in italics)

DESCRIPTION:

Hydrocortisone sodium succinate sterile powder contains hydrocortisone sodium succinate as the active ingredient. Hydrocortisone sodium succinate is a white or nearly white, odorless, hygroscopic amorphous solid. It is very soluble in water and in alcohol, very slightly soluble in acetone and insoluble in chloroform. The chemical name is pregn-4-ene- 3,20-dione,21-(3-carboxy-1-oxopropoxy)-11,17-dihydroxy-, monosodium salt, (11β)- and its molecular weight is 484.52.

Hydrocortisone sodium succinate is an anti-inflammatory adrenocortical steroid. This highly water-soluble sodium succinate ester of hydrocortisone permits the immediate intravenous administration of high doses of hydrocortisone in a small volume of diluent and is particularly useful where high blood levels of hydrocortisone are required rapidly.

Hydrocortisone sodium succinate sterile powder is available in several packages for intravenous or intramuscular administration.

100 mg Plain: Vials containing hydrocortisone sodium succinate equivalent to 100 mg hydrocortisone, also 0.8 mg monobasic sodium phosphate anhydrous, 8.73 mg dibasic sodium phosphate dried (TABLE 1):

TABLE 1 ACT-O-VIAL System (Single-Dose Vial) in four strengths:

	100 mg ACT-O-VIAL Each 2 ml contains: (when mixed)	250 mg ACT-O-VIAL Each 2 ml contains: (when mixed)	500 mg ACT-O-VIAL Each 4 ml contains: (when mixed)	1000 mg ACT-O-VIAL Each 8 ml contains: (when mixed)
Hydrocortisone sodium succinate	equiv. to 100 mg hydrocortisone	equiv. to 250 mg hydrocortisone	equiv. to 500 mg hydrocortisone	equiv. to 1000 mg hydrocortisone
Monobasic sodium phosphate anhydrous	0.8 mg	2 mg	4 mg	8 mg
Dibasic sodium phosphate dried	8.76 mg	21.8 mg	44 mg	87.32 mg
Benzyl alcohol added as preservative	18.1 mg	16.4 mg	33.4 mg	66.9 mg

When necessary, the pH of each formula was adjusted with sodium hydroxide so that the pH of the reconstituted solution is within the USP specified range of 7 to 8.

CLINICAL PHARMACOLOGY:

Hydrocortisone sodium succinate has the same metabolic and anti- inflammatory actions as hydrocortisone. When given parenterally and in equimolar quantities, the two compounds are equivalent in biologic activity. Following the intravenous injection of hydrocortisone sodium succinate, demonstrable effects are evident within one hour and persist for a variable period. Excretion of the administered dose is nearly complete within 12 hours. Thus, if constantly high blood levels are required, injections should be made every 4 to 6 hours. This preparation is also rapidly absorbed when administered intramuscularly and is excreted in a pattern similar to that observed after intravenous injection.

INDICATIONS AND USAGE:

When oral therapy is not feasible, and the strength, dosage form and route of administration of the drug reasonably lend the preparation to the treatment of the condition, hydrocortisone sodium succinate sterile powder is indicated for intravenous or intramuscular use in the following conditions:

Endocrine Disorders: Primary or secondary adrenocortical insufficiency (hydrocortisone or cortisone is the drug of choice; synthetic analogs may be used in conjunction with mineralocorticoids where applicable; in infancy, mineralocorticoid supplementation is of particular importance).

Acute adrenocortical insufficiency (hydrocortisone or cortisone is the drug of choice; mineralocorticoid supplementation may be necessary, particularly when synthetic analogs are used).

Preoperatively, and in the event of serious trauma or illness, in patients with known adrenal insufficiency or when adrenocortical reserve is doubtful.

INDICATIONS AND USAGE: *(cont'd)*

Shock unresponsive to conventional therapy if adrenocortical insufficiency exists or is suspected.

Congenital adrenal hyperplasia

Hypercalcemia associated with cancer

Nonsuppurative thyroiditis

Rheumatic Disorders:

Post-traumatic osteoarthritis
Synovitis of osteoarthritis
Rheumatoid arthritis, including juvenile rheumatoid arthritis (selected cases may require low-dose maintenance therapy)
Acute and subacute bursitis
Ankylosing spondylitis
Epicondylitis
Acute nonspecific tenosynovitis
Acute gouty arthritis
Psoriatic arthritis

Collagen Diseases: During an exacerbation or as maintenance therapy in selected cases of:
Systemic lupus erythematosus
Systemic dermatomyositis (polymyositis)
Acute rheumatic carditis

Dermatologic Diseases
Pemphigus
Severe erythema multiforme (Stevens-Johnson syndrome)
Exfoliative dermatitis
Bullous dermatitis herpetiformis
Severe seborrheic dermatitis
Severe psoriasis
Mycosis fungoides

Allergic States: Control of severe or incapacitating allergic conditions intractable to adequate trials of conventional treatment in:
Bronchial asthma
Contact dermatitis
Atopic dermatitisedema (epinephrine is the seasonal or perennial allergic rhinitis drug of first choice)
Drug hypersensitivity reactions
Urticarial transfusion reactions
Acute noninfectious laryngeal
Serum sickness

Ophthalmic Diseases: Severe acute and chronic allergic and inflammatory processes involving the eye such as:
Herpes zoster ophthalmicus
Iritis, iridocyclitis
Chorioretinitis
Diffuse posterior uveitis and choroiditis
Optic neuritis
Sympathetic ophthalmia
Anterior segment inflammation
Allergic conjunctivitis
Allergic corneal marginal ulcers
Keratitis

Gastrointestinal Diseases: To tide the patient over a critical period of the disease in:
Ulcerative colitis (Systemic therapy)
Regional enteritis (Systemic therapy)

Respiratory Diseases
Symptomatic sarcoidosis
Berylliosis
Fulminating or disseminated pulmonary tuberculosis when used concurrently with appropriate antituberculous chemotherapy.
Loeffler's syndrome not manageable by other means.
Aspiration pneumonitis

Hematologic Disorders
Acquired (autoimmune) hemolytic anemia
Idiopathic thrombocytopenia purpura in adults (IV only; IM administration is contraindicated)
Secondary thrombocytopenia in adults
Erythroblastopenia (RBC anemia)
Congenital (erythroid) hypoplastic anemia
Idiopathic thrombocytopenic purpura hypoplastic anemia (IV only; IM administration is contraindicated)

Neoplastic diseases: For palliative management of:
Leukemias and lymphomas in adults
Acute leukemia of childhood

Edematous states: To induce diuresis or remission of proteinuria in the nephrotic syndrome, without uremia, of the idiopathic type, or that due to lupus erythematosus

Nervous sytem: Acute exacerbations of multiple sclerosis

Miscellaneous: Tuberculous meningitis with subarachnoid block or impending block when used concurrently with appropriate antituberculous chemotherapy, Trichinosis with neurologic or myocardial involvement.

CONTRAINDICATIONS:

The use of hydrocortisone sodium succinate sterile powder is contraindicated in premature infants because the 100 mg, 250 mg, 500 mg and 1000 mg ACT-O-VIAL System contain benzyl alcohol. Benzyl alcohol has been reported to be associated with a fatal "Gasping Syndrome" in premature infants. Hydrocortisone sodium succinate sterile powder is also contraindicated in systemic fungal infections and patients with known hypersensitivity to the product and its constituents.

WARNINGS:

In patients on corticosteroid therapy to unusual stress, increased dosage of rapidly acting corticosteroids before, during, and after the stressful situation is indicated.

Corticosteroids may mask some signs of infection, and new infections may appear during their use. There may be decreased resistance and inability to localize infection when corticosteroids are used.

Prolonged use of corticosteroids may produce posterior subcapsular cataracts, glaucoma with possible damage to the optic nerves, and may enhance the establishment of secondary ocular infections due to fungi or viruses.

Usage In Pregnancy: Since adequate human reproduction studies have not been done with corticosteroids, the use of these drugs in pregnancy, nursing mothers, or women of childbearing potential requires that the possible benefits of the drug be weighted against the potential hazards to the mother and embryo or fetus. Infants born of mothers who have received substantial doses of corticosteroids during pregnancy should be carefully observed for signs of hypoadrenalism.

Average and large doses of hydrocortisone can cause elevation of blood pressure, salt and water retention, and increased excretion of potassium. These effects are less likely to occur with the synthetic derivatives except when used in large doses. Dietary salt restriction and potassium supplementation may be necessary. All corticosteroids increase calcium excretion.

While on corticosteroid therapy patients should not be vaccinated against smallpox. Other immunization procedures should not be undertaken in patients who are on corticosteroids, especially on high dose, because of possible hazards of neurological complications and a lack of antibody response.

The use of hydrocortisone sodium succinate sterile powder in active tuberculosis should be restricted to those cases of fulminating or disseminated tuberculosis in which the corticosteroid is used for the management of the disease in conjunction with appropriate antituberculous regimen.

If corticosteroids are indicated in patients with latent tuberculosis or tuberculin reactivity, close observation is necessary as reactivation of the disease may occur. During prolonged corticosteroid therapy, these patients should receive chemoprophylaxis.

Because rare instances of anaphylactoid reactions (*e.g.,* bronchospasm) have occurred in patients receiving parenteral corticosteroid therapy, appropriate precautionary measures should be taken prior to administration, especially when the patient has a history of allergy to any drug.

WARNINGS: *(cont'd)*

Children who are on immunosuppressant drugs are more susceptible to infections than healthy children. Chickenpox and measles, for example, can have more serious or even fatal course in children on immunosuppressant corticosteroids. In such children, or in adults who have not had these diseases, particular care should be taken to avoid exposure. If exposed, therapy with varicella zoster immune globulin (VZIG) or pooled intravenous immunoglobin (IVIG), as appropriate, may be indicated. If chickenpox develops, treatment with antiviral agents may be considered.

PRECAUTIONS:

GENERAL

Drug-induced secondary adrenocortical insufficiency may be minimized by gradual reduction of dosage. This type of relative insufficiency may persist for months after discontinuation of therapy; therefore, in any situation of stress occurring during that period, hormone therapy should be reinstituted. Since mineralocorticoid secretion may be impaired, salt and/or a mineralocorticoid should be administered concurrently.

There is an enhanced effect of corticosteroids in patients with hypothyroidism and in those with cirrhosis.

Corticosteroids should be used cautiously in patients with ocular herpes simplex for fear of corneal perforation.

The lowest possible dose of corticosteroid should be used to control the condition under treatment, and when reduction in dosage is possible, the reduction must be gradual.

Psychic derangements may appear when corticosteroids are used, ranging from euphoria, insomnia, mood swings, personality changes, and severe depression to frank psychotic manifestations. Also, existing emotional instability or psychotic tendencies may be aggravated by corticosteroids.

Aspirin should be used cautiously in conjunction with corticosteroids in hypoprothrombinemia.

Steroids should be used with caution in nonspecific ulcerative colitis, if there is a probability of impending perforation, abscess or other pyogenic infection, also in diverticulitis, fresh intestinal anastomoses, active or latent peptic ulcer, renal insufficiency, hypertension, osteoporosis, and myasthenia gravis.

Growth and development of infants and children on prolonged corticosteroid therapy should be carefully followed.

Although controlled clinical trials have shown corticosteroids to be effective in speeding the resolution of acute exacerbations of multiple sclerosis, they do not show that corticosteroids affect the ultimate outcome or natural history of the disease. The studies do show that relatively high doses of corticosteroids are necessary to demonstrate a significant effect. (See DOSAGE AND ADMINISTRATION.)

Since complications of treatment with glucocorticoids are dependent on the size of the dose and the duration of treatment, a risk/benefit decision must be made in each individual case as to dose and duration of treatment and as to whether daily or intermittent therapy should be used.

INFORMATION FOR THE PATIENT

Patients who are on immunosuppressant doses of corticosteroids should be warned to avoid exposure to chickenpox or measles and, if exposed, to obtain medical advice.

ADVERSE REACTIONS:

Fluid and Electrolyte Disturbances: Sodium retention, Fluid retention, Congestive heart failure in susceptible patients, Potassium loss, Hypokalemic alkalosis, Hypertension.

Musculoskeletal: Muscle weakness, Steroid myopathy, Loss of muscle mass, Osteoporosis, Vertebral compression fractures, Aseptic necrosis of femoral and humeral heads, Pathologic fracture of long bones.

Gastrointestinal: Peptic ulcer with possible perforation and hemorrhage, Pancreatitis, Abdominal distention, Ulcerative esophagitis.

Dermatologic: Impaired wound healing, Thin fragile skin, Petechiae and ecchymoses, Facial erythema, Increased sweating, May suppress reactions to skin tests.

Neurological: Convulsions, Increased intracranial pressure with papilledema (pseudo-tumor cerebri) usually after treatment, Vertigo, Headache.

Endocrine: Menstrual irregularities; Development of Cushingoid state; Suppression of growth in children; Secondary adrenocortical and pituitary unresponsiveness, particularly in times of stress, as in trauma, surgery or illness;Decreased carbohydrate tolerance; Manifestations of latent diabetes mellitus; Increased requirements for insulin or oral hypoglycemic agents in diabetics,

Ophthalmic: Posterior subcapsular cataracts, Increased intraocular pressure, Glaucoma, Exophthalmos.

Metabolic: Negative nitrogen balance due to protein catabolism

DOSAGE AND ADMINISTRATION:

This preparation may be administered by intravenous injection, by intravenous infusion, or by intramuscular injection, the preferred method for initial emergency use being intravenous injection. Following the initial emergency period, consideration should be given to employing a longer acting injectable preparation or an oral preparation.

Therapy is initiated by administering hydrocortisone sodium succinate sterile powder intravenously over a period of 30 seconds (*e.g.,* 100 mg) to 10 minutes (*e.g.,* 500 mg or more). In general, high dose corticosteroid therapy should be continued only until the patient's condition has stabilized—usually not beyond 48 to 72 hours. Although adverse effects associated with high dose, short-term corticoid therapy are uncommon, peptic ulceration may occur. Prophylactic antacid therapy may be indicated.

When high dose hydrocortisone therapy must be continued beyond 48-72 hours, hypernatremia may occur. Under such circumstances it may be desirable to replace hydrocortisone sodium succinate with a corticoid such as methylprednisolone sodium succinate which causes little or no sodium retention.

The initial dose of hydrocortisone sodium succinate sterile powder is 100 mg to 500 mg, depending on the severity of the condition. This dose may be repeated at intervals of 2, 4 or 6 hours as indicated by the patient's response and clinical condition. While the dose may be reduced for infants and children, it is governed more by the severity of the condition and response of the patient than by age or body weight but should not be less than 25 mg daily.

Patients subjected to severe stress following corticosteroid therapy should be observed closely for signs and symptoms of adrenocortical insufficiency.

Corticoid therapy is an adjunct to, and not a replacement for, conventional therapy.

PREPARATION OF SOLUTIONS

100 mg Plain: For intravenous or intramuscular injection, prepare solution by aseptically adding **not more than 2 ml** of Bacteriostatic Water for Injection or Bacteriostatic Sodium Chloride Injection to the contents of one vial. **For intravenous infusion,** first prepare solution by adding **not more than 2 ml** of Bacteriostatic Water for Injection to the vial; this solution

DOSAGE AND ADMINISTRATION: *(cont'd)*

may then be added to 100 to 1000 ml of the following: 5% dextrose in water (or isotonic saline solution or 5% dextrose in isotonic saline solution if patient is not on sodium restriction).

Directions for Using the Act-O-Vial System

1. Press down on plastic activator to force diluent into the lower compartment.

2. Gently agitate to effect solution.

3. Remove plastic tab covering center of stopper.

4. Sterilize to top of stopper with a suitable germicide.

5. Insert needle **squarely through center** of stopper until tip is just visible. Invert vial and withdraw dose.

Further dilution is not necessary for intravenous or intramuscular injection. For intravenous infusion, first prepare solution as just described. The **100 mg** solution may then be added to 100 to 1000 ml of 5% dextrose in water (or isotonic saline solution or 5% dextrose in isotonic saline solution if patient is not on sodium restriction). The **250 mg** solution may be added to 250 to 1000 ml, the **500 mg** solution may be added to 500 to 1000 ml and the **1000 mg** solution to 1000 ml of the same diluents. In cases where administration of a small volume of fluid is desirable, 100 mg to 3000 mg of Hydrocortisone Sodium Succinate may be added to 50 ml of the above diluents. The resulting solutions are stable for at least 4 hours and may be administered either directly or by IV piggyback.

When reconstituted as directed, pH's of the solutions range from 7 to 8 and the tonicities are: 100 mg ACT-O-VIAL,.36 osmolar; 250 mg ACT-O- VIAL, 500 mg ACT-O-VIAL, and the 1000 mg ACT-O-VIAL,.57 osmolar. (Isotonic saline =.28 osmolar.)

Store at controlled room temperature 15°-30° C (59°-86° F).

HOW SUPPLIED - RATED THERAPEUTICALLY EQUIVALENT:

Injection, Lyphl-Soln - Intramuscular; - 100 mg/vial

1's	$1.90	Hydrocortisone Sod Succinate, Elkins Sinn	00641-2365-41
1's	$3.31	A-HYDROCORT, Abbott	00074-5676-02
1's	**$3.34**	**SOLU-CORTEF, Pharmacia & Upjohn**	**00009-0900-13**
1's	$3.50	Hydrocortisone Sod Succinate, HL Moore Drug Exch	00839-7587-23
1's	$3.75	Hydrocortisone Sod Succinate, Consolidated Midland	00223-7893-02
2 ml	$2.55	A-HYDROCORT, Abbott	00074-5671-02
25's	$46.25	Hydrocortisone Sod Succinate, Fujisawa USA	00469-1070-10
25's	**$83.50**	**SOLU-CORTEF, Pharmacia & Upjohn**	**00009-0900-20**
100 mg	**$3.27**	**SOLU-CORTEF, Pharmacia & Upjohn**	**00009-0825-01**

Injection, Lyphl-Soln - Intramuscular; - 250 mg/2ml

1's	$5.00	Hydrocortisone Sod Succinate, Elkins Sinn	00641-2366-41
1's	**$7.57**	**SOLU-CORTEF, Pharmacia & Upjohn**	**00009-0909-08**
1's	$9.50	Hydrocortisone Sod Succinate, Consolidated Midland	00223-7894-02
2 ml	$5.78	A-HYDROCORT, Abbott	00074-5672-02
25's	$117.50	Hydrocortisone Sod Succinate, Fujisawa USA	00469-1080-10
25's	**$189.21**	**SOLU-CORTEF, Pharmacia & Upjohn**	**00009-0909-16**

Injection, Lyphl-Soln - Intramuscular; - 500 mg/4ml

1's	$8.88	Hydrocortisone Sod Succinate, Fujisawa USA	00469-1090-70
1's	$10.00	Hydrocortisone Sod Succinate, Elkins Sinn	00641-2367-41
1's	**$14.72**	**SOLU-CORTEF, Pharmacia & Upjohn**	**00009-0912-05**
1's	$15.00	Hydrocortisone Sod Succinate, Consolidated Midland	00223-7898-08
4 ml	$11.26	A-HYDROCORT, Abbott	00074-5673-04

Injection, Lyphl-Soln - Intramuscular; - 1000 mg/8ml

1's	$16.90	Hydrocortisone Sod Succinate, Fujisawa USA	00469-1110-08
1's	$20.00	Hydrocortisone Sod Succinate, Elkins Sinn	00641-2368-41
1's	**$29.31**	**SOLU-CORTEF, Pharmacia & Upjohn**	**00009-0920-03**
1's	$30.00	Hydrocortisone Sod Succinate, Consolidated Midland	00223-7899-08
8 ml	$22.91	A-HYDROCORT, Abbott	00074-5674-08

HYDROCORTISONE VALERATE *(001486)*

CATEGORIES: Anti-Inflammatory Agents; Dermatologicals; Dermatoses; Glucocorticoids; Hormones; Skin/Mucous Membrane Agents; Steroids; Topical; Pruritus*; Pregnancy Category C; FDA Approval Pre 1982
* Indication not approved by the FDA

BRAND NAMES: *Hydcort*; **Westcort**
(International brand names outside U.S. in italics)

DESCRIPTION:

Note: This monograph pertains to Hydrocortisone valerate 0.2% Cream and 0.2% Ointment.

Westcort cream/ointment is a topical formulation containing hydrocortisone valerate, a non-fluorinated steroid. It has the chemical name Pregn-4-ene-3,20-dione, 11, 21-dihydroxy-17-((1-oxopentyl) oxy)-,(11β)-; the empirical formula is: $C_{26}H_{36}O_6$; the molecular weight is 446.58, and the CAS registry number is: 57524-89-7.

Each gram of Westcort Cream contains 2.0 mg hydrocortisone valerate in a hydrophilic base composed of white petrolatum, stearyl alcohol, propylene glycol, amphoteric-9, carbomer 940, dried sodium phosphate, sodium lauryl sulfate, sorbic acid and water.

Each gram of Westcort Ointment contains 2.0 mg hydrocortisone valerate in a hydrophilic base composed of white petrolatum, stearyl alcohol, propylene glycol, sorbic acid, sodium lauryl sulfate carbomer 934, dried sodium phosphate, mineral oil, steareth-2, steareth-100, and water.

CLINICAL PHARMACOLOGY:

Topical corticosteroids share anti-inflammatory, anti-pruritic and vasoconstrictive actions.

The mechanism of anti-inflammatory activity of the topical corticosteroids is unclear.[1] Various laboratory methods, including vasoconstrictor assays, are used to compare and predict potencies and/or clinical efficacies of the topical corticosteroids.[2] There is some evidence to suggest that a recognizable correlation exists between vasoconstrictor potency and therapeutic efficacy in man.[3]

Pharmacokinetics: The extent of percutaneous absorption of topical corticosteroids is determined by many factors including the vehicle, the integrity of the epidermal barrier, and the use of occlusive dressings.[4,5,6]

Topical corticosteroids can be absorbed from normal intact skin.[5,6,7] Inflammation and/or other disease processes in the skin increase percutaneous absorption.[8] Occlusive dressings substantially increase the percutaneous absorption of topical corticosteroids.[4,7] Thus, occlusive dressings may be a valuable therapeutic adjunct for treatment of resistant dermatoses (see DOSAGE AND ADMINISTRATION.)

Once absorbed through the skin, topical corticosteroids are handled through pharmacokinetic pathways similar to systemically administered corticosteroids. Corticosteroids are bound to plasma proteins in varying degrees. Corticosteroids are metabolized primarily in the liver and are then excreted by the kidneys. Some of the topical corticosteroids and thier metabolites are also excreted into the bile.

INDICATIONS AND USAGE:

Westcort Cream/Ointment is indicated for the relief of the inflammatory and pruritic manifestations of the corticosteroid-responsive dermatoses.

CONTRAINDICATIONS:

Topical corticosteroids are contraindicated in those patients with a history of hypersensitivity to any of the components of the preparation.

PRECAUTIONS:

GENERAL

Systemic absorption of topical corticosteroids has produced reversible hypothalamic pituitary-adrenal (HPA) axis suppression, manifestations of Cushing's syndrome, hyperglycemia, and glucosuria in some patients.[9]

Conditions which augment systemic absorption include the application of the more potent steroids, use over large surface areas, prolonged use, and the addition of occlusive dressings.[10]

Therefore, patients receiving a large dose of a potent topical steroid applied to a large surface area or under an occlusive dressing should be evaluated periodically for evidence of HPA axis suppression by using the urinary free cortisol and ACTH stimulation tests. If HPA axis suppression is noted, and attempt should be made to withdraw the drug, to reduce the frequency of application, or to substitute a less potent steroid.

Recovery of HPA axis function is generally prompt and complete upon discontinuation of the drug.[10] Infrequently, signs and symptoms of steroid withdrawal may occur, requiring supplemental systemic corticosteroids.[11,12]

Children may absorb proportionally larger amounts of topical corticosteroids and thus be more susceptible to systemic toxicity[13,14] (see PRECAUTIONS, Pediatric Use.)

If irritation develops, topical corticosteroids should be discontinued and appropriate therapy instituted.

In the presence of dermatological infections, the use of an appropriate antifungal or anti-bacterial agent should be instituted. If a favorable response does not occur promptly, the corticosteroid should be discontinued until the infection has been adequately controlled.

INFORMATION FOR THE PATIENT

Patients using topical corticosteroids should receive the following information and instructions:

1. This medication is to be used as directed by physician. It is for external use only. Avoid contact with the eyes.

2. Patients should be advised not to use this medication for any disorder other than for which it was prescribed.

3. The treated skin area should not be bandaged or otherwise covered or wrapped as to be occlusive unless directed by the physician.

4. Patients should report any signs of local adverse reactions especially under occlusive dressing.

5. Parents of pediatric patients should be advised not to use tight- fitting diapers or plastic pants on a child being treated in a diaper area, as these garments may constitute occlusive dressing.

LABORATORY TESTS

The following tests may be helpful in evaluating the HPA axis suppression:

Urinary free cortisol test

ACTH stimulation test

CARCINOGENESIS, MUTAGENESIS, AND IMPAIRMENT OF FERTILITY

Long-term studies have not been performed to evaluate the carcinogenic potential or the effect on fertility of topical corticosteroids.

Studies to determine mutagenicity with prednisolone and hydrocortisone have revealed negative results.[15,16]

PREGNANCY CATEGORY C

Corticosteroids are generally teratogenic in laboratory animals when administered systemically at relatively low dosage levels. The more potent corticosteroids have been shown to be teratogenic after dermal application in laboratory animals. There are no adequate and well-controlled studies in pregnant women on teratogenic effects from topically applied corticosteroids. Therefore, topical corticosteroids should be used during pregnancy only if the potential benefit justifies the potential risk to the fetus. Drugs of this class should not be used extensively on pregnant patients, in large amounts, or for prolonged periods of time.

NURSING MOTHERS

It is not known whether topical administration of corticosteroids could result in sufficient systemic absorption to produce detectable quantities in breast milk. Systemically administered corticosteroids are secreted into breast milk in quantities *not* likely to have a deleterious effect on the infant.[17,18] Nevertheless, caution should be exercised when topical corticosteroids are administered to a nursing woman.

PEDIATRIC USE

Pediatric patients may demonstrate greater susceptibility to topical corticosteroid-induced HPA axis suppression and Cushing's syndrome than mature patients because of a larger skin surface area to body weight ratio.

Hypothalamic-pituitary-adrenal (HPA) axis suppression, Cushing's syndrome, and intracranial hypertension have been reported in children receiving topical corticosteroids. Manifestations of adrenal suppression in children include linear growth retardation, delayed weight gain, low plasma cortisol level, and absence of response to ACTH stimulation. Manifestations of intracranial hypertension include bulging fontanelles, headaches, and bilateral papilledema.

Administration of topical corticosteroids to children should be limited to the least amount compatible with an effective therapeutic regimen. Chronic corticosteroid therapy may interfere with the growth and development of children.

ADVERSE REACTIONS:

The following local adverse reactions are reported infrequently with topical corticosteroids, but may occur more frequently with the use of occlusive dressings. These reactions are listed in an approximate decreasing order of occurrence: burning, itching, irritation, dryness, folliculitis, hypertrichosis, acneiform eruptions, hypopigmentation, perioral dermatitis, allergic contact dermatitis, maceration of the skin, secondary infection, skin atrophy, striae, miliaria.

OVERDOSAGE:

Topically applied corticosteroids can be absorbed in sufficient amounts to produce systemic effects (see PRECAUTIONS.)

DOSAGE AND ADMINISTRATION:

Westcort Cream/Lotion should be applied to the affected area as a thin film two or three times daily depending on the severity of the condition.

Occlusive dressings may be used for management of psoriasis or recalcitrant conditions.

DOSAGE AND ADMINISTRATION: *(cont'd)*

If an infection develops, the use of occlusive dressings should be discontinued and appropriate antimicrobial therapy instituted.

Store below 78°F (26°C).

REFERENCES:

1. Maibach HI, Stoughton RB: *Med Clin N Am* **57**: 1253-64, 1973. **2.** Engel JC, et al: *Arch Dermatol* **109**: 863-5, 1974. **3.** Barry BW: *Dermatologica* **152** (Supplement 1): 47-65, 1976. **4.** McKenzie AW, Stoughton RB: *Arch Dermatol* **86**: 608-10, 1962. **5.** Feldmann RJ, Maibach HI: *J Invest Dermatol* **52**: 89-94, 1969. **6.** Feldmann RJ, Maibach HI: *J Invest Dermatol* **48**: 181-3, 1967. **7.** Feldmann RJ, Maibach HI: *Arch Dermatol* **91**: 661-6, 1965. **8.** Schaefer H, Zesch A, Stuttgen G: *Arch Dermatol Res***258**: 241-9, 1977. **9.** Hendhkse JCM, Moolenaar AJ: *Dermatologica* **144**: 179- 86, 1972. **10.** Monro DD: *Br J Dermatol* **94** (Supplement 12): 67-76, 1976. **11.** Nathan AW, Rose GL: *Lancet* **1**: 207, 1979. **12.** May P, et al: *Arch Intern Med* **136**: 612-3, 1976. **13.** Johns AM, Bower BD: *Br Med J* **1**: 347-8, 1970. **14.** Feiwel M, James VHT, Barnett ES: *Lancet* **1**: 485-7, 1969. **15.** Seino Y, et al: *Cancer Res* **36**: 2148-56, 1978. **16.** Hemmerly J, Demeree M: *Cancer Res* **15** (Supplement 3): 69-75, 1955. **17.** McKenzie SA, Selley JA, Agnew JE: *Arch Dis Child* **50**: 894-6, 1975. **18.** Katz FH, Duncan BR: *N Eng J Med* **293**: 1154, 1975.

HOW SUPPLIED - EQUIVALENTS NOT AVAILABLE:

Cream - Topical - 0.2 %

15 gm	**$12.49**	**WESTCORT, Westwood Squibb**	**00072-8100-15**
45 gm	**$25.91**	**WESTCORT, Westwood Squibb**	**00072-8100-45**
60 gm	**$31.16**	**WESTCORT, Westwood Squibb**	**00072-8100-60**

Ointment - Topical - 2 mg

15 gm	**$12.49**	**WESTCORT, Westwood Squibb**	**00072-7800-15**
45 gm	**$25.91**	**WESTCORT, Westwood Squibb**	**00072-7800-45**
60 gm	**$31.16**	**WESTCORT, Westwood Squibb**	**00072-7800-60**

HYDROCORTISONE; IODOQUINOL *(001068)*

CATEGORIES: Acne; Anti-Infectives; Anti-Inflammatory Agents; Antibacterials; Antifungals; DESI Drugs; Dermatitis; Dermatologicals; Eczema; Intertrigo; Pruritus; Skin/Mucous Membrane Agents; Steroids; Pregnancy Category C; FDA Pre 1938 Drugs

BRAND NAMES: Diiodohydroxyquin; **Vytone**

Prescribing information not available at time of publication.

HOW SUPPLIED - EQUIVALENTS NOT AVAILABLE:

Cream - Topical - 1 %/1 %

28.4 gm	**$24.69**	**VYTONE, Dermik Labs**	**00066-0051-01**

HYDROCORTISONE; LIDOCAINE *(001473)*

CATEGORIES: Dermatologicals; Skin/Mucous Membrane Agents; FDA Pre 1938 Drugs

BRAND NAMES: Lida-Mantle-Hc

Prescribing information not available at time of publication.

HOW SUPPLIED - EQUIVALENTS NOT AVAILABLE:

Cream - Topical - 0.50 %

30 gm	$36.89	LIDA-MANTLE-HC, Bayer	00026-1508-81

HYDROCORTISONE; NEOMYCIN SULFATE *(001489)*

CATEGORIES: Anti-Infectives; Antibiotics; Dermatologicals; Skin/Mucous Membrane Agents; FDA Approved 1984 Jun

BRAND NAMES: Biocort; *Neo*; *Neocort*; *Neocortisun Sterile Eye Ear*
(International brand names outside U.S. in italics)

Prescribing information not available at time of publication.

HOW SUPPLIED - RATED THERAPEUTICALLY EQUIVALENT:

Ointment - Topical - 1 %/0.5 %

20 gm	$2.70	Neomycin Sulfate/Hydrocortisone, Clay Park Labs	45802-0062-02
454 gm	$34.56	Neomycin Sulfate/Hydrocortisone, Clay Park Labs	45802-0062-05

HYDROCORTISONE; NEOMYCIN SULFATE; POLYMYXIN B SULFATE *(001490)*

CATEGORIES: Anti-Infectives; Anti-Inflammatory Agents; Antibacterials; Antibiotics; Burns; Conjunctivitis; Corneal Inflammation; Corneal Injury; Dermatologicals; EENT Drugs; Edema; Eye, Ear, Nose, & Throat Preparations; Inflammatory Conditions; Ocular Infections; Ophthalmics; Otic Hydrocortisones; Otic Preparations; Otologic; Skin/Mucous Membrane Agents; Steroids; Topical; Uveitis; Pregnancy Category C; FDA Approval Pre 1982; Top 200 Drugs

BRAND NAMES: *Aerocortin*; Ak-Spore HC; Antibiotic Ear; Aural Acute; *Auriswell*; Bacticort; Biocot; Biotis; C-Sporin; Cobiron; Cort-Biotic; Cortatrigen; Cortiotic; **Cortisporin**; *Cortisporin Ear*; Cortomycin; *Deltabiox*; Drotic; Ear-Eze; Equi-C-Sporin; Genasporin H.C.; Hydromycin; I-Neocort; Infa-Otic; Lazersporin-C; Masporin Otic; Mayotic; Medisol-Sp; Neo-Otosol-Hc; Neocin Pb-Hc; Neomycin Polymyxin Hc; *Neosporin-H*; Octicair; Octigen; Ocusporin Hc; Ocutricin Hc; Ortega-Otic-M; Oti-Sone; Otic-Care; Oticair; Oticin Hc; Oticrex; Otimar; Otisol Hc; Otitricin; Oto K Plus; Otobione; Otocidin; Otocort; Otomycin-Hpn; *Otosporin*; Pediotic; Phn-Otic; *Pocin-H*; Poly Otic; Qrp Ear Suspension; Spectro-Sporin; Storz H-P-N; Tex Sporin-Hc; Tri-Otic; Triple-Gen; Uad Otic; Visporin
(International brand names outside U.S. in italics)

FORMULARIES: Aetna; BC-BS; DoD; FHP; PCS

DESCRIPTION:

Hydrocortisone acetate neomycin sulfate; Polymyxin B a sterile antibacterial and anti-inflammatory drug product. Each ml contains: polymyxin B sulfate 10,000 units, neomycin sulfate equivalent to 3.5 mg neomycin base, and hydrocortisone 10 mg (1%). The vehicle contains thimerosal 0.01% (added as a preservative) and the inactive ingredients cetyl alcohol, propylene glycol, polysorbate 80, and Water for Injection. Sulfuric acid may be added to adjust

DESCRIPTION: *(cont'd)*

pH. Pediotic suspension has a minimum pH of 3.0.Polymyxin B sulfate is the sulfate salt of polymyxin B_1 and B_2, which are produced by the growth of*Bacillus polymyxa* (Prazmowski) Migula (Fam. Bacillaceae). It has a potency of not less than 6,000 polymyxin B units per mg, calculated on an anhydrous basis.

Neomycin sulfate is the sulfate salt of neomycin B and C, which are produced by the growth of *Streptomyces fradiae*Waksman (Fam.*Streptomycetaceae*). It has a potency equivalent of not less than 600 mcg of neomycin standard per mg, calculated on an anhydrous basis.

Hydrocortisone, 11β,17,21-trihydroxypregn-4-ene-3, 20-dione, is an anti-inflammatory hormone.

OTIC SOLUTION

Hydrocortisone acetate; neomycin sulfate; Polymyxin B a sterile antibacterial and anti-inflammatory drug product. Each ml contains: polymyxin B sulfate 10,000 units, neomycin sulfate equivalent to 3.5 mg neomycin base, and hydrocortisone 10 mg (1%). This vehicle contains potassium metabisulfite 0.1% (added as a preservative and the active ingredients cupric sulfate, glycerin, hydrochloric acid, propylene glycol and water for infection.

CLINICAL PHARMACOLOGY:

Corticoids suppress the inflammatory response to a variety of agents and they may delay healing. Since corticoids may inhibit the body's defense mechanism against infection, a concomitant antimicrobial drug may be used when this inhibition is considered to be clinically significant in a particular case.

The anti-infective components in the combination are included to provide action against specific organisms susceptible to them. Polymyxin B sulfate and neomycin sulfate together are considered active against the following microorganisms: *Staphylococcus aureus, Escherichia coli, Haemophilus influenzae, Klebsiella-Enterobacter* species,*Neisseria* species, and *Pseudomonas aeruginosa*. This product does not provide adequate coverage against *Serratia marcescens* and streptococci, including *Streptococcus pneumonia*.

The relative potency of corticosteroids depends on the molecular structure, concentration, and release from the vehicle.

ADDITIONAL INFORMATION FOR OPHTHALMIC SOLUTION

When used topically, polymyxin B and neomycin are rarely irritating, and absorption from the intact skin or mucous membrane is insignificant. The incidence of skin sensitization to this combination has been shown to be low on normal skin. Since these antibiotics are seldom used systemically, the patient is spared sensitization to those antibiotics which might later be required systemically.

When a decision to administer both a corticoid and antimicrobials is made, the administration of such drugs in combination has the advantage of greater patient compliance and convenience, with the added assurance that the intended dosage of both drugs is administered, plus assured compatibility of ingredients when both types of drugs are in the same formulation and, particularly that the intended volume of each drug is delivered simultaneously, thereby avoiding dilution of either medication by successive instillations.

INDICATIONS AND USAGE:

PEDIOTIC AND SUSPENSION

For the treatment of superficial bacterial infections of the external auditory canal caused by organisms susceptible to the action of the antibiotics, and for the treatment of infections of mastoidectomy and fenestration cavities caused by organisms susceptible to the antibiotics.

OPHTHALMIC SUSPENSION

For steroid-responsive inflammatory ocular conditions for which a corticosteroid is indicated and where bacterial infection or a risk of bacterial ocular infection exists. Ocular steroids are indicated in inflammatory conditions of the palpebral and bulbar conjunctiva, cornea and anterior segment of the globe where the inherent risk of steroid use uncertain infective conjunctivitises is accepted to obtain a diminution in edema and inflammation. They are also indicated in chronic anterior uveitis and corneal injury from chemical, radiation, or thermal burns, or penetration of foreign bodies.

The use of a combination drugs with an anti-infective component is indicated where the risk of infection is high or where there is an expectation that potentially dangerous numbers of bacteria will be present in the eye.

The particular anti-infective drugs in this product are active against the following bacterial eye pathogens: *Staphylococcus aureus, Escherichia coli, Haemophilus influenzae, Klebsiella-Enterobacter* species, *Neisseria* species, and *Pseudomonas aeruginosa*. This product does not provide adequate coverage against *Serratia marcescens* and streptococci, including *Streptococcus pneumonia*.

OTIC SOLUTION

For the treatment of superficial bacterial infections of the external auditory canal caused by organisms susceptible to the action of the antibiotics.

CONTRAINDICATIONS:

OTIC AND PEDIOTIC SUSPENSIONS, OTIC SOLUTION

This product is contraindicated in those individuals who have shown hypersensitivity to any of its components, and in herpes simplex, vaccinia and varicella infections.

OPHTHALMIC SUSPENSION

Epithelial herpes keratitis (dendritic keratitis), vaccinia, varicella, and many other viral diseases of the cornea and conjunctiva. Mycobacterial infection of the eye. Fungal diseases of ocular structures. Hypersensitivity to a component of the medication. (Hypersensitivity to the antibiotic component occurs at a higher rate than for other components). The use of these combinations is always contraindicated after uncomplicated removal of a corneal foreign body.

WARNINGS:

OTIC AND PEDIOTIC SUSPENSION

This product should be used with care in cases of perforated eardrum and in longstanding cases of chronic otitis media because of the possibility of ototoxicity.

Neomycin sulfate may cause cutaneous sensitization. A precise incidence of hypersensitivity reactions (primarily skin rash) due to topical neomycin is not known.

When using neomycin-containing products to control secondary infection in the chronic dermatoses, such as chronic otitis externa or stasis dermatitis, it should be borne in mind that the skin in these conditions is more liable than is normal skin to become sensitized to many substances, including neomycin. The manifestation of sensitization to neomycin is usually a low-grade reddening with swelling, dry scaling and itching; it may be manifest simply as a failure to heal. Periodic examination for such signs is advisable, and the patient should be told to discontinue the product if they are observed. These symptoms regress quickly on withdrawing the medication. Neomycin-containing applications should be avoided for the patient thereafter.

WARNINGS: *(cont'd)*

ADDITIONAL INFORMATION FOR OTIC SOLUTION

Contains potassium metabisulfite, a sulfate that may cause allergic-type reactions including anaphylactic symptoms and life threatening or less severe asthmatic episodes in certain susceptible people. The overall prevalence of sulfite sensitivity in the general population is unknown and probably low. Sulfite sensitivity is seen more frequently in asthmatic than in nonasthmatic people.

OPHTHALMIC SUSPENSION

Prolonged use may result in glaucoma, with damage to the optic nerve, defects in visual acuity and fields of vision, and posterior subcapsular cataract formation. Prolonged use may suppress the host response and thus increase the hazard of secondary ocular infections. In those diseases causing thinning of the cornea or sclera, perforations have been known to occur with the use of topical steroids. In acute purulent conditions of the eye, steroids may mask infection or enhance existing infection. If these products are used for 10 days or longer, intraocular pressure should be routinely monitored even though it may be difficult in children and uncooperative patients.

Employment of steroid medication in the treatment of herpes simplex requires great caution. Neomycin sulfate may cause cutaneous sensitization. A precise incidence of hypersensitivity is not known. The manifestations of sensitization to neomycin are usually itching, reddening and edema of the conjunctiva and eyelid. It may be manifest simply as failure to heal. During long-term use of neomycin-containing products, periodic examination of such signs is advisable, and the patient should be told to discontinue the product if they are observed. These symptoms subside quickly on withdrawing the medication. Neomycin-containing products should be avoided for the patient thereafter.

PRECAUTIONS:

OTIC AND PEDIOTIC SUSPENSION, OTIC SOLUTION

General: As with other antibiotic preparations, prolonged use may result in overgrowth of nonsusceptible organisms, including fungi.

If the infection is not improved after one week, cultures and susceptibility tests should be repeated to verify the identity of the organism and to determine whether therapy should be changed. Treatment should not be continued for longer than ten days.

Allergic cross-reactions may occur which could prevent the use of any or all of the following antibiotics for the treatment of future infections: kanamycin, paromomycin, streptomycin, and possibly gentamicin.

Information for the Patient: Avoid contaminating the dropper with material from the ear, fingers, or other source. This caution is necessary if the sterility of the drops is to be preserved.

If sensitization or irritation occurs, discontinue use immediately and contact your physician.

Do not use in the eyes.

SHAKE WELL BEFORE USING.

Laboratory Tests: Systemic effects of excessive levels of hydrocortisone may include a reduction in the number of circulating eosinophils and a decrease in urinary excretion of 17-hydroxycorticosteroids.

Carcinogenesis, Mutagenesis, Impairment of Fertility: Long-term studies in animals (rats, rabbits, mice) showed no evidence of carcinogenicity attributable to oral administration of corticosteroids.

Pregnancy, Teratogenic Effects, Pregnancy Category C: Corticosteroids have been shown to be teratogenic in rabbits when applied topically at concentrations of 0.5% on days 6 to 18 of gestation and in mice when applied topically at a concentration of 15% on days 10 to 13 of gestation. There are no adequate and well-controlled studies in pregnant women. Corticosteroids should be used during pregnancy only if the potential benefit justifies the potential risk to the fetus.

Nursing Mothers: Hydrocortisone appears in human milk following oral administration of the drug. Since systemic absorption of hydrocortisone may occur when applied topically, caution should be exercised when Cortisporin Otic Suspension is used by a nursing woman.

Pediatric Use: See DOSAGE AND ADMINISTRATION.

OPHTHALMIC SUSPENSION

General: The initial prescription and renewal of the medication beyond 20 ml should be made by a physician only after examination of the patient with the aid of magnification, such as slit lamp biomicroscopy and, where appropriate, fluorescein staining. The possibility of persistent fungal infection should be considered after prolonged steroid dosing. Allergic cross-reactions may occur which could prevent the use of any or all of the following antibiotics for the treatment of future infections: kanamycin, paromomycin, streptomycin, and possibly gentamicin.

Carcinogenesis, Mutagenesis, and Impairment of Fertility: Long-term studies in animals (rats, rabbits, mice) showed no evidence of carcinogenicity attributable to oral administration of corticosteroids.

Pregnancy, Teratogenic Effects, Pregnancy Category C: Corticosteroids have been shown to be teratogenic in rabbits when applied topically at concentrations of 0.5% on days 6 to 18 of gestation and in mice when applied topically at a concentration of 15% on days 10 to 13 of gestation. There are no adequate and well-controlled studies in pregnant women. Corticosteroids should be used during pregnancy only if the potential benefit justifies the potential risk to the fetus.

Nursing Mothers: Hydrocortisone appears in human milk following oral administration of the drug. Since systemic absorption of hydrocortisone may occur when applied topically, caution should be exercised when Cortisporin Otic Suspension is used by a nursing woman.

ADVERSE REACTIONS:

OTIC AND PEDIOTIC SUSPENSION, OTIC SOLUTION

Neomycin occasionally causes skin sensitization. Ototoxicity and nephrotoxicity have also been reported (See WARNINGS.) Adverse reactions have occurred with topical use of antibiotic combinations including neomycin and polymyxin B. Exact incidence figures are not available since no denominator of treated patients is available. The reaction occurring most often is allergic sensitization. In one clinical study, using a 20% neomycin patch, neomycin-induced allergic skin reactions occurred in two of 2,175 (0.09%) individuals in the general population. In another study, the incidence was found to be approximately 1%.

The following local adverse reactions have been reported with topical corticosteroids, especially under occlusive dressings: burning, itching, irritation, dryness, folliculitis, hypertrichosis, acneiform eruptions, hypopigmentation, perioral dermatitis, allergic contact dermatitis, maceration of the skin, secondary infection, skin atrophy, striae and miliaria. Stinging and burning have been reported rarely when this drug has gained access to the middle ear.

OPHTHALMIC SUSPENSION

Adverse reactions have occurred with steroid /anti-infective combination drugs which can be attributed to the steroid component, the anti-infective component, or the combination. Reactions occurring most often from the presence of the anti-infective ingredient are localized

ADVERSE REACTIONS: *(cont'd)*

hypersensitivity, including itching, swelling and conjunctive erythema. Local irritation on instillation has also been reported. Exact incidence figures are not available since no denominator of treated patients is available.

The reactions due to steroid component in decreasing order of frequency are: elevation of intraocular pressure (IOP) with possible development of glaucoma, and infrequent optic nerve damage; posterior subcapsular cataract formation; and delayed wound healing.

Secondary infection: The development of secondary infection has occurred after use of combinations containing steroids and microbials. Fungal infections of the cornea are particularly prone to develop coincidentally with long-term applications of steroid. The possibility of fungal invasion must be considered in any persistent corneal ulceration where steroid treatment has been used. Secondary bacterial ocular infection following suppression of host responses also occurs.

DOSAGE AND ADMINISTRATION:

OTIC AND PEDIOTIC SUSPENSION, OTIC SOLUTION

The external auditory canal should be thoroughly cleansed and dried with a sterile cotton applicator.

For adults, 4 drops of the suspension should be instilled into the affected ear 3 or 4 times daily. For infants and children, 3 drops are suggested because of the smaller capacity of the ear canal. The patient should lie with the affected ear upward and then the drops should be instilled. This position should be maintained for 5 minutes to facilitate penetration of the drops into the ear canal. Repeat, if necessary, for the opposite ear.

If preferred, a cotton wick may be inserted into the canal and then the cotton may be saturated with the suspension. This wick should be kept moist by adding further suspension every four hours. The wick should be replaced at least once every 24 hours.

OPHTHALMIC SUSPENSION

One or two drops in the affected eye every 3 to 4 hours, depending on the severity of the condition. The suspension may be used more frequently if necessary. Not more than 20 ml should be prescribed initially and the prescription should not be refilled without further evaluation.

SHAKE WELL BEFORE USING.

Store at 15 to 25°C (59 to 77°F).

REFERENCES:

1 Leyden JJ, Kligman AM. Contact dermatitis to neomycin sulfate. *JAMA* 1979;242(12):1276-1278. 2 Prystowsky SD, Allen AM, Smith RW, et al: Allergic contact hypersensitivity to nickel, neomycin, ethylenediamine, and benzocaine. *Arch Dermatol* 1979;115:959-962.

PATIENT INFORMATION:

Hydrocortisone; neomycin; polymyxin contains antibiotic and corticosteroid medications used to treat bacterial eye or ear infections and swelling. Notify your physician in you are pregnant or nursing. It is important that this medication is administered using the proper technique. Please obtain detailed administration directions from your pharmacist or physician. Gently shake the ophthalmic and otic suspensions before administering. The ophthalmic suspension may cause temporary blurring of vision or stinging following administration. Notify your physician if stinging, burning or itching becomes severe or if redness, irritation, swelling, decreasing vision or pain persist or worsen. The ophthalmic suspension may cause sensitivity to light. Hold the otic suspension container in your hand for a few minutes to warm it if it has been refrigerated. Notify your physician if burning or itching occurs or persists after using the otic suspension. Avoid touching the dropper or dispensing container to your eye or ear, or to anything else.

HOW SUPPLIED - RATED THERAPEUTICALLY EQUIVALENT:

Solution - Otic - 1 %/3.5 mg/10,0

10 ml	$2.98	CORT-BIOTIC, AF Hauser	52637-0708-10
10 ml	$3.12	Neomycin/Polymyxin/Hydrocortisone, H.C.F.A. F F P	99999-1490-01
10 ml	$3.50	BIO-COT OTIC, C O Truxton	00463-8050-10
10 ml	$7.02	Neomycin Poly Hydro, HL Moore Drug Exch	00839-6490-30
10 ml	$7.50	DROTIC, Ascher	00225-0340-55
10 ml	$7.70	ANTIBIOTIC EAR, Geneva Pharms	00781-7409-70
10 ml	$7.85	ANTIBIOTIC EAR, United Res	00677-0680-21
10 ml	$7.90	Neomycin/Polymyxin/Hydrocortisone, Steris Labs	00402-0708-10
10 ml	$7.90	CORTOMYCIN, Major Pharms	00904-3141-10
10 ml	$8.30	OTOCORT, Teva	00093-0047-43
10 ml	$8.95	CORTATRIGEN, MODIFIED EAR DROPS, Goldline Labs	00182-1388-63
10 ml	$8.95	OTIC CARE EAR, Parmed Pharms	00349-8895-70
10 ml	$8.95	QRP-OTIC, Quality Res Pharms	52765-0708-10
10 ml	$9.18	Neomycin/Polymyxin/Hc, Fougera	00168-0256-10
10 ml	$9.25	LAZERSPORIN-C, Pedinol Pharma	00884-4086-10
10 ml	$9.45	COBIOTIC, IDE-Interstate	00814-1745-40
10 ml	$10.13	AK-SPORE HC OTIC, Akorn	17478-0237-11
10 ml	$11.46	Neomycin/Polymyxin B/Hydroco, Schein Pharm (US)	00364-7300-54
10 ml	$12.38	ANTIBIOTIC EAR, Rugby	00536-4050-70
10 ml	**$21.34**	**CORTISPORIN, Glaxo Wellcome**	**00173-0199-92**
10 ml	$22.00	OTICIN HC, Teral Labs	51234-0114-10

Suspension - Ophthalmic - 1 %/3.5 mg/10,0

7.5 ml	$8.95	CORTOMYCIN, Major Pharms	00904-2994-32
7.5 ml	$10.50	Neomycin/Polymyxin B/Hydroco, Schein Pharm (US)	00364-0842-71
7.5 ml	$10.50	Neomycin/Polymyxin/Hydrocortisone, Steris Labs	00402-0774-07
7.5 ml	$10.89	NEOMYCIN/POLYMAXIN OPHTHALMIC, Rugby	00536-2590-77
7.5 ml	$11.81	Neomycin/Polymyxin/Hydrocortisone, HL Moore Drug Exch	00839-7175-28
7.5 ml	$12.00	AK-SPORE H.C., Akorn	17478-0231-09
7.5 ml	**$17.99**	**CORTISPORIN, Glaxo Wellcome**	**00173-0193-02**
10 ml	$14.21	NEOMYCYN/POLYMIXIN/HYDROCORT, Aligen Independ	00405-6130-07

Suspension - Otic - 1 %/3.5 mg/10,0

7.5 ml	$5.25	Neomycin/Polymyxin/Hydrocortisone, H.C.F.A. F F P	99999-1490-02
7.5 ml	$7.45	PHN-OTIC, Major Pharms	00904-7668-32
7.5 ml	$15.65	PEDIOTIC, Glaxo Wellcome	00173-0910-02
10 ml	$3.12	Neomycin/Polymyxin/Hydrocortisone, H.C.F.A. F F P	99999-1490-04
10 ml	$3.25	Tri-Otic Susp, H & H Labs	46703-0082-10
10 ml	$3.78	ANTIBIOTIC OTIC, Balan	00304-0949-56
10 ml	$3.98	CORT-BIOTIC, AF Hauser	52637-0709-10
10 ml	$4.35	ANTIBIOTIC EAR, Geneva Pharms	00781-7410-70
10 ml	$7.00	Neomycin/Polymyxin/Hydrocortisone, H.C.F.A. F F P	99999-1490-03
10 ml	$7.35	ANTIBIOTIC EAR, United Res	00677-0874-21
10 ml	$7.81	Neomycin/Polymixin/Hydrocort, Aligen Independ	00405-6160-10
10 ml	$7.88	Poly Otic, Poly Pharms	50991-0736-10
10 ml	$7.90	CORTOMYCIN, Major Pharms	00904-3017-10
10 ml	$8.63	COBIOTIC OTIC, IDE-Interstate	00814-1746-40
10 ml	$9.38	AK-SPORE H.C., Akorn	17478-0236-11
10 ml	$9.61	Neomycin/Polymyxin/Hydrocortisone, Steris Labs	00402-0736-10

HOW SUPPLIED - RATED THERAPEUTICALLY EQUIVALENT: *(cont'd)*

10 ml	$9.79	OCTICAIR, HL Moore Drug Exch	00839-6664-90
10 ml	$10.05	ANTIBIOTIC EAR, Rugby	00536-4071-70
10 ml	$10.09	OTOCORT, Teva	00093-0363-43
10 ml	$10.44	Neomycin/Polymyxin/Hc, Fougera	00168-0257-10
10 ml	$10.60	CORTATRIGEN MODIFIED EAR, Goldline Labs	00182-1563-63
10 ml	$10.99	OTIC CARE EAR, Parmed Pharms	00349-8894-70
10 ml	$11.01	Neomycin/Polymixin/Hydrocort, Aligen Independ	00405-6161-10
10 ml	$12.63	Neomycin/Polymyxin/Hydrocortisone, Schein Pharm (US)	00364-7374-54
10 ml	$15.07	UAD OTIC, UAD Labs	00785-9069-10
10 ml	**$21.34**	**CORTISPORIN, Glaxo Wellcome**	**00173-0198-92**
10 ml	$22.00	OTICIN HC, Teral Labs	51234-0115-10

HOW SUPPLIED - NOT RATED EQUIVALENT:

Solution - Otic - 1 %/3.5 mg/10,0

10 ml	$2.15	Infa-Otic Solution, Infinity Pharm	58154-0630-04
10 ml	$3.00	Octigen, Logen Pharm	00820-0114-24
10 ml	$3.05	Oticair, Raway	00686-0630-04
10 ml	$3.30	Equi-C-Sporin, Equipharm	57779-0131-10
10 ml	$6.00	Neocin Pb-Hc, Ocusoft	54799-0600-10
10 ml	$7.88	Poly Otic, Poly Pharms	50991-0708-10
10 ml	$8.71	Ear-Eze Solution, Hyrex Pharms	00314-0020-10

Suspension - Ophthalmic - 1 %/3.5 mg/10,0

7.5 ml	$8.50	Neomycin/Polymyxin/Hc, Consolidated Midland	00223-6752-75
7.5 ml	$10.89	Neomycin/Polymyxin/Hc, United Res	00677-1574-17

Suspension - Otic - 1 %/3.5 mg/10,0

10 ml	$2.15	Infa-Otic Suspension, Infinity Pharm	58154-0635-62
10 ml	$3.00	Octigen, Logen Pharm	00820-0115-24
10 ml	$3.05	Oticair, Raway	00686-7635-62
10 ml	$6.75	Aural Acute, Saron	00834-0004-71
10 ml	$8.95	Qrp Ear Suspension, Quality Res Pharms	52765-0736-10

HYDROCORTISONE; POLYMYXIN B SULFATE *(001492)*

CATEGORIES: Anti-Infectives; Anti-Inflammatory Agents; Antibacterials; Antibiotics; EENT Drugs; Eye, Ear, Nose, & Throat Preparations; Infections; Otic Hydrocortisones; Otic Preparations; Otologic; Steroids; Topical; FDA Approval Pre 1982

BRAND NAMES: Otobiotic; Otofair-B Otic; **Pyocidin**

FORMULARIES: Aetna; FHP

DESCRIPTION:

Each ml contains 10,000 USP units of polymyxin B sulfate and 5 mg hydrocortisone in a vehicle containing propylene glycol and water. Sodium hydroxide or hydrochloric acid may have been added to adjust pH.

CLINICAL PHARMACOLOGY:

Polymyxin B sulfate is effective against the gram-negative Pseudomonas Aeruginosa, one of the most resistant micro-organisms commonly causing otitis externa. The addition of hydrocortisone to the antibiotic affords an anti-inflammatory effect and relief against allergic manifestations and reduces the possibility of sensitivity and tissue reaction.

INDICATIONS AND USAGE:

For the treatment of superficial bacterial infections of the external auditory canal caused by organisms susceptible to the action of the antibiotic.

CONTRAINDICATIONS:

This product is contraindicated in those individuals who have shown hypersensitivity to any of its components, and in herpes simplex, vaccinia and varicella. Perforated tympanic membrane is considered a contraindication to the use of any medication in the external ear canal.

WARNINGS:

Discontinue promptly if sensitization or irritation occurs.

As with other antibiotic preparations, prolonged treatment may result in overgrowth of nonsusceptible organisms and fungi.

If the infection is not improved after one week, cultures and susceptibility tests should be repeated to verify the identity of the organism and to determine whether therapy should be changed.

Patients who prefer to warm the medication before using should be cautioned against heating the solution above body temperature, in order to avoid loss of potency.

PRECAUTIONS:

If sensitization or irritation occurs, medication should be discontinued promptly.

DOSAGE AND ADMINISTRATION:

The external auditory canal should be thoroughly cleaned and dried with a sterile cotton applicator.

For adults, 4 drops of the solution should be instilled into the affected ear 3 or 4 times daily. For infants and children, 3 drops are suggested because of the smaller capacity of the ear canal.

The patient should lie with the affected ear upward and then the drops should be instilled. This position should be maintained for 5 minutes to facilitate penetration of the drops into the ear canal. Repeat, if necessary, for the opposite ear.

If preferred, a cotton wick may be inserted into the canal and then the cotton may be saturated with the solution. This wick should be kept moist by adding further solution every four hours. The wick should be replaced at least once every 24 hours.

HOW SUPPLIED - RATED THERAPEUTICALLY EQUIVALENT:

Solution - Otic - 5 mg/10000 unit

10 ml	$5.90	Tri-Otic Sol, H & H Labs	46703-0051-10
15 ml	$18.00	OTOBIOTIC OTIC, Schering	00085-0847-05

HYDROFLUMETHIAZIDE *(001496)*

CATEGORIES: Antihypertensives; Cardiovascular Drugs; Cirrhosis; Congestive Heart Failure; Diuretics; Edema; Electrolytic, Caloric-Water Balance; Heart Failure; Hypertension; Renal Drugs; Renal Failure; Thiazides; Pregnancy Category C; FDA Approval Pre 1982

BRAND NAMES: *Diademil* (Japan); Diucardin; *Hydravern*; *Hydrenox* (England); *Leodrine*; *Rivosil*; *Rontyl* (Japan); **Saluron**; Sonazide
(International brand names outside U.S. in italics)

FORMULARIES: Medi-Cal

DESCRIPTION:

Hydroflumethiazide is an oral thiazide (benzothiadiazide) diuretic-antihypertensive agent.

Hydroflumethiazide is available as 50 mg tablets for oral administration.

Chemical Name: 3,4-Dihydro-6-(trifluoromethyl)-2H-1,2,4-benzothiadiazine-7-sulfonamide1,1-dioxide.

Hydroflumethiazide is an odorless, white to cream-colored, finely divided, crystalline powder. It has a melting point between 270° and 275°C. Hydroflumethiazide is freely soluble in acetone, soluble in alcohol, and very slightly soluble in water.

The inactive ingredients contained in hydroflumethiazide tablets are: lactose, magnesium stearate, microcrystalline cellulose, povidone, and starch.

CLINICAL PHARMACOLOGY:

Hydroflumethiazide is incompletely but rapidly absorbed from the gastrointestinal tract. It appears to have a biphasic biological half-life with an estimated alpha-phase of about 2 hours and an estimated beta-phase of about 17 hours; it has a metabolite with a longer half-life, which is extensively bound to the red blood cells. Hydroflumethiazide is excreted in the urine; its metabolite has also been detected in the urine.

The mechanism of action results in an interference with the renal tubular mechanism of electrolyte reabsorption. At maximal therapeutic dosage, all thiazides are approximately equal in their diuretic potency. The mechanism whereby thiazides function in the control of hypertension is unknown.

INDICATIONS AND USAGE:

Hydroflumethiazide is indicated as adjunctive therapy in edema associated with congestive heart failure, hepatic cirrhosis, and corticosteroid and estrogen therapy.

Hydroflumethiazide has also been found useful in edema due to various forms of renal dysfunction such as: nephrotic syndrome; acute glomerulonephritis; and chronic renal failure.

Hydroflumethiazide is indicated in the management of hypertension either as the sole therapeutic agent or to enhance the effect of other antihypertensive drugs in the more severe forms of hypertension.

USAGE IN PREGNANCY

The routine use of diuretics in an otherwise healthy woman is inappropriate and exposes mother and fetus to unnecessary hazard. Diuretics do not prevent development of toxemia of pregnancy, and there is no satisfactory evidence that they are useful in the treatment of developed toxemia.

Edema during pregnancy may arise from pathological causes or from the physiologic and mechanical consequences of pregnancy. Thiazides are indicated in pregnancy when edema is due to pathologic causes just as they are in the absence of pregnancy (see PRECAUTIONS, Pregnancy).

Dependent edema in pregnancy, resulting from restriction of venous return by the expanded uterus, is properly treated through elevation of the lower extremities and use of support hose. Use of diuretics to lower intravascular volume in this case is illogical and unnecessary. There is hypervolemia during normal pregnancy which is harmful to neither the fetus nor the mother (in the absence of cardiovascular disease), but which is associated with edema, including generalized edema, in the majority of pregnant women. If this edema produces discomfort, increased recumbency will often provide relief. In rare instances, this edema may cause extreme discomfort which is not relieved by rest. In these cases, a short course of diuretics may provide relief and may be appropriate.

CONTRAINDICATIONS:

Anuria: Hypersensitivity to this or other sulfonamide-derived drugs.

WARNINGS:

Hydroflumethiazide should be used with caution in severe renal disease. In patients with renal disease, thiazides may precipitate azotemia. Cumulative effects of the drug may develop in patients with impaired renal function.

Thiazides should be used with caution in patients with impaired hepatic function or progressive liver disease, since minor alterations of fluid and electrolyte balance may precipitate hepatic coma.

Thiazides may add to or potentiate the action of other antihypertensive drugs. Potentiation occurs with ganglionic or peripheral adrenergic blocking drugs.

Sensitivity reactions may occur in patients with a history of allergy or bronchial asthma.

The possibility of exacerbation or activation of systemic lupus erythematosus has been reported.

PRECAUTIONS:

GENERAL

All patients receiving thiazide therapy should be observed for clinical signs of fluid or electrolyte imbalance; namely, hyponatremia, hypochloremic alkalosis, and hypokalemia. Serum and urine electrolyte determinations are particularly important when the patient is vomiting excessively or receiving parenteral fluids. Medication such as digitalis may also influence serum electrolytes. Warning signs, irrespective of cause, are: dryness of mouth, thirst, weakness, lethargy, drowsiness, restlessness, muscle pains or cramps, muscular fatigue, hypotension, oliguria, tachycardia, and gastrointestinal disturbances such as nausea and vomiting.

Hypokalemia may develop with thiazides as with any other potent diuretic, especially with brisk diuresis, when severe cirrhosis is present, or during concomitant use of corticosteroids or ACTH.

Interference with adequate oral electrolyte intake will also contribute to hypokalemia. Digitalis therapy may exaggerate metabolic effects of hypokalemia, especially with reference to myocardial activity.

PRECAUTIONS: *(cont'd)*

Any chloride deficit is generally mild and usually does not require specific treatment except under extraordinary circumstances (as in liver disease or renal disease). Dilutional hyponatremia may occur in edematous patients in hot weather; appropriate therapy is water restriction, rather than administration of salt, except in rare instances when the hyponatremia is life-threatening. In actual salt depletion, appropriate replacement is the therapy of choice.

Hyperuricemia may occur or frank gout may be precipitated in certain patients receiving thiazide therapy.

Insulin requirements in diabetic patients may be increased, decreased, or unchanged. Latent diabetes mellitus may become manifested during thiazide administration.

The antihypertensive effects of the drug may be enhanced in the post-sympathectomy patient.

If progressive renal impairment becomes evident, as indicated by a rising creatinine or blood urea nitrogen, a careful reappraisal of therapy is necessary with consideration given to withholding or discontinuing diuretic therapy.

Thiazides may decrease serum PBI levels without signs of thyroid disturbance.

Lithium generally should not be given with diuretics because they reduce its renal clearance and increase the risk of lithium toxicity. Read circulars for lithium preparations before use of such concomitant therapy with hydroflumethiazide.

Thiazides have been shown to increase the urinary excretion of magnesium; this may result in hypomagnesemia.

Calcium excretion is decreased by thiazides. Pathological changes in the parathyroid gland with hypercalcemia and hypophosphatemia have been observed in a few patients on prolonged thiazide therapy. The common complications of hyperparathyroidism, such as renal lithiasis, bone resorption, and peptic ulceration, have not been seen.

LABORATORY TESTS

Periodic determination of serum electrolytes to detect possible electrolyte imbalance should be performed at appropriate intervals.

CARCINOGENESIS, MUTAGENESIS, AND IMPAIRMENT OF FERTILITY

No studies have been performed to evaluate carcinogenic or mutagenic potential of hydroflumethiazide or the potential ofazude to impair fertility.

PREGNANCY CATEGORY C

Teratogenic Effects: Animal reproduction studies have not been conducted with hydroflumethiazide. It is also not known whether hydroflumethiazide can cause fetal harm when administered to a pregnant woman or can affect reproduction capacity. Hydroflumethiazide should be given to a pregnant woman only if clearly needed.

Nonteratogenic Effects: Fetal or neonatal jaundice, thrombocytopenia, and possibly other adverse reactions which have occurred in the adult.

NURSING MOTHERS

Thiazides appear in breast milk. If use of the drug is deemed essential, the patient may consider stopping nursing.

PEDIATRIC USE

Safety and effectiveness in children have not been established.

DRUG INTERACTIONS:

Anticoagulants, Oral: (Effects may be decreased when used concurrently with thiazide diuretics; dosage adjustments may be necessary.)

Antigout Medications: (Thiazide diuretics may raise the level of blood uric acid; dosage adjustment of antigout medications may be necessary to control hyperuricemia and gout.)

Antihypertensive medications, other, especially diazoxide, or preanesthetic and anesthetic agents used in surgery or skeletal-muscle relaxants, nondepolarizing, used in surgery

(Effects may be potentiated when used concurrently with thiazide diuretics; dosage adjustments may be necessary.)

Amphotericin B or Corticosteroids or Corticotropin (ACTH): (Concurrent use with thiazide diuretics may intensify electrolyte imbalance, particularly hypokalemia.)

Cardiac Glycosides: (Concurrent use with thiazide diuretics may enhance the possibility of digitalis toxicity associated with hypokalemia.)

Colestipol: (May inhibit gastrointestinal absorption of the thiazide diuretics; administration 1 hour before or 4 hours after colestipol is recommended.)

Hypoglycemics: (Thiazide diuretics may raise blood glucose levels; for adult-onset diabetics, dosage adjustment of hypoglycemic medications may be necessary during and after thiazide diuretic therapy; insulin requirements may be increased, decreased, or unchanged.)

Lithium salts: (Concurrent use with thiazide diuretics is not recommended, as they may provoke lithium toxicity because of reduced renal clearance.)

Methenamine: (Effectiveness may be decreased when used concurrently with thiazide diuretics because of alkalinization of the urine.)

Nonsteroidal Anti-Inflammatory Agents: (In some patients, the steroidal anti-inflammatory agent can reduce the diuretic, natriuretic, and antihypertensive effects of loop, potassium sparing, and thiazide diuretics. Therefore, when hydroflumethiazide and nonsteroidal anti-inflammatory agents are used concomitantly, the patient should be observed closely to determine if the desired effect of the diuretic is obtained.)

Norepinephrine: (Thiazides may decrease arterial responsiveness to norepinephrine. This diminution is not sufficient to preclude effectiveness of the pressor agent for therapeutic use.)

Tubocurarine: (Thiazide drugs may increase the responsiveness to tubocurarine.)

Diagnostic Interference: With expected physiologic effects:

Blood and urine glucose levels (usually only in patients with a predisposition to glucose intolerance) and

Serum bilirubin levels (by displacement from albumin binding) and

Serum calcium levels (thiazide diuretics should be discontinued before parathyroid-function tests are carried out) and

Serum uric acid levels (may be increased)

Serum magnesium, potassium, and sodium levels (may be decreased; serum magnesium levels may increase in uremic patients)

Serum protein-bound iodine (PBI) levels (may be decreased)

Thiazides should be discontinued before carrying out tests for parathyroid function (see PRECAUTIONS, General) Calcium excretion.

ADVERSE REACTIONS:

The following adverse reactions have been observed, but there is not enough systematic collection of data to support an estimate of their frequency.

Gastrointestinal System: Anorexia, gastric irritation, nausea, vomiting, cramping, diarrhea, constipation, jaundice (intrahepatic cholestatic jaundice), pancreatitis, sialadenitis.

CNS: Dizziness, vertigo, paresthesias, headache, xanthopsia.

Hematologic: Leukopenia, agranulocytosis, thrombocytopenia, aplastic anemia, hemolytic anemia.

ADVERSE REACTIONS: *(cont'd)*

Cardiovascular: Orthostatic hypotension (may be aggravated by alcohol, barbiturates, or narcotics).

Dermatologic-Hypersensitivity: Purpura, photosensitivity, rash, urticaria, necrotizing angiitis (vasculitis, cutaneous vasculitis), fever, respiratory distress including pneumonitis, anaphylactic reactions.

Other: Hyperglycemia, glycosuria, hyperuricemia, muscle spasm, weakness, restlessness, transient blurred vision.

Whenever adverse reactions are moderate or severe, thiazide dosage should be reduced or therapy withdrawn.

OVERDOSAGE:

Signs and Symptoms: Diuresis, lethargy progressing to coma, with minimal cardiorespiratory depression and with or without significant serum electrolyte changes or dehydration; GI irritation; hypermotility; transient elevation in BUN level.

Treatment: Empty stomach by gastric lavage, taking care to avoid aspiration. Monitor serum electrolyte levels and renal function, and institute supportive measures, as required to maintain hydration, electrolyte balance, respiration, and cardiovascular and renal function. Treat GI effects symptomatically.

DOSAGE AND ADMINISTRATION:

The average adult diuretic dose is 25 to 200 mg per day. The average adult antihypertensive dose is 50 to 100 mg per day.

Therapy should be individualized according to patient response. This therapy should be titrated to gain maximal therapeutic response as well as the minimal dose possible to maintain that therapeutic response.

Store at room temperature (approximately 25°C).

HOW SUPPLIED - RATED THERAPEUTICALLY EQUIVALENT:

Tablet, Uncoated - Oral - 50 mg

100's	$47.86	DIUCARDIN, Ayerst	00046-0702-81
100's	**$64.60**	**SALURON, Mead Johnson**	**00015-5410-60**

HYDROFLUMETHIAZIDE; RESERPINE *(001497)*

CATEGORIES: Antihypertensives; Cardiovascular Drugs; Diuretics; Hypertension; Renal Drugs; Vascular Disorders, Cerebral/Peripheral; FDA Approval Pre 1982

BRAND NAMES: *Adelfan*; *Diuritens*; Genutensin; Hydro-Fluserpine; Hydropine Hp; Salazide; **Salutensin**; Serflugen
(International brand names outside U.S. in italics)

FORMULARIES: Medi-Cal

> WARNING:
> This fixed combination drug is not indicated for initial therapy of hypertension. Hypertension requires therapy titrated to the individual patient. If the fixed combination represents the dosage so determined, its use may be more convenient in patient management. The treatment of hypertension is not static, but must be preevaluated as conditions in each patient warrant.

DESCRIPTION:

These tablets for oral administration combine two antihypertensive agents: Hydroflumethiazide and reserpine. The chemical name for hydroflumethiazide is 3,4-dihydro-7-sulfamyl-6-trifluoromethyl-2H-1,2,4-benzothiadiazine-1,1-dioxide. Hydroflumethiazide is very slightly soluble in water, soluble in methanol and freely soluble in acetone.

Reserpine (3,4,5-trimethoxybenzoyl methyl reserpate) is a crystalline alkaloid derived from Rauwolfia serpentina. It is very slightly soluble in water, slightly soluble in acetone, methanol and ethanol and freely soluble in chloroform and methylene chloride.

Each Tablet Contains:

Hydroflumethiazide 50 mg
Reserpine 0.125 mg
or
Hydroflumethiazide 25 mg
Reserpine 0.125 mg

Inactive Salutensin Ingredients in the 50 mg Tablets Are: D&C Yellow No. 10 Lake, FD&C Blue 1 Lake 12%, lactose, magnesium stearate, povidone, starch and sucrose.

Inactive Salutensin Ingredients in the 25 mg Tablets Are: D&C Red No. 30 Lake, D&C Yellow No. 10 Lake, lactose, magnesium stearate, povidone, starch and sucrose.

CLINICAL PHARMACOLOGY:

Hydroflumethiazide is incompletely but fairly rapidly absorbed form the gastrointestinal tract. It appears to have a biphasic biological half-life with an estimated alpha-phase of about 2 hours and an estimated beta-phase of about 17 hours; it has a metabolite with a longer half-life, which is extensively bound to the red blood cells. Hydroflumethiazide is excreted in the urine; its metabolite has also been detected in the urine.

Hydroflumethiazide is an oral diuretic-antihypertensive agent. It exerts its effect by inhibiting renal tubular reabsorption, including increased excretion of sodium and chloride and water with variable concomitant loss of potassium and bicarbonate as well. When used alone as an antihypertensive agent, hydroflumethiazide usually induces a gradual but sustained decrease in abnormally elevated blood-pressure - both systolic and diastolic. Hypertensive patients who have been maintained on chlorothiazide or hydrochlorothiazide may also be maintained on hydroflumethiazide.

Reserpine is absorbed from the gastrointestinal tract. About 6% has been reported to be excreted in the urine in the first 24 hours and about 8% in the first 4 days mainly as the metabolite trimethyoxybenzoic acid. Over 60% is excreted in the feces in the first 4 days, mainly unchanged. Reserpine crosses the placental barrier and also appears in breast milk.

The component, reserpine, probably produces its antihypertensive effects through depletion of tissue stores of catecholamines (epinephrine and norepinephrine) from peripheral sites. By contrasts, its sedative and tranquilizing properties are thought to be related to depletion of 5-hydroxytryptamine from the brain.

Reserpine is characterized by slow onset of action and sustained effect. Both its cardiovascular and central nervous system effects may persist following withdrawal of the drug.

Careful observation for changes in blood pressure must be made when hydroflumethiazide w/ reserpine is used with other antihypertensive drugs.

INDICATIONS AND USAGE:

Hypertension: (See BOXED WARNING.)

CONTRAINDICATIONS:

This drug is contraindicated in patients with a history of mental depression because the possibility that it will potentiate depression and increase the possibility of suicide or in patients who have previously demonstrated hypersensitivity to its components. Patients with anuria or oliguria should not be given this medication. The presence of an active peptic ulcer, ulcerative colitis or depression contraindicates the use of reserpine. If electroshock therapy is necessary, treatment with hydroflumethiazide w/reserpine should be discontinued at least seven (7) days prior to this therapy.

WARNINGS:

Azotemia may be precipitated or increased by hydroflumethiazide. Special caution is necessary in patients with impaired renal function to avoid cumulative or toxic effects.

Since in hepatic cirrhosis, minor alterations of fluid and electrolyte balance may precipitate coma, hydroflumethiazide should be given with caution.

The possibility of sensitivity reactions should be considered in patients with a history of allergy or bronchial asthma.

Hydroflumethiazide potentiates the action of other antihypertensive drugs. Therefore, the dosage of these agents, especially the ganglion blockers, must be reduced by at least 50 percent as soon as hydroflumethiazide is added to the regimen.

The possibility of exacerbation or activation of systemic lupus erythematosus has been reported for sulfonamide derivatives (including thiazides) and reserpine.

Reserpine may cause mental depression. Recognition of depression may be difficult because depression may often be disguised by somatic complaints (Masked Depression). The drug should be discontinued at first signs of depression such as despondency, early morning insomnia, loss of appetite, impotence, or self-deprecation. Drug-induced depression may persist for several months after drug withdrawal and may be severe enough to result in suicide.

PRECAUTIONS:

GENERAL

This is a combination product containing hydroflumethiazide and reserpine. Precautions to be observed are associated with the individual components and are listed below.

HYDROFLUMETHIAZIDE

Careful check should be kept for signs of fluid and electrolyte imbalance. Serum and urine electrolyte determinations are particularly important when the patient is vomiting excessively or receiving parenteral fluids. Warnings signs, irrespective of cause are: dryness of mouth, thirst, weakness, lethargy, drowsiness, restlessness, muscle pains or cramps, muscular fatigue, hypotension, oliguria, tachycardia, and gastrointestinal disturbances.

Potassium excretion is usually minimal. However, hypokalemia may develop with hydroflumethiazide as with any other potent diuretic, especially with brisk diuresis, when severe cirrhosis is present, or during concomitant use of steroids or ACTH. Interference with adequate electrolyte intake will contribute to hypokalemia. Digitalis therapy may exaggerate metabolic effects of hypokalemia especially with reference to myocardial activity. If dietary salt is unduly restricted, especially during hot weather, in severely edematous patients with congestive failure or renal disease, a low salt syndrome may complicate therapy with thiazides.

Hypokalemia may be avoided or treated by use of potassium chloride or giving foods with a high potassium content. Any chloride deficit may similarly be corrected by use of ammonium chloride (excepting patients with hepatic disease) and largely prevented by near normal salt intake.

Thiazide drugs may increase the responsiveness to tubocurarine. The antihypertensive effect of the drug may be enhanced in the post-sympathectomy patient. Hydroflumethiazide decreases arterial responsiveness to norepinephrine, as do other thiazides, necessitating due care in surgical patients. It is recommended that thiazide be discontinued 48 hours before elective surgery. Orthostatic hypotension may occur and may be potentiated by alcohol, barbiturates, or narcotics.

Pathological changes in the parathyroid glands with hypercalcemia and hypophosphatemia have been observed in a few patients on prolonged thiazide therapy. The common complications of hyperparathyroidism such as renal lithiasis, bone resorption, and peptic ulceration have not been seen. The effect of discontinuance of thiazide therapy on serum calcium and phosphorus levels may be helpful in assessing the need for parathyroid surgery in such patients. Parathyroidectomy has been followed by subjective clinical improvement in most patients, but is without effect on the hypertension. Following surgery, thiazide therapy may be resumed.

Caution is necessary in patients with hyperuricemia or a history of gout, since gout may be precipitated. Insulin requirements in diabetic patients may be increased, decreased, or unchanged. In latent diabetics, hydroflumethiazide, in common with other benzothiadiazines, may cause hyperglycemia and glycosuria.

RESERPINE

Since reserpine may increase gastric secretion and mobility, it should be used cautiously in patients with a history of peptic ulcer, ulcerative colitis, or other gastrointestinal disorders. This compound may precipitate biliary colic in patients with gallstones, or bronchial asthma in susceptible persons.

Reserpine may cause hypotension including orthostatic hypotension. In hypertensive patients on reserpine therapy significant hypotension and bradycardia may develop during surgical anesthesia. Therefore, the drug should be discontinued two weeks before giving anesthesia. For emergency surgical procedures, it may be necessary to give vagal blocking agents parenterally to prevent or reverse hypotension and/or bradycardia.

Anxiety, depression, as well as psychosis, may develop during reserpine therapy. If depression is present when therapy is begun, it may be aggravated. Mental depression is unusual with reserpine doses of 0.25 mg daily or less. In any case, hydroflumethiazide w/reserpine should be discontinued at the first sign of depression.

As with most antihypertensive therapy, caution should be exercised when treating hypertensive patients with renal insufficiency, since they adjust poorly to lowered blood pressure levels. Use reserpine cautiously with digitalis and quinidine; cardiac arrhythmias have occurred with reserpine preparations. Thiazides may decrease serum P.B.I. levels without signs of thyroid disturbance.

INFORMATION FOR THE PATIENT

If you miss a dose of this medicine, take it as soon as possible. If it is almost time for your next dose, do not take the missed dose at all and do not double the next one. Instead, go back to your regular dosing schedule. If you have any questions about this, check with your doctor.

This Medicine May Cause a Loss of Potassium From Your Body. To help prevent this, you doctor may want you to:

PRECAUTIONS: *(cont'd)*

eat or drink foods that have a high potassium content (for example, orange or citrus fruit juices,) or

take a potassium supplement, or

take another medicine to help prevent the loss of the potassium in the first place.

It is very important to follow these directions. Also, it is important not to change your diet on your own. This is more important if you are already on a special diet (as for diabetes), or if you are taking a potassium supplement or a medicine to reduce potassium loss. Extra potassium may not be necessary and, in some cases, too much potassium could be harmful.

Check with your doctor if you become sick and have severe or continuing vomiting or diarrhea. These problems may cause you to lose additional water and potassium.

Caution: Diabetics-This medicine may raise blood sugar levels. While you are using this medicine, be especially careful in testing for sugar in your urine. If you have any questions about this, check with your doctor.

A few people who take this medicine may become more sensitive to sunlight than they are normally. When you begin to take this medicine, avoid too much sun or use of a sunlamp until you see how you react, especially if you tend to burn easily. If you have a severe reaction, check with your doctor.

This medicine may cause some people to become drowsy or less alert than they are normally. This is more likely to happen when you begin to take it or when you increase the amount of medicine you are taking. **Make sure you know how you react to this medicine before you drive, use machines, or do other jobs that require you to be alert.**

Dizziness, lightheadedness, or fainting may occur, especially when you get up from a lying or sitting position. Getting up slowly may help, but if the problem continues or gets worse, check with your doctor.

In some patients, this medicine may cause mental depression. **Tell Your Doctor Right Away:**

if you or anyone else notices unusual changes in your moods.

if you start having early-morning sleeplessness or unusually vivid dreams or nightmares.

This medicine will add to the effects of alcohol and other medicines (CNS depressants) that slow down the nervous system. Some examples of CNS depressants are antihistamines or medicine for hay fever, other allergies, or colds; sedatives, tranquilizers, or sleeping medicine, prescription pain medicine or narcotics; barbiturates; medicine for seizures; tricyclic antidepressants (medicine for depression); or anesthetics; including dental anesthetics. **Check with your doctor before taking any of the above while you are taking this medicine.**

Before having any kind of surgery (including dental surgery), or emergency treatment, make sure the doctor or dentist in charge knows that you are taking this medicine.

This medicine may cause stuffiness in the nose. However, do not use nasal decongestant medicines without first checking with your doctor or pharmacist.

Do not take other medicines unless they have been discussed with your doctor. This especially includes over-the-counter (nonprescription) medicines for appetite control, asthma, colds, cough, hay fever, or sinus, since that may tend to increase your blood pressure.

Your mouth, nose, and throat may feel very dry while you are taking this medicine. To help relieve mouth dryness; chew sugarless gum or dissolve bits of ice in your mouth.

LABORATORY TESTS

Determination of serum electrolytes to detect possible electrolyte imbalance should be performed at appropriate intervals.

DIAGNOSTIC INTERFERENCE

Reserpine

With diagnostic test results

Urinary steroid colorimetric determinations by modified Glenn-Nelson technique or Holtroff Koch modification of Zimmerman reaction (falsely low because rauwolfia alkaloids slightly decrease absorbance)

With expected physiologic effects

Serum prolactin levels (may be increased)

Urinary catecholamine excretion (large parenteral doses of reserpine may cause an initial increase, although an overall decrease is usually noted chronic administration of rauwolfia alkaloids)

Urinary vanilmandelic acid (VMA) excretion (intramuscular administration of reserpine causes an initial increase of about 40%, followed by a decrease by the end of the second day; chronic or parenteral administration of rauwolfia alkaloids results in an overall decrease)

Hydroflumethiazide

With expected physiologic effects

Blood and urine glucose levels (usually only in patients with a predisposition to glucose intolerance) and

Serum bilirubin levels (by displacement from albumin binding) and

Serum calcium levels (thiazide diuretics should be discontinued before parathyroid function tests are carried out) and

Serum uric acid levels (may be increased)

Serum magnesium, potassium, and sodium levels (may be decreased; serum magnesium levels may increase in uremic patients)

Serum protein-bound iodine (PBI) levels (may be decreased)

ANIMAL TUMORIGENICITY

Rodent studies have shown that reserpine is an animal tumorigen, causing an increased incidence of mammary fibroadenomas in female mice, malignant tumors of the seminal vesicals in male mice, malignant adrenal medullary tumors in male rats. These findings arose in 2-year studies in which the drug was administered in the feed at concentrations of 5 and 10 ppm - about 100 to 300 times the usual human dose. The breast neoplasms are thought to be related to reserpine's prolactin-elevating effect. Several other prolactin elevating drugs have also been associated with an increased incidence of mammary neoplasia in rodents.

The extent to which these findings indicate a risk to humans is uncertain. Tissue culture experiments show that about one-third of human breast tumors are prolactin-dependent *in vitro*, a factor of considerable importance if the use of the drug is contemplated in a patient with previously detected breast cancer. The possibility of an increased risk of breast cancer in reserpine users has been studied extensively; however, no firm conclusion has emerged. Although a few epidemiologic studies have suggested a slightly increased risk (less than two-fold in all studies except one) in women who have used reserpine, other studies of generally similar design have not confirmed this. Epidemiologic studies conducted using other drugs (neuroleptic agents) that, like reserpine, increase prolactin levels and therefore would be considered rodent mammary carcinogens, have not shown an association between chronic administration of the drug and human mammary tumorigenesis. While long-term clinical observation has not suggested such an association, the available evidence is considered too limited to be conclusive at this time. An association of reserpine intake with pheochromocytoma or tumors of the seminal vesicles has not been explored.

PRECAUTIONS: *(cont'd)*

PREGNANCY CATEGORY C

Teratogenic Effects

Animal reproduction studies *have not* been conducted with hydroflumethiazide w/reserpine. It is also not known whether this combination drug can cause fetal harm when administered to a pregnant woman or can affect reproduction capacity. Hydroflumethiazide w/reserpine should be given to a pregnant woman only if clearly indicated.

Nonteratogenic Effects

There is some evidence that side effects such as nasal congestion, lethargy, depressed Moro reflex, and bradycardia may appear in infants born of reserpine treated mothers. Thiazides cross the placental barrier and appear in cord blood. When hydroflumethiazide w/reserpine is used in women of childbearing age, the potential benefits of the drug should be weighed against the possible hazards to the fetus. These hazards included fetal or nonfetal jaundice, thrombocytopenia, and possibly other adverse reactions which have occurred in the adult.

NURSING MOTHERS

Thiazides and reserpine appear in breast milk. If use of the drug is deemed essential, the mother may consider stopping nursing.

PEDIATRIC USE

Safety and effectiveness in children have not been established.

DRUG INTERACTIONS:

RESERPINE

Alcohol or CNS depressants (concurrent use may enhance the CNS depressant effects of either these medications or rauwolfia alkaloids).

Antihypertensives, other, or diuretics (antihypertensive effects may be potentiated when used concurrently with rauwolfia alkaloids; although some combinations are frequently used for therapeutic advantage, when used concurrently, dosage adjustments may be necessary).

Beta-blockers (concurrent administration with beta-blockers may result in additive and possibly excessive beta-adrenergic blockage. Although this effect is largely theoretical, close observations is recommended).

Digitalis glycosides or quinidine (Concurrent use may result in cardiac arrhythmias; although this interaction is controversial and does not appear to be significant with usual doses, caution is recommended, especially when large doses of rauwolfia alkaloids are used in digitalized patients).

Levodopa (since rauwolfia alkaloids may cause dopamine depletion and parkinsonism effects, concurrent use is not recommended).

Methotrimeprazine (concurrent use may result in additive hypotension).

Monamine oxidase (MAO) inhibitors (concurrent use with rauwolfia alkaloids may result in moderate to sudden and severe hypertension and hyperpyrexia which can reach crisis levels).

Sympathomimetic, indirect-acting amines such as amphetamines, ephedrine, methylphenidate, phenylpropanolamine, pseudoephedrine, tyramine (rauwolfia alkaloids inhibit the action of indirect-acting sympathomimetics by depleting catecholamine stores).

Direct-acting amines such as epinephrine, isoproterenol, and norepinephrine (levarterenol), included are metaraminol and phenylephrine which are thought to act both directly and indirectly (rauwolfia alkaloids may theoretically prolong the action of direct-acting sympathomimetics by preventing uptake into storage granules; a "denervation supersensitivity" response is also possible; although concurrent use with rauwolfia alkaloids is not known to produce severe adverse effects, a significant increase in blood pressure has been documented when phenylephrine ophthalmic drops have been administered to patients taking reserpine, and caution and close observation are recommended).

Tricyclic antidepressants (concurrent use may decrease the hypotensive effects of rauwolfia alkaloids and interfere with the antidepressant effects of these medications).

HYDROFLUMETHIAZIDE

Antihypertensive medications, other, especially diazoxide, or

Preanesthetic and anesthetic agents used in surgery or

Skeletal muscle relaxants, nondepolarizing, used in surgery (effects may be potentiated when used concurrently with thiazide diuretics; dosage adjustments may be necessary).

Amphotericin B or

Corticosteroids or

Corticotropin (ACTH) (Concurrent use with thiazide diuretics may intensify electrolyte imbalance, particularly hypokalemia).

Colestipol (may inhibit gastrointestinal absorption of the thiazide diuretics; administrations 1 hour before or 4 hours after colestipol is recommended.)

Hypoglycemics (thiazide diuretics may raise blood glucose levels; for adult onset diabetics, dosage adjustment of hypoglycemic medications may be necessary during and after thiazide diuretic therapy; insulin requirements may be increased, decreased, or unchanged).

Lithium salts (concurrent use with thiazide diuretics is not recommended, as they may provoke lithium toxicity because of reduced renal clearance).

Methenamine (effectiveness may be decreased when used concurrently with thiazide diuretics because of alkalinization of the urine).

Nonsteroidal anti-inflammatories (in some patients, the administration of a non-steroidal anti-inflammatory agent can reduce the diuretic, natriuretic and antihypertensive effects of looped, potassium sparing and thiazide diuretics. Therefore, when hydroflumethiazide w/reserpine and nonsteroidal anti-inflammatory agents are used concomitantly, the patient should be observed closely to determine if the desired effect of the diuretic is obtained).

ADVERSE REACTIONS:

The following adverse reactions have been observed, but there is not enough systematic collection of data to support an estimate of their frequency.

HYDROFLUMETHIAZIDE

A. Gastrointestinal System Reactions: anorexia, gastric irritation, nausea, vomiting, cramping, diarrhea, constipation, jaundice (intrahepatic cholestatic jaundice), pancreatitis, hyperglycemia, and glycosuria.

B. Central Nervous System Reactions: dizziness, vertigo paresthesias, headache, and xanthopsia.

C. Hematologic Reactions: leukopenia, thrombocytopenia, agranulocytosis, and aplastic anemia.

D. Dermatologic-Hypersensitivity Reactions: purpura, photosensitivity rash, urticaria, and necrotizing angitis (vasculitis) (cutaneous vasculitis).

E. Cardiovascular Reaction: orthostatic hypotension may occur and may be aggravated by alcohol, barbiturates or narcotics.

F. Miscellaneous: muscle spasm, weakness, restlessness, fever, respiratory distress including pneumonitis, pulmonary edema and anaphylactic reactions.

Whenever adverse reactions are moderate or severe, thiazide dosage should be reduced or therapy withdrawn.

ADVERSE REACTIONS: *(cont'd)*

RESERPINE

A. Gastrointestinal System Reactions: anorexia nausea, increased intestinal motility, diarrhea, dryness of the mouth, increased salivation, vomiting.

B. Central Nervous System Reactions: excessive sedation, nightmares, headaches, dizziness, blurred vision, syncope, impotence or decreased libido, mental depression, nervousness, paradoxical anxiety, dull sensorium, deafness, glaucoma, uveitis, optic atrophy, parkinson-like syndrome.

C. Hematologic Reactions: epistaxis, purpura due to thrombocytopenia.

D. Dermatological Reactions: conjunctival injection, flushing of the skin, pruritus, rash.

E. Cardiovascular Reactions: bradycardia, dyspnea, angina pectoris and other direct cardiac effects (*e.g.,* premature ventricular contractions, fluid retention, congestive failure).

F. Miscellaneous: nasal congestion, weight gain, muscular aches, enhanced susceptibility to colds, dysuria, non-puerperal lactation.

OVERDOSAGE:

SIGNS AND SYMPTOMS

Hydroflumethiazide-Related Effects: diuresis, lethargy progressing to coma with minimal cardiorespiratory depression, GI irritation, hypermotility, elevated BUN, serum electrolyte changes.

Reserpine-Related Effects: impairment of consciousness ranging from drowsiness to coma, flushing, conjunctival injection, miosis, hypotension, hypothermia, respiratory depression, bradycardia, diarrhea.

TREATMENT

Induce emesis or use gastric lavage, followed by activated charcoal, to empty stomach. Treat hypotension by volume expansion, if possible. If a vasopressor is needed, use phenylephrine, levarterenol, or metaraminol. Treat significant bradycardia with vagal blocking agents, along with other appropriate measures. Monitor serum electrolytes and renal function, and institute supportive measures, as required. Treat GI effects symptomatically. Observe patient for at least 72 hours.

DIALYZABILITY

There is no information on the dialyzability of hydroflumethiazide w/reserpine.

DOSAGE AND ADMINISTRATION:

As determined by individual titration (see BOXED WARNING).

The usual adult dose of hydroflumethiazide w/reserpine is one tablet (50 mg) once or twice daily. If a smaller amount of thiazide diuretic is desired, hydroflumethiazide w/reserpine "Demi" (25 mg) one tablet once or twice daily, can be given. Most patients will respond to this dosage level. In cases where a patient has been previously titrated to a higher dose of reserpine than that contained in 1 or 2 tablets of hydroflumethiazide w/reserpine, reserpine should be added as the single entity alone. Doses of hydroflumethiazide greater than 100 mg a day can significantly increase the incidence of hypokalemia and other adverse effects without any evidence that such doses increase the antihypertensive efficacy of the combination.

Store below 86°F (30°F).

HOW SUPPLIED - EQUIVALENTS NOT AVAILABLE:

Tablet, Uncoated - Oral - 25 mg/0.125 mg

100's	$3.55	HYDROSINE, Major Pharms	00904-2169-60
100's	**$88.17**	**SALUTENSIN-DEMI, Mead Johnson**	**00015-5455-60**
250's	$4.15	HYDROSINE, Major Pharms	00904-2169-70
1000's	$27.75	HYDROSINE, Major Pharms	00904-2169-80

Tablet, Uncoated - Oral - 50 mg/0.125 mg

100's	$20.10	Hydroflumethiazide & Reserpine, United Res	00677-0830-01
100's	**$113.33**	**SALUTENSIN, Roberts Labs**	**54092-0056-01**
1000's	**$1013.65**	**SALUTENSIN, Mead Johnson**	**00015-5436-90**
1000's	**$1099.81**	**SALUTENSIN, Roberts Labs**	**54092-0056-10**

HYDROGEN PEROXIDE *(001499)*

CATEGORIES: Eye, Ear, Nose, & Throat Preparations; Mouthwashes and Gargle; Mucous Membrane Agents; Skin/Mucous Membrane Agents; FDA Pre 1938 Drugs

BRAND NAMES: Perimax Perio Rinse

FORMULARIES: WHO

Prescribing information not available at time of publication.

HYDROMORPHONE HYDROCHLORIDE *(001500)*

CATEGORIES: Analgesics; Antipyretics; Central Nervous System Agents; Narcotic Analgesics; Narcotics, Synthetics & Combinations; Opiate Agonists (Controlled); Pain; Pregnancy Category C; DEA Class CII; FDA Approved 1984 Jan

BRAND NAMES: Dilaudid; *Dilaudid HP* (Canada); **Dilaudid-Hp**; Hydromorphone Hcl; Hydrostat; *Palladone*
(International brand names outside U.S. in italics)

FORMULARIES: Aetna; BC-BS; Medi-Cal; PCS

DESCRIPTION:

HYDROMORPHONE HCL IS HYDROGENATED KETONE OF MORPHINE WHICH IS A NARCOTIC ANALGESIC.

INJECTION

WARNING: HYDROMORPHONE HCl (HIGH POTENCY) IS A HIGHLY CONCENTRATED SOLUTION OF HYDROMORPHONE INTENDED FOR USE IN NARCOTIC-TOLERANT PATIENTS. DO NOT CONFUSE DILAUDID-HIGH POTENCY WITH STANDARD PARENTERAL FORMULATIONS OF DILAUDID OR OTHER NARCOTICS. OVERDOSE AND DEATH COULD RESULT.

High potency dilaudid is available in Amber ampules for subcutaneous (SC) or intramuscular (IM) administration. Each 1 ml of sterile solution contains 10 mg hydromorphone HCl with 0.2% sodium citrate, 0.2% citric acid solution.

TABLETS

Each 8 mg tablet contains dilaudid (hydromorphone HCl). In addition, the tablets include lactose anhydrous, and magnesium stearate. Dilaudid 8 mg tablet may contain traces of sodium bisulfite.

DESCRIPTION: *(cont'd)*

ORAL SOLUTION

Each 5 ml (1 teaspoon) of dilaudid oral liquid contains 5 mg of dilaudid (hydromorphone HCl). In addition, other ingredients include purified water, methylparaben, propylparaben, sucrose, and glycerin. Dilaudid oral liquid may contain traces of sodium bisulfite.

CLINICAL PHARMACOLOGY:

MANY OF THE EFFECTS DESCRIBED BELOW ARE COMMON TO THE CLASS OF NARCOTIC ANALGESICS. IN SOME INSTANCES, DATA MAY NOT EXIST TO DEMONSTRATE THAT HYDROMORPHONE HCL-HIGH POTENCY, HYDROMORPHONE HCL TABLETS, AND HYDROMORPHONE HCL ORAL SOLUTION POSSESSES SIMILAR OR DIFFERENT EFFECTS THAN THOSE OBSERVED WITH OTHER NARCOTIC ANALGESICS. HOWEVER, IN THE ABSENCE OF DATA TO THE CONTRARY, IT IS ASSUMED THAT HYDROMORPHONE HCL WOULD POSSESS THESE EFFECTS.

CENTRAL NERVOUS SYSTEM: Narcotic analgesics have multiple actions but exert their primary effects on the central nervous system and organs containing smooth muscle. The principal actions of therapeutic value are analgesia and sedation. A significant feature of the analgesia is that it occurs without loss of consciousness. Narcotic analgesics also suppress the cough reflex and cause respiratory depression, mood changes, mental clouding, euphoria, dysphonia, nausea, vomiting and electroencephalographic changes.

The precise mode of analgesic action of narcotic analgesics is unknown. However, specific CNS opiate receptors have been identified. Narcotics are believed to express their pharmacological effects by combining with these receptors.

Narcotics depress the cough reflex by direct effect on the cough center in the medulla.

Narcotics produce respiratory depression by direct effect on brain stem respiratory centers. The mechanism of respiratory depression also involves a reduction in the responsiveness of the brain stem respiratory centers to increases in carbon dioxide tension.

Narcotics cause miosis. Pinpoint pupils are a common sign of narcotic overdose but are not pathognomonic (*e.g.,* pontine lesions of hemorrhagic or ischemic origin may produce similar findings) and marked mydriasis occurs when asphyxia intervenes.

Gastrointestinal Tract and Other Smooth Muscle: Gastric, biliary and pancreatic secretions are decreased by narcotics. Narcotics cause a reduction in motility associated with an increase in lone in the antrum portion of the stomach and duodenum. Digestion of food in the small intestine is delayed and propulsive contractions are decreased. Propulsive peristaltic waves in the colon are decreased, and tone may be increased to the point of spasm. The end result is constipation. Narcotics can cause a marked increase in biliary tract pressure as a result of spasm of the sphincter of Oddi.

Cardiovascular System: Certain narcotics produce peripheral vasodilation which may result in orthostatic hypotension. Release of histamine may occur with narcotics and may contribute to narcotic-induced hypotension. Other manifestations of histamine release and/or peripheral vasodilation may include pruritus, flushing, and red eyes.

INJECTION

Effects on the myocardium after IV administration of narcotics are not significant in normal persons, very with different narcotic analgesic agents and vary with the hemodynamic state of the patient, state of hydration and sympathetic drive.

Pharmacokinetics: In normal human volunteers hydromorphone is metabolized primarily in the liver. It is excreted primarily as the glucuronidated conjugate, with small amounts of parent drug and minor amounts of 6-hydroxy reduction metabolites.

Following intravenous administration of hydromorphone HCl to normal volunteers, the mean half-life of eliminating was 2.64 ± 0.88 hours. The mean volume of distribution was 91.5 liters, suggesting extensive tissue uptake. Hydromorphone HCl is rapidly removed from the blood stream and distributed to skeletal muscle, kidneys, liver, intestinal tract, lungs, spleen and brain. Hydromorphone HCl also crosses the placental membranes.

In terms of area under the analgesic time-effect curve, hydromorphone is approximately 8 times more potent than morphine (*i.e.,* 1.3 mg of hydromorphone produces analgesia equal to that produced by 10 mg of morphine). After intramuscular administration, hydromorphone has a slightly more rapid onset and slightly shorter duration of action than morphine. The duration of hydromorphone HCl analgesia in th non-tolerant patient with usual doses may be up to 4-5 hours. However, in tolerant subjects, duration will vary substantially depending on tolerance and dose. Dose should be adjusted so that 3-4 hours of path relief may be achieved.

TABLETS AND ORAL SOLUTION

The dosage of opioid analgesics like hydromorphone should be individualized for any given patient, since adverse events can occur at doses that may not provide complete freedom from pain (see INDIVIDUALIZATION OF DOSAGE).

Pharmacokinetics: In a single-dose crossover study in 27 normal subjects the pharmacokinetics of hydromorphone HCl 8 mg tablets was compared was compared to that of 8 ml of hydromorphone HCl oral liquid (1 mg/ml). Plasma hydromorphone concentration was determined using a sensitive and specific assay. The pharmacokinetic parameters from this study are outlined below.

TABLE 1

Parameter Mean & (CV)	8 mg Tablet	8 ml Oral Liquid (1 mg/ml)
C_{max} (ng/ml)	5.5 (33%)	5.7 (31%)
T^{max} (hr)	0.74 (34%)	0.73 (71%)
AUC_O (ng* hr/ml)	23.7 (28%)	24.6 (29%)
$T_{1/2}$ (hr)	2.6 (18%)	2.8 (20%)

Dose proportionally between the 8 mg hydromorphone HCl tablets and other strengths of hydromorphone HCl tablets has not been established.

In normal human volunteers hydromorphone is metabolized primarily in the liver. It is excreted in the urine primarily as the glucuronidated conjugate, with small amounts of parent drug and minor amounts of 6-hydroxy reduction metabolites. The effects of renal disease on the clearance of hydromorphone are unknown, but caution should be taken to guard against unanticipated accumulation if renal and/or hepatic functions are seriously impaired. Hydromorphone has been shown to cross placental membranes.

CLINICAL STUDIES:

Analgesic effects of single doses of hydromorphone HCl oral liquid administered to patients with post-surgical pain have been studied in double-blind controlled trials. In one study with 61 patients, both 5 mg and 10 mg of hydromorphone HCl provided significantly more analgesia than placebo. In another trial with 80 patients, 5 mg and 10 mg of hydromorphone HCl oral liquid were compared to 30 mg and 60 mg of morphine sulfate oral liquid. The pain relief provided by 5 mg and 10 mg hydromorphone HCl was comparable to 30 mg and 60 mg oral morphine sulfate, respectively.

CLINICAL STUDIES: *(cont'd)*

Individualization of Dosage: Safe and effective administration of opioid analgesics to patients with acute or chronic pain depends upon a comprehensive assessment of the patient. The nature of the pain (severity, frequency, etiology and pathophysiology) as well as the concurrent medical status of the patient will affect selection of the starting dosage.

In non-opioid-tolerant patients, therapy with hydromorphone is typically initiated at an oral dose of 2-4 mg every four hours, but elderly patients may require lower doses (see PRECAUTIONS, Geriatric Use.)

In patients receiving opioids, both the dose and duration of analgesia will vary substantially depending on the patient's opioid tolerance. The dose should be selected and adjusted so that at least 3-4 hours of pain relief may be achieved. In patients taking opioid analgesics, the starting dose of hydromorphone HCl should be based on prior opioid usage. This should be done by converting the total daily usage of the previous opioid to an equivalent total daily dosage of oral hydromorphone HCl using an equianalgesic table (see TABLE 2). For opioids not in the table, first estimate the equivalent total daily usage of oral morphine, then use the table to find the equivalent total daily dosage of hydromorphone HCl.

Once the total daily dosage of hydromorphone HCl has been estimated, it should be divided into the desired number of doses. Since there is individual variation in response to different opioid drugs, only ½ to 2/3 of the estimated dose of hydromorphone HCl calculated from equivalence tables should be given for the first few doses, then increased as needed according to the patient's response.

In chronic pain, doses should be administered around-the-clock. A supplemental dose of 5-15% of the total daily usage may be administered every two hours on an "as needed" basis.

Periodic reassessment after the initial dosing is always required. if pain management is not satisfactory and in the absence of significant opioid-induced adverse events, the hydromorphone dose may be increased gradually. If excessive opioid side effects are observed early in the dosing interval, the hydromorphone dose may be increased gradually. If excessive opioid side effects are observed early in the dosing interval, the hydromorphone dose should be reduced. If this results in breakthrough pain at the end of the dosing interval, the hydromorphone dose should be reduced. If this results in breakthrough pain at the end of the dosing interval, the dosing interval may need to be shortened. Dose titration should be guided more by the need for analgesia than the absolute dose of opioid employed.

TABLE 2 Opioid Analgesic Equivalents With Approximately Equianalgesic Potency*

Nonproprietary Name	IM or SC Dose	Oral Dose
Morphine sulfate	10 mg	40-60 mg
Hydromorphone HCl	1.3-2 mg	6.5-7.5 mg
Oxymorphone HCl	1-1.1 mg	6.6 mg
Levorphanol tartrate	2.2-3 mg	4 mg
Meperidine, pethidine HCl	75-100 mg	300-400 mg
Methadone HCl	10 mg	10-20 mg

* Dosages, ranges of dosages, represented, are a compilation of estimated equipotent dosages from published references comparing opioid analgesics in cancer and severe pain.

INDICATIONS AND USAGE:

INJECTION

Hydromorphone HCl-high potency is indicated for the relief of moderate-to-severe pain in narcotic-tolerant patients who require larger than usual doses of narcotics to provide adequate pain relief. Because hydromorphone HCl-high potency contains 10 mg of hydromorphone per ml, a smaller injection volume can be used than with other parenteral narcotic formulations. Discomfort associated with the intramuscular or subcutaneous injection of an unusually large volume of solution can therefore be avoided.

TABLETS AND ORAL SOLUTION

Hydromorphone HCl oral liquid and 8 mg tablets are indicated for the management of pain in patients where an opioid analgesic is appropriate.

CONTRAINDICATIONS:

Hydromorphone HCl is Contraindicated In: Patients with known hypersensitivity to the drug, patients with respiratory depression in the absence of resuscitative equipment, and in patients with status asthmaticus. Hydromorphone HCl is also contraindicated for use in obstetrical analgesia.

INJECTION

Hydromorphone HCl-high potency is also contraindicated in patients who are not already receiving large amounts of parenteral narcotics.

WARNINGS:

INJECTION, TABLETS, AND ORAL SOLUTION

Drug Dependence: Hydromorphone HCl-high potency, hydromorphone HCl tablets, and hydromorphone HCl oral solution can produce drug dependence of the morphine type and therefore has the potential for being abused. Psychic dependence, physical dependence and tolerance may develop upon repeated administration of hydromorphone HCl-high potency, and it should be prescribed and administered with the same degree of caution appropriate for the use of morphine. Since hydromorphone HCl-high potency is indicated for use in patients who are already tolerant to and hence physically dependent on narcotics, abrupt discontinuance in the administration of hydromorphone HCl-high potency is likely to result in a withdrawal syndrome (See DRUG ABUSE AND DEPENDENCE).

Impaired Respiration: Respiratory depressing is the chief hazard of hydromorphone HCl. Respiratory depression occurs most frequently in the elderly, in the debilitated, and in those suffering from conditions accompanied by hypoxia or hypercapnia when even moderate therapeutic doses may dangerously decrease pulmonary ventilation.

Hydromorphone HCl-high potency, hydromorphone HCl tablets, and hydromorphone HCl oral solution should be used with extreme caution in patients with chronic obstructive pulmonary disease or cor pulmonale, patient having a substantially decreased respiratory reserve, hypoxia, hypercapnia, or preexisting respiratory depression. In such patients even usual therapeutic doses of narcotic analgesics may decrease respiratory drive while simultaneously increasing airway resistance to the point of apnea.

INJECTION

Infants born to mothers physically dependent on hydromorphone HCl-high potency will also be physically dependent and may exhibit respiratory difficulties and withdrawal symptoms (see DRUG ABUSE AND DEPENDENCE).

Head Injury and Increased Intracranial Pressure: The respiratory depressant effect of hydromorphone HCl with carbon dioxide retention and secondary elevation of cerebrospinal fluid pressure may be markedly exaggerated in the presence of head injury, other intracranial lesions, or preexisting increase in intracranial pressure. Narcotic analgesics including hydromorphone HCl may produce effects which can obscure the clinical course and neurologic signs of further increasing pressure in patients with head injuries.

WARNINGS: *(cont'd)*

Hypotensive Effect: Narcotic analgesics, including hydromorphone HCl-high potency, may cause severe hypotension in an individual whose ability to maintain his blood pressure has already been compromised by a depleted blood volume, or a concurrent administration of drugs such as phenothiazines or general anesthetics (see also DRUG INTERACTIONS). Hydromorphone HCl-high potency may produce orthostatic hypotension in ambulatory patients.

Hydromorphone HCl-high potency should be administered with caution to patients in circulatory shock, since vasodilation produced by the drug may further reduce cardiac output and blood pressure.

TABLETS AND ORAL SOLUTION

Sulfites: Contains sodium bisulfite, a sulfite that may cause allergic-type reactions including anaphylactic symptoms and life-threatening or less severe asthmatic episodes in certain susceptible people. The overall prevalence of sulfite sensitivity in the general population is unknown and probably low. Sulfite sensitivity is seen more frequently in asthmatic than in non-asthmatic people.

PRECAUTIONS:

INJECTION, TABLETS, AND ORAL SOLUTION

In general, narcotics should be given with caution and the initial dose should be reduced in the elderly or debilitated and those with severe impairment of hepatic, pulmonary or renal function; myxedema or hypothyroidism; adrenocortical insufficiency (*e.g.*, Addison's Disease); CNS depression or coma; toxic psychoses; prostatic hypertrophy or urethral stricture; gall bladder disease; acute alcoholism; delirium tremens; or kyphoscoliosis.

The administration of narcotic analgesics including hydromorphone HCl may obscure the diagnosis or clinical course in patients with acute abdominal conditions and may aggravate preexisting convulsions in patients with convulsive disorders.

Narcotic analgesics including hydromorphone HCl should also be used with caution in patients about to undergo surgery of the biliary tract since it may cause spasm of the sphincter of Oddi.

Labor and Delivery: Hydromorphone HCl-high potency, hydromorphone HCl tablets, and hydromorphone HCl oral solution are contraindicated in Labor and Delivery (see CONTRAINDICATIONS).

Nursing Mothers: Low levels of narcotic analgesics have been detected in human milk. As a general rule, nursing should not be undertaken while a patient is receiving hydromorphone HCl since they, and other drugs in this class, may be excreted in the milk.

Pediatric Use: Safety and effectiveness in children have not been established.

INJECTION

General: Because of its high concentration, the delivery of precise doses of hydromorphone HCl-high potency may be difficult if low doses of hydromorphone are required. Therefore, hydromorphone HCl-high potency should be used only if the amount of hydromorphone required can be delivered accurately with this formulation.

In the case of hydromorphone HCl-high potency, however, the patient is presumed to be receiving a narcotic to which he or she exhibits tolerance and that initial dose of hydromorphone HCl-high potency selected should be estimated based on the relative potency of hydromorphone and the narcotic previously used by the patient. See DOSAGE AND ADMINISTRATION.

PREGNANCY CATEGORY C

Human: Adequate animal studies on reproduction have not been performed to determine whether hydromorphone affects fertility in males or females. There are no well-controlled studies in women. Reports based on marketing experience do not identity any specific teratogenic risks following routine (short-term) clinical use. Although there is no clearly defined risk, such reports do not exclude the possibility of infrequent of subtle damage to the human fetus. Hydromorphone HCl-high potency should be used in pregnant women only when clearly needed (see Labor and Delivery and DRUG ABUSE AND DEPENDENCE).

Animal: Literature reports of hydromorphone HCl administration to pregnant Syrian hamsters show that hydromorphone HCl is teratogenic at a dose of 20 mg/kg which is 600 times the human dose. A maximal teratogenic effect (50% of fetuses affected) in the Syrian hamster was observed at a dose of 125 mg/kg.

TABLETS AND ORAL SOLUTION

Head Injury and Increased Intracranial Pressure: The respiratory depressant effects of hydromorphone HCl oral liquid and 8 mg tablets with carbon dioxide retention and secondary elevation of cerebrospinal fluid pressure may be markedly exaggerated in the presence of head injury, other intracranial lesions, or preexisting increase in intracranial pressure. Opioid analgesics including hydromorphone HCl oral liquid and hydromorphone HCl 8 mg tablets may produce effects which can obscure the clinical course and neurologic signs of further increase in intracranial pressure in patients with head injuries.

Hypotensive Effect: Opioid analgesics, including hydromorphone HCl oral liquid and 8 mg tablets, may cause severe hypotension in an individual whose ability to maintain blood pressure has already been compromised by a depleted blood volume, or a concurrent administration of drugs such as phenothiazines or general anesthetics (see DRUG INTERACTIONS). Therefore, hydromorphone HCl oral liquid and 8 mg tablets should be administered with caution to patients in circulatory shock, since vasodilation produced by the drug may further reduce cardiac output and blood pressure.

Use in Ambulatory Patients: Hydromorphone HCl oral liquid and 8 mg tablets may impair mental and/or physical ability required for the performance of potentially hazardous tasks (*e.g.*, driving, operating machinery). Patients should be cautioned accordingly. Hydromorphone HCl may produce orthostatic hypotension in ambulatory patients. The addition of other CNS depressants to hydromorphone HCl therapy may produce additive depressant effects, and hydromorphone HCl should not be taken with alcohol.

Use in Drug and Alcohol Dependent Patients: Hydromorphone HCl should be used with caution in patients with alcoholism and other drug dependencies due to the increased frequency of narcotic tolerance, dependence, and risk of addiction observed in these patient populations. Abuse of hydromorphone HCl in combination with other CNS depressant drugs can result in serious risk to the patient.

Carcinogenesis, Mutagenesis, and Impairment of Fertility: Studies in animals to evaluate the drug's carcinogenic and mutagenic potential or the effect on fertility have not been conducted.

Pregnancy Category C: Literature reports of hydromorphone HCl administration to pregnant Syrian hamsters show that hydromorphone HCl is teratogenic at a dose of 20 mg/kg which is 600 times the human dose. A maximal teratogenic effect (50% of fetuses affected) in the Syrian hamster was observed at a dose of 125 mg/kg (738 mg/m2). There are no well-controlled studies in women. Hydromorphone is known to cross placental membranes. Hydromorphone HCl oral liquid and 8 mg tablets should be used in pregnant women only if the potential benefit justifies the potential risk to the fetus (see Labor and Delivery and DRUG ABUSE AND DEPENDENCE).

PRECAUTIONS: *(cont'd)*

Geriatric Use: Hydromorphone HCl has not been studied in geriatric patients. Elderly subjects have been shown to have at least twice the sensitivity (as measured by EEG changes) of young adults for some opioids. When administering hydromorphone HCl to the elderly, the initial dose should be reduced (see Individualization Of Dosage and PRECAUTIONS).

DRUG INTERACTIONS:

The concomitant use of other central nervous system depressants including sedatives or hypnotics, general anesthetics, phenothiazines, tranquilizers and alcohol may produce additive depressant effects. Respiratory depression, hypotension and profound sedation or coma may occur. When such combined therapy is contemplated, the dose of one or both agents should be reduced. Narcotic analgesics, including hydromorphone HCl-high potency, hydromorphone HCl 8 mg tablets, and hydromorphone HCl oral liquid may enhance the action of neuromuscular blocking agents and produce an increased degree of respiratory depression.

ADVERSE REACTIONS:

INJECTION, TABLETS, AND ORAL SOLUTION

The adverse effects of hydromorphone HCl-high potency, hydromorphone HCl tablets and hydromorphone HCl oral liquid are similar to those of other narcotic analgesics, and represent established pharmacological effects of the drug class. The major hazards include respiratory depression and apnea. To a lesser degree, circulatory depression, respiratory arrest, shock and cardiac arrest have occurred.

The most frequently observed adverse effects are lightheadedness, dizziness, sedation, nausea, vomiting, and sweating. These effects seem to be more prominent in ambulatory patients and in those not experiencing severe pain. Some adverse reactions in ambulatory patients may be alleviated if the patient lies down.

Less Frequently Observed With Narcotic Analgesics

General and CNS: Dysphonia, euphoria, weakness, headache, agitation, tremor, uncoordinated muscle movements, alterations of mood (nervousness, apprehension, depression, floating feelings, dreams), muscle rigidity, paresthesia, muscle tremor, blurred vision, nystagmus, diplopia and miosis, transient hallucinations and disorientation, visual disturbances, insomnia and increased intracranial pressure may occur.

Cardiovascular: Chills, tachycardia, bradycardia, palpitation, faintness, syncope, hypotension and hypertension have been reported.

Respiratory: Bronchospasm and laryngospasm have been known to occur.

Gastrointestinal: Constipation, biliary tract spasm, anorexia, diarrhea, cramps and taste alterations have been reported.

Genitourinary: Urinary retention or hesitancy, and antidiuretic effects have been reported.

Dermatologic: Pruritus, urticaria, other skin rashes, and diaphoresis.

INJECTION

General and CNS: Hallucinations, although unusual with pure agonist narcotics, have been observed in one patient following both a 6 mg and a 4 mg hydromorphone HCl-high potency dose. However, the patient was receiving several concomitant medications during the second episode and a causal relationship cannot be established.

Cardiovascular: Flushing of the face.

Gastrointestinal: Dry mouth.

Dermatologic: Wheal and flare over the vein with intravenous injection have been reported with narcotic analgesics.

Other: In clinical trials, neither local tissue irritation nor induration was observed at the site of subcutaneous injection of hydromorphone HCl-high potency; pain at the injection site was rarely observed. However, local irritation and induration have been seen following parenteral injection of other narcotic drug products.

DRUG ABUSE AND DEPENDENCE:

Narcotic analgesics may cause psychological and physical dependence (see WARNINGS). Physical dependence results in withdrawal symptoms in patients who abruptly discontinue the drug. Withdrawal symptoms also may be precipitated in the patient with physical dependence by the administration of a drug with narcotic antagonist activity, (*e.g.*, naloxone) (see also OVERDOSAGE).

Physical dependence usually does not occur to a clinically significant degree until after several weeks of continued narcotic usage. Tolerance, in which increasingly large doses are required in order to produce the same degree of analgesia, is initially manifested by a shortened duration of analgesic effect, and subsequently, by decreases in the intensity of analgesia. In chronic pain patients, and in narcotic-tolerant cancer patients, the dose of hydromorphone HCl-high potency, hydromorphone HCl tablets or hydromorphone HCl oral solution should be guided by the degree of tolerance manifested.

In chronic pain patients in whom narcotic analgesics including hydromorphone HCl-high potency, hydromorphone HCl tablets and hydromorphone HCl oral solution are abruptly discontinued, a severe abstinence syndrome should be anticipated. This may be similar to the abstinence syndrome noted in patients who withdraw from heroin. The latter abstinence syndrome may be characterized by restlessness, lacrimation, rhinorrhea, yawning, perspiration, gooseflesh, restless sleep or "yen" and mydriasis during the first 24 hours. These symptoms may increase in severity and over the next 72 hours may be accompanied by increasing irritability, anxiety, weakness, twitching and spasms of muscles, kicking movements, severe backache, abdominal and leg pains, abdominal and muscle cramps, hot and cold flashes, insomnia, nausea, anorexia, vomiting, intestinal spasm, diarrhea, coryza and repetitive sneezing, increase in body temperature, blood pressure, respiratory rate and heart rate.

Because of excessive loss of fluid through sweating, or vomiting and diarrhea, there is usually marked weight loss, dehydration, ketosis, and disturbances in acid-base balance. Cardiovascular collapse can occur. Without treatment most observable symptoms disappear in 5-14 days; however, there appears to be a phase of secondary or chronic abstinence which may last for 2-6 months characterized by insomnia, irritability, muscular aches, and autonomic instability.

In the treatment of physical dependence on hydromorphone HCl-high potency, hydromorphone HCl tablets or hydromorphone HCl oral solution the patient may be detoxified by gradual reduction of the dosage, although this is unlikely to be necessary in the terminal cancer patient. If abstinence symptoms become severe, the patient may be given methadone. Temporary administration of tranquilizers and sedatives may aid in reducing patient anxiety. Gastrointestinal disturbances or dehydration should be treated accordingly.

OVERDOSAGE:

Serious overdosage with hydromorphone HCl is characterized by respiratory depression, somnolence progressing to stupor or coma, skeletal muscle flaccidity, cold and clammy skin, constricted pupils, and sometimes bradycardia and hypotension. In serious overdosage, particularly following intravenous injection, apnea, circulatory collapse, cardiac arrest and death may occur.

OVERDOSAGE: *(cont'd)*

In the treatment of overdosage primary attention should be given to the reestablishment of adequate respiratory exchange through provision of a patent airway and institution of assisted or controlled ventilation.

Narcotic-Tolerant Patient: Since tolerance to the respiratory and CNS depressant effects of narcotics develops concomitantly with tolerance to their analgesic effects, serious respiratory depression due to an acute overdose is unlikely to be seen in narcotic-tolerant patients receiving hydromorphone HCl for chronic pain.

Note: In such an individual who is physically dependent on narcotics, administration of the usual dose of the antagonist will precipitate an acute withdrawal syndrome. The severity will depend on the degree of physical dependence and the dose of the antagonist administered. Use of a narcotic antagonist in such a person should be avoided. If necessary to treat serious respiratory depression in the physically-dependent patient, the antagonist should be administered with extreme care and by titration with smaller than usual doses of the antagonist.

Non-Tolerant Patient: The narcotic antagonist, naloxone, is a specific antidote against respiratory depression which may result from overdosage, or unusual sensitivity to hydromorphone HCl. A dose of naloxone (usually 0.4 to 2.0 mg) should be administered intravenously, if possibly, simultaneously with respiratory resuscitation. The dose can be repeated in 3 minutes. Naloxone should not be administered in the absence of clinically significant respiratory or circulatory depression. Naloxone should be administered cautiously to persons who are known, or suspected to be physically dependent on hydromorphone HCl. In such cases, an abrupt or complete reversal of narcotic effects may precipitate an acute abstinence syndrome.

Since the duration of action for hydromorphone HCl may exceed that of the antagonist, the patient should be kept under continued surveillance; repeated doses of the antagonist may be required to maintain adequate respiration. Apply other supportive measures when indicated.

Supportive measures (including, oxygen, vasopressors) should be employed in the management of circulatory shock and pulmonary edema accompanying overdose as indicated. Cardiac arrest or arrhythmias may require cardiac massage of defibrillation.

DOSAGE AND ADMINISTRATION:

INJECTION

Parenteral: DILAUDID-HIGH POTENCY SHOULD BE GIVEN ONLY TO PATIENTS WHO ARE ALREADY RECEIVING LARGE DOSES OF NARCOTICS. Hydromorphone HCl-high potency is indicated for relief of moderate-to-severe pain in narcotic-tolerant patients. Thus, these patients will already have been treated with other narcotic analgesics. If the patient is being changed from regular hydromorphone HCl to hydromorphone HCl-high potency, similar doses should be used, depending on the patient's clinical response to the drug. If hydromorphone HCl-high potency is substituted for a different narcotic analgesic, TABLE 2, an equivalency table, should be used as a guide to determine the appropriate starting dose of hydromorphone HCl-high potency (hydromorphone HCl).

TABLE 2 Strong Analgesics And Structurally Related Drugs Used In The Treatment Of Cancer Pain*

Nonproprietary Names	IM or SC Administration Dose, mg Equianalgesic to 10 mg of IM Morphine†	Duration Compared With Morphine
Morphine sulfate	10	Same
Papaveretum	20	Same
Hydromorphone HCl	1.3	Slightly Shorter
Oxymorphone HCl	1.1	Slightly Shorter
Nalbuphine HCl	12	Same
Heroin, diamorphine HCl (NA in U.S.)	4 - 5	Slightly Shorter
Levorphanol tartrate	2.3	Same
Butorphanol tartrate	1.5 - 2.5	Same
Pentazocine lactate or HCl	60	Shorter
Meperidine, pethidine HCl	80	Shorter
Methadone HCl	10	Same

* From Beaver WT, Management of cancer pain with parenteral medication J. Am. Med. Assoc. 244:2653-2657 (1980)
† In terms of the area under the analgesic time-effect curve.

In open clinical trials with hydromorphone HCl-high potency in patients with terminal cancer, doses ranged from 1-14 mg subcutaneously or intramuscularly; one patient received 30 mg subcutaneously on two occasions. In these trials, both subcutaneous and intramuscular injections of hydromorphone HCl-high potency were well-tolerated, with minimal pain and/or burning at the injection site. Mild erythema was rarely noted after intramuscular injection. There was no induration after either intramuscular or subcutaneous administration of hydromorphone HCl-high potency. Subcutaneous injections of hydromorphone HCl-high potency were particularly well accepted when administered with a short, 30-gauge needle.

Experience with administration of hydromorphone HCl-high potency by the intravenous route is limited. Should intravenous administration be necessary, the injection should be given slowly, over at least 2 to 3 minutes. The intravenous route is usually painless. A gradual increase in dose may be required if analgesia is inadequate, tolerance occurs, or if pain severity increases. The first sign of tolerance is usually a reduced duration of effect.

Note: Parenteral drug products should be inspected visually for particulate matter and discoloration prior to administration, whenever solution and container permit. A slight yellowish discoloration may develop in hydromorphone HCl-high potency ampules. No loss of potency has been demonstrated. Hydromorphone HCl injection is physically compatible and chemically stable for at least 24 hours at 25°C protected from light in most common large volume parenteral solutions.

Storage: Parenteral forms of hydromorphone HCl should be stored at 59°-86°F, (15°-30°C). Protect from light.

Tablets: The usual starting dose for hydromorphone HCl 8 mg tablets is 2 mg to 4 mg, orally, every 4 to 6 hours. Appropriate use of the 8 mg tablet must be decided by careful evaluation of each clinical situation.

Oral Solution: The usual adult oral dosage of hydromorphone HCl oral liquid is one-half (2.5 ml) to two teaspoonfuls (10 ml) (2.5 mg-10 mg) every 3 to 6 hours as directed by the clinical situation. Oral dosages higher than the usual dosages may be required in some patients.

TABLETS AND ORAL SOLUTION

A gradual increase in dose may be required if analgesia is inadequate, as tolerance develops, or if pain severity increases. The first sign of tolerance is usually a decreased duration of effect.

Safety and Handling Instructions: Hydromorphone HCl oral liquid and 8 mg tablets pose little risk of direct exposure to health care personnel and should be handled and disposed of prudently in accordance with hospital or institutional policy. Significant absorption from dermal exposure is unlikely; accidental dermal exposure to hydromorphone HCl oral liquid

DOSAGE AND ADMINISTRATION: *(cont'd)*

should be treated by removal of any contaminated clothing and rinsing the affected area with water. Patients and their families should be instructed to flush any hydromorphone HCl oral liquid and 8 mg tablets that are no longer needed.

Access to abusable drugs such as hydromorphone HCl oral liquid and tablets presents an occupational hazard for addiction in the health care industry. Routine procedures for handling controlled substances developed to protect the public may not be adequate to protect health care workers. Implementation of more effective accounting procedures and measures to restrict access to drugs of this class (appropriate to the practice setting) may minimize the risk of self-administration by health care providers.

HOW SUPPLIED:

ORAL SOLUTION

Dilaudid oral liquid is a clear, sweet, slightly viscous liquid.

TABLETS

Dilaudid 8 mg tablets are white and triangular shaped, embossed with a double 'Knoll' triangle on the other side. They are available in:

Oral Form Storage: Dilaudid oral liquid and 8 mg tablets should be stored at 59-77°F (15-25°C). Protect from light.

HOW SUPPLIED - RATED THERAPEUTICALLY EQUIVALENT:

Injection, Solution - Intramuscular; - 10 mg/ml

1 ml x 10	$9.63	Hydromorphone Hcl, Wyeth Labs	00008-0387-03
5 ml x 10	**$151.26**	**DILAUDID-HP, Knoll Labs**	**00044-1017-25**
10's	**$31.85**	**DILAUDID-HP, Knoll Labs**	**00044-1017-10**
50 ml	**$143.71**	**DILAUDID-HP, Knoll Labs**	**00044-1017-06**

HOW SUPPLIED - NOT RATED EQUIVALENT:

Injection, Solution - Intramuscular; - 1 mg/ml

1 ml x 10	$9.07	Hydromorphone, Sanofi Winthrop	00024-0726-02
1 ml x 10	$10.75	DILAUDID, Knoll Labs	00044-1011-01
1 ml x 10	$13.38	Hydromorphone Hcl, Wyeth Labs	00008-0387-50

Injection, Solution - Intramuscular; - 2 mg/ml

1 ml x 10	$9.39	Hydromorphone, Sanofi Winthrop	00024-0728-02
1 ml x 10	$9.94	Hydromorphone Hcl, Wyeth Labs	00008-0295-01
1 ml x 10	$11.85	DILAUDID, Knoll Labs	00044-1012-01
1 ml x 10	$13.69	Hydromorphone Hcl, Wyeth Labs	00008-0295-50
1 ml x 25	$15.63	Hydromorphone Hcl, Elkins Sinn	00641-0121-25
1 ml x 25	$28.21	DILAUDID, Knoll Labs	00044-1012-09
20 ml	$10.63	Hydromorphone Hcl, Elkins Sinn	00641-2341-41
20 ml	$12.50	Hydromorphone Hcl, Steris Labs	00402-0918-20
20 ml	$13.13	Hydromorphone HCl, Schein Pharm (US)	00364-2422-55
20 ml	$18.28	DILAUDID, Knoll Labs	00044-1062-05
20 ml	$57.81	Hydromorphone Hcl, Astra USA	00186-1309-01

Injection, Solution - Intramuscular; - 3 mg/ml

1 ml x 10	$10.34	Hydromorphone Hcl, Wyeth Labs	00008-0388-01

Injection, Solution - Intramuscular; - 4 mg/ml

1 ml x 10	$10.09	Hydromorphone, Sanofi Winthrop	00024-0727-02
1 ml x 10	$10.69	Hydromorphone Hcl, Wyeth Labs	00008-0296-01
1 ml x 10	$14.35	DILAUDID, Knoll Labs	00044-1014-01
1 ml x 10	$14.44	Hydromorphone Hcl, Wyeth Labs	00008-0296-50

Injection, Solution - Intravenous - 250 mg

1's	**$80.00**	**DILAUDID-HP, Knoll Labs**	**00044-1911-01**

Powder

1 gm	$162.50	Hydromorphone Hcl, Mallinckrodt	00406-3245-52
1 gm	$172.61	DILAUDID, Knoll Labs	00044-1040-01

Solution - Oral - 1 mg/ml

480 ml	$84.76	DILAUDID-5, Knoll Labs	00044-1085-01

Suppository - Rectal - 3 mg

6's	$18.78	DILAUDID, Knoll Labs	00044-1053-01

Tablet, Uncoated - Oral - 2 mg

100's	$27.98	Hydromorphone Hcl, Roxane	00054-4392-25
100's	$28.12	Hydromorohone Hcl, Vintage Pharms	00254-3611-28
100's	$28.12	Hydromorphone Hcl, Qualitest Pharms	00603-3925-21
100's	$31.10	Hydromorphone Hcl, Roxane	00054-8392-24
100's	$32.20	HYDROSTAT IR, ORANGE, Richwood Pharm	58521-0002-01
100's	$38.54	DILAUDID, Knoll Labs	00044-1022-02
100's	$48.88	DILAUDID, Knoll Labs	00044-1022-45
500's	$183.04	DILAUDID, Knoll Labs	00044-1022-03

Tablet, Uncoated - Oral - 4 mg

100's	$39.00	Hydromorphone Hcl, Halsey Drug	00879-0717-01
100's	$40.00	HYDROMOPHONE 4, Goldline Labs	00182-9173-01
100's	$45.45	Hydromorohone Hcl, Vintage Pharms	00254-3612-28
100's	$45.45	Hydromorphone Hcl, Qualitest Pharms	00603-3926-21
100's	$46.15	Hydromorphone Hcl, Roxane	00054-4394-25
100's	$47.64	Hydromorphone Hcl, Roxane	00054-8394-24
100's	$52.30	HYDROSTAT IR, YELLOW, Richwood Pharm	58521-0004-01
100's	$52.75	Hydromorphone Hcl, Goldline Labs	00182-9178-01
100's	$63.11	DILAUDID, Knoll Labs	00044-1024-02
100's	$74.33	DILAUDID, Knoll Labs	00044-1024-45
500's	$300.56	DILAUDID, Knoll Labs	00044-1024-03

Tablet, Uncoated - Oral - 8 mg

100's	$114.85	DILAUDID, Knoll Labs	00044-1028-02

HYDROQUINONE *(001503)*

CATEGORIES: Depigmenting/Pigmenting Agents; Dermatologicals; Hyperpigmentation; Pharmaceutical Adjuvants; Pigmenting Agents; Skin Bleaches; Skin/Mucous Membrane Agents; Topical; Pregnancy Category C; FDA Pre 1938 Drugs

BRAND NAMES: *Aida*; *Aldoquin 2*; Banquin; *Crema Blanca Bustillos* (Mexico); *Cremoquinona*; *Domina*; *Eldopaque* (Mexico); Eldopaque Forte; *Eldoquin* (Mexico); *Eldoquin Cream*; **Eldoquin Forte**; *Epocler*; *Esoterica*; Hydroxyquinone; Melanex; Melanol; *Melanox*; Melpaque Hp; Melquin; *Melquine*; Nuquin Hp; *Solaquin*; Solaquin Forte

(International brand names outside U.S. in italics)

FORMULARIES: Aetna; BC-BS

DESCRIPTION:

FOR EXTERNAL USE ONLY.

Solaquin Forte 4% Cream: Each gram of Solaquin Forte 4% cream contains 40 mg of hydroquinone, 80 mg octyl dimethyl-p-aminobenzoate and 30 mg dioxybenzone USP and 20 mg oxybenzone USP in a vanishing cream base of purified water, glyceryl monostearate, octyldodecyl stearoyl stearate, glyceryl dilaurate, quaternium-26, coceth-6, stearyl alcohol, diethylaminoethyl stearate, dimethicone, polysorbate-80, lactic acid, ascorbic acid, hydroxyethylcellulose, quaternium 14, myristylkonium chloride, disodium EDTA, and sodium metabisulfite.

Eldopaque Forte 4% Cream: Each gram of Eldopaque Forte contains 40 mg of hydroquinone in a tinted sunblocking cream base of water, stearic acid, talc, PEG-40 stearate, PEG-25 propylene glycol stearate, propylene glycol, glyceryl stearate, iron oxides, mineral oil, squalene, disodium EDTA, sodium metabisulfite, and potassium sorbate.

Eldoquin Forte 4% Cream: Each gram of Eldoquin Forte contains 40 mg of hydroquinone in a vanishing cream base of purified water, stearic acid, propylene glycol, polyoxyl 40 stearate, propylene glycol monostearate, glyceryl monostearate, mineral oil, squalene, propylparaben, and sodium metabisulfite.

Solaquin Forte 4% Gel: Each gram of Solaquin Forte gel contains 40 mg of hydroquinone USP, 50 mg of octyl dimethyl p-aminobenzoate USP, and 30 mg dioxybenzone USP, in a hydro-alcoholic base of ethyl alcohol, purified water, propylene glycol, tetrahydroxypropyl ethylenediamine, carbomer 940, disodium EDTA, and sodium metabisulfite.

CLINICAL PHARMACOLOGY:

Topical application of hydroquinone produces a reversible depigmentation of the skin by inhibition of the enzymatic oxidation of tyrosine to 3,4-dihydroxyphenylalanine (dopa)[1] and suppression of other melanocyte metabolic processes[2]. Exposure to sunlight or ultraviolet light will cause repigmentation of bleached areas which may be prevented by sun blocking agents contained in hydroquinone 4% cream and by the broad spectrum sunscreen agents contained in Solaquin Forte 4% cream and Solaquin Forte 4% gel.[3].

INDICATIONS AND USAGE:

All forms are indicated for the gradual bleaching of hyperpigmented skin conditions such as chloasma, melasma, freckles, senile lentigines, and other unwanted areas of melanin hyperpigmentation.

Eloquin Forte 4% Cream: This cream is intended for night-time use only since it contains no sunblocking agents. For daytime usage, Solaquin Forte 4% cream, Solaquin Forte 4% gel or Eldopaque Forte 4% cream should be prescribed.

CONTRAINDICATIONS:

Prior history of sensitivity or allergic reaction to these products or any of the ingredients. The safety of topical hydroquinone use during pregnancy or in children (12 years and under) has not been established.

WARNINGS:

A. Caution: Hydroquinone is a skin bleaching agent which may produce unwanted cosmetic effects if not used as directed. The physician should be familiar with the contents of this insert before prescribing or dispensing these medications.

B. Test for skin sensitivity before using these medications by applying a small amount to an unbroken patch of skin and check in 24 hours. Minor redness is not a contraindication, but where there is itching or vesicle formation of excessive inflammatory response further treatment is not advised. Close patient supervision is recommended. Contact with the eyes should be avoided. If no bleaching or lightening effect is noted after 2 months of treatment use, the medication should be discontinued. Hydroquinone 4% cream or gel are formulated for use as a skin bleaching agent and should not be used for the prevention of sunburn.

C. Sunscreen use is an essential aspect of hydroquinone therapy because even minimal sunlight exposure sustains melanocytic activity. The sunscreens in Hydroquinone 4% cream or gel provide the necessary sun protection during skin bleaching therapy. After clearing and during maintenance therapy, sun exposure should be avoided on bleached skin by application of a sunscreen or sunblock agent or protective clothing to prevent repigmentation.

D. Keep this and all medication out of the reach of children. In case of accidental ingestion, call a physician or a poison control center immediately.

E. Warning: Contains sodium metabisulfite, a sulfite that may cause serious allergic type reactions (*e.g.,* hives, itching, wheezing, anaphylaxis, severe asthma attack) in certain susceptible persons.

PRECAUTIONS:

SEE WARNINGS.

A. Pregnancy Category C: Animal reproduction studies have not been conducted with topical hydroquinone. It is also not known whether hydroquinone can cause fetal harm when used topically on a pregnant woman or affect reproductive capacity. It is not known to what degree, if any, topical hydroquinone is absorbed systemically. Topical hydroquinone should be used in pregnant women only when clearly indicated.

B. Nursing Mothers: It is not known whether topical hydroquinone is absorbed or excreted in human milk. Caution is advised when topical hydroquinone is used by a nursing mother.

C. Pediatric Usage: Safety and effectiveness in pediatric patients below the age of 12 years have not been established.

ADVERSE REACTIONS:

No systemic adverse reactions have been reported. Occasional hypersensitivity (localized contact dermatitis) may occur in which case the medication should be discontinued and the physician notified immediately.

OVERDOSAGE:

There have been no systemic reactions from the use of topical hydroquinone in Hydroquinone 4% cream or gel. However, treatment should be limited to relatively small areas of the body at one time since some patients experience a transient skin reddening and a mild burning sensation which does not preclude treatment.

DOSAGE AND ADMINISTRATION:

Solaquin Forte 4% Cream and Solaquin Forte 4% Gel: These forms should be applied to the affected area and rubbed in well twice daily or as directed by a physician to achieve maximum therapeutic potential.

Eldopaque Forte 4% Cream: This form should be applied with a thin application to the affected area twice daily or as directed by a physician. Do not rub in.

Eldoquin Forte 4% Cream: This form is indicated to be used during night hours as the product contains no sunblocking agent. Apply to affected area and rub in well twice daily or as directed by a physician.

DOSAGE AND ADMINISTRATION: *(cont'd)*

There is no recommended dosage for children under 12 years of age except under the advice and supervision of a physician.

Hydroquinone 4% cream and gel should be stored at controlled room temperature (15°-30° C) 59°-86°F.

REFERENCES:

1. Denton, C., A.B. Lerner and A.B. Lerner and T.B. Fitzpatrick, 'Inhibition of Melanin Formation by Chemical Agents', **Journal of Investigative Dermatology, 18:**119-135, 1952. **2.** Jimbow, K., H. Obata, M. Pathak, and T.B. Fitzpatrick, 'Mechanism of Depigmentation by Hydroquinone', **Journal of Investigative Dermatology, 62:**436-449, 1974. **3.** Parrish, J.A., R.R. Anderson, F. Urbach, D. Pitts,**UVA, Biological Effects of Ultraviolet Radiation with Emphasis on Human Responses to Longwave Ultraviolet**. Plenum Press, New York and London, 1978, p. 151.

HOW SUPPLIED - EQUIVALENTS NOT AVAILABLE:

Cream - Topical - 4 %

15 gm	$11.25	Nuquin Hp, Stratus Pharms	58980-0474-05
15 gm	$11.90	Melquin Hp, Stratus Pharms	58980-0472-05
15 gm	$11.90	Melpaque Hp, Stratus Pharms	58980-0473-05
15 gm	$11.90	Nuquin Hp, Stratus Pharms	58980-0574-05
15 gm	**$16.69**	**ELDOQUIN FORTE, ICN Pharms**	**00187-0394-35**
15 gm	$16.69	ELDOPAQUE FORTE, ICN Pharms	00187-0395-35
15 gm	$16.69	SOLAQUIN FORTE, ICN Pharms	00187-0396-35
30 gm	$17.90	Nuquin Hp, Stratus Pharms	58980-0474-10
30 gm	$19.75	Melquin Hp, Stratus Pharms	58980-0472-10
30 gm	$19.75	Melpaque Hp, Stratus Pharms	58980-0473-10
30 gm	$19.75	Nuquin Hp, Stratus Pharms	58980-0574-10
30 gm	**$32.12**	**ELDOQUIN FORTE, ICN Pharms**	**00187-0394-31**
30 gm	$32.12	ELDOPAQUE FORTE, ICN Pharms	00187-0395-31
30 gm	$32.12	SOLAQUIN FORTE, ICN Pharms	00187-0396-31
60 gm	$2.75	Hydroquinone Skin Cream, Consolidated Midland	00223-4330-02
60 gm	$30.30	Nuquin Hp, Stratus Pharms	58980-0474-20
60 gm	$32.13	Nuquin Hp, Stratus Pharms	58980-0574-20

Gel - Topical - 4 %

15 gm	$11.90	NUQUIN HP, Stratus Pharms	58980-0475-05
15 ml	$16.69	SOLAQUIN FORTE, ICN Pharms	00187-0523-35
30 gm	$19.75	NUQUIN HP, Stratus Pharms	58980-0475-10
30 ml	$32.12	SOLAQUIN FORTE, ICN Pharms	00187-0523-31
60 gm	$32.13	NUQUIN HP, Stratus Pharms	58980-0475-20

Solution - Topical - 30 mg/ml

30 ml	$8.70	Melquin-3, Stratus Pharms	58980-0476-10
30 ml	$11.94	MELANEX, Neutrogena	10812-9300-01

HYDROXOCOBALAMIN *(001504)*

CATEGORIES: Blood Formation/Coagulation; Deficiency Anemias; Homeostatic & Nutrient; Vitamin B Complex; Vitamin B12; Vitamins; FDA Approval Pre 1982

BRAND NAMES: Alphamin; Alpharedisol; *Behepan*; *Berubi* (Germany); Codroxomin; *Cohemin Depot*; *Cobalin-H* (England); *Droxofor*; *Duradoce* (Mexico); *Erycytol Depot*; *Forta B 5000*; Hydro-Cobex; Hydro-Cristi; Hydrobexan; Hydrocobalamin; Hydroxo-12; *Hydroxo 5000* (France); *Hydroxocobalamine*; Hydroxomin; La-12; *Neo-Cytamen* (Australia, England); *Neocytamen*; *OH B12*; Primabalt Rp 1000; *Ultrafor*; Vibal La; *Vibeden*

(International brand names outside U.S. in italics)

FORMULARIES: WHO

Prescribing information not available at time of publication.

HOW SUPPLIED - RATED THERAPEUTICALLY EQUIVALENT:

Injection, Solution - Intramuscular - 250 mg/ml

5 ml	$10.90	LA-12, Hyrex Pharms	00314-0678-30

Injection, Solution - Intramuscular - 1000 mcg/ml

10 ml	$4.12	B-12 Hydroxocobalamin, Rugby	00536-2050-70
10 ml	$5.00	Hydroxocobalamin, C O Truxton	00463-1094-10
10 ml	$7.50	Hydroxocobalamin, Consolidated Midland	00223-7912-10
30 ml	$3.49	Hydroxocobalamin, McGuff	49072-0335-30
30 ml	$3.60	Hydroxocobalamin, Americal Pharm	54945-0542-43
30 ml	$5.75	Hydroxocobalamin, Pasadena	00418-0221-61
30 ml	$5.75	Hydroxocobalamin, Harber Pharm	51432-0747-30
30 ml	$6.80	Hydroxocobalamin, Steris Labs	00402-0208-30
30 ml	$8.50	Hydroxocobalamin, Consolidated Midland	00223-7912-30
30 ml	$8.65	Hydroxocobalamin Inj, Major Pharms	00904-0916-30
30 ml	$11.25	B-12 Hydroxocobalamin, Rugby	00536-2050-75
30 ml	$11.85	Hydroxy-Cobal, Merit Pharms	30727-0612-80

HYDROXYAMPHETAMINE HYDROBROMIDE; TROPICAMIDE *(003117)*

CATEGORIES: Cycloplegics/Mydriatics; Diagnostic Agents; EENT Drugs; Eye, Ear, Nose, & Throat Preparations; Mydriasis; Mydriatics; Mydriatics & Cycloplegics; Ophthalmics; Pupil Dilation; Pregnancy Category C; FDA Approved 1992 Jan

BRAND NAMES: **Paremyd**

DESCRIPTION:

Paremyd (Hydroxyamphetamine hydrobromide with tropicamide) sterile ophthalmic solution is a topical mydriatic combination product for ophthalmic use.

Chemical Name: Hydroxyamphetamine hydrobromide: Phenol, 4-(2-aminopropyl)-hydrobromide

Tropicamide: Benzeneacetamide, N-ethyl-α-(hydromethyl)-N-(4-pyridinyl-methyl)-

CONTAINS:

Hydroxyamphetamine hydrobromide, USP 1.0%

Tropicamide, USP 0.25%

with: benzalkonium chloride 0.005%; edetate disodium 0.015%; sodium chloride; and purified water. Hydrochloric acid and/or sodium hydroxide are added to adjust the pH. The pH of Paremyd can range from 4.2 to 5.8 during its shelf life. The osmolality of Paremyd is approximately 307 m0sm/l.

CLINICAL PHARMACOLOGY:

Hydroxyamphetamine hydrobromide with tropicamide solution combines the effects of the adrenergic agent hydroxyamphetamine hydrobromide, and the anticholinergic agent, tropicamide.

Hydroxyamphetamine hydrobromide is an indirectly-acting sympathomimetic agent which, when applied topically to the eye, causes the release of endogenous norepinephrine from intact adrenergic nerve terminals resulting in mydriasis. Since hydroxyamphetamine hydrobromide has little or no direct activity on the receptor site, dilation does not usually occur if there is damage to the presynaptic nerve terminal, (*e.g.,* Horner's Syndrome). However, it is not known whether damage to the presynaptic nerve terminal will influence the extent of mydriasis produced by hydroxyamphetamine hydrobromide with tropicamide. Hydroxyamphetamine hydrobromide has minimal cycloplegic action.

Tropicamide is a parasympatholytic agent which, when applied topically to the eye, blocks the responses of the sphincter muscle of the iris and the ciliary muscle to cholinergic stimulation, producing dilation of the pupil of the pupil and paralysis of the ciliary muscle. Tropicamide produces short-duration mydriasis. Although cycloplegia occurs with higher doses of tropicamide, there is evidence with 0.25% tropicamide that full cycloplegia does not occur.

Since both these agents act on different effector sites, their simultaneous use produces an additive mydriatic effect. Hydroxyamphetamine hydrobromide with tropicamide provides diminished pupil responsiveness to light, facilitating ophthalmoscopy. The onset of action with hydroxyamphetamine hydrobromide with tropicamide occurs within 15 minutes, followed by maximum effect within 60 minutes after instillation of one drop. Clinically significant dilation, inhibition of pupillary light response, and partial cycloplegia last 3 hours, with recovery beginning at approximately 90 minutes and with complete recovery occurring in most patients in 6 to 8 hours. However, in some cases complete recovery may take up to 24 hours. Effectiveness may differ slightly in patients with light and dark irides, with those patients with light irides experiencing a slightly greater mydriasis.

INDICATIONS AND USAGE:

Hydroxyamphetamine hydrobromide with tropicamide solution is indicated for mydriasis in routine diagnostic procedures and in conditions where short term-term pupil dilation is desired. Hydroxyamphetamine hydrobromide with tropicamide provides clinically significant mydriasis with partial cycloplegia.

CONTRAINDICATIONS:

Hydroxyamphetamine hydrobromide with tropicamide solution should not be used in patients with angle-closure glaucoma or in those narrow angles in whom dilation of the pupil may precipitate an attack of angle-closure glaucoma. This product is also contraindicated in patients who are hypersensitive to any of its components.

WARNINGS:

For topical ophthalmic use only; not for injection.

There is evidence that mydriatics may produce a transient elevation of intraocular pressure in patients with open-angle glaucoma.

This preparation rarely may cause CNS disturbances which may be particularly dangerous in infants, children or the aged. Psychotic reactions, behavioral disturbances and vasomotor or cardio-respiratory collapse in children have been reported with the use of anticholinergic drugs.

PRECAUTIONS:

GENERAL

Patients with hypertension, hyperthyroidism, diabetes or cardiac disease (*i.e.,* arrhythmias or chronic ischemic heart disease) should be monitored after instillation. The elderly and others in whom glaucoma or increased intraocular pressure may be encountered following administration of hydroxyamphetamine hydrobromide with tropicamide solution should be monitored closely. To avoid inducing angle-closure glaucoma, an estimation of the depth of the angle of the anterior chamber should be made.

INFORMATION FOR THE PATIENT

Patients should be advised not to touch the dropper tip to any surface since this may contaminate the solution. Patients should be advised to use caution when driving or engaging in other hazardous activities while pupils are dilated. Patients may experience photophobia and/or blurred vision and should protect their eyes in bright illumination while the pupils are dilated. Parents should be warned not to get this preparation in their child's mouth and to wash their own hands and the child's hands following administration.

CARCINOGENESIS, MUTAGENESIS, AND IMPAIRMENT OF FERTILITY

No studies have been performed to evaluate the carcinogenic, mutagenic or impairment of fertility potential of hydroxyamphetamine hydrobromide with tropicamide.

PREGNANCY CATEGORY C

Animal reproduction studies have not been conducted with hydroxyamphetamine hydrobromide with tropicamide. It is also not known whether hydroxyamphetamine hydrobromide with tropicamide can cause fetal harm when administered to a pregnant woman or can effect reproduction capability. Hydroxyamphetamine hydrobromide with tropicamide should be given to a pregnant woman only if clearly needed.

NURSING MOTHERS

It is not known whether this drug is excreted in human milk. Because many drugs are excreted in human milk, caution should be exercised when hydroxyamphetamine hydrobromide with tropicamide is administered to a nursing woman.

PEDIATRIC USE

Safety and effectiveness in children have not been established. Hydroxyamphetamine hydrobromide with tropicamide may rarely cause CNS disturbances which may be dangerous in infants and children. Psychotic reactions, behavioral disturbances and vasomotor or cardio-respiratory collapse in children have been reported with the use of anticholinergic drugs. (See WARNINGS.)

Keep this and all medications out of the reach of children.

ADVERSE REACTIONS:

Increased intraocular pressure has been reported following use of mydriatics. Transient stinging, dryness of the mouth, blurred vision, photophobia with or without corneal staining, tachycardia, headache, allergic reactions, nausea, vomiting, pallor, and muscle rigidity have been reported with the use of tropicamide and/or hydroxyamphetamine hydrobromide, and thus may occur with hydroxyamphetamine hydrobromide with tropicamide solution. Central nervous system disturbances have also been reported. Psychotic reactions, behavioral disturbances, and vasomotor or cardio-respiratory collapse in children have been reported with the use of anticholinergic drugs.

OVERDOSAGE:

Ocular overdosage will cause dilation of the pupils. Systemic overdosage or ingestion of large doses may result in hypertension, cardiac arrhythmias, sub-sternal discomfort, headache, sweating, nausea, vomiting, and gastrointestinal irritation. Patients with systemic overdosage should be carefully monitored and treated symptomatically.

DOSAGE AND ADMINISTRATION:

One of two drops in the conjunctival sac. The onset of action with hydroxyamphetamine hydrobromide with tropicamide solution occurs within 15 minutes, followed by maximum effect within 60 minutes. Clinically significant dilation, inhibition of pupillary light response, and partial cycloplegia last 3 hours.

Mydriasis will reverse spontaneously with time, typically in 6 to 8 hours. However, in some cases, complete recovery may take up to 24 hours.

Note: Protect from light. Store between 15° to 25°C (59° to 77°F).

HOW SUPPLIED - EQUIVALENTS NOT AVAILABLE:

Solution - Ophthalmic - 1 %/0.25 %

15 ml	$7.81	PAREMYD, Allergan-Amer	11980-0289-15

HYDROXYCHLOROQUINE SULFATE *(001506)*

CATEGORIES: Aminoquinolines; Antiarthritics; Anti-Infectives; Antimalarial Agents; Antiprotozoals; Arthritis; Lupus Erythematosus; Malaria; Parasiticidal; FDA Approval Pre 1982

BRAND NAMES: *Ercoquin* (Japan); *Erquin*; *Haloxin*; *Oxiklorin*; **Plaquenil**; *Plaquenil Sulfate* (Canada); *Plaquinol*; *Quensyl* (Germany); *Toremonil* (Japan); *Yuma* *(International brand names outside U.S. in italics)*

FORMULARIES: Aetna; BC-BS; Medi-Cal; PCS

> WARNING:
> PHYSICIANS SHOULD COMPLETELY FAMILIARIZE THEMSELVES WITH THE COMPLETE CONTENTS OF THIS MONOGRAPH BEFORE PRESCRIBING HYDROXYCHLOROQUINE.

DESCRIPTION:

The compound is a colorless crystalline solid, soluble in water to at least 20 percent; chemically the drug is 2-[[4-[(7-Chloro-4-quinolyl)amino]pentyl]ethylamino]ethanol sulfate (1:1). *Inactive Ingredients:* Dibasic calcium phosphate, magnesium stearate, starch.

CLINICAL PHARMACOLOGY:

The drug possesses antimalarial actions and also exerts a beneficial effect in lupus erythematosus (chronic discoid or systemic) and acute or chronic rheumatoid arthritis. The precise mechanism of action is not known.

Malaria: Like chloroquine phosphate, USP, hydroxychloroquine sulfate is highly active against the erythrocytic forms of *P. vivax* and *malariae* and most strains of *P. falciparum* (but not the gametocytes of *P. falciparum*).

Hydroxychloroquine sulfate does not prevent relapses in patients with *vivax* or *malariae* malaria because it is not effective against exo-erythrocytic forms of the parasite, nor will it prevent *vivax* or *malariae* infection when administered as a prophylactic. It is highly effective as a suppressive agent in patients with *vivax* or *malariae* malaria, in terminating acute attacks, and significantly lengthening the interval between treatment and relapse. In patients with *falciparum* malaria, it abolishes the acute attack and effects complete cure of the infection, unless due to a resistant strain of *P. falciparum*.

INDICATIONS AND USAGE:

Hydroxychloroquine sulfate is indicated for the suppressive treatment and treatment of acute attacks of malaria due to *Plasmodium vivax, P. malariae, P. ovale,* and susceptible strains of *P.falciparum*. It is also indicated for the treatment of discoid and systemic lupus erythematosus, and rheumatoid arthritis.

Malaria: Hydroxychloroquine sulfate is indicated for the treatment of acute attacks and suppression of malaria.

Lupus Erythematosus and Rheumatoid Arthritis: Hydroxychloroquine sulfate is useful in patients with the following disorders who have not responded satisfactorily to drugs with less potential for serious side effects: lupus erythematosus (chronic discoid and systemic) and acute or chronic rheumatoid arthritis.

CONTRAINDICATIONS:

Use of this drug is contraindicated (1) in the presence of retinal or visual field changes attributable to any 4-aminoquinoline compound, (2) in patients with known hypersensitivity to 4-aminoquinoline compounds, and (3) for long-term therapy in children.

WARNINGS:

General: Hydroxychloroquine sulfate is not effective against chloroquine-resistant strains of *P.falciparum.*

Children are especially sensitive to the 4-aminoquinoline compounds. A number of fatalities have been reported following the accidental ingestion of chloroquine, sometimes in relatively small doses (0.75 g or 1 g in one 3-year-old child). Patients should be strongly warned to keep these drugs out of the reach of children.

Use of hydroxychloroquine sulfate in patients with psoriasis may precipitate a severe attack of psoriasis. When used in patients with porphyria the condition may be exacerbated. The preparation should not be used in these conditions unless in the judgment of the physician the benefit to the patient outweighs the possible hazard.

Usage in Pregnancy: Usage of this drug during pregnancy should be avoided except in the suppression or treatment of malaria when in the judgment of the physician the benefit outweighs the possible hazard. It should be noted that radioactively-tagged chloroquine administered intravenously to pregnant, pigmented CBA mice passed rapidly across the placenta. It accumulated selectively in the melanin structures of the fetal eyes and was retained in the ocular tissues for five months after the drug had been eliminated from the rest of the body.

Malaria: In recent years, it has been found that certain strains of *P. falciparum* have become resistant to 4-aminoquinoline compounds (including hydroxychloroquine sulfate) as shown by the fact that normally adequate doses have failed to prevent or cure clinical malaria or parasitemia. Treatment with quinine or other specific forms of therapy is therefore advised for patients infected with a resistant strain of parasites.

WARNINGS: *(cont'd)*

Lupus Erythematosus and Rheumatoid Arthritis: Irreversible retinal damage has been observed in some patients who had received long-term or high-dosage 4-aminoquinoline therapy for discoid and systemic lupus erythematosus, or rheumatoid arthritis. Retinopathy has been reported to be dose-related.

When prolonged therapy with any antimalarial compound is contemplated, initial (base line) and periodic (every three months) ophthalmologic examinations (including visual acuity, expert slit-lamp, funduscopic, and visual field tests) should be performed.

If there is any indication of abnormality in the visual acuity, visual field, or retinal macular areas (such as pigmentary changes, loss of foveal reflex), or any visual symptoms (such as light flashes and streaks) which are not fully explainable by difficulties of accommodation or corneal opacities, the drug should be discontinued immediately and the patient closely observed for possible progression. Retinal changes (and visual disturbances) may progress even after cessation of therapy.

All patients on long-term therapy with this preparation should be questioned and examined periodically, including the testing of knee and ankle reflexes, to detect any evidence of muscular weakness. If weakness occurs, discontinue the drug.

In the treatment of rheumatoid arthritis, if objective improvement (such as reduced joint swelling, increased mobility) does not occur within six months, the drug should be discontinued. Safe use of the drug in the treatment of juvenile arthritis has not been established.

PRECAUTIONS:

General: Antimalarial compounds should be used with caution in patients with hepatic disease or alcoholism or in conjunction with known hepatotoxic drugs.

Periodic blood cell counts should be made if patients are given prolonged therapy. If any severe blood disorder appears which is not attributable to the disease under treatment, discontinuation of the drug should be considered. The drug should be administered with caution in patients having G-6-PD (glucose-6-phosphate dehydrogenase) deficiency.

Lupus Erythematosus and Rheumatoid Arthritis: Dermatologic reactions to hydroxychloroquine sulfate may occur and, therefore, proper care should be exercised when it is administered to any patient receiving a drug with a significant tendency to produce dermatitis.

The methods recommended for early diagnosis of "chloroquine retinopathy" consist of (1) funduscopic examination of the macula for fine pigmentary disturbances or loss of the foveal reflex and (2) examination of the central visual field with a small red test object for pericentral or paracentral scotoma or determination of retinal thresholds to red. Any unexplained visual symptoms, such as light flashes or streaks should also be regarded with suspicion as possible manifestations of retinopathy.

If serious toxic symptoms occur from overdosage or sensitivity, it has been suggested that ammonium chloride (8 g daily in divided doses for adults) be administered orally three or four days a week for several months after therapy has been stopped, as acidification of the urine increases renal excretion of the 4-aminoquinoline compounds by 20 to 90 percent. However, caution must be exercised in patients with impaired renal function and/or metabolic acidosis.

ADVERSE REACTIONS:

Malaria: Following the administration in doses adequate for the treatment of an acute malarial attack, mild and transient headache, dizziness, and gastrointestinal complaints (diarrhea, anorexia, nausea, abdominal cramps and, on rare occasions, vomiting) may occur.

Lupus Erythematosus and Rheumatoid Arthritis: Not all of the following reactions have been observed with every 4-aminoquinoline compound during long-term therapy, but they have been reported with one or more and should be borne in mind when drugs of this class are administered. Adverse effects with different compounds vary in type and frequency.

CNS Reactions: Irritability, nervousness, emotional changes, nightmares, psychosis, headache, dizziness, vertigo, tinnitus, nystagmus, nerve deafness, convulsions, ataxia.

Neuromuscular Reactions: Extraocular muscle palsies, skeletal muscle weakness, absent or hypoactive deep tendon reflexes.

OCULAR REACTIONS

Ciliary body: Disturbance of accommodation with symptoms of blurred vision. This reaction is dose-related and reversible with cessation of therapy.

Cornea: Transient edema, punctate to lineal opacities, decreased corneal sensitivity. The corneal changes, with or without accompanying symptoms (blurred vision, halos around lights, photophobia), are fairly common, but reversible. Corneal deposits may appear as early as three weeks following initiation of therapy.

The incidence of corneal changes and visual side effects appears to be considerably lower with hydroxychloroquine than with chloroquine.

Retina: *Macula:* Edema, atrophy, abnormal pigmentation (mild pigment stippling to a "bull's-eye" appearance), loss of foveal reflex, increased macular recovery time following exposure to a bright light (photo-stress test), elevated retinal threshold to red light in macular, paramacular, and peripheral retinal areas.

Other fundus changes include optic disc pallor and atrophy, attenuation of retinal arterioles, fine granular pigmentary disturbances in the peripheral retina and prominent choroidal patterns in advanced stage.

Visual Field Defects: pericentral or paracentral scotoma, central scotoma with decreased visual acuity, rarely field constriction.

The most common visual symptoms attributed to the retinopathy are: reading and seeing difficulties (words, letters, or parts of objects missing), photophobia, blurred distance vision, missing or blacked out areas in the central or peripheral visual field, light flashes and streaks.

Retinopathy appears to be dose related and has occurred within several months (rarely) to several years of daily therapy; a small number of cases have been reported several years after antimalarial drug therapy was discontinued. It has not been noted during prolonged use of weekly doses of the 4-aminoquinoline compounds for suppression of malaria.

Patients with retinal changes may have visual symptoms or may be asymptomatic (with or without visual field changes). Rarely scotomatous vision or field defects may occur without obvious retinal change.

Retinopathy may progress even after the drug is discontinued. In a number of patients, early retinopathy (macular pigmentation sometimes with central field defects) diminished or regressed completely after therapy was discontinued. Paracentral scotoma to red targets (sometimes called "premaculopathy") is indicative of early retinal dysfunction which is usually reversible with cessation of therapy.

A small number of cases of retinal changes have been reported as occurring in patients who received only hydroxychloroquine sulfate. These usually consisted of alteration in retinal pigmentation which was detected on periodic ophthalmologic examination; visual field defects were also present in some instances. A case of delayed retinopathy has been reported with loss of vision starting one year after administration of hydroxychloroquine sulfate had been discontinued.

ADVERSE REACTIONS: *(cont'd)*

Dermatologic Reactions: Bleaching of hair, alopecia, pruritus, skin and mucosal pigmentation, skin eruptions (urticarial, morbilliform, lichenoid, maculopapular, purpuric, erythema annulare centrifugum and exfoliative dermatitis).

Hematologic Reactions: Various blood dyscrasias such as aplastic anemia, agranulocytosis, leukopenia, thrombocytopenia (hemolysis in individuals with glucose-6-phosphate dehydrogenase (G-6-PD) deficiency).

Gastrointestinal Reactions: Anorexia, nausea, vomiting, diarrhea, and abdominal cramps.

Miscellaneous Reactions: Weight loss, lassitude, exacerbation or precipitation of porphyria and nonlight-sensitive psoriasis.

OVERDOSAGE:

The 4-aminoquinoline compounds are very rapidly and completely absorbed after ingestion, and in accidental overdosage, or rarely with lower doses in hypersensitive patients, toxic symptoms may occur within 30 minutes. These consist of headache, drowsiness, visual disturbances, cardiovascular collapse, and convulsions, followed by sudden and early respiratory and cardiac arrest. The electrocardiogram may reveal atrial standstill, nodal rhythm, prolonged intraventricular conduction time, and progressive bradycardia leading to ventricular fibrillation and/or arrest. Treatment is symptomatic and must be prompt with immediate evacuation of the stomach by emesis (at home, before transportation to the hospital) or gastric lavage until the stomach is completely emptied. If finely powdered, activated charcoal is introduced by the stomach tube, after lavage, and within 30 minutes after ingestion of the tablets, it may inhibit further intestinal absorption of the drug. To be effective, the dose of activated charcoal should be at least five times the estimated dose of hydroxychloroquine sulfate ingested. Convulsions, if present, should be controlled before attempting gastric lavage. If due to cerebral stimulation, cautious administration of an ultrashort-acting barbiturate may be tried but, if due to anoxia, it should be corrected by oxygen administration, artificial respiration or, in shock with hypotension, by vasopressor therapy. Because of the importance of supporting respiration, tracheal intubation or tracheostomy, followed by gastric lavage, may also be necessary. Exchange transfusions have been used to reduce the level of 4-aminoquinoline drug in the blood.

A patient who survives the acute phase and is asymptomatic should be closely observed for at least six hours. Fluids may be forced, and sufficient ammonium chloride (8 g daily in divided doses for adults) may be administered for a few days to acidify the urine to help promote urinary excretion in cases of both overdosage and sensitivity.

DOSAGE AND ADMINISTRATION:

Malaria: One tablet of 200 mg of hydroxychloroquine sulfate is equivalent to 155 mg base.

SUPPRESSION

In Adults: 400 mg (=310 mg base) on exactly the same day of each week.

In Infants and Children The weekly suppressive dosage is 5 mg, calculated as base, per kg of body weight, but should not exceed the adult dose regardless of weight.

If circumstances permit, suppressive therapy should begin two weeks prior to exposure. However, failing this, in adults an initial double (loading) dose of 800 mg (=620 mg base), or in children 10 mg base/kg may be taken in two divided doses, six hours apart. The suppressive therapy should be continued for eight weeks after leaving the endemic area.

TREATMENT OF THE ACUTE ATTACK

In Adults: An initial dose of 800 mg (=620 mg base) followed by 400 mg (=310 mg base) in six to eight hours and 400 mg (310 mg base) on each of two consecutive days (total 2 g hydroxychloroquine sulfate or 1.55 g base). An alternative method, employing a single dose of 800 mg (=620 mg base), has also proved effective.

The dosage for adults may also be calculated on the basis of body weight; this method is preferred for infants and children. A total dose representing 25 mg of base per kg of body weight is administered in three days, as follows:

First Dose: 10 mg base per kg (but not exceeding a single dose of 620 mg base).

Second Dose: 5 mg base per kg (but not exceeding a single dose of 310 mg base) 6 hours after first dose.

Third Dose: 5 mg base per kg 18 hours after second dose.

Fourth Dose: 5 mg base per kg 24 hours after third dose.

For radical cure of *vivax* and *malariae* malaria concomitant therapy with an 8-amino-quinoline compound is necessary.

LUPUS ERYTHEMATOSUS AND RHEUMATOID ARTHRITIS

One tablet of hydroxychloroquine sulfate, 200 mg, is equivalent to 155 mg base.

Lupus Erythematosus: Initially, the average *adult* dose is 400 mg (=310 mg base) once or twice daily. This may be continued for several weeks or months, depending on the response of the patient. For prolonged maintenance therapy, a smaller dose, from 200 mg to 400 mg (=155 mg to 310 mg base) daily will frequently suffice.

The incidence of retinopathy has been reported to be higher when this maintenance dose is exceeded.

Rheumatoid Arthritis: The compound is cumulative in action and will require several weeks to exert its beneficial therapeutic effects, whereas minor side effects may occur relatively early. Several months of therapy may be required before maximum effects can be obtained. If objective improvement (such as reduced joint swelling, increased mobility) does not occur within six months, the drug should be discontinued. Safe use of the drug in the treatment of juvenile rheumatoid arthritis has not been established.

Initial Dosage: In adults, from 400 mg to 600 mg (=310 mg to 465 mg base) daily, each dose to be taken with a meal or a glass of milk. In a small percentage of patients, troublesome side effects may require temporary reduction of the initial dosage. Later (usually from five to ten days), the dose may gradually be increased to the optimum response level, often without return of side effects.

Maintenance Dosage: When a good response is obtained (usually in four to twelve weeks), the dosage is reduced by 50 percent and continued at a usual maintenance level of 200 mg to 400 mg (=155 mg to 310 mg base) daily, each dose to be taken with a meal or a glass of milk. The incidence of retinopathy has been reported to be higher when this maintenance dose is exceeded.

Should a relapse occur after medication is withdrawn, therapy may be resumed or continued on an intermittent schedule if there are no ocular contraindications.

Corticosteroids and Salicylates: may be used in conjunction with this compound, and they can generally be decreased gradually in dosage or eliminated after the drug has been used for several weeks. When gradual reduction of steroid dosage is indicated, it may be done by reducing every four to five days the dose of cortisone by no more than from 5 mg to 15 mg; of hydrocortisone from 5 mg to 10 mg; of prednisolone and prednisone from 1 mg to 2.5 mg; of methylprednisolone and triamcinolone from 1 mg to 2 mg; and of dexamethasone from 0.25 mg to 0.5 mg.

HOW SUPPLIED - RATED THERAPEUTICALLY EQUIVALENT:

Tablet - Oral - 200 mg

100's	$108.00	Hydroxychloroquine Sulfate, H.C.F.A. F F P	99999-1506-01

Tablet, Uncoated - Oral - 200 mg

100's	$104.35	Hydroxychloroquine Sulfate, Copley Pharm	38245-0774-10
100's	$109.57	Hydroxychloroquine Sulfate, HL Moore Drug Exch	00839-7963-06
100's	**$115.94**	**PLAQUENIL, Sanofi Winthrop**	**00024-1562-10**
500's	$511.35	Hydroxychloroquine Sulfate, Copley Pharm	38245-0774-50

HYDROXYPROGESTERONE CAPROATE *(001508)*

CATEGORIES: Antineoplastics; Hormones; Oncologic Drugs; Progestins; FDA Approval Pre 1982

BRAND NAMES: Delta-Lutin; *Depolut*; Deprolutin; Dura-Lutin; Gesterol LA; *HPC*; *Hormofort*; Hy-Gestrone; Hylutin; Hyprogest 250; *Lentogest*; *Primolut Depot* (Mexico); Pro-Depo; Pro-Span; Prodrox; *Progesterone-Retard Phalon* (France); *Progestin Depot*; *Proluten Depot* (Germany)
(International brand names outside U.S. in italics)

Prescribing information not available at time of publication.

HOW SUPPLIED - RATED THERAPEUTICALLY EQUIVALENT:

Injection, Solution - Intramuscular - 250 mg/ml

5 ml	$10.49	Hydroxyprogesterone Caproate, Balan	00304-1372-55
5 ml	$12.25	Hydroxyprogesterone Caproate, Harber Pharm	51432-0617-20
5 ml	$13.15	Hydroxyprogesterone Caproate, Major Pharms	00904-0852-05
5 ml	$14.43	Hydroxyprogesteron Caproate, HL Moore Drug Exch	00839-6279-25
5 ml	$15.75	Hydroxyprogesterone Caproate, Goldline Labs	00182-3072-62

HOW SUPPLIED - NOT RATED EQUIVALENT:

Injection, Solution - Intramuscular - 125 mg/ml

10 ml	$7.40	HY-GESTRONE, Pasadena	00418-0521-41

Injection, Solution - Intramuscular - 250 mg/ml

5 ml	$10.54	HY-GESTRONE 250, Pasadena	00418-0521-31
5 ml	$13.50	Hydroxyprogesterone Caproate, Consolidated Midland	00223-7896-05
5 ml	$13.79	HYLUTIN, Hyrex Pharms	00314-0891-75
5 ml	$14.00	DELTA-LUTIN, Bolan Pharm	44437-0598-05
5 ml	$14.45	Hydroxyprogesterone Caproate, Steris Labs	00402-0598-05
5 ml	$15.75	Hydroxyprogesterone Caproate, Rugby	00536-1695-65
5 ml	$16.50	Hydroxyprogesterone Caproate, Schein Pharm (US)	00364-6690-53

HYDROXYPROPYL CELLULOSE *(001509)*

CATEGORIES: Conjunctival Hyperemia; Conjunctivitis; Corneal Erosions; Corneal Sensitivity; EENT Drugs; Eye, Ear, Nose, & Throat Preparations; Keratitis; Keratoconjunctivitis; Ophthalmic Lubricants; Ophthalmics; Photophobia; FDA Approval Pre 1982

BRAND NAMES: **Lacrisert**

DESCRIPTION:

Lacrisert (Hydroxypropyl Cellulose) is a sterile, translucent, rod-shaped, water soluble, ophthalmic insert made of hydroxypropyl cellulose, for administration into the inferior cul-de-sac of the eye.

The chemical name for hydroxypropyl cellulose is cellulose, 2-hydroxypropyl ether. It is an ether of cellulose in which hydroxypropyl groups ($-CH_2CHOHCH_3$) are attached to the hydroxyls present in the anhydroglucose rings of cellulose by ether linkages.

The molecular weight is typically 1×10^6.

Hydroxypropyl cellulose is an off-white, odorless, tasteless powder. It is soluble in water below 38°C, and in many polar organic solvents such as ethanol, propylene glycol, dioxane, methanol, isopropyl alcohol (95%), dimethyl sulfoxide, and dimethyl formamide.

Each Lacrisert is 5 mg of hydroxypropyl cellulose. Lacrisert contains no preservatives or other ingredients. It is about 1.27 mm in diameter by about 3.5 mm long.

Lacrisert is supplied in packages of 60 units, together with illustrated instructions and a special applicator for removing Lacrisert from the unit dose blister and inserting it into the eye. A spare applicator is included in each package.

CLINICAL PHARMACOLOGY:

PHARMACODYNAMICS

Lacrisert acts to stabilize and thicken the precorneal tear film and prolong the tear film breakup time which is usually accelerated in patients with dry eye states. Lacrisert also acts to lubricate and protect the eye.

Lacrisert usually reduces the signs and symptoms resulting from moderate to severe dry eye syndromes, such as conjunctival hyperemia, corneal and conjunctival staining with rose bengal, exudation, itching, burning, foreign body sensation, smarting, photophobia, dryness and blurred or cloudy vision. Progressive visual deterioration which occurs in some patients may be retarded, halted, or sometimes reversed.

In a multicenter crossover study the 5 mg Lacrisert administered once a day during the waking hours was compared to artificial tears used four or more times daily. There was a prolongation of tear film breakup time and a decrease in foreign body sensation associated with dry eye syndrome in patients during treatment with inserts as compared to artificial tears; these findings were statistically significantly different between the treatment groups. Improvement, as measured by amelioration of symptoms, by slit lamp examination and by rose bengal staining of the cornea and conjunctiva, was greater in most patients with moderate to severe symptoms during treatment with Lacrisert. Patient comfort was usually better with Lacrisert than with artificial tears solution, and most patients preferred Lacrisert.

In most patients treated with Lacrisert for over one year, improvement was observed as evidenced by amelioration of symptoms generally associated with keratoconjunctivitis sicca such as burning, tearing, foreign body sensation, itching, photophobia and blurred or cloudy vision.

During studies in healthy volunteers, a thickened precorneal tear film was usually observed through the slit-lamp while Lacrisert was present in the conjunctival sac.

PHARMACOKINETICS AND METABOLISM

Hydroxypropyl cellulose is a physiologically inert substance. In a study of rats fed hydroxypropyl cellulose or unmodified cellulose at levels up to 5% of their diet, it was found that the two were biologically equivalent in that neither was metabolized.

CLINICAL PHARMACOLOGY: *(cont'd)*

Studies conducted in rats fed ^{14}C-labeled hydroxypropyl cellulose demonstrated that when orally administered, hydroxypropyl cellulose is not absorbed from the gastrointestinal tract and is quantitatively excreted in the feces.

Dissolution studies in rabbits showed that hydroxypropyl cellulose inserts became softer within 1 hour after they were placed in the conjunctival sac. Most of the inserts dissolved completely in 14 to 18 hours; with a single exception, all had disappeared by 24 hours after insertion. Similar dissolution of the inserts was observed during prolonged administration (up to 54 weeks).

INDICATIONS AND USAGE:

Lacrisert is indicated in patients with moderate to severe dry eye syndromes, including keratoconjunctivitis sicca. Lacrisert is indicated especially in patients who remain symptomatic after an adequate trial of therapy with artificial tear solutions.

Lacrisert is also indicated for patients with:

Exposure keratitis
Decreased corneal sensitivity
Recurrent corneal erosions

CONTRAINDICATIONS:

Lacrisert is contraindicated in patients who are hypersensitive to hydroxypropyl cellulose.

WARNINGS:

Instructions for inserting and removing Lacrisert should be carefully followed.

PRECAUTIONS:

GENERAL

If improperly placed, Lacrisert may result in corneal abrasion (see DOSAGE AND ADMINISTRATION.)

INFORMATION FOR THE PATIENT

Patients should be advised to follow the instructions for using Lacrisert which accompany the package.

Because this product may produce transient blurring of vision, patients should be instructed to exercise caution when operating hazardous machinery or driving a motor vehicle.

CARCINOGENESIS, MUTAGENESIS, AND IMPAIRMENT OF FERTILITY

Feeding of hydroxypropyl cellulose to rats at levels up to 5% of their diet produced no gross or histopathologic changes or other deleterious effects.

DRUG INTERACTIONS:

Application of hydroxypropyl cellulose inserts to the eyes of unanesthetized rabbits immediately prior to or two hours before instilling pilocarpine, proparacaine HCl (0.5%), or phenylephrine (5%) did not markedly alter the magnitude and/or duration of the miotic, local corneal anesthetic, or mydriatic activity, respectively, of these agents.

Under various treatment schedules, the anti-inflammatory effect of ocularly instilled dexamethasone (0.1%) in unanesthetized rabbits with primary uveitis was not affected by the presence of hydroxypropyl cellulose inserts.

ADVERSE REACTIONS:

The following adverse reactions have been reported in patients treated with Lacrisert, but were in most instances mild and transient:

Transient blurring of vision (See PRECAUTIONS)
Ocular discomfort or irritation
Matting or stickiness of eyelashes
Photophobia
Hypersensitivity
Edema of the eyelids
Hyperemia

DOSAGE AND ADMINISTRATION:

One Lacrisert ophthalmic insert in each eye once daily is usually sufficient to relieve the symptoms associated with moderate to severe dry eye syndromes. Individual patients may require more flexibility in the use of Lacrisert; some patients may require twice daily use for optimal results.

Clinical experience with Lacrisert indicates that in some patients several weeks may be required before satisfactory improvement of symptoms is achieved.

Lacrisert is inserted into the inferior cul-de-sac of the eye beneath the base of the tarsus, not in apposition to the cornea, nor beneath the eyelid at the level of the tarsal plate. If not properly positioned, it will be expelled into the interpalpebral fissure, and may cause symptoms of a foreign body. Illustrated instructions are included in each package. While in the licensed practitioner's office, the patient should read the instructions, then practice insertion and removal of Lacrisert until proficiency is achieved.

NOTE: Occasionally Lacrisert is inadvertently expelled from the eye, especially in patients with shallow conjunctival fornices. The patient should be cautioned against rubbing the eye(s) containing Lacrisert, especially upon awakening, so as not to dislodge or expel the insert. If required, another Lacrisert ophthalmic insert may be inserted. If experience indicates that transient blurred vision develops in an individual patient, the patient may want to remove Lacrisert a few hours after insertion to avoid this. Another Lacrisert ophthalmic insert may be inserted if needed.

If Lacrisert causes worsening of symptoms, the patient should be instructed to inspect the conjunctival sac to make certain Lacrisert is in the proper location, deep in the inferior cul-de-sac of the eye beneath the base of the tarsus. If these symptoms persist, Lacrisert should be removed and the patient should contact the practitioner.

Storage: Store below 30°C (86°F).

(Merck 8/89, 7415108)

HOW SUPPLIED - EQUIVALENTS NOT AVAILABLE:

Insert - Ophthalmic - 5 mg

60's	**$49.29**	**LACRISERT, Merck**	**00006-3380-60**

HYDROXYUREA *(001512)*

CATEGORIES: Antineoplastics; Cancer; Cytotoxic Agents; Leukemia; Melanoma; Oncologic Drugs; Ovarian Carcinoma; Skin Cancer; Tumors; Anemia*; Sickle Cell Disease*; FDA Approval Pre 1982
* Indication not approved by the FDA

BRAND NAMES: **Hydrea**; *Litalir* (Germany); *Onco-Carbide*
(International brand names outside U.S. in italics)

FORMULARIES: Aetna; BC-BS; Medi-Cal

COST OF THERAPY: $643.75 (Ovarian Carcinoma; Capsule; 500 mg; 2/day; 252 days)

DESCRIPTION:

Hydroxyurea is an antineoplastic agent, available for oral use as capsules providing 500 mg hydroxyurea. Inactive ingredients: citric acid, colorants (D&C Yellow No. 10, FD&C Blue No. 1, FD&C Red 40 and D&C Red 28), gelatin, lactose, magnesium stearate, sodium phosphate, and titanium dioxide. Hydroxyurea occurs as an essentially tasteless, white crystalline powder.

CLINICAL PHARMACOLOGY:

Mechanism of Action: The precise mechanism by which hydroxyurea produces its cytotoxic effects cannot, at present, be described. However, the reports of various studies in tissue culture in rats and man lend support to the hypothesis that hydroxyurea causes an immediate inhibition of DNA synthesis without interfering with the synthesis of ribonucleic acid or of protein. This hypothesis explains why, under certain conditions, hydroxyurea may induce teratogenic effects.

Three mechanisms of action have been postulated for the increased effectiveness of concomitant use of hydroxyurea therapy with irradiation on squamous cell (epidermoid) carcinomas of the head and neck. *In vitro* studies utilizing Chinese hamster cells suggest that hydroxyurea (1) is lethal to normally radioresistant S-stage cells, and (2) holds other cells of the cell cycle in the G1 or pre-DNA synthesis stage where they are most susceptible to the effects of irradiation. The third mechanism of action has been theorized on the basis of *in vitro* studies of HeLa cells: it appears that hydroxyurea, by inhibition of DNA synthesis, hinders the normal repair process of cells damaged but not killed by irradiation, thereby decreasing their survival rate; RNA and protein synthesis have shown no alteration.

Absorption, Metabolism, Fate and Excretion: After oral administration in man, hydroxyurea is readily absorbed from the gastrointestinal tract. The drug reaches peak serum concentrations within 2 hours; by 24 hours the concentration in the serum is essentially zero. Approximately 80 percent of an oral or intravenous dose of 7 to 30 mg/kg may be recovered in the urine within 12 hours.

Animal Pharmacology and Toxicology: The oral LD_{50} of hydroxyurea is 7330 mg/kg in mice and 5780 mg/kg in rats, given as a single dose.

In subacute and chronic toxicity studies in the rat, the most consistent pathological findings were an apparent dose-related mild to moderate bone marrow hypoplasia as well as pulmonary congestion and mottling of the lungs. At the highest dosage levels (1260 mg/kg/day for 37 days then 2520 mg/kg/day for 40 days), testicular atrophy with absence of spermatogenesis occurred; in several animals, hepatic cell damage with fatty metamorphosis was noted. In the dog, mild to marked bone marrow depression was a consistent finding except at the lower dosage levels. Additionally, at the higher dose levels (140 to 420 mg or 140 to 1260 mg/kg/week given 3 or 7 days weekly for 12 weeks), growth retardation, slightly increased blood glucose values, and hemosiderosis of the liver or spleen were found; reversible spermatogenic arrest was noted. In the monkey, bone marrow depression, lymphoid atrophy of the spleen, and degenerative changes in the epithelium of the small and large intestines were found. At the higher, often lethal, doses (400 to 800 mg/kg/day for 7 to 15 days), hemorrhage and congestion were found in the lungs, brain, and urinary tract. Cardiovascular effects (changes in heart rate, blood pressure, orthostatic hypotension, EKG changes) and hematological changes (slight hemolysis, slight methemoglobinemia) were observed in some species of laboratory animals at doses exceeding clinical levels.

INDICATIONS AND USAGE:

Significant tumor response to hydroxyurea has been demonstrated in melanoma, resistant chronic myelocytic leukemia, and recurrent, metastatic, or inoperable carcinoma of the ovary.

Hydroxyurea used concomitantly with irradiation therapy is intended for use in the local control of primary squamous cell (epidermoid) carcinomas of the head and neck, excluding the lip.

CONTRAINDICATIONS:

Hydroxyurea is contraindicated in patients with marked bone marrow depression, (*i.e.*, leukopenia (<2500 WBC) or thrombocytopenia (<100,000), or severe anemia).

WARNINGS:

Treatment with hydroxyurea should not be initiated if bone marrow function is markedly depressed (see CONTRAINDICATIONS). Bone marrow suppression may occur, and leukopenia is generally its first and most common manifestation. Thrombocytopenia and anemia occur less often, and are seldom seen without a preceding leukopenia. However, the recovery from myelosuppression is rapid when therapy is interrupted. It should be borne in mind that bone marrow depression is more likely in patients who have previously received radiotherapy or cytotoxic cancer chemotherapeutic agents; hydroxyurea should be used cautiously in such patients.

Patients who have received irradiation therapy in the past may have an exacerbation of postirradiation erythema.

Severe anemia must be corrected with whole blood replacement before initiating therapy with hydroxyurea.

Erythrocytic Abnormalities: megaloblastic erythropoiesis, which is self-limiting, is often seen early in the course of hydroxyurea therapy. The morphologic change resembles pernicious anemia, but is not related to vitamin B_{12} or folic acid deficiency. Hydroxyurea may also delay plasma iron clearance and reduce the rate of iron utilization by erythrocytes, but it does not appear to alter the red blood cell survival time.

Hydroxyurea should be used with caution in patients with marked renal dysfunction.

Elderly patients may be more sensitive to the effects of hydroxyurea, and may require a lower dose regimen.

Usage in Pregnancy: Drugs which affect DNA synthesis, such as hydroxyurea, may be potential mutagenic agents. The physician should carefully consider this possibility before administering this drug to male or female patients who may contemplate conception.

Hydroxyurea is a known teratogenic agent in animals. Therefore, hydroxyurea should not be used in women who are or may become pregnant unless in the judgment of the physician the potential benefits outweigh the possible hazards.

PRECAUTIONS:

Therapy with hydroxyurea requires close supervision. The complete status of the blood, including bone marrow examination, if indicated, as well as kidney function and liver function should be determined prior to, and repeatedly during, treatment. The determination of the hemoglobin level, total leukocyte counts, and platelet counts should be performed at least once a week throughout the course of hydroxyurea therapy. If the white blood cell count

PRECAUTIONS: *(cont'd)*

decreases to less than 2500/mm^3, or the platelet count to less than 100,000/mm^3, therapy should be interrupted until the values rise significantly toward normal levels. Anemia, if it occurs, should be managed with whole blood replacement, without interrupting hydroxyurea therapy.

ADVERSE REACTIONS:

Adverse reactions have been primarily bone marrow depression (leukopenia, anemia, and occasionally thrombocytopenia), and less frequently gastrointestinal symptoms (stomatitis, anorexia, nausea, vomiting, diarrhea, and constipation), and dermatological reactions such as maculopapular rash and facial erythema. Dysuria and alopecia occur very rarely. Large doses may produce moderate drowsiness. Neurological disturbances have occurred extremely rarely and were limited to headache, dizziness, disorientation, hallucinations, and convulsions. Hydroxyurea occasionally may cause temporary impairment of renal tubular function accompanied by elevations in serum uric acid, BUN, and creatinine levels. Abnormal BSP retention has been reported. Fever, chills, malaise, and elevation of hepatic enzymes have also been reported.

Adverse reactions observed with combined hydroxyurea and irradiation therapy are similar to those reported with the use of hydroxyurea alone. These effects primarily include bone marrow depression (anemia and leukopenia), and gastric irritation. Almost all patients receiving an adequate course of combined hydroxyurea and irradiation therapy will demonstrate concurrent leukopenia. Platelet depression (<100,000 cells/mm^3) has occurred rarely and only in the presence of marked leukopenia. Gastric distress has also been reported with irradiation alone and in combination with hydroxyurea therapy.

It should be borne in mind that therapeutic doses of irradiation alone produce the same adverse reactions as hydroxyurea; combined therapy may cause an increase in the incidence and severity of these side effects.

Although inflammation of the mucous membranes at the irradiated site (mucositis) is attributed to irradiation alone, some investigators believe that the more severe cases are due to combination therapy.

The association of hydroxyurea with the development of acute pulmonary reactions consisting of diffuse pulmonary infiltrates, fever and dyspnea has been rarely reported.

DOSAGE AND ADMINISTRATION:

Procedures for proper handling and disposal of antineoplastic drugs should be considered. Several guidelines on this subject have been published.[1-6] There is no general agreement that all of the procedures recommended in the guidelines are necessary or appropriate.

Because of the rarity of melanoma, resistant chronic myelocytic leukemia, carcinoma of the ovary, and carcinomas of the head and neck in children, dosage regimens have not been established.

All dosage should be based on the patient's actual or ideal weight, whichever is less.

Note: If the patient prefers, or is unable to swallow capsules, the contents of the capsules may be emptied into a glass of water and taken immediately. Some inert material used as a vehicle in the capsule may not dissolve, and may float on the surface.

SOLID TUMORS

Intermittent Therapy: 80 mg/kg administered orally as a *single* dose every *third* day

Continuous Therapy: 20 to 30 mg/kg administered orally as a *single* dose *daily*

The intermittent dosage schedule offers the advantage of reduced toxicity since patients on this dosage regimen have rarely required complete discontinuance of therapy because of toxicity.

Concomitant Therapy with Irradiation: *Carcinoma of the Head and Neck:* 80 mg/kg administered orally as a *single* dose every *third* day.

Administration of hydroxyurea should be begun at least seven days before initiation of irradiation and continued during radiotherapy as well as indefinitely afterwards provided that the patient may be kept under adequate observation and evidences no unusual or severe reactions.

Irradiation should be given at the maximum dose considered appropriate for the particular therapeutic situation; adjustment of irradiation dosage is not usually necessary when hydroxyurea is used concomitantly.

RESISTANT CRONIC MYELOCYTIC LEUKEMIA

Until the intermittent therapy regimen has been evaluated, CONTINUOUS therapy (20 to 30 mg/kg administered orally as a *single* dose *daily*) is recommended.

An adequate trial period for determining the antineoplastic effectiveness of hydroxyurea is 6 weeks of therapy. When there is regression in tumor size or arrest in tumor growth, therapy should be continued indefinitely. Therapy should be interrupted if the white blood cell count drops below 2500/mm^3, or the platelet count below 100,000/mm^3. In these cases, the counts should be rechecked after three days, and therapy resumed when the counts rise significantly toward normal values. Since the hematopoietic rebound is prompt, it is usually necessary to omit only a few doses. If prompt rebound has not occurred during combined hydroxyurea and irradiation therapy, irradiation may also be interrupted. However, the need for postponement of irradiation has been rare; radiotherapy has usually been continued using the recommended dosage and technique. Anemia, if it occurs, should be corrected with whole blood replacement, without interrupting hydroxyurea therapy. Because hematopoiesis may be compromised by extensive irradiation or by other antineoplastic agents, it is recommended that hydroxyurea be administered cautiously to patients who have recently received extensive radiation therapy or chemotherapy with other cytotoxic drugs.

Pain or discomfort from inflammation of the mucous membranes at the irradiated site (mucositis) is usually controlled by measures such as topical anesthetics and orally administered analgesics. If the reaction is severe, hydroxyurea therapy may be temporarily interrupted; if it is extremely severe, irradiation dosage may, in addition, be temporarily postponed. However, it has rarely been necessary to terminate these therapies.

Severe gastric distress, such as nausea, vomiting, and anorexia, resulting from combined therapy may usually be controlled by temporary interruption of hydroxyurea administration; rarely has the additional interruption of irradiation been necessary.

Storage: Store at room temperature; avoid excessive heat. Keep tightly closed.

REFERENCES:

1. Recommendations for the Safe Handling of Parenteral Antineoplastic Drugs. NIH Publication No. 83-2621. For sale by the Superintendent of Documents, U.S. Government Printing Office, Washington, DC 20402. **2.** AMA Council Report. Guidelines for Handling Parenteral Antineoplastics. JAMA 1985; March 15. **3.** National Study Commission on Cytotoxic Exposure - Recommendations for Handling Cytotoxic Agents. Available from Louis P. Jeffrey, Sc.D., Chairman, National Study Commission on Cytotoxic Exposure, Massachusetts College of Pharmacy and Allied Health Sciences, 179 Longwood Avenue, Boston, MA 02115. **4.** Clinical Oncological Society of Australia: Guidelines and Recommendations for Safe Handling of Antineoplastic Agents. Med J Australia 1983; 1: 426-428. **5.** Jones RB, *et al:* Safe Handling of Chemotherapeutic Agents: A Report from the Mount Sinai Medical Center, CA - A Cancer Journal for Clinicians 1983; (Sept./Oct.) 258-263. **6.** American Society of Hospital Pharmacists Technical Assistance Bulletin on Handling Cytotoxic and Hazardous Drugs. Am J Hosp Pharm 1990; 47: 1033-1049. **7.** OSHA Work-Practice Guidelines for Personnel Dealing with Cytotoxic (Antineoplastic) Drugs. Am J Hosp Pharm 1986; 43: 1193-1204.

HOW SUPPLIED:

500 mg Capsules: *Identification number:* 830.

HOW SUPPLIED - RATED THERAPEUTICALLY EQUIVALENT:

Capsule, Gelatin - Oral - 500 mg

100's	$127.73	Hydroxyurea, Roxane	00054-2247-25
100's	$132.27	Hydroxyurea, Roxane	00054-8247-25
100's	**$141.93**	**HYDREA, Bristol Myers Squibb**	**00003-0830-50**
100's	**$141.93**	**HYDREA, Immunex**	**58406-0501-01**

HYDROXYZINE HYDROCHLORIDE *(001513)*

CATEGORIES: Alcoholism; Allergies; Anesthesia; Antianxiety Drugs; Antiasthmatics/Bronchodilators; Antihistamines; Antimicrobials; Antiseptics, Urinary Tract; Anxiety; Anxiolytics, Sedatives, Hypnotic; Barbiturates; Central Nervous System Agents; Chemotherapy; Delirium; Dermatitis; Dermatoses; Hypotension/Shock; Hysteria; Nausea; Pruritus; Renal Drugs; Respiratory & Allergy Medications; Respiratory Muscle Relaxant; Smooth Muscle Relaxants; Tension; Tranquilizers; Urticaria; Vertigo/Motion Sickness/Vomiting; Headache*; FDA Approval Pre 1982

* Indication not approved by the FDA

BRAND NAMES: *AH3 N* (Germany); *Abacus*; Adroxazine; Anxanil; *Apo-Hydroxyzine* (Canada); **Atarax**; *Atarax P* (Japan); *Atazina*; *Aterax*; *Bobsule* (Japan); *Calmofilase*; *Cedar*; *Centilax*; *Cerax*; *Disron*; *Disron P* (Japan); *Drazine*; *Hiderax*; *Histan*; *Hizin*; Hydroxacen; Hyzine; *Iremofar*; *Iterax*; *Masmoran* (Germany); *Multipax* (Canada); Neucalm 50; *Novohydroxyzin* (Canada); Orgatrax; *Otarex*; *Paxistil*; *Postarax*; Quiess; Rezine; *Trandozine*; *Tranquijust* (Japan); *Ucerax*; *Ultramax*; Visrex; Vista-Plex 50; Vistacon-50; Vistacot; Vistaject; Vistaril; Vistazine *(International brand names outside U.S. in italics)*

FORMULARIES: Aetna; BC-BS; CIGNA; DoD; FHP; Humana; Kaiser; Medco; Medi-Cal; PCS; PruCare; United

COST OF THERAPY: $3.10 (Rhinitis; Tablet; 25 mg; 3/day; 30 days)

PRIMARY ICD9: 477.9 (Allergic Rhinitis, Cause Unspecified)

DESCRIPTION:

Tablets, Syrup and IM Solution: Hydroxyzine hydrochloride is designated chemically as 1-(p-chlorobenzhydryl) 4-[2-(2-hydroxyethoxy)-ethyl] piperazine dihydrochloride.

Tablets: Inert ingredients for the tablets are: acacia; carnauba wax; dibasic calcium phosphate; gelatin; lactose; magnesium stearate; precipitated calcium carbonate; shellac; sucrose; talc; white wax. The 10 mg tablets also contain: sodium hydroxide; starch; titanium dioxide, Yellow 6 Lake. The 25 mg tablets also contain: starch; velo dark green. The 50 mg tablets also contain: starch; velo yellow. The 100 mg tablets also contain: alginic acid; Blue 1; polyethylene glycol; Red 3.

Syrup: *The inert ingredients for the syrup are:* alcohol; menthol; peppermint oil; sodium benzoate; spearmint oil; sucrose; water.

CLINICAL PHARMACOLOGY:

Tablets, Syrup and IM Solution: Hydroxyzine HCl is unrelated chemically to the phenothiazines, reserpine, meprobamate, or the benzodiazepines.

Hydroxyzine HCl is not a cortical depressant, but its action may be due to a suppression of activity in certain key regions of the subcortical area of the central nervous system. Primary skeletal muscle relaxation has been demonstrated experimentally. Bronchodilator activity, and antihistaminic and analgesic effects have been demonstrated experimentally and confirmed clinically. An antiemetic effect, both by the apomorphine test and the veriloid test, has been demonstrated. Pharmacological and clinical studies indicate that hydroxyzine in therapeutic dosage does not increase gastric secretion or acidity and in most cases has mild antisecretory activity. Hydroxyzine is rapidly absorbed from the gastrointestinal tract and hydroxyzine HCl's clinical effects are usually noted within 15 to 30 minutes after oral administration.

Hydroxyzine has been shown experimentally to have antispasmodic properties, apparently mediated through interference with the mechanism that responds to spasmogenic agents such as serotonin, acetylcholine, and histamine.

INDICATIONS AND USAGE:

Tablets and Syrup: For symptomatic relief of anxiety and tension associated with psychoneurosis and as an adjunct in organic disease states in which anxiety is manifested.

Useful in the management of pruritus due to allergic conditions such as chronic urticaria and atopic and contact dermatoses, and in histamine-mediated pruritus.

As a sedative when used as premedication and following general anesthesia, **Hydroxyzine may potentiate meperidine and barbiturates,** so their use in pre-anesthetic adjunctive therapy should be modified on an individual basis. Atropine and other belladonna alkaloids are not affected by the drug. Hydroxyzine is not known to interfere with the action of digitalis in any way and it may be used concurrently with this agent.

The effectiveness of hydroxyzine as an antianxiety agent for long term use, that is more than 4 months, has not been assessed by systematic clinical studies. The physician should reassess periodically the usefulness of the drug for the individual patient.

IM Solution: The total management of anxiety, tension, and psychomotor agitation in conditions of emotional stress requires in most instances a combined approach of psychotherapy and chemotherapy. Hydroxyzine has been found to be particularly useful for this latter phase of therapy in its ability to render the disturbed patient more amenable to psychotherapy in long term treatment of the psychoneurotic and psychotic, although it should not be used as the sole treatment of psychosis or of clearly demonstrated cases of depression.

Hydroxyzine is also useful in alleviating the manifestations of anxiety and tension as in the preparation for dental procedures and in acute emotional problems. It has also been recommended for the management of anxiety associated with organic disturbances and as adjunctive therapy in alcoholism and allergic conditions with strong emotional overlay, such as in asthma, chronic urticaria, and pruritus.

Hydroxyzine HCl IM Solution is useful in treating the following types of patients when intramuscular administration is indicated:

1. The acutely disturbed or hysterical patient.

2. The acute or chronic alcoholic with anxiety withdrawal symptoms or delirium tremens.

3. As pre- and postoperative and pre- and postpartum adjunctive medication to permit reduction in narcotic dosage, allay anxiety and control emesis.

Hydroxyzine HCl has also demonstrated effectiveness in controlling nausea and vomiting, excluding nausea and vomiting of pregnancy (see CONTRAINDICATIONS).

INDICATIONS AND USAGE: *(cont'd)*

In prepartum states, the reduction in narcotic requirement effected by hydroxyzine if of particular benefit to both mother and neonate.

Hydroxyzine benefits the cardiac patients by its ability to allay the associated anxiety and apprehension attendant to certain types of heart disease. Hydroxyzine is not known to interfere with the action of digitalis in any way and may be used concurrently with this agent.

The effectiveness of hydroxyzine in long term use, that is, more than 4 months, has not been assessed by systemic clinical studies. The physician reassess periodically the usefulness of the drug for the individual patient.

CONTRAINDICATIONS:

Tablets, Syrup and IM Solution: Hydroxyzine, when administered to the pregnant mouse, rat, and rabbit, induced fetal abnormalities in the rat and mouse at doses substantially above the human therapeutic range. Clinical data in human beings are inadequate to establish safety in early pregnancy. Until such data are available, hydroxyzine is contraindicated in early pregnancy.

Hydroxyzine is contraindicated for patients who have shown a previous hypersensitivity to it.

IM Solution: Hydroxyzine HCl intramuscular solution is intended only for intramuscular administration only and should not, under any circumstances, be injected subcutaneously, intra-arterially, or intravenously.

WARNINGS:

TABLETS AND SYRUP

Nursing Mothers: It is not known whether this drug is excreted in human milk. Since many drugs are so excreted, hydroxyzine should not be given to nursing mothers.

Tablets Only: This product is manufactured with 1.1.1-trichloroethane, a substance which harms public health and the environment by destroying ozone in the upper atmosphere.

PRECAUTIONS:

Tablets, Syrup and IM Solution: THE POTENTIATING ACTION OF HYDROXYZINE MUST BE CONSIDERED WHEN THE DRUG IS USED IN CONJUNCTION WITH CENTRAL NERVOUS SYSTEM DEPRESSANTS SUCH AS NARCOTICS, NON-NARCOTIC ANALGESICS AND BARBITURATES. Since drowsiness may occur with use of this drug, patients should be warned of this possibility and cautioned against driving a car or operating dangerous machinery while taking hydroxyzine HCl.

Tablets and Syrup: Therefore when central nervous system depressants are administered concomitantly with hydroxyzine their dosage should be reduced.

Patients should be advised against the simultaneous use of other CNS depressant drugs, and cautioned that the effect of alcohol may be increased.

IM Solution: Rarely, cardiac arrests and death have been reported in association with the combined use of hydroxyzine HCl IM and other CNS depressants. Therefore when central nervous system depressants are administered concomitantly with hydroxyzine their dosage should be reduced up to 50 per cent. The efficacy of hydroxyzine as adjunctive pre- and postoperative sedative medication has been well established, especially as regards to its ability to allay anxiety, control emesis, and reduce the amount of narcotic required

HYDROXYZINE MAY POTENTIATE NARCOTICS AND BARBITURATES, so their use in preanesthetic adjunctive therapy should be modified on an individual basis. Atropine and other belladonna alkaloids are not affected by the drug.

When hydroxyzine is used preoperatively or prepartum, narcotic requirements may be reduced as much as 50 per cent. Thus, when 50 mg of hydroxyzine HCl IM solution is employed, meperidine dosage may be reduced from 100 mg to 50 mg. The administration of meperidine may result in severe hypotension in the postoperative patient or any individual whose ability to maintain blood pressure has been compromised by a depleted blood volume. Meperidine should be used with great caution and in reduced dosage in patients who are receiving other pre- and/or postoperative medications and in whom there is a risk of respiratory depression, hypotension, and profound sedation or coma occurring. Before using any medications concomitant with hydroxyzine, the manufacturer's prescribing information should be read carefully.

Since drowsiness may occur

As with all IM preparations, hydroxyzine HCl IM should be injected well within the body of a relatively large muscle. In advertent subcutaneous injection may result in significant tissue damage.

Adults: The preferred site is the upper outer quadrant of the buttock (*i.e.,* glutenous maximus), or the mid-lateral thigh.

Children: It is recommended that IM injections be given preferably in the mid-lateral muscles of the thigh. In infants and small children the periphery of the upper outer quadrant of the gluteal region should be used only when necessary, such as in burn patients, in order to minimize the possibility of damage to the sciatic nerve.

The deltoid area should be used only if well developed such as in certain adults and older children and then only with caution to avoid radial nerve injury. IM injections should not be made into the lower and mid- third of the upper arm. Aspiration is necessary to help avoid inadvertent injection into a blood vessel.

ADVERSE REACTIONS:

TABLETS, SYRUP AND IM SOLUTION

Side effects reported with the administration of hydroxyzine HCl are usually mild and transitory in nature.

Anticholinergic: Dry mouth.

Central Nervous System: Drowsiness is usually transitory and may disappear in a few days of continued therapy or upon reduction of the dose. Involuntary motor activity including rare instances of tremor and convulsions have been reported, usually with doses considerably higher than those recommended. Clinically significant respiratory depression has not been reported at recommended doses.

IM Solution: Extensive clinical use has substantiated the absence of toxic effects on the liver or bone marrow when administered in the recommended doses for over four years of uninterrupted therapy. The absence of adverse effects has been further demonstrated in experimental studies in which excessively high doses were administered.

OVERDOSAGE:

Tablets and Syrup: The most common manifestation of hydroxyzine HCl overdosage is hypersedation. As in the management of overdosage with any drug, it should be borne in mind that multiple agents may have been taken.

If vomiting has not occurred spontaneously, it should be induced. Immediate gastric lavage is also recommended. General supportive care, including frequent monitoring of the vital signs and close observation of the patient, is indicated. Hypotension, though unlikely, may be controlled with intravenous fluids and Levophed (levarterenol), or Aramine (metaraminol). Do not use epinephrine as hydroxyzine HCl counteracts its pressor action.

OVERDOSAGE: *(cont'd)*

There is no specific antidote. It is doubtful that hemodialysis would be of any value in the treatment of overdosage with hydroxyzine. However, if other agents such as barbiturates have been ingested concomitantly, hemodialysis may be indicated. There is no practical method to quantitate hydroxyzine in body fluids or tissue after its ingestion or administration.

DOSAGE AND ADMINISTRATION:

Oral Forms: For symptomatic relief of anxiety and tension associated with psychoneurosis and as an adjunct in organic disease states in which anxiety is manifested: in adults, 50-100 mg q.i.d.; children under 6 years, 50 mg daily in divided doses and over 6 years, 50-100 mg daily in divided doses.

For use in the management of pruritus due to allergic conditions such as chronic urticaria and atopic and contact dermatoses, and in histamine-mediated pruritus: in adults, 25 mg t.i.d. or q.i.d.; children under 6 years, 50 mg daily in divided doses and over 6 years, 50-100 mg daily in divided doses.

As a sedative when used as a premedication and following general anesthesia: 50-100 mg in adults, and 0.6 mg/kg in children.

When treatment is initiated by the intramuscular route of administration, subsequent doses may be administered orally.

As with all medications, the dosage should be adjusted according to the patient's response to therapy.

IM Solution: The recommended dosages for hydroxyzine HCl IM solution are given in TABLE 1:

TABLE 1

Adult psychiatric and emotional emergencies, including acute alcoholism	IM: 50-100 mg stat., and q. 4-6h., p.r.n.
Nausea and vomiting excluding nausea and vomiting of pregnancy.	Adults: 25-100 mg IM Children: 0.5 mg/lb body weight IM
Pre- and postoperative adjunctive medication	Adults: 25-100 mg IM Children: 0.5 mg/lb body weight IM
Pre- and postpartum adjunctive therapy	25-100 mg IM

As with all potent medications, the dosage should be adjusted according to the patient's response to therapy.

FOR ADDITIONAL INFORMATION OF THE ADMINISTRATION AND SITE OF SELECTION SEE PRECAUTIONS SECTIONS NOTE: Hydroxyzine HCl IM solution may be administered without further dilution.

Patients may be started on IM therapy when indicated. They should be maintained on oral therapy whenever this route is practicable.

HOW SUPPLIED - RATED THERAPEUTICALLY EQUIVALENT:

Injection, Solution - Intramuscular - 25 mg/ml

1 ml	$0.53	Hydroxyzine Hcl, Fujisawa USA	00469-2100-00
1 ml	$14.38	Hydroxyzine Hcl, Solopak Labs	39769-0023-02
1 ml x 10	$6.23	Hydroxyzine HCl, Sanofi Winthrop	00024-0711-02
1 ml x 25	$12.05	Hydroxyzine Hcl, Elkins Sinn	00641-0432-25
1 ml x 25	$18.44	Hydroxyzine Hcl, Am Regent	00517-4201-25
1 ml x 25	$25.00	Hydroxyzine Hcl, Consolidated Midland	00223-7885-01
10 ml	$2.03	Hydroxyzine Hcl, HL Moore Drug Exch	00839-6337-30
10 ml	$2.84	Hydroxyzine Hcl, Balan	00304-1373-56
10 ml	$3.00	Hydroxyzine Hcl, Consolidated Midland	00223-7877-10
10 ml	$3.51	Hydroxyzine Hcl, Steris Labs	00402-0170-10
10 ml	$5.09	Hydroxyzine HCl, Schein Pharm (US)	00364-6718-54
10 ml	$6.38	Hydroxyzine HCl, Rugby	00536-5050-70
10 ml	$9.63	VISTARIL, Roerig	00049-5450-74
10 ml x 25	$54.69	Hydroxyzine Hcl, Am Regent	00517-4210-25

Injection, Solution - Intramuscular - 50 mg/ml

1 ml	$14.38	Hydroxyzine Hcl Inj 50, Solopak Labs	39769-0024-02
1 ml	$15.63	Hydroxyzine Hydrochloride, Fujisawa USA	00469-5100-00
1 ml x 10	$7.19	Hydroxyzine HCl, Sanofi Winthrop	00024-0712-02
1 ml x 25	$12.05	Hydroxyzine Hcl, Elkins Sinn	00641-0433-25
1 ml x 25	$22.19	Hydroxyzine Hcl, Am Regent	00517-5601-25
1 ml x 25	$25.00	Hydroxyzine Hcl, Consolidated Midland	00223-7883-01
2 ml	$14.38	Hydroxyzine Hcl Inj 50, Solopak Labs	39769-0024-06
2 ml	$18.44	Hydroxyzine Hydrochloride, Fujisawa USA	00469-5100-10
2 ml x 10	$8.14	Hydroxyzine HCl, Sanofi Winthrop	00024-0713-02
2 ml x 25	$12.05	Hydroxizine Hydorchloride, Elkins Sinn	00641-0434-25
2 ml x 25	$25.00	Hydroxyzine Hcl, Consolidated Midland	00223-7884-02
2 ml x 25	$32.19	Hydroxyzine Hcl, Am Regent	00517-5602-25
10 ml	$1.66	Hydroxyzine Hcl, Insource	58441-0107-10
10 ml	$2.63	Hydroxyzine Hcl, HL Moore Drug Exch	00839-6338-30
10 ml	$3.50	Hydroxyzine Hcl, Consolidated Midland	00223-7878-10
10 ml	$3.53	Hydroxyzine Hcl, IDE-Interstate	00814-3805-40
10 ml	$3.90	Hydroxyzine Hcl, Goldline Labs	00182-1182-63
10 ml	$3.95	Hydroxyzine Hcl, Steris Labs	00402-0171-10
10 ml	$5.00	VISTAZINE, Bolan Pharm	44437-0171-10
10 ml	$5.50	VISTACOT 50, C O Truxton	00463-1101-10
10 ml	$6.38	Hydroxyzin HCl, Schein Pharm (US)	00364-6719-54
10 ml	$7.13	Hydroxyzine HCl, Rugby	00536-5060-70
10 ml	$7.26	HYZINE, Hyrex Pharms	00314-1400-70
10 ml	$11.60	HYDROXACEN, Schwarz Pharma (US)	00131-1081-05
10 ml	$11.80	VISTAQUEL 50, Pasadena	00418-6911-10
10 ml	$15.10	VISTAJECT-50, Mayrand Pharms	00259-0340-10
10 ml	$15.37	VISTARIL, Roerig	00049-5460-74
10 ml x 1	$3.03	Hydroxyzine Hcl, Elkins Sinn	00641-2518-41
10 ml x 25	$78.44	Hydroxyzine Hcl, Am Regent	00517-5610-25
10 ml x 25	$95.63	Hydroxyzine Hcl, Fujisawa USA	00469-0350-25

Syrup - Oral - 10 mg/5ml

120 ml	$2.00	Hydroxyzine Hcl, H.C.F.A. F F P	99999-1513-01
120 ml	$4.30	Hydroxyzine Hcl, Morton Grove	60432-0150-04
480 ml	$6.76	Hydroxyzine HCl, H.C.F.A. F F P	99999-1513-02
480 ml	$8.01	Hydroxyzine Hydrochloride, United Res	00677-1421-33
480 ml	$8.45	Hydroxyzine Hcl Syrup, Harber Pharm	51432-0608-20
480 ml	$10.44	Hydroxyzine Hcl, Qualitest Pharms	00603-1310-58
480 ml	$11.25	Hydroxyzine HCl, Geneva Pharms	00781-6570-16
480 ml	$11.50	Hydroxyzine Hcl, Consolidated Midland	00223-6525-01
480 ml	$11.55	Hydroxyzine HCl, Schein Pharm (US)	00364-7273-16
480 ml	$11.55	ATOZINE, Major Pharms	00904-0379-16
480 ml	$11.56	Hydroxyzine Hcl, Morton Grove	60432-0150-16
480 ml	$12.00	Hydroxyzine Hcl, Hi Tech Pharma	50383-0796-16
480 ml	$12.20	Hydroxyzine Hcl, Aligen Independ	00405-2900-16
480 ml	$12.45	Hydroxyzine Hcl, Goldline Labs	00182-1376-40
480 ml	$12.79	Hydroxyzine HCl, Rugby	00536-1002-85
480 ml	$12.81	Hydroxyzine HCl, Alpharma	00472-0771-16
480 ml	$13.22	Hydroxyzine Hcl, HL Moore Drug Exch	00839-6476-69

HOW SUPPLIED - RATED THERAPEUTICALLY EQUIVALENT: *(cont'd)*

480 ml	**$46.67**	**ATARAX, Roerig**	**00049-5590-93**
3840 ml	$64.12	Hydroxyzine Hcl, H.C.F.A. F F P	99999-1513-03
3840 ml	$70.20	Hydroxyzine Hcl, Rugby	00536-1002-90
3840 ml	$75.00	Hydroxyzine Hcl, Consolidated Midland	00223-6525-02
3840 ml	$85.57	Hydroxyzine HCl, Alpharma	00472-0771-28

Tablet - Oral - 10 mg

100's	$7.75	Hydroxyzine Hcl, Duramed Pharms	51285-0880-02
1000's	$74.50	Hydroxyzine Hcl, Duramed Pharms	51285-0880-05

Tablet - Oral - 25 mg

100's	$11.85	Hydroxyzine Hcl, Duramed Pharms	51285-0881-02

Tablet - Oral - 50 mg

100's	$12.75	Hydroxyzine Hcl, Duramed Pharms	51285-0882-02
1000's	$102.15	Hydroxyzine Hcl, Duramed Pharms	51285-0882-05

Tablet, Coated - Oral - 10 mg

30's	$1.65	Hydroxyzine, Talbert Phcy	44514-0418-18
100's	$2.21	Hydroxyzine HCl, H.C.F.A. F F P	99999-1513-04
100's	$4.13	Hydroxyzine Hcl, IDE-Interstate	00814-3793-14
100's	$4.25	Hydroxyzine Hcl, US Trading	56126-0012-11
100's	$5.25	Hydroxyzine Hcl, Consolidated Midland	00223-1006-01
100's	$6.47	Hydroxyzine Hcl, HL Moore Drug Exch	00839-7437-06
100's	$6.75	Hydroxyzine Hcl, Major Pharms	00904-0357-60
100's	$6.79	Hydroxyzine Hyrochloride, United Res	00677-0604-01
100's	$6.80	Hydroxyzine Hcl, Qualitest Pharms	00603-3970-21
100's	$6.85	Hydroxyzine HCl 10 Mg, Geneva Pharms	00781-1332-01
100's	$7.00	Hydroxyzine Hcl, Mutual Pharm	53489-0126-01
100's	$7.20	Hydroxyzine Hcl, Goldline Labs	00182-1492-01
100's	$7.20	Hydroxyzine Hcl, Schein Pharm (US)	00364-0494-01
100's	$7.20	HYDROXYZINE HCL SC, Rugby	00536-4567-01
100's	$7.20	Hydroxyzine Hcl, Sidmak Labs	50111-0307-01
100's	$7.44	Hydroxyzine Hcl, Voluntary Hosp	53258-0135-01
100's	$7.55	Hydroxyzine Hcl, Royce	51875-0345-01
100's	$7.55	Hydroxyzine Hcl, Martec Pharms	52555-0557-01
100's	$7.58	Hydroxyzine Hcl, Aligen Independ	00405-4511-01
100's	$15.20	REZINE, Marnel Pharceut	00682-9403-01
100's	$15.55	Hydroxyzine Hcl, Vangard Labs	00615-1525-13
100's	$17.94	Hydroxyzine Hcl, Voluntary Hosp	53258-0135-13
100's	$24.97	Hydroxyzine Hcl, Medirex	57480-0415-01
100's	$31.15	Hydroxyzine Hcl, Major Pharms	00904-0357-61
100's	$36.50	Hydroxyzine Hcl, Goldline Labs	00182-1492-89
100's	**$49.33**	**ATARAX, Roerig**	**00049-5600-66**
100's UD	$35.50	Hydroxyzine HCl, U.D., Schein Pharm (US)	00364-0494-90
250's	$5.52	Hydroxyzine HCl, H.C.F.A. F F P	99999-1513-05
250's	$15.20	Hydroxyzine Hcl 10, Major Pharms	00904-0357-70
500's	$11.05	Hydroxyzine HCl, H.C.F.A. F F P	99999-1513-06
500's	$18.53	Hydroxyzine Hcl, IDE-Interstate	00814-3793-28
500's	$26.99	Hydroxyzine Hcl, HL Moore Drug Exch	00839-7437-12
500's	$27.50	Hydroxyzine Hcl, Consolidated Midland	00223-1006-05
500's	$29.79	Hydroxyzine Hyrochloride, United Res	00677-0604-05
500's	$29.80	Hydroxyzine Hcl, Qualitest Pharms	00603-3970-28
500's	$29.92	Hydroxyzine HCl 10 Mg, Geneva Pharms	00781-1332-05
500's	$30.08	Hydroxyzine Hcl, Aligen Independ	00405-4511-02
500's	$30.50	Hydroxyzine Hcl, Goldline Labs	00182-1492-05
500's	$30.50	Hydroxyzine Hcl, Sidmak Labs	50111-0307-02
500's	$31.40	Hydroxyzine HCl, Schein Pharm (US)	00364-0494-05
500's	$32.25	Hydroxyzine Hcl SC, Rugby	00536-4567-05
500's	$32.70	Hydroxyzine Hcl, Mutual Pharm	53489-0126-05
500's	$35.88	Hydroxyzine Hcl, Royce	51875-0345-02
500's	$35.88	Hydroxyzine Hcl, Martec Pharms	52555-0557-05
500's	**$234.48**	**ATARAX, Roerig**	**00049-5600-73**
600's	$93.40	Hydroxyzine Hcl, Medirex	57480-0415-06
1000's	$22.10	Hydroxyzine Hcl, H.C.F.A. F F P	99999-1513-07
1000's	$24.00	Hydroxyzine Hcl, Sidmak Labs	50111-0307-03
1000's	$47.50	Hydroxyzine Hcl, Consolidated Midland	00223-1006-02
1000's	$55.10	Hydroxyzine Hyrochloride, United Res	00677-0604-10
1000's	$55.25	Hydroxyzine HCl 10 Mg, Geneva Pharms	00781-1332-10
1000's	$55.25	Hydroxyzine Hcl 10, Major Pharms	00904-0357-80
1000's	$57.95	Hydroxyzine Hcl, Mutual Pharm	53489-0126-10
1000's	$58.25	Hydroxyzine Hcl, Goldline Labs	00182-1492-10
1000's	$61.32	Hydroxyzine Hcl, Aligen Independ	00405-4511-03
1000's	$64.88	Hydroxyzine Hcl, Royce	51875-0345-04
1000's	$64.88	Hydroxyzine Hcl, Martec Pharms	52555-0557-10
1000's	$64.90	Hydroxyzine Hydrochloride 10s, Rugby	00536-4567-10

Tablet, Coated - Oral - 25 mg

30's	$2.30	Hydroxyzine Hcl, Talbert Phcy	44514-0419-18
100's	$3.45	Hydroxyzine Hcl, Sidmak Labs	50111-0308-01
100's	$3.45	Hydroxyzine HCl, H.C.F.A. F F P	99999-1513-08
100's	$5.43	Hydroxyzine Hcl, US Trading	56126-0013-11
100's	$5.93	Hydroxyzine Hcl, IDE-Interstate	00814-3794-14
100's	$6.95	Hydroxyzine Hcl, Consolidated Midland	00223-1007-01
100's	$8.50	Hydroxyzine Hcl, Qualitest Pharms	00603-3971-21
100's	$9.17	Hydroxyzine Hcl, HL Moore Drug Exch	00839-7438-06
100's	$9.49	Hydroxyzine Hcl, United Res	00677-0605-01
100's	$9.50	Hydroxyzine Hcl, Major Pharms	00904-0358-60
100's	$9.85	Hydroxyzine Hcl, Goldline Labs	00182-1493-01
100's	$9.95	Hydroxyzine HCl, Geneva Pharms	00781-1334-01
100's	$9.95	Hydroxyzine Hcl, Mutual Pharm	53489-0127-01
100's	$10.37	Hydroxyzine Hcl, Aligen Independ	00405-4512-01
100's	$10.50	Hydroxyzine HCl, Schein Pharm (US)	00364-0495-01
100's	$10.56	ANX, Embrex Economed	38130-0044-01
100's	$10.89	Hydroxyzine Hcl, Voluntary Hosp	53258-0136-01
100's	$11.07	Hydroxyzine Hcl, Royce	51875-0346-01
100's	$11.40	Hydroxyzine Hcl, Martec Pharms	52555-0558-01
100's	$11.90	Hydroxyzine HCl SC, Rugby	00536-4568-01
100's	$21.36	Hydroxyzine Hcl, Voluntary Hosp	53258-0136-13
100's	$21.90	REZINE, Marnel Pharceut	00682-9404-01
100's	$31.12	Hydroxyzine Hcl, Vangard Labs	00615-1526-13
100's	$31.38	Hydroxyzine Hcl, Medirex	57480-0429-01
100's	$37.91	Hydroxyzine Hcl, Major Pharms	00904-0358-61
100's	$43.00	Hydroxyzine Hcl, Goldline Labs	00182-1493-89
100's	**$72.36**	**ATARAX, Roerig**	**00049-5610-66**
100's UD	$34.00	Hydroxyzine HCl, U.D., Schein Pharm (US)	00364-0495-90
250's	$8.62	Hydroxyzine Hcl, H.C.F.A. F F P	99999-1513-09
250's	$21.40	Hydroxyzine Hcl, Major Pharms	00904-0358-70
500's	$17.25	Hydroxyzine HCl, H.C.F.A. F F P	99999-1513-10
500's	$28.28	Hydroxyzine Hcl, IDE-Interstate	00814-3794-28
500's	$32.50	Hydroxyzine Hcl, Consolidated Midland	00223-1007-05
500's	$40.55	Hydroxyzine Hcl, Qualitest Pharms	00603-3971-28
500's	$40.94	Hydroxyzine Hcl, United Res	00677-0605-05
500's	$42.75	Hydroxyzine Hcl, Major Pharms	00904-0358-40

HOW SUPPLIED - RATED THERAPEUTICALLY EQUIVALENT: *(cont'd)*

500's	$43.00	Hydroxyzine HCl, Schein Pharm (US)	00364-0495-05
500's	$44.95	Hydroxyzine HCl, Geneva Pharms	00781-1334-05
500's	$45.50	Hydroxyzine Hcl, Goldline Labs	00182-1493-05
500's	$45.50	Hydroxyzine Hcl, Sidmak Labs	50111-0308-02
500's	$46.20	Hydroxyzine Hcl, Mutual Pharm	53489-0127-05
500's	$48.32	Hydroxyzine Hcl, Aligen Independ	00405-4512-02
500's	$50.15	Hydroxyzine HCl SC, Rugby	00536-4568-05
500's	$52.58	Hydroxyzine Hcl, Royce	51875-0346-02
500's	$52.60	Hydroxyzine Hcl, Martec Pharms	52555-0558-05
500's	**$345.12**	**ATARAX, Roerig**	**00049-5610-73**
1000's	$34.50	Hydroxyzine Hcl, Sidmak Labs	50111-0308-03
1000's	$34.50	Hydroxyzine HCl, H.C.F.A. F F P	99999-1513-11
1000's	$69.50	Hydroxyzine Hcl, Consolidated Midland	00223-1007-02
1000's	$73.91	Hydroxyzine Hcl, HL Moore Drug Exch	00839-7438-16
1000's	$76.77	Hydroxyzine Hcl, Qualitest Pharms	00603-3971-32
1000's	$76.82	Hydroxyzine Hcl, United Res	00677-0605-10
1000's	$76.95	Hydroxyzine Hcl, Major Pharms	00904-0358-80
1000's	$79.95	Hydroxyzine HCl, Geneva Pharms	00781-1334-10
1000's	$82.95	Hydroxyzine Hcl, Mutual Pharm	53489-0127-10
1000's	$87.45	Hydroxyzine Hcl, Goldline Labs	00182-1493-10
1000's	$87.50	Hydroxyzine HCl, Schein Pharm (US)	00364-0495-02
1000's	$87.82	Hydroxyzine Hcl, Aligen Independ	00405-4512-03
1000's	$94.64	Hydroxyzine Hcl, Royce	51875-0346-04
1000's	$94.65	Hydroxyzine Hcl, Martec Pharms	52555-0558-10
1000's	$95.30	Hydroxyzine HCl SC, Rugby	00536-4568-10

Tablet, Coated - Oral - 50 mg

100's	$3.98	Hydroxyzine HCl, H.C.F.A. F F P	99999-1513-12
100's	$7.05	Hydroxyzine Hcl, IDE-Interstate	00814-3795-14
100's	$7.20	Hydroxyzine Hcl, US Trading	56126-0014-11
100's	$7.63	Hydroxyzine Hcl, HL Moore Drug Exch	00839-7439-06
100's	$8.75	Hydroxyzine Hcl, Consolidated Midland	00223-1008-01
100's	$10.10	Hydroxyzine Hcl, Purepac Pharm	00228-2206-10
100's	$10.60	Hydroxyzine Hcl, Qualitest Pharms	00603-3972-21
100's	$10.70	Hydroxyzine Hcl, Major Pharms	00904-0359-60
100's	$10.95	Hydroxyzine Hcl, Goldline Labs	00182-1494-01
100's	$10.95	Hydroxyzine Hcl, Sidmak Labs	50111-0309-01
100's	$11.24	Hydroxyzine Hcl, United Res	00677-0606-01
100's	$12.00	Hydroxyzine Hcl, Mutual Pharm	53489-0128-01
100's	$12.10	Hydroxyzine HCl, Geneva Pharms	00781-1336-01
100's	$12.11	Hydroxyzine Hcl, Aligen Independ	00405-4513-01
100's	$12.30	Hydroxyzine Hcl, Voluntary Hosp	53258-0137-01
100's	$12.59	Hydroxyzine Hcl, Royce	51875-0347-01
100's	$12.60	Hydroxyzine Hcl, Martec Pharms	52555-0559-01
100's	$13.75	Hydroxyzine HCl SC, Rugby	00536-4569-01
100's	$14.86	Hydroxyzine HCl, Schein Pharm (US)	00364-0496-01
100's	$16.87	Hydroxyzine Hcl, Major Pharms	00904-0359-61
100's	$23.25	Hydroxyzine Hcl, Voluntary Hosp	53258-0137-13
100's	$34.44	Hydroxyzine Hcl, Vangard Labs	00615-1527-13
100's	$35.50	Hydroxyzine HCl, Schein Pharm (US)	00364-0496-90
100's	$36.00	Hydroxyzine Hcl, Goldline Labs	00182-1494-89
100's	$36.10	Hydroxyzine Hcl, Medirex	57480-0430-01
100's	**$88.19**	**ATARAX, Roerig**	**00049-5620-66**
100's	**$101.79**	**ATARAX, Roerig**	**00049-5620-41**
250's	$9.95	Hydroxyzine HCl, H.C.F.A. F F P	99999-1513-13
250's	$19.90	Hydroxyzine Hcl, Major Pharms	00904-0359-70
500's	$19.90	Hydroxyzine HCl, H.C.F.A. F F P	99999-1513-14
500's	$33.30	Hydroxyzine Hcl, IDE-Interstate	00814-3795-28
500's	$46.40	Hydroxyzine Hcl, Qualitest Pharms	00603-3972-28
500's	$46.88	Hydroxyzine HCl SC, Rugby	00536-4569-05
500's	$47.50	Hydroxyzine Hcl, Consolidated Midland	00223-1008-05
500's	$49.95	Hydroxyzine Hcl, Mutual Pharm	53489-0128-05
500's	$52.25	Hydroxyzine Hcl, Goldline Labs	00182-1494-05
500's	$52.25	Hydroxyzine Hcl, Sidmak Labs	50111-0309-02
500's	$52.50	Hydroxyzine Hcl, United Res	00677-0606-05
500's	$52.50	Hydroxyzine HCl, Geneva Pharms	00781-1336-05
500's	$56.65	Hydroxyzine Hcl, Royce	51875-0347-02
500's	$56.65	Hydroxyzine Hcl, Martec Pharms	52555-0559-05
500's	$58.85	Hydroxyzine HCl, Schein Pharm (US)	00364-0496-05
500's	**$420.75**	**ATARAX, Roerig**	**00049-5620-73**
600's	$139.00	Hydoxyzine Hcl, Medirex	57480-0430-06
1000's	$39.80	Hydroxyzine HCl, H.C.F.A. F F P	99999-1513-15
1000's	$41.30	Hydroxyzine Hcl, Sidmak Labs	50111-0309-03
1000's	$75.00	Hydroxyzine Hcl, Consolidated Midland	00223-1008-02
1000's	$92.45	Hydroxyzine Hcl, Martec Pharms	52555-0559-10
1000's	$96.75	Hydroxyzine Hcl, United Res	00577-0606-10
1000's	$100.00	Hydroxyzine Hcl, Mutual Pharm	53489-0128-10
1000's	$101.97	Hydroxyzine Hcl, Royce	51875-0347-04
1000's	$112.17	Hydroxyzine Hcl, HL Moore Drug Exch	00839-7439-16

Tablet, Coated - Oral - 100 mg

100's	$22.50	Hydroxyzine Hcl, Consolidated Midland	00223-1009-01
100's	**$108.37**	**ATARAX, Roerig**	**00049-5630-66**
100's	**$122.81**	**ATARAX, Roerig**	**00049-5630-41**

HYDROXYZINE PAMOATE *(001514)*

CATEGORIES: Alcoholism; Allergies; Anesthesia; Antianxiety Drugs; Antiasthmatics/Bronchodilators; Anticonvulsants; Antihistamines; Anxiety; Anxiolytics, Sedatives, Hypnotic; Barbiturates; Central Nervous System Agents; Dermatitis; Dermatoses; Hysteria; Neuromuscular; Pruritus; Respiratory & Allergy Medications; Skeletal Muscle Hyperactivity; Tension; Tranquilizers; Urticaria; Vertigo/Motion Sickness/Vomiting; FDA Approval Pre 1982

BRAND NAMES: Hy-Pam; **Vistaril**

FORMULARIES: Aetna; Medi-Cal

COST OF THERAPY: **$30.81** (Anxiety; Capsule; 50 mg; 4/day; 120 days) vs. Potential Cost of $3,628.44 (Psychoses)

DESCRIPTION:

Hydroxyzine pamoate is designed chemically as 1-(p-chlorobenzhydryl) 4-(2-(2-hydroxyethoxy) ethyl) diethylenediamine salt of 1,1'-methylene bis (2 hydroxy-3-naphthalene carboxylic acid).

Inert ingredients for the capsule formulations are: hard gelatin capsules (which may contain Yellow 10, Green 3, Yellow 6, Red 33, and other inert ingredients); magnesium stearate; sodium lauryl sulfate; starch; sucrose.

Inert ingredients for the oral suspension formulation are: carboxymethylcellulose sodium; lemon flavor; propylene glycol; sorbic acid; sorbitol solution; water.

CLINICAL PHARMACOLOGY:

Hydroxyzine pamoate is unrelated chemically to the phenothiazines, reserpine, meprobamate, or the benzodiazepines.

Hydroxyzine pamoate is not a cortical depressant, but its action may be due to a suppression of activity in certain key regions of the subcortical area of the central nervous system. Primary skeletal muscle relaxation has been demonstrated experimentally. Bronchodilator activity, and antihistaminic and analgesic effects have been demonstrated experimentally and confirmed clinically. An antiemetic effect, both by the apomorphine test and the veriloid test, has been demonstrated. Pharmacological and clinical studies indicate that hydroxyzine in therapeutic dosage does not increase gastric secretion or acidity and in most cases has mild antisecretory activity. Hydroxyzine is rapidly absorbed from the gastrointestinal tract and Hydroxyzine pamoate's clinical effects are usually noted within 15 to 30 minutes after oral administration.

INDICATIONS AND USAGE:

For symptomatic relief of anxiety and tension associated with psychoneurosis and as an adjunct in organic disease states in which anxiety is manifested.

Useful in the management of pruritus due to allergic conditions such as chronic urticaria and atopic and contact dermatoses, and in histamine-mediated pruritus.

As a sedative when used as premedication and following general anesthesia, **Hydroxyzine may potentiate meperidine and barbiturates,** so their use in pre-anesthetic adjunctive therapy should be modified on an individual basis. Atropine and other belladonna alkaloids are not affected by the drug. Hydroxyzine is not known to interfere with the action of digitalis in any way and it may be used concurrently with this agent.

The effectiveness of hydroxyzine as an antianxiety agent for long term use, that is more than 4 months, has not been assessed by systematic clinical studies. The physician should reassess periodically the usefulness of the drug for the individual patient.

CONTRAINDICATIONS:

Hydroxyzine, when administered to the pregnant mouse, rat, and rabbit, induced fetal abnormalities in the rat and mouse at doses substantially above the human therapeutic range. Clinical data in human beings are inadequate to establish safety in early pregnancy. Until such data are available, hydroxyzine is contraindicated in early pregnancy.

Hydroxyzine pamoate is contraindicated for patients who have shown a previous hypersensitivity to it.

WARNINGS:

Nursing Mothers: It is not known whether this drug is excreted in human milk. Since many drugs are so excreted, hydroxyzine should not be given to nursing mothers.

PRECAUTIONS:

THE POTENTIATING ACTION OF HYDROXYZINE MUST BE CONSIDERED WHEN THE DRUG IS USED IN CONJUNCTION WITH CENTRAL NERVOUS SYSTEM DEPRESSANTS SUCH AS NARCOTICS, NON-NARCOTIC ANALGESICS AND BARBITURATES. Therefore, when central nervous system depressants are administered concomitantly with hydroxyzine their dosage should be reduced. Since drowsiness may occur with use of the drug, patients should be warned of this possibility and cautioned against driving a car or operating dangerous machinery while taking Hydroxyzine pamoate. Patients should be advised against the simultaneous use of other CNS depressant drugs, and cautioned that the effect of alcohol may be increased.

ADVERSE REACTIONS:

Side effects reported with the administration of Hydroxyzine pamoate are usually mild and transitory in nature.

Anticholinergic: Dry mouth.

Central Nervous System: Drowsiness is usually transitory and may disappear in a few days of continued therapy or upon reduction of the dose. Involuntary motor activity including rare instances of tremor and convulsions has been reported, usually with doses considerably higher than those recommended. Clinically significant respiratory depression has not been reported at recommended doses.

OVERDOSAGE:

The most common manifestation of overdosage of Hydroxyzine pamoate is hypersedation. As in the management of overdosage with any drug, it should be borne in mind that multiple agents may have been taken.

If vomiting has not occurred spontaneously, it should be induced. Immediate gastric lavage is also recommended. General supportive care, including frequent monitoring of the vital signs and close observation of the patient, is indicated. Hypotension, though unlikely, may be controlled with intravenous fluids and Levophed (levarterenol) or Aramine (metaraminol). Do not use epinephrine as Hydroxyzine pamoate counteracts its pressor action. Caffeine and Sodium Benzoate Injection, U.S.P., may be used to counteract central nervous system depressant effects.

There is no specific antidote. It is doubtful that hemodialysis would be of any value in the treatment of overdosage with hydroxyzine. However, if other agents such as barbiturates have been ingested concomitantly, hemodialysis may be indicated. There is no practical method to quantitate hydroxyzine in body fluids or tissue after its ingestion or administration.

DOSAGE AND ADMINISTRATION:

For symptomatic relief of anxiety and tension associated with psychoneurosis and as an adjunct in organic disease states in which anxiety is manifested: in adults, 50-100 mg q.i.d.; children under 6 years, 50 mg daily in divided doses and over 6 years, 50-100 mg daily in divided doses.

For use in the management of pruritus due to allergic conditions such as chronic urticaria and atopic and contact dermatoses, and in histamine-mediated pruritus: in adults, 25 mg t.i.d. or q.i.d.; children under 6 years, 50 mg daily in divided doses and over 6 years, 50-100 mg daily in divided doses.

As a sedative when used as a premedication and following general anesthesia: 50-100 mg in adults, and 0.6 mg/kg in children.

When treatment is initiated by the intramuscular route of administration, subsequent doses may be administered orally.

As with all medications, the dosage should be adjusted according to the patient's response to therapy.

HOW SUPPLIED - RATED THERAPEUTICALLY EQUIVALENT:

Capsule, Gelatin - Oral - 25 mg

100's	$5.97	Hydroxyzine Pamoate, US Trading	56126-0069-11
100's	$7.95	Hydroxyzine Pamoate, Consolidated Midland	00223-1049-01
100's	$8.33	Hydroxyzine Pamoate, H.C.F.A. F F P	99999-1514-01

HOW SUPPLIED - RATED THERAPEUTICALLY EQUIVALENT: *(cont'd)*

100's	$8.55	Hydroxyzine Pamoate, Voluntary Hosp	53258-0417-01
100's	$10.00	Hydroxyzine Pamoate, Eon Labs Mfg	00185-0613-01
100's	$11.95	Hydroxyzine Pamoate, Harber Pharm	51432-0495-03
100's	$14.38	Hydroxyzine Pamoate, HL Moore Drug Exch	00839-6270-06
100's	$15.10	Hydroxyzine Pamoate, United Res	00677-0596-01
100's	$15.15	Hydroxyzine Pamoate, Major Pharms	00904-0362-60
100's	$15.40	Hydroxyzine Pamoate, Qualitest Pharms	00603-3994-21
100's	$17.38	Hydroxyzine Pamoate, Barr	00555-0323-02
100's	$17.82	Hydroxyzine Pamoate, Martec Pharms	52555-0326-01
100's	$17.82	Hydroxyzine Pamoate, Martec Pharms	52555-0562-01
100's	$18.37	Hydroxyzine Pamoate, Amer Preferred	53445-1098-01
100's	$18.75	Hydroxyzine Pamoate, Zenith Labs	00172-2911-60
100's	$18.75	Hydroxyzine Pamoate, Goldline Labs	00182-1098-01
100's	$18.75	Hydroxyzine Pamoate, Geneva Pharms	00781-2252-01
100's	$18.75	Hydroxyzine Pamoate, Mova Pharms	55370-0517-07
100's	$20.46	Hydroxyzine Pamoate 25, Aligen Independ	00405-4518-01
100's	$20.60	Hydroxyzine Pamoate, Schein Pharm (US)	00364-0483-01
100's	$20.65	Hydroxyzine Pamoate, Rugby	00536-3893-01
100's	$20.95	Hydroxyzine Pamoate, Parmed Pharms	00349-8919-01
100's	$23.31	Hydroxyzine Pamoate, Voluntary Hosp	53258-0417-13
100's	$35.56	Hydroxyzine Pamoate, Major Pharms	00904-0362-61
100's	$44.97	Hydroxyzine Pamoate, Vangard Labs	00615-0331-13
100's	$45.00	Hydroxyzine Pamoate, Goldline Labs	00182-1098-89
100's	**$72.36**	**VISTARIL, Pfizer Labs**	**00069-5410-66**
100's	**$82.19**	**VISTARIL, Pfizer Labs**	**00069-5410-41**
500's	$26.25	Hypam 25, H & H Labs	46703-0055-05
500's	$41.65	Hydroxyzine Pamoate, H.C.F.A. F F P	99999-1514-02
500's	$44.65	Hydroxyzine Pamoate, Eon Labs Mfg	00185-0613-05
500's	$59.75	Hydroxyzine Pamoate, Harber Pharm	51432-0495-05
500's	$64.79	Hydroxyzine Pamoate, HL Moore Drug Exch	00839-6270-12
500's	$70.12	Hydroxyzine Pamoate, Qualitest Pharms	00603-3994-28
500's	$70.48	Hydroxyzine Pamoate, United Res	00677-0596-05
500's	$70.80	Hydroxyzine Pamoate, Major Pharms	00904-0362-40
500's	$82.38	Hydroxyzine Pamoate, Barr	00555-0323-04
500's	$82.52	Hydroxyzine Pamoate, Martec Pharms	52555-0326-05
500's	$82.52	Hydroxyzine Pamoate, Martec Pharms	52555-0562-05
500's	$86.80	Hydroxyzine Pamoate, Zenith Labs	00172-2911-70
500's	$86.80	Hydroxyzine Pamoate, Goldline Labs	00182-1098-05
500's	$86.80	Hydroxyzine Pamoate, Geneva Pharms	00781-2252-05
500's	$86.80	Hydroxyzine Pamoate, Mova Pharms	55370-0517-08
500's	$92.30	Hydroxyzine Pamoate, Schein Pharm (US)	00364-0483-05
500's	$92.40	Hydroxyzine Pamoate, Rugby	00536-3893-05
500's	$101.87	Hydroxyzine Pamoate 25, Aligen Independ	00405-4518-02
500's	**$345.12**	**VISTARIL, Pfizer Labs**	**00069-5410-73**
1000's	$67.50	Hydroxyzine Pamoate, Consolidated Midland	00223-1049-02
1000's	$83.30	Hydroxyzine Pamoate, H.C.F.A. F F P	99999-1514-03
1000's	$132.35	Hydroxyzine Pamoate, Goldline Labs	00182-1098-10
1000's	$132.40	Hydroxyzine Pamoate, Rugby	00536-3893-10

Capsule, Gelatin - Oral - 50 mg

100's	$6.42	Hydroxyzine Pamoate, US Trading	56126-0070-11
100's	$10.28	Hydroxyzine Pamoate, H.C.F.A. F F P	99999-1514-04
100's	$11.25	Hydroxyzine Pamoate, Consolidated Midland	00223-1050-01
100's	$11.97	Hydroxyzine Pamoate, Voluntary Hosp	53258-0418-01
100's	$12.55	Hydroxyzine Pamoate, Eon Labs Mfg	00185-0615-01
100's	$14.65	Hydroxyzine Pamoate, Harber Pharm	51432-0496-03
100's	$15.26	Hydroxyzine Pamoate, HL Moore Drug Exch	00839-6271-06
100's	$18.00	Hydroxyzine Pamoate, United Res	00677-0597-01
100's	$18.01	Hydroxyzine Pamoate, Qualitest Pharms	00603-3995-21
100's	$18.83	Hydroxyzine Pamoate, Martec Pharms	52555-0563-01
100's	$19.97	Hydroxyzine Pamoate, Amer Preferred	53445-1099-01
100's	$19.98	Hydroxyzine Pamoate, Geneva Pharms	00781-2254-01
100's	$20.00	Hydroxyzine Pamoate, Zenith Labs	00172-2909-60
100's	$20.00	Hydroxyzine Pamoate, Goldline Labs	00182-1099-01
100's	$20.00	Hydroxyzine Pamoate, Mova Pharms	55370-0519-07
100's	$21.95	Hydroxyzine Pamoate, Schein Pharm (US)	00364-0484-01
100's	$22.00	Hydroxyzine Pamoate, Parmed Pharms	00349-8920-01
100's	$22.20	Hydroxyzine Pamoate, Rugby	00536-3894-01
100's	$22.79	Hydroxyzine Pamoate 50, Aligen Independ	00405-4519-01
100's	$25.23	Hydroxyzine Pamoate, Voluntary Hosp	53258-0418-13
100's	$41.66	Hydroxyzine Pamoate, Major Pharms	00904-0363-61
100's	$63.60	Hydroxyzine Pamoate, Goldline Labs	00182-1099-89
100's	$63.85	Hydroxyzine Pamoate, Vangard Labs	00615-0332-13
100's	$76.50	Hydroxyzine Pamoate, Major Pharms	00904-0363-40
100's	**$88.19**	**VISTARIL, Pfizer Labs**	**00069-5420-66**
100's	**$99.80**	**VISTARIL, Pfizer Labs**	**00069-5420-41**
500's	$35.75	Hypam 50, H & H Labs	46703-0056-05
500's	$50.00	Hydroxyzine Pamoate, Eon Labs Mfg	00185-0615-05
500's	$51.40	Hydroxyzine Pamoate, H.C.F.A. F F P	99999-1514-05
500's	$68.30	Hydroxyzine Pamoate, HL Moore Drug Exch	00839-6271-12
500's	$73.25	Hydroxyzine Pamoate, Harber Pharm	51432-0496-05
500's	$78.37	Hydroxyzine Pamoate, United Res	00677-0597-05
500's	$78.38	Hydroxyzine Pamoate, Qualitest Pharms	00603-3995-28
500's	$95.00	Hydroxyzine Pamoate, Zenith Labs	00172-2909-70
500's	$95.00	Hydroxyzine Pamoate, Goldline Labs	00182-1099-05
500's	$95.00	Hydroxyzine Pamoate 50, Aligen Independ	00405-4519-02
500's	$95.00	Hydroxyzine Pamoate, Mova Pharms	55370-0519-08
500's	$97.00	Hydroxyzine Pamoate, Schein Pharm (US)	00364-0484-05
500's	$97.61	Hydroxyzine Pamoate, Martec Pharms	52555-0327-05
500's	$97.61	Hydroxyzine Pamoate, Martec Pharms	52555-0563-05
500's	$97.65	Hydroxyzine Pamoate, Rugby	00536-3894-05
500's	**$420.75**	**VISTARIL, Pfizer Labs**	**00069-5420-73**
1000's	$16.50	Hydroxyzine Pamoate, Major Pharms	00904-0363-60
1000's	$97.50	Hydroxyzine Pamoate, Consolidated Midland	00223-1050-02
1000's	$102.80	Hydroxyzine Pamoate, H.C.F.A. F F P	99999-1514-06
1000's	$138.90	Hydroxyzine Pamoate, Rugby	00536-3894-10

Capsule, Gelatin - Oral - 100 mg

100's	$18.25	Hydroxyzine Pamoate, Harber Pharm	51432-0497-03
100's	$18.95	Hydroxyzine Pamoate, Consolidated Midland	00223-1051-01
100's	$22.43	Hydroxyzine Pamoate, H.C.F.A. F F P	99999-1514-07
100's	$29.50	Hydroxyzine Pamoate, HL Moore Drug Exch	00839-6272-06
100's	$32.38	Hydroxyzine Pamoate, Goldline Labs	00182-1991-01
100's	$32.38	Hydroxyzine Pamoate, Barr	00555-0324-02
100's	$33.75	Hydroxyzine Pamoate, Rugby	00536-3896-01
100's	$34.10	Hydroxyzine Pamoate, Qualitest Pharms	00603-3996-21
100's	$41.71	Hydroxyzine Pamoate, Aligen Independ	00405-4520-01
100's	**$108.37**	**VISTARIL, Pfizer Labs**	**00069-5430-66**
500's	$112.15	Hydroxyzine Pamoate, H.C.F.A. F F P	99999-1514-08
500's	**$530.98**	**VISTARIL, Pfizer Labs**	**00069-5430-73**
1000's	$167.50	Hydroxyzine Pamoate, Consolidated Midland	00223-1051-02

HOW SUPPLIED - NOT RATED EQUIVALENT:

Suspension - Oral - 25 mg/5ml

120 ml x 4	**$110.40**	**VISTARIL, Pfizer Labs**	**00069-5440-97**
480 ml	**$110.40**	**VISTARIL, Pfizer Labs**	**00069-5440-93**

HYOSCAMINE; METHENAMINE; METHYLENE BLUE; PHENYL SALICYLATE; SODIUM BIPHOSPHATE *(003178)*

CATEGORIES: Anti-Infectives; Antibacterials; Antimicrobials; Antiseptics, Urinary Tract; Antispasmodics; Cystitis; Inflammation; Relaxants/Stimulants, Urinary Tract; Renal Drugs; Trigonitis; Urethritis; Urinary Anti-Infectives; Urinary Antibacterial; Urinary Tract Infections; Pregnancy Category C; FDA Pre 1938 Drugs

BRAND NAMES: Disurex D/S; **Uro Blue**

Prescribing information not available at time of publication.

HOW SUPPLIED - EQUIVALENTS NOT AVAILABLE:

Tablet, Uncoated - Oral - 0.12 mg/81.6 mg

100's	**$27.40**	**URO BLUE, RA McNeil**	**12830-0301-01**

HYOSCYAMINE SULFATE *(001516)*

CATEGORIES: Abdominal Cramps; Abdominal Distress; Anesthesia; Anticholinergic Agents; Anticholinesterase; Antimuscarinics/Antispasmodics; Antiparkinson Agents; Antispasmodics; Autonomic Drugs; Bradycardia; Colic; Colitis; Cystitis; Diagnostic Agents; Enterocolitis; Gastric Acid Secretion Inhibitors; Gastrointestinal Drugs; Gastrointestinal Hypermotility; Heart Block; Hyperhidrosis; Intubation; Irritable Bowel Syndrome; Pain; Pancreatitis; Parkinsonism; Peptic Ulcer; Poisoning; Relaxants/Stimulants, Urinary Tract; Renal Drugs; Rhinitis; Sialorrhea; Spasm; Tremor; Ulcer; Urinary Tract Infections; Pregnancy Category C; FDA Pre 1938 Drugs

BRAND NAMES: A-Spas S L; Anaspaz; Cystospaz-M; Donnamar; Ed-Spaz; Gastrosed; Hyco; Hyosol Sl; Hyospaz; Levbid; **Levsin**; *Levsin Drops*; *Levsin SL*; Levsinex; Liqui-Sooth; Medispaz; Pasmex; Setamine; Spasdel
(International brand names outside U.S. in italics)

FORMULARIES: Aetna; BC-BS; FHP; Harvard; Humana; Kaiser; PruCare; PCS

COST OF THERAPY: $1,532.63 (Parkinsonism; Tablet; 0.125 mg; 5/day; 365 days)

DESCRIPTION:

Hyoscyamine (hyoscyamine sulfate USP) is one of the principal anticholinergic/antispasmodic components of belladonna alkaloids. The empirical formula is $(C_{17}H_{23}NO_3)^2 \cdot H_2SO_4 \cdot 32H_2O$ and the molecular weight is 712.85. Chemically, it is benzeneacetic acid,alpha-(hydroxymethyl)-,8-methyl-8-azabicyclo[3.2.1.]oct-3-yl ester, (3(S)-endo)-,sulfate (2: 1),dihydrate.

Hyoscyamine sublingual tablets contain 0.125 mg hyoscyamine sulfate formulated for sublingual administration.

However, the tablets may also be chewed or taken orally.

Each tablet also contains as inactive ingredients: colloidal silicon dioxide, dextrates. FD&C Green #3, flavor, mannitol, and stearic acid.

Hyoscyamine tablets contain 0.125 mg hyoscyamine sulfate formulated for oral administration. Each tablet may also contain as inactive ingredients: Acacia, confectioner's sugar, corn starch, lactose, powdered cellulose and stearic acid.

Hyoscyamine elixir contains 0.125 mg hyoscyamine sulfate per 5 ml (teaspoonful) with 20% alcohol for oral use. Hyoscyamine elixir may also contain as inactive ingredients: FD&C Red #40, FD&C Yellow #6, flavor, glycerin, purified water, sorbitol solution and sucrose.

Hyoscyamine drops, oral solution, contain 0.125 mg hyoscyamine sulfate per ml with 5% alcohol.

Hyoscyamine Drops May Also Contain as Inactive Ingredients: FD&C Red #40, FD&C Yellow #6, flavor, glycerin, purified water, sodium citrate, sorbitol solution, and sucrose.

Hyoscyamine injection is a sterile solution containing 0.5 mg hyoscyamine sulfate per ml. The 1 ml ampuls contain as inactive ingredients: water for injection, pH is adjusted with hydrochloric acid when necessary.

Hyoscyamine extended-release contain 0.375 mg hyoscyamine sulfate in a timed-release formulation designed for oral b.i.d. dosage. Each capsule may also contain as inactive ingredients: corn starch, D&C Red #28, FD&C Blue #1, FD&C Blue #2, FD&C Red #40, FD&C Yellow #6, gelatin, sucrose, titanium dioxide and other ingredients.

CLINICAL PHARMACOLOGY:

Hyoscyamine inhibits specifically the actions of acetylcholine on structures innervated by postganglionic cholinergic nerves and on smooth muscles that respond to acetylcholine but lack cholinergic innervation. These peripheral cholinergic receptors are present in the autonomic effector cells of the smooth muscle, cardiac muscle, the sinoatrial node, the atrioventricular node, and the exocrine glands.

It is completely devoid of any action in the autonomic ganglia. Hyoscyamine inhibits gastrointestinal propulsive motility and decreases gastric acid secretion. Hyoscyamine also controls excessive pharyngeal, tracheal and bronchial secretions.

Hyoscyamine is absorbed totally and completely by sublingual administration as well as oral administration. Once absorbed, hyoscyamine disappears rapidly from the blood and is distributed throughout the entire body. The half-life of hyoscyamine is 3 $\frac{1}{2}$ hours. Hyoscyamine is partly hydrolyzed to tropic acid and tropine but the majority of the drug is excreted in the urine unchanged within the first 12 hours. Only traces of this drug are found in breast milk. Hyoscyamine passes the blood brain barrier and the placental barrier.

Hyoscyamine sublingual tablets can be taken orally with the same pharmacological effects occurring; however, the effects may not occur as rapidly as with sublingual administration.

Hyoscyamine extended-release tablet release 0.375 mg hyoscyamine sulfate at a controlled and predictable rate for 12 hours. Peak blood levels occur in 2 $\frac{1}{2}$ hours and the apparent plasma half-life is approximately 7 hours. The urinary excretion from both the immediate-release dosage form and the timed-release dosage form is equal and uniform over a 24 hour period.

INDICATIONS AND USAGE:

Hyoscyamine is effective as adjunctive therapy in the treatment of peptic ulcer. It can also be used to control gastric secretion, visceral spasm, and hypermotility in spastic colitis, spastic bladder, cystitis, pylorospasm, and associated abdominal cramps. May be used in functional intestinal disorders to reduce symptoms such as those seen in mild dysenteries, diverticulitis, and acute enterocolitis. For use as adjunctive therapy in the treatment of irritable bowel syndrome (irritable colon, spastic colon, mucouscolitis) and functional gastrointestinal disorders. Also as adjunctive therapy in the treatment of neurogenic bladder and neurogenic bowel disturbances including the splenic flexure syndrome and neurogenic colon. Also used in the treatment of infant colic (elixir and drops). Hyoscyamine is indicated along with morphine or other narcotics in symptomatic relief of biliary and renal colic; as a "drying agent" in the relief of symptoms of acute rhinitis; in the therapy of parkinsonism to reduce rigidity and tremors and to control associated sialorrhea and hyperhidrosis. May be used in the therapy of poisoning by anticholinesterase agents.

Parenterally administered hyoscyamine is also effective in reducing gastrointestinal motility to facilitate diagnostic procedures such as endoscopy or hypotonic duodenography. Hyoscyamine may be used to reduce pain and hypersecretion in pancreatitis.

Hyoscyamine may also be used in certain cases of partial heart block associated with vagal activity.

In Anesthesia: Hyoscyamine injection is indicated as a pre-operative antimuscarinic to reduce salivary, tracheobronchial, and pharyngeal secretions; to reduce the volume and acidity of gastric secretions, and to block cardiac vagal inhibitory reflexes during induction of anesthesia and intubation. Hyoscyamine protects against the peripheral muscarinic effects such as bradycardia and excessive secretions produced by halogenated hydrocarbons and cholinergic agents such as physostigmine, neostigmine, and pyridostigmine given to reverse the actions of curariform agents.

In Urology: Hyoscyamine injection may also be used intravenously to improve radiologic visibility of the kidneys.

CONTRAINDICATIONS:

Glaucoma; obstructive uropathy (for example, bladder neck obstruction due to prostatic hypertrophy); obstructive disease of the gastrointestinal tract (as in achalasia, pyloroduodenal stenosis); paralytic ileus, intestinal atony of elderly or debilitated patients; unstable cardiovascular status in acute hemorrhage; severe ulcerative colitis; toxic megacolon complicating ulcerative colitis; myasthenia gravis.

WARNINGS:

In the presence of high environmental temperature, heat prostration can occur with drug use (fever and heat stroke due to decreased sweating). Diarrhea may be an early symptom of incomplete intestinal obstruction, especially in patients with ileostomy or colostomy. In this instance, treatment with this drug would be inappropriate and possibly harmful. Like other anticholinergic agents, hyoscyamine may produce drowsiness or blurred vision. In this event, the patient should be warned not to engage in activities requiring mental alertness such as operating a motor vehicle or other machinery or to perform hazardous work while taking this drug.

Psychosis has been reported in sensitive individuals given anticholinergic drugs. CNS signs and symptoms include confusion, disorientation, short term memory loss, hallucinations, dysarthria, ataxia, coma, euphoria, decreased anxiety, fatigue, insomnia, agitation and mannerisms, and inappropriate affect. These CNS signs and symptoms usually resolve within 12-48 hours after discontinuation of the drug.

PRECAUTIONS:

General: Use with caution in patients with: autonomic neuropathy, hyperthyroidism, coronary heart disease, congestive heart failure, cardiac arrhythmias, hypertension and renal disease.

Investigate any tachycardia before giving any anticholinergic drug since they may increase the heart rate. Use with caution in patients with hiatal hernia associated with reflux esophagitis.

Information for the Patient: Hyoscyamine may cause drowsiness, dizziness or blurred vision; patients should observe caution before driving, using machinery or performing other tasks requiring mental alertness.

Use of hyoscyamine may decrease sweating resulting in heat prostration, fever or heat stroke; febrile patients or those who may be exposed to elevated environmental temperatures should use caution.

Carcinogenesis, Mutagenesis, and Impairment of Fertility: No long term studies in animals have been performed to determine the carcinogenic, mutagenic or impairment of fertility potential of hyoscyamine; however, over 30 years of marketing experience shows no demonstrable evidence of a problem.

Pregnancy Category C: Animal reproduction studies have not been conducted with hyoscyamine. It is also not known whether hyoscyamine can cause fetal harm when administered to a pregnant woman or can affect reproduction capacity. Hyoscyamine should be given to a pregnant woman only if clearly needed.

Nursing Mothers: Hyoscyamine is excreted in human milk. Caution should be exercised when hyoscyamine is administered to a nursing woman.

DRUG INTERACTIONS:

Additive adverse effects resulting from cholinergic blockade may occur when hyoscyamine is administered concomitantly with other antimuscarinics, amantadine, haloperidol, phenothiazines, monoamine oxidase (MAO) inhibitors, tricyclic antidepressants or some antihistamines.

Antacids may interfere with the absorption of hyoscyamine; take hyoscyamine before meals and antacids after meals.

ADVERSE REACTIONS:

Not all of the following adverse reactions have been reported with hyoscyamine sulfate. The following adverse reactions have been reported for pharmacologically similar drugs with anti-cholinergic-antispasmodic action. Adverse reactions may include dryness of the mouth; urinary hesitancy and retention; blurred vision; tachycardia; palpitations; mydriasis; cycloplegia, increased ocular tension; loss of taste; headache; nervousness; drowsiness; weakness;dizziness; insomnia; nausea; vomiting; impotence; suppression of lactation; constipation; bloated feeling; allergic reactions or drug idiosyncrasies; urticaria and other dermal manifestations; ataxia; speech disturbance; some degree of mental confusion and/or excitement (especially in elderly persons); and decreased sweating.

OVERDOSAGE:

The signs and symptoms of overdose are headache, nausea, vomiting, blurred vision, dilated pupils, hot dry skin, dizziness, dryness of the mouth, difficulty in swallowing and CNS stimulation.

Measures to be taken are immediate lavage of the stomach and injection of physostigmine 0.5 to 2 mg intravenously and repeated as necessary up to a total of 5 mg. Fever may be treated symptomatically (tepid water sponge baths, hypothermic blanket). Excitement to a

OVERDOSAGE: *(cont'd)*

degree which demands attention may be managed with sodium thiopental 2% solution given slowly intravenously or chloral hydrate (100-200 ml of a 2% solution) by rectal infusion. In the event of progression of the curare-like effect to paralysis of the respiratory muscles, artificial respiration should be instituted and maintained until effective respiratory action returns.

In rats, the LD_{50} for hyoscyamine is 375 mg/kg. Hyoscyamine is dialyzable.

DOSAGE AND ADMINISTRATION:

Dosage may be adjusted according to the conditions and severity of symptoms.

HYOSCYAMINE SUBLINGUAL TABLETS

The tablets may be taken sublingually orally or chewed.

Adults and Pediatric Patients 12 Years of Age and Older: 1 to 2 tablets every four hours or as needed. Do not exceed 12 tablets in 24 hours.

Pediatric Patients 2 to Under 12 Years of Age: $\frac{1}{2}$ to 1 tablet every four hours or as needed. Do not exceed 6 tablets in 24 hours.

HYOSCYAMINE TABLETS

Adults and Pediatric Patients 12 Years of Age and Older: 1 to 2 capsules every 12 hours. Dosage may be adjusted to 1 capsule ever 8 hours if needed. Do not exceed 4 capsules in 24 hours.

HYOSCYAMINE ELIXIR

Adults and Pediatric Patients 12 Years of Age and Older: 1 to 2 teaspoonfuls every four hours or as needed. Do not exceed 12 teaspoonfuls in 24 hours.

Pediatric Patients 2 to Under 12 Years of Age: Please see the following dosage guide based on body weight. The doses may be repeated every four hours or as needed. Do not exceed 6 teaspoonfuls in 24 hours.

TABLE 1

Body Weight	Usual Dose
10 kg (22 lb)	$\frac{1}{4}$ tsp
20 kg (44 lb)	$\frac{1}{2}$ tsp
40 kg (88 lb)	$\frac{3}{4}$ tsp
50 kg (110 lb)	1 tsp

HYOSCYAMINE DROPS

Adults and Pediatric Patients 12 Years of Age and Older: 1 to 2 ml every four hours or as needed. Do not exceed 12 ml in 24 hours.

Pediatric Patients 2 to Under 12 Years of Age: $\frac{1}{4}$ to 1 ml every four hours or as needed. Do not exceed 6 ml in 24 hours.

Pediatric Patients Under 2 Years of Age: The following dosage guide is based upon body weight. The doses may be repeated every four hours or as needed.

TABLE 2

Body Weight	Usual Dose	Do Not Exceed in 24 Hours
3.4 kg (7.5 lb)	4 drops	24 drops
5 kg (11 lb)	5 drops	30 drops
7 kg (15 lb)	6 drops	36 drops
10 kg (22 lb)	8 drops	48 drops

HYOSCYAMINE INJECTION

The dose may be administered subcutaneously, intramuscularly, or intravenously without dilution.

Gastrointestinal Disorders: The usual adult recommended dose is 0.5 to 1.0 ml (0.25 to 0.5 mg). Some patients may need only a single dose; others may require administration two, three, or four times a day at four hour intervals.

Diagnostic Procedures: The usual adult recommended dose is 0.5 to 1.0 ml (0.25 to 0.5 mg) administered intravenously 5 to 10 minutes prior to the diagnostic procedure.

Anesthesia

Adults and Pediatric Patients Over 2 Years of Age: As a pre-anesthetic medication, the recommended dose is 5 mcg (0.005 mg) per kg of body weight. This dose is usually given 30 to 60 minutes prior to the anticipated time of induction of anesthesia or at the time the pre-anesthetic narcotic or sedative is administered.

Hyoscyamine injection may be used during surgery to reduce drug-induced bradycardia. It should be administered intravenously in increments of 0.25 ml and repeated as needed. To achieve reversal of neuromuscular blockade, the recommended dose is 0.2 mg (0.4 ml) hyoscyamine injection for every 1 mg neostigmine or the equivalent dose of physostigmine or pyridostigmine.

Parenteral drug products should be inspected visually for particulate matter and discoloration prior to administration, whenever solution and container permit.

HYOSCYAMINE EXTENDED-RELEASE TABLET

Adults and Pediatric Patients 12 Years of Age and Older: 1 to 2 capsules every 12 hours.

Dosage may be adjusted to 1 capsules every 8 hours if needed. Do not exceed 4 capsules in 24 hours.

HOW SUPPLIED - RATED THERAPEUTICALLY EQUIVALENT:

Capsule, Gelatin, Sustained Action - Oral - 0.375 mg

100's	$48.04	Hyoscyamine Sulfate, Ethex	58177-0017-04

Tablet, Sustained Action - Oral - 0.375 mg

500's	$237.94	LEVBID, Schwarz Pharma (US)	00091-3538-05

HOW SUPPLIED - NOT RATED EQUIVALENT:

Capsule, Gelatin, Sustained Action - Oral - 0.375 mg

100's	$44.06	Hyoscyamine Sulfate, Qualitest Pharms	00603-4004-21
100's	$45.95	Hyoscyamine Sulfate, Major Pharms	00904-7833-60
100's	$47.30	Hyoscyamine Sulfate, United Res	00677-1507-01
100's	$50.20	Hyoscyamine Sulfate, Goldline Labs	00182-1993-01
100's	$51.00	Hyoscyamine Sulfate, Rugby	00536-5592-01
100's	$51.00	Huoscamine Sulfate, HL Moore Drug Exch	00839-7910-06
100's	$51.00	Hyoscyamine Sulfate, Pecos	59879-0109-01
100's	$51.87	LEVBID, Schwarz Pharma (US)	00091-3538-01
100's	**$58.34**	**LEVSINEX TIMECAPS, Schwarz Pharma (US)**	**00091-3537-01**
500's	**$248.12**	**LEVSINEX TIMECAPS, Schwarz Pharma (US)**	**00091-3537-05**

Elixir - Oral - 0.125 mg/5ml

480 ml	$11.45	Hyoscyamine Sulfate, Goldline Labs	00182-6136-40
480 ml	$25.00	Hyco, Hi Tech Pharma	50383-0290-16
480 ml	$25.96	Hyoscyamine Sulfate, Cypress Pharm	60258-0801-16

HOW SUPPLIED - NOT RATED EQUIVALENT: *(cont'd)*

480 ml	$27.00	Liqui-Sooth, Liquipharm	54198-0147-16
480 ml	**$40.26**	**LEVSIN, Schwarz Pharma (US)**	**00091-4532-16**

Injection, Solution - Intramuscular; - 0.5 mg/ml

1 ml x 5	**$35.16**	**LEVSIN, Schwarz Pharma (US)**	**00091-1536-05**

Solution - Oral - 0.125 mg/ml

15 ml	$8.40	Hyoscyamine Sulfate, Rugby	00536-2680-72
15 ml	$9.00	Hyoscyamine Sulfate, Harber Pharm	51432-0751-10
15 ml	$10.00	Hyco, Hi Tech Pharma	50383-0291-15
15 ml	$10.18	Hyoscyamine Sulfate, Cypress Pharm	60258-0802-15
15 ml	$10.25	Hyoscyamine Sulfate, Econolab	55053-0380-15
15 ml	$10.70	LIQUI-SOOTH, Liquipharm	54198-0146-15
15 ml	$10.79	Hyoscyamine Sulfate, Aligen Independ	00405-2910-61
15 ml	**$15.55**	**LEVSIN DROPS, Schwarz Pharma (US)**	**00091-4538-15**
30 ml	$8.00	Spacol I.D., Dayton Labs	52041-0046-26

Tablet, Uncoated - Oral; Sublingua - 0.125 mg

100's	$11.25	Hyoscyamine Sulfate, Alphagen Labs	59743-0026-01
100's	$11.30	DONNAMAR, Marnel Pharceut	00682-0106-01
100's	$11.61	Hyoscyamine Sulfate, Qualitest Pharms	00603-4003-21
100's	$11.94	A-Spas S/L, Hyrex Pharms	00314-0011-01
100's	$11.95	Hyoscyamine Sulfate, Major Pharms	00904-2496-60
100's	$12.37	Hyoscyamine Sulfate, Equipharm	57779-0101-04
100's	$12.84	Hyoscyamine Sulfate, Qualitest Pharms	00603-4002-21
100's	$13.00	Hyoscyamine Sulfate, Contract Pharma	10267-1621-01
100's	$13.25	Hyoscyamine Sulfate, Jerome Stevens	50564-0539-01
100's	$13.50	Hyoscyamine Sulfate, Aligen Independ	00405-4521-01
100's	$13.50	Hyoscyamine Sulfate, Econolab	55053-0130-01
100's	$13.75	Hyoscyamine Sulfate, Goldline Labs	00182-1607-01
100's	$13.75	Hyoscyamine Sulfate, United Res	00677-1419-01
100's	$15.68	Hyoscyamine Sulfate, Rugby	00536-3918-01
100's	$18.00	ED-SPAZ, Edwards Pharms	00485-0056-01
100's	$18.95	Hyosol/Sl, Econolab	55053-0717-01
100's	$19.95	Hyoscyamine Sulfate, Aligen Independ	00405-4523-01
100's	$19.95	Hyoscyamine Sulfate, Pecos	59879-0301-01
100's	$20.22	ANASPAZ, Ascher	00225-0295-15
100's	$20.25	Hyoscyamine Sulfate, Equipharm	57779-0140-04
100's	$20.78	Hyoscyamine Sulfate, HL Moore Drug Exch	00839-7521-06
100's	$20.89	MEDISPAZ, Med Tek Pharms	52349-0240-10
100's	$21.65	Hyoscamine Sulfate, Rugby	00536-5575-01
100's	$22.15	Hyoscyamine Sulfate, Trinity Technologies	61355-0002-10
100's	$22.90	Hyoscyamine Sulfate, United Res	00677-1536-01
100's	$22.94	Hyoscyamine Sulfate, HL Moore Drug Exch	00839-7806-06
100's	**$29.27**	**LEVSIN/SL, Schwarz Pharma (US)**	**00091-3532-01**
100's	**$30.37**	**LEVSIN, Schwarz Pharma (US)**	**00091-3531-01**
100's	$33.25	Hyoscyamine Sulfate, Trinity Technologies	61355-0003-10
500's	$98.58	ANASPAZ, Ascher	00225-0295-20
500's	**$130.23**	**LEVSIN/SL, Schwarz Pharma (US)**	**00091-3532-05**
500's	**$135.05**	**LEVSIN, Schwarz Pharma (US)**	**00091-3531-05**

HYOSCYAMINE SULFATE; PHENOBARBITAL

(001517)

CATEGORIES: Abdominal Cramps; Abdominal Distress; Anesthesia; Anticholinergic Agents; Antimuscarinics/Antispasmodics; Antiparkinson Agents; Autonomic Drugs; Central Nervous System Agents; Colic; DESI Drugs; Enterocolitis; Gastrointestinal Drugs; Gastrointestinal Hypermotility; Hyperhidrosis; Irritable Bowel Syndrome; Parkinsonism; Peptic Ulcer; Relaxants/Stimulants, Urinary Tract; Renal Drugs; Rhinitis; Sedatives/Hypnotics; Sialorrhea; Ulcer; Pregnancy Category C; FDA Pre 1938 Drugs

BRAND NAMES: *Belladenal*; Elixiral; Levsin-PB; Levsin W/Phenobarbital; Sedatans
(International brand names outside U.S. in italics)

FORMULARIES: Aetna; BC-BS; FHP; Harvard; Humana; Kaiser; PruCare

DESCRIPTION:

Tablets: Hyoscyamine sulfate with phenobarbital tablets contain 0.125 mg Hyoscyamine sulfate USP and 15 mg phenobarbital USP (*WARNING:* may be habit forming) for oral administration.

Oral Solution: Hyoscyamine sulfate with phenobarbital drops contain 0.125 mg Hyoscyamine sulfate USP, 15 mg phenobarbital USP (*WARNING:* may be habit forming), and 5% alcohol USP per ml. It is formulated for oral use only.

CLINICAL PHARMACOLOGY:

Hyoscyamine sulfate, one of the principal anticholinergic/antispasmodic components of belladonna alkaloids. Hyoscyamine sulfate inhibits gastrointestinal propulsive motility and decreases gastric acid secretion. Hyoscyamine sulfate also inhibits the action of acetylcholine at the postganglionic nerve endings of the parasympathetic nervous system. A fixed ratio combination with phenobarbital provides mild sedation to protect patients against the physical and emotional stresses often present in conditions causing vagotonia or parasympathotonia.

INDICATIONS AND USAGE:

BASED ON A REVIEW OF THESE DRUGS BY THE NATIONAL ACADEMY OF SCIENCES-NATIONAL RESEARCH COUNCIL AND/OR OTHER INFORMATION, FDA HAS CLASSIFIED THE INDICATION AS FOLLOWS: 'POSSIBLY' EFFECTIVE:
FOR USE AS ADJUNCTIVE THERAPY IN THE TREATMENT OF PEPTIC ULCER.
IT SHOULD BE NOTED AT THIS POINT IN TIME THAT THERE IS A LACK OF CONCURRENCE AS TO THE VALUE OF ANTICHOLINERGICS/ANTISPASMODICS IN THE TREATMENT OF GASTRIC ULCER. IT HAS NOT BEEN SHOWN CONCLUSIVELY WHETHER ANTICHOLINERGIC/ANTISPASMODIC DRUGS AID IN THE HEALING OF A PEPTIC ULCER, DECREASE THE RATE OF RECURRENCES, OR PREVENT COMPLICATION.
MAY ALSO BE USEFUL IN THE IRRITABLE BOWEL SYNDROME

INDICATIONS AND USAGE: *(cont'd)*

(IRRITABLE COLON, SPASTIC COLON, MUCOUS COLITIS), AND ACUTE ENTEROCOLITIS. FINAL CLASSIFICATION OF THE LESS-THAN-EFFECTIVE INDICATIONS REQUIRES FURTHER INVESTIGATION.

CONTRAINDICATIONS:

Glaucoma, obstructive uropathy (for example, bladder neck obstruction due to prostatic hypertrophy); obstructive disease of the gastrointestinal tract (as in achalasia, pyloroduodenal stenosis, etc.); paralytic ileus, intestinal atony of the elderly or debilitated patient; unstable cardiovascular status in acute hemorrhage; severe ulcerative colitis especially if complicated by toxic megacolon; myasthenia gravis; hiatal hernia associated with reflux esophagitis.

Phenobarbital is contraindicated in acute intermittent porphyria. A sensitivity to phenobarbital contraindicates the use of hyoscyamine sulfate with phenobarbital and in patients in whom phenobarbital produces restlessness and/or excitement.

WARNINGS:

Belladonna alkaloids with phenobarbital should be used in pregnancy, lactation, or in women of childbearing age only when, in the judgment of the physician, the expected benefits outweigh the potential hazards to the mother and child.

In the presence of high environmental temperature, heat prostration can occur with the drug use (fever and heatstroke due to decreased sweating).

Diarrhea may be an early symptom of incomplete intestinal obstruction, especially in patients with ileostomy or colostomy. In this instance, treatment with this drug would be inappropriate and possibly harmful.

Hyoscyamine sulfate with phenobarbital may produce drowsiness or blurred vision. In this event, the patient should be warned not to engage in activities requiring mental alertness such as operating a motor vehicle or other machinery, or perform hazardous work while taking this drug.

Phenobarbital in patients taking anticoagulants may decrease the effect of the anticoagulant and thus require larger doses of the anticoagulant for optimal effect. When the phenobarbital is discontinued, the dose of the anticoagulant may have to be decreased. Barbiturates may thus decease the action of anticoagulant drugs.

Phenobarbital may be habit forming and should not be administered to individuals known to be addiction prone or to those with a history of physical and/or psychological dependence upon habit forming drugs. Since barbiturates are metabolized in the liver, use with initial small doses and caution in patients with hepatic dysfunction.

PRECAUTIONS:

General: Use with caution in patients with: autonomic neuropathy, hepatic or renal disease, hyperthyroidism, coronary heart disease, congestive heart failure, cardiac arrhythmias, and hypertension.

It should be noted that the use of anticholinergic/antispasmodic drugs in the treatment of gastric ulcer may produce a delay in gastric emptying time and may complicate such therapy (antral stasis).

Do not rely on the use of the drug in the presence of complications of biliary tract disease.

Investigate any tachycardia before giving anticholinergic (atropine-like) drugs since they may increase the heart rate.

With overdosage, a curare-like action may occur.

ADVERSE REACTIONS:

Adverse reactions may include dryness of the mouth; urinary hesitancy and retention; blurred vision; tachycardia; palpitation; mydriasis; cycloplegia; increased ocular tension; loss of taste; headache; nervousness; drowsiness; weakness; dizziness; insomnia; nausea; vomiting; impotence; suppression of lactation; constipation; bloated feeling; severe allergic reaction or drug idiosyncrasies including anaphylaxis; urticaria and other dermal manifestations; and decreased sweating. Elderly patients may react with symptoms of excitement, agitation, drowsiness, and other untoward manifestations to even small doses of the drug.

Phenobarbital may produce excitement in some patients rather than a sedative effect. An occasional patient may experience musculoskeletal pain. Some patients may acquire a sensitivity to barbiturates and experience allergic phenomena and/or dermatologic response.

In patients habituated to barbiturates, abrupt withdrawal may produce delirium or convulsions.

OVERDOSAGE:

The signs and symptoms of overdose are headache, nausea, vomiting, blurred vision, dilated pupils, hot dry skin, dizziness, dryness of the mouth, difficulty in swallowing, and CNS stimulation. Treatment should consist of gastric lavage, emetics, and activated charcoal. If indicated, parenteral cholinergic agents such as bethanechol chloride USP should be used.

DOSAGE AND ADMINISTRATION:

TABLETS

The dosage may be adjusted to the needs of the individual patient to assure symptomatic control with a minimum of adverse effects.

Adults: 1 or 2 tablets three or four times a day according to conditions and severity of symptoms.

ORAL SOLUTION

The dosage may be adjusted to the needs of the individual patient to assure symptomatic control with a minimum of adverse effects.

Adults: 1-2 ml every four hours or as needed.

Children 1-10 years: $\frac{1}{2}$ to 1 ml every four hours or as needed.

Infants: The following dosage guide is based on body weight. The doses may be repeated every four hours or as needed (TABLE 1):

TABLE 1

Body Weight	Starting Dose
5 lb	3 drops
7.5 lb	4 drops
10 lb	6 drops
15 lb	7 drops
20 lb	9 drops

Store at controlled room temperature 15-30°C (59-86°F).

HOW SUPPLIED - EQUIVALENTS NOT AVAILABLE:

Solution - Oral - 0.125 mg/15 mg

15 ml	$22.44	LEVSIN-PB, Schwarz Pharma (US)	00091-4536-15

Tablet, Plain Coated - Oral - 0.125 mg/15 mg

100's	$49.12	LEVSIN WITH PHENOBARBITAL, Schwarz Pharma (US)	00091-3534-01

HYOSCYAMINE; METHENAMINE MANDELATE *(003172)*

CATEGORIES: Anti-Infectives; Antibacterials; Antiseptics, Urinary Tract; Relaxants/Stimulants, Urinary Tract; Spasm; Sulfonamides; Urinary Anti-Infectives; Urinary Antibacterial; Urinary Tract Infections; Pregnancy Category C; FDA Pre 1938 Drugs

BRAND NAMES: **Urisedamine**

DESCRIPTION:

Methenamine Mandelate 500 mg, Hyoscyamine 0.15 mg

Urisedamine is a light blue, capsule shaped, plain coated tablet for oral administration. It contains the urinary tract antiseptic Methenamine as its mandelate salt and the parasympatholytic agent, *l*-hyoscyamine.

Each Tablet Contains: *Actives:* Methenamine Mandelate 500 mg and *l*-Hyoscyamine 0.15 mg. *Inactives:* Acacia, beeswax, calcium carbonate, carnauba wax, gelatin, magnesium stearate, opalux blue, povidone, shellac, starch, sucrose and talc.

CLINICAL PHARMACOLOGY:

Methenamine mandelate is readily absorbed from the gastrointestinal tract and excreted unchanged, almost quantitatively in the urine. There is little decomposition in the bloodstream and tissues. Methenamine mandelate w/hyoscyamine is therefore virtually nontoxic systemically. Methenamine itself has no antiseptic properties in the urine. It exerts its urinary antiseptic effect on hydrolysis to formaldehyde at urine pH values of 6 or below.[1]

When given as directed and the daily urine volume is 1000 to 1500 ml, a daily dose of 2 grams will yield a urinary concentration of 18 to 60 mcg/ml of free formaldehyde in the urine. This is more than the minimal inhibitory concentration for most urinary tract pathogens. Mandelic Acid is poorly metabolized and excreted relatively unchanged in the urine. Apart from urinary acidification, however, it is bacteriostatic *in vitro*, beyond its effect on pH. Whether this bacteriostatic effect is operative *in vivo*, however, has not been well established. Through parasympatholytic action, *l*-hyoscyamine relaxes smooth muscle spasms resulting from parasympathetic stimulation.[2]

INDICATIONS AND USAGE:

Methenamine mandelate w/hyoscyamine is effectively employed in subacute, as well as milder chronic urinary infections, especially as associated with the bladder and lower urinary tract disorders when painful smooth muscle spasm accompanies infection. It is employed in the management of severe urinary infection to provide symptomatic relief of discomfort and antibacterial action pending laboratory identification of the causative organism.

It is used in the management of mild urinary tract infection caused by such common organisms as *E. Coli*, staphylocci and streptococci. *Enterobacter aerogenes* and *Proteus vulgaris* are usually resistant. It may be used pre- and post-operatively or with instrumentation. It may also be used in conjunction with specific chemotherapeutic agents or antibiotics when indicated but not with sulfonamides.

CONTRAINDICATIONS:

Contraindicated in patients suffering from renal insufficiency or inflammatory disease of the kidneys in which release of formaldehyde might cause irritation.

Also contraindicated in the presence of glaucoma, urinary bladder neck or pyloric obstruction, duodenal obstruction, cardiospasm or hypersensitivity to any of the ingredients.

WARNINGS:

Do not exceed recommended dose. Methenamine may combine with certain sulfonamides in the urine causing mutual antagonism and thus should not be used with sulfonamides.

PRECAUTIONS:

GENERAL

Administer with caution to persons with known idiosyncrasy to atropine-like compounds and to patients suffering from cardiac disease. Bacteriological studies of the urine may be helpful in the following the patient response. No long-term animal studies have been performed to evaluate carcinogenic potential. Drugs and foods which produce an alkaline urine should be restricted.

DRUG/LABORATORY TEST INTERACTIONS

Formaldehyde interferes with fluorometric procedures for determination of urinary catecholamines and vanilmandelic (VMA) causing erroneously high results. Formaldehyde also falsely decreased urine estriol levels by reacting with estriol when acid hydrolysis techniques are used; estriol determinations which use enzymatic hydrolysis are unaffected by formaldehyde. Formaldehyde causes falsely elevated 17-hydroxy-corticoid levels when the Porter-Silber method is used and falsely decreased 5-hydroxy-indoleacetic acid (5HIAA) levels by inhibiting color development when nitrosonaphthol methods are used.

PREGNANCY CATEGORY C

Animal reproduction studies have not been conducted with methenamine mandelate w/hyoscyamine tablets. It also not known whether methenamine mandelate w/hyoscyamine tablets can cause fetal harm when administered to a pregnant woman or can affect reproduction capacity. Methenamine mandelate w/hyoscyamine tablets should be given to a pregnant woman only if clearly needed.

NURSING MOTHERS

It is not known whether this drug is excreted in human milk. Because many drugs are excreted in human milk, caution should be exercised when this drug is administered to a nursing woman.

DRUG INTERACTIONS:

Formaldehyde and sulfamethizole form an insoluble precipitate in acid urine; therefore, mandelamine should not be administered concurrently with sulfamethizole.

ADVERSE REACTIONS:

Prolonged use may result in generalized skin rash, pronounced dryness of the mouth, flushing, difficulty in initiating micturition, rapid pulse, dizziness or blurring of vision. If any of these reactions occur, discontinue use immediately. Acute urinary retention may be precipitated in prostatic hypertrophy. Crystalluria from the mandelate moiety can also occur. Microscopic and gross hematuria have been described. (See OVERDOSAGE.)

OVERDOSAGE:

By exceeding the recommended dosage of methenamine mandelate w/hyoscyamine symptomology related to the overdosage of its active ingredients may be expected as follows:

Methenamine Mandelate: If large amounts of the drug (exceeding 8 g/day) are used over extended periods, bladder and gastrointestinal irritation, painful and frequent micturition, albuminuria and gross hematuria may be expected.

Hyoscyamine: Symptomology associated with an overdosage of methenamine mandelate w/hyoscyamine will most probably be manifested in the symptoms related to overdosage of the alkaloid Hyoscyamine. Such symptoms as dryness of mucous membranes; dilation of pupils; hot, dry, flushed skin; hyperpyrexia; tachycardia; palpitations; elevated blood pressure; coma; circulatory collapse and death from respiratory failure may occur.

DOSAGE AND ADMINISTRATION:

Adults: Two tablets orally four times daily, or less as required, with liberal fluid intake.

Children (12 years and under): Reduce dosage in proportion to age and weight, as recommended by physician.

Note: If testing of the urine indicates the need, additional acidification by means of diet restriction or acidifying agents may be employed.

Storage: Store at room temperature.

REFERENCES:

1. Gollamudi, R., Straughn, A.B., and Meyer, M.C., *Urinary Excretion of Methenamine and Formaldehyde: Evaluation of 10 Methenamine Products in Humans*, J. Pharm. Sci, 70, 596, 1981. **2.** Goodman, L.S. and Gilman G., *The Pharmacological Basis of Therapeutic*, Sixth Edition, MacMilan Publishing Co.

HOW SUPPLIED - EQUIVALENTS NOT AVAILABLE:

Tablet, Coated - Oral - 0.15 mg/500 mg

100's	$57.50	URISEDAMINE, Alcon-PR	00998-2210-10

IBUPROFEN *(001520)*

CATEGORIES: Analgesics; Anti-Inflammatory Agents; Antiarthritics; Antipyretics; Arthritis; Central Nervous System Agents; Common Cold; Dysmenorrhea; Fever; Hay Fever; Headache; Influenza; NSAIDS; Nasal Congestion; Nonsteroidal Anti-Inflammatory; Osteoarthritis; Pain; Pharyngitis; Tonsillitis; Cystic Fibrosis*; Migraine*; Sales > $100 Million; FDA Approval Pre 1982; Top 200 Drugs

* Indication not approved by the FDA

BRAND NAMES: *Act-3* (Australia); *Adex 200*; Advil; *Alaxan*; *Alfam*; *Algofen*; *Amersol* (Canada); *Am-Fam 400*; *Anafen*; *Anco* (Germany); *Andran* (Japan); *Anflagen* (Japan); *Anna Friend*; *Antiflam*; *Apo-Ibuprofen* (Canada); *Apsifen* (England); *Arthrifen*; *Artofen*; *Artril*; *Atril 300*; *Balkaprofen*; *Betaprofen*; *Bloom*; *Bluton* (Japan); *Brofen*; *Brufanic* (Japan); *Brufen* (Australia, Europe, Asia); *Brufen Retard*; *Brufen 400*; *Brufort*; *Bruzon*; *Buburone* (Japan); *Burana*; *Butacortelone* (Mexico); *Carol*; *Clinofen*; *Codral Period Pain* (Australia); *Combiflam*; *Deflem*; *Dibufen* (Mexico); *Dicerfen*; Dolgesic; *Dolgit* (Germany); *Dolocyl*; *Dolofen*; *Dolofen-F*; *Donjust*; *Donjust B* (Japan); *Dorival*; *Drin*; *Dynofen*; *Easifon*; *Ebufac* (England); *Ecofrol*; *Emflam*; *Emflam-200*; *Emodin*; *Epobron* (Japan); *Fenbid* (England); *Fenspan*; *Focus*; *Gofen*; *Hostalgin*; *IB-100* (Japan); *Ibosure*; Ibren; Ibu-Tab; *Ibufen*; *Ibuflamar*; *Ibufug* (Germany); *Ibugen*; *Ibugesic*; *Ibulgan*; *Ibumetin*; *Ibupirac*; Ibupro-600; *Ibuprocin* (Japan); *Ibuprofen*; Ibuprohm; *Ibusal*; *Ibu-slow*; *Ibuslow*; Ibutex; Ifen; *Imbun*; *Inabrin*; *Inberol*; *Inflam*; *Inza*; *Ipren*; *Irfen*; *Isodol*; *Kedvil* (Mexico); *Lamidon* (Japan); *Librofem* (England); *Lidifen* (England); *Liptan* (Japan); *Lopane*; *Magnatex*; *Melfen*; Menadol; *Mensoton* (Germany); **Motrin**; *Mynosedin* (Japan); *Nagifen-D* (Japan); *Namelin*; *Napacetin* (Japan); *Nerofen*; *Nobafon*; *Nobfelon* (Japan); *Nobgen* (Japan); *Noritis*; *Norton*; *Novogent* (Germany); *Novoprofen* (Canada); *Nurofen* (Australia, England, France); *Optifen*; *Opturem* (Germany); *Ostarin*; *Ostofen*; *Paduden*; *Pamored*; *Panafen*; *Pantrop* (Japan); *Paxofen*; Pedia-Profen; *Perofen*; *Proartinal* (Mexico); Profen; *Proflex* (England); *Quadrax* (Mexico); *Prontalgin*; *Rafen* (Australia); *Relcofen* (England); *Remofen*; Ro-Profen; *Roidenin* (Japan); Rufen; Saleto; *Seclodin* (England); *Tabalon*; *Tabalon 200*; *Tabalon 400* (Mexico); *Tarein*; *Tatanal*; *Uprofen*; *Urem* (Germany); *Zofen*

(International brand names outside U.S. in italics)

FORMULARIES: Aetna; BC-BS; CIGNA; DoD; FHP; Foundation; Humana; Kaiser; Medco; Medi-Cal; PCS; PruCare; United; WHO

COST OF THERAPY: $37.01 (Arthritis; Tablet; 400 mg; 3/day; 365 days)

PRIMARY ICD9: 715.99 (Osteoarthritis, Unspecified, Multiple Sites)

DESCRIPTION:

TABLETS AND SUSPENSION

Ibuprofen tablets and ibuprofen children's suspension contains the active ingredient ibuprofen, which is (±)-2-(*p*-isobutylphenyl) propionic acid. Ibuprofen is a white powder with a melting point of 74°-77°C and is very slightly soluble in water (<1 mg/ml) and readily soluble in organic solvents such as ethanol and acetone.

TABLETS

Ibuprofen, a nonsteroidal anti-inflammatory agent, is available in 300 mg, 400 mg, 600 mg, and 800 mg tablets for oral administration. *Inactive ingredients:* **300 mg:** carnauba wax, colloidal silicon dioxide, corn starch, pregelatinized starch, stearic acid, hydroxypropyl methylcellulose, propylene glycol. **400 mg:** carnauba wax, colloidal silicon dioxide, corn starch, pregelatinized starch, stearic acid, titanium dioxide, hydroxypropyl cellulose, hydroxypropyl methylcellulose, propylene glycol. **600 mg:** carnauba wax, colloidal silicon dioxide, corn starch, hydroxypropyl methylcellulose, pregelatinized starch, propylene glycol, stearic acid, titanium dioxide. **800 mg:** carnauba wax, colloidal silicon dioxide, croscarmellose sodium, hydroxypropyl methylcellulose, magnesium stearate, microcrystalline cellulose, propylene glycol, talc, titanium dioxide.

SUSPENSION

Ibuprofen children's suspension is a nonsteroidal anti-inflammatory agent. It is available for oral administration as a sucrose-sweetened, fruit-flavored liquid suspension containing 100 mg of ibuprofen per 5 ml.

DESCRIPTION: *(cont'd)*

Inactive Ingredients: Cellulose gum, citric acid, disodium edta, fd&c red no. 40, flavors, glycerin, microcrystalline cellulose, polysorbate 80, sodium benzoate, sorbitol, sucrose, water, xanthan gum.

CLINICAL PHARMACOLOGY:

TABLETS AND SUSPENSION

Ibuprofen tablets and ibuprofen children's suspension contains ibuprofen which possesses analgesic and antipyretic activities. Its mode of action, like that of other nonsteroidal anti-inflammatory agents, is not completely understood, but may be related to prostaglandin synthetase inhibition.

In clinical studies in patients with rheumatoid arthritis and osteoarthritis, ibuprofen has been shown to be comparable to aspirin in controlling pain and inflammation and to be associated with a statistically significant reduction in the milder gastrointestinal side effects (see ADVERSE REACTIONS). Ibuprofen may be well tolerated in some patients who have had gastrointestinal side effects with aspirin, but these patients, when treated with ibuprofen, should be carefully followed for signs and symptoms of gastrointestinal ulceration and bleeding. Although it is not definitely known whether ibuprofen causes less peptic ulceration than aspirin, in one study involving 885 patients with rheumatoid arthritis treated for up to one year, there were no reports of gastric ulceration with ibuprofen whereas frank ulceration was reported in 13 patients in the aspirin group (statistically significant $p<.001$).

Gastroscopic studies at varying doses show an increased tendency toward gastric irritation at higher doses. However, at comparable doses, gastric irritation is approximately half that seen with aspirin. Studies using ^{51}Cr-tagged red cells indicate that fecal blood loss associated with ibuprofen in doses up to 2400 mg daily did not exceed the normal range, and was significantly less than that seen in aspirin-treated patients.

In clinical studies in patients with rheumatoid arthritis, ibuprofen has been shown to be comparable to indomethacin in controlling the signs and symptoms of disease activity and to be associated with a statistically significant reduction of the milder gastrointestinal (see ADVERSE REACTIONS) and CNS side effects.

Ibuprofen may be used in combination with gold salts and/or corticosteroids.

SUSPENSION

In clinical studies in patients aged 2 to 15 with juvenile arthritis, ibuprofen children's suspension in doses of 20 to 50 mg/kg/day divided into 3 or 4 daily doses, has been shown to be similar to aspirin in controlling the signs and symptoms of their disease. In these trials, there was a significantly lower incidence of liver test abnormalities associated with ibuprofen children's suspension than with aspirin. Although ibuprofen may be better tolerated in terms of liver test abnormalities in children treated with ibuprofen children's suspension, they should be carefully followed for signs and symptoms suggesting liver dysfunction particularly with doses above 30 mg/kg/day, or if abnormal liver tests have occurred with previous NSAID treatment (see PRECAUTIONS).

TABLETS AND SUSPENSION

Controlled studies have demonstrated that ibuprofen is a more effective analgesic than propoxyphene for the relief of episiotomy pain, pain following dental extraction procedures, and for the relief of the symptoms of primary dysmenorrhea.

In patients with primary dysmenorrhea, ibuprofen has been shown to reduce elevated levels of prostaglandin activity in the menstrual fluid and to reduce resting and active intrauterine pressure, as well as the frequency of uterine contractions. The probable mechanism of action is to inhibit prostaglandin synthesis rather than simply to provide analgesia.

SUSPENSION

Controlled clinical trials comparing doses of 5 and 10 mg/kg ibuprofen and 10-15 mg/kg of acetaminophen have been conducted in children 6 months to 12 years of age with fever primarily due to viral illnesses. In these studies there were no differences between treatments in fever reduction for the first hour and maximum fever reduction occurred between 2 and 4 hours. Response after 1 hour was dependent on both the level of temperature elevation as well as the treatment. In children with baseline temperatures at or below 102.5°F, both ibuprofen doses and acetaminophen were equally effective in their maximum effect. In those children with temperatures above 102.5°F, the ibuprofen 10 mg/kg dose was more effective. By 6 hours children treated with ibuprofen 5 mg/kg tended to have recurrence of fever, whereas children treated with ibuprofen 10 mg/kg still had significant fever reduction at 8 hours. In control groups treated with 10 mg/kg acetaminophen, fever reduction resembled that seen in children treated with 5 mg/kg of ibuprofen, with the exception that temperature elevation tended to return 1-2 hours earlier.

In other trials, the antipyretic effect of ibuprofen children's suspension at 10 mg/kg was similar to that of acetaminophen at 15 mg/kg.

PHARMACOKINETICS

Ibuprofen is rapidly absorbed when administered orally. As is true with most tablet and suspension formulations, ibuprofen children's suspension is absorbed somewhat faster than the tablet with a time to peak serum level generally within one hour. Peak serum ibuprofen levels are generally attained one to two hours after administration of ibuprofen tablets and within about 1 hour after the suspension. With single, oral, solid doses up to 800 mg, in adults, a linear relationship exists between the amount of drug administered and the integrated area under the serum drug concentration vs. time curve. Above 800 mg, however, the area under the curve increase is less than proportional to the increase in dose. There is no evidence of age-dependent kinetics in patients 2 to 11 years old. With single doses of ibuprofen children's suspension ranging up to 10 mg/kg, a dose/response relationship exists between the amount of drug administered to febrile children and the serum concentration vs. time curve. There is also a correlation between reduction of fever and drug concentration over time, although the peak reduction in fever occurs 2-4 hours after dosing.

No absorption differences are noticeable when ibuprofen tablets or suspension are given under fasting conditions or immediately before meals. When either product is taken with food, however, the peak levels are somewhat lower (up to 30%) and the time to reach peak levels is slightly prolonged (up to 30 min.) although the extent of absorption is unchanged. A bioavailability study has shown that there was no interference with the absorption of ibuprofen when given in conjunction with an antacid containing both aluminum hydroxide and magnesium hydroxide.

TABLETS

The ibuprofen in ibuprofen tablets is rapidly absorbed. Peak serum ibuprofen levels are generally attained one to two hours after administration. With single doses up to 800 mg, a linear relationship exists between amount of drug administered and the integrated area under the serum drug concentration vs time curve. Above 800 mg, however, the area under the curve increases less than proportional to increases in dose. There is no evidence of drug accumulation or enzyme induction.

The administration of ibuprofen tablets either under fasting conditions or immediately before meals yields quite similar serum ibuprofen concentration-time profiles. When ibuprofen is administered immediately after a meal, there is a reduction in the rate of absorption but no appreciable decrease in the extent of absorption. The bioavailability of the drug is minimally altered by the presence of food.

CLINICAL PHARMACOLOGY: *(cont'd)*

A bioavailability study has shown that there was no interference with the absorption of ibuprofen when ibuprofen was given in conjunction with an antacid containing both aluminum hydroxide and magnesium hydroxide.

TABLETS AND SUSPENSION

Ibuprofen is rapidly metabolized and eliminated in the urine. The excretion of ibuprofen is virtually complete 24 hours after the last dose. The serum half-life is 1.8 to 2.0 hours.

TABLETS

Studies have shown that following ingestion of the drug, 45% to 79% of the dose was recovered in the urine within 24 hours as metabolite A (25%), (+)-2-[*p*-(2 hydroxymethyl-propyl) phenyl] propionic acid and metabolite B (37%), (+)-2-[*p*-(2 carboxypropyl)phenyl] propionic acid; the percentages of free and conjugated ibuprofen were approximately 1% and 14%, respectively.

SUSPENSION

Studies have shown that following ingestion of the drug, 45% to 79% of the dose was recovered in the urine within 24 hours as metabolite A (25%), (+)-2-4'-(2-hydroxy-2-methylpropyl)-phenylpropionic acid and metabolite B (37%), (+)-2-4'-(2-carboxypropyl)-phenylpropionic acid; the percentages of free and conjugated ibuprofen were approximately 1% and 14%, respectively.

INDICATIONS AND USAGE:

TABLETS

Ibuprofen tablets are indicated for relief of the signs and symptoms of rheumatoid arthritis and osteoarthritis.

Ibuprofen is indicated for relief of mild to moderate pain.

Ibuprofen is also indicated for the treatment of primary dysmenorrhea.

Since there have been no controlled clinical trials to demonstrate whether or not there is any beneficial effect or harmful interaction with the use of ibuprofen in conjunction with aspirin, the combination cannot be recommended (see DRUG INTERACTIONS).

Controlled clinical trials to establish the safety and effectiveness of ibuprofen in children have not been conducted.

SUSPENSION

Ibuprofen children's suspension is indicated for relief of the signs and symptoms of juvenile arthritis, rheumatoid arthritis and osteoarthritis.

Ibuprofen children's suspension is indicated for the relief of mild to moderate pain in adults and of primary dysmenorrhea.

Ibuprofen children's suspension is also indicated for the reduction of fever in patients ages 6 months and older.

Since there have been no controlled clinical trials to demonstrate whether there is any beneficial effect or harmful interaction with the use of ibuprofen in conjunction with aspirin, the combination cannot be recommended (See DRUG INTERACTIONS).

CONTRAINDICATIONS:

Ibuprofen tablets or ibuprofen children's suspension should not be used in patients who have previously exhibited hypersensitivity to ibuprofen, or in individuals with all or part of the syndrome of nasal polyps, angioedema, and bronchospastic reactivity to aspirin or other nonsteroidal anti-inflammatory agents. Anaphylactoid reactions have occurred in such patients.

WARNINGS:

RISK OF GI ULCERATION, BLEEDING AND PERFORATION WITH NONSTEROIDAL ANTI-INFLAMMATORY THERAPY

Serious gastrointestinal toxicity such as bleeding, ulceration, and perforation, can occur at any time, with or without warning symptoms, in patients treated chronically with nonsteroidal anti-inflammatory drugs. Although minor upper gastrointestinal problems, such as dyspepsia, are common, usually developing early in therapy, physicians should remain alert for ulceration and bleeding in patients treated chronically with nonsteroidal anti-inflammatory drugs even in the absence of previous GI tract symptoms. In patients observed in clinical trials of several months to two years duration, symptomatic upper GI ulcers, gross bleeding or perforation appear to occur in approximately 1% of patients treated for 3-6 months, and in about 2-4% of patients treated for one year. Physicians should inform patients about the signs and/or symptoms of serious GI toxicity and what steps to take if they occur.

Studies to date have not identified any subset of patients not at risk of developing peptic ulceration and bleeding. Except for a prior history of serious GI events and other risk factors known to be associated with peptic ulcer disease, such as alcoholism, smoking, etc., no risk factors (*e.g.,* age, sex) have been associated with increased risk. Elderly or debilitated patients seem to tolerate ulceration or bleeding less well than other individuals and most spontaneous reports of fatal GI events are in this population. Studies to date are inconclusive concerning the relative risk of various nonsteroidal anti-inflammatory agents in causing such reactions. High doses of any such agents probably carry a greater risk of these reactions, although controlled clinical trials showing this do not exist in most cases. In considering the use of relatively large doses (within the recommended dosage range), sufficient benefit should be anticipated to offset the potential increased risk of GI toxicity.

PRECAUTIONS:

GENERAL

Blurred and/or diminished vision, scotomata, and/or changes in color vision have been reported. If a patient develops such complaints while receiving ibuprofen, the drug should be discontinued, and the patient should have an ophthalmologic examination which includes central visual fields and color vision testing.

Fluid retention and edema have been reported in association with ibuprofen; therefore, the drug should be used with caution in patients with a history of cardiac decompensation or hypertension.

Ibuprofen, like other nonsteroidal anti-inflammatory agents, can inhibit platelet aggregation, but the effect is quantitatively less and of shorter duration than that seen with aspirin. Ibuprofen has been shown to prolong bleeding time (but within the normal range) in normal subjects. Because this prolonged bleeding effect may be exaggerated in patients with underlying hemostatic defects, ibuprofen should be used with caution in persons with intrinsic coagulation defects and those on anticoagulant therapy.

Patients on ibuprofen should report to their physicians signs or symptoms of gastrointestinal ulceration or bleeding, blurred vision or other eye symptoms, skin rash, weight gain, or edema.

In order to avoid exacerbation of disease or adrenal insufficiency, patients who have been on prolonged corticosteroid therapy should have their therapy tapered slowly rather than discontinued abruptly when ibuprofen is added to the treatment program.

PRECAUTIONS: *(cont'd)*

The antipyretic and anti-inflammatory activity of ibuprofen may reduce fever and inflammation, thus diminishing their utility as diagnostic signs in detecting complications of presumed noninfectious, noninflammatory painful conditions.

LIVER EFFECTS

As with other nonsteroidal anti-inflammatory drugs, borderline elevations of one or more liver function tests may occur in up to 15% of patients. These abnormalities may progress, may remain essentially unchanged, or may be transient with continued therapy. The SGPT (ALT) test is probably the most sensitive indicator of liver dysfunction. Meaningful (3 times the upper limit of normal) elevations of SGPT or SGOT (AST) occurred in controlled clinical trials in less than 1% of patients. A patient with symptoms and/or signs suggesting liver dysfunction, or in whom an abnormal liver test has occurred, should be evaluated for evidence of the development of more severe hepatic reactions while on therapy with ibuprofen. Severe hepatic reactions, including jaundice and cases of fatal hepatitis, have been reported with ibuprofen as with other nonsteroidal anti-inflammatory drugs. Although such reactions are rare, if abnormal liver tests persist or worsen, if clinical signs and symptoms consistent with liver disease develop, or if systemic manifestations occur (*e.g.,* eosinophilia, rash, etc), ibuprofen should be discontinued.

HEMOGLOBIN LEVELS

In cross-study comparisons with doses ranging from 1200 mg to 3200 mg daily for several weeks, a slight dose-response decrease in hemoglobin/hematocrit was noted. This has been observed with other nonsteroidal anti-inflammatory drugs; the mechanism is unknown. With daily doses of 3200 mg, the total decrease in hemoglobin may exceed 1 gram; if there are no signs of bleeding, it is probably not clinically important.

In two postmarketing clinical studies with ibuprofen the incidence of a decreased hemoglobin level was greater than previously reported. Decrease in hemoglobin of 1 gram or more was observed in 17.1% of 193 patients on 1600 mg ibuprofen daily (osteoarthritis), and in 22.8% of 189 patients taking 2400 mg of ibuprofen daily (rheumatoid arthritis). Positive stool occult blood tests and elevated serum creatinine levels were also observed in these studies.

ASEPTIC MENINGITIS

Aseptic meningitis with fever and coma has been observed on rare occasions in patients on ibuprofen therapy. Although it is probably more likely to occur in patients with systemic lupus erythematosus and related connective tissue diseases, it has been reported in patients who do not have an underlying chronic disease. If signs or symptoms of meningitis develop in a patient on ibuprofen, the possibility of its being related to ibuprofen should be considered.

RENAL EFFECTS

As with other nonsteroidal anti-inflammatory drugs, long-term administration of ibuprofen to animals has resulted in renal papillary necrosis and other abnormal renal pathology. In humans, there have been reports of acute interstitial nephritis with hematuria, proteinuria, and occasionally nephrotic syndrome.

A second form of renal toxicity has been seen in patients with prerenal conditions leading to a reduction in renal blood flow or blood volume, where the renal prostaglandins have a supportive role in the maintenance of renal perfusion. In these patients administration of a nonsteroidal anti-inflammatory drug may cause a dose dependent reduction in prostaglandin formation and may precipitate overt renal decompensation. Patients at greatest risk of this reaction are those with impaired renal function, heart failure, liver dysfunction, those taking diuretics and the elderly. Discontinuation of nonsteroidal anti-inflammatory drug therapy is typically followed by recovery to the pretreatment state. Those patients at high risk who chronically take ibuprofen should have renal function monitored if they have signs or symptoms which may be consistent with mild azotemia, such as malaise, fatigue, loss of appetite, etc. Occasional patients may develop some elevation of serum creatinine and BUN levels without signs or symptoms.

Since ibuprofen is eliminated primarily by the kidneys, patients with significantly impaired renal function should be closely monitored; and a reduction in dosage should be anticipated to avoid drug accumulation. Prospective studies on the safety of ibuprofen in patients with chronic renal failure have not been conducted.

LABORATORY TESTS

Because serious GI tract ulcerations and bleeding can occur without warning symptoms, physicians should follow chronically treated patients for the signs and symptoms of ulcerations and bleeding and should inform them of the importance of this follow-up (see WARNINGS).

PREGNANCY

Reproductive studies conducted in rats and rabbits at doses somewhat less than the maximal clinical dose did not demonstrate evidence of developmental abnormalities. However, animal reproduction studies are not always predictive of human response. As there are no adequate and well-controlled studies in pregnant women, this drug should be used during pregnancy only if clearly needed. Because of the known effects of nonsteroidal anti-inflammatory drugs on the fetal cardiovascular system (closure of ductus arteriosus), use during late pregnancy should be avoided. As with other drugs known to inhibit prostaglandin synthesis, an increased incidence of dystocia and delayed parturition occurred in rats. Administration of ibuprofen is not recommended during pregnancy.

NURSING MOTHERS

In limited studies, an assay capable of detecting 1 mcg/ml did not demonstrate ibuprofen in the milk of lactating mothers. However, because of the limited nature of the studies, and the possible adverse effects of prostaglandin-inhibiting drugs on neonates, ibuprofen is not recommended for use in nursing mothers.

SUSPENSION

Infants: Safety and efficacy of ibuprofen children's suspension in children below the age of 6 months has not been established.

DRUG INTERACTIONS:

Coumarin-Type Anticoagulants: Several short-term controlled studies failed to show that ibuprofen significantly affected prothrombin times or a variety of other clotting factors when administered to individuals on coumarin-type anticoagulants. However, because bleeding has been reported when ibuprofen and other nonsteroidal anti-inflammatory agents have been administered to patients on coumarin-type anticoagulants, the physician should be cautious when administering ibuprofen to patients on anticoagulants.

Aspirin: Animal studies show that aspirin given with nonsteroidal anti-inflammatory agents, including ibuprofen, yields a net decrease in anti-inflammatory activity with lowered blood levels of the non-aspirin drug. Single dose bioavailability studies in normal volunteers have failed to show an effect of aspirin on ibuprofen blood levels. Correlative clinical studies have not been performed.

Methotrexate: Ibuprofen, as well as other nonsteroidal anti-inflammatory drugs, probably reduces the tubular secretion of methotrexate based on *in vitro* studies in rabbit kidney slices. This may indicate that ibuprofen could enhance the toxicity of methotrexate. Caution should be used if ibuprofen is administered concomitantly with methotrexate.

H-2 Antagonists: In studies with human volunteers, co-administration of cimetidine or ranitidine with ibuprofen had no substantive effect on ibuprofen serum concentrations.

DRUG INTERACTIONS: *(cont'd)*

Furosemide: Clinical studies, as well as random observations, have shown that ibuprofen can reduce the natriuretic effect of furosemide and thiazides in some patients. This response has been attributed to inhibition of renal prostaglandin synthesis. During concomitant therapy with ibuprofen, the patient should be observed closely for signs of renal failure (see PRECAUTIONS, Renal Effects), as well as to assure diuretic efficacy.

Lithium: Ibuprofen produced an elevation of plasma lithium levels and a reduction in renal lithium clearance in a study of eleven normal volunteers. The mean minimum lithium concentration increased 15% and the renal clearance of lithium was decreased by 19% during this period of concomitant drug administration.

This effect has been attributed to inhibition of renal prostaglandin synthesis by ibuprofen. Thus, when ibuprofen and lithium are administered concurrently, patients should be observed carefully for signs of lithium toxicity. (Read circulars for lithium preparation before use of such concurrent therapy).

SUSPENSION

Diabetes: Each 5 ml of ibuprofen children's suspension contains approximately 2.5 grams of sucrose, which should be taken into consideration when treating patients with impaired glucose tolerance. It also contains 350 mg of sorbitol per 5 ml. Although in clinical trials ibuprofen children's suspension was not associated with more diarrhea than control treatments, should a patient develop diarrhea, the physician may wish to review the patient's dietary intake of sorbitol from other sources.

ADVERSE REACTIONS:

TABLETS AND SUSPENSION

The most frequent type of adverse reaction occurring with ibuprofen is gastrointestinal. In controlled clinical trials, the percentage of patients reporting one or more gastrointestinal complaints ranged from 4% to 16%.

In controlled studies when ibuprofen was compared to aspirin and indomethacin in equally effective doses, the overall incidence of gastrointestinal complaints was about half that seen in either the aspirin- or indomethacin-treated patients.

SUSPENSION

In a 12-week comparison of ibuprofen children's suspension (n=45) and aspirin (n=47) in children with juvenile arthritis, the most common adverse experiences were also gastrointestinal in nature, usually of mild severity. Abdominal pain of possible drug relationship was reported in about 25% of patients on ibuprofen and/or aspirin; other possibly drug-related effects associated with the digestive system were reported in 42% of the children taking ibuprofen and in 70% of those taking aspirin.

TABLETS AND SUSPENSION

Adverse reactions observed during controlled clinical trials at an incidence greater than 1% are listed in the tables (TABLE 1A and TABLE 1B). Those reactions listed in column one encompass observations in approximately 3,000 patients. More than 500 of these patients were treated for periods of at least 54 weeks.

Still other reactions occurring less frequently than 1 in 100 were reported in controlled clinical trials and from marketing experience. These reactions have been divided into two categories: column two of the tables lists reactions with therapy with ibuprofen where the probability of a causal relationship exists; for the reactions in column three, a causal relationship with ibuprofen has not been established.

Reported side effects were higher at doses of 3200 mg/day than at doses of 2400 mg or less per day in clinical trials of patients with rheumatoid arthritis. The increases in incidence were slight and still within the ranges reported in the tables below (TABLE 1A and TABLE 1B).

TABLE 1A

Incidence Greater than 1% (but less than 3%) Probable Causal Relationship	Precise Incidence Unknown (but less than 1%) Probable Causal Relationship**	Precise Incidence Unknown (but less than 1%) Causal Relationship Unknown**
GASTROINTESTINAL		
Nausea*, epigastric pain*, heartburn*, diarrhea, abdominal distress, nausea and vomiting, indigestion, constipation, abdominal cramps or pain, fullness of GI tract (bloating and flatulence)	Gastric or duodenal ulcer with bleeding and/or perforation, gastrointestinal hemorrhage, melena, gastritis, hepatitis, jaundice, abnormal liver function tests; pancreatitis	
CENTRAL NERVOUS SYSTEM		
Dizziness*, headache, nervousness	Depression, insomnia, confusion, emotional lability, somnolence, aseptic meningitis with fever and coma (SeePRECAUTIONS)	Paresthesias, hallucinations, dream abnormalities, pseudotumor cerebri
DERMATOLOGIC		
Rash* (including maculopapular type), pruritus	Vesiculobullous eruptions, urticaria, erythema multiforme, Stevens-Johnson syndrome, alopecia	Toxic epidermal necrolysis, photoallergic skin reactions
SPECIAL SENSES		
Tinnitus	Hearing loss, amblyopia (blurred and/or diminished vision, scotomata and/or changes in color vision) (seePRECAUTIONS)	Conjunctivitis, diplopia, optic neuritis, cataracts

* Reactions occurring in 3% to 9% of patients treated with ibuprofen. (Those reactions occurring in less than 3% of the patients are unmarked.)

** Reactions are classified under *"Probable Causal Relationship (PCR)"* if there has been one positive rechallenge or if three or more cases occur which might be causally related. Reactions are classified under *"Causal Relationship Unknown"* if seven or more events have been reported but the criteria for PCR have not been met.

OVERDOSAGE:

Approximately 1 ½ hours after the reported ingestion of from 7 to 10 ibuprofen tablets (400 mg), a 19-month old child weighing 12 kg was seen in the hospital emergency room, apneic and cyanotic, responding only to painful stimuli. This type of stimulus, however, was sufficient to induce respiration. Oxygen and parenteral fluids were given; a greenish-yellow fluid was aspirated from the stomach with no evidence to indicate the presence of ibuprofen. Two hours after ingestion the child's condition seemed stable; she still responded only to painful stimuli and continued to have periods of apnea lasting from 5 to 10 seconds. She was admitted to intensive care and sodium bicarbonate was administered as well as infusions of dextrose and normal saline. By four hours post-ingestion she could be aroused easily, sit by

OVERDOSAGE: *(cont'd)*

TABLE 1B

Incidence Greater than 1% (but less than 3%) Probable Causal Relationship	Precise Incidence Unknown (but less than 1%) Probable Causal Relationship**	Precise Incidence Unknown (but less than 1%) Causal Relationship Unknown**
HEMATOLOGIC		
	Neutropenia, agranulocytosis, aplastic anemia, hemolytic anemia (sometimes Coombs positive), thrombocytopenia with or without purpura, eosinophilia, decreases in hemoglobin and hematocrit (see PRECAUTIONS)	Bleeding episodes (*e.g.*, epistaxis, menorrhagia)
METABOLIC/ ENDOCRINE		
Decreased appetite		Gynecomastia, hypoglycemic reaction, acidosis
CARDIOVASCULAR		
Edema, fluid retention (generally responds promptly to drug discontinuation) (see PRECAUTIONS)	Congestive heart failure in patients with marginal cardiac function, elevated blood pressure, palpitations	Arrhythmias (sinus tachycardia, sinus bradycardia)
ALLERGIC		
	Syndrome of abdominal pain, fever, chills, nausea and vomiting; anaphylaxis; bronchospasm (see CONTRAINDICATIONS)	Serum sickness, lupus erythematosus syndrome, Henoch-Schonlein vasculitis, angioedema
RENAL		
	Acute renal failure (See PRECAUTIONS), decreased creatinine clearance, polyuria, azotemia, cystitis, hematuria	Renal papillary necrosis
MISCELLANEOUS		
	Dry eyes and mouth, gingival ulcer, rhinitis	

** Reactions are classified under *"Probable Causal Relationship (PCR)"* if there has been one positive rechallenge or if three or more cases occur which might be causally related. Reactions are classified under *"Causal Relationship Unknown"* if seven or more events have been reported but the criteria for PCR have not been met.

herself and respond to spoken commands. Blood level of ibuprofen was 102.9 mcg/ml, approximately 8 ½ hours after accidental ingestion. At 12 hours she appeared to be completely recovered.

In two other reported cases where children (each weighing approximately 10 kg) accidentally, acutely ingested approximately 120 mg/kg, there were no signs of acute intoxication or late sequelae. Blood level in one child 90 minutes after ingestion was 700 mcg/ml, about 10 times the peak levels seen in absorption-excretion studies.

A 19-year old male who had taken 8,000 mg of ibuprofen over a period of a few hours complained of dizziness, and nystagmus was noted. After hospitalization, parenteral hydration and three days bed rest, he recovered with no reported sequelae.

In cases of acute overdosage, the stomach should be emptied by vomiting or lavage, though little drug will likely be recovered if more than an hour has elapsed since ingestion. Because the drug is acidic and is excreted in the urine, it is theoretically beneficial to administer alkali and induce diuresis. In addition to supportive measures, the use of oral activated charcoal may help to reduce the absorption and reabsorption of ibuprofen.

DOSAGE AND ADMINISTRATION:

TABLETS

Do not exceed 3200 mg total daily dose. If gastrointestinal complaints occur, administer ibuprofen tablets with meals or milk.

Rheumatoid Arthritis and Osteoarthritis, Including Flare-Ups of Chronic Disease

Suggested Dosage: 1200 mg-3200 mg daily (300 mg qid; 400 mg, 600 mg or 800 mg tid or qid). Individual patients may show a better response to 3200 mg daily, as compared with 2400 mg, although in well-controlled clinical trials patients on 3200 mg did not show a better mean response in terms of efficacy. Therefore, when treating patients with 3200 mg/day, the physician should observe sufficient increased clinical benefits to offset potential increased risk.

The dose should be tailored to each patient, and may be lowered or raised depending on the severity of symptoms either at time of initiating drug therapy or as the patient responds or fails to respond.

In general, patients with rheumatoid arthritis seem to require higher doses of ibuprofen than do patients with osteoarthritis.

The smallest dose of ibuprofen that yields acceptable control should be employed. A linear blood level dose-response relationship exists with single doses up to 800 mg (See CLINICAL PHARMACOLOGY) for effects of food on rate of absorption.

The availability of four tablet strengths facilitates dosage adjustment.

In Chronic Conditions: A therapeutic response to therapy with ibuprofen is sometimes seen in a few days to a week but most often is observed by two weeks. After a satisfactory response has been achieved, the patient's dose should be reviewed and adjusted as required.

Mild to Moderate Pain: 400 mg every 4 to 6 hours as necessary for relief of pain.

In controlled analgesic clinical trials, doses of ibuprofen greater than 400 mg were no more effective than the 400 mg dose.

Dysmenorrhea: For the treatment of dysmenorrhea, beginning with the earliest onset of such pain. Ibuprofen should be given in a dose of 400 mg every 4 hours as necessary for the relief of pain.

Store at controlled room temperature 15° to 30°C (59° to 86°F).

SUSPENSION

Shake well prior to administration.

Do not exceed 3200 mg total daily dose. If gastrointestinal complaints occur, administer ibuprofen with meals or milk.

Juvenile Arthritis: The usual dose is 30 to 40 mg/kg/day divided into 3 or 4 doses. Patients with milder disease may be adequately treated with 20 mg/kg/day.

Doses above 50 mg/kg/day are not recommended because they have not been studied and because side effects appear to be dose related.

DOSAGE AND ADMINISTRATION: *(cont'd)*

Therapeutic response may require from a few days to several weeks to be achieved. Once a clinical response is obtained, dosage should be lowered to the smallest dose of ibuprofen children's suspension needed to maintain adequate control of disease.

Rheumatoid Arthritis and Osteoarthritis, Including Flare-Ups of Chronic Disease: *Suggested Adult Dosage:* 1200-3200 mg daily (3300 mg q.i.d, or 400 mg, 600 mg or 800 mg t.i.d. or q.i.d.). Individual patients may show a better response to 3200 mg daily, as compared with 2400 mg, although in well-controlled clinical trials patients on 3200 mg did not show a better mean response in terms of efficacy. Therefore, when treating patients with 3200 mg/day, the physician should observe sufficient increased clinical benefits to offset potential increased risk.

The dose of ibuprofen children's suspension should be tailored to each patient, and may be lowered or raised from the suggested doses depending on the severity of symptoms either at the time of initiating drug therapy or as the patient responds ot fails to respond.

In general, patients with rheumatoid arthritis seem to require higher doses of ibuprofen than do patients with osteoarthritis.

The smallest dose of ibuprofen children's suspension that yields acceptable control should be employed. A linear blood level dose-response relationship exists with single doses up to 800 mg (see CLINICAL PHARMACOLOGY, Pharmacokinetics for effects of food on rate of absorption).

In chronic conditions, a therapeutic response to ibuprofen therapy is sometimes seen in a few days to a week but most often is observed by two weeks. After a satisfactory response has been achieved, the patient's dose should be reviewed and adjusted as required.

Mild to Moderate Pain: 400 mg every 4 to 6 hours as necessary for the relief of pain in adults.

In controlled analgesic clinical trials, doses of ibuprofen greater than 400 mg were no more effective than the 400 mg dose.

Dysmenorrhea: For the treatment of dysmenorrhea, beginning with the earliest onset of such pain, ibuprofen children's suspension should be given in a dose of 400 mg every 4 hours as necessary for the relief of pain.

Fever Reduction in Children 6 Months to 12 Years of Age: Dosage should be adjusted on the basis of the initial temperature level (see CLINICAL PHARMACOLOGY for a description of the controlled clinical trial results). The recommended dose is 5 mg/kg if the baseline temperature is 102.5°F or below or 10 mg/kg if the baseline temperature is greater than 102.5°F. The duration of fever reduction is generally 6-8 hours and is longer with the higher dose. The recommended maximum daily dose is 40 mg/kg (TABLE 2).

TABLE 2

		5 mg/kg (Fever ≤102.5°F)		10 mg/kg (Fever >102.5°F)	
Age	**Weight (lb)**	**(mg)**	**(tsp)**	**(mg)**	**(tsp)**
6-11 mos	13-17	25	¼	50	½
12-23 mos	18-23	50	½	100	1
2-3 yrs	24-35	75	¾	150	1 ½
4-5 yrs	36-47	100	1	200	2
6-8 yrs	48-59	125	1 ½	250	2 ½
9-10 yrs	60-71	150	1 ½	300	3
11-12 yrs	72-95	200	2	400	4

Fever Reduction in Adults: 400 mg every 4-6 hours as necessary.

Information for Patients

Ibuprofen, like other drugs of its class, is not free of side effects. The side effects of these drugs can cause discomfort and, rarely, there are more serious side effects, such as gastrointestinal bleeding, which may result in hospitalization and even fatal outcomes.

Nonsteroidal anti-inflammatory drugs are often essential agents in the management of arthritis and have a major role in the treatment of pain, but they also may be commonly employed for conditions which are less serious.

Physicians may wish to discuss with their patients the potential risks (see WARNINGS, PRECAUTIONS, and ADVERSE REACTIONS) and likely benefits of nonsteroidal anti-inflammatory drug treatment, particularly when the drugs are used for less serious conditions where treatment without such agents may represent an acceptable alternative to both the patient and physician.

Ibuprofen children's suspension should be stored at controlled room temperature; 20°C to 25°C (68°F to 77°F).

Shake well before use. Keep container tightly closed.

PATIENT INFORMATION:

Ibuprofen is a nonsteroidal anti-inflammatory drug (NSAID) used to relieve pain and inflammation, reduce fever, and treat osteoarthritis, rheumatoid arthritis, and menstrual cramps. Inform your physician if you are pregnant or nursing. Ibuprofen should not be taken during the last three months of pregnancy. Inform your physician if you use alcohol chronically. Ibuprofen should not be taken with aspirin products. This medication should be taken with food, milk or antacids if stomach upset occurs. Ibuprofen may cause dizziness and drowsiness; use caution while driving or operating hazardous machinery. Ibuprofen may cause increased sensitivity to sunlight. Use sunscreens and wear protective clothing until degree of sensitivity is determined. Notify your physician if you develop stomach pain, bloody vomit, bloody or black tarry stools, cloudy urine, trouble breathing, rash or hives.

HOW SUPPLIED - RATED THERAPEUTICALLY EQUIVALENT:

Tablet, Coated - Oral - 300 mg

60's	$5.18	Ibuprofen, Rugby	00536-3976-08
60's	**$11.92**	**MOTRIN, Pharmacia & Upjohn**	**00009-0733-01**
100's	$4.95	Ibuprofen, Harber Pharm	51432-0447-03
100's	$8.58	Ibuprofen, US Trading	56126-0161-11
100's	$18.90	Ibuprofen, Voluntary Hosp	53258-0179-13
500's	$13.50	Ibuprofen, US Trading	56126-0161-05
500's	$36.00	Ibuprofen, Goldline Labs	00182-1770-05

Tablet, Coated - Oral - 400 mg

20's	$2.45	Ibuprofen, Vangard Labs	00615-2525-15
30's	$3.00	Ibuprofen, Talbert Phcy	44514-0574-18
50's	$1.69	Ibuprofen, H.C.F.A. F F P	99999-1520-01
90's	$8.82	Ibuprofen, Talbert Phcy	44514-0574-54
100's	$3.38	Ibuprofen, United Res	00677-1031-01
100's	$3.38	Ibuprofen, H.C.F.A. F F P	99999-1520-02
100's	$4.67	Ibuprofen, US Trading	56126-0162-11
100's	$5.63	Ibuprofen, IDE-Interstate	00814-3813-14
100's	$6.50	Ibuprofen, Consolidated Midland	00223-1091-01
100's	$8.00	Ibuprofen, Raway	00686-0281-20
100's	$9.80	Ibuprofen, Talbert Phcy	44514-0574-88
100's	$10.01	Ibuprofen, Sidmak Labs	50111-0387-01
100's	$10.90	Ibuprofen, Qualitest Pharms	00603-4018-21

HOW SUPPLIED - RATED THERAPEUTICALLY EQUIVALENT: *(cont'd)*

100's	$10.94	Ibuprofen, Rugby	00536-3977-01
100's	$11.00	Ibuprofen, Goldline Labs	00182-1809-01
100's	$11.00	Ibuprofen, H N Norton Co.	50732-0744-01
100's	$11.21	Ibuprofen, Barr	00555-0419-02
100's	$11.60	MORPEN, Major Pharms	00904-1648-60
100's	$11.61	Ibuprofen, Caremark	00339-5915-12
100's	$11.69	Ibuprofen, Purepac Pharm	00228-2124-10
100's	$11.94	Ibuprofen, Rugby	00536-4604-01
100's	$12.00	Ibuprofen, Schein Pharm (US)	00364-0765-01
100's	$12.00	Ibuprofen, Winsor Pharm	59004-0140-50
100's	$12.00	Ibuprofen, Greenstone	59762-7378-01
100's	$12.30	Ibuprofen, Caremark	00339-5161-12
100's	$12.35	Ibu, Knoll Labs	00044-0165-01
100's	$12.38	Ibuprofen, Aligen Independ	00405-4527-01
100's	$12.39	Ibuprofen, Par Pharm	49884-0162-01
100's	$12.39	Ibuprofen, Par Pharm	49884-0467-01
100's	$12.95	Ibuprofen, Geneva Pharms	00781-1352-01
100's	$12.96	Ibuprofen, HL Moore Drug Exch	00839-7112-06
100's	$13.00	IBU-TAB, Alra Labs	51641-0214-01
100's	$13.41	Ibuprofen, Lederle Pharm	00005-3121-23
100's	$13.82	Ibuprofen, Warner Chilcott	00047-0516-24
100's	$15.95	Ibuprofen, Parmed Pharms	00349-8282-01
100's	$16.00	Ibuprofen, Winsor Pharm	59004-0140-55
100's	$16.80	Ibuprofen, Voluntary Hosp	53258-0138-01
100's	$18.50	Ibuprofen, Schein Pharm (US)	00364-0765-90
100's	$18.73	Ibuprofen, Medirex	57480-0336-01
100's	$19.20	Ibuprofen, Voluntary Hosp	53258-0138-13
100's	$19.38	Ibuprofen, Major Pharms	00904-1748-61
100's	**$19.84**	**MOTRIN, Pharmacia & Upjohn**	**00009-7385-01**
100's	$21.12	Ibuprofen, Vangard Labs	00615-2525-13
100's	**$21.57**	**MOTRIN, Pharmacia & Upjohn**	**00009-7385-04**
100's	$22.50	Ibuprofen, Goldline Labs	00182-1809-89
100's	$32.19	IBU-TAB, Alra Labs	51641-0214-11
100's	$49.42	Ibuprofen, Aligen Independ	00405-4527-02
120's	$4.05	Ibuprofen, H.C.F.A. F F P	99999-1520-04
120's	**$23.81**	**MOTRIN, Pharmacia & Upjohn**	**00009-0750-26**
360's	$35.53	Ibuprofen, Rugby	00536-3977-07
500's	$16.90	Ibuprofen, United Res	00677-1031-05
500's	$16.90	Ibuprofen, Sidmak Labs	50111-0387-02
500's	$16.90	Ibuprofen, H.C.F.A. F F P	99999-1520-03
500's	$21.00	Ibuprofen, IDE-Interstate	00814-3813-28
500's	$27.50	Ibuprofen, Consolidated Midland	00223-1091-05
500's	$44.90	Ibuprofen, Barr	00555-0419-04
500's	$46.64	IBU-TAB, Alra Labs	51641-0214-05
500's	$47.00	Ibuprofen, Voluntary Hosp	53258-0138-05
500's	$47.86	Ibuprofen, Purepac Pharm	00228-2124-50
500's	$48.05	Ibuprofen, Qualitest Pharms	00603-4018-28
500's	$48.13	Ibuprofen, Rugby	00536-3977-05
500's	$48.70	MORPEN, Major Pharms	00904-1648-40
500's	$48.70	Ibuprofen, Major Pharms	00904-1748-40
500's	$49.00	Ibuprofen, Winsor Pharm	59004-0140-80
500's	$49.00	Ibuprofen, Greenstone	59762-7378-02
500's	$49.35	Ibu, Knoll Labs	00044-0165-05
500's	$49.95	Ibuprofen, Goldline Labs	00182-1809-05
500's	$49.95	Ibuprofen, H N Norton Co.	50732-0744-05
500's	$53.95	Ibuprofen, Rugby	00536-4604-05
500's	$54.25	Ibuprofen, Parmed Pharms	00349-8282-05
500's	$58.00	Ibuprofen, Par Pharm	49884-0162-05
500's	$58.00	Ibuprofen, Par Pharm	49884-0467-05
500's	$59.72	Ibuprofen, Lederle Pharm	00005-3121-31
500's	$60.89	Ibuprofen, HL Moore Drug Exch	00839-7112-12
500's	$60.89	Ibuprofen, HL Moore Drug Exch	00839-7699-12
500's	$60.95	Ibuprofen, Schein Pharm (US)	00364-0765-05
500's	$60.95	Ibuprofen, Geneva Pharms	00781-1352-05
500's	$62.92	Ibuprofen, Warner Chilcott	00047-0516-30
500's	$62.95	Ibuprofen, Mylan	00378-1401-05
500's	$76.32	Ibuprofen, Voluntary Hosp	53258-0802-05
500's	**$82.27**	**MOTRIN, Pharmacia & Upjohn**	**00009-7385-02**
600's	$113.00	Ibuprofen, Medirex	57480-0336-06
750's	$96.00	Ibuprofen, Glasgow Pharm	60809-0128-55
750's	$96.00	Ibuprofen, Glasgow Pharm	60809-0128-72
1000's	$33.80	Ibuprofen, H.C.F.A. F F P	99999-1520-05
1000's	$60.63	Ibuprofen, Rugby	00536-3977-10
1000's	$69.00	Ibuprofen, Goldline Labs	00182-1809-10
1000's	$89.78	IBU-TAB, Alra Labs	51641-0214-10
1000's	$95.00	Ibuprofen, Parmed Pharms	00349-8282-10
1440's	$98.08	Ibuprofen, Rugby	00536-3977-41
10000's	$338.00	Ibuprofen, H.C.F.A. F F P	99999-1520-06
10000's	**$804.00**	**MOTRIN, Pharmacia & Upjohn**	**00009-7385-03**

Tablet, Coated - Oral - 600 mg

30's	$1.32	Ibuprofen, H.C.F.A. F F P	99999-1520-07
30's	$2.95	Ibuprofen, Major Pharms	00904-1758-46
30's	$4.32	Ibuprofen, Talbert Phcy	44514-0636-18
60's	$2.65	Ibuprofen, H.C.F.A. F F P	99999-1520-08
60's	$4.60	Ibuprofen, Major Pharms	00904-1758-52
60's	$8.64	Ibuprofen, Talbert Phcy	44514-0636-36
90's	$3.98	Ibuprofen, H.C.F.A. F F P	99999-1520-09
90's	$12.96	Ibuprofen, Talbert Phcy	44514-0636-54
90's	**$25.34**	**MOTRIN, Pharmacia & Upjohn**	**00009-7386-05**
100's	$4.43	Ibuprofen, United Res	00677-1032-01
100's	$4.43	Ibuprofen, H.C.F.A. F F P	99999-1520-10
100's	$6.08	Ibuprofen, US Trading	56126-0163-11
100's	$7.20	Ibuprofen, IDE-Interstate	00814-3814-14
100's	$7.75	Ibuprofen, Consolidated Midland	00223-1092-01
100's	$10.00	Ibuprofen, Raway	00686-0282-20
100's	$13.96	IBREN, Embrex Economed	38130-0053-01
100's	$14.40	Ibuprofen, Talbert Phcy	44514-0636-88
100's	$14.75	Ibuprofen, H N Norton Co.	50732-0747-01
100's	$14.80	Ibuprofen, Qualitest Pharms	00603-4019-21
100's	$15.00	Ibuprofen, Goldline Labs	00182-1810-01
100's	$15.00	Ibuprofen, Voluntary Hosp	53258-0139-01
100's	$15.10	Ibuprofen, Mutual Pharm	53489-0132-01
100's	$15.13	Ibuprofen, Sidmak Labs	50111-0388-01
100's	$15.61	Ibuprofen, Purepac Pharm	00228-2125-10
100's	$16.12	Ibuprofen, Caremark	00339-5917-12
100's	$16.50	Ibuprofen, Winsor Pharm	59004-0160-50
100's	$16.50	Ibuprofen, Greenstone	59762-7379-01
100's	$16.54	Ibuprofen, HL Moore Drug Exch	00839-7113-06
100's	$16.70	Ibuprofen, Boots Pharm	00524-0162-01
100's	$16.75	Ibuprofen, Rugby	00536-4605-01
100's	$16.75	MORPEN, Major Pharms	00904-1658-60
100's	$16.75	Ibuprofen, Major Pharms	00904-1758-60

HOW SUPPLIED - RATED THERAPEUTICALLY EQUIVALENT: *(cont'd)*

100's	$16.75	Ibuprofen, Par Pharm	49884-0163-01
100's	$16.75	Ibuprofen, Par Pharm	49884-0468-01
100's	$16.83	Ibuprofen, Aligen Independ	00405-4528-01
100's	$16.85	Ibuprofen, Warner Chilcott	00047-0922-24
100's	$17.55	Ibuprofen, Geneva Pharms	00781-1362-01
100's	$17.77	Ibuprofen, Schein Pharm (US)	00364-0766-01
100's	$18.50	IBU-TAB, Alra Labs	51641-0213-01
100's	$18.79	Ibuprofen, Lederle Pharm	00005-3122-23
100's	$21.00	Ibuprofen, Voluntary Hosp	53258-0139-13
100's	$22.00	Ibuprofen, Winsor Pharm	59004-0160-55
100's	$24.25	Ibuprofen, Parmed Pharms	00349-8425-01
100's	$27.42	Ibuprofen, Medirex	57480-0337-01
100's	**$28.13**	**MOTRIN, Pharmacia & Upjohn**	**00009-7386-01**
100's	$28.30	Ibuprofen, Schein Pharm (US)	00364-0766-90
100's	$28.45	Ibuprofen, Major Pharms	00904-1758-61
100's	$30.10	Ibuprofen, Goldline Labs	00182-1810-89
100's	$31.33	Ibuprofen, Vangard Labs	00615-2526-13
100's	**$31.51**	**MOTRIN, Pharmacia & Upjohn**	**00009-7386-04**
100's	$40.00	IBU-TAB, Alra Labs	51641-0213-11
100's	$79.84	Ibuprofen, Aligen Independ	00405-4528-02
120's	$5.31	Ibuprofen, H.C.F.A. F F P	99999-1520-12
120's	$7.70	Ibuprofen, Major Pharms	00904-1758-18
180's	$7.97	Ibuprofen, H.C.F.A. F F P	99999-1520-13
180's	$12.55	Ibuprofen, Major Pharms	00904-1758-93
360's	$49.74	Ibuprofen, Rugby	00536-3978-07
500's	$22.15	Ibuprofen, United Res	00677-1032-05
500's	$22.15	Ibuprofen, Sidmak Labs	50111-0388-02
500's	$22.15	Ibuprofen, H.C.F.A. F F P	99999-1520-11
500's	$29.63	Ibuprofen, IDE-Interstate	00814-3814-28
500's	$29.75	Ibuprofen, Consolidated Midland	00223-1092-05
500's	$61.90	Ibuprofen, Mova Pharms	55370-0534-08
500's	$64.00	Ibuprofen, Voluntary Hosp	53258-0139-05
500's	$65.32	Ibuprofen, Purepac Pharm	00228-2125-50
500's	$65.65	Ibuprofen, Teva	00093-0492-05
500's	$65.95	Ibuprofen, H N Norton Co.	50732-0747-05
500's	$66.79	IBU-TAB, Alra Labs	51641-0213-05
500's	$67.45	IBREN, Embrex Economed	38130-0053-05
500's	$67.91	Ibuprofen, Qualitest Pharms	00603-4019-28
500's	$68.69	Ibuprofen, Rugby	00536-4605-05
500's	$68.75	Ibuprofen, Goldline Labs	00182-1810-05
500's	$68.75	MORPEN, Major Pharms	00904-1658-40
500's	$68.75	Ibuprofen, Major Pharms	00904-1758-40
500's	$68.90	Ibuprofen, Mutual Pharm	53489-0132-05
500's	$72.00	Ibuprofen, Winsor Pharm	59004-0160-80
500's	$72.00	Ibuprofen, Greenstone	59762-7379-02
500's	$72.15	Ibu, Knoll Labs	00044-0162-05
500's	$75.20	Ibuprofen, HL Moore Drug Exch	00839-7113-12
500's	$79.35	Ibuprofen, Parmed Pharms	00349-8425-05
500's	$83.20	Ibuprofen, Schein Pharm (US)	00364-0766-05
500's	$83.36	Ibuprofen, Geneva Pharms	00781-1362-05
500's	$83.63	Ibuprofen, Lederle Pharm	00005-3122-31
500's	$83.75	Ibuprofen, Par Pharm	49884-0163-05
500's	$83.75	Ibuprofen, Par Pharm	49884-0468-05
500's	$87.95	Ibuprofen, HL Moore Drug Exch	00839-7700-12
500's	$90.00	Ibuprofen, Warner Chilcott	00047-0922-30
500's	$90.95	Ibuprofen, Mylan	00378-1601-05
500's	$112.86	Ibuprofen, Voluntary Hosp	53258-0803-05
500's	**$116.48**	**MOTRIN, Pharmacia & Upjohn**	**00009-7386-02**
600's	$165.00	Ibuprofen, Medirex	57480-0337-06
750's	$97.61	Ibuprofen, Glasgow Pharm	60809-0129-55
750's	$97.61	Ibuprofen, Glasgow Pharm	60809-0129-72
1000's	$44.30	Ibuprofen, H.C.F.A. F F P	99999-1520-14
1000's	$75.94	Ibuprofen, Rugby	00536-4605-10
1000's	$120.00	Ibuprofen, Parmed Pharms	00349-8425-10
1000's	$125.49	IBU-TAB, Alra Labs	51641-0213-10
1080's	$105.18	Ibuprofen, Rugby	00536-3978-11
8000's	$354.40	Ibuprofen, H.C.F.A. F F P	99999-1520-15
8000's	**$1031.28**	**MOTRIN, Pharmacia & Upjohn**	**00009-7386-03**

Tablet, Coated - Oral - 800 mg

30's	$1.84	Ibuprofen, H.C.F.A. F F P	99999-1520-16
30's	$3.95	Ibuprofen, Major Pharms	00904-1760-46
30's	$6.24	Ibuprofen, Talbert Phcy	44514-0637-18
50's	$3.07	Ibuprofen, H.C.F.A. F F P	99999-1520-17
50's	$10.40	Ibuprofen, Talbert Phcy	44514-0637-33
90's	$5.53	Ibuprofen, H.C.F.A. F F P	99999-1520-18
90's	$9.20	Ibuprofen, Major Pharms	00904-1760-89
90's	$18.72	Ibuprofen, Talbert Phcy	44514-0637-54
90's	**$33.25**	**MOTRIN, Pharmacia & Upjohn**	**00009-7387-05**
100's	$6.15	Ibuprofen, United Res	00677-1119-01
100's	$6.15	Ibuprofen, H.C.F.A. F F P	99999-1520-19
100's	$8.79	Ibuprofen, US Trading	56126-0359-11
100's	$9.45	Ibuprofen, IDE-Interstate	00814-3816-14
100's	$13.25	Ibuprofen, Consolidated Midland	00223-1093-01
100's	$14.50	Ibuprofen, Raway	00686-0596-20
100's	$20.71	Ibuprofen, PRL Enterpr	53633-0359-11
100's	$20.80	Ibuprofen, Talbert Phcy	44514-0637-88
100's	$21.45	Ibuprofen, Sidmak Labs	50111-0451-01
100's	$21.50	IBU-TAB, Alra Labs	51641-0212-01
100's	$21.89	Ibuprofen, Lederle Pharm	00005-3221-23
100's	$21.90	Ibuprofen, Qualitest Pharms	00603-4020-21
100's	$21.95	Ibuprofen, Major Pharms	00904-1760-60
100's	$22.07	Ibuprofen, Purepac Pharm	00228-2111-10
100's	$22.63	Ibuprofen, Caremark	00339-5919-12
100's	$22.75	Ibuprofen, Rugby	00536-4606-01
100's	$23.00	Ibuprofen, Goldline Labs	00182-1297-01
100's	$23.00	Ibuprofen, H N Norton Co.	50732-0781-01
100's	$23.00	Ibuprofen, Winsor Pharm	59004-0180-50
100's	$23.00	Ibuprofen, Greenstone	59762-7380-01
100's	$23.05	Ibu, Knoll Labs	00044-0173-01
100's	$23.10	Ibuprofen, Schein Pharm (US)	00364-2137-01
100's	$23.18	Ibuprofen, Aligen Independ	00405-4529-01
100's	$23.89	Ibuprofen, Par Pharm	49884-0216-01
100's	$23.89	Ibuprofen, Par Pharm	49884-0469-01
100's	$24.02	Ibuprofen, HL Moore Drug Exch	00839-7239-06
100's	$24.95	Ibuprofen, Parmed Pharms	00349-8609-01
100's	$25.04	Ibuprofen, HL Moore Drug Exch	00839-7236-06
100's	$25.20	Ibuprofen, Warner Chilcott	00047-0914-24
100's	$25.20	Ibuprofen, Geneva Pharms	00781-1363-01
100's	$27.00	Ibuprofen, Winsor Pharm	59004-0180-55
100's	$28.40	Ibuprofen, Voluntary Hosp	53258-0218-13
100's	$29.00	Ibuprofen, Medirex	57480-0338-01
100's	$30.78	Ibuprofen, Voluntary Hosp	53258-0218-01

HOW SUPPLIED - RATED THERAPEUTICALLY EQUIVALENT: *(cont'd)*

100's	$32.10	Ibuprofen, Goldline Labs	00182-1297-89
100's	$32.53	Ibuprofen, Vangard Labs	00615-2528-13
100's	$33.06	Ibuprofen, Schein Pharm (US)	00364-2137-90
100's	$35.93	Ibuprofen, Major Pharms	00904-1760-61
100's	**$36.93**	**MOTRIN, Pharmacia & Upjohn**	**00009-7387-01**
100's	**$39.92**	**MOTRIN, Pharmacia & Upjohn**	**00009-7387-04**
100's	$46.15	IBU-TAB, Alra Labs	51641-0212-11
100's	$106.89	Ibuprofen, Aligen Independ	00405-4529-02
360's	$76.76	Ibuprofen, Rugby	00536-3979-07
500's	$30.75	Ibuprofen, United Res	00677-1119-05
500's	$30.75	Ibuprofen, Sidmak Labs	50111-0451-02
500's	$30.75	Ibuprofen, H.C.F.A. F F P	99999-1520-20
500's	$44.40	Ibuprofen, IDE-Interstate	00814-3816-28
500's	$44.50	Ibuprofen, Consolidated Midland	00223-1093-05
500's	$46.15	IBU-TAB, Alra Labs	51641-0212-05
500's	$87.54	Ibuprofen, Lederle Pharm	00005-3221-31
500's	$90.40	Ibuprofen, Mova Pharms	55370-0535-08
500's	$103.15	Ibuprofen, Qualitest Pharms	00603-4020-28
500's	$104.00	Ibuprofen, Winsor Pharm	59004-0180-80
500's	$104.00	Ibuprofen, Greenstone	59762-7380-02
500's	$104.10	Ibu, Knoll Labs	00044-0173-05
500's	$104.88	Ibuprofen, Rugby	00536-4606-05
500's	$104.90	Ibuprofen, Major Pharms	00904-1760-40
500's	$108.00	Ibuprofen, Goldline Labs	00182-1297-05
500's	$108.00	Ibuprofen, H N Norton Co.	50732-0781-05
500's	$110.00	Ibuprofen, Parmed Pharms	00349-8609-05
500's	$119.45	Ibuprofen, Par Pharm	49884-0216-05
500's	$119.45	Ibuprofen, Par Pharm	49884-0469-05
500's	$119.70	Ibuprofen, Geneva Pharms	00781-1363-05
500's	$124.00	Ibuprofen, Schein Pharm (US)	00364-2137-05
500's	$125.42	Ibuprofen, HL Moore Drug Exch	00839-7236-12
500's	$125.42	Ibuprofen, HL Moore Drug Exch	00839-7239-12
500's	$127.50	Ibuprofen, Warner Chilcott	00047-0914-30
500's	$127.95	Ibuprofen, Mylan	00378-1801-05
500's	**$147.73**	**MOTRIN, Pharmacia & Upjohn**	**00009-7387-02**
600's	$189.00	Ibuprofen, Medirex	57480-0338-06
750's	$148.91	Ibuprofen, Glasgow Pharm	60809-0130-55
750's	$148.91	Ibuprofen, Glasgow Pharm	60809-0130-72
1000's	$61.50	Ibuprofen, H.C.F.A. F F P	99999-1520-21
1000's	$124.00	Ibuprofen, Rugby	00536-4606-10
1000's	$181.90	Ibuprofen, Parmed Pharms	00349-8609-10
1000's	$185.25	IBU-TAB, Alra Labs	51641-0212-10
1080's	$163.45	Ibuprofen, Rugby	00536-3979-11
8000's	$492.00	Ibuprofen, H.C.F.A. F F P	99999-1520-22
8000's	**$1397.68**	**MOTRIN, Pharmacia & Upjohn**	**00009-7387-03**

HOW SUPPLIED - NOT RATED EQUIVALENT:

Powder - Oral - 40 mg/ml

15 ml	**$4.97**	**MOTRIN, McNeil Lab**	**00045-0446-15**

Suspension - Oral - 100 mg/5ml

120 ml	**$6.18**	**MOTRIN, McNeil Lab**	**00045-0448-04**
120 ml	$6.44	CHILDREN'S ADVIL, Wyeth Labs	00008-0800-01
120 ml x 24	**$148.32**	**MOTRIN, McNeil Lab**	**00045-0448-03**
480 ml	**$20.66**	**MOTRIN, McNeil Lab**	**00045-0448-16**
480 ml	$21.52	CHILDREN'S ADVIL, Wyeth Labs	00008-0800-03
480 ml x 12	**$247.91**	**MOTRIN, McNeil Lab**	**00045-0448-17**

Tablet, Chewable - Oral - 50 mg

100's	**$10.79**	**MOTRIN, McNeil Lab**	**00045-0361-10**

Tablet, Chewable - Oral - 100 mg

100's	**$19.19**	**MOTRIN, McNeil Lab**	**00045-0431-10**

Tablet, Uncoated - Oral - 100 mg

100's	**$16.79**	**MOTRIN, McNeil Lab**	**00045-0445-10**

IBUTILIDE FUMARATE *(003275)*

CATEGORIES: Antiarrhythmic Agents; Arrhythmia; Myocardial Infarction; Tachycardia; FDA Approved 1996 Mar

BRAND NAMES: **Corvert**

DESCRIPTION:

Corvert Injection (ibutilide fumarate injection) is an antiarrhythmic drug with predominantly class III (cardiac action potential prolongation) properties according to the Vaughan Williams Classification. Each milliliter of Corvert Injection contains 0.1 mg of ibutilide fumarate (equivalent to 0.087 mg ibutilide free base), 0.189 mg sodium acetate trihydrate, 8.90 mg sodium chloride, hydrochloric acid to adjust pH to approximately 4.6, and Water for Injection.

Ibutilide fumarate injectionis an isotonic, clear, colorless, sterile aqueous solution.

Ibutilide fumarate has one chiral center, and exists as a racemate of the (+) and (-) enantiomers.

The chemical name for ibutilide fumarate is Methanesulfonamide, N-<4-<4-(ethylheptylamino) -l-hydroxybutyl>phenyl>, (+) (-), (E)-2-butenedioate (1:0.5) (hemifumarate salt). Its molecular formula is $C_{22}H_{38}N_2O_3S$, and its molecular weight is 442.62.

Ibutilide fumarate is a white to off-white powder with an aqueous solubility of over 100 mg/mL at pH 7 or lower.

CLINICAL PHARMACOLOGY:

Mechanism of Action: Ibutilide fumarate prolongs action potential duration in isolated adult cardiac myocytes and increases both atrial and ventricular refractoriness *in vivo*, (*i.e.*, class III electrophysiologic effects). Voltage clamp studies indicate that ibutilide fumarate, at nanomolar concentrations, delays repolarization by activation of a slow, inward current (predominantly sodium), rather than by blocking outward potassium currents, which is the mechanism by which most other class III antiarrhythmics act. These effects lead to prolongation of atrial and ventricular action potential duration and refractoriness, the predominant electrophysiologic properties of ibutilide fumarate in humans that are thought to be the basis for its antiarrhythmic effect.

Electrophysiologic Effects: Ibutilide fumarate produces mild slowing of the sinus rate and atrioventricular conduction. Ibutilide fumarate produces no clinically significant effect on QRS duration at intravenous doses up to 0.03 mg/kg administered over a 10-minute period. Although there is no established relationship between plasma concentration and antiarrhythmic effect, ibutilide fumarate produces dose-related prolongation of the QT interval, which is thought to be associated with its antiarrhythmic activity. (See WARNINGS for relationship between QTc prolongation and torsades de pointes-type arrhythmias.) In a study in healthy

CLINICAL PHARMACOLOGY: *(cont'd)*

volunteers, intravenous infusions of ibutilide fumarate resulted in prolongation of the QT interval that was directly correlated with ibutilide plasma concentration during and after 10-minute and 8-hour infusions. A steep ibutilide concentration/response (QT prolongation) relationship was shown. The maximum effect was a function of both the dose of ibutilide fumarate and the infusion rate.

Hemodynamic Effects: A study of hemodynamic function in patients with ejection fractions both above and below 35% showed no clinically significant effects on cardiac output, mean pulmonary arterial pressure, or pulmonary capillary wedge pressure at doses of ibutilide fumarate up to 0.03 mg/kg.

PHARMACOKINETICS

After intravenous infusion, ibutilide plasma concentrations rapidly decrease in a multiexponential fashion. The pharmacokinetics of ibutilide are highly variable among subjects. Ibutilide has a high systemic plasma clearance that approximates liver blood flow (about 29 mL/min/kg), a large steady-state volume of distribution (about 11 L/kg) in healthy volunteers, and minimal (about 40%) protein binding. Ibutilide is also cleared rapidly and highly distributed in patients being treated for atrial flutter or atrial fibrillation. The elimination half-life averages about 6 hours (range from 2 to 12 hours). The pharmacokinetics of ibutilide are linear with respect to the dose of ibutilide fumarate over the dose range of 0.01 mg/kg to 0.10 mg/kg. The enantiomers of ibutilide fumarate have pharmacokinetic properties similar to each other and to ibutilide fumarate.

The pharmacokinetics of ibutilide fumarate in patients with atrial flutter or atrial fibrillation are similar regardless of the type of arrhythmia, patient age, sex, or the concomitant use of digoxin, calcium channel blockers, or beta blockers.

Metabolism and Elimination: In healthy male volunteers, about 82% of a 0.01 mg/kg dose of [^{14}C] ibutilide fumarate was excreted in the urine (about 7% of the dose as unchanged ibutilide) and the remainder (about 19%) was recovered in the feces. Eight metabolites of ibutilide were detected in metabolic profiling of urine. These metabolites are thought to be formed primarily by ω-oxidation followed by sequential ω-oxidation of the heptyl side chain of ibutilide. Of the eight metabolites, only the ω-hydroxy metabolite possesses class III electrophysiologic properties similar to that of ibutilide in an *in vitro* isolated rabbit myocardium model. The plasma concentrations of this active metabolite, however, are less than 10% of that of ibutilide.

CLINICAL STUDIES:

Treatment with intravenous ibutilide fumarate for acute termination of recent onset atrial flutter/fibrillation was evaluated in 466 patients participating in two randomized, double-blind, placebo-controlled clinical trials. Patients had had their arrhythmias for 3 hours to 90 days, were anticoagulated for at least 2 weeks if atrial fibrillation was present more than 3 days, had serum potassium of at least 4.0 mEq/L and QT_c below 440 msec, and were monitored by telemetry for at least 24 hours. Patients could not be on class I or other class III antiarrhythmics (these had to be discontinued at least 5 half-lives prior to infusion) but could be on calcium channel blockers, beta blockers, or digoxin. In one trial, single 10-minute infusions of 0.005 to 0.025 mg/kg were tested in parallel groups (0.3 to 1.5 mg in a 60 kg person). In the second trial, up to two infusions of ibutilide fumarate were evaluated—the first 1.0 mg, the second given 10 minutes after completion of the first infusion, either 0.5 or 1.0 mg. In a third double blind-study, 319 patients with atrial fibrillation or atrial flutter of 3 hours to 45 days duration were randomized to receive single, 10-minute intravenous infusions of either sotalol (1.5 mg/kg) or ibutilide fumarate (1 mg or 2 mg). Among patients with atrial flutter, 53% receiving 1 mg ibutilide fumarate and 70% receiving 2 mg ibutilide fumarate converted, compared to 18% of those receiving sotalol. In patients with atrial fibrillation, 22% receiving 1 mg ibutilide fumarate and 43% receiving 2 mg ibutilide fumarate converted compared to 10% of patients receiving sotalol.

Patients in clinical trials were hemodynamically stable. Patients with specific cardiovascular conditions such as symptomatic heart failure, recent acute myocardial infarction, and angina were excluded. About two thirds had cardiovascular symptoms, and the majority of patients had left atrial enlargement, decreased left ventricular ejection fraction, a history of valvular disease, or previous history of atrial fibrillation or flutter. Electrical cardioversion was allowed 90 minutes after the infusion was complete. Patients could be given other antiarrhythmic drugs 4 hours postinfusion.

Results of the first two studies are shown in TABLE 1 and TABLE 2. Conversion of atrial flutter/fibrillation usually (70% of those who converted) occurred within 30 minutes of the start of infusion and was dose related. The latest conversion seen was at 90 minutes after the start of the infusion. Most converted patients remained in normal sinus rhythm for 24 hours. Overall responses in these patients, defined as termination of arrhythmias for any length of time during or within 1 hour following completed infusion of randomized dose, were in the range of 43% to 48% at doses above 0.0125 mg/kg (vs 2% for placebo). Twenty-four hour responses were similar. For these atrial arrhythmias, ibutilide was more effective in patients with flutter than fibrillation (>48% vs ≤40%).

TABLE 1 Percent of Patients Who Converted (First Trial)

			Ibutilide			
	n	**Placebo 41**	**0.005 mg/kg 41**	**0.01 mg/kg 40**	**0.015 mg/kg 38**	**0.025 mg/kg 40**
Both	Initially*	2	12	33	45	48
	At 24 hours†	2	12	28	42	43
Atrial flutter	Initially*	0	14	30	58	55
	At 24 hours†	0	14	30	58	50
Atrial fibrillation	Initially*	5	10	35	32	40
	At 24 hours†	5	10	25	26	35

* Percent of patients who converted within 70 minutes after the start of infusion
† Percent of patients who remained in sinus rhythm 24 hours after dosing

TABLE 2 Percent of Patients Who Converted (Second Trial)

			Ibutilide	
	n	**Placebo 86**	**1.0 mg/ 0.5 mg 86**	**1.0 mg/ 1.0 mg 94**
Both	Initially*	2	43	44
	At 24 hours†	2	34	37
Atrial flutter	Initially*	2	48	63
	At 24 hours†	2	45	59
Atrial Fibrillation	Initially*	2	38	25
	At 24 hours†	2	21	17

* Percent of patients who converted within 90 minutes after the start of infusion
† Percent of patients who remained in sinus rhythm 24 hours after dosing

CLINICAL STUDIES: *(cont'd)*

The numbers of patients who remained in the converted rhythm at the end of 24 hours were slightly less than those patients who converted initially, but the difference between conversion rates for ibutilide compared to placebo was still statistically significant. In long-term follow-up, approximately 40% of all patients remained recurrence free, usually with chronic prophylactic treatment, 400 to 500 days after acute treatment, regardless of the method of conversion.

Patients with more recent onset of arrhythmia had a higher rate of conversion. Response rates were 42% and 50% for patients with onset of atrial fibrillation/flutter for less than 30 days in the two efficacy studies compared to 16% and 31% in those with more chronic arrhythmias.

Ibutilide was equally effective in patients below and above 65 years of age and in men and women. Female patients constituted about 20% of patients in controlled studies.

INDICATIONS AND USAGE:

Ibutilide fumarate is indicated for the rapid conversion of atrial fibrillation or atrial flutter of recent onset to sinus rhythm. Patients with atrial arrhythmias of longer duration are less likely to respond to ibutilide fumarate. The effectiveness of ibutilide has not been determined in patients with arrhythmias of more than 90 days in duration.

Life-Threatening Arrhythmias-Appropriate Treatment Environment

Ibutilide fumarate can cause potentially fatal arrhythmias, particularly sustained polymorphic ventricular tachycardia, usually in association with QT prolongation (torsades de pointes), but sometimes without documented QT prolongation. In clinical studies, these arrhythmias, which require cardioversion, occurred in 1.7% of treated patients during, or within a number of hours of, use of ibutilide fumarate. These arrhythmias can be reversed if treated promptly (see WARNINGS, Proarrhythmia). It is essential that ibutilide fumarate be administered in a setting of continuous ECG monitoring and by personnel trained in identification and treatment of acute ventricular arrhythmias, particularly polymorphic ventricular tachycardia. *Patients with atrial fibrillation of more than 2 to 3 days duration must be adequately anticoagulated, generally for at least 2 weeks.*

Choice of Patients

Patients with chronic atrial fibrillation have a strong tendency to revert after conversion to sinus rhythm (see CLINICAL STUDIES) and treatments to maintain sinus rhythm carry risks. Patients to be treated with ibutilide fumarate, therefore, should be carefully selected such that the expected benefits of maintaining sinus rhythm outweigh the immediate risks of ibutilide fumarate, and the risks of maintenance therapy, and are likely to offer an advantage compared with alternative management.

CONTRAINDICATIONS:

Ibutilide fumarate is contraindicated in patients who have previously demonstrated hypersensitivity to ibutilide fumarate or any of the other product components.

WARNINGS:

Proarrhythmia: Like other antiarrhythmic agents, ibutilide fumarate can induce or worsen ventricular arrhythmias in some patients. This may have potentially fatal consequences. Torsades de pointes, a polymorphic ventricular tachycardia that develops in the setting of a prolonged QT interval, may occur because of the effect ibutilide fumarate has on cardiac repolarization, but ibutilide fumarate can also cause polymorphic VT in the absence of excessive prolongation of the QT interval. In general, with drugs that prolong the QT interval, the risk of torsades de pointes is thought to increase progressively as the QT interval is prolonged and may be worsened with bradycardia, a varying heart rate, and hypokalemia. In clinical trials conducted in patients with atrial fibrillation and atrial flutter, those with QT_c intervals >440 msec were not usually allowed to participate, and serum potassium had to be above 4.0 mEq/L. Although change in QT_c was dose dependent for ibutilide, there was no clear relationship between risk of serious proarrhythmia and dose in clinical studies, possibly due to the small number of events. In clinical trials of intravenous ibutilide, patients with a history of congestive heart failure (CHF) or low left ventricular ejection fraction appeared to have a higher incidence of sustained polymorphic ventricular tachycardia (VT), than those without such underlying conditions; for sustained polymorphic VT the rate was 5.4% in patients with a history of CHF and 0.8% without it. There was also a suggestion that women had a higher risk of proarrhythmia, but the sex difference was not observed in all studies and was most prominent for nonsustained ventricular tachycardia. The incidence of sustained ventricular arrhythmias was similar in male (1.8%) and female (1.5%) patients, possibly due to the small number of events. Ibutilide fumarate is not recommended in patients who have previously demonstrated polymorphic ventricular tachycardia (*e.g.,* torsades de pointes).

During clinical trials, 1.7% of patients with atrial flutter or atrial fibrillation treated with ibutilide fumarate developed sustained polymorphic ventricular tachycardia requiring cardioversion. In these clinical trials, many initial episodes of polymorphic ventricular tachycardia occurred after the infusion of ibutilide fumarate was stopped but generally not more than 40 minutes after the start of the first infusion. There were, however, instances of recurrent polymorphic VT that occurred about 3 hours after the initial infusion. In two cases, the VT degenerated into ventricular fibrillation, requiring immediate defibrillation. Other cases were managed with cardiac pacing and magnesium sulfate infusions. Nonsustained polymorphic ventricular tachycardia occurred in 2.7% of patients and nonsustained monomorphic ventricular tachycardias occurred in 4.9% of the patients (see ADVERSE REACTIONS).

Proarrhythmic events must be anticipated. Skilled personnel and proper equipment, including cardiac monitoring equipment, intracardiac pacing facilities, a cardioverter/defibrillator, and medication for treatment of sustained ventricular tachycardia, including polymorphic ventricular tachycardia, must be available during and after administration of ibutilide fumarate. Before treatment with ibutilide fumarate, hypokalemia and hypomagnesemia should be corrected to reduce the potential for proarrhythmia. Patients should be observed with continuous ECG monitoring for at least 4 hours following infusion or until QTc has returned to baseline. Longer monitoring is required if any arrhythmic activity is noted. Management of polymorphic ventricular tachycardia includes discontinuation of ibutilide, correction of electrolyte abnormalities, especially potassium and magnesium, and overdrive cardiac pacing, electrical cardioversion, or defibrillation. Pharmacologic therapies include magnesium sulfate infusions. Treatment with antiarrhythmics should generally be avoided.

PRECAUTIONS:

GENERAL

Antiarrhythmics: Class Ia antiarrhythmic drugs (Vaughan Williams Classification), such as disopyramide, quinidine, and procainamide, and other class III drugs, such as amiodarone and sotalol, should not be given concomitantly with ibutilide fumarate or within 4 hours postinfusion because of their potential to prolong refractoriness. In the clinical trials, class 1 or other class III antiarrhythmic agents were withheld for at least 5 half-lives prior to ibutilide infusion and for 4 hours after dosing, but thereafter were allowed at the physician's discretion.

PRECAUTIONS: *(cont'd)*

Other Drugs That Prolong the QT Interval: The potential for proarrhythmia may increase with the administration of ibutilide fumarate to patients who are being treated with drugs that prolong the QT interval, such as phenothiazines, tricyclic antidepressants, tetracyclic antidepressants, and certain antihistamine drugs (H_1, receptor antagonists).

Heart Block: Of the nine (1.5%) ibutilide-treated patients with reports of reversible heart block, five had first degree, three had second degree, and one had complete heart block.

Laboratory Test Interactions: None known.

Carcinogenesis, Mutagenesis, and Impairment of Fertility: No animal studies have been conducted to determine the carcinogenic potential of ibutilide fumarate; however, it was not genotoxic in a battery of assays, including the Ames assay, mammalian cell forward gene mutation assay, unscheduled DNA synthesis assay, and mouse micronucleus assay. Similarly, no drug-related effects on fertility or mating were noted in a reproductive study in rats.

Pregnancy Category C: Ibutilide administered orally was teratogenic (adactyly, cleft palate, scoliosis) and embryocidal in reproduction studies in rats. On a mg/m^2 basis, corrected for the 3% oral bioavailability, the "no adverse effect dose" (5 mg/kg per day given orally) was approximately the same as the maximum recommended human dose (MRHD); the teratogenic dose (20 mg/kg per day given orally) was about four times the MRHD on a mg/m^2 basis, or 16 times the MRHD on a mg/kg basis. Ibutilide fumarate should not be administered to a pregnant woman unless clinical benefit outweighs potential risk to the fetus.

Nursing Mothers: The excretion of ibutilide into breast milk has not been studied; accordingly, breastfeeding should be discouraged during therapy with ibutilide fumarate.

Pediatric Use: Clinical trials with ibutilide fumarate in patients with atrial fibrillation and atrial flutter did not include anyone under the age of 18. Safety and effectiveness of ibutilide in pediatric patients has not been established.

Geriatric Use: The mean age of patients in clinical trials was 65. No age-related differences were observed in pharmacokinetic, efficacy, or safety parameters for patients less than 65 compared to patients 65 years and older.

Use in Patients With Hepatic or Renal Dysfunction: The safety, effectiveness, and pharmacokinetics of ibutilide fumarate have not been established in patients with hepatic or renal dysfunction. However, it is unlikely that dosing adjustments would be necessary in patients with compromised renal or hepatic function based on the following considerations: (1) ibutilide fumarate is indicated for rapid intravenous therapy (duration ≤30 minutes) and is dosed to a known, well-defined pharmacologic action (termination of arrhythmia) or to a maximum of two 10-minute infusions; (2) less than 10% of the dose of ibutilide fumarate is excreted unchanged in the urine; and (3) drug distribution appears to be one of the primary mechanisms responsible for termination of the pharmacologic effect. Nonetheless, patients with abnormal liver function should be monitored by telemetry for more than the 4-hour period generally recommended.

In 285 patients with atrial fibrillation or atrial flutter who were treated with ibutilide fumarate, the clearance of ibutilide was independent of renal function, as assessed by creatinine clearance (range 21 to 140 ml/min).

DRUG INTERACTIONS:

No specific pharmacokinetic or other formal drug interaction studies were conducted.

Digoxin: Supraventricular arrhythmias may mask the cardiotoxicity associated with excessive digoxin levels. Therefore, it is advisable to be particularly cautious in patients whose plasma digoxin levels are above or suspected to be above the usual therapeutic range. Coadministration of digoxin did not have effects on either the safety or efficacy of ibutilide in the clinical trials.

Calcium Channel Blocking Agents: Coadministration of calcium channel blockers did not have any effect on either the safety or efficacy of ibutilide in the clinical trials.

Beta-adrenergic Blocking Agents: Coadministration of beta-adrenergic blocking agents did not have any effect on either the safety or efficacy of ibutilide in the clinical trials.

ADVERSE REACTIONS:

Ibutilide fumarate injection was generally well tolerated in clinical trials. Of the 586 patients with atrial fibrillation or atrial flutter who received ibutilide fumarate in phase II/III studies, 149 (25%) reported medical events related to the cardiovascular system, including sustained polymorphic ventricular tachycardia (1.7%) and nonsustained polymorphic ventricular tachycardia (2.7%).

Other clinically important adverse events with an uncertain relationship to ibutilide fumarate include the following (0.2% represents one patient): sustained monomorphic ventricular tachycardia (0.2%), nonsustained monomorphic ventricular tachycardia (4.9%), AV block (1.5%), bundle branch block (1.9%), ventricular extrasystoles (5.1%), supraventricular extrasystoles (0.9%), hypotension/postural hypotension (2.0%), bradycardia/sinus bradycardia (1.2%), nodal arrhythmia (0.7%), congestive heart failure (0.5%), tachycardia/sinus tachycardia/supraventricular tachycardia (2.7%), idioventricular rhythm (0.2%), syncope (0.3%), and renal failure (0.3%). The incidence of these events, except for syncope, was greater in the group treated with ibutilide fumarate than in the placebo group.

Another adverse reaction that may be associated with the administration of ibutilide fumarate was nausea, which occurred with a frequency greater than 1% more in ibutilide-treated patients than those treated with placebo.

The medical events reported for more than 1% of the placebo- and ibutilide-treated patients are shown in TABLE 3.

TABLE 3 Treatment-Emergent Medical Events With Frequency of More Than 1% and Higher Than That of Placebo

Event	Placebo N=127 Patients		All Ibutilide N=586 Patients	
	n	%	n	%
Cardiovascular				
Venticular extrasystoles	1	0.8	30	5.1
Nonsustained monomorphic VT	1	0.8	29	4.9
Nonsustained polymorphic VT			16	2.7
Hypotension	2	1.6	12	2.0
Bundle branch block			11	1.9
Sustained polymorphic VT			10	1.7
AV block	1	0.8	9	1.5
Hypertension			7	1.2
QT segment prolonged			7	1.2
Bradycardia	1	0.8	7	1.2
Palpitation	1	0.8	6	1.0
Tachycardia	1	0.8	16	2.7
Gastrointestinal				
Nausea	1	0.8	11	1.9
Central Nervous System				
Headache	4	3.1	21	3.6

OVERDOSAGE:

Acute Experience in Animals: Acute overdose in animals results in CNS toxicity; notably, CNS depression, rapid gasping breathing, and convulsions. The intravenous median lethal dose in the rat was more than 50 mg/kg which is, on a mg/m^2 basis, at least 250 times the maximum recommended human dose.

Human Experience: In the clinical trials with ibutilide fumarate, four patients were unintentionally overdosed. The largest dose was 3.4 mg administered over 15 minutes. One patient (0.025 mg/kg) developed increased ventricular ectopy and monomorphic ventricular tachycardia, another patient (0.032 mg/kg) developed AV block-3rd degree and nonsustained polymorphic VT, and two patients (0.038 and 0.020 mg/kg) had no medical event reports. Based on known pharmacology, the clinical effects of an overdosage with ibutilide could exaggerate the expected prolongation of repolarization seen at usual clinical doses. Medical events (*e.g.*, proarrhythmia, AV block) that occur after the overdosage should be treated with measures appropriate for that condition.

DOSAGE AND ADMINISTRATION:

The recommended dose based on controlled trials (see CLINICAL STUDIES) is outlined in TABLE 4. Ibutilide infusion should be stopped as soon as the presenting arrhythmia is terminated or in the event of sustained or nonsustained ventricular tachycardia, or marked prolongation of QT or QT$_c$.

TABLE 4

Patient Weight	Initial Infusion (over 10 minutes)	Second Infusion
60 kg (132 lb) or more	One vial (1 mg ibutilide fumarate)	If the arrhythmia does not terminate within 10 minutes after the end of the initial infusion, a second 10-minute infusion of equal strength may be administered 10 minutes after completion of the first infusion.
Less than 60 kg (132 lb)	0.1 ml/kg (0.01 mg/kg ibulitide fumarate)	

In a trial comparing ibutilide and sotalol (see CLINICAL STUDIES), 2 mg ibutilide fumarate administered as a single infusion to patients weighing more than 60 kg was also effective in terminating atrial fibrillation or atrial flutter.

Patients should be observed with continuous ECG monitoring for at least 4 hours following infusion or until QTc has returned to baseline. Longer monitoring is required if any arrhythmic activity is noted. Skilled personnel and proper equipment (see WARNINGS, Proarrhythmia), such as a cardioverter/defibrillator, and medication for treatment of sustained ventricular tachycardia, including polymorphic ventricular tachycardia, must be available during administration of ibutilide fumarate and subsequent monitoring of the patient.

Dilution: Ibutilide fumarate may be administered undiluted or diluted in 50 mL of diluent. Ibutilide fumarate may be added to 0.9% sodium chloride injection or 5% dextrose injection before infusion. The contents of one 10-ml vial (0.1 mg/ml) may be added to a 50-ml infusion bag to form an admixture of approximately 0.017 mg/ml ibutilide fumarate. Parenteral drug products should be inspected visually for particulate matter and discoloration prior to administration whenever solution and container permit.

Compatibility and Stability: The following diluents are compatible with ibutilide fumarate injection (0.1 mg/ml):

5% dextrose injection

0.9% sodium chloride injection

The following intravenous solution containers are compatible with admixtures of ibutilide fumarate (0.1 mg/mL):

polyvinyl chloride plastic bags

polyolefin bags

Admixtures of the product, with approved diluents, are chemically and physically stable for 24 hours at room temperature (15° to 30°C or 59° to 86°F) and for 48 hours at refrigerated temperatures (2° to 8°C or 36° to 46°F). Strict adherence to the use of aseptic technique during the preparation of the admixture is recommended in order to maintain sterility.

HOW SUPPLIED:

Corvert Injection (ibutilide fumarate injection) is supplied as an acetate-buffered isotonic solution at a concentration of 0.1 mg/ml that has been adjusted to approximately pH 4.6 in 10-ml clear glass flip-top vials.

Store at controlled room temperature (20° to 25°C or 68° to 77°F). Store vial in carton until used.

ICHTHAMMOL *(001522)*

CATEGORIES: Keratoplastic Agents; Pharmaceutical Adjuvants; Skin/Mucous Membrane Agents; FDA Pre 1938 Drugs

Prescribing information not available at time of publication.

HOW SUPPLIED - EQUIVALENTS NOT AVAILABLE:

Ointment - Topical - 10 %

30 gm	$1.51	Ichthammol, Qualitest Pharms	00603-7791-78

Powder

120 gm	$13.30	Ichthammol, Millgood	53118-0712-04
454 gm	$30.80	Ichthammol, Millgood	53118-0712-10

IDARUBICIN HYDROCHLORIDE *(003013)*

CATEGORIES: Antineoplastics; Cancer; Chemotherapy; Leukemia; Leukemia, Acute Myeloid; Orphan Drugs; Pregnancy Category D; FDA Class 1A ("Important Therapeutic Advantage"); FDA Approved 1990 Sep

BRAND NAMES: **Idamycin**; *Zavedos* (Australia, England, France, Germany)
(International brand names outside U.S. in italics)

WARNING:

1. Idamycin should be given slowly into a freely flowing intravenous infusion. It must never be given intramuscularly or subcutaneously. Severe local tissue necrosis can occur if there is extravasation during administration.
2. As is the case with other anthracyclines the use of idamycin can cause myocardial toxicity leading to congestive heart failure. Cardiac toxicity is more common in patients who have received prior anthracyclines or who have pre-existing cardiac disease.
3. As is usual with antileukemic agents, severe myelosuppression occurs when idamycin is used at effective therapeutic doses.
4. It is recommended that idamycin be administered only under the supervision of a physician who is experienced in leukemia chemotherapy and in facilities with laboratory and supportive resources adequate to monitor drug tolerance and protect and maintain a patient compromised by drug toxicity. The physician and institution must be capable of responding rapidly and completely to severe hemorrhagic conditions and/or overwhelming infection.
5. Dosage should be reduced in patients with impaired hepatic or renal function. (See DOSAGE AND ADMINISTRATION.)

DESCRIPTION:

Idamycin (idarubicin hydrochloride for injection, USP) is a sterile, synthetic antineoplastic anthracycline for intravenous use. Chemically, idarubicin hydrochloride is 5, 12-Naphthacenedione, 9-acetyl-7-[(3-amino-2,3,6-trideoxy-α-l-*lyxo*-hexopyranosyl)oxy]-7,8,9,10-tetrahydro-6, 9, 11-trihydroxy-hydrochloride, (7*S-cis*).

Empirical formula is $C_{26}H_{27}NO_9 \cdot HCl$. Molecular weight is 533.96.

Idamycin, a sterile parenteral, is available in 5 mg, 10 mg and 20 mg single use only vials.

Each 5 mg vial contains 5 mg idarubicin hydrochloride, USP and 50 mg of lactose NF (hydrous) as an orange-red, lyophilized powder.

Each 10 mg vial contains 10 mg idarubicin hydrochloride, USP and 100 mg of lactose NF (hydrous) as an orange-red, lyophilized powder.

Each 20 mg vial contains 20 mg idarubicin hydrochloride, USP and 200 mg of lactose NF (hydrous) as an orange-red, lyophilized powder.

CLINICAL PHARMACOLOGY:

Idamycin is a DNA-intercalating analog of daunorubicin which has an inhibitory effect on nucleic acid synthesis and interacts with the enzyme topoisomerase II. The absence of a methoxy group at position 4 of the anthracycline structure gives the compound a high lipophilicity which results in an increased rate of cellular uptake compared with other anthracyclines.

Pharmacokinetic studies have been performed in adult leukemia patients with normal renal and hepatic function following intravenous administration of 10 to 12 mg/m^2 of idamycin daily for 3 to 4 days, as a single agent or combined with cytarabine (Ara-C). The plasma concentrations of idamycin are best described by a two or three compartment open model. The disposition profile shows a rapid distributive phase with a very high volume of distribution presumably reflecting extensive tissue binding. The plasma clearance is twice the expected hepatic plasma flow indicating extensive extrahepatic metabolism. The drug is eliminated predominately by biliary and to a lesser extent by renal excretion, mostly in the form of the primary metabolite, 13-dihydroidarubicin (idarubicinol).

The elimination rate of idamycin from plasma is slow with an estimated mean terminal half-life of 22 hours (range: 4 to 46 hours) when used as a single agent and 20 hours (range: 7 to 38 hours) when used in combination with cytarabine. The elimination of idarubicinol is considerably slower than that of the parent drug with an estimated mean terminal half-life that exceeds 45 hours; hence its plasma levels are sustained for a period greater than 8 days. As idarubicinol has cytotoxic activity it presumably contributes to the effects of idamycin.

The extent of drug and metabolite accumulation predicted in leukemia patients for Day 2 and 3 of dosing, based on the mean plasma levels and half-life obtained after the first dose, is 1.7- and 2.3-fold, respectively, and suggests no change in kinetics following a daily x 3 regimen.

The pharmacokinetics of idamycin have not been evaluated in leukemia patients with hepatic impairment. It is expected that in patients with moderate or severe hepatic dysfunction, the metabolism of idamycin may be impaired and lead to higher systemic drug levels.

Studies of cellular (nucleated blood and bone marrow cells) drug concentrations in leukemia patients have shown that peak cellular idarubicin concentrations are reached a few minutes after injection. Idarubicin and idarubicinol concentrations in nucleated blood and bone marrow cells are more than a hundred times the plasma concentrations. Idarubicin disappearance rates in plasma and cells were comparable with a terminal half-life of about 15 hours. The terminal half-life of idarubicinol in cells was about 72 hours.

Protein binding was studied *in vitro* by equilibrium dialysis at concentrations of idarubicin and idarubicinol similar to the maximum plasma level obtained in the pharmacokinetic studies. The percentages of idarubicin and idarubicinol bound to human plasma proteins averaged 97% and 94%, respectively. The binding is concentration independent. Idamycin studies in pediatric leukemia patients, at doses of 4.2 to 13.3 mg/m^2/day × 3, suggest dose independent kinetics. There is no difference between the half-lives of the drug following daily × 3 or weekly × 3 administration.

Cerebrospinal fluid (CSF) levels of idarubicin and its active metabolite, idarubicinol, were measured in pediatric leukemia patients treated intravenously. Idarubicin was detected in 2 of 21 CSF samples (0.14 and 1.57 ng/ml), while idarubicinol was detected in 20 of these 21 CSF samples obtained 18 to 30 hours after dosing (mean = 0.51 ng/ml, range 0.22 to 1.05 ng/ml). The clinical relevance of these findings is currently being evaluated.

CLINICAL STUDIES:

Four prospective randomized studies, three U.S. and one Italian, have been conducted to compare the efficacy and safety of idarubicin (IDR) to that of daunorubicin (DNR), each in combination with cytarabine (Ara-C) as induction therapy in previously untreated adult patients with acute myeloid leukemia (AML). These data are summarized in the following table (TABLE 1A and TABLE 1B) and demonstrate significantly greater complete remission rates for the IDR regimen in two of the three U.S. studies and significantly longer overall survival for the IDR regimen in two of the three U.S. studies.

There is no consensus regarding optional regimens to be used for consolidation; however, the following consolidation regimens were used in U.S. controlled trials. Patients received the same anthracycline for consolidation as was used for induction.

Studies 1 and 3 utilized 2 courses of consolidation therapy consisting of idarubicin 12 or 13 mg/m^2 daily for 2 days, respectively (or DNR 50 or 45 mg/m^2 daily for 2 days), and Ara-C, either 25 mg/m^2 by IV bolus followed by 200 mg/m^2 daily by continuous infusion for 4 days (Study 1), or 100 mg/m^2 daily for 5 days by continuous infusion (Study 3). A rest period of 4 to 6 weeks is recommended prior to initiation of consolidation and between the courses. Hematologic recovery is mandatory prior to initiation of each consolidation course.

Study 2 utilized 3 consolidation courses, administered at intervals of 21 days or upon hematologic recovery. Each course consisted of idarubicin 15 mg/m^2 IV for 1 dose (or DNR 50 mg/m^2 IV for 1 dose), Ara-C 100 mg/m^2 every 12 hours for 10 doses and 6-thioguanine 100 mg/m^2 po for 10 doses. If severe myelosuppression occurred, subsequent courses were

CLINICAL STUDIES: *(cont'd)*

TABLE 1A

	Induction[a] Regimen Dose in mg/m^2 - Daily × 3 Days		Complete Remission Rate All Pts Randomized	
	IDR	DNR	IDR	DNR
U.S. (IND Studies)				
1. MSKCC* (Age ≤60 years)	12[b]	50[b]	51/65+ (78%)	38/65 (58%)
2. SEG** (Age ≥15 years)	12[c]	45[c]	76/111+ (69%)	65/119 (55%)
3. U.S. Multicenter (Age ≥18 years)	13[c]	45[c]	68/101 (67%)	66/113 (58%)
Foreign (non-IND study) GIMEMA*** (Age ≥55 years)	12[c]	45[c]	49/124 (40%)	49/125 (39%)

* Memorial Sloan Kettering Cancer Center
** Southeastern Cancer Study Group
*** Gruppo Italiano Malattie Ematologiche Maligne dell' Adulto
+Overall $p < 0.05$, unadjusted for prognostic factors or multiple endpoints.
[a]Patients who had persistent leukemia after the first induction course received a second course.
[b]Ara-C 25 mg/m^2 bolus IV followed by 200 mg/m^2 daily × 5 days by continuous infusion.
[c]Ara-C 100 mg/m^2 daily × 7 days by continuous infusion.

TABLE 1B

	Median Survival (Days) All Pts Randomized	
	IDR	DNR
U.S. (IND Studies) 1. MSKCC* (Age ≤60 years)	508*	435
2. SEG** (Age ≥15 years)	328	277
3. U.S. Multicenter (Age ≥18 years)	393+	281
Foreign (non-IND study) GIMEMA*** (Age ≥55 years)	87	169

* Memorial Sloan Kettering Cancer Center
** Southeastern Cancer Study Group
*** Gruppo Italiano Malattie Ematologiche Maligne dell' Adulto
+Overall $p < 0.05$, unadjusted for prognostic factors or multiple endpoints.
[a]Patients who had persistent leukemia after the first induction course received a second course.
[b]Ara-C 25 mg/m^2 bolus IV followed by 200 mg/m^2 daily × 5 days by continuous infusion.
[c]Ara-C 100 mg/m^2 daily × 7 days by continuous infusion.

given with 25% reduction in the doses of all drugs. In addition, this study included 4 courses of maintenance therapy (2 days of the same anthracycline as was used in induction and 5 days of Ara-C).

Toxicities and duration of aplasia were similar during induction on the 2 arms in the U.S. studies except for an increase in mucositis on the IDR arm in one study. During consolidation, duration of aplasia on the IDR arm was longer in all three studies and mucositis was more frequent in two studies. During consolidation, transfusion requirements were higher on the IDR arm in the two studies in which they were tabulated, and patients on the IDR arm in Study 3 spent more days on IV antibiotics (Study 3 used a higher dose of idamycin).

The benefit of consolidation and maintenance therapy in prolonging the duration of remission and survival is not proven.

Intensive maintenance with idamycin is not recommended in view of the considerable toxicity (including deaths in remission) experienced by patients during the maintenance phase of Study 2.

A higher induction death rate was noted in patients on the IDR arm in the Italian trial. Since this was not noted in patients of similar age in the U.S. trials, one may speculate that it was due to a difference in the level of supportive care.

INDICATIONS AND USAGE:

Idamycin in combination with other approved antileukemic drugs is indicated for the treatment of acute myeloid leukemia (AML) in adults. This includes French-American-British (FAB) classifications M1 through M7.

WARNINGS:

Idamycin is intended for administration under the supervision of a physician who is experienced in leukemia chemotherapy.

Idamycin is a potent bone marrow suppressant. Idamycin should not be given to patients with pre-existing bone marrow suppression induced by previous drug therapy or radiotherapy unless the benefit warrants the risk.

Severe myelosuppression will occur in all patients given a therapeutic dose of this agent for induction, consolidation or maintenance. Careful hematologic monitoring is required. Deaths due to infection and/or bleeding have been reported during the period of severe myelosuppression. Facilities with laboratory and supportive resources adequate to monitor drug tolerability and protect and maintain a patient compromised by drug toxicity should be available. It must be possible to treat rapidly and completely a severe hemorrhagic condition and/or a severe infection.

Pre-existing heart disease and previous therapy with anthracyclines at high cumulative doses or other potentially cardiotoxic agents are co-factors for increased risk of idarubicin-induced cardiac toxicity and the benefit to risk ratio of idarubicin therapy in such patients should be weighed before starting treatment with idamycin.

Myocardial toxicity as manifested by potentially fatal congestive heart failure, acute life-threatening arrhythmias or other cardiomyopathies may occur following therapy with idamycin. Appropriate therapeutic measures for the management of congestive heart failure and/or arrhythmias are indicated.

Cardiac function should be carefully monitored during treatment in order to minimize the risk of cardiac toxicity of the type described for other anthracycline compounds. The risk of such myocardial toxicity may be higher following concomitant or previous radiation to the mediastinal-pericardial area or in patients with anemia, bone marrow depression, infections,

WARNINGS: *(cont'd)*

leukemic pericarditis and/or myocarditis. While there are no reliable means for predicting congestive heart failure, cardiomyopathy induced by anthracyclines is usually associated with a decrease of the left ventricular ejection fraction (LVEF) from pretreatment baseline values.

Since hepatic and/or renal function impairment can affect the disposition of idamycin, liver and kidney function should be evaluated with conventional clinical laboratory tests (using serum bilirubin and serum creatinine as indicators) prior to and during treatment. In a number of Phase III clinical trials, treatment was not given if bilirubin and/or creatinine serum levels exceeded 2 mg%. However, in one Phase III trial, patients with bilirubin levels between 2.6 and 5 mg% received the anthracycline with a 50% reduction in dose. Dose reduction of idamycin should be considered if the bilirubin and/or creatinine levels are above the normal range. (See DOSAGE AND ADMINISTRATION.)

Pregnancy Category D: Idarubicin was embryotoxic and teratogenic in the rat at a dose of 1.2 $mg/m^2/day$ or one tenth the human dose, which was nontoxic to dams. Idarubicin was embryotoxic but not teratogenic in the rabbit even at a dose of 2.4 $mg/m^2/day$ or two tenths the human dose, which was toxic to dams. There is no conclusive information about idarubicin adversely affecting human fertility or causing teratogenesis.

There are no adequate and well-controlled studies in pregnant women. If idamycin is to be used during pregnancy, or if the patient becomes pregnant during therapy, the patient should be apprised of the potential hazard to the fetus. Women of childbearing potential should be advised to avoid pregnancy.

PRECAUTIONS:

General: Therapy with idamycin requires close observation of the patient and careful laboratory monitoring. Hyperuricemia secondary to rapid lysis of leukemic cells may be induced. Appropriate measures must be taken to prevent hyperuricemia and to control any systemic infection before beginning therapy.

Extravasation of idamycin can cause severe local tissue necrosis. Extravasation may occur with or without an accompanying stinging or burning sensation even if blood returns well on aspiration of the infusion needle. If signs or symptoms of extravasation occur the injection or infusion should be terminated immediately and restarted in another vein. (See DOSAGE AND ADMINISTRATION.)

Laboratory Tests: Frequent complete blood counts and monitoring of hepatic and renal function tests are recommended.

Carcinogenesis, Mutagenesis, and Impairment of Fertility: Formal long-term carcinogenicity studies have not been conducted with idamycin. Idamycin and related compounds have been shown to have mutagenic and carcinogenic properties when tested in experimental models (including bacterial systems, mammalian cells in culture and female Sprague-Dawley rats).

In male dogs given 1.8 $mg/m^2/day$ or more idarubicin (3 times/week for 13 weeks), testicular atrophy was observed with inhibition of spermiogenesis and sperm maturation, and few or no mature sperm. Effects were not readily reversible after an eight week recovery period.

Pregnancy Category D: (See WARNINGS.)

Nursing Mothers: It is not known whether this drug is excreted in human milk. Because many drugs are excreted in human milk and because of the potential for serious adverse reactions in nursing infants from idarubicin, mothers should discontinue nursing prior to taking this drug.

Pediatric Use: Safety and effectiveness in children have not been established.

ADVERSE REACTIONS:

Approximately 550 patients with AML have received idamycin in combination with Ara-C in controlled clinical trials worldwide. In addition, over 550 patients with acute leukemia have been treated in uncontrolled trials utilizing idamycin as a single agent or in combination. The table below (TABLE 2) lists the adverse experiences reported in U.S. Study 2 (see CLINICAL STUDIES) and is representative of the experiences in other studies. These adverse experiences constitute all reported or observed experiences, including those not considered to be drug related. Patients undergoing induction therapy for AML are seriously ill due to their disease, are receiving multiple transfusions, and concomitant medications including potentially toxic antibiotics and antifungal agents. The contribution of the study drug to the adverse experience profile is difficult to establish.

TABLE 2

Induction Phase	Percentage of Patients	
Adverse Experiences	IDR (N=110)	DNR (N=118)
Infection	95%	97%
Nausea & Vomiting	82%	80%
Hair Loss	77%	72%
Abdominal Cramps/Diarrhea	73%	68%
Hemorrhage	63%	65%
Mucositis	50%	55%
Dermatologic	46%	40%
Mental Status	41%	34%
Pulmonary-Clinical	39%	39%
Fever (not elsewhere classified)	26%	28%
Headache	20%	24%
Cardiac-Clinical	16%	24%
Neurologic-Peripheral Nerves	7%	9%
Pulmonary Allergy	2%	4%
Seizure	4%	5%
Cerebellar	4%	4%

The duration of aplasia and incidence of mucositis were greater on the IDR arm than the DNR arm, especially during consolidation in some U.S. controlled trials (see CLINICAL STUDIES).

The following information reflects experience based on U.S. controlled clinical trials.

Myelosuppression: Severe myelosuppression is the major toxicity associated with idamycin therapy, but this effect of the drug is required in order to eradicate the leukemic clone. During the period of myelosuppression, patients are at risk of developing infection and bleeding which may be life-threatening or fatal.

Gastrointestinal: Nausea and/or vomiting, mucositis, abdominal pain and diarrhea were reported frequently, but were severe (equivalent to WHO Grade 4) in less than 5% of patients. Severe enterocolitis with perforation has been reported rarely. The risk of perforation may be increased by instrumental intervention. The possibility of perforation should be considered in patients who develop severe abdominal pain and appropriate steps for diagnosis and management should be taken.

Dermatologic: Alopecia was reported frequently and dermatologic reactions including generalized rash, urticaria and a bullous erythrodermatous rash of the palms and soles have occurred. The dermatologic reactions were usually attributed to concomitant antibiotic therapy. Local reactions including hives at the injection site have been reported.

ADVERSE REACTIONS: *(cont'd)*

Hepatic and Renal: Changes in hepatic and renal function tests have been observed. These changes were usually transient and occurred in the setting of sepsis and while patients were receiving potentially hepatotoxic and nephrotoxic antibiotics and antifungal agents. Severe changes in renal function (equivalent to WHO Grade 4) occurred in no more than 1% of patients, while severe changes in hepatic function (equivalent to WHO Grade 4) occurred in less than 5% of patients.

Cardiac: Congestive heart failure (frequently attributed to fluid overload), serious arrhythmias including atrial fibrillation, chest pain, myocardial infarction and asymptomatic declines in LVEF have been reported in patients undergoing induction therapy for AML. Myocardial insufficiency and arrhythmias were usually reversible and occurred in the setting of sepsis, anemia and aggressive intravenous fluid administration. The events were reported more frequently in patients over age 60 years and in those with pre-existing cardiac disease.

OVERDOSAGE:

There is no known antidote to idamycin. Two cases of fatal overdosage in patients receiving therapy for AML have been reported. The doses were 135 mg/m^2 over 3 days and 45 mg/m^2 of idarubicin and 90 mg/m^2 of daunorubicin over a three day period.

It is anticipated that overdosage with idarubicin will result in severe and prolonged myelosuppression and possibly in increased severity of gastrointestinal toxicity. Adequate supportive care including platelet transfusions, antibiotics and symptomatic treatment of mucositis is required. The effect of acute overdose on cardiac function is not fully known, but severe arrhythmia occurred in 1 of the 2 patients exposed. It is anticipated that very high doses of idarubicin may cause acute cardiac toxicity and may be associated with a higher incidence of delayed cardiac failure.

Disposition studies with idarubicin in patients undergoing dialysis have not been carried out. The profound multicompartment behavior, extensive extravascular distribution and tissue binding, coupled with the low unbound fraction available in the plasma pool make it unlikely that therapeutic efficacy or toxicity would be altered by conventional peritoneal or hemodialysis.

DOSAGE AND ADMINISTRATION:

(See WARNINGS).

For induction therapy in adult patients with AML the following dose schedule is recommended:

Idamycin 12 mg/m^2 daily for 3 days by slow (10 to 15 min) intravenous injection in combination with Ara-C. The Ara-C may be given as 100 mg/m^2 daily by continuous infusion for 7 days or as Ara-C 25 mg/m^2 intravenous bolus followed by Ara-C 200 mg/m^2 daily for 5 days continuous infusion. In patients with unequivocal evidence of leukemia after the first induction course, a second course may be administered. Administration of the second course should be delayed in patients who experience severe mucositis, until recovery from this toxicity has occurred, and a dose reduction of 25% is recommended. In patients with hepatic and/or renal impairment, a dose reduction of idamycin should be considered. Idamycin should not be administered if the bilirubin level exceeds 5 mg%. (See WARNINGS.)

The benefit of consolidation in prolonging the duration of remissions and survival is not proven. There is no consensus regarding optional regimens to be used for consolidation. (See CLINICAL STUDIES for doses used in U.S. Clinical studies.)

Preparation of Solution: Caution in handling of the powder and preparation of the solution must be exercised as skin reactions associated with idamycin may occur. Skin accidentally exposed to idamycin should be washed thoroughly with soap and water and if the eyes are involved, standard irrigation techniques should be used immediately. The use of goggles, gloves, and protective gowns is recommended during preparation and administration of the drug.

Idamycin 5 mg, 10 mg and 20 mg vials should be reconstituted with 5 ml, 10 ml and 20 ml, respectively, of Sodium Chloride Injection USP (0.9%) to give a final concentration of 1 mg/ml of idarubicin hydrochloride. Bacteriostatic diluents are not recommended.

The vial contents are under a negative pressure to minimize aerosol formation during reconstitution; therefore, particular care should be taken when the needle is inserted. Inhalation of any aerosol produced during reconstitution must be avoided.

Reconstituted solutions are physically and chemically stable for at least 168 hours (7 days) under refrigeration (2° to 8°C, 36° to 46°F) and 72 hours (3 days) at controlled room temperature, (15° to 30°C, 59° to 86°F). Discard unused solutions in an appropriate manner (see Handling and Disposal).

Care in the administration of idamycin will reduce the chance of perivenous infiltration. It may also decrease the chance of local reactions such as urticaria and erythematous streaking. During intravenous administration of idamycin extravasation may occur with or without an accompanying stinging or burning sensation even if blood returns well on aspiration of the infusion needle. If any signs or symptoms of extravasation have occurred, the injection or infusion should be immediately terminated and restarted in another vein. If it is known or suspected that subcutaneous extravasation has occurred it is recommended that intermittent ice packs ($\frac{1}{2}$ hour immediately, then $\frac{1}{2}$ hour 4 times per day for 3 days) be placed over the area of extravasation and that the affected extremity be elevated. Because of the progressive nature of extravasation reactions, the area of injection should be frequently examined and plastic surgery consultation obtained early if there is any sign of a local reaction such as pain, erythema, edema or vesication. If ulceration begins or if there is severe persistent pain at the site of extravasation, early wide excision of the involved area should be considered.[1]

Idamycin should be administered slowly (over 10 to 15 minutes) into the tubing of a freely running intravenous infusion of sodium chloride injection USP (0.9%) or 5% dextrose injection USP. The tubing should be attached to a Butterfly needle or other suitable device and inserted preferably into a large vein.

Incompatibility: Unless specific compatibility data are available, idamycin should not be mixed with other drugs. Precipitation occurs with heparin. Prolonged contact with any solution of an alkaline pH will result in degradation of the drug.

Parenteral drug products should be inspected visually for particulate matter and discoloration prior to administration whenever solution and containers permit.

Handling and Disposal: Procedures for handling and disposal of anticancer drugs should considered. Several guidelines on this subject have been published.[2-8] There is no general agreement that all of the procedures recommended in the guidelines are necessary or appropriate.

REFERENCES:

1. Rudolph R, Larson DL: Etiology and Treatment of Chemotherapeutic Agent Extravasation Injuries: A Review. J Clin Oncol 5: 1116-1126, 1987. **2.** Recommendations for the Safe Handling of Parenteral Antineoplastic Drugs. NIH Publication No. 83-2621. For sale by the Superintendent of Documents, US Government Printing Office, Washington, DC 20402. **3.** AMA Council Report, Guidelines for Handling Parenteral Antineoplastics, JAMA. 1985; 253 (11): 1590-1592. **4.** National Study Commission on Cytotoxic Exposure- Recommendations for Handling Cytotoxic Agents. Available from Louis P. Jeffrey, Sc.D., Chairman, National Study Commission on Cytotoxic Exposure, Massachusetts College of Pharmacy and Allied Health Sciences, 179 Longwood Avenue, Boston, Massachusetts 02115. **5.** Clinical Oncological Society of Australia. Guidelines and Recommendations for Safe Handling of Antineoplastic Agents. Med J Australia. 1983; 1:426-428. **6.** Jones RB, et al: Safe Handling of Chemotherapeutic Agents: A Report from the Mount Sinai Medical Center. CA-A Cancer Journal for Clinicians.

REFERENCES: *(cont'd)*

1983; (Sept/Oct) 258-263. **7.** American Society of Hospital Pharmacists Technical Assistance Bulletin on Handling Cytotoxic and Hazardous Drugs. Am J Hosp Pharm. 1990; 47:1033-1049. **8.** OSHA Work-Practice Guidelines for Personnel Dealing with Cytotoxic (Antineoplastic) Drugs. Am J Hosp Pharm. 1986; 43:1193-1204.

HOW SUPPLIED:

Idamycin (Idarubicin Hydrochloride for Injection, USP)

5 mg single dose vial. Available in 5 vial packs.

10 mg single dose vial. Available in single vials.

20 mg single dose vial. Available in single vials.

Store at controlled room temperature, 15° to 30°C (59° to 86°F), and protect from light.

HOW SUPPLIED - EQUIVALENTS NOT AVAILABLE:

Injection, Lyphl-Soln - Intravenous - 5 mg/vial

5 mg x 5 $254.15 IDAMYCIN, Pharmacia & Upjohn 00013-2506-94

Injection, Lyphl-Soln - Intravenous - 10 mg/vial

10 mg x 1 $508.30 IDAMYCIN, Pharmacia & Upjohn 00013-2516-86

IDOXURIDINE *(001523)*

CATEGORIES: Anti-Infectives; Antivirals; EENT Drugs; Eye, Ear, Nose, & Throat Preparations; Herpes; Herpes Simplex; Keratitis; Ocular Infections; Ophthalmics; Viral Agents, Ophthalmological; FDA Approval Pre 1982

BRAND NAMES: *Antidep*; *Chrytemin*; *Daypress*; *Dendrid*; *Depsol*; *Dispersidu*; *Ethipramine*; *Fronil*; *Herpidu*; *Herplex*; *Herplex-D*; *Herplex Liquifilm* (Canada); *IDU* (Germany); *IDU Ofteno*; *IDU Opthalmic Solution* (Japan); *Iduridin*; *Idurin*; Imavate; *Imidol*; *Imine*; Imipramine Hcl; *Imiprex*; *Imiprin*; *Impril*; Janimine; *Medipramine*; *Melipramine*; Norfranil; *Novopramine*; *Oftan IDU*; Presamine; *Primonil*; *Ridinox*; *Sermonil*; *Sipramine*; *Stoxil* (Australia, Canada); *Surplix*; *Synmiol* (Germany); Tipramine; *Tofnil*; **Tofranil**; *Virusan*; *Xurin*
(International brand names outside U.S. in italics)

FORMULARIES: Aetna; BC-BS; Medi-Cal; WHO

DESCRIPTION:

Herplex (idoxuridine) 0.1% Liquifilm sterile ophthalmic solution is a topical ophthalmic antiviral chemotherapeutic preparation.

Chemical Name: 2'-Deoxy-5-iodouridine.

Contains: idoxuridine 0.1% with: Liquifilm (polyvinyl alcohol) 1.4%; benzalkonium chloride; sodium chloride; edetate disodium; and purified water.

CLINICAL PHARMACOLOGY:

In chemical structure, idoxuridine closely approximates the configuration of thymidine, one of the four building blocks of DNA—the genetic material of the herpes virus. As a result, idoxuridine is able to replace thymidine in the enzymatic step of viral replication or "growth". The consequent production of faulty DNA results in a pseudostructure which cannot infect or destroy tissue. In short, by preempting a vital building block in the genetic material of the herpes simplex virus, idoxuridine destroys the infective and destructive capacity of the viral material.

INDICATIONS AND USAGE:

Idoxuridine is indicated for the treatment of keratitis caused by the herpes simplex virus.

CONTRAINDICATIONS:

Idoxuridine is contraindicated for those who have a hypersensitivity to the active ingredient or other components of this medication.

PRECAUTIONS:

General: Some strains of herpes simplex virus appear resistant to the action of idoxuridine. If there is no lessening of fluorescein staining in 14 days, another form of therapy should be undertaken.

Carcinogenesis, Mutagenesis, and Impairment of Fertility: The studies performed to date on idoxuridine are inadequate for assessment of carcinogenicity. This cytotoxic drug should be regarded as benign potentially carcinogenic. It can inhibit DNA synthesis or function and is incorporated into the DNA of mammalian cells as well as into the genome of DNA viruses. Idoxuridine has been reported to induce RNA tumor virus (type C particles) production from virus-negative mouse cells. The degree of oncogenic activity of idoxuridine-induced oncornaviruses has not been documented. However, several idoxuridine-activated oncornaviruses have caused *in vitro* cell transformation and induction of specific neoplasms (lymphatic leukemias and carcinomas) upon inoculation into syngeneic mice.

Idoxuridine has been reported to cause chromosome aberrations in mice and to be mutagenic in mammalian cells in culture (*e.g.,* diploid human lymphoblasts and mouse lymphoma cells), Drosophila melanogaster and in host-mediated assay system utilizing mammalian cells.

Pregnancy Category C: Idoxuridine has been reported to cross the placental barrier and to produce fetal malformations in rabbits when administered topically to the eyes of pregnant females in doses similar to those used clinically. Idoxuridine has also been reported to produce fetal malformations in the rat after intraperitoneal and oral administration and in the mouse after subcutaneous administration. There are no adequate and well-controlled studies in pregnant women. Idoxuridine should be used during pregnancy only of the potential benefit justifies the potential risk to the fetus.

Nursing Mothers: It is not known whether this drug is excreted in human milk. Because of the potential for tumorigenicity shown for idoxuridine in animal studies, a decision should be made whether to discontinue nursing or to discontinue the drug, taking into account the importance of the drug to the mother.

Pediatric Use: Safety and effectiveness in children have not been established.

DRUG INTERACTIONS:

Boric acid should not be administered during the course of therapy. The potential exists for interaction between boric acid and ingredients in idoxuridine which may result in precipitate formation.

ADVERSE REACTIONS:

Exact incidence figures are not available since no denominator of treated patients is available.

Adverse reactions associated with topical idoxuridine administration include occasional irritation, pain, pruritus, inflammation, edema of the eyes or lids. allergic reactions, photophobia, occasional corneal clouding, stippling, and punctuate defects of the epithelium.

OVERDOSAGE:

Overdosage will not ordinarily cause acute problems. Should accidental overdosage in the eye (s) occur, flush the eye(s) with water or normal saline. If accidentally ingested, drink fluids to dilute.

DOSAGE AND ADMINISTRATION:

For optimal results, the infected tissues should be kept "saturated" with idoxuridine. Under practical, clinical conditions, one of the following "high frequency" dosage schedules is recommended.

1. Instill one drop in the infected eye(s) every hour during the day. At night the dosage may be reduced to one drop every other hour.

2. Instill one drop every 5 minutes. This schedule should be repeated four hours-night and day.

HOW SUPPLIED:

Herplex (idoxuridine) 0.1% Liquifilm sterile ophthalmic solution is supplied in plastic dropper bottles int he following size: 15 ml

Note: Store at controlled room temperature (59°-86°F). Protect from light.

HOW SUPPLIED - RATED THERAPEUTICALLY EQUIVALENT:

Solution - Ophthalmic; Top - 0.1 %

15 ml $13.21 HERPLEX, Allergan 00023-0033-15

IFOSFAMIDE *(001524)*

CATEGORIES: Antineoplastics; Cancer; Chemotherapy; Cystitis; Cytotoxic Agents; Hemorrhagic Cystitis; Orphan Drugs; Testicular Carcinoma; Pregnancy Category D; FDA Class 1A ("Important Therapeutic Advantage"); FDA Approved 1988 Dec; Patent Expiration 1995 Dec

BRAND NAMES: *Holoxan* (Australia, Asia, Germany, France); **Ifex**; Ifex Mesnex; *Ifoxan* (Mexico); *Mitoxana* (England); *Tronoxal*
(International brand names outside U.S. in italics)

FORMULARIES: BC-BS; Medi-Cal

> **WARNING:**
> Ifosfamide should be administered under the supervision of a qualified physician experienced in the use of cancer chemotherapeutic agents. Urotoxic side effects, especially hemorrhagic cystitis, as well as CNS toxicities such as confusion and coma have been associated with the use of ifosfamide. When they occur, they may require cessation of ifosfamide therapy. Severe myelosuppression has been reported. (See ADVERSE REACTIONS.)

DESCRIPTION:

Ifex (sterile ifosfamide) single-dose vials for constitution and administration by intravenous infusion each contain 1 gram or 3 grams of sterile ifosfamide. Ifosfamide is a chemotherapeutic agent chemically related to the nitrogen mustards and a synthetic analog of cyclophosphamide. Ifosfamide is 3-(2-chloroethyl)-2-[(2-chloroethyl)amino]tetrahydro-2H-1,3,2-oxazaphosphorine 2-oxide. The molecular formula is $C_7H_{15}Cl_2N_2O_2P$ and its molecular weight is 261.1.

Ifosfamide is a white crystalline powder that is soluble in water.

CLINICAL PHARMACOLOGY:

Ifosfamide has been shown to require metabolic activation by microsomal liver enzymes to produce biologically active metabolites. Activation occurs by hydroxylation at the ring carbon atom 4 to form the unstable intermediate 4-hydroxyifosfamide. This metabolite rapidly degrades to the stable urinary metabolite 4-ketoifosfamide. Opening of the ring results in formation of the stable urinary metabolite, 4-carboxyifosfamide. These urinary metabolites have not been found to be cytotoxic. N, N-*bis* (2-chloroethyl)-phosphoric acid diamide (ifosphoramide) and acrolein are also found. Enzymatic oxidation of the chloroethyl side chains and subsequent dealkylation produces the major urinary metabolites, dechloroethyl ifosfamide and dechloroethyl cyclophosphamide. The alkylated metabolites of ifosfamide have been shown to interact with DNA.

In vitro incubation of DNA with activated ifosfamide has produced phosphotriesters. The treatment of intact cell nuclei may also result in the formation of DNA-DNA cross-links. DNA repair most likely occurs in G-1 and G-2 stage cells.

PHARMACOKINETICS

Ifosfamide exhibits dose-dependent pharmacokinetics in humans. At single doses of 3.8-5.0 gm/m^2, the plasma concentrations decay biphasically and the mean terminal elimination half-life is about 15 hours. At doses of 1.6 -2.4 gm/m^2/day, the plasma decay is monoexponential and the terminal elimination half-life is about 7 hours. Ifosfamide is extensively metabolized in humans and the metabolic pathways appear to be saturated at high doses.

After administration of doses of 5 gm/m^2 of ^{14}C-labeled ifosfamide, from 70% to 86% of the dosed radioactivity was recovered in the urine, with about 61% of the dose excreted as parent compound. At doses of 1.6-2.4 g/m^2 only 12% to 18% of the dose was excreted in the urine as unchanged drug within 72 hours.

Two different dechloroethylated derivatives of ifosfamide, 4-carboxyifosfamide, thiodiacetic acid and cysteine conjugates of chloroacetic acid have been identified as the major urinary metabolites of ifosfamide in humans and only small amounts of 4-hydroxyifosfamide and acrolein are present. Small quantities (nmole/ml) of ifosfamide mustard and 4-hydroxyifosfamide are detectable in human plasma. Metabolism of ifosfamide is required for the generation of the biologically active species and while metabolism is extensive, it is also quite variable among patients.

In a study at Indiana University, 50 fully evaluable patients with germ cell testicular cancer were treated with ifosfamide in combination with cisplatin and either vinblastine or etoposide after failing (47 of 50 patients) at least two prior chemotherapy regimens consisting of cisplatin/vinblastine/bleomycin, (PVB), cisplatin/vinblastine/actinomycin D/bleomycin/cyclophosphamide, (VAB6), or the combination of cisplatin and etoposide. Patients were selected for remaining cisplatin sensitivity because they had previously responded to a cisplatin containing regimen and had not progressed while on the cisplatin containing regimen or within 3 weeks of stopping it. Patients served as their own control based on the premise that long term complete responses could not be achieved by retreatment with a regimen to which they had previously responded and subsequently relapsed.

CLINICAL PHARMACOLOGY: *(cont'd)*

Ten of 50 fully evaluable patients were still alive 2 to 5 years after treatment. Four of the 10 long term survivors were rendered free of cancer by surgical resection after treatment with the ifosfamide regimen; median survival for the entire group of 50 fully evaluable patients was 53 weeks.

INDICATIONS AND USAGE:

Ifosfamide, used in combination with certain other approved antineoplastic agents, is indicated for third line chemotherapy of germ cell testicular cancer. It should ordinarily be used in combination with a prophylactic agent for hemorrhagic cystitis, such as mesna.

CONTRAINDICATIONS:

Continued use of ifosfamide is contraindicated in patients with severely depressed bone marrow function (See WARNINGS and PRECAUTIONS). Ifosfamide is also contraindicated in patients who have demonstrated a previous hypersensitivity to it.

WARNINGS:

Urinary System: Urotoxic side effects, especially hemorrhagic cystitis, have been frequently associated with the use of ifosfamide. It is recommended that a urinalysis should be obtained prior to each dose of ifosfamide. If microscopic hematuria, (greater than 10 RBC's per high power field), is present, then subsequent administration should be withheld until complete resolution.

Further administration of ifosfamide should be given with vigorous oral or parenteral hydration.

Hematopoietic System: When ifosfamide is given in combination with other chemotherapeutic agents, severe myelosuppression is frequently observed. Close hematologic monitoring is recommended. White blood cell (WBC) count, platelet count and hemoglobin should be obtained prior to each administration had at appropriate intervals. Unless clinically essential, ifosfamide should not be given to patients with a WBC count below 2000/mcl and/or a platelet count below 50,000/mcl.

Central Nervous System: Neurologic manifestations consisting of somnolence, confusion, hallucinations and in some instances, coma, have been reported following ifosfamide therapy. The occurrence of these symptoms requires discontinuing ifosfamide therapy. The symptoms have usually been reversible and supportive therapy should be maintained until their complete resolution.

Pregnancy: Animal studies indicate that the drug is capable of causing gene mutations and chromosomal damage *in vivo.* Embryotoxic and teratogenic effects have been observed in mice, rats and rabbits at doses 0.05 to 0.075 times the human dose. Ifosfamide can cause fetal damage when administered to a pregnant woman. If ifosfamide is used during pregnancy, or if the patient becomes pregnant while taking this drug, the patient should be apprised of the potential hazard to the fetus.

PRECAUTIONS:

General: Ifosfamide should be given cautiously to patients with impaired renal function as well as to those with compromised bone marrow reserve, as indicated by: leukopenia, granulocytopenia, extensive bone marrow metastases, prior radiation therapy, or prior therapy with other cytotoxic agents.

Laboratory Tests: During treatment, the patient's hematologic profile (particularly neutrophils and platelets) should be monitored regularly to determine the degree of hematopoietic suppression. Urine should also be examined regularly for red cells which may precede hemorrhagic cystitis.

Wound Healing: Ifosfamide may interfere with normal wound healing.

Pregnancy Category D: See WARNINGS.

Nursing Mothers: Ifosfamide is excreted in breast milk. Because of the potential for serious adverse events and the tumorigenicity shown for ifosfamide in animal studies, a decision should be made whether to discontinue nursing or to discontinue the drug, taking into account the importance of the drug to the mother.

Carcinogenesis, Mutagenesis, and Impairment of Fertility: Ifosfamide has been shown to be carcinogenic in rats, with female rats showing a significant incidence of leiomyosarcomas and mammary fibroadenomas.

The mutagenic potential of ifosfamide has been documented in bacterial systems *in vitro* and mammalian cells *in vivo. In vivo,* ifosfamide has induced mutagenic effects in mice and *Drosophila melanogaster* germ cells, and has induced a significant increase in dominant lethal mutations in male mice as well as recessive sex-linked lethal mutations in Drosophila.

In pregnant mice, resorptions increased and anomalies were present at day 19 after 30 mg/m^2 dose of ifosfamide was administered on day 11 of gestation. Embryolethal effects were observed in rats following the administration of 54 mg/m^2 doses of ifosfamide from the sixth through the fifteenth day of gestation and embryotoxic effects were apparent after dams received 18 mg/m^2 doses over the same dosing period. Ifosfamide is embryotoxic to rabbits receiving 88 mg/m^2/day doses from the sixth through the eighteenth day after mating. The number of anomalies was also significantly increased over the control group.

Pediatric Use: Safety and effectiveness in children have not been established.

DRUG INTERACTIONS:

The physician should be alert for possible combined drug actions, desirable or undesirable, involving ifosfamide even though ifosfamide has been used successfully concurrently with other drugs, including other cytotoxic drugs.

ADVERSE REACTIONS:

In patients receiving ifosfamide as a single agent, the dose-limiting toxicities are myelosuppression and urotoxicity. Dose fractionation, vigorous hydration and a protector such as mesna can significantly reduce the incidence of hematuria, especially gross hematuria, associated with hemorrhage cystitis. At a dose of 1.2 gm/m^2 daily for 5 consecutive days, leukopenia, when it occurs, is usually mild to moderate. Other significant side effects include alopecia, nausea, vomiting, and central nervous system toxicities (TABLE 1):

Hematologic Toxicity: Myelosuppression was dose-related and dose-limiting. It consisted mainly of leukopenia and, to a lesser extent, thrombocytopenia. A WBC count <3000/mcl is expected in 50% of the patients treated with ifosfamide single agent at doses of 1.2 gm/m^2 per day for 5 consecutive days. At this dose level, thrombocytopenia (platelets <100,000/mcl) occurred in about 20% of the patients. At higher dosages, leukopenia was almost universal, and at total dosages of 10-12 gm/m^2/cycle, one-half of the patients had a WBC count below 1000/mcl and 8% of patients had platelet counts less than 50,000 mcl. Myelosuppression was usually reversible and treatment can be given every 3 to 4 weeks. When ifosfamide is used in combination with other myelosuppressive agents, adjustments in dosing may be necessary. Patients who experience severe myelosuppression are potentially at increased risk for infection.

Digestive System: Nausea and vomiting occurred in 58% of the patients who received ifosfamide. They were usually controlled by standard antiemetic therapy. Other gastrointestinal side effects include anorexia, diarrhea, and in some cases, constipation.

ADVERSE REACTIONS: *(cont'd)*

TABLE 1

Adverse Reaction	*Incidence (%)
Alopecia	83
Nausea-Vomiting	58
Hematuria	46
Gross Hematuria	12
CNS Toxicity	12
Infection	8
Renal Impairment	6
Liver Dysfunction	3
Phlebitis	2
Fever	1
Allergic Reaction	<1
Anorexia	<1
Cardiotoxicity	<1
Coagulopathy	<1
Constipation	<1
Dermatitis	<1
Diarrhea	<1
Fatigue	<1
Hypertension	<1
Hypotension	<1
Malaise	<1
Polyneuropathy	<1
Pulmonary Symptoms	<1
Salivation	<1
Stomatitis	<1

* Based upon 2,070 patients from the published literature in 30 single agent studies.

Urinary System: Urotoxicity consisted of hemorrhagic cystitis, dysuria, urinary frequency and other symptoms of bladder irritation. Hematuria occurred in 6% to 92% of patients treated with ifosfamide. The incidence and severity of hematuria can be significantly reduced by using vigorous hydration, a fractionated dose schedule and a protector such as mesna. At daily doses of 1.2 gm/m^2 for 5 consecutive days without a protector microscopic hematuria is expected in about one-half of the patients and gross hematuria in about 8% of patients.

Renal toxicity occurred in 6% of the patients treated with ifosfamide as a single agent. Clinical signs, such as elevation in BUN or serum creatinine or decrease in creatinine clearance, were usually transient. They were most likely to be related to tubular damage. One episode of renal tubular acidosis which progressed into chronic renal failure was reported. Proteinuria and acidosis also occurred in rare instances. Metabolic acidosis was reported in 31% of patients in one study when ifosfamide was administered at doses of 2.0-2.5 gm/m^2/day for 4 days. Renal tubular acidosis, Fanconi syndrome and renal rickets have been reported. Close clinical monitoring of serum and urine chemistries including phosphorus, potassium, alkaline phosphatase and other appropriate laboratory studies is recommended. Appropriate replacement therapy should be administered as indicated.

Central Nervous System: CNS side effects were observed in 12% of patients treated with ifosfamide. Those most commonly seen were somnolence, confusion, depressive psychosis, and hallucinations. Other less frequent symptoms include dizziness, disorientation, and cranial nerve dysfunction. Seizures and coma were occasionally reported. The incidence of CNS toxicity may be higher in patients with altered renal function.

Other: Alopecia occurred in approximately 83% of the patients treated with ifosfamide as a single agent. In combination, this incidence may be as high as 100%, depending on the other agents included in the chemotherapy regimen. Increases in liver enzymes and/or bilirubin were noted in 3% of the patients. Other less frequent side effects included phlebitis, pulmonary symptoms, fever of unknown origin, allergic reactions, stomatitis, cardiotoxicity, and polyneuropathy.

OVERDOSAGE:

No specific antidote for ifosfamide is known. Management of overdosage would include general supportive measures to sustain the patient through any period of toxicity that might occur.

DOSAGE AND ADMINISTRATION:

Ifosfamide should be administered intravenously at a dose of 1.2 gm/m^2 per day for five consecutive days. Treatment is repeated every three weeks or after recovery from hematologic toxicity (Platelets ≥100,000/mcl, WBC ≥4,000/mcl). In order to prevent bladder toxicity, ifosfamide should be given with extensive hydration consisting of at least two liters of oral or intravenous fluid per day. A protector, such as mesna, should also be used to prevent haemorrhagia cystitis. Ifosfamide should be administered as a slow intravenous infusion lasting a minimum of 30 minutes. Although ifosfamide has been administered to a small number of patients with compromised hepatic and/or renal function, studies to establish optimal dose schedules of ifosfamide in such patients have not been conducted.

PREPARATION FOR INTRAVENOUS ADMINISTRATION/STABILITY

Injections are prepared for parenteral use by adding *Sterile Water for Injection USP* or *Bacteriostatic Water for Injection USP* (benzyl alcohol or parabens preserved) to the vial and shaking to dissolve. Use the quantity of diluent shown in TABLE 2 to reconstitute the product:

TABLE 2

Dosage Strength	Quantity of Diluent	Final Concentration
1 gram	20 ml	50 mg/ml
3 gram	60 ml	50 mg/ml

Reconstituted solutions are chemically and physically stable for 1 week at 30°C or 3 weeks at 5°C.

Solutions of ifosfamide may be diluted further to achieve concentrations of 0.6 to 20 mg/ml in the following fluids:

5% Dextrose Injection, USP

0.9% Sodium Chloride Injection, USP

Lactated Ringer's Injection, USP

Sterile Water for Injection, USP

Such admixtures, when stored in large volume parenteral glass bottles, Viaflex bags, or PAB bags, are physically and chemically stable for at least one week at 30°C or six weeks at 5°C.

Because essentially identical stability results were obtained for Sterile Water admixtures as for the other admixtures (5% Dextrose Injection, 0.9% Sodium Chloride Injection, and Lactated Ringer's Injection), the use of large volume parenteral glass bottles, Viaflex bags or PAB bags

DOSAGE AND ADMINISTRATION: *(cont'd)*

that contain intermediate concentrations or mixtures of excipients (*e.g.,* 2.5% Dextrose Injection, 0.45% Sodium Chloride Injection, or 5% Dextrose and 0.9% Sodium Chloride Injection) is also acceptable.

The microbiological qualities of the constituted products or prepared admixtures should be considered, particularly where unpreserved vehicles are used.

Dilutions of ifosfamide not prepared by constitution with Bacteriostatic Water for Injection, USP; (benzyl alcohol or parabens preserved), should be refrigerated and within 6 hours.

Parenteral drug products should be inspected visually for particulate matter and discoloration prior to administration.

REFERENCES:

1. Recommendations for the Safe Handling of Parenteral Antineoplastic Drugs. NIH Publication No. 83-2621. For sale by the Superintendent of Documents, U.S. Government Printing Office, Washington, D.C. 20204. **2.** AMA Council Report. Guidelines for Handling Parenteral Antineoplastics. JAMA, March 15, 1985. **3.** National Study Commission on Cytotoxic Exposure—Recommendations for Handling Cytotoxic Agents. Available from Louis P. Jeffrey, Sc.D., Director of Pharmacy Services, Rhode Island Hospital, 595 Eddy St., Providence, Rhode Island 02902. **4.** Clinical Oncological Society of Australia: Guidelines and Recommendations for Safe Handling of Antineoplastic Agents. Med. J. Australia 1:426-428, 1983. **5.** Jones, R. B., et al; Safe Handling of Chemotherapeutic Agents: A report from the Mount Sinai Medical Center, CA-A Cancer Journal for Clinicians Sept/Oct, 258- 263, 1983. **6.** American Society of Hospital Pharmacists Technical Assistance Bulletin on Handling Cytotoxic Drugs in Hospitals. Am. J. Hosp. Pharm, 42:131-137, 1985. **7.** OSHA Work Practice Guidelines for Personnel Dealing with Cytotoxic (Antineoplastic) Drugs. Am. J. Hosp. Pharm. 43:1193-1204, 1986.

HOW SUPPLIED:

Ifex is only available in combination packages with the uroprotective agent Mesnex (mesna) injection.

The dry powder may be stored at room temperature. Storage above 104°F (40°C) should be avoided.

Procedures for proper handling and disposal of anticancer drugs should be considered. Skin reactions associated with accidental exposure to Ifex may occur. The use of gloves is recommended. If Ifex solution contacts the skin or mucosa, immediately wash the skin thoroughly with soap and water or rinse the mucosa with copious amounts of water. Several guidelines on this subject have been published.[1-7] There is no general agreement that all of the procedures recommended in the guidelines are necessary or appropriate.

HOW SUPPLIED - EQUIVALENTS NOT AVAILABLE:

Injection, Lyphl-Soln - Intravenous - 1 gm/vial

combination pac	$740.07	IFEX MESNEX COMBINATION, Mead Johnson	00015-3558-41
20 ml	$103.57	IFEX, Mead Johnson	00015-0556-41

Injection, Lyphl-Soln - Intravenous - 3 gm/vial

3 gm vial 400 m	$888.10	IFEX/MESNEX, Mead Johnson	00015-3559-41
60 ml	$310.74	IFEX, Mead Johnson	00015-0557-41

Kit - Intravenous - 3 mg/1 g

1's	$1072.92	IFEX/MESNEX, Mead Johnson	00015-3564-15

Package - Intravenous - 1 gm/1 gm

1's	$740.07	IFEX/MESNEX, Mead Johnson	00015-3556-26
1's	$1788.30	IFEX/MESNEX, Mead Johnson	00015-3554-27
1's	$1788.30	IFEX/MESNEX COMBO PACK, Mead Johnson	00015-3557-41

IMIGLUCERASE *(003208)*

CATEGORIES: Enzymes; Gaucher's Disease; Orphan Drugs; FDA Class 1P ("Priority Review"); Recombinant DNA Origin; Sales > $100 Million; FDA Approved 1994 May

BRAND NAMES: **Cerezyme**; Glucocerebrosidase

FORMULARIES: Medi-Cal

COST OF THERAPY: $351,130.00 (Gaucher's Disease; Injection; 200 unit; 1.3/day; 365 days)

PRIMARY ICD9: 272.7 (Lipidoses)

DESCRIPTION:

Cerezyme (imiglucerase for injection) is an analogue of the human enzyme, β-glucocerebrosidase produced by recombinant DNA technology. β-Glucocerebrosidase (β-D-glucosyl-N-acylsphingosine glucohydrolase, E.C.3.2.1.45) is a lysosomal glycoprotein enzyme which catalyzes the hydrolysis of the glycolipid glucocerebroside to glucose and ceramide.

Cerezyme is produced by recombinant DNA technology using mammalian cell culture (Chinese hamster ovary). Purified imiglucerase is a monomeric glycoprotein of 497 amino acids, containing 4 N-linked glycosylation sites (Mr=60,430). Imiglucerase differs from placental glucocerebrosidase by one amino acid at position 495 where histidine is substituted for arginine. The oligosaccharide chains at the glycosylation sites have been modified to terminate in mannose sugars. The modified carbohydrate structures on imiglucerase are somewhat different from those on placental glucocerebrosidase. These mannose-terminated oligosaccharide chains of imiglucerase are specifically recognized by endocytic carbohydrate receptors on macrophages, the cells that accumulate lipid in Gaucher disease.

Cerezyme is supplied as a sterile, non-pyrogenic, white to off-white lyophilized product. The quantitative composition of the lyophilized drug per vial is:

Imiglucerase 212 units (total amount)*

Mannitol 155 mg

Sodium Citrates 70 mg (Trisodium Citrate 52 mg and Disodium Hydrogen Citrate 18 mg)

Polysorbate 80, NF 0.53 mg

Citric Acid and/or Sodium Hydroxide may have been added at the time of manufacture to adjust pH.

*This provides a withdrawal dose of 200 units of imiglucerase.

An enzyme unit (U) is defined as the amount of enzyme that catalyzes the hydrolysis of one micromole of the synthetic substrate para-nitrophenyl β-D-glucopyranoside (pNP-Glc) per minute at 37°C. The product is stored at 2°-8°C (36°-46°F.) After reconstitution with 5.1 ml of Sterile Water for Injection, USP, the imiglucerase concentration is 40 U/ml in a final volume of 5.3 ml which provides a withdrawal volume of 5.0 ml (200 enzyme units). Reconstituted solutions have a pH of approximately 6.1.

In addition, Haemaccel (cross-linked gelatin polypeptides), which is used as a stabilizing agent during the manufacturing process, may also be present in very small amounts in the final product.

CLINICAL PHARMACOLOGY:

MECHANISM OF ACTION/PHARMACODYNAMICS

Gaucher disease is characterized by a deficiency of β-glucocerebrosidase activity, resulting in accumulation of glucocerebroside in tissue macrophages which become engorged and are typically found in the liver, spleen, and bone marrow and occasionally in lung, kidney, and intestine. Secondary hematologic sequelae include severe anemia and thrombocytopenia in addition to the characteristic progressive hepatosplenomegaly, skeletal complications, including osteonecrosis and osteopenia with secondary pathological fractures. Imiglucerase for injection catalyzes the hydrolysis of glucocerebroside to glucose and ceramide. In clinical trials, imiglucerase for injection improved anemia and thrombocytopenia, reduced spleen and liver size, and decreased cachexia to a degree similar to that observed with Ceredase.

PHARMACOKINETICS

During one hour intravenous infusions of four doses (7.5, 15, 30, 60 U/kg) of imiglucerase for injection steady-state enzymatic activity declined rapidly with a half-life ranging from 3.6 to 10.4 minutes. Plasma clearance ranged from 9.8 to 20.3 ml/min/kg, (mean ± S.D, 14.5 ± 4.0 ml/min/kg). The volume of distribution corrected for weight ranged from 0.09 to 0.15 L/kg (0.12 ± 0.02 L/kg). These variables do not appear to be influenced by dose or duration of infusion. However, only one or two patients were studied at each dose level and infusion rate. The pharmacokinetics of imiglucerase for injection do not appear to be different from placental-derived alglucerase (Ceredase).

In patients who developed IgG antibody to imiglucerase for injection, an apparent effect on serum enzyme levels resulted in diminished volume of distribution and clearance and increased elimination half-life compared to patients without antibody (see WARNINGS).

INDICATIONS AND USAGE:

Imiglucerase for injection is indicated for long-term enzyme replacement therapy for patients with a confirmed diagnosis of Type 1 Gaucher disease that results in one or more of the following conditions:

a. anemia

b. thrombocytopenia

c. bone disease

d. hepatomegaly or splenomegaly

CONTRAINDICATIONS:

There are no known contraindications to the use of imiglucerase for injection. Treatment with imiglucerase for injection should be carefully re-evaluated if there is significant clinical evidence of hypersensitivity to the product.

WARNINGS:

During the clinical trials (duration 9 months), 4 of 25 patients (16%) treated with imiglucerase for injection developed IgG antibodies reactive with imiglucerase for injection. During the same clinical trial, 6 of 15 patients (40%) treated with placental-derived alglucerase (Ceredase) developed IgG antibodies to Ceredase, and one of these patients has clinical allergic signs and symptoms resulting in withdrawal from the study.

Of those patients treated with imiglucerase for injection, only one patient developed a transient rash. No patients treated with imiglucerase for injection, either initially or after changing over from Ceredase, have exhibited serious symptoms of immediate hypersensitivity, although a risk for such reactions may be present.

Treatment with imiglucerase for injection should be approached with caution in patients who have exhibited symptoms of hypersensitivity to the product.

PRECAUTIONS:

GENERAL

Therapy with imiglucerase for injection should be directed by physicians knowledgeable in the management of patients with Gaucher disease.

Caution may be advisable in administration of imiglucerase for injection to patients previously treated with Ceredase and who have exhibited symptoms of hypersensitivity to Ceredase.

CARCINOGENESIS, MUTAGENESIS, AND IMPAIRMENT OF FERTILITY

Studies have not been conducted in either animals or humans to assess the potential effects of imiglucerase for injection on carcinogenesis, mutagenesis, or impairment of fertility.

TERATOGENIC EFFECTS: PREGNANCY CATEGORY C

Animal reproduction studies have not been conducted with imiglucerase for injection. It is also not known whether imiglucerase for injection can cause fetal harm when administered to a pregnant woman, or can affect reproductive capacity. Imiglucerase for injection should not be administered during pregnancy except when the indication and need are clear and the potential benefit is judged by the physician to substantially justify the risk.

NURSING MOTHERS

It is not known whether this drug is excreted in human milk. Because many drugs are excreted in human milk, caution should be exercised when imiglucerase for injection is administered to a nursing woman.

ADVERSE REACTIONS:

During clinical trials with imiglucerase for injection involving 25 patients with Gaucher disease, the following adverse events were noted that were possibly related to imiglucerase for injection.

Headache was noted in three patients. Nausea, abdominal discomfort, dizziness, pruritus, and rash occurred in one patient each. One patient was noted to have a mild decrease in blood pressure and another a decrease in urinary frequency. None of these events was judged to be serious or to warrant medical intervention or interruption of therapy. All proved transient and did not recur frequently.

Symptoms suggestive of allergic hypersensitivity have been noted in a number of patients treated with Ceredase (see WARNINGS.)

OVERDOSAGE:

Effects of dosages exceeding 120 U/kg per four weeks have not been studied and therefore dosages above 120 U/kg are not recommended.

DOSAGE AND ADMINISTRATION:

Imiglucerase for injection is administered by intravenous infusion over 1-2 hours. Dosage should be individualized to each patient. Initial dosage may be as little as 2.5 units/kg of body weight 3 times a week up to as much as 60 U/kg administered as frequently as once a week or as infrequently as every 4 weeks. 60 units/kg every 2 weeks is the dosage for which the most data is available. Disease severity may dictate that treatment be initiated at a relatively high dose or relatively frequent administration. After patient response is well

DOSAGE AND ADMINISTRATION: *(cont'd)*

established, a reduction in dosage may be attempted for maintenance therapy. Progressive reductions can be made at intervals of 3-6 months while carefully monitoring response parameters.

Imiglucerase for injection should be stored at 2°-8° (36°-46°F). Each vial, after reconstitution with 5.1 ml Sterile Water for Injection, USP, should be inspected visually for particulate matter and discoloration before use. Any vials exhibiting particulate matter or discoloration should not be used. DO NOT USE imiglucerase for injection after the expiration date on the vial.

On the day of use, after the correct amount of imiglucerase for injection to be administered to the patient has been determined, the appropriate number of vials are each reconstituted with 5.1 ml of Sterile Water for Injection, USP, to give a reconstituted volume of 5.3 ml. A nominal 5.0 ml volume is then withdrawn from each vial and pooled with 0.9% sodium chloride injection, USP, to a final volume of 100 to 200 ml. Imiglucerase for injection is administered by intravenous infusion over 1 to 2 hours. Alternatively, the appropriate dose of imiglucerase for injection may be administered such that a rate of no greater than 1 unit per kg body weight per minute is infused. Aseptic techniques should be used when diluting the dose. Since imiglucerase for injection does not contain any preservative, after reconstitution, vials should be promptly diluted and not stored for subsequent use. Imiglucerase for injection, when diluted to 50 ml has been shown to be stable for up to 24 hours when stored at 2°- 8°C (36°-46°F).

Relatively low toxicity, combined with the extended time course of response, allows small dosage adjustments to be made occasionally to avoid discarding partially used bottles. Thus, the dosage administered in individual infusions may be slightly increased or decreased to utilize fully each vial as long as the monthly administered dosage remains substantially unaltered.

HOW SUPPLIED:

Cerezyme (imiglucerase for injection) is supplied as a sterile, non-pyrogenic, lyophilized product.

Store at 2°-8°C (36°-46°F).

HOW SUPPLIED - EQUIVALENTS NOT AVAILABLE:

Injection, Solution - Intravenous - 200 unit

1's	$740.00	CEREZYME, Genzyme	58468-1983-01

IMIPRAMINE HYDROCHLORIDE *(001525)*

CATEGORIES: Antidepressants; Central Nervous System Agents; Cystourethrography; Depression; Enuresis; Psychostimulants; Psychotherapeutic Agents; Tricyclics; Tricyclic Antidepressants; Urinary Incontinence; Panic Disorder*; FDA Approval Pre 1982

* Indication not approved by the FDA

BRAND NAMES: *Antidep*; *Apo-Imipramine* (Canada); *Chrytemin* (Japan); *Daypress* (Japan); *Depsol*; *Depsonil*; *Ethipramine*; *Fronil*; Imavate; *Imidol* (Japan); *Imimine*; *Imine*; *Imipramin*; Imipramine Hcl; *Imiprex*; *Imiprin*; *Impril* (Canada); Janimine; *Medipramine*; *Melipramine*; *Mipralin*; Norfranil; *Novopramine* (Canada); Presamine; *Primonil*; *Pryleugan* (Germany); *Sermonil*; *Sipramine*; *Surplix*; *Talpramin* (Mexico); Tipramine; *Tofnil*; **Tofranil**; *Tofranil-PM* (Mexico); *Venefon*
(International brand names outside U.S. in italics)

FORMULARIES: Aetna; BC-BS; CIGNA; FHP; Humana; Kaiser; Medco; Medi-Cal; PCS; PruCare; United

COST OF THERAPY: $4.19 (Depression; Tablet; 25 mg; 2/day; 90 days)

PRIMARY ICD9: 311 (Depressive Disorder, Not Elsewhere Classified)

DESCRIPTION:

Imipramine hydrochloride, USP, the original tricyclic antidepressant, is a member of the dibenzazepine group of compounds. It is designated 5-(3-dimethylamino)propyl)-10,11-dihydro-5H-dibenz(b,f)azepine monohydrochloride.

Imipramine hydrochloride USP is a white to off-white, odorless, or practically odorless crystalline powder. It is freely soluble in water and in alcohol, soluble in acetone, and insoluble in ether and in benzene. Its molecular weight is 316.87.

Tofranil Inactive Ingredients: (Tablets) Calcium phosphate, cellulose compounds, docusate sodium, iron oxides, magnesium stearate, polyethylene glycol, povidone, sodium starch glycolate, sucrose, talc and titanium dioxide.

Each 2 cc ampul (for IM injection) contains imipramine HCl, USP, 25 mg; ascorbic acid, 2 mg; sodium bisulfite, 1 mg; sodium sulfite, anhydrous, 1 mg.

CLINICAL PHARMACOLOGY:

The mechanism of action of imipramine HCl is not definitely known. However, it does not act primarily by stimulation of the central nervous system. The clinical effect is hypothesized as being due to potentiation of adrenergic synapses by blocking uptake of norepinephrine at nerve endings. The mode of action of the drug in controlling childhood enuresis is thought to be apart from its antidepressant effect.

INDICATIONS AND USAGE:

Depression: For the relief of symptoms of depression. Endogenous depression is more likely to be alleviated than other depressive states. One to three weeks of treatment may be needed before optimal therapeutic effects are evident.

Childhood Enuresis: May be useful as temporary adjunctive therapy in reducing enuresis in children aged 6 years and older, after possible organic causes have been excluded by appropriate tests. In patients having daytime symptoms of frequency and urgency, examination should include voiding cystourethrography and cystoscopy, as necessary. The effectiveness of treatment may decrease with continued drug administration.

CONTRAINDICATIONS:

The concomitant use of monoamine oxidase inhibiting compounds is contraindicated. Hyperpyretic crises or severe convulsive seizures may occur in patients receiving such combinations. The potentiation of adverse effects can be serious, or even fatal. When it is desired to substitute imipramine HCl in patients receiving a monoamine oxidase inhibitor, as long an interval should elapse as the clinical situation will allow, with a minimum of 14 days. Initial dosage should be low and increases should be gradual and cautiously prescribed.

The drug is contraindicated during the acute recovery period after a myocardial infarction. Patients with a known hypersensitivity to this compound should not be given the drug. The possibility of cross-sensitivity to other dibenzazepine compounds should be kept in mind.

WARNINGS:

Children: A dose of 2.5 mg/kg/day of imipramine HCl should not be exceeded in childhood. ECG changes of unknown significance have been reported in pediatric patients with doses twice this amount.

Extreme caution should be used when this drug is given to: patients with cardiovascular disease because of the possibility of conduction defects, arrhythmias, congestive heart failure, myocardial infarction, strokes and tachycardia. These patients require cardiac surveillance at all dosage levels of the drug; patients with increased intraocular pressure, history of urinary retention, or history of narrow-angle glaucoma because of the drug's anticholinergic properties; hyperthyroid patients or those on thyroid medication because of the possibility of cardiovascular toxicity; patients with a history of seizure disorder because this drug has been shown to lower the seizure threshold;

patients receiving guanethidine, clonidine, or similar agents, since imipramine HCl may block the pharmacologic effects of these drugs;

patients receiving methylphenidate hydrochloride. Since methylphenidate hydrochloride may inhibit the metabolism of imipramine HCl, downward dosage adjustment of imipramine hydrochloride may be required when given concomitantly with methylphenidate hydrochloride.

Imipramine HCl may enhance the CNS depressant effects of alcohol. Therefore, it should be borne in mind that the dangers inherent in a suicide attempt of accidental overdosage with the drug may be increased for the patient who uses excessive amounts of alcohol (See PRECAUTIONS).

Since imipramine HCl may impair the mental and/or physical abilities required for the performance of potentially hazardous tasks, such as operating an automobile or machinery, the patient should be cautioned accordingly.

For The Injectable Form Only: Contains sodium sulfite and sodium bisulfite, that may cause allergic-type reactions including anaphylactic symptoms and life-threatening or less severe asthmatic episodes in certain susceptible people. The overall prevalence of sulfite sensitivity in the general population is unknown and probably low. Sulfite sensitivity is seen more frequently in asthmatic than in nonasthmatic people.

PRECAUTIONS:

TABLETS ONLY

An ECG recording should be taken prior to the initiation of larger-than-usual doses of imipramine HCl and at appropriate intervals thereafter until steady state is achieved. (Patients with any evidence of cardiovascular disease require cardiac surveillance at all dosage levels of the drug. See WARNINGS.) Elderly patients and patients with cardiac disease or a prior history of cardiac disease are at special risk of developing the cardiac abnormalities associated with the use of imipramine HCl.

It should be kept in mind that the possibility of suicide in seriously depressed patients is inherent in the illness and may persist until significant remission occurs. Such patients should be carefully supervised during the early phase of treatment with imipramine HCl, and may require hospitalization. Prescriptions should be written for the smallest amount feasible. Hypomanic or manic episodes may occur, particularly in patients with cyclic disorders. Such reactions may necessitate discontinuation of the drug. If needed, imipramine HCl may be resumed in lower dosage when these episodes are relieved.

Administration of a tranquilizer may be useful in controlling such episodes.

An activation of the psychosis may occasionally be observed in schizophrenic patients and may require reduction of dosage and the addition of a phenothiazine.

Concurrent administration of imipramine HCl with electroshock therapy may increase the hazards; such treatment should be limited to those patients for whom it is essential, since there is limited clinical experience.

Usage During Pregnancy and Lactation: Animal reproduction studies have yielded inconclusive results. (See also ANIMAL PHARMACOLOGY).

There have been no well-controlled studies conducted with pregnant women to determine the effect of imipramine HCl on the fetus. However, there have been clinical reports of congenital malformations associated with the use of the drug. Although a casual relationship between these effects and the drug could not be established, the possibility of fetal risk from the maternal ingestion of imipramine HCl cannot be excluded. Therefore, imipramine HCl should be used in women who are or might become pregnant only if the clinical condition clearly justifies potential risk to the fetus.

Limited data suggest that imipramine HCl is likely to be excreted in human breast milk. As a general rule, a woman taking a drug should not nurse since the possibility exists that the drug may be excreted in breast milk and be harmful to the child.

Usage in Children: The effectiveness of the drug in children for conditions other than nocturnal enuresis has not been established.

The safety and effectiveness of the drug as temporary adjunctive therapy for nocturnal enuresis in children less than 6 years of age has not been established.

The safety of the drug for long-term, chronic use as adjunctive therapy for nocturnal enuresis in children 6 years of age or older has not been established; consideration should be given to instituting a drug-free period following an adequate therapeutic trial with a favorable response.

A dose of 2.5 mg/kg/day should not be exceeded in childhood. ECG changes of unknown significance have been reported in pediatric patients with doses twice this amount.

Patients should be warned that imipramine HCl may enhance the CNS depressant effects of alcohol. (See WARNINGS.)

Imipramine HCl should be used with caution in patients with significantly impaired renal or hepatic function.

Patients who develop a fever and sore throat during therapy with imipramine HCl should have leukocyte and differential blood counts performed. Imipramine HCl should be discontinued if there is evidence of pathological neutrophil depression.

Prior to elective surgery, imipramine HCl should be discontinued for as long as the clinical situation will allow.

In occasional susceptible patients or in those receiving anticholinergic drugs (including antiparkinsonism agents) in addition, the atropine-like effects may become more pronounced (*e.g.,* paralytic ileus).

Close supervision and careful adjustment of dosage is required when imipramine HCl is administered concomitantly with anticholinergic drugs.

Avoid the use of preparations, such as decongestants and local anesthetics, which contain any sympathomimetic amine (*e.g.,* epinephrine, norepinephrine), since it has been reported that tricyclic antidepressants can potentiate the effects of catecholamines.

Caution should be exercised when imipramine HCl is used with agents that lower blood pressure.

Imipramine HCl may potentiate the effects of CNS depressant drugs.

PRECAUTIONS: *(cont'd)*

The plasma concentration of imipramine HCl may increase when the drug is given concomitantly with hepatic enzyme inhibitors (*e.g.,* cimetidine, fluoxetine) and decrease by concomitant administration of hepatic enzyme inducers (*e.g.,* barbiturates, phenytoin), and adjustment of the dosage of imipramine HCl may therefore be necessary.

Patients taking imipramine HCl should avoid excessive exposure to sunlight since there have been reports of photosensitization.

Both elevation and lowering of blood sugar levels have been reported with imipramine HCl use.

ADVERSE REACTIONS:

Note: Although the listing which follows includes a few adverse reactions which have not been reported with this specific drug, the pharmacological similarities among the tricyclic antidepressant drugs require that each of the reactions be considered when imipramine HCl is administered.

Cardiovascular: Orthostatic hypotension, hypertension, tachycardia, palpitation, myocardial infarction, arrhythmias, heart block, ECG changes, precipitation of congestive heart failure, stroke.

Psychiatric: Confusional states (especially in the elderly) with hallucinations, disorientation, delusions; anxiety, restlessness, agitation; insomnia and nightmares; hypomania; exacerbation of psychosis.

Neurological: Numbness, tingling, paresthesias of extremities; incoordination, ataxia, tremors; peripheral neuropathy; extrapyramidal symptoms; seizures, alterations in EEG patterns; tinnitus.

Anticholinergic: Dry mouth, and rarely, associated sublingual adenitis; blurred vision, disturbances of accommodation, mydriasis; constipation, paralytic ileus; urinary retention, delayed micturition, dilation of the urinary track.

Allergic: Skin rash, petechiae, urticaria, itching, photosensitization, edema (general or of face and tongue); drug fever; cross-sensitivity with desipramine.

Hematologic: Bone marrow depression including agranulocytosis; eosinophilia; purpura; thrombocytopenia.

Gastrointestinal: Nausea and vomiting, anorexia, epigastric distress, diarrhea; peculiar taste, stomatitis, abdominal cramps, black tongue.

Endocrine: Gynecomastia in the male; breast enlargement and galactorrhea in the female; increased or decreased libido, impotence; testicular swelling; elevation or depression of blood sugar levels; inappropriate antidiuretic hormone (ADH) secretion syndrome.

Other: Jaundice (simulating obstructive); altered liver function; weight gain or loss; perspiration; flushing; urinary frequency; drowsiness; dizziness; weakness and fatigue; headache; parotid swelling; alopecia; proneness to falling.

Withdrawal Symptoms: Though not indicative of addiction, abrupt cessation of treatment after prolonged therapy may produce nausea, headache and malaise.

Note: In enuretic children treated with imipramine HCl the most common adverse reactions have been nervousness, sleep disorders, tiredness, and mild gastrointestinal disturbances. These usually disappear during continued drug administration or when dosage is decreased. Other reactions which have been reported include constipation, convulsions, anxiety, emotional instability, syncope, and collapse. All of the adverse effects reported with adult use should be considered.

OVERDOSAGE:

Children have been reported to be more sensitive than adults to an acute overdosage of imipramine hydrochloride. An acute overdose of any amount in infants or young children, especially, must be considered serious and potentially fatal.

Signs and Symptoms: These may vary in severity depending upon factors such as the amount of drug absorbed, the age of the patient, and the interval between drug ingestion and the start of treatment. Blood and urine levels of imipramine HCl may not reflect the severity of poisoning; they have chiefly a qualitative rather than quantitative value, and are unreliable indicators in the clinical management of the patient.

CNS abnormalities may include drowsiness, stupor, coma, ataxia, restlessness, agitation, hyperactive reflexes, muscle rigidity, athetoid and choreiform movements, and convulsions.

Cardiac abnormalities may include arrhythmia, tachycardia, ECG evidence of impaired conduction, and signs of congestive failure. Respiratory depression, cyanosis, hypotension, shock, vomiting, hyperpyrexia, mydriasis, and diaphoresis may also be present.

Treatment: The recommended treatment for overdosage with tricyclic antidepressants may change periodically. Therefore, it is recommended that the physician contact a poison control center for current information on treatment. Because CNS involvement, respiratory depression and cardiac arrhythmia can occur suddenly, hospitalization and close observation may be necessary, even when the amount ingested is thought to be small or the initial degree of intoxication appears slight or moderate. All patients with ECG abnormalities should have continuous cardiac monitoring and be closely observed until well after cardiac status has returned to normal; relapses may occur after apparent recovery. In the alert patient, empty the stomach promptly by lavage. In the obtunded patient, secure the airway with a cuffed endotracheal tube before beginning lavage (do not induce emesis). Instillation of activated charcoal slurry may held reduce absorption of imipramine.

Minimize external stimulation to reduce the tendency to convulsions. If anticonvulsants are necessary, diazepam and phenytoin may be useful. Maintain adequate respiratory exchange. Do not use respiratory stimulants.

Shock should be treated with supportive measures, such as appropriate position, intravenous fluids, and, if necessary, a vasopressor agent. The use of corticosteroids in shock is controversial and may be contraindicated in cases of overdosage with tricyclic antidepressants. Digitalis may increase conduction abnormalities and further irritate an already sensitized myocardium. If congestive heart failure necessitates rapid digitalization, particular care must be exercised.

Hyperpyrexia should be controlled by whatever external means are available, including ice packs and cooling sponge baths, if necessary.

Hemodialysis, peritoneal dialysis, exchange transfusions and forced diuresis have been generally reported as ineffective because of the rapid fixation of imipramine HCl in tissues. Blood and urine levels of imipramine HCl may not correlate with the degree of intoxication, and are unreliable indicators in the clinical management of the patient.

The slow intravenous administration of physostigmine salicylate has been used as a last resort to reverse severe CNS anticholinergic manifestations of overdosage with tricyclic antidepressants; however, it should not be used routinely, since it may induce seizures and cholinergic crises.

DOSAGE AND ADMINISTRATION:

TABLETS

Depression

Lower dosages are recommended for elderly patients and adolescents. Lower dosages are also recommended for outpatients as compared to hospitalized patients who will be under close supervision. Dosage should be initiated at a low level and increased gradually, noting carefully the clinical response and any evidence of intolerance. Following remission, maintenance, medication may be required for a longer period of time, at the lowest dose that will maintain remission.

Usual Adult Dose

Hospitalized Patients: Initially, 100 mg/day in divided doses gradually increased to 200 mg/day as required. If no response after two weeks, increase to 250-300 mg/day.

Outpatients: Initially 75 mg/day increased to 150 mg/day. Dosages over 200 mg/day are not recommended. Maintenance, 50-150 mg/day.

Adolescent and Geriatric Patients: Initially, 30-40 mg/day; it is generally not necessary to exceed 100 mg/day.

Childhood Enuresis

Initially, an oral dose of 25 mg/day should be tried in children aged 6 and older. Medication should be given one hour before bedtime. If a satisfactory response does not occur within one week, increase the dose to 50 mg nightly in children under 12 years; children over 12 may receive up to 75 mg nightly. A daily dose greater than 75 mg does not enhance efficacy and tends to increase side effects. Evidence suggests that in early night bedwetters, the drug is more effective given earlier and in divided amounts, (*i.e.,* 25 mg in midafternoon), repeated at bedtime. Consideration should be given to instituting a drug-free period following an adequate therapeutic trial with a favorable response. Dosage should be tapered off gradually rather than abruptly discontinued; this may reduce the tendency to relapse. Children who relapse when the drug is discontinued do not always respond to a subsequent course of treatment.

A dose of 2.5 mg/kg/day should not be exceeded. ECG changes of unknown significance have been reported in pediatric patients with doses twice this amount.

The safety and effectiveness of imipramine HCl as temporary adjunctive therapy for nocturnal enuresis in children less than 6 years of age has not been established.

INJECTION

Initially, up to 100 mg/day intramuscularly in divided doses.

Parenteral administration should be used for starting therapy in patients unable or unwilling to use oral medication. The oral form should supplant the injectable as soon as possible.

Lower dosages are recommended for elderly patients and adolescents. Lower dosages are also recommended for outpatients as compared t hospitalized patients who will be under close supervision. Dosage should be initiated at a low level and gradually increased, noting carefully the clinical response and any evidence of intolerance. Following remission, oral maintenance medication may be required for a longer period of time, at the lowest dose that will maintain remission.

Store tablets and ampuls (for injection) between 59°-86° F (15°-30° C).

Dispense tablets in tight container (USP).

Note: Upon storage of ampuls, minute crystals may form. This has no influence on the therapeutic efficacy of the preparation, and the crystals redissolve when the affected ampuls are immersed in hot tap water for 1 minute.

ANIMAL PHARMACOLOGY:

A. Acute: Oral LD_{50} ranges are as follows: Rat - 355 to 682 mg/kg, Dog - 100 to 215 mg/kg. Depending on the dosage in both species, toxic signs proceeded progressively from depression, irregular respiration and ataxia to convulsions and death.

B. Reproduction/Teratogenic: The overall evaluation may be summed up in the following manner:

Oral: Independent studies in three species (rat, mouse and rabbit) revealed that when imipramine HCl is administered orally in doses up to approximately 2 1/2 times the maximum human dose in the first 2 species and up to 25 times the maximum human dose in the third species, the drug is essentially free from teratogenic potential. In the three species studied, only one instance of fetal abnormality occurred (in the rabbit) and in that study there was likewise an abnormality in the control group. However, evidence does exist from the rat studies that some systemic and embryotoxic potential is demonstrable. This is manifested by reduced litter size, a slight increase in the stillborn rate and a reduction in the mean birth weight.

Parenteral: In contradistinction to the oral data, imipramine HCl does exhibit a slight but definite teratogenic potential when administered by the subcutaneous route. Drug effects on both the mother and fetus in the rabbit are manifested in higher resorption rates and decreases in mean fetal birth weights, while teratogenic findings occurred at a level of 5 times the maximum human dose. In the mouse, teratogenicity occurred at $1\frac{1}{2}$ and $6\frac{1}{2}$ the maximum human dose, but no teratogenic effects were seen at levels 3 times the maximum human dose. Thus, in the mouse, the findings are equivocal.

HOW SUPPLIED - RATED THERAPEUTICALLY EQUIVALENT:

Tablet, Sugar Coated - Oral - 10 mg

30's	$.56	Imipramine HCl, H.C.F.A. F F P	99999-1525-01
100's	$1.88	Imipramine HCl, H.C.F.A. F F P	99999-1525-02
100's	$3.07	Imipramine HCl, Teva	00332-2111-09
100's	$3.12	Imipramine Hcl, Qualitest Pharms	00603-4043-21
100's	$3.15	Imipramine Hcl, Major Pharms	00904-0925-60
100's	$3.15	Imipramine Hcl, US Trading	56126-0054-11
100's	$3.85	Imipramine Hcl, Mutual Pharm	53489-0330-01
100's	$4.32	Imipramine Hcl, United Res	00677-0421-01
100's	$4.45	Imipramine HCl, Schein Pharm (US)	00364-0443-01
100's	$4.46	Imipramine Hcl, HL Moore Drug Exch	00839-1370-06
100's	$4.50	Imipramine Hcl, Goldline Labs	00182-0826-01
100's	$4.50	Imipramine Hcl, Rugby	00536-3929-01
100's	$4.60	Imipramine Hcl, Martec Pharms	52555-0254-01
100's	$4.62	Imipramine Hcl, Aligen Independ	00405-4534-01
100's	$4.73	Imipramine Hcl, Par Pharm	49884-0054-01
100's	$4.95	Imipramine Hcl, Parmed Pharms	00349-2079-01
100's	$4.95	Imipramine HCl, Geneva Pharms	00781-1762-01
100's	$8.02	Imipramine Hcl, Vangard Labs	00615-0528-13
100's	$9.85	Imipramine Hcl, Major Pharms	00904-0925-61
100's	**$26.09**	**TOFRANIL, Novartis**	**00028-0032-01**
250's	$4.70	Imipramine HCl, H.C.F.A. F F P	99999-1525-03
250's	$6.70	Imipramine Hcl, Major Pharms	00904-0925-70
750's	$56.86	Imipramine HCl, Glasgow Pharm	60809-0104-55
750's	$56.86	Imipramine HCl, Glasgow Pharm	60809-0104-72
1000's	$18.00	Imipramine Hcl, Major Pharms	00904-0925-80
1000's	$18.80	Imipramine HCl, H.C.F.A. F F P	99999-1525-04
1000's	$21.38	Imipramine Hcl, United Res	00677-0421-10
1000's	$21.40	Imipramine Hcl, Qualitest Pharms	00603-4043-32

HOW SUPPLIED - RATED THERAPEUTICALLY EQUIVALENT:
(cont'd)

1000's	$21.40	Imipramine Hcl, Mutual Pharm	53489-0330-10
1000's	$21.85	Imipramine HCl, Teva	00332-2111-15
1000's	$25.99	Imipramine Hcl, HL Moore Drug Exch	00839-1370-16
1000's	$31.25	Imipramine HCl, Rugby	00536-3929-10
1000's	$31.80	Imipramine Hcl, Martec Pharms	52555-0254-10
1000's	$32.71	Imipramine Hcl, Par Pharm	49884-0054-10
1000's	$32.78	IMIPRAMINE HCL, Aligen Independ	00405-4534-03
1000's	$34.26	Imipramine Hc1, Parmed Pharms	00349-2079-10

Tablet, Sugar Coated - Oral - 25 mg

30's	$.69	Imipramine HCl, H.C.F.A. F F P	99999-1525-05
100's	$2.33	Imipramine HCl, H.C.F.A. F F P	99999-1525-06
100's	$3.15	Imipramine Hcl, Qualitest Pharms	00603-4044-21
100's	$3.42	Imipramine HCl, Teva	00332-2113-09
100's	$3.60	Imipramine Hcl, Major Pharms	00904-0927-60
100's	$4.31	Imipramine Hcl, US Trading	56126-0055-11
100's	$4.59	Imipramine Hcl, United Res	00677-0422-01
100's	$4.60	Imipramine Hcl, Mutual Pharm	53489-0331-01
100's	$4.93	Imipramine Hcl, HL Moore Drug Exch	00839-1371-06
100's	$5.29	Imipramine HCl, Schein Pharm (US)	00364-0406-01
100's	$6.05	Imipramine Hcl, Goldline Labs	00182-0827-01
100's	$6.10	Imipramine Hcl, Aligen Independ	00405-4535-01
100's	$6.17	Imipramine Hcl, Martec Pharms	52555-0255-01
100's	$6.25	Imipramine Hcl, Parmed Pharms	00349-2080-01
100's	$6.36	Imipramine Hcl, Par Pharm	49884-0055-01
100's	$6.37	Imipramine HCl, Geneva Pharms	00781-1764-01
100's	$10.30	Imipramine HCl, Goldline Labs	00182-0827-89
100's	$10.54	Imipramine Hcl, Roxane	00054-8419-25
100's	$11.00	IMAVATE, AH Robins	00031-5625-63
100's	$11.63	Imipramine Hcl, Vangard Labs	00615-0529-13
100's	$11.64	Imipramine HCl, Geneva Pharms	00781-1764-13
100's	$17.23	Imipramine Hcl, Major Pharms	00904-0927-61
100's	**$43.63**	**TOFRANIL, Novartis**	**00028-0140-01**
100's	$49.50	Imipramine Hcl, Rugby	00536-3930-01
250's	$5.82	Imipramine HCl, H.C.F.A. F F P	99999-1525-07
250's	$7.65	Imipramine Hcl, Major Pharms	00904-0927-70
750's	$72.25	Imipramine HCl, Glasgow Pharm	60809-0105-55
750's	$72.25	Imipramine HCl, Glasgow Pharm	60809-0105-72
1000's	$22.30	Imipramine Hcl, Qualitest Pharms	00603-4044-32
1000's	$23.30	Imipramine HCl, H.C.F.A. F F P	99999-1525-08
1000's	$29.00	Imipramine Hcl, Mutual Pharm	53489-0331-10
1000's	$29.25	Imipramine Hcl, Major Pharms	00904-0927-80
1000's	$30.13	Imipramine Hcl, United Res	00677-0422-10
1000's	$33.16	Imipramine HCl, Teva	00332-2113-15
1000's	$40.66	Imipramine Hcl, Lederle Pharm	00005-3216-34
1000's	$43.29	JANIMINE, Abbott	00074-1898-19
1000's	$44.35	Imipramine Hcl, HL Moore Drug Exch	00839-1371-16
1000's	$45.85	Imipramine Hcl, Amer Preferred	53445-0827-00
1000's	$48.64	Imipramine HCl, Schein Pharm (US)	00364-0406-02
1000's	$49.50	Imipramine Hcl, Rugby	00536-3930-10
1000's	$52.63	Imipramine Hcl, Goldline Labs	00182-0827-10
1000's	$52.82	Imipramine Hcl, Aligen Independ	00405-4535-03
1000's	$53.68	Imipramine Hcl, Martec Pharms	52555-0255-10
1000's	$55.26	Imipramine Hcl, Par Pharm	49884-0055-10
1000's	$57.95	Imipramine Hcl, Parmed Pharms	00349-2080-10
1000's	$60.52	Imipramine HCl, Geneva Pharms	00781-1764-10
1000's	$70.53	Imipramine Hcl, Roxane	00054-4419-31
1200's	**$490.34**	**TOFRANIL, Novartis**	**00028-0140-65**

Tablet, Sugar Coated - Oral - 50 mg

30's	$.92	Imipramine HCl, H.C.F.A. F F P	99999-1525-09
100's	$3.08	Imipramine HCl, H.C.F.A. F F P	99999-1525-10
100's	$4.30	Imipramine Hcl, Qualitest Pharms	00603-4045-21
100's	$4.94	Imipramine HCl, Teva	00332-2117-09
100's	$5.09	Imipramine Hcl, US Trading	56126-0056-11
100's	$5.38	Imipramine Hcl, United Res	00677-0423-01
100's	$5.60	Imipramine Hcl, Mutual Pharm	53489-0332-01
100's	$5.93	Imipramine Hcl, HL Moore Drug Exch	00839-1372-06
100's	$5.96	Imipramine Hcl, Aligen Independ	00405-4536-01
100's	$7.00	Imipramine HCl, Schein Pharm (US)	00364-0435-01
100's	$7.50	Imipramine, Parmed Pharms	00349-2081-01
100's	$8.43	Imipramine Hcl, Lederle Pharm	00005-3217-23
100's	$8.55	Imipramine Hcl, Rugby	00536-3931-01
100's	$8.90	Imipramine Hcl, Goldline Labs	00182-0828-01
100's	$9.08	Imipramine Hcl, Martec Pharms	52555-0256-01
100's	$9.19	Imipramine Hcl, Par Pharm	49884-0056-01
100's	$9.20	Imipramine HCl, Geneva Pharms	00781-1766-01
100's	$16.00	Imipramine HCl, Goldline Labs	00182-0828-89
100's	$17.22	Imipramine Hcl, Vangard Labs	00615-0530-13
100's	$17.25	Imipramine HCl, Geneva Pharms	00781-1766-13
100's	$18.10	IMAVATE, AH Robins	00031-5650-63
100's	$18.91	Imipramine Hcl, Roxane	00054-8420-25
100's	$31.55	Imipramine Hcl, Major Pharms	00904-0929-61
100's	**$74.12**	**TOFRANIL, Novartis**	**00028-0136-01**
250's	$7.70	Imipramine HCl, H.C.F.A. F F P	99999-1525-11
250's	$11.10	Imipramine Hcl, Major Pharms	00904-0929-70
1000's	$30.80	Imipramine HCl, Teva	00332-2117-15
1000's	$30.80	Imipramine HCl, H.C.F.A. F F P	99999-1525-12
1000's	$39.80	Imipramine Hcl, Qualitest Pharms	00603-4045-32
1000's	$40.95	Imipramine Hcl, Major Pharms	00904-0929-80
1000's	$42.00	Imipramine Hcl, Mutual Pharm	53489-0332-10
1000's	$44.90	Imipramine Hcl, United Res	00677-0423-10
1000's	$59.33	Imipramine Hcl, HL Moore Drug Exch	00839-1372-16
1000's	$65.00	Imipramine, Parmed Pharms	00349-2081-10
1000's	$67.51	Imipramine HCl, Schein Pharm (US)	00364-0435-02
1000's	$71.22	Imipramine Hcl, Lederle Pharm	00005-3217-34
1000's	$72.47	Imipramine Hcl, Amer Preferred	53445-0828-00
1000's	$74.50	Imipramine HCl, Rugby	00536-3931-10
1000's	$76.84	Imipramine Hcl, Purepac Pharm	00228-2233-96
1000's	$77.43	Imipramine Hcl, Goldline Labs	00182-0828-10
1000's	$77.48	Imipramine Hcl, Aligen Independ	00405-4536-03
1000's	$78.98	Imipramine Hcl, Martec Pharms	52555-0256-10
1000's	$79.09	Imipramine Hcl, Par Pharm	49884-0056-10
1000's	$87.40	Imipramine HCl, Geneva Pharms	00781-1766-10
1000's	$125.61	Imipramine Hcl, Roxane	00054-4420-31

HOW SUPPLIED - NOT RATED EQUIVALENT:

Injection, Solution - Intramuscular - 25 mg

10's	**$22.52**	**TOFRANIL AMPUL 25, Novartis**	**00028-0065-23**

Tablet, Sugar Coated - Oral - 10 mg

100's	$3.25	Imipramine Hcl, Consolidated Midland	00223-1103-01
1000's	$25.95	Imipramine Hcl, Consolidated Midland	00223-1103-02

HOW SUPPLIED - NOT RATED EQUIVALENT: *(cont'd)*

Tablet, Sugar Coated - Oral - 25 mg

100's	$4.50	Imipramine Hcl, Consolidated Midland	00223-1102-01
1000's	$34.50	Imipramine Hcl, Consolidated Midland	00223-1102-02

Tablet, Sugar Coated - Oral - 50 mg

100's	$5.75	Imipramine Hcl, Consolidated Midland	00223-1104-01
1000's	$43.50	Imipramine Hcl, Consolidated Midland	00223-1104-02

IMIPRAMINE PAMOATE *(001526)*

CATEGORIES: Antidepressants; Central Nervous System Agents; Depression; Psychostimulants; Psychotherapeutic Agents; Tricyclics; Tricyclic Antidepressants; FDA Approval Pre 1982

BRAND NAMES: **Tofranil-Pm**

FORMULARIES: Aetna

COST OF THERAPY: $93.30 (Depression; Capsule; 75 mg; 1/day; 90 days)

PRIMARY ICD9: 311 (Depressive Disorder, Not Elsewhere Classified)

DESCRIPTION:

Each 75-mg Tofranil-Pm capsule contains imipramine pamoate equivalent to 75 mg of imipramine hydrochloride. Each 100-mg capsule contains imipramine pamoate equivalent to 100 mg of imipramine hydrochloride. Each 125-mg capsule contains imipramine pamoate equivalent to 125 mg of imipramine hydrochloride. Each 150-mg capsule contains imipramine pamoate equivalent to 150 mg of imipramine hydrochloride. *Inactive Ingredients:* D&C Red No. 28, edetate calcium disodium, FD&C Blue No.1, FD&C Yellow No. 6, gelatin, magnesium stearate, parabens, sodium lauryl sulfate, sodium propionate, starch, talc, and titanium dioxide.

Imipramine pamoate is a tricyclic antidepressant, available as capsules for oral administration. The 75, 100, 125, and 150 mg capsules contain imipramine pamoate equivalent to 75, 100, 125, and 150 mg of imipramine hydrochloride. Imipramine pamoate is 5-(3-(dimethylamino)propyl)-10,11-dihydro-5H-dibenz(b,f)azepine4,4'-methylenebis-(3-hydroxy-2-naphtholate)(2:1).

Imipramine pamoate is a fine, yellow, tasteless, odorless powder. It is soluble in ethanol, in acetone, in ether, in chloroform, and in carbon tetrachloride, and is insoluble in water. Its molecular weight is 949.21.

CLINICAL PHARMACOLOGY:

The mechanism of action of imipramine is not definitely known. However, it does not act primarily by stimulation of the central nervous system. The clinical effect is hypothesized as being due to potentiation of adrenergic synapses by blocking uptake of norepinephrine at nerve endings.

INDICATIONS AND USAGE:

For the relief of symptoms of depression. Endogenous depression is more likely to be alleviated than other depressive states. One to three weeks of treatment may be needed before optimal therapeutic effects are evident.

CONTRAINDICATIONS:

The concomitant use of monoamine oxidase inhibiting compounds is contraindicated. Hyperpyretic crises or severe convulsive seizures may occur in patients receiving such combinations. The potentiation of adverse effects can be serious, or even fatal. When it is desired to substitute imipramine pamoate in patients receiving a monoamine oxidase inhibitor, as long an interval should elapse as the clinical situation will allow, with a minimum of 14 days. Initial dosage should be low and increases should be gradual and cautiously prescribed.

The drug is contraindicated during the acute recovery period after a myocardial infarction. Patients with a known hypersensitivity to this compound should not be given the drug. The possibility of cross-sensitivity to other dibenzazepine compounds should be kept in mind.

WARNINGS:

Extreme caution should be used when this drug is given to: patients with cardiovascular disease because of the possibility of conduction defects, arrhythmias, congestive heart failure, myocardial infarction, strokes, and tachycardia. These patients require cardiac surveillance at all dosage levels of the drug; patients with increased intraocular pressure, history of urinary retention, or history of narrow-angle glaucoma because of the drug's anticholinergic properties: hyperthyroid patients or those on thyroid medication because of the possibility of cardiovascular toxicity; patients with a history of seizure disorder because this drug has been shown to lower the seizure threshold; patients receiving guanethidine, clonidine, or similar agents, since imipramine pamoate may block the pharmacologic effects of these drugs; patients receiving methylphenidate hydrochloride. Since methylphenidate hydrochloride may inhibit the metabolism of imipramine pamoate, downward dosage adjustment of imipramine pamoate may be required when given concomitantly with methylphenidate hydrochloride.

Since imipramine pamoate may impair the mental and/or physical abilities required for the performance of potentially hazardous tasks, such as operating an automobile or machinery, the patient should be cautioned accordingly.

Imipramine pamoate may enhance the CNS depressant effects of alcohol. Therefore, it should be borne in mind that the dangers inherent in a suicide attempt or accidental overdosage with the drug may be increased for the patient who uses excessive amounts of alcohol. (See PRECAUTIONS.)

Usage in Children: Imipramine pamoate should not be used in children of any age because of the increased potential for acute overdosage due to the high unit potency (75 mg, 100 mg, 125 mg, and 150 mg). Each capsule contains imipramine pamoate equivalent to 75 mg, 100 mg, 125 mg or 150 mg imipramine hydrochloride.

PRECAUTIONS:

An ECG recording should be taken prior to the initiation of larger-than-usual doses of imipramine pamoate and at appropriate intervals thereafter until steady state is achieved. (Patients with any evidence of cardiovascular disease require cardiac surveillance at all dosage levels of the drug. See WARNINGS.) Elderly patients and patients with cardiac disease or a prior history of cardiac disease are at special risk of developing the cardiac abnormalities associated with the use of imipramine pamoate. It should be kept in mind that the possibility of suicide in seriously depressed patients is inherent in the illness and may persist until significant remission occurs. Such patients should be carefully supervised during the early phase of treatment with imipramine pamoate and may require hospitalization. Prescriptions should be written for the smallest amount feasible.

PRECAUTIONS: *(cont'd)*

Hypomanic or manic episodes may occur, particularly in patients with cyclic disorders. Such reactions may necessitate discontinuation of the drug. If needed, imipramine pamoate may be resumed in lower dosage when these episodes are relieved. Administration of a tranquilizer may be useful in controlling such episodes.

An activation of the psychosis may occasionally be observed in schizophrenic patients and may require reduction of dosage and the addition of a phenothiazine.

Concurrent administration of imipramine pamoate with electroshock therapy may increase the hazards: such treatment should be limited to those patients for whom it is essential, since there is limited clinical experience.

Usage During Pregnancy and Lactation: Animal reproduction studies have yielded inconclusive results. (See ANIMAL PHARMACOLOGY).

There have been no well-controlled studies conducted with pregnant women to determine the effect of imipramine on the fetus. However, there have been clinical reports of congenital malformations associated with the use of the drug. Although a causal relationship between these effects and the drug could not be established, the possibility of fetal risk from the maternal ingestion of imipramine cannot be excluded. Therefore, imipramine should be used in women who are or might become pregnant only if the clinical condition clearly justifies potential risk to the fetus.

Limited data suggest that imipramine is likely to be excreted in human breast milk. As a general rule, a woman taking a drug should not nurse since the possibility exists that the drug may be excreted in breast milk and be harmful to the child.

Patients should be warned that imipramine pamoate may enhance the CNS depressant effects of alcohol. (See WARNINGS.) Imipramine pamoate should be used with caution in patients with significantly impaired renal or hepatic function.

Patients who develop a fever and a sore throat during therapy with imipramine pamoate should have leukocyte and differential blood counts performed.

Imipramine pamoate should be discontinued if there is evidence of pathological neutrophil depression.

Prior to elective surgery, imipramine pamoate should be discontinued for as long as the clinical situation will allow.

In occasional susceptible patients or in those receiving anticholinergic drugs (including antiparkinsonism agents) in addition, the atropine-like effects may become more pronounced (*e.g.,* paralytic ileus). Close supervision and careful adjustment of dosage is required when imipramine pamoate is administered concomitantly with anticholinergic drugs.

Avoid the use of preparations, such as decongestants and local anesthetics, which contain any sympathomimetic amine (*e.g.,* epinephrine, norepinephrine), since it has been reported that tricyclic antidepressants can potentiate the effects of catecholamines.

Caution should be exercised when imipramine pamoate is used with agents that lower blood pressure.

Imipramine pamoate may potentiate the effects of CNS depressant drugs.

The plasma concentration of imipramine may increase when the drug is given concomitantly with hepatic enzyme inhibitors (*e.g.,* cimetidine, fluoxetine) and decrease by concomitant administration with hepatic enzyme inducers (*e.g.,* barbiturates, phenytoin), and adjustment of the dosage of imipramine may therefore be necessary.

Patients taking imipramine pamoate should avoid excessive exposure to sunlight since there have been reports of photosensitization.

Both elevation and lowering of blood sugar levels have been reported with imipramine pamoate use.

ADVERSE REACTIONS:

Note: Although the listing which follows includes a few adverse reactions which have not been reported with this specific drug, the pharmacological similarities among the tricyclic antidepressant drugs require that each of the reactions be considered when imipramine is administered.

Cardiovascular: Orthostatic hypotension, hypertension, tachycardia, palpitation, myocardial infarction, arrhythmias, heart block, ECG changes, precipitation of congestive heart failure, stroke.

Psychiatric: Confusional states (especially in the elderly) with hallucinations, disorientation, delusions: anxiety, restlessness, agitation; insomnia and nightmares; hypomania; exacerbation of psychosis.

Neurological: Numbness, tingling, paresthesias of extremities; incoordination, ataxia, tremors; peripheral neuropathy; extrapyramidal symptoms; seizures, alterations in EEG patterns; tinnitus.

Anticholinergic: Dry mouth, and, rarely associated sublingual adenitis; blurred vision, disturbances of accommodation, mydriasis; constipation, paralytic ileus; urinary retention, delayed micturition, dilation off the urinary tract.

Allergic: Skin rash, petechiae, urticaria, itching, photosensitization; edema (general or of face and tongue); drug fever; cross sensitivity with desipramine.

Hematologic: Bone marrow depression including agranulocytosis; eosinophilia; purpura; thrombocytopenia.

Gastrointestinal: Nausea and vomiting, anorexia, epigastric distress, diarrhea; peculiar taste, stomatitis abdominal cramps, black tongue.

Endocrine: Gynecomastia in the male; breast enlargement and galactorrhea in the female; increased or decreased libido, impotence; testicular swelling; elevation or depression of blood sugar levels; inappropriate antidiuretic hormone (ADH) secretion syndrome.

Other: Jaundice (simulating obstructive); altered liver function; weight gain or loss; perspiration; flushing; urinary frequency; drowsiness, dizziness weakness and fatigue; headache; parotid swelling; alopecia; proneness to falling.

Withdrawal Symptoms: Though not indicative of addiction, abrupt cessation of treatment after prolonged therapy may produce nausea, headache and malaise.

OVERDOSAGE:

Children have been reported to be more sensitive than adults to an acute overdosage of imipramine pamoate. An acute overdose of any amount in infants or young children, especially, must considered serious and potentially fatal.

Signs and Symptoms: These may vary in severity depending upon factors such as the amount of drug absorbed, the age of the patient, and the interval between drug ingestion and the start of treatment. Blood and urine levels of imipramine may not reflect the severity of poisoning; they have chiefly a qualitative rather than a quantitative value, and are unreliable indicators in the clinical management of the patient.

CNS abnormalities may include drowsiness, stupor, coma, ataxia, restlessness, agitation, hyperactive reflexes, muscle rigidity, athetoid and choreiform movements, and convulsions.

Cardiac abnormalities may include arrhythmia, tachycardia, ECG evidence of impaired conduction, and signs of congestive heart failure.

OVERDOSAGE: *(cont'd)*

Respiratory depression, cyanosis, hypotension, shock, vomiting, hyperpyrexia, mydriasis, and diaphoresis may also be present.

Treatment: The recommended treatment for overdosage with tricyclic antidepressants may change periodically. Therefore, it is recommended that the physician contact a poison control center for current information on treatment. Because CNS involvement, respiratory depression and cardiac arrhythmia can occur suddenly, hospitalization and close observation may be necessary, even when the amount ingested is thought to be small or the initial degree of intoxication appears slight or moderate. All patients with ECG abnormalities should have continuous cardiac monitoring and be closely observed until well after cardiac status has returned to normal; relapses may occur after apparent recovery. In the alert patient, empty the stomach promptly by lavage. In the obtunded patient, secure the airway with a cuffed endotracheal tube before beginning lavage (do not induce emesis). Instillation of activated charcoal slurry may help reduce absorption of imipramine.

Minimize external stimulation to reduce the tendency to convulsions. If anticonvulsants are necessary, diazepam and phenytoin may be useful.

Maintain adequate respiratory exchange. Do not use respiratory stimulants.

Shock should be treated with supportive measures, such as appropriate position, intravenous fluids, and, if necessary, a vasopressor agent. The use of corticosteroids in shock is controversial and may be contraindicated in cases of overdosage with tricyclic antidepressants. Digitalis may increase conduction abnormalities and further irritate an already sensitized myocardium. If congestive heart failure necessitates rapid digitalization, particular care must be exercised.

Hyperpyrexia should be controlled by whatever external means are available, including ice packs and cooling sponge baths, if necessary.

Hemodialysis, peritoneal dialysis, exchange transfusions and forced diuresis have been generally reported as ineffective because of the rapid fixation of imipramine in tissues. Blood and urine levels of imipramine may not correlate with the degree of intoxication, and are unreliable indicators in the clinical management of the patient.

The slow intravenous administration of physostigmine salicylate has been used as a last resort to reverse severe CNS anticholinergic manifestations of overdosage with tricyclic antidepressants; however, it should not be used routinely since it may induce seizures and cholinergic crises.

Do not store above 86°F (30°C)

DOSAGE AND ADMINISTRATION:

The following recommended dosages for imipramine pamoate should be modified as necessary by the clinical response and any evidence of intolerance.

INITIAL ADULT DOSAGE

Outpatients: Therapy should be initiated at 75 mg/day. Dosage may be increased to 150 mg/day which is the dose level at which optimum response is usually obtained. If necessary, dosage may be increased to 200 mg/day.

Dosage higher than 75 mg/day may also be administered on a once-a-day basis after the optimum dosage and tolerance have been determined. The daily dosage may be given at bedtime. In some patients it may be necessary to employ a divided-dose schedule.

As with all tricyclics, the antidepressant effect of imipramine may not be evident for one to three weeks in some patients.

Hospitalized Patients: Therapy should be initiated at 100-150 mg/day and may be increased to 200 mg/day. If there is no response after two weeks, dosage should be increased to 250-300 mg/day.

Dosage higher than 150 mg/day may also be administered on a once-a-day basis after the optimum dosage and tolerance have been determined. The daily dosage may be given at bedtime. In some patients it may be necessary to employ a divided-dose schedule.

As with all tricyclics, the antidepressant effect of imipramine may not be evident for one to three weeks in come patients.

Adult Maintenance Dosage: Following remission, maintenance medication may be required for a longer period of time at the lowest dose that will maintain remission after which the dosage should gradually be decreased.

The usual maintenance dosage is 75-150 mg/day. The total daily dosage can be administered on a once-a-day basis, preferably at bedtime. In some patients it may be necessary to employ a divided-dose schedule.

In cases of relapse due to premature withdrawal of the drug, the effective dosage of imipramine should be reinstituted.

Adolescent and Geriatric Patients: Therapy in these age groups should be initiated with Tofranil, brand of imipramine hydrochloride, tablets at a total daily dosage of 25-50 mg, since imipramine pamoate capsules are not available in these strengths. Dosage may be increased according to response and tolerance, but it is generally unnecessary to exceed 100 mg/day in these patients. Imipramine pamoate capsules may be used when total daily dosage is established at 75 mg or higher.

The total daily dosage can be administered on a once-a-day basis, preferably at bedtime. In some patients it may be necessary to employ a divided-dose schedule.

As with all tricyclics, the antidepressant effect of imipramine may not be evident for to three weeks in some patients.

Adolescent and geriatric patients can usually be maintained at lower dosage. Following remission, maintenance medication may be required for a longer period of time at the lowest dose that will maintain remission after which the dosage should gradually be decreased.

The total daily maintenance dosage can be administered on a once-a-day basis, preferably at bedtime.

In some patients it may be necessary to employ a divided-dose schedule.

In cases of relapse due to premature withdrawal of the drug, the effective dosage of imipramine should be reinstituted.

ANIMAL PHARMACOLOGY:

TOXICOLOGY

A. Acute: *Oral* LD_{50}:Mouse 2185 mg/kg; Rat (F) 1142 mg/kg; (M) 1807 mg/kg; Rabbit 1016 mg/kg; Dog 693 mg/kg (Emesis ED_{50})

B. Subacute: Two three-month studies in dogs gave evidence of an adverse drug effect on the testes, but only at the highest dose level employed, (*i.e.,* 90 mg/kg (10 times the maximum human dose)). Depending on the histological section of the testes examined, the findings consisted of a range of degenerative changes up to and including complete atrophy of the seminiferous tubules, with spermatogenesis usually arrested.

Human studies show no definitive effect on sperm count, sperm motility, sperm morphology or volume of ejaculate.

One three-month study was done in rats at dosage levels comparable to those of the dog studies. No adverse drug effect on the tests was noted in this study, as confirmed by histological examination.

C. Reproduction/Teratogenic:

ANIMAL PHARMACOLOGY: *(cont'd)*

Oral: Imipramine pamoate was fed to male and female albino rats for 28 weeks through two breeding cycles at dose levels of 15 mg/kg/day and 40 mg/kg/day (equivalent 2 1/2 and 7 times the maximum human dose).

No abnormalities which could be related to drug administration were noted in gross inspection. Autopsies performed on pups from the second breeding likewise revealed no pathological changes in organs or tissues; however, a decrease in mean litter size from both matings was noted in the drug-treated groups and significant growth suppression occurred in the nursing pups of both sexes in the high group as well as in the females of the low-level group. Finally, the lactation index (pups weaned divided by number left to nurse) was significantly lower in the second litter of the high-level group.

HOW SUPPLIED - EQUIVALENTS NOT AVAILABLE:

Capsule, Gelatin - Oral - 75 mg

30's	$31.81	TOFRANIL-PM, Novartis	00028-0020-26
100's	$103.67	TOFRANIL-PM, Novartis	00028-0020-01

Capsule, Gelatin - Oral - 100 mg

30's	$41.77	TOFRANIL-PM, Novartis	00028-0040-26
100's	$136.29	TOFRANIL-PM, Novartis	00028-0040-01

Capsule, Gelatin - Oral - 125 mg

30's	$51.93	TOFRANIL-PM, Novartis	00028-0045-26
100's	$169.95	TOFRANIL-PM, Novartis	00028-0045-01

Capsule, Gelatin - Oral - 150 mg

30's	$59.36	TOFRANIL-PM, Novartis	00028-0022-26
100's	$193.73	TOFRANIL-PM, Novartis	00028-0022-01

IMIQUIMOD *(003328)*

CATEGORIES: Condylomata Acuminata; Genital Warts; Immuno Response Modifier; Pregnancy Category B; Perianal Warts; Sexually Transmitted Diseases; Skin/Mucous Membrane Agents; Topical; FDA Approved 1997 Mar

BRAND NAMES: **Aldara**

DESCRIPTION:

Imiquimod is an immune response modifier. Each gram of Aldara 5% cream contains 50 mg of imiquimod in an off-white oil-in-water vanishing cream base consisting of isostearic acid, cetyl alcohol, stearyl alcohol, white petrolatum, polysorbate 60, sorbitan monostearate, glycerin, xanthan gum, purified water, benzyl alcohol, methylparaben, and propylparaben. Chemically, imiquimod is 1-(2-methylpropyl)-1*H*-imidazo(4,5-c)quinolin-4-amine. Imiquimod has a molecular formula of $C_{14}H_{16}N_4$ and a molecular weight of 240.3.

CLINICAL PHARMACOLOGY:

PHARMACODYNAMICS

The mechanisms of action of imiquimod in treating genital/perianal warts is unknown. Imiquimod has no direct antiviral activity in cell culture. Mouse skin studies suggest that imiquimod induces cytokines including interferon-α. However, the clinical relevance of these findings is unknown.

PHARMACOKINETICS

Percutaneous absorption of [^{14}C] imiquimod was minimal in a study involving 6 healthy subjects treated with a single topical application (5 mg) of [^{14}C] imiquimod cream formulation. No radioactivity was detected in the serum (lower limit of quantitation: 1 ng/ml) and <0.9% of the radiolabelled dose was excreted in the urine and feces following topical application.

CLINICAL STUDIES:

In a double-blind, placebo-controlled clinical trial, 209 otherwise healthy patients 18 years of age and older with genital/perianal warts were treated with Imiquimod 5% cream or vehicle control three times a week for a maximum of 16 weeks. The median baseline wart area was 69 mm^2 (range 8 to 5525 mm^2).

Data on complete clearance are listed in TABLE 1. The median time to complete wart clearance was 10 weeks.

TABLE 1 Clearance Study 1004

	Treatment	Patients with Complete Clearance of Warts	Patients Without Follow-up	Patients with Warts Remaining at Week 16
Overall	imiquimod 5% (n=109)	50%	17%	33%
	vehicle (n=100)	11%	27%	62%
Females	imiquimod 5% (n=46)	72%	11%	17%
	vehicle (n=40)	20%	33%	48%
Males	imiquimod 5% (n=63)	33%	22%	44%
	vehicle (n=60)	5%	23%	72%

INDICATIONS AND USAGE:

Imiquimod 5% cream is indicated for the treatment of external genital and perianal warts/condyloma acuminata in adults.

CONTRAINDICATIONS:

None known.

WARNINGS:

Imiquimod cream has not been evaluated for the treatment of urethral, intra-vaginal, cervical, rectal, or intra-anal human papilloma viral disease and is not recommended for these conditions.

PRECAUTIONS:

GENERAL

Local skin reactions such as erythema, erosion, excoriation/flaking, and edema are common. Should severe local skin reaction occur, the cream should be removed by washing the treatment area with mild soap and water. Treatment with imiquimod cream can be resumed after the skin reaction has subsided. There is no clinical experience with imiquimod cream therapy immediately following the treatment of genital/perianal warts with other cutaneously

PRECAUTIONS: *(cont'd)*

applied drugs; therefore, imiquimod cream administration is not recommended until genital/perianal tissue is healed from any previous drug or surgical treatment. Imiquimod has the potential to exacerbate inflammatory conditions of the skin.

INFORMATION FOR PATIENTS

Patients using imiquimod 5% cream should receive the following information and instructions: The effect of imiquimod 5% cream on the transmission of genital/perianal warts is unknown. Imiquimod 5% cream may weaken condoms and vaginal diaphragms. Therefore, concurrent use is not recommended.

1. This medication is to be used as directed by a physician. It is for external use only. Eye contact should be avoided.

2. The treatment area should not be bandaged or otherwise covered or wrapped as to be occlusive.

3. Sexual (genital, anal, oral) contact should be avoided while the cream is on the skin.

4. It is recommended that 6-10 hours following imiquimod 5% cream application the treatment area be washed with mild soap and water.

5. It is common for patients to experience local skin reactions such as erythema, erosion, excoriation/flaking, and edema at the site of application or surrounding areas. Most skins reactions are mild to moderate. Severe skin reactions can occur and should be reported promptly to the prescribing physician.

6. Uncircumcised males treating warts under the foreskin should retract the foreskin and clean the area daily.

7. Patients should be aware that new warts may develop during therapy, as imiquimod is not a cure.

CARCINOGENESIS, MUTAGENESIS, AND IMPAIRMENT OF FERTILITY

Rodent carcinogenicity data are not available. Imiquimod was without effect in a series of eight different mutagenicity assays including Ames, mouse lymphoma, CHO chromosomes aberration, human lymphocyte chromosome aberration, SHE cell transformation, rat and hamster bone marrow cytogenetics, and mouse dominant lethal test. Daily oral administration of imiquimod to rats, at doses up to 8 times the recommended human dose on a mg/m^2 basis throughout mating, gestation, parturition and lactation, demonstrated no impairment of reproduction.

PREGNANCY, TERATOGENIC EFFECTS, PREGNANCY CATEGORY B

There are no adequate and well-controlled studies in pregnant women. Imiquimod was not found to be teratogenic in rat or rabbit teratology studies. In rats at a high maternally toxic dose (28 times human dose on a mg/m^2 basis), reduced pup weights and delayed ossification were observed. In developmental studies with offspring of pregnant rats treated with imiquimod (8 times human dose), no adverse effects were demonstrated.

NURSING MOTHERS

It is not known whether topically applied imiquimod is excreted in breast milk.

PEDIATRIC USE

Safety and efficacy in patients below the age of 18 years have not been established.

ADVERSE REACTIONS:

In controlled clinical trials, the most frequently reported adverse reactions were those of local skin and application site reactions; some patients also reported systemic reactions. These reactions were usually mild to moderate in intensity; however, severe reactions were reported with three times a week application. These reactions were more frequent and more intense with daily application than with three times a week application. Overall, in the three times a week application clinical studies, 1.2% (4/327) of the patients discontinued due to local skin/application site reactions. The incidence and severity of local skin reactions during controlled clinical trials are shown in TABLE 2A and TABLE 2B.

TABLE 2A Three Times a Week Application Wart Site Reaction as Assessed By Investigator

	Mild /Moderate Females	Males	Females	Males
	Imiquimod N=114	Vehicle N=99	Imiquimod N=156	Vehicle N=157
Erythema	61%	21%	54%	22%
Erosion	30%	8%	29%	6%
Excoriation/Flaking	18%	8%	25%	8%
Edema	17%	5%	12%	1%
Induration	5%	2%	7%	2%
Ulceration	5%	1%	4%	1%
Scabbing	4%	0%	13%	3%
Vesicles	3%	0%	2%	0%

TABLE 2B Three Times a Week Application Wart Site Reaction as Assessed By Investigator

	Severe Females	Males	Females	Males
	5% Imiquimod N=114	Vehicle N=99	5% Imiquimod N=156	Vehicle N=157
Erythema	4%	0%	4%	0%
Erosion	1%	0%	1%	0%
Excoriation/Flaking	0%	0%	1%	0%
Edema	1%	0%	0%	0%
Induration	0%	0%	0%	0%
Ulceration	3%	0%	0%	0%
Scabbing	0%	0%	0%	0%
Vesicles	0%	0%	0%	0%

Remote site skin reactions were also reported in female and male patients treated three times a week with imiquimod 5% cream. The severe remote site skin reactions reported for females were erythema (3%), ulceration (2%), and edema (1%); and for males, erosion (2%), and erythema, edema, induration, and excoriation/flaking (each 1%).

Adverse events judged to be probably or possibly related to imiquimod reported by more than 5% of patients are listed in TABLE 3; also included are soreness, influenza-like symptoms and myalgia.

Adverse events judged to be possibly or probably related to imiquimod and reported by more than 1% of patients include:

Application Site Disorders: wart site reactions (burning, hypopigmentation, irritation, itching, pain, rash, sensitivity, soreness, stinging, tenderness); remote site reactions (bleeding, burning, itching, pain, tenderness, tinea cruris);

Body as a Whole: fatigue, fever, influenza-like symptoms;

Central and Peripheral Nervous System: headache;

ADVERSE REACTIONS: *(cont'd)*

TABLE 3 Three Times a Week Application

	Females 5% Imiquimod	Vehicle	Males 5% Imiquimod	Vehicle
	(n=117)	(n=103)	(n=156)	(n=158)
Application Site Disorders:				
Application Site Reaction				
Wart Site:				
Itching	32%	20%	22%	10%
Burning	26%	12%	9%	5%
Pain	8%	2%	2%	1%
Soreness	3%	0%	0%	1%
Fungal Infection*	11%	3%	2%	1%
Systemic Reactions				
Headache	4%	3%	5%	2%
Influenza-like symptoms	3%	2%	1%	0%
Myalgia	1%	0%	1%	1%

* Incidences reported without regard to causality with imiquimod.

Gastro-Intestinal System Disorders: diarrhea;

Musculo-Skeletal System Disorders: myalgia.

OVERDOSAGE:

Overdosage of imiquimod 5% cream in humans is unlikely due to minimal percutaneous absorption. Animal studies reveal a rabbit dermal lethal imiquimod dose of greater than 1600 mg/m^2. Persistent topical overdosing of imiquimod 5% cream could result in severe local skin reactions. The most clinically serious adverse event reported following multiple oral imiquimod doses of >200 mg was hypotension which resolved following oral or intravenous fluid administration.

DOSAGE AND ADMINISTRATION:

Imiquimod cream is to be applied three times per week, prior to normal sleeping hours, and left on the skin for 6-10 hours. Following the treatment period cream should be removed by washing the treated area with mild soap and water. Examples of three times per week application schedules are: Monday, Wednesday, Friday; or Tuesday, Thursday, Saturday application prior to sleeping hours. Imiquimod treatment should continue until there is total clearance of the genital/perianal warts or for a maximum of 16 weeks. Local skin reactions (erythema) at the treatment site are common. A rest period of several days may be taken if required by the patient's discomfort or severity of the local skin reaction. Treatment may resume once the reaction subsides. Non-occlusive dressings such as cotton gauze or cotton underwear may be used in the management of skin reactions. The technique for proper dose administration should be demonstrated by the prescriber to maximize the benefit of imiquimod therapy. Handwashing before and after cream application is recommended. Imiquimod 5% cream is packaged in single-use packets which contain sufficient cream to cover a wart area of up to 20 cm^2; use of excessive amounts of cream should be avoided. Patients should be instructed to apply imiquimod cream to external and/or perianal warts. A thin layer is applied to the wart area and rubbed in until the cream is no longer visible. The application site is not to be occluded.

Do not store above 30°C (86°F). Avoid freezing.

PATIENT INFORMATION:

Imiquidmod is for the treatment of external genital warts. It is not a cure. There is no information regarding pregnancy or breast-feeding. Use only as directed. Avoid getting into eyes. Do not bandage the treatment area. Avoid sexual contact while the drug is on the skin. Wash treated area 6 to 10 hours after application of the cream. May cause redness, irritation, flaking and swelling in and around the treatment area. Report severe skin reactions to your physician. Uncircumcised males treating warts under the foreskin should retract the foreskin and clean the area daily. Wash hands before and after applying the cream.

HOW SUPPLIED - EQUIVALENTS NOT AVAILABLE:

Cream - Topical - 5%

12 x 250 mg $108.00 ALDARA, 3M Pharms 00089-0610-12

IMMUNE SERUM GLOBULIN HUMAN *(001527)*

CATEGORIES: Abortion; AIDS Related Complex; Biologicals; Blood Components/Substitutes; Blood Formation/Coagulation; Bone Marrow Transplantation; Chemotherapy; Hepatitis A; HIV Infection; Immune Globulin; Immunodeficiency; Immunologic; Immunomodulators; Infections; Kawaski Syndrome; Measles; Orphan Drugs; Plasma Fractions, Human; Purpura; Rubella; Serums, Toxoids and Vaccines; Severe Combined Immunodeficiency; Vaccines; Varicella; Pregnancy Category C; FDA Pre 1938 Drugs

BRAND NAMES: *Allerglobuline*; *Aunativ*; *Beriglobin* (Germany); *Beriglobin P*; *Beriglobin-P*; *Beriglobina*; *Citax F* (Mexico); *Endobulin* (England); *Gamafine*; *Gamanate*; Gamastan; *Gamastan Immune Globulin*; *Gamimune N*; Gamimune-N; *Gamma 16*; *Gammabulin*; Gamma Globulin; Gammagard; *Gammagard S D*; **Gammar**; *Gammonativ* (Germany); *Globuman Berna*; *Glogama*; IG; *IG Gamma*; Immune Globulin; IGIM; IGIV; *Intacglobin* (Mexico); *Intraglobin* (Germany); Iveegam; *Pentaglobin* (Germany); *Sando Globulin*; Sandoglobulin; *Sandoglobulina* (Mexico); *Sandoglobuline* (France); Venoglobulin; *Venoglobulin-I*; WinRho SD
(International brand names outside U.S. in italics)

FORMULARIES: WHO

DESCRIPTION:

GAMMAR IV

Immune Globulin Intravenous (Human), Gammar-IV, is a sterile, lyophilized preparation of intact, unmodified, immunoglobulin, primarily IgG, stabilized with Albumin (Human) and Sucrose. The distribution of IgG sub-classes is similar to that present in normal human plasma. It is prepared by cold alcohol fractionation of pooled plasma and is not chemically altered or enzymatically degraded. When reconstituted with the appropriate volume of Sterile Water for Injection USP, Gammar-IV contains 5% IgG, 3% Albumin (Human), 5% sucrose, and 0.5% sodium chloride. The pH of the solution has been adjusted to 6.8 ± 0.4 with citric acid and/or sodium carbonate. Gammar-IV contains no preservative. This product is intended for intravenous administration.

DESCRIPTION: *(cont'd)*

GAMMAR IM

Immune Globulin (Human) (IG) Gammar is a sterile solution of immunoglobulin G (IgG), containing 16.5=1.5% protein. It is prepared by cold alcohol fractionation of pooled plasma. Immune Globulin (Human)-Gammar contains the mercurial preservative thimerosal, at a concentration of 100 mg per liter and is stabilized with 0.3 M glycine. The pH of the solution has been adjusted to 6.8=0.4 with sodium bicarbonate. The product is intended for the intramuscular route of administration

CLINICAL PHARMACOLOGY:

GAMMAR IV

Immune Globulin Intravenous (Human), Gammar-IV provides a broad range of antibodies, capable of opsonization and neutralization of microbes and toxins, against bacterial and viral antigens for prevention or attenuation of infectious diseases. The half-life of Gammar-IV, as reflected in circulating lgG levels, is approximately three weeks, although individual variations have occurred.

Gammar-IV is a native, non-chemically modified lgG fractionated from pooled human donor plasma. The distribution of lgG sub-classes (lgG_1, lgG_2, lgG_3, lgG_4) is similar to that present in Cohn Fraction II. Since the lgG concentrate is prepared from a large pool of at least 1000 donors, it represents the expected diversity of antibodies in that population. The processing steps used in the manufacture of this product have been shown capable of eliminating at least 6.75 logs of added HIV.

Albumin (Human) and sucrose are added to the formulation in order to provide adequate stabilization of the lgG molecules and the reconstituted product. Because sucrose, when given intravenously, is excreted unchanged in the urine, Immune Globulin Intravenous (Human), Gammar-IV, may be given to diabetics without compensatory changes in insulin dosage regimen.

GAMMAR IM

Peak blood levels of immunoglobulin G are obtained approximately 2 days after intramuscular injection of IG. The half-life of IgG in the circulation of individuals with normal IgG levels is 23 days.

Passive immunization with IG modifies hepatitis A, prevents or modifies measles, and provides replacement therapy in persons with hypo- or agammaglobulinemia. IG is not standardized with respect to antibody titers against hepatitis B surface antigen and should not be used for prophylaxis of viral hepatitis type B. Prophylactic treatment to prevent hepatitis B can best be accomplished with the use of Hepatitis B Immune Globulin, often in combination with Hepatitis B Vaccine.

IG may be of benefit in women who have been exposed to rubella in the first trimester of pregnancy and who would not consider a therapeutic abortion. IG may also be considered for use in immunocompromised patients for passive immunization against varicella-Zoster Immune Globulin (Human) is not available.

IG is not indicated for routine prophylaxis or treatment of rubella, poliomyelitis, mumps, or varicella. It is not indicated for allergy or asthma in patients who have normal levels of immunoglobulin.

INDICATIONS AND USAGE:

GAMMAR IV

Indicated for patients with primary defective antibody synthesis such as agammaglobulinemia or hypogammaglobulinemia, who are at increased risk of infection. When high levels or rapid elevation of circulating gamma globulins are desired, intravenous administration is more desirable than intramuscular therapy.

GAMMAR IM

Hepatis A: The Prophylactic value of IG is greatest when given before or soon after exposure to Hepatitis A. IG is not indicated in persons with clinical manifestations of hepatitis A or in those exposed more than two weeks previously.

Measles (Rubeola): IG should be given to prevent or modify measles in a susceptible person exposed less than 6 days previously. (A susceptible person is one who has not been vaccinated and has not had measles previously). IG may be especially indicated for susceptible household contacts under one year of age, for whom the risk of complications is highest. IG and measles vaccine should not be given at the same time. If a child is older than 12 months and has received IG, he should be given measles vaccines about 3 months later, when the measles antibody titer will have disappeared.

If a susceptible child exposed to measles is immunocompromised, IG should be given immediately. Children who are immunocompromised should not receive measles vaccine or any other live viral vaccine.

Immunoglobulin Deficiency: In patients with immunoglobulin deficiencies, IG may prevent serious infection. However, IG may not prevent chronic infections of the external secretory tissues such as the respiratory and gastrointestinal tract.

Prophylactic therapy, especially against infections due to encapsulated bacteria, is effective in Bruton-type, sex linked congenital agammaglobulinemia, agammaglobulinemia and severe combined immunodeficiency.

Varicella: passive immunization against varicella in immunosuppressed patients is best accomplished by use of Varicella-Zoster Immune Globulin (Human) (VZIG). If VZIG is unavailable, IG, promptly given, may also modify varicella.

Rubella: The routine use of IG for prophylaxis of rubella in early pregnancy is of dubious value and cannot be justified. Some studies suggest that the use of IG in exposed susceptible women can lessen the likelihood of infection and fetal damage. IG may benefit those women who will not consider a therapeutic abortion.

CONTRAINDICATIONS:

These products are contraindicated in individuals with a history of anaphylactic or severe systemic response to immune globulin intramuscular or intravenous preparations.

Gammar-IV: should not be given to persons with isolated immunoglobulin A (lgA) deficiency. Such persons have the potential for developing antibodies to lgA and could have anaphylactic reactions to subsequent administration of blood products that contain lgA.

Gammar IM: IG should not be administered to patients who have severe thrombocytopenia or any coagulation disorder that would contraindicate intramuscular injections.

WARNINGS:

GAMMAR IV

If anaphylactic or severe anaphylactoid reactions occur, discontinue infusion immediately. Epinephrine should be available for the treatment of any acute anaphylactoid reactions.

Patients with agammaglobulinemia or extreme hypogammaglobulinemia who have not received immunoglobulin therapy within the preceding 8 weeks may be at risk of developing inflammatory reactions upon the infusion of human immunoglobulins. These reactions are manifested by a rise in temperature, chills, nausea and vomiting, and appear to be related to the rate of infusion.

WARNINGS: *(cont'd)*

Infusion rates and the patient's clinical state should be monitored closely during infusion. (See DOSAGE AND ADMINISTRATION.)

GAMMAR IM

IG should be given with caution to patients with a history of prior systemic allergic reactions following the administration of human immunoglobulin preparations.

IG is for intramuscular injection only.

PRECAUTIONS:

GENERAL

Gammar IV: Epinephrine should be available for treatment of acute allergic reactions. See DOSAGE AND ADMINISTRATIONsection for product compatibility information.

Gammar IM: IG should not be administered intravenously because of the potential for serious reactions. Injections should be made intramuscularly and care should be taken to draw back on the plunger of the syringe before the injection in order to be certain that the needle is not in the blood vessel.

Although systemic reactions to intramuscularly administered immunoglobulin preparations are rare, epinephrine should be available for the treatment of acute symptoms.

Pregnancy Category C: Animal reproduction studies have not been performed with Immune Globulin Intravenous (Human), Gammar-IV. It is also not known whether Gammar-IV can cause fetal harm when administered to a pregnant women or can affect reproduction capacity. Gammar-IV should be given to a pregnant women only if clearly needed.

Pediatric Use: See DOSAGE AND ADMINISTRATIONsection.

DRUG INTERACTIONS:

GAMMAR IV

It is reported that antibodies in immune globulin preparations may interfere with the response by pediatric patients to live viral vaccines such as measles, mumps and rubella. Immunizing physicians should be informed of recent therapy with Immune Globulin Intravenous (Human) so that appropriate precautions may be taken.

GAMMAR IM

Antibodies in the globulin preparation may interfere with the response to live viral vaccines such as measles, mumps, and rubella. Therefore, use of such vaccines should be deferred until approximately three months after IG administration.

ADVERSE REACTIONS:

GAMMAR IV

Adverse reactions which may occur include headache, backache, myalgia, pyrexia, hypotension, chills, flushing and nausea, usually beginning within one hour of the start of the infusion. Symptoms subside in most cases within 30 minutes. The incidence of adverse reactions reported for a twelve month multi-center, repeated administration crossover study was shown to be 16% for Immune Globulin Intravenous (Human), Gammar-IV and 11% for another manufacturer's Immune Globulin Intravenous (Human). Data from this clinical evaluation indicated that the numbers of patients experiencing adverse reactions to each preparation were comparable, and that similar reactions were involved regardless of preparation.

True anaphylactic reactions may occur in patients with a history of prior systemic allergic reactions or seizure following administration of human immunoglobulin preparations. Very rarely an anaphylactoid reaction may occur in patients with no prior history of severe allergic reactions to human immunoglobulin preparations. Patients previously sensitized to certain antigens, most commonly lgA, may be at risk of immediate anaphylactoid and hypersensitivity reactions. Epinephrine should be available for the treatment of any acute anaphylactoid reaction. (See WARNINGS and CONTRAINDICATIONS)

Infusion rates and clinical state should be monitored closely during infusion. If an adverse reaction occurs, the infusion rate should be reduced or the infusion stopped until the symptoms have subsided. (See DOSAGE AND ADMINISTRATION)

GAMMAR IM

Local pain and tenderness at the injection site, urticaria, and angioedema may occur. Anaphylactic reactions, although rare, have been reported following the injection of human immune globulin preparations. Anaphylaxis is more likely to occur if IG is given intravenously; therefore IG must be administered intramuscularly.

DOSAGE AND ADMINISTRATION:

GAMMAR IV

The usual dose of Immune Globulin Intravenous (Human) is directed toward restoration of the immune deficient patient's circulating lgG level to near-normal levels. Use of 100-200 mg/kg body weight every three to four weeks is recommended. An initial loading dose of at least 200 mg/kg at more frequent intervals, proceeding to 100-200 mg/kg at three week intervals once a therapeutic plasma level has been established can be used. However, treatment must be individualized for each patient due to variation among patients in catabolic rate of lgG.

Product Compatibility: It is recommended that Gammar IV be administered by a separate infusion line without admixture with other drugs or medications which the patient may be receiving. However, based upon compatibility studies, Gammar IV may be infused sequentially into a primary iv line containing either 0.9% sodium chloride injection or 5% dextrose injection or flushed with 0.9% sodium chloride injection or 5% dextrose injection. **Do not mix Immune Globulin Intravenous (Human) products of differing formulations.** If several doses of Immune Globulin Intravenous (Human), Gammar IV, are to be administered, several reconstituted vials of identical formulation and diluent may be pooled, using proper aseptic technique. As described under Reconstitution, below, do not shake or cause excessive foaming. Swirl gently to mix. Filtration is acceptable but not required; pore sizes of greater than equal or equal to 15 microns will be less likely to slow infusion.

Reconstitution: Directions must be followed exactly.

1. Bring diluent and lyophilized product vials to room temperature prior to reconstitution.
2. Remove plastic flip-off caps from both vials.
3. Treat rubber stoppers with antiseptic solution and allow to dry.
4. Remove the **clear** guard from the *plastic piercing pin* (with double orifice). Insert *plastic piercing pin*of the transfer spike into the upright **diluent** via first.
5. Remove the **blue** guard from the *plastic needle* (with single orifice). Invert the diluent vial with the attached transfer spike and insert *plastic needle* into the upright **product** vial.
6. The vacuum in the product vial will pull the diluent into the product vial. As soon as all diluent has been transferred the transfer spike will automatically admit filtered air to the product. An additional venting of the product vial after diluent addition is not necessary. Withdraw and discard transfer spike.

DOSAGE AND ADMINISTRATION: *(cont'd)*

7. Do not shake product vial. Solubilize the product by gently swirling it in an upright position. Avoid the formation of foam. *NOTE:*If the product cake is badly broken prior to addition of diluent, allow product vial to remain undisturbed for 2-3 minutes after addition of diluent **before** gently swirling to mix product.

8. Examine solution. Any small particles will dissolve with gentle swirling of vial. The solution should be clear and ready to administer in less than 20 minutes.

9. Product contains no preservative. Use within 3 hours of reconstitution.

Note: If several doses of Immune Globulin Intravenous (Human), Gammar IV, are to be pooled aseptically for administration, avoid excessive formation of foam in the pooling container and gently swirl the pooling container to mix. DO NOT SHAKE THE POOLING CONTAINER.

ADMINISTRATION

Caution: When entering the product stopper with an IV set spike for administration, care should be taken to follow the path made by the *plastic needle* of the transfer spike (see Reconstitution).

Immune Globulin Intravenous (Human) Gammar-IV is to be administered by intravenous infusion. The infusion should begin at a rate of 0.01 ml/kg/minute, increasing to 0.02 ml/kg/minute after 15 to 30 minutes. Most patients tolerate a gradual increase to 0.03-0.06 ml/kg/minute. For the average 70 kg person this is equivalent to 2 to 4 ml/minute. If adverse reactions develop, slowing the infusion rate will usually eliminate the reaction. Discard any unused solution.

Parenteral drug products should be inspected visually for particulate matter and discoloration prior to administration whenever solution and container permit.

GAMMAR IM

Dosage

Hepatitis A: IG in a dose of 0.01 ml/lb (0.02 ml/kg) is recommended for household and institutional hepatitis A contacts.

The following doses of IG are recommended for persons who plan to travel in areas where hepatitis A is common (TABLE 1):

TABLE 1

Length of Stay	Dose Volume
Less than three months	0.02 ml/kg
3 Months or longer	0.06 ml/kg (repeat every 4-6 months)

Measles (Rubeola): IG should be given in a dose of 0.11 ml/lb (0.25 ml/kg) to prevent or modify measles in a susceptible person exposed less than 6 days previously.

If a susceptible child who is also immunocompromised is exposed, IG in a dose of 0.5 ml/kg (maximum 15 ml) should be given immediately.

Immunoglobulin Deficiency: IG may prevent serious infection in patients with immunoglobulin deficiencies if circulating IgG levels are appear 200 mg/100 ml plasma are maintained. The recommended dosage is 0.66 ml/kg (at least 100 mg/kg) given every 3 to 4 weeks. A double dose is given at onset of therapy: some patients may require more frequent injections.

Varicella: If Varicella-Zoster Immune Globulin (Human) is unavailable, IG at a dose of 0.6 to 1.2 ml/kg given promptly, is the recommended dose.

Rubella: The recommended dose of 0.55 ml/kg IG may benefit women who will not consider a therapeutic abortion.

ADMINISTRATION

IG is administered intramuscularly (see PRECAUTIONS), preferably in the gluteal region. Doses over 10 ml should be divided and injected into several muscular sites to reduce local pain and discomfort.

Parenteral drug products should be inspected visually for particulate matter and discoloration prior to administration whenever solution and container permit.

REFERENCES:

1. Fudenberg HH. Sensitization to immunoglobulins and hazards of gamma globulin therapy. *Immunoglobulins, Biologic Aspects and Clinical Uses.* 1970; 211-220. Edited by Merler E. National Academy of Sciences, Washington, D.C. 2. Steele RW, Augustine RA, Tannenbaum AS, Marmer DJ. Intravenous Immune Globulin for Hypogammaglobulinemia: A Comparison of Opsonizing Capacity in Recipient Sera. *Clin. Immunol. Immunopathol.*1985; 34:275-283. 3. Martindale. *The Extra Pharmacopoeia*27th ed. Edited by Wade A. London: The Pharmaceutical Press. 1979;65. 4. Polley MJ, Fischetti VA, Landaburu PH. Native Intravenous IgG Exhibits Greater Biological Activity than Modified IgG. From the XX Cong. Int. Soc. of Hematology; 1984.

HOW SUPPLIED:

GAMMAR IV

Individual Vial Packages: Immune Globulin Intravenous (Human), Gammar IV, is supplied in single dose vials, with diluent and sterile, vented transfer spike for reconstitution. The 10 g dosage form package also contains an administration set.

Bulk Package: Immune Globulin Intravenous (Human), Gammar IV, 5.0 g immune globulin/vial is supplied in a bulk pack of six (6) single dose vials with six (6) sterile vented transfer spikes for reconstitution. Each single dose vial should be reconstituted with 100 ml Sterile Water for Injection, U.S.P. (not supplied).

Storage: When stored at temperatures not exceeding 30°C (86°F), Gammar-IV is stable for the period indicated by the expiration date on its label. Avoid freezing which may damage container for the diluent. For Gammar-IM, Vials should be stored at 2°-8° C (36°-46° F) Do not freeze. Do not use after expiration date.

HOW SUPPLIED - EQUIVALENTS NOT AVAILABLE:

Injection, Lyphl-Soln - Intravenous - 1 gm/vial

1 gm	$70.02	SANDOGLOBULIN, Novartis	00078-0120-58
1.0 gm	**$58.13**	**GAMMAR-IV, Centeon**	**00053-7490-01**

Injection, Lyphl-Soln - Intravenous - 2.5 gm

2.5 gm	**$145.31**	**GAMMAR-IV, Centeon**	**00053-7490-02**

Injection, Lyphl-Soln - Intravenous - 3 gm/vial

3 gm	$133.20	SANDOGLOBULIN, Novartis	00078-0122-59
3 gm	$1305.00	SANDOGLOBULIN, Novartis	00078-0122-19

Injection, Lyphl-Soln - Intravenous - 5 gm

5.0 gm	**$290.63**	**GAMMAR-IV, Centeon**	**00053-7490-05**

Injection, Lyphl-Soln - Intravenous - 6 gm/vial

1's	$252.00	SANDOGLOBULIN, Novartis	00078-0124-96
6 gm	$2484.00	SANDOGLOBULIN, Novartis	00078-0124-19

Injection, Solution - Intramuscular

2 ml	$3.00	Immune Serum Globulin, Baxter Hyland	00944-0442-01
10 ml	$9.00	Immune Serum Globulin, Baxter Hyland	00944-0442-02
10 ml	$16.75	Immune Globulin, Melville	13143-0357-26
10 ml	$18.00	GAMASTAN, Bayer Pharm	00192-0615-12

HOW SUPPLIED - EQUIVALENTS NOT AVAILABLE: *(cont'd)*

Injection, Solution - Intramuscular - 16.5 %

10 ml	**$22.13**	**GAMMAR, Centeon**	**00053-7595-02**

Injection, Solution - Intravenous - 0.5 gm

1's	$54.92	GAMMAGARD S/D, Baxter Hyland	00944-2620-01

Injection, Solution - Intravenous - 1 gm

1's	$65.00	IVEEGAM, Immuno-US	54129-0233-10

Injection, Solution - Intravenous - 2.5 gm

1's	$150.22	VENOGLOBULIN-I, Abbott	00074-1600-20
1's	$152.05	VENOGLOBULIN-I, Alpha Therapeutic	49669-1602-01
1's	$156.62	GAMMAGARD S/D, Baxter Hyland	00944-2620-02
1's	$162.50	IVEEGAM, Immuno-US	54129-0233-25
1's	$166.16	VENOGLOBULIN-I, Abbott	00074-1600-21

Injection, Solution - Intravenous - 5 %

10 ml	$45.60	GAMIMUNE N, Bayer Pharm	00192-0640-12
50 ml	$142.80	GAMIMUNE N, Bayer Pharm	00192-0640-20
50 ml	$190.38	VENOGLOBULIN-S, Alpha Therapeutic	49669-1612-01
100 ml	$285.60	GAMIMUNE N, Bayer Pharm	00192-0640-71
100 ml	$380.75	VENOGLOBULIN-S, Alpha Therapeutic	49669-1613-01
200 ml	$761.50	VENOGLOBULIN-S, Alpha Therapeutic	49669-1614-01
250 ml	$714.00	GAMIMUNE N, Bayer Pharm	00192-0640-25

Injection, Solution - Intravenous - 5 gm

1's	$300.44	VENOGLOBULIN-I, Abbott	00074-1600-30
1's	$304.10	VENOGLOBULIN-I, Alpha Therapeutic	49669-1603-01
1's	$317.98	GAMMAGARD S/D, Baxter Hyland	00944-2620-03
1's	$325.00	IVEEGAM, Immuno-US	54129-0233-50
1's	$325.39	VENOGLOBULIN-I, Abbott	00074-1600-31

Injection, Solution - Intravenous - 10 %

10 ml	$75.00	GAMIMUNE-N, Bayer Pharm	00192-0649-12
50 ml	$375.00	GAMIMUNE N, Bayer Pharm	00192-0649-20
50 ml	$400.00	VENOGLOBULIN-S, Alpha Therapeutic	49669-1622-01
100 ml	$750.00	GAMIMUNE N, Bayer Pharm	00192-0649-71
100 ml	$800.00	VENOGLOBULIN-S, Alpha Therapeutic	49669-1623-01
200 ml	$1500.00	GAMIMUNE N, Bayer Pharm	00192-0649-24
200 ml	$1600.00	VENOGLOBULIN-S, Alpha Therapeutic	49669-1624-01

Injection, Solution - Intravenous - 10 gm

1's	**$581.25**	**GAMMAR IV, Centeon**	**00053-7490-10**
1's	$608.20	VENOGLOBULIN-I, Alpha Therapeutic	49669-1604-01
1's	$640.71	GAMMAGARD S/D, Baxter Hyland	00944-2620-04

Injection, Solution - Intravenous - 12 gm

1's	$504.00	SANDOGLOBULIN, Novartis	00078-0244-93
10's	$4956.00	SANDOGLOBULIN, Novartis	00078-0244-19

INDAPAMIDE *(001529)*

CATEGORIES: Antihypertensives; Cardiovascular Drugs; Congestive Heart Failure; Diuretics; Electrolytic, Caloric-Water Balance; Heart Failure; Hypertension; Indoline Antihypertensives; Renal Drugs; Pregnancy Category B; Sales > $100 Million; FDA Approved 1983 Jul

BRAND NAMES: *Agelan*; *Damide*; *Dapadox*; *Dapa-tabs* (Australia); *Depermide*; *Difierix*; *Dixamid*; *Extur*; *Fludex* (France); *Frumeron*; *Hemidol*; *Ipamix*; *Lorvas*; *Lozide* (Canada); **Lozol**; *Magniton-R*; *Millibar*; *Napamide*; *Naplin*; *Natralix*; *Natrilix* (Australia, England, Germany); *Natrix*; *Pamid*; *Tandix*; *Tertensif*
(International brand names outside U.S. in italics)

FORMULARIES: Aetna; BC-BS; Medi-Cal; PCS

COST OF THERAPY: $240.79 (Hypertension; Tablet; 2.5 mg; 1/day; 365 days)

PRIMARY ICD9: 401.1 (Essential Hypertension, Benign)

DESCRIPTION:

Lozol (indapamide) is an oral antihypertensive/diuretic. Its molecule contains both a polar sulfamoyl chlorobenzamide moiety and a liquid-soluble methylindoline moiety. It differs chemically from the thiazides in that it does not possess the thiazide ring system and contains only one sulfonamide group. The chemical name of indapamide is 1-(4-chloro-3-sulfamoylbenzamido)-2-methylindoline, and its molecular weight is 365.84. The compound is a weak acid, pK_a = 8.8, and is soluble in aqueous solutions of strong bases. It is a white to yellow-white crystalline (tetragonal) powder.

The tablets also contain microcrystalline cellulose, coloring agent, corn starch, pregelatinized starch, hydroxypropyl methylcellulose, lactose, magnesium stearate, polyethylene glycol, and talc.

CLINICAL PHARMACOLOGY:

Indapamide is the first of a new class of antihypertensive/diuretics, the indolines. The oral administration of 2.5 mg (two 1.25 mg tablets) of indapamide to male subjects produced peak concentrations of approximately 115 ng/ml of the drug in the blood within two hours. The oral administration of 5 mg (two 2.5 mg tablets) of indapamide to healthy male subjects produced peak concentrations of approximately 260 ng/ml of the drug in the blood within two hours. A minimum of 70% of a single oral dose is eliminated by the kidneys and an additional 23% by the gastrointestinal tract, probably including the biliary route. The half-life of Indapamide in whole blood is approximately 14 hours.

Indapamide is preferentially and reversibly taken up by the erythrocytes in the peripheral blood. The whole blood/plasma ratio is approximately 6:1 at the time of peak concentration and decreases to 3.5:1 at eight hours. From 71 to 79% of the indapamide in plasma is reversibly bound to plasma proteins.

Indapamide is an extensively metabolized drug, with only about 7% of the total dose administered, recovered in the urine as unchanged drug during the first 48 hours after administration. The urinary elimination of ^{14}C-labeled indapamide and metabolites is biphasic with a terminal half-life of excretion of total radioactivity of 26 hours.

In a parallel design double-blind, placebo controlled trial in hypertension, daily doses of indapamide between 1.25 mg and 10.0 mg produced dose-related antihypertensive effects. Doses of 5.0 and 10.0 mg were not distinguishable from each other although each was differentiated from placebo and 1.25 mg indapamide. At daily doses of 1.25 mg, 5.0 mg and 10.0 mg, a mean decrease of serum potassium of 0.28, 0.61 and 0.76 mEq/L, respectively, was observed and uric acid increased by about 0.69 mg/100 ml.

In other parallel design, dose-ranging clinical trials in hypertension and edema, daily doses of indapamide between 0.5 and 5.0 mg produced dose-related effects. Generally, doses of 2.5 and 5.0 mg were not distinguishable from each other although each was differentiated from

CLINICAL PHARMACOLOGY: *(cont'd)*

placebo and from 0.5 or 1.0 mg indapamide. At daily doses of 2.5 and 5.0 mg a mean decrease of serum potassium of 0.5 and 0.6 mEq/L, respectively, was observed and uric acid increased by about 1.0 mg/100 ml.

At these doses, the effects of indapamide on blood pressure and edema are approximately equal to those obtained with conventional doses of other antihypertensive/diuretics.

In hypertensive patients, daily doses of 1.25, 2.5 and 5.0 mg of indapamide have no appreciable cardiac inotropic or chronotropic effect. The drug decreases peripheral resistance, with little or no effect on cardiac output, rate or rhythm. Chronic administration of indapamide to hypertensive patients has little or no effect on glomerular filtration rate or renal plasma flow.

Indapamide had an antihypertensive effect in patients with varying degrees of renal impairment, although in general, diuretic effects declined as renal function decreased.

In a small number of controlled studies, indapamide taken with other antihypertensive drugs such as hydralazine, propranolol, guanethidine and methyldopa, appeared to have the additive effect typical of thiazide-type diuretics.

INDICATIONS AND USAGE:

Indapamide is indicated for the treatment of hypertension, alone or in combination with other antihypertensive drugs.

Indapamide is also indicated for the treatment of salt and fluid retention associated with congestive heart failure.

Usage in Pregnancy: The routine use of diuretics in an otherwise healthy woman is inappropriate and exposes mother and fetus to unnecessary hazard (see PRECAUTIONS).

Diuretics do not prevent development of toxemia of pregnancy, and there is no satisfactory evidence that they are useful in the treatment of developed toxemia.

Edema during pregnancy may arise from pathologic causes or from the physiologic and mechanical consequences of pregnancy. Indapamide is indicated in pregnancy when edema is due to pathologic causes, just as it is in the absence of pregnancy (see PRECAUTIONS). Dependent edema in pregnancy, resulting from restriction of venous return by the expanded uterus, is properly treated through elevation of the lower extremities and use of support hose; use of diuretics to lower intravascular volume in this case is illogical and unnecessary. There is hypervolemia during normal pregnancy which is not harmful to either the fetus or the mother (in the absence of cardiovascular disease), but which is associated with edema, including generalized edema in the majority of pregnant women. If this edema produces discomfort, increased recumbency will often provide relief. In rare instances, this edema may cause extreme discomfort which is not relieved by rest. In these cases, a short course of diuretics may provide relief and may be appropriate.

CONTRAINDICATIONS:

Anuria. Known hypersensitivity to indapamide or to other sulfonamide-derived drugs.

WARNINGS:

Infrequent cases of severe hyponatremia, accompanied by hypokalemia, have been reported with 2.5 mg and 5.0 mg indapamide primarily in elderly females. Symptoms were reversed by electrolyte replenishment.

Hyponatremia considered possibly clinically significant (<125 mEq/L) has not been observed in clinical trials with the 1.25 mg dosage (see PRECAUTIONS).

Hypokalemia occurs commonly with diuretics (see ADVERSE REACTIONS, Hypokalemia), and electrolyte monitoring is essential, particularly in patients who would be at increased risk from hypokalemia, such as those with cardiac arrhythmias or who are receiving concomitant cardiac glycosides.

In general, diuretics should not be given concomitantly with lithium because they reduce its renal clearance and add a high risk of lithium toxicity. Read prescribing information for lithium preparations before use of such concomitant therapy.

Carcinogenesis, Mutagenesis, Impairment of Fertility: Both mouse and rat lifetime carcinogenicity studies were conducted. There was no significant difference in the incidence of tumors between the indapamide-treated animals and the control groups.

Pregnancy, Teratogenic Effects, Pregnancy Category B: Reproduction studies have been performed in rats, mice and rabbits at doses up to 6,250 times the therapeutic human dose and have revealed no evidence of impaired fertility or harm to the fetus due to indapamide. Postnatal development in rats and mice was unaffected by pretreatment of parent animals during gestation. There are, however, no adequate and well-controlled studies in pregnant women. Moreover, diuretics are known to cross the placental barrier and appear in cord blood. Because animal reproduction studies are not always predictive of human response, this drug should be used during pregnancy only if clearly needed. There may be hazards associated with this use such as fetal or neonatal jaundice, thrombocytopenia, and possibly other adverse reactions that have occurred in the adult.

Nursing Mothers: It is not known whether this drug is excreted in human milk. Because most drugs are excreted in human milk, if use of this drug is seemed essential, the patient should stop nursing.

PRECAUTIONS:

GENERAL

Hypokalemia, Hyponatremia, and Other Fluid and Electrolyte Imbalances: Periodic determinations of serum electrolytes should be performed at appropriate intervals. In addition, patients should be observed for clinical signs of fluid or electrolyte imbalance, such as hyponatremia, hypochloremic alkalosis, or hypokalemia. Warning signs include dry mouth, thirst, weakness, fatigue, lethargy, drowsiness, restlessness, muscle pains or cramps, hypotension, oliguria, tachycardia and gastrointestinal disturbance. Electrolyte determinations are particularly important in patients who are vomiting excessively or receiving parenteral fluids, in patients subject to electrolyte imbalance (including those with heart failure, kidney disease, and cirrhosis), and in patients on a salt-restricted diet.

The risk of hypokalemia secondary to diuresis and natriuresis is increased when larger doses are used, when the diuresis is brisk, when severe cirrhosis is present and during concomitant use of corticosteroids or ACTH. Interference with adequate oral intake of electrolytes will also contribute to hypokalemia. Hypokalemia can sensitize or exaggerate the response of the heart to the toxic effects of digitalis, such as increased ventricular irritability.

Dilutional hyponatremia may occur in edematous patients; the appropriate treatment is restriction of water rather than administration of salt, except in rare instances when the hyponatremia is life threatening. However, in actual salt depletion, appropriate replacement is the treatment of choice. Any chloride deficit that may occur during treatment is generally mild and usually does not require specific treatment except in extraordinary circumstances as in liver or renal disease. Thiazide- like diuretics have been shown to increase the urinary excretion of magnesium; this may result in hypomagnesemia.

PRECAUTIONS: *(cont'd)*

Hyperuricemia and Gout: Serum concentrations of uric acid increased by an average of 0.69 mg/100 ml in patients treated with indapamide 1.25 mg, and by an average of 1.0 mg/100 ml in patients treated with indapamide 2.5 mg and 5.0 mg, and frank gout may be precipitated in certain patients receiving indapamide (see ADVERSE REACTIONS). Serum concentrations of uric acid should therefore be monitored periodically during treatment.

Renal Impairment: Indapamide, like the thiazides, should be used with caution in patients with severe renal disease, as reduced plasma volume may exacerbate or precipitate azotemia. If progressive renal impairment is observed in a patient receiving indapamide, withholding or discontinuing diuretic therapy should be considered. Renal function tests should be performed periodically during treatment with indapamide.

Impaired Hepatic Function: Indapamide, like the thiazides, should be used with caution in patients with impaired hepatic function or progressive liver disease, since minor alterations of fluid and electrolyte balance may precipitate hepatic coma.

Glucose Tolerance: Latent diabetes may become manifest and insulin requirements in diabetic patients may be altered during thiazide administration. A mean increase in glucose of 6.47 mg/dL was observed in patients treated with indapamide 1.25 mg, which was not considered clinically significant in these trials. Serum concentrations of glucose should be monitored routinely during treatment with indapamide.

Calcium Excretion: Calcium excretion is decreased by diuretics pharmacologically related to indapamide. After six to eight weeks of indapamide 1.25 mg treatment and in long-term studies of hypertensive patients with higher doses of indapamide, however, serum concentrations of calcium increased only slightly with indapamide. Prolonged treatment with drugs pharmacologically related to indapamide may in rare instances be associated with hypercalcemia and hypophosphatemia secondary to physiologic changes in the parathyroid gland; however, the common complications of hyperparathyroidism, such as renal lithiasis, bone resorption, and peptic ulcer, have not been seen. Treatment should be discontinued before tests for parathyroid function are performed. Like the thiazides, indapamide may decrease serum PBI levels without signs of thyroid disturbance.

Interaction with Systemic Lupus Erythematosus: Thiazides have exacerbated or activated systemic lupus erythematosus and this possibility should be considered with indapamide as well.

DRUG INTERACTIONS:

1. Other Antihypertensives: Indapamide (indapamide) may add to or potentiate the action of other antihypertensive drugs. In limited controlled trials that compared the effect of indapamide combined with other antihypertensive drugs with the effect of the other drugs administered alone, there was no notable change in the nature or frequency of adverse reactions associated with the combined therapy.

2. Lithium: See WARNINGS.

3. Post-Sympathectomy Patient: The antihypertensive effect of the drug may be enhanced in the postsympathectomized patient.

4. Norepinephrine: Indapamide, like the thiazides, may decrease arterial responsiveness to norepinephrine, but this diminution is not sufficient to preclude effectiveness of the pressor agent for therapeutic use.

ADVERSE REACTIONS:

Most adverse effects have been mild and transient.

The clinical adverse reactions listed in table 1 represent data from Phase II/III placebo-controlled studies (306 patients given indapamide 1.25 mg). The clinical adverse reactions listed in table 2 represent data from Phase II placebo-controlled studies and long-term controlled clinical trials (426 patients given indapamide 2.5 mg or 5.0 mg). The reactions are arranged into two groups: 1) a cumulative incidence equal to or greater than 5%; 2) a cumulative incidence less than 5%. Reactions are counted regardless of relation to drug.

TABLE 1 Adverse Reactions from Studies of 1.25 mg

Incidence ≥5%	Incidence <5%*
Body As A Whole	
Headache	Asthenia
Infection	Flu Syndrome
Pain	Abdominal Pain
Back Pain	Chest Pain
Gastrointestinal System	Constipation
	Diarrhea
	Dyspepsia
	Nausea
Metabolic System	Peripheral Edema
Central Nervous System	Nervousness
Dizziness	Hypertonia
Respiratory System	Cough
Rhinitis	Pharyngitis
	Sinusitis
Special Senses	Conjunctivitis

*** other**
All other clinical adverse reactions occurred at an incidence of <1%.

Approximately 4% of patients given indapamide 1.25 mg compared to 5% of the patients given placebo discontinued treatment in the trials of up to eight weeks because of adverse reactions.

In controlled clinical trials of six to eight weeks in duration, 20% of patients receiving indapamide 1.25 mg, 61% of patients receiving indapamide 5.0 mg, and 80% of patients receiving indapamide 10.0 mg had a least one potassium value below 3.4 mEq/L. In the indapamide 1.25 mg group, about 40% of those patients who reported hypokalemia as a laboratory adverse event returned to normal serum potassium values without intervention. Hypokalemia with concomitant clinical signs or symptoms occurred in 2% of patients receiving indapamide 1.25 mg.

Because most of these data are from long-term studies (up to 40 weeks of treatment), it is probable that many of the adverse experiences reported are due to causes other than the drug. Approximately 10% of patients given indapamide discontinued treatment in long-term trials because of reactions either related or unrelated to the drug.

Hypokalemia with concomitant clinical signs or symptoms occurred in 3% of patients receiving indapamide 2.5 mg q.d. and 7% of patients receiving indapamide 5 mg q.d in long-term controlled clinical trials comparing the hypokalemic effects of daily doses of indapamide and hydrochlorothiazide, however, 47% of patients receiving indapamide 2.5 mg, 72% of patients receiving indapamide 5 mg, and 44% of patients receiving hydrochlorothiazide 50 mg had at least one potassium value (out of a total of 11 taken during the study) below 3.5 mEq/L. In the indapamide 2.5 mg group, over 50% of those patients returned to normal serum potassium values without intervention.

In clinical trials of six to eight weeks, the mean changes in selected values were as shown in the following tables.

ADVERSE REACTIONS: *(cont'd)*

TABLE 2 Adverse Reactions from Studies of 2.5 mg and 5.0 mg

Incidence ≥5%	Incidence <5%
Central Nervous System/Neuromuscular	
Headache	Lightheadedness
Dizziness	Drowsiness
Fatigue, weakness, loss of energy, lethargy, tiredness or malaise	Vertigo
	Insomnia
Muscle cramps or spasm, or numbness of the extremities	Depression
	Blurred Vision
Nervousness, tension, anxiety, irritability, or agitation	
Gastrointestinal System	Constipation
	Nausea
	Vomiting
	Diarrhea
	Gastric irritation
	Abdominal pain or cramps
	Anorexia
Cardiovascular System	Orthostatic hypotension
	Premature ventricular contractions
	Irregular heart beat
	Palpitations
Genitourinary System	Frequency of urination
	Nocturia
	Polyuria
Dermatologic	Rash
Hypersensitivity	Hives
	Pruritus
	Vasculitis
Other	Impotence or reduced libido
	Rhinorrhea
	Flushing
	Hyperuricemia
	Hyperglycemia
	Hyponatremia
	Hypochloremia
	Increase in serum urea nitrogen (BUN) or creatinine
	Glycosuria
	Weight loss
	Dry mouth
	Tingling of extremities

TABLE 3 Mean Changes from Baseline after 8 Weeks of Treatment - 1.25 mg

	Serum Electrolytes (mEq/L) Potassium	Sodium	Chloride	Serum Uric Acid (mg/dl)	BUN (mg/dL)
Indapamide 1.25 mg (n=255-257)	-0.28	-0.63	-2.60	0.69	1.46
Placebo (n=263-266)	0.00	-0.11	-0.21	0.06	0.06

No patients receiving indapamide 1.25 mg experienced hyponatremia considered possibly clinically significant (<125 mEqL).

TABLE 4 Mean Changes from Baseline after 40 Weeks of Treatment - 2.5 and 5.0 mg

	Serum Electrolytes (mEq/L) Potassium	Sodium	Chloride	Serum Uric Acid (mg/dl)	BUN (mg/dl)
Indapamide 2.5 mg (n=76)	-0.4	-0.6	-3.6	0.7	-0.1
Indapamide 5.0 mg (n=81)	-0.6	-0.7	-5.1	1.1	1.4

Other adverse reactions reported with antihypertensive/diuretics are jaundice (intrahepatic cholestatic jaundice), sialadenitis, xanthopsia, photosensitivity, purpura, bullous eruptions, Stevens-Johnson Syndrome, necrotizing angiitis, fever, respiratory distress (including pneumonitis), and anaphylactic reactions; also, agranulocytosis, leukopenia, thrombocytopenia, and aplastic anemia. These reactions should be considered as possible occurrences with clinical usage of indapamide.

OVERDOSAGE:

Symptoms of overdosage include nausea, vomiting, weakness, gastrointestinal disorders and disturbances of electrolyte balance. In severe instances, hypotension and depressed respiration may be observed. If this occurs, support of respiration and cardiac circulation should be instituted. There is no specific antidote. An evacuation of the stomach is recommended by emesis and gastric lavage after which the electrolyte and fluid balance should be evaluated carefully.

DOSAGE AND ADMINISTRATION:

Hypertension: The adult starting indapamide dose for hypertension is 1.25 mg as a single daily dose taken in the morning. If the response to 1.25 mg is not satisfactory after four weeks, the daily dose may be increased to 2.5 mg taken once daily. If the response to 2.5 mg is not satisfactory after four weeks, the daily dose may be increased to 5.0 mg taken once daily, but adding another antihypertensive should be considered.

Edema of Congestive Heart Failure: The adult starting indapamide dose for edema of congestive heart failure is 2.5 as a single daily dose taken in the morning. If the response to 2.5 mg is not satisfactory after one week, the daily dose may be increased to 5.0 mg once daily.

If the antihypertensive response to indapamide is insufficient, indapamide may be combined with other antihypertensive drugs, with careful monitoring of blood pressure. It is recommended that the usual dose of other agents be reduced by 50% during initial combination therapy. As the blood pressure response becomes evident, further dosage adjustments may be necessary.

In general, doses of 5.0 mg and larger have not appeared to provide additional effects on blood pressure or heart failure, but are associated with a greater degree of hypokalemia. There is minimal clinical trial experience in patients with doses greater than 5.0 mg once a day.

HOW SUPPLIED:

Caution: Federal (U.S.A.) law prohibits dispensing without prescription.

Keep tightly closed. Store at controlled room temperature, 15°C-30°C (59°F-86°F). Avoid excessive heat. Dispense in tight containers as defined in USP.

TABLE 5 Lozol

Strength	Color	Shape	Markings
1.25 mg	Orange film-coated	Octagon Shaped*	R and 7
2.5 mg	White film-coated	Octagon Shaped*	R and 8

* The distinctive design of the Lozol tablet is patented by Rhone-Poulenc Rorer Pharmaceuticals Inc. U.S. Pat. No. Des. 300,673.

HOW SUPPLIED - RATED THERAPEUTICALLY EQUIVALENT:

Tablet - Oral - 1.25 mg

100's	$63.95	Indapamide, Mylan	00378-0069-01
500's	$303.76	Indapamide, Mylan	00378-0069-05

Tablet - Oral - 2.5 mg

100's	$80.06	Indapamide, Mylan	00378-0080-01
1000's	$790.29	Indapamide, Mylan	00378-0080-10

Tablet, Plain Coated - Oral - 1.25 mg

100's	**$64.93**	**LOZOL, Rhone-Poulenc Rorer**	**00075-0700-00**
1000's	**$616.82**	**LOZOL, Rhone-Poulenc Rorer**	**00075-0700-99**

Tablet, Plain Coated - Oral - 2.5 mg

30's	$21.89	Indapamide, Zenith Labs	00172-4259-46
100's	$65.97	Indapamide, Qualitest Pharms	00603-4061-21
100's	$65.98	Indapamide, Aligen Independ	00405-4538-01
100's	$67.09	Indapamide, United Res	00677-1577-01
100's	$73.72	Indapamide, Arcola	00070-3000-00
100's	$73.72	Indapamide, Zenith Labs	00172-4259-60
100's	$75.72	Indapamide, Goldline Labs	00182-2610-89
100's	$76.25	Indapamide, Major Pharms	00904-5074-60
100's	$78.40	Indapamide, Rugby	00536-3969-01
100's	**$84.73**	**LOZOL, Rhone-Poulenc Rorer**	**00075-0082-00**
100's	**$84.73**	**LOZOL, Rhone-Poulenc Rorer**	**00075-0082-62**
500's	$364.90	Indapamide, Zenith Labs	00172-4259-70
1000's	$685.58	Indapamide, Aligen Independ	00405-4538-03
1000's	$727.61	Indapamide, Arcola	00070-3000-99
1000's	$727.61	Indapamide, Zenith Labs	00172-4259-80
1000's	**$836.33**	**LOZOL, Rhone-Poulenc Rorer**	**00075-0082-99**

INDECAINIDE HYDROCHLORIDE *(003026)*

CATEGORIES: Antiarrhythmic Agents; Arrhythmia; Myocardial Infarction; Tachycardia; Pregnancy Category B; FDA Approved 1989 Dec

BRAND NAMES: **Decabid**

DESCRIPTION:

.Introduction being delayed by Lilly

For How Supplied Information, Contact Lilly (NDA# 19693)

INDIGOTINDISULFONATE SODIUM *(001530)*

CATEGORIES: Diagnostic Agents; Kidney Function; FDA Pre 1938 Drugs

BRAND NAMES: Indigo Carmine

Prescribing information not available at time of publication.

HOW SUPPLIED - EQUIVALENTS NOT AVAILABLE:

Injection, Solution - Intramuscular; - 8 mg/ml

5 ml x 10	$90.00	INDIGO CARMINE, Am Regent	00517-0375-10
5 ml x 10	$102.00	INDIGO CARMINE, BD Microbiology	00011-8366-09
5 ml x 10	$140.00	Indigo Carmine, Raway	00686-0375-10
5 ml x 10	$150.00	Indigo Carmine, Consolidated Midland	00223-7902-10
10 x 5 ml	$119.00	Indigo Carmine, Pasadena	00418-2501-31

INDINAVIR SULFATE *(003252)*

CATEGORIES: AIDS Related Complex; Anti-Infectives; Antimicrobials; Antivirals; HIV Infection; Infections; Protease Inhibitors; Viral Agents; FDA Approved 1996 Feb

BRAND NAMES: **Crixivan**; MK-639

FORMULARIES: PCS

Indinavir sulfate is indicated for the treatment of HIV infection in adults when antiretroviral therapy is warranted. This indication is based on analyses of surrogate endpoints in studies of up to 24 weeks in duration. At present, there are no results from controlled clinical trials evaluating the effect of therapy with indinavir sulfate on clinical progression of HIV infection, such as survival or the incidence of opportunistic infections.

DESCRIPTION:

Crixivan (indinavir sulfate) is an inhibitor of the human immunodeficiency virus (HIV) protease. Indinavir sulfate capsules are formulated as a sulfate salt and are available for oral administration in strengths of 200 and 400 mg of indinavir (corresponding to 250 and 500 mg indinavir sulfate, respectively). Each capsule also contains the inactive ingredients anhydrous lactose and magnesium stearate. The capsule shell has the following inactive ingredients and dyes: gelatin, titanium dioxide, silicon dioxide and sodium lauryl sulfate.

The chemical name for indinavir sulfate is [1(1*S*,2*R*),5(*S*)] -2,3,5-trideoxy-*N*-(2,3-dihydro-2-hydroxy-1*H*-inden-1-yl)-5-[2-[[(1,1-dimethylethyl)amino]carbonyl]-4-(3-pyridinylmethyl)-1-piperazinyl]-2-(phenylmethyl)-D-erythro-pentonamide sulfate (1:1) salt.

Indinavir sulfate is a white to off-white, hygroscopic, crystalline powder with the molecular formula $C_{36}H_{47}N_5O_4{\cdot}H_2SO_4$ and a molecular weight of 711.88. It is very soluble in water and in methanol.

CLINICAL PHARMACOLOGY:

Mechanism of Action: HIV protease is an enzyme required for the proteolytic cleavage of the viral polyprotein precursors into the individual functional proteins found in infectious HIV. Indinavir binds to the protease active site and inhibits the activity of the enzyme. This inhibition prevents cleavage of the viral polyproteins resulting in the formation of immature noninfectious viral particles.

CLINICAL PHARMACOLOGY: *(cont'd)*

Antiretroviral Activity *In Vitro*: The relationship between in vitro susceptibility of HIV to indinavir and inhibition of HIV replication in humans has not been established. The in vitro activity of indinavir was assessed in cell lines of lymphoblastic and monocytic origin and in peripheral blood lymphocytes. HIV variants used to infect the different cell types include laboratory-adapted variants, primary clinical isolates and clinical isolates resistant to nucleoside analogue and nonnucleoside inhibitors of the HIV reverse transcriptase. The IC_{95} (95% inhibitory concentration) of indinavir in these test systems was in the range of 25 to 100 nM. In drug combination studies with the nucleoside analogues zidovudine and didanosine, as well as with an investigational nonnucleoside (L-697,661), indinavir showed synergistic activity in cell culture.

Drug Resistance: Isolates of HIV with reduced susceptibility to the drug have been recovered from some patients treated with indinavir. Viral resistance was correlated with the accumulation of mutations that resulted in the expression of amino acid substitutions in the viral protease. Eleven amino acid residue positions, at which substitutions are associated with resistance, have been identified. Resistance was mediated by the co-expression of multiple and variable substitutions at these positions. In general, higher levels of resistance were associated with the co-expression of greater numbers of substitutions.

Cross-Resistance to Other Antiviral Agents: Cross-resistance between indinavir and HIV reverse transcriptase inhibitors is unlikely because the enzyme targets involved are different. Cross-resistance was noted between indinavir and the protease inhibitor ritonavir. Varying degrees of cross-resistance have been observed between indinavir and other HIV-protease inhibitors.

PHARMACOKINETICS

Absorption: Indinavir was rapidly absorbed in the fasted state with a time to peak plasma concentration (T_{max}) of 0.8 ± 0.3 hours (mean ± S.D.) (n=11). A greater than dose-proportional increase in indinavir plasma concentrations was observed over the 200-1000 mg dose range. At a dosing regimen of 800 mg every 8 hours, steady-state area under the plasma concentration time curve (AUC) was 30,691 ± 11,407 nM· hour (n=16), peak plasma concentration (C_{max}) was 12,617 ± 4037 nM (n=16), and plasma concentration eight hours post dose (trough) was 251 ± 178 nM (n=16).

Effect of Food on Oral Absorption: Administration of indinavir with a meal high in calories, fat, and protein (784 kcal, 48.6 g fat, 31.3 g protein) resulted in a 77% ± 8% reduction in AUC and an 84% ± 7% reduction in C_{max} (n=10). Administration with lighter meals (*e.g.,* a meal of dry toast with jelly, apple juice, and coffee with skim milk and sugar or a meal of corn flakes, skim milk and sugar) resulted in little or no change in AUC, C_{max} or trough concentration.

Distribution: Indinavir was approximately 60% bound to human plasma proteins over a concentration range of 81 nM to 16,300 nM.

Metabolism: Following a 400-mg dose of ^{14}C-indinavir, 83 ± 1% (n=4) and 19 ± 3% (n=6) of the total radioactivity was recovered in feces and urine, respectively; radioactivity due to parent drug in feces and urine was 19.1% and 9.4%, respectively. Seven metabolites have been identified, one glucuronide conjugate and six oxidative metabolites. *In vitro* studies indicate that cytochrome P-450 3A4 (CYP344) is the major enzyme responsible for formation of the oxidative metabolites.

Elimination: Less than 20% of indinavir is excreted unchanged in the urine. Mean urinary excretion of unchanged drug was 10.4 ± 4.9% (n=10) and 12.0 ± 4.9% (n=10) following a single 700-mg and 1000-mg dose, respectively. Indinavir was rapidly eliminated with a half-life of 1.8 ± 0.4 hours (n=10). Significant accumulation was not observed after multiple dosing at 800 mg every 8 hours.

SPECIAL POPULATIONS

Hepatic Insufficiency: Patients with mild to moderate hepatic insufficiency and clinical evidence of cirrhosis had evidence of decreased metabolism of indinavir resulting in approximately 60% higher mean AUC following a single 400-mg dose (n=12). The half-life of indinavir increased to 2.8 ± 0.5 hours. Indinavir pharmacokinetics have not been studied in patients with severe hepatic insufficiency (see DOSAGE AND ADMINISTRATION, Hepatic Insufficiency).

Renal Insufficiency: The pharmacokinetics of indinavir have not been studied in patients with renal insufficiency.

Gender: Pharmacokinetics of indinavir appear to be comparable in men and women based on pharmacokinetic studies including 32 women (15 HIV-positive).

Race: Pharmacokinetics of indinavir appear to be comparable in Caucasians and Blacks based on pharmacokinetic studies including 42 Caucasians (26 HIV-positive) and 16 Blacks (4 HIV-positive).

CLINICAL STUDIES:

Description of Studies: Study 028 is an ongoing multicenter, double-blind, randomized clinical endpoint trial in patients with no prior antiretroviral therapy. The effects of indinavir sulfate on CD4 cell counts and serum viral RNA were evaluated in a cohort of 224 HIV-1 seropositive adults (75% male, 90% Caucasian) over a 24-week period. At baseline, patients were randomized to one of three treatment groups: indinavir sulfate alone, zidovudine alone, and indinavir sulfate plus zidovudine. The median age for these patients was 34 years (range 20-67 years). The mean baseline CD4 cell count over all patients was 145.0 cells/mm^3, and the serum viral RNA was 4.40 log_{10}copies/ml (25,330 copies/ml).

At 24 weeks of therapy, 22 of 59 (37%) of patients receiving indinavir alone, 21 of 58 (36%) of patients receiving indinavir in combination with zidovudine, and 4 of 62 (7%) of patients receiving zidovudine alone had serum viral RNA levels at or below 500 copies/ml, the limit of detection of the assay; the clinical significance of this finding is unknown.

Study 033 is an ongoing, multicenter, double-blind, randomized clinical trial in patients without prior antiretroviral therapy. The effects of indinavir sulfate on CD4 cell counts and serum viral RNA were evaluated in 266 HIV-1 seropositive adults (91% male, 85% Caucasian) over a 24-week period. At baseline, patients were randomized to one of three treatment groups: indinavir sulfate alone, zidovudine alone, and indinavir sulfate plus zidovudine. The median age for these patients was 37 years (range 22-76 years). The mean baseline CD4 cell count over all patients was 254.4 cells/mm^3, and the mean baseline serum viral RNA was 4.28 log_{10}copies/ml (19,210 copies/ml).

At 24 weeks of therapy, 18 of 49 (37%) of patients receiving indinavir alone, 29 of 52 (56%) of patients receiving indinavir in combination with zidovudine, and 1 of 53 (2%) of patients receiving zidovudine alone had serum viral RNA levels at or below 500 copies/ml, the limit of detection of the assay; the clinical significance of this finding is unknown.

Study 035 is an ongoing multicenter, double-blind, randomized trial in HIV-1 seropositive patients with prior zidovudine experience (median time of zidovudine therapy-30.9 months). The effects of indinavir sulfate on CD4 cell counts and serum viral RNA were evaluated in a cohort of 96 patients (85% male), with zidovudine experience, over a 24-week period. At baseline, patients were randomized to one of three treatment groups: indinavir sulfate, zidovudine plus lamivudine or indinavir sulfate plus zidovudine plus lamivudine. The median age for these patients was 39 years (range 18-67 years), with 72% Caucasian. The mean baseline CD4 cell count over all patients was 174.8 cells/mm^3, and the mean baseline serum viral RNA was 4.58 log_{10}copies/ml (38,400 copies/ml).

CLINICAL STUDIES: *(cont'd)*

At 24 weeks of therapy, 7 of 20 (35%) of patients receiving indinavir alone, 20 of 22 (91%) of patients receiving indinavir in combination with zidovudine and lamivudine, and 0 of 19 (0%) of patients receiving zidovudine plus lamivudine had serum viral RNA levels at or below 500 copies/ml, the limit of detection of the assay; the clinical significance of this finding is unknown.

Additional Studies: In open-label study 020, 78 zidovudine- and didanosine-naive HIV-infected patients were randomized to one of three treatment groups: indinavir sulfate 600 mg every 6 hours, zidovudine plus didanosine, and indinavir sulfate plus zidovudine plus didanosine. At 24 weeks of therapy, all three groups had a significant increase in CD4 cell counts and decrease in serum viral RNA compared to baseline; however, there were no differences in mean CD4 cell count changes between treatment arms. Patients treated with indinavir sulfate plus zidovudine plus didanosine had a greater mean decline in serum viral RNA than those treated with indinavir alone or zidovudine plus didanosine.

Study 021 was a randomized trial in which 70 HIV-seropositive patients received indinavir sulfate at one of three doses (800 mg every 8 hours, 1000 mg every 8 hours and 800 mg every 6 hours). At 24 weeks, changes in CD4 cell counts and serum viral RNA were similar in all three treatment groups.

Genotypic Resistance in Clinical Studies: Study 006 was a dose-ranging study in which patients were initially treated with indinavir sulfate at a dose of <2.4 g/day followed by 2.4 g/day. Study 019 was a randomized comparison of indinavir sulfate 600 mg every 6 hours, indinavir sulfate plus zidovudine, and zidovudine alone. TABLE 1 shows the incidence of genotypic resistance at 24 weeks in these studies.

TABLE 1 Genotypic Resistance at 24 weeks

Treatment Group	Resistance to IDV n/N*	Resistance to ZVD n/N*
IDV	-	-
<2.4g/day	31/37 (84%)	-
2.4g/day	9/21 (43%)	1/17 (6%)
IDV/ZVD	4/22 (18%)	1/22 (5%)
ZVD	1/18 (6%)	11/17 (65%)

* N-includes patients with non-amplifiable virus at 24 weeks who had amplifiable virus at week 0.

INDICATIONS AND USAGE:

Indinavir sulfate is indicated for the treatment of HIV infection in adults when antiretroviral therapy is warranted. This indication is based on analyses of surrogate endpoints in studies of up to 24 weeks in duration evaluating patients who received indinavir sulfate in combination with other antiretroviral agents or alone. At present, there are no results from controlled trials evaluating the effect of therapy with indinavir sulfate on clinical progression of HIV infection, such as survival or the incidence of opportunistic infection.

CONTRAINDICATIONS:

Indinavir sulfate is contraindicated in patients with clinically significant hypersensitivity to any of its components.

WARNINGS:

Nephrolithiasis may occur with indinavir sulfate. If signs and symptoms of nephrolithiasis, including flank pain with or without hematuria (including microscopic hematuria), occur, temporary interruption of therapy (*e.g.,* 1-3 days) during the acute episode of nephrolithiasis may be considered. **Adequate hydration is recommended in all patients treated with indinavir sulfate. (See DOSAGE AND ADMINISTRATION, Nephrolithiasis).**

Indinavir should not be administered concurrently with terfenadine, astemizole, cisapride, triazolam, and midazolam because competition for CYP3A4 by indinavir could result in inhibition of the metabolism of these drugs and create the potential for serious and/or life-threatening events (*i.e.,* cardiac arrhythmias, prolonged sedation).

PRECAUTIONS:

GENERAL

Indirect hyperbilirubinemia has occurred frequently during treatment with indinavir sulfate and has infrequently been associated with increases in serum transaminases (see ADVERSE REACTIONS). It is not known whether indinavir sulfate will exacerbate the physiologic hyperbilirubinemia seen in neonates. (See Nonteratogenic Effects.)

COEXISTING CONDITIONS

Patients With Hepatic Insufficiency Due to Cirrhosis: In these patients, the dosage of indinavir sulfate should be lowered because of decreased metabolism of indinavir sulfate (see DOSAGE AND ADMINISTRATION).

Patients With Renal Insufficiency: Patients with renal insufficiency have not been studied.

INFORMATION FOR THE PATIENT

Indinavir sulfate is not a cure for HIV infection and patients may continue to develop opportunistic infections and other complications associated with HIV disease. Indinavir sulfate has not been shown to reduce the incidence or frequency of such illnesses. The long-term effects of indinavir sulfate are unknown at this time. Indinavir sulfate has not been shown to reduce the risk of transmission of HIV to others through sexual contact or blood contamination.

Patients should be advised to remain under the care of a physician when using indinavir sulfate and should not modify or discontinue treatment without first consulting the physician. Therefore, if a dose is missed, patients should take the next dose at the regularly scheduled time and should not double this dose. Therapy with indinavir sulfate should be initiated and maintained at the recommended dosage.

For optimal absorption, indinavir sulfate should be administered without food but with water 1 hour before or 2 hours after a meal. Alternatively, indinavir sulfate may be administered with other liquids such as skim milk, juice, coffee, or tea, or with a light meal, e.g., dry toast with jelly, juice, and coffee with skim milk and sugar; or corn flakes, skim milk and sugar (see CLINICAL PHARMACOLOGY, Effect of Food on Oral Absorption and DOSAGE AND ADMINISTRATION). Ingestion of indinavir sulfate with a meal high in calories, fat, and protein reduces the absorption of indinavir.

Indinavir sulfate capsules are sensitive to moisture. Patients should be informed that indinavir sulfate should be stored and used in the original container and the desiccant should remain in the bottle.

CARCINOGENESIS, MUTAGENESIS, AND IMPAIRMENT OF FERTILITY

Long-term carcinogenicity studies of indinavir in rats and mice are in progress. No evidence of mutagenicity or genotoxicity was observed in *in vitro* microbial mutagenesis (Ames) tests, in vitro alkaline elusion assays for DNA breakage, *in vitro* and *in vivo* chromosomal aberration studies, and *in vitro* mammalian cell mutagenesis assays. No treatment-related effects on mating, fertility, or embryo survival were seen in female rats and no treatment-related effects on mating performance were seen in male rats at doses providing systemic

PRECAUTIONS: *(cont'd)*

exposure comparable to or slightly higher than that with the clinical dose. In addition, no treatment-related effects were observed in fecundity or fertility of untreated females mated to treated males.

PREGNANCY

Pregnancy Category C: Developmental toxicity studies performed in rats and rabbits (at doses comparable to or slightly greater than human exposure) revealed no evidence of teratogenicity. No treatment-related external or visceral changes were observed in rats. Treatment-related increases over controls in the incidence of supernumerary ribs (at exposures at or below those in humans) and of cervical ribs (at exposures comparable to or slightly greater than those in humans) were seen in rats. No treatment-related external, visceral, or skeletal changes were observed in rabbits. In both species, no treatment-related effects on embryonic/fetal survival or fetal weights were observed. *In utero* exposure to indinavir was significant in rats. Since fetal exposure was low in the rabbit, a developmental toxicity study in dogs is in progress. There are no adequate and well controlled studies in pregnant women. Indinavir sulfate should be used during pregnancy only if the potential benefit justifies the potential risk to the fetus.

NONTERATOGENIC EFFECTS

Hyperbilirubinemia has occurred during treatment with indinavir sulfate (see PRECAUTIONS and ADVERSE REACTIONS). It is unknown whether indinavir sulfate administered to the mother in the perinatal period will exacerbate physiologic hyperbilirubinemia in neonates.

NURSING MOTHERS

Studies in lactating rats have demonstrated that indinavir is excreted in milk. Although it is not known whether indinavir sulfate is excreted in human milk, there exists the potential for adverse effects from indinavir in nursing infants. Mothers should be instructed to discontinue nursing if they are receiving indinavir sulfate. This is consistent with the recommendation by the U.S. Public Health Service Centers for Disease Control and Prevention that HIV-infected mothers not breast-feed their infants to avoid risking postnatal transmission of HIV.

PEDIATRIC USE

Safety and effectiveness in pediatric patients have not been established.

DRUG INTERACTIONS:

Specific drug interaction studies were performed with indinavir and a number of drugs.

DRUGS REQUIRING DOSE MODIFICATION

Rifabutin: Administration of indinavir (800 mg every 8 hours) with rifabutin (300 mg once daily) for 10 days resulted in a 32% ± 19% decrease in indinavir AUC and a 204% ± 142% increase in rifabutin AUC (see DOSAGE AND ADMINISTRATION, Concomitant Therapy).

Due to an increase in the plasma concentrations of rifabutin, a dosage reduction of rifabutin is necessary when it is coadministered with indinavir sulfate. (See DOSAGE AND ADMINISTRATION, Concomitant Therapy ; DRUG INTERACTIONS.)

Ketoconazole: Administration of a 400-mg dose of ketoconazole with a 400-mg dose of indinavir resulted in a 68% ± 48% increase in indinavir AUC (see DOSAGE AND ADMINISTRATION, Concomitant Therapy). The effects of administering a 400- or 800-mg dose of ketoconazole with an 800-mg dose of indinavir are not known.

Due to an increase in the plasma concentrations of indinavir, a dosage reduction of indinavir should be considered when indinavir sulfate and ketoconazole are coadministered (see DOSAGE AND ADMINISTRATION, Concomitant Therapy; DRUG INTERACTIONS).

DRUGS NOT REQUIRING DOSE MODIFICATION

Nucleoside Analogue Antiretroviral Agents: Administration of indinavir (1000 mg every 8 hours) with zidovudine (200 mg every 8 hours) for one week resulted in a 13% ± 48% increase in indinavir AUC and a 17% ± 23% increase in zidovudine AUC. In another study, administration of indinavir (800 mg every 8 hours) with zidovudine (200 mg every 8 hours) in combination with lamivudine (150 mg twice daily) for one week resulted in no change in indinavir AUC, a 36% increase in zidovudine AUC, and a 6% decrease in lamivudine AUC. Administration of indinavir (800 mg every 8 hours) in combination with stavudine (40 mg every 12 hours) for one week resulted in no change in indinavir AUC and a 25 ± 26% increase in stavudine AUC.

ORTHO-NOVUM 1/35:** Administration of indinavir (800 mg every 8 hours) with ORTHO-NOVUM 1/35 for one week resulted in a 24% ± 17% increase in ethinyl estradiol AUC and a 26% ± 14% increase in norethindrone AUC.

Cimetidine, Quinidine, Grapefruit Juice: Administration of a single 400-mg dose of indinavir following six days of cimetidine (600 mg every 12 hours) did not affect indinavir AUC. Administration of a single 400-mg dose of indinavir with 8 oz. of grapefruit juice resulted in a decrease in indinavir AUC (26% ± 18%). Administration of a single 400-mg dose of indinavir with 200 mg of quinidine sulfate resulted in a 10% ± 26% increase in indinavir AUC.

Trimethoprim/Sulfamethoxazole, Fluconazole, Isoniazid Clarithromycin: Administration of indinavir (400 mg every 6 hours) with trimethoprim/sulfamethoxazole (one double strength tablet every 12 hours) for one week resulted in no change in indinavir AUC, a 19% ± 31% increase in trimethoprim AUC, and no change in sulfamethoxazole AUC. Administration of indinavir (1000 mg every 6 hours) with fluconazole (400 mg once daily) for one week resulted in a 19% ± 33% decrease in indinavir AUC and no change in fluconazole AUC. Administration of indinavir (800 mg every 8 hours) with isoniazid (300 mg once daily) for one week resulted in no change in indinavir AUC and a 13% ± 15% increase in isoniazid AUC. Administration of indinavir (800 mg every 8 hours) with clarithromycin (500 mg every 12 hours) for one week resulted in a 29% ± 42% increase in indinavir AUC and a 53% ± 36% increase in clarithromycin AUC.

Rifampin: Because rifampin is a potent inducer of P-450 3A4 which could markedly diminish plasma concentrations of indinavir, coadministration of indinavir sulfate and rifampin is not recommended.

OTHER

If indinavir sulfate and didanosine are administered concomitantly, they should be administered at least one hour apart on an empty stomach; a normal (acidic) gastric pH may be necessary for optimum absorption of indinavir, whereas acid rapidly degrades didanosine which is formulated with buffering agents to increase pH (consult the manufacturer's product circular for didanosine).

Studies were not performed with the CYP3A4 substrates terfenadine, astemizole, cisapride, triazolam, and midazolam. Because competition for CYP3A4 by indinavir could result in inhibition of the metabolism of these drugs and create the potential for serious and/or life-threatening events (*i.e.*, cardiac arrhythmias, prolonged sedation), indinavir sulfate should not be administered concurrently with any of these agents.

ADVERSE REACTIONS:

Nephrolithiasis, including flank pain with or without hematuria (including microscopic hematuria), has been reported in approximately 4% (79/2205) of patients receiving indinavir sulfate in clinical trials. In general, these events were not associated with renal dysfunction

ADVERSE REACTIONS: *(cont'd)*

and resolved with hydration and temporary interruption of therapy (*e.g.*, 1-3 days). Following the acute episode, 9.2% (7/76) of patients discontinued therapy. (See WARNINGS and DOSAGE AND ADMINISTRATION, Nephrolithiasis.)

Asymptomatic hyperbilirubinemia (total bilirubin ≥2.5 mg/dL), reported predominantly as elevated indirect bilirubin, has occurred in approximately 10% of patients treated with indinavir sulfate. In <1% this was associated with elevations in ALT or AST.

Hyperbilirubinemia and nephrolithiasis occurred more frequently at doses exceeding 2.4 g/day compared to doses ≤2.4 g/day.

Drug-related clinical adverse experiences of moderate or severe intensity in ≥2% of patients treated with indinavir sulfate alone, indinavir sulfate in combination with zidovudine, or zidovudine alone are presented in TABLE 2.

TABLE 2 Drug-Related Clinical Adverse Experiences of Moderate or Severe Intensity Reported in ≥2% of Patients (Studies 028 and 033)

Adverse Experience	Indinavir Sulfate % (n=196)	Indinavir Sulfate plus Zidovudine % (n=196)	Zidovudine % (n=195)
Body As A Whole			
Abdominal pain	8.7	8.2	5.1
Anesthesia/fatigue	3.6	9.2	7.7
Flank pain	2.6	1.0	0
Malaise	0.5	2.0	1.5
Digestive System			
Nausea	11.7	32.1	14.4
Diarrhea	4.6	4.1	2.1
Vomiting	4.1	12.2	4.6
Acid regurgitation	2.0	2.0	0.5
Anorexia	0.5	2.0	3.1
Dry mouth	0.5	0	2.1
Musculoskeletal System			
Back pain	2.0	1.0	1.5
Nervous System/ Psychiatric			
Headache	5.6	11.7	5.1
Insomnia	3.1	1.5	0
Dizziness	1.0	3.6	0.5
Somnolence	1.0	1.5	3.6
Special Senses			
Taste perversion	2.6	3.6	2.1

In Phase I and II controlled trials, the following adverse events were reported significantly more frequently by those randomized to indinavir sulfate-containing arms than by those randomized to nucleoside analogues: rash, upper respiratory infection, dry skin, pharyngitis, taste perversion.

Adverse events occurring in less than 2% of patients receiving indinavir sulfate in all Phase II/Phase III studies and considered at least possibly related or of unknown relationship to treatment and of at least moderate intensity are listed below by body system.

Body As A Whole/Site Unspecified: Abdominal distention, chest pain, chills, fever, flank pain, flu-like illness, fungal infection, malaise, pain, syncope

Cardiovascular System: Cardiovascular disorder, palpitation

Digestive System: Acid regurgitation, anorexia, aphthous stomatitis, cheilitis, cholecystitis, cholecystasis, constipation, dry mouth, dyspepsia, eructation, flatulence, gastritis, gingivitis, gingival hemorrhage, increased appetite, infectious gastroenteritis, jaundice, liver cirrhosis,

Hemic and Lymphatic System: Anemia, lymphadenopathy, spleen disorder,

Metabolic/Nutritional/Immune: Food allergy

Musculoskeletal System: Arthralgia, back pain, leg pain, myalgia, muscle cramps, muscle weakness, musculoskeletal pain, shoulder pain, stiffness,

Nervous System and Psychiatric: Agitation, anxiety, anxiety disorder, bruxism, decreased mental acuity, depression, dizziness, dream abnormality, dysesthesia, excitement, fasciculation, hypesthesia, nervousness, neuralgia, neurotic disorder, paresthesia, peripheral neuropathy, sleep disorder, somnolence, tremor, vertigo

Respiratory System: Cough, dyspnea, halitosis, pharyngeal hyperemia, pharyngitis, pneumonia, rales/rhonchi, respiratory failure, sinus disorder, sinusitis, upper respiratory infection

Skin and Skin Appendage: Body odor, contact dermatitis, dermatitis, dry skin, flushing, folliculitis, herpes simplex, herpes zoster, night sweats, pruritus, seborrhea, skin disorder, skin infection, sweating, urticaria

Special Senses: Accomodation disorder, blurred vision, eye pain, eye swelling, orbital edema, taste disorder,

Urogenital System: Dysuria, hematuria, hydronephrosis, nocturia, premenstrual syndrome, proteinuria, renal colic, urinary frequency, urinary tract infection, urine abnormality, urine sediment abnormality, urolithiasis

TABLE 3 Selected Laboratory Abnormalities Reported in Studies 028 and 033

	Indinavir Sulfate Percent (n=196)	Indinavir Sulfate plus Zidovudine Percent (n=196)	Zidovudine Percent (n=195)
Hematology			
Decreased hemoglobin <8.0 g/dL	0.5	1.1	0.5
Decreased platelet count <50 THS/mm^3	0.5	0.5	0
Decreased neutrophils <0.75 THS/mm^3	1.1	1.6	3.8
Blood Chemistry			
Increased ALT >500% ULN*	3.1	3.2	2.1
Increased AST >500% ULN	2.1	2.1	1.1
Total serum bilirubin >2.5 mg/dL	7.8	7.4	0.5
Increased serum amylase >200% ULN	1.0	2.1	0.5

* Upper limit of normal range.

OVERDOSAGE:

No reports are available with regard to overdosage in humans. It is not known whether indinavir sulfate is dialyzable by peritoneal or hemodialysis. Single oral or intraperitoneal doses of indinavir up to 20 times the related human dose in rats and 10 times the related human dose in mice caused no lethality.

DOSAGE AND ADMINISTRATION:

The recommended dosage of indinavir sulfate is 800 mg (two 400-mg capsules) orally every 8 hours. The dosage is the same whether indinavir sulfate is used alone or in combination with other antiretroviral agents. The antiretroviral activity of indinavir sulfate may be increased when used in combination with approved reverse transcriptase inhibitors. (See CLINICAL STUDIES, Description of Studies and Genotypic Resistance in Clinical Studies.)

Indinavir sulfate must be taken at intervals of 8 hours. For optimal absorption, indinavir sulfate should be administered without food but with water 1 hour before or 2 hours after a meal. Alternatively, indinavir sulfate may be administered with other liquids such as skim milk, juice, coffee, or tea, or with a light meal, e.g., dry toast with jelly, juice, and coffee with skim milk and sugar; or corn flakes, skim milk and sugar. (See CLINICAL PHARMACOLOGY, Effect of Food on Oral Absorption.)

To ensure adequate hydration, it is recommended that the patient drink at least 1.5 liters (approximately 48 ounces) of liquids during the course of 24 hours.

CONCOMITANT THERAPY

Dose reduction of rifabutin to half the standard dose is recommended (consult the manufacturer's product circular).

Dose reduction of indinavir sulfate to 600 mg every 8 hours should be considered when administering ketoconazole concurrently.

If indinavir and didanosine are administered concomitantly, they should be administered at least one hour apart on an empty stomach (consult the manufacturer's product circular for didanosine).

HEPATIC INSUFFICIENCY

The dosage of indinavir sulfate should be reduced to 600 mg every 8 hours in patients with mild-to-moderate hepatic insufficiency due to cirrhosis.

NEPHROLITHIASIS

In addition to adequate hydration, medical management in patients who experience nephrolithiasis may include temporary interruption of therapy (*e.g.,* 1-3 days) during the acute episode of nephrolithiasis or discontinuation of therapy.

PATIENT INFORMATION:

Indinavir sulfate is used for the treatment of HIV infection. This agent interacts with many other drugs. Inform your doctor if you are taking any other medications. Notify your doctor or pharmacist if you are pregnant or have kidney disease.

Take with food, 1 hour before or 2 hours after meals. If a dose is missed, take the next dose at the regular time; DO NOT double the dose.

Drink plenty of water, at least 48oz (1.5L) per day.

Indinavir sulfate may cause kidney pain, nausea, stomach ache or headache. Notify your doctor or pharmacist if these occur.

HOW SUPPLIED:

Indinavir sulfate capsules are supplied as follows:

No. 3756-200 mg capsules: white opaque capsules coded "Crixivan 200 mg" in blue.

No. 3758-400 mg capsules: white opaque capsules coded "Crixivan 400 mg" in green.

Storage: Store in a tightly-closed container at room temperature, 15°-30°C (59°-86°F). Protect from moisture.

Indinavir sulfate capsules are sensitive to moisture. Indinavir sulfate should be dispensed and stored in the original container. The desiccant should remain in the original bottle.

HOW SUPPLIED - EQUIVALENTS NOT AVAILABLE:

Capsule - Oral - 400 mg

180's	$360.00	CRIXIVAN, Merck	00006-0573-62

INDOMETHACIN *(001532)*

CATEGORIES: Analgesics; Ankylosing Spondylitis; Anti-Inflammatory Agents; Antianginals; Antiarthritics; Antigout; Antipyretics; Arthritis; Bursitis; Cardiovascular Drugs; Central Nervous System Agents; Ductus Arteriosus; Gouty Arthritis; NSAIDS; Nonsteroidal Anti-Inflammatory; Osteoarthritis; Pain; Respiratory Distress; Spondylitis; Steroids; Alzheimer's Disease*; FDA Approval Pre 1982

* Indication not approved by the FDA

BRAND NAMES: *Ainscrid 75mg LP* (France); *Amuno* (Germany); *Amuno Retard* (Germany); *Antalgin*; *Antalgin Dialicels* (Mexico); *Apo-Indomethacin* (Canada); *Areumatin*; *Argilex*; *Artherexin*; *Arthrexin*; *Articulen*; *Artrinovo*; *Asiamet*; *Bavilon*; *Benocid*; *Betacin*; *Bonidon*; *Boutycin*; *Chrono-Indocid* (France); *Cidalgon*; *Confortid*; *Confortid Retard*; *Confortid Retardkapseln*; *Confortind*; *Dolazal*; *Domecid*; *Dometin*; *Durametacin* (Germany); *Dynametcin*; *Elmetacin* (Germany); *IDC*; *Idicin*; *IM-75*; *Imbrilon* (England); *Imet*; *Inacid*; *Indacin* (Japan); Indameth; *Indecin*; *Indo*; *Indocal*; *Indocap*; *Indocap S.R.*; *Indocen*; *Indocid* (Australia, Canada, Mexico, England, France); *Indocid PDA* (Canada); *Indocid R*; *Indocid-R*; **Indocin**; Indoflex; *Indogesic*; *Indolag*; *Indolar*; *Indolar SR* (England); *Indomed*; *Indomee*; *Indomelan*; *Indometacinum*; *Indometicina*; *Indometicina Gen-Far*; *Indometicina McKesson*; *Indometin*; *Indo-Phlogont* (Germany); *Indorem*; *Indo-Spray*; *Indo-Tablinen* (Germany); *Indotard*; *Indovis*; *Indox*; *Indoy*; *Indozu*; *Indrenin*; *Indylon*; *Inflazon* (Japan); *Inpan*; *Lauzit* (Japan); *Liometacen*; *Malival* (Mexico); *Malival AP* (Mexico); *Metacen*; *Methacin*; *Metindol*; *Metocid*; *Mezolin*; *Mobilan*; *Neotica*; *Novomethacin* (Canada); *Peralgon*; *Reflox*; *Reumacid*; *Reusin*; *Rheumacid*; *Rheumacin*; *Rheumacin SR*; *Rumitard*; *Salinac* (Japan); *Servimeta*; *Servindomet*; *Toshisan*; *Vonum* (Germany)

(International brand names outside U.S. in italics)

FORMULARIES: Aetna; BC-BS; CIGNA; DoD; FHP; Foundation; Humana; Kaiser; Medco; Medi-Cal; PCS; PruCare; United

COST OF THERAPY: $23.57 (Arthritis; Capsule; 25 mg; 2/day; 365 days)

PRIMARY ICD9: 715.99 (Osteoarthritis, Unspecified, Multiple Sites)

DESCRIPTION:

INTRAVENOUS

Sterile indomethacin IV (indomethacin sodium trihydrate) for intravenous administration is lyophilized indomethacin sodium trihydrate. Each vial contains indomethacin sodium trihydrate equivalent to 1 mg indomethacin as a white to yellow lyophilized powder or plug. Variations in the size of the lyophilized plug and the intensity of color have no relationship to the quality or amount of indomethacin present in the vial.

Indomethacin sodium trihydrate is designated chemically as 1-(4-chlorobenzoyl)-5-methoxy-2-methyl-1*H*-indole-3-acetic acid, sodium salt, trihydrate. Its molecular weight is 433.82. Its empirical formula is $C_{19}H_{15}ClNNaO_4 \cdot 3H_2O$.

DESCRIPTION: *(cont'd)*

CAPSULES, ORAL SUSPENSION AND SUPPOSITORIES

Indomethacin cannot be considered a simple analgesic and should not be used in conditions other than those recommended under INDICATIONS AND USAGE.

Indomethacin is supplied in four dosage forms. Indomethacin capsules for oral administration contain either 25 mg or 50 mg of indomethacin and the following inactive ingredients: colloidal silicon dioxide, FD & C Blue 1, FD & C Red 3, gelatin, lactose, lecithin, magnesium stearate, and titanium dioxide. Indomethacin extended—release capsules for sustained release oral administration contain 75 mg of indomethacin and the following inactive ingredients: cellulose, confectioner's sugar, FD & C Blue 1, FD & C Blue 2, FD & C Red 3, gelatin, hydroxypropyl methylcellulose, magnesium stearate, polyvinyl acetate-crotonic acid copolymer, starch, and titanium dioxide. Capsules indomethacin sustained-release conform to the requirements of the USP Drug Release Test 1 for indomethacin Extended-release capsules. Suspension indomethacin for oral use contains 25 mg of indomethacin per 5 ml, alcohol 1%, and sorbic acid 0.1% added as a preservative and the following inactive ingredients: antifoam AF emulsion, flavors, purified water, sodium hydroxide or hydrochloric acid to adjust pH, sorbitol solution, tragacanth. Suppositories indomethacin for rectal use contain 50 mg of indomethacin and the following inactive ingredients: butylated hydroxyanisole, butylated hydroxytoluene, edetic acid, glycerin, polyethylene glycol 3350, polyethylene glycol 8000 and sodium chloride. Indomethacin is a non-steroidal anti-inflammatory indole derivative designated chemically as 1-(4-chlorobenzoyl)-5-methoxy-2-methyl-1*H*-indole-3-acetic acid. Indomethacin is practically insoluble in water and sparingly soluble in alcohol. It has a pKa of 4.5 and is stable in neutral or slightly acidic media and decomposes in strong alkali. The suspension has a pH of 4.0-5.0.

CLINICAL PHARMACOLOGY:

INTRAVENOUS

Although the exact mechanism of action through which indomethacin causes closure of a patent ductus arteriosus is not known, it is believed to be through inhibition of prostaglandin synthesis. Indomethacin has been shown to be a potent inhibitor of prostaglandin synthesis, both *in vitro* and *in vivo*. In human newborns with certain congenital heart malformations, PGE 1 dilates the ductus arteriosus. In fetal and newborn lambs, E type prostaglandins have also been shown to maintain the patency of the ductus, and as in human newborns, indomethacin causes its constriction.

Studies in healthy young animals and in premature infants with patent ductus arteriosus indicated that, after the first dose of intravenous indomethacin, there was a transient reduction in cerebral blood flow velocity and cerebral blood flow. The clinical significance of this effect has not been established.

In double-blind placebo-controlled studies of indomethacin IV in 460 small pre-term infants, weighing 1750 g or less, the infants treated with placebo had a ductus closure rate after 48 hours of 25 to 30 percent, whereas those treated with indomethacin IV had a 75 to 80 percent closure rate. In one of these studies, a multicenter study, involving 405 pre-term infants, later re-opening of the ductus arteriosus occurred in 26 percent of infants treated with indomethacin IV, however, 70 percent of these closed subsequently without the need for surgery or additional indomethacin.

Pharmacokinetics and Metabolism

The disposition of indomethacin following intravenous administration (0.2 mg/kg) in pre-term neonates with patent ductus arteriosus has not been extensively evaluated. Even though the plasma half-life of indomethacin was variable among premature infants, it was shown to vary inversely with postnatal age and weight. In one study, of 28 infants who could be evaluated, the plasma half-life in those infants less than 7 days old averaged 20 hours (range: 3-60 hours, n=18). In infants older than 7 days, the mean plasma half-life of indomethacin was 12 hours (range: 4-38 hours, n=10). Grouping the infants by weight, mean plasma half-life in those weighing less than 1000 g was 21 hours (range: 9-60 hours, n=10); in those infants weighing more than 1000 g, the mean plasma half-life was 15 hours (range: 3-52 hours, n=18).

Following intravenous administration in adults, indomethacin is eliminated via renal excretion, metabolism, and biliary excretion. Indomethacin undergoes appreciable enterohepatic circulation. The mean plasma half-life of indomethacin is 4.5 hours. In the absence of enterohepatic circulation, it is 90 minutes.

In adults, about 99 percent of indomethacin is bound to protein in plasma over the expected range of therapeutic plasma concentrations. The percent bound in neonates has not been studied. In controlled trials in premature infants, however, no evidence of bilirubin displacement has been observed as evidenced by increased incidence of bilirubin encephalopathy (kernicterus).

CAPSULES, ORAL SUSPENSION AND SUPPOSITORIES

Indomethacin is a non-steroidal drug with anti-inflammatory, antipyretic and analgesic properties. Its mode of action, like that of other anti-inflammatory drugs, is not known. However, its therapeutic action is not due to pituitary-adrenal stimulation.

Indomethacin is a potent inhibitor of prostaglandin synthesis *in vitro*. Concentrations are reached during therapy which have been demonstrated to have an effect *in vivo* as well. Prostaglandins sensitize afferent nerves and potentiate the action of bradykinin in inducing pain in animal models. Moreover, prostaglandins are known to be among the mediators of inflammation. Since indomethacin is an inhibitor of prostaglandin synthesis, its mode of action may be due to a decrease of prostaglandins in peripheral tissues.

Indomethacin has been shown to be an effective anti-inflammatory agent, appropriate for long-term use in rheumatoid arthritis, ankylosing spondylitis, and osteoarthritis.

Indomethacin affords relief of symptoms; it does not alter the progressive course of the underlying disease.

Indomethacin suppresses inflammation in rheumatoid arthritis as demonstrated by relief of pain, and reduction of fever, swelling and tenderness. Improvement in patients treated with indomethacin for rheumatoid arthritis has been demonstrated by a reduction in joint swelling, average number of joints involved, and morning stiffness; by increased mobility as demonstrated by a decrease in walking time; and by improved functional capability as demonstrated by an increase in grip strength.

Indomethacin has been reported to diminish basal and CO_2 stimulated cerebral blood flow in healthy volunteers following acute oral and intravenous administration. In one study after one week of treatment with orally administered indomethacin, this effect on basal cerebral blood flow had disappeared. The clinical significance of this effect has not been established.

Indomethacin capsules have been found effective in relieving the pain, reducing the fever, swelling, redness, and tenderness of acute gouty arthritis. Indomethacin capsules rather than indomethacin sustained-release capsules are recommended for treatment of acute gouty arthritis (see INDICATIONS AND USAGE).

Following single oral doses of indomethacin capsules 25 mg or 50 mg, indomethacin is readily absorbed, attaining peak plasma concentrations of about 1 and 2 mcg/ml, respectively, at about 2 hours. Orally administered indomethacin capsules are virtually 100% bioavailable, with 90% of the dose absorbed within 4 hours. A single 50 mg dose of oral suspension indomethacin was found to be bioequivalent to a 50 mg indomethacin capsule when each was administered with food.

CLINICAL PHARMACOLOGY: *(cont'd)*

Indomethacin sustained-release capsules 75 mg are designed to release 25 mg of the drug initially and the remaining 50 mg over approximately 12 hours (90% of dose absorbed by 12 hours). When measured over a 24-hour period, the cumulative amount and time-course of indomethacin absorption from a single capsule indomethacin SR are comparable to those of 3 doses of 25 mg indomethacin capsules given at 4-6 hour intervals.

Plasma concentrations of indomethacin fluctuate less and are more sustained following administration of indomethacin sustained-release capsules than following administration of 25 mg indomethacin capsules given at 4-6 hour intervals. In multiple-dose comparisons, the mean daily steady-state plasma level of indomethacin attained with daily administration of indomethacin sustained-release capsules 75 mg was indistinguishable from that following indomethacin capsules 25 mg given at 0, 6 and 12 hours daily. However, there was a significant difference in indomethacin plasma levels between the two dosage regimens especially after 12 hours.

Controlled clinical studies of safety and efficacy in patients with osteoarthritis have shown that one capsule indomethacin SR was clinically comparable to one 25 mg capsule indomethacin t.i.d.; and in controlled clinical studies in patients with rheumatoid arthritis, one capsule indomethacin SR taken in the morning and one in the evening were clinically indistinguishable from one 50 mg capsule indomethacin t.i.d.

Indomethacin is eliminated via renal excretion, metabolism, and biliary excretion. Indomethacin undergoes appreciable enterohepatic circulation. The mean half-life of indomethacin is estimated to be about 4.5 hours. With a typical therapeutic regimen of 25 or 50 mg t.i.d., the steady-state plasma concentrations of indomethacin are an average 1.4 times those following the first dose.

The rate of absorption is more rapid from the rectal suppository than from indomethacin capsules. Ordinarily, therefore, the total amount absorbed from the suppository would be expected to be at least equivalent to the capsule. In controlled clinical trials, however, the amount of indomethacin absorbed was found to be somewhat less (80-90%) than that absorbed from indomethacin capsules. This is probably because some subjects did not retain the material from the suppository for the one hour necessary to assure complete absorption. Since the suppository dissolves rather quickly rather than melting slowly, it is seldom recovered in recognizable form if the patient retains the suppository for more than a few minutes.

Indomethacin exists in the plasma as the parent drug and its desmethyl, desbenzoyl, and desmethyl-desbenzoyl metabolites, all in the unconjugated form. About 60 percent of an oral dosage is recovered in urine as drug and metabolites (26 percent as indomethacin and its glucuronide), and 33 percent is recovered in feces (1.5 percent as indomethacin).

About 99% of indomethacin is bound to protein in plasma over the expected range of therapeutic plasma concentrations. Indomethacin has been found to cross the blood-brain barrier and the placenta.

In a gastroscopic study in 45 healthy subjects, the number of gastric mucosal abnormalities was significantly higher in the group receiving indomethacin capsules than in the group taking suppositories indomethacin or placebo.

In a double-blind comparative clinical study involving 175 patients with rheumatoid arthritis, however, the incidence of upper gastrointestinal adverse effects with suppositories or indomethacin capsules was comparable. The incidence of lower gastrointestinal adverse effects was greater in the suppository group.

INDICATIONS AND USAGE:

INTRAVENOUS

Indomethacin IV is indicated to close a hemodynamically significant patent ductus arteriosus in premature infants weighing between 500 and 1750 g when after 48 hours usual medical management (*e.g.,* fluid restriction, diuretics, digitalis, respiratory support, etc.) is ineffective. Clear-cut clinical evidence of a hemodynamically significant patent ductus arteriosus should be present, such as respiratory distress, a continuous murmur, a hyperactive precordium, cardiomegaly and pulmonary plethora on chest x-ray.

CAPSULES, ORAL SUSPENSION AND SUPPOSITORIES

Indomethacin has been found effective in active stages of the following:

1. Moderate to severe rheumatoid arthritis including acute flares of chronic disease.

2. Moderate to severe ankylosing spondylitis.

3. Moderate to severe osteoarthritis.

4. Acute painful shoulder (bursitis and/or tendinitis).

5. Acute gouty arthritis.

Indomethacin sustained-release capsules are recommended for all of the indications for indomethacin capsules except acute gouty arthritis.

Indomethacin may enable the reduction of steroid dosage in patients receiving steroids for the more severe forms of rheumatoid arthritis. In such instances the steroid dosage should be reduced slowly and the patients followed very closely for any possible adverse effects.

The use of indomethacin in conjunction with aspirin or other salicylates is not recommended. Controlled clinical studies have shown that the combined use of Indomethacin and aspirin does not produce any greater therapeutic effect than the use of indomethacin alone. Furthermore, in one of these clinical studies, the incidence of gastrointestinal side effects was significantly increased with combined therapy (see DRUG INTERACTIONS).

CONTRAINDICATIONS:

INTRAVENOUS

Indomethacin IV Is Contraindicated In: Infants with proven or suspected infection that is untreated; infants who are bleeding, especially those with active intracranial hemorrhage or gastrointestinal bleeding; infants with thrombocytopenia; infants with coagulation defects; infants with or who are suspected of having necrotizing enterocolitis; infants with significant impairment of renal function; infants with congenital heart disease in whom patency of the ductus arteriosus is necessary for satisfactory pulmonary or systemic blood flow (*e.g.,* pulmonary atresia, severe tetralogy of Fallot, severe coarctation of the aorta).

CAPSULES, ORAL SUSPENSION AND SUPPOSITORIES

Indomethacin should not be used in: Patients who are hypersensitive to this product.

Patients in whom acute asthmatic attacks, urticaria, or rhinitis are precipitated by aspirin or other non-steroidal anti-inflammatory agents.

Suppositories Indomethacin are contraindicated in patients with a history of proctitis or recent rectal bleeding.

WARNINGS:

INTRAVENOUS

Gastrointestinal Effects: In the collaborative study, major gastrointestinal bleeding was no more common in those infants receiving indomethacin than in those infants on placebo. However, minor gastrointestinal bleeding (*i.e.,* chemical detection of blood in the stool) was more commonly noted in those infants treated with indomethacin. Severe gastrointestinal effects have been reported in adults with various arthritic disorders treated chronically with oral indomethacin. (For further information, see package circular for indomethacin capsules).

Central Nervous System Effects: Prematurity per se, is associated with an increased incidence of spontaneous intraventricular hemorrhage. Because indomethacin may inhibit platelet aggregation, the potential for intraventricular bleeding may be increased. However, in the large multi-center study of indomethacin IV (see CLINICAL PHARMACOLOGY), the incidence of intraventricular hemorrhage in babies treated with indomethacin IV was not significantly higher than in the control infants.

Renal Effects: Indomethacin IV may cause significant reduction in urine output (50 percent or more) with concomitant elevations of blood urea nitrogen and creatinine, and reductions in glomerular filtration rate and creatinine clearance. These effects in most infants are transient, disappearing with cessation of therapy with indomethacin IV. However, because adequate renal function can depend upon renal prostaglandin synthesis, indomethacin IV may precipitate renal insufficiency, including acute renal failure, especially in infants with other conditions that may adversely affect renal function (*e.g.,* extracellular volume depletion from any cause, congestive heart failure, sepsis, concomitant use of any nephrotoxic drug, hepatic dysfunction). When significant suppression of urine volume occurs after a dose of indomethacin IV, no additional dose should be given until the urine output returns to normal levels.

Indomethacin IV in pre-term infants may suppress water excretion to a greater extent than sodium excretion. When this occurs, a significant reduction in serum sodium values (*i.e.,* hyponatremia) may result. Infants should have serum electrolyte determinations done during therapy with indomethacin IV. Renal function and serum electrolytes should be monitored (see PRECAUTIONS, DRUG INTERACTIONS, and DOSAGE AND ADMINISTRATION).

CAPSULES, ORAL SUSPENSION AND SUPPOSITORIES

General: Because of the variability of the potential of indomethacin to cause adverse reactions in the individual patient, the following are strongly recommended:

1. The lowest possible effective dose for the individual patient should be prescribed. Increased dosage tends to increase adverse effects, particularly in doses over 150-200 mg/day, without corresponding increase in clinical benefits.

2. Careful instructions to, and observations of, the individual patient are essential to the prevention of serious adverse reactions. As advancing years appear to increase the possibility of adverse reactions, indomethacin should be used with greater care in the aged.

3. Effectiveness of indomethacin in children has not been established. Indomethacin should not be prescribed for children 14 years of age and younger unless toxicity or lack of efficacy associated with other drugs warrants the risk.

In experience with more than 900 children reported in the literature or to Merck Sharp and Dohme who were treated with indomethacin capsules, side effects in children were comparable to those reported in adults. Experience in children has been confined to the use of indomethacin capsules.

If a decision is made to use indomethacin for children two years of age or older, such patients should be monitored closely and periodic assessment of liver function is recommended. There have been cases of hepatotoxicity reported in children with juvenile rheumatoid arthritis, including fatalities. If indomethacin treatment is instituted, a suggested starting dose is 2 mg/kg/day given in divided doses. Maximum daily dosage should not exceed 4 mg/kg/day or 150-200 mg/day, whichever is less. As symptoms subside, the total daily dosage should be reduced to the lowest level required to control symptoms, or the drug should be discontinued.

4. If indomethacin sustained-release capsules are used for initial therapy or during dosage adjustment, observe the patient closely (see DOSAGE AND ADMINISTRATION).

Gastrointestinal Effects: Single or multiple ulcerations, including perforation and hemorrhage of the esophagus, stomach, duodenum or small and large intestine, have been reported to occur with indomethacin. Fatalities have been reported in some instances. Rarely, intestinal ulceration has been associated with stenosis and obstruction.

Gastrointestinal bleeding without obvious ulcer formation and perforation of pre-existing sigmoid lesions (diverticulum, carcinoma, etc.) have occurred. Increased abdominal pain in ulcerative colitis patients or the development of ulcerative colitis and regional ileitis have been reported to occur rarely.

Because of the occurrence, and at times severity, of gastrointestinal reactions to indomethacin, the prescribing physician must be continuously alert for any sign or symptom signaling a possible gastrointestinal reaction. The risks of continuing therapy with indomethacin in the face of such symptoms must be weighed against the possible benefits to the individual patient.

Indomethacin should not be given to patients with active gastrointestinal lesions or with a history of recurrent gastrointestinal lesions except under circumstances which warrant the very high risk and where patients can be monitored very closely.

The gastrointestinal effects may be reduced by giving indomethacin capsules or indomethacin sustained-release capsules immediately after meals, with food, or with antacids.

Risk of GI Ulcerations, Bleeding and Perforation with NSAID Therapy: Serious gastrointestinal toxicity such as bleeding, ulceration, and perforation, can occur at any time, with or without warning symptoms, in patients treated chronically with NSAID therapy. Although minor upper gastrointestinal problems, such as dyspepsia, are common, usually developing early in therapy, physicians should remain alert for ulceration and bleeding in patients treated chronically with NSAIDs even in the absence of previous GI tract symptoms. In patients observed in clinical trials of several months to two years duration, symptomatic upper GI ulcers, gross bleeding or perforation appear to occur in approximately 1% of patients treated for 3-6 months, and in about 2-4% of patients treated for one year. Physicians should inform patients about the signs and/or symptoms of serious GI toxicity and what steps to take if they occur.

Studies to date have not identified any subset of patients not at risk of developing peptic ulceration and bleeding. Except for a prior history of serious GI events and other risk factors known to be associated with peptic ulcer disease, such as alcoholism, smoking, etc., no risk factors (*e.g.,* age, sex) have been associated with increased risk. Elderly or debilitated patients seem to tolerate ulceration or bleeding less well than other individuals and most spontaneous reports of fatal GI events are in this population. Studies to date are inconclusive concerning the relative risk of various NSAIDs in causing such reactions. High doses of any NSAID probably carry a greater risk of these reactions, although controlled clinical trials showing this do not exist in most cases. In considering the use of relatively large doses (within the recommended dosage range), sufficient benefit should be anticipated to offset the potential increased risk of GI toxicity.

Renal Effects: As with other non-steroidal anti-inflammatory drugs, long term administration of indomethacin to animals has resulted in renal papillary necrosis and other abnormal renal pathology. In humans, there have been reports of acute interstitial nephritis with hematuria, proteinuria, and occasionally nephrotic syndrome.

WARNINGS: *(cont'd)*

A second form of renal toxicity has been seen in patients with prerenal and renal conditions leading to a reduction in renal blood flow or blood volume, where the renal prostaglandins have a supportive role in the maintenance of renal perfusion. In these patients administration of an NSAID may cause a dose dependent reduction in prostaglandin formation and may precipitate overt renal decompensation. Patients at greatest risk of this reaction are those with conditions such as renal or hepatic dysfunction, diabetes mellitus, advanced age, extracellular volume depletion from any cause, congestive heart failure, septicemia, pyelonephritis, or concomitant use of any nephrotoxic drug. Indomethacin or other NSAIDs should be given with caution and renal function should be monitored in any patient who may have reduced renal reserve. Discontinuation of NSAID therapy is typically followed by recovery to the pretreatment state.

Increases in serum potassium concentration, including hyperkalemia, have been reported, even in some patients without renal impairment. In patients with normal renal function, these effects have been attributed to a hyporeninemic-hypoaldosteronism state (see PRECAUTIONS and DRUG INTERACTIONS).

Since indomethacin is eliminated primarily by the kidneys, patients with significantly impaired renal function should be closely monitored; a lower daily dosage should be anticipated to avoid excessive drug accumulation.

Ocular Effects: Corneal deposits and retinal disturbances, including those of the macula, have been observed in some patients who had received prolonged therapy with indomethacin. The prescribing physician should be alert to the possible association between the changes noted and indomethacin. It is advisable to discontinue therapy if such changes are observed. Blurred vision may be a significant symptom and warrants a thorough ophthalmological examination. Since these changes may be asymptomatic, ophthalmologic examination at periodic intervals is desirable in patients where therapy is prolonged.

Central Nervous System Effects: Indomethacin may aggravate depression or other psychiatric disturbances, epilepsy, and parkinsonism, and should be used with considerable caution in patients with these conditions. If severe CNS adverse reactions develop, indomethacin should be discontinued.

Indomethacin may cause drowsiness; therefore, patients should be cautioned about engaging in activities requiring mental alertness and motor coordination, such as driving a car. Indomethacin may also cause headache. Headache which persists despite dosage reduction requires cessation of therapy with indomethacin.

Use in Pregnancy and the Neonatal Period: Indomethacin is not recommended for use in pregnant women, since safety for use has not been established, and because of the known effect of drugs of this class on the human fetus (closure of the ductus arteriosus, platelet dysfunction with resultant bleeding, renal dysfunction or failure with oligohydramnios, gastrointestinal bleeding or perforation, and myocardial degenerative changes) during the third trimester of pregnancy.

Teratogenic studies were conducted in mice and rats at dosages of 0.5, 1.0, 2.0, and 4.0 mg/kg/day. Except for retarded fetal ossification at 4 mg/kg/day considered secondary to the decreased average fetal weights, no increase in fetal malformations was observed as compared with control groups. Other studies in mice reported in the literature using higher doses (5 to 15 mg/kg/day) have described maternal toxicity and death, increased fetal resorptions, and fetal malformations. Comparable studies in rodents using high doses of aspirin have shown similar maternal and fetal effects.

As with other non-steroidal anti-inflammatory agents which inhibit prostaglandin synthesis, indomethacin has been found to delay parturition in rats.

In rats and mice, 4.0 mg/kg/day given during the last three days of gestation caused a decrease in maternal weight gain and some maternal and fetal deaths. An increased incidence of neuronal necrosis in the diencephalon in the live-born fetuses was observed. At 2.0 mg/kg/day, no increase in neuronal necrosis was observed as compared to the control groups. Administration of 0.5 or 4.0 mg/kg/day during the first three days of life did not cause an increase in neuronal necrosis at either dose level.

Use in Nursing Mothers: Indomethacin is excreted in the milk of lactating mothers. Indomethacin is not recommended for use in nursing mothers.

PRECAUTIONS:

INTRAVENOUS

General: Indomethacin may mask the usual signs and symptoms of infection. Therefore, the physician must be continually on the alert for this and should use the drug with extra care in the presence of existing controlled infection.

Severe hepatic reactions have been reported in adults treated chronically with oral indomethacin for arthritic disorders. (For further information, see package circular for capsules, indomethacin). If clinical signs and symptoms consistent with liver disease develop in the neonate, or if systemic manifestations occur, indomethacin IV should be discontinued.

Indomethacin IV may inhibit platelet aggregation. In one small study, platelet aggregation was grossly abnormal after indomethacin therapy (given orally to premature infants to close the ductus arteriosus). Platelet aggregation returned to normal by the tenth day. Premature infants should be observed for signs of bleeding.

The drug should be administered carefully to avoid extravascular injection or leakage as the solution may be irritating to tissue.

Neonatal Effects: In rats and mice, oral indomethacin 4.0 mg/kg/day given during the last three days of gestation caused a decrease in maternal weight gain and some maternal and fetal deaths. An increased incidence of neuronal necrosis in the diencephalon in the live-born fetuses was observed. At 2.0 mg/kg/day, no increase in neuronal necrosis was observed as compared to the control groups. Administration of 0.5 or 4.0 mg/kg/day during the first three days of life did not cause an increase in neuronal necrosis at either dose level.

Pregnant rats, given 2.0 mg/kg/day and 4.0 mg/kg/day during the last trimester of gestation, delivered offspring whose pulmonary blood vessels were both reduced in number and excessively muscularized. These findings are similar to those observed in the syndrome of persistent pulmonary hypertension of the newborn.

CAPSULES, ORAL SUSPENSION AND SUPPOSITORIES

General: Non-steroidal anti-inflammatory drugs, including indomethacin, may mask the usual signs and symptoms of infection. Therefore, the physician must be continually on the alert for this and should use the drug with extra care in the presence of existing infection.

Fluid retention and peripheral edema have been observed in some patients taking indomethacin. Therefore, as with other non-steroidal anti-inflammatory drugs, indomethacin should be used with caution in patients with cardiac dysfunction, hypertension, or other conditions predisposing to fluid retention.

In a study of patients with severe heart failure and hyponatremia, indomethacin was associated with significant deterioration of circulatory hemodynamics, presumably due to inhibition of prostaglandin dependent compensator mechanisms.

Indomethacin, like other non-steroidal anti-inflammatory agents, can inhibit platelet aggregation. This effect is of shorter duration than that seen with aspirin and usually disappears within 24 hours after discontinuation of indomethacin. Indomethacin has been shown to prolong bleeding time (but within the normal range) in normal subjects. Because this effect may be exaggerated in patients with underlying hemostatic defects, indomethacin should be used with caution in persons with coagulation defects.

As with other non-steroidal anti-inflammatory drugs, borderline elevation of one or more liver tests may occur in up to 15% of patients. These abnormalities may progress, may remain essentially unchanged, or may be transient with continued therapy. The SGPT (ALT) test is probably the most sensitive indicator of liver dysfunction. Meaningful (3 times the upper limit of normal) elevations of SGPT or SGOT (AST) occurred in controlled clinical trials in less than 1% of patients. A patient with symptoms and/or signs suggesting liver dysfunction, or in whom an abnormal liver test has occurred, should be evaluated for evidence of the development of more severe hepatic reaction while on therapy with indomethacin. Severe hepatic reactions, including jaundice and cases of fatal hepatitis, have been reported with indomethacin as with other non-steroidal anti-inflammatory drugs. Although such reactions are rare, if abnormal liver tests persist or worsen, if clinical signs and symptoms consistent with liver disease develop, or if systemic manifestations occur (*e.g.,* eosinophilia, rash, etc.), indomethacin should be discontinued.

Information for the Patient: Indomethacin, like other drugs of its class, is not free of side effects. The side effects of these drugs can cause discomfort and, rarely, there are more serious side effects such as gastrointestinal bleeding, which may result in hospitalization and even fatal outcomes.

NSAIDs (Non-steroidal Anti-inflammatory Drugs) are often essential agents in the management of arthritis; but they also may be commonly employed for conditions which are less serious.

Physicians may wish to discuss with their patients the potential risks (see WARNINGS, PRECAUTIONS, and ADVERSE REACTIONS) and likely benefits of NSAID treatment, particularly when the drugs are used for less serious conditions where treatment without NSAIDs may represent an acceptable alternative to both the patient and physician.

Laboratory Tests: Because serious GI tract ulceration and bleeding can occur without warning symptoms, physicians should follow chronically treated patients for the signs and symptoms of ulceration and bleeding and should inform them of the importance of this follow-up (see WARNINGS, Risk of GI Ulcerations, Bleeding and Perforation with NSAID Therapy).

Carcinogenesis, Mutagenesis, and Impairment of Fertility: In an 81-week chronic oral toxicity study in the rat at doses up to 1 mg/kg/day, indomethacin had no tumorigenic effect.

Indomethacin produced no neoplastic or hyperplastic changes related to treatment in carcinogenic studies in the rat (dosing period 73-110 weeks) and the mouse (dosing period 62-88 weeks) at doses up to 1.5 mg/kg/day.

Indomethacin did not have any mutagenic effect in *in vitro* bacterial tests (Ames test and *E. coli* with or without metabolic activation) and a series of *in vivo* tests including the host-mediated assay, sex-linked recessive lethals in *Drosophila,* and the micronucleus test in mice.

Indomethacin at dosage levels up to 0.5 mg/kg/day had no effect on fertility in mice in a two generation reproduction study or a two litter reproduction study in rats.

Pediatric Use: Effectiveness in children 14 years of age and younger has not been established (see WARNINGS).

DRUG INTERACTIONS:

INTRAVENOUS

Since renal function may be reduced by indomethacin IV, consideration should be given to reduction in dosage of those medications that rely on adequate renal function for their elimination. Because the half-life of digitalis (given frequently to pre-term infants with patent ductus arteriosus and associated cardiac failure) may be prolonged when given concomitantly with indomethacin, the infant should be observed closely; frequent ECGs and serum digitalis levels may be required to prevent or detect digitalis toxicity early. Furthermore, in one study of premature infants treated with indomethacin IV and also receiving either gentamicin or amikacin, both peak and trough levels of these aminoglycosides were significantly elevated.

Therapy with indomethacin may blunt the natriuretic effect of furosemide. This response has been attributed to inhibition of prostaglandin synthesis by non-steroidal anti-inflammatory drugs. In a study of 19 premature infants with patent ductus arteriosus treated with either indomethacin IV alone or a combination of indomethacin IV and furosemide, results showed that infants receiving both indomethacin IV and furosemide had significantly higher urinary output, higher levels of sodium and chloride excretion, and higher glomerular filtration rates than did those infants receiving indomethacin IV alone. In this study, the data suggested that therapy with furosemide helped to maintain renal function in the premature infant when indomethacin IV was added to the treatment of patent ductus arteriosus.

CAPSULES, ORAL SUSPENSION AND SUPPOSITORIES

In normal volunteers receiving indomethacin, the administration of diflunisal decreased the renal clearance and significantly increased the plasma levels of indomethacin. In some patients, combined use of indomethacin and diflunisal has been associated with fatal gastrointestinal hemorrhage. Therefore, diflunisal and indomethacin should not be used concomitantly.

In a study in normal volunteers, it was found that chronic concurrent administration of 3.6 g of aspirin per day decreases indomethacin blood levels approximately 20%.

Clinical studies have shown that indomethacin does not influence the hypoprothrombinemia produced by anticoagulants. However, when any additional drug, including indomethacin, is added to the treatment of patients on anticoagulant therapy, the patients should be observed for alterations of the prothrombin time.

When indomethacin is given to patients receiving probenecid, the plasma levels of indomethacin are likely to be increased. Therefore, a lower total daily dosage of indomethacin may produce a satisfactory therapeutic effect. When increases in the dose of indomethacin are made, they should be made carefully and in small increments.

Caution should be used if indomethacin is administered simultaneously with methotrexate. Indomethacin has been reported to decrease the tubular secretion of methotrexate and to potentiate its toxicity.

Administration of non-steroidal anti-inflammatory drugs concomitantly with cyclosporine has been associated with an increase in cyclosporine-induced toxicity, possibly due to decreased synthesis of renal prostacyclin. NSAIDs should be used with caution in patients taking cyclosporine, and renal function should be carefully monitored.

Indomethacin capsules 50 mg t.i.d. produced a clinically relevant elevation of plasma lithium and reduction in renal lithium clearance in psychiatric patients and normal subjects with steady state plasma lithium concentrations. This effect has been attributed to inhibition of prostaglandin synthesis. As a consequence, when indomethacin and lithium are given concomitantly, the patient should be carefully observed for signs of lithium toxicity. (Read circulars for lithium preparations before use of such concomitant therapy.) In addition, the frequency of monitoring serum lithium concentration should be increased at the outset of such combination drug treatment.

Indomethacin given concomitantly with digoxin has been reported to increase the serum concentration and prolong the half-life of digoxin. Therefore, when indomethacin and digoxin are used concomitantly, serum digoxin levels should be closely monitored.

DRUG INTERACTIONS: *(cont'd)*

In some patients, the administration of indomethacin can reduce the diuretic, natriuretic, and, antihypertensive effects of loop, potassium-sparing, and thiazide diuretics. Therefore, when indomethacin and diuretics are used concomitantly, the patient should be observed closely to determine if the desired effect of the diuretic is obtained.

Indomethacin reduces basal plasma renin activity (PRA), as well as those elevations of PRA induced by furosemide administration, or salt or volume depletion. These facts should be considered when evaluating plasma renin activity in hypertensive patients.

It has been reported that the addition of triamterene to a maintenance schedule of indomethacin resulted in reversible acute renal failure in two of four healthy volunteers. Indomethacin and triamterene should not be administered together.

Indomethacin and potassium-sparing diuretics each may be associated with increased serum potassium levels. The potential effects of indomethacin and potassium-sparing diuretics on potassium kinetics and renal function should be considered when these agents are administered concurrently.

Most of the above effects concerning diuretics have been attributed, at least in part, to mechanisms involving inhibition of prostaglandin synthesis by indomethacin.

Blunting of the antihypertensive effect of beta-adrenoceptor blocking agents by non-steroidal anti-inflammatory drugs including indomethacin has been reported. Therefore, when using these blocking agents to treat hypertension, patients should be observed carefully in order to confirm that the desired therapeutic effect has been obtained. There are reports that indomethacin can reduce the antihypertensive effect of captopril in some patients.

False-negative results in the dexamethasone suppression test (DST) in patients being treated with indomethacin have been reported. Thus, results of the DST should be interpreted with caution in these patients.

ADVERSE REACTIONS:

INTRAVENOUS

In a double-blind placebo-controlled trial of 405 premature infants weighing less than or equal to 1750 g with evidence of large ductal shunting, in those infants treated with indomethacin (n = 206), there was a statistically significantly greater incidence of bleeding problems, including gross or microscopic bleeding into the gastrointestinal tract, oozing from the skin after needle stick, pulmonary hemorrhage, and disseminated intravascular coagulopathy. There was no statistically significant difference between treatment groups with reference to intracranial hemorrhage.

The infants treated with indomethacin sodium trihydrate also had a significantly higher incidence of transient oliguria and elevations of serum creatinine (greater than or equal to 1.8 mg/dl) than did the infants treated with placebo.

The incidences of retrolental fibroplasia (grades III and IV) and pneumothorax in infants treated with indomethacin IV were no greater than in placebo controls and were statistically significantly lower than in surgically-treated infants.

The following additional adverse reactions in infants have been reported from the collaborative study, anecdotal case reports, and from other studies using rectal, oral, or intravenous indomethacin for treatment of patent ductus arteriosus. The rates are based on the experience of 849 indomethacin-treated infants reported in the medical literature, regardless of the route of administration. One year follow-up is available on 175 infants and shows no long-term sequelae which could be attributed to indomethacin. In controlled clinical studies, only electrolyte imbalance and renal dysfunction (of the reactions listed below) occurred statistically significantly more frequently after indomethacin IV than after placebo.

Renal: renal dysfunction in 41 percent of infants, including one or more of the following: reduced urinary output; reduced urine sodium, chloride, or potassium, urine osmolality, free water clearance, or glomerular filtration rate; elevated serum creatinine or BUN; uremia.

Cardiovascular: intracranial bleeding**, pulmonary hypertension.

Gastrointestinal: gastrointestinal bleeding*, vomiting, abdominal distention, transient ileus, localized perforation(s) of the small and/or large intestine.

Metabolic: hyponatremia*, elevated serum potassium*, reduction in blood sugar, including hypoglycemia, increased weight gain (fluid retention).

Coagulation: decreased platelet aggregation (see PRECAUTIONS).

The following adverse reactions have also been reported in infants treated with indomethacin, however, a causal relationship to therapy with indomethacin IV has not been established:

Cardiovascular: bradycardia.

Respiratory: apnea, exacerbation of pre-existing pulmonary infection.

Metabolic: acidosis/alkalosis.

Hematologic: disseminated intravascular coagulation.

Gastrointestinal: necrotizing enterocolitis.

Ophthalmic: retrolental fibroplasia.**

A variety of additional adverse experiences have been reported in adults treated with oral indomethacin for moderate to severe rheumatoid arthritis, osteoarthritis, ankylosing spondylitis, acute painful shoulder and acute gouty arthritis (see ADVERSE REACTIONS,TABLE 1). Their relevance to the pre-term neonate receiving indomethacin for patent ductus arteriosus is unknown, however, the possibility exists that these experiences may be associated with the use of indomethacin IV in pre-term neonates.

*Incidence 3-9 percent. Those reactions which are unmarked occurred in 1-3 percent of patients.

**Incidence in both indomethacin and placebo-treated infants 3-9 percent. Those reactions which are unmarked occurred in less than 3 percent.

CAPSULES, ORAL SUSPENSION AND SUPPOSITORIES

The adverse reactions for indomethacin capsules listed in the following table have been arranged into two groups: (1) incidence greater than 1%; and (2) incidence less than 1%. The incidence for group (1) was obtained from 33 double-blind controlled clinical trials reported in the literature (1,092 patients). The incidence for group (2) was based on reports in clinical trials, in the literature, and on voluntary reports since marketing. The probability of a causal relationship exists between indomethacin and these adverse reactions, some of which have been reported only rarely.

In controlled clinical trials, the incidence of adverse reactions to indomethacin sustained-release capsules and equal 24-hour doses of indomethacin capsules were similar.

The adverse reactions reported with indomethacin capsules may occur with use of the suppositories. In addition, rectal irritation and tenesmus have been reported in patients who have received the suppositories.

The adverse reactions reported with indomethacin capsules may also occur with use of the suspension (TABLE 1A and TABLE 1B):

Causal Relationship Unknown: Other reactions have been reported but occurred under circumstances where a causal relationship could not be established. However, in these rarely reported events, the possibility cannot be excluded. Therefore, these observations are being listed to serve as alerting information to physicians:

Cardiovascular: Thrombophlebitis

ADVERSE REACTIONS: *(cont'd)*

TABLE 1A

Incidence greater than 1%	Incidence less than 1%	
Gastrointestinal		
nausea* with or without vomiting	anorexia	gastrointestinal bleeding without obvious ulcer formation and perforation of pre-existing sigmoid lesions (diverticulum, carcinoma, etc.) development of ulcerative colitis and regional ileitis
dyspepsia* (including indigestion, heartburn and epigastric pain)	bloating (includes distention)	ulcerative stomatitis
diarrhea	flatulence	toxic hepatitis and jaundice (some fatal cases have been reported)
abdominal distress or pain	peptic ulcer	
constipation	gastroenteritis	
	rectal bleeding	
	proctitis	
	single or multiple ulcerations, including perforation and hemorrhage of the esophagus, stomach, duodenum or small and large intestines	
	intestinal ulceration associated with stenosis and obstruction	
Central Nervous System		
headache (11.7%)	anxiety (includes nervousness)	light-headedness
dizziness*	muscle weakness	syncope
vertigo	involuntary muscle movements	paresthesia
somnolence	insomnia	aggravation of epilepsy and parkinsonism
depression and fatigue (including malaise and listlessness)	muzziness	depersonalization
	psychic disturbances including psychotic episodes	coma
	mental confusion	peripheral neuropathy
	drowsiness	convulsions
		dysarthria
Special Senses		
tinnitus	ocular — corneal deposits and retinal disturbances, including those of the macula, have been reported in some patients on prolonged therapy with Indomethacin	blurred vision
		diplopia
		hearing disturbances, deafness
Cardiovascular		
none	hypertension	congestive heart failure
	hypotension	arrhythmia; palpitations
	tachycardia	
	chest pain	
Metabolic		
none	edema	hyperglycemia
	weight gain	glycosuria
	fluid retention	hyperkalemia
	flushing or sweating	
Integumentary		
none	pruritus	exfoliative dermatitis
	rash; urticaria	erythema nodosum
	petechiae or ecchymosis	loss of hair
		Stevens-Johnson syndrome
		erythema multiforme
		toxic epidermal necrolysis

* Reactions occurring in 3% to 9% of patients treated with Indomethacin. (Those reactions occurring in less than 3% of the patients are unmarked.)

TABLE 1B

Incidence greater than 1%	Incidence less than 1%	
Hematologic		
none	leukopenia	aplastic anemia
	bone marrow depression	hemolytic anemia
	anemia secondary to obvious or occult gastrointestinal bleeding	agranulocytosis
		thrombocytopenic purpura
		disseminated intravascular coagulation
Hypersensitivity		
none	acute anaphylaxis	dyspnea
	acute respiratory distress	asthma purpura
	rapid fall in blood pressure resembling a shock-like state	angiitis
	angioedema	pulmonary edema fever
Genitourinary		
none	hematuria	BUN elevation
	vaginal bleeding	renal insufficiency, including renal failure
	proteinuria	
	nephrotic syndrome	
	interstitial nephritis	
Miscellaneous		
none	epistaxis	
	breast changes, including enlargement and tenderness, or gynecomastia	

ADVERSE REACTIONS: *(cont'd)*

Hematologic: Although there have been several reports of leukemia, the supporting information is weak

Genitourinary: Urinary frequency.

A rare occurrence of fulminant necrotizing fasciitis, particularly in association with Group A β-hemolytic streptococcus, has been described in persons treated with non-steroidal anti-inflammatory agents, including indomethacin, sometimes with fatal outcome (see PRECAUTIONS, General).

OVERDOSAGE:

CAPSULES, ORAL SUSPENSION AND SUPPOSITORIES

The following symptoms may be observed following overdosage: nausea, vomiting, intense headache, dizziness, mental confusion, disorientation, or lethargy. There have been reports of paresthesias, numbness, and convulsions.

Treatment is symptomatic and supportive. The stomach should be emptied as quickly as possible if the ingestion is recent. If vomiting has not occurred spontaneously, the patient should be induced to vomit with syrup of ipecac. If the patient is unable to vomit, gastric lavage should be performed. Once the stomach has been emptied, 25 or 50 g of activated charcoal may be given. Depending on the condition of the patient, close medical observation and nursing care may be required. The patient should be followed for several days because gastrointestinal ulceration and hemorrhage have been reported as adverse reactions of indomethacin. Use of antacids may be helpful.

The oral LD_{50} of indomethacin in mice and rats (based on 14 day mortality response) was 50 and 12 mg/kg, respectively.

DOSAGE AND ADMINISTRATION:

INTRAVENOUS

FOR INTRAVENOUS ADMINISTRATION ONLY.

Dosage recommendations for closure of the ductus arteriosus depends on the age of the infant at the time of therapy. A course of therapy is defined as three intravenous doses of indomethacin IV given at 12-24 hour intervals, with careful attention to urinary output. If anuria or marked oliguria (urinary output <0.6 ml/kg/hr) is evident at the scheduled time of the second or third dose of indomethacin IV, no additional doses should be given until laboratory studies indicate that renal function has returned to normal (see WARNINGS, Renal Effects).

Dosage according to age is as follows (TABLE 2):

TABLE 2

AGE at 1st dose	DOSAGE (mg/kg) 1st	2nd	3rd
Less than 48 hours	0.2	0.1	0.1
2-7 days	0.2	0.2	0.2
over 7 days	0.2	0.25	0.25

If the ductus arteriosus closes or is significantly reduced in size after an interval of 48 hours or more from completion of the first course of indomethacin IV, no further doses are necessary. If the ductus arteriosus re-opens, a second course of 1-3 doses may be given, each dose separated by a 12-24 hour interval as described above.

If the infant remains unresponsive to therapy with indomethacin IV after 2 courses, surgery may be necessary for closure of the ductus arteriosus. If severe adverse reactions occur, STOP THE DRUG.

Directions for Use: Parenteral drug products should be inspected visually for particular matter and discoloration prior to administration whenever solution and container permit.

The solution should be prepared only with 1 to 2 ml of preservative-free sterile sodium chloride injection, 0.9 percent or preservative-free sterile water for injection. Benzyl alcohol as a preservative has been associated with toxicity in newborns. Therefore, all diluents should be preservative-free. If 1 ml of diluent is used, the concentration of indomethacin in the solution will equal approximately 0.1 mg/0.1 ml; if 2 ml of diluent are used, the concentration of the solution will equal approximately 0.05 mg/0.1 ml. Any unused portion of the solution should be discarded because there is no preservative contained in the vial. A fresh solution should be prepared just prior to each administration. Once reconstituted, the indomethacin solution may be injected intravenously over 5-10 seconds.

Further dilution with intravenous infusion solutions is not recommended. Indomethacin IV is not buffered, and reconstitution with solutions at pH values below 6.0 may result in precipitation of the insoluble indomethacin free acid moiety.

Storage: Store below 30°C (86°F). *Protect from light.* Store container in carton until contents have been used.

CAPSULES, ORAL SUSPENSION AND SUPPOSITORIES

Indomethacin is available as 25 and 50 mg indomethacin capsules, 75 mg indomethacin sustained-release capsules for oral use, oral suspension indomethacin, containing 25 mg of indomethacin per 5 ml, and 50 mg suppositories indomethacin for rectal use. Indomethacin sustained-release capsules 75 mg once a day can be substituted for indomethacin capsules 25 mg t.i.d. However, there will be significant differences between the two dosage regimens in indomethacin blood levels, especially after 12 hours (see CLINICAL PHARMACOLOGY). In addition, indomethacin sustained-release capsules 75 mg b.i.d. can be substituted for indomethacin capsules 50 mg t.i.d. Indomethacin sustained-release capsules may be substituted for all the indications for indomethacin capsules except acute gouty arthritis.

Adverse reactions appear to correlate with the size of the dose of indomethacin in most patients but not all. Therefore, every effort should be made to determine the smallest effective dosage for the individual patient.

Always give indomethacin capsules, indomethacin sustained-release capsules, or oral suspension indomethacin with food, immediately after meals, or with antacids to reduce gastric irritation.

Pediatric Use: Indomethacin ordinarily should not be prescribed for children 14 years of age and under (see WARNINGS).

Adult Use: *Dosage Recommendations for Active Stages of the Following:* Moderate to severe rheumatoid arthritis including acute flares of chronic disease; moderate to severe ankylosing spondylitis; and moderate to severe osteoarthritis.

Suggested Dosage: Indomethacin capsules 25 mg b.i.d. or t.i.d. If this is well tolerated, increase the daily dosage by 25 or by 50 mg, if required by continuing symptoms, at weekly intervals until a satisfactory response is obtained or until a total daily dose of 150-200 mg is reached. DOSES ABOVE THIS AMOUNT GENERALLY DO NOT INCREASE THE EFFECTIVENESS OF THE DRUG.

DOSAGE AND ADMINISTRATION: *(cont'd)*

Night Pain and/or Morning Stiffness

In patients who have persistent night pain and/or morning stiffness, the giving of a large portion, up to a maximum of 100 mg, of the total daily dose at bedtime, either orally or by rectal suppositories, may be helpful in affording relief. The total daily dose should not exceed 200 mg. In acute flares of chronic rheumatoid arthritis, it may be necessary to increase the dosage by 25 mg or, if required, by 50 mg daily.

If indomethacin sustained-release capsules 75 mg are used for initiating indomethacin treatment, one capsule daily should be the usual starting dose in order to observe patient tolerance since 75 mg per day is the maximum recommended starting dose for indomethacin. If indomethacin sustained-release capsules are used to increase the daily dose, patients should be observed for possible signs and symptoms of intolerance since the daily increment will exceed the daily increment recommended for the other dosage forms. For patients who require 150 mg of indomethacin per day and have demonstrated acceptable tolerance, indomethacin SR may be prescribed as one capsule twice daily.

If minor adverse effects develop as the dosage is increased, reduce the dosage rapidly to a tolerated dose and OBSERVE THE PATIENT CLOSELY.

If severe adverse reactions occur, STOP THE DRUG. After the acute phase of the disease is under control, an attempt to reduce the daily dose should be made repeatedly until the patient is receiving the smallest effective dose or the drug is discontinued.

Careful instructions to, and observations of, the individual patient are essential to the prevention of serious, irreversible, including fatal, adverse reactions.

As advancing years appear to increase the possibility of adverse reactions, indomethacin should be used with greater care in the aged.

Acute Painful Shoulder (Bursitis and/or Tendinitis).

Initial Dose: 75-150 mg daily in 3 or 4 divided doses.

The drug should be discontinued after the signs and symptoms of inflammation have been controlled for several days. The usual course of therapy is 7-14 days.

Acute Gouty Arthritis

Suggested Dosage: Indomethacin capsules 50 mg t.i.d. until pain is tolerable. The dose should then be rapidly reduced to complete cessation of the drug. Definite relief of pain has been reported within 2 to 4 hours. Tenderness and heat usually subside in 24 to 36 hours, and swelling gradually disappears in 3 to 5 days.

Storage Store oral suspension indomethacin below 30°C (86°F). Avoid temperatures above 50°C (122°F). Protect from freezing.

Store suppositories indomethacin below 30°C (86°F). Avoid transient temperatures above 40°C (104°F).

HOW SUPPLIED - RATED THERAPEUTICALLY EQUIVALENT:

Capsule, Gelatin - Oral - 25 mg

90's	$2.90	Indomethacin, H.C.F.A. F F P	99999-1532-01
90's	$4.15	Indomethacin, Major Pharms	00904-1175-89
100's	$3.23	Indomethacin, United Res	00677-0872-01
100's	$3.23	Indomethacin, Sidmak Labs	50111-0406-01
100's	$3.23	Indomethacin, H.C.F.A. F F P	99999-1532-02
100's	$4.43	Indomethacin, IDE-Interstate	00814-3837-14
100's	$4.61	Indomethacin, US Trading	56126-0067-11
100's	$6.15	Indomethacin, Novopharm (US)	55953-0420-40
100's	$6.50	Indomethacin, Consolidated Midland	00223-1195-01
100's	$8.45	Indomethacin, Watson Labs	52544-0303-01
100's	$9.33	Indomethacin, Novopharm (US)	55953-0420-01
100's	$10.70	Indomethacin, Major Pharms	00904-1175-60
100's	$10.85	Indomethacin, West Point Pharma	59591-0172-68
100's	$10.85	Indomethacin, Endo Labs	60951-0772-70
100's	$11.96	Indomethacin, Caremark	00339-5471-12
100's	$13.32	Indomethacin, Voluntary Hosp	53258-0426-01
100's	$13.94	Indomethacin, Qualitest Pharms	00603-4067-21
100's	$14.90	Indomethacin, Par Pharm	49884-0067-01
100's	$15.90	Indomethacin, Mutual Pharm	53489-0133-01
100's	$16.46	Indomethacin, Aligen Independ	00405-4541-01
100's	$17.25	Indomethacin, Rugby	00536-3981-01
100's	$18.65	Indomethacin, Zenith Labs	00172-4029-60
100's	$18.65	Indomethacin, Goldline Labs	00182-1681-01
100's	$19.96	Indomethacin, Warner Chilcott	00047-0887-24
100's	$19.96	Indomethacin, Schein Pharm (US)	00364-0691-01
100's	$19.96	Indomethacin, HL Moore Drug Exch	00839-6762-06
100's	$20.00	Indomethacin, Bristol Myers Squibb	00003-0280-50
100's	$20.90	Indomethacin, Lederle Pharm	00005-3761-23
100's	$20.90	Indomethacin, Geneva Pharms	00781-2325-01
100's	$20.95	Indomethacin, Mylan	00378-0143-01
100's	$24.56	Indomethacin, Parmed Pharms	00349-8341-01
100's	$27.15	Indomethacin, Voluntary Hosp	53258-0426-13
100's	$29.93	Indomethacin, Major Pharms	00904-1175-61
100's	$32.00	Indomethacin, Medirex	57480-0406-01
100's	$32.30	Indomethacin, Goldline Labs	00182-1681-89
100's	$33.22	Indomethacin, Geneva Pharms	00781-2325-13
100's	$33.27	Indomethacin, Vangard Labs	00615-2516-13
100's	**$53.93**	**INDOCIN, Merck**	**00006-0025-68**
500's	$16.15	Indomethacin, United Res	00677-0872-05
500's	$16.15	Indomethacin, H.C.F.A. F F P	99999-1532-03
500's	$27.12	Indomethacin, Novopharm (US)	55953-0420-70
500's	$29.50	Indomethacin, Consolidated Midland	00223-1195-05
500's	$40.13	Indomethacin, Watson Labs	52544-0303-05
500's	$59.00	Indomethacin, Mutual Pharm	53489-0133-05
500's	$64.83	Indomethacin, Par Pharm	49884-0067-05
500's	$69.25	Indomethacin, Rugby	00536-3981-05
500's	$85.60	Indomethacin, Zenith Labs	00172-4029-70
500's	$85.60	Indomethacin, Goldline Labs	00182-1681-05
500's	$99.49	Indomethacin, Lederle Pharm	00005-3761-31
1000's	$32.30	Indomethacin, United Res	00677-0872-10
1000's	$32.30	Indomethacin, Sidmak Labs	50111-0406-03
1000's	$32.30	Indomethacin, Watson Labs	52544-0303-10
1000's	$32.30	Indomethacin, H.C.F.A. F F P	99999-1532-04
1000's	$48.17	Indomethacin, Novopharm (US)	55953-0420-80
1000's	$63.91	Indomethacin, Qualitest Pharms	00603-4067-32
1000's	$64.00	Indomethacin, Major Pharms	00904-1175-80
1000's	$73.82	Indomethacin, Halsey Drug	00879-0507-10
1000's	$81.80	Indomethacin, West Point Pharma	59591-0172-82
1000's	$81.80	Indomethacin, Endo Labs	60951-0772-90
1000's	$114.00	Indomethacin, Mutual Pharm	53489-0133-10
1000's	$129.63	Indomethacin, Par Pharm	49884-0067-10
1000's	$132.90	Indomethacin, Rugby	00536-3981-10
1000's	$159.90	Indomethacin, Parmed Pharms	00349-8341-10
1000's	$167.85	Indomethacin, Zenith Labs	00172-4029-80
1000's	$167.85	Indomethacin, Goldline Labs	00182-1681-10
1000's	$167.95	Indomethacin, Warner Chilcott	00047-0887-32
1000's	$187.55	Indomethacin, Aligen Independ	00405-4541-03

HOW SUPPLIED - RATED THERAPEUTICALLY EQUIVALENT:
(cont'd)

1000's	$188.00	Indomethacin, Schein Pharm (US)	00364-0691-02
1000's	$188.06	Indomethacin, HL Moore Drug Exch	00839-6762-16
1000's	$193.95	Indomethacin, Bristol Myers Squibb	00003-0280-75
1000's	$200.00	Indomethacin, Lederle Pharm	00005-3761-34
1000's	$200.00	Indomethacin, Geneva Pharms	00781-2325-10
1000's	$204.95	Indomethacin, Mylan	00378-0143-10
1000's	**$523.25**	**INDOCIN, Merck**	**00006-0025-82**

Capsule, Gelatin - Oral - 50 mg

60's	$7.67	Indomethacin, Talbert Phcy	44514-0453-36
100's	$4.88	Indomethacin, United Res	00677-0873-01
100's	$4.88	Indomethacin, H.C.F.A. F F P	99999-1532-05
100's	$6.25	Indoflex, H & H Labs	46703-0070-01
100's	$6.38	Indomethacin, IDE-Interstate	00814-3838-14
100's	$6.92	Indomethacin, US Trading	56126-0068-11
100's	$7.50	Indomethacin, Consolidated Midland	00223-1196-01
100's	$11.54	Indomethacin, Novopharm (US)	55953-0439-40
100's	$14.04	Indomethacin, Novopharm (US)	55953-0439-01
100's	$14.07	Indomethacin, Watson Labs	52544-0304-01
100's	$17.70	Indomethacin, West Point Pharma	59591-0159-68
100's	$17.70	Indomethacin, Endo Labs	60951-0773-70
100's	$18.53	Indomethacin, Halsey Drug	00879-0508-01
100's	$18.87	Indomethacin, Voluntary Hosp	53258-0427-01
100's	$19.40	Indomethacin, Qualitest Pharms	00603-4068-21
100's	$19.55	Indomethacin, Major Pharms	00904-1176-60
100's	$22.40	Indomethacin, Par Pharm	49884-0068-01
100's	$28.75	Indomethacin, Rugby	00536-3982-01
100's	$30.00	Indomethacin, Mutual Pharm	53489-0134-01
100's	$30.25	Indomethacin, Sidmak Labs	50111-0407-01
100's	$31.50	Indomethacin, Zenith Labs	00172-4030-60
100's	$31.50	Indomethacin, Goldline Labs	00182-1682-01
100's	$31.82	Indomethacin, Aligen Independ	00405-4542-01
100's	$31.95	Indomethacin, Warner Chilcott	00047-0888-24
100's	$31.96	Indomethacin, Schein Pharm (US)	00364-0692-01
100's	$31.98	Indomethacin, HL Moore Drug Exch	00839-6763-06
100's	$32.64	Indomethacin, Bristol Myers Squibb	00003-0295-50
100's	$34.35	Indomethacin, Voluntary Hosp	53258-0427-13
100's	$37.65	Indomethacin, Lederle Pharm	00005-3762-23
100's	$37.65	Indomethacin, Geneva Pharms	00781-2350-01
100's	$37.95	Indomethacin, Mylan	00378-0147-01
100's	$39.15	Indomethacin, Amer Preferred	53445-1682-01
100's	$41.03	Indomethacin, Roxane	00054-8441-25
100's	$53.70	Indomethacin, Goldline Labs	00182-1682-89
100's	$53.71	Indomethacin, Geneva Pharms	00781-2350-13
100's	**$88.00**	**INDOCIN, Merck**	**00006-0050-68**
100's	**$89.09**	**INDOCIN, Merck**	**00006-0050-28**
100's	$134.70	Indomethacin, Aligen Independ	00405-4542-02
500's	$24.40	Indomethacin, United Res	00677-0873-05
500's	$24.40	Indomethacin, H.C.F.A. F F P	99999-1532-06
500's	$28.25	Indoflex, H & H Labs	46703-0070-05
500's	$31.95	Indomethacin, Consolidated Midland	00223-1196-05
500's	$45.10	Indomethacin, Novopharm (US)	55953-0439-70
500's	$64.00	Indomethacin, Major Pharms	00904-1176-40
500's	$65.34	Indomethacin, Halsey Drug	00879-0508-05
500's	$65.95	Indomethacin, Watson Labs	52544-0304-05
500's	$89.00	Indomethacin, Mutual Pharm	53489-0134-05
500's	$89.70	Indomethacin, Qualitest Pharms	00603-4068-28
500's	$112.80	Indomethacin, Par Pharm	49884-0068-05
500's	$132.90	Indomethacin, Rugby	00536-3982-05
500's	$134.75	Indomethacin, Sidmak Labs	50111-0407-02
500's	$136.63	Indomethacin, Bristol Myers Squibb	00003-0295-60
500's	$149.60	Indomethacin, Zenith Labs	00172-4030-70
500's	$149.60	Indomethacin, Goldline Labs	00182-1682-05
500's	$149.92	Indomethacin, HL Moore Drug Exch	00839-6763-12
500's	$183.54	Indomethacin, Lederle Pharm	00005-3762-31
500's	$183.54	Indomethacin, Geneva Pharms	00781-2350-05
500's	$184.95	Indomethacin, Mylan	00378-0147-05
1000's	$48.80	Indomethacin, H.C.F.A. F F P	99999-1532-07
1000's	$85.69	Indomethacin, Novopharm (US)	55953-0439-80
1000's	$168.00	Indomethacin, Mutual Pharm	53489-0134-10
1000's	$194.88	Indomethacin, Par Pharm	49884-0068-10

Capsule, Gelatin, Sustained Action - Oral - 75 mg

30's	$15.27	Indomethacin, H.C.F.A. F F P	99999-1532-08
30's	**$43.97**	**INDOCIN SR, Merck**	**00006-0693-31**
60's	$30.55	Indomethacin, United Res	00677-1197-06
60's	$30.55	Indomethacin, H.C.F.A. F F P	99999-1532-09
60's	$56.51	Indomethacin, Inwood Labs	00258-3607-06
60's	$57.80	Indomethacin, Qualitest Pharms	00603-4070-20
60's	$58.50	Indomethacin, West Point Pharma	59591-0157-61
60's	$58.50	Indomethacin, Endo Labs	60951-0774-60
60's	$59.15	Indomethacin, Major Pharms	00904-1178-52
60's	$61.00	Indomethacin, Goldline Labs	00182-1469-26
60's	$62.00	Indomethacin, Teva	00093-0628-06
60's	$63.00	Indomethacin, Warner Chilcott	00047-0875-20
60's	$68.99	Indomethacin, Geneva Pharms	00781-2153-60
60's	$69.95	Indomethacin Sustained Release, Parmed Pharms	00349-8731-60
60's	$71.48	Indomethacin Extended Release, Rugby	00536-4939-08
60's	$71.48	Indomethacin, HL Moore Drug Exch	00839-7374-05
60's	**$87.92**	**INDOCIN SR, Merck**	**00006-0693-61**
60's	$93.30	Indomethacin Sr, Martec Pharms	52555-0069-06
100's	$50.93	Indomethacin, H.C.F.A. F F P	99999-1532-10
100's	$84.18	Indomethacin, Inwood Labs	00258-3607-01
100's	$88.03	Indomethacin, Qualitest Pharms	00603-4070-21
100's	$88.61	Indomethacin, Aligen Independ	00405-4547-01
100's	$92.60	Indomethacin, HL Moore Drug Exch	00839-7374-06
100's	$97.50	Indomethacin, Warner Chilcott	00047-0875-24
100's	$97.50	Indomethacin, West Point Pharma	59591-0157-68
100's	$97.50	Indomethacin, Endo Labs	60951-0774-70
100's	$97.51	Indomethacin, Schein Pharm (US)	00364-2211-01
100's	$99.80	Indomethacin, Major Pharms	00904-1178-60
100's	$99.95	Indomethacin Sustained Release, Parmed Pharms	00349-8731-01
100's	$99.95	Indomethacin Extended Release, Rugby	00536-4939-01
1000's	$88.20	Indomethacin, Goldline Labs	00182-1469-01

Suppository - Rectal - 50 mg

12's	$35.00	Indomethacin, Raway	00686-0176-30
30's	$30.62	Indomethacin, GW Labs	00713-0176-30
30's	$40.45	Indomethacin, Goldline Labs	00182-7031-17
30's	$40.85	Indomethacin, Qualitest Pharms	00603-8132-16
30's	$40.85	Indomethacin, HL Moore Drug Exch	00839-7901-19
30's	**$46.43**	**INDOCIN, Merck**	**00006-0150-30**

HOW SUPPLIED - RATED THERAPEUTICALLY EQUIVALENT:
(cont'd)

Suspension - Oral - 25 mg/5ml

237 ml	**$40.50**	**INDOCIN, Merck**	**00006-3376-66**
500 ml	$61.89	Indomethacin, Roxane	00054-3423-63

HOW SUPPLIED - NOT RATED EQUIVALENT:

Injection, Lyphl-Soln - Intravenous - 1 mg/vial

2 ml x 3	**$77.69**	**INDOCIN I.V., Merck**	**00006-3406-17**

Powder

100 gm	$72.10	Indomethacin, Paddock Labs	00574-0590-01

INFLUENZA VIRUS VACCINE *(001533)*

CATEGORIES: Biologicals; Influenza; Serums, Toxoids and Vaccines; Vaccines; Pregnancy Category C; FDA Pre 1938 Drugs

BRAND NAMES: *Agrippal*; *Alorbat* (Germany); *Begrivac* (Germany); *Begrivac F*; Flu Shield; **Fluimmune**; Fluogen; Flushield; *Fluvax* (Australia); Fluvirin; *Fluvirine* (France); Fluzone; *Inflexal*; *Inflexal Berna*; *Inflexal Berna Polyvalent Vaccine*; *Influvac*; *Mutagrip* (Germany, France); *Sandovac*; *Vaxigrip* (France); *X-Flu* *(International brand names outside U.S. in italics)*

FORMULARIES: Medi-Cal; WHO

DESCRIPTION:

Influenza Virus Vaccine, Trivalent, Types A and B (chromatograph- and filter-purified subvirion antigen)

1993-94 FORMULA

DO NOT INJECT INTRAVENOUSLY FluShield (influenza virus vaccine, trivalent, types A and B (purified subvirion)) is a sterile injectable for administration intramuscularly.

Influenza virus vaccine, trivalent, types A and B (purified subvirion) is prepared from the allantoic fluids of chick embryos inoculated with a specific type of influenza virus. During processing, not more than 5 mcg of gentamicin sulfate per ml is added. The harvested virus is inactivated with formaldehyde and is concentrated and purified.

Influenza virus vaccine, trivalent, types A and B (purified subvirion) is concentrated and refined by a column-chromatographic procedure. At the same time, addition of tri(n)butylphosphate and polysorbate 80, USP, to the column-eluting fluids effects disruption and inactivation of a significant proportion of the virus to smaller subunit particles. The recovered subvirion (split-virus) suspension is freed of substantial portions of the disrupting agents by dialysis and of other undesirable materials by selective filtration through membranes of controlled pore size.

The viral antigen content has been standardized by immunodiffusion tests, according to current U.S. Public Health Service requirements. Each dose (0.5 ml) contains the proportions and not less than the microgram amounts of hemagglutinin antigens (mcg HA) representative of the specific components recommended for the 1993-1994 season: 15 mcg HA of A/Texas 36/91 (H1N1), 15 mcg HA of A/Beijing/32/92 (H3N2), and 15 mcg HA of B/Panama/45/90.

The vaccine contains 1:10,000 thimerosal (mercury derivative) as a preservative. Gentamicin sulfate is used during manufacturing but is not detectable in the final product by current assay procedures.

CLINICAL PHARMACOLOGY:

The administration of inactivated influenza vaccine to high-risk persons each year before the influenza season is the single most important influenza-control measure.[1]

The injection of antigens prepared from inactivated influenza virus stimulates the production of specific antibodies. Protection is afforded only against those strains of virus from which the vaccine is prepared or closely related strains. With the passing of time, there may be major antigenic changes in the prevalent strains, or there may be continuous and progressive antigenic variation within a given virus subtype over time (antigenic drift), so that infection or immunization with one strain may not induce immunity to distantly related strains. Field studies of influenza vaccines conducted on many occasions since the 1940's have shown marked variation in efficacy, as measured by protection from disease, ranging from undemonstrable to 70-80%. The PHS regularly reviews the antigenic characteristics of current strains in order to select those to be included in the contemporary vaccine.

Based upon the epidemiological data available through the early months of 1993, the Federal Government determined, after consultation with advisory groups, that the influenza vaccines to be distributed in 1993-1994 will be trivalent including 15 mcg HA each of strains that are antigenically similar to A/Texas 36/91, A/Beijing/32/92 (H3N2), and B/Panama/45/90.

INDICATIONS AND USAGE:

Influenza virus vaccine is recommended for 1) high-risk persons 6 months of age or older and for their medical-care providers or household contacts; 2) for children and teenagers receiving long-term aspirin therapy who, therefore, may be at increased risk of developing Reye's syndrome after an influenza virus infection; and 3) for other persons who wish to reduce their chances of acquiring influenza.

Guidelines for the use of vaccine among different groups are given below.

TARGET GROUPS FOR VACCINATION

Groups at Increased Risk for Influenza-Related Complications:

1. Otherwise healthy persons 65 years of age or older.

2. Residents of nursing homes and other chronic-care facilities housing patients of any age with chronic medical conditions.

3. Adults and children with chronic disorders of the pulmonary or cardiovascular systems requiring regular medical follow-up or hospitalization during the preceding year, including children with asthma.

4. Adults and children who have required regular medical follow-up or hospitalization during the preceding year because of chronic metabolic diseases (including diabetes mellitus), renal dysfunction, hemoglobinopathies, or immunosuppression (including immunosuppression caused by medications).

5. Children and teenagers (aged 6 months to 18 years) who are receiving long-term aspirin therapy and, therefore, may be at risk of developing Reye's syndrome after influenza infection.

Elderly persons and persons with certain chronic diseases may develop lower post-vaccination antibody titers than healthy young adults and thus may remain susceptible to influenza upper-respiratory-tract infections. Nevertheless, even if such persons develop influenza illness, the vaccine has been shown to be effective in preventing lower-respiratory-tract involvement or other complications, thereby reducing the risk of hospitalization and death.

INDICATIONS AND USAGE: *(cont'd)*

GROUPS POTENTIALLY CAPABLE OF NOSOCOMIAL TRANSMISSION OF INFLUENZA TO HIGH-RISK PERSONS

Individuals attending high-risk persons can transmit influenza infections to them while they are themselves incubating infection, undergoing subclinical infection, or working despite the existence of symptoms. Some high-risk persons, (*e.g.,* the elderly, transplant recipients, persons with acquired immunodeficiency syndrome (AIDS)), can have relatively low antibody responses to influenza vaccine. Efforts to protect them against influenza may be improved by reducing the chances that their care providers may expose them to influenza. Therefore, the following groups should be vaccinated:

1. Physicians, nurses, and other personnel in both hospital and outpatient settings.

2. Providers of home care to high-risk persons (*e.g.,* visiting nurses, volunteer workers) as well as all household members of high-risk persons, including children, whether or not they provide care.

VACCINATION OF OTHER GROUPS

General Population: Physicians should administer influenza vaccine to any person who wishes to reduce his/her chances of acquiring influenza infection. Persons who provide essential community services and students or other healthy individuals in institutional settings (*i.e.,* schools and colleges) should be encouraged to receive vaccine to minimize the disruption of routine activity during outbreaks.

Pregnant Women: Influenza-associated excess mortality among pregnant women has not been documented, except in the largest pandemics of 1918-19 and 1957-58. However, pregnant women who have medical conditions increasing their risks of complications from influenza should be vaccinated, as the vaccine is considered safe for pregnant women. Administering the vaccine after the first trimester is a reasonable precaution to minimize any concern over the theoretical possibility of teratogenicity. However, it is undesirable to delay vaccination of pregnant women with high-risk conditions who will still be in the first trimester of pregnancy when the influenza season begins.

Persons Infected With Human Immunodeficiency Virus (HIV): Little information exists regarding the frequency and severity of influenza illness in human immunodeficiency virus (HIV)-infected persons, but recent reports suggest that symptoms may be prolonged and the risk of complications increased for this high-risk group. Because influenza may result in serious illness and complications, vaccination is a prudent precaution and will result in protective antibody levels in many recipients. However, the antibody response to vaccine may be low in persons with advanced HIV-related illnesses; a booster dose of vaccine has not improved the immune response for these individuals.

Foreign Travelers: The risk of exposure to influenza during foreign travel varies, depending on, among other factors, season of travel and destination. Influenza can occur throughout the year in the tropics; the season of greatest influenza activity in the Southern Hemisphere is April-September. Because of the short incubation period for influenza, exposure to the virus during travel will often result in clinical illness that begins during travel, an inconvenience or potential danger, especially for persons at increased risk for complications. Persons preparing to travel to the tropics at any time of year or to the Southern Hemisphere during April-September should review their vaccination histories. If not vaccinated the previous fall/winter, they should be considered for influenza vaccination prior to travel. Persons in the high-risk categories especially should be encouraged to receive the vaccine. The most current available vaccine should be used. High-risk persons given the previous season's vaccine prior to travel should be revaccinated in the fall/winter with current vaccine.[1]

IMMUNIZATION PROGRAMS

If this product is to be used in an immunization program sponsored by an organization WHERE A TRADITIONAL PHYSICIAN/PATIENT RELATIONSHIP DOES NOT EXIST, each participant (or legal guardian) should be made aware of the possible risks that have been associated with the use of influenza virus vaccines, including the possible risk of a form of paralysis sometimes known as Guillain-Barre syndrome. Information about possible side effects and adverse reactions is presented below, and consent, preferably written, should be obtained from the intended recipient (or legal guardian) before vaccine administration.

Simultaneous Administration of Pneumoccal or Pediatric Vaccines: Pneumococcal vaccine and influenza vaccine can be given at the same time at different sites without increased side effects. However, it should be emphasized that whereas influenza vaccine is given annually, it is currently recommended that, with few exceptions, pneumococcal vaccine be given only once.[1]

It may be desirable to simultaneously administer influenza vaccine, if indicated, with routine pediatric vaccine but at different sites. Although studies have not been done, no diminution of immunogenicity or enhancement of adverse reactions should be expected.[1] Influenza vaccine should not be given within 3 days of vaccination with pertussis vaccine.

CONTRAINDICATIONS:

INFLUENZA VIRUS VACCINE SHOULD NOT BE ADMINISTERED TO INDIVIDUALS WITH A HISTORY OF HYPERSENSITIVITY (ALLERGY) TO CHICKEN EGG OR OTHER COMPONENTS OF INFLUENZA VIRUS VACCINES WITHOUT FIRST CONSULTING A PHYSICIAN (SEE ADVERSE REACTIONS). Before being vaccinated, persons known to be hypersensitive to egg protein should be given a skin test or other allergy-evaluating test, using the Influenza Virus Vaccine as the antigen. Persons with adverse reactions to such testing should not be vaccinated. Chemoprophylaxis may be indicated for prevention of influenza A in such persons. However, persons with a history of anaphylactic hypersensitivity to vaccine components but who are also at highest risk for complications of influenza infections may benefit from vaccine after appropriate evaluation and desensitization.[1]

Although gentamicin sulfate is not detectable in the final product by current assay procedures, the vaccine should not be administered to persons with known sensitivity to gentamicin or other aminoglycosides.

Persons with a past history of Guillain-Barre syndrome (GBS) should not be given influenza virus vaccine.

Persons with acute febrile illnesses usually should not be vaccinated until their symptoms have abated. However, minor illness with or without fever should not contraindicate the use of influenza vaccine, particularly in children with a mild upper-respiratory-tract infection or allergic rhinitis.[3]

WARNINGS:

Patients with impaired immune responsiveness, whether due to the use of immunosuppressive therapy (including irradiation, large amounts of corticosteroids, antimetabolites, alkylating agents, and cytotoxic agents), a genetic defect, human immunodeficiency virus (HIV) infection, leukemia, lymphoma, generalized malignancy, or other causes, may have a reduced antibody response to active immunization procedures.[1] Short-term (less than 2 weeks) corticosteroid therapy or intra-articular, bursal, or tendon injections with corticosteroids should not be immunosuppressive. Inactivated vaccines are not a risk to immunocompromised individuals, although their efficacy may be substantially reduced. Because patients with immunodeficiencies may not have an adequate response to immunizing agents, they may remain susceptible despite having received an appropriate vaccine. If feasible, specific serum

WARNINGS: *(cont'd)*

antibody titers or other immunologic responses may be determined after immunization to assess immunity.[3] Chemoprophylaxis may be indicated for high-risk persons who are expected to have a poor antibody response to influenza vaccine.[1]

PRECAUTIONS:

GENERAL

Influenza virus is remarkably capricious antigenically, and significant changes may occur from time to time. *It is known definitely that Influenza vaccine, as now constituted, is not effective against all possible strains of influenza virus. Protection is afforded most people only against those strains of virus from which the vaccine is prepared or against closely related strains.*

Influenza vaccine often contains one or more antigens used in previous years. However, immunity declines during the year following immunization. Therefore, revaccination on a yearly basis is necessary to provide optimal protection for the current season. REMAINING 1992-1993 VACCINE SHOULD NOT BE USED.

Epinephrine injection (1:1000) must be immediately available should an acute anaphylactoid reaction occur due to any component of the vaccine.

A separate sterile syringe and needle should be used for each patient to prevent transmission of hepatitis B virus or other infectious agents from one person to another. Reusable glass syringes and needles should be heat-sterilized.

PREGNANCY CATEGORY C

Animal reproduction studies have not been conducted with Influenza Virus Vaccine. It is also not known whether influenza virus vaccine can cause fetal harm when administered to a pregnant woman or can affect reproduction capacity. Influenza virus vaccine should be given to a pregnant woman only if clearly needed. (See INDICATIONS AND USAGE).

DRUG INTERACTIONS:

There have been conflicting reports[4-13] on the effects of influenza virus vaccine on the elimination of some drugs metabolized by the hepatic cytochrome P-450 system. Hypoprothrombinemia in patients receiving warfarin and elevated theophylline serum concentrations have occurred. Most studies have failed to show any adverse effects of influenza vaccine in patients receiving these drugs. Nevertheless, observation for possible enhanced drug effect or toxicity is indicated for those persons taking theophylline preparations or warfarin sodium.

Individuals receiving therapy with immunosuppressive agents (large amounts of corticosteroids, antimetabolites, alkylating agents, cytotoxic agents) may not respond optimally to active immunization procedures. (See WARNINGS.)

ADVERSE REACTIONS:

Side effects of influenza vaccine are generally inconsequential in adults and occur at low frequency, but at younger ages side effects may be more common.

BECAUSE INFLUENZA VACCINE CONTAINS ONLY NONINFECTIOUS VIRUSES, IT CANNOT CAUSE INFLUENZA. Occasional cases of respiratory disease following vaccination represent coincidental illnesses unrelated to influenza vaccination.

The most frequent side effect of vaccination is soreness around the vaccination site for up to 2 days; this occurs in less than one-third of vaccinees.

In addition, the following three types of systemic reactions have occurred:

1. Fever, malaise, myalgia, and other systemic symptoms occur infrequently and most often affect persons who have had no exposure to the influenza virus antigens in the vaccine (*e.g.,* young children). These reactions begin 6 to 12 hours after vaccination and can persist for 1 or 2 days.

2. Immediate, presumably allergic, reactions such as hives; angioedema, allergic asthma, or systemic anaphylaxis occur extremely rarely after influenza vaccination. These reactions probably result from hypersensitivity to some vaccine component - the majority are most likely residual egg protein. Although current influenza vaccines contain only a small quantity of egg protein, this protein may induce immediate hypersensitivity reactions in persons with severe egg allergy. Persons who have developed those who have developed hives, have had swelling of the lips or tongue, or experienced acute respiratory distress or collapse after eating eggs should consult a physician for appropriate evaluation to assist in determining whether vaccination may proceed or should be deferred. Persons with a documented immunoglobulin E (IgE)-mediated hypersensitivity to eggs, including those who have experienced occupational asthma or other allergic responses from occupational exposure to egg protein, may also be at increased risk for reactions from influenza vaccine, and similar consultation should be considered. The protocol for influenza vaccination developed by Murphy and Strunk may be considered for patients who have egg allergies and medical conditions that place them at increased risk for influenza infection or its complications.[15] The potential exists for hypersensitivity reactions to any vaccine component. Although exposure to vaccines containing thimerosal can lead to induction of hypersensitivity, most patients do not develop reactions to thimerosal administered as a component of vaccines even when patch or intradermal tests for thimerosal indicate hypersensitivity. When it has been reported, hypersensitivity to thimerosal has usually consisted of local delayed type hypersensitivity reactions.[1]

3. Guillain-Barre syndrome (GBS). This is an uncommon illness characterized by ascending paralysis which is usually self-limited and reversible. Though most persons with GBS recover without residual weakness, approximately 5% of cases are fatal. Before 1976, no association of GBS with influenza vaccine use was recognized.

Except for the 1976-77 swine influenza vaccine, subsequent vaccines prepared from other virus strains have not been clearly associated with an increased frequency of Guillain-Barre syndrome.[1, 16-19] Although, in 1990-91, there may have been a small increase in GBS cases in vaccinated persons 18 to 64 years of age, the epidemiologic features of the possible association of the 1990-91 vaccine with GBS were not as convincing as those found with the swine influenza vaccine. It is difficult to make a precise estimate of risk for a rare condition such as GBS.[1] Therefore, candidates for influenza virus vaccine should be made aware of the possible risks, including GBS, and the benefits of administration.

Other neurologic disorders, including encephalopathies, not defined as GBS, have been temporarily associated with influenza vaccination.[20]

DOSAGE AND ADMINISTRATION:

Although influenza virus vaccine often contains one or more antigens used in previous years, immunity declines during the year following vaccination. Therefore, a history of vaccination in any previous year with a vaccine containing one or more antigens included in the current vaccine does NOT preclude the need for revaccination for the 1993-1994 influenza season to provide optimal protection. REMAINING 1992-1993 VACCINE SHOULD NOT BE USED.

Influenza vaccine may be offered to high-risk persons presenting for routine care or hospitalization beginning in September, but not until new vaccine is available (see INDICATIONS AND USAGE, Vaccination of Other Groups for foreign travel, related exceptions). Opportunities to vaccinate persons at high risk for complications of influenza should not be missed. In the United States, influenza activity generally peaks between late December and early March, and high levels of influenza activity infrequently occur in the contiguous 48 states before December. Therefore, the optimal time for organized vaccination campaigns for high-

DOSAGE AND ADMINISTRATION: *(cont'd)*

risk persons usually is the period between mid-October and mid-November. In facilities such as nursing homes it is particularly important to avoid administering vaccine too far in advance of the influenza season because antibody may begin to decline within a few months. Such vaccination programs may be undertaken as soon as current vaccine is available in September or October if regional influenza activity is expected to begin earlier than normal.

Children less than 9 years of age who have not been vaccinated previously should receive two doses with at least 1 month between doses to maximize the chance of a satisfactory antibody response to all three vaccine antigens. The second dose should be given before December if possible. Vaccine should continue to be offered to both children and adults up to and even after influenza virus activity is documented in a community which may be as late as April in some years.

Parenteral drug products should be inspected visually for particulate matter and discoloration, whenever solution and container permit.

DO NOT INJECT INTRAVENOUSLY. Injections of FluShield are recommended to be given intramuscularly. The recommended site is the deltoid muscle for adults and older children. The preferred site for infants and young children is the anterolateral aspect of the thigh musculature. Because of lack of adequate evaluation of other route in high-risk persons, the preferred route of vaccination is intramuscularly whenever possible. Before injection, the skin over the site to be injected should be cleansed with a suitable germicide. After insertion of the needle, aspirate to help avoid inadvertent injection into a blood vessel (TABLE 1).

TABLE 1

AGE GROUP	DOSAGE SCHEDULE
9 years and older	0.5 ml (one dose)
3 to 8 years	0.5 ml (1 or 2 doses)*
6 to 35 months	0.25 ml (1 or 2 doses)*
For those under 13 years, only split-virus (subvirion) vaccine is recommended.	

* A single dose is considered sufficient for those under 9 years who have received at least 1 dose of influenza virus vaccine. With the 2-dose regimen, allow 4 weeks or more between doses. Both doses are recommended for maximum protection.

Immunogenicity and reactogenicity of split- and whole-virus vaccines are similar in adults when used according to the recommended dosage.[1]

Storage: Store between 2°-8°C (35°-46° F). Potency is destroyed by freezing; do not use Influenza Virus Vaccine that has been frozen.

REFERENCES:

1. Recommendations of the Advisory Committee on Immunization Practices — Prevention and Control of Influenza: Part 1, vaccines. MMWR 1993: *42 (no. RR-7)*.**2.** ACIP. Pneumococcal polysaccharride vaccine. MMWR 1989: *38:* 64- 8, 73-6. **3.** American Academy of Pediatrics: Report of the Committee on Infectious Diseases, 22nd ed. Elk Grove Village, IL, American Academy of Pediatrics, 1991. **4.** KRAMER, P. and McCLAIN, C.: Depression of aminopyrine metabolism by influenza vaccination. NEJM *305:* 1262, 1981. **5.** RENTON, K. et al: Decreased elimination of theophylline after influenza vaccination. Canadian Med. Assoc. J. *123:*288, 1980. **6.** GOLDSTEIN, R. S. et al: Decreased elimination of theophylline after influenza vaccination. Canadian Med. Assoc. J. *126:* 470, 1982. **7.** BRITTON, L. and RUBEN, F. L.: Serum and theophylline levels after influenza vaccination. Canadian Med. Assoc. J. *126:* 1375, 1982. **8.** FISCHER, R. G. et al: Influence of trivalent influenza vaccine on serum theophylline levels. Canadian Med. Assoc. J. *126:*1312-1313, 1982. **9.** SAN JOAQUIN, V. H., REYES, S., and MARKS, M. I.: Influenza vaccination in asthmatic children on maintenance theophylline therapy. Clin. Pediatrics *21:* 724-726, 1982. **10.** STULTS, B. and HASISAKI, P.: Influenza vaccination and theophylline pharmacokinetics in patients with chronic obstructive lung disease. West J. Med. *139:* 651-654, 1983. **11.** PATRIARCA, P.A. et al: Influenza vaccination and warfarin or theophylline toxicity in nursing-home residents. New Eng. J. Med.*308:* 1601, 1983. **12.** MEREDITH, C. G. et al: Effects of influenza virus vaccine on hepatic drug metabolism. Clin. Pharm. Ther. *37:*396-401, 1985. **13.** LIPSKY, B. A. et al: Influenza vaccination and warfarin anticoagulation. Ann. Int. Med. *100:* 835-837, 1984. **14.** KRAMER, P. et al: Effect of Influenza vaccine on warfarin anticoagulation. Clin. Pharmacol. Ther. *35:* 416, 1984. **15.** MURPHY, K. R. and STRUNK, R. L.: Safe administration of Influenza vaccine in asthmatic children hypersensitive to egg proteins. J. Pediatr.*106:* 931-3, 1985. **16.** SCHONBERGER, L. et al: Guillain-Barre syndrome following vaccination in the National Influenza Immunization Program, United States 1976-1977. Am. J. Epidemiol. *110:* 105, 1979. **17.** SCHONBERGER, L. et al: Guillain-Barre syndrome: Its epidemiology and associations with influenza vaccination. Ann. Neurol. *9* (Supplement: 31, 1981). **18.** HURWITZ, E. et al: Guillain-Barre syndrome and the 1978-1979 influenza vaccine. New Eng. J. Med. *304:* 1557, 1981. **19.** KAPLAN, J. et al: Guillain-Barre syndrome in the United States, 1979-1980 and 1980-1981. Lack of association with influenza vaccination. JAMA *248:* 698, 1982. **20.** RETAILLIAU, H. et al: Illness after influenza vaccination reported through a nation-wide surveillance system, 1976-1977. Am. J. Epidemiol.*111:* 170, 1980.

HOW SUPPLIED - EQUIVALENTS NOT AVAILABLE:

Injection, Solution - Intramuscular

0.5 ml x 10	$38.75	FLUZONE, Bristol Myers Squibb	00003-1342-31
0.5 ml x 10	$42.75	FLUZONE, Connaught Labs	49281-0344-11
0.5 ml x 10	$47.55	Flushield, Wyeth Labs	00008-0848-02
0.5 ml x 10	$47.55	Flushield, Wyeth Labs	00008-0848-45
0.5 ml x 10	$48.94	FLUZONE, Connaught Labs	49281-0350-11
0.5 ml x 10	$48.95	FLUOGEN, Parke-Davis	00071-4091-40
0.5 ml x 10	$48.95	FLUOGEN, Parke-Davis	00071-4092-40
0.5 ml x 10	$48.95	FLUOGEN, Parke-Davis	00071-4095-40
5 ml	$34.75	FLUZONE, Bristol Myers Squibb	00003-1341-10
5 ml	$34.75	FLUZONE, Bristol Myers Squibb	00003-1342-15
5 ml	$36.50	FLUZONE, Connaught Labs	49281-0343-10
5 ml	$36.50	FLUZONE, Connaught Labs	49281-0344-10
5 ml	$36.50	FLUZONE, Connaught Labs	49281-0344-15
5 ml	$36.68	Flushield, Wyeth Labs	00008-0848-01
5 ml	$36.68	Flushield, Wyeth Labs	00008-0848-35
5 ml	$39.88	Fluzone, Connaught Labs	49281-0349-10
5 ml	$39.88	Fluzone, Connaught Labs	49281-0350-15
5 ml	$42.00	Fluvirin, Medeva Pharms	53014-0100-10
5 ml	$44.44	FLUOGEN, Parke-Davis	00071-4091-08
5 ml	$44.44	FLUOGEN, Parke-Davis	00071-4092-08
5 ml	$46.66	FLUOGEN, Parke-Davis	00071-4095-08

INSULIN (ANIMAL SOURCE) *(001540)*

CATEGORIES: Antidiabetic Agents; Blood Glucose Regulators; Diabetes; Hormones; Sales > $100 Million; FDA Pre 1938 Drugs

BRAND NAMES: Iletin I Lente; Iletin I Nph; Iletin I Protamine,Zinc; Iletin I Regular; Iletin I Semilente; Iletin I Ultralente; Iletin Lente; Iletin Nph; Iletin Pzi; Iletin Regular; Iletin Semilente; Iletin Ultralente; Lente Iletin I; Nph Iletin I; Protamine, Zinc & Iletin I; Regular Iletin I

FORMULARIES: WHO

ANY CHANGE OF INSULIN SHOULD BE MADE CAUTIOUSLY AND ONLY UNDER MEDICAL SUPERVISION. CHANGES IN PURITY, STRENGTH, BRAND (MANUFACTURER), TYPE (REGULAR, NPH, LENTE, ETC), SPECIES (BEEF, PORK, BEEF-PORK, HUMAN), AND/OR METHOD OF MANUFACTURE (RECOMBINANT DNA VERSUS ANIMAL-SOURCE INSULIN) MAY RESULT IN THE NEED FOR A CHANGE IN DOSAGE. IF AN ADJUSTMENT IS NEEDED, IT MAY OCCUR WITH THE FIRST DOSE OR DURING THE FIRST SEVERAL WEEKS OR MONTHS.

PATIENT PACKAGE INSERT:

DIABETES

Insulin is a hormone produced by the pancreas, a large gland that lies near the stomach. This hormone is necessary for the body's correct use of food, especially sugar. Diabetes occurs when the pancreas does not make enough insulin to meet your body's needs.

To control your diabetes, your doctor has prescribed injections of insulin to keep your blood glucose at a nearly normal level. Proper control of your diabetes requires close and constant cooperation with your doctor. In spite of diabetes, you can lead an active, healthy, and useful life if you eat a balanced diet daily, exercise regularly, and take your insulin injections as prescribed.

You have been instructed to test your blood and/or your urine regularly for glucose. If your blood tests consistently show above- or below-normal glucose levels or your urine tests consistently show the presence of glucose, your diabetes is not properly controlled and you must lt your doctor know.

Always keep an extra supply of insulin as well as a spare syringe and needle on hand. Always wear diabetic identification so that appropriate treatment can be given if complications occur away from home.

DESCRIPTION

Regular beef-pork insulin is obtained from beef and pork pancreas.

Regular Iletin I (insulin, Lilly) consists of zinc-insulin crystals dissolved in a clear fluid. Regular Iletin I has nothing added to change the speed or length of its action. It takes effect rapidly and has a relatively short duration of activity (4 to 12 hours) as compared with other insulins.

NPH beef-pork insulin is obtained from beef and pork pancreas.

NPH Iletin I (insulin, Lilly) is a crystalline suspension of insulin with protamine and zinc providing an intermediate-acting insulin with a slower onset of action and a longer duration of activity (slightly more than 24 hours) than that of regular insulin.

Lente beef-pork insulin is obtained from beef and pork pancreas.

Lente Iletin I (insulin, Lilly) is an amorphous and crystalline suspension of insulin with zinc providing an intermediate acting insulin with a slower onset and a longer duration of activity (slightly more than 24 hours) than regular insulin.

Regular pork insulin is obtained from pork pancreas.

Regular Iletin II (purified insulin, Lilly) consists of zinc-insulin crystals dissolved in a clear fluid Regular Iletin II has had nothing added to change the speed or length of its action. It takes effect rapidly and has a relatively short duration of activity (4 to 12 hours) as compared to other insulins.

NPH pork insulin is obtained from pork pancreas.

NPH Iletin II (purified insulin, Lilly) is a crystalline suspension of insulin with protamine and zinc providing an intermediate-acting insulin with a slower onset of action and a longer duration of activity (slightly more than 24 hours) than that of regular insulin.

Lente pork insulin is obtained from pork pancreas.

Lente Iletin II (purified insulin, Lilly) is an amorphous and crystalline suspension of human insulin with zinc providing an intermediate-acting insulin with a slower onset and a longer duration of activity (slightly more than 24 hours) than regular insulin.

The time course of action of any insulin may vary considerably in different individuals or at different times in the same individual. As with all insulin preparations, the duration of action of Iletin I is dependent on dose, site of injection, blood supply, temperature, and physical activity. Iletin I is a sterile solution and is for subcutaneous injection. It should not be used intravenously or intramuscularly. The concentration of Iletin I and Iletin II is 100 units/ml (U-100).

IDENTIFICATION

This insulin, manufactured by Eli Lilly and Company, has the trademark Iletin I and Iletin II and is available in various types—Regular, NPH, and Lente. (Iletin I is also available in Semilente and Ultralente). Your doctor has prescribed the type of insulin that he/she believes is best for you. **DO NOT USE ANY OTHER INSULIN EXCEPT ON HIS/HER ADVICE AND DIRECTION.**

Always check the carton and the bottle label for the name and letter designation of the insulin you receive from your pharmacy to make sure it is the same as that your doctor has prescribed.

Always examine the appearance of your bottle of insulin before withdrawing each dose.

Regular Iletin I and Iletin II is a clear and colorless liquid with a water-like appearance and consistency. Do not use if it appears cloudy, thickened, or slightly colored or if solid particles are visible. Always check the appearance of your bottle of insulin before using, and if you note anything unusual in the appearance of your insulin or notice your insulin requirements changing markedly, consult your doctor.

A bottle of NPH or Lente Iletin I or II must be carefully shaken or rotated before each injection so that the contents are uniformly mixed. NPH and Lente Iletin I should look uniformly cloudy or milky after mixing. Do not use it if the insulin substance (the white material) remains at the bottom of the bottle after mixing.

Always check the appearance of your bottle of insulin before using, and if you note anything unusual in the appearance of your insulin or notice your insulin requirements changing markedly, consult your doctor.

STORAGE

Insulin should be stored in a refrigerator but not in the freezer. If refrigeration is not possible, the bottle of insulin that you are currently using can be kept unrefrigerated as long as it is kept as cool as possible (below 86°F [30°]) and away from heat and light. Do not use insulin if it has been frozen. Do not use a bottle of insulin after the expiration date stamped on the label.

INJECTION PROCEDURES

Correct Syringe

Doses of insulin are measured in **units**. U-100 insulin contains 100 units/ml (1 m/l = 1 cc). With Iletin I, it is important to use a syringe that is marked for U-100 insulin preparations. Failure to use the proper syringe can lead to a mistake in dosage, causing serious problems for you, such as a blood glucose level that is too low or too high.

Syringe Use

To help avoid contamination and possible infection, follow these instructions exactly.

Disposable syringes and needles should be used only once and then discarded. **NEEDLES AND SYRINGES MUST NOT BE SHARED.**

Reusable syringes and needles must be sterilized before each injection. **Follow the package directions supplied with your syringe.** Described below are 2 methods of sterilizing.

Boiling

1. Put syringe, plunger, and needle in strainer, place in saucepan, and cover with water. Boil for 5 minutes.

2. Remove articles from water. When they have cooled, insert plunger into barrel, and fasten needle to syringe with a slight twist.

PATIENT PACKAGE INSERT: *(cont'd)*

3. Push plunger in and out several times until water is completely removed.

Isopropyl Alcohol

If the syringe, plunger, and needle cannot be boiled, as when you are traveling, they may be sterilized by immersion for at least 5 minutes in Isopropyl Alcohol, 91%. Do not use bathing, rubbing, or medicated alcohol for this sterilization. If the syringe is sterilized with alcohol, it must be absolutely dry before use.

Preparing the Dose

1. Wash your hands.

2. *(NPH and Lente insulins only.)* Carefully shake or rotate the insulin bottle several times to completely mix the insulin.

3. Inspect the insulin.

Regular Iletin I and II should look clear and colorless. Do not use Regular Iletin I or II if it appears cloudy, thickened, or slightly colored or if solid particles are present.

NPH Iletin I and II and Lente Iletin I and II should look uniformly cloudy or milky. Do not use if you notice anything unusual in the appearance.

4. If using a new bottle, flip off the plastic protective cap, but **do not** remove the stopper. When using a new bottle, wipe the top of the bottle with an alcohol swab.

5. If you are mixing insulins, refer to the Warnings below.

6. Draw air into the syringe equal to your insulin dose. Put the needle through the rubber top of the insulin bottle and inject the air into the bottle.

7. Turn the bottle and syringe upside down. Hold the bottle and syringe firmly in 1 hand and shake gently.

8. Making sure the tip of the needle is in the insulin, withdraw the correct dose of insulin into the syringe.

9. Before removing the needle from the bottle, check your syringe for air bubbles which reduce the amount of insulin in it. If bubbles are present, hold the syringe straight up and tap its side until the bubbles float to the top. Push them out with the plunger and withdraw the correct dose.

10. Remove the needle from the bottle and lay the syringe down so that the needle does not touch anything.

WARNINGS: SEE ADDITIONAL WARNINGS ABOVE

Patients who have been directed by their doctors to mix 2 types of insulin should be aware that insulin hypodermic syringes of different manufacturers may vary in the amount of space between the bottom line and the needle.

Because Of This, Do Not Change:

1. The order of mixing that your doctor has prescribed or

2. The model and brand of syringe or needle without first consulting your doctor.

The mixing should be done immediately prior to injection. Failure to heed this warning could result in a dosage error.

Injection

Cleanse the skin with alcohol where the injection is to be made. Stabilize the skin by spreading it or pinching up a large area. Insert the needle as instructed by your doctor. Push the plunger in as far as it will go. Pull the needle out and apply gentle pressure over the injection site for several seconds. **Do not rub the area.** To avoid tissue damage, give the next injection at a site at least $\frac{1}{2}$" from the previous site.

DOSAGE

Your doctor has told you which insulin to use, how much, and when and how often to inject it. Because each patient's case of diabetes is different, this schedule has been individualized for you.

Your usual insulin dose may be affected by changes in your food, activity, or work schedule. Carefully follow your doctor's instructions to allow for these changes. Other things that may affect your insulin dose are:

ILLNESS

Illness, especially with nausea and vomiting, may cause your insulin requirements to change. Even if you are not eating, you will still require insulin. You and your doctor should establish a sick day plan for you to use in case of illness. When you are sick, test your blood/urine frequently and call your doctor as instructed.

PREGNANCY

Good control of diabetes is especially important for you and your unborn baby. Pregnancy may make managing your diabetes more difficult. If you are planning to have a baby, are pregnant, or are nursing, consult your doctor.

MEDICATION

Insulin requirements may be increased if you are taking other drugs with hyperglycemic activity, such as oral contraceptives, corticosteroids, or thyroid replacement therapy. Insulin requirements may be reduced in the presence of drugs with hypoglycemic activity, such as oral hypoglycemics, salicylates (for example, aspirin), sulfa antibiotics, and certain antidepressants. Always discuss any medications you are taking with your doctor.

EXERCISE

Exercise may lower your body's need for insulin during and for some time after the activity. Exercise may also speed up the effect of an insulin dose, especially if the exercise involves the area of injection site (for example, the leg should not be used for injection just prior to running). Discuss with your doctor how you should adjust your regimen to accommodate exercise.

TRAVEL

Persons traveling across more than 2 time zones should consult their doctor concerning adjustments in their insulin schedule.

COMMON PROBLEMS OF DIABETES

Hypoglycemia (Insulin Reaction)

Hypoglycemia (too little glucose in the blood) is one of the most frequent adverse events experienced by insulin users. It can be brought about by:

1. Taking too much insulin

2. Missing or delaying meals

3. Exercising or working more than usual

4. An infection or illness (especially with nausea or vomiting)

5. A change in the body's need for insulin

6. Diseases of the adrenal, pituitary, or thyroid gland, or progression of kidney or liver disease

7. Interactions with other drugs that lower blood glucose, such as oral hypoglycemics, salicylates (for example, aspirin), sulfa antibiotics, and certain antidepressants

8. Consumption of alcoholic beverages

Symptoms of mild to moderate hypoglycemia may occur suddenly and can include:

PATIENT PACKAGE INSERT: *(cont'd)*

sweating; dizziness; palpitation; tremor; hunger; restlessness; tingling in the hands, feet, lips, or tongue; lightheadedness; inability to concentrate; headache; drowsiness; sleep disturbances; anxiety; blurred vision; slurred speech; depressive mood; irritability; abnormal behavior; unsteady movement; personality changes; seizures; death

Signs of severe hypoglycemia can include:

disorientation; unconsciousness; seizures; death

Therefore, it is important that assistance be obtained immediately.

Early warning symptoms of hypoglycemia may be different or less pronounced under certain conditions, such as long duration of diabetes, diabetic nerve disease, medications such as beta-blockers, change in insulin preparations, or intensified control (3 or more insulin injections per day) of diabetes.

Without recognition of early warning symptoms, you may not be able to take steps to avoid more serious hypoglycemia. Be alert for all of the various types of symptoms that may indicate hypoglycemia. Patients who experience hypoglycemia without early warning symptoms should monitor their blood glucose frequently, especially prior to activities such as driving. If the blood glucose is below your normal fasting glucose, you should consider eating or drinking sugar-containing foods to treat your hypoglycemia.

Mild to moderate hypoglycemia may be treated by eating foods or taking drinks that contain sugar. Patients should always carry a quick source of sugar, such as candy mints or glucose tablets. More severe hypoglycemia may require the assistance of another person. Patients who are unable to take sugar orally or who are unconscious require an injection of glucagon or should be treated with intravenous administration of glucose at a medical facility.

You should learn to recognize your own symptoms of hypoglycemia. If you are uncertain about these symptoms, you should monitor your blood glucose frequently to help you learn to recognize the symptoms that you experience with hypoglycemia.

If you have frequent episodes of hypoglycemia or differently in recognizing the symptoms, you should consult your doctor to discuss possible changes in therapy, meal plans, and/or exercise programs to help you avoid hypoglycemia.

Hyperglycemia and Diabetic Acidosis

Hyperglycemia (too much glucose in the blood) may develop if your body has too little insulin. Hyperglycemia can be brought about by:

1. Omitting your insulin or taking less than the doctor has prescribed

2. Eating significantly more than your meal plan suggests

3. Developing a fever or infection

In patients with insulin-dependent diabetes, prolonged hyperglycemia can result in diabetic acidosis. The first symptoms of diabetic acidosis usually come on gradually, over a period of hours or days, and include a drowsy feeling, flushed face, thirst, loss of appetite, and fruity odor on the breath. With acidosis, urine tests show large amounts of glucose and acetone. Heavy breathing and a rapid pulse are more severe symptoms. If uncorrected, prolonged hyperglycemia or diabetic acidosis can result in loss of consciousness or death. Therefore, it is important that you obtain medical assistance immediately.

Lipodystrophy

Rarely, administration of insulin subcutaneously can result in lipoatrophy (depression in the skin) or lipohypertrophy (enlargement or thickening of tissue). If you notice either of these conditions, consult your doctor. A change in your injection technique may help alleviate the problem.

Allergy to Insulin

Local Allergy: Patients occasionally experience redness, swelling, and itching at the site of injection of insulin. This condition, called local allergy, usually clears up in a few days to a few weeks. In some instances, this condition may be related to factors other than insulin, such as irritants in the skin cleansing agent or poor injection technique. If you have local reactions, contact your doctor.

Systemic Allergy: Less common, but potentially more serious, is generalized allergy to insulin, which may cause rash over the whole body, shortness of breath, wheezing, reduction in blood pressure, fast pulse, or sweating. Severe cases of generalized allergy may be life threatening. If you think you are having a generalized allergic reaction to insulin, notify a doctor immediately.

ADDITIONAL INFORMATION

Additional information about diabetes may be obtained from your diabetes educator.

Diabetes Forecast is a national magazine designed especially for patients with diabetes and their families and is available by subscription from the American Diabetes Association, National Service Center, 1660 Duke Street, Alexandria, Virginia 22314.

Another publication, *Diabetes Countdown*, is available from the Juvenile Diabetes Association, 432 Park Avenue South, New York, New York 10016-8013.

HOW SUPPLIED - EQUIVALENTS NOT AVAILABLE:

Injection, Solution - Subcutaneous - 100 unit/ml

10 ml	$13.72	ULTRALENTE ILETIN I, Lilly	00002-8610-01
10 ml	$14.34	INSULIN REGULAR PORK, Novo Nordisk Pharm	00169-3512-15
10 ml	$22.27	Insulin Regular Purified Pork, Novo Nordisk Pharm	00169-2440-10
10 ml	$22.27	Insulin Lente Purified Pork, Novo Nordisk Pharm	00169-2442-10
10 ml	$22.27	Insulin Nph Purified Pork, Novo Nordisk Pharm	00169-2447-10
10 ml	$23.42	REGULAR ILETIN II PORK, Lilly	00002-8211-01
10 ml	$23.42	NPH ILETIN II PORK, Lilly	00002-8311-01
10 ml	$23.42	LENTE ILETIN II PORK, Lilly	00002-8411-01
20 ml	$125.51	REGULAR ILETIN II, Lilly	00002-8500-01

Injection, Susp - Subcutaneous - 40 unit/ml

10 ml	$5.79	PROTAMINE ZINC AND ILETIN I, Lilly	00002-8140-01
10 ml	$5.79	REGULAR ILETIN I, Lilly	00002-8240-01
10 ml	$5.79	NPH ILETIN I, Lilly	00002-8340-01
10 ml	$5.79	ULTRALENTE ILETIN I, Lilly	00002-8640-01
10 ml x 1	$5.79	LENTE ILETIN I, Lilly	00002-8440-01
10 ml x 1	$5.79	SEMILENTE ILETIN I, Lilly	00002-8540-01

Injection, Susp - Subcutaneous - 100 unit/ml

10 ml	$12.68	PROTAMINE ZINC & ILETIN, Lilly	00002-8110-01
10 ml	$13.72	SEMILENTE ILETIN I, Lilly	00002-8510-01
10 ml	$14.34	REGULAR ILETIN I, Lilly	00002-8210-01
10 ml	$14.34	NPH ILETIN I, Lilly	00002-8310-01
10 ml	$14.34	LENTE ILETIN I, Lilly	00002-8410-01
10 ml	$20.72	PROTAMINE ZINC & ILETIN II PORK, Lilly	00002-8111-01

INSULIN (BEEF) *(000378)*

CATEGORIES: Antidiabetic Agents; Blood Glucose Regulators; Diagnostic Agents; Hormones; FDA Pre 1938 Drugs

BRAND NAMES: Iletin II Lente Beef; Iletin II Lente(Beef); Iletin II Nph Beef; Iletin II Nph(Beef); Iletin II Protamine,Zinc(Beef); Iletin II Pzi Beef; Iletin II Reg. Beef; Iletin II Regular(Beef); Insulin Lente Beef; Insulin Nph Beef; Insulin Semi-lente Beef; Insulin Ultralente Beef

Prescribing information not available at time of publication.

HOW SUPPLIED - EQUIVALENTS NOT AVAILABLE:

Injection, Solution - Subcutaneous - 100 unit/ml

10 ml	$18.87	REGULAR ILETIN II, Lilly	00002-8212-01

Injection, Susp - Subcutaneous - 100 unit/ml

10 ml	$14.34	INSULIN NPH BEEF, Novo Nordisk Pharm	00169-3522-15
10 ml	$14.34	INSULIN LENTE BEEF, Novo Nordisk Pharm	00169-3528-15
10 ml	$17.44	PROTAMINE ZINC ILETIN II, Lilly	00002-8112-01
10 ml	$18.87	NPH ILETIN II, Lilly	00002-8312-01
10 ml	$18.87	LENTE ILETIN II, Lilly	00002-8412-01

INSULIN (HUMAN RECOMBINANT) *(001544)*

CATEGORIES: Antidiabetic Agents; Blood Glucose Regulators; Diabetes; Hormones; Recombinant DNA Origin; Sales > $500 Million; FDA Approved 1982 Oct; Top 200 Drugs

BRAND NAMES: *Actrapid* (Australia); *Actrapid HM* (France, Germany); *Actrapid Human*; *Berlinsulin Actrapid Normal U-40* (Germany); *Berlinsulin H Basal U-40* (Germany); *Human Actrapid*; *Human Nordisulin*; *Huminsulin "Lilly" Normal*; *Huminsulin Normal* (Germany); **Humulin**; *Humulina Regular*; Humulin Br; *Humulin C*; Humulin R; *Humulin-R* (Canada); *Humulin Regular*; *Humulin (Regular)*; *Humuline Regular*; *Insulina*; *Insulina Actrapid HM*; *Insulina Velosulin HM*; *Insulin Hoechst-Rapid U-100*; Insulin Human; *Insulin Human Actrapid* (England); *Insulin Actrapid HM*; *Insulin "Novo Nordisk" Actrapid HM*; *Insulin "Novo Nordisk" Velosulin HM*; *Insulin Velosulin HM*; *Insuline*; *Insuline Actrapid*; *Insuline Humuline Regular*; *Insuline Velosulin Humaan*; *Insuman* (France); Mixtard Human 70 30; Novolin 70 30 Penfill; Novolin N Penfill; Novolin R; *Novolin-Toronto* (Canada); *Velosulin*; Velosulin Human; Velosulin Human R; *Velosuline Humaine* (France)
(International brand names outside U.S. in italics)

FORMULARIES: BC-BS; FHP

THIS LILLY HUMAN INSULIN PRODUCT DIFFERS FROM ANIMAL-SOURCE INSULINS BECAUSE IT IS STRUCTURALLY IDENTICAL TO THE INSULIN PRODUCED BY YOUR BODY'S PANCREAS AND BECAUSE OF ITS UNIQUE MANUFACTURING PROCESS.

ANY CHANGE OF INSULIN SHOULD BE MADE CAUTIOUSLY AND ONLY UNDER MEDICAL SUPERVISION. CHANGES IN PURITY, STRENGTH, BRAND (MANUFACTURER), TYPE (REGULAR, NPH, LENTE, ETC), SPECIES (BEEF, PORK, BEEF-PORK, HUMAN), AND/OR METHOD OF MANUFACTURE (RECOMBINANT DNA VERSUS ANIMAL-SOURCE INSULIN) MAY RESULT IN THE NEED FOR A CHANGE IN DOSAGE.

SOME PATIENTS TAKING HUMULIN (HUMAN INSULIN, RECOMBINANT DNA ORIGIN, LILLY) MAY REQUIRE A CHANGE IN DOSAGE FROM THAT USED WITH ANIMAL-SOURCE INSULINS. IF AN ADJUSTMENT IS NEEDED, IT MAY OCCUR WITH THE FIRST DOSE OR DURING THE FIRST SEVERAL WEEKS OR MONTHS.

PATIENT PACKAGE INSERT:

DIABETES

Insulin is a hormone produced by the pancreas, a large gland that lies near the stomach. This hormone is necessary for the body's correct use of food, especially sugar. Diabetes occurs when the pancreas does not make enough insulin to meet your body's needs.

To control your diabetes, your doctor has prescribed injections of insulin to keep your blood glucose at a nearly normal level. Proper control of your diabetes, you can lead an active, healthy, and useful life if you eat a balanced diet daily, exercise regularly, and take your insulin injections as prescribed.

You have been instructed to test your blood and/or your urine regularly for glucose. If your blood tests consistently show above- or below-normal glucose levels or your urine tests consistently show the presence of glucose, your diabetes is not properly controlled and you must let your doctor know.

Always keep an extra supply of insulin as well as a spare syringe and needle on hand. Always wear diabetic identification so that appropriate treatment can be given if complications occur away from home.

DESCRIPTION

Humulin is synthesized in a special non-disease-producing special laboratory strain of *Escherichia coli* bacteria that has been genetically altered by the addition of the gene for human insulin production.

Humulin R consists of zinc-insulin crystals dissolved in a clear fluid. Humulin R has nothing added to change the speed or length of its action. It takes effect rapidly and has a relatively short duration of activity (4 to 12 hours) as compared with other insulins.

Humulin N is a crystalline suspension of human insulin with protamine and zinc providing an intermediate-acting insulin with a slower onset of action and a longer duration of activity (up to 24 hours) than that of regular insulin.

Humulin L is an amorphous and crystalline suspension of human insulin with a slower onset and a longer duration of activity (up to 24 hours) than regular insulin.

Humulin U is a crystalline suspension of human insulin with zinc providing a slower onset and a longer and less intense duration of activity (up to 28 hours) than regular insulin or the intermediate-acting insulins (NPH and Lente).

Humulin 50/50 is a mixture of 50% Human Insulin Isophane Suspension and 50% Human Insulin Injection. It is an intermediate-acting insulin combined with the more rapid onset of action than regular insulin. The duration of activity may last up to 24 hours following injection.

Humulin 70/30 is a mixture of 70% Human Insulin Isophane Suspension and 30% Human Insulin Injection. It is an intermediate-acting insulin combined with the more rapid onset of action of regular insulin. The duration of activity may last up to 24 hours following injection.

PATIENT PACKAGE INSERT: *(cont'd)*

The time course of action of any insulin may vary considerably in different individuals or at different times in the same individual. As with all insulin preparation, the duration of action of all forms of Humulin is dependent on dose, site of injection, blood supply, temperature, and physical activity. Humulin is a sterile solution and is for subcutaneous injection. It should not be used intravenously or intramuscularly. The concentration of all forms of Humulin is 100 units/ml (U-100).

IDENTIFICATION

Human insulin manufactured by Eli Lilly and Company has the trademark Humulin and is available in 7 formulations—Regular (R), Buffered Regular (BR), NPH (N), Lente (L), Ultralente (U), 50% Human Insulin Isophane Suspension [buffered regular] (50/50), and 70% Human Insulin Isophane Suspension [NPH]/30% Human Insulin Injection [buffered regular] (70/30). Your doctor has prescribed the type of insulin that he/she believes is best for you. **DO NOT USE ANY OTHER INSULIN EXCEPT ON HIS/HER ADVICE AND DIRECTION.**

Always check the carton and the bottle label for the name and letter designation of the insulin you receive from your pharmacy to make sure it is the same as that your doctor has prescribed. Always examine the appearance of your bottle of insulin before withdrawing each dose.

Humulin R can be identified as follows: Humulin R is a clear and colorless liquid with a water-like appearance and consistency. Do not use if it appears cloudy, thickened, or slightly colored or if solid particles are visible.

Humulin N can be identified as follows: A bottle of Humulin N must be carefully shaken or rotated before each injection so that the contents are uniformly mixed. Humulin N should look uniformly cloudy or milky after mixing. Do not use it if the insulin substance (the white material) remains at the bottom of the bottle after mixing. Do not use a bottle of Humulin N if there are clumps in the insulin after mixing. Do not use a bottle of Humulin N if solid white particles stick to the bottom or wall of the bottle, giving it a frosted appearance.

Humulin L can be identified as follows: A bottle of Humulin L must be carefully shaken or rotated before each injection so that the contents are uniformly mixed. Humulin L should look uniformly cloudy or milky after mixing. Do not use it if the insulin substance (the white material) remains at the bottom of the bottle after mixing. Do not use a bottle of Humulin L if there are clumps in the insulin after mixing.

Humulin U can be identified as follows: A bottle of Humulin U must be carefully shaken or rotated before each injection so that the contents are uniformly mixed. Humulin U should look uniformly cloudy or milky after mixing Do not use it if the insulin substance (the white material) remains at the bottom of the bottle after mixing. Do not use a bottle of Humulin U if there are clumps in the insulin after mixing.

Humulin 50/50 can be identified as follows: A bottle of Humulin 50/50 must be carefully shaken or rotated before each injection so that the contents are uniformly mixed. Humulin 50/50 should look uniformly cloudy or milky after mixing. Do not use it if the insulin substance (the white material) remains at the bottom of the bottle after mixing. Do not use a bottle of Humulin 50/50 if there are clumps in the insulin after mixing. Do not use a bottle of Humulin 50/50 if solid white particles stick to the bottom or wall of the bottle, giving it a frosted appearance.

Humulin 70/30 can be identified as follows: A bottle of Humulin 70/30 must be carefully shaken or rotated before each injection so that the contents are uniformly mixed. Humulin 70/30 should look uniformly cloudy or milky after mixing. Do not use it if the insulin substance (the white material) remains at the bottom of the bottle after mixing. Do not use a bottle of Humulin 70/30 if there are clumps in the insulin after mixing. Do not use a bottle of Humulin 70/30 if solid white particles stick to the bottom or wall of the bottle, giving it a frosted appearance.

Always check the appearance of your bottle of insulin before using, and if you note anything unusual in the appearance of your insulin or notice your insulin requirements changing markedly, consult your doctor.

STORAGE

Insulin should be stored in a refrigerator but not in the freezer. If refrigeration is not possible, the bottle of insulin that you are currently using can be kept unrefrigerated as long as it is kept cool as possible (below 86°F [30°]) and away from heat and light. Do not use insulin if it has been frozen. Do not use a bottle of insulin after the expiration date on the label.

INJECTION PROCEDURES

Correct Syringe

Doses of insulin are measured in **units**. U-100 insulin contains 100 units/ml (1 ml = 1 cc). With Humulin, it is important to use a syringe that is marked for U-100 insulin preparations. Failure to use the proper syringe can lead to a mistake in dosage, causing serious problems for you, such as a blood glucose level that is too low or too high.

Syringe Use

To help avoid contamination and possible infection, follow these instructions exactly.

Disposable syringes and needles should be used only once and then discarded. **NEEDLES AND SYRINGES MUST NOT BE SHARED.**

Reusable syringes and needles must be sterilized before each injection.**Follow the package directions supplied with your syringe.**Described below are 2 methods of sterilizing.

Boiling

1. Put syringe, plunger, and needle in strainer, place in saucepan, and cover with water. Boil for 5 minutes.

2. Remove articles from water. When they have cooled, insert plunger into barrel, and fasten needle to syringe with a slight twist.

3. Push plunger in and out several times until water is completely removed.

Isopropyl Alcohol

If the syringe, plunger, and needle cannot be boiled, as when you are traveling, they may be sterilized by immersion for at least 5 minutes in Isopropyl Alcohol, 91%. Do not use bathing, rubbing, or medicated alcohol for this sterilization. If the syringe is sterilized with alcohol, it must be absolutely dry before use.

PREPARING THE DOSE OF HUMULIN R

1. Wash your hands.

2. Inspect the insulin. Humulin R should look clear and colorless. Do not use Humulin R if it appears cloudy, thickened, or slightly colored or if solid particles are visible.

3. If using a new bottle, flip off the plastic protective cap, but **do not** remove the stopper. When using a new bottle, wipe the top of the bottle with an alcohol swab.

4. If you are mixing insulins, refer to the instructions for mixing that follow.

5. Draw air into the syringe equal to your insulin dose. Put the needle through rubber top of the insulin bottle and inject the air into the bottle.

6. Turn the bottle and syringe upside down. Hold the bottle and syringe firmly in 1 hand and shake gently.

7. Making sure the tip of the needle is in the insulin, withdraw the correct dose of insulin into the syringe.

PATIENT PACKAGE INSERT: *(cont'd)*

8. Before removing the needle from the bottle, check your syringe for air bubbles which reduce the amount of insulin in it. If bubbles are present, hold the syringe straight up and tap its side until the bubbles float to the top. Push them out with the plunger and withdraw the correct dose.

9. Remove the needle from the bottle and lay the syringe down so that the needle does not touch anything.

PREPARING THE DOSE OF HUMULIN N, L, U, 50/50, OR 70/30

1. Wash your hands.

2. Carefully shake or rotate the insulin bottle several times to completely mix the insulin.

3. Inspect the insulin. The Humulin should look uniformly cloudy or milky. Do not use it if you notice anything unusual in the appearance.

4. If using a new bottle, flip off the plastic protective cap, but **do not** remove the stopper. When using a new bottle, wipe the top of the bottle with an alcohol swab.

5. If you are mixing insulins, refer to the instructions for mixing that follow.

6. Draw air into the syringe equal to your insulin dose. Put the needle through rubber top of the insulin bottle and inject the air into the bottle.

7. Turn the bottle and syringe upside down. Hold the bottle and syringe firmly in 1 hand and shake gently.

8. Making sure the tip of the needle is in the insulin, withdraw the correct dose of insulin into the syringe.

9. Before removing the needle from the bottle, check your syringe for air bubbles which reduce the amount of insulin in it. If bubbles are present, hold the syringe straight up and tap its side until the bubbles float to the top. Push them out with the plunger and withdraw the correct dose.

10. Remove the needle from the bottle and lay the syringe down so that the needle does not touch anything.

MIXING HUMULIN R WITH LONGER-ACTING HUMAN INSULINS

1. Regular human insulin should be mixed with longer-acting human insulins only on the advice of your doctor.

2. Draw air into your syringe equal to the amount of longer-acting insulin you are taking. Insert the needle into the longer-acting insulin bottle and and inject the air. Withdraw the needle.

3. Now inject air into your regular human insulin bottle in the same manner, but **do notwithdraw** the needle.

4. Turn the bottle and syringe upside down.

5. Making sure the tip of the needle is in the insulin, withdraw the correct dose of regular insulin into the syringe.

6. Before removing the needle from the bottle, check your syringe for air bubbles which reduce the amount of insulin in it. If bubbles are present, hold the syringe straight up and tap its side until the bubbles float to the top. Push them out with the plunger and withdraw the correct dose.

7. Remove the needle from the bottle of regular insulin and insert it into the bottle of the longer-acting insulin. Turn the bottle and syringe upside down. Hold the bottle and syringe firmly in 1 hand and shake gently. Making sure the tip of the needle is in the insulin, withdraw your dose of longer-acting insulin.

8. Remove the needle and lay the syringe down so that the needle does not touch anything.

MIXING HUMULIN N AND REGULAR HUMAN INSULIN

1. NPH human insulin should be mixed only with regular human insulin.

2. Draw air into your syringe equal to the amount of Humulin N you are taking. Insert the needle into the Humulin N bottle and inject the air. Withdraw the needle.

(For remaining instructions, see **Mixing Humulin with Longer-acting Human Insulins**, numbers 3-8.)

MIXING HUMAN INSULINS

Follow your doctor's instructions on whether to mix your insulins ahead of time or just before giving your injection. It is important to be consistent in your method.

Syringes from different manufacturers may vary in the amount of space between the bottom line and the needle. Because of this, do not change:

the sequence of mixing, or

the model and brand of syringe or needle that the doctor has prescribed.

INJECTION

Cleanse the skin with alcohol where the injection is to be made. Stabilize the skin by spreading it or pinching up a large area. Insert the needle as instructed by your doctor. Push the plunger in as far as it will go. Pull the needle out and apply gentle pressure over the injection site for several seconds. **Do not rub the area.** To avoid tissue damage, give the next injection at a site at least 1/2" from the previous site.

DOSAGE

Your doctor has told you which insulin to use, how much, and when and how often to inject it. Because each patient's case of diabetes is different, this schedule has been individualized for you.

Your usual insulin dose may be affected by changes in your food, activity, or work schedule. Carefully follow your doctor's instructions to allow for these changes. Other things that may affect your insulin dose are:

ILLNESS

Illness, especially with nausea and vomiting, may cause your insulin requirements to change. Even if you are not eating, you will still require insulin. You and your doctor should establish a sick day plan for you to use in case of illness. When you are sick, test your blood/urine frequently and call your doctor as instructed.

PREGNANCY

Good control of diabetes is especially important for you and your unborn baby. Pregnancy may make managing your diabetes more difficult. If you are planning to have a baby, are pregnant, or are nursing a baby, consult your doctor.

MEDICATION

Insulin requirements may be increased if you are taking other drugs with hyperglycemic activity, such as oral contraceptives, corticosteroids, or thyroid replacement therapy. Insulin requirements may be reduced in the presence of drugs with hypoglycemic activity, such as oral hypoglycemics, salicylates (for example, aspirin), sulfa antibiotics, and certain antidepressants. Always discuss any medications you are taking with your doctor.

EXERCISE

Exercise may lower your body's need for insulin during and for some time after the activity. Exercise may also help speed up the effect of an insulin dose, especially if the exercise involved the area of injection site (for example, the leg should not be used for injection just prior to running). Discuss with your doctor how you should adjust your regimen to accommodate exercise.

PATIENT PACKAGE INSERT: *(cont'd)*

TRAVEL

Persons traveling across more than 2 time zones should consult their doctor concerning adjustments in their insulin schedule.

COMMON PROBLEMS OF DIABETES

Hypoglycemia (Insulin Reaction)

Hypoglycemia (too little glucose in the blood) is one of the most frequent adverse events experienced by insulin users. It can be brought about by:

1. Taking too much insulin

2. Missing or delaying meals

3. Exercising or working more than usual

4. An infection or illness (especially with diarrhea or vomiting)

5. A change in the body's need for insulin

6. Diseases of the adrenal, pituitary, or thyroid gland, or progression of kidney or liver disease

7. Interactions with other drugs that lower blood glucose such as oral hypoglycemics, salicylates (for example, aspirin), sulfa antibiotics, and certain antidepressants

8. Consumption of alcoholic beverages

Symptoms of mild to moderate hypoglycemia may occur suddenly and can include:

sweating; dizziness; palpitation; tremor; hunger; restlessness; tingling in the hands, feet, lips, or tongue; lightheadedness; inability to concentrate; headache; drowsiness; sleep disturbances; anxiety; blurred vision; slurred speech; depressive mood; irritability; abnormal behavior; unsteady movement; personality changes

Signs of severe hypoglycemia can include:

disorientation; unconsciousness; seizures; death

Therefore, it is important that assistance be obtained immediately.

Early warning symptoms of hypoglycemia may be different or less pronounced under certain conditions, such as long duration of diabetes, diabetic nerve disease, medications such as beta-blockers, change in insulin preparations, or intensified control (3 or more insulin injections per day) of diabetes.

A few patients who have experienced hypoglycemic reactions after transfer from animal-source insulin to human insulin have reported that the early warning symptoms of hypoglycemia were less pronounced or different from those experienced with their previous insulin.

Without recognition of early warning symptoms, you may not be able to take steps to avoid more serious hypoglycemia. Be alert for all of the various types of symptoms that may indicate hypoglycemia. Patients who experience hypoglycemia without early warning symptoms should monitor their blood glucose frequently, especially prior to activities such as driving. If the blood glucose is below your normal fasting glucose, you should consider eating or drinking sugar-containing foods to treat your hypoglycemia.

Mild to moderate hypoglycemia may be treated by eating foods or drinks that contain sugar. Patients should always carry a quick source of sugar, such as candy mints or glucose tablets. More severe hypoglycemia may require the assistance of another person. Patients who are unable to take sugar orally or who are unconscious require an injection of glucagon or should be treated with intravenous administration of glucose at a medical facility.

You should learn to recognize your own symptoms of hypoglycemia. If you are uncertain about these symptoms, you should monitor your blood glucose frequently to help you learn to recognize the symptoms that you experience with hypoglycemia.

If you have frequent episodes of hypoglycemia or experience difficultly in recognizing the symptoms, you should consult your doctor to discuss possible changes in therapy, meal plans, and/or exercise programs to help you avoid hypoglycemia.

Hyperglycemia and Diabetic Acidosis

Hyperglycemia (too much glucose in the blood) may develop if your body has too little insulin. Hyperglycemia can be brought about by:

1. Omitting your insulin or taking less than the doctor has prescribed

2. Eating significantly more than your meal plan suggests

3. Developing a fever or infection

In patients with insulin-dependent diabetes, prolonged hyperglycemia can result in diabetic acidosis. The first symptoms of diabetic acidosis usually come on gradually, over a period of hours or days, and include a drowsy feeling, flushed face, thirst, loss of appetite, and fruity odor on the breath. With acidosis, urine tests show large amounts of glucose and acetone. Heavy breathing and a rapid pulse are more severe symptoms. If uncorrected, prolonged hyperglycemia or diabetic acidosis can result in loss of consciousness or death. Therefore, it is important that you obtain medical assistance immediately.

Lipodystrophy

Rarely, administration of insulin subcutaneously can result in lipoatrophy (depression in the skin) or lipohypertrophy (enlargement or thickening of tissue). If you notice either of these conditions, consult your doctor. A change in your injection technique may help alleviate the problem.

Allergy to Insulin

Local Allergy: Patients occasionally experience redness, swelling, and itching at the site of injection of insulin. This condition, called local allergy, usually clears up in a few days to a few weeks. In some instances, this condition may be related to factors other than insulin, such as irritants in the skin cleansing agent or poor injection technique. If you have local reactions, contact your doctor.

Systemic Allergy: Less common, but potentially more serious, is generalized allergy to insulin, which may cause rash over the whole body, shortness of breath, wheezing, reduction in blood pressure, fast pulse, or sweating. Severe cases of generalized allergy may be life threatening. If you think you are having a generalized allergic reaction to insulin, notify a doctor immediately.

ADDITIONAL INFORMATION

Additional information about diabetes may be obtained from your diabetes educator.

Diabetes Forecast is a national magazine designed especially for patients with diabetes and their families and is available by subscription from the American Diabetes Association, National Service Center, 1660 Duke Street, Alexandria, Virginia 22314.

Another publication, *Diabetes Countdown*, is available from the Juvenile Diabetes Foundation, 432 Park Avenue South, New York, New York 10016-8013.

HOW SUPPLIED - EQUIVALENTS NOT AVAILABLE:

Injection, Solution - Intramuscular; - 100 unit/ml

1.5 ml x 5	$15.95	NOVOLIN R REGULAR HUMAN INSULIN INJECTIO, Bristol Myers Squibb	00003-1833-15
1.5 ml x 5	$18.32	NOVOLIN R, Novo Nordisk Pharm	00169-1833-17
10 ml	$15.95	NOVOLIN R REGULAR HUMAN INSULIN INJECTIO, Bristol Myers Squibb	00003-1833-10

HOW SUPPLIED - EQUIVALENTS NOT AVAILABLE: *(cont'd)*

10 ml	$17.42	NOVOLIN R, Novo Nordisk Pharm	00169-1833-11
10 ml	$18.68	VELOSULIN HUMAN R, Novo Nordisk Pharm	00169-0111-01

Injection, Solution - Subcutaneous - 1 ml

10 ml x 1	$17.42	HUMULIN 70/30 100 UNITS/ML, Lilly	00002-8715-01

Injection, Solution - Subcutaneous - 100 unit

10 ml	$17.42	HUMULIN N, Lilly	00002-8315-01
10 ml x 1	$16.83	HUMULIN BR, Lilly	00002-8216-01

Injection, Solution - Subcutaneous - 100 unit/ml

10 ml	$17.42	HUMULIN U, Lilly	00002-8615-01
10 ml	$17.42	NOVOLIN L, Novo Nordisk Pharm	00169-1835-11
10 ml x 1	$17.42	HUMULIN R, Lilly	00002-8215-01
10 ml x 1	$17.42	HUMULIN L 100 UNITS/ML, Lilly	00002-8415-01

Injection, Susp - Intramuscular; - 100 unit/ml

1.5 ml x 5	$15.95	NOVOLIN N, Bristol Myers Squibb	00003-1834-15
1.5 ml x 5	$15.95	NOVOLIN 70/30, Bristol Myers Squibb	00003-1837-15
1.5 ml x 5	$18.32	NOVOLIN N, Novo Nordisk Pharm	00169-1834-17
1.5 ml x 5	$18.32	NOVOLIN 70/30, Novo Nordisk Pharm	00169-1837-17
1.5 ml x 5	$19.78	NOVOLIN 70/30, Novo Nordisk Pharm	00169-0017-71
10 ml	$15.95	NOVOLIN N NPH HUMAN INSULIN ISOPHANE SUS, Bristol Myers Squibb	00003-1834-10
10 ml	$15.95	NOVOLIN L LENTE HUMAN INSULIN ZINC SUSPE, Bristol Myers Squibb	00003-1835-10
10 ml	$15.95	NOVOLIN 70/30 (SQUIBB-NOVO), Bristol Myers Squibb	00003-1837-10
10 ml	$17.42	HUMULIN 50/50, Lilly	00002-9515-01
10 ml	$17.42	NOVOLIN N, Novo Nordisk Pharm	00169-1834-11
10 ml	$17.42	NOVOLIN 70/30, Novo Nordisk Pharm	00169-1837-11

INSULIN LISPRO (HUMAN ANALOG) *(003293)*

CATEGORIES: Antidiabetic Agents; Blood Glucose Regulators; Diabetes; Hormones; FDA Approved 1996 Jun

BRAND NAMES: **Humalog**; *Humalog Lispro*; *Insuline Lispro Humalog* (France) *(International brand names outside U.S. in italics)*

FORMULARIES: PCS

DESCRIPTION:

Humalog (insulin lispro, rDNA origin) is a human insulin analog that is a rapid-acting, parenteral blood glucose-lowering agent. Chemically, it is Lys(B28), Pro(B29) human insulin analog, created when the amino acids at positions 28 and 29 on the insulin B-chain are reversed. Humalog is synthesized in a special non-pathogenic laboratory strain of *Escherichia coli* bacteria that has been genetically altered by the addition of the gene for insulin lispro.

Humalog has the empirical formula $C_{257}H_{383}N_{65}O_{77}S_6$ and a molecular weight of 5808, both identical to that of human insulin.

The vials and cartridges contain a sterile solution of humalog for use as an injection. Humalog injection consists of zinc-insulin lispro crystals dissolved in a clear aqueous fluid.

Each milliliter of humalog injection contains insulin lispro 100 Units, 16 mg glycerin, 1.88 mg dibasic sodium phosphate, 3.15 mg *m*-cresol, zinc oxide content adjusted to provide 0.0197 mg zinc ion, trace amounts of phenol, and water for injection. Insulin lispro has a pH of 7.0–7.8. Hycrochloric acid 10% and/or sodium hydroxide 10% may be added to adjust pH.

CLINICAL PHARMACOLOGY:

ANTIDIABETIC ACTIVITY

The primary activity of insulin, including insulin lispro, is the regulation of glucose metabolism. In addition, all insulins have several anabolic and anti-catabolic actions on many tissues in the body. In muscle and other tissues (except the brain), insulin causes rapid transport of glucose and amino acids intracellularly, promotes anabolism, and inhibits protein catabolism. In the liver, insulin promotes the uptake and storage of glucose in the form of glycogen, inhibits gluconeogenesis, and promotes the conversion of excess glucose into fat.

Insulin lispro has been shown to be equipotent to human insulin on a molar basis. One unit of insulin lispro has the same glucose-lowering effect as one unit of human regular insulin, but its effect is more rapid and of shorter duration. The glucose-lowering activity of insulin lispro and human regular insulin is comparable when administered to normal volunteers by the intravenous route.

PHARMACOKINETICS

Absorption and Bioavailability: Insulin lispro is as bioavailable as human regular insulin, with absolute bioavailability ranging between 55%-77% with doses between 0.1-0.2 U/kg, inclusive. Studies in normal volunteers and patients with type I (insulin-dependent) diabetes demonstrated that insulin lispro is absorbed faster than human regular insulin (U100). In normal volunteers given subcutaneous doses of insulin lispro ranging from 0.1-0.4 U/kg, peak serum levels were seen 30-90 minutes after dosing. When normal volunteers received equivalent doses of human regular insulin, peak insulin doses occurred between 50-120 minutes after dosing. Similar results were seen in patients with type I diabetes. The pharmacokinetic profiles of insulin lispro and human regular insulin are comparable to one another when administered to normal volunteers by the intravenous route. Insulin lispro was absorbed at a consistently faster rate than human regular insulin in healthy male volunteers given 0.2 U/kg human regular insulin or insulin lispro at abdominal, deltoid, or femoral sites, the three sites often used by patients with diabetes. After abdominal administration of insulin lispro, serum drug levels are higher and the duration of action is slightly shorter than after deltoid or thigh administration (see DOSAGE AND ADMINISTRATION). Insulin lispro has less intra- and inter-patient variability compared to human regular insulin.

Distribution: The volume of distribution for insulin lispro is identical to that of human regular insulin, with a range of 0.26-0.36 L/kg.

Metabolism: Human metabolism studies have not been conducted. However, animal studies indicate that the metabolism of humalog is identical to that of human regular insulin.

Elimination: When insulin lispro is given subcutaneously, its $t_{\frac{1}{2}}$ is shorter than that of human regular insulin (1 vs 1.5 hours, respectively). When given intravenously, humalog and human regular insulin show identical dose-dependent elimination, with a $t_{\frac{1}{2}}$ of 26 and 52 minutes at 0.1 U/kg and 0.2 U/kg, respectively.

PHARMACODYNAMICS

Studies in normal volunteers and patients with diabetes demonstrated that insulin lispro has a more rapid onset of glucose lowering activity, an earlier peak for glucose lowering, and a shorter duration of glucose-lowering activity than human regular insulin. The earlier onset of activity of insulin lispro is directly related to its more rapid rate of absorption. The time course of action of insulin and insulin analogs such as insulin lispro may vary considerably in different individuals or within the same individual. The rate of insulin absorption and consequently the onset of activity is known to be affected by the site of injection, exercise, and other variables (see CLINICAL PHARMACOLOGY, Absorption and Bioavailability).

CLINICAL PHARMACOLOGY: *(cont'd)*

In open-label, crossover studies of 1008 patients with type I diabetes and 722 patients with type II (non-insulin-dependent) diabetes, insulin lispro reduced postprandial glucose compared with human regular insulin (see TABLE 1). The clinical significance of improvement in postprandial hyperglycemia has not been established.

TABLE 1 Comparison of Means of Glycemic Parameters at the End of Combined Treatment Periods. All Randomized Patients in Cross-Over Studies (3 months for each treatment)

Type I, N=1008 Glycemic Parameter, (mmol/L)[†]	Insulin lispro[a]	Humulin Ra*	*P*-value
Premeal Blood Glucose	11.64 ± 5.09	11.34 ± 4.96	.274
1-Hour Postprandial	12.91 ± 5.43	13.89 ± 5.37	<.001
2-Hour Postprandial	11.16 ± 5.30	12.87 ± 5.77	<.001
HbA1c (%)	8.24 ± 1.49	8.17 ± 1.46	.089
Type II, N=722 Glycemic Parameter, (mmol/l)[†]	**Insulin lispro[a]**	**Humulin R[a]**	***P*-value**
Premeal Blood Glucose	10.67 ± 3.77	10.17 ± 3.67	.002
1-Hour Postprandial	13.23 ± 4.43	13.89 ± 4.18	<.001
2-Hour Postprandial	12.08 ± 4.62	13.14 ± 4.48	<.001
HbA1c (%)	8.18 ± 1.30	8.18 ± 1.38	.924

[a]Mean ± Standard Deviation
* Humulin (Regular insulin human injection, USP, [recombinant DNA origin])
[†]mg/dl=mmol/L × 18.0

In 12-month parallel studies of type I and type II patients, hemoglobin A_{1c} did not differ between patients treated with human regular insulin and those treated with insulin lispro.

While the overall rate of hypoglycemia did not differ between patients with type I and type II diabetes treated with insulin lispro compared with human regular insulin, patients with type I diabetes treated with insulin lispro had fewer hypoglycemic episodes between midnight and 6 a.m. The lower rate of hypoglycemia in the humalog-treated group may have been related to higher nocturnal blood glucose levels, as reflected by a small increase in mean fasting blood glucose levels.

SPECIAL POPULATIONS

Age and Gender: Information on the effect of age and gender on the pharmacokinetics of insulin lispro is unavailable. However, in large clinical trials, subgroup analysis based on age and gender did not indicate any difference in postprandial glucose parameters between insulin lispro and human regular insulin.

Smoking: The effect of smoking on the pharmacokinetics and glucodynamics of insulin lispro has not been studied.

Pregnancy: The effect of pregnancy on the pharmacokinetics and glucodynamics of insulin lispro has not been studied.

Obesity: The effect of obesity and/or subcutaneous fat thickness on the pharmacokinetics and glucodynamics of insulin lispro has not been studied. In large clinical trials, which included patients with Body-Mass-Index up to and including 35 kg/m^2, no consistent differences were seen between insulin lispro and Humulin R with respect to postprandial glucose parameters.

Renal Impairment: Some studies with human insulin have shown increased circulating levels of insulin in patients with renal failure. Information on the effect of renal impairment on the pharmacokinetics of insulin lispro is limited. Careful glucose monitoring and dose adjustments of insulin, including insulin lispro, may be necessary in patients with renal dysfunction.

Hepatic Impairment: Some studies with human insulin have shown increased circulating levels of insulin in patients with hepatic failure. Careful glucose monitoring and dose adjustments of insulin, including insulin lispro, may be necessary in patients with hepatic dysfunction.

INDICATIONS AND USAGE:

Insulin lispro is an insulin analog that is indicated in the treatment of patients with diabetes mellitus for the control of hyperglycemia. Insulin lispro has a more rapid onset and a shorter duration of action than human regular insulin. Therefore, insulin lispro should be used in regimens including a longer-acting insulin.

CONTRAINDICATIONS:

Insulin lispro is contraindicated during episodes of hypoglycemia and in patients sensitive to insulin lispro or one of its excipients.

WARNINGS:

This human insulin analog differs from human regular insulin by its rapid onset of action as well as a shorter duration of activity. When used as a mealtime insulin, the dose of insulin lispro should be given within 15 minutes before the meal. Because of the short duration of action of insulin lispro, patients with type I diabetes also require a longer-acting insulin to maintain glucose control.

Hypoglycemia is the most common adverse effect of insulins, including insulin lispro. As with all insulins, the timing of hypoglycemia may differ among various insulin formulations. Glucose monitoring is recommended for all patients with diabetes[†].

Any change of insulin should be made cautiously and only under medical supervision. Changes in insulin strength, manufacturer, type (*e.g.*, regular, NPH, analog), species (animal, human), or method of manufacture (rDNA versus animal-source insulin) may result in the need for a change in dosage.

PRECAUTIONS:

GENERAL

Hypoglycemia and hypokalemia are among the potential clinical adverse effects associated with the use of all insulins. Because of differences in the action of insulin lispro and other insulins, care should be taken in patients in whom such potential side effects might be clinically relevant (*e.g.*, patients who are fasting, have autonomic neuropathy, or are using potassium-lowering drugs). Lipodystrophy and hypersensitivity are among other potential clinical adverse effects associated with the use of all insulins.

As with all insulin preparations, the time course of insulin lispro action may vary in different individuals or at different times in the same individual and is dependent on site of injection, blood supply, temperature, and physical activity.

Adjustment of dosage of any insulin may be necessary if patients change their physical activity or their usual meal plan. Insulin requirements may be altered during illness, emotional disturbances, or other stress.

HYPOGLYCEMIA

As with all insulin preparations, hypoglycemic reactions may be associated with the administration of insulin lispro. Rapid changes in serum glucose levels may induce symptoms of hypoglycemia in persons with diabetes, regardless of the glucose value. Early warning symp-

PRECAUTIONS: *(cont'd)*

toms of hypoglycemia may be different or less pronounced under certain conditions, such as long duration of diabetes, diabetic nerve disease, use of medications such as beta-blockers, or intensified diabetes control.

RENAL IMPAIRMENT

Although there are no specific data in patients with diabetes, insulin lispro requirements may be reduced in the presence of renal impairment, similar to observations found with other insulins.

HEPATIC IMPAIRMENT

Although studies have not been performed in diabetes patients with hepatic disease, insulin lispro requirements may be reduced in the presence of impaired hepatic function, similar to observations found with other insulins.

Allergy

Local Allergy: As with any insulin therapy, patients may experience redness, swelling, or itching at the site of injection. These minor reactions usually resolve in a few days to a few weeks. In some instances, these reactions may be related to factors other than insulin, such as irritants in a skin cleansing agent or poor injection technique.

Systemic Allergy: Less common, but potentially more serious, is generalized allergy to insulin, which may cause rash (including pruritus) over the whole body, shortness of breath, wheezing, reduction in blood pressure, rapid pulse, or sweating. Severe cases of generalized allergy, including anaphylactic reaction, may be life threatening. In controlled clinical trials, pruritus (with or without rash) was seen in 17 patients receiving Humulin R (N=2969) and 30 patients receiving insulin lispro (N=2944) (p=.053). Localized reactions and generalized myalgias have been reported with the use of cresol as an injectable excipient.

Antibody Production: In large clinical trials, antibodies that cross react with human insulin and insulin lispro were observed in both Humulin R- and insulin lispro-treatment groups. As expected, the largest increase in the antibody levels during the 12-month clinical trials was observed with patients new to insulin therapy.

Information for the Patient: Patients should be informed of the potential risks and advantages of insulin lispro and alternative therapies. Patients should also be informed about the importance of proper insulin storage, injection technique, timing of dosage, adherence to meal planning, regular physical activity, regular blood glucose monitoring, periodic glycosylated hemoglobin testing, recognition and management of hypo- and hyperglycemia, and periodic assessment for diabetes complications.

Patients should be advised to inform their physician if they are pregnant or intend to become pregnant.

Refer patients to the Information for the Patient circular for information on proper injection technique, timing of insulin lispro dosing (≤15 minutes before a meal), storing and mixing insulin, and common adverse effects.

Laboratory Tests: As with all insulins, the therapeutic response to insulin lispro should be monitored by periodic blood glucose tests. Periodic measurement of glycosylated hemoglobin is recommended for the monitoring of long-term glycemic control.

MIXING OF INSULINS

Care should be taken when mixing all insulins as a change in peak action may occur. The American Diabetes Association warns in its Position Statement on Insulin Administration, "On mixing, physiochemical changes in the mixture may occur (either immediately or over time). As a result, the physiological response to the insulin mixture may differ from that of the injection of the insulins separately."[1] A decrease in the absorption rate, but not total bioavailability, was seen when insulin lispro was mixed with Humulin N. This decrease in absorption rate was not seen when insulin lispro was mixed with Humulin U. When insulin lispro is mixed with either Humulin U or Humulin N, the mixture should be given within 15 minutes before a meal.

The effects of mixing insulin lispro with insulins of animal source or insulin preparations produced by other manufacturers have not been studied(see WARNINGS).

If insulin lispro is mixed with a longer-acting insulin, insulin lispro should be drawn into the syringe first to prevent clouding of the insulin lispro by the longer-acting insulin. Injection should be made immediately after mixing. Mixtures should not be administered intravenously.

Carcinogenesis, Mutagenesis, and Impairment of Fertility: Long-term studies in animals have not been performed to evaluate the carcinogenic potential of insulin lispro. Insulin lispro was not mutagenic in a battery of *in vitro* and *in vivo* genetic toxicity assays (bacterial mutation tests, unscheduled DNA synthesis, mouse lymphoma assay, chromosomal aberration tests, and a micronucleus test). There is no evidence from animal studies of insulin lispro-induced impairment of fertility.

Pregnancy, Teratogenic Effects, Pregnancy Category B: Reproduction studies have been performed in pregnant rats and rabbits at parenteral doses up to 4 and 0.3 times, respectively, the average human dose (40 units/day) based on body surface area. The results have revealed no evidence of impaired fertility or harm to the fetus due to insulin lispro. There are, however, no adequate and well-controlled studies in pregnant women. Because animal reproduction studies are not always predictive of human response, this drug should be used during pregnancy only if clearly needed.

Although there are no clinical studies of the use of insulin lispro in pregnancy, published studies with human insulins suggest that optimizing overall glycemic control, including postprandial control, before conception and during pregnancy improves fetal outcome. Although the fetal complications of maternal hyperglycemia have been well documented, fetal toxicity also has been reported with maternal hypoglycemia. Insulin requirements usually fall during the first trimester and increase during the second and third trimesters. Careful monitoring of the patient is required throughout pregnancy. During the perinatal period, careful monitoring of infants born to mothers with diabetes is warranted.

Nursing Mothers: It is unknown whether insulin lispro is excreted in significant amounts in human milk. Many drugs, including human insulin, are excreted in human milk. For this reason, caution should be exercised when insulin lispro is administered to a nursing woman. Patients with diabetes who are lactating may require adjustments in insulin lispro dose, meal plan, or both.

Pediatric Use: Safety and effectiveness in patients less than 12 years of age have not been established.

DRUG INTERACTIONS:

(See CLINICAL PHARMACOLOGY) Insulin requirements may be increased by medications with hyperglycemic activity such as corticosteroids, isoniazid, certain lipid-lowering drugs (*e.g.*, niacin), estrogens, oral contraceptives, phenothiazines, and thyroid replacement therapy.

Insulin requirements may be decreased in the presence of drugs with hypoglycemic activity, such as oral hypoglycemic agents, salicylates, sulfa antibiotics, and certain antidepressants (monoamine oxidase inhibitors), certain angiotensin-converting-enzyme inhibitors, beta-adrenergic blockers, inhibitors of pancreatic function (*e.g.*, octreotide), and alcohol. Beta-adrenergic blockers may mask the symptoms of hypoglycemia in some patients.

ADVERSE REACTIONS:

Clinical studies comparing insulin lispro with human regular insulin did not demonstrate a difference in frequency of adverse events between the two treatments.

Adverse events commonly associated with human insulin therapy include the following:

Body as a Whole: allergic reactions (see PRECAUTIONS).

Skin and Appendages: injection site reaction, lipodystrophy, pruritus, rash.

Other: hypoglycemia (see WARNINGS) and PRECAUTIONS).

OVERDOSAGE:

Hypoglycemia may occur as a result of an excess of insulin relative to food intake, energy expenditure, or both. Mild episodes of hypoglycemia usually can be treated with oral glucose. Adjustments in drug dosage, meal patterns, or exercise, may be needed. More severe episodes with coma, seizure, or neurologic impairment may be treated with intramuscular/subcutaneous glucagon or concentrated intravenous glucose. Sustained carbohydrate intake and observation may be necessary because hypoglycemia may recur after apparent clinical recovery.

DOSAGE AND ADMINISTRATION:

Insulin lispro is intended for subcutaneous administration. Dosage regimens of insulin lispro will vary among patients and should be determined by the health care professional familiar with the patient's metabolic needs, eating habits, and other lifestyle variables. Pharmacokinetic and pharmacodynamic studies showed insulin lispro to be equipotent to human regular insulin (*i.e.*, one unit of insulin lispro has the same glucose-lowering capability as one unit of human regular insulin), but with more rapid activity. The quicker glucose-lowering effect of insulin lispro is related to the more rapid absorption rate from subcutaneous tissue. An adjustment of dose or schedule of basal insulin may be needed when a patient changes from other insulins to insulin lispro, particularly to prevent pre-meal hyperglycemia.

When used as a meal-time insulin, insulin lispro should be given within 15 minutes before a meal. Human regular insulin is best given 30-60 minutes before a meal. To achieve optimal glucose control, the amount of longer acting insulin being given may need to be adjusted when using insulin lispro.

The rate of insulin absorption and consequently the onset of activity is known to be affected by the site of injection, exercise, and other variables. Insulin lispro was absorbed at a consistently faster rate than human regular insulin in healthy male volunteers given 0.2 U/kg human regular insulin or insulin lispro at abdominal, deltoid, or femoral sites, the three sites often used by patients with diabetes. When not mixed in the same syringe with other insulins, insulin lispro maintains its rapid onset of action and has less variability in its onset of action among injection sites compared with human regular insulin (see PRECAUTIONS). After abdominal administration, insulin lispro concentrations are higher than those following deltoid or thigh injections. Also, the duration of action of insulin lispro is slightly shorter following abdominal injection, compared with deltoid and femoral injections. As with all insulin preparations, the time course of action of insulin lispro may vary considerably in different individuals or within the same individual. Patients must be educated to use proper injection techniques.

Parenteral drug products should be inspected visually prior to administration whenever the solution and the container permit. If the solution is cloudy, contains particulate matter, is thickened, or is discolored, the contents must not be injected. insulin lispro should not be used after its expiration date.

Storage: Insulin lispro should be stored in a refrigerator (2° to 8°C [36° to 46°F]), but not in the freezer. If refrigeration is impossible, the vial or cartridge of insulin lispro in use can be unrefrigerated for up to 28 days, as long as it is kept as cool as possible (not greater than 86°F [30°C]) and away from direct heat and light. Unrefrigerated vials and cartridges must be used within this time period or be discarded. Do not use insulin lispro if it has been frozen.

REFERENCES:

1. American Diabetes Association: Clinical Practice Recommendations 1996, Insulin Administration. *Diabetes Care*, 1996; 19(Supp 1):31-34.

HOW SUPPLIED - EQUIVALENTS NOT AVAILABLE:

Injection - Intravenous - 100 u/ml

5 x 1.500 ml	$29.99	HUMALOG, Lilly	00002-7515-59
10 ml	$24.98	HUMALOG, Lilly	00002-7510-01

INTERFERON ALFA-2A, RECOMBINANT

(001545)

CATEGORIES: AIDS Related Complex; Antimetabolites; Antimicrobials; Antineoplastics; Antivirals; Biologicals; Cytotoxic Agents; HIV Infection; Immunomodulators; Kaposi's Sarcoma; Lesions; Leukemia; Oncologic Drugs; Orphan Drugs; Renal Cell Carcinoma; Melanoma*; Pregnancy Category C; Recombinant DNA Origin; FDA Approved 1986 Jun
* Indication not approved by the FDA

BRAND NAMES: *Roceron-A*; *Roferon A* (Canada); **Roferon-A**; *Green-Alpha*; *Laroferon* (France)
(International brand names outside U.S. in italics)

FORMULARIES: Aetna; BC-BS; Medi-Cal

COST OF THERAPY: $59,200.09 (AIDS Kaposi's Sarcoma; Injection; 36000000 iv/ml; 0.429/day; 365 days)

DESCRIPTION:

Roferon-A (interferon alfa-2a, recombinant) is a sterile protein product for use by injection. Roferon-A is manufactured by recombinant DNA technology that employs a genetically engineered *E. coli* bacterium containing DNA that codes for the human protein. Interferon alfa-2a, recombinant is a highly purified protein containing 165 amino acids, and it has an approximate molecular weight of 19,000 daltons. The purification procedure includes affinity chromatography using a murine monoclonal antibody. Fermentation is carried out in a defined nutrient medium containing the antibiotic tetracycline hydrochloride, 5 mg/l. However, the presence of the antibiotic is not detectable in the final product. Roferon-A is supplied as an injectable solution or as a sterile powder for injection with its accompanying diluent.

Injectable Solution: *3 million IU Roferon-A Per Vial:* The solution is colorless and each ml contains 3 million IU of interferon alfa-2a, recombinant, 9 mg sodium chloride, 5 mg Albumin (Human) and 3 mg phenol as a preservative.

9 million IU Roferon-A Per Vial: The solution is colorless and each 0.9 ml contains 9 million IU of interferon alfa-2a, recombinant, 8.1 mg sodium chloride, 4.5 mg albumin (human) and 2.7 mg phenol as a preservative. This dosage form should not be used for the treatment of hairy cell leukemia.

DESCRIPTION: *(cont'd)*

18 million IU Roferon-A Per Vial: The solution is colorless and each ml contains 6 million IU of interferon alfa-2a, recombinant, 9 mg sodium chloride, 5 mg albumin (human) and 3.3 mg phenol as a preservative. Each 0.5 ml contains 3 million IU of interferon alfa-2a, recombinant.

36 million IU Roferon-A Per Vial: The solution is colorless and each ml contains 36 million IU of interferon alfa-2a, recombinant, 9 mg sodium chloride, 5 mg albumin (human) and 3 mg phenol as a preservative. This dosage form should not be used for hairy cell leukemia.

Sterile Powder for Injection: 18 million IU Roferon-A Per Vial: The powder is white to beige and when reconstituted with Diluent for sterile powder for injection each 1 ml of reconstituted solution contains 6 million IU of interferon alfa-2a, recombinant, 9 mg sodium chloride, 1.67 mg albumin (human) and 3.3 mg phenol as a preservative. Each 0.5 ml contains 3 million IU of interferon alfa-2a, recombinant.

Diluent for Sterile Powder for Injection: *3 ml Per Vial:* Each ml contains 6 mg sodium chloride and 3.3 mg phenol as a preservative.

The specific activity of interferon alfa-2a, recombinant is 2×10^8 IU/mg protein. The route of administration is subcutaneous or intramuscular.

CLINICAL PHARMACOLOGY:

The mechanism by which interferon alfa-2a, recombinant, or any other interferon, exerts antitumor activity is not clearly understood. However, it is believed that direct antiproliferative action against tumor cells and modulation of the host immune response play important roles in the antitumor activity.

The biological activities of interferon alfa-2a, recombinant are species-restricted, i.e., they are expressed in a very limited number of species other than humans. As a consequence, preclinical evaluation of interferon alfa-2a, recombinant has involved *in vitro* experiments with human cells and some *in vivo* experiments.[1] Using human cells in culture, interferon alfa-2a, recombinant has been shown to have antiproliferative and immunomodulatory activities that are very similar to those of the mixture of interferon alfa subtypes produced by human leukocytes. *In vivo,* interferon alfa-2a, recombinant has been shown to inhibit the growth of several human tumors growing in immunocompromised (nude) mice. Because of its species-restricted activity, it has not been possible to demonstrate antitumor activity in immunologically intact syngeneic tumor model systems, where effects on the host immune system would be observable. However, such antitumor activity has been repeatedly demonstrated with, for example, mouse interferon-alfa in transplantable mouse tumor systems. The clinical significance of these findings is unknown.

The metabolism of interferon alfa-2a, recombinant is consistent with that of alfa interferons in general. Alfa interferons are totally filtered through the glomeruli and undergo rapid proteolytic degradation during tubular reabsorption, rendering a negligible reappearance of intact alfa interferon in the systemic circulation. Small amounts of radiolabeled interferon alfa-2a, recombinant appear in the urine of isolated rat kidneys, suggesting near complete reabsorption of interferon alfa-2a, recombinant catabolites. Liver metabolism and subsequent biliary excretion are considered minor pathways of elimination for alfa interferons.

The serum concentrations of interferon alfa-2a, recombinant reflected a large intersubject variation in both healthy volunteers and patients with disseminated cancer.

In healthy people, interferon alfa-2a, recombinant exhibited an elimination half-life of 3.7 to 8.5 hours (mean 5.1 hours), volume of distribution at steady-state of 0.223 to 0.748 l/kg (mean 0.400 l/kg) and a total body clearance of 2.14 to 3.62 ml/min/kg (mean 2.79 ml/min/kg) after a 36 million IU (2.2×10^8 pg) intravenous infusion. After intramuscular and subcutaneous administrations of 36 million IU, peak serum concentrations ranged from 1500 to 2580 pg/ml (mean 2020 pg/ml) at a mean time to peak of 3.8 hours and from 1250 to 2320 pg/ml (mean 1730 pg/ml) at a mean time to peak of 7.3 hours, respectively. The apparent fraction of the dose absorbed after intramuscular injection was greater than 80%.

The pharmacokinetics of interferon alfa-2a, recombinant after single intramuscular doses to patients with disseminated cancer were similar to those found in healthy volunteers. Dose proportional increases in serum concentrations were observed after single doses up to 198 million IU. There were no changes in the distribution or elimination of interferon alfa-2a, recombinant during twice daily (0.5 to 36 million IU), once daily (1 to 54 million IU), or three times weekly (1 to 136 million IU) dosing regimens up to 28 days of dosing. Multiple intramuscular doses of interferon alfa-2a, recombinant resulted in an accumulation of two to four times the single dose serum concentrations. There is no pharmacokinetic information in patients with hairy cell leukemia, AIDS-related Kaposi's sarcoma and chronic myelogenous leukemia.

Serum neutralizing activity, determined by a highly sensitive enzyme immunoassay, and a neutralization bioassay, was detected in approximately 25% of all patients who received Roferon-A.[2] Antibodies to human leukocyte interferon may occur spontaneously in certain clinical conditions (cancer, systemic lupus erythematosus, herpes zoster) in patients who have never received exogenous interferon.[3] The significance of the appearance of serum neutralizing activity is not known.

CLINICAL STUDIES:

Studies have shown that Roferon-A can produce clinically meaningful tumor regression or disease stabilization in patients with hairy cell leukemia or in patients with AIDS-related Kaposi's sarcoma.[4-6] In Ph positive Chronic Myelogenous Leukemia, interferon alfa-2a, recombinant supplemented with intermittent chemotherapy has been shown to prolong overall survival and to delay disease progression compared to patients treated with chemotherapy alone.[7] In addition, interferon alfa-2a, recombinant has been shown to produce sustained complete cytogenetic responses in a small subset of patients with CML in chronic phase. The activity of interferon alfa-2a, recombinant in Ph *negative* CML has not been determined.

Effects on Hairy Cell Leukemia: A multicenter US phase II study (N2752) enrolled 218 patients; 75 were evaluable for efficacy in a preliminary analysis; 218 patients were evaluable for safety. Patients were to receive a starting dose of interferon alfa-2a, recombinant up to 6 MIU/m²/day, for an induction period of 4 to 6 months. Responding patients were to receive 12 months maintenance therapy.

During the first one to two months of treatment of patients with hairy cell leukemia, significant depression of hematopoiesis was likely to occur. Subsequently, there was improvement in circulating blood cell counts. Of the 75 patients who were evaluable for efficacy following at least 16 weeks of therapy, 46 (61%) achieved complete or partial response. Twenty-one patients (28%) had a minor remission, eight (11%) remained stable, and none had worsening of disease. All patients who achieved either a complete or partial response had complete or partial normalization of all peripheral blood elements including hemoglobin level, white blood cell, neutrophil, monocyte and platelet counts with a concomitant decrease in peripheral blood and bone marrow hairy cells. Responding patients also exhibited a marked reduction in red blood cell and platelet transfusion requirements, a decrease in infectious episodes and improvement in performance status. The probability of survival for two years in patients receiving interferon alfa-2a, recombinant (94%) was statistically increased compared to a historical control group (75%).

CLINICAL STUDIES: *(cont'd)*

Effects on AIDS-Related Kaposi's Sarcoma: In six studies with interferon alfa-2a, recombinant, doses of 3 to 54 million IU daily were evaluated for the treatment of AIDS-related Kaposi's sarcoma in more than 350 patients. Four dosage regimens of interferon alfa-2a, recombinant were evaluated for initial induction. Thirty-nine patients received 3 million IU daily; 99 patients received an escalating regimen of 3 million, 9 million and 18 million IU each daily for 3 days, followed by 36 million IU daily; 119 patients received 36 million IU daily; and 16 patients received doses greater than 36 million IU to a maximum of 54 million IU daily. An additional 91 patients received interferon alfa-2a, recombinant in combination with vinblastine. The best response rate associated with acceptable toxicity was observed when interferon alfa-2a, recombinant was administered as a single agent at a dose of 36 million IU daily. The escalating regimen of 3 to 36 million IU daily provided equivalent therapeutic benefit with some amelioration of acute toxicity in some patients. In AIDS-related Kaposi's sarcoma, lower doses were less effective in inducing tumor regression and doses higher than 36 million IU daily were associated with unacceptable toxicity.

As summarized in TABLE 1, the likelihood of response to interferon alfa-2a, recombinant varied with the clinical manifestations of human immunodeficiency virus (HIV) infection. Patients with prior opportunistic infection or B symptoms are unlikely to respond to treatment with interferon alfa-2a, recombinant.

TABLE 1 Likelihood of Response to Interferon Alfa-2a, Recombinant in Patients with AIDS-Related Kaposi's Sarcoma

		Objective Response Rate (%)		
No. Pts.*	**CD_4 (T_4) Lymphocyte Count (cells/mm³)**	**CR**	**PR**	**Total**
83	0-200	3.6	3.6	7.2
51	201-400	15.7	11.8	27.5
33	>400	24.2	21.2	45.4

In the 28 patients evaluated who had prior opportunistic infection or B symptoms, the response rate was 3.6%.

* Patients had no prior opportunistic infection or B symptoms. B symptoms include night sweats, weight loss of greater than 10% of body weight or 15 lbs., or fever greater than 100°F without an identifiable source of infection.

Patients who were otherwise asymptomatic, with no prior opportunistic infection and near-normal levels of CD_4 lymphocytes, experienced higher response rates. Responding patients with a baseline CD_4 lymphocyte count greater than 200 cells/mm³ had a distinct survival advantage over both responding patients with a baseline CD_4 lymphocyte count of 200 cell/mm³ or less and nonresponding patients regardless of their baseline CD_4 lymphocyte count. Median survival for responding patients with CD_4 lymphocyte counts of greater than 200 to 400 cells/mm³ had not been reached but was greater than 32.7 months from the initiation of therapy. For responding patients with CD_4 lymphocyte counts of greater than 400 cells/mm³, the median survival had not been reached but was greater than 29.5 months.

A classification system for staging AIDS-related Kaposi's sarcoma has been described based on location and extent of disease. In studies of interferon alfa-2a, recombinant, no difference was noted in response rates for patients with different stages of Kaposi's sarcoma. Likelihood of response was related to manifestations of HIV infection (baseline CD_4 lymphocyte count, prior opportunistic infection or B symptoms) and not to extent of tumor involvement. The median time to response was 2.7 months. The median duration of response for patients achieving a partial or complete response was 6.3 and 20.7 months, respectively. Complete and partial responses lasting in excess of three years have been observed. Therapy was discontinued because of progression of Kaposi's sarcoma, development of severe opportunistic infection or severe adverse effects. The median time to discontinuation of treatment was 12.5 months for responding patients and 2.3 months for patients who did not respond.

Effects on pH Positive Chronic Myelogenous Leukemia(CML): Interferon alfa-2a, recombinant was evaluated in two trials of patients with chronic phase CML. Study DM84-38 was a single center phase II study conducted at the MD Anderson Cancer Center, which enrolled 91 patients, 81% were previously treated, 82% were Ph positive, and 63% received interferon alfa-2a, recombinant within 1 year of diagnosis. Study MI400 was a multicenter randomized phase III study conducted in Italy by the Italian Cooperative Study Group on CML in 335 patients; 226 interferon alfa-2a, recombinant and 109 chemotherapy. Patients with Ph positive, newly diagnosed or minimally treated CML were randomized (ratio 2:1) to either interferon alfa-2a, recombinant or conventional chemotherapy with either hydroxyurea or busulfan. In study DM84-38, patients started interferon alfa-2a, recombinant at 9 MIU/day, whereas in study MI400, it was progressively escalated from 3 to 9 MIU/day over the first month. In both trials, dose escalation for insufficient hematologic response, and dose attenuation or interruption for toxicity was permitted. No formal guidelines for dose attenuation were given in the chemotherapy arm of study MI400. In addition, in the interferon alfa-2a, recombinant arm, the MI400 protocol allowed the addition of intermittent single agent chemotherapy for insufficient hematologic response to interferon alfa-2a, recombinant alone. In this trial, 44% of the interferon alfa-2a, recombinant treated patients also received intermittent single agent chemotherapy at some time during the study.

The two studies were analyzed according to uniform response criteria. For hematologic response: complete response (WBC $<90.10^9$/l), normalization of the differential with no immature forms in the peripheral blood, disappearance of splenomegaly), partial response (>50% decrease from baseline of WBC to $<20.10^9$/l). For cytogenetic response: complete response (0% Ph-positive metaphases), partial response (1-34% Ph-positive metaphases).

In study DM84-38, the median survival from initiation of interferon alfa-2a, recombinant was 47 months. In study MI400, the median survival for the patients on the interferon arm was 69 months, which was significantly better than the 55 months seen in the chemotherapy control group (48 patients in study MI400 proceeded to BMT and in study DM84-38, 15 patients proceeded to BMT). Interferon alfa-2a, recombinant treatment significantly delayed disease progression to blastic phase as evidenced by a median time to disease progression of 69 months compared to 46 months with chemotherapy.

By multivariate analysis of prognostic factors associated with all 335 patients entered into the randomized study, treatment with interferon alfa-2a, recombinant (with or without intermittent additional chemotherapy; $p=0.006$), Sokal index[8] ($p=0.006$) and WBC ($p=0.023$) were the three variables associated with an improved survival, independent of other baseline characteristics (Karnofsky performance status and hemoglobin being the other factors entered into the model).

In study MI400, overall hematologic responses, [complete responses (CR) and partial responses (PR)], were observed in approximately 60% of patients treated with interferon alfa-2a, recombinant (40% CR, 20% PR), compared to 70% with chemotherapy (30% CR, 40% PR). The median time to reach a complete hematologic response was 5 months in the interferon alfa-2a, recombinant arm and 4 months in the chemotherapy arm. The overall cytogenetic response rate (CR+PR), in patients receiving interferon alfa-2a, recombinant, was 10% and 12% in studies MI400 and DM84-38, respectively, according to the intent-to-treat principle. In contrast, only 2% of the patients in the chemotherapy arm of study MI400 achieved a cytogenetic response (with no complete responses). Cytogenetic responses were observed only in patients who had complete hematologic responses. In study DM84-38, hematologic and cytogenetic response rates were higher in the subset of patients treated with

CLINICAL STUDIES: *(cont'd)*

interferon alfa-2a, recombinant within 1 year of diagnosis (76% and 17%, respectively) compared to the subset initiating interferon alfa-2a, recombinant therapy more than 1 year from diagnosis (29% and 4%, respectively). In an exploratory analysis, patients who achieve a cytogenetic response live longer than those who did not.

Severe adverse events were observed in 66% and 31% of patients on study DM84-38 and MI400, respectively. Dose reduction and temporary cessation of therapy was required frequently. Permanent cessation of interferon alfa-2a, recombinant, due to intolerable side effects, was required in 15% and 23% of patients on studies DM84-38 and MI400, respectively (see ADVERSE REACTIONS).

Limited data are available on the use of interferon alfa-2a, recombinant in children with Ph positive, adult type CML. A published report on 15 children with CML suggest a safety profile similar to that seen in adult CML; clinical responses were also observed[9] (see DOSAGE AND ADMINISTRATION).

INDICATIONS AND USAGE:

Interferon alfa-2a, recombinant is indicated for the treatment of hairy cell leukemia and AIDS-related Kaposi's sarcoma in patients 18 years of age or older. In addition, it is indicated for chronic phase, Philadelphia chromosome (Ph) positive chronic myelogenous leukemia (CML) patients who are minimally pretreated (within 1 year of diagnosis).

For Patients with AIDS-Related Kaposi's Sarcoma: Interferon alfa-2a, recombinant is useful for the treatment of AIDS-related Kaposi's sarcoma in a select group of patients. In determining whether a patient should be treated, the physician should assess the likelihood of response based on the clinical manifestations of HIV infection, including prior opportunistic infections, presence of B symptoms, and CD_4 count, and the manifestations of Kaposi's sarcoma requiring treatment (see CLINICAL PHARMACOLOGY).

CONTRAINDICATIONS:

Interferon alfa-2a, recombinant is contraindicated in patients with known hypersensitivity to alfa interferon, mouse immunoglobulin or any component of the product.

WARNINGS:

Interferon alfa-2a, recombinant should be administered under the guidance of a qualified physician (see DOSAGE AND ADMINISTRATION). Appropriate management of the therapy and its complications is possible only when adequate diagnostic and treatment facilities are readily available.

DEPRESSION, AND SUICIDAL BEHAVIOR INCLUDING SUICIDAL IDEATION, SUICIDAL ATTEMPTS AND SUICIDES HAVE BEEN REPORTED IN ASSOCIATION WITH TREATMENT WITH ALFA INTERFERONS, INCLUDING INTERFERON ALFA-2A, RECOMBINANT. Patients to be treated with interferon alfa-2a, recombinant should be informed that depression and suicidal ideation may be side effects of treatment and should be advised to report these side effects immediately to the prescribing physician. Patients receiving interferon alfa-2a, recombinant therapy should receive close monitoring for the occurrence of depressive symptomatology. Cessation of treatment should be considered for patients experiencing depression. Although dose reduction or treatment cessation may lead to resolution of the depressive symptomatology, depression may persist and suicides have occurred after withdrawing therapy (see PRECAUTIONS and ADVERSE REACTIONS).

Interferon alfa-2a, recombinant should not be used for the treatment of visceral AIDS-related Kaposi's sarcoma associated with rapidly progressive or life-threatening disease.

Interferon alfa-2a, recombinant should be used with caution in patients with severe preexisting cardiac disease, severe renal or hepatic disease, seizure disorders and/or compromised central nervous system function.

Infrequently, severe or fatal gastrointestinal hemorrhage has been reported in association with alfa interferon therapy.

Because of the possibility of severe or even fatal adverse reactions, patients should be informed not only of the benefits of therapy but also of the risks involved.

Interferon alfa-2a, recombinant should be administered with caution to patients with cardiac disease or with any history of cardiac illness. It is likely that acute, self-limited toxicities (*i.e.*, fever, chills) frequently associated with interferon alfa-2a, recombinant administration may exacerbate preexisting cardiac conditions. Rarely, myocardial infarction has occurred in patients receiving interferon alfa-2a, recombinant. Cases of cardiomyopathy have been observed on rare occasions in patients treated with alfa-interferons.

Caution should be exercised when administering interferon alfa-2a, recombinant to patients with myelosuppression or when interferon alfa-2a, recombinant is used in combination with other agents that are known to cause myelosuppression. Synergistic toxicity has been observed when interferon alfa-2a, recombinant is administered in combination with zidovudine (AZT).[10] The effects of interferon alfa-2a, recombinant when combined with other drugs used in the treatment of AIDS-related disease are not known.

Central nervous system adverse reactions have been reported in a number of patients. These reactions included decreased mental status, dizziness, impaired memory, agitation, manic behavior and psychotic reactions. More severe obtundation and coma have been rarely observed. Most of these abnormalities were mild and reversible within a few days to three weeks upon dose reduction or discontinuation of interferon alfa-2a, recombinant therapy. Careful periodic neuropsychiatric monitoring of all patients is recommended.

Leukopenia and elevation of hepatic enzymes occurred frequently but were rarely dose-limiting. Thrombocytopenia occurred less frequently. Proteinuria and increased cells in urinary sediment were also seen infrequently. Dose-limiting hepatic or renal toxicities were unusual. Infrequently, severe renal toxicities, sometimes requiring renal dialysis, have been reported with alfa interferon therapy alone or in combination with IL-2 (see PRECAUTIONS).

PRECAUTIONS:

GENERAL

In all instances where the use of interferon alfa-2a, recombinant is considered for chemotherapy, the physician must evaluate the need and usefulness of the drug against the risk of adverse reactions. Most adverse reactions are reversible if detected early. If severe reactions occur, the drug should be reduced in dosage or discontinued and appropriate corrective measures should be taken according to the clinical judgment of the physician. Reinstitution of interferon alfa-2a, recombinant therapy should be carried out with caution and with adequate consideration of the further need for the drug, and alertness to possible recurrence of toxicity. The minimum effective doses of interferon alfa-2a, recombinant for treatment of hairy cell leukemia, AIDS-related Kaposi's sarcoma, and chronic myelogenous leukemia have not been established.

Variations in dosage and adverse reactions exist among different brands of interferon. Therefore, do not use different brands of interferon in a single treatment regimen.

INFORMATION FOR THE PATIENT

Patients should be cautioned not to change brands of interferon without medical consultation, as a change in dosage may result. Patients should be informed regarding the potential benefits and risks attendant to the use of interferon alfa-2a, recombinant. If home use is

PRECAUTIONS: *(cont'd)*

determined to be desirable by the physician, instructions on appropriate use should be given, including review of the contents of the enclosed Patient Information Sheet. Patients should be well hydrated, especially during the initial stages of treatment.

Patients should be thoroughly instructed in the importance of proper disposal procedures and cautioned against reusing syringes and needles. If home use is prescribed, a puncture resistant container for the disposal of used syringes and needles should be supplied to the patient. The full container should be disposed of according to directions provided by the physician.

Patients receiving high dose alfa-interferon should be cautioned against performing tasks that require complete mental alertness such as operating machinery or driving a motor vehicle. Patients to be treated with interferon alfa-2a, recombinant should be informed that depression and suicidal ideation may be side effects of treatment and should be advised to report these side effects immediately to the prescribing physician.

LABORATORY TESTS

Complete blood counts and clinical chemistry tests should be performed before initiation of interferon alfa-2a, recombinant therapy and at appropriate periods during therapy. Since responses of hairy cell leukemia, AIDS-related Kaposi's sarcoma, and chronic myelogenous leukemia are not generally observed for one to three months after initiation of treatment, very careful monitoring for severe depression of blood cell counts is warranted during the initial phase of treatment.

Those patients who have preexisting cardiac abnormalities and/or are in advanced stages of cancer should have electrocardiograms taken before and during the course of treatment.

CARCINOGENESIS, MUTAGENESIS AND IMPAIRMENT OF FERTILITY

Carcinogenesis: Interferon alfa-2a, recombinant has not been tested for its carcinogenic potential.

Mutagenesis: *Internal Studies:* Ames tests using six different tester strains, with and without metabolic activation, were performed with interferon alfa-2a, recombinant up to a concentration of 1920 mcg/plate. There was no evidence of mutagenicity.

Human lymphocyte cultures were treated *in vitro* with interferon alfa-2a, recombinant at noncytotoxic concentrations. No increase in the incidence of chromosomal damage was noted.

Published studies. There are no published studies on the mutagenic potential of interferon alfa-2a, recombinant. However, a number of studies on the genotoxicity of human leukocyte interferon have been reported.

A chromosomal defect following the addition of human leukocyte interferon to lymphocyte cultures from a patient suffering from a lymphoproliferative disorder has been reported.

In contrast, other studies have failed to detect chromosomal abnormalities following treatment of lymphocyte cultures from healthy volunteers with human leukocyte interferon.

It has also been shown that human leukocyte interferon protects primary chick embryo fibroblasts from chromosomal aberrations produced by gamma rays.

Impairment of Fertility: Interferon alfa-2a, recombinant has been studied for its effect on fertility in Macaca mulatta (rhesus monkeys). Nonpregnant rhesus females treated with interferon alfa-2a, recombinant at doses of 5 and 25 million IU/kg/day have shown menstrual cycle irregularities, including prolonged or shortened menstrual periods and erratic bleeding; these cycles were considered to be anovulatory on the basis that reduced progesterone levels were noted and that expected increases in preovulatory estrogen and luteinizing hormones were not observed. These monkeys returned to a normal menstrual rhythm following discontinuation of treatment.

PREGNANCY CATEGORY C

Teratogenic Effects: Interferon alfa-2a, recombinant has been shown to demonstrate a statistically significant increase in abortifacient activity in rhesus monkeys when given at approximately 20 to 500 times the human dose. A study in pregnant rhesus monkeys treated with 1, 5 or 25 million IU/kg/day of interferon alfa-2a, recombinant in their early to midfetal period (days 22 to 70 of gestation) has failed to demonstrate teratogenic activity for interferon alfa-2a, recombinant.

There are no adequate and well-controlled studies in pregnant women.

Nonteratogenic Effects: Dose-related abortifacient activity was observed in pregnant rhesus monkeys treated with 1, 5 or 25 million IU/kg/day of interferon alfa-2a, recombinant in their early to midfetal period (days 22 to 70 of gestation). A late-fetal period study (days 79 to 100 of gestation) is in progress and as yet there have been no reports of any increased rate of abortion.

Usage in Pregnancy: Safe use in human pregnancy has not been established. Therefore, interferon alfa-2a, recombinant should be used during pregnancy only if the potential benefit justifies the potential risk to the fetus. Information from primate studies showed dose-related menstrual irregularities and an increased incidence of spontaneous abortions. Decreases in serum estradiol and progesterone concentrations have been reported in women treated with human leukocyte interferon.[13] Therefore, fertile women should not receive interferon alfa-2a, recombinant unless they are using effective contraception during the therapy period.

Male fertility and teratologic evaluations have yielded no significant adverse effects to date.

NURSING MOTHERS

It is known whether this drug is excreted in human milk. Because many drugs are excreted in human milk and because of the potential for serious adverse reactions in nursing infants from interferon alfa-2a, recombinant, a decision should be made whether to discontinue nursing or to discontinue the drug, taking into account the importance of the drug to the mother.

PEDIATRIC USE

Use of interferon alfa-2a, recombinant in children with Ph-positive adult-type CML is supported by evidence from adequate and well-controlled studies of interferon alfa-2a, recombinant in adults with additional data from the literature on the use of alfa interferon in children with CML. A published report on 15 children with Ph-positive adult-type CML suggests a safety profile similar to that seen in adult CML; clinical responses were also observed[9] (see DOSAGE AND ADMINISTRATION).

DRUG INTERACTIONS:

Interferon alfa-2a, recombinant, apparently through an unknown effect on certain microsomal enzyme systems, has been reported to reduce the clearance of theophylline.[11,12] The clinical relevance of this interaction is presently unknown. Interactions between interferon alfa-2a, recombinant and other drugs have not been fully evaluated. Caution should be exercised when administering interferon alfa-2a, recombinant in combination with other potentially myelosuppressive agents (see WARNINGS).

Other Drug Interactions: Alfa-interferons may affect the oxidative metabolic process by reducing the activity of hepatic microsomal cytochrome enzymes in the P450 group. Although the clinical relevance is still unclear, this should be taken into account when prescribing concomitant therapy with drugs metabolized by this route. Reduced clearance of theophylline following the concomitant administration of alfa-interferons has been reported.

It has been observed that the neurotoxic, hematotoxic or cardiotoxic effects of previously or concurrently administered drugs may be increased by interferons. Interactions could occur following concurrent administration of centrally-acting drugs. Use of interferon alfa-2a, recombinant in conjunction with interleukin-2 may potentiate risks of renal failure.

ADVERSE REACTIONS:

Depressive illness and suicidal behavior, including suicidal ideation and suicides, have been reported in association with the use of alfa interferon products. The incidence of reported depression has varied substantially among trials, possibly related to the underlying disease, dose, duration of therapy, and degree of monitoring, but has been reported to be 15% or higher (see WARNINGS).

FOR PATIENTS WITH HAIRY CELL LEUKEMIA

Constitutional (100%): Fever (92%), fatigue (86%), headache (64%), chills (64%), weight loss (33%), dizziness (21%) and flu-like symptoms (16%).

Integumentary (79%): Skin rash (44%), diaphoresis (22%), partial alopecia (17%), dry skin (17%) and pruritus (13%).

Musculoskeletal (73%): Myalgia (71%), joint or bone pain (25%) and arthritis or polyarthritis (5%).

Gastrointestinal (69%): Anorexia (43%), nausea/vomiting (39%) and diarrhea (34%).

Head and neck (45%): Throat irritation (21%), rhinorrhea (12%) and sinusitis (11%).

Pulmonary (40%): Coughing (16%), dyspnea (12%) and pneumonia (11%).

Central nervous system (39%): Dizziness (21%), depression (16%), sleep disturbance (10%), decreased mental status (10%), anxiety (6%), lethargy (6%), visual disturbance (6%) and confusion (5%).

Cardiovascular (39%): Chest pain (11%), edema (11%) and hypertension (11%).

Pain (34%): Pain (24%) and pain in back (16%).

Peripheral Nervous System (23%): Paresthesia (12%) and numbness (12%).

Rarely (<5%), central nervous system effects including gait disturbance, nervousness, syncope and vertigo, as well as cardiac adverse events including murmur, thrombophlebitis and hypotension were reported. Adverse experiences that occurred rarely, and may have been related to underlying disease, included ecchymosis, epistaxis, bleeding gums and petechiae. Urticaria and inflammation at the site of injection were also rarely observed.

FOR PATIENTS WITH AIDS-RELATED KAPOSI'S SARCOMA

Flu-Like Symptoms: Fatigue (95%), fever (74%), myalgia (69%), headache (66%), chills (41%) and arthralgia (24%).

Gastrointestinal: Anorexia (65%), nausea (51%), diarrhea (42%), emesis (17%) and abdominal pain (15%).

Central and Peripheral Nervous System: Dizziness (40%), decreased mental status (17%), depression (16%), paresthesia (8%), confusion (8%), diaphoresis (7%), visual disturbances (5%), sleep disturbances (5%) and numbness (3%).

Pulmonary and Cardiovascular: Coughing (27%), dyspnea (11%), edema (9%), chest pain (4%) and hypotension (4%).

Skin: Partial alopecia (22%), rash (11%) and dry skin or pruritus (5%).

Other: Weight loss (25%), change in taste (25%), dryness or inflammation of the oropharynx (14%), night sweats (8%) and rhinorrhea (4%).

Occasionally (<3%) nervous system effects including anxiety, nervousness, emotional lability, vertigo and forgetfulness, as well as cardiac adverse events, including palpitations and arrhythmia, were reported. Other adverse experiences that occurred occasionally (<3%) and may have been related to underlying disease, included sinusitis, constipation, chest congestion, pneumonia, urticaria, and flatulence. Adverse experiences which occurred rarely (<1%) included ataxia, seizures, cyanosis, gastric distress, bronchospasm, pain at injection site, earache, eye irritation and rhinitis. Miscellaneous adverse experiences such as poor coordination, lethargy, muscle contractions, neuropathy, tremor, involuntary movement, syncope, aphasia, aphonia, dysarthria, amnesia, weakness, and flushing of skin were observed in less than 0.5% of patients. Cases of cardiomyopathy have been observed on rare occasions in patients treated with alfa-interferons.

For Patients with Chronic Myelogenous Leukemia: For patients with chronic myelogenous leukemia, the percentage of adverse events, whether related to drug therapy or not, experienced by patients treated with rIFNα-2a is given below. Severe adverse events were observed in 66% and 31% of patients on study DM84-38 and MI400, respectively. Dose reduction and temporary cessation of therapy was required frequently. Permanent cessation of interferon alfa-2a, recombinant, due to intolerable side effects, was required in 15% and 23% of patients on studies DM84-38 and MI400, respectively.

Flu-Like Symptoms: Fever (92%), asthenia or fatigue (88%), myalgia (68%), chills (63%), arthralgia/bone pain (47%) and headache (44%).

Gastrointestinal: Anorexia (48%), nausea/vomiting (37%) and diarrhea (37%).

Central and Peripheral Nervous System: Headache (44%), depression (28%), decreased mental status (16%), dizziness (11%), sleep disturbances (11%), paresthesia (8%), involuntary movements (7%) and visual disturbance (6%).

Pulmonary and Cardiovascular: Coughing (19%), dyspnea (8%) and dysrhythmia (7%).

Skin: Hair changes (including alopecia) (18%), skin rash (18%), sweating (15%), dry skin (7%) and pruritus (7%).

Uncommon adverse events (<4%) reported in clinical studies included chest pain, syncope, hypotension, impotence, alterations in taste or hearing, confusion, seizures, memory loss, disturbances of libido, bruising and coagulopathy. Miscellaneous adverse events which were rarely observed included Coombs' positive hemolytic anemia, aplastic anemia, hypothyroidism, cardiomyopathy, hypertriglyceridemia, and bronchospasm.

In Other Investigational Studies of Interferon Alpha-2a Recombinant: The following infrequent adverse events have been reported in one or more of the approved clinical indications as well as with the investigational use of Roferon-A (<5%): pancreatitis, colitis, gastrointestinal hemorrhage, stomatitis, thyroid dysfunction (including hypothyroidism and hyperthyroidism), diabetes (in some patients requiring insulin therapy), and pneumonitis (some cases responding to interferon cessation and corticosteroid therapy). In addition to the adverse experiences noted above, other adverse experiences that occurred included: abdominal fullness, hypermotility, hepatitis, gait disturbance, hallucinations, encephalopathy, psychomotor retardation, coma, stroke, transient ischemic attacks, dysphasia, sedation, apathy, irritability, hyperactivity, claustrophobia, loss of libido, congestive heart failure, myocardial infarction, Raynaud's phenomenon, hot flashes, tachypnea, ischemic retinopathy, excessive salivation, and anaphylactic reactions. These adverse experiences occurred rarely (<1%).

The following events have been rarely observed (<3%) in some patients receiving interferon alfa-2a, recombinant: vasculitis, arthritis, hemolytic anemia, and lupus erythematosus syndrome. The mechanism by which these events develop and their relationship to interferon alfa-2a, recombinant therapy are unclear. Similar events have been reported for other types of interferon.

Abnormal Laboratory Test Values: The percentage of patients with Hairy Cell Leukemia, with AIDS-related Kaposi's Sarcoma, and with Chronic Myelogenous Leukemia who experienced a severe or life-threatening abnormal laboratory test value at least once during their treatment with interferon alfa-2a, recombinant is shown in the following table (TABLE 2):

ADVERSE REACTIONS: *(cont'd)*

TABLE 2 Severe Or Life-Threatening Abnormal Laboratory Test Values

	Hairy Cell Leukemia (n=218)	AIDS-related Kaposi's Sarcoma (n=241)	Chronic Myelogenous Leukemia***	
			US study (n=91)	non-US study (n=219)
Leukopenia	45%*	49%	20%	3%
Neutropenia	68%*	52%	22%	0%
Thrombocytopenia	62%*	35%	27%	5%
Anemia (Hb)	31%*	27%	15%	4%
SGOT	9%	46%	5%	1%
Alk. Phosphatase	3%	11%	3%	1%
LDH	<1%	10%	NA	NA
Bilirubin	<1%	<1%	0%	0%
BUN	<1%	0%	0%	0%
Serum Creatinine	<1%	<1%	0%	0%
Proteinuria	10%**	<1%	NA	NA

* In the majority of patients, initial hematologic laboratory test values were abnormal due to their underlying disease.
** Ten percent of the patients experienced a proteinuria >1+ at least once.
*** Patients enrolled in the two clinical studies receiving at least one dose of Roferon-A.
NA = Not Assessed.

Hairy Cell Leukemia: Increases in serum phosphorus (≥1.6 mmol/l) and serum uric acid (≥9.1 mg/dl) were observed in 9% and 10% of patients, respectively. The increase in serum uric acid is likely to be related to the underlying disease. Decreases in serum calcium (≤1.9 mmol/l) and serum phosphorus (≤0.9 mmol/l) were seen in 28% and 22% of patients, respectively.

Chronic Myelogenous Leukemia: In the two clinical studies, a severe or life-threatening anemia was seen in up to 15% of patients. A severe or life-threatening leukopenia and thrombocytopenia were observed in up to 20% and 27% of patients, respectively. Changes were usually reversible when therapy was discontinued. One case of aplastic anemia and one case of Coombs' positive hemolytic anemia were seen in 310 patients treated with rIFNα-2a in clinical studies. Severe cytopenias led to discontinuation of therapy in 4% of all interferon alfa-2a, recombinant treated patients.

Transient increases in liver transaminases or alkaline phosphatase of any intensity were seen in up to 50% of patients during treatment with interferon alfa-2a, recombinant. Only 5% of patients had a severe or life-threatening increase in SGOT. In the clinical studies, such abnormalities required termination of therapy in less than 1% of patients.

DOSAGE AND ADMINISTRATION:

The recommended dosages of interferon alfa-2a, recombinant differ for hairy cell leukemia, AIDS-related Kaposi's sarcoma and chronic myelogenous leukemia. See indication-specific dosages below.

Note: Parenteral drug products should be inspected visually for particulate matter and discoloration before administration, whenever solution and container permit.

Hairy Cell Leukemia: Prior to initiation of therapy, tests should be performed to quantitate peripheral blood hemoglobin, platelets, granulocytes and hairy cells and bone marrow hairy cells. These parameters should be monitored periodically (*e.g.,* monthly) during treatment to determine whether response to treatment has occurred. If a patient does not respond within six months, treatment should be discontinued. If a response to treatment does occur, treatment should be continued until no further improvement is observed and these laboratory parameters have been stable for about three months. Patients with hairy cell leukemia have been treated for up to 24 consecutive months. The optimal duration of treatment for this disease has not been determined.

The induction dose of interferon alfa-2a, recombinant is 3 million IU daily for 16 to 24 weeks, administered as a subcutaneous or intramuscular injection. Subcutaneous administration is particularly suggested for, but not limited to, thrombocytopenic patients (platelet count <50,000) or for patients at risk for bleeding. The recommended maintenance dose is 3 million IU, three times per week. Dose reduction by one-half or withholding of individual doses may be needed when severe adverse reactions occur. The use of doses higher than 3 million IU is not recommended in hairy cell leukemia. The 9 and 36 million IU dosage forms should not be used for the treatment of hairy cell leukemia.

AIDS-Related Kaposi's Sarcoma: Interferon alfa-2a, recombinant is useful for the treatment of AIDS-related Kaposi's sarcoma in a select group of patients. In determining whether a patient should be treated, the physician should assess the likelihood of response based on the clinical manifestations of HIV infection and the manifestations of Kaposi's sarcoma requiring treatment (see CLINICAL PHARMACOLOGY).

Indicator lesion measurements and total lesion count should be performed before initiation of therapy. These parameters should be monitored periodically (*e.g.,* monthly) during treatment to determine whether response to treatment or disease stabilization has occurred. When disease stabilization or a response to treatment occurs, treatment should continue until there is no further evidence of tumor or until discontinuation is required because of a severe opportunistic infection or adverse effects. The optimal duration of treatment for this disease has not been determined.

The recommended induction dose of interferon alfa-2a, recombinant is 36 million IU daily for 10 to 12 weeks, administered as an intramuscular or subcutaneous injection. Subcutaneous administration is particularly suggested for, but not limited to, patients who are thrombocytopenic (platelet count <50,000) or who are at risk for bleeding. The recommended maintenance dose is 36 million IU, three times per week. If severe reactions occur, the dose should be modified (50% reduction) or therapy should be temporarily discontinued until the adverse reactions abate. An escalating schedule of 3 million IU, 9 million IU and 18 million IU each daily for 3 days followed by 36 million IU daily for the remainder of the 10- to 12-week induction period has also produced equivalent therapeutic benefit with some amelioration of the acute toxicity in some patients.

Chronic Myelogenous Leukemia: For patients with Ph positive CML in chronic phase: Prior to initiation of therapy, a diagnosis of Philadelphia chromosome positive CML in chronic phase by the appropriate peripheral blood, bone marrow and other diagnostic testing should be made. Monitoring of hematologic parameters should be done regularly (*e.g.,* monthly). Since significant cytogenetic changes are not readily apparent until after hematologic response has occurred, and usually not until several months of therapy have elapsed, cytogenetic monitoring may be performed at less frequent intervals. Achievement of complete cytogenetic response has been observed up to 2 years following the start of interferon alfa-2a, recombinant treatment.

The recommended initial dose of interferon alfa-2a, recombinant is 9 million units daily administered as a subcutaneous or intramuscular injection. Based on clinical experience[3], short-term tolerance may be improved by gradually increasing the dose of interferon alfa-2a, recombinant over the first week of administration from 3 MIU daily for 3 days to 6 MIU daily for 3 days to the target dose of 9 MIU daily for the duration of the treatment period.

DOSAGE AND ADMINISTRATION: *(cont'd)*

The optimal dose and duration of therapy have not yet been determined. Even though the median time to achieve a complete hematologic response was 5 months in study MI400, hematologic responses have been observed up to 18 months after treatment start. Treatment should be continued until disease progression. If severe side effects occur, a treatment interruption or a reduction in either the dose or the frequency of injections may be necessary to achieve the individual maximally tolerated dose (see PRECAUTIONS).

Limited data are available on the use of interferon alfa-2a, recombinant in children with CML. In one report of 15 children with Ph-positive, adult-type CML doses between 2.5 to 5 MIU/m²/day given intramuscularly were tolerated.[9] In another study, severe adverse effects including deaths were noted in children with previously untreated, Ph-negative, juvenile CML, who received interferon doses of 30 MIU/m²/day.[14]

REFERENCES:

1. Trown PW *et al: Cancer 57* (Suppl.):1648-1656, 1986. **2.** Itri LM *et al: Cancer 59*:668-674, 1987. **3.** Jones GJ, Itri LM: *Cancer 57* (Suppl.):1709-1715, 1986. **4.** Foon KA *et al: Blood 64* (Suppl. 1):164a, 1984. **5.** Quesada Jr *et al: Cancer 57* (Suppl.):1678-1680, 1986. **6.** Krown SE *et al: N Eng J Med 308*:1071-1076, 1983. **7.** The Italian Cooperative Study Group on CML, *N Engl J Med 330*:820-825, 1994. **8.** Sokal JE *et al: Blood 63 (4)*:789-799, 1984. **9.** Dow LW *et al: Cancer 68*:1678-1684, 1991. **10.** Krown SE *et al: Proc Am Soc Clin Oncol 7*:1, 1988. **11.** Williams SJ *et al: Lancet 2*:939-941, 1987. **12.** Jonkman JHG*et al: Br J Clin Pharmacol 2(27)*:795-802, 1989. **13.** Kauppila A *et al: Int J Cancer 29*:291-294, 1982. **14.** Maybee D *et al: Proc Annu Meet Am Soc Clin Oncol 11*: A950, 1992.

HOW SUPPLIED:

Injectable Solution: *3 million IU Roferon-A Per Vial:* Each 1 ml contains 3 million IU of interferon alfa-2a, recombinant, 9 mg sodium chloride, 5 mg albumin (human) and 3 mg phenol as a preservative.

9 million IU Roferon-A Per Vial: Each 0.9 ml contains 9 million IU of interferon alfa-2a, recombinant, 8.1 mg sodium chloride, 4.5 mg albumin (human) and 2.7 mg phenol as a preservative. This dosage form should not be used for the treatment of hairy cell leukemia.

18 million IU Roferon-A Per Vial: Each 1 ml contains 6 million IU of interferon alfa-2a, recombinant, 9 mg sodium chloride, 5 mg albumin (human) and 3.3 mg phenol as a preservative. Each 0.5 ml contains 3 million IU of Interferon alfa-2a, recombinant.

36 million IU Roferon-A Per Vial: Each 1 ml contains 36 million IU of interferon alfa-2a, recombinant, 9 mg sodium chloride, 5 mg albumin (human) and 3 mg phenol as a preservative. This dosage form should not be used for the treatment of hairy cell leukemia.

Sterile Powder for Injection: 18 million IU Roferon-A Per Vial: Reconstitute with 3 ml diluent and swirl gently to dissolve. When reconstituted with accompanying diluent for roferon-A, each 1 ml of reconstituted solution contains 6 million IU interferon alfa-2a, recombinant, 9 mg sodium chloride, 1.67 mg albumin (human) and 3.3 mg phenol as a preservative. Each 0.5 ml contains 3 million IU of interferon alfa-2a, recombinant. Once the powder is reconstituted, it must be used within 30 days.

Storage: The sterile powder and its accompanying diluent, the reconstituted solution and the injectable solution should be stored in the refrigerator at 36° to 46°F (2° to 8°C). Do *not* freeze or shake.

HOW SUPPLIED - RATED THERAPEUTICALLY EQUIVALENT:

Injection, Dry-Soln - Intramuscular; - 18000000 iu

18000000 iu $189.04 ROFERON-A STERILE, Roche 00004-1993-09

HOW SUPPLIED - NOT RATED EQUIVALENT:

Injection, Dry-Soln - Intramuscular; - 9 mmunit/0.9 ml

1 ml $88.76 ROFERON-A, Roche 00004-6900-09

Injection, Solution - Intramuscular - 36000000 iv/ml

1 ml $378.07 ROFERON-A INJECTABLE, Roche 00004-2005-09

Injection, Solution - Intramuscular; - 3000000 unit/0.

0.5 ml $189.04 ROFERON-A, Roche 00004-1988-09

Injection, Solution - Intramuscular; - 3000000 unit/ml

1 ml $31.51 ROFERON-A, Roche 00004-1987-09

INTERFERON ALFA-2B, RECOMBINANT

(001546)

CATEGORIES: AIDS Related Complex; Antimetabolites; Antineoplastics; Antivirals; Biologicals; Condylomata Acuminata; Cytotoxic Agents; Genital Warts; Hairy Cell Leukemia; Hepatitis; Hepatitis B; Hepatitis C; Immunomodulators; Kaposi's Sarcoma; Leukemia; Oncologic Drugs; Orphan Drugs; Bladder Carcinoma*; Brain Carcinoma*; Cervical Carcinoma*; Melanoma*; Multiple Sclerosis*; Ovarian Carcinoma*; Renal Cell Carcinoma*; Pregnancy Category C; Recombinant DNA Origin; Sales > $500 Million; FDA Approved 1986 Jun

* Indication not approved by the FDA

BRAND NAMES: **Intron A**; *Intron-A* (Canada, Mexico); *Introna* (France); *Introne*; *Roferon*

(International brand names outside U.S. in italics)

FORMULARIES: BC-BS; Medi-Cal

COST OF THERAPY: $16,445.33 (AIDS Kaposi's Sarcoma; Kit; 10m unit/vial; 0.429/day; 365 days)

DESCRIPTION:

Intron A interferon alfa-2b, recombinant for intramuscular, subcutaneous, or intralesional Injection is a purified sterile recombinant interferon product.

Powder for Injection: The 3 million, 5 million, 18 million, 25 million, and 50 million IU packages are for use by intramuscular or subcutaneous injection or intravenous infusion. The 10 million IU package is for intramuscular, subcutaneous, or intralesional injection. (See WARNINGS and PRECAUTIONS.)

Solution for Injection: The 10 million, 18 million multidose, and 25 million IU packages are for use by intramuscular or subcutaneous injection, and not for intralesional use. (See WARNINGS and PRECAUTIONS.)

Interferon alfa-2b, recombinant for Injection has been classified as an alpha interferon and is a water soluble protein with a molecular weight of 19,271 daltons produced by recombinant DNA techniques. It is obtained from the bacterial fermentation of a strain of *Escherichia coli* bearing a genetically engineered plasmid containing an interferon alfa-2b gene from human leukocytes. The fermentation is carried out in a defined nutrient medium containing the antibiotic tetracycline hydrochloride at a concentration of 5 to 10 mg/l; the presence of this antibiotic is not detectable in the final product. The specific activity of Interferon alfa-2b, recombinant is approximately 2×10^8 IU/mg protein.

DESCRIPTION: *(cont'd)*

Powder for Injection: After reconstitution, the 3 million, 5 million, 10 million (1 ml), 18 million, 25 million, and 50 million IU vials contain, respectively, per ml either 3 million, 5 million, 10 million, 18 million, 5 million, or 50 million IU of interferon alfa-2b, recombinant. Each ml also contains 20 mg glycine, 2.3 mg sodium phosphate dibasic, 0.55 mg sodium phosphate monobasic, and 1.0 mg human albumin. Based on the specific activity of approximately 2×10^8 IU/mg protein, the corresponding quantities of interferon alfa-2b, recombinant in the vials described above are approximately 0.015 mg, 0.025 mg, 0.05 mg, 0.90 mg, 0.125 mg, and 0.25 mg protein, respectively. Prior to administration, the interferon alfa-2b powder for injection is to be reconstituted with the provided Diluent for interferon alfa-2b, recombinant for injection (bacteriostatic water for injection) containing 0.9% benzyl alcohol as a preservative. (See DOSAGE AND ADMINISTRATION). Interferon alfa-2b powder for injection is a white to cream colored powder.

Solution for Injection: Each interferon alfa-2b vial contains either 10 million IU of interferon alfa-2b, recombinant per 2 ml (5 million IU/ml), 22.8 million IU of interferon alfa-2b, recombinant per 3.8 ml (6 million IU/ml), or 25 million IU of interferon alfa-2b, recombinant per 5 ml (5 million IU/ml). Each ml also contains 20 mg glycine, 2.3 mg sodium phosphate dibasic, 0.55 mg sodium phosphate monobasic, 1.0 mg human albumin, and 1.2 mg methylparaben and 0.12 mg propylparaben as preservatives. The 18 million IU multidose vial contains a total of 22.8 million IU of interferon alfa-2b, recombinant per 3.8 ml in order to provide the delivery of six 0.5 ml doses, each containing 3 million IU of interferon alfa-2b, recombinant for Injection (for a label strength of 18 million IU). Based on the specific activity of approximately 2×10^8 IU/mg protein, the corresponding quantities of interferon alfa-2b, recombinant in the vials described above are approximately 0.05 mg, 0.114 mg, and 0.125 mg protein, respectively. These packages do not require reconstitution prior to administration. (See DOSAGE AND ADMINISTRATION). Interferon alfa-2b solution for injection is a colorless to light yellow solution.

CLINICAL PHARMACOLOGY:

General: The interferons are a family of naturally occurring small proteins and glycoproteins with molecular weights of approximately 15,000 to 27,600 daltons produced and secreted by cells in response to viral infections and to synthetic or biological inducers.

Preclinical Pharmacology: Interferons exert their cellular activities by binding to specific membrane receptors on the cell surface. Once bound to the cell membrane, interferons initiate a complex sequence of intracellular events. *In vitro* studies demonstrated that these include the induction of certain enzymes, suppression of cell proliferation, immunomodulating activities such as enhancement of the phagocytic activity of macrophages and augmentation of the specific cytotoxicity of lymphocytes for target cells, and inhibition of virus replication in virus-infected cells.

In a study using human hepatoblastoma cell line, HB 611, the *in vitro* antiviral activity of alpha interferon was demonstrated by its inhibition of hepatitis B virus (HBV) replication.

The correlation between these *in vitro* data and the clinical results is unknown. Any of these activities might contribute to interferon's therapeutic effects.

Pharmacokinetics: The pharmacokinetics of interferon alfa-2b, recombinant for Injection were studied in 12 healthy male volunteers following single doses of 5 million IU/m² administered intramuscularly, subcutaneously, and as a 30-minute intravenous infusion in a crossover design. Interferon alfa-2b concentrations were determined using a radioimmunoassay (RIA) with a detection limit equal to 10 IU/ml.

The mean serum interferon alfa-2b concentrations following intramuscular and subcutaneous injections were comparable. The maximum serum concentrations obtained via these routes were approximately 18 to 116 IU/ml and occurred 3 to 12 hours after administration. The elimination half-life of interferon alfa-2b, recombinant for Injection following both intramuscular and subcutaneous injections was approximately 2 to 3 hours. Serum concentrations were below the detection limit by 16 hours after the injections.

After intravenous administration, serum Intron A concentrations peaked (135 to 273 IU/ml) by the end of the 30-minute infusion, then declined at a slightly more rapid rate than after intramuscular or subcutaneous drug administration, becoming undetectable 4 hours after the infusion. The elimination half-life was approximately 2 hours.

Urine Intron A concentrations following a single dose (5 million IU/m²) were not detectable after any of the parenteral routes of administration. This result was expected since preliminary studies with isolated and perfused rabbit kidneys have shown that the kidney may be the main site of interferon catabolism.

There are no pharmacokinetic data available for the intralesional route of administration.

Serum Neutralizing Antibodies: In interferon alfa-2b treated patients tested for antibody activity in clinical trials, serum anti-interferon neutralizing antibodies were detected in 0% (0/90) of patients with hairy cell leukemia, 0.8% (2/260) of patients treated intralesionally for condylomata acuminata, and 4% (1/24) of patients with AIDS-Related Kaposi's Sarcoma. Serum neutralizing antibodies have been detected in <3% of patients treated with higher Intron A doses in malignancies other than hairy cell leukemia or AIDS-Related Kaposi's Sarcoma. The clinical significance of the appearance of serum anti-interferon neutralizing activity in these indications is not known.

Serum anti-interferon neutralizing antibodies were detected in 15% (7/46) of patients with chronic hepatitis NANB/C and in 13% (6/48) of patients who received Intron A therapy for chronic hepatitis B at 5 million IU QD for 4 months, and in 3% (1/33) of patients treated at 10 million IU TIW. In patients with chronic hepatitis the titers detected were low (≤1:40) and the appearance of serum anti-interferon neutralizing activity did not appear to affect safety or efficacy.

Hairy Cell Leukemia: In clinical trials in patients with hairy cell leukemia, there was depression of hematopoiesis during the first 1 to 2 months of Intron A treatment, resulting in reduced numbers of circulating red and white blood cells, and platelets. Subsequently, both splenectomized and non-splenectomized patients achieved substantial and sustained improvements in granulocytes, platelets, and hemoglobin levels in 75% of treated patients and at least some improvement (minor responses) occurred in 90%. Interferon alfa-2b treatment resulted in a decrease in bone marrow hypercellularity and hairy cell infiltrates. The hairy cell index (HCI), which represents the percent of bone marrow cellularity times the percent of hairy cell infiltrate, was greater than or equal to 50% at the beginning of the study in 87% of patients. The percentage of patients with such an HCI decreased to 25% after 6 months and to 14% after 1 year. These results indicate that even though hematologic improvement had occurred earlier, prolonged interferon alfa-2b treatment may be required to obtain maximal reduction in tumor cell infiltrates in the bone marrow.

The percentage of patients with hairy cell leukemia who required red blood cell or platelet transfusions decreased significantly during treatment and the percentage of patients with confirmed and serious infections declined as granulocyte counts improved. Reversal of splenomegaly and of clinically significant hypersplenism was demonstrated in some patients.

A study was conducted to assess the effects of extended interferon alfa-2b treatment on duration of response for patients who responded to initial therapy. In this study, 126 responding patients were randomized to receive additional interferon alfa-2b treatment for 6 months or observation for a comparable period, after 12 months of initial interferon alfa-2b therapy. During this 6-month period, 3% (2/66) of interferon alfa-2b treated patients relapsed compared with 18% (11/60) who were not treated. This represents a significant difference in

CLINICAL PHARMACOLOGY: *(cont'd)*

time to relapse in favor of continued interferon alfa-2b treatment (p=0.006/0.01, Log Rank/Wilcoxon). Since a small proportion of the total population had relapsed, median time to relapse could not be estimated in either group. A similar pattern in relapses was seen when all randomized treatment, including that beyond 6 months, and available follow-up data were assessed. The 15% (10/66) relapses among interferon alfa-2b patients occurred over a significantly longer period of time than the 40% (24/60) with observation (p=0.0002/0.0001, Log Rank/Wilcoxon). Median time to relapse was estimated, using the Kaplan-Meier method, to be 6.8 months in the observation group but could not be estimated in the interferon alfa-2b group.

Subsequent follow-up with a median time of approximately 40 months demonstrated an overall survival of 87.8%. In a comparable historical control group followed for 24 months, overall median survival was approximately 40%.

Malignant Melanoma: The safety and efficacy of interferon alfa-2b, recombinant for injection was evaluated as adjuvant to surgical treatment in patients with melanoma who were free of disease (post-surgery) but at high risk for systemic recurrence. These included patients with lesions of Breslow thickness >4 mm, or patients with lesions of any Breslow thickness with primary or recurrent nodal involvement. In a randomized controlled trial in 280 patient, 143 patients received interferon alfa-2b therapy at 20 million IU/m^2 intravenously five times per week for 4 weeks (induction phase) followed by 10 million IU/m^2 subcutaneously three times per week for 48 weeks (maintenance phase). Interferon alfa-2b therapy was begun ≤56 days after surgical resection. The remaining 137 patients were observed.

Interferon alfa-2b therapy produced a significant increase in relapse-free and overall survival. Median time to relapse for the interferon alfa-2b treated patients was 1.72 years *versus* 0.98 years (p<0.01, stratified Log Rank). The estimated 5-year relapse-free survival rate, using the Kaplan-Meier method, was 37% for interferon alfa-2b treated patients *versus* 26% for observation patients. Median overall survival time for Intron A treated patients *versus* observation patients was 3.82 years *versus* 2.78 years (p=0.47, stratified Log Rank). The estimated 5–year overall survival rate, using the Kaplan-Meier method, was 46% for the interferon alfa-2b treated patients *versus* 37% for observation patients.

Condylomata Acuminata: Condylomata acuminata (venereal or genital warts) are associated with infections of the human papilloma virus (HPV). The safety and efficacy of interferon alfa-2b, recombinant for Injection in the treatment of condylomata acuminata were evaluated in three controlled double-blind clinical trials. In these studies interferon alfa-2b doses of 1 million IU per lesion were administered intralesionally three times a week (TIW), in ≤5 lesions per patient for 3 weeks. The patients were observed for up to 16 weeks after completion of the full treatment course.

Interferon alfa-2b treatment of condylomata was significantly more effective than placebo, as measured by disappearance of lesions, decreases in lesion size, and by an overall change in disease status. Of 192 interferon alfa-2b treated patients and 206 placebo treated patients who were evaluable for efficacy at the time of best response during the course of the study, 42% of interferon alfa-2b patients *versus* 17% of placebo patients experienced clearing of all treated lesions. Likewise 24% of interferon alfa-2b patients *versus* 8% of placebo patients experienced marked (≥75% to <100%) reduction in lesion size, 18% *versus* 9% experienced moderate (≥50% to ≤75%) reduction in lesion size, 10% *versus* 42% had a slight (<50%) reduction in lesion size, 5% *versus* 24% had no change in lesion size and 0% *versus* 1% experienced exacerbation (p<0.001).

In one of these studies, 43% (54/125) of patients in whom multiple (≤3) lesions were treated, experienced complete clearing of all treated lesions during the course of the study. Of these patients, 81% remained cleared 16 weeks after treatment was initiated.

Patients who did not achieve total clearing of all their treated lesions had these same lesions treated with a second course of therapy. During this second course of treatment, 38% to 67% of patients had clearing of all treated lesions. The overall percentage of patients who had cleared all their treated lesions after 2 courses of treatment ranged from 57% to 85%.

Interferon alfa-2b treated lesions showed improvement within 2 to 4 weeks after the start of treatment in the above study; maximal response to interferon alfa-2b therapy was noted 4 to 8 weeks after initiation of treatment.

The response to interferon alfa-2b therapy was better in patients who had condylomata for shorter durations than in patients with lesions for a longer duration.

Another study involved 97 patients in whom three lesions were treated with either an intralesional injection of 1.5 million IU of interferon alfa-2b, recombinant for Injection per lesion followed by a topical application of 25% podophyllin, or a topical application of 25% podophyllin alone. Treatment was given once a week for 3 weeks. The combined treatment of interferon alfa-2b, recombinant for Injection and podophyllin was shown to be significantly more effective than podophyllin alone, as determined by the number of patients whose lesions cleared. This significant difference in response was evident after the second treatment (week 3) and continued through 8 weeks posttreatment. At the time of the patient's best response, 67% (33/49) of the interferon alfa-2b, recombinant for Injection and podophyllin treated patients had all three treated lesions clear while 42% (20/48) of the podophyllin treated patients had all three clear (p=0.003).

AIDS-Related Kaposi's Sarcoma: The safety and efficacy of interferon alfa-2b, recombinant for Injection in the treatment of Kaposi's Sarcoma (KS), a common manifestation of the Acquired Immune Deficiency Syndrome (AIDS), were evaluated in clinical trials in 144 patients.

In one study, interferon alfa-2b doses of 30 million IU/m^2 were administered subcutaneously three times per week (TIW), to patients with AIDS-Related KS. Doses were adjusted for patient tolerance. The average weekly dose delivered in the first 4 weeks was 150 million IU; at the end of 12 weeks this averaged 110 million IU/week; and by 24 weeks averaged 75 million IU/week.

Forty-four percent of asymptomatic patients responded *versus* 7% of symptomatic patients. The median time to response was approximately 2 months and 1 month, respectively, for asymptomatic and symptomatic patients. The median duration of response was approximately 3 months and 1 month, respectively, for the asymptomatic and symptomatic patients. Baseline T4/T8 ratios were 0.46 for responders *versus* 0.33 for nonresponders.

In another study, interferon alfa-2b doses of 35 million IU were administered subcutaneously, daily (QD), for 12 weeks. Maintenance treatment, with every other day dosing (QOD), was continued for up to 1 year in patients achieving antitumor and antiviral responses. The median time to response was 2 months and median duration of response was 5 months in the asymptomatic patients.

In all studies, the likelihood of response was greatest in patients with relatively intact immune systems as assessed by baseline CD4 counts (interchangeable with T4 counts). Results at doses of 30 million IU/m^2 TIW and 35 million IU/QD, subcutaneously were similar and are provided together in (TABLE 1). This table demonstrates the relationship of response to baseline CD4 count in both asymptomatic and symptomatic patients in the 30 million IU/m^2 TIW and the 35 million IU/QD treatment groups.

In the 30 million IU study group, 7% (5/72) of patients were complete responders and 22% (16/72) of the patients were partial responders. The 35 million IU study had 13% (3/23 patients) complete responders and 17% (4/23) partial responders.

CLINICAL PHARMACOLOGY: *(cont'd)*

TABLE 1 Response By Baseline CD4 Count* In AIDS-Related Ks Patients

	TIW, SC and 35 million IU QD, SC Asymptomatic		Symptomatic	
CD4<200	4/14	(29%)	0/19	(0%)
200≤CD4≤400	6/12	(50%)	0/5	(0%)
CD4>400	5/7	(71%)	0/0	(0%)

* Data for CD4, and asymptomatic and symptomatic classification were not available for all patients.

For patients who received 30 million IU TIW, the median survival time was longer in patients with CD4 greater than 200 (30.7 months) than in patients with CD4 less than or equal to 200 (8.9 months). Among responders, the median survival time was 22.6 months *versus* 9.7 months in nonresponders.

Chronic Hepatitis Non-A, Non-B/C (NANB/C): The safety and efficacy of Intron A Interferon alfa-2b, recombinant for Injection in the treatment of chronic hepatitis NANB/C were evaluated in 4 randomized controlled clinical studies in which Intron A doses of 1, 2, or 3 million IU three times a week (TIW), were administered subcutaneously for 6 months (23 or 24 weeks). The patients were 18 years of age or older and had compensated liver disease. Of the 332 patients evaluable for efficacy, 81% had a history of blood or blood product exposure, 8% had a history of intravenous drug abuse, 2% had a history of surgery without blood products, and the remainder had other exposure. Retrospectively, 86% (172/199) of the patients with blood or blood product exposure who were tested were found to be positive for antibody to hepatitis C virus (HCV).

In each of 3 clinical studies, interferon alfa-2b therapy at 3 million IU, TIW, resulted in a reduction in serum alanine aminotransferase (ALT) in a statistically significantly greater proportion of patients *verus* control patients (see TABLE 2).

TABLE 2 Alt Responses† In Chronic Hepatitis NANB/C Patients

Study Number	Treatment Group - Number of Patients (%) Intron A 3 million IU		Controls‡		P(S) Value
1[1]	29/55	(53%)	5/55	(9%)	<0.001
2[2]	10/23	(43%)	3/25	(12%)	0.02
3[3]	12/17	(71%)	3/17	(18%)	0.005
All Studies	51/95	(54%)	11/97	(11%)	<0.001

† Includes reduction in serum ALT to: normal. near normal (≤1.5 times the upper limit of normal), or partial response (>50% decrease in serum ALT).
‡ Untreated or Placebo (S)Intron A 3 million IU TIW. 6 months versus control.

Of the 54% of patients responding to interferon alfa-2b therapy at a dose of 3 million IU, 70% achieved reductions in ALT levels to normal, 18% achieved reductions to near normal levels, and 12% achieved partial responses.

Histological improvement was evaluated by comparison of pre- and posttreatment liver biopsies using the semi-quantitative Knodell Histology Activity Index (HAI).[4]

In one of the three studies there was histological improvement in a statistically significantly greater proportion of interferon alfa-2b treated patients compared to controls (see TABLE 3). A similar, but not statistically significant trend for improvement was observed in the other two studies.

TABLE 3 Histological Improvement‡ In Chronic Hepatitis NANB/C Patients

Study Number	Treatment Group - Number of Patients (%) Intron A 3 million IU		Controls**		P § Value
1	29/45	(64%)	18/36	(50%)	0.26
2	12/19	(63%)	10/18	(56%)	0.75
3	14/16	(88%)	8/15	(53%)	0.054
All Studies	55/80	(69%)	36/69	(52%)	0.04

‡ Assessed by the Knodell Histology Activity Index which includes: Category I - Periportal necrosis Category II - Intralobular degeneration and necrosis Category III - Portal inflammation Category IV - Fibrosis
** Untreated or Placebo
§ Intron A 3 million IU, TIW, 6 months compared to control for improvement versus no improvement.

Subsequent combined analysis of results for the 3 studies showed histological improvement in a statistically significantly greater proportion of patients treated with Intron A doses of 3 million IU than in control patients (p=0.04). The improvement was due primarily to decreases in severity of necrosis and degeneration in the lobular and periportal regions (Knodell HAI Categories I + II), which were observed in 65% (52/80) of patients treated at 3 million IU compared to 46% (32/70) of controls. Diminution of disease activity in these regions of the liver was accompanied by a reduction or normalization of serum ALT in many patients. Disease activity increased in these regions in only 3% of all interferon alfa-2b treated patients, whereas an increase was observed in 16% of the controls. No patient achieving an ALT response with 3 million IU interferon alfa-2b therapy showed increased periportal or lobular necrosis and degeneration.

Patients were followed for 6 months after the end of interferon alfa-2b therapy. During this period the ALT response was maintained in 51% (26/51) of patients who responded at the 3 million IU TIW dose. Of patients who relapsed during the follow-up period and were retreated at this dose, 83% (15/18) responded to retreatment.

Chronic Hepatitis B: The safety and efficacy of interferon alfa-2b, recombinant for Injection in the treatment of chronic hepatitis B were evaluated in three clinical trials in which interferon alfa-2b doses of 30 to 35 million IU per week were administered subcutaneously (SC), as either 5 million IU daily (QD), or 10 million IU three times a week (TIW) for 16 weeks *versus* no treatment. All patients were 18 years of age or older with compensated liver disease, and had chronic hepatitis B virus (HBV) infection (serum HBsAg positive for at least 6 months) and HBV replication (serum HBeAg positive). Patients were also serum HBV-DNA positive, an additional indicator of HBV replication, as measured by a research assay.[5,6] All patients had elevated serum alanine aminotransferase (ALT) and liver biopsy findings compatible with the diagnosis of chronic hepatitis. Patients with the presence of antibody to human immunodeficiency virus (anti-HIV) or antibody to hepatitis delta virus (anti-HDV) in the serum were excluded from the studies.

Virologic response to treatment was defined in these studies as a loss of serum markers of HBV replication (HBeAg and HBV DNA). Secondary parameters of response included loss of serum HBsAg, decreases in serum ALT, and improvement in liver histology.

CLINICAL PHARMACOLOGY: *(cont'd)*

In each of two randomized controlled studies, a significantly greater proportion of Intron A treated patients exhibited a virologic response compared with untreated control patients (see TABLE 4). In a third study without a concurrent control group, a similar response rate to interferon alfa-2b therapy was observed. Pretreatment with prednisone, evaluated in two of the studies, did not improve the response rate and provided no additional benefit.

TABLE 4 Virologic Response* In Chronic Hepatitis B Patients

Study Number	Treatment Group† - Number of Patients (%): Interferon alfa-2b 5 million IU QD		Interferon alfa-2b 10 million IU TIW		Untreated Controls		P** Value
1[5]	15/38	(39%)	-	-	3/42	(7%)	0.0009
2	-	-	10/24	(42%)	1/22	(5%)	0.005
3[6]	-	-	13/24‡	(54%)	2/27	(7%)‡	NA‡
All Studies	15/38	(39%)	23/48	(48%)	6/91	(7%)	-

* Loss of HBeAg and HBV DNA by 6 months posttherapy.
† Patients pretreated with prednisone not shown.
** Intron A treatment group versus untreated control.
‡ Untreated control patients evaluated after 24 week observation period. A subgroup subsequently received interferon alfa-2b therapy. A direct comparison is not applicable (NA).

The response to interferon alfa-2b therapy was durable. No patient responding to interferon alfa-2b therapy at a dose of 5 million IU QD or 10 million IU TIW, relapsed during the follow-up period which ranged from 2 to 6 months after treatment ended. The loss of serum HBeAg and HBV DNA was maintained 100% of 19 responding patients followed for 3.5 to 36 months after the end of therapy.

In a proportion of responding patients, loss of HBeAg was followed by the loss of HBsAg. HBsAg was lost in 27% (4/15) of patients who responded to interferon alfa-2b therapy at a dose of 5 million IU QD, and 35% (8/23) of patients who responded to 10 million IU TIW. No untreated control patient lost HBsAg in these studies.

In a pilot study, 12 patients responding to interferon alfa-2b therapy were followed for 3.8 to 6.6 years after treatment; 100% (12/12) remained serum HBeAg negative and 58% (7/12) loss serum HBsAg.

Interferon alfa-2b therapy resulted in normalization of serum ALT in a significantly greater proportion of treated patients compared to untreated patients in each of two controlled studies (see TABLE 5). In a third study without a concurrent control group, normalization of serum ALT was observed in 50% (12/24) of patients receiving Intron A therapy.

TABLE 5 Alt Responses* In Chronic Hepatitis B Patients

Study Number	Treatment Group - Number of Patients (%): Interferon alfa-2b 5 million IU QD		Interferon alfa-2b 10 million IU TIW		Untreated Controls		P** Value
1	16/38	(42%)	-	-	8/42	(19%)	0.03
2	-	-	10/24	(42%)	1/22	(5%)	0.0034
3	-	-	12/24†	(50%)	2/27	(7%)†	NA†
All Studies	16/38	(42%)	22/48	(46%)	11/91	(12%)	-

* Reduction in serum ALT to normal by 6 months posttherapy.
** Interferon alfa-2b treatment group versusuntreated control.
† Untreated control patients evaluated after 24 week observation period. A subgroup subsequently received interferon alfa-2b therapy. A direct comparison is not applicable (NA).

Virologic response was associated with a reduction in serum ALT to normal or near normal (≤1.5 times the upper limit of normal) in 87% (13/15) of patients responding to Intron A therapy at 5 million IU QD, and 100% (23/23) of patients responding to 10 million IU TIW.

Improvement in liver histology was evaluated in Studies 1 and 3 by comparison of pre- and 6 month posttreatment liver biopsies using the semi-quantitative Knodell Histology Activity Index.[4] No statistically significant difference in liver histology was observed in treated patients compared to control patients in Study 1. Although statistically significant histological improvement from baseline was observed in treated patients in Study 3 ($p \leq 0.01$), there was no control group for comparison. Of those patients exhibiting a virologic response following treatment with 5 million IU QD or 10 million IU TIW, histological improvement was observed in 85% (17/20) compared to 36% (9/25) of patients who were not virologic responders. The histological improvement was due primarily to decreases in severity of necrosis, degeneration, and inflammation in the periportal, lobular, and portal regions of the liver (Knodell Categories I + II + III). Continued histological improvement was observed in four responding patients who lost serum HBsAg and were followed 2 to 4 years after the end of Intron A therapy.[7]

INDICATIONS AND USAGE:

General: Interferon alfa-2b, recombinant for Injection is indicated in patients 18 years of age or older for the treatment of hairy cell leukemia, selected cases of condylomata acuminata involving external surfaces of the genital and perianal areas, selected patients with AIDS-Related Kaposi's Sarcoma, chronic hepatitis Non-A, Non-B/C (NANB/C) in patients with compensated liver disease who have a history of blood or blood product exposure and/or are HCV antibody positive, and chronic hepatitis B in patients with compensated liver disease and HBV replication (serum HBeAg positive).

Hairy Cell Leukemia: Interferon alfa-2b, recombinant for Injection is indicated for the treatment of patients 18 years of age or older with hairy cell leukemia. Studies have shown that interferon alfa-2b therapy can produce clinically meaningful regression or stabilization of this disease, both in previously splenectomized and non-splenectomized patients.

Prior to initiation of therapy, tests should be performed to quantitate peripheral blood hemoglobin, platelets, granulocytes and hairy cells and bone marrow hairy cells. These parameters should be monitored periodically during treatment to determine whether response to treatment has occurred. If a patient does not respond within 6 months, treatment should be discontinued. If a response to treatment does occur, treatment usually should be continued until no further improvement is observed and these laboratory parameters have been stable for about 3 months (see DOSAGE AND ADMINISTRATION). Responding patients may benefit from continued treatment after that time point with fewer relapses and a longer relapse-free interval. If treatment with Intron A therapy has been interrupted, it should be noted that re-treatment with Intron A therapy has led to response in greater than 90% of patients.

Malignant Melanoma: Interferon alfa-2b, recombinant for injection is indicated as adjuvant to surgical treatment in patients 18 years of age or older with malignant melanoma who are free of disease but at high risk for systemic recurrence, within 56 days of surgery.

INDICATIONS AND USAGE: *(cont'd)*

Condylomata Acuminata: Interferon alfa-2b, recombinant for Injection is indicated for intralesional treatment of selected patients 18 years of age or older with condylomata acuminata involving external surfaces of the genital and perianal areas (see DOSAGE AND ADMINISTRATION).

In selecting patients for interferon alfa-2b treatment, the physician should consider the nature of the patient's lesion and the patient's past treatment history, in addition to the patient's ability to comply with the treatment regimen. Interferon alfa-2b therapy offers an additional approach to treatment in condylomata and is particularly useful for those patients who do not respond satisfactorily to other treatment modalities (*e.g.,* podophyllin resin, surgery, cryotherapy, chemotherapy, and laser therapy), or whose lesions are more readily treatable by interferon alfa-2b, recombinant for Injection than by other treatments.

The use of this product in adolescents has not been studied. Interferon alfa has been shown to affect the menstrual cycle in nonhuman primates and to decrease serum estradiol and progesterone levels in women. Consideration should be given as to whether the adolescent patient should be treated.

AIDS-Related Kaposi's Sarcoma: Interferon alfa-2b, recombinant for Injection is indicated for the treatment of selected patients 18 years of age or older with AIDS-Related Kaposi's Sarcoma. Studies have demonstrated a greater likelihood of response to interferon alfa-2b therapy in patients who are without systemic symptoms, who have limited lymphadenopathy and who have a relatively intact immune system.

Lesion measurements and blood counts should be performed prior to initiation of therapy and should be monitored periodically during treatment to determine whether response to treatment or disease stabilization has occurred.

When disease stabilization or a response to treatment occurs, treatment should continue until there is no further evidence of tumor or until discontinuation is required by evidence of a severe opportunistic infection or adverse effect (see DOSAGE AND ADMINISTRATION).

Chronic Hepatitis Non-A, Non-B/C (NANB/C): Interferon alfa-2b, recombinant for Injection is indicated for the treatment of chronic hepatitis Non-A, Non-B/C (NANB/C) in patients 18 years of age or older with compensated liver disease who have a history of blood or blood product exposure and/or are HCV antibody positive. Studies in these patients demonstrated that interferon alfa-2b therapy can produce clinically meaningful effects on this disease, manifested by normalization of serum alanine aminotransferase (ALT) and reduction in liver necrosis and degeneration.

A liver biopsy should be performed to establish the diagnosis of chronic hepatitis. Patients should be tested for the presence of antibody to HCV. Patients with other causes of chronic hepatitis, including autoimmune hepatitis, should be excluded. Prior to initiation of interferon alfa-2b therapy, the physician should establish that the patient has compensated liver disease. The following patient entrance criteria for compensated liver disease were used in the clinical studies and should be considered before interferon alfa-2b treatment of patients with chronic hepatitis NANB/C:

No history of hepatic encephalopathy, variceal bleeding, ascites, or other clinical signs of decompensation

Bilirubin ≤2 mg/dl

Albumin =Stable and within normal limits

Prothrombin Time <3 seconds prolonged

WBC ≥3000/mm^3

Platelets ≥70,000/mm^3

Serum creatinine should be normal or near normal.

Prior to initiation of interferon alfa-2b therapy, CBC and platelet counts should be evaluated in order to establish baselines for monitoring potential toxicity. These tests should be repeated at weeks 1 and 2 following initiation of interferon alfa-2b therapy, and monthly thereafter. Serum ALT should be evaluated after 2, 16, and 24 weeks of therapy to assess response to treatment (see DOSAGE AND ADMINISTRATION).

Patients with preexisting thyroid abnormalities may be treated if thyroid stimulating hormone (TSH) levels can be maintained in the normal range by medication. TSH levels must be within normal limits upon initiation of interferon alfa-2b treatment and TSH testing should be repeated at 3 and 6 months (see PRECAUTIONS, Laboratory Tests).

Chronic Hepatitis B: Interferon alfa-2b, recombinant for Injection is indicated for the treatment of chronic hepatitis B in patients 18 years of age or older with compensated liver disease and HBV replication. Patients must be serum HBsAg positive for at least 6 months and have HBV replication (serum HBeAg positive) with elevated serum ALT. Studies in these patients demonstrated that interferon alfa-2b therapy can produce virologic remission of this disease (loss of serum HBeAg), and normalization of serum aminotransferases. Interferon alfa-2b therapy resulted in the loss of serum HBsAg in some responding patients.

Prior to initiation of interferon alfa-2b therapy, it is recommended that a liver biopsy be performed to establish the presence of chronic hepatitis and the extent of liver damage. The physician should establish that the patient has compensated liver disease. The following patient entrance criteria for compensated liver disease were used in the clinical studies and should be considered before interferon alfa-2b treatment of patients with chronic hepatitis B:

No history of hepatic encephalopathy, variceal bleeding, ascites, or other signs of clinical decompensation

Bilirubin Normal

Albumin Stable and within normal limits

Prothrombin Time <3 seconds prolonged

WBC ≥4000/mm^3

Platelets ≥100,000/mm^3

Patients with causes of chronic hepatitis other than chronic hepatitis B or chronic hepatitis NANB/C should be treated with interferon alfa-2b, recombinant for Injection. CBC and platelet counts should be evaluated prior to initiation of interferon alfa-2b therapy in order to establish baselines for monitoring potential toxicity. These tests should be repeated at treatment weeks 1, 2, 4, 8, 12, and 16. Liver function tests, including serum ALT, albumin, and bilirubin, should be evaluated at treatment weeks 1, 2, 4, 8, 12, and 16. HBeAg, HBsAg, and ALT should be evaluated at the end of therapy, as well as 3 and 6 months posttherapy, since patients may become virologic responders during the 6-month period following the end of treatment. In clinical studies, 39% (15/38) of responding patients lost HBeAg 1 to 6 months following the end of interferon alfa-2b therapy. Of responding patients who lost HBsAg, 58% (7/12) did so 1 to 6 months posttreatment.

A transient increase in ALT ≥2 times baseline value (flare) can occur during Intron A therapy for chronic hepatitis B. In clinical trials, this flare generally occurred 8 to 12 weeks after initiation of therapy and was more frequent in responders (63%, 24/38) than in nonresponders (27%, 13/48). However, elevations in bilirubin ≥3 mg/dl occurred infrequently (2%, 2/86) during therapy. When ALT flare occurs, in general, interferon alfa-2b therapy should be continued unless signs and symptoms of liver failure are observed. During ALT flare, clinical symptomatology and liver function tests including ALT, prothrombin time, alkaline phosphatase, albumin, and bilirubin, should be monitored at approximately 2-week intervals (see WARNINGS).

CONTRAINDICATIONS:

Interferon alfa-2b, recombinant for Injection is contraindicated in patients with a history of hypersensitivity to interferon alfa or any component of the injection.

WARNINGS:

General: Moderate to severe adverse experiences may require modification of the patient's dosage regimen, or in some cases termination of interferon alfa-2b therapy. Because of the fever and other "flu-like" symptoms associated with interferon alfa-2b administration, it should be used cautiously in patients with debilitating medical conditions, such as those with a history of pulmonary disease (*e.g.,* chronic obstructive pulmonary disease), or diabetes mellitus prone to ketoacidosis. Caution should also be observed in patients with coagulation disorders (*e.g.,* thrombophlebitis, pulmonary embolism) or severe myelosuppression.

Patients with platelet counts of less than 50,000/mm^3 should not be administered Interferon alfa-2b, recombinant for Injection intramuscularly, but instead by subcutaneous administration.

Interferon alfa-2b therapy should be used cautiously in patients with a history of cardiovascular disease such as unstable angina or uncontrolled congestive heart failure. Those patients with a recent history of myocardial infarction and/or previous or current arrhythmic disorder who require interferon alfa-2b therapy should be closely monitored (see PRECAUTIONS, Laboratory Tests). Cardiovascular adverse experiences, which include hypotension, arrhythmia, or tachycardia of 150 beats per minute or greater, and transient reversible cardiomyopathy have been observed in some interferon alfa-2b treated patients. Transient reversible cardiomyopathy was reported in approximately 2% of the AIDS-Related Kaposi's Sarcoma patients treated with interferon alfa-2b, recombinant for Injection. The incidence of these complications in patients with preexisting heart disease is unknown. Hypotension may occur during interferon alfa-2b administration, or up to 2 days posttherapy, and may require supportive therapy including fluid replacement to maintain intravascular volume. Supraventricular arrhythmias occurred rarely and appeared to be correlated with preexisting conditions and prior therapy with cardiotoxic agents. These adverse experiences were controlled by modifying the dose or discontinuing treatment, but may require specific additional therapy.

DEPRESSION AND SUICIDAL BEHAVIOR INCLUDING SUICIDAL IDEALATION, SUICIDAL ATTEMPTS, AND COMPLETED SUICIDES HAVE BEEN REPORTED IN ASSOCIATION WITH TREATMENT WITH ALFA INTERFERONS, INCLUDING INTERFERON ALFA-2B THERAPY. Patients with a preexisting psychiatric condition, especially depression, or a history of severe psychiatric disorder should not be treated with interferon alfa-2b, recombinant for injection.[8] Interferon alfa-2b therapy should be discontinued for any patient developing severe depression or other psychiatric disorder during treatment. Obtundation and coma have also been observed in some patients, usually elderly, treated at higher doses. While these effects are usually rapidly reversible upon discontinuation of therapy, full resolution of symptoms has taken up to 3 weeks in a few severe episodes. Narcotics, hypnotics, or sedatives may be used concurrently with caution and patients should be closely monitored until the adverse effects have resolved.

Patients with a preexisting psychiatric condition, especially depression, or a history of severe psychiatric disorder should not be treated with interferon alfa-2b, recombinant for Injection.[8]

Interferon alfa-2b therapy should be discontinued for any patient developing severe depression or other psychiatric disorder during treatment. Central nervous system effects manifested by depression, confusion, and other alterations of mental status have been observed in some interferon alfa-2b treated patients, and suicidal ideation and attempted suicide have been observed rarely. These adverse effects have occurred in patients treated with recommended doses as well as in patients treated with higher interferon alfa-2b doses. More significant obtundation and coma have also been observed in some patients, usually elderly, treated at higher doses. While these effects are usually rapidly reversible upon discontinuation of therapy, full resolution of symptoms has taken up to 3 weeks in a few severe episodes. Narcotics, hypnotics, or sedatives may be used concurrently with caution and patients should be closely monitored until the adverse effects have resolved.

Patients with preexisting thyroid abnormalities whose thyroid function cannot be maintained in the normal range by medication should not be treated with interferon alfa-2b, recombinant for Injection. Therapy should be discontinued for patients developing thyroid abnormalities during treatment whose thyroid function cannot be normalized by medication.

Hepatotoxicity, including fatality, has been observed rarely in interferon alfa-2b treated patients. Any patient developing liver function abnormalities during treatment should be monitored closely and if appropriate, treatment should be discontinued.

Pulmonary infiltrates, pneumonitis and pneumonia, including fatality, have been observed rarely in interferon alfa treated patients, including those treated with interferon alfa-2b, recombinant for Injection. The etiologic explanation for these pulmonary findings has yet to be established. Any patient developing fever, cough, dyspnea, or other respiratory symptoms should have a chest X-ray taken. If the chest X-ray shows pulmonary infiltrates or there is evidence of pulmonary function impairment, the patient should be closely monitored, and, if appropriate, interferon alfa treatment should be discontinued. While this has been reported more often in patients with chronic hepatitis NANB/C treated with interferon alfa, it has also been reported in patients with oncologic diseases treated with interferon alfa.

Retinal hemorrhages, cotton-wool spots, and retinal artery or vein obstruction have been observed rarely in patients treated with interferon alfa, including those treated with interferon alfa-2b, recombinant for Injection. The etiologic explanation for these findings has not yet been established. These events appear to occur after use of the drug for several months, but also have been reported after shorter treatment periods. Diabetes mellitus or hypertension have been present in some patients. Any patient complaining of changes in visual acuity or visual fields, or reporting other ophthalmologic symptoms during treatment with interferon alfa-2b, recombinant for Injection, should have an eye examination. Because the retinal events may have to be differentiated from those seen with diabetic or hypertensive retinopathy, a baseline ocular examination is recommended prior to treatment with interferon in patients with diabetes mellitus or hypertension.

The 50 million IU strength of the interferon alfa-2b Powder for Injection is not to be used for the treatment of hairy cell leukemia, condylomata acuminata, chronic hepatitis NANB/C, or chronic hepatitis B. The 3 million, 5 million, 18 million multidose, and 25 million IU strengths of the Intron A Powder for Injection are not to be used for the intralesional treatment of condylomata acuminata since the dilution required for the intralesional use would result in hypertonic solution.

The 10 million, 18 million multidose, and 25 million IU strengths of the interferon alfa-2b Solution for Injection are not to be used for the treatment of condylomata acuminata or AIDS-Related Kaposi's Sarcoma.

AIDS-Related Kaposi's Sarcoma: Interferon alfa-2b therapy should not be used for patients with rapidly progressive visceral disease (see CLINICAL PHARMACOLOGY). Also of note, there may be synergistic adverse effects between interferon alfa-2b, recombinant for Injection and zidovudine. Patients receiving concomitant zidovudine have had a higher incidence of neutropenia than that expected with zidovudine alone. Careful monitoring of the WBC count is indicated in all patients who are myelosuppressed and in all patients receiving other myelosuppressive medications. The effects of interferon alfa-2b, recombinant for injection when combined with other drugs used in the treatment of AIDS-Related disease are unknown.

WARNINGS: *(cont'd)*

Chronic Hepatitis Non-A, Non-B/C (NANB/C) and Chronic Hepatitis B: Patients with decompensated liver disease, autoimmune hepatitis or a history of autoimmune disease, and patients who are immunosuppressed transplant recipients should not be treated with interferon alfa-2b, recombinant for Injection. There are reports of worsening liver disease, including jaundice, hepatic encephalopathy, hepatic failure and death following interferon alfa-2b therapy in such patients. Therapy should be discontinued for any patient developing signs and symptoms of liver failure.

Chronic hepatitis B patients with evidence of decreasing hepatic synthetic functions, such as decreasing albumin levels or prolongation of prothrombin time, who nevertheless meet the entry criteria to start therapy, may be at increased risk of clinical decompensation if a flare of aminotransferases occurs during interferon alfa-2b treatment. In such patients, if increases in ALT occur during interferon alfa-2b therapy for chronic hepatitis B, they should be followed carefully including close monitoring of clinical symptomatology and liver function tests, including ALT, prothrombin time, alkaline phosphatase, albumin, and bilirubin. In considering these patients for interferon alfa-2b therapy, the potential risks must be evaluated against the potential benefits of treatment.

PRECAUTIONS:

General: Acute serious hypersensitivity reactions (*e.g.,* urticaria, angioedema, bronchoconstriction, anaphylaxis) have been observed rarely in interferon alfa-2b treated patients; if such an acute reaction develops, the drug should be discontinued immediately and appropriate medical therapy instituted. Transient rashes have occurred in some patients following injection, but have not necessitated treatment interruption.

While fever may be related to the flu-like syndrome reported commonly in patients treated with interferon, other causes of persistent fever should be ruled out.

There have been reports of interferon exacerbating preexisting psoriasis; therefore, Intron A therapy should be used in these patients only if the potential benefit justifies the potential risk.

Variations in dosage, routes of administration, and adverse reactions exist among different brands of interferon. Therefore, do not use different brands of interferon in any single treatment regimen.

Information for Patients: Patients receiving interferon alfa-2b treatment should be directed in its appropriate use, informed of benefits and risks associated with treatment, and referred to the Patient Information Sheet. This information is intended to aid in the safe and effective use of this medication. It is not a disclosure of all possible adverse or intended effects.

If home use is prescribed, a puncture-resistant container for the disposal of used syringes and needles should be supplied to the patient. Patients should be thoroughly instructed in the importance of proper disposal and cautioned against any reuse of needles and syringes. The full container should be disposed of according to the directions provided by the physician. For detailed instructions see Patient Information Sheet.

Patients should be cautioned not to change brands of interferon without medical consultation as a change in dosage may result.

Patients receiving high interferon alfa-2b doses should be cautioned against performing tasks that would require complete mental alertness, such as operating machinery or driving a motor vehicle.

The most common adverse experiences occurring with interferon alfa-2b therapy are "flu-like" symptoms, such as fever, headache, fatigue, anorexia, nausea, or vomiting (see ADVERSE REACTIONS) and appear to decrease in severity as treatment continues. Some of these "flu-like" symptoms may be minimized by bedtime administration. Acetaminophen may be used to prevent or partially alleviate the fever and headache. Another common adverse experience is thinning of the hair.

It is advised that patients be well hydrated, especially during the initial stages of treatment.

Laboratory Tests: In addition to those tests normally required for monitoring patients, the following laboratory tests are recommended for all patients on Intron A therapy, prior to beginning treatment and then periodically thereafter.

Standard Hematologic Tests: including hemoglobin, complete and differential white blood cell counts, and platelet count.

Blood Chemistries: electrolytes, liver function tests, and TSH.

Those patients who have preexisting cardiac abnormalities and/or are in advanced stages of cancer should have electrocardiograms taken prior to and during the course of treatment.

Mild to moderate leukopenia and elevated serum liver enzyme (SGOT) levels have been reported with intralesional administration of interferon alfa-2b, recombinant for Injection (see ADVERSE REACTIONS); therefore, the monitoring of these laboratory parameters should be considered.

Baseline chest X-rays are suggested and should be repeated if clinically indicated.

For malignant melanoma patients, differential WBC count and liver function tests should be monitored weekly during the induction phase of therapy and monthly during the maintenance phase of therapy.

For specific recommendations in chronic hepatitis NANB/C and chronic hepatitis B, (see INDICATIONS AND USAGE).

Carcinogenesis, Mutagenesis, Impairment of Fertility: Studies with interferon alfa-2b, recombinant for Injection have not been performed to determine carcinogenicity.

Interferon may impair fertility. In studies of interferon administration in nonhuman primates, menstrual cycle abnormalities have been observed. Decreases in serum estradiol and progesterone concentrations have been reported in women treated with human leukocyte interferon.[9] Therefore, fertile women should not receive interferon alfa-2b therapy unless they are using effective contraception during the therapy period. Interferon alfa-2b therapy should be used with caution in fertile men.

Mutagenicity studies have demonstrated that interferon alfa-2b, recombinant for Injection is not mutagenic.

Studies in mice (0.1, 1.0 million IU/day), rats (4, 20, 100 million IU/kg/day), and cynomolgus monkeys (1.1 million IU/kg/day; 0.25, 0.75, 2.5 million IU/kg/day) injected with interferon alfa-2b, recombinant for Injection for up to 9 days, 3 months, and 1 month, respectively, have revealed no evidence of toxicity. However, in cynomolgus monkeys (4, 20, 100 million IU/kg/day) injected daily for 3 months with interferon alfa-2b, recombinant for injection toxicity was observed at the mid- and high-doses and mortality was observed at the high dose.

However, due to the known species-specificity of interferon, the effects in animals are unlikely to be predictive of those in man.

Pregnancy Category C: Interferon alfa-2b, recombinant for injection has been shown to have abortifacient effects in *Macaca mulatta* (rhesus monkeys) at 7.5, 15, and 30 million IU/kg (90, 180, and 360 times the intramuscular or subcutaneous dose of 2 million IU/m^2). Although abortion was observed in all dose groups, it was only statistically significant at the mid- and high-dose groups. There are no adequate and well-controlled studies in pregnant women. Interferon alfa-2b therapy should be used during pregnancy only if the potential benefit justifies the potential risk to the fetus.

PRECAUTIONS: *(cont'd)*

Nursing Mothers: It is not known whether this drug is excreted in human milk. However, studies in mice have shown that mouse interferons are excreted into the milk. Because of the potential for serious adverse reactions from the drug in nursing infants, a decision should be made whether to discontinue nursing or to discontinue interferon alfa-2b therapy, taking into account the importance of the drug to the mother.

Pediatric Use: Safety and effectiveness have not been established in patients below the age of 18 years.

DRUG INTERACTIONS:

Interactions between interferon alfa-2b, recombinant for injection and other drugs have not been fully evaluated. Caution should be exercised when administering interferon alfa-2b therapy in combination with other potentially myelosuppressive agents such as zidovudine.

ADVERSE REACTIONS:

The adverse experiences listed below (TABLE 6 and TABLE 6A) were reported to be possibly or probably related to interferon alfa-2b therapy during clinical trials. Most of these adverse reactions were mild to moderate in severity and were manageable. Some were transient and most diminished with continued therapy.

The most frequently reported adverse reactions were flu-like symptoms, particularly fever, headache, chills, myalgia, and fatigue. More severe toxicities are observed generally at higher doses and may be difficult for patients to tolerate.

TABLE 6 Treatment-Related Adverse Experiences By Indication Dosing Regimens-Percentage (%) of Patients

Adverse Experience	Hairy Cell Leukemia 2 million IU/m^2 TIW/SC N=145	Condylomata Acuminata 1 million IU/lesion N=352
Application-Site Disorders	20	
injection site inflammation	-	-
other (<5%) burning, injection site bleeding, injection site pain, injection site reaction, itching		
Blood Disorders (<5%) anemia, granulocytopenia, hemolytic anemia, leukopenia, thrombocytopenia		
Body as a Whole		
facial edema	-	<1
weight decrease	<1	<1
other (<5%) cachexia, dehydration, earache, hypercalcemia, lymphadenopathy, periorbital edema, peripheral edema, thirst, weakness		
Cardiovascular System Disorders (<5%) arrhythmia, atrial fibrillation, bradycardia, cardiac failure, cardiomyopathy, extrasystoles, hypertension, hypotension, palpitations, postural hypotension, tachycardia		
Endocrine System Disorders (<5%) aggravation of diabetes mellitus, gynecomastia, thyroid disorder, virilism		
Flu-like Symptoms		
fever	68	56
headache	39	47
chills	46	45
myalgia	39	44
fatigue	61	18
increased sweating	8	2
asthenia	7	-
rigors	-	-
arthralgia	8	9
dizziness	12	9
influenza-like symptoms	37	-
back pain	19	6
dry mouth	19	-
chest pain	<1	<1
malaise	-	14
pain (unspecified)	18	3
other (<5%) chest pain substernal, rhinitis, rhinorrhea		
Gastrointestinal System Disorders		
diarrhea	18	2
anorexia	19	1
nausea	21	17
taste alteration	13	<1
abdominal pain	<5	1
loose stools	-	<1
vomiting	6	2
constipation	<1	-
gingivitis	-	-
dyspepsia	-	2
other (<5%) abdominal distention, dysphagia, eructation, esophagitis, flatulence, gastric ulcer, gastrointestinal hemorrhage, gastrointestinal mucosal discoloration, gingival bleeding, gum hyperplasia, increased appetite, increased saliva, melena, oral leukoplakia, rectal bleeding after stool, rectal hemorrhage, stomatitis, stomatitis ulcerative, taste loss		

Hairy Cell Leukemia: The adverse reactions most frequently reported during clinical trials in 145 patients with hairy cell leukemia were the flu-like symptoms of fever (68%), fatigue (61%), and chills (46%).

Condylomata Acuminata: Eighty-eight percent (311/352) of patients treated with interferon alfa-2b, recombinant for injection for condylomata acuminata who were evaluable for safety, reported an adverse reaction during treatment. The incidence of the adverse reactions reported increased when the number of treated lesions increased from 1 to 5. All 40 patients who had 5 warts treated, reported some type of adverse reaction during treatment.

Adverse reactions and abnormal laboratory test values reported by patients who were retreated were qualitatively and quantitatively similar to those reported during the initial Intron A treatment period.

AIDS-Related Kaposi's Sarcoma: In patients with AIDS-Related Kaposi's Sarcoma, patients some type of adverse reaction occurred in 100% of the 74 patients treated with 30 million IU/m^2 three times a week and in 97% of the 29 patients treated with 35 million IU per day.

Of these adverse reactions, those classified as severe (World Health Organization grade 3 or 4) were reported in 27% to 55% of patients. Severe adverse reactions in the 30 million IU/m^2 TIW study included: fatigue (20%), influenza-like symptoms (15%), anorexia (12%), dry mouth (4%), headache (4%), confusion (3%), fever (3%), myalgia (3%), and nausea and

ADVERSE REACTIONS: *(cont'd)*

vomiting (1% each). Severe adverse reactions for patients who received the 35 million IU QD included: fever (24%), fatigue (17%), influenza-like symptoms (14%), dyspnea (14%), headache (10%), pharyngitis (7%), and ataxia, confusion, dysphagia, GI hemorrhage, abnormal hepatic function, increased SGOT, myalgia, cardiomyopathy, face edema, depression, emotional lability, suicide attempt, chest pain, and coughing (1 patient each). Overall, the incidence of severe toxicity was higher among patients who received the 35 million IU per day dose.

Chronic Hepatitis Non-A, Non-B/C (NANB/C): In patients with chronic hepatitis NANB/C, alopecia, injection site reactions, rash, depression, and irritability apparently increased in incidence with continued treatment; residual mild alopecia persisted posttreatment.

TABLE 6A

Adverse Experience	Hairy Cell Leukemia 2 million IU/m^2 TIW/SC N=145	Condylomata Acuminata 1 million IU/lesion N=352
Liver and Biliary System Disorders (<5%) abnormal hepatic function tests, bilirubinemia, increased transaminases, jaundice, right upper quadrant pain and very rarely, hepatic encephalopathy, hepatic failure, and death		
Musculoskeletal System Disorders		
musculoskeletal pain	-	-
other (<5%) arthritis, arthrosis, bone pain, leg cramps, muscle weakness		
Nervous System and Psychiatric Disorders		
depression	6	3
paresthesia	6	1
impaired concentration	-	<1
amnesia	<5	-
confusion	<5	4
hypoesthesia	<5	1
irritability	-	-
somnolence	<5	3
anxiety	5	<1
insomnia	-	<1
nervousness	-	1
decreased libido	<5	-
other (<5%) abnormal coordination, abnormal dreaming, abnormal gait, abnormal thinking, aggravated depression, aggressive reaction, agitation, apathy, aphasia, ataxia, CNS dysfunction, coma, convulsions, dysphonia, emotional lability, extrapyramidal disorder, feeling of ebriety, flushing, hearing disorder, hot flashes, hyperesthesia, hyperkinesia, hypertonia, hypokinesia, impaired consciousness, migraine, neuropathy, neurosis, paresis, paroniria, parosmia, personality disorder, polyneuropathy, speech disorder, suicide attempt, syncope, tinnitus, tremor, vertigo		
Reproduction System Disorders (<5%) amenorrhea, impotence, leukorrhea, menorrhagia, uterine bleeding		
Resistance Mechanism Disorders		
moniliasis	-	<1
herpes simplex	-	1
other (<5%) abscess, conjunctivitis, sepsis, stye		
Respiratory System Disorders		
dyspnea	<1	-
coughing	<1	-
pharyngitis	<5	1
sinusitis	-	-
nonproductive coughing	-	-
nasal congestion	-	1
other (<5%) bronchospasm, cyanosis, epistaxis, pleural pain, pneumonia, sneezing, wheezing		
Skin and Appendages Disorders		
dermatitis	8	-
alopecia	8	-
pruritus	11	1
rash	25	-
dry skin	9	-
other (<5%) abnormal hair texture, acne, cyanosis of the hand, cold and clammy skin, dermatitis lichenoides, epidermal necrolysis, erythema, furunculosis, increased hair growth, lacrimal gland disorder, melanosis, nail disorders, nonherpetic cold sores, peripheral ischemia, photosensitivity, purpura, skin depigmentation, skin discoloration, caria, vitiligo		
Urinary System Disorders (<5%) increased BUN, hematuria, micturition disorder, micturition frequency, nocturia, polyuria		
Vision Disorders (<5%) abnormal vision, blurred vision, diplopia, dry eyes, eye pain, photophobia		

* Dash (-) indicates not reported

Infrequently, patients receiving interferon alfa-2b therapy for chronic hepatitis NANB/C developed thyroid abnormalities, either hypothyroid or hyperthyroid. In clinical trials <1% (4/426) developed thyroid abnormalities. The abnormalities were controlled by conventional therapy for thyroid dysfunction. The mechanism by which interferon alfa-2b, recombinant for injection may alter thyroid status is unknown. Prior to initiation of interferon alfa-2b therapy for the treatment of chronic hepatitis NANB/C, serum TSH should be evaluated. Patients developing symptoms consistent with possible thyroid dysfunction during the course of interferon alfa-2b therapy should have their thyroid function evaluated and appropriate treatment instituted. Interferon alfa-2b treatment may be continued if TSH levels can be maintained in the normal range by medication. Discontinuation of Intron A therapy has not always reversed thyroid dysfunction occurring during treatment.

Chronic Hepatitis B: In patients with chronic hepatitis B, some type of adverse reaction occurred in 98% of the 101 patients treated at 5 million IU QD and 90% of the 78 patients treated at 10 million IU TIW. Most of these adverse reactions were mild to moderate in severity, were manageable, and were reversible following the end of therapy.

Adverse reactions classified as severe (causing a significant interference with normal daily activities or clinical state) were reported in 21% to 44% of patients. The severe adverse reactions reported most frequently were the flu-like symptoms of fever (28%), fatigue (15%), headache (5%), myalgia (4%), and rigors (4%), and other severe flu-like symptoms which occurred in 1% to 3% of patients. Other severe adverse reactions occurring in more than one patient were alopecia (8%), anorexia (6%), depression (3%), nausea (3%), and vomiting (2%).

To manage side effects, the dose was reduced, or interferon alfa-2b therapy was interrupted in 25% to 38% of patients. Five percent of patients discontinued treatment due to adverse experiences.

DOSAGE AND ADMINISTRATION:

IMPORTANT: Interferon alfa-2b, recombinant for Injection dosing regimens are different for each of the following indications described in this section of the product information sheet.

Hairy Cell Leukemia: The recommended dosage of interferon alfa-2b, recombinant for injection for the treatment of hairy cell leukemia is 2 million IU/m^2 administered intramuscularly (see WARNINGS) or subcutaneously 3 times a week. The 50 million IU strength of the interferon alfa-2b Powder for Injection is not to be used for the treatment of hairy cell leukemia. Higher doses are not recommended. The normalization of one or more hematologic variables usually begins within 2 months of initiation of therapy. Improvement in all three hematologic variables may require 6 months or more of therapy.

This dosage regimen should be maintained unless the disease progresses rapidly, or severe intolerance is manifested. If severe adverse reactions develop, the dosage should be modified (50% reduction) or therapy should be temporarily discontinued until the adverse reactions abate. If persistent or recurrent intolerance develops following adequate dosage adjustment, or disease progresses, interferon alfa-2b treatment should be discontinued. The minimum effective interferon alfa-2b dose has not been established.

TABLE 6C AIDS-Related Kaposi's Sarcoma Treatment-Related Adverse Experiences Dosing Regimens-Percentage (%) of Patients

Application-Site Disorders		
injection site inflammation	-	-
other (<5%) burning, injection site bleeding, injection site pain, injection site reaction, itching		
Blood Disorders (<5%) anemia, granulocytopenia, hemolytic anemia, leukopenia, thrombocytopenia		
Body as a Whole		
facial edema	-	10
weight decrease	5	3
other (<5%) cachexia, dehydration, earache, hypercalcemia, lymphadenopathy, periorbital edema, peripheral edema, thirst, weakness		
Cardiovascular System Disorders (<5%) arrhythmia, atrial fibrillation, bradycardia, cardiac failure, cardiomyopathy, extrasystoles, hypertension, hypotension, palpitations, postural hypotension, tachycardia		
Endocrine System Disorders (<5%) aggravation of diabetes mellitus, gynecomastia, thyroid disorder, virilism		
Flu-like Symptoms		
fever	47	55
headache	36	21
chills	-	-
myalgia	34	28
fatigue	84	48
increased sweating	4	21
asthenia	11	-
rigors	30	14
arthralgia	-	3
dizziness	7	24
influenza-like symptoms	45	79
back pain	1	3
dry mouth	22	28
chest pain	1	28
malaise	5	-
pain (unspecified)	3	3
other (<5%) chest pain substernal, rhinitis, rhinorrhea		

TABLE 6D

Adverse Experience	AIDS-Related Kaposi's Sarcoma 30 million IU/m^2 TIW/SC N=74	35 million IU/QD/SC N=29
Gastrointestinal System Disorders		
diarrhea	18	45
anorexia	38	41
nausea	28	21
taste alteration	5	7
abdominal pain	5	21
loose stools	-	10
vomiting	11	14
constipation	1	10
gingivitis	-	14
dyspepsia	4	-
other (<5%) abdominal distention, dysphagia, eructation, esophagitis, flatulence, gastric ulcer, gastrointestinal hemorrhage, gastrointestinal mucosal discoloration, gingival bleeding, gum hyperplasia, increased appetite, increased saliva, melena, oral leukoplakia, rectal bleeding after stool, rectal hemorrhage, stomatitis, stomatitis ulcerative, taste loss		
Liver and Biliary System Disorders (<5%) abnormal hepatic function tests, bilirubinemia, increased transaminases, jaundice, right upper quadrant pain and very rarely, hepatic encephalopathy, hepatic failure, and death		
Musculoskeletal System Disorders		
musculoskeletal pain	-	-
other (<5%) arthritis, arthrosis, bone pain, leg cramps, muscle weakness		
Nervous System and Psychiatric Disorders		
depression	9	28
paresthesia	3	21
impaired concentration	3	14
amnesia	-	14
confusion	12	10
hypoesthesia	-	10
irritability	-	-
somnolence	3	-
anxiety	1	3
insomnia	3	3
nervousness	-	3
decreased libido	-	-
other (<5%) abnormal coordination, abnormal dreaming, abnormal gait, abnormal thinking, aggravated depression, aggressive reaction, agitation, apathy, aphasia, ataxia, CNS dysfunction, coma, convulsions, dysphonia, emotional lability, extrapyramidal disorder, feeling of ebriety, flushing, hearing disorder, hot flashes, hyperesthesia, hyperkinesia, hypertonia, hypokinesia, impaired consciousness, migraine, neuropathy, neurosis, paresis, paroniria, parosmia, personality disorder, polyneuropathy, speech disorder, suicide attempt, syncope, tinnitus, tremor, vertigo		

DOSAGE AND ADMINISTRATION: *(cont'd)*

TABLE 6E

Adverse Experience	AIDS-Related Kaposi's Sarcoma 30 million IU/m^2 TIW/SC N=74	35 million IU/QD/SC N=29
Reproduction System Disorders (<5%) amenorrhea, impotence, leukorrhea, menorrhagia, uterine bleeding		
Resistance Mechanism Disorders		
moniliasis	-	17
herpes simplex	-	3
other (<5%) abscess, conjunctivitis, sepsis, stye		
Respiratory System Disorders		
dyspnea	1	34
coughing	-	31
pharyngitis	1	31
sinusitis	-	21
nonproductive coughing	-	14
nasal congestion	-	10
other (<5%) bronchospasm, cyanosis, epistaxis, pleural pain, pneumonia, sneezing, wheezing		
Skin and Appendages Disorders		
dermatitis	-	-
alopecia	12	31
pruritus	7	-
rash	9	10
dry skin	9	10
other (<5%) abnormal hair texture, acne, cyanosis of the hand, cold and clammy skin, dermatitis lichenoides, epidermal necrolysis, erythema, furunculosis, increased hair growth, lacrimal gland disorder, melanosis, nail disorders, nonherpetic cold sores, peripheral ischemia, photosensitivity, purpura, skin depigmentation, skin discoloration, urticaria, vitiligo		
Urinary System Disorders (<5%) increased BUN, hematuria, micturition disorder, micturition frequency, nocturia, polyuria		
Vision Disorders (<5%) abnormal vision, blurred vision, diplopia, dry eyes, eye pain, photophobia		

* Dash (-) indicates not reported

TABLE 6F

Adverse Experience	Chronic Hepatitis NANB/C 3 million IU TIW N=159	Malgignant Melanoma 20MIU/m2 Induction IV 10 MIU/m^2 Maintenance (SC) N=143
Application-Site Disorders		
injection site inflammation	7	-
other (<5%) burning, injection site bleeding, injection site pain, injection site reaction, itching		
Blood Disorders (<5%) anemia, granulocytopenia, hemolytic anemia, leukopenia, thrombocytopenia		
Body as a Whole		
facial edema	1	-
weight decrease	<1	3
other (<5%) cachexia, dehydration, earache, hypercalcemia, lymphadenopathy, periorbital edema, peripheral edema, thirst, weakness		
Cardiovascular System Disorders (<5%) arrhythmia, atrial fibrillation, bradycardia, cardiac failure, cardiomyopathy, extrasystoles, hypertension, hypotension, palpitations, postural hypotension, tachycardia		
Endocrine System Disorders (<5%) aggravation of diabetes mellitus, gynecomastia, thyroid disorder, virilism		
Flu-like Symptoms		
fever	43	81
headache	43	62
chills	-	54
myalgia	42	75
fatigue	19	96
increased sweating	3	6
asthenia	24	-
rigors	27	2
arthralgia	19	6
dizziness	9	23
influenza-like symptoms	9	10
back pain	3	-
dry mouth	4	1
chest pain	1	2
malaise	3	6
pain (unspecified)	-	15
other (<5%) chest pain substernal, rhinitis, rhinorrhea		

Malignant Melanoma: The recommended interferon alfa-2b treatment regimen includes induction treatment 5 consecutive days per week as an intravenous (IV) infusion at a dose of 20 million IU/m^2, followed by maintenance treatment 3 times per week for 48 weeks as a subcutaneous (SC) injection, at a dose of 10 million IU/m^2.

In the clinical trial, the median daily interferon alfa-2b doses administered to patients were 19.1 million IU/m^2 during the maintenance phase.

Regular laboratory testing should be performed to monitor laboratory abnormalities for the purposes of dose modification (see PRECAUTIONS, Laboratory Tests). If adverse reactions develop during interferon alfa-2b treatment, particularly if granulocytes decrease to <500/mm^3 or SGPT/SGOT rises to >5 × upper limit of normal, treatment should be temporarily discontinues until the adverse reactions abate. Interferon alfa-2b treatment should be restarted at 50% of the previous dose if intolerance persists after dose adjustments for if granulocytes decrease to <250/mm^3 or SGPT/SGOT rises to 10 × upper limit of normal, interferon alfa-2b therapy should be discontinued. In the clinical trial, patients were able to achieve clinical benefit in conjunction with appropriate dose modifications. Therapy should be maintained for 1 year unless there is progression of disease.

DOSAGE AND ADMINISTRATION: *(cont'd)*

TABLE 6G

Adverse Experience	Chronic Hepatitis NANB/C 3 million IU TIW N=159	Malgignant Melanoma 20MIU/m2 Induction IV 10 MIU/m^2 Maintenance (SC) N=143
Gastrointestinal System Disorders		
diarrhea	13	35
anorexia	13	69
nausea	23	66
taste alteration	1	24
abdominal pain	6	2
loose stools	3	-
vomiting	3	†
constipation	<1	1
gingivitis	-	2‡
dyspepsia	3	-
other (<5%) abdominal distention, dysphagia, eructation, esophagitis, flatulence, gastric ulcer, gastrointestinal hemorrhage, gastrointestinal mucosal discoloration, gingival bleeding, gum hyperplasia, increased appetite, increased saliva, melena, oral leukoplakia, rectal bleeding after stool, rectal hemorrhage, stomatitis, stomatitis ulcerative, taste loss		
Liver and Biliary System Disorders (<5%) abnormal hepatic function tests, bilirubinemia, increased transaminases, jaundice, right upper quadrant pain and very rarely, hepatic encephalopathy, hepatic failure, and death		
Musculoskeletal System Disorders		
musculoskeletal pain	-	-
other (<5%) arthritis, arthrosis, bone pain, leg cramps, muscle weakness		
Nervous System and Psychiatric Disorders		
depression	8	40
paresthesia	1	13
impaired concentration	4	-
amnesia	-	**
confusion	1	8
hypoesthesia	-	-
irritability	4	1
somnolence	1	1
anxiety	1	1
insomnia	4	5
nervousness	-	1
decreased libido	1	1
other (<5%) abnormal coordination, abnormal dreaming, abnormal gait, abnormal thinking, aggravated depression, aggressive reaction, agitation, apathy, aphasia, ataxia, CNS dysfunction, coma, convulsions, dysphonia, emotional lability, extrapyramidal disorder, feeling of ebriety, flushing, hearing disorder, hot flashes, hyperesthesia, hyperkinesia, hypertonia, hypokinesia, impaired consciousness, migraine, neuropathy, neurosis, paresis, paroniria, parosmia, personality disorder, polyneuropathy, speech disorder, suicide attempt, syncope, tinnitus, tremor, vertigo		

TABLE 6H

Adverse Experience	Chronic Hepatitis NANB/C 3 million IU TIW N=159	Malgignant Melanoma 20MIU/m2 Induction IV 10 MIU/m^2 Maintenance (SC) N=143
Reproduction System Disorders (<5%) amenorrhea, impotence, leukorrhea, menorrhagia, uterine bleeding		
Resistance Mechanism Disorders		
moniliasis	-	-
herpes simplex	-	1
other (<5%) abscess, conjunctivitis, sepsis, stye		
Respiratory System Disorders		
dyspnea	<1	15
coughing	<1	6
pharyngitis	1	2
sinusitis	-	1
nonproductive coughing	-	2
nasal congestion	-	1
other (<5%) bronchospasm, cyanosis, epistaxis, pleural pain, pneumonia, sneezing, wheezing		
Skin and Appendages Disorders		
dermatitis	-	1
alopecia	17	29
pruritus	6	-
rash	6	19
dry skin	<1	1
other (<5%) abnormal hair texture, acne, cyanosis of the hand, cold and clammy skin, dermatitis lichenoides, epidermal necrolysis, erythema, furunculosis, increased hair growth, lacrimal gland disorder, melanosis, nail disorders, nonherpetic cold sores, peripheral ischemia, photosensitivity, purpura, skin depigmentation, skin discoloration, urticaria, vitiligo		
Urinary System Disorders (<5%) increased BUN, hematuria, micturition disorder, micturition frequency, nocturia, polyuria		
Vision Disorders (<5%) abnormal vision, blurred vision, diplopia, dry eyes, eye pain, photophobia		

* Dash (-) indicates not reported

Condylomata Acuminata: The 10 million IU vial of interferon alfa-2b powder for injection must be reconstituted with 1 ml of Diluent for interferon alfa-2b, recombinant for injection (bacteriostatic water for injection). Do not reconstitute the 10 million IU vial of interferon alfa-2b powder for injection with more than 1 ml of diluent since the injection would be subpotent. Do not use the 3 million, 5 million, 18 million multidose, 25 million, or 50 million IU vials of interferon alfa-2b powder for injection for the treatment of condylomata acuminata since the resulting reconstituted solution would be either hypertonic or an inappropriate concentration. Do not use the 10 million, 18 million multidose, or 25 million IU vials of interferon alfa-2b solution for injection for the intralesional treatment of condylomata acuminata since the concentrations are inappropriate for such use.

DOSAGE AND ADMINISTRATION: *(cont'd)*

TABLE 6I

Adverse Experience	Chronic Hepatitis B 5 million IU QD N=101	10 million IU TIW N=78
Application-Site Disorders		
injection site inflammation	3	-
other (<5%) burning, injection site bleeding, injection site pain, injection site reaction, itching		
Blood Disorders (<5%) anemia, granulocytopenia, hemolytic anemia, leukopenia, thrombocytopenia		
Body as a Whole		
facial edema	3	1
weight decrease	2	5
other (<5%) cachexia, dehydration, earache, hypercalcemia, lymphadenopathy, periorbital edema, peripheral edema, thirst, weakness		
Cardiovascular System Disorders (<5%) arrhythmia, atrial fibrillation, bradycardia, cardiac failure, cardiomyopathy, extrasystoles, hypertension, hypotension, palpitations, postural hypotension, tachycardia		
Endocrine System Disorders (<5%) aggravation of diabetes mellitus, gynecomastia, thyroid disorder, virilism		
Flu-like Symptoms		
fever	66	86
headache	61	44
chills	-	-
myalgia	59	40
fatigue	75	69
increased sweating	1	1
asthenia	5	15
rigors	38	42
arthralgia	19	8
dizziness	13	10
influenza-like symptoms	5	-
back pain	-	-
dry mouth	6	5
chest pain	4	-
malaise	9	6
pain (unspecified)	-	-
other (<5%) chest pain substernal, rhinitis, rhinorrhea		

TABLE 6J

Adverse Experience	Chronic Hepatitis B 5 million IU QD N=101	10 million IU TIW N=78
Gastrointestinal System Disorders		
diarrhea	19	8
anorexia	43	53
nausea	50	33
taste alteration	10	-
abdominal pain	5	4
loose stools	2	-
vomiting	7	10
constipation	5	-
gingivitis	1	-
dyspepsia	3	8
other (<5%) abdominal distention, dysphagia, eructation, esophagitis, flatulence, gastric ulcer, gastrointestinal hemorrhage, gastrointestinal mucosal discoloration, gingival bleeding, gum hyperplasia, increased appetite, increased saliva, melena, oral leukoplakia, rectal bleeding after stool, rectal hemorrhage, stomatitis, stomatitis ulcerative, taste loss		
Liver and Biliary System Disorders (<5%) abnormal hepatic function tests, bilirubinemia, increased transaminases, jaundice, right upper quadrant pain and very rarely, hepatic encephalopathy, hepatic failure, and death		
Musculoskeletal System Disorders		
musculoskeletal pain	9	1
other (<5%) arthritis, arthrosis, bone pain, leg cramps, muscle weakness		
Nervous System and Psychiatric Disorders		
depression	17	6
paresthesia	6	3
impaired concentration	8	5
amnesia	-	-
confusion	-	-
hypoesthesia	-	-
irritability	16	12
somnolence	14	9
anxiety	2	-
insomnia	11	6
nervousness	3	-
decreased libido	5	1
other (<5%) abnormal coordination, abnormal dreaming, abnormal gait, abnormal thinking, aggravated depression, aggressive reaction, agitation, apathy, aphasia, ataxia, CNS dysfunction, coma, convulsions, dysphonia, emotional lability, extrapyramidal disorder, feeling of ebriety, flushing, hearing disorder, hot flashes, hyperesthesia, hyperkinesia, hypertonia, hypokinesia, impaired consciousness, migraine, neuropathy, neurosis, paresis, paroniria, parosmia, personality disorder, polyneuropathy, speech disorder, suicide attempt, syncope, tinnitus, tremor, vertigo		
Reproduction System Disorders (<5%) amenorrhea, impotence, leukorrhea, menorrhagia, uterine bleeding		
Resistance Mechanism Disorders		
moniliasis	-	-
herpes simplex	5	-
other (<5%) abscess, conjunctivitis, sepsis, stye		

DOSAGE AND ADMINISTRATION: *(cont'd)*

TABLE 6K

Adverse Experience	Chronic Hepatitis B 5 million IU QD N=101	10 million IU TIW N=78
Respiratory System Disorders		
dyspnea	5	-
coughing	4	-
pharyngitis	7	1
sinusitis	-	-
nonproductive coughing	1	-
nasal congestion	4	-
other (<5%) bronchospasm, cyanosis, epistaxis, pleural pain, pneumonia, sneezing, wheezing		
Skin and Appendages Disorders		
dermatitis	1	-
alopecia	26	38
pruritus	6	4
rash	8	1
dry skin	3	-
other (<5%) abnormal hair texture, acne, cyanosis of the hand, cold and clammy skin, dermatitis lichenoides, epidermal necrolysis, erythema, furunculosis, increased hair growth, lacrimal gland disorder, melanosis, nail disorders, nonherpetic cold sores, peripheral ischemia, photosensitivity, purpura, skin depigmentation, skin discoloration, urticaria, vitiligo		
Urinary System Disorders (<5%) increased BUN, hematuria, micturition disorder, micturition frequency, nocturia, polyuria		
Vision Disorders (<5%) abnormal vision, blurred vision, diplopia, dry eyes, eye pain, photophobia		

* Dash (-) indicates not reported

TABLE 7A Abnormal Laboratory Test Values
Dosing Regimens-Percentage (%) of Patients

Laboratory Tests	Hairy Cell Leukemia 2 million IU/m^2 TIW/SC N=145	Condylomata Acuminata 1 million IU/lesion N=352
Hemoglobin	NA	-
White Blood Cell Count	NA	17%
Platelet Count	NA	-
Serum Creatinine	0%	-
Alkaline Phosphatase	4%	-
Lactase Dehydrogenase	0%	-
Serum Urea Nitrogen	0%	-
SGOT	4%	12%
SGPT	13%	-
Granulocyte Count		
• Total	NA	-
• 1000 - $<1500/mm^3$	-	-
• 750 - $<1000/mm^3$	-	-
• 500 - $<750/mm^3$	-	-
• $<500/mm^3$	-	-

NA - Not Applicable - Patients' initial hematologic laboratory test values were abnormal due to their condition.
* Decrease of ≥ 2 g/dl
‡ Decrease to $<70,000/mm^3$
† Decrease to $<3000/mm^3$
S Neutrophils plus bands

TABLE 7B

Laboratory Tests	AIDS-Related Kaposi's Sarcoma 30 million IU/m^2 TIW/SC N=69-73	35 million IU/QD/SC N=26-28
Hemoglobin	1%	15%
White Blood Cell Count	10%	22%
Platelet Count	0%	8%
Serum Creatinine	-	-
Alkaline Phosphatase	-	-
Lactase Dehydrogenase	-	-
Serum Urea Nitrogen	-	-
SGOT	11%	41%
SGPT	10%	15%
Granulocyte Count		
• Total	31%	39%
• 1000 - $<1500/mm^3$	-	-
• 750 - $<1000/mm^3$	-	-
• 500 - $<750/mm^3$	-	-
• $<500/mm^3$	-	-

NA - Not Applicable - Patients' initial hematologic laboratory test values were abnormal due to their condition.
* Decrease of ≥ 2 g/dl
‡ Decrease to $<70,000/mm^3$
† Decrease to $<3000/mm^3$
S Neutrophils plus bands

Inject 1.0 million IU of interferon alfa-2b, recombinant for Injection (0.1 ml of reconstituted interferon alfa-2b solution) into each lesion three times per week on alternate days, for 3 weeks. The injection should be administered intralesionally using a Tuberculin or similar syringe and a 25-30 gauge needle. The needle should be directed at the center of the base of the wart and at an angle almost parallel to the plane of the skin (approximating that in the commonly used PPD test). This will deliver the interferon to the dermal core of the lesion, infiltrating the lesion and causing a small wheal. Care should be taken not to go beneath the lesion too deeply; subcutaneous injection should be avoided, since this area is below the base of the lesion. Do not inject too superficially since this will result in possible leakage, infiltrating only the keratinized layer, and not the dermal core. As many as 5 lesions can be treated at one time. To reduce side effects, interferon alfa-2b injections may be administered in the evening, when possible. Additionally, acetaminophen may be administered at the time of injection to alleviate some of the potential side effects.

DOSAGE AND ADMINISTRATION: *(cont'd)*

TABLE 7C

Laboratory Tests	Chronic Hepatitis NANB/C 3 million IU TIW N=87-158	Malignant Melanoma 20 MIU/m2 Induction (IV), 10 MIU/m2 Maintenance (SC) N=143
Hemoglobin	15%	22%
White Blood Cell Count	18%	**
Platelet Count	9%	15%
Serum Creatinine	2%	3%
Alkaline Phosphatase	3%	13%
Lactase Dehydrogenase	-	1%
Serum Urea Nitrogen	1%	12%
SGOT	-	63%
SGPT	-	2%
Granulocyte Count		
• Total	37% S	92%
• 1000 - $<1500/mm^3$	-	66%
• 750 - $<1000/mm^3$	-	25%
• 500 - $<750/mm^3$	-	25%
• $<500/mm^3$	-	1%

NA - Not Applicable - Patients' initial hematologic laboratory test values were abnormal due to their condition.
* Decrease of ≥ 2 g/dl
‡ Decrease to $<70,000/mm^3$
† Decrease to $<3000/mm^3$
S Neutrophils plus bands

TABLE 7D

Laboratory Tests	Chronic Hepatitis 5 million IU QD N=96-101	10 million IU TIW N=75-103
Hemoglobin	32%*	23%*
White Blood Cell Count	68%†	34%†
Platelet Count	12%‡	5%‡
Serum Creatinine	3%	0%
Alkaline Phosphatase	8%	4%
Lactase Dehydrogenase	-	-
Serum Urea Nitrogen	2%	0%
SGOT	-	-
SGPT	-	-
Granulocyte Count		
• Total	75%S	61%S
•1000 - $<1500/mm^3$	30%	32%
• 750 - $<1000/mm^3$	24%	18%
• 500 - $<750/mm^3$	17%	9%
• $<500/mm^3$	4%	2%

NA - Not Applicable - Patients' initial hematologic laboratory test values were abnormal due to their condition.
* Decrease of ≥ 2 g/dl
‡ Decrease to $<70,000/mm^3$
† Decrease to $<3000/mm^3$
S Neutrophils plus bands

The maximum response usually occurs 4 to 8 weeks after initiation of the first treatment course. If results at 12 to 16 weeks after the initial treatment course has concluded are not satisfactory, a second course of treatment using the above dosage schedule may be instituted providing that clinical symptoms and signs, or changes in laboratory parameters (liver function tests, WBC, and platelets) do not preclude such a course of action.

Patients with six to ten condylomata may receive a second (sequential) course of treatment at the above dosage schedule, to treat up to five additional condylomata per course of treatment. Patients with greater than ten condylomata may receive additional sequences depending on how large a number of condylomata are present.

AIDS-Related Kaposi's Sarcoma: The recommended interferon alfa-2b dosage is 30 million IU/m^2 three times a week administered subcutaneously or intramuscularly. The 10 million, 18 million multidose, and 25 million IU vials of the interferon alfa-2b Solution for Injection are not to be used for the treatment of condylomata acuminata or AIDS-Related Kaposi's Sarcoma.

The selected dosage regimen should be maintained unless the disease progresses rapidly or severe intolerance is manifested. If severe adverse reactions develop, the dosage should be modified (50% reduction) or therapy should be temporarily discontinued until the adverse reactions abate. When patients initiate therapy at 30 million IU/m^2 TIW, the average dose tolerated at the end of 12 weeks of therapy is 110 million IU/week and 75 million IU/week at the end of 24 weeks of therapy.

When disease stabilization or a response to treatment occurs, treatment should continue until there is no further evidence of tumor or until discontinuation is required by evidence of a severe opportunistic infection or adverse effect.

Chronic Hepatitis Non-A, Non-B/C (NANB/C): The recommended dosage of interferon alfa-2b, recombinant for Injection for the treatment of chronic hepatitis NANB/C is 3 million IU three times a week (TIW) administered subcutaneously or intramuscularly.

Normalization of serum alanine aminotransferase (ALT) may occur in some patients as early as 2 weeks after initiation of treatment; however, current experience suggests that patients responding to interferon alfa-2b therapy with a reduction in serum ALT should complete 6 months (24 weeks) of treatment. The optimal dose and duration of therapy are currently under investigation.

In clinical trials, 54% (51/95) of the patients at a dose of 3 million IU TIW responded with a reduction in serum ALT after 6 months of interferon alfa-2b therapy. Since most of these patients (49/51) responded within the first 16 weeks of treatment, consideration could be given to discontinuing interferon alfa-2b therapy in patients who fail to respond after 16 weeks. The effect of dose escalation in these patients is under investigation.

If severe adverse reactions develop during interferon alfa-2b treatment, the dose should be modified (50% reduction) or therapy should be temporarily discontinued until the adverse reactions abate. If intolerance persists after dose adjustment, interferon alfa-2b therapy should be discontinued.

DOSAGE AND ADMINISTRATION: *(cont'd)*

Patients who relapse following interferon alfa-2b therapy may be retreated with the same dosage regimen to which they had previously responded.

Chronic Hepatitis B: The recommended dosage of interferon alfa-2b, recombinant for Injection for the treatment of chronic hepatitis B is 30 to 35 million IU per week, administered subcutaneously or intramuscularly, either as 5 million IU daily (QD) or as 10 million IU three times a week (TIW) for 16 weeks.

If severe adverse reactions or laboratory abnormalities develop during interferon alfa-2b therapy the dose should be modified (50% reduction), or discontinued if appropriate, until the adverse reactions abate. If intolerance persists after dose adjustment, interferon alfa-2b therapy should be discontinued.

For patients with decreases in granulocyte or platelet counts, the guidelines found in TABLE 8 for dose modification were used in the clinical trials.

TABLE 8

Intron A Dose	Granulocyte Count	Platelet Count
Reduce 50%	<750/mm³	<50,000/mm³
Interrupt	<500/mm³	<30,000/mm³

Intron A therapy was resumed at up to 100% of the initial dose when granulocyte and/or platelet counts returned to normal or baseline values.

At the discretion of the physician, the patient may self-administer the medication. For detailed instructions see Patient Information Sheet.

PREPARATION AND ADMINISTRATION OF INTRON A INTERFERON ALFA- 2B, RECOMBINANT POWDER FOR INJECTION

Reconstitution of Interferon Alfa-2b Powder for Injection: Inject the amount of Diluent for interferon alfa-2b, recombinant for Injection (bacteriostatic water for injection) stated in the appropriate chart below (diluent is supplied in either a vial or syringe, see HOW SUPPLIED), into the interferon alfa-2b vial. Swirl gently to hasten complete dissolution of the powder. The appropriate interferon alfa-2b dose should then be withdrawn and injected intramuscularly, subcutaneously, or intralesionally. For detailed instructions see Patient Information Sheet.

After preparation and administration of the interferon alfa-2b injection, it is essential to follow the procedure for proper disposal of syringes and needles. For detailed instructions see Patient Information Sheet.

TABLE 9A Hairy Cell Leukemia

Vial Strength	ml Diluent	Final Concentration
3 million IU	1	3 million IU/ml
5 million IU	1	5 million IU/ml
10 million IU	2	5 million IU/ml
‡18 million IU multidose	3.8	6 million IU/ml
25 million IU	5	5 million IU/ml

‡ This is a multidose vial which contains a total of 22.8 million IU of interferon alfa-2b, recombinant in order to provide the delivery of six 0.5 ml doses, each containing 3 million IU of Intron A Interferon alfa-2b, recombinant for Injection (for a label strength of 18 million IU), when reconstituted with 3.8 ml of the diluent provided.

TABLE 9B Condylomata Acuminata

Vial Strength	ml Diluent	Final Concentration
*10 million IU	1	10 million IU/ml

* IMPORTANT: For patients with condylomata acuminata reconstitute the 10 million IU vial with only1 ml of the diluent provided to reach a final concentration of 10 million IU/ml to be administered intralesionally (see DOSAGE AND ADMINISTRATION, Condylomata Acuminata).

TABLE 9C AIDS-Related Kaposi's Sarcoma

Vial Strength	ml Diluent	Final Concentration
50 million IU	1	50 million IU/ml

IMPORTANT: This vial size is to be used onlyfor treatment of patients with AIDS-Related Kaposi's Sarcoma (see DOSAGE AND ADMINISTRATION, AIDS-Related Kaposi's Sarcoma).

TABLE 9D Malignant Melanoma

Vial Strength	mL Diluent	Final Concentration
Induction Phase		
3 million IU	1	3 million IU/ml
5 million IU	1	5 million IU/ml
10 million IU	1	10 million IU/ml
18 million IU	1	18 million IU/ml
25 million IU	5	5 million IU/ml
*50 million IU	1	50 million IU/ml
Maitenance Phase		
3 million IU	1	3 million IU/ml
5 million IU	1	5 million IU/ml
10 million IU	1	10 million IU/ml
18 million IU	1	18 million IU/ml
*50 million IU	1	50 million IU/ml

DOSAGE AND ADMINISTRATION: *(cont'd)*

TABLE 9E Chronic Hepatitis Non-A, Non-B/C

Vial Strength	mL Dilutent	Final Concentration
3 million IU	1	3 million IU/ml
†18 million IU multidose	3.8	6 million IU/ml

† This is a multidose vial which contains a total of 22.8 million IU of interferon alfa-2b, recombinant in order to provide the delivery of six 0.5 ml doses, each containing 3 million IU of intron A interferon alfa-2b, recombinant for injection (for a label strength of 18 million IU), when reconstituted with 3.8 ml of the diluent provided.

TABLE 9F Chronic Hepatitis B

Vial Strength	ml Diluent	Final Concentration
5 million IU	1	5 million IU/ml
10 million IU	1	10 million IU/ml

Stability: Interferon alfa-2b, recombinant Powder for Injection provided in vials ranging from 3 to 50 million IU per vial, is stable at 45°C (113°F) for up to 7 days. After reconstitution with Diluent for interferon alfa-2b, recombinant for injection (bacteriostatic water for Injection) the solution is stable for 1 month at 2° to 8°C (36° to 46°F). The reconstituted solution is clear and colorless to light yellow.

PREPARATION AND ADMINISTRATION OF INTRON A INTERFERON ALFA-2B, RECOMBINANT SOLUTION FOR INJECTION

The 10 million IU vials of interferon alfa-2b Solution for Injection are supplied in 2 ml vials. The 18 million multidose and 25 million IU vials of interferon alfa-2b Solution for Injection are supplied in 5 ml vials. The solution is colorless to light yellow. These packages do not require reconstitution prior to administration. The appropriate interferon alfa-2b dose should be withdrawn from the vial and injected intramuscularly or subcutaneously. For detailed instructions see Patient Information Sheet. After administration of interferon alfa-2b Solution for Injection, it is essential to follow the procedure for proper disposal of syringes and needles. For detailed instructions see Patient Information Sheet.

TABLE 10A Hairy Cell Leukemia

Vial Strength	ml Solution	Final Concentration
10 million IU	2 ml	5 million IU/ml
‡18 million IU multidose	3.8 ml	6 million IU/ml
25 million IU	5 ml	5 million IU/ml

‡ This is a multidose vial which contains a total of 22.8 million IU of interferon alfa-2b, recombinant per 3.8 ml in order to provide the delivery of six 0.5 ml doses, each containing 3 million IU of Intron A Interferon alfa-2b, recombinant for Injection (for a label strength of 18 million IU).

TABLE 10B Chronic Hepatitis Non-A, Non-B/C

Vial Strength	ml Solution	Final Concentration
10 million IU	2 ml	5 million IU/ml
†18 million IU multidose	3.8 ml	6 million IU/ml
25 million IU	5 ml	5 million IU/ml

† This is a multidose vial which contains a total of 22.8 million IU of interferon alfa-2b, recombinant per 3.8 ml in order to provide the delivery of six 0.5 ml doses, each containing 3 million IU of intron A interferon alfa-2b, recombinant for injection (for a label strength of 18 million IU).

TABLE 10C Chronic Hepatitis B

Vial Strength	ml Solution	Final Concentration
10 million IU	2 ml	5 million IU/ml
25 million IU	5 ml	5 million IU/ml

IMPORTANT: The 10 million, 18 million multidose, and 25 million IU strengths of Intron A Solution for Injection are not to be used for condylomata acuminata or for AIDS-Related Kaposi's Sarcoma. (See DOSAGE AND ADMINISTRATION, Condylomata Acuminata ; DOSAGE AND ADMINISTRATION, AIDS-Related Kaposi's Sarcoma).

Parenteral drug products should be inspected visually for particulate matter and discoloration prior to administration, whenever solution and container permit. Interferon alfa-2b, recombinant for Injection may be administered using either sterilized glass or plastic disposable syringes.

REFERENCES:

1. Davis G, et al. *N Engl J Med.*1989;321:1501-1506. 2. Causse X, et al. *Gastroenterology.*1991;101:497-502. 3. Marcellin P, et al. *Hepatology.*1991;13:393-397. 4. Knodell R, et al. *Hepatology.*1981;1:431-435. 5. Perrillo R, et al. *N Engl J Med.*1990;323:295-301. 6. Perez V, et al. *J Hepatol.* 1990;11:S113-S117. 7. Perrillo R, et al. *Ann Intern Med.*1991;115:113-115. 8. Renault P, et al. *Arch Intern Med.*1987;147:1577-1580. 9. Kauppila A, et al. *Int J Cancer.*1982;29:291-294.

HOW SUPPLIED:

Intron A Interferon alfa-2b, Recombinant Powder for Injection: Intron A interferon alfa-2b, recombinant powder for injection, 3 million IU per vial and diluent for intron A interferon alfa-2b, recombinant for Injection (bacteriostatic water for injection) 1 ml per vial or syringe; boxes containing 1 intron A vial and 1 vial of intron A diluent; boxes containing 1 intron A vial and 1 syringe of intron A diluent.

HOW SUPPLIED: *(cont'd)*

Intron A interferon alfa-2b, recombinant powder for injection intron A, Pak-3, containing 6 intron A vials, 3 million IU per vial, and 6 syringes of diluent for intron A interferon alfa-2b, recombinant for injection (bacteriostatic water for injection) 1 ml per syringe for chronic hepatitis non-A, non-B/C.

Intron A interferon alfa-2b, recombinant powder for injection, 5 million IU per vial and diluent for intron A interferon alfa-2b, recombinant for injection (bacteriostatic water for injection) 1 ml per vial or syringe; boxes containing 1 intron A vial and 1 vial of intron A diluent; boxes containing 1 intron A vial and 1 syringe of intron A diluent.

Intron A interferon alfa-2b, recombinant powder for injection intron A, Pak-5, containing 14 intron A vials, 5 million IU per vial, and 14 syringes of diluent for intron A interferon alfa-2b, recombinant for injection (bacteriostatic water for injection) 1 ml per syringe for chronic hepatitis B.

Intron A interferon alfa-2b, recombinant powder for injection, 10 million IU per vial and diluent for intron A interferon alfa-2b, recombinant for injection (bacteriostatic water for injection) 2 ml per vial; boxes containing 1 intron A vial and 1 vial of intron A diluent.

Intron A interferon alfa-2b, recombinant powder for injection intron A, pak-10, containing 6 Intron A vials, 10 million IU per vial, and 6 syringes of Diluent for Intron A Interferon alfa-2b, recombinant for Injection (bacteriostatic water for injection) 1 ml per syringe for Chronic Hepatitis B.

Intron A Interferon alfa-2b, recombinant Powder for Injection, 18 million IU multidose vial (22.8 million IU per vial) and Diluent for Intron A Interferon alfa-2b, recombinant for Injection (bacteriostatic water for injection) 3.8 ml per vial; boxes containing 1 Intron A multidose vial and 1 vial of Intron A Diluent.

Intron A interferon alfa-2b, recombinant powder for injection, 25 million IU per vial and diluent for intron A interferon alfa-2b, recombinant for injection (bacteriostatic water for injection) 5 ml per vial; boxes containing 1 intron A vial and 1 vial of intron A diluent.

Intron A interferon alfa-2b, recombinant powder for injection, 50 million IU per vial and diluent for intron A interferon alfa-2b, recombinant for injection (bacteriostatic water for injection) 1 ml per vial; boxes containing 1 Intron A vial and 1 vial of intron A diluent.

Store Intron A Interferon alfa-2b, recombinant Powder for Injection both before and after reconstitution between 2° and 8°C (36° and 46°F).

Intron A Interferon alfa-2b, recombinant Solution for Injection: Intron A interferon alfa-2b, recombinant solution for injection, 10 million IU per 2 ml per vial; boxes containing 1 vial of intron A solution for injection.

Intron A interferon alfa-2b, recombinant solution for injection, 18 million IU multidose vial (22.8 million IU per 3.8 ml per vial); boxes containing 1 vial of Iintron A solution for injection.

Intron A interferon alfa-2b, recombinant solution for injection, 25 million IU per 5 ml per vial; boxes containing 1 vial of intron A solution for injection.

Store Intron A Interferon alfa-2b, recombinant Solution for Injection between 2° and 8°C (36° and 46°F).

HOW SUPPLIED - EQUIVALENTS NOT AVAILABLE:

Injection, Conc-Soln - Intramuscular - 5m unit
2 ml $52.51 INTRON A, Schering 00085-0120-02

Injection, Conc-Soln - Intramuscular - 25m unit/vial
6 ml $262.57 INTRON A 25 MILLION I.U., Schering 00085-0285-02

Injection, Conc-Soln - Intramuscular; - 50m unit/vial
2 ml $525.12 INTRON A, Schering 00085-0539-01

Injection, Lyphl-Soln - Intramuscular - 3m unit
2 ml $31.51 INTRON A, Schering 00085-0647-03
2 ml $31.51 INTRON A, Schering 00085-0647-04

Injection, Lyphl-Soln - Intravenous - 10m unit/vial
1's $105.03 INTRON A, Schering 00085-0571-02

Injection, Solution - Intravenous - 5 mmunit/ml
2 ml $105.02 INTRON A, Schering 00085-0923-01
5 ml $262.57 INTRON A, Schering 00085-0769-01

Injection, Solution - Intravenous - 6 mmunit/ml
3 ml $189.04 INTRON A, Schering 00085-0953-01

Injection, Solution - Intravenous - 18m unit
1's $189.04 INTRON A, Schering 00085-0689-01

Kit - Intravenous - 3m unit
6's $189.04 INTRON A, Schering 00085-0647-05

Kit - Intravenous - 5m unit
1's $52.51 INTRON A, Schering 00085-0120-03
14's $735.19 INTRON A, Schering 00085-0120-04

Kit - Intravenous - 10m unit/vial
6's $630.15 INTRON A, Schering 00085-0571-06

INTERFERON ALFA-N3 *(003048)*

CATEGORIES: Antineoplastics; Antivirals; Condylomata Acuminata; Genital Warts; Lesions; Viral Agents; Warts; Pregnancy Category C; FDA Approved 1990 Jun

BRAND NAMES: **Alferon N**

DESCRIPTION:

Alferon N Injection (Interferon alfa-n3 (Human Leukocyte Derived)) is a sterile aqueous formulation of purified, natural, human interferon alpha proteins for use by injection. Alferon N Injection consists of interferon alpha proteins comprising approximately 166 amino acids ranging in molecular weights from 16,000 to 27,000 daltons. The specific activity of Interferon alfa-n3 is approximately equal to, or greater than 2×10^4 IU/mg of protein.

Alferon N Injection is manufactured from pooled units of human leukocytes which have been induced by incomplete infection with an avian virus (Sendai virus) to produce Interferon alfa-n3. The manufacturing process includes immunoaffinity chromatography with a murine monoclonal antibody, acidification (pH 2) for 5 days at 4°C, and ge filtration chromatography.

Since Alferon N Injection is manufactured using source leukocytes, human, donor screening is performed to minimize the risk that the leukocytes could contain infectious agents. In addition, the manufacturing process contains steps which have been shown to inactivate viruses, and there has been no evidence of infection transmission to recipients in clinical

DESCRIPTION: *(cont'd)*

trials. The laboratory and clinical data obtained support the conclusion that Alferon N Injection is equivalent to other products derived from human blood or plasma which are free of risk of transmission of infectious agents, such as immunoglobulin and albumin.

Each unit of leukocytes used in the production of Alferon N Injection is from a donor whose serum is tested and found negative for hepatitis B surface antigen (HBsAg) and antibodies to human immunodeficiency virus (HIV-1) and human T lymphotropic virus-1 (HTLV-1) by FDA approved tests: the donor's serum has also been screened for ALT (alanine aminotransferase) levels. All donors are screened to eliminate those in high risk groups for transmission of diseases caused by retroviruses and hepatitis viruses.

The Alferon N Injection manufacturing process was evaluated for quantitative removal or inactivation of model pathogenic viruses. The viruses were deliberately added to the leukocytes in amounts far exceeding those present in contaminated blood, (*i.e.,* $\geq 10^9$ infectious units per milliliter. The manufacturing process yielded a cumulative reduction of $\geq 10^{14}$ of infectious HIV-1, i.e., $\geq 10^{6.5}$ removal by acid inactivation and $\geq 10^{7.9}$ removal by the purification process. In the validation studies, there was 10^8 reduction in the titer of hepatitis B virus as determined by HBsAg assay, and a 10^9 reduction in the infectious titer of herpes simplex virus-1 (HSV-1). Cultivation of Alferon N Injection Purified Drug Concentrate with human indicator cells, (*i.e.,* MRC-5 cells, peripheral blood leukocytes in the presence of Cyclosporin A, and fetal cord blood cells), did not defect the presence of infectious viruses.

As part of a validation study, Alferon N Injection (Interferon alfa-(Human Leukocyte Derived)) was examined for the presence of the following viruses: Sendai virus (SV), HIV-1, HTLV-I, HBV, HSV-1, CMV, and EBV. Alferon N Injection contained no detectable quantities of these viruses. In addition other studies. i.e. Polymerase Chain Reaction (PCR) and Dot Blot Hybridization (DBH), have shown no detectable genetic material from these viruses in Alferon N Injection. The sensitivity of the PCR was 10 copies for HIV-1 (envgene probe) and 10 copies for HBV (S/P gene probe). The sensitivity of the DBH was 1 pg for EBV, <10 pg for CMV, <10 pg for HSV-1, and <2 pg for SV. Furthermore, sera from 105 patients treated with Alferon N Injection (95 with condylomata acuminata and 10 with cancer) were tested for antibody to HIV-1 and HIV p24 antigen. there was no evidence to suggest transmission of HIV-1 by Alferon N Injection. Sera from 135 patients with condylomata acuminata treated with Alferon N Injection were tested to determine abnormal SGOT laboratory values. There was no evidence to suggest transmission of hepatitis by Alferon N Injection based on both SGOT results and patient data collected during clinical trials.

Alferon N Injection has been extensively purified using immunoaffinity chromatography with a murine monoclonal antibody, acidification (pH 2) for 5 days at 4°C, and gel filtration chromatography. Alferon N Injection has been subjected to the acid treatment for five days during its manufacture in order to reduce the risk of viral transmission. Subsequent analyses of the Alferon N Injection Purified Drug Concentrate confirm the absence of detectable infectious or non-infectious viral particles.

The leukocyte nutrient medium contains the antibiotic neomycin sulfate at a concentration of 35 mg/l: however, neomycin sulfate is not detectable in the final product, (*i.e.* <0.64 mcg/ml).

Murine immunoglobulin (IgG) is detected in the Alferon N Injection Purified Drug Concentrate at levels below 0.15% of the Interferon alfa-n3 protein. This equates to levels less than 8 ng of murine IgG per million IU Interferon alfa-n3 (range of 0.9 to 5.6 ng typically found).

Alferon N Injection (Interferon alfa-n3 (Human Leukocyte Derived) is available in an injectable solution containing 5 million IU Alferon N Injection per vial for intralesional injection. The solution is clear and colorless. Each milliliter (ml) contains five million IU of Interferon alfa-n3 in phosphate buffered saline (8.0 mg sodium chloride, 1.74 mg sodium phosphate dibasic, 0.20 mg potassium phosphate monobasic, and 0.20 mg potassium chloride) containing 3.3 mg phenol as a preservative and 1 mg Albumin (Human) as a stabilizer.

CLINICAL PHARMACOLOGY:

GENERAL

Interferons are naturally occurring proteins with both antiviral and antiproliferative properties. They are produced and secreted in response to viral infections and to a variety of other synthetic and biological inducers. Three major families of interferons have been identified: alpha, beta, and gamma. The interferon alpha family contains at least 15 different molecular species. Their molecular weights range from 16,000 to 27,000 daltons.

Interferons bind to specific membrane receptors on cell surfaces. Interferon alfa-n3 has been shown to bind to the same receptors as Interferon alfa-2b. The receptors have a high degree of selectivity for the binding of human but not mouse interferon. This correlates with the high species specificity found in laboratory studies.

Binding of interferon to membrane receptors initiates a series of events including induction of protein synthesis. These actions are followed by a variety of cellular responses, including inhibition of virus replication and suppression of cell proliferation. Immunomodulation, including enhancement of phagocytosis by macrophages, augmentation of the cytotoxicity of lymphocytes and enhancement of human leukocyte antigen expression occurs in response to exposure to interferons. One or more of these activities may contribute to the therapeutic effect of interferon.

Pharmacokinetics: In a study of intralesional use of Alferon N Injection (Interferon alfa-n3 (Human Leukocyte Derived)) for the treatment of condylomata acuminata, plasma concentrations of interferon were below the detection limit of the assay. (*i.e.,* ≤3 IU/ml). Minor systemic effects (*e.g.,* myalgias, fever, and headaches) were noted, indicating that some of the injected interferon entered the systemic circulation (See ADVERSE REACTIONS).

Condylomata Acuminata: Condylomata acuminata (venereal or genital warts) are associated with infections of human papilloma virus (HPV), especially HPV type-6 and possibly type-11. Given the antiviral and antiproliferative activities of interferons and the viral etiology of condylomata, a placebo-controlled clinical trial was conducted to evaluate the safety and efficacy of intralesional injection of Alferon N Injection in the treatment of condylomata acuminata.

In a multicenter randomized double-blind, placebo-controlled clinical trial, intralesional administration of Alferon N Injection was an effective treatment for condylomata acuminata.[1-4] One hundred fifty-six patients were evaluable for efficacy (81 Alferon N Injection patients and 75 placebo patients). Patients had a mean of five warts (range was 2-14) and all warts were treated. Patients were injected intralesionally with a mean of 225,000 IU of Alferon N Injection per wart 2 times a week for up to 8 weeks.

Overall, 80% (65/81) of patients treated with Alferon N Injection had a complete or partial resolution of warts compared with 44% (33/75) of placebo-treated patients (p<0.001). Alferon N Injection was significantly more effective than placebo in producing a complete resolution of warts (p<0.001), as shown in TABLE 1.

Of the patients who had a complete resolution of warts, approximately half (21/44) the patients had complete resolution of warts by the end of treatment, and half (23/44) had complete resolution of warts during the three months after the cessation of treatment.

CLINICAL PHARMACOLOGY: *(cont'd)*

TABLE 1 Degree of Resolution as Measured By Total Wart Volume per Patient

	Percent of Patients with:			
	Complete Resolution	Partial Resolution (≥50% resolution)	Minor Resolution (<50% resolution)	Progression/ No change
Alferon (n=81)	54%	26%	15%	5%
Placebo (n=75)	20%	24%	13%	43%

Patients with complete resolution of warts were followed for a median of 48 weeks. Overall, 76% (31/41) of Alferon N Injection (Interferon alfa-n3 (Human Leukocyte Derived))-treated patients who achieved complete resolution of warts remained clear of all treated lesions during follow-up, while 79% (11/14) of the placebo-treated patients remained clear of all treated lesions during follow-up.

A total of 762 evaluable warts were injected in this trial. Of the 407 Alferon N Injection-treated warts, 73% (297/407) completely resolved, as compared to 35% (125/355) of the placebo-treated warts (p<0.0001). Alferon N Injection was effective in treating lesions of all sizes, and there was no difference in resolution for perianal, penile, or vulvar lesions.

There was no difference in resolution for patients who had received prior treatment of their warts and for those who had not. Among patients with recalcitrant warts (*i.e.*, warts that were refractory to previous treatment or recurring), 82% (58/71) of the evaluable patients had complete or partial resolution of warts due to intralesional administration of Alferon N Injection as compared to 43% (29/67) of placebo patients (p<0.001). Fifty-four percent (38/71) of the evaluable Alferon N Injection patients had complete resolution of warts as compared to 18% (12/67) of placebo patients (p<0.001). Patients with primary occurrence of genital warts (*i.e.*, no prior treatment of warts) had a similar resolution rate compared to the patients with recalcitrant warts: 70% (7/10) had complete or partial resolution of warts due to Alferon N Injection treatment and 60% (6/10) had complete resolution of warts, as compared to 50% (4/8) of placebo recipients who had complete or partial resolution of warts and 38% (3/8) who had complete resolution. Overall, 83% (5/6) of Alferon N Injection (Interferon alfa-n3 (Human Leukocyte Derived))-treated patients with primary occurrence, who achieved complete resolution of warts, remained clear of all treated lesions during a median follow-up of 52 weeks. Because the number of patient with primary occurrence of warts was small (10 Alferon N Injection recipients and 8 placebo recipients), the difference between Alferon N Injection and placebo treatment was not statistically significant. However, when the resolution of primary warts was examined, 75% (33/44) of the Alferon N Injection-treated primary warts resolved completely as compared to 39% (11/28) of the placebo-treated primary warts (p=0.003).

In an open clinical trial using a once a week treatment schedule for up to 16 weeks, 28 patients were evaluable for efficacy. Eighty-nine percent (25/28) of patients had a complete or partial resolution of warts following treatment with Alferon N Injection. The condylomata acuminata resolved completely in 46% (13/28) of the patients. Of the 154 warts treated, 77% (118/154) resolved completely.

After injections of Alferon N Injection, side effects were minor and transient. After 4 weeks of treatment, the frequency of adverse reactions was similar in Alferon N Injection and placebo treatment groups. The most frequent side effects were myalgias, fever, and headache (See ADVERSE REACTIONS).

ANTIGENICITY

1. Alferon N Injection: One hundred and five (105) patients treated with alferon N injection during clinical trials were tested for the presence of anti-interferon antibodies using three different antibody assays: Immunoradiometric Assay (IRMA), Enzyme Linked Immunosorbent Assay (ELISA), and neutralization by the Cytopathic Effect Assay (CPE). To date, no antibodies to Interferon alfa-n3 have been detected in any of the patients.

2. Mouse Proteins: No hypersensitivity reactions to the components in alferon N injection (Interferon alfa-n3 (Human Leukocyte Derived)) have been observed. Alferon N Injection uses a murine monoclonal antibody in one of the purification procedures. A possibility exists that patients treated with Alferon N Injection may develop hypersensitivity to the mouse proteins. However, none of the patients receiving Alferon N Injection during clinical trials developed antibodies or hypersensitivity to mouse proteins (See CONTRAINDICATIONS.)

3. Egg Protein: The initial stage in the manufacture of Alferon N Injection uses Sendai virus which was grown in chicken eggs as the specific Interferon alfa-n3 inducer. Although no egg protein (ovalbumin) has been detected in the initial stage of interferon manufacture using an ELISA (sensitivity of 16 ng/ml) a possibility exists that patients treated with Alferon N Injection may develop hypersensitivity to egg protein (See CONTRAINDICATIONS).

INDICATIONS AND USAGE:

Alferon N Injection is indicated for the intralesional treatment of refractory or recurring external condylomata acuminata in patients 18 years of age or older (See DOSAGE AND ADMINISTRATION).

The physician should select patients for treatment with Alferon N Injection after consideration of a number of factors: the locations and sizes of the lesions, past treatment and response thereto, and the patient's ability to comply with the treatment regimen. Alferon N Injection is particularly useful for patients who have not responded satisfactorily to other treatment modalities, (*e.g.*, podophyllin resin, surgery, laser or cryotherapy).

There have been no studies with this product in adolescents. This product is not recommended for use in patients less than 18 years of age.

CONTRAINDICATIONS:

Alferon N Injection is contraindicated in patients with known hypersensitivity to human interferon alpha or any component of the product. The product also is contraindicated in patients who have anaphylactic sensitivity to mouse immunoglobulin (IgG), egg protein or neomycin.

WARNINGS:

Because of the fever and other "flu-like" symptoms associated with Alferon N Injection (Interferon alfa-n3 (Human Leukocyte Derived)) (See ADVERSE REACTIONS). It should be used cautiously in patients with debilitating medical conditions such as cardiovascular disease (*e.g.*, unstable angina and uncontrolled congestive heart failure), severe pulmonary disease (*e.g.*, chronic obstructive pulmonary disease), or diabetes mellitus with ketoacidosis. Alferon N Injection should be used cautiously in patients with coagulation disorders (*e.g.*, thrombophlebitis, pulmonary embolism and hemophilia), severe myelosuppression, or seizure disorders. Acute, serious hypersensitivity reactions (*e.g.*, urticaria, angioedema, bronchoconstriction, and anaphylaxis) have not been observed in patients receiving Alferon N Injection. However, if such reactions develop, drug administration should be discontinued immediately and appropriate medical therapy should be instituted.

PRECAUTIONS:

GENERAL

Patients being treated with Alferon N Injection should be informed of the benefits and risks associated with the treatment. Because the manufacturing process, strength, and type of interferon (*e.g.*, natural, human leukocyte interferon versus single-subspecies recombinant interferon) may vary for different interferon formulations, changing brands may require a change in dosage. Therefore, physicians are cautioned not to change from one interferon product to another without considering these factors.

INFORMATION FOR THE PATIENT

Patients should be informed of the early signs of hypersensitivity reactions including hives, generalized urticaria, tightness of the chest, wheezing, hypotension and anaphylaxis, and should be advised to contact their physician if these symptoms occur.

Patients being treated with Alferon N Injection should be informed of benefits and risks associated with treatment.

Patients should be cautioned not to change brands of interferon without medical consultation, as a change in dosage may occur.

CARCINOGENESIS, MUTAGENESIS, AND IMPAIRMENT OF FERTILITY

Studies with Alferon N Injection (Interferon alfa-n3 (Human Leukocyte Derived)) have not been performed to determine carcinogenicity, mutagenicity, or the effect on fertility. In studies with adult females, interferon alpha has been shown to affect the menstrual cycle and decrease serum estradiol and progesterone levels[5].

Alferon N Injection should be used with caution in fertile men. Fertile women should be cautioned to use effective contraception while being treated with Alferon N Injection.

Changes in the menstrual cycle and abortions have been reported to occur in non-human primates given extremely high doses of recombinant interferon alpha[4]. In these studies, Macaca mulatto (rhesus monkeys) were given interferon daily by intramuscular injection. When given at daily intramuscular doses 326 times the average intralesional dose of Alferon N Injection (120 times the maximum recommended dose), this recombinant interferon formulation produced menstrual cycle changes in the monkeys.

In human clinical trials with Alferon N Injection, menstrual cycle data were reported by 51 patients (36 Alferon N Injection and 15 placebo). There was no significant difference between Alferon N Injection and placebo treatment groups with regard to menstrual cycle changes.

PREGNANCY CATEGORY C

Animal reproduction studies have not been conducted with Alferon N Injection. It is also not known whether Alferon N Injection can cause fetal harm when administered to a pregnant woman or can affect reproductive capacity. Alferon N Injection should be given to a pregnant woman only if clearly needed.

Changes in the menstrual cycle and abortions have been reported to occur in non-human primates given extremely high doses of recombinant interferon alpha. In these studies, Macaca mulatto (rhesus monkeys) were given interferon daily by intramuscular injection. Abortifacient effects were noted when the recombinant interferon alpha was given daily during early to mid-gestation at intramuscular doses of 978 times the average intralesional dose of Alferon N Injection (Interferon alfa-n3 (Human Leukocyte Derived)) (360 times the maximum recommended dose).

NURSING MOTHERS

It is not known whether Alferon N Injection is excreted in human milk. Studies in mice have shown that mouse interferons are excreted in milk. Because many drugs are excreted in human milk and because of the potential for serious adverse reactions in nursing infants, a decision should be made whether to discontinue nursing or to not initiate drug treatment, taking into account the importance of the drug to the mother and the potential risks to the infant.

Pediatric Use: Safety and effectiveness have not been established in patients below the age of 18 years.

ADVERSE REACTIONS:

Adverse reactions were evaluated in 202 patients with condylomata acuminata receiving Alferon N Injection by intralesional administration and in 31 patients with cancer receiving Alferon N Injection by systemic administration. In the double-blind efficacy trial for the treatment of condylomata acuminata, 104 patients were treated with doses of Alferon N Injection of 0.05 million to 2.5 million IU per treatment session (average dose=0.92 million IU per treatment session) by intralesional injection. In open trials, an additional 98 patients received a dose range of 0.05 to 4.6 million IU of Alferon N Injection per treatment session (average dose=1.12 million IU per treatment session). Patients with cancer were given doses of Alferon N Injection of 3 million, 9 million, or 15 million IU per day for ten days by intramuscular injection.

ADVERSE REACTIONS IN PATIENTS WITH CONDYLOMATA ACUMINATA

A total of 104 patients with condylomata acuminata was treated with Alferon N Injection during the double-blind clinical trial. Adverse reactions were reported to be likely, unlikely, or not known to be related to Alferon N Injection. Adverse reactions consisted primarily of "flu-like" symptoms (myalgias, fever, and/or headache) which were in most cases mild or moderate, and transient, and did not interfere with treatment.

The "flu-like" adverse reactions, consisting of fever, myalgias, and/or headache, occurred primarily after the first treatment session and were reported by 30% of the patients. The frequency of "flu-like" adverse reactions abated with repeated dosing of Alferon N Injection (Interferon alfa-n3 (Human Leukocyte Derived) so that the incidences due to Alferon N Injection and placebo were similar after three to four weeks of treatment (after six to eight treatment sessions). "Flu-like" symptoms were relieved by administration of acetaminophen.

Adverse reactions were reported at least once during the course of treatment in the percentages of patients in each treatment group (TABLE 2).

Most of the systemic adverse reactions were mild or moderate. Severe systemic adverse reactions were reported by 18% of Alferon N Injection (Interferon alfa-n3 (Human Leukocyte Derived))-treated patients and 13% of placebo-treated patients (not statistically significant difference). Most of the severe systemic adverse reactions reported were "flu-like". Other severe systemic adverse reactions included back pain, insomnia and sensitivity to allergens. Those adverse reactions which were reported by 1% of patients treated with Alferon N Injection in the double-blind trial include: left groin lymph node swelling, tongue hyperaesthesia, thirst, tingling of legs/feet, hot sensation on bottom of feet, strange taste in mouth, increased salivation, heat intolerance, visual disturbances, pharyngitis, sensitivity to allergens, muscle cramps, nose bleed, throat tightness, and papular rash on neck. Additional adverse reactions which were reported by 1% of patients treated with placebo include: pharyngitis, oral pain, penile discharge, cold, knuckle stiffness, herpes outbreak, cough, disorientation, and weight/appetite loss.

Additional adverse reactions which occurred only in open clinical trials of intralesional use of Alferon N Injection for treatment of condylomata acuminata were herpes labialis, hot flashes, nervousness, decrease in concentration, dysuria, photosensitivity, and swollen lymph nodes. These reactions occurred in 1% of the patients. One patient with a history of epilepsy, who

ADVERSE REACTIONS: *(cont'd)*

TABLE 2 Percent of Patients with Adverse Reactions

Adverse Reactions:	Alferon (n=104)	Placebo (n=85)
Autonomic Nervous System		
Sweating	2%	1%
Vasovagal Reaction	2%	0%
Body as a Whole		
Fever	40%	19%
Chills	14%	2%
Fatigue	14%	6%
Malaise	9%	9%
Skin		
Generalized Pruritus	2%	0%
Central & Peripheral Nervous System		
Dizziness	9%	4%
Insomnia	2%	1%
Gastrointestinal System		
Nausea	4%	7%
Vomiting	3%	0%
Dyspepsia/Heartburn	3%	1%
Diarrhea	2%	2%
Musculoskeletal System		
Arthralgia	5%	1%
Back Pain	4%	1%
Myalgias	45%	15%
Headache	31%	15%
Psychiatric Disorders		
Depression	2%	1%
Nasopharyngeal		
Nose/sinus drainage	2%	2%

was not taking anticonvulsant medication, had a grand mal seizure while being treated with Alferon N Injection: this seizure was judged to be unrelated to Alferon N Injection administration.

APPLICATION SITE DISORDERS

The frequency of application site disorders (such as itching and pain) for patients treated with Alferon N Injection was significantly less than that reported with placebo (12% versus 26%). No severe application site disorders were reported by patients treated with Alferon N Injection, while 7% of placebo-treated patients reported severe disorders.

LABORATORY TEST VALUES

Abnormalities were seen with statistically equivalent frequencies in both the Alferon N Injection and placebo groups. None of the laboratory abnormalities were considered clinically significant. The abnormalities in the Alferon N Injection (Interferon alfa-n3 (Human Leukocyte Derived)-treated patients consisted primarily of decreased WBC (11%). Decreases also occurred in 4% of the placebo patients (not a statistically significant difference). The abnormalities in Alferon N Injection-treated patients involved increases of only one WHO grade.

ADVERSE REACTIONS IN PATIENTS WITH CANCER

Thirty-one patients with cancer were treated with a maximum of ten intramuscular injections of Alferon Injection in doses of 3 million IU. 9 million IU, or 15 million IU per treatment session. The occurrence of adverse reactions was judged to be unrelated to the dose of Alferon N Injection. The following adverse reactions were reported at least once (the percentage of patients experiencing the reaction is indicated in parentheses): chills (87%), fever (81%), anorexia (68%), malaise (65%), nausea (48%), vomiting (29%), myalgias (16%), arthralgia (10%), chest pains (10%), soreness at injection site (10%), sleepiness (10%), headache (10%), diarrhea (6%), fatigue (6%), low blood pressure (6%), sore mouth/stomatitis (6%), and blurred vision (6%). Those adverse reactions which were each reported by only one patient treated with Alferon N Injection include: stiff shoulders, face flushed, edema, dry mouth, mucositis, coughing, numbness, numbness in hands, numbness in fingers, pain on ocular rotation, shakes/shivers, ringing in ears, cramps, constipation, muscle soreness, confusion, light-headedness, depression, upset stomach, and sweating. The following adverse reactions were reported as severe by at least one patient (the percentage of patients experiencing the reaction is indicated in parentheses): fever (55%), malaise (54%), anorexia (45%), chills (45%), nausea (16%), myalgias (13%), vomiting (10%), fatigue (6%), low blood pressure (6%), chest pains (6%), sore mouth/stomatitis (6%), headache (3%), diarrhea (3%), sleepiness (3%), arthralgia (3%), blurred vision (3%), stiff shoulders (3%), numbness (3%), pain on ocular rotation (3%), muscle soreness (3%), confusion (3%), lightheadedness (3%), depression (3%), and sweating (3%).

The number and percentage of patients with cancer who experienced a significant abnormal laboratory test value (values that changed from WHO Grades 0.1 or 2 at baseline to WHO Grades 3 or 4 during or after treatment) at least once during the trials are shown in TABLE 3.

TABLE 3 Abnormal Laboratory Test Values

	Cancer (n = 31)
Hemoglobin Level	2 (7%)
White Blood Cell Count	1 (3%)
Platelet Count	1 (3%)
GGT	1 (6%)
SGOT	1 (3%)
Alkaline Phosphatase	2 (8%)
Total Bilirubin	1 (4%)

DOSAGE AND ADMINISTRATION:

The recommended dose of Alferon N Injection (Interferon alfa-n3 (Human Leukocyte Derived)) for the treatment of condylomata acuminata is 0.05 ml (250,000 IU) per wart. Alferon N Injection should be administered twice weekly for up to 8 weeks. The maximum recommended dose per treatment session is 0.5 ml (2.5 million IU). Alferon N Injection should be injected into the base of each wart, preferably using a 30 gauge needle. For large warts, Alferon N Injection may be injected at several points around the periphery of the wart, using a total dose of 0.05 ml per wart.

The minimum effective dose of Alferon N Injection for the treatment of condylomata acuminata has not been established. Moderate to severe adverse experiences may require modification of the dosage regimen or, in some cases, termination of therapy with Alferon N Injection.

Genital warts usually begin to disappear after several weeks of treatment with Alferon N Injection. Treatment should continue for a maximum of 8 weeks. In clinical trials with Alferon N Injection, many patients who had partial resolution of warts during treatment

DOSAGE AND ADMINISTRATION: *(cont'd)*

experienced further resolution of their warts after cessation of treatment. Of the patients who had complete resolution of warts due to treatment, half the patients had complete resolution of warts by the end of the treatment and half had complete resolution of warts during the 3 months after cessation of treatment. Thus, it is recommended that no further therapy (Alferon N Injection or conventional therapy) be administered for 3 months after the initial 8-week course of treatment unless the warts enlarge or new warts appear. Studies to determine the safety and efficacy of a second course of treatment with Alferon N Injection (Interferon alfa-n3 (Human Leukocyte Derived)) have not been conducted.

Parenteral drug products should be inspected visually for particulate matter and discoloration prior to administration, whenever solution and container permit.

Storage: Alferon N Injection should be stored at 2° to 8°C (36° to 46°F). Do not freeze. Do not shake.

REFERENCES:

1. Friedman-Kien, AE, Eron, L.I. Conant. M, et al. *JAMA, 259*:533-538, 1988. 2. Kirby. P. (editorial comment). *JAMA, 259*:570-572, 1988. 3. Friedman-Kien, AE, Plasse, TF, et al., *Papilloma Viruses: Molecular and Clinical Aspects* (Howley, PM, Broker, TR (eds)), New York, Alan R. Liss,Inc., 1986, pp. 217-233. 4. Geffen, JR, Klein, R.I. Friedman-Kien, AE, *J. Infect. Dis., 150*:612-615, 1984. 5. Kauppila, A, et al., *Int. J. Cancer, 29*:291-294, 1982. 6. Trown, PW, et al., *Cancer, 57 (Suppl)*: 1648-1656, 1986. 7. Schafer, TW, et al., *Science, 176*:1326-1327, 1972.

HOW SUPPLIED - EQUIVALENTS NOT AVAILABLE:

Injection, Solution - Intradermal; Su - 250000 unit/.05

1 ml $141.62 ALFERON N, Purdue Frederick 00034-1019-01

INTERFERON BETA-1A *(003287)*

CATEGORIES: Autonomic Drugs; Biologicals; Multiple Sclerosis; Neuromuscular; Recombinant DNA Origin; Pregnancy Category C; FDA Approved 1996 May

BRAND NAMES: **Avonex**

PRIMARY ICD9: 340 (Multiple Sclerosis)

DESCRIPTION:

Interferon beta-1a is produced by recombinant DNA technology. Interferon beta-1a is a 166 amino acid glycoprotein with a predicted molecular weight of approximately 22,500 daltons. It is produced by mammalian cells (Chinese Hamster Ovary cells) into which the human interferon beta gene has been introduced. The amino acid sequence of interferon beta-1a is identical to that of natural human interferon beta.

Using the World Health Organization (WHO) natural interferon beta standard, Second International Standard for Interferon, Human Fibroblast (Gb-23-902-531), interferon beta-1a has a specific activity of approximately 200 million international units (IU) of antiviral activity per mg; 30 mcg of interferon beta-1a contains 6 million IU of antiviral activity. The activity against other standards is not known.

Interferon beta-1a is formulated as a sterile, white to off-white lyophilized powder for intramuscular injection after reconstitution with supplied diluent or Sterile Water for Injection, USP, preservative-free.

Each 1.0 ml (1.0 cc) of reconstituted avonex contains 30 mcg of Interferon beta-1a, 15 mg albumin human, USP, 5.8 mg sodium chloride, USP, 5.7 mg dibasic sodium phosphate, USP and 1.2 mg monobasic sodium phosphate, USP at a pH of approximately 7.3.

CLINICAL PHARMACOLOGY:

GENERAL

Interferons are a family of naturally occurring proteins and glycoproteins that are produced by eukaryotic cells in response to viral infection and other biological inducers. Interferon beta, one member of this family, is produced by various cell types including fibroblasts and macrophages. Natural interferon beta and Interferon beta-1a are glycosylated, with each containing a single N-linked complex carbohydrate moiety. Glycosylation of other proteins is known to affect their stability, activity, biodistribution and half-life in blood. However, the effects of glycosylation of interferon beta on these properties have not been fully defined.

BIOLOGIC ACTIVITIES

Interferons are cytokines that mediate antiviral, antiproliferative and immunomodulatory activities in response to viral infection and other biological inducers. Three major interferons have been distinguished: alpha, beta and gamma. Interferons alpha and beta form the Type I class of interferons, and interferon gamma is a Type II interferon. These interferons have overlapping but clearly distinct biological activities.

Interferon beta exerts its biological effects by binding to specific receptors on the surface of human cells. This binding initiates a complex cascade of intracellular events that leads to the expression of numerous interferon-induced gene products and markers. These include 2', 5'-oligoadenylate synthetase, β_2-microglobulin and neopterin. These products have been measured in the serum and cellular fractions of blood collected from patients treated with interferon beta-1a.

The specific interferon-induced proteins and mechanisms by which interferon beta-1a exerts its effects in multiple sclerosis have not been fully defined.

PHARMACOKINETICS

Pharmacokinetics of interferon beta-1a in multiple sclerosis patients have not been evaluated. The pharmacokinetic and pharmacodynamic profiles of interferon beta-1a in healthy subjects following doses of 30 mcg through 75 mcg have been investigated. Serum levels of interferon beta-1a as measured by antiviral activity are slightly above detectable limits following a 30 mcg intramuscular (IM) dose, and increase with higher doses.

TABLE 1 compares general pharmacokinetic parameters for interferon beta-1a following administration of a 60 mcg dose by IM and subcutaneous (SC) routes to healthy volunteers. After an IM dose, serum levels of interferon beta-1a typically peak between 3 and 15 hours and then decline at a rate consistent with a 10 hour elimination half-life. Serum levels of interferon beta-1a may be sustained after IM administration due to prolonged absorption from the IM site. Systemic exposure, as determined by AUC and C_{max} values, is greater following IM than SC administration.

TABLE 1 Mean Single Dose Pharmacokinetic Parameters Following 60 mcg Administration

Route of Administration	AUC (IU·h/ml)	C_{max} (IU/ml)	T_{max}(Range) (h)	Elimination Half-life (h)
IM	1352	45	9.8 (3-15)	10.0
SC	478	30	7.8 (3-18)	8.6

Biological response markers (*e.g.*, neopterin and β_2-microglobulin) are induced by interferon beta-1a following parenteral doses of 15 mcg through 75 mcg in healthy subjects and treated patients. Biological response marker levels increase within 12 hours of dosing and remain

CLINICAL PHARMACOLOGY: *(cont'd)*

elevated for at least 4 days. Peak biological response marker levels are typically observed 48 hours after dosing. The relationship of serum interferon beta-1a levels or levels of these induced biological response markers to the mechanisms by which interferon beta-1a exerts its effects in multiple sclerosis is unknown.

CLINICAL STUDIES:

Effects in Multiple Sclerosis: The clinical effects of interferon beta-1a in multiple sclerosis were studied in a randomized, multicenter, double-blind, placebo-controlled study in patients with relapsing (stable or progressive) multiple sclerosis[1]. In this study, 301 patients received either 6 million IU (30 mcg) of interferon beta-1a (n=158) or placebo (n=143) by IM injection once weekly. Patients were entered into the trial over a $2\frac{1}{2}$ year period, received injections for up to 2 years, and continued to be followed until study completion. Two hundred eighty-two patients completed 1 year on study, and 172 patients completed 2 years on study. There were 144 patients treated with interferon beta-1a for more than 1 year, 115 patients for more than 18 months and 82 patients for 2 years.

All patients had a definite diagnosis of multiple sclerosis of at least 1 year duration and had at least two exacerbations in the 3 years prior to study entry (or one per year if the duration of disease was less than 3 years). At entry, study participants were without exacerbation during the prior 2 months and had Kurtzke Expanded Disability Status Scale (EDSS2) scores ranging from 1.0 to 3.5. Patients with chronic progressive multiple sclerosis were excluded from this study.

The primary outcome assessment was time to progression in disability, measured as an increase in the EDSS of at least 1.0 point that was sustained for at least 6 months. An increase in EDSS score reflects accumulation of disability. This endpoint was used to assure that progression reflected permanent increase in disability rather than a transient effect due to an exacerbation. Secondary outcomes included exacerbation frequency and results of magnetic resonance imaging (MRI) scans including gadolinium (Gd)-enhanced lesion number and volume and T2-weighted (proton density) lesion volume. Additional secondary endpoints included two upper limb (tested in both arms) and three lower limb function tests.

Twenty-three of the 301 patients (8%) discontinued treatment prematurely. Of these, one patient treated with placebo (1%) and six patients treated with interferon beta-1a (4%) discontinued treatment due to adverse events. Thirteen of these 23 patients remained on study and were evaluated for clinical endpoints.

Time to onset of sustained progression in disability was significantly longer in patients treated with interferon beta-1a than in patients receiving placebo (p=0.02). The Kaplan-Meier plots of these data are presented in Figure 1 of manufacturer's original package insert. The Kaplan-Meier estimate of the percentage of patients progressing by the end of 2 years was 34.9% for placebo-treated patients and 21.9% for interferon beta-1a-treated patients, indicating a slowing of the disease process. This represents a 37% reduction in the risk of accumulating disability in the interferon beta-1a-treated group compared to the placebo-treated group.

The distribution of confirmed EDSS change from study entry (baseline) to the end of the study is shown in Figure 2. There was a statistically significant difference between treatment groups in confirmed change for patients with at least two scheduled visits (136 placebo-treated and 150 interferon beta-1a-treated patients; p=0.006; see TABLE 2) Confirmed EDSS change was calculated as the difference between the EDSS score at study entry and one of the scores determined at the last two scheduled visits. If the EDSS score at either of the last two scheduled visits showed improvement (reduction in score), the higher score was used. Otherwise, the lower score was used. Nineteen patients had one score higher and one score lower than baseline; the higher score was used. The last two scheduled visits occurred at varying time points among patients.

The rate and frequency of exacerbations were determined as secondary outcomes. For all patients included in the study, irrespective of time on study, the annual exacerbation rate was 0.67 per year in the interferon beta-1a-treated group and 0.82 per year in the placebo-treated group (p=0.04).

TABLE 2 Major Clinical Endpoints

Endpoint	Placebo	Interferon beta-1a	*P*-value
Primary Endpoint			
Time to sustained progression in disability (N: 143, 158)[1]		0.02[2]	
Percentage of patients progressing in diability at 2 years (Kaplan-Meier estimate)[1]	34.9%	21.9%	
Secondary Endpoints: Disability			
Mean confirmed change in EDSS[1]	0.50	0.20	0.006[3]
Exacerbations			
Number of exacerbations in subset completing 2 years (N: 87, 85)			
0	26%	38%	0.03[3]
1	30%	31%	
2	11%	18%	
3	14%	7%	
≥4	18%	7%	
Percentage of patients exacerbation-free in subset completing 2 years (N: 87, 85)	26%	38%	0.10[4]
MRI			
Number of Gd-enhanced lesions:			
At study entry (N: 132, 141)			
Mean (Median)	2.3 (1.0)	3.2 (1.0)	
Range	0-23	0-56	
Year 1 (N:			
Mean (Median)	1.6 (0)	1.0 (0)	0.02[3]
Range	0-22	0-28	
Year 2 (N: 82, 83)			
Mean (Median)	1.6 (0)	0.8 (0)	0.05[3]
Range	0-34	0-13	
TS lesion volume:			
Percentage change from study entry to year 1 (N: 116, 123)			
Median	-3.3%	-13.1%	0.02[3]
Percentage change from study entry to year 2 (N: 83, 81)			
Median	-6.5%	-13.2%	0.36[3]

Note: (N:,) denotes the number of evaluable placebo and interferon beta-1a patients, respectively.
[1]Patient data included in this analysis represent variable periods of time on study.
[2]Analyzed by Mantel-Cox (logrank) test.
[3]Analyzed by Mann-Whitney rank-sum test.
[4]Analyzed by Cochran-Mantel-Haenszel test.
[5]Analyzed by likelihood ratio test.

Interferon beta-1a treatment significantly decreased the frequency of exacerbations in the subset of patients who were enrolled in the study for at least 2 years (87 placebo-treated patients and 85 interferon 1–a-treated patients; p = 0.03; see TABLE 2)

CLINICAL STUDIES: *(cont'd)*

Gd-enhanced and T2-weighted (proton density) MRI scans of the brain were obtained in most patients at baseline and at the end of 1 and 2 years of treatment. Gd-enhancing lesions seen on brain MRI scans represent areas of breakdown of the blood brain barrier thought to be secondary to inflammation. Patients treated with interferon beta-1a demonstrated significantly lower Gd-enhanced lesion number after 1 and 2 years of treatment ($p \leq 0.05$; see Table 2). The volume of Gd-enhanced lesions was also analyzed, and showed similar treatment effects ($p \leq 0.03$). Percentage change in T2-weighted lesion volume from study entry to year 1 was significantly lower in interferon beta-1a-treated than placebo-treated patients (p=0.02). A significant difference in T2-weighted lesion volume change was not seen between study entry and year 2.

The exact relationship between MRI findings and the clinical status of patients is unknown. Changes in lesion area often do not correlate with changes in disability progression. The prognostic significance of the MRI findings in this study has not been evaluated.

Of the limb function tests, only one demonstrated a statistically significant difference between treatment groups (favoring interferon beta-1a). A summary of the effects of interferon beta-1a on the primary and major secondary endpoints of this study is presented in Table 2. Safety and efficacy of treatment with interferon beta-1a beyond 2 years are not known.

INDICATIONS AND USAGE:

Interferon beta-1a is indicated for the treatment of relapsing forms of multiple sclerosis to slow the accumulation of physical disability and decrease the frequency of clinical exacerbations. Safety and efficacy in patients with chronic progressive multiple sclerosis have not been evaluated.

CONTRAINDICATIONS:

Interferon beta-1a is contraindicated in patients with a history of hypersensitivity to natural or recombinant interferon beta, human albumin, or any other component of the formulation.

WARNINGS:

Interferon beta-1a should be used with caution in patients with depression. Depression and suicide have been reported to occur in patients receiving other interferon compounds. Depression and suicidal ideation are known to occur at an increased frequency in the multiple sclerosis population. A relationship between occurrence of depression and/or suicidal ideation and the use of Avonex has not been established. An equal incidence of depression was seen in the placebo-treated and interferon beta-1a-treated patients in the placebo-controlled multiple sclerosis study. Patients treated with interferon beta-1a should be advised to report immediately any symptoms of depression and/or suicidal ideation to their prescribing physicians. If a patient develops depression, cessation of interferon beta-1a therapy should be considered.

PRECAUTIONS:

GENERAL

Caution should be exercised when administering Interferon beta-1a to patients with pre-existing seizure disorder. In the placebo-controlled study, four patients receiving interferon beta-1a experienced seizures, while no seizures occurred in the placebo group. Three of these four patients had no prior history of seizure. It is not known whether these events were related to the effects of multiple sclerosis alone, to interferon beta-1a, or to a combination of both. For patients with no prior history of seizure who develop seizures during therapy with interferon beta-1a, an etiologic basis should be established and appropriate anti-convulsant therapy instituted prior to considering resumption of interferon beta-1a treatment. The effect of interferon beta-1a administration on the medical management of patients with seizure disorder is unknown.

Patients with cardiac disease, such as angina, congestive heart failure or arrhythmia, should be closely monitored for worsening of their clinical condition during initiation of therapy with interferon beta-1a. Interferon beta-1a does not have any known direct-acting cardiac toxicity; however, symptoms of flu syndrome seen with interferon beta-1a therapy may prove stressful to patients with severe cardiac conditions.

INFORMATION FOR THE PATIENT

Patients should be informed of the most common adverse events associated with interferon beta-1a administration, including symptoms associated with flu syndrome (see ADVERSE REACTIONS and PRECAUTIONS). Symptoms of flu syndrome are most prominent at the initiation of therapy and decrease in frequency with continued treatment. In the placebo-controlled study, patients were instructed to take 650 mg acetaminophen immediately prior to injection and for an additional 24 hours after each injection to modulate acute symptoms associated with interferon beta-1a administration.

Patients should be cautioned to report depression or suicidal ideation (see WARNINGS).

Patients should be advised about the abortifacient potential of interferon beta (see Pregnancy, Teratogenic Effects, Pregnancy Category C).

When a physician determines that interferon beta-1a can be used outside of the physician's office, persons who will be administering interferon beta-1a should receive instruction in reconstitution and injection, including the review of the injection procedures (see DOSAGE AND ADMINISTRATION). If a patient is to self-administer, the physical ability of that patient to self-inject intramuscularly should be assessed. The first injection should be performed under the supervision of a qualified health care professional. A puncture-resistant container for disposal of needles and syringes should be used. Patients should be instructed in the technique and importance of proper syringe and needle disposal and be cautioned against reuse of these items.

LABORATORY TESTS

In addition to those laboratory tests normally required for monitoring patients with multiple sclerosis, complete blood and differential white blood cell counts, platelet counts, and blood chemistries, including liver function tests, are recommended during interferon beta-1a therapy. During the placebo-controlled study, these tests were performed at least every 6 months. There were no significant differences between the placebo and interferon beta-1a groups in the incidence of liver enzyme elevation, leukopenia or thrombocytopenia. However, these are known to be dose-related laboratory abnormalities associated with the use of interferons. Patients with myelosuppression may require more intensive monitoring of complete blood cell counts, with differential and platelet counts.

CARCINOGENESIS, MUTAGENESIS, AND IMPAIRMENT OF FERTILITY

Carcinogenesis: No carcinogenicity data for interferon beta-1a are available in animals or humans.

Mutagenesis: Interferon beta-1a was not mutagenic when tested in the Ames bacterial test and in an *in vitro* cytogenetic assay in human lymphocytes in the presence and absence of metabolic activation. These assays are designed to detect agents that interact directly with and cause damage to cellular DNA. Interferon beta-1a is a glycosylated protein that does not directly bind to DNA.

Impairment of Fertility: No studies were conducted to evaluate the effects of interferon beta on fertility in normal women or women with multiple sclerosis. It is not known whether interferon beta-1a can affect human reproductive capacity. Menstrual irregularities were

PRECAUTIONS: *(cont'd)*

observed in monkeys administered interferon beta at a dose 100 times the recommended weekly human dose (based upon a body surface area comparison). Anovulation and decreased serum progesterone levels were also noted transiently in some animals. These effects were reversible after discontinuation of drug. Treatment of monkeys with interferon beta at 2 times the recommended weekly human dose (based upon a body surface area comparison) had no effects on cycle duration or ovulation. The accuracy of extrapolating animal doses to human doses is not known. In the placebo-controlled study, 6% of patients receiving placebo and 5% of patients receiving interferon beta-1a experienced menstrual disorder. If menstrual irregularities occur in humans, it is not known how long they will persist following treatment.

PREGNANCY, TERATOGENIC EFFECTS, PREGNANCY CATEGORY C

The reproductive toxicity of interferon beta-1a has not been studied in animals or humans. In pregnant monkeys given interferon beta at 100 times the recommended weekly human dose (based upon a body surface area comparison), no teratogenic or other adverse effects on fetal development were observed. Abortifacient activity was evident following 3 to 5 doses at this level. No abortifacient effects were observed in monkeys treated at 2 times the recommended weekly human dose (based upon a body surface area comparison). Although no teratogenic effects were seen in these studies, it is not known if teratogenic effects would be observed in humans. There are no adequate and well-controlled studies with interferons in pregnant women. If a woman becomes pregnant or plans to become pregnant while taking interferon beta-1a, she should be informed of the potential hazards to the fetus, and it should be recommended that the woman discontinue therapy.

NURSING MOTHERS

It is not known whether interferon beta-1a is excreted in human milk. Because of the potential of serious adverse reactions in nursing infants, a decision should be made to either discontinue nursing or to discontinue interferon beta-1a.

PEDIATRIC USE

Safety and effectiveness in pediatric patients below the age of 18 years have not been established.

DRUG INTERACTIONS:

No formal drug interaction studies have been conducted with interferon beta-1a. In the placebo-controlled study, corticosteroids or ACTH were administered for treatment of exacerbations in some patients concurrently receiving interferon beta-1a. In addition, some patients receiving interferon beta-1a were also treated with anti-depressant therapy and/or oral contraceptive therapy. No unexpected adverse events were associated with these concomitant therapies.

Other interferons have been noted to reduce cytochrome P-450 oxidase-mediated drug metabolism. Formal hepatic drug metabolism studies with interferon beta-1a in humans have not been conducted. Hepatic microsomes isolated from interferon beta-1a-treated rhesus monkeys showed no influence of interferon beta-1a on hepatic P-450 enzyme metabolism activity. As with all interferon products, proper monitoring of patients is required if interferon beta-1a is given in combination with myelosuppressive agents.

ADVERSE REACTIONS:

The safety data describing the use of interferon beta-1a in multiple sclerosis patients are based on the placebo-controlled trial in which 158 patients randomized to interferon beta-1a were treated for up to 2 years (seeCLINICAL STUDIES).

The five most common adverse events associated (at p≤0.075) with interferon beta-1a treatment were flu-like symptoms (otherwise unspecified), muscle ache, fever, chills and asthenia. The incidence of all five adverse events diminished with continued treatment.

One patient in the placebo group attempted suicide; no interferon beta-1a-treated patient attempted suicide. The incidence of depression was equal in the two treatment groups. However, since depression and suicide have been reported with other interferon products, interferon beta-1a should be used with caution in patients with depression (see WARNINGS.)

In the placebo-controlled study, four patients receiving interferon beta-1a experienced seizures, while no seizures occurred in the placebo group. Three of these four patients had no prior history of seizure. It is not known whether these events were related to the effects of multiple sclerosis alone, to interferon beta-1a, or to a combination of both (see PRECAUTIONS.)

TABLE 3 enumerates adverse events and selected laboratory abnormalities that occurred at an incidence of 2% or more among the 158 multiple sclerosis patients treated with 30 mcg of interferon beta-1a once weekly by IM injection. Reported adverse events have been classified using standard COSTART terms. Terms so general as to be uninformative and those events that were equal in incidence or more common in the placebo-treated patients have been excluded.

Interferon beta-1a has also been evaluated in 290 patients with illnesses other than multiple sclerosis. The majority of these patients were enrolled in studies to evaluate interferon beta-1a treatment of chronic viral hepatitis B and C, in which the doses studied ranged from 15 mcg to 75 mcg, given SC, 3 times a week, for up to 6 months. The incidence of common adverse events in these studies was generally seen at a frequency similar to that seen in the placebo-controlled multiple sclerosis study. In these non-multiple sclerosis studies, inflammation at the site of the SC injection was seen in 52% of treated patients. In contrast, injection site inflammation was seen in 3% of multiple sclerosis patients receiving interferon beta-1a, 30 mcg by IM injection. Subcutaneous injections were also associated with the following local reactions: injection site necrosis, injection site atrophy, injection site edema and injection site hemorrhage. None of the above was observed in the multiple sclerosis patients participating in the placebo-controlled study.

Other events observed during premarket evaluation of interferon beta-1a, administered either SC or IM in all patient populations studied, are listed in the paragraph that follows. Because most of the events were observed in open and uncontrolled studies, the role of interferon beta-1a in their causation cannot be reliably determined.

Body as a Whole: abscess, ascites, cellulitis, facial edema, hernia, injection site fibrosis, injection site hypersensitivity, lipoma, neoplasm, photosensitivity reaction, sepsis, sinus headache, toothache;

Cardiovascular System: arrhythmia, arteritis, heart arrest, hemorrhage, hypotension, palpitation, pericarditis, peripheral ischemia, peripheral vascular disorder, postural hypotension, pulmonary embolus, spider angioma, telangiectasia, vascular disorder;

Digestive System: blood in stool, colitis, constipation, diverticulitis, dry mouth, gallbladder disorder, gastritis, gastrointestinal hemorrhage, gingivitis, gum hemorrhage, hepatoma, hepatomegaly, increased appetite, intestinal perforation, intestinal obstruction, periodontal abscess, periodontitis, proctitis, thirst, tongue disorder;

Endocrine System: hypothyroidism;

Hemic and Lymphatic System: coagulation time increased, ecchymosis, lymphadenopathy, petechia;

Metabolic and Nutritional Disorders: abnormal healing, dehydration, hypoglycemia, hypomagnesemia, hypokalemia;

Musculoskeletal System: arthritis, bone pain, myasthenia, osteonecrosis, synovitis;

ADVERSE REACTIONS: *(cont'd)*

TABLE 3 Adverse Events and Selected Laboratory Abnormalities in the Placebo-Controlled Study

Adverse Event	Placebo (N=143)	Interferon beta-1a (N=158)
Body As A Whole		
Headache	57%	67%
Flu-like symptoms (otherwise unspecified)*	40%	61%
Pain	20%	24%
Fever*	13%	23%
Asthenia	13%	21%
Chills*	7%	21%
Infection	6%	11%
Abdominal pain	6%	9%
Chest pain	4%	6%
Injection site reaction	1%	4%
Malaise	3%	4%
Injection site inflammation	0%	3%
Hypersensitivity reaction	0%	3%
Ovarian cyst	0%	3%
Cardiovascular System		
Syncope	2%	4%
Vasodilation	1%	4%
Digestive System		
Nausea	23%	33%
Diarrhea	10%	16%
Dyspepsia	7%	11%
Anorexia	6%	7%
Hemic And Lymphatic System		
Anemia*	3%	8%
Eosinophils ≥10%	4%	5%
HCT (%) ≤32 (females) or ≤37 (males)	1%	3%
Ecchymosis injection site	1%	2%
Metabolic And Nutritional Disorders		
SGOT ≥3 × ULN	1%	3%
Musculoskeletal System		
Muscle ache*	15%	34%
Arthralgia	5%	9%
Nervous System		
Sleep difficult	16%	19%
Dizziness	13%	15%
Muscle spasm	6%	7%
Suicidal tendency	1%	4%
Seizure	0%	3%
Speech disorder	0%	3%
Ataxia	0%	2%
Respiratory System		
Upper respiratory tract infection	28%	31%
Sinusitis	17%	18%
Dyspnea	3%	6%
Skin And Appendages		
Urticaria	2%	5%
Alopecia	1%	4%
Nevus	0%	3%
Herpes zoster	2%	3%
Herpes simplex	1%	2%
Special Senses		
Otitis media	5%	6%
Hearing decreased	0%	3%
Urogenital		
Vaginitis	2%	4%

* Significantly associated with interferon beta-1a treatment (p ≤0.05).

Nervous System: abnormal gait, amnesia, Bell's Palsy, clumsiness, depersonalization, drug dependence, facial paralysis, hyperesthesia, increased libido, neurosis, psychosis;

Respiratory System: emphysema, hemoptysis, hiccup, hyperventilation, laryngitis, pharyngeal edema, pneumonia;

Skin and Appendages: basal cell carcinoma, blisters, cold clammy skin, contact dermatitis, erythema, furunculosis, genital pruritus, nevus, seborrhea, skin ulcer, skin discoloration;

Special Senses: abnormal vision, conjunctivitis, earache, eye pain, labyrinthitis, vitreous floaters;

Urogenital: breast fibroadenosis, breast mass, dysuria, epididymitis, fibrocystic change of the breast, fibroids, gynecomastia, hematuria, kidney calculus, kidney pain, leukorrhea, menopause, nocturia, pelvic inflammatory disease, penis disorder, Peyronies Disease, polyuria, postmenopausal hemorrhage, prostatic disorder, pyelonephritis, testis disorder, urethral pain, urinary urgency, urinary retention, urinary incontinence, vaginal hemorrhage.

SERUM NEUTRALIZING ACTIVITY

Throughout the placebo-controlled multiple sclerosis study, serum samples from patients were monitored for the development of interferon beta-1a neutralizing activity. During the study, 24% of interferon beta-1a-treated patients were found to have serum neutralizing activity at one or more time points tested. Fifteen percent of interferon beta-1a-treated patients tested positive for neutralizing activity at a level at which no placebo patient tested positive. The significance of the appearance of serum neutralizing activity is unknown.

DRUG ABUSE AND DEPENDENCE:

There is no evidence that abuse or dependence occurs with interferon beta-1a therapy. However, the risk of dependence has not been systematically evaluated.

DOSAGE AND ADMINISTRATION:

The recommended dosage of interferon beta-1a for the treatment of relapsing forms of multiple sclerosis is 30 mcg injected intramuscularly once a week (see Figure 3 in the manufacturer's original package insert).

Interferon beta-1a is intended for use under the guidance and supervision of a physician. Patients may self-inject only if their physician determines that it is appropriate and with medical follow-up, as necessary, after proper training in intramuscular injection technique.

REFERENCES:

1. Jacobs LD, et al. Ann Neurol 1996; 39: 285-294. **2.** Kurtzke JF. Neurol 1983; 33: 1444-1452.

PATIENT INFORMATION:

Interferon beta-1a is intended for use under the guidance and supervision of a physician. If your physician recommends self-injection, you should be instructed in the preparation of interferon beta-1a for administration and in the technique of self-injection. Do not attempt self-administration until you are sure that you understand the requirements for preparing the product and giving an injection to yourself.

Interferon beta-1a must be used as prescribed by your physician. However, if you miss a dose, take it as soon as you remember. You may resume your regular schedule, but two injections should not be administered within 2 days of each other. While using interferon beta-1a, please keep in mind the following facts:

Interferon beta-1a) must be kept cold. Be sure to store it in a refrigerator before and after reconstitution. Do not freeze. If refrigeration is not available, interferon beta-1a can be stored before reconstitution at 25°C (77°F) for up to 30 days. When storing outside of a refrigerator, do not allow interferon beta-1a to be exposed to high temperatures as may occur in a glove compartment or on a window sill.

For treatment of multiple sclerosis, interferon beta-1a must be injected into the muscle (intramuscular injection).

Keep syringes and needles away from children. Do not reuse needles or syringes. Discard used syringes and needles in a syringe disposal unit as instructed by your health care professional.

Women: Interferon beta-1a should not be used during pregnancy or if you are trying to become pregnant. If you wish to become pregnant while using interferon beta-1a, discuss the matter with your doctor. While using interferon beta-1a, women of childbearing age should use birth control measures. If you do become pregnant you should discontinue treatment and contact your doctor immediately.

Flu-like symptoms are common. They include fever, chills, fatigue and muscle ache. Your physician may recommend taking acetaminophen to help lessen the impact of flu-like symptoms.

Depression has been reported by patients treated with interferon drugs. If you experience such symptoms, contact your physician promptly.

As with any prescription medication, side effects related to therapy can occur. Consult with your physician if you have any problems, whether or not you think they may be related to interferon beta-1a.

RECONSTITUTION AND ADMINISTRATION

Read through entire instructions prior to starting procedure.

Wash hands prior to preparing medication and after the medication has been administered. Allow the vial of Avonex (interferon beta-1a) and the vial of diluent to reach room temperature. Reconstitute Avonex using sterile technique, as discussed below.

The following supplies will be needed:

vial of Avonex
vial of diluent, single-use (Sterile Water for Injection, USP, preservative-free)
syringe
blue MICRO PIN
sterile needle
alcohol wipes
syringe disposal container
adhesive bandage

Reconstitution with diluent vial

1. Remove the cap from the vial of Avonex and vial of diluent, and clean the rubber stopper of each vial with an alcohol wipe.
2. Remove the small protective cover from the syringe with a counterclockwise turn.
3. Attach the blue MICRO PIN (vial access pin) to the syringe with a half turn clockwise.
4. Remove the MICRO PIN cover. Save for later use.
5. Pull back the syringe plunger to the 1.1 cc mark.
6. Push the MICRO PIN down through the center of the rubber stopper of the diluent vial.
7. Inject air into the diluent vial by pushing down on the plunger until it cannot be pushed any further.
8. Turn the diluent vial and syringe upside down.
9. Keeping the MICRO PIN in the fluid, withdraw 1.1 cc of diluent into the syringe by pulling back on the plunger.
10. Tap the syringe gently to make any air bubbles rise to the top. If bubbles are present, press the plunger until the diluent is at the top of the syringe. Make sure there is still 1.1 cc of diluent in the syringe.
11. Pull the MICRO PIN out of the diluent vial.
12. Insert the MICRO PIN through the center of the rubber stopper of the vial of Avonex.
13. Slowly inject the diluent. CAUTION: Rapid addition of the diluent may cause foaming, making it difficult to withdraw Avonex.
14. Without removing the syringe, gently swirl the vial until the white cake of Avonex is dissolved. *CAUTION:*DO NOT SHAKE.
15. Check to see that all of the Avonex cake is dissolved.
16. Turn the vial and syringe upside down. Slowly withdraw 1.0 cc of Avonex. If bubbles appear, push solution slowly back into the vial and withdraw the solution again.
17. Check the contents of the syringe. If you see areas of discoloration (other than a slightly yellow solution) or solid particles do not use the syringe. Get a new set of materials, including syringe, and start again with Step 1.
18. With the vial still upside down, tap the syringe gently to make any air bubbles rise to the top. Then press the plunger until the Avonex is at the top of the syringe. Check the volume (should be 1.0 cc) and withdraw more medication if necessary. Withdraw the MICRO PIN and syringe from the vial.
19. Replace the cover on the MICRO PIN and remove from the syringe with a counterclockwise turn.
20. Attach a needle to the syringe with a ½ turn clockwise until the needle is secure.

Injection

1. Use a new alcohol wipe to clean the skin at one of the recommended intramuscular injection sites. Pull the protective cover off the needle.
2. With one hand stretch the skin taut around the injection site. Hold the syringe with the other hand, making sure it is horizontal, until ready for injection. Insert the needle with a quick dart-like thrust at a 90° angle, through the skin and into the muscle. Expect to feel some resistance.
3. Once inserted, release the stretched skin and gently pull back slightly on the plunger and check for blood. If there is blood in the syringe, do not use it. Get a new set of materials, and go to Step 1 of the Reconstitution section and begin again.
4. If you do not see blood, slowly push the plunger until the syringe is empty.

PATIENT INFORMATION: *(cont'd)*

5. Hold an alcohol wipe near the needle at the injection site and pull the needle straight out. Use the wipe to apply pressure to the site for a few seconds or rub gently in a circular motion.
6. If there is bleeding at the site, wipe it off and, if necessary, apply an adhesive bandage.
7. Dispose of all supplies properly, including the diluent.

HOW SUPPLIED:

Avonex (interferon beta-1a) is supplied as a lyophilized powder in a single-use vial containing 33 mcg (6.6 million IU) of Interferon beta-1a, 16.5 mg Albumin Human, USP, 6.4 mg Sodium Chloride, USP, 6.3 mg Dibasic Sodium Phosphate, USP, and 1.3 mg Monobasic Sodium Phosphate, USP, and is preservative-free. Diluent is supplied in a single-use vial (Sterile Water For Injection, USP, preservative-free). Reconstitute Avonex with 1.1 mL (cc) of diluent and swirl gently to dissolve (approximate pH 7.3). Withdraw 1.0 mL (cc) for administration.

Avonex is available in the following package configuration: Package (Administration Pack) containing 4 Administration Dose Packs (each containing one vial of Avonex, one 10 mL (10 cc) diluent vial, two alcohol wipes, one 3 cc syringe, one Micro Pin vial access pin, one needle and one adhesive bandage).

Stability and Storage Vials of Avonex (interferon beta-1a) must be stored in a 2°-8°C (36°-46°F) refrigerator. Should refrigeration be unavailable, Avonex can be stored at 25°C (77°F) for a period of up to 30 days. DO NOT EXPOSE TO HIGH TEMPERATURES. DO NOT FREEZE. Do not use beyond the expiration date stamped on the vial. Following reconstitution, it is recommended the product be used as soon as possible within 6 hours stored at 2°-8°C (36°-46°F). DO NOT FREEZE.

HOW SUPPLIED - EQUIVALENTS NOT AVAILABLE:

Injectable - Intravenous - 33 g

33 g x 4 $710.00 AVONEX, Biogen **59627-0001-03**

INTERFERON BETA-1B, RECOMBINANT

(003154)

CATEGORIES: Autonomic Drugs; Biologicals; Multiple Sclerosis; Neuromuscular; Skeletal Muscle Hyperactivity; Spasticity; Recombinant DNA Origin; Sales > $500 Million; FDA Approved 1993 Jul

BRAND NAMES: **Betaseron**

FORMULARIES: Medi-Cal

COST OF THERAPY: $13,140.00 (Multiple Sclerosis; Injection; 0.3 mg/vial; 0.5/ day; 365 days)

DESCRIPTION:

Betaseron (interferon beta-1b) is a purified, sterile, lyophilized protein product produced by recombinant DNA techniques and formulated for use by injection. Interferon beta-1b is manufactured by bacterial fermentation of a strain of *Escherichia coli* that bears a genetically engineered plasmid containing the gene for human interferon beta $_{ser17}$. The native gene was obtained from human fibroblasts and altered in a way that substitutes serine for the cysteine residue found at position 17. Interferon beta-1b is a highly purified protein that has 165 amino acids and an approximate molecular weight of 18,500 daltons. It does not include the carbohydrate side chains found in the natural material.

The specific activity of interferon beta-1b, recombinant is approximately 32 million international units (IU)/mg Interferon beta-1b. Each vial contains 0.3 mg (9.6 million IU) of Interferon beta-1b. The unit measurement is derived by comparing the antiviral activity of the product to the World Health Organization (WHO) reference standard of recombinant human interferon beta. Dextrose and Albumin Human, USP (15 mg each/vial) are added as stabilizers. Prior to 1993, a different analytical standard was used to determine potency. It assigned 54 million IU to 0.3 mg Interferon beta- 1b.

Lyophilized interferon beta-1b, recombinant is a sterile, white to off-white powder intended for subcutaneous injection after reconstitution with the diluent supplied (Sodium Chloride, 0.54% Solution).

CLINICAL PHARMACOLOGY:

General: Interferons are a family of naturally occurring proteins, which have molecular weights ranging from 15,000 to 21,000 daltons. Three major classes of interferons have been identified: alfa, beta, and gamma. Interferon beta-1b, interferon alfa, and interferon gamma have overlapping yet distinct biologic activities.[1-5] The activities of Interferon beta-1b are species-restricted and, therefore, the most pertinent pharmacologic information on interferon beta-1b, recombinant is derived from studies of human cells in culture and in humans.

Biologic Activities: Interferon beta-1b has been shown to possess both antiviral and immunoregulatory activities. The mechanisms by which interferon beta-1b, recombinant exerts its actions in multiple sclerosis (MS) are not clearly understood. However, it is known that the biologic response-modifying properties of Interferon beta-1b are mediated through its interactions with specific cell receptors found on the surface of human cells. The binding of Interferon beta-1b to these receptors induces the expression of a number of interferon-induced gene products (*e.g.,* 2',5'-oligoadenylate synthetase, protein kinase, and indoleamine 2,3-dioxygenase) that are believed to be the mediators of the biological actions of Interferon beta-1b.[1,3,6-10] A number of these interferon-induced products have been readily measured in the serum and cellular fractions of blood collected from patients treated with Interferon beta-1b.[11,12]

Pharmacokinetics: Because serum concentrations of Interferon beta-1b are low or not detectable following subcutaneous administration of 0.25 mg (8 million IU) or less of interferon beta-1b, recombinant, pharmacokinetic information in patients with MS receiving the recommended dose of interferon beta-1b, recombinant is not available. Following single and multiple daily subcutaneous administrations of 0.5 mg (16 million IU) interferon beta-1b, recombinant to healthy volunteers (N=12), serum Interferon beta-1b concentrations were generally below 100 IU/ml. Peak serum Interferon beta-1b concentrations occurred between 1 to 8 hours, with a mean peak serum interferon concentration of 40 IU/ml. Bioavailability, based on a total dose of 0.5 mg (l6 million IU) interferon beta-1b, recombinant given as two subcutaneous injections at different sites, was approximately 50%.

After intravenous administration of interferon beta-1b, recombinant (0.006 mg [0.2 million IU] to 2.0 mg [64 million IU)], similar pharmacokinetic profiles were obtained from healthy volunteers (N=12) and from patients with diseases other than MS (N=142). In patients receiving single intravenous doses up to 2.0 mg (64 million IU), increases in serum concentrations were dose proportional. Mean serum clearance values ranged from 9.4 ml/min°kg^{-1} to 28.9 ml/min°kg^{-1} and were independent of dose. Mean terminal elimination half-life values ranged from 8.0 minutes to 4.3 hours and mean steady-state volume of distribution values ranged from 0.25 L/kg to 2.88 L/kg. Three-times-a-week intravenous dosing for 2 weeks

CLINICAL PHARMACOLOGY: *(cont'd)*

resulted in no accumulation of Interferon beta-1b in the serum of patients. Pharmacokinetic parameters after single and multiple intravenous doses of interferon beta-1b, recombinant were comparable.

CLINICAL STUDIES:

The effectiveness of interferon beta-1b, recombinant in relapsing-remitting MS was evaluated in a double-blind, multiclinic (11 sites: 4 Canadian and 7 United States), randomized, parallel, placebo-controlled clinical investigation of 2 years duration. The study enrolled MS patients, aged 18 to 50, who were ambulatory (Kurtzke expanded disability status scale [EDSS] of ≤5.5), exhibited a relapsing-remitting clinical course, met Poser's criteria[13] for clinically definite and/or laboratory supported definite MS and had experienced at least two exacerbations over 2 years preceding the trial without exacerbation in the preceding month. Patients who had received prior immunosuppressant therapy were excluded.

An exacerbation was defined, per protocol, as the appearance of a new clinical sign/symptom or the clinical worsening of a previous sign/symptom (one that had been stable for at least 30 days) that persisted for a minimum of 24 hours.

Patients selected for study were randomized to treatment with either placebo (N=123), 0.05 mg (1.6 million IU) of interferon beta-1b, recombinant (N=125), or 0.25 mg (8 million IU) of interferon beta-1b, recombinant (N=124) self-administered subcutaneously every other day. Outcome based on the 372 randomized patients was evaluated after 2 years.

Patients who required more than three 28-day courses of corticosteroids were removed from the study. Minor analgesics (acetaminophen, codeine), antidepressants, and oral baclofen were allowed ad libitum but chronic nonsteroidal anti-inflammatory drug (NSAID) use was not allowed.

The primary, protocol defined, outcome assessment measures were 1) frequency of exacerbations per patient and 2) proportion of exacerbation free patients. A number of secondary outcome measures were also employed as described in TABLE 1A and TABLE 1B.

In addition to clinical measures, annual magnetic resonance imaging (MRI) was performed and quantitated for extent of disease as determined by changes in total area of lesions. In a substudy of patients (N=52) at one site, MRIs were performed every 6 weeks and quantitated for disease activity as determined by changes in size and number of lesions.

Results at the protocol designated endpoint of 2 years (see TABLE 1A and TABLE 1B): In the 2-year analysis, there was a 31% reduction in annual exacerbation rate, from 1.31 in the placebo group to 0.9 in the 0.25 mg (8 million IU) group. The p-value for this difference was 0.0001. The proportion of patients free of exacerbations was 16% in the placebo group, compared with 25% in the interferon beta-1b, recombinant 0.25 mg (8 million IU) group.

TABLE 1A 2 Year Study Results: Primary and Secondary Clinical Endpoints

Efficacy Parameters / Primary Endpoints	Placebo (N=123)	Treatment Groups: 0.05 mg (1.6 mIU) (N=125)	0.25 mg (8mIU) (N=124)
Annual exacerbation rate	1.31	1.14	0.90
Proportion of exacerbation-free patients†	16%	18%	25%
Exacerbation frequency per patient 0†	20	22	29
1	32	31	39
2	20	28	17
3	15	15	14
4	15	7	9
≥5	21	16	8
Secondary Endpoints††			
Median number of months to first on-study exacerbation	5	6	9
Rate of moderate or severe exacerbations per year	0.47	0.29	0.23
Mean number of moderate or severe exacerbation days per patient	44.1	33.2	19.5
Mean change in EDSS score‡ at endpoint	0.21	0.21	-0.07
Mean change in Scripps score‡‡ at endpoint	-0.53	-0.50	0.66
Median duration in days per exacerbation	36	33	35.5
% change in mean MRI lesion area at endpoint	21.4%	9.8%	-0.9%

† 14 exacerbation-free patients (0 from placebo, 6 from 0.05 mg,and 8 from 0.25 mg) dropped out of the study before completing 6 months of therapy. These patients are excluded from this analysis.
†† Sequelae and Functional Neurologic Status, both required by protocol, were not analyzed individually but are included as a function of the EDSS.
‡ EDSS scores range from 0-10, with higher scores reflecting greater disability.
‡‡ Scripps neurologic rating scores range from 0-100, with smaller scores reflecting greater disability.

Of the 372 patients randomized, 72 (19%) failed to complete 2 full years on their assigned treatments. The reasons given for withdrawal varied with treatment assignment. Excessive use of steroids accounted for 11 of the 26 placebo withdrawals, but only 2 of the 21 withdrawals from the 0.05 mg (1.6 million IU) assigned group and 1 of the 25 withdrawals from the 0.25 mg (8 million IU) assigned group. Withdrawals for adverse events attributed to study article, however, were more common among interferon beta-1b, recombinant-treated patients: 1, 5, and 10 withdrew from the placebo, 0.05 mg (l.6 million IU), and 0.25 mg (8 million IU) groups, respectively.

Over the 2-year period, there were 25 MS-related hospitalizations in the 0.25 mg (8 million IU) Betaseron-treated group compared to 48 hospitalizations in the placebo group. In comparison, non-MS hospitalizations were evenly distributed among the groups, with 16 in the 0.25 mg (8 million IU) interferon beta-1b, recombinant group and 15 in the placebo group. The average number of days of MS-related steroid use was 41 days in the 0.25 mg (8 million IU) interferon beta-1b, recombinant group and 55 days in the placebo group (p=0.004).

MRI data were also analyzed for patients in this study. A frequency distribution of the observed percent changes in MRI area at the end of 2 years was obtained by grouping the percentages in successive intervals of equal width. Figure 1 (which can be found in the original manufacturer's package insert) displays a histogram of the proportions of patients who fell into each of these intervals. The median percent change in MRI area for the 0.25 mg (8 million IU) group was -1.1% which was significantly smaller than the 16.5% observed for the placebo group (p=0.0001).

In an evaluation of frequent MRI scans (every 6 weeks) on 52 patients at one site, the percent of scans with new or expanding lesions was 29% in the placebo group and 6% in the 0.25 mg (8 Million IU) treatment group (p=0.006).

CLINICAL STUDIES: *(cont'd)*

TABLE 1B 2 Year Study Results: Primary and Secondary Clinical Endpoints

Efficacy Parameters / Primary Endpoints	Statistical Comparisons p-value: Placebo vs 0.05 mg (1.6 mIU)	0.05 mg (1.6 mIU) vs 0.25 mg (8 mIU)	Placebo vs 0.25 mg (8 mIU)
Annual exacerbation rate	0.005	0.113	0.0001
Proportion of exacerbation-free patients†	0.609	0.288	0.094
Exacerbation frequency per patient	0.151	0.077	0.001
Secondary Endpoints††			
Median number of months to first on-study exacerbation	0.299	0.097	0.010
Rate of moderate or severe exacerbations per year	0.020	0.257	0.001
Mean number of moderate or severe exacerbation days per patient	0.229	0.064	0.001
Mean change in EDSS score‡ at endpoint	0.995	0.108	0.144
Mean change in Scripps score‡‡ at endpoint	0.641	0.051	0.126
Median duration in days per exacerbation	ND	ND	ND
% change in mean MRI lesion area at endpoint	0.015	0.019	0.0001

† 14 exacerbation-free patients (0 from placebo, 6 from 0.05 mg,and 8 from 0.25 mg) dropped out of the study before completing 6 months of therapy. These patients are excluded from this analysis.
†† Sequelae and Functional Neurologic Status, both required by protocol. were not analyzed individually but are included as a function of the EDSS.
‡ EDSS scores range from 0-10, with higher scores reflecting greater disability.
‡‡ Scripps neurologic rating scores range from 0-100, with smaller scores reflecting greater disability.
ND Not done.

MRI scanning is viewed as a useful means to visualize changes in white matter that are believed to be a reflection of the pathologic changes that, appropriately located within the central nervous system (CNS), account for some of the signs and symptoms that typify relapsing-remitting MS. The exact relationship between MRI findings and the clinical status of patients is unknown. Changes in lesion area often do not correlate with clinical exacerbations probably because many of the lesions affect so-called "silent" regions of the CNS. Moreover, it is not clear what fraction of the lesions seen on MRI become foci of irreversible demyelinization (*i.e.*, classic white matter plaques). The prognostic significance of the MRI findings in this study has not been evaluated.

At the end of 2 years on assigned treatment, patients in the study had the option of continuing on treatment under blinded conditions. Approximately 80% of patients under each treatment accepted. Although there was a trend toward patient benefit in the interferon beta-1b, recombinant groups during the third year, particularly in the 0.25 mg (8 million IU) group, there was no statistically significant difference between the interferon beta-1b, recombinant-treated vs. placebo-treated patients in exacerbation rate, or in any of the secondary endpoints described in TABLES 1A and 1B. As noted above, in the 2-year analysis, there was a 31% reduction in exacerbation rate in the 0.25 mg (8 million IU) group, compared with placebo. The p-value for this difference was 0.0001. In the analysis of the third year alone, the difference between treatment groups was 28%. The p-value was 0.065. The lower number of patients may account for the loss of statistical significance, and lack of direct comparability among the patient groups in this extension study make the interpretation of these results difficult. The third year MRI data did not show a trend toward additional benefit in the interferon beta-1b, recombinant arm compared with the placebo arm.

Throughout the clinical trial, serum samples from patients were monitored for the development of antibodies to Interferon beta-1b. In patients receiving 0.25 mg (8 million IU) of interferon beta-1b, recombinant (N=124) every other day in the clinical trial, 45% were found to have serum neutralizing activity at one or more of the time points tested. The relationship between antibody formation and clinical efficacy is not known.

INDICATIONS AND USAGE:

Interferon beta-1b, recombinant is indicated for use in ambulatory patients with relapsing-remitting multiple sclerosis to reduce the frequency of clinical exacerbations. (See CLINICAL STUDIES.) Relapsing-remitting MS is characterized by recurrent attacks of neurologic dysfunction followed by complete or incomplete recovery. The safety and efficacy of interferon beta-1b, recombinant in chronic-progressive MS has not been evaluated.

CONTRAINDICATIONS:

Interferon beta-1b, recombinant is contraindicated in patients with a history of hypersensitivity to natural or recombinant interferon beta, Albumin Human USP, or any other component of the formulation.

WARNINGS:

One suicide and 4 attempted suicides were observed among 372 study patients during a 3-year period. All five patients received interferon beta-1b, recombinant (three in the 0.05 mg [1.6 million IU] group and two in the 0.25 mg [8 million IU] group). There were no attempted suicides in patients on study who did not receive interferon beta-1b, recombinant. Depression and suicide have been reported to occur in patients receiving interferon alfa, a related compound. Patients to be treated with interferon beta-1b, recombinant should be informed that depression and suicidal ideation may be a side effect of the treatment and should report these symptoms immediately to the prescribing physician. Patients exhibiting depression should be monitored closely and cessation of therapy should be considered.

PRECAUTIONS:

General: Patients should be instructed in injection techniques to assure the safe self-administration of interferon beta-1b, recombinant. (See PRECAUTIONS, Information to patients, and interferon beta-1b, recombinant Patient Information sheet.)

Information to Patients: *Instruction on Self-Injection Technique and Procedures:* Patients should be instructed in the use of aseptic technique when administering interferon beta-1b, recombinant. Appropriate instruction for reconstitution of interferon beta-1b, recombinant and self-injection should be given including careful review of the interferon beta-1b, recombinantPatient Information sheet. If possible, the first injection should be performed under the supervision of an appropriately qualified health care professional.

Patients should be cautioned against the re-use of needles or syringes and instructed in safe disposal procedures. A puncture resistant container for disposal of used needles and syringes should be supplied to the patient along with instructions for safe disposal of full containers.

PRECAUTIONS: *(cont'd)*

Eighty-five percent of patients in the controlled MS trial reported injection site reactions at one or more times during therapy. In general, these were transient and did not require discontinuation of therapy, but the nature and severity of all reported reactions should be carefully assessed. Patient understanding and use of aseptic self-injection technique and procedures should be periodically reevaluated.

Flu-like symptoms are not uncommon following initiation of therapy with interferon beta-1b, recombinant. In the controlled MS clinical trial, acetaminophen was permitted for relief of fever or myalgia.

Patients should be cautioned not to change the dosage or the schedule of administration without medical consultation.

Awareness of Adverse Reactions: Patients should be advised about the common adverse events associated with the use of interferon beta-1b, recombinant, particularly, injection site reactions and the flu-like symptom complex (see ADVERSE REACTIONS).

Patients should be cautioned to report depression or suicidal ideation (see WARNINGS).

Patients should be advised about the abortifacient potential of interferon beta-1b, recombinant (see PRECAUTIONS, Pregnancy, Teratogenic effects).

Laboratory Tests: The following laboratory tests are recommended prior to initiating interferon beta-1b, recombinant therapy and at periodic intervals thereafter: hemoglobin, complete and differential white blood cell counts, platelet counts and blood chemistries including liver function tests. In the controlled MS trial, patients were monitored every 3 months. The study protocol stipulated that interferon beta-1b, recombinant therapy be discontinued in the event the absolute neutrophil count fell below $750/mm^3$. When the absolute neutrophil count had returned to a value greater than $750/mm^3$, therapy could be restarted at a 50% reduced dose. No patients were withdrawn or dose reduced for neutropenia or lymphopenia.

Similarly, if hepatic transaminase (SGOT/SGPT) levels exceeded 10 times the upper limit of normal, or if the serum bilirubin exceeded 5 times the upper limit of normal, therapy was discontinued. In each instance during the controlled MS trial, hepatic enzyme abnormalities returned to normal following discontinuation of therapy. When measurements had decreased to below these levels, therapy could be restarted at a 50% dose reduction, if clinically appropriate. Two patients were dose reduced for increased liver enzymes; one continued on treatment and one was ultimately withdrawn.

Carcinogenesis: The carcinogenic potential of interferon beta-1b, recombinant was evaluated by studying its effect on the morphological transformation of the mammalian cell line BALBc-3T3. No significant increases in transformation frequency were noted. No carcinogenicity data are available in animals or humans.

Interferon beta-1b, recombinant was not mutagenic when assayed for genotoxicity in the Ames bacterial test in the presence or absence of metabolic activation.

Impairment of Fertility: Studies in rhesus monkeys at doses up to 0.33 mg (10.7 million IU)/kg/day (32 times the recommended human dose based on body surface area comparison)* in normal cycling rhesus female monkeys had no apparent adverse effects on the menstrual cycle or on associated hormonal profiles (progesterone and estradiol) when administered over 3 consecutive menstrual cycles. The extrapolability of animal doses to human doses is not known. Effects of interferon beta-1b, recombinant on normal cycling human females are not known.

*body surface dose based on 70 kg female

Pregnancy, Teratogenic Effects, Pregnancy Category C: Interferon beta-1b, recombinant was not teratogenic at doses up to 0.42 mg (13.3 million IU)/kg/day in rhesus monkeys, but demonstrated a dose-related abortifacient activity when administered at doses ranging from 0.028 mg (0.89 million IU)/kg/day (2.8 times the recommended human dose based on body surface area comparison) to 0.42 mg (13.3 million IU)/kg/day (40 times the recommended human dose based on body surface area comparison). The extrapolability of animal doses to human doses is not known. Lower doses were not studied in monkeys. Spontaneous abortions while on treatment were reported in patients (N=4) who participated in the interferon beta-1b, recombinant MS clinical trial. Interferon beta-1b, recombinant given to rhesus monkeys on gestation days 20 to 70 did not cause teratogenic effects, however, it is not known if teratogenic effects exist in humans. There are no adequate and well-controlled studies in pregnant women. If the patient becomes pregnant or plans to become pregnant while taking interferon beta-1b, recombinant, the patient should be apprised of the potential hazard to the fetus and it should be recommended that the patient discontinue therapy.

Nursing Mothers: It is not known whether interferon beta-1b, recombinant is excreted in human milk. Because many drugs are excreted in human milk and because of the potential for serious adverse reactions in nursing infants from interferon beta-1b, recombinant, a decision should be made as to whether either to discontinue nursing or discontinue the drug, taking into account the importance of drug to the mother.

Pediatric Use: Safety and efficacy in children under 18 years of age have not been established.

DRUG INTERACTIONS:

Interactions between interferon beta-1b, recombinant and other drugs have not been fully evaluated. Although studies designed to examine drug interactions have not been done, it was noted that corticosteroid or ACTH treatment of relapses for periods of up to 28 days has been administered to patients (N=180) receiving interferon beta-1b, recombinant.

Interferon beta-1b, recombinant administration to three cancer patients over a dose range of 0.025 mg (0.8 million IU) to 2.2 mg (71 million IU) led to a dose-dependent inhibition of antipyrine elimination.[14] The effect of alternate-day administration of 0.25 mg (8 million IU) of interferon beta-1b, recombinant on drug metabolism in MS patients is unknown.

ADVERSE REACTIONS:

Experience with interferon beta-1b, recombinant in patients with MS is limited to a total of 147 patients at the recommended dose of 0.25 mg (8 million IU) every other day or more. Consequently, adverse events that are associated with the use of interferon beta-1b, recombinant in MS patients at a low incidence may not have been observed in pre-marketing studies. Clinical experience with interferon beta-1b, recombinant in other populations (patients with cancer, HIV positive patients, etc.) provides additional data regarding adverse reactions; however, experience in non-MS populations may not be fully applicable to the MS population.

Injection site reactions (85%) and injection site necrosis (5%) occurred after administration of interferon beta-1b, recombinant. Inflammation, pain, hypersensitivity, necrosis, and non-specific reactions were significantly associated ($p<0.05$) with the 0.25 mg (8 million IU) interferon beta-1b, recombinant-treated group. Only inflammation, pain, and necrosis were reported as severe events. The incidence rate for injection site reactions was calculated over the course of 3 years. This incidence rate decreased over time, with 79% of patients experiencing the event during the first 3 months of treatment compared to 47% during the last 6 months. The median time to the first occurrence of an injection site reaction was 7 days. Patients with injection site reactions reported these events 183.7 days per year. Three patients withdrew from the 0.25 mg (8 million IU) interferon beta-1b, recombinant-treated group for injection site pain.

ADVERSE REACTIONS: *(cont'd)*

Flu-like symptom complex was reported in 76% of the patients treated with 0.25 (8 million IU) interferon beta-1b, recombinant. A patient was defined as having a flu-like symptom complex if flu-like symptoms or at least two of the following symptoms were concurrently reported: fever, chills, myalgia, malaise, or sweating. Only myalgia, fever, and chills were reported as severe in more than 5% of the patients. The incidence rate for flu-like symptom complex was also calculated over the course of 3 years. The incidence rate of these events decreased over time, with 51% of patients experiencing the event during the first 3 months of treatment compared to 4% during the last 6 months. The median time to the first occurrence of flu-like symptom complex was 3 days and the median duration per patient was 10.4 days per year.

Laboratory abnormalities included absolute neutrophil count less than $1500/mm^3$ (18%) (no patients had absolute neutrophil counts less than $500/mm^3$), WBC less than $3000/mm^3$ (16%), SGPT greater than 5 times baseline value (19%), and total bilirubin greater than 2.5 times baseline value (6%). Three patients were withdrawn from treatment with 0.25 mg (8 million IU) interferon beta-1b, recombinant for abnormal liver enzymes including one following dose reduction (see PRECAUTIONS, Laboratory Tests).

Twenty-one (28%) of the 76 premenopausal females treated at 0.25 mg (8 million IU) interferon beta-1b, recombinant and 10 (13%) of the 76 premenopausal females treated with placebo reported menstrual disorders. All of these reports were of mild to moderate severity and included: intermenstrual bleeding and spotting, early or delayed menses, decreased days of menstrual flow, and clotting and spotting during menstruation.

Mental disorders have been observed in patients in this study. Symptoms included depression, anxiety, emotional lability, depersonalization, suicide attempts, confusion, etc. In the treatment group, two patients withdrew for confusion. One suicide and four attempted suicides were also reported. It is not known whether these symptoms may be related to the underlying neurological basis of MS, to interferon beta-1b, recombinant treatment, or to a combination of both. Some similar symptoms have been noted in patients receiving interferon alfa and both interferons are thought to act through the same receptor. Patients who experience these symptoms should be closely monitored and cessation of therapy considered.

Additional common adverse clinical and laboratory events associated with the use of interferon beta-1b, recombinant are listed in the following paragraphs. These events occurred at an incidence of 5% or more in the 124 MS patients treated with 0.25 mg (8 million IU) of interferon beta-1b, recombinant every other day for periods of up to 3 years in the controlled trial, and at an incidence that was at least twice that observed in the 123 placebo patients. Common adverse clinical and laboratory events associated with the use of interferon beta-1b, recombinant were: injection site reaction (85%), injection site necrosis (5%), flu-like symptoms (53%), palpitation (8%), hypertension (7%), tachycardia (6%), peripheral vascular disorders (5%), gastrointestinal disorders (6%), absolute neutrophil count $<1500/mm^3$ (18%), WBC $<3000/mm^3$ (16%), SGPT >5 times baseline value (19%), total bilirubin >2.5 times baseline value (6%), somnolence (6%), dyspnea (8%), laryngitis (6%), menstrual disorder (17%), cystitis (8%), breast pain (7%), pelvic pain (6%), and menorrhagia (6%).

A total of 277 MS patients have been treated with interferon beta-1b, recombinant in doses ranging from 0.025 mg (0.8 million IU) to 0.5 mg (16 million IU). During the first 3 years of treatment, withdrawals due to clinical adverse events or laboratory abnormalities not mentioned above included: fatigue (2%, 6 patients), cardiac arrhythmia (<1%, 1 patient), allergic urticarial skin reaction to injections (<1%, 1 patient), headache (<1%, 1 patient), unspecified adverse events (<1%, 1 patient), and "felt sick" (<1%, 1 patient).

The tables that follow (TABLES 2A and 2B) enumerates adverse events and laboratory abnormalities that occurred at an incidence of 2% or more among the 124 MS patients treated with 0.25 (8 million IU) interferon beta-1b, recombinant every other day for periods of up to 3 years in the controlled trial and at an incidence that was at least 2% more than that observed in the 123 placebo patients. Reported adverse events have been reclassified using the standard COSTART glossary to reduce the total number of terms employed in the table. In the following tables (TABLES 2A and 2B), terms so general as to be uninformative, and those events where a drug cause was remote have been excluded.

TABLE 2A Adverse Reactions and Laboratory Abnormalities

Adverse Reaction	Placebo N=123	0.25 mg (8 mIU) N=124
Body as a Whole		
Injection site reaction*	37%	85%
Headache	77%	84%
Fever*	41%	59%
Flu-like symptom complex*	56%	76%
Pain	48%	52%
Asthenia*	35%	49%
Chills*	19%	46%
Abdominal pain	24%	32%
Malaise*	3%	15%
Generalized edema	6%	8%
Pelvic pain	3%	6%
Injection site necrosis*	0%	5%
Cyst	2%	4%
Necrosis	0%	2%
Suicide attempt	0%	2%
Cardiovascular System		
Migraine	7%	12%
Palpitation*	2%	8%
Hypertension	2%	7%
Tachycardia	3%	6%
Peripheral vascular disorder	2%	5%
Hemorrhage	1%	3%
Digestive System		
Diarrhea	29%	35%
Constipation	18%	24%
Vomiting	19%	21%
Gastrointestinal disorder	3%	6%
Endocrine System		
Goiter	0%	2%
Hemic and Lymphatic System		
Lymphocytes $<1500/mm^3$	67%	82%
ANC $<1500/mm^3$*	6%	18%
WBC $<3000/mm^3$*	5%	16%
Lymphadenopathy	11%	14%

* Significantly associated with betaseron treatment.

It should be noted that the figures cited in the tables (TABLES 2A and 2B) cannot be used to predict the incidence of side effects in the course of usual medical practice where patient characteristics and other factors differ from those that prevailed in the clinical trials. The cited figures do provide the prescribing physician with some basis for estimating the relative contribution of drug and nondrug factors to the side effect incidence rate in the population studied.

ADVERSE REACTIONS: *(cont'd)*

TABLE 2B

Adverse Reaction	Placebo N=123	0.25 mg (8 mIU) N=124
Metabolic and Nutritional Disorders		
SGPT >5 times baseline*	6%	19%
Glucose <55 mg/dl	13%	15%
Total bilirubin >2.5 times baseline	2%	6%
Urine protein > 1+	3%	5%
SGOT >5 times baseline*	0%	4%
Weight gain	0%	4%
Weight loss	2%	4%
Musculoskeletal System		
Myalgia*	28%	44%
Myasthenia	10%	13%
Nervous System		
Dizziness	28%	35%
Hypertonia	24%	26%
Anxiety	13%	15%
Nervousness	5%	8%
Somnolence	3%	6%
Confusion	2%	4%
Speech disorder	1%	3%
Convulsion	0%	2%
Hyperkinesia	0%	2%
Amnesia	0%	2%
Respiratory System		
Sinusitis	26%	36%
Dyspnea*	2%	8%
Laryngitis	2%	6%
Skin and Appendages		
Sweating*	11%	23%
Alopecia	2%	4%
Special Senses		
Conjunctivitis	10%	12%
Abnormal vision	4%	7%
Urogenital System		
Dysmenorrhea	11%	18%
Menstrual disorder*	8%	17%
Metrorrhagia	8%	15%
Cystitis	4%	8%
Breast pain	3%	7%
Menorrhagia	3%	6%
Urinary urgency	2%	4%
Fibrocystic breast	1%	3%
Breast neoplasm	0%	2%

* Significantly associated with Betaseron treatment.

Other events observed during premarketing evaluation of various doses of interferon beta-1b, recombinant in 1440 patients are listed in the paragraph that follows. Because most of the events were observed in open and uncontrolled studies, the role of interferon beta-1b, recombinant in their causation cannot be reliably determined. *Body as a Whole:* abscess, adenoma, anaphylactoid reaction, ascites, cellulitis, hernia, hydrocephalus, hypothermia, infection, peritonitis, photosensitivity, sarcoma, sepsis, and shock;*Cardiovascular System:* angina pectoris, arrhythmia, atrial fibrillation, cardiomegaly, cardiac arrest, cerebral hemorrhage, cerebral ischemia, endocarditis, heart failure, hypotension, myocardial infarct, pericardial effusion, postural hypotension, pulmonary embolus, spider angioma, subarachnoid hemorrhage, syncope, thrombophlebitis, thrombosis, varicose vein, vasospasm, venous pressure increased, ventricular extrasystoles, and ventricular fibrillation; *Digestive System:* aphthous stomatitis, cardiospasm, cheilitis, cholecystitis, cholelithiasis, duodenal ulcer, dry mouth, enteritis, esophagitis, fecal impaction, fecal incontinence, flatulence, gastritis, gastrointestinal hemorrhage, gingivitis, glossitis, hematemesis, hepatic neoplasia, hepatitis, hepatomegaly, ileus, increased salivation, intestinal obstruction, melena, nausea, oral leukoplakia, oral moniliasis, pancreatitis, periodontal abscess, proctitis, rectal hemorrhage, salivary gland enlargement, stomach ulcer, and tenesmus; *Endocrine System:* Cushing's Syndrome, diabetes insipidus, diabetes mellitus, hypothyroidism, and inappropriate ADH; *Hemic and Lymphatic System:* chronic lymphocytic leukemia, hemoglobin less than 9.4 g/100 ml, petechia, platelets less than 75,000/mm^3, and splenomegaly;*Metabolic and Nutritional Disorders:* alcohol intolerance, alkaline phosphatase greater than 5 times baseline value, BUN greater than 40 mg/dl, calcium greater than 11.5 mg/dl, cyanosis, edema, glucose greater than 160 mg/dl, glycosuria, hypoglycemic reaction, hypoxia, ketosis, and thirst; *Musculoskeletal System:* arthritis, arthrosis, bursitis, leg cramps, muscle atrophy, myopathy, myositis, ptosis, and tenosynovitis; *Nervous System:* abnormal gait, acute brain syndrome, agitation, apathy, aphasia, ataxia, brain edema, chronic brain syndrome, coma, delirium, delusions, dementia, depersonalization, diplopia, dystonia, encephalopathy, euphoria, facial paralysis, foot drop, hallucinations, hemiplegia, hypalgesia, hyperesthesia, incoordination, intracranial hypertension, libido decreased, manic reaction, meningitis, neuralgia, neuropathy, neurosis, nystagmus, oculogyric crises, ophthalmoplegia, papilledema, paralysis, paranoid reaction, psychosis, reflexes decreased, stupor, subdural hematoma, torticollis, tremor, and urinary retention; *Respiratory System:* apnea, asthma, atelectasis, carcinoma of lung, hemoptysis, hiccup, hyperventilation, hypoventilation, interstitial pneumonia, lung edema, pleural effusion, pneumonia, and pneumothorax; *Skin and Appendages:* contact dermatitis, erythema nodosum, exfoliative dermatitis, furunculosis, hirsutism, leukoderma, lichenoid dermatitis, maculopapular rash, psoriasis, seborrhea, skin benign neoplasm, skin carcinoma, skin hypertrophy, skin necrosis, skin ulcer, urticaria, and vesiculobullous rash; *Special Senses:* blepharitis, blindness, deafness, dry eyes, ear pain, iritis, keratoconjunctivitis, mydriasis, otitis externa, otitis media, parosmia, photophobia, retinitis, taste loss, taste perversion, and visual field defect; *Urogenital System:* anuria, balanitis, breast engorgement, cervicitis, epididymitis, gynecomastia, hematuria, impotence, kidney calculus, kidney failure, kidney tubular disorder, leukorrhea, nephritis, nocturia, oliguria, polyuria, salpingitis, urethritis, urinary incontinence, uterine fibroids enlarged, uterine neoplasm, and vaginal hemorrhage.

DRUG ABUSE AND DEPENDENCE:

No evidence or experience suggests that abuse or dependence occurs with interferon beta-1b, recombinant therapy; however, the risk of dependence has not been systematically evaluated.

DOSAGE AND ADMINISTRATION:

The recommended dose of interferon beta-1b, recombinant for the treatment of ambulatory relapsing-remitting MS is 0.25 mg (8 million IU) injected subcutaneously every other day. Limited data regarding the activity of a lower dose are presented above (see CLINICAL STUDIES.)

Evidence of efficacy beyond 2 years is not known since the primary evidence of efficacy derives from a 2-year, double-blind, placebo-controlled clinical trial (see CLINICAL STUDIES). Safety data are not available beyond the third year. Patients were discontinued from this trial due to unremitting disease progression of 6 months or greater.

DOSAGE AND ADMINISTRATION: *(cont'd)*

To reconstitute lyophilized interferon beta-1b, recombinant for injection, use a sterile syringe and needle to inject 1.2 ml of the diluent supplied, Sodium Chloride, 0.54% Solution, into the interferon beta-1b, recombinant vial. Gently swirl the vial of interferon beta-1b, recombinant to dissolve the drug completely; do not shake. Inspect the reconstituted product visually and discard the product before use if it contains particulate matter or is discolored. After reconstitution with accompanying diluent, interferon beta-1b, recombinant vials contain 0.25 mg (8 million IU) Interferon beta-1b/ml of solution.

Withdraw 1 ml of reconstituted solution from the vial into a sterile syringe fitted with a 27-gauge needle and inject the solution subcutaneously. Sites for self-injection include arms, abdomen, hips, and thighs. A vial is suitable for single use only; unused portions should be discarded. See interferon beta-1b, recombinant PATIENT INFORMATION sheet for SELF, INJECTION PROCEDURE.

Stability: The reconstituted product contains no preservative. Before and after reconstitution with diluent, store at 2° to 8°C (36° to 46°F). Product should be used within 3 hours of reconstitution.

REFERENCES:

1. Ruzicka FJ, et al. J Biol Chem, 1987; 262: 16142-16149. **2.** Uze G, et al. Cell, 1990; 60: 225-234. **3.** DeMaeyer E, et al. In: Interferons and other regulatory cytokines, NY, Wiley 1988. **4.** Colby CB, et al. J Immunol 1984; 133: 3091-3095. **5.** Pestka S, et al. Annu Rev Biochem 1987; 56: 727-777. **6.** Lengyel P. Annu Rev Biochem 1982; 51: 251-282. **7.** Witt PL, et al. J Interferon Res 1990; 10: 393-402. **8.** Schiller JH, et al. J Biol Resp Mod 1990; 9: 377-386. **9.** Rosenblum MG, et al. J Interferon Res 1990; 10: 141-151. **10.** Carlin JM, et al. J Immuno 1987; 130(7): 2414-2418. **11.** Witt PL, et al. J Immunotherapy 1993; 13: 191-200. **12.** Goldstein D, et al. J Natl Cancer Inst 1989; 81: 1061-1068. **13.** Poser CM, et al. Ann Neurol 1983; 13(3): 227-231. **14.** Blaschke TF, et al. Clinical Research 1985; 33(1): 19A.

PATIENT PACKAGE INSERT:

Interferon beta-1b is intended for use under the guidance and supervision of a physician. Your physician or his/her delegate should instruct you in the preparation of interferon beta-1b, recombinant for administration and in the technique of self injection. Do not attempt self-administration until you are sure that you understand the requirements for mixing the product and giving an injection to yourself.

Interferon beta-1b, recombinant should be used as prescribed by your physician. However, if you miss a dose, take it as soon as you remember. Your next injection, however, should be scheduled about 48 hours later. While using interferon beta-1b, recombinant, please keep in mind the following facts:

Interferon beta-1b, recombinant must be kept cold. Be sure to store it in a refrigerator before and after reconstitution. Do not freeze. Keep syringes and needles away from children. Do not reuse needles or syringes. Discard used syringes and needles in a syringe disposal unit as instructed by your physician.

Women: Interferon beta-1b, recombinant should not be used during pregnancy or if you are trying to become pregnant. If you wish to become pregnant while using interferon beta-1b, recombinant, discuss the matter with your doctor. While using interferon beta-1b, recombinant, women of childbearing age should use birth control measures. If you do become pregnant you should discontinue treatment and contact your doctor immediately.

Injection site reactions are common. They include redness, pain and swelling, and discoloration. To minimize the chances for a reaction, ask your doctor to suggest a series of injection sites so that you will not have to use the same one repeatedly. Do not make an injection into skin that is tender, red, or hard.

Flu-like symptoms are also common. They include fever, chills, sweating, fatigue, and muscle aches. Taking interferon beta-1b, recombinant at night may help lessen the impact of flu-like symptoms.

Depression, including suicide attempts, has been reported by patients. If you experience such symptoms, contact your physician promptly.

As with any medication, side effects related to therapy can occur. Consult with your physician if you have any problems, whether or not you think they may be related to interferon beta-1b, recombinant.

SELF-INJECTION PROCEDURE

To Mix The Contents Of One Vial: Only the vial of diluent (liquid) that comes inside your prescription package should be used to dissolve the white cake of drug in the interferon beta-1b, recombinant vial.

1. Wash your hands thoroughly with soap and water.

2. Collect all your equipment before you begin the process.

You'll need:

vial of Diluent for interferon beta-1b, recombinant (Sodium Chloride 0.54%)

vial of interferon beta-1b, recombinant

3-ml syringe with 21-gauge needle (1)

1-ml syringe with 27-gauge needle (1)

alcohol wipes

disposal unit (an opaque, puncture-resistant, sealable container for used syringes/needles)

Note: Be sure needle guards are on the needles tightly.

3. Remove the protective caps from both vials.

4. Use alcohol wipes to clean the tops of the vials—move in one direction and use one wipe per vial.

Note: Leave an alcohol wipe on top of each vial until you are ready to use it.

5. Resting your hands on a stable surface, remove the needle cover on the 3-ml syringe by pulling the cover straight off the needle.

6. Pull back the plunger (on the 3-ml syringe) to the 1.2 ml mark.

Note: Read the labels on the vials—find the Diluent for interferon beta-1b, recombinant vial and throw away the alcohol wipe on top of it.

7. Holding the vial of Diluent for interferon beta-1b, recombinant on a stable surface, slowly insert the needle straight through the stopper, into the top of the vial.

Note: When inserting and removing needles from vials, be sure not to touch the needles or the rubber stoppers on the vials with your hands.

If you do touch a stopper, clean it with a fresh alcohol wipe.

If you touch a needle, throw away the entire syringe into the disposal unit and start over with a new syringe.

If the needle touches any surface, throw away the entire syringe into the disposal unit and start over with a new syringe.

8. Push in the plunger all the way to gently inject air into the vial (leave the needle in the vial of Diluent for interferon beta-1b, recombinant).

9. Turn the vial of Diluent for interferon beta-1b, recombinant upside down.

Note: Keep the needle tip in the liquid.

10. Resting your hands on a stable surface, hold the vial and syringe in one hand and slowly pull back the plunger on the syringe to the 1.2 ml mark (to draw up that amount of liquid) with your other hand.

PATIENT PACKAGE INSERT: *(cont'd)*

11. Keeping the vial upside down, gently tap the syringe until any air bubbles that formed rise to the top of the barrel of the syringe.

12. Carefully push in the plunger to eject ONLY THE AIR through the needle.

13. Remove the needle/syringe from the vial of Diluent for interferon beta-1b, recombinant.

Note: Find the interferon beta-1b, recombinant vial and throw away the alcohol wipe on top of it.

14. Holding the interferon beta-1b, recombinant vial on a stable surface, slowly insert the needle of the syringe (containing 1.2 ml of liquid) all the way through the stopper of the vial.

15. Push the plunger down slowly, directing the needle toward the side of the vial to allow the liquid to run down the inside wall (injecting Diluent for interferon beta-1b, recombinant directly onto the cake of drug will cause excess foaming).

16. Remove the needle/syringe from the interferon beta-1b, recombinant vial.

17. Throw away the 3 ml syringe into the disposal unit.

Note: Double-check that you are throwing away the correct syringe into the disposal unit.

18. Roll the vial between your hands gently to completely dissolve the white cake of interferon beta-1b, recombinant (DO NOT SHAKE).

19. Look closely at the solution (it should be clear).

Note: If the mixture contains particles or is discolored, discard it and start again.

PREPARING THE INJECTION

1. Remove the needle guard of the 1 ml syringe and pull back the plunger to the 1 ml mark.

2. Insert the needle of the 1 ml syringe through the stopper of the vial of interferon beta-1b, recombinant solution.

3. Gently push the plunger all the way down to inject air into the vial (leave the needle in the vial).

4. Turn the vial of interferon beta-1b, recombinant solution upside down.

Note: Keep the needle tip in the liquid.

5. Pull back the plunger to withdraw 1 ml of liquid into the syringe.

6. Hold the syringe with the needle pointing upward.

7. Tap the syringe gently until any air bubbles that formed rise to the top of the barrel of the syringe.

8. Carefully push in the plunger to eject ONLY THE AIR through the needle.

9. Remove the needle/syringe from the vial.

10. Recap the needle on the syringe.

Note: The injection should be administered immediately after mixing (if the injection is delayed, refrigerate the solution and inject it within 3 hours).

Do not freeze.

11. Throw away unused portion of the solution remaining in the vial.

GIVING THE INJECTION

Subcutaneous (Under The Skin) Self-Administration

1. Choose an injection site (see INJECTION SITES diagram in package insert); you may want to hold the syringe like a pencil or dart. Use a different site each day you inject:

Arms (upper back portion)

Abdomen (except around navel and waistline)

Hips (upper, outer rear quadrant)

Thighs (front and sides except at groin and knee)

Note: Do not use any areas in which you feel lumps, firm knots, depressions, pain, or discoloration; talk to your doctor or healthcare professional about anything you find.

2. Use an alcohol wipe to clean the skin at the injection site; let it air dry.

3. Throw away the wipe.

4. Uncap the needle.

5. Gently pinch the skin together around the site (to lift it up a bit).

6. Resting your wrist on the skin near the site, stick the needle straight into the skin at a 90° angle with a quick, firm motion.

7. Inject the drug by using a slow, steady push (push the plunger all the way in until the syringe is empty).

8. Hold a swab on the injection site. Remove the needle from the skin.

9. Gently massage the injection site with a dry cotton ball or gauze.

10. Throw away the 1 ml syringe in the disposal unit.

INJECTION SITE

Picking An Injection Site: Interferon beta-1b therapy should be injected into subcutaneous tissue (between the fat layer just under the skin and the muscles beneath). The best areas for injection are loose and soft (flabby), away from joints and nerves.

Each therapy day you can choose an injection site from the ones identified in the diagrams. It's a good idea to know where your injection will be given before you prepare your syringe.

If there are any sites that are difficult for you to reach, you can ask your support person (or someone who has been trained to give injections) to help you.

Rotating Injection Sites: Changing sites each time helps prevent injection reactions: it gives the site time to "bounce back" from the last injection. Today's injection should not be given in the same areas as the last one. Keep a record of where and when you last gave yourself an injection. One way to do that is to note the injection site on a calendar.

You may use a site again after waiting 1 week. If all areas become tender, talk to the doctor about choosing other injection sites.

HOW SUPPLIED:

Betaseron is supplied as a lyophilized powder containing 0.3 mg (9.6 million IU) of Interferon beta-1b, 15 mg Albumin Human USP, and 15 mg dextrose, USP. Drug is packaged in a clear glass, single-use vial (3 ml capacity); a separate vial containing 2 ml of diluent (Sodium Chloride, 0.54% solution) is included for each vial of drug. Store under refrigeration, between 2° to 8°C (36° to 46°F).

HOW SUPPLIED - EQUIVALENTS NOT AVAILABLE:

Injection, Lyphl-Soln - Subcutaneous - 0.3 mg/vial

1's	$72.00	BETASERON, Berlex Labs	50419-0521-15
5's	$360.00	BETASERON, Berlex Labs	50419-0521-05

INTERFERON GAMMA-1B, RECOMBINANT

(003049)

CATEGORIES: Antineoplastics; Antivirals; Granulomatous Disease; Immune Interferon; Immunoregulator; Infections; Orphan Drugs; Pregnancy Category C; Recombinant DNA Origin; FDA Approved 1990 Dec

BRAND NAMES: **Actimmune**; *Imufor* (Germany); *Imukin*; *Imukin Cream & Ointment*; *Imukin Inj.*
(International brand names outside U.S. in italics)

FORMULARIES: Aetna

DESCRIPTION:

Actimmune (Interferon gamma-1b), a biologic response modifier, is a single-chain polypeptide containing 140 amino acids. Production of Actimmune is achieved by fermentation of a genetically engineered *Escherichia coli* bacterium containing the DNA which encodes for the human protein. Purification of the product is achieved by conventional column chromatography. Actimmune is a highly purified sterile solution consisting of non-covalent dimers of two identical 16,465 dalton monomers; with a specific activity of 30 million U/mg.

Actimmune (Interferon gamma-1b) is a sterile, clear, colorless solution filled in a single-dose vial for subcutaneous injection. Each 0.5 ml of Actimmune contains: **100 mcg (3 million U)** of Interferon gamma-1b, formulated in 20 mg mannitol, 0.36 mg sodium succinate, 0.05 mg polysorbate 20 and Sterile Water for Injection.

CLINICAL PHARMACOLOGY:

General: Interferons are a family of functionally related, species-specific, proteins synthesized by eukaryotic cells in response to viruses and a variety of natural and synthetic stimuli. The most striking differences between interferon-gamma and other classes of interferon concern the immunomodulatory properties of this molecule. While gamma, alpha and beta interferons share certain properties, interferon-gamma has potent phagocyte-activating effects not seen with other interferon preparations. These effects include the generation of toxic oxygen metabolites within phagocytes, which are capable of mediating the killing of microorganisms such as *Staphylococcus aureus, Toxoplasma gondii, Leishmania donovani, Listeria monocytogenes,* and *Mycobacterium avium intracellulare.*

Clinical studies in patients using interferon-gamma, have revealed a broad range of biological activities including the enhancement of the oxidative metabolism of tissue macrophages, enhancement of antibody-dependent cellular cytotoxicity (ADCC) and natural killer (NK) cell activity. Additionally, effects on Fc receptor expression on monocytes and major histocompatibility antigen expression have been noted.[1,2]

To the extent that interferon-gamma is produced by antigen-stimulated T lymphocytes and regulates the activity of immune cells, it is appropriate to characterize interferon-gamma as a lymphokine of the interleukin type. There is growing evidence that interferon-gamma interacts functionally with other interleukin molecules such as interleukin-2 and that all of the interleukins form part of a complex, lymphokine regulatory network.[3] For example, interferon-gamma and interleukin-4 appear to reciprocally interact to regulate murine IgE levels; interferon-gamma can suppress IgE levels in humans.[4,5] Interferon-gamma also inhibits the production of collagen at the transcription level in human systems.[6]

More specifically, with respect to Chronic Granulomatous Disease (an inherited disorder characterized by deficient phagocyte oxidative metabolism), pilot clinical trials of the systemic administration of Actimmune in patients with Chronic Granulomatous Disease were initiated which provided evidence for a treatment-related enhancement of phagocyte function including elevation of superoxide levels and improved killing of *Staphylococcus aureus.*[7,8] Based on this evidence, a randomized, double-blind, placebo-controlled clinical study was initiated to further delineate the effects of Actimmune in Chronic Granulomatous Disease.

Pharmacokinetics: The intravenous, intramuscular, and subcutaneous pharmacokinetics of Actimmune (Interferon gamma-1b) have been investigated in 24 healthy male subjects following single-dose administration of 100 mcg/square m^2. Actimmune is rapidly cleared after intravenous administration (1.4 liters/minute) and slowly absorbed after intramuscular or subcutaneous injection. After intramuscular or subcutaneous injection, the apparent fraction of dose absorbed was greater than 89%. The mean elimination half-life after intravenous administration of 100 mcg/m^2 in healthy male subjects was 38 minutes. The mean elimination half-lives for intramuscular and subcutaneous dosing with 100 mcg/m^2 were 2.9 and 5.9 hours, respectively. Peak plasma concentrations, determined by ELISA, occurred approximately 4 hours (1.5 ng/ml) after intramuscular dosing and 7 hours (0.6 ng/ml) after subcutaneous dosing. Multiple dose subcutaneous pharmacokinetic studies were conducted in 38 healthy male subjects. There was no accumulation of Actimmune after 12 consecutive daily injections of 100 mcg/m^2. Pharmacokinetic studies in patients with Chronic Granulomatous Disease have not been performed.

Excretion studies of Actimmune have been performed. Trace amounts of interferon-gamma were detected in the urine of squirrel monkeys following intravenous administration of 500 mcg/kg. Interferon-gamma was not detected in the urine of healthy human volunteers following administration of 100 mcg/m^2 of Actimmune by the intravenous, intramuscular and subcutaneous routes. *In vitro* perfusion studies utilizing rabbit livers and kidneys demonstrate that these organs are capable of clearing interferon-gamma from perfusate. Studies of the administration of interferon-gamma to nephrectomized mice and squirrel monkeys demonstrate a reduction in clearance of interferon-gamma from blood; however, prior nephrectomy did not prevent elimination.

Effects on Chronic Granulomatous Disease: A randomized, double-blind, placebo-controlled study of Actimmune in patients with Chronic Granulomatous Disease, was performed to determine whether Actimmune administered subcutaneously on a three times weekly schedule could decrease the incidence of serious infectious episodes and improve existing infectious and inflammatory conditions in patients with Chronic Granulomatous Disease. One hundred twenty-eight eligible patients were enrolled on this study including patients with different patterns of inheritance. Most patients received prophylactic antibiotics. Patients ranged in age from 1 to 44 years with the mean age being 14.6 years. The study was terminated early following demonstration of a highly statistically significant benefit of Actimmune therapy compared to placebo with respect to time to serious infection ($p=0.0036$), the primary endpoint of the investigation. Serious infection was defined as a clinical event requiring hospitalization and the use of parenteral antibiotics. The final analysis provided further support for the primary endpoint ($p=0.0006$). There was a 67 percent reduction in relative risk of serious infection in patients receiving Actimmune ($n=63$) compared to placebo ($n=65$). Additional supportive evidence of treatment benefit included a twofold reduction in the number of primary serious infections in the Actimmune group (30 on placebo versus 14 on Actimmune, $p=0.002$) and the total number and rate of serious infections including recurrent events (56 on placebo versus 20 on Actimmune, $p=<0.0001$). Moreover, the length of hospitalization for the treatment of all clinical events provided evidence highly supportive of an Actimmune treatment benefit. Placebo patients required three times as many inpatient hospitalization days for treatment of clinical events compared to patients receiving Actimmune (1493 versus 497 total days, $p=0.02$). An Actimmune treatment benefit with respect to time to serious infection was consistently demonstrated in all subgroup analyses according to

CLINICAL PHARMACOLOGY: *(cont'd)*

stratification factors, including pattern of inheritance, use of prophylactic antibiotics, as well as age. There was a 67 percent reduction in relative risk of serious infection in patients receiving Actimmune compared to placebo across all groups. The beneficial effect of Actimmune therapy was observed throughout the entire study, in which the mean duration of Actimmune administration was 8.9 months/patient.

INDICATIONS AND USAGE:

Actimmune (Interferon gamma-1b) is indicated for reducing the frequency and severity of serious infections associated with Chronic Granulomatous Disease. Safety and effectiveness in children under the age of 1 year has not been established.

CONTRAINDICATIONS:

Actimmune is contraindicated in patients who develop or have known hypersensitivity to interferon-gamma, *E. coli* derived products, or any component of the product.

WARNINGS:

Actimmune should be used with caution in patients with pre-existing cardiac disease, including symptoms of ischemia, congestive heart failure or arrhythmia. No direct cardiotoxic effect has been demonstrated but it is possible that acute and transient "flu-like" or constitutional symptoms such as fever, and chills frequently associated with Actimmune administration at doses of 250 mcg/m²/day or higher may exacerbate preexisting cardiac conditions.

Caution should be exercised when treating patients with known seizure disorders and or compromised central nervous system function. Central nervous system adverse reactions including decreased mental status, gait disturbance and dizziness have been observed, particularly in patients receiving doses greater than 250 mcg/m²/day. Most of these abnormalities were mild and reversible within a few days upon dose reduction or discontinuation of therapy.

Caution should be exercised when administering Actimmune to patients with myelosuppression. Reversible neutropenia and elevation of hepatic enzymes can be dose limiting at doses above 250 mcg/m²/day. Thrombocytopenia and proteinuria have also been seen rarely.

PRECAUTIONS:

General: Acute serious hypersensitivity reactions have not been observed in patients receiving Actimmune, however, if such an acute reaction develops the drug should be discontinued immediately and appropriate medical therapy instituted. Transient cutaneous rashes have occurred in some patients following injection but have rarely necessitated treatment interruption.

Information for the Patient: Patients being treated with Actimmune and/or their parents should be informed regarding the potential benefits and risks associated with treatment. If home use is determined to be desirable by the physician, instructions on appropriate use should be given, including review of the contents of the Patient Information Insert. This information is intended to aid in the safe and effective use of the medication. It is not a disclosure of all possible adverse or intended effects.

If home use is prescribed, a puncture resistant container for the disposal of used syringes and needles should be supplied to the patient. Patients should be thoroughly instructed in the importance of proper disposal and cautioned against any reuse of needles and syringes. The full container should be disposed of according to the directions provided by the physician.

The most common adverse experiences occurring with Actimmune therapy are "flu-like" or constitutional symptoms such as fever, headache, chills, myalgia or fatigue (see ADVERSE REACTIONS) which may decrease in severity as treatment continues. Some of the "flu-like" symptoms may be minimized by bedtime administration. Acetaminophen may be used to prevent or partially alleviate the fever and headache.

The long-term effects of Actimmune therapy on growth, development or other parameters, are not known.

Laboratory Tests: In addition to those tests normally required for monitoring patients with Chronic Granulomatous Disease, the following laboratory tests are recommended for all patients on Actimmune (Interferon gamma-1b) therapy prior to the beginning of and at three month intervals during treatment.

Hematologic Tests: Including complete blood counts, differential and platelet counts.

Blood Chemistries: Including renal and liver function tests.

Urinalysis.

Carcinogenesis, Mutagenesis, and Impairment of Fertility: *Carcinogenesis:* Actimmune has not been tested for its carcinogenic potential.

Mutagenesis: Ames tests using five different tester strains of bacteria with and without metabolic activation revealed no evidence of mutagenic potential. Actimmune was tested in a micronucleus assay for its ability to induce chromosomal damage in bone marrow cells of mice following two intravenous doses of 20 mg/kg. No evidence of chromosomal damage was noticed.

Impairment of Fertility: Female cynomolgus monkeys treated with daily subcutaneous doses of 150 mcg/kg Actimmune (approximately 100 times the human dose) exhibited irregular menstrual cycles or absence of cyclicity during treatment. Similar findings were not observed in animals treated with 3 or 30 mcg/kg Actimmune. No studies have been performed assessing any potential effects of Actimmune on male fertility.

Pregnancy, Teratogenic Effects, Pregnancy Category C: Actimmune has shown an increased incidence of abortions in primates when given in doses approximately 100 X the human dose. A study in pregnant primates treated with intravenous doses, 2-100 X the human dose failed to demonstrate teratogenic activity for Actimmune. There are no adequate and well-controlled studies in pregnant women. Actimmune should be used during pregnancy only if the potential benefit justifies the potential risk to the fetus. In addition, studies evaluating recombinant murine interferon-gamma in pregnant mice, revealed increased incidences of uterine bleeding and abortifacient activity and decreased neonatal viability at maternally toxic doses. The clinical significance of this latter observation with recombinant murine interferon-gamma tested in a homologous system is uncertain.

Nursing Mothers: It is not known whether Actimmune is excreted in human milk. Because many drugs are excreted in human milk and because of the potential for serious adverse reactions in nursing infants from Actimmune, a decision should be made whether to discontinue nursing or to discontinue the drug, dependent upon the importance of the drug to the mother.

Pediatric Use: Safety and effectiveness in children under the age of 1 year has not been established.

DRUG INTERACTIONS:

Interactions between Actimmune and other drugs have not been fully evaluated. Caution should be exercised when administering Actimmune in combination with other potentially myelosuppressive agents (see WARNINGS).

DRUG INTERACTIONS: *(cont'd)*

Preclinical studies in rodents using species-specific interferon-gamma have demonstrated a decrease in hepatic microsomal cytochrome P-450 concentrations. This could potentially lead to a depression of the hepatic metabolism of certain drugs that utilize this degradative pathway.

ADVERSE REACTIONS:

The following data on adverse reactions are based on the subcutaneous administration of Actimmune at a dose of 50 mcg/m², three times weekly, in 63 patients with Chronic Granulomatous Disease during an investigational trial in the United States and Europe. Sixty-five additional patients with Chronic Granulomatous Disease received placebo on this study. The following (TABLE 1) represents the percentage of patients experiencing common adverse reactions observed on this study.

TABLE 1

Clinical Toxicity	Percent of Patients Actimmune	Placebo
Fever	52	28
Headache	33	9
Rash	17	6
Chills	14	0
Injection site erythema or tenderness	14	2
Fatigue	14	11
Diarrhea	14	12
Vomiting	13	5
Nausea	10	2
Weight loss	6	6
Myalgia	6	0
Anorexia	3	5
Arthralgia	2	0
Injection site pain	0	2

Miscellaneous adverse events which occurred infrequently and may have been related to underlying disease included back pain (2 percent versus 0 percent), abdominal pain (8 percent versus 3 percent) and depression (3 percent versus 0 percent) for Actimmune (Interferon gamma-1b) and placebo treated patients, respectively.

Actimmune has also been evaluated in additional disease states in studies in which patients have generally received higher doses (>100 mcg/m²/day) administered by intramuscular injection or intravenous infusion. All of the previously described adverse reactions which occurred in patients with Chronic Granulomatous Disease have also been observed in patients receiving higher doses. Adverse reactions not observed in patients with Chronic Granulomatous Disease receiving doses less than 100 mcg/m²/day but seen rarely in patients receiving Actimmune in other studies include: *Cardiovascular:* hypotension, syncope, tachyarrhythmia, heart block, heart failure, and myocardial infarction. *Central Nervous System:* confusion, disorientation, gait disturbance, Parkinsonian symptoms, seizure, hallucinations, and transient ischemic attacks.*Gastrointestinal:* hepatic insufficiency, gastrointestinal bleeding, and pancreatitis. *Renal:* reversible renal insufficiency. *Hematologic:* deep venous thrombosis and pulmonary embolism. *Pulmonary:* tachypnea, bronchospasm, and interstitial pneumonitis. *Metabolic*—hyponatremia and hyperglycemia.*Other:* exacerbation of dermatomyositis.

Abnormal Laboratory Test Values: No statistically significant differences between the Actimmune and placebo treatment groups were observed with regard to effect of treatment on hematologic, coagulation, hepatic and renal laboratory studies.

No neutralizing antibodies to Actimmune have been detected in any Chronic Granulomatous Disease patient receiving Actimmune.

DOSAGE AND ADMINISTRATION:

The recommended dosage of Actimmune (Interferon gamma-1b) for the treatment of patients with Chronic Granulomatous Disease is 50 mcg/m² (1.5 million U/m²) for patients whose body surface area is greater than 0.5 m² and 1.5 mcg/kg/dose for patients whose body surface area is equal to or less than 0.5 m². Injections should be administered subcutaneously three times weekly (for example, Monday, Wednesday, Friday). The optimum sites of injection are the right and left deltoid and anterior thigh. Actimmune can be administered by a physician, nurse, family member or patient when trained in the administration of subcutaneous injections. Parenteral drug products should be inspected visually for particulate matter and discoloration prior to administration, whenever solution and container permit.

The formulation does not contain a preservative. A vial of Actimmune is suitable for a single dose only. The unused portion of any vial should be discarded.

Higher doses are not recommended. Safety and efficacy has not been established for Actimmune (Interferon gamma-1b) given in doses greater or less than the recommended dose of 50 mcg/m². The minimum effective dose of Actimmune has not been established.

If severe reactions occur, the dosage should be modified (50 percent reduction) or therapy should be discontinued until the adverse reaction abates.

Actimmune (Interferon gamma-1b) may be administered using either sterilized glass or plastic disposable syringes.

Stability and Storage: Vials of Actimmune (Interferon gamma-1b) must be placed in a 2°-8°C (36°-46°F) refrigerator immediately upon receipt to insure optimal retention of physical and biochemical integrity. DO NOT FREEZE. Avoid excessive or vigorous agitation. DO NOT SHAKE. An unentered vial of Actimmune should not be left at room temperature for a total time exceeding 12 hours prior to use. Vials exceeding this time period should not be returned to the refrigerator; such vials should be discarded.

Do not use beyond the expiration date stamped on the vial.

REFERENCES:

1. Maluish AE, Urba WJ, Longo DL, *et al.*: The determination of an immunologically active dose of interferon gamma in patients with melanoma. J Clin Onc *6*:434-445, 1988. **2.** Nathan CF, Kaplan G, Levis W, *et al.*: Local and systemic effects of intradermal recombinant interferon gamma in patients with lepromatous leprosy. NEJM *315*:6-11, 1986. **3.** Fauci AS, Rosenberg SA, Sherwin SA, *et al.*: Immunomodulators in clinical medicine. Ann Internal Med *106*:421-433, 1987. **4.** Snapper CM, Paul WE: Interferon-gamma and B cell stimulatory factor-1 reciprocally regulate Ig isotype production. Science *236*:944-947, 1987. **5.** King CL, Gallin JI, Malech HL, *et al.*: Regulation of immunoglobulin production in hyperimmunoglobulin E recurrent-infection syndrome by interferon gamma. PNAS USA *86*:10085-10089, 1989. **6.** Rosenbloom J, Feldman G, Freundlich B, Jimenez SA: Inhibition of excessive scleroderma fibroblast collagen production by recombinant gamma-interferon. Arth Rheum *29*:851-856, 1986. **7.** Ezekowitz RAB, Dinauer MC, Jaffe HS, *et al.*: Partial correction of the phagocyte defect in patients with X-linked chronic granulomatous disease by subcutaneous interferon gamma. NEJM *319*:146-151, 1988. **8.** Sechler JMG, Malech HL, White CJ, Gallin JI: Recombinant human interferon-gamma reconstitutes defective phagocyte function in patients with chronic granulomatous disease of childhood. PNAS USA *85*:4874-4878, 1988.

HOW SUPPLIED:

Actimmune (Interferon gamma-1b) is a sterile, clear, colorless solution filled in a single-dose vial for subcutaneous injection. *Each 0.5 Ml Of Actimmune Contains:* **100 mcg (3 million U)** of Interferon gamma-1b, formulated in 20 mg mannitol, 0.36 mg sodium succinate, 0.05 mg polysorbate 20 and Sterile Water for Injection.

HOW SUPPLIED - EQUIVALENTS NOT AVAILABLE:

Injection, Solution - Subcutaneous - 100 mcg/0.5

1's	$140.00	ACTIMMUNE, Genentech	50242-0052-14
12's	$1526.00	ACTIMMUNE, Genentech	50242-0052-23

INULIN *(001549)*

CATEGORIES: Diagnostic Agents; Kidney Function; FDA Approval Pre 1982

BRAND NAMES: Inulin And Sodium Chloride

Prescribing information not available at time of publication.

HOW SUPPLIED - EQUIVALENTS NOT AVAILABLE:

Injection, Solution - Intravenous - 100 mg/ml

50 ml	$52.00	Inulin (w/ Sodium), Iso-Tex Dxs	50914-7730-03

IODINATED GLYCEROL *(001555)*

CATEGORIES: Airway Obstruction; Antitussives/Expectorants/Mucolytics; Asthma; Atelectasis; Bronchitis; Congestion; Cough Preparations; Cystic Fibrosis; Decongestants; Expectorants; Iodide Salts; Mucolytic Agents; Perioperative Prophylaxis; Pulmonary Emphysema; Respiratory & Allergy Medications; Sinusitis; Pregnancy Category X; FDA Pre 1938 Drugs

BRAND NAMES: Bestadin; Biophen; *Desputum*; Glycerol, Iodinated; *IPG*; Iocen; Iodrol; Iodur; Iogan; Iophen; *Ipol*; *Mucorama*; Myodine; Organ-I; Organic-I; **Organidin**; Oridol; R-Gen; Sil-O-Tuss; *Tandin*; Trinidin
(International brand names outside U.S. in italics)

FORMULARIES: Aetna; BC-BS; FHP

COST OF THERAPY: $311.27 (Asthma; Tablet; 30 mg; 8/day; 365 days)

PRIMARY ICD9: 493.90 (Asthma, Unspecified, Without Mention of Status Asthmaticus)

DESCRIPTION:

Iodinated glycerol, a mucolytic-expectorant, is an isomeric mixture formed by the interaction of iodine and glycerol, whose active ingredient is thought to be iodopropylidene glycerol but whose structural and chemical formulas have not been precisely established.

Iodinated glycerol is a viscous, amber liquid stable in acid media, including gastric juice, which contains virtually no inorganic iodide and no free iodine. Iodinated glycerol is available for oral administration as:

Solution: 5%, containing 50 mg iodinated glycerol (25 mg organically bound iodine) per ml. *Other Ingredients:* caramel, glycerin, purified water.

Tablets: each containing 30 mg iodinated glycerol (15 mg organically bound iodine). *Other Ingredients:* corn starch, dibasic calcium phosphate, FD&C Red No. 40, magnesium stearate, microcrystalline cellulose, tribasic calcium phosphate.

Elixir: 1.2%, containing 60 mg iodinated glycerol (30 mg organically bound iodine) per 5 ml (teaspoonful); and alcohol, 21.75% by volume. *Other Ingredients:* flavors (natural and artificial), liquid glucose, purified water, saccharin sodium.

CLINICAL PHARMACOLOGY:

Iodinated glycerol increases the output of thin respiratory tract fluid and helps liquefy tenacious mucus in the bronchial tree. Iodines are readily absorbed from the gastrointestinal tract and concentrated primarily in the secretions of the respiratory tract, but their mechanism of action as mucolytic-expectorants is not clear.

INDICATIONS AND USAGE:

Iodinated glycerol is indicated for adjunctive treatment as a mucolytic-expectorant in respiratory tract conditions such as bronchitis, bronchial asthma, pulmonary emphysema, cystic fibrosis, chronic sinusitis, or after surgery to help prevent atelectasis.

CONTRAINDICATIONS:

History of marked sensitivity to inorganic iodides; hypersensitivity to any of the ingredients or related compounds; pregnancy; newborns; and nursing mothers.

The human fetal thyroid begins to concentrate iodine in the 12th to 14th week of gestation and the use of inorganic iodides in pregnant women during this period and thereafter has rarely been reported to induce fetal goiter (with or without hypothyroidism) with the potential for airway obstruction. If the patient becomes pregnant while taking iodinated glycerol, the drug should be discontinued and the patient should be apprised of the potential risk to the fetus.

WARNINGS:

Discontinue use if rash or other evidence of hypersensitivity appears. Use with caution or avoid use in patients with history or evidence of thyroid disease.

PRECAUTIONS:

General: Iodides have been reported to cause a flare-up of adolescent acne. Children with cystic fibrosis appear to have an exaggerated susceptibility to the goitrogenic effect of iodides.

Dermatitis and other reversible manifestations of iodism have been reported with chronic use of inorganic iodides. Although these have not been reported to be a problem clinically with iodinated glycerol, they should be kept in mind in patients receiving these preparations for prolonged periods.

Carcinogenesis, Mutagenesis, and Impairment of Fertility: No long-term animal studies have been performed with iodinated glycerol.

Pregnancy, Teratogenic Effects, Pregnancy Category X: (see CONTRAINDICATIONS.)

Nursing Mothers: Iodinated glycerol should not be administered to a nursing woman.

DRUG INTERACTIONS:

Iodides may potentiate the hypothyroid effect of lithium and other antithyroid drugs.

ADVERSE REACTIONS:

Reports of gastrointestinal irritation, rash, hypersensitivity, thyroid gland enlargement, and acute parotitis have been rare.

OVERDOSAGE:

Acute overdosage experience with iodinated glycerol has been rare and there have been no reports of any serious problems.

DOSAGE AND ADMINISTRATION:

Note: Add solution to fruit juice or other liquid.

One drop solution equals approximately 3 mg iodinated glycerol.

ADULTS

Solution: 20 drops 4 times a day.

Tablets: 2 tablets 4 times a day, with liquid.

Elixir: 1 teaspoonful 4 times a day.

CHILDREN

Up to one-half the adult dosage based on the child's weight.

HOW SUPPLIED - EQUIVALENTS NOT AVAILABLE:

Elixir - Oral - 60 mg/5ml

5 ml x 40	$17.58	Iodinated Glycerol, Roxane	00054-8395-16
30 ml	$2.15	Biophen, Bio Pharm	59741-0133-30
30 ml	$5.50	ORGANIC-I, Major Pharms	00904-1547-30
30 ml	$5.60	Iogan, Hi Tech Pharma	50383-0773-01
30 ml	$5.80	IOCEN, HR Cenci	00556-0459-30
30 ml	$16.62	ORIDOL, H N Norton Co.	50732-0819-30
120 ml	$1.25	Biophen, Bio Pharm	59741-0132-04
120 ml	$3.60	Iogan, Hi Tech Pharma	50383-0776-04
120 ml	$3.70	IOCEN, HR Cenci	00556-0458-04
120 ml	$6.93	ORIDOL, H N Norton Co.	50732-0777-04
480 ml	$3.45	Biophen, Bio Pharm	59741-0132-16
480 ml	$11.00	Iogan, Hi Tech Pharma	50383-0776-16
480 ml	$11.25	IODUR, Duramed Pharms	51285-0707-57
480 ml	$11.40	IOCEN, HR Cenci	00556-0458-16
480 ml	$11.75	Iodinated Glycerol, Aligen Independ	00405-2950-16
480 ml	$14.50	Iodinated Glycerol, Geneva Pharms	00781-6305-16
480 ml	$20.23	ORIDOL, H N Norton Co.	50732-0777-16
500 ml	$7.07	Iodinated Glycerol, Roxane	00054-3395-63
3840 ml	$144.35	ORIDOL, H N Norton Co.	50732-0777-28

Tablet, Uncoated - Oral - 30 mg

	$31.80	ORGANIC-1, Major Pharms	00904-1553-70
100's	$10.66	Iodinated Glycerol Mucolytic, HL Moore Drug Exch	00839-7545-06
100's	$12.00	Iodinated Glycerol, Invamed	52189-0258-24
100's	$12.50	Iodinated Glycerol, Harber Pharm	51432-0877-03
100's	$13.10	Iodinated Glycerol Tablets 30 Mg, Able Labs	53265-0143-10
100's	$14.65	Iodinated Glycerol, Geneva Pharms	00781-1467-01
100's	$14.95	ORGANIC-1, Major Pharms	00904-1553-60
100's	$15.59	ORIDOL, H N Norton Co.	50732-0839-01
100's	$15.75	Iodinated Glycerol, Goldline Labs	00182-1907-01
250's	$30.00	Iodinated Glycerol, Able Labs	53265-0143-26
500's	$54.10	ORGANIC-I, Major Pharms	00904-1553-40
500's	$70.49	ORIDOL, H N Norton Co.	50732-0839-05

IODINATED GLYCEROL; THEOPHYLLINE *(001556)*

CATEGORIES: Airway Obstruction; Antiasthmatics/Bronchodilators; Antitussives/Expectorants/Mucolytics; Asthma; Bronchial Dilators; Bronchospasm; Decongestants; Expectorants; Iodide Salts; Mucolytic Agents; Pulmonary Emphysema; Respiratory & Allergy Medications; Respiratory Muscle Relaxant; Smooth Muscle Relaxants; Wheezing; Xanthine Derivatives; FDA Pre 1938 Drugs

BRAND NAMES: Iophylline; **Theo-Organidin**; Theo-Oridol; Theo-R; Theo-R-Gen

Prescribing information not available at time of publication.

HOW SUPPLIED - EQUIVALENTS NOT AVAILABLE:

Liquid - Oral - 30 mg/120 mg

480 ml	$16.50	THEO-ORIDOL, H N Norton Co.	50732-0891-16
480 ml	$18.00	THEO-R-GEN, Goldline Labs	00182-1372-40
3840 ml	$103.99	THEO-ORIDOL, H N Norton Co.	50732-0891-28

IODINE *(001557)*

CATEGORIES: Anti-Infectives; Electrolytic, Caloric-Water Balance; Homeostatic & Nutrient; Local Infections; Pharmaceutical Adjuvants; Replacement Solutions; Skin/Mucous Membrane Agents; Vitamins; FDA Pre 1938 Drugs

BRAND NAMES: *Aqueous Iodine*; Iodopen; Strong Iodine
(International brand names outside U.S. in italics)

FORMULARIES: WHO

Prescribing information not available at time of publication.

HOW SUPPLIED - EQUIVALENTS NOT AVAILABLE:

Injection, Solution - Intravenous - 100 mcg/ml

10 ml	$195.31	IODOPEN, Fujisawa USA	00469-1900-30

IODIPAMIDE MEGLUMINE *(001562)*

CATEGORIES: Cholangiography; Cholecystectomy; Cholecystography; Diagnostic Agents; Roentgenography; FDA Approval Pre 1982

BRAND NAMES: **Cholografin Meglumine**

DESCRIPTION:

Iodipamide meglumine is a radiopaque contrast agent for rapid intravenous cholangiography and cholecystography, supplied as a sterile, aqueous solution. Each ml provides 520 mg iodipamide meglumine with 3.2 mg sodium citrate as a buffer and 0.4 mg edetate disodium as a sequestering agent; pH has been adjusted between 6.5 and 7.7 with meglumine. Each ml of solution also contains approximately 0.91 mg (0.039 mEq) sodium (18.2 mg/20 ml) and 257 mg organically bound iodine (5.2 g/20 ml). At the time of manufacture, the air in the container is replaced by nitrogen.

The appearance of the solution may vary from essentially colorless to light amber. Solutions which have become substantially darker, however, should not be used.

CLINICAL PHARMACOLOGY:

Following intravenous administration of iodipamide meglumine, iodipamide is carried to the liver where it is rapidly secreted. The contrast medium appears in the bile within 10 to 15 minutes after injection, thus permitting visualization of the hepatic and common bile ducts, even in cholecystectomized patients. The biliary ducts are readily visualized within about 25 minutes after administration, except in patients with impaired liver function. The gallbladder begins to fill within an hour after injection; maximum filling is reached after two to two and one-half hours. The contrast medium is finally eliminated in the feces without passing through the enterohepatic circulation, except for approximately 10 percent of the intravenously administered dose which is excreted through the kidneys.

The LD 50 for intravenous administration of a 52% iodipamide meglumine solution in mice is 6.2 ± 0.3 ml/kg (equivalent to 3224 ± 156 mg iodipamide meglumine/kg).

INDICATIONS AND USAGE:

Iodipamide meglumine is indicated for intravenous cholangiography and cholecystography as follows:

(a) Visualization of the gallbladder and biliary ducts in the differential diagnosis of acute abdominal conditions.

(b) Visualization of the biliary ducts, especially in patients with symptoms after after cholecystectomy.

(c) Visualization of the gallbladder in patients unable to take oral contrast media or to absorb contrast media from the gastrointestinal tract.

CONTRAINDICATIONS:

Iodipamide meglumine is contraindicated in patients with a hypersensitivity to salts of iodipamide or who exhibit sensitivity reactions to the test dose. It is also contraindicated in patients with concomitant severe impairment of renal and liver function.

WARNINGS:

Administration of radiopaque materials to patients known or suspected to have pheochromocytoma should be performed with extreme caution. If, in the opinion of the physician, the possible benefits of such procedures outweigh the considered risks, the procedures may be performed; however, the amount of radiopaque medium injected should be kept to an absolute minimum. The blood pressure should be assessed throughout the procedure and measures for treatment of a hypertensive crisis should be available.

Contrast media have been shown to promote the phenomenon of sickling in individuals who are homozygous for sickle cell disease when the material is injected intravenously or intra-arterially.

Since iodine-containing contrast agents may alter the results of thyroid function tests, such tests, if indicated, should be performed prior to the administration of this preparation.

A history of sensitivity to iodine per se or to other contrast agents is not an absolute contraindication to the use of iodipamide meglumine, but calls for extreme caution in administration.

PRECAUTIONS:

Diagnostic procedures which involve the use of radiopaque contrast agents should be carried out under the direction of personnel with the prerequisite training and with a thorough knowledge of the particular procedure to be performed. Appropriate facilities should be available for coping with situations which may arise as a result of the procedure, as well as for emergency treatment of severe reactions to the contrast agent itself.

After intravascular administration of a radiopaque agent, competent personnel and emergency facilities should be available for at least 30 to 60 minutes, since severe delayed reactions have been known to occur.

These severe, life-threatening reactions suggest hypersensitivity to the radiopaque agent, which has prompted the use of several pretesting methods, none of which can be relied upon to predict severe reactions. Many authorities question the value of any pretest. A history of bronchial asthma or allergy, a family history of allergy, or a previous reaction to a contrast agent warrant special attention. Such a history, by suggesting histamine sensitivity and a consequent proneness to reactions, may be more accurate than pretesting in predicting the likelihood of a reaction, although not necessarily the severity or type of reaction in the individual case.

The sensitivity test most often performed is the slow injection of 0.5 to 1.0 ml of the radiopaque medium, administered intravenously, prior to injection of the full diagnostic dose. It should be noted that the absence of a reaction to the test dose does not preclude the possibility of a reaction to the full diagnostic dose. If the test dose causes an untoward response of any kind, the necessity for continuing with the examination should be carefully reevaluated and, if it is deemed essential, the examination should be conducted with all possible caution. In rare instances reactions to the test dose itself may be extremely severe; therefore, close observation of the patient, and facilities for emergency treatment, appear indicated.

Caution should be exercised with the use of radiopaque media in severely debilitated patients and in those with marked hypertension. The possibility of thrombosis should be borne in mind when intravenous techniques are employed.

Contrast agents may interfere with some chemical determinations made on urine specimens; therefore, urine should be collected before administration of the contrast media or two or more days afterwards.

Some clinicians feel it may be advisable to have a continuous intravenous infusion running prior to and during administration of the drug.

The admixture of benadryl (R) (diphenhydramine hydrochloride injection) with iodipamide meglumine injection USP 52% may cause a precipitate which may form in the syringe or tubing. If antihistamines are administered concomitantly, they should not be mixed with the contrast agent but administered at another site.

Pregnancy: The safety of iodipamide meglumine for use during pregnancy has not been established; therefore it should be used in pregnant patients, only when, in the judgement of the physician, its use is deemed essential to the welfare of the patient.

ADVERSE REACTIONS:

Local reactions at the site of injection are not observed, unless excessive amounts are extravasated during injection. After too rapid administration, mild transient symptoms such as restlessness, sensations of warmth, sneezing, perspiration, salivation, flushing, pressure in the upper abdomen, dizziness, nausea, vomiting, chills, fever, headache, pallor and tremors may occur. These symptoms disappear when the injection has been completed. Rarely, swollen eyelids, laryngospasm, respiratory difficulties, hypotension, cardiac reactions and cyanosis have been reported. Hypersensitivity reactions may occur. In rare instances, despite the most careful sensitivity testing, anaphylactoid reactions may occur.

Renal function tests may be altered and renal failure may occur.

DOSAGE AND ADMINISTRATION:

Iodipamide meglumine injection USP, 52% is for intravenous use only.

DIRECTIONS FOR USE

Preparation Of The Patient: For best results, the usual preliminary measures for cholecystography are recommended, particularly in cholecystectomized patients, (*i.e.,* a low residue diet on the day before examination and administration of castor oil the night before or neostigmine at the time of examination to dispel excess intestinal gas). Cholecystography is preferably carried out in the morning with the patient fasting.

Dose: The usual adult dose is 20 ml. For infants and children, the suggested dose is 0.3 to 0.6 ml/kg of body weight; the dosage for infants and children should not exceed 20 ml.

Note: The dose should not be repeated for 24 hours.

Administration: After warming to body temperature, iodipamide meglumine should be given by slow intravenous injection, following the usual precautions of intravenous administrations. it is important that the preparation be injected slowly over a period of 10 minutes. Use of a narrow bore hypodermic needle will ensure a slow rate of injection. During the injection, the patient should be watched for untoward reactions such as a feeling of warmth, flushing and occasionally nausea. Nausea indicates that the injection rate is too rapid.

Radiography: A scout film should be exposed routinely before the intravenous injection is made.

Position Of The Patient: With the patient prone and the right side elevated, radiographs are made in the posterior-anterior projection. Some radiologists prefer the supine position with the left side elevated. Serial 10-minute exposures should be started 10 minutes after the injection is made and continued until optimal visualization of the biliary ducts is obtained. Wet films should be examined immediately by the radiologist. In some cases a 15-degree rotation or the upright position may prove helpful.

Depending on the situation revealed by the roentgenograms in which the duct is first seen, the position of the subject should be changed to displace the shadow of the common bile duct from that of the spine. Tomography is a useful technique for enhancing bile duct visualization after administration of the radiopaque medium.

Examination of the gallbladder should be started about two hours after administration. The standard positions in routine examination of the gallbladder should be used unless otherwise indicated. There is no need for the patient to remain quiet awaiting the time for the gallbladder film to be exposed. Moderate activity on the part of the patient will, in most cases, preclude "stratification" of the contrast agent in the gallbladder. If the contrast medium should stratify in the gallbladder, decubitus as well as upright films should be obtained. Additional exposures may be made after the ingestion of a fatty meal.

If visualization is not achieved after two and one half hours, the patient should be returned for a 24-hour film, whenever possible. Occasionally, delayed opacification of the gallbladder will occur in 24 hours.

In infants and children, gallbladder visualization may be expected to occur 30 minutes to four hours after administration.

Note: In the presence of liver disease (BSP retention greater than 30 to 40 percent), the contrast medium is not excreted efficiently by the liver and visualization is usually not achieved. Visualization is rarely achieved in the presence of a serum bilirubin of 3.0 mg per 100 ml if the elevated bilibrium level is due to mechanical obstruction or hepatocellular damage. In the presence of severe liver damage, the contrast agent is excreted by the kidneys.

Interpretation: When intravenous cholecystography and cholangiography are used as an aid in the differential diagnosis of acute abdominal conditions, visualization of the gallbladder is considered strong evidence against a diagnosis of acute cholecystitis, while nonvisualization of the gallbladder two and one-half hours after administration with visualization of the bile ducts is considered strong evidence in favor of a diagnosis of acute cholecystitis (if the bile ducts are only faintly visualized, gallbladder films four hours after administration may occasionally show visualization of the gallbladder). When neither the bile ducts nor the gallbladder is visualized, the study provides no definitive information with regard to determining the presence or absence of acute cholecystitis.

Storage: Protect from light; store at room temperature; avoid excessive heat.

In the event that crystallization occurs, the solution may be clarified by placing the viual hot water and shaking gently for several minutes or until the solids redissolve. If cloudiness persists, discard the preparation. Allow the solution to cool to body temperature before administering.

HOW SUPPLIED - EQUIVALENTS NOT AVAILABLE:

Injection, Solution - Intravenous - 10.3 %

100 ml x 10	**$608.81**	**CHOLOGRAFIN MEGLUMINE, Bristol Myers Squibb**	**00003-0393-30**

Injection, Solution - Intravenous - 52 %

20 ml	$51.08	CHOLOGRAFIN, Bristol Myers Squibb	00003-0265-20

IODOQUINOL *(001067)*

CATEGORIES: Amebiasis; Amebicides; Anti-Infectives; Antiparasitics; Antiprotozoals; Parasiticidal; Protozoal Agents; FDA Pre 1938 Drugs

BRAND NAMES: Diiodohydroxyquin; *Diodoquin*; Diquinol; *Direxiode*; *Dysetrin*; **Yodoxin**

(International brand names outside U.S. in italics)

FORMULARIES: BC-BS

DESCRIPTION:

Iodoquinol is a light yellowish to tan color, nearly odorless and stable in air. The compound is practically insoluble in water, and sparingly soluble in most other solvents. It contains 64 per cent organically bound iodine.

CLINICAL PHARMACOLOGY:

Iodoquinol is amebicidal against Entamoeba histolytica & is considered effective against the trophozoite and cyst forms.

INDICATIONS AND USAGE:

Iodoquinol is used in the treatment of intestinal amebiasis. Iodoquinol is not recommended for the treatment of non-specific diarrhea.

CONTRAINDICATIONS:

Known hypersensitivity to iodine and 8-hydroxyquinolines. Contraindicated in patients with hepatic damage.

WARNINGS:

Optic neuritis, optic atrophy, and peripheral neuropathy have been reported following prolonged high dosage therapy with halogenated 8-hydroxyquinolines. Long term use of this drug should be avoided.

PRECAUTIONS:

iodoquinol should be used with caution in patients with thyroid disease.

Protein-bound serum iodine levels may be increased during treatment with iodoquinol and therefore interfere with certain thyroid function tests. These effects may persist for as long as six months after discontinuation of therapy. Discontinue the drug if hypersensitivity reactions occur.

Use in Pregnancy: Safety for use in pregnancy or during lactation has established.

ADVERSE REACTIONS:

Skin: Various forms of skin eruptions (acneiform papular and pustular; bullae; vegetating or tuberous iododerma), urticaria and pruritus.

Gastrointestinal: Nausea, vomiting, abdominal cramps, diarrhea, and pruritus ani. Fever, chills, headache, vertigo, and enlargement of thyroid have been reported.

Optic neuritis, Optic atrophy and peripheral neuropathy have been reported in association with prolonged high-dosage 8-hydroxyquinoline therapy.

DOSAGE AND ADMINISTRATION:

Usual Adult Dose: (210 mg each) 3 tablets three time daily, after meals for 20 days.

Children 6 to 12 Years: (210 mg each) 2 tablets three time daily. Children under 6 (210 mg each) one tablet per 15 pounds of body weight.

Usual Adult Dose: (650 mg each) one tablet three times a day for twenty days, to be taken after meals.

Children (650 mg. Each): For twenty days, 40 mg per kg of body weight daily divided into three doses, not to exceed 1.95 grams in 24 hours, for 20 days.

HOW SUPPLIED:

Storage: store at controlled room temperature 15°-30°C (59°- 86°F).

HOW SUPPLIED - EQUIVALENTS NOT AVAILABLE:

Powder - Oral

25 gm	**$27.98**	**YODOXIN, Glenwood**	**00516-0091-26**

Tablet, Uncoated - Oral - 210 mg

100's	**$32.80**	**YODOXIN, Glenwood**	**00516-0092-01**
1000's	**$233.26**	**YODOXIN, Glenwood**	**00516-0092-10**

Tablet, Uncoated - Oral - 650 mg

100's	$37.50	Diquinol, Consolidated Midland	00223-0850-01
100's	$37.50	Iodoquinol, Consolidated Midland	00223-0851-01
100's	**$40.29**	**YODOXIN, Glenwood**	**00516-0093-01**
500's	$175.00	Diquinol, Consolidated Midland	00223-0850-05
500's	$175.00	Iodoquinol, Consolidated Midland	00223-0851-05
1000's	**$313.46**	**YODOXIN, Glenwood**	**00516-0093-10**

IOHEXOL *(001566)*

CATEGORIES: Angina; Angiocardiography; Angiography; Cerebral Angiography; Diagnostic Agents; Endoscopic Retrograde Pancreatography; Excretory Urography; Herniography; Hysterosalpingography; Myelography; Pediatric Angiocardiography; Peripheral Angiography; Peripheral Arteriography; Roentgenography; Urography; Pregnancy Category B; Sales > $500 Million; FDA Approved 1985 Dec; Patent Expiration 1998 Dec

BRAND NAMES: Myelo-Kit; **Omnipaque**; Omnipaque 140; Omnipaque 180; Omnipaque 210; Omnipaque 240; Omnipaque 300; Omnipaque 350

Prescribing information not available at time of publication.

HOW SUPPLIED - EQUIVALENTS NOT AVAILABLE:

Injection, Solution - Intravenous - 140 mg/ml

50 ml x 10	**$389.41**	**OMNIPAQUE, Nycomed**	**00407-1401-50**
50 ml x 10	**$389.41**	**OMNIPAQUE, Nycomed**	**00407-1401-51**

Injection, Solution - Intravenous - 180 mg/ml

10 ml x 5	**$246.16**	**OMNIPAQUE, Nycomed**	**00407-1411-07**
10 ml x 10	**$480.54**	**OMNIPAQUE, Nycomed**	**00407-1411-10**
20 ml x 5	**$274.32**	**OMNIPAQUE, Nycomed**	**00407-1411-08**
20 ml x 10	**$536.95**	**OMNIPAQUE, Nycomed**	**00407-1411-20**

Injection, Solution - Intravenous - 210 mg/ml

15 ml x 10	**$529.18**	**OMNIPAQUE, Nycomed**	**00407-1402-15**

Injection, Solution - Intravenous - 240 mg/ml

10 ml x 5	**$267.09**	**OMNIPAQUE, Nycomed**	**00407-1412-07**
10 ml x 10	**$522.47**	**OMNIPAQUE, Nycomed**	**00407-1412-10**
20 ml x 10	**$552.20**	**OMNIPAQUE, Nycomed**	**00407-1412-20**
50 ml x 10	**$456.47**	**OMNIPAQUE, Nycomed**	**00407-1412-50**
50 ml x 10	**$456.47**	**OMNIPAQUE, Nycomed**	**00407-1412-51**
75 ml x 10	**$670.59**	**OMNIPAQUE, Nycomed**	**00407-1412-52**
100 ml x 10	**$782.30**	**OMNIPAQUE, Nycomed**	**00407-1412-70**
100 ml x 10	**$888.41**	**OMNIPAQUE, Nycomed**	**00407-1412-60**
125 ml x 10	**$1088.23**	**OMNIPAQUE, Nycomed**	**00407-1412-53**
150 ml x 10	**$1052.19**	**OMNIPAQUE, Nycomed**	**00407-1412-75**
150 ml x 10	**$1207.05**	**OMNIPAQUE, Nycomed**	**00407-1412-49**
200 ml x 10	**$1428.50**	**OMNIPAQUE, Nycomed**	**00407-1412-72**
200 ml x 10	**$1646.34**	**OMNIPAQUE, Nycomed**	**00407-1412-17**

Injection, Solution - Intravenous - 300 mg/ml

10 ml x 10	**$482.41**	**OMNIPAQUE, Nycomed**	**00407-1413-10**
30 ml x 10	**$485.18**	**OMNIPAQUE, Nycomed**	**00407-1413-30**
50 ml x 10	**$540.00**	**OMNIPAQUE, Nycomed**	**00407-1413-50**
50 ml x 10	**$540.00**	**OMNIPAQUE, Nycomed**	**00407-1413-51**
75 ml x 10	**$811.76**	**OMNIPAQUE, Nycomed**	**00407-1413-52**
100 ml x 10	**$932.50**	**OMNIPAQUE, Nycomed**	**00407-1413-80**
100 ml x 10	**$1058.12**	**OMNIPAQUE, Nycomed**	**00407-1413-60**
125 ml x 10	**$1308.81**	**OMNIPAQUE, Nycomed**	**00407-1413-53**
150 ml x 10	**$1342.10**	**OMNIPAQUE, Nycomed**	**00407-1413-85**
150 ml x 10	**$1543.29**	**OMNIPAQUE, Nycomed**	**00407-1413-90**

Injection, Solution - Intravenous - 350 mg/ml

50 ml x 10	**$588.12**	**OMNIPAQUE, Nycomed**	**00407-1414-50**
50 ml x 10	**$588.12**	**OMNIPAQUE, Nycomed**	**00407-1414-51**

HOW SUPPLIED - EQUIVALENTS NOT AVAILABLE: *(cont'd)*

75 ml x 10	**$880.12**	**OMNIPAQUE, Nycomed**	**00407-1414-75**
100 ml x 10	**$1019.70**	**OMNIPAQUE, Nycomed**	**00407-1414-61**
100 ml x 10	**$1175.76**	**OMNIPAQUE, Nycomed**	**00407-1414-60**
125 ml x 10	**$1389.65**	**OMNIPAQUE, Nycomed**	**00407-1414-76**
150 ml x 10	**$1424.90**	**OMNIPAQUE, Nycomed**	**00407-1414-65**
150 ml x 10	**$1623.18**	**OMNIPAQUE, Nycomed**	**00407-1414-03**
175 ml x 10	**$1801.40**	**OMNIPAQUE, Nycomed**	**00407-1414-77**
200 ml x 10	**$1765.20**	**OMNIPAQUE, Nycomed**	**00407-1414-62**
200 ml x 10	**$1999.52**	**OMNIPAQUE, Nycomed**	**00407-1414-04**
250 ml x 10	**$2411.75**	**OMNIPAQUE, Nycomed**	**00407-1414-80**

Kit - Intravenous - 180 mg/ml

5's	$310.94	MYELO-KIT, Nycomed	00407-1415-05
5's	$338.97	MYELO-KIT, Nycomed	00407-1415-06

Kit - Intravenous - 240 mg/ml

5's	$331.84	MYELO-KIT, Nycomed	00407-1416-05

IPRATROPIUM BROMIDE *(001578)*

CATEGORIES: Airway Obstruction; Antiasthmatics/Bronchodilators; Anticholinergic Agents; Antimuscarinics/Antispasmodics; Autonomic Drugs; Bronchial Dilators; Bronchitis; Bronchospasm; Chronic Bronchitis; Common Cold; Emphysema; Pulmonary Disease; Respiratory & Allergy Medications; Rhinitis; Rhinorrhea; Sympathomimetic Agents; Asthma*; FDA Approved 1986 Dec; Patent Expiration 1991 Aug; Top 200 Drugs

* Indication not approved by the FDA

BRAND NAMES: *Aerovent*; *Atem*; *Atronase*; **Atrovent**; *Atrovent Aerosol* (Australia); *Atrovent Nasal* (Australia); *Disne-Asmol*; *Itrop*; *Narilet*; *Tropium*
(International brand names outside U.S. in italics)

FORMULARIES: Aetna; BC-BS; CIGNA; FHP; Humana; Kaiser; Medco; Medi-Cal; PCS; PruCare; United

DESCRIPTION:

The active ingredient in Atrovent (ipratropium bromide) is ipratropium bromide monohydrate. It is an anticholinergic bronchodilator chemically described as 8-azoniabicyclo[3.2.1]-octane,3-(3-hydroxy-1-oxo-2-phenylpropoxy)-8-methyl-8-(1-methylethyl)-,bromide, monohydrate*(endo, syn)*-, (±)-; a synthetic quaternary ammonium compound, chemically related to atropine.

Ipratropium bromide is a white crystalline substance, freely soluble in water and lower alcohols. It is a quaternary ammonium compound and thus exists in an ionized state in aqueous solutions. It is relatively insoluble in non-polar media.

Atrovent Inhalation Aerosol is an inhalation aerosol for oral administration. The net weight is 14 grams; it yields 200 inhalations. Each actuation of the valve delivers 18 mcg of ipratropium bromide from the mouthpiece. The inert ingredients are dichlorodifluoromethane, dichlorotetrafluoroethane, and trichlorofluoromethane as propellants and soya lecithin.

Atrovent Inhalation Solution is administered by oral inhalation with the aid of a nebulizer. It contains ipratropium bromide 0.02% (anhydrous basis) in a sterile, preservative-free, isotonic saline solution, pH-adjusted to 3.4 (3 to 4) with hydrochloric acid.

CLINICAL PHARMACOLOGY:

Atrovent (ipratropium bromide) is an anticholinergic (parasympatholytic) agent that, based on animal studies, appears to inhibit vagally-mediated reflexes by antagonizing the action of acetylcholine, the transmitter agent released from the vagus nerve.

Anticholinergics prevent the increases in intracellular concentration of cyclic guanosine monophosphate (cyclic GMP) that are caused by interaction of acetylcholine with the muscarinic receptor on bronchial smooth muscle.

The bronchodilation following inhalation of Atrovent is primarily a local, site-specific effect, not a systemic one. Much of an administered dose is swallowed but not absorbed, as shown by fecal excretion studies.

Following nebulization of a 2 mg dose, a mean 7% of the dose was absorbed into the systemic circulation either from the surface of the lung or from the gastrointestinal tract. The half-life of elimination is about 1.6 hours after intravenous administration. Ipratropium bromide is minimally (0 to 9% *in vitro*) bound to plasma albumin and α_1-acid glycoproteins. It is partially metabolized. Autoradiographic studies in rats have shown that Atrovent does not penetrate the blood-brain barrier. Atrovent has not been studied in patients with hepatic or renal insufficiency. It should be used with caution in those patient populations.

In controlled 12-week studies in patients with bronchospasm associated with chronic obstructive pulmonary disease (chronic bronchitis and emphysema) significant improvements in pulmonary function (FEV_1 increases of 15% or more) occurred within 15 to 30 minutes, reached a peak in 1-2 hours, and persisted for periods of 4-5 hours in the majority of patients, with about 25-38% of the patients demonstrating increases of 15% or more for at least 7-8 hours. Continued effectiveness of atrovent inhalation solution was demonstrated throughout the 12-week period. In addition, significant increases in forced vital capacity (FVC) have been demonstrated. However, Atrovent did not consistently produce significant improvement in subjective symptom scores nor in quality of life scores over the 12-week duration of study.

Additional controlled 12-week studies were conducted to evaluate the safety and effectiveness of Atrovent Inhalation Solution administered concomitantly with the beta adrenergic bronchodilator solutions metaproterenol and albuterol compared with the administration of each of the beta agonists alone. Combined therapy produced significant additional improvement in FEV_1 and FVC. On combined therapy, the median duration of 15% improvement in FEV_1 was 5-7 hours, compared with 3-4 hours in patients receiving a beta agonist alone.

INDICATIONS AND USAGE:

Ipratropium bromide inhalation solution administered either alone or with other bronchodilators, especially beta adrenergics, is indicated as a bronchodilator for maintenance treatment of bronchospasm associated with chronic obstructive pulmonary disease, including chronic bronchitis and emphysema.

CONTRAINDICATIONS:

Ipratropium bromide inhalation aerosol is contraindicated in patients with a history of hypersensitivity to soya lecithin or related food products such as soybean and peanut.

Ipratropium bromide is contraindicated in known or suspected cases of hypersensitivity to ipratropium bromide, or to atropine and its derivatives.

WARNINGS:

The use of ipratropium bromide inhalation solution as a single agent for the relief of bronchospasm in acute COPD exacerbation has not been adequately studied. Drugs with faster onset of action may be preferable as initial therapy in this situation. Combination of ipratropium bromide and beta agonists has not been shown to be more effective than either drug alone in reversing the bronchospasm associated with acute COPD exacerbation.

PRECAUTIONS:

General: Ipratropium bromide should be used with caution in patients with narrow-angle glaucoma, prostatic hypertrophy or bladder-neck obstruction.

Information for the Patient: Patients should be advised that temporary blurring of vision, precipitation or worsening of narrow-angle glaucoma or eye pain may result if the solution comes into direct contact with the eyes. Use of a nebulizer with mouthpiece rather than face mask may be preferable, to reduce the likelihood of the nebulizer solution reaching the eyes. Patients should be advised that ipratropium bromide inhalation solution can be mixed in the nebulizer with albuterol if used within one hour. Compatibility data are not currently available with other drugs. Patients should be reminded that ipratropium bromide Inhalation Solution should be used consistently as prescribed throughout the course of therapy.

Carcinogenesis, Mutagenesis, and Impairment of Fertility: Two-year oral carcinogenicity studies in rats and mice have revealed no carcinogenic potential at dietary doses up to 6 mg/kg/day of ipratropium bromide.

Results of various mutagenicity studies (Ames test, mouse dominant lethal test, mouse micronucleus test and chromosome aberration of bone marrow in Chinese hamsters) were negative.

Fertility of male or female rats at oral doses up to 50 mg/kg/day was unaffected by ipratropium bromide administration. At doses above 90 mg/kg, increased resorption and decreased conception rates were observed.

Pregnancy, Teratogenic Effects, Pregnancy Category B: Oral reproduction studies performed in mice, rats and rabbits at doses 10, 100, and 125 mg/kg respectively, and inhalation reproduction studies in rats and rabbits at doses of 1.5 and 1.8 mg/kg (or approximately 38 and 45 times the recommended human daily dose) respectively, have demonstrated no evidence of teratogenic effects as a result of ipratropium bromide. However, no adequate or well-controlled studies have been conducted in pregnant women. Because animal reproduction studies are not always predictive of human response, ipratropium bromide should be used during pregnancy only if clearly needed.

Nursing Mothers: It is not known whether ipratropium bromide is excreted in human milk. Although lipid-insoluble quaternary bases pass into breast milk, it is unlikely that ipratropium bromide would reach the infant to a significant extent, especially when taken by inhalation since ipratropium bromide is not well absorbed systematically after inhalation or oral administration. However, because many drugs are excreted in human milk, caution should be exercised when ipratropium bromide is administered to a nursing woman.

Pediatric Use: Safety and effectiveness in children below the age of 12 have not been established.

DRUG INTERACTIONS:

Ipratropium bromide has been shown to be a safe and effective bronchodilator when used in conjunction with beta adrenergic bronchodilators. Ipratropium bromide has also been used with other pulmonary medications, including methylxanthines and corticosteroids, without adverse drug interactions.

ADVERSE REACTIONS:

Adverse reaction information concerning ipratropium bromide inhalation solution is derived from 12-week active-controlled clinical trials. Additional information is derived from foreign post-marketing experience and the published literature.

All adverse events, regardless of drug relationship, reported by three percent or more patients in the 12-week controlled clinical trials appear in Table 1A, B, and C below.

Additional adverse reactions reported in less than three percent of the patients treated with ipratropium bromide include tachycardia, palpitations, eye pain, urinary retention, urinary tract infection and urticaria. A single case of anaphylaxis thought to be possibly related to ipratropium bromide has been reported. Cases of precipitation or worsening of narrow-angle glaucoma and acute eye pain have been reported.

Lower respiratory adverse reactions (bronchitis, dyspnea and bronchospasm) were the most common events leading to discontinuation of ipratropium bromide therapy in the 12-week trials. Headache, mouth dryness and aggravation of COPD symptoms are more common when the total daily dose of ipratropium bromide equals or exceeds 2,000 mcg.

OVERDOSAGE:

Acute systemic overdosage by inhalation is unlikely since ipratropium bromide is not well absorbed after inhalation at up to four-fold the recommended dose, or after oral administration at up to forty-fold the recommended dose. The oral LD_{50} of ipratropium bromide ranged between 1001 and 2010 mg/kg in mice; between 1667 and 4000 mg/kg in rats; and between 400 and 1300 mg/kg in dogs.

DOSAGE AND ADMINISTRATION:

The usual dosage of ipratropium bromide inhalation solution is 500 mcg (1 Unit-Dose Vial) administered three to four times a day by oral nebulization, with doses 6 to 8 hours apart. Ipratropium bromide inhalation solution unit-dose vials contain 500 mcg ipratropium bromide anhydrous in 2.5 ml normal saline. Ipratropium bromide inhalation solution can be mixed in the nebulizer with albuterol if used within one hour. Compatibility data are not currently available with other drugs.

PATIENT INFORMATION:

Ipratropium widens the passageways in the lungs and is used to treat asthma, bronchitis, emphysema, and other lung diseases. This medication should not be used to treat an acute attack of asthma. Full effects of ipratropium may not occur for up to 15 minutes after administration. It is important that this medication is administered using the proper technique. Please obtain detailed administration directions from your pharmacist or physician. Inform your physician if you are pregnant or nursing. Avoid spraying this medication in the eye; temporary blurring of vision may occur. Notify your physician if your condition does not improve or gets worse within 30 minutes after administering ipratropium. If the ipratropium aerosol canister floats in a bowl of cold water, it is empty.

HOW SUPPLIED:

Ipratropium bromide inhalation solution unit dose vial is supplied as a 0.02% clear, colorless solution containing 2.5 ml with 25 vials per foil pouch.

TABLE 1A All Adverse Events, from a Double-Blind, Parallel, 12-Week Study of Patients with COPD*

	PERCENT OF PATIENTS Atrovent (500 mcg t.i.d.) n=219	Alupent (15 mg t.i.d) n=212
Body as a Whole-General Disorders		
Headache	6.4	5.2
Pain	4.1	3.3
Influenza-like symptoms	3.7	4.7
Back pain	3.2	1.9
Chest pain	3.2	4.2
Cardiovascular Disorders		
Hypertension/Hypertension Aggravated	0.9	1.9
Central & Peripheral Nervous System		
Dizziness	2.3	3.3
Insomnia	0.9	0.5
Tremor	0.9	7.1
Nervousness	0.5	4.7
Gastrointestinal System Disorders		
Mouth Dryness	3.2	0.0
Nausea	4.1	3.8
Constipation	0.9	0.0
Musculo-skeletal System Disorders		
Arthritis	0.9	1.4
Respiratory System Disorders (Lower)		
Coughing	4.6	8.0
Dyspnea	9.6	13.2
Bronchitis	14.6	24.5
Bronchospasm	2.3	2.8
Sputum Increased	1.4	1.4
Respiratory Disorder	0.0	6.1
Respiratory System Disorders (Upper)		
Upper Respiratory Tract Infection	13.2	11.3
Pharyngitis	3.7	4.2
Rhinitis	2.3	4.2
Sinusitis	2.3	2.8

* All adverse events, regardless of drug relationship, reported by three percent or more patients in the 12-week controlled clinical trials.

TABLE 1B Ipratropium Bromide, Adverse Reactions
All Adverse Events, from a Double-Blind, Parallel, 12-Week Study of Patients with COPD*

	PERCENT OF PATIENTS Atrovent/Alupent (500 mcg t.i.d./ 15 mg t.i.d.) n=108	Albuterol (2.5 mg t.i.d.) n=205
Body as a Whole-General Disorders		
Headache	6.5	6.3
Pain	0.9	2.9
Influenza-like symptoms	6.5	0.5
Back pain	1.9	2.4
Chest pain	5.6	2.0
Cardiovascular Disorders		
Hypertension/Hypertension Aggravated	0.9	1.5
Central & Peripheral Nervous System		
Dizziness	1.9	3.9
Insomnia	4.6	1.0
Tremor	8.3	1.0
Nervousness	6.5	1.0
Gastrointestinal System Disorders		
Mouth Dryness	1.9	2.0
Nausea	1.9	2.9
Constipation	3.7	1.0
Musculo-skeletal System Disorders		
Arthritis	0.9	0.5
Respiratory System Disorders (Lower)		
Coughing	6.5	5.4
Dyspnea	16.7	12.7
Bronchitis	15.7	16.6
Bronchospasm	4.6	5.4
Sputum Increased	4.6	3.4
Respiratory Disorder	6.5	2.0
Respiratory System Disorders (Upper)		
Upper Respiratory Tract Infection	9.3	12.2
Pharyngitis	5.6	2.9
Rhinitis	1.9	2.4
Sinusitis	0.9	5.4

* All adverse events, regardless of drug relationship, reported by three percent or more patients in the 12-week controlled clinical trials.

Each vial is made from a low density polyethylene (LDPE) resin.

Store between 59°F (15°C) and 86°F (30°C). Protect from light. Store unused vials in the foil pouch.

Ipratropium bromide inhalation aerosol is supplied as a metered dose inhaler with a white mouthpiece which has a clear, colorless sleeve and a green protective cap. Ipratropium bromide inhalation aerosol with mouthpiece, net contents 14 g. Ipratropium bromide inhalation aerosol refill, net contents 14 g. Each 14 gram vial provides sufficient medication for 200 inhalations. Each actuation delivers 18 mcg of ipratropium bromide from the mouthpiece.

HOW SUPPLIED: *(cont'd)*

Note: The statement below is required by the federal Clean Air Act for all products containing chlorofluorocarbons (CFCs), including products such as this one:

Warning: Contains trichloromonofluoromethane (CFC-11), dichlorodifluoromethane (CFC-12) and dichlorotetrafluoroethane (CFC-114), substances which harm public health and the environment by destroying ozone in the upper atmosphere.

A notice similar to the above WARNING has been placed in the "Instructions for Use" portion of this package insert pursuant to regulations of the United States Environmental Protection Agency.

Store between 59°F (15°C) and 86°F (30°C). Avoid excessive humidity.

Caution: Federal law prohibits dispensing without prescription.

HOW SUPPLIED - RATED THERAPEUTICALLY EQUIVALENT:

Solution - Inhalation - 0.2%

25 x 2.500 ml	$44.06	IPRATROPIUM BROMIDE, Roxane	00054-8402-11
30 x 2.500 ml		IPRATROPIUM BROMIDE, Roxane	00054-8402-13
UD	$52.87		

HOW SUPPLIED - NOT RATED EQUIVALENT:

Aerosol - Inhalation - 18 mcg

200's	**$26.64**	**ATROVENT, REFILL, Boehringer Pharms**	**00597-0082-18**
200's	**$29.12**	**ATROVENT INHALER, Boehringer Pharms**	**00597-0082-14**

Solution - Inhalation - 0.2 mg/ml

2.5 ml x 25	**$48.96**	**ATROVENT, Boehringer Pharms**	**00597-0080-62**

TABLE 1C All Adverse Events, from a Double-Blind, Parallel, 12-week Study of Patients with COPD*

	PERCENT OF PATIENTS Atrovent/Albuterol (500 mcg t.i.d./2.5 mg t.i.d.) n=100
Body as a Whole-General Disorders	
Headache	9.0
Pain	5.0
Influenza-like symptoms	1.0
Back pain	0.0
Chest pain	1.0
Cardiovascular Disorders	
Hypertension/Hypertension Aggravated	4.0
Central & Peripheral Nervous System	
Dizziness	4.0
Insomnia	1.0
Tremor	0.0
Nervousness	1.0
Gastrointestinal System Disorders	
Mouth Dryness	3.0
Nausea	2.0
Constipation	1.0
Musculo-skeletal System Disorders	
Arthritis	3.0
Respiratory System Disorders (Lower)	
Coughing	6.0
Dyspnea	9.0
Bronchitis	20.0
Bronchospasm	5.0
Sputum Increased	0.0
Respiratory Disorder	4.0
Respiratory System Disorders (Upper)	
Upper Respiratory Tract Infection	16.0
Pharyngitis	4.0
Rhinitis	0.0
Sinusitis	4.0

* All adverse events, regardless of drug relationship, reported by three percent or more patients in the 12-week controlled clinical trials.

IRINOTECAN HYDROCHLORIDE *(003296)*

CATEGORIES: Antineoplastics; Chemotherapy; Camptothecin Derivative; Colon Cancer; Oncologic Drugs; Pregnancy Category D; FDA Approved 1996 Jun

BRAND NAMES: *Campto* (France, Japan); **Camptosar**; *Topotecin* (Japan) *(International brand names outside U.S. in italics)*

PRIMARY ICD9: 154.0 (Malignant Neoplasm of the Colon or Rectum)

WARNING:

1. Irinotecan injection should be administered only under the supervision of a physician who is experienced in the use of cancer chemotherapeutic agents. Appropriate management of complications is possible only when adequate diagnostic and treatment facilities are readily available.
2. Irinotecan injection can induce both early and late forms of diarrhea that appear to be mediated by different mechanisms. Both forms of diarrhea may be severe. Early diarrhea (occurring during or within 24 hours of administration of irinotecan) may be preceded by complaints of diaphoresis and abdominal cramping and may be ameliorated by atropine. Late diarrhea (occurring more than 24 hours after administration of irinotecan) can be prolonged, may lead to dehydration and electrolyte imbalance, and can be life-threatening. Late diarrhea should be treated promptly with loperamide; patients with severe diarrhea should be carefully monitored and given fluid and electrolyte replacement if they become dehydrated (see WARNINGS section). Administration of irinotecan should be interrupted if severe diarrhea occurs.
3 Severe myelosuppression may occur (see WARNINGS section).

DESCRIPTION:

Irinotecan hydrochloride injection is an antineoplastic agent of the topoisomerase I inhibitor class. Irinotecan hydrochloride was clinically investigated as CPT-11.

Camptosar is supplied as a sterile, pale yellow, clear, aqueous solution. It is available in 100 mg, single-dose, 5 ml vials. Each milliliter of solution contains 20 mg of irinotecan HCl (on the basis of the trihydrate salt), 45 mg of sorbitol NF powder, and 0.9 mg of lactic acid, USP. The pH of the solution has been adjusted to 3.5 (range, 3.0 to 3.8) with sodium hydroxide or hydrochloric acid. Camptosar is intended for dilution with 5% Dextrose Injection, USP (D5W), or 0.9% Sodium Chloride Injection, USP, prior to intravenous infusion. The preferred diluent is 5% Dextrose Injection, USP.

Irinotecan HCl is a semisynthetic derivative of camptothecin, an alkaloid extract from plants such as *Camptotheca acuminata*. The chemical name is (4*S*)-4, 11-diethyl-4-hydroxy-9-[(4-piperi-dinopiperidino)carbony-loxy]-1*H*-pyrano[3',4' :6, 7] indolizino [1,2-*b*]quinoline-3, 14(4*H*, 12*H*)dione hydrochloride.

Irinotecan HCl is a pale yellow to yellow crystalline powder, with the empirical formula $C_{33}H_{38}N_4O_6 \cdot HCl \cdot 3H_2O$ and a molecular weight of 677.19. It is slightly soluble in water and organic solvents.

CLINICAL PHARMACOLOGY:

Irinotecan is a derivative of camptothecin. Camptothecins interact specifically with the enzyme topoisomerase I which relieves torsional strain in DNA by inducing reversible single-strand breaks. Irinotecan and its active metabolite SN-38 bind to the topoisomerase I-DNA complex and prevent religation of these single-strand breaks. Current research suggests that the cytotoxicity of irinotecan is due to double-strand DNA damage produced during DNA synthesis when replication enzymes interact with the ternary complex formed by topoisomerase I, DNA, and either irinotecan or SN-38. Mammalian cells cannot efficiently repair these double-strand breaks.

Irinotecan serves as a water-soluble precursor of the lipophilic metabolite SN-38 is formed from irinotecan by carboxylesterase-mediated cleavage of the carbamate bond between the camptothecin moiety and the dipiperidino side chain. SN-38 is approximately 1000 times as potent as irinotecan as an inhibitor of topoisomerase I purified from human and rodent tumor cell lines. *In vitro* cytotoxicity assays show that potency of SN-38 relative to irinotecan varies from 2- to 2000-fold. However, the plasma area under the concentration versus time curve (AUC) values for SN-38 are 2% to 8% of irinotecan and SN-38 is 95% bound to plasma proteins compared to approximately 50% bound to plasma proteins for irinotecan (see Pharmacokinetics).

The precise contribution of SN-38 to the activity of irinotecan HCl is thus unknown. Both irinotecan and SN-38 exist in an active lactone form and an inactive hydroxy acid anion form. A pH-dependent equilibrium exists between the two forms such that an acid pH promotes the formation of the lactone, while a more basic pH favors the hydroxy acid anion form.

Administration of irinotecan has resulted in antitumor activity in mice bearing cancers of rodent origin and in human carcinoma xenografts of various histological types.

PHARMACOKINETICS

After intravenous infusion of irinotecan HCl in humans, irinotecan plasma concentrations decline in a multiexponential manner, with a mean terminal elimination half-life of about 6 hours. The mean terminal elimination half-life of the active metabolite SN-38 is about 10 hours. The half-lives of the lactone (active) forms of irinotecan and SN-38 are similar to those of total irinotecan and SN-38, as the lactone and hydroxy acid forms are in equilibrium.

Over the dose range of 50 to 350 mg/m^2, the AUC of irinotecan increases linearly with dose; the AUC of SN-38 increases less than proportionally with dose. Maximum concentrations of the active metabolite SN-38 are generally seen within 1 hour following the end of a 90-minute infusion of irinotecan.

Irinotecan exhibits moderate plasma protein binding (30% to 68% bound). SN-38 is highly bound to human plasma proteins (approximately 95% bound). The plasma protein to which irinotecan and SN-38 predominately binds is albumin.

TABLE 1 Summary of Mean (± Standard Deviation) Irinotecan and SN-38 Pharmacokinetic Parameters in Patients with Metastatic Carcinoma of the Colon and Rectum

	Irinotecan					SN-38		
Dose (mg/m^2)	C_{max} (ng/mL)	AUC_{0-24} (ng·hr/mL)	$t_{1/2}$ (hr)	V_{area} (L/m^2)	CL (L/hr/m^2)	C_{max} (ng/mL)	AUC_{0-24} (ng·hr/mL)	$t_{1/2}$ (hr)
125 (N=64)	1,660 ± 797	10,200 – 3,270	5.8 ± 0.7	110 ± 48.5	13.3 ± 6.01	26.3 – 11.9	229 – 108	10.4 – 3.1

C_{max} Maximum plasma concentration
AUC_{0-24} Area under the plasma concentration-time curve from time 0 to 24 hours after the end of the 90-minute infusion.
$t_{1/2}$ Terminal elimination half-life.
V_{area} Volume of distribution of terminal elimination phase.
CL Total systemic clearance.

Metabolism and Excretion: The metabolic conversion or irinotecan to the active metabolite SN-38 is mediated by carboxylesterase enzymes and primarily occurs in the liver. SN-38 subsequently undergoes conjugation to form a glucuronide metabolite. SN-38 glucuronide had 1/50 to 1/100 the activity of SN-38 in cytotoxicity assays using two cell lines *in vitro*. The disposition of irinotecan has not been fully elucidated in humans. The urinary excretion of irinotecan is 11% to 20%; SN-38, <1%; and SN-38 glucuronide, 3%. The cumulative biliary and urinary excretion of irinotecan and its metabolites (SN-38 and SN-38 glucuronide) over a period of 48 hours following administration of irinotecan in two patients ranged from approximately 25% (100 mg/m^2) to 50% (300 mg/m^2).

PHARMACOKINETICS IN SPECIAL POPULATIONS

Geriatric: The terminal half-life of irinotecan was 6.0 hours in patients who were 65 years or older and 5.5 hours in patients younger than 65 years. Dose-normalized AUC_{0-24} for SN-38 in patients who were at least 65 years of age was 11% higher than in patients younger than 65 years of age. No change in dosage and administration is recommended for geriatric patients.

CLINICAL PHARMACOLOGY: *(cont'd)*

Pediatric: The pharmacokinetics of irinotecan have not been studied in the pediatric population.

Gender: The pharmacokinetics of irinotecan do not appear to be influenced by gender.

Race: The influence of race on the pharmacokinetics of irinotecan has not been evaluated.

Hepatic Insufficiency: The influence of hepatic insufficiency on the pharmacokinetic characteristics of irinotecan and its metabolites has not been formally studied. Among patients with known hepatic tumor involvement (a majority of patients), irinotecan and SN-38 AUC values were somewhat higher than values for patients without liver metastases. For patients having liver metastases without decreased hepatic function, no change in dosage and administration is recommended.

Renal Insufficiency: The influence of renal insufficiency on the pharmacokinetics of irinotecan has not been evaluated.

DRUG-DRUG INTERACTIONS

Possible pharmacokinetic interactions of irinotecan with other concomitantly administered medications have not been formally investigated.

CLINICAL STUDIES:

In phase 1 studies of irinotecan injection, the maximum-tolerated dose as a single agent in the treatment of patients with solid tumors was 120 to 150 mg/m^2 when administered once weekly for 4 weeks, followed by a 2-week rest period. The dose-limiting toxicities were diarrhea and neutropenia. In one study, use of granulocyte colony-stimulating factor (G-CSF) appeared to increase the tolerated dose from 120 to 145 mg/m^2.

Data from three open-label, phase 2, single-agent clinical studies, involving a total of 304 patients in 59 centers, support the use of irinotecan in the treatment of patients with metastatic cancer of the colon or rectum that has recurred or progressed following treatment with fluorouracil (5–FU)-based therapy. These studies were designed to evaluate tumor response rate and do not provide information on actual clinical benefit, such as effect on survival and disease-related symptoms. In each study, Irinotecan was administered in repeated 6-week courses consisting of a 90-minute intravenous infusion once weekly for 4 weeks, followed by a 2 week rest period. Starting doses of irinotecan in these trials were 100, 125, or 150 mg/m^2, but the 150 mg/m^2 dose proved poorly tolerated (unacceptably high rates of grade 4 late diarrhea and febrile neutropenia). Study 1 enrolled 48 patients and was conducted under the auspices of a single investigator at several regional hospitals. Study 2 was a multicenter study conducted by the North Central Cancer Treatment Group. All 90 patients enrolled in Study 2 received a starting dose of 125 mg/m^2. Study 3 was a multicenter study that enrolled 166 patients from 30 institutions. The initial dose in Study 3 was 125 mg/m^2 but was reduced to 100 mg/m^2 because the toxicity seen at the 125 mg/m^2 dose was perceived to be greater than that seen in previous studies. All patients in these studies had metastatic colorectal cancer, and the majority had disease that recurred or progressed following a 5-FU-based regimen administered for metastatic disease.

The results of the individual studies are shown in TABLE 2.

In the intent-to-treat analysis of the pooled data across all three studies, 193 of the 304 patients began therapy at the recommended starting dose of 125 mg/m^2. Among these 193 patients, 2 complete and 27 partial responses were observed, for an overall response rate of 15.0% (95% Confidence Interval [CI], 10.0% to 20.1%) at this starting dose. A considerably lower response rate was seen with a starting dose of 100 mg/m^2. The majority of responses were observed within the first two courses of therapy, and all but one of the responses were observed by the fourth course of therapy (one response was observed after the eighth course). The response duration (median) for patients beginning therapy at 125 mg/m^2 was 5.8 months (range, 2.6 to 15.1 months).

Response rates to irinotecan were similar in males and females and among patients older and younger than 65 years. Rates were also similar in patients with cancer of the colon or cancer of the rectum and in patients with single and multiple metastatic sites. Response rate was 18.5 % in patients with a performance status of 0 and 7.6% in patients with a performance status of 1 or 2. Patients with a performance status of 3 or 4 have not been studied. Over half of the patients responding to irinotecan had not responded to prior 5-FU-based treatment given for metastatic disease. Patients who had received previous irradiation to the pelvis also responded to irinotecan at approximately the same rate as those who had not previously received irradiation.

INDICATIONS AND USAGE:

Irinotecan injection is indicated for the treatment of patients with metastatic carcinoma of the colon or rectum whose disease has recurred or progressed following 5-FU-based therapy.

CONTRAINDICATIONS:

Irinotecan injection is contraindicated in patients with a known hypersensitivity to the drug.

WARNINGS:

DIARRHEA

Irinotecan injection can induce both early and late forms of diarrhea that appear to be mediated by different mechanisms. Early diarrhea (occurring during or within 24 hours of administration of irinotecan) is cholinergic in nature. It can be severe but is usually transient. It may be preceded by complaints of diaphoresis and abdominal cramping. Early diarrhea may be ameliorated by administration of atropine (see PRECAUTIONS, General, for dosing recommendations for atropine).

Late diarrhea (occurring more than 24 hours after administration of irinotecan) can be prolonged, may lead to dehydration and electrolyte imbalance, and can be life threatening. Late diarrhea should be treated promptly with loperamide (see PRECAUTIONS, Information for Patients, for dosing recommendations for loperamide). Patients with severe diarrhea should be carefully monitored and given fluid and electrolyte replacement if they become dehydrated. National Cancer Institute (NCI) grade 3 diarrhea is defined as an increase of 7 to 9 stools daily, or incontinence, or severe cramping and NCI grade 4 diarrhea is defined as an increase of ≥10 stools daily, or grossly bloody stool, or need for parenteral support. If grade 3 or 4 late diarrhea occurs, administration of irinotecan should be delayed until the patient recovers and subsequent doses should be decreased (see DOSAGE AND ADMINISTRATION).

WARNINGS: *(cont'd)*

TABLE 2

	1	2	3	
Number of Patients	48	90	64	102
Dose (mg/m^2/wk × 4)	125*	125	125	100
Male (%)	54	64	50	49
Age < 65 yr (%)	54	54	64	54
Ethnic Origin (%) White	79.2	95.6	81.3	91.2
African American	12.5	4.4	10.9	4.9
Hispanic	8.3	0.0	7.8	2.0
Oriental /Asian	0.0	0.0	0.0	2.0
Performance Status 0 (%)	60	38	59	44
Performance Status 1 (%)	38	48	33	51
Performance Status 2 (%)	2	14	8	5
Prior 5-FU Therapy (%)				
For Metastatic Disease	81.3	65.5	73.4	67.7
≤ 6 months after Adjuvant	14.6	6.7	26.6	27.5
> 6 months after Adjuvant	2.1	15.6	0.0	2.0
Classification Unknown	2.1	12.2	0.0	2.9
Primary Tumor (%)				
Colon	100	71	89	87
Rectum	0	29	11	8
Number of Courses of Irinotecan (median)	3.5	3.0	3.0	3.0
Median Dose Intensity† (mg/m^2/wk)	62	56	61	54
Objective Response Rate (%) ‡	20.8	13.3	14.1	7.8
[95% CI]	[9.3, 32.3]	[6.3, 20.4]	[5.5, 22.6]	[2.6,13.1]
Time to Response (median, months)	2.6	2.1	2.8	2.8
Response Duration (median, months)	6.4	5.9	5.6	6.2
Survival (median, months)	10.4	8.1	10.7	9.3

* Nine patients received 150 mg/m^2 as a starting dose; 2 (22.2%) responded to irinotecan.
† Total dose administered in a course ÷ 6 (number of weeks in a course).
‡ There were 2/304 complete responses; the remainder were partial responses.

MYELOSUPPRESSION

Deaths due to sepsis following severe myelosuppression have been reported in patients treated with irinotecan. Therapy with irinotecan should be temporarily discontinued if neutropenic fever occurs or if the absolute neutrophil count drops below 500/mm^3. The dose of irinotecan should be reduced if there is a clinically significant decrease in the total white blood cell count (<2000/mm^3), neutrophil count (<1000/mm^3), hemoglobin (<8 gm/dl), or platelet count (<100,000/mm^3) (see DOSAGE AND ADMINISTRATION). Routine administration of a colony-stimulating factor (CSF) is not necessary, but physicians may wish to consider CSF use in individual patients experiencing significant neutropenia.

PREGNANCY

Irinotecan injection may cause fetal harm when administered to a pregnant woman. Radioactivity related to ^{14}C-irinotecan crosses the placenta of rats following intravenous administration of 10 mg/kg (which in separate studies produced an irinotecan C_{max} and AUC about 3 and 0.5 times, respectively, the corresponding values in patients administered 125 mg/m^2). Administration of 6 mg/kg/day intravenous irinotecan to rats (which in separate studies produced an irinotecan C_{max} and AUC about 2 and 0.2 times, respectively, the corresponding values in patients administered 125 mg/m^2) and rabbits (about one-half the recommended human dose on mg/m^2 basis) during the period of organogenesis, is embryotoxic as characterized by increased post-implantation loss and decreased numbers of live fetuses. Irinotecan was teratogenic in rats at doses greater than 1.2 mg/kg/day (which in separate studies produced an irinotecan C_{max} and AUC about 2/3 and 1/40th respectively, of the corresponding values in patients administered 125 mg/m^2) and in rabbits at 6.0 mg/kg/day (about one-half the recommended weekly human dose on a mg/m^2 basis). Teratogenic effects included a variety of external, visceral, and skeletal abnormalities. Irinotecan administered to rat dams for the period following organogenesis through weaning at doses of 6 mg/kg/day caused decreased learning ability and decreased female body weights in the offspring. There are no adequate and well-controlled studies of irinotecan in pregnant women. If the drug is used during pregnancy, or if the patient becomes pregnant while receiving this drug, the patient should be apprised of the potential hazard to the fetus. Women of childbearing potential should be advised to avoid becoming pregnant while receiving treatment with irinotecan.

PRECAUTIONS:

GENERAL

Care of Intravenous Site: Irinotecan is administered by intravenous infusion. Care should be taken to avoid extravasation, and the infusion site should be monitored for signs of inflammation. Should extravasation occur, flushing the site with sterile water and application of ice are recommended.

PRECAUTIONS: *(cont'd)*

Premedication with Antiemetics: Irinotecan is emetigenic. It is recommended that patients receive premedication with antiemetic agents. In clinical studies, the majority of patients received 10 mg of dexamethasone given in conjunction with another type of antiemetic agent, such as 5-HT_3 blocker (*e.g.*, ondansetron or granisetron). Antiemetic agents should be given on the day of treatment, starting at least 30 minutes before administration of irinotecan. Physicians should also consider providing patients with an antiemetic regimen (*e.g.* prochlorperazine) for subsequent use as needed.

Treatment of Early Diarrhea: Administration of 0.25 to 1 mg of intravenous atropine should be considered (unless clinically contraindicated) in patients experiencing diaphoresis, abdominal cramping, or early diarrhea (diarrhea occurring during or within 24 hours following administration of irinotecan).

Patients at Particular Risk: Physicians should exercise particular caution in monitoring the effects of irinotecan in the elderly (≥65 years of age) and in patients who had previously received pelvic/abdominal irradiation (see ADVERSE REACTIONS).

INFORMATION FOR THE PATIENT

Patients and patient's caregivers should be informed of the expected toxic effects of irinotecan, particularly of its gastrointestinal manifestations, such as nausea, vomiting, and diarrhea. Each patient should be instructed to have loperamide readily available and to begin treatment for late diarrhea (occurring more than 24 hours after administration of irinotecan) at the first episode of poorly formed or loose stools, or the earliest onset of bowel movements more frequent than normally expected for the patient. One dosage regimen for loperamide used in clinical trials consisted of the following (Note: This dosage regimen exceeds the usual dosage recommendations for loperamide.): 4 mg at the first onset of late diarrhea and then 2 mg every 2 hours until the patient is diarrhea-free for at least 12 hours. During the night, the patient may take 4 mg of loperamide every 4 hours. The patient should also be instructed to notify the physician if diarrhea occurs. Premedication with loperamide is not recommended.

The use of drugs with laxative properties should be avoided because of the potential for exacerbation of diarrhea. Patients should be advised to contact their physician to discuss any laxative use.

Patients should consult their physician if vomiting occurs, fever, or evidence of infection develops, or if symptoms of dehydration, such as fainting, light-headedness, or dizziness, are noted following therapy with irinotecan.

Patients should be alerted to the possibility of alopecia.

LABORATORY TESTS

Careful monitoring of the white blood cell count with differential, hemoglobin, and platelet count is recommended before each dose of irinotecan.

CARCINOGENESIS, MUTAGENESIS, AND IMPAIRMENT OF FERTILITY

Long-term carcinogenicity studies with irinotecan were not conducted. Rats were, however, administered intravenous doses of 2 mg/kg or 25 mg/kg irinotecan once per week for 13 weeks (in separate studies, the 25 mg/kg dose produced an irinotecan C_{max} and AUC that were about 7.0 times and 1.3 times the respective values in patients administered 125 mg/m^2) and were then allowed to recover for 91 weeks. Under these conditions, there was a significant linear trend with dose for the incidence of combined uterine horn endometrial stromal polyps and endometrial stromal sarcomas. Neither irinotecan or SN-38 was mutagenic in the *in vitro* Ames assay. Irinotecan was clastogenic both *in vitro* (chromosome aberrations in Chinese hamster ovary cells) and *in vivo* (micronucleus test in mice). No significant adverse effects on fertility and general reproductive performance were observed after intravenous administration of irinotecan in doses of up to 6 mg/kg/day to rats and rabbits. However, atrophy of male reproductive organs was observed after multiple daily irinotecan doses both in rodents at 20 mg/kg (which in separate studies produced an irinotecan C_{max} and AUC about 5 and 1 times, respectively, the corresponding values in patients administered 125 mg/m^2) and dogs at 0.4 mg/kg (which in separate studies produced an irinotecan C_{max} and AUC about one-half and 1/15th, respectively, the corresponding values in patients administered 125 mg/m^2).

PREGNANCY CATEGORY D

See WARNINGS.

NURSING MOTHERS

Radioactivity appeared in rat milk within 5 minutes of intravenous administration of radiolabeled irinotecan and was concentrated up to 65-fold at 4 hours after administration relative to plasma concentrations. Because many drugs are excreted in human milk and because of the potential for serious adverse reactions in nursing infants, it is recommended that nursing be discontinued when receiving therapy with irinotecan.

PEDIATRIC USE

The safety and effectiveness of irinotecan in pediatric patients have not been established.

DRUG INTERACTIONS:

The adverse effects of irinotecan, such as myelosuppression and diarrhea, would be expected to be exacerbated by other antineoplastic agents having similar adverse effects.

Patients who have previously received pelvic/abdominal irradiation are at increased risk of severe myelosuppression following the administration of irinotecan. The concurrent administration of irinotecan with irradiation has not been adequately studied and is not recommended.

Lymphocytopenia has been reported in patients receiving irinotecan, and it is possible that the administration of dexamethasone as antiemetic prophylaxis may have enhanced the likelihood of this effect. However, serious opportunistic infections have not been observed, and no complications have specifically been attributed to lymphocytopenia.

Hyperglycemia has also been reported in patients receiving irinotecan. Usually, this has been observed in patients with a history of diabetes mellitus or evidence of glucose intolerance prior to administration of irinotecan. It is probable that dexamethasone, given as antiemetic prophylaxis, contributed to hyperglycemia in some patients.

The incidence of akathsia in clinical trials was greater (8.5%, 4/47 patients) when prochlorperazine was administered on the same day as irinotecan than when these drugs were given on separate days (1.3%, 1/80 patients). The 8.5% incidence of akathsia, however, is within the range reported for use of prochlorperazine when given as a premedication for other chemotherapies.

It would be expected that laxative use during therapy with irinotecan would worsen the incidence or severity of diarrhea, but this has not been studied.

DRUG INTERACTIONS: *(cont'd)*

In view of the potential risk of dehydration secondary to vomiting and/or diarrhea induced by irinotecan, the physician may wish to withhold diuretics during dosing with irinotecan, and certainly, during periods of active vomiting or diarrhea.

DRUG-LABORATORY TEST INTERACTIONS

There are no known interactions between irinotecan and laboratory tests.

ADVERSE REACTIONS:

US CLINICAL TRIALS

In three clinical studies, 304 patients with metastatic carcinoma of the colon or rectum that had recurred or progressed following 5-FU-based therapy were treated with irinotecan. Seventeen of the patients died within 30 days of the administration of irinotecan; in five cases (1.6%, 5/304), the deaths were potentially drug-related. These five patients experienced a constellation of medical events that included known effects of irinotecan. One of these patients died of neutropenic sepsis without fever. Neutropenic fever, defined as NCI grade 4 neutropenia and grade 2 or greater fever, occurred in nine (3.0%) other patients; these patients recovered with supportive care. One hundred and nineteen (39.1%) of the 304 patients were hospitalized a total of 156 times because of adverse events; 81 (26.6%) patients were hospitalized for events judged to be related to administration of irinotecan. The primary reasons for drug-related hospitalization were diarrhea, with or without nausea and/or vomiting (18.4%); neutropenia/leukopenia, with or without diarrhea and/or fever (8.2%); and nausea and/or vomiting (4.9%). Adjustments in the dose of irinotecan were made during the course of treatment and for subsequent courses based on individual patient tolerance. The first dose of at least one course of irinotecan was reduced for 67% of patients who began the studies at the 125 mg/m^2 starting dose. Within-course dose reductions were required for 32% of the courses initiated at the 125 mg/m^2 dose level. The most common reasons for dose reduction were late diarrhea, neutropenia, and leukopenia. Thirteen (4.3%) patients discontinued treatment with irinotecan because of adverse events. The adverse events in TABLE 3 are based on the experience of the 304 patients enrolled in the three studies described in the CLINICAL STUDIES section.

TABLE 3 Adverse Events Occurring in >10% of 304 Previously Treated Patients with Metastatic Carcinoma of the Colon or Rectum

Body System and Event	% of Patients Reporting NCI Grades 1-4	NCI Grades 3 & 4
GASTROINTESTINAL		
Diarrhea (late)*	87.8	30.6
7-9 stools/day (grade 3)	-	(16.4)
≥10 stools/day (grade 4)	-	(14.1)
Nausea	86.2	16.8
Vomiting	66.8	12.5
Anorexia	54.9	5.9
Diarrhea (early)†	50.7	7.9
Constipation	29.9	2.0
Flatulence	12.2	0
Stomatitis	11.8	0.7
Dyspepsia	10.5	0
HEMATOLOGIC		
Leukopenia	63.2	28.0
Anemia	60.5	6.9
Neutropenia	53.9	26.3
500 to < 1000/mm^3 (grade 3)	-	(14.8)
<500/mm^3 (grade 4)	-	(11.5)
BODY AS A WHOLE		
Asthenia	75.7	12.2
Abdominal Cramping/Pain	56.9	16.4
Fever	45.4	0.7
Pain	23.7	2.3
Headache	16.8	0.7
Back Pain	14.5	1.6
Chills	13.8	0.3
Minor Infection‡	14.5	0
Edema	10.2	1.3
Abdominal Enlargement	10.2	0.3
METABOLIC & NUTRITIONAL		
↓ Body Weight	30.3	0.7
Dehydration	14.8	4.3
↑ Alkaline Phosphatase	13.2	3.9
↑SGOT	10.5	1.3
DERMATOLOGIC		
Alopecia	60.5	NA§
Sweating	16.4	0
Rash	12.8	0.7
RESPIRATORY		
Dyspnea	22.0	3.6
↑ Coughing	17.4	0.3
Rhinitis	15.5	0
NEUROLOGIC		
Insomnia	19.4	0
Dizziness	14.8	0
CARDIOVASCULAR		
Vasodilation (Flushing)	11.2	0

* Occurring >24 hours after administration of irinotecan.
† Occurring ≤24 hours after administration of irinotecan.
‡ Primarily upper respiratory infections.
§ Not applicable; complete hair loss = NCI grade 2.

Gastrointestinal: Diarrhea, nausea, and vomiting were common adverse events following treatment with irinotecan and could be severe. These events occurred early (during or within 24 hours of administration of irinotecan) or late (more than 24 hours after administration of irinotecan). The median time to onset of late diarrhea was 11 days following administration of irinotecan. For patients starting treatment at the 125 mg/m^2 dose, the median duration of any grade of diarrhea was 3 days. Among those patients treated at the 125 mg/m^2 dose who experienced grade 3 or 4 diarrhea, the median duration of the entire episode of diarrhea was 7 days. The frequency of grade 3 or 4 late diarrhea was somewhat greater in patients starting treatment at 125 mg/m^2 than in patients given a 100 mg/m^2 starting dose (34% versus 24%). The frequency of grade 3 and 4 late diarrhea was significantly greater in patients ≥65 years than in patients <65 years of age (39.8% versus 23.4%; p=0.0025). In Study 2, the frequency of grade 3 and

ADVERSE REACTIONS: *(cont'd)*

4 late diarrhea was significantly greater in male than in female patients (43.1% versus 15.6%; p=0.01). However, there were no gender differences in the frequency of grade 3 and 4 late diarrhea in the other two studies.

Hematology: Irinotecan commonly caused neutropenia, leukopenia (including lymphocytopenia), and anemia. Serious thrombocytopenia was uncommon. Neutropenic fever (concurrent NCI grade 4 neutropenia and fever of grade 2 or greater) occurred in 3.0% of the patients; 5.6% of patients received G-CSF for the treatment of neutropenia. NCI grade 3 or 4 anemia was noted in 6.9% of the patients. Blood transfusions were given to 9.9% of the patients. The frequency of grade 3 and 4 neutropenia was significantly higher in patients who received previous pelvic/abdominal irradiation than in those who had not received irradiation (48.1% versus 24.1%; p=0.0356). There were no significant differences in the frequency of grade 3 and 4 neutropenia by age or gender.

Body as a Whole: Asthenia, fever, and abdominal pain were the most common events of this type.

Hepatic: NCI grade 3 or 4 liver enzyme abnormalities were observed in fewer than 10% of the patients. These events typically occurred in patients with known hepatic metastases.

Dermatologic: Alopecia was reported during treatment with irinotecan. Rashes have also been reported but did not result in discontinuation of treatment.

Respiratory: Severe pulmonary events were infrequent; NCI grade 3 or 4 dyspnea was reported in 3.6% of patients. Over half the patients with dyspnea had lung metastases; the extent to which malignant pulmonary involvement or other pre-existing lung disease may have contributed to dyspnea in these patients is unknown.

Neurologic: Insomnia and dizziness were observed, but were not usually considered to be directly related to the administration of irinotecan. Dizziness may sometimes have represented symptomatic evidence of orthostatic hypotension in patients with dehydration.

Cardiovascular: Vasodilation (flushing) has been observed during administration of irinotecan but has not required intervention.

NON-U.S. CLINICAL TRIALS

Irinotecan has been studied in over 1100 patients in Japan and in over 400 patients in France. Patients in these studies had a variety of tumor types, including cancer of the colon or rectum, and were treated with several different doses and schedules. In general, the types of toxicities observed were similar to those seen in U.S. trials with irinotecan. There is some information from Japanese trials that patients with considerable ascites or pleural effusions were at increased risk for neutropenia or diarrhea. A potentially life-threatening pulmonary syndrome, consisting of dyspnea, fever, and a reticulonodular pattern on chest x-ray, was observed in a small percentage of patients in early Japanese studies. The contribution of irinotecan to these preliminary events was difficult to assess because these patients also had lung tumors and some had pre-existing nonmalignant pulmonary disease. As a result of the these observations, however, clinical studies in the United States have enrolled few patients with compromised pulmonary function, significant ascites, or pleural effusions.

OVERDOSAGE:

In U.S. phase 1 trials, single doses of up to 345 mg/m^2 of irinotecan injection were administered to patients with various cancers. Single doses of up to 750 mg/m^2 of irinotecan have been given in non-U.S. trials. The adverse events in these patients were similar to those reported with the recommended dosage and regimen. There is no known antidote for overdosage of irinotecan. Maximum supportive care should be instituted to prevent dehydration due to diarrhea and to treat any infectious complications.

Lethality was observed after single intravenous irinotecan doses of approximately 111 mg/kg in mice and 73 mg/kg in rats (approximately 2.6 and 3.4 times the recommended human dose of 125 mg/m^2, respectively). Death was preceded by cyanosis, tremors, respiratory distress, and convulsions.

DOSAGE AND ADMINISTRATION:

STARTING DOSE AND DOSE MODIFICATIONS

The recommended starting dose of irinotecan injection is 125 mg/m^2. All doses should be administered as an intravenous infusion over 90 minutes (see Preparation of Infusion Solution). The recommended treatment regimen (one treatment course) is 125 mg/m^2 administered once weekly for 4 weeks, followed by a 2-week rest period. Thereafter, additional courses of treatment may be repeated every 6 weeks (4 weeks on therapy, followed by 2 weeks off therapy). Subsequent doses should be adjusted to as high as 150 mg/m^2 or to as low as 50 mg/m^2 in 25 to 50 mg/m^2 increments depending upon individual patient tolerance of treatment (see Recommended Dose Modifications table). Provided intolerable toxicity does not develop, treatment with additional courses of irinotecan may be continued indefinately in patients who attain a response or in patients whose disease remains stable. Patients should be carefully monitored for toxicity.

TABLE 4 describes the recommended dose modifications during a course of therapy and at the start of each subsequent course of therapy. These recommendations are based on toxicities commonly observed with the administration of irinotecan. Therapy with irinotecan should be interrupted when grade 3 or 4 late diarrhea occurs (see PRECAUTIONS, Information for Patients) or when other intolerable toxicity is observed. Dose modifications for hematological toxicities other than neutropenia (*e.g.*, leukopenia, anemia or thrombocytopenia, and platelets) during a course of therapy and at the start of a subsequent course of therapy are the same as recommended for neutropenia. Dose modifications for nonhematologic toxicities other than diarrhea (nausea, vomiting, etc.) during a course of therapy are the same as those recommended for diarrhea. At the start of a subsequent course of therapy, the dose of irinotecan should be decreased by 25 mg/m^2, compared to the initial dose of the previous course, for other NCI grade 2 or by 50 mg/m^2 for other grade 3 or 4 nonhematologic toxicities. All dose modifications should be based on the worst preceding toxicity. A new course of therapy should not begin until the granulocyte count has recovered to ≥1500/mm^3 and the platelet count has recovered to ≥100,000/mm^3 and treatment-related diarrhea is fully resolved. Treatment should be delayed 1 to 2 weeks to allow for recovery from treatment-related toxicity. If the patient has not recovered after a 2-week delay, consideration should be given to discontinuing irinotecan.

It is recommended that patients receive premedication with antiemetic agents (see PRECAUTIONS, General).

DOSAGE AND ADMINISTRATION: *(cont'd)*

TABLE 4 Recommended Dose Modifications†

A new course of therapy should not begin until the granulocyte count has recovered to ≥1500/mm^3, and the platelet count has recovered to ≥100,000/mm^3, and the treatment–related diarrhea is fully resolved. Treatment should be delayed 1 to 2 weeks to allow for recovery from treatment-related toxicities. If the patient has not recovered after a 2-week delay, consideration should be given to discontinuing irinotecan.

Toxicity NCI Grade * (Value)	During a Course of Therapy†	At the Start of the Next Courses of Therapy† (After Adequate Recovery), Compared to the Starting Dose in the Previous Course
No toxicity	**Maintain dose level**	**↑ 25 mg/m^2 up to a maximum dose of 150 mg/m^2**
Neutropenia		
1 (1500 to 1900/mm^3)	Maintain dose level	Maintain dose level
2 (1000 to 1400/mm^3)	↓25 mg/m^2	Maintain dose level
3 (500 to 900/mm^3)	Omit dose, then ↓25 mg/m^2 when resolved to ≤ grade 2	↓25 mg/m^2
4 (<500/mm^3)	Omit dose, then ↓50 mg/m^2 when resolved to ≤ grade 2	↓50 mg/m^2
Neutropenic Fever (grade 4 neutropenia & ≥grade 2 fever)	Omit dose, then ↓50 mg/m^2 when resolved	↓50 mg/m^2
Other Hematologic Toxicities	Dose modifications for leukopenia, thrombocytopenia, and anemia during a course of therapy and at the start of subsequent courses of therapy are also based on NCI toxicity criteria and are the same as recommended for neutropenia above.	
Diarrhea		
1 (2-3 stools/day > pretx‡	Maintain dose level	Maintain dose level
2 (4-6 stools/day > pretx)	↓25 mg/m^2	Maintain, if the only grade 2 tox§
3 (7-9 stools/day > pretx)	Omit dose, then ↓25 mg/m^2 when resolved to ≤ grade 2	↓25 mg/m^2, if the only grade 3 tox
4 (≥10 stools/day > pretx)	Omit dose, then ↓50mg/m^2 when resolved to ≤ grade 2	↓50mg/m^2
Other Nonhematologic Toxicities		
1	Maintain dose level	Maintain dose level
2	↓25 mg/m^2	↓25 mg/m^2
3	Omit dose, then ↓25 mg/m^2 when resolved to ≤ grade 2	↓50mg/m^2
4	Omit dose, then ↓50 mg/m^2 when resolved to ≤ grade 2	↓50mg/m^2

* National Cancer Institute Common Toxicity Criteria.
† All dose modifications should be based on the worst preceding toxicity.
‡ Pretreatment.
§ Toxicity

PREPARATION & ADMINISTRATION PRECAUTIONS

As with other potentially toxic anticancer agents, care should be exercised in the handling and preparation of infusion solutions prepared from irinotecan injection. The use of gloves is recommended. If a solution of irinotecan contacts the skin, wash the skin immediately and thoroughly with soap and water. If irinotecan contacts the mucous membranes, flush thoroughly with water. Several published guidelines for handling and disposal of anticancer agents are available.[1-7]

PREPARATION OF INFUSION SOLUTION

Inspect vial contents for particulate matter and repeat inspection when drug product is withdrawn from vial into syringe.

Irinotecan injection must be diluted prior to infusion. Irinotecan should be diluted in 5% Dextrose Injection, USP, (preferred) or 0.9% Sodium Chloride Injection, USP, to a final concentration range of 0.12 to 1.1 mg/ml. In most clinical trials, irinotecan was administered in 500 ml of 5% Dextrose Injection, USP.

The solution is physically and chemically stable for up to 24 hours at room temperature (approximately 25°C) and in ambient fluorescent lighting. Solutions diluted in 5% Dextrose Injection, USP, and stored at refrigerated temperatures (approximately 2° to 8°C), and protected from light are physically and chemically stable for 48 hours. Refrigeration of admixtures using 0.9% Sodium Chloride Injection, USP, is not recommended due to a low and sporadic incidence of visible particulates. **Freezing irinotecan and admixtures of irinotecan may result in precipitation of the drug and should be avoided.** Because of the possible microbial contamination during dilution, it is advisable to use the admixture within 24 hours if refrigerated (2° to 8°C, 36° to 46°F) or within 6 hours if kept at room temperature (15° to 30°C, 59° to 86°F).

Other drugs should not be added to the infusion solution. Parenteral drug products should be inspected visually for particulate matter and discoloration prior to administration whenever solution and container permit.

REFERENCES:

1. Recommendations for the Safe Handling of Parenteral Antineoplastic Drugs. NIH Publication, No. 83–2621. For sale by the Superintendent of Documents, U.S. Government Printing Office, Washington, D.C. 20402. **2.** AMA Council Report. Guidelines for handling parenteral antineoplastics. JAMA 1985; 253(11): 1590–2. **3.** National Study Commission on Cytotoxic Exposure. Recommendations for handling cytotoxic agents. Available from Louis P Jeffrey, ScD, Chairman, National Study Commission on Cytotoxic Exposure, Massachusetts College of Pharmacy and Allied Health Sciences, 179 Longwood Avenue, Boston, MA 02115. **4.** Clinical Oncological Society of Australia. Guideline and recommendations for safe handling of antineoplastic agents. Med J Australia 1983;1:426-8. **5.** Jones RB, et. al. Safe handling of chemotherapeutic agents: A report from the Mount Sinai Medical Center. CA-A Cancer J for Clinicians, 1983; Sept./Oct., 258–63. **6.** American Society of Hospital Pharmacists Technical Assistance Bulletin on Handling Cytotoxic and hazardous drugs. Am J Hosp Pharm 1990; 47:1033-49. **7.** OSHA work-practice guidelines for personnel dealing with cytotoxic (antineoplastic) drugs. Am J Hosp Pharm 1986; 43:1193-1204.

HOW SUPPLIED:

Each ml of Camptosar Injection contains 20 mg irinotecan (on the basis of the trihydrate salt); 45 mg sorbitol; and 0.9 mg lactic acid. When necessary, pH has been adjusted to 3.5 (range, 3.0 to 3.8) with sodium hydroxide or hydrochloric acid.

Camptosar Injection is available as single-dose vials in the following package size:

5 ml amber glass vial, packaged in a backing/plastic blister to protect against inadvertent breakage and leakage. **The vial should be inspected for damage and visible signs of leaks before removing the backing/plastic blister. If damaged, incinerate the unopened package.**

Store at controlled room temperature 15° to 30°C (59° to 86°F). Protect from light. It is recommended that the vial (and backing/plastic blister) should remain in the carton until the time of use.

For How Supplied Information, Contact Pharmacia & Upjohn (NDA# 020571)

IRON DEXTRAN *(001579)*

CATEGORIES: Anemia; Antianemia Drugs; Blood Formation/Coagulation; Deficiency Anemias; Hematinics; Homeostatic & Nutrient; Iron Deficiency; Iron Preparations; Vitamins; Pregnancy Category C; FDA Approval Pre 1982

BRAND NAMES: Feostat; Hematran; **Imferon**; Infed; Irodex; Norefmi; Norferan; Pri-Dextra; Proferdex

FORMULARIES: BC-BS; Medi-Cal; WHO

WARNING:
THE PARENTERAL USE OF COMPLEXES OF IRON AND CARBOHYDRATES HAS RESULTED IN ANAPHYLACTIC-TYPE REACTIONS. DEATHS ASSOCIATED WITH SUCH ADMINISTRATION HAVE BEEN REPORTED. THEREFORE, IRON DEXTRAN SHOULD BE USED ONLY IN THOSE PATIENTS IN WHOM THE INDICATIONS HAVE BEEN CLEARLY ESTABLISHED AND LABORATORY INVESTIGATIONS CONFIRM AN IRON DEFICIENT STATE NOT AMENABLE TO ORAL IRON THERAPY.

DESCRIPTION:

Infed (iron dextran injection, USP) is a dark brown, slightly viscous sterile liquid complex of ferric hydroxide and dextran for intravenous or intramuscular use.

Each ml contains the equivalent of 50 mg of elemental iron (as an iron dextran complex), approximately 0.9% sodium chloride, in water for injection. Sodium hydroxide and/or hydrochloric acid may have been used to adjust pH. The pH of the solution is between 5.2 and 6.5.

Therapeutic Class: Hematinic.

CLINICAL PHARMACOLOGY:

General: After intramuscular injection, iron dextran is absorbed from the injection site into the capillaries and the lymphatic system. Circulating iron dextran is removed from the plasma by cells of the reticuloendothelial system, which split the complex into its components of iron and dextran. The iron is immediately bound to the available protein moieties to form hemosiderin or ferritin, the physiological forms of iron, or to a lesser extent to transferrin. This iron which is subject to physiological control replenishes hemoglobin and depleted iron stores.

Dextran, a polyglucose, is either metabolized or excreted. Negligible amounts of iron are lost via the urinary or alimentary pathways after administration of iron dextran.

The major portion of intramuscular injections of iron dextran is absorbed within 72 hours; most of the remaining iron is absorbed over the ensuing 3 to 4 weeks.

Various studies involving intravenously administered ^{59}Fe iron dextran to iron deficient subjects, some of whom had coexisting diseases, have yielded half-life values ranging from 5 hours to more than 20 hours. The 5-hour value was determined for ^{59}Fe iron dextran from a study that used laboratory methods to separate the circulating ^{59}Fe iron dextran from the transferrin-bound ^{59}Fe. The 20-hour value reflects a half-life determined by measuring total ^{59}Fe, both circulating and bound. It should be understood that these half-life values do not represent clearance of iron from the body. Iron is not easily eliminated from the body and accumulation of iron can be toxic.

INDICATIONS AND USAGE:

Intravenous or intramuscular injections of iron dextran are indicated for treatment of patients with documented iron deficiency in whom oral administration is unsatisfactory or impossible.

CONTRAINDICATIONS:

Hypersensitivity to the product. All anemias not associated with iron deficiency.

WARNINGS:

See BOXED WARNING.

A risk of carcinogenesis may attend the intramuscular injection of iron-carbohydrate complexes. Such complexes have been found under experimental conditions to produce sarcoma when large doses or small doses injected repeatedly at the same site were given to rats, mice, and rabbits, and possibly in hamsters.

The long latent period between the injection of a potential carcinogen and the appearance of a tumor makes it impossible to measure accurately the risk in man. There have, however, been several reports in the literature describing tumors at the injection site in humans who had previously received intramuscular injections of iron-carbohydrate complexes.

Large intravenous doses, such as used with total dose infusions (TDI), have been associated with an increased incidence of adverse effects. The adverse effects frequently are delayed (1-2 days) reactions typified by one or more of the following symptoms: arthralgia, backache, chills, dizziness, moderate to high fever, headache, malaise, myalgia, nausea, and vomiting. The onset is usually 24-48 hours after administration and

WARNINGS: *(cont'd)*

symptoms generally subside within 3-4 days. These symptoms have also been reported following intramuscular injection and generally subside within 3-7 days. The etiology of these reactions is not known. The potential for a delayed reaction must be considered when estimating the risk/benefit of treatment.

The maximum daily dose should not exceed 2 ml undiluted iron dextran.

This preparation should be used with extreme care in patients with serious impairment of liver function.

It should not be used during the acute phase of infectious kidney disease.

Adverse reactions experienced following administration of iron dextran may exacerbate cardiovascular complications in patients with pre-existing cardiovascular disease.

PRECAUTIONS:

General: Unwarranted therapy with parenteral iron will cause excess storage of iron with the consequent possibility of exogenous hemosiderosis. Such iron overload is particularly apt to occur in patients with hemoglobinopathies and other refractory anemias that might be erroneously diagnosed as iron deficiency anemias.

Iron dextran should be used with caution in individuals with histories of significant allergies and/or asthma.

Anaphylaxis and other hypersensitivity reactions have been reported after uneventful test doses as well as therapeutic doses of iron dextran injection. Therefore, administration of subsequent test doses during therapy should be considered. (See DOSAGE AND ADMINISTRATION, Administration).

Epinephrine should be immediately available in the event of acute hypersensitivity reactions. (*Usual Adult Dose:* 0.5 ml of a 1:1000 solution, by subcutaneous or intramuscular injection.)

Note: Patients using beta-blocking agents may not respond adequately to epinephrine. Isoproterenol or similar beta-agonist agents may be required in these patients.

Patients with rheumatoid arthritis may have an acute exacerbation of joint pain and swelling following the administration of iron dextran.

Reports in the literature from countries outside the United States (in particular, New Zealand) have suggested that the use of intramuscular iron dextran in neonates has been associated with an increased incidence of gram-negative sepsis, primarily due to *E. Coli*.

Information for the Patient: Patients should be advised of the potential adverse reactions associated with the use of iron dextran.

Drug/Laboratory Test Interactions: Large doses of iron dextran (5 ml or more) have been reported to give a brown color to serum from a blood sample drawn 4 hours after administration.

The drug may cause falsely elevated values of serum bilirubin and falsely decreased values of serum calcium.

Serum iron determinations (especially by colorimetric assays) may not be meaningful for 3 weeks following the administration of iron dextran. Serum ferritin peaks approximately 7 to 9 days after an intravenous dose of iron dextran and slowly returns to baseline after about 3 weeks.

Examination of the bone marrow for iron stores may not be meaningful for prolonged periods following iron dextran therapy because residual iron dextran may remain in the reticuloendothelial cells.

Bone scans involving 99m Tc-disphosphonate have been reported to show a dense, crescentic area of activity in the buttocks, following the contour of the iliac crest, 1 to 6 days after intramuscular injections of iron dextran.

Bone scans with 99m Tc-labeled bone seeking agents, in the presence of high serum ferritin levels or following iron dextran infusions, have been reported to show reduction of bony uptake, marked renal activity, and excessive blood pool and soft tissue accumulation.

Carcinogenesis, Mutagenesis, and Impairment of Fertility: See WARNINGS.

Pregnancy Category C: Iron dextran has been shown to be teratogenic and embryocidal in mice, rats, rabbits, dogs, and monkeys when given in doses of about 3 times the maximum human dose.

No consistent adverse fetal effects were observed in mice, rats, rabbits, dogs and monkeys at doses of 50 mg iron/kg or less. Fetal and maternal toxicity has been reported in monkeys at a total intravenous dose of 90 mg iron/kg over a 14 day period. Similar effects were observed in mice and rats on administration of a single dose of 125 mg iron/kg. Fetal abnormalities in rats and dogs were observed at doses of 250 mg iron/kg and higher. The animals used in these tests were not iron deficient. There are no adequate and well-controlled studies in pregnant women. Iron dextran should be used during pregnancy only if the potential benefit justifies the potential risks to the fetus.

Placental Transfer: Various animal studies and studies in pregnant humans have demonstrated inconclusive results with respect to the placental transfer of iron dextran as iron dextran. It appears that some iron does reach the fetus, but the form in which it crosses the placenta is not clear.

Nursing Mothers: Caution should be exercised when iron dextran is administered to a nursing woman. Traces of unmetabolized iron dextran are excreted in human milk.

Pediatric Use: Not recommended for use in infants under 4 months of age (see DOSAGE AND ADMINISTRATION).

ADVERSE REACTIONS:

Severe/Fatal: Anaphylactic reactions have been reported with the use of iron dextran injection; on occasions these reactions have been fatal. Such reactions, which occur most often within the first several minutes of administration, have been generally characterized by sudden onset of respiratory difficult and/or cardiovascular collapse. (see BOXED WARNINGand PRECAUTIONS: General, pertaining to immediate availability of epinephrine)

Cardiovascular: Chest pain, chest tightness, shock, hypotension, hypertension, tachycardia, flushing, arrhythmias. (Flushing and hypotension may occur from too rapid injections by the intravenous route).

Dermatologic: Urticaria, pruritus, purpura, rash.

ADVERSE REACTIONS: *(cont'd)*

Gastrointestinal: Abdominal pain, nausea, vomiting, diarrhea.

Hematologic/lymphatic: Leucocytosis, lymphadenopathy.

Musculoskeletal/soft tissue : Arthralgia, arthritis (may represent reactivation in patients with quiescent rheumatoid arthritis (see PRECAUTIONS, General), myalgia; backache; sterile abscess, atrophy/fibrosis (intramuscular injection site); brown skin and/or underlying tissue discoloration (staining), soreness or pain at or near intramuscular injection sites; cellulitis; swelling; inflammation; local phlebitis at or near intravenous injection site.

Neurologic: Convulsions, seizures, syncope, headache, weakness, unresponsiveness, paresthesia, febrile episodes, chills, dizziness, disorientation, numbness.

Respiratory: Respiratory arrest, dyspnea, bronchospasm.

Urologic: Hematuria.

Delayed reactions: Arthralgia, backache, chills, dizziness, fever, headache, malaise, myalgia, nausea, vomiting (see WARNINGS).

Miscellaneous: Febrile episodes, sweating, shivering, chills, malaise, altered taste.

OVERDOSAGE:

Overdosage with iron dextran is unlikely to be associated with any acute manifestations. Dosages of iron dextran in excess of the requirements for restoration of hemoglobin and replenishment of iron stores may lead to hemosiderosis. Periodic monitoring of serum ferritin levels may be helpful in recognizing a deleterious progressive accumulation of iron resulting from impaired uptake of iron from the reticuloendothelial system in concurrent medical conditions such as chronic renal failure. Hodgkins disease, and rheumatoid arthritis. The LD_{50} of iron dextran is not less than 500 mg/kg in the mouse.

DOSAGE AND ADMINISTRATION:

Oral iron should be discontinued prior to administration of iron dextran.

DOSAGE

1. Iron Deficiency Anemia: Periodic hematologic determination (hemoglobin and hematocrit) is a simple and accurate technique for monitoring hematological response, and should be used as a guide in therapy. It should be recognized that iron storage may lag behind the appearance of normal blood morphology. Serum iron, total iron binding capacity (TIBC) and percent saturation of transferrin are other important tests for detecting and monitoring the iron deficient state.

After administration of iron dextran complex, evidence of a therapeutic response can be seen in a few days as an increase in the reticulocyte count.

Although serum ferritin is usually a good guide to body iron stores, the correlation of body iron stores and serum ferritin may not be valid in patients on chronic renal dialysis who are also receiving iron dextran complex.

Although there are significant variations in body build and weight distribution among males and females, the accompanying table and formula represent a convenient means for estimating the total iron required. This total iron requirement reflects the amount of iron needed to restore hemoglobin concentration to normal or near normal levels plus an additional allowance to provide adequate replenishment of iron stores in most individuals with moderately or severely reduced levels of hemoglobin. It should be remembered that iron deficiency anemia will not appear until essentially all iron stores have been depleted. Therapy, thus, should aim at not only replenishment of hemoglobin iron but iron stores as well.

$$\frac{\text{mg blood iron}}{\text{lb in body weight}} = \frac{\text{ml blood}}{\text{lb in body weight}} \times \frac{\text{g hemoglobin}}{\text{ml blood}} \times \frac{\text{mg iron}}{\text{g hemoglobin}}$$

a) Blood volume... 65 ml/kg of body weight

b) Normal hemoglobin (males and females):...

over 15 kg (33 lbs)... 14.8 g/dl

15 kg (33 lbs) or less... 12.0 g/dl

c)Iron content of hemoglobin... 0.34%

d) Hemoglobin deficit

e) Weight

Based on the above factors, individuals with normal hemoglobin levels will have approximately 33 mg of blood iron per kilogram of body weight (15 mg/lb).

Note: The table and accompanying formula are applicable for dosage determinations only in patients with iron deficiency anemia; they are not to be used for dosage determinations in patients requiring iron replacement for blood loss.

The total amount of iron dextran in ml required to treat the anemia and replenish iron stores may approximated as follows:

Adults and Children over 15 kg (33 lbs): See Dosage Table.

Alternatively the Total Dose May be Calculated: Dose (ml) = 0.0442 (Desired Hb - Observed Hb) × LBW + (0.26 × LBW)

Based On: Desired Hb = the target Hb in g/dl.

Observed Hb = the patient's current hemoglobin in g/dl.

LBW = lean body weight in kg. A patient's lean body weight (or actual weight if less than lean body weight) should be utilized when determining dosage.

For Males: LBW = 50 kg + 2.3 kg for each inch of patient's height over 5 feet

For Females: LBW = 45.5 kg + 2.3 kg for each inch of patient's height over 5 feet

To calculate a patient's weight in kg when lbs are known:

$$\frac{\text{patient's weight in pounds}}{2.2} = \text{weight in kilograms}$$

Children 5-15 kg (11-33 lbs): See Dosage Table.

DOSAGE AND ADMINISTRATION: *(cont'd)*

TABLE 2 TOTAL IRON DEXTRAN REQUIREMENT FOR HEMOGLOBIN RESTORATION AND IRON STORES REPLACEMENT*

PATIENT LEAN BODY WEIGHT kg	lb	Milliliter Requirement of Infed Based On Observed Hemoglobin of 3 (g/dl)	4 (g/dl)	5 (g/dl)	6 (g/dl)	7 (g/dl)	8 (g/dl)	9 (g/dl)	10 (g/dl)
5	11	3	3	3	3	2	2	2	2
10	22	7	6	6	5	5	4	4	3
15	33	10	9	9	8	7	7	6	5
20	44	16	15	14	13	12	11	10	9
25	55	20	18	17	16	15	14	13	12
30	66	23	22	21	19	18	17	15	14
35	77	27	26	24	23	21	20	18	17
40	88	31	29	28	26	24	22	21	19
45	99	35	33	31	29	27	25	23	21
50	110	39	37	35	32	30	28	26	24
55	121	43	41	38	36	33	31	28	26
60	132	47	44	42	39	36	34	31	28
65	143	51	48	45	42	39	36	34	31
70	154	55	52	49	45	42	39	36	33
75	165	59	55	52	49	45	42	39	35
80	176	63	59	55	52	48	45	41	38
85	187	66	63	59	55	51	48	44	40
90	198	70	66	62	58	54	50	46	42
95	209	74	70	66	62	57	53	49	45
100	220	78	74	69	65	60	56	52	47
105	231	82	77	73	68	63	59	54	50
110	242	86	81	76	71	67	62	57	52
115	253	90	85	80	75	70	64	59	54
120	264	94	88	83	78	73	67	62	57

* Table values were calculated based on a normal adult hemoglobin of 14.8 g/dl for weights less than or equal to 15 kg (33 lbs) and a hemoglobin of 12.0 g/dl for weights less than or equal to 15 kg (33 lbs).

Iron dextran should not normally be given in the first four months of life. (See PRECAUTIONS, Pediatric Use).

Alternatively the Total Dose May be Calculated: Dose (ml) = 0.0442 (Desired Hb - Observed Hb) x W + (0.26 × W)

Based On: Desired Hb = the target Hb in g/dl. (Normal Hb for Children 15 kg or less is 12 g/dl)

W = Weight in kg.

2. Iron Replacement for Blood Loss: Some individuals sustain blood losses oN an intermittent or repetitive basis. Such blood losses may occur periodically in patients with hemorrhagic diatheses (familial telangiectasia; hemophilia; gastrointestinal bleeding) and on a repetitive basis from procedures such as renal hemodialysis.

Iron therapy in these patients should be directed toward replacement of the equivalent amount of iron represented in the blood loss. The table and formula described under **I. *Iron Deficiency Anemia*** are ***not*** applicable for simple iron replacement values.

Quantitative estimates of the individual's periodic blood loss and hematocrit during the bleeding episode provide a convenient method for the calculation of the required iron dose.

The formula shown is based on the approximation that 1 ml of normochromic red cells contains 1 mg of elemental iron: (see TABLE 3)

TABLE 3

Replacement iron (in mg) =Blood loss (in ml) × hematocrit
Example: Blood loss of 500 ml with 20% hematocrit
Replacement Iron = 500 × 0.20 = 100 mg
Infed dose = 100 mg ÷ 50 = 2 ml

ADMINISTRATION

The total amount of iron dextran required for the treatment of iron deficiency anemia or iron replacement for blood loss is determined from the table or appropriate formula (see DOSAGE AND ADMINISTRATION).

1. Intravenous Injection: PRIOR TO RECEIVING THEIR FIRST IRON DEXTRAN THERAPEUTIC DOSE, ALL PATIENTS SHOULD BE GIVEN AN INTRAVENOUS TEST DOSE OF 0.5 ml (see PRECAUTIONS, General). THE TEST DOSE SHOULD BE ADMINISTERED AT A GRADUAL RATE OVER AT LEAST 30 SECONDS. Although anaphylactic reactions known to occur following iron dextran administration are usually evident within a few minutes, or sooner, it is recommended that a period of an hour or longer elapse before the remainder of the initial therapeutic dose is given.

Individual doses of 2 ml or less may be given on a daily basis until the calculated total amount required has been reached. Iron dextran is given undiluted at a **slow gradual rate** not to exceed 50 mg (1 ml) per minute.

2. Intramuscular Injection: PRIOR TO RECEIVING THEIR FIRST IRON DEXTRAN THERAPEUTIC DOSE, ALL PATIENTS SHOULD BE GIVEN AN INTRAMUSCULAR TEST DOSE OF 0.5 ml (see PRECAUTIONS, General). The test dose should be administered in the same recommended test site and by the same technique as described in the last paragraph of this section. Although anaphylactic reactions known to occur following iron dextran administration are usually evident within a few minutes or sooner, it is recommended that at least an hour or longer elapse before the remainder of the initial therapeutic dose is given.

DOSAGE AND ADMINISTRATION: *(cont'd)*

If no adverse reactions are observed, iron dextran can be given according to the following schedule until the calculated total amount required has been reached. Each day's dose should ordinarily not exceed 0.5 ml (25 mg of iron) for infants under 5 kg (11 lbs); 1.0 ml (50 mg of iron) for children under 10 kg (22 lbs); and 2.0 ml (100 mg of iron) for other patients.

Iron dextran should be injected only into the muscle mass of the upper outer quadrant of the buttock - never into the arm or other exposed areas - and should be injected deeply, with a 2-inch or 3-inch 19 or 20 gauge needle. If the patient is standing, he/she should be bearing his/her weight on the leg opposite the injection site, or if in bed, he/she should be in the lateral position with injection site uppermost. To avoid injection or leakage into the subcutaneous tissue, a Z-track technique (displacement of the skin laterally prior to injection) is recommended.

Note: Do not mix iron dextran with other medications or add to parenteral nutrition solutions for intravenous infusion.

Parenteral drug products should be inspected visually for particulate matter and discoloration prior to administration, whenever the solution and container permit.

HOW SUPPLIED:

Infed (Iron Dextran Injection, USP) containing 50 mg of elemental iron per ml, is available in 2 ml single dose amber vials (for intramuscular or intravenous use) in cartons of 10.

Store at controlled room temperature 15°-30°C (59°-86°F).

HOW SUPPLIED - EQUIVALENTS NOT AVAILABLE:

Injection, Solution - Intramuscular; - 50 mg/ml

2 ml x 10	$377.04	Infed, Schein Pharm (US)	00364-3012-47

ISOETHARINE HYDROCHLORIDE *(001582)*

CATEGORIES: Antiasthmatics/Bronchodilators; Asthma; Autonomic Drugs; Beta Adrenergic Stimulators; Bronchial Dilators; Bronchitis; Bronchospasm; Emphysema; Respiratory & Allergy Medications; Sympathomimetic Agents; Sympathomimetics, Beta Agonist; Pregnancy Category C; FDA Approval Pre 1982

BRAND NAMES: Arm-A-Med; *Asthmalitan* (Germany); Beta-2; Bisorine; **Bronkosol**; Dey-Lute; *Numotac*
(International brand names outside U.S. in italics)

FORMULARIES: Aetna

PRIMARY ICD9: 493.90 (Asthma, Unspecified, Without Mention of Status Asthmaticus)

DESCRIPTION:

BRONCHODILATOR SOLUTION FOR ORAL INHALATION

Isoetharine hydrochloride, USP, 1% also contains: Acetone Sodium Bisulfite, Glycerin, Parabens, Purified Water, Sodium Chloride, and Sodium Citrate.

CLINICAL PHARMACOLOGY:

Isoetharine is a sympathomimetic amine with preferential affinity for $Beta_2$ adrenergic receptor sites of bronchial and certain arteriolar musculature and a lower order of affinity for $Beta_1$ adrenergic receptors. Its activity in symptomatic relief of bronchospasm is rapid and of relatively long duration. By relieving bronchospasm, isoetharine helps give prompt relief and significantly increases vital capacity.

INDICATIONS AND USAGE:

Isoetharine hydrochloride is indicated for use as a bronchodilator for bronchial asthma and for reversible bronchospasm that may occur in association with bronchitis and emphysema.

CONTRAINDICATIONS:

Isoetharine inhalation solution should not be administered to patients who are hypersensitive to any of its ingredients.

WARNINGS:

Contains acetone sodium bisulfite, a sulfite that may cause allergic-type reactions including anaphylactic symptoms and life-threatening or less severe asthmatic episodes in certain susceptible people. The overall prevalence of sulfite sensitivity in the general population is unknown and probably low. Sulfite sensitivity is seen more frequently in asthmatic than in nonasthmatic people.

Excessive use of an adrenergic aerosol should be discouraged as it may lose its effectiveness. Occasional patients have been reported to develop severe paradoxical airway resistance with repeated excessive use of an aerosol adrenergic inhalation preparation. The cause of this refractory state is unknown. It is advisable that in such instances the use of the aerosol adrenergic be discontinued immediately and alternative therapy instituted, since in the reported cases the patients did not respond to other forms of therapy until the drug was withdrawn. Cardiac arrest has been noted in several instances.

Isoetharine hydrochloride should not be administered along with epinephrine or other sympathomimetic amines, since these drugs are direct cardiac stimulants and may cause excessive tachycardia. They may, however, be alternated if desired.

Usage in Pregnancy: Although there has been no evidence of teratogenic effects with this drug, use of any drug in pregnancy, lactation, or in women of childbearing potential requires that the potential benefit of the drug be weighed against its possible hazard to the mother or child.

PRECAUTIONS:

General: Dosage must be carefully adjusted in patients with hyperthyroidism, hypertension, acute coronary disease, cardiac asthma, limited cardiac reserve and in individuals sensitive to sympathomimetic amines since overdosage may result in tachycardia, palpitations, nausea, headache or epinephrine like side effects.

ADVERSE REACTIONS:

Although isoetharine hydrochloride is relatively free of toxic side effects, too frequent use may cause tachycardia, palpitation, nausea, headache, changes in blood pressure, anxiety, tension, restlessness, insomnia, tremor, weakness, dizziness, and excitement, as is the case with other sympathomimetic amines.

DOSAGE AND ADMINISTRATION:

Isoetharine hydrochloride can be administered by hand nebulizer, oxygen aerosolization, or intermittent positive pressure breathing (IPPB). Usually treatment need not be repeated more often than every four hours, although in severe cases more frequent administration may be necessary. (TABLE 1).

TABLE 1

Method Of Administration	Usual Dose (1% Solution)*	Range
Oxygen aerosolization**	0.50 ml	0.25-0.50 ml
IPPB†	0.50 ml	0.25-1 ml

*The doses given are for the 1% solution which must be suitably diluted prior to administration. Below are the dose equivalents for the entire prediluted and ready-to-use line:

Product Strength(%)	Volume (mL)	Equivalent to - mL of Isoetharine HCl 1%
0.062%	4 ml	0.25 ml
0.125%	4 ml	0.5 ml
0.167%	3 ml	0.5 ml
0.2%	2.5 ml	0.5 ml
0.25%	2 ml	0.5 ml

** Administered with oxygen flow adjusted to 4 to 6 liters/minuter over a period of 15 to 20 minutes

† Usually an inspiratory flow rate of 15 liters/minute at a cycling pressure of 15 cm H_2O is recommended. It may be necessary, according to patient and type of IPPB apparatus to adjust flow rate to 6 to 30 liters per minute, cycling pressure to 10 to 15 cm H_2O and further dilution according to needs of patient.

Store at controlled room temperature, 15 - 30° C (59- 86° F).

PROTECT FROM LIGHT. Store vial in pouch until time of use. Do not use solution if its color is pinkish or darker than slightly yellow or if it contains a precipitate.

HOW SUPPLIED - RATED THERAPEUTICALLY EQUIVALENT:

Solution - Inhalation - 0.08 %

3 ml x 25	$19.90	ISOETHARINE S/F, Dey Labs	49502-0661-03

Solution - Inhalation - 0.1 %

2.5 ml x 100	$99.35	Isoetharine Hcl, Roxane	00054-8429-25
5 ml x 25	$19.90	ISOETHARINE S/F, Dey Labs	49502-0664-05

Solution - Inhalation - 0.125 %

4 ml x 100	$99.35	Isoetharine Hcl, Roxane	00054-8430-25

Solution - Inhalation - 0.167 %

3 ml x 100	$99.35	Isoetharine Hcl, Roxane	00054-8432-25

Solution - Inhalation - 0.17 %

3 ml x 25	$19.90	ISOETHARINE S/F, Dey Labs	49502-0660-03

Solution - Inhalation - 0.2 %

2.5 ml x 100	$57.38	ARM-A-MED, Astra USA	00186-4113-01
2.5 ml x 100	$99.35	Isoetharine Hcl, Roxane	00054-8431-25

Solution - Inhalation - 0.25 %

2 ml x 25	$19.90	ISOETHARINE S/F, Dey Labs	49502-0659-02
2 ml x 100	$99.35	Isoetharine Hcl, Roxane	00054-8434-25

Solution - Inhalation - 1 %

10 ml	$5.00	BETA-2, Nephron	00487-7601-00
10 ml	$6.10	Isoetharine Hcl, Roxane	00054-3408-40
10 ml	$7.50	Isoetharine Hcl, H.C.F.A. F F P	99999-1582-01
10 ml	**$17.49**	**BRONKOSOL, Sanofi Winthrop**	**00024-1071-10**
30 ml	$10.00	BETA-2, Nephron	00487-7601-01
30 ml	$17.65	Isoetharine Hcl, Roxane	00054-3408-44
30 ml	$22.50	Isoetharine Hcl, H.C.F.A. F F P	99999-1582-02
30 ml	$23.10	BISORINE, Major Pharms	00904-2353-30
30 ml	**$47.96**	**BRONKOSOL, Sanofi Winthrop**	**00024-1071-30**

ISOETHARINE MESYLATE *(001583)*

CATEGORIES: Airway Obstruction; Antiasthmatics/Bronchodilators; Asthma; Autonomic Drugs; Beta Adrenergic Stimulators; Bronchial Dilators; Bronchitis; Bronchospasm; Emphysema; Respiratory & Allergy Medications; Sympathomimetic Agents; Sympathomimetics, Beta Agonist; FDA Approval Pre 1982

BRAND NAMES: **Bronkometer**

FORMULARIES: Medi-Cal

COST OF THERAPY: $204.98 (Asthma; Aerosol; 0.61 %; 0.3/day; 365 days)

PRIMARY ICD9: 493.90 (Asthma, Unspecified, Without Mention of Status Asthmaticus)

DESCRIPTION:

Bronkometer is a complete pocket nebulizer containing isoetharine mesylate 0.61% (w/w) with alcohol 30% (w/w), ascorbic acid 0.1% (w/w), (as a preservative), fluorochlorohydrocarbons (as gaseous propellants), menthol and saccharin.

The Bronkometer unit is designed to contain 20 metered doses per ml of solution (*e.g.,* 200 doses per 10 ml) and to deliver 340 mcg isoetharine mesylate at the mouthpiece per actuation.

Isoetharine mesylate is a sympathomimetic amine which provides therapeutic bronchodilation in a metered dose inhaler.

Chemically, isoetharine mesylate is 3,4-Dihydroxy-α-[1-(isopropylamino) propyl]benzylalcoholmethanesulfonate (salt).

CLINICAL PHARMACOLOGY:

Isoetharine is a sympathomimetic amine with preferential affinity for $Beta_2$ adrenergic receptor sites of bronchial and certain arteriolar musculature, and a lower order of affinity for $Beta_1$ adrenergic receptors. Its activity in symptomatic relief of bronchospasm is rapid and of relatively long duration. By relieving bronchospasm, Bronkometer helps give prompt relief and significantly increases the FVC, FEV_1, and $FEF_{25\%-75\%}$.

Recent studies in laboratory animals (minipigs, rodents, and dogs) recorded the occurrence of cardiac arrhythmias and sudden death (with histologic evidence of myocardial necrosis) when beta agonists and methylxanthines were administered concurrently. The significance of these findings when applied to humans is currently unknown.

INDICATIONS AND USAGE:

Bronkometer is indicated for use as a bronchodilator for bronchial asthma and for reversible bronchospasm that may occur in association with bronchitis and emphysema.

CONTRAINDICATIONS:

Bronkometer should not be administered to patients who are hypersensitive to any of its ingredients.

WARNINGS:

Excessive use of an adrenergic aerosol should be discouraged as it may lose its effectiveness. Occasional patients have been reported to develop severe paradoxical airway resistance with repeated excessive use of an aerosol adrenergic inhalation preparation. The cause of this refractory state is unknown. It is advisable that in such instances the use of the aerosol adrenergic be discontinued immediately and alternative therapy instituted, since in the reported cases the patients did not respond to other forms of therapy until the drug was withdrawn. Cardiac arrest has been noted in several instances.

Bronkometer should not be administered along with epinephrine or other sympathomimetic amines, since these drugs are direct cardiac stimulants and may cause excessive tachycardia. They may, however, be alternated if desired.

PRECAUTIONS:

Dosage must be carefully adjusted in patients with hyperthyroidism, hypertension, acute coronary disease, cardiac asthma, limited cardiac reserve, and in individuals sensitive to sympathomimetic amines, since overdosage may result in tachycardia, palpitations, nausea, headache, or epinephrine-like side effects.

Information for the Patient: Do not inhale more often than directed by your physician. Read the instructions before using. (See PATIENT PACKAGE INSERT.) Do not exceed the dose prescribed by your physician. If difficulty in breathing persists, contact your physician immediately. Avoid spraying in eyes. Contents under pressure. Do not break or incinerate. Store at controlled room temperature 15° C to 30° C (59° F to 86° F). Keep out of reach of children.

Carcinogenesis, Mutagenesis, and Impairment of Fertility: Chronic toxicity studies up to twelve months in dogs with doses up to 20 mg/kg/day (equivalent to approximately 200 times the human dose based on a 70 kg individual) and chronic toxicity studies in rats with the doses up to 45 mg/kg/day (equivalent to approximately 450 times the human dose, based on a 70 kg individual) revealed no evidence of carcinogenicity due to isoetharine. No animal studies have been conducted for evaluating the potential for mutagenesis and impairment of fertility of Bronkometer.

Pregnancy Category C: Animal reproduction studies have not been conducted with isoetharine mesylate. It is also not known whether isoetharine mesylate can cause fetal harm when administered to a pregnant woman or can affect reproduction capacity, although there is no evidence of such harm or effects. Isoetharine mesylate should be given to a pregnant woman only if clearly needed.

Nursing Mothers: It is not known whether this drug is excreted in human milk. Because many drugs are excreted in human milk, caution should be exercised when isoetharine mesylate is administered to a nursing woman.

Pediatric Use: The safety and efficacy of this product in children under the age of 12 have not been established.

DRUG INTERACTIONS:

Bronkometer should not be administered along with epinephrine or other sympathomimetic amines, since these drugs are direct cardiac stimulants and may cause excessive tachycardia. They may, however, be alternated if desired.

ADVERSE REACTIONS:

Although Bronkometer is relatively free of toxic side effects, too frequent use may cause the following reactions, as is the case with other sympathomimetic amines:

Cardiovascular: Tachycardia, palpitations, changes in blood pressure.

Gastrointestinal: Nausea.

CNS: Headache, restlessness, insomnia, anxiety, tension, dizziness, excitement.

Other: Tremor, weakness.

OVERDOSAGE:

Overdosage of Bronkometer may produce signs and symptoms typical of excessive sympathomimetic effects, including tachycardia, palpitations, nausea, headache, blood pressure changes, anxiety, restlessness, insomnia, tremor, weakness, dizziness and excitation. Excessive use of adrenergic aerosols may result in loss of effectiveness or severe paradoxical airway resistance. Cardiac arrest has been noted in several instances. In all cases of overdose or excessive use of Bronkometer, the drug should be discontinued immediately and vital functions supported until the patient is stabilized. It is not known whether isoetharine mesylate is dialyzable.

The single dose amount of drug that may be toxic or life threatening is highly variable according to patient characteristics and drug history. The acute oral LD_{50} in mice is 2000 mg/kg.

DOSAGE AND ADMINISTRATION:

The average adult dose is one or two inhalations. Occasionally, more may be required. It is important, however, to wait one full minute after the initial one or two inhalations in order to be certain whether another is necessary. In most cases, inhalations need not be repeated more often than every four hours, although more frequent administration may be necessary in severe cases.

PATIENT PACKAGE INSERT:

HOW TO USE YOUR BRONKOMETER WITH ORAL NEBULIZER AND REFILL

1. Remove cap and mouthpiece from nebulizer bottle.

2. Separate protective cap from mouthpiece.

3. Turn mouthpiece sideways and fit metal stem of nebulizer into hole in flattened end of mouthpiece.

4. Hold Bronkometer upside down between thumb and forefinger and close lips loosely around end of mouthpiece.

5. Breathe out completely. Start slow inhalation.

6. While inhaling, squeeze the bottle and mouthpiece firmly between thumb and forefinger. Inhale deeply.

7. Hold deep breath for a moment to allow maximum absorption. Exhale slowly through pursed lips.

8. WARNING: Do not exceed the dose prescribed by your physician. If difficulty in breathing persists, contact your physician immediately.

9. Always keep the plastic mouthpiece clean. When possible, rinse with tap water after each use, and wash thoroughly each day.

WARNING: Avoid spraying in eyes. Contents under pressure. Do not break or incinerate. Do not store at temperature above 120° F. Keep out of reach of children.

HOW SUPPLIED:

The Bronkometer unit is designed to contain 20 metered doses per ml of solution (*e.g.,* 200 doses per 10 ml) and to deliver 340 mcg isoetharine mesylate at the mouthpiece per actuation.

The bronchodilator isoetharine is also available in a convenient solution for use with conventional nebulizers by oxygen aerosolization and in IPPB machines as Bronkosol brand of isoetharine inhalation solution, 1%.

Store at controlled room temperature 15° C to 30° C (59° F to 86° F).

WARNING: Contains dichlorodifluoromethane and dichlorotetrafluoroethane, substances which harm public health and environment by destroying ozone in the upper atmosphere.

HOW SUPPLIED - EQUIVALENTS NOT AVAILABLE:

Aerosol - Inhalation - 0.61 %

10 ml	**$21.75**	**BRONKOMETER, Sanofi Winthrop**	**00024-1041-01**
10 ml	**$23.20**	**BRONKOMETER, Sanofi Winthrop**	**00024-1040-01**
15 ml	**$28.08**	**BRONKOMETER, Sanofi Winthrop**	**00024-1041-03**
15 ml	**$30.84**	**BRONKOMETER, Sanofi Winthrop**	**00024-1040-03**

ISOFLUROPHATE *(001584)*

CATEGORIES: EENT Drugs; Esotropia; Eye, Ear, Nose, & Throat Preparations; Glaucoma; Iridectomy; Miotics; Ophthalmics; Pregnancy Category X; FDA Approval Pre 1982

BRAND NAMES: **Floropryl**; *DFP* (Japan)
(International brand names outside U.S. in italics)

FORMULARIES: Medi-Cal

DESCRIPTION:

FOR TOPICAL APPLICATION INTO THE CONJUNCTIVAL SAC

Isoflurophate is available as a 0.025% sterile ophthalmic ointment on polyethylene mineral oil gel. Isoflurophate has a molecular weight of 184.15 and is known chemically as bis (1-methylethyl) phosphorofluoridate. Its empirical formula is $C_6H_{14}FO_3P$.

CLINICAL PHARMACOLOGY:

Isoflurophate is a cholinesterase inhibitor with sustained activity. Application to the eye produces intense miosis and ciliary muscle contraction due to inhibition of cholinesterase, allowing acetylcholine to accumulate at sites of cholinergic transmission.

Isoflurophate *irreversibly* inactivates cholinesterase. Thus, following use of isoflurophate in the eye, cholinesterase must be either regenerated or supplied from depots elsewhere in the body before ophthalmic action dependent on cholinesterase returns.

If given systemically in sufficient amounts, isoflurophate reduces plasma cholinesterase to zero. However, when applied locally to the eye, plasma cholinesterase is usually reduced only slightly.

INDICATIONS AND USAGE:

Open-angle glaucoma (isoflurophate should be used in glaucoma only when shorter-acting miotics have proved inadequate.)

Conditions obstructing aqueous outflow, such as synechial formation, that are amenable to miotic therapy

Following iridectomy

Accommodative esotropia (accommodative convergent strabismus)

CONTRAINDICATIONS:

Hypersensitivity to any component of this product.

Because of the toxicity of cholinesterase inhibitors in general, isoflurophate is contraindicated in women who are or may become pregnant. If this drug is used during pregnancy, or if the patient becomes pregnant while taking this drug, the patient should be apprised of the potential hazard to the fetus.

Because miotics may aggravate inflammation, isoflurophate should not be used in active uveal inflammation and/or glaucoma associated with iridocyclitis.

WARNINGS:

In patients receiving cholinesterase inhibitors such as isoflurophate, succinylcholine should be administered with extreme caution before and during general anesthesia because of possible respiratory and cardiovascular collapse.

WARNINGS: *(cont'd)*

Because of possible adverse additive effects, isoflurophate should be administered only with extreme caution to patients with myasthenia gravis who are receiving systemic anticholinesterase therapy; conversely, extreme caution should be exercised in the use of an anticholinesterase drug for the treatment of myasthenia gravis patients who are already undergoing topical therapy with cholinesterase inhibitors.

PRECAUTIONS:

GENERAL

Isoflurophate should be used with caution in patients with chronic angle-closure (narrow-angle) glaucoma or in patients with narrow angles, because of the possibility of producing pupillary block and increasing angle blockage.

Gonioscopy is recommended prior to medication with isoflurophate.

When an intraocular inflammatory process is present, the intensity and persistence of miosis and ciliary muscle contraction that result from anticholinesterase therapy require abstention from, or cautious use of, isoflurophate.

Systemic effects are infrequent when isoflurophate is applied carefully. The hands should be washed immediately following application.

Discontinue isoflurophate if salivation, urinary incontinence, diarrhea, profuse sweating, muscle weakness, respiratory difficulties, shock, or cardiac irregularities occur.

Persons receiving cholinesterase inhibitors who are exposed to organophosphate-type insecticides and pesticides (gardeners, organophosphate plant or warehouse workers, farmers, residents of communities which are undergoing insecticide spraying or dusting, etc.) should be warned of the added systemic effects possible from absorption through the respiratory tract or skin. Wearing of respiratory masks, frequent washing, and clothing changes may be advisable.

Anticholinesterase drugs should be used with extreme caution, if at all, in patients with marked vagotonia, bronchial asthma, spastic gastrointestinal disturbances, peptic ulcer, pronounced bradycardia and hypotension, recent myocardial infarction, epilepsy, parkinsonism, and other disorders that may respond adversely to vagotonic effects.

After long-term use of isoflurophate, dilation of blood vessels and resulting greater permeability increase the possibility of hyphema during ophthalmic surgery. Therefore, this drug should be discontinued before surgery.

Despite observance of all precautions and the use of only the recommended dose, there is some evidence that repeated administration may cause depression of the concentration of cholinesterase in the serum and erythrocytes, with resultant systemic effects.

There have been reports of bacterial keratitis associated with the use of multiple dose containers of topical ophthalmic products. These containers had been inadvertently contaminated by patients who, in most cases, had a concurrent corneal disease or a disruption of the ocular epithelial surface. (See PRECAUTIONS, Information for the Patient).

INFORMATION FOR THE PATIENT

Patients should be instructed to avoid allowing the tip of the dispensing container to contact the eye or surrounding structures.

Patients should also be instructed that ocular preparations, if handled improperly, can become contaminated by common bacteria known to cause ocular infections. Serious damage to the eye and subsequent loss of vision may result from using contaminated preparations. (See PRECAUTIONS, General)

Patients should also be advised that if they develop an intercurrent ocular condition (*e.g.*, trauma, ocular surgery or infection), they should immediately seek their physician's advice concerning the continued use of the present multidose container.

CARCINOGENESIS, MUTAGENESIS, AND IMPAIRMENT OF FERTILITY

Long-tern studies in animals have not been performed to evaluate the effects of isoflurophate on fertility or carcinogenic potential.

PREGNANCY CATEGORY X

See CONTRAINDICATIONS.

NURSING MOTHERS

It is not known whether this drug is excreted in human milk. Because of the potential for serious adverse reactions in nursing infants from isoflurophate, a decision should be made whether to discontinue nursing or to discontinue the drug, taking into account the importance of the drug to the mother.

PEDIATRIC USE

The occurrence of iris cysts is more frequent in children (see ADVERSE REACTIONS and DOSAGE AND ADMINISTRATION).

Extreme caution should be exercised in children receiving isoflurophate who may require general anesthesia (see WARNINGS).

Since isoflurophate is a potent cholinesterase inhibitor it should be kept out of the reach of children.

DRUG INTERACTIONS:

See WARNINGS regarding possible drug interactions of isoflurophate with succinylcholine or with other anticholinesterase agents.

ADVERSE REACTIONS:

Stinging, burning, lacrimation, lid muscle twitching, conjunctival and ciliary redness, brow ache, headache, and induced myopia with visual blurring may occur.

As with all miotic therapy, retinal detachment has been reported occasionally.

Activation of latent iritis or uveitis may occur.

Iris cysts may form, enlarge, and obscure vision. Occurrence is more frequent in children. The iris cyst usually shrinks upon discontinuance of the miotic. Rarely, the cyst may rupture or break free into the aqueous. Frequent examination for this occurrence is advised.

Prolonged use may cause conjunctival thickening and obstruction of nasolacrimal canals.

Systemic effects, which occur rarely, are suggestive of increased cholinergic activity. Such effects may include nausea, vomiting, abdominal cramps, diarrhea, urinary incontinence, salivation, difficulty in breathing, bradycardia, or cardiac irregularities. Medical management of systemic effects may be indicated (see Treatment Of Adverse Effects).

Lens opacities have been reported in patients on miotic therapy. Routine slitlamp examinations, including the lens, should accompany prolonged use.

Paradoxical increase in intraocular pressure may follow anticholinesterase application. This may be alleviated by pupil-dilating medication.

TREATMENT OF ADVERSE EFFECTS

If isoflurophate is taken systemically by accident, or if systemic effects occur after topical application in the eye or from accidental skin contact, atropine sulfate in a dose (for adults) of 0.4 to 0.6 mg or more should be given parenterally (intravenously if necessary). The recommended dosage of atropine in infants and children up to 12 years of age is 0.01 mg/kg repeated every two hours as needed until the desired effect is obtained, or adverse effects of atropine preclude further usage. The maximum single dose should not exceed 0.4 mg.

ADVERSE REACTIONS: *(cont'd)*

The use of much larger doses of atropine in treating anticholinesterase intoxication in adults has been reported in the literature. Initially 2 to 6 mg may be given followed by 2 mg every hour or more often, as long as muscarinic effects continue. The greater possibility of atropinization with large doses, particularly in sensitive individuals, should be borne in mind.

Pralidoxime (Protopam) chloride has been reported to be useful in treatment of systemic effects due to cholinesterase inhibitors. However, its use is recommended in addition to and not as a substitution for atropine.

A short-acting barbiturate is indicated if convulsions occur that are not entirely relieved by atropine. Barbiturate dosage should be carefully adjusted to avoid central respiratory depression. Marked weakness or paralysis of muscles of respiration should be treated promptly by artificial respiration and maintenance of a clean airway.

The oral LD_{50} of isoflurophate is 37 mg/kg in the mouse, 5-10 mg/kg in the rat, and 4-10 mg/kg in the rabbit.

DOSAGE AND ADMINISTRATION:

Isoflurophate *is intended solely for topical use in the conjunctival sac.*

Isoflurophate hydrolyzes in the presence of water to form hydrofluoric acid. To prevent absorption of moisture and loss of potency, the ointment tube should be kept tightly closed; the tip of the tube should not be washed or allowed to touch the eyelid or other moist surface.

Whenever possible, isoflurophate should be applied at night before retiring to lessen blurring of vision. As it is an extremely potent drug, it should be used with great care and only by those familiar with its use and thoroughly indoctrinated in the technic of application.

The required dose is applied in the conjunctival sac, with the patient supine, care being taken not to touch the cornea with the tip of the tube. *Wash the hands immediately after administration.*

ISOFLUROPHATE SHOULD NOT BE USED MORE OFTEN THAN DIRECTED. CAUTION IS NECESSARY TO AVOID OVERDOSAGE.

Keep frequency of use to a minimum in all patients, but especially in children, to reduce the chance of iris cyst development (see ADVERSE REACTIONS). If tolerance develops, another miotic should be used. Isoflurophate may be resumed later.

GLAUCOMA

For initial therapy ¼ inch strip of ophthalmic ointment isoflurophate 0.025 percent is placed in the glaucomatous eye every 8 to 72 hours. A decrease in intraocular pressure should occur within a few hours. During this period, keep the patient under supervision and make tonometric examinations at least hourly for 3 or 4 hours to be sure that no immediate rise in pressure occurs (see ADVERSE REACTIONS).

STRABISMUS

Essentially equal visual acuity of both eyes is a prerequisite to successful treatment. For initial evaluation, isoflurophate may be used as a diagnostic aid to determine if an accommodative factor exists. This is especially useful preoperatively in young children and in patients with normal hypermetropic refractive errors. Not more than ¼ inch strip of ointment is administered every night for 2 weeks. If the eyes become straighter, an accommodative factor is demonstrated. This technic may supplement or complement standard testing with atropine and trial with glasses for the accommodative factor.

In esotropia uncomplicated by amblyopia or anisometropia, ophthalmic ointment isoflurophate may be used in both eyes, not more than ¼ inch strip at a time every night for 2 weeks, as too severe a degree of miosis may interfere with vision. The dosage is then reduced from ¼ inch strip every other day to ¼ inch strip once a week for 2 months, after which the patient's status should be reevaluated.

If benefit can not be maintained with a dosage interval of at least 48 hours, therapy with isoflurophate should be stopped. Frequency of administration and duration of maintenance therapy depend on how long the eyes remain straight without medication. Intervals between administration should be gradually increased to the greatest length compatible with good results. Therapy may need to be continued for many years in some patients; in others, it has been possible to discontinue therapy after several months.

Storage: Protect from moisture, freezing and excessive heat.

HOW SUPPLIED - EQUIVALENTS NOT AVAILABLE:

Ointment - Ophthalmic - 0.025 %

3.5 gm	$8.14	FLOROPRYL, Merck	00006-7742-04

ISONIAZID *(001585)*

CATEGORIES: Anti-Infectives; Antibiotics; Antimicrobials; Antimycobacterials; Antituberculosis Agents; Chemotherapy; Tuberculosis; Hepatitis B*; FDA Approval Pre 1982

* Indication not approved by the FDA

BRAND NAMES: *Abdizide*; *Cemidon*; *Dianicotyl*; *Diazid* (Japan); *Dipicin*; *Eutizon*; *Fetefu*; *Hidrazida*; *Hydra* (Japan); *Hydrazide* (Japan); *Hydrazin*; Hyzyd; INH; *Iscotin* (Japan); *Isokin*; *Isonex*; *Isoniazid* (Australia); *Isoniazid Atlantic*; *Isoniazida N.T.*; *Isonicid*; *Isonin*; *Isotamine* (Canada); *Isozid* (Germany); Laniazid; *Medic Aid Isoniazid*; Niazid; *Nicotibine*; *Nicozid*; Nydrazid; *PMS Isoniazid* (Canada); *Rimicid*; Rimifon; Stanozide; *Tibinide*; *Tubilysin*; Tubizid; *Yuhan-Zid*
(International brand names outside U.S. in italics)

FORMULARIES: Aetna; BC-BS; DoD; FHP; Medi-Cal; PCS; WHO

COST OF THERAPY: $4.46 (Tuberculosis; Tablet; 300 mg; 1/day; 180 days)

PRIMARY ICD9: 011.93 (Pulmonary Tuberculosis, Unspecified, Tubercle Bacilli Found)

WARNING:
Severe and sometimes fatal hepatitis associated with isoniazid therapy may occur and may develop even after many months of treatment. The risk of developing hepatitis is age related. Approximate case rates by age are: 0 per 1,000 for persons under 20 years of age, 3 per 1,000 for persons in the 20-34 year age group, 12 per 1,000 for persons in the 35-49 year age group, 23 per 1,000 for persons in the 50-64 year age group, and 8 per 1,000 for persons over 65 years of age.
The risk of hepatitis is increased with daily consumption of alcohol. Precise data to provide a fatality rate for isoniazid-related hepatitis is not available; however, in a U.S. Public Health Service Surveillance Study of 13,838 persons taking isoniazid, there were 8 deaths among 174 cases of hepatitis.
Therefore, patients given isoniazid should be carefully monitored and

interviewed at monthly intervals. Serum transaminase concentration becomes elevated in about 10-20 percent of patients, usually during the first few months of therapy but it can occur at any time. Usually enzyme levels return to normal despite continuance of drug but in some cases progressive liver dysfunction occurs.

Patients should be instructed to report immediately any of the prodromal symptoms of hepatitis, such as fatigue, weakness, malaise, anorexia, nausea, or vomiting. If these symptoms appear or if signs suggestive of hepatic damage are detected, isoniazid should be discontinued promptly, since continued use of the drug in these cases has been reported to cause a more severe form of liver damage.

Patients with tuberculosis should be given appropriate treatment with alternative drugs. If isoniazid must be reinstituted, it should be reinstituted only after symptoms and laboratory abnormalities have cleared. The drug should be restarted in very small and gradually increasing doses and should be withdrawn immediately if there is any indication of recurrent liver involvement.

Preventive treatment should be deferred in persons with acute hepatic diseases.

DESCRIPTION:

Oral Tablets: Isoniazid USP, is an antibiotic available as 100 mg and 300 mg tablets for oral administration. Isoniazid is isonicotinic acid hydrazide.

Isoniazid USP is colorless or white crystals or white crystalline powder. It is odorless and slowly affected by exposure to air and light. It is freely soluble in water, sparingly soluble in alcohol, and slightly soluble in chloroform and in ether. Its molecular weight is 137.14.

Injection: Isoniazid Injection provides 100 mg isoniazid per ml with 0.25% chlorobutanol (chloral derivative) as a preservative; the pH has been adjusted to 6.0 to 7.0 with sodium hydroxide or hydrochloric acid. At the time of manufacture, the air in the container is replaced by nitrogen.

Syrup: This product produced by Carolina is an orange flavored syrup containing 50 mg of Isoniazid per 5 ml of syrup. Sorbitol Solution USP, (containing 70% Sorbitol) is used as the vehicle.

CLINICAL PHARMACOLOGY:

Isoniazid acts against actively growing tubercle bacilli.

Within one to two hours after oral administration isoniazid produces peak blood levels which decline to 50% or less within six hours. It diffuses readily into all body fluids (cerebrospinal, pleural, and ascitic), tissues, organs, and excreta (saliva, sputum, and feces). The drug also passes through the placental barrier and into milk in concentrations comparable to those in the plasma. From 50 to 70% of a dose of isoniazid is excreted in the urine in 24 hours.

Isoniazid is metabolized primarily by acetylation and dehydrazination. The rate of acetylation is genetically determined. Approximately 50% of Blacks and Caucasians are "slow acetylators" and the rest are rapid acetylators; the majority of Eskimos and Orientals are "rapid acetylators."

The rate of acetylation does not significantly alter the effectiveness of isoniazid. However, slow acetylation may lead to higher blood levels of the drug, and thus an increase in toxic reactions.

Pyridoxine (B_6) deficiency is sometimes observed in adults with high doses of isoniazid and is considered probably due to its competition with pyridoxal phosphate for the enzyme apotryptophanase.

INDICATIONS AND USAGE:

For all forms of tuberculosis in which organisms are susceptible.

For preventive therapy for the following groups, in order of priority:

1. Household members and other close associates of persons with recently diagnosed tuberculous disease.

2. Positive tuberculin skin test reactors with findings on the chest roentgenogram consistent with nonprogressive tuberculous disease, in whom there are neither positive bacteriologic findings nor a history of adequate chemotherapy.

3. Newly infected persons.

4. Positive tuberculin skin test reactors in the following special clinical situations: prolonged therapy with adrenocorticosteroids; immunosuppressive therapy; some hematologic and reticuloendothelial diseases, such as leukemia or Hodgkin's disease; diabetes mellitus; silicosis; after gastrectomy.

5. Other positive tuberculin reactors under 35 years of age. The risk of hepatitis must be weighed against the risk of tuberculosis in positive tuberculin reactors over the age of 35. However, the use of isoniazid is recommended for those with the additional risk factors listed above (1-4) and on an individual basis in situations where there is likelihood of serious consequences to contacts who may become infected.

CONTRAINDICATIONS:

Isoniazid is contraindicated in patients who develop severe hypersensitivity reactions, including drug-induced hepatitis. Previous isoniazid-associated hepatic injury: severe adverse reactions to isoniazid, such as drug fever, chills, and arthritis; acute liver disease of any etiology.

WARNINGS:

See BOXED WARNING.

PRECAUTIONS:

All drugs should be stopped and an evaluation made at the first sign of a hypersensitivity reaction. If isoniazid therapy must be reinstituted, the drug should be given only after symptoms have cleared. The drug should be restarted in very small and gradually increasing doses and should be withdrawn immediately if there is any indication of recurrent hypersensitivity reaction.

Use of isoniazid should be carefully monitored in the following:

1. Patients who are receiving phenytoin concurrently. Isoniazid may decrease the excretion of phenytoin or may enhance its effects. To avoid phenytoin intoxication, appropriate adjustment of the anticonvulsant should be made.

2. Daily users of alcohol. Daily ingestion of alcohol may be associated with a higher incidence of isoniazid hepatitis.

3. Patients with current chronic liver disease or severe renal dysfunction.

Ophthalmologic examinations (including ophthalmoscopy) should be done*before* Isoniazid is started and periodically thereafter, even without occurrence of visual symptoms.

PRECAUTIONS: *(cont'd)*

Usage in Pregnancy and Lactation: It has been reported that in both rats and rabbits, isoniazid may exert an embryocidal effect when administered orally during pregnancy, although no isoniazid-related congenital anomalies have been found in reproduction studies in mammalian species (mice, rats, and rabbits). Isoniazid should be prescribed during pregnancy only when therapeutically necessary. The benefit of preventive therapy should be weighed against a possible risk to the fetus. Preventive treatment generally should be started after delivery because of the increased risk of tuberculosis for new mothers.

Since isoniazid is known to cross the placental barrier and to pass into maternal breast milk, neonates and breast-fed infants of isoniazid-treated mothers should be carefully observed for any evidence of adverse effects.

Carcinogenesis: Isoniazid has been reported to induce pulmonary tumors in a number of strains of mice.

ADVERSE REACTIONS:

The most frequent reactions are those affecting the nervous system and the liver.

Nervous System Reactions: Peripheral neuropathy is the most common toxic effect. It is dose-related, occurs most often in the malnourished and in those predisposed to neuritis (*e.g.,* alcoholics and diabetics), and is usually preceded by paresthesias of the feet and hands. The incidence is higher in "slow inactivators."

Other neurotoxic effects, which are uncommon with conventional doses, are convulsions, toxic encephalopathy, optic neuritis and atrophy, memory impairment, and toxic psychosis.

Gastrointestinal Reactions: Nausea, vomiting, epigastric distress.

Hepatic Reactions: Elevated serum transaminases (SGOT; SGPT), bilirubinemia, bilirubinuria, jaundice and occasionally severe and sometimes fatal hepatitis. The common prodromal symptoms are anorexia, nausea, vomiting, fatigue, malaise, and weakness. Mild and transient elevation of serum transaminase levels, occurs in 10 to 20 percent of persons taking isoniazid. The abnormality usually occurs in the first 4 to 6 months of treatment but can occur at any time during therapy. In most instances, enzyme levels return to normal with no necessity to discontinue medication. In occasional instances, progressive liver damage occurs, with accompanying symptoms. In these cases, the drug should be discontinued immediately. The frequency of progressive liver damage increases with age. It is rare in persons under 20, but occurs in up to 2.3 percent of those over 50 years of age.

Hematologic Reactions: Agranulocytosis; hemolytic, sideroblastic, or aplastic anemia; thrombocytopenia; and eosinophilia.

Hypersensitivity Reactions: Fever, skin eruptions (morbilliform, maculopapular, purpuric, or exfoliative), lymphadenopathy and vasculitis.

Metabolic and Endocrine Reactions: Pyridoxine deficiency, pellagra, hyperglycemia, metabolic acidosis, and gynecomastia.

Miscellaneous Reactions: Rheumatic syndrome and systemic lupus erythematosus-like syndrome. Local irritation has been observed at the site of intramuscular injection.

OVERDOSAGE:

Signs and Symptoms: Isoniazid overdosage produces signs and symptoms within 30 minutes to 3 hours after ingestion. Nausea, vomiting, dizziness, slurring of speech, blurring of vision, and visual hallucinations (including bright colors and strange designs), are among the early manifestations. With marked overdosage, respiratory distress and CNS depression, progressing rapidly from stupor to profound coma, are to be expected, along with severe, intractable seizures. Severe metabolic acidosis, acetonuria, and hyperglycemia are typical laboratory findings.

Treatment: Untreated or inadequately treated cases of gross isoniazid overdosage can terminate fatally, but good response has been reported in most patients brought under adequate treatment within the first few hours after drug ingestion.

Secure the airway and establish adequate respiratory exchange. Gastric lavage within the first 2 to 3 hours is advised, but should not be attempted until convulsions are under control. To control convulsions administer IV shortacting barbiturates and IV pyridoxine (usually 1 mg/1 mg isoniazid ingested).

Obtain blood samples for immediate determination of gases, electrolytes, BUN, glucose, etc.; type and crossmatch blood in preparation for possible hemodialysis.

Rapid Control of Metabolic Acidosis is Fundamental to Management: Give IV sodium bicarbonate at once and repeat as needed, adjusting subsequent dosage on the basis of laboratory findings (*i.e.,* serum sodium, pH, etc.).

Forced osmotic diuresis must be started early and should be continued for some hours after clinical improvement to hasten renal clearance of drug and help prevent relapse; monitor fluid intake and output.

Hemodialysis is advised for severe cases; if this is not available, peritoneal dialysis can be used along with forced diuresis.

Along with measures based on initial and repeated determination of blood gases and other laboratory tests as needed, utilize meticulous respiratory and other intensive care to protect against hypoxia, hypotension, aspiration pneumonitis, etc.

Note: For preventive therapy of tuberculous infection it is recommended that physicians be familiar with the joint recommendations of the American Thoracic Society, American Lung Association, and the Center for Disease Control, as published in the American Review of Respiratory Disease, Vol. 110, No.3, September, 1974, or CDC's Morbidity and Mortality Weekly Report, Vol. 24, No. 8, February 22, 1975.

DOSAGE AND ADMINISTRATION:

ORAL TABLETS AND SYRUP

For Treatment of Active Tuberculosis: Isoniazid is used in conjunction with other effective antituberculous agents.

If the bacilli become resistant, therapy must be changed to agents to which the bacilli are susceptible.

Usual Oral Dosage

Adults: 5 mg/kg up to 300 mg daily in a single dose.

Infants and children: 10-20 mg/kg depending on severity of infection, (up to 300-500 mg daily) in a single dose.

For Preventive Therapy

Adults: 300 mg per day in a single dose.

Infants and Children: 10 mg/kg (up to 300 mg daily) in a single dose.

Continuous administration of isoniazid for a sufficient period is an essential part of the regimen because relapse rates are higher if chemotherapy is stopped prematurely. In the treatment of tuberculosis, resistant organisms may multiply and the emergence of resistant organisms during the treatment may necessitate a change in the regimen.

Concomitant administration of pyridoxine (B_6) is recommended in the malnourished and in those predisposed to neuropathy (*e.g.,* alcoholics and diabetics).

DOSAGE AND ADMINISTRATION: *(cont'd)*

INJECTION

Isoniazid injection is used in conjunction with other effective antituberculosis agents. If the bacilli become resistant, therapy must be changed to agents to which the bacilli are susceptible.

Usual Parenteral Dosage

For Treatment of Tuberculosis: *Adults:* 5 mg/kg up to 300 mg daily in a single dose. *Infants and Children:* 10 to 20 mg/kg depending on severity of infection (up to 300 to 500 mg daily) in a single dose.

For Preventive Therapy: *Adults:* 300 mg per day in a single. *Infants and Children:* 10 mg/kg (up to 300 mg daily) in a single dose.

Continuous administration of isoniazid for a sufficient period of time is an essential part of the regimen because relapse rate are higher if chemotherapy is stopped prematurely. In the treatment of tuberculosis, resistant organisms may multiply and their emergence during the treatment may necessitate a change in the regimen.

Concomitant administration of pyridoxine (B_6) is recommended in the malnourished and in those predisposed to neuropathy (*e.g.,* alcoholics and diabetics).

Storage: Store at room temperature.

Isoniazid for injection may crystallize at low temperatures. If this occurs, warm the vial to room temperature before use to redissolve the crystals.

HOW SUPPLIED - RATED THERAPEUTICALLY EQUIVALENT:

Syrup - Oral - 50 mg/ml

480 ml	$17.50	Isoniazid Syrup, Carolina Med	46287-0009-01

Tablet, Uncoated - Oral - 100 mg

30's	$.78	Isoniazid, H.C.F.A. F F P	99999-1585-01
30's	$1.95	Isoniazid, Eon Labs Mfg	00185-4351-30
100's	$1.18	LANIAZID, Lannett	00527-1092-01
100's	$1.25	Isoniazid, Anabolic	00722-5212-01
100's	$1.25	Niazid, Apotheca	12634-0129-01
100's	$2.63	Isoniazid, H.C.F.A. F F P	99999-1585-02
100's	$3.50	Isoniazid, United Res	00677-0077-01
100's	$4.00	Isoniazid, Eon Labs Mfg	00185-4351-01
100's	$4.20	Isoniazid, Paddock Labs	00574-0100-01
100's	$4.25	Tubizid, Consolidated Midland	00223-1150-01
100's	$4.45	Isoniazid, Raway	00686-1260-25
100's	$5.16	Isoniazid, Barr	00555-0066-02
100's	$5.61	Isoniazid, Rugby	00536-3948-01
100's	$5.70	IZONID, Major Pharms	00904-2095-60
100's	$5.80	Isoniazid, Goldline Labs	00182-0559-01
100's	$5.92	Isoniazid 100, Aligen Independ	00405-4552-01
100's	$6.45	Isoniazid, US Trading	56126-0264-11
100's	$6.60	Isoniazid, Halsey Drug	00879-0113-01
100's	$7.55	NYDRAZID, Bristol Myers Squibb	00003-0637-50
100's	$10.00	Isoniazid, Raway	00686-0082-20
1000's	$4.70	Niazid, Apotheca	12634-0129-10
1000's	$6.40	Isoniazid, Anabolic	00722-5212-03
1000's	$7.90	LANIAZID, Lannett	00527-1092-10
1000's	$23.50	Isoniazid, Eon Labs Mfg	00185-4351-10
1000's	$24.50	Tubizid, Consolidated Midland	00223-1150-02
1000's	$26.30	Isoniazid, H.C.F.A. F F P	99999-1585-03
1000's	$28.73	Isoniazid, Barr	00555-0066-05
1000's	$32.20	IZONID, Major Pharms	00904-2095-80
1000's	$43.25	Isoniazid, Rugby	00536-3948-10
1000's	$57.65	Isoniazid, Halsey Drug	00879-0113-10
1000's	$61.48	NYDRAZID, Bristol Myers Squibb	00003-0637-80
1000's	$67.30	Isoniazid, Schein Pharm (US)	00364-0150-02

Tablet, Uncoated - Oral - 300 mg

30's	$1.57	Isoniazid, H.C.F.A. F F P	99999-1585-04
30's	$1.95	Isoniazid, Major Pharms	00904-2096-46
30's	$2.25	Isoniazid, Vangard Labs	00615-0654-30
30's	$2.90	Isoniazid, Dixon Shane	17236-0182-30
30's	$2.95	Isoniazid, Eon Labs Mfg	00185-4350-30
30's	$3.75	Isoniazid, Paddock Labs	00574-0300-03
30's	$4.00	Isoniazid, US Trading	56126-0265-07
30's	$5.20	Isoniazid, Duramed Pharms	51285-0277-30
30's	$7.45	Isoniazid, Barr	00555-0071-01
35's	$1.83	Isoniazid, H.C.F.A. F F P	99999-1585-05
35's	$3.10	Isoniazid, Dixon Shane	17236-0182-35
35's	$5.55	Isoniazid, Halsey Drug	00879-0341-35
100's	$2.48	LANIAZID, Lannett	00527-1109-01
100's	$4.25	Isoniazid, United Res	00677-0664-01
100's	$4.95	Isoniazid, Vangard Labs	00615-0654-01
100's	$5.21	Isoniazid, US Trading	56126-0265-11
100's	$5.25	Isoniazid, H.C.F.A. F F P	99999-1585-06
100's	$5.75	Isoniazid, Eon Labs Mfg	00185-4350-01
100's	$6.95	Tubizid, Consolidated Midland	00223-1151-01
100's	$7.00	Isoniazid, Dixon Shane	17236-0182-01
100's	$8.02	Isoniazid, Duramed Pharms	51285-0277-02
100's	$8.43	Isoniazid 300, Aligen Independ	00405-4553-01
100's	$8.55	Isoniazid, Barr	00555-0071-02
100's	$8.57	Isoniazid, Schein Pharm (US)	00364-0151-01
100's	$8.58	Isoniazid, Rugby	00536-3941-01
100's	$8.70	IZONID, Major Pharms	00904-2096-60
100's	$9.00	Isoniazid, Goldline Labs	00182-1356-01
100's	$10.75	Isoniazid, Halsey Drug	00879-0341-01
100's	$12.00	Isoniazid, Raway	00686-0083-20
100's	$13.98	Isoniazid, Voluntary Hosp	53258-0143-13
500's	$26.25	Isoniazid, H.C.F.A. F F P	99999-1585-07
1000's	$13.90	LANIAZID, Lannett	00527-1109-10
1000's	$49.95	Isoniazid, Eon Labs Mfg	00185-4350-10
1000's	$52.50	Isoniazid, H.C.F.A. F F P	99999-1585-08
1000's	$59.50	Tubizid, Consolidated Midland	00223-1151-02
1000's	$68.00	Isoniazid, Goldline Labs	00182-1356-10
1000's	$68.07	Isoniazid, Rugby	00536-3941-10
1000's	$68.65	Isoniazid, Barr	00555-0071-05
1000's	$68.72	Isoniazid, Duramed Pharms	51285-0277-05
1000's	$69.75	Isoniazid, Halsey Drug	00879-0341-10
1000's	$69.90	IZONID, Major Pharms	00904-2096-80

HOW SUPPLIED - NOT RATED EQUIVALENT:

Injection, Solution - Intramuscular - 100 mg/ml

10 ml	$15.85	NYDRAZID, Bristol Myers Squibb	00003-0643-50

ISONIAZID; PYRAZINAMIDE; RIFAMPIN

(003210)

CATEGORIES: Anti-Infectives; Antibiotics; Antimicrobials; Antimycobacterials; Antituberculosis Agents; Orphan Drugs; Tuberculosis; FDA Class 4S ("Standard Review"); FDA Approved 1994 May

BRAND NAMES: **Rifater**; *Rimactazide + Z*
(International brand names outside U.S. in italics)

FORMULARIES: Medi-Cal; WHO

COST OF THERAPY: $1,620.00 (Tuberculosis; Tablet; 50 mg/300 mg/120 mg; 5/day; 180 days)

PRIMARY ICD9: 011.93 (Pulmonary Tuberculosis, Unspecified, Tubercle Bacilli Found)

DESCRIPTION:

FOR COMPLETE PRESCRIBING INFORMATION, REFER TO THE INDIVIDUAL DRUG MONOGRAPHS (ISONIAZID; PYRAZINAMIDE; RIFAMPIN).

INDICATIONS AND USAGE:

This combination drug is indicated in the initial phase of the short-course treatment of pulmonary tuberculosis. During this phase, which should last 2 months, Rifater should be administered on a daily, continuous basis.

Following and initial phase and treatment with this combination drug, treatment should be continued with rifampin and isoniazid (*e.g.,* Rifamate) for at least 4 months. Treatment should be continued for a longer period of time if the patient is still sputum or culture positive, if resistant organisms are present, or if the patient is HIV positive.

In the treatment of tuberculosis, the small number of cells present within large populations of susceptible cells can rapidly become the predominant type. Since resistance can emerge rapidly, susceptibility tests should be performed in the event of persistent positive cultures during the course of treatment. Bacteriologic smears or cultures should be obtained before the start of therapy to confirm the susceptibility of the organism to rifampin, isoniazid, and pyrazinamide and they should be repeated throughout therapy to monitor response to the treatment. If test results show resistance to any of the components of this combination drug and the patient is not responding to therapy, the drug regimen should be modified.

DOSAGE AND ADMINISTRATION:

Adults: Patients should be given the following single daily dose of Rifater either 1 hour before or 2 hours after a meal with a full glass of water.

Patients weighing ≤44 kg - 4 tablets

Patients weighing between 45-54 kg - 5 tablets

Patients weighing ≥55 kg - 6 tablets

Children: The ratio of the drugs in this combination may not be appropriate in children or adolescents under the age of 15 (*e.g.,* higher mg/kg doses of isoniazid are usually given in children than adults).

This combination drug is recommended in the initial phase of short-course therapy which is usually continued for 2 months. The Advisory Council for the Elimination of Tuberculosis, the American Thoracic Society, and the Centers for Disease Control and Prevention recommend that either streptomycin or ethambutol be added as a fourth drug in a regimen containing isoniazid (INH), rifampin and pyrazinamide for initial treatment of tuberculosis unless the likelihood of INH or rifampin resistance is very low. The need for fourth drug should be reassessed when the results of susceptibility testing are known. If community rates of INH resistance are currently less than 4%, an initial treatment regimen with less than four drugs maybe considered.

Following the initial phase, treatment should be continued with rifampin and isoniazid (*e.g.,* Rifamate) for at least 4 months. Treatment should be continued for longer if the patient is still sputum or culture positive, if resistant organisms are present, or if the patient is HIV positive. Concomitant administration of pyridoxine (B_6) is recommended in the malnourished, in those predisposed to neuropathy (*e.g.,* alcoholics and diabetics), and in adolescents.

HOW SUPPLIED:

Rifater tablets are light beige, smooth, round, and shiny sugar-coated tablets imprinted with "RIFATER" in black ink and contain 120 mg rifampin, 50 mg isoniazid, and 300 mg pyrazinamide, and are supplied as:

Bottles of 60 tablets.

Unit dose blister packages of 100 tablets.

Storage Conditions: Store at controlled room temperature 59°-86°F (15°-30°C). Protect from excessive humidity.

HOW SUPPLIED - EQUIVALENTS NOT AVAILABLE:

Tablet, Uncoated - Oral - 50 mg/300 mg/12

60's	**$108.00**	**RIFATER, Hoechst Marion Roussel**	**00088-0576-41**

ISONIAZID; RIFAMPIN *(001587)*

CATEGORIES: Anti-Infectives; Antibiotics; Antimicrobials; Antimycobacterials; Antituberculosis Agents; Tuberculosis; FDA Approval Pre 1982

BRAND NAMES: *Dipicin-INH; Iso-Ramp 300; Ramicin-ISO; Refinah; Refinah 300; Ricinis; Rif Plus; Rifaina;* Rifamate; *Rifamiso; Rifazida; Rifinah* (England, Germany, France); *Rifinah 300; Rifoldin 300MG + INH;* **Rimactane INH**; *Rimactazid* (England); *Rimactazid 300; Rimactizid; Rimpazid 450*
(International brand names outside U.S. in italics)

FORMULARIES: WHO

COST OF THERAPY: $1,019.88 (Tuberculosis; Capsule; 300 mg/300 mg; 2/day; 180 days)

PRIMARY ICD9: 011.93 (Pulmonary Tuberculosis, Unspecified, Tubercle Bacilli Found)

DESCRIPTION:

FOR COMPLETE PRESCRIBING INFORMATION, REFER TO THE INDIVIDUAL DRUG MONOGRAPHS (ISONIAZID; RIFAMPIN).

INDICATIONS AND USAGE:

For pulmonary tuberculosis in which organisms are susceptible, and when the patient has been titrated on the individual components and it has therefore been established that this fixed dosage is therapeutically effective.

This fixed-dosage combination drug is not recommended for initial therapy of tuberculosis or for preventive therapy.

In the treatment of tuberculosis, small numbers of resistant cells, present within large populations of susceptible cells, can rapidly become the predominating type. Since rapid emergence of resistance can occur, culture and susceptibility tests should be performed in the event of persistent positive cultures.

This drug is not indicated for the treatment of meningococcal infections or asymptomatic carriers of *N. meningitidis* to eliminate meningococci from the nasopharynx.

DOSAGE AND ADMINISTRATION:

In general, therapy should be continued until bacterial conversion and maximal improvement have occurred.

Adults: Two rifampin-isoniazid capsules (600 mg rifampin, 300 mg isoniazid) once daily, administered one hour before or two hours after a meal.

Concomitant administration of pyridoxine (B_6) is recommended in the malnourished, in those predisposed to neuropathy (*e.g.,* diabetics) and in adolescents.

SUSCEPTIBILITY TESTING-RIFAMPIN

Rifampin susceptibility powders are available for both direct and indirect methods of determining the susceptibility of strains of mycobacteria. The MIC's of susceptible clinical isolates when determined in 7H10 or other non-egg-containing media have ranged from 0.1 to 2 mcg/ml.

Quantitative methods that require measurement of zone diameters give the most precise estimates of antibiotic susceptibility. One such procedure has been recommended for use with discs for testing susceptibility to rifampin. Interpretations correlate zone diameters from the disc test with MIC (minimal inhibitory concentration) values for rifampin.

(Marion Merrell Dow, 5/91)

HOW SUPPLIED - EQUIVALENTS NOT AVAILABLE:

Capsule, Gelatin - Oral - 150 mg/300 mg

60's $145.92 RIFAMATE, Hoechst Marion Roussel 00068-0509-60

Capsule, Gelatin - Oral - 300 mg/300 mg

30's $84.99 RIMACTANE/INH, DUAL PACKS, Novartis 00083-8912-23

ISOPROTERENOL HYDROCHLORIDE *(001590)*

CATEGORIES: Adams-Stokes Syndrome; Airway Obstruction; Antiarrhythmic Agents; Antiasthmatics/Bronchodilators; Arrhythmia; Asthma; Autonomic Drugs; Beta Adrenergic Stimulators; Bronchial Dilators; Bronchitis; Bronchospasm; Cardiac Output; Cardiogenic Shock; Cardiovascular Drugs; Chronic Bronchitis; Congestive Heart Failure; Emphysema; Heart Block; Heart Failure; Hypotension/Shock; Hypovolemic Shock; Respiratory & Allergy Medications; Shock; Sympathomimetic Agents; Sympathomimetics, Beta Agonist; Pregnancy Category C; FDA Approval Pre 1982

BRAND NAMES: Aerolone; Dispos-A-Med Isoproterenol HCC; Isopro Aerometer ; **Isuprel**; *Isuprel Mistometer* (Canada); *Isuprel Nebulimetro*; Medihaler-Iso; Norisodrine; *Saventrine* (England); Vapo-Iso

(International brand names outside U.S. in italics)

FORMULARIES: Medi-Cal; WHO

PRIMARY ICD9: 493.90 (Asthma, Unspecified, Without Mention of Status Asthmaticus)

DESCRIPTION:

Chemically, isoproterenol hydrochloride is 3,4-Dihydroxy-α-[(isopropylamino) methyl]-benzyl alcohol hydrochloride, a synthetic sympathomimetic amine that is structurally related to epinephrine but acts almost exclusively on beta receptors.

Isoproterenol hydrochloride is a racemic compound with a molecular weight of 247.72 and the molecular formula $C_{11}H_{17}NO_3 \cdot HCl$.

INJECTION

Each milliliter of the sterile 1:5000 Isuprel solution contains:

Isoproterenol hydrochloride injection, USP 0.2 mg

Lactic Acid 0.12 mg

Sodium Chloride 7.0 mg

Sodium Lactate 1.8 mg

Sodium Metabisulfite (as preservative) 1.0 mg

Water for Injection qs ad 1.0 ml

The pH is adjusted between 3.5 and 4.5 with hydrochloric acid. The air in the ampuls has been displaced by nitrogen gas.

The sterile 1:5000 solution can be administered by intravenous, intramuscular, subcutaneous, or intracardiac routes.

INHALATION AEROSOL

Isuprel Mistometer is a beta agonist sympathomimetic bronchodilator. It is a complete nebulizing unit consisting of a plastic-coated vial of aerosol solution, detachable plastic mouthpiece with built-in nebulizer, and protective cap. The vial contains isoproterenol hydrochloride 0.25% (w/w) with inert ingredients of alcohol 33% (w/w) and ascorbic acid 0.1% (w/w) and, as propellants, dichlorodifluoromethane and dichlorotetrafluoroethane.

The contents permit the delivery of not less than 200 actuations from the 11.2 g (10 ml) vial and not less than 300 actuations from the 16.8 (15 ml) vial. The Mistometer delivers a measured dose of 131 mcg of the bronchodilator in a fine, even mist for inhalation.

INHALATION SOLUTION

Isuprel hydrochloride, brand of isoproterenol inhalation solution, is a beta agonist sympathomimetic bronchodilator.

Solution 1:200: Contains isoproterenol hydrochloride 5 mg/ml.

Inactive Ingredients: Chlorobutanol 0.5 percent and sodium metabisulfite 0.3 percent as preservatives, citric acid, glycerin, purified water, and sodium chloride.

Solution 1:100: Contains isoproterenol hydrochloride 10 mg/ml.

Inactive Ingredients: Chlorobutanol 0.5 percent and sodium metabisulfite 0.3 percent as preservatives, citric acid, purified water, saccharin sodium, sodium chloride, and sodium citrate.

DESCRIPTION: *(cont'd)*

Isoproterenol hydrochloride is soluble in water (1 g isoproterenol hydrochloride dissolves in 3 ml H_2O). The solutions have a pH range of 3 to 4.5.

The air in the bottles has been displaced by nitrogen gas.

CLINICAL PHARMACOLOGY:

INJECTION

Isoproterenol hydrochloride injection acts primarily on the heart and on smooth muscle of bronchi, skeletal muscle vasculature, and alimentary tract. The positive inotropic and chronotropic actions of the drug result in an increase in minute blood flow. There is an increase in heart rate, an approximately unchanged stroke volume, and an increase in ejection velocity. The rate of discharge of cardiac pacemakers is increased with isoproterenol hydrochloride injection. Venous return to the heart is increased through a decreased compliance of the venous bed. Systemic resistance and pulmonary vascular resistance are decreased, and there is an increase in coronary and renal blood flow. Systolic blood pressure may increase and diastolic blood pressure may decrease. Mean arterial blood pressure is usually unchanged or reduced. The peripheral and coronary vasodilating effects of the drug may aid tissue perfusion.

Isoproterenol hydrochloride injection relaxes most smooth muscle, the most pronounced effect being on bronchial and gastrointestinal smooth muscle. It produces marked relaxation in the smaller bronchi and may even dilate the trachea and main bronchi past the resting diameter.

Isoproterenol hydrochloride injection is metabolized primarily in the liver by COMT. The duration of action of isoproterenol hydrochloride injection may be longer than epinephrine, but it is still brief.

INHALATION AEROSOL AND INHALATION SOLUTION

Isoproterenol HCl relaxes bronchial spasm and facilitates expectoration of pulmonary secretions by acting almost exclusively on beta receptors. It is frequently effective when epinephrine and other drugs fail, and it has a wide margin of safety.

Isoproterenol HCl is readily absorbed when given as an aerosol. It is metabolized primarily in the liver and other tissues by catechol-0-methyltransferase (COMT).

Recent studies in laboratory animals (minipigs, rodents, and dogs) recorded the occurrence of cardiac arrhythmias and sudden death (with histologic evidence of myocardial necrosis) when beta agonists and methylxanthines were concomitantly administered. The significance of these findings when applied to human usage is currently unknown.

INDICATIONS AND USAGE:

Injection: Isoproterenol hydrochloride injection is indicated:

For mild or transient episodes of heart block that do not require electric shock or pacemaker therapy.

For serious episodes of heart block and Adams-Stokes attacks (except when caused by ventricular tachycardia or fibrillation). (See CONTRAINDICATIONS.)

For use in cardiac arrest until electric shock or pacemaker therapy, the treatments of choice, is available. (See CONTRAINDICATIONS.)

For bronchospasm occurring during anesthesia.

As an adjunct to fluid and electrolyte replacement therapy and the use of other drugs and procedures in the treatment of hypovolemic and septic shock, low cardiac output (hypoperfusion) states, congestive heart failure, and cardiogenic shock. (See WARNINGS.)

Inhalation Aerosol and Inhalation Solution: Isoproterenol HCl is indicated for the relief of bronchospasm associated with acute and chronic asthma and reversible bronchospasm which may be associated with chronic bronchitis or emphysema.

CONTRAINDICATIONS:

Injection: Use of isoproterenol hydrochloride injection is contraindicated in patients with tachyarrhythmias; tachycardia or heart block caused by digitalis intoxication; ventricular arrhythmias which require inotropic therapy; and angina pectoris.

Inhalation Aerosol and Inhalation Solution: Use of isoproterenol in patients with preexisting cardiac arrhythmias associated with tachycardia is generally considered contraindicated because the cardiac stimulant effect of the drug may aggravate such disorders. The use of this medication is contraindicated in those patients who have a known hypersensitivity to isoproterenol or to any of the other components of this drug.

WARNINGS:

Injection: Isoproterenol hydrochloride injection, by increasing myocardial oxygen requirements while decreasing effective coronary perfusion, may have a deleterious effect on the injured or failing heart. Most experts discourage its use as the initial agent in treating cardiogenic shock following myocardial infarction. However, when a low arterial pressure has been elevated by other means, isoproterenol hydrochloride injection may produce beneficial hemodynamic and metabolic effects.

In a few patients, presumably with organic disease of the AV node and its branches, isoproterenol hydrochloride injection has paradoxically been reported to worsen heart block or to precipitate Adams-Stokes attacks during normal sinus rhythm or transient heart block.

Injection and Inhalation Solution: Contains sodium metabisulfite, a sulfite that may cause allergic-type reactions including anaphylactic symptoms and life-threatening or less severe asthmatic episodes in certain susceptible people. The overall prevalence of sulfite sensitivity in the general population is unknown and probably low. Sulfite sensitivity is seen more frequently in asthmatic than in nonasthmatic people.

Inhalation Aerosol and Inhalation Solution: Excessive use of an adrenergic aerosol should be discouraged as it may lose its effectiveness.

Inhalation Aerosol: In patients with status asthmaticus and abnormal blood gas tensions, improvement in vital capacity and in blood gas tensions may not accompany apparent relief of bronchospasm. Facilities for administering oxygen mixtures and ventilatory assistance are necessary for such patients.

Occasional patients have been reported to develop severe paradoxical airway resistance with repeated, excessive use of isoproterenol inhalation preparations. The cause of this refractory state is unknown. It is advisable that in such instances the use of this preparation be discontinued immediately and alternative therapy instituted, since in the reported cases the patients did not respond to other forms of therapy until the drug was withdrawn.

Inhalation Solution: Isoproterenol administration as a solution for nebulization has been associated with a decrease in arterial pO_2 in asthmatic patients as a result of ventilation-perfusion abnormalities despite improvement in airway obstruction. The clinical significance of this relative hypoxemia is unclear.

As with other inhaled beta adrenergic agonists, isoproterenol HCl can produce paradoxical bronchospasm, that can be life threatening. If this occurs, the product should be discontinued immediately and alternative therapy instituted.

WARNINGS: *(cont'd)*

Inhalation Aerosol and Inhalation Solution: Deaths have been reported following excessive use of isoproterenol inhalation preparations and the exact cause is unknown. Cardiac arrest was noted in several instances. It is therefore essential that the physician instruct the patient in the need for further evaluation if his/her asthma worsens.

PRECAUTIONS:

GENERAL

Injection: Isoproterenol hydrochloride injection should generally be started at the lowest recommended dose. This may be gradually increased if necessary while carefully monitoring the patient. Doses sufficient to increase the heart rate to more than 130 beats per minute may increase the likelihood of inducing ventricular arrhythmias. Such increases in heart rate will also tend to increase cardiac work and oxygen requirements which may adversely affect the failing heart or the heart with a significant degree of arteriosclerosis.

Particular caution is necessary in administering isoproterenol hydrochloride injection to patients with coronary artery disease, coronary insufficiency, diabetes, hyperthyroidism, and sensitivity to sympathomimetic amines.

Adequate filling of the intravascular compartment by suitable volume expanders is of primary importance in most cases of shock and should precede the administration of vasoactive drugs. In patients with normal cardiac function, determination of central venous pressure is a reliable guide during volume replacement. If evidence of hypoperfusion persists after adequate volume replacement, isoproterenol hydrochloride injection may be given.

In addition to the routine monitoring of systemic blood pressure, heart rate, urine flow, and the electrocardiograph, the response to therapy should also be monitored by frequent determination of the central venous pressure and blood gases. Patients in shock should be closely observed during isoproterenol hydrochloride injection administration. If the heart rate exceeds 110 beats per minute, it may be advisable to decrease the infusion rate or temporarily discontinue the infusion. Determinations of cardiac output and circulation time may also be helpful. Appropriate measures should be taken to ensure adequate ventilation. Careful attention should be paid to acid-base balance and to the correction of electrolyte disturbances. In cases of shock associated with bacteremia, suitable antimicrobial therapy is, of course, imperative.

Inhalation Aerosol: Isoproterenol should be used with caution in patients with cardiovascular disorders including coronary insufficiency, diabetes, or hyperthyroidism, and in persons sensitive to sympathomimetic amines.

A single treatment with the isoproterenol HCl aerosol is usually sufficient for controlling isolated attacks of asthma.

Inhalation Solution: Isoproterenol HCl, as with all sympathomimetic amines, should be used with caution in patients with cardiovascular disorders, especially coronary insufficiency, cardiac arrhythmias, and hypertension; in patients with convulsive disorders, hyperthyroidism, or diabetes mellitus; and in patients who are unusually responsive to sympathomimetic amines. Clinically significant changes in systolic and diastolic blood pressure have been seen in some patients after use of any beta adrenergic bronchodilator.

When compressed oxygen is employed as the aerosol propellant, the percentage of oxygen used should be determined by the patient's individual requirements to avoid depression of respiratory drive.

Inhalation Aerosol and Inhalation Solution: Any patient who requires more than three aerosol treatments within a 24-hour period should be under the close supervision of a physician. Further therapy with the bronchodilator aerosol alone is inadvisable when three to five treatments within six to twelve hours produce minimal or no relief.

CARCINOGENESIS, MUTAGENESIS, AND IMPAIRMENT OF FERTILITY

Long-term studies in animals to evaluate the carcinogenic potential of isoproterenol hydrochloride have not been done. Mutagenic potential and effect on fertility have not been determined. There is no evidence from human experience that isoproterenol hydrochloride injection may be carcinogenic or mutagenic or that it impairs fertility.

PREGNANCY CATEGORY C

Animal reproduction studies have not been conducted with isoproterenol hydrochloride. It is also not known whether isoproterenol hydrochloride can cause fetal harm when administered to a pregnant woman or can affect reproduction capacity. Isoproterenol hydrochloride should be given to a pregnant woman only if clearly needed.

NURSING MOTHERS

It is not known whether this drug is excreted in human milk. Because many drugs are excreted in human milk, caution should be exercised when isoproterenol hydrochloride is administered to a nursing woman.

INFORMATION FOR THE PATIENT

Inhalation Aerosol: Do not inhale more often than directed by your physician. Read enclosed instructions before using (see attachment to insert.) Do not exceed the dose prescribed by your physician. If difficulty in breathing persists, contact your physician immediately. Avoid spraying in eyes. Contents under pressure. Do not break or incinerate. Do not store at temperatures above 120°F. Keep out of reach of children.

PEDIATRIC USE

Inhalation Aerosol and Inhalation Solution: In general, the technique of isoproterenol HCl aerosol and isoproterenol hydrochloride solution in administration to children is similar to that of adults, since children's smaller ventilatory exchange capacity automatically provides proportionally smaller aerosol intake. However, it is generally recommended that the 1:200 solution (rather than the 1:100) be used for an acute attack of bronchospasm, and no more than 0.25 ml of the 1:200 solution should be used for each 10 to 15 minute programmed treatment in chronic bronchospastic disease.

DRUG INTERACTIONS:

Injection: Isoproterenol hydrochloride injection and epinephrine should not be administered simultaneously because both drugs are direct cardiac stimulants and their combined effects may induce serious arrhythmias. The drugs may, however, be administered alternately provided a proper interval has elapsed between doses.

Isoproterenol HCl should be used with caution, if at all, when potent inhalational anesthetics such as halothane are employed because of potential to sensitize the myocardium to effects of sympathomimetic amines.

Inhalation Aerosol: Epinephrine should not be administered concomitantly with isoproterenol HCl, as both drugs are direct cardiac stimulants and their combined effects may induce serious arrhythmia. If desired they may, however, be alternated, provided an interval of at least four hours has elapse.

Inhalation Solution: Other sympathomimetic aerosol bronchodilators or epinephrine should not be used concomitantly with isoproterenol HCl. If additional adrenergic drugs are to be administered by any route to the patient using isoproterenol HCl, they should be used with caution to avoid deleterious cardiovascular effects.

Beta adrenergic agonists should be administered with caution to patients being treated with MAO inhibitors or tricyclic antidepressants since the action of the beta adrenergic agonists on the vascular system may be potentiated.

DRUG INTERACTIONS: *(cont'd)*

Beta receptor blocking agents and isoproterenol HCl inhibit the effects of each other.

ADVERSE REACTIONS:

INJECTION

The following reactions to isoproterenol hydrochloride have been reported:

CNS: Nervousness, headache, dizziness.

Cardiovascular: Tachycardia, palpitations, angina, Adams-Stokes attacks, pulmonary edema, hypertension, hypotension, ventricular arrhythmias, tachyarrhythmias.

In a few patients, presumably with organic disease of the AV node and its branches, isoproterenol hydrochloride injection has been reported to precipitate Adams-Stokes seizures during normal sinus rhythm or transient heart block.

Other: Flushing of the skin, sweating, mild tremors, weakness.

INHALATION AEROSOL AND INHALATION SOLUTION

The mist from the isoproterenol HCl aerosol contains alcohol but is generally very well tolerated. An occasional patient may experience some transient throat irritation which has been attributed to the alcohol content.

Serious reactions to isoproterenol HCl are infrequent. The following reactions, however, have been reported:

CNS: Nervousness, headache, dizziness, weakness.

Gastrointestinal: Nausea, vomiting.

Cardiovascular: Tachycardia, palpitations, precordial distress, angina-type pain.

Other: Flushing of the skin, tremor, and sweating.

The inhalation route is usually accompanied by a minimum of side effects. These untoward reactions disappear quickly and do not as a rule, inconvenience the patient to the extent that the drug must be discontinued. No cumulative effects have been reported.

OVERDOSAGE:

Injection: The acute toxicity of isoproterenol hydrochloride in animals is much less than that of epinephrine. Excessive doses in animals or man can cause a striking drop in blood pressure, and repeated large doses in animals may result in cardiac enlargement and focal myocarditis.

In case of accidental overdosage as evidenced mainly by tachycardia or other arrhythmias, palpitations, angina, hypotension, or hypertension, reduce rate of administration or discontinue isoproterenol hydrochloride injection until patient's condition stabilizes. Blood pressure, pulse, respiration, and EKG should be monitored.

It is not known whether isoproterenol hydrochloride is dialyzable.

The oral LD_{50} of isoproterenol hydrochloride in mice is 3,850 mg/kg ± 1,190 mg/kg of pure drug in solution.

Inhalation Aerosol and Inhalation Solution: Overdosage of isoproterenol HCl may produce signs and symptoms typical of excessive sympathomimetic effects, including tachycardia, palpitations, nervousness, nausea, and vomiting. Excessive use of adrenergic aerosols may result in loss of effectiveness or severe paradoxical airway resistance. Cardiac arrest has been noted in several instances. In all cases of overdose or excessive use of isoproterenol HCl, the drug should be discontinued immediately and vital functions supported until the patient is stabilized. It is not known whether isoproterenol hydrochloride is dialyzable.

The acute oral LD_{50} in mice is 3,850 mg/kg ± 1,190 mg/kg of pure drug in solution (isoproterenol hydrochloride). In dogs, the toxic dose is 1,000 times the therapeutic dose. Converted to the amount used clinically in man, this would be about 2,500 times the therapeutic dose.

DOSAGE AND ADMINISTRATION:

INJECTION

Isoproterenol HCl injection 1:5000 should generally be started at the lowest recommended dose and the rate of administration gradually increased if necessary while carefully monitoring the patient. The usual route of administration is by intravenous infusion or bolus intravenous injection. In dire emergencies, the drug may be administered by intracardiac injection. If time is not of the utmost importance, initial therapy by intramuscular or subcutaneous injection is preferred (TABLE 1).

TABLE 1 Recommended dosage for adults with heart block, Adams-Stokes attacks, and cardiac arrest:

Route of Administration	Preparation of Dilution	Initial Dose	Subsequent Dose Range*
Bolus intravenous injection	Dilute 1 ml (0.2 mg) to 10 ml with Sodium Chloride Injection, USP, or 5% Dextrose Injection, USP	0.02 mg to 0.06 mg (1 ml to 3 ml of diluted solution)	0.01 mg to 0.2 mg (0.5 ml to 10 ml of diluted solution)
Intravenous infusion	Dilute 10 ml (2 mg) in 500 ml of 5% Dextrose Injection, USP	5 mcg/min. (1.25 ml of diluted solution per minute)	
Intramuscular	Use Solution 1:5000 undiluted	0.2 mg (1 ml)	0.02 mg to 1 mg (0.1 ml to 5 ml)
Subcutaneous	Use Solution 1:5000 undiluted	0.2 mg (1 ml)	0.15 mg to 0.2 mg (0.75 ml to 1 ml)
Intracardiac	Use Solution 1:5000 undiluted	0.02 mg (0.1 ml)	

* Subsequent dosage and method of administration depend on the ventricular rate and the rapidity with which the cardiac pacemaker can take over when the drug is gradually withdrawn.

There are no well-controlled studies in children to establish appropriate dosing; however, the American Heart Association recommends an initial infusion rate of 0.1 mcg/kg/min, with the usual range being 0.1 mcg/kg/min to 1.0 mcg/kg/min (TABLE 2).

Parenteral drug products should be inspected visually for particulate matter and discoloration prior to administration, whenever solution and container permit. Such solution should not be used.

Store in a cool place between 8°C to 15°C (46°F to 50°F).

Do not use if the injection is pinkish to brownish in color or contains a precipitate.

INHALATION AEROSOL

Acute Bronchial Asthma: Hold the aerosol in an inverted position. Close lips and teeth around open end of mouthpiece. Breathe out, expelling as much air from the lungs as possible; then inhale deeply while pressing down on the bottle to activate spray mechanism. Try to

DOSAGE AND ADMINISTRATION: *(cont'd)*

TABLE 2 Recommended dosage for adults with shock and hypoperfusion states:

Route of Administration	Preparation of Dilution†	Infusion Rate††
Intravenous infusion	Dilute 5 ml (1 mg) in 500 ml of 5% Dextrose Injection, USP	0.5 mcg to 5 mcg per minute (0.25 ml to 2.5 ml of diluted solution)

† Concentrations up to 10 times greater have been used when limitation of volume is essential.
†† Rates over 30 mcg per minute have been used in advanced stages of shock. The rate of infusion should be adjusted on the basis of heart rate, central venous pressure, systemic blood pressure, and urine flow. If the heart rate exceeds 110 beats per minute, it may be advisable to decrease or temporarily discontinue the infusion (TABLE 3).

TABLE 3 Isoproterenol Hydrochloride, DOSAGE AND ADMINISTRATION
Recommended dosage for adults with bronchospasm occurring during anesthesia:

Route of Administration	Preparation of Dilution	Initial Dose	Subsequent Dose
Bolus intravenous injection	Dilute 1 ml (0.2 mg) to 10 ml with Sodium Chloride Injection, USP, or 5% Dextrose Injection, USP	0.01 mg to 0.02 mg (0.5 ml to 1 ml of diluted solution)	The initial dose may be repeated when necessary

hold breath for a few seconds before exhaling. Wait one full minute in order to determine the effect before considering a second inhalation. A treatment may be repeated up to 5 times daily if necessary. (See PRECAUTIONS.) If carefully instructed, children quickly learn to keep the stream of mist clear of the teeth and tongue, thereby assuring inhalation into the lungs. Occlusion of the nares of very young children may be advisable to make inhalation certain.

Warm water should be run through the mouthpiece once daily to wash it and prevent clogging.

The mouthpiece may also be sanitized by immersion in alcohol.

Bronchospasm in Chronic Obstructive Lung Disease: The aerosol provides a convenient aerosol method for delivering isoproterenol HCl. The treatment described above for Acute Bronchial Asthma may be repeated at not less than 3 to 4 hour intervals as part of a programmed regimen of treatment of obstructive lung disease complicated by a reversible bronchospastic component. One application from the aerosol may be regarded as equivalent in effectiveness to 5 to 7 operations of a hand- bulb nebulizer using a 1:100 solution.

Children's Dosage: In general, the technique of isoproterenol HCl aerosol in administration to children is similar to that of adults, since children's smaller ventilatory exchange capacity automatically provides proportionally smaller aerosol intake.

Store at controlled room temperature 15°C to 30°C (59°F to 86°F).

INHALATION SOLUTION

Isoproterenol HCl hydrochloride solutions can be administered as an aerosol mist by hand-bulb nebulizer, compressed air or oxygen operated nebulizer, or by intermittent positive pressure breathing (IPPB) devices. The method of delivery, and the treatment regimen employed in the management of the reversible bronchospastic element accompanying bronchial asthma, chronic bronchitis, and chronic obstructive lung diseases, will depend on such factors as the severity of the bronchospasm, patient age, tolerance to the medication, complicating cardiopulmonary conditions, and whether therapy is for an intermittent acute attack of bronchospasm or is part of a programmed treatment regimen for constant bronchospasm.

Acute Bronchial Asthma Hand-Bulb Nebulizer: Depending on the frequency of treatment and the type of nebulizer used, a volume of solution of isoproterenol HCl, sufficient for not more than one day's treatment, should be placed in the nebulizer using the dropper provided. In time, the patient can learn to adjust the volume required. For adults and children, the 1:200 solution is administered by hand-bulb nebulization in a dosage of 5 to 15 deep inhalations (using an all glass or plastic nebulizer). In adults, the 1:100 solution may be used if a stronger solution seems to be indicated. The dose is 3 to 7 deep inhalations. If after about 5 to 10 minutes inadequate relief is observed, these doses may be repeated one more time. If the acute attack recurs, treatments may be repeated up to 5 times daily if necessary. (See PRECAUTIONS.)

Bronchospasm in Chronic Obstructive Lung Disease Hand-Bulb Nebulizer: A solution of 1:200 or 1:100 of isoproterenol HCl may be administered daily at not less than 3 to 4 hour intervals for subacute bronchospastic attacks or as part of a programmed treatment regimen in patients with chronic obstructive lung disease with a reversible bronchospastic component. An adequate dose is usually 5 to 15 deep inhalations, using the 1:200 solution. Some patients with severe attacks of bronchospasm may require 3 to 7 deep inhalations using the 1:100 solution of isoproterenol HCl.

Nebulization by Compressed Air or Oxygen: A method often used in patients with severe chronic obstructive lung disease is to deliver the isoproterenol mist *in more dilute form over a longer period of time.* The purpose is, not so much to increase the dose supplied, as to achieve progressively deeper bronchodilation and thus insure that the mist achieves maximum penetration of the finer bronchioles. In this method, 0.5 ml of a 1:200 solution of isoproterenol HCl is diluted to 2 ml to 2.5 ml with water or isotonic saline to achieve a use concentration of 1:800 to 1:1000. If desired, 0.25 ml of the 1:100 solution may be similarly diluted to achieve the same use concentration. The diluted solution is placed in a nebulizer (*e.g.,* DeVilbiss #640 unit) connected to either a source of compressed air or oxygen. The flow rate is regulated to suit the particular nebulizer so that the diluted solution of isoproterenol HCl will be delivered over approximately 10 to 20 minutes. A treatment may be repeated up to 5 times daily if necessary. Although the total delivered dose of isoproterenol HCl is somewhat higher than with the treatment regimen employing the hand-bulb nebulizer, patients usually tolerate it well because of the greater dilution and longer application-time factors.

Intermittent Positive Pressure Breathing (IPPB): Diluted solutions of 1:200 or 1:100 of isoproterenol HCl are used in a programmed regimen for the treatment of reversible bronchospasm in patients with chronic obstructive lung disease who require intermittent positive pressure breathing therapy. These devices generally have a small nebulizer, usually of 3 ml to 5 ml capacity, on a patient-operated side arm. The effectiveness of IPPB therapy is greatly enhanced by the simultaneous use of aerosolized bronchodilators. As with compressed air or oxygen operated nebulizers, the usual regimen is to place 0.5 ml of 1:200 solution of isoproterenol HCl diluted to 2 ml to 2.5 ml with water or isotonic saline in the nebulizer cup and follow the IPPB manufacturer's operating instructions. IPPB-bronchodilator treatments are usually administered over 15 to 20 minutes, up to 5 times if necessary.

Children's Dosage: In general, the technique of isoproterenol hydrochloride solution in administration to children is similar to that of adults, since children's smaller ventilatory exchange capacity automatically provides proportionally smaller aerosol intake. However, it is

DOSAGE AND ADMINISTRATION: *(cont'd)*

generally recommended that the 1:200 solution (rather than the 1:100) be used for an acute attack of bronchospasm, and no more than 0.25 ml of the 1:200 solution should be used for each 10 to 15 minute programmed treatment in chronic bronchospastic disease.

Protect from light. Do not use the inhalation solution of their color are pinkish to brownish or if they contain a precipitate. Although solutions of isoproterenol HCl left in nebulizers will remain clear and potent for many days, for sanitary reasons it is recommended that they be changed daily.

Store at controlled room temperature 15°C to 30°C (59°F to 86°F).

HOW SUPPLIED - RATED THERAPEUTICALLY EQUIVALENT:

Injection, Solution - Intravenous - 0.2 mg/ml

1 ml x 25	**$127.54**	**ISUPREL, Sanofi Winthrop**	**00024-0866-25**
5 ml	$12.99	Isoproterenol Hcl, Abbott	00074-4978-15
5 ml x 10	**$184.49**	**ISUPREL, Sanofi Winthrop**	**00024-0866-02**
5 ml x 25	$89.43	Isoproterenol Hcl, Elkins Sinn	00641-1438-35
5 ml x 25	$125.00	Isoproterenol Hcl, Consolidated Midland	00223-7910-05
10 ml	$17.55	Isoproterenol Hcl, Abbott	00074-4977-18

HOW SUPPLIED - NOT RATED EQUIVALENT:

Aerosol - Inhalation - 0.25 %

15 ml	$15.30	Isoproterenol Hcl, Harber Pharm	51432-0614-10
15 ml	$19.27	NORISODRINE AEROTROL, Abbott	00074-6869-03
15 ml	**$27.12**	**ISUPREL, Sanofi Winthrop**	**00024-0879-01**
15 ml	**$30.60**	**ISUPREL, Sanofi Winthrop**	**00024-0878-01**

Aerosol, Spray - Inhalation - 0.25 %

15 ml	$13.49	Isoproterenol Hcl, HL Moore Drug Exch	00839-6403-61
15 ml	$16.60	Isoproterenol Hydrochloride, Alpharma	00472-0994-99
15 ml	$19.85	Isoproterenol Hcl Inhalation Aeroso, Rugby	00536-1060-72

Aerosol, Spray - Inhalation - 2 mg/ml

15 ml	$20.52	MEDIHALER-ISO, 3M Pharms	00089-0785-11
15 ml	$26.16	MEDIHALER-ISO, 3M Pharms	00089-0785-21

Injection, Solution - Intravenous - 0.02 mg/ml

10 ml	$13.24	ISOPROTERENOL HCL, Abbott	00074-4905-18

Solution - Inhalation - 0.5 %

10 ml	**$22.69**	**ISUPREL, Sanofi Winthrop**	**00024-0871-01**
60 ml	**$93.21**	**ISUPREL, Sanofi Winthrop**	**00024-0871-03**

Solution - Inhalation - 1 %

10 ml	**$23.98**	**ISUPREL, Sanofi Winthrop**	**00024-0873-01**

ISOPROTERENOL HYDROCHLORIDE; PHENYLEPHRINE BITARTRATE *(001591)*

CATEGORIES: Antiasthmatics/Bronchodilators; Asthma; Autonomic Drugs; Bronchitis; Bronchospasm; Chronic Bronchitis; Emphysema; Respiratory & Allergy Medications; Sympathomimetic Agents; Pregnancy Category C; FDA Approval Pre 1982

BRAND NAMES: **Duo-Medihaler**; *Medihaler-Duo* (England)
(International brand names outside U.S. in italics)

COST OF THERAPY: $113.58 (Asthma; Aerosol; 4 mg/6 mg; 0.2/day; 365 days)

PRIMARY ICD9: 493.90 (Asthma, Unspecified, Without Mention of Status Asthmaticus)

DESCRIPTION:

This Combination Drug is Abbreviated Here as: isoproterenol/phenylephrine.

Isoproterenol/phenylephrine is a combination of two sympathomimetics administered by oral inhalation for the treatment of bronchoconstriction. Each metered dose of the aerosol delivers through the oral adapter 0.16 mg isoproterenol hydrochloride and 0.24 mg phenylephrine bitartrate of appropriate particle size (the majority less than 5 micro). This drug product also contains cetylpyridinium chloride, dichlorodifluoromethane, dichlorotetrafluoroethane, sorbitan trioleate, and trichloromonofluoromethane. Chemically, isoproterenol hydrochloride is 4-((1-hydroxy-2-((1-methylethyl)amino)ethyl)-1,2-benzenediol hydrochloride and phenylephrine bitartrate is (-)-m-hydroxy-a-((methylamino)methyl)benzyl alcohol bitartrate.

Isoproterenol Hydrochloride: $C_{11}H_{17}NO_3$. HCl. M.W. = 247.72.

Phenylephrine Bitartrate: $C_9H_{13}NO_2{\cdot}C_4H_6O_6$.

CLINICAL PHARMACOLOGY:

Isoproterenol acts directly on beta-adrenergic receptors and phenylephrine acts directly on alpha-adrenergic receptors. The beta-adrenergic effects stem from the release of cyclic AMP following activation of the enzyme adenyl cyclase. Alpha-adrenergic effects probably result from inhibition of adenyl cyclase. Isoproterenol produces bronchodilatation, systemic vasodilation, mild hypotension, and tachycardia. Phenylephrine produces mild bronchodilatation, systemic vasoconstriction, mild hypertension, and bradycardia. These two drugs appear to act synergistically to allow the expression of each product's ability to relax bronchial smooth muscle. The vasoconstrictor effect of phenylephrine reduces bronchiolar blood flow thereby producing a decongestant effect, promotes retention of the drug in the bronchial mucosa, and blocks the tachycardia of isoproterenol. After oral inhalation of the combination, the pulmonary effects occur within a few minutes and persist up to three hours.

Studies demonstrate that the ventilatory effects of isoproterenol-phenylephrine are superior to those obtained with the administration of isoproterenol alone. Because isoproterenol is a potent vasodilator that lowers blood pressure and acts upon the heart to increase cardiac output and pulse rate, its combination with phenylephrine results in a product with fewer cardiovascular effects. Studies have shown the absence of tachycardia and hypotension.

Isoproterenol alone often lowers arterial blood oxygen (PO2). Several studies have shown that the combination of isoproterenol and phenylephrine rarely produces a significant drop in arterial oxygen tension while usually producing an increase in PaO2 in asthmatic patients.

Pharmacokinetics: The average half-life for isoproterenol administered by aerosol was five minutes. A plasma concentration of 0.03 ng/ml was found within minutes following an inhalation dose of 500 mcg isoproterenol.

Isoproterenol excretion following oral or inhalation administration is primarily renal. When given by inhalation, the major metabolite is the sulfate conjugate of the drug. When the drug is administered directly into the bronchial tree, it is inactivated by the enzyme catechol-o-methyl transferase, and the predominant metabolite is 3-o-methylisoproterenol sulfate. The explanation for this difference is supported by the observation that most (90%) of an aerosol dose is deposited in the mouth, swallowed, and converted to is sulfate conjugate in the gut

CLINICAL PHARMACOLOGY: *(cont'd)*

wall, and to a lesser extent in the liver. The remaining isoproterenol is excreted as follows: 1% to 2% unchanged, 1% to 2% free methylated metabolite, and small amounts of metabolites in the bile.

Plasma levels following inhalation of phenylephrine have not been reported. Following oral and intravenous administrations, the average half-life was about 2.5 hours. Phenylephrine is metabolized in the liver and intestine by the enzyme monoamine oxidase. About 80% of a dose is recovered in the urine, primarily as phenolic conjugates and m-hydroxymandelic acid. About 16% of a dose is excreted as unchanged drug following intravenous administration and, due to first pass metabolism, less than 3% is excreted unchanged following oral dosing.

Recent studies in laboratory animals (minipigs, rodents, and dogs) recorded the occurrence of cardiac arrhythmias and sudden death (with histologic evidence of myocardial necrosis) when beta agonists and methylxanthines were concomitantly administered. The significance of these findings when applied to human usage is currently unknown.

INDICATIONS AND USAGE:

Isoproterenol/phenylephrine is indicated for the treatment of bronchospasm associated with acute and chronic asthma and reversible bronchospasm which may be associated with chronic bronchitis or emphysema.

CONTRAINDICATIONS:

Isoproterenol/phenylephrine must not be used by patients with known hypersensitivity to sympathomimetics. The use of isoproterenol in patients with pre-existing cardiac arrhythmias associated with tachycardia is contraindicated because the cardiac stimulant effects of the drug may aggravate such disorders.

WARNINGS:

Excessive use of an adrenergic aerosol should be discouraged, as it may lose effectiveness. Occasional patients have been reported to develop severe paradoxical airway resistance with repeated, excessive use of isoproterenol inhalation preparations (See ADVERSE REACTIONS). The cause of this is unknown. It is advisable that in such instances the use of this preparation be discontinued immediately and alternative therapy instituted, since in the reported cases the patients did not respond to other forms of therapy until the drug was withdrawn. Deaths have been reported following excessive use of isoproterenol inhalation preparations, and the exact cause is unknown. Cardiac arrest was noted in several instances (See ADVERSE REACTIONS).

PRECAUTIONS:

General: As with all sympathomimetic drugs, isoproterenol/phenylephrine should be used with great caution in the presence of coronary insufficiency, hypertension, hyperthyroidism, and diabetes.

Information for the Patient: Patients who are being treated with DUO-MEDIHALER should be informed adequately of the dangers of overusage, tolerance and rebound bronchospasm (See WARNINGS and ADVERSE REACTIONS). They should be instructed to take no more than two inhalations at any one time, nor more than six in any one hour during a 24-hour period, unless advised by the physician (See DOSAGE AND ADMINISTRATION).

Isoproterenol may cause the patient's saliva to turn pinkish to red in color. Proper use of isoproterenol/phenylephrine oral inhaler should be demonstrated and discussed. Patient Instructions for Use are available with the package insert and should be provided when the medication is dispensed.

As with any drug, patients should be advised against the ingestion of alcohol during treatment.

Drug/Laboratory Test Interactions: Isoproterenol causes false elevations of bilirubin as measured in vitro by sequential multiple analyzer. An effect on serum bilirubin determinations in patients receiving the drug has not been determined. One case of surreptitious self-administration of a 500 mg subcutaneous dose of isoproterenol resulted in increased urinary excretion of epinephrine, norepinephrine, and vanilmandelic acid.Isoproterenol inhalation may result in enough absorption of the drug to produce increased values for urinary epinephrine. This effect is probably small with standard doses, but is likely to increase with larger doses.

Carcinogenesis, Mutagenesis and Impairment of Fertility: Isoproterenol hydrochloride, phenylephrine bitartrate, or DUO-MEDIHALER have not been evaluated for carcinogenicity, mutagenicity or impairment of fertility.

Pregnancy, Teratogenic Effects, Pregnancy Category C: Reproduction studies have not been done with isoproterenol/phenylephrine. Reproduction studies with isoproterenol have been performed in rats and rabbits with aerosol doses (30 minutes per day for 12 days) up to 15 times the human dose and have revealed no evidence of impaired fertility or harm to the fetus. It is also not known whether isoproterenol/phenylephrine can cause fetal harm when administered to a pregnant woman or can affect reproduction capacity. Isoproterenol/phenylephrine should be given to a pregnant woman only if clearly needed.

Labor and Delivery: Isoproterenol/phenylephrine has no recognized use during labor and delivery. Phenylephrine administration during late pregnancy or labor may cause fetal anoxia and bradycardia by increasing uterine contractility and decreasing uterine blood flow.

Nursing Mothers: It is not know whether isoproterenol/phenylephrine is excreted in human milk. Because many drugs are excreted in human milk, caution should be exercised when isoproterenol/phenylephrine is administered to a nursing woman.

Pediatric Use: Safe and effective use of isoproterenol/phenylephrine in children below the age of 12 has not been established.

Geriatric Use: Lower doses in elderly patients may be required due to increased sympathomimetic sensitivity (See DOSAGE AND ADMINISTRATION.)

DRUG INTERACTIONS:

A monoamine oxidase (MAO) inhibitor, a tricyclic antidepressant, or guanethidine may increase the cardiac and pressor effects of phenylephrine and isoproterenol; however, normal volunteers given isoproterenol by inhalation along with an MAO inhibitor or a tricyclic antidepressant had no adverse cardiovascular effects.

Arrhythmias may result from the concurrent administration of DUO- MEDIHALER to patients who are receiving digitalis, epinephrine, cyclopropane, or halogenated hydrocarbon anesthetics.

Beta-adrenergic blocking drugs such as propranolol antagonize the cardiac, bronchodilating, and vasodilating effects of isoproterenol and the stimulating effects of phenylephrine.

Ergot alkaloids may increase blood pressure in patients receiving isoproterenol or phenylephrine. Phentolamine mesylate (Regitine), an alpha-adrenergic blocker, may decrease the pressor response to phenylephrine.

Phenothiazine drugs have some alpha-adrenergic blocking activity and may reduce the pressor effects and duration of action of phenylephrine.

ADVERSE REACTIONS:

The following adverse effects, listed by organ system in decreasing frequency have been associated with the use of isoproterenol/phenylephrine and are similar to those produced by other sympathomimetic agents:

TABLE 1 Isoproterenol HCl; Phenylephrine Bitartrate, Adverse Reactions

	ISOPROTERENOL	PHENYLEPHRINE
CARDIOVASCULAR:	palpitation	bradycardia
	tachycardia	decreased cardiac output
	coronary insufficiency	
	flushing of skin	blanching of skin
	blood pressure changes	peripheral and visceral vasoconstriction
	cardiac arrhythmias	cardiac irregularities
	cardiac arrest	anginal pain
	anginal pain	
PULMONARY:	paradoxical airway resistance	respiratory distress
	rebound bronchospasm	
CENTRAL NERVOUS SYSTEM:	headache	tremor
	tremor	dizziness
	vertigo	central excitation
	central excitation	pilomotor response
	insomnia	
GASTROINTESTINAL:	nausea	

DRUG ABUSE AND DEPENDENCE:

Drug abuse and dependence have not been reported with DUO- MEDIHALER.

OVERDOSAGE:

Isoproterenol: The oral LD50 values are as follows: mouse, 1260 mg/kg; rabbit, 3070 mg/kg; male rat, 2230 mg/kg; female rat, 2840 mg/kg; and dog, 600 mg/kg. The intravenous LD50 values are as follows: mouse, 126 mg/kg; rabbit, 27 mg/kg; male rat, 96 mg/kg; female rat, 112 mg/kg; and dog, 50 mg/kg.

Phenylephrine: The oral LD50 values are as follows: rat, 350 mg/kg; and mouse, 120 mg/kg. The intravenous LD50 values are as follows: rat, 6.8 mg/kg; and mouse, 21 mg/kg.

Symptoms: The individual patient's sensitivity to either drug will dictate the overdosage signs. There is reason to believe, however, that the overdosage effects of either drug are antagonized by the other drug in the combination. Severe symptoms of overdosage are more likely to result from parenteral administration of isoproterenol rather than from oral inhalation of isoproterenol and phenylephrine in an aerosol.

Manifestations of acute overdosage include chest pain, dizziness, headache, irregular heartbeat, fast or pounding heartbeat, bradycardia, nausea or vomiting, restlessness, weakness flushing, decreased diastolic pressure, convulsions, cerebral hemorrhage, or hypertension.

Treatment: Discontinued dosing allows rapid reversal of adverse effects. Blood pressure and ECG may be monitored and the following treatment used, as appropriate: Tachycardia in asthmatic patients may be treated with cardioselective betablockers (metoprolol or atenolol, but use cautiously since cardioselectivity may not be absolute) and in nonasthmatics with propranolol; bradycardia may be treated with atropine; blood pressure may be regulated with rapid- acting vasodilators (nitrites, sodium nitroprusside) or alpha-blocking agents (quinidine, phentolamine).

It is not known if isoproterenol or phenylephrine are dialyzable.

DOSAGE AND ADMINISTRATION:

Adults: The usual dose for the relief of dyspnea caused by acute bronchospasm is one or two inhalations. Start with a single inhalation. If no relief is evident after two to five minutes, a second inhalation may be taken. For daily maintenance, use one or two inhalations four to six times daily or as directed by the physician. The physician should be careful to instruct the patient in the proper technique of administration so that the number of inhalations per treatment and the frequency of retreatment may be titrated to the patient's response.

No more than two inhalations should be taken at any one time, nor more than six inhalations in any one hour during a 24-hour period, unless advised by the physician. Lower doses in elderly patients may be required due to increased sympathomimetic sensitivity. Each depression of the valve delivers through the oral adapter 0.16 mg isoproterenol hydrochloride and 0.24 mg phenylephrine bitartrate.

Children: Safety and effectiveness for children under 12 years have not yet been established (see Pediatric Use.)

Store at room temperature between 15°C and 30°C (59°F and 86°F).

HOW SUPPLIED - EQUIVALENTS NOT AVAILABLE:

Aerosol - Inhalation - 4 mg/6 mg

15 ml	$23.34	DUO-MEDIHALER, 3M Pharms	00089-0735-11
15 ml	$26.34	DUO-MEDIHALER, 3M Pharms	00089-0735-21

ISOSORBIDE *(001592)*

CATEGORIES: Antiglaucomatous Agents; Diuretics; EENT Drugs; Electrolytic, Caloric-Water Balance; Eye, Ear, Nose, & Throat Preparations; Glaucoma; Hyperosmotic Agents; Ocular Hypertension; Ophthalmics; Pregnancy Category B; FDA Approval Pre 1982

BRAND NAMES: **Ismotic**

FORMULARIES: Aetna

DESCRIPTION:

Ismotic is a 45% w/v solution of isosorbide in a vanilla-mint flavored vehicle. Ismotic is a caramel colored aqueous solution that is chemically stable at room temperature.

Each ml contains:

Isosorbide 45% w/v (Isosorbide Concentrate 60.6%), Alcohol 0.3 w/v, Caramel, Creme de Menthe, Malic Acid, Potassium Citrate, Potassium Sorbate, Saccharin Calcium, Sodium Citrate, Sorbitol Solution, Vanilla Concentrate Imitation #20, Potassium Hydroxide (to adjust pH), and Purified Water.

Typical analysis of electrolyte content:

4.6 meq of Sodium/220 ml Ismotic Solution

0.9 meq of Potassium/220 ml Ismotic Solution

Isosorbide, the osmotic agent in Ismotic, is a dihydric alcohol with the formula $C_6H_{10}O_4$.

CLINICAL PHARMACOLOGY:

Isosorbide is rapidly absorbed after oral administration. It is essentially non-metabolized, and in the circulation, it contributes to the tonicity of the blood until it is eliminated by the kidney unchanged. While in the blood, isosorbide acts as an osmotic agent to promote redistribution of water toward the circulation with ultimate elimination in the urine. The physical action of Ismotic is similar to that of other osmotic drugs.

INDICATIONS AND USAGE:

For the short-term reduction of intraocular pressure. May be used prior to and after intraocular surgery. May be used prior to interrupt an acute attack of glaucoma. Use where less risk of nausea and vomiting than that posed by other oral hyperosmotic agents is needed.

CONTRAINDICATIONS:

1. Well-established anuria
2. Severe dehydration.
3. Frank or impending acute pulmonary edema
4. Severe cardiac decompensation
5. Hypersensitivity to any component of this preparation

WARNINGS:

1. With repeated doses, consideration should be given to maintenance of adequate fluid and electrolyte balance.

2. If urinary output continues to decrease, the patient's clinical status should be closely reviewed. Accumulation of Ismotic may result in overexpansion of the extracellular fluid.

As with all medications, keep out of the reach of children.

PRECAUTIONS:

For oral use only — not for injection.

Repetitive doses should be used with caution particularly in patients with diseases associated with salt retention. Ensure that patient's bladder has been emptied prior to surgery.

Usage In Pregnancy: Pregnancy Category B: Reproduction studies have been preformed in rats and rabbits and there was no evidence of impaired fertility or harm to animal fetus due to isosorbide. There are no adequate or well controlled studies on whether this drug may affect fertility in human males or females or have a teratogenic potential or other adverse effect on the fetus. Because animal reproduction studies are not always predictive of human responses, this drug should be used during pregnancy only if clearly needed.

ADVERSE REACTIONS:

Nausea, vomiting, headache, confusion, and disorientation may occur. Occurrences of syncope, gastric discomfort, lethargy, vertigo, thirst, dizziness, hiccups, hypernatremia, hyperosmolarity, irritability, rash and light-headedness have been reported.

DOSAGE AND ADMINISTRATION:

The recommended initial dose 1.5 gm/kg body weight of isosorbide (equivalent to 1.5 ml/lb of body weight). The onset of action is usually within 30 minutes while the maximum effect is expected at 1 to 1 1/2 hours. The useful dose range is 1 to 3 gm/kg body weight and the drug effect will persist up to 5 to 6 hours. Use two to four times a day as indicated. Palatability may be improved if the medication is poured over cracked ice and sipped. (TABLE 1)

TABLE 1 RECOMMENDED DOSAGES ARE:

POUNDS	MILLILITERS	POUNDS	MILLILITERS
100	150	155	235
105	155	160	240
110	165	165	250
115	170	170	255
120	180	175	265
125	190	180	270
130	195	185	280
135	205	190	285
140	210	195	295
145	220	200	300
150	225		

Storage: Store at room temperature.

HOW SUPPLIED:

Disposable plastic bottle of 220 ml (100 gm of isosorbide/220 ml) for oral use only.
NDC 0065-0034-08

HOW SUPPLIED - EQUIVALENTS NOT AVAILABLE:

Solution - Oral - 45 %

220 ml $306.72 ISMOTIC, Alcon 00065-0034-08

ISOSORBIDE DINITRATE *(001593)*

CATEGORIES: Angina; Antianginals; Antimicrobials; Cardiovascular Drugs; Fatigue; Nitrates; Pain; Sulfonamides; Vasodilating Agents; Glaucoma*; Pregnancy Category C; FDA Approved 1986 Sep
* Indication not approved by the FDA

BRAND NAMES: *Acordin*; *Angitrit*; *APO-ISDN* (Canada); *Caranil* (Japan); *Cardio*; *Cardioguard SR*; *Cardopax*; *Cardopax Retard*; *Carsodil*; *Carvasin*; *Cedocarb*; *Cedocard* (England); *Cedocard Retard* (England); *Cedocard SR* (Canada); *Conducil*; *Cordil*; *Cordil 40 SR*; *Cornilat*; *Coronex* (Canada); *Corosorbide*; *Corovliss* (Germany); *Corovliss Retard* (Germany); *Difutrat*; *Dilanid*; Dilatrate-Sr; *Dinisor*; *Duranitrat* (Germany); *Eurecor* (Germany); *Insucar*; Isd; *ISDN* (Germany); *Ismo 20*; *Isobar*; Iso-Bid; *Isobid*; *Isobide*; *Isobinate*; *Isocard*; *Isocard Retard*; *Isocardide*; *Isocord*; *Isoday 40*; *Isoket* (Germany); *Isoket Retard* (England, Germany); *Isoket Spray*; *Isomack*; *Iso-Mack*; *Iso Mack* (Germany); *Isomack Retard*; *Isomack Spray*; *Iso-Mack Retard*; *Iso Mack Retard*; Isonate; *Isonit*; Iso-Par; *Iso-Puren* (Germany); Isorbid; *Isorbide*; *Isordil* (Canada, England); **Isorem**; *Isostenase* (Germany); *Isotard 20*; *Isotard 40*; Isotrate; *Isovis*; *Izodinit*; *Izonit*; *Langoran* (France); *Lomilan*; *Maycor* (Germany); *Maycor Retard*; *Mono Mack*; *Nitorol*; *Nitrol* (Japan); *Nitrol R* (Japan); *Nitrosid*; *Nitrosid Retard*; *Nitrosorbide*; *Nitrosorbon* (Germany); *Nosim*; *Novosorbide* (Canada); *Pensordil*; *Rigedal*; *Risordan* (France); *Sigillum*; *Soni-Slo* (England); *Sorbangil*; *Sorbichew* (England); *Sorbidilat* (Germany); *Sorbidilat Retard* (Germany); *Sorbidilat SR*; *Sorbidin*; Sorbitrate; *Sorbonit*; *Storo* (Japan); *Surantol*; *Tinidil*; *U-Sorbide*; *Vascardin*; *Vasodilat*
(International brand names outside U.S. in italics)

FORMULARIES: Aetna; BC-BS; CIGNA; DoD; FHP; Humana; Kaiser; Medco; Medi-Cal; PruCare; United; WHO

COST OF THERAPY: $19.12 (Angina; Tablet; 10 mg; 4/day; 365 days)

DESCRIPTION:

(In order to avoid confusion, the brand name for this product has been included in the prescribing information).

Isosorbide dinitrate, an organic nitrate, is a vasodilator with effects on both arteries and veins. Sorbitrate is available as 2.5 mg, 5 mg, and 10 mg sublingual tablets; 5 mg, 10 mg, 20 mg, 30 mg, and 40 mg oral tablets; and 5 mg and 10 mg chewable tablets.

Sorbitrate sublingual tablets 2.5 mg, 5 mg, or 10 mg contain isosorbide dinitrate. The inactive ingredients present are corn starch, lactose (hydrous), magnesium stearate, and pregelatinized starch. The 5 mg dosage strength also contains red 7. The 10 mg dosage strength also contains yellow 10.

Sorbitrate oral tablets 5 mg, 10 mg, 20 mg, 30 mg or 40 mg contain isosorbide dinitrate. The inactive ingredients present are corn starch, lactose (hydrous), magnesium stearate, pregelatinized starch. The 5 mg dosage strength also contains blue 1 and yellow 10. the 10 mg dosage strength also contains yellow 10; and the 20 mg and 40 mg contain blue 1.

Isosorbide dinitrate is available as 40 mg extended-release tablets.

The chemical name for isosorbide dinitrate is 1,4,3,6-dianhydrosorbitol-2,5-dinitrate.

Isosorbide dinitrate is a white, crystalline, odorless compound which is stable in air and in solution, has a melting point of 70° C and has an optical rotation of + 134° (c = 1.0, alcohol, 20° C). Isosorbide dinitrate is freely soluble in organic solvents such as acetone, alcohol, and ether; but is only sparingly soluble in water.

CLINICAL PHARMACOLOGY:

The principal pharmacological action of isosorbide dinitrate is relaxation of vascular smooth muscle, producing a vasodilatory effect on both peripheral arteries and veins, with predominant effects on the latter. Dilation of the post-capillary vessels, including large veins, promotes peripheral pooling of blood and decreases venous return to the heart, thereby reducing left-ventricular end-diastolic pressure (pre-load). Arteriolar relaxation reduces systemic vascular resistance and arterial pressure (after-load).

Dosing regimens for most chronically used drugs are designed to provide plasma concentrations that are continuously greater than a minimally effective concentration This strategy is inappropriate for organic nitrates. Several well-controlled clinical trials have used exercise testing to assess the anti-anginal efficacy of continuously delivered nitrates. In the large majority of these trials, active agents were no more effective than placebo after 24 hours (or less) of continuous therapy. Attempts to overcome nitrate tolerance by dose escalation, even to doses far in excess those used acutely, have consistently failed. Only after nitrates have been absent from the body for several hours has their anti-anginal efficacy been restored.

Pharmacokinetics: Once absorbed, the distribution volume of isosorbide dinitrate is 2-4 L/kg, and this volume is cleared at the rate of 2-4 L/min, so ISDN's half-life in serum is about an hour. Since the clearance exceeds hepatic blood flow, considerable extrahepatic metabolism must also occur. Clearance is effected primarily by denitration to the 2-mononitrate (15%-25%) and the 5 mononitrate (75%-55%).

Both metabolites have biological activity, especially the 5-mononitrate. With an overall half-life of about 5 hours, the 5-mononitrate is cleared from the serum by denitration to isosorbide; glucuronidation to the 5-mononitrate glucuronide; and denitration/hydration to sorbitol. The 2–mononitrate has been less well studied, but it appears to participate in the same metabolic pathways, with a half-life of about 2 hours.

The daily dose-free interval sufficient to avoid tolerance to organic nitrates has not been well defined. Studies of nitroglycerin (an organic nitrate with a very short half-life) have shown that daily dose-free intervals of 10–12 hours are usually sufficient to minimize tolerance. Daily dose-free intervals that have succeeded in avoiding tolerance during trials of moderate doses (*e.g.*, 30 mg) of immediate release ISDN have generally been somewhat longer (at least 14 hours), but this is consistent with the longer half-lives of ISDN and its active metabolites.

Few well-controlled clinical trials of organic nitrates have been designed to detect rebound or withdrawal effects. In one such trial, however, subjects receiving nitroglycerin had less exercise tolerance at the end of the daily dose-free interval than the parallel group receiving placebo. The incidence, magnitude, and clinical significance of similar phenomena in patients receiving ISDN have not been studied.

Bioavailability of ISDN after single sublingual doses is 40%-50%. Multiple-dose studies of sublingual ISDN pharmacokinetics have not been reported; multiple-dose studies of ingested ISDN have observed progressive increases in bioavailability during chronic therapy. Serum levels of ISDN reach their maxima 10-15 minutes after sublingual dosing.

Absorption of isosorbide dinitrate after oral dosing is nearly complete, but bioavailability is highly variable (10%-90%), with extensive first-pass metabolism in the liver. Serum levels reach their maxima about an hour after ingestion. The average bioavailability of ISDN is about 25%; most studies have observed progressive increases in bioavailability during chronic therapy.

The absorption kinetics of chewable isosorbide dinitrate tablets have not been studied. Absorption of ingested ISDN is known to be nearly complete, although bioavailability is highly variable. Ingested ISDN undergoes extensive first-pass metabolism in the liver; it is not known what portion of this first-pass effect is avoided by buccal absorption of the chewable formulation. Kinetic studies of absorption of immediate-release formulations of ISDN have found highly variable bioavailability with extensive first-pass metabolism in the liver. Most such studies have observed progressive increases in bioavailability during chronic therapy.

CLINICAL STUDIES:

In a controlled trial in which 0.4 mg of sublingual nitroglycerin took 1.9 minutes to begin to produce an anti-anginal effect, 5 mg of sublingual ISDN took 3.4 minutes to begin to produce a similar effect. In the same trial, the anti-anginal effect of the sublingual nitroglycerin was evident for about an hour, while that of the sublingual ISDN lasted about 2 hours.

In other controlled trials, the anti-anginal efficacy of sublingual ISDN has persisted for periods ranging from 30 minutes up to 4 hours. Multiple-dose trials of sublingual ISDN have not been reported.

Multiple-dose trials of ingested formulations of ISDN have shown that ISDN's anti-anginal efficacy is substantially attenuated by tolerance unless the daily regimen does not include at least one interdosing interval of at least 14 hours. The daily interdosing interval necessary in any chronic regimen using sublingual ISDN is not known.

In clinical trials, immediate-release oral isosorbide dinitrate has been administered in a variety of regimens, with total daily doses ranging from 30 mg to 480 mg. Controlled trials of single oral doses of isosorbide dinitrate have demonstrated effective reductions in exercise related angina for up to 8 hours. Anti-anginal activity is present about 1 hour after dosing.

CLINICAL STUDIES: *(cont'd)*

Most controlled trials of multiple-dose oral ISDN taken every 12 hours (or more frequently) for several weeks have shown statistically significant anti-anginal efficacy for only 2 hours after dosing. Once-daily regimens, and regimens with at least one daily interval of at least 14 hours (eg. a regimen providing doses at 0800, 1400 and 1800) have shown efficacy after the first dose of each day that was similar to that shown in the single dose studies cited above.

In controlled trials in which sublingual nitroglycerin took 1 ½-2 minutes to begin to produce an anti-anginal effect, chewable ISDN tablets took 2 ½-3 minutes to begin to produce a similar effect. In these same trials the anti-anginal effect of sublingual nitroglycerin was evident for about 1-1 ½ hours, while that of chewable ISDN lasted about an hour longer.

Clinical trials of chewable ISDN have used doses of 5 and 10 mg. It is not known whether lower doses would be equally effective.

Multiple-dose trials of chewable ISDN have not been reported. Multiple dose trials of ingested formulations of ISDN have shown that ISDN's anti-anginal efficacy is substantially attenuated by tolerance unless the daily regimen does not include at least one interdosing interval of at least 14 hours. The daily interdosing interval necessary in any chronic regimen using chewable ISDN is, because of the rapid onset of action of this formulation, probably somewhat longer.

From large, well-controlled studies of other nitrates it is reasonable to believe that the maximal achievable daily duration of anti-anginal effect from isosorbide dinitrate is about 12 hours. No dosing regimen for isosorbide dinitrate has, however, ever actually been shown to achieve this duration of effect. In the absence of data from multiple-dose trials, and considering the capacity of organic nitrates to induce tolerance, it is not reasonable to assume that multiple sublingual ISDN tablets taken during the course of a day will all have similar effects.

INDICATIONS AND USAGE:

Sorbitrate is indicated for the treatment and prevention of angina pectoris. Controlled clinical trials have demonstrated that the sublingual, chewable, immediate-release, and controlled-release oral dosage forms of isosorbide dinitrate are effective in improving exercise tolerance in patients with angina pectoris. When single sublingual or chewable doses (5 mg) of isosorbide dinitrate were administered prophylactically to patients with angina pectoris in various clinical studies, duration of exercise until chest pain or fatigue was significantly improved for at least 45 minutes (and as long as 2 hours in some studies) following dosing. Similar studies after single oral (15 to 120 mg) and oral controlled-release (40 to 80 mg) doses of isosorbide dinitrate have shown significant improvement in exercise tolerance for up to 8 hours following dosing. The exercise electrocardiographic evidence suggests that improved exercise tolerance with isosorbide dinitrate is not at the expense of greater myocardial ischemia. All dosage forms of isosorbide dinitrate may therefore be used prophylactically to decrease frequency and severity of anginal attacks and can be expected to decrease the need for sublingual nitroglycerin.

The sublingual and chewable forms of the drug are indicated for acute prophylaxis of angina pectoris are when taken a few minutes before situations likely to provoke anginal attacks. Because of a slower onset of effect, the oral forms of isosorbide dinitrate are not indicated for acute prophylaxis.

In controlled clinical trials, chewable and sublingual isosorbide dinitrate were effective in relieving an acute attack of angina pectoris. Relief occurred with a mean time of 2.9 and 3.4 minutes (chewable and sublingual respectively) compared to relief of angina with a mean time of 1.9 minutes following sublingual nitroglycerin. Because of the more rapid relief of chest pain with sublingual nitroglycerin, the use of sublingual or chewable isosorbide dinitrate for aborting an acute anginal attack should be limited to patients intolerant or unresponsive to sublingual nitroglycerin.

CONTRAINDICATIONS:

Isosorbide dinitrate is contraindicated in patients who have shown purported hypersensitivity or idiosyncrasy to it or other nitrates or nitrites.

Isosorbide dinitrate is contraindicated in patients with marked low blood pressure, shock and/or acute myocardial infarction with low left ventricular filling pressure.

WARNINGS:

The benefits of Sorbitrate during the early days of an acute myocardial infarction have not been established. If one elects to use organic nitrates in early infarction, hemodynamic monitoring and frequent clinical assessment should be used because of the potential deleterious effects of hypotension. Because the effects of oral and chewable ISDN tablets are so difficult to terminate rapidly, this formulation is not recommended in these settings.

PRECAUTIONS:

GENERAL

Severe hypotensive response, particularly with upright posture, may occur with even small doses of sorbitrate. The drug should therefore be used with caution in subjects who may have blood volume depletion from diuretic therapy or in subjects who have low systolic blood pressure (*e.g.,* below 90 mm Hg). Paradoxical bradycardia and increased angina pectoris may accompany nitrate-induced hypotension.

Nitrate therapy may aggravate the angina caused by hypertrophic cardiomyopathy. Tolerance to this drug and cross-tolerance to other nitrates and nitrites may occur.

Marked symptomatic, orthostatic hypotension has been reported when calcium channel blockers and organic nitrates were used in combination. Dose adjustment of either class of agents may be necessary.

Tolerance to the vascular and antianginal effects of isosorbide dinitrate or nitroglycerin has been demonstrated in clinical trials, experience through occupational exposure, and in isolated tissue experiments in the laboratory. The importance of tolerance to the appropriate use of isosorbide dinitrate in the management of patients with angina pectoris has not been determined. However, one clinical trial using treadmill exercise tolerance (as an endpoint) found an 8-hour duration of action of oral isosorbide dinitrate following the first dose (after a 2-week placebo washout) and only a 2-hour duration of effect of the same dose after 1 week of repetitive dosing at conventional dosing intervals. On the other hand, several trials have been able to differentiate isosorbide dinitrate from placebo after 4 weeks of therapy, and in open trials an effect seems detectable for as long as several months.

Tolerance clearly occurs in industrial workers continuously exposed to nitroglycerin. Moreover, physical dependence also occurs, since chest pain, acute myocardial infarction, and even sudden death have occurred during temporary withdrawal of nitroglycerin from the workers. In clinical trials in angina patients, there are reports of anginal attacks being more easily provoked and of rebound in the hemodynamic effects soon after nitrate withdrawal. The relative importance of these observations to the routine, clinical use of isosorbide dinitrate is not known. However, it seems prudent to gradually withdraw patients from isosorbide dinitrate when the therapy is being terminated, rather than stopping the drug abruptly.

PRECAUTIONS: *(cont'd)*

INFORMATION FOR THE PATIENT

Pateints should be told that the anti-anginal efficacy of isodorbide dinitrate is strongly related to its dosing regimen, so the prescribed schedule of dosing should be followed carefully. In particular, daily headaches sometimes accompany treatment with isosorbide dinitrate. In patients who get these headaches, the headaches are a marker of the activity of the drug. Patients should resist the temptation to avoid headaches by altering the schedule of their treatment with isosorbide dinitrate, since loss of headache may be associated with simultaneous loss of anti-anginal efficacy. Aspirin and/or acetaminophen, on the other hand, often sucessfully releive isosorbide dinitrate-induced headaches with no deterious effect on isosorbide dinitrate's anti-anginal efficacy.

Treatment with isosorbide dinitrate may be associated with lightheadedness on standing, especially just after rising from a recumbent or seated positiion. This effect may be more frequent in patients who have consumed alcohol.

CARCINOGENESIS, MUTAGENESIS, AND IMPAIRMENT OF FERTILITY

No long-term studies in animals have been performed to evaluate the carcinogenic potential of this drug. A modified two-litter reproduction study in rats fed isosorbide dinitrate at 25 or 100 mg/kg/day did not reveal any effects on fertility or gestation or any remarkable gross pathology in any parent or offspring fed isosorbide dinitrate as compared with rats fed a basal-controlled diet.

PREGNANCY CATEGORY C

Isosorbide dinitrate has been shown to cause a dose-related increase in embryotoxicity (increase in mummified pups) in rabbits at oral doses 35 and 150 times the maximum recommended human daily dose. There are no adequate and well-controlled studies in pregnant women. Sorbitrate should be used during pregnancy only if the potential benefit justifies the potential risk to the fetus.

NURSING MOTHERS

It is not known whether this drug is excreted in human milk. Because many drugs are excreted in human milk, caution should be exercised when sorbitrate is administered to a nursing woman.

PEDIATRIC USE

The safety and effectiveness of sorbitrate in children has not been established.

DRUG INTERACTIONS:

Alcohol may enhance any marked sensitivity to the hypotensive effect of nitrates.

Isosorbide dinitrate acts directly on vascular smooth muscle; therefore, any other agent that depends on vascular smooth muscle as the final common path can be expected to have decreased or increased effect, depending on the agent.

Marked symptomatic, orthostatic hypotension has been reported when calcium channel blockers and organic nitrates were used in combination. Dose adjustment of either class of agents may be necessary.

ADVERSE REACTIONS:

Adverse reactions, particularly headache and hypotension, are dose-related. In clinical trials at various doses, the following have been observed.

Headache is the most common adverse reaction and may be severe and persistent; reported incidence varies widely, apparently being dose-related, with an average occurrence of about 25%.

Cutaneous vasodilation with flushing may occur.

Transient episodes of dizziness and weakness, as well as other signs of cerebral ischemia associated with postural hypotension, may occasionally develop (the incidence of reported symptomatic hypotension ranges from 2% to 36%). An occasional individual will exhibit marked sensitivity to the hypotensive effects of nitrates, and severe responses (nausea, vomiting, weakness, restlessness, pallor, perspiration, and collapse) may occur even with the usual therapeutic dose. Drug rash and/or exfoliative dermatitis may occasionally occur. Nausea and vomiting appear to be uncommon.

OVERDOSAGE:

SIGNS AND SYMPTOMS

These may include the following: a prompt fall in blood pressure, persistent and throbbing headache, vertigo, palpitation, visual disturbances, flushed and perspiring skin (later becoming cold and cyanotic), nausea and vomiting (possible with colic and even bloody diarrhea), syncope (especially in the upright position), methemoglobinemia with cyanosis and anoxia, initial hyperpnea, dyspnea and slow breathing, slow pulse (dicrotic and intermittent), heart block, increased intracranial pressure with cerebral symptoms of confusion and moderate fever, paralysis and coma followed by clonic convulsions and possibly death due to circulatory collapse.

It is not known what dose of the drug is associated with symptoms of overdosing or what dose of the drug would be life-threatening. The acute oral LD_{50} of isosorbide dinitrate in rats was found to be approximately 1100 mg/kg of body weight. These animal experiments indicate that approximately 500 times the usual therapeutic dose would be required to produce such toxic symptoms in humans. It is not known whether the drug is dialyzable.

TREATMENT

Prompt removal of the ingested material by gastric lavage is reasonable, but not documented to be useful. Keep the patient recumbent in a shock position and comfortably warm. Passive movements of the extremities may aid venous return. Administer oxygen and artificial respiration if necessary. If methemoglobinemia is present, administer methylene blue (1% solution), 1 to 2 mg/kg intravenously.

No data are available to suggest physiological maneuvers (eg, maneuvers to change pH of the urine) that might accelerate elimination of isosorbide dinitrate and its active metabolites. Similarly, it is not known which-if any-of these substances can usefully be removed from the body by hemodialysis.

No specific antagonist to the vasodilator effects of isosorbide dinitrate is known, and no intervention has been subject to controlled study as a therapy of isosorbide dinitrate overdose. Because the hypotension associated with isosorbide dinitrate overdose is the result of venodilatation and arterial hypovolemia, prudent therapy in this situation should be directed toward increase in central fluid volume. Passive elevation of the patient's legs and passive movement of extremities may be sufficient, but intravenous infusion of normal saline or similar fluid may also be necessary.

The use epinephrine or other arterial vasoconstrictors in this setting is likely to do more harm than good.

In patients with renal disease or congestive heart failure, therapy resulting in central volume expansion is not without hazard. Treatment of isosorbide dinitrate overdose in these patients may be subtle and difficult, and invasive monitoring may be required.

OVERDOSAGE: *(cont'd)*

METHEMOGLOBIN

Nitrate ions liberated during metabolism of isosorbide dinitrate can oxidize hemoglobin into methemoglobin. Even in patients totally without cytochrome b_5 reductase activity however, and even assuming that the nitrate moieties of isosorbide dinitrate are quantitatively applied to oxidation of hemoglobin about 1 mg/kg of isosorbide dinitrate should be required before any of these patients manifests clinically significant (≥10%) methemoglobinemia. In patients with normal reductase function significant production of rnethemoglobin should require even larger doses of isosorbide dinitrate. In one study in which 36 patients received 2-4 weeks of continuous nitroglycerin therapy at 3.1 to 4.4 mg/hr (equivalent in total administered dose of nitrate ions to 4.8-6.9 mg of bioavailable isosorbide dinitrate per hour) the average methemoglobln level measured was 0.2%; this was comparable to that observed in parallel patients who received placebo.

Not withstanding these observations there are case reports of significant methemoglobinemia in association with moderate overdoses of organic nitrates. None of the affected patients had been thought to be unusually susceptible.

Methemoglobin levels are available from most clinical laboratories. The diagnosis should be suspected in patients who exhibit signs of impaired oxygen delivery despite adequate cardiac output and adequate arterial pO_2. Classically, methemoglobinemic blood is described as chocolate brown, without color change on exposure to air.

When methemoglobinemia is diagnosed, the treatment of choice is methylene blue, 1–2 mg/kg intravenously.

WARNING: Epinephrine is ineffective in reversing the severe hypotensive events associated with overdose. It and related compounds are contraindicated in this situation.

DOSAGE AND ADMINISTRATION:

As noted above (CLINICAL STUDIES), multiple studies with ISDN and other nitrates have sown that maintenance of continuous 24–hour plasmas levels results in refractory tolerance. To achieve the necessary nitrate-free interval with immediate release oral ISDN, it appears that at least one of the daily dose-free intervals must be at least 14 hours long. In case of sublingual and chewable tablets, it is probably true that one of the daily dose-free intervals must be somewhat longer than 14 hours.

As also noted above (CLINICAL STUDIES) the effects of the second and later doses have been smaller and shorter lasting than the effects of the first.

Large controlled studies with other nitrates suggest that no dosing regimen with isosorbide dinitrate should be expected to provide more than about 12 hours of continuous anti-anginal efficacy per day.

A patient anticipating activity likely to cause angina should take one isosorbide dinitrate chewable tablets, 5 mg, about 15 minutes before activity is expected to begin. Isosorbide sublingual tablet, 2.5 mg to 5 mg, may be used to abort an acute anginal episode, but this use is recommended only in patients who fail to respond to sublingual nitroglycerin.

In clinical trials, immediate-release oral isosorbide dinitrate has been administered in a variety of regimens, with total daily dosing ranging from 30 mg to 480 mg.

As with all titratable drugs, it is important to administer the minimum dose that produces the desired effect. The usual starting dose of isosorbide dinitrate oral tablets is 5 mg to 20 mg, two or three times daily. For maintenance therapy, 10 mg to 40 mg, two to three times daily is recommended. Some patients may require higher doses. A daily dose-free interval of at least 14 hours is advisable to minimize tolerance. The optimal interval will vary with the individual patient, dose and regimen.

HOW SUPPLIED:

SORBITRATE SUBLINGUAL TABLETS

2.5 mg Sublingual Tablets: White, round tablets (identified front "S", reverse "853") are supplied in bottles of 100.

5 mg Sublingual Tablets: Pink, round tablets (identified front "S", reverse "760") are supplied in bottles of 100.

10 mg Sublingual Tablets: Yellow, round tablets (identified front "S", reverse "761") are supplied in bottles of 100.

SORBITRATE CHEWABLE TABLETS

5 mg Chewable Tablets: Green, round, scored tablets (identified front "S", reverse "810") are supplied in bottles of 100 and 500.

10 mg Chewable Tablets: Yellow, round, scored tablets (identified front "S", reverse "815") are supplied in bottles of 100.

SORBITRATE ORAL (SWALLOWED) TABLETS

5 mg Oral Tablets: Green, oval-shaped, scored tablets (identified front "S," reverse "770") are supplied in bottles of 100, 500, and Unit Dose 100.

10 mg Oral Tablets: Yellow, oval-shaped, scored tablets (identified front "S", reverse "780") are supplied in bottles of 100, 500, and Unit Dose 100.

20 mg Oral Tablets: Blue, oval-shaped, scored tablets (identified front "S", reverse "820") are supplied in bottles of 100 and Unit Dose 100.

30 mg Oral Tablets: White, oval-shaped, scored tablets (identified front "S", reverse "773") are supplied in bottles of 100 and Unit Dose 100.

40 mg Oral Tablets: Light blue, oval-shaped, scored tablets (identified front "S", reverse "774") are supplied in bottles of 100 and Unit Dose 100.

GENEVA EXTENDED-RELEASE TABLETS

40 mg: Round, yellow-green, scored tablets, debossed GG 229 on one side and plain on the reverse in bottles of 100 and 1000.

HOW SUPPLIED - RATED THERAPEUTICALLY EQUIVALENT:

Tablet, Sublingual - Sublingual - 2.5 mg

100's	$3.50	Isosorbide Dinitrate, West Ward Pharm	00143-1765-01
100's	$3.68	Isosorbide Dinitrate, H.C.F.A. F F P	99999-1593-01
100's	$4.13	Isosorbide Dinitrate, Caremark	00339-5655-12
100's	$4.15	Isosorbide Dinitrate, Major Pharms	00904-2342-60
100's	$4.25	Isosorbide Dinitrate, Qualitest Pharms	00603-4122-21
100's	$4.30	Isosorbide Dinitrate, United Res	00677-0408-01
100's	$4.44	Isosorbide Dinitrate, HL Moore Drug Exch	00839-5044-06
100's	$5.67	Isosorbide Dinitrate, Schein Pharm (US)	00364-0367-01
100's	$6.25	Isosorbide Dinitrate Sublingual, Rugby	00536-3928-01
500's	$18.40	Isosorbide Dinitrate, H.C.F.A. F F P	99999-1593-02
1000's	$13.50	Isosorbide Dinitrate, West Ward Pharm	00143-1765-10
1000's	$14.20	Isosorbide Dinitrate, Schein Pharm (US)	00364-0367-02
1000's	$14.21	Isosorbide Dinitrate, Aligen Independ	00405-4569-03
1000's	$15.10	Isosorbide Dinitrate, Major Pharms	00904-2342-80
1000's	$18.30	Isosorbide Dinitrate, Qualitest Pharms	00603-4122-32
1000's	$20.39	Isosorbide Dinitrate, HL Moore Drug Exch	00839-5044-16
1000's	$25.50	Isosorbide Dinitrate Sublingual, Rugby	00536-3928-10
1000's	$36.80	Isosorbide Dinitrate, H.C.F.A. F F P	99999-1593-03

HOW SUPPLIED - RATED THERAPEUTICALLY EQUIVALENT: *(cont'd)*

Tablet, Sublingual - Sublingual - 5 mg

100's	$3.53	Isosorbide Dinitrate, H.C.F.A. F F P	99999-1593-04
100's	$3.53	Isosorbide Dinitrate, H.C.F.A. F F P	99999-1593-05
100's	$3.60	Isosorbide Dinitrate, West Ward Pharm	00143-1767-01
100's	$4.00	Isosorbide Dinitrate, Rugby	00536-3967-01
100's	$4.32	Isosorbide Dinitrate, Caremark	00339-5657-12
100's	$4.45	ISONATE, Major Pharms	00904-2343-60
100's	$4.50	Isosorbide Dinitrate, Qualitest Pharms	00603-4123-21
100's	$4.60	Isosorbide Dinitrate Sublingual, United Res	00677-0409-01
100's	$5.06	Isosorbide Dinitrate, HL Moore Drug Exch	00839-5043-06
100's	$5.57	Isosorbide Dinitrate, Schein Pharm (US)	00364-0368-01
100's	$5.92	Isosorbide Dinitrate Sublingual, Aligen Independ	00405-4570-01
100's	$6.25	Isosorbide Dinitrate, Rugby	00536-3944-01
500's	$17.65	Isosorbide Dinitrate, H.C.F.A. F F P	99999-1593-06
1000's	$13.75	Isosorbide Dinitrate, West Ward Pharm	00143-1767-10
1000's	$14.50	Isosorbide Dinitrate, Aligen Independ	00405-4570-03
1000's	$15.00	Isosorbide Dinitrate, Schein Pharm (US)	00364-0368-02
1000's	$17.10	Isosorbide Dinitrate, Major Pharms	00904-2343-80
1000's	$18.56	Isosorbide Dinitrate, HL Moore Drug Exch	00839-5043-16
1000's	$19.86	Isosorbide Dinitrate, Qualitest Pharms	00603-4123-32
1000's	$23.50	Isosorbide Dinitrate, Rugby	00536-3967-10
1000's	$27.95	Isosorbide Dinitrate, Rugby	00536-3944-10
1000's	$35.30	Isosorbide Dinitrate, H.C.F.A. F F P	99999-1593-07
1000's	$35.30	Isosorbide Dinitrate, H.C.F.A. F F P	99999-1593-08

Tablet, Uncoated - Oral - 5 mg

100's	$2.64	Isosorbide Dinitrate, West Ward Pharm	00143-1769-01
100's	$2.96	Isosorbide Dinitrate, HL Moore Drug Exch	00839-1378-06
100's	$3.00	Isosorbide Dinitrate, Goldline Labs	00182-0550-01
100's	$3.00	Isosorbide Dinitrate, United Res	00677-0572-01
100's	$3.00	Isosorbide Dinitrate, Caraco Pharm	57664-0102-08
100's	$3.10	Isosorbide Dinitrate, Major Pharms	00904-2150-60
100's	$3.15	Isosorbide Dinitrate, Qualitest Pharms	00603-4116-21
100's	$3.52	Isosorbide Dinitrate, Caremark	00339-5572-12
100's	$3.53	Isosorbide Dinitrate, H.C.F.A. F F P	99999-1593-09
100's	$4.10	Isosorbide Dinitrate, Raway	00686-0084-20
100's	$4.35	Isosorbide Dinitrate, Aligen Independ	00405-4558-01
100's	$4.65	Isosorbide Dinitrate, Par Pharm	49884-0020-01
100's	$4.80	Isosorbide Dinitrate, Schein Pharm (US)	00364-0340-01
100's	$4.95	Isosorbide Dinitrate, Geneva Pharms	00781-1635-01
100's	$8.00	Isosorbide Dinitrate, West Ward Pharm	00143-1769-25
100's	$8.75	Isosorbide Dinatrate, Medirex	57480-0339-01
100's	$12.31	Isosorbide Dinitrate, Geneva Pharms	00781-1635-13
100's	$15.20	Isosorbide Dinitrate, Goldline Labs	00182-0550-89
100's	$15.69	Isosorbide Dinitrate, Major Pharms	00904-2150-61
100's	$15.79	Isosorbide Dinitrate, Vangard Labs	00615-1564-13
100's	**$25.79**	**ISORDIL, Wyeth Labs**	**00008-4152-01**
100's	**$27.84**	**ISORDIL, Wyeth Labs**	**00008-4152-05**
500's	$17.65	Isosorbide Dinitrate, H.C.F.A. F F P	99999-1593-10
500's	**$122.98**	**ISORDIL, Wyeth Labs**	**00008-4152-02**
600's	$65.80	Isosorbide Dinitrate, Medirex	57480-0339-06
750's	$112.50	Isosorbide Dinitrate, Glasgow Pharm	60809-0142-55
750's	$112.50	Isosorbide Dinitrate, Glasgow Pharm	60809-0142-72
1000's	$10.68	Isosorbide Dinitrate, West Ward Pharm	00143-1769-10
1000's	$10.95	I S D Oral 5 Mg, H & H Labs	46703-0059-10
1000's	$12.14	Isosorbide Dinitrate, HL Moore Drug Exch	00839-1378-16
1000's	$12.50	Isosorbide Dinitrate, Major Pharms	00904-2150-80
1000's	$16.00	Isosorbide Dinitrate, Goldline Labs	00182-0550-10
1000's	$16.00	Isosorbide Dinitrate, United Res	00677-0572-10
1000's	$16.85	Isosorbide Dinitrate, Qualitest Pharms	00603-4116-32
1000's	$16.95	Isosorbide Dinitrate, Geneva Pharms	00781-1635-10
1000's	$27.84	Isosorbide Dinitrate, Aligen Independ	00405-4558-03
1000's	$27.84	Isosorbide Dinitrate, Par Pharm	49884-0020-10
1000's	$27.85	Isosorbide Dinitrate, Schein Pharm (US)	00364-0340-02
1000's	$35.30	Isosorbide Dinitrate, H.C.F.A. F F P	99999-1593-11
1000's	**$242.00**	**ISORDIL, Wyeth Labs**	**00008-4152-03**

Tablet, Uncoated - Oral - 10 mg

100's	$1.31	Isosorbide Dinitrate, Talbert Phcy	44514-0465-88
100's	$2.06	Isosorbide Dinitrate, H.C.F.A. F F P	99999-1593-12
100's	$2.75	Isosorbide Dinitrate, Qualitest Pharms	00603-4117-21
100's	$2.95	Isosorbide Dinitrate, Consolidated Midland	00223-1096-01
100's	$3.15	Isosorbide Dinitrate, Goldline Labs	00182-0514-01
100's	$3.15	Isosorbide Dinitrate, Caraco Pharm	57664-0106-08
100's	$3.90	Isosorbide Dinitrate, Caremark	00339-5573-12
100's	$4.15	Isosorbide Dinitrate, United Res	00677-0348-01
100's	$4.17	Isosorbide Dinitrate, HL Moore Drug Exch	00839-1381-06
100's	$4.35	Isosorbide Dinitrate, Raway	00686-0029-20
100's	$4.40	Isosorbide Dinitrate, Major Pharms	00904-2151-60
100's	$4.85	Isosorbide Dinitrate, Aligen Independ	00405-4559-01
100's	$4.85	Isosorbide Dinitrate, Par Pharm	49884-0021-01
100's	$4.85	Isosorbide Dinitrate, Mova Pharms	55370-0807-07
100's	$4.90	Isosorbide Dinitrate, Rugby	00536-3943-01
100's	$4.90	Isosorbide Dinitrate, Geneva Pharms	00781-1556-01
100's	$5.13	Isosorbide Dinitrate, Schein Pharm (US)	00364-0341-01
100's	$9.50	Isosorbide Dinitrate, West Ward Pharm	00143-1771-25
100's	$9.83	Isosorbide Dinitrate, Medirex	57480-0340-01
100's	$14.81	Isosorbide Dinitrate, Geneva Pharms	00781-1556-13
100's	$18.50	Isosorbide Dinitrate, Goldline Labs	00182-0514-89
100's	$19.21	Isosorbide Dinitrate, Vangard Labs	00615-1560-13
100's	$19.56	Isosorbide Dinitrate, Major Pharms	00904-2151-61
100's	**$28.84**	**ISORDIL, Wyeth Labs**	**00008-4153-01**
100's	**$31.45**	**ISORDIL, Wyeth Labs**	**00008-4153-05**
120's	$1.58	Isosorbide Dinitrate, Talbert Phcy	44514-0465-90
500's	$10.30	Isosorbide Dinitrate, H.C.F.A. F F P	99999-1593-13
500's	$17.19	Isosorbide Dinitrate, Geneva Pharms	00781-1556-05
500's	**$137.09**	**ISORDIL, Wyeth Labs**	**00008-4153-02**
600's	$75.00	Isosorbide Dinitrate, Medirex	57480-0340-06
600's	$110.00	Isosorbide Dinitrate, Medirex	57480-0341-06
750's	$144.07	Isosorbide Dinitrate, Glasgow Pharm	60809-0143-55
750's	$144.07	Isosorbide Dinitrate, Glasgow Pharm	60809-0143-72
1000's	$8.75	I.S.D. 10 Mg Oral, H & H Labs	46703-0060-10
1000's	$11.03	Isosorbide Dinitrate, West Ward Pharm	00143-1771-10
1000's	$11.25	Isosorbide Dinitrate, Consolidated Midland	00223-1096-02
1000's	$17.00	Isosorbide Dinitrate, Caraco Pharm	57664-0106-18
1000's	$18.21	Isosorbide Dinitrate, HL Moore Drug Exch	00839-1381-16
1000's	$18.99	Isosorbide Dinitrate, United Res	00677-0348-10
1000's	$19.00	Isosorbide Dinitrate, Goldline Labs	00182-0514-10
1000's	$19.20	Isosorbide Dinitrate, Qualitest Pharms	00603-4117-32
1000's	$20.60	Isosorbide Dinitrate, H.C.F.A. F F P	99999-1593-14
1000's	$22.00	Isosorbide Dinitrate, Parmed Pharms	00349-2327-10
1000's	$22.10	Isosorbide Dinitrate, Major Pharms	00904-2151-80
1000's	$24.06	Isosorbide Dinitrate, Geneva Pharms	00781-1556-10

HOW SUPPLIED - RATED THERAPEUTICALLY EQUIVALENT: *(cont'd)*

1000's	$27.50	Isosorbide Dinitrate, Schein Pharm (US)	00364-0341-02
1000's	$27.50	Isosorbide Dinitrate, Rugby	00536-3943-10
1000's	$32.19	Isosorbide Dinitrate, Aligen Independ	00405-4559-03
1000's	$32.19	Isosorbide Dinitrate, Par Pharm	49884-0021-10
1000's	$32.19	Isosorbide Dinitrate, Mova Pharms	55370-0807-09
1000's	**$271.20**	**ISORDIL, Wyeth Labs**	**00008-4153-03**

Tablet, Uncoated - Oral - 20 mg

90's	$1.96	Isosorbide Dinitrate, H.C.F.A. F F P	99999-1593-15
90's	$3.05	Isosorbide Dinitrate, Major Pharms	00904-2154-89
100's	$1.88	Isosorbide Dinitrate, Talbert Phcy	44514-0477-88
100's	$2.18	Isosorbide Dinitrate, H.C.F.A. F F P	99999-1593-16
100's	$2.91	Isosorbide Dinitrate, West Ward Pharm	00143-1772-01
100's	$3.16	Isosorbide Dinitrate, Qualitest Pharms	00603-4118-21
100's	$3.90	Isosorbide Dinitrate, Goldline Labs	00182-0868-01
100's	$4.25	Isosorbide Dinitrate, Consolidated Midland	00223-1099-01
100's	$4.30	Isosorbide Dinitrate, United Res	00677-0689-01
100's	$4.31	Isosorbide Dinitrate, HL Moore Drug Exch	00839-6017-06
100's	$4.44	Isosorbide Dinitrate, Caremark	00339-5574-12
100's	$4.60	Isosorbide Dinitrate, Major Pharms	00904-2154-60
100's	$5.50	Isosorbide Dinitrate, Aligen Independ	00405-4560-01
100's	$5.50	Isosorbide Dinitrate, Mova Pharms	55370-0808-07
100's	$5.61	Isosorbide Dinitrate, Schein Pharm (US)	00364-0509-01
100's	$5.89	Isosorbide Dinitrate, Par Pharm	49884-0022-01
100's	$5.95	Isosorbide Dinitrate, Rugby	00536-3927-01
100's	$5.99	Isosorbide Dinitrate, Geneva Pharms	00781-1695-01
100's	$12.85	Isosorbide Dinitrate, Medirex	57480-0341-01
100's	$14.00	Isosorbide Dinitrate, Vangard Labs	00615-1575-13
100's	$17.00	Isosorbide Dinitrate, West Ward Pharm	00143-1772-25
100's	$21.92	Isosorbide Dinitrate, Major Pharms	00904-2154-61
100's	$22.45	Isosorbide Dinitrate, Goldline Labs	00182-0868-89
100's	$22.45	Isosorbide Dinitrate, Geneva Pharms	00781-1695-13
100's	$36.49	SORBITRATE, Zeneca Pharms	00310-0820-10
100's	$42.04	SORBITRATE, Zeneca Pharms	00310-0820-39
100's	**$46.53**	**ISORDIL, Wyeth Labs**	**00008-4154-01**
100's	**$50.24**	**ISORDIL, Wyeth Labs**	**00008-4154-05**
120's	$2.26	Isosorbide Dinitrate, Talbert Phcy	44514-0477-90
120's	$2.61	Isosorbide Dinitrate, H.C.F.A. F F P	99999-1593-17
120's	$3.60	Isosorbide Dinitrate, Major Pharms	00904-2154-18
180's	$3.92	Isosorbide Dinitrate, H.C.F.A. F F P	99999-1593-18
180's	$4.65	Isosorbide Dinitrate, Major Pharms	00904-2154-93
360's	$14.22	Isosorbide Dinitrate, Major Pharms	00904-2154-58
500's	$10.90	Isosorbide Dinitrate, H.C.F.A. F F P	99999-1593-19
500's	**$221.20**	**ISORDIL, Wyeth Labs**	**00008-4154-02**
1000's	$12.80	Isosorbide Dinitrate, West Ward Pharm	00143-1772-10
1000's	$18.75	Isosorbide Dinitrate, Consolidated Midland	00223-1099-02
1000's	$19.50	Isosorbide Dinitrate, Goldline Labs	00182-0868-10
1000's	$20.80	Isosorbide Dinitrate, Qualitest Pharms	00603-4118-32
1000's	$21.19	Isosorbide Dinitrate, United Res	00677-0689-10
1000's	$21.80	Isosorbide Dinitrate, H.C.F.A. F F P	99999-1593-20
1000's	$22.20	Isosorbide Dinitrate, Schein Pharm (US)	00364-0509-02
1000's	$23.25	Isosorbide Dinitrate, Major Pharms	00904-2154-80
1000's	$23.34	Isosorbide Dinitrate, HL Moore Drug Exch	00839-6017-16
1000's	$25.50	Isosorbide Dinitrate, Rugby	00536-3927-10
1000's	$27.16	Isosorbide Dinitrate, Geneva Pharms	00781-1695-10
1000's	$28.00	Isosorbide Dinitrate, Parmed Pharms	00349-2348-10
1000's	$37.85	Isosorbide Dinitrate, Par Pharm	49884-0022-10
1000's	$37.85	Isosorbide Dinitrate, Mova Pharms	55370-0808-09
1000's	$37.88	Isosorbide Dinitrate, Aligen Independ	00405-4560-03

Tablet, Uncoated - Oral - 30 mg

100's	$2.93	Isosorbide Dinitrate, United Res	00677-0786-01
100's	$2.93	Isosorbide Dinitrate, H.C.F.A. F F P	99999-1593-21
100's	$4.15	Isosorbide Dinitrate, Major Pharms	00904-2682-60
100's	$4.81	Isosorbide Dinitrate, Qualitest Pharms	00603-4119-21
100's	$5.25	Isosorbide Dinitrate, Rugby	00536-3938-01
100's	$5.45	Isosorbide Dinitrate, Caremark	00339-5653-12
100's	$6.48	Isosorbide Dinitrate, Aligen Independ	00405-4561-01
100's	$6.75	Isosorbide Dinitrate, HL Moore Drug Exch	00839-6618-06
100's	$6.90	Isosorbide Dinitrate, Par Pharm	49884-0009-01
100's	$40.60	SORBITRATE, Zeneca Pharms	00310-0773-10
100's	$46.63	SORBITRATE, Zeneca Pharms	00310-0773-39
100's	**$52.36**	**ISORDIL TITRADOSE, Wyeth Labs**	**00008-4159-01**
100's	**$56.49**	**ISORDIL, Wyeth Labs**	**00008-4159-04**
500's	$14.65	Isosorbide Dinitrate, H.C.F.A. F F P	99999-1593-22
500's	**$248.55**	**ISORDIL TITRADOSE, Wyeth Labs**	**00008-4159-02**
1000's	$28.43	Isosorbide Dinitrate, Rugby	00536-3938-10
1000's	$29.30	Isosorbide Dinitrate, United Res	00677-0786-10
1000's	$29.30	Isosorbide Dinitrate, H.C.F.A. F F P	99999-1593-23
1000's	$30.25	Isosorbide Dinitrate, Major Pharms	00904-2682-80
1000's	$46.11	Isosorbide Dinitrate, Par Pharm	49884-0009-10
1000's	$48.40	Isosorbide Dinitrate, HL Moore Drug Exch	00839-6618-16

Tablet, Uncoated - Oral - 40 mg

100's	$6.30	Isosorbide Dinitrate, Harber Pharm	51432-0755-03
100's	$6.47	Isosorbide Dinitrate, Mova Pharms	55370-0809-07
100's	$24.96	Isosorbide Dinitrate, Jerome Stevens	50564-0533-01
100's	$42.72	SORBITRATE, Zeneca Pharms	00310-0774-10
100's	$49.10	SORBITRATE, Zeneca Pharms	00310-0774-39
100's	**$56.84**	**ISORDIL TITRADOSE, Wyeth Labs**	**00008-4192-01**
100's	**$61.28**	**ISORDIL, Wyeth Labs**	**00008-4192-04**
1000's	$53.99	Isosorbide Dinitrate, Mova Pharms	55370-0809-09
1000's	$63.00	Isosorbide Dinitrate, Harber Pharm	51432-0755-06
1000's	$199.68	Isosorbide Dinitrate, Jerome Stevens	50564-0533-10

HOW SUPPLIED - NOT RATED EQUIVALENT:

Capsule, Gelatin, Sustained Action - Oral - 40 mg

60's	$29.87	DILATRATE-SR, Schwarz Pharma (US)	00091-0920-02
100's	$5.83	Isosorbide Dinitrate Td, Parmed Pharms	00349-2083-01
100's	$17.88	Isosorbide Dinitrate, Inwood Labs	00258-3575-01
100's	$26.99	Isosorbide Dinitrate, HL Moore Drug Exch	00839-5037-06
100's	$37.12	Isosorbide Dinitrate, Rugby	00536-3949-01
100's	$47.35	DILATRATE-SR, Schwarz Pharma (US)	00091-0920-01
100's	**$55.09**	**ISORDIL, Wyeth Labs**	**00008-4140-01**
500's	**$261.78**	**ISORDIL, Wyeth Labs**	**00008-4140-02**
1000's	$66.02	Isosorbide Dinitrate Td, Parmed Pharms	00349-2083-10

Tablet, Chewable - Oral - 5 mg

100's	$19.99	CHEWABLE SORBITRATE, Zeneca Pharms	00310-0810-10
500's	$96.92	CHEWABLE SORBITRATE, Zeneca Pharms	00310-0810-50

Tablet, Chewable - Oral - 10 mg

100's	$22.96	CHEWABLE SORBITRATE, Zeneca Pharms	00310-0815-10

HOW SUPPLIED - NOT RATED EQUIVALENT: *(cont'd)*

Tablet, Coated, Sustained Action - Oral - 40 mg

90's	$8.70	Isosorbide Dinitrate, Major Pharms	00904-2149-89
100's	$4.95	Isosorbide Dinitrate, Consolidated Midland	00223-1097-01
100's	$6.21	Isosorbide Dinitrate, Aligen Independ	00405-4564-01
100's	$6.75	Isosorbide Dinitrate, HL Moore Drug Exch	00839-6188-06
100's	$7.45	Isosorbide Dinitrate, Major Pharms	00904-2149-60
100's	$8.00	Isosorbide, Schein Pharm (US)	00364-0401-01
100's	$8.80	Isosorbide Dinitrate, Qualitest Pharms	00603-4120-21
100's	$10.00	Isosorbide Dinitrate, United Res	00677-0473-01
100's	$10.05	Isosorbide Dinitrate Tablets 40 Mg, Goldline Labs	00182-0879-01
100's	$10.05	Isosorbide Dinitrate, Rugby	00536-4296-01
100's	$10.33	Isosorbide Dinitrate, Caremark	00339-5833-12
100's	$10.52	Isosorbide Dinitrate, Geneva Pharms	00781-1417-01
100's	$12.69	Isosorbide Dinitrate, Major Pharms	00904-2153-61
100's	$21.25	Isosorbide Dinitrate, Bristol Myers Squibb	00003-0279-50
100's	$24.35	Isosorbide Dinitrate, Major Pharms	00904-2149-61
100's	$24.96	Isosorbide Dinitrate, Pecos	59879-0221-01
100's	**$55.09**	**ISORDIL, Wyeth Labs**	**00008-4125-01**
500's	**$261.78**	**ISORDIL, Wyeth Labs**	**00008-4125-02**
1000's	$33.57	Isosorbide Dinitrate, Rugby	00536-3940-10
1000's	$34.00	Isosorbide Dinitrate, Consolidated Midland	00223-1097-02
1000's	$49.82	Isosorbide Dinitrate, Inwood Labs	00258-3549-10
1000's	$55.35	Isosorbide Dinitrate, Aligen Independ	00405-4564-03
1000's	$57.16	Isosorbide Dinitrate, HL Moore Drug Exch	00839-6188-16
1000's	$65.95	Isosorbide Dinitrate, Major Pharms	00904-2149-80
1000's	$71.40	Isosorbide Dinitrate, Qualitest Pharms	00603-4120-32
1000's	$76.50	Isosorbide Dinitrate, Goldline Labs	00182-0879-10
1000's	$78.98	Isosorbide, Schein Pharm (US)	00364-0401-02
1000's	$78.98	Isosorbide Dinitrate, United Res	00677-0473-10
1000's	$79.03	Isosorbide Dinitrate, Rugby	00536-4296-10
1000's	$92.27	Isosorbide Dinitrate, Geneva Pharms	00781-1417-10
1000's	$199.68	Isosorbide Dinitrate, Pecos	59879-0221-10
1000's	$200.00	Isosorbide Dinitrate, Bristol Myers Squibb	00003-0279-75
1000's	**$515.32**	**ISORDIL, Wyeth Labs**	**00008-4125-03**

Tablet, Sublingual - Sublingual - 2.5 mg

100's	$18.62	SORBITRATE, Zeneca Pharms	00310-0853-10
100's	**$24.04**	**ISORDIL, Wyeth Labs**	**00008-4139-01**
100's	**$25.91**	**ISORDIL, Wyeth Labs**	**00008-4139-05**
500's	**$114.01**	**ISORDIL, Wyeth Labs**	**00008-4139-03**
1000's	$8.75	Isosorbide Dinitrate, Consolidated Midland	00223-1091-02

Tablet, Sublingual - Sublingual - 5 mg

100's	$2.50	Isosorbide Dinitrate, Consolidated Midland	00223-1094-01
100's	$19.99	SORBITRATE, Zeneca Pharms	00310-0760-10
100's	**$25.69**	**ISORDIL, Wyeth Labs**	**00008-4126-01**
100's	**$27.71**	**ISORDIL, Wyeth Labs**	**00008-4126-07**
500's	**$122.38**	**ISORDIL, Wyeth Labs**	**00008-4126-03**
1000's	$11.00	Isosorbide Dinitrate, Consolidated Midland	00223-1094-02

Tablet, Sublingual - Sublingual - 10 mg

100's	**$29.99**	**ISORDIL SUBLINGUAL, Wyeth Labs**	**00008-4161-01**

Tablet, Uncoated - Oral - 5 mg

100's	$19.99	SORBITRATE, Zeneca Pharms	00310-0770-10
100's	$22.96	SORBITRATE, Zeneca Pharms	00310-0770-39
500's	$96.92	SORBITRATE, Zeneca Pharms	00310-0770-50

Tablet, Uncoated - Oral - 10 mg

100's	$22.96	SORBITRATE, Zeneca Pharms	00310-0780-10
100's	$26.41	SORBITRATE, Zeneca Pharms	00310-0780-39
500's	$111.35	SORBITRATE, Zeneca Pharms	00310-0780-50

ISOSORBIDE MONONITRATE *(003106)*

CATEGORIES: Angina; Antianginals; Cardiovascular Drugs; Nitrates; Vasodilating Agents; Pregnancy Category C; FDA Class 1C ("Little or No Therapeutic Advantage"); FDA Approved 1991 Dec; Top 200 Drugs

BRAND NAMES: *Corangin*; *Elan*; *Elantan* (Germany, England, Mexico); *Elantan Long* (Germany); *Elantan Retard*; Imdur; *Imdur Durules*; *ISMN* (Germany); *Ismexin*; **Ismo**; *Ismo-20*; *Ismo 20*; *Ismox*; *Isomon*; *Isomonat*; *Isomonit* (Germany); *Medocor 5-MNIS*; *Monicor* (France); *Monis*; *Monit 20*; *Monocinque*; *Monocinque Retard*; *Monocord 20*; *Monocord 40*; *Monocord 50 SR*; Monoket; *Monoket OD*; *Monoket Retard*; *Monolong* (Germany); *Monolong 40*; *Monolong 60*; *Mono-Mack*; *Mono Mack* (Mexico); *Mononit*; *Monopront*; *Monosorbitrate*; *Monosordil*; *Monotrate*; *Monotrate OD*; *Monovas*; *Mononit 20*; *Mononit 40*; *Mononit Retard 50*; *Nitramin*; *Pentacard*; *Pentacard 20*; *Vasotrate*
(International brand names outside U.S. in italics)

COST OF THERAPY: $421.35 (Angina; Tablet; 20 mg; 2/day; 365 days)

DESCRIPTION:

Isosorbide mononitrate is 1,4:3,6-dianhydro-D-glucitol,5-nitrate, an organic nitrate and whose molecular weight is 191.14. The organic nitrates are vasodilators, active on both arteries and veins.

Each Ismo tablet contains 20 mg of isosorbide mononitrate. The inactive ingredients in each tablet are D&C Yellow 10 Aluminum Lake, FD&C Yellow 6 Aluminum Lake, hydroxypropyl methylcellulose, lactose, magnesium stearate, microcrystalline cellulose, polyethylene glycol, polysorbate 20, povidone, silicon dioxide, sodium starch glycolate, titanium dioxide and hydroxypropyl cellulose.

CLINICAL PHARMACOLOGY:

Isosorbide mononitrate is the major active metabolite of isosorbide dinitrate (ISDN), and most of the clinical activity of the dinitrate is attributable to the mononitrate.

The principal pharmacological action of isosorbide mononitrate is relaxation of vascular smooth muscle and consequent dilatation of peripheral arteries and veins, especially the latter. Dilation of the veins promotes peripheral pooling of blood and decreases venous return to the heart, thereby reducing left ventricular end-diastolic pressure and pulmonary capillary wedge pressure (preload). Arteriolar relaxation reduces systemic vascular resistance, systolic arterial pressure, and mean arterial pressure (afterload). Dilatation of the coronary arteries also occurs. The relative importance of preload reduction, afterload reduction, and coronary dilatation remains undefined.

Pharmacodynamics: Dosing regimens for most chronically used drugs are designed to provide plasma concentrations that are continuously greater than a minimally effective concentration. This strategy is inappropriate for organic nitrates. Several well-controlled clinical trials have used exercise testing to assess the antianginal efficacy of continuously-delivered nitrates. In the large majority of these trials, active agents were indistinguishable from placebo after 24

CLINICAL PHARMACOLOGY: *(cont'd)*

hours (or less) of continuous therapy. Attempts to overcome tolerance by dose escalation, even to doses far in excess of those used acutely, have consistently failed. Only after nitrates have been absent from the body for several hours has their antianginal efficacy been restored.

The drug-free interval sufficient to avoid tolerance to isosorbide mononitrate has not been completely defined. In the only regimen of twice-daily isosorbide mononitrate that has been shown to avoid development of tolerance, the two doses of Ismo tablets are given 7 hours apart, so there is a gap of 17 hours between the second dose of each day and the first dose of the next day. Taking account of the relatively long half-life of isosorbide mononitrate this result is consistent with those obtained for other organic nitrates.

The same twice-daily regimen of Ismo tablets successfully avoided significant rebound/withdrawal effects. The incidence and magnitude of such phenomena have appeared, in studies of other nitrates, to be highly dependent upon the schedule of nitrate administration.

Pharmacokinetics: In humans, isosorbide mononitrate is not subject to first pass metabolism in the liver. The absolute bioavailability of isosorbide mononitrate from Ismo tablets is nearly 100%. Maximum serum concentrations of isosorbide mononitrate are achieved 30 to 60 minutes after ingestion of Ismo.

The volume of distribution of isosorbide mononitrate is approximately 0.6 L/Kg, and less than 4% is bound to plasma proteins. It is cleared from the serum by denitration to isosorbide; glucuronidation to the mononitrate glucuronide; and denitration/hydration to sorbitol. None of these metabolites is vasoactive. Less than 1% of administered isosorbide mononitrate is eliminated in the urine.

The overall elimination half-life of isosorbide mononitrate is about 5 hours; the rate of clearance is the same in healthy young adults, in patients with various degrees of renal, hepatic, or cardiac dysfunction, and in the elderly. In a single-dose study, the pharmacokinetics of isosorbide mononitrate were dose-proportional up to at least 60 mg.

CLINICAL STUDIES:

Controlled trials of single doses of Ismo tablets have demonstrated that antianginal activity is present about 1 hour after dosing, with peak effect seen from 1-4 hours after dosing.

In placebo-controlled trials lasting 2-3 weeks, Ismo tablets were administered twice daily, in asymmetric regimens (with interdosing intervals of 7 and 17 hours) designed to avoid tolerance. One trial tested doses of 10 mg and 20 mg; one trial tested doses of 20 mg, 40 mg, and 60 mg; and three trials tested only doses of 20 mg. In each trial, the subjects were persons with known chronic stable angina, and the primary measure of efficacy was exercise tolerance on a standardized treadmill test. After initial dosing and for at least three weeks, exercise tolerance in patients treated with Ismo 20 mg tablets was significantly greater than that seen in patients treated with placebo, although there was some attenuation of effect with time. Treatment with Ismo tablets was superior to placebo for at least 12 hours after the first dose (*i.e.,* 5 hours after the second dose) of each day. Significant tolerance and rebound phenomena were not observed.

The 10-mg dose was not unequivocally superior to placebo, while the effect of the 40-mg dose was similar to that of the 20-mg dose. The 60-mg dose appeared to be less effective, and it was associated with a rebound phenomenon (early-morning worsening).

INDICATIONS AND USAGE:

Ismo tablets are indicated for the prevention of angina pectoris due to coronary artery disease. The onset of action of oral isosorbide mononitrate is not sufficiently rapid for this product to be useful in aborting an acute anginal episode.

CONTRAINDICATIONS:

Allergic reactions to organic nitrates are extremely rare, but they do occur. Isosorbide mononitrate is contraindicated in patients who are allergic to it.

WARNINGS:

The benefits of isosorbide mononitrate in patients with acute myocardial infarction or congestive heart failure have not been established. Because the effects of isosorbide mononitrate are difficult to terminate rapidly, this drug is not recommended in these settings.

If isosorbide mononitrate is used in these conditions, careful clinical or hemodynamic monitoring must be used to avoid the hazards of hypotension and tachycardia.

PRECAUTIONS:

General: Severe hypotension, particularly with upright posture, may occur with even small doses of isosorbide mononitrate. This drug should therefore be used with caution in patients who may be volume depleted or who, for whatever reason, are already hypotensive. Hypotension induced by isosorbide mononitrate may be accompanied by paradoxical bradycardia and increased angina pectoris.

Nitrate therapy may aggravate the angina caused by hypertrophic cardiomyopathy.

In industrial workers who have had long-term exposure to unknown (presumably high) doses of organic nitrates, tolerance clearly occurs. Chest pain, acute myocardial infarction, and even sudden death have occurred during temporary withdrawal of nitrates from these workers, demonstrating the existence of true physical dependence. The importance of these observations to the routine, clinical use of oral isosorbide mononitrate is not known.

Information for the Patient: Patients should be told that the antianginal efficacy of Ismo tablets can be maintained by carefully following the prescribed schedule of dosing (two doses taken seven hours apart). For most patients, this can be accomplished by taking the first dose on awakening and the second dose 7 hours later.

As with other nitrates, daily headaches sometimes accompany treatment with isosorbide mononitrate. In patients who get these headaches, the headaches are a marker of the activity of the drug. Patients should resist the temptation to avoid headaches by altering the schedule of their treatment with isosorbide mononitrate, since loss of headache may be associated with simultaneous loss of antianginal efficacy. Aspirin and/or acetaminophen, on the other hand, often successfully relieve isosorbide mononitrate-induced headaches with no deleterious effect on isosorbide mononitrate's antianginal efficacy.

Treatment with isosorbide mononitrate may be associated with light-headedness on standing, especially just after rising from a recumbent or seated position. This effect may be more frequent in patients who have also consumed alcohol.

Carcinogenesis, Mutagenesis, and Impairment of Fertility: No carcinogenic effects were observed in mice exposed to oral isosorbide mononitrate for 104 weeks at doses of up to 900 mg/kg/day (102 X the human exposure comparing body surface area). Rats treated with 900 mg/kg/day for 26 weeks (225 X the human exposure comparing body surface area) and 500 mg/kg/day for the remaining 95-111 weeks (males and females, respectively) showed no evidence of tumors.

No mutagenic activity was seen in a variety of *in vitro* and *in vivo* assays.

No adverse effects on fertility were observed when isosorbide mononitrate was administered to male and female rats at doses of up to 500 mg/kg/day (125 X the human exposure comparing body surface area).

PRECAUTIONS: *(cont'd)*

Pregnancy Category C: Isosorbide mononitrate has been shown to be associated with stillbirths and neonatal death in rats receiving 500 mg/kg/day of isosorbide mononitrate (125 X the human exposure comparing body surface area). At 250 mg/kg/day, no adverse effects on reproduction and development were reported.

In rats and rabbits receiving isosorbide mononitrate at up to 250 mg/kg/day, no developmental abnormalities, fetal abnormalities, or other effects upon reproductive performance were detected; these doses are larger than the maximum recommended human dose by factors between 70 (body-surface-area basis in rabbits) and 310 (body-weight basis, either species). In rats receiving 500 mg/kg/day, there were small but statistically significant increases in the rates of prolonged gestation, prolonged parturition, stillbirth, and neonatal death; and there were small but statistically significant decreases in birth weight, live litter size, and pup survival.

There are no adequate and well-controlled studies in pregnant women. Isosorbide mononitrate should be used during pregnancy only if the potential benefit justifies the potential risk to the fetus.

Nursing Mothers: It is not known whether isosorbide mononitrate is excreted in human milk. Because many drugs are excreted in human milk, caution should be exercised when isosorbide mononitrate is administered to a nursing woman.

Pediatric Use: Safety and effectiveness of isosorbide mononitrate in children have not been established.

DRUG INTERACTIONS:

The vasodilating effects of isosorbide mononitrate may be additive with those of other vasodilators. Alcohol, in particular, has been found to exhibit additive effects of this variety.

Marked symptomatic orthostatic hypotension has been reported when calcium channel blockers and organic nitrates were used in combination. Dose adjustments of either class of agents may be necessary.

ADVERSE REACTIONS:

The table below shows the frequencies of the adverse reactions observed in more than 1% of the subjects (a) in 6 placebo-controlled domestic studies in which patients in the active-treatment arm received 20 mg of isosorbide mononitrate twice daily, and (b) in all studies in which patients received isosorbide mononitrate in a variety of regimens. In parentheses, the same table shows the frequencies with which these adverse reactions led to discontinuation of treatment. Overall, eleven percent of the patients who received isosorbide mononitrate in the six controlled U.S. studies discontinued treatment because of adverse reactions. Most of these discontinued because of headache. "Dizziness" and nausea were also frequently associated with withdrawal from these studies (TABLE 1):

TABLE 1 Frequency of Adverse Reactions (Discontinuations) *

Dose	6 Controlled Studies: Placebo	6 Controlled Studies: 20 mg	92 Clinical Studies (varied)
Patients	204	219	3344
Headache	9% (0%)	38% (9%)	19% (4.3%)
Dizziness	1% (0%)	5% (1%)	3% (0.2%)
Nausea, Vomiting	<1% (0%)	4% (3%)	2% (0.2%)

* Some individuals discontinued for multiple reasons.

Other adverse reactions, each reported by fewer than 1% of exposed patients, and in many cases of uncertain relation to drug treatment, were:

Cardiovascular: angina pectoris, arrhythmias, atrial fibrillation, hypotension, palpitations, postural hypotension, premature ventricular contractions, supraventricular tachycardia, syncope.

Dermatologic: pruritus, rash.

Gastrointestinal: abdominal pain, diarrhea, dyspepsia, tenesmus, tooth disorder, vomiting.

Genitourinary: dysuria, impotence, urinary frequency.

Miscellaneous: asthenia, blurred vision, cold sweat, diplopia, edema, malaise, neck stiffness, rigors.

Musculoskeletal: arthralgia.

Neurologic: agitation, anxiety, confusion, dyscoordination, hypoesthesia, hypokinesia, increased appetite, insomnia, nervousness, nightmares.

Respiratory: bronchitis, pneumonia, upper respiratory tract infection.

Extremely rarely, ordinary doses of organic nitrates have caused methemoglobinemia in normal-seeming patients; for further discussion of its diagnosis and treatment, see OVERDOSAGE.

OVERDOSAGE:

Hemodynamic Effects: The ill effects of isosorbide mononitrate overdose are generally the results of isosorbide mononitrate's capacity to induce vasodilatation, venous pooling, reduced cardiac output, and hypotension. These hemodynamic changes may have protean manifestations, including increased intracranial pressure, with any or all of persistent throbbing headache, confusion, and moderate fever; vertigo; palpitations; visual disturbances; nausea and vomiting (possibly with colic and even bloody diarrhea); syncope (especially in the upright posture); air hunger and dyspnea, later followed by reduced ventilatory effort; diaphoresis, with the skin either flushed or cold and clammy; heart block and bradycardia; paralysis; coma; seizures and death.

Laboratory determinations of serum levels of isosorbide mononitrate and its metabolites are not widely available, and such determinations have, in any event, no established role in the management of isosorbide mononitrate overdose.

There are no data suggesting what dose of isosorbide mononitrate is likely to be life-threatening in humans. In rats and mice, there is significant lethality at doses of 2000 mg/kg and 3000 mg/kg, respectively.

No data are available to suggest physiological maneuvers (*e.g.,* maneuvers to change the pH of the urine) that might accelerate elimination of isosorbide mononitrate. In particular, dialysis is known to be ineffective in removing isosorbide mononitrate from the body.

No specific antagonist to the vasodilator effects of isosorbide mononitrate is known, and no intervention has been subject to controlled study as a therapy of isosorbide mononitrate overdose. Because the hypotension associated with isosorbide mononitrate overdose is the result of venodilatation and arterial hypovolemia, prudent therapy in this situation should be directed toward an increase in central fluid volume. Passive elevation of the patient's legs may be sufficient, but intravenous infusion of normal saline or similar fluid may also be necessary.

The use of epinephrine or other arterial vasoconstrictors in this setting is likely to do more harm than good.

OVERDOSAGE: *(cont'd)*

In patients with renal disease or congestive heart failure, therapy resulting in central volume expansion is not without hazard. Treatment of isosorbide mononitrate overdose in these patients may be subtle and difficult, and invasive monitoring may be required.

Methemoglobinemia: Methemoglobinemia has been reported in patients receiving other organic nitrates, and it probably could also occur as a side effect of isosorbide mononitrate. Certainly nitrate ions liberated during metabolism of isosorbide mononitrate can oxidize hemoglobin into methemoglobin. Even in patients totally without cytochrome b_5 reductase activity, however, and even assuming that the nitrate moiety of isosorbide mononitrate is quantitatively applied to oxidation of hemoglobin, about 2 mg/kg of isosorbide mononitrate should be required before any of these patients manifests clinically significant ($\geq$ 10%) methemoglobinemia. In patients with normal reductase function, significant production of methemoglobin should require even larger doses of isosorbide mononitrate. In one study in which 36 patients received 2-4 weeks of continuous nitroglycerin therapy at 3.1 to 4.4 mg/hr (equivalent, in total administered dose of nitrate ions, to 7.8-11.1 mg of isosorbide mononitrate per hour), the average methemoglobin level measured was 0.2%; this was comparable to that observed in parallel patients who received placebo.

Notwithstanding these observations, there are case reports of significant methemoglobinemia in association with moderate overdoses of organic nitrates. None of the affected patients had been thought to be unusually susceptible.

Methemoglobin levels are available from most clinical laboratories. The diagnosis should be suspected in patients who exhibit signs of impaired oxygen delivery despite adequate cardiac output and adequate arterial pO_2. Classically, methemoglobinemic blood is described as chocolate brown, without color change on exposure to air.

When methemoglobinemia is diagnosed, the treatment of choice is methylene blue, 1-2 mg/kg intravenously.

DOSAGE AND ADMINISTRATION:

The recommended regimen of Ismo tablets is 20 mg (one tablet) twice daily, with the two doses given seven hours apart. For most patients, this can be accomplished by taking the first dose on awakening and the second dose 7 hours later. Dosage adjustments are not necessary for elderly patients or patients with altered renal or hepatic function.

As noted in CLINICAL PHARMACOLOGY, multiple studies of organic nitrates have shown that maintenance of continuous 24-hour plasma levels results in refractory tolerance. The dosing regimen for Ismo tablets provides a daily nitrate-free interval to avoid the development of this tolerance.

As also noted in CLINICAL PHARMACOLOGY, well-controlled studies have shown that tolerance to Ismo tablets is avoided when using the twice-daily regimen in which the two doses are given seven hours apart. This regimen has been shown to have antianginal efficacy beginning one hour after the first dose and lasting at least five hours after the second dose. The duration (if any) of antianginal activity beyond twelve hours has not been studied; large controlled studies with other nitrates suggest that no dosing regimen should be expected to provide more than about twelve hours of continuous antianginal efficacy per day.

In clinical trials, Ismo tablets have been administered in a variety of regimens. Single doses less than 20 mg have not been adequately studied, while single doses greater than 20 mg have demonstrated no greater efficacy than doses of 20 mg.

Store at controlled room temperature between 15 and 30°C (59 and 86°F).

PATIENT INFORMATION:

Isosorbide mononitrate is used to prevent chest pain in patients with a heart condition known as angina. This medication is normally taken twice a day. The first dose should be taken in the morning and second dose should be taken 7 hours later. This medication works by dilating blood vessels throughout the body. This can cause dizziness and lightheadedness when standing quickly and during the first days of therapy. This medication can cause headache - which also indicates the drug is working. These headaches are relieved with aspirin or acetaminophen. For this drug to be most effective it should be taken as prescribed, separating doses by 7 hours. Missed doses should not be doubled up.

HOW SUPPLIED - RATED THERAPEUTICALLY EQUIVALENT:

Tablet, Uncoated - Oral - 20 mg

60's	$34.62	MONOKET, Schwarz Pharma (US)	00091-3620-60
100's	$57.72	MONOKET, Schwarz Pharma (US)	00091-3620-01
100's	$63.48	MONOKET, Schwarz Pharma (US)	00091-3620-11
100's	**$69.04**	**ISMO, Wyeth Labs**	**00008-0771-01**
100's	**$75.93**	**ISMO, Wyeth Labs**	**00008-0771-02**
180's	$103.89	MONOKET, Schwarz Pharma (US)	00091-3620-18

HOW SUPPLIED - NOT RATED EQUIVALENT:

Tablet, Coated, Sustained Action - Oral - 60 mg

100's	$103.50	IMDUR, Schering	00085-4110-03
100's	$113.85	IMDUR, Schering	00085-4110-01

Tablet, Coated, Sustained Action - Oral - 120 mg

100's	$144.90	IMDUR, Schering	00085-1153-03
100's	$159.37	IMDUR, Schering	00085-1153-04

Tablet, Uncoated - Oral - 10 mg

100's	$54.84	MONOKET, Schwarz Pharma (US)	00091-3610-01

ISOTRETINOIN *(001595)*

CATEGORIES: Acne; Antibiotics; Dermatologicals; Mucous Membrane Agents; Skin/Mucous Membrane Agents; Vitamin A; Cervical Carcinoma*; Leukemia*; Pregnancy Category X; FDA Approved 1982 May
* Indication not approved by the FDA

BRAND NAMES: **Accutane**; *Accutane Roche* (Canada); *Isotrex*; *Isotrex Gel*; *Roaccutane* (Australia, England, France); *Roaccutan* (Germany); *Roacutan*; *Roacuttan* *(International brand names outside U.S. in italics)*

FORMULARIES: Aetna; BC-BS; PCS

WARNING:
Avoid Pregnancy
Contraindications And Warning: Accutane must not be used by females who are pregnant or who may become pregnant while undergoing treatment. Although not every fetus exposed to Accutane has resulted in a deformed child, there is an extremely high risk that a deformed infant can result if pregnancy occurs while taking Accutane in any amount even for short periods. Potentially any fetus exposed during pregnancy can be affected. Presently, there is no accurate means of determining after Accutane exposure which fetus has been affected and which fetus has not been affected.

Accutane is contraindicated in women of childbearing potential unless the PATIENT MEETS ALL OF THE FOLLOWING CONDITIONS:
has severe disfiguring nodular acne that is recalcitrant to standard therapies (see INDICATIONS AND USAGE for definition)
is reliable in understanding and carrying out instructions
is capable of complying with the mandatory contraceptive measures
has received both oral and written warnings of the hazards of taking Accutane during pregnancy and the exposing a fetus to the drug
has received both oral and written warnings of the risk of possible contraception failure and of the need to use two reliable forms of contraception simultaneously, unless abstinence is the chosen method, or the patient has undergone a hysterectomy and has acknowledged in writing her understanding of these warnings and of the need for using dual contraceptive methods
has had a negative serum pregnancy test with a sensitivity of at least 50 mIU/ml within one week prior to beginning therapy
will begin therapy only on the second or third day of the next normal menstrual period

It is recommended that a prescription for Accutane should not be issued by the physician until a report of a negative pregnancy test has been obtained and the patient has begun her menstrual period. It is also recommended that pregnancy testing and contraception counseling be repeated on a monthly basis. To encourage compliance with this recommendation, the physician should prescribe no more than a 1 month supply of the drug.

Major human fetal abnormalities related to Accutane administration have been documented: CNS abnormalities (including cerebral abnormalities, cerebellar malformation, hydrocephalus, microcephaly, cranial nerve deficit); skull abnormality; external ear abnormalities (including anotia, micropinna, small or absent external auditory canals); eye abnormalities (including microphthalmia); cardiovascular abnormalities; facial dysmorphia; thymus gland abnormality; parathyroid hormone deficiency. In some cases death has occurred with certain of the abnormalities previously noted. Cases of IQ scores less than 85 with or without obvious CNS abnormalities have also been reported. There is an increased risk of spontaneous abortion. In addition, premature births have been reported.

Effective contraception must be used for at least 1 month before beginning Accutane therapy, during therapy and for 1 month following discontinuation of therapy even where there has been a history of infertility, unless due to hysterectomy. It is recommended that two reliable forms of contraception be used simultaneously unless abstinence is the chosen method.

If pregnancy does occur during treatment, the physician and patient should discuss the desirability of continuing the pregnancy.

Accutane should be prescribed only by physicians who have special competence in the diagnosis and treatment of severe recalcitrant nodular acne, are experienced in the use of systemic retinoids and understand the risk of teratogenicity if Accutane is used during pregnancy.

DESCRIPTION:

Accutane (isotretinoin), a retinoid which inhibits sebaceous gland function and keratinization, is available in 10-mg, 20-mg and 40-mg soft gelatin capsules for oral administration. Each capsule also contains beeswax, butylated hydroxyanisole, edetate disodium, hydrogenated soybean oil flakes, hydrogenated vegetable oil and soybean oil. Gelatin capsules contain glycerin and parabens (methyl and propyl), with the following dye systems: 10 mg-iron oxide (red) and titanium dioxide; 20 mg—FD&C Red No. 3, FD&C Blue No. 1 and titanium dioxide; 40 mg—FD&C Yellow No. 6, D&C Yellow No. 10 and titanium dioxide.

Chemically, isotretinoin is 13-*cis*-retinoic acid and is related to both retinoic acid and retinol (vitamin A). It is a yellow-orange to orange crystalline powder with a molecular weight of 300.44.

CLINICAL PHARMACOLOGY:

The exact mechanism of action of Accutane is unknown.

Nodular Acne: Clinical improvement in nodular acne patients occurs in association with a reduction in sebum secretion. The decrease in sebum secretion is temporary and is related to the dose and duration of treatment with Accutane, and reflects a reduction in sebaceous gland size and an inhibition of sebaceous gland differentiation.[1]

Clinical Pharmacokinetics: The pharmacokinetic profile of isotretinoin is predictable and can be described using linear pharmacokinetic theory.

After oral administration of 80 mg (two 40-mg capsules), peak blood concentrations ranged from 167 to 459 ng/ml (mean 256 ng/ml) and mean time to peak was 3.2 hours in normal volunteers, while in acne patients peak concentrations ranged from 98 to 535 ng/ml (mean 262 ng/ml) with a mean time to peak of 2.9 hours. The drug is 99.9% bound in human plasma almost exclusively to albumin. The terminal elimination half-life of isotretinoin ranged from 10 to 20 hours in volunteers and patients. Following an 80-mg liquid suspension oral dose of ^{14}C-isotretinoin, ^{14}C-activity in blood declined with a half-life of 90 hours. Relatively equal amounts of radioactivity were recovered in the urine and feces with 65% to 83% of the dose recovered.

The major identified metabolite in blood is 4-*oxo*-isotretinoin. The mean elimination half-life of this metabolite is 25 hours (range 17-50 hours). Tretinoin and 4-*oxo*-tretinoin were also observed. After two 40-mg capsules of isotretinoin, maximum concentrations of the metabolite of 87 to 399 ng/ml occurred at 6 to 20 hours. The blood concentration of the major metabolite generally exceeded that of isotretinoin after 6 hours.

When taken with food or milk, the oral absorption of isotretinoin is increased.

The mean $\pm$ SD minimum steady-state blood concentration of isotretinoin was 160 $\pm$ 19 ng/ml in ten patients receiving 40-mg *b.i.d.* doses. After single and multiple doses, the mean ratio of areas under the blood concentration:time curves of 4-*oxo*-isotretinoin to isotretinoin was 3 to 3.5.

Tissue Distribution in Animals: Tissue distribution of ^{14}C-isotretinoin in rats after oral dosing revealed high concentrations of radioactivity in many tissues after 15 minutes, with a maximum in 1 hour, and declining to nondetectable levels by 24 hours in most tissues. After 7 days, however, low levels of radioactivity were detected in the liver, ureter, adrenal, ovary and lacrimal gland.

INDICATIONS AND USAGE:

Severe recalcitrant nodular acne: Accutane is indicated for the treatment of severe recalcitrant nodular acne. Nodules are inflammatory lesions with a diameter of 5 mm or greater. The nodules may become suppurative or hemorrhagic. "Severe," by definition,[2] means "many" as opposed to "few or several" nodules. Because of significant adverse effects associated with its use, Accutane should be reserved for patients with severe nodular acne who are unresponsive to conventional therapy, including systemic antibiotics.

A single course of therapy has been shown to result in complete and prolonged remission of disease in many patients.[1,3,4] If a second course of therapy is needed, it should not to be initiated until at least 8 weeks after completion of the first course, because experience has shown that patients may continue to improve while off Accutane.

CONTRAINDICATIONS:

PREGNANCY CATEGORY X

See BOXED WARNING. Accutane should not be given to patients who are sensitive to parabens, which are used as preservatives in the gelatin capsule.

WARNINGS:

Pseudotumor cerebri: Accutane use has been associated with a number of cases of pseudotumor cerebri (benign intracranial hypertension). Early signs and symptoms of pseudotumor cerebri include papilledema, headache, nausea and vomiting, and visual disturbances. Patients with these symptoms should be screened for papilledema and, if present, they should be told to discontinue Accutane immediately and be referred to a neurologist for further diagnosis and care.

Decreased Night Vision: A number of cases of decreased night vision have occurred during Accutane therapy. Because the onset in some patients was sudden, patients should be advised of this potential problem and warned to be cautious when driving or operating any vehicle at night. Visual problems should be carefully monitored.

Corneal Opacities: Corneal opacities have occurred in patients receiving Accutane for acne and more frequently when higher drug dosages were used in patients with disorders of keratinization. All Accutane patients experiencing visual difficulties should discontinue the drug and have an ophthalmological examination. The corneal opacities that have been observed in patients treated with Accutane have either completely resolved or were resolving at follow-up 6 to 7 weeks after discontinuation of the drug. See ADVERSE REACTIONS.

Inflammatory Bowel Disease: Accutane has been temporally associated with inflammatory bowel disease (including regional ileitis) in patients without a prior history of intestinal disorders. Patients experiencing abdominal pain, rectal bleeding or severe diarrhea should discontinue Accutane immediately.

Lipids: Blood lipid determinations should be performed before Accutane is given and then at intervals until the lipid response to Accutane is established, which usually occurs within 4 weeks. See PRECAUTIONS.

Approximately 25% of patients receiving Accutane experienced an elevation in plasma triglycerides. Approximately 15% developed a decrease in high density lipoproteins and about 7% showed an increase in cholesterol levels. These effects on triglycerides, HDL and cholesterol were reversible upon cessation of Accutane therapy.

Patients with increased tendency to develop hypertriglyceridemia include those with diabetes mellitus, obesity, increased alcohol intake and familial history.

The cardiovascular consequences of hypertriglyceridemia are not well understood, but may increase the patient's risk status. In addition, elevation of serum triglycerides in excess of 800 mg/dl has been associated with acute pancreatitis. Therefore, every attempt should be made to control significant triglyceride elevation.

Some patients have been able to reverse triglyceride elevation by reduction in weight, restriction of dietary fat and alcohol, and reduction in dose while continuing Accutane.[5]

An obese male patient with Darier's disease developed elevated triglycerides and subsequent eruptive xanthomas.[6]

Hyperostosis: In clinical trials of disorders of keratinization with a mean dose of 2.24 mg/kg/day, a high prevalence of skeletal hyperostosis was noted. Two children showed x-ray findings suggestive of premature closure of the epiphysis. Additionally, skeletal hyperostosis was noted in 6 of 8 patients in a prospective study of disorders of keratinization.[7] Minimal skeletal hyperostosis has also been observed by x-rays in prospective studies of nodular acne patients treated with a single course of therapy at recommended doses.

Hepatotoxicity: Several cases of clinical hepatitis have been noted which are considered to be possibly or probably related to Accutane therapy. Additionally, mild to moderate elevations of liver enzymes have been observed in approximately 15% of individuals treated during clinical trials, some of which normalized with dosage reduction or continued administration of the drug. If normalization does not readily occur or if hepatitis is suspected during treatment with Accutane, the drug should be discontinued and the etiology further investigated.

Animal Studies: In rats given 32 or 8 mg/kg/day of isotretinoin for 18 months or longer, the incidences of focal calcification, fibrosis and inflammation of the myocardium, calcification of coronary, pulmonary and mesenteric arteries and metastatic calcification of the gastric mucosa were greater than in control rats of similar age. Focal endocardial and myocardial calcifications associated with calcification of the coronary arteries were observed in two dogs after approximately 6 to 7 months of treatment with isotretinoin at a dosage of 60 to 120 mg/kg/day.

In dogs given isotretinoin chronically at a dosage of 60 mg/kg/day, corneal ulcers and corneal opacities were encountered at a higher incidence than in control dogs. In general, these ocular changes tended to revert toward normal when treatment with isotretinoin was stopped, but did not completely clear during the observation period.

In rats given isotretinoin at a dosage of 32 mg/kg/day for approximately 15 weeks, long bone fracture has been observed.

PRECAUTIONS:

Information for the Patient: Women of childbearing potential should be instructed that they must not be pregnant when Accutane therapy is initiated, and that they should use effective contraception while taking Accutane and for 1 month after Accutane has been stopped. They should also sign a consent form prior to beginning Accutane therapy. See boxed CONTRAINDICATIONS AND WARNING.

Because of the relationship of Accutane to vitamin A, patients should be advised against taking vitamin supplements containing vitamin A to avoid additive toxic effects.

Patients should be informed that transient exacerbation of acne has been seen, generally during the initial period of therapy.

Patients should be informed that they may experience decreased tolerance to contact lenses during and after therapy.

PRECAUTIONS: *(cont'd)*

It is recommended that patients not donate blood during therapy and for at least 1 month following discontinuance of the drug.

Laboratory Tests: The incidence of hypertriglyceridemia is 1 patient in 4 on Accutane therapy. Pretreatment and follow-up blood lipids should be obtained under fasting conditions. After consumption of alcohol at least 36 hours should elapse before these determinations are made. It is recommended that these tests be performed at weekly or biweekly intervals until the lipid response to Accutane is established.

Since elevations of liver enzymes have been observed during clinical trials, pretreatment and follow-up liver function tests should be performed at weekly or biweekly intervals until the response to Accutane has been established.

Certain patients receiving Accutane have experienced problems in the control of their blood sugar. In addition, new cases of diabetes have been diagnosed during Accutane therapy, although no causal relationship has been established. Some patients undergoing vigorous physical activity while on Accutane therapy have experienced elevated CPK levels; however, the clinical significance is unknown.

Carcinogenesis, Mutagenesis, and Impairment of Fertility: In Fischer 344 rats given isotretinoin at dosages of 8 or 32 mg/kg/day for greater than 18 months, there was an increased incidence of pheochromocytoma. The incidence of adrenal medullary hyperplasia was also increased at the higher dosage. The relatively high level of spontaneous pheochromocytomas occurring in the Fischer 344 rat makes it a poor model for study of this tumor, since the increase in adrenal medullary proliferative lesions following chronic treatment with relatively high dosages of isotretinoin may be an accentuation of a genetic predisposition in the Fischer 344 rat, and its relevance to the human population is not clear. In addition, a decreased incidence of liver adenomas, liver angiomas and leukemia was noted at the dose levels of 8 and 32 mg/kg/day.

The Ames test was conducted in two laboratories. The results of the tests in one laboratory were negative while in the second laboratory a weakly-positive response (less than 1.6 x background) was noted in *S. typhimurium* TA100 when the assay was conducted with metabolic activation. No dose-response effect was seen and all other strains were negative. Additionally, other tests designed to assess genotoxicity (Chinese hamster cell assay, mouse micronucleus test, *S. cerevisiae* D7 assay, *in vitro* clastogenesis assay in human-derived lymphocytes and unscheduled DNA synthesis assay) were all negative.

No adverse effects on gonadal function, fertility, conception rate, gestation or parturition were observed at dose levels of 2, 8 or 32 mg/kg/day in male and female rats.

In dogs, testicular atrophy was noted after treatment with isotretinoin for approximately 30 weeks at dosages of 20 or 60 mg/kg/day. In general, there was microscopic evidence for appreciable depression of spermatogenesis but some sperm were observed in all testes examined and in no instance were completely atrophic tubules seen. In studies in 66 human males, 30 of whom were patients with nodular acne, no significant changes were noted in the count or motility of spermatozoa in the ejaculate. In a study of 50 men (ages 17 to 32 years) receiving Accutane (isotretinoin) therapy for nodular acne, no significant effects were seen on ejaculate volume, sperm count, total sperm motility, morphology or seminal plasma fructose.

Pregnancy: Category X. See BOXED WARNING.

Nursing Mothers: It is not known whether this drug is excreted in human milk. Because of the potential for adverse effects, nursing mothers should not receive Accutane.

ADVERSE REACTIONS:

Clinical: Many of the side effects and adverse reactions seen or expected in patients receiving Accutane are similar to those described in patients taking high doses of vitamin A.

The percentages of adverse reactions listed below reflect the total experience in Accutane studies, including investigational studies of disorders of keratinization, with the exception of those pertaining to dry skin and mucous membranes. These latter reflect the experience only in patients with nodular acne because reactions relating to dryness are more commonly recognized as adverse reactions in this disease. Included in this category are dry skin, skin fragility, pruritus, epistaxis, dry nose and dry mouth, which may be seen in up to 80% of nodular acne patients.

The most frequent adverse reaction to Accutane is cheilitis, which occurs in over 90% of patients. A less frequent reaction was conjunctivitis (about 2 patients in 5).

Skeletal hyperostosis has been observed on x-rays of patients treated with Accutane. See WARNINGS. Other types of bone abnormalities have also been reported; however, no causal relationship has been established.

Approximately 16% of patients treated with Accutane developed musculoskeletal symptoms (including arthralgia) during treatment. In general, these were mild to moderate and have occasionally required discontinuation of drug. Less frequently, transient pain in the chest has also been reported. These symptoms generally cleared rapidly after discontinuation of Accutane but in rare cases have persisted.

Less than 1 patient in 10 experienced rash (including erythema, seborrhea and eczema); thinning of hair, which in rare cases has persisted.

Approximately 1 patient in 20 experienced peeling of palms and soles, skin infections, nonspecific urogenital findings, nonspecific gastrointestinal symptoms, fatigue, headache and increased susceptibility to sunburn.

Accutane has been associated with a number of cases of pseudotumor cerebri, some of which involved concomitant use of tetracyclines. See WARNINGS.

The following CNS reactions have been reported and may bear no relationship to therapy-seizures, emotional instability, dizziness, nervousness, drowsiness, malaise, weakness, insomnia, lethargy and paresthesias.

Depression has been reported in some patients on Accutane therapy. In some of these patients, this has subsided with discontinuation of therapy and recurred with reinstitution of therapy.

The following reactions have been reported in less than 1% of patients and may bear no relationship to therapy—changes in skin pigment (hypo- and hyperpigmentation), flushing, urticaria, bruising, disseminated herpes simplex, edema, hair problems (other than thinning), hirsutism, respiratory infections, weight loss, erythema nodosum, paronychia, nail dystrophy, bleeding and inflammation of the gums, abnormal menses, optic neuritis, photophobia, eye lid inflammation, arthritis, anemia, palpitation, tachycardia, lymphadenopathy, sweating, tinnitus and voice alteration.

A few isolated reports of vasculitis, including Wegener's granulomatosis, have been received, but no causal relationship to Accutane therapy has been established.

In Accutane studies to date, of 72 patients who had normal pretreatment ophthalmological examinations, 5 developed corneal opacities while on Accutane (all 5 patients had a disorder of keratinization). Corneal opacities have also been reported in nodular acne patients treated with Accutane. See WARNINGS. Dry eyes and decrease in night vision have been reported and in rare instances have persisted. See WARNINGS. Cataracts and visual disturbances have also been reported.

Accutane has been temporally associated with inflammatory bowel disease. See WARNINGS.

ADVERSE REACTIONS: *(cont'd)*

As may be seen with healing nodular acne lesions, an occasional exaggerated healing response, manifested by exuberant granulation tissue with crusting, has been reported in patients receiving therapy with Accutane. Pyogenic granuloma has also been diagnosed in a number of cases.

Laboratory: Accutane therapy induces change in serum lipids in a significant number of treated subjects. Approximately 25% of patients had elevation of plasma triglycerides. Five out of 135 patients treated for nodular acne and 32 out of 298 total subjects treated for all diagnoses showed an elevation of triglycerides above 500 mg percent. About 16% of patients showed a mild to moderate decrease in serum high density lipoprotein (HDL) levels while receiving treatment with Accutane and about 7% of patients experienced minimal elevations of serum cholesterol during treatment. Abnormalities of serum triglycerides, HDL and cholesterol were reversible upon cessation of Accutane therapy.

Approximately 40% of patients receiving Accutane developed elevated sedimentation rates, often from elevated baseline values.

From 1 in 10 to 1 in 5 patients showed decreases in red blood cell parameters and white blood cell counts, elevated platelet counts, white cells in the urine, increased alkaline phosphatase, SGOT, SGPT, GGTP or LDH. See WARNINGS, Hepatotoxicity.

Less than 1 in 10 patients showed proteinuria, microscopic or gross hematuria, elevated fasting blood sugar, elevated CPK, hyperuricemia or thrombocytopenia.

Dose Relationship and Duration: Cheilitis and hypertriglyceridemia are usually dose-related.

Most adverse reactions were reversible when therapy was discontinued; however, some have persisted after cessation of therapy. (See WARNINGS and ADVERSE REACTIONS.)

OVERDOSAGE:

The oral LD_{50} of isotretinoin is greater than 4000 mg/kg in rats and mice and is approximately 1960 mg/kg in rabbits. Overdose has been associated with transient headache, vomiting, facial flushing, cheilosis, abdominal pain, headache, dizziness and ataxia. All symptoms quickly resolved without apparent residual effects.

DOSAGE AND ADMINISTRATION:

The recommended dosage range for Accutane is 0.5 to 2 mg/kg given in 2 divided doses daily for 15 to 20 weeks. In studies comparing 0.1, 0.5 and 1 mg/kg/day,[7] it was found that all doses provided initial clearing of disease but there was a greater need for retreatment with the lower dose(s).

It is recommended that for most patients the initial dose of Accutane be 0.5 to 1 mg/kg/day. Patients whose disease is very severe or is primarily manifest on the body may require up to the maximum recommended dose, 2 mg/kg/day. During treatment, the dose may be adjusted according to response of the disease and/or the appearance of clinical side effects-some of which may be dose-related.

If the total nodule count has been reduced by more than 70% prior to completing 15 to 20 weeks of treatment, the drug may be discontinued. After a period of 2 months or more off therapy, and if warranted by persistent or recurring severe nodular acne, a second course of therapy may be initiated. Contraceptive measures must be followed for any subsequent course of therapy.

Accutane should be administered with food.

TABLE 1 Accutane Dosing By Body Weight

Body Weight kilograms	pounds	0. 5 mg/kg	Total mg/Day 1 mg/kg	2 mg/kg
40	88	20	40	80
50	110	25	50	100
60	132	30	60	120
70	154	35	70	140
80	176	40	80	160
90	198	45	90	180
100	220	50	100	200

PATIENT PACKAGE INSERT:

Accutane must not be used by females who are pregnant or who may become pregnant while undergoing treatment.

IMPORTANT INFORMATION AND WARNING:

Accutane can cause severe birth defects if it is taken when a woman is pregnant. There is an extremely high risk that you will have a severely deformed baby if:

you are pregnant when you start taking Accutane,

you become pregnant while you are taking Accutane,

you do not wait at least 1 month after you stop taking Accutane before becoming pregnant.

It is recommended that you and your doctor schedule an appointment every month to repeat the pregnancy test and check your body's response to Accutane. For your health and well-being, be sure to keep your appointments as scheduled.

THE CONSENT:

My treatment with Accutane has been personally explained to me by my doctor.

The following points of information, among others, have been specifically discussed and made clear:

1. I, (Patient's Name) understand that Accutane is a very powerful medicine used to treat severe nodular acne that did not get better with other treatments including oral antibiotics.

2. I understand that I must not take Accutane if I am or may become pregnant during treatment.

3. I understand that severe birth defects have occurred in babies of women who took Accutane during pregnancy. I have been warned by my doctor that there is an extremely high risk of severe damage to my unborn baby if I am or become pregnant while taking Accutane.

4. I have been told by my doctor that effective birth control (contraception) must be used for at least 1 month before starting Accutane, all during Accutane therapy and for at least 1 month after Accutane treatment has stopped. My doctor has recommended that I either abstain from sexual intercourse or use two reliable kinds of birth control at the same time. I have also been told that any method of birth control can fail. I must use two forms of reliable birth control simultaneously even if I think I cannot become pregnant, unless I abstain from sexual intercourse or have had a hysterectomy.

5. I know that I must have a blood or urine test that shows I am not pregnant within two weeks before starting Accutane, and I understand that I must wait until the second or third day of my next normal menstrual period before starting Accutane.

6. My doctor has told me that I can participate in the "Patient Referral" program for an initial free pregnancy test and birth control counseling session by a consulting physician.

PATIENT PACKAGE INSERT: *(cont'd)*

7. I also know that I must immediately stop taking Accutane if I become pregnant while taking the drug and immediately contact my doctor to discuss the desirability of continuing the pregnancy. I also know that I must immediately contact my doctor if I become pregnant during the month after stopping Accutane.

8. I have carefully read the Accutane patient brochure, "Important information concerning your treatment with Accutane,"given to me by my doctor. I understand all of its contents and have talked over any questions I have with my doctor.

9. I am not now pregnant, nor do I plan to become pregnant for at least 30 days after I have completely finished taking Accutane.

10. My doctor has told me that I can participate in a survey concerning Accutane use in women by completing an additional form.

I now authorize my doctor to begin my treatment with Accutane.

(Record of patient's name, address, phone number, and signature)

I have fully explained to the patient the nature and purpose of the treatment described above and the risks to women of childbearing potential. I have asked the patient if she has any questions regarding her treatment with Accutane and have answered those questions to the best of my ability.

(Record of the physician's name, signature, and date)

HOW SUPPLIED:

Soft gelatin capsules, 10 mg (light pink), imprinted ACCUTANE 10 ROCHE. Boxes of 100 containing 10 Prescription Paks of 10 capsules

Soft gelatin capsules, 20 mg (maroon), imprinted ACCUTANE 20 ROCHE. Boxes of 100 containing 10 Prescription Paks of 10 capsules

Soft gelatin capsules, 40 mg (yellow), imprinted ACCUTANE 40 ROCHE. Boxes of 100 containing 10 Prescription Paks of 10 capsules

Store at 59° to 86°F; 15° to 30°C. Protect from light.

REFERENCES:

1. Peck GL, Olsen TG, Yoder FW, Strauss JS, Downing DT, Pandya M, Butkus D, Arnaud-Battandier J: Prolonged remissions of cystic and conglobate acne with 13-*cis*-retinoic acid. *N Engl J Med300*:329-333, 1979. **2.** Farrell LN, Strauss JS, Stranieri AM: The treatment of severe cystic acne with 13-*cis*-retinoic acid. Evaluation of sebum production and the clinical response in a multiple-dose trial. *J Am Acad Dermatol 3*:602-611, 1980. **3.** Jones H, Blanc D, Cunliffe WJ: 13-*cis*-retinoic acid and acne. *Lancet 2*:1048-1049, 1980. **4.** Katz RA, Jorgensen H, Nigra TP: Elevation of serum triglyceride levels from oral isotretinoin in disorders of keratinization. *Arch Dermatol 116*:1369-1372, 1980. **5.** Dicken CH, Connolly SM: Eruptive xanthomas associated with isotretinoin (13-*cis*-retinoic acid).*Arch Dermatol 116*:951-952, 1980. **6.** Ellis CN, Madison KC, Pennes DR, Martel W, Voorhees JJ: Isotretinoin therapy is associated with early skeletal radiographic changes. *J Am Acad Dermatol 10*: 1024-1029, 1984. **7.** Strauss JS, Rapini RP, Shalita AR, Konecky E, Pochi PE, Comite H, Exner JH: Isotretinoin therapy for acne: Results of a multicenter dose-response study. *J Am Acad Dermatol 10*:490-496, 1984.

HOW SUPPLIED - EQUIVALENTS NOT AVAILABLE:

Capsule, Elastic - Oral - 10 mg

100's $332.99 ACCUTANE, Roche 00004-0155-49

Capsule, Elastic - Oral - 20 mg

100's $394.89 ACCUTANE, Roche 00004-0169-49

Capsule, Elastic - Oral - 40 mg

100's $458.78 ACCUTANE, Roche 00004-0156-49

ISOXSUPRINE HYDROCHLORIDE *(001596)*

CATEGORIES: Analgesics; Cardiovascular Drugs; DESI Drugs; Pain; Peripheral Vasodilators; Renal Drugs; Vascular Disease; Vascular Disorders, Cerebral/Peripheral; Vasodilating Agents; FDA Pre 1938 Drugs

BRAND NAMES: *Dilator*; *Dilavase*; *Dilum*; *Dilum Retard*; *Duvadilan* (France, Germany, Japan); *Duvadilan Retard*; *Isoxilan*; *Isoxine*; *Pervadil*; *Sentra*; *Sincen*; *Synzedrin* (Japan); *Vadosilan*; *Vadosilan 20* (Mexico); *Vahodilan* (Japan); **Vasodilan**; *Vasolan*; *Vasosuprina*; *Vasotran*; *Xuprin*
(International brand names outside U.S. in italics)

FORMULARIES: Aetna

DESCRIPTION:

Isoxsuprine Hydrochloride (abbreviated here as Isoxsuprine HCl) is available in 10 mg and 20 mg tablets. These tablets contain the following inactive ingredients: acacia, dibasic calcium phosphate, lactose, magnesium stearate, starch (corn), and talc.

INDICATIONS AND USAGE:

Based on a review of this drug by the National Academy of Sciences-National Research Council and/or other information, the FDA has classified the indications as follows:
Possibly Effective:

1. For the relief of symptoms associated with cerebrovascular insufficiency.

2. In the peripheral vascular disease of arteriosclerosis obliterans, thromboangiitis obliterans (Buerger's disease) and Raynaud's disease.

Final classification of the less-than-effective indications requires further investigation.

CONTRAINDICATIONS:

ORAL

There are no known contraindications to oral use when administered to recommended doses. Isoxsuprine HCl should not be given immediately postpartum or in the presence of arterial bleeding.

PRECAUTIONS:

See CONTRAINDICATIONS.

ADVERSE REACTIONS:

On rare occasions oral administration of the drug has been associated in time with the occurrence of hypotension, tachycardia, chest pain, nausea, vomiting, dizziness, abdominal distress, and severe rash. If rash appears, the drug should be discontinued.

Although available evidence suggests a temporal association of these reactions with Isoxsuprine, a casual relationship can neither be confirmed nor refuted.

ADVERSE REACTIONS: *(cont'd)*

β-Adrenergic receptor stimulants such as Isoxsuprine HCl have been used to inhibit preterm labor. Maternal and fetal tachycardia may occur under such use. Hypocalcemia, hypoglycemia, hypotension and ileus have been reported to occur in infants whose mothers received Isoxsuprine. Pulmonary edema has been reported in mothers treated with β-stimulants. Isoxsuprine HCl is neither approved nor recommended for use in the treatment of premature labor.

DOSAGE AND ADMINISTRATION:

ORAL

10 to 20 mg, three or four times daily.

(Mead Johnson, BMS, P1393-03, March 1991)

HOW SUPPLIED - EQUIVALENTS NOT AVAILABLE:

Tablet, Uncoated - Oral - 10 mg

100's	$4.30	Isoxsuprine Hcl, Eon Labs Mfg	00185-0530-01
100's	$5.55	Isoxsuprine Hcl, Goldline Labs	00182-1055-01
100's	$5.78	Isoxsuprine Hcl, Rugby	00536-3935-01
100's	$5.79	Isoxsuprine Hcl, Qualitest Pharms	00603-4146-21
100's	$5.80	Isoxsuprine Hcl, Major Pharms	00904-0635-60
100's	$5.81	Isoxsuprine HCl, Geneva Pharms	00781-1840-01
100's	$5.81	Isoxsuprine Hcl, HL Moore Drug Exch	00839-1382-06
100's	$5.83	Isoxsuprine Hcl, Aligen Independ	00405-4575-01
100's	$6.44	Isoxsuprine Hcl, Voluntary Hosp	53258-0180-13
100's	$25.38	Isoxsuprine Hcl, Geneva Pharms	00781-1840-13
100's	**$30.10**	**VASODILAN, Bristol Myers Squibb**	**00087-0543-01**
100's	**$248.45**	**VASODILAN, Bristol Myers Squibb**	**00087-0543-53**
1000's	$23.94	Isoxsuprine Hcl, Rugby	00536-3935-10
1000's	$27.37	Isoxsuprine Hcl, Aligen Independ	00405-4575-03
1000's	$31.30	Isoxsuprine Hcl, Major Pharms	00904-0635-80
1000's	$34.45	Isoxsuprine Hcl, Eon Labs Mfg	00185-0530-10
1000's	$34.95	Isoxsuprine Hcl, Goldline Labs	00182-1055-10
1000's	$39.81	Isoxsuprine Hcl, HL Moore Drug Exch	00839-1382-16
1000's	**$275.18**	**VASODILAN, Bristol Myers Squibb**	**00087-0543-02**

Tablet, Uncoated - Oral - 20 mg

100's	$5.45	Isoxsuprine Hcl, Eon Labs Mfg	00185-0531-01
100's	$8.02	Isoxsuprine Hcl, Aligen Independ	00405-4576-01
100's	$8.08	Isoxsuprine, Qualitest Pharms	00603-4147-21
100's	$8.10	Isoxsuprine Hcl, Goldline Labs	00182-1056-01
100's	$8.17	Isoxsuprine Hcl, HL Moore Drug Exch	00839-6182-06
100's	$8.18	Isoxsuprine HCl, Rugby	00536-3936-01
100's	$8.25	Isoxsuprine Hcl, Major Pharms	00904-0636-60
100's	$8.95	Isoxsuprine HCl, Geneva Pharms	00781-1842-01
100's	$10.50	Isoxsuprine Hcl, Voluntary Hosp	53258-0181-13
100's	$13.78	Isoxsuprine Hcl, Major Pharms	00904-0636-61
100's	$40.10	Isoxsuprine Hcl, Geneva Pharms	00781-1842-13
100's	**$48.23**	**VASODILAN, Bristol Myers Squibb**	**00087-0544-01**
100's	**$53.45**	**VASODILAN, Bristol Myers Squibb**	**00087-0544-03**
500's	$24.69	Isoxsuprine Hcl, Rugby	00536-3936-05
500's	**$211.63**	**VASODILAN, Bristol Myers Squibb**	**00087-0544-02**
1000's	$43.10	Isoxsuprine Hcl, Eon Labs Mfg	00185-0531-10
1000's	$47.32	Isoxsuprine Hcl, Aligen Independ	00405-4576-03
1000's	$48.75	Isoxsuprine Hcl 20, Major Pharms	00904-0636-80
1000's	$53.31	Isoxsuprine Hcl, HL Moore Drug Exch	00839-6182-16
1000's	$60.75	Isoxsuprine Hcl, Goldline Labs	00182-1056-10
1000's	$60.84	Isoxsuprine HCl, Geneva Pharms	00781-1842-10
1000's	**$426.54**	**VASODILAN, Bristol Myers Squibb**	**00087-0544-06**
5000's	**$1778.05**	**VASODILAN, Bristol Myers Squibb**	**00087-0544-47**

ISRADIPINE *(003014)*

CATEGORIES: Antihypertensives; Calcium Channel Blockers; Cardiovascular Drugs; Hypertension; Pregnancy Category C; FDA Class 1C ("Little or No Therapeutic Advantage"); FDA Approved 1990 Dec

BRAND NAMES: **Dynacirc**; *Dynacirc SRO*; *Lomir* (Germany); *Lomir Retard*; *Lomir SRO*; *Prescal* (England); *Vascal*
(International brand names outside U.S. in italics)

FORMULARIES: Aetna; BC-BS; Medi-Cal; PCS

COST OF THERAPY: $380.62 (Hypertension; Capsule; 2.5 mg; 2/day; 365 days)

PRIMARY ICD9: 401.1 (Essential Hypertension, Benign)

DESCRIPTION:

Isradipine is a calcium antagonist available for oral administration in capsules containing 2.5 mg or 5 mg.

Chemically, isradipine is 3,5-Pyridinedicarboxylic acid, 4-(4-benzofurazanyl) -1,4-dihydro-2,6-dimethyl-,methyl 1-methylethyl ester. Isradipine is a yellow, fine crystalline powder which is odorless or has a faint characteristic odor. Isradipine is practically insoluble in water (<10 mg/L at 37°C), but is soluble in ethanol and freely soluble in acetone, chloroform and methylene chloride.

Active Ingredient: isradipine

Dynacirc Inactive Ingredients: colloidal silicon dioxide, D&C Red No. 7 Calcium Lake, FD&C Red No. 40 (5 mg capsule only), FD&C Yellow No. 6 Aluminum Lake, gelatin, lactose, starch, titanium dioxide and other ingredients.

The 2.5 mg and 5 mg capsules may also contain: benzyl alcohol, butylparaben, edetate calcium disodium, methylparaben, propylparaben, sodium propionate.

CLINICAL PHARMACOLOGY:

Mechanism of Action: Isradipine is a dihydropyridine calcium channel blocker. It binds to calcium channels with high affinity and specificity and inhibits calcium flux into cardiac and smooth muscle. The effects observed in mechanistic experiments *in vitro* and studied in intact animals and man are compatible with this mechanism of action and are typical of the class.

Except for diuretic activity, the mechanism of which is not clearly understood, the pharmacodynamic effects of isradipine observed in whole animals can also be explained by calcium channel blocking activity, especially dilating effects in arterioles which reduce systemic resistance and lower blood pressure, with a small increase in resting heart rate. Although like other dihydropyridine calcium channel blockers, isradipine has negative inotropic effects *in vitro*, studies conducted in intact anesthetized animals have shown that the vasodilating effect occurs at doses lower than those which affect contractility. In patients with normal ventricular function, isradipine's afterload reducing properties lead to some increase in cardiac output.

CLINICAL PHARMACOLOGY: *(cont'd)*

Effects in patients with impaired ventricular function have not been fully studied.

Clinical Effects: Dose-related reductions in supine and standing blood pressure are achieved within 2-3 hours following single oral doses of 2.5 mg, 5 mg, 10 mg, and 20 mg isradipine, with a duration of action (at least 50% of peak response) of more than 12 hours following administration of the highest dose.

Isradipine has been shown in controlled, double blind clinical trials to be an effective antihypertensive agent when used as monotherapy, or when added to therapy with thiazide-type diuretics. During chronic administration, divided doses (b.i.d.) in the range of 5-20 mg daily have shown to be effective, with response at trough(prior to next dose) over 50% of the peak blood pressure effect. The response is dose-related between 5-10 mg daily. Isradipine is equally effective in reducing supine, sitting and standing blood pressure.

On chronic administration, increases in resting pulse rate averaged about 3-5 beats/min. These increases were not dose-related.

Hemodynamics: In man, peripheral vasodilation produced by isradipine is reflected by decreased systemic vascular resistance and increased cardiac output. Hemodynamic studies conducted in patients with normal left ventricular function produced, following intravenous isradipine administration, increases in cardiac index, stroke volume index, coronary sinus blood flow, heart rate, and peak positive left ventricular dP/dt. Systemic, coronary, and pulmonary vascular resistance were decreased. These studies were conducted with doses of isradipine which produced clinically significant decreases in blood pressure. The clinical consequences of these hemodynamic effects, if any, have not been evaluated.

Effects on heart rate are variable, dependent upon rate of administration and presence of underlying cardiac condition. While increases in both peak positive dP/dt and LV ejection fraction are seen when intravenous isradipine is given, it is impossible to conclude that these represent a positive inotropic effect due to simultaneous changes in preload and afterload. In patients with coronary artery disease, undergoing atrial pacing during cardiac catheterization, intravenous isradipine diminished abnormalities of systolic performance. In patients with moderate left ventricular dysfunction, oral and intravenous isradipine in doses which reduce blood pressure by 12%-30% percent, resulted in improvement in cardiac index without increase in heart rate, and with no change or reduction in pulmonary capillary wedge pressure, Combination of isradipine and propranolol did not significantly effect left ventricular dP/dt max. The clinical consequences of these effects have not been evaluated.

Electrophysiologic Effects: In general, no detrimental effects on the cardiac conduction system were seen with the use of isradipine. Electrophysiologic studies were conducted on patients with normal sinus and atrioventricular node function. Intravenous isradipine in doses which reduce systolic blood pressure did not effect PR, QRS, AH* or HV* intervals.

No changes were seen in Wenckebach cycle length, atrial, and ventricular refractory periods. Slight prolongation of QT_c interval of 3% was seen in one study. Effects on sinus node recovery time (CSNRT) were mild or not seen.

In patients with sick sinus syndrome, at doses which significantly reduced blood pressure, intravenous isradipine resulted in no depressant effect on sinus and atrioventricular node function.

*AH= conduction time from low right atrium to His bundle deflection, or AV nodal conduction time;

HV= conduction time through the His bundle and the bundle branch-Purkinje system.

Pharmacokinetics and Metabolism: Isradipine is 90%-95% absorbed and is subject to extensive first-pass metabolism, resulting in a bioavailability of about 15%-24%. Isradipine is detectable in plasma within 20 minutes after administration of single oral doses of 2.5-20 mg, and peak concentrations of approximately 1 ng/ml/mg dosed occur about 1.5 hours after drug administration. Administration of isradipine with food significantly increases the time to peak by about an hour, but has no effect on the total bioavailability (area under the curve)of the drug. Isradipine is 95% bound to plasma proteins. Both peak plasma concentration and AUC exhibit a linear relationship to dose over the 0-20 mg dose range. The elimination of isradipine is biphasic with an early half-life of 1.5-2 hours, and a terminal half-life of about 8 hours. The total body clearance of isradipine is 1.4 L/min and the apparent volume of distribution is 3 L/kg.

Isradipine is completely metabolized prior to excretion and no unchanged drug is detected in the urine. Six metabolites have been characterized in blood and urine, with the mono acids of the pyridine derivative and a cyclic lactone product accounting for >75% of the material identified. Approximately 60%-65% of an administered dose is excreted in the urine and 25%-30% in the feces. Mild renal impairment (creatinine clearance 30-80 mL/min) increases the bioavailability (AUC) of isradipine by 45%. Progressive deterioration reverses this trend, and patients with severe renal failure (creatinine clearance <10mL/min) who have been on hemodialysis show a 20%-50% lower AUC than healthy volunteers. No pharmacokinetic information is available on drug therapy during hemodialysis. In elderly patients, $C_{max}$and AUC are increased by 13% and 40%, respectively; in patients with hepatic impairment, C_{max} and AUC are increased by 32% and 52%, respectively (see DOSAGE AND ADMINISTRATION.)

INDICATIONS AND USAGE:

Hypertension: Isradipine is indicated in the management of hypertension. It may be used alone or concurrently with thiazide-type diuretics.

CONTRAINDICATIONS:

Isradipine is contraindicated in individuals who have shown hypersensitivity to any of the ingredients in the formulation.

WARNINGS:

None

PRECAUTIONS:

GENERAL

Blood Pressure: Because isradipine decreases peripheral resistance, like other calcium blockers isradipine may occasionally produce symptomatic hypotension. However, symptoms like syncope and severe dizziness have rarely been reported in hypertensive patients administered isradipine, particularly at the initial recommended doses (see DOSAGE AND ADMINISTRATION.)

Use in Patients with Congestive Heart Failure: Although acute hemodynamic studies in patients with congestive heart failure have shown that isradipine reduced afterload without impairing myocardial contractility, it has a negative inotropic effect at high doses *in vitro*, and possibly in some patients. Caution should be exercised when using the drug in congestive heart failure patients, particularly in combination with a beta-blocker.

CARCINOGENESIS, MUTAGENESIS, AND IMPAIRMENT OF FERTILITY

Treatment of male rats for 2 years with 2.5, 12.5, or 62.5 mg/kg/day isradipine admixed with the diet (approximately 6, 31, and 156 times the maximum recommended daily dose based on a 50 kg man) resulted in dose dependent increases in the incidence of benign Leydig cell tumors and testicular hyperplasia relative to untreated control animals. These findings, which were replicated in a subsequent experiment, may have been indirectly related to an effect of

PRECAUTIONS: *(cont'd)*

isradipine on circulating gonadotropin levels in the rats; a comparable endocrine effect was not evident in male patients receiving therapeutic doses of the drug on a chronic basis. Treatment of mice for two years with 2.5, 15, or 80 mg/kg/day isradipine in the diet (approximately 6, 38, and 200 times the maximum recommended daily dose based on a 50 kg man)showed no evidence of oncogenicity. There was no evidence of mutagenic potential based on the results of a battery of mutagenicity tests. No effect on fertility was observed in male and female rats treated with up to 60 mg/kg/day isradipine.

PREGNANCY CATEGORY C

Isradipine was administered orally to rats and rabbits during organogenesis. Treatment of pregnant rats with doses of 6, 20, or 60 mg/kg/day produced a significant reduction in material weight gain during treatment with the highest dose (150 times the maximum recommended human daily dose) but with no lasting effects on the mother or the offspring. Treatment of pregnant rabbits with doses of 1, 3, or 10 mg/kg/day (2.5, 7.5, and 25 times the maximum recommended human daily dose) produced decrements in maternal body weight gain and increased fetal resorptions at the two higher doses. There was no evidence of embryotoxicity at doses which were not maternotoxic and no evidence of teratogenicity at any dose tested. In a peri/postnatal administration study in rats, reduced maternal body weight gain during late pregnancy at oral doses of 20 and 60 mg/kg/day isradipine was associated with reduced birth weights and decreased peri and postnatal pup survival.

There are no adequate and well controlled studies in pregnant women. The use of isradipine during pregnancy should only be considered if the potential benefit outweighs potential risks.

NURSING MOTHERS

It is not known whether isradipine is excreted in human milk. Because many drugs are excreted in human milk, and because of the potential for adverse effects of isradipine on nursing infants, a decision should be made as to whether to discontinue nursing or discontinue the drug, taking into account the importance of the drug to the mother.

PEDIATRIC USE

Safety and effectiveness have not been established in children.

DRUG INTERACTIONS:

Nitroglycerin: Isradipine has been safely coadministered with nitroglycerin.

Hydrochlorothiazide: A study in normal healthy volunteers has shown that concomitant administration of isradipine and hydrochlorothiazide does not result in altered pharmacokinetics of either drug. In a study in hypertensive patients, addition of isradipine to existing hydrochlorothiazide therapy did not result in any unexpected adverse effects, and isradipine had an additional antihypertensive effect.

Propranolol: In a single dose study in normal volunteers, coadministration of propranolol had a small effect on the rate but no effect on the extent of isradipine bioavailability. Significant increases in AUC (27%) and C_{max} (58%) and decreases in t_{max} (23%) of propranolol were noted in this study. However, concomitant administration of 5 mg b.i.d. isradipine and 40 mg b.i.d. propranolol, to healthy volunteers under steady-state conditions had no relevant effect on either drug's bioavailability. AUC and C_{max} differences were <20% between isradipine given singly and in combination with propanolol, and between propranolol given singly and in combination with isradipine.

Cimetidine: In a study in healthy volunteers, a one-week course of cimetidine at 400 mg b.i.d. with a single 5 mg dose of isradipine on the sixth day showed an increase in isradipine mean peak plasma concentrations (36%) and significant increase in area under the curve (50%). If isradipine therapy is initiated in a patient currently receiving cimetidine, careful monitoring for adverse reactions is advised and downward dose adjustment may be required.

Rifampicin: In a study in healthy volunteers, a six-day course of rifampicin at 600 mg/day followed by a single 5 mg dose of isradipine resulted in a reduction in isradipine levels to below detectable limits. If rifampicin therapy is required, isradipine concentrations and therapeutic effects are likely to be markedly reduced or abolished as a consequence of increased metabolism and higher clearance of isradipine.

Warfarin: In a study in healthy volunteers, no clinically relevant pharmacokinetic or pharmacodynamic interaction between isradipine and racemic warfarin was seen when two single oral doses of warfarin (0.7 mg/kg body weight) were administered during 11 days of multiple-dose treatment with 5 mg b.i.d. isradipine. Neither racemic warfarin nor isradipine binding to plasma proteins *in vitro* was altered by the addition of the other drug.

Digoxin: The concomitant administration of DynaCirc (isradipine) and digoxin in a single-dose pharmacokinetic study did not affect renal, non-renal and total body clearance of digoxin.

Fentanyl Anesthesia: Severe hypotension has been reported during fentanyl anesthesia with concomitant use of a beta blocker and a calcium channel blocker. Even though such interactions have not been seen in clinical studies with DynaCirc (isradipine), an increased volume of circulating fluids might be required if such an interaction were to occur.

ADVERSE REACTIONS:

In multiple dose U.S. studies in hypertension, 1228 patients received Isradipine alone or in combination with other agents, principally a thiazide diuretic, 934 of them in controlled comparisons with placebo or active agents. An additional 652 patients (which includes 374 normal volunteers) received isradipine in U.S. studies of conditions other than hypertension, and 1321 patients received isradipine in non-U.S. studies. About 500 patients received isradipine in long-term hypertension studies, 410 of them for at least 6 months. The adverse reaction rates given below are principally based on controlled hypertension studies, but rarer serious events are derived from all exposures to isradipine, including foreign marketing experience.

Most adverse reactions were mild and related to the vasodilatory effects of isradipine (dizziness, edema, palpitations, flushing, tachycardia) and many were transient. About 5% of isradipine patients left studies prematurely because of adverse reactions (vs. 3% of placebo patients and 6% of active control patients), principally due to headache, edema, dizziness, palpitations and gastrointestinal disturbances.

The following table below shows the most common adverse reactions, volunteered or elicited, considered by the investigator to be at least possibly drug related. The results for the isradipine treated patients are presented for all doses pooled together (reported by 1% or greater of patients receiving any dose of isradipine, and also for the two treatment regimens most applicable to the treatment of hypertension with Isradipine: (1) initial and maintenance dose of 2.5 mg b.i.d., and (2) initial dose of 2.5 mg b.i.d. followed by maintenance dose of 5.0 mg b.i.d.

Except for headache, which is not clearly drug-related (see TABLE 1), the more frequent adverse reactions listed above show little change, or increase slightly, in frequency over time, as shown in the following table:

Edema, palpitations, fatigue, and flushing appear to be dose-related, especially at the higher doses of 15-20 mg/day.

ADVERSE REACTIONS: *(cont'd)*

TABLE 1

	All Doses	**2.5 mg b.i.d.**	**5 mg b.i.d.†**	**10 mg b.i.d.††**	**Placebo**	**Active Controls***
N=	**934**	**199**	**150**	**59**	**297**	**414**
Adverse Experience	**%**	**%**	**%**	**%**	**%**	**%**
Headache	13.7	12.6	10.7	22.0	14.1	9.4
Dizziness	7.3	8.0	5.3	3.4	4.4	8.2
Edema	7.2	3.5	8.7	8.5	3.0	2.9
Palpitations	4.0	1.0	4.7	5.1	1.4	1.5
Fatigue	3.9	2.5	2.0	8.5	0.3	6.3
Flushing	2.6	3.0	2.0	5.1	0.0	1.2
Chest Pain	2.4	2.5	2.7	1.7	2.4	2.9
Nausea	1.8	1.0	2.7	5.1	1.7	3.1
Dyspnea	1.8	0.5	2.7	3.4	1.0	2.2
Abdominal Discomfort	1.7	0.0	3.3	1.7	1.7	3.9
Tachycardia	1.5	1.0	1.3	3.4	0.3	0.5
Rash	1.5	1.5	2.0	1.7	0.3	0.7
Pollakiuria	1.5	2.0	1.3	3.4	0.0	<1.0
Weakness	1.2	0.0	0.7	0.0	0.0	1.2
Vomiting	1.1	1.0	1.3	0.0	0.3	0.2
Diarrhea	1.1	0.0	2.7	3.4	2.0	1.9

† Initial dose of 2.5 mg b.i.d. followed by maintenance dose of 5.0 mg b.i.d.
†† Initial dose of 2.5 mg bid followed by sequential titration to 5.0 mg b.i.d., 7.5 mg bid, and maintenance dose of 10.0 mg b.i.d.
* Propranolol, prazosin, hydrochlorothiazide, enalapril, captopril.

TABLE 2 Incidence Rates for Isradipine (All Doses) by Week (%)

Week	**1**	**2**	**3**	**4**	**5**	**6**
N	**694**	**906**	**649**	**847**	**432**	**494**
Adverse Reaction						
Headache	6.5	6.1	5.2	5.2	5.8	4.5
Dizziness	1.6	1.9	1.7	2.2	2.3	2.0
Edema	1.2	2.5	3.2	3.2	5.3	5.5
Palpitations	1.2	1.3	1.4	1.9	2.1	1.4
Fatigue	0.4	1.0	1.4	1.2	1.2	1.6
Flushing	1.2	1.3	2.0	1.4	2.1	1.4
Week	**7**	**8**	**9**	**10**	**11**	**12**
N	**153**	**377**	**261**	**362**	**107**	**105**
Headache	20.	2.7	1.9	2.8	2.8	3.8
Dizziness	2.0	1.9	2.3	3.9	4.7	3.8
Edema	5.9	5.0	4.6	4.7	3.8	3.8
Palpitations	1.3	0.8	0.8	1.7	1.9	2.9
Fatigue	2.0	2.7	1.5	1.4	0.9	1.9
Flushing	3.3	1.3	1.1	0.8	0.0	0.0

In open-label, long-term studies of up to two years in duration, the adverse events reported were generally the same as those reported in the short-term controlled trials. The overall frequencies of these adverse events were slightly higher in the long-term than in the controlled studies, but as in the controlled trials most adverse reactions were mild and transient.

The following adverse events were reported in 0.5-1.0% of the isradipine treated patients in hypertension studies, or are rare. More serious events from this and other data sources, including postmarketing exposure, are shown in italics. The relationship of these adverse events to isradipine administration is uncertain.

Skin: pruritus, *urticaria*

Musculoskeletal: cramps of legs/feet

Respiratory: cough

Cardiovascular: shortness of breath, hypotension, *atrial fibrillation, ventricular fibrillation, myocardial infarction, heart failure*

Gastrointestinal: abdominal discomfort, constipation, diarrhea

Urogenital: nocturia

Nervous System: drowsiness, insomnia, lethargy, nervousness, impotence, decreased libido, depression, *syncope, paresthesia* (which includes numbness and tingling), *transient ischemic attack, stroke*

Autonomic: hyperhidrosis, visual disturbance, dry mouth, numbness

Miscellaneous: throat discomfort, *leukopenia, elevated liver function tests*

OVERDOSAGE:

Minimal empirical data are available on isradipine overdosage. Three individual suicide attempts with dosages of isradipine reported to be from 20 mg up to 100 mg resulted in lethargy, sinus tachycardia and, in the case of the person ingesting 100 mg, transient hypotension which responded to fluid therapy. A foreign report of the ingestion of 200 mg of isradipine with ethanol resulted only in flushing, tachycardia with ST depression on ECG, and hypotension, all of which were reversible. The ingestion of 5 mg of isradipine by a 22-month old child and the accidental ingestion of 100 mg of isradipine by a 58-year old female did not result in any sequelae.

Available data suggest that, as with other dihropyridines, overdosage with isradipine might result in excessive peripheral vasodilatation with subsequent marked and probably prolonged systemic hypotension, and tachycardia. Emesis, gastric lavage, administration of activated charcoal followed in 30 minutes by a saline cathartic would be reasonable therapy. Isradipine is highly protein-bound and *not*removed by hemodialysis. Overdosage characterized by clinically significant hypotension should be treated with active cardiovascular support including monitoring of cardiac and respiratory function, elevation of lower extremities, and attention to circulating fluid volume and urine output. A vasoconstrictor (such as epinephrine, norepinephrine, or levarterenol) may be helpful in restoring a normotensive state, provided that there is no contraindication to its use.

Refractory hypotension or AV conduction disturbances may be treated with intravenous calcium salts, or glucagon. Cimetidine should be withheld in such instances due to the risk of further increasing plasma isradipine levels.

Significant lethality was observed in mice given oral doses of over 200 mg/kg and rabbits given about 50 mg/kg of isradipine. Rats tolerated doses of over 2000 mg/kg without effects on survival.

DOSAGE AND ADMINISTRATION:

The dosage of isradipine should be individualized. The recommended initial dose of isradipine is 2.5 mg b.i.d. alone or in combination with a thiazide diuretic. An antihypertensive response usually occurs within 2-3 hours. Maximal response may require 2-4 weeks. If a

DOSAGE AND ADMINISTRATION: *(cont'd)*

satisfactory reduction in blood pressure does not occur after this period, the dose may be adjusted in increments of 5 mg/day at 2-4 week intervals up to a maximum of 20 mg per day. Most patients, however, show no additional response to doses above 10 mg/day, and adverse effects are increased in frequency above 10 mg/day.

The bioavailability of increased AUC is increased in elderly patients (above 65 years of age), patients with hepatic functional impairment, and patients with mild renal impairment. Ordinarily, the starting dose should still be 2.5 mg b.i.d. in these patients.

HOW SUPPLIED:

DynaCirc Capsules 2.5 mg: White, imprinted twice with the DynaCirc (isradipine) logo and "DynaCirc" on one end, and "2.5" and "S" (within a triangle) on the other.

DynaCirc Capsules 5 mg: Light pink, imprinted twice with the DynaCirc (isradipine) logo and "DynaCirc" on one end, and "5" and "S" (within a triangle) on the other.

Store and Dispense: Below 86°F (30°C) in a tight container. Protect from light.

HOW SUPPLIED - EQUIVALENTS NOT AVAILABLE:

Capsule, Gelatin - Oral - 2.5 mg

60's	$34.44	DYNACIRC, Novartis	00078-0226-44
100's	$52.14	DYNACIRC, Novartis	00078-0226-06
100's	$56.04	DYNACIRC, Novartis	00078-0226-05
640's	$367.44	DYNACIRC, Novartis	00078-0226-65

Capsule, Gelatin - Oral - 5 mg

60's	$50.16	DYNACIRC, Novartis	00078-0227-44
100's	$82.20	DYNACIRC, Novartis	00078-0227-05
640's	$528.12	DYNACIRC, Novartis	00078-0227-65

ITRACONAZOLE *(003133)*

CATEGORIES: AIDS Related Complex; Anti-Infectives; Antibiotics; Antifungals; Antimicrobials; Antimycotics; Aspergillosis; Blastomycosis; Fungal Agents; Fungal Infections; Histoplasmosis; HIV Infection; Immunodeficiency; Infections; Onychomycosis; Pulmonary Disease; Candidiasis*; Coccidioidomycosis*; Meningitis*; Sporotrichosis*; Pregnancy Category C; FDA Class 1P ("Priority Review"); FDA Approved 1992 Sep

* Indication not approved by the FDA

BRAND NAMES: *Isox* (Mexico); *Itranax* (Mexico); *Sopranox*; *Sporacid*; *Sporal*; **Sporanox**; *Sporanox 15 D* (Mexico)

(International brand names outside U.S. in italics)

FORMULARIES: Medi-Cal; PCS

COST OF THERAPY: $970.85 (Histoplasmosis; Capsule; 100 mg; 2/day; 90 days)

WARNING:

Coadministration of terfenadine with itraconazole is contraindicated. Serious cardiovascular adverse events, including death, ventricular tachycardia, and torsades de pointes have occurred in patients taking itraconazole concomitantly with terfenadine. This is due to elevated terfenadine concentrations caused by itraconazole. See CONTRAINDICATIONS, WARNINGS and PRECAUTIONS.

Another oral azole antifungal, ketoconazole, inhibits the metabolism of astemizole, resulting in elevated plasma concentrations of astemizole and its active metabolite desmethylastemizole, which may prolong QT intervals. Based on results of an in vitro study and the chemical resemblance of itraconazole and ketoconazole, coadministration of astemizole and itraconazole is contraindicated. See CONTRAINDICATIONS, WARNINGS and PRECAUTIONS.

Coadministration of cisapride with itraconazole is contraindicated. Serious cardiovascular adverse events including death, ventricular tachycardia, and torsades de pointes have occurred in patients taking itraconazole concomitantly with cisapride. See CONTRAINDICATIONS, WARNINGS and PRECAUTIONS.

DESCRIPTION:

Sporanox is the brand name of itraconazole, a synthetic triazole antifungal agent. Itraconazole is a 1:1:1:1 racemic mixture of four diastereomers (two enantiomeric pairs), each possessing three chiral centers. It may be represented by the following nomenclature: (±)-1-[(R*)-sec-butyl]-4-[p-[4-[p- [[(2R*,4S*)-2-(2,4-dichlorophenyl)-2-(1H-1,2,4- triazol-1-ylmethyl)-1,3-dioxolan-4-yl]methoxy]phenyl]-1-piperazinyl]phenyl]-Δ²-1,2,4-triazolin-5-one mixture with (±)-1-[(R*)-sec-butyl]-4-[p-[4-[p- [[(2S*4R*)-2-(2,4,-dichlorophenyl)-2-(1H-1,2,4- triazol-1-yl-methyl)-1,3-dioxolan-4-yl]methoxy]phenyl]-1-piperazinyl]phenyl]-Δ²-1,2,4-triazolin-5-one or (±)-1-[(RS)-sec-butyl]-4-[p-[4-[p- [[(2R,4S)-2-(2,4-dichlorophenyl)-2-(1H-1,2,4- triazol-1-yl-methyl)-1,3,-dioxolan-4-yl]methoxy]phenyl]-1-piperazinyl]phenyl]-Δ²-1,2,4-triazolin-5-one

Itraconazole has a molecular formula of $C_{35}H_{38}Cl_2N_8O_4$ and a molecular weight of 705.64. It is a white to slightly yellowish powder. It is insoluble in water, very slightly soluble in alcohols, and freely soluble in dichloromethane. It has a pKa of 3.70 (based on extrapolation of values obtained from methanolic solutions) and a log (n-octanol/water) partition coefficient of 5.66 at pH 8.1.

Sporanox contains 100 mg of itraconazole coated on sugar spheres. Inactive ingredients are gelatin, hydroxypropyl methylcellulose, polyethylene glycol (PEG) 20,000, starch, sucrose, titanium dioxide, FD&C Blue No. 1, FD&C Blue No. 2, D&C Red No. 22 and D&C Red No. 28.

CLINICAL PHARMACOLOGY:

Mode of Action: *In vitro* studies have demonstrated that itraconazole inhibits the cytochrome P-450-dependent synthesis of ergosterol, which is a vital component of fungal cell membranes.

Pharmacokinetics and Metabolism: *NOTE:* The plasma concentrations reported below were measured by high performance liquid chromatography (HPLC) specific for itraconazole. When itraconazole in plasma is measured by a bioassay, values reported are approximately 3.3 times higher than those obtained by HPLC due to the presence of the bioactive metabolite, hydroxyitraconazole. See CLINICAL PHARMACOLOGY, Microbiology.

CLINICAL PHARMACOLOGY: *(cont'd)*

The pharmacokinetics of itraconazole after intravenous administration and its absolute oral bioavailability from an oral solution were studied in a randomized cross-over study using six healthy male volunteers. The total plasma clearance averaged 381 ± 95 ml/min and the apparent volume of distribution averaged 796 ± 185 l. The observed absolute oral bioavailability of itraconazole was 55%.

The oral bioavailability of itraconazole is maximal when itraconazole is taken with a full meal. The pharmacokinetics of itraconazole were studied using six healthy male volunteers who received, in a cross-over design, single 100 mg doses of itraconazole as a polyethylene glycol capsule, with or without a full meal. The same six volunteers also received 50 mg or 200 mg with a full meal in a cross-over design. In this study, only itraconazole plasma concentrations were measured. Presented in TABLE 1 are the respective pharmacokinetic parameters for itraconazole:

TABLE 1

	50 mg (fed)	100 mg (fed)	100 mg (fasted)	200 mg (fed)
C_{max} (ng/ml)	45 ± 16	132 ± 67	38 ± 20	289 ± 100
T_{max} (hours)	3.2 ± 1.3	4.0 ± 1.1	3.3 ± 1.0	4.7 ± 1.4
$AUC_{0-\infty}$ (ng°h/ml)	567 ± 264	1899 ± 838	722 ± 289	5211 ± 2116

Values are means ± standard deviation

Doubling the itraconazole dose results in approximately a three-fold increase in the itraconazole plasma concentrations.

Values given in TABLE 2 represent data from a cross-over pharmacokinetics study in which 27 healthy male volunteers each took a single 200 mg dose of itraconazole with or without a full meal:

TABLE 2

	Itraconazole		Hydroxyitraconazole	
	Fed	Fasted	Fed	Fasted
C_{max} (ng/ml)	239 ± 85	140 ± 65	397 ± 103	286 ± 101
T_{max} (hours)	4.5 ± 1.1	3.9 ± 1.0	5.1 ± 1.6	4.5 ± 1.1
$AUC_{0-\infty}$ (ng·h/ml)	3423 ± 1154	2094 ± 905	7978 ± 2648	5191 ± 2489
$t_{1/2}$ (hours)	21 ± 5	21 ± 7	12 ± 3	12 ± 3

Values are means ± standard deviation

Absorption of itraconazole under fasted conditions in individuals with relative or absolute achlorhydria, such as patients with AIDS or volunteers taking gastric acid secretion suppressors (*e.g.*, H_2 inhibitors), was increased when itraconazole was administered with a cola beverage. Eighteen males with AIDS received single 200 mg doses of itraconazole under fasted conditions with 8 ounces of water or 8 ounces of a cola beverage in a crossover design. The absorption of itraconazole was increased when itraconazole was coadministered with a cola beverage with AUC_{0-24} and C_{max} increasing 75 ± 121% and 95 ± 128%, respectively. Thirty healthy males received single 200 mg doses of itraconazole under fasted conditions either 1) with water; 2) with water, after ranitidine 150 mg b.i.d. for 3 days; or 3) with cola, after ranitidine 150 mg b.i.d. for 3 days. When itraconazole was administered after ranitidine pretreatment, itraconazole was absorbed to a lesser extent than when itraconazole was administered alone, with decreases in AUC_{0-24} and C_{max} of 39 ± 37% and 42 ± 39%, respectively. When itraconazole was administered with cola after ranitidine pretreatment, itraconazole absorption was comparable to that observed when itraconazole was administered alone.

Steady-state concentrations were reached within 15 days following oral doses of 50-400 mg daily. Values given in the table below (TABLE 3) are data at steady-state from a pharmacokinetics study in which 27 healthy male volunteers took 200 mg itraconazole b.i.d. (with a full meal) for 15 days:

TABLE 3

	Itraconazole	Hydroxyitraconazole
C_{max} (ng/ml)	2282 ± 514	3488 ± 742
C_{min} (ng/ml)	1855 ± 535	3349 ± 761
T_{max} (hours)	4.6 ± 1.8	3.4 ± 3.4
AUC_{0-12h} (ng°h/ml)	22569 ± 5375	38572 ± 8450
$t_{1/2}$ (hours)	64 ± 32	56 ± 24

Values are means ± standard deviation

Results of the pharmacokinetics study suggest that itraconazole may undergo saturation metabolism with multiple dosing.

Itraconazole is extensively metabolized by the liver into a large number of metabolites, including hydroxyitraconazole, the major metabolite. Fecal excretion of the parent drug varies between 3-18% of the dose. Renal excretion of the parent drug is less than 0.03% of the dose. About 40% of the dose is excreted as inactive metabolites in the urine. No single excreted metabolite represents more than 5% of a dose. The main metabolic pathways are oxidative scission of the dioxolane ring, aliphatic oxidation at the 1-methylpropyl substituent, N-dealkylation of this 1-methylpropyl substituent, oxidative degradation of the piperazine ring and triazolone scission.

Plasma concentrations of itraconazole in subjects with renal insufficiency were comparable to those obtained in healthy subjects. The effect of hepatic impairment on the plasma concentration of itraconazole is unknown. It is recommended that plasma concentrations of itraconazole in patients with hepatic impairment be carefully monitored.

The plasma protein binding of itraconazole is 99.8% and that of hydroxyitraconazole is 99.5%. Itraconazole is not removed by hemodialysis.

In animal studies, itraconazole is extensively distributed into lipophilic tissues. Concentrations of itraconazole in fatty tissues, omentum, liver, kidney and skin tissues are 2-20 times the corresponding plasma concentrations. Aqueous fluids such as cerebrospinal fluid and saliva contain negligible amounts of the drug.

Microbiology: Itraconazole exhibits *in vitro* activity against *Blastomyces dermatitidis, Histoplasma capsulatum, Histoplasma duboisii, Aspergillus flavus, Aspergillus fumigatus* and *Cryptococcus neoformans.* Itraconazole also exhibits varying *in vitro* activity against *Sporothrix schenckii,* Trichophyton spp., *Candida albicans* and Candida spp. The bioactive metabolite, hydroxyitraconazole, has not been evaluated against *Histoplasma capsulatum* and *Blastomyces dermatitidis.*Correlation between*in vitro* minimum inhibitory concentration (MIC) results and clinical outcome has yet to be established for azole antifungal agents.

Itraconazole administered orally was active in a variety of animal models of fungal infection using standard laboratory strains of fungi. Fungistatic activity has been demonstrated against disseminated fungal infections caused by *Blastomyces dermatitidis, Histoplasma duboisii,*

CLINICAL PHARMACOLOGY: *(cont'd)*

Aspergillus fumigatus, Coccidioides immitis, Cryptococcus neoformans, Paracoccidioides brasiliensis, Sporothrix schenckii, Trichophyton rubrum and *Trichophyton mentagrophytes.* Itraconazole administered at 2.5 mg/kg and 5.0 mg/kg via the oral and parenteral routes increased survival rates and sterilized organ systems in normal and immunosuppressed guinea pigs with disseminated *Aspergillus fumigatus* infections. Oral itraconazole administered daily at 40 mg/kg and 80 mg/kg increased survival rates in normal rabbits with disseminated disease and immunosuppressed rats with pulmonary*Aspergillus fumigatus* infection, respectively. Itraconazole has demonstrated antifungal activity in a variety of animal models infected with *Candida albicans* and other Candida species.

In vivo studies suggest that the activity of amphotericin B may be suppressed by azole antifungal therapy. As with other azoles, ketoconazole and itraconazole inhibit the ^{14}C-demethylation step in the synthesis of ergosterol, a cell wall component of fungi. Ergosterol is the active site for amphotericin B. In one study the antifungal activity of amphotericin B against *Aspergillus fumigatus* infections in mice was inhibited by ketoconazole therapy. The clinical significance of test results obtained in this study is unknown.

INDICATIONS AND USAGE:

Itraconazole is indicated for the treatment of the following fungal infections in immunocompromised and non- immunocompromised patients:

1. Blastomycosis, pulmonary and extrapulmonary;

2. Histoplasmosis, including chronic cavitary pulmonary disease and disseminated, non-meningeal histoplasmosis;

3. Aspergillosis, pulmonary and extrapulmonary, in patients who are intolerant of or who are refractory to amphotericin B therapy; and

4. Onychomycosis due to dermatophytes (tinea unguium) of the toenail with or without fingernail involvement.

Specimens for fungal cultures and other relevant laboratory studies (wet mount, histopathology, serology) should be obtained prior to therapy to isolate and identify causative organisms. Therapy may be instituted before the results of the cultures and other laboratory studies are known; however, once these results become available, anti-active therapy should be adjusted accordingly.

Blastomycosis: Analyses were conducted on data from two open-label, non-currently controlled studies (n=73 combined) in patients with normal or abnormal immune status. The median dose was 200 mg/day. A response for most signs and symptoms was observed within the first two weeks, and all cleared between 3 and 6 months. Results of these two studies demonstrated substantial evidence of the effectiveness of itraconazole, for the treatment of blastomycosis, compared to the natural history of untreated cases.

Histoplasmosis: Analyses were conducted on data from two open-label, non-currently controlled studies (n=34 combined) in patients with normal or abnormal immune status (not including HIV-infected patients). The median dose was 200 mg/day. A response for most signs and symptoms was observed within the first 2 weeks, and all cleared between 3 and 12 months. Results of these two studies demonstrated substantial evidence of the effectiveness of itraconazole, for the treatment of histoplasmosis, compared to the natural history of untreated cases.

Histoplasmosis in HIV-infected patients: Data from a small number of HIV-infected patients suggested that the response rate of histoplasmosis in HIV-infected patients is similar to non-HIV-infected patients. The clinical course of histoplasmosis in HIV-infected patients is more severe and usually requires maintenance therapy to prevent relapse. Studies to investigate the efficacy and safety of itraconazole in HIV-infected patients, including optimal dosage regimens for treatment and maintenance therapies, are ongoing.

Aspergillosis: Analyses were conducted on data from an open-label, "single-patient-use" protocol designed to make itraconazole available in the U.S. for patients who either failed or were intolerant to amphotericin B therapy (n=190). The findings were corroborated by two smaller open-label studies (n=31 combined) in the same patient population. Most adult patients were treated with a daily dose of 200 to 400 mg with a median duration of 3 months. Results of these studies demonstrated substantial evidence of effectiveness of itraconazole, as a second-line therapy for the treatment of aspergillosis, compared to the natural history of the disease in patients who either failed or were intolerant to amphotericin B therapy.

Onychomycosis: Analyses were conducted on data from three double-blind, placebo-controlled studies (n=214 total) in which patients with onychomycosis of the toenails received 200 mg once daily for 12 consecutive weeks. Results of these studies demonstrated mycological cure in 54% of patients, defined as simultaneous occurrence of negative KOH plus negative culture. Thirty-five (35) percent of patients were considered an overall success (mycological cure plus clear or minimal nail involvement with significantly decreased signs); 14% of patients demonstrated mycological cure plus clinical cure (clearance of all signs, with or without residual nail deformity). The mean time to overall success was approximately 10 months. Twenty-one (21) percent of the overall success group had a relapse (worsening of the global score or conversion of KOH or culture from negative to positive).

CONTRAINDICATIONS:

Coadministration of terfenadine, astemizole or cisapride with itraconazole is contraindicated. (See BOXED WARNING, WARNINGS, and PRECAUTIONS.)

Concomitant administration of itraconazole with oral triazolam or with oral midazolam is contraindicated. (See PRECAUTIONS).

Itraconazole should not be administered for the treatment of onychomycosis to pregnant patients or to women contemplating pregnancy.

Itraconazole is contraindicated in patients who have shown hypersensitivity to the drug or its excipients. There is no information regarding cross hypersensitivity between itraconazole and other azole antifungal agents. Caution should be used in prescribing itraconazole to patients with hypersensitivity to other azoles.

WARNINGS:

In U.S. clinical trials prior to marketing, there have been three cases of reversible idiosyncratic hepatitis reported among more than 2500 patients taking itraconazole. One patient outside the U.S. developed fulminant hepatitis and died during itraconazole administration. Since this patient was on multiple medications, the casual association with itraconazole is uncertain. If clinical signs and symptoms consistent with liver disease develop that may be attributable to itraconazole, itraconazole should be discontinued.

Prior to U.S. marketing, there have been three cases of life-threatening cardiac dysrhythmias and one death reported in patients receiving terfenadine and itraconazole. (See BOXED WARNING), CONTRAINDICATIONS, and PRECAUTIONS.

Coadministration of astemizole with itraconazole is contraindicated. (See BOXED WARNING, CONTRAINDICATIONS, and PRECAUTIONS.)

Concomitant administration of oral ketoconazole with cisapride has resulted in markedly elevated cisapride plasma concentrations, prolonged QT intervals, and has rarely been associated with ventricular arrhythmias and torsades de pointes. Due to potent *in vitro* inhibition of the hepatic enzyme system mainly responsible for the metabolism of cisapride

WARNINGS: *(cont'd)*

(cytochrome P450 3A4), itraconazole is also expected to markedly raise cisapride plasma concentrations; therefore, concomitant use of cisapride with itraconazole is contraindicated. (See BOXED WARNING, CONTRAINDICATIONS, and PRECAUTIONS).

PRECAUTIONS:

General: Hepatic enzyme test values should be monitored in patients with preexisting hepatic function abnormalities.

Hepatic enzyme test values should be monitored periodically in all patients receiving continuous treatment for more than one month or at any time a patient develops signs or symptoms suggestive of liver dysfunction.

Itraconazole should be administered after a full meal. See CLINICAL PHARMACOLOGY, Pharmacokinetics and Metabolism.

Under fasted conditions, itraconazole absorption was decreased in the presence of decreased gastric acidity. The absorption of itraconazole may be decreased with the concomitant administration of antacids or gastric acid secretion suppressors. Studies conducted under fasted conditions demonstrated that administration with 8 ounces of a cola beverage resulted in increased absorption of itraconazole in AIDS patients with relative or absolute achlorhydria. This increase relative to the effects of a full meal is unknown. (See Pharmacokinetics and Metabolism.)

Information for the Patient: Patients should be instructed to take itraconazole with a full meal.

Patients should be instructed to report any signs and symptoms that may suggest liver dysfunction so that the appropriate laboratory testing can be done. Such signs and symptoms may include unusual fatigue, anorexia, nausea and/or vomiting, jaundice, dark urine or pale stool.

Carcinogenesis, Mutagenesis and Impairment of Fertility: Itraconazole showed no evidence of carcinogenicity potential in mice treated orally for 23 months at dosage levels up to 80 mg/kg/day [approximately 10x the maximum recommended human dose (MRHD)]. Male rats treated with 25 mg/kg/day (3.1 x MRHD) had a slightly increased incidence of soft tissue sarcoma. These sarcomas may have been a consequence of hypercholesterolemia, which is a response of rats, but not dogs or humans, to chronic itraconazole administration. Female rats treated with 50 mg/kg/day (6.25x MRHD) had an increased incidence of squamous cell carcinoma of the lung (2/50) as compared to the untreated group. Although the occurrence of squamous cell carcinoma in the lung is extremely uncommon in untreated rats, the increase in this study was not statistically significant.

Itraconazole produced no mutagenic effects when assayed in appropriate bacterial, non-mammalian and mammalian test systems.

Itraconazole did not affect the fertility of male or female rats treated orally with dosage levels of up to 40 mg/kg/day (5x MRHD) even though parental toxicity was present at this dosage level. More severe signs of parental toxicity, including death, were present in the next higher dosage level, 160 mg/kg/day (20x MRHD).

Pregnancy, Teratogenic Effects, Pregnancy Category C: Itraconazole was found to cause a dose-related increase in maternal toxicity, embryotoxicity and teratogenicity in rats at dosage levels at approximately 40-160 mg/kg/day (5-20x MRHD) and in mice at dosage levels of approximately 80 mg/kg/day (10x MRHD). In rats, the teratogenicity consisted of major skeletal defects; in mice it consisted of encephaloceles and/or macroglossia.

There are no studies in pregnant women. Itraconazole should be used for the treatment of systemic fungal infections in pregnancy only if the benefit outweighs the potential risk. Itraconazole should not be administered for the treatment of onychomycosis to pregnant patients or to women contemplating pregnancy. Itraconazole should not be administered to women of child-bearing potential for the treatment of onychomycosis unless they are taking effective measures to prevent pregnancy and the patient begins therapy on the second or third day of the next normal menstrual period. Effective contraception should be continued throughout itraconazole therapy and for 2 months following treatment.

Nursing Mothers: Itraconazole is excreted in human milk; therefore, itraconazole should not be administered to nursing women.

Pediatric Use: The efficacy and safety of itraconazole have not been established in pediatric patients. No pharmacokinetic data are available in children. A small number of patients from age 3 to 16 years have been treated with 100 mg/day of itraconazole for systemic fungal infections and no serious unexpected adverse effects have been reported.

In three toxicology studies using rats, itraconazole induced bone defects at dosage levels as low as 20 mg/kg/day (2.5x MRHD). The induced defects included reduced bone plate activity, thinning of the zona compacta of the large bones and increased bone fragility. At a dosage level of 80 mg/kg/day (10x MRHD) over one year or 160 mg/kg/day (20x MRHD) for six months, itraconazole induced small tooth pulp with hypocellular appearance in some rats.

While no such bone toxicity has been reported in adult patients, the long term effect of itraconazole in pediatric patients is unknown.

HIV-infected Patients: Because hypochlorhydria has been reported in HIV-infected individuals, the absorption of itraconazole in these patients may be decreased.

The results from a study in which eight HIV-infected individuals were treated with zidovudine, 8 ± 0.4 mg/kg/day, showed that the pharmacokinetics of zidovudine were not affected during concomitant administration of itraconazole, 100 mg b.i.d.

DRUG INTERACTIONS:

Both itraconazole and its major metabolite, hydroxyitraconazole, are inhibitors of the cytochrome P450 3A4 enzyme system. Coadministration of itraconazole and drugs primarily metabolized by the cytochrome P450 3A4 enzyme system may result in increased plasma concentrations of the drugs that could increase or prolong both therapeutic and adverse effects. Therefore, unless otherwise specified, appropriate dosage adjustments may be necessary.

Coadministration of terfenadine with itraconazole has led to elevated plasma concentrations of terfenadine, resulting in rare instances of life- threatening cardiac dysrhythmias and one death. See BOXED WARNING, CONTRAINDICATIONS, and WARNINGS.

Another oral azole antifungal, ketoconazole, inhibits the metabolism of astemizole, resulting in elevated plasma concentrations of astemizole and its active metabolite desmethylastermizole which may prolong QT intervals. *In vitro* data suggest that itraconazole, when compared to ketoconazole, has a less pronounced effect on the biotransformation system responsible for the metabolism of astemizole. Based on the chemical resemblance of itraconazole and ketoconazole, coadministration of astemizole with itraconazole is contraindicated. See BOXED WARNING, CONTRAINDICATIONS, and WARNINGS.

Human pharmacokinetics data indicate that oral ketoconazole potently inhibits the metabolism of cisapride resulting in an eight-fold increase in the mean AUC of cisapride. Data suggest that coadministration of oral ketoconazole and cisapride can result in prolongation of the QT interval on the ECG. *In vitro* data suggest that itraconazole also markedly inhibits the biotransformation system mainly responsible for the metabolism of cisapride; therefore concomitant administration of itraconazole with cisapride is contraindicated. See BOXED WARNING, CONTRAINDICATIONS, and WARNINGS.

DRUG INTERACTIONS: *(cont'd)*

Coadministration of itraconazole with oral midazolam or triazolam has resulted in elevated plasma concentrations of the latter two drugs. This may potentiate and prolong hypnotic and sedative effects. These agents should not be used in patients treated with itraconazole. If midazolam is administered parenterally, special precaution is required since the sedative effect may be prolonged. (See CONTRAINDICATIONS.)

Coadministration of itraconazole and cyclosporine, tacrolimus or digoxin has led to increased plasma concentrations of the latter three drugs. Cyclosporine, tacrolimus and digoxin concentrations should be monitored at the initiation of itraconazole therapy and frequently thereafter, and the dose of these three drug products adjusted appropriately.

There have been rare reports of rhabdomyolysis involving renal transplant patients receiving the combination of itraconazole, cyclosporine, and the HMG-CoA reductase inhibitors lovastatin or simvastatin. Rhabdomyolysis has been observed in patients receiving HMG-CoA reductase inhibitors administered alone (at recommended dosages) or concomitantly with immunosuppressive drugs including cyclosporine.

When itraconazole was coadministered with phenytoin, rifampin, or H_2antagonists, reduced plasma concentrations of itraconazole were reported. The physician is advised to monitor the plasma concentrations of itraconazole when any of these drugs is taken concurrently, and to increase the dose of itraconazole if necessary. Although no studies have been conducted, concomitant administration of itraconazole and phenytoin may alter the metabolism of phenytoin; therefore, plasma concentrations of phenytoin should also be monitored when it is given concurrently with itraconazole.

It has been reported that itraconazole enhances the anticoagulant effect of coumarin-like drugs. Therefore, prothrombin time should be carefully monitored in patients receiving itraconazole and coumarin-like drugs simultaneously.

Plasma concentrations of azole antifungal agents are reduced when given concurrently with isoniazid. Itraconazole plasma concentrations should be monitored when itraconazole and isoniazid are coadministered.

Severe hypoglycemia has been reported in patients concomitantly receiving azole antifungal agents and oral hypoglycemic agents. Blood glucose concentrations should be carefully monitored when itraconazole and oral hypoglycemic agents are coadministered.

Tinnitus and decreased hearing have been reported in patients concomitantly receiving itraconazole and quinidine. Edema has been reported in patients concomitantly receiving itraconazole and dihydropyridine calcium channel blockers. Appropriate dosage adjustments may be necessary.

The results from a study in which eight HIV-infected individuals were treated with zidovudine, 8 ± 0.4 mg/kg/day, showed that the pharmacokinetics of zidovudine were not affected during concomitant administration of itraconazole, 100 mg b.i.d.

ADVERSE REACTIONS:

In U.S. clinical trials prior to marketing, there have been three cases of reversible idiosyncratic hepatitis reported among more than 2500 patients. One patient outside the U.S. developed fulminant hepatitis and died during itraconazole administration. Because this patient was on multiple medications, the causal association with itraconazole is uncertain. (See WARNINGS.)

Onychomycosis: Adverse events in TABLE 4 led to either temporary or permanent discontinuation of treatment:

TABLE 4

Body System/Adverse Event	Incidence (%) (n=112)
Elevated Liver Enzymes (>2x normal range)	4%
Gastrointestinal Disorders	4%
Rash	3%
Hypertension	2%
Orthostatic Hypotension	1%
Headache	1%
Malaise	1%
Myalgia	1%
Vasculitis	1%
Vertigo	1%

Systemic Fungal Infections: Adverse experience data in the following table (TABLE 5) are derived from 602 patients treated for systemic fungal disease in U.S. clinical trials, who were immunocompromised or receiving multiple concomitant medications. Of these patients, treatment was discontinued in 10.5% of patients due to adverse events. The median duration before discontinuation of therapy was 81 days, with a range of 2-776 days. The TABLE 5 lists adverse events reported by at least 1% of patients.

TABLE 5

Body System/Adverse Event (Incidence ≥ 1%)	Incidence (%)
Gastrointestinal Disorders	
Nausea	10.6
Vomiting	5.1
Diarrhea	3.3
Abdominal Pain	1.5
Anorexia	1.2
Body as a Whole	
Edema	3.5
Fatigue	2.8
Fever	2.5
Malaise	1.2
Skin and Appendages	
Rash	8.6*
Pruritus	2.5
Central and Peripheral Nervous System	
Headache	3.8
Dizziness	1.7
Psychiatric Disorders	
Libido decreased	1.2
Somnolence	1.2
Cardiovascular Disorders	
Hypertension	3.2
Metabolic and Nutritional Disorders	
Hypokalemia	2.0
Urinary System Disorders	
Albuminuria	1.2
Liver and Biliary System Disorders	
Hepatic function abnormal	2.7
Reproductive Disorders, Male Impotence	1.2

* Rash tends to occur more frequently in immunocompromised patients receiving immunosuppressive medications.

ADVERSE REACTIONS: *(cont'd)*

Adverse events infrequently reported in all studies indicated: constipation, gastritis, depression, insomnia, tinnitus, menstrual disorder, adrenal insufficiency, gynecomastia and male breast pain.

In worldwide postmarketing experience with itraconazole, allergic reactions including rash, pruritus, urticaria, angioedema and in rare instances, anaphylaxis and Stevens-Johnson syndrome, have been reported. Marketing experiences have also included reports of elevated liver enzymes and rare hepatitis. Although the causal association with itraconazole is uncertain, rare hypertriglyceridemia and isolated cases of neuropathy have also been reported.

OVERDOSAGE:

Itraconazole is not removed by dialysis. In the event of accidental overdosage, supportive measures, including gastric lavage with sodium bicarbonate, should be employed.

No significant lethality was observed when itraconazole was administered orally to mice and rats at dosage levels of 320 mg/kg or to dogs at 200 mg/kg.

DOSAGE AND ADMINISTRATION:

itraconazole should be taken with a full meal to ensure maximal absorption.

Treatment of blastomycosis and histoplasmosis: The recommended dose is 200 mg once daily (2 capsules). If there is no obvious improvement or there is evidence of progressive fungal disease, the dose should be increased in 100 mg increments to a maximum of 400 mg daily. Doses above 200 mg per day should be given in two divided doses.

Treatment of aspergillosis: A daily dose of 200 to 400 mg of itraconazole is recommended.

In life-threatening situations: Although these studies did not provide for a loading dose, it is recommended, based on pharmacokinetic data, that a loading dose of 200 mg (2 capsules) t.i.d. (600 mg/day) be given for the first three days.

Treatment should be continued for a minimum of three months and until clinical parameters and laboratory tests indicate that the active fungal infection has subsided. An inadequate period of treatment may lead to recurrence of active infection. The above recommendations for the treatment of blastomycosis and histoplasmosis are based on the results of two open-label studies of patients with blastomycosis (n=73) and histoplasmosis (n=34) where results were compared to the expected outcome for untreated patients from historical controls. The recommendation for the treatment of aspergillosis is based primarily on the results of an open-label, single-patient use protocol designed to make itraconazole available in the U.S. for patients who either failed or were intolerant to amphotericin B therapy (n=190), and is supported by two smaller open- label studies (n=31 combined) in the same patient population.

Onychomycosis: The recommended dose is 200 mg once daily for 12 consecutive weeks.

HOW SUPPLIED:

Sporanox is available as capsules containing 100 mg of itraconazole, with a blue opaque cap and pink transparent body, imprinted with "Janssen" and "Sporanox 100".

Store at room temperature (59°-86°F/15°- 30°C). Protect from light and moisture.

HOW SUPPLIED - EQUIVALENTS NOT AVAILABLE:

Capsule, Gelatin - Oral - 100 mg

30's	$161.81	SPORANOX, Janssen Phar	50458-0290-01
30's	$161.81	SPORANOX, Janssen Phar	50458-0290-04

IVERMECTIN *(003134)*

CATEGORIES: Anthelmintics; Antiparasitics; FDA Approved 1996 Nov; FDA Veterinary Approval; Onchocerciasis; Parasiticidal; River Blindness; Strongyloidiasis; Pregnancy Category C

BRAND NAMES: **Mectizan**; Stromectol

FORMULARIES: WHO

DESCRIPTION:

Ivermectin is a semisynthetic, anthelmintic agent for oral administration. Ivermectin is derived from the avermectins, a class of highly active broad-spectrum anti-parasitic agents isolated from the fermentation products of *Streptomyces avermitilis*. Ivermectin is a mixture containing at least 90% 5-*O*-demethyl-22,23-dihydroavermectin A_{1a} and less than 10% 5-*O*-demethyl-25-de(1-methylpropyl)-22,23-dihydro-25-(1-methylethyl)avermectin A_{1a}, generally referred to as 22,23-dihydroavermectin B_{1a} and B_{1b}, respectively. The respective empirical formulas are $C_{48}H_{74}O_{14}$ and $C_{47}H_{72}O_{14}$, with molecular weights of 875.10 and 861.07, respectively.

Ivermectin is a white to yellowish-white, nonhygroscopic, crystalline powder with a melting point of about 155°C. It is insoluble in water but is freely soluble in methanol and soluble in 95% ethanol.

Ivermectin is available in 6 mg scored tablets. Each tablet contains the following inactive ingredients: microcrystalline cellulose, pregelatinized starch, magnesium stearate, butylated hydroxyanisole, and the citric acid powder (anhydrous).

CLINICAL PHARMACOLOGY:

PHARMACOKINETICS

Following oral administration of ivermectin, plasma concentrations are approximately proportional to the dose. In two studies, after single 12 mg doses of ivermectin (2×6 mg) in fasting healthy volunteers (representing a mean dose of 165 mcg/kg), the mean peak plasma concentrations of the major component (H_2B_{1a}) were 46.6 (±21.9) (range: 16.4-101.1) and 30.6 (±16.6) (range: 13.9-68.4) ng/ml respectively at approximately 4 hours after dosing. Ivermectin is metabolized in the liver, and invermectin and/or its metabolites are excreted almost exclusively in the feces over an estimated 12 days, with less than 1% of the administered dose excreted in the urine. The apparent plasma half-life of ivermectin is approximated at least 16 hours following oral administration.

The effect(s) of food on the systemic availability of ivermectin has not been studied.

MICROBIOLOGY

Ivermectin is a member of the avermectin class of broad-spectrum anti-parasitic agents which have a unique mode of action. Compounds of the class bind selectively and with high affinity to glutamate-gated chloride ion channels which occur in invertebrate nerve and muscle cells. This leads to an increase in the permeability of the cell membrane to chloride ions with hyperpolarization of the nerve or muscle cell, resulting in paralysis and death of the parasite. Compounds of this class may also interact with other ligand-gated chloride channels, such as those gated by the neurotransmitter gamma-aminobutyric acid (GABA).

The selective activity of compounds of this class is attributable to the facts that some mammals do not have glutamate-gated chloride channels and that the avermectins have a low affinity for mammalian ligand-gated chloride channels. In addition, ivermectin does not readily cross the blood-brain barrier in humans.

CLINICAL PHARMACOLOGY: *(cont'd)*

Ivermectin is active against various life-cycle stages of many but not all nematodes. It is active against the tissue microfilariae of *Onchocerca volvulus* but not against the adult form. Its activity against *Strongyloides stercoralis* is limited to the intestinal stages.

CLINICAL STUDIES:

STRONGYLOIDIASIS

Two controlled clinical studies using albendazole as the comparative agent were carried out in international sites where albendazole is approved for the treatment of strongyloidiasis of the gastrointestinal tract, and three controlled studies were carried out in the US and internationally using thiabendazole as the comparative agent. Efficacy, as measured by cure rate, was defined as the absence of larvae in at least two follow-up stool examinations 3 to 4 weeks post-therapy. Based on this criterion, efficacy was significantly greater for ivermectin (a single dose of 170 to 200 mcg/kg) than for albendazole (200 mg b.i.d. for 3 days). Ivermectin administered as a single dose of 200 mcg/kg for 1 day was as efficacious as thiabendazole administered at 25 mg/kg b.i.d. for 3 days.

TABLE 1 Summary of Cure Rates for Ivermectin Versus Comparative Agents in the Treatment of Stongyloidiasis

	Cure Rate* (%) Ivermectin†	Comparative Agent
Albendazole‡ Comparative		
International Study	24/26 (92)	12/22 (55)
WHO Study	126/152 (83)	67/149 (45)
Thiabendazole§ Comparative		
International Study	9/14 (64)	13/15 (13/15)
US Studies	14/14 (100)	16/17 (94)

* Number and % of evaluable patients.
† 170-200 mcg/kg.
‡ 200 mg bid for 3 days.
§ 25 mg/kg bid for 3 days.

In one study conducted in France, a non-endemic area where there was no possibility of reinfection, several patients were observed to have recrudescence of *Strongyloides* larvae in the their stool as long as 106 days following ivermectin therapy. Therefore, at least three stool examinations should be conducted over the three months following treatment to ensure eradication. If recrudescence of larvae is observed, retreatment with ivermectin is indicated. Concentration techniques (such as using a Baermann apparatus) should be employed when performing these stool examinations, as the number of *Strongyloides* larvae per gram of feces may be very low.

ONCHOCERCIASIS

The evaluation of ivermectin in the treatment of onchocerciasis is based on the results of clinical studies involving 1278 patients. In a double-blind, placebo-controlled study involving adult patients with moderate to severe onchocercal infection, patients who received a single dose of 150 mcg/kg ivermectin experienced an 83.2% and 99.5% decrease in skin microfilariae count (geometric mean) 3 days and 3 months after the dose, respectively. A marked reduction of >90% was maintained for up to 12 months after the single dose. As with other microfilaricidal drugs, there was an increase in the microfilariae count in the anterior chamber of the eye at day 3 after treatment in some patients. However, at 3 and 6 months after the dose, a significantly greater percentage of patients treated with ivermectin had decreases in microfilariae count in the anterior chamber than patients treated with placebo.

In a separate open study involving pediatric patients ages 6 to 13 (n=103; weight range: 17-41kg), similar decreases in skin microfilariae counts were observed for up to 12 months after dosing.

INDICATIONS AND USAGE:

Ivermectin is indicated for the treatment of the following infections:

Strongyloidiasis of the Intestinal Tract: Ivermectin is indicated for the treatment of intestinal (*i.e.,* nondisseminated) strongyloidiasis due to the nematode parasite *Strongyloides stercoralis.*

This indication is based on clinical studies of both comparative and open-label designs, in which from 64-100% of infected patients were cured following a single 200 mcg/kg dose of ivermectin. (See CLINICAL STUDIES.)

Onchocerciasis: Ivermectin is indicated for the treatment of onchocerciasis due to the nematode parasite *Onchocerca volvulus.*

This indication is based on randomized, double-blind, placebo-controlled and comparative studies conducted in 1427 patients in onchocerciasis-endemic areas of West Africa. The comparative studies used diethylcarbamazine citrate (DEC-C).

Note: Ivermectin has no activity against adult *Onchocerca volvulus* parasites. The adult parasites reside in subcutaneous nodules which are infrequently palpable. Surgical excision of these nodules (nodulectomy) may be considered in the management of patients with onchocerciasis, since this procedure will eliminate the microfilariae-producing adult parasites.

CONTRAINDICATIONS:

Ivermectin is contraindicated in patients who are hypersensitive to any component of this product.

WARNINGS:

Historical data have shown that microfilaricidal drugs, such as diethylcarbamazine citrate (DEC-C), might cause cutaneous and/or systemic reactions of varying severity (the Mazzotti reaction) and ophthalmological reactions in patients with onchocerciasis. These reactions are probably due to allergic and inflammatory responses to the death of microfilariae. Patients treated with ivermectin for onchocerciasis may experience these reactions in addition to clinical adverse reactions possibly, probably, or definitely related to the drug itself. (See ADVERSE REACTIONS, Onchocerciasis.) The treatment of severe Mazzotti reactions has not been subjected to controlled clinical trials. Oral hydration, recumbency, intravenous normal saline, and/or parenteral corticosteroids have been used to treat postural hypotension. Antihistamines and /or aspirin have been used for most mild to moderate cases.

PRECAUTIONS:

General: After treatment with microfilaricidal drugs, patients with hyperreactive onchodermatitis (sowda) may be more likely than others to experience severe adverse reactions, especially edema and aggravation of onchodermatitis.

Carcinogenesis, Mutagenesis, Impairment of Fertility: Long-term studies in animals have not been performed to evaluate the carcinogenic potential of ivermectin.

Ivermectin was not genotoxic in vitro in the Ames microbial mutagenicity assay of *Salmonella typhimurium* strains TA1535, TA1537, TA98, and TA100 with and without rat liver enzyme activation, the Mouse Lymphoma Cell Line L5178Y (cytotoxicity and mutagenicity) assays, or the unscheduled DNA synthesis assay in human fibroblasts.

PRECAUTIONS: *(cont'd)*

Ivermectin has no adverse effects on the fertility in rats in studies at repeated doses of up to 3 times the maximum recommended human dose of 200 mcg/kg (on a mg/m^2/day basis).

Information for Patients: Ivermectin should be taken with water. *Strongyloidiasis:* The patient should be reminded of the need for repeated stool examinations to document clearance of infection with *Strongyloides stercoralis. Onchocerciasis:* The patient should be reminded that treatment with ivermectin does not kill the adult *Onchocerca parasites*, and therefore repeated follow-up retreatment is usually required.

Pregnancy, Teratogenic Effects, Pregnancy Category C: Ivermectin has been shown to be teratogenic in mice, rats, and rabbits when given in repeated doses of 0.2, 8.1, and 4.5 times the maximum recommended human dose, respectively (on a mg/m^2/day basis). Teratogenicity was characterized in the three species tested by cleft palate; clubbed forepaws were additionally observed in rabbits. These development effects were found only at or near doses that were maternotoxic to the pregnant female. Therefore, ivermectin does not appear to be selectively fetotoxic to the developing fetus. There are, however, no adequate and well-controlled studies in pregnant women. Ivermectin should not be used during pregnancy since safety in pregnancy has not been established.

Nursing Mothers: Ivermectin is excreted in human milk in low concentrations. Treatment of mothers who intend to breast feed should only be undertaken when the risk of delayed treatment to the mother outweighs the possible risk to the newborn.

Pediatric Use: Safety and effectiveness in pediatric patients weighing less than 15 kg have not been established.

Strongyloidiasis in Immunocompromised Hosts: In immunocompromised (including HIV-infected) patients being treated for intestinal strongyloidiasis, repeated courses of therapy may be required. Adequate and well-controlled clinical studies have not been conducted in such patients to determine the optimal dosing regimen. Several treatments, (*i.e.,* at 2 week intervals), may be required, and cure may not be achievable. Control of extra-intestinal strongyloidiasis in these patients is difficult, and suppressive therapy, (*i.e.,* once per month may be helpful).

ADVERSE REACTIONS:

STRONGYLOIDIASIS

In four clinical studies involving a total of 109 patients given either one or two doses of 170-200 mcg/kg of ivermectin, the following adverse reactions were reported as possibly, probably, or definitely related to ivermectin:

Body as a Whole: asthenia/fatigue (0.9%), abdominal pain (0.9%)

Gastrointestinal: anorexia (0.9%), constipation (0.9%), diarrhea (1.8%), nausea (1.8%), vomiting (0.9%)

Nervous System/Psychiatric: dizziness (2.8%), somnolence (0.9%), vertigo (0.9%), tremor (0.9%)

Skin: pruritus (2.8%), rash (0.9%), and urticaria (0.9%)

In comparative trials, patients treated with ivermectin experienced more abdominal distention and chest discomfort than patients treated with albendazole. However, ivermectin was better tolerated than thiabendazole in comparative studies involving 37 patients treated with thiabendazole.

The Mazzotti-type and ophthalmologic reactions associated with the treatment of onchocerciasis or the disease itself would not be expected to occur in strongyloidiasis patients treated with ivermectin. (See ADVERSE REACTIONS, Onchocerciasis.)

Laboratory Test Findings: In clinical trials involving 109 patients given either one or two doses of 170-200 mcg/kg ivermectin, the following laboratory abnormalities were seen irrespective of drug relationship: elevation in ALT and/or AST (2%), decrease in leukocyte count (3%). Leukopenia and anemia were seen in one patient.

ONCHOCERCIASIS

In clinical trials involving 963 adult patients treated with 100 to 200 mcg/kg ivermectin, worsening of the following Mazzotti reactions during the first 4 days post-treatment were reported: arthralgia/synovitis (9.3%), axillary lymph node enlargement and tenderness (11.0%) and 4.4%, respectively), cervical lymph node enlargement and tenderness (5.3% and 1.2%, respectively), inguinal lymph node enlargement and tenderness (12.6% and 13.9%, respectively), other lymph node enlargement and tenderness (3.0% and 1.9%, respectively), pruritus (27.5%), skin involvement including edema, papular and pustular or frank urticarial rash (22.7%), and fever (22.6%). (See WARNINGS.)

In clinical trials, ophthalmological conditions were examined in 963 adult patients before treatment, at day 3, and months 3 and 6 after treatment with 100 to 200 mcg/kg ivermectin. Changes observed were primarily deterioration from baseline 3 days post-treatment. Most changes either returned to baseline condition or improved over baseline severity at the month 3 and 6 visits. The percentages of patients with worsening of the following conditions at day 3, month 3 and 6, respectively were: limbitis: 5.5%, 4.8%, and 3.5% and punctate opacity: 1.8%, 1.8%, and 1.4%. The corresponding percentages for patients treated with placebo were: limbitis: 6.2%, 9.9%, and 9.4% and punctate opacity: 2.0%, 6.4%, and 7.2%. (See WARNINGS.)

In clinical trials involving 963 adult patients who received 100 to 200 mcg/kg ivermectin, the following clinical adverse reactions were reported as possibly, probably, or definitely related to the drug ≥1% of the patients: facial edema (1.2%), peripheral edema (3.2%), orthostatic hypotension (1.1%), and tachycardia (3.5%). Drug-related headache and myalgia occurred in <1% of patients (0.2%, and 0.4%, respectively). However, these were the most common adverse experiences reported overall during these trials regardless of causality (22.3% and 19.7%, respectively).

A similar safety profile was observed in an open study in pediatric patients ages 6 to 13.

Additionally, hypotension (mainly orthostatic hypotension) and worsening of bronchial asthma have been reported since the drug was registered overseas.

The following ophthalmological side effects do occur due to the disease itself but have also been reported after treatment with ivermectin: abnormal sensation in the eyes, eyelid edema, anterior uveitis, conjunctivitis, limbitis, keratitis, and chorioretinitis or choroiditis. These have rarely been severe or associated with loss of vision and have generally resolved without corticosteroid treatment.

Laboratory Test Findings: In controlled clinical trials, the following laboratory adverse experiences were reported as possibly, probably, or definitely related to the drug in ≥1% of the patients: eosinophilia (3%) and hemoglobin increase (1%).

OVERDOSAGE:

Significant lethality was observed in mice and rats after single oral doses of 25 to 50 mg/kg and 40 to 50 mg/kg, respectively. No significant lethality was observed in dogs after single oral doses of up to 10 mg/kg. At these doses, the treatment related signs that were observed in these animals include ataxia, bradypnea, tremors, ptosis, decreased activity, emesis, and mydriasis.

In accidental intoxication with or significant exposure to unknown quantities of veterinary formulations of ivermectin in humans, either by ingestion, inhalation, injection, or exposure to body surfaces, the following adverse effects have been reported most frequently: rash,

OVERDOSAGE: *(cont'd)*

edema, headache, dizziness, asthenia, nausea, vomiting, and diarrhea. Other adverse effects that have been reported include: seizure, ataxia, dyspnea, abdominal pain, paresthesia, and urticaria.

In case of accidental poisoning, supportive therapy, if indicated, should include parenteral fluids and electrolytes, respiratory support (oxygen and mechanical ventilation if necessary) and pressor agents if clinically significant hypotension is present. Induction of emesis and/or gastric lavage as soon as possible, followed by purgatives and other routine anti-poison measures, may be indicated if needed to prevent absorption of ingested material.

DOSAGE AND ADMINISTRATION:

Strongyloidiasis: The recommended dosage of ivermectin for the treatment of strongyloidiasis is a single oral dose designed to provide approximately 200 mcg of ivermectin per kg of body weight. See TABLE 2 for dosage guidelines. Patients should take tablets with water. In general, additional doses are not necessary. However, follow-up stool examinations should be performed to verify eradication of infection (see CLINICAL STUDIES).

TABLE 2 Dosage Guidelines for Ivermectin for Strongyloidiasis

Body Weight (kg)	Single Oral Dose
15-24	½ tablet
25-35	1 tablet
36-50	1½ tablets
51-65	2 tablets
66-79	2½ tablets
≥80	200 mcg/kg

Onchocerciasis: The recommended dosage of ivermectin for the treatment of onchocerciasis is a single oral dose designed to provide approximately 150 mcg of ivermectin per kg of body weight. See TABLE 3 for dosage guidelines. Patients should take tablets with water. In mass distribution campaigns in international treatment programs, the most commonly use dose interval is 12 months. For the treatment of individual patients, retreatment may be considered at intervals as short as 3 months.

TABLE 3 Dosage Guidelines for Ivermectin for Onchocerciasis

Body Weight (kg)	Single Oral Dose
15-24	½ tablet
25-35	1 tablet
36-50	1½ tablets
51-65	2 tablets
66-79	2½ tablets
≥80	150 mcg/kg

PATIENT INFORMATION:

Take ivermectin with plenty of water. At least three follow-up office visits for stool sample examinations will be needed over a period of three months to ensure clearance of infection.

HOW SUPPLIED:

Tablets: Stromectol 6mg are white, scored, round, flat, beveled-edged tablets coded MSD 139 on one side and scored on the other.

Storage: Store at temperatures below 30°C (86°F).

KANAMYCIN SULFATE *(001597)*

CATEGORIES: Aminoglycosides; Anti-Infectives; Antibiotics; Antimicrobials; Antimycobacterials; Infections; Tuberculosis*; Pregnancy Category D; FDA Approval Pre 1982
* Indication not approved by the FDA

BRAND NAMES: *Kamycine* (France); *Kanacin*; *Kanamed*; *Kanamicina*; *Kanamicina Gen-Far*; *Kanamicina McKesson*; *Kanamin*; *Kanamycin*; *Kanamycin Capsules Meiji*; *Kanamycin Meiji*; *Kanamycin Novo*; *Kanamycin Sanbe*; *Kanamytrex*; *Kanarco*; *Kancin*; *Kanescin*; *Kannasyn* (England); *Kanoxin*; **Kantrex**; Klebcil; *Randikan* (Mexico)
(International brand names outside U.S. in italics)

FORMULARIES: Medi-Cal

WARNING:

Patients treated with aminoglycosides by any route should be under close clinical observation because of the potential toxicity associated with their use. As with other aminoglycosides, the major toxic effects of kanamycin sulfate are its action on the auditory and vestibular branches of the eighth nerve and the renal tubules. Neurotoxicity is manifested by bilateral auditory toxicity which often is permanent and, sometimes, by vestibular ototoxicity. Loss of high frequency perception usually occurs before there is noticeable clinical hearing loss and can be defected by audiometric testing. There may not be clinical symptoms to warn of developing cochlear damage. Vertigo may occur and may be evidence of vestibular injury. Other manifestations of neurotoxicity may include numbness, skin tingling, muscle twitching, and convulsions. The risk of hearing loss increases with the degree of exposure to either high peak or high trough serum concentrations and continues to progress after drug withdrawal.

Renal impairment may be characterized by decreased creatinine clearance, the presence of cells or casts, oliguria, proteinuria, decreased urine specific gravity, or evidence of increasing nitrogen retention (increasing BUN, NPN, or serum creatinine).

The risks of severe ototoxic and nephrotoxic reactions are sharply increased in patients with impaired renal function and in those with normal renal function who receive high doses or prolonged therapy.

Renal and eighth nerve function should be closely monitored, especially in patients with known or suspected reduced renal function at the onset of therapy, and also in those whose renal function in initially normal but who develop signs of renal dysfunction during therapy. Serum concentrations of parenterally administered aminoglycosides should be monitored when feasible to assure adequate levels and to avoid potentially toxic levels. Urine should be examined for decreases specific gravity, increased excretion of protein, and the presence of cells or casts. Blood urea nitrogen, serum creatinine, or creatinine clearance should be measured periodically. Serial audiograms should be obtained when feasible in patients old enough to be tested, particularly high risk patients. Evidence of ototoxicity (dizziness, vertigo, tinnitus, roaring in the ears, and hearing loss) or nephrotoxicity requires dosage adjustment of discontinuance of the drug.

Neuromuscular blockade with respiratory paralysis may occur when kanamycin sulfate is instilled intraperitoneally concomitantly with anesthesia and muscle-relaxing drugs. Neuromuscular blockade has been reported following parenteral injection and the oral use of aminoglycosides. The possibility of the occurrence of neuromuscular blockade and respiratory paralysis should be considered it aminoglycosides are administered by any route, especially in patients receiving anesthetics, neuromuscular-blocking agents such as tubocurarine, succinylcholine, decamethonium or in patients massive transfusions of citrate-anticoagulated blood. It blockage occurs, calcium salts may reduce these phenomenal but mechanical respiratory assistance may be necessary.

The concurrent and/or sequential systemic, oral, or topical use of kanamycin and other potentially nephrotoxic, and/or neurotoxic drugs, particularly polymyxin B, bacitracin, colistin, amphotericin B, cisplatin, vancomycin, and all other aminoglycosides (including paromomycin) should be avoided because the toxicity may be additive. Other factors which may increase patient risk of toxicity are advanced age and dehydration.

Kanamycin sulfate should not be given concurrently with potent diuretics (ethacrynic acid, furosemide, meralluride sodium, sodium mercaptomerin or mannitol). Some diuretics themselves cause ototoxicity, and intravenously administered diuretics may enhance aminoglycoside toxicity by altering antibiotic concentrations in serum and tissue.

DESCRIPTION:

Kanamycin sulfate is an aminoglycoside antibiotic produced by *Streptomyces kanamyceticus*. It is $C_{18}H_{36}N_4O_{11}\cdot 2H_2SO_4$. D-Streptamine, 0-3-amino -3-deoxy-α -D-glucopyranosyl - (1→6)-o-(6-amino -6-deoxy- α-D-glucopyranosyl-(1→4))-2-deoxy, sulfate 1:2 (salt). It consists of two amino sugars glycosidically linked to deoxystreptamine.

Kanamycin sulfate Injection, USP, sterile solution for parenteral administration, contains respectively, kanamycin sulfate 75 mg, 500 mg, and 1.0 g; sodium bisulfite, an antioxidant, 0.099%, 0.66%, and 0.45%; and sodium citrate, 0.33%, 2.2%, and 2.2% with pH of each dosage form adjusted to 4.5 with sulfuric acid.

Vial headspace contains nitrogen.

CLINICAL PHARMACOLOGY:

The drug is rapidly absorbed after intramuscular injection and peak serum levels are generally reached within approximately one hour. Doses of 7.5 mg/kg given mean levels of 22 mcg/ml. At 8 hours following a 7.5 mg/kg dose, mean serum levels are 3.2 mcg/ml. The serum half-life is 2 1/2 hours. Intravenous administration kanamycin over a period of one hour resulted in serum concentrations similar to those obtained by intramuscular administration.

Kanamycin diffuses rapidly into most body fluids including synovial and peritoneal fluids and bile. Significant levels of the drug appear in cord blood and amniotic fluids following intramuscular administration to pregnant patients. Spinal fluid concentrations in normal infants are approximately 10 to 20 percent serum levels and may reach 50 percent when the meninges are inflamed.

Studies in normal adult patients have shown only trace levels of kanamycin in spinal fluid. No data are available on adults with meningitis.

The drug is excreted almost entirely by glomerular filtration and is not reabsorbed by the renal tubules. Hence, high concentrations are attained in the nephron, and the urine may contain levels 10 to 20 times higher than those in serum. Little, if any, metabolic transformation occurs. Renal excretion is extremely rapid. In patients with normal renal function, approximately one-half of the administered dose is cleared within 4 hours and excretion is complete with 24 to 48 hours. Patients with impaired renal function or with diminished glomerular filtration pressure excrete kanamycin more slowly. Such patients may build up excessively high blood levels which greatly increase the risk of ototoxic reactions. In severely burned patients half-life may be significantly decreased and resulting serum concentration may be lower than anticipated from the mg per kg dose.

MICROBIOLOGY

Kanamycin sulfate is bactericidal antibiotic which acts by inhibiting the synthesis of protein in susceptible microorganisms. Kanamycin sulfate is active *in vitro* against many strains of *Staphylococcus aureus* (including penicillinase and non penicillinase-producing strains), *Staphylococcus epidermidis, N. gonorrhoeae, H. influenzae, E. coli, Enterobacter aerogenes, Shigella* a nd *Salmonella* species, *K pneumoniae, Serratia marcescens Providencia* species, *Acinetobacter* species and *Citrobacter freundii* and *Citrobacter* species, and many strains of both indole-positive and indole-negative *Proteus* strains that are frequently resistant to other antibiotic.

Aminoglycosides have a low order of activity against most gram-positive organisms including *Streptococcus pyogenes, Streptococcus pneumoniae* and *enterococci. In vitro* studies have demonstrated that an aminoglycoside combined with an antibiotic which interferes with cell wall synthesis (*i.e.,* Penicillin G or ampicillin) affects some Group D streptococcal strains synergistically. Bacteriological testing and tests for antibiotic synergism are necessary.

Enzymatic inactivation of deoxystreptamine is the principal mechanism of resistance.

Susceptibility Testing: Quantitative methods for susceptibility testing that require measurement of zone diameters give the most precise estimates of antibiotic susceptibility. One such procedure has been recommended for use with discs to tests susceptibility to kanamycin. Interpretation involves correlation of the diameters obtained in the disc test that minimal inhibitory concentration (MIC) values of kanamycin.

Reports from the laboratory give results of the standardized single disc susceptibility tests (Bauer, et al. Am. J. Clin. Path. 1966; 45:493 and Federal Register 37:20529, 1972), using a 30-mcg kanamycin disc should be interpreted according to the following criteria:

Organisms producing zones of 18 mm or greater, or MIC's of 16 mcg or less are considered susceptible, indicating that the test organism is likely to respond to therapy.

Resistant organisms produce zones of 14 mm or less or MIC's of 16 mcg or greater. A report of "resistant" from the laboratory indicates that the infection organism is not likely to respond to therapy.

Zones greater than 14 mm and less than 18 mm, or MIC's of greater than 16 mcg and less than 65 mcg, indicate intermediate susceptibility. A report of "intermediate" susceptibility suggests that the organism would be susceptible if the infection is confined to tissues and fluids (*e.g.,* urine), in which high antibiotic levels are attained.

CLINICAL PHARMACOLOGY: *(cont'd)*

Control organisms are recommended for susceptibility testing. Each time the test is performed one or more of the following organisms should be included: *Escherichia coli* ATCC 15922, *Staphylococcus aureus* ATCC 25923 and *Pseudomonas aeruginosa* ATCC 27853. The control organisms should produce zones of inhibition with the following ranges:

Escherichia coli (ATCC 15922)—22-30 mm

Staphylococcus aureus (ATCC 25923)—22-31 mm

Pseudomonas aeruginosa (ATCC 27853)—17-23 mm

INDICATIONS AND USAGE:

Kanamycin is indicated in the short term treatment of serious infections caused by susceptible strains of the designated microorganisms below. Bacteriological studies to identify the causative organisms and to determine their susceptibility to kanamycin should be performed. Therapy may be instituted prior to obtaining the results of susceptibility testing.

Kanamycin may be considered as initial therapy in the treatment of infection where one or more of the following are the known or suspected pathogens. *E. coli, Proteus* species (both indole-positive and indole-negative), *Enterobacter aerogenes, Klebsiella pneumoniae, Serratia marcescens, Acinetobacter* species. The decision to continue therapy with the drug should be based on results of the susceptibility tests, the response of the infection to therapy, and the important additional concepts contained in the BOXED WARNING.

In serious infections when the causative organisms are unknown, kanamycin sulfate may be administered as initial therapy in conjunction with an penicillin or cephalosporin-type drug before obtaining results of susceptibility testing. If anaerobic organisms are suspected, consideration should be given to using other suitable antimicrobial therapy in conjunction with kanamycin.

Although kanamycin is not the drug of choice for staphylococcal infections, it may be indicated under certain conditions for the treatment of known or suspected staphylococcal disease. These situations include the initial therapy of server infections where the organism is thought to be either a Gram-negative bacterium or a staphylococcus, infections due to susceptible strains of staphylococci in patients allergic to other antibiotics, and mixed staphylococcal/Gram-negative infections.

CONTRAINDICATIONS:

A history of hypersensitivity or toxic reactions to one aminoglycoside may also contraindicate the use of any other aminoglycoside, because of the known cross-sensitivity and cumulative effects of drugs in this category.

THIS DRUG IS NOT INDICATED IN LONG-TERM THERAPY (*e.g.,* Tuberculosis) BECAUSE OF THE TOXIC HAZARD ASSOCIATED WITH EXTENDED ADMINISTRATION.

WARNINGS:

See BOXED WARNING.

Aminoglycosides can cause fetal harm when administered to pregnant women. Aminoglycoside antibiotics cross the placenta and there have been several reports of total, irreversible, bilateral congenital deafness in children whose mothers received streptomycin during pregnancy. Although serious side effects to fetus or new born have not been reported in treatment of pregnant women with other aminoglycosides, the potential for harm exists.

Reproductive studies have been performed in rats and rabbits and have revealed no evidence of impaired fertility or teratogenic effects. Dosages of 200 mg/kg/day in pregnant rats and pregnant cayenne pigs led to hearing impairment in the off-spring. There are not well-controlled studies in pregnant women but clinical experience does not include any positive evidence of adverse effects on the fetus. However, if the drug is used during pregnancy, or if the patient becomes pregnant while taking this drug, the patient should be apprised of the potential hazard on the fetus.

Contains sodium bisulfite, a sulfite that may cause allergic-type reactions including anaphylactic symptoms and life-threatening or less severe asthmatic episodes in certain susceptible people. The overall prevalence of sulfite sensitivity in the general population is unknown and probably low. Sulfite sensitivity is seen more frequently in asthmatic than in nonasthmatic people.

PRECAUTIONS:

GENERAL

Neurotoxic and nephrotoxic antibiotics may be almost completely absorbed from body surfaces (except that urinary bladder) after local irrigation and after topical application during surgical procedures. The potential toxic effects of antibiotics administered in this fashion (oto-and nephrotoxicity, neuromuscular blockade, respiratory paralysis) should be considered. (See BOXED WARNING.)

Increased nephrotoxicity has been reported following concomitant administration of aminoglycoside antibiotics with some cephalosporins.

Aminoglycosides should be used with caution in patients with neuromuscular disorders such as myasthenia gravis, Parkinsonism, or infant botulism, since these drugs may aggravate muscle weakness because of their potential curare-like effect on neuromuscular junction.

Elderly patients may have a decrease in renal function which may not be evident in the results of routine screening tests, such as BUN or serum creatine levels. Measurement of creatinine clearance or an estimate based on published nomograms or equations may be more useful. Monitoring of renal function during treatment with kanamycin as with other aminoglycosides, is particularly important in such patients.

Because of high concentrations of kanamycin sulfate in the urinary excretory system, patients should be well hydrated before treatment to prevent irritation of the renal tubules.

NOTE : The risk of toxic reactions is low in well-hydrated patients with normal kidney function, who receive a total dose of 15 g of kanamycin or less. Treatment with kanamycin may result in overgrowth of nonsusceptible organisms. If this occurs kanamycin should be discontinued and appropriate therapy initiated.

LABORATORY TESTS

Tests of eighth cranial nerve functions: Serial audiometric tests are suggested, particularly when renal function is impaired and/or prolonged aminoglycoside therapy is required; such tests should also be repeated periodically after treatment if there is evidence of a hearing deficit or vestibular abnormalities before or during therapy or when consecutive or concomitant use of other potentially ototoxic drug is unavoidable.

Test of renal functio:n It should be emphasized that since renal function may after appreciably during therapy, renal function should be tested daily or more frequently. Urine should be examined for increased excretion of protein and for presence of cells and casts, keeping in mind the effects of the primary illness on these tests. One or more of the following laboratory measurements should be obtained at the onset of therapy, frequently during therapy, and at, or shortly after, the end of therapy:

Creatinine clearance rate (either carefully measured or estimated from published nomograms or equations based on patient's age, sex, body weight, and serial creatinine concentrations) (preferred over BUN).

PRECAUTIONS: *(cont'd)*

Serum creatinine concentration (preferred over BUN).

Blood urea nitrogen (BUN).

More frequent testing is desirable if renal function is changing. If sings of renal irritation appear, such as casts, white or red cells, and albumin, hydration should be increased and a reduction in dosage may be desirable (see DOSAGE AND ADMINISTRATION.) These signs usually disappear when treatment is completed. However, if azotemia or a progressive decrease of urine output occurs, treatment should be stopped.

LABORATORY TEST INTERACTIONS

Concomitant cephalosporin therapy may spuriously elevate creatinine determinations.

The inactivation between aminoglycosides and beta-lactam antibiotics described in DRUG INTERACTIONS may continue in specimens of body fluids collected for assay, resulting in inaccurate, false low aminoglycoside readings. Such specimens should be properly handled, i.e. assayed promptly, frozen, or treated with beta-lactamase.

CARCINOGENESIS, MUTAGENESIS, AND IMPAIRMENT OF FERTILITY

Studies have not been performed with kanamycin to determine its effect in carcinogenesis, mutagenesis, or impairment of fertility.

PREGNANCY CATEGORY D

See WARNINGS.

NURSING MOTHERS

Kanamycin sulfate is excreted in minute amounts in human milk. Because of the potential for serious adverse reactions from aminoglycosides in nursing infants, a decision should be made whether to discontinue nursing or to discontinue the drug taking into account the importance of the drug to the mother.

PEDIATRIC USE

Aminoglycosides should be used with caution in prematures and neonates because of the renal immaturity of these patients and the resulting prolongation of serum half-life of these drugs.

DRUG INTERACTIONS:

In vitro mixing of an aminoglycoside with beta-lactam-type antibiotics (penicillins or cephalosporins) may result in a significant mutual inactivation. Even when an aminoglycoside and a penicillin-type drug are administered separately by different routes, a reduction in aminoglycoside serum half-life or serum levels has been reported in patients with impaired renal function and in some patients with normal renal function. Usually, such inactivation of the aminoglycoside is clinically significant only in patients with severely impaired renal function. (See Laboratory Test Interactions). See BOXED WARNING regarding concurrent use of potent diuretics, concurrent and/or sequential use of other neurotoxic and/or nephrotoxic antibiotics, and for other essential information.

ADVERSE REACTIONS:

Kanamycin has the potential to induce auditory and sometimes vestibular toxicity, renal toxicity, and neuromuscular blockade. The risks are higher for patients with a present or past history of renal impairment (especially if hemodialysis is required), for those receiving concomitant or sequential treatment with other ototoxic or nephrotoxic drugs or rapid acting diuretic agents given intravenously (ethacrynic acid, furosemide, and mannitol), and for patients treated for longer periods and/or with higher doses than recommended.

Ototoxicity: Toxic effects of kanamycin on the eighth cranial never can result in partially reversible or irreversible bilateral loss of hearing, loss of balance, or both. Tinnitus or vertigo may or may not be experienced. Cochlear damage is usually manifested initially by small changes in audiometric test results at the high frequencies and may not be associated with subjective hearing loss. Vestibular dysfunction is usually manifested by nystagmus, vertigo, nausea, vomiting, or acute Meniere's syndrome.

Nephrotoxicity: Albuminuria, presence of red and white cells, and granular casts: azotemia and oliguria have been reported. Renal function changes are usually reversible when the drug is discontinued. Renal impairment may be characterized by a rise in serum creatinine and may be accompanied by oliguria, presence of casts, cells, and protein in the urine, by rising levels of BUN or by decrease in creatinine clearance.

Neuromuscular Blockade: Acute muscular paralysis and apnea can occur following treatment with aminoglycoside antibiotics. Neurotoxicity can occur after intrapleural and interperitoneal instillation of large doses of an aminoglycoside; however, the reaction has followed intravenous, intramuscular, and even the oral administration of these agents.

Other: Some local irritation or pain may follow the intramuscular injection of kanamycin. Other adverse reactions of the drug reported on rare occasions are skin rash, drug fever, headache, paresthesia, nausea, vomiting, and diarrhea. The "malabsorption syndrome" characterized by an increase in fecal fat, decrease in serum carotene, and fall in xylose absorption, reportedly has occurred with prolonged therapy.

OVERDOSAGE:

In the event of overdosage or toxic reaction, hemodialysis or peritoneal dialysis will aid in the removal of kanamycin from the blood. In the newborn infant, exchange transfusion may also be considered.

DOSAGE AND ADMINISTRATION:

Kanamycin Injection may be given intramuscularly or intravenously. The patient's pretreatment body weight should be obtained for calculation of the correct dosage. The dosage of an aminoglycoside in obese patients should be based on an estimate of the lean body mass. The status of renal function should be determined by measurement of serum creatinine concentration or calculation of the endogenous creatinine clearance rate. The blood urea nitrogen (BUN) level is much less reliable for this purpose. Renal function should be reassessed frequently during therapy.

It is desirable to measure both peak and trough serum concentrations intermittently during therapy since both concentrations are used to determine the adequacy and safety of the dose and to adjust the dosage during treatment. Peak serum concentrations (30 to 90 minutes after injection) above 35 mcg per ml and trough concentrations (just prior to the next dose) above 10 mcg per ml should be avoided.

Intramuscular Route: Inject deeply into the upper outer quadrant of e gluteal muscle. The recommended dose for adults or children is 15 mg/kg/day in two equally divided dosages administered at equally divided intervals; i.e. 7.5 mg/kg g 12h. If continuously high blood levels are desired, the daily dose of 15 mg/kg may be given in equally divided doses every 6 or 8 hours. Treatment of patients in the heavier weight classes, i.e. 100 kg, should not exceed 1.5 g/day.

In patients with impaired renal function, it is desirable to follow therapy by appropriate serum assays. If this is not feasible, a suggested method is to reduce the frequency of administration in patients with renal dysfunction. The interval between doses may be calculated with the following formula:

DOSAGE AND ADMINISTRATION: *(cont'd)*

Serum creatinine (mg/100 ml) x 9 = Dosage Interval (in hours); e.g., if the serum creatinine is 2 mg, the recommended dose (7.5 mg/kg) should be administered every 18 hours. Changes in creatinine concentration during therapy would, of course, necessitate changes in the dosage frequency.

It is desirable to limit the duration of treatment with kanamycin to short term. The usual duration of treatment is 7 to 10 days. Total daily dose by all routes of administration should not exceed 1.5 g/day. If longer therapy is required, measurement of kanamycin peak and trough serum concentrations is particularly important as a basis for determining the adequacy and safety of the dose. These patients should be carefully monitored for changes in renal, auditory, and vestibular function. Dosage should be adjusted as needed. The risks of toxicity multiply as the length of treatment increases.

At the recommended dosage level, uncomplicated infections due to kanamycin-susceptible organisms should respond to therapy in 24 to 48 hours. If definite clinical response dose not occur within 3 to 5 days, therapy should be stopped and the antibiotic susceptibility pattern of the invading organism should be rechecked. Failure of the infection to respond may be due to resistance of the organism or to the presence of septic foci requiring surgical drainage.

Intravenous Administration: The dose should not exceed 15 mg/kg per day and must be administered slowly. The solution for intravenous use is prepared by adding the contents of a 500-mg vial to 100 to 200 ml of sterile diluent such as Normal Saline or 5% Dextrose in Water, or the contents of a 1.0-g vial to 200 to 400 ml of sterile diluent. The appropriate dose is administered over a 30- to 60-minute period. The total daily dose should be divided into 2 or 3 equally divided doses.

In pediatric patients the amount of diluent used should be sufficient to infuse the kanamycin sulfate over a 30- to 60-minute period.

Kanamycin sulfate injection. USP should both be physically mixed with other antibacterial agents but each should be administered separately in accordance with its recommended route of administration and dosage schedule.

Intraperitoneal Use: (Following exploration for established peritonitis or after peritoneal contamination due to fecal spill during surgery).

Adults: 500 mg diluted in 20 ml sterile distilled water may be instilled through a polyethylene catheter sutured into the wound at closure. If possible, instillation should be postponed until the patient has fully recovered from the effects of anesthesia and muscle-relaxing drugs (see duration of treatmentBOXED WARNING.) Serum levels should be carefully monitored during treatment.

Aerosol Treatment: 250 mg 2 to 4 times a day. Withdraw 250 mg (1.0 ml) from a 500-mg vial and dilute it with 3 ml Physiological Saline and nebulize. Serum levels should be carefully monitored during treatment.

Other Routes of Administration: Kanamycin sulfate Injection in concentrations of 0.25 percent (2.5 mg/ml) has been used as an irrigating solution in abscess cavities, pleural space, peritoneal and ventricular cavities. Possible absorption of Kanamycin sulfate by such routes must be taken into account and dosage adjustments should be arranged so that a maximum total dose of 1.5 g/day by all routes of administration is not exceeded. Serum levels should be carefully monitored during treatment (TABLE 1):

TABLE 1 Pediatric Dosage Guide For Kanamycin Sulfate Pediatric Injection, 75 mg/2 ml - Amount Per 24 Hours To Be Given In Divided Doses

Weight in pounds	Weight in Kilograms	Daily Dosage in Milligrams	Daily Dosage in Milliliters
2.2	1.00	15.0	0.4
2.8	1.25	18.8	0.5
3.3	1.50	22.5	0.6
3.9	1.75	26.2	0.7
4.4	2.00	30.0	0.8
5.0	2.25	33.8	0.9
5.5	2.50	37.5	1.0
6.0	2.75	41.2	1.1
6.6	3.00	45.0	1.2
7.7	3.50	52.5	1.4
8.8	4.00	60.0	1.6
9.9	4.50	67.5	1.8
11.0	5.00	75.0	2.0

STABILITY

Occasionally, some vials may darken during the shelf life of the product, but this does not indicate a loss of potency.

Parenteral drug products should be inspected visually for particulate matter and discoloration prior to administration, whenever container and solution permit.

(Apothecon, 6/90, 3502DIM-13

HOW SUPPLIED - RATED THERAPEUTICALLY EQUIVALENT:

Injection, Solution - Intramuscular; - 1 gm/3ml

3 ml	**$9.49**	**KANTREX, Mead Johnson**	**00015-3503-20**
3 ml	$238.13	Kanamycin Sulfate Inj 1, Solopak Labs	39769-0063-05

Injection, Solution - Intramuscular; - 75 mg/2ml

2 ml	**$3.04**	**KANTREX PEDIATRIC, Mead Johnson**	**00015-3512-20**
2 ml x 10	$15.00	Kanamycin Sulfate, Voluntary Hosp	53258-9600-01
2 ml x 10	$50.63	PEDIATRIC KANAMYCIN SULFATE INJ 75, Solopak Labs	39769-0065-02

Injection, Solution - Intramuscular; - 500 mg/2ml

2 ml	**$4.80**	**KANTREX, Mead Johnson**	**00015-3502-20**
2 ml	**$11.39**	**KANTREX, Mead Johnson**	**00015-3502-94**
2 ml	$111.25	Kanamycin Sulfate Inj 500, Solopak Labs	39769-0064-02

HOW SUPPLIED - NOT RATED EQUIVALENT:

Capsule, Gelatin - Oral - 0.5 gm

20's	**$41.30**	**KANTREX, Mead Johnson**	**00015-3506-25**
100's	**$198.29**	**KANTREX, Mead Johnson**	**00015-3506-60**

KETAMINE HYDROCHLORIDE *(001604)*

CATEGORIES: Anesthesia; Anxiolytics, Sedatives, Hypnotic; Central Nervous System Agents; General Anesthetics; Injectable Anesthetics; FDA Approval Pre 1982

BRAND NAMES: *Calypsol*; *Ketalin* (Mexico); **Ketalar**; *Ketamax*; *Ketanest* (Germany); *Ketava*; *Ketmin*; *Ketolar*, *Petar*, *Soon-Soon*
(International brand names outside U.S. in italics)

FORMULARIES: WHO **SPECIAL NOTE**

EMERGENCE REACTIONS HAVE OCCURRED IN APPROXIMATELY 12 PERCENT OF PATIENTS.

THE PSYCHOLOGICAL MANIFESTATIONS VARY IN SEVERITY BETWEEN PLEASANT DREAM-LIKE STATES, VIVID IMAGERY, HALLUCINATIONS, AND EMERGENCE DELIRIUM. IN SOME CASES THESE STATES HAVE BEEN ACCOMPANIED BY CONFUSION, EXCITEMENT, AND IRRATIONAL BEHAVIOR WHICH A FEW PATIENTS RECALL AS AN UNPLEASANT EXPERIENCE. THE DURATION ORDINARILY IS NO MORE THAN A FEW HOURS; IN A FEW CASES, HOWEVER, RECURRENCES HAVE TAKEN PLACE UP TO 24 HOURS POSTOPERATIVELY. NO RESIDUAL PSYCHOLOGICAL EFFECTS ARE KNOWN TO HAVE RESULTED FROM USE OF KETALAR.

THE INCIDENCE OF THESE EMERGENCE PHENOMENA IS LEAST IN THE YOUNG (15 YEARS OF AGE OR LESS) AND ELDERLY (OVER 65 YEARS OF AGE) PATIENT. ALSO, THEY ARE LESS FREQUENT WHEN THE DRUG IS GIVEN INTRAMUSCULARLY AND THE INCIDENCE IS REDUCED AS EXPERIENCE WITH THE DRUG IS GAINED.

THE INCIDENCE OF PSYCHOLOGICAL MANIFESTATIONS DURING EMERGENCE, PARTICULARLY DREAM-LIKE OBSERVATIONS AND EMERGENCE DELIRIUM, MAY BE REDUCED BY USING LOWER RECOMMENDED DOSAGES OF KETALAR IN CONJUNCTION WITH INTRAVENOUS DIAZEPAM DURING INDUCTION AND MAINTENANCE OF ANESTHESIA. (See DOSAGE AND ADMINISTRATION.) ALSO, THESE REACTIONS MAY BE REDUCED IF VERBAL, TACTILE AND VISUAL STIMULATION OF THE PATIENT IS MINIMIZED DURING THE RECOVERY PERIOD. THIS DOES NOT PRECLUDE THE MONITORING OF VITAL SIGNS.

IN ORDER TO TERMINATE A SEVERE EMERGENCE REACTION THE USE OF A SMALL HYPNOTIC DOSE OF A SHORT-ACTING OR ULTRASHORT-ACTING BARBITURATE MAY BE REQUIRED.

WHEN KETALAR IS USED ON AN OUTPATIENT BASIS, THE PATIENT SHOULD NOT BE RELEASED UNTIL RECOVERY FROM ANESTHESIA IS COMPLETE AND THEN SHOULD BE ACCOMPANIED BY A RESPONSIBLE ADULT.

DESCRIPTION:

KETALAR IS A NONBARBITURATE ANESTHETIC CHEMICALLY DESIGNATED *DL*2-(O-CHLOROPHENYL)-2-(METHYLAMINO) CYCLOHEXANONE HYDROCHLORIDE. IT IS FORMULATED AS A SLIGHTLY ACID (PH 3.5-5.5) STERILE SOLUTION FOR INTRAVENOUS OR INTRAMUSCULAR INJECTION IN CONCENTRATIONS CONTAINING THE EQUIVALENT OF EITHER 10, 50 OR 100 MG KETAMINE BASE PER MILLILITER AND CONTAINS NOT MORE THAN 0.1 MG/ML PHEMEROL (BENZETHONIUM CHLORIDE) ADDED AS A PRESERVATIVE. THE 10 MG/ML SOLUTION HAS BEEN MADE ISOTONIC WITH SODIUM CHLORIDE.

CLINICAL PHARMACOLOGY:

Ketalar is a rapid-acting general anesthetic producing an anesthetic state characterized by profound analgesia, normal pharyngeal-laryngeal reflexes, normal or slightly enhanced skeletal muscle tone, cardiovascular and respiratory stimulation, and occasionally a transient and minimal respiratory depression.

A patient airway is maintained partly by virtue of unimpaired pharyngeal and laryngeal reflexes. See WARNINGS and PRECAUTIONS.

The biotransformation of Ketalar includes N-dealkylation (metabolite I), hydroxylation of the cyclohexone ring (metabolites III and IV), conjugation with glucuronic acid and dehydration of the hydroxylated metabolites to form the cyclohexene derivative (metabolite II).

Following intravenous administration, the ketamine concentration has an initial slope (alpha phase) lasting about 45 minutes with a half-life of 10 to 15 minutes. This first phase corresponds clinically to the anesthetic effect of the drug. The anesthetic action is terminated by a combination of redistribution from the CNS to slower equilibrating peripheral tissues and by hepatic biotransformation to metabolite I. This metabolite is about as active as ketamine in reducing halothane requirements (MAC) of the rat. The later half-life of ketamine (beta phase) is 2.5 hours.

The anesthetic state produced by Ketalar has been termed "dissociative anesthesia" in that it appears to selectively interrupt association pathways of the brain before producing somesthetic sensory blockade. It may selectively depress the thalamoneocortical system before significantly obtunding the more ancient cerebral centers and pathways (reticular-activating and limbic systems).

Elevation of blood pressure begins shortly after injection, reaches a maximum within a few minutes and usually returns to preanesthetic values within 15 minutes after injection. In the majority of cases, the systolic and diastolic blood pressure peaks from 10% to 50% above preanesthetic levels shortly after induction of anesthesia, but the elevation can be higher or longer in individual cases (see CONTRAINDICATIONS).

Ketamine has a wide margin of safety; several instances of unintentional administration of overdoses of Ketalar (up to ten times that usually required) have been followed by prolonged but complete recovery.

Ketalar has been studied in over 12,000 operative and diagnostic procedures, involving over 10,000 patients from 105 separate studies. During the course of these studies Ketalar was administered as the sole agent, as induction for other general agents, or to supplement low-potency agents.

Specific areas of application have included the following:

1. debridement, painful dressings, and skin grafting in burn patients, as well as other superficial surgical procedures.

2. neurodiagnostic procedures such as pneumoencephalograms, ventriculograms, myelograms, and lumbar punctures. See also Precaution concerning increased intracranial pressure.

3. diagnostic and operative procedures of the eye, ear, nose, and mouth, including dental extractions.

4. diagnostic and operative procedures of the pharynx, larynx, or bronchial tree. NOTE: Muscle relaxants, with proper attention to respiration, may be required (see PRECAUTIONS).

5. sigmoidoscopy and minor surgery of the anus and rectum, and circumcision.

6. extraperitoneal procedures used in gynecology such as dilatation and curettage.

7. orthopedic procedures such as closed reductions, manipulations, femoral pinning, amputations, and biopsies.

8. as an anesthetic in poor-risk patients with depression of vital functions.

9. in procedures where the intramuscular route of administration is preferred.

10. in cardiac catheterization procedures.

In these studies, the anesthesia was rated either "excellent" or "good" by the anesthesiologist and the surgeon at 90% and 93%, respectively; rated "fair" at 6% and 4%, respectively; and rated "poor" at 4% and 3%, respectively. In a second method of evaluation, the anesthesia was rated "adequate" in at least 90%, and "inadequate" in 10% or less of the procedures.

INDICATIONS AND USAGE:

Ketalar is indicated as the sole anesthetic agent for diagnostic and surgical procedures that do not require skeletal muscle relaxation. Ketalar is best suited for short procedures but it can be used, with additional doses, for longer procedures.

Ketalar is indicated for the induction of anesthesia prior to the administration of other general anesthetic agents.

Ketalar is indicated to supplement low-potency agents, such as nitrous oxide.

Specific areas of application are described in the Clinical Pharmacology section.

CONTRAINDICATIONS:

Ketamine hydrochloride is contraindicated in those in whom a significant elevation of blood pressure would constitute a serious hazard and in those who have shown hypersensitivity to the drug.

WARNINGS:

Cardiac function should be continually monitored during the procedure in patients found to have hypertension or cardiac decompensation.

Postoperative confusional states may occur during the recovery period. (See Special Note.)

Respiratory depression may occur with overdosage or too rapid a rate of administration of Ketalar, in which case supportive ventilation should be employed. Mechanical support of respiration is preferred to administration of analeptics.

PRECAUTIONS:

GENERAL

Ketalar should be used by or under the direction of physicians experienced in administering general anesthetics and in maintenance of an airway and in the control of respiration.

Because pharyngeal and laryngeal reflexes are usually active, Ketalar should not be used alone in surgery or diagnostic procedures of the pharynx, larynx, or bronchial tree. Mechanical stimulation of the pharynx should be avoided, whenever possible, if Ketalar is used alone. Muscle relaxants, with proper attention to respiration, may be required in both of these instances.

Resuscitative equipment should be ready for use.

The incidence of emergence reactions may be reduced if verbal and tactile stimulation of the patient is minimized during the recovery period. This does not preclude the monitoring of vital signs (see Special Note).

The intravenous dose should be administered over a period of 60 seconds. More rapid administration may result in respiratory depression or apnea and enhanced pressor response.

In surgical procedures involving visceral pain pathways, Ketalar should be supplemented with an agent which obtunds visceral pain.

Use with caution in the chronic alcoholic and the acutely alcohol-intoxicated patient.

An increase in cerebrospinal fluid pressure has been reported following administration of ketamine hydrochloride. Use with extreme caution in patients with preanesthetic elevated cerebrospinal fluid pressure.

INFORMATION FOR THE PATIENT

As appropriate, especially in cases where early discharge is possible, the duration of Ketalar and other drugs employed during the conduct of anesthesia should be considered. The patients should be cautioned that driving an automobile, operating hazardous machinery or engaging in hazardous activities should not be undertaken for 24 hours or more (depending upon the dosage of Ketalar and consideration of other drugs employed) after anesthesia.

PREGNANCY

Since the safe use in pregnancy, including obstetrics (either vaginal or abdominal delivery), has not been established, such use is not recommended (see Animal Reproduction).

DRUG INTERACTIONS:

Prolonged recovery time may occur if barbiturates and/or narcotics are used concurrently with Ketalar.

Ketalar is clinically compatible with the commonly used general and local anesthetic agents when an adequate respiratory exchange is maintained.

ADVERSE REACTIONS:

Cardiovascular: Blood pressure and pulse rate are frequently elevated following administration of Ketalar alone. However, hypotension and bradycardia have been observed. Arrhythmia has also occurred.

Respiration: Although respiration is frequently stimulated, severe depression of respiration or apnea may occur following rapid intravenous administration of high doses of Ketalar. Laryngospasms and other forms of airway obstruction have occurred during Ketalar anesthesia.

Eye: Diplopia and nystagmus have been noted following Ketalar administration.

It also may cause a slight elevation in intraocular pressure measurement.

Psychological: (See Special Note.)

Neurological: In some patients, enhanced skeletal muscle tone may be manifested by tonic and clonic movements sometimes resembling seizures (see DOSAGE AND ADMINISTRATION).

Gastrointestinal: Anorexia, nausea and vomiting have been observed; however this is not usually severe and allows the great majority of patients to take liquids by mouth shortly after regaining consciousness (see DOSAGE AND ADMINISTRATION).

General: Local pain and exanthema at the injection site have infrequently been reported. Transient erythema and/or morbilliform rash have also been reported.

OVERDOSAGE:

Respiratory depression may occur with overdosage or too rapid a rate of administration of Ketalar, in which case supportive ventilation should be employed. Mechanical support of respiration is preferred to administration of analeptics.

DOSAGE AND ADMINISTRATION:

Note: Barbiturates and Ketalar, being chemically incompatible because of precipitate formation, *should not* be injected from the same syringe.

If the Ketalar dose is augmented with diazepam, the two drugs must be given separately. Do not mix Ketalar and diazepam in syringe or infusion flask. For additional information on the use of diazepam, refer to the Warnings and DOSAGE AND ADMINISTRATIONSections of the diazepam insert.

PREOPERATIVE PREPARATIONS

1. While vomiting has been reported following Ketalar administration, some airway protection may be afforded because of active laryngeal-pharyngeal reflexes. However, since aspiration may occur with Ketalar and since protective reflexes may also be diminished by

DOSAGE AND ADMINISTRATION: *(cont'd)*

supplementary anesthetics and muscle relaxants, the possibility of aspiration must be considered. Ketalar is recommended for use in the patient whose stomach is not empty when, in the judgment of the practitioner, the benefits of the drug outweigh the possible risks.

2. Atropine, scopolamine, or another drying agent should be given at an appropriate interval prior to induction.

ONSET AND DURATION

Because of rapid induction following the initial intravenous injection, the patient should be in a supported position during administration.

The onset of action of Ketalar is rapid; an intravenous dose of 2 mg/kg (1 mg/lb) of body weight usually produces surgical anesthesia within 30 seconds after injection, with the anesthetic effect usually lasting five to ten minutes. If a longer effect is desired, additional increments can be administered intravenously or intramuscularly to maintain anesthesia without producing significant cumulative effects.

Intramuscular doses, from experience primarily in children, in a range of 9 to 13 mg/kg (4 to 6 mg/lb) usually produce surgical anesthesia within 3 to 4 minutes following injection, with the anesthetic effect usually lasting 12 to 25 minutes.

DOSAGE

As with other general anesthetic agents, the individual response to Ketalar is somewhat varied depending on the dose, route of administration, and age of patient, so that dosage recommendation cannot be absolutely fixed. The drug should be titrated against the patient's requirements.

INDUCTION

Intravenous Route: The initial dose of Ketalar administered intravenously may range from 1 mg/kg to 4.5 mg/kg (0.5 to 2 mg/lb). The average amount required to produce five to ten minutes of surgical anesthesia has been 2 mg/kg (1 mg/lb).

Alternatively, in adult patients an induction dose of 1 mg to 2 mg/kg intravenous ketamine at a rate of 0.5 mg/kg/min may be used for induction of anesthesia. In addition, diazepam in 2 mg to 5 mg doses, administered in a separate syringe over 60 seconds, may be used. In most cases, 15 mg of intravenous diazepam *or less* will suffice. The incidence of psychological manifestations during emergence, particularly dream-like observations and emergence delirium, may be reduced by this induction dosage program.

Note: The 100 mg/ml concentration of Ketalar *should not* be injected intravenously without proper dilution. It is recommended the drug be diluted with an equal volume of either Sterile Water for Injection, USP, Normal Saline, or 5% Dextrose in Water.

Rate of Administration: It is recommended that Ketalar be administered slowly (over a period of 60 seconds). More rapid administration may result in respiratory depression and enhanced pressor response.

Intramuscular Route: The initial dose of Ketalar administered intramuscularly may range from 6.5 to 13 mg/kg (3 to 6 mg/lb). A dose of 10 mg/kg (5 mg/lb) will usually produce 12 to 25 minutes of surgical anesthesia.

MAINTENANCE OF ANESTHESIA

The maintenance dose should be adjusted according to the patient's anesthetic needs and whether an additional anesthetic agent is employed.

Increments of one-half to the full induction dose may be repeated as needed for maintenance of anesthesia. However, it should be noted that purposeless and tonic-clonic movements of extremities may occur during the course of anesthesia. These movements do not imply a light plane and are not indicative of the need for additional doses of the anesthetic.

It should be recognized that the larger the total dose of Ketalar administered, the longer will be the time to complete recovery.

Adult patients induced with Ketalar augmented with intravenous diazepam may be maintained on Ketalar given by slow microdrip infusion technique at a dose of 0.1 to 0.5 mg/minute, augmented with diazepam 2 to 5 mg administered intravenously as needed. In many cases 20 mg *or less*of intravenous diazepam total for combined induction and maintenance will suffice. However, slightly more diazepam may be required depending on the nature and duration of the operation, physical status of the patient, and other factors. The incidence of psychological manifestations during emergence, particularly dream-like observations and emergence delirium, may be reduced by this maintenance dosage program.

Dilution: To prepare a dilute solution containing 1 mg of ketamine per ml, aseptically transfer 10 ml (50 mg per ml Steri-Vial) or 5 ml (100 mg per ml Steri-Vial) to 500 ml of 5% Dextrose Injection, USP or Sodium Chloride (0.9%) Injection, USP (Normal Saline) and mix well. The resultant solution will contain 1 mg of ketamine per ml.

The fluid requirements of the patient and duration of anesthesia must be considered when selecting the appropriate dilution of Ketalar. If fluid restriction is required, Ketalar can be added to a 250 ml infusion as described above to provide a Ketalar concentration of 2 mg/ml.

Ketalar Steri-Vials, 10 mg/ml are not recommended for dilution.

SUPPLEMENTARY AGENTS

Ketalar is clinically compatible with the commonly used general and local anesthetic agents when an adequate respiratory exchange is maintained.

The regimen of a reduced dose of Ketalar supplemented with diazepam can be used to produce balanced anesthesia by combination with other agents such as nitrous oxide and oxygen.

ANIMAL PHARMACOLOGY:

Toxicity: The acute toxicity of Ketalar has been studied in several species. In mature mice and rats, the intraperitoneal LD_{50} values are approximately 100 times the average human intravenous dose and approximately 20 times the average human intramuscular dose. A slightly higher acute toxicity observed in neonatal rats was not sufficiently elevated to suggest an increased hazard when used in children. Daily intravenous injections in rats of five times the average human intravenous dose and intramuscular injections in dogs at four times the average human intramuscular dose demonstrated excellent tolerance for as long as 6 weeks. Similarly, twice weekly anesthetic sessions of one, three, or six hours' duration in monkeys over a four- to six-week period were well tolerated.

Interaction With Other Drugs Commonly Used For Preanesthetic Medication: Large doses (three or more times the equivalent effective human dose) of morphine, meperidine, and atropine increased the depth and prolonged the duration of anesthesia produced by a standard anesthetizing dose of Ketalar in Rhesus monkeys. The prolonged duration was not of sufficient magnitude to contraindicate the use of these drugs for preanesthetic medication in human clinical trials.

Blood Pressure: Blood pressure responses to Ketalar vary with the laboratory species and experimental conditions. Blood pressure is increased in normotensive and renal hypertensive rats with and without adrenalectomy and under pentobarbital anesthesia.

Intravenous Ketalar produces a fall in arterial blood pressure in the Rhesus monkey and a rise in arterial blood pressure in the dog. In this respect the dog mimics the cardiovascular effect observed in man. The pressor response to Ketalar injected into intact, unanesthetized dogs is accompanied by a tachycardia, rise in cardiac output and a fall in total peripheral

ANIMAL PHARMACOLOGY: *(cont'd)*

resistance. It causes a fall in perfusion pressure following a large dose injected into an artificially perfused vascular bed (dog hindquarters), and it has little or no potentiating effect upon vasoconstriction responses of epinephrine or norepinephrine. The pressor response to Ketalar is reduced or blocked by chlorpromazine (central depressant and peripheral α-adrenergic blockade), by β-adrenergic blockade, and by ganglionic blockade. The tachycardia and increase in myocardial contractile force seen in intact animals does not appear in isolated hearts (Langendorff) at a concentration of 0.1 mg of Ketalar nor in Starling dog heart-lung preparations at a Ketalar concentration of 50 mg/kg of HLP. These observations support the hypothesis that the hypertension produced by Ketalar is due to selective activation of central cardiac stimulating mechanisms leading to an increase in cardiac output. The dog myocardium is not sensitized to epinephrine and Ketalar appears to have a weak antiarrhythmic activity.

Metabolic Disposition: Ketalar is rapidly absorbed following parenteral administration. Animal experiments indicated that Ketalar was rapidly distributed into body tissues, with relatively high concentrations appearing in body fat, liver, lung, and brain; lower concentrations were found in the heart, skeletal muscle, and blood plasma. Placental transfer of the drug was found to occur in pregnant dogs and monkeys. No significant degree of binding to serum albumin was found with Ketalar.

Balance studies in rats, dogs, and monkeys resulted in the recovery of 85% to 95% of the dose in the urine, mainly in the form of degradation products. Small amounts of drug were also excreted in the bile and feces. Balance studies with tritium-labeled Ketalar in human subjects (1 mg/lb given intravenously) resulted in the mean recovery of 91% of the dose in the urine and 3% in the feces. Peak plasma levels averaged about 0.75 mcg/ml, and CSF levels were about 0.2 mcg/ml, 1 hour after dosing.

Ketalar undergoes N-demethylation and hydroxylation of the cyclohexanone ring, with the formation of water-soluble conjugates which are excreted in the urine. Further oxidation also occurs with the formation of a cyclohexanone derivative. The unconjugated N-demethylated metabolite was found to be less than one-sixth as potent as Ketalar. The unconjugated demethyl cyclohexanone derivative was found to be less than one-tenth as potent as Ketalar. Repeated doses of Ketalar administered to animals did not produce any detectable increase in microsomal enzyme activity.

Reproduction: Male and female rats, when given five times the average human intravenous dose of Ketalar for three consecutive days about one week before mating, had a reproductive performance equivalent to that of saline-injected controls. When given to pregnant rats and rabbits intramuscularly at twice the average human intramuscular dose during the respective periods of organogenesis, the litter characteristics were equivalent to those of saline-injected controls. A small group of rabbits was given a single large dose (six times the average human dose) of Ketalar on Day 6 of pregnancy to simulate the effect of an excessive clinical dose around the period of nidation. The outcome of pregnancy was equivalent in control and treated groups.

To determine the effect of Ketalar on the perinatal and postnatal period, pregnant rats were given twice the average human intramuscular dose during Days 18 to 21 of pregnancy. Litter characteristics at birth and through the weaning period were equivalent to those of the control animals. There was a slight increase in incidence of delayed parturition by one day in treated dams of this group. Three groups each of mated beagle bitches were given 2.5 times the average human intramuscular dose twice weekly for the three weeks of the first, second, and third trimesters of pregnancy, respectively, without the development of adverse effects in the pups.

HOW SUPPLIED - EQUIVALENTS NOT AVAILABLE:

Injection, Solution - Intramuscular; - 10 mg

20 ml	$96.29	KETALAR, Parke-Davis	00071-4581-12
50 ml	$156.58	KETALAR, Parke-Davis	00071-4581-15

Injection, Solution - Intramuscular; - 50 mg/ml

10 ml	$198.22	KETALAR, Parke-Davis	00071-4582-10

Injection, Solution - Intramuscular; - 100 mg

5 ml	$194.39	KETALAR 100, Parke-Davis	00071-4585-08

KETOCONAZOLE *(001605)*

CATEGORIES: Anti-Infectives; Antibiotics; Antifungals; Antimicrobials; Blastomycosis; Candidiasis; Candiduria; Coccidioidomycosis; Dandruff; Dermatitis; Dermatologicals; Fungal Agents; Fungal Infections; Histoplasmosis; Infections; Skin Infections; Skin/Mucous Membrane Agents; Thrush; Tinea Corporis; Tinea Cruris; Tinea Pedis; Tinea Versicolor; Topical; Cushing's Syndrome*; Prostatic Carcinoma*; Pregnancy Category C; Sales > $100 Million; FDA Approval Pre 1982; Patent Expiration 1999 Dec

* Indication not approved by the FDA

BRAND NAMES: *Akorazol* (Mexico); *Anfuhex*; *Aquarius*; *Conazol* (Mexico); *Formyco*; *Funazole*; *Funazole Tabs*; *Fungarest*; *Fungazol*; *Fungazol Tabs*; *Fungicide*; *Fungicide Tabs*; *Funginox*; *Funginox Tabs*; *Fungoral*; *Kenazol*; *Ketoconazol*; *Ketoderm* (France); *Ketoisdin*; *Ketomicon*; *Ketozol*; *Mycofebrin*; *Nazoltec* (Mexico); *Niz Creme*; *Niz Shampoo*; **Nizoral**; *Nizoral 2% Cream* (Australia); *Nizoral Cream and Tablets* (England, Mexico); *Nizoral Shampoo* (Australia, Germany); *Nizoral Tablets* (Australia, France, Mexico); *Nizoral Tabs and Cream*; *Panfungol*; *Pasalen*; *Spike*; *Sporozol*; *Termizol* (Mexico); *Unidox*; *Zoralin*; *Zoralin Tabs*
(International brand names outside U.S. in italics)

FORMULARIES: Aetna; BC-BS; Medi-Cal; PCS; WHO

COST OF THERAPY: $18.96 (Candidiasis; Tablet; 200 mg; 1/day; 7 days)

When used orally, ketoconazole has been associated with hepatic toxicity, including some fatalities. Patients receiving this drug should be informed by the physician of the risk and should be closely monitored. See WARNINGS and PRECAUTIONS.

Coadministration of terfenadine with ketoconazole tablets is contraindicated. Rare cases of serious cardiovascular adverse events including death, ventricular tachycardia and torsades de pointes have been observed in patients taking ketoconazole concomitantly with terfenadine, due to increased terfenadine concentrations induced by ketoconazole tablets. See CONTRAINDICATIONS, WARNINGS and PRECAUTIONS.

Pharmacokinetic data indicate that oral ketoconazole inhibits the metabolism of astemizole, resulting in elevated plasma levels of astemizole and its active metabolite desmethylastemizole which may prolong QT intervals. Coadministration of astemizole with ketoconazole tablets is therefore contraindicated. See CONTRAINDICATIONS, WARNINGS and PRECAUTIONS.

DESCRIPTION:

Ketoconazole is cis-1-acetyl-4-[4-[[2-(2,4-dichlorophenyl)-2-(1H-imidazol-1-ylmethyl)-1,3-dioxolan-4-yl]methoxyl]phenyl] piperazine.

DESCRIPTION: *(cont'd)*

Ketoconazole is a white to slightly beige, odorless powder, soluble in acids, with a molecular weight of 531.44.

Tablets: Ketoconazole is a synthetic broad-spectrum antifungal agent available in scored white tablets, each containing 200 mg ketoconazole base for oral administration. Inactive ingredients are colloidal silicon dioxide, corn starch, lactose, magnesium stearate, microcrystalline cellulose, and povidone.

Shampoo: Ketoconazole 2% Shampoo is a red-orange liquid for topical application, containing the broad-spectrum synthetic antifungal agent ketoconazole in a concentration of 2% in an aqueous suspension. It also contains: coconut fatty acid diethanolamide, disodium monolauryl ether sulfosuccinate, FD&C Red No. 40, hydrochloric acid, imidurea, laurdimonium hydrolyzed animal collagen, macrogol 120 methyl glucose dioleate, perfume bouquet, sodium chloride, sodium hydroxide, sodium lauryl ether sulphate, and purified water.

Cream: Ketoconazole 2% cream contains the broad-spectrum synthetic antifungal agent ketoconazole 2% formulated in an aqueous cream vehicle consisting of propylene glycol, stearyl and cetyl alcohols, sorbitan monostearate, polysorbate 60, isopropyl myristate, sodium sulfite anhydrous, polysorbate 80 and purified water.

CLINICAL PHARMACOLOGY:

TABLETS

Mean peak plasma levels of approximately 3.5 mcg/ml are reached within 1 to 2 hours, following oral administration of a single 200 mg dose taken with a meal. Subsequent plasma elimination is biphasic with half-life of 2 hours during the first 10 hours and 8 hours thereafter. Following absorption from the gastrointestinal tract, ketoconazole is converted into several inactive metabolites. The major identified metabolic pathways are oxidation and degradation of the imidazole and piperazine rings, oxidative O-dealkylation and aromatic hydroxylation. About 13% of the dose is excreted in the urine, of which 2 to 4% is unchanged drug. The major route of excretion is through the bile into the intestinal tract. *In vitro*, the plasma protein binding is about 99%, mainly to the albumin fraction. Only a negligible proportion of ketoconazole reaches the cerebral-spinal fluid. Ketoconazole is weak dibasic agent and thus requires acidity for dissolution and absorption.

Ketoconazole Tablets are active against clinical infections with*Blastomyces dermatitidis, Candida spp., Coccidioides immitis, Histoplasma capsulatum, Paracoccidioides brasiliensis,* and *Phialophora spp.* Ketoconazole Tablets are also active against*Trichophyton spp., Epidermophyton spp.,* and *Microsporum spp.* Ketoconazole is also active *in vitro* against a variety of fungi and yeast. In animal models, activity has been demonstrated against *Candida spp., Blastomyces dermatitidis, Histoplasma capsulatum, Malassezia furfur, Coccidioides immitis,* and *Cryptococcus neoformans.*

Mode of Action: *In vitro* studies suggest that Ketoconazole impairs the synthesis of ergosterol, which is a vital component of fungal cell membranes.

SHAMPOO

When ketoconazole 2% shampoo was applied dermally to intact or abraded skin of rabbits for 28 days at doses up to 50 mg/kg and allowed to remain one hour before being washed away, there were no detectable plasma ketoconazole levels using an assay method having a lower detection limit of 5 ng/ml. Ketoconazole was not detected in plasma in 39 patients who shampooed 4-10 times per week for 6 months or in 33 patients who shampooed 2-3 times per week for 3-26 months (mean: 16 months).

Twelve hours after a single shampoo, hair samples taken from six patients showed that high amounts of ketoconazole were present on the hair but only about 5% had penetrated into the hair keratin. Chronic shampooing (twice weekly for two months) increased the ketoconazole levels in the hair keratin to 20%, but did not increase levels on the hair. There were no detectable plasma levels.

An exaggerated use washing test on the sensitive antecubital skin of 10 subjects twice daily for five consecutive days showed that the irritancy potential of ketoconazole 2% shampoo was significantly less than that of 2.5% selenium sulfide shampoo.

A human sensitization test, a phototoxicity study, and a photoallergy study conducted in 38 male and 22 female volunteers showed no contact sensitization of the delayed hypersensitivity type, no phototoxicity and no photoallergic potential due to ketoconazole 2% shampoo.

Mode of Action: Interpretations of *in vivo* studies suggest that ketoconazole impairs the synthesis of ergosterol, which is a vital component of fungal cell membranes. It is postulated that the therapeutic effect of ketoconazole in dandruff is due to the reduction of*Pityrosporum ovale (Malassezia ovale)*, but this has not been proven. Support for this hypothesis comes from a 4-week double-blind, placebo controlled clinical trial in which the decrease in *P. ovale* on the scalp was significantly greater with ketoconazole (36 patients) than with placebo (20 patients) and was comparable to that with selenium sulfide (42 patients). In the same study, ketoconazole and selenium sulfide reduced the severity of adherent dandruff significantly more than placebo did. Ketoconazole produced significantly higher proportions of patients with at least 50% reductions in adherent dandruff (50% vs. 15%) and in loose dandruff (67% vs. 15%) than did the placebo.

Microbiology: Ketoconazole is a broad-spectrum synthetic antifungal agent which inhibits the growth of the following common dermatophytes and yeasts by altering the permeability of the cell membrane: dermatophytes: *Trichophyton rubrum, T. mentagrophytes, T. tonsurans, Microsporum canis, M. audouini, M. gypseum* and *Epidermophyton floccosum*; yeasts: *Candida albicans, C. tropicalis, Pityrosporum ovale (Malassezia ovale)* and *Pityrosporum orbiculare (M. furfur).* Development of resistance by these microorganisms to ketoconazole has not been reported.

CREAM

When ketoconazole 2% cream was applied dermally to intact or abraded skin of Beagle dogs for 28 consecutive days at a dose of 80 mg, there were no detectable plasma levels using an assay method having a lower detection limit of 2 ng/ml.

After a single topical application to the chest, back and arms of normal volunteers, systemic absorption of ketoconazole was not detected at the 5 ng/ml level in blood over a 72-hour period.

Two dermal irritancy studies, a human sensitization test, a phototoxicity study and a photoallergy study conducted in 38 male and 62 female volunteers showed no contact sensitization of the delayed hypersensitivity type, no irritation, no phototoxicity and no photoallergic potential due to ketoconazole 2% cream.

Microbiology: Ketoconazole is a broad spectrum synthetic antifungal agent which inhibits the *in vitro* growth of the following common dermatophytes and yeast by altering the permeability of the cell membrane: dermatophytes: *Trichophyton rubrum, T. mentagrophytes, T. tonsurans, Microsporum canis, M. audouini, M. gypseum* and *Epidermophyton floccosum;* yeasts: *Candida albicans, Malassezia ovale (pityrosporum ovale)* and *C. tropicalis;* and the organism responsible for tinea versicolor,*Malassezia furfur (Pityrosporum orbiculare).* Only those organisms listed in the INDICATIONS AND USAGE have been proven to be clinically affected. Development of resistance to ketoconazole has not been reported.

Mode of Action: *In vitro* studies suggest that ketoconazole impairs the synthesis of ergosterol, which is a vital component of fungal cell membranes. It is postulated that the therapeutic effect of ketoconazole in seborrheic dermatitis is due to the reduction of M. ovale, but this has not been proven.

INDICATIONS AND USAGE:

Tablets: Ketoconazole tablets are indicated for the treatment of the following systemic fungal infections: candidiasis, chronic mucocutaneous candidiasis, oral thrush, candiduria, blastomycosis, coccidioidomycosis, histoplasmosis, chromomycosis, and paracoccidioidomycosis. Ketoconazole should not be used for fungal meningitis because it penetrates poorly into the cerebral-spinal fluid.

Ketoconazole tablets are also indicated for the treatment of patients with severe recalcitrant cutaneous dermatophyte infections who have not responded to topical therapy or oral griseofulvin, or who are unable to take griseofulvin.

Shampoo: Ketoconazole 2% shampoo is indicated for the reduction of scaling due to dandruff.

Cream: Ketoconazole 2% cream is indicated for the topical treatment of tinea corporis, tinea cruris and tinea pedis caused by *Trichophyton rubrum, T. mentagrophytes,* (efficacy for this organism in this organ system was studied in fewer than ten infections), and *Epidermophyton floccosum;* in the treatment of tinea (pityriasis) versicolor caused by *Malassezia furfur (Pityrosporum orbiculare);* in the treatment of cutaneous candidiasis caused by *Candida spp.* and in the treatment of seborrheic dermatitis.

CONTRAINDICATIONS:

Tablets, Shampoo and Cream: Ketoconazole is contraindicated in patients who have shown hypersensitivity to the drug or excipients of the formulation(s).

Tablets: Coadministration of terfenadine or astemizole with ketoconazole tablets is contraindicated. (See BOXED WARNING, WARNINGS, and PRECAUTIONS.)

WARNINGS:

Tablets: Hepatotoxicity, primarily of the hepatocellular type, has been associated with the use of Ketoconazole Tablets, including rare fatalities. The reported incidence of hepatotoxicity has been about 1:10,000 exposed patients, but this probably represents some degree of under-reporting, as is the case for most reported adverse reactions to drugs. The median duration of ketoconazole therapy in patients who developed symptomatic hepatotoxicity was about 28 days, although the range extended to as low as 3 days. The hepatic injury has usually, but not always, been reversible upon discontinuation of ketoconazole treatment. Several cases of hepatitis have been reported in children.

Prompt recognition of liver injury is essential. Liver function tests (such as SGGT, alkaline phosphatase, SGPT, SGOT and bilirubin) should be measured before starting treatment and at frequent intervals during treatment. Patients receiving ketoconazole concurrently with other potentially hepatotoxic drugs should be carefully monitored, particularly those patients requiring prolonged therapy or those who have had a history of liver disease.

Most of the reported cases of hepatic toxicity have to date been in patients treated for onychomycosis. Of 180 patients worldwide developing idiosyncratic liver dysfunction during ketoconazole tablet therapy, 61.3% had onychomycosis and 16.8% had chronic recalcitrant dermatophytoses.

Transient minor elevations in liver enzymes have occurred during ketoconazole treatment. The drug should be discontinued if these persist, if the abnormalities worsen, or if the abnormalities become accompanied by symptoms of possible liver injury.

In rare cases anaphylaxis has been reported after the first dose. Several cases of hypersensitivity reactions including urticaria have also been reported.

Coadministration of ketoconazole tablets and terfenadine has led to elevated plasma concentrations of terfenadine which may prolong QT intervals, sometimes resulting in life-threatening cardiac dysrhythmias. Cases of torsades de pointes and other serious ventricular dysrhythmias, in rare cases leading to fatality, have been reported among patients taking terfenadine concurrently with ketoconazole tablets. Coadministration of ketoconazole tablets and terfenadine is contraindicated.

Coadministration of astemizole with ketoconazole tablets is contraindicated. (See BOXED WARNING, CONTRAINDICATIONS, and PRECAUTIONS.)

In European clinical trials involving 350 patients with metastatic prostatic cancer, eleven deaths were reported within two weeks of starting treatment with high dose of ketoconazole (1200 mg/day). It is not possible to ascertain from the information available whether death was related to ketoconazole therapy in these patients with serious underlying disease. However, high doses of ketoconazole tablets are known to suppress adrenal corticosteroid secretion.

In female rats treated three to six months with ketoconazole at dose levels of 80 mg/kg and higher, increased fragility of long bones, in some cases leading to fracture, was seen. The maximum "no effect" dose level in these studies was 20 mg/kg (2.5 times the maximum recommended human dose). The mechanisms responsible for this phenomenon is obscure. Limited studies in dogs failed to demonstrated such an effect on the metacarpals and ribs.

Cream: Ketoconazole 2% cream is not for ophthalmic use.

Ketoconazole 2% cream contains sodium sulfite anhydrous, a sulfite that may cause allergic-type reactions including anaphylactic symptoms and life-threatening or less severe asthmatic episodes in certain susceptible people. The overall prevalence of sulfite sensitivity in the general population is unknown, and probably low. Sulfite sensitivity is seen more frequently in asthmatic than in nonasthmatic people.

PRECAUTIONS:

GENERAL

Shampoo: If a reaction suggesting sensitivity or chemical irritation should occur, use of the medication should be discontinued.

Tablets: Ketoconazole tablets have been demonstrated to lower serum testosterone. Once therapy with ketoconazole has been discontinued, serum testosterone levels return to baseline values. Testosterone levels are impaired with doses of 800 mg per day and abolished by 1600 mg per day. Ketoconazole also decrease ACTH induced corticosteroid serum levels at similar high doses. The recommended dose of 200 mg - 400 mg daily should be followed closely.

In four subjects with drug-induced achlorhydria, a marked reduction in ketoconazole absorption was observed. Ketoconazole tablets require acidity for dissolution. If concomitant antacids, anticholinergics, and H_2-blockers are needed, they should be given at least two hours after administration of ketoconazole Tablets. In cases of achlorhydria, the patients should be instructed to dissolve each tablet in 4 ml aqueous solution of 0.2 N HCl. For ingesting the resulting mixture, they should use a drinking straw so as to avoid contact with the teeth. This administration should be followed with a cup of tap water.

INFORMATION FOR THE PATIENT

Shampoo: May be irritating to mucous membranes of the eyes and contact with this area should be avoided.

There have been reports that use of the shampoo resulted in removal of the curl from permanently waved hair.

Tablet: Patients should be instructed to report any signs and symptoms which may suggest liver dysfunction so that appropriate biochemical testing can be done. Such signs and symptoms may include unusual fatigue, anorexia, nausea and/or vomiting, jaundice, dark urine or pale stools (see WARNINGS.)

PRECAUTIONS: *(cont'd)*

CARCINOGENESIS, MUTAGENESIS, AND IMPAIRMENT OF FERTILITY

The dominant lethal mutation test in male and female mice revealed that single oral doses of ketoconazole as high as 80 mg/kg produce no mutation in any stage of germ cell development. The *Ames Salmonella* microsomal activator assay was also negative. A long term feeding study in Swiss Albino mice and in Wistar rats showed no evidence of oncogenic activity.

PREGNANCY, TERATOGENIC EFFECTS, PREGNANCY CATEGORY C

Ketoconazole has been shown to be teratogenic (syndactylia and oligodactylia) in the rate when given in the diet at 80 mg/kg/day, (10 times the maximum recommended human dose). However, these effects may be related to maternal toxicity, evidence of which also was seen at this and higher dose levels.

There are no adequate and well controlled studies in pregnant women.

Ketoconazole should be used during pregnancy only if the potential benefit justifies the potential risk to the fetus.

Shampoo: Ketoconazole is not detected in plasma after chronic shampooing.

Tablets: *Nonteratogenic Effects:* Ketoconazole has also been found to be embryotoxic in the rat when given in the diet at doses higher than 80 mg/kg during the first trimester of gestation.

In addition, dystocia (difficult labor) was noted in rats administered oral ketoconazole during the third trimester of gestation. This occurred when ketoconazole was administered at doses higher than 10 mg/kg (higher than 1.25 times the maximum human dose).

It is likely that both the malformations and the embryotoxicity resulting from the administration of oral ketoconazole during gestation are a reflection of the particular sensitivity of the female rat to this drug. For example, the oral LD_{50}, of ketoconazole given by gavage to the female rat is 166 mg/kg whereas in the male rat the oral LD_{50} is 287 mg/kg.

NURSING MOTHERS

Cream: It is not known whether ketoconazole 2% cream administered topically could result in sufficient systemic absorption to produce detectable quantities in breast milk. Nevertheless, a decision should be made whether to discontinue nursing or discontinue the drug, taking into account the importance of the drug to the mother.

Shampoo: Ketoconazole is not detected in plasma after chronic shampooing. Nevertheless, caution should be exercised when ketoconazole 2% shampoo is administered to a nursing woman.

Tablets: Since ketoconazole is probably excreted in the milk, mothers who are under treatment should not breast feed.

PEDIATRIC USE

Cream: Safety and effectiveness in children have not been established.

Shampoo: Safety and effectiveness in children have not been established.

Tablets: Ketoconazole Tablets have not been systematically studied in children of any age, and essentially no information is available on children under 2 years. Ketoconazole should not be used in pediatric patients unless the potential benefit outweighs the risks.

DRUG INTERACTIONS:

Tablets When taken orally, imidazole compounds like ketoconazole may enhance the anticoagulant effect of coumarin-like drugs. In simultaneous treatment with imidazole drugs and coumarin drugs, the anticoagulant effect should be carefully titrated and monitored.

Concomitant administration of rifampin with ketoconazole reduces the blood levels of the latter. INH (isoniazid) is also reported to affect ketoconazole concentrations adversely. These drugs should not be given concomitantly.

Ketoconazole tablets may alter the metabolism of cyclosporine and methylprednisolone, resulting in elevated plasma concentrations of the latter drugs. Dosage adjustment may be required if cyclosporine or methylprednisolone are given concomitantly with ketoconazole tablets.

Concomitant administration of ketoconazole with phenytoin may alter the metabolism of one or both of the drugs. It is suggested to monitor both ketoconazole and phenytoin.

Because severe hypoglycemia has been reported in patients concomitantly receiving oral miconazole (an imidazole) and oral hypoglycemic agents, such a potential interaction involving the latter agents when used concomitantly with ketoconazole (an imidazole) can not be ruled out.

Ketoconazole tablets inhibit the metabolism of terfenadine, resulting in an increased plasma concentration of terfenadine ad a delay in the elimination of its acid metabolite. Increased plasma concentration of terfenadine or its acid metabolite may result in prolonged QT intervals. (See BOXED WARNING, CONTRAINDICATIONS, and WARNINGS.)

Pharmacokinetic data indicate that oral ketoconazole inhibits the metabolism of astemizole, resulting in elevated plasma levels of astemizole and its active metabolite desmethylastemizole which may prolong QT intervals. Coadministration of astemizole with ketoconazole tablets is therefore contraindicated. (See BOXED WARNING, CONTRAINDICATIONS, and WARNINGS.)

After the coadministration of 200 mg oral ketoconazole twice daily and one 20 mg dose of loratadine to 11 subjects, the AUC and C_{max} of loratadine averaged 302% ($\pm$ 142 S.D.) and 251% ($\pm$ 68 S.D.), respectively, of those obtained after co-treatment with placebo. The AUC and C_{max} of descarboethoxyloratadine, an active metabolite, averaged 155% ($\pm$ 27 S.D.) and 141% ($\pm$ 35 S.D.), respectively. However, no related changes were noted in the QT_0 on ECG taken at 2, 6, and 24 hours after the coadministration. Also, there were no clinically significant differences in adverse events when loratadine was administered with or without ketoconazole.

Rare cases of a disulfiram-like reaction to alcohol have been reported. These experiences have been characterized by flushing, rash, peripheral edema, nausea, and headache. Symptoms resolved within a few hours.

ADVERSE REACTIONS:

Tablets: In rare cases anaphylaxis has been reported after the first dose. Several cases of hypersensitivity reactions including urticaria have also been reported. However, the most frequent adverse reactions were nausea and/or vomiting in approximately 3%, abdominal pain in 1.2%, pruritus in 1.5%, and the following in less than 1% of the patients: headache, dizziness, somnolence, fever and chills, photophobia, diarrhea, gynecomastia, impotence, thrombocytopenia, leukopenia, hemolytic anemia, and bulging fontanelles. Oligospermia has been reported in investigational studies with the drug at dosages above those currently approved. Oligospermia has not been reported at dosages up to 400 mg daily, however, sperm counts have been obtained infrequently in patients treated with these dosages. Most of these reactions were mild and transient and rarely required discontinuation of ketoconazole tablets. In contrast, the rare occurrences of hepatic dysfunction require special attention (see WARNINGS.)

Neuropsychiatric disturbances, including suicidal tendencies and severe depression, have occurred rarely in patients using ketoconazole Tablets.

ADVERSE REACTIONS: *(cont'd)*

Ventricular dysrhythmias (prolonged QT intervals) have occurred with the concomitant use of terfenadine with ketoconazole tablets. (See BOXED WARNING, CONTRAINDICATIONS, and WARNINGS.)

Shampoo: In 11 double-blind trials in 264 patients using ketoconazole 2% shampoo, an increase in normal hair loss and irritation occurred in less than 1% of patients. In three open-label safety trials in which 41 patients shampooed 4-10 times weekly for six months, the following adverse experiences each occurred once: abnormal hair texture, scalp pustules, mild dryness of the skin, and itching. As with other shampoos, oiliness and dryness of hair and scalp have been reported.

Cream: During clinical trials 45 (5.0%) of 905 patients treated with ketoconazole 2% Cream and 5 (2.4%) of 208 patients treated with placebo reported side effects consisting mainly of severe irritation, pruritus and stinging. One of the patients treated with ketoconazole Cream developed a painful allergic reaction.

OVERDOSAGE:

Tablets: In the event of accidental overdosage, supportive measures, including gastric lavage with sodium bicarbonate, should be employed.

Shampoo: Ketoconazole 2% Shampoo is intended for external use only. In the event of ingestion, supportive measures, including gastric lavage with sodium bicarbonate, should be employed.

DOSAGE AND ADMINISTRATION:

TABLETS

Adults: The recommended starting dose of ketoconazole Tablets is a single daily administration of 200 mg (one tablet). In very serious infections or if clinical responsiveness is insufficient within the expected time, the dose of ketoconazole may be increased to 400 mg (two tablets) once daily.

Children: In small numbers of children over 2 years of age, a single daily dose of 3.3 to 6.6 mg/kg has been used. Ketoconazole tablets have not been studied in children under 2 years of age.

There should be laboratory as well as clinical documentation of infection prior to starting ketoconazole therapy. Treatment should be continued until tests indicate that active fungal infection has subsided. Inadequate periods of treatment may yield poor response and lead to early recurrence of clinical symptoms. Minimum treatment for candidiasis is one or two weeks. Patients with chronic mucocutaneous candidiasis usually require maintenance therapy. Minimum treatment for the other indicated systemic mycoses is six months.

Minimum treatment for recalcitrant dermatophyte infections is four weeks in cases involving glabrous skin. Palmar and plantar infections may respond more slowly. Apparent cures may subsequently recur after discontinuation of therapy in some cases.

SHAMPOO

1. Moisten hair and scalp thoroughly with water.
2. Apply sufficient shampoo to produce enough lather to wash the scalp and hair gently massage it over the entire scalp area for approximately one minute.
3. Rinse the hair thoroughly with warm water.
4. Repeat, leaving the shampoo on the scalp for an additional 3 minutes.
5. After the second thorough rinse, dry the hair with a towel or warm air flow.

Shampoo twice a week for four weeks with at least three days between each shampooing and then intermittently as needed to maintain control.

CREAM

Cutaneous candidiasis, tinea corporis, tinea cruris, and tinea (pityriasis) versicolor: It is recommended that ketoconazole 2% cream be applied once daily to cover the affected and immediate surrounding area. Clinical improvement may be seen fairly soon after treatment is begun; however, candidal infections and tinea cruris and corporis should be treated for two weeks in order to reduce the possibility of recurrence. Patients with tinea versicolor usually require two weeks of treatment. Patients with tinea pedis require six weeks of treatment.

Seborrheic Dermatitis: Ketoconazole 2% cream should be applied to the affected area twice daily for four weeks or until clinical clearing.

If a patient shows no clinical improvement after the treatment period, the diagnosis should be redetermined.

HOW SUPPLIED:

Tablets: Nizoral is available as white, scored tablets containing 200 mg of ketoconazole debossed "JANSSEN" and on the reverse side debossed "NIZORAL". *Storage:* Store at room temperature (59°-86°F/15°-30°C). Protect from moisture.

Shampoo: Nizoral 2% shampoo is a red-orange liquid supplied in a 4-fluid ounce non-breakable plastic bottle. *Storage:* Store at a temperature not above 25°C (77°F). Protect from light.

Cream: Nizoral 2% cream is supplied in 15, 30 and 60 gm tubes.

HOW SUPPLIED - EQUIVALENTS NOT AVAILABLE:

Cream - Topical - 20 mg/gm

15 gm	$13.46	NIZORAL, Janssen Phar	50458-0221-15
30 gm	$22.63	NIZORAL, Janssen Phar	50458-0221-30
60 gm	$34.39	NIZORAL, Janssen Phar	50458-0221-60

Shampoo - Topical - 2 %

120 ml	$16.64	NIZORAL, Janssen Phar	50458-0223-04

Tablet, Uncoated - Oral - 200 mg

100's	$270.92	NIZORAL, Janssen Phar	50458-0220-10
100's	$297.91	NIZORAL, Janssen Phar	50458-0220-01

KETOPROFEN *(001606)*

CATEGORIES: Analgesics; Anti-Inflammatory Agents; Antiarthritics; Antipyretics; Arthritis; Central Nervous System Agents; Dysmenorrhea; NSAIDS; Nonsteroidal Anti-Inflammatory; Osteoarthritis; Pain; Pregnancy Category B; Sales > $100 Million; FDA Approved 1986 Jan; Top 200 Drugs

BRAND NAMES: *Alrheumat* (England); *Alrheumun* (Germany); *Alrhumat*; *Aneol* (Japan); *Apo-Keto* (Canada); *Arcental*; *Bi-Profenid* (France); *Bi-Rofenid*; *Dexal*; *Epatec* (Japan); *Fastum*; *Gabrilen Retard* (Germany); *Kapren*; *Kaprofen*; *Keduril* (Mexico); *Kefen*; *Kefenid*; *Keprofen* (Japan); *Ketofen*; *Ketomex*; *Ketonal*; *Ketorin*; *Ketosolan*; *Kevadon*; *Knavon*; *K-Profen* (Mexico); *Naxal* (Japan); *Novo-Keto-EC* (Canada); *Orucote*; **Orudis**; *Orudis E-100*; *Orudis EC*; *Orudis R-PR*; *Orudis SR* (Australia); Oruvail; *Oruvail EC*; *Oruvail SR* (Australia); *Ostofen*; *Profenid* (France, Mexico); *Profenid 50*; *Profenil*; *Rofenid*; *Topren*; *Treosin* (Japan)
(International brand names outside U.S. in italics)

FORMULARIES: Aetna; BC-BS; Medi-Cal

COST OF THERAPY: $981.88 (Arthritis; Capsule; 75 mg; 3/day; 365 days)

PRIMARY ICD9: 715.99 (Osteoarthritis, Unspecified, Multiple Sites)

DESCRIPTION:

Ketoprofen is a nonsteroidal anti-inflammatory drug. The chemical name for ketoprofen is 2-(3-benzoylphenyl)-propionic acid.

Its empirical formula is $C_{16}H_{14}O_3$, with a molecular weight of 254.29. It has a pKa of 5.94 in methanol:water (3:1) and an n-octanol:water partition coefficient of 0.97 (buffer pH 7.4).

Ketoprofen is a white or off-white, odorless, non-hygroscopic, fine to granular powder, melting at about 95° C. It is freely soluble in ethanol, chloroform, acetone, ether and soluble in benzene and strong alkali, but practically insoluble in water at 20° C.

Ketoprofen capsules contain 25 mg, 50 mg, or 75 mg of ketoprofen for oral administration. The inactive ingredients present are D&C Yellow 10, FD&C Blue 1, FD&C Yellow 6, gelatin, lactose, magnesium stearate, and titanium dioxide. The 25 mg dosage strength also contains D&C Red 28 and FD&C Red 40.

Each ketoprofen 100 mg, 150 mg, or 200 mg capsule contains ketoprofen in the form of hundreds of coated pellets. The dissolution of the pellets is pH dependent with optimum dissolution occurring at pH 6.5 -7.5. There is no dissolution at pH 1.

In addition to the active ingredient, each 100 mg, 150 mg, or 200 mg capsule of Orudis contains the following inactive ingredients: D&C Red 22, D&C Red 28, FD&C Blue 1, ethyl cellulose, gelatin, shellac, silicon dioxide, sodium lauryl sulfate, starch, sucrose, talc, titanium dioxide, and other proprietary ingredients. The 100 and 150 mg capsules also contain D&C Yellow 10 and FD&C Green 3.

CLINICAL PHARMACOLOGY:

Ketoprofen is a nonsteroidal anti-inflammatory drug with analgesic and antipyretic properties.

The anti-inflammatory, analgesic, and antipyretic properties of ketoprofen have been demonstrated in classical animal and *in vitro* test systems. In anti-inflammatory models ketoprofen has been shown to have inhibitory effects on prostaglandin and leukotriene synthesis, to have antibradykinin activity, as well as to have lysosomal membrane-stabilizing action. However, its mode of action, like that of other nonsteroidal anti-inflammatory drugs, is not fully understood.

PHARMACODYNAMICS

Ketoprofen is a racemate with only the S enantiomer possessing pharmacological activity. The enantiomers have similar concentration time curves and do not appear to interact with one another.

An analgesic effect-concentration relationship for ketoprofen was established in an oral surgery pain study with ketoprofen capsules. The effect-site rate constant (k_{eo}) was estimated to be 0.9 hour^{-1} (95% confidence limits: 0 to 2.1), and the concentration (Ce_{50}) of ketoprofen that produced one-half the maximum PID (pain intensity difference) was 0.3 mcg/ml (95% confidence limits: 0.1 to 0.5). Thirty-three (33) to 68% of patients had an onset of action (as measured by reporting some pain relief) within 30 minutes following a single oral dose in post-operative pain and dysmenorrhea studies. Pain relief (as measured by remedication) persisted for up to 6 hours in 26 to 72% of patients in these studies.

PHARMACOKINETICS

General: Ketoprofen capsules and ketoprofen extended-release capsules differ only in their release characteristics. Ketoprofen capsules release drug in the stomach whereas the pellets in ketoprofen extended-release capsules are designed to resist dissolution in the low pH of gastric fluid but release drug at a controlled rate in the higher pH environment of the small intestine (see DESCRIPTION).

Irrespective of the pattern of release, the systemic availability (F_s) when either oral formulation is compared with IV administration is approximately 90% in humans. For 75 to 200 mg single doses, the area under the curve has been shown to be dose proportional.

Ketoprofen is > 99% bound to plasma proteins, mainly to albumin.

Separate sections follow which delineate differences between ketoprofen capsules and ketoprofen extended-release capsules.

Absorption: Ketoprofen capsules—Ketoprofen is rapidly and well-absorbed, with peak plasma levels occurring within 0.5 to 2 hours.

Ketoprofen extended-release capsules—Ketoprofen is also well-absorbed from this dosage form, although an observable increase in plasma levels does not occur until approximately 2 to 3 hours after taking the formulation. Peak plasma levels are usually reached 6 to 7 hours after dosing. (See TABLE 1.)

When ketoprofen is administered with food, its total bioavailability (AUC) is not altered; however, the rate of absorption from either dosage form is slowed.

Ketoprofen capsules—Food intake reduces C_{max} by approximately one-half and increases the mean time to peak concentration (t_{max}) from 1.2 hours for fasting subjects (range, 0.5 to 3 hours) to 2.0 hours for fed subjects (range, 0.75 to 3 hours). The fluctuation of plasma peaks may also be influenced by circadian changes in the absorption process.

Concomitant administration of magnesium hydroxide and aluminum hydroxide does not interfere with absorption of ketoprofen from ketoprofen capsules.

Ketoprofen extended-release capsules—Administration of ketoprofen extended-release capsules with a high-fat meal causes a delay of about 2 hours in reaching the C_{max}; neither the total bioavailability (AUC) nor the C_{max} is affected. Circadian changes in the absorption process have not been studied.

The administration of antacids or other drugs which may raise stomach pH would not be expected to change the rate or extent of absorption of ketoprofen from ketoprofen extended-release capsules.

Multiple Dosing: Steady-state concentrations of ketoprofen are attained within 24 hours after commencing treatment with either formulation. In studies with healthy male volunteers, trough levels at 24 hours following administration of ketoprofen extended-release capsules were 0.4 mg/l compared with 0.07 mg/ml at 24 hours following administration of ketoprofen 50 mg capsules QID (12 hours) or 0.13 mg/l following administration of ketoprofen 75 mg capsules TID for 12 hours. Thus, relative to the peak plasma concentration, the accumulation of ketoprofen after multiple doses of either formulation is minimal.

Metabolism: The metabolism fate of ketoprofen is glucuronide conjugation to form an unstable acyl-glucuronide. The glucuronic acid moiety can be converted back to the parent compound. Thus, the metabolite serves as a potential reservoir for parent drug, and this may be important in persons with renal insufficiency, whereby the conjugate may accumulate in the serum and undergo deconjugation back to the parent drug (see Special Populations, Renally Impaired). The conjugates are reported to appear only in trace amounts in plasma in healthy adults, but are higher in elderly subjects—presumably because of reduced renal clearance. It has been demonstrated that in elderly subjects following multiple doses (50 mg every 6 h), the ratio of conjugated to parent ketoprofen AUC was 30% and 3%, respectively for the S & R enantiomers.

CLINICAL PHARMACOLOGY: *(cont'd)*

TABLE 1 Comparison Of Pharmacokinetic Parameters # For Ketoprofen Capsules And Ketoprofen Extended-Release Capsules

Kinetic Parameters	Ketoprofen capsules (4 x 50 mg)	Ketoprofen extended-release capsules (1 x 200 mg)
Extent of oral absorption (bioavailability F_s (%)	~90	~90
Peak plasma levels C_{max} (mg/l)		
Fasted	3.9 ± 1.3	3.1 ± 1.2
Fed	2.4 ± 1.0	3.4 ± 1.3
Time to peak concentration t_{max} (h)		
Fasted	1.2 ± 0.6	6.8 ± 2.1
Fed	2.0 ± 0.8	9.2 ± 2.6
Fasted	32.1 ± 7.2	30.1 ± 7.9
Fed	36.6 ± 8.1	31.3 ± 8.1
Oral-dose clearance Cl/F (l/h)	6.9 ± 0.8	6.8 ± 1.8
Half-life $t_{1/2}$ (h) [See footnote 1]	2.1 ± 1.2	5.4 ± 2.2

># Values expressed are mean ± standard deviation

[1] **In the case of ketoprofen extended-release capsules, absorption is slowed, intrinsic clearance is unchanged, but because the rate of elimination is dependent on absorption, the half-life is prolonged.**

There are no known active metabolites of ketoprofen. Ketoprofen has been shown not to induce drug-metabolizing enzymes.

Elimination: The plasma clearance of ketoprofen is approximately 0.08 l/kg/h with a V_d of 0.1 l/kg after IV administration. The elimination half-life of ketoprofen has been reported to be 2.05 ± 0.58 h (Mean ± S.D.) following IV administration, from 2 to 4 h following administration of ketoprofen capsules, and 5.4 ± 2.2 h after administration of ketoprofen extended-release capsules. In cases of slow drug absorption, the elimination rate is dependent on the absorption rate and thus $t_{1/2}$ relative to an IV dose appears prolonged.

After a single 200 mg dose of ketoprofen extended-release capsules, the plasma levels decline slowly, the average 0.4 mg/l after 24 hours.

In a 24-hour period, approximately 80% of an administered dose of ketoprofen is excreted in the urine, primarily as the glucuronide metabolite.

Enterohepatic recirculation of the drug has been postulated, although biliary levels have never measured to confirm this.

SPECIAL POPULATIONS

Elderly: *Clearance and unbound fraction:* The plasma and renal clearance of ketoprofen is reduced in the elderly (mean age, 73 years) compared to a younger normal population (mean age, 27 years). Hence, ketoprofen peak concentration and AUC increase with increasing age. In addition, there is a corresponding increase in unbound fraction with increasing age. Data from one trial suggest that the increase is greater in women than in men. It has not been determined whether age-related changes in absorption among the elderly contribute to the changes in bioavailability of ketoprofen.

Ketoprofen capsules—In a study conducted with young and elderly men and women, results for subjects older than 75 years of age showed that free drug AUC increased by 40% and C_{max} increased by 60% as compared with estimates of the same parameters in young subjects (those younger than 35 years of age; see Individualization of Dosage).

Also in the elderly, the rate of intrinsic clearance/availability decreased by 35% and plasma half-life was prolonged by 26%. This reduction is thought to be due to a decrease in hepatic extraction associated with aging.

Ketoprofen extended-release capsules—The effects of age and gender on ketoprofen disposition were investigated in 2 small studies in which elderly male and female subjects received ketoprofen extended-release capsules. The results were compared with those from another study conducted in healthy young men.

Compared to the younger subject group, the elimination half-life in the elderly was prolonged by 54% and total drug C_{max} and AUC were 40% and 70% higher, respectively. Plasma concentrations in the elderly after single doses and at steady state were essentially the same. Thus, no drug accumulation occurs.

In comparison to younger subjects taking the immediate-release formulation, there was a decrease of 16% and 25% in the total drug C_{max} and AUC, respectively, among the elderly. Free drug data are not available for ketoprofen extended-release capsules.

Renally Impaired: Studies of the effects of renal-function impairment have been small. They indicate a decrease in clearance in patients with impaired renal function. In 23 patients with renal impairment, free ketoprofen peak concentration was not significantly elevated, but free ketoprofen clearance was reduced from 15 l/kg/h for normal subjects to 7 l/kg/h in patients with mildly impaired renal function, and to 4 l/kg/h in patients with moderately to severely impaired renal function. The elimination $t_{1/2}$ was prolonged from 1.6 hours in normal subjects to approximately 3 hours in patients with mild renal impairment, and to approximately 5 to 9 hours in patients with moderately to severely impaired renal function.

No studies have been conducted in patients with renal impairment taking ketoprofen extended-release capsules. It is recommended that only the immediate-release formulation of ketoprofen be used to treat patients with significant renal impairment (see Individualization of Dosage).

Hepatically Impaired: For patients with alcoholic cirrhosis, no significant changes in the kinetic disposition of ketoprofen capsules were observed relative to age-matched normal subjects: the plasma clearance of drug was 0.07 l/kg/h in 26 hepatically impaired patients. The elimination half-life was comparable to that observed for normal subjects. However, the unbound (biologically active) fraction was approximately doubled, probably due to hypoalbuminemia and high variability which was observed in the pharmacokinetics for cirrhotic patients. Therefore, these patients should be carefully monitored and daily doses of ketoprofen kept at the minimum providing the desired therapeutic effect.

No studies have been conducted in patients with hepatic impairment taking ketoprofen extended-release capsules. It is recommended that only the immediate-release formulation of ketoprofen be used to treat patients who have hepatic impairment and serum albumin levels below 3.5 g/dl (see Individualization of Dosage).

CLINICAL STUDIES:

Rheumatoid Arthritis And Osteoarthritis: The efficacy of ketoprofen has been demonstrated in patients with rheumatoid arthritis and osteoarthritis. Using standard assessments of therapeutic response, there were no detectable differences in effectiveness or in the incidence of adverse events in crossover comparison of ketoprofen capsules and ketoprofen extended-release capsules. In other trials, ketoprofen demonstrated effectiveness comparable to aspirin, ibuprofen, naproxen, piroxicam, diclofenac and indomethacin. In some of these studies there were more dropouts due to gastrointestinal side effects among patients on ketoprofen than among patients on other NSAIDs.

CLINICAL STUDIES: *(cont'd)*

In studies with patients with rheumatoid arthritis, ketoprofen was administered in combination with gold salts, antimalarials, low-dose methotrexate, d-penicillamine, and/or corticosteroids with results comparable to those seen with control nonsteroidal drugs.

Management Of Pain: The effectiveness of ketoprofen capsules as a general-purpose analgesic has been studied in standard pain models which have shown the effectiveness of doses of 25 to 150 mg. Doses of 25 mg were superior to placebo. Doses larger than 25 mg generally could not be shown to be significantly more effective, but there was a tendency toward faster onset and greater duration of action with 50 mg, and, in the case of dysmenorrhea, a significantly greater effect overall with 75 mg. Doses greater than 50 to 75 mg did not have increased analgesic effect. Studies in postoperative pain have shown that ketoprofen capsules in doses of 25 to 100 mg were comparable to 650 mg of acetaminophen with 60 mg of codeine, or 650 mg of acetaminophen with 10 mg of oxycodone. Ketoprofen tended to be somewhat slower in onset; peak pain relief was about the same and the duration of the effect tended to be 1 to 2 hours longer, particularly with the higher doses of ketoprofen.

The use of ketoprofen extended-release capsules in patients with acute pain is not recommended, since, in comparison to the immediate-release formulation, ketoprofen extended-release capsules would be expected to have a delayed analgesic response due to their controlled-release characteristics.

Individualization of Dosage: The recommended starting dose of ketoprofen in otherwise healthy patients is ketoprofen capsules, 75 mg three times or 50 mg four times a day, or ketoprofen extended-release capsules, 200 mg administered once a day. Smaller doses of ketoprofen capsules or ketoprofen extended-release capsules should be utilized initially in small individuals or in debilitated or elderly patients. The recommended maximum daily dose of ketoprofen is 300 mg/day for ketoprofen capsules or 200 mg/day for ketoprofen extended-release capsules is not recommended.

If minor side effects appear, they may disappear at a lower dose which may still have an adequate therapeutic effect. If well tolerated but not optimally effective, the dosage may be increased. Individual patients may show a better response to 300 mg of ketoprofen daily as compared to 200 mg, although in well-controlled clinical trials patients on 300 mg did not show greater mean effectiveness. They did, however, show an increased frequency of upper- and lower-GI distress and headaches. It is of interest that women also had an increased frequency of these adverse effects compared to men. When treating patients with 300 mg/day, the physician should observe sufficient increased clinical benefit to offset potential increased risk.

In patients with mildly impaired renal function, the maximum recommended total daily dose of ketoprofen capsules or ketoprofen extended-release capsules is 150 mg. In patients with a more severe renal impairment (GFR less than 25 ml/min/1.73a^2 or end-stage renal impairment), the maximum daily dose of ketoprofen capsules or ketoprofen extended-release capsules should not exceed 100 mg.

In elderly patients, renal function may be reduced with apparently normal serum creatinine and/or BUN levels. Therefore, it is recommended that the initial dosage of ketoprofen capsules or ketoprofen extended-release capsules should be reduced for patients over 75 years of age.

It is recommended that for patients with impaired liver function and serum albumin concentration less than 3.5 g/dl, the maximum initial total daily dose of ketoprofen capsules and ketoprofen extended-release capsules should be 100 mg. All patients with metabolic impairment, particularly those with both hypoalbuminemia and reduced renal function, may have increased levels of free (biologically active) ketoprofen and should be closely monitored. The dosage may be increased to the range recommended for the general population, if necessary, only after good individual tolerance has been ascertained.

Because hypoalbuminemia and reduced renal function both increase the fraction of free drug (biologically active form), patients who have both conditions may be at greater risk of adverse effects. Therefore, it is recommended that such patients also be started on lower doses of ketoprofen capsules and ketoprofen extended-release capsules and closely monitored.

As with other nonsteroidal anti-inflammatory drugs, the predominant adverse effects of ketoprofen are gastrointestinal. To attempt to minimize these effects, physicians may wish to prescribe that ketoprofen capsules or ketoprofen extended-release capsules be taken with antacids, food, or milk. Although food delays the absorption of both formulations (see CLINICAL PHARMACOLOGY), in most of the clinical trials ketoprofen was taken with food or milk.

Physicians may want to make specific recommendations to patients about when they should take ketoprofen capsules or ketoprofen extended-release capsules in relation to food and/or what patients should do if they experience minor GI symptoms associated with either formulation.

INDICATIONS AND USAGE:

Ketoprofen capsules or ketoprofen extended-release capsules are indicated for the management of the signs and symptoms of rheumatoid arthritis and osteoarthritis. Ketoprofen extended-release capsules are not recommended for treatment of acute pain because of their controlled-release characteristics (see Pharmacokinetics).

Ketoprofen capsules are indicated for the management of pain. Ketoprofen capsules are also indicated for treatment of primary dysmenorrhea.

CONTRAINDICATIONS:

Ketoprofen is contraindicated in patients who have shown hypersensitivity to it. Ketoprofen should not be given to patients in whom aspirin or other nonsteroidal anti-inflammatory drugs induce asthma, urticaria, or other allergic-type reactions, because severe, rarely fatal, anaphylactic reactions to ketoprofen have been reported in such patients.

WARNINGS:

Risk Of GI Ulceration, Bleeding And Perforation With Nsaid Therapy: Serious gastrointestinal toxicity, such as bleeding, ulceration, and perforation, can occur at any time with or without warning symptoms, in patients treated chronically with NSAID therapy. Although minor upper-gastrointestinal problems, such as dyspepsia, are common, usually developing early in therapy, physicians should remain alert for ulceration and bleeding in patients treated chronically with NSAIDs even in the absence of previous GI-tract symptoms. In patients observed in clinical trials of several months to two years' duration, symptomatic upper-GI ulcers, gross bleeding, or perforation appear to occur in approximately 1% of patients treated for 3 to 6 months, and in about 2-4% of patients treated for one year. Physicians should inform patients about the signs and/or symptoms of serious GI toxicity and what steps to take if they occur.

Studies to date have not identified any subset of patients not at risk of developing peptic ulceration and bleeding. Except for a prior history of serious GI events and other risk factors known to be associated with peptic ulcer disease, such as alcoholism, smoking, etc., no other risk factors (*e.g.,* age, sex) have been associated with increased risk. Elderly or debilitated patients seem to tolerate ulceration or bleeding less well than other individuals, and most spontaneous reports of fatal GI events are in this population. Studies to date are inconclusive concerning the relative risk of various NSAIDs in causing such reactions. High doses of any NSAID probably carry a greater risk of these reactions, although controlled clinical trials

WARNINGS: *(cont'd)*

showing this do not exist in most cases. In considering the use of relatively large doses (within the recommended dosage range), sufficient benefit should be anticipated to offset the potential increased risk of GI toxicity.

PRECAUTIONS:

General: Ketoprofen and other nonsteroidal anti-inflammatory drugs cause nephritis in mice and rats associated with chronic administration. Rare cases of interstitial nephritis or nephrotic syndrome have been reported in humans with ketoprofen since it has been marketed.

A second form of renal toxicity has been seen in patients with conditions leading to a reduction in renal blood flow or blood volume, where renal prostaglandins have a supportive role in the maintenance of renal blood flow. In these patients, administration of a nonsteroidal anti-inflammatory drug results in a dose-dependent decrease in prostaglandin synthesis and, secondarily, in renal blood flow which may precipitate overt renal failure. Patients at greatest risk of this reaction are those with impaired renal function, heart failure, liver dysfunction, those taking diuretics, and the elderly. Discontinuation of nonsteroidal anti-inflammatory drug therapy is typically followed by recovery to the pretreatment state.

Since ketoprofen is primarily eliminated by the kidneys and its pharmacokinetics are altered by renal failure (see CLINICAL PHARMACOLOGY), patients with significantly impaired renal function should be closely monitored, and a reduction of dosage should be anticipated to avoid accumulation of ketoprofen and/or its metabolites (see Individualization of Dosage).

As with other nonsteroidal anti-inflammatory drugs, borderline elevations of one or more liver function tests may occur in up to 15% of patients. These abnormalities may progress, may remain essentially unchanged, or may disappear with continued therapy. The ALT (SGPT) test is probably the most sensitive indicator of liver dysfunction. Meaningful (3 times the upper limit of normal) elevations of ALT or AST (SGOT) occurred in controlled clinical trials in less than 1% of patients. A patient with symptoms and/or signs suggesting liver dysfunction, or in whom an abnormal liver test has occurred, should be evaluated for evidence of the development of a more severe hepatic reaction while on therapy with ketoprofen. Serious hepatic reactions, including jaundice, have been reported from post-marketing experience with ketoprofen as well as with other nonsteroidal anti-inflammatory drugs.

In patients with chronic liver disease with reduced serum albumin levels, ketoprofen's pharmacokinetics are altered (see CLINICAL PHARMACOLOGY). Such patients should be closely monitored, and a reduction of dosage should be anticipated to avoid high blood levels of ketoprofen and/or its metabolites (see Individualization of Dosage).

If steroid dosage is reduced or eliminated during therapy, it should be reduced slowly and the patients observed closely for any evidence of adverse effects, including adrenal insufficiency and exacerbation of symptoms of arthritis.

Anemia is commonly observed in rheumatoid arthritis and is sometimes aggravated by nonsteroidal anti-inflammatory drugs, which may produce fluid retention or significant gastrointestinal blood loss in some patients. Patients on long-term treatment with NSAIDs, including ketoprofen capsules or ketoprofen extended-release capsules, should have their hemoglobin or hematocrit checked if they develop signs or symptoms of anemia.

Peripheral edema has been observed in approximately 2% of patients taking ketoprofen. Therefore, as with other nonsteroidal anti-inflammatory drugs, ketoprofen should be used with caution in patients with fluid retention, hypertension, or heart failure.

Information for the Patient: The capsules and extended-release capsules contain ketoprofen. Like other drugs of its class, ketoprofen, is not free of side effects. The side effects of these drugs can cause discomfort and, rarely, there are more serious side effects, such as gastrointestinal bleeding, which may result in hospitalization and even fatal outcomes.

NSAIDs are often essential agents in the management of arthritis and have a major role in the treatment of pain, but they also may be commonly employed for conditions which are less serious. Physicians may wish to discuss with their patients the potential risks (see WARNINGS, PRECAUTIONS, and ADVERSE REACTIONS) and likely benefits of NSAID treatment, particularly when the drugs are used for less serious conditions where treatment without NSAIDs might represent an acceptable alternative to both the patient and physician.

Because aspirin causes an increase in the level of unbound ketoprofen, patients should be advised not to take aspirin while taking ketoprofen (see DRUG INTERACTIONS). It is possible that minor adverse symptoms of gastric intolerance may be prevented by administering ketoprofen capsules with antacids, food, or milk. Ketoprofen extended-release capsules have not been studied with antacids. Because food and milk do affect the rate but not the extent of absorption (see CLINICAL PHARMACOLOGY), physicians may want to make specific recommendations to patients about when they should take ketoprofen in relation to food and/or what patients should do if they experience minor GI symptoms associated with ketoprofen therapy.

Laboratory Tests: Because serious GI-tract ulceration and bleeding can occur without warning symptoms, physicians should follow chronically treated patients for the signs and symptoms of ulceration and bleeding and should inform them of the importance of this follow-up (see WARNINGS, Risk Of Gi Ulceration, Bleeding And Perforation With Nsaid Therapy).

Drug/Laboratory Test Interactions: Effect On Blood Coagulation: Ketoprofen decreases platelet adhesion and aggregation. Therefore, it can prolong bleeding time by approximately 3 to 4 minutes from baseline values. There is no significant change in platelet count, prothrombin time, partial thromboplastin time, or thrombin time.

Carcinogenesis, Mutagenesis, and Impairment of Fertility: Chronic oral toxicity studies in mice (up to 32 mg/kg/day; 96 mg/m^2/day) did not indicate a carcinogenic potential for ketoprofen. The maximum recommended human therapeutic dose is 300 mg/day for a 60 kg patient with a body surface area of 1.6 m^2, which is 5 mg/kg/day or 185 mg/m^2/day. Thus the mice were treated at 0.5 times the maximum human daily dose based on surface area.

A 2-year carcinogenicity study in rats, using doses up to 6.0 mg/kg/day (36 mg/m^2/day), showed no evidence of tumorigenic potential. All groups were treated for 104 weeks except the females receiving 6.0 mg/kg/day (36 mg/m^2/day) where the drug treatment was terminated in week 81 because of low survival; the remaining rats were sacrificed after week 87. Their survival in the groups treated for 104 weeks was within 6% of the control group. An earlier 2-year study with doses up to 12.5 mg/kg/day (75 mg/m^2/day) also showed no evidence of tumorigenicity, but the survival rate was low and the study was therefore judged inconclusive. Ketoprofen did not show mutagenic potential in the Ames Test. Ketoprofen administered to male rats (up to 9 mg/kg/day; or 54 mg/m^2/day) had no significant effect on reproductive performance or fertility. In female rats administered 6 or 9 mg/kg/day (36 or 54 mg/m^2/day), a decrease in the number of implantation sites has been noted. The dosages of 36 mg/m^2/day in rats represent 0.2 times the maximum recommended human dose of 185 mg/m^2/day.

Abnormal spermatogenesis or inhibition of spermatogenesis developed in rats and dogs at high doses, and a decrease in the weight of the testes occurred in dogs and baboons at high doses.

Pregnancy, Teratogenic Effects, Pregnancy Category B: In teratology studies ketoprofen administered to mice at doses up to 12 mg/kg/day (36 mg/m^2/day) and rats at doses up to 9 mg/kg/day (54 mg/m^2/day), the approximate equivalent of 0.2 times the maximum recommended

PRECAUTIONS: *(cont'd)*

therapeutic dose of 185 mg/m^2/day, showed no teratogenic or embryotoxic effects. In separate studies in rabbits, maternally toxic doses were associated with embryotoxicity but not teratogenicity.

There are no adequate and well-controlled studies in pregnant women. Because animal teratology studies are not always predictive of the human response, ketoprofen should be used during pregnancy only if the potential benefit justifies the risk.

Labor and Delivery: The effects of ketoprofen on labor and delivery in pregnant women are unknown. Studies in rats have shown ketoprofen at doses of 6 mg/kg (36 mg/m^2/day, approximately equal to 0.2 times the maximum recommended human dose) prolong pregnancy when given before the onset of labor. Because of the known effects of prostaglandin-inhibiting drugs on the fetal cardiovascular system (closure of ductus arteriosus), use of ketoprofen during late pregnancy should be avoided.

Nursing Mothers: Data on secretion in human milk after ingestion of ketoprofen do not exist. In rats, ketoprofen at doses of 9 mg/kg (54 mg/m^2/day; approximately 0.3 times the maximum human therapeutic dose) did not affect perinatal development. Upon administration to lactating dogs, the milk concentration of ketoprofen was found to be 4 to 5% of the plasma drug level. As with other drugs that are excreted in milk, ketoprofen is not recommended for use in nursing mothers.

Pediatric Use: Ketoprofen is not recommended for use in children, because its safety and effectiveness have not been studied in children.

DRUG INTERACTIONS:

The following drug interactions were studied with ketoprofen doses of 200 mg/day. The possibility of increased interaction should be kept in mind when doses of ketoprofen capsules greater than 50 mg as a single dose or 200 mg of ketoprofen per day are used concomitantly with highly bound drugs.

1. Antacids: Concomitant administration of magnesium hydroxide and aluminum hydroxide does not interfere with the rate or extent of the absorption of ketoprofen administered as ketoprofen capsules.

2. Aspirin: Ketoprofen does not alter aspirin absorption; however, in a study of 12 normal subjects, concurrent administration of aspirin decreased ketoprofen protein binding and increased ketoprofen plasma clearance from 0.07 l/kg/h without aspirin to 0.11 l/kg/h with aspirin. The clinical significance of these changes has not been adequately studied. Therefore, concurrent use of aspirin and ketoprofen is not recommended.

3. Diuretic: Hydrochlorothiazide, given concomitantly with ketoprofen, produces a reduction in urinary potassium and chloride excretion compared to hydrochlorothiazide alone. Patients taking diuretics are at greater risk of developing renal failure secondary to a decrease in renal blood flow caused by prostaglandin inhibition (see PRECAUTIONS, General).

4. Digoxin: In a study in 12 patients with congestive heart failure where ketoprofen and digoxin were concomitantly administered, ketoprofen did not alter the serum levels of digoxin.

5. Warfarin: In a short-term controlled study in 14 normal volunteers, ketoprofen did not significantly interfere with the effect of warfarin on prothrombin time. Bleeding from a number of sites may be a complication of warfarin treatment and GI bleeding a complication of ketoprofen treatment. Because prostaglandins play an important role in hemostasis and ketoprofen has an effect on platelet function as well (see Drug/Laboratory Test Interactions, Effect on Blood Coagulation), concurrent therapy with ketoprofen and warfarin requires close monitoring of patients on both drugs.

6. Probenecid: Probenecid increases both free and bound ketoprofen by reducing the plasma clearance of ketoprofen to about one-third, as well as decreasing its protein binding. Therefore, the combination of ketoprofen and probenecid is not recommended.

7. Methotrexate: Ketoprofen, like other NSAIDs, may cause changes in the elimination of methotrexate leading to elevated serum levels of the drug and increased toxicity.

8. Lithium: Nonsteroidal anti-inflammatory agents have been reported to increase steady-state plasma lithium levels. It is recommended that plasma lithium levels be monitored when ketoprofen is co-administered with lithium.

ADVERSE REACTIONS:

The incidence of common adverse reactions (above 1%) was obtained from a population of 835 patients treated with ketoprofen capsules in double-blind trials lasting from 4 to 54 weeks and in 622 ketoprofen extended-release capsules (200 mg/day) patients in trials lasting from 4 to 16 weeks.

Minor gastrointestinal side effects predominated; upper gastrointestinal symptoms were more common than lower gastrointestinal symptoms. In crossover trials in 321 patients with rheumatoid arthritis or osteoarthritis, there was no difference in either upper or lower gastrointestinal symptoms between patients treated with 200 mg of ketoprofen extended-release capsules once a day or 75 mg of ketoprofen capsules TID (225 mg/day). Peptic ulcer or GI bleeding occurred in controlled clinical trials in less than 1% of 1,076 patients; however, in open label continuation studies in 1,292 patients the rate was greater than 2%.

The incidence of peptic ulceration in patients on NSAIDs is dependent on many risk factors including age, sex, smoking, alcohol use, diet, stress, concomitant drugs such as aspirin and corticosteroids, as well as the dose and duration of treatment with NSAIDs (see WARNINGS).

Gastrointestinal reactions were followed in frequency by central nervous system side effects, such as headache, dizziness, or drowsiness. The incidence of some adverse reactions appears to be dose-related (see DOSAGE AND ADMINISTRATION). Rare adverse reactions (incidence less than 1%) were collected from foreign reports to manufacturers and regulatory agencies, publications, and U.S. clinical trials.

Reactions are listed below under body system, then by incidence or number of cases in decreasing incidence.

Incidence Greater Than 1% (Probable Causal Relationship)

Digestive: Dyspepsia (11%), nausea*, abdominal pain*, diarrhea*, constipation*, flatulence*, anorexia, vomiting, stomatitis.

Nervous System: Headache*, dizziness, CNS inhibition (*i.e.,* pooled reports of somnolence, malaise, depression, etc.) or excitation (*i.e.,* insomnia, nervousness, dreams, etc.).*

Special Senses: Tinnitus, visual disturbance.

Skin and Appendages: Rash.

Urogenital: Impairment of renal function (edema, increased BUN)*, signs or symptoms of urinary-tract irritation. * Adverse events occurring in 3 to 9% of patients.

Incidence Less Than 1% (Probable Causal Relationship)

Body as a Whole: Chills, facial edema, infection, pain, allergic reaction, anaphylaxis.

Cardiovascular: Hypertension, palpitation, tachycardia, congestive heart failure, peripheral vascular disease, vasodilation.

Digestive: Appetite increased, dry mouth, eructation, gastritis, rectal hemorrhage, melena, fecal occult blood, salivation, peptic ulcer, gastrointestinal perforation, hematemesis, intestinal ulceration.

ADVERSE REACTIONS: *(cont'd)*

Hemic: Hypocoagulability, agranulocytosis, anemia, hemolysis, purpura, thrombocytopenia.

Metabolic and Nutritional: Thirst, weight gain, weight loss, hepatic dysfunction, hyponatremia.

Musculoskeletal: Myalgia.

Nervous System: Amnesia, confusion, impotence, migraine, paresthesia, vertigo.

Respiratory: Dyspnea, hemoptysis, epistaxis, pharyngitis, rhinitis, bronchospasm, laryngeal edema.

Skin and Appendages: Alopecia, eczema, pruritus, purpuric rash, sweating, urticaria, bullous rash, exfoliative dermatitis, photosensitivity, skin discoloration, onycholysis.

Special Senses: Conjunctivitis, conjunctivitis sicca, eye pain, hearing impairment, retinal hemorrhage and pigmentation change, taste perversion.

Urogenital: Menometrorrhagia, hematuria, renal failure, interstitial nephritis, nephrotic syndrome.

Incidence Less Than 1% (Causal Relationship Unknown): The following rare adverse reactions, whose causal relationship to ketoprofen is uncertain, are being listed to serve as alerting information to the physician.

Body as a Whole: Septicemia, shock.

Cardiovascular: Arrhythmias, myocardial infarction.

Digestive: Buccal necrosis, ulcerative colitis, microvesicular steatosis, jaundice, pancreatitis.

Endocrine: Diabetes mellitus (aggravated).

Nervous System: Dysphoria, hallucination, libido disturbance, nightmares, personality disorder, aseptic meningitis.

Urogenital: Acute tubulopathy, gynecomastia.

OVERDOSAGE:

Signs and symptoms following acute NSAID overdose are usually limited to lethargy, drowsiness, nausea, vomiting, and epigastric pain, which are generally reversible with supportive care. Respiratory depression, coma, or convulsions have occurred following large ketoprofen overdoses. Gastrointestinal bleeding, hypotension, hypertension, or acute renal failure may occur, bur are rare.

Patients should be managed by symptomatic and supportive care following an NSAID overdose. There are no specific antidotes. Gut decontamination may be indicated in patients with symptoms seen within 4 hours (longer for sustained-release products) or following a large overdose (5 to 10 times the usual dose). This should be accomplished via emesis and/or activated charcoal (60 to 100 g in adults, 1 to 2 g/kg in children) with a saline cathartic or sorbitol added to the first dose. Forced diuresis, alkalinization of the urine, hemodialysis or hemoperfusion would probably not be useful due to ketoprofen's high protein binding.

Case reports include twenty-six overdoses: 6 were in children, 16 in adolescents, and 4 in adults. Five of these patients had minor symptoms (vomiting in 4, drowsiness in 1 child). A 12-year-old girl had tonic- clonic convulsions 1-2 hours after ingesting an unknown quantity of ketoprofen and 1 or 2 tablets of acetaminophen with hydrocodone. Her ketoprofen level was 1128 mg/l (56 times the upper therapeutic level of 20 mg/l) 3-4 hours post ingestion. Full recovery ensued 18 hours after ingestion following management with intubation, diazepam, and activated charcoal. A 45-year-old woman ingested twelve 200 mg ketoprofen extended-release capsules and 375 ml vodka, was treated with emesis and supportive measurers 2 hours after ingestion, and recovered completely with her only complaint being mild epigastric pain.

DOSAGE AND ADMINISTRATION:

Rheumatoid Arthritis And Osteoarthritis: The recommended starting dose of ketoprofen in otherwise healthy patients is for ketoprofen capsules 75 mg three times or 50 mg four times a day or for ketoprofen extended-release capsules 200 mg administered once a day. Smaller doses of ketoprofen capsules and ketoprofen extended-release capsules should be utilized initially in small individuals or in debilitated or elderly patients. The recommended maximum daily dose of ketoprofen is 300 mg/day for ketoprofen or 200 mg/day for ketoprofen extended-release capsules (see Individualization of Dosage).

Dosage higher than 300 mg/day of ketoprofen capsules or 200 mg/day of ketoprofen extended-release capsules are not recommended because the have not been studied.

Concomitant use of ketoprofen capsules and ketoprofen extended-release capsules is not recommended. Relatively smaller people may need smaller doses (see Individualization of Dosage).

Management Of Pain And Dysmenorrhea: The usual dose of ketoprofen capsules recommended for mild-to-moderate pain and dysmenorrhea is 25 to 50 mg every 6 to 8 hours as necessary. A smaller dose should be utilized initially in small individuals, in debilitated or elderly patients, or in patients with renal or liver disease (see PRECAUTIONS, General). A larger dose may be tried if the patient's response to a previous dose was less than satisfactory, but doses above 75 mg have not been shown to give added analgesia. Daily doses above 300 mg are not recommended because they have not been adequately studied. Because of its typical nonsteroidal anti-inflammatory drug-side-effect profile, including as its principal adverse effect GI side effects (see WARNINGS and ADVERSE REACTIONS), higher doses of ketoprofen capsules should be used with caution and patients receiving them observed carefully (see Individualization of Dosage).

Ketoprofen extended-release capsules are not recommended for use in treating acute pain because of their controlled-release characteristics.

Keep tightly closed. Store at room temperature, approximately 25° C (77° F). Dispense in a tight container.

PATIENT INFORMATION:

Ketoprofen is a nonsteroidal anti-inflammatory drug (NSAID) used to relieve pain and inflammation, treat osteoarthritis, rheumatoid arthritis, and menstrual cramps. Inform your physician if you are pregnant or nursing. Ketoprofen should not be taken with aspirin products. Avoid alcoholic beverages while taking ketoprofen. This medication should be taken with food, milk or antacids if stomach upset occurs. Extended-release capsules must be swallowed whole; they should not be crushed or chewed. Ketoprofen may cause dizziness, drowsiness, or blurred vision; use caution while driving or operating hazardous machinery. Ketoprofen may cause increased sensitivity to sunlight. Use sunscreens and wear protective clothing until degree of sensitivity is determined. Notify your physician if you develop stomach pain, bloody vomit, bloody or black tarry stools, cloudy urine, trouble breathing, rash or hives.

HOW SUPPLIED - RATED THERAPEUTICALLY EQUIVALENT:

Capsule - Oral - 50 mg

100's	$91.95	Ketoprofen, Mylan	00378-4070-01

Capsule - Oral - 75 mg

100's	$102.23	Ketoprofen, Mylan	00378-5750-01

HOW SUPPLIED - RATED THERAPEUTICALLY EQUIVALENT: *(cont'd)*

Capsule, Gelatin - Oral - 25 mg

100's	$65.68	Ketoprofen, Goldline Labs	00182-1958-01
100's	$65.68	Ketoprofen, Teva	00332-3191-09
100's	$67.49	Ketoprofen, HL Moore Drug Exch	00839-7768-06
100's	$69.50	Ketoprofen, Harber Pharm	51432-0791-03
100's	$72.15	Ketoprofen, West Point Pharma	59591-0001-68
100's	$74.35	Ketoprofen, Lederle Pharm	00005-3284-43
100's	$78.50	Ketoprofen, Aligen Independ	00405-4578-01
100's	**$80.66**	**ORUDIS, Wyeth Labs**	**00008-4186-01**

Capsule, Gelatin - Oral - 50 mg

100's	$80.62	Ketoprofen, Teva	00332-3193-09
100's	$80.62	Ketoprofen, Qualitest Pharms	00603-4177-21
100's	$88.00	Ketoprofen, Goldline Labs	00182-1959-01
100's	$89.11	Ketoprofen, Rugby	00536-5564-01
100's	$89.11	Ketoprofen, United Res	00677-1463-01
100's	$89.15	Ketoprofen, West Point Pharma	59591-0002-68
100's	$89.20	Ketoprofen, Schein Pharm (US)	00364-2571-01
100's	$89.25	Ketoprofen, Major Pharms	00904-7711-60
100's	$90.44	Ketoprofen, HL Moore Drug Exch	00839-7769-06
100's	$91.91	Ketoprofen, Lederle Pharm	00005-3285-43
100's	$92.20	Ketoprofen, Aligen Independ	00405-4579-01
100's	$95.00	Ketoprofen, Harber Pharm	51432-0792-03
100's	**$99.01**	**ORUDIS, Wyeth Labs**	**00008-4181-01**

Capsule, Gelatin - Oral - 75 mg

100's	$89.67	Ketoprofen, Teva	00332-3195-09
100's	$98.00	Ketoprofen, Goldline Labs	00182-1960-01
100's	$98.40	Ketoprofen, HL Moore Drug Exch	00839-7770-06
100's	$98.90	Ketoprofen, Qualitest Pharms	00603-4178-21
100's	$99.00	Ketoprofen, Rugby	00536-5565-01
100's	$99.11	Ketprofen, United Res	00677-1464-01
100's	$99.15	Ketoprofen, West Point Pharma	59591-0003-68
100's	$99.29	Ketoprofen, Aligen Independ	00405-4580-01
100's	$99.30	Ketoprofen, Major Pharms	00904-7712-60
100's	$99.32	Ketoprofen, Schein Pharm (US)	00364-2572-01
100's	$100.00	Ketoprofen, Harber Pharm	51432-0793-03
100's	$102.21	Ketoprofen, Lederle Pharm	00005-3286-43
100's	**$110.13**	**ORUDIS, Wyeth Labs**	**00008-4187-01**
100's	**$114.41**	**ORUDIS, Wyeth Labs**	**00008-4187-04**
500's	$427.12	Ketoprofen, Teva	00332-3195-13
500's	$427.12	Ketoprofen, Aligen Independ	00405-4580-02
500's	$427.12	Ketoprofen, Qualitest Pharms	00603-4178-28
500's	$440.00	Ketoprofen, Rugby	00536-5565-05
500's	$458.99	Ketoprofen, HL Moore Drug Exch	00839-7770-12
500's	$464.00	Ketoprofen, Goldline Labs	00182-1960-05
500's	$472.40	Ketoprofen, Major Pharms	00904-7712-40
500's	$500.00	Ketoprofen, Harber Pharm	51432-0793-05
500's	**$524.60**	**ORUDIS, Wyeth Labs**	**00008-4187-02**

HOW SUPPLIED - NOT RATED EQUIVALENT:

Capsule, Gelatin, Sustained Action - Oral - 100 mg

100's	$162.50	ORUVAIL, Wyeth Labs	00008-0821-01
100's	$165.75	ORUVAIL, Wyeth Labs	00008-0821-03

Capsule, Gelatin, Sustained Action - Oral - 150 mg

100's	$197.50	ORUVAIL, Wyeth Labs	00008-0822-01
100's	$201.45	ORUVAIL, Wyeth Labs	00008-0822-03

Capsule, Gelatin, Sustained Action - Oral - 200 mg

100's	$235.25	ORUVAIL, Wyeth Labs	00008-0690-01
100's	$235.25	ORUVAIL, Wyeth Labs	00008-0690-02

KETOROLAC TROMETHAMINE *(001607)*

CATEGORIES: Allergies; Analgesics; Anti-Inflammatory Agents; Antipyretics; Central Nervous System Agents; Conjunctivitis; EENT Drugs; Eye, Ear, Nose, & Throat Preparations; NSAIDS; Nonsteroidal Anti-Inflammatory; Ophthalmics; Pain; Pregnancy Category B; FDA Class 1B ("Modest Therapeutic Advantage"); Sales > $100 Million; FDA Approved 1989 Nov

BRAND NAMES: Acular; *Dolac* (Mexico); *Kelac*; *Ketanov*; *Ketonic*; *Ketowin*; *Nodine*; *Tarasyn*; *Topadol*; **Toradol**; *Torolac*; *Torvin*
(International brand names outside U.S. in italics)

FORMULARIES: BC-BS; PCS

COST OF THERAPY: $24.49 (Pain; Tablet; 10 mg; 4/day; 5 days)

WARNING:
Ketorolac tromethamine, a nonsteroidal anti-inflammatory drug (NSAID) is indicated for the short-term (up to 5 days) management of moderately severe, acute pain, that requires analgesia at the opioid level. It is NOT indicated for minor or chronic painful conditions. Ketorolac tromethamine is a potent NSAID analgesic, and its administration carries many risks. The resulting NSAID-related adverse events can be serious in certain patients for whom ketorolac tromethamine is indicated, especially when the drug is used inappropriately. Increasing the dose of ketorolac tromethamine beyond the label recommendations will not provide better efficacy but will result in increasing the risk of developing serious adverse events.

Gastrointestinal Effects: Ketorolac tromethamine can cause peptic ulcers, gastrointestinal bleeding, and/or perforation. Therefore, ketorolac tromethamine is CONTRAINDICATED in patients with active peptic ulcer disease, in patients with active peptic ulcer disease, in patients with recent gastrointestinal bleeding or perforation, and in patients with a history of peptic ulcer disease or gastrointestinal bleeding.

Renal Effects: Ketorolac tromethamine is CONTRAINDICATED in patients with advanced renal impairment and in patients at risk for renal failure due to volume depletion (see WARNINGS).

Risk of Bleeding: Ketorolac tromethamine inhibits platelet function and is, therefore, CONTRAINDICATED in patients with suspected or confirmed cerebrovascular bleeding, patients with hemorrhagic diathesis, incomplete hemostasis, and those at high risk of bleeding (see WARNINGS and PRECAUTIONS).

Ketorolac tromethamine is CONTRAINDICATED as prophylactic an-

analgesic before any major surgery, and it is CONTRAINDICATED intra-operatively when hemostasis is critical because of the increased risk of bleeding.

Hypersensitivity: Hypersensitivity reactions, ranging from bronchospasm to anaphyl- actic shock, have occurred and appropriate counteractive measures must be available when administering the first dose of ketorolac tromethamine IV/IM (see CONTRAINDICATIONS and WARNINGS). Ketorolac tromethamine is CONTRAINDICATED in patients with previously demonstrated hypersensitivity to ketorolac tromethamine or allergic manifestations to aspirin or other nonsteroidal anti-inflammatory drugs (NSAIDs).

Intrathecal or Epidural Administration: Ketorolac tromethamine is CONTRAINDICATED for intrathecal or epidural administra- tion due to its alcohol content.

Labor, Delivery, and Nursing: The use of ketorolac tromethamine in labor and delivery is CONTRAINDICATED because it may adversely affect fetal circulation and inhibit uterine contractions.

The use of ketorolac tromethamine is CONTRAINDICATED in nursing mothers because of the potential adverse effects of prostaglandin-inhibiting drugs on neonates.

Concomittant Use with NSAIDs: Ketorolac tromethamine is CONTRAINDICATED in patients currently receiving ASA or NSAIDs because of the cumulative risk of inducing serious NSAID- related side effects.

Dosage and Administration: Oral ketorolac tromethamine is indicated only as continuation therapy to ketorolac tromethamine IV/IM, and the combined duration of use of ketorolac tromethamine IV/IM and oral ketorolac tromethamine is not to exceed 5 (five) days because of the increased risk of serious adverse events.

The recommended total daily dose of oral ketorolac tromethamine (maximum 40 mg) is significantly lower than for ketorolac tromethamine IV/IM (maximum 120 mg) (see DOSAGE AND ADMINISTRATION and Transition from Ketorolac Tromethamine IV/IM to Ketorolac Tromethamine Oral).

Special Populations: Dosage should be adjusted for patients 65 years or older, for patients under 50 kg (110 lbs) of body weight (see DOSAGE AND ADMINISTRATION), and for patients with moderately elevated serum creatinine (see WARNINGS). Doses of ketorolac tromethamine IV/IM are not to exceed 60 mg (total dose per day) in these patients.

DESCRIPTION:

Ketorolac tromethamine is a member of the pyrrolo-pyrrole group of nonsteroidal anti-inflammatory drugs (NSAIDs). The chemical name for ketorolac tromethamine is (±)-5-benzoyl-2,3-dihydro-1H-pyrrolizine-1-carboxylic acid, 2-amino-2-(hydroxymethyl)-1,3-propanediol.

Toradol is a racemic mixture of [-]S and [+]R ketorolac tromethamine. Ketorolac tromethamine may exist in three crystal forms. All forms are equally soluble in water. Ketorolac tromethamine has a pKa of 3.5 and an n-octanol/water partition coefficient of 0.26. The molecular weight of ketorolac tromethamine is 376.41.

Toradol is available for intravenous (IV) or intramuscular (IM) administration as: 15 mg in 1 ml (1.5%), and 30 mg in 1 ml (3%) in sterile solution; 60 mg in 2 ml (3%) of ketorolac tromethamine in sterile solution is available for IM administration only. The solutions contain 10% (w/v) alcohol, USP, and 6.68 mg, 4.35 mg, and 8.70 mg, respectively, of sodium chloride in sterile water. The pH is adjusted with sodium hydroxide or hydrochloric acid and the solutions are packaged with nitrogen. The sterile solutions are clear and slightly yellow in color.

Toradol oral is available as round, white, film-coated, red-printed tablets. Each tablet contains 10 mg ketorolac tromethamine, the active ingredient, with added lactose, magnesium stearate, and microcrystalline cellulose. The white film-coating contains hydroxypropyl methylcellulose, polyethylene glycol, and titanium dioxide.

The tablets are printed with red ink which includes FD&C Red #40 Aluminum lake as the colorant. There is a large T printed on both sides of the tablet, as well as the word Toradol on one side, and the word SYNTEX on the other.

Ophthalmic Solution: Acular (ketorolac tromethamine) is a member of the pyrrolo-pyrrole group of nonsteroidal anti-inflammatory drugs (NSAIDs). The chemical name for ketorolac tromethamine is (±)-5-benzoyl-2,3-dihydro-1H-pyrrolizine-1-carboxylic acid, 2-amino-2-(hydroxymethyl)-1,3-propanediol (1:1).

Acular (ketorolac tromethamine) is supplied as a sterile isotonic aqueous 0.5% solution, with a pH of 7.4. Acular is a racemic mixture of R-(+)- and S-(-)-ketorolac tromethamine. Ketorolac tromethamine may exist in three crystal forms. All forms are equally soluble in water. Ketorolac tromethamine has a pKa of 3.5. The white to off-white crystalline substance discolors on prolonged exposure to light. The molecular weight of ketorolac tromethamine is 376.41.

CLINICAL PHARMACOLOGY:

Pharmacodynamics: Ketorolac is a nonsteroidal anti-inflammatory drug (NSAID). Ketorolac tromethamine inhibits synthesis of prostaglandins and may be considered a peripherally-acting analgesic. The biological activity of ketorolac is associated with the S-form. Ketorolac tromethamine possesses no sedative or anxiolytic properties.

Pain relief was statistically different after ketorolac tromethamine dosing from that of placebo at 1/2 hour (the first time point at which it was measured) following the largest recommended doses of ketorolac tromethamine, and by 1 hour following the smallest recommended doses. The peak analgesic effect occurred within 2 to 3 hours and was not statistically significantly different over the recommended dosage range of ketorolac tromethamine. The greatest difference between large and small doses of ketorolac tromethamine by either route was in the duration of analgesia.

Pharmacokinetics: Ketorolac tromethamine is a racemic mixture of [-]S- and [+]R-enantiomeric forms, with the S-form having analgesic activity.

Comparison of IV, IM, and Oral Pharmacokinetics: The pharmacokinetics of ketorolac tromethamine following IV, IM, and oral doses of ketorolac tromethamine, are compared in TABLE 1. The extent of bioavailability following administration of the oral and IM forms of ketorolac tromethamine was equal to that following an IV bolus.

Linear Kinetics: Following administration of single oral, IM or IV doses of ketorolac tromethamine, in the recommended dosage ranges, the clearance of the racemate does not change. This implies that the pharmacokinetics of ketorolac tromethamine in humans, following single or multiple IM, IV, or recommended oral doses of ketorolac tromethamine, are linear. At the higher recommended doses, there is a proportional increase in the concentrations of free and bound racemate.

CLINICAL PHARMACOLOGY: *(cont'd)*

Binding and Distribution: The ketorolac tromethamine racemate has been shown to be highly protein-bound (99%). Nevertheless, even plasma concentrations as high as 10 mcg/ml will only occupy approximately 5% of the albumin binding sites. Thus, the unbound fraction for each enantiomer will be constant over the therapeutic range. A decrease in serum albumin, however, will result in increased free drug concentrations.

The mean apparent volume (V_β) of ketorolac tromethamine following complete distribution was approximately 13 liters. This parameter was determined from single-dose data.

Metabolism: Ketorolac tromethamine is largely metabolized in the liver. The metabolic products are hydroxylated and conjugated forms of the parent drug. The products of metabolism, and some unchanged drug, are excreted in the urine.

Clearance and Excretion: A single-dose study with 10 mg ketorolac tromethamine (n=9) demonstrated that the S-enantiomer is cleared approximately two times faster than the R-enantiomer, and that the clearance was independent of the route of administration. This means that the ratio of S/R plasma concentrations decreases with time after each dose. There is little or no inversion of the R- to S- form in humans. The clearance of the racemate in normal subjects, elderly individuals, and in hepatically and renally impaired patients, is outlined in TABLE 2.

The half-life of the ketorolac tromethamine S-enantiomer was approximately 2.5 hours (SD ± 0.4) compared with 5 hours (SD ± 1.7) for the R-enantiomer. In other studies, the half-life for the racemate has been reported to lie within the range of 5-6 hours.

Accumulation: Ketorolac tromethamine administered as an IV bolus, every 6 hours, for 5 days, to healthy subjects (n=13), showed no significant difference in C_{max} on Day 1 and Day 5. Trough levels averaged 0.29 mcg/ml (SD ± 0.13) on Day 1 and 0.55 mcg/ml (SD ± 0.23) on Day 6. Steady-state was approached after the fourth dose.

Accumulation of ketorolac tromethamine has not been studied in special populations (elderly patients, renal failure patients, or hepatic disease patients).

Effects of Food: Oral administration of ketorolac tromethamine after a high-fat meal resulted in decreased peak and delayed time-to-peak concentrations of ketorolac tromethamine by about 1 hour. Antacids did not affect the extent of absorption.

Kinetics in Special Populations Elderly Patients: Based on single-dose data only, the half-life of the ketorolac tromethamine racemate increased from 5 to 7 hours in the elderly (65-78 years) compared with young healthy volunteers (24-35 years) (see TABLE 2). There was little difference in the C_{max} for the two groups (elderly, 2.52 mcg/,l ± 1.03) (see PRECAUTIONS, Use in the Elderly.

Renally Impaired Patients: Based on single-dose data only, the mean half-life of ketorolac tromethamine in renally impaired patients in between 6 and 19 hours, and is dependent on the extent of the impairment. There is poor correlation between creatine clearance and total ketorolac tromethamine clearance in the elderly and populations with renal impairment (r=0.5).

In patients with renal disease, the AUC_∞ of each enantiomer increased by approximately 100% compared with healthy volunteers. The volume of distribution doubles for the S-enantiomer and increases by 1/5th for the R-enantiomer. The increase in volume of distribution of ketorolac tromethamine implies an increase in unbound fraction.

The AUC_∞ ratio of the ketorolac tromethamine enantiomers in healthy subjects and patients remained similar, indicating there was no selective excretion of either enantiomer in patients compared to healthy subjects (see PRECAUTIONS, Hepatic Effects).

Hepatic Effects: There was no significant difference in estimates of half-life AUC_∞, C_{max}, in 7 patients with liver disease compared to healthy volunteers (see PRECAUTIONS, Hepatic Effects).

TABLE 1A Table of Approximate Average Pharmacokinetic Parameters (Mean ± SD) Oral, Intramuscular and Intravenous Doses of Ketorolac Tromethamine

Pharmacokinetic Parameter (units)	Oral† 10 mg
Bioavailability (extent)	100%
T_{max} [1] (min)	44 ± 34
C_{max} [2] (mcg/ml)[single dose]	0.87 ± 0.22
C_{max} (mcg/ml)[steady state qid]	1.05 ± 0.26**
C_{min} [3] (mcg/ml)[steady state qid]	0.29 ± 0.07**
C_{avg} [4] (mcg/ml)[steady state qid]	0.59 ± 0.20**
V_β [5] (L/kg)	—0.175 ± 0.039—

TABLE 1B Table of Approximate Average Pharmacokinetic Parameters (Mean ± SD) Oral, Intramuscular and Intravenous Doses of Ketorolac Tromethamine

Pharmacokinetic Parameter (units)	Intramuscular* 15 mg	30 mg	60 mg
Bioavailability (extent)			— 100% —
T_{max} [1] (min)	33 ± 21**	44 ± 29	33 ± 21**
C_{max} [2] (mcg/ml)[single dose]	1.14 ± 0.32**	2.42 ± 0.68	4.55 ± 1.27**
C_{max} (mcg/ml)[steady state qid]	1.56 ± 0.44**	3.11 ± 0.87**	N/A††
C_{min} [3] (mcg/ml)[steady state qid]	0.47 ± 0.13**	0.93 ± 0.26**	N/A
C_{avg} [4] (mcg/ml)[steady state qid]	0.94 ± 0.29**	1.88 ± 0.59**	N/A
V_β [5] (L/kg)			— 0.175-0.039—

CLINICAL STUDIES:

The analgesic efficacy of intramuscularly, intravenously and orally administered ketorolac tromethamine was investigated in two postoperative pain models: general surgery (orthopedic, gynecologic and abdominal) and oral surgery (removal of impacted third molars). The studies were primarily double-blind, single- and multi-dose, parallel trial designs, in patients with moderate to severe pain at baseline. Ketorolac tromethamine IV/IM was compared as follows: IM to meperidine or morphine administered intramuscularly, and IV to morphine administered either directly IV or through a PCA (Patient-Controlled Analgesia) pump.

Short Term Use (up to 5 days): In the comparisons of intramuscular administration during the first hour, the onset of analgesic action was similar for ketorolac tromethamine and the narcotics, but the duration of analgesia was longer with ketorolac tromethamine than with the opioid comparators meperidine or morphine.

In a multi-dose, postoperative (general surgery) double-blind trial of ketorolac tromethamine IM 30 mg versus morphine 6 and 12 mg IM, each drug given on an "as needed" basis for up to 5 days, the overall analgesic effect of ketorolac tromethamine IM 30 mg was in between that of morphine 6 and 12 mg. Ketorolac tromethamine 30 mg caused less drowsiness, nausea and vomiting than morphine 12 mg. The majority of patients treated with either ketorolac tromethamine or morphine were dosed for up to 3 days; a small percentage of patients received 5 days of dosing.

CLINICAL STUDIES: *(cont'd)*

TABLE 1C Table of Approximate Average Pharmacokinetic Parameters (Mean ± SD) Oral, Intramuscular and Intravenous Doses of Ketorolac Tromethamine

Pharmacokinetic Parameter (units)	Intravenous Bolus‡ 15 mg	30 mg
Bioavailability (extent)	100%	
T_{max}[1] (min)	1.1 ± 0.7**	2.9 ± 1.8
C_{max}[2] (mcg/ml)[single dose]	2.47 ± 0.51**	4.65 ± 0.96
C_{max} (mcg/ml)[steady state qid]	3.09 ± 1.17**	6.85 ± 2.61
C_{min}[3] (mcg/ml)[steady state qid]	0.61 ± 0.21**	1.04 ± 0.35
C_{avg}[4] (mcg/ml)[steady state qid]	1.09 ± 0.30**	2.17 ± 0.59
V_β[5] (L/kg)	0.210 ± 0.044	
% Dose metabolized = <50	% Dose excreted in feces = 6	
% Dose excreted in urine = 91	% Plasma protein binding = 99	

† Derived from PO pharmacokinetic studies in 77 normal fasted volunteers.
* Derived from IM pharmacokinetic studies in 54 normal volunteers.
†† Not applicable because 60 mg is only recommended as a single dose.
‡ Derived from IV pharmacokinetic studies in 24 normal volunteers.
** Mean value was simulated from observed plasma concentration data and standard deviation was simulated from percent coefficient of variation for observed C_{max} and T_{max} data

[1] Time-to-peak plasma concentration
[2] Peak plasma concentration
[3] Trough plasma concentration
[4] Average plasma concentration
[5] Volume of distribution

TABLE 2 The Influence of Age, Liver and Kidney Function, on the Clearance and Terminal Half-life of Ketorolac Tromethamine (IM [1] and ORAL[2])

Type of Subjects	Total Clearance [in l/h/kg][3] IM Mean (range)	Oral Mean (range)	Terminal Half-life [in hours] IM Mean (range)	Oral Mean (range)
Normal Subjects IM (n=54)	0.023 (0.010-0.046)	0.025 (0.013-0.050)	5.3 (3.5-9.2)	5.3 (2.4-9.0)
mean range=32, range=18-60, (n=77), mean age=32, range=20-60				
Healthy Elderly Subjects IM (n=13),	0.019 (0.013-0.034)	0.024 (0.018-0.034)	7.0 (4.7-8.6)	6.1 (4.3-7.6)
Oral (n=12) (mean age=72, range=65-78)				
Patients with Hepatic Dysfunction IM	0.029 (0.013-0.066)	0.033 (0.019-0.051)	5.4 (2.2-6.9)	4.5 (1.6-7.6)
Oral (n=7) (mean age=51, range=43-64)				
Patients with Renal Impairment IM and Oral (n=9) serum creatinine 1.9-5.0mg/dl	0.015 (0.005-0.043)	0.016 (0.007-0.052)	10.3 (5.9-19.2)	10.8 (3.4-18.9)
(mean age (IM)=54, range=35-71 mean age (Oral)=5, range=39-70)				
Renal Dialysis Patients IM and Oral	0.016 (0.003-0.036)	-	13.6 (8.0-39.1)	- -
(n=9) mean age=40, range=27-63				

[1] Estimated from 30 mg single IM doses of ketorolac tromethamine
[2] Estimated from 10 mg single oral doses of ketorolac tromethamine
[3] Liters/hour/kilogram IV-Administration: In normal studies (n=37), the total clearance of 30 mg IV-administered ketorolac tromethamine was 0.030 (0.017-0.051) l/h/kg. The terminal half-life was 5.6 (4.0-7.9) hours.

In clinical settings where perioperative morphine was allowed, ketorolac tromethamine IV 30 mg, given once or twice as needed, provided analgesia comparable to morphine 4 mg IV once or twice as needed.

There was relatively limited experience with 5 consecutive days of ketorolac tromethamine IV use in controlled clinical trials, as most patients were given the drug for 3 days or less. The adverse events seen with IV- administered ketorolac tromethamine were similar to those observed with IM-administered ketorolac tromethamine, as would be expected based on the similar pharmacokinetics and bioequivalence (AUC, clearance, plasma half-life) of IV and IM routes of ketorolac tromethamine administration.

Clinical Studies with Concomitant Use of Opioids: Clinical studies in postoperative pain management have demonstrated that ketorolac tromethamine IV/IM, when used in combination with opioids, significantly reduced opioid consumption. This combination may be useful in the subpopulation of patients especially prone to opioid-related complications. Ketorolac tromethamine and narcotics should not be administered in the same syringe.

In postoperative study, where all patients received morphine by a PCA device, patients treated with ketorolac tromethamine IV as fixed intermittent boluses (*e.g.,* 30 mg initial dose followed by 15 mg q3h), required significantly less morphine (26%) than the placebo group. Analgesia was significantly superior, at various postdosing pain assessment times, in the patients receiving ketorolac tromethamine IV plus PCA morphine as compared to patients receiving PCA administered morphine.

Postmarketing Surveillance Study: A large postmarketing observational, non-randomized study, involving approximately 10,000 patients receiving ketorolac tromethamine, demonstrated that the risk of clinically serious gastrointestinal (G.I.) bleeding was dose-dependent (see TABLE 3A and 3B). This was particularly true in elderly patients who received an average daily dose greater than 60 mg/day of ketorolac tromethamine (TABLE 3A).

TABLE 3A Incidence of Clinically Serious G.I. Bleeding as Related to Age, Total Daily Dose, and History of G.I. Perforation, Ulcer, Bleeding (PUB) after up to 5 Days of Treatment with Ketorolac Tromethamine IV/IM A. Patients without History of PUB

Age of Patients	Total Daily Dose of Ketorolac Tromethamine IV/IM ≤60 mg	>60 to 90 mg	>90 to 120 mg	>120 mg
<65 years of age	0.4%	0.4%	0.9%	4.6%
≥65 years of age	1.2%	2.8%	2.2%	7.7%

Ophthalmic Solution: Ocular administration of ketorolac tromethamine reduces the prostaglandin E_2 levels in aqueous humor. The mean concentration of PGE_2 was 80 pg/ml in the aqueous humor of the eyes receiving vehicle and 28 pg/ml in the eyes receiving 0.5% Acular (ketorolac tromethamine) ophthalmic solution.

CLINICAL STUDIES: *(cont'd)*

TABLE 3B Incidence of Clinically Serious G.I. Bleeding as Related to Age, Total Daily Dose, and History of G.I. Perforation, Ulcer, Bleeding (PUB) after up to 5 Days of Treatment with Ketorolac Tromethamine IV/IM B. Patients with History of PUB

Age of Patients	Total Daily Dose of ketorolac tromethamine IV/IM ≤60 mg	>60 to 90 mg	>90 to 120 mg	>120 mg
<65 years of age	2.1%	4.6%	7.8%	15.4%
≥65 years of age	4.7%	3.7%	2.8%	25.0%

Ketorolac tromethamine given systemically does not cause pupil constriction.

Results from clinical studies indicate that Acular ophthalmic solution has no significant effect upon intraocular pressure.

Two controlled studies showed that Acular (ketorolac tromethamine) ophthalmic solution was significantly more effective than its vehicle in receiving ocular itch caused by seasonal allergic conjunctivitis. Two drops (0.1 ml) of 0.5% Acular (ketorolac tromethamine) ophthalmic solution instilled into the patient 12 hours and 1 hour prior to cataract extraction achieved measurable levels in 8 of 9 patients' eyes (mean ketorolac concentration 95 ng/ml aqueous humor, range 40 to 170 ng/ml).

One drop (0.05 ml) of 0.5% of Acular ophthalmic solution was instilled into one eye and one drop of vehicle into the other eye tid in 26 normal subjects. Only 5 of 26 subjects had a detectable amount of ketorolac in their plasma (range 10.7 to 22.5 ng/ml) at Day 10 during topical ocular treatment. When ketorolac tromethamine 10 mg is administered systemically every 6 hours, peak plasma levels at steady state are round 960 ng/ml.

Acular ophthalmic solution has been safely administered in conjunction with other ophthalmic medications, such as antibiotics, beta blockers, carbonic anhydrase inhibitors, cycloplegics, and mydriatics.

INDICATIONS AND USAGE:

Ketorolac tromethamine is indicated for the short-term (≤5 days) management of moderately severe, acute pain that requires analgesia at the opioid level, usually in a postoperative setting. Therapy should always be initiated with ketorolac tromethamine IV/IM and oral ketorolac tromethamine is to be used only as continuation treatment, if necessary. Combined use of ketorolac tromethamine IV/IM and oral ketorolac tromethamine is not to exceed 5 days of use because of the potential of increasing the frequency and severity of adverse reactions associated with the recommended doses (see WARNINGS, PRECAUTIONS, DOSAGE AND ADMINISTRATION, and ADVERSE REACTIONS). Patients should be switched to alternative analgesics as soon as possible, but ketorolac tromethamine therapy is not to exceed 5 days.

Ketorolac tromethamine IV/IM has been used concomitantly with morphine and meperidine, and has shown an opioid-sparing effect. For breakthrough pain, it is recommended to supplement the lower end of the ketorolac tromethamine IV/IM dosage range with low doses of narcotics prn, unless otherwise contraindicated. Ketorolac tromethamine IV/IM and narcotics should not be administered in the same syringe (see DOSAGE AND ADMINISTRATION), Pharmaceutical Information for ketorolac tromethamine IV/IM.

Ophthalmic Solution: Acular ophthalmic solution is indicated for the relief of ocular itching due to seasonal allergic conjunctivitis.

CONTRAINDICATIONS:

(see also BOXED WARNING)

Ketorolac tromethamine is CONTRAINDICATED in patients with active peptic ulcer disease, in patients with recent gastrointestinal bleeding or perforation, and in patients with a history of peptic ulcer disease or gastrointestinal bleeding.

Ketorolac tromethamine is CONTRAINDICATED in patients with advanced renal impairment, or in patients at risk of renal failure due to volume depletion (see WARNINGS for correction of volume depletion).

Ketorolac tromethamine is CONTRAINDICATED in labor and delivery because, through its prostaglandin synthesis inhibitory effect, it may adversely affect fetal circulation and inhibit uterine contraindications, thus increasing the risk of uterine hemorrhage.

The use of ketorolac tromethamine is CONTRAINDICATED in nursing mothers because of the potential adverse effects of prostaglandin-inhibiting drugs on neonates.

Ketorolac tromethamine is CONTRAINDICATED in patients with previously demonstrated hypersensitivity to ketorolac tromethamine, or allergic manifestations to aspirin or other non-steroidal anti-inflammatory drugs (NSAIDs).

Ketorolac tromethamine is CONTRAINDICATED as prophylactic analgesic before any major surgery is critical because of the increased risk of bleeding.

Ketorolac tromethamine inhibits platelet function and is, therefore, CONTRAINDICATED in patients with suspected or confirmed cerebrovascular bleeding, hemorrhagic diathesis, incomplete hemostasis and those at high risk of bleeding (see WARNINGS and PRECAUTIONS).

Ketorolac tromethamine is CONTRAINDICATED in patients currently receiving ASA or NSAIDs because of the cumulative risks of inducing serious NSAID related adverse events.

Ketorolac tromethamine IV/IM is CONTRAINDICATED for neuraxial (epidural or intrathecal) administration due to its alcohol content.

The concomitant use of ketorolac tromethamine and probenecid is CONTRAINDICATED.

Ophthalmic Solution: Acular (ketorolac tromethamine) ophthalmic solution is contraindicated in patients while wearing soft contact lenses and in patients with previously demonstrated hypersensitivity to any of the ingredients in the formulation.

WARNINGS:

(see also BOXED WARNING)

The combined use of ketorolac tromethamine IV/IM and oral ketorolac tromethamine is not to exceed 5 days.

The most serious risks associated ketorolac tromethamine are:

Gastrointestinal Ulcerations-Bleeding and Perforation: Ketorolac tromethamine is CONTRAINDICATED in patients with previously documented peptic ulcers and/or G.I. bleeding. Serious gastrointestinal toxicity, such as bleeding ulceration, and perforation, can occur at any time, with or without warning symptoms, in patients treated with ketorolac tromethamine. Studies to date with NSAIDs have not identified any subset of patients not at risk of developing peptic ulceration and bleeding. Elderly or debilitated patients seem to tolerate ulceration or bleeding less well than other individuals, and most spontaneous reports of fatal GI events are in this population. Postmarketing experience with parenterally administered ketorolac tromethamine suggests that there may be a greater risk of gastrointestinal ulcerations, bleeding and perforation in the elderly.

WARNINGS: *(cont'd)*

The incidence and severity of gastrointestinal compilations increases with increasing dose of, and duration of treatment with, ketorolac tromethamine. In a non-randomized, in-hospital postmarketing surveillance study, comparing parental ketorolac tromethamine to parental opioids, higher rates of clinically serious G.I. bleeding were seen in patients <65 years of age who received an average total daily dose of more than 90 mg of ketorolac tromethamine IV/IM per day (see CLINICAL PHARMACOLOGY, Postmarketing Surveillance Study.

The same study showed that elderly (≥65 years of age), and debilitated patients are more susceptible to gastrointestinal complications. A history of peptic ulcer disease was revealed as another risk factor that increases the possibility of developing serious gastrointestinal complications during ketorolac tromethamine therapy (see TABLES 3A and B).

Impaired Renal Function: *Ketorolac tromethamine should be with caution in patients with impaired renal function, or a history of kidney disease because it is a potent inhibitor of prostaglandin synthesis.*

Renal toxicity with ketorolac tromethamine has been seen in patients with conditions leading to a reduction in blood volume and/or renal blood flow, where renal prostaglandins have a supportive role in the maintenance of renal perfusion. In these patients, administration of ketorolac tromethamine may cause a dose- dependent reduction in renal prostaglandin formation and may precipitate acute renal failure. Patients at greatest risk of this reaction are those with impaired renal function, dehydration, heart failure, liver dysfunction, those taking diuretics and the elderly. Discontinuation of ketorolac tromethamine therapy is usually followed by recovery to the pretreatment state.

Renal Effects: Ketorolac tromethamine and its metabolites are eliminated primarily by the kidneys, which, in patients with reduced creatinine clearance, will result in diminished clearance of the drug (see CLINICAL PHARMACOLOGY). Therefore, ketorolac tromethamine should be used with caution in patients with impaired renal function (see DOSAGE AND ADMINISTRATION) and such patients should be followed closely. With the use of ketorolac tromethamine, there have been reports of acute renal failure, nephritis, and nephrotic syndrome.

Because patients with underlying renal insufficiency are at increased risk of developing acute renal failure, the risks and benefits should be assessed prior to giving ketorolac tromethamine to these patients. Hence, in patients with moderately elevated serum creatinine, it is recommended that the daily dose of ketorolac tromethamine IV/IM be reduced by half, not to exceed 60 mg/day. **KETOROLAC TROMETHAMINE IS CONTRAINDICATED IN PATIENTS WITH SERUM CREATININE CONCENTRATIONS INDICATING ADVANCED RENAL IMPAIRMENT** (see CONTRAINDICATIONS).

Hypovolemia should be corrected before treatment with ketorolac tromethamine is initiated.

Fluid Retention and Edema: Fluid Retention, edema, retention of NaCl, oliguria, elevations of serum urea nitrogen and creatine have been reported in clinical trials with ketorolac tromethamine. Therefore, ketorolac tromethamine should be used only very cautiously in patients with cardiac decompensation, hypertension, or similar conditions.

Hemorrhage: Because prostaglandins play an important role in hemostasis, and NSAIDs affect platelet aggregation as well, use of ketorolac tromethamine in patients who have coagulation disorders should be undertaken very cautiously, and those patients should be carefully monitored. Patients on therapeutic doses of anticoagulants (*e.g.,* heparin or dicumarol derivatives) have an increased risk of bleeding complications if given ketorolac tromethamine concurrently; therefore, physicians should administer such concomitant therapy only extremely cautiously. The concurrent use of ketorolac tromethamine and prophylactic low-dose heparin (2500-5000 units q12h), warfarin and dextrans have not been studied extensively, but may also be associated with an increased risk of bleeding. Until data from such studies are available, physicians should carefully weigh the benefits against the risks, and use such concomitant therapy in these patients only extremely cautiously. In patients who receive anticoagulants for any reason, there is an increased risk of intramuscular hematoma formation from administered ketorolac tromethamine IM (see DRUG INTERACTIONS). Patients receiving therapy that affects hemostasis should be monitored closely.

In postmarketing experience, postoperative hematomas and other signs of wound bleeding have been reported in association with the perioperative use of ketorolac tromethamine IV/IM. Therefore, perioperative use of ketorolac tromethamine should be avoided and postoperative use be undertaken with caution when hemostasis is critical (see WARNINGS and PRECAUTIONS).

Anaphylactoid Reactions: Anaphylactoid reactions may occur in patients without a known previous exposure or hypersensitivity to aspirin, ketorolac tromethamine, or other NSAIDs, or in individuals with a history of angioedema, bronchospastic reactivity (*e.g.,* asthma), and nasal polyps. Anaphylactoid reactions, like anaphylaxis, may have a fatal outcome.

Ophthalmic Solution: There is potential for cross sensitivity to acetylsalicylic acid, phenylacetic acid derivatives, and other nonsteroidal anti-inflammatory agents. Therefore, caution should be used when treating individuals who have previously exhibited sensitivities to these drugs.

PRECAUTIONS:

Hepatic Effects: Ketorolac tromethamine should be used with caution in patients with impaired hepatic function, or a history of liver disease. Treatment with ketorolac tromethamine may cause elevations of liver enzymes, and in patients with pre-existing liver dysfunction it may lead to the development of a more severe hepatic reaction. The administration of ketorolac tromethamine should be discontinued in patients in whom an abnormal liver test has occurred as a result of ketorolac tromethamine therapy.

Hematologic Effects: Ketorolac tromethamine inhibits platelet aggregation and may prolong bleeding time; therefore, it is contraindicated as a preoperative medication and caution should be used when hemostasis is critical. Unlike aspirin, the inhibition of platelet function by ketorolac tromethamine disappears within 24 to 48 hours after the drug is discontinued. Ketorolac tromethamine does not appear to affect platelet count, prothrombin time (PT) or partial thromboplastin time (PTT). In controlled clinical studies, where ketorolac tromethamine was administered intramuscularly or intravenously postoperatively, the incidence of clinically significant postoperative bleeding was 0.4% for ketorolac tromethamine compared to 0.2% in the control groups receiving narcotic analgesics.

Information for Patients: Ketorolac tromethamine is a potent NSAID and may cause serious side effects such as gastrointestinal bleeding or kidney failure, which may result in hospitalization and even fatal outcome.

Physicians, when prescribing ketorolac tromethamine should inform their patients of the potential risks of ketorolac tromethamine treatment (see BOXED WARNING, WARNINGS, PRECAUTIONS, and ADVERSE REACTIONS). *Advise patients not to give oral ketorolac tromethamine to other family members and to discard any unused drug.* Remember that the total duration of ketorolac tromethamine therapy is not to exceed 5 (five) days.

Carcinogenesis Mutagenesis, and Impairment of Fertility: (For ALL forms including Ophthalmic Solution) An 18-month study in mice with oral doses of ketorolac tromethamine at 2 mg/kg/day (0.9 times the human systemic exposure at the recommended IM or IV dose of 30 mg qid, based on area-under-the plasma-concentration curve <AUC>, and a 24-month study in rats at 5 mg/kg/day (0.5 times the human AUC), showed no evidence of tumorigenicity.

PRECAUTIONS: *(cont'd)*

Ketorolac tromethamine was not mutagenic in Ames test, unscheduled DNA synthesis and repair, and in forward mutation assays. Ketorolac tromethamine did not cause chromosome breakage in the *in vivo*mouse micronucleus assay. At 1590 mcg/ml and at higher concentrations, ketorolac tromethamine increased the incidence of chromosomal aberrations in Chinese hamster ovarian cells.

Impairment of fertility did not occur in male or female rats at oral doses of 9 mg/kg (0.9 times the human AUC) and 16 mg/kg (1.6 times the human AUC) of ketorolac tromethamine, respectively.

Pregnancy Category C Reproduction studies have been performed during organogenesis, using daily oral doses of ketorolac tromethamine at 3.6 mg/kg (0.37 times the human AUC) in rabbits and at 10 mg/kg (1.0 times the human AUC) in rats. Results of these studies did not reveal evidence of teratogenicity to the fetus. Oral doses of ketorolac tromethamine at 1.5 mg/kg (0.14 times the human AUC), administered after gestation day 17, caused dystocia and higher pup mortality in rats. There are no adequate and well-controlled studies of ketorolac tromethamine in pregnant women. Ketorolac tromethamine should be used during pregnancy only if the potential benefit justifies the potential risk to the fetus.

Labor and Delivery: The use of ketorolac tromethamine is contraindicated in labor and delivery because, through its prostaglandin synthesis inhibitory effect, it may adversely affect fetal circulation and inhibit uterine contractions, thus increasing the risk of uterine hemorrhage (see CONTRAINDICATIONS).

Lactation and Nursing: After a single administration of 10 mg of oral ketorolac tromethamine to humans, the maximum milk concentration observed was 7.3 ng/ml and the maximum milk-to-plasma ratio was 0.037. After one day of dosing (qid), the maximum milk concentration was 7.9 ng/ml and the maximum milk-to-plasma ratio was 0.025. Because of the possible adverse effects of prostaglandin-inhibiting drugs on neonates, use in nursing mothers is contraindicated.

Pediatric Use: (For ALL forms including Ophthalmic Solution)

Safety and efficacy in children (less than 16 years of age) have not been established. Therefore, use of ketorolac tromethamine is not recommended for use in children is not recommended.

Acular: Safety and efficacy in children have not been established.

Use in the Elderly (≥65 YEARS OF AGE): Because ketorolac tromethamine may be cleared more slowly by the elderly (see CLINICAL PHARMACOLOGY) who are also more sensitive to the adverse effects of NSAIDs (see WARNINGS, Renal Effects), extra caution and reduced dosages (see DOSAGE AND ADMINISTRATION) must be used when treating the elderly with ketorolac tromethamine$^{IV/IM}$. The lower dosage range is recommended for patients over 65 years of age and total daily dose is not to exceed 60 mg. The incidence and severity of gastrointestinal complications increases with increasing dose of, and duration of treatment with, ketorolac tromethamine.

Additional Precautions for the Ophthalmic Solution: It is recommended that Acular (ketorolac tromethamine) 0.5% Sterile Ophthalmic Solution be used with caution in patients with known bleeding tendencies or who are receiving other medication which may prolong bleeding time.

DRUG INTERACTIONS:

Ketorolac is highly bound to human plasma proteins (mean 99.2%).

The *in vitro* binding of ***warfarin***to plasma proteins is only slightly reduced by ketorolac tromethamine (99.5% control vs 99.3%) when ketorolac plasma concentrations reach 5 to 10 mcg/ml. Ketorolac does not alter ***digoxin***protein binding. *In vitro* studies indicate that, at therapeutic concentrations of ***salicylate***(300 mcg/ml), the binding of ketorolac was reduced from approximately 99.2% to 97.5%, representing a potential two-fold increase in unbound ketorolac plasma levels. Therapeutic concentrations of ***digoxin, warfarin, ibuprofen, naproxen, piroxicam, acetaminophen, phenytoin,*** and ***tolbutamide***did not alter ketorolac tromethamine protein binding.

In a study involving 12 volunteers, oral ketorolac tromethamine was co-administered with a single dose of 25 mg ***warfarin***, causing no significant changes in pharmacokinetics or pharmacodynamics of warfarin. In another study, ketorolac tromethamine IV/IM was given with two doses of 5000 U of ***heparin***to 11 healthy volunteers, resulting in a mean template bleeding time of 6.4 minutes (3.2-11.4 min) compared to a mean of 6.0 minutes (3.4-7.5 min) for heparin alone and 5.1 minutes (3.5-8.5 min) for placebo. Although these results do not indicate a significant interaction between ketorolac tromethamine and warfarin or heparin, the administration of ketorolac tromethamine to patients taking anticoagulants should be done extremely cautiously and patients should be closely monitored. (See WARNINGS and PRECAUTIONS).

Ketorolac tromethamine IV/IM reduced the diuretic response to ***furosemide***in normovolemic healthy subjects by approximately 20% (mean sodium and urinary output decreased 17%).

Concomitant administration of oral ketorolac tromethamineand ***probenecid***resulted in decreased clearance of ketorolac and significant increases in ketorolac plasma levels (total AUC increased approximately 3-fold from 5.4 to 17.8 mcg/h/ml) and terminal half-life increased approximately 2-fold from 6.6 to 15.1 hours. Therefore, concomitant use of ketorolac tromethamine and probenecid is contraindicated.

Inhibition of renal ***lithium***clearance, leading to an increase in plasma lithium concentration, has been reported with some prostaglandin synthesis-inhibiting drugs. The effect of ketorolac tromethamine on plasma lithium has not been studied, but cases of increased lithium plasma levels during ketorolac tromethamine therapy have been reported.

Concomitant administration of ***methotrexate***and some NSAIDs has been reported to reduce the clearance of methotrexate, enhancing the toxicity of methotrexate. The effect of ketorolac tromethamine on methotrexate clearance has not been studied.

In postmarketing experience, there have been three reports of a possible interaction between ketorolac tromethamine IV/IM and ***non-depolarizing muscle relaxants***, that resulted in apnea. The concurrent use of ketorolac tromethamine with muscle relaxants has not been formally studied.

Concomitant use of **ACE inhibitors** may increase the risk of renal impairment, particularly in volume-depleted patients.

Sporadic cases of seizures have been reported during concomitant use of ketorolac tromethamine and ***antiepilectic drugs***(Dilantin, Tegretol).

Hallucinations have been reported when ketorolac tromethamine was used in patients taking ***psychoactive drugs***(Prozac, Navane, Xanax).

Ketorolac tromethamine IV/IM has been administered concurrently with ***morphine***in several clinical trials of postoperative pain without evidence of adverse interactions. Do not mix ketorolac tromethamine and morphine in the same syringe.

There is no evidence, in animal or human studies, that ketorolac tromethamine induces or inhibits hepatic enzymes capable of metabolizing itself or other drugs.

ADVERSE REACTIONS:

Adverse reaction rates increase with higher doses of ketorolac tromethamine. Practitioners should be alert for the severe complications of treatment with ketorolac tromethamine, such as G.I. ulceration, bleeding and perforation, postoperative bleeding, acute renal failure, anaphylactic and anaphylactoid reactions, and liver failure (see BOXED WARNING, WARNINGS, PRECAUTIONS, and DOSAGE AND ADMINISTRATION. These NSAID-related complications can be serious in certain patients for whom ketorolac tromethamine is indicated, especially when the drug is used inappropriately.

The adverse reactions listed below were reported in clinical trials as probably related to ketorolac tromethamine.

Incidence Greater Than 1%

Body as a Whole: Edema (4%).

Cardiovascular: hypertension.

Dermatologic: pruritus, rash.

Gastrointestinal: nausea (12%), dyspepsia (12%), gastrointestinal pain (13%), diarrhea (7%), constipation, flatulence, gastrointestinal fullness, vomiting, stomatitis.

Hemic and Lymphatic: purpura.

Nervous System: headache (17%), drowsiness (6%), dizziness (7%), sweating.

Injection-site pain: was reported by 2% of patients in multi-dose studies.

[Percentage of incidence in parentheses for those events reported in 3% or more patients]

Incidence 1% Or Less

Body as a Whole: weight gain, fever, infections, asthenia.

Cardiovascular: palpitation, pallor, syncope.

Dermatologic: urticaria.

Gastrointestinal: gastritis, rectal bleeding, eructation, anorexia, increased appetite.

Hemic and Lymphatic: epistaxis, anemia, eosinophilia.

Nervous System: tremors, abnormal dreams, hallucinations, euphoria, extrapyramidal symptoms, vertigo, paresthesia, depression, insomnia, nervousness, excessive thirst, dry mouth, abnormal vision, inability to concentrate, hyperkinesis, stupor.

Respiratory: dyspnea, pulmonary edema, rhinitis, cough.

Special Senses: abnormal taste, abnormal vision, blurred vision, tinnitus, hearing loss.

Urogenital: hematuria, proteinuria, oliguria, urinary retention, polyuria, increased urinary frequency.

The following adverse events were reported from postmarketing experience.

Body as a Whole: hypersensitivity reactions such as anaphylaxis, anaphylactoid reaction, laryngeal edema, tongue edema (see BOXED WARNING, WARNINGS), myalgia.

Cardiovascular: hypotension and flushing.

Dermatologic: Lyell's syndrome, Stevens-Johnson syndrome, exfoliative dermatitis, maculopapular rash, urticaria.

Gastrointestinal: peptic, ulceration, GI hemorrhage, GI perforation (see BOXED WARNING, WARNINGS), melena, acute pancreatitis.

Hemic and Lymphatic: postoperative wound hemorrhage (rarely requiring blood transfusion-see BOXED WARNING, WARNINGS and PRECAUTIONS), thrombocytopenia, leukopenia.

Hepatic: hepatitis, liver failure, cholestatic, jaundice.

Nervous System: convulsions, psychosis, aseptic meningitis.

Respiratory: asthma, bronchospasm.

Urogenital : acute renal failure (see BOXED WARNING, WARNINGS), flank pain with or without hematuria and/or azotemia, nephritis, hyponatremia, hyperkalemia, hemolytic, uremic syndrome.

Ophthalmic Solution: In patients with allergic conjunctivitis, the most adverse events reported with the use of Acular (ketorolac tromethamine) ophthalmic solution have been transient stinging and burning on instillation. These events were reported by approximately 40% of the patients treated with Acular ophthalmic solution. In all development studies conducted, other adverse events reported during treatment with Acular include ocular irritation (3%), allergic reactions (3%), superficial ocular infections (0.5%) and superficial keratitis (1%).

OVERDOSAGE:

In controlled overdosage, daily doses of 360 mg of ketorolac tromethamine IV/IMgiven for five days (3 times the highest recommended dose), caused abdominal pain and peptic ulcers which healed after discontinuation of doses. Metabolic acidosis has been reported following intentional overdosage.

Dialysis does not significantly clear ketorolac tromethamine from the blood stream.

DOSAGE AND ADMINISTRATION:

THE COMBINED DURATION OF USE OF KETOROLAC TROMETHAMINE IV/IM AND KETOROLAC TROMETHAMINE ORAL IS NOT TO EXCEED FIVE (5) DAYS.

THE USE OF KETOROLAC TROMETHAMINE ORAL IS ONLY INDICATED AS CONTINUATION THERAPY TO KETOROLAC TROMETHAMINE IV/IM.

Ketorolac Tromethamine IV/IM: Ketorolac tromethamine IV/IM may be used as a single or multiple dose, on a regular or "pm" schedule for the management of moderately severe, acute pain that requires analgesia at the opioid level, usually in a postoperative setting. Hypovolemia should be corrected prior to the administration of ketorolac tromethamine (see WARNINGS, Renal Effects). Patients should be switched to alternative analgesics as soon as possible, but ketorolac tromethamine therapy is not to exceed 5 days.

When administering ketorolac tromethamine IV/IM, the IV bolus must be given over no less than 15 seconds. The IM administration should be given slowly and deeply into the muscle. The analgesic effect begins in ~30 minutes with maximum effect 1 to 2 hours after dosing IV or IM. Duration of analgesic effect is usually 4 to 6 hours.

SINGLE-DOSE TREATMENT: THE FOLLOWING REGIMEN SHOULD BE LIMITED TO SINGLE ADMINISTRATION USE ONLY

IM Dosing

Patients <65 years of age: One dose of 60 mg.

Patients ≥65 years of age, renally impaired and/or less than 50 kg **(110 lbs) of body weight:** One dose of 30 mg.

IV Dosing

Patients <65 years of age: One dose of 30 mg.

Patients ≥65 years of age, renally impaired and/or less than 50 kg **(110 lbs) of body weight:** One dose of 15 mg.

MULTIPLE-DOSE TREATMENT (IV OR IM)

Patients <65 years of age: The recommended dose is 30 mg ketorolac tromethamine IV/IM every 6 hours. The maximum daily dose should not exceed 120 mg.

DOSAGE AND ADMINISTRATION: *(cont'd)*

For patients ≥65 years of age, renally impaired patients (see WARNINGS), and patients less than 50 kg (110 lbs): The recommended dose is 15 mg ketorolac tromethamine IV/IM every 6 hours. The maximum daily dose for these populations should not exceed 60 mg.

For breakthrough pain, do not increase the dose or the frequency of ketorolac tromethamine. Consideration should be given to supplementing these regiments with low doses of opioids "pm" unless otherwise contraindicated.

Pharmaceutical Information for Ketorolac Tromethamine IV/IM: Parenteral drug products should be inspected visually for particulate matter and discoloration prior to administration, whenever solution and container permit.

Ketorolac tromethamine IV/IM should not be mixed in a small volume (*e.g.,* in a syringe) with morphine sulfate, meperidine hydrochloride, promethazine hydrochloride or hydroxyzine hydrochloride; this will result in precipitation of ketorolac from solution.

Ketorolac Tromethamine Oral: Oral ketorolac tromethamine is indicated ONLY as continuation therapy to ketorolac tromethamine IV/IM for the management of moderately severe, acute pain that requires analgesia at the opioid level. See also PRECAUTIONS, Information for Patients.

Transition from Ketorolac Tromethamine IV/IM to Ketorolac Tromethamine Oral: The recommended oral ketorolac tromethamine dose is as follows:

Patients <65 years of age: Two (2) tablets as a first oral dose for patients who received **60 mg IM single dose, 30 mg IV single dose** or 30 **mg multiple dose** ketorolac tromethamine IV/IM followed by one (1) tablet oral ketorolac tromethamine every 4 to 6 hours, not to exceed 40 mg/24 h of oral ketorolac tromethamine.

Patients ≥65 years of age, renally impaired and/or less than 50 kg (110 lbs) of body weight: One (1) tablet as a first oral dose for patients who received **30 mg IM single dose, 15 mg IV single dose** or **15 mg multiple dose** ketorolac tromethamine IV/IM followed by one (1) tablet oral ketorolac tromethamine every 4 to 6 hours, not to exceed 40 mg/24 h of oral ketorolac tromethamine.

Shortening the recommended dosing intervals may result in increased frequency and severity of adverse reactions.

THE MAXIMUM COMBINED DURATION OF USE (PARENTERAL AND ORAL KETOROLAC TROMETHAMINE) IS LIMITED TO 5 DAYS.

OPHTHALMIC SOLUTION: The recommended dose of Acular is one drop (0.25 mg) four times a day for relief of ocular itching due to seasonal allergic conjunctivitis. The efficacy of Acular (ketorolac tromethamine) ophthalmic solution has not been established beyond one week of therapy.

ANIMAL PHARMACOLOGY:

Ophthalmic Solution Only: Ketorolac tromethamine prevented the development of increased intraocular pressure induced in rabbits with topically applied arachidonic acid. Ketorolac did not inhibit rabbit lens aldose reductase *in vivo.*

Ketorolac tromethamine ophthalmic solution did not enhance the spread of ocular infections induced in rabbits with *Candida albicans, Herpes Simplex virus type one,* or *pseudomonas aeruginosa.*

HOW SUPPLIED:

Store injectionables at controlled room temperature 15° to 30°C (59° to 86° F) with protection from light.

Store oral tablets at controlled room temperature, 15° to 30°C (59° to 86°F). Store blister packages at controlled room temperature, 15° to 30°C (59° to 86°F). Protect from excessive humidity and light.

Acular Ophthalmic Solution: Store at controlled room temperature, 15- 30°C (59-86°F) with protection from light.

(Roche Laboratories, 02-2435-42-00, 12/94)

HOW SUPPLIED - EQUIVALENTS NOT AVAILABLE:

Injection, Solution - Intramuscular - 15 mg/ml

1 ml x 10	$70.52	TORADOL INJECTABLE, Syntex Labs	00033-2443-40
1 ml x 10	$78.51	TORADOL, Roche	00004-6921-06
1 ml x 10	$81.56	TORADOL, Roche	00004-6920-06

Injection, Solution - Intramuscular - 30 mg/ml

1 ml x 10	$72.43	TORADOL INJECTABLE, Syntex Labs	00033-2434-40
1 ml x 10	$82.22	TORADOL, Syntex Labs	00033-2434-50
1 ml x 10	$85.42	TORADOL, Roche	00004-6922-06
2 ml x 10	$86.23	TORADOL, Syntex Labs	00033-2444-01

Injection, Solution - Intramuscular - 60 mg

2 ml disposable	$74.34	TORADOL, Syntex Labs	00033-2444-40

Solution - Ophthalmic - 0.5 %

5 ml	$27.78	ACULAR, Allergan	00023-2181-05
5 ml x 3	$76.50	ACULAR, Allergan	00023-2181-35

Tablet, Uncoated - Oral - 10 mg

100's	$122.45	TORADOL, Syntex Labs	00033-2435-42

KETOTIFEN FUMARATE *(003081)*

CATEGORIES: Airway Obstruction; Antiasthmatics/Bronchodilators; Asthma; Respiratory & Allergy Medications; Sympathomimetic Agents; FDA Unapproved

BRAND NAMES: *Asmafen*; *Asmanoc*; *Asthafen*; *Astifen*; *Demetofrin*; *Denerel*; *Dhatifen*; *Difen*; *Eucycline*; *Fin-A* (Mexico); *K-Asmal* (Mexico); *Ketasma*; *Ketifen*; *Keto*; *Ketoben* (Mexico); *Ketofar*; *Ketonal*; *Ketotisin*; *Ketovent*; *Orpidix*; *Prevas*; *Profiten*; *Scanditen*; *Sykofen*; *Zadec*; *Zadec SRO*; **Zaditen**; *Zaditen SRO*; *Zasten*; *Zerosma*

(International brand names outside U.S. in italics)

Prescribing information not available at time of publication.

L-CYSTEINE HYDROCHLORIDE *(001609)*

CATEGORIES: Caloric Agents; Electrolyte Solutions; Electrolytic, Caloric-Water Balance; Homeostatic & Nutrient; Vitamins; FDA Pre 1938 Drugs

BRAND NAMES: Cysteine Hydrochloride; L-Cysteine

Prescribing information not available at time of publication.

HOW SUPPLIED - EQUIVALENTS NOT AVAILABLE:

Injection, Conc-Soln - Intravenous - 50 mg/ml

10 ml	$8.88	L-Cysteine, Am Regent	00517-2064-05
10 ml	$17.77	L-CYSTEINE, Abbott	00074-8975-18
10 ml x 10	$10.80	Cysteine Hcl, McGaw	00264-6000-03
10 ml x 10	$102.00	L-Cysteine, Gensia Labs	00703-5324-03
50 ml x 10	$510.00	L-Cysteine, Gensia Labs	00703-5328-03

L-TRYPTOPHAN *(003224)*

CATEGORIES: Antidepressants; Depression; Electrolytic, Caloric-Water Balance; Hypnotics; Insomnia; FDA Pre 1938 Drugs

BRAND NAMES: *Amifan* (Japan); Amino Acids; *Eltrip* (Japan)
(International brand names outside U.S. in italics)

Prescribing information not available at time of publication.

LABETALOL HYDROCHLORIDE *(001613)*

CATEGORIES: Antihypertensives; Beta Adrenergic Blocking Agents; Beta Blockers; Cardiovascular Drugs; Hypertension; Pregnancy Category C; FDA Approved 1984 Aug; Patent Expiration 1994 Aug

BRAND NAMES: *Abetol*; *Albetol*; *Amipress*; *Coreton*; *Hybloc*; *Ipolab*; *Labelol*; *Labrocol* (England); *Lamitol*; *Liondox*; *Normadate*; **Normodyne**; *Presolol*; *Pressalolo*; *Salmagne*; *Tramin*; Trandate
(International brand names outside U.S. in italics)

FORMULARIES: Aetna; BC-BS; Medi-Cal; PCS

COST OF THERAPY: $324.41 (Hypertension; Tablet; 100 mg; 2/day; 365 days)

PRIMARY ICD9: 401.1 (Essential Hypertension, Benign)

DESCRIPTION:

Labetalol HCl is an adrenergic receptor blocking agent that has both selective alpha$_1$- and nonselective beta-adrenergic receptor blocking actions in a single substance.

Labetalol HCl is a racemate, chemically designated as 5-[1-hydroxy-2-[(1-methyl-3-phenylpropyl) amino] ethyl]salicylamide monohydrochloride.

Labetalol HCl has the empirical formula $C_{19}H_{24}N_2O_3 \cdot HCl$ and a molecular weight of 364.9. It has two asymmetric centers and therefore exists as a molecular complex of two diastereoisomeric pairs. Dilevalol, the R,R' stereoisomer, makes up 25% of racemic labetalol.

Labetalol HCl is a white or off-white crystalline powder, soluble in water.

Injection: Labetalol HCl injection is a clear, colorless to light yellow aqueous sterile isotonic solution for intravenous injection. It has a pH range of 3.0 to 4.0. Each ml contains 5 mg labetalol HCl, USP, 45 mg anhydrous dextrose, 0.10 mg edetate disodium; 0.80 mg methylparaben and 0.10 mg propylparaben as preservatives; citric acid monohydrate and sodium hydroxide, as necessary, to bring the solution into the pH range.

Tablets: Labetalol HCl tablets contain 100 mg, 200 mg, or 300 mg labetalol HCl, USP, and are taken orally.

The inactive ingredients for labetalol HCl tablets, 100 mg, include: corn starch, FD&C Blue No. 2 Al Lake, FD&C Yellow No. 6 Al Lake, hydroxypropyl methylcellulose, lactose, magnesium stearate, methylparaben, PEG, and propylparaben. May also contain: potato starch and wheat starch.

The inactive ingredients for labetalol HCl tablets, 200 mg, include: corn starch, hydroxypropyl methylcellulose, lactose, magnesium stearate, methylparaben, PEG, propylparaben, and titanium dioxide. May also contain: potato starch and wheat starch.

The inactive ingredients for labetalol HCl tablets, 300 mg, include: corn starch, FD&C Blue No. 2 Al Lake, hydroxypropyl methylcellulose, lactose, magnesium stearate, methylparaben, PEG, and propylparaben. May also contain: potato starch and wheat starch.

CLINICAL PHARMACOLOGY:

Labetalol HCl combines both selective, competitive alpha$_1$- adrenergic blocking and nonselective, competitive beta-adrenergic blocking activity in a single substance. In man, the ratios of alpha- to beta-blockade have been estimated to be approximately 1:3 and 1:7 following oral and intravenous administration, respectively. Beta$_2$-agonist activity has been demonstrated in animals with minimal beta$_1$-agonist (ISA) activity detected. In animals, at doses greater than those required for alpha- or beta-adrenergic blockade, a membrane-stabilizing effect has been demonstrated.

Pharmacodynamics: The capacity of labetalol HCl to block alpha receptors in man has been demonstrated by attenuation of the pressor effect of phenylephrine and by a significant reduction of the pressor response caused by immersing the hand in ice-cold water ("cold-pressor test"). Labetalol HCl's beta$_1$-receptor blockade in man was demonstrated by a small decrease in the resting heart rate, attenuation of tachycardia produced by isoproterenol or exercise, and by attenuation of the reflex tachycardia to the hypotension produced by amyl nitrite. Beta$_2$-receptor blockade was demonstrated by inhibition of the isoproterenol-induced fall in diastolic blood pressure. Both the alpha- and beta-blocking actions of orally administered labetalol HCl contribute to a decrease in blood pressure in hypertensive patients. Labetalol HCl consistently, in dose-related fashion, blunted increases in exercise-induced blood pressure and heart rate, and in their double product. The pulmonary circulation during exercise was not affected by labetalol HCl dosing.

Single oral doses of labetalol HCl administered in patients with coronary artery disease had no significant effect on sinus rate, intraventricular conduction, or QRS duration. The AV conduction time was modestly prolonged in 2 of 7 patients. In another study, intravenous labetalol HCl slightly prolonged AV nodal conduction time and atrial effective refractory period with only small changes in heart rate. The effects on AV nodal refractoriness were inconsistent.

Labetalol HCl produces dose-related falls in blood pressure without reflex tachycardia and without significant reduction in heart rate, presumably through a mixture of its alpha-blocking and beta-blocking effects. Hemodynamic effects are variable with small nonsignificant changes in cardiac output seen in some studies but not others, and small decreases in total peripheral resistance. Elevated plasma renins are reduced.

CLINICAL PHARMACOLOGY: *(cont'd)*

Doses of labetalol HCl that controlled hypertension did not affect renal function in mild to severe hypertensive patients with normal renal function.

INJECTION

Due to the alpha$_1$-receptor blocking activity of labetalol HCl, blood pressure is lowered more in the standing than in the supine position, and symptoms of postural hypotension can occur. During dosing with intravenous labetalol HCl, the contribution of the postural component should be considered when positioning patients for treatment, and patients should not be allowed to move to an erect position unmonitored until their ability to do so is established.

In a clinical pharmacologic study in severe hypertensives, an initial 0.25 mg/kg injection of labetalol HCl, administered to patients in the supine position, decreased blood pressure by an average of 11/7 mmHg. Additional injections of 0.5 mg/kg at 15-minute intervals up to a total cumulative dose of 1.75 mg/kg of labetalol HCl caused further dose- related decreases in blood pressure. Some patients required cumulative doses of up to 3.25 mg/kg. The maximal effect of each dose level occurred within 5 minutes. Following discontinuation of intravenous treatment with labetalol HCl, the blood pressure rose gradually and progressively, approaching pretreatment baseline values within an average of 16-18 hours in the majority of patients.

Similar results were obtained in the treatment of patients with severe hypertension requiring urgent blood pressure reduction with an initial dose of 20 mg (which corresponds to 0.25 mg/kg for an 80 kg patient) followed by additional doses of either 40 or 80 mg at 10-minute intervals to achieve the desired effect or up to a cumulative dose of 300 mg.

Labetalol HCl administered as a continuous intravenous infusion, with a mean dose of 136 mg (27 to 300 mg) over a period of 2 to 3 hours (mean of 2 hours and 39 minutes) lowered the blood pressure by an average of 60/35 mmHg.

TABLETS

Due to the alpha$_1$-receptor blocking activity of labetalol HCl, blood pressure is lowered more in the standing than in the supine position, and symptoms of postural hypotension (2%), including rare instances of syncope, can occur. Following oral administration, when postural hypotension has occurred, it has been transient and is uncommon when the recommended starting dose and titration increments are closely followed (see DOSAGE AND ADMINISTRATION.) Symptomatic postural hypotension is more likely to occur 2 to 4 hours after a dose, especially following the use of large initial doses or upon large changes in dose.

The peak effects of single oral doses of labetalol HCl occur within 2 to 4 hours. The duration of effect depends upon dose, lasting at least 8 hours following single oral doses of 100 mg and more than 12 hours following single oral doses of 300 mg. The maximum, steady-state blood pressure response upon oral, twice-a-day dosing occurs within 24 to 72 hours.

The antihypertensive effect of labetalol has a linear correlation with the logarithm of labetalol plasma concentration, and there is also a linear correlation between the reduction in exercise-induced tachycardia occurring at 2 hours after oral administration of labetalol HCl and the logarithm of the plasma concentration.

About 70% of the maximum beta-blocking effect is present for 5 hours after the administration of a single oral dose of 400 mg, with suggestion that about 40% remains at 8 hours.

The anti-anginal efficacy of labetalol HCl has not been studied. In 37 patients with hypertension and coronary artery disease, labetalol HCl did not increase the incidence or severity of angina attacks.

INJECTION AND TABLETS

Exacerbation of angina and, in some cases, myocardial infarction and ventricular dysrhythmias have been reported after abrupt discontinuation of therapy with beta-adrenergic blocking agents in patients with coronary artery disease. Abrupt withdrawal of these agents in patients without coronary artery disease has resulted in transient symptoms, including tremulousness, sweating, palpitation, headache, and malaise. Several mechanisms have been proposed to explain these phenomena, among them increased sensitivity to catecholamines because of increased numbers of beta receptors.

Although beta-adrenergic receptor blockade is useful in the treatment of angina and hypertension, there are also situations in which sympathetic stimulation is vital. For example, in patients with severely damaged hearts, adequate ventricular function may depend on sympathetic drive. Beta-adrenergic blockade may worsen AV block by preventing the necessary facilitating effects of sympathetic activity on conduction. Beta$_2$-adrenergic blockade results in passive bronchial constriction by interfering with endogenous adrenergic bronchodilator activity in patients subject to bronchospasm and may also interfere with exogenous bronchodilators in such patients.

PHARMACOKINETICS AND METABOLISM

The metabolism of labetalol is mainly through conjugation to glucuronide metabolites. These metabolites are present in plasma and are excreted in the urine and, via the bile, into the feces. Approximately 55% to 60% of a dose appears in the urine as conjugates or unchanged labetalol within the first 24 hours of dosing.

Labetalol has been shown to cross the placental barrier in humans. Only negligible amounts of the drug crossed the blood-brain barrier in animal studies. Labetalol is approximately 50% protein bound. Neither hemodialysis nor peritoneal dialysis removes a significant amount of labetalol HCl from the general circulation (<1%).

Injection: Following intravenous infusion, the elimination half-life is about 5.5 hours and the total body clearance is approximately 33 ml/min/kg. The plasma half-life of labetalol following oral administration is about 6 to 8 hours. In patients with decreased hepatic or renal function, the elimination half-life of labetalol is not altered; however, the relative bioavailability in hepatically impaired patients is increased due to decreased "first-pass" metabolism.

Tablets: Labetalol HCl is completely absorbed from the gastrointestinal tract with peak plasma levels occurring 1 to 2 hours after oral administration. The relative bioavailability of labetalol HCl tablets compared to an oral solution is 100%. The absolute bioavailability (fraction of drug reaching systemic circulation) of labetalol when compared to an intravenous infusion is 25%; this is due to extensive "first-pass" metabolism. Despite "first-pass" metabolism there is a linear relationship between oral doses of 100 to 3000 mg and peak plasma levels. The absolute bioavailability of labetalol is increased when administered with food.

The plasma half-life of labetalol following oral administration is about 6 to 8 hours. Steady-state plasma levels of labetalol during repetitive dosing are reached by about the third day of dosing. In patients with decreased hepatic or renal function, the elimination half-life of labetalol is not altered; however, the relative bioavailability in hepatically impaired patients is increased due to decreased "first-pass" metabolism.

INDICATIONS AND USAGE:

Injection: Labetalol HCl injection is indicated for control of blood pressure in severe hypertension.

Tablets: Labetalol HCl tablets are indicated in the management of hypertension. Labetalol tablets may be used alone or in combination with other antihypertensive agents, especially thiazide and loop diuretics.

CONTRAINDICATIONS:

Labetalol HCl injection and tablets are contraindicated in bronchial asthma, overt cardiac failure, greater than first degree heart block, cardiogenic shock, severe bradycardia, other conditions associated with severe and prolonged hypotension, and in patients with a history of hypersensitivity to any component of the product (see WARNINGS.)

WARNINGS:

Hepatic Injury: Severe hepatocellular injury, confirmed by rechallenge in at least one case, occurs rarely with labetalol therapy. The hepatic injury is usually reversible, but hepatic necrosis and death have been reported. Injury has occurred after both short- and long-term treatment and may be slowly progressive despite minimal symptomatology. Similar hepatic events have been reported with a related compound, dilevalol HCl, including two deaths. Dilevalol HCl is one of the four isomers of labetalol HCl. Thus, for patients taking labetalol, periodic determination of suitable hepatic laboratory tests would be appropriate. Laboratory testing should also be done at the very first symptom or sign of liver dysfunction (*e.g.,* pruritus, dark urine, persistent anorexia, jaundice, right upper quadrant tenderness, or unexplained "flu-like" symptoms). If the patient has jaundice or laboratory evidence of liver injury, labetalol HCl should be stopped and not restarted.

Cardiac Failure: Sympathetic stimulation is a vital component supporting circulatory function in congestive heart failure. Beta blockade carries a potential hazard of further depressing myocardial contractility and precipitating more severe failure. Although beta- blockers should be avoided in overt congestive heart failure, if necessary, labetalol HCl can be used with caution in patients with a history of heart failure who are well-compensated. Congestive heart failure has been observed in patients receiving labetalol HCl. Labetalol HCl does not abolish the inotropic action of digitalis on heart muscle.

In Patients Without a History of Cardiac Failure: In patients with latent cardiac insufficiency, continued depression of the myocardium with beta-blocking agents over a period of time can, in some cases, lead to cardiac failure. At the first sign or symptom of impending cardiac failure, patients should be fully digitalized and/or be given a diuretic, and the response observed closely. If cardiac failure continues, despite adequate digitalization and diuretic, labetalol HCl therapy should be withdrawn (gradually if possible).

Pheochromocytoma: Labetalol HCl has been shown to be effective in lowering the blood pressure and relieving symptoms in patients with pheochromocytoma; higher than usual doses may be required-(Injection). However, paradoxical hypertensive responses have been reported in a few patients with this tumor; therefore, use caution when administering labetalol HCl to patients with pheochromocytoma.

Diabetes Mellitus and Hypoglycemia: Beta-adrenergic blockade may prevent the appearance of premonitory signs and symptoms (*e.g.,* tachycardia) of acute hypoglycemia. This is especially important with labile diabetics. Beta-blockade also reduces the release of insulin in response to hyperglycemia; it may therefore be necessary to adjust the dose of antidiabetic drugs.

Major Surgery: The necessity of desirability of withdrawing beta- blocking therapy prior to major surgery is controversial. Protracted severe hypotension and difficulty in restarting or maintaining a heartbeat have been reported with beta-blockers. The effect of labetalol HCl's alpha-adrenergic activity has not been evaluated in this setting.

A synergism between labetalol HCl and halothane anesthesia has been shown (see DRUG INTERACTIONS.)

INJECTION

Ischemic Heart Disease: Angina pectoris has not been reported upon labetalol HCl discontinuation. However, following abrupt cessation of therapy with some beta-blocking agents in patients with coronary artery disease, exacerbations of angina pectoris and, in some cases, myocardial infarction have been reported. Therefore, such patients should be cautioned against interruption of therapy without the physician's advice. Even in the presence of overt angina pectoris, when discontinuation of labetalol HCl is planned, the patient should be carefully observed and should be advised to limit physical activity. If angina markedly worsens or acute coronary insufficiency develops, labetalol HCl administration should be reinstituted promptly, at least temporarily, and other measures appropriate for the management of unstable angina should be taken.

Nonallergic Bronchospasm (*e.g.,* chronic bronchitis and emphysema): Since labetalol HCl injection at the usual intravenous therapeutic doses has not been studied in patients with nonallergic bronchospastic disease, it should not be used in such patients.

TABLETS

Exacerbation of Ischemic Heart Disease Following Abrupt Withdrawal: Angina pectoris has not been reported upon labetalol HCl discontinuation. However, hypersensitivity to catecholamines has been observed in patients withdrawn from beta-blocker therapy; exacerbation of angina and, in some cases, myocardial infarction have occurred after *abrupt* discontinuation of such therapy. When discontinuing chronically administered labetalol HCl, particularly in patients with ischemic heart disease, the dosage should be gradually reduced over a period of 1 to 2 weeks and the patient should be carefully monitored. If angina markedly worsens or acute coronary insufficiency develops, labetalol HCl administration should be reinstituted promptly, at least temporarily, and other measures appropriate for the management of unstable angina should be taken. Patients should be warned against interruption or discontinuation of therapy without the physician's advice. Because coronary artery disease is common and may be unrecognized, it may be prudent not to discontinue labetalol HCl therapy abruptly even in patients treated only for hypotension.

Nonallergic bronchospasm (*e.g.,* chronic bronchitis and emphysema) patients with bronchospastic disease should, in general, not receive beta-blockers: Labetalol HCl may be used with caution, however, in patients who do not respond to, or cannot tolerate, other antihypertensive agents. It is prudent, if labetalol HCl is used, to use the smallest effective dose, so that inhibition of endogenous or exogenous beta-agonists is minimized.

PRECAUTIONS:

GENERAL

Impaired Hepatic Function: Labetalol HCl tablets should be used with caution in patients with impaired hepatic function since metabolism of the drug may be diminished.

Jaundice or Hepatic Dysfunction: (see WARNINGS.)

Injection

Following Coronary Artery Bypass Surgery: In one uncontrolled study, patients with low cardiac indices and elevated systemic vascular resistance following intravenous labetalol HCl experienced significant declines in cardiac output with little change in systemic vascular resistance. One of these patients developed hypotension following labetalol treatment. Therefore, use of labetalol HCl should be avoided in such patients.

High-Dose Labetalol HCl: Administration of up to 3 g/d as an infusion for up to 2 to 3 days has been anecdotally reported; several patients experienced hypotension or bradycardia (see DOSAGE AND ADMINISTRATION.)

Hypotension: Symptomatic postural hypotension (incidence 58%) is likely to occur if patients are tilted or allowed to assume the upright position within 3 hours of receiving labetalol HCl injection. Therefore, the patients's ability to tolerate an upright position should be established before permitting any ambulation.

PRECAUTIONS: *(cont'd)*

INFORMATION FOR PATIENTS

As with all drugs with beta-blocking activity, certain advice to patients being treated with labetalol HCl is warranted. This information is intended to aid in the safe and effective use of this medication. It is not a disclosure of all possible adverse or intended effects. While no incident of the abrupt withdrawal phenomenon (exacerbation of angina pectoris) has been reported with labetalol HCl, dosing with labetalol HCl tablets should not be interrupted or discontinued without a physician's advice. Patients being treated with labetalol HCl tablets should consult a physician at any signs or symptoms of impending cardiac failure or hepatic dysfunction (see WARNINGS.) Also, transient scalp tingling may occur, usually when treatment with labetalol HCl tablets is initiated (see ADVERSE REACTIONS.)

Injection: The following information is intended to aid in the safe and effective use of this medication. It is not a disclosure of all possible adverse or intended effects. During and immediately following (for up to 3 hours) labetalol HCl injection, the patient should remain supine. Subsequently, the patient should be advised on how to proceed gradually to become ambulatory, and should be observed at the time of first ambulation.

When the patient is started on labetalol HCl tablets, following adequate control of blood pressure with labetalol HCl injection, appropriate directions for titration of dosage should be provided (see DOSAGE AND ADMINISTRATION.)

LABORATORY TESTS

Injection: Routine laboratory tests are ordinarily not required before or after intravenous labetalol HCl. In patients with concomitant illnesses, such as impaired renal function, appropriate tests should be done to monitor these conditions.

Tablets: As with any new drug given over prolonged periods, laboratory parameters should be observed over regular intervals. In patients with concomitant illnesses, such as impaired renal function, appropriate tests should be done to monitor these conditions.

DRUG/LABORATORY TEST INTERACTIONS

The presence of labetalol metabolites in the urine may result in falsely elevated levels of urinary catecholamines, metanephrine, normetanephrine, and vanillylmandelic acid (VMA) when measured by fluorimetric or photometric methods. In screening patients suspected of having a pheochromocytoma and being treated with labetalol HCl, a specific method, such as a high performance liquid chromatographic assay with solid phase extraction (*e.g., J Chromatogr* 385:241, 1987) should be employed in determining levels of catecholamines.

Labetalol HCl has also been reported to produce a false-positive test for amphetamine when screening urine for the presence of drugs using the commercially available assay methods Toxi-Lab A (thin-layer chromatographic assay) and Emit-d.a.u. (radioenzymatic assay). When patients being treated with labetalol HCl have a positive urine test for amphetamine using these techniques, confirmation should be made by using more specific methods, such as a gas chromatographic-mass spectrometer technique.

CARCINOGENESIS, MUTAGENESIS, IMPAIRMENT OF FERTILITY

Long-term oral dosing studies with labetalol HCl for 18 months in mice and for 2 years in rats showed no evidence of carcinogenesis. Studies with labetalol HCl, using dominant lethal assays in rats and mice, and exposing microorganisms according to modified Ames tests, showed no evidence of mutagenesis.

PREGNANCY CATEGORY C

Teratogenic studies have been performed with labetalol HCl in rats and rabbits at oral doses up to approximately 6 and 4 times the maximum recommended human dose (MRHD), respectively. No reproducible evidence of fetal malformations was observed. Increased fetal resorptions were seen in both species at doses approximating the MRHD. A teratology study performed with labetalol HCl in rabbits at intravenous doses up to 1.7 times the MRHD revealed no evidence of drug- related harm to the fetus. There are no adequate and well-controlled studies in pregnant women. Labetalol HCl should be used during pregnancy only if the potential benefit justifies the potential risk to the fetus.

Nonteratogenic Effects: Hypotension, bradycardia, hypoglycemia, and respiratory depression have been reported in infants of mothers who were treated with labetalol HCl for hypertension during pregnancy. Oral administration of labetalol to rats during late gestation through weaning at doses of 2 to 4 times the MRHD caused a decrease in neonatal survival.

LABOR AND DELIVERY

Labetalol HCl given to pregnant women with hypertension did not appear to affect the usual course of labor and delivery.

NURSING MOTHERS

Small amounts of labetalol (approximately 0.004% of the maternal dose) are excreted in human milk. Caution should be exercised when labetalol HCl injection or tablets are administered to a nursing woman.

PEDIATRIC USE

Safety and effectiveness in children have not been established.

DRUG INTERACTIONS:

In one survey, 2.3% of patients taking labetalol HCl orally in combination with tricyclic antidepressants experienced tremor as compared to 0.7% reported to occur with labetalol HCl alone. The contribution of each of the treatments to this adverse reaction is unknown but the possibility of a drug interaction cannot be excluded.

Drugs possessing beta-blocking properties can blunt the bronchodilator effect of beta-receptor agonist drugs in patients with bronchospasm; therefore, doses greater than the normal anti-asthmatic dose of beta- agonist bronchodilator drugs may be required.

Cimetidine has been shown to increase the bioavailability of labetalol HCl administered orally. Since this could be explained either by enhanced absorption or by an alteration of hepatic metabolism of labetalol HCl, special care should be used in establishing the dose required for blood pressure control in such patients.

Synergism has been shown between halothane anesthesia and intravenously administered labetalol HCl. During controlled hypotensive anesthesia using labetalol HCl in association with halothane, high concentrations (3% or above) of halothane should not be used because the degree of hypotension will be increased and because of the possibility of a large reduction in cardiac output and an increase in central venous pressure. The anesthesiologist should be informed when a patient is receiving labetalol HCl.

Labetalol HCl blunts the reflex tachycardia produced by nitroglycerin without preventing its hypotensive effect. If labetalol HCl is used with nitroglycerin in patients with angina pectoris, additional antihypertensive effects may occur.

Care should be taken if labetalol HCl is used concomitantly with calcium antagonists of the verapamil type.

Risk of Anaphylactic Reaction: While taking beta-blockers, patients with a history of severe anaphylactic reactions to a variety of allergens may be more reactive to repeated challenge, either accidental, diagnostic, or therapeutic. Such patients may be unresponsive to the usual doses of epinephrine used to treat allergic reaction.

DRUG INTERACTIONS: *(cont'd)*

INJECTION ONLY

Since labetalol HCl injection may be administered to patients already being treated with other medications, including other antihypertensive agents, careful monitoring of these patients is necessary to detect and treat promptly any undesired effect from concomitant administration.

When drug products that are alkaline, such as furosemide, have been administered in combination with labetalol, a white precipitate has been noted. Therefore, these drugs should not be administered in the same infusion line.

ADVERSE REACTIONS:

INJECTION

Labetalol HCl injection is usually well tolerated. Most adverse effects have been mild and transient and in controlled trials involving 92 patients did not require labetalol HCl withdrawal. Symptomatic postural hypotension (incidence 58%) is likely to occur if patients are tilted or allowed to assume the upright position within 3 hours of receiving labetalol HCl injection. Moderate hypotension occurred in 1 of 100 patients while supine. Increased sweating was noted in 4 of 100 patients, and flushing occurred in 1 of 100 patients.

The following also were reported with labetalol HCl injection with the incidence per 100 patients as noted:

Cardiovascular System: Ventricular arrhythmia in 1.

Central and Peripheral Nervous Systems: Dizziness in 9; tingling of the scalp/skin 7; hypoesthesia (numbness) and vertigo, 1 each.

Gastrointestinal System: Nausea in 13; vomiting 4; dyspepsia and taste distortion, 1 each.

Metabolic Disorders: Transient increases in blood urea nitrogen and serum creatinine levels occurred in 8 of 100 patients; these were associated with drops in blood pressure, generally in patients with prior renal insufficiency.

Psychiatric Disorders: Somnolence/yawning in 3.

Respiratory System: Wheezing in 1.

Skin: Pruritus in 1.

The incidence of adverse reactions depends upon the dose of labetalol HCl. The largest experience is with oral labetalol HCl (see labetalol HCl tablet product information for details.) Certain of the side effects increased with increasing oral dose as shown in the table below which depicts the entire U.S. therapeutic trials data base for adverse reactions that are clearly or possibly dose related (TABLE 1).

TABLE 1

Daily Dose (mg)	200	300	400	600	800	900	1200	1600	2400
Number of Patients	522	181	606	608	503	117	411	242	175
Dizziness (%)	2	3	3	3	5	1	9	13	16
Fatigue	2	1	4	4	5	3	7	6	10
Nausea	<1	0	1	2	4	0	7	11	19
Vomiting	0	0	<1	<1	<1	0	1	2	3
Dyspepsia	1	0	2	1	1	0	2	2	4
Paresthesias	2	0	2	2	1	1	2	5	5
Nasal Stuffiness	1	1	2	2	2	2	4	5	6
Ejaculation Failure	0	2	1	2	3	0	4	3	5
Impotence	1	1	1	1	2	4	3	4	3
Edema	1	0	1	1	1	0	1	2	2

In addition, a number of other less common adverse events have been reported:

Cardiovascular: Hypotension, and rarely, syncope, bradycardia, heart block.

Liver and Biliary System: Hepatic necrosis, hepatitis, cholestatic jaundice, elevated liver function tests.

Hypersensitivity: Rare reports of hypersensitivity (*e.g.,* rash, urticaria, pruritus, angioedema, dyspnea) and anaphylactoid reactions.

The oculomucocutaneous syndrome associated with the beta-blocker practolol has not been reported with labetalol HCl during investigational use and extensive foreign marketing experience.

Clinical Laboratory Tests: Among patients dosed with labetalol HCl tablets, there have been reversible increases of serum transaminases in 4% of patients tested, and more rarely, reversible increases in blood urea.

TABLETS

Most adverse effects are mild, transient and occur early in the course of treatment. In controlled clinical trials of 3 to 4 months duration, discontinuation of labetalol HCl tablets due to one or more adverse effects was required in 7% of all patients. In these same trials, beta- blocker control agents led to discontinuation in 8% to 10% of patients, and a centrally acting alpha-agonist in 30% of patients.

The incidence rates of adverse reactions listed in the following table (TABLE 2) were derived from multicenter controlled clinical trials, comparing labetalol HCl, placebo, metoprolol, and propranolol, over treatment periods of 3 and 4 months. Where the frequency of adverse effects for labetalol HCl and placebo is similar, causal relationship is uncertain. The rates are based on adverse reactions considered probably drug related by the investigator. If all reports are considered, the rates are somewhat higher (*e.g.,* dizziness 20%, nausea 14%, fatigue 11%), but the overall conclusions are unchanged.

The adverse effects were reported spontaneously and are representative of the incidence of adverse effects that may be observed in a properly selected hypertensive patient population, i.e., a group excluding patients with bronchospastic disease, overt congestive heart failure, or other contraindications to beta-blocker therapy.

Clinical trials also included studies utilizing daily doses up to 2400 mg in more severely hypotensive patients. Certain of the side effects increased with increasing dose as shown in TABLE 3 which depicts the entire U.S. therapeutic trials data base for adverse reactions that are clearly or possibly drug related.

In addition, a number of the less common adverse events have been reported:

Body as a Whole : Fever.

Cardiovascular: Hypotension, and rarely, syncope, bradycardia, heart block.

Central and Peripheral Nervous Systems: Paresthesia, most frequently described as scalp tingling. In most cases, it was mild, transient and usually occurred at the beginning of treatment.

Collagen Disorders: Systemic lupus erythematosus; positive antinuclear factor (ANF).

Eyes: Dry eyes.

Immunological System: Antimitochondrial antibodies.

ADVERSE REACTIONS: *(cont'd)*

TABLE 2

	Labetalol HCl	Placebo	Propranolol	Metoprolol
(N=227) %	(N=98) %	(N=84) %	(N=49) %	
Body as a Whole				
fatigue	5	0	12	12
asthenia	1	1	1	0
headache	2	1	1	2
Gastrointestinal				
nausea	6	1	1	2
vomiting	<1	0	0	0
dyspepsia	3	1	1	0
abdominal pain	0	0	1	2
diarrhea	<1	0	2	0
taste distortion	1	0	0	0
Central and Peripheral Nervous System				
dizziness	11	3	4	4
paresthesias	<1	0	0	0
drowsiness	<1	2	2	2
Autonomic Nervous System				
nasal stuffiness	3	0	0	0
ejaculation failure	2	0	0	0
impotence	1	0	1	3
increased sweating	<1	0	0	0
Cardiovascular				
edema	1	0	0	0
postural hypotension	1	0	0	0
bradycardia	0	0	5	12
Respiratory				
dyspnea	2	0	1	2
Skin				
rash	1	0	0	0
Special Senses				
vision abnormality	1	0	0	0
vertigo	2	1	0	0

TABLE 3

Daily Dose (mg)	200	300	400	600	800
Number of patients	522	181	606	608	503
Dizziness (%)	2	3	3	3	5
Fatigue	2	1	4	4	5
Nausea	<1	0	1	2	4
Vomiting	0	0	<1	<1	<1
Dyspepsia	1	0	2	1	1
Paresthesias	2	0	2	2	1
Nasal Stuffiness	1	1	2	2	2
Ejaculation Failure	0	2	1	2	3
Impotence	1	1	1	1	2
Edema	1	0	1	1	1
Daily Dose (mg)	**900**	**1200**	**1600**	**2400**	
Number of Patients	117	411	242	175	
Dizziness (%)	1	9	13	16	
Fatigue	3	7	6	10	
Nausea	0	7	11	19	
Vomiting	0	1	2	3	
Dyspepsia	0	2	2	4	
Paresthesias	1	2	5	5	
Nasal Stuffiness	2	4	5	6	
Ejaculation Failure	0	4	3	5	
Impotence	4	3	4	3	
Edema	0	1	2	2	

Liver and Biliary System: Hepatic necrosis; hepatitis; cholestatic jaundice; elevated liver function tests.

Musculoskeletal System: Muscle cramps; toxic myopathy.

Respiratory System: Bronchospasm.

Skin and Appendages: Rashes of various types, such as generalized maculopapular; lichenoid; urticarial; bullous lichen planus; psoriaform; facial erythema; Peyronie's disease; reversible alopecia.

Urinary System: Difficulty in micturition, including acute urinary bladder retention.

Hypersensitivity: Rare reports of hypersensitivity (*e.g.,* rash, urticaria, pruritus, angioedema, dyspnea) and anaphylactoid reactions.

Following approval for marketing in the United Kingdom, a monitored release survey involving approximately 6,800 patients was conducted for further safety and efficacy evaluation of this product. Results of this survey indicate that the type, severity, and incidence of adverse effects were comparable to those cited above.

Potential Adverse Effects: In addition, other adverse effects not listed above have been reported with other beta-adrenergic blocking agents.

Central Nervous System: Reversible mental depression progressing to catatonia; an acute reversible syndrome characterized by disorientation for time and place, short-term memory loss, emotional lability, slightly cloudy sensorium, and decreased performance on neuropsychometrics.

Cardiovascular: Intensification of AV block (see CONTRAINDICATIONS.)

Allergic: Fever combined with aching and sore throat; laryngospasm; respiratory distress.

Hematologic: Agranulocytosis; thrombocytopenic or nonthrombocytopenic purpura.

Gastrointestinal: Mesenteric artery thrombosis; ischemic colitis.

The oculomucocutaneous syndrome associated with the beta-blocker practolol has not been reported with labetalol HCl.

Clinical Laboratory Tests: There have been reversible increases of serum transaminases in 4% of patients treated with labetalol HCl and tested, and more rarely, reversible increases in blood urea.

OVERDOSAGE:

Overdosage with labetalol HCl injection or tablets causes excessive hypotension that is posture sensitive, and sometimes, excessive bradycardia. Patients should be placed supine and their legs raised if necessary to improve the blood supply to the brain. If overdosage with labetalol HCl follows oral ingestion, gastric lavage or pharmacologically induced emesis (using syrup of ipecac) may be useful for removal of the drug shortly after ingestion. The following additional measures should be employed if necessary: *Excessive bradycardia:* administer atropine or epinephrine. *Cardiac failure:* administer a digitalis glycoside and a diuretic. Dopamine or dobutamine may also be useful. *Hypotension:* administer vasopressors, e.g.,

OVERDOSAGE: *(cont'd)*

norepinephrine. There is pharmacological evidence that norepinephrine may be the drug of choice. *Bronchospasm:* administer epinephrine and/or an aerosolized $beta_2$-agonist. *Seizures:* administer diazepam.

In severe beta-blocker overdose resulting in hypotension and/or bradycardia, glucagon has been shown to be effective when administered in large doses (5 to 10 mg rapidly over 30 seconds, followed by continuous infusion of 5 mg/hr that can be reduced as the patient improves).

Neither hemodialysis nor peritoneal dialysis removes a significant amount of labetalol HCl from the general circulation (<1%).

The oral LD_{50} value of labetalol HCl in the mouse is approximately 600 mg/kg and in the rat is greater than 2 g/kg. The intravenous LD_{50} in these species is 50 to 60 mg/kg.

DOSAGE AND ADMINISTRATION:

INJECTION

Labetalol HCl injection is intended for intravenous use in hospitalized patients. DOSAGE MUST BE INDIVIDUALIZED depending upon the severity of hypertension and the response of the patient during dosing.

Patients should always be kept in a supine position during the period of intravenous drug administration. A substantial fall in blood pressure on standing should be expected in these patients. The patient's ability to tolerate an upright position should be established before permitting any ambulation, such as using toilet facilities.

Either of two methods of administration of labetalol HCl injection may be used: a) repeated intravenous injections, b) slow continuous infusion.

Repeated Intravenous Injection: Initially, labetalol HCl injection should be given in a dose of 20 mg labetalol HCl (which corresponds to 0.25 mg/kg for an 80 kg patient) by slow intravenous injection over a 2-minute period.

Immediately before the injection and at 5 and 10 minutes after injection, supine blood pressure should be measured to evaluate response. Additional injections of 40 mg or 80 mg can be given at 10-minute intervals until a desired supine blood pressure is achieved or a total of 300 mg labetalol HCl has been injected. The maximum effect usually occurs within 5 minutes of each injection.

Slow Continuous Infusion: Labetalol HCl injection is prepared for intravenous continuous infusion by diluting the contents with commonly used intravenous fluids (see below). Examples of methods of preparing the infusion solution are: The contents of either two 20 ml vials (40 ml), or one 40 ml vial, are added to 160 ml of a commonly used intravenous fluid such that the resultant 200 ml of solution contains 200 mg of labetalol HCl, 1 mg/ml. The diluted solution should be administered at a rate of 2 ml/min to deliver 2 mg/min.

Alternatively, the contents of either two 20 ml vials (40 ml), or one 40 ml vial, of labetalol HCl injection are added to 250 ml of a commonly used intravenous fluid. The resultant solution will contain 200 mg of labetalol HCl, approximately 2 mg/3 ml. The diluted solution should be administered at a rate of 3 ml/min to deliver approximately 2 mg/min.

The rate of infusion of the diluted solution may be adjusted according to the blood pressure response, at the discretion of the physician. To facilitate a desired rate of infusion, the diluted solution can be infused using a controlled administration mechanism, e.g., graduated burette or mechanically driven infusion pump.

Since the half life of labetalol is 5 to 8 hours, steady-state blood levels (in the face of a constant rate of infusion) would not be reached during the usual infusion time period. The infusion should be continued until a satisfactory response is obtained and should then be stopped and oral labetalol HCl started (see below). The effective intravenous dose is usually in the range of 50 to 200 mg. A total dose of up to 300 mg may be required in some patients.

Blood Pressure Monitoring: The blood pressure should be monitored during and after completion of the infusion or intravenous injections. Rapid or excessive falls in either systolic or diastolic blood pressure during intravenous treatment should be avoided. In patients with excessive systolic hypertension, the decrease in systolic pressure should be used as indicator of effectiveness in addition to the response of the diastolic pressure.

Initiation of Dosing with Labetalol HCl Tablets: Subsequent oral dosing with labetalol HCl tablets should begin when it has been established that the supine diastolic blood pressure has begun to rise. The recommended initial dose is 200 mg, followed in 6-12 hours by an additional dose of 200 or 400 mg, depending on the blood pressure response. Thereafter, inpatient titration with labetalol HCl tablets may proceed as follows (TABLE 4):

TABLE 4 Inpatient Titration Instructions

Regimen	Daily Dose*
200 mg b.i.d.	400 mg
400 mg b.i.d.	800 mg
800 mg b.i.d.	1600 mg
1200 mg b.i.d.	2400 mg

* If needed, the total daily dose may be given in three divided doses.

While in the hospital, the dosage of labetalol HCl tablets may be increased at 1-day intervals to achieve the desired blood pressure reduction.

For subsequent outpatient titration or maintenance dosing see labetalol HCl tablets Product Information DOSAGE AND ADMINISTRATION for additional recommendations.

Compatibility with commonly used intravenous fluids: Parenteral drug products should be inspected visually for particulate matter and discoloration prior to administration, whenever solution and container permit.

Labetalol HCl injection was tested for compatibility with commonly used intravenous fluids at final concentrations of 1.25 mg to 3.75 mg labetalol HCl per ml of the mixture. Labetalol HCl injection was found to be compatible with and stable (for 24 hours refrigerated or at room temperature) in mixtures with the following solutions:

Ringers Injection, USP; Lactated Ringers Injection, USP; 5% Dextrose and Ringers Injection; 5% Lactated Ringers and 5% Dextrose Injection; 5% Dextrose Injection, USP; 0.9% Sodium Chloride Injection, USP; 5% Dextrose and 0.2% Sodium Chloride Injection, USP; 2.5% Dextrose and 0.45% Sodium Chloride Injection, USP; 5% Dextrose and 0.9% Sodium Chloride Injection, USP; 5% Dextrose and 0.33% Sodium Chloride Injection, USP

Labetalol HCl injection was NOT compatible with 5% Sodium Bicarbonate Injection, USP.

Store between 2° and 30°C (36° and 86°F). Protect from freezing. Protect syringe from light.

Note: To ensure patient safety, the needle and the pre-filled syringes should be handled with care and should be destroyed and discarded if damaged in any manner. If the cannula is bent, no attempt should be made to straighten it. To prevent needle-stick injuries, needles should not be recapped, purposely bent, or broken by hand.

DOSAGE AND ADMINISTRATION: *(cont'd)*

TABLETS

DOSAGE MUST BE INDIVIDUALIZED. The recommended initial dose is 100 mg twice daily whether used alone or added to a diuretic regimen. After 2 or 3 days, using standing blood pressure as an indicator, dosage may be titrated in increments of 100 mg b.i.d. every 2 or 3 days. The usual maintenance dosage of labetalol HCl is between 200 and 400 mg twice daily.

Since the full antihypertensive effect of labetalol HCl is usually seen within the first 1 to 3 hours of the initial dose or dose increment, the assurance of a lack of an exaggerated hypotensive response can be clinically established in the office setting. The antihypertensive effects of continued dosing can be measured at subsequent visits, approximately 12 hours after a dose, to determine whether future titration is necessary.

Patients with severe hypertension may require from 1200 mg to 2400 mg per day, with or without thiazide diuretics. Should side effects (principally nausea or dizziness) occur with these doses administered b.i.d., the same total daily dose administered t.i.d. may improve tolerability and facilitate further titration. Titration increments should not exceed 200 mg b.i.d.

When a diuretic is added, an additive antihypertensive effect can be expected. In some cases this may necessitate a labetalol HCl dosage adjustment. As with most antihypertensive drugs, optimal dosages of labetalol HCl tablets are usually lower in patients also receiving a diuretic.

When transferring patients from other antihypertensive drugs, labetalol HCl tablets should be introduced as recommended and the dosage of the existing therapy progressively decreased.

Labetalol HCl tablets should be stored between 2° and 30°C (36° and 86°F). Labetalol HCl tablets in the unit-dose boxes should be protected from excessive moisture.

HOW SUPPLIED - RATED THERAPEUTICALLY EQUIVALENT:

Injection, Solution - Intravenous - 5 mg/ml

4 ml	**$13.93**	**NORMODYNE, Schering**	**00085-0362-08**
8 ml	**$20.90**	**NORMODYNE, Schering**	**00085-0362-09**
20 ml	**$32.27**	**NORMODYNE, Schering**	**00085-0362-07**
20 ml	$33.98	TRANDATE, Glaxo Wellcome	00173-0350-58
40 ml	**$62.51**	**NORMODYNE, Schering**	**00085-0362-06**
40 ml	$65.84	TRANDATE, Glaxo Wellcome	00173-0350-57

Tablet, Coated - Oral - 100 mg

100's	**$44.44**	**NORMODYNE, Schering**	**00085-0244-04**
100's	**$47.19**	**NORMODYNE, Schering**	**00085-0244-08**
100's	$48.89	TRANDATE, Glaxo Wellcome	00173-0346-43
100's	$51.92	TRANDATE, Glaxo Wellcome	00173-0346-47
500's	**$210.82**	**NORMODYNE, Schering**	**00085-0244-05**
500's	$232.00	TRANDATE, Glaxo Wellcome	00173-0346-44
1000's	**$388.78**	**NORMODYNE, Schering**	**00085-0244-07**

Tablet, Coated - Oral - 200 mg

100's	**$63.04**	**NORMODYNE, Schering**	**00085-0752-04**
100's	**$65.78**	**NORMODYNE, Schering**	**00085-0752-08**
100's	$69.36	TRANDATE, Glaxo Wellcome	00173-0347-43
100's	$72.40	TRANDATE, Glaxo Wellcome	00173-0347-47
500's	**$299.44**	**NORMODYNE, Schering**	**00085-0752-05**
500's	$329.52	TRANDATE, Glaxo Wellcome	00173-0347-44
1000's	**$552.00**	**NORMODYNE, Schering**	**00085-0752-07**

Tablet, Coated - Oral - 300 mg

100's	**$83.84**	**NORMODYNE, Schering**	**00085-0438-03**
100's	**$86.61**	**NORMODYNE, Schering**	**00085-0438-06**
100's	$92.26	TRANDATE, Glaxo Wellcome	00173-0348-43
100's	$95.32	TRANDATE, Glaxo Wellcome	00173-0348-47
500's	**$398.18**	**NORMODYNE, Schering**	**00085-0438-05**
500's	$438.17	TRANDATE, Glaxo Wellcome	00173-0348-44

LACTIC ACID *(001617)*

CATEGORIES: Emollients; Keratolytic Agents; Pharmaceutical Adjuvants; Skin/Mucous Membrane Agents; FDA Pre 1938 Drugs

BRAND NAMES: **Lac-Hydrin**; Lactinol; Lactinol-E

FORMULARIES: Aetna; BC-BS

Prescribing information not available at time of publication.

HOW SUPPLIED - EQUIVALENTS NOT AVAILABLE:

Cream - Topical - 10 %

113.4 gm	$12.00	LACTINOL-E, Pedinol Pharma	00884-4990-04

Lotion - Topical - 10 %

226.8 ml	$13.25	LACTINOL, Pedinol Pharma	00884-5292-08

LACTIC ACID; SALICYLIC ACID *(001619)*

CATEGORIES: Dermatologicals; Keratolytic Agents; Skin/Mucous Membrane Agents; Vitamins; Warts; FDA Pre 1938 Drugs

BRAND NAMES: Bifilm; Co-Flex; **Duofilm**; *Duofilm Solution*; Gordofilm; *Kusmin*; Lactisol; Salactic Film; *Salatac Gel* (England); Tiflex; Verukan; Viranol
(International brand names outside U.S. in italics)

Prescribing information not available at time of publication.

HOW SUPPLIED - RATED THERAPEUTICALLY EQUIVALENT:

Solution - Topical - 16.7 %/16.7 %

15 ml	$7.15	Salicylic Acid/La/Collod, Harber Pharm	51432-0439-10

HOW SUPPLIED - NOT RATED EQUIVALENT:

Liquid - Topical - 16.7 %/16.7 %

15 ml	**$8.39**	**DUOFILM, Stiefel Labs**	**00145-6788-05**

Solution - Topical - 16.7 %/16.7 %

15 ml	$6.25	Salactic Film, Pedinol Pharma	00884-2592-15

LACTOSE *(001620)*

CATEGORIES: Pharmaceutical Adjuvants; FDA Pre 1938 Drugs

BRAND NAMES: Cebocap #1; Cebocap #2; Cebocap #3; Placebo

Prescribing information not available at time of publication.

HOW SUPPLIED - EQUIVALENTS NOT AVAILABLE:

Capsule, Gelatin - Oral - 500 mg

100's	$30.73	CEBOCAP 1, Forest Pharms	00456-0707-01
100's	$30.73	CEBOCAP 2, Forest Pharms	00456-0708-01
100's	$30.73	CEBOCAP 3, Forest Pharms	00456-0709-01
1000's	$29.50	Placebo, Consolidated Midland	00223-1465-02
1000's	$35.00	Placebo, Consolidated Midland	00223-1468-02

Tablet, Uncoated - Oral - 325 mg

1000's	$22.50	Placebo, Consolidated Midland	00223-1470-02

Tablet, Uncoated - Oral - 330 mg

1000's	$22.50	Placebo, Consolidated Midland	00223-1469-02

Tablet, Uncoated - Oral - 440 mg

1000's	$25.00	Placebo, Consolidated Midland	00223-1453-02

Tablet, Uncoated - Oral - 500 mg

1000's	$25.00	Placebo, Consolidated Midland	00223-1464-02

LACTULOSE *(001621)*

CATEGORIES: Ammonia Detoxicants; Cathartics & Laxatives; Coma; Constipation; Electrolyte Solutions; Electrolytic, Caloric-Water Balance; Encephalopathy; Fecal Softeners; Gastrointestinal Drugs; Homeostatic & Nutrient; Hyperammonia Reduction; Laxatives; Pregnancy Category B; FDA Approval Pre 1982

BRAND NAMES: *Acilac*; *Actilax*; *Alpha-Lactulose*; *Avilac*; *B-Cut*; *Bifinorma* (Germany); *Bifiteral* (Germany); C-Cephulose; C-Chronulose; **Cephulac**; Cholac; *Chronulac* (Canada); Constilac; *Constipen*; Constulose; *Dia-Colon*; Duphalac; Enulose; Generlac; *Hepalac*; *Lacson*; *Lactocur* (Germany); *Lactuverlan* (Germany); *Laevolac*; *Laxette*; *Levolac*; *Livo Luk*; *Monilac* (Japan); Portalac; *Sirolax* *(International brand names outside U.S. in italics)*

FORMULARIES: Aetna; BC-BS; PCS

DESCRIPTION:

This monograph contains information for both Cephulac and Chronulac where noted.

Cephulac: Cephulac (lactulose) is a synthetic disaccharide in solution form for oral or rectal administration. Cephulac is a colonic acidifier for treatment and prevention of portal-systemic encephalopathy.

Chronulac: Chronulac (lactulose) is a synthetic disaccharide in solution form for oral administration. Chronulac is a colonic acidifier that promotes laxation. The pH range is 3.0 to 7.0.

Both Forms: Each 15 ml of lactulose contains: 10 g lactulose (and less than 2.2 g galactose, less than 1.2 g lactose, and 1.2 g or less of other sugars). Also contains FD&C Blue No. 1, FD&C Yellow No. 6, water, and flavoring. A minimal quantity of sodium hydroxide is used to adjust pH when necessary.

The chemical name for lactulose is 4-*O*-β-D-galactopyranosyl-D-fructofuranose.

The molecular weight is 342.30. It is freely soluble in water.

CLINICAL PHARMACOLOGY:

Cephulac: Lactulose causes a decrease in blood ammonia concentration and reduces the degree of portalsystemic encephalopathy. These actions are considered to be results of the following:

Bacterial degradation of lactulose in the colon acidifies the colonic contents.

This acidification of colonic contents results in the retention of ammonia in the colon as the ammonium ion. Since the colonic contents are then more acid than the blood, ammonia can be expected to migrate from the blood into the colon to form the ammonium ion.

The acid colonic contents convert NH_3 to the ammonium ion $(NH_4)^+$, trapping it and preventing its absorption.

The laxative action of the metabolites of lactulose then expels the trapped ammonium ion from the colon.

Experimental data indicate that lactulose is poorly absorbed. Lactulose given orally to man and experimental animals resulted in only small amounts reaching the blood. Urinary excretion has been determined to be 3% or less and is essentially complete within 24 hours.

When incubated with extracts of human small intestinal mucosa, lactulose was not hydrolyzed during a 24-hour period and did not inhibit the activity of these extracts on lactose. Lactulose reaches the colon essentially unchanged. There it is metabolized by bacteria with the formation of low molecular weight acids that acidify the colon contents.

Chronulac: Chronulac is poorly absorbed from the gastrointestinal tract and no enzyme capable of hydrolysis of this disaccharide is present in human gastrointestinal tissue. As a result, oral doses of Chronulac reach the colon virtually unchanged. In the colon, Chronulac is broken down primarily to lactic acid, and also to small amounts of formic and acetic acids, by the action of colonic bacteria, which results in an increase in osmotic pressure and slight acidification of the colonic contents. This in turn causes an increase in stool water content and softens the stool.

Since Chronulac does not exert its effect until it reaches the colon, and since transit time through the colon may be slow, 24 to 48 hours may be required to produce the desired bowel movement.

Chronulac given orally to man and experimental animals resulted in only small amounts reaching the blood. Urinary excretion has been determined to be 3% or less and is essentially complete within 24 hours.

INDICATIONS AND USAGE:

Cephulac: For the prevention and treatment of portal-systemic encephalopathy, including the stages of hepatic pre-coma and coma.

Controlled studies have shown that lactulose solution therapy reduces the blood ammonia levels by 25-50%; this is generally paralleled by an improvement in the patients' mental state and by an improvement in EEG patterns. The clinical response has been observed in about 75% of patients, which is at least as satisfactory as that resulting from neomycin therapy. An increase in patients' protein tolerance is also frequently observed with lactulose therapy. In the treatment of chronic portal-systemic encephalopathy, Cephulac has been given for over 2 years in controlled studies.

INDICATIONS AND USAGE: *(cont'd)*

Chronulac: For the treatment of constipation. In patients with a history of chronic constipation, lactulose solution (Chronulac) therapy increases the number of bowel movements per day and the number of days on which bowel movements can occur.

CONTRAINDICATIONS:

Since Cephulac and Chronulac contain galactose (less than 2.2 g/15 ml), it is contraindicated in patients who require a low galactose diet.

WARNINGS:

A theoretical hazard may exist for patients being treated with lactulose solution who may be required to undergo electrocautery procedures during proctoscopy or colonoscopy. Accumulation of H_2 gas in significant concentration in the presence of an electrical spark may result in an explosive reaction. Although this complication has not been reported with lactulose, patients on lactulose therapy undergoing such procedures should have a thorough bowel cleansing with a nonfermentable solution. Insufflation of CO_2 as an additional safeguard may be pursued but is considered to be a redundant measure.

PRECAUTIONS:

GENERAL

Since Cephulac and Chronulac contains galactose (less than 2.2 g/15 ml) and lactose (less than 1.2 g/15 ml), it should be used with caution in diabetics.

Cephulac: In the overall management of portal-systemic encephalopathy, it should be recognized that there is serious underlying liver disease with complications such as electrolyte disturbance (*e.g.*, hypokalemia) for which other specific therapy may be required.

INFORMATION FOR THE PATIENT

Chronulac: In the event that an unusual diarrheal condition occurs, contact your physician.

LABORATORY TESTS

Chronulac: Elderly, debilitated patients who receive Chronulac for more than six months should have serum electrolytes (potassium, chloride, carbon dioxide) measured periodically.

Infants receiving lactulose may develop hyponatremia and dehydration.

CARCINOGENESIS, MUTAGENESIS, AND IMPAIRMENT OF FERTILITY

There are no known human data on long-term potential for carcinogenicity, mutagenicity, or impairment of fertility.

There are no known animal data on long-term potential for mutagenicity.

Administration of lactulose solution in the diet of mice for 18 months in concentrations of 3 and 10% (V/W) did not produce any evidence of carcinogenicity.

In studies in mice, rats, and rabbits, doses of lactulose solution up to 6 or 12 ml/kg/day produced no deleterious effects on breeding, conception, or parturition.

PREGNANCY, TERATOGENIC EFFECTS, PREGNANCY CATEGORY B

Reproduction studies have been performed in mice, rats, and rabbits at doses up to 2 or 4 times the usual human oral dose (Cephulac) and 3 or 6 times the usual human oral dose (Chronulac) and have revealed no evidence of impaired fertility or harm to the fetus due to Cephulac. There are, however, no adequate and well-controlled studies in pregnant women. Because animal reproduction studies are not always predictive of human response, this drug should be used during pregnancy only if clearly needed.

NURSING MOTHERS

It is not known whether this drug is excreted in human milk. Because many drugs are excreted in human milk, caution should be exercised when Cephulac is administered to a nursing woman.

PEDIATRIC USE

Cephulac: Very little information on the use of lactulose in young children and adolescents has been recorded. (See DOSAGE AND ADMINISTRATION.)

Chronulac: Safety and effectiveness in pediatric patients have not been established.

DRUG INTERACTIONS:

Cephulac: There have been conflicting reports about the concomitant use of neomycin and lactulose solution. Theoretically, the elimination of certain colonic bacteria by neomycin and possibly other anti-infective agents may interfere with the desired degradation of lactulose and thus prevent the acidification of colonic contents. Thus the status of the lactulose-treated patient should be closely monitored in the event of concomitant oral anti-infective therapy.

Results of preliminary studies in humans and rats suggest that nonabsorbable antacids given concurrently with lactulose may inhibit the desired lactulose-induced drop in colonic pH. Therefore, a possible lack of desired effect of treatment should be taken into consideration before such drugs are given concomitantly with Cephulac.

Other laxatives should not be used, especially during the initial phase of therapy for portal-systemic encephalopathy, because the loose stools resulting from their use may falsely suggest that adequate Cephulac dosage has been achieved.

Chronulac: Results of preliminary studies in humans and rats suggest that nonabsorbable antacids given concurrently with lactulose may inhibit the desired lactulose-induced drop in colonic pH. therefore, a possible lack of desired effect of treatment should be taken into consideration before such drugs are given concomitantly with Chronulac.

ADVERSE REACTIONS:

Precise frequency data are not available.

Excessive dosage can lead to diarrhea with potential complications such as loss of fluids, hypokalemia, and hypernatremia. Nausea and vomiting have been reported.

Cephulac: Cephulac may produce gaseous distention with flatulence or belching and abdominal discomfort such as cramping in about 20% of patients.

Chronulac: Initial dosing of Chronulac may produce flatulence and intestinal cramps, which are usually transient.

OVERDOSAGE:

Signs and Symptoms: There have been no reports of accidental overdosage. In the event of overdosage, it is expected that diarrhea and abdominal cramps would be the major symptoms. Medication should be terminated.

Oral LD_{50} : The acute oral LD_{50} of the drug is 48.8 ml/kg in mice and greater than 30 ml/kg in rats.

Dialysis: Dialysis data are not available for lactulose. Its molecular similarity to sucrose, however, would suggest it should be dialyzable.

DOSAGE AND ADMINISTRATION:

ORAL CEPHULAC

Adult: The usual adult, oral dosage is 2 to 3 tablespoonfuls (30 to 45 ml, containing 20 g to 30 g of lactulose) three or four times daily. The dosage may be adjusted every day or two to produce 2 or 3 soft stools daily.

DOSAGE AND ADMINISTRATION: *(cont'd)*

Hourly doses of 30 to 45 ml of Cephulac may be used to induce the rapid laxation indicated in the initial phase of the therapy of portal-systemic encephalopathy. When the laxative effect has been achieved, the dose of Cephulac may then be reduced to the recommended daily dose. Improvement in the patient's condition may occur within 24 hours but may not begin before 48 hours or even later.

Continuous long-term therapy is indicated to lessen the severity and prevent the recurrence of portal-systemic encephalopathy. The dose of Cephulac for this purpose is the same as the recommended daily dose.

Pediatric: Very little information on the use of lactulose in pediatric patients has been recorded. As with adults, the subjective goal in proper treatment is to produce 2 to 3 soft stools daily. On the basis of information available, the recommended initial daily oral dose in infants is 2.5 to 10 ml in divided doses. For older children and adolescents, the total daily dose is 40 to 90 ml. If the initial dose causes diarrhea, the dose should be reduced immediately. If diarrhea persists, lactulose should be discontinued.

RECTAL CEPHULAC

When the adult patient is in the impending coma or coma stage of portal-systemic encephalopathy and the danger of aspiration exists, or when the necessary endoscopic or intubation procedures physically interfere with the administration of the recommended oral doses, Cephulac may be given as a retention enema via a rectal balloon catheter. Cleansing enemas containing soapsuds or other alkaline agents should not be used.

Three hundred ml of Cephulac should be mixed with 700 ml of water or physiologic saline and retained for 30 to 60 minutes. Cephulac enema may be repeated every 4 to 6 hours. If the enema is inadvertently evacuated too promptly, it may be repeated immediately.

The goal of treatment is reversal of the coma stage in order that the patient may be able to take oral medication. Reversal of coma may take place within 2 hours of the first enema in some patients. Cephulac, given orally in the recommended doses, should be started before Cephulac by enema is stopped entirely.

CHRONULAC

The usual dose is 1 to 2 tablespoonfuls (15 to 30 ml, containing 10 g to 20 g of lactulose) daily. The dose may be increased to 60 ml daily if necessary. Twenty-four to 48 hours may be required to produce a normal bowel movement.

Note: Some patients have found that Chronulac may be more acceptable when mixed with fruit juice, water, or milk.

STORAGE

Store at room temperature, 59-86°F (15-30°C).

Under recommended storage conditions, a normal darkening of color may occur. Such darkening is characteristic of sugar solutions and does not affect therapeutic action. Prolonged exposure to temperatures above 86°F (30°C) or to direct light may cause extreme darkening and turbidity which may be pharmaceutically objectionable. If this condition develops, do not use.

Prolonged exposure to freezing temperatures may cause change to a semisolid, too viscous to pour. Viscosity will return to normal upon warming to room temperature.

(Cephulac: Marion Merrell Dow, 4/92)(Chronulac: Marion Merrell Dow, 2/95)

HOW SUPPLIED - RATED THERAPEUTICALLY EQUIVALENT:

Solution - Oral - 10 gm/15 ml

8 oz	$14.10	Lactulose, Mylan	00378-3331-70
480 ml	$12.43	Lactulose, H.C.F.A. F F P	99999-1621-01

Solution - Oral - 10 gm/15ml

32 oz	$52.10	Laculose, Mylan	00378-3331-74

Syrup - Oral - 10 gm/15ml

2 quarts	$97.77	ENULOSE, Alpharma	00472-1360-64
15 ml x 50	$63.09	Lactulose, Xactdose	50962-0032-15
15 ml x 100	$106.55	Lactulose, Xactdose	50962-0031-15
30 ml	$2.09	CONSTILAC, Alra Labs	51641-0224-61
30 ml	$2.09	CHOLAC, Alra Labs	51641-0225-61
30 ml x 10	$28.91	DUPHALAC, Solvay Pharms	00032-1602-84
30 ml x 10	**$366.84**	**CEPHULAC, Hoechst Marion Roussel**	**00068-0413-39**
30 ml x 40	$115.60	Lactulose, Roxane	00054-8486-16
30 ml x 50	$99.32	Lactulose, Xactdose	50962-0032-30
30 ml x 100	$224.77	Lactulose, Xactdose	50962-0031-30
237 ml	$13.50	Lactulose Syrup, Goldline Labs	00182-6075-44
237 ml	$14.05	CONSTULOSE, Alpharma	00472-1358-08
237 ml	$15.19	Lactulose Syrup 10G/15 Ml, HL Moore Drug Exch	00839-7199-66
240 ml	$10.80	Constulose, Harber Pharm	51432-0534-19
240 ml	$12.60	CATULAC, Major Pharms	00904-2117-09
240 ml	$13.50	Lactulose, Schein Pharm (US)	00364-2519-76
240 ml	$13.70	CONSTILAC, Alra Labs	51641-0224-68
240 ml	$13.70	CHOLAC, Alra Labs	51641-0225-68
240 ml	$13.73	Lactulose, Rugby	00536-1418-59
240 ml	$13.95	Lactulose, Qualitest Pharms	00603-1378-56
240 ml	$14.51	DUPHALAC 10G/15ML SYRUP, Solvay Pharms	00032-1602-08
240 ml	$15.50	Lactulose, Copley Pharm	38245-0661-19
240 ml	$18.60	CHRONULAC SYRUP, Hoechst Marion Roussel	00068-0409-08
473 ml	$30.95	Lactulose, Copley Pharm	38245-0670-07
480 ml	$12.43	ENULOSE SYRUP, United Res	00677-1098-33
480 ml	$12.43	CHOLAC, Alra Labs	51641-0225-76
480 ml	$19.50	CONSTILAC, Alra Labs	51641-0224-76
480 ml	$21.50	Enulose, Harber Pharm	51432-0536-20
480 ml	$25.75	Lactulose, Schein Pharm (US)	00364-2347-16
480 ml	$25.90	CALULOSE SYRUP, Major Pharms	00904-2115-16
480 ml	$26.00	LACTTULOSE SYRUP 10, Goldline Labs	00182-6072-40
480 ml	$26.05	R-O-LACTULOSE, Qualitest Pharms	00603-1648-58
480 ml	$26.11	ENULOSE, Alpharma	00472-1360-16
480 ml	$26.47	Lactulose Syrup, Geneva Pharms	00781-6405-16
480 ml	$27.05	DUPHALAC 10G/15ML SYRUP, Solvay Pharms	00032-1602-78
480 ml	$30.38	Lactulose Syrup 10, HL Moore Drug Exch	00839-7196-69
480 ml	$30.38	Lactulose, HL Moore Drug Exch	00839-7199-69
480 ml	$34.40	Lactulose, Rugby	00536-1417-85
480 ml	**$37.14**	**CEPHULAC, Hoechst Marion Roussel**	**00068-0413-16**
500 ml	$25.95	Lactulose, Roxane	00054-3486-63
946 ml	$45.00	Lactulose Syrup, Goldline Labs	00182-6075-58
946 ml	$46.44	CATULAC, Major Pharms	00904-2117-69
946 ml	$50.28	Lactulose Syrup 10G/15 Ml, HL Moore Drug Exch	00839-7199-62
946 ml	$66.41	CHRONULAC SYRUP, Hoechst Marion Roussel	00068-0409-32
960 ml	$24.86	CONSTILAC, Alra Labs	51641-0224-82
960 ml	$38.45	Lactulose, Harber Pharm	51432-0534-22
960 ml	$48.52	Lactulose, Qualitest Pharms	00603-1378-59
960 ml	$48.90	Lactulose, Schein Pharm (US)	00364-2519-32
960 ml	$50.39	Lactulose, Geneva Pharms	00781-6406-62
960 ml	$50.45	CONSTULOSE, Alpharma	00472-1358-32
960 ml	$52.47	DUPHALAC 10G/15ML SYRUP, Solvay Pharms	00032-1602-80
960 ml	$55.39	Lactulose, Copley Pharm	38245-0661-13
960 ml	$62.70	Lactulose, Rugby	00536-1418-86

HOW SUPPLIED - RATED THERAPEUTICALLY EQUIVALENT: *(cont'd)*

1000 ml	$47.00	Lactulose, Roxane	00054-3486-68
1920 ml	$67.75	CHOLAC, Alra Labs	51641-0225-94
1920 ml	$76.74	Enulose, Harber Pharm	51432-0536-23
1920 ml	$89.49	CALULOSE SYRUP, Major Pharms	00904-2115-74
1920 ml	$89.97	ENULOSE, Balan	00304-2031-94
1920 ml	$89.99	LACTTULOSE SYRUP 10, Goldline Labs	00182-6072-97
1920 ml	$97.75	Lactulose, Schein Pharm (US)	00364-2347-64
1920 ml	$110.65	Lactulose, Copley Pharm	38245-0670-83
1920 ml	**$132.77**	**CEPHULAC, Hoechst Marion Roussel**	**00068-0413-64**
3785 ml	$67.75	CONSTILAC, Alra Labs	51641-0224-97
3785 ml	$99.45	CHOLAC, Alra Labs	51641-0225-97

syrup - Oral - 10 g per 15 ml

250 ml	$15.80	CHRONULAC, UDL	51079-0636-44

syrup - oral - 10 g per 15 ml

1,000 ml	$56.50	CHRONULAC, UDL	51079-0636-39

LAMIVUDINE *(003253)*

CATEGORIES: AIDS Related Complex; Anti-Infectives; Antimicrobials; Antivirals; HIV Infection; Infections; Nucleoside Analogue Drugs; Viral Agents; FDA Approved 1995 Nov

BRAND NAMES: 3TC; **Epivir**

FORMULARIES: PCS

WARNING:

Lamivudine is indicated for use in combination with zidovudine for the treatment of human immunodeficiency virus (HIV) infection when antiretroviral therapy is warranted based on clinical and/or immunological evidence of disease progression. This indication is based on analyses of surrogate endpoints. At present, there are no results from controlled clinical trials evaluating the effect of therapy with lamivudine plus zidovudine on the clinical progression of HIV infection, such as the incidence of opportunistic infections or survival.

Patients receiving lamivudine plus zidovudine may continue to develop opportunistic infections and other complications of HIV infection, and therefore should remain under close observation by physicians experienced in the treatment of patients with HIV-associated diseases.

DESCRIPTION:

Lamivudine is a synthetic nucleoside analogue with activity against HIV. The chemical name of lamivudine is (2R,cis)-4-amino-1-(2-hydroxymethyl-1,3-oxathiolan- 5-yl)-(1H)-pyrimidin-2-one. Lamivudine is the (-)enantiomer of a dideoxy analogue of cytidine. Lamivudine has also been referred to as (-)2',3'-dideoxy, 3'-thiacytidine. It has a molecular formula of $C_8H_{11}N_3O_3S$ and a molecular weight of 229.3.

Lamivudine is a white to off-white crystalline solid with a solubility of approximately 70 mg/ml in water at 20°C.

Epivir tablets are for oral administration. Each tablet contains 150 mg of lamivudine and the inactive ingredients magnesium stearate, microcrystalline cellulose, and sodium starch glycolate. Opadry YS-1-7706-G White is the coloring agent in the tablet coating.

Epivir Oral Solution is for oral administration. One milliliter (1 ml) of lamivudine oral solution contains 10 mg of lamivudine (10 mg/ml) in an aqueous solution and the inactive ingredients artificial strawberry and banana flavors, citric acid (anhydrous), edetate disodium, ethanol (6% v/v), methylparaben, propylene glycol, propylparaben, and sucrose.

CLINICAL PHARMACOLOGY:

MECHANISM OF ACTION

Lamivudine is a synthetic nucleoside analogue. *In vitro* studies have shown that, intracellularly, lamivudine is phosphorylated to its active 5'-triphosphate metabolite (L-TP), which has an intracellular half-life of 10.5 to 15.5 hours. The principle mode of action of L-TP is inhibition of HIV reverse transcription via viral DNA chain termination. L-TP also inhibits the RNA- and DNA-dependent DNA polymerase activities of reverse transcriptase (RT). L-TP is a weak inhibitor of mammalian α-, β-, and γ-DNA polymerases.

MICROBIOLOGY

Antiviral Activity *In Vitro*: The relationship between *in vitro* susceptibility of HIV to lamivudine and the inhibition of HIV replication in humans has not been established. *In vitro* activity of lamivudine against HIV-1 was assessed in a number of cell lines (including monocytes and fresh human peripheral blood lymphocytes) using standard susceptibility assays. IC_{50}values (50% inhibitory concentrations) were in the range of 2 nM to 15 μM. Lamivudine had anti-HIV-1 activity in all acute virus-cell infections tested. In HIV-1-infected MT-4 cells, lamivudine in combination with zidovudine had synergistic antiretroviral activity. Synergistic activity of lamivudine/zidovudine was also shown in a variable-ratio study.

Drug Resistance: Lamivudine-resistant isolates of HIV-1 have been selected *in vitro*. The resistant isolates showed reduced susceptibility to lamivudine and genotypic analysis showed that the resistance was due to specific substitution mutations in the HIV-1 reverse transcriptase at codon 184 from methionine to either isoleucine or valine. HIV-1 strains resistant to both lamivudine and zidovudine have been isolated.

Susceptibility of clinical isolates to lamivudine and zidovudine was monitored in controlled clinical trials. In patients receiving lamivudine monotherapy or combination therapy with lamivudine plus zidovudine, HIV-1 isolates from most patients became phenotypically and genotypically resistant to lamivudine within 12 weeks. In some patients harboring zidovudine-resistant virus, phenotypic sensitivity to zidovudine by 12 weeks of treatment was restored. Combination therapy with lamivudine plus zidovudine delayed the emergence of mutations conferring resistance to zidovudine.

PHARMACOKINETICS IN ADULTS

The pharmacokinetic properties of lamivudine have been studied in asymptomatic, HIV-infected adult patients after administration of single intravenous (IV) doses ranging from 0.25 to 8 mg/kg, as well as single and multiple (twice daily regimen) oral doses ranging from 0.25 to 10 mg/kg.

Absorption and Bioavailability: Lamivudine was rapidly absorbed after oral administration in HIV-infected patients. Absolute bioavailability in 12 adult patients was 86% ± 16% (mean ± S.D.) for the tablet and 87% ± 13% for the oral solution. After oral administration of 2 mg/kg twice a day to nine adults with HIV, the peak serum lamivudine concentration (C_{max})

CLINICAL PHARMACOLOGY: *(cont'd)*

was 1.5 ± 0.5 mcg/ml (mean ± S.D.). The area under the plasma concentration versus time curve (AUC) and C_{max} increased in proportion to oral dose over the range from 0.25 to 10 mg/kg.

An investigational 25 mg dosage form of lamivudine was administered orally to 12 asymptomatic, HIV-infected patients on two occasions, once in the fasted state and once with food (1,099 kcal; 75 grams fat, 34 grams protein, 72 grams carbohydrate). Absorption of lamivudine was slower in the fed state (T_{max}: 3.2 ± 1.3 hours) compared with the fasted state (T_{max}: 0.9 ± 0.3 hours); C_{max} in the fed state was 40% ± 23% (mean ± S.D.) lower than in the fasted state. There was no significant difference in systemic exposure (AUC∞) in the fed and fasted states; therefore, lamivudine tablets and oral solution may be administered with or without food.

The accumulation ratio of lamivudine in HIV-positive asymptomatic adults with normal renal function was 1.50 following 15 days of oral administration of 2 mg/kg twice daily.

Distribution: The apparent volume of distribution after IV administration of lamivudine to 20 patients was 1.3 ± 0.4 L/kg, suggesting that lamivudine distributes into extravascular spaces. Volume of distribution was independent of dose and did not correlate with body weight.

Binding of lamivudine to human plasma proteins is low (<36%). *In vitro* studies showed that, over the concentration range of 0.1 to 100 mcg/ml, the amount of lamivudine associated with erythrocytes ranged from 53% to 57% and was independent of concentration.

Metabolism: Metabolism of lamivudine is a minor route of elimination. In man, the only known metabolite of lamivudine is the trans-sulfoxide metabolite. Within 12 hours after a single oral dose of lamivudine in six HIV-infected adults, 5.2% ± 1.4% (mean ± S.D.) of the dose was excreted as the trans-sulfoxide metabolite in the urine. Serum concentrations of this metabolite have not been determined.

Elimination: The majority of lamivudine is eliminated unchanged in urine. In 20 patients given a single IV dose, renal clearance was 0.22 ± 0.06 L/hr*kg (mean ± S.D.) representing 71% ± 16% (mean ± S.D.) of total clearance of lamivudine.

In most single-dose studies in HIV-infected patients with serum sampling for 24 hours after dosing, the observed mean elimination half-life ($T_{1/2}$) ranged from 5 to 7 hours. Total clearance was 0.37 ± 0.05 L/hr*kg (mean ± S.D.). Oral clearance and elimination half-life were independent of dose and body weight over an oral dosing range from 0.25 to 10 mg/kg.

SPECIAL POPULATIONS

Adults With Impaired Renal Function: The pharmacokinetic properties of lamivudine have been determined in a small group of HIV-infected adults with impaired renal function, as summarized in TABLE 1.

TABLE 1 Pharmacokinetic Parameters (Mean ± S.D.) After a Single 300-mg Oral Dose of Lamivudine in Three Groups of Adults With Varying Degrees of Renal Function (CrCl>60 ml/min, CrCl = 10-30 ml/min, and CrCl<10 ml/min)

Number of subjects	6	4	6
Creatinine clearance criterion	>60 ml/min	10-30 ml/min	<10 ml/min
Creatinine clearance (ml/min)	111 ± 14	28 ± 8	6 ± 2
C_{max} (mcg/ml)	2.6 ± 0.5	3.6 ± 0.8	5.8 ± 1.2
AUC∞ (mcg·h/ml)	11.0 ± 1.7	48.0 ± 19	157 ± 74
Cl/F (ml/min)	464 ± 76	114 ± 34	36 ± 11

Exposure (AUC∞), C_{max}, and half-life increased with diminishing renal function (as expressed by creatinine clearance). Apparent total oral clearance (Cl/F) of lamivudine decreased as creatinine clearance decreased. T_{max} was not significantly affected by renal function. Based on these observations, it is recommended that the dosage of lamivudine be modified in patients with renal impairment (see DOSAGE AND ADMINISTRATION.) The effects of renal impairment on lamivudine pharmacokinetics in pediatric patients are not known.

Pediatric Patients: For pharmacokinetic properties of lamivudine in pediatric patients, see PRECAUTIONS: Pediatric Use.

Geriatric Patients: Lamivudine pharmacokinetics have not been specifically studied in patients over 65 years of age.

Gender: The pharmacokinetics of lamivudine with respect to gender have not been evaluated.

Race: The pharmacokinetics of lamivudine with respect to race have not been evaluated.

INDICATIONS AND USAGE:

Lamivudine in combination with zidovudine is indicated for the treatment of HIV infection when therapy is warranted based on clinical and/or immunological evidence of disease progression. This indication is based on analyses of surrogate endpoints. At present, there are no results from controlled trials evaluating the effect of lamivudine plus zidovudine on clinical progression of HIV infection, such as the incidence of opportunistic infections or survival.

Description of Clinical Studies: *Adults Without Prior Antiretroviral Therapy:* Two studies were conducted in patients who received up to 4 weeks of prior antiretroviral therapy. A3001 was a randomized, double-blind study comparing lamivudine 150 mg twice daily plus zidovudine 200 mg three times daily; lamivudine 300 mg twice daily plus zidovudine; lamivudine 300 mg twice daily; and zidovudine. 366 adults enrolled with the following demographics: male (87%), Caucasian (61%), median age of 34 years, asymptomatic HIV infection (80%), and baseline CD4 cell counts of 200 to 500 cells/mm^3 (median = 352 cells/mm^3). B3001 was a randomized, double-blind study comparing lamivudine 300 mg twice daily plus zidovudine 200 mg three times daily versus zidovudine. 129 adults enrolled with the following demographics: male (74%), Caucasian (82%), median age of 33 years, asymptomatic HIV infection (64%), and baseline CD4 cell counts of 100 to 400 cells/mm^3 (median = 260 cells/mm^3).

Adults With Prior Zidovudine Therapy: Two studies were conducted in patients who received at least 24 weeks of prior zidovudine therapy. A3002 was a randomized, double-blind study comparing lamivudine 150 mg twice daily plus zidovudine 200 mg three times daily; lamivudine 300 mg twice daily plus zidovudine; and zidovudine plus zalcitabine 0.75 mg three times daily 254 adults enrolled with the following demographics: male (83%), Caucasian (63%), median age of 37 years, asymptomatic HIV infection (58%), median duration of prior zidovudine use of 24 months, and baseline CD4 cell counts of 100 to 300 cells/mm^3 (median = 211 cells/mm^3). B3002 was a randomized, double-blind study comparing lamivudine 150 mg twice daily plus zidovudine, lamivudine 300 mg twice daily plus zidovudine, and zidovudine, 223 adults enrolled with the following demographics: male (83%), Caucasian (96%), median age of 36 years, asymptomatic HIV infection (53%), median duration of prior zidovudine use of 23 months, and baseline CD4 cell counts of 100 to 400 cells/mm^3 (median = 241 cells/mm^3).

HIV RNA: Mean changes from baseline HIV RNA are summarized in TABLE 2A and 2B.

CONTRAINDICATIONS:

Lamivudine tablets and oral solution are contraindicated in patients with previously demonstrated clinically significant hypersensitivity to any of the components of the products.

TABLE 2A Mean Changes in log 10 HIV RNA From Baseline in Studies A3001 and A3002 at 24 Weeks of Treatment

	Mean (± S.D.) Changes in log 10 HIV RNA From Baseline*		
	Lamivudine 150 mg twice daily + Zidovudine	Zidovudine	Lamivudine 300 mg twice daily
Study A3001 (antiretroviral-naive adults)	-0.9 ± 0.8	-0.3 ± 0.8	-0.4 ± 0.8
Study A3002 (antiretroviral-experienced adults)	-0.7 ± 0.8	not applicable	not applicable

*** THE CLINICAL SIGNIFICANCE OF CHANGES IN HIV RNA DURING THERAPY IS UNKNOWN.**

TABLE 2B Mean Changes in log 10 HIV RNA From Baseline in Studies A3001 and A3002 at 24 Weeks of Treatment

	Mean (± S.D.) Changes in log 10 HIV RNA From Baseline*	
	Lamivudine 300 mg twice daily + Zidovudine	Zidovudine + Zalcitabine
Study A3001 (antiretroviral-naive adults)	-1.0 ± 0.8	not applicable
Study A3002 (antiretroviral-experienced adults)	-0.7 ± 0.8	-0.7 ± 0.8

*** THE CLINICAL SIGNIFICANCE OF CHANGES IN HIV RNA DURING THERAPY IS UNKNOWN.**

WARNINGS:

PANCREATITIS IN PEDIATRIC PATIENTS: IN PEDIATRIC PATIENTS WITH A HISTORY OF PANCREATITIS OR OTHER SIGNIFICANT RISK FACTORS FOR THE DEVELOPMENT OF PANCREATITIS, THE COMBINATION OF LAMIVUDINE AND ZIDOVUDINE SHOULD BE USED WITH EXTREME CAUTION AND ONLY IF THERE IS NO SATISFACTORY ALTERNATIVE THERAPY. TREATMENT WITH LAMIVUDINE SHOULD BE STOPPED IMMEDIATELY IF CLINICAL SIGNS, SYMPTOMS, OR LABORATORY ABNORMALITIES SUGGESTIVE OF PANCREATITIS OCCUR (SEE ADVERSE REACTIONS.)

The complete prescribing information for zidovudine should be consulted before combination therapy with lamivudine and zidovudine is initiated.

PRECAUTIONS:

Patients With Impaired Renal Function: Reduction of the dosage of lamivudine is recommended for patients with impaired renal function (see CLINICAL PHARMACOLOGY) and DOSAGE AND ADMINISTRATION.

Information for the Patient: Lamivudine is not a cure for HIV infection and patients may continue to experience illnesses associated with HIV infection, including opportunistic infections. Treatment with lamivudine has not been shown to reduce the frequency of such illnesses and patients should remain under the care of a physician when using lamivudine. Patients should be advised that the use of lamivudine has not been shown to reduce the risk of transmission of HIV to others through sexual contact or blood contamination.

Patients should be advised that the long-term effects of lamivudine are unknown at this time.

Lamivudine tablets and oral solution are for oral ingestion only.

Patients should be advised of the importance of taking lamivudine exactly as it is prescribed.

Parents or guardians should be advised to monitor pediatric patients for signs and symptoms of pancreatitis.

Carcinogenesis, Mutagenesis, and Impairment of Fertility: Long-term carcinogenicity studies of lamivudine in animals have not yet been completed. Lamivudine was not active in a microbial mutagenicity screen or an *in vitro* cell transformation assay, but showed weak *in vitro* mutagenic activity in a cytogenetic assay using cultured human lymphocytes and in the mouse lymphoma assay. However, lamivudine showed no evidence of *in vivo*genotoxic activity in the rat at oral doses of up to 2,000 mg/kg (approximately 65 times the recommended human dose based on body surface area comparisons). In a study of reproductive performance, lamivudine, administered to rats at doses up to 130 times the usual adult dose based on body surface area comparisons, revealed no evidence of impaired fertility and no effect on the survival, growth, and development to weaning of the offspring.

Pregnancy Category C: Reproduction studies have been performed in rats and rabbits at orally administered doses up to approximately 130 and 60 times, respectively, the usual adult dose and have revealed no evidence of harm to the fetus due to lamivudine. Some evidence of early embryolethality was seen in the rabbit at doses similar to those produced by the usual adult dose and higher, but there was no indication of this effect in the rat at orally administered doses up to 130 times the usual adult dose. Studies in pregnant rats and rabbits showed that lamivudine is transferred to the fetus through the placenta. There are no adequate and well-controlled studies in pregnant women. Because animal reproductive toxicity studies are not always predictive of human response, lamivudine should be used during pregnancy only if the potential benefits outweigh the risks.

Antiretroviral Pregnancy Registry: To monitor maternal-fetal outcomes of pregnant women exposed to lamivudine, an Antiretroviral Pregnancy Registry has been established. Physicians are encouraged to register patients by calling (800) 722-9292, ext. 58465.

Nursing Mothers: A study in which lactating rats were administered 45 mg/kg of lamivudine showed that lamivudine concentrations in milk were slightly greater than those in plasma. Although it is not known if lamivudine is excreted in human milk, there is the potential for adverse effects from lamivudine in nursing infants. Mothers should be instructed to discontinue nursing if they are receiving lamivudine. This instruction is consistent with the Centers for Disease Control recommendation that HIV-infected mothers not breast-feed their infants to avoid risking postnatal transmission of HIV infection.

Pediatric Use: THERE ARE NO DATA ON THE USE OF LAMIVUDINE IN COMBINATION WITH ZIDOVUDINE IN PEDIATRIC PATIENTS.

Lamivudine monotherapy was studied in one open-label, uncontrolled trial (study A2002) in 97 pediatric patients with the following demographics: male (56%), Caucasian (57%), median age of 7.7 years (range: 0.4 to 17.3 years), symptomatic HIV (84%), median duration of prior antiretroviral therapy of 148 weeks, and median baseline CD4 of 132 cells/mm^3.

Pharmacokinetic properties of lamivudine were assessed in a subset of 57 patients (age range: 4.8 months to 16 years, weight range: 5 to 66 kg) after oral and IV administration of 1, 2, 4, 8, 12, and 20 mg/kg per day. In the 9 infants and children receiving 8 mg/kg per day (the usual recommended pediatric dose), absolute bioavailability was 66% ± 26% (mean ±

PRECAUTIONS: *(cont'd)*

S.D.), which is less than the 86% ± 16% (mean ± S.D.) observed in adolescents and adults. The mechanism for the diminished absolute bioavailability of lamivudine in infants and children is unknown.

Systemic clearance decreased with increasing age in pediatric patients.

After oral administration of 8 mg/kg per day of lamivudine to 11 pediatric patients ranging from 4 months to 14 years of age, C_{max} was 1.1 ± 0.6 mcg/ml and half-life was 2.0 ± 0.6 hours, (In adults with similar blood sampling, the half-life was 3.7 ± 1 hours.) Total exposure to lamivudine, as reflected by mean AUC values, was comparable between pediatric patients receiving an 8 mg/kg/day dose and adults receiving a 4 mg/kg/day dose.

Distribution of lamivudine into cerebrospinal fluid (CSF) was assessed in 38 pediatric patients after multiple oral dosing with lamivudine. CSF samples were collected between 2 and 4 hours postdose. At the dose of 8 mg/kg/day, CSF lamivudine concentrations in eight patients ranged from 5.6% to 30.9% (mean ± S.D. of 14.2% ± 7.9%) of the concentration in a simultaneous serum sample, with CSF lamivudine concentrations ranging from 0.04 to 0.3 mcg/ml. (See INDICATIONS AND USAGE, Description of Clinical Studies), WARNINGS, ADVERSE REACTIONS, and DOSAGE AND ADMINISTRATION.

DRUG INTERACTIONS:

Lamivudine and zidovudine were coadministered to 12 asymptomatic HIV-positive adult patients in a single-center, open-label, randomized, crossover study. No significant differences were observed in AUC∞ or total clearance for lamivudine or zidovudine when the two drugs were administered together. Coadministration of lamivudine with zidovudine resulted in an increase of 39% ± 62% (mean ± S.D.) in C_{max} of zidovudine.

Lamivudine and trimethoprim/sulfamethoxazole (TMP/SMX) were coadministered to 14 HIV-positive patients in a single-center, open-label, randomized, crossover study. Each patient received treatment with a single 300-mg dose of lamivudine and TMP 160 mg/SMX 800 mg once a day for 5 days with concomitant administration of lamivudine 300 mg with the fifth dose in a crossover design. Coadministration of TMP/SMX with lamivudine resulted in an increase of 44% ± 23% (mean ± S.D.) in lamivudine AUC∞, a decrease of 29% ± 13% in lamivudine oral clearance, and a decrease of 30% ± 36% in lamivudine renal clearance. The pharmacokinetic properties of TMP and SMX were not altered by coadministration with lamivudine.

TMP 160 mg/SMX 800 mg once daily has been shown to increase lamivudine exposure (AUC). The effect of higher doses of TMP/SMX on lamivudine pharmacokinetics has not been investigated.

ADVERSE REACTIONS:

Adults: Selected clinical adverse events with a ≥5% frequency during therapy with lamivudine 150 mg twice daily plus zidovudine 200 mg three times daily compared with zidovudine are listed in TABLE 3.

TABLE 3 Selected Clinical Adverse Events (≥5% Frequency) in Four Controlled Clinical Trials (A3001, A3002, B3001, B3002)

Adverse Event	Lamivudine 150 mg twice daily plus Zidovudine (n = 251)	Zidovudine (n = 230)
Body as a whole		
Headache	35%	27%
Malaise & fatigue	27%	23%
Fever or chills	10%	12%
Digestive		
Nausea	33%	29%
Diarrhea	18%	22%
Nausea & vomiting	13%	12%
Anorexia and/or decreased appetite	10%	7%
Abdominal pain	9%	11%
Abdominal cramps	6%	3%
Dyspepsia	5%	5%
Nervous System		
Neuropathy	12%	10%
Insomnia & other sleep disorders	11%	7%
Dizziness	10%	4%
Depressive disorders	9%	4%
Respiratory		
Nasal signs & symptoms	20%	11%
Cough	18%	13%
Skin		
Skin rashes	9%	6%
Musculoskeletal		
Musculoskeletal pain	12%	10%
Myalgia	8%	6%
Arthralgia	5%	5%

Pancreatitis was observed in 3 of the 656 adult patients (<0.5%) who received lamivudine in controlled clinical trials.

Selected laboratory abnormalities observed during therapy are listed in TABLE 4.

TABLE 4 Frequencies of Selected Laboratory Abnormalities Among Adults in Four Controlled Clinical Trials (A3001, A3002, B3001, B3002)*

Test (Abnormal Level)	Lamivudine 150 mg twice daily plus Zidovudine % (n)	Zidovudine % (n)
Neutropenia (ANC<750/mm^3)	7.2% (237)	5.4% (222)
Anemia (Hgb<8.0 g/dl)	2.9% (241)	1.8% (218)
Thrombocytopenia (platelets <50,000/mm^3)	0.4% (240)	1.3% (223)
ALT (>5.0 x ULN)	3.7% (241)	3.6% (224)
AST (>5.0 x ULN)	1.7% (241)	1.8% (223)
Bilirubin (>2.5 ULN)	0.8% (241)	0.4% (220)
Amylase (>2.0 ULN)	4.2% (72)	1.5% (133)

* Frequencies of these laboratory abnormalities were higher in patients with mild laboratory abnormalities at baseline.
ULN=Upper limit of normal
ANC=absolute neutrophil count
n =Number of patients assessed

Pediatric Patients: Limited information on the incidence of adverse events in children receiving lamivudine monotherapy is available from one open-label, uncontrolled study (see PRECAUTIONS, Pediatric Use) section for description of study A2002. **Of 97 pediatric patients, 14 patients (14%) developed pancreatitis while receiving monotherapy with lamivudine.**

ADVERSE REACTIONS: *(cont'd)*

In a second ongoing study in 47 pediatric patients (age range: 3 months to 18 years) enrolled in an open-label evaluation of lamivudine/didanosine, lamivudine/zidovudine, and lamivudine/zidovudine/didanosine, 7 patients (15%) developed pancreatitis. (see WARNINGS)

Paresthesias and peripheral neuropathies were reported in 13 patients (13%) in study A2002 and resulted in treatment discontinuation in 3 patients.

Selected laboratory abnormalities during lamivudine therapy in children are listed in TABLE 5A and 5B.

TABLE 5A Frequencies of Selected Laboratory Abnormalities in an Uncontrolled Phase I/II Clinical Trial of Lamivudine in 97 Pediatric Patients

Test (Abnormal Level)	Patients With Normal Baselines % (n)
Neutropenia (ANC<750/mm_3	22% (55)
Anemia (Hgb<8.0 g/dl)	2% (50)
Thrombocytopenia (platelets <40,000/mm^3	0% (68)
ALT (>5.0 x ULN)	4% (51)
AST (>5.0 x ULN)	0% (29)
Amylase (>2.0 ULN)	3% (69)

ULN=Upper limit of normal
ANC=absolute neutrophil count
n=Number of patients assessed

TABLE 5B Frequencies of Selected Laboratory Abnormalities in an Uncontrolled Phase I/II Clinical Trial of Lamivudine in 97 Pediatric Patients

Test (Abnormal Level)	Patients With Abnormal Baselines % (n)
Neutropenia (ANC<750/mm^3)	45% (33)
Anemia (Hgb<8.0 g/dl)	24% (46)
Thrombocytopenia (platelets <40,000/mm^3)	25% (12)
ALT (>5.0 x ULN)	29% (42)
AST (>5.0 x ULN)	19% (57)
Amylase (>2.0 ULN)	23% (13)

ULN=Upper limit of normal
ANC=absolute neutrophil count
n=Number of patients assessed

OVERDOSAGE:

There is no known antidote for lamivudine. One case of an adult ingesting 6 g of lamivudine was reported; there were no clinical signs or symptoms noted and hematologic tests remained normal. It is not known whether lamivudine can be removed by peritoneal dialysis or hemodialysis.

DOSAGE AND ADMINISTRATION:

Adults and Adolescents (12 to 16 years): The recommended oral dose of lamivudine for adults and adolescents is 150 mg twice daily administered in combination with zidovudine. The complete prescribing information for zidovudine should be consulted for information on its dosage and administration.

For adults with low body weights (less than 50 kg or 110 lbs), the recommended oral dose of lamivudine is 2 mg/kg twice daily administered in combination with zidovudine. No data are available to support a dosage recommendation for adolescents with low body weight (less than 50 kg).

Pediatric Patients: The recommended oral dose of lamivudine for pediatric patients 3 months to up to 12 years of age is 4 mg/kg twice daily (up to a maximum of 150 mg twice a day) administered in combination with zidovudine. The complete prescribing information for zidovudine should be consulted for information on its dosage and administration.

Dose Adjustment: It is recommended that doses of lamivudine be adjusted in accordance with renal function in patients older than age 16 years as in TABLE 6, (See CLINICAL PHARMACOLOGY.)

TABLE 6 Adjustment of Dosage of Lamivudine in Accordance With Creatinine Clearance

Creatinine Clearance (ml/min)	Recommended Dosage of Lamivudine
≥ 50	150 mg twice daily
30-49	150 mg once daily
15-29	150 mg first dose, then 100 mg once daily
5-14	150 mg first dose, then 50 mg once daily
< 5	50 mg first dose, then 25 mg once daily

Insufficient data are available to recommend a dosage of lamivudine in patients undergoing dialysis.

HOW SUPPLIED:

Epivir tablets, 150 mg, are white, modified diamond-shaped, film-coated tablets imprinted with "150" on one side and "GXCJ7" on the reverse side. **Store between 2° and 30°C (36° and 86°F) in tightly closed bottles.**

Epivir Oral Solution, a clear, colorless to pale yellow, strawberry-banana flavored, liquid. This product does not require reconstitution. **Store between 2° and 25°C (36° and 77°F) in tightly closed bottles.**

HOW SUPPLIED - EQUIVALENTS NOT AVAILABLE:

Solution - Oral - 10 mg/ml

240 ml	$61.44	EPIVIR, Glaxo Wellcome	00173-0471-00

Tablet - Oral - 150 mg

60's	$230.41	EPIVIR, Glaxo Wellcome	00173-0470-01

LAMOTRIGINE *(003155)*

CATEGORIES: Anticonvulsants; Antiepileptics; Central Nervous System Agents; Convulsions; Epilepsy; Neuromuscular; Seizures; FDA Class 1P ("Priority Review"); FDA Approved 1994 Dec

BRAND NAMES: **Lamictal**

FORMULARIES: Medi-Cal; PCS

COST OF THERAPY: $1,346.36 (Epilepsy; Tablet; 150 mg; 2/day; 365 days)

PRIMARY ICD9: 345.90 (Epilepsy, Unspecified, Without Mention of Intractable)

WARNING:
SEVERE, POTENTIALLY LIFE-THREATENING RASHES HAVE BEEN REPORTED IN ASSOCIATION WITH THE USE OF LAMOTRIGINE. THESE REPORTS, OCCURRING IN APPROXIMATELY ONE IN EVERY THOUSAND ADULTS, HAVE INCLUDED STEVENS-JOHNSON SYNDROME (SJS) AND, RARELY, TOXIC EPIDERMAL NECROLYSIS (TEN). RARE DEATHS HAVE BEEN REPORTED, BUT THEIR NUMBERS ARE TOO FEW TO PERMIT A PRECISE ESTIMATE OF THE RATE.
THE INCIDENCE OF SEVERE, POTENTIALLY LIFE-THREATENING RASH IN PEDIATRIC PATIENTS, HOWEVER, IS VERY MUCH HIGHER THAN THAT REPORTED IN ADULTS USING LAMOTRIGINE; SPECIFICALLY, REPORTS FROM CLINICAL TRIALS SUGGEST AS MANY AS 1 IN 50 TO 1 IN 100 PEDIATRIC PATIENTS DEVELOP A POTENTIALLY LIFE-THREATENING RASH. IT BEARS EMPHASIS, ACCORDINGLY, THAT LAMOTRIGINE IS NOT APPROVED FOR USE IN PATIENTS BELOW THE AGE OF 16 (SEE INDICATIONS AND USAGE).
OTHER THAN AGE, THERE ARE AS YET NO FACTORS IDENTIFIED THAT ARE KNOWN TO PREDICT THE RISK OF OCCURRENCE OR THE SEVERITY OF RASH ASSOCIATED WITH LAMOTRIGINE. THERE ARE SUGGESTIONS, YET TO BE PROVEN, THAT THE RISK OF RASH MAY ALSO BE INCREASED BY 1) COADMINISTRATION OF LAMOTRIGINE WITH VALPROIC ACID (VPA), 2) EXCEEDING THE RECOMMENDED INITIAL DOSE OF LAMOTRIGINE, OR 3) EXCEEDING THE RECOMMENDED DOSE ESCALATION FOR LAMOTRIGINE. HOWEVER, CASES HAVE BEEN REPORTED IN THE ABSENCE OF THESE FACTORS.
NEARLY ALL CASES OF LIFE-THREATENING RASHES ASSOCIATED WITH LAMOTRIGINE HAVE OCCURRED WITHIN 2 TO 8 WEEKS OF TREATMENT INITIATION. HOWEVER, ISOLATED CASES HAVE BEEN REPORTED AFTER PROLONGED TREATMENT (*E.G.,* 6 MONTHS). ACCORDINGLY, DURATION OF THERAPY CANNOT BE RELIED UPON AS A MEANS TO PREDICT THE POTENTIAL RISK HERALDED BY THE FIRST APPEARANCE OF A RASH.
ALTHOUGH BENIGN RASHES ALSO OCCUR WITH LAMOTRIGINE, IT IS NOT POSSIBLE TO PREDICT RELIABLY WHICH RASHES WILL PROVE TO BE LIFE-THREATENING. ACCORDINGLY, LAMOTRIGINE SHOULD BE DISCONTINUED AT THE FIRST SIGN OF RASH, UNLESS THE RASH IS CLEARLY NOT DRUG RELATED. DISCONTINUATION OF TREATMENT MAY NOT PREVENT A RASH FROM BECOMING LIFE-THREATENING OR PERMANENTLY DISABLING OR DISFIGURING.

DESCRIPTION:

Lamictal, an antiepileptic drug of the phenyltriazine class, is chemically unrelated to existing antiepileptic drugs(AED's). Its chemical name is 6-(2,3-dichlorophenyl)-1,2,4-triazine-3,5-diamine, its molecular formula is $C_9H_7Cl_2N_5$ and its molecular weight is 256.09. Lamotrigine is a white to pale cream-colored powder and has a Pka of 5.7. Lamotrigine is very slightly soluble in water (0.17 mg/ml at 25°C) and slightly soluble in 0.1 M HCl (4.1 mg/ml at 25°C).

Lamictal is supplied for oral administration as 25 mg (white), 100 mg (peach), 150 mg (cream), and 200 mg (blue) tablets. Each tablet contains the labeled amount of lamotrigine and the following inactive ingredients: lactose; magnesium stearate; microcrystalline cellulose; povidone; sodium starch glycolate; FD&C Yellow No. 6 Lake (100 mg tablet only); ferric oxide; yellow (150 mg tablet only); FD&C Blue No. 2 Lake (200 mg tablet only).

CLINICAL PHARMACOLOGY:

Mechanism of Action: The precise mechanism(s) by which lamotrigine exerts its anticonvulsant action are unknown. In animal models designed to detect anticonvulsant activity, lamotrigine was effective in preventing seizure spread in the maximum electroshock (MES) and pentylenetetrazol (scMet) tests, and prevented seizures in the visually and electrically evoked after-discharge (EEAD) tests for antiepileptic activity. The relevance of these models to human epilepsy, however, is not known.

One proposed mechanism of action of Lamotrigine, the relevance of which remains to be established in humans, involves an effect on sodium channels. *In vitro* pharmacological studies suggest that lamotrigine inhibits voltage-sensitive sodium channels thereby stabilizing neuronal membranes and consequently modulating presynaptic transmitter release of excitatory amino acids, (*e.g.,* glutamate and aspartate).

Pharmacological Properties: Although the relevance for human use is unknown, the following data characterize the performance of Lamotrigine in receptor binding assays. Lamotrigine had a weak inhibitory effect on the serotonin 5-HT_3 receptor (IC_{50}= 18 μM). It does not exhibit high affinity binding (IC_{50}>100 μM) to the following neurotransmitter receptors: adenosine $A_1$and A_2, adrenergic $_{1}$ · $_{2}$, and β; dopamine $D_1$and D_2; γ-aminobutyric acid (GABA) A and B; histamine H_1; kappa opioid; muscarinic acetylcholine; and serotonin 5- HT_2. Studies have failed to detect an effect of lamotrigine on dihydropyridine-sensitive calcium channels. It had weak effects at sigma opioid receptors (IC_{50}= 145 μM). Lamotrigine did not inhibit the uptake of norepinephrine, dopamine, serotonin, or aspartic acid (IC_{50}> 100 μM).

Effect of lamotrigine on NMDA-mediated activity: Lamotrigine did not inhibit NMDA-induced depolarizations in rat cortical slices or NMDA- induced cyclic GMP formation in immature rat cerebellum nor did lamotrigine displace compounds that are either competitive or non-competitive ligands at this glutamate receptor complex (CNQX, CGS, TCHP). The IC_{50} for lamotrigine effects on NMDA-induced currents (in the presence of 3 μM glycine) in cultured hippocampal neurons exceeded 100 μM.

Folate Metabolism: *In vitro,* lamotrigine was a shown to be an inhibitor of dihydrofolate reductase, the enzyme that catalyzes the reduction of dihydrofolate to tetrahydrofolate. Inhibition of this enzyme may interfere with the biosynthesis of nucleic acids and proteins. When oral daily doses of lamotrigine were given to pregnant rats during organogenesis, fetal, placental, and maternal folate concentrations were reduced. Significantly reduced concentrations of folate are associated with teratogenesis (see PRECAUTIONS, Pregnancy). Folate concentrations were also reduced in male rats given repeated oral doses of lamotrigine. Reduced concentrations were partially returned to normal when supplemented with folic acid.

Accumulation in Kidneys: Lamotrigine was found to accumulate in the kidney of the male rat causing chronic progressive nephrosis, necrosis, and mineralization. These findings are attributed to α-2 microglobulin, a species and sex specific protein that has not been detected in humans or other animal species.

CLINICAL PHARMACOLOGY: *(cont'd)*

Melanin Binding: Lamotrigine binds to melanin-containing tissues, *e.g.,* in the eye and pigmented skin. It has been found in the uveal tract up to 52 weeks after a single dose in rodents.

Cardiovascular: In dogs, lamotrigine is extensively metabolized to a 2-N-methyl metabolite. This metabolite causes dose-dependent prolongations of the PR interval, widening of the QRS complex, and, at higher doses, complete AV conduction block. Similar cardiovascular effects are not anticipated in humans because only trace amounts of the 2-N-methyl metabolite (<0.6% of lamotrigine dose) have been found in human urine (see Drug Disposition). However, it is conceivable that plasma concentrations of this metabolite could be increased in patients with a reduced capacity to glucuronidase lamotrigine (*e.g.,* in patients with liver disease).

Pharmacokinetics and Drug Metabolism: The pharmacokinetics of lamotrigine have been studied in patients with epilepsy, healthy young and elderly volunteers, and volunteers with chronic renal failure. Lamotrigine pharmacokinetic parameters for adult patients and healthy normal volunteers are summarized in TABLE 1.

TABLE 1 Pharmacokinetic Parameters In Adult Patients With Epilepsy Of Healthy Volunteers Mean [1]

Adult Study Population	Number of Subjects	T_{max}:Time of Maximum Plasma Concentration (hours)	t 1/2 Elimination Half-Life (hours)	CL/F Plasma Clearance (ml/min/kg)
Patients Taking Enzyme-Inducing Antiepileptic Drugs[2]:				
Single-Dose Lamotrigine	24	2.3 (0.5-5.0)	14.4 (6.4-30.4)	1.10 (0.51-2.22)
Multiple-Dose Lamotrigine	17	2.0 (0.75-5.93)	12.6 (7.5-23.1)	1.21 (0.66-1.82)
Patients Taking Enzyme-Inducing Antiepileptic Drugs + Valproic Acid:				
Single-Dose Lamotrigine	25	3.8 (1.0-10.0)	27.2 (11.2-51.6)	0.53 (0.27-1.04)
Patients Taking Valproic Acid Only:				
Single-Dose Lamotrigine	4	4.8 (1.8-8.4)	58.8 (30.5-88.8)	0.28 (0.16-0.40)
Healthy Volunteers Taking Valproic Acid:				
Single-Dose Lamotrigine	6	1.8 (1.0-4.0)	48.3 (31.5-88.6)	0.30 (0.14-0.42)
Multiple-Dose Lamotrigine	18	1.9 (0.5-3.5)	70.3 (41.9-113.5)	0.18 (0.12-0.33)
Healthy Volunteers Taking No Other Medications:				
Single-Dose Lamotrigine	179	2.2 (0.25-12.0)	32.8 (14.0-103.0)	0.44 (0.12-1.10)
Multiple-Dose Lamotrigine	36	1.7 (0.5-4.0)	25.4 (11.6-61.6)	0.58 (0.24-1.15)

[1] The majority of parameter means determined in each study had coefficients of variation between 20% and 40% for $t_{1/2}$ and plasma clearance, and between 30% and 70% for T_{max}. The overall mean values were calculated from individual study means that were weighted based on the number of volunteers in each study. The numbers in parentheses below each parameter mean represent the range of individual volunteer/patient values across studies.
[2] Examples of enzyme-inducing antiepileptic drugs (EIAEDs) are carbamazepine, phenobarbital, phenytoin, and primidone.

The clearance of lamotrigine is affected by the co-administration of antiepileptic drugs: Lamotrigine is eliminated more rapidly in patients who have been taking hepatic enzyme inducing antiepileptic drugs (EIAEDs), including carbamazepine, phenytoin, phenobarbital, and primidone. Most clinical experience is derived from this population.

Valproic acid (VPA), however, actually decreases the clearance of lamotrigine (*i.e.,* more than doubles the elimination $1_{1/2}$ of lamotrigine), whether given with or without EIAEDs. Accordingly, if lamotrigine is to be administered to a patient receiving VPA, lamotrigine must be given at a reduced dosage, less than half the dose used in patients not receiving VPA (see DOSAGE AND ADMINISTRATION and DRUG INTERACTIONS).

ABSORPTION

Lamotrigine is rapidly and completely absorbed after oral administration with negligible first-pass metabolism (absolute bioavailability is 98%). The bioavailability is not affected by food. Peak plasma concentrations occur anywhere from 1.4 to 4.8 hours following drug administration.

DISTRIBUTION

Estimates of the mean apparent volume of distribution (Vd/F) of lamotrigine following oral administration ranged from 0.9 to 1.3 L/kg. Vd/F is independent of dose and is similar following single and multiple doses in both patients with epilepsy and in healthy volunteers.

PROTEIN BINDING

Data from *in vitro* studies indicate that lamotrigine is approximately 55% bound to human plasma proteins at plasma lamotrigine concentrations from 1 to 10 mcg/ml (10 mcg/ml is 4 to 6 times the trough plasma concentration observed in the controlled efficacy trials). Because lamotrigine is not highly bound to plasma proteins, clinically significant interactions with other drugs through completion for protein binding sites are unlikely. The binding of lamotrigine to plasma proteins did not change in the presence of therapeutic concentrations of phenytoin, phenobarbital, or valproic acid. Lamotrigine did not displace other antiepileptic drugs (carbamazepine, phenytoin, phenobarbital) from protein binding sites.

DRUG DISPOSITION

Lamotrigine is metabolized predominantly by glucuronic acid conjugation; the major metabolite is an inactive 2-N-glucuronide conjugate. After oral administration of 240 mg ^{14}C-lamotrigine (15 μCi) to six healthy volunteers, 94% was recovered in the urine and 2% was recovered in the feces. The radioactivity in the urine consisted of unchanged lamotrigine (10%), the 2-N-glucuronide (76%), a 5-N-glucuronide (10%), a 2-N- methyl metabolite (0.14%), and other unidentified minor metabolites (4%).

ENZYME INDUCTION

The effects of lamotrigine on specific families of mixed-function oxidase isozymes have not been systematically evaluated.

Following multiple administrations (150 mg b.i.d.) to normal volunteers taking no other medications, lamotrigine induced its own metabolism resulting in a 25% decrease in t 1/2 and a 37% increase in CL/F at steady state compared to values obtained in the same volunteers following a single dose. Evidence gathered from other sources suggests that self- induction by lamotrigine may not occur when lamotrigine is given as adjunctive therapy in patients receiving EIAEDs.

CLINICAL PHARMACOLOGY: *(cont'd)*

DOSE PROPORTIONALITY

In healthy volunteers not receiving any other medications and given single doses, the plasma concentrations of lamotrigine increased in direct proportion to the dose administered over the range of 50 to 400 mg. In two small studies (n = 7 and 8) of patients with epilepsy who were maintained on other antiepileptic drugs there also was a linear relationship between dose and lamotrigine plasma concentrations at steady state following doses of 50 mg to 350 mg b.i.d.

Elimination: (See TABLE 1)

SPECIAL POPULATIONS

Patients with renal insufficiency: Twelve volunteers with chronic renal failure (mean creatinine clearance = 13 ml/min; range 6 to 23) and another six individuals undergoing hemodialysis were each given a single 100 mg dose of Lamotrigine. The mean plasma half-lives determined in the study were 42.9 hours (chronic renal failure), 13.0 hours (during hemodialysis), and 57.4 hours (between hemodialysis) compared to 26.2 hours in healthy volunteers. On average, approximately 20% (range = 5.6 to 35.1) of the amount of lamotrigine present in the body was eliminated during a 4-hour hemodialysis session.

Hepatic disease: The pharmacokinetic parameters of lamotrigine in patients with impaired liver function have not been studied.

Elderly: In a single dose study (150 mg Lamotrigine), the pharmacokinetics of lamotrigine in twelve elderly volunteers between the ages of 65 and 76 years (mean creatinine clearance = 61 ml/min, range 33 to 108) were similar to those of young healthy volunteers in other studies.

Gender: The clearance of lamotrigine is not affected by gender.

Race: The apparent oral clearance of lamotrigine was 25% lower in noncaucasians than caucasians.

CLINICAL STUDIES:

The effectiveness of Lamotrigine as adjunctive therapy (added to other antiepileptic drugs) was established in three multi-center placebo controlled double blind clinical trials in 355 adults with refractory partial seizures. The patients had a history of at least 4 partial seizures per month in spite of receiving one or more antiepileptic drugs at therapeutic concentrations and, in 2 of the studies, were observed on their established antiepileptic drug regimen during baselines that varied between 8 to 12 weeks. In the third, patients were not observed in a prospective baseline. In patients continuing to have at least 4 seizures per month during the baseline, Lamotrigine or placebo was then added to existing therapy. In all three studies, change from baseline in seizure frequency was the primary measure of effectiveness. The results given below are for all partial seizures in the intent to treat (all patients who received at least one dose of treatment) population in each study, unless otherwise indicated. The median seizure frequency at baseline was 3 per week while the mean was 6.6 per week for all patients enrolled in efficacy studies.

One study (n=216) was a double-blind placebo-controlled parallel trial consisting of a 24-week treatment period. Patients could not be on more than two other anticonvulsants and valproic acid was not allowed. Patients were randomized to receive placebo, a target dose of 300 mg/day of Lamotrigine, or a target dose of 500 mg/day of Lamotrigine. The median reductions in the frequency of all partial seizures relative to baseline were 8% in patients receiving placebo, 20% in patients receiving 300 mg/day of Lamotrigine, and 36% in patients receiving 500 mg/day of Lamotrigine. The seizure frequency reduction was statistically significant in the 500 mg/day group compared to the placebo group, but not in the 300 mg/day group.

A second study (n=98) was a double-blind, placebo-controlled, randomized crossover trial consisting of two 14-week treatment periods (the last 2 weeks of which consisted of dose tapering), separated by a 4-week washout period. Patients could not be on more than two other anticonvulsants and valproic acid was not allowed. The target dose of Lamotrigine was 400 mg/day. When the first twelve weeks of the treatment periods were analyzed, the median change in seizure frequency was a 25% reduction on Lamotrigine compared to placebo ($p<0.001$).

The third study (n=41) was a double-blind placebo-controlled crossover trial consisting of two 12-week treatment periods, separated by a 4-week washout period. Patients could not be on more than two other anticonvulsants. Thirteen patients were on concomitant valproic acid; these patients received 150 mg/day of Lamotrigine. The 28 other patients had a target dose of 300 mg/day of Lamotrigine. The median change in seizure frequency was a 26% reduction on Lamotrigine compared to placebo ($p<0.01$).

No differences in efficacy based on age, sex, or race, as measured by change in seizure frequency, were detected.

INDICATIONS AND USAGE:

Lamotrigine is indicated as adjunctive therapy in the treatment of partial seizures in adults with epilepsy. Safety and effectiveness in pediatric patients below the age of 16 have not been established (see BOXED WARNING).

CONTRAINDICATIONS:

Lamotrigine is contraindicated in patients who have demonstrated hypersensitivity to the drug or its ingredients.

WARNINGS:

See BOXED WARNING REGARDING THE RISK OF SEVERE, POTENTIALLY LIFE-THREATENING RASH ASSOCIATED WITH THE USE OF LAMOTRIGINE.

Rash In The Pediatric Population: The incidence of severe, potentially life-threatening rash in pediatric patients is very much higher than that reported in adults using lamotrigine. Specifically, reports from clinical trials suggest as many as 1 in 50 to 1 in 100 pediatric patients develop a potentially life-threatening rash. It bears emphasis, accordingly, that lamotrigine is not approved for use in patients below the age of 16 (see INDICATIONS AND USAGE).

Hypersensitivity Reactions: Hypersensitivity reactions, some fatal or life threatening, have also occurred. Some of these reactions have included clinical features of multiorgan dysfunction such as hepatic abnormalities and evidence of disseminated intravascular coagulation. It is important to note that early manifestations of hyposensitivity (*e.g.,* fever, lymphadenopathy) may be present even though a rash is not evident. If such signs or symptoms are present, the patient should be evaluated immediately. Lamotrigine should be discontinued if an alternative etiology for the signs or symptoms cannot be established.

Prior initiation of treatment with lamotrigine, the patient should be instructed that a rash or other signs or symptoms oh hypersensitivity (e.g., fever, lymphadenopathy) may herald a serious medical event and that the patient should report any such occurrence to a physician immediately.

Acute Multiorgan Failure: Fatalities associated with multiorgan failure and various degrees of hepatic failure have been reported in five patients from among 7000 exposed during premarketing development of lamotrigine. These cases occurred in association with other serious medical events (e.g., status epilepticus, overwhelming sepsis), making it impossible to identify the initiating cause.

WARNINGS: *(cont'd)*

Dermatologic Events: In clinical trials, approximately 10% of all Lamotrigine exposed individuals develop a rash. However, not all cases of rash can be attributed to Lamotrigine; five percent (5%) of patients exposed to placebo developed a rash. The overall rate of discontinuation due to rash in patients participating in clinical trials (n=3501) was 3.8%. The incidence of rash appears to be increased among patients being treated with a multi-drug regimen that includes both VPA and EIAEDs. When VPA and Lamotrigine have been used as a two-drug combination, the incidence of rash is further increased; NOTE: dosing recommendations for the use of Lamotrigine and VPA alone cannot be provided because of insufficient experience with that combination (see DOSAGE AND ADMINISTRATION). The incidence of rash also appears to increase with the magnitude of the initial dose and the subsequent rate of dose escalation (see DOSAGE AND ADMINISTRATION).

Lamotrigine associated rashes do not appear to have unique identifying features. Typically, rash occurs in the first 2 to 8 weeks following treatment initiation. A benign initial appearance of a rash cannot predict an entirely benign outcome (see BOXED WARNING).

SERIOUS RASH LEADING TO HOSPITALIZATION

Rash resulting in hospitalization occurred in 0.3% of the approximately 3400 subjects who participated in premarketing clinical trials. No fatalities occurred among these individuals, but rash has been associated with a fatal outcome in reports from post-marketing experience.

Among the rashes leading to hospitalization were Stevens-Johnson syndrome, toxic epidermal necrolysis, angioedema, and a rash associated with a variable number of the following systemic manifestations: fever, lymphadenopathy, facial swelling, hematologic, and hepatologic abnormalities.

There is evidence that the inclusion of valproate in a multi-drug regimen increases the risk of serious, potentially life-threatening rash. Specifically, of 584 patients administered Lamotrigine with VPA in clinical trials, 6 (1%) were hospitalized in association with rash; in contrast, 4 (0.16%) of 2398 clinical trial patients and volunteers administered Lamotrigine in the absence of VPA were hospitalized.

Other examples of serious and potentially life-threatening rash that did not lead to hospitalization also occurred in pre-marketing development. Among these, one case was reported to be Stevens-Johnson like.

RASH LEADING TO LAMOTRIGINE WITHDRAWAL

Although not a certain indicator of severity, the clinician's decision to withdraw a patient from Lamotrigine in the face of rash provides some insight into the clinical importance attributed to the finding. Rash leading to withdrawal was more common in patients on drug regimens including valproate as a component and has been reported to be even more common when Lamotrigine is co-administered with valproate alone (see DOSAGE AND ADMINISTRATION).

Because rash occurs frequently in association with a number of other signs and symptoms, it is impossible to discern reliably in what proportion of patients withdrawn with rash, the rash was the primary reason for withdrawal. The overall rate of discontinuation due to rash in patients participating in clinical trials (n=3501) was 3.8%.

In assessing the importance of a rash, consideration should be given to the fact that a substantial number of patients with rash were continued on treatment and had an uneventful course.

ACUTE HEPATIC FAILURE/MULTIORGAN FAILURE

A case of fulminant hepatic failure has been reported in non-domestic post-marketing use. A 23 year-old woman receiving concomitant valproic acid and carbamazepine developed headache, fever, and a maculopapular rash 3 weeks after starting Lamotrigine. Hepatic coma followed within 3 days; despite apparent subsequent clinical improvement, the patient died unexpectedly from pulmonary embolus 2 months later.

Fatalities associated with multiorgan failure and various degrees of hepatic failure have been reported in five patients among 7000 exposed during pre-marketing development of Lamotrigine. These cases occurred in association with other serious medical events (*e.g.,*status epilepticus, overwhelming sepsis) making it impossible to identify the initiating cause.

Additionally, in the absence of any obvious precipitating event, a 45 year-old woman treated with carbamazepine and clonazepam developed DIC, rhabdomyolysis, renal failure, rash, ataxia, and elevated AST fourteen days after Lamotrigine was added to her antiepileptic drug regimen. She subsequently recovered with supportive care after Lamotrigine treatment was discontinued.

SUDDEN UNEXPLAINED DEATH IN EPILEPSY (SUDEP)

During the premarketing development of Lamotrigine, 20 sudden and unexplained deaths were recorded among a cohort of 4700 patients with epilepsy (5747 patient-years of exposure).

Some of these could represent seizure-related deaths in which the seizure was not observed, e.g., at night. This represents an incidence of.0035 deaths per patient-year. Although this rate exceeds that expected in a healthy population matched for age and sex, it is within the range of estimates for the incidence of sudden unexplained deaths in patients with epilepsy not receiving Lamotrigine (ranging from 0.0005 for the general population of patients with epilepsy, to 0.004 for a recently studied clinical trial population similar to that in the clinical development program for Lamotrigine, to 0.005 for patients with refractory epilepsy). Consequently, whether these figures are reassuring or suggest concern depends on the comparability of the populations reported upon to the cohort receiving Lamotrigine and the accuracy of the estimates provided. Probably most reassuring is the similarity of estimated SUDEP rates in patients receiving Lamotrigine and those receiving another antiepileptic drug that underwent clinical testing in a similar population at about the same time. Importantly, that drug is chemically unrelated to Lamotrigine. This evidence suggests, although it certainly does not prove, that the high SUDEP rates reflect population rates, not a drug effect.

WITHDRAWAL SEIZURES

As a rule, antiepileptic drugs should not be abruptly discontinued because of the possibility of increasing seizure frequency. Unless safety concerns require a more rapid withdrawal, the dose of Lamotrigine should be tapered over a period of at least two weeks (see DOSAGE AND ADMINISTRATION).

STATUS EPILEPTICUS

Valid estimates of treatment emergent status epilepticus among Lamotrigine treated patients are difficult to obtain because reported participating in clinical trials did not all employ identical rules for identifying cases. At a minimum, 7 of 2343 adult patients had episodes that could unequivocally be described as status. In addition, a number of reports of variably defined episodes of seizure exacerbation (*e.g.,*seizure clusters, seizure flurries, etc.) were made.

PRECAUTIONS:

GENERAL

Dermatologic Events (seeBOXED WARNING and WARNINGS: Severe, potentially life-threatening rashes have been reported in association with therapy with lamotrigine. Rare deaths have been reported, but their numbers are too few to permit a precise estimate of the rate. There are suggestions, yet to be proven, that the risk of rash may also be increased by 1)

PRECAUTIONS: *(cont'd)*

coadministration of lamotrigine with valproic acid, 2) exceeding the recommended dose of lamotrigine, or 3) exceeding the recommended dose escalation for lamotrigine. However, cases have been reported in the absence of these factors.

Addition of Lamotrigine to a multi-drug regimen that includes VPA: dosage reduction: Because VPA reduces the clearance of lamotrigine, the dosage of lamotrigine in the presence of VPA is less than half of that required in its absence. (See DOSAGE AND ADMINISTRATION.)

Use in Patients with Concomitant Illness: Clinical experience with Lamotrigine in patients with concomitant illness is limited. Caution is advised when using Lamotrigine in patients with diseases or conditions that could affect metabolism or elimination of the drug, such as renal, hepatic, or cardiac functional impairment.

Hepatic metabolism to the glucuronide followed by renal excretion is the principal route of elimination of lamotrigine (see CLINICAL PHARMACOLOGY).

A study in individuals with severe chronic renal failure (mean creatinine clearance = 13 ml/min) not receiving other AEDs indicated that the elimination half-life of unchanged lamotrigine is prolonged relative to individuals with normal renal function. Until adequate numbers of patients with severe renal impairment have been evaluated during chronic treatment with Lamotrigine, it should be used with caution in these patients, generally using a reduced maintenance dose for patients with significant impairment.

Because there is no experience with the use of Lamotrigine in patients with impaired liver function, the use in such patients may be associated with as yet unrecognized risks.

Binding in the Eye and other Melanin Containing Tissues: Because lamotrigine binds to melanin, it could accumulate in melanin rich tissues over time. This raises the possibility that lamotrigine may toxicity in these tissues after extended use. Although ophthalmological testing was performed in one controlled clinical trial, the testing was inadequate to exclude subtle effects or injury occurring after long-term exposure. Moreover, the capacity of available tests to detect potentially adverse consequences, if any, of lamotrigine's binding to melanin is unknown.

Accordingly, although there are no specific recommendations for periodic ophthalmological monitoring, prescribers should be aware of the possibility of long-term ophthalmologic effects.

INFORMATION FOR THE PATIENT

Prior to initiation of treatment with lamotrigine, the patient should be instructed that a rash or other signs or symptoms of hypersensitivity (e.g., fever, lymphadenopathy) may herald a serious medical event and that the patient should report any such occurrence to a physician immediately. In addition, the patient should notify his/her physician if worsening of seizure control occurs.

Patients should be advised to notify their physician immediately if they develop a skin rash while taking Lamotrigine, or if they acutely develop any worsening of seizure control.

Patients should be advised that Lamotrigine may cause dizziness, somnolence and other symptoms and signs of CNS depression. Accordingly, they should be advised neither to drive a car nor to operate other complex machinery until they have gained sufficient experience on Lamotrigine to gauge whether or not it affects their mental and/or motor performance adversely.

Patients should be advised to notify their physician if they become pregnant or intend to become pregnant during therapy. Patients should be advised to notify their physician if they intend to breast-feed or are breast-feeding an infant.

LABORATORY TESTS

The value of monitoring plasma concentrations of Lamotrigine has not been established. Because of the possible pharmacokinetic interactions between Lamotrigine and other AEDs been taken concomitantly (see TABLE 2), monitoring of the plasma levels of Lamotrigine and concomitant AEDs may be indicated, particularly during dosage adjustments. In general, clinical judgement should be exercised regarding monitoring of plasma levels of Lamotrigine and other anti-seizure drugs and whether or not dosage adjustments are necessary.

DRUG/LABORATORY TEST INTERACTIONS

None known.

CARCINOGENESIS, MUTAGENESIS, AND IMPAIRMENT OF FERTILITY

No evidence of carcinogenicity was seen in one mouse study or two rat studies following oral administration of lamotrigine for up to 2 years at maximum tolerated doses (30 mg/kg/day for mice and 10 to 15 mg/kg/day for rats, doses which are equivalent to 90 mg/m^2 and 60 to 90 mg/m^2, respectively). Steady state plasma concentrations ranged from 1 to 4 mcg/ml in the mouse study and 1 to 10 mcg/ml in the rat study. Plasma concentrations associated with the recommended human dose of 300 to 500 mg/day are generally in the range of 2 to 5 mcg/ml, but concentrations as high as 19 mcg/ml have been recorded.

Lamotrigine was not mutagenic in the presence or absence of metabolic activation when tested in two gene mutation assays (the Ames test and the*in vitro* rat bone marrow assay). In two cytogenetic assays (the*in vitro* human lymphocyte assay and the *in vivo* rat bone marrow assay), lamotrigine did not increase the incidence of structural or numerical chromosomal abnormalities.

No evidence of impairment of fertility was detected in rats given oral doses of lamotrigine up to 2.4 times the highest usual human maintenance dose of 8.33 mg/kg/day or 0.4 times the human dose on a mg/m^{2}basis. The effect of lamotrigine on human fertility is unknown.

PREGNANCY CATEGORY C

No evidence of teratogenicity was found in mice, rats, or rabbits when lamotrigine was orally administered to pregnant animals during the period of organogenesis at doses up to 1.2, 0.5, and 1.1 times, respectively, on a mg/m^2 basis, the highest usual human maintenance dose (*i.e.*, 500 mg/day). However, maternal toxicity and secondary fetal toxicity producing fetal weight and/or delayed ossification were seen in mice and rats, but not in rabbits at these doses. Teratology studies were also conducted using bolus intravenous (IV) administration of the isethionate salt of lamotrigine rats and rabbits. In rat dams administered an IV dose at 0.6 times the highest usual human maintenance dose, the incidence of intrauterine death without signs of teratogenicity was increased.

A behavioral teratology study was conducted in rats dosed during the period of organogenesis. At day 21 postpartum offspring of dams receiving 5 mg/kg/day or higher displayed a significantly longer latent period for open field exploration and a lower frequency of rearing. In a swimming maze test performed on days 39 to 44 postpartum, time to completion was increased in offspring of dams receiving 25 mg/kg/day. These doses represent 0.1 and 0.5 times the clinical dose on a mg/m^2 basis, respectively.

Lamotrigine did not affect fertility, teratogenesis, or postnatal development when rats were dosed prior to and during mating, and throughout gestation and lactation at doses equivalent to 0.4 times the highest usual human maintenance dose on a mg/m^2 basis.

When pregnant rats were orally dosed at 0.1, 0.14, or 0.3 times the highest human maintenance dose (on a mg/m^2 basis) during the latter part of gestation (days 15 to 20), maternal toxicity and fetal death were seen. In dams, food consumption and weight gain were reduced, and the gestation period was slightly prolonged (22.6 vs. 22.0 days in the control group). Stillborn pups were found in all three drug-treated groups with the highest number in the high dose group. Post-natal death was also seen but only in the two highest doses and

PRECAUTIONS: *(cont'd)*

occurred between day 1 and 20. Some of these deaths appear to be drug-related and not secondary to the maternal toxicity. A no observed effect level (NOEL) could not be determined for this study.

Although Lamotrigine was not found to be teratogenic in the above studies, lamotrigine decreases fetal folate concentrations in rats, an effect known to be associated with teratogenesis in animals and humans. There are no adequate and well-controlled studies in pregnant women. Because animal reproduction studies are not always predictive of human response, this drug should be used during pregnancy only if the potential benefit justifies the potential risk to the fetus.

Pregnancy Exposure Registry: To facilitate monitoring fetal outcomes of pregnant women exposed to lamotrigine, physicians are encouraged to register patients in the Antiepileptic Drug Pregnancy Registry by calling (800) 233-2334 (toll free).

LABOR AND DELIVERY

The effect of Lamotrigine on labor and delivery in humans is unknown.

NURSING MOTHERS

Preliminary data indicate that lamotrigine passes into human milk. Because the effects on the infant exposed to Lamotrigine by this route are unknown, breast-feeding while taking Lamotrigine is not recommended.

PEDIATRIC USE

Safety and effectiveness in children below the age of 16 have not been established (see BOXED WARNING.

GERIATRIC USE

Because few patients over the age of 65 (approximately 20) were exposed to Lamotrigine during its premarket evaluation, no specific statements about the safety or effectiveness of Lamotrigine in this age group can be made.

DRUG INTERACTIONS:

Antiepileptic Drugs (AEDs): The use of AEDs in combination is complicated by the potential for pharmacokinetic interactions.

The interaction of lamotrigine with phenytoin, carbamazepine, and VPA has been characterized. With the exception of VPA, the addition of lamotrigine to these AEDs does not affect their steady state plasma concentrations. The net effects of these various AED combinations on individual AED plasma concentrations are summarized in TABLE 2.

TABLE 2 Summary Of Antiepileptic Drug (AED) Interactions With Lamotrigine

Antiepileptic Drug (AED)	AED Plasma Concentration with Adjunctive Lamotrigine[a]	Lamotrigine Plasma Concentration with Adjunctive AEDS[b]
Phenytoin (PHT)	↔	↓
Carbamazepine (CBZ)	↔	↓
CBZ epoxide[c]	?[d]	
Valproic Acid (VPA)	↓	↑
VPA + PHT and/or CBZ	NE[e]	↔

No significant effect
a From adjunctive clinical trials and volunteer studies
b Net effects were estimated by comparing the mean clearance values obtained in adjunctive clinical trials and volunteers studies.
c Not administered, but an active metabolite of carbamazepine
d Conflicting data
e NE = not evaluated

SPECIFIC EFFECTS OF LAMOTRIGINE ON THE PHARMACOKINETICS OF OTHER ANTIEPILEPTIC DRUG PRODUCTS

Lamotrigine Added To Phenytoin: Lamotrigine has no appreciable effect on steady state phenytoin plasma concentration.

Lamotrigine Added To Carbamazepine: Lamotrigine has no appreciable effect on steady state carbamazepine plasma concentration. Limited clinical data suggest there is a higher incidence of dizziness, diplopia, ataxia, and blurred vision in patients receiving carbamazepine with Lamotrigine than in patients receiving other enzyme-inducing AEDs with Lamotrigine (see ADVERSE REACTIONS). The mechanism of this interaction is unclear. The effect of lamotrigine on plasma concentrations of carbamazepine-epoxide is unclear. In a small subset of patients (n=7) studied in a placebo-controlled trial, lamotrigine had no effect on carbamazepine-epoxide plasma concentrations, but in a small uncontrolled study (n=9), carbamazepine-epoxide levels were seen to increase.

Lamotrigine added to valproic acid: When Lamotrigine was administered to healthy volunteers already receiving valproic acid (VPA), the trough steady-state VPA concentrations in plasma decreased by an average of 25% over a 3-week period, and then stabilized.

Lamotrigine added to valproic acid + phenytoin and/or carbamazepine: Although the effects of Lamotrigine on plasma levels of these AEDs given in combination has not been systematically evaluated, it is expected that the effects would be similar to those when Lamotrigine is added to each independently (*e.g.*, valproic levels decrease, phenytoin and carbamazepine do not change).

SPECIFIC EFFECTS OF OTHER ANTIEPILEPTIC DRUG PRODUCTS ON THE PHARMACOKINETICS OF LAMOTRIGINE

Phenytoin added to Lamotrigine: The addition of phenytoin decreases lamotrigine steady-state concentrations by approximately 45% to 54% depending upon the total daily dose of phenytoin (*i.e.*, from 100 to 400 mg).

Carbamazepine added to Lamotrigine: The addition of carbamazepine decreases lamotrigine steady-state concentrations by approximately 40%.

Phenobarbital or primidone added to Lamotrigine: The addition of phenobarbital or primidone decreases lamotrigine steady-state concentrations by approximately 40%.

Valproic acid added to Lamotrigine: The addition of valproic acid (VPA) increases lamotrigine steady-state concentrations in volunteers by slightly more than two-fold.

INTERACTIONS WITH DRUG PRODUCTS OTHER THAN ANTIEPILEPTICS

Folate Inhibitors: Lamotrigine is an inhibitor of dihydrofolate reductase. Prescribers should be aware of this action when prescribing other medications which inhibit folate metabolism.

ADVERSE REACTIONS:

SEVERE, POTENTIALLY LIFE-THREATENING RASHES, INCLUDING STEVENS-JOHNSON SYNDROME AND TOXIC EPIDERMAL NECROLYSIS HAVE OCCURRED IN ASSOCIATION WITH THERAPY WITH LAMOTRIGINE. RARE DEATHS HAVE BEEN REPORTED, BUT THEIR NUMBERS ARE TOO FEW TO PERMIT A PRECISE ESTIMATE OF THE RATE (SEE BOXED WARNING).

The most commonly observed adverse experiences associated with the use Lamotrigine in combination with other antiepileptic drugs, not seen at equivalent frequency among placebo-treated patients, were: dizziness, ataxia, somnolence, headache, diplopia, blurred vision,

ADVERSE REACTIONS: *(cont'd)*

nausea, vomiting and rash. Dizziness, diplopia, ataxia, blurred vision, nausea and vomiting were dose-related. Dizziness, diplopia, ataxia, and blurred vision occurred more commonly in patients receiving carbamazepine with Lamotrigine than in patients receiving other enzyme-inducing AEDs with Lamotrigine. Clinical data suggest a higher incidence of rash, including serious rash, in patients receiving concomitant valproic acid than in patients not receiving valproic acid (see WARNINGS).

Approximately 10% of the 3015 individuals who received Lamotrigine in premarketing clinical trials discontinued treatment because of an adverse experience. The adverse events most commonly associated with discontinuation were: rash (3%), dizziness (1.4%), and headache (1.1%).

In a dose response study, the rate of discontinuation of Lamotrigine for dizziness, ataxia, diplopia, blurred vision, nausea, and vomiting was dose-related.

Incidence in Controlled Clinical Studies: TABLE 3 lists treatment-emergent signs and symptoms that occurred in at least 1% of patients with epilepsy treated with Lamotrigine participating in placebo- controlled trials and were numerically more common in the patients treated with Lamotrigine. In these studies, either Lamotrigine or placebo was added to the patient's current antiepileptic drug therapy. Adverse events were usually mild to moderate in intensity.

The prescriber should be aware that these figures, obtained when Lamotrigine was added to concurrent antiepileptic drug therapy, cannot be used to predict the frequency of adverse experiences in the course of usual medical practice where patient characteristics and other factors may differ from those prevailing during clinical studies. Similarly, the cited frequencies cannot be directly compared with figures obtained from other clinical investigations involving different treatments, uses, or investigators. An inspection of these frequencies, however does provide the prescriber with one basis to estimate the relative contribution of drug and non-drug factors to the adverse events incidences in the population studied.

In a randomized parallel study comparing placebo, 300 mg, and 500 mg per day of Lamotrigine, some of the more common drug-related adverse events were dose-related (see TABLE 4).

Other events which occurred in more than 1% of patients but equally or more frequently in the placebo group included: asthenia, back pain, chest pain, flatulence, menstrual disorder, myalgia, paresthesia, respiratory disorder, and urinary tract infection.

The overall adverse experience profile for Lamotrigine was similar between females and males, and was independent of age. Because the largest non- white racial subgroup was only 6% of patients exposed to Lamotrigine (46/711) in placebo-controlled trials, there are insufficient data to support a statement regarding the distribution of adverse experience reports by race. Generally, females receiving either add-on Lamotrigine or placebo were more likely to report adverse experiences than males. The only adverse experience for which the reports on Lamotrigine were greater than 10% more frequent in females than males (without a corresponding difference by gender on placebo) was dizziness (difference=16.5%). There was little difference between females and males in the rates of discontinuation of Lamotrigine for individual adverse experiences.

OTHER ADVERSE EVENTS OBSERVED DURING ALL CLINICAL TRIALS

Other Adverse Events: Lamotrigine has been administered to 3015 individuals during all clinical trials, only some of which were placebo-controlled. During these trials, all adverse events were recorded by the clinical investigators using terminology of their own choosing. To provide a meaningful estimate of the proportion of individuals having adverse events, similar types of events were grouped into a smaller number of standardized categories using modified COSTART dictionary terminology. The frequencies presented represent the proportion of the 3015 individuals exposed to Lamotrigine who experienced an event of the type cited on at least one occasion while receiving Lamotrigine. All reported events are included except those already listed in the previous table, those too general to be informative, and those not reasonably associated with the use of the drug.

Events are further classified within body system categories and enumerated in order of decreasing frequency using the following definitions: *frequent* adverse events are defined as those occurring in at least 1/100 patients; *infrequent*adverse events are those occurring in 1/100 to 1/1000 patients; rare adverse events are those occurring in fewer than 1/1000 patients.

Body as a Whole: *Infrequent:* face edema and halitosis.*Rare:* abdomen enlarged, photosensitivity, and suicide attempt.

Cardiovascular System: *Infrequent:* flushing, migraine, syncope, tachycardia, and vasodilation. *Rare:* angina pectoris, atrial fibrillation, deep thrombophlebitis, hemorrhage, hypertension, myocardial infarction, and postural hypotension.

Dermatological: *Infrequent:* dry skin, eczema, erythema, hirsutism, maculopapular rash, sweating, and urticaria. *Rare:* angioedema, fungal dermatitis, herpes zoster, leukoderma, petechial rash, pustular rash, seborrhea, skin discoloration, Stevens-Johnson syndrome, and vesiculobullous rash.

Digestive System: *Infrequent:* dysphagia, flatulence, gingivitis, gum hyperplasia, increased appetite, increased salivation, liver function tests abnormal, mouth ulceration, stomatitis, and thirst.*Rare:* eructation, gastritis, gastrointestinal hemorrhage, glossitis, gum hemorrhage, hemorrhagic colitis, hepatitis, stomach ulcer, and tongue edema.

Endocrine System: *Rare:* goiter and hyperthyroidism.

Hematologic and Lymphatic System: *Infrequent:* anemia, ecchymosis, leukocytosis, leukopenia, lymphadenopathy, and petechia.*Rare:* allergic reactions, eosinophilia, fibrin decrease, iron deficiency anemia, and thrombocytopenia.

Metabolic and Nutritional Disorders: *Frequent:* weight gain. *Infrequent:* weight loss. *Rare:* hyperglycemia, and peripheral edema.

Musculoskeletal System: *Infrequent:* twitching.*Rare:* arthritis, bursitis, leg cramps, tendinous contracture, and pathological fracture.

Nervous System: *Frequent:* amnesia, nervousness, thinking abnormality. *Infrequent:* abnormal dreams, abnormal gait, agitation, akathisia, aphasia, CNS depression, depersonalization, dyskinesia, dysphoria, euphoria, faintness, hallucinations, hostility, hyperkinesia, hypesthesia, myoclonus, panic attack, paranoid reaction, personality disorder, psychosis, and stupor. *Rare:* apathy, cerebrovascular accident, cerebellar syndrome, cerebral sinus thrombosis, choreoathetosis, CNS stimulation, delirium, delusions, dystonia, grand mal convulsions, hemiplegia, hyperalgesia, hyperesthesia, hypertonia, hypokinesia, hypomania, hypotonia, libido decreased, libido increased, manic depression reaction, movement disorder, neuralgia, neurosis, paralysis, and suicidal ideation.

Respiratory System: *Infrequent:* epistaxis and hyperventilation. *Rare:* bronchospasm, hiccup, and pneumonia.

Special Senses: *Infrequent:* abnormality of accommodation, conjunctivitis, oscillopsia, photophobia, and taste perversion.*Rare:* deafness, dry eyes, lacrimation disorder, parosmia, ptosis, strabismus, and taste loss.

Urogenital System: *Infrequent:* female lactation, hematuria, polyuria, urinary frequency, urinary incontinence, urinary tract infection, and vaginal moniliasis. *Rare:* abnormal ejaculation, acute kidney failure, breast pain, breast abscess, cystitis, dysuria, breast neoplasm, creatinine increase, epididymitis, impotence, kidney pain, menorrhagia, urine abnormality, and urinary retention.

ADVERSE REACTIONS: *(cont'd)*

TABLE 3 Treatment-Emergent Adverse Event Incidence In Placebo-Controlled Adjunctive Trials [1] (Events In At Least 1% Of Patients Treated With Lamotrigine And Numerically More Frequent Than In The Placebo Group.)

Body System/Adverse Experience[2]	Percent of Patients Receiving Lamictal (n = 711)	Percent of Patients Receiving Placebo (n = 419)
Body As A Whole		
Headache	29.1	19.1
Accidental Injury	9.1	8.6
Flu Syndrome	7.0	5.5
Fever	5.5	3.6
Abdominal Pain	5.2	3.6
Infection	4.4	4.1
Neck Pain	2.4	1.2
Malaise	2.3	1.9
Reaction Aggravated (Seizure Exacerbation)	2.3	0.5
Chills	1.3	0.5
Cardiovascular		
Hot Flashes	1.3	0.0
Palpitations	1.0	0.5
Digestive		
Nausea	18.6	9.5
Vomiting	9.4	4.3
Diarrhea	6.3	4.1
Dyspepsia	5.3	2.1
Constipation	4.1	3.1
Tooth Disorder	3.2	1.7
Anorexia	1.8	1.4
Dry Mouth	1.0	0.2
Musculoskeletal		
Arthralgia	2.0	0.2
Joint Disorder	1.3	1.0
Myasthenia	1.3	0.0
Nervous		
Dizziness	38.4	13.4
Ataxia	21.7	5.5
Somnolence	14.2	6.9
Incoordination	6.0	2.1
Insomnia	5.6	1.9
Tremor	4.4	1.4
Depression	4.2	2.6
Anxiety	3.8	2.6
Convulsion	3.2	1.2
Irritability	3.0	1.9
Speech Disorder	2.5	0.2
Memory Decreased	2.4	1.9
Confusion	1.8	1.7
Concentration Disturbance	1.7	0.7
Sleep Disorder	1.4	0.5
Emotional Lability	1.3	0.2
Vertigo	1.1	0.2
Mind Racing	1.0	0.5
Nystagmus	1.0	0.5
Dysarthria	1.0	0.2
Muscle Spasm	1.0	0.2
Respiratory		
Rhinitis	13.6	9.3
Pharyngitis	9.8	8.8
Cough Increased	7.5	5.7
Dyspnea	1.1	0.2
Skin And Appendages		
Rash	10.0	5.0
Pruritus	3.1	1.7
Alopecia	1.3	1.2
Acne	1.3	0.5
Special Senses		
Diplopia	27.6	6.7
Blurred Vision	15.5	4.5
Vision Abnormality	3.4	1.0
Ear Pain	1.8	1.7
Tinnitus	1.1	1.0
Urogenital		
Female Patients Only	(n=365)	(n=207)
Dysmenorrhea	6.6	6.3
Vaginitis	4.1	0.5
Amenorrhea	1.9	0.5

[1] Patients in these adjunctive studies were receiving 1 to 3 concomitant enzyme-inducing antiepileptic drugs in addition to Lamictal or placebo. Patients may have reported multiple adverse experiences during the study or at discontinuation; thus, patients may be included in more than one category.

[2] Adverse Experiences reported by at least 1% of patients treated with Lamictal are included.

TABLE 4 Dose-Related Adverse Events from a Randomized Placebo-Controlled Trial

Adverse Experience (AE)	Percent of Patients Experiencing AE: Placebo (n=73)	Lamictal 300 mg (n=71)	Lamictal 500 mg (n=72)
Ataxia	10	10	28[1,2]
Blurred Vision	10	11	25[1,2]
Diplopia	8	24[1]	49[1,2]
Dizziness	27	31	54[1,2]
Nausea	11	18	25[1]
Vomiting	4	11	18[1]

[1] Significantly greater than placebo group ($p < 0.05$)
[2] Significantly greater than group receiving Lamictal 300 mg ($p < 0,05$)

Postmarketing and Other Experience: In addition to the adverse experiences reported during clinical testing of Lamotrigine, the following adverse experiences have been reported in patients receiving marketed Lamotrigine in other countries and from worldwide non-controlled investigational use. These adverse experiences have not been listed above and data are insufficient to support an estimate of their incidence or to establish causation. The listing is alphabetized: Aplastic anemia, apnea, erythema multiforme, esophagitis, hematemesis, hemolytic anemia, pancreatitis, pancytopenia and progressive immunosuppression.

DRUG ABUSE AND DEPENDENCE:

The abuse and dependence potential of Lamotrigine have not been evaluated in human studies.

OVERDOSAGE:

Human Overdose Experience: Experience with single or daily dose greater than 700 mg is limited. During the clinical development of Lamotrigine, the highest known overdoses were in two women who each ingested doses greater than 4000 mg. The plasma concentration of lamotrigine in one woman was 52 mcg/ml four hours after the ingestion (a value more than 10 times greater than that seen in clinical trials). She became comatose and remained comatose for 8 to 12 hours; no electrocardiographic abnormalities were detected. The other patient had dizziness, headache and somnolence. Both women recovered without sequelae.

Management of Overdose: There are no specific antidotes for Lamotrigine. Following a suspected overdose, hospitalization of the patient is advised. General supportive care is indicated, including frequent monitoring of vital signs and close observation of the patient. If indicated, emesis should be induced or gastric lavage should be performed; usual precautions should be taken to protect the airway. It should be kept in mind that lamotrigine is rapidly absorbed (see CLINICAL PHARMACOLOGY). It is uncertain whether hemodialysis is an effective means of removing lamotrigine from the blood. In six renal failure patients about 20% of the amount of lamotrigine in the body was removed during 4 hours of hemodialysis. A Poison Control Center should be contacted for information on the management of overdosage of Lamotrigine.

DOSAGE AND ADMINISTRATION:

Lamotrigine is recommended as adjunctive therapy in adults. Safety and effectiveness in pediatric patients below the age of 16 have not been established (see BOXED WARNING).

GENERAL DOSING CONSIDERATIONS

The risk of nonserious rash is increased when the recommended initial dose and/or the rate of dose escalation of lamotrigine is exceeded. There are suggestions, yet to be proven, that the risk of severe, potentially life-threatening rash may be increased by 1) coadministration of lamotrigine with valproic acid, 2) exceeding the recommended initial dose of lamotrigine, or 3) exceeding the recommended dose escalation of lamotrigine. However, cases have been reported in the absence of these factors (see BOXED WARNING). Therefore, it is important that the dosing recommendations be followed closely.

Patients Receiving VPA As One Component Of A Combination Regimen Also Including EIAEDs: In patients taking valproic acid as one component of a combination regimen also including enzyme inducing anti epileptic drugs, the initial dose of Lamotrigine is 25 mg every other day for two weeks, followed by 25 mg once a day for two weeks. Because the clearance of lamotrigine is decreased about 50% in the presence of valproate, the daily dose of Lamotrigine should ordinarily be no more than 150 mg a day, and should be administered on a b.i.d. schedule. To achieve maintenance, doses may be increased by 25 to 50 mg every 1 to 2 weeks (see TABLE 5).

Note: The efficacy of adjunctive lamotrigine in patients taking VPA alone has not been evaluated in controlled trials although it has been used in some patients. Consequently, an effective and safe dosing recommendation for the use of lamotrigine and VPA as a two-drug regimen cannot be offered. If this regimen is nonetheless used, it should be noted that blood concentrations of lamotrigine appear to be twice those associated with the use of lamotrigine, in a regimen containing both EIAEDs and VPA.

Patients Receiving EIAEDs, But Not VPA: The initial dose of Lamotrigine in patients not taking valproic acid is 50 mg once a day for two weeks, followed by 100 mg/day given in two divided doses for two weeks. Thereafter, the usual maintenance dose is 300 to 500 mg/day given in two divided doses (see TABLE 5).

TABLE 5 Lamotrigine Dose Recommendations (mg/day) for Adults (over 16 years)

	Weeks 1 and 2	Weeks 3 and 4	Usual Maintenance Dose
With EIAEDs & valproic acid (VPA)	25 mg every other day	25 mg (once a day)	100 mg-150 mg/day (in two divided doses) To acheive maintenance, doses may be increased by 25-50 mg every 1 to 2 weeks.
With EIAEDs & no valproic acid	50 mg (once a day)	100 mg (two divided doses)	300 mg-500 mg/day (two divided doses) To acheive maintenance, dose may be increased by 100 mg/day every 1 to 2 weeks.

* *e.g.*, phenytoin, carbamazepine, phenobarbital, and primidone

Because of an increased risk of rash, the recommended initial dose and subsequent dose escalations of Lamotrigine should not be exceeded (see BOXED WARNING).

The Usual Maintenance Doses identified in the table above are derived from dosing regimens employed in the placebo controlled add-on studies in which the efficacy of Lamotrigine was established. In patients receiving multidrug regimens employing EIAEDs without VPA, maintenance doses of Lamotrigine as high as 200 mg/day have been used. The advantage of using doses above those recommended in the table above has not been established in controlled trials.

Patients with Renal Functional Impairment: Initial doses of Lamotrigine should be based on patients' AED regimen (see DOSAGE AND ADMINISTRATION, General Dosing Considerations); reduced maintenance doses may be effective for patients with significant renal functional impairment (see CLINICAL PHARMACOLOGY). Few patients with severe renal impairment have been evaluated during chronic treatment with Lamotrigine. Because there is an inadequate experience in this population, Lamotrigine should be used with caution in these patients.

Discontinuation Strategy: For patients receiving Lamotrigine in combination with other AEDs, a re-evaluation of all AEDs in the regimen should be considered if a change in seizure control or an appearance or worsening of adverse experiences is observed.

If a decision is made to discontinue therapy with Lamotrigine, a step-wise reduction of dose over at least two weeks (approximately 50% per week) is recommended unless safety concerns require a more rapid withdrawal (see PRECAUTIONS).

Discontinuing an EIAED should prolong the half-life of lamotrigine; discontinuing valproic acid should shorten the half-life of lamotrigine.

Target Plasma Levels: A therapeutic plasma concentration range has not been established for lamotrigine. Dosing of Lamotrigine should be based on therapeutic response.

HOW SUPPLIED:

25 mg (white) scored, shield-shaped tablets engraved with "LAMICTAL" and "25".

100 mg (peach) scored, shield-shaped tablets engraved with "LAMICTAL" and "100".

150 mg (cream) scored, shield-shaped tablets engraved with "LAMICTAL" and "150".

HOW SUPPLIED: *(cont'd)*

200 mg (blue) scored, shield-shaped tablets engraved with "LAMICTAL" and "200".

Store at 15° to 25°C (59° to 77°F) in a dry place and protect from light.

HOW SUPPLIED - EQUIVALENTS NOT AVAILABLE:

Tablet, Uncoated - Oral - 100 mg

100's $175.54 LAMICTAL, Glaxo Wellcome 00173-0642-55

Tablet, Uncoated - Oral - 150 mg

60's $110.66 LAMICTAL, Glaxo Wellcome 00173-0643-60

Tablet, Uncoated - Oral - 200 mg

60's $116.00 LAMICTAL, Glaxo Wellcome 00173-0644-60

LANSOPRAZOLE *(003230)*

CATEGORIES: Antiulcer Drugs; Duodenal Ulcer; Esophagitis; GERD; Gastric Acid Secretion Inhibitors; Gastroesophagael Reflux Disease; Gastrointestinal Drugs; Hypersecretory Conditions; Proton Pump Inhibitors; Reflux; Ulcer; Zollinger-Ellison Syndrome; FDA Class 1S ("Standard Review"); FDA Approved 1995 May; Top 200 Drugs; Top 200 Drugs

BRAND NAMES: **Prevacid**

DESCRIPTION:

The active ingredient in Prevacid (lansoprazole) Delayed-Release Capsules is a substituted benzimidazole, 2-[[[3-methyl-4-(2,2,2 tri- fluroethoxy)-2-pyridyl]methyl]sulfinyl] benzimidazole, a compound that inhibits gastric acid secretion. Its empirical formula is $C_{16}H_{14}F_3N_3O_2S$ with a molecular weight of 369.37.

Lansoprazole is a white to brownish-white odorless, crystalline powder which melts with decomposition at approximately 166°C. Lansoprazole is freely soluble in dimethylformamide; soluble in methanol; sparingly soluble in ethanol; slightly soluble in ethyl acetate, dichloromethane and acetonitrile; very slightly soluble in ether; and practically insoluble in hexane and water.

Lansoprazole is stable when exposed to light for up to two months. The compound degrades in aqueous solution, the rate of degradation increasing with decreasing pH. At 25°C the $t_{1/2}$ is approximately 0.5 hour at pH 5.0 and approximately 18 hours at pH 7.0.

Prevacid is supplied in delayed-release capsules for oral administration. The delayed-release capsules contain the active ingredient, lansoprazole, in the form of enteric-coated granules and are available in two dosage strengths: 15 mg and 30 mg of lansoprazole per capsule. Each delayed- release capsule contains enteric-coated granules consisting of lansoprazole, hydroxypropyl cellulose, low substituted hydroxypropyl cellulose, colloidal silicon dioxide, magnesium carbonate, methacrylic acid copolymer, starch, talc, sugar sphere, sucrose, polyethylene glycol, polysorbate 80, and titanium dioxide. Components of the gelatin capsule include gelatin, titanium dioxide, D&C Red No. 28, FD&C Blue No. 1, FD&C Green No. 3*, and FD&C Red No. 40.

* Prevacid 15 mg capsules only.

CLINICAL PHARMACOLOGY:

PHARMACOKINETICS AND METABOLISM

Prevacid Delayed-Release Capsules contain an enteric-coated granule formulation of lansoprazole. Absorption of lansoprazole begins only after the granules leave the stomach. Absorption is rapid, with mean peak plasma levels of lansoprazole occurring after approximately 1.7 hours. Peak plasma concentrations of lansoprazole (C_{max}) and the area under plasma concentration curve (AUC) of lansoprazole are approximately proportional in doses from 15 mg to 60 mg after single-oral administration. Lansoprazole does not accumulate and its pharmacokinetics are unaltered by multiple dosing.

Absorption: The absorption of lansoprazole is rapid, with mean C_{max} occurring approximately 1.7 hours after oral dosing, and relatively complete with absolute bioavailability over 80%. In healthy subjects, the mean (± SD) plasma half-life was 1.5 (± 1.0) hours. Both C_{max} and AUC are diminished by about 50% if the drug is given 30 minutes after food as opposed tot he fasting condition. There is no significant food effect if the drug is given before meals.

Distribution: Lansoprazole is 97% bound plasma proteins. Plasma protein binding is constant over the concentration range of 0.05 to 5.0 mcg/ml.

Metabolism: Lansoprazole is extensively metabolized in the liver. Two metabolites have been identified in measurable quantities in plasma (the hydroxylated sulfinyl and sulfone derivatives of lansoprazole). These metabolites have very little or no antisecretory activity. Lansoprazole is thought to be transformed into two active species which inhibit acid secretion by (H^+,K^+)-ATPase within the parietal cell canaliculus, but are not present in the systemic circulation. The plasma elimination half-life of lansoprazole does not reflect its duration of suppression of gastric acid secretion. Thus, the plasma elimination half-life is less than two hours while the acid inhibitory effect lasts more than 24 hours.

Elimination: Following single-dose oral administration of lansoprazole, virtually no unchanged lansoprazole was excreted in the urine. In one study, after a single oral dose of ^{14}C-lansoprazole, approximately one-third of the administered radiation was excreted in the urine and two-thirds was recovered in the feces. This implies a significant biliary excretion of the metabolites of lansoprazole.

SPECIAL POPULATIONS

Geriatric: The clearance of lansoprazole is decreased in the elderly, with elimination half-life increased approximately 50% to 100%. Because the mean half-life in the elderly remains between 1.9 to 2.9 hours, repeated once daily dosing does not result in accumulation of lansoprazole. Peak plasma levels were not increased in the elderly.

Pediatric: The pharmacokinetics of lansoprazole has not been investigated in patients < 18 years of age.

Gender: In a study comparing 12 male and six female human subjects, no gender differences were found in pharmacokinetics and intragastric pH results (also see Use in Women).

Renal Insufficiency: In patients with severe renal insufficiency, plasma protein binding decreased by 1.0%-1.5% after administration of 60 mg of lansoprazole. Patients with renal insufficiency had a shortened elimination half-life and decreased total AUC (free and bound). AUC for free lansoprazole in plasma, however, was not related to the degree of renal impairment, and C_{max} and T_{max} were not different from subjects with healthy kidneys.

Hepatic Insufficiency: In patients with various degrees of chronic hepatic disease, the mean plasma half-life of the drug was prolonged from 1.5 hours to 3.2-7.2 hours. An increase in mean AUC of up to 500% was observed at steady state in hepatically-impaired patients compared to healthy subjects. Dose reduction in patients with severe hepatic disease should be considered.

PHARMACODYNAMICS

Mechanism of Action: Lansoprazole belongs to a class of antisecretory compounds, the substituted benzimidazoles, that do not exhibit anticholinergic or histamine H_2-receptor antagonist properties, but that suppress gastric acid secretion by specific inhibition of the

CLINICAL PHARMACOLOGY: *(cont'd)*

(H^+,K^+)-ATPase enzyme system at the secretory surface of the gastric parietal cell. Because this enzyme system is regarded as the acid (proton) pump within the parietal cell, lansoprazole has been characterized as a gastric acid- pump inhibitor, in that it blocks the final step of acid production. This effect is dose-related and lead to inhibition of both basal and stimulated gastric acid secretion irrespective of the stimulus.

Antisecretory Activity: After oral administration lansoprazole was shown to significantly decrease the basal acid output and significantly increase the mean gastric pH and percent of time the gastric pH was >3 and >4. Lansoprazole also significantly reduced meal- stimulated gastric acid output and secretion volume, as well as pentagastrin-stimulated acid output. In patients with hypersecretion of acid, lansoprazole significantly reduced basal and pentagastrin- stimulated gastric acid secretion. Lansoprazole inhibited the normal increases in secretion volume, acidity and acid output induced by insulin.

In a crossover study comparing lansoprazole 15 and 30 mg with omeprazole 20 mg for five days, the following effects on intragastric pH were noted: (TABLE 1)

TABLE 1 Mean Antisecretory Effects after Single and Multiple Daily Dosing

		Prevacid				Omeprazole	
	Baseline	15 mg		30 mg		20 mg	
Parameter	Value	Day 1	Day 5	Day 1	Day 5	Day 1	Day 5
Mean 24hr pH	2.1	2.7⁺	4.0⁺	3.6*	4.9*	2.5	4.2⁺
Mean Nighttime pH	1.9	2.4	3.0⁺	2.6	3.8*	2.2	3.0⁺
% Time Gastric pH>3	18	33⁺	59⁺	51*	72*	30⁺	61⁺
% Time Gastric pH>4	12	22⁺	49⁺	41*	66*	19	51⁺

* (p<0.05) versus baseline, lansoprazole 15 mg and omeprazole 20 mg.
⁺(p<005) versus baseline only.
NOTE: An intragastric pH of >4 reflects a reduction in gastric acid by 99%.

After the initial dose in this study, increased gastric pH was seen within 1-2 hours with lansoprazole 30 mg, 2-3 hours with lansoprazole 15 mg, and 3-4 hours with omeprazole 20 mg. After multiple daily dosing, increased gastric pH was seen within the first hour post-dosing with lansoprazole 30 mg and within 1-2 hours postdosing with lansoprazole 15 mg and omeprazole 20 mg.

The inhibition of gastric acid secretion as measured by intragastric pH returns gradually to normal over two to four days after multiple doses. There is no indication of rebound gastric acidity.

Enterochromaffin-Like (ECL) Cell Effects: During lifetime exposure of rates with up to 150 mg/kg/day of lansoprazole dosed seven days per week, marked hypergastrinemia was observed followed by ECL cell proliferation and formation of carcinoid tumors, especially in female rats (see PRECAUTIONS, Carcinogenesis, Mutagenesis, and Impairment of Fertility).

Gastric biopsy specimens from the body of the stomach from approximately 150 patients treated continuously with lansoprazole for at least one year have not shown evidence of ECL cell effects similar to those seen on rat studies. Longer term data are needed to rule out the possibility of an increased risk of the development of gastric tumors in patients receiving long-term therapy with lansoprazole.

Other Gastric Effects In Humans: Lansoprazole did not significantly affect mucosal blood flow in the fundus stomach. Due to the normal, physiologic effect caused by the inhibition of gastric acid secretion, a decrease of about 17% in blood flow in the antrum, pylorus and duodenal bulb was seen. Lansoprazole significantly slowed the gastric emptying of digestible solids. Lansoprazole increased serum pepsinogen levels and decreased pepsin activity under basal conditions and in response to meal stimulation or insulin injection. As with other agents that elevate intragastric pH, increases in gastric pH were associated with increases in nitrate concentration in gastric juice in patients with gastric ulcer. No significant increase in nitrosamine concentrations was observed.

Serum Gastrin Effects: In over 2100 patients, median fasting serum gastrin levels increased 50% to 100% from baseline, but remained within normal range after treatment with lansoprazole given orally in doses of 15 mg to 60 mg. These elevations reached a plateau within two months of therapy and returned to pretreatment levels within four weeks after discontinuation of therapy.

Endocrine Effects: Human studies for up to eight weeks have not detected any clinically significant effects in the endocrine system. Hormones studied include testosterone, luteinizing hormone (LH), follicle stimulating hormone (FSH), sex hormone binding globulin (SHBG), dehydroepiandrosterone sulfate (DHEA-S), prolactin, cortisol, estradiol, insulin. aldosterone, parathormone, glucagon, thyroid stimulating hormone (TSH), tri-iodothyronine (T_3), thyroxine (T_4), and somatotropic hormone (STH). Lansoprazole in oral doses of 15 to 60 mg for up to one year, had no clinically significant effect on sexual function. In addition, lansoprazole in oral doses of 15 to 60 mg for two to eight weeks had no clinically significant effect on thyroid function.

In 24-month carcinogenicity studies on Sprague-Dawley rats with daily dosages up to 150 mg/kg, proliferative changes in the Leydig cells of the testes, including benign neoplasm, were increased compared to control rates.

Other Effects: No systemic effects of lansoprazole on the central nervous system, lymphoid, hematopoietic, renal, hepatic, cardiovascular or respiratory systems have been found in humans. No visual toxicity was observed among 56 patients who had extensive baseline eye evaluations, were treated with up to 180 mg/day of lansoprazole and were observed for up to 58 months. Other rat-specific findings after lifetime exposure included focal pancreatic atrophy, diffuse lymphoid hyperplasia in the thymus, and spontaneous retinal atrophy.

CLINICAL STUDIES:

Duodenal Ulcer: In a U.S. multicenter, double- blind, placebo-controlled, dose-response (15, 30, and 60 mg of lansoprazole once daily) study of 284 patients with endoscopically documented duodenal ulcer, the percentage of patients healed after two and four weeks was significantly higher with all doses of lansoprazole than with placebo. There was no evidence of a greater or earlier response with the two higher doses compared with lansoprazole 15 mg. Based on this study and the second study described below, the recommended dose of lansoprazole in duodenal ulcer is 15 mg per day. (TABLE 2)

TABLE 2 Duodenal Ulcer Healing Rates

		Prevacid		
Week	15 mg qd (N=68)	30 mg qd (N=74)	60 mg qd (N=70)	Placebo (N=72)
2	42.4%*	35.6%*	39.1%*	11.3%
4	89.4%*	91.7%*	89.9%*	46.1%

* (p≤0.001) versus placebo.

CLINICAL STUDIES: *(cont'd)*

lansoprazole 15 mg was significantly more effective than placebo in relieving day and nighttime abdominal pain and in decreasing the amount of antacid taken per day.

In a second U.S. multicenter study, also double-blind, placebo-, dose-comparison (15 and 30 mg of lansoprazole once daily), and including a comparison with ranitidine, in 280 patients with endoscopically documented duodenal ulcer, the percentage of patients healed after four weeks was significantly higher with both doses of lansoprazole than with placebo. There was no evidence of a greater or earlier response with the higher dose of lansoprazole. Although the 15 mg dose of lansoprazole was superior to ranitidine at 4 weeks, the lack of significant difference at 2 weeks and the absence of a difference between 30 mg of lansoprazole and ranitidine leaves the comparative effectiveness of the two agents undetermined. (TABLE 3).

TABLE 3 Duodenal Ulcer Healing Rates

	Prevacid			
Week	15 mg qd (N=80)	30 mg qd (N=77)	Ranitidine 300 mg hs (N=82)	Placebo (N=41)
2	35.0%	44.2%	30.5%*	34.2%
4	92.3%**	80.3%*	70.5%*	47.5%

* (p≤0.001) versus placebo.
** (p≤0.05) versus placebo and ranitidine.

Erosive Esophagitis: In a U.S. multicenter, double-blind, placebo- controlled study 269 patients entering with an endoscopic diagnosis of esophagitis with mucosal grading of 2 or more and grades 3 and 4 signifying erosive disease, the percentages of patients with healing are in (TABLE 4).

TABLE 4 Erosive Esophagitis Healing Rates

		Prevacid		
Week	15 mg qd (N=69)	30 mg qd (N=65)	60 mg qd (N=72)	Placebo (N=63)
4	67.6%*	81.3%**	80.6%**	32.8%
6	87.7%*	95.4%*	94.3%*	52.5%
8	90.9%*	95.4%*	94.4%*	52.5%

* (p≤0.001) versus placebo.
** (p≤0.05) versus Prevacid 15 mg and placebo.

In this study, all lansoprazole groups reported significantly greater relief of heartburn and less day and night abdominal pain along with fewer days of antacid use and fewer antacid tablets taken per day than the placebo group.

Although all doses were effective, the earlier healing in the higher two doses suggest 30 mg qd as the recommended dose.

lansoprazole was also compared in a U.S. multicenter, double-blind study to a low dose of ranitidine in 242 patients with erosive reflux esophagitis. Lansoprazole at a dose of 30 mg was significantly more effective than ranitidine 150 mg bid as shown below. (TABLE 5)

TABLE 5 Erosive Esophagitis Healing Rates

Week	Prevacid 30 mg qd (N=115)	Ranitidine 150 mg bid (N=127)
2	66.7%*	38.7%
4	82.5%*	52.0%
6	93.0%*	67.8%
8	92.1%*	69.9%

* (p≤0.001) versus ranitidine.

In addition, patients treated with lansoprazole reported less day and nighttime heartburn and took less antacid tablets for fewer days than patients taking ranitidine 150 mg bid.

Although this study demonstrates effectiveness of lansoprazole in healing erosive esophagitis, it does not represent an adequate comparison with ranitidine because the recommended ranitidine dose for esophagitis is 150 mg qid, twice the dose used in this study.

In the two trials described and in several smaller studies involving patients with moderate to severe erosive esophagitis, lansoprazole produced healing rates similar to those shown above.

In a U.S. multicenter, double-blind, active-controlled study, 30 mg of lansoprazole was compared with ranitidine 150 mg bid in 151 patients with erosive reflux esophagitis that was poorly responsive to a minimum of 12 weeks of treatment with at least one H_2-receptor antagonist given at the dose indicated for symptom relief or greater, namely cimetidine 800 mg/day, ranitidine 300 mg/day, famotidine 40 mg/day or nizatidine 300 mg/day. Lansoprazole 30 mg was more effective than ranitidine 150 mg bid in healing reflux esophagitis and the percentage of patients with healing were as follows. This study does not constitute a comparison of the effectiveness of histamine H_2-receptor antagonists with lansoprazole as all patients had demonstrated unresponsiveness to the histamine H_2-receptor antagonist mode of treatment. It does indicate, however, that lansoprazole may be useful in patients failing on a histamine H_2-receptor antagonist. (TABLE 6).

TABLE 6 Reflux Esophagitis Healing Rates in Patients Poorly Responsive to Histamine H 2-Receptor Antagonist Therapy

Week	Prevacid 30 mg gd (N=100)	Ramitidine 150 mg bid (N=51)
4	74.7%*	42.6%
8	83.7%*	32.0%

* (p≤0.001) versus ranitidine.

Pathological Hypersecretory Conditions Including Zollinger-Ellison Syndrome: In open studies of 57 patients with pathological hypersecretory conditions, such as Zollinger-Ellison (ZE) syndrome with or without multiple endocrine adenomas, lansoprazole significantly inhibited gastric acid secretion and controlled associated symptoms of diarrhea, anorexia and pain. Doses ranging from 15 mg every other day to 180 mg per day maintained basal acid secretion below 10 mEq/hr in patients without prior gastric surgery, and below 5 m/Eq/hr in patients with prior gastric surgery.

Initial dose were titrated to the individual patient need, and adjustments were necessary with time in some patients (see DOSAGE AND ADMINISTRATION). Lansoprazole was well tolerated at these high dose levels for prolonged periods (greater than four years in some patients). In most ZE patients, serum gastrin levels were not modified by lansoprazole. However, in some patients serum gastrin increased to levels greater than those present prior to initiation of lansoprazole therapy.

INDICATIONS AND USAGE:

Short-Term Treatment of Active Duodenal Ulcer: Lansoprazole is indicated for short-term treatment (up to 4 weeks) for healing and symptom relief active duodenal ulcer.

INDICATIONS AND USAGE: *(cont'd)*

LANSOPRAZOLE SHOULD NOT BE USED AS MAINTENANCE THERAPY FOR TREATMENT OF PATIENTS WITH DUODENAL ULCER DISEASE.

Short-Term Treatment of Erosive Esophagitis: Lansoprazole are indicated for short-term treatment (up to 8 weeks) for healing and symptom relief of all grades of erosive esophagitis.

For patients who do not heal with lansoprazole for 8 weeks (5-10%) it may be helpful to give an additional 8 weeks of treatment.

If there is a recurrence of erosive esophagitis an additional 8 week course of lansoprazole may be considered.

LANSOPRAZOLE SHOULD NOT BE USED AS MAINTENANCE THERAPY.

Pathological Hypersecretory Conditions Including Zollinger-Ellison Syndrome: Lansoprazole are indicated for the long-term treatment of pathological hypersecretory conditions, including Zollinger-Ellison syndrome.

CONTRAINDICATIONS:

Llansoprazole is contraindicated in patients with known hypersensitivity to any component of the formulation.

PRECAUTIONS:

General: Symptomatic response to therapy with lansoprazole does not preclude the presence of gastric malignancy.

Information for the Patient: Lansoprazole should be taken before eating.

Patients should be cautioned that lansoprazole should not be opened, chewed or crushed. Capsules should be swallowed whole.

Carcinogenesis, Mutagenesis, and Impairment of Fertility: In two 24-month carcinogenicity studies, Sprague-Dawley rats were treated orally with doses of 5 to 150 mg/kg/day, about 1 to 40 times the exposure on a body surface (mg/m^2) basis, of a 50 kg person of average height (1.46 m^2 body surface area) given the recommended human dose of 30 mg/day (22.2 mg/m^2). Lansoprazole produced dose-related gastric enterochromaffin like (ECL) cell hyperplasia and ECL cell carcinoids in both male and female rats. It also increased the incidence of intestinal metaplasia of the gastric epithelium in both sexes. In male rats, lansoprazole produced a dose-related increase of testicular interstitial cell adenomas. The incidence of these adenomas in rats receiving doses of 15 to 150 mg/kg/day (4 to 40 times the recommended human dose based on body surface area) exceeded the low background incidence (range = 1.4 to 10%) for this strain of rat. Testicular interstitial cell adenoma also occurred in 1 of 30 rats treated with 50 mg/kg/day (13 times the recommended human dose based on body surface area) in a 1-year toxicity study.

In a 24-month carcinogenicity study, CD-1 mice were treated orally with doses of 15 to 600 mg/kg/day, 2 to 80 times the recommended human dose based on body surface area. Lansoprazole produced as dose related increased incidence of gastric ECL cell hyperplasia. It also produced an increased incidence of liver tumors (hepatocellular adenoma plus carcinoma). The tumor incidences in male mice treated with 300 and 600 mg/kg/day (40 to 80 times the recommended human dose based on body surface area) and female mice treated with 150 to 600 mg/kg/day (20 to 80 times the recommended human dose based on body surface area) exceeded the ranges of background incidences in historical controls for this strain of mice. Lansoprazole treatment produced adenoma of rete testis in male mice receiving 75 to 600 mg/kg/day (10 to 80 times the recommended human dose based on the body surface area).

Lansoprazole was not genotoxic in the Ames test, the *ex vivo* rat hepatocyte unscheduled DNA synthesis (UDS) test, the *in vivo*mouse micronucleus test or the rat bone marrow cell chromosomal aberration test. It was positive in *in vitro* human lymphocyte chromosomal aberration assays.

Lansoprazole oral doses up to 150 mg/kg/day (40 times the recommended human dose based on body surface area) was found to have no effect on fertility and reproductive performance of male and female rats.

Pregnancy, Teratogenic Effects, Pregnancy Category B: Teratology studies have been performed in pregnant rats at oral doses up to 150 mg/kg/day (40 times the recommended human dose based on body surface area) and pregnant rabbits at oral doses up to 30 mg/kg/day (16 times the recommended human dose based on body surface area) and have revealed no evidence of impaired fertility or harm to the fetus due to lansoprazole.

There are, however, no adequate or well-controlled studies in pregnant women. Because animal reproduction studies are not always predictive of human response, this drug should be used during pregnancy only if clearly needed.

Nursing Mothers: Lansoprazole or its metabolites are excreted in the milk of rats. It is not known whether lansoprazole is excreted in human milk. Because many drugs are excreted in human milk, because of the potential for serious adverse reactions in nursing infants from lansoprazole in rat carcinogenicity studies, a decision should be made whether to discontinue nursing or to discontinue the drug, taking into account the importance of the drug to the mother.

Pediatric Use: Safety and effectiveness in children have not been established.

Use in Women: Over 800 women were treated with lansoprazole. Ulcer healing rates in females are similar to those in males. The incidence rates of adverse events are also similar to those seen in males.

Geriatric Use: Ulcer healing rates in elderly patients are similar to those in a younger age group. The incidence rates of adverse events and laboratory test abnormalities are also similar to those seen in younger patients. The initial dosing regimen need not be altered for elderly patients, but subsequent doses higher than 30 mg per day should not be administered unless additional gastric acid suppression is necessary.

DRUG INTERACTIONS:

Lansoprazole is metabolized through the cytochrome P_{450} system, specifically through the CYP3A and CYP2C19 isozymes. Studies have shown that lansoprazole does not have clinically significant interactions with other drugs metabolized by the cytochrome P_{450} system, such as warfarin, antipyrine, indomethacin, ibuprofen, phenytoin, propranolol, prednisone, or diazepam in healthy subjects. These compounds are metabolized through various cytochrome P_{450} isozymes including CYP1A2, CYP2C9, CYP2C19, CYP2D6, and CYP3A. When lansoprazole was administered concomitantly with theophylline (CYP1A2, CYP3A), a minor increase (10%) in the clearance of theophylline was seen. Because the small magnitude and the direction of the effect on theophylline clearance, this interaction is unlikely to be clinical concern. Nonetheless, individual patients may require additional titration of their theophylline dosage when lansoprazole is started or stopped to ensure clinically effective blood levels.

Coadministration of lansoprazole with sucralfate delayed absorption and reduced lansoprazole bioavailability by approximately 30%. Therefore, lansoprazole should be taken at least 30 minutes prior to sucralfate. In clinical trials, antacids were administered concomitantly with lansoprazole; this did not interfere with its effect.

Lansoprazole causes a profound and long lasting inhibition of gastric acid secretion; therefore, it is theoretically possible that lansoprazole may interfere with the absorption of drugs where gastric pH is an important determinant of bioavailability (*e.g.,* ketoconazole, ampicillin esters, iron salts, digoxin).

ADVERSE REACTIONS:

Worldwide, over 6100 patients have been treated with lansoprazole in Phase II-III clinical trials involving various dosages and duration of treatment. In general, lansoprazole treatment has been well tolerated in both short-term and long-term trials.

Incidence in Clinical Trials: The following adverse events were reported by the treating physician to have a possible or probable relationship to drug in 1% or more of lansoprazole treated patients and occurred at a greater rate in lansoprazole-treated patients than placebo-treated patients: (TABLE 7)

TABLE 7 Incidence of Possibly or Probably Treated-Related Averse Events in Short-term, Placebo-Controlled Studies

Body System/ Adverse Event	Prevacid (N=1457) %	Placebo (N=467) %
Body as a Whole		
Abdominal Pain	1.8	1.3
Digestive System		
Diarrhea	3.6	2.6
Nausea	1.4	1.3

Headache was also seen at greater than 1% incidence but was more common on placebo. The incidence of diarrhea is similar between placebo and lansoprazole 15 mg and 30 mg patients, but higher in the lansoprazole 60 mg patients (2.9%, 1.4%, 4.2, and 7.4%, respectively).

The most commonly reported possibly or probably treatment-related adverse event during maintenance therapy was diarrhea.

In short-term and long-term studies, the following adverse events were reported in <1% of the lansoprazole-treated patients:

Body as a Whole: asthenia, candidiasis, chest pain (not otherwise specified), edema, fever, flu syndrome, halitosis, infection (not otherwise specified), malaise; *Cardiovascular System:* angina, cerebrovascular accident, hypertension/hypotension, myocardial infarction, palpitations, shock, (circulatory failure), vasodilation;*Digestive System:* melena, anorexia, bezoar, cardiospasm, cholelithiasis, constipation, dry mouth/thirst, dyspepsia, dysphagia, eructation, esophageal stenosis, esophageal ulcer, esophagitis, fecal discoloration, flatulence, gastric nodules/fundic gland polyps, gastroenteritis, gastrointestinal hemorrhage, stomatitis, tenesmus, ulcerative colitis; *Endocrine System:* diabetes, mellitus, goiter, hyperglycemia/hypoglycemia. *Hematologic and Lymphatic System:* anemia, hemolysis; *Metabolic and Nutritional Disorders:* gout, weight gain/loss; *Musculoskeletal System*arthritis/arthralgia, musculoskeletal pain, myalgia; *Nervous System:* agitation, amnesia, anxiety, apathy, confusion, depression, dizziness/syncope, hallucinations, hemiplegia, hostility aggravated, libido decreased, nervousness, paresthesia, thinking abnormality;*Respiratory System:* asthma, bronchitis, cough increased, dyspnea, epistaxis, hemoptysis, hiccup, pneumonia, upper respiratory inflammation/infection; *Skin and Appendages:* acne, alopecia, pruritis, rash, urticaria; *Special Senses:* amblyopia, deafness, eye pain, visual field defect, otitis media, taste perversion, tinnitus;*Urogenital System:* abnormal menses, albuminuria, breast enlargement/gynecomastia, breast tenderness, glycosuria, hematuria, impotence, kidney calculus.

Laboratory Values: The following changes in laboratory parameters were reported as adverse events.

Abnormal liver function tests, increased SGOT (AST), increased SGPT (ALT), increased creatinine, increased alkaline phosphatase, increased globulins, increased GGTP, increased/decreased/abnormal WBC, abnormal AG ratio, abnormal RBC, bilirubinemia, eosinophilia, hyperlipemia, increased/decreased electrolytes, increased/decreased cholesterol, increased glucocorticoids, increased LDH, increase/decreased/abnormal platelets and increased gastrin levels. Additional isolated laboratory abnormalities were reported.

In the placebo controlled studies, when SGOT (ALT) and SGPT (AST) were evaluated 0.4% (1/250) placebo patients and 0.3% (2/795) lansoprazole patients had enzyme elevations greater than three times the upper limit of normal range at the first final treatment visit. None of these patients reported jaundice at any time during the study.

OVERDOSAGE:

Oral doses up to 5000 mg/kg in rats (approximately 1300 times the recommended human dose based on body surface area) and mice (about 675.7 times the recommended human dose based on body surface area) did not produce deaths or any clinical signs.

Lansoprazole is not removed from the circulation by hemodialysis. In one reported case of overdose, the patient consumed 600 mg of lansoprazole with no adverse reaction.

DOSAGE AND ADMINISTRATION:

Treatment of Duodenal Ulcer: The recommended adult oral dose is 15 mg daily before eating for 4 weeks. (See INDICATIONS AND USAGE.)

Treatment of Erosive Esophagitis: The recommended adult oral dose is 30 mg daily before eating for up to 8 weeks. For patients who do not heal with lansoprazole for 8 weeks (5-10%) it may be helpful to give an additional 8 weeks of treatment.

(See INDICATIONS AND USAGE)

If there is a recurrence of erosive esophagitis, an additional 8 week course of lansoprazole may be considered.

Pathological Hypersecretory Conditions Including Zollinger-Ellison Syndrome: The dosage of lansoprazole in patients with pathologic hypersecretory conditions varies with the individual patient. The recommended adult oral starting dose 60 mg once a day. Doses should be adjusted to individual patient needs and should continue for as long as clinically indicated. Dosages up to 90 mg bid have been administered. Daily dosages of greater than 120 mg should be administered in divided doses. Some patients with Zollinger-Ellison syndrome have been treated continuously with lansoprazole for more than four years.

No dosage adjustment is necessary in patients with renal insufficiency or the elderly. For patients with severe liver disease, dosage adjustment should be considered.

PATIENT INFORMATION:

Lansprazole is used short-term (4-8 weeks) to treat duodenal ulcer and erosive esophagitis. It may used long term to treat Zollinger-Ellison syndrome, a problem with too much acid being secreted. Lansoprazole capsules should be taken before eating. The capsules are delayed release' meaning they work over time. The capsules should be swallowed whole and not crushed, opened or chewed. If you are taking theophylline, you may need your dosage checked when you start and stop lansoprazole to ensure your dose is effective. If you are taking sucralfate, it should be taken 30 minutes after taking lansoprazole. The most common side effects reported were diarrhea, nausea and abdominal pain. These occurred in fewer than 5% of patients. If your symptoms return after completing your course of therapy, talk to your physician for further evaluation.

HOW SUPPLIED:

Prevacid Delayed-Release Capsules, 15 mg, are opaque, hard gelatin, colored pink and green. The 30 mg are opaque, hard gelatin, pink and black colored capsules.

HOW SUPPLIED: *(cont'd)*

Storage: Prevacid capsules should be stored in a tight container protected from moisture. Store between 59°F and 86°F

(TAP Pharmaceuticals Inc., MS-P97-1233)

HOW SUPPLIED - EQUIVALENTS NOT AVAILABLE:

Capsule, Gelatin, Sustained Action - Oral - 15 mg

30's	$97.51	PREVACID, TAP Pharm	00300-1541-30
100's	$325.00	PREVACID, TAP Pharm	00300-1541-11

Capsule, Gelatin, Sustained Action - Oral - 30 mg

100's	$325.00	PREVACID, TAP Pharm	00300-3046-11
100's	$325.00	PREVACID, TAP Pharm	00300-3046-13

LATANOPROST *(003299)*

CATEGORIES: Antiglaucomatous Agents; Antihypertensives; EENT Drugs; Eye, Ear, Nose, & Throat Preparations; Glaucoma; Hypertension; Intraocular Pressure; Ocular Hypertension; Ophthalmics; Pregnancy Category C; FDA Approved 1996 Aug

BRAND NAMES: **Xalatan**

PRIMARY ICD9: 365.04 (Ocular Hypertension, Unspecified)

DESCRIPTION:

Latanoprost is a prostaglandin $F_{2\alpha}$ analogue. Its chemical name is isopropyl-(Z) 7[(1R, 2R, 3R, 5S)3, 5-dihydroxy-2-[(3R)-3 hydroxy-5-phenylpentyl]cyclopentyl]-5 heplenoate. Its molecular formula is $C_{26}H_{40}O_5$and its molecular weight is 432.58.

Latanoprost is a colorless to slightly yellow oil which is very soluble in acetonitrite and freely soluble in acetone, ethanol, ethyl acetate, isopropanol, methanol, and octanol. It is practically insoluble in water.

Xalatan Sterile Ophthalmic Solution is supplied as sterile, isotonic, buffered aqueous solution of latanoprost with a pH of approximately 6.7. Each ml of Xalatan contains 50 micrograms of latanoprost. Benzalkonium chloride, 0.02% is added as a preservative. The inactive ingredients are: sodium chloride, sodium dihydrogen phosphate monohydrate, disodium hydrogen phosphate anhydrous and water for injection. One drop contains approximately 1.5 mcg of latanoprost.

CLINICAL PHARMACOLOGY:

MECHANISM OF ACTION

Latanoprost is a prostanoid selective FP receptor agonist which is believed to reduce the intraocular pressure by increasing the outflow of aqueous humor. Studies in animals and humans suggest that the main mechanism of action is increased uveoscleral outflow.

PHARMACOKINETICS / PHARMACODYNAMICS

Absorption: Latanoprost is absorbed through the cornea where the isopropyl ester prodrug is hydrolyzed to the acid form to become biologically active. Studies in humans indicate that the peak concentration in the aqueous humor is reached about 2 hours after topical administration.

Distribution: The distribution volume in humans is 0.16 ± 0.02 L/kg. The acid of latanoprost could be measured in aqueous humor during the first four hours, and in plasma only during the first hour after local administration.

Metabolism: Latanoprost, an isopropyl ester prodrug, is hydrolyzed by esterases in the cornea to the biologically active acid. The active acid of latanoprost reaching the systemic circulation is primarily metabolized by the liver to the 1,2-dinor and 1,2,3,4-tetranor metabolites via fatty acid β-oxidation.

Excretion: The elimination of the acid of latanoprost from human plasma was rapid ($t_{1/2}$ = 17 min) after both intravenous and topical administration. Systemic clearance is approximately 7 ml/min/kg. Following hepatic β-oxidation, the metabolites are mainly eliminated via the kidneys. Approximately 88% and 98% of the administered dose is recovered in the urine after topical and intravenous dosing, respectively.

ANIMAL STUDIES

In monkeys, latanoprost has been shown to induce increased pigmentation of the iris. The results from the preclinical program demonstrated that the increased pigmentation unlikely to be associated with proliferation of melanocytes. It appears that the mechanism of increased pigmentation is stimulation of melanin production in melanocytes of the iris stroma.

In ocular toxicity studies, administration of latanoprost at a dose of 6 mcg/eye/day (4 times the daily human dose) to cynomolgus monkeys has also been shown to induce increased palpebral fissure. This effect has been reversible and occurred at doses above the standard clinical dose level.

CLINICAL STUDIES:

Patients with mean baseline intraocular pressure of 24-25 who were treated for 6 months in multicenter, randomized, controlled trials demonstrated 6-8 mmHg reductions in intraocular pressure. This IOP reduction latanoprost 0.005% dosed once daily was equivalent to the effect of timolol 0.5% dosed twice daily.

INDICATIONS AND USAGE:

Latanoprost is indicated for the reduction of elevated intraocular pressure in patients with open-angle glaucoma and ocular hypertension who are intolerant of other intraocular pressure lowering medications or insufficiently responsive (failed to achieve target IOP determined after multiple measurements over time) to another intraocular pressure lowering medication.

CONTRAINDICATIONS:

Known hypersensitivity to latanoprost, benzalkonium chloride or any other ingredients in this product.

WARNINGS:

Latanoprost may gradually change eye color, increasing the amount of brown pigment in the iris by increasing the number of melanosomes (pigment granules) in melanocytes. The long term effects on the melanocyles and the consequences of potential injury to the melanocytes and/or deposition of pigment granules to other areas of the eye is currently unknown.

The change in iris color occurs slowly and may not be noticeable for several months to years. Patients should be informed of the possibility of iris color change. Patients who are expected to receive treatment in only one eye should be informed about the potential for increased brown pigmentation in the treated eye and thus, heterochromia between the eyes. The increased pigmentation may be permanent.

PRECAUTIONS:

GENERAL

Latanoprost is hydrolyzed in the cornea The effect of continued administration of latanoprost on the corneal endothelium has not been fully evaluated.

There have been reports of bacterial keratitis associated with the use of multiple-dose containers of topical ophthalmic products. These containers had been inadvertently contaminated by patients who, in most cases, had a concurrent corneal disease or a disruption of the ocular epithelial surface (see Information for the Patient).

Patients may slowly develop increased brown pigmentation of the iris. This change may not be noticeable for several months to years (see WARNINGS.) Typically the brown pigmentation around the pupil spreads concentrically towards the periphery in affected eyes, but the entire iris or parts of it may also become more brownish. Until more information about increased brown pigmentation is available, patients should be examined regularly and, depending on the clinical situation, treatment may be stopped if increased pigmentation ensues. During clinical trials, the increase in brown iris pigment has not been shown to progress further upon discontinuation of treatment, but the resultant color change may be permanent. Neither nevi nor freckles of the iris have been affected by treatment.

There is no experience with latanoprost in the treatment of angle closure, inflammatory or neovascular glaucoma and only limited experience in pseudophakic patients.

Latanoprost has not been studied in patients with renal or hepatic impairment and should therefore be used with caution in such patients.

Latanoprost should not be administered while wearing contact lenses.

INFORMATION FOR THE PATIENT

Patients should be informed about the possibility of iris color change due to an increase of the brown pigment and resultant cosmetically different eye coloration that may occur when only one eye is treated.

Iris pigmentation changes may be more noticeable in patients with green-brown, blue/gray-brown or yellow-brown irises.

Patients should be instructed to avoid allowing the tip of the dispensing container to contact the eye or surrounding structures because this could cause the lip to become contaminated by common bacteria known to cause ocular infections. Serious damage to the eye and subsequent loss of vision may result from using contaminated solutions. Patients also should be advised that if they develop an intercurrent ocular condition (*e.g.,* trauma, or infection) or have ocular surgery, they should immediately seek their physicians advice concerning the continued use of the multidose container they had been using. Patients should be advised that if they develop any ocular reactions, particularly conjunctivitis and lid reactions, they should immediately seek their physicians advice.

Patients should also be advised that latanoprost contains benzalkonium chloride which may be absorbed by contact lenses. Contact lenses should be removed prior to administration of the solution. Lenses may be reinserted 15 minutes following latanoprost administration. If more than one topical ophthalmic drug is being used, the drugs should be administered at least five (5) minutes apart.

DRUG INTERACTIONS

In vitro studies have shown that precipitation occurs when eye drops containing theomersal are mixed with latanoprost. If such drugs are used they should be administered with an interval of at least five (5) minutes between applications.

CARCINOGENESIS, MUTAGENESIS, AND IMPAIRMENT OF FERTILITY

Latanoprost was not mutagenic in bacteria, in mouse lymphoma or in mouse micronucleus tests. Chromosome aberrations were observed *in vitro* with human lymphocytes Latanoprost was not carcinogenic in either mice or rats when administered by oral gavage at doses of up to 170 mcg/kg/day (approximately 2,800 times the recommended human dose) for up to 20 and 24 months, respectively. Additional *in vitro* and *in vivo* studies on unscheduled DNA synthesis in rats were negative. Latanoprost has not been found to have any effect on male or female fertility in animal studies.

PREGNANCY, TERATOGENIC EFFECTS, PREGNANCY CATEGORY C

Reproduction studies have been performed in rats and rabbits. In rabbits an incidence of 4 of 16 dams had no viable fetuses at a dose that was approximately 80 times the maximum human dose, and the highest nonembryocidal dose in rabbits was approximately 15 times the maximum human dose There are no adequate and well-controlled studies in pregnant women. Latanoprost should be used during pregnancy only if the potential benefit justifies the potential risk to the fetus.

NURSING MOTHERS

It is not known whether this drug or its metabolites are excreted in human milk. Because many drugs are excreted in human milk, caution should be exercised when latanoprost is administered to a nursing woman.

PEDIATRIC PATIENTS

Safety and effectiveness in pediatric patients have not been established.

ADVERSE REACTIONS:

The ocular adverse events and ocular signs and symptoms reported in 5 to 15% of the patients on latanoprost in the 6 month, multi-center, double-masked, active-controlled trials were blurred vision, burning and stinging, conjunctival hyperemia, foreign body sensation, itching, increased pigmentation of the iris, and punctate epithelial keratopathy.

Local conjunctiva hyperemia was observed; however, less than 1% of the latanoprost treated patients required discontinuation of therapy because of intolerance to conjunctiva hyperemia.

In addition to the above listed ocular events/signs and symptoms, the following were reported in 1 to 4% of the patients: dry eye, excessive tearing, eye pain, lid crusting, lid edema, lid erythema, lid discomfort/pain and photophobia.

The following events were reported in less than 1% of the patients: conjunctivitis, diplopia and discharge from the eye.

During clinical studies, there were extremely rare reports of the following: retinal artery embolus, retinal detachment, and vitreous hemorrhage from diabetic retinopathy.

The most common systemic adverse events seen with latanoprost were upper respiratory tract infection/cold/flu which occurred at a rate of approximately 4%. Pain in muscle/joint/back, chest pain/angina pectoris and rash/allergic skin reaction each occurred at a ratio of 1 to 2%.

OVERDOSAGE:

Apart from ocular irritation and conjunctival or episcleral hyperemia, the ocular effects of latanoprost administered at high doses are not known. Intravenous administration of large doses of latanoprost in monkeys has been associated with transient bronchoconstriction; however, in 11 patients with bronchial asthma treated with latanoprost, bronchoconstriction was not induced. Intravenous infusion of up to 3 mcg/kg in healthy volunteers produced mean plasma concentrations 200 times higher than during clinical treatment and no adverse reactions were observed. Intravenous dosages of 5.5 to 10 mcg/kg caused abdominal pain dizziness fatigue, hot flushes, nausea, and sweating.

If overdosage with latanoprost occurs, treatment should be symptomatic.

DOSAGE AND ADMINISTRATION:

The recommended dosage is one drop (1.5 mcg) in the affected eye(s) once daily in the evening.

The dosage of latanoprost should not exceed once daily since it has been shown that more frequent administration may decrease the intraocular pressure lowering effect.

Reduction of the intraocular pressure starts approximately 3 to 4 hours after administration and the maximum effect is reached after 8 to 12 hours.

Latanoprost may be used concomitantly with other topical ophthalmic drug products to lower intraocular pressure. If more than one topical ophthalmic drug is being used, the drugs should be administered at least five (5) minutes apart.

PATIENT INFORMATION:

This drug is used to lower elevated intraocular pressure in patients who have open-angle glaucoma or ocular hypertension.

This medication may change light eye color to a brown color. The change happens very slowly, over a period of months or years, but may be permanent.

Report any eye reactions, especially conjunctivitis or lid reaction, to your physician.

Remove contact lenses before using the solution; re-insert after a period of not less than 15 minutes.

Do not allow dropper tip to touch the eye.

This medication may cause blurred vision, burning and stinging, foreign body sensation, red or inflamed eyes, and/or itching. Inform your doctor if any of these symptoms occur.

HOW SUPPLIED:

Xalatan (Latanoprost Solution) Sterile Ophthalmic Solution is a clear, isotonic, buffered, preserved, colorless, solution supplied in plastic ophthalmic dispenser bottles with a dropper tip and tamper evident overcap.

The solution is supplied as: 2.5 ml fill, 0.005% (50 mcg/ml), in cartons of 1 & 6.

Storage: Protect from light. Store unopened bottle under refrigeration at 2° to 8°C (36° to 46°F).

Once opened the container may be stored at room temperature up to 25°C (77°F) for 6 weeks.

HOW SUPPLIED - EQUIVALENTS NOT AVAILABLE:

Solution - Ophthalmic - 0.005%

2.5 ml	$31.99	XALATAN, Pharmacia & Upjohn	00013-8303-04

LEUCOVORIN CALCIUM *(001630)*

CATEGORIES: Anemia; Antagonists and Antidotes; Anti-Folic Acid Antagonists; Antidotes; Antineoplastics; Blood Formation/Coagulation; Deficiency Anemias; Orphan Drugs; Vitamins; Colon Carcinoma*; Pregnancy Category C; FDA Approval Pre 1982; Patent Expiration 1995 Aug

* Indication not approved by the FDA

BRAND NAMES: *Antrex*; *Calciumfolinat-Ebewe*; *Calcium Folinate*; *Calcium Leucovorin*; *Citrec*; *Lederfolin* (England); *Lederfoline* (France); *Lederle Leucovorin* (Canada); *Ledervorin-Calcium*; *Ledervorin Calcium*; *Lerderfoline*; *Leucovorin* (England, Germany); *Leucovorin Calcium* (Australia); *Leucovorina Calcica*; *Leucovorine Abic*; *Medsavorin* (Mexico); *Refolinon* (England); *Rescufolin*; *Rescuvolin* (Germany); Wellcovorin

(International brand names outside U.S. in italics)

FORMULARIES: Aetna; BC-BS; Medi-Cal; WHO

DESCRIPTION:

Leucovorin is one of several active, chemically reduced derivatives of folic acid. It is useful as an antidote to drugs which act as folic acid antagonists. Also known as folinic acid, Citrovorum factor, or 5-formyl-5,6,7,8-tetrahydrofolic acid, this compound has the chemical designation of L-Glutamic acid, N-[4-[[(2-amino- 5-formyl-1,4,5,6,7,8-hexahydro-4-oxo-6-pteridinyl)methyl]amino]benzoyl]-,calcium salt (1:1). The formula weight is 511.51.

Tablets: Leucovorin calcium tablets, 5 mg, contain 5 mg of leucovorin (equivalent to 5.40 mg of anhydrous leucovorin calcium) and the following inactive ingredients: Corn Starch, Dibasic Calcium Phosphate, Magnesium Stearate, and Pregelatinized Starch.

Leucovorin calcium tablets, 15 mg, contain 15 mg of leucovorin (equivalent to 16.20 mg of anhydrous leucovorin calcium) and the following inactive ingredients: Lactose, Magnesium Stearate, Microcrystalline Cellulose, Pregelatinized Starch, and Sodium Starch Glycolate.

Leucovorin calcium tablets are indicated for oral administration only.

Injection: Leucovorin calcium for injection is indicated for intravenous or intramuscular administration and is supplied as a sterile lyophilized powder. The 50, 100 and 350 mg vials are preservative free. The inactive ingredient is sodium chloride 40 mg/vial for the 50 mg vial, 80 mg/vial for the 100 mg vial, and 140 mg/vial for 350 mg vial. Sodium hydroxide and/or hydrochloric acid are used to adjust the pH to approximately 8.1 during manufacture. There is 0.004 mEq of calcium per mg of leucovorin in each dosage form.

CLINICAL PHARMACOLOGY:

Leucovorin is a mixture of the diastereoisomers of the 5-formyl derivative of tetrahydrofolic acid (THF). The biologically active component of the mixture is the (-)-*l*-isomer, known as Citrovorum factor, or (-)-folinic acid. Leucovorin does *not*require reduction by the enzyme dihydrofolate reductase in order to participate in reactions utilizing folates as a source of "one-carbon" moieties.

Tablets: Following oral administration, leucovorin is rapidly absorbed and enters the general body pool of reduced folates.

The increase in plasma and serum folate activity (determined microbiologically with *Lactobacillus casei*) seen after oral administration of leucovorin is predominantly due to 5-methyltetrahydrofolate.

Following a 20 mg dose of leucovorin calcium, the mean maximum serum total reduced folate concentrations were:

Tablet 364 ± 12.1 ng/ml at 2.0 ± 0.07 hours

Oral Solution 375 ± 12.8 ng/ml at 2.1 ± 0.11 hours

Parenteral 355 ± 17.2 ng/ml at 0.96 ± 0.10 hours

The half-life of plasma 5-formyltetrahydrofolate was 1.5 ± 0.08 hours and that of the methyltetrahydrofolate was 3.0 ± 0.09 hours.

CLINICAL PHARMACOLOGY: *(cont'd)*

Oral tablets produced equivalent bioavailability (8% difference) when compared to the parenteral administration. The parenteral solution also provided equal bioavailability to the tablets when administered orally (2% difference). Oral absorption of leucovorin is saturable at doses above 25 mg. The apparent bioavailability of leucovorin was 97% for 25 mg, 75% for 50 mg and 37% for 100 mg.

Injection: *l*-Leucovorin (*l*-5- formyltetrahydrofolate) is rapidly metabolized (via 5,10- methyltetrahydrofolate then 5,10-methylenetetrahydrofolate) to *l*- 5-methyltetrahydrofolate. *l*-5-Methyltetrahydrofolate can in turn be metabolized via other pathways back to 5,10 methylenetetrahydrofolate, which is converted to 5-methyltetrahydrofolate by an irreversible, enzyme catalyzed reduction using the cofactors $FADH_2$ and NADPH.

Administration of leucovorin can counteract the therapeutic and toxic effects of folic acid antagonists such as methotrexate, which act by inhibiting dihydrofolate reductase.

In contrast, leucovorin can enhance the therapeutic and toxic effects of fluoropyrimidines used in cancer therapy, such as 5-fluorouracil. Concurrent administration of leucovorin does not appear to alter the plasma pharmacokinetics of 5-fluorouracil. 5-Fluorouracil is metabolized to fluorodeoxyuridylic acid, which binds to and inhibits the enzyme thymidylate synthase (an enzyme important in DNA repair and replication).

Leucovorin is readily converted to another reduced folate, 5,10- methylenetetrahydrofolate, which acts to stabilize the binding of fluorodeoxyuridylic acid to thymidylate synthase and thereby enhances the inhibition of this enzyme.

The pharmacokinetics after intravenous, intramuscular, and oral administration of a 25 mg dose of leucovorin were studied in male volunteers. After intravenous administration, serum total reduced folates (as measured by *Lactobacillus casei* assay) reached a mean peak of 1259 ng/ml (range 897-1625). The mean time to peak was 10 minutes. This initial rise in total reduced folates was primarily due to the parent compound 5-formyl-THF (measured by *Streptococcus faecalis* assay) which rose to 1206 ng/ml at 10 minutes. A sharp drop in parent compound followed and coincided with the appearance of the active metabolite 5- methyl-THF which became the predominant circulating form of the drug.

The mean peak of 5-methyl-THF was 258 ng/ml and occurred at 1.3 hours. The terminal half-life for total reduced folates was 6.2 hours. The area under the concentration versus time curves (AUCs) for *l*-leucovorin,*d*-leucovorin and 5-methyltetrahydrofolate were 28.4 ± 3.5, 956 ± 97 and 129 ± 12 (mg/min/L ± S.E.). When a higher dose of*d,l*-leucovorin (200 mg/m^2) was used, similar results were obtained. The *d*-isomer persisted in plasma at concentrations greatly exceeding those of the *l*-isomer.

After intramuscular injection, the mean peak of serum total reduced folates was 436 ng/ml (range 240-725) and occurred at 52 minutes. Similar to IV administration, the initial sharp rise due to the parent compound. The mean peak of 5-formyl-THF was 360 ng/ml and occurred at 28 minutes. The level of the metabolite 5-methyl-THF increased subsequently over time until at 1.5 hours it represented 50% of the circulating total folates. The mean peak of 5-methyl was 226 ng/ml at 2.8 hours. The terminal half- life of total reduced folates was 6.2 hours. There was no difference of statistical significance between IM and IV administration in the AUC for total reduced folates, 5-formyl-THF or 5 Methyl-THF.

After oral administration of leucovorin reconstituted with aromatic elixir, the mean peak concentration of serum total reduced folates was 393 ng/ml (range 160-550) The mean time to peak was 2.3 hours and the terminal half-life was 5.7 hours. The major component was the metabolite 5- methyltetrahydrofolate to which leucovorin is primarily converted in the intestinal mucosa. The mean peak of 5-methyl-THF was 367 ng/ml at 2.4 hours. The peak level of the parent compound was 51 ng/ml at 1.2 hours. The AUC of total reduced folates after oral administration of the 25 mg dose was 92% of the AUC after intravenous administration.

Following oral administration, leucovorin is rapidly absorbed and expands the serum pool of reduced folates. At a dose of 25 mg, almost 100% of the*l*-isomer but only 20% of the *d*-isomer is absorbed. Oral absorption of leucovorin is saturable at doses above 25 mg. The apparent bioavailability of leucovorin was 97% for 25 mg, 75% for 50 mg, and 37% for 100 mg.

In a randomized clinical study conducted by the Mayo Clinic and the North Central Cancer Treatment Group (Mayo/NCCTG) in patients with advanced metastatic colorectal cancer three treatment regimens were compared: Leucovorin (LV) 200 mg/m^2 and 5-fluorouracil (5-FU) 370 mg/m^2 versus LV 20 mg/m^2 and 5-FU 425 mg/m^2 versus 5-FU 500 mg/m^2. All drugs were by slow intravenous infusion daily for 5 days repeated every 28-35 days. Response rates were 26% (p = 0.04 versus 5-FU alone), 43% (p = 0.001 versus 5-FU alone) and 10% for the high dose leucovorin, low dose leucovorin and 5-FU alone groups respectively. Respective median survival times were 12.2 months (p = 0.037), 12 months (p = 0.050), and 7.7 months. The low dose LV regimen gave a statistically significant improvement in weight gain of more than 5%, relief of symptoms, and improvement in performance status. The high dose LV regimen gave a statistically significant improvement in weight gain and in relief of symptoms but these were not statistically significant.[1]

In a second Mayo/NCCTGF randomized clinical study the 5-FU alone arm was replaced by a regimen of sequentially administered methotrexate (MTX), 5- FU, and LV. Response rates with LV 200 mg/$m^2$and 5-FU 370 mg/m^2 versus LV 20 mg/m^2 and 5-FU 425 mg/m^2 versus sequential MTX and 5-FU and LV were respectively 31% (p = <.01), 42% (p = <.04), and 14%. Respective median survival times were 12.7 months (p = <.01), and 8.4 months. No statistically significant difference in weight gain of more than 5% or in improvement in performance status was seen between the treatment arms.[2]

INDICATIONS AND USAGE:

Leucovorin calcium rescue is indicated after high-dose methotrexate therapy in osteosarcoma. Leucovorin calcium is also indicated to diminish the toxicity and counteract the effects of impaired methotrexate elimination and of inadvertent overdosages of folic acid antagonists.

Injection: Leucovorin calcium is indicated in the treatment of megaloblastic anemias due to folic acid deficiency when oral therapy is not feasible.

Leucovorin is also indicated for use in combination with 5-fluorouracil to prolong survival in the palliative treatment of patients with advanced colorectal cancer. Leucovorin should not be mixed in the same infusion as 5-fluorouracil because a precipitate may form.

CONTRAINDICATIONS:

Leucovorin is improper therapy for pernicious anemia and other megaloblastic anemias secondary to the lack of vitamin B_{12}. A hematologic remission may occur while neurologic manifestations remain progressive.

WARNINGS:

In the treatment of accidental overdosage of folic acid antagonists, leucovorin should be administered as promptly as possible. As the time interval between antifolate administration [e.g., methotrexate (MTX)] and leucovorin rescue increases, leucovorin's effectiveness in counteracting hematologic toxicity decreases. Do not administer leucovorin intrathecally.

Monitoring of serum MTX concentration is essential in determining the optimal dose and duration of treatment with leucovorin.

WARNINGS: *(cont'd)*

Delayed MTX excretion may be caused by a third space fluid accumulation (*i.e.,* ascites, pleural effusion), renal insufficiency, or inadequate hydration. Under such circumstances, higher doses of leucovorin or prolonged administration may be indicated. Doses higher than those recommended for oral use must be given intravenously.

Tablets: Leucovorin may enhance the toxicity of fluorouracil. Deaths from severe enterocolitis, diarrhea, and dehydration have been reported in elderly patients receiving leucovorin and fluorouracil.[7] Concomitant granulocytopenia and fever were present in some but not all of the patients.

Injection Because of the benzyl alcohol contained in certain diluents used for leucovorin calcium for Infection, when doses greater than 10 mg/m^2 are administered, leucovorin calcium for injection should be reconstituted with Sterile Water for Injection, USP, and used immediately (see DOSAGE AND ADMINISTRATION.)

Because of the calcium content of the leucovorin solution, no more than 160 mg of leucovorin should be injected intravenously per minute (16 ml of a 10 mg/ml, or 8 ml of a 20 mg/ml solution per minute).

Leucovorin enhances the toxicity of 5-fluorouracil. When these drugs are administered concurrently in the palliative therapy of advanced colorectal cancer, the dosage of 5-fluorouracil must be lower than usually administered. Although the toxicities observed in patients treated with the combination of leucovorin plus 5-fluorouracil are qualitatively similar to those observed in patients treated with 5-fluorouracil alone, gastrointestinal toxicities (particularly stomatitis and diarrhea are observed more commonly and may be more severe and of prolonged duration in patients treated with the combination.

In the first Mayo/NCCTG controlled trial, toxicity, primarily gastrointestinal, resulted in 7% of patients requiring hospitalization when treated with 5-fluorouracil alone or 5-fluorouracil in combination with 200 mg/m^2 of leucovorin and 20% when treated with 5- fluorouracil in combination with 20 mg/m^2 of leucovorin. In the second Mayo/NCCTG trial, hospitalizations related to treatment toxicity also appeared to occur more often in patients treated with the low dose leucovorin/5-fluorouracil combination than in patients treated with the high dose combination—11% versus 3%. Therapy with leucovorin/5- fluorouracil must not be initiated or continued in patients who have symptoms of gastrointestinal toxicity of any severity, until those symptoms have completely resolved. Patients with diarrhea must be monitored with particular care until the diarrhea has resolved, as rapid clinical deterioration leading to death can occur. In an additional study utilizing higher weekly doses of 5-FU and leucovorin, elderly and/or debilitated patients were found to be at greater risk for severe gastrointestinal toxicity.[3]

PRECAUTIONS:

General: Parenteral administration is preferable to oral dosing if there is a possibility that the patient may vomit or not absorb the leucovorin. Leucovorin has no effect on other established toxicities of MTX such as the nephrotoxicity resulting from drug and/or metabolite precipitation in the kidney.

Pregnancy, Teratogenic Effects, Pregnancy Category C: Adequate animal reproduction studies have not been conducted with leucovorin. It is also not known whether leucovorin can cause fetal harm when administered to a pregnant woman or can affect reproduction capacity. Leucovorin should be given to a pregnant woman only if clearly needed.

Nursing Mothers: It is not known whether this drug is excreted in human milk. Because many drugs are excreted in human milk, caution should be exercised when leucovorin is administered to a nursing mother.

Pediatric Use: See DRUG INTERACTIONS.

Geriatric Use: *Injection:* **Since leucovorin enhances the toxicity of fluorouracil, leucovorin/5 fluorouracil combination therapy for advanced colorectal cancer should be administered under the supervision of a physician experienced in the use of antimetabolite cancer chemotherapy. Particular care should be taken in the treatment of elderly or debilitated colorectal cancer patients, as these patients may at increased risk of severe toxicity.**

Laboratory Tests: Patients being treated with the leucovorin/5-fluorouracil combination should have a CBC with differential and platelets prior to each treatment. During the first two courses a CBC with differential and platelets has to be repeated weekly and thereafter once each cycle at the time of anticipated WBC nadir. Electrolytes and liver function tests should be performed prior to each treatment for the first three cycles then prior to every other cycle. Dosage modifications of fluorouracil should be instituted as follows, based on the most severe toxicities (TABLE 1).

TABLE 1

Diarrhea and/or Stomatitis	WBC/mm^3 Nadir	Platelets/mm^3 Nadir	5-FU Dose
Moderate	1,000-1,900	25-75,000	decrease 20%
Severe	<1,000	<25,000	decrease 30%

If no toxicity occurs, the 5-fluorouracil dose may increase 10%.

Treatment should be deferred until WBC's are 4,000/mm^3 and platelets 130,000/mm^3. If blood counts do not reach these levels within two weeks, treatment should be discontinued. Patients should be followed up with physical examination prior to each treatment course and appropriate radiological examination as needed. Treatment should be discontinued when there is clear evidence of tumor progression.

DRUG INTERACTIONS:

Folic acid in large amounts may counteract the antiepileptic effect of phenobarbital, phenytoin and primidone, and increase the frequency of seizures in susceptible children.

Preliminary animal and human studies have shown that small quantities of systemically administered leucovorin enter the CSF primarily as 5- methyltetrahydrofolate and, in humans, remain 1-3 orders of magnitude lower than the usual methotrexate concentrations following intrathecal administration. However, high doses of leucovorin may reduce the efficacy of intrathecally administered methotrexate.

Leucovorin may enhance the toxicity of 5-fluorouracil (see WARNINGS.)

ADVERSE REACTIONS:

Allergic sensitization, including anaphylactoid reactions and urticaria, has been reported following administration of both oral and parenteral leucovorin. No other adverse reactions have been attributed to the use of leucovorin *per se.*

Injection: The following tables (TABLES 2A, 2B, 2C) summarize significant adverse events occurring in 316 patients treated with the leucovorin-5-fluorouracil combinations compared against 70 patients treated with 5-fluorouracil alone for advanced colorectal carcinoma. These data are taken from the Mayo/NCCTG large multicenter prospective trial evaluating the efficacy and safety of the combination regimen.

TABLE 2A Percentage Of Patients Treated With Leucovorin/Fluorouracil For Advanced Colorectal Carcinoma Reporting Adverse Experiences Or Hospitalized For Toxicity

	(High LV)/5-FU (N = 155) Any (%)	Grade 3+ (%)
Leukopenia	69	14
Thrombocytopenia	8	2
Infection	8	1
Nausea	74	10
Vomiting	46	8
Diarrhea	66	18
Stomatitis	75	27
Constipation	3	0
Lethargy/Malaise/Fatigue	13	3
Alopecia	42	5
Dermatitis	21	2
Anorexia	14	1
Hospitalization for Toxicity	5%	

High LV = Leucovorin 200 mg/m^2
Any = percentage of patients reporting toxicity of any severity
Grade 3+ = percentage of patients reporting toxicity of Grade 3 or higher

TABLE 2B

	(Low LV)/5-FU (N = 161) Any (%)	Grade 3+ (%)
Leukopenia	83	23
Thrombocytopenia	8	1
Infection	3	1
Nausea	80	9
Vomiting	44	9
Diarrhea	67	14
Stomatitis	84	29
Constipation	4	0
Lethargy/Malaise/Fatigue	12	2
Alopecia	43	6
Dermatitis	25	1
Anorexia	22	4
Hospitalization for Toxicity	15%	

LV = Leucovorin 20 mg/m^2
Any = percentage of patients reporting toxicity of any severity
Grade 3+ = percentage of patients reporting toxicity of Grade 3 or higher

TABLE 2C

	5-FU Alone (N = 70) Any (%)	Grade 3+ (%)
Leukopenia	93	48
Thrombocytopenia	18	3
Infection	7	2
Nausea	60	6
Vomiting	40	7
Diarrhea	43	11
Stomatitis	59	16
Constipation	1	-
Lethargy/Malaise/Fatigue	6	3
Alopecia	37	7
Dermatitis	13	-
Anorexia	14	-
Hospitalization for Toxicity	7%	

Any = percentage of patients reporting toxicity of any severity
Grade 3+ = percentage of patients reporting toxicity of Grade 3 or higher

OVERDOSAGE:

Excessive amounts of leucovorin may nullify the chemotherapeutic effect of folic acid antagonists.

DOSAGE AND ADMINISTRATION:

Leucovorin Rescue After High-Dose Methotrexate Therapy: The recommendations for leucovorin rescue are based on a methotrexate dose of 12-15 grams/m^2 administered by intravenous infusion over 4 hours (see methotrexate package insert for full prescribing information).[4]

Leucovorin rescue at a dose of 15 mg (approximately 10 mg/m^2) every 6 hours for 10 doses starts 24 hours after the beginning of the methotrexate infusion. In the presence of gastrointestinal toxicity, nausea or vomiting, leucovorin should be administered parenterally. Do not administer leucovorin intrathecally. Serum creatinine and methotrexate levels should be determined at least once daily. Leucovorin administration, hydration, and urinary alkalinization (pH of 7.0 or greater) should be continued until the methotrexate level is below 5×10^{-8} M (0.05 micromolar). The leucovorin dose should be adjusted or leucovorin rescue extended based on the following guidelines (TABLE 3):

Patients who experience delayed early methotrexate elimination are likely to develop reversible renal failure. In addition to appropriate leucovorin therapy, these patients require continuing hydration and urinary alkalinization, and close monitoring of fluid and electrolyte status, until the serum methotrexate level has fallen to below 0.05 micromolar and the renal failure has resolved.

Some patients will have abnormalities in methotrexate elimination or renal function following methotrexate administration, which are significant but less severe than the abnormalities described in the table above. These abnormalities may or may not be associated with significant clinical toxicity. If significant clinical toxicity is observed, leucovorin rescue should be extended for an additional 24 hours (total of 14 doses over 84 hours) in subsequent courses of therapy. The possibility that the patient is taking other medications which interact with methotrexate (*e.g.,* medications which may interfere with methotrexate elimination or binding to serum albumin) should always be reconsidered when laboratory abnormalities or clinical toxicities are observed.

TABLETS

Leucovorin calcium tablets are intended for oral administration. Because absorption is saturable, oral administration of doses greater than 25 mg is not recommended.

Impaired Methotrexate Elimination or Inadvertent Overdosage: The same dosage and administration guidelines may be used. However, leucovorin administration should begin as soon as possible after an Inadvertent overdosage is recognized.

DOSAGE AND ADMINISTRATION: *(cont'd)*

TABLE 3
Do Not Administer Leucovorin Intrathecally

Clinical Situation	Laboratory Findings	Leucovorin Dosage and Duration
Normal Methotrexate Elimination	Serum methotrexate level approximately 10 micromolar at 24 hours after administration, 1 micromolar at 48 hours, and less than 0.2 micromolar at 72 hours.	15 mg PO, IM, or IV q 6 hours for 60 hours (10 doses starting at 24 hours after start of methotrexate infusion).
Delayed Late Methotrexate Elimination	Serum methotrexate level remaining above 0.2 micromolar at 72 hours, and more than 0.05 micromolar at 96 hours after administration.	Continue 15 mg PO, IM, or IV q 6 hours, until methotrexate level is less than 0.05 micromolar.
Delayed Early Methotrexate Elimination and/or Evidence of Acute Renal Injury		150 mg IV q 3 hours, until methotrexate level is less than 1 micromolar; then 15 mg IV q 3 hours until methotrexate level is less than 0.05 micromolar.
level of 1 mg/dl or more).		

STORE BETWEEN 15°-30°C (59°-86°F). PROTECT FROM LIGHT.

INJECTION

Advanced Colorectal Cancer: Leucovorin should not be mixed in the same infusion as 5-fluorouracil because a precipitate may form. Either of the following two regimens is recommended:

1. Leucovorin is administered at 200 mg/m² by slow intravenous injection over a minimum of 3 minutes, followed by 5-fluorouracil at 370 mg/m² by intravenous injection.

2. Leucovorin is administered at 20 mg/m² by intravenous injection followed by 5-fluorouracil at 425 mg/m² by intravenous injection.

Treatment is repeated daily for five days. This five-day treatment course may be repeated at 4 week (28-day) intervals, for 2 courses and then repeated at 4-5 week (28-35 day) intervals provided that the patient has completely recovered from the toxic effects of the prior treatment course.

In subsequent treatment courses, the dosage of 5-fluorouracil should be adjusted based on patient tolerance of the prior treatment course. The daily dosage of 5-fluorouracil should be reduced by 20% for patients who experienced moderate hematologic or gastrointestinal toxicity in the prior treatment course, and by 30% for patients who experienced severe toxicity (see PRECAUTIONS, Laboratory Tests.) For patients who experienced no toxicity in the prior treatment course, 5-fluorouracil dosage may be increased by 10%. Leucovorin dosages are not adjusted for toxicity.

Several other doses and schedules of leucovorin/5-fluorouracil therapy have also been evaluated in patients with advanced colorectal cancer; some of these alternative regimens may also have efficacy in the treatment of this disease. However, further clinical research will be required to confirm the safety and effectiveness of these alternative leucovorin/5- fluorouracil treatment regimens.

Impaired Methotrexate Elimination or Inadvertent Overdosage: Leucovorin rescue should begin as soon as possible after an inadvertent overdosage and within 24 hours of methotrexate administration when there is delayed excretion (see WARNINGS.) Leucovorin 10 mg/m² should be administered IV, IM, or PO every 6 hours until the serum methotrexate level is less than 10^{-8} M. In the presence of gastrointestinal toxicity, nausea, or vomiting, leucovorin should be administered parenterally.

Serum creatinine and methotrexate levels should be determined at 24 hour intervals. If the 24 hour serum creatinine has increased 50% over baseline or if the 24 hour methotrexate level is greater than 5×10^{-6} M or the 48 hour level is greater than 9×10^{-7} M, the dose of leucovorin should be increased to 100 mg/m² IV every 3 hours until the methotrexate level is less than 10^{-8} M.

Hydration (3 L/d) and urinary alkalinization with sodium bicarbonate solution should be applied concomitantly. The bicarbonate dose should be adjusted to maintain the urine pH at 7.0 or greater.

Megaloblastic Anemia Due to Folic Acid Deficiency: Up to 1 mg daily. There is no evidence that doses greater than 1 mg/day have greater efficacy than those of 1 mg; additionally, loss of folate in urine becomes roughly logarithmic as the amount administered exceeds 1 mg.

Each 50 and 100 mg vial of leucovorin calcium for injection when reconstituted with 5 and 10 ml, respectively, of sterile diluent yields a leucovorin concentration of 10 mg per ml. Each 350 mg vial of leucovorin calcium for injection when reconstituted with 17 ml of sterile diluent yields a leucovorin concentration of 20 mg leucovorin per ml. Leucovorin calcium for injection contains no preservative. Reconstitute with Bacteriostatic Water for Injection, USP, which contains benzyl alcohol, or with Sterile Water for Injection, USP. When reconstituted with Bacteriostatic Water for Injection, USP, the resulting solution must be used within 7 days. If the product is reconstituted with Sterile Water for Injection, USP, it must be used immediately.

Because of the benzyl alcohol contained in Bacteriostatic Water for Injection, USP, when doses greater than 10 mg/m² are administered leucovorin calcium for injection should be reconstituted with Sterile Water for Injection, USP, and used immediately (see WARNINGS.) Because of the calcium content of the leucovorin solution, no more than 160 mg of leucovorin should be injected intravenously per minute (16 ml of a 10 mg/ml, or 8 ml of a 20 mg/ml solution per minute).

Parenteral drug products should be inspected visually for particulate matter and discoloration prior to administration, whenever solution and container permit.

STORE BETWEEN 15°-25°C (59°-77°F).

PROTECT FROM LIGHT.

(Tablets, Immunex, 5/94, 0164-00) (Injection, Immunex, 6/94, 0163-00)

REFERENCES:

Tablets 1. Grem, JL, Shoemaker, DD, Petrelli, NJ, Douglas, HO, "Severe and Fatal Toxic Effects Observed in Treatment with High- and Low-Dose Leucovorin Plus 5-Fluorouracil for Colorectal Carcinoma," *Cancer Treat Rep* 1987; 71:1122. **2.** Link, MP, Goorin, AM, Miser, AW, et al, "The Effect of Adjuvant Chemotherapy on Relapse-Free Survival in Patients with Osteosarcoma of the Extremity," *N Engl J Med* 1986; 314:1600-1606. **Injection 1.** Poon MA, et al. Biochemical Modulation of Fluorouracil: Evidence of Significant Improvement of Survival and Quality of Life in patients with Advanced Colorectal Carcinoma, *J Clin Oncol* 1989; 7:1407-1418. **2.** Poon MA, et al, Biochemical Modulation of Fluorouracil with Leucovorin: Confirmatory Evidence of Improved Therapeutic Efficacy in Advanced Colorectal Cancer, *J Clin Oncol* 1991; 9, 11:1967-1972. **3.** Grem JL, Shoemaker DD, Petrelli NJ, Douglas HO. "Severe and Fatal Toxic Effects Observed in Treatment with High-

REFERENCES: *(cont'd)*

and Low-Dose Leucovorin Plus 5-Fluorouracil for Colorectal Carcinoma," *Cancer Treat Rep* 1987; 71:1122. **4.** Link MP, Goorin AM, Miser AW, et al. "The Effect of Adjuvant Chemotherapy on Relapse-Free Survival in Patients with Osteosarcoma of the Extremity." *N Engl J Med* 1986; 314:1600-1606.

HOW SUPPLIED - RATED THERAPEUTICALLY EQUIVALENT:

Injection, Lyphl-Soln - Intramuscular; - 50 mg/vial

1's	$19.74	Leucovorin Calcium, Gensia Labs	00703-5130-01
1's	$88.75	Leucovorin Calcium, Fujisawa USA	00469-1370-30
1's	$119.00	Leucovorin Calcium, Harber Pharm	51432-0557-10
50 mg vial	$56.25	Leucovorin Calcium, Elkins Sinn	00641-2369-41
50 mg x 25	$538.13	Leucovorin Calcium, Lederle Parenterals	00205-5330-19

Injection, Lyphl-Soln - Intramuscular; - 100 mg/vial

1's	$39.00	Leucovorin Calcium, Gensia Labs	00703-5140-01
1's	$41.51	WELLCOVORIN, STERILE, Glaxo Wellcome	00173-0638-93
1's	$56.25	LEUCOVORIN CALCIUM, Elkins Sinn	00641-2364-41

Injection, Solution - Intravenous - 350 mg

10's	$1103.50	LEUCOVORIN CALCIUM, Immunex	58406-0623-33

Tablet, Uncoated - Oral - 5 mg

20's	$41.98	Leucovorin Calcium, H.C.F.A. F F P	99999-1630-01
20's	$59.24	WELLCOVORIN, Glaxo Wellcome	00173-0631-20
30's	$61.48	Leucovorin Calcium, Roxane	00054-4496-13
30's	$62.97	Leucovorin Calcium, Geneva Pharms	00781-1220-31
30's	$62.97	Leucovorin Calcium, H.C.F.A. F F P	99999-1630-02
30's	$70.81	Leucovorin Calcium, Barr	00555-0484-01
30's	$122.50	Leucovorin Calcium, Rugby	00536-4148-07
30's	$149.00	Leucovorin Calcium, Goldline Labs	00182-1869-17
50's	$104.96	Leucovorin Calcium, H.C.F.A. F F P	99999-1630-03
50's	$148.66	WELLCOVORIN, Glaxo Wellcome	00173-0631-35
100's	$202.68	Leucovorin Calcium, Roxane	00054-4496-25
100's	$209.93	Leucovorin Calcium, Geneva Pharms	00781-1220-01
100's	$209.93	Leucovorin Calcium, H.C.F.A. F F P	99999-1630-04
100's	$235.20	Leucovorin Calcium, Barr	00555-0484-02
100's	$297.33	WELLCOVORIN, Glaxo Wellcome	00173-0631-55
100's	$472.43	Leucovorin Calcium, HL Moore Drug Exch	00839-7463-06
100's	$493.45	Leucovorin Calcium, Major Pharms	00904-2315-60
100's	$551.87	Leucovorin Calcium, Qualitest Pharms	00603-4183-21
100's	$566.30	Leucovorin Calcium, Goldline Labs	00182-1869-01

Tablet, Uncoated - Oral - 10 mg

5 x 10	$349.84	Leucovorin Calcium, Lederle Pharm	00005-4525-64
12's	$69.86	LEUCOVORIN CALCIUM, Roxane	00054-4497-05
12's	$84.13	Leucovorin Calcium, Lederle Pharm	00005-4525-83
24's	$138.33	LEUCOVORIN CALCIUM, Roxane	00054-4497-10
24's	$168.11	Leucovorin Calcium, Lederle Pharm	00005-4525-90

Tablet, Uncoated - Oral - 15 mg

5 x 10	$430.80	LEUCOVERIN CALCIUM, Lederle Pharm	00005-4501-64
12's	$100.56	LEUCOVORIN CALCIUM, Immunex	58406-0626-68
12's	$104.81	LEUCOVORIN CALCIUM, Roxane	00054-4498-05
24's	$160.77	LEUCOVORIN CALCIUM, Immunex	58406-0626-74
24's	$195.62	LEUCOVORIN CALCIUM, Roxane	00054-4498-10

Tablet, Uncoated - Oral - 25 mg

10's	$210.18	WELLCOVORIN, Glaxo Wellcome	00173-0632-13
20 (2 x 10)	$273.75	Leucovorin Calcium, UDL	51079-0582-05
20's	$295.00	Leucovorin Calcium, Raway	00686-0582-05
25's	$475.07	Leucovorin Calcium, Roxane	00054-4499-11
25's	$525.45	WELLCOVORIN, Glaxo Wellcome	00173-0632-25
25's	$593.93	Leucovorin Calcium, HL Moore Drug Exch	00839-7464-08
25's	$600.00	Leucovorin Calcium, Barr	00555-0485-27
25's	$603.00	Leucovorin Calcium, Geneva Pharms	00781-1222-63
25's	$666.79	Leucovorin Calcium, Rugby	00536-4149-04
25's	$675.00	Leucovorin Calcium, Goldline Labs	00182-1870-24
25's	$680.34	Leucovorin Calcium, Qualitest Pharms	00603-4184-35

HOW SUPPLIED - NOT RATED EQUIVALENT:

Injection, Lyphl-Soln - Intramuscular; - 5 mg/ml

10 ml	$9.74	Leucovorin Calcium, Balan	00304-2177-56

Injection, Lyphl-Soln - Intramuscular; - 50 mg/vial

10's	$172.20	Leucovorin Calcium, Immunex	58406-0621-37

Injection, Lyphl-Soln - Intramuscular; - 100 mg/vial

10's	$315.30	Leucovorin Calcium, Immunex	58406-0622-35

Injection, Solution - Intramuscular - 3 mg/ml

1 ml x 6	$22.44	Leucovorin Calcium, Lederle Parenterals	00205-4004-51

Tablet, Uncoated - Oral - 5 mg

30's	$68.43	Leucovorin Calcium, Immunex	58406-0624-62
50's	$142.56	Leucovorin Calcium, Lederle Pharm	00005-4536-40
50's	$175.00	Leucovorin Calcium, Raway	00686-0561-06
100's	$494.99	Leucovorin Calcium, Balan	00304-1910-01

LEUPROLIDE ACETATE *(001631)*

CATEGORIES: Androgen Inhibitors; Anemia; Anterior Pituitary/Hypothalmic Function; Antineoplastics; Cancer; Gonadotropin Releasing; Hormones; Lh-Rh Analog; Oncologic Drugs; Orphan Drugs; Precocious Puberty; Prostatic Carcinoma; Pregnancy Category X; Sales > $500 Million; FDA Approved 1985 Apr; Patent Expiration 1996 Dec

BRAND NAMES: *Carcinil* (Germany); *Enanton Depot*; *Enantone* (France, Germany); *Enantone Depot*; *Enantone LP*; *Enantone SR*; *Leuplin*; *Leuplin Depot*; *Lucrin* (Australia, France, Mexico); *Lucrin Depot* (Mexico); *Lucrin Depot Inj* (Australia); *Luprolex*; **Lupron**; Lupron Depot; *Procren*; *Procren Depot*; *Procrin*; *Procrin Depot*; *Tapros*
(International brand names outside U.S. in italics)

FORMULARIES: Aetna; BC-BS; Medi-Cal

DESCRIPTION:

Lupron, Lupron Depot, and Lupron Depot-Ped (leuprolide acetate) are a synthetic nonapeptide analog of naturally occurring gonadotropin releasing hormone (GnRH or LH-RH). The analog possesses greater potency than the natural hormone. The chemical name is 5-Oxo-L-prolyl-L-histidyl-L-tryptophyl-L-seryl-L-tyrosyl-D-leucyl-L-leucyl-L-arginyl-N-ethyl-L-prolinamide acetate (salt).

DESCRIPTION: *(cont'd)*

Lupron Injection: Lupron is a sterile, aqueous solution intended for subcutaneous injection. It is available in a 2.8 ml multiple-dose vial containing 5 mg/ml of leuprolide acetate, sodium chloride for tonicity adjustment, 9 mg/ml of benzyl alcohol as a preservative and water for injection. The pH may have been adjusted with sodium hydroxide and/or acetic acid.

Lupron Injection (For Pediatric Use): Lupron Injection is a sterile, aqueous solution intended for daily subcutaneous injection.

A 2.8 ml multiple dose vial containing leuprolide acetate (5 mg/ml), sodium chloride (6.3 mg/ml) for tonicity adjustment, benzyl alcohol as a preservative (9 mg/ml), and water for injection. The pH may have been adjusted with sodium hydroxide and/or acetic acid.

Lupron Depot 3.75 mg and Lupron Depot 7.5 mg: Lupron Depot is supplied in a vial containing sterile lyophilized microspheres, which when mixed with diluent, become a suspension, which is intended as a monthly intramuscular injection.

Lupron Depot 3.75 mg: The single-dose vial of Lupron Depot contains leuprolide acetate (3.75 mg), purified gelatin (0.65 mg), DL-lactic and glycolic acids copolymer (33.1 mg), and D-mannitol (6.6 mg). The accompanying ampule of diluent contains carboxymethylcellulose sodium (7.5 mg), D-mannitol (75 mg), polysorbate 80 (1.5 mg), water for injection, USP, and glacial acetic acid, USP to control pH.

During the manufacturing process of Lupron Depot, acetic acid is lost, leaving the peptide.

Lupron Depot 7.5 mg: The single-dose vial of Lupron Depot contains leuprolide acetate (7.5 mg), purified gelatin (1.3 mg), DL-lactic and glycolic acids copolymer (66.2 mg), and D-mannitol (13.2 mg). The accompanying ampule of diluent contains carboxymethylcellulose sodium (7.5 mg), D-mannitol (75 mg), polysorbate 80 (1.5 mg), water for injection, USP, and acetic acid, NF to control pH.

During the manufacture of Lupron Depot, acetic acid is lost leaving the peptide.

Lupron Depot-Ped: Lupron Depot-Ped is supplied in a vial containing sterile lyophilized microspheres, which when mixed with diluent, become a suspension, intended as a single intramuscular injection.

The single-dose vial of Lupron Depot-Ped contains, respectively for each dosage strength, leuprolide acetate (7.5/11.25/15 mg), purified gelatin (1.3/1.95/2.6 mg), DL-lactic and glycolic acids copolymer (66.2/99.3/132.4 mg), and D-mannitol (13.2/19.8/26.4 mg). The accompanying ampule of diluent contains carboxymethylcellulose sodium (7.5 mg), D-mannitol (75 mg), polysorbate 80 (1.5 mg), water for injection, USP, and acetic acid, NF to control pH.

During the manufacture of Lupron Depot-Ped, acetic acid is lost leaving the peptide.

CLINICAL PHARMACOLOGY:

LUPRON INJECTION AND LUPRON DEPOT 7.5 MG

Leuprolide acetate, an LH-RH agonist, acts as a potent inhibitor of gonadotropin secretion when given continuously and in therapeutic doses. Animal and human studies indicate that following an initial stimulation, chronic administration of leuprolide acetate results in suppression of ovarian and testicular steroidogenesis. This effect is reversible upon discontinuation of drug therapy. Administration of leuprolide acetate has resulted in inhibition of the growth of certain hormone dependent tumors (prostatic tumors in Noble and Dunning male rats and DMBA-induced mammary tumors in female rats) as well as atrophy of the reproductive organs.

Lupron Injection: In humans, subcutaneous administration of single daily doses of leuprolide acetate results in an initial increase in circulation levels of luteinizing hormone (LH) and follicle stimulating hormone (FSH), leading to a transient increase in levels of the gonadal steroids (testosterone and dihydrotestosterone in males, and estrone and estradiol in pre-menopausal females). However, continuous daily administration of leuprolide acetate results in decreased levels of LH and FSH in all patients. In males, testosterone is reduced to castrate levels. In pre- menopausal females, estrogens are reduced to post-menopausal levels. These decreases occur within two to four weeks after initiation of treatment, and castrate levels of testosterone in prostatic cancer patients have been demonstrated for periods of up to five years.

Leuprolide acetate is not active when given orally. Bioavailability by subcutaneous administration is comparable to that by intravenous administration. Leuprolide acetate has a plasma half-life of approximately three hours. The metabolism, distribution and excretion of leuprolide acetate in man have not been determined.

Lupron Depot 7.5 mg: In humans, administration of leuprolide acetate results in an initial increase in circulating levels of luteinizing hormone (LH) and follicle stimulating hormone (FSH), leading to a transient increase in levels of the gonadal steroids (testosterone and dihydrotestosterone in males, and estrone and estradiol in pre-menopausal females). However, continuous administration of leuprolide acetate results in decreased levels of LH and FSH. In males, testosterone is reduced to castrate levels. In pre- menopausal females, estrogens are reduced to post-menopausal levels. These decreases occur within two to four weeks after initiation of treatment, and castrate levels of testosterone in prostatic cancer patients have been demonstrated for periods of up to five years.

Leuprolide acetate is not active when given orally. Following a single Lupron Depot injection to patients, mean peak leuprolide plasma concentration was almost 20 ng/ml at 4 hours and 0.36 ng/ml at 4 weeks. Nondetectable leuprolide plasma concentrations have been observed during chronic Lupron Depot administration, but testosterone levels appear to be maintained at castrate levels. The metabolism, distribution, and excretion of leuprolide in humans have not been determined.

LUPRON INJECTION (FOR PEDIATRIC USE) AND LUPRON DEPOT-PED

Leuprolide acetate, a GnRH agonist, acts as a potent inhibitor of gonadotropin secretion when given continuously and in therapeutic doses. Human studies indicate that following an initial stimulation of gonadotropins, chronic stimulation with leuprolide acetate results in suppression or "downregulation" of these hormones and consequent suppression of ovarian and testicular steroidogenesis. These effects are reversible on discontinuation of drug therapy.

In children with central precocious puberty (CPP), stimulated and basal gonadotropins are reduced to prepubertal levels. Testosterone and estradiol are reduced to prepubertal levels in males and females respectively. Reduction of gonadotropins will allow for normal physical and psychological growth and development. Natural maturation occurs when gonadotropins return to pubertal levels following discontinuation of leuprolide acetate.

The following physiologic effects have been noted with the chronic administration of leuprolide acetate in this patient population.

1. Skeletal Growth: A measurable increase in body length can be noted since the epiphyseal plates will not close prematurely.

2. Organ growth: Reproductive organs will return to a prepubertal state.

3. Menses: Menses, if present, will cease.

Lupron Injection (For Pediatric Use): Leuprolide acetate is not active when given orally. In adults, bioavailability by subcutaneous administration is comparable to that by intravenous administration; and leuprolide acetate has a plasma half-life of approximately three hours. The metabolism, distribution and excretion of leuprolide acetate in humans have not been determined. A pharmacokinetic study of leuprolide acetate in children has not been performed.

CLINICAL PHARMACOLOGY: *(cont'd)*

Lupron Depot-Ped: Leuprolide acetate is not active when given orally. In adults, intramuscular injection of the depot formulation provides plasma concentrations of leuprolide over a period of one month. The metabolism, distribution and excretion of leuprolide in humans have not been determined.

In a study of 22 children with central precocious puberty, doses of Lupron Depot were given every 4 weeks and plasma levels were determined according to weight categories as summarized below (TABLE 1):

TABLE 1

Patient Weight Range (kg)	Group Weight Average (kg)	Dose (mg)	Trough Plasma Leuprolide Level Mean ± SD (ng/ml)*
20.2 - 27.0	22.7	7.5	0.77 ± 0.033
28.4 - 36.8	32.5	11.25	1.25 ± 1.06
39.3 - 57.5	44.2	15.0	1.59 ± 0.65

* Group average values determined at Week 4 immediately prior to leuprolide injection. Drug levels at 12 and 24 weeks were similar to respective 4 week levels.

LUPRON DEPOT 3.75 MG

Leuprolide acetate is a long-acting GnRH analog. A single monthly injection of Lupron Depot results in an initial stimulation followed by a prolonged suppression of pituitary gonadotropins. Repeated dosing at monthly intervals results in decreased secretion of gonadal steroids; consequently, tissues and functions that depend on gonadal steroids for their maintenance become quiescent. This effect is reversible on discontinuation of drug therapy.

Leuprolide acetate is not active when given orally. Intramuscular injection of the depot formulation provides plasma concentrations of leuprolide over a period of one month.

Pharmacokinetics

Absorption: A single dose of Lupron Depot 3.75 mg was administered by intramuscular injection to healthy female volunteers. The absorption of leuprolide was characterized by an initial increase in plasma concentration, with peak concentration ranging from 4.6 to 10.2 ng/ml at four hours postdosing. However, intact leuprolide and an inactive metabolite could not be distinguished by the assay used in the study. Following the initial rise, leuprolide concentrations started to plateau within two days after dosing and remained relatively stable for about four to five weeks with plasma concentrations of about 0.30 ng/ml.

Distribution: The mean steady-state volume of distribution of leuprolide following intravenous bolus administration to healthy male volunteers was 27 l. *In vitro* binding to human plasma proteins ranged from 43% to 49%.

Metabolism: In healthy male volunteers, a 1 mg bolus of leuprolide administered intravenously revealed that the mean systemic clearance was 7.6 l/h, with a terminal elimination half-life of approximately 3 hours based on two compartment model.

In rats and dogs, administration of ^{14}C-labeled leuprolide was shown to be metabolized to smaller inactive peptides, pentapeptide (Metabolite I), tripeptide (Metabolite II and III) and dipeptide (Metabolite IV). These fragments may be further catabolized.

The major metabolite (M-I) plasma concentrations measured in 5 prostate cancer patients reached mean maximum concentration 2 to 6 hours after dosing and were approximately 6% of the peak parent drug concentration. One week after dosing, mean plasma M-I concentrations were approximately 20% of leuprolide concentrations.

Excretion: Following administration of Lupron Depot 3.75 mg to 3 patients, less than 5% of the dose was recovered as parent and M-I metabolite in the urine.

Special Populations: The pharmacokinetics of the drug in hepatically and renally impaired patients have not been determined.

CLINICAL STUDIES:

Endometriosis: In controlled clinical studies, Lupron Depot 3.75 mg monthly for six months was shown to be comparable to danazol 800 mg/day in relieving the clinical symptoms of endometriosis (pelvic pain, dysmenorrhea, dyspareunia, pelvic tenderness, and induration) and in reducing the size of endometrial implants as evidenced by laparoscopy. The clinical significance of a decrease in endometriotic lesions is not known at this time, and in addition laparoscopic staging of endometriosis does not necessarily correlate with the severity of symptoms.

Lupron Depot 3.75 mg monthly induced amenorrhea in 74% and 98% of the patients after the first and second treatment months respectively. Most of the remaining patients reported episodes of only light bleeding or spotting. In the first, second and third post-treatment months, normal menstrual cycles resumed in 7%, 71% and 95% respectively, of those patients who did not become pregnant.

Uterine Leiomyomata (Fibroids): In controlled clinical trials, administration of Lupron Depot 3.75 mg for a period of three or six months was shown to decrease uterine and fibroid volume, thus allowing for relief of clinical symptoms (abdominal bloating, pelvic pain, and pressure). Excessive vaginal bleeding (menorrhagia and menometorrhagia) decreased, resulting in improvement in hematologic parameters.

In three clinical trials, enrollment was not based on hematologic status. Mean uterine volume decreased by 41% and myoma volume decreased by 37% at final visit as evidenced by ultrasound or MRI. These patients also experienced a decrease in symptoms including excessive vaginal bleeding and pelvic discomfort. Benefit occurred by three months of therapy, but additional gain was observed with an additional three months of Lupron Depot 3.75 mg. Ninety-five percent of these patients became amenorrheic with 61%, 25%, and 4% experiencing amenorrhea during the first, second, and third treatment months respectively.

Post-treatment follow-up was carried out for a small percentage of Lupron Depot 3.75 mg patients among the 77% who demonstrated a ≥ 25% decrease in uterine volume while on therapy. Menses usually returned within two months of cessation of therapy. Mean time to return to pretreatment uterine size was 8.3 months. Regrowth did not appear to be related to pretreatment uterine volume.

In another controlled clinical study, enrollment was based on hematocrit ≤ 30% and/or hemoglobin ≤ 10.2 g/dl. Administration of Lupron Depot 3.75 mg, concomitantly with iron, produced an increase ≥ 6% hematocrit and ≥ 2 g/dl hemoglobin in 77% of patients at three months of therapy. The mean change in hematocrit was 10.1% and the mean change in hemoglobin was 4.2 g/dl. Clinical response was judged to be a hematocrit of ≥ 36% and hemoglobin of ≥ 12 g/dl, thus allowing for autologous blood donation prior to surgery. At three months, 75% of patients met this criterion.

At three months, 80% of patients experienced relief from either menorrhagia or menometorrhagia. As with the previous studies, episodes of spotting and menstrual-like bleeding were noted in some patients.

In this same study, a decrease of ≥ 25% was seen in uterine and myoma volumes in 60% and 54% of patients respectively. Lupron Depot 3.75 mg was found to relieve symptoms of bloating, pelvic pain, and pressure.

There is no evidence that pregnancy rates are enhanced or adversely affected by the use of Lupron Depot.

INDICATIONS AND USAGE:

LUPRON INJECTION AND LUPRON DEPOT 7.5 MG

Lupron (leuprolide acetate) is indicated in the palliative treatment of advanced prostatic cancer. It offers an alternative treatment of prostatic cancer when orchiectomy or estrogen administration are either not indicated or unacceptable to the patient.

Lupron Injection: In a controlled study comparing Lupron 1 mg/day given subcutaneously to DES (diethylstilbestrol), 3 mg/day, the survival rate for the two groups was comparable after two years treatment. The objective response to treatment was also similar for the two groups.

Lupron Depot 7.5 mg: In clinical trials, the safety and efficacy of Lupron Depot does not differ from that of the original daily subcutaneous injection.

LUPRON INJECTION (FOR PEDIATRIC USE) AND LUPRON DEPOT-PED

Lupron is indicated in the treatment of children with central precocious puberty. Children should be selected using the following criteria:

1. Clinical diagnosis of CPP (idiopathic or neurogenic) with onset of secondary sexual characteristics earlier than 8 years in females and 9 years in males.

2. Clinical diagnosis should be confirmed prior to initiation of therapy:

Confirmation of diagnosis by a pubertal response to a GnRH stimulation test. The sensitivity and methodology of this assay must be understood.

Bone age advanced one year beyond the chronological age.

3. Baseline evaluation should also include:

Height and weight measurements.

Sex steroid levels.

Adrenal steroid level to exclude congenital adrenal hyperplasia.

Beta human chorionic gonadotropin level to rule out a chorionic gonadotropic secreting tumor.

Pelvic/adrenal/testicular ultrasound to rule out a steroid secreting tumor.

Computerized tomography of the head to rule out intracranial tumor.

LUPRON DEPOT 3.75 MG

Endometriosis: Experience with Lupron Depot in females has been limited to women 18 years of age and older treated for 6 months.

Lupron Depot 3.75 mg is indicated for management of endometriosis, including pain relief and reduction of endometriotic lesions.

Uterine Leiomyomata (Fibroids): Experience with Lupron Depot in females has been limited to women 18 years of age and older.

Lupron Depot 3.75 mg and iron therapy are indicated for the preoperative hematologic improvement of patients with anemia caused by uterine leiomyomata. The clinician may wish to consider a one-month trial period on iron alone in as much as some of the patients will respond to iron alone (see CLINICAL STUDIES.) Lupron may be added if the response to iron alone is considered inadequate. Recommended duration of therapy with Lupron Depot is **up to** 3 months (TABLE 2).

TABLE 2 Percentage Of Patients Achieving Hemoglobin ≥ 12 gm/dl

Treatment Group	Week 4	Week 8	Week 12
Lupron Depot 3.75 mg with Iron	41*	71**	79*
Iron Alone	17	40	56

* P-Value < 0.01
** P-Value < 0.001

CONTRAINDICATIONS:

LUPRON INJECTION AND LUPRON DEPOT 7.5 MG

A report of an anaphylactic reaction to synthetic GnRH (Factrel) has been reported in the medical literature.[1]

Lupron is contraindicated in women who are or may become pregnant while receiving the drug. When administered on day 6 of pregnancy at test dosages of 0.00024, 0.0024, and 0.024 mg/kg (1/600 to 1/6 the human dose) to rabbits, Lupron produced a dose-related increase in major fetal abnormalities. Similar studies in rats failed to demonstrate an increase in fetal malformations. There was increased fetal mortality and decreased fetal weights with the two higher doses of Lupron in rabbits and with the highest dose in rats. The effects on fetal mortality are logical consequences of the alterations in hormonal levels brought about by this drug. Therefore, the possibility exists that spontaneous abortion may occur if the drug is administered during pregnancy.

LUPRON INJECTION (FOR PEDIATRIC USE) AND LUPRON DEPOT-PED

Lupron is contraindicated in women who are or may become pregnant while receiving the drug. When administered on day 6 of pregnancy at test dosages of 0.00024, 0.0024, and 0.024 mg/kg (1/1200 to 1/12 the human pediatric dose) to rabbits, Lupron produced a dose-related increase in major fetal abnormalities. Similar studies in rats failed to demonstrate an increase in fetal malformations. There was increased fetal mortality and decreased fetal weights with the two higher doses of Lupron in rabbits and with the highest dose in rats. The effects on fetal mortality are logical consequences of the alterations in hormonal levels brought about by this drug. Therefore, the possibility exists that spontaneous abortion may occur if the drug is administered during pregnancy.

Leuprolide acetate is contraindicated in children demonstrating hypersensitivity to GnRH, GnRH agonist analogs, or any of the excipients.

A report of an anaphylactic reaction to synthetic GnRH (Factrel) has been reported in the medical literature.[1]

LUPRON DEPOT 3.75 MG

1. Hypersensitivity to GnRH, GnRH agonist analogs or any of the excipients in Lupron Depot.

2. Undiagnosed abnormal vaginal bleeding.

3. Lupron Depot is contraindicated in women who are or may become pregnant while receiving the drug. Lupron Depot may cause fetal harm when administered to a pregnant woman. Major fetal abnormalities were observed in rabbits but not in rats after administration of Lupron Depot throughout gestation. There was increased fetal mortality and decreased fetal weights in rats and rabbits (see PRECAUTIONS, Pregnancy.) The effects on fetal mortality are expected consequences of the alterations in hormonal levels brought about by the drug. If this drug is used during pregnancy or if the patient becomes pregnant while taking this drug, she should be apprised of the potential hazard to the fetus.

4. Use in women who are breast feeding (see PRECAUTIONS, Nursing Mothers.)

5. A report of an anaphylactic reaction to synthetic GnRH (Factrel) has been reported in the medical literature.[1]

WARNINGS:

LUPRON INJECTION

Isolated cases of worsening of signs and symptoms during the first weeks of treatment have been reported. Worsening of symptoms may contribute to paralysis with or without fatal complications.

LUPRON INJECTION (FOR PEDIATRIC USE) AND LUPRON DEPT-PED

During the early phase of therapy, gonadotropins and sex steroids rise above baseline because of the natural stimulatory effect of the drug. Therefore, an increase in clinical signs and symptoms may be observed (see CLINICAL PHARMACOLOGY.)

Noncompliance with drug regimen or inadequate dosing may result in inadequate control of the pubertal process. The consequences of poor control include the return of pubertal signs such as menses, breast development, and testicular growth. The long-term consequences of inadequate control of gonadal steroid secretion are unknown, but may include a further compromise of adult stature.

LUPRON DEPOT 3.75 MG

Safe use of leuprolide acetate in pregnancy has not been established clinically. Before starting treatment with Lupron Depot, pregnancy must be excluded.

When used monthly at the recommended dose, Lupron Depot usually inhibits ovulation and stops menstruation. Contraception is not insured, however, by taking Lupron Depot. Therefore, patients should use nonhormonal methods of contraception. Patients should be advised to see their physician if they believe they may be pregnant. If a patient becomes pregnant during treatment, the drug must be discontinued and the patient must be apprised of the potential risk to the fetus.

During the early phase of therapy, sex steroids temporarily rise above baseline because of the physiologic effect of the drug. Therefore, an increase in clinical signs and symptoms may be observed during the initial days of therapy, but these will dissipate with continued therapy.

LUPRON DEPOT 7.5 MG

Isolated cases of worsening of signs and symptoms during the first weeks of treatment have been reported with LH-RH analogs. Worsening of symptoms may contribute to paralysis with or without fatal complications. For patients at risk, the physician may consider initiating therapy with daily Lupron (leuprolide acetate) Injection for the first two weeks to facilitate withdrawal of treatment if that is considered necessary.

PRECAUTIONS:

GENERAL

Lupron Injection and Lupron Depot 7.5 mg: Patients with metastatic vertebral lesions and/or with urinary tract obstruction should be closely observed during the first few weeks of therapy [see ADVERSE REACTIONS - (Lupron Injection) section] and [see WARNINGS - (Lupron Depot 7.5 mg) section].

LABORATORY TESTS

Lupron Injection and Lupron Depot 7.5 mg: Response to leuprolide acetate should be monitored by measuring serum levels of testosterone and acid phosphatase. In the majority of patients, testosterone levels increased above baseline during the first week, declining thereafter to baseline levels or below by the end of the second week of treatment. Castrate levels were reached within two to four weeks and once achieved were maintained for as long as drug administration continued or for as long as the patients received their monthly injection on time. Transient increases in acid phosphatase levels may occur sometime early in treatment. However, by the fourth week, the elevated levels usually can be expected to decrease to values at or near baseline.

Lupron Injection (For Pediatric Use) and Lupron Depot-Ped Response to leuprolide acetate should be monitored 1-2 months after the start of therapy with a GnRH stimulation test and sex steroid levels. Measurement of bone age for advancement should be done every 6-12 months.

Sex steroids may increase or rise above prepubertal levels if the dose is inadequate (see WARNINGS.) Once a therapeutic dose has been established, gonadotropin and sex steroid levels will decline to prepubertal levels.

DRUG/LABORATORY TEST INTERACTIONS

Lupron Injection (For Pediatric Use) and Lupron Depot-Ped: Administration of leuprolide acetate in therapeutic doses results in suppression of the pituitary-gonadal system. Normal function is usually restored within 4 to 12 weeks after treatment is discontinued.

Lupron Depot 3.75 mg Administration of Lupron Depot in therapeutic doses results in suppression of the pituitary-gonadal system. Normal function is usually restored within one to three months after treatment is discontinued. Therefore, diagnostic tests of pituitary gonadotropic and gonadal functions conducted during treatment and up to one to two months after discontinuation of Lupron Depot therapy may be misleading.

INFORMATION FOR PATIENTS

Lupron Injection: NOTE: Be sure to consult your physician with any questions you may have or for information about Lupron (leuprolide acetate) Injection and its use.

Lupron Injection (For Pediatric Use): Prior to starting therapy with Lupron Injection, the parent or guardian must be aware of the importance of continuous therapy. Adherence to daily drug administration schedules must be accepted if therapy is to be successful.

Lupron Depot-Ped: Prior to starting therapy with Lupron Depot-Ped, the parent or guardian must be aware of the importance of continuous therapy. Adherence to 4 week drug administration schedules must be accepted if therapy is to be successful.

Lupron Injection and Lupron Injection (For Pediatric Use): Patients with known allergies to benzyl alcohol, an ingredient of the drug's vehicle, may present symptoms of hypersensitivity, usually local, in the form of erythema and induration at the injection site.

Lupron Injection (For Pediatric Use) and Lupron Depot-Ped

During the first 2 months of therapy, a female may experience menses or spotting. If bleeding continues beyond the second month, notify the physician.

Any irritation at the injection site should be reported to the physician immediately.

Report any unusual signs or symptoms to the physician.

Lupron Depot 3.75 mg: An information pamphlet for patients is included with the product. Patients should be aware of the following information:

1. Since menstruation should stop with effective doses of Lupron Depot, the patient should notify her physician if regular menstruation persists. Patients missing successive doses of Lupron Depot may experience breakthrough bleeding.

2. Patients should not use Lupron Depot if they are pregnant, breast feeding, have undiagnosed abnormal vaginal bleeding, or are allergic to any of the ingredients in Lupron Depot.

3. Safe use of the drug in pregnancy has not been established clinically. Therefore, a nonhormonal method of contraception should be used during treatment. Patients should be advised that if they miss successive doses of Lupron Depot, breakthrough bleeding or ovulation may occur with the potential for contraception. If a patient becomes pregnant during treatment, she should discontinue treatment and consult her physician.

PRECAUTIONS: *(cont'd)*

4. Adverse events occurring in clinical studies with Lupron Depot that are associated with hypoestrogenism include: hot flashes, headaches, emotional lability, decreased libido, acne, myalgia, reduction in breast size, and vaginal dryness. Estrogen levels returned to normal after treatment was discontinued.

5. The induced hypoestrogenic state **also** results in a small loss in bone density over the course of treatment, some of which may not be reversible. For a period up to six months, this bone loss should not be important. In patients with major risk factors for decreased bone mineral content such as chronic alcohol and/or tobacco use, strong family history of osteoporosis, or chronic use of drugs that can reduce bone mass such as anticonvulsants or corticosteroids, Lupron Depot therapy may pose an additional risk. In these patients, the risks and benefits must be weighed carefully before therapy with Lupron Depot is instituted. Repeated courses of therapy with gonadotropin-releasing hormone analogs beyond six months are not advisable in patients with major risk factors for loss of bone mineral content.

6. Retreatment cannot be recommended since safety data beyond six months are not available.

CARCINOGENESIS, MUTAGENESIS, IMPAIRMENT OF FERTILITY

Lupron Injection (For Pediatric Use) and Lupron Depot-Ped: Although no clinical studies have been completed in children to assess the full reversibility of fertility suppression, animal studies (prepubertal and adult rats and monkeys) with leuprolide acetate and other GnRH analogs have shown functional recovery. However, following a study with leuprolide acetate, immature male rats demonstrated tubular degeneration in the testes even after a recovery period. In spite of the failure to recover histologically, the treated males proved to be as fertile as the controls. Also, no histologic changes were observed in the female rats following the same protocol. In both sexes, the offspring of the treated animals appeared normal. The effect of the treatment of the parents on the reproductive performance of the F1 generation was not tested. The clinical significance of these findings is unknown.

Lupron Injection (For Pediatric Use), Lupron Depot 3.75 mg, and Lupron Depot-Ped: A two-year carcinogenicity study was conducted in rats and mice. In rats, a dose- related increase of benign pituitary hyperplasia and benign pituitary adenomas was noted at 24 months when the drug was administered subcutaneously at high daily doses (0.6 to 4 mg/kg). There was a significant but not dose-related increase of pancreatic islet-cell adenomas in females and of testicular interstitial cell adenomas in males (highest incidence in the low dose group). In mice, no leuprolide acetate-induced tumors or pituitary abnormalities were observed at a dose as high as 60 mg/kg for two years. Adult patients have been treated with leuprolide acetate for up to three years with doses as high as 10 mg/day and for two years with doses as high as 20 mg/day without demonstrable pituitary abnormalities.

Lupron Depot 3.75 mg: Mutagenicity studies have been performed with leuprolide acetate using bacterial and mammalian systems. These studies provided no evidence of a mutagenic potential.

Clinical and pharmacologic studies in adults with leuprolide acetate and similar analogs have shown full reversibility of fertility suppression when the drug is discontinued after continuous administration for periods of up to six months. Although no clinical studies have been completed in children to assess the full reversibility of fertility suppression, animal studies (prepubertal and adult rats and monkeys) with leuprolide acetate and other GnRH analogs have shown functional recovery.

Two-year carcinogenicity studies were conducted in rats and mice. In rats, a dose- related increase of benign pituitary hyperplasia and benign pituitary adenomas was noted at 24 months when the drug was administered subcutaneously at high daily doses (0.6 to 4 mg/kg). In mice no pituitary abnormalities were observed at a dose as high as 60 mg/kg for two years. Patients have been treated with leuprolide acetate for up to three years with doses as high as 10 mg/day and for two years with doses as high as 20 mg/day without demonstrable pituitary abnormalities.

Mutagenicity studies have been performed with leuprolide acetate using bacterial and mammalian systems. These studies provided no evidence of a mutagenic potential.

Clinical and pharmacologic studies with leuprolide acetate and similar analogs have shown full reversibility of fertility suppression when the drug is discontinued after continuous administration for periods of up to 24 weeks.

Lupron Injection: However, no clinical studies have been conducted with leuprolide acetate to assess the reversibility of fertility suppression.

PREGANACY

Lupron Injection, Lupron Injection (For Pediatric Use), Lupron Depot 7.5 mg, and Lupron Depot-Ped: Pregnancy Category X. See CONTRAINDICATIONS.

Lupron Depot 3.75 mg: Pregnancy, Teratogenic Effects: Pregnancy Category X. (See CONTRAINDICATIONS.) When administered on day 6 of pregnancy at test dosages of 0.00024, 0.0024, and 0.024 mg/kg (1/300 to 1/3 the human dose) to rabbits, Lupron Depot produced a dose-related increase in major fetal abnormalities. Similar studies in rats failed to demonstrate an increase in fetal malformations. There was increased fetal mortality and decreased fetal weights with the two higher doses of Lupron Depot in rabbits and with the highest dose (0.024 mg/kg) in rats.

NURSING MOTHERS

Lupron Depot 3.75 mg: It is not known whether Lupron Depot is excreted in human milk. Because many drugs are excreted in human milk, and because the effects of Lupron Depot on lactation and/or the breastfed child have not been determined, Lupron Depot should not be used by nursing mothers.

Lupron Injection (For Pediatric Use) and Lupron Depot-Ped It is not known whether leuprolide acetate is excreted in human milk. Lupron should not be used by nursing mothers.

PEDIATRIC USE

Lupron Depot 3.75 mg: See Lupron Depot-Ped (leuprolide acetate for depot suspension) labeling for the safety and effectiveness in children with central precocious puberty.

DRUG INTERACTIONS:

Lupron Injection and Lupron Depot 7.5 mg: None have been reported.

Lupron Injection (For Pediatric Use), Lupron Depot 3.75 mg, and Lupron Depot-Ped: No pharmacokinetic-based drug-drug interaction studies have been conducted. However, because leuprolide acetate is a peptide that is primarily degraded by peptidase and not by cytochrome P-450 enzymes as noted in specific studies, and the drug is only about 46% bound to plasma proteins, drug interactions would not be expected to occur.

ADVERSE REACTIONS:

LUPRON INJECTION

In the majority of patients testosterone levels increased above baseline during the first week, declining thereafter to baseline levels or below by the end of the second week of treatment. This transient increase was occasionally associated with a temporary worsening of signs and symptoms, usually manifested by an increase in bone pain (See WARNINGS.) In a few cases a temporary worsening of existing hematuria and urinary tract obstruction occurred during the first week. Temporary weakness and paresthesia of the lower limbs have been reported in a few cases.

ADVERSE REACTIONS: *(cont'd)*

Potential exacerbations of signs and symptoms during the first few weeks of treatment is a concern in patients with vertebral metastases and/or urinary obstruction which, if aggravated, may lead to neurological problems or increase the obstruction.

In a comparative trial of Lupron (leuprolide acetate) Injection versus DES, in 5% or more of the patients receiving either drug, the following adverse reactions were reported to have a possible or probable relationship to drug as ascribed by the treating physician. Often, causality is difficult to assess in patients with metastatic prostate cancer. Reactions considered not drug related are excluded (TABLE 3).

TABLE 3

	LUPRON (N=98)	DES (N=101)
	Number of Reports	
Cardiovascular System		
Congestive heart failure	1	5
ECG changes/ischemia	19	22
High blood pressure	8	5
Murmur	3	8
Peripheral edema	12	30
Phlebitis/thrombosis	2	10
Gastrointestinal System		
Anorexia	6	5
Constipation	7	9
Nausea/vomiting	5	17
Endocrine System		
*Decreased testicular size	7	11
*Gynecomastia/breast tenderness or pain	7	63
*Hot flashes	55	12
*Impotence	4	12
Hemic And Lymphatic System		
Anemia	5	5
Musculoskeletal System		
Bone pain	5	2
Myalgia	3	9
Central/Peripheral Nervous System		
Dizziness/lightheadedness	5	7
General pain	13	13
Headache	7	4
Insomnia/sleep disorders	7	5
Respiratory System		
Dyspnea	2	8
Sinus congestion	5	6
Integumentary System		
Dermatitis	5	8
Urogenital System		
Frequency/urgency	6	8
Hematuria	6	4
Urinary tract infection	3	7
Miscellaneous		
Asthenia	10	10

*Physiologic effect of decreased testosterone.

In this same study, the following adverse reactions were reported in less than 5% of the patients on Lupron.

Cardiovascular System: Angina, Cardiac arrhythmias, Myocardial infarction, Pulmonary emboli; *Gastrointestinal System:* Diarrhea, Dysphagia, Gastrointestinal bleeding, Gastrointestinal disturbance, Peptic ulcer, Rectal polyps; *Endocrine System:* Libido decrease, Thyroid enlargement; *Musculoskeletal System:* Joint pain;*Central/Peripheral Nervous System:* Anxiety, Blurred vision, Lethargy, Memory disorder, Mood swings, Nervousness, Numbness, Paresthesia, Peripheral neuropathy, Syncope/blackouts, Taste disorders;*Respiratory System:* Cough, Pleural rub, Pneumonia, Pulmonary fibrosis; *Integumentary System:* Carcinoma of skin/ear, Dry skin, Ecchymosis, Hair loss, Itching, Local skin reactions, Pigmentation, Skin lesions; *Urogenital System:* Bladder spasms, Dysuria, Incontinence, Testicular pain, Urinary obstruction;*Miscellaneous:* Depression, Diabetes, Fatigue, Fever/chills, Hypoglycemia, Increased BUN, Increased calcium, Increased creatinine, Infection/inflammation, Ophthalmologic disorders, Swelling (temporal bone).

The following additional adverse reactions have been reported with Lupron or Lupron Depot (leuprolide acetate for depot suspension) during other clinical trials and/or during postmarketing surveillance. Reactions considered as nondrug related by the treating physician are excluded.

Cardiovascular System: Hypotension, Transient ischemic attack/stroke; *Gastrointestinal System:* Hepatic dysfunction;*Endocrine System:* Libido increase; *Hemic and Lymphatic System:* Decreased WBC, Hemoptysis; *Musculoskeletal System:* Ankylosing spondylosis, Pelvic fibrosis; *Central/Peripheral Nervous System:* Hearing disorder, Peripheral neuropathy, Spinal fracture/paralysis; *Respiratory System:* Pulmonary infiltrate, Respiratory disorders; *Integumentary System:* Hair growth;*Urogenital System:* Penile swelling, Prostate pain;*Miscellaneous:* Hypoproteinemia, Hard nodule in throat, Weight gain, Increased uric acid.

LUPRON DEPOT 7.5 MG

In the majority of patients testosterone levels increased above baseline during the first week, declining thereafter to baseline levels or below by the end of the second week of treatment.

Potential exacerbations of signs and symptoms during the first few weeks of treatment is a concern in patients with vertebral metastases and/or urinary obstruction or hematuria which, if aggravated, may lead to neurological problems such as temporary weakness and/or paresthesia of the lower limbs or worsening of urinary symptoms (see WARNINGS.)

In a clinical trial of Lupron Depot (leuprolide acetate for depot suspension), the following adverse reactions were reported to have a possible or probable relationship to drug as ascribed by the treating physician in 5% or more of the patients receiving the drug. Often, causality is difficult to assess in patients with metastatic prostate cancer. Reactions considered not drug related are excluded (TABLE 4).

Laboratory: Elevations of certain parameters were observed, but it is difficult to assess these abnormalities in this population (TABLE 5).

In this same study, the following adverse reactions were reported in less than 5% of the patients on Lupron Depot.

Cardiovascular System: Angina, Cardiac arrhythmia

Gastrointestinal System: Anorexia, Diarrhea

Endocrine System: Gynecomastia, Libido decrease

Musculoskeletal System: Bone pain, Myalgia

Central/Peripheral Nervous System: Paresthesia, Insomnia

Respiratory System: Hemoptysis

Integumentary System: Dermatitis, Local skin reactions, Hair growth

Urogenital System: Dysuria, Frequency/urgency, Hematuria, Testicular pain

ADVERSE REACTIONS: *(cont'd)*

TABLE 4

	LUPRON DEPOT (N=56)	(Percent)
Cardiovascular System		
Edema	7	(12.5%)
Gastrointestinal System		
Nausea/vomiting	3	(5.4%)
Endocrine System		
*Decreased testicular size	3	(5.4%)
*Hot flashes/sweats	33	(58.9%)
*Impotence	3	(5.4%)
Central/Peripheral Nervous System		
General pain	4	(7.1%)
Respiratory System		
Dyspnea	3	(5.4%)
Miscellaneous		
Asthenia	3	(5.4%)

* Physiologic effect of decreased testosterone.

TABLE 5

SGOT (>2N)	4	(5.4%)
LDH (>2N)	11	(19.6%)
Alkaline phos (>1.5 N)	4	(5.4%)

Miscellaneous: Diabetes, Fever/chills, Hard nodule in throat, Increased calcium, Weight gain, Increased uric acid.

The following additional adverse reactions have been reported with Lupron (leuprolide acetate) Injection. Reactions considered by the treating physician as nondrug related are not included.

Cardiovascular System: Congestive heart failure, ECG changes/ischemia, High blood pressure, Hypotension, Myocardial infarction, Murmur, Phlebitis/thrombosis, Pulmonary emboli, Transient ischemic attack/stroke

Gastrointestinal System: Constipation, Dysphagia, Gastrointestinal bleeding, Gastrointestinal disturbance, Hepatic dysfunction, Peptic ulcer, Rectal polyps

Endocrine System: Breast tenderness or pain, Libido increase, Thyroid enlargement

Hemic and Lymphatic System: Anemia, Decreased WBC

Musculoskeletal System: Ankylosing spondylosis, Joint pain, Pelvic fibrosis

Central/Peripheral Nervous System: Anxiety, Blurred vision, Dizziness/light-headedness, Headache, Hearing disorder, Sleep disorders, Lethargy, Memory disorder, Mood swings, Nervousness, Numbness, Peripheral neuropathy, Spinal fracture/paralysis, Syncope/blackouts, Taste disorders

Respiratory System: Cough, Pleural rub, Pneumonia, Pulmonary fibrosis, Pulmonary infiltrate, Respiratory disorders, Sinus congestion

Integumentary System: Carcinoma of the skin/ear, Dry skin, Ecchymosis, Hair loss, Itching, Pigmentation, Skin lesions

Urogenital System: Bladder spasms, Incontinence, Penile swelling, Prostrate pain, Urinary obstruction, Urinary tract infection

Miscellaneous: Depression, Hypoglycemia, Hypoproteinemia, Increased BUN, Increased creatinine, Infection/inflammation, Ophthalmologic disorders, Swelling (temporal bone).

LUPRON INJECTION (FOR PEDIATRIC USE) AND LUPRON DEPOT-PED

Potential exacerbation of signs and symptoms during the first few weeks of treatment (See PRECAUTIONS) is a concern in patients with rapidly advancing central precocious puberty.

In two studies of children with central precocious puberty, in 2% or more of the patients receiving the drug, the following adverse reactions were reported to have a possible or probable relationship to drug as ascribed by the treating physician. Reactions considered not drug related are excluded (TABLE 6).

TABLE 6

	Number of Patients N = 395	(Percent)
Body as a Whole		
General Pain	7	(2)
Integumentary System Acne/Seborrhea	7	(2)
Injection Site Reactions Including Abscess	21	(5)
Rash Including Erythema Multiforme	8	(2)
Urogenital System		
Vaginitis/Bleeding/Discharge	7	(2)

In those same studies, the following adverse reactions were reported in less than 2% of the patients. *Body as a Whole:* Body Odor, Fever, Headache, Infection;*Cardiovascular System:* Syncope, Vasodilation; *Digestive System:* Dysphagia, Gingivitis, Nausea/Vomiting; *Endocrine System:* Accelerated Sexual Maturity; *Metabolic and Nutritional Disorders:* Peripheral Edema, Weight Gain; *Nervous System:* Nervousness, Personality Disorder, Somnolence, Emotional Lability;*Respiratory System:* Epistaxis; *Integumentary System:* Alopecia, Skin Striae; *Urogenital System:* Cervix Disorder, Gynecomastia/Breast Disorders, Urinary Incontinence.

See other leuprolide package inserts for adverse events reported in other patient populations.

LUPRON DEPOT 3.75 MG

Estradiol levels may increase during the first weeks following the initial injection, but then decline to menopausal levels. This transient increase in estradiol can be associated with a temporary worsening of signs and symptoms (see WARNINGS.)

As would be expected with a drug that lowers serum estradiol levels, the most frequently reported adverse reactions were those related to hypoestrogenism.

Endometriosis: In controlled studies comparing Lupron Depot, 3.75 mg monthly and danazol (800 mg/day), or placebo, adverse reactions most frequently reported and thought to be possibly or probably drug- related. *Cardiovascular System:* Palpitations, Syncope, Tachycardia;*Gastrointestinal System:* Dry mouth, Thirst, Appetite changes;*Central/Peripheral Nervous System:* Anxiety,* Personality disorder, Memory disorder, Delusions; *Integumentary System:* Ecchymosis, Alopecia, Hair disorder; *Urogenital System:* Dysuria,* Lactation; *Miscellaneous:* Ophthalmologic disorders,* Lymphadenopathy.

Uterine Leiomyomata (Fibroids): In controlled clinical trials comparing Lupron Depot 3.75 mg and placebo, adverse events reported in >5% of patients and thought to be potentially related to drug are noted in the following table (TABLE 7).

Symptoms reported in < 5% of patients included: *Body as Whole :* Body odor, Flu syndrome, Injection site reactions; *Cardiovascular System:* Tachycardia; *Digestive System:* Appetite changes, Dry mouth, GI disturbances, Nausea/vomiting; *Metabolic and Nutritional Disorders:* Weight changes; *Musculoskeletal System* :Myalgia; *Nervous System:* Anxiety, Decreased libido,* Dizziness, Insomnia, Nervousness,* Neuromuscular disorders,* Paresthesias; *Respiratory System:* Rhinitis; *Integumentary System:* Androgen-like effects, Nail disorder, Skin reactions;*Special Senses:* Conjunctivitis, Taste perversion;*Urogenital System:* Breast changes,* Menstrual disorders.

* = Physiologic effect of the drug.

ADVERSE REACTIONS: *(cont'd)*

TABLE 7

	Lupron Depot N=166 (%)	Placebo N=163 (%)
Body as a Whole		
Asthenia	14 (8.4)	8 (4.9)
General pain	14 (8.4)	10 (6.1)
Headache*	43 (25.9)	29 (17.8)
Cardiovascular System		
Hot flashes/sweats*	121 (72.9)	29 (17.8)
Metabolic and Nutritional Disorders		
Edema	9 (5.4)	2 (1.2)
Musculoskeletal System		
Joint disorder*	13 (7.8)	5 (3.1)
Nervous System		
Depression/emotional lability*	18 (10.8)	7 (4.3)
Urogenital System		
Vaginitis*	19 (11.4)	3 (1.8)

In one controlled clinical trial, patients received a higher dose (7.5 mg) of Lupron Depot. Events seen with this dose that were thought to be potentially related to drug and were not seen at the lower dose included palpitations, syncope, glossitis, ecchymosis, hypesthesia, confusion, lactation, pyelonephritis, and urinary disorders. Generally, a higher incidence of hypoestrogenic effects was observed at the higher dose.

In other clinical trials involving patients with prostate cancer and during postmarketing surveillance, the following adverse reactions were reported to have a possible, probable, or unknown relationship to Lupron as ascribed by the treating physician. Often, it is difficult to assess causality in patients with prostate cancer. Reactions considered not drug related have been excluded. *Cardiovascular System:* Congestive heart failure, ECG changes/ischemia, High blood pressure, Murmur, Phlebitis/thrombosis, Angina, Cardiac arrhythmias, Myocardial infarction, Pulmonary emboli, Hypotension, Transient ischemic attack/stroke; *Gastrointestinal System:* Dysphagia, Gastrointestinal bleeding, Peptic ulcer, Rectal polyps, Hepatic dysfunction; *Endocrine System:* Decreased testicular size, gynecomastia, Impotence, Libido increase, Thyroid enlargement; *Hemic and Lymphatic System:* Anemia, Decreased WBC, Hemoptysis; *Musculoskeletal System:*Bone pain;*Central/Peripheral Nervous System:* Peripheral neuropathy, Syncope/blackouts, Hearing disorder, Spinal fracture/paralysis;*Respiratory System:* Dyspnea, Sinus congestion, Cough, Pleural rub, Pneumonia, Pulmonary fibrosis, Respiratory disorders;*Urogenital System:* Frequency/urgency, Hematuria, Urinary tract infection, Bladder spasm, Incontinence, Testicular pain, Urinary obstruction, Penile swelling, Prostrate pain; *Miscellaneous:* Diabetes, Fever, Hypoglycemia, Increased BUN, Increased calcium, Increased creatinine, Inflammation.

CHANGES IN BONE DENSITY

Endometriosis: A controlled study in endometriosis patients showed that vertebral bone density as measured by dual energy x-ray absorptiometry (DEXA) decreased by an average of 3.9% at six months compared with the pretreatment value. Earlier studies in endometriosis patients, utilizing quantitative computed tomography (QCT), demonstrated that in the few patients who were retested at six and 12 months, partial to complete recovery of bone density was recorded in the post-treatment period. Use of Lupron Depot for longer than six months or in the presence of other known risk factors for decreased bone mineral content may cause additional bone loss.

Uterine Leiomyomata (Fibroids): In one study, vertebral trabecular bone mineral density as assessed by quantitative digital radiography (QDR) revealed a mean decrease of 2.7% at three months compared with the pretreatment value. It would be anticipated that this loss of bone mineral density would be complete to partially reversible following discontinuation of therapy. Use of Lupron Depot 3.75 mg for uterine leiomyomata for longer than three months or in the presence of other known risk factors for decreased bone mineral content may cause additional bone loss **and is not recommended.**

CHANGES IN LABORATORY VALUES DURING TREATMENT

Plasma Enzymes

Endometriosis: During clinical trials with Lupron Depot, regular laboratory monitoring revealed that SGOT levels were more than twice the upper limit of normal in only one patient. There was no other clinical or laboratory evidence of abnormal liver function.

Uterine Leiomyomata (Fibroids): In clinical trials with Lupron Depot 3.75 mg, five (3%) patients had a post-treatment transaminase value that was at least twice the baseline value and above the upper limit of the normal range. None of the laboratory increases were associated with clinical symptoms.

Lipids

Endometriosis: At enrollment, 4% of the Lupron Depot patients and 1% of the danazol patients had total cholesterol values above the normal range. These patients also had cholesterol values above the normal range at the end of treatment.

Of those patients whose pretreatment cholesterol values were in the normal range, 7% of the Lupron Depot patients and 9% of the danazol patients had post-treatment values above the normal range.

The mean ($\pm$SEM) pretreatment values for total cholesterol from all patients were 178.8 (2.9) mg/dl in the Lupron Depot groups and 175.3 (3.0) mg/dl in the danazol group. At the end of treatment, the mean values for total cholesterol from all patients were 193.3 mg/dl in the Lupron Depot group and 194.4 mg/dl in the danazol group. These increases from the pretreatment values were statistically significant ($p<0.03$) in both groups.

Triglycerides were increased above the upper limit of normal in 12% of the patients who received Lupron Depot and in 6% of the patients who received danazol.

At the end of treatment, HDL cholesterol fractions decreased below the lower limit of the normal range in 2% of the Lupron Depot patients compared with 54% of those receiving danazol. LDL cholesterol fractions increased above the upper limit of the normal range in 6% of the patients receiving Lupron Depot compared with 23% of those receiving danazol. There was no increase in the LDL/HDL ratio in patients receiving Lupron Depot but there was approximately a two-fold increase in the LDL/HDL ratio in patients receiving danazol.

Uterine Leiomyomata (Fibroids): In patients receiving Lupron Depot 3.75 mg, mean changes in cholesterol (+11 mg/dl to +29 mg/dl), LDL cholesterol (+8 mg/dl to +22 mg/dl), HDL cholesterol (0 to 6 g/dl), and the LDL/HDL ratio (-0.1 to +0.5) were observed across studies. In the one study in which triglyceride levels were determined, the mean increase from baseline was 32 mg/dl.

ADVERSE REACTIONS: *(cont'd)*

Other Changes

Endometriosis: In comparative studies, the following changes were seen in approximately 5% to 8% of patients. Lupron Depot was associated with elevations of LDH and phosphorus, and deceases in WBC counts. Danazol therapy was associated with increases in hematocrit, platelet count, and LDH.

Uterine Leiomyomata (Fibroids): Hematology: (See CLINICAL STUDIES.) In Lupron Depot treated patients, although there were statistically significant mean decreases in platelet counts from baseline to final visit, the last mean platelet counts were within the normal range. Decreases in total WBC count and neutrophils, were observed, but were not clinically significant.

Chemistry

Slight to moderate mean increases were noted for glucose, uric acid, BUN, creatinine, total protein, albumin, bilirubin, alkaline phosphatase, LDH, calcium, and phosphorus. None of these increases were clinically significant.

OVERDOSAGE:

LUPRON INJECTION AND LUPRON DEPOT 7.5 MG

In rats subcutaneous administration of 250 to 500 times the recommended human dose, expressed on a per body weight basis, resulted in dyspnea, decreased activity, and local irritation at the injection site. There is no evidence at present that there is a clinical counterpart of this phenomenon. In early clinical trials with leuprolide acetate doses as high as 20 mg/day for up to two years caused no adverse effects differing from those observed with the 1 mg/day dose.

LUPRON INJECTION (FOR PEDIATRIC USE) AND LUPRON DEPOT-PED

In rats, subcutaneous administration of 125 to 250 times the recommended human pediatric dose, expressed on a per body weight basis, resulted in dyspnea, decreased activity, and local irritation at the injection site. There is no evidence at present that there is a clinical counterpart of this phenomenon. In early clinical trials using leuprolide acetate in adult patients, doses as high as 20 mg/day for up to two years caused no adverse effects differing from those observed with the 1 mg/day dose.

LUPRON DEPOT 3.75 MG

In rats subcutaneous administration of 250 to 500 times the recommended human dose, expressed on a per body weight basis, resulted in dyspnea, decreased activity, and local irritation at the injection site. There is no evidence at present that there is a clinical counterpart of this phenomenon. In early clinical trials using daily subcutaneous leuprolide acetate in patients with prostate cancer, doses as high as 20 mg/day for up to two years caused no adverse effects differing from those observed with the 1 mg/day dose.

DOSAGE AND ADMINISTRATION:

LUPRON INJECTION

The recommended dose is 1 mg (0.2 ml) administered as a single daily subcutaneous injection. As with other drugs administered chronically by subcutaneous injection, the injection site should be varied periodically.

NOTE: As with all parenteral products, inspect container's solution for discoloration and particulate matter before each use.

LUPRON INJECTION (FOR PEDIATRIC USE)

Lupron Injection can be administered by a patient/parent or health care professional.

LUPRON DEPOT-PED

Lupron Depot-Ped must be administered under the supervision of a physician.

LUPRON INJECTION (FOR PEDIATRIC USE) AND LUPRON DEPOT-PED

The dose of Lupron must be individualized for each child. The dose is based on a mg/kg ratio of drug to body weight. Younger children require higher doses on a mg/kg ratio.

For either dosage form, after 1-2 months of initiating therapy or changing doses, the child must be monitored with a GnRH stimulation test, sex steroids, and Tanner staging to confirm downregulation. Measurements of bone age for advancement should be monitored every 6-12 months. The dose should be titrated upward until no progression of the condition is noted either clinically and/or by laboratory parameters.

The first dose found to result in adequate downregulation can probably be maintained for the duration of therapy in most children. However, there are insufficient data to guide dosage adjustment as patients move into higher weight categories after beginning therapy at very young ages and low dosages. It is recommended that adequate downregulation be verified in such patients whose weight has increased significantly while on therapy.

As with other drugs administered by injection, the injection site should be varied periodically.

Discontinuation of Lupron should be considered before age 11 for females and age 12 for males.

LUPRON INJECTION (FOR PEDIATRIC USE)

The recommended starting dose is 50 mcg/kg/day administered as a single subcutaneous injection. If total downregulation is not achieved, the dose should be titrated upward by 10 mcg/kg/day. This dose will be considered the maintenance dose.

NOTE: As with all parenteral products, inspect container's solution for discoloration and particulate matter before each use.

LUPRON DEPOT-PED

The recommended starting dose is 0.3 mg/kg/4 weeks (minimum 7.5 mg) administered as a single intramuscular injection. The starting dose will be dictated by the child's weight (TABLE 8).

TABLE 8

≤ 25 kg	7.5 mg
> 25-37.5 kg	11.25 mg
> 37.5 kg	15 mg

If total downregulation is not achieved, the dose should be titrated upward in increments of 3.75 mg every 4 weeks. This dose will be considered the maintenance dose.

The lyophilized microspheres are to be reconstituted and administered as a single intramuscular injection, in accord with the following directions:

1. Using a syringe with a 22 gauge needle, withdraw 1 ml of diluent from the ampule, and inject it into the vial. (Extra diluent is provided; any remaining should be discarded.)

2. Shake well to thoroughly disperse particles to obtain a uniform suspension. The suspension will appear milky.

3. Withdraw the entire contents of the vial into the syringe and inject it at the time of reconstitution.

Although the suspension has been shown to be stable for 24 hours following reconstitution, since the product does not contain a preservative, the suspension should be discarded if not used immediately.

DOSAGE AND ADMINISTRATION: *(cont'd)*

LUPRON DEPOT 3.75 MG

Lupron Depot Must Be Administered Under The Supervision Of A Physician.

The recommended dose of Lupron Depot is 3.75 mg, incorporated in a depot formulation. The lyophilized microspheres are to be reconstituted and administered monthly as a single intramuscular injection, in accord with the following directions:

1. Using a syringe with a 22 gauge needle, withdraw 1 ml of diluent from the ampule, and inject it into the vial. (Extra diluent is provided; any remaining should be discarded.)

2. Shake well to thoroughly disperse particles to obtain a uniform suspension. The suspension will appear milky.

3. Withdraw the entire contents of the vial into the syringe and inject it at the time of reconstitution.

Although the suspension has been shown to be stable for 24 hours following reconstitution, since the product does not contain a preservative, the suspension should be discarded if not used immediately.

Endometriosis: The recommended duration of administration is six months. Retreatment cannot be recommended since safety data for retreatment are not available. If the symptoms of endometriosis recur after a course of therapy, and further treatment with Lupron Depot is contemplated, it is recommended that bone density be assessed before retreatment begins to ensure that values are within normal limits.

Uterine Leiomyomata (Fibroids): Recommended duration of therapy with Lupron Depot is **up to** 3 months. The symptoms associated with uterine leiomyomata will recur following discontinuation of therapy. If additional treatment with Lupron Depot 3.75 mg is contemplated, bone density should be assessed prior to initiation of therapy to ensure that values are within normal limits.

As with other drugs administered by injection, the injection site should be varied periodically.

The vial of Lupron Depot and the ampule of diluent may be stored at room temperature.

LUPRON DEPOT 7.5 MG

Lupron Depot Must Be Administered Under The Supervision Of A Physician.

The recommended dose of Lupron Depot (leuprolide acetate for depot suspension) is 7.5 mg, incorporated in a depot formulation. The lyophilized microspheres are to be reconstituted and administered monthly as a single intramuscular injection, in accord with the following directions:

1. Using a syringe with a 22 gauge needle, withdraw 1 ml of diluent from the ampule, and inject it into the vial. (Extra diluent is provided; any remaining should be discarded.)

2. Shake well to thoroughly disperse particles to obtain a uniform suspension. The suspension will appear milky.

3. Withdraw the entire contents of the vial into the syringe and inject it at the time of reconstitution.

Although the solution has been shown to be stable for 24 hours following reconstitution, since the product does not contain a preservative, the suspension should be discarded if not used immediately.

As with other drugs administered by injection, the injection site should be varied periodically.

The vial of Lupron Depot and the ampule of diluent may be stored at room temperature.

REFERENCES:

Lupron Injection, Lupron Injection (For Pediatric Use), Lupron Depot 3.75 mg, Lupron Depot 7.5 mg, and Lupron Depot-Ped1. MacLeod TL, Eisen A, Sussman GL, et al: Anaphylactic reaction to synthetic luteinizing hormone-releasing hormone. *Fertil Steril* 1987 Sept;48(3):500-502.

PATIENT PACKAGE INSERT:

LUPRON INJECTION

WHAT IS LUPRON? Lupron (leuprolide acetate) Injection is chemically similar to gonadotropin releasing hormone (GnRH or LH-RH) a hormone which occurs naturally in your body.

Normally, your body releases small amounts of LH-RH and this leads to events which stimulate the production of sex hormones.

However, when you inject Lupron (leuprolide acetate) Injection, the normal events that lead to sex hormone production are interrupted and testosterone is no longer produced by the testes.

Lupron must be injected because, like insulin which is injected by diabetics, Lupron is inactive when taken by mouth.

If you were to discontinue the drug for any reason, your body would begin making testosterone again.

DIRECTIONS FOR USING LUPRON

1. Wash hands thoroughly with soap and water.

2. If using a new bottle for the first time, flip off the plastic cover to expose the gray rubber stopper. Wipe metal ring and rubber stopper with an alcohol wipe each time you use Lupron. Check the liquid in the container. If it is not clear or has particles in it, DO NOT USE IT. Exchange it at your pharmacy for another container.

3. Remove outer wrapping from one syringe. Pull plunger back until the tip of the plunger is at the.2 or 20 unit mark.

4. Take cover off needle. Push the needle through the center of the rubber stopper on the Lupron bottle.

5. Push the plunger all the way in to inject air into the bottle.

6. Keep the needle in the bottle and turn the bottle upside down. Check to make sure the tip of the needle is in the liquid. Slowly pull back on the plunger, until the syringe fills to the.2 or 20 unit mark.

7. Toward the end of a two-week period, the amount of Lupron left in the bottle will be small. Take special care to hold the bottle straight and to keep the needle tip in liquid while pulling back on the plunger.

8. Keeping the needle in the bottle and the bottle upside down, check for air bubbles in the syringe. If you see any, push the plunger *slowly* in to push the air bubble back into the bottle. Keep the tip of the needle in the liquid and pull the plunger back again to fill to the.2 or 20 unit mark.

9. Do this again if necessary to eliminate air bubbles. Remove needle from bottle and lay syringe down. DO NOT TOUCH THE NEEDLE OR ALLOW THE NEEDLE TO TOUCH ANY SURFACE.

10. To protect your skin, inject each daily dose at a different body spot.

11. Choose an injection spot. Cleanse the injection spot with another alcohol wipe.

12. Hold the syringe in one hand. Hold the skin taut, or pull up a little flesh with the other hand, as you were instructed.

13. Holding the syringe as you would a pencil, thrust the needle all the way into the skin at a 90° angle.

PATIENT PACKAGE INSERT: *(cont'd)*

14. Hold an alcohol wipe down on your skin where the needle is inserted and withdraw the needle at the same angle it was inserted.

15. Use the disposable syringe only once and dispose of it properly as you were instructed. Needles thrown into a garbage bag could accidentally stick someone. NEVER LEAVE SYRINGES, NEEDLES OR DRUGS WHERE CHILDREN CAN REACH THEM.

SOME SPECIAL ADVICE

You may experience hot flashes when using Lupron (leuprolide acetate) Injection. During the first few weeks of treatment you may experience increased bone pain, increased difficulty in urinating, and less commonly but most importantly, you may experience the onset or aggravation of nerve symptoms. In any of these events, discuss the symptoms with your doctor.

You may experience some irritation at the injection site, such as burning, itching or swelling. These reactions are usually mild and go away. If they do not, tell your doctor.

Do not stop taking your injections because you feel better. You need an injection every day to make sure Lupron keeps working for you.

If you need to use an alternate to the syringe supplied with Lupron, insulin syringes should be utilized.

When the drug level gets low, take special care to hold the bottle straight up and down and to keep the needle tip in liquid while pulling back on the plunger.

Do not try to get every last drop out of the bottle. This will increase the possibility of drawing air into the syringe and getting an incomplete dose. Some extra drug has been provided so that you can withdraw the recommended number of doses.

Tell your pharmacist when you will need Lupron so it will be at the pharmacy when you need it.

Store below 77°F (25°C). Do not store near a radiator or other very warm place. Avoid freezing. Protect from light - store vial in carton until use.

Do not leave your drug or hypodermic syringes where anyone can pick them up.

Keep this and all other medications out of reach of children.

HOW SUPPLIED:

LUPRON INJECTION

Lupron (leuprolide acetate) Injection is a sterile solution supplied in a 2.8 ml multiple-dose vial. Store below 77°F (25°C). Avoid freezing. Protect from light.

Store vial in carton until use.

Each 0.2 ml contains 1 mg of leuprolide acetate, sodium chloride for tonicity adjustment, 1.8 mg of benzyl alcohol as preservative and water for injection. The pH may have been adjusted with sodium hydroxide and/or acetic acid.

LUPRON INJECTION (FOR PEDIATRIC USE)

Lupron (leuprolide acetate) Injection is a sterile solution.

A 2.8 ml multiple dose vial (NDC 0300-3626-28) contains leuprolide acetate (5 mg/ml), sodium chloride (6.3 mg/ml) for tonicity adjustment, benzyl alcohol as a preservative (9 mg/ml), and water for injection. The pH may have been adjusted with sodium hydroxide and/or acetic acid.

Store below 77°F (25°C). Avoid freezing. Protect from light - store vial in carton until use.

Use the syringes supplied with Lupron Injection. Insulin syringes may be substituted for use with Lupron Injection. The volume of drug for the dose will vary depending on the syringe used and the concentration of drug.

LUPRON DEPOT 3.75 MG

Lupron Depot is available in a vial containing sterile lyophilized microspheres which is leuprolide acetate incorporated in a biodegradable copolymer of lactic and glycolic acids.

The single-dose vial of Lupron Depot contains leuprolide acetate (3.75 mg), purified gelatin (0.65 mg), DL-lactic and glycolic acids copolymer (33.1 mg), and D-mannitol (6.6 mg). The accompanying ampule of diluent contains carboxymethylcellulose sodium (7.5 mg), D-mannitol (75 mg), polysorbate 80 (1.5 mg), and water for injection, USP, and glacial acetic acid, USP to control pH. When mixed with 1 ml of diluent, Lupron Depot (leuprolide acetate for depot suspension) is administered as a single monthly IM injection.

Lupron Depot 3.75 mg is available in a single use kit and in a six pack of drug only.

LUPRON DEPOT 7.5 MG

Lupron Depot is available in a vial containing sterile lyophilized microspheres which is leuprolide acetate incorporated in a biodegradable copolymer of lactic and glycolic acids.

The single-dose vial of Lupron Depot contains leuprolide acetate (7.5 mg), purified gelatin (1.3 mg), DL-lactic and glycolic acids copolymer (66.2 mg), and D-mannitol (13.2 mg). The accompanying ampule of diluent contains carboxymethylcellulose sodium (7.5 mg), D-mannitol (75 mg), polysorbate 80 (1.5 mg), water for injection, USP, and acetic acid, NF to control pH. When mixed with 1 ml of diluent, Lupron Depot is administered as a single monthly IM injection.

No refrigeration necessary. Protect from freezing.

LUPRON DEPOT-PED

Lupron Depot-Ped is available in three packages providing a dose of 7.5 mg, 11.25 mg or 15 mg. Each vial contains sterile lyophilized microspheres which is leuprolide acetate incorporated in a biodegradable copolymer of lactic and glycolic acids.

The single-dose vial of Lupron Depot-Ped contains, respectively for each dosage strength, leuprolide acetate (7.5/11.25/15 mg), purified gelatin (1.3/1.95/2.6 mg), DL-lactic and glycolic acids copolymer (66.2/99.3/132.4 mg), and D-mannitol (13.2/19.8/26.4 mg). The accompanying ampule of diluent contains carboxymethylcellulose sodium (7.5 mg), D-mannitol (75 mg), polysorbate 80 (1.5 mg), water for injection, USP, and acetic acid, NF to control pH.

The vial of Lupron Depot-Ped and the ampule of diluent may be stored at room temperature. Keep from freezing.

Use the syringes supplied in the Lupron Depot-Ped kits. Any 22-gauge needle may be used with Lupron Depot-Ped.

HOW SUPPLIED - EQUIVALENTS NOT AVAILABLE:

Injection, Solution - Intramuscular - 3.75 mg/vial

6's	$2381.25	LUPRON DEPOT, TAP Pharm	00300-3639-06

Injection, Solution - Subcutaneous - 1 mg/0.2ml

2.8 ml	$278.12	LUPRON, TAP Pharm	00300-3626-28
2.8 ml x 6	$1668.72	LUPRON, TAP Pharm	00300-3626-24

Injection, Susp - Intramuscular - 7.5 mg/vial

1's	$496.25	LUPRON DEPOT, TAP Pharm	00300-3629-01
6's	$2977.50	LUPON DEPOT, TAP Pharm	00300-3629-06

Kit - Intramuscular - 3.75 mg/vial

1's	$396.87	LUPRON DEPOT, TAP Pharm	00300-3639-01

HOW SUPPLIED - EQUIVALENTS NOT AVAILABLE: *(cont'd)*

Kit - Intramuscular - 7.5 mg/vial

1's	$496.25	LUPRON DEPOT-PED, TAP Pharm	00300-2106-01

Kit - Intramuscular - 11.25 mg/vial

1's	$893.12	LUPRON DEPOT-PED, TAP Pharm	00300-2270-01

Kit - Intramuscular - 15 mg/vial

1's	$992.50	LUPRON DEPOT-PED, TAP Pharm	00300-2437-01

LEVAMISOLE HYDROCHLORIDE *(001632)*

CATEGORIES: Antineoplastics; Cancer; Colon Carcinoma; Pregnancy Category C; FDA Class 1A ("Important Therapeutic Advantage"); FDA Approved 1990 Jun

BRAND NAMES: *Ascaridil*; *Ascaryl*; *Decaris*; *Decas*; *Detrax 40*; *Dewormis*; *Dewormis 50*; **Ergamisol**; *Immunol*; *Ketrax*; *Levazole*; *Solaskil* (France); *Termizole*; *Vermisol*
(International brand names outside U.S. in italics)

FORMULARIES: Aetna; BC-BS; Medi-Cal; WHO

COST OF THERAPY: $1,267.35 (Colon Cancer; Tablet; 50 mg; 0.643/day; 365 days)

DESCRIPTION:

Levamisole hydrochloride is an immunomodulator available in tablets for oral administration containing the equivalent of 50 mg as levamisole base. Fifty-nine (59) mg of levamisole HCl is equivalent to 50 mg of levamisole base. Inactive ingredients are colloidal silicon dioxide, hydrogenated vegetable oil, hydroxypropyl methylcellulose, lactose, microcrystalline cellulose, polyethylene glycol 6000, polysorbate 80, and talc.

Levamisole hydrochloride is (-)-(S)-2,3,5,6-tetrahydro-6-phenylimidazo [2,1-b] thiazole monohydrochloride.

Levamisole hydrochloride is a white to pale cream colored crystalline powder which is almost odorless and is freely soluble in water. It is quite stable in acid aqueous media but hydrolyzes in alkaline or neutral solutions. It has a molecular weight of 240.75.

CLINICAL PHARMACOLOGY:

Two clinical trials having essentially the same design have demonstrated an increase in survival and a reduction in recurrence rate in the subset of patients with resected Dukes' C colon cancer treated with a regimen of Levamisole hydrochloride plus fluorouracil[1,2]. After surgery, patients were randomized to no further therapy, levamisole HCl alone, or levamisole HCl plus fluorouracil.

In one clinical trial in which 408 Dukes' B and C colorectal cancer patients were studied, 262 Dukes' C patients were evaluated for a minimum follow-up of five years[1]. A subset analysis of these Dukes' C patients showed the estimated reduction in death rate was 27% for levamisole HCl plus fluorouracil ($p = 0.11$) and 28% for levamisole HCl alone ($p = 0.11$)[3]. The estimated reduction in recurrence rate was 36% for levamisole HCl plus fluorouracil ($p = 0.025$) and 28% for levamisole HCl alone ($p = 0.11$)[3]. In another clinical trial designed to confirm the above results, 929 Dukes' C colon cancer patients were evaluated for a minimum follow-up of 2 years[2]. The estimated reduction in recurrence rate was 41% for levamisole HCl plus fluorouracil ($p<0.0001$). The levamisole HCl alone group did not show advantage over no treatment on improving recurrence or survival rates. There are presently insufficient data to evaluate the effect of the combination of levamisole HCl plus fluorouracil in Dukes'B patients. There are also insufficient data to evaluate the effect of levamisole HCl plus fluorouracil in patients with rectal cancer because only 12 patients with rectal cancer were treated with the combination in the first study and none in the second study.

The mechanism of action of levamisole HCl in combination with fluorouracil is unknown. The effects of levamisole on the immune system are complex. The drug appears to restore depressed immune function rather than to stimulate response to above-normal levels. Levamisole can stimulate formation of antibodies to various antigens, enhance T-cell responses by stimulating T-cell activation and proliferation, potentiate monocyte and macrophage functions including phagocytosis and chemotaxis, and increase neutrophil mobility, adherence, and chemotaxis. Other drugs have similar short-term effects and the clinical relevance is unclear.

Besides its immunomodulatory function, levamisole has other mammalian pharmacologic activities, including inhibition of alkaline phosphatase, and cholinergic activity.

The pharmacokinetics of levamisole HCl have not been studied in the dosage regimen recommended with fluorouracil not in patients with hepatic insufficiency. After administration of a single oral dose of 50 mg of a research formulation of levamisole HCl, it appears that levamisole is rapidly absorbed from the gastrointestinal tract. Mean peak plasma concentrations of 0.13 mcg/ml are attained within 1.5 to 2 hours. The plasma elimination half-life of levamisole is between 3-4 hours. Following a 150-mg radio-labelled dose, levamisole is extensively metabolized by the liver in humans and the metabolites excreted mainly by the kidneys (70% over 3 days). The elimination half-life of metabolite excretion is 16 hours. Approximately 5% is excreted in the feces. Less than 5% is excreted unchanged in the urine and less than 0.2% in the feces. Approximately 12% is recovered in the urine as the glucuronide of p-hydroxy-levamisole. The clinical significance of these data are unknown since a 150-mg dose may not be proportional to a 50-mg dose.

INDICATIONS AND USAGE:

Levamisole hydrochloride is only indicated as adjuvant treatment in combination with fluorouracil after surgical resection in patients with Dukes' stage C colon cancer.

CONTRAINDICATIONS:

Levamisole hydrochloride is contraindicated in patients with a known hypersensitivity to the drug or its components.

WARNINGS:

Levamisole hydrochloride has been associated with agranulocytosis, sometimes fatal. The onset of agranulocytosis is frequently accompanied by a flu-like syndrome (fever, chills, etc.); however, in a small number of patients it is asymptomatic. A flu-like syndrome may also occur in the absence of agranulocytosis. It is essential that appropriate hematological monitoring be done routinely during therapy with levamisole HCl and fluorouracil. Neutropenia is usually reversible following discontinuation of therapy. Patients should be instructed to report immediately any flu-like symptoms.

Higher than recommended doses of levamisole HCl may be associated with an increased incidence of agranulocytosis, so the recommended dose should not be exceeded.

The combination of levamisole HCl and fluorouracil has been associated with frequent neutropenia, anemia and thrombocytopenia.

PRECAUTIONS:

Before beginning this combination adjuvant treatment, the physician should become familiar with the labeling for fluorouracil.

Information for the Patient: The patient should be informed that if flu-like symptoms or malaise occurs, the physician should be notified immediately.

Laboratory Tests: On the first day of therapy with levamisole HCl fluorouracil, patients should have a CBC with differential and platelets, electrolytes and liver function tests performed. Thereafter, a CBC with differential and platelets should be performed weekly prior to each treatment with fluorouracil with electrolytes and liver function tests performed every 3 months for a total of one year. Dosage modifications should be instituted as follows: If WBC is 2500-3500/mm^3 defer the fluorouracil dose until WBC is >3500/mm^3. If WBC is <2500/mm^3, defer the fluorouracil dose until WBC is >3500/mm^3; then resume the fluorouracil dose reduced by 20%. If WBC remains <2500/mm^3 for over 10 days despite deferring fluorouracil, discontinue administration of levamisole HCl. Both drugs should be deferred unless enough platelets are present (≥100,000/mm^3).

Carcinogenesis, Mutagenesis, and Impairment of Fertility: Adequate animal carcinogenicity studies have not been conducted with levamisole. Studies of levamisole administered in drinking water at 5, 20, and 80 mg/kg/day to mice for up to 18 months or administered to rats in the diet at 5, 20, and 80 mg/kg/day for 24 months showed no evidence of neoplastic effects. These studies were not conducted at the maximum tolerated dose, therefore the animals may not have been exposed to a reasonable drug challenge. No mutagenic effects were demonstrated in dominant lethal studies in male and female mice, in an Ames test, and in a study to detect chromosomal aberrations in cultured peripheral human lymphocytes.

Adverse effects were not observed on male or female fertility when levamisole was administered to rats in the diet at doses of 2.5, 10, 40 and 160 mg/kg. In a rat gavage study at doses of 20, 60, and 180 mg/kg, the copulation period was increased, the duration of pregnancy was slightly increased, and fertility, pup viability and weight, lactation index, and number of fetuses were decreased at 60 mg/kg. No negative reproductive effects were present when the offspring were allowed to mate and litter.

Pregnancy Category C: Teratogenicity studies have been performed in rats and rabbits at oral doses up to 180 mg/kg. Fetal malformations were not observed. In rats, embryotoxicity was present at 160 mg/kg and in rabbits, significant embryotoxicity was observed at 180 mg/kg. There are no adequate and well-controlled studies in pregnant women and levamisole HCl should not be administered unless the potential benefits outweigh the risks. Women taking the combination of levamisole HCl and fluorouracil should be advised not to become pregnant.

Nursing Mothers: It is not known whether levamisole HCl is excreted in human milk; it is excreted in cows' milk. Because of the potential for serious adverse reactions in nursing infants from levamisole HCl, a decision should be made whether to discontinue nursing or to discontinue the drug, taking into account the importance of the drug to the mother.

Pediatric Use: Safety and effectiveness of levamisole HCl in children have not been established.

DRUG INTERACTIONS:

Levamisole hydrochloride has been reported to produce "Antabuse" -like side effects when given concomitantly with alcohol. Concomitant administration of phenytoin and levamisole HCl plus fluorouracil has led to increased plasma levels of phenytoin. The physician is advised to monitor plasma levels of phenytoin and to decrease the dose if necessary.

Because of reports of prolongation of the prothrombin time beyond the therapeutic range in patients taking concurrent levamisole and warfarin sodium, it is suggested that the prothrombin time be monitored carefully, and the dose of warfarin sodium and other coumarin-like drugs should be adjusted accordingly, in patients taking both drugs.

ADVERSE REACTIONS:

Almost all patients receiving Levamisole hydrochloride and fluorouracil reported adverse experiences. Tabulated in TABLE 1 is the incidence of adverse experiences that occurred in at least 1% of patients enrolled in two clinical trials who were adjuvantly treated with either levamisole HCl or levamisole HCl plus fluorouracil following colon surgery. In the larger clinical trial, 66 of 463 patients (14%) discontinued the combination of levamisole HCl plus fluorouracil because of adverse reactions. Forty-three of these patients (9%) developed isolated or a combination of gastrointestinal toxicities (*e.g.*, nausea, vomiting, diarrhea, stomatitis and anorexia). Ten patients developed rash and/or pruritus. Five patients discontinued therapy because of flu-like symptoms or fever with chills; ten patients developed central nervous system symptoms such as dizziness, ataxia, depression, confusion, memory loss, weakness, inability to concentrate, and headache; two patients developed reversible neutropenia and sepsis; one patient because of thrombocytopenia; one patient because of hyperbilirubinemia. One patient in the levamisole HCl plus fluorouracil group developed agranulocytosis and sepsis and died.

In the levamisole HCl alone arm of the trial, 15 of 310 patients (4.8%) discontinued therapy because of adverse experiences. Six of these (2%) discontinued because of rash, six because of arthralgia/myalgia, and one each for fever and neutropenia, urinary infection, and cough (TABLE 1):

In worldwide experience with levamisole HCl, less frequent adverse experiences included exfoliative dermatitis, periorbital edema, vaginal bleeding, anaphylaxis, confusion, convulsions, hallucinations, impaired concentration, renal failure, pancreatitis, elevated serum creatinine, and increased alkaline, phosphatase.

Reports of hyperlipidemia have been observed in patients receiving combination therapy of levamisole HCl and fluorouracil; elevations of triglyceride levels have been greater than increases in cholesterol levels.

Cases of an encephalopathy-like syndrome associated with demyelination have been reported in patients treated with levamisole HCl. Worldwide postmarketing experience with the combination therapy of levamisole HCl and fluorouracil has also included several reports of neurological changes associated with demyelination and several reports of peripheral neuropathy. The onset of symptoms and the clinical presentation in these cases are quite varied. Symptoms may include confusion, speech disturbances, muscle weakness, lethargy, and paresthesia. If an acute neurological syndrome occurs, immediate discontinuation of levamisole HCl and fluorouracil therapy should be considered.

The following additional adverse experiences have been reported for fluorouracil alone: esophagopharyngitis, pancytopenia, myocardial ischemia, angina, gastrointestinal ulceration and bleeding, anaphylaxis and generalized allergic reactions, acute cerebellar syndrome, nystagmus, dry skin, fissuring, photosensitivity, lacrimal duct stenosis, photophobia, euphoria, thrombophlebitis, and nail changes.

OVERDOSAGE:

Fatalities have been reported in a three-year-old child who ingested 15 mg/kg and in an adult who ingested 32 mg/kg. No further clinical information is available. In cases of overdosage, gastric lavage is recommended together with symptomatic and supportive measures.

TABLE 1

Adverse Experience	Levamisole HCl N = 440 %	Levamisole HCl plus fluorouracil N = 599 %
Gastrointestinal		
Nausea	22	65
Diarrhea	13	52
Stomatitis	3	39
Vomiting	6	20
Anorexia	2	6
Abdominal pain	2	5
Constipation	2	3
Flatulence	<1	2
Dyspepsia	<1	1
Hematological		
Leukopenia		
<2000/mm^3	<1	1
≥2000 to <4000/mm^3	4	19
≥4000/mm^3	2	33
unscored category	0	<1
Thrombocytopenia		
<50,000/mm^3	0	0
≥50,000 to <130,000/mm^3	1	8
≥130,000/mm^3	1	10
Anemia	0	6
Granulocytopenia	<1	2
Epistaxis	0	1
Skin and Appendages		
Dermatitis	8	23
Alopecia	3	22
Pruritus	1	2
Skin discoloration	0	2
Urticaria	<1	0
Body as a Whole		
Fatigue	6	11
Fever	3	5
Rigors	3	5
Chest pain	<1	1
Edema	1	1
Resistance Mechanisms		
Infection	5	12
Special Sense		
Taste Perversion	8	8
Altered sense of smell	1	1
Musculoskeletal System		
Arthralgia	5	4
Myalgia	3	2
Central and peripheral nervous system		
Dizziness	3	4
Headache	3	4
Paresthesia	2	3
Ataxia	0	2
Psychiatric		
Somnolence	3	2
Depression	1	2
Nervousness	1	2
Insomnia	1	1
Anxiety	1	1
Forgetfulness	0	1
Vision		
Abnormal tearing	0	4
Blurred vision	1	2
Conjunctivitis	<1	2
Liver and biliary system		
Hyperbilirubinemia	<1	1

DOSAGE AND ADMINISTRATION:

The adjuvant use of Levamisole hydrochloride and fluorouracil is limited to the following dosage schedule:

INITIAL THERAPY:

Levamisole HCl: 50 mg p.o. q8h for 3 days (starting 7-30 days post-surgery)

Fluorouracil: 450 mg/m^2/day IV for 5 days concomitant with a 3-day course of levamisole HCl (starting 21-34 days post-surgery)

MAINTENANCE:

Levamisole HCl: 50 mg p.o. q8h for 3 days every 2 weeks.

Fluorouracil: 450 mg/m^2/day IV once a week beginning 28 days after the initiation of the 5-day course.

Treatment: levamisole HCl, administered orally, should be initiated no earlier than 7 and no later than 30 days post surgery at a dose of 50 mg q8h X 3 days repeated every 14 days for 1 year. Fluorouracil therapy should be initiated no earlier than 21 days and no later than 35 days after surgery providing the patient is out of the hospital, ambulatory, maintaining normal oral nutrition, has well-healed wounds, and is fully recovered from any postoperative complications. If levamisole HCl has been initiated from 7 to 20 days after surgery, initiation of fluorouracil therapy should be coincident with the second course of levamisole HCl, i.e., at 21 to 34 days. If levamisole HCl is initiated from 21 to 30 days after surgery, fluorouracil should be initiated simultaneously with the first course of levamisole HCl.

Fluorouracil should be administered by rapid IV push at a dosage of 450 mg/m^2/day for 5 consecutive days. Dosage calculation is based on actual weight (estimated dry weight if there is evidence of fluid retention). *This course should be discontinued before the full 5 doses are administered if the patient develops any stomatitis or diarrhea* (5 or more loose stools). Twenty-eight days after initiation of this course, weekly fluorouracil should be instituted at a dosage of 450 mg/m^2/week and continued for a total treatment time of 1 year. If stomatitis or diarrhea develop during weekly therapy, the next dose of fluorouracil should be deferred until these side effects have subsided. If these side effects are moderate to severe, the fluorouracil dose should be reduced 20% when it is resumed.

Dosage modifications should be instituted as follows: If WBC is 2500-3500/mm^3 defer the fluorouracil dose until WBC is >3500mm^3. If WBC is <2500/mm^3, defer the fluorouracil dose until WBC is >3500/mm^3; then resume the fluorouracil dose, reduced by 20%. If WBC remains <2500/mm^3 for over 10 days despite deferring fluorouracil, discontinue administration of levamisole HCl. Both drugs should be deferred unless platelets are adequate (≥100,000/mm^3).

Levamisole HCl should not be used at doses exceeding the recommended dose or frequency. Clinical studies suggest a relationship between levamisole HCl adverse experiences and increasing dose, and since some of these, e.g., agranulocytosis, may be life-threatening, the recommended dosage regimen should not be exceeded (see WARNINGS.)

DOSAGE AND ADMINISTRATION: *(cont'd)*

Before beginning this combination adjuvant treatment, the physician should become familiar with the labeling for fluorouracil.

REFERENCES:

1. Laurie JA, Moertel CG, Fleming TR, et al. Surgical adjuvant therapy of large-bowel carcinoma: An evaluation of levamisole and the combination of levamisole and fluorouracil. *J Clin Oncol.* 1989; 7:1447-1456. 2. Moertel CG, Fleming TR, Macdonald JS, et al. Levamisole and fluorouracil for adjuvant therapy of resected colon carcinoma. *New Engl J Med.* 1990; 322:352-358. 3. Data on file, Janssen Pharmaceutica Inc.

HOW SUPPLIED:

Ergamisol (levamisole hydrochloride) is available in white, coated tablets containing the equivalent of 50 mg of levamisole base, debossed "JANSSEN" and "L" "50."

Store at room temperature, 15°-30°C (59°-86°F). Protect from moisture.

HOW SUPPLIED - EQUIVALENTS NOT AVAILABLE:

Tablet, Coated - Oral - 50 mg

36's $194.40 ERGAMISOL, Janssen Phar 50458-0270-36

LEVOBUNOLOL HYDROCHLORIDE *(001633)*

CATEGORIES: Antiglaucomatous Agents; Beta Adrenergic Blocking Agents; Beta Blockers; Compliance Aids; EENT Drugs; Eye, Ear, Nose, & Throat Preparations; Glaucoma; Intraocular Pressure; Ocular Hypertension; Ophthalmics; Pregnancy Category C; FDA Approved 1985 Dec; Patent Expiration 1991 Mar

BRAND NAMES: **Betagan**; *Bunolgan*; *Gotensin* (Japan); Levobunolol HCl; *Vistagan* (Germany); *Vistagen* (Japan)
(International brand names outside U.S. in italics)

FORMULARIES: Aetna; BC-BS; CIGNA; FHP; Humana; Kaiser; Medco; Medi-Cal; PCS; PruCare; United

COST OF THERAPY: $103.78 (Glaucoma; Solution; 0.5 %; 0.1/day; 365 days) vs. Potential Cost of $1,851.63 (Iredectomy)

PRIMARY ICD9: 365.11 (Primary Open-Angle Glaucoma)

DESCRIPTION:

Levobunolol HCl sterile ophthalmic solution is a noncardioselective beta-adrenoceptor blocking agent for ophthalmic use.

Chemical Name: (-)-5-(3-(*tert*-Butylamino)-2-hydroxypropoxy)-3, 4-dihydro-)(*2H*)-naphthalenone hydrochloride.

Contains: Betagan 0.25% and 0.5% contains:

levobunolol HCl 0.25%, 0.5%; with: Liquifilm (polyvinyl alcohol) 1.4%; benzalkonium chloride 0.004%; edetate disodium; sodium metabisulfite; sodium phosphate; dibasic; potassium phosphate; monobasic; sodium chloride; hydrochloric acid or sodium hydroxide to adjust pH; and purified water.

CLINICAL PHARMACOLOGY:

Levobunolol HCl is a noncardioselective beta-adrenoceptor blocking agent, equipotent at both $beta_1$, and $beta_2$ receptors. Levobunolol HCl is greater than 60 times more potent than its dextro isomer in its beta-blocking activity, yet equipotent in its potential for direct myocardial depression. Accordingly, the levo isomer, levobunolol HCl, is used. Levobunolol HCl does not have significant local anesthetic (membrane-stabilizing) or intrinsic sympathomimetic activity.

Beta-adrenergic receptor blockage reduces cardiac output in both healthy subjects and patients with heart disease in patients with severe impairment of myocardial function, beta-adrenergic receptor blockade may inhibit the stimulatory effect of the sympathetic nervous system necessary to maintain adequate cardiac function.

Beta-adrenergic receptor blockade in the bronchi and bronchioles results in increased airway resistance from unopposed para-sympathetic activity. Such an effect in patients with asthma or other bronchospastic conditions is potentially dangerous.

Levobunolol HCl has been shown to be an active agent in lowering elevated as well as normal intraocular pressure (IOP) whether or not accompanied by glaucoma. Elevated IOP presents a major risk factor in glaucomatous field loss. The higher the level of IOP, the greater the likelihood of optic nerve damage and visual field loss.

The onset of action with one drop of levobunolol HCl can be detected within one hour after treatment, with maximum effect seen between 2 and 6 hours.

A significant decrease in IOP can be maintained for up to 24 hours following a single dose.

In two, separate, controlled studies (one three month and one up to 12 months duration) levobunolol HCl 0.25% b.i.d. controlled the IOP of approximately 64% and 70% of the subjects. The overall mean decrease from baseline was 5.4 mm Hg and 5.1 mm Hg respectively. In an open-label study, levobunolol HCl 0.25% q.d. controlled the IOP of 72% of the subjects while achieving an overall mean decrease of 5.9 mm Hg.

In controlled clinical studies of approximately two years duration, intraocular pressure was well-controlled in approximately 80% of subjects treated with levobunolol HCl 0.5% b.i.d. The mean IOP decrease from baseline was between 6.87 mm Hg and 7.81 mm Hg. No significant effects on pupil size, tear production or corneal sensitivity were observed. Levobunolol HCl at the concentrations tested, when applied topically, decreased heart rate and blood pressure in some patients. The IOP-lowering effect of levobunolol HCl was well maintained over the course of these studies.

In a three month clinical study, a single daily application of levobunolol HCl 0.5% controlled the IOP of 72% of subjects achieving an overall mean decrease in IOP of 7.0 mm Hg.

The primary mechanism of the ocular hypotensive action of levobunolol HCl in reducing IOP is most likely a decrease in aqueous humor production. Levobunolol HCl reduces IOP with little or no effect on pupil size or accommodation in contrast to the miosis which cholinergic agents are known to produce. The blurred vision and night blindness often associated with miotics would not be expected and have not been reported with the use of levobunolol HCl. This is particularly important in cataract patients with central lens opacities who would experience decreased visual acuity with pupillary constriction.

INDICATIONS AND USAGE:

Levobunolol HCl has been shown to be effective in lowering intraocular pressure and may be used in patients with chronic open-angle glaucoma or ocular hypertension.

CONTRAINDICATIONS:

Levobunolol HCl is contraindicated in those individuals with bronchial asthma or with a history of bronchial asthma, or severe chronic obstructive pulmonary disease (see WARNINGS); sinus bradycardia; second and third degree atrioventricular block; overt cardiac failure (see WARNINGS); cardiogenic shock; or hypersensitivity to any component of these products.

WARNINGS:

As with other topically applied ophthalmic drugs, levobunolol HCl may be absorbed systemically. The same adverse reactions found with systemic administration of beta-adrenergic blocking agents may occur with topical administration. For example, severe respiratory reactions and cardiac reactions, including death due to bronchospasm in patients with asthma, and rarely death in association with cardiac failure, have been reported with topical application of beta-adrenergic blocking agents (see CONTRAINDICATIONS.)

Cardiac Failure: Sympathetic stimulation may be essential for support of the circulation in individuals with diminished myocardial contractility, and its inhibition by beta-adrenergic receptor blockade may precipitate more severe failure.

In Patients Without a History of Cardiac Failure: Continued depression of the myocardium with beta-blocking agents over a period of time can, in some cases, lead to cardiac failure. At the first sign or symptom of cardiac failure, levobunolol HCl should be discontinued.

Obstructive Pulmonary Disease: PATIENTS WITH CHRONIC OBSTRUCTIVE PULMONARY DISEASE (*e.g.*, CHRONIC BRONCHITIS, EMPHYSEMA) OF MILD OR MODERATE SEVERITY, BRONCHOSPASTIC DISEASE OR A HISTORY OF BRONCHOSPASTIC DISEASE (OTHER THAN BRONCHIAL ASTHMA OR A HISTORY OF BRONCHIAL ASTHMA, IN WHICH LEVOBUNOLOL HCl IS CONTRAINDICATED, SEE CONTRAINDICATIONS), SHOULD IN GENERAL NOT RECEIVE BETA BLOCKERS, INCLUDING LEVOBUNOLOL HCl. However, if LEVOBUNOLOL HCl is deemed necessary in such patients, then it should be administered cautiously since it may block bronchodilation produced by endogenous and exogenous catecholamine stimulation of $beta_2$ receptors.

Major Surgery: The necessity or desirability of withdrawal of beta-adrenergic blocking agents prior to major surgery is controversial. Beta-adrenergic receptor blockade impairs the ability of the heart to respond to beta-adrenergically mediated reflex stimuli. This may augment the risk of general anesthesia in surgical procedures. Some patients receiving beta-adrenergic receptor blocking agents have been subject to protracted severe hypotension during anesthesia. Difficulty in restarting and maintaining the heartbeat has also been reported. For these reasons, in patients undergoing elective surgery, gradual withdrawal of beta-adrenergic receptor blocking agents may be appropriate.

If necessary during surgery, the effects of beta-adrenergic blocking agents may be reversed by sufficient doses of such agonists as isoproterenol, dopamine, dobutamine or levarterenol (see OVERDOSAGE.)

Diabetes Mellitus: Beta-adrenergic blocking agents should be administered with caution in patients subject to spontaneous hypoglycemia or to diabetic patients (especially those with labile diabetes) who are receiving insulin or oral hypoglycemic agents. Beta-adrenergic receptor blocking agents may mask the signs and symptoms of acute hypoglycemia.

Thyrotoxicosis: Beta-adrenergic blocking agents may mask certain clinical signs (*e.g.*, tachycardia) of hyperthyroidism. Patients suspected of developing thyrotoxicosis should be managed carefully to avoid abrupt withdrawal of beta-adrenergic blocking agents which might precipitate a thyroid storm.

These products contain sodium metabisulfite, a sulfite that may cause allergic-type reactions including anaphylactic symptoms and life-threatening or less severe asthmatic episodes in certain susceptible people. The overall prevalence of sulfite sensitivity in the general population is unknown and probably low. Sulfite sensitivity is seen more frequently in asthmatic than in nonasthmatic people.

PRECAUTIONS:

GENERAL

Levobunolol HCl should be used with caution in patients with known hypersensitivity to other beta-adrenoceptor blocking agents.

Use with caution in patients with known diminished pulmonary function.

Levobunolol HCl should be used with caution in patients who are receiving a beta- adrenergic blocking agent orally, because of the potential for additive effects on systemic beta-blockade or on intraocular pressure. Patients should not typically use two or more topical ophthalmic beta-adrenergic blocking agents simultaneously.

Because of the potential effects of beta-adrenergic blocking agents on blood pressure and pulse rates, these medications must be used cautiously in patients with cerebrovascular insufficiency. Should signs or symptoms develop that suggest reduced cerebral blood flow while using levobunolol HCl, alternative therapy should be considered.

In patients with angle-closure glaucoma, the immediate objective of treatment is to reopen the angle. This requires, in most cases, constricting the pupil with a miotic. Levobunolol HCl Liquifilm sterile ophthalmic solution has little or no effect on the pupil. When levobunolol HCl is used to reduce elevated intraocular pressure in angle-closure glaucoma, it should be followed with a miotic and not alone.

Muscle Weakness: Beta-adrenergic blockade has been reported to potentiate muscle weakness consistent with certain myasthenic symptoms (*e.g.*, diplopia, ptosis and generalized weakness).

Animal Studies: No adverse ocular effects were observed in rabbits administered levobunolol HCl topically in studies lasting one year in concentrations up to 10 times the human dose concentration.

CARCINOGENESIS, MUTAGENESIS, AND IMPAIRMENT OF FERTILITY

In a lifetime oral study in mice, there were statistically significant ($p \leq 0.05$) increases in the incidence of benign leiomyomas in female mice at 200 mg/kg/day (14,000 times the recommended human dose for glaucoma), but not at 12 or 50 mg/kg/day (850 and 3,500 times the human dose). In a two-year oral study of levobunolol HCl in rats, there was a statistically significant ($p \leq 0.05$) increase in the incidence of benign hepatomas in male rats administered 12,800 times the recommended human dose for glaucoma. Similar differences were not observed in rats administered oral doses equivalent to 350 times to 2,000 times the recommended human dose for glaucoma.

Levobunolol did not show evidence of mutagenic activity in a battery of microbiological and mammalian *in vitro* and *in vivo* assays.

Reproduction and fertility studies in rats showed no adverse effect on male or female fertility at doses up to 1,800 times the recommended human dose for glaucoma.

PREGNANCY CATEGORY C

Fetotoxicity (as evidenced by a greater number of resorption sites) has been observed in rabbits when doses of levobunolol HCl equivalent to 200 and 700 times the recommended dose for the treatment of glaucoma were given. No fetotoxic effects have been observed in similar studies with rats at up to 1,800 times the human dose for glaucoma. Teratogenic studies with levobunolol in rats at doses up to 25 mg/kg/day (1,800 times the recommended human dose for glaucoma) showed no evidence of fetal malformations. There were no

PRECAUTIONS: *(cont'd)*

adverse effects on postnatal development of offspring. It appears when results from studies using rats and studies with other beta-adrenergic blockers are examined, that the rabbit may be a particularly sensitive species. There are no adequate and well-controlled studies in pregnant women. Levobunolol HCl should be used during pregnancy only if the potential benefit justifies the potential risk to the fetus.

NURSING MOTHERS

It is not known whether this drug is excreted in human milk. Systemic beta-blockers and topical timolol maleate are known to be excreted in human milk. Caution should be exercised when levobunolol HCl is administered to a nursing woman.

PEDIATRIC USE

Safety and effectiveness in children have not been established.

DRUG INTERACTIONS:

Although levobunolol HCl used alone has little or no effect on pupil size, mydriasis resulting from concomitant therapy with levobunolol HCl and epinephrine may occur.

Close observation of the patient is recommended when a beta-blocker is administered to patients receiving catecholamine-depleting drugs such as reserpine, because of possible additive effects and the production of hypotension and/or marked bradycardia, which may produce vertigo, syncope, or postural hypotension.

Patients receiving beta-adrenergic blocking agents along with either oral or intravenous calcium antagonists should be monitored for possible atrioventricular conduction disturbances, left ventricular failure and hypotension. In patients with impaired cardiac function, simultaneous use should be avoided altogether.

The concomitant use of beta-adrenergic blocking agents with digitalis and calcium antagonists may have additive effects on prolonging atrioventricular conduction time.

Phenothiazine-related compounds and beta-adrenergic blocking agents may have additive hypotensive effects due to the inhibition of each other's metabolism.

Risk of Anaphylactic Reaction: While taking beta-blockers, patients with a history of severe anaphylactic reaction to a variety of allergens may be more reactive to repeated challenge, either accidental, diagnostic, or therapeutic. Such patients may be unresponsive to the usual doses of epinephrine used to treat allergic reaction.

ADVERSE REACTIONS:

In clinical trials the use of levobunolol HCl has been associated with transient ocular burning and stinging in up to 1 in 3 patients, and with blepharoconjunctivitis in up to 1 in 20 patients. Decreases in heart rate and blood pressure have been reported (see CONTRAINDICATIONS and WARNINGS).

The following adverse effects have been reported rarely with the use of levobunolol HCl: iridocyclitis, headache, transient ataxia, dizziness, lethargy, urticaria and pruritus.

Decreased corneal sensitivity has been noted in a small number of patients. Although levobunolol has minimal membrane-stabilizing activity, there remains a possibility of decreased corneal sensitivity after prolonged use.

The following additional adverse reactions have been reported either with levobunolol HCl or ophthalmic use of other beta-adrenergic receptor blocking agents: *Body As A Whole:* Headache, asthenia, chest pain.*Cardiovascular:* Bradycardia, arrhythmia, hypotension, syncope, heart block, cerebral vascular accident, cerebral ischemia, congestive heart failure, palpitation, cardiac arrest. *Digestive:* Nausea, diarrhea. *Psychiatric:* Depression, increase in signs and symptoms of myasthenia gravis, paresthesia. *Skin:* Hypersensitivity, including localized and generalized rash. *Respiratory:* Bronchospasm (predominantly in patients with pre-existing bronchospastic disease), respiratory failure, dyspnea, nasal congestion.*Endocrine:* Masked symptoms of hypoglycemia in insulin-dependent diabetics (see WARNINGS.) *Special Senses:* Signs and symptoms of keratitis, blepharoptosis, visual disturbances including refractive changes (due to withdrawal of miotic therapy in some cases), diplopia, ptosis.

Other reactions associated with the oral use of non-selective adrenergic receptor blocking agents should be considered potential effects with ophthalmic use of these agents.

OVERDOSAGE:

No data are available regarding overdosage in humans. Should accidental ocular overdosage occur, flush eye(s) with water or normal saline. If accidentally ingested, efforts to decrease further absorption may be appropriate (gastric lavage).

The most common signs and symptoms to be expected with overdosage with administration of a systemic beta-adrenergic blocking agent are symptomatic bradycardia, hypotension, bronchospasm, and acute cardiac failure. Should these symptoms occur, discontinue levobunolol HCl therapy and initiate appropriate supportive therapy. The following supportive measures should be considered:

1. Symptomatic Bradycardia: Use atropine sulfate intravenously in a dosage of 0.25 mg to 2 mg to induce vagal blockade. If bradycardia persists, intravenous isoproterenol hydrochloride should be administered cautiously. In refractory cases the use of a transvenous cardiac pacemaker should be considered.

2. Hypotension: Use sympathomimetic pressor drug therapy, such as dopamine, dobutamine or levarterenol. In refractory cases the use of glucagon hydrochloride may be useful.

3. Bronchospasm: Use isoproterenol hydrochloride. Additional therapy with aminophylline may be considered.

4. Acute Cardiac Failure: Conventional therapy with digitalis, diuretics and oxygen should be instituted immediately. In refractory cases the use of intravenous aminophylline is suggested. This may be followed, if necessary, by glucagon hydrochloride which may be useful.

5. Heart Block (second or third degree): Use isoproterenol hydrochloride or a transvenous cardiac pacemaker.

DOSAGE AND ADMINISTRATION:

The recommended starting dose is one to two drops of levobunolol HCl 0.5% in the affected eye(s) once a day. Typical dosing with levobunolol HCl 0.25% is one to two drops twice daily. In patients with more severe or uncontrolled glaucoma, levobunolol HCl 0.5% can be administered b.i.d. As with any new medication, careful monitoring of patients is advised.

Dosages above one drop of levobunolol HCl 0.5% b.i.d. are not generally more effective. If the patient's IOP is not at a satisfactory level on this regimen, concomitant therapy with dipivefrin and/or epinephrine, and/or pilocarpine and other miotics, and/or systemically administered carbonic anhydrase inhibitors, such as acetazolamide, can be instituted. Patients should not typically use two or more topical ophthalmic beta-adrenergic blocking agents simultaneously.

HOW SUPPLIED:

NOTE: Protect from light. Store at controlled room temperature 15°-30°C (59°-86°F). (Allergan, Inc., 2/92, 70354 30-3/T)

HOW SUPPLIED - RATED THERAPEUTICALLY EQUIVALENT:

Solution - Ophthalmic - 0.25 %

5 ml	$12.52	Levobunolol Hcl, Goldline Labs	00182-7003-62
5 ml	$13.37	Akbeta, Akorn	17478-0286-10
5 ml	$13.38	Levobunolol HCl, Schein Pharm (US)	00364-3053-53
5 ml	**$14.53**	**BETAGAN, Allergan-Amer**	**11980-0469-25**
10 ml	$24.83	Levobunolol Hcl, Goldline Labs	00182-7003-63
10 ml	$26.60	Akbeta, Akorn	17478-0286-11
10 ml	$26.62	Levobunolol HCl, Schein Pharm (US)	00364-3053-54
10 ml	**$28.80**	**BETAGAN, Allergan-Amer**	**11980-0469-20**

Solution - Ophthalmic - 0.5 %

2 ml	**$9.04**	**BETAGAN, Allergan-Amer**	**11980-0252-02**
5 ml	$14.95	Levobunolol, Major Pharms	00904-7887-05
5 ml	$14.98	Levobunolol Hcl, Goldline Labs	00182-7002-62
5 ml	$15.35	Levobunolol Hcl, Qualitest Pharms	00603-7168-37
5 ml	$16.11	Levobunolol Hcl, Aligen Independ	00405-6065-05
5 ml	$16.27	Levobunolol HCl, Schein Pharm (US)	00364-3039-53
5 ml	$16.80	Akbeta, Akorn	17478-0287-10
5 ml	$16.86	Levobunolol Hcl, HL Moore Drug Exch	00839-7929-85
5 ml	**$17.38**	**BETAGAN, Allergan-Amer**	**11980-0252-25**
5 ml	**$17.38**	**BETAGAN, Allergan-Amer**	**11980-0252-65**
10 ml	$29.25	Levobunolol, Major Pharms	00904-7887-10
10 ml	$29.28	Levobunolol Hcl, Goldline Labs	00182-7002-63
10 ml	$29.28	Levobunolol HCl, Rugby	00536-2509-70
10 ml	$29.90	Levobunolol Hcl, Qualitest Pharms	00603-7168-39
10 ml	$31.50	Akbeta, Akorn	17478-0287-11
10 ml	$31.51	Levobunolol HCl, Schein Pharm (US)	00364-3039-54
10 ml	$31.51	Levobunolol Hcl, Aligen Independ	00405-6065-10
10 ml	$32.93	Levobunolol Hcl, HL Moore Drug Exch	00839-7929-90
10 ml	**$33.95**	**BETAGAN, Allergan-Amer**	**11980-0252-20**
10 ml	**$33.95**	**BETAGAN, Allergan-Amer**	**11980-0252-60**
15 ml	$42.65	Levobunolol HCl, Major Pharms	00904-7887-35
15 ml	$42.67	Levobunolol Hcl, Goldline Labs	00182-7002-64
15 ml	$42.67	Levobunolol Hcl, Rugby	00536-2509-72
15 ml	$43.60	Levobunolol Hcl, Qualitest Pharms	00603-7168-41
15 ml	$45.80	Levobunolol HCl, Schein Pharm (US)	00364-3039-72
15 ml	$45.92	Levobunolol Hcl, Aligen Independ	00405-6065-15
15 ml	$46.20	Akbeta, Akorn	17478-0287-12
15 ml	$47.99	Levobunolol, HL Moore Drug Exch	00839-7929-61
15 ml	**$49.50**	**BETAGAN, Allergan-Amer**	**11980-0252-21**
15 ml	**$49.50**	**BETAGAN, Allergan-Amer**	**11980-0252-61**

HOW SUPPLIED - NOT RATED EQUIVALENT:

Solution - Ophthalmic - 0.25 %

5 ml	$12.84	Levobunolol Hcl, Caremark	00339-5931-50
10 ml	$25.51	Levobunolol Hcl, Caremark	00339-5931-51

Solution - Ophthalmic - 0.5 %

5 ml	$15.54	Levobunolol Hcl, Caremark	00339-5933-50
5 ml	$15.54	Levobunolol Hcl, Caremark	00339-5935-50
10 ml	$30.10	Levobunolol Hcl, Caremark	00339-5933-51
10 ml	$30.10	Levobunolol Hcl, Caremark	00339-5935-51
15 ml	$43.90	Levobunolol Hcl, Caremark	00339-5933-52
15 ml	$43.90	Levobunolol Hcl, Caremark	00339-5935-52

LEVOCABASTINE HYDROCHLORIDE *(003187)*

CATEGORIES: Allergies; Antihistamines; Conjunctivitis; EENT Drugs; Eye, Ear, Nose, & Throat Preparations; Ophthalmic Decongestants; Ophthalmics; Respiratory & Allergy Medications; FDA Class 1P ("Priority Review"); FDA Approved 1993 Nov

BRAND NAMES: **Livostin**

DESCRIPTION:

Levocabastine HCl is a selective histamine H_1-receptor antagonist for topical ophthalmic use. Each ml contains 0.54 mg levocabastine hydrochloride equivalent to 0.5 mg levocabastine; 0.15 mg benzalkonium chloride; propylene glycol; polysorbate 80; dibasic sodium phosphate, monohydrate; disodium edetate; hydroxypropyl methylcellulose; and purified water. It has a pH of 6.0 to 8.0.

The chemical name for levocabastine hydrochloride is (-)-*trans*-1-(*cis*-4-Cyano-4-(p-fluorophenyl)cyclohexyl)-3-methyl-4- phenylisonipecotic acid monohydrochloride.

CLINICAL PHARMACOLOGY:

Levocabastine is a potent, selective histamine H_1-antagonist.

Antigen challenge studies performed two to four hours after initial drug instillation indicated activity was maintained for at least two and four hours.

In an environmental study, levocabastine HCl instilled four times daily was shown to be significantly more effective than its vehicle in reducing ocular itching associated with seasonal allergic conjunctivitis.

After instillation in the eye, levocabastine is systemically absorbed. However, the amount of systemically absorbed levocabastine after therapeutic ocular doses is low (mean plasma concentrations in the range of 1-2 ng/ml).

INDICATIONS AND USAGE:

Levocabastine HCl is indicated for the temporary relief of the signs and symptoms of seasonal allergic conjunctivitis.

CONTRAINDICATIONS:

This product is contraindicated in persons with known or suspected hypersensitivity to any of its components. It should not be used' while soft contact lenses are being worn.

WARNINGS:

For topical use only. Not for injection.

PRECAUTIONS:

Information for Patients: SHAKE WELL BEFORE USING. To prevent contaminating the dropper tip and suspension, care should be taken not to touch the eyelids or surrounding areas with the dropper tip of the bottle. Keep bottle tightly closed when not in use. Do not use if the suspension has discolored. Store at controlled room temperature. Protect from freezing.

Carcinogenesis, Mutagenesis, and Impairment of Fertility: Levocabastine was not carcinogenic in male or female rats or in male mice when administered in the diet for up to 24 months. In female mice, levocabastine doses of 5,000 and 21,500 times the maximum recommended ocular human use level resulted in an increased incidence of pituitary gland adenoma and

PRECAUTIONS: *(cont'd)*

mammary gland adenocarcinoma possibly produced by increased prolactin levels. The clinical relevance of this finding is unknown with regard to the interspecies differences in prolactin physiology and the very low plasma concentrations of levocabastine following ocular administration.

Mutagenic potential was not demonstrated for levocabastine when tested in Ames' Salmonella Reversion test or in *Escherichia coli*, *Drosophila melanogaster*, a mouse Dominant Lethal Assay or in rat Micronucleus test.

In reproduction studies in rats, levocabastine showed no effects on fertility at oral doses of 20 mg/kg/day (8,300 times the maximum recommended human ocular dose).

Teratogenic Effects: Pregnancy Category C. Levocabastine has been shown to be teratogenic (polydactyly) in rats when given in doses 16,500 times the maximum recommended human ocular dose. Teratogenicity (polydactyly, hydrocephaly, brachygnathia), embryotoxicity, and maternal toxicity were observed in rats at 66,000 times the maximum recommended ocular human dose. There are no adequate and well-controlled studies in pregnant women. Levocabastine should be used during pregnancy only if the potential benefit justifies the potential risk to the fetus.

Nursing Mothers: Based on determinations of levocabastine in breast milk after ophthalmic administration of the drug to one nursing woman, it was calculated that the daily dose of levocabastine in the infant was about 0.5 mcg.

Pediatric Use: Safety and effectiveness in children below the age of 12 have not been established.

ADVERSE REACTIONS:

The most frequent complaint with the use of levocabastine HCl is that of mild, transient stinging and burning (15%) and headache (5%).

Other adverse experiences which have been reported in approximately 1-3% of patients treated with Livostin include visual disturbances, dry mouth, fatigue, pharyngitis, eye pain/dryness, somnolence, red eyes, lacrimation/discharge, cough, nausea, rash/erythema, eyelid edema, and dyspnea.

DOSAGE AND ADMINISTRATION:

Shake Well Before Using. The usual dose is one drop instilled in affected eyes four times per day. Treatment may be continued for up to 2 weeks.

HOW SUPPLIED:

Livostin 0.05% 2.5 ml, 5 ml and 10 ml, is provided in white, polyethylene dropper tip squeeze bottles.

Keep tightly closed when not in use. Do not use if the suspension has discolored. Store at controlled room temperature 15 to 30°C (59 to 86°F). Protect from freezing.

HOW SUPPLIED - EQUIVALENTS NOT AVAILABLE:

Solution - Ophthalmic - 0.05 %

5 ml	$23.94	LIVOSTIN, Ciba Vision	00058-2610-05
10 ml	$37.80	LIVOSTIN, Ciba Vision	58768-0610-10

LEVOCARNITINE *(001634)*

CATEGORIES: Caloric Agents; Carnitine Deficiency, Primary Systemic; Dietary Supplements; Electrolytic, Caloric-Water Balance; Gastrointestinal Drugs; Muscular Energy Production; Orphan Drugs; Vitamins; Pregnancy Category B; FDA Approved 1985 Dec

BRAND NAMES: *Abedine* (Japan); *Bicarnesine*; *Biocarn* (Germany); *Cardiogen*; *Carnicor*, *Carnil*; *Carnitin*; *Carnitene*; *Carnitolo*; **Carnitor**; *Entomin* (Japan); *Entomine*; *L-Carn* (Germany); *L-Carnitin*; *L-Carnitina*; *Monocamin* (Japan); Vitacarn
(International brand names outside U.S. in italics)

FORMULARIES: Medi-Cal

DESCRIPTION:

LEVOCARNITINE IS (R)-3-CARBOXY-2-HYDROXY-N,N,N-TRIMETHYL-1-PROPANANMINIUM HYDROXIDE, INNER SALT. LEVOCARNITINE IS A CARRIER MOLECULE IN THE TRANSPORT OF LONG CHAIN FATTY ACROSS THE INNER MITOCHONDRIAL MEMBRANE. AS A BULK DRUG SUBSTANCE IT IS A WHITE POWDER WITH A MELTING POINT OF 196-197œC AND IS READILY SOLUBLE IN WATER, HOT ALCOHOL, AND INSOLUBLE IN ACETONE. THE PH OF A SOLUTION (1 IN 20) IS BETWEEN 6-8 AND ITS PKA VALUE IS 3.8. THE EMPIRICAL FORMULA IS $C_7H_{15}NO_3$ and the molecular weight is 161.20.

Tablets: Each Carnitor tablet contains 330 mg of levocarnitine and the inactive ingredients magnesium stearate, microcrystalline cellulose and povidone.

Oral Solution: Each 118 ml container of the Carnitor oral solution contains 1 g of levocarnitine/10 ml. Also contains: Artificial Cherry Flavor, D&C Red No. 33, D,L-Malic Acid, FD&C Red No. 40, Purified Water, Sucrose Syrup. Methylparaben NF and Propylparaben NF are added as preservatives. The Ph is approximately 5.

CLINICAL PHARMACOLOGY:

Levocarnitine is a naturally occurring substance required in mammalian energy metabolism. It has been shown to facilitate long-chain fatty acid entry into cellular mitochondria, therefor delivering substrate for oxidation & subsequent energy production. Fatty acids are utilized as an energy substrate in all tissues except the brain. In skeletal and cardiac muscle they serve as major fuel. Primary systemic carnitine deficiency is characterized by low plasma, RBC, and/or tissue levels. It has not been possible to determine which symptoms are due to carnitine deficiency and which are due to the underlying organic acidemia, as symptoms of both abnormalities may be expected to improve with carnitine. The literature reports that carnitine can promote the excretion of excess organic or fatty acids in patients with defects in fatty acid metabolism and/or specific organic acidopathies that bioaccumulate acyl CoA esters.[1-6]

Secondary levocarnitine deficiency can be a consequence of inborn errors of metabolism. Levocarnitine may alleviate the metabolic abnormalities of patients with inborn errors that result in accumulation of toxic organic acids. Conditions for which this effect was demonstrated are: glutaric aciduria II, methyl malonic aciduria, propionic acidemia, and medium chain fatty acyl CoA dehydrogenase deficiency.[7,8] Autointoxication occurs in these patients due to the accumulations of acyl CoA compounds that disrupt intermediary metabolism. The subsequent hydrolysis of the acyl CoA compound to its free acid results in acidosis that can be life threatening. Levocarnitine clears the acyl CoA compound by formation of acyl carnitine which is quickly excreted. Levocarnitine deficiency is defined biochemically as abnormally low plasma levels of free carnitine, less than 20 mcm/L at age greater than one week post term and may be associated with low tissue and/or urine levels. Further, this condition may be associated with a ratio of plasma ester/free levocarnitine levels greater than

CLINICAL PHARMACOLOGY: *(cont'd)*

0.4 or abnormally elevated levels of esterified levocarnitine in the urine. In premature infants and newborns, secondary deficiency is defined as plasma free levocarnitine levels below age related normal levels.

BIOAVAILABILITY/PHARMACOKINETICS

In a relative bioavailability study in 15 healthy adult male volunteers levocarnitine tablets were found to be bio-equivalent to levocarnitine oral solution. Following the administration of 1980 mg b.i.d., the maximum plasma concentration level (C_{max}) was 80 nmol/ml and the time to maximum concentration (T_{max}) occurred at 3.3 hours. There were no significant differences for AUC and urinary excretion observed between these two formulations.

In the same bioavailability study of 15 healthy adult males, levocarnitine injection administered as a slow 3 minute bolus intravenous injection at a dose of 20 mg/kg showed that free levocarnitine plasma profiles are best fit by a two compartment model. Approximately 76% of free levocarnitine is eliminated in the urine. Using plasma levels uncorrected for endogenous levocarnitine, the mean distribution half life was 0.585 hours and the mean apparent terminal elimination half life was 17.4 hours following a single intravenous dose.

The absolute bioavailability of L-carnitine from levocarnitine tablets and oral solution was determined compared to the bioavailability of L-carnitine from levocarnitine intravenous injection in 15 healthy male volunteers. After correction for circulating endogenous levels of L-carnitine in the plasma, absolute bioavailability was 15.1% ± 5.3% for L-carnitine from levocarnitine tablets and 15.9% ± 4.9% from the oral solution.

Total body clearance of L-carnitine (Dose/AUC including endogenous baseline levels) was a mean of 4.00 L/hr. Endogenous baseline levels were not subtracted since total body clearance of levocarnitine does not distinguish between exogenous sources of levocarnitine and endogenously synthesized levocarnitine. Volume of distribution of the intravenously administered dose above baseline endogenous levels was calculated to be a mean of 29.0 ± 7.1 L (approximately 0.39 L/kg) which is an underestimate of the true volume of distribution since plasma L-carnitine is known to equilibrate slowly with, for instance, muscle L-carnitine.

L-carnitine was not bound to plasma protein or albumin when treated at any concentration or with any species including the human.[9]

METABOLISM AND EXCRETION

Five normal adult male volunteers, administered a dose of (^{3}H-methyl)-L-carnitine following 15 days of a high carnitine diet and additional carnitine supplement, excreted 58-65% of administered radioactive dose in 5 to 11 days in the urine and feces. Maximum concentration of (^{3}H-methyl)-L-carnitine in serum occurred from 2.0 to 4.5 hr after drug administration. Major metabolites found were trimethylamine N-oxide, primarily in urine (8% to 49% of the administered dose) and (^{3}H)-butyrobetaine, primarily in feces (0.44% to 45% of the administered dose). Urinary excretion of carnitine was 4% to 8% of the dose. Fecal excretion of total carnitine was less than 1% of total carnitine excretion.[10]

After attainment of steady state following 4 days of oral administration of L-carnitine with levocarnitine tablets (1980 mg q12h) oral solution (2000 mg q12h) to 15 healthy male volunteers, urinary excretion of L-carnitine was a mean of 2107 and 2339 mcmoles, respectively, equivalent to 8.6% and 9.4%, respectively, of the orally administered doses (uncorrected for endogenous urinary excretion). After a single intravenous dose (20 mg/kg) prior to multiple oral doses, urinary excretion of L-carnitine was 6974 mcmoles equivalent to 75.6% of the intravenously administered dose (uncorrected for endogenous urinary excretion).

INDICATIONS AND USAGE:

For the acute and chronic treatment of patients with an inborn error of metabolism that results in secondary carnitine deficiency.

Tablets And Oral Solution: Levocarnitine is indicated in the treatment of primary systemic carnitine deficiency. In the reported cases, the clinical presentation consisted of recurrent episodes of Reye-like encephalopathy, hypoketotic hypoglycemia, and/or cardiomyopathy. Associated symptoms included hypotonia, muscle weakness and failure to thrive. A diagnosis of primary carnitine deficiency requires that serum, red cell and/or tissue carnitine levels be low and that the patient does not have a primary defect in fatty acid or organic acid oxidation (see CLINICAL PHARMACOLOGY.) In some patients, particularly those presenting with cardiomyopathy, carnitine supplementation rapidly alleviated signs and symptoms. Treatment should include, in addition to carnitine, supportive and other therapy as indicated by the condition of the patient.

CONTRAINDICATIONS:

None known.

WARNINGS:

None.

PRECAUTIONS:

GENERAL

Oral Solution: Levocarnitine oral solution is for oral/internal use only.

Not for parenteral use.

Gastrointestinal reactions may result from too rapid consumption of carnitine. Levocarnitine oral solution may be consumed alone, or dissolved in drinks or other liquid foods to reduce taste fatigue. It should be consumed slowly and doses should be spaced evenly throughout the day to maximize tolerance.

CARCINOGENESIS, MUTAGENESIS, AND IMPAIRMENT OF FERTILITY

Mutagenicity tests have been performed in *Salmonella typhimurium*, *Saccharomyces cerevisiae*, and *Schizosaccharomyces pombe* that do not indicate that levocarnitine is mutagenic. Long-term animal studies have not been conducted to evaluate the carcinogenicity of the compound.

PREGNANCY CATEGORY B

Reproductive studies have been performed in rats and rabbits at doses up to 3.8 times the human dose on the basis of surface area and have revealed no evidence of impaired fertility or harm to the fetus due to levocarnitine. There are, however, no adequate and well controlled studies in pregnant women. Because animal reproduction studies are not always predictive of human response, this drug should be used during pregnancy only if clearly needed.

NURSING MOTHERS

It is not whether this drug is excreted in human milk. Because many drugs are excreted in human milk, a decision should be made whether to discontinue the drug, taking into account the importance of the drug to the mother.

PEDIATRIC USE

See DOSAGE AND ADMINISTRATION.

ADVERSE REACTIONS:

Tablets And Oral Solution: Various gastrointestinal complaints have been reported during the long-term administration of oral L - or D,L-carnitine; these include transient nausea and vomiting; abdominal cramps, and diarrhea. Mild myasthenia has been described only in

ADVERSE REACTIONS: *(cont'd)*

uremic patients receiving D,L-carnitine. Gastrointestinal adverse reactions with levocarnitine oral solution dissolved in liquids might be avoided by a slow consumption of the solution or by a greater dilution. Decreasing the dosage often diminishes or eliminates drug-related patient body odor or gastrointestinal symptoms when present. Tolerance should be monitored very closely during the first week of administration, and after any dosage increases.

OVERDOSAGE:

There have been no reports of toxicity from carnitine overdosage. The oral LD_{50} of levocarnitine in mice is 19.2 g/kg. Carnitine may cause diarrhea.

Tablets And Oral Solution Only: Overdosage should be treated with supportive care.

DOSAGE AND ADMINISTRATION:

TABLETS

Adults: The recommended oral dosage for adults is 990 mg two or three times a day using the 330 mg tablets, depending on clinical response.

Infants and children: The recommended oral dosage for infants and children is between 50 and 100 mg/kg/day in divided doses, with a maximum of 3 g/day. Dosage should begin at 50 mg/kg/day. The exact dosage will depend on clinical response.

Monitoring should include periodic blood chemistries, vital signs, plasma carnitine concentrations and overall clinical condition.

Store at room temperature (25°C/77°F).

ORAL SOLUTION

For oral use only. **Not for parenteral use.**

Adults: The recommended dosage of levocarnitine is 1 to 3 g/day for a 50 kg subject which is equivalent to 10 to 30 ml/day of levocarnitine oral solution. Higher doses should be administered only with caution and only where clinical and biochemical considerations make it seem likely that higher doses will be of benefit. Dosage should start at 1 g/day, (10ml/day), and be increased slowly while assessing tolerance and therapeutic response. Monitoring should include periodic blood chemistries, vital signs, plasma carnitine concentrations, and overall clinical condition.

Infants and children: The recommended dosage of levocarnitine is 50 to 100 mg/kg/day which is equivalent to 0.5 ml/kg/day levocarnitine oral solution. Higher doses should be administered only with caution and only where clinical and biochemical considerations make it seem likely that higher doses will be of benefit. Dosage should start at 50 mg/kg/day, and be increased slowly to a maximum of 3 g/day (30 ml/day) while assessing tolerance and therapeutic response. Monitoring should include periodic blood chemistries, vital signs, plasma carnitine concentrations, and overall clinical condition.

Levocarnitine oral solution may be consumed alone or dissolved in drink or other liquid food. Doses should be spaced evenly throughout the day (every three or four hours) preferably during or following meals and should be consumed slowly in order to maximize tolerance.

Store at room temperature (25°C/77°F).

INJECTION

Levocarnitine injection is administered intravenously. The recommended dose is 50 mg/kg given as a slow 2-3 minute bolus injection or by infusion. Often a loading dose is given in patients with severe metabolic crisis followed by an equivalent dose over the following 24 hours. It should be administered q3h or q4h, and never less than q6h either by infusion or by intravenous injection. All subsequent daily doses are recommended to be in the range of 50 mg/kg or as therapy may require. The highest dose administered has been 300 mg/kg.

It is recommended that a plasma carnitine level be obtained prior to beginning this parenteral therapy. Weekly and monthly monitoring is recommended as well. This monitoring should include blood chemistries; vital signs, plasma carnitine concentrations (the plasma free carnitine level should be between 35 and 60 micromoles/liter) and overall clinical condition.

Parenteral drug products should be inspected visually for particulate matter and discoloration prior to administration, whenever solution and container permit.

Store ampoules at room temperature (25°C/77°F) in carton until their use to protect from light. Discard unused portion of an opened ampoule, as they contain no preservative.

(Tablets and Oral Solution: Sigma-Tau, 1/93, ST-N18-948) (Injection: Sigma-Tau, 1/93, ST-N20-182)

HOW SUPPLIED - RATED THERAPEUTICALLY EQUIVALENT:

Solution - Oral - 1 gm/10ml

120 ml	$31.80	VITACARN, McGaw	00264-6802-66

HOW SUPPLIED - NOT RATED EQUIVALENT:

Injection, Solution - Intravenous - 1 gm/5ml

5 ml x 5	**$180.00**	**CARNITOR, Sigma Tau Pharms**	**54482-0146-09**

Solution - Oral - 1 gm/10ml

118 ml	**$677.39**	**CARNITOR, Sigma Tau Pharms**	**54482-0145-08**

Tablet, Uncoated - Oral - 330 mg

90's	**$71.07**	**CARNITOR, Sigma Tau Pharms**	**54482-0144-07**

LEVODOPA *(001635)*

CATEGORIES: Anticholinergic Agents; Antiparkinson Agents; Autonomic Drugs; Extrapyramidal Movement Disorders; Parkinsonism; FDA Approval Pre 1982

BRAND NAMES: *Bidopal*; *Brocadopa* (England); *Brocadopa Retard*; *Ceredopa*; *Dopaflex* (Germany); Dopar; *Doparkin*; *Doparkine*; *Dopari* (Japan); *Dopasol* (Japan); *Dopastan* (Japan); *Dopaston*; *Dopastral*; *Eldopal*; *Eldopal Retard*; L-Dopa; *Laradopa*; **Larodopa**; *Levodopa-Woelm* (Germany); *Levopa*; *Levotrifar*, *Medidopa*
(International brand names outside U.S. in italics)

FORMULARIES: Medi-Cal

COST OF THERAPY: $263.38 (Parkinsonism; Tablet; 250 mg; 2/day; 365 days)

In order to reduce the high incidence of adverse reactions, it is necessary to individualize the therapy and to gradually increase the dosage to the desired therapeutic level.

DESCRIPTION:

Larodopa Tablets contain 100 mg, 250 mg or 500 mg levodopa. Each tablet also contains corn starch, magnesium stearate, microcrystalline cellulose, povidone, talc and D&C Red No. 7 lake dye.

Dopar Capsules, 100 mg, 250 mg, 500 mg, levodopa. Inactive ingredients: Each capsule contains edible black ink, FD&C Blue # 1, gelatin, lactose, talc, titanium dioxide, and FD&C yellow # 5.

DESCRIPTION: *(cont'd)*

Chemically, levodopa is (-)-3-(3,4-dihydroxyphenyl)-*L*-alanine. It is a colorless, crystalline compound, slightly soluble in water and insoluble in alcohol, with a molecular weight of 197.2.

CLINICAL PHARMACOLOGY:

Evidence indicates that the symptoms of Parkinson's disease are related to depletion of striatal dopamine. Since dopamine apparently does not cross the blood-brain barrier, its administration is ineffective in the treatment of Parkinson's disease. However, levodopa, the levo-rotatory isomer of dihydroxyphenylalanine (dopa) which is the metabolic precursor of dopamine, does cross the blood-brain barrier. Presumably it is converted into dopamine in the basal ganglia. This is generally thought to be the mechanism whereby oral levodopa acts in relieving the symptoms of Parkinson's disease.

The major urinary metabolites of levodopa in man appear to be dopamine and homovanillic acid (HVA). In 24-hour urine samples, HVA accounts for 13 to 42 percent of the ingested dose of levodopa.

INDICATIONS AND USAGE:

Levodopa is indicated in the treatment of idiopathic Parkinson's disease (Paralysis Agitans), postencephalitic parkinsonism, symptomatic parkinsonism which may follow injury to the nervous system by carbon monoxide intoxication, and manganese intoxication. It is indicated in those elderly patients believed to develop parkinsonism in association with cerebral arteriosclerosis.

CONTRAINDICATIONS:

Monoamine oxidase (MAO) inhibitors and Levodopa should not be given concomitantly and these inhibitors must be discontinued two weeks prior to initiating therapy with Levodopa. Levodopa is contraindicated in patients with known hypersensitivity to the drug and in narrow angle glaucoma.

Because levodopa may activate a malignant melanoma, it should not be used in patients with suspicious, undiagnosed skin lesions or a history of melanoma.

WARNINGS:

Levodopa should be administered cautiously to patients with severe cardiovascular or pulmonary disease, bronchial asthma, renal, hepatic or endocrine disease.

Care should be exercised in administering Levodopa to patients with a history of myocardial infarction who have residual atrial, nodal or ventricular arrhythmias. If Levodopa is necessary in this type of patient, it should be used in a facility with a coronary care unit or an intensive care unit.

One must be on the alert for the possibility of upper gastrointestinal hemorrhage in those patients with a past history of active peptic ulcer disease.

All patients should be carefully observed for the development of depression with concomitant suicidal tendencies. Psychotic patients should be treated with caution.

Pyridoxine hydrochloride (vitamin B_6) in oral doses of 10 to 25 mg rapidly reverses the toxic and therapeutic effects of Levodopa. This should be considered before recommending vitamin preparations containing pyridoxine hydrochloride (vitamin B_6).

USAGE IN PREGNANCY:

The safety of Levodopa in women who are or who may become pregnant has not been established; hence it should be given only when the potential benefits have been weighed against possible hazards to mother and child. Studies in rodents have shown that levodopa at dosages in excess of 200 mg/kg/day has an adverse effect on fetal and postnatal growth and viability.

Levodopa should not be used in nursing mothers.

USAGE IN CHILDREN:

The safety of Levodopa under the age of 12 has not been established.

PRECAUTIONS:

Periodic evaluations of hepatic, hematopoietic, cardiovascular and renal function are recommended during extended therapy in all patients.

Patients with chronic wide angle glaucoma may be treated cautiously with Levodopa, provided the intraocular pressure is well controlled and the patient monitored carefully for changes in intraocular pressure during therapy.

Postural hypotensive episodes have been reported as adverse reactions. Therefore, Levodopa should be administered to patients on antihypertensive drug cautiously (for patients receiving pargyline, see note on MAO inhibitors contraindications), and it may be necessary to adjust the dosage of the antihypertensive drugs.

Dopar Capsules contain FD&C Yellow No. 5 (tartrazine) which may cause allergic type reactions (including bronchial asthma) in certain susceptible individuals. Although the overall incidence of FD&C Yellow No. 5 (tartrazine) sensitivity in the general population is low, it is frequently seen in patients who also have aspirin hypersensitivity

ADVERSE REACTIONS:

The most serious adverse reactions associated with the administration of Levodopa having frequent occurrences are: adventitious movements such as choreiform and/or dystonic movements. Other serious adverse reactions with a lower incidence are: cardiac irregularities and/or palpitations, orthostatic hypotensive episodes, bradykinetic episodes (the "on-off" phenomena), mental changes including paranoid ideation and psychotic episodes, depression with or without the development of suicidal tendencies, dementia, and urinary retention.

Rarely, gastrointestinal bleeding, development of duodenal ulcer, hypertension, phlebitis, hemolytic anemia, agranulocytosis, and convulsions have been observed. (The causal relationship between convulsions and Levodopa has not been established.)

Adverse reactions of a less serious nature having a relatively frequent occurrence are the following: anorexia, nausea and vomiting with or without abdominal pain and distress, dry mouth, dysphagia, sialorrhea, ataxia, increased hand tremor, headache, dizziness, numbness, weakness and faintness, bruxism, confusion, insomnia, nightmares, hallucinations and delusions, agitation and anxiety, malaise, fatigue and euphoria. Occurring with a lesser order of frequency are the following: muscle twitching and blepharospasm (which may be taken as an early sign of overdosage; consideration of dosage reduction may be made at this time), trismus, burning sensation of the tongue, bitter taste, diarrhea, constipation, flatulence, flushing, skin rash, increased sweating, bizarre breathing patterns, urinary incontinence, diplopia, blurred vision, dilated pupils, hot flashes, weight gain or loss, dark sweat and/or urine.

Rarely, oculogyric crises, sense of stimulation, hiccups, development of edema, loss of hair, hoarseness, priapism and activation of latent Horner's syndrome have been observed.

Elevations of blood urea nitrogen, SGOT, SGPT, LDH, bilirubin, alkaline phosphatase or protein-bound iodine have been reported; and the significance of this is not known. Occasional reductions in WBC, hemoglobin, and hematocrit have been noted.

ADVERSE REACTIONS: *(cont'd)*

Leukopenia has occurred and requires cessation, at least temporarily, of Levodopa administration. The Coombs test has occasionally become positive during extended therapy. Elevations of uric acid have been noted when colorimetric method was used but not when uricase method was used.

OVERDOSAGE:

For acute overdosage general supportive measures should be employed, along with immediate gastric lavage. Intravenous fluids should be administered judiciously and an adequate airway maintained.

Electrocardiographic monitoring should be instituted and the patient carefully observed for the possible development of arrhythmias; if required, appropriate antiarrhythmic therapy should be given. Consideration should be given to the possibility of multiple drug ingestion by the patient. To date, no experience has been reported with dialysis; hence its value in Levodopa overdosage is not known. Although pyridoxine hydrochloride (vitamin B_6) has been reported to reverse the antiparkinson effects of Levodopa, its usefulness in the management of acute overdosage has not been established.

DOSAGE AND ADMINISTRATION:

The optimal daily dose of Levodopa, i.e., the dose producing maximal improvement with tolerated side effects, must be determined and *carefully titrated for each individual patient.* The usual initial dosage is 0.5 to 1 gm daily, divided in two or more doses with food.

The total daily dosage is then increased gradually in increments not more than 0.75 g every three to seven days as tolerated. The usual optimal therapeutic dosage *should not exceed 8 g.* The exceptional patient may carefully be given more than 8 gms as required. In some patients, a significant therapeutic response may not be obtained until six months of treatment.

In the event general anesthesia is required, Levodopa therapy may be continued as long as the patient is able to take fluids and medication by mouth. If therapy is temporarily interrupted, the usual daily dosage may be administered as soon as the patient is able to take oral medication. Whenever therapy has been interrupted for longer periods, dosage should again be adjusted gradually; however, in many cases the patient can be rapidly titrated to his previous therapeutic dosage.

HOW SUPPLIED - EQUIVALENTS NOT AVAILABLE:

Capsule, Gelatin - Oral - 100 mg
100's $27.99 DOPAR, Roberts Labs 54092-0060-01

Capsule, Gelatin - Oral - 250 mg
100's $49.48 DOPAR, Roberts Labs 54092-0061-01

Capsule, Gelatin - Oral - 500 mg
100's $74.69 DOPAR, Roberts Labs 54092-0062-01

Tablet, Uncoated - Oral - 100 mg
100's $22.60 LARODOPA, Roche 00004-0072-01

Tablet, Uncoated - Oral - 250 mg
100's $36.08 LARODOPA, Roche 00004-0057-01

Tablet, Uncoated - Oral - 500 mg
100's $61.98 LARODOPA, Roche 00004-0056-01

LEVOMETHADYL ACETATE HYDROCHLORIDE *(003174)*

CATEGORIES: Analgesics; Central Nervous System Agents; Narcotic Addiction; Narcotic Detoxification; Narcotics, Synthetics & Combinations; Opiate Agonists (Controlled); Orphan Drugs; Pain; DEA Class CII; FDA Class 1P ("Priority Review"); FDA Approved 1993 Jul

BRAND NAMES: LAAM; Levo-Alpha-Acetylmethadol; **Orlaam**

WARNING:
Warning: May be habit forming.
CONDITIONS FOR DISTRIBUTION AND USE OF ORLAAM (21 CFR 291.505)
Levomethadyl acetate HCl used for the treatment of narcotic addiction shall be dispensed only by treatment programs approved by FDA, DEA and the designated State authority. Approved treatment programs shall dispense and use levomethadyl acetate HCl in oral form only and according to the treatment requirements stipulated in Federal regulations. Failure to abide by these requirements may result in injunction precluding operation of the program, seizure of the drug supply, revocation of the program approval, and possible criminal prosecution.
Levomethadyl acetate HCl has no recommended used outside of the treatment of opiate addiction.

DESCRIPTION:

LEVOMETHADYL ACETATE HCL IS A SYNTHETIC OPIATE AGONIST. CHEMICALLY, IT IS LEVO-ALPHA-6-DIMETHYLAMINO-4, 4- DIPHENYL-3-HEPTYL ACTETATE HYDROCHLORIDE, $C_{23}H_{31}NO_2$·HCl. It is also known as levo-alpha- acetylmethadol hydrochloride (LAAM).

THE COMPOUND IS WHITE CRYSTALLINE POWDER, SOLUBLE IN WATER (> 15 MG/ML), ETHANOL, AND METHYL ETHYL KETON. THE OCTANOL:WATER PARTITION COEFFICIENT OF LAAM IS 405:1 AT PHYSIOLOGIC PH. DOSES OF LEVOMETHADYL ACETATE HCL (LAAM) ARE ALWAYS EXPRESSED AS THE WEIGHT OF THE HYDROCHLORIDE SALT (MOLECULAR WEIGHT 389.95).

ORLAAM IS AN AQUEOUS SOLUTION WHICH IS DILUTED FOR ORAL ADMINISTRATION. EACH ONE ML OF ORLAAM CONTAINS:

LEVOMETHADYL ACETATE HYDROCHLORIDE (LAAM) 10 MG; *Inactive ingredients:* Methylparaben: 1.8 mg; Propylparaben: 0.2 mg.

CLINICAL PHARMACOLOGY:

LAAM is a synthetic opioid agonist with actions quantitatively similar to morphine (a prototypic mu agonist) and affecting the central nervous system (CNS) and smooth muscle. Principal actions include analgesia and sedation. Tolerance to these effects develops with repeated use. An abstinence syndrome generally occurs upon cessation of chronic administration similar to that observed with other opiates, but with slower onset, more prolonged course, and less severe symptoms.

CLINICAL PHARMACOLOGY: *(cont'd)*

LAAM exerts its clinical effects in the treatment of opiate abuse through two mechanisms. First, LAAM cross-substitutes for opiates of the morphine-type, suppressing symptoms of withdrawal in opiate-dependent individuals. Second, chronic oral administration of LAAM can produce sufficient tolerance to block the subjective "high" of usual doses of parenterally administered opiates.

LAAM is metabolized by N-demethylation to nor-LAAM and dinor-LAAM, which are also opioid agonists. These metabolites are more potent than the parent drug. The opioid effect which occurs when LAAM is administered is slower in onset and longer in duration (72 hours) than that of methadone (24 hours). The extended duration of action allows three-times-weekly administration (see CLINICAL STUDIES.)

PHARMACODYNAMICS

The duration of action of a single dose of LAAM is due to the sum of the opioid activity of the parent drug and its metabolites. A single dose of orally administered LAAM has an onset of opioid effects averaging 2 to 4 hours after ingestion and a duration of action of 48 to 72 hours (as measured by pupillary constriction and suppression of abstinence signs). LAAM cross-substitutes for opiates like morphine in opiate-dependent individuals, suppressing symptoms of withdrawal from these compounds. Single oral doses of 30 to 60 mg of LAAM eliminate signs of abstinence for 24 to 48 hours in individuals maintained on high doses of morphine who are abruptly withdrawn. At higher doses (80 mg and above), suppression of withdrawal can increase to 48-72 hours in most individuals.

Repeated oral administration of LAAM can produce sufficient tolerance to block the effects of parenterally administered opiates. Chronic oral administration of 70 to 100 mg of LAAM three times weekly produces tolerance which blocks the "high" of a 25 mg dose of intravenously administered heroin for up to 72 hours; maintenance on lower doses (50 mg) of LAAM produces only partial blockade for the same period.

PHARMACOKINETICS

Absorption: LAAM is rapidly absorbed from an oral solution. Plasma levels are detectable within 15 to 30 minutes after ingestion and reach their peak within 1.5 to 2 hours at steady-state. LAAM undergoes first-pass metabolism to its demethylated metabolite nor-LAAM, which is sequentially N-demethylated to dinor-LAAM. Both metabolites are active and contribute to the extent and duration of levomethadyl acetate HCl's clinical activity (see Pharmacodynamics).

PHARMACOKINETIC MODEL

The steady-state pharmacokinetics of LAAM were modeled from a study in 25 healthy adult addicts using three-times-a-week dosing over a 15-day observation period. LAAM and its metabolites were found to follow a multi-compartment model with extensive tissue distribution (Vd - 20 l/kg). LAAM had a clearance of about 0.22 l/kg/hr, mostly by conversion to nor-LAAM. Kinetic studies of the pure metabolites in man have not yet provided accurate estimated of their clearance in the absence of the precursor, but the half-lives observed in this study were 2.6 days for LAAM, approximately 2 days for nor-LAAM, and approximately 4 days for dinor-LAAM.

The pharmacokinetic model used to estimate steady-state plasma levels for each subject in this study assumed a common 3 mg/kg/wk dosage regimen (0.94 mg/kg on Mon. and Wed., 1.125 mg/kg on Fri.). The estimates (which fit the observed data with a correlation of better than 0.95) revealed a large inter-patient variability. There was at least a 5-fold range in peak plasma concentrations for LAAM and its metabolites across the 25 subjects over the 72-hour interval from Friday to Monday on a 3-times-a- week dosage regimen. TABLE 1 contains these estimates of peal and trough plasma concentrations of LAAM, nor-LAAM, and dinor-LAAM.

TABLE 1 Peak and Trough Estimated Steady-State Plasma Concentrations During the 72 Hour Interval (Friday to Monday) for a 65-kg Patient Given 3 mg/kg/Week on Mon./Wed./Fri.

Mean & (CV)	LAAM	Nor-LAAM	Dinor-LAAM
Cmax (ng/ml)*	204 (34%)	173 (34%)	114 (28%)
Cmin(ng/ml)**	36 (62%)	85 (58%)	96 (34%)

* Following Friday Morning Dose
** Prior to Monday Morning Dose

METABOLISM AND ELIMINATION

As noted above, the formation of nor-LAAM and dinor-LAAM is by sequential demethylation, such that dinor-LAAM is formed from nor-LAAM, not directly from LAAM. While N-demethylation is the primary route of metabolism, minor pathways of elimination include direct excretion and deacetylation to methadol, nor-methanol, and dinor-methadol.

SPECIAL POPULATIONS

Gender: An analysis of the data from the above study showed some difference in the plasma clearance of LAAM in 8 females versus 17 males. Males showed a trend toward a slower conversion of LAAM to nor-LAAM, which may alter the plasma concentration profile of LAAM and its active opioid metabolites. Although this effect was much smaller than the observed inter-individual differences, physicians should be alert to a possible gender difference(see CLINICAL STUDIES, Individualization Of Dosage.)

Hepatic and Renal Disease: At the present time no pharmacokinetics studies have been carried out in subjects with clinically significant hepatic insufficiency or serious renal impairment. Since both the pharmacokinetics and pharmacodynamics of opiate agonists may be altered in these subjects, and any additional risks of levomethadyl acetate HCl therapy are not well understood in such patients, physicians may choose to manage such patients with methadone due to its simpler metabolic profile.

CLINICAL STUDIES:

Levomethadyl acetate HCl has been studied in 2666 street addicts and 3319 methadone maintenance patients, including 5697 males and 288 females. During the course of 27 studies, 4610 patients received orally administered levomethadyl acetate HCl for up to three years in thrice-weekly doses ranging from 10 to 140 mg. Twenty-one studies provide the primary evidence upon which the dosing recommendations for levomethadyl acetate HCl are based.

The vast majority of patients who received levomethadyl acetate HCl were treated on a thrice-weekly basis, typically on Mondays, Wednesdays, and Fridays (Mon./Wed./Fri.), although every-other-day dosing schedules were used in some settings. Most of the sites dosing patients with LAAM on a 3-times- a-week (Mon./Wed./Fri. or Tues./Thurs./Sat.) schedule increased the dose prior too the 72-hour inter-dose interval by 20 to 40% to obtain coverage for the full 72 hours.

In controlled clinical trials, treatment with levomethadyl acetate HCl was found to be comparable to treatment with methadone with respect to reduction in use of illicit opioids. Levomethadyl acetate HCl doses in the range of 60 to 100 mg 3-times-a- week reduced the average frequency of urine samples positive for opiates to 15-20%, as did therapy with 50 to 100 mg a day of methadone. There was a trend for more patients to drop out of levomethadyl acetate HCl therapy than methadone therapy in the first 4 weeks of treatment (16% dropouts for levomethadyl acetate HCl v. 12% for methadone), but the dropout rates

CLINICAL STUDIES: *(cont'd)*

for both treatments rapidly declined and both were in the range of 1 to 2% per week for the remaining patients by the end of the third month of the studies. Global ratings of patient acceptability and response to treatment were similar for both LAAM and methadone.

In the Phase III studies, levomethadyl acetate HCl tended to be more effective in patients perceived by staff to benefit from a reduced frequency of clinic visits and less effective in patients perceived as needing the added support of daily clinic visits.

Four independent studies were concerned with other research objectives, including induction regimens, methadone-to-levomethadyl acetate HCl (and levomethadyl acetate HCl-to- methadone) crossover ratios, and detoxification. This research involved 800 adults (including 11 females), approximately 440 of whom were methadone maintenance patients. The results of these studies,as well as the results of a nationwide Phase III usage study of 623 patients (including 204 females) in 25 representative clinics across the country, are reflected in the dosing recommendations.

INDIVIDUALIZATION OF DOSAGE

Levomethadyl acetate HCl is intended for use as part of a comprehensive treatment plan for narcotic dependence of the opioid type. Supplying narcotic drugs to narcotic addicts for the treatment of an addiction without appropriate medical evaluation, treatment planning, and counseling has not been shown to be effective, and is a violation of law except in special circumstances.

The therapeutic goal early in treatment with levomethadyl acetate HCl is to reduce illicit opioid use. The dose of levomethadyl acetate HCl should be chosen and adjusted as needed to provide a dose that is high enough to suppress drug withdrawal, illicit drug seeking and usage, and related high-risk behavior. If opioid side effects persist once illicit drug use is controlled, the dose of levomethadyl acetate HCl may require further adjustment later in treatment to minimize adverse effects.

Physicians should be alert to patient differences in levels of opioid tolerance and inter-patient variability in the absorption, distribution and metabolism of both levomethadyl acetate HCl and its metabolites. As with methadone, an important contribution to continued abuse of illicit drugs is an inadequate dose of the treatment medication.

Initial dosage adjustment with levomethadyl acetate HCl is complex due to its delayed onset of action. If the starting dose is too high or if the dose is escalated too rapidly for the patient's level of tolerance, symptoms characteristic of excessive opioid effect may occur, i.e., poor concentrations, sedation and orthostatic hypotension. Patients should be watched for such symptoms, and the dose should be lowered if they appear. In rare instances, serious symptoms of narcotic overdosage may occur, leading to profound CNS and respiratory depression.

Levomethadyl acetate HCl and its metabolites quickly accumulate to toxic levels if the does intended for 3-times-a-week dosing are given too frequently. The recommended doses are intended for every-other-day or 3-times-a-week dosing and <u>should not be given daily.</u>

The recommended initial dose for patients with low or unknown tolerance to opioids is 20 to 40 mg <u>three times a week</u> or <u>every-other-day.</u> Successive doses may be increased by 5 or 10 mg. At least two weeks are needed to achieve a clinical plateau after a dosage adjustment. Adjustment to a dosing schedule is dependent upon the rate at which an individual develops tolerance to the increasing level of levomethadyl acetate HCl (and its metabolites) as well as the time required for levomethadyl acetate HCl and its metabolites to accumulate to steady-state levels.

The goal of dosage titration is to suppress narcotic withdrawal while avoiding excessive opioid effects due to the build-up of long-acting metabolites. It may be safer to provide extra counseling and support rather than to attempt to completely suppress a patient's withdrawal or narcotic hunger during the first week or two of therapy. On the other hand, there is the ever-present danger that patients who receive sub- therapeutic starting doses will supplement with street drugs, resulting in overdose. Patients should be strongly warned against this practice. Later in the titration process, dosage adjustments are better made on a weekly basis whenever possible.

For patients on methadone maintenance whose level of tolerance is known, the recommended initial dose of levomethadyl acetate HCl is 1.2 to 1.3 times the patient's daily dose of methadone, not to exceed 120 mg. Care should be taken not to adjust the dose too frequently thereafter (usually 5 to 10 mg changes every second or third dose) since increasing the dose too rapidly may result in oversedation.

One major advantage of levomethadyl acetate HCl therapy is reduction in the need for daily clinic visits and for take-home medication. In some patients, levomethadyl acetate HCl may not provide adequate suppression of withdrawal for a full 72 hours. For such individuals, several therapeutic options are available: (1) extra support and an explanation of the reasons for the effect, (2) increasing the dose given prior to the 72-hour interval, (3) switching to an every- other-day dosage schedule, (4) dispensing a supplemental methadone dose.

Most patients do not experience withdrawal during the 72-hour inter-dose interval after reaching pharmacological steady-state <u>with or without</u> adjustment of the Friday dose. If additional opioids are required, small <u>doses of supplemental</u> methadone should be given rather than giving levomethadyl acetate HCl on two consecutive days. Take-home doses of methadone always pose a risk in this setting and physicians should carefully weigh the potential therapeutic benefit against the risk of diversion (see DOSAGE AND ADMINISTRATION.)

Patients should receive extra support and counseling and be warned against supplementing with street drugs as they make the switch from methadone to levomethadyl acetate HCl. The variability in the clearance of LAAM, nor-LAAM, and dinor-LAAM and clinical experience suggest that there will be a small number of patients who require either lower or higher doses than those recommended.

DURATION OF LEVOMETHADYL ACETATE HCL THERAPY

There is no information from controlled clinical trials as to the appropriate duration of levomethadyl acetate HCl therapy. There are reports from investigators that some patients on levomethadyl acetate HCl may experience less variation in opioid effect and have less drug craving than with methadone, so levomethadyl acetate HCl should be considered for patients who need long-term maintenance during social and vocational rehabilitation.

When a patient has eliminated illicit drug use, achieved social and occupational stability, and made lifestyle changes to reduce the risk of relapse, consideration may be given to discontinuation of levomethadyl acetate HCl therapy. Such a decision should be carefully considered as part of an individualized treatment plan. Stable long-term levomethadyl acetate HCl therapy is preferable to repeated cycles of premature discontinuation of medication followed by relapse to uncontrolled addiction.

A patient is most likely to remain abstinent if discontinuation of medication is attempted after the achievement of behavioral objectives and is accompanied by appropriate non-pharmacological support. The rate of dose reduction should very according to the patient's response. Discontinuation of levomethadyl acetate HCl therapy for administrative reasons or because of adverse reactions to the drug should be managed as described below under DOSAGE AND ADMINISTRATION.

INDICATIONS AND USAGE:

Levomethadyl acetate HCl is indicated for the management of opiate dependence.

CONTRAINDICATIONS:

The only known contraindication in the treatment of opiate dependence is hypersensitivity to LAAM. Levomethadyl acetate HCl is not recommended for any use other than for the treatment of opioid dependence (see WARNINGS.)

WARNINGS:

Administration of levomethadyl acetate HCl on a daily basis has led to excessive drug accumulation and risk of fatal overdose.
Levomethadyl acetate HCl has only been studied on a thrice-weekly or every-other-day dosing regimen. Routine daily dosing after a patient has been inducted onto levomethadyl acetate HCl treatment is not allowed by current treatment regulations.
Any decision to administer levomethadyl acetate HCl more frequently than every other day FOR ANY REASON should be approached with extreme caution. Even then only very small doses (5 to 10 mg) should be considered.

Risk of Overdose: Analysis of some of the deaths from overdose observed in the development of levomethadyl acetate HCl has shown that when levomethadyl acetate HCl is diverted into channels of abuse, the uninformed addict can become impatient with the slow onset of levomethadyl acetate HCl (2 to 4 hours) and take illicit drugs, resulting in a potentially lethal combined overdose when the peak levomethadyl acetate HCl effect develops. Due to these risks of diversion and accidental death. Levomethadyl acetate HCl has been approved for use only when <u>dispensed</u> by a licensed facility and is not given in take-home doses.

Use of Narcotic Antagonists: In an individual receiving levomethadyl acetate HCl, the administration of the usual dose of a narcotic antagonist may precipitate an acute withdrawal syndrome. The severity of this syndrome depends on the dose of the antagonist administered and the patient's level of physical dependence. Narcotic antagonists should be used in patients receiving levomethadyl acetate HCl only if needed. If a narcotic antagonist is used to treat respiratory depression in the physically dependent patient, it should be administered with care and titration should begin with much smaller-than-usual doses (0.1 - 0.2 mg recommended). If the desired effect is not achieved, escalating doses may be administered every 2 to 3 minutes. If a cumulative dose of 10 mg of naloxone has been given without effect, further administration is unlikely to be of benefit (see OVERDOSAGE.)

If the patient does respond to narcotic agonists, physicians should remember that naloxone has a much shorter duration of action than levomethadyl acetate HCl. Such patients should remain under prolonged observation rather than being allowed to leave emergency treatment, since levomethadyl acetate HCl's action will outlast naloxone-induced reversal, putting the unsupervised patient at risk of relapse, a return of respiratory depression and possible death if continuing medical attention is not available. Use of other parenteral opioid antagonists may be appropriate in some cases, but only of the dosage of such drugs can be readily titrated. Oral naltrexone would not be appropriate for the treatment of levomethadyl acetate HCl overdose, as it has been associated with the precipitation of prolonged opioid withdrawal symptoms when used in overdose settings.

Warnings to Patients: Patients must be warned that the peak activity of levomethadyl acetate HCl is not immediate, and that the use or abuse of other psychoactive drugs, including alcohol, may result in FATAL overdose, especially with the first few doses of levomethadyl acetate HCl, either during initiation of of treatment or after a lapse in treatment.

Use in High-Risk Patients: Suicide attempts with opiates, especiallly in combination with tricyclic antidepressants, alcohol, and other CNS active agents, are part of the clinical pattern of addiction. Although outpatient therapy with levomethadyl acetate HCl and other drugs of this class is usually associated with a reduction in the risk of suicide, such risk is not eliminated. Individualized evaluation and treatment planning, inlcuding hospitalization, should be considered for patients who continue to exhibit uncontrolled drug use and persistent high-risk behavior despite adequate pharmacotherapy.

PRECAUTIONS:

GENERAL

Initial Dosage Adjustment: Due to the long half-lives of levomethadyl acetate HCl and its metabolites, patients will not feel the full effects of the medication for at least several days. Consequently, extra care is needed when starting patients on levomethadyl acetate HCl and when making initial dosage adjustments (see CLINICAL STUDIES, Individualization Of Dosageand DOSAGE AND ADMINISTRATION.)

Use in Ambulatory Patients: Initiation of therapy or excessive doses of levomethadyl acetate HCl may impair the mental and/or physical abilities required for performance of potentially hazardous tasks, such as driving a car or operating machinery. Patients should be warned not to engage in such activities if their alertness and behavior are affected. Most patients show no detectable impairment at ordinary tasks on levomethadyl acetate HCl therapy.

Head Injury and Increased Intracranial Pressure: The respiratory depressant effects of narcotics and their capacity to elevate cerebrospinal fluid pressure may be markedly exaggerated in the presence of increased intracranial pressure. Furthermore, narcotics produce side effects that may make it difficult to evaluate the clinical course of patients with head injuries. In view of LAAM's profile as a mu agonist, it should be used with extreme caution an only if deemed essential in such patients.

Asthma and Other Respiratory Conditions: Levomethadyl acetate HCl, as with other opioids, should be used with caution in patients with asthma, in those with chronic obstructive pulmonary disease or cor pulmonale, and in individuals with a substantially decreased respiratory reserve, preexisting respiratory depression, hypoxia, or hypercapnea. In such patients, even usual therapeutic doses of narcotics may decrease regulatory drive while simultaneously increasing airway resistance to the point of apnea.

Special Risk Patients: Opioids should be given with caution and at reduced initial dose in certain patients, such as the elderly or debilitated and those with significant hepatic or renal dysfunction, hypothyroidism, Addison's Disease, prostatic hypertrophy, or urethral stricture.

Effects on Cardiac Conduction: Levomethadyl acetate HCl has been shown to prolong the ST segment of the electrocardiogram in beagle dogs dosed five days a week. Serial EKGs performed in a pharmacokinetics study showed a prolongation of the QTc interval in some patients which was not associated with dose.

Such a prolongation of the QTc interval has been seen with other opioids, and is not known if this is an effect specific to LAAM or if it is also seen with methadone. In either case, careful monitoring is recommended when using levomethadyl acetate HCl in patients with a history of known cardiac conduction defects, those taking medications affecting cardiac conduction, and in other cases where an unusual risk of dysrhythmia is suggested by history or physical examination. This information is provided to alert the prescribing physician, and is not intended to deter the appropriate use of opioid agonists in patients with a history of

PRECAUTIONS: *(cont'd)*

cardiac disease. No adverse cardiac events have been associated with levomethadyl acetate HCl therapy in the clinical study of the drug, and the risk of morbidity from treatment with either methadone or LAAM is less than the risk of morbidity from untreated addiction.

Acute Abdominal Conditions: As with other mu agonists, treatment with levomethadyl acetate HCl may obscure the diagnosis or clinical course in patients with acute abdominal conditions.

INFORMATION FOR THE PATIENT

Patients should be provided the patient package insert for levomethadyl acetate HCl if they are new to the drug, and in addition should be advised that:

Levomethadyl acetate HCl, unlike methadone, is not to be taken daily, and daily use of the usual doses will lead to serious overdose.

Levomethadyl acetate HCl is slow acting and patients should be alerted to the risk of abusing any psychoactive drug, including alcohol, while on levomethadyl acetate HCl therapy. This is particularly important during the first 7 to 10 days of treatment, before levomethadyl acetate HCl has had time to exert its full pharmacologic effect.

In addition to being warned of the delay in onset of levomethadyl acetate HCl, patients who are transferring from levomethadyl acetate HCl to methadone should be informed that: they should wait 48 hours after the last dose of levomethadyl acetate HCl before ingesting their first dose of methadone or other narcotic (See DOSAGE AND ADMINISTRATION.)

Patients should inform their adult family members that, in the event of overdose, the treating physician or emergency room staff should be told that the patient is being treated with levomethadyl acetate HCl, a long-acting opioid which is likely to outlast naloxone-induced reversal and which requires prolonged observation and careful monitoring. In addition, the treatment physician or emergency room staff should be informed that the patient is physically dependent on narcotics and that naloxone should be administered with care so as to minimize an precipitated abstinence syndrome.

As with most mu agonists, levomethadyl acetate HCl may interact with other CNS depressants and should be used with caution, and in reduced dosage, in patients concurrently receiving other narcotic analgesics, antihistamines, benzodiazepines, phenothiazines or other major tranquilizers, anxiolytics, sedative-hypnotics, tricyclic antidepressants, and other CNS depressants, including alcohol. Patients should be warned of the importance of reporting the use of any of these compounds to their physicians, as serious side effects could result, including respiratory depression, hypotension, profound sedation or coma.

CARCINOGENESIS, MUTAGENESIS AND IMPAIRMENT OF FERTILITY

Two-year carcinogenicity studies with LAAM in rats at 13 mg/kg (77 mg/m^2) and in mice at 30 mg/kg (90 mg/m^2) given orally in the diet did not show carcinogenic changes. LAAM is not mutagenic in the Ames test, the unscheduled DNA synthesis and repair test, mouse lymphoma cells *in vitro*, or chromosomal aberration tests in rats *in vivo*. LAAM tested positive in the forward mutation assay in N. crassa at 150 mcg/ml *in vitro* and in the heritable translocation assay in mice at 21 mg/kg (63 mg/m^2). The clinical significance of these findings is not known.

Chronic treatment with LAAM at 80 mg three times a week did not produce chromosomal aberrations in peripheral human lymphocytes. Effects of LAAM on fertility in animals has not been fully evaluated.

PREGNANCY CATEGORY C

Animal reproduction studies are not complete and there are no clinical data on the safety of levomethadyl acetate HCl in pregnancy. For these reasons, levomethadyl acetate HCl is not recommended for use in pregnancy. Women who may become pregnant should be advised of the risks of levomethadyl acetate HCl therapy and of the desirability of discontinuing levomethadyl acetate HCl prior to a planned pregnancy. Current regulations mandate monthly pregnancy tests in female patients of childbearing potential who are using levomethadyl acetate HCl.

If a female patient becomes pregnant on levomethadyl acetate HCl despite these precautions, it is recommended she be transferred to methadone for the remainder of the pregnancy (see DOSAGE AND ADMINISTRATION, TRANSFER FROM LEVOMETHADYL ACETATE HCL TO METHADONE.) If it appears wiser to continue a specific patient on levomethadyl acetate HCl, the physician should be alert to possible respiratory depression of the newborn and other perinatal complications (see Labor and Delivery.)

LABOR AND DELIVERY

The effects of levomethadyl acetate HCl on labor and delivery are not known. Like other mu agonist opioids, however, levomethadyl acetate HCl is expected to produce respiratory depression and a possible neonatal dependence syndrome with a delayed emergence of withdrawal symptoms. Use of levomethadyl acetate HCl in labor and delivery is not recommended unless, in the opinion of the treating physician, the potential benefits outweigh the possible hazards.

PEDIATRIC USE

The use of levomethadyl acetate HCl in addicts under 18 years of age has not been studied. Its use is not recommended and is contrary to current regulations.

DRUG INTERACTIONS:

Polydrug and Alcohol Abusers: Patients who are known to abuse sedatives, tranquilizers, propoxyphene, antidepressants, benzodiazepines, and alcohol should be warned of the risk of serious overdose if these substances are taken while on levomethadyl acetate HCl maintenance.

Interaction With Narcotic Antagonists, Mixed Agonists/Antagonists, Partial Agonists, and Pure Agonists: As with other mu agonists, patients maintained on levomethadyl acetate HCl may experience withdrawal symptoms when administered pure narcotic antagonists, mixed agonists/antagonists or partial agonists, such as naloxone, naltrexone, pentazocine, nalbuphine, butorphanol, and buprenorphine.

In addition, agonists such as meperidine and propoxyphene, which are N- demethylated to long-acting, excitatory metabolites, should not be used by patients taking levomethadyl acetate HCl because they would be ineffective unless given in such high doses that the risk of toxic effects of the metabolites becomes unacceptable.

Anesthesia and Analgesia: Patients receiving levomethadyl acetate HCl will develop a similar level of tolerance for opioids as patients receiving methadone. Anesthetists and other practitioners should be prepared to adjust their management of these patients accordingly.

Other Drug Interactions: The anti-tuberculosis drug rifampin has been found to produce a marked (50%) reduction in serum methadone levels, leading to the appearance of symptoms of withdrawal in well-stabilized methadone maintenance patients. Similar effects on serum methadone levels have been observed for carbamazepine, phenobarbital, and phenytoin. The presumed mechanism for this effect is the induction of methadone metabolizing enzymes. Since levomethadyl acetate HCl is metabolized into a <u>more</u> active metabolite, (nor-LAAM), administration of these drugs may <u>increase</u> levomethadyl acetate HCl's peak activity and/or <u>shorten</u> its duration of action.

DRUG INTERACTIONS: *(cont'd)*

Conversely, drugs like erythromycin, cimetidine, and anti-fungal drugs like a ketoconazole that inhibit hepatic metabolism, may <u>slow</u> the onset, <u>lower</u> the activity, and/or <u>increase</u> the duration of action or levomethadyl acetate HCl. Caution and close observation of patients receiving these drugs are advised to allow early detection of any need to adjust the dose or dosing interval.

ADVERSE REACTIONS:

Physicians should be alert to palpitations, syncope, or other symptoms suggestive of episodes of an irregular cardiac rhythm in patients taking levomethadyl acetate HCl and promptly evaluate such cases (see PRECAUTIONS, Effects on Cardiac Conduction).

HEROIN OR METHADONE WITHDRAWAL REACTIONS

Patients presenting for levomethadyl acetate HCl treatment are frequently in withdrawal from heroin or other opiates. They may display typical withdrawal symptoms which should be differentiated from levomethadyl acetate HCl's side effects. Patients may exhibit some or all of the following signs and symptoms associated with withdrawal from opiates: lacrimation, rhinorrhea, sneezing, yawning, perspiration, gooseflesh, fever, chilliness alternating with flushing, restlessness, irritability, insomnia, weakness, anxiety, depression, dilated pupils, tremors, tachycardia, abdominal cramps, body aches, anorexia, nausea, vomiting, diarrhea, and weight loss. Control of such symptoms is a primary goal of therapy. However, because of the slow onset and long half-lives of levomethadyl acetate HCl, nor- LAAM, and dinor-LAAM, overly aggressive increases in dosage to control these withdrawal symptoms with levomethadyl acetate HCl may result in overdose (see CLINICAL STUDIES, Individualization Of Dosage.)

SIGNS AND SYMPTOMS OF LEVOMETHADYL ACETATE HCL EXCESS

The interaction between the development and maintenance of opioid tolerance and levomethadyl acetate HCl dose can be complex. Dose reduction is recommended in cases where patients develop signs and symptoms of excessive levomethadyl acetate HCl effects, characterized by complaints of "feeling wired", poor concentration, drowsiness, and possibly dizziness on standing.

LEVOMETHADYL ACETATE HCL WITHDRAWAL

Patient may experience withdrawal symptoms (nasal congestion, abdominal symptoms, diarrhea, muscle aches, anxiety) over the 72-hour dosing interval if the dose of levomethadyl acetate HCl is too low. This may managed as described under CLINICAL STUDIES, Individualization Of Dosage, but physicians should be alert to the possible need for dose or dose schedule adjustments if patients complain of weekend withdrawal symptoms in the last day of the 72-hour dosing interval.

ADVERSE REACTIONS ON STABLE THERAPY

The following adverse evens were observed in the 25-site, 623 patient usage study in male and female opiate addicts (see CLINICAL STUDIES.) These signs and symptoms were reported during the second and third months of treatment with levomethadyl acetate HCl, and were considered severe enough to require medical evaluation. In this study, both questionnaires and spontaneous reports were used to gather information. Questionnaire-elicited symptom frequencies were about five times as frequent as the spontaneous reporting frequencies given below.

Incidence greater than 1%, Probably Causally Related

Body as a Whole: Asthenia, back pain, chills, edema, hot flashes (males 2:1), flu syndrome and malaise.

Cardiovascular: Bradycardia.

Gastrointestinal: Abdominal pain, constipation, diarrhea, dry mouth, nausea and vomiting.

Musculoskeletal: Arthralgia.

Nervous System: Abnormal dreams, anxiety, decreased sex drive, depression, euphoria, headache, hypesthesia, insomnia, nervousness, somnolence

Respiratory: Cough, rhinitis, and yawning.

Skin/appendage: Rash, sweating.

Special Senses: Blurred vision.

Urogenital: Difficult ejaculation, impotence.

*Reactions in 3-9% of patients; reactions in 1-3% are unmarked.

Incidence less than 1%, Probably Causally Related

Cardiovascular: Postural hypotension.

Musculo-skeletal: Myalgia.

Special senses: Tearing.

CAUSAL RELATIONSHIP UNKNOWN

These reactions were reported with low frequency in controlled and uncontrolled studies of LAAM, are not known to be causally related to the administration of the drug, and are provided as alerting information for physicians.

Cardiovascular: Hypertension, prolongation of the QT interval, non- specific ST-T wave Changes.

Hepatic: Hepatitis and abnormal liver function tests.

Urogenital: Amenorrhea, pyuria.

DRUG ABUSE AND DEPENDENCE:

Levomethadyl acetate HCl is a Schedule II controlled substance under the Federal Controlled Substances Act. Levomethadyl acetate HCl produces dependence of the morphine-type and has potential for abuse. Tolerance and physical dependence will develop upon repeated administration. As with methadone and any other narcotic administered to narcotic addicts, levomethadyl acetate HCl is at risk for diversion and illicit use, and should be handled accordingly (see WARNINGS.)

OVERDOSAGE:

SIGNS AND SYMPTOMS

All but a few cases of levomethadyl acetate HCl overdose have involved multiple drugs. Overdose on levomethadyl acetate HCl alone is rare and has always been the result of too frequent (daily) dosing. Overdose is primarily of concern in persons not tolerant to opiates, since in such individuals a dose of 20 to 40 mg of levomethadyl acetate HCl may cause somnolence, and a larger initial dose may cause serious overdose. Tolerant individuals will generally not show symptoms unless higher doses are administered.

In levomethadyl acetate HCl overdose, as with other mu agonists opioids, the following signs and symptoms should be anticipated: respiratory depression (decrease in respiratory rate and/or tidal volume. Cheyne-Stokes respiration, cyanosis), extreme somnolence progressing to stupor or coma, maximally constricted pupils, skeletal muscle flaccidity, cold and clammy skin, bradycardia, and hypotension, In severe overdose, apnea, circulatory collapse, pulmonary edema, cardiac arrest and death may occur.

TREATMENT

In the case or levomethadyl acetate HCl overdose, protect the patient's airways and support ventilation and circulation. Absorption of levomethadyl acetate HCl from the gastrointestinal tract may be decreased by gastric emptying and/or administration of activated charcoal.

OVERDOSAGE: *(cont'd)*

(Safeguard the patient's airway when employing gastric emptying or administering charcoal in any patient with diminished consciousness). Forced diuresis, peritoneal dialysis, hemodialysis, or charcoal hemoperfusion are unlikely to be beneficial for levomethadyl acetate HCl overdose due its high lipid solubility and large volume of distribution.

In managing levomethadyl acetate HCl overdose, the physician should consider the possibility of multiple drugs, the interaction between drugs, and any unusual drug kinetics in the patient. Naloxone may be given to antagonize opiate effects, but the airway must be secured as vomiting may ensue. If possible, naloxone should be titrated to clinical effect rather than given as a large single bolus, since rapid reversal of opioid effects by large naloxone doses can cause severe precipitated withdrawal effects that may include cardiac instability. If a patient has received a total of 10 mg of naloxone without clinical response, the diagnosis of opioid overdose is unlikely.

If the patient dose respond to naloxone, the physician should remember that the duration of levomethadyl acetate HCl activity is much longer (days) than that of naloxone (minutes) and repeated dosing with or continuous intravenous infusion of naloxone is likely to be required. Use of oral naltrexone in this setting is not recommended because it may precipitate prolonged opioid withdrawal symptoms (see Use of Narcotic Antagonists.)

DOSAGE AND ADMINISTRATION:

Levomethadyl acetate HCl produces opioid effects and a high degree of opioid tolerance that inhibits drug-seeking behavior and blocks the euphoria produced by the usual doses of heroin. The dose of levomethadyl acetate HCl in each patient should be adjusted to achieve the optimal therapeutic benefit with acceptable adverse opioid effects (see CLINICAL STUDIES, Individualization Of Dosage.)

Levomethadyl acetate HCl must always be diluted before administration, and should be mixed with diluent prior to dispensing. To avoid confusion between prepared doses of levomethadyl acetate HCl and methadone, the liquid used to dilute levomethadyl acetate HCl should be a different color from that used to dilute methadone in any specific clinic setting.

LEVOMETHADYL ACETATE HCL DOSING

Dosing Schedules

Levomethadyl acetate HCl is usually administered three times a week, either on Monday, Wednesday, and Friday, or on Tuesday, Thursday, and Saturday. If withdrawal is a problem during the 72-hour inter-dose interval, the preceding dose may be increased. In some cases, an every-other-day schedule may be appropriate (see CLINICAL STUDIES, Individualization Of Dosage.)

The usual doses of levomethadyl acetate HCl must not be given on consecutive days because of the risk of fatal overdose. No dose mentioned in this label isever meant to be given as a daily dose (see WARNINGS.)

Induction

The initial dose of levomethadyl acetate HCl for street addicts should be 20 to 40 mg. Each subsequent dose, administered at 48- or 72-hour intervals, may be adjusted in increments of 5 to 10 mg until a pharmacokinetic and pharmacodynamic steady-state is reached, usually within 1 or 2 weeks (see CLINICAL STUDIES, Individualization Of Dosage.)

Patients dependent on methadone may require higher initial doses of levomethadyl acetate HCl. The suggested initial 3-times-a-week dose of levomethadyl acetate HCl for such patients is 1.2 to 1.3 times the daily methadone maintenance dose being replaced. This initial dose should not exceed 120 mg and subsequent doses, administered at 48- or 72-hour intervals, should be adjusted according to clinical response.

Most patients can tolerate the 72-hour inter-dose interval during the induction period. Some patients may require additional intervention (see CLINICAL STUDIES, Individualization Of Dosage.) If additional opioids are required, supplemental methadone in small doses should be given rather than giving levomethadyl acetate HCl on two consecutive days. Take-home doses of methadone always pose a risk in this setting and physicians should carefully weigh the potential therapeutic benefit against the risk of diversion.

In some cases, where the degree of tolerance is unknown, patients can be started on methadone to facilitate more rapid titration to an effective dose, then converted to levomethadyl acetate HCl after a few weeks of methadone therapy.

The crossover from methadone to levomethadyl acetate HCl should be accomplished in a single dose; complete transfer to levomethadyl acetate HCl is simpler and preferable to more complex regimens involving escalating doses of levomethadyl acetate HCl and decreasing doses of methadone.

Dosage should be carefully titrated to the individual; induction too rapid for the patient's level of tolerance may result in overdose. Serious hazards, as seen in association with all narcotic analgesics, are respiratory depression and, to a lesser extent, circulatory depression.

Maintenance:

Most patients will be stabilized on doses in the range of 60 to 90 mg, 3- times-a-week. Doses as low as 10 mg and as high as 140 three times a week have been given in clinical studies.

Supplemental dosing over the 72-hour inter-dose interval (weekend) is rarely needed. For example, if a patient on a Mon./Wed./Fri. schedule complains of withdrawal on Sundays, the recommended dosage adjustment is to increase the Friday dose in 5 to 10 mg increments up to 40% over the Mon./Wed. dose or to a maximum of 140 mg.

If withdrawal symptoms persist after adjustment of dose, consideration may be given to every-other-day dosing if clinic hours permit. If the clinic is not open seven days a week and every-other-day dosing is not practical, the patient's schedule may be adjusted so the 72-hour interval occurs during the week and the patient can come to the clinic to receive a supplemental dose of methadone (see CLINICAL STUDIES, Individualization Of Dosage.)

The maximum total amount of levomethadyl acetate HCl recommended for any patient is 140-140-140 or 130-130-180 mg on a thrice-weekly schedule or 140 mg every other day.

PLANNED TEMPORARY INTERRUPTION OF LEVOMETHADYL ACETATE HCL MAINTENANCE

Levomethadyl acetate HCl take-home doses are not permitted by regulation. Thus, several circumstances may cause the planned temporary discontinuation of treatment with levomethadyl acetate HCl. Patients eligible for one or more take-home doses of methadone, who are unable to attend the clinic for their next regularly scheduled levomethadyl acetate HCl dose because of illness, personal or family crisis, other hardships, travel and/or state/federal holidays, may be temporarily transferred directly to methadone.

Patients meeting these criteria may receive one or more methadone doses. Methadone doses should be 80% of the patient's Monday/Wednesday levomethadyl acetate HCl dose (*e.g.,* patients receiving 80-80-100 mg of levomethadyl acetate HCl on a Monday/Wednesday/ Friday regimen would be transferred to a daily methadone dose of 64 mg). The first dose of methadone should be ingested no sooner than 48 hours after the last levomethadyl acetate HCl dose. The number of take-home methadone doses should be two less than the number of days expected absence and should not exceed, in any case, the number of take- homes allowed in the methadone regulations.

DOSAGE AND ADMINISTRATION: *(cont'd)*

Upon return to clinic, patients should resume levomethadyl acetate HCl maintenance following the same dosage regimen prior to the temporary interruption See DOSAGE AND ADMINISTRATION, Maintenance. If more than 48 hours has elapsed since their last methadone dose, patients should be reinducted on levomethadyl acetate HCl at a dose determined by clinical and/or toxicological evaluation of the patient by the physician.

REINDUCTION AFTER AN UNPLANNED LAPSE IN DOSING

Following a lapse of one Levomethadyl Acetate HCl dose: 1) If a patient comes to the clinic to be dosed on the day following a missed scheduled dose (misses Monday, arrives Tuesday), the regular Monday dose should be administered on Tuesday, with the scheduled Wednesday dose administered on Thursday and the Friday dose given on Saturday. The patient's regular schedule may be resumed the following Monday (misses Wednesday, receives the regular dose on Thursday and Saturday, and returns to the regular Monday/Wednesday/Friday dosing schedule the next week).

2) If a patient misses one dose and comes to the clinic on the day of the next schedule dose (missed Monday, arrives Wednesday), the usual dose will be well tolerated in most instances, although a reduced dose may be appropriate in selected cases.

Following a lapse of more than one Levomethadyl Acetate HCl dose: Patients should be reinducted at an initial dose of 1/2 to 3/4 their previous levomethadyl acetate HCl dose, followed by increases of 5 to 10 mg every dosing day (48- or 72-hour intervals) until their previous maintenance dose is achieved. Patients who have been off of levomethadyl acetate HCl treatment for more than a week should be reinducted.

TRANSFER FROM LEVOMETHADYL ACETATE HCL TO METHADONE

Patients maintained on levomethadyl acetate HCl may be transferred directly to methadone. Because of the difference between the two compounds' metabolites and their pharmacological half-lives, it is recommended that methadone be started on a daily dose at 80% of the levomethadyl acetate HCl dose being replaced; the initial methadone dose must be given no sooner than 48 hours after the last levomethadyl acetate HCl dose. Subsequent increases or decreases of 5 to 10 mg in the daily methadone dose may be given to control symptoms of withdrawal or, less likely, symptoms of excessive sedation, in accordance with clinical observations.

DETOXIFICATION FROM LEVOMETHADYL ACETATE HCL

There is limited experience with detoxifying patients from levomethadyl acetate HCl in a systematic manner, with both gradual reduction (5 to 10% a week) and abrupt withdrawal schedules have been used successfully. The decision to discontinue levomethadyl acetate HCl therapy should be made as part of a comprehensive treatment plan (see CLINICAL STUDIES, Individualization Of Dosage.)

SAFETY AND HANDLING

Levomethadyl acetate HCl is a solution of a potent narcotic (LAAM). There are no known specific hazards associated with dermal and aerosol exposure to levomethadyl acetate HCl. In case of accidental dermal exposure, promptly remove contaminated clothing and rinse the affected skin with cool water.

For the first six to twelve months, sales of levomethadyl acetate HCl will be restricted to clinics that have received training in its use, until there is general knowledge about how to use the drug safely. Since levomethadyl acetate HCl can be potential dangerous if diverted, appropriate security measures should be taken to safeguard stock of levomethadyl acetate HCl as required by 21 CFR 1301.74 & 1304.28.

Store at controlled room temperature, 15-30° (59-86°F).

Levomethadyl acetate HCl is compatible with the materials used in most dispensing systems. Information about obtaining appropriate dispensing systems suitable for use with levomethadyl acetate HCl is available from the manufacturer upon request.

HOW SUPPLIED - EQUIVALENTS NOT AVAILABLE:

Solution - Oral - 10 mg/ml

474 ml $240.00 ORLAAM, Roxane 00054-3649-62

LEVONORDEFRIN; PROCAINE HYDROCHLORIDE; PROPOXYCAINE HYDROCHLORIDE

(003119)

CATEGORIES: Anesthesia; Dental; Local Anesthetics; Pregnancy Category C; FDA Approval Pre 1982

BRAND NAMES: *Ravocaine; Ravocaine And Novocain with Levophed*; **Ravocaine And Novocain W Neo-Cobefrin**
(International brand names outside U.S. in italics)

DESCRIPTION:

Propoxycaine hydrochloride is 2-(diethylamino)-ethyl 4-amino-2-propoxy-benzoate monohydrochloride.

It is an odorless white or slightly yellow crystalline solid which is readily soluble in water but incompatible with alkalies.

Procaine hydrochloride is 2-(diethylamino)ethyl *p*-aminobenzoate monohydrochloride.

It is an odorless white crystalline solid which is readily soluble in water but incompatible with alkalies, iodides, and mercurial compounds.

Levonordefrin is (-)-α-(1-aminoethyl)-3,4-dihydroxybenzyl alcohol.

It is a white or buff-colored crystalline solid, freely soluble in aqueous solutions of mineral acids, but practically insoluble in water (TABLE 1):

TABLE 1 Dental Cartridges May Not Be Autoclaved

Contents:	Per ml	Per cartridge
Propoxycaine hydrochloride	4 mg	7.2 mg
Procaine hydrochloride	20 mg	36 mg
Levonordefrin	0.05 mg	0.09 mg
Sodium chloride	3.0 mg	5.4 mg
Acetone sodium bisulfite, not more than	2.0 mg	3.6 mg
Water for Injection, q.s. ad	1.0 ml	1.8 ml
pH is adjusted between 3.5 and 5.0 with NaOH or HCl.		

CLINICAL PHARMACOLOGY:

This solution stabilizes the neuronal membrane and prevents the initiation and transmission of nerve impulses, thereby effecting local anesthesia. The onset of action is usually 2 to 5 minutes and the duration of action is from 2 to 3 hours.

Para-aminobenzoic acid esters are rapidly metabolized through hydrolysis by plasma cholinesterase with some metabolism occurring in the liver.

CLINICAL PHARMACOLOGY: *(cont'd)*

Levonordefrin is a sympathomimetic amine used as a vasoconstrictor in local anesthetic solutions. It has pharmacologic activity similar to that of epinephrine but it is more stable than epinephrine. In equal concentrations, levonordefrin is less potent than epinephrine in raising blood pressure, and as a vasoconstrictor.

INDICATIONS AND USAGE:

This solution is indicated for the production of local anesthesia for dental procedures by infiltration injection or nerve block in adults and children.

CONTRAINDICATIONS:

This solution in contraindicated in patients with a known hypersensitivity to local anesthetics of the para-aminobenzoic acid ester group.

WARNINGS:

DENTAL PRACTITIONERS WHO EMPLOY LOCAL ANESTHETICS IN THEIR OFFICES SHOULD BE WELL VERSED IN DIAGNOSIS AND MANAGEMENT OF EMERGENCIES WHICH MIGHT ARISE FROM THEIR USE. RESUSCITATIVE EQUIPMENT, OXYGEN AND OTHER RESUSCITATIVE DRUGS SHOULD BE AVAILABLE FOR IMMEDIATE USE.

Reactions resulting in fatality have occurred on rare occasions with the use of local anesthetics, even in the absence of a history of hypersensitivity.

Solutions which contain a vasoconstrictor should be used with extreme caution for patients whose medical history and physical evaluation suggest the existence of hypertension, arteriosclerotic heart disease, cerebral vascular insufficiency, heart block, thyrotoxicosis, diabetes, etc.

Contains acetone sodium bisulfite, a sulfite that may cause allergic-type reactions including anaphylactic symptoms and life-threatening or less severe asthmatic episodes in certain susceptible people. The overall prevalence of sulfite sensitivity is seen more frequently in asthmatic than in non-asthmatic people.

PRECAUTIONS:

The safety and effectiveness of this solution depend upon proper dosage, correct technique, adequate precautions, and readiness for emergencies.

RESUSCITATIVE EQUIPMENT, OXYGEN AND OTHER RESUSCITATIVE DRUGS SHOULD BE AVAILABLE FOR IMMEDIATE USE (SEE WARNINGS).

The lowest dose that results in effective anesthesia should be used to avoid high plasma levels and serious undesirable systemic side effects. Repeated administrations may result in accumulation of the anesthetics in plasma.

INJECTIONS SHOULD ALWAYS BE MADE SLOWLY WITH ASPIRATION TO AVOID INTRAVASCULAR INJECTION AND THEREFORE SYSTEMIC REACTION TO BOTH LOCAL ANESTHETIC AND VASOCONSTRICTOR.

Tolerance varies with the status of the patient. Debilitated, elderly patients, acutely ill patients, and children should be given reduced doses commensurate with their weight and physical status.

If sedatives are employed to reduce patient apprehension, use reduced doses, since local anesthetic agents, like sedatives, are central nervous system depressants which in combination may have an additive effect. Young children should be given minimal doses of each agent.

Changes in sensorium such as excitation, disorientation, drowsiness may be early indications of a high blood level of the local anesthetic agents and may occur following inadvertent intravascular administration or rapid absorption.

USAGE IN CHILDREN:

Great care must be exercised in adhering to safe concentrations and dosages for pediatric administration (see DOSAGE AND ADMINISTRATION.)

PREGNANCY CATEGORY C:

Animal reproduction studies have not been conducted with this solution. It is also not known whether this solution can cause fetal harm when administered to a pregnant woman or can affect reproduction capacity. This solution should be given to a pregnant woman only if clearly needed.

NURSING MOTHER:

It is not known whether this drug is excreted in human milk. Because many drugs are excreted in human milk, caution should be exercised when this solution is administered to a nursing woman.

Local anesthetic procedures should be used with caution when there is inflammation and/or sepsis in the region of the proposed injection.

This solution should be used with caution in patients with history of hypertension, arteriosclerotic heart disease, cerebral vascular insufficiency or heart block. Bradycardia may follow administration of this solution.

DRUG INTERACTIONS:

Solutions which contain a vasoconstrictor should also be used with extreme caution in patients receiving drugs known to produce blood pressure alterations (*i.e.,* MAO inhibitors, tricyclic antidepressants, phenothiazines, etc) as either sustained hypertension or hypotension may occur.

Solutions containing a vasoconstrictor should be used cautiously in the presence of diseases which may adversely affect the patient's cardiovascular system. Serious cardiac arrhythmias may occur if preparations containing a vasoconstrictor are employed in patients during or following the administration of potent general anesthetics.

Caution should be used in administering local anesthetics to patients with a history of drug sensitivity or allergy. A thorough history of the patient's prior experience with this and other local anesthetics as well as concomitant or recent drug use should be taken (see CONTRAINDICATIONS.) Patients with known sensitivity to the para-aminobenzoic acid ester-type of local anesthetics have not shown cross sensitivity to amide-type drugs.

ADVERSE REACTIONS:

Systemic reactions involving the central nervous system and the cardiovascular system usually result from high plasma levels due to excessive dosage, rapid absorption, or inadvertent intravascular injection.

A small number of reactions may result from hypersensitivity, idiosyncrasy, or diminished tolerance to normal dosage on the part of the patient.

Central nervous system reactions are characterized by excitation and/or depression. Nervousness, dizziness, blurred vision, or tremors may occur followed by drowsiness, convulsions, unconsciousness, and possibly respiratory arrest.

Cardiovascular system reactions may result either from the local anesthetic or from the vasoconstrictor employed, and may include depression of the myocardium, hypotension, profound bradycardia, and cardiac arrest. Cardiovascular reactions may be the result of drugs employed or may result from vasovagal reaction particularly in the sitting position. Early

ADVERSE REACTIONS: *(cont'd)*

recognition and management of premonitory signs such as sweating, feeling of faintness, changes in heart rate, will avoid resultant cerebral hypoxia which may progress to seizure or cardiovascular catastrophe. Management consists of placing the patient in the recumbent position and administration of oxygen. Should symptoms persist, vasoactive drugs such as ephedrine or methoxamine should be administered intravenously.

Allergic reactions are characterized by cutaneous lesions of delayed onset, or urticaria, edema, and other manifestations of allergy. The detection of sensitivity by skin testing is of limited value. As with other local anesthetics, hypersensitivity, idiosyncrasy, anaphylactoid reactions to this solution have occurred rarely. The reactions may be abrupt and severe, and is not usually dose related.

OVERDOSAGE:

Treatment of a patient with toxic manifestations consists of assuring and maintaining a patent airway and supporting ventilation with oxygen and assisted or controlled ventilation (respiration) as required. This usually will be sufficient in the management of most reactions. Should a convulsion persist despite ventilatory therapy, small increments of anticonvulsive agents may be given intravenously, such as benzodiazepine (*e.g.,* diazepam) or ultra-short acting barbiturates (*e.g.,* pentobarbital or secobarbital). Cardiovascular depression may require circulatory assistance with intravenous fluids and/or vasopressor (*e.g.,* ephedrine) as dictated by the clinical situation. Allergic reactions are rare and may occur as a result of sensitivity to the local anesthetic and are characterized by cutaneous lesions, urticaria, edema, and anaphylactoid type symptomatology. These allergic reactions should be managed by conventional means. The detection of potential sensitivity by skin testing is of limited value.

DOSAGE AND ADMINISTRATION:

As with all local anesthetics the dose varies and depends upon the area to be anesthetized, vascularity of the tissues, individual tolerance and the technique of anesthesia. The lowest dose needed to provide effective anesthesia should be administered. For specific techniques and procedures, refer to standard dental manuals and textbooks.

For infiltration and block injections in the upper or lower jaw, the average dose of 1 cartridge will usually suffice.

The 1.8 ml cartridge contains 43.2 mg of the anesthetics (7.2 mg propoxycaine HCl and 36 mg procaine HCl).

Adults: Five cartridges (216 mg of the anesthetics) are usually adequate to effect anesthesia of the entire oral cavity. However, a dose of up to 3 mg per pound of body weight may be administered for one procedure.

Children: Based on a dose of 3 mg per pound of body weight, 5 cartridges maximum are usually adequate for any procedure.

Using infiltration or regional block anesthesia, injections should always be made slowly and with frequent aspiration.

Any unused portion of a cartridge should be discarded.

DISINFECTION OF CARTRIDGES

As in the case of any cartridge, the diaphragm should be disinfected before needle puncture. The diaphragm should be thoroughly swabbed with either pure 91% isopropyl alcohol or 70% ethyl alcohol, USP, just prior to use. Many commercially available alcohol solutions contain ingredients which are injurious to container components, and therefore, should not be used. Cartridges should not be immersed in any solution.

Store at controlled room temperature between 15 and 30°C (59 and 86°F). **Protect from light.**

LEVONORGESTREL *(003015)*

CATEGORIES: Contraceptives; Hormones; Pregnancy Category X; Sales > $100 Million; FDA Approved 1990 Dec

BRAND NAMES: **Norplant**; *Norplant 36*
(International brand names outside U.S. in italics)

FORMULARIES: WHO

COST OF THERAPY: $1.00 (Contraceptive; Kit; 216 mg; 1/day; 1 days) vs. Potential Cost of $2,351.94 (DRG 372, Pregnancy)

DESCRIPTION:

PATIENTS SHOULD BE COUNSELED THAT THIS PRODUCT DOES NOT PROTECT AGAINST HIV INFECTION (AIDS) AND OTHER SEXUALLY TRANSMITTED DISEASES.

THE NORPLANT SYSTEM KIT CONTAINS LEVONORGESTREL IMPLANTS, A SET OF SIX FLEXIBLE CLOSED CAPSULES MADE OF SILASTIC (DIMETHYLSILOXANE/METHYLVINYLSILOXANE COPOLYMER), EACH CONTAINING 36 MG OF THE PROGESTIN LEVONORGESTREL CONTAINED IN AN INSERTION KIT TO FACILITATE IMPLANTATION. THE CAPSULES ARE SEALED WITH SILASTIC (POLYDIMETHYLSILOXANE) ADHESIVE AND STERILIZED. EACH CAPSULE IS 2.4 MM IN DIAMETER AND 34 MM IN LENGTH. THE CAPSULES ARE INSERTED IN A SUPERFICIAL PLANE BENEATH THE SKIN OF THE UPPER ARM.

INFORMATION CONTAINED HEREWITH REGARDING SAFETY AND EFFICACY WAS DERIVED FROM STUDIES WHICH USED TWO SLIGHTLY DIFFERENT SILASTIC TUBING FORMULATIONS. THE FORMULATION BEING USED IN THE NORPLANT SYSTEM HAS SLIGHTLY HIGHER RELEASE RATES OF LEVONORGESTREL AND AT LEAST COMPARABLE EFFICACY.

EVIDENCE INDICATES THAT THE DOSE OF LEVONORGESTREL PROVIDED BY THE NORPLANT SYSTEM IS INITIALLY ABOUT 85 MCG/DAY FOLLOWED BY A DECLINE TO ABOUT 50 MCG/DAY BY 9 MONTHS AND TO ABOUT 35 MCG/DAY BY 18 MONTHS WITH A FURTHER DECLINE THEREAFTER TO ABOUT 30 MCG/DAY. THE NORPLANT SYSTEM IS A PROGESTIN-ONLY PRODUCT AND DOES NOT CONTAIN ESTROGEN.

LEVONORGESTREL, (D)(-)-13-BETA-ETHYL-17-ALPHA -ETHINYL-17-BETA-HYDROXYGON -4-EN-3-ONE), THE ACTIVE INGREDIENT IN THE NORPLANT SYSTEM, HAS A MOLECULAR WEIGHT OF 312.46.

CLINICAL PHARMACOLOGY:

Levonorgestrel is a totally synthetic and biologically active progestin which exhibits no significant estrogenic activity and is highly progestational. The absolute configuration conforms to that of D-natural steroids. Levonorgestrel is not subjected to a "first-pass" effect and is virtually 100% bioavailable. Plasma concentrations average approximately 0.30 ng/ml over 5 years but are highly variable as a function of individual metabolism and body weight.

Diffusion of levonorgestrel through the wall of each capsule provides a continuous low dose of the progestin. Resulting blood levels are substantially below those generally observed among users of combination oral contraceptives containing the progestins norgestrel or

CLINICAL PHARMACOLOGY: *(cont'd)*

levonorgestrel. Because of the range of variability in blood levels and variation in individual response, blood levels alone are not predictive of the risk of pregnancy in an individual woman.

At least two mechanisms are active in preventing pregnancy: ovulation inhibition and thickening of the cervical mucus. Other mechanisms may add to these contraceptive effects.

Levonorgestrel concentrations among women show considerable variation depending on individual clearance rates, body weight, and possibly other factors. Levonorgestrel concentrations reach a maximum, or near maximum, within 24 hours after placement with mean values of 1600 ± 1100 pg/ml. They decline rapidly over the first month partially due to a circulating protein, SHBG, that binds levonorgestrel and which is depressed by the presence of levonorgestrel. At 3 months, mean levels decline to values of around 400 pg/ml while concentrations normalized to a 60 kg body weight were 327 ± 119 (SD) pg/ml at 12 months with further decline by 1.4 pg/ml/month to reach 258 ± 95 (SD) pg/ml at 60 months. Concentrations decreased with an increasing body weight by a mean of 3.3 pg/ml/kg. After capsule removal, mean concentrations drop to below 100 pg/ml by 96 hours and to below assay sensitivity (50 pg/ml) by 5 to 14 days. Fertility rates return to levels comparable to those seen in the general population of women using no method of contraception. Circulating concentrations can be used to forecast the risk of pregnancy only in a general statistical sense. Mean concentrations associated with pregnancy have been 210 ± 60 (SD) pg/ml. However, in clinical studies, 20 percent of women had one or more values below 200 pg/ml but an average annual gross pregnancy rate of less than 1.0 per 100 women through 5 years.

Although lipoprotein levels were altered in several clinical studies with the Norplant System, the long-term clinical effects of these changes has not been determined. A decrease in total cholesterol levels has been reported in all lipoprotein studies and reached statistical significance in several. Both increases and decreases in high-density lipoprotein (HDL) levels have been reported in clinical trials. No statistically significant increases have been reported in the ratio of total cholesterol to HDL-cholesterol. Low-density lipoprotein (LDL) levels decreased during Norplant System use. Triglyceride levels also decreased from pretreatment values.

INDICATIONS AND USAGE:

The Norplant System is indicated for the prevention of pregnancy and is a long-term (up to 5 years) reversible contraceptive system. The capsules should be removed by the end of the 5th year. New capsules may be inserted at that time if continuing contraceptive protection is desired.

In multicenter trials with the Norplant System, involving 2470 women, the relationship between body weight and efficacy was investigated. Tabulated below is the pregnancy experience as a function of body weight. Because Norplant System is a long-term method of contraception, this is reported over five years of use.

TABLE 1 Annual And Five-Year Cumulative Pregnancy Rates Per 100 Users By Weight Class

Weight class	Year 1	Year 2	Year 3	Year 4	Year 5	Cumulative
<50 kg (<110 lbs)	0.2	0	0	0	0	0.2
50-59 kg (110-130 lbs)	0.2	0.5	0.4	2.0	0.4	3.4
60-69 kg (131-153 lbs)	0.4	0.5	1.6	1.7	0.8	5.0
≥70 kg (≥154 lbs)	0	1.1	5.1	2.5	0	8.5
All	0.2	0.5	1.2	1.6	0.4	3.9

Typically, pregnancy rates with contraceptive methods are reported only for the first year of use as shown below. The efficacy of these contraceptive methods, except the IUD and sterilization, depends in part on the reliability of use. The efficacy of the Norplant System does not depend on patient compliance. However no contraceptive method is 100% effective.

TABLE 2 Lowest Expected and Typical Failure Rates (%) During the First Year of Use of a Contraceptive Method

Method	Lowest Expected	Typical
Norplant System	0.09	0.09
Male Sterilization	0.1	0.15
Female Sterilization	0.4	0.4
DMPA (injectable progestogen)	0.3	0.3
Oral Contraceptives		3
Combined	0.1	N/A
Progestin Only	0.5	N/A
IUD		
Progesterone	1.5	2.0
Copper T 380A	0.6	0.8
Condom (male) without spermicide	3	12
Cervical Cap		
nulliparous	9	18
parous	26	36
Diaphragm With Spermicide cream or jelly	6	18
Vaginal Sponge		
nulliparous	9	18
parous	20	36
Spermicides Alone (Foam, Creams, Jellies, And Vaginal Suppositories)	6	21
Periodic Abstinence (all methods)	1-9*	20
Withdrawal	4	19
No Contraception No contraception(planned pregnancy)	85	85

N/A—not available.

* Depending on method (calendar, ovulation, symptothermal, post-ovulation) Adapted from Hatcher, RA et al. *Contraceptive Technology* 1994-1996. New York, NY: Irvington Publishers, 1994.

Norplant System gross annual discontinuation and continuation rates are summarized in TABLE 3.

CONTRAINDICATIONS:

1. Active thrombophlebitis or thromboembolic disorders. There is insufficient information regarding women who have had previous thromboembolic disease.
2. Undiagnosed abnormal genital bleeding.
3. Known or suspected pregnancy.
4. Acute liver disease; benign or malignant liver tumors.
5. Known or suspected carcinoma of the breast.

TABLE 3 Annual and Five-Year Cumulative Rates per 100 users

Annual and Five-Year Cumulative Rates per 100 users	Year 1	Year 2	Year 3	Year 4	Year 5	Cumulative
Pregnancy	0.2	0.5	1.2	1.6	0.4	3.9
Bleeding Irregularities	9.1	7.9	4.9	3.3	2.9	25.1
Medical (excl. bleeding irreg.)	6.0	5.6	4.1	4.0	5.1	22.4
Personal	4.6	7.7	11.7	10.7	11.7	38.7
Continuation	81.0	77.4	79.2	76.7	77.6	29.5

WARNINGS:

WARNINGS BASED ON EXPERIENCE WITH THE NORPLANT SYSTEM

Bleeding Irregularities

Most women can expect some variation in menstrual bleeding patterns. Irregular menstrual bleeding, intermenstrual spotting, prolonged episodes of bleeding and spotting, and amenorrhea occur in some women. Irregular bleeding patterns associated with the Norplant System could mask symptoms of cervical or endometrial cancer. Overall, these irregularities diminish with continuing use. Since some Norplant System users experience periods of amenorrhea, missed menstrual periods cannot serve as the only means of identifying early pregnancy. Pregnancy tests should be performed whenever a pregnancy is suspected. Six (6) weeks or more of amenorrhea after a pattern of regular menses may signal pregnancy. If pregnancy occurs, the capsules must be removed.

Although bleeding irregularities have occurred in clinical trials, proportionately more women had increases rather than decreases in hemoglobin concentrations, a difference that was highly statistically significant. This finding generally indicates that reduced menstrual blood loss is associated with the use of the Norplant System. In rare instances, blood loss did result in hemoglobin values consistent with anemia.

Delayed Follicular Atresia

If follicular development occurs with the Norplant System, atresia of the follicle is sometimes delayed, and the follicle may continue to grow beyond the size it would attain in a normal cycle. These enlarged follicles cannot be distinguished clinically from ovarian cysts. In the majority of women, enlarged follicles will spontaneously disappear and should not require surgery. Rarely, they may twist or rupture, sometimes causing abdominal pain, and surgical intervention may be required.

Ectopic Pregnancies

Ectopic pregnancies have occurred among Norplant System users, although clinical studies have shown no increase in the rate of ectopic pregnancies per year among Norplant System users as compared with users of no method or of IUDs. The incidence among Norplant System users was 1.3 per 1000 women-years, a rate significantly below the rate that has been estimated for noncontraceptive users in the United States (2.7 to 3.0 per 1000 woman-years). The risk of ectopic pregnancy may increase with the duration of Norplant System use and possibly with increased weight of the user. Physicians should be alert to the possibility of an ectopic pregnancy among women using the Norplant System who become pregnant or complain of lower-abdominal pain. Any patient who presents with lower-abdominal pain must be evaluated to rule out ectopic pregnancy.

Foreign-body Carcinogenesis

Rarely, cancers have occurred at the site of foreign-body intrusions or old scars. None has been reported in the Norplant System clinical trials. In rodents, which are highly susceptible to such cancers, the incidence decreases with decreasing size of the foreign body. Because of the resistance of human beings to these cancers and because of the small size of the capsules, the risk to users of the Norplant System is judged to be minimal.

Thromboembolic Disorders and Other Vascular Problems

An increased risk of thromboembolic and thrombotic disease (pulmonary embolism, superficial venous thrombosis, and deep-vein thrombosis) has been found to be associated with the use of combination oral contraceptives. The relative risk has been estimated to be 4- to 11-fold higher for users than for nonusers. There have also been post-marketing reports of these events coincident with Norplant System use. The reports of thrombophlebitis and superficial phlebitis have more commonly occurred in the arm of insertion. Some of these cases have been associated with trauma to that arm.

Cerebrovascular Disorders: Combination oral contraceptives have been shown to increase both the relative and attributable risks of cerebrovascular events (thrombotic and hemorrhagic strokes), although, in general, the risk is greatest among older (>35 years) hypertensive women who also smoke. Hypertension was found to be a risk factor for both users and nonusers for both types of strokes, while smoking interacted to increase the risk for hemorrhagic strokes. There have been post-marketing reports of stroke coincident with Norplant System use.

Myocardial Infarction: An increased risk of myocardial infarction has been attributed to combination oral-contraceptive use. This is thought to be primarily thrombotic in origin and is related to the estrogen component of combination oral contraceptives. This increased risk occurs primarily in smokers or in women with other underlying risk factors for coronary-artery disease, such as family history of coronary-artery disease, hypertension, hypercholesterolemia, morbid obesity, and diabetes. The current relative risk of heart attack for combination oral-contraceptive users has been estimated as 2 to 6 times the risk for nonusers. The absolute risk is very low for women under 30 years of age.

Studies indicate a significant trend toward higher rates of myocardial infarctions and strokes with increasing doses of progestin in combination oral contraceptives. However, a recent study showed no increased risk of myocardial infarction associated with the past use of levonorgestrel-containing combination oral contraceptives. There have been post-marketing reports of myocardial infarction coincident with Norplant System use.

Patients who develop active thrombophlebitis or thromboembolic disease should have the Norplant System capsules removed. Removal should also be considered in women who will be subjected to prolonged immobilization due to surgery or other illnesses.

Use Before or During Early Pregnancy

Extensive epidemiological studies have revealed no risk of birth defects in women who have used oral contraceptives prior to pregnancy. Studies also do not suggest a teratogenic effect, particularly insofar as cardiac anomalies and limb-reduction defects are concerned, when taken inadvertently during early pregnancy. There is no evidence suggesting that the risk associated with Norplant System use is different.

There have been rare reports of congenital anomalies in offspring of women who were using the Norplant System inadvertently during early pregnancy. A cause and effect relationship is not believed to exist.

WARNINGS BASED ON EXPERIENCE WITH COMBINATION (PROGESTIN PLUS ESTROGEN) ORAL CONTRACEPTIVES

WARNINGS: *(cont'd)*

Cigarette Smoking

Cigarette smoking increases the risk of serious cardiovascular side effects from the use of combination oral contraceptives. This risk increases with age and heavy smoking (15 or more cigarettes per day) and is quite marked in women over 35 years old. While this is believed to be an estrogen-related effect, it is not known whether a similar risk exists with progestin-only methods such as the Norplant System; however, women who use the Norplant System should be advised not to smoke.

Elevated Blood Pressure

Increased blood pressure has been reported in users of combination oral contraceptives. The prevalence of elevated blood pressure increases with long exposure. Although there were no statistically significant trends among Norplant System users in clinical trials, physicians should be aware of the possibility of elevated blood pressure with the Norplant System.

Carcinoma

Numerous epidemiological studies have been performed to determine the incidence of breast, endometrial, ovarian, and cervical cancer in women using combination oral contraceptives. Recent evidence in the literature suggests that use of combination oral contraceptives is not associated with an increased risk of developing breast cancer in the overall population of users. The Cancer and Steroid Hormone (CASH) study also showed no latent effect on the risk of breast cancer for at least a decade following long-term use. However, some of these same recent studies have shown an increased relative risk of breast cancer in certain subgroups of combination oral- contraceptives users, although no consistent pattern of findings has been identified. This information should be considered when prescribing the Norplant System.

Some studies suggest that combination oral-contraceptive use has been associated with an increase in the risk of cervical intraepithelial neoplasia in some populations of women. However, there continues to be controversy about the extent to which such findings may be due to differences in sexual behavior and other factors. In spite of many studies of the relationship between combination oral-contraceptive use and breast and cervical cancers, a cause-and-effect relationship has not been established.

Evidence indicates that combination oral contraceptives may decrease the risk of ovarian and endometrial cancer. Irregular bleeding patterns associated with the Norplant System could mask symptoms of cervical or endometrial cancer.

Hepatic Tumors

Hepatic adenomas have been found to be associated with the use of combination oral contraceptives with an estimated incidence of about 3 occurrences per 100,000 users per year, a risk that increases after 4 or more years of use. Although benign, hepatic adenomas may rupture and cause death through intra-abdominal hemorrhage. The contribution of the progestin component of oral contraceptives to the development of hepatic adenomas is not known.

Ocular Lesions

There have been clinical case reports of retinal thrombosis associated with the use of oral contraceptives. Although it is believed that this adverse reaction is related to the estrogen component of oral contraceptives, the Norplant System capsules should be removed if there is unexplained partial or complete loss of vision; onset of proptosis or diplopia; papilledema; or retinal vascular lesions. Appropriate diagnostic and therapeutic measures should be undertaken immediately.

Gallbladder Disease

Earlier studies have reported an increased lifetime relative risk of gallbladder surgery in users of oral contraceptives and estrogens. More recent studies, however, have shown that the relative risk of developing gallbladder disease among oral-contraceptive users may be minimal. The recent findings of minimal risk may be related to the use of oral-contraceptive formulations containing lower hormonal doses of estrogens and progestins. The association of this risk with the use of the Norplant System progestin-only method is not known.

PRECAUTIONS:

GENERAL

Patients should be counseled that this product does not protect against HIV infection (AIDS) and other sexually transmitted diseases.

1. Physical Examination and Follow-Up: A complete medical history and physical examination should be taken prior to the implantation or reimplantation of Norplant System capsules and at least annually during its use. These physical examinations should include special reference to the implant site, blood pressure, breasts, abdomen and pelvic organs, including cervical cytology and relevant laboratory tests. In case of undiagnosed, persistent or recurrent abnormal vaginal bleeding, appropriate diagnostic measures should be conducted to rule out malignancy. Women with a strong family history of breast cancer or who have breast nodules should be monitored with particular care.

2. Carbohydrate and Lipid Metabolism: An altered glucose tolerance characterized by decreased insulin sensitivity following glucose loading has been found in some users of combination and progestin-only oral contraceptives. The effects of the Norplant System on carbohydrate metabolism appear to be minimal. In a study in which pretreatment serum-glucose levels were compared with levels after 1 and 2 years of Norplant System use, no statistically significant differences in mean serum-glucose levels were evident 2 hours after glucose loading. The clinical significance of these findings is unknown, but diabetic and prediabetic patients should be carefully observed while using the Norplant System. Women who are being treated for hyperlipidemias should be followed closely if they elect to use the Norplant System. Some progestins may elevate LDL levels and may render the control of hyperlipidemias more difficult. (See WARNINGS, Thromboembolic Disorders and Other Vascular Problems.)

3. Liver Function: If jaundice develops in any women while using the Norplant System, consideration should be given to removing the capsules. Steroid hormones may be poorly metabolized in patients with impaired liver function.

4. Fluid Retention: Steroid contraceptives may cause some degree of fluid retention. They should be prescribed with caution, and only with careful monitoring, in patients with conditions which might be aggravated by fluid retention.

5. Emotional Disorders: Consideration should be given to removing Norplant System capsules in women who become significantly depressed since the symptom may be drug-related. Women with a history of depression should be carefully observed and removal considered if depression recurs to a serious degree.

6. Contact Lenses: Contact-lens wearers who develop visual changes or changes in lens tolerance should be assessed by an ophthalmologist.

7. Idiopathic Intracranial Hypertension: Idiopathic intracranial hypertension (pseudotumor cerebri, benign intracranial hypertension) is a disorder of unknown etiology which is seen most commonly in obese females of reproductive age. There have been reports of idiopathic intracranial hypertension in Norplant System users; however, a causal relationship is unclear. A cardinal sign of idiopathic intracranial hypertension is papilledema; early symptoms may include headache (associated with a change in the frequency, pattern, severity, or persistence; of particular importance are those headaches that are unremitting in nature) and visual

PRECAUTIONS: *(cont'd)*

disturbances. Patients with these symptoms should be screened for papilledema and, if present, the patient should be referred to a neurologist for further diagnosis and care. Norplant System should be removed from patients experiencing this disorder.

8. Autoimmune Disease: Autoimmune diseases such as scleroderma, systemic lupus erythematosus and rheumatoid arthritis occur in the general population and more frequently among women of childbearing age. There have been rare reports of various autoimmune diseases, including the above, in Norplant System users; however, the rate of reporting is significantly less than the expected incidence for these diseases. Studies have raised the possibility of developing antibodies against silicone-containing devices; however, the specificity and clinical relevance of these antibodies are unknown. While it is believed that the occurrence of autoimmune disease among Norplant System users is coincidental, health-care providers should be alert to the earliest manifestations.

9. Insertion and Removal: To be sure that the woman is not pregnant at the time of capsule placement and to assure contraceptive effectiveness during the first cycle of use, it is advisable that insertion be done during the first 7 days of the menstrual cycle or immediately following an abortion. However, Norplant System capsules may be inserted at any time during the cycle provided pregnancy has been excluded and a nonhormonal contraceptive method is used for the remainder of the cycle. Insertion is not recommended before 6 weeks postpartum in breast-feeding women. Insertion and removal are not difficult procedures but instructions must be followed closely. It is strongly advised that all health-care professionals who insert and remove Norplant System capsules be instructed in the procedures before they attempt them. A proper insertion just under the skin will facilitate removals. Proper Norplant System insertion and removal should result in minimal scarring. If the capsules are placed too deeply, they can be harder to remove. There have been infrequent reports of the use of general anesthesia during the removal procedure; it is generally not required. Before initiating the removal procedure, all Norplant System capsules should be located via palpation. If all six capsules cannot be palpated, they may be localized via ultrasound (7 MHz) or X ray (soft tissue). If all capsules cannot be removed at the first attempt, removal should be attempted later when the site has healed. Bruising may occur at the implant site during insertion or removal. Other cutaneous reactions that have been reported include blistering, ulcerations and sloughing. There have been reports of arm pain, numbness and tingling following these procedures. In some women, hyperpigmentation occurs over the implantation site but is usually reversible following removal. See detailed Insertion and Removal Instructions below.

10. Infections: Infection at the implant site, including cellulitis, has been uncommon. Attention to aseptic technique and proper insertion and removal of the Norplant System capsules reduces the possibility of infection. If infection occurs, suitable treatment should be instituted. If infection persists, the capsules should be removed.

11. Expulsion: Expulsion of capsules was uncommon. It occurred more frequently when placement of the capsules was extremely shallow, too close to the incision, or when infection was present. Replacement of an expelled capsule must be accomplished using a new sterile capsule. If infection is present, it should be treated and cured before replacement. Contraceptive efficacy may be inadequate with fewer than 6 capsules.

12. Provisions for Removal Women should be advised that the capsules will be removed at any time for any reason. The removal should be done on such request or at the end of 5 years of usage by personnel instructed in the removal technique.

Upon removal, Norplant System capsules should be disposed of in accordance with Center for Disease Control Guidelines for the handling of biohazardous waste.

DRUG/LABORATORY TEST INTERACTIONS

Certain endocrine tests may be affected by Norplant System use:

1. Sex-hormone-binding globulin concentrations are decreased.

2. Thyroxine concentrations may be slightly decreased and triiodothyronine uptake increased.

CARCINOGENESIS

See WARNINGS.

PREGNANCY CATEGORY X

See WARNINGS.

NURSING MOTHERS

Steroids are not considered the contraceptives of first choice for lactating women. Levonorgestrel has been identified in the breast milk of lactating women. No significant effects were observed on the growth or health of infants whose mothers used the Norplant System beginning 6 weeks after parturition in comparative studies with mothers using IUDs or barrier methods. Eighty (80) infants were monitored for three years. No information is available beyond that time. No data are available on use in breast-feeding mothers earlier than 6 weeks after parturition.

INFORMATION FOR THE PATIENT

Patient Labeling is included to help describe the characteristics of the Norplant System to the patient. One copy should be provided to the patient. Patients should also be advised that the Prescribing Information is available to them at their request. It is recommended that prospective users be fully informed about the risks and benefits associated with the use of the Norplant System, with other forms of contraception, and with no contraception at all. It is also recommended that prospective users be fully informed about the insertion and removal procedures. Health-care providers may wish to obtain informed consent from all patients in light of the techniques involved with insertion and removal.

DRUG INTERACTIONS:

Reduced efficacy (pregnancy) has been reported for Norplant System users taking phenytoin and carbamazepine. Norplant System users should be warned of the possibility of decreased efficacy with use of any related drugs.

ADVERSE REACTIONS:

The following adverse reactions have been associated with the Norplant System during the first year of use. They include:

TABLE 4

Many bleeding days or prolonged bleeding	27.6%
Spotting	17.1%
Amenorrhea	9.4%
Irregular (onsets of) bleeding	7.6%
Frequent bleeding onsets	7.0%
Scanty bleeding	5.2%
Pain or itching near implant site (usually transient)	3.7%
Infection at implant site	0.7%

In addition, removal difficulties have been reported with a frequency of 6.2%, which is based on 849 removals occurring through 5 years of use.

Clinical studies comparing Norplant System users with other contraceptive method users suggest that the following adverse reactions occurring during the first year are probably associated with Norplant System use. These adverse reactions have also been reported postmarketing:

ADVERSE REACTIONS: *(cont'd)*

Headache; Nervousness/Anxiety; Nausea/Vomiting; Dizziness; Adnexal enlargement; Dermatitis/Rash; Acne; Change of appetite; Mastalgia; Weight gain; Hirsutism, hypertrichosis, and scalp-hair loss

In addition, the following adverse reactions have been reported with a frequency of 5% or greater during the first year and possibly may be related to Norplant System use:

Breast discharge; Cervicitis; Musculoskeletal pain; Abdominal discomfort; Leukorrhea; Vaginitis

The following adverse reactions have been reported post-marketing with an incidence of less than 1%. These events occurred under circumstances where a causal relationship to the Norplant System is unknown. These reactions are listed as information for physicians:

Emotional lability; Congenital anomalies; Pulmonary embolism; Superficial venous thrombosis; Deep-vein thrombosis; Myocardial infarction; Thrombotic thrombocytopenic purpura (TTP); Idiopathic intracranial hypertension (IIH, pseudotumor cerebri); Stroke; Pruritus; Urticaria; Dysmenorrhea; Migraine; Arm Pain; Numbness; Tingling

OVERDOSAGE:

Overdosage can result if more than six capsules of the Norplant System are *in situ.* All implanted Norplant System capsules should be removed before inserting a new set of Norplant System capsules. Overdosage may cause fluid retention with its associated effects and uterine bleeding irregularities.

DOSAGE AND ADMINISTRATION:

The Norplant System consists of six Silastic capsules, each containing 36 mg of the progestin, levonorgestrel. The total administered (implanted) dose is 216 mg. Implantation of all six capsules should be performed during the first 7 days of the onset of menses by a health-care professional instructed in the Norplant System insertion technique. Insertion is subdermal in the midportion of the upper arm about 8 to 10 cm above the elbow crease. Distribution should be in a fanlike pattern, about 15 degrees apart, for a total of 75 degrees. Proper insertion will facilitate later removal.

Instructions For Insertion And Removal: The Norplant System consists of six levonorgestrel-releasing capsules that are inserted subdermally in the medial aspect of the upper arm.

The Norplant System provides up to 5 years of effective contraceptive protection.

The basis for successful use and subsequent removal of Norplant System capsules is a correct and carefully performed subdermal insertion of the six capsules. It is recommended that health-care professionals performing insertions or removals of Norplant System capsules avail themselves of instruction and supervision in the proper technique prior to attempting these procedures. During insertion, special attention should be given to the following:

asepsis

correct subdermal placement of the capsules

careful technique to minimize tissue trauma

Insertion Procedure: Insertion should be performed within seven days from the onset of menses. However, Norplant System capsules may be inserted at any time during the cycle provided pregnancy has been excluded and a nonhormonal contraceptive method is used for the remainder of the cycle. A gynecological examination should be performed before the insertion of Norplant System capsules, as would be the case before initiating any hormonal contraception. Determine if the subject has any allergies to the antiseptic or anesthetic to be used or contraindications to progestin-only contraception. If none are found, the capsules are inserted using the procedure outlined below.

One Norplant System set consists of six capsules in a sterile pouch. The insertion is performed under aseptic conditions using a trocar to place the capsules under the skin.

The following equipment is recommended for the insertion:

an examining table for the patient to lie on.

sterile surgical drapes, sterile gloves (free of talc), antiseptic solution.

local anesthetic, needles, and syringe.

#11 scalpel, #10 trocar forceps.

skin closure, sterile gauze, and compresses.

The plastic cover and tray are NOT STERILE.

2. Have the patient lie on her back on the examination table with her left arm (if the patient is left-handed, the right arm) flexed at the elbow and externally rotated so that her hand is lying by her head. The capsules will be inserted subdermally through a small 2-mm incision and positioned in a fanlike manner with the fan opening towards the shoulder.

3. Prep the patient's upper arm with antiseptic solution; cover the arm above and below the insertion area with a sterile cloth. The optimal insertion area is in the inside of the upper arm about 8 to 10 cm above the elbow crease.

4. Open the sterile Norplant System package carefully by pulling apart the sheets of the pouch, allowing the capsules to fall onto a sterile drape. Count the six capsules.

5. After determining the absence of known allergies to the anesthetic agent of related drugs, fill a 5-ml syringe with the local anesthetic. Since blood loss is minimal with this procedure, use of epinephrine-containing anesthetics is not considered necessary. Anesthetize the insertion area by first inserting the needle under the skin and injecting a small amount of anesthetic. Then anesthetize six areas about 4 to 4.5 cm long, to mimic the fanlike position of the implanted capsules.

6. Use the scalpel to make a small incision (about 2 mm) just through the dermis of the skin.

7. The trocar has two marks on it. The first mark is closer to the hub and indicates how far the trocar should be introduced under the skin before the loading of each capsule. The second mark is close to the tip and indicates how much of the trocar should remain under the skin following the insertion of each implant.

8. Insert the tip of the trocar through the incision beneath the skin at a shallow angle. Once the trocar is inserted, it should be oriented with the bevel up toward the skin to keep the capsules in a superficial plane. It is important to keep the trocar subdermal by tenting the skin with the trocar, as failure to do so may result in deep placement of the capsules and could make removal more difficult.

Advance the trocar gently under the skin to the first mark near the hub of trocar. The tip of the trocar is now at a distance of about 4 to 4.5 cm from the incision.

Do not force the trocar, and if resistance is felt, try another direction.

9. When the trocar has been inserted the appropriate distance, remove the obturator and load the first capsule into the trocar using the thumb and forefinger.

10. Gently advance the capsule with the obturator towards the tip of the trocar until you feel resistance. Never force the obturator.

11. Hold the obturator steady, and bring the trocar back until it touches the handle of the obturator.

12. The capsule should have been released under the skin when the mark close to the tip of the trocar is visible in the incision. Release of the capsule can be checked by palpitation. It is important to keep the obturator steady and not to push the capsule into the tissue.

DOSAGE AND ADMINISTRATION: *(cont'd)*

13. Do not remove the trocar from the incision until all capsules have been inserted. The trocar is withdrawn only to the mark close to its tip. Each succeeding capsule is always inserted next to the previous one, to form a fanlike shape. Fix the position of the previous capsule with the forefinger and middle finger of the free hand, and advance the trocar along the tips of the fingers. This will ensure a suitable distance of about 15 degrees between capsules and keep the trocar from puncturing any of the previously inserted capsules. Leave a distance of about 5 mm between the incision and the tips of the capsules. This will help avoid spontaneous expulsions. The correct position of the capsules can be ensured by feeling them with the fingers after the insertion has been completed.

14. After the insertion of the sixth capsule, palpate the capsules to make sure that all six have been inserted.

15. Press the edges of the incision together, and close the incision with a skin closure. Suturing the incision should not be necessary.

16. Cover the insertion area with a dry compress, and wrap gauze around the arm to ensure hemostasis.

Observe the patient for a few minutes for signs of syncope or bleeding from the incision before shew is discharged.

Advise the patient to keep the insertion area dry for 2 to 3 days.. The gauze may be removed after 1 day, and the butterfly bandage as soon as the incision has healed (*i.e.,* normally in 3 days).

Removal Procedure: Described below is a removal procedure which was developed and used during the clinical trials for the Norplant System. As with many surgical procedures, variations of the technique have appeared and some have been published. No one particular procedure routinely appears to have any advantage over another.

It is recommended that removals be prescheduled so that preparations for carrying out the procedure can be facilitated.

Removal of the capsules should be performed very gently and will usually take more time than insertion. Capsules are sometimes nicked or cut during removal. The incidence of overall removal difficulties, including damage to capsules, has been 13.2 percent. Less than half of these removal difficulties have caused inconvenience to the patient. If the removal of some of the capsules proves difficult, have the patient return for another visit. The remaining capsule(s) will be easier to remove after the area is healed. If contraception is still desired, a barrier method should be advised until all capsules are removed.

The position of the patient and the asepsis are the same as for insertion.

1. The following equipment is needed for the removal:

an examining table for the patient to lie on.

sterile surgical drapes, sterile gloves, (free of talc), antiseptic solution.

local anesthetic, needles, and syringe.

#11 scalpel, forceps (straight and curved mosquito).

skin closure, sterile gauze, and compresses.

2. Palpate the capsules to make sure that all six capsules have been located, marketing their position with a sterile marker. If all six capsules cannot be palpated, they may be localized via ultrasound (7 MHz) or X ray (soft tissue).

3. Once all six capsules are located apply a small amount of local anesthetic *under* the capsule ends nearest the original incision site. This will serve to raise the ends of the capsules. Anesthetic injected over the capsules will obscure them and make removal more difficult. Additional small amounts of the anesthetic can be used for the removal of each of the capsules, if required.

4. Make a 4-mm incision with the scalpel close to the ends of the capsules. Do not make a large incision.

5. Push each capsule gently towards the incision with the fingers. When the tip is visible or near to the incision, grasp it with a mosquito forceps.

6. Use the scalpel very gently to open the tissue sheath that has formed around the capsule.

7. Remove the capsule from the incision with the second forceps.

8. After the procedure is completed, the incision is closed and bandaged as with insertion. The upper arm should be kept dry for a few days. Following removal, a return to the previous level of fertility is usually prompt, and a pregnancy may occur at any time. If the patient wishes to continue using the method, a new set of Norplant System capsules can be inserted through the same incision in the same or opposite direction.

INSERTION

Hints: Counselling of the patient of the benefits and side effects of the method prior to insertion will greatly increase patient satisfaction.

Correct subdermal placement of the capsules will facilitate removal.

Before insertion, apply the anesthetic just beneath the skin so as to raise the dermis above the underlying tissue.

Never force the trocar.

To ensure subdermal placement, the trocar with bevel up, should be supported by the index finger and should visibly raise the skin at all times during insertion.

To avoid damaging the previous implanted capsule, stabilize the capsule with your forefinger and middle finger and advance the trocar alongside the finger tips at an angle of 15 degrees.

After insertion, make a drawing for the patient's file showing the location of the 6 capsules and describe any variations in placement. This will greatly aid removal.

Removal: Alternative removal techniques have developed.

The removal of the implanted capsules will usually take a little more time than insertion.

Before initiating removal, all capsules should be located by palpation. If all six capsules cannot be palpated, they may be localized via ultrasound (7 MHz) or X ray (soft tissue).

Before removal, apply the anesthetic *under* the capsule ends nearest the original incision sites.

If the removal of some of the capsules proves difficult, interrupt the procedure and have the patient return for another visit. The remaining capsule(s) will be easier to remove after the area is healed.

HOW SUPPLIED:

The Norplant System Kit includes the following items: 1 Norplant System (levonorgestrel implants), a set of six implants (capsules); 1 Norplant System trocar; 1 Package of skin closures; 1 Scalpel; 3 Packages of gauze sponges; 1 Forceps; 1 Stretch bandage; 1 Syringe; 1 Surgical drape (fenestrated); 2 Syringe needles; 2 Surgical drapes.

Store at room temperature away from excess heat and moisture.

Note: The indented statement below is required by the Federal government's Clean Air Act for all products containing or manufactured with chlorofluorocarbons (CFC's).

WARNING: Manufactured with dichlorodifluoromethane, a substance which harms public health and environment by destroying ozone in the upper atmosphere.

A notice similar to the above WARNING has been placed in the patient information leaflet of this product pursuant to EPA regulations.

HOW SUPPLIED: *(cont'd)*

Dichlorodifluoromethane is a chemical used in the sterilization process of the Norplant System and is not contained on the product itself.

HOW SUPPLIED - EQUIVALENTS NOT AVAILABLE:

Kit - Misc - 216 mg

1 kit	$456.25	**NORPLANT SYSTEM KIT, Wyeth Labs**	**00008-2564-01**

LEVORPHANOL TARTRATE *(001636)*

CATEGORIES: Analgesics; Cancer; Central Nervous System Agents; Colic; Myocardial Infarction; Narcotic Analgesics; Narcotics, Synthetics & Combinations; Opiate Agonists (Controlled); Pain; DEA Class CII; FDA Approved 1991 Dec

BRAND NAMES: *Dromoran* (Japan); **Levo-Dromoran**
(International brand names outside U.S. in italics)

FORMULARIES: Aetna; Medi-Cal

DESCRIPTION:

Levorphanol tartrate is available as 1-ml ampuls containing 2 mg levorphanol tartrate compounded with 0.2% parabens (methyl and propyl) as preservatives and sodium hydroxide to adjust pH to approximately 4.3; as 10-ml vials containing 2 mg levorphanol tartrate per ml, compounded with 0.45% phenol as preservative and sodium hydroxide to adjust pH to approximately 4.3; and as scored tablets, each containing 2 mg levorphanol tartrate plus lactose, corn starch, stearic acid and talc.

Levorphanol tartrate is a highly potent synthetic analgesic with properties and actions similar to those of morphine. It produces a degree of analgesia at least equal to that of morphine and greater than that of meperidine at far smaller doses than either. It is longer acting than either; from 6 to 8 hours of pain relief can be expected with levorphanol tartrate whether given orally or by injection. It is almost as effective orally as it is parenterally. Its safety margin is about equal to that of morphine, but it is less likely to produce nausea, vomiting and constipation.

INDICATIONS AND USAGE:

Levorphanol tartrate is recommended whenever a narcotic-analgesic is required. It is recommended for the relief of pain whether moderate or severe. For example, it may be used in alleviating pain due to biliary and renal colic, myocardial infarction, and severe trauma; intractable pain due to cancer and other tumors; and for postoperative pain relief. Used preoperatively, it allays apprehension, provides prolonged analgesia, reduces thiopental requirements and shortens recovery-room time. Levorphanol tartrate is compatible with a wide range of anesthetic agents. It is a useful supplement to nitrous oxide-oxygen anesthesia. It has been given by slow intravenous injection for special indications.

CONTRAINDICATIONS:

As with the use of morphine, levorphanol tartrate is contraindicated in acute alcoholism, bronchial asthma, increased intracranial pressure, respiratory depression and anoxia.

WARNINGS:

May be habit forming. Levorphanol tartrate is a narcotic with an addiction liability similar to that of morphine, and for this reason the same precautions should be taken in administering the drug as with morphine. As with all narcotics, levorphanol tartrate should be used in early pregnancy only when expected benefits outweigh risks.

PRECAUTIONS:

To counteract narcotic-induced respiratory depression, a narcotic antagonist, such as Naloxone Hydrochloride (Narcan), is recommended and should be readily available whenever levorphanol tartrate is used by parenteral administration.

ADVERSE REACTIONS:

As is true with the use of any narcotic-analgesic, nausea, emesis and dizziness are not uncommon in the ambulatory patient. Respiratory depression, hypotension, urinary retention and various cardiac arrhythmias have been infrequently reported following the use of levorphanol tartrate, primarily in surgical patients. Occasional allergic reactions in the form of skin rash or urticaria have been reported. Pruritus or sweating are rarely observed.

OVERDOSAGE:

In the event of overdosage of levorphanol tartrate, an appropriate dose of a narcotic antagonist, such as Naloxone HCl (Narcan), should be administered; consult the prescribing information of the specific narcotic antagonist for details about use.

DOSAGE AND ADMINISTRATION:

Good medical practice dictates that the dose of any narcotic-analgesic be appropriate to the degree of pain to be relieved. This is especially important during the postoperative period because (a) residual CNS-depressant effects of anesthetic agents may still be present, and (b) later, gradual lessening of pain may not warrant full narcotizing doses. The average adult dose is 2 mg orally or subcutaneously. The dosage may be increased to 3 mg, if necessary.

(Roche, 9/85, 13-06-72201-0591)

HOW SUPPLIED - EQUIVALENTS NOT AVAILABLE:

Injection, Solution - Subcutaneous - 2 mg/ml

1 ml x 10	$28.28	**LEVO-DROMORAN, Roche**	**00004-1910-06**
10 ml	$21.92	**LEVO-DROMORAN, Roche**	**00004-1911-06**

Tablet, Uncoated - Oral - 2 mg

100's	$54.68	Levorphanol Tartrate, Roxane	00054-4494-25
100's	$59.84	**LEVO-DROMORAN, Roche**	**00004-0044-01**
100's	$72.94	Levorphanol Tartrate, Roxane	00054-8494-24

LEVOTHYROXINE SODIUM *(001612)*

CATEGORIES: Goiter; Hormones; Hypothyroidism; Myxedema; Synthetic Thyroid Hormone; Thyroid Agents; Thyroid Carcinoma; Thyroid Function; Thyroid Preparations; Pregnancy Category A; Sales > $500 Million; FDA Pre 1938 Drugs; Top 200 Drugs

BRAND NAMES: *Berlthyrox* (Germany); *Droxine* (Australia); *Eferox* (Germany); *Elthyrone*; *Eltroxin* (Asia, England, Canada); *Euthyrox* (Germany); *Eutirox* (Mexico); L-Thyroxine; *Letter*; *Levaxin*; Levo-T; *Levotirox*; Levothroid; *Levothyrox* (France); *Levotrix*; Levoxyl; *Oroxine* (Australia); **Synthroid**; Synthrox; *T4KP*; *Thevier* (Germany); *Throxinique*; *Thyradin*; *Thyradin S* (Japan); *Thyrax*; *Thyrax Duotab*; *Thyrex*; *Thyro-4*; *Thyrosit*; *Thyroxin*; *Thyroxin-Natrium*; *Thyroxine*; *Tiroidine* (Mexico)
(International brand names outside U.S. in italics)

FORMULARIES: Aetna; BC-BS; CIGNA; DoD; FHP; Humana; Kaiser; Medco; Medi-Cal; PCS; PruCare; United; WHO

COST OF THERAPY: $60.88 (Hypothyroidism; Tablet; 0.1 mg; 1/day; 365 days)

Thyroid hormones, either alone or together with other therapeutic agents, should not be used for the treatment of obesity. In euthyroid patients, doses within the range of daily hormonal requirements are ineffective for weight reduction. Larger doses may produce serious or even life threatening manifestations of toxicity, particularly when given in association with sympathomimetic amines such as those used for their anorectic effects.

The use of levothyroxine sodium in the treatment of obesity, either alone or in combination with other drugs, is unjustified. The use of levothyroxine is also unjustified in the treatment of male or female infertility unless this condition is associated with hypothyroidism.

DESCRIPTION:

Each levothyroxine sodium, USP tablet contains synthetic crystalline levothyroxine sodium (L-thyroxine). L-thyroxine is the principal hormone secreted by the normal thyroid gland. Chemically, L-thyroxine is designated as L-tyrosine, O-(4-hydroxy-3, 5-diiodophenyl) - 3,5-diiodo -, monosodium salt, hydrate. The empirical formula is $C_{15}H_{10}I_4N$ Na O_4 x H_2O, molecular weight of 798.86 (anhydrous).

Synthroid Inactive Ingredients: acacia, confectioner's sugar, lactose, magnesium stearate, povidone, and talc. The following are the color additives by tablet strength: *25mcg:* FD&C Yellow No. 6; *50mcg:* None; *75mcg:* FD&C Red No. 40, FD&C Blue No. 2; *88mcg:* FD&C Blue No. 1, FD&C Yellow No. 6, D&C Yellow No. 10; *100mcg:* D&C Yellow No.10, FD&C Yellow No. 6; *112mcg:* D&C Red No. 27 & 30; *125mcg:* FD&C Yellow No. 6, FD&C Red No. 40, FD&C Blue No. 1; *150mcg:* FD&C Blue No. 2; *175mcg:* FD&C Blue No. 1, D&C Red No. 27 & 30; *200mcg:* FD&C Red No. 40; *300mcg:* D&C Yellow No. 10, FD&C Yellow No. 6, FD&C Blue No. 1.

CLINICAL PHARMACOLOGY:

The synthesis and secretion of the major thyroid hormones L-thyroxine (T_4) and L-triiodothyronine (T_3) from the normally functioning thyroid gland are regulated by complex feedback mechanisms of the hypothalamic-pituitary-thyroid axis. The thyroid gland is stimulated to secrete thyroid hormones by the action of thyrotropin (thyroid stimulating hormone, TSH) which is produced in the anterior pituitary gland. TSH secretion is in turn controlled by thyrotropin-releasing hormone (TRH) produced in the hypothalamus, circulating thyroid hormones, and possibly other mechanisms. Thyroid hormones circulating in the blood act as feedback inhibitors of both TSH and TRH secretion. Thus, when serum concentrations of T_3 and T_4 are increased, secretion of TSH and TRH is increased Administration of exogenous thyroid hormones to euthyroid individuals results in suppression of endogenous thyroid hormone secretion.

The mechanisms by which thyroid hormones exert their physiologic actions have not been completely elucidated. T_4 and T_3 are transported into cells by passive and active mechanisms. T_3 in cell cytoplasm and T_3 generated from T_4 within the cell diffuse into the nucleus and bind to thyroid receptor proteins, which appear to be primarily attached to DNA. Receptor binding leads to activation or repression of DNA transcription, thereby altering the amounts of mRNA and resultant proteins. Changes in protein concentrations are responsible for the metabolic changes observed in organs and tissues.

Thyroid hormones enhance oxygen consumption of most body tissues and increase the basal metabolic rate and metabolism of carbohydrates, lipids, and proteins. Thus, they exert a profound influence on every organ system and are of particular importance in the development of the central nervous system. Thyroid hormones also appear to have direct effects on tissues, such as increased myocardial contractility and decreased systemic vascular resistance.

The physiologic effects of thyroid hormones are produced primarily by T_3, a large portion of which is derived from the from the deiodination of T_4 in peripheral tissues. About 70 to 90 percent of peripheral T_3 is produced by monodeoidination of T_4 at the 5' position (outer ring). Peripheral monodeiodination of T_4 at the 5 position (inner ring) results in the formation of reverse triiodothyronine (rT_3), which is calorigenically inactive.

PHARMACOKINETICS

Few clinical studies have evaluated the kinetics of orally administered thyroid hormone. In animals, the most active sites of absorption appear to be the proximal and mid-jejunum. T_4 is not absorbed from the stomach and little, if any, drug is absorbed from the duodenum. There seems to be no absorption of the T_4 from the distal colon in animals. A number of human studies have confirmed the importance of an intact jejunum dileum for T_4 absorption and have shown some absorption from the duodenum. Studies involving radioiodinated T_4 fecal tracer excretion methods, equilibration, and AUC methods have shown that absorption varies from 48 to 80 percent of the administered dose. The extent of absorption is increased in the fasting state and decreased in malabsorption syndromes, such as sprue. Absorption may also decrease with age. The degree of T_4 absorption is dependent on the product formulation as well as on the character of the intestinal contents, including plasma protein and soluble dietary factors, which bind thyroid hormone making it unavailable for diffusion. Decreased absorption may result from administration of infant soybean formula, ferrous sulfate, sodium polystyrene sulfonate, aluminum hydroxide sucralfate, or bile acid sequestrants. T_4 absorption following intramuscular administration.

Distribution of thyroid hormones in human body tissues and fluids has not been fully elucidated. More than percent of circulating hormones is bound to serum proteins, including thyroxine-binding globulin(TGB), thyroxine-binding prealbumin (TBPA), and albumin (TBA). T_4 is more extensively and firmly bound to serum proteins than is T_3. Only unbound thyroid hormone is metabolically active. The higher affinity of TGB and TBPA for T_4 partly explains the higher serum levels, slower metabolic clearance, and longer serum elimination half-life of this hormone.

Certain drugs and physiologic conditions can alter the binding of thyroid hormones to serum proteins and/or the concentrations of the serum proteins available for thyroid hormone binding. These effects must be considered when interpreting the results of thyroid function tests. (See DRUG INTERACTIONSand Laboratory Test Interactions.)

T_4 is eliminated slowly from the body, with a half-life of 6 to 7 days. T_3 has a half-life of 1 to 2 days. The liver is the major site of degradation for both hormones. T_4 and T_3 are conjugated with glucuronic and sulfuric acids and excreted in the bile. There is an enterohepatic circulation of thyroid hormones, as they are liberated by hydrolysis in the intestine and reabsorbed. A portion of the conjugated material reaches the colon unchanged, id hydrolyzed there, and is eliminated as free compounds in the feces. In man, approximately 20 to 40 percent of T_4 is eliminated in the stool. About 70 percent of the T_4 secreted daily is deiodonated to yield equal amounts of T_3 and rT_3. Subsequent deiodination of T_3 and rT_3 yields multiple forms of diiodothyronine. A number of other minor T_4 metabolites have also been identified. Although some of the metabolites have biological activity, their overall contribution to the therapeutic effect of T_4 is minimal.

INDICATIONS AND USAGE:

Levothyroxine sodium is indicated:

1. As replacement or supplemental therapy in patients of any age or state (including pregnancy) with hypothyroidism of any etiology except transient hypothyroidism during the recovery phase of subacute thyroiditis: primary hypothyroidism resulting from thyroid dysfunction, primary atrophy, or partial or total absence of the thyroid gland, or from the effects of surgery, radiation or drugs, with or without the presence of goiter, including subclinical hypothyroidism; secondary (pituitary) hypothyroidism; and tertiary (hypothalamic) hypothyroidism (see CONTRAINDICATIONS and PRECAUTIONS). Levothyroxine sodium Injection can be used intravenously when rapid repletion is required, and either intravenously or intramuscularly when the oral route is precluded.

2. As a pituitary TSH supressant in the treatment or prevention of various types of euthyroid goiters, including thyroid nodules, subacute or chronic lymphocytic thydroiditis (Hashimoto's), multinodular goiter, and in conjunction with surgery and radioactive iodine therapy in the management of thyrotropin-dependent well differentiated papillary or follicular carcinoma of the thyroid.

CONTRAINDICATIONS:

Levothyroxine sodium therapy is contraindicated in patients with untreated thyrotoxicosis of any etiology or an apparent hypersensitivity to thyroid hormones or any of the inactive product constituents. (The 50 mcg tablet is formulated without color additives for patients who are sensitive to dyes.) There is no well-documented evidence of true allergic or idiosyncratic reactions to thyroid hormone. Levothyroxine sodium is also contraindicated in the patients with uncorrected adrenal insufficiency, as thyroid hormones increase tissue demands, for adrenocortical hormones and may thereby precipitate acute adrenal crisis (see PRECAUTIONS).

PRECAUTIONS:

GENERAL

Levothyroxine should be used with caution in patients with cardiovascular disorders, including angina, coronary artery disease, and hypertension, and in the elderly who have a greater likelihood of occult cardiac disease. Concomitant administration of thyroid hormone and sympathomimetic agents to patients with coronary artery disease may increase the risk of coronary insufficiency.

Use of levothyroxine in patients with concomitant diabetes mellitus, diabetes insipidus or adrenal cortical insufficiency may aggravate the intensity of their symptoms. Appropriate adjustments of the various therapeutic measures directed at these concomitant endocrine diseases may therefore be required. Treatment of myxedema coma may require simultaneous administration of glucocorticoids (see DOSAGE AND ADMINISTRATION).

T_4 enhances the response to anticoagulant therapy. Prothrombin time should be closely monitored in patients taking both levothyroxine and oral anticoagulants, and the dosage of anticoagulant adjusted accordingly.

Seizures have been reported rarely in association with the initiation of levothyroxine sodium therapy, and may be related to the effect of thyroid hormone on seizure threshold.

Lithium blocks the TSH-mediated release of $T_4$and T_3. Thyroid function should therefore be carefully monitored during lithium initiation, stabilization, and maintenance. If hypothyroidism occurs during lithium treatment, a higher than usual levothyroxine sodium dose may be required.

INFORMATION FOR THE PATIENT

1. Levothyroxine sodium is intended to replace a hormone that is normally produced by your thyroid gland. It is generally taken for life, except in cases of temporary hypothyroidism associated with an inflammation of the thyroid gland.

2. Before, or at any time while, using levothyroxine sodium, you should tell your doctor if you are allergic to any foods or medicines, are pregnant or intend to become pregnant, are breast-feeding, are taking or start taking any other prescription or non-prescription (OTC) medications, or have any other medical problems (especially hardening of the arteries, heart disease, high blood pressure, or history of thyroid, adrenal or pituitary gland problems).

3. Use levothyroxine sodium only as prescribed by your doctor. Do not discontinue levothyroxine sodium or change the amount you take or how often you take it except as directed by your doctor.

4. Levothyroxine sodium, like all medicines obtained from your doctor, must be used only by you and for the condition determined appropriate by your doctor.

5. It may take a few weeks for levothyroxine sodium to begin working. Until it begins working, you may not notice any change in your symptoms.

6. You should notify your doctor if you experience any of the following symptoms, or if you experience any other unusual medical event: chest pain, shortness of breath, hives or skin rash, rapid or irregular heartbeat, headache, irritability, nervousness, sleeplessness, diarrhea, excessive sweating, heat intolerance, changes in appetite, vomiting, weight gain or loss, changes in menstrual periods, fever, hand tremors, leg cramps.

7. You should inform your doctor or dentist that you are taking levothyroxine sodium before having any kind of surgery

8. You should notify your doctor if you become pregnant while taking levothyroxine sodium. Your dose of this medicine will likely have to be increased while you are pregnant

9. If you have diabetes, your dose of insulin or oral antidiabetic agent may need to be changed after starting levothyroxine sodium. You should monitor your blood or urinary glucose levels as directed by your doctor and report any changes to your doctor immediately.

10. If you are taking an oral anticoagulant drug such as warfarin, your dose may need to be changed after starting levothyroxine sodium. Your coagulation status should be checked often to determine if a change in dose is required.

11. Partial hair loss may occur rarely during the first few months of levothyroxine sodium therapy, but it is usually temporary.

12. SYNTHROID is the trade name for tablets containing the thyroid hormone levothyroxine, manufactured by Knoll Pharmaceutical Company. Other manufactures also make tablets containing levothyroxine. You should not change to another manufacture's product without discussing that change with your doctor first. Repeat blood tests and a change in the amount of levothyroxine sodium you take may be required.

13. Keep levothyroxine sodium out of the reach of children. Store away from heat and moisture.

LABORATORY TESTS

Treatment of patients with levothyroxine requires periodic assessment of thyroid status by appropriate laboratory tests and clinical evaluation. Selection of appropriate tests for the diagnosis and management of thyroid disorders depends on patient variables such as presenting signs and symptoms, pregnancy, and concomitant medications. A combination of sensitive TSH assay and free T_4 estimate (free T_4index, FT_4I) are recommended to confirm a diagnosis of thyroid disease. TSH alone or initially may be useful for thyroid disease screening and for monitoring therapy for primary hypothyroidism as a linear inverse correlation exists between serum TSH and free T_4. Measurement of total serum T_4 and T_3, resin T_3 uptake, and free T_3concentrations may also be useful. Antithyroid microsomal antibodies are an indicator of autoimmune thyroid disease. The combination of an increased TSH and positive microsomal antibodies in an euthyroid patient is a major risk factor for the future development of clinical hypothyroidism. An elevated serum TSH in the presence of normal T_4 may indicate subclinical hypothyroidism. Intracellular resistance to thyroid hormone is quite rare, and is suggested by clinical signs and symptoms of hypothyroidism in the presence of high serum T_4 levels. Adequacy of levothyroxine sodium therapy for hypothyroidism of pituitary or hypothalamic origin should be assessed by measuring FT_4I, which should be maintained in the upper half of the normal range. Measurement of TSH is not a reliable indicator of response to therapy for this condition.

LABORATORY TEST INTERACTIONS

A number of drugs or moieties are known to alter serum levels of TSH, T_4 and T_3 and may thereby influence the interpretation of laboratory tests of thyroid function (see DRUG INTERACTIONS).

1. Changes in TBG concentration should be taken into consideration in the interpretation of T_4 and T_3values. In such cases, the unbound (free) hormone should be measured. Pregnancy, estrogens, and estrogen-containing oral contraceptives increase TBG concentrations. TBG may also be increased during infectious hepatitis. Decreases in TBG concentrations are observed in nephrosis, acromegaly, and after androgen or corticosteroid therapy. Familial hyper- or hypo-thyroxine-binding-globulinemias have been described. The incidence of TBG deficiency approximates 1 in 9000. The binding of thyroxine of thyroid-binding prealbumin (TBPA) is inhibited by salicylates.

2. Medical or dietary iodine interferes with all in vivo tests of radioiodine uptake, producing low uptakes which may not be reflective of a true decrease in hormone synthesis.

3. The persistence of clinical and laboratory evidence of hypothyroidism in spite of adequate dosage replacement indicates either poor patient compliance, poor absorption, excessive fecal loss, or inactivity of the preparation. Intracellular resistance to thyroid hormone is quite rare.

CARCINOGENESIS, MUTAGENESIS, AND IMPAIRMENT OF FERTILITY

A reported association between prolonged thyroid therapy and breast cancer has not been confirmed and patients on thyroid for established indications should not discontinue therapy. Although no confirmatory long-term studies in animals have been performed to evaluate carcinogenic potential, mutagenicity, or impairment of fertility in either males or females, synthetic T_4 is identical to that produced by the human thyroid gland.

PREGNANCY CATEGORY A

Studies in pregnant women have not shown that levothyroxine sodium increases the risk of fetal abnormalities if administered during pregnancy. If levothyroxine sodium is used during pregnancy, the possibility of fetal harm appears remote. Because the studies cannot rule out the possibility of harm, levothyroxine sodium should be used during pregnancy only if clearly needed.

Thyroid hormones cross the placental barrier to some extent. T_4 levels in the cord blood of athyroid fetuses have been shown to be about one-third of maternal levels. Nevertheless, maternal-fetal transfer of T_4 may not prevent *in utero* hypothyroidism.

Hypothyroidism during pregnancy is associated with a higher rate of complications, including spontaneous abortion and preeclampsia, and has been reported to have an adverse effect on fetal and childhood development. On the basis of current knowledge, levothyroxine sodium, USP should therefore not be discontinued during pregnancy, and hypothyroidism diagnosed during pregnancy should be treated. Studies have shown that during pregnancy T_4 concentrations may decrease and TSH concentrations may increase to values outside normal ranges. Postpartum values are similar to preconception values. Elevations in TSH may occur as early as at 4 weeks gestation.

Pregnant women who are maintained on levothyroxine sodium should have their TSH measured periodically. An elevated TSH should be corrected by an increase in levothyroxine sodium dose. After pregnancy, the dose can be decreased to the optimal preconception dose.

NURSING MOTHERS

Minimal amounts of thyroid hormones are excreted in human milk. Thyroid hormones are not associated with serious adverse reactions and do not have known tumorigenic potential. While caution should be exercised when levothyroxine sodium is administered to a nursing woman, adequate replacement doses of levothyroxine sodium are generally needed to maintain normal lactation.

PEDIATRIC USE

Pregnant mothers provide little or no thyroid hormone to the fetus. The incidence of congenital hypothyroidism is relatively high (1 in 4,000) and the hypothyroid fetus would not derive any benefit from the small amounts of hormone crossing the placental barrier. Routine determinations of serum (T_4) and/or TSH is strongly advised in neonates in view of the deleterious effects of thyroid deficiency on growth and development.

Treatment should be initiated immediately upon diagnosis, and maintained for life, unless transient hypothyroidism is suspected; in which case, therapy may be interrupted for 30 days after the age of 3 years to reassess the condition. If T_4 is low and TSH is elevated after that time, permanent hypothyroidism is confirmed and therapy should be reinstituted. If the T_4 and TSH remain in the normal range, a preliminary diagnosis of transient hypothyroidism can be made. Nevertheless, continued close observation with periodic thyroid function testing is warranted.

DRUG INTERACTIONS:

The magnitude and relative importance of the effects noted below are likely to be patient specific and may vary by such factors as age, gender, race, intercurrent illnesses, dose of either agent, additional concomitant medications, and timing of drug administration. Any agent that alters thyroid hormone synthesis, secretion, distribution, effect on target tissues, metabolism, or elimination may alter the optimal therapeutic dose of levothyroxine sodium:

Levothyroxine sodium absorption: The following agents may bind and decrease absorption of levothyroxine sodium from the gastrointestinal tract: aluminum hydoxide, cholestyramine resin, colestipol hydrochloride, ferrous sulfate, sodium polystyrene sulfonate, soybean flour (*e.g.,* infant formula), sucralfate.

Thyroid physiology: The following agents may alter thyroid hormone or TSH levels, generally by effects on thyroid hormone synthesis, secretion, distribution, metabolism, hormone action, or elimination, or altered TSH secretion: aminoglutethimide, p-aminosalicylic acid, amiodarone, androgens and related anabolic hormones, complex anions (thiocyanate, perchlorate, pertechnetate), antithyroid drugs, β-adrenergic blocking agents, carbamazepine, chloral hydrate, diazepam, dopamine and dopamine agonists, ethionamide, glucocorticoids, heparin, hepatic enzyme inducers, insulin, iodinated cholestographic agents, iodine- containing compounds, levodopa, lovastatin, lithium, 6-mercaptopurine, metoclopramide, mitotane, nitroprusside, phenobarbital, phenytoin, resorcinol, rifampin, somatostatin analogs, sulfonamides, sulfonylureas, thiazide diuretics.

Adrenocorticoids: Metabolic clearance of adrenocorticoids is decreased in hypothyroid patients and increased in hyperthyroid patients, and may therefore change with changing thyroid status.

Amiodarone: Amiodarone therapy alone can cause hypothyroidism or hyperthyroidism.

DRUG INTERACTIONS: *(cont'd)*

Anticoagulants (oral): The hypoprothrombinemic effect of anticoagulants may be potentiated, apparently by increased catabolism of vitamin K-dependent clotting factors.

Antidiabetic agents (insulin, sulfonylureas): Requirements for insulin or oral antidiabetic agents may be reduced in hypothyroid patients with diabetes mellitus and may subsequently increase with the initiation of thyroid hormone replacement therapy.

β-Adrenergic blocking agents: Actions of some of beta-blocking agents may be impaired when hypothyroid patients become euthyroid.

Digitalis glycosides: Therapeutic effects of digitalis glycosides may be reduced. Serum digitalis levels may be decreased in hyperthyroidism or when a hypothyroid patient becomes euthyroid.

Ketamine: Marked hypertension and tachycardia have been reported in association with concomitant administration of levothyroxine sodium and ketamine.

Maprotiline: Risk of cardiac arrhythmias may increase.

Sodium Iodide (^{123}I and ^{131}I), sodium pertechnetate Tc99m: Uptake of radiolabeled ions may be decreased.

Somatrem/somatropin: Excessive concurrent use of thyroid hormone may accelerate epiphyseal closure. Untreated hypothyroidism may interfere with the growth response to somatrem or somatropin.

Theophylline: Theophylline clearance may decrease in hypothyroid patients and return toward normal when a euthyroid state is achieved.

Tricyclic antidepressants: Concurrent use may increase the therapeutic and toxic effects of both drugs, possibly due to increased catecholamine sensitivity. Onset of action of tricyclics may be accelerated.

Sympathomimetic agents: Possible increased risk of coronary insufficiency in patients with coronary artery disease.

ADVERSE REACTIONS:

Adverse reactions other than those indicative of thyrotoxicosis as a result of therapeutic overdosage, either initially or during the maintenance periods, are rare (see OVERDOSAGE). Craniosynostosis has been associated with iatrogenic hyperthyroidism in infants receiving thyroid hormone replacement therapy. Inadequate doses of levothyroxine sodium may produce or fail to resolve symptoms of hypothyroidism. Hypersensitivity reactions to the product excipients, such as rash and urticaria, may occur. Partial hair loss may occur during the initial months of therapy, but is generally transient. The incidence of continued hair loss is unknown. Pseudotumor cerebri has been reported in pediatric patients receiving thyroid hormone replacement therapy.

OVERDOSAGE:

Signs and Symptoms: Excessive doses of thyroid medication may result in a hypermetabolic state indistinguishable from thyrotoxicosis of endogenous origin. Signs and symptoms of thyrotoxicosis include weight loss, increased appetite, palpitations, nervousness, diarrhea, abdominal cramps, sweating, tachycardia, increased pulse and blood pressure, cardiac arrhythmias, tremors, insomnia, heat intolerance, fever, and menstrual irregularities. Symptoms are not always evident or may not appear until several days after ingestion.

Treatment: Levothyroxine sodium should be reduced in dose or temporarily discontinued if signs and symptoms of overdosage appear.

In the treatment of acute massive levothyroxine sodium overdosage, symptomatic and supportive therapy should be instituted immediately. Treatment is aimed at reducing gastrointestinal absorption and counteracting central and peripheral effects, mainly those of increased sympathetic activity. The stomach should be emptied immediately by emesis or gastric lavage if not otherwise indicated (*e.g.,* coma, convulsions, or loss of gag reflex). Cholestyramine and activated charcoal have also been used to decrease levothyroxine sodium absorption. Oxygen should be administered and ventilation maintained as necessary. β-receptor antagonists, particularly propranolol, are useful in counteracting many of the effects of increased sympathetic activity. Propranolol may be administered intravenously at a dosage of 1 to 3 mg over a ten minute period or orally, 80 to 160 mg/day, especially when no contraindications exist for its use. Cardiac glycosides may be administered if congestive heart failure develops. Measures to control fever, hypoglycemia, or fluid loss should be initiated as necessary. Glucocorticoids may be administered to inhibit the conversion of T_4 to T_3.

Since T_4 is extensively protein bound, very little drug will be removed by dialysis.

DOSAGE AND ADMINISTRATION:

The dosage and rate of administration of levothyroxine sodium is determined by the indication, and must in every case be individualized according to patient response and laboratory findings.

HYPOTHYROIDISM

The goal of therapy for primary hypothyroidism is to achieve and maintain a clinical and biochemical euthyroid state with consequent resolution of hypothyroid signs and symptoms. The starting dose of levothyroxine sodium, the frequency of dose titration, and the optimal full replacement dose must be individualized for every patient, and will be influenced by such factors as age, weight, cardiovascular status, presence of other illness, and the severity and duration of hypothyroid symptoms.

The usual full replacement dose of levothyroxine sodium for younger, healthy adults is approximately 1.6 mcg/kg/day administered once daily. In the elderly, the full replacement dose may be altered by decreases in T_4 metabolism and levothyroxine sodium absorption. Older patients may require less than 1 mcg/kg/day. Children generally require higher doses (see Pediatric Dosage). Women who are maintained on levothyroxine sodium during pregnancy may require increased doses (see PRECAUTIONS, Pregnancy).

Therapy is usually limited in younger, healthy adults at the anticipated full replacement dose. Clinical and laboratory evaluations should be performed at 6 to 8 week intervals (2 to 3 weeks in severely hypothyroid patients), and the dosage adjusted by 12.5 to 25 mcg increments until the serum TSH concentration is normalized and signs and symptoms resolve. In older patients or in younger patients with a history of cardiovascular disease, the starting dose should be 12.5 to 50 mcg once daily with adjustments of 12.5 to 25 mcg every 3 to 6 weeks until TSH is normalized. If cardiac symptoms develop or worsen the cardiac disease should be evaluated and the dose of levothyroxine sodium reduced. Rarely, worsening angina or other signs of cardiac ischema may prevent achieving a TSH in the normal range.

Treatment of subclinical hypothyroidism, when indicated, may require lower than usual replacement doses, e.g., 1.0 mcg/kg/day. Patients for whom treatment is not initiated should be monitored yearly for changes in clinical status, TSH, and thyroid antibodies.

In patients with hypothyroidism resulting from pituitary or hypothalamic disease, the possibility of secondary adrenal insufficiency should be considered, and if present, treated with glucocorticoids prior to initiation of levothyroxine sodium. The adequacy of levothyroxine sodium therapy should be assessed in these patients by measuring FT_4I, which should be maintained in the upper half of the normal range, in addition to clinical assessment. Measurement of TSH is not a reliable indicator of response to therapy for this condition.

DOSAGE AND ADMINISTRATION: *(cont'd)*

Few patients require doses greater than 200 mcg/day. An inadequate response to daily doses of 300 to 400 mcg/day is rare, and may suggest malabsorption, poor patient compliance, and/or drug interactions.

Once optimal replacement is achieved, clinical and laboratory evaluations should be conducted at least annually or whenever warranted by a change in patient status. Levothyroxine sodium products from different manufacturers should not be used interchangeably unless retesting of the patient and retitration of the dosage, as necessary, accompanies the product switch.

Levothyroxine sodium injection by the intravenous or intramuscular route can be substituted for the oral dosage form when the oral administration is precluded. The initial parenteral dosage should be approximately one-half the previously established oral dosage of levothyroxine tablets. Close observation of the patient is recommended, with adjustment of the dosage as needed. Administration of levothyroxine sodium injection by the subcutaneous route is not recommended as studies have shown that the influx of T_4 from the subcutaneous site is very slow, and depends on many factors such as volume of injectate, the anatomic site of injection, ambient temperature, and presence of venospasm.

MYXEDEMA COMA

Myxedema coma represents the extreme expression of severe hypothyroidism and is considered a medical emergency. It is characterized by hypothermia, hypotension, hypoventilation, hyponatremia, and bradycardia. In addition to restoration of normal thyroid hormone levels, therapy should be directed at the correction of electrolyte disturbances and possible infection. Because the mortality rate of patients with untreated myxedema coma is high, treatment must be started immediately, and should include appropriate supportive therapy and corticosteroids to prevent adrenal insufficiency. Possible precipitating factors should also be identified and treated. Levothyroxine sodium may be given via nasogastric tube, but the preferred route of administration is intravenous. A bolus dose of levothyroxine sodium is given immediately to replete the peripheral pool of T_4, usually 300 to 500 mcg. Although such a dose is usually well-tolerated even in the elderly, the rapid intravenous administration of large doses of levothyroxine sodium to patients with cardiovascular disease is clearly not without risks. Under such circumstances, intravenous therapy should not be undertaken without weighing the alternate risks of myxedema coma and the cardiovascular disease. Clinical judgement in this situation may dictate smaller intravenous doses of levothyroxine sodium. The initial dose is followed by daily intravenous doses of 75 to 100 mcg until the patient is stable and oral administration is feasible. Normal T_4 levels are usually achieved in 24 hours, followed by progressive increases in T_3. Improvement in cardiac output, blood pressure, temperature, and mental status generally occur within 24 hours, with improvement in many manifestations of hypothyroidism in 4 to 7 days.

TSH SUPPRESSION IN THYROID CANCER AND THYROID NODULES

The rationale for TSH suppression therapy is that a reduction in TSH secretion may decrease the growth and function of abnormal thyroid tissue. Exogenous thyroid hormone may inhibit recurrence of tumor growth and may produce regression of metastases from well-differentiated (follicular and papillary) carcinoma of the thyroid. It is used an ancillary therapy of these conditions following surgery or radioactive iodine therapy. Medullary and anaplastic carcinoma of the thyroid is unresponsive to TSH suppression therapy. TSH suppression is also used in treating nontoxic solitary nodules and multinodular goiters.

No controlled studies have compared the various degrees of TSH suppression in the treatment of either benign or malignant thyroid nodular disease. Further, the effectiveness of TSH suppression for benign nodular disease is controversial. The dose of levothyroxine sodium used for TSH suppression should therefore be individualized by the nature of the disease, the patient being treated, and the desired clinical response, weighing the potential benefits of therapy against the risks of iatrogenic thyrotoxicosis. In general, levothyroxine sodium should be given in the smallest dose that will achieve the desired clinical response.

For well differentiated thyroid cancer, TSH is generally suppressed to less than 0.1 mU/L. Doses of levothyroxine sodium greater than 2 mcg/kg/day are usually required. The efficacy of TSH suppression in reducing the size of benign thyroid nodules and in preventing nodule regrowth after surgery are controversial. Nevertheless, when treatment with levothyroxine sodium is considered warranted, TSH is generally suppressed to a higher target range (*e.g.,* 0.1 to 0.3 mU/L) than that employed for the treatment of thyroid cancer. Levothyroxine sodium therapy may also be considered for patients with nontoxic multinodular goiter who have a TSH in the normal range, to moderately suppress TSH (*e.g.,* 0.1 to 0.3 mU/L).

Levothyroxine sodium should be administered with caution to patients in whom there is a suspicion of thyroid gland autonomy, in view of the fact that the effects of exogenous hormone administration will be additive to endogenous thyroid hormone production.

PEDIATRIC DOSAGE

The aim of therapy for congenital hypothyroidism is to achieve and maintain normal growth and development. During the first three years of life, serum T_4 concentrations should be maintained in the upper half of the normal range with a serum TSH in the normal range (usually less than 10 mU/L). Normalization of TSH may lag significantly behind T_4 in some infants. In general, despite the smaller body size of children, the dosage (on a weight basis) required to sustain full development and general thriving is higher than in adults. See TABLE 1 The average initial oral dose of levothyroxine sodium at the start of treatment is 10 to 15 mcg/kg/day. Infants with very low (less than 5 mU/L) or undetectable serum T_4 levels should be started at 50 mcg daily. A lower dose (*e.g.,* 25 mcg daily) should be considered for premature neonates weighing less than 2 kg and neonates at risk of cardiac failure, increasing to 37.7 or 50 mcg daily after 4 to 6 weeks.

TABLE 1 Recommended Pediatric Dosage For Congenital Hypothyroidism

Age	Daily Dose*	Levothyroxine Sodium Tablets, USP Daily dose per kg of body weight
0 - 6 months	25-50 mcg	10-15 mcg
6 - 12 months	50 -75 mcg	6-8 mcg
1 - 5 years	75 - 100 mcg	5-6 mcg
6 - 12 years	100 - 150 mcg	4-5 mcg
Older than 12 years	> 150 mcg	2-3 mcg

*To be adjusted on the basis of clinical response and laboratory tests (see Laboratory Tests.)

Evaluation of the infants response to levothyroxine sodium by determination of the serum T_4 and TSH should be performed 2 to 4 weeks after initiation of therapy and after any change in dosage. Additional evaluations should be performed every 1 to 2 months in the first year, every 2 to 3 months between ages 1 and 3, and every 3 to 12 months thereafter until growth is complete. More frequent intervals are indicated when compliance is questioned or abnormal laboratory values are obtained. Levothyroxine sodium may be given to infants and children who cannot swallow intact tablets by crushing the tablet and suspending the freshly crushed tablet in a small amount of water (5 to 10 mL), breast milk, or non-soybean based formula. The suspension can be given by spoon or dropper. DO NOT STORE THE SUSPENSION FOR ANY PERIOD OF TIME. The crushed tablet may also be sprinkled over a small amount of food, such as cooked cereal, or apple sauce.

PATIENT INFORMATION:

Levothyroxine is a synthetic thyroid hormone used for the treatment of hypothyroidism (low thyroid hormone secretion). Inform your physician if you are pregnant or nursing. Take this medication on an empty stomach at approximately the same time each morning. Do not stop taking levothyroxine without talking with your physician. Do not change from one brand of this medication to another without talking with your pharmacist or physician. Notify your physician if headache, nervousness, diarrhea, excessive sweating, chest pain, increased pulse rate, or palpitations occur.

HOW SUPPLIED:

Synthroid tablets are round, color coded, scored, and debossed with "FLINT" and potency.

Directions for Reconstitution: Reconstitute the lyophilized levothyroxine sodium by aseptically adding 5 mL of 0.9% Sodium Chloride Injection, USP or Bacteriostatic Sodium Chloride Injection, USP with Benzyl Alcohol (final volume approximately 5 mL). Shake vial to insure complete mixing. Do not add to other intravenous fluids. Discard any unused portion.

Store at controlled room temperature 15°-30°C (59°-86°F).

HOW SUPPLIED - RATED THERAPEUTICALLY EQUIVALENT:

Injection, Lyphl-Soln - Intramuscular; - 0.2 mg/vial

10 ml	$12.69	Levothyroxine Sodium, UDL	51079-0706-01

Injection, Lyphl-Soln - Intramuscular; - 0.5 mg/vial

10 ml	$12.69	Levothyroxine Sodium, UDL	51079-0707-01

Tablet - Oral - 0.05 mg

100	$13.38	Levothyroxine Sodium, Duramed Pharms	51285-0861-02
1000	$113.01	Levothyroxine Sodium, Duramed Pharms	51285-0861-05

Tablet - Oral - 0.075 mg

100	$14.92	Levothyroxine Sodium, Duramed Pharms	51285-0862-02
1000	$126.00	Levothyroxine Sodium, Duramed Pharms	51285-0862-05

Tablet - Oral - 0.1 mg

100's	$16.68	Levothyroxine Sodium, Duramed Pharms	51285-0863-02
1000's	$142.56	Levothyroxine Sodium, Duramed Pharms	51285-0863-05

Tablet - Oral - 0.125 mg

100's	$18.03	Levothyroxine Sodium, Duramed Pharms	51285-0864-02
1000's	$153.04	Levothyroxine Sodium, Duramed Pharms	51285-0864-05

Tablet - Oral - 0.15 mg

100's	$20.34	Levothyroxine Sodium, Duramed Pharms	51285-0865-02
1000's	$173.08	Levothyroxine Sodium, Duramed Pharms	51285-0865-05

Tablet - Oral - 0.2 mg

100's	$24.54	Levothyroxine Sodium, Duramed Pharms	51285-0866-02
1000's	$207.31	Levothyroxine Sodium, Duramed Pharms	51285-0866-05

Tablet - Oral - 0.3 mg

100's	$33.56	Levothyroxine Sodium, Duramed Pharms	51285-0867-02
1000's	$283.18	Levothyroxine Sodium, Duramed Pharms	51285-0867-05

Tablet, Uncoated - Oral - 0.125 mg

100's	$12.15	L-Thyroxine, Harber Pharm	51432-0241-03

Tablet, Uncoated - Oral - 0.15 mg

100's	$12.25	L-Thyroxine, Harber Pharm	51432-0243-03

Tablet, Uncoated - Oral - 0.3 mg

100's	$15.40	L-Thyroxine, Harber Pharm	51432-0247-03

HOW SUPPLIED - NOT RATED EQUIVALENT:

Injection, Lyphl-Soln - Intramuscular; - 0.2 mg/vial

1's	$5.00	Levothyroxine Sodium, Astra USA	00186-1855-01
5 ml	**$47.88**	**SYNTHROID, Knoll Pharms**	**00048-1014-99**
10 ml	$9.75	Levothyroxine Sodium, Bedford Labs	55390-0880-10
10 ml	$16.50	Levothyroxine Sodium, Gensia Labs	00703-5408-01
10 ml	$17.25	Levothyroxine Sodium, Schein Pharm (US)	00364-2248-54
10 ml	$17.25	Levothyroxine Sodium, Steris Labs	00402-0835-10
10 ml	$34.94	Levothyroxine Sodium, Fujisawa USA	00469-2470-30
10 ml	$62.56	LEVOTHROID, Forest Pharms	00456-0140-88

Injection, Lyphl-Soln - Intramuscular; - 0.5 mg/vial

1's	$11.88	Levothyroxine Sodium, Astra USA	00186-1856-01
1's	$12.50	Levothyroxine Sodium, Consolidated Midland	00223-7921-05
5 ml	**$52.74**	**SYNTHROID, Knoll Pharms**	**00048-1012-99**
10 ml	$11.25	Levothyroxine Sodium, Bedford Labs	55390-0881-10
10 ml	$17.48	Levothyroxine Sodium, Schein Pharm (US)	00364-6772-54
10 ml	$17.48	Levothyroxine Sodium, Steris Labs	00402-0732-10
10 ml	$17.94	Levothyroxine Sodium, Gensia Labs	00703-5418-01
10 ml	$38.43	Levothyroxine Sodium, Fujisawa USA	00469-2480-30
10 ml	$89.50	LEVOTHROID, Forest Pharms	00456-0141-88

Tablet, Uncoated - Oral - 0.025 mg

100's	$3.89	Levothyroxine Sodium, Jerome Stevens	50564-0513-01
100's	$6.88	Levoxyl, Jones Medical	00689-1117-01
100's	$10.10	Levoxyl, Jones Medical	00689-1117-05
100's	$11.86	Levothyroxine Sodium, Duramed Pharms	51285-0860-02
100's	$12.29	LEVOTHROID, Forest Pharms	00456-0320-01
100's	$12.30	Levothyroxine Sodium, Warner Chilcott	00047-0334-24
100's	$12.35	Levothyroxine Sodium, Mova Pharms	55370-0125-07
100's	$12.74	Levo-T, Lederle Parenterals	00205-3610-43
100's	$12.75	L-Thyroxine, Caremark	00339-5923-12
100's	$14.48	Eltroxin, Roberts Labs	54092-0104-01
100's	**$17.64**	**SYNTHROID, Knoll Pharms**	**00048-1020-03**
100's	**$22.14**	**SYNTHROID, Knoll Pharms**	**00048-1050-03**
100's	**$23.76**	**SYNTHROID, Knoll Pharms**	**00048-1050-13**
1000's	$19.86	Levothyroxine Sodium, Vintage Pharms	00254-3911-38
1000's	$19.86	Levothyroxine Sodium, Qualitest Pharms	00603-4192-32
1000's	$28.07	L-Thyroxine (Orange), HL Moore Drug Exch	00839-7672-16
1000's	$28.07	L-Thyroxine, HL Moore Drug Exch	00839-7823-16
1000's	$38.55	Levothyroxine Sodium, Rugby	00536-5684-10
1000's	$57.00	Levotabs, Pecos	59879-0201-10
1000's	$60.40	Levoxyl, Jones Medical	00689-1117-10
1000's	$101.06	Levothyroxine Sodium, Goldline Labs	00182-1529-10
1000's	$101.06	Levothyroxine Sodium, Duramed Pharms	51285-0860-05
1000's	$104.97	Levothyroxine Sodium, Mova Pharms	55370-0125-09
1000's	**$149.76**	**SYNTHROID, Knoll Pharms**	**00048-1020-05**
1000's	**$186.60**	**SYNTHROID, Knoll Pharms**	**00048-1050-05**

Tablet, Uncoated - Oral - 0.05 mg

100's	$4.39	Levothyroxine Sodium, Jerome Stevens	50564-0514-01
100's	$7.78	Levoxyl, Jones Medical	00689-1118-01
100's	$8.66	Levothyroxine Sodium, Talbert Phcy	44514-0502-88
100's	$11.02	Levoxyl, Jones Medical	00689-1118-05
100's	$12.98	LEVOTHROID, Forest Pharms	00456-0321-01

HOW SUPPLIED - NOT RATED EQUIVALENT: *(cont'd)*

100's	$12.98	LEVOTHROID, Forest Pharms	00456-0321-63
100's	$13.80	Levothyroxine Sodium, Warner Chilcott	00047-0336-24
100's	$13.84	L-Thyroxine, Caremark	00339-5925-12
100's	$13.89	Levothyroxine Sodium, Mova Pharms	55370-0126-07
100's	$14.31	Levo-T, Lederle Parenterals	00205-3611-43
100's	$14.48	Eltroxin, Roberts Labs	54092-0105-01
100's	**$19.98**	**SYNTHROID, Knoll Pharms**	**00048-1040-03**
100's	**$21.24**	**SYNTHROID, Knoll Pharms**	**00048-1040-13**
1000's	$20.15	Levothyroxine Sodium, Vintage Pharms	00254-3912-38
1000's	$20.15	Levothyroxine Sodium, Qualitest Pharms	00603-4193-32
1000's	$28.34	L-Thyroxine (White), HL Moore Drug Exch	00839-7673-16
1000's	$28.34	L-Thyroxine, HL Moore Drug Exch	00839-7824-16
1000's	$32.57	Levothyroxine Sodium, Geneva Pharms	00781-1074-10
1000's	$36.56	Levothyroxine Sodium, Jerome Stevens	50564-0514-10
1000's	$41.40	Levothyroxine Sodium, Rugby	00536-5685-10
1000's	$57.20	Levotabs, Pecos	59879-0202-10
1000's	$64.75	Levoxyl, Jones Medical	00689-1118-10
1000's	$113.01	Levothyroxine Sodium, Goldline Labs	00182-1511-10
1000's	$117.28	Levothyroxine Sodium, Mova Pharms	55370-0126-09
1000's	$120.90	Levo-T, Lederle Parenterals	00205-3611-34
1000's	**$167.40**	**SYNTHROID, Knoll Pharms**	**00048-1040-05**
50000's	$4332.00	LEVOTHROID, Forest Pharms	00456-0321-69

Tablet, Uncoated - Oral - 0.075 mg

100's	$8.60	Levoxyl, Jones Medical	00689-1119-01
100's	$10.85	Levothyroxine Sodium, Jerome Stevens	50564-0515-01
100's	$11.93	Levoxyl, Jones Medical	00689-1119-05
100's	$14.48	Eltroxin, Roberts Labs	54092-0106-01
100's	$15.36	LEVOTHROID, Forest Pharms	00456-0322-01
100's	$15.43	Levothyroxine Sodium, Mova Pharms	55370-0127-07
100's	$15.50	L-Thyroxine, Caremark	00339-5927-12
100's	$15.90	Levo-T, Lederle Parenterals	00205-3612-43
1000's	$20.35	Levothyroxine Sodium, Vintage Pharms	00254-3913-38
1000's	$20.35	Levothyroxine Sodium, Qualitest Pharms	00603-4194-32
1000's	$28.47	L-Thyroxine (Violet), HL Moore Drug Exch	00839-7674-16
1000's	$28.47	L-Thyroxine, HL Moore Drug Exch	00839-7825-16
1000's	$41.15	Levothyroxine Sodium, Jerome Stevens	50564-0515-10
1000's	$44.25	Levothyroxine Sodium, Rugby	00536-5686-10
1000's	$57.40	Levotabs, Pecos	59879-0203-10
1000's	$72.87	Levoxyl, Jones Medical	00689-1119-10
1000's	$126.00	Levothyroxine Sodium, Goldline Labs	00182-1527-10
1000's	$131.15	Levothyroxine Sodium, Mova Pharms	55370-0127-09

Tablet, Uncoated - Oral - 0.088 mg

100's	$8.75	Levoxyl, Jones Medical	00689-1132-01
100's	$12.05	Levoxyl, Jones Medical	00689-1132-05
100's	$14.48	Eltroxin, Roberts Labs	54092-0117-01
100's	$15.19	LEVOTHROID, Forest Pharms	00456-0329-01
100's	**$22.50**	**SYNTHROID, Knoll Pharms**	**00048-1060-03**
1000's	$73.92	Levoxyl, Jones Medical	00689-1132-10

Tablet, Uncoated - Oral - 0.1 mg

100's	$5.63	Levothyroxine Sodium, Vangard Labs	00615-2522-13
100's	$7.37	Levothyroxine Sodium.1, Major Pharms	00904-2236-61
100's	$8.87	Levoxyl, Jones Medical	00689-1110-01
100's	$9.75	Levothyroxine Sodium, US Trading	56126-0468-11
100's	$9.82	Levothyroxine Sodium, Talbert Phcy	44514-0504-88
100's	$12.17	Levoxyl, Jones Medical	00689-1110-05
100's	$14.48	Eltroxin, Roberts Labs	54092-0108-01
100's	$15.71	Levothyroxine Sodium, Warner Chilcott	00047-0341-24
100's	$15.78	LEVOTHROID, Forest Pharms	00456-0323-01
100's	$15.78	LEVOTHROID, Forest Pharms	00456-0323-63
100's	$16.31	Levo-T, Lederle Parenterals	00205-3613-43
100's	$16.42	Levothyroxine Sodium, Caremark	00339-5579-12
100's	$16.80	Levothyroxine Sodium, Mova Pharms	55370-0129-07
100's	**$22.68**	**SYNTHROID, Knoll Pharms**	**00048-1070-03**
100's	**$24.54**	**SYNTHROID, Knoll Pharms**	**00048-1070-13**
500's	$66.66	Eltroxin, Roberts Labs	54092-0108-05
1000's	$17.00	Levothyroxine Sodium, Jerome Stevens	50564-0516-10
1000's	$17.81	L-Thyroxin Sodium, HL Moore Drug Exch	00839-1384-16
1000's	$20.75	Levothyroxine Sodium, Vintage Pharms	00254-3914-38
1000's	$20.75	Levothyroxine Sodium, Qualitest Pharms	00603-4195-32
1000's	$22.50	L-Thyroxin, Goldline Labs	00182-0638-10
1000's	$28.74	L-Thyroxine (Yellow), HL Moore Drug Exch	00839-7675-16
1000's	$28.74	L-Thyroxine, HL Moore Drug Exch	00839-7826-16
1000's	$34.25	Levothyroxine Sodium.1, Major Pharms	00904-2236-80
1000's	$39.85	Levothyroxine Sodium, Aligen Independ	00405-4581-03
1000's	$41.90	L Thyroxine Sodium, Geneva Pharms	00781-1905-10
1000's	$42.00	Levothyroxine Sodium, United Res	00677-0078-10
1000's	$42.75	Levothyroxine Sodium, Rugby	00536-3952-10
1000's	$57.60	Levotabs, Pecos	59879-0204-10
1000's	$75.00	Levoxyl, Jones Medical	00689-1110-10
1000's	$134.79	Levothyroxine Sodium, Mova Pharms	55370-0129-09
1000's	$138.95	Levo-T, Lederle Parenterals	00205-3613-34
1000's	$142.56	Levothyroxine Sodium, Goldline Labs	00182-1116-10
1000's	$162.01	Levothyroxine Sodium, Warner Chilcott	00047-0341-32
1000's	**$192.42**	**SYNTHROID, Knoll Pharms**	**00048-1070-05**
50000's	$4910.00	LEVOTHROID, Forest Pharms	00456-0323-69

Tablet, Uncoated - Oral - 0.112 mg

100's	$9.62	Levoxyl, Jones Medical	00689-1130-01
100's	$12.97	Levoxyl, Jones Medical	00689-1130-05
100's	$14.31	Levothyroxine Sodium, Mova Pharms	55370-0161-07
100's	$14.48	Eltroxin, Roberts Labs	54092-0118-01
100's	$17.75	LEVOTHROID, Forest Pharms	00456-0330-01
100's	**$26.28**	**SYNTHROID, Knoll Pharms**	**00048-1080-03**
1000's	$78.80	Levoxyl, Jones Medical	00689-1130-10
1000's	**$223.20**	**SYNTHROID, Knoll Pharms**	**00048-1080-05**

Tablet, Uncoated - Oral - 0.125 mg

100's	$5.83	Levothyroxine Sodium, Jerome Stevens	50564-0519-01
100's	$10.32	Levoxyl, Jones Medical	00689-1120-01
100's	$13.73	Levoxyl, Jones Medical	00689-1120-05
100's	$14.48	Eltroxin, Roberts Labs	54092-0110-01
100's	$18.33	Levothyroxine Sodium, Warner Chilcott	00047-0343-24
100's	$18.46	LEVOTHROID, Forest Pharms	00456-0324-01
100's	$18.46	LEVOTHROID, Forest Pharms	00456-0324-63
100's	$18.53	Levothyroxine Sodium, Mova Pharms	55370-0130-07
100's	$18.82	L-Thyroxine, Caremark	00339-5929-12
100's	$19.10	Levo-T, Lederle Parenterals	00205-3614-43
100's	**$26.52**	**SYNTHROID, Knoll Pharms**	**00048-1130-03**
100's	**$28.62**	**SYNTHROID, Knoll Pharms**	**00048-1130-13**
1000's	$32.79	L-Thyroxine (Green), HL Moore Drug Exch	00839-7676-16
1000's	$32.79	L-Thyroxine, HL Moore Drug Exch	00839-7827-16
1000's	$43.56	Levothyroxine Sodium, Geneva Pharms	00781-1088-10
1000's	$46.66	Levothyroxine Sodium, Jerome Stevens	50564-0519-10

HOW SUPPLIED - NOT RATED EQUIVALENT: *(cont'd)*

1000's	$47.55	Levothyroxine Sodium, Rugby	00536-5506-10
1000's	$66.60	Levotabs, Pecos	59879-0205-10
1000's	$82.63	Levoxyl, Jones Medical	00689-1120-10
1000's	$153.04	Levothyroxine Sodium, Goldline Labs	00182-1516-10
1000's	$157.50	Levothyroxine Sodium, Mova Pharms	55370-0130-09
1000's	**$223.92**	**SYNTHROID, Knoll Pharms**	**00048-1130-05**

Tablet, Uncoated - Oral - 0.137 mg

100's	$10.47	Levoxyl, Jones Medical	00689-1135-01
100's	$13.88	Levoxyl, Jones Medical	00689-1135-05
100's	$18.11	LEVOTHROID, Forest Pharms	00456-0331-01
1000's	$86.43	Levoxyl, Jones Medical	00689-1135-10

Tablet, Uncoated - Oral - 0.15 mg

100's	$5.75	Levothyroxine Sodium, Vangard Labs	00615-2523-13
100's	$10.62	Levoxyl, Jones Medical	00689-1111-01
100's	$11.97	Levothyroxine Sodium, Talbert Phcy	44514-0503-88
100's	$12.15	Levothyroxine Sodium, Jerome Stevens	50564-0520-01
100's	$14.03	Levoxyl, Jones Medical	00689-1111-05
100's	$14.48	Eltroxin, Roberts Labs	54092-0112-01
100's	$19.10	Levothyroxine Sodium, Mova Pharms	55370-0131-07
100's	$19.18	LEVOTHROID, Forest Pharms	00456-0325-01
100's	$19.18	LEVOTHROID, Forest Pharms	00456-0325-63
100's	$19.69	Levo-T, Lederle Parenterals	00205-3615-43
100's	$20.07	Levothyroxine Sodium, Caremark	00339-5813-12
100's	$22.39	Levothyroxine Sodium, Warner Chilcott	00047-0344-24
100's	**$27.30**	**SYNTHROID, Knoll Pharms**	**00048-1090-03**
100's	**$29.28**	**SYNTHROID, Knoll Pharms**	**00048-1090-13**
1000's	$20.50	Levothyroxine Sodium, Jerome Stevens	50564-0520-10
1000's	$20.78	Levothyroxine Sodium, HL Moore Drug Exch	00839-7048-16
1000's	$24.56	Levothyroxine Sodium, Vintage Pharms	00254-3915-38
1000's	$24.56	Levothyroxine Sodium, Qualitest Pharms	00603-4196-32
1000's	$27.00	L-Thyroxine Sodium, Goldline Labs	00182-1829-10
1000's	$33.87	L-Thyroxine (Blue), HL Moore Drug Exch	00839-7679-16
1000's	$35.22	L-Thyroxine, HL Moore Drug Exch	00839-7828-16
1000's	$38.95	Levothyroxine Sodium, Major Pharms	00904-2234-80
1000's	$45.11	L-Thyroxin Sodium, Geneva Pharms	00781-1908-10
1000's	$46.57	Levothyroxine Sodium, Aligen Independ	00405-4582-03
1000's	$49.00	Levothyroxine Sodium, United Res	00677-0992-10
1000's	$51.30	Levothyroxine Sodium, Rugby	00536-4380-10
1000's	$67.40	Levotabs, Pecos	59879-0206-10
1000's	$90.22	Levoxyl, Jones Medical	00689-1111-10
1000's	$151.80	Levothyroxine Sodium, Warner Chilcott	00047-0344-32
1000's	$161.83	Levothyroxine Sodium, Mova Pharms	55370-0131-09
1000's	$166.83	Levo-T, Lederle Parenterals	00205-3615-34
1000's	$173.06	Levothyroxine Sodium, Goldline Labs	00182-1117-10
1000's	**$231.06**	**SYNTHROID, Knoll Pharms**	**00048-1090-05**
50000's	$5986.80	LEVOTHROID, Forest Pharms	00456-0325-69

Tablet, Uncoated - Oral - 0.175 mg

100's	$11.72	Levoxyl, Jones Medical	00689-1122-01
100's	$14.48	Eltroxin, Roberts Labs	54092-0120-01
100's	$15.23	Levoxyl, Jones Medical	00689-1122-05
100's	$15.90	Levothyroxine Sodium, Mova Pharms	55370-0162-07
100's	$21.84	LEVOTHROID, Forest Pharms	00456-0326-01
100's	**$32.46**	**SYNTHROID, Knoll Pharms**	**00048-1100-03**
1000's	$102.78	Levoxyl, Jones Medical	00689-1122-10

Tablet, Uncoated - Oral - 0.2 mg

100's	$5.81	Levothyroxine Sodium, Vangard Labs	00615-2524-13
100's	$7.37	Levothyroxine Sodium.2, Major Pharms	00904-2237-61
100's	$12.20	Levothyroxine Sodium, Jerome Stevens	50564-0522-01
100's	$12.77	Levoxyl, Jones Medical	00689-1112-01
100's	$13.01	Levothyroxine Sodium, US Trading	56126-0451-11
100's	$14.48	Eltroxin, Roberts Labs	54092-0113-01
100's	$14.70	L-Thyroxine, Harber Pharm	51432-0260-03
100's	$16.28	Levoxyl, Jones Medical	00689-1112-05
100's	$17.25	L-Thyroxine, RID	54807-0760-01
100's	$22.36	Levothyroxine Sodium, Warner Chilcott	00047-0347-24
100's	$22.49	LEVOTHROID, Forest Pharms	00456-0327-01
100's	$22.49	LEVOTHROID, Forest Pharms	00456-0327-63
100's	$22.87	Levothyroxine Sodium, Mova Pharms	55370-0132-07
100's	$23.50	Levothyroxine Sodium, Caremark	00339-5815-12
100's	$23.58	Levo-T, Lederle Parenterals	00205-3616-43
100's	$24.79	L-Thyroxine, RID	54807-0761-01
100's	**$32.64**	**SYNTHROID, Knoll Pharms**	**00048-1140-03**
100's	**$35.28**	**SYNTHROID, Knoll Pharms**	**00048-1140-13**
1000's	$21.50	Levothyroxine Sodium, Jerome Stevens	50564-0522-10
1000's	$21.59	L-Thyroxin Sodium, HL Moore Drug Exch	00839-1386-16
1000's	$27.40	Levothyroxine Sodium, Vintage Pharms	00254-3916-38
1000's	$27.40	Levothyroxine Sodium, Qualitest Pharms	00603-4197-32
1000's	$31.50	L-Thyroxin, Goldline Labs	00182-0639-10
1000's	$34.95	L-Thyroxine (Pink), HL Moore Drug Exch	00839-7677-16
1000's	$34.95	L-Thyroxine, HL Moore Drug Exch	00839-7829-16
1000's	$36.43	Levothyroxine Sodium, Martec Pharms	52555-0360-10
1000's	$41.95	Levothyroxine Sodium.2, Major Pharms	00904-2237-80
1000's	$49.50	Levothyroxine Sodium, Aligen Independ	00405-4583-03
1000's	$50.85	Levothyroxine Sodium, Rugby	00536-4381-10
1000's	$50.85	Levothyroxine Sodium, United Res	00677-0079-10
1000's	$51.25	L Thyroxine Sodium, Geneva Pharms	00781-1910-10
1000's	$69.20	Levotabs, Pecos	59879-0207-10
1000's	$108.02	Levoxyl, Jones Medical	00689-1112-10
1000's	$183.75	Levothyroxine Sodium, Warner Chilcott	00047-0347-32
1000's	$193.85	Levothyroxine Sodium, Mova Pharms	55370-0132-09
1000's	$199.83	Levo-T, Lederle Parenterals	00205-3616-34
1000's	$207.31	Levothyroxine Sodium, Goldline Labs	00182-1118-10
1000's	**$276.66**	**SYNTHROID, Knoll Pharms**	**00048-1140-05**
50000's	$7210.80	LEVOTHROID, Forest Pharms	00456-0327-69

Tablet, Uncoated - Oral - 0.3 mg

100's	$7.26	L-Thyroxine, Geneva Pharms	00781-1913-01
100's	$12.30	Levothyroxine Sodium, Jerome Stevens	50564-0523-01
100's	$14.48	Eltroxin, Roberts Labs	54092-0114-01
100's	$17.18	Levoxyl, Jones Medical	00689-1121-01
100's	$20.83	Levoxyl, Jones Medical	00689-1121-05
100's	$29.74	LEVOTHROID, Forest Pharms	00456-0328-01
100's	$29.74	LEVOTHROID, Forest Pharms	00456-0328-63
100's	$30.33	Levothyroxine Sodium, Warner Chilcott	00047-0348-24
100's	$30.95	Levothyroxine Sodium, Mova Pharms	55370-0134-07
100's	$31.38	Levothyroxine Sodium, Caremark	00339-5817-12
100's	$31.90	Levo-T, Lederle Parenterals	00205-3617-43
100's	**$44.22**	**SYNTHROID, Knoll Pharms**	**00048-1170-03**
1000's	$22.00	Levothyroxine Sodium, Jerome Stevens	50564-0523-10
1000's	$22.46	Levothyroxine Sodium, HL Moore Drug Exch	00839-6765-16
1000's	$29.36	Levothyroxine Sodium, Vintage Pharms	00254-3917-38
1000's	$29.36	Levothyroxine Sodium, Qualitest Pharms	00603-4198-32

HOW SUPPLIED - NOT RATED EQUIVALENT: *(cont'd)*

1000's	$32.50	Levothyroxine Sodium, Harber Pharm	51432-0261-06
1000's	$36.00	Levothyroxine Sodium, Goldline Labs	00182-1498-10
1000's	$36.44	L-Thyroxine, HL Moore Drug Exch	00839-7678-16
1000's	$36.44	L-Thyroxine, HL Moore Drug Exch	00839-7830-16
1000's	$37.70	Levothyroxine Sodium, Martec Pharms	52555-0361-10
1000's	$40.50	Levothyroxine Sodium, United Res	00677-0769-10
1000's	$44.65	CYRONINE, Major Pharms	00904-2235-80
1000's	$53.25	L-Thyroxin Sodium, Rugby	00536-3958-10
1000's	$53.49	Levothyroxine Sodium 0.3, Aligen Independ	00405-4584-03
1000's	$54.50	L-Thyroxine, Geneva Pharms	00781-1913-10
1000's	$71.80	Levotabs, Pecos	59879-0208-10
1000's	$145.92	Levoxyl, Jones Medical	00689-1121-10
1000's	$263.07	Levothyroxine Sodium, Mova Pharms	55370-0134-09
1000's	$283.18	Levothyroxine Sodium, Goldline Labs	00182-1119-10
1000's	**$373.86**	**SYNTHROID, Knoll Pharms**	**00048-1170-05**

LIDOCAINE *(001638)*

CATEGORIES: Anesthesia; Antipruritics/Local Anesthetics; Burns; Dental; Dermatologicals; EENT Drugs; Endotracheal Intubation; Eye, Ear, Nose, & Throat Preparations; Insect Bites; Intubation; Local Anesthetics; Pain; Pharmaceutical Adjuvants; Pruritus; Skin/Mucous Membrane Agents; Sunburn; Topical; Topical Anesthetics; Urethritis; Pregnancy Category B; FDA Approval Pre 1982

BRAND NAMES: *Aeroderm*; Alphacaine; *Cuivasil Spray*; *Esracain*; *Esracain Jelly*; *Esracain Ointment*; *Gesicain Jelly*; *Gesicain Ointment*; *Gesicain Viscous*; *Leostesin*; *Leostesin Jelly*; *Leostesin Ointment*; *Lidocain Gel* (Germany); *Lidocain Ointment*; *Lidocain Spray*; *Lidonest*; *Lignocaine Gel* (Australia); *Remicaine Gel*; *Rucaina*; *Rucaina Pomada* (Mexico); *Rucaina Spray*; *Xilocaina Viscosa*; *Xilonest Pomada*; *Xilotane Gel*; *Xilotane Oral*; *Xylocain Aerosol*; *Xylocain Creme*; *Xylocain Gargle*; *Xylocain Gel* (Germany); *Xylocain Liniment*; *Xylocain Ointment* (Germany); *Xylocain Salve*; *Xylocain Spray* (Germany); *Xylocain Viscous*; *Xylocain Viskos* (Germany); *Xylocain Visks*; *Xylocaina*; *Xylocaina Aerosol*; *Xylocaina Gel*; *Xylocaina Ointment* (Mexico); *Xylocaina Pomada*; *Xylocaina Pomada AL 5%*; *Xylocaina Spray* (Mexico); **Xylocaine**; *Xylocaine Adhesive Ointment*; *Xylocaine Aerosol* (France, Canada); *Xylocaine Gel* (England, France); *Xylocaine Jelly*; *Xylocaine Ointment* (Australia); *Xylocaine Solution* (France); *Xylocaine Spray* (France); *Xylocaine Topical Solution* (Canada); *Xylocaine Viscous*; *Xylocaine Viscous Topical Solution* (England, Canada); *Xylocaine Viscus*; *Xylocaine Viskeus Topical Solution*; *Xylocaine Visquese* (France); *Xylocaine Visqueuse*
(International brand names outside U.S. in italics)

FORMULARIES: Aetna; BC-BS; WHO

DESCRIPTION:

See INDICATIONS AND USAGE for specific uses.

ORAL SPRAY

WARNING—CONTENTS UNDER PRESSURE

10% Lidocaine Oral Spray contains a local anesthetic agent and is administered topically in the oral cavity. See INDICATIONS AND USAGE for specific uses.

Lidocaine 10% Oral Spray contains lidocaine, which is chemically designated as acetamide, 2-(diethylamino)-N-(2,5-dimethylphenyl)-.

Composition of Lidocaine 10% Oral Spray: Each actuation of the metered dose valve delivers a solution containing lidocaine, 10 mg, cetylpyridinium chloride, absolute alcohol, saccharin, flavor, and polyethylene glycol. And as propellants: trichlorofluoromethane/dichlorodifluoromethane (65%/35%).

5% LIDOCAINE OINTMENT

Composition of Lidocaine 5% Ointment: Each gram of the lain and flavored ointments contains lidocaine, 50 mg, polyethylene glycol 1500, polyethylene glycol 4000 and propylene glycol. The flavored ointment contains sodium saccharin, peppermint and spearmint oil.

5% LIDOCAINE LIQUID, FLAVORED

Each ml contains: Lidocaine, 50, mg, propylene glycol, glycerin, saccharin, and flavor.

NOT FOR INJECTION

4% LIDOCAINE HCL TOPICAL SOLUTION

The 50 ml screw-cap bottle should not be autoclaved, because the closure employed cannot withstand autoclaving temperatures and pressures. Composition: Each ml contains Lidocaine HCl, 40 mg, methylparaben, and sodium hydroxide and/or hydrochloric acid to adjust pH to 6.0 - 7.0. An aqueous solution. NOT FOR INJECTION.

2% LIDOCAINE VISCOUS SOLUTION

Composition: Each ml contains 20 mg of lidocaine HCl, flavoring, sodium saccharin, methylparaben, propylparaben and sodium carboxymethylcellulose in purified water. The pH is adjusted to 6.0 - 7.0 by means of sodium hydroxide and/or hydrochloric acid.

2% LIDOCAINE JELLY

Composition: Each ml contains 20 mg of lidocaine HCl. The formulation contains methylparaben, propylparaben, hydroxymethylcellulose, and sodium hydroxide and/or hydrochloric acid to adjust pH to 6.0 to 7.0

CLINICAL PHARMACOLOGY:

Mechanism of Action: Lidocaine stabilizes the neuronal membrane by inhibiting the ionic fluxes required for the initiation and conduction of impulses, thereby effecting local anesthetic action.

Onset and duration of action

Lidocaine 10% Oral Spray acts on intact mucous membranes to produce local anesthesia. Anesthesia occurs usually within 1-2 minutes and persists for approximately 10-15 minutes.

Lidocaine 5% ointment effects local, topical anesthesia. The onset of action is 3-5 minutes. It is ineffective when applied to intact skin.

Lidocaine 5% Liquid (Flavored. Local anesthesia appears within 1-2 minutes after application. and persists for 15-20 minutes in soft tissue.

Lidocaine 2% Jelly. The onset of action is 3 - 5 minutes. It is ineffective when applied to intact skin.

Hemodynamics: Excessive blood levels may cause changes in cardiac output, total peripheral resistance, and mean arterial pressure. These changes may be attributable to a direct depressant effect of the local anesthetic agent on various components of the cardiovascular system.

Pharmacokinetics and Metabolism: Lidocaine may be absorbed following topical administration to mucous membranes, its rate of absorption and percent of dose absorbed depending upon concentration and total dose administered, the specific site of application and duration of exposure. In general, the rate of absorption of local anesthetic agents following topical

CLINICAL PHARMACOLOGY: *(cont'd)*

application occurs most rapidly after intratracheal administration. Lidocaine is well-absorbed from the gastrointestinal tract, but little intact drug appears in the circulation because of biotransformation in the liver.

Lidocaine is metabolized rapidly by the liver, and metabolites and unchanged drug are excreted by the kidney. Biotransformation includes oxidative N-dealkylation, ring hydroxylation, cleavage of the amide linkage, and conjugation. N-dealkylation, a major pathway of biotransformation, yields the metabolites monoethylglycinexylidide and glycinexylidide. The pharmacological/toxicological actions of these metabolites are similar to, but less potent than, those of lidocaine. Approximately 90% of lidocaine administered is excreted in the form of various metabolites, and less than 10% is excreted unchanged. The primary metabolite in urine is a conjugate of 4-hydroxy -2, 6-dimethylaniline.

The plasma binding of lidocaine is dependent on drug concentration, and the fraction bound decreases with increasing concentration. At concentrations of 1 to 4 mcg of free base per ml, 60 to 80 percent of lidocaine is protein bound. Binding is also dependent on the plasma concentration of the alpha-1-acid glycoprotein.

Lidocaine crosses the blood-brain and placental barriers, presumably by passive diffusion.

Studies of lidocaine metabolism following intravenous bolus injections have shown that the elimination half-life of this agent is typically 1.5 to 2 hours. Because of the rapid rate at which lidocaine is metabolized, any condition that affects liver function may alter lidocaine kinetics. The half-life may be prolonged two-fold or more in patients with liver dysfunction. Renal dysfunction does not affect lidocaine kinetics but may increase the accumulation of metabolites.

Factors such as acidosis and the use of CNS stimulants and depressants affect the CNS levels of lidocaine required to produce overt systemic effects. Objective adverse manifestations become increasingly apparent with increasing venous plasma levels above 6 mcg free base per ml. In the rhesus monkey arterial blood levels of 18-21 mcg/ml have been shown to be threshold for convulsive activity.

INDICATIONS AND USAGE:

10% Lidocaine Oral Spray is indicated for the production of topical anesthesia of the accessible mucous membranes of the mouth and oropharynx.

5% Lidocaine Ointment is indicated for the production of anesthesia of accessible mucous membranes of the oropharynx.

It is also useful as an anesthetic lubricant for intubation and for the temporary relief of pain associated with minor burns, including sunburn, abrasions of the skin, and insect bites.

5% Lidocaine Liquid is indicated for the symptomatic relief of painful, irritated or inflamed mucous membranes of the mouth and for anesthesia of these membranes for the performance of minor dental surgical procedures.

4%Lidocaine Topical Solution is indicated for the production of topical anesthesia of accessible mucous membranes of the oral and nasal cavities and proximal portions of the digestive tract.

2% Lidocaine Viscous Solution is indicated for the production of topical anesthesia of irritated or inflamed mucous membranes of the mouth and pharynx. It is also useful for reducing gagging during the taking of X-ray pictures and dental impressions.

2% Lidocaine Jelly is indicated for the prevention and control of pain in procedures involving the male and female urethra, for topical treatment of painful urethritis, and as an anesthetic lubricant for endotracheal intubation (oral and nasal).

CONTRAINDICATIONS:

Lidocaine is contraindicated in patients with a known history of hypersensitivity to local anesthetics of the amide type or to other components of the various topical products.

WARNINGS:

EXCESSIVE DOSAGE, OR SHORT INTERVALS BETWEEN DOSES, CAN RESULT IN HIGH PLASMA LEVELS AND SERIOUS ADVERSE EFFECTS, PATIENTS SHOULD BE INSTRUCTED TO STRICTLY ADHERE TO THE RECOMMENDED DOSAGE AND ADMINISTRATION GUIDELINES AS SET FORTH IN THIS PACKAGE INSERT.

IN ORDER TO MANAGE POSSIBLE ADVERSE REACTIONS, RESUSCITATIVE EQUIPMENT, OXYGEN AND OTHER RESUSCITATIVE DRUGS MUST BE IMMEDIATELY AVAILABLE WHEN LOCAL ANESTHETIC AGENTS, SUCH AS LIDOCAINE, ARE ADMINISTERED TO MUCOUS MEMBRANES.

Lidocaine should be used with extreme caution if there is sepsis or extremely traumatized mucosa in the area of application, since under such conditions there is the potential for rapid systemic absorption.

2% LIDOCAINE JELLY

When used for endotracheal tube lubrication care should be taken to avoid introducing the product into the lumen of the tube. Do not use the jelly to lubricate the endotracheal stylettes. If allowed into the inner lumen, the jelly may dry on the inner surface leaving a residue which tends to clump with flexion, narrowing the lumen. There have been rare reports in which this residue has caused the lumen to occlude. See also ADVERSE REACTIONS and DOSAGE AND ADMINISTRATION.

PRECAUTIONS:

GENERAL

The safety and effectiveness of lidocaine depend on proper dosage, correct technique, adequate precautions, and readiness for emergencies. Resuscitative equipment, oxygen, and other resuscitative drugs should be available for immediate use. (See WARNINGS and ADVERSE REACTIONS.) The lowest dosage that results in effective anesthesia should be used to avoid high plasma levels and serious adverse effects. Repeated doses of lidocaine may cause significant increases in blood levels with each repeated dose because of slow accumulation of the drug or its metabolites. Tolerance varies with the status of the patient. Debilitated, elderly patients, acutely ill patients, and children should be given reduced doses commensurate with their age and physical status. Lidocaine should also be used with caution in patients with severe shock or heart block.

Lidocaine should be used with caution in patients with known drug sensitivities. Patients allergic to para-amino-benzoic acid derivatives (procaine, tetracaine, benzocaine, etc.) have not shown cross sensitivity to lidocaine.

Many drugs used during the conduct of anesthesia are considered potential triggering agents for familiar malignant hyperthermia. Since it is not known whether amide-type local anesthetics may trigger this reaction and since the need for supplemental general anesthesia cannot be predicted in advance, it is suggested that a standard protocol for management should be available. Early unexplained signs of tachycardia, tachypnea, labile blood pressure and metabolic acidosis may precede temperature elevation. Successful outcome is dependent on early diagnosis, prompt discontinuance of the suspect triggering agents(s) and institution of treatment, including oxygen therapy, indicated supportive measures and dantrolene (consult dantrolene sodium intravenous package insert before using).

PRECAUTIONS: *(cont'd)*

INFORMATION FOR THE PATIENT

When topical anesthetics are used in the mouth, the patient should be aware that the production of topical anesthesia may impair swallowing and thus enhance the danger of aspiration. For this reason, food should not be ingested for 60 minutes following use of local anesthetic preparations in the mouth or throat area. This is particularly important in children because of their frequency of eating.

Numbness of the tongue or buccal mucosa may enhance the danger of unintentional biting trauma. Food and chewing gum should not be taken while the mouth or throat area is anesthetized.

CARCINOGENESIS, MUTAGENESIS, AND IMPAIRMENT OF FERTILITY

Studies of lidocaine in animals to evaluate the carcinogenic and mutagenic potential or the effect on fertility have not been conducted.

PREGNANCY, TERATOGENIC EFFECTS, PREGNANCY CATEGORY B

Reproduction studies have been performed in rats at doses up to 6.6 times the human dose and have revealed no evidence of harm to the fetus caused by lidocaine. There are, however, no adequate and well-controlled studies in pregnant women. Animal reproduction studies are not always predictive of human response. General consideration should be given to this fact before administering lidocaine to women of childbearing potential, especially during early pregnancy when maximum organogenesis takes place.

LABOR AND DELIVERY

Lidocaine is not contraindicated in labor and delivery. Should Lidocaine be used concomitantly with other products containing lidocaine, the total dose contributed by all formulations must be kept in mind.

NURSING MOTHERS

It is not known whether this drug is excreted in human milk. Because many drugs are excreted in human milk, caution should be exercised when lidocaine is administered to a nursing woman.

PEDIATRIC USE

10% Oral Spray: Safety and effectiveness in children below the age of 12 years have not been established.

Other Forms: Dosages in children should be reduced, commensurate with age, body weight and physical condition. Caution must be taken to avoid overdosage when applying Lidocaine Ointment to large areas of injured or abraded skin, since the systemic absorption of lidocaine may be increased under such conditions. See DOSAGE AND ADMINISTRATION.

ADVERSE REACTIONS:

Adverse experiences following the administration of lidocaine are similar in nature to those observed with other amide local anesthetic agents. These adverse experiences are, in general, dose-related and may result from high plasma levels caused by excessive dosage or rapid absorption, or may result from a hypersensitivity, idiosyncrasy or diminished tolerance on the part of the patient. Serious adverse experiences are generally systemic in nature. The following types are those most commonly reported:

Central Nervous System: CNS manifestations are excitatory and/or depressant and may be characterized by lightheadedness, nervousness, apprehension, euphoria, confusion, dizziness, drowsiness, tinnitus, blurred or double vision, vomiting, sensations of heat, cold or numbness, twitching, tremors, convulsions, unconsciousness, respiratory depression and arrest. The excitatory manifestations may be very brief or may not occur at all, in which case the first manifestation of toxicity may be drowsiness merging into unconsciousness and respiratory arrest.

Drowsiness following the administration of lidocaine is usually an early sign of a high blood level of the drug and may occur as a consequence of rapid absorption.

Cardiovascular system: Cardiovascular manifestations are usually depressant and are characterized by bradycardia, hypotension, and cardiovascular collapse, which may lead to cardiac arrest.

Allergic: Allergic reactions are characterized by cutaneous lesions, urticaria, edema or anaphylactoid reactions. Allergic reactions may occur as a result of sensitivity either to the local anesthetic agent or to other ingredients in the formulation. Allergic reactions as a result of sensitivity to lidocaine are extremely rare and, if they occur, should be managed by conventional means. The detection of sensitivity by skin testing is of doubtful value.

2% Lidocaine Jelly: There have been rare reports of endotracheal tube occlusion associated with the presence of dried jell residue in the inner lumen of the tube. See also WARNINGS and DOSAGE AND ADMINISTRATION.

OVERDOSAGE:

Acute emergencies from local anesthetics are generally related to high plasma levels encountered during therapeutic use of local anesthetics.(See ADVERSE REACTIONS, WARNINGS, and PRECAUTIONS.)

Management Of Local Anesthetic Emergencies: The first consideration is prevention, best accomplished by careful and constant monitoring of cardiovascular and respiratory vital signs and the patient's state of consciousness after each local anesthetic administration. At the first sign of change, oxygen should be administered.

The first step in the management of convulsions consists of immediate attention to the maintenance of a patent airway and assisted or controlled ventilation with oxygen and a delivery system capable of permitting immediate positive airway pressure by mask. Immediately after the institution of these ventilatory measures, the adequacy of the circulation should be evaluated, keeping in mind that drugs used to treat convulsions sometimes depress the circulation when administered intravenously. Should convulsions persist despite adequate respiratory support, and if the status of the circulation permits, small increments of an ultra-short acting barbiturate (such as thiopental or thiamylal) or a benzodiazepine (such as diazepam) may be administered intravenously. The clinician should be familiar, prior to use of local anesthetics, with these anticonvulsant drugs. Supportive treatment of circulatory depression may require administration of intravenous fluids and, when appropriate, a vasopressor as directed by the clinical situation (*e.g.,* ephedrine).

If not treated immediately, both convulsions and cardiovascular depression can result in hypoxia, acidosis, bradycardia, arrhythmias and cardiac arrest. If cardiac arrest should occur, standard cardiopulmonary resuscitative measures should be instituted.

Dialysis is of negligible value in the treatment of acute overdosage with lidocaine.

The intravenous LD_{50} of lidocaine HCl in female mice is 26(21-31) mg/kg and the subcutaneous LD_{50} is 264(203-304) mg/kg.

The oral LD_{50} of Lidocaine HCl in non-fasted female rats is 459 (346-73) mg/kg (as the salt) and 214 (159-324) mg/kg (as the salt) in fasted female rats.

DOSAGE AND ADMINISTRATION:

When Lidocaine is used concomitantly with other products containing lidocaine, the total dose contributed hy all formulations must be kept in mind.

DOSAGE AND ADMINISTRATION: *(cont'd)*

10% LIDOCAINE ORAL SPRAY

Two metered doses per quadrant are recommended as the upper limit and,*under no circumstances* should one exceed three metered doses per quadrant of oral mucosa over a one-half hour period to produce the desired anesthetic effect. Experience in children is inadequate to recommend a pediatric dose at this time.

STORE AT CONTROLLED ROOM TEMPERATURE 15°-30°C (59°-86°F).

5% LIDOCAINE OINTMENT

Adult: A single application should not exceed 5 g of Lidocaine 5% Ointment, containing 250 mg of Lidocaine base (equivalent chemically to approximately 300 mg of Lidocaine HCl). This is roughly equivalent to squeezing a six (6) inch length of ointment from the tube. In a 70 kg adult this dose equals 3.6 mg/kg (1.6 mg/lb) lidocaine base. No more than one-half tube, approximately 17-20 g of ointment or 850-1000 mg Lidocaine base, should be administered in any one day.

Although the incidence of adverse effects with Lidocaine 5% Ointment is quite low, caution should be exercised, particularly when employing large amounts, since the incidence of adverse effects is directly proportional to the total dose of local anesthetic agent administered.

Dosage for Children: It is difficult to recommend a maximum dose of any drug for children since this varies as a function of age and weight. For children less than ten years who have a normal lean body mass and a normal lean body development, the maximum dose may be determined by the application of one of the standard pediatric drug formulas (*e.g.,* Clark's rule). For example, in a child of five years, weighing 50 lbs., the dose of lidocaine should not exceed 75-100 mg when calculated according to clark's rule. In any case, the maximum amount of Lidocaine administered should not exceed 4.5 mg/kg (2.0 mg/lb) of body weight.

Administration: For medical use, apply topically for adequate control of symptoms. The use of a sterile gauze pad is suggested for application to broken skin tissue. Apply to the tube prior to intubation.

In dentistry, apply to previously dried oral mucosa. Subsequent removal of excess saliva with cotton rolls or saliva ejector minimizes dilution of the ointment, permits maximum penetration, and minimizes the possibility of swallowing the topical ointment.

For use in connection with the insertion of new dentures, apply to all denture surfaces contacting mucosa.

IMPORTANT: Patients should consult a dentist at intervals not exceeding 48 hours throughout the fitting period.

KEEP CONTAINER TIGHTLY CLOSED AT ALL TIMES WHEN NOT IN USE.

Store at controlled room temperature 15 - 30°C)59 - 86°F).

5% LIDOCAINE LIQUID (FLAVORED)

Adult: The maximum recommended single adult dose of lidocaine HCl, administered parenterally, is 300 mg (equivalent to 260 mg of lidocaine.) In a 70 kg adult this dose of lidocaine equals 3.7 mg/kg or 1.7 mg/lb. Thus, a single application of 5% Lidocaine Liquid should not exceed a total of 5 ml for all quadrants. In general, however, much smaller volumes are adequate to produce the desired anesthesia. The maximum recommended single adult dose (5 ml) should not be exceeded within any 3-hour interval.

Pediatric: It is difficult to recommend a maximum dose of any drug for children, since this varies as a function of age and weight. For children over 3 years of age who have a normal lean body mass and normal body development, the maximum dose is determined by the child's weight and age. For example, in a child of 5 years weighing 50 lbs., the dose of Lidocaine should not exceed 75-100 (1.5 - 2.0 mg/lb.).

Administration: This product is for *topical use only*. The solution should be applied with a swab, which should be discarded after single use.

CAUTION: DO NOT INJECT

Store at controlled room temperature.

4% LIDOCAINE HCL TOPICAL SOLUTION

The dosage varies and depends upon the area to be anesthetized, vascularity of the tissues, individual tolerance, and the technique of the anesthesia. The lowest dosage needed to provide effective anesthesia should be administered. Dosages should be reduced for children and for elderly and debilitated patients. The maximum dose should not exceed 4.5 mg/kg (2 mg/lb.) of body weight. Although the incidence of adverse affects with 4% Lidocaine Topical Solution is quite low, caution should be exercised, particularly when employing large volumes, since the incidence of adverse affects is directly proportional to the total dose of local anesthetic agent administered.

The dosages recommended below are for normal, healthy adults:

When used as a spray, or when applied by means of cotton applicators or packs, as when instilled into a cavity, the suggested dosage of 4% Lidocaine Topical Solution is 1-5 ml (40-200 mg lidocaine HCl), i.e., 0.6 - 3.0 mg/kg or 0.3 - 1.5 mg/lb. body weight.

NOTE: The solution may be applied with a sterile swab which is discarded after a single use. When spraying, transfer the solution from the original container to an atomizer.

Maximum Recommended Dosages: Normal healthy adults: The maximum recommended dose of 4% Lidocaine Topical Solution should be such that the dose of Lidocaine HCl is kept below 300 mg and in any case should not exceed 4.5 mg/kg (2 mg/lb) body weight.

Children: It is difficult to recommend a maximum dose of any drug for children since this varies as a function of age and weight. For children of less than ten years who have a normal lean body mass and normal body development, the maximum dose may be determined by the application of one of the standard pediatric drug formulas (*e.g.,* Clark's rule). For example, in a child of five years weighing 50 lbs., the dose of Lidocaine HCl should not exceed 7 mg/kg (3.2 mg/lb) of body weight. When used without epinephrine, the amount of Lidocaine solution administered should be such that the dose is kept below 300 mg and in any case should not exceed 4.5 mg/kg (2.0 mg/lb) of body weight.

NOT FOR INJECTION.

Store at controlled room temperature.

2% LIDOCAINE HCL VISCOUS SOLUTION

Adult: The maximum recommended single dose of Lidocaine HCl 2% Viscous Solution for healthy adults should be such that the dose of lidocaine HCl does not exceed 4.5 mg/kg or 2 mg/lb. body weight and does not in any case exceed a total of 300 mg.

For symptomatic treatment of irritated or inflamed mucous membranes of the mouth and pharynx, the usual adult dose is one 15 ml tablespoonful undiluted. For use in the mouth, the solution should be swished around in the mouth and spit out. For use in the pharynx, the undiluted solution should be gargled and may be swallowed. This dose should not be administered at intervals of less than three hours, and not more than eight doses should be given in a 24-hour period.

This dosage should be adjusted commensurate with the patient's age, weight and physical condition (See PRECAUTIONS.)

Pediatric: It is difficult to recommend a maximum dose of any drug for children since this varies as a function of age and maximum dose is determined by the child's weight or age. For example: in a child of 5 years weighing 50 lbs., the dose of lidocaine HCl should not exceed 75 - 1000 mg (3/4 to 1 teaspoonful).

DOSAGE AND ADMINISTRATION: *(cont'd)*

For infants and in children under three years of age, 1/4 teaspoon of the solution should be accurately measured and applied to the immediate area with a cotton-tipped applicator. This dose should not be administered at intervals of less than three hours. Not more than four doses should be given in a 12-hour period.

The solutions should be stored at controlled room temperatures.

2% LIDOCAINE JELLY

The dosage varies and depends upon the area to be anesthetized, vascularity of the tissues, individual tolerance, and the technique of anesthesia. The lowest dosage needed to provide effective anesthesia should be administered. Dosages should be reduced for children and fr elderly and debilitated patients. Although the incidence of adverse effects with 2% Lidocaine Jelly is quite low, caution should be exercised, particularly when employing large amounts, since the incidence if adverse effect is directly proportional to the total dose of local anesthetic agent administered.

For Surface Anesthesia Of The Male Adult Urethra: The plastic cone is sterilized for 5 minutes in boiling water, cooled, and attached to the tube. The cone may be gas sterilized or cold sterilized, as preferred. The jelly is instilled slowly into the urethra by gently expressing the contents of the tube until the patient has a feeling of tension or until almost half the tube (15 ml, *i.e.,* 300 mg of lidocaine HCl) is emptied. A penile clamp is then applied for several minutes at the corona and then the remaining contents of the tube are instilled.

Prior to sounding or cytoscopy, a penile clamp should be applied for 5 to 10 minutes to obtain adequate anesthesia. The contents of one tube (30 ml, i.e. 600 mg) are usually required to fill and dilate the male urethra.

Prior to catheterization, smaller volumes (5-10 ml, *i.e.,* 100-200 mg) are usually adequate for lubrication.

For Surface Anesthesia Of The Female Adult Urethra: The plastic cone is sterilized for 5 minutes in boiling water, cooled, and attached to the tube. The cone may be gas sterilized or cold sterilized, as preferred. Three to five ml of the jelly is instilled slowly into the urethra by gently expressing approximately 10-20% of the contents of the tube. If desired, some jelly may be deposited on a cotton swab and introduced into the urethra. In order to obtain adequate anesthesia, several minutes should be allowed prior to performing urological procedures.

Lubrication For Endotracheal Intubation: Apply a moderate amount of jelly to the external surface of the endotracheal tube shortly before use. Care should be taken to avoid introducing the product in to lumen of the tube. Do not use jelly to lubricate endotracheal stylettes. See WARNINGS and ADVERSE REACTIONSconcerning rare reports of lumen occlusion. it is also recommended that use of endotracheal tubes with dried jelly on the external surface be avoided for lack of lubricating effect.

Maximum Dosage: No more than one tube (600 mg of lidocaine HCl) should be given in any 12 hour period.

Children: It is difficult to recommend a maximum dose of any drug for children since this varies as a function of age and weight. For children less than years who have a normal lean body mass and a normal lean body development, the maximum dose may be determined by the application of one of the standard pediatric drug formulas (*e.g.,* Clark's rule). For example, in a child of five years weighing 50 lbs., the dose of lidocaine hydrochloride should not exceed 75-100 mg when calculated according to Clark's rule. In any case, the maximum amount of Lidocaine administered should not exceed 4.5 mg/kg (2.0 mg/lb.) of body weight.

A detachable applicator cone and a key for expressing the contents are included in each package.

Store at controlled room temperature.

HOW SUPPLIED - RATED THERAPEUTICALLY EQUIVALENT:

Jelly - Topical - 2 %

5 ml	$7.19	Lidocaine Hcl, Intl Medication	00548-3012-00
10 ml	$8.01	Lidocaine Hcl, Intl Medication	00548-3013-00
20 ml	$9.65	Lidocaine Hcl, Intl Medication	00548-3015-00
30 ml	**$14.34**	**XYLOCAINE, Astra USA**	**00186-0330-01**

Ointment - Topical - 5 %

.50 gm	$2.93	Lidocaine, IDE-Interstate	00814-4410-96
3.5 gm x 10	**$27.10**	**XYLOCAINE, FLAVORED, Astra USA**	**00186-0350-03**
35 gm	$6.25	Lidocaine, Fougera	00168-0204-37
35 gm	**$12.21**	**XYLOCAINE, Astra USA**	**00186-0315-21**
35 gm x 1	**$13.13**	**XYLOCAINE, FLAVORED, Astra USA**	**00186-0350-01**
50 gm	$2.30	Lidocaine, Thames Pharma	49158-0130-19

Solution - Topical - 4 %

4 ml	$8.85	Lidocaine Hcl Laryng-O-Jet Kit, Intl Medication	00548-6300-00
4 ml	$13.45	Lta Ii Kit, Abbott	00074-1001-01
50 ml	$7.04	Lidocaine Hcl, Roxane	00054-3505-47
50 ml	**$15.04**	**XYLOCAINE, Astra USA**	**00186-0320-01**
100 ml	$16.00	Lidocaine, Geneva Pharms	00781-6706-46

Solution - Topical; Oral - 2 %

15 ml	$5.44	ANESTACON, Alcon-PR	00998-0300-10
20 ml x 25	**$47.96**	**XYLOCAINE VISCOUS, Astra USA**	**00186-0361-78**
20 ml x 40	$46.76	Lidocaine Viscous, Roxane	00054-8500-16
100 ml	$2.44	Lidocaine Viscous, Roxane	00054-3500-49
100 ml	$3.15	Lidocaine Viscous, United Res	00677-1015-27
100 ml	$3.65	Lidocaine Hcl, HL Moore Drug Exch	00839-6502-40
100 ml	$4.05	Lidocaine Hcl Viscous, Qualitest Pharms	00603-1392-64
100 ml	$4.12	Lidocaine HCl, Rugby	00536-1331-82
100 ml	$4.62	Lidocaine HCl, Alpharma	00472-0996-33
100 ml	$6.15	Lidocaine Hcl, Goldline Labs	00182-1360-70
100 ml	$6.15	Lidocaine HCl, Geneva Pharms	00781-6190-46
100 ml	**$15.74**	**XYLOCAINE VISCOUS, Astra USA**	**00186-0360-01**
240 ml	$24.37	ANESTACON, Alcon-PR	00998-0300-20
450 ml	**$52.63**	**XYLOCAINE VISCOUS, Astra USA**	**00186-0360-11**

HOW SUPPLIED - NOT RATED EQUIVALENT:

Aerosol, Spray - Oral; Topical - 10 %

30 ml	**$44.82**	**XYLOCAINE, Astra USA**	**00186-0356-01**
50 x 1	**$26.15**	**XYLOCAINE, CANNULA'S FOR SPRAY, Astra USA**	**00186-9035-05**

Powder

25 gm	$13.90	LIDOCAINE BASE, Paddock Labs	00574-0613-25
25 gm	$13.90	LIDOCAINE HCL, Paddock Labs	00574-0617-25
30 gm	$13.30	Lidocaine Base, Millgood	53118-0510-01
120 gm	$33.00	Lidocaine Base, Millgood	53118-0510-04
454 gm	$105.00	Lidocaine Base, Millgood	53118-0510-10

Solution - Topical; Oral - 2 %

30 ml	**$13.13**	**XYLOCAINE, FLAVORED, Astra USA**	**00186-0325-01**

LIDOCAINE HYDROCHLORIDE *(001639)*

CATEGORIES: Anesthesia; Antiarrhythmic Agents; Antipruritics/Local Anesthetics; Arrhythmia; Cardiac Surgery; Cardiovascular Drugs; Cathartics & Laxatives; Caudal; Dermatologicals; EENT Drugs; Electrolyte Solutions; Epidural; Eye, Ear, Nose, & Throat Preparations; Gag Reflex; Gastrointestinal Drugs; Injectable Anesthetics; Local Anesthetics; Myocardial Infarction; Pharmaceutical Adjuvants; Pruritus; Skin/Mucous Membrane Agents; Pregnancy Category B; FDA Approval Pre 1982

BRAND NAMES: Alphacaine HCl; Anestacon; D-Caine; Dalcaine; Dilocaine; Duo-Trach; *Esracain*; *Gesicain*; L-Caine; Laryng-O-Jet Kit; *Leostein*; *Leostesin*; Lido-Storz; Lidocaine HCl Injectable; Lidocaine Hcl; Lidoject; Lidomar; *Lidonest*; Lidopen; Lta II Kit; Mylocaine; Nervocaine; Newcaine; Norocaine; *Rucaina*; Shocaine; Truxacaine; *Xylocaina*; **Xylocaine Injectable**
(International brand names outside U.S. in italics)

FORMULARIES: FHP

DESCRIPTION:

These solutions contain lidocaine HCl, which is chemically designated as acetamide, 2-(diethylamino)-N-(2,6-dimethylphenyl)-, monohydrochloride and has the molecular wt. 270.8. Lidocaine HCl ($C_{14}H_{22}N_2O$°HCl).

Epinephrine is (-)-3,4-Dihydroxy-α-((methylamino) methyl) benzyl alcohol and has the molecular wt. 183.21. Epinephrine ($C_9H_{13}NO_3$).

For Infiltration and Nerve Block: Lidocaine HCl Injections are sterile, non pyrogenic, aqueous solutions that contain a local anesthetic agent with or without epinephrine and are administered parenterally by injection. See INDICATIONS AND USAGE for specific uses.

Dosage forms listed as Lidocaine HCl-MPF indicate single dose solutions that are Methyl P araben Free (MPF).

Lidocaine HCl MPF is a sterile, non pyrogenic, isotonic solution containing sodium chloride. Lidocaine HCl in multiple dose vials, each ml also contains 1 mg methylparaben as antiseptic preservative. The pH of these solutions is adjusted to approximately 6.5 (5.0-7.0) with sodium hydroxide and/or hydrochloric acid.

Lidocaine HCl MPF with Epinephrine is a sterile, non pyrogenic, isotonic solution containing sodium chloride. Each ml contains lidocaine hydrochloride and epinephrine, with 0.5 mg sodium metabisulfite as an antioxidant and 0.2 mg citric acid as a stabilizer. Lidocaine HCl with Epinephrine in multiple dose vials, each ml also contains 1 mg methylparaben as antiseptic preservative. The pH of these solutions is adjusted to approximately 4.5 (3.3-5.5) with sodium hydroxide and/or hydrochloric acid. Filled under nitrogen.

For Ventricular Arrhythmias: Lidocaine HCl injection is a sterile and non-pyrogenic solution of an antiarrhythmic agent administered intravenously by either direct injection or continuous infusion. The specific quantitative for each available solution appears in TABLE 1.

TABLE 1 Composition of available solutions

	Dosage Form	Composition* Lidocaine HCl (mg/ml)	Sodium Chloride (mg/ml)
For Direct IV Injection	5 ml (50 mg) prefilled syringe	10	7
	5 ml (100 mg) prefilled syringe	20	6
	5 ml (100 mg) ampule	20	6
For Preparation of IV Infusion Solutions	25 ml (One Gram) single use vile	40	None
	5 ml (One Gram) additive syringe	200	None
	10 ml (Two Grams) additive syringe	200	None

* pH of all solutions adjusted to 5.0-7.0 with sodium hydroxide and/or hydrochloric acid. All containers are for single use: solutions do contain preservatives.

Spinal Anesthesia: Xylocaine-MPF 5% with Glucose 7.5% (lidocaine HCl and dextrose Injection, USP) is a sterile hyperbaric solution that contains a local anesthetic agent and is administered into the spinal subarachnoid space by injection. See INDICATIONS AND USAGE for specific uses.

Xylocaine-MPF 5% with Glucose 7.5% contains lidocaine HCl, which is chemical designated as acetamide, 2-(diethylamino)-N-(2,6- dimethylphenyl)-, monohydrochloride, and dextrose (D-Glucose, anhydrous).

Xylocaine-MPF 5% with Glucose 7.5% may be autoclaved at 15 lbs pressure at 121°C (250°F) for 15 minutes (USP Standard). Since this preparation contains glucose, caramelization may occur under prolonged heating and, in some instances, prolonged storage. Therefore, this preparation should not be autoclaved more than once, according to the above instructions, and should not be permitted to remain in the autoclave any longer than necessary. The solution should not be used if it is discolored or a precipitate is present.

Composition of Xylocaine-MPF 5% with Glucose 7.5%:

Each ml contains lidocaine HCl, 50 mg; dextrose (D-Glucose, anhydrous), 75 mg; sodium hydroxide and/or hydrochloric acid to adjust pH to 5.5- 7.0.

Specific gravity, 1.032-1.037.

CLINICAL PHARMACOLOGY:

FOR INFILTRATION AND NERVE BLOCK

Mechanism of Action: Lidocaine stabilizes the neuronal membrane by inhibiting the ionic fluxes required for the initiation and conduction of impulses thereby effecting local anesthetic action.

Hemodynamics: Excessive blood levels may cause changes in cardiac output, total peripheral resistance, and mean arterial pressure. With central neural blockade these changes may be attributable to block of autonomic fibers, a direct depressant effect of the local anesthetic agent on various components of the cardiovascular system, and/or the beta-adrenergic receptor stimulating action of epinephrine when present. The net effect is normally a modest hypotension when the recommended dosages are not exceeded.

FOR VENTRICULAR ARRHYTHMIAS

Mechanism of action and electrophysiology: Studies of the effects of therapeutic concentrations of lidocaine on the electrophysiological properties of mammalian Purkinje fibers have shown that lidocaine attenuates phase 4 diagnostic depolarization, decreases automatically, and causes a decrease or no change in excitability and membrane responsiveness. Action potential duration and effective refractory period of Purkinje fibers are decreased, while the ratio of effective refractory period to action potential duration is increased. Action potential duration and effective refractory period of ventricular muscle are also decreased. Effective refractory period of the AV node may increase, decrease, or remain unchanged, and atrial

CLINICAL PHARMACOLOGY: *(cont'd)*

effective refractory period is unchanged. Lidocaine raises the ventricular fibrillation threshold. No significant interactions between lidocaine and the autonomic nervous system have been described and consequently, lidocaine has little or no effect on autonomic tone.

Clinical electrophysiological studies with lidocaine have demonstrated no change in sinus node recovery time or sinoatrial conduction time. AV nodal conduction time is unchanged or shortened, and His-Purkinje, conduction time is unchanged.

Hemodynamics: At therapeutic doses, lidocaine has minimal hemodynamic effects in normal subjects and in patients with heart disease. Lidocaine has been shown to cause no, or minimal, decrease in ventricular contractility, cardiac output, arterial pressure or heart rate.

PHARMACOKINETICS AND METABOLISM

Lidocaine is rapidly metabolized by the liver, and less than 10% of a dose is excreted unchanged in the urine. Oxidative N-dealkylation, a major pathway of metabolism, results in the metabolites monoethylglycinexylidide and glycinexylidide. The pharmacological/toxicological activities of these metabolites are a similar to, but less potent than, lidocaine. The primary metabolite in urine is a conjugate of 4-hydroxy -2,6-dimethylaniline.

The elimination half-life of lidocaine following an intravenous bolus injection is typically 1.5 to 2 hours. There are data that indicate that the half-life may be 3 hours or longer following infusions of greater than 24 hours.

Because of the rapid rate at which lidocaine is metabolized, any condition that alters liver function, including changes in liver blood flow, which could result from severe congestive heart failure or shock, may alter lidocaine kinetics. The half-life may be two-fold or more greater in patients with liver dysfunction. Renal dysfunction does not affect lidocaine kinetics, but may increase rhe accumulation of metabolites.

Therapeutics effects of lidocaine are generally associated with plasma levels of 6 to 25 µmole/L (1.5 to 6 mcg free base per ml). The blood to plasma distribution ratio is approximately 0.84. Objective adverse manifestations become increasingly apparent with increasing plasma levels above 6 mcg free base per ml.

The plasma protein binding of lidocaine is dependent on drug concentration, and the fraction bound decreases with increasing concentration. At concentrations of 1 to 4 mcg free base per ml, 60 to 80 percent of lidocaine is protein bound. In addition to lidocaine concentration, the binding is dependent on the plasma concentration of the α-1-acid glycoprotein.

Lidocaine readily crosses the placental and blood-brain barriers. Dialysis has negligible effects on the kinetics of lidocaine.

SPINAL ANESTHESIA

Mechanism of Action: Lidocaine stabilizes the neuronal membrane by inhibiting the ionic fluxes required for the initiation and conduction of impulses, thereby effecting local anesthetic action.

Onset and Duration of Anesthesia: The onset of action is rapid. The duration of perineal anesthesia provided by 1 ml (50 mg) Xylocaine- MPF 5% with Glucose 7.5% averages 100 minutes, with analgesia continuing for an additional 40 minutes. The duration of surgical anesthesia provided by 1.5 to 2 ml (75-100 mg) of this agent is approximately two hours.

Hemodynamics: Excessive blood levels may cause changes in cardiac output, total peripheral resistance, and mean arterial pressure. With central neural blockade these changes may be attributable to block of autonomic fibers, or a direct depressant effect of the local anesthetic agent on various components of the cardiovascular system. The net effect is normally a modest hypotension when recommended dosages are not exceeded.

FOR INFILTRATION AND NERVE BLACK AND SPINAL ANESTHESIA

Pharmacokinetics and Metabolism: Information derived from diverse formulations, concentrations and usages reveals that lidocaine is completely absorbed following parenteral administration, its rate of absorption depending, for example, upon various factors such as the site of administration and the presence or absence of a vasoconstrictor agent. Except for intravascular administration, the highest blood levels are obtained following intercostal nerve block and the lowest after subcutaneous administration.

The plasma binding of lidocaine is dependent on drug concentration, and the fraction bound decreases with increasing concentration. At concentrations of 1 to 4 mcg of free base per ml 60 to 80 percent of lidocaine is protein bound. Binding is also dependent on the plasma concentration of the alpha-1-acid glycoprotein.

Lidocaine crosses the blood-brain and placental barriers, presumably by passive diffusion.

Lidocaine is metabolized rapidly by the liver, and metabolites and unchanged drug are excreted by the kidneys. Biotransformation includes oxidative N-dealkylation, ring hydroxylation, cleavage of the amide linkage, and conjugation. N-dealkylation, a major pathway of biotransformation, yields the metabolites monoethylglycinexylidide and glycinexylidide. The pharmacological/toxicological actions of these metabolites are similar to, but less potent than, those of lidocaine. Approximately 90% of lidocaine administered is excreted in the form of various metabolites, and less than 10% is excreted unchanged. The primary metabolite in urine is a conjugate of 4-hydroxy-2,6-dimethylaniline.

The elimination half-life of lidocaine following an intravenous bolus injection is typically 1.5 to 2.0 hours. Because of the rapid rate at which lidocaine is metabolized, any condition that affects liver function may alter lidocaine kinetics. The half-life may be prolonged two-fold or more in patients with liver dysfunction. Renal dysfunction does not affect lidocaine kinetics but may increase the accumulation of metabolites.

Factors such as acidosis and the use of CNS stimulants and depressants affect the CNS levels of lidocaine required to produce overt systemic effects. Objective adverse manifestations become increasingly apparent with increasing venous plasma levels above 6 mcg free base per ml. In the rhesus monkey arterial blood levels of 18-21 mcg/ml have been shown to be threshold for convulsive activity.

INDICATIONS AND USAGE:

For Infiltration and Nerve Block: Lidocaine HCl Injections are indicated for production of local or regional anesthesia by infiltration techniques such as percutaneous injection and intravenous regional anesthesia by peripheral nerve block techniques such as brachial plexus and intercostal and by central neural techniques such as lumbar and caudal epidural blocks, when the accepted procedures for these techniques as described in standard textbooks are observed.

For Ventricular Arrhythmias: Lidocaine HCl Injection administered intravenously as specifically indicated in the acute management of ventricular arrhythmias such as those occurring in relation to acute myocardial infarction, or during cardiac manipulation, such as cardiac surgery.

Spinal Anesthesia: Xylocaine-MPF 5% with Glucose 7.5% (lidocaine HCl and dextrose Injection, USP) is indicated for this production of spinal anesthesia when the accepted procedures for this technique as described in standard textbooks are observed.

CONTRAINDICATIONS:

Lidocaine is contraindicated in patients with a known history of hypersensitivity to local anesthetics of the amide type.

CONTRAINDICATIONS: *(cont'd)*

For Ventricular Arrhythmias: Lidocaine HCl Injection should not be used in patients with Stoke-Adams syndrome, Wolff- Parkinson-White syndrome, or with severe degrees of sinoatrial, atrioventricular, or intraventricular block in the absence of an artificial pacemaker.

Spinal Anesthesia: The following conditions preclude the use of spinal anesthesia:

1. Severe hemorrhage, shock or heart block
2. Local infection at the site of proposed puncture
3. Septicemia
4. Known sensitivity to the local anesthetic agent.

WARNINGS:

For Infiltration and Nerve Block: LIDOCAINE HCL INJECTIONS FOR INFILTRATION AND NERVE BLOCK SHOULD BE EMPLOYED ONLY BY CLINICIANS WHO ARE WELL VERSED IN DIAGNOSIS AND MANAGEMENT OF DOSE-RELATED TOXICITY AND OTHER ACUTE EMERGENCIES THAT MIGHT ARISE FROM THE BLOCK TO BE EMPLOYED AND THEN ONLY AFTER ENSURING THE *IMMEDIATE* AVAILABILITY OF OXYGEN, OTHER RESUSCITATIVE DRUGS, CARDIOPULMONARY EQUIPMENT AND THE PERSONNEL NEEDED FOR PROPER MANAGEMENT OF TOXIC REACTIONS AND RELATED EMERGENCIES. (See also ADVERSE REACTIONS and PRECAUTIONS.) DELAY IN PROPER MANAGEMENT OF DOSE-RELATED TOXICITY, UNDERVENTILATION FROM ANY CAUSE AND/OR ALTERED SENSITIVITY MAY LEAD TO THE DEVELOPMENT OF ACIDOSIS, CARDIAC ARREST AND, POSSIBLY, DEATH.

To avoid intravascular injection, aspiration should be performed before the local anesthetic solution is injected. The needle must be repositioned until no return of blood can be elicited by aspiration. Note, however, that the absence of blood in the syringe does not guarantee that intravascular injection has been avoided.

Local anesthetic solutions containing antimicrobial preservatives, (*e.g.,* methylparaben) should not be used for epidural or spinal anesthesia because the safety of these agents has not been established with regard to intrathecal injection, either intentional or accidental.

Lidocaine HCl with epinephrine solutions contain sodium metabisulfite, a sulfite that may cause allergic-type reactions including anaphylactic symptoms and life-threatening or less severe asthmatic episodes in certain susceptible people. The overall prevalence of sulfite sensitivity in the general population is unknown and probably low. Sulfite sensitivity is seen more frequently in asthmatic than in non-asthmatic people.

For Ventricular Arrhythmias: IN ORDER TO MANAGE POSSIBLE ADVERSE REACTIONS, RESUSCITATIVE EQUIPMENT, OXYGEN AND OTHER RESUSCITATIVE DRUGS SHOULD BE IMMEDIATELY AVAILABLE WHEN LIDOCAINE HYDROCHLORIDE INJECTION IS USED.

Systemic toxicity may result in manifestations of central nervous system depression (sedation) or irritability (twitching), which may progress to frank convulsions accompanied by respiratory depression and or arrest. Early recognition of premonitory signs, assurance of adequate oxygenation, and, where necessary, establishment of artificial airway with ventilatory support are essential to management of this problem. Should convulsions persist despite ventilatory therapy with oxygen,*small* increments of anticonvulsant drugs may be used intravenously. Examples of such agents include benzodiazepines (*e.g.,* diazepam), ultra short-acting barbiturates (*e.g.,* thiopental or thiamylal), or a short acting barbiturate (*e.g.,* pentobarbital or secobarbital). If a patient is under anesthesia, a short acting muscle relaxant (*e.g.,* succinylcholine) may be used. Longer acting drugs should be used only when recurrent convulsions are evidenced.

Should circulatory depression occur, vasopressors may be used.

Constant electrocardiographic monitoring is essential to the proper administration of Lidocaine HCl Injections. Signs of excessive depression of cardiac electrical activity such as sinus node dysfunction, prolongation of the P-R interval and ORS complex or the appearance or aggravation of arrhythmias, should be followed by flow adjustment and, if necessary, prompt cessation of the intravenous infusion of this agent. Occasionally, acceleration of ventricular rate may occur when Lidocaine Injection is administered to patients with atrial flutter or fibrillation.

Spinal Anesthesia: XYLOCAINE-MPF 5% WITH GLUCOSE 7.5% FOR SPINAL ANESTHESIA SHOULD BE EMPLOYED ONLY BY CLINICIANS WHO ARE WELL VERSED IN DIAGNOSIS AND MANAGEMENT OF DOSE-RELATED TOXICITY AND OTHER ACUTE EMERGENCIES THAT MIGHT ARISE FROM SPINAL ANESTHESIA AND THEN ONLY AFTER ENSURING THE *IMMEDIATE* AVAILABILITY OF OXYGEN, OTHER RESUSCITATIVE DRUGS, CARDIOPULMONARY EQUIPMENT, AND THE PERSONNEL NEEDED FOR PROPER MANAGEMENT OF TOXIC REACTIONS AND RELATED EMERGENCIES. (See also ADVERSE REACTIONS and PRECAUTIONS.) DELAY IN PROPER MANAGEMENT OF DOSE-RELATED TOXICITY, UNDERVENTILATION FROM ANY CAUSE AND/OR ALTERED SENSITIVITY MAY LEAD TO THE DEVELOPMENT OF ACIDOSIS, CARDIAC ARREST, AND POSSIBLY, DEATH.

To avoid intravascular injection, aspiration should be performed before the local anesthetic solution is injected. The needle must be repositioned until no return of blood can be elicited by aspiration. Note, however, that the absence of blood in the syringe does not guarantee that intravascular injection has been avoided.

Spinal anesthetics should not be injected during uterine contractions since spinal fluid current may carry the drug farther cephalad than desired.

PRECAUTIONS:

FOR INFILTRATION AND NERVE BLOCK

General: The safety and effectiveness of lidocaine depend on proper dosage, correct technique, adequate precautions, and readiness for emergencies. Standard text-books should be consulted for specific techniques and precautions for various regional anesthetic procedures.

Resuscitative equipment, oxygen, and other resuscitative drugs should be available for immediate use. (See WARNINGS and ADVERSE REACTIONS.) The lowest dosage that results in effective anesthesia should be used to avoid high plasma levels and serious adverse effects. Syringe aspirations should also be performed before and during each supplemental injection when using indwelling catheter techniques.

During the administration of epidural anesthesia, it is recommend that a test dose be administered initially and that the patient be monitored for central nervous system toxicity and cardiovascular toxicity, as well as for signs of unintended intrathecal administration, before proceeding. When clinical conditions permit, consideration should be given to employing local anesthetic solutions that contain epinephrine for the test dose because circulatory changes compatible with epinephrine may also serve as a warning sign of unintended intravascular injection. An intravascular injection is still possible even if aspirations for blood are negative. Repeated doses of lidocaine may cause significant increases in blood levels with each repeated dose because of slow accumulation of the drug or its metabolites. Tolerance to elevated blood levels varies with the status of the patient. Debilitated, elderly patients, acutely ill patients, and children should be given reduced doses commensurate with their age and physical condition. Lidocaine should also be used with caution in patients with severe shock or heart block.

PRECAUTIONS: *(cont'd)*

Lumber and caudal epidural anesthesia should be used with extreme caution in persons with the following conditions: existing neurological disease, spinal deformities, septicemia, and severe hypertension.

Local anesthetic solutions containing a vasoconstrictor should be used cautiously and in carefully circumscribed quantities in areas of the body supplied by end arteries or having otherwise compromised blood supply. Patients with peripheral vascular disease and those with hypertensive vascular disease may exhibit exaggerated vasoconstrictor response. Ischemic injury or necrosis may result. Preparations containing a vasoconstrictor should be used with caution in patients during or following the administration of potent general anesthetic agents, since cardiac arrhythmias may occur under such conditions.

Careful and constant monitoring of cardiovascular and respiratory (adequacy of ventilation) vital signs and the patient's state of consciousness should be accomplished after each local anesthetic injection. It should be kept in mind at such times that restlessness, anxiety, tinnitus, dizziness, blurred vision, tremors, depression or drowsiness may be early warning signs of central nervous system toxicity.

Since amide-type local anesthetics are metabolized by the liver, Lidocaine HCl Injection should be used with caution in patients with hepatic disease. Patients with severe hepatic disease, because of their inability to metabolize local anesthetics normally, are at greater risk of developing toxic plasma concentrations. Lidocaine HCl Injection should also be used with caution in patients with impaired cardiovascular function since they may be less able to compensate for functional changes associated with the prolongation of A-V conduction produced by these drugs.

Many drugs used during the conduct of anesthesia are considered potential triggering agents for familiar malignant hyperthermia. Since it is not known whether amide-type local anesthetics may trigger this reaction and since the need for supplemental general anesthesia cannot be predicted in advance, it is suggested that a standard protocol for the management of malignant hyperthermia should be available. Early unexplained signs of tachycardia, tachypnea, labile blood pressure and metabolic acidosis may precede temperature elevation. Successful outcome is dependent on early diagnosis, prompt discontinuance of the suspect triggering agent(s) and institution of treatment, including oxygen therapy, indicated supportive measures and dantrolene (consult dantrolene sodium intravenous package insert before using).

Proper tourniquet technique, as described in publications and standard textbooks, is essential in the performance of intravenous regional anesthesia. Solutions containing epinephrine or other vasoconstrictors should not be used for this technique.

Lidocaine should be used with caution in persons with known drug sensitivities. Patients allergic to para-aminobenzoic acid derivatives (procaine, tetracaine, benzocaine, etc.) have not shown cross sensitivity to lidocaine.

Use in the Head and Neck Area: Small doses of local anesthetics injected into the head and neck area, including retrobulbar, dental and stellate ganglion blocks, may produce adverse reactions similar to systemic toxicity seen with unintentional intravascular injections of larger doses. Confusion, convulsions, respiratory depression and/or respiratory arrest, and cardiovascular stimulation or depression have been reported. These reactions may be due to intra-arterial injection of the local anesthetic with retrograde flow to the cerebral circulation. Patients receiving these blocks should have their circulation and respiration monitored are be constantly observed. Resuscitative equipment and personnel for treating adverse reactions should be immediately available. Dosage recommendations should not be exceeded. (See DOSAGE AND ADMINISTRATION.)

Information for the Patient: When appropriate, patients should be informed in advance that they may experience temporary loss of sensation and motor activity, usually in the lower half of the body, following pooper administration of epidural anesthesia.

Drug/Laboratory Test Interactions: The intramuscular injection of lidocaine may result in an increase in creatine phosphokinase levels. Thus, the use of this enzyme determination, without isoenzyme separation, as a diagnostic test for the presence of acute myocardial infarction may be compromised by the intramuscular injection of lidocaine.

Carcinogenesis, Mutagenesis, and Impairment of Fertility: Studies of lidocaine in animals to evaluate the carcinogenic and mutagenic potential or the effect on fertility have not been conducted.

Pregnancy, Teratogenic Effects: Pregnancy Category B. Reproduction studies have been performed in rats at doses up to 6.6 times the human dose and have revealed no evidence of harm to the fetus caused by lidocaine. There are, however, no adequate and well-controlled studies in pregnant women. Animal reproduction studies are not always predictive of human response. General consideration should be given to this fact before administering lidocaine to women of childbearing potential, especially during early pregnancy when maximum organogenesis takes place.

Labor and Delivery: Local anesthetics rapidly cross the placenta and when used for epidural, paracervical, pudendal or caudal block anesthesia, can cause varying degrees of maternal, fetal and neonatal toxicity. See CLINICAL PHARMACOLOGY, Pharmacokinetics.The potential for toxicity depends upon the procedure performed, the type and amount of drug used, and the technique of drug administration. Adverse reactions in the parturient, fetus and neonate involve alterations of the central nervous system, peripheral vascular tone and cardiac function.

Maternal hypotension has resulted from regional anesthesia. Local anesthetics produce vasodilation by blocking sympathetic nerves. Elevating the patient's legs and positioning her on her left side will help prevent decreases in blood pressure. The fetal heart rate also should be monitored continuously, and electronic fetal monitoring is highly advisable.

Epidural, spinal, paracervical, or pudendal anesthesia may alter the forces of parturition through changes in uterine contractility or maternal expulsive efforts. In one study, paracervical block anesthesia was associated with a decrease in the mean duration of first stage labor and facilitation of cervical dilation. However, spinal and epidural anesthesia have also been reported to prolong the second stage of labor by removing the parturient's reflex urge to bear down or by interfering with motor function. The use of obstetrical anesthesia may increase the need for forceps assistance.

The use of some local anesthetic drug products during labor and delivery may be followed by diminished muscle strength and tone for the first day or two of life. The long-term significance of these observations is unknown. Fetal bradycardia may occur in 20 to 30 percent of patients receiving paracervical nerve block anesthesia with the amide-type local anesthetics and may be associated with fetal acidosis. Fetal heart rate should always be monitored during paracervical anesthesia. The physician should weigh the possible advantages against risks when considering a paracervical block in prematurity, toxemia of pregnancy, and fetal distress. Careful adherence to recommended dosage is of the utmost importance in obstetrical paracervical block. Failure to achieve adequate analgesia with recommended doses should arouse suspicion of intravascular or fetal intracranial injection. Cases compatible with unintended fetal intracranial injection of local anesthetic solution have been reported following intended paracervical or pudendal block or both. Babies so affected present with unexplained neonatal depression at birth, which correlates with high local

PRECAUTIONS: *(cont'd)*

anesthetic serum levels, and often manifest seizures within six hours. Prompt use of supportive measures combined with forced urinary excretion of the local anesthetic has been used successfully to manage this complication.

Case reports of maternal convulsions and cardiovascular collapse following use of some local anesthetics for paracervical block in early pregnancy (as anesthesia for elective abortion) suggest that systemic absorption under these circumstances may be rapid. The recommended maximum dose of each drug should not be exceeded. Injection should be made slowly and with frequent aspiration. Allow a 5-minute interval between sides.

Nursing Mothers: It is not known whether this drug is excreted in human milk. Because many drugs are excreted in human milk, caution should be exercised when lidocaine is administered to a nursing woman.

Pediatric Use: Dosages in children should be reduced, commensurate with age, body weight and physical condition. See DOSAGE AND ADMINISTRATION.

FOR VENTRICULAR ARRHYTHMIAS

General: Caution should be employed in the use of Lidocaine Injection in patients with severe liver or kidney disease because accumulation of the drug or metabolites may occur.

Lidocaine HCl Injection should be used with caution in the treatment of patients with hypovolemia, severe congestive heart failure, shock, and all forms of heart block. In patients with sinus bradycardia, or incomplete heart block, the administration of Lidocaine HCl Injection intravenously for the elimination of ventricular ectopic beats, without prior acceleration in heart rate (*e.g.,* by atropine, isoproterenol or electric pacing), may promote more frequent and serious ventricular arrhythmias or complete heart block (See CONTRAINDICATIONS.)

Dosage should be reduced for children and for debilitated and/or elderly patients, commensurate with their age and physical status.

The safety of amide local anesthetic agents in patients with genetic predisposition to malignant hypothermia has not been fully assessed; therefore, lidocaine should be used with caution in such patients.

In hospital environments where drugs known to be triggering agents for malignant hypothermia (fulminant hypermetabolism) are administered, it is suggested that a standard protocol for management should be available.

It is not known whether lidocaine may trigger this reaction; however, large doses resulting in significant plasma concentrations, as may be achieved by intravenous infusion, pose potential risk to these individuals. Recognition of early unexplained signs of tachycardia, tachypnea, labile blood pressure and metabolic acidosis may precede temperature elevation. Successful outcome is dependent on early diagnosis, prompt discontinuance of the triggering agent and institution of treatment including oxygen therapy, supportive measures and dantrolene (for details see dantrolene prescribing information/package insert).

Patient Information: The patient should be advised of the possible occurrence of the experiences listed under ADVERSE REACTIONS.

Laboratory Tests: None known.

Carcinogenesis, Mutagenesis, and Impairment of Fertility: Long term studies in animals to evaluate the carcinogenic and mutagenic potential or the effect on fertility of Lidocaine HCl Injection have not been conducted.

Pregnancy, Teratogenic Effects, Pregnancy Category B Reproduction studies have been performed in rats at doses of up to 6.6 times the maximum human doses and have revealed no significant findings. There are, however, no adequate and well-controlled studies in pregnant women. Because animal reproduction studies are not always predictive of human response, this drug should be used during pregnancy only if clearly needed.

Labor and Delivery: The effects of Lidocaine HCl Injection on the mother and the fetus, when used in the management of cardiac arrhythmias during labor and delivery, are not known. Lidocaine readily crosses the placental barrier.

Nursing Mothers: It is not known whether this drug is excreted in human milk. Because many drugs are excreted in human milk, caution should be exercised when lidocaine is administered to a nursing woman.

Pediatric Use: Safety and effectiveness in children have not been established by controlled clinical studies. (See DOSAGE AND ADMINISTRATION.)

SPINAL ANESTHESIA

General: The safety and effectiveness of lidocaine depend on proper dosage, correct technique, adequate precautions, and readiness for emergencies. Standard textbooks should be constituted for specific techniques and precautions for spinal anesthetic procedures. Resuscitative equipment, oxygen and other resuscitative drugs should be available for immediate use. (See WARNINGS and ADVERSE REACTIONS.) The lowest dosage that results in effective anesthesia should be used to avoid high plasma levels and serious adverse effects. Repeated doses of lidocaine may cause significant increases in blood levels with each repeated dose because of slow accumulation of the drug or its metabolites. Tolerance to elevated blood levels varies with the physical condition of the patient. Debilitated, elderly patients, acutely ill patients, and children should be given reduced doses commensurate with their age and physical status. Lidocaine should also be used with caution in patients with severe shock or heart block.

Neurologic deficits have been reported with the use of small bore needles and microcatheters for spinal anesthesia. It has been postulated, based on *in vitro* models, that these deficits were due to pooling and non-uniform distribution of concentrated local anesthetic within the subarachnoid space. Animal studies suggest mixing the 5% Xylocaine with an equal volume of CSF or preservative-free 0.9% saline solution anesthetic. (See DOSAGE AND ADMINISTRATION.)

The following conditions may preclude the use of spinal anesthesia, depending upon the physician's ability to deal with the complications or complaints that may occur:

a. pre-existing diseases of the central nervous system such as those attributable to poliomyelitis, pernicious anemia, paralysis from nerve injuries, and syphilis.

b. Disturbance in blood morphology and/or anticoagulant therapy. In these conditions, trauma to a blood vessel during needle puncture may result in uncontrollable hemorrhage into the epidural or subarachnoid space. Also profuse hemorrhage into the soft tissue may occur.

c. Extremes of age.

d. Chronic backache and preoperative headache.

e. Hypotension and hypertension.

f. Arthritis or spinal deformity.

g. Technical problems (persistent paresthesias, persistent bloody tap).

h. Psychotic or uncooperative patients.

CONSULT STANDARD TEXTBOOKS FOR SPECIFIC TECHNIQUES AND PRECAUTIONS FOR SPINAL ANESTHETIC PROCEDURES.

PRECAUTIONS: *(cont'd)*

Careful and constant monitoring of cardiovascular and respiratory (adequacy of ventilation) vital signs and the patient's state of consciousness should be accomplished after each local anesthetic injection. It should be kept in mind at such times that restlessness, anxiety, tinnitus, dizziness, blurred vision, tremors, depression or drowsiness may be early warning signs of central nervous system toxicity.

Since amide-type local anesthetics are metabolized by the liver, lidocaine should be used with caution in patients with hepatic disease. Patients with severe hepatic disease, because of their inability to metabolize local anesthetics normally, are at greater risk of developing toxic plasma concentrations. Lidocaine should also be used with caution in patients with impaired cardiovascular function since they may be less able to compensate for functional changes associated with the prolongation of A-V conduction produced by these drugs.

Many drugs used during the conduct of anesthesia are considered potential triggering agents for familial malignant hyperthermia. Since it is not known whether amide-type local anesthetics may trigger this reaction and since the need for supplemental general anesthesia cannot be predicted in advance, it is suggested that a standard protocol for management should be available. Early unexplained signs of tachycardia, tachypnea, labile blood pressure and metabolic acidosis may precede temperature elevation. Successful outcome is dependent on early diagnosis, prompt discontinuance of the suspect triggering agent(s) and institution of treatment, including oxygen therapy, indicated supportive measures and dantrolene (consult dantrolene sodium intravenous package insert before using).

Lidocaine should be used with caution in persons with known drug sensitivities. Patients allergic to para-aminobenzoic acid derivatives (procaine, tetracaine, benzocaine, etc.) have not shown cross sensitivity to lidocaine.

Information for the Patient: When appropriate, patients should be informed in advance that they may experience temporary loss of sensation and motor activity, usually in the lower half of the body, following proper administration of spinal anesthesia.

Carcinogenesis, Mutagenesis, and Impairment of Fertility: Studies of lidocaine in animals to evaluate the carcinogenic and mutagenic potential or the effect on fertility have not been conducted.

Use in Pregnancy: Teratogenic Effects: Pregnancy Category B: Reproduction studies have been performed in rats at doses up to 6.6 times the human dose and have revealed no evidence of harm to the fetus caused by lidocaine. There are, however, no adequate and well- controlled studies in pregnant women. Animal reproduction studies are not always predictive of human response. General consideration should be given to this fact, before administering lidocaine to women of childbearing potential, especially during early pregnancy when maximum organogenesis takes place.

Labor and Delivery: Maternal hypotension has resulted from regional anesthesia. Local anesthetics produce vasodilation by blocking sympathetic nerves. Elevating the patient's legs and positioning her on her left side will prevent decreases in blood pressure. The fetal heart rate also should be monitored continuously, and electronic fetal monitoring is highly advisable.

Spinal anesthesia may alter the forces of parturition through changes in uterine contractility or maternal expulsive efforts. However, spinal anesthesia has also been reported to prolong the second stage of labor by removing the parturient's reflex urge to bear down or by interfering with motor function. The use of obstetrical anesthesia may increase the need for forceps assistance.

Nursing Mothers: It is not known whether this drug is excreted in human milk. Because many drugs are excreted in human milk, caution should be exercised when lidocaine is administered to a nursing woman.

Pediatric Use: Safety and effectiveness in children below the age of 16 years have not been established.

DRUG INTERACTIONS:

For Infiltration and Nerve Block: The administration of local anesthetic solutions containing epinephrine or norepinephrine to patients receiving monoamine oxidase inhibitors or tricyclic antidepressants may produce severe, prolonged hypertension.

Phenothiazines and butyrophenones may reduce or reverse the pressor effect of epinephrine.

Concurrent use of these agents should generally be avoided. In situations when concurrent therapy is necessary, careful patient monitoring is essential.

Concurrent administration of vasopressor drugs (for the treatment of hypotension related to obstetric blocks) and ergot-type oxytocic drugs may cause severe, persistent hypertension or cerebrovascular accidents.

For Ventricular Arrhythmias: Lidocaine HCl Injections should be used with caution in patients with digitalis toxicity accompanied by atrioventricular block. Concomitant use of beta-blocking agents or cimetidine may reduce hepatic blood flow and thereby reduce lido clearance.

Lidocaine and tocainide are pharmacodynamically similar. The concomitant use of these two agents may cause an increased incidence of adverse reactions, including central nervous system adverse reactions such as seizure.

Spinal Anesthesia: The administration of local anesthetic solutions containing epinephrine or norepinephrine to patients receiving monoamine oxidase inhibitors, tricyclic antidepressants or phenothiazines may produce severe, prolonged hypotension or hypertension. Concurrent use of these agents should be generally avoided. In situations when concurrent therapy is necessary, careful patient monitoring is essential.

Concurrent administration of vasopressor drugs (for the treatment of hypotension related to spinal blocks) and ergot-type oxytocic drugs may cause severe, persistent hypertension or cerebrovascular accidents.

ADVERSE REACTIONS:

Systemic: Adverse experiences following the administration of lidocaine are similar in nature to those observed with other amide local anesthetic agents. These adverse experiences are, in general, dose- related and may result from high plasma levels caused by excessive dosage, rapid absorption of inadvertent intravascular injection, or may result from a hypersensitivity, idiosyncrasy or diminished to tolerance on the part of the patient. Serious adverse experiences are generally systemic in nature. The following types are those most commonly reported.

FOR INFILTRATION AND NERVE BLOCK

Central Nervous System: CNS manifestations are excitatory and/or depressant and may be characterized by lightheadedness, nervousness, apprehension, euphoria, confusion, dizziness, drowsiness, tinnitus, blurred or double vision, vomiting, sensations of heat, cold or numbness, twitching, tremors, convulsions, unconsciousness, respiratory depression and arrest. The excitatory manifestation may be very brief or may not occur at all, in which case the first manifestation of toxicity may be drowsiness merging into unconsciousness and respiratory arrest.

Drowsiness following the administration of lidocaine is usually an early sign of a high blood level of the drug and may occur as consequence of rapid absorption.

ADVERSE REACTIONS: *(cont'd)*

Cardiovascular System: Cardiovascular manifestations are usually depressant and are characterized by bradycardia, hypotension, and cardiovascular collapse, which may lead to cardiac arrest.

Allergic: Allergic reactions are characterized by cutaneous lesions, urticaria, edema or anaphylactoid reactions. Allergic reactions may occur as a result of sensitivity either to local anesthetic agents or to the methylparaben used as a preservative in the multiple dose vials. Allergic reactions as a result of sensitivity to lidocaine are extremely rare and, if they occur, should be managed by conventional means. The detection of sensitivity by skin testing is of doubtful value.

Neurologic: The incidences of adverse reactions associated with the use of local anesthetics may be related to the total dose of local anesthetic administered and are also dependent upon the particular drug used, the route of administration and the physical status of the patient. In a prospective review of 10,440 patients who received lidocaine for spinal anesthesia, the incidences of adverse reactions were reported to be about 3 percent each for positional headaches, hypotension and backache; 2 percent for shivering; and less than 1 percent each for peripheral nerve symptoms, nausea, respiratory inadequacy and double vision. Many of these observations may be related to local anesthetic techniques, with or without a contribution from the local anesthetic.

In the practice of caudal or lumbar epidural block, occasional unintentional penetration of the subarachnoid space by the catheter may occur. Subsequent adverse effects may depend partially on the amount of drug administered subdurally. These may include spinal block or varying magnitude (including total spinal block), hypotension secondary to spinal block, loss of bladder and bowel control, and loss of perineal sensation and sexual function. Persistent motor, sensory and/or autonomic (sphincter control) deficit of some lower spinal segments with slow recovery (several months) or incomplete recovery have been reported in rare instances when caudal or lumbar epidural block has been attempted. Backache and headache have also been noted following use of these anesthetic procedures.

FOR VENTRICULAR ARRHYTHMIAS

Central Nervous System: CNS reactions are excitatory and/or depressant, and may be characterized by lightheadedness, nervousness, apprehension, euphoria, confusion, dizziness, drowsiness, tinnitus, blurred or double vision, vomiting, sensations of heat, cold or numbness, twitching, tremors, convulsions, unconsciousness, respiratory depression and arrest. The excitatory reactions may be very brief or may not occur at all, in which case, the first manifestation of toxicity may be drowsiness, merging in unconsciousness and respiratory arrest.

Cardiovascular system: Cardiovascular reactions are usually depressant in nature and are characterized by bradycardia, hypotension, and cardiovascular collapse, which may lead to cardiac arrest.

Allergic reactions as a result of sensitivity to lidocaine are extremely rare and, if they occur, should be managed by conventional means.

SPINAL ANESTHESIA

Central Nervous System: CNS manifestations are excitatory and/or depressant and may be characterized by lightheadness nervousness, apprehension, euphoria, confusion, dizziness, drowsiness, tinnitus, blurred or double vision, vomiting, sensations of heat, cold or numbness, twitching, tremors, convulsions, unconsciousness, respiratory depression and arrest. The excitatory manifestations may be very brief or may not occur at all, in which case the first manifestation of toxicity may be drowsiness merging into unconsciousness and respiratory arrest.

Drowsiness following the administration of lidocaine is usually an early sign of a high blood level of the drug and may occur as a consequence of rapid absorption.

Cardiovascular System: Cardiovascular manifestations are usually depressant and are characterized by bradycardia, hypotension, and cardiovascular collapse, which may lead to cardiac arrest.

Allergic: Allergic reactions are characterized by cutaneous lesions, urticaria, edema or anaphylactoid reactions. Allergic reactions as a result of sensitivity to lidocaine are extremely rare and, if they occur, should be managed by conventional means. The detection of sensitivity by skin testing is of doubtful value.

Neurologic: The incidences of adverse reactions associated with the use of local anesthetics may be related to the total dose of local anesthetic administered and are also dependent upon the particular drug used, the route of administration and the physical status of the patient. In a prospective review of 10,440 patients who received lidocaine for spinal anesthesia, the incidences of adverse reactions were reported to be about 3 percent each for positional headaches, hypotension and backache; 2 percent for shivering; and less than 1 percent each for peripheral nerve symptoms, nausea, respiratory inadequacy and double vision. Many of these observations may be related to local anesthetic techniques with or without a contribution from the local anesthetic.

Neurologic effects following spinal anesthesia may include loss of perineal sensation and sexual function; persistent anesthesia, paresthesia, weakness and paralysis of the lower extremities, and loss of sphincter control all of which may have slow, incomplete, or no recovery; hypotension; high or total spinal block; urinary retention; headache; backache; septic meningitis; meningismus, arachnoiditis; slowing of labor; increased incidence of forceps delivery; shivering; cranial nerve palsies due to traction on nerves from loss of cerebrospinal fluid; and fecal and urinary incontinence.

DRUG ABUSE AND DEPENDENCE:

Although specific studies have not been conducted, Lidocaine HCl Injection has been used clinically without evidence of abuse of this drug or of psychological or physical dependence as a result of its use.

OVERDOSAGE:

FOR INFILTRATION AND NERVE BLOCK AND SPINAL ANESTHESIA

Acute emergencies from local anesthetics are generally related to high plasma levels encountered during therapeutic use of local anesthetics or to unintended subarachnoid injection of local anesthetic solution (see ADVERSE REACTIONS, WARNINGS, and PRECAUTIONS).

Management of Local Anesthetic Emergencies: The first step in the management of convulsions, as well as underventilation or apnea due to unintended subarachnoid injection of drug solution, consists of immediate attention to the maintenance of a patient airway and assisted or controlled ventilation with oxygen and delivery system capable of permitting immediate positive airway pressure by mask. Immediately after the institution of these ventilatory measures, the adequacy of the circulation should be evaluated, keeping in mind that drugs used to treat convulsions sometimes depress the circulation when administered intravenously. Should convulsions persist dispirit adequate respiratory support, and if the status of the circulations permits, small increments of an ultra-short acting barbiturate (such as thiopental or thiamylal) or a benzodiazepine (such as diazepam) may be administered intravenously. The clinician should be familiar, prior to the use of local anesthetics, with these anticonvulsant drugs. Supportive treatment of circulatory depression may require administration on intravenous fluids, and, when appropriate, a vasopressor as directed by the clinical situation (*e.g.,* ephedrine).

OVERDOSAGE: *(cont'd)*

If not treated immediately, both convulsions and cardiovascular depression can result in hypoxia, acidosis, bradycardia, arrhythmias and cardiac arrest. Underventilation or apnea due to unintentional subarachnoid injection of local anesthetic solution may produce these same signs and also lead to cardiac arrest if ventilatory support is not instituted. If cardiac arrest should occur, standard cardiopulmonary resuscitative measures should be instituted.

Endotracheal intubation, employing drugs and techniques familiar to the clinician, may be indicated, after initial administration of oxygen by mask, if difficulty is encountered in the maintenance of patent airway or if prolonged ventilatory support (assisted or controlled) is indicated.

FOR INFILTRATION AND NERVE BLOCK

Management of Local Anesthetic Emergencies: The first consideration is prevention, best accomplished by careful and constant monitoring of cardiovascular and respiratory vital signs and the patient's state of consciousness after each local anesthetic injection. At the first sign of change, oxygen should be administered.

Dialysis is of negligible value in the treatment of acute overdosage with lidocaine. The oral LD_{50} of lidocaine HCl in non-fasted female rats is 459 (346- 773) mg/kg (as the salt) and 214 (159-324) mg/kg (as the salt) in fasted female rats.

SPINAL ANESTHESIA

The intravenous LD_{50} of lidocaine HCl in female mice is 26 (21-31) mg/kg and subcutaneous LD_{50} is 264 (203-304) mg/kg.

FOR VENTRICULAR ARRHYTHMIAS

Overdosage of Lidocaine HCl Injection usually results in signs of central nervous system or cardiovascular toxicity. See ADVERSE REACTIONS.

Should convulsions or signs of respiratory depression and arrest develop, the patency of the air way and adequacy of ventilation must be assured immediately. Should convulsions persist despite ventilatory therapy with oxygen, small with oxygen, small increments of anticonvulsive agents may be given intravenously. Examples of such agents include a benzodiazepine (*e.g.,* diazepam), an ultrashort-acting barbiturate (*e.g.,* thiopental or thiamylal), or a short-acting barbiturate (*e.g.,* pentobarbital or secobarbital). If the patient is under general anesthesia, a short-acting muscle relaxant (*e.g.,* succinylcholine) may be administered.

Should circulatory depression occur, vasopressors may be used. Should cardiac arrest occur, standard CPR procedures should be instituted.

Dialysis is of negligible value in the treatment of acute overdosage from Lidocaine HCl Injection.

DOSAGE AND ADMINISTRATION:

For Infiltration and Nerve Block: TABLE 3 (Recommended Dosages) summarizes the recommended volumes and concentrations of Lidocaine HCl Injection for various types of anesthetic procedures. The dosages suggested in this table are for normal healthy adults and refer to the use of epinephrine-free solutions. When larger volumes are required, only solutions containing epinephrine should be used except in those cases where vasopressor drugs may be contraindicated.

These recommended doses serve only as a guide to the amount of anesthetic required for most routine procedures. The actual volumes and concentrations to be used depend on a number of factors such as type and extent of surgical procedure, depth of anesthesia and degree of muscular relaxation required, duration of anesthesia required, and the physical condition of the patient. In all cases the lowest concentration and smallest dose that will produce the desired result should be given. Dosages should be reduced for children and for the elderly and debilitated patients and patients with cardiac and/or liver disease.

The onset of anesthesia, the duration of anesthesia and the degree of muscular relaxation are proportional to the volume and concentration (*i.e.,* total dose) of local anesthetic used. Thus, an increase in volume and concentration of Lidocaine HCl Injection will decrease the onset of anesthesia, prolong the duration anesthesia, provide a greater degree of muscular relaxation and increase the segmental spread of anesthesia. However, increasing the volume and concentration of Lidocaine HCl Injection may be result in a more profound fall in blood pressure when used in epidural anesthesia. Although the incidence of side effects with lidocaine is quite low, caution should be exercised when employing large volumes and concentrations, since the incidence of side effects is directly proportional to the total dose of local anesthetic agent injected.

For intravenous regional anesthesia, only the 50 ml single dose vial containing Lidocaine HCl (lidocaine HCl) 0.5% Injection should be used.

Epidural Anesthesia: For epidural anesthesia, only the following dosage forms of Lidocaine HCl Injection are recommended (TABLE 2):

TABLE 2

1% without epinephrine	30 ml ampules 30 ml single dose vials
1% with epinephrine 1:200,000	30 ml ampules 30 ml single dose vials
1.5% without epinephrine	20 ml ampules 20 ml single dose vials
1.5% with epinephrine 1:200,000	30 ml ampules 30 ml single dose vials
2% without epinephrine	10 ml ampules 10 ml single dose vials
2% with epinephrine 1:200,000	20 ml ampules 20 ml single dose vials

Although these solutions are intended specifically for epidural anesthesia, they may also be used for infiltration and peripheral nerve block, provided they are employed as single dose units. These solutions contain no bacteriostatic agent.

In epidural anesthesia, the dosage varies with the number of dermatomes to be anesthetized (generally 2-3 ml of the indicated concentration per dermatome).

Caudal and Lumbar Epidural Block: As a precaution against the adverse experience sometimes observed following unintentional penetration of the subarachnoid space, a test dose such as 2-3 ml of 1.5% lidocaine should be administered at least 5 minutes prior to injecting the total volume required for a lumbar or caudal epidural block. The test dose should be repeated if the patient is moved in a manner that may have displaced the catheter. Epinephrine, if contained in the test dose, (10- 15 mcg have been suggested), may serve as a warning of unintentional intravascular injection. If injected into a blood vessel, this amount of epinephrine is likely to produce a transient "epinephrine response" with 45 seconds, consisting of an increase in heart rate and systolic blood pressure, circumoral pallor, palpitations and nervousness in the unsedated patient. The sedated patient may exhibit only a pulse rate increase of 20 or more beats per minute for 15 or more seconds. Patients on beta blockers may not manifest changes in heart rate, but blood pressure monitoring can detect an evanescent rise in systolic blood pressure. Adequate time should be allowed for onset of anesthetic after administration of each test dose. The rapid injection of a large volume of Lidocaine HCl Injection through the catheter should be avoided, and when feasible, fractional doses should be administered.

In the event of the known injection of a large volume of local anesthetic solution into the subarachnoid space, after suitable resuscitation and if the catheter is in place, consider attempting the recovery of drug by draining a moderate amount of cerebrospinal fluid (such as 10 ml) through the epidural catheter.

DOSAGE AND ADMINISTRATION: *(cont'd)*

MAXIMUM RECOMMENDED DOSAGES

Adults: For normal healthy adults, the individual maximum recommended dose of lidocaine HCl with epinephrine should not exceed 7 mg/kg (3.5 mg/lb) of body weight, and in general it is recommended that the maximum total dose not exceed 500 mg. When used without epinephrine the maximum individual dose should not exceed 4.5 mg/kg (2 mg/lb) of body weight, and in general it is recommended that the maximum total dose does not exceed 300 mg. For continuous epidural or caudal anesthesia, the maximum recommended dosage should not be administered at intervals of less than 90 minutes. When continuous lumbar or caudal epidural anesthetic is used for non-obstetrical procedures, more drug may be administered if required to produce adequate anesthesia.

The maximum recommended dose per 90 minute period of lidocaine hydrochloride for paracervical block in obstetrical patients and non- obstetrical patients is 200 mg total. One half of the total dose is usually administered to each side. Inject slowly, five minutes between sides. (See also discussion of paracervical block in PRECAUTIONS).

For intravenous regional anesthesia, the dose administered should not exceed 4 mg/kg in adults.

Children: It is difficult to recommend a maximum dose of any drug of children, since this varies as a function of age and weight. For children over 3 years of age who have a normal lean body development, the maximum dose is determined by the child's age and weight. For example, in a child of 5 years weighing 50 lbs the dose of lidocaine HCl should not exceed 75-100 mg (1.5-2 mg/lb). The use of even more dilute solutions (*i.e.,* 0.25-0.5%) and total dosages not to exceed 3 mg/kg (1.4 mg/kg/lb) are recommended for induction of intravenous regional anesthesia in children.

In order to guard against systemic toxicity, the lowest effective concentration and lowest effective dose should be used at all times. In some cases it will be necessary to dilute available concentrations with 0.9% sodium chloride injection in order to obtain the required final concentration.

NOTE: Parenteral drug products should be inspected visually for particulate matter and discoloration prior to administration whenever the solution and container permit. The Injection is not to be used if its color is pinkish or darker than slightly yellow or if it contains a precipitate.

TABLE 3 Recommended Dosages

Procedure	Lidocaine Hydrochloride Injection (without epinephrine) Cone (%)	Vol (ml)	Total Dose (mg)
Infiltration			
Percutaneous	0.5 or 1	1-60	5-300
Intravenous regional	0.5	10-60	50-300
Peripheral Nerve Blocks, e.g.,			
Brachial	1.5	15-20	225-300
Dental	2	1-5	20-100
Intercostal	1	3	30
Paravertebral	1	3-5	30-50
Pudendal (each side)	1	10	100
Paracervical			
Obstetrical analgesia (each side)	1	10	100
Sympathetic Nerve Blocks, e.g.,			
Cervical (stellate ganglion)	1	5	50
Lumbar	1	5-10	50-100
Central Neural Blocks			
Epidural*			
Thoracic	1	20-30	200-300
Lumbar			
Analgesia	1	25-30	250-300
Anesthesia	1.5	15-20	225-300
	2	10-15	200-300
Caudal			
Obstetrical analgesia	1	20-30	200-300
Surgical anesthesia	1.5	15-20	225-300

* Dose determined by number of dermatomes to be anesthetized (2-3 ml/dermatome).

THE ABOVE SUGGESTED CONCENTRATIONS AND VOLUMES SERVE ONLY AS A GUIDE. OTHER VOLUMES AND CONCENTRATIONS MAY BE USED PROVIDED THE TOTAL MAXIMUM RECOMMENDED DOSE IS NOT EXCEED.

STERILIZATION, STORAGE AND TECHNICAL PROCEDURES

Disinfecting agents containing heavy, meals, which cause release of respective ions (mercury, zinc, copper, etc.) should not be used for skin or mucous membrane disinfection as they have been related to incidents of swelling and edema. When chemical disinfection of multi-dose vials is desired, either isopropyl alcohol (91%) or ethyl alcohol (70%) is recommended. Many commercially available brands of rubbing alcohol, as well as solutions of ethyl alcohol not of U.S.P. grade, contains denaturants which are injurious to rubber and therefore are not to be used.

Dosage forms listed as Lidocaine HCl-MPF indicates single dose solutions that are Methyl P araben Free (MPF).

All solutions should be stored at room temperature, approximately (25°C (77°F). Protect from light.

For Ventricular Arrhythmias: ADULTS Single Direct Intravenous Injection (bolus): ONLY THE 5 ML, 50 MG or 100 MG DOSAGE SIZES should be used for direct intravenous injection. The usual dose is 50 to 100 mg of lidocaine hydrochloride (0.70 to 1.4 mg/kg; 0.32 to 0.63 mg/lb) administered intravenously under ECG monitoring. This dose may be administered at the rate of approximately 25 to 50 mg/min (0.35 to 0.70 mg/kg/min; 0.16 to 0.32 mg/lb/min). Sufficient time should be allowed to enable a slow circulation to carry the drug to the site of action. If the initial injection of 50 to 100 mg does not produce a desired response, a second dosage may be injected after 5 minutes. The syringe should be activated immediately prior to the injection. NO MORE THAN 200 TO 300 MG OF LIDOCAINE HYDROCHLORIDE SHOULD BE ADMINISTERED DURING A ONE HOUR PERIOD.

Continuous Intravenous Infusion: Following bolus administration, intravenous infusions of Lidocaine HCl Injection may be initiated at the rate of 1 to 4 mg/min of lidocaine hydrochloride (0.014 to 0.057 mg/kg/min; 0.006 to 0.026 mg/lb/min). The rate of intravenous infusions should be reassessed as soon as the patient's basic cardiac rhythm appears to be stable or at the earliest signs of toxicity. It should rarely be necessary to continue intravenous infusions of lidocaine for prolonged periods.

Solutions for intravenous infusion may be prepared by the addition of one gram (or two grams) of lidocaine hydrochloride to one liter of 5% dextrose in water using aseptic technique. Approximately a 0.1% (or 0.2%) solution will result from this procedure; that is, each milliliter will contain approximately 1 (or 2 mg) of lidocaine hydrochloride. In those cases in which fluid restriction is medically appropriate, a more concentrated solution may be prepared.

DOSAGE AND ADMINISTRATION: *(cont'd)*

Lidocaine HCl Injection has been found to be chemically stable for 24 hours after dilution in 5% dextrose in water. However, as with all intravenous dilution of the solution should be made just prior to its administration.

Parenteral drug products should be inspected visually for particulate matter and discoloration prior to administration whenever the solution and container permit. Do not use if solution is discolored or cloudy.

PEDIATRIC

Although controlled clinical studies to establish pediatric dosing schedules have not been conducted, the American Heart Association's *Standards and Guidelines*recommends a bolus dose of 1 mg/kg followed by an infusion rate of 30 mcg/kg/min.

Note regarding prolonged infusions: There are data that indicate the half-life may be 3 hours longer following infusions greater than 24 hours in duration.

Solutions should be stored at controlled room temperature 15-30° (59-86°F)

Spinal Anesthesia: Spinal anesthesia with Xylocaine-MPF 5% with Glucose 7.5% (lidocaine HCl and dextrose injection, USP) may be induced in the right or left lateral recumbent or the sitting position. Since this is a hyperbaric solution, the anesthetic will tend to move in the direction in which the table is tilted. After the desired level of anesthesia is obtained and the anesthetic has become fixed, usually in 5- 10 minutes with lidocaine, the patient may be positioned according to the requirement of the surgeon or obstetrician.

In clinical trials, the safety of hyperbaric Xylocaine for single injection spinal anesthesia was demonstrated using 22 or 25 gauge spinal needles. In these studies, free flow of CSF was visible before injection of Xylocaine.

Neurologic deficits have been reported with the use of small bore needles and microcatheters for spinal anesthesia. It has been postulated, based on *in vitro* models, that these deficits were caused by pooling and non-uniform distribution of concentrated local anesthetic within the subarachnoid space. Animal studies suggest that mixing 5% Xylocaine with an equal volume of CSF or preservative-free 0.9% saline solution may reduce the risk of nerve injury due to pooling of concentrated local anesthetic.

Intrathecal distribution of anesthetic may be facilitated by using a spinal needle of sufficient gauge to insure adequate withdrawal of CSF through the needle prior to and after anesthetic administration. If the technique is properly performed and the drug is properly placed in the subarachnoid space, a separate injection is seldom necessary.

An incomplete or patchy block not responsive to patient repositioning may indicate misplacement or inadequate distribution of drug. To avoid excessive drug pooling, additional doses of xylocaine should not be administered with the same needle placement.

INJECTIONS SHOULD BE MADE SLOWLY. Consult standard textbooks for specific techniques for spinal anesthetic procedures.

RECOMMENDED DOSAGES

Normal Healthy Adults: The following recommended dosages are for normal healthy adults and serve only as a guide to the amount of anesthetic required for most routine procedures. In all cases, the smallest dose that will produce the desired result should be given.

If the technique is properly performed, and the needle is properly placed in the subarachnoid space, it should not be necessary to administer more than one ampule (100 mg).

Obstetrical Low Spinal or "Saddle Block" Anesthesia—The dosage recommended for normal vaginal delivery is approximately 1 ml (50 mg). For Caesarean section and those deliveries requiring intrauterine manipulations, 1.5 (75 mg) is usually adequate.

Surgical Anesthesia—The dosage recommended for abdominal anesthesia is 1.5-2 ml (75-100 mg).

Children: The dosage recommendations in healthy adolescents, 16 years of age and older, is the same as for normal healthy adults. There is insufficient data in children below the age of 16 years to make dosage recommendations (see PRECAUTIONS.)

NOTE: Parenteral drug products should be inspected visually for particulate matter and discoloration prior to administration whenever the solution and container permit. Solutions that are discolored and/or contain particulate matter should not be used.

REFERENCES:

(Spinal Anesthesia: Astra, 4/95, 021564R12)

HOW SUPPLIED - RATED THERAPEUTICALLY EQUIVALENT:

Injection, Solution - 0.5 %

50 ml	$3.22	0.5% Lidocaine Hcl Injecti, Abbott	00074-4275-01
50 ml	$3.22	0.5% Lidocaine Hcl, Abbott	00074-4278-01
50 ml	$3.79	XYLOCAINE, Astra USA	00186-0135-01
50 ml	$9.44	XYLOCAINE, Astra USA	00186-0137-01

Injection, Solution - 1 %

2 ml x 10	$14.56	XYLOCAINE, Astra USA	00186-0210-03
2 ml x 10	$14.61	XYLOCAINE, Astra USA	00186-0276-13
2 ml x 10	$20.74	XYLOC, Astra USA	00186-0241-13
2 ml x 25	$24.38	Lidocaine Hcl 1%, Fujisawa USA	00469-1201-15
5 ml	$1.51	1% Lidocaine Hcl, Abbott	00074-4713-01
5 ml	$2.08	Lidocaine Hcl, Abbott	00074-4713-02
5 ml	$4.75	Lidocaine Hcl, Intl Medication	00548-1111-00
5 ml	$4.84	Lidocaine Hcl, Intl Medication	00548-1192-00
5 ml	$9.99	LIDOCAINE HCL, Abbott	00074-4904-15
5 ml	$9.99	LIDOCAINE HCL, Abbott	00074-4924-15
5 ml	$10.79	1% Lidocaine Hcl, Abbott	00074-8026-01
5 ml	$10.89	Lidocaine Hcl, Abbott	00074-4904-23
5 ml	$11.33	LIDOCAINE HCL, Abbott	00074-4904-34
5 ml	$23.24	XYLOCAINE, Astra USA	00186-0615-01
5 ml x 10	$18.73	XYLOCAINE, Astra USA	00186-0277-13
5 ml x 10	$19.68	XYLOCAINE, Astra USA	00186-0230-03
5 ml x 10	$32.40	Lidocaine Hcl, Voluntary Hosp	53258-9149-08
5 ml x 10	$72.63	Lidocaine Hcl, Fujisawa USA	00469-9149-87
5 ml x 25	$16.15	Lidocaine Hcl, Elkins Sinn	00641-0436-25
5 ml x 25	$30.00	Lidocaine Hcl, Consolidated Midland	00223-7936-05
10 ml	$4.43	Lidocaine Hcl, Intl Medication	00548-1193-00
10 ml	$5.39	Lidocaine Hcl, Intl Medication	00548-1115-00
10 ml	$72.63	Lidocaine Hcl, Fujisawa USA	00469-9161-87
10 ml x 5	$8.51	XYLOCAINE, Astra USA	00186-0275-12
10 ml x 5	$24.25	XYLOCAINE, Astra USA	00186-0278-12
10 ml x 10	$45.00	Lidocaine Hcl, Voluntary Hosp	53258-9161-08
10 ml x 25	$21.25	Lidocaine Hcl Inj 1 %, Fujisawa USA	00469-2201-25
20 ml	$2.11	XYLOCAINE 1%, Astra USA	00186-0110-01
20 ml	$2.24	1% Lidocaine Hcl, Abbott	00074-4276-01
20 ml	$2.28	XYLOCAINE, Astra USA	00186-0120-01
20 ml	$8.04	Lidocaine Hcl, Intl Medication	00548-1078-00
20 ml	$9.48	Lidocaine Hcl Inj 1%, Intl Medication	00548-1080-00
30 ml	$1.56	1% Lidocaine Hcl, Abbott	00074-4279-02
30 ml	$1.88	Lidocaine Hcl, HL Moore Drug Exch	00839-5599-36
30 ml	$7.68	1% Lidocaine Hcl, Abbott	00074-4270-01
30 ml	$7.71	XYLOCAINE, Astra USA	00186-0112-01
30 ml	$8.51	Lidocaine Hcl, Intl Medication	00548-1079-00

HOW SUPPLIED - RATED THERAPEUTICALLY EQUIVALENT: *(cont'd)*

30 ml	$10.70	Lidocaine Hcl, Intl Medication	00548-1081-00
30 ml x 5	$41.89	XYLOCAINE, Astra USA	00186-0112-91
30 ml x 5	$45.04	XYLOCAINE, Astra USA	00186-0255-02
30 ml x 5	$49.85	XYLOCAINE, Astra USA	00186-0255-92
30 ml x 25	$15.00	Lidocaine Hcl, Elkins Sinn	00641-2380-45
30 ml x 25	$28.75	Lidocaine Hcl, Consolidated Midland	00223-7933-30
50 ml	$1.75	Lidocaine Hcl, Consolidated Midland	00223-7953-50
50 ml	$1.79	Lidocaine Hcl, Balan	00304-2012-51
50 ml	$2.05	Lidocaine Hcl, HL Moore Drug Exch	00839-5597-38
50 ml	$2.10	Lidocaine Hcl, Pasadena	00418-1141-50
50 ml	$2.50	TRUXACAINE 1%, C O Truxton	00463-1077-50
50 ml	$2.79	1% Lidocaine Hcl, Abbott	00074-4276-02
50 ml	$2.85	L-CAINE, Century Pharms	00436-0226-79
50 ml	$2.90	Lidocaine Hcl, United Res	00677-0281-24
50 ml	$2.95	UAD CAINE, UAD Labs	00785-9065-55
50 ml	$3.00	Lidocaine Hcl 1%, Goldline Labs	00182-0565-67
50 ml	$3.05	Lidocaine Hcl, Steris Labs	00402-0055-50
50 ml	$3.25	Lidocaine, Schein Pharm (US)	00364-6549-57
50 ml	$3.25	Lidocaine HCl, Forest Pharms	00456-0779-83
50 ml	$3.48	XYLOCAINE, Astra USA	00186-0145-01
50 ml	$3.50	Lidocaine Hcl, Hyrex Pharms	00314-0679-50
50 ml	$4.88	Lidocaine HCl, Rugby	00536-1450-80
50 ml	$6.60	LIDOJECT-1, Mayrand Pharms	00259-0325-50
50 ml x 25	$20.63	Lidocaine Hcl, Elkins Sinn	00641-2390-45
50 ml x 25	$27.19	Lidocaine Hcl, Am Regent	00517-0625-25
50 ml x 25	$36.25	Lidocaine Hcl, Fujisawa USA	00469-3201-25

Injection, Solution - 1.5 %

10 ml x 5	$26.66	XYLOCAINE, Astra USA	00186-0244-12
20 ml	$5.96	1.5% Lidocaine Hcl, Abbott	00074-4056-01
20 ml	$8.43	1.5% Lidocaine Hcl Inj., Abbott	00074-4776-01
20 ml	$10.46	XYLOCAINE, Astra USA	00186-0118-01
20 ml x 5	$47.20	XYLOCAINE, Astra USA	00186-0245-02
20 ml x 5	$52.81	XYLOCAINE, Astra USA	00186-0118-91

Injection, Solution - 2 %

1.8 ml cartridg	$35.00	XYLOCAINE, Astra USA	00186-0170-14
2 ml	$1.51	2% Lidocaine Hcl, Abbott	00074-4282-01
2 ml x 10	$18.24	XYLOCAINE, Astra USA	00186-0215-03
2 ml x 25	$21.25	Lidocaine Hcl 2%, Fujisawa USA	00469-1202-25
5 ml	$4.75	Lidocaine Hcl, Intl Medication	00548-1112-00
5 ml	$5.03	Lidocaine Hcl, Intl Medication	00548-1190-00
5 ml	$9.30	2% Lidocaine Hcl, Abbott	00074-8027-01
5 ml	$10.45	LIDOCAINE HCL, Abbott	00074-4923-15
5 ml	$10.48	Lidocaine Hcl, Intl Medication	00548-2190-00
5 ml	$11.33	Lidocaine Hcl, Abbott	00074-4903-23
5 ml	$11.53	Lidocaine Hcl, Intl Medication	00548-3190-00
5 ml x 10	$19.56	XYLOCAINE, Astra USA	00186-0242-13
5 ml x 10	$22.83	XYLOCAINE, Astra USA	00186-0611-01
5 ml x 10	$40.20	Lidocaine Hcl, Voluntary Hosp	53258-9142-08
5 ml x 10	$43.19	XYLOCAINE, Astra USA	00186-0232-03
5 ml x 25	$16.15	Lidocaine Hcl, Elkins Sinn	00641-0437-25
5 ml x 25	$30.00	Lidocaine Hcl, Consolidated Midland	00223-7937-05
5 ml x 25	$30.94	Lidocaine Hcl, Fujisawa USA	00469-1208-25
5 x 10 ml.	$28.83	XYLOCAINE, Astra USA	00186-0240-02
10 ml	$2.51	2% Lidocaine Hcl, Abbott	00074-4282-02
10 ml x 5	$10.01	XYLOCAINE, Astra USA	00186-0243-12
10 ml x 5	$29.13	XYLOCAINE, Astra USA	00186-0240-12
20 ml	$2.24	2% Lidocaine Hcl, Abbott	00074-4277-01
30 ml	$2.60	2% Lidocaine Hcl, Abbott	00074-4281-02
30 ml x 25	$15.94	Lidocaine Hcl, Elkins Sinn	00641-2400-45
30 ml x 25	$31.75	Lidocaine Hcl, Consolidated Midland	00223-7935-30
50 ml	$2.00	Lidocaine Hcl, Consolidated Midland	00223-7952-00
50 ml	$2.20	Lidocaine Hcl, Pasadena	00418-1201-50
50 ml	$2.21	Lidocaine Hcl, HL Moore Drug Exch	00839-5598-38
50 ml	$2.50	TRUXACAINE 2%, C O Truxton	00463-1078-50
50 ml	$2.69	Lidocaine Hcl, Balan	00304-1318-51
50 ml	$2.75	Lidocaine Hcl, UAD Labs	00785-8050-55
50 ml	$2.85	Lidocaine Hcl, Major Pharms	00904-0865-50
50 ml	$3.00	Lidocaine Hcl 2%, Goldline Labs	00182-0566-67
50 ml	$3.10	Lidocaine Hcl, Steris Labs	00402-0056-50
50 ml	$3.22	2% Lidocaine Hcl, Abbott	00074-4277-02
50 ml	$3.25	Lidocaine HCl, Forest Pharms	00456-0782-83
50 ml	$3.33	Lidocaine HCl, Schein Pharm (US)	00364-6551-57
50 ml	$3.50	Lidocaine Hcl, Hyrex Pharms	00314-0680-50
50 ml	$4.36	XYLOCAINE, Astra USA	00186-0155-01
50 ml	$6.60	LIDOJECT-2, Mayrand Pharms	00259-0326-50
50 ml x 25	$21.56	Lidocaine Hcl, Elkins Sinn	00641-2410-45
50 ml x 25	$30.94	Lidocaine Hcl, Am Regent	00517-0626-25
50 ml x 25	$40.00	Lidocaine Hcl, Consolidated Midland	00223-7952-25

Injection, Solution - 4 %

5 ml	$2.98	4% Lidocaine Hcl, Abbott	00074-4283-01
25 ml	$1.59	XYLOCAINE, Astra USA	00186-0166-01
25 ml	$2.25	XYLOCAINE, Astra USA	00186-0167-01
25 ml x 10	$40.00	Lidocaine Hcl, Voluntary Hosp	53258-9179-08
25 ml x 10	$118.13	Lidocaine Hcl, Fujisawa USA	00469-9179-87
25 ml x 12	$18.14	Lidocaine Hcl, Fujisawa USA	00469-2214-01
50 ml	$2.03	XYLOCAINE, Astra USA	00186-0169-01
50 ml	$2.53	XYLOCAINE, Astra USA	00186-0168-01
50 ml x 10	$40.00	Lidocaine Hcl, Voluntary Hosp	53258-9140-09
50 ml x 10	$165.50	Lidocaine Hcl, Fujisawa USA	00469-9140-90
50 ml x 12	$21.70	Lidocaine Hcl, Fujisawa USA	00469-2215-01

Injection, Solution - 10 %

10 ml	$8.65	10% Lidocaine Hcl, Abbott	00074-6254-01

Injection, Solution - 20 %

5 ml	$10.45	LIDOCAINE HCL, Abbott	00074-4903-15
5 ml	$11.78	LIDOCAINE HCL, Abbott	00074-4903-34
5 ml	$12.40	20% Lidocaine Hcl, Abbott	00074-6249-01
5 ml x 10	$72.63	Lidocaine Hcl, Fujisawa USA	00469-9151-87
5 ml x 10	$122.00	Lidocaine Hcl, Fujisawa USA	00469-9142-87
10 ml	$11.93	20% Lidocaine Hcl, Abbott	00074-6248-01
10 ml	$15.77	20% Lidocaine Hcl, Abbott	00074-6217-02
10 ml	$18.13	20% Lidocaine Hcl, Abbott	00074-6250-01
10 ml x 10	$176.13	Lidocaine Hcl, Fujisawa USA	00469-9143-87
500 ml	$10.27	0.2% Lidocaine Hcl In 5% Dextrose I, Abbott	00074-1516-03

Injection, Solution - Intravenous - 50 mg

2 ml	$5.53	Lidocaine Hcl & Dextrose 7.5%, Abbott	00074-4712-01

Jel - Topical; Oral - 2 %

5 ml x 100	**$65.63**	**XYLOCAINE, Astra USA**	**00186-0330-36**
30 gm	$12.85	Lidocaine Hcl, Copley Pharm	38245-0200-11

HOW SUPPLIED - RATED THERAPEUTICALLY EQUIVALENT: *(cont'd)*

Kit - Intracavity; In - 4 %

5 kits	$38.23	XYLOCAINE, Astra USA	00186-0235-72
5 ml x 10	$58.85	XYLOCAINE, Astra USA	00186-0235-03

Ointment - Topical - 5 %

50 gm	$2.36	Lidocaine HCl, HL Moore Drug Exch	00839-5474-81

Solution - Topical; Oral - 2 %

20 ml	$0.63	Lidocaine Hcl, H.C.F.A. F F P	99999-1639-03
50 ml	$4.10	Lidocaine Hcl 2% Viscous, Major Pharms	00904-0863-04
100 ml	$2.85	Lidocaine Hcl Viscous, Raway	00686-0996-33
100 ml	$3.15	Lidocaine HCl, H.C.F.A. F F P	99999-1639-01
100 ml	$3.64	Lidocaine Hcl Viscous, Morton Grove	60432-0464-00
100 ml	$3.95	Lidocaine Hcl Viscous, Harber Pharm	51432-0622-14
100 ml	$4.02	Lidocaine Hcl Viscous, Aligen Independ	00405-3150-60
100 ml	$4.35	Lidocaine HCl Viscous, Schein Pharm (US)	00364-7282-61
450 ml	$14.18	Lidocaine Hcl, H.C.F.A. F F P	99999-1639-02

HOW SUPPLIED - NOT RATED EQUIVALENT:

Injection, Solution - 1.5 %

2 ml x 10	$91.73	XYLOCAINE 1.5%, WITH DEXTROSE 7.5%, Astra USA	00186-0212-03

Ointment - Topical - 5 %

35 gm	$2.50	Lidocaine Hcl, Consolidated Midland	00223-4351-35

Powder

30 gm	$11.90	Lidocaine Hcl, Millgood	53118-0511-01
120 gm	$32.00	Lidocaine Hcl, Millgood	53118-0511-04
454 gm	$91.00	Lidocaine Hcl, Millgood	53118-0511-10

LIDOCAINE; OXYTETRACYCLINE HYDROCHLORIDE *(001640)*

CATEGORIES: Acne; Amebiasis; Anti-Infectives; Antibiotics; Antimicrobials; Antiprotozoals; Conjunctivitis; EENT Drugs; Eye, Ear, Nose, & Throat Preparations; Granuloma; Lyme Disease; Lymphogranuloma; Parasiticidal; Pneumonia; Rickettsial Disease; Rocky Mountain Fever; Tetracyclines; Typhoid Fever; FDA Pre 1938 Drugs

BRAND NAMES: **Terramycin**

Prescribing information not available at time of publication.

HOW SUPPLIED - EQUIVALENTS NOT AVAILABLE:

Injection, Solution - Intramuscular - 100 mg/2ml

5's	**$39.73**	**TERRAMYCIN, Roerig**	**00049-0750-77**

LIDOCAINE; PRILOCAINE *(003146)*

CATEGORIES: Anesthesia; Antipruritics/Local Anesthetics; Dermatologicals; Local Anesthetics; Pain; Skin/Mucous Membrane Agents; Topical Anesthetics; Pregnancy Category B; FDA Approved 1992 Dec

BRAND NAMES: **Emla**; *Emla Cream*
(International brand names outside U.S. in italics)

DESCRIPTION:

Lidocaine 2.5% and prilocaine 2.5% is an emulsion in which the oil phase is a eutectic mixture of lidocaine and prilocaine in a ratio of 1:1 by weight. A eutectic mixture has a melting point below room temperature and therefore both local anesthetics exist as a liquid oil rather than as crystals.

Lidocaine is chemically designated as acetamide, 2-(diethylamino)-N(2,6-dimethylphenyl), has an octanol:water partition ratio of 43 at pH 7.4.

Prilocaine is chemically designated as propanamide, N-(2-methyl-phenyl)-2-(propylamino) and has an octanol:water partition ratio of 25 at pH 7.4.

Each gram of EMLA Cream contains lidocaine 25 mg, prilocaine 25 mg, polyoxyethylene fatty acid esters (as emulsifiers), carboxypolymethylene (as a thickening agent), sodium hydroxide to adjust to a pH approximating 9, and purified water (about 92%) to 1 gram. Lidocaine 2.5% and prilocaine 2.5% cream contains no preservative, however it passes the USP antimicrobial effectiveness test due to the pH. The specific gravity of this drug is 1.00.

CLINICAL PHARMACOLOGY:

MECHANISM OF ACTION

Lidocaine 2.5% and prilocaine 2.5%, applied to intact skin under occlusive dressing, provides dermal analgesia by the release of lidocaine and prilocaine from the cream into the epidermal and dermal layers of the skin and the accumulation of lidocaine and prilocaine in the vicinity of dermal pain receptors and nerve endings. Lidocaine and prilocaine are amide-type local anesthetic agents. Both lidocaine and prilocaine stabilize neuronal membranes by inhibiting the ionic fluxes required for the initiation and conduction of impulses, thereby effecting local anesthetic action.

The onset, depth and duration of dermal analgesia provided by Lidocaine 2.5% and prilocaine 2.5% cream depends primarily on the duration of application. To provide sufficient analgesia for clinical procedures such as IV catheter placement and venipuncture, Lidocaine 2.5% and prilocaine 2.5% cream should be applied under an occlusive dressing for at least 1 hour. To provide dermal analgesia for clinical procedures such as split skin graft harvesting, Lidocaine 2.5% and prilocaine 2.5% cream should be applied under occlusive dressing for at least 2 hours. Satisfactory dermal analgesia is achieved 1 hour after application, reaches maximum at 2 to 3 hours, and persists for 1 to 2 hours after removal.

Dermal application of Lidocaine 2.5% and prilocaine 2.5% cream may cause a transient, local blanching followed by a transient, local redness or erythema.

Pharmacokinetics: Lidocaine 2.5% and prilocaine 2.5% cream is a eutectic mixture of lidocaine 2.5% and prilocaine 2.5% formulated as an oil in water emulsion. As a eutectic mixture, both anesthetics are liquid at room temperature (see DESCRIPTION) and the penetration and subsequent systemic absorption of both prilocaine and lidocaine are enhanced over that which would be seen if each component in crystalline form was applied separately as 2.5% topical cream.

The amount of lidocaine and prilocaine systemically absorbed from lidocaine 2.5% and prilocaine 2.5% cream is directly related to both the duration of application and the area over which it is applied. In two pharmacokinetic studies, 60 g of EMLA Cream (1.5 g lidocaine and 1.5 g prilocaine) was applied to 400 cm^2 of intact skin on the lateral thigh and then

CLINICAL PHARMACOLOGY: *(cont'd)*

covered by an occlusive dressing. The subjects were then randomized such that one-half of the subjects had the occlusive dressing and residual cream removed after 3 hours, while the remainder left the dressing in place for 24 hours. The results from these studies are summarized in TABLE 1.

TABLE 1 Absorption of Lidocaine and Prilocaine from EMLA Cream Normal Volunteers (N=16)

EMLA(g)	Area (cm²)	Time on (hrs)	Drug Content (mg)	Absorbed (mg)	C_{max} (mcg/ml)	T_{max}(hr)
60	400	3	lidocaine 1500	54	0.12	4
			prilocaine 1500	92	0.07	4
60	400	24*	lidocaine 1500	243	0.28	10
			prilocaine 1500	503	0.14	10

* Maximum recommended duration of exposure is 4 hours.

When Lidocaine 2.5% and prilocaine 2.5% cream is used according to the recommended dosing instructions, peak blood levels of lidocaine are approximately 1/20 the systemic toxic level. Likewise, the maximum prilocaine level is about 1/36 the toxic level. The application of Lidocaine 2.5% and prilocaine 2.5% cream to broken or inflamed skin, or to 2,000 cm²or more of skin where more of both anesthetics are absorbed, could result in higher plasma levels that could, in susceptible individuals, produce a systemic pharmacologic response. When each drug is administered intravenously, the steady-state volume of distribution is 1:1 to 2:1 l/kg (mean 1.5 ± 0.3 SD, n=13) for lidocaine and 0.7 to 4.4 l/kg (mean 2.6, ± 1.3 SD,n=13) for prilocaine. The larger distribution volume for prilocaine produces the lower plasma concentrations of prilocaine observed when equal amounts of prilocaine and lidocaine are administered. At concentrations produced by application of Lidocaine 2.5% and prilocaine 2.5% cream, lidocaine is approximately 70% bound to plasma proteins, primary alpha-1-acid glycoprotein. At much higher plasma concentrations (1 to 4 mcg/ml of free base) the plasma protein binding of lidocaine is concentration dependent. Prilocaine is 55% bound to plasma proteins. Both lidocaine and prilocaine cross the placental and blood brain barrier, presumably by passive diffusion.

It is not known if lidocaine or prilocaine are metabolized in the skin. Lidocaine is metabolized rapidly by the liver to a number of metabolites including monoethylglycinexylidide (MEGX) and glycinexylidide (GX), both of which have pharmacologic activity similar to, but less potent than that of lidocaine. The metabolite 2,6-xylidine, has unknown pharmacologic activity but is carcinogenic in rats (see PRECAUTIONS, Carcinogenesis). Following IV administration, MEGX and GX concentrations in serum range from 11 to 36% and from 5 to 11% of lidocaine concentrations, respectively. Prilocaine is metabolized in both the liver and kidneys by amidases to various metabolites including *ortho*-toluidine and N-n-propylalanine. It is not metabolized by plasma esterases. The *ortho*-toluidine metabolite has been shown to be carcinogenic in several animal modes. (see PRECAUTIONS, Carcinogenesis). In addition, ortho-toluidine can produce methemoglobinemia following systemic doses of prilocaine approximating 8 mg/kg (see ADVERSE REACTIONS). Very young patients, patients with glucose-6-phosphate deficiencies, and patients taking oxidizing drugs such as antimalarials and sulfonamides are more susceptible to methemoglobinemia (see PRECAUTIONS, Methemoglobinemia).

The half-life of lidocaine elimination from the plasma following IV administration is approximately 65 to 150 minutes (mean 110 ± 24 SD, n=13). This half-life may be increased in cardiac or hepatic dysfunction. More than 98% of an absorbed dose of lidocaine can be recovered in the urine as metabolites or parent drug. The systemic clearance is 10 to 20 ml/min/kg (mean 13, ± 3 SD, n=13). The elimination half-life of prilocaine is approximately 10 to 150 minutes (mean 70, ± 48 SD, n=13). The systemic clearance is 18 to 64 ml/min/kg (mean 38, ± 15 SD, n=13). Prilocaine's half-life may also be increased in hepatic or renal dysfunction since both of these organs are involved in prilocaine metabolism.

Individualization of Dose: The dose of Lidocaine 2.5% and prilocaine 2.5% cream which provides effective analgesia depends on the duration of the application over the treated area.

All pharmacokinetic and clinical studies employed a thick layer of Lidocaine 2.5% and prilocaine 2.5% cream (1-2 g/10 cm²). The duration of application prior to venipuncture was 1 hour. The duration of application prior to taking split thickness skin grafts was 2 hours. Although a thinner application may be efficacious, such has not been studied and may result in less complete analgesia or a shorter duration of adequate analgesia.

The systemic absorption of lidocaine and prilocaine is a side effect of the desired local effect. The amount of drug absorbed depends on surface area and duration of application. The systemic blood levels depend on the amount absorbed and patient size (weight) and rate of systemic drug elimination. Long duration of application, large treatment area, small patients, or impaired elimination may result in high blood levels. The systemic blood levels are typically a small fraction (1/20 to 1/50) of the blood levels which produce toxicity. TABLE 2 gives the maximum recommended application areas for infants and children.

TABLE 2 Recommended Application Area* For Infants and Children Based on Application to Intact Skin

Body Weight (kg)	Maximum Skin Area (cm²)**
up to 10 kg	100
10 to 20 kg	600
above 20 kg	2000

* These are broad guidelines for avoiding systemic toxicity in applying EMLA Cream to patients with normal intact skin and with normal renal and hepatic function.
** For more individualized calculation of how much lidocaine and prilocaine may be absorbed, physicians can use the following estimates of lidocaine and prilocaine absorption for children and adults:
The estimated mean (± SD) absorption of lidocaine is 0.045 (± 0.016) mg/cm²/hr.
The estimated mean (± SD) absorption of prilocaine is 0.077 (± 0.036) mg/cm²/hr.

An IV antiarrhythmic dose of lidocaine is 1 mg/kg (70 mg/70 kg) and gives a blood level of about 1 mcg/ml. Toxicity would be expected at blood levels above 5 mcg/ml. Smaller areas of treatment are recommended in a debilitated patient, a small child or a patient with impaired elimination. Decreasing the duration of application is likely to decrease the analgesic effect.

CLINICAL STUDIES:

Lidocaine 2.5% and prilocaine 2.5% cream application in adults prior to IV cannulation or venipuncture was studied in 200 patients in four clinical studies in Europe. Application for at least 1 hour provided significantly more dermal analgesia than placebo cream or ethyl chloride. Lidocaine 2.5% and prilocaine 2.5% cream was comparable to subcutaneous lidocaine, but was less efficacious than intradermal lidocaine. Most patients found lidocaine 2.5% and prilocaine 2.5% cream treatment preferable to lidocaine infiltration or ethyl chloride spray.

Lidocaine 2.5% and prilocaine 2.5% cream was compared with 0.5% lidocaine infiltration prior to skin graft harvesting in one open label study in 80 adult patients in England. Application of lidocaine 2.5% and prilocaine 2.5% cream for 2 to 5 hours provided dermal analgesia comparable to lidocaine infiltration.

Lidocaine 2.5% and prilocaine 2.5% cream application in children was studied in seven non-US studies (320 patients) and one US study (100 patients). In controlled studies, application of Lidocaine 2.5% and prilocaine 2.5% cream for at least 1 hour with or without presurgical medication prior to needle insertion provided significantly more pain reduction than placebo. In children under the age of seven years, lidocaine 2.5% and prilocaine 2.5% cream was less effective than in older children or adults.

Lidocaine 2.5% and prilocaine 2.5% cream was compared with placebo in the laser treatment of facial port-wine stains in 72 pediatric patients (ages 5-16). Lidocaine 2.5% and prilocaine 2.5% cream was effective in providing pain relief during laser treatment.

Local dermal effects associated with lidocaine 2.5% and prilocaine 2.5% cream application in these studies on intact skin included paleness, redness and edema and were transient in nature (see ADVERSE REACTIONS).

INDICATIONS AND USAGE:

A eutectic mixture of lidocaine 2.5% and prilocaine 2.5% is indicated as a topical anesthetic for use on **normal, intact skin** for local analgesia.

Lidocaine 2.5% and prilocaine 2.5% cream is not recommended for use on mucous membranes because limited studies show much greater absorption of lidocaine and prilocaine than through intact skin. Safe dosing recommendations for use on mucous membranes cannot be made because it has not been studied adequately.

Lidocaine 2.5% and prilocaine 2.5% cream is not recommended in any clinical situation in which penetration or migration beyond the tympanic membrane into the middle ear is possible because of the ototoxic effects observed in animal studies (see WARNINGS).

CONTRAINDICATIONS:

Lidocaine 2.5% and prilocaine 2.5% is contraindicated in patients with a known history of sensitivity to local anesthetics of the amide type or to any other component of the product.

WARNINGS:

Application of Lidocaine 2.5% and prilocaine 2.5% cream to larger areas or for longer times than those recommended could result in sufficient absorption of lidocaine and prilocaine resulting in serious adverse effects (see CLINICAL PHARMACOLOGY, Individualization of Dose).

Studies in laboratory animals (guinea pigs) have shown that lidocaine 2.5% and prilocaine 2.5% cream has an ototoxic effect when instilled into the middle ear. In these same studies, animals exposed to lidocaine 2.5% and prilocaine 2.5% cream in the external auditory canal only, showed no abnormality. Lidocaine 2.5% and prilocaine 2.5% cream should not be used in any clinical situation in which its penetration or migration beyond the tympanic membrane into the middle ear is possible.

METHEMOGLOBINEMIA

Lidocaine 2.5% and prilocaine 2.5% cream should not be used in those rare patients with congenital or idiopathic methemoglobinemia and in infants under the age of twelve months who are receiving treatment with methemoglobin-inducing agents.

Very young patients or patients with glucose-6-phosphate deficiencies are more susceptible to methemoglobinemia.

Patients taking drugs associated with drug-induced methemoglobinemia such as sulfonamides, acetaminophen, acetanilid, aniline dyes, benzocaine, chloroquine, dapsone, naphthalene, nitrates and nitrites, nitrofurantoin, nitroglycerin, nitroprusside, pamaquine, para-aminosalicylic acid, phenacetin, phenobarbital, phenytoin, primaquine, quinine, are also at greater risk for developing methemoglobinemia.

A Methemoglobinemia value of 28% (of total hemoglobin) developed in a three-month old male infant (5.3 kg) who had 5 grams of Lidocaine 2.5% and prilocaine 2.5% cream under an occlusive dressing applied to the back of the hands and in the cubital regions for 5 hours. The methemoglobinemia was successfully treated with IV methylene blue. The patient was concomitantly receiving trimethoprim (16 mg/day) and sulfamethoxazole (80 mg/day) for a urinary tract infection.

PRECAUTIONS:

GENERAL

Repeated doses of Lidocaine 2.5% and prilocaine 2.5% cream may increase blood levels of lidocaine and prilocaine. Lidocaine 2.5% and prilocaine 2.5% cream should be used with caution in patients who may be more sensitive to the systemic effects of lidocaine and prilocaine including acutely ill, debilitated, or elderly patients.

Lidocaine 2.5% and prilocaine 2.5% cream coming in contact with the eye should be avoided because animal studies have demonstrated severe eye irritation. Also the loss of protective reflexes can permit corneal irritation and potential abrasions. Absorption of Lidocaine 2.5% and prilocaine 2.5% cream in conjunctival tissues has not yet been determined. If eye contact occurs, immediately wash out the eye with water or saline and protect the eye until sensitization returns.

Patients allergic to para-aminobenzoic acid derivatives (procaine, tetracaine, benzocaine, etc.) have not shown cross sensitivity to lidocaine or prilocaine, however, Lidocaine 2.5% and prilocaine 2.5% cream should be used with caution in patients with a history of drug sensitivities, especially if the etiologic agent is uncertain.

Patients with severe hepatic disease, because of their inability to metabolize local anesthetics normally, are at greater risk of developing toxic plasma concentrations of lidocaine and prilocaine

INFORMATION FOR PATIENTS

When Lidocaine 2.5% and prilocaine 2.5% cream is used, the patient should be aware that the production of dermal analgesia may be accompanied by the block of all sensations in the treated skin. For this reason, the patient should avoid inadvertent trauma to the treated area by scratching, rubbing, or exposure to extreme hot or cold temperatures until complete sensation has returned.

Prilocaine may contribute to the formation of methemoglobin in patients treated with other drugs known to cause this condition. (See WARNINGS, Methemoglobinemia.)

CARCINOGENESIS, MUTAGENESIS, IMPAIRMENT OF FERTILITY

Carcinogenesis: Metabolites of both lidocaine and prilocaine have been shown to be carcinogenic in laboratory animals. In the animal studies reported below, doses or blood levels are compared to the Single Dermal Administration (SDA) of 60 g of Lidocaine 2.5% and

PRECAUTIONS: *(cont'd)*

prilocaine 2.5% cream to 400 cm^2 for 3 hours to a small person (50 kg). The typical application for one or two treatments for venipuncture sites (2.5 or 5 g) would be 1/24 or 1/12 of that dose in an adult or about the same mg/kg dose in an infant.

A two-year oral toxicity study of 2,6-xylidine, a metabolite of lidocaine, has shown that in both male and female rats 2,6-xylidine in daily doses of 900 mg/m^2 (60 times SDA) resulted in carcinomas and adenomas of the nasal cavity. With daily doses of 300 mg/m^2 (20 times SDA) the increase in incidence of nasal carcinomas and/or adenomas in each sex of that rat were not statistically greater than the control group. In the low dose (90 mg/m^2, 6 times SDA) and control groups, no nasal tumors were observed. A rhabdomyosarcoma, a rare tumor, was observed in the nasal cavity of both male and female rats at the high dose of 900 mg/m^2. In addition, the compound caused subcutaneous fibromas and/or fibrosarcomas in both male and female rats and neoplastic nodules of the liver in the female rats with a significantly positive trend test; pairwise comparisons using Fisher's Exact Test showed significance only at the high dose of 900 mg/m^2. The animal study was conducted at oral doses of 15, 50, and 150 mg/kg/day. The dosages have been converted to mg/m^2 for the SDA calculations above.

Chronic oral toxicity studies of *ortho*-toluidine, a metabolite of prilocaine, in mice (900 to 14,000 mg/m^2, 60 to 960 times SDA) and rats (900 to 4,800 mg/m^2, 60 to 320 times SDA) have shown that *ortho*-toluidine is a carcinogen in both species. The tumors included hepatocarcinomas/adenomas in female mice, multiple occurrences of hemangiosarcomas/hemangiomas in both sexes of mice, sarcomas of multiple organs, transitional-cell carcinomas/papillomas of urinary bladder in both sexes of rats, subcutaneous fibromas/fibrosarcomas and mesotheliomas in male rats, and mammary gland fibroadenomas/adenomas in female rats. The lowest dose tested (900 mg/m^2, 60 times SDA) was carcinogenic in both species. Thus the no-effect dose must be less than 60 times SDA. The animal studies were conducted at 150 to 2,400 mg/kg in mice and at 150 to 800 mg/kg in rats. The dosages have been converted to mg/m^2 for the SDA calculations above.

Mutagenesis: The mutagenic potential of lidocaine HCl has been tested in the Ames Salmonella/mammalian microsome test and by analysis of structural chromosome aberrations in human lymphocytes *in vitro*, and by the mouse micronucleus test *in vivo*. There was no indication in these three tests of any mutagenic effects.

The mutagenicity of 2,6-xylidine, a metabolite of lidocaine, has been studied in different tests with mixed results. The compound was found to be weakly mutagenic in the Ames test only under metabolic activation conditions. In addition, 2,6-xylidine was observed to be mutagenic at the thymidine kinase locus, with or without activation, and induced chromosome aberrations and sister chromatid exchanges at concentrations at which the drug precipitated out of the solution (1.2 mg/ml). No evidence of genotoxicity was found in the *in vivo* assays measuring unscheduled DNA synthesis in rat hepatocytes, chromosome damage in polychromatic erythrocytes or preferential killing of DNA repair-deficient bacteria in liver, lung, kidney, testes and blood extracts from mice. However, covalent binding studies of DNA from liver and ethmoid turbinates in rats indicate that 2,6-xylidine may be genotoxic under certain conditions *in vivo*.

Ortho-toluidine, a metabolite of prilocaine, (0.5 mcg/ml) showed positive results in *Escherichia coli* DNA repair and phage-induction assays. Urine concentrates from rats treated with *ortho*-toluidine (300 mg/kg orally; 300 times SDA) were mutagenic for *Salmonella typhimurium* with metabolic activation. Several other tests on *ortho-* toluidine, including, reverse mutations in five different *Salmonella typhimurium* strains with or without metabolic activation and with single strand breaks in DNA of V79 Chinese hamster cells, were negative.

Impairment of Fertility: See Pregnancy.

PREGNANCY, TERATOGENIC EFFECTS, PREGNANCY CATEGORY B

Reproduction studies with lidocaine have been performed in rats and have revealed no evidence of harm to the fetus (30 mg/kg subcutaneously; 22 times SDA). Reproduction studies with prilocaine have been performed in rats and have revealed no evidence of impaired fertility or harm to the fetus (300 mg/kg intramuscularly; 188 times SDA). There are, however, no adequate and well-controlled studies in pregnant women. Because animal reproduction studies are not always predictive of human response, EMLA Cream should be used during pregnancy only if clearly needed.

Reproduction studies have been performed in rats receiving subcutaneous administration of an aqueous mixture containing lidocaine HCl and prilocaine HCl at 1:1 (w/w). At 40 mg/kg each, a dose equivalent to 29 times SDA lidocaine and 25 times SDA prilocaine, no teratogenic, embryotoxic or fetotoxic effects were observed.

LABOR AND DELIVERY

Neither lidocaine nor prilocaine are contraindicated in labor and delivery. Should Lidocaine 2.5% and prilocaine 2.5% cream be used concomitantly with other products containing lidocaine and/or prilocaine, total doses contributed by all formulations must be considered.

NURSING MOTHERS

Lidocaine, and probably prilocaine, are excreted in human milk. Therefore, caution should be exercised when Lidocaine 2.5% and prilocaine 2.5% cream is administered to a nursing mother since the milk:plasma ratio of lidocaine is 0.4 and is not determined for prilocaine.

PEDIATRIC USE

Controlled studies of lidocaine 2.5% and prilocaine 2.5% cream in children under the age of seven years have shown less overall benefit than in older children or adults. These results illustrate the importance of emotional and psychological support of younger children undergoing medical or surgical procedures.

Lidocaine 2.5% and prilocaine 2.5% cream should be used with care in patients with conditions or therapy associated with methemoglobinemia (see WARNINGS, Methemoglobinemia.)

When using lidocaine 2.5% and prilocaine 2.5% cream in young children, care must be taken to insure that application of the cream is limited to the intended site (see DOSAGE AND ADMINISTRATION.) Accidental ingestion may lead to dose related toxicity.

In children weighing less than 20 kg, the area and duration should be limited (see TABLE 2).

DRUG INTERACTIONS:

Lidocaine 2.5% and prilocaine 2.5% cream should be used with caution in patients receiving Class I antiarrhythmic drugs (such as tocainide and mexiletine) since the toxic effects are additive and potentially synergistic.

ADVERSE REACTIONS:

Localized Reactions: During or immediately after treatment with Lidocaine 2.5% and prilocaine 2.5% cream, the skin at the site of treatment may develop erythema or edema or may be the locus of abnormal sensation. In clinical studies involving over 1,300 lidocaine 2.5% and prilocaine 2.5% cream-treated subjects, one or more such local reactions were noted in 56% of patients, and were generally mild and transient, resolving spontaneously within 1 or 2 hours. There were no serious reactions which were ascribed to lidocaine 2.5% and prilocaine 2.5% cream.

In patients treated with lidocaine 2.5% and prilocaine 2.5% cream, local effects observed in the trials included: paleness (pallor or blanching) 37%, redness (erythema) 30%, alterations in temperature sensations 7%, edema 6%, itching 2% and rash, less than 1%.

ADVERSE REACTIONS: *(cont'd)*

Allergic Reactions: Allergic and anaphylactoid reactions associated with lidocaine or prilocaine can occur. They are characterized by urticaria, angioedema, bronchospasm, and shock. If they occur they should be managed by conventional means. The detection of sensitivity by skin testing is of doubtful value.

Systemic (Dose Related) Reactions: Systemic adverse reactions following appropriate use of Lidocaine 2.5% and prilocaine 2.5% cream are unlikely due to the small dose absorbed (see CLINICAL PHARMACOLOGY, Pharmacokinetics). Systemic adverse effects of lidocaine and/or prilocaine are similar in nature to those observed with other amide local anesthetic agents including CNS excitation and/or depression (light-headedness, nervousness, apprehension, euphoria, confusion, dizziness, drowsiness, tinnitus, blurred or double vision, vomiting, sensations of heat, cold or numbness, twitching, tremors, convulsions, unconsciousness, respiratory depression and arrest). Excitatory CNS reactions may be brief or not occur at all, in which case the first manifestation may be drowsiness merging into unconsciousness. Cardiovascular manifestations may include bradycardia, hypotension and cardiovascular collapse leading to arrest.

OVERDOSAGE:

Peak blood levels following a 60 g application to 400 cm^2 for 3 hours are 0.05 to 0.16 μ/ml for lidocaine and 0.02 to 0.10 μ/ml for prilocaine. Toxic levels of lidocaine (>5μ/ml) and/or prilocaine (>6 μ/ml) cause decreases in cardiac output, total peripheral resistance and mean arterial pressure. These changes may be attributable to direct depressant effects of these local anesthetic agents on the cardiovascular system. In the absence of massive topical overdosage or oral ingestion, evaluation should include evaluation of other etiologies for the clinical effects or overdosage from other sources of lidocaine, prilocaine or other local anesthetics. Consult the package inserts for parenteral xylocaine (lidocaine HCl) or Citanest (prilocaine HCl) for further information for the management of overdose.

DOSAGE AND ADMINISTRATION:

A thick layer of lidocaine 2.5% and prilocaine 2.5% cream is applied to intact skin and covered with an occlusive dressing.

Minor Dermal Procedures: For minor procedures such as IV cannulation and venipuncture, apply 2.5 grams of lidocaine 2.5% and prilocaine 2.5% cream (1/2 the 5 g tube) over 20 to 25 cm^2 of skin surface for at least 1 hour. In controlled clinical trials, two sites were usually prepared in case there was a technical problem with cannulation or venipuncture at the first site.

Major Dermal Procedures: For more painful dermatological procedures involving a larger skin area such as split thickness skin graft harvesting, apply 2 grams if lidocaine 2.5% and prilocaine 2.5% cream per 10 cm^2 of skin and allow to remain in contact with the skin for at least 2 hours.

Dermal analgesia can be expected to increase for up to 3 hours under occlusive dressing and persist for 1 to 2 hours after removal of the cream. The amount of lidocaine and prilocaine absorbed during the period of application can be estimated from the information in TABLE 2, ** footnote, in Individualization of Dose.

A single application of Lidocaine 2.5% and prilocaine 2.5% cream in a child weighing less than 10 kg should not be applied over an area larger than 100 cm^2. A single application of Lidocaine 2.5% and prilocaine 2.5% cream in children weighing between 10 kg and 20 kg should not be applied over an area larger than 600 cm^2(see TABLE 2).

Lidocaine 2.5% and prilocaine 2.5% cream should not be used in infants under the age of one month or in infants, under the age of twelve months, who are receiving treatment with methemoglobin-inducing agents (see WARNINGS, Methemoglobinemia).

When lidocaine 2.5% and prilocaine 2.5% cream is used concomitantly with other products containing local anesthetic agents, the amount absorbed from all formulations must be considered (see CLINICAL PHARMACOLOGY, Individualization of Dose.) The amount absorbed in the case of Lidocaine 2.5% and prilocaine 2.5% cream is determined by the area over which it is applied and the duration of application under occlusion (see TABLE 2 **, footnote CLINICAL PHARMACOLOGY, Individualization of Dose).

Although the incidence of systemic adverse reactions with Lidocaine 2.5% and prilocaine 2.5% cream is very low, caution should be exercised, particularly when applying it over large areas and leaving it on for longer than two hours. The incidence of systemic adverse reactions can be expected to be directly proportional to the area and time of exposure (see CLINICAL PHARMACOLOGY, Individualization of Dose.)

HOW SUPPLIED:

KEEP CONTAINER TIGHTLY CLOSED AT ALL TIMES WHEN NOT IN USE. NOT FOR OPHTHALMIC USE.

Store at controlled room temperature 15 - 30°C (59 - 86°F).

Note: For illustrations on Instructions for Application, please see manufacturer's original package insert.

HOW SUPPLIED - EQUIVALENTS NOT AVAILABLE:

Cream - Topical - 2.5% mg/2.5 %

30 gm	$33.47	EMLA, Astra USA	00186-1516-01

Kit - Topical - 2.5% mg/2.5 %

5 gm	$7.23	EMLA, Astra USA	00186-1515-01
5 gm x 5	$34.79	EMLA, Astra USA	00186-1515-03

LINCOMYCIN HYDROCHLORIDE *(001641)*

CATEGORIES: Anti-Infectives; Antibiotics; Antimicrobials; Infections; Lincosamides/Macrolides; FDA Approval Pre 1982

BRAND NAMES: *Albiotic* (Germany); *Biolincom*; *Cillimicina*; *Cillimycin*; *Frademicina*; L-Mycin; *Lincobiotic*; **Lincocin**; *Lincocine* (France); Lincoject; *Lincomec*; *Lincophar*; Lincorex; *Linmycin*; *Princol* (Mexico); *Zumalin*
(International brand names outside U.S. in italics)

WARNING:
Lincomycin therapy has been associated with severe colitis which may end fatally. Therefore, it should be reserved for serious infections where less toxic antimicrobial agents are inappropriate, as described in the Indications Section. It should not be used in patients with nonbacterial infections, such as most upper respiratory tract infections. Studies indicate a toxin(s) produced by Clostridia is one primary cause of antibiotic associated colitis.[1-5] (See WARNINGS.) The colitis is usually characterized by severe, persistent diarrhea and severe abdominal cramps and may be associated with the passage of blood and mucus. Endoscopic examination may reveal pseudomembranous colitis.

> When significant diarrhea occurs, the drug should be discontinued or, if necessary, continued only with close observation of the patient. Large bowel endoscopy has been recommended.
> Antiperistaltic agents such as opiates and diphenoxylate with atropine (Lomotil) may prolong and/or worsen the condition. Vancomycin has been found to be effective in the treatment of antibiotic associated pseudomembranous colitis produced by Clostridium difficile. The usual adult dose is 500 milligrams to 2 grams of vancomycin orally per day in three to four divided doses administered for 7 to 10 days. Cholestyramine or colestipol resins bind vancomycin in vitro. If both a resin and vancomycin are to be administered concurrently it may be advisable to separate the time of administration of each drug.
> Diarrhea, colitis, and pseudomembranous colitis have been observed to begin up to several weeks following cessation of therapy with lincomycin.

DESCRIPTION:

Lincocin Capsules and Lincocin Sterile Solution contain lincomycin hydrochloride which is the monohydrated salt of lincomycin, a substance produced by the growth of a member of the *lincolnensis* group of *Streptomyces lincolnensis(EI> (Fam. Streptomycetaceae)*. It is a white or practically white, crystalline powder and is odorless or has a faint odor. Its solutions are acid and are dextrorotatory. Lincomycin hydrochloride is freely soluble in water; soluble in dimethylformamide and very slightly soluble in acetone.

Lincocin Capsules contain the following inactive ingredients: erythrosine sodium, FD&C blue No. 1, gelatin, lactose, magnesium stearate, talc and titanium dioxide.

CLINICAL PHARMACOLOGY:

Microbiology: Lincomycin has been shown to be effective against most of the common gram-positive pathogens. Depending on the sensitivity of the organism and concentration of the antibiotic, it may be either bactericidal or bacteriostatic. Cross resistance has not been demonstrated with penicillin, chloramphenicol, ampicillin, cephalosporins or the tetracyclines. Despite chemical differences, lincomycin exhibits antibacterial activity similar but not identical to the macrolide antibiotics (*e.g.,* erythromycin). Some cross resistance (with erythromycin) including a phenomenon known as dissociated cross resistance or macrolide effect has been reported. Microorganisms have not developed resistance to lincomycin rapidly when tested by *in vitro* or *in vivo* methods. Staphylococci develop resistance to lincomycin in a slow, stepwise manner based on *in vitro,* serial subculture experiments. This pattern of resistance development is unlike that shown for streptomycin.

STUDIES INDICATE THAT LINCOMYCIN DOES NOT SHARE ANTIGENICITY WITH PENICILLIN COMPOUNDS.

BIOLOGICAL STUDIES: *In vitro* studies indicate that the spectrum of activity includes *Staphylococcus aureus, Staphylococcus albus, β-hemolytic Streptococcus, Streptococcus viridans, Diplococcus pneumoniae, Clostridium tetani, Clostridium perfringens, Corynebacterium diphtheriae and Corynebacterium acnes.*

NOTE: This drug is not active against most strains of*Streptococcus faecalis,* nor against *Neisseria gonorrhoeae, Neisseria meningitidis, Hemophilus influenzae,* or other gram-negative organisms or yeasts.

Human Pharmacology: Lincomycin is absorbed rapidly after a 500 mg oral dose, reaching peak levels in 2 to 4 hours. Levels are maintained above the MIC (minimum inhibitory concentration) for most gram-positive organisms for 6 to 8 hours. Urinary recovery of drug in a 24-hour period ranges from 1.0 to 31 percent (mean: 4.0) after a single oral dose of 500 mg of lincomycin. Tissue level studies indicate that bile is an important route of excretion. Significant levels have been demonstrated in the majority of body tissues. Although the drug is not present in significant amounts in the spinal fluid of normal volunteers, it has been demonstrated in the spinal fluid of one patient with pneumococcal meningitis.

Intramuscular administration of a single dose of 600 mg of lincomycin produces a peak serum level at 30 minutes with detectable levels persisting for 24 hours. Urinary excretion after this dose ranges from 1.8 to 24.8 percent (mean: 17.3).

The intravenous infusion over a 2-hours interval of 600 mg of lincomycin in 500 ml of 5 percent glucose in distilled water yields therapeutic levels for 14 hours. Urinary excretion ranges from 4.9 to 30.3 percent (mean: 13.8).

The biological half-life, after oral, intramuscular or intravenous administration is 5.4 ± 1.0 hours.

Hemodialysis and peritoneal dialysis do not effectively remove lincomycin from the blood.

CLINICAL STUDIES:

Experience with 345 obstetrical patients receiving this drug revealed no ill effects related to pregnancy.

INDICATIONS AND USAGE:

Lincocin Capsules and Lincocin Sterile Solution are indicated in the treatment of serious infections due to susceptible strains of streptococci, pneumococci, and staphylococci. Its use should be reserved for penicillin-allergic patients or other patients for whom, in the judgment of the physician, a penicillin is inappropriate. Because of the risk of colitis, as described in the BOXED WARNING, before selecting lincomycin the physician should consider the nature of the infection and suitability of less toxic alternatives (*e.g.,* erythromycin).

Lincomycin has been demonstrated to be effective in the treatment of staphylococcal infections resistant to other antibiotics and susceptible to lincomycin. Staphylococcal strains resistant to Lincocin have been recovered; culture and susceptibility studies should be done in conjunction with therapy with Lincocin. In the case of macrolides, partial but not complete cross resistance may occur (see CLINICAL PHARMACOLOGY, Microbiology.) The drug may be administered concomitantly with other antimicrobial agents when indicated.

CONTRAINDICATIONS:

This drug is contraindicated in patients previously found to be hypersensitive to lincomycin or clindamycin. It is not indicated in the treatment of minor bacterial infections or viral infections.

WARNINGS:

(See BOXED WARNING.) Studies indicate a toxin(s) produced by*Clostridia* is one primary cause of antibiotic associated colitis.[1-5] Mild cases of colitis may respond to drug discontinuance alone. Moderate to severe cases should be managed promptly with fluid, electrolyte and protein supplementation as indicated. Vancomycin has been found to be effective in the treatment of antibiotic associated pseudomembranous colitis produced by *Clostridium difficile.* The usual adult dose is 500 milligrams to 2 grams of vancomycin orally per day in three to four divided doses administered for 7 to 10 days. Cholestyramine or colestipol resins bind vancomycin *in vitro.* If both a resin and vancomycin are to be administered concurrently, it may be advisable to separate the time of administration of each drug. Systemic corticoids and corticoid retention enemas may help relieve the colitis. Other causes of colitis should also be considered.

A careful inquiry should be made concerning previous sensitivities to drugs and other allergens.

Usage in Pregnancy: Safety for use in pregnancy has not been established.

Usage in Newborn: Until further clinical experience is obtained, Lincocin preparations (lincomycin) are not indicated in the newborn.

Nursing Mothers: Lincomycin has been reported to appear in breast milk in ranges of 0.5 to 2.4 mcg/ml.

Lincocin Sterile Solution contains benzyl alcohol which has been associated with a fatal gasping syndrome in infants.

PRECAUTIONS:

Review of experience to date suggests that a subgroup of older patients with associated severe illness may tolerate diarrhea less well. When Lincocin preparations (lincomycin) are indicated in these patients, they should be carefully monitored for change in bowel frequency.

Lincocin should be prescribed with caution in individuals with a history of gastrointestinal disease, particularly colitis.

Lincocin like any drug, should be used with caution in patients with a history of asthma or significant allergies.

The use of antibiotics occasionally results in overgrowth of nonsusceptible organisms-particularly yeasts. Should superinfections occur, appropriate measures should be taken. When patients with pre-existing monilial infections require therapy with Lincocin, concomitant antimonilial treatment should be given.

During prolonged therapy with Lincocin, periodic liver and renal function studies and blood counts should be performed.

Since adequate data are not yet available in patients with pre-existing liver disease, its use in such patients is not recommended at this time unless special clinical circumstances so indicate.

Lincomycin has been shown to have neuromuscular blocking properties that may enhance the action of other neuromuscular blocking agents. Therefore, it should be used with caution in patients receiving such agents.

Indicated surgical procedures should be performed in conjunction with antibiotic therapy.

ADVERSE REACTIONS:

Gastrointestinal: Glossitis, stomatitis, nausea, vomiting. Persistent diarrhea, enterocolitis and pruritus ani. (See BOXED WARNING.)

Hematopoietic: Neutropenia, leukopenia, agranulocytosis and thrombocytopenic purpura have been reported. There have been rare reports of aplastic anemia and pancytopenia in which Lincocin could not be ruled out as the causative agent.

Hypersensitivity Reactions: Hypersensitivity reactions such as angioneurotic edema, serum sickness and anaphylaxis have been reported, some of these in patients known to be sensitive to penicillin. Rare instances of erythema multiforme, some resembling Stevens-Johnson syndrome, have been associated with Lincocin preparations. If an allergic reaction should occur, the drug should be discontinued and the usual agents (epinephrine, corticosteroids, antihistamines) should be available for emergency treatment.

Skin and Mucous Membranes: Skin rashes, urticaria and vaginitis and rare instances of exfoliative and vesiculobullous dermatitis have been reported.

Liver: Although no direct relationship of Lincocin to liver dysfunction has been established, jaundice and abnormal liver function tests (particularly elevations of serum transaminase) have been observed in a few instances.

Renal: Although no direct relationship of lincomycin to renal damage has been established, renal dysfunction as evidenced by azotemia, oliguria, and/or proteinuria has been observed in rare instances.

Cardiovascular: After too rapid intravenous administration, rare instances of cardiopulmonary arrest and hypotension have been reported. (See DOSAGE AND ADMINISTRATION.)

Special Senses: Tinnitus and vertigo have been reported occasionally.

Local Reactions: Patients have demonstrated excellent local tolerance to intramuscularly administered Lincocin. Reports of pain following injection have been infrequent. Intravenous administration of Lincocin in 250 to 500 ml of 5 percent glucose in distilled water or normal saline produced no local irritation or phlebitis.

DOSAGE AND ADMINISTRATION:

If significant diarrhea occurs during therapy, this antibiotic should be discontinued. (See BOXED WARNING.)

ORAL

Adults: *Serious infections:* 500 mg 3 times per day (500 mg approximately every 8 hours). *More severe infections:* 500 mg or more 4 times per day (500 mg or more approximately every 6 hours).

Children over 1 month of age: *Serious infections:* 30 mg/kg/day (15 mg/lb/day) divided into 3 or 4 equal doses. *More severe infections:* 60 mg/kg/day (30 mg/lb/day) divided into 3 or 4 equal doses.

With β-hemolytic streptococcal infections, treatment should continue for at least 10 days to diminish the likelihood of subsequent rheumatic fever or glomerulonephritis.

Note: For optimal absorption it is recommended that nothing be given by mouth except water for a period of one to two hours before and after oral administration of Lincocin preparations (lincomycin).

INTRAMUSCULAR

Adults: *Serious infections:* 600 mg (2 ml) intramuscularly every 24 hours. *More severe infections:* 600 mg (2 ml) intramuscularly every 12 hours or more often.

Children over 1 month of age: *Serious infections:* one intramuscular injection of 10 mg/kg (5 mg/lb) every 24 hours or more often. *More severe infections:* one intramuscular injection of 10 mg/kg (5 mg/lb) every 12 hours or more often.

INTRAVENOUS

Adults: The intravenous dose will be determined by the severity of the infection. For serious infections doses of 600 mg of lincomycin (2 ml of Lincocin) to 1 gram are given every 8-12 hours. For more severe infections these doses may have to be increased. In life-threatening situations daily intravenous doses of as much as 8 grams have been given. **Intravenous doses are given on the basis of 1 gram of lincomycin diluted in not less than 100 ml of appropriate solution** (See PHYSICAL COMPATIBILITIES)**and infused over a period of not less than one hour.** (TABLE 1):

These doses may be repeated as often as required to the limit of the maximum recommended daily dose of 8 grams of lincomycin.

DOSAGE AND ADMINISTRATION: *(cont'd)*

TABLE 1

Dose	Vol. Diluent	Time
600 mg	100 ml	1 hr
1 gram	100 ml	1 hr
2 grams	200 ml	2 hr
3 grams	300 ml	3 hr
4 grams	400 ml	4 hr

Children over 1 month of age: 10-20 mg/kg/day (5-10 mg/lb/day) depending on the severity of the infection may be infused in divided doses as described above for adults.

NOTE: Severe cardiopulmonary reactions have occurred when this drug has been given at greater than the recommended concentration and rate.

Subconjunctival Injection: 0.25 ml (75 mg) injected subconjunctivally will result in ocular fluid levels of antibiotic (lasting for at least 5 hours) with MIC's sufficient for most susceptible pathogens.

Patients with diminished renal function: *When therapy with Lincocin is required in individuals with severe impairment of renal function, an appropriate dose is 25 to 30% of that recommended for patients with normally functioning kidneys.*

PHYSICAL COMPATIBILITIES

Physically compatible for 24 hours at room temperature unless otherwise indicated.

Infusion Solutions

Dextrose in Water, 5% and 10%
Dextrose in Saline, 5% and 10%
Ringer's Solution
Sodium Lactate 1/6 Molar
Travert 10%—Electrolyte No. 1
Dextran in Saline 6% w/v

Vitamins in Infusion Solutions

B-Complex

B-Complex with Ascorbic Acid

Antibiotics in Infusion Solutions

Penicillin G Sodium (Satisfactory for 4 hours)
Cephalothin
Tetracycline HCl
Cephaloridine
Colistimethate (Satisfactory for 4 hours)
Ampicillin
Methicillin
Chloramphenicol
Polymyxin B Sulfate

Physically Incompatible with:

Novobiocin

Kanamycin

IT SHOULD BE EMPHASIZED THAT THE COMPATIBLE AND INCOMPATIBLE DETERMINATIONS ARE PHYSICAL OBSERVATIONS ONLY, NOT CHEMICAL DETERMINATIONS. ADEQUATE CLINICAL EVALUATION OF THE SAFETY AND EFFICACY OF THESE COMBINATIONS HAS NOT BEEN PERFORMED.

Store at controlled room temperature 15°-30° C (59°-86° F).

ANIMAL PHARMACOLOGY:

In vivo experimental animal studies demonstrated the effectiveness of Lincocin preparations (lincomycin) in protecting animals infected with *Streptococcus viridans, β-hemolytic Streptococcus, Staphylococcus aureus, Diplococcus pneumoniae* and *Leptospira pomona.* It was ineffective in *Klebsiella, Pasteurella, Pseudomonas, Salmonella and Shigella* infections.

REFERENCES:

1. Bailey, WR, Scott, EG, *Diagnostic Microbiology* CV Mosby Company, St.Louis, 1978. 2. Bartlett, JG, et al,"Clindamycin-associated Colitis due to Toxin-producing Species of *Clostridium in Hamsters*" *J.inf.Dis.***136** (5): 701-705, (November) 1977. 3. Larson, HE, Price, AB,"Pseudomembranous Colitis: Presence of Clostridial Toxin," *Lancet*, 1312-1314 (December) 24 and 31, 1977. 4. Lusk, RH, et al,"Clindamycin-Induced Enterocolitis in Hamsters" *J.inf.Dis.* 137 (4):464-474 (April) 1978. 5. "Antibiotic-associated Colitis: A Progress Report", *British Med.J.* **1**:669-671 (March 18) 1978.

HOW SUPPLIED - RATED THERAPEUTICALLY EQUIVALENT:

Injection, Solution - Intramuscular; - 300 mg/ml

2 ml	**$5.37**	**LINCOCIN, Pharmacia & Upjohn**	**00009-0555-01**
10 ml	$10.33	Lincomycin Hcl, Insource	58441-0119-10
10 ml	$11.50	LAMBDA-MYCIN, Bolan Pharm	44437-0908-10
10 ml	$12.45	LINCOREX, Hyrex Pharms	00314-0804-10
10 ml	$13.08	Lincomycin Hcl, HL Moore Drug Exch	00839-7688-30
10 ml	$14.25	Lincomycin Hcl, IDE-Interstate	00814-4415-40
10 ml	$16.12	Lincomycin HCl, Rugby	00536-3987-70
10 ml	$16.95	Lincoject, Llorens Pharm	54859-0402-10
10 ml	$19.00	Lincomycin Hcl, Goldline Labs	00182-3031-63
10 ml	$19.95	Lincomycin Hcl, Steris Labs	00402-0908-10
10 ml	**$24.11**	**LINCOCIN, Pharmacia & Upjohn**	**00009-0555-02**

HOW SUPPLIED - NOT RATED EQUIVALENT:

Capsule, Gelatin - Oral - 500 mg

100's	**$132.26**	**LINCOCIN, Pharmacia & Upjohn**	**00009-0500-02**

LINDANE *(001642)*

CATEGORIES: Anti-Infectives; Antiseptics/Disinfectants; Dermatologicals; Lice; Parasiticidal; Pediculosis; Scabicides/Pediculicides; Skin/Mucous Membrane Agents; Topical; Pregnancy Category B; FDA Approval Pre 1982

BRAND NAMES: *Aphtiria*; *Benhex Cream*; *Bicide*; Bio-Well; *Delice*; *Delitex* (Germany); *Desintan*; *Elentol* (France); *GAB*; G-Well; *Gamabenceno*; *Gambex*; Gamene; *Gammalin*; Gbh; *Herklin* (Mexico); *Hexicid*; *Jacutin* (Germany); Kildane; **Kwell**; *Kwellada* (Canada); *Lencid*; *Locion-V*; *Locion Y Shampoo Dual*; *Lorexane*; *Naledyn Champu-Medicado*; *PMS Lindane* (Canada); *Quellada*; *Quellada Cream*; *Quellada Creme Rinse*; *Quellada-H* (Germany); *Quellada Head Lice Treatment*; *Quellada Lotion* (Australia); *Sarconyl*; *Scabecid* (France); Scabene; *Scabex*; *Scabexyl*; *Scabi*; *Scabisan* (Mexico); Thionex; *Varsan* (Japan)
(International brand names outside U.S. in italics)

FORMULARIES: Aetna; BC-BS; CIGNA; FHP; Humana; Kaiser; Medco; Medi-Cal; PCS; PruCare; United

DESCRIPTION:

Lindane cream 1% is an ectoparasiticide and ovicide effective against Sarcoptes scabiei (scabies) and their ova. Inert ingredients: 99% in a pleasantly scented water dispersible cream containing stearic acid, glycerin, lanolin, 2-amino-2-methyl-1-propanol, perfume and purified water.

DESCRIPTION: *(cont'd)*

Lindane shampoo 1% is an ectoparasiticide and ovicide effective against Pediculosis capitis (head lice), Pediculosis pubis (crab lice) and their ova. In addition to the active ingredients, lindane, it contains Trolamine Lauryl Sulfate, Polysorbate 60, acetone and purified water to form a cosmetically pleasant shampoo.

Lindane, which is the highly purified gamma isomer of 1, 2, 3, 4, 5, 6, hexachlorocyclohexane.

CLINICAL PHARMACOLOGY:

Lindane exerts its parasiticidal action by being directly absorbed into the parasites and their ova. Feldmann and Maibach reported approximately 10% absorption of a lindane acetone solution applied to the forearm and left in place to 24 hours. Dale, et al reported a blood level of 290 ng/ml associated with convulsions following the accidental ingestion of a lindane containing product. Ginsburg found a mean peak blood level of 28 ng/ml 6 hours after total body application of Lindane Lotion to scabietic infants and children. The half-life was determined to be 18 hours.

Analysis of blood taken from subjects before and after the use of Lindane shampoo showed a mean peak blood level of only 3 ng/ml which appeared at six hours and disappeared at eight hours after the shampoo was applied.

INDICATIONS AND USAGE:

Lindane cream is indicated for the treatment of patients infested with Sarcoptes scabiei (scabies).

Lindane shampoo is indicated for the treatment of patients infested with Pediculus capitis (head lice), Pediculus pubis (crab lice) and their ova.

CONTRAINDICATIONS:

Lindane cream is contraindicated for premature neonates because their skin may be more permeable than full term infants and their liver enzymes may not be sufficiently developed. It is also contraindicated for patients with known seizure disorders and for individuals with a known sensitivity to the product or any of its components.

WARNINGS:

LINDANE PENETRATES HUMAN SKIN AND HAS THE POTENTIAL FOR CNS TOXICITY (SEE CLINICAL PHARMACOLOGY). LINDANE CREAM SHOULD BE USED ACCORDING TO RECOMMENDED DOSAGE (SEE DIRECTIONS FOR USE) ESPECIALLY ON INFANTS, PREGNANT WOMEN AND NURSING MOTHERS. ANIMAL STUDIES INDICATE THAT POTENTIAL TOXIC EFFECTS OF TOPICALLY APPLIED LINDANE ARE GREATER IN THE YOUNG. Seizures have been reported after excessive use or oral ingestion of lindane. No residual effects of Lindane treatment have been demonstrated, therefore, this product should not be used to ward off a possible infestation.

If accidental ingestion occurs prompt gastric lavage is indicated. Because oils may enhance absorption, saline rather than oily cathartics should be used. Central nervous excitation can be controlled by the administration of pentobarbital, phenobarbital or diazepam.

PRECAUTIONS:

General: Care should be taken to avoid contact with the eyes. If such contact occurs, eyes should be immediately flushed with water. If irritation or sensitization occurs, the patient should be advised to consult a physician.

Information for the Patient: Patients should be instructed on the proper use of the medication. Directions for Use should accompany the prescription.

Laboratory Tests: No laboratory tests are needed for the proper use of this medication.

Carcinogenesis: Although no studies have been conducted with Lindane cream or shampoo, numerous long term feeding studies have been conducted in mice and rats to evaluate the carcinogenic potential of the technical grade of hexachlorocyclohexane (BHC) as well as the alpha, beta, gamma lindane) and delta isomers. Both oral and topical applications have been evaluated. Nagasaki Goto and Hanada found varying amounts of benign and malignant hepatomas associated with BHC and the alpha, delta and epsilon isomers. None reported a carcinogenic potential for lindane. Tumors were found only in the animals which had received the alpha isomer. Weisse and Herbst also evaluated the carcinogenic potential of lindane in mice but could find no evidence of lindane in mice but could find no evidence of lindane carcinogenicity. The National Cancer Institute also found no evidence of carcinogenicity.

Thorpe and Walker compared beta BHC with lindane, dieldrin, DDT and hexobarbital in mice.

Despite the unusually high incidence of tumors in the control group, they concluded that 600 ppm of lindane was associated with a significant increase in the incidence of hepatoma and thus considered it a tumorigen.

Orr and Kashyap, et al evaluated the carcinogenic potential in mice of topically carcinogenic potential in mice of topically applied BHC. In neither study was there any evidence of a tumorigenic or carcinogenic potential associated with topical application of BHC.

Mutagenicity tests have been used as predictive information about the carcinogenicity of various chemical compounds. Numerous types of mutagenicity tests have been performed with lindane. The results of these tests do not indicate that lindane is mutagenic.

Pregnancy, Teratogenic Effects, Pregnancy Category B: Reproduction, including multigeneration, studies have been performed in mice, rats, rabbits, pigs, and dogs at doses up to 10 times the human dose and have revealed no evidence of impaired fertility or harm to the fetus due to administered lindane. There are, however, no adequate and well controlled studies in pregnant women. Because animal reproduction studies are not always predictive of human response, the recommended dosage should not be exceeded on pregnant women. They should be treated no more than twice during a pregnancy.

Nursing Mothers: Lindane is secreted in human milk in low concentrations. Studies conducted in the United States as well as Europe and South America found levels of lindane in human milk ranging from 0 to 113 ppb, as the result of ingestion of foods which had been treated with lindane. There appeared to be no difference in concentrations between country and urban dwellers. Although the levels of lindane found in blood after topical application with Lindane cream and shampoo make it unlikely that amounts of lindane sufficient to cause serious adverse reactions will be excreted in the milk of nursing mothers who have used Lindane cream, if there is any concern, an alternate method of feeding may be used for 2 days.

Pediatric Use: Refer to CONTRAINDICATIONS and WARNINGS.

DRUG INTERACTIONS:

Oils may enhance absorption, therefore, simultaneous use of creams, ointments or oils should be avoided. If an oil-based hair dressing is used, it is recommended that the hair be shampooed, rinsed and dried before application of lindane shampoo.

ADVERSE REACTIONS:

Lindane has been reported to cause central nervous stimulation ranging from dizziness to convulsions. Cases of convulsions have been reported in connection with Lindane cream therapy.

However, these incidents were almost always associated with accidental oral ingestion or misuse of the product. Eczematous eruptions due to irritation from this product have also been reported. Incidence of these adverse reactions is relatively infrequent, occurring in less than 1 in 100,000 patients.

DRUG ABUSE AND DEPENDENCE:

Lindane cream is not subject to abuse, nor is there any dependence on the drug.

OVERDOSAGE:

Overdosage or oral ingestion of Lindane cream can cause central nervous system excitation and, if taken in sufficient quantities, convulsions may occur.

If accidental ingestion occurs, prompt gastric lavage should be instituted. However, since oils favor absorption, saline cathartics for intestinal evacuation should be given rather than oil laxatives. If central nervous system manifestations occur they can be antagonized by the administration of pentobarbital, phenobarbital or diazepam.

DOSAGE AND ADMINISTRATION:

CAUTION: USE ONLY AS DIRECTED. DO NOT EXCEED RECOMMENDED DOSAGE

No residual effects of Lindane treatment have been demonstrated therefore, this product should not be used to ward off a possible infestation.

NOTE: PLEASE READ CAREFULLY.

DIRECTIONS FOR USE-CREAM

Scabies (sarcoptes Scabiei)—The cream should be applied to dry skin in a thin layer and rubbed in thoroughly. If crusted lesions are present, a tepid bath preceding the medication is helpful.

If a bath is used, allow the skin to dry before applying the cream. Usually two ounces are sufficient for an adult. A total body application should be made from the neck down including the soles of the feet. Scabies rarely affects the head of children or adults but may occur in infants.

The cream should be left on for 8-12 hours and should then be removed by thorough washing. ONE APPLICATION IS USUALLY CURATIVE.

Sexual contacts should be treated simultaneously.

Avoid unnecessary skin contact. Particularly when applying to more than one patient, those assisting in lindane therapy (especially pregnant and/or nursing women) should wear rubber gloves.

Avoid use on open cuts and extensive excoriations.

Many patients exhibit persistent pruritus after treatment; this is rarely a sign of treatment failure and is not an indication for retreatment unless living mites can be demonstrated.

DIRECTIONS FOR USE-SHAMPOO

Pediculosis capitis (head lice) - 1) Apply a sufficient quantity of the shampoo to the dry hair. Approximately 1 oz. (30 ml) for short, 1.5 oz. (45 ml) for medium, and 2 oz. (60 ml) for long hair. 2) Work thoroughly into the hair and allow to remain in place four minutes. 3) Add small quantities of water until a good lather forms. 4) Rinse thoroughly. Towel briskly. Nits should be removed using a nit comb or tweezers.

Retreatment is usually not necessary. Demonstrable living organisms after 7 days indicate that retreatment is necessary.

Note

1. If a person to be treated uses an oil-based hair dressing, it is recommended that their hair be shampooed and dried before applying Lindane shampoo.

2. Avoid unnecessary skin contact. Particularly when applying to more than one patient, those assisting in lindane therapy (especially pregnant and/or nursing women) should wear rubber gloves.

3. Avoid use on open cuts and extensive excoriations. Sexual contacts should be treated simultaneously.

HOW SUPPLIED - RATED THERAPEUTICALLY EQUIVALENT:

Lotion - Topical - 1 %

59 ml	$3.35	G-WELL, Goldline Labs	00182-1475-43
59 ml	$4.94	Lindane, Alpharma	00472-0570-02
60 ml	$1.80	Lindane, Raway	00686-0570-02
60 ml	$2.03	Lindane, Stafford Miller	55372-4670-00
60 ml	$2.61	Lindane, H.C.F.A. F F P	99999-1642-01
60 ml	$2.65	Lindane, Harber Pharm	51432-0623-17
60 ml	$2.75	Lindane, Consolidated Midland	00223-6546-01
60 ml	$3.31	Lindane, Qualitest Pharms	00603-1404-49
60 ml	$3.50	Lindane, Aligen Independ	00405-3175-56
60 ml	$3.95	Lindane, Rugby	00536-1262-96
60 ml	$4.10	Lindane, Schein Pharm (US)	00364-7326-58
60 ml	$4.20	Lindane, Morton Grove	60432-0546-60
60 ml	$4.94	Lindane, Major Pharms	00904-0690-03
60 ml	$5.60	Lindane, HL Moore Drug Exch	00839-6571-64
60 ml	$5.95	Lindane, Geneva Pharms	00781-7150-02
480 ml	$11.90	Lindane, H.C.F.A. F F P	99999-1642-02
480 ml	$12.95	Lindane, Stafford Miller	55372-4670-01
480 ml	$13.45	Lindane, Qualitest Pharms	00603-1404-58
480 ml	$15.40	Lindane, Harber Pharm	51432-0623-20
480 ml	$15.75	G-WELL, Goldline Labs	00182-1475-40
480 ml	$16.10	KWILDANE, Major Pharms	00904-0690-16
480 ml	$16.50	Lindane, Consolidated Midland	00223-6546-02
480 ml	$18.20	Lindane, Aligen Independ	00405-3175-16
480 ml	$18.63	Lindane, Morton Grove	60432-0546-16
480 ml	$19.00	Lindane, Schein Pharm (US)	00364-7326-16
480 ml	$19.76	Lindane, Alpharma	00472-0570-16
480 ml	$20.88	Lindane, United Res	00677-0808-33
480 ml	$24.10	Lindane, Rugby	00536-1262-85
480 ml	$31.15	Lindane, Geneva Pharms	00781-7150-16
480 ml	$31.32	Lindane, HL Moore Drug Exch	00839-6571-69
3785 ml	$123.90	Lindane, Alpharma	00472-0570-28
3840 ml	$95.23	Lindane, H.C.F.A. F F P	99999-1642-03
3840 ml	$97.88	KWILDANE, Major Pharms	00904-0690-28
3840 ml	$104.99	Lindane, Consolidated Midland	00223-6546-03

Shampoo - Topical - 1 %

1 gal	$116.08	Lindane, Rugby	00536-1270-90
1 pint	$23.13	Lindane Shampoo, United Res	00677-0809-33
1 pint	$32.98	Lindane Shampoo, Geneva Pharms	00781-7160-16
1 pt	$18.90	Lindane Shampoo, Schein Pharm (US)	00364-7327-16
1 pt	$28.55	Lindane, Rugby	00536-1270-85

HOW SUPPLIED - RATED THERAPEUTICALLY EQUIVALENT: *(cont'd)*

2 oz	$4.85	Lindane, Rugby	00536-1270-96
2 oz	$5.15	Lindane Shampoo, Schein Pharm (US)	00364-7327-58
2 oz	$5.60	Lindane, HL Moore Drug Exch	00839-6572-64
2 oz	$6.47	SCABENE, Stiefel Labs	00145-7066-02
2 oz	$6.95	Lindane Shampoo, Geneva Pharms	00781-7160-02
16 oz	$31.32	Lindane, HL Moore Drug Exch	00839-6572-69
16 oz	**$76.12**	**KWELL, Reed & Carnrick**	**00021-0610-16**
59 ml	$4.05	G-WELL SHAMPOO, Goldline Labs	00182-1476-43
59 ml	$5.81	Lindane, Alpharma	00472-0572-02
60 ml	$2.10	Lindane, Raway	00686-1572-02
60 ml	$2.21	Lindane, Stafford Miller	55372-4660-00
60 ml	$2.61	Lindane, Qualitest Drugs	52446-0946-52
60 ml	$2.89	Lindane, H.C.F.A. F F P	99999-1642-06
60 ml	$2.90	Lindane, Harber Pharm	51432-0625-17
60 ml	$2.95	Lindane, Consolidated Midland	00223-6562-01
60 ml	$3.47	Lindane, Qualitest Pharms	00603-1406-49
60 ml	$4.00	Lindane, Aligen Independ	00405-3200-56
60 ml	$5.20	Lindane, Morton Grove	60432-0547-60
60 ml	$5.95	Lindane, Major Pharms	00904-0692-03
473 ml	$19.40	G-WELL SHAMPOO, Goldline Labs	00182-1476-40
473 ml	$23.24	Lindane Shampoo, Alpharma	00472-0572-16
480 ml	$6.50	Lindane, Consolidated Midland	00223-6562-02
480 ml	$13.44	Lindane, H.C.F.A. F F P	99999-1642-05
480 ml	$14.22	Lindane, Stafford Miller	55372-4660-01
480 ml	$16.78	Lindane, Qualitest Pharms	00603-1406-58
480 ml	$18.05	Lindane, Harber Pharm	51432-0625-20
480 ml	$18.40	Lindane, Major Pharms	00904-0692-16
480 ml	$21.77	Lindane, Morton Grove	60432-0547-16
480 ml	$22.10	Lindane, Aligen Independ	00405-3200-16
3785 ml	$144.40	Lindane Shampoo 1%, Alpharma	00472-0572-28
3840 ml	$107.52	Lindane, H.C.F.A. F F P	99999-1642-04
3840 ml	$115.47	Lindane, Major Pharms	00904-0692-28
3840 ml	$124.99	Lindane, Consolidated Midland	00223-6562-03

HOW SUPPLIED - NOT RATED EQUIVALENT:

Cream - Topical - 1 %

60 gm	**$12.88**	**KWELL, Reed & Carnrick**	**00021-0601-02**

LIOTHYRONINE SODIUM *(001645)*

CATEGORIES: Diagnostic Agents; Goiter; Hormones; Hyperthyroidism; Hypothyroidism; Myxedema; Pituitary; Synthetic Thyroid Hormone; Thyroid Agents; Thyroid Function; Thyroid Preparations; Thyroiditis; Pregnancy Category A; FDA Approval Pre 1982

BRAND NAMES: *Cynomel* (France, Mexico); **Cytomel**; *Cytomel 25*; *T3*; *Tertroxin* (Australia); *Thyronine* (Japan); *Trijodthyronin*; *Trijodthyronin BC N* (Germany); Triostat

(International brand names outside U.S. in italics)

FORMULARIES: Aetna; BC-BS; FHP

DESCRIPTION:

Thyroid hormone drugs are natural or synthetic preparations containing tetraiodothyronine (T_4, levothyroxine) sodium or triiodothyronine (T_3, liothyronine) sodium or both. T_4 and T_3 are produced in the human thyroid gland by the iodination and coupling of the amino acid tyrosine. T_4 contains four iodine atoms and is formed by the coupling of two molecules of diiodotyrosine (DIT). T_3contains three atoms of iodine and is formed by the coupling of one molecule of DIT with one molecule of monoiodotyrosine (MIT). Both hormones are stored in the thyroid colloid as thyroglobulin.

Thyroid Hormone Preparations Belong To Two Categories: (1) natural hormonal preparations derived from animal thyroid, and (2) synthetic preparations. Natural preparations include desiccated thyroid and thyroglobulin. Desiccated thyroid is derived from domesticated animals that are used for food by man (either beef or hog thyroid), and thyroglobulin is derived from thyroid glands of the hog. The United States Pharmacopeia (USP) has standardized the total iodine content of natural preparations. Thyroid USP contains not less than (NLT) 0.17 percent and not more than (NMT) 0.23 percent iodine, and thyroglobulin contains not less than (NLT) 0.7 percent of organically bound iodine. Iodine content is only an indirect indicator of true hormonal biologic activity.

Tablets: Cytomel (liothyronine sodium) Tablets contain liothyronine (L-triiodothyronine or LT_3), a synthetic form of a natural thyroid hormone, and is available as the sodium salt.

The empirical formula of liothyronine sodium is $C_{15}H_{11}I_3NNaO_4$. The molecular weight is 672.96.

L-Tyrosine, *O*-(4-hydroxy-3-iodophenyl) -3,5 -diiodo, monosodium salt

Twenty-five mcg of liothyronine is equivalent to approximately 1 grain of desiccated thyroid or thyroglobulin and 0.1 mg of L-thyroxine.

Each round, white to off-white Cytomel (liothyronine sodium) tablet contains liothyronine sodium equivalent to liothyronine as follows: 5 mcg debossed SKF and D14; 25 mcg scored and debossed. SKF and D16:50 mcg scored and debossed SKF and D17. Inactive ingredients consist of calcium sulfate, gelatin, starch, stearic acid, sucrose and talc.

Injection: The major source of T_3 has been shown to be peripheral deiodination of T_4. T_3 is bound less firmly than T_4 in the serum, enters peripheral tissues more readily, and binds to specific nuclear receptor(s) to initiate hormonal, metabolic effects. T_4 is the prohormone which is deiodinated for T_3 for hormone activity.

Triostat (liothyronine sodium injection) (T_3) contains liothyronine (L-tri-iodothyronine or L-T_3) a synthetic form of a natural thyroid hormone, as the sodium salt.

In euthyroid patients, 25 mcg of liothyronine is equivalent to approximately 1 grain of desiccated thyroid or thyroglobulin and 0.1 mg of L-thyroxine.

Each ml of Triostat in amber-glass vials contains, in sterile non- pyrogenic aqueous solution, sodium liothyronine equivalent to 10 mcg of liothyronine; alcohol, 6.8% by volume; anhydrous citric acid, 0.175 mg; ammonia, 2.19 mg as ammonium hydroxide.

CLINICAL PHARMACOLOGY:

Tablets: The mechanisms by which thyroid hormones exert their physiologic action are not well understood. These hormones enhance oxygen consumption by most tissues of the body, increase the basal metabolic rate and the metabolism of carbohydrates, lipids and proteins. Thus, they exert a profound influence on every organ system in the body and are of particular importance in the development of the central nervous system.

Injection: Thyroid hormones enhance oxygen consumption by most tissues of the body and increase the basal metabolic rate and the metabolism of carbohydrates, lipids and proteins. *In vitro* studies indicate that T_3 increases aerobic mitochondrial function, thereby increasing the

CLINICAL PHARMACOLOGY: *(cont'd)*

rates of synthesis and utilization of myocardial high-energy phosphates. This, in turn, stimulates myosin ATPase and reduces tissue lactic acidosis. Thus, thyroid hormones exert a profound influence on virtually every organ system in the body and are of particular importance in the development of the central nervous system.

While the source of levothyroxine (T_4) and some triiodothyronine (T_3) is via secretion from the thyroid gland, it is now well- established that approximately 80% of circulating T_3 arises predominantly by way of the extrathyroidal conversion of T_4. The membrane-bound enzyme responsible for this reaction is iodothyronine 5'- deiodinase. Activity of the enzyme is greatest in the liver and kidney. A second pathway to T_4 to T_3 conversion occurs via a PTU-insensitive 5'-deiodinase located primarily in the pituitary and central nervous system.

The prohormone T_4 must be converted to T_3 in the body before it can exert biological effects. During periods of illness or stress, this conversion is often inhibited and can be diverted to the inactive reverse T_3 (rT_3) moiety. Therefore, correction of the hypothyroid condition in patients with myxedema coma is facilitated by the parenteral administration of triiodothyronine (T_3). T_3 is bound much less firmly to serum binding proteins and therefore penetrates into the cells much more rapidly than T_4. Also, the binding of T_3 to a nuclear thyroid hormone in tissues. Although most thyroid hormone analogs, both natural and synthetic, will bind to this protein, the affinity of T_3 for this receptor is roughly 10-fold higher than that of T_4. Thus $T_3$is the biologically active thyroid hormone.

PHARMACODYNAMICS

Injection: The clinical features of myxedema coma include depression of the cardiovascular, respiratory, gastrointestinal and central nervous system, impaired diuresis, and hypothermia. Administration of thyroid reverses or attenuates these conditions. Thyroid hormones increase heart rate, ventricular contractility and cardiac output, as well as decrease total systemic vascular resistance. They also increase the rate of respiration, motility of the gastrointestinal tract, rapidity of cerebration, and vasodilation. Thyroid hormones correct hypothermia by markedly increasing the basal metabolic rate, as well as the number and activity of mitochondria in almost all cells of the body.

PHARMACOKINETICS

Since liothyronine sodium (T_3) is not firmly bound to serum protein, it is readily available to body tissues. The onset of activity of liothyronine sodium is rapid, occurring within a few hours. Maximum pharmacologic response occurs within two or three days, providing early clinical response. The biological half-life is about 2 1/2 days.

T_3 is almost totally absorbed, 95 percent in four hours. The hormones contained in the natural preparations are absorbed in a manner similar to the synthetic hormones.

Liothyronine sodium has a rapid cutoff of activity which permits quick dosage adjustment and facilitates control of the effects of overdosage, should they occur.

The higher affinity of levothyroxine (T_4) for both thyroid-binding globulin and thyroid-binding prealbumin as compared to triiodothyronine (T_3) partially explains the higher serum levels and longer half-life of the former hormone. Both protein-bound hormones exist in reverse equilibrium with minute amounts of free hormone, the latter accounting for the metabolic activity.

Injection: A single dose of liothyronine sodium administered intravenously produces a detectable metabolic response in as little as two to four hours and a maximum therapeutic response within two days. However, no pharmacokinetic studies have been performed with intravenous liothyronine (T_3) in myxedema coma or precoma patients.

INDICATIONS AND USAGE:

Tablets: Thyroid hormone drugs are indicated:

1. As replacement of supplemental therapy in patients with hypothyroidism of any etiology, except transient hypothyroidism during the recovery phase of subacute thyroiditis. This category includes cretinism, myxedema and ordinary hypothyroidism in patients of any age (children, adults, the elderly), or state (including pregnancy); primary hypothyroidism resulting from functional deficiency, primary atrophy, partial or total absence of thyroid gland, or the effects of surgery, radiation, or drugs, with or without the presence of goiter; and secondary (pituitary) or tertiary (hypothalamic) hypothyroidism (See WARNINGS.)

2. As pituitary thyroid-stimulating hormone (TSH) suppressants, in the treatment or prevention of various types of euthyroid goiters, including thyroid nodules, subacute or chronic lymphocytic thyroiditis (Hashimoto's) and multinodular goiter.

3. As diagnostic agents in suppression tests to differentiate suspected mild hyperthyroidism or thyroid gland autonomy.

Cytomel (liothyronine sodium) Tablets can be used in patients allergic to desiccated thyroid or thyroid extract derived from pork or beef.

Injection: Triostat (liothyronine sodium injection)(T_3) is indicated in the treatment of myxedema coma/precoma.

Triostat can be used in patients allergic to desiccated thyroid or thyroid extract derived from pork or beef.

CONTRAINDICATIONS:

Thyroid hormone preparations are generally contraindicated in patients with diagnosed but as yet uncorrected adrenal cortical insufficiency, untreated thyrotoxicosis and apparent hypersensitivity to any of their active or extraneous constituents. There is no well-documented evidence from the literature, however, of true allergic or idiosyncratic reactions to thyroid hormone.

WARNINGS:

Drugs with thyroid hormone activity, alone or together with other therapeutic agents, have been used for the treatment of obesity. In euthyroid patients, doses within the range of daily hormonal requirements are ineffective for weight reduction. Larger doses may produce serious or even life-threatening manifestations of toxicity, particularly when given in association with sympathomimetic amines such as those used for their anorectic effects.

The use of thyroid hormones in the therapy of obesity, alone or combined with other drugs, is unjustified and has been shown to be ineffective. Neither is their use justified for the treatment of male or female infertility unless this condition is accompanied by hypothyroidism.

Thyroid hormones should be used with great caution in a number of circumstances where the integrity of the cardiovascular system, particularly the coronary arteries, is suspected. These include patients with angina pectoris or the elderly, in whom there is a greater likelihood of occult cardiac disease. In these patients, liothyronine sodium therapy should be initiated with low doses, with due consideration for its relatively rapid onset of action.

Morphologic hypogonadism and nephrosis should be ruled out before the drug is administered. If hypopituitarism is present, the adrenal deficiency must be corrected prior to starting the drug.

WARNINGS: *(cont'd)*

Myxedematous patients are very sensitive to thyroid; dosage should be started at a very low level and increased gradually as acute changes may precipitate adverse cardiovascular events.

Severe and prolonged hypothyroidism can lead to a decreased level of adrenocortical activity commensurate with the lowered metabolic state. When thyroid-replacement therapy is administered, the metabolism increases at a greater rate than adrenocortical activity. This can precipitate adrenocortical insufficiency. Therefore, in severe and prolonged hypothyroidism, supplemental adrenocortical steroids may be necessary.

In rare instances the administration of thyroid hormone may precipitate a hyperthyroid state or may aggravate existing hyperthyroidism.

Tablets: In patients with angina pectoris or the elderly, liothyronine sodium therapy should be initiated in low doses, with due consideration for its relatively rapid onset of action. Starting dosage of Cytomel (liothyronine sodium) Tablets is 5 mcg daily, and should be increased by no more than 5 mcg increments at 2-week intervals. When, in such patients, a euthyroid state can only be reached at the expense of an aggravation of the cardiovascular disease, thyroid hormone dosage should be reduced. Morphologic hypogonadism and nephrosis should be ruled out before the drug administered. If hypopituitarism is present, the adrenal deficiency must be corrected prior to starting the drug.

Injection: Therefore, in patients with compromised cardiac function, use thyroid hormones in conjunction with careful cardiac monitoring. Although the specific dosage of Triostat depends upon individual circumstances, in patients with known or suspected cardiovascular disease the extremely rapid onset of action of Triostat may warrant initiating therapy at a dose of 10 mcg to 20 mcg. (See DOSAGE AND ADMINISTRATION.)

Extreme caution is advised when administering thyroid hormones with digitalis or vasopressors. (See DRUG INTERACTIONS.)

Fluid therapy should be administered with great care to prevent cardiac decompensation. (See PRECAUTIONS, Adjunctive Therapy.)

PRECAUTIONS:

GENERAL

Thyroid hormone therapy in patients with concomitant diabetes mellitus (see DRUG INTERACTIONS, Insulin or Oral Hypoglycemics regarding interaction and dose adjustment with insulin) or insipidus or adrenal cortical insufficiency aggravates the intensity of their symptoms. Appropriate adjustments of the various therapeutic measures directed at these concomitant endocrine diseases are required.

The therapy of myxedema coma requires simultaneous administration of glucocorticoids. (See PRECAUTIONS, Adjunctive Therapy.)

Hypothyroidism decreases and hyperthyroidism increases the sensitivity to oral anticoagulants. Prothrombin time should be closely monitored in thyroid-treated patients on oral anticoagulants and dosage of the latter agents adjusted on the basis of frequent prothrombin time determinations.

Injection

General: Oral therapy should be resumed as soon as the clinical situation has been stabilized and the patient is able to take oral medication. If L-thyroxine rather than liothyronine sodium is used in initiating oral therapy, the physician should bear in mind that there is a delay of several days in the onset of L-thyroxine activity and that intravenous therapy should be discontinued gradually.

Adjunctive Therapy: Many investigators recommend that corticosteroids be administered routinely in the initial emergency treatment for all patients with myxedema coma. Patients with pituitary myxedema should receive adrenocortical hormone replacement therapy at or before the start of Triostat therapy. Similarly, patients with primary myxedema may also require adrenocortical hormone replacement therapy since a rapid return to normal body metabolism from a severely hypothyroid state may result in acute adrenocortical insufficiency and shock.

In considering the need to elevate blood pressure, it should be kept in mind that tissue metabolic requirements are markedly reduced in the hypothyroid patient. Because arrhythmias and circulatory collapse have infrequently occurred following the concomitant administration of thyroid hormones and vasopressor therapies, use caution when administering these therapies consistently (see DRUG INTERACTIONS, Vasopressors).

Hyponatremia is frequently present in myxedema coma, but usually resolves without specific therapy as the metabolic status of the patient is improved with thyroid hormone treatment. Fluid therapy should be administered with great care to prevent cardiac decompensation. In addition, some patients with myxedema have inappropriate secretion of ADH and are susceptible to water intoxication.

In some patients, respiratory depression has been a significant factor in the development or the persistence of the comatose state. Decreased oxygen saturation and elevated $C0_2$ levels respond quickly to artificial respiration.

Infection is often present in myxedema coma and should be looked for and treated appropriately.

Concomitant use of Triostat and artificial rewarming of patients is contraindicated. Although patients in myxedema coma are often hypothermic, most investigators believe that the artificial warming is of little value or may be harmful. The peripheral vasodilation produced by external heat serves to further decrease circulation to vital internal organs and to increase shock if present. It has been reported that the administration of liothyronine sodium will restore a normal body temperature in 24 to 48 hours if heat loss is prevented by keeping the patient covered with blankets in a warm room.

DRUG/LABORATORY TEST INTERACTIONS

The following drugs or moieties are known to interfere with laboratory tests performed in patients on thyroid hormone therapy: androgens, corticosteroids, estrogens, oral contraceptives containing estrogens, iodine-containing preparations and the numerous preparations containing salicylates.

Tablets

1. Changes in TBG concentration should be taken into consideration in the interpretation of $T_4$and T_3 values. In such cases, the unbound (free) hormone should be measured. Pregnancy, estrogens and estrogen- containing oral contraceptives increase TBG concentrations. TBG may also be increased during infectious hepatitis. Decreases in TBG concentrations are observed in nephrosis, acromegaly and after androgen or corticosteroid therapy. Familial hyper- or hypo-thyroxine-binding globulinemias have been described. The incidence of TBG deficiency approximates 1 in 9000. The binding of thyroxine by thyroxine-binding prealbumin (TBPA) is inhibited by salicylates.

2. Medicinal or dietary iodine interferes with all *in vivo* tests of radioiodine uptake, producing low uptakes which may not be reflective of a true decrease in hormone synthesis.

3. The persistence of clinical and laboratory evidence of hypothyroidism in spite of adequate dosage replacement indicates either poor patient compliance, poor absorption, excessive fecal loss, or inactivity of the preparation. Intracellular resistance to thyroid hormone is quite rare.

PRECAUTIONS: *(cont'd)*

CARCINOGENESIS, MUTAGENESIS, AND IMPAIRMENT OF FERTILITY

A reportedly apparent association between prolonged thyroid therapy and breast cancer has not been confirmed and patients on thyroid for established indications should not discontinue therapy. No confirmatory long-term studies in animals have been performed to evaluate carcinogenic potential, mutagenicity, or impairment of fertility in either males or females.

PREGNANCY CATEGORY A

Thyroid hormones do not readily cross the placental barrier. The clinical experience to date does not indicate any adverse effect on fetuses when thyroid hormones are administered to pregnant women. On the basis of current knowledge, thyroid replacement therapy to hypothyroid women should not be discontinued during pregnancy.

NURSING MOTHERS

Minimal amounts of thyroid hormones are excreted in human milk. Thyroid is not associated with serious adverse reactions and does not have a known tumorigenic potential. However, caution should be exercised when thyroid is administered to a nursing woman.

Tablets: In infants, excessive doses of thyroid hormone preparations may produce craniosynostosis.

INFORMATION FOR THE PATIENT

Patients on thyroid hormone preparations and parents of children on thyroid therapy should be informed that:

1. Replacement therapy is to be taken essentially for life, with the exception of cases of transient hypothyroidism, usually associated with thyroiditis, and in those patients receiving a therapeutic trial of the drug.

2. They should immediately report during the course of therapy any signs or symptoms of thyroid hormone toxicity, e.g., chest pain, increased pulse rate, palpitations, excessive sweating, heat intolerance, nervousness, or any other unusual event.

3. In case of concomitant diabetes mellitus, the daily dosage of antidiabetic medication may need readjustment as thyroid hormone replacement is achieved. If thyroid medication is stopped, a downward readjustment of the dosage of insulin or oral hypoglycemic agent may be necessary to avoid hypoglycemia. At all times, close monitoring of urinary glucose levels is mandatory in such patients.

4. In case of concomitant oral anticoagulant therapy, the prothrombin time should be measured frequently to determine if the dosage of oral anticoagulants is to be readjusted.

5. Partial loss of hair may be experienced by children in the first few months of thyroid therapy, but this is usually a transient phenomenon and later recovery is usually the rule.

LABORATORY TESTS

Treatment of patients with thyroid hormones requires the periodic assessment of thyroid status by means of appropriate laboratory tests besides the full clinical evaluation. The TSH suppression test can be used to test the effectiveness of any thyroid preparation, bearing in mind the relative insensitivity of the infant pituitary to the negative feedback effect of thyroid hormones. Serum T_4 levels can be used to test the effectiveness of all thyroid medications except products containing liothyronine sodium. When the total serum $T_4$is low but TSH is normal, a test specific to assess unbound (free) T_4 levels is warranted. Specific measurements of T_4 and T_3 by competitive protein binding or radioimmunoassay are not influenced by blood levels of organic or inorganic iodine and have essentially replaced older tests of thyroid hormone measurements, *i.e.*, PBI, BEI and T_4 by column.

Injection: Treatment of patients with thyroid hormones requires the periodic assessment of thyroid status by means of appropriate laboratory tests besides the full clinical evaluation. Serum T_3 and TSH levels should be monitored to assess dosage adequacy and biologic effectiveness.

PEDIATRIC USE

Pregnant mothers provide little or no thyroid hormone to the fetus. The incidence of congenital hypothyroidism is relatively high (1:4000) and the hypothyroid fetus would not derive any benefit from the small amounts of hormone crossing the placental barrier. Routine determinations of serum T_4 and/or TSH is strongly advised in neonates in view of the deleterious effects of thyroid deficiency on growth and development.

Treatment should be initiated immediately upon diagnosis and maintained for life, unless transient hypothyroidism is suspected, in which case, therapy may be interrupted for 2 to 8 weeks after the age of 3 years to reassess the condition. Cessation of therapy is justified in patients who have maintained a normal TSH during those 2 to 8 weeks.

Injections: There is limited experience with Triostat in children. Safety and effectiveness have not been established.

DRUG INTERACTIONS:

Oral Anticoagulants: Thyroid hormones appear to increase catabolism of vitamin K-dependent clotting factors. If oral anticoagulants are also being given, compensatory increases in clotting factor synthesis are impaired. Patients stabilized on oral anticoagulants who are found to require thyroid replacement therapy should be watched very closely when thyroid is started. If a patient is truly hypothyroid, it is likely that a reduction in anticoagulant dosage will be required. No special precautions appear to be necessary when oral anticoagulant therapy is begun in a patient already stabilized on maintenance thyroid replacement therapy.

Insulin or Oral Hypoglycemics: Initiating thyroid replacement therapy may cause increases in insulin or oral hypoglycemic requirements. The effects seen are poorly understood and depend upon a variety of factors such as dose and type of thyroid preparations and endocrine status of the patient. Patients receiving insulin or oral hypoglycemics should be closely watched during initiation of thyroid replacement therapy.

Estrogen, Oral Contraceptives: Estrogens tend to increase serum thyroxine-binding globulin (TBG). In a patient with a nonfunctioning thyroid gland who is receiving thyroid replacement therapy, free levothyroxine may be decreased when estrogens are started thus increasing thyroid requirements. However, if the patient's thyroid gland has sufficient function, the decreased free thyroxine will result in a compensatory increase in thyroxine output by the thyroid. Therefore, patients without a functioning thyroid gland who are on thyroid replacement therapy may need to increase their thyroid dose if estrogens or estrogen-containing oral contraceptives are given.

Tricyclic Antidepressants: Use of thyroid products with imipramine and other tricyclic antidepressants may increase receptor sensitivity and enhance antidepressant activity; transient cardiac arrhythmias have been observed. Thyroid hormone activity may also be enhanced.

Digitalis: Thyroid preparations may potentiate the toxic effects of digitalis. Thyroid hormonal replacement increases metabolic rate, which requires an increase in digitalis dosage.

Ketamine: When administered to patients on a thyroid preparation, this parenteral anesthetic may cause hypertension and tachycardia. Use with caution and be prepared to treat hypertension, if necessary.

DRUG INTERACTIONS: *(cont'd)*

Vasopressors: Thyroid hormones increase the adrenergic effect of catecholamines such as epinephrine and norepinephrine. Therefore, use of vasopressors in patients receiving thyroid hormone preparations may increase the risk of precipitating coronary insufficiency, especially in patients with coronary artery disease. Therefore, use with caution when administering vasopressors with liothyronine (T_3)

TABLETS

Cholestyramine: Cholestyramine binds both T_4 and T_3in the intestine, thus impairing absorption of these thyroid hormones. *In vitro* studies indicate that the binding is not easily removed. Therefore, 4 to 5 hours should elapse between administration of cholestyramine and thyroid hormones.

ADVERSE REACTIONS:

Tablets: Adverse reactions, other than those indicative of hyperthyroidism because of therapeutic overdosage, either initially or during the maintenance period are rare (See OVERDOSAGE.)

In rare instances, allergic skin reactions have been reported with Cytomel (liothyronine sodium) Tablets.

Injection: The most frequently reported adverse events when arrhythmia (6% of patients) and tachycardia (3%). Cardiopulmonary arrest, hypotension and myocardial infarction occurred in approximately 2% of patients. The following events occurred in approximately 1% or fewer of patients: angina, congestive heart failure, fever, hypotension, phlebitis, and twitching.

In rare instances, allergic skin reactions have been reported with liothyronine sodium tablets.

OVERDOSAGE:

SIGNS AND SYMPTOMS

Headache, irritability, nervousness, sweating, tachycardia, increased bowel motility and menstrual irregularities. Angina pectoris or congestive heart failure may be induced or aggravated. Shock may also develop if there is untreated pituitary or adrenocortical failure. Massive overdosage may result in symptoms resembling thyroid storm. Chronic excessive dosage will produce the signs and symptoms of hyperthyroidism.

TREATMENT

Dosage should be reduced or therapy temporarily discontinued if signs and symptoms of overdosage appear. Treatment may be reinstituted at a lower dosage. In normal individuals, normal hypothalamic-pituitary-thyroid axis function is restored in six to eight weeks after thyroid suppression.

TABLETS

Treatment of acute massive thyroid hormone overdosage is aimed at reducing gastrointestinal absorption of the drugs and counteracting central and peripheral effects, mainly those of increased sympathetic activity. Vomiting may be induced initially if further gastrointestinal absorption can reasonably be prevented and barring contraindications such as coma, convulsions, or loss of the gagging reflex. Treatment is symptomatic and supportive. Oxygen may be administered and ventilation maintained. Cardiac glycosides may be indicated if congestive heart failure develops. Measures to control fever, hypoglycemia, or fluid loss should be instituted if needed. Antiadrenergic agents, particularly propranolol, have been used advantageously in the treatment of increased sympathetic activity. Propranolol may be administered intravenously at a dosage of 1 to 3 pf over a 10-minute period or orally, 80 to 160 mg/day, especially when no contraindications exist for its use.

INJECTION

Treatment is symptomatic and supportive. Oxygen may be administered and ventialtion maintained. Cardiac glycosides may be indicated if congestive heart failure develops. Beta-adrenergic antagonists have been used advantageously in the treatment of increased sympathetic activity. Measures to control fever, hypoglycemia or fluid loss should be instituted if needed.

DOSAGE AND ADMINISTRATION:

Tablets: The dosage of thyroid hormones is determined by the indication and must in every case be individualized according to patient response and laboratory findings.

Cytomel (liothyronine sodium) Tablets are intended for oral administration; once-a-day dosage is recommended. Although liothyronine sodium has a rapid cutoff, its metabolic effects persist for a few days following discontinuance.

Mild Hypothyroidism: Recommended starting dosage is 25 mcg daily. Daily dosage then may be increased by 12.5 or 25 mcg every 1 or 2 weeks. Usual maintenance dose is 25 to 75 mcg daily. Smaller doses may be fully effective in some patients, while dosage of 100 mcg daily may be required in others.

The rapid onset and dissipation of action of liothyronine sodium (T_3), as compared with levothyroxine sodium (T_4), has led some clinicians to prefer its use in patients who might be more susceptible to the untoward effects of thyroid medication. However, the wide swings in serum T_3 levels that follow its administration and the possibility of more pronounced cardiovascular side effects tend to counterbalance the stated advantages.

Cytomel (liothyronine sodium) Tablets may be used in preference to levothyroxine (T_4) during radioisotope scanning procedures, since induction of hypothyroidism in those cases is more abrupt and can be of shorter duration. It may also be preferred when impairment of peripheral conversion of T_4 and T_3 is suspected.

Myxedema: Recommended starting dosage is 5 mcg daily. This may be increased by 5 to 10 mcg daily every 1 or 2 weeks. When 25 mcg daily is reached, dosage may often be increased by 12.5 or 25 mcg every one or two weeks. Usual maintenance dose is 50 to 100 mcg daily.

Myxedema Coma: Myxedema coma is usually precipitated in the hypothyroid patient of long standing by intercurrent illness or drugs such as sedatives and anesthetics and should be considered a medical emergency. *Congenital Hypothyroidism:* Recommended starting dosage is 5 mcg daily, with a 5 mcg increment every 3 to 4 days until the desired response is achieved. Infants a few months old may require only 20 mcg daily for maintenance. At 1 year, 50 mcg daily may be required. Above 3 years, full adult dosage may be necessary (See PRECAUTIONS, Pediatric Use.)

Simple (non-toxic) Goiter: Recommended starting dosage is 5 mcg daily. This dosage may be increased by 5 to 10 mcg daily every 1 or 2 weeks. When 25 mcg daily is reached, dosage may be increased every week or two by 12.5 or 25 mcg. Usual maintenance dosage is 75 mcg daily.

In the elderly or in children , therapy should be started with 5 mcg daily and increased only by 5 mcg increments at the recommended intervals.

When switching a patient to Cytomel (liothyronine sodium) Tablets from thyroid, L-thyroxine or thyroglobulin, discontinue the other medication, initiate Cytomel at a low dosage, and increase gradually according to the patient's response. When selecting a starting dosage, bear in mind that this drug has a rapid onset of action, and that residual effects of the other thyroid preparation may persist for the first several weeks of therapy.

Thyroid Suppression Therapy: Administration of thyroid hormone in doses higher than those produced physiologically be be the gland results in suppression of the production of endogenous hormone. This is the basis for the thyroid suppression test and is used as an aid in the diagnosis of patients with signs of mild hyperthyroidism in whom baseline laboratory tests

DOSAGE AND ADMINISTRATION: *(cont'd)*

appear normal or to demonstrate thyroid gland autonomy in patients with Graves' ophthalmopathy. ^{131}I uptake is determined before and after the administration of the exogenous hormone. A 50% or greater suppression of uptake indicates a normal thyroid-pituitary axis and thus rules out thyroid gland autonomy.

Cytomel (liothyronine sodium) Tablets are given in doses of 75 to 100 mcg/day for 7 days, and radioactive iodine uptake is determined before and after administration of the hormone. If thyroid function is under normal control, the radioiodine uptake will drop significantly after treatment. Cytomel (liothyronine sodium) Tablets should be administered cautiously to patients in whom there is a strong suspicion of thyroid gland autonomy, in view of the fact that the exogenous hormone effects will be additive to the endogenous source.

Injection: *Adults:* Myxedema coma is usually precipitated in the hypothyroid patient of long standing by intercurrent illness or drugs such as sedatives and anesthetics and should be considered a medical emergency. Therapy should be directed at the correction of electrolyte disturbances, possible infection, or other intercurrent illness in addition to the administration of intravenous liothyronine (T_3). Simultaneous glucorticosteroids are required.

Triostat (liothyronine sodium injection (T_3) is for intravenous administration only. It should not be given intramuscularly or subcutaneously.

Prompt administration of an adequate dose of intravenous liothyronine (T_3) is important in determining clinical outcome.

Initial and subsequent doses of Triostat should be based on continuous monitoring of the patient's clinical status and response to therapy.

Triostat doses should normally be administered at least four hours- and not more than 12 hours-apart.

Administration of at least 65 mcg/day of intravenous liothyronine (T_3) in the initial days of therapy was associated with lower mortality.

There is limited clinical experience with intravenous liothyronine.

(T_3) at total daily doses exceeding 100 mcg/day.

No controlled clinical studies have been done with Triostat. The following dosing guidleines have been derived from data analysis of myxedema coma/precoma case reports collected by SmithKline Beecham Pharmaceuticals since 1963 and from scientific literature since 1956.

An initial intravenous Triostat dose ranging from 25 mcg to 50 mcg is recommended in the emergency treatment of myxedema coma/precoma in adults. In patients with known or suspected cardiovascular disease, an initial dose of 10 mcg to 20 mcg is suggested (see WARNINGS.) However, both the initial dose and subsequent doses should be determined on the basis of continuous monitoring of the patient's clinical condition and response to Triostat therapy. Normally at least four hours should be allowed between doses to adequately assess therapeutic response and no more than 12 hours should elapse between doses to avoid fluctuation in hormone levels. Caution should be exercised in adjusting the dose due to the potential of large changes in precipitate adverse cardiovascular events. Review of the myxedema case reports indicate decreased mortality in patients receiving at least 65 mcg/day in the initial days of treatment. However, there is limited clinical experience at total daily doses above 100 mcg. See DRUG INTERACTIONSfor potential interactions between thyroid hormones and digitalis and vasopressors.

Pediatric Use: There is limited experience with Triostat in children. Safety and effectiveness have not been established.

Switching to Oral Therapy: Oral therapy should be resumed as soon as the clinical situation has been stabilized and the patient is able to take oral medication. When switching a patient to liothyronine sodium tablets from Triostat, discontinue Triostat, initiate oral therapy at a low dosage, and increase gradually according to the patient's response.

If L-thyroxine rather than liothyronine sodium is used in initiating oral therapy, the physician should bear in mind that there is a delay of several days in the onset of L-thyroxine activity and that intravenous therapy should be discontinued gradually.

HOW SUPPLIED:

Tablet: Cytomel (liothyronine sodium) Tablets: 5 mcg in bottles of 100; 25 mcg in bottles of 100; and 50 mcg in bottles of 100.

Injection: In packages of six 1 ml vials at a concentration of 10 mcg/ml.

Store between 2 and 8°C.

HOW SUPPLIED - EQUIVALENTS NOT AVAILABLE:

Injection, Solution - Intravenous - 10 mcg/ml

1 ml x 6 $1373.00 TRIOSTAT, SKB Pharms 00007-5210-06

Tablet, Uncoated - Oral - 5 mcg

100's $14.50 CYTOMEL, SKB Pharms 00007-3414-20

Tablet, Uncoated - Oral - 25 mcg

100's $17.55 CYTOMEL, SKB Pharms 00007-3416-20

Tablet, Uncoated - Oral - 50 mcg

100's $26.80 CYTOMEL, SKB Pharms 00007-3417-20

LIOTRIX (T3 AND T4) *(001646)*

CATEGORIES: Hormones; Hypothyroidism; Myxedema; Synthetic Thyroid Hormone; Thyroid Agents; Thyroid Preparations; Thyroiditis; Pregnancy Category A; FDA Approval Pre 1982

BRAND NAMES: *Cynoplus 3* (Mexico); **Euthroid**; *Euthroid 2*; *Eutroid*; *Proloid S-1* (Mexico); *Proloid S-2* (Mexico); *Thyreotom*; *Thyreotom Forte*; Thyrolar
(International brand names outside U.S. in italics)

FORMULARIES: Aetna; BC-BS

DESCRIPTION:

Liotrix tablets, USP is synthetic microcrystalline levothyroxine sodium (T_4) USP and synthetic microcrystalline liothyronine sodium (T_3) USP combined in a constant 4:1 ratio. Each Liotrix-1 tablet contains 60 mcg levothyroxine (T_4) and 15 mcg liothyronine (T_3).

Each Liotrix-1 tablet will give a dose benefit approximately equivalent to 1 grain of desiccated thyroid, 100 mcg T_4 (levothyroxine sodium), 25 mcg T_3 (liothyronine sodium), or 60 mcg T_4/15 mcg T_3 (liotrix).

See Conversion Table at end of insert.

Liotrix tablets also contain calcium phosphate, USP; cellulose, NF; corn starch, NF; hydrogenated vegetable oil, NF; magnesium stearate, NF; mannitol, USP; and silicon dioxide, NF. In addition, Liotrix-1/2 contains D&C red No. 30 lake and FD&C yellow No. 5 lake. Liotrix-1 and Liotrix-3 contain D&C red No. 30 lake, FD&C blue No. 2 lake and FD&C yellow No. 5 lake. Liotrix-2 contains D&C red No. 30 lake and FD&C blue No. 2 lake.

DESCRIPTION: *(cont'd)*

Thyroid hormone drugs are natural or synthetic preparations containing tetraiodothyronine (T_4, levothyroxine) sodium or triiodothyronine (T_3, liothyronine) sodium or both. $T_4$and T_3 are produced in the human thyroid gland by the iodination and coupling of the amino acid tyrosine. T_4contains four iodine atoms and is formed by the coupling of two molecules of diiodotyrosine (DIT). T_3contains three atoms of iodine and is formed by the coupling of one molecule of DIT with one molecule of monoiodotyrosine (MIT). Both hormones are stored in the thyroid colloid as thyroglobulin.

Thyroid hormone preparations belong to two categories: (1) natural hormonal preparations derived from animal thyroid, and (2) synthetic preparations. Natural preparations include desiccated thyroid and thyroglobulin. Desiccated thyroid is derived from domesticated animals that are used for food by man (either beef or hog thyroid), and thyroglobulin is derived from thyroid glands of the hog.

There are five (5) preparations in the USP. They are: (1) Thyroid Tablets, (21) Thyroglobulin Tablets, (3) Levothyroxine Sodium Tablets, (4) Liothyronine Sodium Tablets, and (5) Liotrix Tablets (a ratio, by weight, of 4 to 1, of the sodium salts of T_4 and T_3, respectively).

The empirical formulas, molecular weights, and Chemical Abstract Service (CAS) registry numbers of the synthetic sodium salts T4 and T3 are given below.

Liothyronine (T_3) Sodium

$C_{15}H_{11}I_3NNaO_4$ MW 672.96 (CAS 55-06-1)

L-Tyrosine, *O*-(4-hydroxy -3-iodophenyl)-3,5 -diiodo-monosodium salt

Levothyroxine (T_4) Sodium

$C_{15}H_{10}I_4NNaO_4\text{-}xH_2O$ (CAS 25416-65-3)

MW 798.86(anhydrous) (CAS 55-03-8)

L-Tyrosine, *O*-(4-hydroxy -3,5-diiodophenyl)-3,5-diiodo-monosodium salt, hydrate

CLINICAL PHARMACOLOGY:

The steps in the synthesis of the thyroid hormones are controlled by thyrotropin (Thyroid Stimulating Hormone, TSH) secreted by the anterior pituitary. This hormone's secretion is in turn controlled by a feedback mechanism effected by the thyroid hormones themselves and by thyrotropin releasing hormone (TRH), a tripeptide of hypothalamic origin. Endogenous thyroid hormone secretion is suppressed when exogenous thyroid hormones are administered to euthyroid individuals in excess of the normal gland's secretion.

The mechanisms by which thyroid hormones exert their physiologic action are not well understood. These hormones enhance oxygen consumption by most tissues of the body, increase the basal metabolic rate, and the metabolism of carbohydrates, lipids, and proteins. Thus, they exert a profound influence on every organ system in the body and are of particular importance in the development of the central nervous system.

The normal thyroid gland contains approximately 200 mcg of levothyroxine (T_4) per gram of gland, and 15 mcg of triiodothyronine (T_3) per gram. The ratio of these two hormones in the circulation does not represent the ratio in the thyroid gland, since about 80 percent of peripheral triiodothyronine comes from monodeiodination of levothyroxine. Peripheral monodeiodination of levothyroxine at the 5 position (inner ring) also results in the formation of reverse triiodothyronine (rT_3), which is calorigenically inactive. These facts would seem to advocate levothyroxine as the treatment of choice for the hypothyroid patient and to militate against the administration of hormone combinations, which while normalizing thyroxine levels may produce triiodothyronine levels in the thyrotoxic range.

Triiodothyronine (T_3) level is low in the fetus and newborn, in old age, in chronic caloric deprivation, hepatic cirrhosis, renal failure, surgical stress, and chronic illnesses representing what has been called the "low triiodothyronine syndrome."

Pharmacokinetics: Animal studies have shown that T_4 is only partially absorbed from the gastrointestinal tract. The degree of absorption is dependent on the vehicle used for its administration and by the character of the intestinal contents, the intestinal flora, including plasma protein, soluble dietary factors, all of which bind thyroid and thereby make it unavailable for diffusion. Only 41 percent is absorbed when given in a gelatin capsule as opposed to a 74 percent absorption when given with an albumin carrier.

Depending on the other factors, absorption has varied from 48 to 79 percent of the administered dose. Fasting increases absorption. Malabsorption syndromes, as well as dietary factors (children's soybean formula, concomitant use of anionic exchange resins such as cholestyramine), cause excessive fecal loss. T_3 is almost totally absorbed, 95 percent in 4 hours. The hormones contained in the natural preparations are absorbed in a manner similar to the synthetic hormones.

More than 99 percent of circulating hormones are bound to serum proteins, including thyroid-binding globulin (TBg), thyroid-binding prealbumin (TBPA), and albumin (TBa), whose capacities and affinities vary for the hormones. The higher affinity of levothyroxine (T_4) for both TBg and TBPA as compared to triiodothyronine (T_3) partially explains the higher serum levels and longer half-life of the former hormone. Both protein-bound hormones exist in reverse equilibrium with minute amounts of free hormone, the latter accounting for the metabolic activity.

Deiodination of levothyroxine (T_4) occurs at a number of sites, including liver, kidney, and other tissues. The conjugated hormone, in the form of glucuronide or sulfate, is found in the bile and gut where it may complete an enterohepatic circulation. Eighty-five percent of levothyroxine (T_4) metabolized daily is deiodinated.

INDICATIONS AND USAGE:

Thyroid hormone drugs are indicated:

As replacement or supplemental therapy in patients with hypothyroidism of any etiology, except transient hypothyroidism during the recovery phase of subacute thyroiditis. This category includes cretinism, myxedema, and ordinary hypothyroidism in patients of any age (children, adults, the elderly), or state (including pregnancy); primary hypothyroidism resulting from functional deficiency, primary atrophy, partial or total absence of thyroid gland, or the effects of surgery, radiation, or drugs, with or without the presence of goiter; and secondary (pituitary) or tertiary (hypothalamic) hypothyroidism (see WARNINGS.)

CONTRAINDICATIONS:

Thyroid hormone preparations are generally contraindicated in patients with diagnosed but as yet uncorrected adrenal cortical insufficiency, untreated thyrotoxicosis, and apparent hypersensitivity to any of their active or extraneous constituents. There is no well-documented evidence from the literature, however, of true allergic or idiosyncratic reactions to thyroid hormone.

WARNINGS:

Drugs with thyroid hormone activity, alone or together with other therapeutic agents, have been used for the treatment of obesity. In euthyroid patients, doses within the range of daily hormonal requirements are ineffective for weight reduction. Larger doses may produce serious or even life-threatening manifestations of toxicity, particularly when given in association with sympathomimetic amines such as those used for their anorectic effects.

The use of thyroid hormones in the therapy of obesity, alone or combined with other drugs, is unjustified and has been shown to be ineffective. Neither is their use justified for the treatment of male or female infertility unless this condition is accompanied by hypothyroidism.

PRECAUTIONS:

General: Thyroid hormones should be used with great caution in a number of circumstances where the integrity of the cardiovascular system, particularly the coronary arteries, is suspect. These include patients with angina pectoris or the elderly, in whom there is a greater likelihood of occult cardiac disease. In these patients, therapy should be initiated with low doses, i.e., 25-50 mcg levothyroxine (T_4) or its isocaloric equivalents (see Conversion Table at end of insert). When, in such patients, a euthyroid state can only be reached at the expense of an aggravation of the cardiovascular disease, thyroid hormone dosage should be reduced.

Thyroid hormone therapy in patients with concomitant diabetes mellitus or insipidus or adrenal cortical insufficiency aggravates the intensity of their symptoms. Appropriate adjustments of the various therapeutic measures directed at these concomitant endocrine diseases are required. The therapy of myxedema coma requires simultaneous administration of glucocorticoids (see DOSAGE AND ADMINISTRATION.)

Hypothyroidism decreases and hyperthyroidism increases the sensitivity to oral anticoagulants. Prothrombin time should be closely monitored in thyroid-treated patients on oral anticoagulants and dosage of the latter agents adjusted on the basis of frequent prothrombin time determination. In infants, excessive doses of thyroid hormone preparations may produce craniosynostosis.

Liotrix-1/2, -1, -3 contain FD&C Yellow No. 5 (tartrazine) which may cause allergic-type reactions (including bronchial asthma) in certain susceptible individuals. Although the overall incidence of FD&C Yellow No 5 (tartrazine) sensitivity in the general population is low, it is frequently seen in patients who also have aspirin hypersensitivity.

Information for the Patient: Patients on thyroid hormone preparations and parents of children on thyroid therapy should be informed that:

1. Replacement therapy is to be taken essentially for life, with the exception of cases of transient hypothyroidism, usually associated with thyroiditis, and in those patients receiving a therapeutic trial of the drug.

2. They should immediately report during the course of therapy any signs or symptoms of thyroid hormone toxicity, e.g., chest pain, increased pulse rate, palpitations, excessive sweating, heat intolerance, nervousness, or any other unusual event.

3. In case of concomitant diabetes mellitus, the daily dosage of antidiabetic medication may need readjustment as thyroid hormone replacement is achieved. If thyroid medication is stopped, a downward readjustment of the dosage of insulin or oral hypoglycemic agent may be necessary to avoid hypoglycemia. At all times, close monitoring of urinary glucose levels is mandatory in such patients.

4. In case of concomitant oral anticoagulant therapy, the prothrombin time should be measured frequently to determine if the dosage of oral anticoagulants is to be readjusted.

5. Partial loss of hair may be experienced by children in the first few months of thyroid therapy, but this is usually a transient phenomenon and later recovery is usually the rule.

Laboratory Tests: Treatment of patients with thyroid hormones requires the periodic assessment of thyroid status by means of appropriate laboratory tests besides the full clinical evaluation. The TSH suppression test can be used to test the effectiveness of any thyroid preparation, bearing in mind the relative insensitivity of the infant pituitary to the negative feedback effect of thyroid hormones. Serum T_4 levels can be used to test the effectiveness of all thyroid medications except T_3. When the total serum T_4 is low but TSH is normal, a test specific to assess unbound (free) T_4levels is warranted. Specific measurements of T_4 and T_3 by competitive protein binding or radioimmunoassay are not influenced by blood levels of organic or inorganic iodine and have essentially replaced older tests of thyroid hormone measurements, i.e., PBI, BEI, and T_4 by column.

Drug/Laboratory Test Interactions: The following drugs or moieties are known to interfere with laboratory tests performed in patients on thyroid hormone therapy: androgens, corticosteroids, estrogens, oral contraceptives containing estrogens, iodine-containing preparations, and the numerous preparations containing salicylates.

1. Changes in TBg concentration should be taken into consideration in the interpretation of $T_4$and T_3 values. In such cases, the unbound (free) hormones should be measured. Pregnancy, estrogens, and estrogen-containing oral contraceptives increase TBg concentrations. TBg may also be increased during infectious hepatitis. Decreases in TBg concentrations are observed in nephrosis, acromegaly, and after androgen or corticosteroid therapy. Familial hyper-or hypothyroxine-binding-globulinemias have been described. The incidence of TBg deficiency approximates 1 in 9000. The binding of thyroxine by TBPA is inhibited by salicylates.

2. Medicinal or dietary iodine interferes with all *in vivo* tests of radioiodine uptake, producing low uptakes which may not be reflective of a true decrease in hormone synthesis.

3. The persistence of clinical and laboratory evidence of hypothyroidism in spite of adequate dosage replacement indicates poor patient compliance, poor absorption, excessive fecal loss, or inactivity of the preparation. Intracellular resistance to thyroid hormone is quite rare.

Carcinogenesis, Mutagenesis, and Impairment of Fertility: A reportedly apparent association between prolonged thyroid therapy and breast cancer has not been confirmed and patients on thyroid for established indications should not discontinue therapy. No confirmatory long-term studies in animals have been performed to evaluate carcinogenic potential, mutagenicity, or impairment of fertility in either males or females.

Pregnancy Category A: Thyroid hormones do not readily cross the placental barrier. The clinical experience to date does not indicate any adverse effect on fetuses when thyroid hormones are administered to pregnant women. On the basis of current knowledge, thyroid replacement therapy to hypothyroid women should not be discontinued during pregnancy.

Nursing Mothers: Minimal amounts of thyroid hormones are excreted in human milk. Thyroid is not associated with serious adverse reactions and does not have a known tumorigenic potential. However, caution should be exercised when thyroid is administered to a nursing woman.

Pediatric Use: Pregnant mothers provide little or no thyroid hormone to the fetus. The incidence of congenital hypothyroidism is relatively high (1:4000) and the hypothyroid fetus would not derive any benefit from the small amounts of hormone crossing the placental barrier. Routine determinations of serum T_4 and/or TSH are strongly advised in neonates in view of the deleterious effects of thyroid deficiency on growth and development.

PRECAUTIONS: *(cont'd)*

Treatment should be initiated immediately upon diagnosis and maintained for life, unless transient hypothyroidism is suspected; in which case, therapy may be interrupted for 2 to 8 weeks after the age of 3 years to reassess the condition. Cessation of therapy is justified in patients who have maintained a normal TSH during those 2 to 8 weeks.

DRUG INTERACTIONS:

Oral Anticoagulants: Thyroid hormones appear to increase catabolism of vitamin-K-dependent clotting factors. If oral anticoagulants are also being given, compensatory increases in clotting factor synthesis are impaired. Patients stabilized on oral anticoagulants who are found to require thyroid replacement therapy should be watched very closely when thyroid is started. If a patient is truly hypothyroid, it is likely that a reduction in anticoagulant dosage will be required. No special precautions appear to be necessary when oral anticoagulant therapy is begun in a patient already stabilized on maintenance thyroid replacement therapy.

Insulin or Oral Hypoglycemics: Initiating thyroid replacement therapy may cause increases in insulin or oral hypoglycemic requirements. The effects seen are poorly understood and depend upon a variety of factors such as dosage and type of thyroid preparations and endocrine status of the patient. Patients receiving insulin or oral hypoglycemics should be closely watched during initiation of thyroid replacement therapy.

Cholestyramine: Cholestyramine binds both T_4 and T_3 in the intestine, thus impairing absorption of these thyroid hormones. *In vitro* studies indicate that the binding is not easily removed. Therefore, four to five hours should elapse between administration of cholestyramine or similar resins, such as colestipol, and thyroid hormones.

Estrogen, Oral Contraceptives: Estrogens tend to increase serum thyroxine-binding globulin (TBg). In a patient with a nonfunctioning thyroid gland who is receiving thyroid replacement therapy, free levothyroxine may be decreased when estrogens are started, thus increasing thyroid requirements. However, if the patient's thyroid gland has sufficient function, the decreased free thyroxine will result in a compensatory increase in thyroxine output by the thyroid. Therefore, patients without a functioning thyroid gland who are on thyroid replacement therapy may need to increase their thyroid dose if estrogens or estrogen-containing oral contraceptives are given.

ADVERSE REACTIONS:

Adverse reactions other than those indicative of hyperthyroidism because of therapeutic overdosage, either initially or during the maintenance period, are rare (see OVERDOSAGE.)

OVERDOSAGE:

Signs and Symptoms: Excessive doses of thyroid result in a hypermetabolic state resembling in every respect the condition of endogenous origin. The condition may be self-induced.

Treatment: Dosage should be reduced or therapy temporarily discontinued if signs and symptoms of overdosage appear. Treatment may be reinstituted at a lower dosage. In normal individuals, normal hypothalamic-pituitary-thyroid axis function is restored in 6 to 8 weeks after thyroid suppression.

Treatment of acute massive thyroid hormone overdosage is aimed at reducing gastrointestinal absorption of the drugs and counteracting central and peripheral effects, mainly those of increased sympathetic activity. Vomiting may be induced initially if further gastrointestinal absorption can reasonably be prevented and barring contraindications such as coma, convulsions, or loss of the gagging reflex. Treatment is symptomatic and supportive. Oxygen may be administered and ventilation maintained. Cardiac glycosides may be indicated if congestive heart failure develops. Measures to control fever, hypoglycemia, or fluid loss should be instituted if needed. Antiadrenergic agents, particularly propranolol, have been used advantageously in the treatment of increased sympathetic activity. Propranolol may be administered intravenously at a dosage of 1 to 3 mg over a 10 minute period or orally, 80 to 160 mg/day initially, especially when no contraindications exist for its use.

DOSAGE AND ADMINISTRATION:

The dosage of thyroid hormones is determined by the indication and must in every case be individualized according to patient response and laboratory findings.

Thyroid hormones are given orally. In acute, emergency conditions, injectable sodium levothyroxine may be given intravenously when oral administration is not feasible or desirable, as in the treatment of myxedema coma, or during total parenteral nutrition. Injectable sodium liothyronine is also available upon request from the manufacture, under investigational status, for the treatment of myxedema coma. Intramuscular administration of these two preparations is not advisable because of reported poor absorption.

Hypothyroidism: Therapy is usually instituted using low doses, with increments which depend on the cardiovascular status of the patient. The usual starting dose is 50 mcg of levothyroxine (T_4) or its isocaloric equivalent (Liotrix-1/2), with increments of 25 mcg every 2 to 3 weeks. A lower starting dosage, 25 mcg/day of levothyroxine (T_4) or its isocaloric equivalent, is recommended in patients with longstanding myxedema, particularly if cardiovascular impairment is suspected, in which case extreme caution is recommended. The appearance of angina is an indication for a reduction in dosage. The 200 to 400 mcg levothyroxine (T_4) recommended in the early trials are now considered excessive and most patients require 100 to 200 mcg/day or the caloric equivalent. Failure to respond to doses of 300 mcg suggests lack of compliance or malabsorption. Maintenance dosages of 100-200 mcg/day (Liortrix-1 or Liotrix-2) usually result in normal serum levothyroxine (T_4) and triiodothyronine (T_3) levels. Adequate therapy usually results in normal TSH and T_4 levels after 2 to 3 weeks of therapy.

Readjustment of thyroid hormone dosage should be made within the first four weeks of therapy, after proper clinical and laboratory evaluations, including serum levels of T_4, bound and free, and TSH.

The rapid onset and dissipation of action of sodium liothyronine (T_3), as compared with sodium levothyroxine (T_4), has led some clinicians to prefer its use in patients who might be more susceptible to the untoward effects of thyroid medication. However, the wide swings in serum T_3 levels that follow its administration and the possibility of more pronounced cardiovascular side effects tend to counterbalance the stated advantages. Many physicians continue to use thyroid tablets, USP, a T_3/T4 combination, or a newer synthetic combination.

T_3 may be used in preference to levothyroxine (T_4) during radioisotope scanning procedures, since induction of hypothyroidism in those cases is more abrupt and can be of shorter duration. It may also be preferred when impairment of peripheral conversion of T_4 and T_3 is suspected.

Myxedema Coma: Myxedema coma is usually precipitated in the hypothyroid patient of long standing by intercurrent illness or drugs such as sedatives and anesthetics and should be considered a medical emergency. Therapy should be directed at the correction of electrolyte disturbances and possible infection besides the administration of thyroid hormones. Corticosteroids should be administered routinely. $T_4$and T_3 may be administered via a nasogastric tube, but the preferred route of administration of both hormones is intravenous. Sodium levothyroxine (T_4) is given at a starting dose of 400 mcg (100 mcg/ml) given rapidly and is usually well tolerated, even in the elderly. This initial dose is followed by daily supplements of 100 to 200 mcg given IV. Normal T_4 levels are achieved in 24 hours followed in 3 days by threefold elevation of T_3. Triiodothyronine (T_3) (which is obtained only by special request

DOSAGE AND ADMINISTRATION: *(cont'd)*

from the manufacturer) is given at doses of 200 mcg IV followed by 25 mcg supplements at 8-hour intervals. Oral therapy with either hormone would be resumed as soon as the clinical situation has been stabilized and the patient is able to take oral medication.

Thyroid Cancer: Exogenous thyroid hormone may produce regression of metastases from follicular and papillary carcinoma of the thyroid and is used as ancillary therapy of these conditions with radioactive iodine. TSH should be suppressed to low or undetectable levels. Therefore, larger amounts of thyroid hormone than those used for replacement therapy are required. Medullary carcinoma of the thyroid is usually unresponsive to this therapy.

Thyroid Suppression Therapy: Administration of thyroid hormone in doses higher than those produced physiologically by the gland results in suppression of the production of endogenous hormone. This is the basis for the thyroid suppression test and is used as an aid in the diagnosis of patients with signs of mild hyperthyroidism in whom baseline laboratory tests appear normal or to demonstrate thyroid gland autonomy in patients with Graves' ophthalmopathy. Radioiodine uptake is determined before and after the administration of the exogenous hormone. A fifty percent or greater suppression of uptake indicates a normal thyroid-pituitary axis and thus rules out thyroid gland autonomy.

For adults, the usual suppressive dose of levothyroxine (T_4) is 2.6 mcg/kg of body weight per day given for 7 to 10 days. These doses usually yield normal serum T_4 and T_3 levels and lack of response to TSH.

T_3 is given in doses of 75-100 mcg/day for 7 days and radioactive iodine uptake is determined before and after administration of the hormone. If thyroid function is under normal control, the radioiodine uptake will drop significantly after treatment with either hormone.

Either hormone or combination therapy should be administered cautiously to patients in whom there is a strong suspicion of thyroid gland autonomy, in view of the fact that the exogenous hormone effects will be additive to the endogenous source.

Pediatric Dosage: Pediatric dosage should follow the recommendations summarized in TABLE 1. In infants with congenital hypothyroidism, therapy with full doses should be instituted as soon as the diagnosis has been made.

TABLE 1 Recommended Pediatric Dosage for Congenital Hypothyroidism

Age	Tetraiodothyronine (T_4, levothyroxine) sodium Dose per day	Daily dose per kg of body weight
0-6 mos	25-50 mcg	8-10 mcg
6-12 mos	50-75 mcg	6-8 mcg
1-5 yrs	75-100 mcg	5-6 mcg
6-12 yrs	100-150 mcg	4-5 mcg
over 12 yrs	over 150 mcg	2-3 mcg

TABLE 2 Conversion Table

Tablet	(Liotrix tablets, USP) T4*/T3** mcg	Color	Natural Thyroid USP	Synthetic T4*	T3**
Liotrix -1/2	(30/7.5)	pale orange	1/2 grain	0.05 mg	12.5 mcg
Liotrix -1	(60/15)	light brown	1 grain	0.1 mg	25.0 mcg
Liotrix -2	(120/30)	violet	2 grains	0.2 mg	50.0 mcg
Liotrix -3	(180/45)	gray	3 grains	0.3 mg	75.0 mcg

* T4 =levothyroxine sodium (l-thyroxine)
** T3 = liothyronine sodium (*l*-triiodothyronine)

Following a change from one type of thyroid hormone preparation to another, patients may still require fine adjustment of dosage because the equivalents are only estimates.

Store between 15° and 25°C (59 and 77°F).

HOW SUPPLIED - EQUIVALENTS NOT AVAILABLE:

Tablet, Uncoated - Oral - 30 mcg/7.5 mcg

100's	**$12.35**	**EUTHROID 1/2, Parke-Davis**	**00071-0260-24**
100's	$39.28	THYROLAR-1/2, Forest Pharms	00456-0045-01

Tablet, Uncoated - Oral - 60 mcg/15 mcg

100's	**$17.70**	**EUTHROID-1, Parke-Davis**	**00071-0261-24**
100's	$35.38	THYROLAR-1/4, Forest Pharms	00456-0040-01
100's	$49.09	THYROLAR-1, Forest Pharms	00456-0050-01

Tablet, Uncoated - Oral - 120 mcg/30 mcg

100's	**$22.44**	**EUTHROID-2, Parke-Davis**	**00071-0262-24**
100's	$57.71	THYROLAR-2, Forest Pharms	00456-0055-01

Tablet, Uncoated - Oral - 180 mcg/45 mcg

100's	**$26.83**	**EUTHROID-3, Parke-Davis**	**00071-0263-24**
100's	$70.57	THYROLAR-3, Forest Pharms	00456-0060-01

LISINOPRIL *(001647)*

CATEGORIES: ACE Inhibitors; Angiotensin Converting Enzyme Inhibitors; Antihypertensives; Cardiovascular Drugs; Congestive Heart Failure; Heart Failure; Hypertension; Pregnancy Category D; Sales > $1 Billion; FDA Approved 1987 Dec; Patent Expiration 2001 Dec; Top 200 Drugs

BRAND NAMES: *Acerbon* (Germany); *Alapril*; *Carace* (England); *Cipril*; *Coric* (Germany); *Linvas*; *Lipril*; *Lisipril*; *Lisoril*; *Lispril*; *Listril*; *Noperten*; *Novatec*; *Prinil*; Prinivil; *Prinvil*; *Tensopril*; *Vivatec*; **Zestril**
(International brand names outside U.S. in italics)

FORMULARIES: Aetna; BC-BS; CIGNA; FHP; Foundation; Humana; Kaiser; Medco; Medi-Cal; PCS; PruCare; United

COST OF THERAPY: $296.70 (Hypertension; Tablet; 10 mg; 1/day; 365 days)

PRIMARY ICD9: 401.1 (Essential Hypertension, Benign)

WARNING:
Use In Pregnancy: When used in pregnancy during the second and third trimesters, ACE inhibitors can cause injury and even death to the developing fetus. When pregnancy is detected, Lisinopril should be discontinued as soon as possible. See WARNINGS, Fetal/Neonatal Morbidity and Mortality.

DESCRIPTION:

Lisinopril is an oral long-acting angiotensin converting enzyme inhibitor. Lisinopril, a synthetic peptide derivative, is chemically described as (*S*)-1-[N^2-(1-carboxy-3- phenylpropyl)-L-lysyl]-L-proline dihydrate. Its empirical formula is $C_{21}H_{31}N_3O_5 \cdot 2H_2O$.

Lisinopril is a white to off-white, crystalline powder, with a molecular weight of 441.52. It is soluble in water and sparingly soluble in methanol and practically insoluble in ethanol.

Lisinopril is supplied as 2.5 mg, 5 mg, 10 mg, 20 mg and 40 mg tablets for oral administration. In addition to the active ingredient lisinopril, each tablet contains the following inactive ingredients: calcium phosphate, mannitol, magnesium stearate, and starch. The 10 mg, 20 mg and 40 mg tablets also contain iron oxide.

CLINICAL PHARMACOLOGY:

Mechanism of Action: Lisinopril inhibits angiotensin- converting enzyme (ACE) in human subjects and animals. ACE is a peptidyl dipeptidase that catalyzes the conversion of angiotensin I to the vasoconstrictor substance, angiotensin II. Angiotensin II also stimulates aldosterone secretion by the adrenal cortex. The beneficial effects of lisinopril in hypertension and heart failure appear to result primarily from suppression of the renin-angiotensin-aldosterone system. Inhibition of ACE results in decreased plasma angiotensin II which leads to decreased vasopressor activity and to decreased aldosterone secretion. The latter decrease may result in a small increase of serum potassium. In hypertensive patients with normal renal function treated with lisinopril alone for up to 24 weeks, the mean increase in serum potassium was approximately 0.1 mEq/l; however, approximately 15 percent of patients had increases greater than 0.5 mEq/l and approximately six percent had a decrease greater than 0.5 mEq/l. In the same study, patients treated with lisinopril and hydrochlorothiazide for up to 24 weeks had a mean decrease in serum potassium of 0.1 mEq/l; approximately 4 percent of patients had increases greater than 0.5 mEq/l and approximately 12 percent had a decrease greater than 0.5 mEq/l. (See PRECAUTIONS.) Removal of angiotensin II negative feedback on renin secretion leads to increased plasma renin activity.

ACE is identical to kininase, an enzyme that degrades bradykinin. Whether increased levels of bradykinin, a potent vasodepressor peptide, play a role in the therapeutic effects of lisinopril remains to be elucidated.

While the mechanism through which lisinopril lowers blood pressure is believed to be primarily suppression of the renin-angiotensin-aldosterone system, lisinopril is antihypertensive even in patients with low-renin hypertension. Although lisinopril was antihypertensive in all races studied, black hypertensive patients (usually a low-renin hypertensive population) had a smaller average response to monotherapy than non-black patients.

Concomitant administration of lisinopril and hydrochlorothiazide further reduced blood pressure in black and non-black patients and any racial difference in blood pressure response was no longer evident.

Pharmacokinetics and Metabolism: Following oral administration of lisinopril, peak serum concentrations of lisinopril occur within about 7 hours. Declining serum concentrations exhibit a prolonged terminal phase which does not contribute to drug accumulation. This terminal phase probably represents saturable binding to ACE and is not proportional to dose. Lisinopril does not appear to be bound to other serum proteins.

Lisinopril does not undergo metabolism and is excreted unchanged entirely in the urine. Based on urinary recovery, the mean extent of absorption of lisinopril is approximately 25 percent, with large inter-subject variability (6-60 percent) at all doses tested (5-80 mg). Lisinopril absorption is not influenced by the presence of food in the gastrointestinal tract. The absolute bioavailability of lisinopril is reduced to about 16% in patients with stable NYHA Class II-IV congestive heart failure, and the volume of distribution appears to be slightly smaller than that in normal subjects.

Upon multiple dosing, lisinopril exhibits an effective half-life of accumulation of 12 hours.

Impaired renal function decreases elimination of lisinopril, which is excreted principally through the kidneys, but this decrease becomes clinically important only when the glomerular filtration rate is below 30 ml/min. Above this glomerular filtration rate, the elimination half-life is little changed. With greater impairment, however, peak and trough lisinopril levels increase, time to peak concentration increases and time to attain steady state is prolonged. Older patients, on average, have (approximately doubled) higher blood levels and area under the plasma concentration time curve (AUC) than younger patients. (See DOSAGE AND ADMINISTRATION.) Lisinopril can be removed by hemodialysis.

Studies in rats indicate that lisinopril crosses the blood-brain barrier poorly. Multiple doses of lisinopril in rats do not result in accumulation in any tissues. Milk of lactating rats contains radioactivity following administration of ^{14}C lisinopril. By whole body autoradiography, radioactivity was found in the placenta following administration of labeled drug to pregnant rats, but none was found in the fetuses.

PHARMACODYNAMICS AND CLINICAL EFFECTS

Hypertension: Administration of lisinopril to patients with hypertension results in a reduction of supine and standing blood pressure to about the same extent with no compensatory tachycardia. Symptomatic postural hypotension is usually not observed although it can occur and should be anticipated in volume and/or salt-depleted patients. (See WARNINGS.) When given together with thiazide-type diuretics, the blood pressure lowering effects of the two drugs are approximately additive.

In most patients studied, onset of antihypertensive activity was seen at one hour after oral administration of an individual dose of lisinopril, with peak reduction of blood pressure achieved by six hours. Although an antihypertensive effect was observed 24 hours after dosing with recommended single daily doses, the effect was more consistent and the mean effect was considerably larger in some studies with doses of 20 mg or more than with lower doses. However, at all doses studied, the mean antihypertensive effect was substantially smaller 24 hours after dosing than it was six hours after dosing.

In some patients achievement of optimal blood pressure reduction may require two to four weeks of therapy.

The antihypertensive effects of lisinopril are maintained during long-term therapy. Abrupt withdrawal of lisinopril has not been associated with a rapid increase in blood pressure or a significant increase in blood pressure compared to pretreatment levels.

Two dose-response studies utilizing a once daily regimen were conducted in 438 mild to moderate hypertensive patients not on a diuretic. Blood pressure was measured 24 hours after dosing. An antihypertensive effect of lisinopril was seen with 5 mg in some patients. However, in both studies blood pressure reduction occurred sooner and was greater in patients treated with 10, 20 or 80 mg of lisinopril. In controlled clinical studies, lisinopril 20-80 mg has been compared in patients with mild to moderate hypertension to hydrochlorothiazide 12.5-50 mg and with atenolol 50-200 mg; and in patients with moderate to severe hypertension to metoprolol 100-200 mg. It was superior to hydrochlorothiazide in effects on systolic and diastolic blood pressure in a population that was 3/4 Caucasian. Lisinopril was approximately equivalent to atenolol and metoprolol in effects on diastolic blood pressure and had somewhat greater effects on systolic blood pressure.

Lisinopril had similar effectiveness and adverse effects in younger and older (>65 years) patients. It was less effective in blacks than in Caucasians.

CLINICAL PHARMACOLOGY: *(cont'd)*

In hemodynamic studies in patients with essential hypertension, blood pressure reduction was accompanied by a reduction in peripheral arterial resistance with little or no change in cardiac output and in heart rate. In a study in nine hypertensive patients, following administration of lisinopril, there was an increase in mean renal blood flow that was not significant. Data from several small studies are inconsistent with respect to the effect of lisinopril on glomerular filtration rate in hypertensive patients with normal renal function, but suggest that changes, if any, are not large.

In patients with renovascular hypertension lisinopril has been shown to be well tolerated and effective in controlling blood pressure. (See PRECAUTIONS.)

Heart Failure: During baseline-controlled clinical trials, in patients receiving digitalis and diuretics, single doses of lisinopril resulted in decreases in pulmonary capillary wedge pressure, systemic vascular resistance and blood pressure accompanied by an increase in cardiac output and no change in heart rate.

In two placebo controlled, 12-week clinical studies, lisinopril as adjunctive therapy to digitalis and diuretics improved the following signs and symptoms due to congestive heart failure: edema, rales, paroxysmal nocturnal dyspnea and jugular venous distention. In one of the studies beneficial response was also noted for: orthopnea, presence of third heart sound and the number of patients classified as NYHA Class III and IV. Exercise tolerance was also improved in this one study. The effect of lisinopril on mortality in patients with heart failure has not been evaluated.

INDICATIONS AND USAGE:

Hypertension: Lisinopril is indicated for the treatment of hypertension. It may be used alone as initial therapy or concomitantly with other classes of antihypertensive agents.

Heart Failure: Lisinopril is indicated as adjunctive therapy in the management of heart failure in patients who are not responding adequately to diuretics and digitalis.

In considering use of Lisinopril, it should be noted that in controlled trials, ACE inhibitors have an effect on blood pressure that is less in black patients than in non-blacks. In addition, ACE inhibitors have been associated with a higher rate of angioedema in black than in non-black patients (see WARNINGS, Angioedema).

In using lisinopril, consideration should be given to the fact that another angiotensin converting enzyme inhibitor, captopril, has caused agranulocytosis, particularly in patients with renal impairment or collagen vascular disease, and that available data are insufficient to show that lisinopril does not have a similar risk. (See WARNINGS.)

CONTRAINDICATIONS:

Lisinopril is contraindicated in patients who are hypersensitive to this product and in patients with a history of angioedema related to previous treatment with an angiotensin converting enzyme inhibitor. Patients with a history of angioedema unrelated to ACE inhibitor therapy may be at increased risk of angioedema while receiving an ACE inhibitor.

WARNINGS:

Anaphylactoid and Possibly Related Reactions: Presumably because angiotensin-converting enzyme inhibitors affect the metabolism of eicosanoids and polypeptides, including endogenous bradykinin, patients receiving ACE inhibitors (including lisinopril) may be subject to a variety of adverse reactions, some of them serious.

Angioedema: Angioedema of the face, extremities, lips, tongue, glottis and/or larynx has been reported in patients treated with angiotensin converting enzyme inhibitors, including lisinopril. This may occur at any time during treatment. ACE inhibitors have been associated with a higher rate of angioedema in black than in non-black patients. In such cases, lisinopril should be promptly discontinued and appropriate therapy and monitoring should be provided until complete and sustained resolution of signs and symptoms has occurred. In instances where swelling has been confined to the face and lips the condition has generally resolved without treatment, although antihistamines have been useful in relieving symptoms. Angioedema associated with laryngeal edema may be fatal. **Where there is involvement of the tongue, glottis or larynx, likely to cause airway obstruction, appropriate therapy, e.g., subcutaneous epinephrine solution 1:1000 (0.3 ml to 0.5 ml) and/or measures necessary to ensure a patent airway, should be promptly provided.** (See ADVERSE REACTIONS.)

Patients with a history of angioedema unrelated to ACE inhibitor therapy may be at increased risk of angioedema while receiving an ACE inhibitor (see also CONTRAINDICATIONS).

Anaphylactoid reactions during desensitization: Two patients undergoing desensitizing treatment with hymenoptera venom while receiving ACE inhibitors sustained life-threatening anaphylactoid reactions. In the same patients, these reactions were avoided when ACE inhibitors were temporarily withheld, but they reappeared upon inadvertent rechallenge.

Anaphylactoid reactions during membrane exposure: Sudden and potentially life-threatening anaphylactoid reactions have been reported in patients dialyzed with high-flux membranes and treated concomitantly with an ACE inhibitor. In such patients, dialysis must be stopped immediately, and aggressive therapy for anaphylactoid reactions be initiated. Symptoms have not been relieved by antihistamines in these situations. In these patients, consideration should be given to using a different type of dialysis membrane or a different class of antihypertensive. Anaphylactoid reactions have also been reported in patients undergoing low-density lipoprotein apheresis with dextran sulfate absorption (a procedure dependent upon devices not approved in the United States).

Hypotension: Excessive hypotension is rare in patients with uncomplicated hypertension treated with lisinopril alone.

Patients with heart failure given lisinopril commonly have some reduction in blood pressure with peak blood pressure reduction occurring 6 to 8 hours post dose, but discontinuation of therapy because of continuing symptomatic hypotension usually is not necessary when dosing instructions are followed; caution should be observed when initiating therapy. (See DOSAGE AND ADMINISTRATION.)

Patients at risk of excessive hypotension, sometimes associated with oliguria and/or progressive azotemia, and rarely with acute renal failure and/or death, include those with the following conditions or characteristics: heart failure with systolic blood pressure below 100 mmHg, hyponatremia, high dose diuretic therapy, recent intensive diuresis or increase in diuretic dose, renal dialysis, or severe volume and/or salt depletion of any etiology. It may be advisable to eliminate the diuretic (except in patients with heart failure), reduce the diuretic dose or increase salt intake cautiously before initiating therapy with lisinopril in patients at risk for excessive hypotension who are able to tolerate such adjustments. (See DRUG INTERACTIONS and ADVERSE REACTIONS.)

In patients at risk of excessive hypotension, therapy should be started under very close medical supervision and such patients should be followed closely for the first two weeks of treatment and whenever the dose of lisinopril and/or diuretic is increased. Similar considerations may apply to patients with ischemic heart or cerebrovascular disease, in whom an excessive fall in blood pressure could result in a myocardial infarction or cerebrovascular accident.

WARNINGS: *(cont'd)*

If excessive hypotension occurs, the patient should be placed in the supine position and, if necessary, receive an intravenous infusion of normal saline. A transient hypotensive response is not a contraindication to further doses of lisinopril which usually can be given without difficulty once the blood pressure has stabilized. If symptomatic hypotension develops, a dose reduction or discontinuation of lisinopril or concomitant diuretic may be necessary.

Leukopenia/Neutropenia/Agranulocytosis: Another angiotensin converting enzyme inhibitor, captopril, has been shown to cause agranulocytosis and bone marrow depression, rarely in uncomplicated patients but more frequently in patients with renal impairment especially if they also have a collagen vascular disease. Available data from clinical trials of lisinopril are insufficient to show that lisinopril does not cause agranulocytosis at similar rates. Marketing experience has revealed rare cases of leukopenia/neutropenia and bone marrow depression in which a causal relationship to lisinopril cannot be excluded. Periodic monitoring of while blood cell counts in patients with collagen vascular disease and renal disease should be considered.

Hepatic Failure: Rarely, ACE inhibitors have been associated with a syndrome that starts with cholestatic jaundice and progresses to fulminant hepatic necrosis, and (sometimes) death. The mechanism of this syndrome is not understood. Patients receiving ACE inhibitors who develop jaundice or marked elevations of hepatic enzymes should discontinue the ACE inhibitor and receive appropriate medical follow-up.

Fetal/Neonatal Morbidity and Mortality: ACE inhibitors can cause fetal and neonatal morbidity and death when administered to pregnant women. Several dozen cases have been reported in the world literature. When pregnancy is detected, ACE inhibitors should be discontinued as soon as possible.

The use of ACE inhibitors during the second and third trimesters of pregnancy has been associated with fetal and neonatal injury, including hypotension, neonatal skull hypoplasia, anuria, reversible or irreversible renal failure, and death. Oligohydramnios has also been reported, presumably resulting from decreased fetal renal function; oligohydramnios in this setting has been associated with fetal limb contractures, craniofacial deformation, and hypoplastic lung development. Prematurity, intrauterine growth retardation, and patent ductus arteriosus have also been reported, although it is not clear whether these occurrences were due to the ACE-inhibitor exposure.

These adverse effects do not appear to have resulted from intrauterine ACE-inhibitor exposure that has been limited to the first trimester. Mothers whose embryos and fetuses are exposed to ACE inhibitors only during the first trimester should be so informed. Nonetheless, when patients become pregnant, physicians should make every effort to discontinue the use of lisinopril as soon as possible.

Rarely (probably less often than once in every thousand pregnancies), no alternative to ACE inhibitors will be found. In these rare cases, the mothers should be apprised of the potential hazards to their fetuses, and serial ultrasound examinations should be performed to assess the intraamniotic environment.

If oligohydramnios is observed, lisinopril should be discontinued unless it is considered lifesaving for the mother. Contraction stress testing (CST), a non-stress test (NST), or biophysical profiling (BPP) may be appropriate, depending upon the week of pregnancy. Patients and physicians should be aware, however, that oligohydramnios may not appear until after the fetus has sustained irreversible injury.

Infants with histories of *in utero* exposure to ACE inhibitors should be closely observed for hypotension, oliguria, and hyperkalemia. If oliguria occurs, attention should be directed toward support of blood pressure and renal perfusion. Exchange transfusion or dialysis may be required as means of reversing hypotension and/or substituting for disordered renal function. Lisinopril, which crosses the placenta, has been removed from neonatal circulation by peritoneal dialysis with some clinical benefit, and theoretically may be removed by exchange transfusion, although there is no experience with the latter procedure.

No teratogenic effects of lisinopril were seen in studies of pregnant rats, mice, and rabbits. On a mg/kg basis, the doses used were up to 625 times (in mice), 188 times (in rats), and 0.6 times (in rabbits) the maximum recommended human dose.

PRECAUTIONS:

GENERAL

General Impaired Renal Function: As a consequence of inhibiting the renin-angiotensin-aldosterone system, changes in renal function may be anticipated in susceptible individuals. In patients with severe congestive heart failure whose renal function may depend on the activity of the renin-angiotensin-aldosterone system, treatment with angiotensin converting enzyme inhibitors, including lisinopril, may be associated with oliguria and/or progressive azotemia and rarely with acute renal failure and/or death.

In hypertensive patients with unilateral or bilateral renal artery stenosis, increases in blood urea nitrogen and serum creatinine may occur. Experience with another angiotensin converting enzyme inhibitor suggests that these increases are usually reversible upon discontinuation of lisinopril and/or diuretic therapy. In such patients renal function should be monitored during the first few weeks of therapy.

Some patients with hypertension or heart failure with no apparent pre-existing renal vascular disease have developed increases in blood urea nitrogen and serum creatinine, usually minor and transient, especially when lisinopril has been given concomitantly with a diuretic. This is more likely to occur in patients with pre-existing renal impairment. Dosage reduction and/or discontinuation of the diuretic may be required.

Evaluation of patients with hypertension or heart failure should always include assessment of renal function: (See DOSAGE AND ADMINISTRATION.)

Hyperkalemia: In clinical trials hyperkalemia (serum potassium greater than 5.7 mEq/l) occurred in approximately 2.2 percent of hypertensive patients and 4.8 percent of patients with heart failure. In most cases these were isolated values which resolved despite continued therapy. Hyperkalemia was a cause of discontinuation of therapy in approximately 0.1 percent of hypertensive patients and 0.6 percent of patients with heart failure. Risk factors for the development of hyperkalemia include renal insufficiency, diabetes mellitus, and the concomitant use of potassium-sparing diuretics, potassium supplements and/or potassium-containing salt substitutes, which should be used cautiously, if at all, with lisinopril. (See DRUG INTERACTIONS.)

Cough: Presumably due to the inhibition of the degradation of endogenous bradykinin, persistent nonproductive cough has been reported with all ACE inhibitors, almost always resolving after discontinuation of therapy. ACE inhibitor-induced cough should be considered in the differential diagnosis of cough.

Surgery/Anesthesia: In patients undergoing major surgery or during anesthesia with agents that produce hypotension, lisinopril may block angiotensin II formation secondary to compensatory renin release. If hypotension occurs and is considered to be due to this mechanism, it can be corrected by volume expansion.

INFORMATION FOR PATIENTS

Information for Patients Angioedema: Angioedema, including laryngeal edema, may occur at any time during treatment with angiotensin converting enzyme inhibitors, including lisinopril. Patients should be so advised and told to report immediately any signs or symptoms

PRECAUTIONS: *(cont'd)*

suggesting angioedema (swelling of face, extremities, eyes, lips, tongue, difficulty in swallowing or breathing) and to take no more drug until they have consulted with the prescribing physician.

Symptomatic Hypotension: Patients should be cautioned to report lightheadedness especially during the first few days of therapy. If actual syncope occurs, the patient should be told to discontinue the drug until they have consulted with the prescribing physician.

All patients should be cautioned that excessive perspiration and dehydration may lead to an excessive fall in blood pressure because of reduction in fluid volume. Other causes of volume depletion such as vomiting or diarrhea may also lead to a fall in blood pressure; patients should be advised to consult with their physician.

Hyperkalemia: Patients should be told not to use salt substitutes containing potassium without consulting their physician.

Leukopenia/Neutropenia: Patients should be told to report promptly any indication of infection (*e.g.,* sore throat, fever) which may be a sign of leukopenia/neutropenia.

Pregnancy: Female patients of childbearing age should be told about the consequences of second- and third-trimester exposure to ACE inhibitors, and they should also be told that these consequences do not appear to have resulted from intrauterine ACE-inhibitor exposure that has been limited to the first trimester. These patients should be asked to report pregnancies to their physicians as soon as possible.

NOTE: As with many other drugs, certain advice to patients being treated with lisinopril is warranted. This information is intended to aid in the safe and effective use of this medication. It is not a disclosure of all possible adverse or intended effects.

CARCINOGENESIS, MUTAGENESIS, IMPAIRMENT OF FERTILITY

There was no evidence of a tumorigenic effect when lisinopril was administered for 105 weeks to male and female rats at doses up to 90 mg/kg/day (about 56 times† the maximum recommended daily human dose) or when lisinopril was administered for 92 weeks to (male and female) mice at doses up to 135 mg/kg/day (about 84 times† the maximum recommended daily human dose).

†Based on patient weight of 50 kg

Lisinopril was not mutagenic in the Ames microbial mutagen test with or without metabolic activation. It was also negative in a forward mutation assay using Chinese hamster lung cells. Lisinopril did not produce single strand DNA breaks in an *in vitro* alkaline elution rat hepatocyte assay. In addition, lisinopril did not produce increases in chromosomal aberrations in an *in vitro* test in Chinese hamster ovary cells or in an *in vivo* study in mouse bone marrow.

There were no adverse effects on reproductive performance in male and female rats treated with up to 300 mg/kg/day of lisinopril. This dose is 188 times and 30 times the maximum human dose when based on mg/kg and mg/m^2, respectively.

PREGNANCY

Pregnancy Categories C (first trimester) and D (second and third trimesters): (See WARNINGS, Fetal/Neonatal Morbidity and Mortality.)

NURSING MOTHERS

Milk of lactating rats contains radioactivity following administration of ^{14}C lisinopril. It is not known whether this drug is secreted in human milk. Because many drugs are secreted in human milk, caution should be exercised when lisinopril is given to a nursing mother.

PEDIATRIC USE

Safety and effectiveness in children have not been established.

DRUG INTERACTIONS:

Hypotension-Patients on Diuretic Therapy: Patients on diuretics, and especially those in whom diuretic therapy was recently instituted, may occasionally experience an excessive reduction of blood pressure after initiation of therapy with lisinopril. The possibility of hypotensive effects with lisinopril can be minimized by either discontinuing the diuretic or increasing the salt intake prior to initiation of treatment with lisinopril. If it is necessary to continue the diuretic, initiate therapy with lisinopril at a dose of 5 mg daily, and provide close medical supervision after the initial dose until blood pressure has stabilized. See WARNINGS, and DOSAGE AND ADMINISTRATION. When a diuretic is added to the therapy of a patient receiving lisinopril, an additional antihypertensive effect is usually observed. Studies with ACE inhibitors in combination with diuretics indicate that the dose of the ACE inhibitor can be reduced when it is given with a diuretic. (See DOSAGE AND ADMINISTRATION.)

Indomethacin: In a study in 36 patients with mild to moderate hypertension where the antihypertensive effects of lisinopril alone were compared to lisinopril given concomitantly with indomethacin, the use of indomethacin was associated with a reduced effect, although the difference between the two regimens was not significant.

Other Agents: Lisinopril has been used concomitantly with nitrates and/or digoxin without evidence of clinically significant adverse interactions. No clinically important pharmacokinetic interactions occurred when lisinopril was used concomitantly with propranolol or hydrochlorothiazide. The presence of food in the stomach does not alter the bioavailability of lisinopril.

Agents Increasing Serum Potassium: Lisinopril attenuates potassium loss caused by thiazide-type diuretics. Use of lisinopril with potassium-sparing diuretics (*e.g.,* spironolactone, triamterene, or amiloride), potassium supplements, or potassium-containing salt substitutes may lead to significant increases in serum potassium. Therefore, if concomitant use of these agents is indicated because of demonstrated hypokalemia, they should be used with caution and with frequent monitoring of serum potassium. Potassium sparing agents should generally not be used in patients with heart failure who are receiving lisinopril.

Lithium: Lithium toxicity has been reported in patients receiving lithium concomitantly with drugs which cause elimination of sodium, including ACE inhibitors. Lithium toxicity was usually reversible upon discontinuation of lithium and the ACE inhibitor. It is recommended that serum lithium levels be monitored frequently if lisinopril is administered concomitantly with lithium.

ADVERSE REACTIONS:

Lisinopril has been found to be generally well tolerated in controlled clinical trials involving 1969 patients. For the most part, adverse experiences were mild and transient.

In clinical trials in patients with hypertension treated with lisinopril, discontinuation of therapy due to clinical adverse experiences occurred in 5.7 percent of patients. The overall frequency of adverse experiences could not be related to total daily dosage within the recommended therapeutic dosage range.

In patients with heart failure treated with lisinopril for up to four years, discontinuation of therapy due to clinical adverse experiences occurred in 11.0 percent of patients. In controlled studies in patients with heart failure, therapy was discontinued in 8.1 percent of patients treated with lisinopril for 12 weeks, compared to 7.7 percent of patients treated with placebo for 12 weeks.

ADVERSE REACTIONS: *(cont'd)*

Hypertension: For adverse experiences occurring in greater than one percent of patients with hypertension treated with lisinopril or lisinopril plus hydrochlorothiazide in controlled clinical trials, comparative incidence data are listed in TABLE 1 below:

TABLE 1 Percent of Patients in Controlled Studies

	Lisinopril (n = 1349) Incidence (discontinuation)	Lisinopril/ Hydrochlorothiazide (n = 629) Incidence (discontinuation)	Placebo (n = 207) Incidence (discontinuation)
Body As A Whole:			
Fatigue	2.5 (0.3)	4.0 (0.5)	1.0 (0.0)
Asthenia	1.3 (0.5)	2.1 (0.2)	1.0 (0.0)
Chest Pain	1.2 (0.1)	1.3 (0.2)	1.4 (0.0)
Orthostatic Effects	1.2 (0.0)	3.5 (0.2)	1.0 (0.0)
Cardiovascular			
Hypotension	1.2 (0.5)	1.6 (0.5)	0.5 (0.5)
Digestive			
Diarrhea	2.7 (0.2)	2.7 (0.3)	2.4 (0.0)
Nausea	2.0 (0.4)	2.5 (0.2)	2.4 (0.0)
Vomiting	1.1 (0.2)	1.4 (0.1)	0.5 (0.0)
Dyspepsia	0.9 (0.0)	1.9 (0.0)	0.0 (0.0)
Musculoskeletal			
Back Pain	0.6 (0.0)	1.1 (0.1)	1.4 (0.0)
Muscle Cramps	0.5 (0.0)	2.9 (0.8)	0.5 (0.0)
Nervous/ Psychiatric			
Headache	5.7 (0.2)	4.5 (0.5)	1.9 (0.0)
Dizziness	5.4 (0.4)	9.2 (1.0)	1.9 (0.0)
Paresthesia	0.8 (0.1)	2.1 (0.2)	0.0 (0.0)
Decreased Libido	0.4 (0.1)	1.3 (0.1)	0.0 (0.0)
Vertigo	0.2 (0.1)	1.1 (0.2)	0.0 (0.0)
Respiratory			
Cough	3.5 (0.7)	4.6 (0.8)	1.0 (0.0)
Upper Respiratory			
Infection	2.1 (0.1)	2.7 (0.1)	0.0 (0.0)
Common Cold	1.1 (0.1)	1.3 (0.1)	0.0 (0.0)
Nasal Congestion	0.4 (0.1)	1.3 (0.1)	0.0 (0.0)
Influenza	0.3 (0.1)	1.1 (0.1)	0.0 (0.0)
Skin			
Rash	1.3 (0.4)	1.6 (0.2)	0.5 (0.5)
Urogenital:			
Impotence	1.0 (0.4)	1.6 (0.5)	0.0 (0.0)

Heart Failure: TABLE 2 lists those adverse experiences which occurred in greater than one percent of patients with heart failure treated with lisinopril or placebo for up to 12 weeks in controlled clinical trials. Also listed are those adverse experiences occurring in greater than one percent of patients with heart failure treated with lisinopril for up to four years.

TABLE 2

	Controlled Trials Incidence (discontinuation) Lisinopril	12 weeks Placebo	All Trials up to 4 years Lisinopril
	(n = 407)	(n = 155)	(n = 620)
Body As A Whole			
Chest Pain	3.4 (0.2)	1.3 (0.0)	7.3 (0.3)
Asthenia	3.2 (0.2)	3.2 (0.0)	6.9 (0.3)
Abdominal Pain	2.2 (0.7)	1.9 (0.0)	4.0 (0.5)
Edema	1.0 (0.0)	0.6 (0.0)	2.4 (0.2)
Syncope	1.0 (0.0)	0.6 (0.6)	1.8 (0.0)
Orthostatic Effects	1.0 (0.2)	0.0 (0.0)	1.1 (0.2)
Fever	0.5 (0.0)	0.6 (0.0)	1.1 (0.0)
Malaise	1.0 (0.2)	0.0 (0.0)	1.1 (0.3)
Cardiovascular			
Hypotension	4.4 (1.7)	0.6 (0.6)	5.3 (1.8)
Angina Pectoris	1.5 (0.2)	3.2 (1.3)	3.7 (0.3)
Worsening of Heart Failure	0.0 (0.0)	3.2 (1.9)	2.9 (0.6)
Orthostatic Hypotension	1.0 (0.2)	0.0 (0.0)	1.9 (0.3)
Palpitation	1.0 (0.0)	0.0 (0.0)	1.9 (0.0)
CVA	0.2 (0.0)	0.0 (0.0)	1.6 (0.2)
Myocardial Infarction	0.5 (0.2)	0.6 (0.0)	1.3 (0.5)
Digestive			
Diarrhea	3.7 (0.5)	1.9 (0.0)	6.1 (0.6)
Nausea	2.7 (0.5)	5.2 (0.0)	5.0 (0.5)
Vomiting	1.0 (0.5)	0.6 (0.0)	2.4 (0.3)
Dyspepsia	0.2 (0.2)	0.0 (0.0)	1.8 (0.2)
Anorexia	0.7 (0.2)	1.3 (0.0)	1.5 (0.3)
Increased Salivation	0.0 (0.0)	1.3 (0.0)	0.2 (0.0)
Metabolic			
Gout	0.5 (0.2)	0.0 (0.0)	1.5 (0.2)
Musculoskeletal			
Muscle Cramps	0.5 (0.0)	1.3 (0.0)	2.1 (0.0)
Back Pain	0.5 (0.0)	1.9 (0.0)	1.6 (0.0)
Leg Pain	0.5 (0.0)	0.6 (0.0)	1.3 (0.2)
Myalgia	0.5 (0.0)	1.9 (0.6)	0.6 (0.0)
Nervous/ Psychiatric			
Dizziness	11.8 (1.2)	4.5 (1.3)	14.0 (1.8)
Headache	4.4 (0.2)	3.9 (0.0)	4.5 (0.2)
Paresthesia	1.0 (0.0)	0.0 (0.0)	2.6 (0.0)
Insomnia	0.7 (0.0)	0.6 (0.0)	2.3 (0.0)
Depression	0.0 (0.0)	1.3 (0.0)	1.1 (0.0)
Respiratory			
Dyspnea	2.7 (0.2)	4.5 (0.6)	7.6 (0.3)
Cough	1.7 (0.0)	2.6 (0.0)	6.1 (0.2)
Upper Respiratory Infection	1.5 (0.0)	1.3 (0.0)	4.5 (0.0)
Bronchitis	0.5 (0.0)	0.0 (0.0)	1.6 (0.0)
Chest Sound Abnormalities	0.0 (0.0)	1.3 (0.0)	0.3 (0.0)
Pulmonary Edema	0.2 (0.0)	1.3 (0.0)	0.3 (0.0)
Skin			
Rash	1.7 (0.5)	0.6 (0.6)	4.8 (1.0)
Pruritus	1.2 (0.2)	1.9 (0.6)	1.5 (0.2)
Urogenital			
Urinary Tract Infection	0.5 (0.0)	0.0 (0.0)	1.5 (0.0)

Other clinical adverse experiences occurring in 0.3 to 1.0 percent of patients with hypertension or heart failure treated with lisinopril in controlled trials and rarer, serious, possibly drug-related events reported in uncontrolled studies or marketing experience are listed below, and within each category, are in order of decreasing severity:

ADVERSE REACTIONS: *(cont'd)*

Body as a Whole: Anaphylactoid reactions (see WARNINGS, Anaphylactoid, Reactions During Membrane Exposure), chest discomfort, pain, pelvic pain, flank pain, facial edema, peripheral edema, virus infection, chills.

Cardiovascular: Cardiac arrest; myocardial infarction or cerebrovascular accident, possibly secondary to excessive hypotension in high risk patients (see WARNINGS, Hypotension) ; pulmonary embolism and infarction, arrhythmias, (including ventricular tachycardia, atrial tachycardia, atrial fibrillation, bradycardia and premature ventricular contractions), transient ischemic attacks, paroxysmal nocturnal dyspnea, decreased blood pressure, peripheral edema, vasculitis.

Digestive: Pancreatitis, hepatitis (hepatocellular or cholestatic jaundice) (see WARNINGS, Hepatic Failure), gastritis, heartburn, gastrointestinal cramps, constipation, flatulence, dry mouth.

Hematologic: Rare cases of bone marrow depression, leukopenia/neutropenia, and thrombocytopenia.

Endocrine: Diabetes mellitus.

Metabolic: Weight loss, dehydration, fluid overload, weight gain.

Musculoskeletal: Arthritis, arthralgia, neck pain, hip pain, low back pain, joint pain, knee pain, shoulder pain, arm pain, lumbago.

Nervous System/Psychiatric: Stroke, ataxia, memory impairment, tremor, peripheral neuropathy, (*e.g.,* dysesthesia), spasm, confusion, somnolence, hypersomnia, irritability, and nervousness.

Respiratory System: Malignant lung neoplasms, hemoptysis, pulmonary infiltrates, bronchospasm, asthma, pleural effusion, pneumonia, wheezing, orthopnea, painful respiration, epistaxis, laryngitis, sinusitis, pharyngeal pain, pharyngitis, rhinitis, rhinorrhea.

Skin: Urticaria, alopecia, herpes zoster, photosensitivity, skin lesions, skin infections, erythema, flushing, diaphoresis.

Other severe skin reactions have been reported rarely; causal relationship has not been established.

Special Senses: Visual loss, diplopia, blurred vision, tinnitus, photophobia.

Urogenital System: Acute renal failure, oliguria, anuria, uremia, progressive azotemia, renal dysfunction (see PRECAUTIONSand DOSAGE AND ADMINISTRATION), pyelonephritis, dysuria, breast pain.

Miscellaneous: A symptom complex has been reported which may include a positive ANA, an elevated erythrocyte sedimentation rate, arthralgia/arthritis, myalgia, fever, vasculitis, leukocytosis, eosinophilia, photosensitivity, rash, and other dermatological manifestations.

Angioedema: Angioedema has been reported in patients receiving lisinopril (0.1 percent). Angioedema associated with laryngeal edema may be fatal. If angioedema of the face, extremities, lips, tongue, glottis and/or larynx occurs, treatment with lisinopril should be discontinued and appropriate therapy instituted immediately. (See WARNINGS.)

Hypotension: In hypertensive patients, hypotension occurred in 1.2 percent and syncope occurred in 0.1 percent of patients. Hypotension or syncope was a cause for discontinuation of therapy in 0.5 percent of hypertensive patients. In patients with heart failure, hypotension occurred in 5.3 percent and syncope occurred in 1.8 percent of patients. These adverse experiences were causes for discontinuation of therapy in 1.8 percent of these patients. (See WARNINGS.)

Fetal/Neonatal Morbidity and Mortality: (See WARNINGS, Fetal/Neonatal Morbidity and Mortality.)

Cough: See PRECAUTIONS, Cough.

Clinical Laboratory Test Findings Serum Electrolytes: Hyperkalemia (see PRECAUTIONS, hyponatremia.

Creatinine, Blood Urea Nitrogen: Minor increases in blood urea nitrogen and serum creatinine, reversible upon discontinuation of therapy, were observed in about 2.0 percent of patients with essential hypertension treated with lisinopril alone. Increases were more common in patients receiving concomitant diuretics and in patients with renal artery stenosis. (See PRECAUTIONS.) Reversible minor increases in blood urea nitrogen and serum creatinine were observed in approximately 11.6 percent of patients with heart failure on concomitant diuretic therapy. Frequently, these abnormalities resolved when the dosage of the diuretic was decreased.

Hemoglobin and Hematocrit: Small decreases in hemoglobin and hematocrit (mean decreases of approximately 0.4 g percent and 1.3 vol percent, respectively) occurred frequently in patients treated with lisinopril but were rarely of clinical importance in patients without some other cause of anemia. In clinical trials, less than 0.1 percent of patients discontinued therapy due to anemia. Hemolytic anemia has been reported; a causal relationship to lisinopril cannot be excluded.

Liver Function Tests: Rarely, elevations of liver enzymes and/or serum bilirubin have occurred (see WARNINGS, Hepatic Failure).

In hypertensive patients, 2.0 percent discontinued therapy due to laboratory adverse experiences, principally elevations in blood urea nitrogen (0.6 percent), serum creatinine (0.5 percent) and serum potassium (0.4 percent). In the heart failure trials, 3.4 percent of patients discontinued therapy due to laboratory adverse experiences, 1.8 percent due to elevations in blood urea nitrogen and/or creatinine and 0.6 percent due to elevations in serum potassium.

OVERDOSAGE:

The oral LD_{50} of lisinopril is greater than 20 g/kg in mice and rats. The most likely manifestation of overdosage would be hypotension, for which the usual treatment would be intravenous infusion of normal saline solution.

Lisinopril can be removed by hemodialysis.

DOSAGE AND ADMINISTRATION:

HYPERTENSION

Initial Therapy: In patients with uncomplicated essential hypertension not on diuretic therapy, the recommended initial dose is 10 mg once a day. Dosage should be adjusted according to blood pressure response. The usual dosage range is 20 to 40 mg per day administered in a single daily dose. The antihypertensive effect may diminish toward the end of the dosing interval regardless of the administered dose, but most commonly with a dose of 10 mg daily. This can be evaluated by measuring blood pressure just prior to dosing to determine whether satisfactory control is being maintained for 24 hours. If it is not, an increase in dose should be considered. Doses up to 80 mg have been used but do not appear to give a greater effect. If blood pressure is not controlled with lisinopril alone, a low dose of a diuretic may be added. Hydrochlorothiazide, 12.5 mg has been shown to provide an additive effect. After the addition of a diuretic, it may be possible to reduce the dose of lisinopril.

Diuretic Treated Patients: In hypertensive patients who are currently being treated with a diuretic, symptomatic hypotension may occur occasionally following the initial dose of lisinopril. The diuretic should be discontinued, if possible, for two to three days before beginning therapy with lisinopril to reduce the likelihood of hypotension. (See WARNINGS.)

DOSAGE AND ADMINISTRATION: *(cont'd)*

The dosage of lisinopril should be adjusted according to blood pressure response. If the patient's blood pressure is not controlled with lisinopril alone, diuretic therapy may be resumed as described above.

If the diuretic cannot be discontinued, an initial dose of 5 mg should be used under medical supervision for at least two hours and until blood pressure has stabilized for at least an additional hour. See WARNINGSand PRECAUTIONS, DRUG INTERACTIONS.

Concomitant administration of lisinopril with potassium supplements, potassium salt substitutes, or potassium-sparing diuretics may lead to increases of serum potassium (see PRECAUTIONS.)

Dosage Adjustment in Renal Impairment: The usual dose of lisinopril (10 mg) is recommended for patients with a creatinine clearance > 30 ml/min (serum creatinine of up to approximately 3 mg/dl). For patients with creatinine clearance ≥ 10 ml/min ≤ 30 ml/min (serum creatinine ≥ 3 mg/dl), the first dose is 5 mg once daily. For patients with creatinine clearance < 10 ml/min (usually on hemodialysis) the recommended initial dose is 2.5 mg. The dosage may be titrated upward until blood pressure is controlled or to a maximum of 40 mg daily (TABLE 3):

TABLE 3 Lisinopril, DOSAGE AND ADMINISTRATION

Renal Status	Creatinine-Clearance ml/min	Initial Dose mg/day
Normal Renal Function to Mild Impairment	> 30 ml/min	10 mg
Moderate to Severe Impairment	≥ 10 ≤ 30 ml/min	5 mg
Dialysis Patients*	< 10 ml/min	2.5 mg**

* See WARNINGS, Anaphylactoid reactions during membrane exposure
** Dosage or dosing interval should be adjusted depending on the blood pressure response.

Heart Failure: Lisinopril is indicated as adjunctive therapy with diuretics and digitalis. The recommended starting dose is 5 mg once a day.

When initiating treatment with lisinopril in patients with heart failure, the initial dose should be administered under medical observation, especially in those patients with low blood pressure (systolic blood pressure below 100 mm Hg). The mean peak blood pressure lowering occurs six to eight hours after dosing. Observations should continue until blood pressure is stable. The concomitant diuretic dose should be reduced, if possible, to help minimize hypovolemia which may contribute to hypotension. See WARNINGSand PRECAUTIONS, DRUG INTERACTIONS. The appearance of hypotension after the initial dose of lisinopril does not preclude subsequent careful dose titration with the drug, following effective management of the hypotension.

The usual effective dosage range is 5 to 20 mg per day administered as a single daily dose.

Dosage Adjustment in Patients with Heart Failure and Renal Impairment or Hyponatremia: In patients with heart failure who have hyponatremia (serum sodium <130 mEq/l) or moderate to severe renal impairment (creatinine clearance ≤30 ml/min or serum creatinine >3 mg/dl), therapy with lisinopril should be initiated at a dose of 2.5 mg once a day under close medical supervision. See WARNINGSand PRECAUTIONS, DRUG INTERACTIONS.

Use in Elderly: In general, blood pressure response and adverse experiences were similar in younger and older patients given similar doses of lisinopril. Pharmacokinetic studies, however, indicate that maximum blood levels and area under the plasma concentration time curve (AUC) are doubled in older patients, so that dosage adjustments should be made with particular caution.

Storage: Store at controlled room temperature, 15 - 30°C (59 - 86°F), and protect from moisture. Dispense in a tight container, if product package is subdivided.

PATIENT INFORMATION:

Lisinopril is an angiotensin-converting enzyme (ACE) inhibitor used for the treatment of high blood pressure or heart failure. Notify your physician if you are pregnant or nursing. The use of lisinopril during months four through nine of pregnancy may permanently injure or cause the death of the developing fetus. Avoid using potassium containing salt substitutes without notifying your physician. Lisinopril may be taken with or without food. Dizziness, lightheadedness or fainting may occur after the first dose or during the first week of therapy. Avoid sudden changes in posture. A persistent dry cough or taste alterations may occur while taking lisinopril. Notify your physician if these become bothersome. Notify your physician if you develop trouble swallowing or breathing; swelling of the face, lips, or tongue; irregular heartbeat; rash, hives or severe itching; unexplained fever; or easy bruising.

HOW SUPPLIED - RATED THERAPEUTICALLY EQUIVALENT:

Tablet - Oral - 2.5 mg

100's	**$54.60**	**ZESTRIL, Zeneca Pharms**	**00310-0135-10**

Tablet, Uncoated - Oral - 2.5 mg

30's	$15.74	PRINIVIL, Merck	00006-0015-31
100's	$52.50	PRINIVIL, Merck	00006-0015-28
100's	$52.50	PRINIVIL, Merck	00006-0015-58

Tablet, Uncoated - Oral - 5 mg

30's	**$22.37**	**Zestril, Talbert Phcy**	**44514-0480-18**
100's	$78.62	PRINIVIL, Merck	00006-0019-28
100's	$78.62	PRINIVIL, Merck	00006-0019-58
100's	**$78.62**	**Zestril, Zeneca Pharms**	**00310-0130-10**
100's	**$78.62**	**Zestril, Zeneca Pharms**	**00310-0130-39**
1000's	**$776.96**	**Zestril, Zeneca Pharms**	**00310-0130-34**
1000's	$786.24	Prinivil, Merck	00006-0019-82
1080's	$849.14	PRINIVIL, 90 X 12, Merck	00006-0019-94
5000's	$3931.20	Prinivil, Merck	00006-0019-86
10000's	$7862.40	PRINIVIL, Merck	00006-0019-87

Tablet, Uncoated - Oral - 10 mg

30's	**$23.12**	**Zestril, Talbert Phcy**	**44514-0481-18**
30's	$24.38	PRINIVIL, Merck	00006-0106-31
100's	$81.29	PRINIVIL, Merck	00006-0106-28
100's	$81.29	PRINIVIL, Merck	00006-0106-58
100's	**$81.29**	**Zestril, Zeneca Pharms**	**00310-0131-10**
100's	**$81.29**	**Zestril, Zeneca Pharms**	**00310-0131-39**
1000's	**$803.20**	**Zestril, Zeneca Pharms**	**00310-0131-34**
1000's	$812.88	Prinivil, Merck	00006-0106-82
1080's	$877.89	PRINIVIL, 90 X 12, Merck	00006-0106-94
3000's	**$2385.03**	**Zestril, Zeneca Pharms**	**00310-0131-73**
5000's	$4064.40	Prinivil, Merck	00006-0106-86
10000's	$8128.80	PRINIVIL, Merck	00006-0106-87

Tablet, Uncoated - Oral - 20 mg

30's	**$24.75**	**Zestril, Talbert Phcy**	**44514-0482-18**
30's	$26.10	PRINIVIL, Merck	00006-0207-31
100's	$87.00	PRINIVIL, Merck	00006-0207-28
100's	$87.00	PRINIVIL, Merck	00006-0207-58

HOW SUPPLIED - RATED THERAPEUTICALLY EQUIVALENT: *(cont'd)*

100's	**$87.00**	**Zestril, Zeneca Pharms**	**00310-0132-10**
100's	**$87.00**	**Zestril, Zeneca Pharms**	**00310-0132-39**
1000's	**$859.61**	**Zestril, Zeneca Pharms**	**00310-0132-34**
1000's	$870.00	Prinivil, Merck	00006-0207-82
1080's	$939.60	PRINIVIL, 90 X 12, Merck	00006-0207-94
3000's	**$2552.58**	**Zestril, Zeneca Pharms**	**00310-0132-73**
5000's	$4350.00	Prinivil, Merck	00006-0207-86
10000's	$8700.00	PRINIVIL, Merck	00006-0207-87

Tablet, Uncoated - Oral - 40 mg

30's	**$36.59**	**Zestril, Talbert Phcy**	**44514-0483-18**
100's	$127.08	PRINIVIL, Merck	00006-0237-58
100's	**$127.08**	**Zestril, Zeneca Pharms**	**00310-0134-10**

LITHIUM CARBONATE *(001648)*

CATEGORIES: Antidepressants; Antimanic Agents; Antipsychotics/Antimanics; Bipolar Disorder; Central Nervous System Agents; Depression; Lithium Salts; Mania; Neuroleptics; Psychotherapeutic Agents; Neutropenia, Chemotherapy*; FDA Approval Pre 1982
* Indication not approved by the FDA

BRAND NAMES: *Calith*; *Camcolit* (England); *Carbolit* (Mexico); *Carbolith* (Canada); *Ceglution*; *Ceglution 300*; *Duralith* (Canada); **Eskalith**; Eskalith-Cr; *Hypnorex*; *Hynorex Retard* (Germany); *Hyponrex*; *Lentolith*; *Licab*; *Licarb*; *Licarbium*; *Lidin*; *Lilipin*; *Lilitin*; *Limas* (Japan); *Liskonum*; *Lithan*; Lithane; *Litheum*; *Litheum 300* (Mexico); *Lithicarb* (Australia); *Lithionate*; *Lithizine* (Canada); Lithobid; *Lithocarb*; *Lithocap*; Lithonate; *Lithosun SR*; Lithotabs; *Lithuril*; *Litilent*; *Manialit*; *Maniprex*; *Phanate*; *Phasal*; *Plenur*; *Priadel* (England); *Priadel Retard*; *Quilonium-R*; *Quilonorm Retardtabletten*; *Quilonum Retard* (Germany); *Teralithe* (France); *Theralite*; *Theralite 300*
(International brand names outside U.S. in italics)

FORMULARIES: Aetna; BC-BS; CIGNA; FHP; Humana; Kaiser; Medco; Medi-Cal; PCS; PruCare; United; WHO

COST OF THERAPY: $14.17 (Depression; Capsule; 300 mg; 3/day; 90 days) vs. Potential Cost of $2,456.15 (Depression)

PRIMARY ICD9: 311 (Depressive Disorder, Not Elsewhere Classified)

> WARNING:
> Lithium toxicity is closely related to serum lithium levels, and can occur at doses close to therapeutic levels. Facilities for prompt and accurate serum lithium determinations should be available before initiating therapy (see DOSAGE AND ADMINISTRATION.)

DESCRIPTION:

Lithium carbonate is a white, light alkaline powder with molecular formula Li_2CO_3 and molecular weight 73.89. Lithium is an element of the alkali-metal group with atomic number 3, atomic weight 6.94 and an emission line at 671 nm on the flame photometer.

Eskalith Capsules: Each capsule, with opaque gray cap and opaque yellow body, is imprinted with the product nameESKALITH and SKF and contains lithium carbonate, 300 mg. Inactive ingredients consist of benzyl alcohol, cetylpyridinium chloride, D&C Yellow No. 10, FD&C Green No. 3, FD&C Red No. 40, FD&C Yellow No. 6, gelatin, lactose, magnesium stearate, povidone, sodium lauryl sulfate, titanium dioxide and trace amounts of other inactive ingredients.

Eskalith Controlled Release Tablets: Each round, buff, scored tablet contains lithium carbonate, 450 mg. Inactive ingredients consist of alginic acid, gelatin, iron oxide, magnesium stearate and sodium starch glycolate.

Lithobid Tablets: 300 mg lithium carbonate *Inactive Ingredients:* Calcium stearate, carnauba wax, cellulose compounds, FD&C Blue No.2 Aluminum Lake, FD&C Red No. 40 Aluminum Lake, FD&C Yellow No. 6 Aluminum Lake, povidone, propylene glycol, sodium chloride, sodium lauryl sulfate, sodium starch glycolate, sorbitol, and titanium dioxide.

Lithium carbonate controlled release tablets 450 mg are designed to release a portion of the dose initially and the remainder gradually; the release pattern of the controlled release tablets reduces the variability in lithium blood levels seen with the immediate release dosage forms.

CLINICAL PHARMACOLOGY:

Preclinical studies have shown that lithium alters sodium transport in nerve and muscle cells and effects a shift toward intraneuronal metabolism of catecholamines, but the specific biochemical mechanism of lithium action in mania is unknown.

INDICATIONS AND USAGE:

Lithium carbonate is indicated in the treatment of manic episodes of manic-depressive illness. Maintenance therapy prevents or diminishes the intensity of subsequent episodes in those manic-depressive patients with a history of mania.

Typical symptoms of mania include pressure of speech, motor hyperactivity, reduced need for sleep, flight of ideas, grandiosity, elation, poor judgment, aggressiveness, and possibly hostility. When given to a patient experiencing a manic episode, lithium carbonate may produce a normalization of symptomatology within 1 to 3 weeks.

WARNINGS:

Lithium should generally not be given to patients with significant renal or cardiovascular disease, severe debilitation or dehydration, or sodium depletion, since the risk of lithium toxicity is very high in such patients. If the psychiatric indication is life-threatening, and if such a patient fails to respond to other measures, lithium treatment may be undertaken with extreme caution, including daily serum lithium determinations and adjustment to the usually low doses ordinarily tolerated by these individuals. In such instances, hospitalization is a necessity.

Chronic lithium therapy may be associated with diminution of renal concentrating ability, occasionally presenting as nephrogenic diabetes insipidus, with polyuria and polydipsia. Such patients should be carefully managed to avoid dehydration with resulting lithium retention and toxicity. This condition is usually reversible when lithium is discontinued.

WARNINGS: *(cont'd)*

Morphologic changes with glomerular and interstitial fibrosis and nephron atrophy have been reported in patients on chronic lithium therapy. Morphologic changes have also been seen in manic-depressive patients never exposed to lithium. The relationship between renal functional and morphologic changes and their association with lithium therapy have not been established.

When kidney function is assessed, for baseline data prior to starting lithium therapy or thereafter, routine urinalysis and other tests may be used to evaluate tubular function (*e.g.*, urine specific gravity or osmolality following a period of water deprivation, or 24-hour urine volume) and glomerular function (*e.g.*, serum creatinine or creatinine clearance). During lithium therapy, progressive or sudden changes in renal function, even within the normal range, indicate the need for reevaluation of treatment.

An encephalopathic syndrome (characterized by weakness, lethargy, fever, tremulousness and confusion, extrapyramidal symptoms, leukocytosis, elevated serum enzymes, BUN and FBS) has occurred in a few patients treated with lithium plus a neuroleptic. In some instances, the syndrome was followed by irreversible brain damage. Because of a possible causal relationship between these events and the concomitant administration of lithium and neuroleptics, patients receiving such combined therapy should be monitored closely for early evidence of neurologic toxicity and treatment discontinued promptly if such signs appear. This encephalopathic syndrome may be similar to or the same as neuroleptic malignant syndrome (NMS).

Lithium toxicity is closely related to serum lithium levels, and can occur at doses close to therapeutic levels (see DOSAGE AND ADMINISTRATION.)

Outpatients and their families should be warned that the patient must discontinue lithium carbonate therapy and contact his physician if such clinical signs of lithium toxicity as diarrhea, vomiting, tremor, mild ataxia, drowsiness, or muscular weakness occur.

Lithium carbonate may impair mental and/or physical abilities. Caution patients about activities requiring alertness (*e.g.*, operating vehicles or machinery).

Lithium may prolong the effects of neuromuscular blocking agents. Therefore, neuromuscular blocking agents should be given with caution to patients receiving lithium.

Usage in Pregnancy: Adverse effects on implantation in rats, embryo viability in mice, and metabolism *in vitro* of rat testes and human spermatozoa have been attributed to lithium, as have teratogenicity in submammalian species and cleft palates in mice.

In humans, lithium carbonate may cause fetal harm when administered to a pregnant woman. Data from lithium birth registries suggest an increase in cardiac and other anomalies, especially Ebsteins anomaly. If this drug is used in women of childbearing potential, or during pregnancy, or if a patient becomes pregnant while taking this drug, the patient should be apprised of the potential hazard to the fetus.

Usage in Nursing Mothers: Lithium is excreted in human milk. Nursing should not be undertaken during lithium therapy except in rare and unusual circumstances where, in the view of the physician, the potential benefits to the mother outweigh possible hazards to the child.

Usage in Children: Since information regarding the safety and effectiveness of lithium carbonate in children under 12 years of age is not available, its use in such patients is not recommended at this time.

There has been a report of a transient syndrome of acute dystonia and hyperreflexia occurring in a 15 kg. child who ingested 300 mg. of lithium carbonate.

Usage in the Elderly: Elderly patients often require lower lithium dosages to achieve therapeutic serum levels. They may also exhibit adverse reactions at serum levels ordinarily tolerated by younger patients.

PRECAUTIONS:

The ability to tolerate lithium is greater during the acute manic phase and decreases when manic symptoms subside (see DOSAGE AND ADMINISTRATION.)

Caution should be used when lithium and diuretics are used concomitantly because diuretic-induced sodium loss may reduce the renal clearance of lithium and increase serum lithium levels with risk of lithium toxicity. Patients receiving such combined therapy should have serum lithium levels monitored closely and the lithium dosage adjusted if necessary.

The distribution space of lithium approximates that of total body water. Lithium is primarily excreted in urine with insignificant excretion in feces. Renal excretion of lithium is proportional to its plasma concentration. The half-life of elimination of lithium is approximately 24 hours. Lithium decreases sodium reabsorption by the renal tubules which could lead to sodium depletion. Therefore, it is essential for the patient to maintain a normal diet, including salt, and an adequate fluid intake (2500-3000 ml.) at least during the initial stabilization period. Decreased tolerance to lithium has been reported to ensue from protracted sweating or diarrhea and, if such occur, supplemental fluid and salt should be administered under careful medical supervision and lithium intake reduced or suspended until the condition is resolved.

In addition to sweating and diarrhea, concomitant infection with elevated temperatures may also necessitate a temporary reduction or cessation of medication.

Previously existing underlying thyroid disorders do not necessarily constitute a contraindication to lithium treatment, where hypothyroidism exists, careful monitoring of thyroid function during lithium stabilization and maintenance allows for correction of changing thyroid parameters, if any; where hypothyroidism occurs during lithium stabilization and maintenance, supplemental thyroid treatment may be used.

DRUG INTERACTIONS:

Indomethacin and piroxicam have been reported to increase significantly, steady state plasma lithium levels. In some cases, lithium toxicity has resulted from such interactions. There is also some evidence that other nonsteroidal anti-inflammatory agents may have a similar effect. When such combinations are used, increased plasma lithium level monitoring is recommended. Concurrent use of metronidazole with lithium may provoke lithium toxicity due to reduced renal clearance. Patients receiving such combined therapy should be monitored closely.

There is evidence that angiotensin-converting enzyme inhibitors, such as enalapril and captopril, may substantially increase steady-state plasma lithium levels, sometimes resulting in lithium toxicity. When such combinations are used, lithium dosage may need to be decreased, and plasma lithium levels should be measured more often.

Concurrent use of calcium channel blocking agents with lithium may increase the risk of neurotoxicity in the form of ataxia, tremors, nausea, vomiting, diarrhea and/or tinnitus. Caution is recommended.

The following drugs can lower serum lithium concentrations by increasing urinary lithium excretion acetazolamide, urea, xanthine preparations and alkalinizing agents such as sodium bicarbonate.

ADVERSE REACTIONS:

The occurrence and severity of adverse reactions are generally directly related to serum lithium concentrations as well as to individual patient sensitivity to lithium, and generally occur more frequently and with greater severity at higher concentrations.

ADVERSE REACTIONS: *(cont'd)*

Adverse reactions may be encountered at serum lithium levels below 1.5 mEq./l. Mild to moderate adverse reactions may occur at levels from 1.5 to 2.5 mEq./l., and moderate to severe reactions may be seen at levels of 2.0 mEq./l. and above.

Fine hand tremor, polyuria, and mild thirst may occur during initial therapy for the acute manic phase, and may persist throughout treatment. Transient and mild nausea and general discomfort may also appear during the first few days of lithium administration.

These side effects usually subside with continued treatment or a temporary reduction or cessation of dosage. If persistent, cessation of lithium therapy may be required.

Diarrhea, vomiting, drowsiness, muscular weakness, and lack of coordination may be early signs of lithium intoxication, and can occur at lithium levels below 2.0 mEq./l. At higher levels, ataxia, giddiness, tinnitus, blurred vision, and a large output of dilute urine may be seen. Serum lithium levels above 3.0 mEq./l may produce a complex clinical picture, involving multiple organs and organ systems. Serum lithium levels should not be permitted to exceed 2.0 mEq./l during the acute treatment phase.

The following reactions have been reported and appear to be related to serum lithium levels, including levels within the therapeutic range:*Neuromuscular/Central Nervous System:* tremor, muscle hyperirritability (fasciculations, twitching, clonic movements of whole limbs), hypertonicity, ataxia, choreo-athetotic movements, hyperactive deep tendon reflex, extrapyramidal symptoms including acute dystonia, cogwheel rigidity, blackout spells, epileptiform seizures, slurred speech, dizziness, vertigo, downbeat nystagmus, incontinence of urine or feces, somnolence, psychomotor retardation, restlessness, confusion, stupor, coma, tongue movements, tics, tinnitus, hallucinations, poor memory, slowed intellectual functioning, startled response, worsening of organic brain syndromes; *Cardiovascular:* cardiac arrhythmia, hypotension, peripheral circulatory collapse, bradycardia, sinus node dysfunction with severe bradycardia (which may result in syncope);*Gastrointestinal:* anorexia, nausea, vomiting, diarrhea, gastritis, salivary gland swelling, abdominal pain, excessive salivation, flatulence, indigestion; *Genitourinary:* glycosuria, decreased creatinine clearance, albuminuria, oliguria, and symptoms of nephrogenic diabetes insipidus including polyuria, thirst, and polydipsia;*Dermatologic:* drying and thinning of hair, alopecia, anesthesia of skin, acne, chronic folliculitis, xerosis cutis, psoriasis or its exacerbation, generalized pruritus with of without rash, cutaneous ulcers, angioedema; *Autonomic:* blurred vision, dry mouth, impotence/sexual dysfunction; *Thyroid Abnormalities:* euthyroid goiter and/or hypothyroidism (including myxedema) accompanied by lower $T_3$and T_4.I^{131} uptake may be elevated. (See PRECAUTIONS.) Paradoxically, rare cases of hyperthyroidism have been reported; *EEG Changes:* diffuse slowing, widening of the frequency spectrum, potentiation and disorganization of background rhythm; *EKG Changes:* reversible flattening, isoelectricity or inversion of T-waves; *Miscellaneous:* fatigue, lethargy, transient scotomata, dehydration, weight loss, leukocytosis, headache, transient hyperglycemia, hypercalcemia, hyperparathyroidism, excessive weight gain, edematous swelling of ankles or wrists, metallic taste, dysgeusia/ taste distortion, salty taste, thirst, swollen lips, tightness in chest, swollen and/or painful joints, fever, polyarthralgia, dental caries.

Some reports of nephrogenic diabetes insipidus, hyperparathyroidism and hypothyroidism which persist after lithium discontinuation have been received.

A few reports have been received of the development of painful discoloration of fingers and toes and coldness of the extremities within one day of the starting of treatment with lithium. The mechanism through which these symptoms (resembling Raynaud's syndrome) developed is not known. Recovery followed discontinuance.

Cases of pseudotumor cerebri (increased intracranial pressure and papilledema) have been reported with lithium use. If undetected, this condition may result in enlargement of the blind spot, constriction of visual fields and eventual blindness due to optic atrophy.

Lithium should be discontinued, if clinically possible, if this syndrome occurs.

OVERDOSAGE:

The toxic levels for lithium are close to the therapeutic levels. It is therefore important that patients and their families be cautioned to watch for early toxic symptoms and to discontinue the drug and inform the physician should they occur. Toxic symptoms are listed in detail under ADVERSE REACTIONS.

Treatment: No specific antidote for lithium poisoning is known. Early symptoms of lithium toxicity can usually be treated by reduction or cessation of dosage of the drug and resumption of the treatment at a lower dose after 24 to 48 hours. In severe cases of lithium poisoning, the first and foremost goal of treatment consists of elimination of this ion from the patient. Treatment is essentially the same as that used in barbiturate poisoning: 1) gastric lavage, 2) correction of fluid and electrolyte imbalance, and 3) regulation of kidney function. Urea, mannitol, and aminophylline all produce significant increases in lithium excretion. Hemodialysis is an effective and rapid means of removing the ion from the severely toxic patient. Infection prophylaxis, regular chest X-rays, and preservation of adequate respiration are essential.

DOSAGE AND ADMINISTRATION:

Immediate release capsules and tablets are usually given t.i.d. or q.i.d. Doses of controlled release tablets are usually given b.i.d. (approximately 12-hour intervals). When initiating therapy with immediate release or controlled release lithium, dosage must be individualized according to serum levels and clinical response.

When switching a patient from immediate release capsules or tablets to the lithium carbonate controlled release tablets, give the same total daily dose when possible. Most patients on maintenance therapy are stabilized on 900 mg daily (*e.g.,* 450 mg lithium carbonate controlled release b.i.d). When the previous dosage of immediate release lithium is not a multiple of 450 mg, for example, 1500 mg, initiate lithium carbonate controlled release dosage at the multiple of 450 mg nearest to, but below, the original daily dose (*i.e.,* 1350 mg). When the two doses are unequal, give the larger dose in the evening. In the above example, with a total daily dosage of 1350 mg, generally 450 mg lithium carbonate controlled release should be given in the morning and 900 mg lithium carbonate controlled release in the evening. If desired, the total daily dosage of 1350 mg can be given in three equal 450 mg lithium carbonate controlled release doses. These patients should be monitored at 1 to 2 week intervals, and dosage adjusted if necessary, until stable and satisfactory serum levels and clinical state are achieved.

When patients require closer titration than that available with lithium carbonate controlled release doses in increments of 450 mg, immediate release capsules should be used.

Acute Mania: Optimal patient response to lithium carbonate can usually be established and maintained with 1800 mg per day in divided doses. Such doses will normally produce the desired serum lithium level ranging between 1.0 and 1.5 mEq/l.

Dosage must be individualized according to serum levels and clinical response. Regular monitoring of the patient's clinical state and serum lithium levels is necessary. Serum levels should be determined twice per week during the acute phase, and until the serum level and clinical condition of the patient have been stabilized.

Long-Term Control: The desirable serum lithium levels are 0.6 to 1.2 mEq/l. Dosage will vary from one individual to another, but usually 900 mg to 1200 mg per day in divided doses will maintain this level. Serum lithium levels in uncomplicated cases receiving maintenance therapy during remission should be monitored at least every two months.

DOSAGE AND ADMINISTRATION: *(cont'd)*

Patients unusually sensitive to lithium may exhibit toxic signs at serum levels below 1.0 mEq/l.

N.B.: Blood samples for serum lithium determinations should be drawn immediately prior to the next dose when lithium concentrations are relatively stable (*i.e.,* 8-12 hours after the previous dose). Total reliance must not be placed on serum levels alone. Accurate patient evaluation requires both clinical and laboratory analysis.

Elderly patients often respond to reduced dosage, and may exhibit signs of toxicity at serum levels ordinarily tolerated by younger patients.

HOW SUPPLIED - RATED THERAPEUTICALLY EQUIVALENT:

Capsule, Gelatin - Oral - 300 mg

90's	$5.70	Lithium Carbonate, Major Pharms	00904-2912-89
100's	$5.25	Lithium Carbonate, United Res	00677-1092-01
100's	$5.25	Lithium Carbonate, H.C.F.A. F F P	99999-1648-01
100's	$5.50	Lithium Carbonate, Solvay Pharms	00032-4160-06
100's	$7.25	Lithium Carbonate, Major Pharms	00904-2912-60
100's	$7.80	Lithium Carbonate, Schein Pharm (US)	00364-0855-01
100's	$7.98	Lithium Carbonate, Caremark	00339-5771-12
100's	$8.13	Lithium Carbonate, Roxane	00054-2527-25
100's	$8.40	LITHONATE, Solvay Pharms	00032-7512-01
100's	$8.40	Lithium Carbonate, Intl Labs	00665-4160-06
100's	$8.48	Lithium Carbonate, Qualitest Pharms	00603-4220-21
100's	$8.50	Lithium Carbonate, Goldline Labs	00182-1781-01
100's	$8.51	Lithium Carbonate, Geneva Pharms	00781-2100-01
100's	$8.67	Lithium Carbonate, Rugby	00536-3739-01
100's	$8.71	Lithium Carbonate, HL Moore Drug Exch	00839-7149-06
100's	$9.05	LITHONATE, Solvay Pharms	00032-7512-11
100's	$10.42	Lithium Carbonate, Roxane	00054-8527-25
100's	$13.25	Lithium Carbonate, Major Pharms	00904-2912-61
100's	**$16.90**	**ESKALITH, SKB Pharms**	**00007-4007-20**
120's	$6.30	Lithium Carbonate, H.C.F.A. F F P	99999-1648-02
120's	$7.10	Lithium Carbonate, Major Pharms	00904-2912-18
500's	$26.25	Lithium Carbonate, H.C.F.A. F F P	99999-1648-03
500's	$42.45	Lithium Carbonate, Rugby	00536-3739-05
500's	**$78.40**	**ESKALITH, SKB Pharms**	**00007-4007-25**
1000's	$49.50	Lithium Carbonate, Solvay Pharms	00032-4160-09
1000's	$52.50	Lithium Carbonate, United Res	00677-1092-10
1000's	$52.50	Lithium Carbonate, H.C.F.A. F F P	99999-1648-04
1000's	$60.45	Lithium Carbonate, Major Pharms	00904-2912-80
1000's	$68.90	Lithium Carbonate, Intl Labs	00665-4160-09
1000's	$69.24	Lithium Carbonate, Roxane	00054-2527-31
1000's	$69.35	LITHONATE, Solvay Pharms	00032-7512-10
1000's	$69.49	Lithium Carbonate, Qualitest Pharms	00603-4220-32
1000's	$69.50	Lithium Carbonate, Goldline Labs	00182-1781-10
1000's	$69.51	Lithium Carbonate, Geneva Pharms	00781-2100-10
1000's	$72.20	Lithium Carbonate, Rugby	00536-3739-10
1000's	$82.15	Lithium Carbonate, HL Moore Drug Exch	00839-7149-16

Tablet, Uncoated - Oral - 300 mg

100's	$7.41	Lithium Carbonate, Roxane	00054-4527-25
100's	$9.11	Lithium Carbonate, Caremark	00339-5773-12
100's	$10.23	LITHOTABS, Solvay Pharms	00032-7516-01
100's	$10.42	Lithium Carbonate, Roxane	00054-8528-25
100's	$11.05	LITHOTABS, Solvay Pharms	00032-7516-11
1000's	$66.00	Lithium Carbonate, Roxane	00054-4527-31
1000's	$91.11	LITHOTABS, Solvay Pharms	00032-7516-10

HOW SUPPLIED - NOT RATED EQUIVALENT:

Capsule, Gelatin - Oral - 150 mg

100's	$7.63	Lithium Carbonate, Roxane	00054-2526-25
100's	$9.95	Lithium Carbonate, Roxane	00054-8526-25

Capsule, Gelatin - Oral - 600 mg

100's	$13.23	Lithium Carbonate, Roxane	00054-2531-25
100's	$17.58	Lithium Carbonate, Roxane	00054-8531-25
1000's	$112.52	Lithium Carbonate, Roxane	00054-2531-31

Tablet, Coated, Sustained Action - Oral - 300 mg

100's	$15.53	LITHOBID, Novartis	00083-0065-30
100's	$17.72	LITHOBID, Novartis	00083-0065-32
100's	$25.38	LITHOBID, Solvay Pharms	00032-4492-01
1000's	$153.52	LITHOBID, Novartis	00083-0065-40
1000's	$248.72	LITHOBID, Solvay Pharms	00032-4492-10

Tablet, Coated, Sustained Action - Oral - 450 mg

100's	**$35.80**	**ESKALITH CR, SKB Pharms**	**00007-4010-20**

LITHIUM CITRATE *(001649)*

CATEGORIES: Antidepressants; Antimanic Agents; Antipsychotics/Antimanics; Bipolar Disorder; Central Nervous System Agents; Depression; Lithium Salts; Mania; Psychotherapeutic Agents; FDA Approval Pre 1982

BRAND NAMES: **Cibalith-S**

FORMULARIES: Aetna; Medi-Cal

COST OF THERAPY: $33.75 (Depression; Syrup; 300 mg/5ml; 15/day; 90 days) vs. Potential Cost of $2,456.15 (Depression)

PRIMARY ICD9: 311 (Depressive Disorder, Not Elsewhere Classified)

> **WARNING:**
> Lithium toxicity is closely related to serum lithium levels, and can occur at doses close to therapeutic levels. Facilities for prompt and accurate serum lithium determinations should be available before initiating therapy.

DESCRIPTION:

Lithium Citrate Syrup is an antimanic medication for oral administration. Lithium Carbonate is a film-coated, slow-release, 300-mg lithium carbonate tablet. This slowly dissolving, film-coated tablet is designed to give lower serum lithium peaks than obtained with conventional oral lithium dosage forms.

Lithium citrate syrup contains 8 mEq of lithium per 5 ml, equivalent to the amount in 300 mg of lithium carbonate.

Lithium citrate is prepared in solution from lithium hydroxide and citric acid in a ratio approximating dilithium citrate.

DESCRIPTION: *(cont'd)*

Cibalith-S: Citric acid, raspberry flavor, alcohol 0.3% v/v, purified water sodium benzoate, sodium saccharin, and sorbitol.

INDICATIONS AND USAGE:

Lithium is indicated in treatment of manic episodes of manic-depressive illness. Maintenance therapy prevents or diminishes the intensity of subsequent episodes in those manic-depressive patients with a history of mania.

Typical symptoms of mania include pressure of speech, motor hyperactivity, reduced need for sleep, flight of ideas, grandiosity, elation, poor judgement, aggressiveness, and possibly hostility. When given to a patient experiencing a manic episode, lithium may produce a normalization of symptomatology within 1 to 3 weeks.

WARNINGS:

Lithium should generally not be given to patients with significant renal or cardiovascular disease, severe debilitation or dehydration, or sodium depletion, and to patients receiving diuretics, since the risk of lithium toxicity is very high in such patients. If the psychiatric indication is life-threatening, and if such a patient fails to respond to other measures, lithium treatment may be undertaken with extreme caution, including daily serum lithium determinations and adjustment to the usually low doses ordinarily tolerated by these individuals. In such instances, hospitalization is a necessity.

Lithium toxicity is closely related to serum lithium levels, and can occur at doses close to therapeutic (see DOSAGE AND ADMINISTRATION.)

Lithium therapy has been reported in some cases to be associated with morphologic changes in the kidneys. The relationship between such changes and renal function has not been established.

Outpatients and their families should be warned that the patient must discontinue lithium therapy and contact his physician if such clinical signs of lithium toxicity as diarrhea, vomiting, tremor, mild ataxia, drowsiness, or muscular weakness occur.

Lithium may impair mental and/or physical abilities. Caution patients about activities requiring alertness (*e.g.,* operating vehicles or machinery).

Lithium may prolong or potentiate the effects of neuromuscular blocking agents, such as decamethonium, pancuronium, and succinylcholine. Therefore, neuromuscular blocking agents should be given with caution to patients receiving lithium.

Combined Use Of Haloperidol And Lithium: An encephalopathic syndrome (characterized by weakness; lethargy; fever; tremulousness and confusion; extrapyramidal symptoms; leukocytosis; elevated serum enzymes, BUN, and fasting blood sugar), followed by irreversible brain damage, has occurred in a few patients treated with lithium plus haloperidol. A causal relationship between these events and the concomitant administration of lithium and haloperidol has not been established. However, patients receiving such combined therapy should be monitored closely for early evidence of neurological toxicity, and treatment discontinued promptly if such signs appear. The possibility of similar adverse interactions with other antipsychotic medications exists. In addition, concurrent use of lithium with chlorpromazine and possibly other phenothiazines decreases serum chlorpromazine levels as much as 40%.

Usage in Pregnancy: Adverse effects on nidation in rats, embryo viability in mice, and metabolism in vitro of rat testis and human spermatozoa have ben attributed to lithium, as have teratogenicity in submammalian species and cleft palates in mice.

They are lithium birth registries in the United States and elsewhere; however there are at the present time insufficient data to determine the effects of lithium on human fetuses. Therefore, at this point, lithium should not be used in pregnancy, especially the first trimester, unless in the opinion of the physician, the potential benefits outweigh the possible hazards.

Usages in Nursing Mothers: Lithium is excreted in human milk. Nursing should not be undertaken during lithium therapy except in rare and unusual circumstances where, in the view of the physician, the potential benefits to the mother outweigh possible hazards to the child.

Usage in Children: Since information regarding the safety and effectiveness of lithium in children under 12 years of age is not available, its use in such patients is not recommended at this time (see OVERDOSAGE.)

PRECAUTIONS:

The ability to tolerate lithium is greater during the acute manic phase and decreases when manic symptoms subside (see DOSAGE AND ADMINISTRATION.)

The distribution space of lithium approximates that of total body water. Lithium is primarily excreted in urine with insignificant excretion in feces. Renal excretion of lithium is proportional to its plasma concentration. The half-elimination time of lithium is approximately 24 hours. Lithium decreases sodium reabsorption by the renal tubules which could lead to sodium depletion. Therefore, it is essential for the patient to maintain a normal diet, including salt, and an adequate fluid intake (2500-3000 ml) at least during the initial stabilization period. Decreased tolerance to lithium has been reported to ensure from protracted sweating or diarrhea and, if such occur, supplemental fluid and salt should be administered.

In addition to sweating and diarrhea, concomitant infection with elevated temperatures may also necessitate a temporary reduction or cessation of medication.

Previously existing underlying disorders do not necessarily constitute a contraindication to lithium treatment; where hypothyroidism exists, careful monitoring of thyroid function during lithium stabilization and maintenance allows for correction of changing thyroid parameters, if any, where hypothyroidism occurs during lithium stabilization and maintenance, supplemental thyroid treatment may be used.

DRUG INTERACTIONS:

Concomitant administration of carbamazepine and lithium may increase the risk of neurotoxic side effects.

Aminophylline, caffeine, dyphylline, oxtriphylline, sodium bicarbonate, or theophylline used concurrently may decrease the therapeutic effect of lithium because of its increased urinary excretion.

Concurrent use of diuretics, especially thiazides, with lithium may provoke lithium toxicity due to reduced renal clearance.

Concurrent extended use of iodide preparations, especially potassium iodide, with lithium may produce hypothyroidism.

Indomethacin and piroxicam have been reported to increase significantly steady state plasma lithium levels. In some cases, lithium toxicity has resulted from such interactions. There is also some evidence that other nonsteroidal, and-inflammatory agents may have a similar effect. When such combinations are used, increased monitoring of plasma lithium levels is recommended (see WARNINGS.)

There is evidence that angiotensin-converting enzyme inhibitors, such as enalapril and captopril, may substantially increase steady-state plasma lithium levels, sometimes resulting in lithium toxicity. When such combinations are used, lithium dosage may need to be decreased, and plasma lithium levels should be measured more often.

ADVERSE REACTIONS:

Adverse reactions are seldom encountered at serum lithium levels below 1.5 mEq/l, except in the occasional patient sensitive to lithium. Mild-to-moderate toxic reactions may occur at levels from 1.5-2.5 mEq/l, and moderate-to-severe reactions may be seen at levels from 2.0-2.5 mEq/l, depending upon individual response to the drug.

Fine hand tremor, polyuria and mild thirst may occur during initial therapy for the acute manic phase, and may persist throughout treatment. Transient and mild nausea and general discomfort may also appear during the first few days of lithium administration.

These side effects are an inconvenience rather than a disabling condition, and usually subside with continued treatment or a temporary reduction or cessation of dosage. If persistent, a cessation of dosage is indicated.

Diarrhea, vomiting, drowsiness, muscular weakness and lack of coordination may be early signs of lithium intoxication, and can occur at lithium levels below 2.0 Meq/l. At higher levels, giddiness, ataxia, blurred vision, tinnitus and a large output of dilute urine may seen. Serum lithium levels above 3.0 Meq/l may produce a complex clinical picture involving multiple organs and organ systems. Serum lithium levels should not be permitted to exceed 2.0 mEq/l during thr acute treatment phase.

The following toxic reactions have been reported and appear to be related to serum lithium levels, including levels within the therapeutic range.

Neuromuscular: tremor, muscle hyperirritability (fasciculations, twitching, clonic movements of whole limbs), ataxia, choreoathetotic movements, hyperactive deep tendon reflexes.

Central Nervous System: blackout spells, epileptiform seizures, downbeat nystagmus, acute dystonia, slurred speech, dizziness, vertigo, incontinence of urine or feces, somnolence, psychomotor retardation, restlessness, confusion, stupor, coma. Cases of pseudotumor cerebri (increased intracranial pressure and papilledema) have been reported with lithium use. If undetected, this condition may result in enlargement of the blind spot, constriction of visual fields, and eventual blindness due to optic atrophy. If this syndrome occurs, lithium should be discontinued if clinically possible.

Cardiovascular: cardiac arrhythmia, hypotension, peripheral circulatory collapse.

Gastrointestinal: anorexia, nausea, vomiting, diarrhea.

Genitourinary: albuminuria, oliguria, polyuria, glycosuria.

Dermatologic: drying and thinning of hair, anesthesia of skin, chronic folliculitis, xerosis cutis, alopecia, exacerbation of psoriasis.

Autonomic Nervous System: blurred vision, dry mouth.

Miscellaneous: fatigue, lethargy, tendency to sleep, dehydration, weight loss, transient scotomata.

Thyroid Abnormalities: euthyroid goiter and/or hypothyroidism (including myxedema) accompanied by lower T_3 and T_4. I_{131} iodine uptake may be elevated (see PRECAUTIONS.) Paradoxically, rare cases of hyperthyroidism have been reported.

EEG Changes: diffuse slowing, widening of frequency spectrum, potentiation and disorganization of background rhythm.

EKG Changes: reversible flattening, isoelectricity or inversion of T-waves.

Miscellaneous reactions unrelated to dosage are: transient electroencephalographic and electrocardiographic changes, leukocytosis, headache, diffuse nontoxic goiter with or without hypothyroidism, transient hyperglycemia, generalized pruritus with or without rash, cutaneous ulcers, albuminuria, worsening or organic brain syndromes, excessive weight gain, edematous swelling of ankles or wrists, metallic taste, and thirst or polyuria, sometimes resembling diabetes insipidus.

A single report has been received of the development of painful discoloration of fingers and toes and coldness of the extremities within one day of the starting of treatment of lithium. The mechanism through which these symptoms (resembling Raynaud's Syndrome) developed is not known. Recovery followed discontinuance.

OVERDOSAGE:

The toxic levels for lithium are close to the therapeutic levels. It is therefore important that patients and their families be cautioned to watch for early toxic symptoms and to discontinue the drug and inform the physician should they occur. There has been a report of a transient syndrome of acute dystonia and hyperreflexia occurring in a 15 kg child who ingested 300 mg of lithium carbonate. Toxic symptoms are listed in detail under ADVERSE REACTIONS.

Treatment: No specific antidote for lithium poisoning is known. Early symptoms of lithium toxicity can usually be treated by reduction or cessation of dosage of the drug and resumption of the treatment at a lower dose after 24 to 48 hours. In severe cases of lithium poisoning, the first and foremost goal of treatment consists of elimination of this ion from the patient.

Treatment is essentially the same as that used in barbiturate poisoning:1) gastric lavage 2) correction of fluid and electrolyte imbalance and 3) regulation of kidney functioning. Urea, mannitol, and aminophylline all produce significant increases in lithium excretion. Hemodialysis is an effective and rapid means of removing the ion from the severely toxic patient. Infection prophylaxis, regular chest X rays, and preservation of adequate respiration are essential.

DOSAGE AND ADMINISTRATION:

Acute Mania: Optimal patient response can usually be established and maintained with the following dosages: 10 ml (2 teaspoons) (16 mEq of lithium) t.i.d.

Such doses will normally produce an effective serum lithium level ranging between 1.0 and 1.5 mEq/l. Dosage must be individualized according to serum levels and clinical response. Regular monitoring of the patient's clinical state and of serum lithium levels is necessary. Serum levels should be determined twice per week during the acute phase, and until the serum level and clinical condition of the patient have been stabilized.

Long-Term Control: The desirable serum lithium levels are 0.6 to 1.2 mEq/l. Dosage will vary from one individual to another, but usually the following dosages will maintain this level: 5 ml (1 teaspoon) (8 mEq of lithium) t.i.d. or q.i.d.

Serum lithium levels in uncomplicated cases receiving maintenance therapy during remission should be monitored at least every two months. Patients abnormally sensitive to lithium may exhibit toxic signs at serum levels of 1.0 to 1.5 mEq/l. Elderly patients often respond to reduced dosage, and may exhibit signs of toxicity at serum levels ordinarily tolerated by other patients.

N.B.: Blood samples for serum lithium determinations should be drawn immediately prior to the next dose when lithium concentrations are relatively stable (*i.e.,* 8-12 hours after previous dose). Total reliance must not be placed on serum levels alone. Accurate patient evaluation requires both clinical and laboratory analysis.

Lithium Carbonate slow-release tablets must be swallowed whole and never crushed or chewed.

Store between 59 - 89° F (15 - 30° C). Protect from light.

Dispense in tight, light-resistant, child-resistant container (USP).

HOW SUPPLIED - RATED THERAPEUTICALLY EQUIVALENT:

Syrup - Oral - 300 mg/5ml

5 ml x 50	$34.00	Lithium Citrate, Raway	00686-0652-10
5 ml x 100	$61.33	Lithium Citrate, Xactdose	50962-0525-05
5 ml x 100	$66.26	Lithium Citrate, Roxane	00054-8529-04
10 ml x 50	$30.00	Lithium Citrate, Raway	00686-0653-10
10 ml x 100	$71.67	Lithium Citrate, Xactdose	50962-0525-10
10 ml x 100	$77.86	Lithium Citrate, Roxane	00054-8530-04
480 ml	$12.00	Lithium Citrate, Harber Pharm	51432-0739-20
480 ml	$13.44	Lithium Citrate, H.C.F.A. F F P	99999-1649-01
480 ml	$14.95	Lithium Citrate, Major Pharms	00904-2914-16
480 ml	$16.15	Lithium Citrate, Qualitest Pharms	00603-1410-58
480 ml	$16.20	Lithium Citrate, Goldline Labs	00182-6148-40
480 ml	$16.23	Lithium Citrate, Aligen Independ	00405-3223-16
480 ml	$16.25	Lithium Citrate, Geneva Pharms	00781-6100-16
480 ml	$16.35	Lithium Citrate, Schein Pharm (US)	00364-2140-16
480 ml	$19.29	Lithium Citrate, Morton Grove	60432-0616-16
500 ml	$14.00	Lithium Citrate, H.C.F.A. F F P	99999-1649-02
500 ml	$18.35	Lithium Citrate, Roxane	00054-3527-63

LIVER DERIVATIVE COMPLEX *(001653)*

CATEGORIES: Acne; Acne Vulgaris; Anti-Inflammatory Agents; Blood Formation/Coagulation; Chronic Fatigue Syndrome; Deficiency Anemias; Dermatitis; Eczema; Edema; Herpes; Herpes Zoster; Inflammation; Keloids; Pityriasis Rosea; Rosacea; Seborrhea; Skin/Mucous Membrane Agents; Sunburn; Urticaria; FDA Pre 1938 Drugs

BRAND NAMES: Kutapressin

DESCRIPTION:

Kutapressin Injection (liver derivative complex) is a sterile solution containing 25.5 mg liver derivative complex per ml in water for injection.

Kutapressin Injection is composed of peptides and amino acids. The product contains no protein, is virtually non-allergenic, and does not exhibit anti-anemia activity.

Kutapressin Injection also contains as inactive ingredients: phenol 0.5%, water for injection, pH is adjusted with hydrochloric acid or sodium hydroxide when necessary.

CLINICAL PHARMACOLOGY:

The specific action of Kutapressin is to enhance the resolution of inflammation and edema. In the late 1920s it was demonstrated that liver was of benefit to patients suffering from acne vulgaris.[1] As a consequence, various techniques were employed for isolating the active "factor" from liver. Studies published in the late 1930s and early 1940s[2,3,4] showed activity in a specially purified liver fraction. During subsequent years refinement as in the isolation of the active material led to the marketing of Kutapressin.

Initially it was thought that the primary action of Kutapressin was on the capillaries and precapillary sphincters. However, it is now believed that this effect is a secondary one and that the primary action of Kutapressin is in response to injury at the cellular level. The capillary changes observed following administration of Kutapressin appear to be part of a more fundamental anti-inflammatory effect. In the normal animal no consistent pharmacodynamic action has been demonstrated for Kutapressin. In particular there is no effect on the systemic blood pressure, no action on the autonomic nervous system and no alteration in prothrombin, coagulation or bleeding times. It is concluded that the specific action of the product is only apparent when tissues have been subjected to injury and when inflammation and edema are present.

INDICATIONS AND USAGE:

A wide variety of dermatological clinical conditions benefit from Kutapressin therapy. The common denominator in these varied conditions is the presence of inflammation and edema. Favorable response to administration of Kutapressin in patients with acne vulgaris,[5,6,7,8] herpes zoster, "poison ivy" dermatitis, pityriasis rosea, seborrheic dermatitis, urticaria and eczema[9,10,11] severe sunburn,[12] and rosacea[13] have been reported.

CONTRAINDICATIONS:

Contraindicated in patients with hypersensitivity or intolerance to liver or pork products.

WARNINGS:

Use with caution in patients suspected of being hypersensitive to liver or with other allergic diatheses.

PRECAUTIONS:

CARCINOGENESIS, MUTAGENESIS, AND IMPAIRMENT OF FERTILITY:

No long-term animal studies have examined the carcinogenic or mutagenic potential of Kutapressin. Kutapressin's effect upon reproductive capacity is similarly unknown.

PREGNANCY CATEGORY C:

Animal reproduction studies have not been conducted with Kutapressin. It is also not known whether Kutapressin can cause fetal harm when administered to a pregnant woman or can affect reproduction capacity. Kutapressin should be given to a pregnant woman only if clearly needed.

NURSING MOTHERS:

It is not known whether this drug is excreted in human milk. Because many drugs are excreted in human milk, caution should be exercised when Kutapressin is administered to a nursing woman.

DRUG INTERACTIONS:

No clinically significant drug interactions have been reported.

ADVERSE REACTIONS:

As with all injectable medications, local reactions may occur. Local reactions may include pain, swelling, and erythema.

DRUG ABUSE AND DEPENDENCE:

The information on drug abuse and dependence is limited to uncontrolled data derived from marketing experience. Such experience has revealed no evidence of drug abuse and dependence associated with Kutapressin injection.

DOSAGE AND ADMINISTRATION:

For the management of skin disorders the usual dose of Kutapressin is 2 ml administered daily or as indicated. The product is given by intramuscular or subcutaneous injection only.

DOSAGE AND ADMINISTRATION: *(cont'd)*

As with all parenteral drug products, Kutapressin should be inspected visually for particulate matter and discoloration prior to administration, whenever solution and container permit.

Store at controlled room temperature 15-30°C (59-86°F).

REFERENCES:

1. Sutton, R. L.: Liver Diets in Acne Vulgaris and in Furunculosis, Arch. Derm. & Syph., 18:887, 1928. See also Sutton, R. L., and Sutton, Jr., R. L.: Disease of the Skin, C. V. Mosby Co., St. Louis, 1939. **2.** Marshall, W.: Further Studies on the Therapy of Acne Vulgaris with Modified Liver Extract, J. Invest. Derm. 2:205, 1939. **3.** Lichtenstein, M. R. and Stillians, A. W.: Liver Extract in Treatment of Acne Vulgaris in Tuberculosis Patients, Arch. Derm. & Syph., 45:959, 1942. **4.** Boreen, C. A.: Boiled Liver in the Treatment of Acne Vulgaris, Minn. Med., 25:276, 1942. **5.** Nierman, M. M.: Treatment of Cystic Acne Vulgaris with a Cutaneous Vasoconstrictor (Kutapressin), The Jour. of Ind. State Med. Assn., 45:497, 1952. **6.** Knox, J. M.: Treatment of Cystic Acne with Kutapressin, U.S.N. News Letter, 20:9, 1952. **7.** Lubowe, I.: Modern Treatment of Acne Vulgaris, Clin. Med. 59: 8, 1952. **8.** Pensky, N. and Goldberg, N.: Treatment of Refractory Acne with a Fractionated Type of Liver Extract, N. Y. State Jour. of Med. 53:2238, Oct. 1953. **9.** Burks, J. W., Jr.: The Modern Treatment of Acne Vulgaris, Jour. La. State Med. Soc., 106:92, 1954. **10.** Burks, J. W. and Knox, J. M.: S-Factor of Liver Extract in Acne Vulgaris, A.M.A. Archives of Derm. & Syphil., 70:508, 1954. **11.** Barksdale, Edwin E.: The Use of S-Factor of Liver Extract (Kutapressin) in Dermatology, South. Med. Jour., 50:1524, 1957. **12.** Heywood, Howard W.: Use of Kutapressin in the Treatment of Severe Sunburn, Clin. Med. 3:8, 1956. **13.** Barrock, J. J.: Rosacea, Medical Times, 86:968, 1958.

HOW SUPPLIED - EQUIVALENTS NOT AVAILABLE:

Injection, Solution - Intramuscular; - 25.5 mg/ml

20 ml	$96.64	KUTAPRESSIN, Schwarz Pharma (US)	00091-1510-21

LIVER EXTRACT *(001654)*

CATEGORIES: Antianemia Drugs; Blood Formation/Coagulation; Deficiency Anemias; Homeostatic & Nutrient; Liver/Stomach Preparations; Vitamins; FDA Pre 1938 Drugs

FORMULARIES: Medi-Cal

Prescribing information not available at time of publication.

HOW SUPPLIED - EQUIVALENTS NOT AVAILABLE:

Injection, Solution - Intramuscular - 2 mcg/ml

10 ml	$0.78	Liver, Lannett	00527-0109-55
30 ml	$1.48	Liver, Lannett	00527-0109-58
30 ml	$16.95	LIVER, Merit Pharms	30727-0335-80

Injection, Solution - Intramuscular - 10 mcg/ml

10 ml	$0.96	Liver, Lannett	00527-0110-55
30 ml	$2.00	Liver, Lannett	00527-0110-58

Injection, Solution - Intramuscular - 20 mcg/ml

10 ml	$1.44	Liver Extract, Lannett	00527-0111-55
30 ml	$3.00	Liver Extract, Lannett	00527-0111-58

Injection, Solution - Intramuscular - 100 mcg/0.4 mg

10 ml	$6.40	Liver-Folic Acid-B12, Major Pharms	00904-0878-10

LODOXAMIDE TROMETHAMINE *(003184)*

CATEGORIES: Allergies; Anti-Inflammatory Agents; Broad Spectrum Penicillins; Conjunctivitis; EENT Drugs; Eye, Ear, Nose, & Throat Preparations; Keratitis; Keratoconjunctivitis; Lacrimation; Ophthalmics; Orphan Drugs; FDA Class 1S ("Standard Review"); FDA Approved 1993 Sep

BRAND NAMES: Alomide

FORMULARIES: Medi-Cal; PCS

DESCRIPTION:

Lodoxamide tromethamin is a sterile ophthalmic solution containing the mast cell stabilizer lodoxamide tromethamine for topical administration to the eyes. Lodoxamide tromethamine is a white, crystalline, water-soluble powder with a molecular weight of 553.91.

Chemical Name: N,N'-(2-chloro-5-cyano-m-phenylene)dioxamic acid tromethamine salt.

Empirical Formula: $C_{19}H_{26}O_{12}N_5Cl$

Each ml of Alomide Ophthalmic Solution contains: *Active* 1.78 mg lodoxamide tromethamine equivalent to 1 mg lodoxamide.*Preservative:* benzalkonium chloride 0.007%. *Inactive:* mannitol, hydroxypropyl methylcellulose 2910, sodium citrate, citric acid, edetate disodium, tyloxapol, hydrochloric acid and/or sodium hydroxide (adjust pH), and purified water. DM-00

CLINICAL PHARMACOLOGY:

Lodoxamide tromethamine is a mast cell stabilizer that inhibits the *in vivo* Type I immediate hypersensitivity reaction. Lodoxamide therapy inhibits the increases in cutaneous vascular permeability that are associated with reagin or IgE and antigen-mediated reactions.

In vitro studies have demonstrated the ability of lodoxamide to stabilize rodent mast cells and prevent antigen-stimulated release of histamine. In addition, lodoxamide prevents the release of other mast cell inflammatory mediators (*i.e.,* SRS-A, a slow-reacting substances of anaphylaxis, also known as the peptido-leukotrienes) and inhibits eosinophil chemotaxis. Although lodoxamide's precise mechanism of action is unknown, the drug has been reported to prevent calcium influx into mast cells upon antigen stimulation.

Lodoxamide has no intrinsic vasoconstrictor, antihistaminic, cyclooxygenase inhibition, or other anti-inflammatory activity.

The disposition of ^{14}C-lodoxamide was studied in six healthy adult volunteers receiving a 3 mg (50 mcCi) oral dose of lodoxamide. Urinary excretion was the major route of elimination. The elimination half-life of ^{14}C-lodoxamide was 8.5 hours in the urine. In a study conducted in twelve healthy adult volunteers, topical administration of Alomide 0.1% (Lodoxamide Tromethamine Ophthalmic Solutions), one drop in each eye four times per day for ten days, did not result in any measurable lodoxamide plasma levels at a detention limit of 2.5 ng/ml.

INDICATIONS AND USAGE:

Lodoxamide tromethamine is indicated in the treatment of the ocular disorders referred to by the terms vernal keratoconjunctivitis, vernal conjunctivitis, and vernal keratitis.

CONTRAINDICATIONS:

Hypersensitivity to any component of this product.

WARNINGS:

Not for injection. As with all ophthalmic preparations containing benzalkonium chloride, patients should be instructed not to wear soft contact lenses during treatment with Alomide Ophthalmic Solution.

PRECAUTIONS:

General: Patients may experience a transient burning or stinging upon instillation of Alomide Ophthalmic Solution. Should these symptoms persist, the patient should be advised to contact the prescribing physician.

Carcinogenesis, Mutagenesis, and Impairment of Fertility: A long-term study with lodoxamide tromethamine in rats (two-year oral administration) showed no neoplastic or tumorigenic effects at doses 100 mg/kg/day (more than 5000 times the proposed human clinical dose). No evidence of mutagenicity or genetic damage was seen in the Ames *Salmonella* Assay, Chromosomal Aberration in CHO Cells Assay, or Mouse Forward Lymphoma Assay. In the BALB/c-3T3 Cells Transformation Assay, some increase in the number of transformation foci was seen at high concentrations (greater than 4000 mcg/ml). No evidence of impairment of reproductive function was shown in laboratory animal studies.

Pregnancy Category B: Reproduction studies with lodoxamide tromethamine administered orally to rats and rabbits in doses of 100 mg/kg/day (more than 5000 times the proposed human clinical dose) produced no evidence of developmental toxicity. There are, however, no adequate and well-controlled studied in pregnant women. Because animal reproduction studies are not always predictive of human response, Alomide 0.1% (Lodoxamide Tromethamine Ophthalmic Solution) should be used during pregnancy only if clearly needed.

Nursing Mothers: It is not known whether lodoxamide tromethamine is excreted in human milk. Because many drugs are excreted in human milk, caution should be exercised when lodoxamide tromethamine is administered to nursing women.

Pediatric Use: Safety and effectiveness in children younger than 2 years of age have not been established.

ADVERSE REACTIONS:

During clinical studies of lodoxamide tromethamine, the most frequently reported ocular adverse experiences were transient burning, stinging, or discomfort upon instillation, which occurred in approximately 15% of the subjects. Other ocular events occurring in 1 to 5% of the subjects included ocular itching/pruritus, blurred vision, dry eye, tearing/discharge, hyperemia, crystalline deposits, and foreign body sensation. Events that occurred in less than 1% of the subjects included corneal erosion/ulcer, scales on lid/lash, eye pain, ocular edema/swelling, ocular warming sensation, ocular fatigue, chemosis, corneal abrasion, anterior chamber cells, keratopathy/keratitis, blepharitis, allergy, sticky sensation, and epitheliopathy.

Nonocular events reported were headache (1.5%) and (at less than 1%) heat sensation, dizziness, somnolence, nausea, stomach discomfort, sneezing, dry nose, and rash.

OVERDOSAGE:

There have been no reports of lodoxamide tromethamine ophthalmic solution overdosage following topical ocular application. Accidental overdose of an oral preparation of 120 to 180 mg of lodoxamide resulted in a temporary sensation of warmth, profuse sweating, diarrhea, light-headedness, and a feeling of stomach distension; no permanent adverse effects were observed. Side effects reported following systemic oral administration of 0.1 mg to 10.0 mg of lodoxamide include a feeling of warmth or flushing, headache, dizziness, fatigue, sweating, nausea, loose stools, and urinary frequency/urgency. The physician may consider emesis in the event of accidental ingestion.

DOSAGE AND ADMINISTRATION:

The dose for adults and children greater than two years of age is one to two drops in each affected eye four times daily for up to 3 months.

HOW SUPPLIED:

Alomide Ophthalmic Solution 0.1% is supplied as 10 ml in plastic ophthalmic DROP-TAINER dispenser.

Storage: Store at 15-27°C (59-80°F).

HOW SUPPLIED - EQUIVALENTS NOT AVAILABLE:

Solution - Ophthalmic - 0.1 %

10 ml $36.25 ALOMIDE, Alcon 00065-0345-10

LOMEFLOXACIN HYDROCHLORIDE *(003114)*

CATEGORIES: Anti-Infectives; Antibacterials; Antibiotics; Bronchitis; Chronic Bronchitis; Fluoroquinolones; Infections; Perioperative Prophylaxis; Quinolones; Respiratory Tract Infections; Transurethral Surgery; Urinary Tract Infections; Pregnancy Category C; FDA Class 1S ("Standard Review"); FDA Approved 1992 Feb

BRAND NAMES: *Logiflox (France)*; **Maxaquin**; *Ontop*
(International brand names outside U.S. in italics)

COST OF THERAPY: $44.87 (Urinary Infections; Tablet; 400 mg; 1/day; 7 days)

DESCRIPTION:

Lomefloxacin HCl is a synthetic broad-spectrum antimicrobial agent for oral administration. Lomefloxacin HCl, a difluoroquinolone, is the monohydrochloride salt of (±)-1-ethyl-6,8-difluoro-1,4-dihydro-7-(3-methyl-1-piperazinyl)-4-oxo-3-quinolinecarboxylic acid. its empirical formula is $C_{17}H_{19}F_2N_3O_3$·HCl,

Lomefloxacin HCl is a white to pale yellow powder with a molecular weight of 387.8. It is slightly soluble in water and practically insoluble in alcohol. Lomefloxacin HCl is stable to heat and moisture but is sensitive to light in dilute aqueous solution.

Maxaquin is available as a film-coated tablet formulation containing 400 mg of lomefloxacin base, present as the hydrochloride salt. The base content of the hydrochloride salt is 90.6%. The inactive ingredients are carboxymethylcellulose calcium, hydroxypropyl cellulose, hydroxypropyl methylcellulose, lactose, magnesium stearate, polyethylene glycol, polyoxyl 40 stearate, and titanium dioxide.

CLINICAL PHARMACOLOGY:

Pharmacokinetics in healthy volunteers: In 6 fasting healthy male volunteers, approximately 95% to 98% of a single oral dose of lomefloxacin was absorbed. Absorption was rapid following single doses of 200 and 400 mg (T_{max} 0.8 to 1.4 hours). Mean plasma concentration increased proportionally between 100 and 400 mg as shown below (TABLE 1):

TABLE 1

Dose (mg)	Mean Plasma*Concentration* (mcg/ml)	Area Under Curve*(AUC)* (mcg.h/ml)
100	0.8	5.6
200	1.4	10.9
400	3.2	26.1

CLINICAL PHARMACOLOGY: *(cont'd)*

In 6 healthy male volunteers administered 400 mg of lomefloxacin on an empty stomach q.d. for 7 days, the following means pharmacokinetic parameter values were obtained (TABLE 2):

TABLE 2

C_{max}	2.8 mcg/ml
C_{min}	0.27 mcg/ml
$AUC_{o\text{-}24\ h}$	25.9 mcg*h/ml
T_{max}	1.5 h
$t_{1/2}$	7.75 h

The elimination half-life in 8 subjects with normal renewal function was approximately 8 hours. At 24 hours post dose, subjects with normal renal function receiving single doses of 200 or 400 mg had mean plasma lomefloxacin concentrations of 0.10 and 0.24 mcg/ml, respectively. Steady-state concentrations were achieved within 48 hours of initiating therapy with once-a-day dosing. There was no drug accumulation with single daily dosing in patients with normal renal function.

Approximately 65% of an orally administered dose was excreted in the urine as unchanged drug in patients with normal renal function. Following a 400-mg dose of lomefloxacin administered q.d. for 7 days, the mean urine concentration was in excess of 300 mcg/ml 4 hours post dose. The mean urine concentration exceeded 35 mcg/ml for at least 24 hours after dosing.

Following a single 400-mg dose, lomefloxacin's solubility in urine usually exceeded its peak urinary concentration 2 to 6 fold. In this study, urine pH affected the solubility of lomefloxacin with solubilities ranging from 7.8 mg/ml at pH 5.2, to 2.4 mg/ml at pH 6.5, and 3.03 mg/ml at pH 8.12.

The urinary excretion of lomefloxacin was virtually complete within 72 hours after cessation of dosing, with approximately 65% of the dose being recovered as parent drug and 9% as its glucuronide metabolite. The mean renal clearance was 145 ml/min in subjects with normal renal function (GFR = 120 ml/min). This may indicate tubular secretion.

Food effect: When lomefloxacin and food were administered concomitantly, the rate of drug absorption was delayed (T_{max}increased to 2 hours (delayed by 41%)m C_{max} decreased by 18%), and the extent of absorption (AUC) was decreased by 12%.

Pharmacokinetics in the geriatric population: In 16 healthy elderly volunteers (61 to 76 years of age) with normal renal function for their age, lomefloxacin's half-life (mean of 8 hours) and peak plasma concentration (mean of 4.2 mcg/ml) following a single 400-mg dose were similar to those in 8 younger subjects dosed with a single 400-mg dose. Thus, drug absorption appears unaffected in the elderly. Plasma clearance was, however, reduced in this elderly population by approximately 25%, and the AUC was increased by approximately 33%. This slower elimination most likely reflects the decreased renal function normally observed in the geriatric population.

Pharmacokinetics in the renally impaired patients: In 8 patients with creatinine clearance (Cl_{cr}) between 10 and 40 ml/min/1.73 m^2, the mean AUC after a single 400-mg dose of lomefloxacin increased 335% over the AUC demonstrated in patients with a Cl_{cr}> 80 ml/min/1.73 m^2. Also, in these patients, the mean $t_{1/2}$increased to 21 hours. In 8 patients with Cl_{cr} < 10 ml/min/1.73 m^2, the mean AUC after a single 400-mg dose of lomefloxacin increased 700% over the AUC demonstrated in patients with a Cl_{cr} > 80 ml/min/1.73 m^2. In these patients with Cl_{cr} < 10 ml/min/1.73 m^2, the mean $t_{1/2}$ increased to 45 hours. The plasma clearance of lomefloxacin was closely correlated with creatinine clearance, ranging from 31 ml/min/1.73 m^2 when creatinine clearance was zero to 271 ml/min/1.73 m^{2}at a normal creatinine clearance of 110 ml/min/1.73 m^2. Peak lomefloxacin concentrations were not affected by the degree of renal function when single doses of lomefloxacin were administered. Adjustment of dosage schedules for patients with such decreases in renal function is warranted. (See DOSAGE AND ADMINISTRATION.)

Pharmacokinetics in patients with cirrhosis: In 12 patients with histologically confirmed cirrhosis, no significant changes in rate or extend of lomefloxacin exposure (C_{max}, T_{max}, $t_{1/2}$or AUC) were observed when they were administered 400 mg of lomefloxacin as a single dose. No date are available in cirrhotic patients treated with multiple doses of lomefloxacin. There does not appear to be a need for a dosage reduction in cirrhotic patients, provided adequate renal function is present.

Metabolism and pharmacodynamics of lomefloxacin: Lomefloxacin is minimally metabolized although 5 metabolites have been identified in human urine. The glucuronide metabolite is found in the highest concentration and accounts for approximately 9% of the administered dose. The other 4 metabolites together account for <0.5% of the dose.

Approximately 10% of an oral dose was recovered as unchanged drug in the feces.

Serum protein binding of lomefloxacin is approximately 10%.

The following are means tissue of fluid to plasma ratios of lomefloxacin following oral administration. Studies have not been conducted to assess the penetration of lomefloxacin into human cerebrospinal fluid (TABLE 3).

TABLE 3

Tissue or Body Fluid	Mean Tissue-or-Fluid-to-Plasma Ratio
Bronchial mucosa	2.1
Bronchial secretions	0.6
Prostatic tissue	2
Sputum	1.3
Urine	140.0

Microbiology: Lomefloxacin is a bactericidal agent with *in vitro* activity against a wide range of gram-negative and gram-positive organisms. The bactericidal action of lomefloxacin results from interference with the activity of the bacterial enzyme DNA gyrase. Which is needed for the transcription and replication of bacterial DNA. The minimum bactericidal concentration (MBC) generally does not exceed the minimum inhibitory concentration (MIC) by more than a factor of 2, except for staphylococci, which usually have MBC's 2 to 4 times the MIC.

Lomefloxacin has been shown to be active against most strains of the following organisms both *in vitro* and in clinical infections: (See INDICATIONS AND USAGE.)

GRAM-POSITIVE AEROBES

Staphylococcus saprophyticus

GRAM-NEGATIVE AEROBES

Citrobacter diversus
Enterobacter cloacae
Escherichia coli
Haemophilus influenzae
Klebsiella pneumoniae
Moraxella(Branhamella) catarrhalis
Proteus mirabilis
Pseudomonas aeruginosa (urinary tract only — see INDICATIONS AND USAGE and WARNINGS)

The following *in vitro* data are available: however, their clinical significance is unknown.

Lomefloxacin exhibits *in vitro* MIC's of 2 mcg/ml or less against most strains of the following organisms; however, the safety and effectiveness of lomefloxacin in treating clinical infections due to these organisms have not been established in adequate and well-controlled trials:

CLINICAL PHARMACOLOGY: *(cont'd)*

GRAM-POSITIVE AEROBES

Staphylococcus aureus (including methicillin-resistant strains)
Staphylococcus epidermidis (including methicillin-resistant strains)

GRAM-NEGATIVE AEROBES

Aeromonas hydrophila
Citrobacter freundii
Enterobacter aerogenes
Enterobacter agglomerans
Haemophilus parainfluenzae
Hafnia alvei
Klebsiella oxytoca
Klebsiella ozaenae
Morganella morganii
Proteus vulgaris
Providencia alcalifaciens
Providencia rettgeri
Serratia liquefaciens
Serratia marcescens

OTHER ORGANISMS

Legionella pneumophila

Beta-lactamase production should have no effect on the *in vitro* activity of lomefloxacin.

Most group A, B, D and G streptococci, *Streptococcus pneumoniae, Pseudomonas cepacia, Ureaplasma urealyticum, Mycoplasma hominis,* and anaerobic bacteria are resistant to lomefloxacin.

Lomefloxacin appears slightly less active *in vitro* when tested at acidic pH. An increase in inoculum size has little effect on the *in vitro* activity of lomefloxacin. *In vitro* resistance to lomefloxacin develops slowly (multiple-step mutation). Rapid one-step development of resistance occurs only rarely ($<10^{-9}$) *in vitro*.

Cross-resistance between lomefloxacin and other quinolone-class antimicrobial agents has been reported; however, cross-resistance between lomefloxacin and members of other classes of antimicrobial agents, such as aminoglycosides, penicillins, tetracyclines, cephalosporins, or sulfonamides has not yet been reported. Lomefloxacin is active *in vitro* against some strains of cephalosporin-and aminoglycoside-resistant gram-negative bacteria.

SUSCEPTIBILITY TESTING

Diffusion Techniques: Quantitative methods that require measurement of zone diameters give the most precise estimate of the susceptibility of bacteria to antimicrobial agents. One such standardized procedure[1] that has been recommended for use with disks to test the susceptibility of organisms to lomefloxacin uses the 10-mcg lomefloxacin disk. Interpretation involves correlation of the diameter obtained in the disk test with the MIC for lomefloxacin.

Reports from the laboratory giving results of the standard single disk susceptibility test with a 10-mcg lomefloxacin disk should be interpreted according to the following criteria (TABLE 4):

TABLE 4

Zone Diameter (mm)	Interpretation
≥22	Susceptible (S)
19-21	Intermediate (I)
≤18	Resistant (R)

A report of "Susceptible" indicates that the pathogen is likely to be inhibited by generally achievable drug concentrations. A report of "Intermediate" indicates that the result should be considered equivocal, and, if the organism is not fully susceptible to alternative clinically feasible drugs, the test should be repeated. This category provides a buffer zone that prevents small uncontrolled technical factors from causing major discrepancies in interpretation. A report of "Resistant" indicates that achievable drug concentrations are unlikely to be inhibitory, and other therapy should be selected.

Standardized susceptibility test procedures require the use of laboratory control organisms. The 10-mcg lomefloxacin disk should give the following zone diameters (TABLE 5):

TABLE 5

Organism	Zone Diameter(mm)
S.aureus (ATCC 25923)	23-29
E. coli (ATCC 25922)	27-33
P. aeruginosa (ATCC 27853)	22-28

Dilution Techniques: Use a standardized dilution method[2](broth, agar, or microdilution) or equivalent with lomefloxacin powder. The MIC values obtained should be interpreted according to the following criteria (TABLE 6):

TABLE 6

MIC (mcg/ml)	Interpretation
≤2	Susceptible (S)
4	Intermediate (I)
≥8	Resistant (R)

As with standard diffusion techniques, dilution methods require the use of laboratory control organisms. Standard lomefloxacin powder should provide the following MIC values (TABLE 7):

TABLE 7

Organism	MIC (mcg/ml)
S. aureus (ATCC 29213)	0.25-2.0
E. coli (ATCC 25922)	0.03-0.12
P. aeruginosa (ATCC 27853)	1.0 -4.0

INDICATIONS AND USAGE:

TREATMENT

Lomefloxacin HCl film-coated tablets are indicated for the treatment of adults with mild to moderate infections caused by susceptible strains of the designated microorganisms in the conditions listed below: (See DOSAGE AND ADMINISTRATION for specific dosing recommendations.)

INDICATIONS AND USAGE: *(cont'd)*

LOWER RESPIRATORY TRACT

Acute Bacterial Exacerbation of Chronic Bronchitis caused by*Haemophilus influenzae* or *Moraxella (Branhamella) catarrhalis**.

NOTE: LOMEFLOXACIN HCl IS NOT INDICATED FOR THE EMPIRIC TREATMENT OF ACUTE BACTERIAL EXACERBATION OF CHRONIC BRONCHITIS WHEN IT IS PROBABLE THAT *S. PNEUMONIAE* IS A CAUSATIVE PATHOGEN. *S. PNEUMONIAE* EXHIBITS *IN VITRO* RESISTANCE TO LOMEFLOXACIN, AND THE SAFETY AND EFFICACY OF LOMEFLOXACIN IN THE TREATMENT OF PATIENTS WITH ACUTE BACTERIAL EXACERBATION OF CHRONIC BRONCHITIS CAUSED BY *S. PNEUMONIAE* HAVE NOT BEEN DEMONSTRATED. IF LOMEFLOXACIN IS TO BE PRESCRIBED FOR GRAM-STAIN GUIDED EMPIRIC THERAPY OF ACUTE BACTERIAL EXACERBATION OF CHRONIC BRONCHITIS, IT SHOULD BE USED ONLY IF SPUTUM GRAM STAIN DEMONSTRATES AN ADEQUATE QUALITY OF SPECIMEN (>25 PMN/LPF) AND THERE IS BOTH A PREDOMINANCE OF GRAM NEGATIVE ORGANISMS AND NOT A PREDOMINANCE OF GRAM POSITIVE ORGANISMS.

URINARY TRACT

Uncomplicated Urinary Tract Infections (cystitis) caused by*Escherichia coli, Klebsiella pneumoniae, proteus mirabilis,* or *Staphylococcus saprophyticus.*

Complicated Urinary Tract Infections caused by *Escherichia coli, Klebsiella pneumoniae, proteus mirabilis, Pseudomonas aeruginosa, Citrobacter diversus**, or *Enterobacter cloacae**.

NOTE: In clinical trials of complicated urinary tract infections due to *P. aeruginosa*, 12 of 16 patients had the organism eradicated from the urine after therapy with lomefloxacin. No patients had concomitant bacteremia. Serum levels of lomefloxacin do not reliably exceed the MIC of *Pseudomonas* isolates. THE SAFETY AND EFFICACY OF LOMEFLOXACIN IN TREATING PATIENTS WITH *PSEUDOMONAS* BACTEREMIA HAS NOT BEEN ESTABLISHED.

*Although treatment of infections due to this organism in this organ system demonstrated a clinically acceptable overall outcome, efficacy was studied in fewer than 10 infections.

Appropriate culture and susceptibility tests should be performed before antimicrobial treatment in order to isolate and identify organisms causing infection and to determine their susceptibility to lomefloxacin. In patients with urinary tract infections, therapy with lomefloxacin HCl film coated tablets may be initiated before results of these tests are known; once these results become available, appropriate therapy should be continued. In patients with an acute bacterial exacerbation of chronic bronchitis, therapy should not be started empirically with lomefloxacin when there is a probability the causative pathogen is *S. pneumoniae.*

Beta-lactamase production should have no effect on lomefloxacin activity.

PROPHYLAXIS

Lomefloxacin HCl film-coated tablets are indicated perioperatively to reduce the incidence of UTIs in the early post-operative period (3-5 days post-surgery) in patients undergoing transurethral surgical procedures. Efficacy in decreasing the incidence of infections other than urinary tract infections in the early postoperative period has not been established. Lomefloxacin HCl, like all drugs for prophylaxis of transurethral surgical procedures, usually should not be used in minor urologic procedures for which prophylaxis is not indicated (*e.g.*, simple cystoscopy or retrograde pyelography).

CONTRAINDICATIONS:

Lomefloxacin is contraindicated in patients with a history of hypersensitivity to lomefloxacin or to any of the quinolone group of antimicrobial agents.

WARNINGS:

MODERATE TO SEVERE PHOTOTOXIC REACTIONS HAVE OCCURRED IN PATIENTS EXPOSED TO DIRECT OR INDIRECT SUNLIGHT OR TO ARTIFICIAL ULTRAVIOLET LIGHT (*e.g.,* sunlamps) DURING OR FOLLOWING TREATMENT WITH LOMEFLOXACIN. THESE REACTIONS HAVE ALSO OCCURRED IN PATIENTS EXPOSED TO SHADED OR DIFFUSED LIGHT, INCLUDING EXPOSURE THROUGH GLASS. PATIENTS SHOULD BE ADVISED TO DISCONTINUE LOMEFLOXACIN THERAPY AT THE FIRST SIGNS OR SYMPTOMS OF A PHOTOTOXICITY REACTION SUCH AS A SENSATION OF SKIN BURNING, REDNESS, SWELLING, BLISTERS, RASH, ITCHING, OR DERMATITIS.

These phototoxic reactions have occurred with and without the use of sunscreens or sunblocks. Single doses of lomefloxacin have been associated with these types of reactions. In a few cases, recovery was prolonged for several weeks. As with some other types of phototoxicity, there is the potential for exacerbation of the reaction on re-exposure to sunlight or artificial ultraviolet light prior to complete recovery from the reaction. In rare cases, reactions have recurred up to several weeks after stopping lomefloxacin therapy.

EXPOSURE TO DIRECT OR INDIRECT SUNLIGHT (EVEN WHEN USING SUNSCREENS OR SUNBLOCKS) SHOULD BE AVOIDED WHILE TAKING LOMEFLOXACIN AND FOR SEVERAL DAYS FOLLOWING THERAPY. LOMEFLOXACIN THERAPY SHOULD BE DISCONTINUED IMMEDIATELY AT THE FIRST SIGNS OR SYMPTOMS OF PHOTOTOXICITY.

THE SAFETY AND EFFICACY OF LOMEFLOXACIN IN CHILDREN, ADOLESCENTS (UNDER THE AGE OF 18 YEARS), PREGNANT WOMEN, AND LACTATING WOMEN HAVE NOT BEEN ESTABLISHED. (See PRECAUTIONS, Pregnancy, Nursing Mothers, and Pediatric Use.) The oral administration of multiple doses of lomefloxacin to juvenile dogs at 0.3 and to rats at 5.4 times the recommended adult human dose based on mg/m^2 (0.6 and 34 times the recommended adult human dose based on mg/kg, respectively) caused arthropathy and lameness. Histopathological examination of the weight-bearing joints of these animals revealed permanent lesions of the cartilage. Other quinolones also produce erosions of cartilage of weight-bearing joints and other sings of arthropathy in juvenile animals of various species. (See ANIMAL PHARMACOLOGY.)

The safety and efficacy of lomefloxacin in the treatment of acute bacterial exacerbation of chronic bronchitis due to *S. pneumoniae* have not been demonstrated. This product should not be used empirically in the treatment of acute bacterial exacerbation of chronic bronchitis when it is probable that *S. pneumoniae* is a causative pathogen.

In clinical trials of complicated UTIs due to *P. aeruginosa*, 12 of 16 patients had the organism eradicated from the urine after therapy with lomefloxacin. No patients had concomitant bacteremia. Serum levels of lomefloxacin do not reliably exceed the MIC of *Pseudomonas isolates.* THE SAFETY AND EFFICACY OF LOMEFLOXACIN IN TREATING PATIENTS WITH *PSEUDOMONAS* BACTEREMIA HAS NOT BEEN ESTABLISHED.

Serious and occasionally fatal hypersensitivity (anaphylactoid or anaphylactic) reactions, some following the first dose, have been reported in patients receiving quinolone therapy. Some reactions were accompanied by cardiovascular collapse, loss of consciousness, tingling, pharyngeal or facial edema, dyspnea, urticaria, or itching. Only a few of these patients had a history of previous hypersensitivity reactions. Serious hypersensitivity reactions have also been reported following treatment with lomefloxacin. If an allergic reaction to lomefloxacin occurs, discontinue the drug. Serious acute hypersensitivity reactions may require immediate

WARNINGS: *(cont'd)*

emergency treatment with epinephrine. Oxygen, intravenous fluids, antihistamines, corticosteroids, pressor amines, and airway management, including intubation, should be administered as indicated.

Convulsions have been reported in patients receiving lomefloxacin. Whether the convulsions were directly related to lomefloxacin administration has not yet been established. However, convulsions, increased intracranial pressure, and toxic psychoses have been reported in patients receiving other quinolones. Quinolones may also cause central nervous system stimulation, which may lead to tremors, restlessness, lightheadedness, confusion, and hallucinations. If any of these reactions occurs in patients receiving lomefloxacin, the drug should be discontinued and appropriate measures instituted. No evidence of an effect of lomefloxacin on the electrical activity of the brain has been demonstrated. Lomefloxacin does not after cerebral blood flow or cerebral glucose uptake in the central nervous system based on positron emission tomography. However, until more information becomes available, lomefloxacin, like all other quinolones, should be used with caution in patients with known or suspected central nervous system disorders, such as severe cerebral arteriosclerosis, epilepsy, or other factors that predispose to seizures. (See ADVERSE REACTIONS.)

Pseudomembranous colitis has been reported with nearly all antibacterial agents, including quinolones, and may range from mild to life-threatening in severity. Therefore, it is important to consider this diagnosis in patients who present with diarrhea subsequent to the administration of antibacterial agents. Treatment with broad-spectrum antibiotics alters the normal flora of the colon and may permit overgrowth of clostridia. Studies indicate that a toxin produced by*Clostridium difficile* is a primary cause of "antibiotic associated colitis." After the diagnosis of pseudomembranous colitis has been established, therapeutic measures should be initiated. Mild cases of pseudomembranous colitis usually respond to discontinuation of drug alone. In moderate to severe cases, consideration should be given to management with fluid and electrolytes, protein supplementation, and treatment with an antibacterial drug clinically effective against *C. difficile* colitis.

PRECAUTIONS:

GENERAL

Alteration ot the dosage regimen is recommended for patients with impairment of renal function (Cl_{cr} < 40 ml/min/1.73 m^2). (See DOSAGE AND ADMINISTRATION.)

Moderate to severe phototoxicity reactions have been observed in patients exposed to excessive sunlight or artificial ultraviolet light while receiving lomefloxacin or some other quinolones. Excessive sunlight and artificial ultraviolet light should be avoided while taking lomefloxacin. Lomefloxacin therapy should be discontinued if phototoxicity occurs.

INFORMATION FOR THE PATIENT

Patients should be advised

to drink fluids liberally,

that lomefloxacin can be taken without regard to meals,

that mineral supplements or vitamins with iron or minerals should not be taken within the 2-hour period before or after taking lomefloxacin (see DRUG INTERACTIONS),

that sucralfate or antacids containing magnesium or aluminum should not be taken within 4 hours before or 2 hours after taking lomefloxacin (see DRUG INTERACTIONS),

that lomefloxacin can cause dizziness and lightheadedness and therefore, patients should know how they react to lomefloxacin before they operate an automobile or machinery or engage in activities requiring mental alertness and coordination,

that lomefloxacin may be associated with hypersensitivity reactions, even following the first dose, and to discontinue the drug at the first sign of a skin rash or other allergic reaction, and

to avoid excessive sunlight and artificial ultraviolet light while receiving lomefloxacin and to discontinue therapy if phototoxicity occurs.

CARCINOGENESIS, MUTAGENESIS, AND IMPAIRMENT OF FERTILITY

Carcinogenesis: Hairless (Skh-1) mice were exposed to UVA light for 3.5 hours five times every two weeks for up to 52 weeks while concurrently being administered lomefloxacin. The lomefloxacin doses used in this study caused a phototoxic response. In mice treated with both UVA and lomefloxacin concomitantly, the time to development of skin tumors was 16 weeks. In mice treated concomitantly in this model with both UVA and other quinolones, the times to development of skin tumors ranged from 28 to 52 weeks.

Ninety-two percent (92%) of the mice treated concomitantly with both UVA and lomefloxacin developed well-differentiated squamous cell carcinomas of the skin. These squamous cell carcinomas of the skin. These squamous cell carcinomas were nonmetastatic and endophytic in character. Two- thirds of these squamous cell carcinomas contained large central keratinous inclusion masses and were thought to arise from the vestigial hair follicles in these hairless animals.

In this model, mice treated with lomefloxacin alone did not develop skin or systemic tumors.

There are no data from similar models using pigmented mice and/or fully haired mice.

The clinical significance of these findings to humans is unknown.

Mutagenesis: One *in vitro* mutagenicity test (CHO/HGPRT assay) was weakly positive at lomefloxacin concentrations of 226 mcg/ml and greater and negative at concentrations less than 226 mcg/ml. Two other *in vitro*mutagenicity tests (chromosomal aberrations in Chinese hamster ovary cells, chromosomal aberrations in human lymphocytes) and two *in vivo* mouse micronucleus mutagenicity tests were all negative.

Impairment of Fertility: Lomefloxacin did not affect the fertility of male and female rats at oral doses up to 8 times the recommended human dose based on mg/m^2(34 times the recommended human dose based on mg/kg).

PREGNANCY, TERATOGENIC EFFECTS, PREGNANCY CATEGORY C

Reproductive function studies have been performed in rats at doses up to 8 times the recommended human dose based on mg/m^2(34 times the recommended human dose based on mg/kg), and no impaired fertility or harm to the fetus was reported due to lomefloxacin. Increased incidence of fetal loss in monkeys has been observed at approximately 3 to 6 times the recommended human dose based on mg/m^2 (6 to 12 times the recommended human dose based on mg/kg). No teratogenicity has been observed in rats and monkeys at up to 16 times the recommended human dose exposure. In the rabbit, maternal toxicity and associated fetotoxicity, decreased placental weight, and variations of the coccygeal vertebrae occurred at doses 2 times the recommended human exposure based on mg/m^2. There are, however, no adequate and well-controlled studies in pregnant women. Lomefloxacin should be used during pregnancy only if the potential benefit justifies the potential risk to the fetus.

NURSING MOTHERS

It is not known whether lomefloxacin is excreted in human milk. However, it is known that other drugs of this class are excreted in human milk and that lomefloxacin is excreted in the milk of lactating rats. Because of the potential for serious adverse reactions from lomefloxacin in nursing infants, a decision should be made whether to discontinue nursing or to discontinue the drug, taking into account the importance of the drug to the mother.

PRECAUTIONS: *(cont'd)*

PEDIATRIC USE

The safety and effectiveness of lomefloxacin in children and adolescents below the age of 18 years have not been established. Lomefloxacin causes arthropathy in juvenile animals of several species. (See WARNINGSand ANIMAL PHARMACOLOGY.)

GERIATRIC USE

Of the total number of patients in clinical studies of lomefloxacin, 26% were ≥65 years of age. No overall differences in effectiveness or safety were observed between these patients and younger patients. (See CLINICAL PHARMACOLOGY, Pharmacokinetics in the Geriatric Population.)

DRUG INTERACTIONS:

Theophylline: In 3 pharmacokinetic studies including 46 normal, healthy subjects, theophylline clearance and concentration were not significantly altered by the addition of lomefloxacin. In clinical studies where patients were on chronic theophylline therapy, lomefloxacin had no measurable effect on the mean distribution of theophylline concentrations or the mean estimates of theophylline clearance. Though individual theophylline levels fluctuated, there were no clinically significant symptoms of drug interaction.

Antacids and sucralfate: Sucralfate and antacids containing magnesium or aluminum form chelation complexes with lomefloxacin and interfere with its bioavailability. Sucralfate administered 2 hours before lomefloxacin resulted in a slower rate of absorption (mean C_{max} decreased by 30% and mean T_{max}increased by 1 hour) and a lesser extent of absorption (mean AUC decreased by approximately 25%). Magnesium and aluminum-containing antacids, administered concomitantly with lomefloxacin, significantly decreased the bioavailability (48%) of lomefloxacin. Separating the doses of antacid and lomefloxacin minimizes this decrease in bioavailability: therefore, administration of these agents should precede lomefloxacin dosing by 4 hours or follow lomefloxacin dosing by at least 2 hours.

Caffeine: One hundred mg of caffeine (equivalent to 1 to 3 cups of American coffee) was administered to 16 normal, healthy volunteers who had achieved steady-state blood concentrations of lomefloxacin after being dosed at 400 mg q.d. This did not result in any statistically or clinically relevant changes in the pharmacokinetic parameters of either caffeine or lomefloxacin. No data are available on potential interactions in individuals who consume greater than 100 mg of caffeine per day or in those, such as the geriatric population, who are generally believed to be more susceptible to the development of drug-induced central nervous system-related adverse effects. Other quinolones have demonstrated moderate to marked interference with metabolism of caffeine, resulting in a reduced clearance, a prolongation of plasma half-life, and an increase in symptoms that accompany high levels of caffeine.

Cimetidine: Cimetidine has been demonstrated to interfere with the elimination of other quinolones. This interference has resulted in significant increases in half-life and AUC. Interaction between lomefloxacin and cimetidine has not been studied.

Cyclosporine: Elevated serum levels of cyclosporine have been reported with concomitant use of cyclosporine with other members of the quinolone class. Interaction between lomefloxacin and cyclosporine has not been studied.

Non-steroidal anti-inflammatory drugs (NSAID's): Concomitant administration of the NSAID fenbufen with some quinolones has been reported to increase the risk of CNS stimulation and convulsive seizures.

There was an increase in the incidence of seizures in mice treated with fenbufen, when fenbufen was administered to mice that had been concomitantly treated with a dose of lomefloxacin equivalent to the recommended human dose on a mg/m^2 basis (10 times the recommended human dose on a mg/kg basis). Fenbufen is not presently an approved drug in the United States. (See ANIMAL PHARMACOLOGY.)

Probenecid: Probenecid slows the renal elimination of lomefloxacin. An increase of 63% in the mean AUC and increases of 50% and 4%, respectively, in the mean $T_{max}$and mean C_{max} were noted in 1 study of 6 individuals.

Warfarin: Quinolones may enhance the effects of the oral anticoagulant, warfarin, or its derivatives. When these products are administered concomitantly, prothrombin or other suitable coagulation test should be monitored closely.

ADVERSE REACTIONS:

In clinical trials, most of the adverse events reported were mild to moderate in severity and transient in nature. During these clinical investigations, 2869 patients received lomefloxacin HCl. In 2.6% of the patients, lomefloxacin was discontinued because of adverse events, primarily involving the gastrointestinal system (0.7%), skin (1.0%), or CNS (0.5%).

ADVERSE CLINICAL EVENTS

The events with the highest incidence (≥1%) in patients, regardless of relationship to drug, were nausea (3.7%), headache (3.2%) photosensitivity (2.4%) (see WARNINGS), dizziness (2.3%), and diarrhea (1.4%).

Additional clinical events reported in less than 1% of patients treated with lomefloxacin HCl, regardless of relationship to drug, are listed below:

Autonomic: dry mouth, flushing, increased sweating.

Body as a Whole: fatigue, back pain, malaise, asthenia, chest pain, chills, allergic reaction, face edema, influenza-like symptoms, decreased heat tolerance.

Cardiovascular: hypotension, hypertension, edema, syncope, tachycardia, bradycardia, arrhythmia, extrasystoles, cyanosis, cardiac failure, angina pectoris, myocardial infarction, pulmonary embolism, cerebrovascular disorder, cardiomyopathy, phlebitis.

Central nervous system: Convulsions, coma, hyperkinesia, tremor, vertigo, paresthesias.

Gastrointestinal: abdominal pain, dyspepsia, vomiting, flatulence, constipation, gastrointestinal inflammation, dysphagia, gastrointestinal bleeding, tongue discoloration.

Hearing: earache, tinnitus.

Hematologic: thrombocytopenia, thrombocythemia, purpura, lymphadenopathy, increased fibrinolysis.

Metabolic: thirst, gout, hypoglycemia.

Musculoskeletal: leg cramps, arthralgia, myalgia.

Ophthalmologic: abnormal vision, conjunctivitis, eye pain.

Psychiatric: somnolence, insomnia, nervousness, anorexia, confusion, anxiety, depression, agitation, increased appetite, depersonalization, paroniria.

Reproductive System: Female: vaginitis, leukorrhea, intermenstrual bleeding, perineal pain, vaginal moniliasis, Male: orchitis, epididymitis.

Respiratory: dyspnea, respiratory infection, epistaxis, respiratory disorder, bronchospasm, cough, increased sputum, stridor.

Skin/Allergic: pruritus, rash, urticaria, eczema, skin exfoliation, skin disorder.

Special Senses: taste perversion.

Urinary: dysuria, hematuria, strangury, micturition disorder, anuria.

ADVERSE LABORATORY EVENTS

Changes in laboratory parameters, listed as adverse events, without regard to drug relationship include:

ADVERSE REACTIONS: *(cont'd)*

Hepatic: elevations of ALT (SGPT)(0.4%), AST (SGOT) (0.3%), bilirubin (0.1%), alkaline phosphatase (0.1%).

Hematologic: monocytosis (0.3%), evaluated ESR (0.1%).

Renal: elevated BUN (0.1%), decreased potassium (0.1%).

Additional laboratory changed occurring in ≤0.1% in the clinical studies included: elevation of serum gamma glutamyl transferase, decrease in total protein or albumin, prolongation of prothrombin time, anemia, decrease in hemoglobin, leukopenia, eosinophilia, thrombocytopenia, abnormalities of urine specific gravity of serum electrolytes, decrease in blood glucose.

QUINOLONE-CLASS ADVERSE EVENTS

Although not reported in completed clinical studies with lomefloxacin HCl, a variety of adverse events have been reported with other quinolones.

Clinical adverse events include: anaphylactoid reactions, erythema nodosum, Stevens-Johnson syndrome, exfoliative dermatitis, toxic epidermal necrolysis, hepatic necrosis, possible exacerbation of myasthenia gravis, dysphasia, nystagmus, pseudomembranous colitis, painful oral mucosa, intestinal perforation, hallucinations, manic reaction, ataxia, phobia, hyperpigmentation, diplopia, interstitial nephritis, renal failure, renal calculi, polyuria, urinary retention, acidosis, cardiopulmonary arrest, cerebral thrombosis, laryngeal or pulmonary edema, hiccough, dysgeusia, and photophobia.

Laboratory adverse events include: agranulocytosis, elevation of serum triglycerides, elevation of serum cholesterol, elevation of blood glucose, elevation of serum potassium, albuminuria, candiduria, and crystalluria.

OVERDOSAGE:

Information on overdosage in humans is limited. In the event of acute overdosage, the stomach should be emptied by inducing vomiting or by gastric lavage, and the patient should be carefully observed and given supportive treatment. Adequate hydration must be maintained. Hemodialysis or peritoneal dialysis is unlikely to aid in the removal of lomefloxacin as less than 3% is removed by these modalities.

Clinical signs of acute toxicity in rodents progressed from salivation to tremors, decreased activity, dyspnea, and clonic convulsions prior to death. These signs were noted in rats and mice as lomefloxacin doses were increased.

DOSAGE AND ADMINISTRATION:

Lomefloxacin HCl may be taken without regard to meals. (See CLINICAL PHARMACOLOGY.)

See INDICATIONS AND USAGE for information on appropriate pathogens and patient populations.

TREATMENT

Patients with Normal Renal Function: The recommended daily dose of lomefloxacin HCl is described in TABLE 8.

TABLE 8

Body System	Infection	Unit Dose	Frequency	Daily Duration	Dose
Lower respiratory tract	Acute bacterial exacerbation of chronic bronchitis	400 mg	q.d	10 days	400 mg
Urinary tract	Cystitis	400 mg	q.d.	10 days	400 mg
	Complicated Urinary Tract Infections	400 mg	q.d.	14 days	400 mg

Elderly Patients: No dosage adjustment is needed for elderly patients with normal renal function ($Cl_{cr} \geq 40$ ml/min/1.73 m_2).

Patients with impaired renal function: Lomefloxacin is primarily eliminated by renal excretion. (See CLINICAL PHARMACOLOGY.) Modification of dosage is recommended in patients with renal dysfunction. In patients with a creatinine clearance greater than 10 but less than 40 ml/min/1.73 m^2, the recommended dosage is an initial loading dose of 400 mg followed by daily maintenance doses of 200 mg (1/2 tablet) once daily for the duration of treatment. It is suggested that serial determinations of lomefloxacin levels be performed to determine any necessary alteration in the appropriate next dosing interval.

If only the serum creatinine is known, the following formula may be used to estimate creatinine clearance (TABLE 9).

TABLE 9

Men: [(weight in kg) × (140 - age)] ÷ [72 × serum creatinine (mg/dl)]
Women: 0.85 × (calculated value for men)

Dialysis patients: Hemodialysis removes only a negligible amount of lomefloxacin (3% in 4 hours). Hemodialysis patients should receive an initial loading dose of 400 mg followed by daily maintenance doses of 200 mg (1/2 tablet) once daily for the duration of treatment.

Patients with Cirrhosis: Cirrhosis does not reduce the non-renal clearance of lomefloxacin. The need for a dosage reduction in this population should be based on the degree of renal function of the patient and on the plasma concentration. (See CLINICAL PHARMACOLOGY and DOSAGE AND ADMINISTRATION, Patients with impaired renal function.)

PROPHYLAXIS

A single dose of 400 mg of lomefloxacin HCl should be administered orally 2 to 6 hours prior to surgery when oral pre-operative prophylaxis for transurethral surgical procedures is considered appropriate.

ANIMAL PHARMACOLOGY:

Lomefloxacin and other quinolones have been shown to cause arthropathy in juvenile animals. Arthropathy, involving multiple diarthrodial joints, was observed in juvenile dogs administered lomefloxacin at doses as low as 4.5 mg/kg for 7 to 8 days (0.3 times the recommended human dose based on mg/kg). In juvenile rats, no changes were observed in the joints with doses up to 91 mg/kg for 7 days (2 times the recommended human dose based on mg/m^2 or 11 times the recommended human dose based on mg/kg). (See WARNINGS.)

In a 13-week oral rat study, gamma globulin decreased when lomefloxacin was administered at less than the recommended human exposure. Beta globulin decreased when lomefloxacin was administered at 0.6 to 2 times the recommended human dose based on mg/m^2. The A/G ration increased when lomefloxacin was administered at 6 to 20 times the human dose. Following a 4-week recovery period, beta globulins in the females and A/G ratios in the female s returned to control values. Gamma globulin values in the females and beta and gamma globulins and A/G ratios in the males were still statistically significantly different from control values. No effects on globulins were seen in oral studies in dogs or monkeys in the limited number of specimens collected.

ANIMAL PHARMACOLOGY: *(cont'd)*

Twenty-seven NSAID's, administered concomitantly with lomefloxacin, were tested for seizure induction in mice at approximately 2 times the recommended human dose based on mg/m^2. At a dose of lomefloxacin equivalent to the recommended human exposure based on mg/m^2 (10 times the human dose based on mg/kg), only fenbufen, when so-administered, produced an increase in seizures.

Crystalluria and ocular toxicity, seen with some related quinolones, were not observed in any lomefloxacin-treated animals, either in studies designed to look for these effects specifically or in subchronic and chronic toxicity studies in rats, dogs, and monkeys.

long-term, high-dose systemic use of other quinolones in experimental animals has caused lenticular opacities; however, this finding was not observed with lomefloxacin.

HOW SUPPLIED:

Maxaquin is supplied as a scored, film-coated tablet containing the equivalent of 400 mg of lomefloxacin base present as the hydrochloride. The tablet is oval, white, and film-coated with "MAXAQUIN 400" debossed on one side and scored on the other side.

Store at 59 to 86°F (15 to 30°C).

REFERENCES:

1. National Committee for Clinical Laboratory Standards,*Performance Standards for Antimicrobial Disk Susceptibility Tests*—Fourth Edition. Approved Standard NCCLS Document M2-A4, Vol. 10, No. 7, NCCLS, Villanova, PA, 1990. **2.** National Committee for Clinical Laboratory Standards, *Methods for Dilution Antimicrobial Susceptibility Tests for Bacteria that Grow Aerobically*—Second Edition. Approved Standard NCCLS Document M7-A2, Vol. 10, No. 8, NCCLS, Villanova, PA, 1990.

HOW SUPPLIED - EQUIVALENTS NOT AVAILABLE:

Tablet, Uncoated - Oral - 400 mg

20's	$122.13	MAXAQUIN, Searle	00025-1651-20
100's	$641.13	MAXAQUIN, Searle	00025-1651-34

LOMUSTINE *(001660)*

CATEGORIES: Antineoplastics; Brain Carcinoma; Cancer; Chemotherapy; Cytotoxic Agents; Hodgkin's Disease; Oncologic Drugs; Tumors; Pregnancy Category D; FDA Approval Pre 1982

BRAND NAMES: *Belustine* (France); *CCNU* (England); *Cecenu* (Germany); **CeeNU**; *CEENU* (Mexico); *CiNU*; *Lomeblastin* (Germany); *Lomustine*; *Lucostin*; *Lucostine*; *Lumustine*; *Lundbeck* (England)
(International brand names outside U.S. in italics)

FORMULARIES: Aetna; BC-BS; Medi-Cal

CeeNU (lomustine [CCNU] Capsules) should be administered under the supervision of a qualified physician experienced in the use of cancer chemotherapeutic agents.

Bone marrow suppression, notably thrombocytopenia and leukopenia, which may contribute to bleeding and overwhelming infections in an already compromised patient, is the most common and severe of the toxic effects of CeeNU (see WARNINGS and ADVERSE REACTIONS).

Since the major toxicity is delayed bone marrow suppression, blood counts should be monitored weekly for at least 6 weeks after a dose (see ADVERSE REACTIONS.) At the recommended dosage, courses of CeeNU should not be given more frequently than every 6 weeks.

The bone marrow toxicity of CeeNU is cumulative and therefore dosage adjustment must be considered on the basis of nadir blood counts from prior dose (see TABLE 1).

DESCRIPTION:

CeeNU (lomustine [CCNU]) Capsules is one of the nitrosoureas used in the treatment of certain neoplastic diseases. It is 1-(2-chloroethyl)-3-cyclohexyl-1-nitrosourea. It is a yellow powder with the empirical formula of $C_9H_{16}ClN_3O_2$ and a molecular weight of 233.71

CeeNU is soluble in 10% ethanol (0.05 mg per ml) and in absolute alcohol (70 mg per ml). CeeNU is relatively insoluble in water (<0.05 mg per ml).

It is relatively unionized at a physiological pH.

Inactive ingredients in CeeNU capsules are: magnesium stearate and mannitol.

CeeNU is available in 10 mg, 40 mg, and 100 mg capsules for oral administration.

CLINICAL PHARMACOLOGY:

Although it is generally agreed that CeeNU alkylates DNA and RNA, it is not cross resistant with other alkylators. As with other nitrosoureas, it may also inhibit several key enzymatic processes by carbamoylation of amino acids in proteins.

CeeNU may be given orally. Following oral administration of radioactive CeeNU at doses ranging from 30 mg/m^2 to 100 mg/m^2 about half of the radioactivity given was excreted within 24 hours.

The serum half-life of the drug and or metabolites ranges from 16 hours to 2 days. Tissue levels are comparable to plasma levels at 15 minutes after intravenous administration.

Because of the high lipid solubility and the relative lack of ionization at a physiological pH, CeeNU crosses the blood brain barrier quite effectively. Levels of radioactivity in the CSF are 50% or greater than those measured concurrently in plasma.

INDICATIONS AND USAGE:

CeeNU has been shown to be useful as a single agent in addition to other modalities, or in established combination therapy with other approved chemotherapeutic agents in the following.

Brain tumors: both primary and metastatic, in patients who have already received appropriate surgical and/or radiotherapeutic procedures;

Hodgkin's Disease: secondary therapy in combination with other approved drugs in patients who relapse while being treated with primary therapy, or who fail to respond to primary therapy.

CONTRAINDICATIONS:

CeeNU should not be given to individuals who have demonstrated a previous hypersensitivity to it.

WARNINGS:

Since the major toxicity is delayed bone marrow suppression, blood counts should be monitored weekly for at least 6 weeks after a dose (see ADVERSE REACTIONS.) At the recommended dosage, courses of CeeNU should not be given more frequently than every 6 weeks.

The bone marrow toxicity of CeeNU is cumulative and therefore dosage adjustment must be considered on the basis of nadir blood counts from prior dose (see TABLE 1).

WARNINGS: *(cont'd)*

Pulmonary toxicity from CeeNU appears to be dose related (see ADVERSE REACTIONS.)

Long term use of nitrosoureas has been reported to be possibly associated with the development of secondary malignancies.

Liver and renal function tests should be monitored periodically (see ADVERSE REACTIONS.)

Pregnancy Category D: CeeNU can cause fetal harm when administered to a pregnant woman. CeeNU is embryotoxic and teratogenic in rats and embryotoxic in rabbits at dose levels equivalent to the human dose. There are no adequate and well controlled studies in pregnant women. If this drug is used during pregnancy, or if the patient becomes pregnant while taking (receiving) this drug, the patient should be apprised of the potential hazard to the fetus. Women of childbearing potential should be advised to avoid becoming pregnant.

PRECAUTIONS:

General: In all instances where the use of CeeNU is considered for chemotherapy, the physician must evaluate the need and usefulness of the drug against the risks of toxic effects or adverse reactions. Most such adverse reactions are reversible if detected early. When such effects or reactions do occur, the drug should be reduced in dosage or discontinued and appropriate corrective measures should be taken according to the clinical judgement of the physician. Re institution of CeeNU therapy should be carried out with caution and with adequate consideration of the further need for the drug and alertness as to possible recurrence of toxicity.

Laboratory Tests: Due to delayed bone marrow suppression, blood counts should be monitored weekly for at least 6 weeks after a dose.

Baseline pulmonary function studies should be conducted along with frequent pulmonary function tests during treatment. Patients with a baseline below 70% of the predicted Forced Vital Capacity (FVC) or Carbon Monoxide Diffusing Capacity (DL_{co}) are particularly at risk.

Since CeeNU (lomustine [CCNU]) Capsules may cause liver dysfunction, it is recommended that liver function tests be monitored periodically.

Carcinogenesis, Mutagenesis, and Impairment of Fertility: CeeNU is carcinogenic in rats and mice, producing a marked increase in tumor incidence in doses approximating those employed clinically. Nitrosourea therapy does have carcinogenic potential in humans (see ADVERSE REACTIONS.) CeeNU also affects fertility in male rats at doses somewhat higher than the human dose.

Pregnancy Category D: See WARNINGS.

Nursing Mothers: It is not known whether this drug is excreted in human milk. Because many drugs are excreted in human milk and because of the potential for serious adverse reactions in nursing infants from CeeNU, a decision should be made whether to discontinue nursing or to discontinue the drug, taking into account the importance of the drug to the mother.

Information for the Patient: Patients receiving CeeNU should be given the following information and instructions by the physician:

1. Patients should be told that CeeNU is an anticancer drug and belongs to the group of medicines known as alkylating agents.

2 In order to provide the proper dose of CeeNU, patients should be aware that there may be two or more different types and colors of capsules in the container dispensed by the pharmacist.

3. Patients should be told that CeeNU is given as a single oral dose and will not be repeated for at least 8 weeks.

4. Patients should be told that nausea and vomiting usually last less than 24 hours, although loss of appetite may last for several days.

5 If any of the following reactions occur, notify the physician: fever, chills, sore throat, unusual bleeding or bruising, shortness of breath, dry cough, swelling of feet or lower legs, mental confusion, or yellowing of eyes and skin.

ADVERSE REACTIONS:

Hematologic Toxicity: The most frequent and most serious toxicity of CeeNU in delayed myelosuppression. It usually occurs 4 to 6 weeks after drug administration and is dose related. Thrombocytopenia occurs at about 4 weeks postadministration and persists for 1 to 2 weeks. Approximately 65% of patients receiving 130 mg/m^{2}develop white blood counts below 5000 wbc/mm^2. Thirty-six percent develop white blood counts below 3000 wbc/mm^2. Thrombocytopenia is generally more severe than leukopenia. However, both may be dose-limiting toxicities.

CeeNU may produce cumulative myelosuppression, manifested by more depressed indices or longer duration of suppression after repeated doses.

The occurrence of acute leukemia and bone marrow dysplasias have been reported in patients following long term nitrosourea therapy.

Anemia also occurs, but is less frequent than thrombocytopenia or leukopenia.

Pulmonary Toxicity: Pulmonary toxicity characterized by pulmonary infiltrates and/or fibrosis has been reported rarely with CeeNU. Onset of toxicity has occurred after an interval of 6 months or longer from the start of therapy with cumulative doses of CeeNU usually greater then 1100 mg/m^2 There is one report of pulmonary toxicity at a cumulative dose of only 600 mg.

Delayed onset pulmonary fibrosis occurring up to 15 years after treatment has been reported in patients who received related nitrosoureas in childhood and early adolescence combined with cranial radiotherapy for intracranial tumors.

Gastrointestinal Toxicity: Nausea and vomiting may occur 3 to 6 hours after an oral dose and usually last less than 24 hours. Prior administration of antiemetics is effective in diminishing and sometimes preventing this side effect. Nausea and vomiting can also be reduced if CeeNU is administered to fasting patients.

Hepatotoxicity: A reversible type of hepatic toxicity, manifested by increased transaminase, alkaline phosphatase and bilirubin levels, has been reported in a small percentage of patients receiving CeeNU.

Nephrotoxicity: Renal abnormalities consisting of progressive azotemia, decrease in kidney size and renal failure have been reported in patients who received large cumulative doses after prolonged therapy with CeeNU. Kidney damage has also been reported occasionally in patients receiving lower total doses.

Other Toxicities: Stomatitis and alopecia have been reported infrequently. Neurological reactions such as disorientation, lethargy, ataxia, and dysarthria have been noted in some patients receiving CeeNU. However, the relationship to medication in these patients is unclear.

OVERDOSAGE:

No proven antidotes have been established for CeeNU overdosage.

DOSAGE AND ADMINISTRATION:

The recommended dose of CeeNU in adults and children as a single agent in previously untreated patients is 130 mg/m^2 as a single dose by mouth every 6 weeks. In individuals with compromised bone marrow function, the dose should be reduced to 100 mg/m^{2}every 6 weeks. When CeeNU is used in combination with other myelosuppressive drugs, the doses should be adjusted accordingly.

Doses subsequent to the initial dose should be adjusted according to the hematologic response of the patient to the preceding dose. The following schedule is suggested as a guide to dosage adjustment (TABLE 1):

TABLE 1

Nadir After Prior Dose: Leukocytes	Platelets	Percentage of Prior Base to be Given
>4000	>100,000	100%
3000-3999	75,000-99,999	100%
2000-2999	25,000-74,999	70%
<2000	<25,000	50%

A repeat course of CeeNU should not be given until circulating blood elements have returned to acceptable levels (platelets above 100,000 cm; leukocytes above 4,000/cm). Blood counts should be monitored weekly and repeat courses should not be given before 6 weeks because the hematologic toxicity is delayed and cumulative.

HOW SUPPLIED:

The dose pack of CeeNU (lomustine [CCNU]) Capsules contains:

2—100 mg capsules (Green/Green)

2—40 mg capsules (White/Green)

2—10 mg capsules (White/White)

Stability: CeeNU are stable for the lot life indicated on package labeling when stored at room temperature in well closed containers. Avoid excessive heat (over 40°C).

Directions to the Pharmacist: The dose pack contains a total of 300 mg and will provide enough medication for titration of a single dose. The total dose prescribed by the physician can be obtained (to within 10 mg) by determining the appropriate combination of the enclosed capsule strengths.

The appropriate number of capsules of each size should be placed in a single vial to which the patient information label (gummed label provided) explaining the differences in the appearance of the capsules is affixed. Each color-coded capsule is imprinted with the dose in milligrams.

A patient information sticker, to be placed on dispensing container, is enclosed.

Procedures for proper handling and disposal of anticancer drugs should be considered. Several guidelines on this subject have been published.[1-7] There is no general agreement that all of the procedures recommended in the guidelines are necessary or appropriate.

REFERENCES:

1. Recommendations for the Safe Handling of Parenteral Antineoplastic Drugs. NIH Publication No. 83-2621. For sale by the Superintendent of Documents, US Government Printing Office, Washington, DC 20402. 2. AMA Council Report. Guidelines for Handling Parenteral Antineoplastics. JAMA 1985: 253 (11):1590-1592. 3. National Study Commission on Cytotoxic Exposure-Recommendations for Handling Cytotoxic Agents. Available from Louis P. Jeffrey, ScD, Chairman, National Study Commission on Cytotoxic Exposure, Massachusetts College of Pharmacy and Allied Health Sciences, 179 Longwood Avenue, Boston, Massachusetts 02115. 4. Clinical Oncological Society of Australia. Guidelines and Recommendations for Safe Handling of Antineoplastic Agents. Med J Australia 1983: 1:426-428. 5. Jones RB, et al: Safe Handling of Chemotherapeutic Agents: A Report from the Mount Sinai Medical Center. CA—A Cancer Journal for Clinicians 1983; (Sept/Oct)258-263. 6. American Society of Hospital Pharmacists Technical Assistance Bulletin on Handling Cytotoxic and Hazardous Drugs. Am J Hosp Pharm 1990:47:1033-1049. 7. OSHA Work-Practice Guidelines for Personnel Dealing with Cytotoxic (Antineoplastic) Drugs. Am J Hosp Pharm 1988; 43:1193-1204.(Bristol Laboratories: 12/90, P8047-02)

HOW SUPPLIED - EQUIVALENTS NOT AVAILABLE:

Capsule, Gelatin - Oral - 10 mg

20's $84.42 CEENU, Mead Johnson 00015-3030-20

Capsule, Gelatin - Oral - 40 mg

20's $254.24 CEENU, Mead Johnson 00015-3031-20

Capsule, Gelatin - Oral - 100 mg

20's $483.27 CEENU, Mead Johnson 00015-3032-20

Capsule, Gelatin - Oral - 300 mg

3 x 2 $77.98 CEENU, Mead Johnson 00015-3034-10

LOPERAMIDE HYDROCHLORIDE *(001661)*

CATEGORIES: Antidiarrhea Agents; Bowel Disease; Diarrhea; Gastrointestinal Drugs; Pregnancy Category B; FDA Approval Pre 1982

BRAND NAMES: *Acanol* (Mexico); *Alomide*; *Amerol*; *Arret*; *Beamodium*; *Betaperamide*; *Binaldan*; *Brek*; *Chisen*; *Colifilm*; *Desitin*; *Diacure*; *Diarlop*; *Diamide*; *Diarent*; *Diarin*; *Diarodil*; *Diarstop-L* (Germany); *Diastop*; *Dicap*; *Dissenten*; *Donafan*; *Elcoman*; *Fortasec*; *Gastron*; *Gastro-Stop*; *Hocular*; *IMD*; *Imode*; **Imodium**; *Imosec*; *Imosen*; *Imossel* (France); *Lilizin*; *Lodia*; *Lomy*; *Lopamide*; *Lop-Dia* (Germany); *Lopedin*; *Lopedium*; *Lopemid*; *Lopemin* (Japan); *Loperastat*; *Loperhoe* (Germany); *Loperin*; *Loperium*; *Lopermide*; *Loperol*; *Loperyl*; *Lopestal*; *Lorico*; *Loridin*; *Motilen*; *Motilex*; *Motilix*; *Novadiar*; *Opox*; *Oramide*; *Orulop*; *Plenterox*; *Pramidal* (Mexico); *Prodium*; *Prosulex*; *Raxedin* (Mexico); *Regulane*; *Regulene*; *Rodderhea*; *Seldiar*; *Stopit*; *Suprasec*; *Tanitril*; *Tebloc*; *Toban*; *Undiarrhea*; *Vacontil* *(International brand names outside U.S. in italics)*

FORMULARIES: Aetna; BC-BS; DoD; PCS

DESCRIPTION:

Loperamide hydrochloride, 4-(p-chlorophenyl)-4-hydroxy-N,N-dimethyl-α,α-diphenyl-1-piperidinebutyramide monohydrochloride, is a synthetic antidiarrheal for oral use.

Loperamide HCl is available in 2 mg capsules.

The inactive ingredients are: Lactose, cornstarch, talc, and magnesium stearate. Loperamide HCl capsules contain FD&C Yellow No. 6.

CLINICAL PHARMACOLOGY:

In vitro and animal studies show that loperamide HCl acts by slowing intestinal motility and by affecting water and electrolyte movement through the bowel. Loperamide HCl inhibits peristaltic activity by a direct effect on the circular and longitudinal muscles of the intestinal wall.

CLINICAL PHARMACOLOGY: *(cont'd)*

In man, loperamide HCl prolongs the transit time of the intestinal contents. It reduces the daily fecal volume, increases the viscosity and bulk density, and diminishes the loss of fluid and electrolytes. Tolerance to the antidiarrheal effect has not been observed.

Clinical studies have indicated that the apparent elimination half-life of loperamide in man is 10.8 hours with a range of 9.1 - 14.4 hours. Plasma levels of unchanged drug remain below 2 nanograms per ml after the intake of a 2 mg capsule of loperamide HCl. Plasma levels are highest approximately five hours after administration of the capsule and 2.5 hours after the liquid. The peak plasma levels of loperamide were similar for both formulations. Of the total excreted in urine and feces, most of the administered drug was excreted in feces.

In those patients in whom biochemical and hematological parameters were monitored during clinical trials no trends toward abnormality during loperamide HCl therapy were noted. Similarly, urinalysis, EKG and clinical ophthalmological examinations did not show trends toward abnormality.

INDICATIONS AND USAGE:

Loperamide HCl is indicated for the control and symptomatic relief of acute nonspecific diarrhea and of chronic diarrhea associated with inflammatory bowel disease. Loperamide HCl is also indicated for reducing the volume of discharge from ileostomies.

CONTRAINDICATIONS:

Loperamide HCl is contraindicated in patients with known hypersensitivity to the drug and in those in whom constipation must be avoided.

WARNINGS:

Loperamide HCl should not be used in the case of acute dysentery, which is characterized by blood in stools and elevated temperatures.

Fluid and electrolyte depletion often occur in patients who have diarrhea. In such cases, administration of appropriate fluid and electrolytes is very important. The use of loperamide HCl does not preclude the administration of appropriate fluid and electrolyte therapy.

In some patients with acute ulcerative colitis, and in pseudomembranous colitis associated with broad-spectrum antibiotics, agents which inhibit intestinal motility or delay intestinal transit time have been reported to induce toxic megacolon.

Loperamide HCl therapy should be discontinued promptly if abdominal distention, constipation, or ileus occurs.

Loperamide HCl should be used with special caution in young children because of the greater variability of response in this age group. Dehydration, particularly in younger children, may further influence the variability of response to loperamide HCl.

PRECAUTIONS:

General: In acute diarrhea, if clinical improvement is not observed in 48 hours, the administration of loperamide HCl should be discontinued. Patients with hepatic dysfunction should be monitored closely for signs of CNS toxicity because of the apparent large first pass biotransformation.

Information for the Patient: Patients should be advised to check with their physician if their diarrhea does not improve after a few days or if they note blood in their stools or develop a fever.

Carcinogenesis, Mutagenesis, and Impairment of Fertility: In an 18-month rat study with doses up to 133 times the maximum human dose (on a mg/kg basis), there was no evidence of carcinogenesis. Mutagenicity studies were not conducted. Reproduction studies in rats indicated that high doses (150-200 times the human dose) could cause marked female infertility and reduced male fertility.

Pregnancy, Teratogenic Effects, Pregnancy Category B: Reproduction studies in rats and rabbits have revealed no evidence of impaired fertility or harm to the fetus at doses up to 30 times the human dose. Higher doses impaired the survival of mothers and nursing young. The studies offered no evidence of teratogenic activity. There are, however, no adequate and well controlled studies in pregnant women. Because animal reproduction studies are not always predictive of human response, this drug should be used during pregnancy only if clearly needed.

Nursing Mothers: It is not known whether this drug is excreted in human milk. Because many drugs are excreted in human milk, caution should be exercised when loperamide HCl is administered to a nursing woman.

Pediatric Use: See the WARNINGS for information on the greater variability of response in this age group.

In case of accidental overdosage of loperamide HCl by children, see OVERDOSAGE for suggested treatment.

DRUG INTERACTIONS:

There was no evidence in clinical trials of drug interactions with concurrent medications.

ADVERSE REACTIONS:

The adverse effects reported during clinical investigations of loperamide HCl are difficult to distinguish from symptoms associated with the diarrheal syndrome. Adverse experiences recorded during clinical studies with loperamide HCl were generally of a minor and self-limiting nature. They were more commonly observed during the treatment of chronic diarrhea.

The following patient complaints have been reported and are listed in decreasing order of frequency with the exception of hypersensitivity reactions which is listed first since it may be the most serious.

Hypersensitivity reactions (including skin rash) have been reported with loperamide HCl use.

Abdominal pain, distention or discomfort

Nausea and vomiting

Constipation

Tiredness

Drowsiness or dizziness

Dry mouth

In postmarketing experiences, there have been rare reports of paralytic ileus associated with abdominal distention. Most of these reports occurred in the setting of acute dysentery, overdosage, and with very young children of less than two years of age.

DRUG ABUSE AND DEPENDENCE:

Abuse: A specific clinical study designed to assess the abuse potential of loperamide at high doses resulted in a finding of extremely low abuse potential.

Dependence: Studies in morphine-dependent monkeys demonstrated that loperamide hydrochloride at doses above those recommended for humans prevented signs of morphine withdrawal. However, in humans, the naloxone challenge pupil test, which when positive indicates opiate-like effects, performed after a single high dose, or after more than two years

DRUG ABUSE AND DEPENDENCE: *(cont'd)*

of therapeutic use of loperamide HCl, was negative. Orally administered loperamide HCl (loperamide formulated with magnesium stearate) is both highly insoluble and penetrates the CNS poorly.

OVERDOSAGE:

In cases of overdosage, paralytic ileus and CNS depression may occur. Children may be more sensitive to CNS effects than adults. Clinical trials have demonstrated that a slurry of activated charcoal administered promptly after ingestion of loperamide hydrochloride can reduce the amount of drug which is absorbed into the systemic circulation by as much as ninefold. If vomiting occurs spontaneously upon ingestion, a slurry of 100 gms of activated charcoal should be administered orally as soon as fluids can be retained.

If vomiting has not occurred, gastric lavage should be performed followed by administration of 100 gms of the activated charcoal slurry through the gastric tube. In the event of overdosage, patients should be monitored for signs of CNS depression for at least 24 hours. Children may be more sensitive to central nervous system effects than adults. If CNS depression is observed, naloxone, may be administered. If responsive to naloxone, vital signs must be monitored carefully for recurrence of symptoms of drug overdose for at least 24 hours after the last dose of naloxone.

In view of the prolonged action of loperamide and the short duration (one to three hours) of naloxone, the patient must be monitored closely and treated repeatedly with naloxone as indicated. Since relatively little drug is excreted in the urine, forced diuresis is not expected to be effective for loperamide HCl overdosage.

In clinical trials an adult who took three 20 mg doses within a 24 hour period was nauseated after the second dose and vomited after the third dose. In studies designed to examine the potential for side effects, intentional ingestion of up to 60 mg of loperamide hydrochloride in a single dose to healthy subjects resulted in no significant adverse effects.

DOSAGE AND ADMINISTRATION:

(1 capsule = 2 mg)

Patients should receive appropriate fluid and electrolyte replacement as needed.

Acute Diarrhea Adults: The recommended initial dose is 4 mg (two capsules) followed by 2 mg (one capsule) after each unformed stool. Daily dosage should not exceed 16 mg (eight capsules). Clinical improvement is usually observed within 48 hours.

Children: Loperamide HCl use is not recommended for children under 2 years of age. In children 2 to 5 years of age (20 kg or less), the non-prescription liquid formulation (Imodium A-D 1 mg/5 ml) should be used; for ages 6 to 12, either loperamide HCl Capsules or loperamide HCl A-D Liquid may be used.

For children 2 to 12 years of age, the following schedule for capsules or liquid will usually fulfill initial dosage requirements:

RECOMMENDED FIRST DAY DOSAGE AND SCHEDULE

Two to five years: 1 mg t.i.d. (3 mg daily dose)
(13 to 20 kg)

Six to eight years: 2 mg b.i.d. (4 mg daily dose)
(20 to 30 kg)

Eight to twelve years: 2 mg t.i.d. (6 mg daily dose)
(greater than 30 kg)

Recommended Subsequent Daily Dosage: Following the first treatment day, it is recommended that subsequent loperamide HCl doses (1 mg/10 kg body weight) be administered only after a loose stool. Total daily dosage should not exceed recommended dosages for the first day.

Chronic Diarrhea Children: Although loperamide HCl has been studied in a limited number of children with chronic diarrhea, the therapeutic dose for the treatment of chronic diarrhea in a pediatric population has not been established.

Adults: The recommended initial dose is 4 mg (two capsules) followed by 2 mg (one capsule) after each unformed stool until diarrhea is controlled, after which the dosage of loperamide HCl should be reduced to meet individual requirements. When the optimal daily dosage has been established, this amount may then be administered as a single dose or in divided doses.

The average daily maintenance dosage in clinical trials was 4 to 8 mg (two to four capsules). A dosage of 16 mg (eight capsules) was rarely exceeded. If clinical improvement is not observed after treatment with 16 mg per day for at least 10 days, symptoms are unlikely to be controlled by further administration. Loperamide HCl administration may be continued if diarrhea cannot be adequately controlled with diet or specific treatment.

Store at room temperature 15°-30°C (59°-86°F).

HOW SUPPLIED - RATED THERAPEUTICALLY EQUIVALENT:

Capsule, Gelatin - Oral - 2 mg

100's	$24.75	Loperamide Hcl, United Res	00677-1422-01
100's	$24.75	Loperamide HCl, H.C.F.A. F F P	99999-1661-01
100's	$34.55	Loperamide Hcl, Roxane	00054-2537-25
100's	$36.23	Loperamide Hcl, Roxane	00054-8537-25
100's	$55.10	Loperamide Hcl, Major Pharms	00904-7617-60
100's	$55.67	Loperamide Hcl, Goldline Labs	00182-1505-01
100's	$55.67	Loperamide Hcl, Mova Pharms	55370-0169-07
100's	$55.67	Loperamide Hcl, Novopharm (US)	55953-0020-40
100's	$55.75	Loperamide HCl, Schein Pharm (US)	00364-2481-01
100's	$56.78	Loperamide Hcl, Martec Pharms	52555-0519-01
100's	$57.96	Loperamide Hcl, Qualitest Pharms	00603-4235-21
100's	$58.46	Loperamide Hcl, HL Moore Drug Exch	00839-7623-06
100's	$58.60	Loperamide Hcl, Aligen Independ	00405-4592-01
100's	$60.00	Loperamide Hcl, Dupont Pharma	00056-0200-70
100's	$61.10	Loperamide, Teva	00093-0311-01
100's	$62.47	Loperamide Hcl, Vangard Labs	00615-0362-13
100's	$64.97	Loperamide HCl, Rugby	00536-3974-01
100's	$64.97	Loperamide HCl, Geneva Pharms	00781-2761-01
100's	$65.25	Loperamide Hcl, Mylan	00378-2100-01
100's	**$71.39**	**IMODIUM, Janssen Phar**	**50458-0400-10**
100's	**$79.70**	**IMODIUM, Janssen Phar**	**50458-0400-01**
500's	$123.75	Loperamide Hcl, United Res	00677-1422-05
500's	$123.75	Loperamide HCl, H.C.F.A. F F P	99999-1661-02
500's	$163.36	Loperamide Hcl, Roxane	00054-2537-29
500's	$266.47	Loperamide Hcl, Rugby	00536-3974-10
500's	$277.67	Loperamide Hcl, Mova Pharms	55370-0169-08
500's	$277.67	Loperamide Hcl, Novopharm (US)	55953-0020-70
500's	$280.00	Loperamide Hcl, Rugby	00536-3974-05
500's	$290.00	Loperamide Hcl, Dupont Pharma	00056-0200-85
500's	$291.59	Loperamide Hcl, HL Moore Drug Exch	00839-7623-12
500's	$292.28	Loperamide Hcl, Aligen Independ	00405-4592-02
500's	$298.10	Loperamide, Teva	00093-0311-05
500's	$298.95	Loperamide Hcl, Mylan	00378-2100-05
500's	**$349.06**	**IMODIUM, Janssen Phar**	**50458-0400-50**
1000's	$247.50	Loperamide HCl, H.C.F.A. F F P	99999-1661-03
1000's	$516.17	Loperamide Hcl, Novopharm (US)	55953-0020-80

LORACARBEF *(003107)*

CATEGORIES: Anti-Infectives; Antibiotics; Beta-Lactam Antibiotics; Bronchitis; Carbacephems; Chronic Bronchitis; Cystitis; Otitis Media; Pharyngitis; Pneumonia; Pyelonephritis; Respiratory Tract Infections; Sinusitis; Skin Infections; Streptococcal Infection; Tonsillitis; Urinary Tract Infections; Rheumatic Fever*; FDA Class 1C ("Little or No Therapeutic Advantage"); Sales > $100 Million; FDA Approved 1991 Dec; Top 200 Drugs

* Indication not approved by the FDA

BRAND NAMES: Lorabid

FORMULARIES: PCS

COST OF THERAPY: $176.12 (Respiratory Infections; Capsule; 200 mg; 4/day; 14 days)

DESCRIPTION:

Loracarbef is a synthetic β-lactam antibiotic of the carbacephem class for oral administration. Chemically, carbacephems differ from cephalosporin-class antibiotics in the dihydrothiazine ring where a methylene group has been substituted for a sulfur atom.

The chemical name for loracarbef is: (6*R*, 7*S*)-7-[(*R*)-2-amino-2-phenylacetamido]-3-chloro-8-oxo-1-azabicyclo[4.2.0]oct-2-ene-2- carboxylic acid, monohydrate. It is a white to off-white solid with a molecular weight of 367.8. The empirical formula is $C_{16}H_{16}ClN_3O_4 \cdot H_2O$.

Lorabid Pulvules and Lorabid for Oral Suspension are intended for oral administration only.

Each Pulvule contains loracarbef equivalent to 200 mg (0.57 mmol) or 400 mg (1.14 mmol) anhydrous loracarbef activity. They also contain cornstarch, dimethicone, F D & C Blue No. 2, gelatin, iron oxides, magnesium stearate, titanium dioxide, and other inactive ingredients.

After reconstitution, each 5 ml of Lorabid for Oral Suspension contains loracarbef equivalent to 100 mg (0.286 mmol) or 200 mg (0.57 mmol) anhydrous loracarbef activity. The suspensions also contain cellulose, F D & C Red No. 40, flavors, methylparaben, propylparaben, simethicone emulsion, sodium carboxymethylcellulose, sucrose, and xanthan gum.

CLINICAL PHARMACOLOGY:

Loracarbef, after oral administration, was approximately 90% absorbed from the gastrointestinal tract. When capsules were taken with food, peak plasma concentrations were 50% to 60% of those achieved when the drug was administered to fasting subjects and occurred from 30 to 60 minutes later. Total absorption, as measured by urinary recovery and area under the plasma concentration versus time curve (AUC), was unchanged. The effect of food on the rate and extent of absorption of the suspension formulation has not been studied to date.

The pharmacokinetics of loracarbef were linear over the recommended dosage range of 200 to 400 mg, with no accumulation of the drug noted when it was given twice daily.

Average peak plasma concentrations after administration of 200-mg or 400-mg single doses of loracarbef as capsules to fasting subjects were approximately 8 to 14 mcg/ml, respectively, and were obtained within 1.2 hours after dosing. The average peak plasma concentration in adults following a 400-mg single dose of suspension was 17 mcg/ml and was obtained within 0.8 hour after dosing (see TABLE 1.)

TABLE 1

Dosage (mg)	Mean Plasma Loracarbef Concentrations (mcg/ml) Peak Cmax	Time to Peak Tmax
Capsule (single dose)		
200 mg	8	1.2 h
400 mg	14	1.2 h
Suspension (single dose)		
400 mg (adult)	17	0.8 h
7.5 mg/kg (pediatric)	13	0.8 h
15 mg/kg (pediatric)	19	0.8 h

Following administration of 7.5 and 15 mg/kg single doses of oral suspension to children, average peak plasma concentrations were 13 and 19 mcg/ml, respectively, and were obtained within 40 to 60 minutes.

This increased rate of absorption (suspension > capsule) should be taken into consideration if the oral suspension is to be substituted for the capsule, and capsules should not be substituted for the oral suspension in the treatment of otitis media (see DOSAGE AND ADMINISTRATION.)

The elimination half-life was an average of 1.0 h in patients with normal renal function. Concomitant administration of probenecid decreased the rate of urinary excretion and increased the half-life to 1.5 hours.

In subjects with moderate impairment of renal function (creatinine clearance 10 to 50 ml/min/1.73 m^2), following a single 400-mg dose, the plasma half-life was prolonged to approximately 5.6 hours. In subjects with severe renal impairment (creatinine clearance <10 ml/min/1.73 m^2), the half-life was increased to approximately 32 hours. During hemodialysis the half-life was approximately 4 hours. In patients with severe renal impairment, the C_{max} increased from 15.4 mcg/ml to 23 mcg/ml (see PRECAUTIONS and DOSAGE AND ADMINISTRATION).

In single-dose studies, plasma half-life and AUC were not significantly altered in healthy elderly subjects with normal renal function.

There is no evidence of metabolism of loracarbef in humans.

Approximately 25% of circulating loracarbef is bound to plasma proteins.

Middle-ear fluid concentrations of loracarbef were approximately 48% of the plasma concentration 2 hours after drug administration in children. The peak concentration of loracarbef in blister fluid was approximately half that obtained in plasma. Adequate data on CSF levels of loracarbef are not available.

Microbiology: Loracarbef exerts its bactericidal action by binding to essential target proteins of the bacterial cell wall, leading to inhibition of cell-wall synthesis. It is stable in the presence of some bacterial β-lactamases. Loracarbef has been shown to be active against most strains of the following organisms both *in vitro* and in clinical infections (see INDICATIONS AND USAGE):

Gram-positive aerobes:

Staphylococcus aureus(including penicillinase-producing strains)

NOTE: Loracarbef (like most β-lactam antimicrobials) is inactive against methicillin-resistant staphylococci.

Staphylococcus saprophyticus

Streptococcus pneumoniae

Streptococcus pyogenes

Gram-negative aerobes:

Escherichia coli; Haemophilus influenzae (including β-lactamase-producing strains)

CLINICAL PHARMACOLOGY: *(cont'd)*

Moraxella (Branhamella) catarrhalis(including β-lactamase-producing strains)

The following *in vitro* data are available; however, their clinical significance is unknown.

Loracarbef exhibits *in vitro* minimum inhibitory concentrations (MIC) of 8 mcg/ml or less against most strains of the following organisms; however, the safety and efficacy of loracarbef in treating clinical infections due to these organisms have not been established in adequate and well-controlled trials.

Gram-positive aerobes:

Staphylococcus epidermidis

Streptococcus agalactiae (group B streptococci)

Streptococcus bovis

Streptococci groups C, F, and G; viridans group streptococci

Gram-negative aerobes:

Citrobacter diversus

Haemophilus parainfluenzae

Klebsiella pneumoniae

Neisseria gonorrhoeae (including penicillinase-producing strains)

Pasteurella multocida

Proteus mirabilis

Salmonella species

Shigella species

Yersinia enterocolitica

NOTE: Loracarbef is inactive against most strains of *Acinetobacter, Enterobacter, Morganella morganii, Proteus vulgaris, Providencia, Pseudomonas,* and *Serratia.*

Anaerobic organisms:

Clostridium perfringens

Fusobacterium necrophorum

Peptococcus niger, Peptostreptococcus intermedius

Propionibacterium acnes

SUSCEPTIBILITY TESTING

Diffusion Techniques: Quantitative methods that require measurement of zone diameters give the most precise estimate of the susceptibility of bacteria to antimicrobial agents. One such standardized method[1] has been recommended for use with the 30-mcg loracarbef disk. Interpretation involves the correlation of the diameter obtained in the disk test with MIC for loracarbef.

Reports from the laboratory giving results of the standard single-disk susceptibility test with a 30 mcg loracarbef disk should be interpreted according to the following criteria (TABLE 2):

TABLE 2

Zone diameter (mm)	Interpretation
≥ 18	(S) Susceptible
15-17	(MS) Moderately Susceptible
≤ 14	(R) Resistant

A report of "susceptible" implies that the pathogen is likely to be inhibited by generally achievable blood concentrations. A report of "moderately susceptible" indicates that inhibitory concentrations of the antibiotic may be achieved if high dosage is used or if the infection is confined to tissues and fluids (*e.g.,* urine) in which high antibiotic concentrations are attained. A report of "resistant" indicates that achievable concentrations of the antibiotic are unlikely to be inhibitory and other therapy should be selected.

Standardized procedures require the use of laboratory control organisms. The 30-mcg loracarbef disk should give the following zone diameters with the NCCLS approved procedure (TABLE 3):

TABLE 3

Organism	Zone Diameter (mm)
E. coli ATCC 25922	23-29
S. aureus ATCC 25923	23-31

Dilution Techniques: Use a standardized dilution method[2](broth, agar, or microdilution) or equivalent with loracarbef powder. The MIC values obtained should be interpreted according to the following criteria (TABLE 4):

TABLE 4

MIC (mcg/ml)	Interpretation
≤8	(S) Susceptible
16	(MS) Moderately Susceptible
≥32	(R) Resistant

As with standard diffusion methods, dilution procedures require the use of laboratory control organisms. Standard loracarbef powder should give the following MIC values with the NCCLS approved procedure (TABLE 5):

TABLE 5

Organism	MIC Range (mcg/ml)
E. coli ATCC 25922	0.5-2
S. aureus ATCC 29213	0.5-2

CLINICAL STUDIES:

ACUTE OTITIS MEDIA:

Study 1: In a controlled clinical study of acute otitis media performed in the United States where significant rates of β-lactamase-producing organisms were found, loracarbef was compared to an oral antimicrobial agent that contained a specific β-lactamase inhibitor. In this study, using very strict evaluability criteria and microbiologic and clinical response criteria at the 10- to 16-day post therapy follow-up, the following presumptive bacterial eradication/clinical cure outcomes (*i.e.,* clinical success) and safety results were obtained (TABLE 12):

Safety: The incidences of the following adverse events were clinically and statistically significantly higher in the control arm versus the loracarbef arm (TABLE 13):

Study 2: In a controlled clinical study of acute otitis media performed in Europe, loracarbef was compared to amoxicillin. As expected in a European population, this study population had a lower incidence of β- lactamase-producing organisms than usually seen in U.S. trials. In

CLINICAL STUDIES: *(cont'd)*

TABLE 12 U.S. Acute Otitis Media Study Loracarbef vs β-lactamase inhibitor-containing control drug

Efficacy: Pathogen	% of Cases With Pathogens (n=204)	Outcome
S. pneumoniae	42.6%	Loracarbef equivalent to control
H. influenzae	30.4%	Loracarbef success rate 9% less than control
M. catarrhalis	20.6%	Loracarbef success rate 19% less than control
S. pyogenes	6.4%	Loracarbef equivalent to control
Overall	100.0%	Loracarbef success rate 12% less than control

TABLE 13

Event	Loracarbef	Control
Diarrhea	15%	26%
Rash*	8%	15%

* The majority of these involved the diaper area in young children.

this study, using very strict evaluability criteria and microbiologic and clinical response criteria at the 10- to 16-day post therapy follow-up, the following presumptive bacterial eradication/clinical cure outcomes (*i.e.*, clinical success) were obtained (TABLE 14):

TABLE 14 European Acute Otitis Media Study: Loracarbef vs Amoxicillin

Efficacy: Pathogen	% of Cases With Pathogens (n=291)	Outcome
S. pneumoniae	51.5%	Loracarbef equivalent to amoxicillin
H. influenzae	29.2%	Loracarbef success rate 14% greater than amoxicillin
M. catarrhalis	15.8%	Loracarbef success rate 31% greater than amoxicillin
S. pyogenes	3.4%	Loracarbef equivalent to amoxicillin
Overall	100.0%	Loracarbef equivalent to amoxicillin

Acute Maxillary Sinusitis: In a controlled clinical study of acute maxillary sinusitis performed in Europe, loracarbef was compared to doxycycline. In this study there were 210 sinus-puncture evaluable patients. As expected in a European population, this study population had a lower incidence of β-lactamase-producing organisms than usually seen in U.S. trials. In this study, using very strict evaluability criteria and microbiologic and clinical response criteria at the 1- to 2-week post therapy follow-up, the following presumptive bacterial eradication/clinical cure outcomes (*i.e.*, clinical success) were obtained (TABLE 15):

TABLE 15 European Acute Maxillary Sinusitis Study: Loracarbef vs Doxycycline

Efficacy: Pathogen	% of Cases With Pathogens (n=210)	Outcome
S. pneumoniae	47.6%	Loracarbef equivalent to doxycycline
H. influenzae	41.4%	Loracarbef equivalent to doxycycline
M. catarrhalis	11.0%	Loracarbef equivalent to doxycycline
Overall	100.0%	Loracarbef equivalent to doxycycline

CYSTITIS

Study 1: In a controlled clinical study of cystitis performed in the United States, loracarbef was compared to cefaclor. In this study, using very strict evaluability criteria and microbiologic and clinical response criteria at the 5- to 9-day post therapy follow-up, the following bacterial eradication rates were obtained (TABLE 16):

TABLE 16 U.S. Uncomplicated Cystitis Study: Loracarbef vs Cefaclor

Efficacy: Pathogen	% of Cases With Pathogens (n=186)	Outcome
E. coli	77.4%	Loracarbef eradication rate 4% greater than cefaclor (loracarbef eradication rate 80%)
Other major *Enterobacteriaceae*	12.5%	Loracarbef equivalent to cefaclor (loracarbef eradication rate 61%)
S. saprophyticus	3.8%	Loracarbef equivalent to cefaclor

Study 2: In a second controlled clinical study of cystitis, performed in Europe, loracarbef was compared to an oral quinolone. In this study, using very strict evaluability criteria and microbiologic and clinical response criteria at the 5- to 9-day post therapy follow-up, the following bacterial eradication rates were obtained (TABLE 17):

TABLE 17 European Uncomplicated Cystitis Study: Loracarbef vs Quinolone

Efficacy: Pathogen	% of Cases With Pathogens (n=189)	Outcome
E. coli	82.0%	Loracarbef eradication rate 7% less than quinolone (loracarbef eradication rate 81%)
Other major *Enterobacteriaceae*	10.1%	Loracarbef eradication rate 32% less than quinolone (loracarbef eradication rate 50%)

INDICATIONS AND USAGE:

Loracarbef is indicated in the treatment of patients with mild to moderate infections caused by susceptible strains of the designated microorganisms in the conditions listed below. (As recommended dosages, durations of therapy, and applicable patient populations vary among these infections, please see DOSAGE AND ADMINISTRATIONfor specific recommendations.)

Lower Respiratory Tract *Secondary Bacterial Infection of Acute Bronchitis* caused by *S. pneumoniae, H. influenzae*(including β-lactamase-producing strains), or *M. catarrhalis* (including β-lactamase-producing strains).

Acute Bacterial Exacerbations of Chronic Bronchitis caused by *S. pneumoniae, H. influenzae* (including β-lactamase-producing strains), or *M. catarrhalis* (including β-lactamase-producing strains).

INDICATIONS AND USAGE: *(cont'd)*

Pneumonia caused by *S. pneumoniae or H. influenzae* (non-β-lactamase-producing strains only). Data are insufficient at this time to establish efficacy in patients with pneumonia caused by β-lactamase-producing strains of *H. influenzae.*

Upper Respiratory Tract Otitis Media†*caused by S. pneumoniae, H. influenzae* (including β-lactamase-producing strains), *M. catarrhalis* (including β-lactamase-producing strains), or *S. pyogenes.*

Acute Maxillary Sinusitis† caused by *S. pneumoniae, H. influenzae* (non-β-lactamase-producing strains only), or *M. catarrhalis* (including β-lactamase-producing strains). Data are insufficient at this time to establish efficacy in patients with acute maxillary sinusitis caused by β-lactamase-producing strains of *H. influenzae.*

† NOTE: In a patient population with significant numbers of β-lactamase-producing organisms, loracarbef's clinical cure and bacteriological eradication rates were somewhat less than those observed with a product containing a β-lactamase inhibitor. Loracarbef's decreased potential for toxicity compared to products containing β-lactamase inhibitors along with the susceptibility patterns of the common microbes in a given geographic area should be taken into account when considering the use of an antimicrobial (see CLINICAL STUDIES.)

Pharyngitis and Tonsillitis caused by *S. pyogenes.*(The usual drug of choice in the treatment and prevention of streptococcal infections, including the prophylaxis of rheumatic fever, is penicillin administered by the intramuscular route. Loracarbef is generally effective in the eradication of *S. pyogenes* from the nasopharynx; however, data establishing the efficacy of loracarbef in the subsequent prevention of rheumatic fever are not available at present.)

Skin and Skin Structure *Uncomplicated Skin and Skin Structure Infections* caused by *S. aureus*(including penicillinase-producing strains) or *S. pyogenes.*Abscesses should be surgically drained as clinically indicated.

Urinary Tract *Uncomplicated Urinary Tract Infections* (cystitis) caused by *E. coli* or *S. saprophyticus**.

NOTE: In considering the use of loracarbef in the treatment of cystitis, loracarbef's lower bacterial eradication rates and lower potential for toxicity should be weighed against the increased eradication rates and increased potential for toxicity demonstrated by some other classes of approved agents (see CLINICAL STUDIES.)

Uncomplicated Pyelonephritis caused by *E. coli.*

* Although treatment of infections due to this organism in this organ system demonstrated a clinically acceptable overall outcome, efficacy was studied in fewer than 10 infections.

Culture and susceptibility testing should be performed when appropriate to determine the causative organism and its susceptibility to loracarbef. Therapy may be started while awaiting the results of these studies. Once these results become available, antimicrobial therapy should be adjusted accordingly.

CONTRAINDICATIONS:

Loracarbef is contraindicated in patients with known allergy to loracarbef or cephalosporin-class antibiotics.

WARNINGS:

BEFORE THERAPY WITH LORACARBEF IS INSTITUTED, CAREFUL INQUIRY SHOULD BE MADE TO DETERMINE WHETHER THE PATIENT HAS HAD PREVIOUS HYPERSENSITIVITY REACTIONS TO LORACARBEF, CEPHALOSPORINS, PENICILLINS, OR OTHER DRUGS. IF THIS PRODUCT IS TO BE GIVEN TO PENICILLIN-SENSITIVE PATIENTS, CAUTION SHOULD BE EXERCISED BECAUSE CROSS-HYPERSENSITIVITY AMONG β-LACTAM ANTIBIOTICS HAS BEEN CLEARLY DOCUMENTED AND MAY OCCUR IN UP TO 10% OF PATIENTS WITH A HISTORY OF PENICILLIN ALLERGY. IF AN ALLERGIC REACTION TO LORACARBEF OCCURS, DISCONTINUE THE DRUG. SERIOUS ACUTE HYPERSENSITIVITY REACTIONS MAY REQUIRE THE USE OF EPINEPHRINE AND OTHER EMERGENCY MEASURES, INCLUDING OXYGEN, INTRAVENOUS FLUIDS, INTRAVENOUS ANTIHISTAMINES, CORTICOSTEROIDS, PRESSOR AMINES, AND AIRWAY MANAGEMENT, AS CLINICALLY INDICATED.

Pseudomembranous colitis has been reported with nearly all antibacterial agents and may range from mild to life-threatening. Therefore, it is important to consider this diagnosis in patients who present with diarrhea subsequent to the administration of antibacterial agents.

Treatment with broad-spectrum antibiotics alters the normal flora of the colon and may permit overgrowth of clostridia. Studies indicate that a toxin produced by *Clostridium difficile* is a primary cause of "antibiotic-associated colitis."

After the diagnosis of pseudomembranous colitis has been established, therapeutic measures should be initiated. Mild cases of pseudomembranous colitis usually respond to discontinuation of drug alone. In moderate to severe cases, consideration should be given to management with fluids and electrolytes, protein supplementation, and treatment with an antibacterial drug effective against *C. difficile*-associated colitis.

PRECAUTIONS:

General: In patients with known or suspected renal impairment (see DOSAGE AND ADMINISTRATION), careful clinical observation and appropriate laboratory studies should be performed prior to and during therapy. The total daily dose of loracarbef should be reduced in these patients because high and/or prolonged plasma antibiotic concentrations can occur in such individuals administered the usual doses. Loracarbef, like cephalosporins, should be given with caution to patients receiving concurrent treatment with potent diuretics because these diuretics are suspected of adversely affecting renal function.

As with other broad-spectrum antimicrobials, prolonged use of loracarbef may result in the overgrowth of nonsusceptible organisms. Careful observation of the patient is essential. If superinfection occurs during therapy, appropriate measures should be taken.

Loracarbef, as with other broad-spectrum antimicrobials, should be prescribed with caution in individuals with a history of colitis.

Information for the Patient: Loracarbef should be taken either at least 1 hour prior to eating or at least 2 hours after eating a meal.

Carcinogenesis, Mutagenesis, and Impairment of Fertility: Although life-time studies in animals have not been performed to evaluate carcinogenic potential, no mutagenic potential was found for loracarbef in standard tests of genotoxicity, which included bacterial mutation tests and *in vitro* and *in vivo* mammalian systems. In rats, fertility and reproductive performance were not affected by loracarbef at doses up to 33 times the maximum human exposure in mg/kg (10 times the exposure based on mg/m^2).

Usage in Pregnancy—Pregnancy Category B: Reproduction studies have been performed in mice, rats, and rabbits at doses up to 33 times the maximum human exposure in mg/kg (4, 10, and 4 times the exposure, respectively, based on mg/m^2) and have revealed no evidence of impaired fertility or harm to the fetus due to loracarbef. There are, however, no adequate and well-controlled studies in pregnant women. Because animal reproduction studies are not always predictive of human response, this drug should be used during pregnancy only if clearly needed.

PRECAUTIONS: *(cont'd)*

Labor and Delivery: Loracarbef has not been studied for use during labor and delivery. Treatment should be given only if clearly needed.

Nursing Mothers: It is not known whether this drug is excreted in human milk. Because many drugs are excreted in human milk, caution should be exercised when loracarbef is administered to a nursing woman.

Pediatric Use: Efficacy and safety in infants less than 6 months of age have not been established.

Geriatric Use: Healthy geriatric volunteers (≥65 years old) with normal renal function who received a single 400-mg dose of loracarbef had no significant differences in AUC or clearance when compared to healthy adult volunteers 20 to 40 years of age. In clinical studies, when geriatric patients received the usual recommended adult doses, clinical efficacy and safety were comparable to results in nongeriatric adult patients. Because significant numbers of elderly patients have decreased renal function, evaluation of renal function in this population is recommended (see DOSAGE AND ADMINISTRATION.)

DRUG INTERACTIONS:

Probenecid: As with other β-lactam antibiotics, renal excretion of loracarbef is inhibited by probenecid and resulted in an approximate 80% increase in the AUC for loracarbef (see CLINICAL PHARMACOLOGY.)

ADVERSE REACTIONS:

The nature of adverse reactions to loracarbef are similar to those observed with orally administered β-lactam antimicrobials. The majority of adverse reactions observed in clinical trials were of a mild and transient nature; 1.5% of patients discontinued therapy because of drug-related adverse reactions. No one reaction requiring discontinuation accounted for >0.03% of the total patient population; however, of those reactions resulting in discontinuation, gastrointestinal events (diarrhea and abdominal pain) and skin rashes predominated.

All Patients: The following adverse events, irrespective of relationship to drug, have been reported following the use of loracarbef in clinical trials. Incidence rates (combined for all dosing regimens and dosage forms) were less than 1% for the total patient population, except as otherwise noted:

Gastrointestinal: The most commonly observed adverse reactions were related to the gastrointestinal system. The incidence of gastrointestinal adverse reactions increased in patients treated with higher doses. Individual event rates included diarrhea, 4.1%; nausea, 1.9%; vomiting 1.4%; abdominal pain, 1.4%; and anorexia.

Hypersensitivity: Hypersensitivity reactions including, skin rashes (1.2%), urticaria, pruritus, and erythema multiforme.

Central Nervous System: Headache (2.9%), somnolence, nervousness, insomnia, and dizziness.

Hemic and Lymphatic Systems: Transient thrombocytopenia, leukopenia, and eosinophilia.

Hepatic: Transient elevations in AST (SGOT), ALT (SGPT), and alkaline phosphatase.

Renal: Transient elevations in BUN and creatinine.

Cardiovascular System: Vasodilatation.

Genitourinary: Vaginitis (1.3%), vaginal moniliasis (1.1%).

As with other β-lactam antibiotics, the following potentially severe adverse experiences have been reported rarely with loracarbef in worldwide post-marketing surveillance: anaphylaxis, hepatic dysfunction including cholestasis, prolongation of the prothrombin time with clinical bleeding in patients taking anticoagulants, and Stevens-Johnson syndrome.

Pediatric Patients: The incidences of several adverse events, irrespective of relationship to drug, following treatment with loracarbef were significantly different in the pediatric population and the adult population as follows (TABLE 6):

TABLE 6

Event	Pediatric	Adult
Diarrhea	5.8%	3.6%
Headache	0.9%	3.2%
Rhinitis	6.3%	1.6%
Nausea	0.0%	2.5%
Rash	2.9%	0.7%
Vomiting	3.3%	0.5%
Somnolence	2.1%	0.4%
Anorexia	2.3%	0.3%

β-Lactam Antimicrobial Class Labeling: The following adverse reactions and altered laboratory test results have been reported in patients treated with β-lactam antibiotics:

Adverse Reactions: Allergic reactions, aplastic anemia, hemolytic anemia, hemorrhage, agranulocytosis, toxic epidermal necrolysis, renal dysfunction, toxic nephropathy. As with other β-lactam antibiotics, serum sickness-like reactions have been reported rarely with loracarbef.

Several β-lactam antibiotics have been implicated in triggering seizures, particularly in patients with renal impairment when the dosage was not reduced. If seizures associated with drug therapy should occur, the drug should be discontinued. Anticonvulsant therapy can be given if clinically indicated.

Altered Laboratory Tests: Increased prothrombin time, positive direct Coombs' test, elevated LDH, pancytopenia, and neutropenia.

OVERDOSAGE:

Signs and Symptoms: The toxic symptoms following an overdose of β-lactams may include nausea, vomiting, epigastric distress, and diarrhea.

Loracarbef is eliminated primarily by the kidneys. Forced diuresis, peritoneal dialysis, hemodialysis, or hemoperfusion have not been established as beneficial for an overdose of loracarbef. Hemodialysis has been shown to be effective in hastening the elimination of loracarbef from plasma in patients with chronic renal failure.

DOSAGE AND ADMINISTRATION:

Loracarbef is administered orally either at least 1 hour prior to eating or at least 2 hours after eating. The recommended dosages, durations of treatment, and applicable patient populations are described in the following chart (TABLE 7): **Population/Infection**

Dosage for Impaired Renal Function: Loracarbef may be administered to patients with impaired renal function. The usual dose and schedule may be employed in patients with creatinine clearance levels of 50 ml/min or greater. Patients with creatinine clearance between 10 and 49 ml/min may be given half of the recommended dose at the usual dosage interval, or the normal recommended dose at twice the usual dosage interval. Patients with creatinine clearance levels less than 10 ml/min may be treated with the recommended dose given every 3 to 5 days; patients on hemodialysis should receive another dose following dialysis.

When only the serum creatinine is available, the following formula (based on sex, weight, and age of the patient) may be used to convert this value into creatinine clearance (CL_{cr}, ml/min). The equation assumes the patient's renal function is stable (TABLE 10):

DOSAGE AND ADMINISTRATION: *(cont'd)*

TABLE 7

Population/ Infection	Dosage (mg)	Duration (days)
ADULTS (13 years and older)		
Lower Respiratory Tract		
Secondary Bacterial Infection of Acute Bronchitis	200-400 q12h	7
Acute Bacterial Exacerbation of Chronic Bronchitis	400 q12h	7
Pneumonia	400 q12h	14
Upper Respiratory Tract‡		
Pharyngitis/Tonsillitis	200 q12h	10*
Sinusitis	400 q12h	10
Skin and Skin Structure		
Uncomplicated Skin and Skin Structure Infections	200 q12h	7
Urinary Tract		
Uncomplicated cystitis	200 q24h	7
Uncomplicated pyelonephritis	400 q12h	14
INFANTS AND CHILDREN (6 months to 12 years)		
Upper Respiratory Tract		
Acute Otitis Media†	30 mg/kg/day in divided doses q12h	10
Pharyngitis/Tonsillitis	15 mg/kg/day in divided doses q12h	10*
Skin and Skin Structure		
Impetigo	15 mg/kg/day in divided doses q12h	7

* In the treatment of infections due to *S. pyogenes,* Lorabid should be administered for at least 10 days.
† Otitis media should be treated with the suspension. Clinical studies of otitis media were conducted with the suspension formulation only. The suspension is more rapidly absorbed than the capsules, resulting in higher peak plasma concentrations when administered at the same dose. Therefore, the capsule should not be substituted for the suspension in the treatment of otitis media (see CLINICAL PHARMACOLOGY).
‡ ([Ss]ee CLINICAL STUDIES) and INDICATIONS AND USAGE for further information.)

TABLE 8 Pediatric Dosage Chart Daily Dose 15 mg/kg/day

Weight		100 mg/5 ml Suspension Dose given twice daily		200 mg/5 ml Suspension Dose given twice daily	
lb	kg	ml	tsp	ml	tsp
15	7	2.6	0.5	—	—
29	13	4.9	1.0	2.5	0.5
44	20	7.5	1.5	3.8	0.75
57	26	9.8	2.0	4.9	1.0

TABLE 9 Pediatric Dosage Chart Daily Dose 30 mg/kg/day

Weight		100 mg/5 ml Suspension Dose given twice daily		200 mg/5 ml Suspension Dose given twice daily	
lb	kg	ml	tsp	ml	tsp
15	7	5.2	1.0	2.6	0.5
29	13	9.8	2.0	4.9	1.0
44	20	—	—	7.5	1.5
57	26	—	—	9.8	2.0

TABLE 10

Males = [(weight in kg) × (140 - age)] ÷ [72 × serum creatinine (mg/100 ml)]
Females = (0.85) × (above value)

TABLE 11 Reconstitution Directions for Oral Suspension

Bottle Size	Reconstitution Directions
100 ml	Add 60 ml of water in 2 portions to the dry mixture in the bottle. Shake well after each addition.
50 ml	Add 30 ml of water in 2 portions to the dry mixture in the bottle. Shake well after each addition.

After mixing, the suspension may be kept at room temperature, 59° to 86°F (15° to 30°C), for 14 days without significant loss of potency.

Keep tightly closed. Discard unused portion after 14 days.

REFERENCES:

1. National Committee for Clinical Laboratory Standards, M2-A4 performance standards for antimicrobial disk susceptibility tests. ed 4, Villanova, PA, April, 1990. 2. National Committee for Clinical Laboratory Standards, M7-A2 methods for dilution antimicrobial susceptibility tests for bacteria that grow aerobically, ed 2, Villanova, PA, April, 1990.

PATIENT INFORMATION:

Loracarbef is an antibiotic used to treat infections such as bronchitis, sinusitis, pneumonia and tonsillitis. This drug should not be used by those with allergies to the cephalosporin antibiotics. You should also consult with your pharmacist or physician if you are allergic to penicillin before taking this medication. This medication shold be taken at least one hour prior to eating or at least 2 hours after eating. The most common side effects are rash, diarrhea and abdominal pain. You should discontinue the medication if you develop a skin rash.

HOW SUPPLIED:

Pulvules: 200 mg, (blue and gray) (No. 3170) (Identi-Code* 3170)

400 mg, (blue and pink) (No. 3171) (Identi-Code 3171)

Keep tightly closed. Store at controlled room temperature, 59° to 86°F (15° to 30°C). Protect from heat.

For Oral Suspension (strawberry bubble gum flavor)

*Identi-Code (formula identification code, Lilly).

HOW SUPPLIED - EQUIVALENTS NOT AVAILABLE:

Capsule, Gelatin - Oral - 200 mg

30's $94.35 LORABID, Lilly 00002-3170-30

HOW SUPPLIED - EQUIVALENTS NOT AVAILABLE: *(cont'd)*

Capsule, Gelatin - Oral - 400 mg

30's	$118.50	LORABID, Lilly	00002-3171-30

Suspension - Oral - 100 mg/5ml

50 ml	$13.66	LORABID, Lilly	00002-5135-87
100 ml	$24.34	LORABID, Lilly	00002-5135-48

Suspension - Oral - 200 mg/5ml

50 ml	$22.80	LORABID, Lilly	00002-5136-87
100 ml	$36.51	LORABID, Lilly	00002-5136-48

LORATADINE *(003161)*

CATEGORIES: Allergies; Antihistamines; Lacrimation; Non-Sedating Antihistamines; Respiratory & Allergy Medications; Rhinitis; Rhinorrhea; Sneezing; Urticaria; Pregnancy Category B; FDA Class 1S ("Standard Review"); Sales > $500 Million; FDA Approved 1993 Apr; Patent Expiration 1998 Aug; Top 200 Drugs

BRAND NAMES: *Civeran*; *Claratyne* (Australia); **Claritin**; *Claritine*; *Clarityn* (England); *Clarityne* (France, Mexico); *Fristamin*; *Lisino* (Germany); *Lorastine*; *Lorfast*; *Lowadina* (Mexico); *Optimin*; *Sensibit* (Mexico); *Velodan*; *Zeos*
(International brand names outside U.S. in italics)

FORMULARIES: BC-BS; Medi-Cal; PCS

COST OF THERAPY: $58.06 (Rhinitis; Tablet; 10 mg; 1/day; 30 days)

PRIMARY ICD9: 477.9 (Allergic Rhinitis, Cause Unspecified)

DESCRIPTION:

Loratadine is a white to off-white powder not soluble in water, but very soluble in acetone, alcohol, and chloroform. It has a molecular weight of 382.89, and empirical formula of $C_{22}H_{23}ClN_2O_2$; its chemical name is ethyl 4-(8-chloro-5, 6 -dihydro-11*H*-benzo(5,6)cyclohepta [1,2-*b*]pyridin-11-ylidene)-1-piperidinecarboxylate.

Claritin Tablets: contain 10 mg micronized loratadine, an antihistamine, to be administered orally. They also contain the following inactive ingredients: corn starch, lactose, and magnesium stearate.

Claritin Syrup: contains 1 mg/ml micronized loratadine, an antihistamine, to be administered orally. It also contains the following inactive ingredients: citric acid, artificial flavor, glycerin, propylene glycol, sodium benzoate, sugar and water. The pH is between 2.5 and 3.1.

CLINICAL PHARMACOLOGY:

Loratadine is a long-acting tricyclic antihistamine with selective peripheral histamine H_1-receptor antagonistic activity.

Human histamine skin wheal studies following single and repeated 10 mg oral doses of loratadine tablets have shown that the drug exhibits an antihistaminic effect beginning within 1 to 3 hours, reaching a maximum at 8 to 12 hours and lasting in excess of 24 hours. There was no evidence of tolerance to this effect after 28 days of dosing with loratadine.

Whole body autoradiographic studies in rats and monkeys, radiolabeled tissue distribution studies in mice and rats, an *in vivo* radioligand studies in mice have shown that neither loratadine nor its metabolites readily cross the blood-brain barrier. Radioligand binding studies with guinea pig pulmonary and brain H_1-receptors indicate that there was preferential binding to peripheral versus central nervous system H_1-receptors.

PHARMACOKINETICS

Loratadine was rapidly absorbed following oral administration of 10 mg tablets, once daily for 10 days to healthy adult volunteers with times to maximum concentration (T_{max}) of 1.3 hours for loratadine and 2.5 hours for its major active metabolite, descarboethoxyloratadine. Based on a cross-study comparison of single doses of loratadine syrup and tablets given to healthy adult volunteers, the plasma concentration profile of descarboethoxyloratadine for the two formulations is comparable. The pharmacokinetics of loratadine and descarboethoxyloratadine are independent of dose over the dose range of 10 to 40 mg and are not altered by the duration of treatment. In a single-dose study, food increased the systemic bioavailability (AUC) of loratadine and descarboethoxyloratadine by approximately 40% and 15%, respectively. The time to peak plasma concentration (T_{max}) of loratadine and descarboethoxyloratadine was delayed by 1 hour. Peak plasma concnetrations (C_{max}) were not affected by food.

Approximately 80% of the total dose administered can be found equally distributed between urine and feces in the form of metabolic products within 10 days. In nearly all patients, exposure (AUC) to the metabolite is greater than to the parent loratadine. The mean elimination half-lives in normal adult subjects (n=54) were 8.4 hours (range=3 to 20 hours) for loratadine and 28 hours (range = 8.8 to 92 hours) for descarboethoxyloratadine. Loratadine and descarboethoxyloratadine reached steady-state in most patients by approximately the fifth dosing day. There was considerable variability in the pharmacokinetic data in all studies of loratadine tablets and syrup, probably due to the extensive first pass metabolism.

In vitro studies with human liver microsomes indicate that loratadine is metabolized to descarboethoxyloratadine predominantly by P450 3A4 (CYP3A4) and, to a lesser extent, by P450 2D6 (CYP2D6). In the presence of a CYP3A4 inhibitor ketoconazole, loratadine is metabolized to descarboethoxyloratadine predominantly by CYP2D6. Concurrent administration of loratadine with either ketoconazole, erythromycin (both CYP3A4 inhibitors), or cimetidine (CYP2D6 and CYP3A4 inhibitor) to healthy volunteers was associated with significantly increased plasma concentrations of loratadine (see DRUG INTERACTIONS).

The pharmacokinetic profile of loratadine in children in the 6- to 12-year age group is similar to that of adults. In a single-dose pharmacokinetic study of 13 pediatric volunteers (aged 8-12 years) given 10 ml of loratadine syrup containing 10 mg loratadine, the ranges of individual subject values of pharmacokinetic parameters (AUC and C_{max}) were comparable to those following administration of a 10 mg tablet or syrup to adult volunteers.

SPECIAL POPULATIONS

In a study involving twelve healthy geriatric subjects (66 to 78 years old), the AUC and peak plasma levels (C_{max}) of both loratadine and descarboethoxyloratadine were approximately 50% greater than those observed in studies of younger subjects. The mean elimination half-lives for the geriatric subjects were 18.2 hours (range=6.7 to 37 hours) for loratadine and 17.5 hours (range=11 to 38 hours) for descarboethoxyloratadine.

In a study involving 12 subjects with chronic renal impairment (creatinine clearance ≤30 ml/min) both the AUC and peak plasma levels (C_{max}) increased on average by approximately 73% for loratadine and by 120% for descarboethoxyloratadine, as compared to 6 subjects with normal renal function (creatinine clearance ≥80 ml/min). The mean elimination half-lives of loratadine (7.6 hours) and descarboethoxyloratadine (23.9 hours) were not substantially different from that observed in normal subjects. Hemodialysis does not have an effect on the pharmacokinetics of loratadine or descarboethoxyloratadine in subjects with chronic renal impairment.

CLINICAL PHARMACOLOGY: *(cont'd)*

In seven patients with chronic alcoholic liver disease, the AUC and peak plasma levels (C_{max}) of loratadine were double while the pharmacokinetic profile of descarboethoxyloratadine was not substantially different from that observed in other trials enrolling normal subjects. The elimination half-lives for loratadine and descarboethoxyloratadine were 24 hours and 37 hours, respectively, and increased with increasing severity of liver disease.

CLINICAL STUDIES:

Clinical trials of loratadine tablets involved over 10,700 patients, 12 years of age and older, who received either loratadine tablets or another antihistamine and/or placebo in double-blind randomized comtrolled studies. In placebo-controlled trials, 10 mg once daily of loratadine tablets was superior to placebo and similar to clemastine (1mg 2 times daily) or terfenadine (60 mg 2 times daily) in effects on nasal and non-nasal symptoms of allergic rhinitis. In these studies, somnolence occurred less frequently with loratadine tablets than with clemastine and at about the same frequency as terfenadine or placebo. In studies with loratadine tablets at doses 2 to 4 times higher than the recommended dose of 10 mg, a dose-related increase in the incidence of somnolence was observed. Therrefore, some patients, particularly those with hepatic or renal impairment and the elderly, or those on medications that impair clearance of loratadine and its metabolites may experience somnolence. In addition, three placebo-controlled, double-blind, 2 week trials in 188 pediatric patients with seasonal allergic rhinitis aged 6 to 12 years, were conducted at doses of loratadine syrup up to 10 mg once daily.

Among those patients involved in double-blind, randomized, controlled studies of loratadine tablets, approximately 1000 patients (age 12 and older) were enrolled in studies of chronic idiopathic urticaria. In placebo-controlled clinical trials, loratadine tablets 10 mg once daily were superior to placebo in the management of chronic idiopathic urticaria, as demonstrated by reduction of associated itching, erythema, and hives. In these studies, the incidence of somnolence seen with loratadine tablets was similar to that seen with placebo.

In a study in which loratadine tablets were administered to adults at 4 times the clinical dose for 90 days, no clinicallly significant increase in the QT_c was seen on ECGs.

INDICATIONS AND USAGE:

Loratadine is indicated for the relief of nasal and non-nasal symptoms of seasonal allergic rhinitis and for the treatment of idiopathic chronic urticaria in patients 6 years of age or older.

CONTRAINDICATIONS:

Loratadine is contraindicated in patients who are hypersensitive to this medication or to any of its ingredients.

PRECAUTIONS:

General: Patients with liver impairment or renal insufficiency (GFR <30 ml/min) should be given a lower initial dose (10 mg every other day)(see CLINICAL PHARMACOLOGY,Special Populations).

Carcinogenesis, Mutagenesis, and Impairment of Fertility: In an 18-month carcinogenicity study in mice and a 2-year study in rats, loratadine was administered in the diet at doses up to 40 mg/kg (mice) and 25 mg/kg (rats). In the carcinogenicity studies, pharmacokinetic assessments were carried out to determine animal exposure to the drug. AUC data demonstrated that the exposure of mice given 40 mg/kg of loratadine was 3.6 (loratadine) and 18 (descarboethoxyloratiadine) times higher than humans given the maximum recommended daily dose. Exposure of rats given 25 mg/kg of loratadine was 28 (loratadine) and 67 (descarboethoxyloratiadine) times higher than a human given the maximum recommended daily dose. Male mice given 40 mg/kg had a significantly higher incidence of hepatocellular tumors (combined adenomas and carcinomas) than concurrent controls. In rats, a significantly higher incidence of hepatocellular tumors (combined adenomas and carcinomas) was observed in males given 10 mg/kg and males and females given 25 mg/kg. The clinical significance of these findings during long-term use of loratadine is not known.

In mutagenicity studies, there was no evidence of mutagenic potential in reverse (Ames) or forward point mutation (CHO-HGPRT) assays, or in the assay for DNA damage (Rat Primary Hepatocyte Unscheduled DNA Assay) or in two assays for chromosomal aberrations (Human Peripheral Blood Lymphocyte Clastogenesis Assay and the Mouse Bone Marrow Erythrocyte Micronucleus Assay). In the Mouse Lymphoma Assay, a positive finding occurred in the nonactivated but not the activated phase of the study.

Decreased fertility in male rats, shown by lower female conception rates, occurred at an oral dose of 64 mg/kg (approximately 50 times the maximum recommended human daily oral dose on a mg/m² basis) and was reversible with cessation of dosing. Loratadine had no effect on male or female fertility or reproduction in the rat at an oral dose of 24 mg/kg (approximately 20 times the maximum recommended human daily oral dose on a mg/m² basis).

Pregnancy Category B: There was no evidence of animal teratogenicity in studies performed in rats and rabbits at oral doses up to 96 mg/kg (75 times and 150 times, respectively, the maximum recommended human daily oral dose on a mg/m² basis). There are, however, no adequate and well-controlled studies in pregnant women. Because animal reproduction studies are not always predictive of human response, loratadine tablets should be used during pregnancy only if clearly needed.

Nursing Mothers: Loratadine and its metabolite, descarboethoxyloratadine, pass easily into breast milk and achieve concentrations that are equivalent to plasma levels with an AUC_{milk}/AUC_{plasma} ratio of 1.17 and 0.85 for loratadine and descarboethoxyloratadine, respectively. Following a single oral dose of 40 mg, a small amount of loratadine and descarboethoxyloratadine was excreted into the breast milk (approximately 0.03% of 40 mg over 48 hours). A decision should be made whether to discontinue nursing or to discontinue the drug, taking into account the importance of the drug to the mother. Caution should be exercised when loratadine tablets are administered to a nursing woman.

Pediatric Use: The safety of loratadine syrup at a dialy dose of 10 mg has been demonstrated in 188 pediatric patients 6-12 years of age in placebo-controlled 2-week trials. The effectiveness of loratadine for the treatement of seasonal allergic rhinitis and chronic idiopathic urticaria in this pediatric age group is based on an extrapolation of the demonstrated efficacy of loratadine in adults in these conditions and the likelihood that the disease course, pathophysiology, and the drug's effect are substantially similar to that of the adults. The recommended dose for the pediatric population is based on cross-study comparison of the pharmacokinetics of loratadine in adults and pediatric subjects and on the safety profile of loratadine in both adults and pediatric patients at doses equal to or higher than the recommended doses. The safety and effectiveness of loratadine in pediatric patients under 6 years of age have not been established.

DRUG INTERACTIONS:

Loratadine (10 mg once daily) has been safely coadministered with therapeutic doses of erythromycin, cimetidine, and ketoconazole in controlled clinical pharmacology studies in adult volunteers. Although increased plasma concentrations (AUC 0-24 hrs) of loratadine and/or descarboethoxyloratadine were observed following coadministration of loratadine with each of these drugs in normal volunteers (n=24 in each study), there were no clinically

DRUG INTERACTIONS: *(cont'd)*

relevant changes in the safety profile of loratadine, as assessed by electrocardiographic parameters, clinical laboratory tests, vital signs, and adverse events. There were no significant effects on QT_c intervals, and no reports of sedation or syncope. No effects on plasma concentrations of cimetidine or ketoconazole were observed. Plasma concentrations (AUC 0-24 hrs) of erythromycin decreased 15% with coadministration of loratadine relative to that observed with erythromycin alone. The clinical relevance of this difference is unknown. These above findings are summarized in TABLE 1.

TABLE 1 Effects on Plasma Concentrations (AUC 0-24 hrs) of Loratadine and Descarboethoxyloratadine After 10 Days of Coadministration (Loratadine 10 mg) in Normal Volunteers

	Loratadine	Descarboethoxyloratadine
Erythromycin (500 mg q8h)	+ 40%	+ 46%
Cimetidine (300 mg qid)	+ 103%	+ 6%
Ketoconazole(200 mg q12h)	+ 307%	+ 73%

There does not appear to be an increase in adverse events in subjects who received oral contraceptives and loratadine.

ADVERSE REACTIONS:

Tablets: Approximately 90,000 patients, aged 12 years or older, received loratadine tablets 10 mg once daily in controlled and uncontrolled studies. Placebo-controlled clinical trials at the recommended dose of 10 mg once a day varied from 2 weeks' to 6 months' duration. The rate of premature withdrawal from these trials was approximately 2% in both the treated and placebo groups (TABLE 2).

TABLE 2 Reported Adverse Events with an Incidence of More Than 2% in Placebo-Controlled Allergic Rhinitis Clinical Trials in Patients 12 Years of Age and Older Percent of Patients Reporting

	Loratadine10 mg qd n=1926	Placebo n=2545	Clemastine 1 mg bid n=536	Terfenadine 60 mg bid n=684
Headache	12	11	8	8
Somnolence	8	6	22	9
Fatigue	4	3	10	2
Dry Mouth	3	2	4	3

Adverse events reported in placebo-controlled idiopathic chronic urticaria trials were similar to those reported in allergic rhinitis studies.

Adverse event rates did not appear to differ significantly based on age, sex, or race, although the number of non-white subjects was relatively small.

Syrup: Approximately 300 pediatric patients 6 to 12 years of age received 10 mg loratadine once daily in controlled clinical trials for a period of 8-15 days. Among these, 188 children were treated with 10 mg loratadine syrup once daily in placebo-controlled trials. Adverse events in these pediatric patients were observed to occur with type and frequency similar to those seen in the adult populaiton. The rate of premature discontinuance due to adverse events among pediatric patients receiving loratadine 10 mg daily was less than 1%.

TABLE 3 Adverse Events Occurring With a Frequency of ≥2% in Loratadine Syrup-Treated Patients (6-12 Years Old) in Placebo-Controlled Trials, and More Frequently Than in The Placebo Group Percent of Patients Reporting

	Loratadine 10 mg Daily n=188	Placebo n=262	Chlorpheniramine 2-4 mg bid/tid n=170
Nervousness	4	2	2
Wheezing	4	2	5
Fatigue	3	2	5
Hyperkinesia	3	1	1
Abdominal Pain	2	0	0
Conjunctivitis	2	<1	1
Dysphoria	2	<1	0
Malaise	2	0	1
Upper Respiratory Tract Infection	2	<1	0

In addition to those adverse events reported above (≥2%), the following adverse events have been reported in at least one patient in loratadine clinical trials in adult and pediatric patients:

Autonomic Nervous System: Altered lacrimation, altered salivation, flushing, hypoesthesia, impotence, increased sweating, thirst.

Body As A Whole: Angioneurotic edema, asthenia, back pain, blurred vision, chest pain, earache, eye pain, fever, leg cramps, malaise, rigors, tinnitus, viral infection, weight gain.

Cardiovascular System: Hypertension, hypotension, palpitations, syncope, tachycardia.

Central and Peripheral Nervous System: Blepharospasm, dizziness, dysphonia, hypertonia, migraine, paresthesia, tremor, vertigo.

Gastrointestinal System: Altered taste, anorexia, constipation, diarrhea, dyspepsia, flatulence, gastritis, hiccup, increased appetite, nausea, stomatitis, toothache, vomiting.

Musculoskeletal System: Arthralgia, myalgia.

Psychiatric: Agitation, amnesia, anxiety, confusion, decreased libido, depression, impaired concentration, insomnia, irritability, paroniria.

Reproductive System: Breast pain, dysmenorrhea, menorrhagia, vaginitis.

Respiratory System: Bronchitis, bronchospasm, coughing, dyspnea, epistaxis, hemoptysis, laryngitis, nasal dryness, pharyngitis, sinusitis, sneezing.

Skin and Appendages: Dermatitis, dry hair, dry skin, photosensitivity reaction, pruritus, purpura, rash, urticaria.

Urinary System: Altered micturition, urinary discoloration, urinary incontinece, urinary retention.

In addition, the following spontaneous adverse events have been reported rarely during the marketing of loratadine: abnormal hepatic function, including jaundice, hepatitis, and hepatic necrosis; alopecia; anaphylaxis; breast enlargement; erythema multiforme; peripheral edema; seizures; and supraventricular tachyarrhythmias.

DRUG ABUSE AND DEPENDENCE:

There is no information to indicate that abuse or dependency occurs with loratadine.

OVERDOSAGE:

In adults, somnolence, tachycardia, and headache have been reported with overdoses greater than 10 mg with the tablet formulation (40 to 180 mg). Extrapyramidal signs and palpitations have been reported in children with overdoses of greater than 10 mg of loratadine syrup. In the event of overdosage, general symptomatic and supportive measures should be instituted promptly and maintained for as long as necessary.

Treatment of overdosage would reasonably consist of emesis (ipecac syrup), except in patients with impaired consciousness, followed by the administration of activated charcoal to absorb any remaining drug. If vomiting is unsuccessful, or contraindicated, gastric lavage should be performed with normal saline. Saline cathartics may also be of value for rapid dilution of bowel contents. Loratadine is not eliminated by hemodialysis. It is not known if loratadine is eliminated by peritoneal dialysis.

No deaths occurred at oral doses up to 5000 mg/kg in rats and mice (greater than 2400 and 1200 times, respectively, the maximum recommended human daily oral dose on a mg/m^2 basis). Single oral doses of loratadine showed no effects in rats, mice, and monkeys at doses as high as 10 times the maximum recommended human daily oral dose on a mg/m^2 basis.

DOSAGE AND ADMINISTRATION:

Adults And Children 12 Years Of Age And Over: The recommmended dose of loratadine is 10 mg once daily.

Children 6-11 Years Of Age: The recommended dose of loratadine is 10 mg (2 teaspoonsful) once daily.

In patients with liver failure or renal insufficiency (GFR <30 ml/min), one tablet or two teaspoonsful every other day should be the starting dose.

PATIENT INFORMATION:

Loratidine is a non-sedating antihistamine used treat the symptoms of seasonal allergies and to manage itching of unknown origins. Headache and sleepiness were the most common reported side effects. Very few patients discontinued therapy as a result. Safety of loratidine has not been fully established in pregnant women, nursing women, or children under the age of 12. Loratidine should be used only when the benefits outweigh any risks. Antihistamines are most effective when taken prior to the development of symptoms. They can be used in conjunction with decongestants. Please consult your pharmacist or physician for specific product selections.

HOW SUPPLIED:

Claritin Tablets: 10 mg, white to off-white compressed tablets; impressed with the product identification number "458" on one side; and "Claritin 10" on the other. Store between 2° C and 30° C (36° F and 86° F).

Claritin Syrup: Clear, colorless to light yellow liquid, containing 1 mg loratadine per ml. Store between 2°C and 25°C (36°F and 77°F).

HOW SUPPLIED - EQUIVALENTS NOT AVAILABLE:

Syrup - Oral - 1 mg/ml

bottle	$116.50	CLARITIN, Schering	00085-0612-02

Tablet, Uncoated - Oral - 10 mg

14's	$36.04	CLARITIN, Schering	00085-0458-01
30's	$58.06	CLARITIN, Schering	00085-0458-05
100's	$193.54	CLARITIN, Schering	00085-0458-03
100's	$193.54	CLARITIN, Schering	00085-0458-04
500's	$967.67	CLARITIN, Schering	00085-0458-06

LORATADINE; PSEUDOEPHEDRINE SULFATE *(003236)*

CATEGORIES: Allergies; Antihistamines; Decongestants; Lacrimation; Non-Sedating Antihistamines; Respiratory & Allergy Medications; Rhinitis; Rhinorrhea; Sneezing; Pregnancy Category B; FDA Class 4S ("Standard Review"); FDA Approved 1994 Nov

BRAND NAMES: *Claratyne Cold*; *Claratyne Decongestant*; *Clarinase*; **Claritin-D**; *Clarityne-D*; *Clarityne D Repetabs* (Mexico)
(International brand names outside U.S. in italics)

FORMULARIES: PCS

COST OF THERAPY: $65.43 (Rhinitis; Tablet; 5 mg/120 mg; 2/day; 30 days)

PRIMARY ICD9: 477.9 (Allergic Rhinitis, Cause Unspecified)

DESCRIPTION:

Claritin-D long-acting antihistamine/extended release decongestant tablets contain 5 mg loratadine in the tablet coating for immediate release and 120 mg pseudoephedrine sulfate, USP equally distributed between the tablet coating for immediate release and the barrier-coated extended release core.

Loratadine is a white to off-white powder, not soluble in water, but very soluble in acetone, alcohol, and chloroform. Loratadine has a molecular weight of 382.89 and empirical formula of $C_{22}H_{23}ClN_2O_2$; the chemical name, ethyl 4-(8-chloro-5,6-dihydro-11*H*-benzo[5,6]cyclohepta[1,2-*b*]pyridin-11-ylidene)-1-piperidinecarboxylate.

Pseudoephedrine sulfate is the synthetic salt of one of the naturally occurring dextrorotatory diastereomers of ephedrine and is classified as an indirect sympathomimetic amine. The empirical formula for pseudoephedrine sulfate is $(C_{10}H_{15}NO)_2 \cdot H_2SO_4$; the chemical name is [S-(R*,R*)]-α-[1(methylamino)ethyl] benzenemethanol sulfate (2:1) (salt).

The molecular weight of pseudoephedrine sulfate is 428.54. It is a white powder, freely soluble in water and methanol and sparingly soluble in chloroform.

The inactive ingredients for Claritin-D tablets are acacia, butylparaben, calcium sulfate, carnauba was, corn starch, lactose, magnesium stearate, microcrystalline cellulose, neutral soap, oleic acid, povidone, rosin, sugar, talc, titanium dioxide, white wax, and zein.

CLINICAL PHARMACOLOGY:

The following information is based upon studies of loratadine alone or pseudoephedrine alone, expect as indicated.

Loratadine is a long-acting tricyclic antihistamine with selective peripheral histamine H_1-receptor antagonistic activity.

Human histamine skin wheal studies following single and repeated oral doses of loratadine have shown that the drug exhibits an antihistaminic effect beginning within 1 to 3 hours, reaching a maximum at 8 to 12 hours and lasting in excess of 24 hours. There was no evidence of tolerance to this effect developing after 28 days of dosing with loratadine.

CLINICAL PHARMACOLOGY: *(cont'd)*

Pharmacokinetic studies following single and multiple oral doses of loratadine in 115 volunteers showed that loratadine is rapidly absorbed and extensively metabolized to an active metabolite (descarbethoxyloratadine). Approximately 80% of the total dose administered can be found equally distributed between urine and feces in the form of metabolic products after 10 days. The mean elimination half-lives found in studies in normal adult subjects (n=54) were 8.4 hours (range = 3 to 20 hours) for loratadine and 28 hours (range = 8.8 to 92 hours) for the major active metabolite (descarboethoxyloratadine). In nearly all patients, exposure (AUC) is greater than exposure to parent loratadine. Loratadine and descarboethoxyloratadine reached steady-state in most patients by approximately the fifth dosing day. The pharmacokinetics of loratadine and descarboethoxyloratadine are dose independent over the dose range of 10 to 40 mg and are not significantly altered by the duration of treatment.

In vitro studies with human liver microsomes indicate that loratadine is metabolized to descarboethoxyloratadine predominantly by P450 CYP3A4 and, to a lesser extent, by P450 CYP2D6. In the presence of a CYP3A4 and, to a lesser extent, by P450 CYP2D6. In the presence of a CYP3A4 inhibitor ketoconazole, loratadine with either ketoconazole, erythromycin (both CYP3A4 inhibitors), or cimetidine (CYP2D6 and CYP3A4 inhibitors), or cimetidine (CYP2D6 and CYP3A4 inhibitor) to healthy volunteers was associated with significantly increased plasma concentrations of loratadine (see DRUG INTERACTIONS).

In a study involving twelve healthy geriatric subjects (66 to 78 years old), the AUC and peak plasma levels (C_{max}) of both loratadine and descarboethoxyloratadine were significantly (approximately 50% increased) than in studies of younger subjects. The mean elimination half-lives for the elderly subjects were 18.2 hours (range = 6.7 to 37 hours) for loratadine and 17.5 hours (range = 11 to 38 hours) for the active metabolite.

In clinical efficacy studies, loratadine was administered before meals. In a single-dose study, food increased the AUC of loratadine by approximately 40% and of descarboethoxyloratadine by approximately 15%. The time of peak plasma concentration (T_{max}) of loratadine and descarboethoxyloratadine was delayed by 1 hour with a meal. Although these differences would not be expected to be clinically important, loratadine should be administered on an empty stomach.

In patients with chronic renal impairment (creatinine clearance ≤30 ml/min) both are AUC and peak plasma levels (C_{max}) increased average by approximately 73% for loratadine; and approximately by 120% for descarboethoxyloratadine, compared to individuals with normal renal function. The mean elimination half-lives of loratadine (7.6 hours) and descarboethoxyloratadine (23.9 hours) were not significantly different from that observed in normal subjects. Hemodialysis does not have an effect on the pharmacokinetics of loratadine or its active metabolite (descarboethoxyloratadine) in subjects with chronic renal impairment.

In patients with chronic alcoholic liver disease with the AUC and peak plasma levels (C_{max}) of loratadine were double while the pharmacokinetic profile of the active metabolite (descarboethoxyloratadine) was not significantly changed from that in normals. The elimination half-lives for loratadine and descarboethoxyloratadine were 24 and 37 hours, respectively, and increased with increasing severity of liver disease.

There was considerable variability in the pharmacokinetic data in all studies of loratadine, probably due to the extensive first-pass metabolism. Individual histograms of area under the curve, clearance, and volume of distribution showed a log normal distribution with a 25-fold range in distribution in healthy subjects.

Loratadine is about 97% bound to plasma proteins at the expected concentrations 2.5 to 100 ng/ml) after therapeutic dose. Loratadine does not affect the plasma proteins binding of warfarin and digoxin. The metabolite descarboethoxyloratadine is 73% to 77% bound to plasma proteins (at 0.5 to 100 ng/ml).

Whole body autoradiographic studies in rats and monkeys, radiolabeled tissue distribution studies mice and rats, and *in vivo* radioligand studies in mice have shown that neither loratadine nor its metabolites readily cross the blood-brain barrier. Radioligand binding studies with guinea pig pulmonary and bran H_1-receptors indicate that there was preferential binding to peripheral versus central nervous system H_1-receptors.

In a study in which loratadine alone was administered at four times the clinical dose for 90 days, no clinically significant increase in the QT_c was seen om ECGs.

Pseudoephedrine sulfate (d-isoephedrine sulfate) is on an orally active sympathomimetic amine which exerts a decongestant action on the nasal mucosa. It is recognized as an effective agent for the relief of nasal congestion due to allergic rhinitis. Pseudoephedrine produces peripheral effects similar to those of ephedrine and central effects similar to, but less intense than, amphetamines. It has the potential for excitatory side effects. The pseudoephedrine component of loratadine; pseudoephedrine tablets was absorbed at a similar rate and was equally available from the combination tablet as from a pseudoephedrine sulfate repetabs 120 mg tablet. Mean (%CV) steady-state peak plasma concentration of 464 ng/ml (22) was attained at 3.9 hours (50). The terminal half-life of pseudoephedrine from the combination tablet administered twice daily was 6.3 hours (23). The ingestion of food was found not to affect the absorption of pseudoephedrine from loratadine; pseudoephedrine tablets. Loratadine and pseudoephedrine sulfate do not influence the pharmacokinetics of each other when administered concomitantly.

Clinical Studies: Clinical trials of loratadine; pseudoephedrine tablets in seasonal allergic rhinitis involved approximately 3700 patients who received either the combination product, a comparative treatment, or placebo, in double-blind, randomized controlled studies. Four of the largest studies involved approximately 1600 patients in comparisons of the combination product, loratadine (5 mg bid), pseudoephedrine sulfate (120 mg bid), and placebo. Improvement in symptoms of seasonal allergic rhinitis for patients receiving loratadine; pseudoephedrine tablets was significantly greater than the improvement in those patients who received the individual components or placebo. The combination reduced the intensity of sneezing, rhinorrhea, nasal pruritus, and eye tearing more than pseudoephedrine and reduced the intensity of nasal congestion more than loratadine, demonstrating a contribution of each of the components. The onset of antihistamine and nasal decongestant actions occurred after the first dose of loratadine; pseudoephedrine tablets. Loratadine; pseudoephedrine tablets were well tolerated, with a frequency of sedation similar to that seen with placebo, and an adverse event profile clinically similar to that of pseudoephedrine.

INDICATIONS AND USAGE:

Loratadine; pseudoephedrine tablets are indicated for the relief of symptoms of seasonal allergic rhinitis. Loratadine; pseudoephedrine tablets should be administered when both the antihistaminic properties of loratadine and the nasal decongestant activity of pseudoephedrine are desired (see CLINICAL PHARMACOLOGY).

CONTRAINDICATIONS:

Loratadine; pseudoephedrine tablets are contraindicated in patients who are hypersensitive to this medication or to any of its ingredients.

This product, due to its pseudoephedrine component, is contraindicated in patients with narrow-angle glaucoma or urinary retention, and in patients receiving monoamine oxidase (MAO) inhibitor therapy or within fourteen (14) days of stopping such treatment (see DRUG INTERACTIONS). It is also contraindicated in patients with severe hypertension, severe coronary artery disease, and in those who have shown hypersensitivity or idiosyncrasy to its

CONTRAINDICATIONS: *(cont'd)*

components, to adrenergic agents, or to other drugs of similar chemical structures. Manifestations of patient idiosyncrasy to adrenergic agents include: insomnia, dizziness, weakness, tremor, or arrhythmias.

WARNINGS:

Loratadine; pseudoephedrine tablets should be used with caution in patients with hypertension, diabetes, mellitus, ischemic heart disease, increased intraocular pressure, hyperthyroidism, renal impairment, or prostatic hypertrophy. Central nervous system stimulation with convulsions or cardiovascular collapse with accompanying hypotension may be produced by sympathomimetic amines.

Use in Patients Approximately 60 Years and Older: The safety and efficacy of loratadine; pseudoephedrine tablets in patients greater than 60 years old have not been investigated in placebo-controlled clinical trials. The elderly are more likely to have adverse reactions to sympathomimetic amines.

PRECAUTIONS:

General: Because the doses of this fixed combination product cannot be individually titrated and hepatic insufficiency results in a reduced clearance of loratadine to a much greater extent than pseudoephedrine, loratadine; pseudoephedrine tablets should generally be avoided in patients with hepatic insufficiency. Patients with renal insufficiency (GFR <30 ml/min) should be given a lower initial dose (one tablet per day) because they have reduced clearance of loratadine and pseudoephedrine.

Information for the Patient: Patients taking loratadine; pseudoephedrine tablets should receive the following information: loratadine; pseudoephedrine tablets are prescribed for the relief symptoms of seasonal allergic rhinitis. Patients should be instructed to take loratadine; pseudoephedrine tablets only as prescribed and not to exceed the prescribed dose. Patients should also be advised against the concurrent use of loratadine; pseudoephedrine tablets with over-the-counter antihistamines and decongestants.

This product should not be used by patients who are hypersensitive to it or to any of its ingredients. Due to its pseudoephedrine component, this product should not be used by patients with narrow-angle glaucoma, urinary retention, or by patients receiving a monoamine oxidase (MAO) inhibitor or within 14 days of stopping use of an MAO inhibitor. It also should not be used by patients with severe hypertension or severe coronary artery disease.

Patients who are or may become pregnant should be told that this product should be used in pregnancy or during lactation only if the potential benefit justifies the potential risk to the fetus or nursing infant.

Patients should be instructed not to break or chew the tablet.

Drug/Laboratory Test Interactions: The *in vitro* addition of pseudoephedrine to sera containing the cardiac isoenzyme MB of serum creatinine phosphokinase progressively inhibits the activity of the enzyme. The inhibition becomes complete over 6 hours.

Carcinogenesis, Mutagenesis, Impairment Fertility: There are no animal or laboratory studies of the combination product loratadine and pseudoephedrine sulfate to evaluate carcinogenesis, mutagenesis, or impairment of fertility.

In an 18-month oncogenicity study in mice and a 2-year study in rats loratadine was administered in the diet at doses up to 40 mg/kg (mice) and 25 mg/kg (rats). In the carcinogenicity studies pharmacokinetic assessments were carried out to determine animal exposure to the drug. AUC data demonstrated that the exposure of mice given 40 mg/kg of loratadine was 3.6 (loratadine) and 18 (active metabolite) times higher than a human given 10 mg/day. Exposure of rats given 25 mg/kg of loratadine was 28 (loratadine) and 67 (active metabolite) times higher than a human given 10 mg/dat. Male mice given 40 mg/kg had a significantly higher incidence of hepatocellular tumors (combined adenomas and carcinomas) than concurrent controls. In rats, a significantly higher incidence of hepatocellular tumors (combined adenomas and carcinomas) was observed in males given 10 mg/kg and males and females given to 25 mg/kg. The clinical significance of these findings during long-term use of loratadine is not known.

In mutagenicity studies with loratadine alone, there was no evidence of mutagenic potential in reverse (Ames) or forward point mutation (CHO-HGRPT) assays, or in the assay for DNA damage (Rat Primary Hepatocyte Unscheduled DNA Assay) or in two assays for chromosomal aberrations (Human Peripheral Blood Lymphocyte Clastogenesis Assay and the Mouse Bone Marrow Erythrocyte Micronucleus Assay). In the Mouse Lymphoma Assay, a positive finding occurred in the nonactivated but not the activated phase of the study.

Loratadine administration produced hepatic microsomal enzyme induction in the mouse at 40 mg/kg and rat at 25 mg/kg, but not at lower doses.

Decreased fertility in male rats, shown by lower female conception rats, occurred at approximately 64 mg/kg of loratadine and was reversible with cessation of dosing. Loratadine had no effect on male or female fertility of reproduction in the rat at doses approximately 24 mg/kg.

Pregnancy Category B: There was no evidence of animal teratogenicity in reproduction studies performed on rats and rabbits with this combination at oral doses up to 150 mg/kg (885 mg/m^2 or 5 times the recommended daily human dosage of 250 mg or 185 mg/m^2), and 120 mg/kg (1416 mg/m^2 or 8 times the recommended daily human dosage), respectively. There are, however, no adequate and well-controlled studies in pregnant women. Because animal reproduction studies are not always predictive of human response, loratadine; pseudoephedrine tablets should be used during pregnancy only if clearly needed.

Nursing Mothers: It is not known if this combination product is excreted in human milk. However, loratadine when administered alone and its metabolite descarboethoxyloratadine pass easily into breast milk and achieve concentrations that are equivalent to plasma levels with an AUC_{milk}/AUC_{plasma} ratio of 1.17 and 0.85 for the parent and active metabolite respectively. Following a single oral dose of 40 mg, a small amount of loratadine and metabolite was excreted into the breast milk (approximately 0.03% of 40 mg after 48 hours). Pseudoephedrine administered alone also distributes into breast milk of the lactating human female. Pseudoephrine concentrations in milk are consistently higher than those in plasma. The total amount of drug in milk as judged by the area under the curve (AUC) is 2 to 3 times greater than in plasma. The fraction of a pseudoephedrine dose excreted in milk is estimated to be 0.4% to 0.7%. A decision should be made whether to discontinue nursing or to discontinue the drug, taking into account the importance of the drug to a nursing mother.

Caution should be exercised in loratadine; pseudoephedrine tablets are administered to a nursing woman.

Pediatric Use: Safety and effectiveness in children below the age of 12 years have not been established.

DRUG INTERACTIONS:

No specific interaction studies have been conducted with loratadine; pseudoephedrine tablets. However, loratadine (10 mg once daily) has been safely coadministered with therapeutic doses of erythromycin, cimetidine, and ketoconazole in controlled clinical pharmacology studies. Although increased plasma concentrations (AUC 0-24 hrs) of loratadine and/or descarboethoxyloratadine were observed following coadministration of loratadine with each of these drugs in normal volunteers (n=24 in each study), there were no clinically relevant changes in the safety profile of loratadine, as assessed by electrocardiographic parameters,

DRUG INTERACTIONS: *(cont'd)*

clinical laboratory tests, vital signs, and adverse events. There was no significant effects on QT_c intervals, and no reports of sedation of syncope. No effects on plasma concentrations of cimetidine or ketoconazole were observed. Plasma concentrations (AUC 0-24 hrs) of erythromycin decreased 15% with coadministration of loratadine relative to that observed with erythromycin alone. The clinical relevance of this difference is unknown. These above findings are summarized in TABLE 1:

TABLE 1 Loratadine; Pseudoephedrine Sulfate, Drug Interactions
Effects on Plasma Concentrations (AUC 0-24 hrs) of Loratadine and Descarboethoxyloratadine After 10 Days of Coadministration (Loratadine 10 mg) in Normal Volunteers

	Loratadine	Descarboethoxyloratadine
Erythromycin (500 mg Q8h)	+ 40%	+46%
Cimetidine (300 mg QID)	+103%	+ 6%
Ketoconazole (200 mg Q12h)	+307%	+73%

There does not appear to be an increase in adverse events in subjects who received oral contraceptives and loratadine.

Loratadine; pseudoephedrine tablets (pseudoephedrine component) are contraindicated in patients taking monoamine oxidase inhibitors and for 2 weeks after stopping use of an MAO inhibitor. The antihypertensive effects of beta-adrenergic blocking agents, methyldopa, mecamylamine, reserpine, and veratrum alkaloids may be reduced by sympathomimetics. Increased ectopic pacemaker activity can occur when pseudoephedrine is used concomitantly with digitalis.

ADVERSE REACTIONS:

Experience from controlled and uncontrolled clinical studies involving approximately 10,000 patients who received the combination of loratadine and pseudoephedrine sulfate for a period of up to 1 month provides information on adverse reactions. The usual dose was one tablet every 12 hours for up to 28 days.

In controlled clinical trials using the recommended dose of one tablet every 12 hours, the incidence of reported adverse events was similar to those reported with placebo, with the exception of insomnia (16%) and dry mouth (14%). See TABLE 2:

TABLE 2 Loratadine; Pseudoephedrine Sulfate, Adverse Reactions
Reported Adverse Events With An Incidence Of ≥2% On Loratadine; Pseudoephedrine Tablets In Placebo-Controlled CLINICAL STUDIES Percent Of Patients Reporting

	Claritin-D n=1023	Loratadine n=543	Pseudo-ephedrine n=548	Placebo n=922
Headache	19	18	17	19
Insomnia	16	4	19	3
Dry Mouth	14	4	9	3
Somnolence	7	8	5	4
Nervousness	5	3	7	2
Dizziness	4	1	5	2
Fatigue	4	6	3	3
Dyspepsia	3	2	3	1
Nausea	3	2	3	2
Pharyngitis	3	3	2	3
Anorexia	2	1	2	1
Thirst	2	1	2	1

Adverse event rates did not appear to differ significantly based on age, sex, or race, although the number of non-white subjects was relatively small.

In addition to those adverse events reported above (≥2%), the following less frequent adverse events have been reported in at least one loratadine; pseudoephedrine tablets treated patient:

Autonomic Nervous System: Abnormal lacrimation, dehydration, flushing, hypoesthesia, increased sweating, mydriasis.

Body As A Whole: Asthenia, back pain, blurred vision, chest pain, conjunctivitis, earache, ear infection, eye pain, fever, flu-like symptoms, leg cramps, lymphadenopathy, malaise, photophobia, rigors, tinnitus, viral infection, weight gain.

Cardiovascular System: Hypertension, hypotension, palpitations, peripheral edema, syncope, tachycardia, ventricular extrasystoles.

Central and Peripheral Nervous System: Dysphonia, hyperkinesia, hypertonia, migraine, paresthesia, tremors, vertigo.

Gastrointestinal System: Abdominal distention, abdominal distress, abdominal pain, altered taste, constipation, diarrhea, eructation, flatulence, gastritis, gingival bleeding, hemorrhoids, increased appetite, stomatitis, taste loss, tongue discoloration, toothache, vomiting.

Liver and Biliary System: Hepatic function abnormal.

Musculoskeletal System: Arthralgia, myalgia, torticollis.

Psychiatric: Aggressive reaction, agitation, anxiety, apathy, confusion, decreased libido, depression, emotional lability, euphoria, impaired concentration, irritability, paroniria.

Reproductive System: Dysmenorrhea, impotence, intermenstrual bleeding, vaginitis.

Respiratory System: Bronchitis, Bronchospasm, chest congestion, coughing, dry throat, dyspnea, epistaxis, halitosis, nasal congestion, nasal irritation, sinusitis, sneezing, sputum increased, upper respiratory infection, wheezing.

Skin and Appendages: Acne, bacterial skin infection, dry skin, eczema, edema, epidermal necrolysis, erythema, hematoma, pruritus, rash, urticaria.

Urinary System: Dysuria, micturition frequency, nocturia, polyuria, urinary retention.

The following additional adverse events have been reported with the use of loratadine; pseudoephedrine tablets: alopecia, altered salivation, amnesia, anaphylaxis, angioneurotic edema, blepharospasm, breast enlargement, breast pain, dermatitis, dry hair, erythema multiforme, hemoptysis, hepatic necrosis, hepatitis, jaundice, laryngitis, menorrhagia, nasal dryness, photosensitivity reaction, purpura, seizures, supraventricular tachyarrhythmias, and urinary discoloration.

Pseudoephedrine may cause mild CNS stimulation in hypersensitive patients. Nervousness, excitability, restlessness, dizziness, weakness, or insomnia may occur. Headache, drowsiness, tachycardia, palpitation, pressor activity, and cardiac arrhythmias have been reported. Sympathomimetic drugs have also been associated with other untoward effects, such as fear, anxiety, tenseness, tremor, hallucinations, seizures, pallor, respiratory difficulty, dysuria, and cardiovascular collapse.

DRUG ABUSE AND DEPENDENCE:

There is no information to indicate that abuse or dependency occurs with loratadine or combination of loratadine and pseudoephedrine. Pseudoephedrine, like other central nervous system stimulants, has been abused. At high doses, subjects commonly experience an elevation of mood, a sense of increased energy and alertness, and decreased appetite. Some individuals anxious, irritable, and loquacious. In addition to the marked euphoria, the user experiences a sense of markedly enhanced physical strength and mental capacity. With continued use, tolerance develops, the user increases the dose, and toxic signs and symptoms appear. Depression may follow rapid withdrawal.

OVERDOSAGE:

Somnolence, tachycardia, and headache have been reported with doses of 40 to 180 mg of loratadine; pseudoephedrine tablets. In the event of overdosage, general symptomatic and supportive measures should be instituted promptly and maintained for as long as necessary. Treatment of overdosage would reasonably consist of emesis (ipecac syrup), except in patients with impaired consciousness, followed by the administration of activated charcoal to absorb any remaining drug. If vomiting is unsuccessful, or contraindicated, gastric lavage should be performed with normal saline. Saline cathartics may also be of value for rapid dilution of bowel contents. Loratadine is not eliminated by hemodialysis. It is not known if loratadine is eliminated by peritoneal dialysis.

In large doses, sympathomimetics may give rise to giddiness, headache, nausea, vomiting, sweating, thirst, tachycardia, precordial pain, palpitations, difficulty in micturition, muscular weakness and tenseness, anxiety, restlessness, and insomnia. Many patients can present a toxic psychosis with delusions and hallucinations. Some may develop cardiac arrhythmias, circulatory collapse, convulsions, coma, and respiratory failure.

The oral LD_{50} values for the mixture of the two drugs were greater than 525 and 1839 mg/kg in mice and rats, respectively. Oral LD_{50} values for loratadine were greater than 5000 mg/kg in rats and mice. Doses of loratadine as high as 10 times the recommended daily clinical dose showed no effect in rats, mice, and monkeys.

DOSAGE AND ADMINISTRATION:

Adults and children 12 years of age and over: one tablet twice a day (every 12 hours) on an empty stomach. Because the doses of this fixed combination product cannot be individually titrated and hepatic insufficiency results in a reduced clearance of loratadine to a much greater extent than pseudoephedrine, loratadine; pseudoephedrine tablets should generally be avoided in patients with hepatic insufficiency. Patients with renal insufficiency (GFR <30 ml/min) should be given a lower initial dose (one tablet per day) because they have reduced clearance of loratadine and pseudoephedrine.

HOW SUPPLIED:

Claritin-D tablets contain 5 mg loratadine and 120 mg pseudoephedrine sulfate. Claritin-D tablets are white tablets branded in green with "Claritin-D", which are supplied in high density polyethylene bottles of 100. Also available are Claritin-D unit-of-use packages of 10 tablets and packages of 30 tablets (3 packs of 10 tablets each); and 10 × 10 tablets unit dose-hospital pack.

Keep Unit-of-Use packaging and Unit Dose-Hospital Pack in a dry place.

Store between 2° and 25°C (36° and 77°F).

HOW SUPPLIED - EQUIVALENTS NOT AVAILABLE:

Tablet, Coated, Sustained Action - Oral - 5 mg/120 mg

30's	$32.71	CLARITIN-D, Schering	00085-0635-05
100's	$109.06	CLARITIN-D, Schering	00085-0635-01
100's	$109.06	CLARITIN-D, Schering	00085-0635-04

LORAZEPAM *(001662)*

CATEGORIES: Anesthesia; Antianxiety Drugs; Antiarthritics; Antipsychotics/Antimanics; Anxiety; Anxiolytics, Sedatives, Hypnotic; Benzodiazepines; Central Nervous System Agents; Sedation; Sedatives; Sedatives/Hypnotics; Tranquilizers; Nausea and Vomiting*; DEA Class CIV; Sales > $500 Million; FDA Approval Pre 1982; Patent Expiration 1994 Apr; Top 200 Drugs

* Indication not approved by the FDA

BRAND NAMES: *Almazine*; *Anxiedin*; *Anxira*; *Anzepam*; *Aplacasse*; *Aplacassee*; *Apo-Lorazepam* (Canada); *Aripax*; **Ativan**; *Azurogen* (Japan); *Bonatranquan* (Germany); *Bonton*; *Control*; *Duralozam* (Germany); *Efasedan*; *Emotion*; *Emotival*; *Kalmalin*; *Larpose*; *Laubeel* (Germany); *Lopam*; *Lorabenz*; *Loram*; *Lorans*; *Lorapam*; *Lorat*; *Lorax*; *Lorazene*; *Lorazep*; *Lorazepam*; *Lorazin*; *Lorazon*; *Lorenin*; *Loridem*; *Lorivan*; *Lorsedal*; *Lorzem*; *Lozepam*; *Merlit*; *Nervistop L*; *Nervistopl*; *NIC*; *Novhepar*; *Novolorazem* (Canada); *Orfidal*; *Punktyl* (Germany); *Renaquil*; *Rocosgen* (Japan); *Sedatival*; *Sedizepan*; *Sidenar*; *Silence*; *Sinestron* (Mexico); *Somnium*; *Stapam*; *Tavor* (Germany); *Temesta* (France); *Titus*; *Tranqipam*; *Trapax*; *Trapex*; *Upan* (Japan); *Wintin*; *Wypax* (Japan)

(International brand names outside U.S. in italics)

FORMULARIES: Aetna; BC-BS; FHP; Foundation; PCS

COST OF THERAPY: $4.96 (Anxiety; Tablet; 1 mg; 2/day; 120 days)

DESCRIPTION:

Lorazepam, an antianxiety agent, has the chemical formula, 7-chloro-5-(*o*-chlorophenyl)-1,3-dihydro-3-hydroxy-2*H*-1,4-benzodiazepin-2-one.

Tablets: It is a nearly white powder almost insoluble in water. Each lorazepam tablet, to be taken orally, contains 0.5 mg, 1 mg, or 2 mg of lorazepam. The inactive ingredients present are lactose and other ingredients.

Injection: Lorazepam injection, a benzodiazepine with antianxiety and sedative effects, is intended for intramuscular or intravenous route of administration. Lorazepam is a nearly white powder almost insoluble in water. Each ml of sterile injection contains either 2.0 or 4.0 mg of lorazepam, 0.18 ml polyethylene glycol 400 in propylene glycol with 2.0% benzyl alcohol as preservative.

CLINICAL PHARMACOLOGY:

TABLETS

Studies in healthy volunteers show that in single high doses lorazepam has a tranquilizing action on the central nervous system with no appreciable effect on the respiratory or cardiovascular systems.

Lorazepam is readily absorbed with an absolute bioavailability of 90 percent. Peak concentrations in plasma occur approximately 2 hours following administration. The peak plasma level of lorazepam from a 2 mg dose is approximately 20 ng/ml.

CLINICAL PHARMACOLOGY: *(cont'd)*

The mean half-life of unconjugated lorazepam in human plasma is about 12 hours and for its major metabolite, lorazepam glucuronide, about 18 hours. At clinically relevant concentrations, lorazepam is approximately 85% bound to plasma proteins. Lorazepam is rapidly conjugated at its 3-hydroxy group into lorazepam glucuronide which is then excreted in the urine. Lorazepam glucuronide has no demonstrable CNS activity in animals.

The plasma levels of lorazepam are proportional to the dose given. There is no evidence of accumulation of lorazepam on administration up to six months.

Studies comparing young and elderly subjects have shown that the pharmacokinetics of lorazepam remain unaltered with advancing age.

INJECTION

Intravenous or intramuscular administration of the recommended dose of 2 mg to 4 mg of lorazepam injection to adult patients is followed by dose-related effects of sedation (sleepiness or drowsiness), relief of preoperative anxiety, and lack of recall of events related to the day of surgery in the majority of patients. The clinical sedation (sleepiness or drowsiness) thus noted is such that the majority of patients are able to respond to simple instructions whether they are give the appearance of being awake or asleep. The lack of recall is relative rather than absolute, as determined under conditions of careful patient questioning and testing, using props designed to enhance recall. The majority of events or recognizing props from before surgery. The lack of recall and recognition was optimum within 2 hours following intramuscular administration and 15 to 20 minutes after intravenous injection.

The intended effects of the recommended adult dose of lorazepam injection usually last 6 to 8 hours. In rare instances and where patients received greater than the recommended dose, excessive sleepiness and prolonged lack of recall were noted. As with other benzodiazepines, unsteadiness, enhanced sensitivity to CNS-depressant effects of ethyl alcohol and other drugs were noted in isolated and rare cases for greater than 24 hours.

Studies in healthy adult volunteers reveal that intravenous lorazepam in doses up to 3.5 mg/70 kg does not alter sensitivity to the respiratory stimulating effect of carbon dioxide and does not enhance the respiratory depressant effects of doses of meperidine up to 100 mg/70 mg (also determined by carbon dioxide challenge) as long as patients remain sufficiently awake to undergo testing. Upper airway obstruction has been observed in rare instances where the patient received greater than the recommended dose and was excessively sleepy and difficult to arouse. (See WARNINGS and ADVERSE REACTIONS.)

Clinically employed doses or lorazepam injectable do not greatly affect the circulatory system in the supine position or employing a 70-degree tilt test. Doses of 8 to 10 mg of intravenous lorazepam (2 to 2.5 times the maximum recommended dosage) will produce loss of lid reflexes within 15 minutes.

Studies in six (6) healthy young adults who lorazepam injection and no other drugs revealed that visual tracking (the ability to keep a moving line centered) was impaired for a mean of eight (8) hours following administration of 4 mg of intramuscular lorazepam and four (4) hours following administration of 2 mg intramuscularly with considerable subject variation. Similar findings were noted with pentobarbital, 150 mg and 75 mg. Although this study showed that both lorazepam and pentobarbital interfered with eye-hand coordination, the data are insufficient to predict when it would be safe to operate a motor vehicle or engage in a hazardous occupation or sport.

PHARMACOKINETICS

Injectable lorazepam is readily absorbed when given intramuscularly. Peak plasma concentrations occur approximately 60 to 90 minutes following administration and appear to be dose-related, e.g., a 2.0 mg dose provides a level of approximately 20 ng/ml and a 4.0 mg dose approximately 40 ng/ml in plasma. The mean half-life or lorazepam is about 16 hours when given intravenously or intramuscularly. Lorazepam is rapidly conjugated at the 3-hydroxyl group into its major metabolite, lorazepam glucuronide, which is then excreted in the urine. Lorazepam glucuronide has no demonstrable CNS activity in animals. When 5 mg of intravenous lorazepam was administered to volunteers once a day for four consecutive days, a steady state of free lorazepam was achieved by the second day (approximately 52 ng/ml of plasma three hours after the first dose and approximately 62 ng/ml three hours after each subsequent dose, one day apart). At clinically relevant concentrations, lorazepam is bound 85% to plasma proteins.

INDICATIONS AND USAGE:

Tablets: Lorazepam is indicated for the management of anxiety disorders or for the short-term relief of the symptoms of anxiety or anxiety associated with depressive symptoms. Anxiety or tension associated with the stress of everyday life usually does not require treatment with an anxiolytic.

The effectiveness of lorazepam in long-term use, that is, more than 4 months, has not been assessed by systematic clinical studies. The physician should periodically reassess the usefulness of the drug for the individual patient.

Injection: Lorazepam injection is indicated in adult patients for preanesthetic medication, producing sedation (sleepiness or drowsiness), relief of anxiety, and a decreased ability to recall events related to the day of surgery. It is most useful in those patients who are anxious about their surgical procedure and who would prefer to have diminished recall of the events of the day of surgery (see Information for Patients).

CONTRAINDICATIONS:

Tablets: Lorazepam is contraindicated in patients with known sensitivity to the benzodiazepines or with acute narrow-angle glaucoma.

Injection: Lorazepam injection is indicated in adult patients for preanesthetic medication, producing sedation (sleepiness or drowsiness), relief of anxiety, and a decreased ability to recall events related to the day of surgery. It is most useful in those patients who are anxious about their surgical procedure and who would prefer to have diminished recall of the day of surgery (Information for Patients).

WARNINGS:

TABLETS

Lorazepam is not recommended for use in patients with a primary depressive disorder or psychosis. As with all patients on CNS-acting drugs, patients receiving lorazepam should be warned not to operate dangerous machinery or motor vehicles and that their tolerance for alcohol and other CNS depressants will be diminished.

Physical And Psychological Dependence

Withdrawal symptoms, similar in character to those noted with barbiturates and alcohol (convulsions, tremor, abdominal and muscle cramps, vomiting, and sweating), have occurred following abrupt discontinuance of lorazepam. The more severe withdrawal symptoms have usually been limited to those patients who received excessive doses over an extended period of time. Generally milder withdrawal symptoms (*e.g.,* dysphoria and insomnia) have been reported following abrupt discontinuance of benzodiazepines taken continuously at therapeutic levels for several months. Consequently, after extended therapy, abrupt discontinuation should generally be avoided and a gradual dosage-tapering schedule followed. Addiction-prone individuals (such as drug addicts or alcoholics) should be under careful surveillance when receiving lorazepam or other psychotropic agents because of the predisposition of such patients to habituation and dependence.

INJECTION

PRIOR TO INTRAVENOUS USE, ATIVAN INJECTION MUST BE DILUTED WITH AN EQUAL AMOUNT OF COMPATIBLE DILUENT (SEE DOSAGE AND ADMINISTRATION). INTRAVENOUS INJECTION SHOULD BE MADE SLOWLY AND WITH REPEATED ASPIRATION. CARE SHOULD BE TAKEN TO DETERMINE THAT ANY INJECTION WILL NOT BE INTRAARTERIAL AND THAT PERIVASCULAR EXTRAVASATION WILL NOT TAKE PLACE.

PARTIAL AIRWAY OBSTRUCTION MAY OCCUR IN HEAVILY SEDATED PATIENTS. INTRAVENOUS LORAZEPAM, WHEN GIVEN ALONE IN GREATER THAN THE RECOMMENDED DOSE, OR AT THE RECOMMENDED DOSE AND ACCOMPANIED BY OTHER DRUGS USED DURING THE ADMINISTRATION OF ANESTHESIA, MAY PRODUCE HEAVY SEDATION; THEREFORE, EQUIPMENT NECESSARY TO MAINTAIN A PATENT AIRWAY AND TO SUPPORT RESPIRATION/VENTILATION SHOULD BE AVAILABLE.

There is no evidence to support the use of lorazepam injection in coma, shock or acute alcohol intoxication at this time. Since the liver os the most likely site of conjugation of lorazepam and since excretion of conjugated lorazepam (glucuronide) is a renal function, this drug is not recommended for use in patients with hepatic and/or renal failure. This does not preclude use of the drug in patients with mild-to-moderate hepatic or renal disease, the lowest effective dose should be considered since drug effect may be prolonged. Experience with other benzodiazepines and limited experience with parenteral lorazepam has demonstrated that tolerance to alcoholic beverages and other central nervous system depressants is diminished when used concomitantly.

As is true of similar CNS-acting drugs, patients receiving injectable lorazepam should not operate machinery or engage in hazardous occupations or drive a motor vehicle for a period of 34 to 48 hours. Impairment of performance may persist for greater intervals because of extremes of age, concomitant use of other drugs, stress of surgery, or the general condition of the patient.

Clinical trials have shown that patients over the age of 50 years may have a more profound and prolonged sedation with intravenous lorazepam. Ordinarily, an initial dose of 2 mg may be adequate unless a greater degree of lack of recall is desired.

As with all central nervous system depressant drugs, care should be exercised in patients given injectable lorazepam that premature ambulation may result in injury from falling.

There is no added beneficial effect to the addition of scopolamine to injectable lorazepam, and their combined effect may result in an increased incidence of sedation, hallucination, and irrational behavior.

Pregnancy

LORAZEPAM MAY CAUSE FETAL DAMAGE WHEN ADMINISTERED TO PREGNANT WOMEN. An increased risk of congenital malformations associated with the use of minor tranquilizers (chlordiazepoxide, diazepam, and meprobamate) during the first trimester of pregnancy has been suggested in several studies. In humans, blood levels obtained from umbilical cord blood indicate placental transfer of lorazepam and lorazepam glucuronide.

Lorazepam injection should not be used during pregnancy. There are insufficient date regarding obstetrical safety of parenteral lorazepam, including use in cesarean section. Such use, therefore,is not recommended.

Reproductive studies in animals were performed in mice, rats, and two strains of rabbits. Occasional anomalies (reduction of tarsals, tibia, metatarsals, malrotated limbs, gastroschisis, malformed skull, and microphthalmia) were seen in drug-related rabbits without relationship to dosage. Although all of these anomalies were not present in the concurrent control group, they have all been reported to occur randomly in historical controls. At doses of 40 mg/kg orally or 4 mg/kg intravenously and higher, there was evidence of fetal resorption and increased fetal loss in rabbits which was not seen at lower doses.

Endoscopic Procedures

The are insufficient data to support the use of lorazepam injection for outpatient endoscopic procedures. Inpatient endoscopic procedures require adequate recovery room observations.

Pharyngeal reflexes are not impaired when lorazepam injection is used for peroral endoscopic procedures; therefore, adequate topical or regional anesthesia is recommended to minimize reflex activity associated with such procedures.

PRECAUTIONS:

TABLETS

In patients with depression accompanying anxiety, a possibility for suicide should be borne in mind.

For elderly or debilitated patients, the initial daily dosage should not exceed 2 mg in order to avoid oversedation.

The usual precautions for treating patients with impaired renal or hepatic function should be observed.

In patients where gastrointestinal or cardiovascular disorders coexist with anxiety, it should be noted that lorazepam has not been shown to be of significant benefit in treating the gastrointestinal or cardiovascular component.

Esophageal dilation occurred in rats treated with lorazepam for more than one year at 6 mg/kg/day. The no-effect dose was 1.25 mg/kg/day (approximately 6 times the maximum human therapeutic dose of 10 mg per day). The effect was reversible only when the treatment was withdrawn within two months of first observation of the phenomenon. The clinical significance of this is unknown. However, use of lorazepam for prolonged periods and in geriatric patients requires caution, and there should be frequent monitoring for symptoms of upper G.I. disease.

Safety and effectiveness of lorazepam in children of less than 12 years have not been established.

Information for the Patient: To assure the safe and effective use of lorazepam, patients should be informed that, since benzodiazepines may produce psychological and physical dependence, it is advisable that they consult with their physician before either increasing the dose or abruptly discontinuing this drug.

Essential Laboratory Tests: Some patients on lorazepam have developed leukopenia, and some have had elevations of LDH. As with other benzodiazepines, periodic blood counts and liver-function tests are recommended for patients on long-term therapy.

Carcinogenesis And Mutagenesis: No evidence of carcinogenic potential emerged in rats during an 18-month study with lorazepam. No studies regarding mutagenesis have been performed.

Pregnancy: Reproductive studies in animals were performed in mice, rats, and two strains of rabbits. Occasional anomalies (reduction of tarsals, tibia, metatarsals, malrotated limbs, gastroschisis, malformed skull, and microphthalmia) were seen in drug-treated rabbits without relationship to dosage. Although all of these anomalies were not present in the concurrent

PRECAUTIONS: *(cont'd)*

control group, they have been reported to occur randomly in historical controls. At doses of 40 mg/kg and higher, there was evidence of fetal resorption and increased fetal loss in rabbits which was not seen at lower doses.

The clinical significance of the above findings is not known. However, an increased risk of congenital malformations associated with the use of minor tranquilizers (chlordiazepoxide, diazepam, and meprobamate) during the first trimester of pregnancy has been suggested in several studies. Because the use of these drugs is rarely a matter of urgency, the use of lorazepam during this period should almost always be avoided. The possibility that a woman of childbearing potential may be pregnant at the time of institution of therapy should be considered. Patients should be advised that if they become pregnant, they should communicate with their physician about the desirability of discontinuing the drug.

In humans, blood levels obtained from umbilical cord blood indicate placental transfer of lorazepam and lorazepam glucuronide.

Nursing Mothers: It is not known whether oral lorazepam is excreted in human milk like the other benzodiazepine tranquilizers. As a general rule, nursing should not be undertaken while a patient is on a drug, since many drugs are excreted in human milk.

Pediatric Use: Safety and effectiveness of lorazepam in children of less than 12 years of age have not been established.

DRUG INTERACTIONS:

TABLETS

Clinically Significant Drug Interactions: The benzodiazepines, including lorazepam, produce CNS-depressant effects when administered with such medications as barbiturates or alcohol.

INJECTION

Lorazepam injection, like other injectable benzodiazepines, produces depression of the central nervous system when administered with ethyl alcohol, phenothiazines, barbiturates, MAO inhibitors, and other antidepressants.When scopolamine is used concomitantly with injectable lorazepam, an increased incidence of sedation, hallucinations, and irrational behavior has been observed.

ADVERSE REACTIONS:

Adverse reactions, if they occur, are usually observed at the beginning of therapy and generally disappear on continued medication or upon decreasing the dose. In a sample of about 3,500 anxious patients, the most frequent adverse reaction to lorazepam is sedation (15.9%), followed by dizziness (6.9%), weakness (4.2%), and unsteadiness (3.4%). Less frequent adverse reactions are disorientation, depression, nausea, change in appetite, headache, sleep disturbance, agitation, dermatological symptoms, eye-function disturbance, together with various gastrointestinal symptoms and autonomic manifestations. The incidence of sedation and unsteadiness increased with age.

Small decreases in blood pressure have been noted but are not clinically significant, probably being related to the relief of anxiety produced by lorazepam.

Transient amnesia or memory impairment has been reported in association with the use of benzodiazepines.

OVERDOSAGE:

TABLETS

In the management of overdosage with any drug, it should be borne in mind that multiple agents may have been taken.

Symptoms: Overdosage of benzodiazepines is usually manifested by varying degrees of central nervous system depression ranging from drowsiness to coma. In mild cases, symptoms include drowsiness, mental confusion, and lethargy. In more serious cases, and especially when other drugs or alcohol were ingested, sypmtoms may include ataxia, hypotonia, hypotension, hypnotic state, stage one (1) to three (3) coma, and very rarely, death.

Management: Induced vomiting and/or gastric lavage should be undertaken, followed by general supportive care, monitoring of vital signs, and close observation of the patient. Hypotension, though unlikely, usually may be controlled with Levarterenol Bitartrate Injection, USP. The usefulness of dialysis has not been determined.

Flumazenil: The benzodiazepine antagonist flumazenil may be used in hospitalized patients as an adjunct to, not as a substitute for, proper management of benzodiazepine overdose. Prior to administration of flumazenil, necessary measures should be instutited to secure airway, ventilation, and intravenous access. Patients treated with flumazenil should be monitored for re-sedation, respiratory depression, and other residual benzodiazepine effects for an appropriate period after treatment.

The prescriber should be aware of a risk of seizure in association with flumazenil treatment, particularly in long-term benzodiazepine users and in cyclic antidepressant overdose. The complete flumazenil package insert including **CONTRAINDICATIONS, WARNINGS,** and PRECAUTIONS should be constituted prior to use.

INJECTION

Symptoms: Overdosage of benzodiazepines is usually manifested by varying degrees of central nervous system depression, ranging from drowsiness to coma. In mild cases symptoms include drowsiness, mental confusion, and lethargy. In more serious examples, symptoms may include ataxia, hypotonia, hypotension, hypnosis, stages one (1) to three (3) coma, and very rarely death.

Management: Treatment of overdosage is mainly supportive until the drug is eliminated from the body. Vital signs and fluid balance should be carefully monitored. An adequate airway should be maintained and assisted respiration used as needed. With normally functioning kidneys, forced diureses with intravenous fluids and electrolytes may accelerate elimination of benzodiazepines from the body. In addition, osmotic diuretics, such as mannitol, may be effective as adjunctive measures. In more critical situations, renal dialysis and exchange blood transfusions may be indicated.

DOSAGE AND ADMINISTRATION:

TABLETS

Lorazepam is administered orally. For optimal results, dose, frequency of administration, and duration of therapy should be individualized according to patient response. To facilitate this, 0.5 mg, 1 mg, and 2 mg tablets are available.

The usual range is 2 to 6 mg/day given in divided doses, the largest dose being taken before bedtime, but the daily dosage may vary from 1 to 10 mg/day. •

For anxiety, most patients require an initial dose of 2 to 3 mg/day given b.i.d. or t.i.d.

For insomnia due to anxiety or transient situational stress, a single daily dose of 2 to 4 mg may be given, usually at bedtime.

For elderly or debilitated patients, an initial dosage of 1 to 2 mg/day in divided doses is recommended, to be adjusted as needed and tolerated.

The dosage of lorazepam should be increased gradually when needed to help avoid adverse effects. When higher dosage is indicated, the evening dose should be increased before the daytime doses.

DOSAGE AND ADMINISTRATION: *(cont'd)*

INJECTION

Intramuscular Injection: For the designated indications as a premedicant, the usual recommended dose of lorazepam for intramuscular injection is 0.05 mg/kg up to a maximum of 4 mg. As with all premedicant drugs, the dose should be individualized. See also CLINICAL PHARMACOLOGY, and WARNINGS. Doses of other central nervous system depressant drugs should be ordinarily reduced. *For optimum effect, measured as lack of recall, intramuscular lorazepam should be administered at least two hours before the anticipated operative procedure.* Narcotic analgesics should be administered at their usual preoperative time. There are insufficient data to support efficacy to make dosage recommendations for intramuscular lorazepam in patients less than 18 years of age; therefore, such use is not recommended.

INTRAVENOUS INJECTION

For the primary purpose of sedation and relief of anxiety, the usual recommended initial dose of lorazepam for intravenous injection is 2 mg total, or 0.02 mg/lb (0.044 mg/kg), whichever is smaller. This dose will suffice for sedating most adult patients and should not ordinarily be exceeded in patients over 50 years of age. In those patients in whom a greater likelihood of lack of recall for perioperative events would be beneficial, larger doses as high as 0.05 mg/kg up to a total of 4 mg may be administered. (See CLINICAL PHARMACOLOGY and WARNINGS). Doses of other injectable central nervous system depressant drugs should ordinarily be reduced (see PRECAUTIONS). *For optimum effect, measured as lack of recall, intravenous lorazepam should be administered 15 to 20 minutes before the anticipated operative procedure.*

EQUIPMENT NECESSARY TO MAINTAIN A PATENT AIRWAY SHOULD BE IMMEDIATELY AVAILABLE PRIOR TO INTRAVENOUS ADMINISTRATION OF LORAZEPAM (see WARNINGS).

There are insufficient data to support efficacy or make dosage recommendations for intravenous lorazepam in patients less than 18 years of age; therefore, such use is not recommended.

ADMINISTRATION

When given intramuscularly, lorazepam injection, undiluted, should be injected deep in the muscle mass.

Injectable lorazepam can be used with atropine sulfate, narcotic analgesics, other parenterally used analgesics, commonly used anesthetics, and muscle relaxants.

Immediately prior to intravenous use, lorazepam injection must be diluted with an equal volume of compatible solution. When properly diluted the drug may be injected directly into a vein or into the tubing of an existing intravenous infusion. The rate of injection should not exceed 2.0 mg per minute.

Parenteral drug products should be inspected visually for particulate matter and discoloration prior to administration, whenever solution and container permit. Do not use if solution is discolored or contains a precipitate.

Lorazepam injection is compatible for dilution purposes with the following solutions: sterile water for injection, USP; sodium chloride injection, USP; 5% dextrose injection, USP.

PATIENT INFORMATION:

Lorazepam is a benzodiazepine used for the treatment of anxiety, anxiety with depression, and insomnia. Inform your physician if you are pregnant or nursing. Lorazepam may cause dizziness and drowsiness; use caution while driving or operating hazardous machinery. Do not take any other sedating drugs or drink alcohol while taking this medication. Lorazepam may be habit forming. Withdrawal symptoms may occur after you stop taking it. This medication may be taken with or without food.

HOW SUPPLIED:

Lorazepam tablets are available in the following dosage strengths:

0.5 mg, white, five-sided tablet with a raised "A" on one side and "WYETH" and "81" on reverse side.

1 mg, white, five-sided tablet with a raised "A" on one side and "WYETH" and "64" on scored reversed side.

2 mg, white, five-sided tablet with a raised "A" on one side and "WYETH" and "65" on scored reverse side.

Store at controlled room temperature. Keep tightly closed. Dispense in tight container. Protect from light. Use carton to protect contents from light.

For IM or IV injection. Protect from light. Keep in a refrigerator.

HOW SUPPLIED - RATED THERAPEUTICALLY EQUIVALENT:

Injection, Solution - Intramuscular; - 2 mg/ml

0.5 ml x 10	**$126.69**	**ATIVAN, Wyeth Labs**	**00008-0581-05**
0.5 ml x 10	**$126.69**	**ATIVAN, Wyeth Labs**	**00008-0581-07**
1 ml	$9.27	Lorazepam, Sanofi Winthrop	00024-1155-06
1 ml	$9.78	Lorazepam, Marsam	00209-4578-20
1 ml	$9.78	Lorazepam, Steris Labs	00402-1013-01
1 ml	**$12.01**	**ATIVAN, Wyeth Labs**	**00008-0581-04**
1 ml	$277.88	Lorazepam, Abbott	00074-6776-01
1 ml x 10	$53.82	Lorazepam, Sanofi Winthrop	00024-1155-30
1 ml x 10	$95.76	Lorazepam, Sanofi Winthrop	00024-1155-10
1 ml x 10	**$126.69**	**ATIVAN, Wyeth Labs**	**00008-0581-02**
1 ml x 10	**$126.69**	**ATIVAN, Wyeth Labs**	**00008-0581-06**
1 ml x 10	**$126.69**	**ATIVAN, Wyeth Labs**	**00008-0581-52**
1 ml x 10	**$126.69**	**ATIVAN, Wyeth Labs**	**00008-0581-53**
2 ml	$247.00	Lorazepam, Abbott	00074-6778-01
2 ml x 10	$80.94	Lorazepam, Sanofi Winthrop	00024-1156-30
10 ml	$81.91	Lorazepam, Sanofi Winthrop	00024-1155-07
10 ml	$90.59	Lorazepam, Schein Pharm (US)	00364-3048-54
10 ml	$90.59	Lorazepam, Steris Labs	00402-1013-10
10 ml	**$107.00**	**ATIVAN, Wyeth Labs**	**00008-0581-01**
10 ml x 25	$1852.50	Lorazepam, Abbott	00074-6780-01

Injection, Solution - Intramuscular; - 4 mg/ml

1 ml	$11.49	Lorazepam, Schein Pharm (US)	00364-3049-51
1 ml	$11.49	Lorazepam, Steris Labs	00402-1014-01
1 ml	**$14.69**	**ATIVAN, Wyeth Labs**	**00008-0570-04**
1 ml	$277.88	Lorazepam, Abbott	00074-6779-01
1 ml	$339.63	Lorazepam, Abbott	00074-6777-01
1 ml x 10	$109.88	Lorazepam, Sanofi Winthrop	00024-1156-10
1 ml x 10	**$126.69**	**ATIVAN, Wyeth Labs**	**00008-0570-50**
1 ml x 10	**$126.69**	**ATIVAN, Wyeth Labs**	**00008-0570-51**
1 ml x 10	**$152.06**	**ATIVAN, Wyeth Labs**	**00008-0570-02**
1 ml x 10	**$152.06**	**ATIVAN, Wyeth Labs**	**00008-0570-05**
10 ml	$98.80	Lorazepam, Abbott	00074-6781-01
10 ml	$114.05	Lorazepam, Schein Pharm (US)	00364-3049-54
10 ml	$114.05	Lorazepam, Steris Labs	00402-1014-10
10 ml	**$133.74**	**ATIVAN, Wyeth Labs**	**00008-0570-01**

HOW SUPPLIED - RATED THERAPEUTICALLY EQUIVALENT: *(cont'd)*

Tablet - Oral - 0.5 mg

100's	$16.25	Lorazepam, Duramed Pharms	51285-0647-02
500's	$58.00	Lorazepam, Duramed Pharms	51285-0647-04

Tablet - Oral - 1 mg

100's	$23.00	Lorazepam, Duramed Pharms	51285-0648-02
500's	$84.00	Lorazepam, Duramed Pharms	51285-0648-04

Tablet - Oral - 2 mg

100's	$30.00	Lorazepam, Duramed Pharms	51285-0649-02
500's	$92.00	Lorazepam, Duramed Pharms	51285-0649-04

Tablet, Uncoated - Oral - 0.5 mg

30's	$6.97	Lorazepam, Talbert Phcy	44514-0098-18
100's	$1.73	Lorazepam, United Res	00677-1056-01
100's	$1.73	Lorazepam, Geneva Pharms	00781-1403-01
100's	$1.73	Lorazepam, Mutual Pharm	53489-0357-01
100's	$1.73	Lorazepam, H.C.F.A. F F P	99999-1662-01
100's	$4.81	Lorazepam, Martec Pharms	52555-0485-01
100's	$9.35	Lorazepam, Elkins Sinn	00641-4000-86
100's	$11.02	Lorazepam, Halsey Drug	00879-0565-01
100's	$11.38	Lorazepam, Watson Labs	52544-0332-01
100's	$12.05	Lorazepam, Qualitest Pharms	00603-4243-21
100's	$12.70	Lorazepam, Purepac Pharm	00228-2057-10
100's	$13.10	Lorazepam, Major Pharms	00904-1500-60
100's	$13.22	Lorazepam, Schein Pharm (US)	00364-0793-01
100's	$13.36	Lorazepam, Aligen Independ	00405-0108-01
100's	$13.43	Lorazepam, HL Moore Drug Exch	00839-7145-06
100's	$13.43	Lorazepam, HL Moore Drug Exch	00839-7902-06
100's	$13.50	Lorazepam, Royce	51875-0240-01
100's	$13.72	Lorazepam, Caremark	00339-4017-12
100's	$14.50	Lorazepam, Geneva Pharms	50752-0293-05
100's	$15.84	Lorazepam, Bristol Myers Squibb	00003-0298-50
100's	$15.95	Lorazepam, Goldline Labs	00182-1806-01
100's	$16.50	Lorazepam, Warner Chilcott	00047-0431-24
100's	$16.55	Lorazepam, Rugby	00536-3959-01
100's	$16.95	Lorazepam, Mylan	00378-0321-01
100's	$24.84	Lorazepam, Parmed Pharms	00349-8461-01
100's	$28.66	Lorazepam, Vangard Labs	00615-0450-47
100's	$32.70	Lorazepam, Geneva Pharms	00781-1403-13
100's	$33.05	Lorazepam, Goldline Labs	00182-1806-89
100's	$35.69	Lorazepam, Vangard Labs	00615-0450-13
100's	**$63.41**	**ATIVAN, Wyeth Labs**	**00008-0081-02**
250's	$4.32	Lorazepam, H.C.F.A. F F P	99999-1662-02
250's	$40.55	Lorazepam, Rugby	00536-3959-02
500's	$8.65	Lorazepam, United Res	00677-1056-05
500's	$8.65	Lorazepam, Geneva Pharms	00781-1403-05
500's	$8.65	Lorazepam, Mutual Pharm	53489-0357-05
500's	$8.65	Lorazepam, H.C.F.A. F F P	99999-1662-03
500's	$31.50	Lorazepam, Major Pharms	00904-1500-40
500's	$34.30	Lorazepam, Watson Labs	52544-0332-05
500's	$40.00	Lorazepam, Elkins Sinn	00641-4000-88
500's	$47.16	Lorazepam, Halsey Drug	00879-0565-05
500's	$48.53	Lorazepam, HL Moore Drug Exch	00839-7145-12
500's	$49.81	Lorazepam, Qualitest Pharms	00603-4243-28
500's	$55.98	Lorazepam, Purepac Pharm	00228-2057-50
500's	$55.99	Lorazepam, Aligen Independ	00405-0108-02
500's	$56.45	Lorazepam, Geneva Pharms	50752-0293-08
500's	$56.50	Lorazepam, Schein Pharm (US)	00364-0793-05
500's	$57.60	Lorazepam, Royce	51875-0240-02
500's	$59.50	Lorazepam, Martec Pharms	52555-0485-05
500's	$59.95	Lorazepam, Warner Chilcott	00047-0431-30
500's	$75.75	Lorazepam, Goldline Labs	00182-1806-05
500's	$75.95	Lorazepam, Mylan	00378-0321-05
500's	$76.99	Lorazepam, Bristol Myers Squibb	00003-0298-60
500's	**$308.20**	**ATIVAN, Wyeth Labs**	**00008-0081-03**
750's	$232.35	Lorazepam, Glasgow Pharm	60809-0505-55
750's	$232.35	Lorazepam, Glasgow Pharm	60809-0505-72
1000's	$17.30	Lorazepam, H.C.F.A. F F P	99999-1662-04
1000's	$50.40	Lorazepam, Major Pharms	00904-1500-80
1000's	$67.22	Lorazepam, Watson Labs	52544-0332-10
1000's	$75.90	Lorazepam, Geneva Pharms	50752-0293-09
1000's	$79.00	Lorazepam, Royce	51875-0240-04
1000's	$79.95	Lorazepam, Halsey Drug	00879-0565-10
1000's	$120.00	Lorazepam, Rugby	00536-3959-10
1000's	$124.19	Lorazepam, HL Moore Drug Exch	00839-7902-16
1000's	$153.70	Lorazepam, Bristol Myers Squibb	00003-0298-75

Tablet, Uncoated - Oral - 1 mg

30's	$4.92	Lorazepam, Talbert Phcy	44514-0099-18
100's	$2.07	Lorazepam, United Res	00677-1057-01
100's	$2.07	Lorazepam, Geneva Pharms	00781-1404-01
100's	$2.07	Lorazepam, Mutual Pharm	53489-0358-01
100's	$2.07	Lorazepam, H.C.F.A. F F P	99999-1662-05
100's	$14.51	Lorazepam, Halsey Drug	00879-0572-01
100's	$15.15	Lorazepam, Watson Labs	52544-0333-01
100's	$15.95	Lorazepam, Qualitest Pharms	00603-4244-21
100's	$16.30	Lorazepam 1, Major Pharms	00904-1501-60
100's	$18.25	Lorazepam, Royce	51875-0241-01
100's	$18.43	Lorazepam, Caremark	00339-4019-12
100's	$19.05	Lorazepam, Schein Pharm (US)	00364-0794-01
100's	$19.26	Lorazepam, Purepac Pharm	00228-2059-10
100's	$19.91	Lorazepam, HL Moore Drug Exch	00839-7146-06
100's	$19.91	Lorazepam, HL Moore Drug Exch	00839-7903-06
100's	$19.95	Lorazepam, Geneva Pharms	50752-0294-05
100's	$19.98	Lorazepam, Aligen Independ	00405-0109-01
100's	$20.40	Lorazepam, Martec Pharms	52555-0486-01
100's	$21.10	Lorazepam, Bristol Myers Squibb	00003-0408-50
100's	$21.95	Lorazepam, Goldline Labs	00182-1807-01
100's	$23.26	Lorazepam, Warner Chilcott	00047-0432-24
100's	$23.95	Lorazepam, Mylan	00378-0457-01
100's	$23.95	Lorazepam, Rugby	00536-3960-01
100's	$34.81	Lorazepam, Vangard Labs	00615-0451-47
100's	$35.10	Lorazepam, Geneva Pharms	00781-1404-13
100's	$35.45	Lorazepam, Goldline Labs	00182-1807-89
100's	$35.76	Lorazepam 1, Major Pharms	00904-1501-61
100's	$35.96	Lorazepam, Parmed Pharms	00349-8462-01
100's	$38.29	Lorazepam, Vangard Labs	00615-0451-13
100's	**$82.58**	**ATIVAN, Wyeth Labs**	**00008-0064-02**
500's	$10.35	Lorazepam, United Res	00677-1057-05
500's	$10.35	Lorazepam, Geneva Pharms	00781-1404-05
500's	$10.35	Lorazepam, Mutual Pharm	53489-0358-05
500's	$10.35	Lorazepam, H.C.F.A. F F P	99999-1662-06
500's	$42.47	Lorazepam, Watson Labs	52544-0333-05

HOW SUPPLIED - RATED THERAPEUTICALLY EQUIVALENT: *(cont'd)*

500's	$47.90	Lorazepam, Elkins Sinn	00641-4001-88
500's	$53.26	Lorazepam, Aligen Independ	00405-0109-02
500's	$54.35	Lorazepam, Qualitest Pharms	00603-4244-28
500's	$59.25	Lorazepam, Geneva Pharms	50752-0294-08
500's	$64.34	Lorazepam, Halsey Drug	00879-0572-05
500's	$82.00	Lorazepam, Royce	51875-0241-02
500's	$84.85	Lorazepam, Martec Pharms	52555-0486-05
500's	$88.72	Lorazepam, Lederle Pharm	00005-3172-31
500's	$96.30	Lorazepam, Purepac Pharm	00228-2059-50
500's	$96.50	Lorazepam, Schein Pharm (US)	00364-0794-05
500's	$102.01	Lorazepam, Bristol Myers Squibb	00003-0408-60
500's	$104.24	Lorazepam, Goldline Labs	00182-1807-05
500's	$104.25	Lorazepam, Warner Chilcott	00047-0432-30
500's	$104.25	Lorazepam, Mylan	00378-0457-05
500's	$104.25	Lorazepam, Rugby	00536-3960-05
500's	**$399.55**	**ATIVAN, Wyeth Labs**	**00008-0064-03**
750's	$249.38	Lorazepam, Glasgow Pharm	60809-0504-55
750's	$249.38	Lorazepam, Glasgow Pharm	60809-0504-72
1000's	$20.70	Lorazepam, United Res	00677-1057-10
1000's	$20.70	Lorazepam, Geneva Pharms	00781-1404-10
1000's	$20.70	Lorazepam, Watson Labs	52544-0333-10
1000's	$20.70	Lorazepam, H.C.F.A. F F P	99999-1662-07
1000's	$84.55	Lorazepam, Elkins Sinn	00641-4001-89
1000's	$87.78	Lorazepam, Qualitest Pharms	00603-4244-32
1000's	$89.90	Lorazepam 1, Major Pharms	00904-1501-80
1000's	$97.50	Lorazepam, Royce	51875-0241-04
1000's	$98.50	Lorazepam, Geneva Pharms	50752-0294-09
1000's	$100.91	Lorazepam, Halsey Drug	00879-0572-10
1000's	$126.29	Lorazepam, HL Moore Drug Exch	00839-7146-16
1000's	$145.13	Lorazepam, HL Moore Drug Exch	00839-7903-16
1000's	$165.54	Lorazepam, Lederle Pharm	00005-3172-34
1000's	$179.55	Lorazepam, Goldline Labs	00182-1807-10
1000's	$179.95	Lorazepam, Mylan	00378-0457-10
1000's	$179.95	Lorazepam, Rugby	00536-3960-10
1000's	$200.46	Lorazepam, Bristol Myers Squibb	00003-0408-75
1000's	**$785.17**	**ATIVAN, Wyeth Labs**	**00008-0064-05**

Tablet, Uncoated - Oral - 2 mg

30's	$8.37	Lorazepam, Talbert Phcy	44514-0100-18
100's	$2.28	Lorazepam, United Res	00677-1058-01
100's	$2.28	Lorazepam, Geneva Pharms	00781-1405-01
100's	$2.28	Lorazepam, Mutual Pharm	53489-0359-01
100's	$2.28	Lorazepam, H.C.F.A. F F P	99999-1662-08
100's	$18.70	Lorazepam, Elkins Sinn	00641-4002-86
100's	$21.43	Lorazepam, Halsey Drug	00879-0573-01
100's	$22.73	Lorazepam, Watson Labs	52544-0334-01
100's	$23.40	Lorazepam, Qualitest Pharms	00603-4245-21
100's	$23.70	Lorazepam 2, Major Pharms	00904-1502-60
100's	$25.15	Lorazepam, Royce	51875-0242-01
100's	$26.20	Lorazepam, Lederle Pharm	00005-3173-23
100's	$26.85	Lorazepam, Geneva Pharms	50752-0295-05
100's	$26.93	Lorazepam, HL Moore Drug Exch	00839-7147-06
100's	$26.93	Lorazepam, HL Moore Drug Exch	00839-7904-06
100's	$27.17	Lorazepam, Caremark	00339-4021-12
100's	$27.40	Lorazepam, Martec Pharms	52555-0487-01
100's	$27.70	Lorazepam, Schein Pharm (US)	00364-0795-01
100's	$27.90	Lorazepam, Purepac Pharm	00228-2063-10
100's	$27.98	Lorazepam, Aligen Independ	00405-0110-01
100's	$29.95	Lorazepam, Goldline Labs	00182-1808-01
100's	$30.95	Lorazepam, Warner Chilcott	00047-0433-24
100's	$31.79	Lorazepam, Bristol Myers Squibb	00003-0487-50
100's	$31.95	Lorazepam, Mylan	00378-0777-01
100's	$31.95	LORAZEPAM, Rugby	00536-3961-01
100's	$49.26	Lorazepam, Parmed Pharms	00349-8463-01
100's	$53.54	Lorazepam, Vangard Labs	00615-0452-47
100's	$59.50	Lorazepam, Geneva Pharms	00781-1405-13
100's	$60.00	Lorazepam, Goldline Labs	00182-1808-89
100's	$60.57	Lorazepam, Vangard Labs	00615-0452-13
100's	**$120.40**	**ATIVAN, Wyeth Labs**	**00008-0065-02**
100's	**$131.34**	**ATIVAN, Wyeth Labs**	**00008-0065-09**
250's	$5.70	Lorazepam, H.C.F.A. F F P	99999-1662-09
250's	$78.25	LORAZEPAM, Rugby	00536-3961-02
500's	$11.40	Lorazepam, United Res	00677-1058-05
500's	$11.40	Lorazepam, Geneva Pharms	00781-1405-05
500's	$11.40	Lorazepam, H.C.F.A. F F P	99999-1662-10
500's	$43.01	Lorazepam, Martec Pharms	52555-0432-05
500's	$66.97	Lorazepam, Watson Labs	52544-0334-05
500's	$74.60	Lorazepam, Geneva Pharms	50752-0295-08
500's	$82.25	Lorazepam, Qualitest Pharms	00603-4245-28
500's	$83.70	Lorazepam, Elkins Sinn	00641-4002-88
500's	$85.75	Lorazepam, Mutual Pharm	53489-0359-05
500's	$89.20	Lorazepam 2, Major Pharms	00904-1502-40
500's	$90.81	Lorazepam, Royce	51875-0242-02
500's	$91.19	Lorazepam, HL Moore Drug Exch	00839-7147-12
500's	$94.21	Lorazepam, Halsey Drug	00879-0573-05
500's	$107.75	Lorazepam, Martec Pharms	52555-0487-05
500's	$127.83	Lorazepam, Lederle Pharm	00005-3173-31
500's	$127.85	Lorazepam, Schein Pharm (US)	00364-0795-05
500's	$128.90	Lorazepam, Aligen Independ	00405-0110-02
500's	$139.50	Lorazepam, Purepac Pharm	00228-2063-50
500's	$142.25	Lorazepam, Warner Chilcott	00047-0433-30
500's	$142.25	Lorazepam, Goldline Labs	00182-1808-05
500's	$142.25	Lorazepam, Mylan	00378-0777-05
500's	$154.64	Lorazepam, Bristol Myers Squibb	00003-0487-60
500's	$189.31	Lorazepam, Parmed Pharms	00349-8463-05
500's	**$585.76**	**ATIVAN, Wyeth Labs**	**00008-0065-03**
1000's	$22.80	Lorazepam, Mutual Pharm	53489-0359-10
1000's	$22.80	Lorazepam, H.C.F.A. F F P	99999-1662-11
1000's	$117.60	Lorazepam, Watson Labs	52544-0334-10
1000's	$122.50	Lorazepam, Geneva Pharms	50752-0295-09
1000's	$123.75	Lorazepam 2, Major Pharms	00904-1502-80
1000's	$130.40	Lorazepam, Qualitest Pharms	00603-4245-32
1000's	$135.40	Lorazepam, Elkins Sinn	00641-4002-89
1000's	$139.04	Lorazepam, HL Moore Drug Exch	00839-7904-16
1000's	$156.00	Lorazepam, Royce	51875-0242-04
1000's	$168.95	Lorazepam, Halsey Drug	00879-0573-10
1000's	$198.90	Lorazepam, Purepac Pharm	00228-2063-96
1000's	$198.90	LORAZEPAM, Rugby	00536-3961-10
1000's	$301.93	Lorazepam, Bristol Myers Squibb	00003-0487-75
1000's	**$1143.67**	**ATIVAN, Wyeth Labs**	**00008-0065-05**

HOW SUPPLIED - NOT RATED EQUIVALENT:

Solution - Oral - 2 mg/ml

30 ml $36.56 LORAZEPAM INTENSOL, Roxane 00054-3532-44

LOSARTAN POTASSIUM *(003231)*

CATEGORIES: Angiotensin II Inhibitors; Antihypertensives; Cardiovascular Drugs; Hypertension; FDA Class 1S ("Standard Review"); FDA Approved 1995 Apr; Top 200 Drugs; Top 200 Drugs

BRAND NAMES: **Cozaar**

WARNING:
Use In Pregnancy: When used in pregnancy during the second and third trimesters, drugs that act directly on the renin-angiotensin system can case injury and even death to the developing fetus. When pregnancy is detected, losartan potassium should be discontinued as soon as possible. See WARNINGS, Fetal/Neonatal/Morbidity and Mortality.

DESCRIPTION:

Losartan potassium, the first of a new class of antihypertensives, is an angiotensin II receptor (type AT_1) antagonist.

Losartan potassium, a non-peptide molecule, is chemically described as 2-butyl-4-chloro-1[*p*-(*o*-1*H*-tetrazol-5- ylphenyl)benzyl]imidazole-5-methanol monopotassium salt.

Its empirical formula is $C_{22}H_{22}ClKN_6O$.

Losartan potassium is a white to off-white free flowing crystalline powder with a molecular weight of 461.01. It is freely soluble in water, soluble in alcohols, and slightly soluble in common organic solvents, such as acetonitrile and methyl ethyl ketone. Oxidation of the 5-hydroxymethyl group on the imidazole ring results in the active metabolite of losartan.

Cozaar is available for oral administration containing either 25 mg or 50 mg of losartan potassium and the following inactive ingredients: microcrystalline cellulose, lactose hydrous, pregelatinized starch, magnesium stearate, hydroxypropyl cellulose, hydroxypropyl methylcellulose, titanium dioxide, D&C yellow No. 10 aluminum lake and FD&C blue No. 2 aluminum lake.

Cozaar 25 mg and 50 mg contain potassium in the following amounts: 2.12 mg (0.054 mEq) and 4.24 mg (0.108 mEq) respectively.

CLINICAL PHARMACOLOGY:

MECHANISM OF ACTION

Angiotensin II [formed from angiotensin I in a reaction catalyzed by angiotensin converting enzyme (ACE, kininase II), is a potent vasoconstrictor, the primary vasoactive hormone of the renin-angiotensin system and an important component in the pathophysiology of hypertension. It also stimulates aldosterone secretion by the adrenal cortex. Losartan and its principal active metabolite block the vasoconstrictor and aldosterone-secreting effects of angiotensin II by selectively blocking the binding of angiotensin II to the AT_1 receptor found in many tissues, (*e.g.*, vascular smooth muscle, adrenal gland). There is also an AT_2 receptor found in many tissues but it is not known to be associated with cardiovascular homeostasis. Both losartan and its principal active metabolite do not exhibit any partial agonist activity at the AT_1 receptor and have much greater affinity (about 1000-fold) for the AT_1 receptor than for the AT_2 receptor. *In vitro* binding studies indicate that losartan is a reversible, competitive inhibitor of the AT_1 receptor. The active metabolite is 10 to 40 times more potent by weight than losartan and appears to be a reversible, non-competitive inhibitor of the AT_1 receptor.

Neither losartan nor its active metabolite inhibits ACE (kininase II, the enzyme that converts angiotensin I to angiotensin II and degrades bradykinin); nor do they bind to or block other hormone receptors or ion channels known to be important in cardiovascular regulation.

PHARMACOKINETICS

General: Losartan is an orally active agent that undergoes substantial first-pass metabolism by cytochrome P450 enzymes. It is converted, in part, to an active carboxylic acid metabolite that is responsible for most of the angiotensin II receptor antagonism that follows losartan treatment. The terminal half-life of losartan is about 2 hours and of the metabolite is about 6-9 hours. The pharmacokinetics of losartan and its active metabolite are linear with oral losartan doses up to 200 mg and do not change over time. Neither losartan nor its metabolite accumulate in plasma upon repeated once-daily dosing.

Following oral administration, losartan is well absorbed (based on absorption of radiolabeled losartan) and undergoes substantial first-pass metabolism; the systemic bioavailability of losartan is approximately 33%. About 14% of an orally-administered dose of losartan is converted to the active metabolite. Mean peak concentrations of losartan and its active metabolite are reached in 1 hour and in 3-4 hours, respectively. While maximum plasma concentrations of losartan id its active metabolite are approximately equal, the AUC of the metabolite is about 4 times great as that of losartan. A meal slows absorption of losartan and decreases its C_{max} but has only minor effects on losartan AUC or on the AUC of the metabolite (about 10% decreased).

Both losartan and its active metabolite are highly bound to plasma proteins, primarily albumin, with plasma free fractions of 1.3% and 0.2% respectively. Plasma protein binding is constant over the concentration range achieved with recommended doses. Studies in rats indicate that losartan crosses the blood-brain barrier poorly, if at all.

Losartan metabolites have been identified in human plasma and urine. In addition to the active carboxylic acid metabolite, several inactive metabolites are formed. Following oral and intravenous administration of ^{14}C-labeled losartan potassium, circulating plasma radioactivity is primarily attributed to losartan and its active metabolite. *In vitro* studies indicate that cytochrome P450 2C9 and 3A4 are involved in the biotransformation of losartan to its metabolites. Minimal conversion of losartan to the active metabolite (less than 1% of the dose compared to 14% of the dose in normal subjects) was seen in about one percent of individuals studied.

The volume of distribution of losartan is about 34 liters and of the active metabolite is about 12 liters. Total plasma clearance of losartan and the active metabolite is about 600 ml/min and 50 ml/min, respectively, with renal clearance of about 75 ml/min and 25 ml/min, respectively. When losartan is administered orally, about 4% of the dose is excreted unchanged in the urine and about 6% is excreted in urine as active metabolite. Biliary excretion contributes to the elimination of losartan and its metabolites. Following oral ^{14}C-labeled losartan, about 35% of radioactivity is recovered in the urine and about 60% in the feces. Following an intravenous dose of ^{14}C-labeled losartan, about 45% of radioactivity is recovered in the urine and 50% in the feces.

CLINICAL PHARMACOLOGY: *(cont'd)*

SPECIAL POPULATIONS

Pediatric: Losartan pharmacokinetics have not been investigated in patients <18 years of age.

Geriatric and Gender: Losartan pharmacokinetics have been investigated in the elderly (65-75 years) and in both genders. Plasma concentrations of losartan and its active metabolite are similar in elderly and young hypertensives. Plasma concentrations of losartan were about twice as high in female hypertensives as male hypertensives, but concentrations of the active metabolite were similar in males and females. No dosage adjustment is necessary (see DOSAGE AND ADMINISTRATION).

Race: Pharmacokinetic differences due to race have not been studied.

Renal Insufficiency: Plasma concentrations of losartan are not altered in patients with creatinine clearance above 30 ml/min. In patients with lower creatinine clearance, AUCs are about 50% greater and they are doubled in hemodialysis patients. Plasma concentrations of the active metabolite are not significantly altered in patients with renal impairment or in hemodialysis patients. Neither losartan nor its active metabolite can be removed by hemodialysis. No dosage adjustment is necessary for patients with renal impairment unless they are volume-depleted (see WARNINGS, Hypotension - Volume Depleted Patients, and DOSAGE AND ADMINISTRATION).

Hepatic Insufficiency: Following oral administration in patients with mild to moderate alcoholic cirrhosis of the liver, plasma concentrations of losartan and its active metabolite were, respectively, 5-times and about 1.7-times those in young male volunteers. Compared to normal subjects the total plasma clearance of losartan in patients with hepatic insufficiency was about 50% lower and the oral bioavailability was about 2-times higher. A lower starting dose is recommended for patients with a history of hepatic impairment (see DOSAGE AND ADMINISTRATION).

PHARMACODYNAMICS AND CLINICAL EFFECTS

Losartan inhibits the pressor effect of angiotensin II (as well as angiotensin I) infusions. A dose of 100 mg inhibits the pressor effect by about 85% at peak with 25-40% inhibition persisting for 24 hours. Removal of the negative feedback of angiotensin II causes a 2-3 fold rise in plasma renin activity and consequent rise in angiotensin II plasma concentration in hypertensive patients. Losartan does not affect the response to bradykinin, whereas ACE inhibitors increase the response to bradykinin. Aldosterone plasma concentrations fall following losartan administration. In spite of the effect of losartan on aldosterone secretion, very little effect on serum potassium was observed.

In a single-dose study in normal volunteers, losartan had no effects on glomerular filtration rate, renal plasma flow or filtration fraction. In multiple dose studies in hypertensive patients, there were no notable effects on systemic or renal prostaglandin concentrations, fasting triglycerides, total cholesterol or HDL-cholesterol or fasting glucose concentrations. There was a small uricosuric effect leading to a minimal decrease in serum uric acid (mean decrease <0.4 mg/dl) during chronic oral administration.

The antihypertensive effects of losartan potassium were demonstrated principally in 4 placebo-controlled 6-12 week trials of dosages from 10 to 150 mg per day in patients with baseline diastolic blood pressures of 95-115. The studies allowed comparisons of two doses (50-100 mg/day) as once-daily or twice-daily regimens, comparisons of peak and trough effects, and comparisons of response by gender, age, and race. Three additional studies examined the antihypertensive effects of losartan and hydrochlorothiazide in combination.

The 4 studies of losartan monotherapy included a total of 1075 patients randomized to several doses of losartan and 334 to placebo. The 10 and 25 mg doses produced some effect at peak (6 hours after dosing) but small and inconsistent trough (24 hour) responses. Doses of 50, 100 and 150 mg once daily gave statistically significant systolic/diastolic mean decreases in blood pressure, compared to placebo in the range of 5.5- 10.5/3.5-7.5 mmHg, with 150 mg dose giving no greater effect than 50-100 mg. Twice-daily dosing at 50-100 mg/day gave consistently larger trough responses than once-daily dosing at the same total dose. Peak (6 hour) effects were uniformly, but moderately, larger than trough effects, with the trough-to-peak ratio for systolic and diastolic responses 50-95% and 60-90%, respectively.

Addition of a low dose of hydrochlorothiazide (12.5 mg) to losartan 50 mg once daily resulted in placebo-adjusted blood pressure reductions of 15.5/9.2 mmHg.

Analysis of age gender, and race subgroups of patients showed that men and women, and patients over and under 65, had generally similar responses. Black patients, however, had notably smaller responses to losartan monotherapy.

The effect of losartan is substantially present within one week but in some studies the maximal effect occurred in 3-6 weeks. In long-term, follow-up studies (without placebo control) the effect of losartan appeared to be maintained for up to a year. There is no apparent rebound effect after abrupt withdrawal of losartan. There was essentially no change in average heart rate in losartan-treated patients in controlled trials.

INDICATIONS AND USAGE:

Losartan potassium is indicated for the treatment of hypertension. It may be used alone or in combination with other antihypertensive agents. In considering the use of monotherapy with losartan potassium, it should be noted that in controlled trials losartan potassium had an effect on blood pressure that was notably less in black patients than in non-blacks, a finding similar to the small effect of angiotensin converting enzyme inhibitors in blacks.

CONTRAINDICATIONS:

Losartan potassium is contraindicated in patients who are hypersensitive to any component of this product.

WARNINGS:

FETAL/NEONATAL MORBIDITY AND MORTALITY

Drugs that act directly on the renin-angiotensin can cause fetal and neonatal morbidity and death when administered to pregnant women. Several dozen cases have been reported in the world literature in patients who were taking angiotensin converting enzyme inhibitors. When pregnancy is detected, losartan potassium should be discontinued as soon as possible.

The use of drugs that act directly on the renin-angiotensin system during the second and third trimesters of pregnancy has been associated with fetal and neonatal injury, including hypotension, neonatal skull hypoplasia, anuria, reversible or irreversible renal failure, and death. Oligohydramnios has also been reported, presumably resulting from decreased fetal renal function; oligohydramnios in this setting has been associated with fetal limb contractures, craniofacial deformation, and hypoplastic lung development. Prematurity, intrauterine growth retardation, and patent ductus arteriosus have also been reported, although it is not clear whether these occurrences were due to exposure to the drug.

These adverse effects do not appear to have resulted from intrauterine drug exposure that has been limited to the first trimester.

Mothers whose embryos and fetuses are exposed to an angiotensin II receptor antagonist only during the first trimester should be so informed. Nonetheless, when patients become pregnant, physicians should have the patient discontinue the use of losartan potassium as soon as possible.

WARNINGS: *(cont'd)*

Rarely (probably less often than once in every thousand pregnancies), no alternative to an angiotensin II receptor antagonist will be found. In these rare cases, the mothers should be apprised of the potential hazards to their fetuses, and serial ultrasound examinations should be performed to assess the intraamniotic environment.

If oligohydramnios is observed, losartan potassium should be discontinued unless it is considered life-saving for the mother. Contraction stress testing (CST), a non-stress test (NST), or biophysical profiling (BPP) may be appropriate, depending upon the week of pregnancy. Patients and physicians should be aware, however, that oligohydramnios may not appear until after the fetus has sustained irreversible injury.

Infants with histories of *in utero* exposure to an angiotensin II receptor antagonist should be closely observed for hypotension, oliguria, and hyperkalemia, If oliguria occurs, attention should be directed toward support of blood pressure and renal perfusion. Exchange transfusion or dialysis may be required as means of reversing hypotension and/or substituting for disordered renal function.

Losartan potassium has been shown to produce adverse effects in rat fetuses and neonates, including decreased body weight, delayed physical and behavioral development, mortality and renal toxicity. With the exception of neonatal weight (which was affected at doses as low as 10 mg/kg/day), doses associated with these effects exceeded 25 mg/kg/day (approximately three times the maximum recommended human dose of 100 mg on a mg/m^2 basis). These findings are attributed to drug exposure in late gestation and during lactation. Significant levels of losartan and its active metabolite were shown to be present in rat fetal plasma during late gestation and in rat milk.

HYPOTENSION - VOLUME DEPLETED PATIENTS

In patients who are intravascularly volume-depleted (*e.g.,* those treated with diuretics), symptomatic hypotension may occur after initiation of therapy with losartan potassium. These conditions should be corrected prior to administration of losartan potassium, or a lower starting dose should be used (see DOSAGE AND ADMINISTRATION).

PRECAUTIONS:

GENERAL

Based on pharmacokinetic data which demonstrates significantly increased plasma concentrations of losartan in cirrhotic patients, a lower dose should be considered for patients with impaired liver function (see DOSAGE AND ADMINISTRATION and CLINICAL PHARMACOLOGY, Pharmacokinetics).

IMPAIRED RENAL FUNCTION

As a consequence of inhibiting the renin-angiotensin-aldosterone system, changes in renal function may be anticipated in susceptible individuals. In patients whose renal function may depend on the activity of the renin-angiotensin-aldosterone system (*e.g.,* patients with severe congestive heart failure), treatment with angiotensin converting enzyme inhibitors has been associated with oliguria and/or progressive azotemia and (rarely) with acute renal failure and/or death. Losartan potassium would be expected to behave similarly. In studies of ACE inhibitors in patients with unilateral or bilateral renal artery stenosis, increases in serum creatinine or BUN have been reported. There has been no known use of losartan potassium in patients with unilateral or bilateral renal artery stenosis, but a similar effect should be anticipated.

CARCINOGENESIS, MUTAGENESIS, AND IMPAIRMENT OF FERTILITY

Losartan potassium was not carcinogenic when administered at maximally tolerated dosages to rats and mice for 105 and 92 weeks, respectively. Female rats given the highest dose (270 mg/kg/day) had a slightly higher incidence of pancreatic acinar adenoma. The maximally tolerated dosages (270 mg/kg/day in rats, 200 mg/kg/day in mice) provided systemic exposures for losartan and its pharmacologically active metabolite that were approximately 160- and 90-times (rats) and 30- and 15-times (mice) the exposure of a 50 kg human given 100 mg per day.

Losartan potassium was negative in the microbial mutagenesis and V-79 mammalian cell mutagenesis assays and in the *in vitro* alkaline elution and *in vitro* and *in vivo* chromosomal aberration assays. In addition, the active metabolite showed no evidence of genotoxicity in the microbial mutagenesis, *in vitro* alkaline elution, and *in vitro* chromosomal aberration assays.

Fertility and reproductive performance were not affected in studies with male rats given oral doses of losartan potassium up to approximately 150 mg/kg/day. The administration of toxic dosage levels in females (300/200 mg/kg/day) was associated with a significant ($p < 0.05$) decrease in the number of corporalutea/female, implants/female, and live fetuses/female at C-section. At 100 mg/kg/day only a decrease in the certain number of corpora lutea/female was observed. The relationship of these findings to drug-treatment is uncertain since there was no effect at these dosage levels on implants/pregnant female, percent post-implantation loss, or live animals/litter at parturition. In nonpregnant rats dosed at 135 mg/kg/day for 7 days, systemic exposure (AUCs) for losartan and its active metabolite were approximately 66 and 26 times the exposure achieved in man at the maximum recommended human daily dosage (100 mg).

PREGNANCY

Pregnancy Categories C (first trimester) and D (second and third trimesters). See WARNINGS, Fetal/Neonatal Morbidity and Mortality.

NURSING MOTHERS

It is not known whether losartan is excreted in human milk, but significant levels of losartan and its active metabolite were shown to be present in rat milk. Because of the potential for adverse effects on the nursing infant, a decision should be made whether to discontinue nursing or discontinue the drug, taking into account the importance of the drug to the mother.

PEDIATRIC USE

Safety and effectiveness in pediatric patients have not been established.

USE IN THE ELDERLY

Of the total number of patients receiving losartan potassium in controlled clinical studies, 391 patients (19%) were 65 years and over, whole 37 patients (2%) were 75 years and over. No overall differences in effectiveness or safety were observed between these patients and younger patients, but greater sensitivity of some older individuals cannot be ruled out.

DRUG INTERACTIONS:

Losartan, administered for 12 days, did not affect the pharmacokinetics or pharmacodynamics of a single dose of warfarin. Losartan did not affect the pharmacokinetics of oral and intravenous digoxin. Coadministration of losartan and cimetidine led to an increase of about 18% in AUC of losartan but did not affect the pharmacokinetics of its active metabolite. Coadministration of losartan and phenobarbital led to reduction of about 20% in the AUC of losartan and that of its active metabolite. There is no pharmacokinetic interaction between losartan and hydrochlorothiazide.

No significant drug-drug pharmacokinetic interactions have been found in interaction studies with hydrochlorothiazide, digoxin, warfarin, cimetidine and phenobarbital. Potent inhibitors of cytochrome P450 3A4 and 2C9 have not been studied clinically but *in vitro* studies show significant inhibition of the formation of the active metabolite by inhibitors of P450 3A4 (ke-

DRUG INTERACTIONS: *(cont'd)*

toconazole, troleandomycin, gestodene) or P450 2C9 (sulfaphenazole) and nearly complete inhibition by the combination of sulfaphenazole and ketoconazole. The pharmacodynamic consequences of concomitant use of losartan and these inhibitors have not been examined.

ADVERSE REACTIONS:

Losartan potassium has been evaluated for safety in more than 3300 patients treated for essential hypertension and 4058 patients/subjects overall. Over 1200 patients were treated for over 6 months and more than 800 for over one year. In general, treatment with losartan potassium was well-tolerated. The overall incidence of adverse experiences reported with losartan potassium was similar to placebo.

In controlled clinical trials, discontinuation of therapy due to clinical adverse experiences was required in 2.3 percent of patients treated with losartan potassium and 3.7 percent of patients given placebo.

The following table of adverse events is based on four 6-12 week placebo controlled trials involving over 1000 patients on various doses (10-150 mg) of losartan and over 300 patients given placebo. All doses of losartan are grouped because none of the adverse events appeared to have a dose-related frequency. The table includes all adverse events, whether or not attributed to the treatment, occurring in at least 1% of patients treated with losartan and that were more frequent in losartan than placebo. (TABLE 1)

TABLE 1

	Losartan Incidence (n=1075)	Placebo Incidence (n=334)
Digestive		
Diarrhea	2.4	2.1
Dyspepsia	1.3	1.2
Musculoskeletal		
Cramp, muscle	1.1	0.3
Myalgia	1.0	0.9
Pain, back	1.8	1.2
Pain, leg	1.0	0.0
Nervous System/Psychiatric		
Dizziness	3.5	2.1
Insomnia	1.4	0.6
Respiratory		
Congestion, nasal	2.0	1.2
Cough	3.4	3.3
Infection, upper respiratory	7.9	6.9
Sinus disorder	1.5	1.2
Sinusitis	1.0	0.3

The following adverse events were also reported at a rate 1% or greater in patients treated with losartan, but were as, or more frequent, in the placebo group: asthenia/fatigue, edema/swelling, abdominal pain, chest pain, nausea, headache, pharyngitis.

Adverse events occurred at about the same rates in men and women, older and younger patients, and black and non-black patients.

A patient with known hypersensitivity to aspirin and penicillin, when treated with losartan potassium, was withdrawn from study due to swelling of the lips and eyelids and facial rash, reported as angioedema, which returned to normal 5 days after therapy was discontinued.

Superficial peeling of palms and hemolysis was reported in one subject.

In addition to the adverse events, above potentially important events that occurred in at least two patients/subjects exposed to losartan or other adverse events occurred in <1% of patients in clinical studies are listed below. It cannot be determined whether these events were casually related to losartan: *Body as a Whole:* facial edema, fever, orthostatic effects, syncope; *Cardiovascular:* angina pectoris, second degree AV block, CVA, hypotension, myocardial infarction, arrhythmias including atrial fibrillation, palpitation, sinus bradycardia, tachycardia, ventricular tachycardia, ventricular fibrillation; *Digestive:* anorexia, constipation, dental pain, dry mouth, flatulence, gastritis, vomiting; *Hematologic:* anemia; *Metabolic:* gout; *Musculoskeletal:* arm pain, hip pain, joint swelling, knee pain, musculoskeletal pain, shoulder pain, stiffness, arthralgia, arthritis, fibromyalgia, muscle weakness;*Nervous System/Psychiatric:* anxiety, anxiety disorder, ataxia, confusion, depression, dream abnormality, hypesthesia, decreased libido, memory impairment, migraine, nervousness, paresthesia, peripheral neuropathy, panic disorder, sleep disorder, somnolence, tremor, vertigo;*Respiratory:* dyspnea, bronchitis, pharyngeal discomfort, epistaxis, rhinitis, respiratory congestion; *Skin:* alopecia, dermatitis, dry skin, ecchymosis, erythema, flushing, photosensitivity, pruritus, rash, sweating, urticaria; *Special Senses:* blurred vision, burning/stinging in the eye, conjunctivitis, taste perversion, tinnitus, decrease in visual acuity; *Urogenital:* impotence, nocturia, urinary frequency, urinary tract infection.

Laboratory Test Findings: In controlled clinical trials, clinically important changes in standard laboratory parameters were rarely associated with administration of losartan potassium.

Creatinine, Blood Urea Nitrogen: Minor increases in blood urea nitrogen (BUN) or serum creatinine were observed in less than 0.1 percent of patients with essential hypertension treated with losartan potassium alone. No patient discontinued taking losartan potassium alone due to increased BUN or serum creatinine (see PRECAUTIONS, Impaired Renal Function).

Hemoglobin and Hematocrit: Small decreases in hemoglobin and hematocrit (mean decreases of approximately 0.11 grams percent and 0.09 volume percent, respectively) occurred frequently in patients treated with losartan potassium alone, but were rarely of clinical importance. No patients were discontinued due to anemia.

Liver Function Tests: Occasional elevations of liver enzymes and/or other serum bilirubin have occurred. In patients with essential hypertension treated with losartan potassium alone, one patient (<0.1%) was discontinued to these laboratory adverse experiences.

OVERDOSAGE:

Significant lethality was observed in mice and rats after oral administration of 1000 mg/kg and 2000 mg/kg, respectively, about 44 and 170 times the maximum recommended human dose on a mg/m^2 basis.

Limited data are available in regard to overdosage in humans. The most likely manifestation of overdosage would be hypotension and tachycardia; bradycardia could occur from parasympathetic (vagal) stimulation. If symptomatic hypotension should occur, supportive treatment should be instituted.

Neither losartan nor its active metabolite can be removed by hemodialysis.

DOSAGE AND ADMINISTRATION:

The usual starting dose of losartan potassium is 50 mg once daily, with 25 mg used in patients with possible depletion of intravascular volume (*e.g.,* patients treated with diuretics) (see WARNINGS, Hypotension - Volume, Depleted Patients) and patients with a history of hepatic impairment (see PRECAUTIONS, General). Losartan potassium can be administered once or twice daily with total daily doses ranging from 25 mg to 100 mg.

DOSAGE AND ADMINISTRATION: *(cont'd)*

If the antihypertensive effect measured at trough using once-a-day dosing is inadequate, a twice-a-day regimen at the same total daily dose or an increase in dose may give a more satisfactory response.

If blood pressure is not controlled by losartan potassium alone, a low dose of a diuretic may be added. Hydrochlorothiazide has been shown to have an additive effect (see CLINICAL PHARMACOLOGY, Pharmacodynamics and Clinical Effects).

No initial dosage adjustment is necessary for elderly patients or for patients with renal impairment, including patients in dialysis.

Losartan potassium may be administered with other antihypersensitive agents.

Losartan potassium may be administered with or without food.

INFORMATION FOR PATIENTS

Pregnancy: Female patients of childbearing age should be told about the consequences of second- and third-trimester exposure to drugs that act on the renin-angiotensin system, and they should also be told that these consequences do not appear to have resulted from intrauterine drug exposure that has been limited to the first trimester. These patients should be asked to report pregnancies to their physicians as soon as possible.

PATIENT INFORMATION:

Losartan potassium is used to treat high blood pressure. It may be used alone or with other medications for high blood pressure. This medication should, generally, not be used during pregnancy. If you are pregnant or considering becoming pregnant, inform your physician immediately to discuss the risks versus benefits. There are few side effects associated with losartan potassium. Those most frequently reported, cough, upper respiratory infection and dizziness, occurred no more frequently than in patients who did not take this medication. You may take this medication with or without food. You should have your blood pressure checked regularly.

HOW SUPPLIED:

Tablets Cozaar, 25 mg, are light green, tear-drop shaped, film-coated tablets with code MRK on one side and 951 on the other.

HOW SUPPLIED - EQUIVALENTS NOT AVAILABLE:

Tablet, Uncoated - Oral - 25 mg

90's	**$99.00**	**COZAAR, Merck**	**00006-0951-54**
100's	**$110.00**	**COZAAR, Merck**	**00006-0951-28**
100's	**$110.00**	**COZAAR, Merck**	**00006-0951-58**

Tablet, Uncoated - Oral - 50 mg

30's	**$33.00**	**COZAAR, Merck**	**00006-0952-31**
90's	**$99.00**	**COZAAR, Merck**	**00006-0952-54**
100's	**$110.00**	**COZAAR, Merck**	**00006-0952-28**
100's	**$110.00**	**COZAAR, Merck**	**00006-0952-58**

LOVASTATIN *(001664)*

CATEGORIES: Antilipemic Agents; Atherosclerosis; Cardiovascular Drugs; Cholesterol; HMG-COA Reductase Inhibitors; Heart Disease; Hypercholesterolemia; Hyperlipidemia; Hyperlipoproteinemia; Hypolipidemics; Vascular Disease; Pregnancy Category X; Sales > $1 Billion; FDA Approved 1987 Aug; Patent Expiration 1999 Nov; Top 200 Drugs

BRAND NAMES: *Lovalip*; **Mevacor**; *Mevinacor* (Germany); *Nergadan*; *Rovacor*; *Taucor*
(International brand names outside U.S. in italics)

FORMULARIES: Aetna; BC-BS; Kaiser; Medi-Cal

COST OF THERAPY: $774.38 (Hypercholesterolemia; Tablet; 20 mg; 1/day; 365 days)

DESCRIPTION:

Mevacor* (Lovastatin) is a cholesterol lowering agent isolated from a strain of *Aspergillus terreus*. After oral ingestion, lovastatin, which is an inactive lactone, is hydrolyzed to the corresponding β-hydroxyacid form. This is a principal metabolite and an inhibitor of 3-hydroxy-3-methylglutaryl-coenzyme A (HMG-CoA) reductase. This enzyme catalyzes the conversion of HMG-CoA to mevalonate, which is an early and rate limiting step in the biosynthesis of cholesterol.

Lovastatin is [1*S*-[1α(*R**),3α,7β;8β(2*S**,4*S**),8aβ]] -1,2,3,7,8, 8a-hexahydro -3,7-dimethyl-8 -[2-(tetrahydro-4 -hydroxy- 6-oxo-2*H*-pyran-2-yl) ethyl]-1- naphthalenyl 2-methylbutanoate. The empirical formula of lovastatin is $C_{24}H_{36}O_5$ and its molecular weight is 404.55.

Lovastatin is a white, nonhygroscopic crystalline powder that is insoluble in water and sparingly soluble in ethanol, methanol, and acetonitrile.

Mevacor Tablets are supplied as 10 mg, 20 mg and 40 mg tablets for oral administration. In addition to the active ingredient lovastatin, each tablet contains the following inactive ingredients: cellulose, lactose, magnesium stearate, and starch. Butylated hydroxyanisole (BHA) is added as a preservative. Tablets Mevacor 10 mg also contain red ferric oxide and yellow ferric oxide. Tablets Mevacor 20 mg also contain FD&C Blue 2. Tablets Mevacor 40 mg also contain D&C Yellow 10 and FD&C Blue 2.

CLINICAL PHARMACOLOGY:

The involvement of low-density lipoprotein (LDL) cholesterol in atherogenesis has been well-documented in clinical and pathological studies, as well as in many animal experiments. Epidemiological studies have established that high LDL (low-density lipoprotein) cholesterol and low HDL (high-density lipoprotein) cholesterol are both risk factors for coronary heart disease. The Lipid Research Clinics Coronary Primary Prevention Trial (LRC-CPPT), coordinated by the National Institutes of Health (NIH) studied men aged 35-59 with total cholesterol levels 265 mg/dl (6.8 mmol/L) or greater, LDL cholesterol values 175 mg/dl (4.5 mmol/L) or greater and triglyceride levels not more than 300 mg/dl (3.4 mmol/L). This seven-year, double-blind, placebo-controlled study demonstrated that lowering LDL cholesterol with diet and cholestyramine decreased the combined rate of coronary heart disease death plus non-fatal myocardial infarction.

Lovastatin has been shown to reduce both normal and elevated LDL cholesterol concentrations. The effect of lovastatin-induced changes in lipoprotein levels, including reduction of serum cholesterol, on cardiovascular morbidity or mortality has not been established.

LDL is formed from VLDL and is catabolized predominantly by the high affinity LDL receptor. The mechanism of the LDL-lowering effect of lovastatin may involve both reduction of VLDL cholesterol concentration, and induction of the LDL receptor, leading to reduced production and/or increased catabolism of LDL cholesterol. Apolipoprotein B also falls substantially during treatment with lovastatin. Since each LDL particle contains one molecule of apolipoprotein B, and since little apolipoprotein B is found in other lipoproteins,

CLINICAL PHARMACOLOGY: *(cont'd)*

this strongly suggests that lovastatin does not merely cause cholesterol to be lost from LDL, but also reduces the concentration of circulating LDL particles. In addition, lovastatincan produce increases of variable magnitude in HDL cholesterol, and modestly reduces VLDL cholesterol and plasma triglycerides (see TABLE 1 and TABLE 4 under Clinical Studies). The effects of lovastatin on Lp(a), fibrinogen, and certain other independent biochemical risk markers for coronary heart disease are unknown.

Lovastatin is a specific inhibitor of HMG-CoA reductase, the enzyme which catalyzes the conversion of HMG-CoA to mevalonate. The conversion of HMG-CoA to mevalonate is an early step in the biosynthetic pathway for cholesterol.

PHARMACOKINETICS

Lovastatin is a lactone which is readily hydrolyzed *in vivo* to the corresponding β-hydroxyacid, a potent inhibitor of HMG-CoA reductase. Inhibition of HMG-CoA reductase is the basis for an assay in pharmacokinetic studies of the β-hydroxyacid metabolites (active inhibitors) and, following base hydrolysis, active plus latent inhibitors (total inhibitors) in plasma following administration of lovastatin.

Following an oral dose of ^{14}C-labeled lovastatin in man, 10% of the dose was excreted in urine and 83% in feces. The latter represents absorbed drug equivalents excreted in bile, as well as any unabsorbed drug. Plasma concentrations of total radioactivity (lovastatin plus ^{14}C-metabolites) peaked at 2 hours and declined rapidly to about 10% of peak by 24 hours postdose. Absorption of lovastatin, estimated relative to an intravenous reference dose, in each of four animal species tested, averaged about 30% of an oral dose. In animal studies, after oral dosing, lovastatin had high selectivity for the liver, where it achieved substantially higher concentrations than in non-target tissues. Lovastatin undergoes extensive first-pass extraction in the liver, its primary site of action, with subsequent excretion of drug equivalents in the bile. As a consequence of extensive hepatic extraction of lovastatin, the availability of drug to the general circulation is low and variable. In a single dose study in four hypercholesterolemic patients, it was estimated that less than 5% of an oral dose of lovastatin reaches the general circulation as active inhibitors. Following administration of lovastatin tablets the coefficient of variation, based on between-subject variability, was approximately 40% for the area under the curve (AUC) of total inhibitory activity in the general circulation.

Both lovastatin and its β-hydroxyacid metabolite are highly bound (>95%) to human plasma proteins. Animal studies demonstrated that lovastatin crosses the blood-brain and placental barriers.

The major active metabolites present in human plasma are the β-hydroxyacid of lovastatin, its 6'-hydroxy derivative, and two additional metabolites. Peak plasma concentrations of both active and total inhibitors were attained within 2 to 4 hours of dose administration. While the recommended therapeutic dose range is 20 to 80 mg/day, linearity of inhibitory activity in the general circulation was established by a single dose study employing lovastatin tablet dosages from 60 to as high as 120 mg. With a once-a-day dosing regimen, plasma concentrations of total inhibitors over a dosing interval achieved a steady state between the second and third days of therapy and were about 1.5 times those following a single dose. When lovastatin was given under fasting conditions, plasma concentrations of total inhibitors were on average about two-thirds those found when lovastatin was administered immediately after a standard test meal.

In a study of patients with severe renal insufficiency (creatinine clearance 10-30 ml/min), the plasma concentrations of total inhibitors after a single dose of lovastatin were approximately two-fold higher than those in healthy volunteers.

CLINICAL STUDIES:

Lovastatin has been shown to be highly effective in reducing total and LDL cholesterol in heterozygous familial and non-familial forms of primary hypercholesterolemia and in mixed hyperlipidemia. A marked response was seen within 2 weeks, and the maximum therapeutic response occurred within 4-6 weeks. The response was maintained during continuation of therapy. Single daily doses given in the evening were more effective than the same dose given in the morning, perhaps because cholesterol is synthesized mainly at night.

In multicenter, double-blind studies in patients with familial or non-familial hypercholesterolemia, lovastatin, administered in doses ranging from 20 mg q.p.m. to 40 mg b.i.d., was compared to placebo. Lovastatin consistently and significantly decreased total plasma cholesterol (TOTAL-C), LDL cholesterol (LDL-C), total cholesterol/HDL cholesterol (TOTAL-C/HDL-C) ratio and LDL cholesterol/HDL cholesterol (LDL-C/HDL-C) ratio. In addition, lovastatin produced increases of variable magnitude in HDL cholesterol (HDL-C), and modestly decreased VLDL cholesterol (VLDL-C) and plasma triglycerides (TRIG.) (see TABLE 1 and TABLE 4 for dose response results.)

TABLE 1 Familial Hypercholesterolemia Study Dose Response Of Lovastatin (Percent Change from Baseline After 6 Weeks)

Dosage	N	Total-C (mean)	LDL-C (mean)	HDL-C (mean)	LDL-C/HDL-C (mean)	Total-C/HDL-C (mean)	TRIG (median)
Placebo	21	-1	-2	+1	-1	0	+3
Lovastatin							
20 mg q.p.m.	20	-18	-19	+10	-26	-24	-7
40 mg q.p.m.	21	-24	-27	+10	-32	-29	-22
10 mg b.i.d.	19	-22	-25	+6	-28	-25	-11
20 mg b.i.d.	20	-27	-31	+12	-38	-34	-18
40 mg b.i.d.	20	-34	-39	+8	-43	-38	-12

Lovastatin was compared to cholestyramine in a randomized open parallel study and to probucol in a double-blind, parallel study. Both studies were performed with patients with hypercholesterolemia who were at high risk of myocardial infarction. Summary results of these two comparative studies are presented in TABLE 2 and TABLE 3.

TABLE 2 Lovastatin vs. Cholestyramine (Percent Change from Baseline After 12 Weeks)

Treatment	N	Total-C (mean)	LDL-C (mean)	HDL-C (mean)	LDL-C/HDL-C (mean)	Total-C/HDL-C (mean)	VLDL-C (median)	TRIG (median)
Lovastatin								
20 mg b.i.d.	85	-27	-32	+9	-36	-31	-34	-21
40 mg b.i.d.	88	-34	-42	+8	-44	-37	-31	-27
Cholestyramine								
12 g b.i.d.	88	-17	-23	+8	-27	-21	+2	+11

CLINICAL STUDIES: *(cont'd)*

TABLE 3 Lovastatin vs. Prubucol (Percent Change from Baseline After 14 Weeks)

Treatment	N	Total-C (mean)	LDL-C (mean)	HDL-C (mean)	LDL-C/ HDL-C (mean)	Total-C/ HDL-C (mean)	VLDL-C (median)	TRIG (median)
Lovastatin								
40 mg q.p.m.	47	-25	-32	+9	-38	-31	-37	-18
80 mg q.p.m.	49	-30	-37	+11	-42	-36	-27	-17
40 mg b.i.d.	47	-33	-40	+12	-45	-39	-40	-25
Probucol								
500 mg b.i.d.	97	-10	-8	-23	+26	+23	-13	+1

Lovastatin was studied in controlled trials in hypercholesterolemic patients with well-controlled non-insulin dependent diabetes mellitus with normal renal function. The effect of lovastatin on lipids and lipoproteins and the safety profile of lovastatin were similar to that demonstrated in studies in nondiabetics. Lovastatin had no clinically important effect on glycemic control or on the dose requirement of oral hypoglycemic agents.

Expanded Clinical Evaluation of Lovastatin (Excel) Study: Lovastatin was compared to placebo in 8,245 patients with hypercholesterolemia (total cholesterol 240-300 mg/dl [6.2 mmol/L-7.6 mmol/L], LDL cholesterol >160 mg/dl [4.1 mmol/L]) in the randomized, double-blind, parallel, 48-week Excel study. All changes in the lipid measurements (TABLE 4) in lovastatin treated patients were dose-related and significantly different from placebo (p≤0.001). These results were sustained throughout the study.

TABLE 4 Lovastatin vs. Placebo (Percent Change from Baseline—Average Values Between Weeks 12 and 48)

Dosage	N*	Total-C (mean)	LDL-C (mean)	HDL-C (mean)	LDL-C/ HDL-C (mean)	Total-C/ HDL-C (mean)	TRIG (median)
Placebo	1683	+0.7	+0.4	+2.0	+0.2	+0.6	+4
Lovastatin							
20 mg q.p.m.	1642	-17	-24	+6.6	-27	-21	-10
40 mg q.p.m.	1645	-22	-30	+7.2	-34	-26	-14
20 mg b.i.d.	1646	-24	-34	+8.6	-38	-29	-16
40 mg b.i.d.	1649	-29	-40	+9.5	-44	-34	-19

* Patients enrolled

Atherosclerosis: In the Canadian Coronary Atherosclerosis Intervention Trial (CCAIT), the effect of therapy with lovastatin on coronary atherosclerosis was assessed by coronary angiography in hyperlipidemic patients. In this randomized, double-blind, controlled clinical trial, patients were treated with conventional measures (usually diet and 325 mg of aspirin every other day) and either lovastatin 20-80 mg daily or placebo. Angiograms were evaluated at baseline and at two years by computerized quantitative coronary angiography (QCA). Lovastatin significantly slowed the progression of lesions as measured by the mean change per-patient in minimum lumen diameter (the primary endpoint) and percent diameter stenosis, and decreased the proportions of patients categorized with disease progression (33% vs. 50%) and with new lesions (16% vs. 32%).

In a similar designed trial, the Monitored Atherosclerosis Regression Study (MARS), patients were treated with diet and either lovastatin 80 mg daily or placebo. No statistically significant difference between lovastatin and placebo was seen for the primary endpoint (mean change per patient in percentage diameter stenosis of all lesions), or for most secondary QCA endpoints. Visual assessment by angiographers who formed a consensus opinion of overall angiographic change (Global Change Score) was also a secondary endpoint. By this endpoint, significant slowing of disease was seen, with regression in 23% of patients treated with lovastatin compared to 11% of placebo patients.

In the Familial Atherosclerosis Treatment Study (FATS), either lovastatin or niacin in combination with a bile acid sequestrant for 2.5 years in hyperlipidemic subjects significantly reduced the frequency of progression and increased the frequency of regression of coronary atherosclerotic lesions by QCA compared to diet and, in some cases, low-dose resin.

Eye: There was a high prevalence of baseline lenticular opacities in the patient population included in the early clinical trials with lovastatin. During these trials the appearance of new opacities was noted in both the lovastatin and placebo groups. There was no clinically significant change in visual acuity in the patients who had new opacities reported nor was any patient, including those with opacities noted at baseline, discontinued from therapy because of a decrease in visual acuity.

A three-year, double-blind, placebo-controlled study in hypercholesterolemic patients to assess the effect of lovastatin on the human lens demonstrated that there were no clinically or statistically significant differences between the lovastatin and placebo groups in the incidence, type or progression of lenticular opacities. There are no controlled clinical data assessing the lens available for treatment beyond three years.

INDICATIONS AND USAGE:

Therapy with lipid-altering agents should be a component of multiple risk factor intervention in those individuals at significantly increased risk for atherosclerotic vascular disease due to hypercholesterolemia. Lovastatin is indicated as an adjunct to diet for the reduction of elevated total and LDL cholesterol levels in patients with primary hypercholesterolemia (Types IIa and IIb[1]), when the response to diet restricted in saturated fat and cholesterol and to other nonpharmacological measures alone has been inadequate.

Lovastatin is also indicated to slow the progression of coronary atherosclerosis in patients with coronary heart disease as part of a treatment strategy to lower total and LDL cholesterol to target levels. Most subjects in the angiographic studies were middle-aged men; therefore, it is not clear to what extent these data can be extrapolated to women and the elderly (see CLINICAL STUDIES).

Prior to initiating therapy with lovastatin, secondary causes for hypercholesterolemia (*e.g.,* poorly controlled diabetes mellitus, hypothyroidism, nephrotic syndrome, dysproteinemias, obstructive liver disease, other drug therapy, alcoholism) should be excluded, and a lipid profile performed to measure TOTAL-C, HDL-C, and triglycerides (TG). For patients with TG less than 400 mg/dl (<4.5 mmol/L), LDL-C can be estimated using the following equation:

INDICATIONS AND USAGE: *(cont'd)*

LDL-C = Total cholesterol - [0.2 × (triglycerides) + HDL-C]

For TG levels >400 mg/dl (>4.5 mmol/l), this equation is less accurate and LDL-C concentrations should be determined by ultracentrifugation. In hypertriglyceridemic patients, LDL-C may be low or normal despite elevated TOTAL-C. In such cases, Mevacor is not indicated.

The effect of lovastatin-induced changes in lipoprotein levels, including reduction of serum cholesterol, on cardiovascular morbidity or mortality has not been established.

The National Cholesterol Education Program (NCEP) Treatment Guidelines are summarized below (TABLE 5):

TABLE 5

Define Atherosclerotic Disease*	Two or More Other Risk Factors**	LDL - Cholesterol mg/dl (mmol/l) Initiation Level	Goal
NO	NO	≥190 (≥4.9)	<160 (<4.1)
NO	YES	≥160 (≥4.1)	<130 (<3.4)
YES	YES or NO	≥130 (≥3.4)	≤100 (≤2.6)

* Coronary heart disease or peripheral vascular disease (including symptomatic carotid artery disease).

** Other risk factors for coronary heart disease (CHD) include: age (males: ≥45 years; females: ≥55 years or premature menopause without estrogen replacement therapy); family history of premature CHD; current cigarette smoking; hypertension; confirmed HDL-C <35 mg/dl (<0.91 mmol/l); and diabetes mellitus. Subtract one risk factor if HDL-C is ≥60 mg/dl (≥1.6 mmol/l).

Since the goal of treatment is to lower LDL-C, the NCEP recommends that LDL-C levels be used to initiate and assess treatment response. Only if LDL-C levels are not available, should the TOTAL-C be used to monitor therapy.

Although lovastatin may be useful to reduce elevated LDL cholesterol levels in patients with combined hypercholesterolemia and hypertriglyceridemia where hypercholesterolemia is the major abnormality (Type IIb hyperlipoproteinemia), it has not been studied in conditions where the major abnormality is elevation of chylomicrons, VLDL or IDL (*i.e.,* hyperlipoproteinemia types I, III, IV, or V).[1]

CONTRAINDICATIONS:

Hypersensitivity to any component of this medication.

Active liver disease or unexplained persistent elevations of serum transaminases (see WARNINGS) (TABLE 6).

TABLE 6 [1]Classification of Hyperlipoproteinemias

Type	Lipoproteins elevated	Lipid Elevations major	minor
I (rare)	chylomicrons	TG	↑→C
IIa	LDL	C	—
IIb	LDL, VLDL	C	TG
III (rare)	IDL	C/TG	—
IV	VLDL	TG	↑→C
V (rare)	chylomicrons, VLDL	TG	↑→C

C = cholesterol, TG = triglycerides,
LDL = low-density lipoprotein
VLDL = very low-density lipoprotein
IDL = intermediate-density lipoprotein

Pregnancy and lactation: Atherosclerosis is a chronic process and the discontinuation of lipid-lowering drugs during pregnancy should have little impact on the outcome of long-term therapy of primary hypercholesterolemia. Moreover, cholesterol and other products of the cholesterol biosynthesis pathway are essential components for fetal development, including synthesis of steroids and cell membranes. Because of the ability of inhibitors of HMG-CoA reductase such as lovastatin to decrease the synthesis of cholesterol and possibly other products of the cholesterol biosynthesis pathway, lovastatin may cause fetal harm when administered to a pregnant woman. Therefore, lovastatin is contraindicated during pregnancy. **Lovastatin should be administered to women of childbearing age only when such patients are highly unlikely to conceive.** If the patient becomes pregnant while taking this drug, lovastatin should be discontinued and the patient should be apprised of the potential hazard to the fetus.

WARNINGS:

Liver Dysfunction: Marked persistent increases (to more than 3 times the upper limit of normal) in serum transaminases occurred in 1.9% of adult patients who received lovastatin for at least one year in early clinical trials (see ADVERSE REACTIONS).

When the drug was interrupted or discontinued in these patients, the transaminase levels usually fell slowly to pretreatment levels. The increases usually appeared 3 to 12 months after the start of therapy with lovastatin, and were not associated with jaundice or other clinical signs or symptoms. There was no evidence of hypersensitivity. In the Excel study (see CLINICAL STUDIES), the incidence of marked persistent increases in serum transaminases over 48 weeks was 0.1% for placebo, 0.1% at 20 mg/day, 0.9% at 40 mg/day, and 1.5% at 80 mg/day in patients on lovastatin. However, in post-marketing experience with Mevacor, symptomatic liver disease has been reported rarely at all dosages (see ADVERSE REACTIONS).

It is recommended that liver function tests be performed before the initiation of treatment, at 6 and 12 weeks after initiation of therapy or elevation in dose, and periodically thereafter (*e.g.,* semiannually). Patients who develop increased transaminase levels should be monitored with a second liver function evaluation to confirm the finding and be followed thereafter with frequent liver function tests until the abnormality(ies) return to normal. Should an increase in AST or ALT of three times the upper limit of normal or greater persist, withdrawal of Mevacor therapy is recommended.

The drug should be used with caution in patients who consume substantial quantities of alcohol and/or have a past history of liver disease. Active liver disease or unexplained transaminase elevations are contraindications to the use of lovastatin.

As with other lipid-lowering agents, moderate (less than three times the upper limit of normal) elevations of serum transaminases have been reported following therapy with lovastatin (see ADVERSE REACTIONS). These changes appeared soon after initiation of therapy with lovastatin, were often transient, were not accompanied by any symptoms and interruption of treatment was not required.

WARNINGS: *(cont'd)*

Skeletal Muscle: Rhabdomyolysis has been associated with lovastatin therapy alone, when combined with immunosuppressive therapy including cyclosporine in cardiac transplant patients, and when combined in non-transplant patients with either gemfibrozil or lipid-lowering doses (≥1 g/day) of nicotinic acid. Some of the affected patients had pre-existing renal insufficiency, usually as a consequence of long-standing diabetes. Acute renal failure from rhabdomyolysis has been seen more commonly with the lovastatin-gemfibrozil combination, and has also been reported in transplant patients receiving lovastatin plus cyclosporine.

Rhabdomyolysis with renal failure has been reported in a renal transplant patient receiving cyclosporine and lovastatin shortly after a dose increase in the systemic antifungal agent itraconazole. Another transplant patient on cyclosporine and a different HMG CoA reductase inhibitor experienced muscle weakness accompanied by marked elevation of creatine phosphokinase following the initiation of systemic itraconazole therapy. The HMG CoA reductase inhibitors and the azole derivative antifungal agents inhibit cholesterol biosynthesis at different points in the biosynthetic pathway. In patients receiving cyclosporine, lovastatin should be temporarily discontinued if systemic azole derivative antifungal therapy is required; patients not taking cyclosporine should be carefully monitored if systemic azole derivative antifungal therapy is required.

Rhabdomyolysis with or without renal impairment has been reported in seriously ill patients receiving erythromycin concomitantly with lovastatin. Therefore, patients receiving concomitant lovastatin and erythromycin should be carefully monitored.

Fulminant rhabdomyolysis has been seen as early as three weeks after initiation of combined therapy with gemfibrozil and lovastatin, but may be seen after several months. For these reasons, it is felt that, in most subjects who have had an unsatisfactory lipid response to either drug alone, the possible benefits of combined therapy with lovastatin and gemfibrozil do not outweigh the risks of severe myopathy, rhabdomyolysis, and acute renal failure. While it is not known whether this interaction occurs with fibrates other than gemfibrozil, myopathy and rhabdomyolysis have occasionally been associated with the use of other fibrates alone, including clofibrate. Therefore, the combined use of lovastatin with other fibrates should generally be avoided.

Physicians contemplating combined therapy with lovastatin and lipid-lowering doses of nicotinic acid or with immunosuppressive drugs should carefully weigh the potential benefits and risks and should carefully monitor patients for any signs and symptoms of muscle pain, tenderness, or weakness, particularly during the initial months of therapy and during any periods of upward dosage titration of either drug. Periodic CPK determinations may be considered in such situations, but there is no assurance that such monitoring will prevent the occurrence of severe myopathy. The monitoring of lovastatin drug and metabolite levels may be considered in transplant patients who are treated with immunosuppressives and lovastatin.

Lovastatin therapy should be temporarily withheld or discontinued in any patient with an acute, serious condition suggestive of a myopathy or having a risk factor predisposing to the development of renal failure secondary to rhabdomyolysis, including: severe acute infection, hypotension, major surgery, trauma, severe metabolic, endocrine and electrolyte disorders, and uncontrolled seizures.

Myalgia has been associated with lovastatin therapy. Transient, mildly elevated creatine phosphokinase levels are commonly seen in lovastatin-treated patients. However, in early clinical trials, approximately 0.5% of patients developed a myopathy, *i.e.*, myalgia or muscle weakness associated with markedly elevated CPK levels. In the Excel study (see CLINICAL STUDIES), five (0.1%) patients taking lovastatin alone (one at 40 mg q.p.m., and four at 40 mg b.i.d.) developed myopathy (muscle symptoms and CPK levels >10 times the upper limit of normal). Myopathy should be considered in any patient with diffuse myalgias, muscle tenderness or weakness, and/or marked elevation of CPK. Patients should be advised to report promptly unexplained muscle pain, tenderness or weakness, particularly if accompanied by malaise or fever. Lovastatin therapy should be discontinued if markedly elevated CPK levels occur or myopathy is diagnosed or suspected.

Most of the patients who have developed myopathy (including rhabdomyolysis) while taking lovastatin were receiving concomitant therapy with immunosuppressive drugs, gemfibrozil or lipid-lowering doses of nicotinic acid. In clinical trials, about 30 percent of patients on concomitant immunosuppressive therapy including cyclosporine developed myopathy; the corresponding percentages for gemfibrozil and niacin were approximately 5 percent and 2 percent respectively.

In six patients with cardiac transplants taking immunosuppressive therapy including cyclosporine concomitantly with lovastatin 20 mg/day, the average plasma level of active metabolites derived from lovastatin was elevated to approximately four times the expected levels. Because of an apparent relationship between increased plasma levels of active metabolites derived from lovastatin and myopathy, the daily dosage in patients taking immunosuppressants should not exceed 20 mg/day (see DOSAGE AND ADMINISTRATION). Even at this dosage, the benefits and risks of using lovastatin in patients taking immunosuppressants should be carefully considered.

PRECAUTIONS:

GENERAL

Before instituting therapy with lovastatin, an attempt should be made to control hypercholesterolemia with appropriate diet, exercise, weight reduction in obese patients, and to treat other underlying medical problems (see INDICATIONS AND USAGE).

Lovastatin may elevate creatine phosphokinase and transaminase levels (see WARNINGS and ADVERSE REACTIONS). This should be considered in the differential diagnosis of chest pain in a patient on therapy with lovastatin.

Homozygous Familial Hypercholesterolemia: Lovastatin is less effective in patients with the rare homozygous familial hypercholesterolemia, possibly because these patients have no functional LDL receptors. Lovastatin appears to be more likely to raise serum transaminases (see ADVERSE REACTIONS) in these homozygous patients.

INFORMATION FOR THE PATIENT

Patients should be advised to report promptly unexplained muscle pain, tenderness or weakness, particularly if accompanied by malaise or fever.

Endocrine Function: HMG-CoA reductase inhibitors interfere with cholesterol synthesis and as such might theoretically blunt adrenal and/or gonadal steroid production. Results of clinical trials with drugs in this class have been inconsistent with regard to drug effects on basal and reserve steroid levels. However, clinical studies have shown that lovastatin does not reduce basal plasma cortisol concentration or impair adrenal reserve, and does not reduce basal plasma testosterone concentration. Another HMG-CoA reductase inhibitor has been shown to reduce the plasma testosterone response to HCG. In the same study, the mean testosterone response to HCG was slightly but not significantly reduced after treatment with lovastatin 40 mg daily for 16 weeks in 21 men. The effects of HMG-CoA reductase inhibitors on male fertility have not been studied in adequate numbers of male patients. The effects, if any, on the pituitary-gonadal axis in pre-menopausal women are unknown. Patients treated with lovastatin who develop clinical evidence of endocrine dysfunction should be evaluated appropriately. Caution should also be exercised if an HMG-CoA reductase inhibitor or other agent used to lower cholesterol levels is administered to patients also receiving other drugs (*e.g.*, ketoconazole, spironolactone, cimetidine) that may decrease the levels or activity of endogenous steroid hormones.

PRECAUTIONS: *(cont'd)*

CNS Toxicity: Lovastatin produced optic nerve degeneration (Wallerian degeneration of retinogeniculate fibers) in clinically normal dogs in a dose-dependent fashion starting at 60 mg/kg/day, a dose that produced mean plasma drug levels about 30 times higher than the mean drug level in humans taking the highest recommended dose (as measured by total enzyme inhibitory activity). Vestibulocochlear Wallerian-like degeneration and retinal ganglion cell chromatolysis were also seen in dogs treated for 14 weeks at 180 mg/kg/day, a dose which resulted in a mean plasma drug level (C_{max}) similar to that seen with the 60 mg/kg/day dose.

CNS vascular lesions, characterized by perivascular hemorrhage and edema, mononuclear cell infiltration of perivascular spaces, perivascular fibrin deposits and necrosis of small vessels, were seen in dogs treated with lovastatin at a dose of 180 mg/kg/day, a dose which produced plasma drug levels (C_{max}) which were about 30 times higher than the mean values in humans taking 80 mg/day.

Similar optic nerve and CNS vascular lesions have been observed with other drugs of this class.

Cataracts were seen in dogs treated for 11 and 28 weeks at 180 mg/kg/day and 1 year at 60 mg/kg/day.

CARCINOGENESIS, MUTAGENESIS, AND IMPAIRMENT OF FERTILITY

In a 21-month carcinogenic study in mice, there was a statistically significant increase in the incidence of hepatocellular carcinomas and adenomas in both males and females at 500 mg/kg/day. This dose produced a total plasma drug exposure 3 to 4 times that of humans given the highest recommended dose of lovastatin (drug exposure was measured as total HMG-CoA reductase inhibitory activity in extracted plasma). Tumor increases were not seen at 20 and 100 mg/kg/day, doses that produced drug exposures of 0.3 to 2 times that of humans at the 80 mg/day dose. A statistically significant increase in pulmonary adenomas was seen in female mice at approximately 4 times the human drug exposure. (Although mice were given 300 times the human dose [HD] on a mg/kg body weight basis, plasma levels of total inhibitory activity were only 4 times higher in mice than in humans given 80 mg of Mevacor.)

There was an increase in incidence of papilloma in the non-glandular mucosa of the stomach of mice beginning at exposures of 1 to 2 times that of humans. The glandular mucosa was not affected. The human stomach contains only glandular mucosa.

In a 24-month carcinogenicity study in rats, there was a positive dose response relationship for hepatocellular carcinogenicity in males at drug exposures between 2-7 times that of human exposure at 80 mg/day (doses in rats were 5, 30 and 180 mg/kg/day).

An increased incidence of thyroid neoplasms in rats appears to be a response that has been seen with other HMG CoA reductase inhibitors.

A chemically similar drug in this class was administered to mice for 72 weeks at 25, 100, and 400 mg/kg body weight, which resulted in mean serum drug levels approximately 3, 15, and 33 times higher than the mean human serum drug concentration (as total inhibitory activity) after a 40 mg oral dose. Liver carcinomas were significantly increased in high dose females and mid- and high dose males, with a maximum incidence of 90 percent in males. The incidence of adenomas of the liver was significantly increased in mid- and high dose females. Drug treatment also significantly increased the incidence of lung adenomas in mid- and high dose males and females. Adenomas of the Harderian gland (a gland of the eye of rodents) were significantly higher in high dose mice than in controls.

No evidence of mutagenicity was observed in a microbial mutagen test using mutant strains of *Salmonella typhimurium* with or without rat or mouse liver metabolic activation. In addition, no evidence of damage to genetic material was noted in an *in vitro* alkaline elution assay using rat or mouse hepatocytes, a V-79 mammalian cell forward mutation study, an *in vitro* chromosome aberration study in CHO cells, or an *in vivo* chromosomal aberration assay in mouse bone marrow.

Drug-related testicular atrophy, decreased spermatogenesis, spermatocytic degeneration and giant cell formation were seen in dogs starting at 20 mg/kg/day. Similar findings were seen with another drug in this class. No drug-related effects on fertility were found in studies with lovastatin in rats. However, in studies with a similar drug in this class, there was decreased fertility in male rats treated for 34 weeks at 25 mg/kg body weight, although this effect was not observed in a subsequent fertility study when this same dose was administered for 11 weeks (the entire cycle of spermatogenesis, including epididymal maturation). In rats treated with this same reductase inhibitor at 180 mg/kg/day, seminiferous tubule degeneration (necrosis and loss of spermatogenic epithelium) was observed. No microscopic changes were observed in the testes from rats of either study. The clinical significance of these findings is unclear.

PREGNANCY CATEGORY X

(See CONTRAINDICATIONS.)

Safety in pregnant women has not been established. Lovastatin has been shown to produce skeletal malformations at plasma levels 40 times the human exposure (for mouse fetus) and 80 times the human exposure (for rat fetus) based on mg/m² surface area (doses were 800 mg/kg/day). No drug-induced changes were seen in either species at multiples of 8 times (rat) or 4 times (mouse) based on surface area. No evidence of malformations was noted in rabbits at exposures up to 3 times the human exposure (dose of 15 mg/kg/day, highest tolerated dose). Rare reports of congenital anomalies have been received following intrauterine exposure to HMG-CoA reductase inhibitors. There has been one report of severe congenital bony deformity, tracheo-esophageal fistula, and anal atresia (VATER association) in a baby born to a woman who took lovastatin with dextroamphetamine sulfate during the first trimester of pregnancy. Lovastatin should be administered to women of child-bearing potential only when such patients are highly unlikely to conceive and have been informed of the potential hazards. If the woman becomes pregnant while taking lovastatin, it should be discontinued and the patient advised again as to the potential hazards to the fetus.

NURSING MOTHERS

It is not known whether lovastatin is excreted in human milk. Because a small amount of another drug in this class is excreted in human breast milk and because of the potential for serious adverse reactions in nursing infants, women taking Mevacor should not nurse their infants (see CONTRAINDICATIONS).

PEDIATRIC USE

Safety and effectiveness in children and adolescents have not been established. Because children and adolescents are not likely to benefit from cholesterol lowering for at least a decade and because experience with this drug is limited (no studies in subjects below the age of 20 years), treatment of children with lovastatin is not recommended at this time.

DRUG INTERACTIONS:

Immunosuppressive Drugs, Itraconazole, Gemfibrozil, Niacin (Nicotinic Acid), Erythromycin: See WARNINGS, Skeletal Muscle.

Coumarin Anticoagulants: In a small clinical trial in which lovastatin was administered to warfarin treated patients, no effect on prothrombin time was detected. However, another HMG-CoA reductase inhibitor has been found to produce a less than two seconds increase in prothrombin time in healthy volunteers receiving low doses of warfarin. Also, bleeding and/or increased prothrombin time have been reported in a few patients taking coumarin anticoag-

DRUG INTERACTIONS: *(cont'd)*

ulants concomitantly with lovastatin. It is recommended that in patients taking anticoagulants, prothrombin time be determined before starting lovastatin and frequently enough during early therapy to insure that no significant alteration of prothrombin time occurs. Once a stable prothrombin time has been documented, prothrombin times can be monitored at the intervals usually recommended for patients on coumarin anticoagulants. If the dose of lovastatin is changed, the same procedure should be repeated. Lovastatin therapy has not been associated with bleeding or with changes in prothrombin time in patients not taking anticoagulants.

Antipyrine: Because lovastatin had no effect on the pharmacokinetics of antipyrine or its metabolites, interactions of other drugs metabolized via the same cytochrome isozymes are not expected.

Propranolol: In normal volunteers, there was no clinically significant pharmacokinetic or pharmacodynamic interaction with concomitant administration of single doses of lovastatin and propranolol.

Digoxin: In patients with hypercholesterolemia, concomitant administration of lovastatin and digoxin resulted in no effect on digoxin plasma concentrations.

Oral Hypoglycemic Agents: In pharmacokinetic studies of lovastatin in hypercholesterolemic non-insulin dependent diabetic patients, there was no drug interaction with glipizide or with chlorpropamide (See CLINICAL STUDIES).

Other Concomitant Therapy: Although specific interaction studies were not performed, in clinical studies, lovastatin was used concomitantly with beta blockers, calcium channel blockers, diuretics and nonsteroidal anti-inflammatory drugs (NSAIDs) without evidence of clinically significant adverse interactions.

ADVERSE REACTIONS:

Lovastatin is generally well tolerated; adverse reactions usually have been mild and transient. Less than 1% of patients were discontinued from controlled clinical studies of up to 14 weeks due to adverse experiences attributable to lovastatin. About 3% of patients were discontinued from extensions of these studies due to adverse experiences attributable to lovastatin; about half of these patients were discontinued due to increases in serum transaminases. The median duration of therapy in these extensions was 5.2 years.

In the Excel study (see CLINICAL STUDIES), 4.6% of the patients treated up to 48 weeks were discontinued due to clinical or laboratory adverse experiences which were rated by the investigator as possibly, probably or definitely related to therapy with lovastatin. The value for the placebo group was 2.5%.

CLINICAL ADVERSE EXPERIENCES

Adverse experiences reported in patients treated with lovastatin in controlled clinical studies are shown in the table below (TABLE 7):

TABLE 7

	Lovastatin (N = 613) %	Placebo (N = 82) %	Cholestyramine (N = 88) %	Probucol (N = 97) %
Gastrointestinal				
Constipation	4.9	—	34.1	2.1
Diarrhea	5.5	4.9	8.0	10.3
Dyspepsia	3.9	—	13.6	3.1
Flatus	6.4	2.4	21.6	2.1
Abdominal pain/cramps	5.7	2.4	5.7	5.2
Heartburn	1.6	—	8.0	—
Nausea	4.7	3.7	9.1	6.2
Musculoskeletal				
Muscle cramps	1.1	—	1.1	—
Myalgia	2.4	1.2	—	—
Nervous System/Psychiatric				
Dizziness	2.0	1.2	—	1.0
Headache	9.3	4.9	4.5	8.2
Skin				
Rash/pruritus	5.2	—	4.5	—
Special Senses				
Blurred vision	1.5	—	1.1	3.1
Dysgeusia	0.8	—	1.1	—

LABORATORY TESTS

Marked persistent increases of serum transaminases have been noted (see WARNINGS).

About 11% of patients had elevations of creatine phosphokinase (CPK) levels of at least twice the normal value on one or more occasions. The corresponding values for the control agents were cholestyramine, 9 percent and probucol, 2 percent. This was attributable to the noncardiac fraction of CPK. Large increases in CPK have sometimes been reported (see WARNINGS, Skeletal Muscle).

EXPANDED CLINICAL EVALUATION OF LOVASTATIN (EXCEL) STUDY

Clinical Adverse Experiences: Lovastatin was compared to placebo in 8,245 patients with hypercholesterolemia (total cholesterol 240-300 mg/dl [6.2-7.8 mmol/l]) in the randomized, double-blind, parallel, 48-week Excel study. Clinical adverse experiences reported as possibly, probably or definitely drug-related in ≥1% in any treatment group are shown in the table (TABLE 8). For no event was the incidence on drug and placebo statistically different.

Other clinical adverse experiences reported as possibly, probably or definitely drug-related in 0.5 to 1.0 percent of patients in any drug-treated group are listed below. In all these cases the incidence on drug and placebo was not statistically different.

Body as a Whole: chest pain;

Gastrointestinal: acid regurgitation, dry mouth, vomiting;

Musculoskeletal: leg pain, shoulder pain, arthralgia;

Nervous System/Psychiatric: insomnia, paresthesia;

Skin: alopecia, pruritus;

Special Senses: eye irritation.

Concomitant Therapy: In controlled clinical studies in which lovastatin was administered concomitantly with cholestyramine, no adverse reactions peculiar to this concomitant treatment were observed. The adverse reactions that occurred were limited to those reported previously with lovastatin or cholestyramine. Other lipid-lowering agents were not administered concomitantly with lovastatin during controlled clinical studies. Preliminary data suggests that the addition of either probucol or gemfibrozil to therapy with lovastatin is not associated with greater reduction in LDL cholesterol than that achieved with lovastatin alone. In uncontrolled clinical studies, most of the patients who have developed myopathy were receiving concomitant therapy with immunosuppressive drugs, gemfibrozil or niacin (nicotinic acid) (see WARNINGS, Skeletal Muscle).

The following effects have been reported with drugs in this class. Not all the effects listed below have necessarily been associated with lovastatin therapy.

ADVERSE REACTIONS: *(cont'd)*

TABLE 8

	Placebo (N=1663) %	Lovastatin 20 mg q.p.m. (N=1642) %	Lovastatin 40 mg q.p.m. (N=1645) %	Lovastatin 20 mg b.i.d. (N=1646) %	Lovastatin 40 mg b.i.d. (N=1649) %
Body As a Whole					
Asthenia	1.4	1.7	1.4	1.5	1.2
Gastrointestinal					
Abdominal pain	1.6	2.0	2.0	2.2	2.5
Constipation	1.9	2.0	3.2	3.2	3.5
Diarrhea	2.3	2.6	2.4	2.2	2.6
Dyspepsia	1.9	1.3	1.3	1.0	1.6
Flatulence	4.2	3.7	4.3	3.9	4.5
Nausea	2.5	1.9	2.5	2.2	2.2
Musculoskeletal					
Muscle cramps	0.5	0.6	0.8	1.1	1.0
Myalgia	1.7	2.6	1.8	2.2	3.0
Nervous System/ Psychiatric					
Dizziness	0.7	0.7	1.2	0.5	0.5
Headache	2.7	2.6	2.8	2.1	3.2
Skin					
Rash	0.7	0.8	1.0	1.2	1.3
Special Senses					
Blurred vision	0.8	1.1	0.9	0.9	1.2

Skeletal: muscle cramps, myalgia, myopathy, rhabdomyolysis, arthralgias.

Neurological: dysfunction of certain cranial nerves (including alteration of taste, impairment of extra-ocular movement, facial paresis), tremor, dizziness, vertigo, memory loss, paresthesia, peripheral neuropathy, peripheral nerve palsy, anxiety, insomnia, depression.

Hypersensitivity Reactions: An apparent hypersensitivity syndrome has been reported rarely which has included one or more of the following features: anaphylaxis, angioedema, lupus erythematous-like syndrome, polymyalgia rheumatica, vasculitis, purpura, thrombocytopenia, leukopenia, hemolytic anemia, positive ANA, ESR increase, eosinophilia, arthritis, arthralgia, urticaria, asthenia, photosensitivity, fever, chills, flushing, malaise, dyspnea, toxic epidermal necrolysis, erythema multiforme, including Stevens-Johnson syndrome.

Gastrointestinal: pancreatitis, hepatitis, including chronic active hepatitis, cholestatic jaundice, fatty change in liver; and rarely, cirrhosis, fulminant hepatic necrosis, and hepatoma; anorexia, vomiting.

Skin: alopecia, pruritus. A variety of skin changes (*e.g.*, nodules, discoloration, dryness of skin/mucous membranes, changes to hair/nails) have been reported.

Reproductive: gynecomastia, loss of libido, erectile dysfunction.

Eye: progression of cataracts (lens opacities), ophthalmoplegia.

Laboratory Abnormalities: elevated transaminases, alkaline phosphatase, γ-glutamyl transpeptidase, and bilirubin; thyroid function abnormalities.

OVERDOSAGE:

After oral administration of lovastatin to mice the median lethal dose observed was >15 g/m^2.

Five healthy human volunteers have received up to 200 mg of lovastatin as a single dose without clinically significant adverse experiences. A few cases of accidental overdosage have been reported; no patients had any specific symptoms, and all patients recovered without sequelae. The maximum dose taken was 5-6 g.

Until further experience is obtained, no specific treatment of overdosage with Mevacor can be recommended.

The dialyzability of lovastatin and its metabolites in man is not known at present.

DOSAGE AND ADMINISTRATION:

The patient should be placed on a standard cholesterol-lowering diet before receiving lovastatin and should continue on this diet during treatment with lovastatin (see NCEP Treatment Guidelines for details on dietary therapy.) Lovastatin should be given with meals.

The usual recommended starting dose is 20 mg once a day given with the evening meal. The recommended dosing range is 10-80 mg/day in single or divided doses; the maximum recommended dose is 80 mg/day. Adjustments of dosage should be made at intervals of 4 weeks or more. Doses should be individualized according to the patient's response (see TABLE 1 and TABLE 4 for dose response results).

In patients taking immunosuppressive drugs concomitantly with lovastatin (see WARNINGS, Skeletal Muscle), therapy should begin with 10 mg of lovastatin and should not exceed 20 mg/day.

Cholesterol levels should be monitored periodically and consideration should be given to reducing the dosage of lovastatin if cholesterol levels fall below the targeted range.

Concomitant Therapy: Preliminary evidence suggests that the cholesterol-lowering effects of lovastatin and the bile acid sequestrant, cholestyramine, are additive.

Dosage in Patients with Renal Insufficiency: In patients with severe renal insufficiency (creatinine clearance <30 ml/min), dosage increases above 20 mg/day should be carefully considered and, if deemed necessary, implemented cautiously (see CLINICAL PHARMACOLOGY and WARNINGS, Skeletal Muscle).

PATIENT INFORMATION:

Lovastatin is used to lower high cholesterol levels. This medication should not be taken if you are pregnant, nursing, or have liver disease. Lovastatin should be taken with the evening meal. This medication may cause increased sensitivity to sunlight. Use sunscreens and wear protective clothing until degree of sensitivity is determined. Notify your physician if you develop blurred vision; skin rash; muscle pain, weakness, or cramps; unexplained fever, or yellowing of the skin or eyes.

HOW SUPPLIED:

Tablets Mevacor 10 mg are peach, octagonal tablets, coded MSD 730.

Tablets Mevacor 20 mg are light blue, octagonal tablets, coded MSD 731.

HOW SUPPLIED: *(cont'd)*

Tablets Mevacor 40 mg are green, octagonal tablets, coded MSD 732.

Storage: Store between 5°-30°C (41°-86°F). Tablets Mevacor must be protected from light and stored in a well-closed, light-resistant container.

HOW SUPPLIED - EQUIVALENTS NOT AVAILABLE:

Tablet, Uncoated - Oral - 10 mg

60's	$73.69	MEVACOR, Merck	00006-0730-61

Tablet, Uncoated - Oral - 20 mg

60's	$125.05	MEVACOR, Merck	00006-0731-61
100's	$212.16	MEVACOR, Merck	00006-0731-28
360's	$750.32	MEVACOR, 30 X 12, Merck	00006-0731-37
1000's	$2084.42	MEVACOR, Merck	00006-0731-82
1080's	$2251.34	MEVACOR, 90 X 12, Merck	00006-0731-94
1200's	$2501.50	MEVACOR, 100 X 12, Merck	00006-0731-78
2160's	$4503.19	MEVACOR, 180 X 12, Merck	00006-0731-98
10000's	$19197.91	MEVACOR, Merck	00006-0731-87

Tablet, Uncoated - Oral - 40 mg

60's	$225.09	MEVACOR, Merck	00006-0732-61
1000's	$3751.73	MEVACOR, Merck	00006-0732-82
1080's	$4052.05	MEVACOR, 90 X 12, Merck	00006-0732-94
10000's	$34554.16	MEVACOR, Merck	00006-0732-87

LOXAPINE SUCCINATE *(001666)*

CATEGORIES: Analeptics; Anesthesia; Antipsychotics/Antimanics; Tricyclic Antidepressants; Central Nervous System Agents; Neuroleptics; Psychotherapeutic Agents; Psychotic Disorders; Schizophrenia; Tranquilizers; Tricyclics; FDA Approval Pre 1982

BRAND NAMES: *Desconex*; *Loxapac* (France, England, Canada); **Loxitane**; Loxapine Hydrochloride
(International brand names outside U.S. in italics)

FORMULARIES: Aetna

COST OF THERAPY: $713.30 (Schizophrenia; Liquid; 25 mg/ml; 1/day; 365 days) vs. Potential Cost of $3,628.44 (Psychoses)

DESCRIPTION:

Loxapine, a dibenzoxazepine compound, represents a new subclass of tricyclic antipsychotic agent, chemically distinct from the thioxanthenes, butyrophenones, and phenothiazines. Chemically, it is 2-Chloro-11-(4-methyl-1-piperazinyl)-dibenz[*b,f*][1,4]oxazepine. It is present in capsules as the succinate salt, and in the concentrate and parenteral primarily as the hydrochloride salt.

Capsules: Each Loxitane capsule contains loxapine succinate equivalent to 5, 10, 25 or 50 mg of loxapine base and the following inactive ingredients: Blue 1, Gelatin, Lactose, Magnesium Stearate, Titanium Dioxide and Yellow 10. Additionally, the 5 mg capsule contains Red 33 and the 10 mg capsule contains Red 28 and Red 33 and the 25 mg capsule contains FD&C Yellow No. 6.

Oral Concentrate: Each ml of Loxitane contains loxapine hydrochloride equivalent to 25 mg of loxapine base and propylene glycol as an inactive ingredient. Hydrochloric acid and, if necessary, sodium hydroxide are used to adjust pH to approximately 5.8 during manufacture.

Intramuscular (Sterile): Not for Intravenous Use. Each ml of Loxitane contains loxapine hydrochloride equivalent to 50 mg of loxapine base. Inactive ingredients: Polysorbate 80 NF 5% w/v, Propylene Glycol 70% v/v, and Water for Injection qs ad 100% v.

Hydrochloric acid and, if necessary, sodium hydroxide are used to adjust pH to approximately 5.5 during manufacture.

CLINICAL PHARMACOLOGY:

PHARMACODYNAMICS

Pharmacologically, loxapine is a tranquilizer for which the exact mode of action has not been established. However, changes in the level of excitability of subcortical inhibitory areas have been observed in several animal species in association with such manifestations of tranquilization as calming effects and suppression of aggressive behavior.

In normal human volunteers, signs of sedation were seen within 20 to 30 minutes after administration, were most pronounced within 1 1/2 to three hours, and lasted through 12 hours. Similar timing of primary pharmacologic effects was seen in animals.

ABSORPTION, DISTRIBUTION, METABOLISM, AND EXCRETION

After administration of loxapine as an oral solution, systemic bioavailability of the parent drug was only about one third that after an equivalent intramuscular dose (25 mg base) in male volunteers. C_{max} for the parent drug was similar for the IM and oral administrations, whereas T_{max} was significantly longer for the IM administration than the oral administration (approximately 5 vs one hour). The lower systemic availability of the parent drug after oral administration as compared to the IM administration may be due to first pass metabolism of the oral form. This is supported by the finding that two metabolites found in serum (8-hydroxyloxapine and 8-hydroxydesmethylloxapine) were formed to a lesser extent after IM administration of loxapine as compared to oral administration.

The apparent half-life of loxapine after oral and IM administration is approximately four hours (range, one-14 hours) and 12 hours (range, eight-23 hours) respectively. The extended half-life for the IM administration as compared to the oral administration may be explained by prolonged absorption of loxapine from the muscle during the concurrent elimination process.

Loxapine is extensively metabolized, and urinary recovery over 48 hours resulted in recoveries of approximately 30% and 40% of an IM and orally administered loxapine dose as five metabolites.

INDICATIONS AND USAGE:

Loxapine is indicated for the management of the manifestations of psychotic disorders. The antipsychotic efficacy of loxapine was established in clinical studies which enrolled newly hospitalized and chronically hospitalized acutely ill schizophrenic patients as subjects.

CONTRAINDICATIONS:

Loxapine is contraindicated in comatose or severe drug-induced depressed states (alcohol, barbiturates, narcotics, etc.).

Loxapine is contraindicated in individuals with known hypersensitivity to dibenzoxazepines.

WARNINGS:

Tardive Dyskinesia: Tardive dyskinesia, a syndrome consisting of potentially irreversible, involuntary, dyskinetic movements may develop in patients treated with neuroleptic (antipsychotic) drugs. Although the prevalence of the syndrome appears to be highest among the elderly, especially elderly women, it is impossible to rely upon prevalence estimates to predict, at the inception of neuroleptic treatment, which patients are likely to develop the syndrome. Whether neuroleptic drug products differ in their potential to cause tardive dyskinesia is unknown.

Both the risk of developing the syndrome and the likelihood that it will become irreversible are believed to increase as the duration of treatment and the total cumulative dose of neuroleptic drugs administered to the patient increase. However, the syndrome can develop, although much less commonly, after relatively brief treatment periods at low doses.

There is no known treatment for established cases of tardive dyskinesia, although the syndrome may remit, partially or completely, if neuroleptic treatment is withdrawn. Neuroleptic treatment, itself, however, may suppress (or partially suppress) the signs and symptoms of the syndrome and thereby may possibly mask the underlying disease process. The effect that symptomatic suppression has upon the long-term course of the syndrome is unknown.

Given these considerations, neuroleptics should be prescribed in a manner that is most likely to minimize the occurrence of tardive dyskinesia. Chronic neuroleptic treatment should generally be reserved for patients who suffer from a chronic illness that, (1) is known to respond to neuroleptic drugs, and, (2) for whom alternative, equally effective, but potentially less harmful treatments are *not* available or appropriate. In patients who do require chronic treatment, the smallest dose and the shortest duration of treatment producing a satisfactory clinical response should be sought. The need for continued treatment should be reassessed periodically.

If signs and symptoms of tardive dyskinesia appear in a patient on neuroleptics, drug discontinuation should be considered. However, some patients may require treatment despite the presence of the syndrome. (See ADVERSE REACTIONS and Information for the Patient.)

NEUROLEPTIC MALIGNANT SYNDROME (NMS)

A potentially fatal symptom complex sometimes referred to as Neuroleptic Malignant Syndrome (NMS) has been reported in association with antipsychotic drugs. Clinical manifestations of NMS are hyperpyrexia, muscle rigidity, altered mental status and evidence of autonomic instability (irregular pulse or blood pressure, tachycardia, diaphoresis, and cardiac dysrhythmias).

The diagnostic evaluation of patients with this syndrome is complicated. In arriving at a diagnosis, it is important to identify cases where the clinical presentation includes both serious medical illness (*e.g.*, pneumonia, systemic infection, etc.) and untreated or inadequately treated extrapyramidal signs and symptoms (EPS). Other important considerations in the differential diagnosis include central anticholinergic toxicity, heat stroke, drug fever and primary central nervous system (CNS) pathology.

The management of NMS should include: (1) immediate discontinuation of antipsychotic drugs and other drugs not essential to concurrent therapy, (2) intensive symptomatic treatment and medical monitoring, and (3) treatment of any concomitant serious medical problems for which specific treatments are available. There is no general agreement about specific pharmacological treatment regimens for uncomplicated NMS.

If a patient requires antipsychotic drug treatment after recovery from NMS, the potential reintroduction of drug therapy should be carefully considered. The patient should be carefully monitored, since recurrences of NMS have been reported.

Loxapine, like other tranquilizers, may impair mental and/or physical abilities, especially during the first few days of therapy. Therefore, ambulatory patients should be warned about activities requiring alertness (*e.g.*, operating vehicles or machinery) and about concomitant use of alcohol and other CNS depressants.

Loxapine has not been evaluated for the management of behavioral complications in patients with mental retardation, and therefore, it cannot be recommended.

PRECAUTIONS:

GENERAL

Loxapine should be used with extreme caution in patients with a history of convulsive disorders since it lowers the convulsive threshold. Seizures have been reported in patients receiving loxapine at antipsychotic dose levels, and may occur in epileptic patients even with maintenance of routine anticonvulsant drug therapy.

Loxapine has an antiemetic effect in animals. Since this effect may also occur in man, loxapine may mask signs of overdosage of toxic drugs and may obscure conditions such as intestinal obstruction and brain tumor.

Loxapine should be used with caution in patients with cardiovascular disease. Increased pulse rates have been reported in the majority of patients receiving antipsychotic doses; transient hypotension has been reported in the presence of severe hypotension requiring vasopressor therapy, the preferred drugs may be norepinephrine or angiotensin. Usual doses of epinephrine may be ineffective because of inhibition of its vasopressor effect by loxapine.

The possibility of ocular toxicity from loxapine cannot be excluded at this time. Therefore, careful observation should be made for pigmentary retinopathy and lenticular pigmentation since these have been observed in some patients receiving certain other antipsychotic drugs for prolonged periods.

Because of possible anticholinergic action, the drug should be used cautiously in patients with glaucoma or a tendency to urinary retention, particularly with concomitant administration of anticholinergic-type antiparkinson medication.

Experience to date indicates the possibility of a slightly higher incidence of extrapyramidal effects following intramuscular administration that normally anticipated with oral formulations. The increase may be attributable to higher plasma levels following intramuscular injection.

Neuroleptic drugs elevate prolactin levels; the elevation persists during chronic administration. Tissue culture experiments indicate that approximately one third of human breast cancers are prolactin dependent*in vitro*, a factor of potential importance if the prescription of these drugs is contemplated in a patient with a previously detected breast cancer. Although disturbances such as galactorrhea, amenorrhea, gynecomastia, and impotence have been reported, the clinical significance of elevated serum prolactin levels is unknown for most patients. An increase in mammary neoplasms has been found in rodents after chronic administration of neuroleptic drugs. Neither clinical studies nor epidemiologic studies conducted to date, however, have shown an association between chronic administration of these drugs and mammary tumorigenesis; the available evidence is considered too limited to be conclusive at this time.

INFORMATION FOR THE PATIENT

Given the likelihood that some patients exposed chronically to neuroleptics will develop tardive dyskinesia, it is advised that all patients in whom chronic use is contemplated be given, if possible, full information about this risk. The decision to inform patients and/or their guardians must obviously take into account the clinical circumstances and the competency of the patient to understand the information provided.

PRECAUTIONS: *(cont'd)*

USAGE IN PREGNANCY

Safe use of loxapine during pregnancy or lactation has not been established; therefore, its use in pregnancy, in nursing mothers, or in women of child-bearing potential requires that the benefits of treatment be weighed against the possible risks to mother and child. No embryotoxicity or teratogenicity was observed in studies in rats, rabbits or dogs although, with the exception of one rabbit study, the highest dosage was only two times the maximum recommended human dose and in some studies it was below this dose. Perinatal studies have shown renal papillary abnormalities in offspring of rats treated from midpregnancy with doses of 0.6 and 1.8 mg/kg, doses which approximate the usual human dose but which are considerably below the maximum recommended human dose.

NURSING MOTHERS

The extent of the excretion of loxapine or its metabolites in human milk is not known. However, loxapine and its metabolites have been shown to be transported into the milk of lactating dogs. Loxapine administration to nursing women should be avoided if clinically possible.

USAGE IN CHILDREN

Studies have not been performed in children; therefore, this drug is not recommended for use in children below the age of 16.

ADVERSE REACTIONS:

CNS Effects: Manifestations of adverse effects on the central nervous system, other than extrapyramidal effects, have been seen infrequently. Drowsiness, usually mild, may occur at the beginning of therapy or when dosage is increased. It usually subsides with continued loxapine therapy. The incidence of sedation has been less than that of certain aliphatic phenothiazines and slightly more than the piperazine phenothiazines. Dizziness, faintness, staggering gait, shuffling gait, muscle twitching, weakness, insomnia, agitation, tension, seizures, akinesia, slurred speech, numbness and confusional states have been reported. Neuroleptic malignant syndrome (NMS) has been reported (see WARNINGS.)

Extrapyramidal Reactions: Neuromuscular (extrapyramidal) reactions during the administration of loxapine have been reported frequently, often during the first few days of treatment. In most patients, these reactions involved parkinsonian-like symptoms such as tremor, rigidity, excessive salivation, and masked facies. Akathisia (motor restlessness) also has been reported relatively frequently. These symptoms are usually not severe and can be controlled by reduction of loxapine dosage or by administration of antiparkinson drugs in usual dosage. Dystonic and dyskinetic reactions have occurred less frequently, but may be more severe. Dystonias include spasms of muscles of the neck and face, tongue protrusion, and oculogyric movement. Dyskinetic reactions have been described in the form of choreoathetoid movements. These reactions sometimes require reduction or temporary withdrawal of loxapine dosage in addition to appropriate counteractive drugs.

Persistent Tardive Dyskinesia: As with all antipsychotic agents, tardive dyskinesia may appear in some patients on long-term therapy or may appear after drug therapy has been discontinued. The risk appears to be greater in elderly patients on high-dose therapy, especially females. The symptoms are persistent and in some patients appear to be irreversible. The syndrome is characterized by rhythmical involuntary movement of the tongue, face, mouth, or jaw (*e.g.,* protrusion of tongue, puffing of cheeks, puckering of mouth, chewing movements). Sometimes these may be accompanied by involuntary movements of extremities.

There is no known effective treatment for tardive dyskinesia, antiparkinson agents usually do not alleviate the symptoms of this syndrome. It is suggested that all antipsychotic agents be discontinued if these symptoms appear. Should it be necessary to reinstitute treatment, or increase the dosage of the agent, or switch to a different antipsychotic agent, the syndrome may be masked. It has been suggested that fine vermicular movements of the tongue may be an early sign of the syndrome, and if the medication is stopped at that time the syndrome may not develop.

Cardiovascular Effects: Tachycardia, hypotension, hypertension, orthostatic hypotension, lightheadedness, and syncope have been reported. A few cases of ECG changes similar to those seen with phenothiazines have been reported. It is not known whether these were related to loxapine administration.

Hematologic: Rarely, agranulocytosis, thrombocytopenia, leukopenia.

Skin: Dermatitis, edema (puffiness of face), pruritus, rash, alopecia and seborrhea have been reported with loxapine.

Anticholinergic Effects: Dry mouth, nasal congestion, constipation, blurred vision, urinary retention and paralytic ileus have occurred.

Gastrointestinal: Nausea and vomiting have been reported in some patients. Hepatocellular injury (*i.e.,* SGOT/SGPT elevation) has been reported in association with loxapine administration and rarely, jaundice and/or hepatitis questionably related to loxapine treatment.

Other Adverse Reactions: Weight gain, weight loss, dyspnea, ptosis, hyperpyrexia, flushed facies, headache, paresthesia, and polydipsia have been reported in some patients. Rarely, galactorrhea, amenorrhea, gynecomastia and menstrual irregularity of uncertain etiology have been reported.

OVERDOSAGE:

Signs and symptoms of overdosage will depend on the amount ingested and individual patient tolerance. As would be expected from the pharmacologic actions of the drug, the clinical findings may range from mild depression of the CNS and cardiovascular systems to profound hypotension, respiratory depression, and unconsciousness. The possibility of occurrence of extrapyramidal symptoms and/or convulsive seizures should be kept in mind. Renal failure following loxapine overdosage has also been reported.

The treatment of overdosage is essentially symptomatic and supportive. Early gastric lavage and extended dialysis might be expected to be beneficial. Centrally acting emetics may have little effect because of the antiemetic action of loxapine. In addition, emesis should be avoided because of the possibility of aspiration of vomitus. Avoid analeptics, such as pentylenetetrazol, which may cause convulsions. Severe hypotension might be expected to respond to the administration of levarterenol or phenylephrine. EPINEPHRINE SHOULD NOT BE USED SINCE ITS USE IN A PATIENT WITH PARTIAL ADRENERGIC BLOCKADE MAY FURTHER LOWER THE BLOOD PRESSURE. Severe extrapyramidal reactions should be treated with anticholinergic antiparkinson agents of diphenhydramine hydrochloride, and anticonvulsant therapy should be initiated as indicated. Additional measures include oxygen and intravenous fluids.

DOSAGE AND ADMINISTRATION:

Loxapine is administered usually in divided doses, two to four times a day. Daily dosage (in terms of base equivalents) should be adjusted to the individual patient's needs as assessed by the severity of the symptoms and previous history of response to antipsychotic drugs.

ORAL ADMINISTRATION

Initial dosage of 10 mg twice daily is recommended, although in severely disturbed patients initial dosage up to a total of 50 mg daily may be desirable. Dosage should then be increased fairly rapidly over the first seven to ten days until there is effective control of psychotic symptoms. The usual therapeutic and maintenance range is 60 to 100 mg daily. However, as with other antipsychotic drugs, some patients respond to lower dosage and other require higher dosage for optimal benefit. Daily dosage higher than 250 mg is not recommended.

Loxapine C Oral Concentrate should be mixed with orange or grapefruit juice shortly before administration. Use only the enclosed calibrated (10 mg, 15 mg, 25 mg, 50 mg) dropper for dosage.

MAINTENANCE THERAPY

For maintenance therapy, dosage should be reduced to the lowest level compatible with symptom control; many patients have been maintained satisfactorily at dosages in the range of 20 to 60 mg daily.

INTRAMUSCULAR ADMINISTRATION

Loxapine IM is utilized for prompt symptomatic control in the acutely agitated patient and in patients whose symptoms render oral medication temporarily impractical. During clinical trial there were only rare reports of significant local tissue reaction.

Loxapine IM is administered by intramuscular (not intravenous) injection in doses of 12.5 mg (1/4 ml) to 50 mg (1 ml) at intervals of four to six hours or longer, both dose and interval depending on patient response. Many patients have responded satisfactorily to twice-daily dosage. As described above for oral administration, attention is directed to the necessity for dosage adjustment on an individual basis over the early days of loxapine administration.

Once the desired symptomatic control is achieved and the patient is above to take medication orally, loxapine should be administered in capsule or oral concentrate form. Usually this should occur within five days.

Store at Controlled Room Temperature 15-30°C (59-86°F).
DO NOT FREEZE.

HOW SUPPLIED - RATED THERAPEUTICALLY EQUIVALENT:

Capsule, Gelatin - Oral - 5 mg

10's	**$87.12**	**LOXITANE, Lederle Pharm**	**00005-5359-60**
100's	$36.24	Loxapine Succinate, Bristol Myers Squibb	00003-0117-50
100's	$44.00	Loxapine Succinate, Raway	00686-0677-20
100's	$46.20	Loxapine Succinate, H.C.F.A. F F P	99999-1666-01
100's	$47.25	Loxapine Succinate, Major Pharms	00904-2310-60
100's	$49.30	Loxapine Succinate, Qualitest Pharms	00603-4268-21
100's	$66.89	Loxapine Succinate, Parmed Pharms	00349-8839-01
100's	$67.20	Loxapine Succinate, Geneva Pharms	50752-0296-05
100's	$67.21	Loxapine Succinate, Goldline Labs	00182-1305-01
100's	$67.21	Loxapine Succinate, Aligen Independ	00405-5120-01
100's	$67.21	Loxapine Succinate, Watson Labs	52544-0369-01
100's	$67.22	Loxapine, HL Moore Drug Exch	00839-7495-06
100's	$69.25	Loxapine Succinate, Schein Pharm (US)	00364-2303-01
100's	$69.30	Loxapine Succinate, Geneva Pharms	00781-2710-01
100's	**$79.07**	**LOXITANE, Lederle Pharm**	**00005-5359-23**
1000's	$462.00	Loxapine Succinate, H.C.F.A. F F P	99999-1666-02
1000's	$638.50	Loxapine Succinate, Watson Labs	52544-0369-10

Capsule, Gelatin - Oral - 10 mg

10's	**$110.26**	**LOXITANE, Lederle Pharm**	**00005-5360-60**
100's	$46.83	Loxapine Succinate, Bristol Myers Squibb	00003-0123-50
100's	$63.53	Loxapine Succinate, H.C.F.A. F F P	99999-1666-03
100's	$67.00	Loxapine Succinate, Raway	00686-0678-20
100's	$68.20	Loxapine Succinate, Qualitest Pharms	00603-4269-21
100's	$69.45	Loxapine Succinate, Major Pharms	00904-2311-60
100's	$86.80	Loxapine Succinate, Geneva Pharms	50752-0297-05
100's	$86.85	Loxapine Succinate, Goldline Labs	00182-1306-01
100's	$86.85	Loxapine Succinate, Aligen Independ	00405-5121-01
100's	$86.85	Loxapine Succinate, Watson Labs	52544-0370-01
100's	$87.81	Loxapine Succinate, HL Moore Drug Exch	00839-7496-06
100's	$88.54	Loxapine Succinate, Parmed Pharms	00349-8836-01
100's	$89.50	Loxapine Succinate, Schein Pharm (US)	00364-2304-01
100's	$89.50	Loxapine Succinate, Rugby	00536-4834-01
100's	$89.55	Loxapine Succinate, Geneva Pharms	00781-2711-01
100's	$95.48	Loxapine Succinate, Warner Chilcott	00047-0632-24
100's	**$102.17**	**LOXITANE, Lederle Pharm**	**00005-5360-23**
1000's	$635.30	Loxapine Succinate, H.C.F.A. F F P	99999-1666-04
1000's	$820.66	Loxapine Succinate, Watson Labs	52544-0370-10
1000's	**$965.47**	**LOXITANE, Lederle Pharm**	**00005-5360-34**

Capsule, Gelatin - Oral - 25 mg

10's	**$162.46**	**LOXITANE, Lederle Pharm**	**00005-5361-60**
100's	$70.74	Loxapine Succinate, Bristol Myers Squibb	00003-0145-50
100's	$89.25	Loxapine Succinate, United Res	00677-1320-01
100's	$89.93	Loxapine Succinate, H.C.F.A. F F P	99999-1666-05
100's	$105.00	Loxapine Succinate, Raway	00686-0679-20
100's	$108.05	Loxapine Succinate, Qualitest Pharms	00603-4270-21
100's	$108.68	Loxapine Succinate, Warner Chilcott	00047-0650-24
100's	$108.90	Loxapine Succinate, Major Pharms	00904-2312-60
100's	$131.20	Loxapine Succinate, Geneva Pharms	50752-0298-05
100's	$131.23	Loxapine Succinate, Goldline Labs	00182-1307-01
100's	$131.23	Loxapine Succinate, Aligen Independ	00405-5122-01
100's	$131.23	Loxapine Succinate, Watson Labs	52544-0371-01
100's	$131.29	Loxapine Succinate, HL Moore Drug Exch	00839-7497-06
100's	$133.78	Loxapine Succinate, Parmed Pharms	00349-8837-01
100's	$135.20	Loxapine Succinate, Schein Pharm (US)	00364-2305-01
100's	$135.30	Loxapine Succinate, Rugby	00536-4835-01
100's	$135.30	Loxapine Succinate, Geneva Pharms	00781-2712-01
100's	**$154.39**	**LOXITANE, Lederle Pharm**	**00005-5361-23**
1000's	$899.30	Loxapine Succinate, H.C.F.A. F F P	99999-1666-06
1000's	$1246.19	Loxapine Succinate, Watson Labs	52544-0371-10
1000's	**$1466.10**	**LOXITANE, Lederle Pharm**	**00005-5361-34**

Capsule, Gelatin - Oral - 50 mg

100's	$94.38	Loxapine Succinate, Bristol Myers Squibb	00003-0153-50
100's	$118.73	Loxapine Succinate, United Res	00677-1321-01
100's	$121.13	Loxapine Succinate, H.C.F.A. F F P	99999-1666-07
100's	$135.00	Loxapine Succinate, Raway	00686-0680-20
100's	$138.65	Loxapine Succinate, Qualitest Pharms	00603-4271-21
100's	$139.95	Loxapine Succinate, Major Pharms	00904-2313-60
100's	$175.00	Loxapine Succinate, Geneva Pharms	50752-0299-05
100's	$175.08	Loxapine Succinate, Goldline Labs	00182-1308-01
100's	$175.08	Loxapine Succinate, Aligen Independ	00405-5123-01
100's	$175.08	Loxapine Succinate, Watson Labs	52544-0372-01
100's	$178.48	Loxapine Succinate, Parmed Pharms	00349-8838-01
100's	$180.55	Loxapine Succinate, Geneva Pharms	00781-2713-01
100's	$181.50	Loxapine Succinate, Schein Pharm (US)	00364-2306-01
100's	$185.08	Loxapine, HL Moore Drug Exch	00839-7498-06
100's	$192.35	Loxapine Succinate, Warner Chilcott	00047-0651-24
100's	$192.35	Loxapine Succinate, Rugby	00536-4836-01
100's	**$205.98**	**LOXITANE, Lederle Pharm**	**00005-5362-23**
100's	**$213.98**	**LOXITANE, Lederle Pharm**	**00005-5362-60**

HOW SUPPLIED - RATED THERAPEUTICALLY EQUIVALENT: *(cont'd)*

1000's	$1211.30	Loxapine Succinate, H.C.F.A. F F P	99999-1666-08
1000's	$1680.54	Loxapine Succinate, Watson Labs	52544-0372-10
1000's	**$1977.10**	**LOXITANE, Lederle Pharm**	**00005-5362-34**

HOW SUPPLIED - NOT RATED EQUIVALENT:

Injection, Solution - Intramuscular - 50 mg/ml

1 ml x 10	**$105.46**	**LOXITANE, Lederle Parenterals**	**00205-5385-55**
10 ml	**$96.34**	**LOXITANE, Lederle Parenterals**	**00205-5385-34**

Liquid - Oral - 25 mg/ml

120 ml	**$234.51**	**LOXITANE C, Lederle Pharm**	**00005-5387-58**

LYMPHOCYTE IMMUNE GLOBULIN *(001671)*

CATEGORIES: Anemia; Biologicals; Bone Marrow Transplantation; Immunologic; Immunomodulators; Neoplastic Disease; Renal Transplantation; Serums, Toxoids and Vaccines; Transplantation; Pregnancy Category C; FDA Pre 1938 Drugs

BRAND NAMES: Atgam

> WARNING:
> Only physicians experienced in immunosuppressive therapy in the management of renal transplant or aplastic anemia patients should use Atgam.
> Patients receiving Atgam should be managed in facilities equipped and staffed with adequate laboratory and supportive medical resources.

DESCRIPTION:

FOR INTRAVENOUS USE ONLY

Atgam Sterile Solution contains lymphocyte immune globulin, anti-thymocyte globulin (equine). It is the purified, concentrated, and sterile gamma globulin, primarily monomeric lgG, from hyperimmune serum of horses immunized with human thymus lymphocytes. Atgam is a transparent to slightly opalescent aqueous protein solution. It may appear colorless to faintly pink or brown and is nearly odorless. It may develop a slight granular or flaky deposit during storage. (For information about in-line filters, see Infusion Instructions in the DOSAGE AND ADMINISTRATION.)

Before release for clinical use, each lot of Atgam is tested to assure its ability to inhibit rosette formation between human peripheral lymphocytes and sheep red blood cells *in vitro*. In each lot, antibody activity against human red blood cells and platelets is also measured and determined to be within acceptable limits. Only lots that test negative for antihuman serum protein antibody, antiglomerular basement membrane antibody and pyrogens are released.

Each milliliter of Atgam contains 50 mg of horse gamma globulin stabilized in 0.3 molar glycine to a pH of approximately 6.8; preserved with thimerosal (mercury derivative) 1: 10,000 (0.01%).

CLINICAL PHARMACOLOGY:

Atgam Sterile Solution is a lymphocyte-selective immunosuppressant as is demonstrated by its ability to reduce the number of circulating, thymus-dependent lymphocytes that form rosettes with sheep erythrocytes. This antilymphocytic effect is believed to reflect an alteration of the function of the T-lymphocytes, which are responsible in part for cell-mediated immunity and are involved in humoral immunity. In addition to its antilymphocytic activity, Atgam contains low concentrations of antibodies against other formed elements of the blood. In rhesus and cynomolgus monkeys, Atgam reduces lymphocytes in the thymus-dependent areas of the spleen and lymph nodes. It also decreases the circulating sheep-erythrocyte-rosetting lymphocytes that can be detected, but ordinarily Atgam does not cause severe lymphopenia.

In general, when Atgam is given with other immunosuppressive therapy, such as antimetabolites and corticosteroids, the patient's own antibody response to horse gamma globulin is minimal. In a small clinical study, Atgam administered with other immunosuppressive therapy and measured as horse lgG had a serum half-life of 5.7 ± 3 days.

INDICATIONS AND USAGE:

RENAL TRANSPLANTATION

Atgam Sterile Solution is indicated for the management of allograft rejection in renal transplant patients. When administered with conventional therapy at the time of rejection, it increases the frequency of resolution of the acute rejection episode. The drug has also been administered as an adjunct to other immunosuppressive therapy to delay the onset of the first rejection episode. Data accumulated to date have not consistently demonstrated improvement in functional graft survival associated with therapy to delay the onset of the first rejection episode.

APLASTIC ANEMIA

Atgam is indicated for the treatment of moderate to severe aplastic anemia in patients who are unsuitable for bone marrow transplantation.

When administered with a regimen of supportive care, Atgam may induce partial or complete hematologic remission. In a controlled trial, patients receiving Atgam showed a statistically significant higher improvement rate compared to standard supportive care at 3 months. Improvement was defined in terms of sustained increase in peripheral blood counts and reduced transfusion needs.

Clinical trials conducted at two centers evaluated the one year survival rate for patients with severe and moderate to severe aplastic anemia. Seventy-four of the 83 patients enrolled were evaluable based on response to treatment. The treatment groups studied consisted of: 1) Atgam and supportive care, 2) Atgam administered following 3 months of supportive care alone, 3) Atgam, mismatched marrow infusion, androgens and supportive care, or 4) Atgam, androgens and supportive care. There were no statistically significant differences between the treatment groups. The one year survival rate for the pooled treatment groups was 69%. These survival results can be compared to a historical survival rate of about 25% for patients receiving standard supportive care alone.

The usefulness of Atgam has not been demonstrated in patients with aplastic anemia who are suitable candidates for bone marrow transplantation or in patients with aplastic anemia secondary to neoplastic disease, storage disease, myelofibrosis, Fanconi's syndrome or in patients known to have been exposed to myelotoxic agents or radiation.

To date, safety and efficacy have not been established in circumstances other than renal transplantation and aplastic anemia.

INDICATIONS AND USAGE: *(cont'd)*

SKIN TESTING

Before the first infusion of Atgam, The Upjohn Company strongly recommends that patients be tested with an intradermal injection of 0.1 ml of a 1:1000 dilution (5 mcg horse lgG) of Atgam in Sodium Chloride Injection, USP and a contralateral Sodium Chloride Injection control. Use only freshly diluted Atgam for skin testing. The patient and specifically the skin test should be observed every 15 to 20 minutes over the first hour after intradermal injection. A local reaction of 10 mm or greater with a wheal or erythema or both with or without pseudopod formation and itching or a marked local swelling should be considered a positive test. Note: The predictive value of this test has not been proven clinically. Allergic reactions such as anaphylaxis have occurred in patients whose skin test is negative. In the presence of a locally positive skin test to Atgam, serious consideration to alternative forms of therapy should be given. The risk to benefit ration must be carefully weighed. If therapy with Atgam is deemed appropriate following a locally positive skin test, treatment should be administered in a setting where intensive life support facilities are immediately available and with a physician familiar with the treatment of potentially life threatening allergic reactions in attendance.

A systemic reaction such as a generalized rash, tachycardia, dyspnea, hypotension, or anaphylaxis precludes any additional administration of Atgam.

See WARNINGS, PRECAUTIONS and ADVERSE REACTIONS.

CONTRAINDICATIONS:

Do not administer Atgam Sterile Solution to a patient who has had a severe systemic reaction during prior administration of Atgam or any other equine gamma globulin preparation.

WARNINGS:

> **Only physicians experienced in immunosuppressive therapy in the management of renal transplant or aplastic anemia patients should use Atgam. Patients receiving Atgam should be managed in facilities equipped and staffed with adequate laboratory and supportive medical resources.**

Precise methods of determining the potency of Atgam have not been established, thus activity may potentially vary from lot to lot.

Discontinue treatment with Atgam if any of the following occurs:

1. Symptoms of anaphylaxis (See ADVERSE REACTIONS)

2. Severe and unremitting thrombocytopenia in renal transplant patients

3. Severe and unremitting leukopenia in renal transplant patients

In common with products derived from, or purified with human blood components, the possibility of transmission of infectious agents exists.

PRECAUTIONS:

Because Atgam Sterile Solution is an immunosuppressive agent ordinarily given with corticosteroids and antimetabolites, watch patients carefully for signs of leukopenia, thrombocytopenia or concurrent infection. Several studies have suggested an increase in the incidence of cytomegalovirus infection in patients receiving Atgam. In one study it has been found that it may be possible to reduce this risk by decreasing the dosage of other immunosuppressive agents administered concomitantly with Atgam. If infection occurs, institute appropriate adjunctive therapy promptly. On the basis of the clinical circumstances, a physician should decide whether or not therapy with Atgam will. continue.

Pregnancy Category C: Atgam has not been evaluated in either pregnant or lactating women. Animal reproduction studies have not been conducted with Atgam. It is also not known whether Atgam can cause fetal harm when administered to a pregnant woman or can affect reproduction capacity. Atgam administration to pregnant women is not recommended and should be considered only under exceptional circumstances.

The safety and effectiveness of Atgam have been demonstrated only in renal transplant patients who received concomitant immunosuppressive therapy.

Experience with children has been limited. Atgam has been administered safely to a small number of pediatric renal allograft recipients and pediatric aplastic anemia patients at dosage levels comparable to those in adults.

Dilution of Atgam in Dextrose Injection, USP, is not recommended, as low salt concentrations may result in precipitation. The use of highly acidic infusion solutions is also not recommended because of possible physical instability over time.

DRUG INTERACTIONS:

We do not recommend the dilution of Atgam Sterile Solution in Dextrose Injection, USP, as low salt concentrations may cause precipitation. The use of highly acidic infusion solutions is also not recommended because of possible physical instability over time. When the dose of corticosteroids and other immunosuppressants is being reduced, some previously masked reactions to Atgam may appear. Under these circumstances, observe patients especially carefully during therapy with Atgam.

ADVERSE REACTIONS:

RENAL TRANSPLANTATION

The primary clinical experience with Atgam Sterile Solution has been in renal allograft patients who were also receiving concurrent standard immunosuppressive therapy (azathioprine, corticosteroids). In controlled trials, investigators frequently reported the following adverse reactions: fever in 1 patient in 3; chills in 1 patient in 7; leukopenia in 1 patient in 7; thrombocytopenia in 1 patient in 9; and dermatological reactions, such as rash, pruritus, urticaria, wheal, and flare, in 1 patient in 8. The following reactions were reported in more than 1% but less than 5% of the patients: arthralgia, chest or back pain or both, clotted A/V fistula, diarrhea, dyspnea, headache, hypotension, nausea or vomiting or both, night sweats, pain at the infusion site, peripheral thrombophlebitis, and stomatitis.

Reactions reported in less than 1% of the patients in the controlled trials were anaphylaxis, dizziness, weakness or faintness, edema, herpes simplex reactivation, hiccoughs or epigastric pain, hyperglycemia, hypertension, iliac vein obstruction, laryngospasm, localized infection, lymphadenopathy, malaise, myalgia, paresthesia, possible serum sickness, pulmonary edema, renal artery thrombosis, seizures, systemic infection, tachycardia, toxic epidermal necrosis, and would dehiscence.

APLASTIC ANEMIA

In premarketing clinical trials with Atgam in the treatment of aplastic anemia, patients were also being concurrently managed with support therapy (transfusions, steroids, antibiotic (antihistamines).

In these trials most patients experienced fever and skin reactions. Other frequently reported adverse reactions were chills, 1 patient in 2; arthralgia, 1 patient in 2; headache, 1 patient in 6; myalgia, 1 patient in 10; nausea, 1 patient in 15; chest pain, 1 patient in 15 and phlebitis, 1 patient in 20.

ADVERSE REACTIONS: *(cont'd)*

The following reactions were reported by at least 1 patient, and less than 5% of the total patients: diaphoresis, joint stiffness, periorbital edema, aches, edema, muscle ache, vomiting, agitation/lethargy, listlessness, lightheadedness, seizures, diarrhea, bradycardia, myocarditis, cardiac irregularity, hepatosplenomegaly, possible encephalitis or post viral encephalopathy, hypotension, congestive heart failure, hypertension, burning soles/palms, foot sole pain, lymphadenopathy, post-cervical lymphadenopathy, tender lymph nodes, bilateral pleural effusion, respiratory distress, anaphylactic reaction, and proteinuria.

In other support studies in patients with aplastic anemia and other hematologic abnormalities who have received Atgam, abnormal tests of liver function (SGOT, SGPT, alkaline phosphatase) and renal function (serum creatinine) have been observed. In some trials, clinical and laboratory findings of serum sickness were seen in a majority of patients.

POST-MARKETING EXPERIENCE

During approximately five years of post-approval marketing experience, the frequency of adverse reactions in voluntarily reported cases is an follows: fever 51%; chills 16%; thrombocytopenia 30%; leukopenia 14%; rashes 27%; systemic infection 13%. Events reported in 5 to 10% of reported cases include: abnormal renal function tests, serum sickness-like symptoms, dyspnea/apnea, arthralgia, chest, back or flank pain, diarrhea and nausea and/or vomiting. Events reported with a frequency of less than 5% include: hypertension, Herpes Simplex infection, pain, swelling or redness at infusion site, eosinophilia, headache, myalgias or leg pains, hypotension, anaphylaxis, tachycardia, edema, localized infection, malaise, seizures, GI bleeding or perforation, deep vein thrombosis, sore mouth/throat, hyperglycemia, acute renal failure, abnormal liver function tests, confusion or disorientation,cough, neutropenia or granulocytopenia, anemia, thrombophlebitis, dizziness, epigastric or stomach pain, lymphadenopathy, pulmonary edema or congestive heart failure, abdominal pain, nosebleed, vasculitis, aplasia or pancytopenia, abnormal involuntary movement or tremor, rigidity, sweating, laryngospasm/edema, hemolysis or hemolytic anemia, viral hepatitis, faintness, enlarged or reputed kidney, paresthesias and renal artery thrombosis.

The recommended management for some of the adverse reactions that could occur with treatment with Atgam follows:

1. Anaphylaxis: is uncommon but serious and may occur at any time during therapy with Atgam. Stop infusion of Atgam immediately; administer 0.3 ml aqueous epinephrine (1:1000 solution) intramuscularly. Administer sterids, assist respiration, and provide other resuscitative measures. DO NOT resume therapy with Atgam.

2. Hemolysis: can usually be detected only in the laboratory. Clinically significant hemolysis has been reported rarely. Appropriate treatment of hemolysis may include transfusion of erythrocytes; if necessary, administer intravenous mannitol; furosemide, sodium bicarbonate, and fluids. Severe and unremitting hemolysis may require discontinuation of therapy with Atgam.

3. Thrombocytopenia is usually transient in renal transplant patients; platelet counts generally return to adequate levels without discontinuing therapy with Atgam. Platelet transfusions may be necessary in patients with aplastic anemia. (See PRECAUTIONS, WARNINGS, and DOSAGE AND ADMINISTRATION.)

4. Respiratory Distress: may indicate an anaphylactoid reaction. Discontinue infusion of Atgam. If distress persists, administer an antihistamine or epinephrine or corticosteroids or some combination of the three.

5. Pain in Chest, Flank, or Back: may indicate anaphylaxis or hemolysis. Treatment is that indicated above for those conditions.

6. Hypotension: may indicate anaphylaxis. Stop infusion of Atgam and stabilize blood pressure with pressors if necessary.

7. Chills and Fever: occur frequently in patients receiving Atgam. Atgam may release endogenous leukocyte pyrogens. Prophylactic and/or therapeutic administration of antihistamines, antipyretics or corticosteroids generally controls this reaction.

8. Chemical Phlebitis: can be caused by infusion of Atgam through peripheral veins. This can often be avoided by administering the infusion solution into a high-flow vein. A subcutaneous arterialized vein produced by a Brescia fistula is also a useful administration site.

9. Itching and Erythema: probably result from the effect of Atgam on blood elements. Antihistamines generally control the symptoms.

10. Serum Sickness-Like Symptoms: in aplastic anemia patients have been treated with oral or IV corticosteroids. Resolution of symptoms has generally been prompt and long-term sequelae have not been observed. Prophylactic administration of corticosteroids may decrease the frequency of this reaction.

OVERDOSAGE:

Because of its mode of action and because it is a biologic substance, the maximal tolerated dose of Atgam Sterile Solution would be expected to vary from patient to patient. To date, the largest single daily dose administered to a patient, a renal transplant recipient, was 7000 mg administered at a concentration of approximately 10 mg/ml Sodium Chloride Injection, USP, approximately 7 times the recommended total dose and infusion concentration. In this patient, administration of Atgam was not associated with any signs of acute intoxication.

The greatest number of doses (10 to 20 mg/kg/dose) that can be administered to a single patient has not yet been determined. Some renal transplant patients have received up to 50 doses in 4 months, and others have received 28-day courses of 21 doses followed by as many as 3 more courses for the treatment of acute rejection. The incidence of toxicologic manifestations did not increase with any of these regimens.

ANIMAL TOXICOLOGY

During the development of Atgam Sterile Solution, aliquots of the various clinical lots were infused intravenously in either *Macaca mulatta or Macaca irus* monkeys. The dosage used was 100 mg/kg on day 0,200 mg/kg on day 2 and 400 mg/kg on day 4. A 3-week observation period followed. Currently, all marketed lots are similarly tested using a dosage of 50 mg/kg on days 0, 2, 4 and 7 followed by a 3-week observation period.

Many of the changes observed could have been anticipated on the basis of the antilymphocytic activity of Atgam. They are decreased peripheral blood lymphocytes and increased total leukocyte and neutrophil counts occurring within 24 hours after infusion, decreased thymus size with involution or atrophy or both, and decreased lymphocyte populations in the thymus-dependent areas of the spleen and lymph nodes. The atrophy was particularly common in the animals receiving the higher doses. In animals receiving either dosage regimen, packed cell volume, total erythrocyte counts, and hemoglobin concentrations have decreased and reticulocytes and nucleated erythrocytes have increased enough to be classified as anemia. An occasional animal death believed to have resulted from anemia has occurred. Transient decreases in blood platelet counts have also occurred. Thrombus formation occurred frequently along the routes of infusion, i.e. the saphenous and femoral veins. However, the incidence of thrombi has dropped since in-line filters have been used during infusion. In these animals, definitive evidence of DIC (disseminated intravascular coagulation) has not been observed.

DOSAGE AND ADMINISTRATION:

RENAL ALLOGRAFT RECIPIENTS

Adult renal allograft patients have received Atgam Sterile Solution at the dosage of 10 to 30 mg/kg of body weight daily. The few children studied received 5 to 25 mg/kg daily. Atgam has been used to delay the onset of the first rejection episode[1-4] and at the time of the first rejection episode.[5-9] Most patients who received Atgam for the treatment of acute rejection had not received it starting at the time of transplantation.

Usually, Atgam is used concomitantly with azathioprine and corticosteroids, which are commonly used to suppress the immune response. Exercise caution during repeat courses of Atgam; carefully observe patients for signs of allergic reactions.

Delaying the Onset of Allograft Rejection: Give a fixed dose of 15 mg/kg daily for 14 days, then every other day for 14 days for a total of 21 doses in 28 days. Administer the 14 days, then every other day for 14 days for a total of 21 doses in 28 days. Administer the first dose within 24 hours before or after the transplant.

Treatment of Rejection: The first dose of Atgam can be delayed until the diagnosis of the first rejection episode. The recommended dose is 10 to 15 mg/kg daily for 14 days. Additional alternate-day therapy up to a total of 21 doses can be given.

APLASTIC ANEMIA

The recommended dosage regimen is 10 to 20 mg/kg daily for 8 to 14 days. Additional alternate-day therapy up to a total of 21 doses can be administered[10-12]. Because thrombocytopenia can be associated with the administration of Atgam, patients receiving it for the treatment of aplastic anemia may need prophylactic platelet transfusions to maintain platelets at clinically acceptable levels.

PREPARATION OF SOLUTION

Parenteral drug products should be inspected visually for particulate matter and discoloration prior to administration whenever solution and container permit. However, because Atgam is a gamma globulin product, it can be transparent to slightly opalescent, colorless to faintly pink or brown and may develop a slight granular or flaky deposit during storage. Atgam (diluted or undiluted) should not be shaken because excessive foaming and/or denaturation of the protein may occur.

Dilute Atgam for intravenous infusion in an inverted bottle of sterile vehicle so the undiluted Atgam does not contact the air inside. Add the total daily dose of Atgam to the sterile vehicle (see Compatibility and Stability.) The concentration should not exceed 4 mg of Atgam per ml. The diluted solution should be gently rotated or swirled to effect thorough mixing.

ADMINISTRATION

The diluted Atgam should be allowed to reach room temperature before infusion. Atgam is appropriately administered into a vascular shunt, arterial venous fistula, or a high-flow central vein through an in-line filter with a pore size of 0.2 to 1.0 micron. The in-line filter should be used with all infusions of Atgam to prevent the administration of any insoluble material that may develop in the product during storage. The use of high-flow veins will minimize the occurrence of phlebitis and thrombosis. Do not infuse a dose of Atgam in less than 4 hours. Always keep appropriate resuscitation equipment at the patient's bedside while Atgam is being administered. Observe the patient continuously for possible allergic reactions throughout the infusions (See ADVERSE REACTIONS).

COMPATIBILITY AND STABILITY

Atgam, once diluted, has been shown to be physically and chemically stable for up to 24 hours at concentrations of up to 4 mg per ml in the following diluents: 0.9% sodium chloride injection, 5% dextrose and 0.22% sodium chloride injection, and 5% dextrose and 0.45% sodium chloride injection.

Adding Atgam to dextrose injection is not recommended, as low salt concentrations can cause precipitation. Highly acidic infusion solutions can also contribute to physical instability over time. It is recommended that diluted Atgam be stored in a refrigerator if it is prepared prior to the time of infusion. Even if it is stored in a refrigerator, the total time in dilution should not exceed 24 hours (including infusion time).

STORAGE

Store in a refrigerator at 2° to 8°C. **DO NOT FREEZE.**

REFERENCES:

1. Cosimi AB, Wortis HH, Delmonico FL, Russell PS: Randomized clinical trial of antithymocyte globulin in cadaver renal allograft recipients: importance of T cell monitoring. Surg 80: 155- 163 (1976) **2.** Wechter WJ, Brodie JA, Morrell RM, M, Schultz JR: Antithymocyte globulin (Atgam) in renal allograft recipients. Trans 28(4): 294-302 (1976) **3.** Kountz SL, Butt KHM, Rao TKS, Zielinski CM, Rafi M, Schultz JR: Antithymocyte globulin (ATG) dosage and graft survival in renal transplantation. Trans Proc 9:1023-1025 (1977) **4.** Butt KMH, Zielinski CM, Parsa l, Elberg AJ, Wechter WJ, Kountz SL: Trends in immunosuppression for kidney transplantation. Kidney Int 13(Suppl 8): S95-S98 (1978) **5.** Filo RS, Smith EJ, Leapman SB: Reversal of acute renal allograft rejection with adjunctive ATG therapy. Trans Proc 13(1): 482-490 (1981) **6.** Nowygrod R, Appel G, Hardy M: Use of ATG for reversal of acute allograft rejection. Trans Proc 13(1): 469-472 (1981) **7.** Hardy MA, Nowygrod R, Elberg A, Appel G: Use of ATG in treatment of steroid-resistant rejection. Trans 29: 162-164 (1980) **8.** Shield CH, Cosimi AB, Tolkoff-Rubin N, Rubin R, Herrin J, Russell PS: Use of antithymocyte globulin for reversal of acute allograft rejection. Trans 28(6): 461-464 (1979) **9.** Cosimi AB: The clinical value of antilymphocyte antibodies. Trans Proc 13(1): 462-468 (1981) **10.** Cosimi AB, Peters C, Harmon D, Ellman L: Treatment of severe aplastic anemia with a prolonged course of antithymocyte globulin, Trans Proc 14:761-764 (1982) **11.** Champlin R, Ho W, Gate R: Antithymocyte globulin treatment in patients with aplastic anemia. NEJM 308(3): 113-118 (1983) **12.** Doney K, Dahlberg S, Monroe D et al: Therapy of severe aplastic anemia with antihuman thymocyte globulin and androgens: The effect of HLA-haploidentical marrow infusion. Blood 63(2): 342-348 (1984) **13.** Rubin RH, Cosimi AB, Hirsch MS, Herrin JT: Effects of antithymocyte globulin on cytomegalovirus infection in renal transplant recipients. Trans 31 (2):143-145 (1981)

HOW SUPPLIED - EQUIVALENTS NOT AVAILABLE:

Injection, Solution - Intravenous - 50 mg/ml

5 ml	$262.45	ATGAM, Pharmacia & Upjohn	00009-0926-04

M-CRESYL ACETATE *(001674)*

CATEGORIES: Anti-Infectives; EENT Drugs; Eye, Ear, Nose, & Throat Preparations; Otic Preparations; Otologic; FDA Pre 1938 Drugs

BRAND NAMES: Cresylate

Prescribing information not available at time of publication.

HOW SUPPLIED - EQUIVALENTS NOT AVAILABLE:

Solution - Otic

15 ml x 12	$7.50	CRESYLATE OTIC, Recsei Labs	10952-0035-13
480 ml	$120.00	CRESYLATE OTIC, Recsei Labs	10952-0035-17

MAFENIDE ACETATE *(001675)*

CATEGORIES: Anti-Infectives; Antibacterials; Burns; Dermatologicals; Local Infections; Skin/Mucous Membrane Agents; Sulfonamides; Topical; Pregnancy Category C; FDA Approval Pre 1982

BRAND NAMES: *Mafylon*; **Sulfamylon**

(International brand names outside U.S. in italics)

Prescribing information not available at time of publication.

HOW SUPPLIED - EQUIVALENTS NOT AVAILABLE:

Cream - Topical - 11.2 mg/g

60 gm	**$18.50**	**Sulfamylon Cream, Dow Hickam**	**00514-0101-50**
120 gm	**$34.00**	**Sulfamylon Cream, Dow Hickam**	**00514-0101-51**
452 gm	**$126.00**	**SULFAMYLON, Dow Hickam**	**00514-0101-54**

MAGNESIUM CHLORIDE *(001681)*

CATEGORIES: Anticonvulsants; Central Nervous System Agents; Electrolyte Solutions; Electrolytic, Caloric-Water Balance; Homeostatic & Nutrient; Mineral Supplements; Replacement Solutions; Vitamins; FDA Pre 1938 Drugs

BRAND NAMES: Chlor-3

Prescribing information not available at time of publication.

HOW SUPPLIED - EQUIVALENTS NOT AVAILABLE:

Crystals - Oral

240 gm	$5.25	CHLOR-3, Fleming	00256-0183-01

Injection, Solution - Intravenous - 200 mg/ml

30 ml	$4.00	Magnesium Chloride, Pegasus Med Svs	10974-0082-30
50 ml	$2.65	Magnesium Chloride, Americal Pharm	54945-0574-44
50 ml	$4.19	Magnesium Chloride, McGuff	49072-0473-50
50 ml	$5.95	Magnesium Chloride, Pasadena	00418-5740-44
50 ml x 1	$4.38	Magnesium Chloride, Am Regent	00517-5034-01

MAGNESIUM SALICYLATE *(001688)*

CATEGORIES: Analgesics; Antiarthritics; Antipyretics; Arthritis; Bursitis; Central Nervous System Agents; Nonsteroidal Anti-Inflammatory; Osteoarthritis; Pain; Salicylates; Pregnancy Category C; FDA Pre 1938 Drugs

BRAND NAMES: Agesic; **Magan**; Mobidin; Reosyn-500

DESCRIPTION:

Each Magnesium Salicylate uncoated, pink, (or yellow) capsule-shaped tablet for oral administration contains 545 mg of magnesium salicylate equivalent to 500 mg of salicylate. Magnesium salicylate is a non-steroidal, antiinflammatory agent with antipyretic and analgesic properties.

Magnesium salicylate is a white, odorless, crystalline powder with a sweet taste. It is soluble in water and alcohol.

CLINICAL PHARMACOLOGY:

Salicylic acid is the active moiety released into the plasma by Magnesium Salicylate.

Salicylic acid is enzymatically biotransformed through two pathways to salicyluric acid and salicylphenolic glucuronide and eliminated in the urine.

Oral salicylates are absorbed rapidly, partly from the stomach but mostly from the upper intestine. Salicylic acid is rapidly distributed throughout all body tissues and most transcellular fluids, mainly by pH-dependent passive processes. It can be detected in synovial, spinal and peritoneal fluid, in saliva and in milk. It readily crosses the placental barrier. From 50% to 90% of salicylic acid is bound to plasma proteins, especially albumin.

Following the ingestion of a single dose of 524 mg of magnesium salicylate, a peak concentration of 3.6 mg/dl salicylic acid is reached in 1.5 hours with a T $\frac{1}{2}$ of 2 hours. The major biotransformation paths for the elimination of salicylic acid from the plasma become saturated by low doses of salicylic acid. As a result, repeated doses of magnesium salicylate increase the plasma concentration and markedly prolong the plasma half-time. The plasma concentration of salicylic acid is increased by conditions that reduce the glomerular filtration rate or tubular secretion such as renal disease or the presence of inhibitors that compete for the transport system such as probenecid.

Therapeutic plasma concentrations of salicylic acid for an adequate antiinflammatory effect needed for the treatment of rheumatoid arthritis range between 20-30 mg/dl. Effective analgesia is achieved at lower concentrations. Salicylates relieve pain by both a peripheral and a CNS effect. Salicylates inhibit the synthesis of prostaglandins; the importance of this mechanism in analgesia and antiinflammation has not been fully elucidated. Salicylates have an antipyretic effect in febrile patients but little in subjects with normal temperatures. This appears to be due to the inhibition of the synthesis of prostaglandins which are powerful pyrogens that affect the hypothalamus. Higher therapeutic concentrations cause reversible tinnitus and high tone hearing loss. Full therapeutic doses of salicylates increase oxygen consumption and CO2 production. They cause an extracellular and intracellular respiratory alkalosis which is rapidly compensated. Salicylates irritate the gastric mucosa and frequently lead to blood loss in the stool; this effect is more pronounced with aspirin than magnesium salicylate.

Salicylates in large doses (over 6 g/day) reduce the plasma prothrombin level. In contrast to aspirin, magnesium salicylate does not affect platelets. Salicylic acid increases the urinary excretion of urates at higher doses but may decrease excretion at lower doses.

INDICATIONS AND USAGE:

Magnesium salicylate is indicated for the relief of the signs and symptoms of rheumatoid arthritis, osteoarthritis, bursitis and other musculoskeletal disorders.

CONTRAINDICATIONS:

Magnesium salicylate is contraindicated in patients with advanced chronic renal insufficiency. It may counteract the effect of uricosuric agents and should not be prescribed for patients on such drugs.

WARNINGS:

As with all salicylates, magnesium salicylate should be avoided or administered with caution to patients with liver damage, pre-existing hypoprothrombinemia, vitamin K deficiency and before surgery.

PRECAUTIONS:

General: Appropriate precautions should be taken in prescribing magnesium salicylate for persons known to be sensitive to salicylates and in patients with erosive gastritis or peptic ulcer. If a reaction develops, the drug should be discontinued. Magnesium salicylate should be used with caution, if at all, concomitantly with anticoagulants. Appropriate precautions should be taken in administering magnesium salicylate to patients with any impairment of renal function including discontinuing other drugs containing magnesium and monitoring serum magnesium levels if dosage levels of magnesium salicylate are high.

PRECAUTIONS: *(cont'd)*

Carcinogenesis, Mutagenesis, and Impairment of Fertility: There have been no studies in animals or humans to evaluate the carcinogenesis, mutagenesis or impairment of fertility for magnesium salicylate.

Aspirin causes testicular atrophy and inhibition of spermatogenesis in animals.

Pregnancy Category C:

1. Teratogenic Effects: Aspirin has been shown to be teratogenic in animals and to increase the incidence of still births and neonatal deaths in women. There are no adequate or well-controlled studies of magnesium salicylate in pregnant women. Magnesium salicylate should be used during pregnancy only if the potential benefit justifies the potential risk to the fetus.

2. Nonteratogenic Effects: Chronic, high dose salicylate therapy of pregnant women increases the length of gestation and the frequency of post maturity and prolongs spontaneous labor.

It is recommended magnesium salicylate be taken during the last three months of pregnancy only under the close supervision of a physician.

Nursing Mothers: Since salicylates are excreted in human milk, caution should be exercised when magnesium salicylate is administered to a nursing woman.

Pediatric Use: Safety and effectiveness of magnesium salicylate in children have not been established.

DRUG INTERACTIONS:

Even small doses of magnesium salicylate should not be given with uricosuric agents such as probenecid that decrease tubular reabsorption because it counteracts their effect. Large doses of magnesium salicylate cause hypoprothrombinemia. Lower doses enhance the effects of anticoagulants such as coumadin and must be used with caution in patients receiving anticoagulants that affect the prothrombin time. Caution should also be exercised in patients concurrently treated with a sulfonylurea hypoglycemic agent or methotrexate because of the drug's capability of displacing them from the plasma protein binding sites, resulting in enhanced action of these agents. A similar displacement of barbiturates and diphenylhydantoin may occur; diphenylhydantoin intoxication has been precipitated by the consumption of aspirin. Salicylates inhibit the diuretic action of spironolactone.

ADVERSE REACTIONS:

Magnesium salicylate in large doses has a hypoprothrombinemic effect and should be given with caution in patients receiving anticoagulant drugs, patients with liver damage, pre-existing hypoprothrombinemia, vitamin K deficiency or before surgery.

Salicylates given in overdose produce stimulation (often manifested as tinnitus) followed by depression of the central nervous system. The dosage should be lowered at the onset of tinnitus.

Salicylates may cause gastric mucosal irritation and bleeding. However, fecal blood loss in patients taking magnesium salicylate is significantly less than in those taking aspirin.

Magnesium salicylate should not be given to patients with severe renal damage because of the possibility of hypermagnesemia.

In moderate to high doses, salicylates lower the blood glucose in diabetics. Aspirin-induced hypoglycemia has been described in adults undergoing hemodialysis.

Unlike aspirin, magnesium salicylate is not known to affect the platelet adhesiveness involved in the clotting mechanism; and therefore, does not prolong bleeding time. Magnesium salicylate has not been associated with reactions causing asthmatic attacks in susceptible people.

OVERDOSAGE:

Acute overdosage results in salicylate toxicity.

Early signs and symptoms from repeated larger doses as well as a large single dose consist of headache, dizziness, tinnitus (which may be absent in children or the elderly), difficulty in hearing, dimness of vision, mental confusion, lassitude, drowsiness, sweating, thirst, hyperventilation, nausea, vomiting and occasionally diarrhea. More severe salicylate poisoning is manifested by CNS disturbances including EEG abnormalities. Hyperventilation occurs producing initial respiratory alkalosis. This is followed by severe metabolic acidosis with dehydration and loss of potassium.

Restlessness, garrulity, incoherent speech, apprehension, vertigo, tremor, diplopia, maniacal delirium, hallucinations, generalized convulsions and coma may occur. Toxic symptoms may occur at serum levels greater than 20 mg/dl in patients over 60 years of age.

Hyperventilation may occur at plasma salicylate levels over 35 mg/dl. Death may result from salicylate levels between 45-75 mg/dl. As with other salicylates, 10 to 30 g of the drug may be fatal. Renal or hepatic insufficiency and fever and dehydration in children enhance the acute toxicity of salicylate overdoses. Treatment of acute poisoning is a medical emergency and should be undertaken in a hospital. Serum Na, K, Cl, CO2 levels, pH, BUN, blood glucose and urine pH and specific gravity should be obtained.

Emesis should be induced or gastric lavage performed. Activated charcoal may be administered. Hyperthermia should be controlled with tepid water sponging. Dehydration should be treated and acid-base imbalance corrected. A high concentration of salicylic acid in the brain may be fatal. Correction of acidosis shifts salicylate from the brain to the plasma.

A bicarbonate solution should be infused to maintain an alkaline diuresis. Care should be taken to avoid pulmonary edema. The blood pH, plasma pCO2 and plasma glucose level should be monitored frequently. Ketosis and hypoglycemia may be corrected by glucose infusions and hypokalemia by potassium chloride added to the intravenous infusate. Avoid respiratory depressants. Shock may be combatted by plasma infusions. Hemorrhagic phenomena may necessitate whole blood transfusions or vitamin K1. In severe intoxication, exchange transfusion, peritoneal dialysis, hemodialysis or hemoperfusion should be performed to remove plasma salicylic acid. Dialysis should be seriously considered if the patient's condition is worsening despite appropriate therapy.

DOSAGE AND ADMINISTRATION:

The dosage for magnesium salicylate in the treatment of musculoskeletal disorders such as arthritis should be adjusted according to individual patient's needs. The recommended initial regimen is two tablets three times per day. Dosage may be increased, if necessary, to achieve the desired therapeutic effect. In adjusting the dosage, the physician should monitor the dose limiting parameters such as tinnitus and/or serum salicylate over 30 mg/dl.

HOW SUPPLIED - EQUIVALENTS NOT AVAILABLE:

Capsule, Gelatin - Oral - 500 mg

100's	$58.00	REOSYN-500, Alba Pharma	10023-0222-90

Tablet, Uncoated - Oral - 545 mg

100's	**$50.95**	**MAGAN, Savage Labs**	**00281-4121-17**

Tablet, Uncoated - Oral - 600 mg

100's	$23.22	MOBIDIN, Ascher	00225-0310-15
500's	$113.16	MOBIDIN, Ascher	00225-0310-20

MAGNESIUM SALICYLATE; PHENYLTOLOXAMINE *(001687)*

CATEGORIES: Analgesics; Antiarthritics; Antipyretics; Central Nervous System Agents; Nonsteroidal Anti-Inflammatory; Pain; Salicylates; FDA Pre 1938 Drugs

BRAND NAMES: Argesic; Arthrogesic; Magsal Tablets; Myogesic

Prescribing information not available at time of publication.

HOW SUPPLIED - EQUIVALENTS NOT AVAILABLE:

Tablet, Uncoated - Oral - 600 mg/25 mg

100's	$110.00	MYOGESIC, AJ Bart	49326-0182-90

MAGNESIUM SULFATE *(001689)*

CATEGORIES: Antiarrhythmic Agents; Anticonvulsants; Caloric Agents; Central Nervous System Agents; Electrolyte Solutions; Electrolytic, Caloric-Water Balance; Gastrointestinal Drugs; Homeostatic & Nutrient; Hypomagnesemia; Labor; Laxatives; Mineral Supplements; Neuromuscular; Pregnancy; Renal Drugs; Replacement Solutions; Uterine Relaxants; Vitamins; FDA Approved 1986 Sep

BRAND NAMES: Pro-Mag-Sul; Sulfa Mag; **Tis U Sol**

FORMULARIES: WHO

DESCRIPTION:

50%
4.06 mEq/ml
4.06 mOsm/ml
10%
0.8 mEq/ml
0.8 mOsm/ml

Magnesium Sulfate Injection, USP is a sterile, non-pyrogenic solution of magnesium sulfate in water for injection.

Each ml of the 50% solution contains 500 mg of magnesium sulfate heptahydrate.

Each ml of the 10% solution contains 100 mg of magnesium sulfate heptahydrate.

The pH of either solution may be adjusted with sodium hydroxide and/or sulphuric acid to between 5.5-7.0 when diluted to a 5% concentration (w/v).

The solution contains no bacteriostatic agent or other preservatives.

Magnesium sulfate heptahydrate is chemically designated $MgSO_4 \circ 7H_2O$ and occurs as a white, bitter, crystalline powder which is freely soluble in water.

CLINICAL PHARMACOLOGY:

Magnesium is the second most plentiful cation of the intracellular fluids. It is essential for the activity of many enzyme systems and plays an important role with regard to neurochemical transmission and muscular excitability. Deficits are accompanied by a variety of structural and functional disturbances.

Some of the effects of magnesium on the nervous system are similar to those of calcium. An increased concentration of magnesium in the extracellular fluid causes depression of the central nervous system (CNS). Magnesium has a direct depressant effect on skeletal muscle.

Abnormally low concentrations of magnesium in the extracellular fluid result in increased acetylcholine release and increased muscle excitability that can produce tetany.

Magnesium slows the rate of S-A nodal impulse formation. Higher concentrations of magnesium (greater than 15 mEq/L) produce cardiac arrest in diastole.

Excess magnesium causes vasodilatation by both a direct action on blood vessels and ganglionic blockade.

Magnesium is excreted principally by the kidney by glomerular filtration.

INDICATIONS AND USAGE:

Magnesium sulfate may be of therapeutic value in the following conditions:

As a CNS depressant, primarily in preeclampsia and eclampsia of pregnancy.

As an electrolyte replenisher for hypomagnesemia and magnesium deficiency to maintain normal neuromuscular irritability.

CONTRAINDICATIONS:

Magnesium sulfate should not be administered parenterally in patients with heart block or myocardial damage.

WARNINGS:

The principal hazard in parenteral magnesium therapy is the production of abnormally high levels of magnesium in the plasma. The most immediate danger to life is respiratory depression. A preparation of calcium, such as the gluconate or gluceptate, should be at hand for intravenous administration as an antidote.

Magnesium sulfate can cause fetal harm when administered to a pregnant woman. When magnesium sulfate is administered to a toxic mother, the newborn is usually not compromised. When Magnesium Sulfate, USP is administered intravenously by a continuous infusion for longer than 24 hours before delivery, the possibility of the baby's showing signs of neuromuscular or respiratory depression of the newborn should be considered, since fetal toxicity can occur. A baby with hypermagnesemia my require resuscitation and assisted ventilation. If this drug is used during pregnancy, or if the patient becomes pregnant while taking this drug, the patient should be apprised of the potential hazard to the fetus.

PRECAUTIONS:

GENERAL

Administer with caution if flushing and sweating occurs.

When barbiturates, narcotics or other hypnotics (or systemic anesthetics) are to be given in conjunction with magnesium, their dosage should be adjusted with caution because of additive CNS depressant effects of magnesium. A preparation of calcium salt should be readily available for intravenous injection to counteract potential serious signs of magnesium intoxication.

Since Magnesium is excreted almost entirely by the kidneys, it should be given very cautiously in the presence of serious impairment of renal function.

PRECAUTIONS: *(cont'd)*

LABORATORY TESTS

Magnesium sulfate should not be given unless hypomagnesemia has been confirmed and the serum concentration of magnesium is monitored. The normal serum level is 1.5 to 2.4 mEq/L.

PREGNANCY CATEGORY D

See WARNINGS.

NURSING MOTHERS

It is not known whether this drug is excreted in human milk. Because many drugs are excreted in human milk, caution should be exercised when magnesium sulfate is administered to a nursing woman.

PEDIATRIC USE

Safety and effectiveness in children have not been established.

DRUG INTERACTIONS:

When barbiturates, narcotics, hypnotics (or systemic anesthetics), or other central nervous system depressants are to be given in conjunction with magnesium, their dosage should be adjusted with caution because of the additive central nervous system depressant effects of magnesium.

Central nervous system depression and peripheral transmission defects produced by magnesium may be antagonized by calcium.

ADVERSE REACTIONS:

Principal adverse reactions are related to the high plasma levels of magnesium and include flushing, sweating, hypotension, circulatory collapse, and cardiac and central nervous system depression. Respiratory depression os the most life-threatening effect.

OVERDOSAGE:

Hypermagnesemia is manifested by muscle weakness, hypotension, ECG changes, sedation, and confusion. As plasma concentrations of magnesium begin to exceed 4 mEq/L, the deep-tendon reflexes are decreased and may be absent at levels approaching 10 mEq/L. At 12 to 15 mEq/L respiratory paralysis is a potential hazard; the respiratory effects can be antagonized to some extent by the intravenous administration of calcium salts. In cases of severe renal impairment, symptomatic hypermagnesemia may be an indication for dialysis. Although man usually tolerates high concentrations of magnesium in plasma, there are occasional instances when cardiac consequences may be seen in the form of complete heart block at concentrations well below 10 mEq/L.

Before the parenteral administration of each dose, the respiratory rate should be at least 16 per minute and urinary function should be adequate. In the event of overdosage, assisted ventilation must be provided until calcium can be given intravenously. Peritoneal dialysis or hemodialysis may be required in cases of extreme hypermagnesemia.

When magnesium sulfate is administered parenterally in doses that are sufficient to induce hypermagnesemia, the drug has a depressant effect on the central nervous system and, via the peripheral neuromuscular junction, on muscle.

DOSAGE AND ADMINISTRATION:

Intramuscular: Adults and older children for severe hypomagnesemia 1-5 g (2-10 ml of 50% solution) daily in divided doses; administration is repeated daily until serum levels have returned to normal. If deficiency is not severe 1 g (2 ml of 50% solution) can be given once or twice daily. Serum magnesium levels should serve as a guide to continued dosage.

Intravenous: 1 to 4 g magnesium sulfate 50% may be given intravenously in 10% to 20% solution, but only with great caution; the rate should not exceed 1.5 ml of 10% solution or equivalent per minute until relaxation is obtained.

Intravenous Infusion: 4 g in 150 ml of 5% Dextrose Injection, USP at a rate not exceeding 3 ml per minute.

Usual Dose Range: 1 to 40 g daily.

Electrolyte Replenisher: Intramuscular 1 to 2 g in 50% solution four times a day until serum magnesium is within normal limits.

Usual Pediatric Dose: Intramuscular 20 to 40 mg/kg of body weight in a 20% solution repeated as necessary.

For Eclampsia: Initially 1 to 2 g in 25% or 50% solution is given intramuscularly. Subsequently, 1 g is given every 30 minutes until relief is obtained. The blood pressure should be monitored after each injection.

Parenteral drug products should be visually inspected for particulate matter and discoloration prior to administration, whenever solution and container permit.

HOW SUPPLIED - EQUIVALENTS NOT AVAILABLE:

Injection, Conc-Soln - Intramuscular; - 12.5 %

8 ml	$2.85	12.5% MAGNESIUM SULFATE, Abbott	00074-4943-01

Injection, Conc-Soln - Intramuscular; - 500 mg/ml

2 ml	$1.73	50% MAGNESIUM SULFATE, Abbott	00074-4075-02
2 ml	$16.25	Magnesium Sulfate, Solopak Labs	39769-0042-01
2 ml x 25	$10.50	50% Magnesium Sulfate, Astra USA	00186-1209-04
2 ml x 25	$14.69	Magnesium Sulfate, Am Regent	00517-2602-25
2 ml x 25	$15.60	Magnesium Sulfate, Gensia Labs	00703-5372-04
2 ml x 25	$21.25	Magnesium Sulfate, Pasadena	00418-2061-22
2 ml x 25	$26.56	Magnesium Sulfate, Fujisawa USA	00469-6400-15
2 ml x 100	$68.75	Magnesium Sulfate, Am Regent	00517-0291-72
5 ml	$12.48	MAGNESIUM SULFATE, Abbott	00074-4913-15
5 ml x 10	$30.00	50% Magnesium Sulfate, Astra USA	00186-0684-01
10 ml	$1.91	50% MAGNESIUM SULFATE, Abbott	00074-2168-01
10 ml	$6.66	Magnesium Sulfate, Intl Medication	00548-1034-00
10 ml	$14.57	MAGNESIUM SULFATE, Abbott	00074-4914-18
10 ml	$18.44	Magnesium Sulfate, Solopak Labs	39769-0042-03
10 ml x 10	$46.88	50% Magnesium Sulfate, Astra USA	00186-0685-01
10 ml x 10	$81.13	Magnesium Sulfate, Fujisawa USA	00469-9266-87
10 ml x 25	$13.75	50% Sulfate, Astra USA	00186-1210-04
10 ml x 25	$23.44	Magnesium Sulfate, Am Regent	00517-2610-25
10 ml x 25	$24.60	Magnesium Sulfate, Gensia Labs	00703-5374-04
10 ml x 25	$33.13	Magnesium Sulfate, Fujisawa USA	00469-6401-15
10 ml x 25	$42.19	50% Magnesium Sulfate, Astra USA	00186-1211-04
10 ml x 100	$44.37	Magnesium Sulfate, Am Regent	00517-0291-70
20 ml	$4.00	50% MAGNESIUM SULFATE, Abbott	00074-2168-02
20 ml	$138.13	Magnesium Sulfate, Fujisawa USA	00469-6400-40
20 ml x 25	$53.52	Magnesium Sulfate, Gensia Labs	00703-5375-04
25 x 50 ml	$270.00	Magnesium Sulfate, Pasadena	00418-2081-50
50 ml	$2.90	Magnesium Sulfate, Americal Pharm	54945-0544-44
50 ml	$3.49	Magnesium Sulfate, McGuff	49072-0475-50
50 ml	$8.85	50% MAGNESIUM SULFATE, Abbott	00074-2168-03
50 ml	$309.38	Magnesium Sulfate, Fujisawa USA	00469-6400-60
50 ml x 10	$53.52	Magnesium Sulfate, Gensia Labs	00703-5377-03

HOW SUPPLIED - EQUIVALENTS NOT AVAILABLE: *(cont'd)*

50 ml x 24	$176.70	MAGNESIUM SULFATE, Abbott	00074-6730-13
50 ml x 25	$60.94	Magnesium Sulfate, Am Regent	00517-2650-25
100 ml x 24	$176.69	MAGNESIUM SULFATE, Abbott	00074-6729-23

Injection, Solution - Intramuscular; - 100 mg/ml

20 ml x 25	$30.00	10% Magnesium Sulfate, Astra USA	00186-1203-04
20 ml x 25	$143.75	MAGNESIUM SULFATE, Consolidated Midland	00223-8071-20
25 x 20 ml	$79.00	Magnesium Sulfate, Pasadena	00418-2041-66
50 ml x 25	$92.50	10% Magnesium Sulfate, Astra USA	00186-1204-04

Injection, Solution - Intravenous - 2 meq/ml

150 ml x 12	$13.77	MAGNESIUM SULFATE, McGaw	00264-1953-30

Solution - Intravenous - 1 %

100 ml	$7.15	MAGNESIUM SULFATE IN DEXTROSE, Abbott	00074-3758-11
1000 ml	$7.50	MAGNESIUM SULFATE IN DEXTROSE, Abbott	00074-3758-05

Solution - Intravenous - 2 %

500 ml	$7.51	MAGNESIUM SULFATE IN DEXTROSE, Abbott	00074-3759-03
1000 ml	$8.34	MAGNESIUM SULFATE IN DEXTROSE, Abbott	00074-3759-05

Solution - Intravenous - 4 %

100 ml	$7.08	Magnesium Sulfate, Abbott	00074-3760-11
500 ml	$8.35	Magnesium Sulfate, Abbott	00074-3760-03
500 ml x 24	$200.28	MAGNESIUM SULFATE, Abbott	00074-6729-03
1000 ml	$9.84	Magnesium Sulfate, Abbott	00074-3760-05
1000 ml x 12	$118.08	MAGNESIUM SULFATE, Abbott	00074-6729-09

Solution - Intravenous - 8 %

50 ml	$7.08	Magnesium Sulfate, Abbott	00074-3761-01

MANGANESE *(001695)*

CATEGORIES: Electrolytic, Caloric-Water Balance; Homeostatic & Nutrient; Mineral Supplements; Replacement Solutions; Vitamins; FDA Pre 1938 Drugs

BRAND NAMES: Manga-Pak

Prescribing information not available at time of publication.

HOW SUPPLIED - EQUIVALENTS NOT AVAILABLE:

Injection, Solution - Intravenous - 0.1 mg/ml

50 ml	$17.27	MANGANESE 0.1, Abbott	00074-4527-05

MANGANESE CHLORIDE *(001696)*

CATEGORIES: Electrolytic, Caloric-Water Balance; Homeostatic & Nutrient; Mineral Supplements; Replacement Solutions; Vitamins; FDA Approved 1986 Jun

BRAND NAMES: Manganese

Prescribing information not available at time of publication.

HOW SUPPLIED - EQUIVALENTS NOT AVAILABLE:

Injection, Conc-Soln - Intravenous - 0.1 mg/ml

10 ml	$4.26	Manganese 0.1, Abbott	00074-4091-01

MANGANESE SULFATE *(001697)*

CATEGORIES: Electrolytic, Caloric-Water Balance; Homeostatic & Nutrient; Mineral Supplements; Replacement Solutions; Vitamins; Pregnancy Category C; FDA Approved 1987 May

DESCRIPTION:

Manganese sulfate injection, USP, is a sterile, nonpyrogenic solution of manganese sulfate in Water for injection. It is intended for use as an additive to solutions for total parenteral nutrition (TPN). (See TABLE 1 for ingredients.)

TABLE 1

Each ml contains:	**10 ml Vial (One Withdrawal Only)**	**30 ml Vial (Multiple Dose)**
Manganese Sulfate monohydrate, USP (equivalent to Manganese)	0.308 mg (0.1 mg)	0.308 mg (0.1 mg)
Benzyl Alcohol, NF	—	0.9%
Water for Injection, USP	q.s.	q.s.

Sulfuric acid and/or sodium hydroxide for pH adjustment (2.0-3.5).

Manganese sulfate is chemically designated $MnSO_4$, a pale red, slightly efflorescent, compound soluble in water. Benzyl alcohol is chemically designated $C_6H_5CH_2OH$, a clear liquid with a faint aromatic odor and miscible with water.

CLINICAL PHARMACOLOGY:

Manganese is an essential nutrient that serves as an activator for enzymes such as polysaccharide polymerase, liver arginase, cholinesterase, and pyruvate carboxylase.

Providing manganese during TPN helps prevent development of deficiency symptoms such as nausea and vomiting, weight loss, dermatitis, and changes in growth and color of hair. Under conditions of minimal intake, 20 mcg manganese/day is retained. Manganese is bound to a specific transport protein, transmanganin, a beta-1-globulin. Manganese is widely distributed but concentrates in the mitochondria-rich tissues such as brain, kidney, pancreas, and liver. Assays for manganese in whole blood result in concentrations ranging from 6 to 12 mcg manganese/liter. Excretion of manganese occurs mainly through the bile, but in the event of obstruction, ancillary excretion routes include pancreatic juice, or return into the lumen of duodenum, jejunum, or ileum. Urinary excretion of manganese is negligible.

INDICATIONS AND USAGE:

Manganese sulfate injection is indicated for use as a supplement to intravenous solutions given for TPN. Administration helps to maintain manganese serum levels and to prevent depletion of endogenous stores and subsequent deficiency symptoms.

CONTRAINDICATIONS:

Direct intramuscular or intravenous injection of manganese sulfate injection is contraindicated, as the acidic pH of the solution (2.0-3.5) may cause considerable tissue irritation.

WARNINGS:

Manganese is eliminated via the bile. In patients with severe liver dysfunction and/or biliary tract obstruction, decreasing or omitting manganese supplements entirely may be necessary.

PRECAUTIONS:

1. Do not use unless the solution is clear and the seal is intact and undamaged.

2. The solution is hypotonic and must not be given by direct intramuscular or intravenous route.

3. Do not use syringes equipped with aluminum needles or hubs, as the solution is acidic.

CARCINOGENESIS, MUTAGENESIS, AND IMPAIRMENT OF FERTILITY

Long-term animal studies have not been performed to evaluate the carcinogenic potential or the effect on fertility of manganese sulfate injection.

PREGNANCY CATEGORY C

Animal reproduction studies have not been conducted with manganese sulfate. It is also not known whether manganese sulfate can cause fetal harm when administered to a pregnant woman or can affect reproductive capacity. Manganese sulfate should be given to a pregnant woman only if clearly indicated.

ADVERSE REACTIONS:

None known.

DRUG ABUSE AND DEPENDENCE:

None known.

OVERDOSAGE:

Manganese toxicity in TPN patients has not been reported with the prescribed dosage.

DOSAGE AND ADMINISTRATION:

Manganese Sulfate Injection provides 0.1 mg manganese/ml. It is administered intravenously only after dilution. Make only one withdrawal from the 10 ml vial. Discard unused portions immediately.

Aseptic addition of Manganese Sulfate Injection to TPN solutions under a laminar flow hood is recommended (see Directions For Dispensing.) Manganese sulfate is physically compatible with the electrolytes and vitamins usually present in the amino acid/dextrose solutions used for TPN.

ADULT

For the metabolically stable adult receiving TPN, the suggested additive dosage for manganese is 0.15 to 0.8 mg (1.5 to 8 ml Manganese Sulfate Injection) per day.

PEDIATRIC

For pediatric patients, a dosage of 2 to 10 mcg (0.02 to 0.1 ml Manganese Sulfate Injection)/kg/day is recommended. Periodic monitoring of manganese plasma levels is suggested as a guideline for subsequent administration.

Parenteral drug products should be inspected visually for particulate matter and discoloration prior to administration, whenever solution and container permit (See PRECAUTIONS).

DIRECTIONS FOR DISPENSING IN HOSPITAL PHARMACY

1. Arrange syringes, vials and TPN solutions in the laminar flow hood.

2. Suspend the TPN bags from the hole in the flat plastic extension at the top.

3. Remove the flip-top seal from the vial and swab the exposed rubber stopper with an antiseptic solution.

4. Withdraw the contents of the vial using the sterile syringe and transfer the required volumes through the medication port into the TPN bags. Unused portions in the 10 ml vial should be discarded immediately.

5. Shake the bag gently to distribute the drug.

6. Check solution for particulate matter.

7. Identify the bag.

Store at controlled room temperature 15°-30° C (59°-86° F). Do not permit to freeze.

HOW SUPPLIED - EQUIVALENTS NOT AVAILABLE:

Injection, Solution - Intravenous - 0.1 mg/ml

10 ml x 25	$62.19	Manganese Sulfate, Am Regent	00517-6410-25
30 ml x 5	$26.56	Manganese Sulfate, Am Regent	00517-7430-05

MANNITOL *(001698)*

CATEGORIES: Antianginals; Diagnostic Agents; Diuresis; Diuretics; Electrolytic, Caloric-Water Balance; Glaucoma; Glomerular Filtration; Intracranial Pressure; Intraocular Pressure; Ocular Infections; Ophthalmics; Pharmaceutical Adjuvants; Renal Drugs; Renal Failure; Pregnancy Category C; FDA Approval Pre 1982

BRAND NAMES: *Acrosmosol*; *D-Mannitol*; *Manitol*; *Manitol Pisa* (Mexico); *Mannitol*; Osmitrol; Resectisol; *Soluciones Diuretico Osmotico*
(International brand names outside U.S. in italics)

FORMULARIES: WHO

DESCRIPTION:

Composition - Each 100 ml contains:

TABLE 1

Solution	**Mannitol USP**	**Calculated Osmolarity mOsmol/liter pH**	**pH**
5% Mannitol Injection USP	5.0 g	275	5.3 (4.5-7.0)
10% Mannitol Injection USP	10.0 g	550	5.3 (4.5-7.0)
15% Mannitol Injection USP	15.0 g	825	5.3 (4.5-7.0)
20% Mannitol Injection USP	20.0 g	1100	5.3 (4.5-7.0)
Water for Injection USP qs			

Mannitol injections USP function as osmotic diuretics. They are sterile and nonpyrogenic solutions of mannitol in water for injection. Mannitol is a 6-carbon sugar alcohol prepared commercially by the reduction of dextrose. Although inert metabolically in humans, it occurs naturally in fruits and vegetables.

Molecular Weight: 182.17

DESCRIPTION: *(cont'd)*

The plastic container is made from a multilayered film specifically developed for parenteral drugs. It contains no plasticizers. The solution contact layer is a rubberized copolymer of ethylene and propylene. Solutions in contact with the plastic container may leach out certain chemical components from the plastic in very small amounts; however, biological testing was supportive of the safety of the plastic container materials. The container-solution unit is a closed system and is not dependent upon entry of external air during administration. The container is overwrapped to provide protection from the physical environment and to provide an additional moisture barrier when necessary. Exposure to temperatures above 25°C/77°F during transport and storage will lead to minor losses in moisture content. Higher temperatures lead to greater losses. It is unlikely that these minor losses will lead to clinically significant changes within the expiration period.

The closure system has two ports; the one for the administration set has a tamper evident plastic protector and the other is a medication addition site. Refer to the Directions for Use of the container.

CLINICAL PHARMACOLOGY:

Mannitol is an obligatory osmotic diuretic. When administered parenterally, mannitol is confined to the extracellular space, only slightly metabolized, and rapidly excreted by the kidney. Approximately 80 percent of a typical dose appears in the urine within 3 hours. Mannitol is freely filtered by the glomeruli with less than 10 percent tubular reabsorption; it is not secreted by tubular cells. It induces diuresis by elevating the osmolarity of the glomerular filtrate and thereby hindering tubular reabsorption of water. Excretion of sodium and chloride is also enhanced.

INDICATIONS AND USAGE:

Mannitol injections USP are indicated for:

Reduction of diuresis in the prevention and/or treatment of the oliguric phase of acute renal failure before irreversible renal failure becomes established.

Reduction of intracranial pressure and treatment of cerebral edema by reducing brain mass.

Reduction of elevated intraocular pressure when the pressure cannot be lowered by other means.

Promotion of urinary excretion of toxins.

CONTRAINDICATIONS:

Mannitol injections are contraindicated in:

Well established anuria due to severe renal disease.

Severe pulmonary congestion or frank pulmonary edema.

Active intracranial bleeding except during craniotomy.

Severe dehydration.

Progressive renal damage or dysfunction after institution of mannitol therapy, including increasing oliguria and azotemia.

Progressive heart failure or pulmonary congestion after institution of mannitol therapy.

WARNINGS:

A test dose should be utilized in patients with severe impairment of renal function. A second test dose may be tried if there is an inadequate response, but no more than two test doses should be attempted.

If urine output continues to decline during mannitol infusion, the patient's clinical status should be closely reviewed and mannitol infusion suspended if necessary. Accumulation of mannitol may result in overexpansion of the extracellular fluid which may intensify existing or latent congestive heart failure.

Excessive loss of water and electrolytes may lead to serious imbalances. With rapid or prolonged administration of mannitol, loss of water in excess of electrolytes can cause hypernatremia. Electrolyte measurements including sodium and potassium are therefore of vital importance in monitoring the infusion of mannitol.

Osmotic nephrosis, a reversible vacuolization of the tubules of no known clinical significance, may proceed to severe irreversible nephrosis, requiring close monitoring during mannitol infusion.

Electrolyte-free mannitol solutions should not be given conjointly with blood.

PRECAUTIONS:

GENERAL

Clinical evaluation and periodic laboratory determinations are necessary to monitor changes in fluid balance, electrolyte concentrations, and acid-base balance during parenteral therapy with mannitol solutions.

These solutions should be used with care in patients with hypervolemia, renal insufficiency, urinary tract obstruction, or impending or frank cardiac decompensation.

The cardiovascular status of the patient should be carefully evaluated before rapidly administering mannitol since sudden expansion of the extracellular fluid may lead to fulminating congestive heart failure.

Shifting of sodium-free intracellular fluid into the extracellular compartment following mannitol infusion may lower serum sodium concentration and aggravate preexisting hyponatremia.

Mannitol administration may obscure and intensify inadequate hydration or hypovolemia by sustaining diuresis.

If it is essential that blood be given simultaneously, at least 20 mEq of sodium chloride should be added per liter of mannitol solution to avoid agglomeration of erythrocytes. In no other instance should additions be made to Mannitol Injections USP. The addition of sodium chloride to 20% mannitol solutions may result in precipitation of mannitol. The final infusate should therefore be inspected for cloudiness or precipitation immediately after mixing, prior to administration, and periodically during administration.

Solutions of mannitol may crystallize when exposed to low temperatures.

Concentrations greater than 15% have a greater tendency to crystallization. If crystals are observed, the container should be warmed by appropriate means to not greater than 60°C, shaken, then cooled to body temperature before administering. If all crystals cannot be completely redissolved, the container must be rejected.

Do not use plastic container in series connection.

If administration is controlled by a pumping device, care must be taken to discontinue pumping action before the container runs dry or air embolism may result.

These solutions are intended for intravenous administration using sterile equipment. It is recommended that intravenous administration apparatus be replaced at least once every 24 hours.

Use only if solution is clear and container and seals are intact.

CARCINOGENESIS, MUTAGENESIS, AND IMPAIRMENT OF FERTILITY

Long term studies in animals to evaluate the carcinogenic and mutagenic potential or the effect on fertility of mannitol injection USP have not been conducted.

PRECAUTIONS: *(cont'd)*

PREGNANCY CATEGORY C

Animal reproduction studies have not been conducted with mannitol injections USP. It is also not known whether mannitol injections USP can cause fetal harm when administered to a pregnant woman or can affect reproduction capacity. Mannitol injections USP should be given to a pregnant woman only if clearly needed.

NURSING MOTHERS

It is not known whether this drug is excreted in human milk. Because many drugs are excreted in human milk, caution should be exercised when mannitol injections USP are administered to a nursing mother.

PEDIATRIC USE

Safety and effectiveness in children below the age of 12 years have not been established.

ADVERSE REACTIONS:

Reactions which may occur because of the solution or the technique of administration include febrile response, infection at the site of injection, venous thrombosis or phlebitis extending from the site of injection, extravasation and hypervolemia.

Isolated cases of adverse reactions, such as pulmonary congestion, fluid and electrolyte imbalance, acidosis, electrolyte loss, dryness of mouth, thirst, marked diuresis, urinary retention, edema, headache, blurred vision, convulsions, nausea, vomiting, rhinitis, arm pain, skin necrosis, thrombophlebitis, chills, dizziness, urticaria, dehydration, hypotension, tachycardia, fever and angina-like chest pains have been reported during or following mannitol infusion.

Too rapid infusion of hypertonic solutions may cause local pain and venous irritation. Rate of administration should be adjusted according to tolerance. Use of the largest peripheral vein and a small bore needle is recommended. (See DOSAGE AND ADMINISTRATION.)

The physician should also be alert to the possibility of adverse reactions to drug additives. Prescribing information for drug additives to be administered in this manner should be consulted.

If an adverse reaction does occur, discontinue the infusion, evaluate the patient, institute appropriate therapeutic countermeasures and save the remainder of the fluid for examination if deemed necessary.

OVERDOSAGE:

In the event of a fluid or solute overload during parenteral therapy, reevaluate the patient's condition, and institute appropriate corrective treatment.

Larger doses than recommended may result in increased electrolyte excretion, particularly sodium, chloride, and potassium. Sodium depletion can result in orthostatic tachycardia and/or hypotension and decreased central venous pressure. Chloride metabolism closely follows that of sodium. Potassium deficit can impair neuromuscular function and cause intestinal dilation and ileus.

Mannitol may cause pulmonary edema or water intoxication if urine flow is inadequate. See WARNINGS.

DOSAGE AND ADMINISTRATION:

These solutions are for intravenous use only.

The total dosage, concentration and rate of administration should be governed by the nature and severity of the condition being treated, fluid requirement and urinary output. The usual adult dosage ranges from 50 to 200 g in a 24-hour period, but in most cases an adequate response will be achieved at a dosage of approximately 100 g/24 hours. The rate of administration is usually adjusted to maintain a urine flow of at least 30 to 50 ml/hr. This outline of dosage and administration is only a general guide to therapy.

Dosage requirements for patients 12 years of age and under have not been established. As with adults, dose is dependent on weight, clinical condition, and laboratory results. Follow recommendations of appropriate pediatric reference text.

TEST DOSE

A test dose of mannitol should be given prior to instituting therapy for patients with marked oliguria or those believed to have inadequate renal function. Such test doses may be approximately 0.2 g/kg of body weight (about 75 ml of a 20% solution, or 100 ml of a 15% solution) infused in a period of 3 to 5 minutes to produce a urine flow of at least 30 to 50 ml/hr. If urine flow does not increase, a second test dose may be given; but if there is an inadequate response, the patient should be reevaluated.

PREVENTION OF ACUTE RENAL FAILURE (OLIGURIA)

When used during cardiovascular and other types of surgery, 50 to 100 g of mannitol as a 5%, 10% or 15% solution may be given. The concentration will depend upon the fluid requirements of the patient. Generally, a concentrated solution is given initially followed by a 5% or 10% solution.

TREATMENT OF OLIGURIA

The usual dose for treatment of oliguria is 100 g administered as a 15% or 20% solution.

REDUCTION OF INTRACRANIAL AND INTRAOCULAR PRESSURE

A dose of 1.5 to 2 g/kg as a 20% solution (7.5 to 10 ml/kg) or as a 15% solution (10 to 13 ml/kg) may be given over a period as short as 30 minutes in order to obtain a prompt and maximal effect. When used preoperatively, the dose should be given one to one and one-half hours before surgery to achieve maximal reduction of pressure before operation.

ADJUNCTIVE THERAPY FOR INTOXICATIONS

As an agent to promote diuresis in intoxications, 5%, 10%, 15% or 20% mannitol is indicated. The concentration will depend upon the fluid requirement and the urinary output of the patient. Generally, a bolus dose of 15% or 20% mannitol is given followed by a slower infusion of 5% mannitol (with electrolytes) to maintain urine output at the desired level.

It is recommended that 20% mannitol injection USP be administered through a blood filter set to ensure against infusion of mannitol crystals.

When a hypertonic solution is to be administered peripherally, it should be slowly infused through a small bore needle, placed well within the lumen of a large vein to minimize venous irritation. Carefully avoid infiltration.

Parenteral drug products should be inspected visually for particulate matter and discoloration prior to administration, whenever solution and container permit.

DIRECTIONS FOR USE OF EXCEL CONTAINER

Do not admix with other drugs.

Caution: Do not use plastic container in series connection.

To Open

Tear overwrap down at notch and remove solution container. Check for minute leaks by squeezing solution container firmly. If leaks are found, discard solution as sterility may be impaired.

Note: Before use, perform the following checks:

Inspect each container. Read the label. Ensure solution is the one ordered and is within the expiration date.

DOSAGE AND ADMINISTRATION: *(cont'd)*

Invert container and carefully inspect the solution in good light for cloudiness, haze, or particulate matter. Any container which is suspect should not be used.

Use only if solution is clear and container and seals are intact.

Preparation for Administration

1. Remove plastic protector from sterile set port at bottom of container.

2. Attach administration set. Refer to complete directions accompanying set.

HOW SUPPLIED - RATED THERAPEUTICALLY EQUIVALENT:

Injection, Solution - Intravenous - 5 %

1000 ml	$32.70	OSMITROL, Baxter Hlthcare	00338-0351-04
1000 ml	$33.68	Mannitol, Abbott	00074-1559-05
1000 ml	$51.51	MANNITOL, Abbott	00074-7712-09
1000 ml	$72.36	MANNITOL, McGaw	00264-7570-00
1000 ml x 6	$27.33	5% MANNITOL, McGaw	00264-1170-00

Injection, Solution - Intravenous - 10 %

100 ml	$73.31	MANNITOL, Abbott	00074-7713-09
500 ml	$37.63	OSMITROL, Baxter Hlthcare	00338-0353-03
500 ml	$53.92	MANNITOL, McGaw	00264-7573-10
1000 ml	$48.67	Mannitol, Abbott	00074-1560-05
1000 ml	$72.36	Mannitol, McGaw	00264-7573-00
1000 ml x 6	$72.50	10% MANNITOL, McGaw	00264-1173-00

Injection, Solution - Intravenous - 15 %

150 ml x 12	$12.57	15% MANNITOL, McGaw	00264-1176-30
500 ml	$49.40	15% MANNITOL I.V., Abbott	00074-1562-04
500 ml	$60.09	OSMITROL, Baxter Hlthcare	00338-0355-03
500 ml	$63.08	Mannitol, Abbott	00074-7714-03
500 ml	$71.68	MANNITOL, McGaw	00264-7576-01

Injection, Solution - Intravenous - 20 %

250 ml	$54.43	Mannitol, McGaw	00264-7578-20
250 ml	$55.34	Mannitol, Abbott	00074-7715-02
250 ml	$56.33	OSMITROL, Baxter Hlthcare	00338-0357-02
250 ml x 12	$54.53	20% MANNITOL, McGaw	00264-1178-20
500 ml	$54.43	Mannitol, McGaw	00264-7578-10
500 ml	$58.37	20% MANNITOL I.V., Abbott	00074-1563-04
500 ml	$70.28	OSMITROL, Baxter Hlthcare	00338-0357-03
500 ml	$73.79	Mannitol, Abbott	00074-7715-03
500 ml x 12	$54.53	20% MANNITOL, McGaw	00264-1178-10

Injection, Solution - Intravenous - 25 %

50 ml	$5.05	25% MANNITOL, Abbott	00074-4031-01
50 ml	$8.51	Mannitol, Intl Medication	00548-1003-00
50 ml x 10	$100.46	Mannitol, Astra USA	00186-0652-01
50 ml x 25	$53.44	Mannitol, Fujisawa USA	00469-0024-25
50 ml x 25	$56.56	Mannitol, Fujisawa USA	00469-0014-25
50 ml x 25	$66.25	Mannitol, Astra USA	00186-1168-04
50 ml x 25	$85.94	Mannitol, Am Regent	00517-4050-25

HOW SUPPLIED - NOT RATED EQUIVALENT:

Injection, Solution - Intravenous - 25 %

25 x 50 ml	$62.50	Mannitol, Pasadena	00418-0014-50
50 ml	$5.50	Mannitol, Consolidated Midland	00223-8105-50
50 ml x 25	$137.50	Mannitol, Consolidated Midland	00223-8105-25

MANNITOL; SORBITOL *(001699)*

CATEGORIES: Electrolytic, Caloric-Water Balance; Irrigating Solutions; Pharmaceutical Aids; Transurethral Surgery; FDA Approval Pre 1982

DESCRIPTION:

Sorbitol-mannitol irrigation is a sterile, nonpyrogenic, hypotonic, aqueous solution for urologic nonelectrolyte irrigation during transurethral surgical procedures. Each 100 ml contains sorbitol 2.70 g and mannitol 0.54 g in water for injection. The solution is nonelectrolytic and hypotonic (178 mOsm/liter calc.); approx. pH 4.9.

The solution contains no bacteriostat, antimicrobial agent or added buffer and is intended for use as a single-dose irrigation. When smaller volumes are required the unused portion should be discarded.

Sorbitol-mannitol irrigation is a nonelectrolyte urologic irrigant.

Sorbitol, NF is chemically designated D-glucitol ($C_6H_{14}O_6$), white powder, granules or flakes very soluble in water.

Mannitol, USP is chemically designated D-mannitol ($C_6H_{14}O_6$), white crystalline powder or free-flowing granules, freely soluble in water.

Water for injection, USP is chemically designated H_2O.

The flexible plastic container is fabricated from a specifically formulated polyvinylchloride. Water can permeate from inside the container into the overwrap but not in amounts sufficient to affect the solution significantly. Solutions inside the plastic container also can leach out certain of its chemical components in very small amounts before the expiration period is attained. However, the safety of the plastic has been confirmed by tests in animals according to USP biological standards for plastic containers.

The semi-rigid container is fabricated from a specially formulated polyolefin. It is a copolymer of ethylene and propylene. The safety of the plastic has been confirmed by tests in animals according to USP biological standards for plastic containers. The container requires no vapor barrier to maintain the proper drug concentration.

CLINICAL PHARMACOLOGY:

Sorbitol and mannitol are hexitols and are nonelectrolytes. A solution of these constituents in water is therefore nonconductive and suitable for urologic irrigation during electrosurgical procedures. A 3% (approx.) total concentration of sorbitol-mannitol contains sufficient solute to minimize the risk if intravascular hemolysis which can occur from absorption of plain water through open prostatic veins during transurethral resection (TUR). Any solution that is absorbed intravascularly during transurethral prostatic or bladder surgery, although variable in amount depending primarily on the extent of surgery, will be excreted by the kidney. When absorbed intravascularly, sorbitol and mannitol act as osmotic diuretics.

Intravascular absorption of sorbitol has been shown to produce elevations of serum lactate after TUR above preoperative values owing to sorbitol's favored metabolism to lactate from pyruvate. Increased lactate levels were not sufficient to produce evidence of metabolic acidosis. Mannitol is only slightly metabolized and rapidly excreted by the kidney.

INDICATIONS AND USAGE:

Sorbitol-mannitol irrigation is indicated for use as a urologic irrigating fluid during transurethral prostatic resection and other transurethral surgical procedures.

CONTRAINDICATIONS:

NOT FOR INJECTION BY USUAL PARENTERAL ROUTES.

Do not use in patients with anuria.

WARNINGS:

FOR UROLOGIC IRRIGATION ONLY.

Solutions for urologic irrigation must be used with caution in patients with severe cardiopulmonary or renal dysfunction.

Irrigating fluids used during transurethral prostatectomy have been demonstrated to enter the systemic circulation in relatively large volumes; thus, sorbitol-mannitol irrigant must be regarded as a systemic drug. Absorption of large amounts of fluids containing sorbitol-mannitol and the osmotic diuretics it produces may significantly alter cardiopulmonary and renal dynamics.

Hypercalcemia from metabolism of sorbitol may occur in patients with diabetes mellitus.

Hyperlactatemia from metabolism of sorbitol may potentially produce a significant lactic acidemia in metabolically compromised patients.

The contents of an opened container should be used promptly to minimize the possibility of bacterial growth or pyrogen formation.

Discard the unused portion of irrigating solution since it contains no preservatives. Do not heat container over 66 deg. C (150 deg. F).

PRECAUTIONS:

Cardiovascular status, especially of the patient with cardiac disease, should be carefully observed before and during transurethral resection of the prostate when using sorbitol-mannitol irrigation, because the quantity of fluid absorbed into the systemic circulation by opened prostatic veins may produce significant expansion of the extracellular fluid and lead to fulminating congestive heart failure.

Shift of sodium-free intracellular fluid into the extracellular compartment following systemic absorption of solution may lower serum sodium concentration and aggravate pre-existing hyponatremia.

Excessive loss of water and electrolytes may lead to serious imbalances. With continuous irrigation, loss of water may occur in excess of electrolytes, producing hypernatremia.

Sustained diuresis that results from transurethral irrigation with sorbitol-mannitol irrigation may obscure and intensify inadequate hydration or hypovolemia.

Aseptic technique is essential for the use of sterile solutions for irrigation. The administration set should be attached promptly. Unused portions should be discarded and a fresh container of appropriate size used for the start-up of each cycle or repeat procedure.

Do not administer unless solution is clear, seal is intact and container is undamaged. Discard unused portion.

ADVERSE REACTIONS:

Adverse reactions may result from intravascular absorption of sorbitol and mannitol. The literature reports occasional adverse reactions from intravenous sorbitol-mannitol infusions. Consequences if absorption of urologic irrigating solutions include fluid and electrolyte disturbances such as acidosis, electrolyte loss, marked diuresis, urinary retention, edema, dryness of mouth, thirst and dehydration; cardiovascular disorders such as hypotension, tachycardia, angina-like pains; pulmonary disorders such as pulmonary congestion; and other general reactions such as blurred vision, convulsions, nausea, vomiting, diarrhea, rhinitis, chills, vertigo, backache, urticaria. Allergic reactions from sorbitol-mannitol have also been reported.

Should any adverse reaction occur, discontinue the irrigant, evaluate the patient, institute appropriate therapeutic countermeasures and save the remainder of the fluid for examination if deemed necessary.

OVERDOSAGE:

In the event of dehydration, fluid or solute overload, discontinue the irrigation, evaluate the patient and institute corrective measures as indicated. (See WARNINGS, PRECAUTIONS, and ADVERSE REACTIONS.)

DOSAGE AND ADMINISTRATION:

Sorbitol-mannitol irrigation should be administered only by transurethral instillation with appropriate urologic instrumentation. A disposable administration set should be used. The total volume of solution used for irrigation is solely at the discretion of the surgeon.

Height of container(s) above the operating table in excess of 60 cm (approx. 2 ft.) has been reported to increase the intravascular absorption of the irrigating fluid.

Parenteral drug products should be inspected visually for particulate matter and discoloration prior to administration, whenever container and solution permit. (See PRECAUTIONS.)

Exposure of pharmaceutical products to heat should be minimized. Avoid excessive heat. Protect from freezing. It is recommended that the product be stored at room temperature (25 deg. C); however, brief exposure up to 40 deg. C does not adversely affect the product.

HOW SUPPLIED - RATED THERAPEUTICALLY EQUIVALENT:

Solution - Irrigation - 0.54 gm/2.7 gm

1500 ml	$28.50	SORBITOL-MANNITOL, Abbott	00074-6144-06
3000 ml	$21.33	SORBITOL-MANNITOL, Abbott	00074-7981-08

MAPROTILINE HYDROCHLORIDE *(001700)*

CATEGORIES: Antidepressants; Antipsychotics/Antimanics; Anxiety; Central Nervous System Agents; Depression; Depressive Neurosis; Psychotherapeutic Agents; Tetracyclics; Pregnancy Category B; FDA Approval Pre 1982

BRAND NAMES: *Delgian* (Germany); *Klimastress*; **Ludiomil**; *Maprostad* (Germany); *Melodil*; *Mirpan* (Germany); *Psymion* (Germany); *Retinyl*
(International brand names outside U.S. in italics)

COST OF THERAPY: $36.79 (Depression; Tablet; 75 mg; 1/day; 90 days)

PRIMARY ICD9: 311 (Depressive Disorder, Not Elsewhere Classified)

DESCRIPTION:

Maprotiline HCl USP, is a tetracyclic antidepressant, available as 25 mg, 50 mg and 75 mg tablets for oral administration. Its chemical name is N-methyl-9,10-ethanoanthracene-9(10H)-propylamine hydrochloride.

Maprotiline HCl USP is a fine, white to off-white, practically odorless crystalline powder. It is freely soluble in methanol and in chloroform, slightly soluble in water, and practically insoluble in isooctane. Its molecular weight is 313.87.

DESCRIPTION: *(cont'd)*

Inactive Ingredients: Calcium phosphate, cellulose compounds, colloidal silicon dioxide, FD&C Yellow No. 6 Aluminum Lake (25-mg and 50-mg tablets), lactose, magnesium stearate, povidone, shellac, starch, stearic acid, talc, and titanium dioxide.

CLINICAL PHARMACOLOGY:

The mechanism of action of maprotiline HCl is not precisely known. It does not act primarily by stimulation of the central nervous system and is not a monoamine oxidase inhibitor. The postulated mechanism of maprotiline HCl is that it acts primarily by potentiation of central adrenergic synapses by blocking reuptake of norepinephrine at nerve endings. This pharmacologic action is thought to be responsible for the drug's antidepressant and anxiolytic effects.

The mean time to peak is 12 hours. The half-life of elimination averages 51 hours.

Steady-state levels measured prior to the morning dose on a one-dosage regimen are summarized as follows (TABLE 1):

TABLE 1 Maprotiline HCl, Clinical Pharmacology

Regimen	Average Minimum Concentration ng/ml	95% Confidence Limits ng/ml
50 mg x 3 daily	238	181-295

INDICATIONS AND USAGE:

Maprotiline HCl is indicated for the treatment of depressive illness in patients with depressive neurosis (dysthymic disorder) and manic-depressive illness, depressed type (major depressive disorder). Maprotiline HCl is also effective for the relief of anxiety associated with depression.

CONTRAINDICATIONS:

Maprotiline HCl is contraindicated in patients hypersensitive to maprotiline and in patients with known or suspected seizure disorders. It should not be given concomitantly with monoamine oxidase (MAO) inhibitors. A minimum of 14 days should be allowed to elapse after discontinuation of MAO inhibitors before treatment with maprotiline is initiated. Effects should be monitored with gradual increase in dosage until optimum response is achieved. The drug is not recommended for use during the acute phase of myocardial infarction.

WARNINGS:

Seizures Have Been Associated With The Use Of Maprotiline HCl : Most of the seizures have occurred in patients without a known history of seizures. However, in some of these cases, other confounding factors were present, including concomitant medications known to lower the seizure threshold, rapid escalation of the dosage of maprotiline, and dosage that exceeded the recommended therapeutic range. The incidence of direct reports is less than 1/10th of 1%. The risk of seizures may be increased when maprotiline is taken concomitantly with phenothiazines, when the dosage of benzodiazepines is rapidly tapered in patients receiving maprotiline or when the recommended dosage of maprotiline is exceeded. While a cause-and-effect relationship has not been established, the risk of seizures in patients treated with maprotiline may be reduced by (1) initiating therapy at a low dosage, (2) maintaining the initial dosage for 2 weeks before raising it gradually in small increments as necessitated by the long half-life of maprotiline (average 51 hours), and (3) keeping the dosage at the minimally effective level during maintenance therapy. (See DOSAGE AND ADMINISTRATION.)

Extreme Caution Should Be Used When This Drug is Given to:

patients with a history of myocardial infarction

patients with a history of presence of cardiovascular disease because of the possibility of conduction defects, arrhythmias, myocardial infarction, strokes and tachycardia

PRECAUTIONS:

GENERAL

The possibility of suicide in seriously depressed patients is inherent in their illness and may persist until significant remission occurs. Therefore, patients must be carefully supervised during all phases of treatment with maprotiline HCl and prescriptions should be written for the smallest number of tablets consistent with good patient management.

Hypomanic or manic episodes have been known to occur in some patients taking tricyclic antidepressant drugs, particularly in patients with cyclic disorders. Such occurrences have also been noted, rarely, with maprotiline.

Prior to elective surgery, maprotiline should be discontinued for as long as clinically feasible, since little is known about the interaction between maprotiline and general anesthetics. Maprotiline should be administered with caution in patients with increased intraocular pressure, history of urinary retention, or history of narrow-angle glaucoma because of the drug's anticholinergic properties.

INFORMATION FOR THE PATIENT

Patients should be warned of the association between seizures and the use of maprotiline. Moreover they should be informed that this association is enhanced in patients with a known history of seizures and in those patients who are taking certain other drugs. (See WARNINGS.)

Warn patients to exercise caution about potentially hazardous tasks, or operating automobiles or machinery since the drug may impair mental and/or physical abilities.

Maprotiline may enhance the response to alcohol, barbiturates, and other CNS depressants, requiring appropriate caution of administration.

LABORATORY TESTS

Maprotiline HCl should be discontinued if there is evidence of pathologic neutrophil depression. Leukocyte and differential counts should be performed in patients who develop fever and sore throat during therapy.

CARCINOGENESIS, MUTAGENESIS, AND IMPAIRMENT OF FERTILITY

Carcinogenicity and chronic toxicity studies have been conducted in laboratory rats and dogs. No drug- or dose-related occurrence of carcinogenesis was evident in rats receiving daily oral doses up to 60 mg/kg of maprotiline HCl for eighteen months or in dogs receiving daily oral doses up to 30 mg/kg of maprotiline HCl for one year. In addition, no evidence of mutagenic activity was found in offspring of female mice mated with males treated with up to 60 times the maximum daily human dose.

PREGNANCY CATEGORY B

Reproduction studies have been performed in female laboratory rabbits, mice, and rats at doses up to 1.3, 7, and 9 times the maximum daily human dose respectively and have revealed no evidence of impaired fertility or harm to the fetus due to maprotiline HCl. There are, however, no adequate and well-controlled studies in pregnant women. Because animal reproduction studies are not always predictive of human response, this drug should be used during pregnancy only if clearly needed.

PRECAUTIONS: *(cont'd)*

LABOR AND DELIVERY

Although the effect of maprotiline HCl on labor and delivery is unknown, caution should be exercised as with any drug with CNS depressant action.

NURSING MOTHERS

Maprotiline is excreted in breast milk. At steady state, the concentrations in milk correspond closely to the concentrations in whole blood. Caution should be exercised when maprotiline is administered to a nursing woman.

PEDIATRIC USE

Safety and effectiveness in children below the age of 18 have not been established.

DRUG INTERACTIONS:

Close supervision and careful adjustment of dosage are required when administering maprotiline concomitantly with anticholinergic or sympathomimetic drugs because of the possibility of additive atropine-like effects.

Concurrent administration of maprotiline with electroshock therapy should be avoided because of the lack of experience in this area.

Caution should be exercised when administering maprotiline to hyperthyroid patients or those on thyroid medication because of the possibility of enhanced potential for cardiovascular toxicity of maprotiline.

Maprotiline should be used with caution in patients receiving guanethidine or similar agents since it may block the pharmacologic effects of these drugs.

The risk of seizures may be increased when maprotiline is taken concomitantly with phenothiazines or when the dosage of benzodiazepines is rapidly tapered in patients receiving maprotiline.

Because of the pharmacologic similarity of maprotiline to the tricyclic antidepressants, the plasma concentration of maprotiline may be increased when the drug is given concomitantly with cimetidine, as has occurred with tricyclic antidepressants. Adjustment of the dosage of maprotiline may therefore be necessary in such cases. (See PRECAUTIONS, Information for the Patient.)

ADVERSE REACTIONS:

The following adverse reactions have been noted with maprotiline HCl and are generally similar to those observed with tricyclic antidepressants.

Cardiovascular: Rare occurrences of hypotension, hypertension, tachycardia, palpitation, arrhythmia, heart block, and syncope have been reported with maprotiline HCl.

Psychiatric: Nervousness (6%), anxiety (3%), insomnia (2%), and agitation (2%); rarely, confusional states (especially in the elderly), hallucinations, disorientation, delusions, restlessness, nightmares, hypomania, mania, exacerbation of psychosis, decrease in memory, and feelings of unreality.

Neurological: Drowsiness (16%), dizziness (8%), tremor (3%), and, rarely, numbness, tingling, motor hyperactivity, akathisia, seizures, EEG alterations, tinnitus, extrapyramidal symptoms, ataxia, and dysarthria.

Anticholinergic: Dry mouth (22%), constipation (6%), and blurred vision (4%); rarely, accommodation disturbances, mydriasis, urinary retention, and delayed micturition.

Allergic: Rare instances of skin rash, petechiae, itching, photosensitization, edema, and drug fever.

Gastrointestinal: Nausea (2%) and, rarely, vomiting, epigastric distress, diarrhea, bitter taste, abdominal cramps and dysphagia.

Endocrine: Rare instances of increased or decreased libido, impotence, and elevation or depression of blood sugar levels.

Other: Weakness and fatigue (4%) and headache (4%); rarely, altered liver function, jaundice, weight loss or gain, excessive perspiration, flushing, urinary frequency, increased salivation, nasal congestion and alopecia.

Note: Although there have been only isolated reports of the following adverse reactions with maprotiline HCl, its pharmacologic similarity to tricyclic antidepressants requires that each reaction be considered when administering maprotiline HCl.

Bone marrow depression, including agranulocytosis, eosinophilia, purpura, and thrombocytopenia, myocardial infarction, stroke, peripheral neuropathy, sublingual adenitis, black tongue, stomatitis, paralytic ileus, gynecomastia in the male, breast enlargement and galactorrhea in the female, and testicular swelling.

OVERDOSAGE:

Animal Oral LD_{50}: The oral LD_{50} of maprotiline HCl is 600-750 mg/kg in mice, 760-900 mg/kg in rats, >1000 mg/kg in rabbits, >300 mg/kg in cats, and >30 mg/kg in dogs.

Signs and Symptoms: Data dealing with overdosage in humans are limited with only a few cases on record. Symptoms are drowsiness, tachycardia, ataxia, vomiting, cyanosis, hypotension, shock, restlessness, agitation, hyperpyrexia, muscle rigidity, athetoid movements, mydriasis, cardiac arrhythmias, impaired cardiac condition. In severe cases, loss of consciousness and generalized convulsions may occur. Since congestive heart failure has been seen with overdosages of tricyclic antidepressants, it should be considered with maprotiline HCl overdosage.

Treatment: The recommended treatment for overdosage with heterocyclics may change periodically. Therefore, it is recommended that the physician contact a poison control center for current information on treatment. Because CNS involvement, respiratory depression, and cardiac arrhythmia can occur suddenly, hospitalization and close observation may be necessary, even when the amount ingested is thought to be small or the initial degree of intoxication appears slight or moderate. All patients with ECG abnormalities should have continuous cardiac monitoring and be closely observed until well after the cardiac status has returned to normal; relapses may occur after apparent recovery.

In the alert patient, the stomach should be emptied promptly by lavage. In the obtunded patient, the airway should be secured with a cuffed endotracheal tube before beginning lavage (do not induce emesis). Installation of an activated charcoal slurry may help reduce the absorption of maprotiline. The room should be darkened, allowing only minimal external stimulation to reduce the tendency to convulsions. If anticonvulsants are necessary, diazepam and phenytoin may be useful. Adequate respiratory exchange should be maintained, including intubation and artificial respiration, if necessary.

Since it has been reported that physostigmine increases the risk of seizures, its use is not recommended in cases of overdosage with maprotiline.

Shock (circulatory collapse) should be treated with supportive measures such as appropriate position, intravenous fluids, and vasopressors if necessary.

Hyperpyrexia should be controlled by whatever means available, including ice packs if necessary.

Digitalis may increase conduction abnormalities and further irritate an already sensitized myocardium. If congestive heart failure necessitates rapid digitalization, particular care must be exercised.

OVERDOSAGE: *(cont'd)*

Dialysis is of little value because of the low plasma concentration of this drug.

DOSAGE AND ADMINISTRATION:

A single daily dose is an alternative to divided daily doses. Therapeutic effects are sometimes seen within 3 to 7 days, although as long as 2 to 3 weeks are usually necessary.

Initial Adult Dosage: An initial dosage of 75 mg daily is suggested for outpatients with mild-to-moderate depression. However, in some patients, particularly the elderly, an initial dosage of 25 mg daily may be used. Because of the long half-life of maprotiline HCl, the initial dosage should be maintained for two weeks. The dosage may then be increased gradually in 25-mg increments as required and tolerated. In most outpatients a maximum dose of 150 mg daily will result in therapeutic efficacy. It is recommended that this dose not be exceeded except in the most severely depressed patients. In such patients, dosage may be gradually increased to a maximum of 225 mg.

More severely depressed, hospitalized patients should be given an initial daily dose of 100 mg to 150 mg which may be gradually increased as required and tolerated. Most hospitalized patients with moderate-to-severe depression respond to a daily dosage of 150 mg although dosages as high as 225 mg may be required in some cases. Daily dosage of 225 mg should not be exceeded.

Elderly Patients: In general, lower dosages are recommended for patients over 60 years of age. Dosages of 50 mg to 75 mg daily are usually satisfactory as maintenance therapy for elderly patients who do not tolerate higher amounts.

Maintenance: Dosage during prolonged maintenance therapy should be kept at the lowest effective level. Dosage may be reduced to levels of 75 mg to 150 mg daily during such periods, with subsequent adjustment depending on therapeutic response.

Storage: Do not store above 86°F (30°C). *Dispense in a tight container (USP).*

HOW SUPPLIED - RATED THERAPEUTICALLY EQUIVALENT:

Tablet, Coated - Oral - 25 mg

30's	$5.82	Maprotiline HCl, H.C.F.A. F F P	99999-1700-01
100's	$19.43	Maprotiline HCl, H.C.F.A. F F P	99999-1700-02
100's	$20.82	Maprotiline Hcl, United Res	00677-1214-01
100's	$26.95	Maprotiline Hcl, Harber Pharm	51432-0277-03
100's	$27.56	Maprotiline, Major Pharms	00904-3320-61
100's	$27.56	Maprotiline Hcl 25, Major Pharms	00904-3323-61
100's	$27.95	Maprotiline HCl, Geneva Pharms	00781-1631-01
100's	$30.00	Maprotiline Hcl, Raway	00686-0493-20
100's	$30.06	Maprotiline Hcl, Qualitest Pharms	00603-4294-21
100's	$30.70	Maprotiline Hcl, Major Pharms	00904-3323-60
100's	$33.10	Maprotiline Hcl, Schein Pharm (US)	00364-2294-01
100's	$33.20	Maprotiline, Rugby	00536-3902-01
100's	$33.61	Maprotiline Hcl, Vangard Labs	00615-3521-13
100's	$35.18	Maprotiline Hcl, Goldline Labs	00182-1882-01
100's	$35.18	Maprotiline Hcl, Watson Labs	52544-0373-01
100's	$35.20	Maprotiline Hcl, Aligen Independ	00405-4594-01
100's	$35.95	Maprotiline Hcl, Parmed Pharms	00349-8879-01
100's	$35.95	Maprotiline Hcl, Martec Pharms	52555-0355-01
100's	$37.19	Maprotiline Hcl, HL Moore Drug Exch	00839-7448-06
100's	$37.50	Maprotiline Hcl, Mylan	00378-0060-01
100's	**$44.34**	**LUDIOMIL, Novartis**	**00083-0110-30**

Tablet, Coated - Oral - 50 mg

30's	$8.73	Maprotiline HCl, H.C.F.A. F F P	99999-1700-03
100's	$29.10	Maprotiline HCl, H.C.F.A. F F P	99999-1700-04
100's	$30.75	Maprotiline Hcl, United Res	00677-1215-01
100's	$36.00	Maprotiline Hcl, Raway	00686-0494-20
100's	$39.49	Maprotiline Hcl, Qualitest Pharms	00603-4295-21
100's	$40.95	Maprotiline HCl, Geneva Pharms	00781-1632-01
100's	$42.82	Maprotiline, Major Pharms	00904-3321-61
100's	$47.55	Maprotiline Hcl, Vangard Labs	00615-3522-13
100's	$47.70	Maprotiline Hcl, Major Pharms	00904-3324-60
100's	$49.00	Maprotiline Hcl, Parmed Pharms	00349-8880-01
100's	$51.00	Maprotiline, Rugby	00536-3903-01
100's	$52.06	Maprotiline Hcl, Goldline Labs	00182-1883-01
100's	$52.06	Maprotiline Hcl, Watson Labs	52544-0374-01
100's	$52.10	Maprotiline Hcl, Aligen Independ	00405-4595-01
100's	$52.52	Maprotiline Hcl, HL Moore Drug Exch	00839-7449-06
100's	$52.80	Maprotiline Hcl, Martec Pharms	52555-0356-01
100's	$55.10	Maprotiline Hcl, Mylan	00378-0087-01
100's	**$65.61**	**LUDIOMIL, Novartis**	**00083-0026-30**

Tablet, Coated - Oral - 75 mg

100's	$40.88	Maprotiline Hcl, United Res	00677-1216-01
100's	$40.88	Maprotiline HCl, H.C.F.A. F F P	99999-1700-05
100's	$54.48	Maprotiline, Major Pharms	00904-3322-61
100's	$54.75	LIPOLINE, Major Pharms	00904-3322-60
100's	$62.65	Maprotiline Hcl, Major Pharms	00904-3325-60
100's	$63.63	Maprotiline Hcl, Vangard Labs	00615-3523-13
100's	$71.43	Maprotiline Hcl, Qualitest Pharms	00603-4296-21
100's	$71.48	Maprotiline Hcl, HL Moore Drug Exch	00839-7450-06
100's	$71.50	Maprotiline Hcl, Goldline Labs	00182-1884-01
100's	$71.50	Maprotiline Hcl, Watson Labs	52544-0375-01
100's	$71.62	Maprotiline Hcl, Aligen Independ	00405-4596-01
100's	$71.70	Maprotiline Hcl, Martec Pharms	52555-0357-01
100's	$74.85	Maprotiline Hcl, Mylan	00378-0092-01
100's	**$90.10**	**LUDIOMIL, Novartis**	**00083-0135-30**

MASOPROCOL *(003142)*

CATEGORIES: Antineoplastics; Dermatologicals; Keratoses; Topical; FDA Class 1S ("Standard Review"); FDA Approved 1992 Sep

BRAND NAMES: **Actinex**

DESCRIPTION:

For Dermatologic Use Only.

Not for Ophthalmic Use.

Actinex cream contains masoprocol 10%, in an emollient cream base. Chemically, masoprocol is (R*, S*)-4,4'-(2,3-dimethyl-1.4- butanediyl)bis(1.2-benzendiol). It has a molecular formular of $C_{18}H_{22}O_4$ and has a molecular weight of 302.37. Masoprocol (also known as meso-nordihydroguaiaretic acid) is a white to off-white crystalline powder.

Each gram of beige-colored cream contains 100 mg of masoprocol in an emollient cream base consisting of citric acid, isostearyl alcohol, light mineral oil, methyl paraben, polyethylene glycol 400, propylene glycol, propylparaben, purified water, sodium metabisulfite (a sulfite), steareth-21, steareth-2, stearyl alcohol, synthetic beeswax and xanthan gum.

CLINICAL PHARMACOLOGY:

The mechanism of action of ^{14}C-labeled masoprocol in the cream fomulation demonstrated low absorption (<1.0%) as measured by ^{14}C content of plasma, urine, and feces over the 96-hour period after application. In a separate study, 6 patients who were treated with unlabeled Actinex cream twice daily for 28 days demonstrated up to 2% absorption after application of ^{14}C-labeled masoprocol in the cream formulation on day 29, as measured by ^{14}C content of plasma, urinem and feces over the 96-hour period after application.

INDICATIONS AND USAGE:

Masoprocol cream is indicated for the topical treatment of actinic (solar) keratoses.

CONTRAINDICATIONS:

Masoprocol cream is contraindicated in patients with known hypersensitivity to masoprocol or other ingredients in this formulation.

WARNINGS:

OCCLUSIVE DRESSINGS SHOULD NOT BE USED WITH THIS PRODUCT

Masoprocol cream contains sodium metabisulfite, a sulfite that may cause allergic-type reactions including anaphylactic symptoms and life-threatening or less severe asthmatic episodes in certain susceptible people. The overall prevalence of sulfite sensitivity in the general population is unknown and probably low. Sulfite sensitivity is seen more frequently in asthmatic than in nonasthmatic people.

PRECAUTIONS:

GENERAL

Masoprocol Frequently Induces Sensitiziation (Allergic Contact Dermatitis): When patients treated with 5% or 10% masoprocol cream in clinical trials were patch tested with a 1% masoprocol cream, 9% had reactions indicative of sensitization. In patients rechallenged with 10% masoprocol cream, dermal reactions were nore frequent and more severe. Use of masoprocol should be discontinued if sensitivity is noted. Masoprocol does not appear to cause photosensitization. However, because solar keratoses are related to exposure to sunlight, the patient should avoid undue sun exposure.

If applying the product near the eyes, nose, or mouth, patients should be advised to do so with special care. If masoprocol comes into contact with the eyes (conjunctiva), itching, irritation, or transient pain may occur. In case of contact with the eye, wash the eye with water promptly. If masoprocol is applied with fingers, the hands should be washed immediately after use.

Masoprocol cream may stain clothing or fabrics.

INFORMATION FOR PATIENTS

1. Special care should be taken if masoprocol cream is to be applied near the eyes, nose, or mouth.

2. In case of contact with the eye, wash the eye with water promptly.

3. If masoprocol cream is applied with fingers, the hands should be washed immediately after use.

4. Contact physician immediately if a severe reaction occurs, including, for example, oozing or blistering.

5. While using this product, other skin care products or make-up should not be used without the advice of a physician.

CARCINOGENESIS. MUTAGENESIS, IMPAIRMENT OF FERTILITY

Animal studies have not been performed to evaluate the effect on fertility or the carcinogenic potential of masoprocol.

Masoprocol produced mutagenic results in the Ames assay. It was negative with three strains of *Salmonella* and positive with one. In an*in vivo* mouse estrogenic activity assay conducted using masoprocol subcutaneously at 2 mg/kg/day for 4 days, treated mice demonstrated no more effects of estrogenic activity than did vehicle controls.

PREGNANCY CATEGORY B

Teratology studies have been perfomred in rabbits and rats at doses up to 6 and 16 times the human dose, based on a mg/m^2 basis, respectively. No adverse fetal effects were observed. There are no adequate and well-controlled studies in pregnant women. Because animal reproduction studies are not always predictive of human response, this drug should be used during pregnancy only if clearly needed.

NURSING MOTHERS

It is not known whether this drug is excreted in human milk. Because many drugs are excreted in human milk, caution should be exercised when Actinex cream is administered to a nursing woman.

PEDIATRIC USE

Safety and effectiveness in children have not been established.

ADVERSE REACTIONS:

The frequently occurring adverse reactions considered related or possibly related to masoprocol cream and their frequency of occurrence are: erythema (46%), flaking (46%), itching (32%), dryness (27%), edema (14%), burning (12%), and soreness (5%). While local skin reactions are frequent, they usually resolve within two weeks of discontinuation. The presence or absence of local skin reactions does not correlate with successful ultimate therapeutic outcome. Reactions reported in 1% to 5% of patients include: bleeding, crusting, eye irritation, oozing, rash, skin irritation, soreness, stinging, tightness, and tingling. Less frequently reported reactions (less than 1%) include: blistering, eczema, excoriation, fissuring, leathery feeling to the the skin, skin roughness, and wrinkling. No necrosis, scarring, or ulceration was observed during the initial course of therapy.

OVERDOSAGE:

There are no reports of human ingestion overdosage. In animals receiving high oral doses of masoprocol, the commonly affected systems were the gastrointestinal and hepatic systems. If ingested, evacuate stomach contents, taking care to prevent aspiration.

DOSAGE AND ADMINISTRATION:

Wash and dry areas where actinic keratoses are present. Gently massage masoprocol cream into the area where actinic keratoses are present until it is evenly distributed, avoiding the eyes and mucous membranes of the nose and mouth. Application should be repeated each morning and evening for 28 days.

OCCLUSIVE DRESSINGS SHOULD NOT BE USED WITH THIS PRODUCT

Immediately after applying masoprocol, the patient might experience a transient local burning sensation.

STORAGE

Masoprocol cream should be stored at controlled room temperature, 15° to 30°C (59° to 86°F).

HOW SUPPLIED - EQUIVALENTS NOT AVAILABLE:

Cream - Topical - 100 mg/gm

30 gm	$44.27	ACTINEX, Schwarz Pharma (US)	00091-4520-37

MAZINDOL *(001701)*

CATEGORIES: Amphetamines; Anorexients/CNS Stimulants; Appetite Suppressants; Central Nervous System Agents; Obesity; Psychostimulants; Respiratory/Cerebral Stimulant; DEA Class CIV; FDA Approval Pre 1982

BRAND NAMES: *Diestet* (Mexico); *Liofindol* (Mexico); Mazanor; **Sanorex**; *Solucaps* (Mexico); *Teronac* (England)
(International brand names outside U.S. in italics)

DESCRIPTION:

Mazindol is an imidazoisoindole anorectic agent. It is chemically designated as 5-(4-chlorophenyl)-2,5-dihydro-3*H*-imidazol(2,1-*a*)isoindol-5-ol, a tautomeric form of 2-(2)'-(p-chlorobenzoyl) phenyl)-2-imidazoline.

Sanorex 1 mg, and 2 mg Tablets: *Active Ingredient:* Mazindol, USP *Inactive Ingredients:* calcium sulfate dihydrate, lactose, magnesium stearate, povidone, starch, and talc, USP.

CLINICAL PHARMACOLOGY:

Mazindol, although an isoindole, has pharmacologic activity similar in many ways to the prototype drugs used in obesity, the amphetamines. Actions include central nervous system stimulation in humans-like effects in animals as the production of stereotyped behavior. Animal experiments also suggest certain differences from phenethylamine anorectic drugs, e.g. amphetamine, with respect to site and mechanism of action; for example, mazindol appears to exert its primary effects on the limbic system. The significance of these differences for humans in uncertain. It does not cause brain norepinephrine depletion in animals; on the other hand, it does appear to inhibit storage site uptake of norepinephrine as is suggested by its marked potentiation of the effect of exogenous norepinephrine on blood pressure in dogs (*see WARNINGS*) and on smooth muscle contraction *in vitro*.

Tolerance has been demonstrated with all drugs of this class in which this phenomenon has been studied.

Drugs used in obesity are commonly known as "anorectics." It has not been established, however, that the action of such drugs in treating obesity is exclusively one of appetite suppression. Other central nervous system actions, or metabolic effects may be involved as well.

Adult obese subjects instructed in dietary management and treated with anorectic drugs, lose more weight on the average than those treated with placebo and diet, as determined in relatively short-term clinical trials.

The average magnitude of increased weight loss of drug-treated patients over placebo-treated patients in studies of anorectics in general is ordinarily only a fraction of a pound a week. The rate of weight loss is greatest in the first weeks of therapy for both drug and placebo subjects and tends to decrease in succeeding weeks.

The amount of weight loss associated with the use of mazindol, as with other anorectic drugs, varies from trial to trial, and the increased weight loss appears to be related in part to variables other than the drugs prescribed, such as the interaction between physician-investigator and the patient, the population treated, and the diet prescribed.

The importance of non-drug factors in such weight loss has not been elucidated.

The natural history of obesity is measured in years, whereas, most studies cited are restricted to a few weeks' duration; thus, the total impact of drug-induced weight loss over that of diet alone must be considered clinically limited.

INDICATIONS AND USAGE:

Mazindol is indicated in the management of exogenous obesity as a short-term (a few weeks) adjunct in a regimen of weight reduction based on caloric restriction. The limited usefulness of agents of this class (see CLINICAL PHARMACOLOGY) should be measured against possible risk factors inherent in their use, such as those described below.

CONTRAINDICATIONS:

Glaucoma; hypersensitivity or idiosyncrasy to mazindol.

Agitated states.

Patients with a history of drug abuse.

During of within 14 days following the administration of monoamine oxidase inhibitors, (hypertensive crises may result).

WARNINGS:

Tolerance to the effect of many anorectic drugs may develop within a few weeks; if this occurs, the recommended dose should not be exceeded in an attempt to increase the effect; rather, the drug should be discontinued.

Mazindol is not recommended for severely hypertensive patients or for patients with sympathomimetic cardiovascular disease including arrhythmias.

PRECAUTIONS:

GENERAL

Mazindol may impair the ability of the patient to engage in potentially hazardous activities such as operating machinery or driving a motor vehicle; the patient should therefore be cautioned accordingly.

PREGNANCY

Mazindol was studied in reproduction experiments in rats and rabbits and an increase in neonatal mortality and a possible increased incidence of rib anomalies in rats were observed at relatively high doses.

Although these studies have not indicated important adverse effects, use of mazindol by women who are or many become pregnant requires that the potential benefit be weighed against the possible hazard to mother and infant.

NURSING MOTHERS

The extent to which mazindol may be transferred in breast milk is not known. Therefore, mothers who are nursing should not receive this drug.

PEDIATRIC USE

Safety and effectiveness in children below the age of 12 years have not yet been established.

DRUG INTERACTIONS:

Mazindol may decrease the hypotensive effect of guanethidine or similar substance; patients should be monitored accordingly.

DRUG INTERACTIONS: *(cont'd)*

Mazindol may markedly potentiate the pressor effect of exogenous catecholamines. If it should be necessary to give a pressor amine agent (*e.g.*, levarterenol or isoproterenol) to a patient in shock (*e.g.*, from a myocardial infarction) who has recently been taking mazindol, extreme care should be taken in monitoring blood pressure at frequent intervals and initiating pressor therapy with a low initial dose and careful titration.

It should be recognized that reduction in carbohydrate intake may require reduced insulin dosage. However, in diabetic patients treated with insulin and given mazindol for 12 weeks, no change in insulin requirement was noted.

Mazindol may potentiate blood pressure increases in those patients taking sympathomimetic medications.

ADVERSE REACTIONS:

The most common adverse effects of mazindol are dry mouth, tachycardia, constipation, nervousness and insomnia.

Cardiovascular: Palpitation, tachycardia, edema.

Central Nervous System: Overstimulation, restlessness, dizziness, insomnia, dysphoria, tremor, headache, depression, drowsiness, weakness.

Gastrointestinal: Dryness of the mouth, unpleasant taste, diarrhea, constipation, nausea, vomiting, abdominal discomfort.

Skin: Rash, excessive sweating, clamminess.

Endocrine: Impotence, changes in libido have rarely been observed with mazindol.

Eye: Treatment of dogs with high doses of mazindol for long periods resulted in some corneal opacities, reversible on cessation of medication. No such effect has been observed in humans.

Automatic: Blurred vision, fainting sensation, hot/cold flashes, hyperdipsia, paresthesia.

Genitourinary: Dysuria, pollakiuria.

DRUG ABUSE AND DEPENDENCE:

Controlled Substance: Mazindol is controlled by the Drug Enforcement Administration and is classified under schedule IV.

Abuse or Dependence: In preliminary chronic safety studies in humans, dosages of 2 mg mazindol t.i.d. were administered for 24 consecutive weeks. Two to three days following abrupt withdrawal of medication the subjects were interviewed and no subject requested of required reinstitution of active medication, and no evidence suggestive of dependence was observed.

In widespread clinical uses of mazindol in the United States since 1973, Sandoz Pharmaceuticals has received no reports of development of physical or psychological dependence, drug tolerance, habituation, chronic abuse, or symptoms of withdrawl or abstinence.

OVERDOSAGE:

The minimum lethal dose for humans is not known. The oral LD_{50}, expressed in mg/kg, is 106 for the mouse, 180-320 for the rat, 98 for the rabbit, and 9-20 for the dog. Fewer than 2 dozen cases of mazindol overdosage in humans have been reported, and all but 1 of these recovered completely. A 25 year-old female died after having ingesting a massive dose of 200 mg of mazindol and an undetermined amount of ethanol.

The maximum overdosage of mazindol on record from which the patient recovered is 80 mg. A 20 year old female ingested 40 mazindol tablets (2 mg each) and 75-125 mg phenmetrazine in a suicide attempt. The patient was alert during hospitalization and the only clinical findings was frequent premature ventricular contractions. The patient was treated with Lidocaine and recovered completely.

Approximately half of the overdosage cases involved accidental ingestion in children 1-4 years of age. The reported doses ingested ranged from 4-40 mg. All recovered.

In cases in which overdosages have been reported, the symptoms listed below were cited: irritability, agitation, hyperactivity, tachycardia, arrhythmia (premature ventricular contractions occurred in the patient also taking phenmetrazine), tachypnea.

The following symptomatic treatment may include:

Emesis: If the patient is conscious, vomiting should be induced with ipecac syrup (15-30) cc.

Gastric Lavage: Patients should have pharyngeal and laryngeal reflexes. In unconscious patients gastric lavage should not be attempted unless cuffed endotracheal intubation has been performed to prevent aspiration and pulmonary complications.

Sedation: Chlorproethazine (0.5-1 mg/kg, IM) may be given every 30 minutes as needed to control symptoms of central nervous (CNS) overstimulation. A short acting barbiturate is generally considered the second best choice. Lidocaine may be administered to counteract cardiac arrhythmias.

Forced Acid Diuresis: Sufficient fluids should be given to maintain a urine output of 5-7 L/m^2/day or 2-4 times normal excretion. A 15% solution of mannitol (2.5 mg/kg) given IV every 4-6 hours or whenever the urine specific gravity falls below 1.025 is usually sufficient to produce an acid urine in young people. If necessary, methenamine mandelate or ammonium chloride can be used to acidify the urine. During prolonged forced diuresis, serum electrolytes must be evaluated frequently to avoid hyponatremia or hypokalemia.

Data about treating acute mazindol overdosage with hemodialysis or peritoneal dialysis are not available. However, mazindol is soluble only in acid so dialysis with basic or neutral solvents would not remove the drug.

DOSAGE AND ADMINISTRATION:

To determine the lowest effective dose, therapy with mazindol may be initiated at 1 mg, once a day, and adjusted to the need and response of the patient. Dosage may be increased to a maximum of 3 mg/day given in divided doses with meals.

HOW SUPPLIED - EQUIVALENTS NOT AVAILABLE:

Tablet, Uncoated - Oral - 1 mg

30's	$30.90	MAZANOR, Wyeth Labs	00008-0071-03
100's	**$124.98**	**SANOREX, Novartis**	**00078-0071-05**

Tablet, Uncoated - Oral - 2 mg

100's	**$198.30**	**SANOREX, Novartis**	**00078-0066-05**

MEASLES VIRUS VACCINE LIVE *(001703)*

CATEGORIES: Biologicals; Immune Globulin; Immunologic; Measles; Serums, Toxoids and Vaccines; Vaccines; Pregnancy Category C; FDA Pre 1938 Drugs

BRAND NAMES: **Attenuvax**; *Diplovax*; *Ervevax* (Mexico); *Lirugen*; *Lirugen Measles*; *M-VAC*; *Mevilin-L*; *Morbilvax*; *Rimevax*; *Rouvax* (France)
(International brand names outside U.S. in italics)

FORMULARIES: WHO

DESCRIPTION:

Attenuvax (Measles Virus Vaccine Live) is a live virus vaccine for immunization against measles (rubeola).

Attenuvax is a sterile lyophilized preparation of a more attenuated line of measles virus derived from Enders' attenuated Edmonston strain. The further modification of the virus in Attenuvax was achieved in the Merck Institute for Therapeutic Research by multiple passage of Edmonston strain virus in cell cultures of chick embryo at low temperature.

The reconstituted vaccine is for subcutaneous administration. When reconstituted as directed, the dose for injection is 0.5 ml and contains not less than the equivalent of 1,000 $TCID_{50}$ (tissue culture infectious doses) of the U.S. Reference Measles Virus. Each dose also contains approximately 25 mcg of neomycin. The product contains no preservative. Sorbitol and hydrolized gelatin are added as stabilizers.

CLINICAL PHARMACOLOGY:

Measles virus vaccine produces a modified measles infection in susceptible persons. Fever and rash may appear. Extensive clinical trials have demonstrated that measles virus vaccine is highly immunogenic and generally well tolerated.[1-5] A single injection of the vaccine has been shown to induce measles hemagglutination-inhibiting (HI) antibodies in 97 percent or more of susceptible persons. Vaccine-induced antibody levels have been shown to persist for at least 13 years without substantial decline.[6] Continued surveillance will be necessary to determine further duration of antibody persistence.

INDICATIONS AND USAGE:

Measles virus vaccine is indicated for immunization against measles (rubeola) in persons 15 months of age or older. A second dose of measles virus vaccine is recommended (see Revaccination).[7,8,9] Infants who are less than 15 months of age may fail to respond to the vaccine due to presence in the circulation of residual measles antibody of maternal origin; the younger the infant, the lower the likelihood of seroconversion. In geographically isolated or other relatively inaccessible populations for whom immunization programs are logistically difficult, and in population groups in which natural measles infection may occur in a significant proportion of infants before 15 months of age, it may be desirable to give the vaccine to infants at an earlier age. Infants vaccinated under these conditions at less than 12 months of age should be revaccinated after reaching 15 months of age. There is some evidence to suggest that infants immunized at less than one year of age may not develop sustained antibody levels when later reimmunized. The advantage of early protection must be weighed against the chance for failure to respond adequately on reimmunization.[10,11]

According to ACIP recommendations, most persons born in 1956 or earlier are likely to have been infected naturally and generally need not be considered susceptible. All children, adolescents, and adults born after 1956 are considered susceptible and should be vaccinated, if there are no contraindications. This includes persons who may be immune to measles but who lack adequate documentation of immunity as evidenced by: (1) physician-diagnosed measles, (2) laboratory evidence of measles immunity, or (3) adequate immunization with live measles vaccine on or after the first birthday.[12]

Measles virus vaccine given immediately after exposure to natural measles may provide some protection. If, however, the vaccine is given a few days before exposure, substantial protection may be provided.

Individuals planning travel outside the United States, if not immune, can acquire measles, mumps or rubella and import these diseases to the United States. Therefore, prior to International travel, individuals known to be susceptible to one or more of these diseases can receive either a single antigen vaccine (measles, mumps or rubella), or a combined antigen vaccine as appropriate. However, M-M-R* II (Measles, Mumps, and Rubella Virus Vaccine Live) is preferred for persons likely to be susceptible to mumps and rubella; and if single-antigen measles vaccine is not readily available, travelers should receive M-M-R II (Measles, Mumps, and Rubella Virus Vaccine Live) regardless of their immune status to mumps or rubella.[13,14,15]

Revaccination: Children first vaccinated when younger than 12 months of age should be revaccinated at 15 months of age, particularly if vaccine was administered with immune serum globulin or measles immune globulin, a standardized globulin preparation.

The American Academy of Pediatrics (AAP), the Immunization Practices Advisory Committee (ACIP), and some state and local health agencies have recommended guidelines for routine measles revaccination and to help control measles outbreaks.[16,17]*

Vaccines available for revaccination include monovalent measles vaccine and polyvalent vaccines containing measles (*e.g.,* M-M-R II (Measles, Mumps, and Rubella Virus Vaccine Live), M-R-VAX II (Measles and Rubella Virus Vaccine Live)). If the prevention of sporadic measles outbreaks is the sole objective, revaccination with a monovalent measles vaccine should be considered. If concern also exists about immune status regarding mumps or rubella, revaccination with appropriate monovalent or polyvalent vaccines should be considered after consulting the appropriate product circulars. Unnecessary doses of a vaccine are best avoided by ensuring that written documentation of vaccination is preserved and a copy given to each vaccinee's parent or guardian.

Despite the risk of reactions (see ADVERSE REACTIONS), persons born since 1956 who have previously been given inactivated vaccine alone or followed by live vaccine within 3 months should be revaccinated with live vaccine to reduce the risk of the severe atypical form of natural measles that may occur.[10,12]

Use with other Vaccines: Routine administration of DTP (diphtheria, tetanus, pertussis) and/or OPV (oral poliovirus vaccine) concomitantly with measles, mumps and rubella vaccines is not recommended because there are insufficient data relating to the simultaneous administration of these antigens. However, the American Academy of Pediatrics has noted that in some circumstances, particularly when the patient may not return, some practitioners prefer to administer all these antigens on a single day. If done, separate sites and syringes should be used for DTP and measles virus vaccine.[18]

Measles virus vaccine should not be given less than one month before or after administration of other virus vaccines.

CONTRAINDICATIONS:

Do not give measles virus vaccine to pregnant females; the possible effects of the vaccine on fetal development are unknown at this time. If vaccination of postpubertal females is undertaken, pregnancy should be avoided for three months following vaccination (see PRECAUTIONS, Pregnancy).

Anaphylactic or anaphylactoid reactions to neomycin (each dose of reconstituted vaccine contains approximately 25 mcg of neomycin).

History of anaphylactic or anaphylactoid reactions to eggs (see Hypersensitivity To Eggs).

Any febrile respiratory illness or other active febrile infection.

Active untreated tuberculosis.

Patients receiving immunosuppressive therapy. This contraindication does not apply to patients who are receiving corticosteroids as replacement therapy, (*e.g.,* for Addison's disease).

Individuals with blood dyscrasias, leukemia, lymphomas of any type, or other malignant neoplasms affecting the bone marrow or lymphatic systems.

CONTRAINDICATIONS: *(cont'd)*

Primary and acquired immunodeficiency states, including patients who are immunosuppressed in association with AIDS or other clinical manifestations of infection with human immunodeficiency viruses;[19,20] cellular immune deficiencies; and hypogammaglobulinemic and dysgammaglobulinemic states.

Individuals with a family history of congenital or hereditary immunodeficiency, until the immune competence of the potential vaccine recipient is demonstrated.[21]

*NOTE: A primary difference among these recommendations is the timing of revaccination: the ACIP recommends routine revaccination at entry into kindergarten or first grade, whereas the AAP recommends routine revaccination at entrance to middle school or junior high school. In addition, some public health jurisdictions mandate the age for revaccination. The complete text of applicable guidelines should be consulted.[16,17]

HYPERSENSITIVITY TO EGGS

Live measles vaccine is produced in chick embryo cell culture. Persons with a history of anaphylactic, anaphylactoid or other immediate reactions (*e.g.,* hives, swelling of the mouth and throat, difficulty breathing, hypotension and shock) subsequent to egg ingestion should not be vaccinated. Evidence indicates that persons are not at increased risk if they have egg allergies that are not anaphylactic or anaphylactoid in nature. Such persons should be vaccinated in the usual manner. There is no evidence to indicate that persons with allergies to chickens or feathers are at increased risk of reaction to the vaccine.[12]

PRECAUTIONS:

GENERAL

Adequate treatment provisions including epinephrine, should be available for immediate use should an anaphylactic or anaphylactoid reaction occur.

Due caution should be employed in administration of measles vaccine to persons with a history of cerebral injury, individual or family histories of convulsions, or of any other condition in which stress due to fever should be avoided. The physician should be alert to the temperature elevation which may occur following vaccination. (See ADVERSE REACTIONS.)

Children and young adults who are known to be infected with human immunodeficiency viruses but without overt clinical manifestations of immunosuppression may be vaccinated; however, the vaccinees should be monitored closely for vaccine-preventable diseases because immunization may be less effective than for uninfected persons.[19,20]

Vaccination should be deferred for at least 3 months following blood or plasma transfusions, or administration of human immune serum globulin.

There are no reports of transmission of live attenuated measles virus from vaccinees to susceptible contacts.

It has been reported that attenuated measles virus vaccine live, may result in a temporary depression of tuberculin skin sensitivity.[10] Therefore, if a tuberculin test is to be done, it should be administered either before or simultaneously with measles virus vaccine.

Children under treatment for tuberculosis have not experienced exacerbation of the disease when immunized with live measles virus vaccine;[22] no studies have been reported to date of the effect of measles virus vaccines on untreated tuberculous children.

As for any vaccine, vaccination with measles virus vaccine may not result in seroconversion in 100% of susceptible persons given the vaccine.

PREGNANCY CATEGORY C

Animal reproduction studies have not been conducted with measles virus vaccine. It is also not known whether measles virus vaccine can cause fetal harm when administered to a pregnant woman or can affect reproduction capacity. Therefore, the vaccine should not be administered to pregnant females; furthermore, pregnancy should be avoided for three months following vaccination (see CONTRAINDICATIONS).

Reports have indicated that contracting of natural measles during pregnancy enhances fetal risk. Increased rates of spontaneous abortion, stillbirth, congenital defects and prematurity have been observed subsequent to natural measles during pregnancy. There are no adequate studies of the attenuated (vaccine) strain of measles virus in pregnancy. However, it would be prudent to assume that the vaccine strain of virus is also, capable of inducing adverse fetal effects for up to three months following vaccination.

Vaccine administration to postpubertal females entails a potential for inadvertent immunization during pregnancy. Theoretical risks involved should be weighed against the risks that measles poses to the unimmunized adolescent or adult. Advisory committees reviewing this matter have recommended vaccination of postpubertal females who are presumed to be susceptible to measles and not known to be pregnant. If a measles exposure occurs during pregnancy, one should consider the possibility of providing temporary passive immunity through the administration of immune globulin (human).

NURSING MOTHERS

It is not known whether measles vaccine virus is secreted in human milk. Therefore, because many drugs are excreted in human milk, caution should be exercised when measles virus vaccine is administered to a nursing woman.

ADVERSE REACTIONS:

Burning and/or stinging of short duration at the injection site have been reported.

Anaphylaxis and anaphylactoid reactions have been reported.

OCCASIONAL

Moderate fever (101° - 102.9°F (38.3° - 39.4°C)) may occur during the month after vaccination. Generally, fever, rash, or both appear between the 5th and the 12th days. Cough and rhinitis have also been reported. Rash, when it occurs, is usually minimal, but rarely may be generalized. Erythema multiforme has also been reported rarely.

LESS COMMON

High fever (over 103°F (39.4°C)).

Mild lymphadenopathy has been reported.

RARE

Reactions at injection site. Allergic reactions such as wheal and flare at the injection site or urticaria have been reported.

Diarrhea has been reported after vaccination with measles-containing vaccines.

Children developing fever may, on rare occasions, exhibit febrile convulsions. Afebrile convulsions or seizures have occurred rarely following vaccination with live attenuated measles vaccine. Syncope, particularly at the time of mass vaccination, has been reported.

Thrombocytopenia and purpura have occurred rarely.

Vasculitis has been reported rarely.

Forms of optic neuritis, including retrobulbar neuritis, papillitis, and retinitis may infrequently follow viral infections, and have been reported to occur 1 to 3 weeks following inoculation with some live virus vaccines.

Experience from more than 80 million doses of all live measles vaccines given in the U.S. through 1975 indicates that significant central nervous system reactions such as encephalitis and encephalopathy occurring within 30 days after vaccination, have been temporally asso-

ADVERSE REACTIONS: *(cont'd)*

ciated with measles vaccine very rarely.[23] In no case has it been shown that reactions were actually caused by vaccine.[24] The Center for Disease Control has pointed out that "a certain number of cases of encephalitis may be expected to occur in a large childhood population in a defined period of time even when no vaccines are administered".[25] However the data suggest the possibility that some of these cases may have been caused by measles vaccines. The risk of such serious neurological disorders following live measles virus vaccine administration remains far less than that for encephalitis and encephalopathy with natural measles (one per two thousand reported cases).[26]

There have been rare reports of ocular palsies, Guillain-Barre syndrome, or ataxia occurring after immunization with vaccines containing live attenuated measles virus. The ocular palsies have occurred approximately 3-24 days following vaccination. No definite causal relationship has been established between these events and vaccination.

There have been reports of subacute sclerosing panencephalitis (SSPE) in children who did not have a history of natural measles but did receive measles vaccine. Some of these cases may have resulted from unrecognized measles in the first year of life or possibly from the measles vaccination. Based on estimated nationwide measles vaccine distribution, the association of SSPE cases to measles vaccination is about one case per million vaccine doses distributed. This is far less than the association with natural measles, 6-22 cases of SSPE per million cases of measles. The results of a retrospective case-controlled study conducted by the Center for Disease Control suggest that the overall effect of measles vaccine has been to protect against SSPE by preventing measles with its inherent higher risk of SSPE.[27]

Local reactions characterized by marked swelling, redness and vesiculation at the injection site of attenuated live virus measles vaccines, and systemic reactions including atypical measles, have occurred in persons who have previously received killed measles vaccine. Rarely, more severe reactions that require hospitalization, including prolonged high fevers, panniculitis, and extensive local reactions, have been reported.[12,28]

DOSAGE AND ADMINISTRATION:

FOR SUBCUTANEOUS ADMINISTRATION

Do not inject intravenously

The dosage of vaccine is the same for all persons. Inject the total volume of the single dose vial (about 0.5 ml) or 0.5 ml of the multiple dose vial of reconstituted vaccine subcutaneously, preferably into the outer aspect of upper arm. *Do not give immune globulin (IG) concurrently with* measles virus vaccine.

During shipment, to insure that there is no loss of potency, the vaccine must be maintained at a temperature of 10°C (50°F) or less.

Before reconstitution, store measles virus vaccine at 2° - 8°C (36° - 46°F). *Protect from light.*

Caution: A sterile syringe free of preservatives, antiseptics, and detergents should be used for each injection and/or reconstitution of the vaccine because these substances may inactivate the live virus vaccine. A 25 gauge, 5/8" needle is recommended.

To reconstitute, use only the diluent supplied, since it is free of preservatives or other antiviral substances which might inactivate the vaccine.

Single Dose Vial: First withdraw the entire volume of diluent into the syringe to be used for reconstitution. Inject all the diluent in the syringe into the vial of lyophilized vaccine, and agitate to mix thoroughly. Withdraw the entire contents into a syringe and inject the total volume of restored vaccine subcutaneously.

It is important to use a separate sterile syringe and needle for each individual patient to prevent transmission of hepatitis B and other infectious agents from one person to another.

10 DOSE VIAL (AVAILABLE ONLY TO GOVERNMENT AGENCIES/INSTITUTIONS)

Withdraw the entire contents (7 ml) of the diluent vial into the sterile syringe to be used for reconstitution, and introduce into the 10 dose vial of lyophilized vaccine. Agitate to ensure thorough mixing. The outer labeling suggests "For Jet Injector or Syringe Use". Use with separate sterile syringes is permitted for containers of 10 doses or less. The vaccine and diluent do not contain preservatives; therefore, the user must recognize the potential contamination hazards and exercise special precautions to protect the sterility and potency of the product. The use of aseptic techniques and proper storage prior to and after restoration of the vaccine and subsequent withdrawal of the individual doses is essential. Use 0.5 ml of the reconstituted vaccine for subcutaneous injection.

It is important to use a separate sterile syringe and needle for each individual patient to prevent transmission of hepatitis B and other infectious agents from one person to another.

50 DOSE VIAL (AVAILABLE ONLY TO GOVERNMENT AGENCIES/INSTITUTIONS)

Withdraw the entire contents (30 ml) of diluent vial into the sterile syringe to be used for reconstitution and introduce into the 50 dose vial of lyophilized vaccine. Agitate to ensure thorough mixing. With full aseptic precautions, attach the vial to the sterilized multidose jet injector apparatus. Use 0.5 ml of the reconstituted vaccine for subcutaneous injection.

Each dose of measles virus vaccine contains not less than 1,000 $TCID_{50}$(tissue culture infectious doses) of measles virus vaccine expressed in terms of the assigned titer of the U.S. Reference Measles Virus.

Parenteral drug products should be inspected visually for particulate matter and discoloration prior to administration. Measles virus vaccine, when reconstituted, is clear yellow.

STORAGE

It is recommended that the vaccine be used as soon as possible after reconstitution. Protect vaccine from light at all times, since such exposure may inactivate the virus. Store reconstituted vaccine in the vaccine vial in a dark place at 2° - 8°C (36° - 46°F) and discard if not used within 8 hours.

REFERENCES:

1) Hilleman, M. R.; Buynak, E. B.; Weibel, R. E.; Stokes, J., Jr.; Whitman, J. E., Jr.; Leagus, M. B.: Development and evaluation of the Moraten measles virus vaccine, J. Amer. Med. Ass. *206:* 587-590, Oct. 14, 1968. 2) Swartz, T.; Klingberg, W.; Nishmi, M.; Goldblum, N.; Gerichter, C.; Yofe, Y.; Cockburn, W. C.: A comparative study of four live measles vaccines in Israel, Bull. WHO *39:* 285-292, 1968. 3) Krugman, S.; Constantinides, P.; Medovy, H.; Giles, J. P.: Comparison of two further attenuated live measles-virus vaccines, Amer. J. Dis. Child.*117:* 137-138, Feb. 1969. 4) Studies conducted under the direction of Dr. Conrado Ristori, National Health Service, Santiago, Chile (Unpublished Data). 5) Studies conducted under the direction of Dr. Victor Villarejos, Louisiana State University International Center of Medical Research and Training, San Jose, Costa Rica (Unpublished Data). 6) Unpublished data: Files of Merck Sharp & Dohme Research Laboratories. 7) Bottiger, M.; Christenson, B.; Romanus, V.; Taranger, J.; Strandell, A.: Swedish experience of two dose vaccination programme aiming at eliminating measles, mumps, and rubella, Brit. Med. J. *295* (14): 1264-1267, November 1987. 8) Markowitz, L. E.; Preblud, S. R.; Orenstein, W. A.; et al: Patterns of transmission in measles outbreaks in the United States, 1985-1986, N. Engl. J. Med. *320* (2): 75-81, January 12, 1989. 9) Peltola, H.; Heinonen, O. P.; Valle, M.; et al: Five-year experience in elimination of indigenous measles, mumps, and rubella in Finland, Abstracts of the 29th ICAAC, Houston, Texas, Abstract #179, 130, September 1989. 10) American Academy of Pediatrics: Report of the Committee on Infectious Disease, Evanston, III., 1982, p. 136, 137. 11) Wilkins, J.; Wehrle, P. F.: Additional evidence against measles vaccine administration to infants less than 12 months of age: Altered immune response following active/passive immunization, J. Pediatric *94* (6): 865-869, June 1979. 12) Recommendation of the Immunization Practices Advisory Committee (ACIP), Measles Prevention, Morbidity and Mortality Weekly Report, *31* (17): 217-224, 229-231, May 7, 1982. 13) Recommendations of the Immunization Practices Advisory Committee (ACIP), Measles Prevention, MMWR *36* (26): 409-425, July 10, 1987. 14) Jong, E. C., The Travel and Tropical Medicine Manual, W. B. Saunders Company, p. 12-16, 1987. 15) Committee on Immunization Council of Medical Societies, American College of Physicians, Phila. PA, Guide for Adult Immunization, First Edition, 1985. 16) American Academy of Pediatrics, Committee on Infectious Diseases, Measles: Reassessment of the Current Immunization Policy, Pediatrics *84* (6): 1110-1113, Dec.1989. 17) Measles Prevention: Recommendations of the Immunization Practices Advisory Committee (ACIP), Morbidity and Mortality Weekly Report *38* (S-9): 5-22, December 29, 1989. 18) American Academy of Pediatrics:

REFERENCES: *(cont'd)*

Report of the Committee on Infectious Disease, Evanston,III., p. 17, 1982. 19) Center for Disease Control: Immunization of Children Infected with Human T-Lymphotropic Virus Type III/Lymphadenopathy-Associated Virus, Annals of Internal Medicine, *106:* 75-78, 1987. 20) Krasinski, K.; Borkowsky, W.; Krugman, S.: Antibody following measles immunization in children infected with human T-cell lymphotropic virus-type III/lymphadenopathy associated virus (HTLV-III/LAV) (Abstract). In: Program and abstracts of the International Conference on Acquired Immunodeficiency Syndrome, Paris, France, June 23-25, 1986. 21) Recommendation of the Immunization Practices Advisory Committee (ACIP), General Recommendation on Immunization, Morbidity and Mortality Weekly Report *32* (1): 13, January 14, 1983. 22) Starr, S.; Berkovich, S.: The effect of measles, gamma globulin modified measles, and attenuated measles vaccine on the course of treated tuberculosis in children, Pediatrics *35:* 97-102, Jan. 1965. 23) CDC. Important Information about Measles, Mumps, and Rubella, and Measles, Mumps, and Rubella Vaccines. 1980. 1983. 24) Recommendation of the Public Health Service Advisory Committee on Immunization Practices, Morbidity and Mortality Weekly Report, *21* (25): 11-13, June 24, 1972. 25) CDC, Measles Surveillance, Report No. 8, p. 23, December 1971. 26) CDC, Encephalitis Surveillance, p. 16, May 1981. 27) CDC, Measles Surveillance Report No. 11, p. 14, September 1982. 28) Buck, B. E.; Yang, L. C.; Caleb, M. H.; Greene, J. M.; South, M. A.: Measles virus panniculitis subsequent to vaccine administration, J.Pediatrics *101* (3): 366-373, September, 1982.

HOW SUPPLIED - EQUIVALENTS NOT AVAILABLE:

Injection, Lyphl-Soln - Subcutaneous - 1 unit/0.5ml

0.5 ml	**$10.95**	**ATTENUVAX, Merck**	**00006-4709-00**
0.5 ml x 10	**$86.79**	**ATTENUVAX, Merck**	**00006-4589-00**

MEASLES AND RUBELLA VIRUS VACCINE LIVE *(001702)*

CATEGORIES: Biologicals; Immunologic; Measles; Rubella; Serums, Toxoids and Vaccines; Vaccines; Pregnancy Category C; FDA Pre 1938 Drugs

BRAND NAMES: **M-R-Vax II**; *Rudi-Rouvax* (France)
(International brand names outside U.S. in italics)

DESCRIPTION:

M-R-VAX II (Measles and Rubella Virus Vaccine Live) is a live virus vaccine for immunization against measles (rubeola) and rubella (German measles).

M-R-VAX II is a sterile lyophilized preparation of (1) Attenuvax (Measles Virus Vaccine Live), a more attenuated line of measles virus, derived from Enders' attenuated Edmonston strain and grown in cell cultures of chick embryo; and (2) Meruvax II (Rubella Virus Vaccine Live), the Wistar RA 27/3 strain of live attenuated rubella virus grown in human diploid cell (WI-38) culture.[1,2] The vaccine viruses are the same as those used in the manufacture of Attenuvax (Measles Virus Vaccine Live) and Meruvax II (Rubella Virus Vaccine Live). The two viruses are mixed before being lyophilized. The product contains no preservative.

The reconstituted vaccine is for subcutaneous administration. When reconstituted as directed, the dose for injection is 0.5 ml and contains not less than the equivalent of 1,000 $TCID_{50}$ (tissue culture infectious doses) of the U.S. Reference Measles Virus; 1,000 $TCID_{50}$ of the U.S. Reference Rubella Virus. Each dose contains approximately 25 mcg of neomycin. The product contains no preservative. Sorbitol and hydrolyzed gelatin are added as stabilizers.

CLINICAL PHARMACOLOGY:

Clinical studies of 237 double seronegative children, 10 months to 10 years of age, demonstrated that M-R-VAX II is highly immunogenic and generally well tolerated. In these studies, a single injection of the vaccine induced measles hemagglutination-inhibition (HI) antibodies in 95 percent and rubella HI antibodies in 99 percent of susceptible persons.

The RA 27/3 rubella strain in M-R-VAX II elicits higher immediate postvaccination HI, complement-fixing and neutralizing antibody levels than other strains of rubella vaccine[3-9] and has been shown to induce a broader profile of circulating antibodies including anti-theta and anti-iota precipitating antibodies.[10,11] The RA 27/3 rubella strain immunologically simulates natural infection more closely than other rubella vaccine viruses.[11-13] The increased levels and broader profile of antibodies produced by RA 27/3 strain rubella virus vaccine appear to correlate with greater resistance to subclinical reinfection with the wild virus,[11,13-15] and provide greater confidence for lasting immunity.

Vaccine induced antibody levels following administration of M-R-VAX II have been shown to persist up to 11 years without substantial decline.[16,41] Continued surveillance will be necessary to determine further duration of antibody persistence.

INDICATIONS AND USAGE:

M-R-VAX II is indicated for simultaneous immunization against measles and rubella in persons 15 months of age or older. A second dose of M-R-VAX II or monovalent measles vaccine is recommended (see Revaccination.)[17,18,19]

Infants who are less than 15 months of age may fail to respond to the measles component of the vaccine due to presence in the circulation of residual measles antibody of maternal origin; the younger the infant, the lower the likelihood of seroconversion. In geographically isolated or other relatively inaccessible populations for whom immunization programs are logistically difficult, and in population groups in which natural measles infection may occur in a significant proportion of infants before 15 months of age, it may be desirable to give the vaccine to infants at an earlier age. Infants vaccinated under these conditions at less than 12 months of age should be revaccinated after reaching 15 months of age. There is some evidence to suggest that infants immunized at less than one year of age may not develop sustained antibody levels when later reimmunized. The advantage of early protection must be weighed against the chance for failure to respond adequately on reimmunization.[20]

Previously unimmunized children of susceptible pregnant women should receive live attenuated rubella vaccine, because an immunized child will be less likely to acquire natural rubella and introduce the virus into the household.

Individuals planning travel outside the United States, if not immune, can acquire measles, mumps or rubella and import these diseases to the United States. Therefore, prior to International travel, individuals known to be susceptible to one or more of these diseases can receive either a single antigen vaccine (measles, mumps or rubella), or a combined antigen vaccine as appropriate. However, M-M-R† II (Measles, Mumps, and Rubella Virus Vaccine Live) is preferred for persons likely to be susceptible to mumps and rubella; and if a single-antigen measles vaccine is not readily available, travelers should receive M-M-R II (Measles, Mumps, and Rubella Virus Vaccine Live) regardless of their immune status to mumps or rubella.[21,22,23]

Non-Pregnant Adolescent and Adult Females: Immunization of susceptible non-pregnant adolescent and adult females of childbearing age with live attenuated rubella virus vaccine is indicated if certain precautions are observed (see PRECAUTIONS). Vaccinating susceptible postpubertal females confers individual protection against subsequently acquiring rubella infection during pregnancy, which in turn prevents infection of the fetus and consequent congenital rubella injury.[24]

Women of childbearing age should be advised not to become pregnant for three months after vaccination and should be informed of the reason for this precaution.*

It is recommended that rubella susceptibility be determined by serologic testing prior to immunization.** If immune, as evidenced by a specific rubella antibody titer of 1:8 or greater (hemagglutination-inhibition test), vaccination is unnecessary. Congenital malformations do

INDICATIONS AND USAGE: *(cont'd)*

occur in up to seven percent of all live births.[25] Their chance appearance after vaccination could lead to misinterpretation of the cause, particularly if the prior rubella-immune status of vaccinees is unknown.

Postpubertal females should be informed of the frequent occurrence of generally self-limited arthralgia and/or arthritis beginning 2 to 4 weeks after vaccination (see ADVERSE REACTIONS).

Postpartum Women: It has been found convenient in many instances to vaccinate rubella-susceptible women in the immediate postpartum period. See PRECAUTIONS, Nursing Mothers.

Revaccination: Children first vaccinated when younger than 12 months of age should be revaccinated at 15 months of age.

The American Academy of Pediatrics (AAP), the Immunization Practices Advisory Committee (ACIP), and some state and local health agencies have recommended guidelines for routine measles revaccination and to help control measles outbreaks.[26,27]***

Vaccines available for revaccination include monovalent measles vaccine (Measles Virus Vaccine Live) and polyvalent vaccines containing measles (*e.g.,* M-M-R II (Measles, Mumps, and Rubella Virus Vaccine Live) M-R-VAX II). If the prevention of sporadic measles outbreaks is the sole objective, revaccination with a monovalent measles vaccine should be considered (see appropriate product circular). If concern also exists about immune status regarding mumps or rubella, revaccination with appropriate monovalent or polyvalent vaccines should be considered after consulting the appropriate product circulars. Unnecessary doses of a vaccine are best avoided by ensuring that written documentation of vaccination is preserved and a copy given to each vaccinee's parent or guardian.

***NOTE:** The Immunization Practices Advisory Committee (ACIP) has recommended "In view of the importance of protecting this age group against rubella, reasonable precautions in a rubella immunization program include asking females if they are pregnant, excluding those who say they are, and explaining the theoretical risks to the others."[24]

****NOTE:** The Immunization Practices Advisory Committee (ACIP) has stated "When practical, and when reliable laboratory services are available, potential vaccinees of childbearing age can have serologic tests to determine susceptibility to rubella.... However, routinely performing serologic tests for all females of childbearing age to determine susceptibility so that vaccine is given only to proven susceptibles is expensive and has been ineffective in some areas. Accordingly, the ACIP believes that rubella vaccination of a woman who is not known to be pregnant and has no history of vaccination is justifiable without serologic testing."[24]

*****NOTE:** A primary difference among these recommendations is the timing of revaccination: the ACIP recommends routine revaccination at entry into Kindergarten or first grade, whereas the AAP recommends routine revaccination at entrance to middle school or junior high school. In addition, some public health jurisdictions mandate the age for revaccination. The complete text of applicable guidelines should be consulted.[26,27]

Use With Other Vaccines: Routine administration of DTP (diphtheria, tetanus, pertussis) and/or OPV (oral poliovirus vaccine) concomitantly with measles, mumps, and rubella vaccines is not recommended because there are insufficient data relating to the simultaneous administration of these antigens. However, the American Academy of Pediatrics has noted that in some circumstances, particularly when the patient may not return, some practitioners prefer to administer all these antigens on a single day. If done, separate sites and syringes should be used for DTP and M-R-VAX II.[28]

M-R-VAX II should not be given less than one month before or after administration of other virus vaccines.

CONTRAINDICATIONS:

Do not give M-R-VAX II to pregnant females; the possible effects of the vaccine on fetal development are unknown at this time. If vaccination of postpubertal females is undertaken, pregnancy should be avoided for three months following vaccination. See PRECAUTIONS, Pregnancy.

Anaphylactic or anaphylactoid reactions to neomycin (each dose of reconstituted vaccine contains approximately 25 mcg of neomycin).

History of anaphylactic or anaphylactoid reactions to eggs (see HYPERSENSITIVITY TO EGGS).

Any febrile respiratory illness or other active febrile infection.

Active untreated tuberculosis.

Patients receiving immunosuppressive therapy. This contraindication does not apply to patients who are receiving corticosteroids as replacement therapy, e.g., for Addison's disease.

Individuals with blood dyscrasias, leukemia, lymphomas of any type, or other malignant neoplasms affecting the bone marrow or lymphatic systems.

Primary and acquired immunodeficiency states, including patients who are immunosuppressed in association with AIDS or other clinical manifestations of infection with human immunodeficiency viruses;[29,30] cellular immune deficiencies; and hypogammaglobulinemic and dysgammaglobulinemic states.

Individuals with a family history of congenital or hereditary immunodeficiency, until the immune competence of the potential vaccine recipient is demonstrated.[31]

HYPERSENSITIVITY TO EGGS

Live measles vaccine is produced in chick embryo cell culture. Persons with a history of anaphylactic, anaphylactoid, or other immediate reactions (*e.g.,* hives, swelling of the mouth and throat, difficulty breathing, hypotension, or shock) subsequent to egg ingestion should not be vaccinated. Evidence indicates that persons are not at increased risk if they have egg allergies that are not anaphylactic or anaphylactoid in nature. Such persons may be vaccinated in the usual manner. There is no evidence to indicate that persons with allergies to chickens or feathers are at increased risk of reaction to the vaccine.[20]

PRECAUTIONS:

GENERAL

Adequate treatment provisions including epinephrine, should be available for immediate use should an anaphylactic or anaphylactoid reaction occur.

Due caution should be employed in administration of M-R-VAX II to persons with a history of cerebral injury, individual or family histories of convulsions, or any other condition in which stress due to fever should be avoided. The physician should be alert to the temperature elevation which may occur following vaccination. (See ADVERSE REACTIONS.)

Children and young adults who are known to be infected with human immunodeficiency viruses but without overt clinical manifestations of immunosuppression may be vaccinated; however, the vaccinees should be monitored closely for vaccine-preventable diseases because immunization may be less effective than for uninfected persons.[29,30]

Vaccination should be deferred for at least 3 months following blood or plasma transfusions, or administration of human immune serum globulin.

PRECAUTIONS: *(cont'd)*

Excretion of small amounts of the live attenuated rubella virus from the nose or throat has occurred in the majority of susceptible individuals 7-28 days after vaccination. There is no confirmed evidence to indicate that such virus is transmitted to susceptible persons who are in contact with the vaccinated individuals. Consequently, transmission through close personal contact, while accepted as a theoretical possibility, is not regarded as a significant risk.[24] However, transmission of the rubella vaccine virus to infants via breast milk has been documented (see Nursing Mothers.)

There are no reports of transmission of live attenuated measles virus from vaccinees to susceptible contacts.

It has been reported that live attenuated measles and rubella virus vaccines given individually may result in a temporary depression of tuberculin skin sensitivity. Therefore, if a tuberculin test is to be done it should be administered either before or simultaneously with M-R-VAX II.

Children under treatment for tuberculosis have not experienced exacerbation of the disease when immunized with live measles virus vaccine;[32] no studies have been reported to date of the effect of measles virus vaccines on untreated tuberculous children.

As for any vaccine, vaccination with M-R-VAX II may not result in seroconversion in 100% of susceptible persons given the vaccine.

PREGNANCY CATEGORY C

Animal reproduction studies have not been conducted with M-R-VAX II. It is also not known whether M-R-VAX II can cause fetal harm when administered to a pregnant woman or can affect reproduction capacity. Therefore, the vaccine should not be administered to pregnant females; furthermore, pregnancy should be avoided for three months following vaccination (see CONTRAINDICATIONS).

In counseling women who are inadvertently vaccinated when pregnant or who become pregnant within 3 months of vaccination, the physician should be aware of the following: (1) In a 10 year survey involving over 700 pregnant women who received rubella vaccine within 3 months before or after conception, (of whom 189 received the Wistar RA 27/3 strain), none of the newborns had abnormalities compatible with congenital rubella syndrome;[33] (2) Reports have indicated that contracting of natural measles during pregnancy enhances fetal risk. Increased rates of spontaneous abortion, stillbirth, congenital defects and prematurity have been observed subsequent to natural measles during pregnancy. There are no adequate studies of the attenuated (vaccine) strain of measles virus in pregnancy. However, it would be prudent to assume that the vaccine strain of virus is also capable of inducing adverse fetal effects.

NURSING MOTHERS

It is not known whether measles vaccine virus is secreted in human milk. Recent studies have shown that lactating postpartum women immunized with live attenuated rubella vaccine may secrete the virus in breast milk and transmit it to breast-fed infants.[34] In the infants with serological evidence of rubella infection, none exhibited severe disease; however, one exhibited mild clinical illness typical of acquired rubella.[35,36] Caution should be exercised when M-R-VAX II is administered to a nursing woman.

ADVERSE REACTIONS:

Burning and/or stinging of short duration at the injection site have been reported.

The adverse clinical reactions associated with the use of M-R-VAX II are those expected to follow administration of the monovalent vaccines given separately. These may include malaise, sore throat, cough, rhinitis, headache, dizziness, fever, rash, nausea, vomiting or diarrhea; mild local reactions such as erythema, induration, tenderness and regional lymphadenopathy; thrombocytopenia and purpura; allergic reactions such as wheal and flare at the injection site or urticaria; polyneuritis, and arthralgia and/or arthritis (usually transient and rarely chronic).

Anaphylaxis and anaphylactoid reactions have been reported.

Vasculitis has been reported rarely.

Moderate fever (101°-102.9°F (38.3°-39.4°C)) occurs occasionally, and high fever (above 103°F (39.4°C)) occurs less commonly. On rare occasions, children developing fever may exhibit febrile convulsions. Afebrile convulsions or seizures have occurred rarely following vaccination with live attenuated measles vaccine. Syncope, particularly at the time of mass vaccination, has been reported. Rash occurs infrequently and is usually minimal, but rarely may be generalized. Erythema multiforme has also been reported rarely.

Forms of optic neuritis, including retrobulbar neuritis, papillitis, and retinitis may infrequently follow viral infections, and have been reported to occur 1 to 3 weeks following inoculation with some live virus vaccines.

Clinical experience with live attenuated measles and rubella virus vaccines given individually indicates that encephalitis and other nervous system reactions have occurred very rarely. These might occur also with M-R-VAX II.

Experience from more than 80 million doses of all live measles vaccines given in the U.S. through 1975 indicates that significant central nervous system reactions such as encephalitis and encephalopathy, occurring within 30 days after vaccination, have been temporally associated with measles vaccine very rarely.[37] In no case has it been shown that reactions were actually caused by vaccine. The Center for Disease Control has pointed out that "a certain number of cases of encephalitis may be expected to occur in a large childhood population in a defined period of time even when no vaccines are administered". However, the data suggest the possibility that some of these cases may have been caused by measles vaccines. The risk of such serious neurological disorders following live measles virus vaccine administration remains far less than that for encephalitis and encephalopathy with natural measles (one per two thousand reported cases).

There have been rare reports of ocular palsies, Guillain-Barre syndrome, or ataxia occurring after immunization with vaccines containing live attenuated measles virus. The ocular palsies have occurred approximately 3-24 days following vaccination. No definite causal relationship has been established between these events and vaccination. Isolated reports of polyneuropathy including Guillain-Barre syndrome have also been reported after immunization with rubella-containing vaccines.

There have been reports of subacute sclerosing panencephalitis (SSPE) in children who did not have a history of natural measles but did receive measles vaccine. Some of these cases may have resulted from unrecognized measles in the first year of life or possibly from the measles vaccination. Based on estimated nationwide measles vaccine distribution, the association of SSPE cases to measles vaccination is about one case per million vaccine doses distributed. This is far less than the association with natural measles, 6-22 cases of SSPE per million cases of measles. The results of a retrospective case-controlled study conducted by the Center for Disease Control suggest that the overall effect of measles vaccine has been to protect against SSPE by preventing measles with its inherent higher risk of SSPE.[38]

Local reactions characterized by marked swelling, redness and vesiculation at the injection site of attenuated live measles virus vaccines, and systemic reactions including atypical measles, have occurred in persons who received killed measles vaccine previously. M-R-VAX II was not given under this condition in clinical trials. Rarely, more severe reactions that

ADVERSE REACTIONS: *(cont'd)*

require hospitalization, including prolonged high fevers and extensive local reactions, have been reported.[39] Panniculitis has been reported rarely following administration of measles vaccine.[40]

Arthralgia and/or arthritis (usually transient and rarely chronic), and polyneuritis are features of natural rubella and vary in frequency and severity with age and sex, being greatest in adult females and least in prepubertal children. This type of involvement as well as myalgia and paresthesia have also been reported following administration of Meruvax II (Rubella Virus Vaccine Live).

Chronic arthritis has been associated with natural rubella infection and has been related to persistent virus and/or viral antigen isolated from body tissues. Only rarely have vaccine recipients developed chronic joint symptoms.

Following vaccination in children, reactions in joints are uncommon and generally of brief duration. In women, incidence rates for arthritis and arthralgia are generally higher than those seen in children (children: 0-3%; women: 12-20%)[41], and the reactions tend to be more marked and of longer duration. Symptoms may persist for a matter of months or on rare occasions for years. In adolescent girls, the reactions appear to be intermediate in incidence between those seen in children and in adult women. Even in older women (35-45 years), these reactions are generally well tolerated and rarely interfere with normal activities.

DOSAGE AND ADMINISTRATION:

FOR SUBCUTANEOUS ADMINISTRATION

Do not inject intravenously

The dosage of vaccine is the same for all persons. Inject the total volume of the single dose vial (about 0.5 ml) or 0.5 ml of the multiple dose vial of reconstituted vaccine subcutaneously, preferably into the outer aspect of upper arm. *Do not give immune globulin (IG) concurrently with* M-R-VAX II.

During shipment, to insure that there is no loss of potency, the vaccine must be maintained at a temperature of 10°C (50°F) or less.

Before reconstitution, store M-R-VAX II at 2° - 8°C (36° - 46°F). *Protect from light.*

Caution: A sterile syringe free of preservatives, antiseptics, and detergents should be used for each injection and/or reconstitution of the vaccine because these substances may inactivate the live virus vaccine. A 25 gauge, 5/8" needle is recommended.

To reconstitute, use only the diluent supplied, since it is free of preservatives or other antiviral substances which might inactivate the vaccine.

Single Dose Vial: First withdraw the entire volume of diluent into the syringe to be used for reconstitution. Inject all the diluent in the syringe into the vial of lyophilized vaccine, and agitate to mix thoroughly. Withdraw the entire contents into a syringe and inject the total volume of restored vaccine subcutaneously.

It is important to use a separate sterile syringe and needle for each individual patient to prevent transmission of hepatitis B and other infectious agents from one person to another.

10 Dose Vial (available Only To Government Agencies/Institutions): Withdraw the entire contents (7 ml) of the diluent vial into the sterile syringe to be used for reconstitution, and introduce into the 10 dose vial of lyophilized vaccine. Agitate to ensure thorough mixing. The outer labeling suggests "For Jet Injector or Syringe Use". Use with separate sterile syringes is permitted for containers of 10 doses or less. The vaccine and diluent do not contain preservatives; therefore, the user must recognize the potential contamination hazards and exercise special precautions to protect the sterility and potency of the product. The use of aseptic techniques and proper storage prior to and after restoration of the vaccine and subsequent withdrawal of the individual doses is essential. Use 0.5 ml of the reconstituted vaccine for subcutaneous injection.

It is important to use a separate sterile syringe and needle for each individual patient to prevent transmission of hepatitis B and other infectious agents from one person to another.

50 Dose Vial (Available Only To Government Agencies/Institutions): Withdraw the entire contents (30 ml) of diluent vial into the sterile syringe to be used for reconstitution and introduce into the 50 dose vial of lyophilized vaccine. Agitate to ensure thorough mixing. With full aseptic precautions, attach the vial to the sterilized multidose jet injector apparatus. Use 0.5 ml of the reconstituted vaccine for subcutaneous injection.

Each dose contains not less than the equivalent of 1,000 $TCID_{50}$ of the U.S. Reference Measles Virus and 1,000 $TCID_{50}$ of the U.S. Reference Rubella Virus.

Parenteral drug products should be inspected visually for particulate matter and discoloration prior to administration. M-R-VAX II, when reconstituted, is clear yellow.

STORAGE

It is recommended that the vaccine be used as soon as possible after reconstitution. Protect vaccine from light at all times, since such exposure may inactivate the virus. Store reconstituted vaccine in the vaccine vial in a dark place at 2° - 8°C (36° - 46°F) and discard if not used within 8 hours.

REFERENCES:

1. Plotkin, S. A.; Cornfeld, D.; Ingalls, T. H.: Studies of immunization with living rubella virus: Trials in children with a strain cultured from an aborted fetus, Am. J. Dis. Child. *110:* 381-389, 1965. **2.** Plotkin, S. A.; Farquhar, J.; Katz, M.; Ingalls; T. H.: A new attenuated rubella virus grown in human fibroblasts: Evidence for reduced nasopharyngeal excretion, Am. J. Epidemiol. *86:* 468-477, 1967. **3.** Fogel, A.; Moshkowitz, A.; Rannon, L.; Gerichter, Ch. B.: Comparative trials of RA 27/3 and Cendehill rubella vaccines in adult and adolescent females, Am. J. Epidemiol. *93:* 392-393, 1971. **4.** Andzhaparidze, O. G.; Desyatskova, R. G.; Chervonski, G. I.; Pryanichnikova, L. V.: Immunogenicity and reactogenicity of live attenuated rubella virus vaccines, Am. J. Epidemiol. *91:* 527-530, 1970. **5.** Freestone, D. S.; Reynolds, G. M.; McKinnon, J. A.; Prydie, J.: Vaccination of schoolgirls against rubella. Assessment of serological status and a comparative trial of Wistar RA 27/3 and Cendehill strain live attenuated rubella vaccines in 13-year-old schoolgirls in Dudley, Br. J. Prev. Soc. Med. *29:* 258-261, 1975. **6.** Grillner, L.; Hedstrom, C. E.; Bergstrom, H.; Forssman, L.; Rigner, A.; Lycke, E.: Vaccination against rubella of newly delivered women, Scand. J. Infect. Dis. *5:* 237-241, 1973. **7.** Grillner, L.: Neutralizing antibodies after rubella vaccination of newly delivered women: a comparison between three vaccines, Scand. J. Infect. Dis. *7:* 169-172, 1975. **8.** Wallace, R. B.; Isacson, P.: Comparative trial of HPV-77, DE-5 and RA 27/3 live-attenuated rubella vaccines, Am. J. Dis. Child. *124:* 536-538, 1972. **9.** Lalla, M.; Vesikari, T.; Virolainen, M.: Lymphoblast proliferation and humoral antibody response after rubella vaccination, Clin. Exp.Immunol. *15:* 193-202, 1973. **10.** LeBouvier, G. L.; Plotkin, S. A.: Precipitin responses to rubella vaccine RA 27/3, J. Infect. Dis. *123:* 220-223, 1971. **11.** Horstmann, D. M.: Rubella: The challenge of its control, J. Infect. Dis.*123:* 640-654, 1971. **12.** Ogra, P. L.; Kerr-Grant, D.; Umana, G.; Dzierba, J.; Weintraub, D.: Antibody response in serum and nasopharynx after naturally acquired and vaccine-induced infection with rubella virus, N. Engl. J. Med. *285:* 1333-1339, 1971. **13.** Plotkin, S. A.; Farquhar, J. D.; Ogra, P. L.: Immunologic properties of RA 27/3 rubella virus vaccine, J. Am. Med. Assoc.*225:* 585-590, 1973. **14.** Liebhaber, H.; Ingalls, T. H.; LeBouvier, G. L.; Horstmann, D. M.: Vaccination with RA 27/3 rubella vaccine. Persistence of immunity and resistance to challenge after two years, Am. J. Dis. Child. *123:* 133-136, 1972. **15.** Farquhar, J. D.: Follow-up on rubella vaccinations and experience with subclinical reinfection, J. Pediatr. *81:* 460-465, 1972. **16.** Weibel, R. E.; Carlson, A. J.; Villarejos, V. M.; Buynak, E. B.; McLean, A. A.; Hilleman, M. R.: Clinical and Laboratory Studies of Combined Live Measles, Mumps, and Rubella Vaccines Using the RA 27/3 Rubella Virus, Proc. Soc. Exp. Biol. Med. *165:* 323-326, 1980. **17.** Bottiger, M.; Christenson, B.; Romanus, V.; Taranger, J.; Strandell, A.: Swedish experience of two dose vaccination programme aiming at eliminating measles, mumps, and rubella, Brit. Med. J.*295* (14):1264-1267, November 1987. **18.** Markowitz, L. E.; Preblud, S. R.; Orenstein, W. A.; et al: Patterns of transmission in measles outbreaks in the United States, 1985-1986, N. Engl. J. Med.*320* (2): 75-81, January 12, 1989. **19.** Peltola, H.; Heinonen, O. P.; Valle, M.; et al: Five-year experience in elimination of indigenous measles, mumps, and rubella in Finland, Abstracts of the 29th ICAAC, Houston, Texas, Abstract #179, 130, September 1989. **20.** American Academy of Pediatrics: Report of the Committee on Infectious Disease, Evanston, III., AAP, p. 136-137, 1982. **21.** Recommendations of the Immunization Practices Advisory Committee (ACIP), Measles Prevention, MMWR *36* (26): 409-425, July 10, 1987. **22.** Jong, E. C., The Travel and Tropical Medicine Manual, W. B. Saunders Company, p. 12-16, 1987. **23.** Committee on Immunization Council of Medical Societies, American College of Physicians, Phila., PA, Guide for Adult Immunization, First Edition, 1985. **24.** Recommendation of the Immunization Practices Advisory Committee (ACIP), Morbidity and Mortality Weekly Report *33* (22): 301-310,315-318, June 8, 1984. **25.** McIntosh, R.; Merritt, K. K.; Richards, M.

REFERENCES: *(cont'd)*

R.; Samuels, M. H.; Bellows, M. T.: The incidence of congenital malformations: A study of 5,964 pregnancies, Pediatr. *14:* 505-521, 1954. **26.** American Academy of Pediatrics, Committee on Infectious Diseases, Measles: Reassessment of the Current Immunization Policy, Pediatrics *84* (6): 1110-1113, December 1989. **27.** Measles Prevention: Recommendations of the Immunization Practices Advisory Committee (ACIP), Morbidity and Mortality Weekly Report*38* (S-9): 5-22, December 29, 1989. **28.** American Academy of Pediatrics: Report of the Committee on Infectious Disease, Evanston, III., 1982, p. 17. **29.** Center for Disease Control: Immunization of Children Infected with Human T-Lymphotropic Virus Type III/Lymphadenopathy-Associated Virus, Annals of Internal Medicine,*106:* 75-78, 1987. **30.** Krasinski, K.; Borkowsky, W.; Krugman, S.: Antibody following measles immunization in children infected with human T-cell lymphotropic virus-type III/lymphadenopathy associated virus (HTLV-III/LAV) (Abstract). In: Program and abstracts of the International Conference on Acquired Immunodeficiency Syndrome, Paris, France, June 23-25, 1986. **31.** Recommendation of the Immunization Practices Advisory Committee (ACIP), General Recommendations on Immunization, Morbidity and Mortality Weekly Report*32* (1): 13, January 14, 1983. **32.** Starr, S.; Berkovich, S.: The effect of measles, gamma globulin modified measles, and attenuated measles vaccine on the course of treated tuberculosis in children, Pediatrics *35:* 97-102, January, 1965. **33.** Rubella vaccination during pregnancy — United States, 1971-1981. Morbidity and Mortality Weekly Report *31* (35): 477-481, September 10, 1982. **34.** Losonsky, G. A.; Fishaut, J. M.; Strussenber, J.; Ogra, P. L.: Effect of immunization against rubella on lactation products. II. Maternal-neonatal interactions, J. Infect. Dis.*145:* 661-666, 1982. **35.** Landes, R. D.; Bass, J. W.; Millunchick, E. W.; Oetgen, W. J.: Neonatal rubella following postpartum maternal immunization, J. Pediatr. *97:* 465-467, 1980. **36.** Lerman, S. J.: Neonatal rubella following postpartum maternal immunization, J. Pediatr. *98:* 668, 1981. (Letter) **37.** CDC. Important Information about Measles, Mumps, and Rubella, and Measles, Mumps, and Rubella Vaccines. 1980. 1983. **38.** CDC, Measles Surveillance, Report No. 11, p. 14, September, 1982. **39.** Recommendation of the Immunization Practices Advisory Committee (ACIP), Measles Prevention, Morbidity and Mortality Weekly Report *31* (17): 217-224, 229-231, May 7, 1982. **40.** Buck, B. E.; Yang, L. C.; Caleb, M. H.; Green, J. M.; South, M. A.: Measles virus panniculitis subsequent to vaccine administration, J.Pediatrics*101* (3): 366-373, 1982. **41.** Unpublished data from the files of Merck Sharp and Dohme Research Laboratories.

HOW SUPPLIED - EQUIVALENTS NOT AVAILABLE:

Injection, Lyphl-Soln - Subcutaneous - 1000 unit/1000

0.5 ml	$17.72	M-R-VAX II, Merck	00006-4751-00
0.5 ml x 10	$146.00	M-R-VAX II, Merck	00006-4677-00

MEASLES, MUMPS AND RUBELLA VIRUS VACCINE LIVE *(001704)*

CATEGORIES: Biologicals; Immunologic; Measles; Mumps; Rubella; Serums, Toxoids and Vaccines; Vaccines; Pregnancy Category C; FDA Pre 1938 Drugs

BRAND NAMES: *Imovax-ROR*; *MMR II*; *M.M.R. II*; *M.M.R. Vaccine*; **M-M-R II**; *M-M-R Vax* (Germany); *Morupar*; *Mumeru Vax*; *Pluserix* (Germany); *R.O.R. Vax* (France); *Trimovax*; *Triviraten Berna*
(International brand names outside U.S. in italics)

FORMULARIES: WHO

DESCRIPTION:

M-M-R II (Measles, Mumps, and Rubella Virus Vaccine Live) is a live virus vaccine for immunization against measles (rubeola), mumps and rubella (German measles).

M-M-R II is a sterile lyophilized preparation of (1) Attenuvax (Measles Virus Vaccine Live), a more attenuated line of measles virus, derived from Enders' attenuated Edmonston strain and grown in cell cultures of chick embryo; (2) Mumpsvax (Mumps Virus Vaccine Live), the Jeryl Lynn (B level) strain of mumps virus grown in cell cultures of chick embryo; and (3) Meruvax II (Rubella Virus Vaccine Live), the Wistar RA 27/3 strain of live attenuated rubella virus grown in human diploid cell (WI-38) culture.[1,2] The vaccine viruses are the same as those used in the manufacture of Attenuvax (Measles Virus Vaccine Live), Mumpsvax (Mumps Virus Vaccine Live) and Meruvax II (Rubella Virus Vaccine Live). The three viruses are mixed before being lyophilized. The product contains no preservative.

The reconstituted vaccine is for subcutaneous administration. When reconstituted as directed, the dose for injection is 0.5 ml and contains not less than the equivalent of 1,000 $TCID_{50}$ (tissue culture infectious doses) of the U.S. Reference Measles Virus; 20,000 $TCID_{50}$ of the U.S. Reference Mumps Virus; and 1,000 $TCID_{50}$ of the U.S. Reference Rubella Virus. Each dose contains approximately 25 mcg of neomycin. The product contains no preservative. Sorbitol and hydrolyzed gelatin are added as stabilizers.

CLINICAL PHARMACOLOGY:

Clinical studies of 279 triple seronegative children, 11 months to 7 years of age, demonstrated that M-M-R II is highly immunogenic and generally well tolerated. In these studies, a single injection of the vaccine induced measles hemagglutination-inhibition (HI) antibodies in 95 percent, mumps neutralizing antibodies in 96 percent, and rubella HI antibodies in 99 percent of susceptible persons.

The RA 27/3 rubella strain in M-M-R II elicits higher immediate postvaccination HI, complement-fixing and neutralizing antibody levels than other strains of rubella vaccine[3-9] and has been shown to induce a broader profile of circulating antibodies including anti-theta and anti-iota precipitating antibodies.[10,11] The RA 27/3 rubella strain immunologically simulates natural infection more closely than other rubella vaccine viruses.[11-13] The increased levels and broader profile of antibodies produced by RA 27/3 strain rubella virus vaccine appear to correlate with greater resistance to subclinical reinfection with the wild virus,[11,13-15] and provide greater confidence for lasting immunity.

Vaccine induced antibody levels following administration of M-M-R II have been shown to persist up to 11 years without substantial decline.[16,43] Continued surveillance will be necessary to determine further duration of antibody persistence.

INDICATIONS AND USAGE:

M-M-R II is indicated for simultaneous immunization against measles, mumps, and rubella in persons 15 months of age or older. A second dose of M-M-R II or monovalent measles vaccine is recommended (see Revaccination.)[17,18,19]

Infants who are less than 15 months of age may fail to respond to the measles component of the vaccine due to presence in the circulation of residual measles antibody of maternal origin, the younger the infant, the lower the likelihood of seroconversion. In geographically isolated or other relatively inaccessible populations for whom immunization programs are logistically difficult, and in population groups in which natural measles infection may occur in a significant proportion of infants before 15 months of age, it may be desirable to give the vaccine to infants at an earlier age. Infants vaccinated under these conditions at less than 12 months of age should be revaccinated after reaching 15 months of age. There is some evidence to suggest that infants immunized at less than one year of age may not develop sustained antibody levels when later reimmunized. The advantage of early protection must be weighed against the chance for failure to respond adequately on reimmunization.[20]

Previously unimmunized children of susceptible pregnant women should receive live attenuated rubella vaccine, because an immunized child will be less likely to acquire natural rubella and introduce the virus into the household.

Individuals planning travel outside the United States, if not immune, can acquire measles, mumps or rubella and import these diseases to the United States. Therefore, prior to International travel, individuals known to be susceptible to one or more of these diseases can receive either a single antigen vaccine (measles, mumps or rubella), or a combined antigen

INDICATIONS AND USAGE: *(cont'd)*

vaccine as appropriate. However, M-M-R II is preferred for persons likely to be susceptible to mumps and rubella; and if single-antigen measles vaccine is not readily available, travelers should receive M-M-R II regardless of their immune status to mumps or rubella.[21,22,23]

Non-Pregnant Adolescent and Adult Females: Immunization of susceptible non-pregnant adolescent and adult females of childbearing age with live attenuated rubella virus vaccine is indicated if certain precautions are observed (see below and PRECAUTIONS). Vaccinating susceptible postpubertal females confers individual protection against subsequently acquiring rubella infection during pregnancy, which in turn prevents infection of the fetus and consequent congenital rubella injury.[24]

Women of childbearing age should be advised not to become pregnant for three months after vaccination and should be informed of the reasons for this precaution.*

It is recommended that rubella susceptibility be determined by serologic testing prior to immunization.** If immune, as evidenced by a specific rubella antibody titer of 1:8 or greater (hemagglutination-inhibition test), vaccination is unnecessary. Congenital malformations do occur in up to seven percent of all live births.[25] Their chance appearance after vaccination could lead to misinterpretation of the cause, particularly if the prior rubella-immune status of vaccinees is unknown.

Postpubertal females should be informed of the frequent occurrence of generally self-limited arthralgia and/or arthritis beginning 2 to 4 weeks after vaccination (see ADVERSE REACTIONS.)

Postpartum Women: It has been found convenient in many instances to vaccinate rubella susceptible women in the immediate postpartum period. (See Nursing Mothers.)

Revaccination: Children first vaccinated when younger than 12 months of age should be revaccinated at 15 months of age.

The American Academy of Pediatrics (AAP), the Immunization Practices Advisory Committee (ACIP), and some state and local health agencies have recommended guidelines for routine measles revaccination and to help control measles outbreaks.[26,27]***

*NOTE: The Immunization Practices Advisory Committee (ACIP) has recommended "In view of the importance of protecting this age group against rubella, reasonable precautions in a rubella immunization program include asking females if they are pregnant, excluding those who say they are, and explaining the theoretical risk to the others."[24]

**NOTE: The Immunization Practices Advisory Committee (ACIP)) has stated "When practical, and when reliable laboratory services are available, potential vaccinees of childbearing age can have serologic tests to determine susceptibility to rubella.... However, routinely performing serologic tests for all females of childbearing age to determine susceptibility so that vaccine is given only to proven susceptibles is expensive and has been ineffective in some areas. Accordingly, the ACIP believes that rubella vaccination of a woman who is not known to be pregnant and has no history of vaccination is justifiable without serologic testing."[24]

***NOTE: A primary difference among these recommendations is the timing of revaccination: the ACIP recommends routine revaccination at entry into kindergarten or first grade, whereas the AAP recommends routine revaccination at entrance to middle school or junior high school. In addition, some public health jurisdictions mandate the age for revaccination. The complete text of applicable guidelines should be consulted.[26,27]

Vaccines available for revaccination include monovalent measles vaccine (Attenuvax (Measles Virus Vaccine Live)) and polyvalent vaccines containing measles (*e.g.*, M-M-R II, M-R-VAX II (Measles and Rubella Virus Vaccine Live)). If the prevention of sporadic measles outbreaks is the sole objective, revaccination with a monovalent measles vaccine should be considered (see appropriate product circular). If concern also exists about immune status regarding mumps or rubella, revaccination with appropriate monovalent or polyvalent vaccine should be considered after consulting the appropriate product circulars. Unnecessary doses of a vaccine are best avoided by ensuring that written documentation of vaccination is preserved and a copy given to each vaccinee's parent or guardian.

USE WITH OTHER VACCINES

Routine administration of DTP (diphtheria, tetanus, pertussis) and/or OPV (oral poliovirus vaccine) concomitantly with measles, mumps, and rubella vaccines is not recommended because there are limited data[28] relating to the simultaneous administration of these antigens. M-M-R II should be given one month before or after administration of other vaccines.

However, other schedules have been used. For example, the American Academy of Pediatrics has noted that when the patient may not return, some practitioners prefer to administer DTP, OPV, and M-M-R II on a single day. If done, separate sites and syringes should be used for DTP and M-M-R II.[29] The Immunization Practices Advisory Committee (ACIP) recommends routine simultaneous administration of M-M-R II, DTP and OPV or inactivated polio vaccine (IPV) to all children ≥ 15 months who are eligible to receive these vaccines on the basis that there are equivalent antibody responses and no clinically significant increases in the frequency of adverse events when DTP, M-M-R II and OPV (or IPV are administered either simultaneously at different sites or separately.* Administration of M-M-R II at 15 months followed by DTP and OPV (or IPV) at 18 months remains an acceptable alternative, especially for children with caregivers known to be generally compliant with other health-care recommendations.

*NOTE: The Immunization Practices Advisory Committee (ACIP) recommends administering M-M-R II concomitantly with the fourth dose of DTP and the third dose of OPV to children 15 months of age or older providing that 6 months have elapsed since DTP-3; or, if fewer than three DTPs have been received, at least 6 weeks have elapsed since the last dose of DTP and OPV.

CONTRAINDICATIONS:

Do not give M-M-R II to pregnant females; the possible effects of the vaccine on fetal development are unknown at this time. If vaccination of postpubertal females is undertaken, pregnancy should be avoided for three months following vaccination. See PRECAUTIONS, Pregnancy.

Anaphylactic or anaphylactoid reactions to neomycin (each dose of reconstituted vaccine contains approximately 25 mcg of neomycin).

History of anaphylactic or anaphylactoid reactions to eggs (see WARNINGS, Hypersensitivity To Eggs.)

Any febrile respiratory illness or other active febrile infection.

Active untreated tuberculosis.

Patients receiving immunosuppressive therapy. This contraindication does not apply to patients who are receiving corticosteroids as replacement therapy, e.g., for Addison's disease.

Individuals with blood dyscrasias, leukemia, lymphomas of any type, or other malignant neoplasms affecting the bone marrow or lymphatic systems.

Primary and acquired immunodeficiency states, including patients who are immunosuppressed in association with AIDS or other clinical manifestations of infection with human immunodeficiency viruses;[30,31] cellular immune deficiencies; and hypogammaglobulinemic and dysgammaglobulinemic states.

Individuals with a family history of congenital or hereditary immunodeficiency, until the immune competence of the potential vaccine recipient is demonstrated.[32]

WARNINGS:

HYPERSENSITIVITY TO EGGS

Live measles vaccine and live mumps vaccine are produced in chick embryo cell culture. Persons with a history of anaphylactic, anaphylactoid, or other immediate reactions (*e.g.*, hives, swelling of the mouth and throat, difficulty breathing, hypotension, or shock) subsequent to egg ingestion should not be vaccinated. Evidence indicates that persons are not at increased risk if they have egg allergies that are not anaphylactic or anaphylactoid in nature. Such persons may be vaccinated in the usual manner. There is no evidence to indicate that persons with allergies to chickens or feathers are at increased risk of reaction to the vaccine.[20]

PRECAUTIONS:

GENERAL

Adequate treatment provisions including epinephrine, should be available for immediate use should an anaphylactic or anaphylactoid reaction occur.

Due caution should be employed in administration of M-M-R II to persons with a history of cerebral injury, individual or family histories of convulsions, or any other condition in which stress due to fever should be avoided. The physician should be alert to the temperature elevation which may occur following vaccination. (See ADVERSE REACTIONS.)

Children and young adults who are known to be infected with human immunodeficiency viruses but without overt clinical manifestations of immunosuppression may be vaccinated; however, the vaccinees should be monitored closely for vaccine-preventable diseases because immunization may be less effective than for uninfected persons.[30,31]

Vaccination should be deferred for at least 3 months following blood or plasma transfusions, or administration of human immune serum globulin.

Excretion of small amounts of the live attenuated rubella virus from the nose or throat has occurred in the majority of susceptible individuals 7-28 days after vaccination. There is no confirmed evidence to indicate that such virus is transmitted to susceptible persons who are in contact with the vaccinated individuals. Consequently, transmission through close personal contact, while accepted as a theoretical possibility, is not regarded as a significant risk.[24] However, transmission of the rubella vaccine virus to infants via breast milk has been documented (see Nursing Mothers.)

There are no reports of transmission of live attenuated measles on mumps viruses from vaccinees to susceptible contacts.

It has been reported that live attenuated measles, mumps and rubella virus vaccines given individually may result in a temporary depression of tuberculin skin sensitivity. Therefore, if a tuberculin test is to be done it should be administered either before or simultaneously with M-M-R II.

Children under treatment for tuberculosis have not experienced exacerbation of the disease when immunized with live measles virus vaccine;[33] no studies have been reported to date of the effect of measles virus vaccines on untreated tuberculous children.

As for any vaccine, vaccination with M-M-R II may not result in seroconversion in 100% of susceptible persons given the vaccine.

PREGNANCY CATEGORY C

Animal reproduction studies have not been conducted with M-M-R II. It is also not known whether M-M-R II can cause fetal harm when administered to a pregnant woman or can affect reproduction capacity. Therefore, the vaccine should not be administered to pregnant females; furthermore, pregnancy should be avoided for three months following vaccination (see CONTRAINDICATIONS.)

In counseling women who are inadvertently vaccinated when pregnant or who become pregnant within 3 months of vaccination, the physician should be aware of the following: (1) In a 10 year survey involving over 700 pregnant women who received rubella vaccine within 3 months before or after conception (of whom 189 received the Wistar RA 27/3 strain), none of the newborns had abnormalities compatible with congenital rubella syndrome;[34] (2) Although mumps virus is capable of infecting the placenta and fetus, there is no good evidence that it causes congenital malformations in humans. Mumps vaccine virus also has been shown to infect the placenta, but the virus has not been isolated from the fetal tissues from susceptible women who were vaccinated and underwent elective abortions;[35] and (3) Reports have indicated that contracting of natural measles during pregnancy enhances fetal risk. Increased rates of spontaneous abortion, stillbirth, congenital defects and prematurity have been observed subsequent to natural measles during pregnancy. There are no adequate studies of the attenuated (vaccine) strain of measles virus in pregnancy. However, it would be prudent to assume that the vaccine strain of virus is also capable of inducing adverse fetal effects.

NURSING MOTHERS

It is not known whether measles or mumps vaccine virus is secreted in human milk. Recent studies have shown that lactating postpartum women immunized with live attenuated rubella vaccine may secrete the virus in breast milk and transmit it to breast-fed infants.[36] In the infants with serological evidence of rubella infection, none exhibited severe disease; however, one exhibited mild clinical illness typical of acquired rubella.[37,38] Caution should be exercised when M-M-R II is administered to a nursing woman.

ADVERSE REACTIONS:

Burning and/or stinging of short duration at the injection site have been reported.

The adverse clinical reactions associated with the use of M-M-R II are those expected to follow administration of the monovalent vaccines given separately. These may include malaise, sore throat, cough, rhinitis, headache, dizziness, fever, rash, nausea, vomiting or diarrhea; mild local reactions such as erythema, induration, tenderness and regional lymphadenopathy; parotitis, orchitis, nerve deafness, thrombocytopenia and purpura; allergic reactions such as wheal and flare at the injection site or urticaria; polyneuritis; and arthralgia and/or arthritis (usually transient and rarely chronic).

Anaphylaxis and anaphylactoid reactions have been reported.

Vasculitis has been reported rarely.

Otitis media and conjunctivitis have been reported.

Moderate fever (101-102.9°F (38.3-39.4°C)) occurs occasionally, and high fever (above 103°F (39.4°C)) occurs less commonly. On rare occasions, children developing fever may exhibit febrile convulsions. Afebrile convulsions or seizures have occurred rarely following vaccination with live attenuated measles vaccine. Syncope, particularly at the time of mass vaccination, has been reported. Rash occurs infrequently and is usually minimal, but rarely may be generalized. Erythema multiforme has also been reported rarely.

Forms of optic neuritis, including retrobulbar neuritis, papillitis, and retinitis may infrequently follow viral infections, and have been reported to occur 1 to 3 weeks following inoculation with some live virus vaccines.

Clinical experience with live attenuated measles, mumps and rubella virus vaccines given individually indicates that encephalitis and other nervous system reactions have occurred very rarely. These might occur also with M-M-R II.

Experience from more than 80 million doses of all live measles vaccines given in the U.S. through 1975 indicates that significant central nervous system reactions such as encephalitis and encephalopathy, occurring within 30 days after vaccination, have been temporally

ADVERSE REACTIONS: *(cont'd)*

associated with measles vaccine very rarely.[39] In no case has it been shown that reactions were actually caused by vaccine. The Center for Disease Control has pointed out that "a certain number of cases of encephalitis may be expected to occur in a large childhood population in a defined period of time even when no vaccines are administered". However, the data suggest the possibility that some of these cases may have been caused by measles vaccines. The risk of such serious neurological disorders following live measles virus vaccine administration remains far less than that for encephalitis and encephalopathy with natural measles (one per two thousand reported cases).

There have been rare reports of ocular palsies, Guillain-Barre syndrome, or ataxia occurring after immunization with vaccines containing live attenuated measles virus. The ocular palsies have occurred approximately 3-24 days following vaccination. No definite causal relationship has been established between these events and vaccination. Isolated reports of polyneuropathy including Guillain-Barre syndrome have also been reported after immunization with rubella-containing vaccines.

There have been reports of subacute sclerosing panencephalitis (SSPE) in children who did not have a history of natural measles but did receive measles vaccine. Some of these cases may have resulted from unrecognized measles in the first year of life or possibly from the measles vaccination. Based on estimated nationwide measles vaccine distribution, the association of SSPE cases to measles vaccination is about one case per million vaccine doses distributed. This is far less than the association with natural measles, 6-22 cases of SSPE per million cases of measles. The results of a retrospective case-controlled study conducted by the Center for Disease Control suggest that the overall effect of measles vaccine has been to protect against SSPE by preventing measles with its inherent higher risk of SSPE.[40]

Local reactions characterized by marked swelling, redness and vesiculation at the injection site of attenuated live measles virus vaccines, and systemic reactions including atypical measles, have occurred in persons who received killed measles vaccine previously. M-M-R II was not given under this condition in clinical trials. Rarely, more severe reactions that require hospitalization, including prolonged high fevers and extensive local reactions, have been reported.[41] Panniculitis has been reported rarely following administration of measles vaccine.[42]

Arthralgia and/or arthritis (usually transient and rarely chronic), and polyneuritis are features of natural rubella and vary in frequency and severity with age and sex, being greatest in adult females and least in prepubertal children. This type of involvement as well as myalgia and paresthesia, have also been reported following administration of Meruvax II (Rubella Virus Vaccine Live).

Chronic arthritis has been associated with natural rubella infection and has been related to persistent virus and/or viral antigen isolated from body tissues. Only rarely have vaccine recipients developed chronic joint symptoms.

Following vaccination in children, reactions in joints are uncommon and generally of brief duration. In women, incidence rates for arthritis and arthralgia are generally higher than those seen in children (children: 0-3%; women: 12-20%),[43] and the reactions tend to be more marked and of longer duration. Symptoms may persist for a matter of months or on rare occasions for years. In adolescent girls, the reactions appear to be intermediate in incidence between those seen in children and in adult women. Even in older women (35-45 years), these reactions are generally well tolerated and rarely interfere with normal activities.

DOSAGE AND ADMINISTRATION:

FOR SUBCUTANEOUS ADMINISTRATION

Do not inject intravenously

The dosage of vaccine is the same for all persons. Inject the total volume of the single dose vial (about 0.5 ml) or 0.5 ml of the 10 dose vial of reconstituted vaccine subcutaneously, preferably into the outer aspect of upper arm. *Do not give immune globulin (IG) concurrently with* M-M-R II.

During shipment, to insure that there is no loss of potency, the vaccine must be maintained at a temperature of 10°C (50°F) or less.

Before reconstitution, store M-M-R II at 2-8°C (36-46°F).*Protect from light.*

CAUTION: A sterile syringe free of preservatives, antiseptics, and detergents should be used for each injection and/or reconstitution of the vaccine because these substances may inactivate the live virus vaccine. A 25 gauge, 5/8" needle is recommended.

To reconstitute, use only the diluent supplied, since it is free of preservatives or other antiviral substances which might inactivate the vaccine.

Single Dose Vial—First withdraw the entire volume of diluent into the syringe to be used for reconstitution. Inject all the diluent in the syringe into the vial of lyophilized vaccine, and agitate to mix thoroughly. Withdraw the entire contents into a syringe and inject the total volume of restored vaccine subcutaneously.

It is important to use a separate sterile syringe and needle for each individual patient to prevent transmission of hepatitis B and other infectious agents from one person to another.

10 Dose Vial (available only to government agencies/institutions) Withdraw the entire contents (7 ml) of the diluent vial into the sterile syringe to be used for reconstitution, and introduce into the 10 dose vial of lyophilized vaccine. Agitate to ensure thorough mixing. The outer labeling suggests "For Jet Injector or Syringe Use". Use with separate sterile syringes is permitted for containers of 10 doses or less. The vaccine and diluent do not contain preservatives; therefore, the user must recognize the potential contamination hazards and exercise special precautions to protect the sterility and potency of the product. The use of aseptic techniques and proper storage prior to and after restoration of the vaccine and subsequent withdrawal of the individual doses is essential. Use 0.5 ml of the reconstituted vaccine for subcutaneous injection.

It is important to use a separate sterile syringe and needle for each individual patient to prevent transmission of hepatitis B and other infectious agents from one person to another.

Each dose contains not less than the equivalent of 1,000 $TCID_{50}$ of the U.S. Reference Measles Virus, 20,000 $TCID_{50}$ of the U.S. Reference Mumps Virus and 1,000 $TCID_{50}$ of the U.S. Reference Rubella Virus.

Parenteral drug products should be inspected visually for particulate matter and discoloration prior to administration. M-M-R II, when reconstituted, is clear yellow.

STORAGE

It is recommended that the vaccine be used as soon as possible after reconstitution. Protect vaccine from light at all times, since such exposure may inactivate the virus. Store reconstituted vaccine in the vaccine vial in a dark place at 2 - 8°C (36 - 46°F) and discard if not used within 8 hours.

REFERENCES:

1) Plotkin, S. A.; Cornfeld, D.; Ingalls, T. H.: Studies of immunization with living rubella virus: Trials in children with a strain cultured from an aborted fetus, Am. J. Dis. Child. *110:*381-389, 1965. 2) Plotkin, S. A.; Farquhar, J.; Katz, M.; Ingalls, T. H.: A new attenuated rubella virus grown in human fibroblasts: Evidence for reduced nasopharyngeal excretion, Am. J. Epidemiol. *86:*468-477,1967. 3) Fogel, A.; Moshkowitz, A.; Rannon, L.; Gerichter, Ch. B.: Comparative trials of RA 27/3 and Cendehill rubella vaccines in adult and adolescent females, Am. J. Epidemiol. *93:* 392-393, 1971. 4) Andzhaparidze, O. G.; Desyatskova, R. G.; Chervonski, G. I.; Pryanichnikova, L. V.: Immunogenicity and reactogenicity of live attenuated rubella virus vaccines, Am. J. Epidemiol. *91:* 527-530, 1970. 5) Freestone, D. S.; Reynolds, G. M.; McKinnon, J. A.; Prydie, J.: Vaccination of schoolgirls against rubella. Assessment of serological status and a comparative trial of Wistar RA 27/3 and

REFERENCES: *(cont'd)*

Cendehill strain live attenuated rubella vaccines in 13-year-old schoolgirls in Dudley, Br. J. Prev. Soc. Med. *29:* 258-261, 1975. 6) Grillner. L.; Hedstrom, C. E.; Bergstrom, H.; Forssman, L.; Rigner, A.; Lycke, E.: Vaccination against rubella of newly delivered women,Scand. J. Infect. Dis. *5:*237-241, 1973. 7) Grillner, L.: Neutralizing antibodies after rubella vaccination of newly delivered women: a comparison between three vaccines, Scand. J. Infect. Dis. *7:* 169-172, 1975. 8) Wallace, R. B.; Isacson, P.: Comparative trial of HPV-77, DE-5 and RA 27/3 live-attenuated rubella vaccines, Am. J. Dis. Child. *124:*536-538, 1972. 9) Lalla, M.; Vesikari, T.; Virolainen, M.: Lymphoblast proliferation and humoral antibody response after rubella vaccination, Clin. Exp.Immunol. *15:* 193-202, 1973. 10) LeBouvier, G. L.; Plotkin, S. A.: Precipitin responses to rubella vaccine RA 27/3, J. Infect. Dis. *123:* 220-223, 1971. 11) Horstmann, D. M.: Rubella: The challenge of its control, J. Infect. Dis. *123:* 640-654, 1971. 12) Ogra, P. L.; Kerr-Grant, D.; Umana, G.; Dzierba, J.; Weintraub, D.: Antibody response in serum and nasopharynx after naturally acquired and vaccine-induced infection with rubella virus, N. Engl. J. Med.*285:* 1333-1339, 1971. 13) Plotkin, S. A.; Farquhar, J. D.; Ogra, P. L.: Immunologic properties of RA 27/3 rubella virus vaccine, J. Am. Med. Assoc. *225:* 585-590, 1973. 14) Liebhaber, H.; Ingalls, T. H.; LeBouvier, G. L.; Horstmann, D.M.: Vaccination with RA 27/3 rubella vaccine. Persistence of immunity and resistance to challenge after two years, Am. J. Dis. Child. *123:*133-136, 1972. 15) Farquhar, J. D.: Follow-up on rubella vaccinations and experience with subclinical reinfection, J. Pediatr. *81:* 460-465, 1972. 16) Weibel, R. E.; Carlson, A. J.; Villarejos, V. M.; Buynak, E. B.; McLean, A. A.; Hilleman, M. R.: Clinical and Laboratory Studies of Combined Live Measles, Mumps, and Rubella Vaccines Using the RA 27/3 Rubella Virus, Proc. Soc. Exp. Biol. Med. *165:* 323-326, 1980. 17) Bottiger, M.; Christenson, B.; Romanus, V.; Taranger, J.; Strandell, A.: Swedish experience of two dose vaccination programme aiming at eliminating measles, mumps, and rubella, Brit. Med. J. *295* (14): 1264-1267, November, 1987. 18) Markowitz, L. E.; Preblud, S. R.; Orenstein, W. A.; et al: Patterns of transmission in measles outbreaks in the United States, 1985-1986, N. Engl. J. Med. *320* (2): 75-81, January 12, 1989. 19) Peltola, H.; Heinonen, O. P.; Valle, M.; et al: Five-year experience in elimination of indigenous measles, mumps, and rubella in Finland, Abstracts of the 29th ICAAC, Houston, Texas, Abstract #179, 130, September, 1989. 20) American Academy of Pediatrics: Report of the Committee on Infectious Disease, Evanston, III., AAP, p. 136-137, 1982. 21) Recommendations of the Immunization Practices Advisory Committee (ACIP), Measles Prevention, MMWR *36* (26): 409-425, July 10, 1987. 22) Jong, E. C., The Travel and Tropical Medicine Manual, W. B. Saunders Company, p. 12-16, 1987. 23) Committee on Immunization Council of Medical Societies, American College of Physicians, Phila., PA, Guide for Adult Immunization, First Edition, 1985. 24) Recommendation of the Immunization Practices Advisory Committee (ACIP), Morbidity and Mortality Weekly Report *33* (22): 301-310, 315-318, June 8, 1984. 25) McIntosh, R,; Merritt, K. K.; Richards, M. R.; Samuels, M. H.; Bellows, M. T.: The incidence of congenital malformations: A study of 5,964 pregnancies, Pediatr. *14:* 505-521, 1954. 26) American Academy of Pediatrics, Committee on Infectious Diseases, Measles: Reassessment of the Current Immunization Policy, Pediatrics *84* (6): 1110-1113, December, 1989. 27) Measles Prevention: Recommendations of the Immunization Practices Advisory Committee (ACIP), Morbidity and Mortality Weekly Report*38* (S-9): 5-22, December 29, 1989. 28) Recommendations of the Immunization Practices Advisory Committee (ACIP), General Recommendations on Immunization, MMWR *38* (13) 205-228, April 7, 1989. 29) American Academy of Pediatrics: Report of the Committee on Infectious Disease, Evanston, III., 1982, p. 17. 30) Center for Disease Control: Immunization of Children Infected with Human T-Lymphotropic Virus Type III/Lymphadenopathy-Associated Virus, Annals of Internal Medicine,*106:* 75-78, 1987. 31) Krasinski, K.; Borkowsky, W.; Krugman, S.: Antibody following measles immunization in children infected with human T-cell lymphotropic virus type III/lymphadenopathy associated virus (HTLV-III/LAV) (Abstract). In: Program and abstracts of the International Conference on Acquired Immunodeficiency Syndrome, Paris, France, June 23-25, 1986. 32) Recommendation of the Immunization Practices Advisory Committee (ACIP), General Recommendations on Immunization, Morbidity and Mortality Weekly Report *32* (1): 13, January 14, 1983. 33) Starr, S.; Berkovich, S.: The effect of measles, gamma globulin modified measles, and attenuated measles vaccine on the course of treated tuberculosis in children, Pediatrics *35:*97-102, January, 1965. 34) Rubella vaccination during pregnancy—United States, 1971-1981. Morbidity and Mortality Weekly Report *31* (35): 477-481, September 10, 1982. 35) Recommendation of the Immunization Practices Advisory Committee (ACIP), Mumps Vaccine, Morbidity and Mortality Weekly Report*31* (46): 617-620, 625, November 26, 1982. 36) Losonsky, G. A.; Fishaut, J. M.; Strussenber, J.; Ogra, P. L.: Effect or immunization against rubella on lactation products. II. Maternal-neonatal interactions, J. Infect. Dis. *145:* 661-666, 1982. 37) Landes, R. D.; Bass, J. W.; Millunchick, E. W.; Oetgen, W. J.: Neonatal rubella following postpartum maternal immunization, J. Pediatr. *97:*465-467, 1980. 38) Lerman, S. J.: Neonatal rubella following postpartum maternal immunization, J. Pediatr. *98:*668, 1981. (Letter) 39) CDC. Important Information about Measles, Mumps, and Rubella, and Measles, Mumps, and Rubella Vaccines. 1980. 1983. 40) CDC, Measles Surveillance, Report No. 11, p. 14, September, 1982. 41) Recommendation of the Immunization Practices Advisory Committee (ACIP), Measles Prevention, Morbidity and Mortality Weekly Report *31* (17): 217-224, 229-231, May 7, 1982. 42) Buck, B. E.; Yang, L. C.; Caleb, M. H.; Green, J. M.; South, M. A.: Measles virus panniculitis subsequent to vaccine administration, J. Pediatrics *101* (3): 366-373, 1982. 43) Unpublished data from the files of Merck Sharp and Dohme Research Laboratories.

HOW SUPPLIED - EQUIVALENTS NOT AVAILABLE:

Injection, Lyphl-Soln - Subcutaneous - 1000 unit/5000

0.5 ml	$36.47	M-M-R II, Merck	00006-4749-00
0.5 ml x 10	$320.88	M-M-R II, Merck	00006-4681-00

MEBENDAZOLE *(001705)*

CATEGORIES: Anthelmintics; Anti-Infectives; Antiparasitics; Ascaris; Enterobius; Helminths; Hookworm; Infections; Parasiticidal; Pinworm; Roundworm; Trichuris; Whipworm; Pregnancy Category C; FDA Approval Pre 1982

BRAND NAMES: *Amycil* (Mexico); *Anelmin*; *Anthex*; *Antiox*; *Astriun*; *Bantenol*; *Benda*; *Bendosan*; *Benex*; *Benzalmin*; *Conquer*; *Damaben*; *Drivermide*; *D-Worm*; *Elmetin*; *Fugacar*; *Gamax*; *Helminzole* (Mexico); *Idibend*; *Kaizole*; *Lomper*; *Mebasol*; *Mebex*; *Mendazole*; *Meforasol*; *Mindol*; *Nemasol* (Canada); *Noverme*; *Ovex*; *Oxibem*; *Pantelmin*; *Penalcol*; *Pharaxis M*; *Revapol* (Mexico); *Soltric* (Mexico); *Thelmox*; *Toloxim*; *Vagaka*; *Vercid*; *Vermona*; *Vermoran*; *Vermorex*; **Vermox**; *Wormgo*; *Wormin*; *Wormox*; *Zadomen*; *Zumin*

(International brand names outside U.S. in italics)

FORMULARIES: Aetna; BC-BS; DoD; Medi-Cal; PCS; WHO

DESCRIPTION:

Mebendazole is a (synthetic) broad-spectrum anthelmintic available as chewable tablets, each containing 100 mg of mebendazole. Inactive ingredients are: colloidal silicon dioxide, corn starch, hydrogenated vegetable oil, magnesium stearate, microcrystalline cellulose, sodium lauryl sulfate, sodium saccharin, sodium starch glycolate, talc, tetrarome orange, and FD&C yellow No. 6.

Mebendazole is methyl 5-benzoylbenzimidazole-2-carbamate.

Mebendazole is a white to slightly yellow powder with a molecular weight of 295.29. It is less than 0.05% soluble in water, dilute mineral acid solutions, alcohol, ether and chloroform, but is soluble in formic acid.

CLINICAL PHARMACOLOGY:

Following administration of 100 mg twice daily for three consecutive days, plasma levels of mebendazole and its primary metabolite, the 2-amine, do not exceed 0.03 mcg/ml and 0.09 mcg/ml, respectively. All metabolites are devoid of anthelmintic activity. In man, approximately 2% of administered mebendazole is excreted in urine and the remainder in the feces as unchanged drug or a primary metabolite.

Mode of Action: Mebendazole inhibits the formation of the worms' microtubules and causes the worms' glucose depletion.

INDICATIONS AND USAGE:

Mebendazole is indicated for the treatment of *Enterobius vermicularis* (pinworm), *Trichuris trichiura* (whipworm), *Ascaris lumbricoides* (common roundworm), *Ancylostoma duodenale* (common hookworm), *Necator americanus* (American hookworm) in single or mixed infections.

Efficacy varies as a function of such factors as pre-existing diarrhea and gastrointestinal transit time, degree of infection, and helminth strains. Efficacy rates derived from various studies are shown in the table below (TABLE 1).:

CONTRAINDICATIONS:

Mebendazole is contraindicated in persons who have shown hypersensitivity to the drug.

TABLE 1	Pinworm (enterobiasis)	Whipworm (trichuriasis)	Common Roundworm (ascariasis)	Hookworm
Cure rates mean	95%	68%	98%	96%
Egg reduction mean	—	93%	99%	99%

WARNINGS:

There is no evidence that mebendazole, even at high doses, is effective for hydatid disease. There have been rare reports of neutropenia and liver function elevations, including hepatitis, when mebendazole is taken for prolonged periods and at dosages substantially above those recommended.

PRECAUTIONS:

Information for the Patient: Patients should be informed of the potential risk to the fetus in women taking mebendazole during pregnancy, especially during the first trimester (see Use in Pregnancy).

Patients should also be informed that cleanliness is important to prevent reinfection and transmission of the infection.

Carcinogenesis, Mutagenesis: In carcinogenicity tests of mebendazole in mice and rats, no carcinogenic effects were seen at doses as high as 40 mg/kg given daily over two years. Dominant lethal mutation tests in mice showed no mutagenicity at single doses as high as 640 mg/kg. Neither the spermatocyte test, the F_1 translocation test, not the Ames test indicated mutagenic properties.

Impairment Fertility: Doses up to 40 mg/kg in mice, given to males for 60 days and to females for 14 days prior to gestation, had no effect upon fetuses and offspring, though there was slight maternal toxicity.

Usage in Pregnancy: Pregnancy Category C. Mebendazole has shown embryotoxic and teratogenic activity in pregnant rats at single oral doses as low as 10 mg/kg. In view of these findings the use of mebendazole is not recommended in pregnant women. In humans, a post-marketing survey has been done of a limited number of women who inadvertently had consumed mebendazole during the first trimester of pregnancy. The incidence of spontaneous abortion and malformation did not exceed that in the general population. In 170 deliveries on term, no teratogenic risk of mebendazole was identified. During pregnancy, especially during the first trimester, mebendazole should be used only if the potential benefit justifies the potential risk to the fetus.

Nursing Mothers: It is not known whether mebendazole is excreted in human milk. Because many drugs are excreted in human milk, caution should be exercised when mebendazole is administered to a nursing woman.

Pediatric Use: The drug has not been extensively studied in children under two years; therefore, in the treatment of children under two years the relative benefit/risk should be considered.

ADVERSE REACTIONS:

Transient symptoms of abdominal pain and diarrhea have occurred in cases of massive infection and expulsion of worms. Hypersensitivity reactions such as rash, urticaria and angioedema have been observed on rare occasions. Very rare cases of convulsions have been reported.

OVERDOSAGE:

In the event of accidental overdosage gastrointestinal complaints lasting up to a few hours may occur. Vomiting and purging should be induced. Activated charcoal may be given.

DOSAGE AND ADMINISTRATION:

The same dosage schedule applies to children and adults. The tablet may be chewed, swallowed, or crushed and mixed with food (TABLE 2).

TABLE 2	Pinworm (enterobiasis)	Whipworm (trichuriasis)	Common Roundworm (ascariasis)	Hookworm
Dose	1 tablet, once	1 tablet morning and evening for 3 consecutive days.	1 tablet morning and evening for 3 consecutive days.	1 tablet morning and evening for 3 consecutive days.

If the patient is not cured three weeks after treatment, a second course of treatment is advised. No special procedures, such as fasting or purging, are required.

HOW SUPPLIED:

Vermox is available as chewable tablets, each containing 100 mg of mebendazole, and is supplied in boxes of twelve tablets.

Store at room temperature 15°-30°C (59°-86°F).

HOW SUPPLIED - RATED THERAPEUTICALLY EQUIVALENT:

Tablet, Chewable - Oral - 100 mg

12's	$52.20	Mebendazole, Copley Pharm	38245-0107-08
12's	**$58.00**	**VERMOX, Janssen Phar**	**50458-0110-01**

MECAMYLAMINE HYDROCHLORIDE *(001706)*

CATEGORIES: Antihypertensives; Cardiovascular Drugs; Hypertension; Renal Drugs; Pregnancy Category C; FDA Approval Pre 1982

BRAND NAMES: **Inversine**; *Mevasine* (Japan)
(International brand names outside U.S. in italics)

DESCRIPTION:

Inversine (mecamylamine HCl) is a potent, oral antihypertensive agent and ganglion blocker, and is a secondary amine. It is *N*,2,3,3-tetramethylbicyclo (2.2.1) heptan-2-amine hydrochloride. Its empirical formula is $C_{11}H_{21}N°4$. It is a white odorless, or practically odorless, crystalline powder, is highly stable, soluble in water and has a molecular weight of 203.75.

DESCRIPTION: *(cont'd)*

Inversine is supplied as tablets for oral use, each containing 2.5 mg mecamylamine HCl. Inactive ingredients are acacia, calcium phosphate, D&C Yellow 10, FD&C Yellow 6, lactose, magnesium stearate, starch, and talc.

CLINICAL PHARMACOLOGY:

Mecamylamine reduces blood pressure in both normotensive & hypertensive individuals. It has a gradual onset of action (30 minutes to 2 hours) and a long-lasting effect (usually 6 to 12 hours or more). A small oral dosage often produces a smooth and predictable reduction of blood pressure. Although this antihypertensive effect is predominantly orthostatic, the supine blood pressure is also significantly reduced.

PHARMACOKINETICS AND METABOLISM

Mecamylamine is almost completely absorbed from the gastrointestinal tract, resulting in consistent lowering of blood pressure in most patients with hypertensive cardiovascular disease. Mecamylamine is excreted slowly in the urine in the unchanged form. The rate of its renal elimination is influenced markedly by urinary pH. Alkalinization of the urine reduces, and acidification promotes, renal excretion of mecamylamine.

Mecamylamine crosses the blood-brain and placental barriers.

INDICATIONS AND USAGE:

For the management of moderately severe to severe essential hypertension and in uncomplicated cases of malignant hypertension.

CONTRAINDICATIONS:

Mecamylamine HCl should not be used in mild, moderate, labile hypertension and may prove unsuitable in uncooperative patients. It is contraindicated in coronary insufficiency or recent myocardial infarction.

Inversine should be given with great discretion, if at all, when renal insufficiency is manifested by a rising or elevated BUN. The drug is contraindicated in uremia. Patients receiving antibiotics and sulfonamides should generally not be treated with ganglion blockers. Other contraindications are glaucoma, organic pyloric stenosis or hypersensitivity to the product.

WARNINGS:

Mecamylamine, a secondary amine, readily penetrates into the brain and thus may produce central nervous system effects. Tremor, choreiform movements, mental aberrations, and convulsions may occur rarely. These have occurred most often when large doses of Inversine were used, especially in patients with cerebral or renal insufficiency.

When ganglion blockers or other potent antihypertensive drugs are discontinued suddenly, hypertensive levels return. In patients with malignant hypertension and others, this may cause fatal cerebral vascular accidents or acute congestive heart failure. When mecamylamine HCl is withdrawn, this should be done gradually and other antihypertensive therapy usually must be substituted. On the other hand, the effects of Inversine sometimes last from hours to days after therapy is discontinued.

PRECAUTIONS:

GENERAL

The patient's condition should be evaluated carefully, particularly as to renal and cardiovascular function. When renal, cerebral, or coronary blood flow id deficient, any additional impairment, which might result from added hypotension, must be avoided. The use of mecamylamine HCl in patients with marked cerebral and coronary arteriosclerosis or after a recent cerebral accident requires caution.

The action of mecamylamine HCl may be potentiated by excessive heat, fever, infection, hemorrhage, pregnancy, anesthesia, surgery, vigorous exercise, other antihypertensive drugs, alcohol, and salt depletion as a result of diminished intake or increased excretion due to diarrhea, vomiting, excessive sweating, or diuretics.

During therapy with mecamylamine HCl, sodium intake should not be restricted, but, if necessary, the dosage of the ganglion blocker must be adjusted.

Since urinary retention may occur in patients on ganglion blockers, caution is required in patients with prostatic hypertrophy, bladder neck obstruction, and urethral stricture.

Frequent loose bowel movements with abdominal distension and decreased borborygmi may be the first signs of paralytic ileus. If these are present, mecamylamine HCl should be discontinued immediately and remedial steps taken.

INFORMATION FOR THE PATIENT

Mecamylamine HCl may cause dizziness, lightheadedness, or fainting, especially when rising from a lying or sitting position. This effect may be increased by alcoholic beverages, exercise, or during hot weather. Getting up slowly may help alleviate such a reaction.

CARCINOGENESIS, MUTAGENESIS, AND IMPAIRMENT OF FERTILITY

Long-term studies in animals have not been performed to evaluate the effects upon fertility, mutagenic or carcinogenic potential of Inversine.

PREGNANCY

Pregnancy Category C: Animal reproduction studies have not been conducted with mecamylamine HCl. It is not known whether Inversine can cause fetal harm when given to a pregnant woman or can effect reproductive capacity. Inversine should be given to a pregnant woman only if clearly needed.

NURSING MOTHERS

Because of the potential for serious adverse reactions in nursing infants from mecamylamine HCl, a decision should be made whether to discontinue nursing or to discontinue the drug, taking into account the importance of the drug to the mother.

DRUG INTERACTIONS:

Patients receiving antibiotics and sulfonamides generally should not be treated with ganglion blockers.

The action of mecamylamine HCl may be potentiated by anesthesia, other antihypertensive drugs and alcohol.

ADVERSE REACTIONS:

The following adverse reactions have been reported and within each category are listed in order of decreasing severity.

Gastrointestinal: Ileus, constipation (sometimes preceded by small frequent liquid stools), vomiting, nausea, anorexia, glossitis and dryness of mouth.

Cardiovascular: Orthostatic dizziness and syncope, postural hypotension.

Nervous System/Psychiatric: Convulsions, choreiform movements, mental aberrations, tremor, and paresthesias (see WARNINGS).

Respiratory: Interstitial pulmonary edema and fibrosis.

Urogenital: Urinary retention, impotence, decreased libido.

Special Senses: Blurred vision, dilated pupils.

ADVERSE REACTIONS: *(cont'd)*

Miscellaneous: Weakness, fatigue, sedation.

OVERDOSAGE:

Signs of overdosage include: hypotension (which may progress to peripheral vascular collapse), postural hypotension, nausea, vomiting, diarrhea, constipation, paralytic ileus, urinary retention, dizziness, anxiety, dry mouth, mydriasis, blurred vision, or palpitations. A rise in intraocular pressure may occur.

Pressor amines may be used to counteract excessive hypotension. Since patients being treated with ganglion blockers are more than normally reactive to pressor amines, small doses of the later are recommended to avoid excessive response.

The oral LD_{50} of mecamylamine in the mouse is 92 mg/kg.

DOSAGE AND ADMINISTRATION:

Therapy is usually started with one 2.5 mg tablet of mecamylamine HCl twice a day. This initial dosage should be modified by increments of one 2.5 mg tablet at intervals of not less than 2 days until the desired blood pressure response occurs (the criterion being a dosage just under that which causes signs of mild postural hypotension).

The average total daily dosage of mecamylamine HCl is 25 mg, usually in three divided doses. However, as little as 2.5 mg daily may be sufficient to control hypertension in some patients. A range of two to four or even more doses may be required in severe cases when smooth control is difficult to obtain. In severe or urgent cases, larger increments at smaller intervals may be needed. Partial tolerance may develop in certain patients, requiring an increase in the daily dosage of Inversine.

Administration of mecamylamine HCl after meals may cause a more gradual absorption and smoother control of excessively high blood pressure. The timing of doses in relation to meals should be consistent. Since the blood pressure response to antihypertensive drugs is increased in the early morning, the larger dose should be given at noontime and perhaps in the evening. The morning dose, as a rule, should be relatively small and in some instances may even be omitted.

The *initial regulation dosage* should be determined by blood pressure readings in the erect position at the time of maximal effect of the drug, as well as by other signs and symptoms of orthostatic hypertension.

The *effective maintenance dosage* should be regulated by blood pressure readings in the erect position and by limitation of dosage to that which causes slight faintness or dizziness in this position. If the patient or a relative can use a sphygmomanometer, instructions may be given to reduce or omit a dose if readings fall below a designated level ir if faintness or lightheadedness occurs. *However, no change should be instituted without the knowledge of a physician.*

Close supervision and education of the patient, as well as critical adjustment of dosage, are essential to successful therapy.

OTHER ANTIHYPERTENSIVE AGENTS

When mecamylamine HCl is given with other antihypertensive drugs, the dosage of these other agents, as well as that of Inversine, should be reduced to avoid excessive hypotension. However, thiazides should be continued in their usual dosage, while that of Inversine is decreased by at least 50 percent.

HOW SUPPLIED - EQUIVALENTS NOT AVAILABLE:

Tablet, Uncoated - Oral - 2.5 mg

100's	$13.03	INVERSINE, Merck	00006-0052-68

MECHLORETHAMINE HYDROCHLORIDE

(001707)

CATEGORIES: Antineoplastics; Cancer; Hodgkin's Disease; Leukemia; Lymphosarcoma; Mycosis Fungoides; Nitrogen Mustard Derivatives; Oncologic Drugs; Polycythemia Vera; Pregnancy Category D; FDA Approval Pre 1982

BRAND NAMES: **Mustargen**; *Mustine*; *Mustine Hydrochloride Boots*
(International brand names outside U.S. in italics)

FORMULARIES: BC-BS; WHO

> **WARNING:**
> Extravasation of the drug into subcutaneous tissues results in a painful inflammation. The area usually becomes indurated and and sloughing may occur. If leakage of drug is obvious, prompt infiltration of the area with sterile isotonic sodium thiosulfate (1/6 molar) and application of an ice compress for 6 to 12 hours may minimize the local reaction. For a 1/6 molar solution of sodium thiosulfate, use 4.14 g of sodium thiosulfate per 100 ml of Sterile Water for Injection or 2.64 g of anhydrous sodium thiosulfate per 100 ml or dilute 4 ml of Sodium Thiosulfate Injection (10%) with 6 ml of Sterile Water for Injection.

DESCRIPTION:

Mustargen (mechlorethamine HCl), an antineoplastic nitrogen mustard also known as HN2 hydrochloride, is a nitrogen analog of sulfur mustard. It is a white, crystalline, hygroscopic powder that is very soluble in water and also soluble in alcohol.

Mechlorethamine hydrochloride is designated chemically as 2-chloro-*N*-(2-chlorethyl)-*N*-methylethanamine hydrochloride. The molecular weight is 192.52 and the melting point is 108°-111°C. The empirical formula is:

$C_5H_{11}Cl_2N{\cdot}HCl$, and the structural formula is: $CH_3N(CH_2CH_2Cl)_2{\cdot}HCl$.

Trituration of mechlorethamine HCl is a sterile, white crystalline powder for injection by the intravenous or intracavitary routes after dissolution. Each vial of mechlorethamine HClcontains 10 mg of mechlorethamine hydrochloride triturated with sodium chloride q.s. 100 mg. When dissolved with 10 ml Sterile Water for Injection or 0.9% Sodium Chloride Injection, the resulting solution had a pH of 3-5 at a concentration of 1 mg mechlorethamine HCl per ml.

CLINICAL PHARMACOLOGY:

Mechlorethamine, a biologic alkylating agent, has a cytotoxic action which inhibits rapidly proliferating cells.

PHARMACOKINETICS AND METABOLISM

In water or body fluids, mechlorethamine undergoes rapid chemical transformation and combines with water or reactive compounds of cells, so that the drug is no longer present in active form a few minutes after administration.[1]

INDICATIONS AND USAGE:

Before using mechlorethamine HCl see CONTRAINDICATIONS,WARNINGS, PRECAUTIONS, ADVERSE REACTIONS, DOSAGE AND ADMINISTRATION, and Special Handling.

Mechlorethamine HCl, administered intravenously, is indicated for the palliative treatment of Hodgkin's disease (Stages III and IV), lymphosarcoma, chronic myelocytic or chronic lymphocytic leukemia, polycythemia vera, mycosis fungoides, and bronchogenic carcinoma.

Mechlorethamine HCl, administered intrapleurally, intraperitoneally, or intrapericardially, is indicated for the palliative treatment of metastatic carcinoma resulting in effusion.

CONTRAINDICATIONS:

The use of mechlorethamine HCl is contraindicated in the presence of known infectious diseases and in patients who have had previous anaphylactic reactions to mechlorethamine HCl.

WARNINGS:

Before using mechlorethamine HCl, an accurate histologic diagnosis of the disease, a knowledge of its natural course, and an adequate clinical history are important. The hematologic status of the patient must first be determined. It is essential to understand the hazards and therapeutic effects to be expected. Careful clinical judgement must be exercised in selecting patients. If the indication for its use is not clear, the drug should not be used.

As nitrogen mustard therapy may contribute to extensive and rapid development of amyloidosis, it should be used only if foci of acute and chronic suppurative inflammation are absent.

USAGE IN PREGNANCY

Mechlorethamine HCl can cause fetal harm when administered to a pregnant woman. Mechlorethamine has been shown to produce fetal malformations in the rat and ferret when given as single subcutaneous injections of 1 mg/kg (2-3 times the maximum recommended human dose). There are no adequate and well controlled studies in pregnant women. If this drug is used during pregnancy, or if the patient becomes pregnant while taking this drug, the patient should be apprised of the potential hazard to the fetus. Women of childbearing potential should be advised to avoid becoming pregnant.

PRECAUTIONS:

GENERAL

This drug is highly toxic and both powder and solution must be handled and administered with care. Since mechlorethamine HCl is a powerful vesicant, it is intended primarily for intravenous use, and in most instances is given by this route. Inhalation of dust or vapors and contact with skin or mucous membranes, especially those of the eyes, must be avoided. Rubber gloves should be worn when handling mechlorethamine HCl. (see DOSAGE AND ADMINISTRATION and Special Handling.)

Because of the toxicity of mechlorethamine HCl, and the unpleasant side effects following its use, the potential risk and discomfort from the use of this drug in patients with inoperable neoplasms or in the terminal stage of the disease must be balanced against the limited gain obtainable. These gains will vary with the nature and the status of the disease under treatment. The routine use of mechlorethamine HCl in all cases of widely disseminated neoplasms is to be discouraged.

The use of mechlorethamine HCl in patients with leukopenia, thrombocytopenia, and anemia, due to invasion of the bone marrow by tumor carries a greater risk. In such patients a good response to treatment with disappearance of the tumor from the bone marrow may be associated with improvement of bone marrow function. However, in the absence of a good response or in patients who have been previously treated with chemotherapeutic agents, hematopoiesis may be further compromised, and leukopenia, thrombocytopenia and anemia may become more severe and lead to the demise of the patient.

Tumors of bone and nervous tissue have responded poorly to therapy. Results are unpredictable in disseminated and malignant tumors of different types.

Precautions must be observed with the use of mechlorethamine HCl and x-ray therapy or other chemotherapy in alternating courses. Hematopoietic function is characteristically depressed by either form of therapy, and neither mechlorethamine HCl following x-ray therapy nor x-ray therapy subsequent to the drug should be given until bone marrow function has recovered. In particular, irradiation of such areas as sternum, ribs, and vertebrae shortly after a course of nitrogen mustard may lead to hematologic complications.

Mechlorethamine HCl has been reported to have immunosuppressive activity. Therefore, it should be borne in mind that use of the drug may predispose the patient to bacterial, viral or fungal infection.

Hyperuricemia may develop during therapy with mechlorethamine HCl. The problem of urate precipitation should be anticipated, particularly in the treatment of the lymphomas, and adequate methods for control of hyperuricemia should be instituted and careful attention directed toward adequate fluid intake before treatment.

Since drug toxicity, especially sensitivity to bone marrow failure, seems to be more common in chronic lymphatic leukemia than in other conditions, the drug should be given in this condition with great caution, if at all.

Extreme caution must be used in exceeding the average recommended dose. (See OVERDOSAGE).

LABORATORY TESTS

Many abnormalities of renal, hepatic, and bone marrow function have been reported in patients with neoplastic disease and receiving mechlorethamine. It is advisable to check renal, hepatic and bone marrow functions frequently.

CARCINOGENESIS, MUTAGENESIS, AND IMPAIRMENT OF FERTILITY

Therapy with alkylating agents such as mechlorethamine HCl may be associated with an increased incidence of a second malignant tumor, especially when such therapy is combined with other antineoplastic agents or radiation therapy.

Young-adult female RF mice were injected intravenously with four doses of 2.4 mg/kg of mechlorethamine (0.1% solution) at 2-week intervals with observations for up to 2 years. An increased incidence of thymic lymphomas and pulmonary adenomas was observed. Painting mechlorethamine on the skin of mice for period sup to 33 weeks resulted in squamous cell tumors in 9 of 33 mice.

Mechlorethamine induced mutations in the Ames test, in *E. Coli*, and *Neurospora Crassa*. Mechlorethamine caused chromosome aberration in a variety of plant and mammalian cells. Dominant lethal mutations were produced in ICR/Ha Swiss mice.

Mechlorethamine impaired fertility in the rat at a daily dose of 500 mg/kg intravenously for two weeks.

PREGNANCY CATEGORY D

See WARNINGS.

PRECAUTIONS: *(cont'd)*

NURSING MOTHERS

It is not known whether this drug is excreted in human milk. Because many drugs are excreted in human milk and because of the potential for serious adverse reactions in nursing infants from mechlorethamine HCl, a decision should be made whether to discontinue nursing or discontinue the drug, taking into the importance of the drug to the mother.

PEDIATRIC USE

Safety and effectiveness in children have not been established by well-controlled studies. Use of mechlorethamine HCl in children has been quite limited. Mechlorethamine HCl has been used in Hodgkin's disease, stages III and IV, in combination with other oncolytic agents (MOPP schedule). The MOPP chemotherapy combination includes mechlorethamine, vincristine, procarbazine, and prednisone or prednisolone.[2,3]

ADVERSE REACTIONS:

Clinical use of mechlorethamine HCl *usually is accompanied by toxic manifestations.*

LOCAL TOXICITY

Thrombosis and thrombophlebitis may result from direct contact of the drug with the intima of the injected vein. Avoid high concentrations and prolonged contact with the drug, especially in cases of elevated pressure in the antebrachial vein (*e.g.,* in mediastinal tumor compression from severe vena cava syndrome).

SYSTEMIC TOXICITY

General: Hypersensitivity reactions, including anaphylaxis, have been reported. Nausea, vomiting and depression of formed elements in the circulating blood are dose-limiting side effects and usually occur with the use of full doses of mechlorethamine HCl. Jaundice, alopecia, vertigo, tinnitus and diminished hearing may occur infrequently. Rarely, hemolytic anemia associated with such diseases as the lymphomas and chronic lymphocytic leukemia may be precipitated by treatment with alkylating agents including mechlorethamine HCl. Also, various chromosomal abnormalities have been reported in association with nitrogen mustard therapy.

Mechlorethamine HCl is given preferably at night in case sedation for side effects is required. Nausea and vomiting usually occur 1 to 3 hours after use of the drug. Emesis may disappear in the first 8 hours, but nausea may persist for 24 hours. Nausea and vomiting may be so severe as to precipitate vascular accidents in patients with a hemorrhagic tendency. Premedication with antiemetics, in addition to sedatives, may help control severe nausea and vomiting. Anorexia, weakness and diarrhea may also occur.

Hematologic: The usual course of mechlorethamine HCl (total dose of 0.4 mg/kg either given as single intravenous dose or divided into two or four daily doses of 0.2 or 0.1 mg/kg respectively) generally produces a lymphocytopenia within 24 hours after the first injection; significant granulocytopenia occurs within 6 to 8 days and lasts for 10 days day to 3 weeks. Agranulocytosis appears to be relatively infrequent and recovery from leukopenia in most cases is complete within two weeks of the maximum reduction. Thrombocytopenia is variable but the time course of the appearance and recovery from reduced platelet counts generally parallels the sequence of granulocyte levels. In some cases severe thrombocytopenia may lead to bleeding from the gums and gastrointestinal tract, petechiae, and small subcutaneous hemorrhages; these symptoms appear to be transient and in most cases disappear with return to a normal platelet count. However, a severe and even uncontrollable depression of the hematopoietic system occasionally may follow the usual dose of mechlorethamine HCl, particularly in patients with widespread disease and debility and in patients previously treated with other antineoplastic agents or x-ray. Persistent pancytopenia has been reported. In rare instances, hemorrhagic complications may be due to hyper-heparinemia. Erythrocyte and hemoglobin levels may decline during the first 2 weeks after therapy but rarely significantly. Depression of the hematopoietic system may be found up to 50 days or more after starting therapy.

Integumentary: Occasionally, a maculopapular skin eruption occurs, but this may be idiosyncratic and does not necessarily recur with subsequent courses of the drug. Erythema multiforme has been observed. Herpes zoster, a common complicating infection in patients with lymphomas, may first appear after therapy is instituted and on occasion may be precipitated by treatment. Further treatment should be discontinued during the acute phase of this illness to avoid progression to generalized herpes zoster.

Reproductive: Since the gonads are susceptible to mechlorethamine HCl, treatment may be followed by delayed catamenia, oligomenorrhea, or temporary or permanent amenorrhea. Impaired spermatogenesis, azoospermia, and total germinal aplasia have been reported in male patients treated with alkylating agents, especially in combination with other drugs. In some instances spermatogenesis may return in patients in remission, but this may occur only several years after intensive chemotherapy has been discontinued. Patients should be warned of the potential risk to their reproductive capacity.

OVERDOSAGE:

With total doses exceeding 0.4 mg/kg of body weight for a single course, severe leukopenia, anemia, thrombocytopenia and a hemorrhagic diathesis with subsequent delayed bleeding may develop. Death may follow. The only treatment in instances of excessive dosage appears to be repeated blood product transfusions, antibiotic treatment of complicating infections and general supportive measures.

The intravenous LD_{50} of mechlorethamine HCl is 2 mg/kg and 1.6 mg/kg in the mouse and rat, respectively.

DOSAGE AND ADMINISTRATION:

INTRAVENOUS ADMINISTRATION

The dosage of mechlorethamine HCl varies with the clinical situation, the therapeutic response and the magnitude of hematologic depression. A total dose of 0.4 mg/kg of body weight for each course usually is given either as a single dose or in divided doses of 0.1 to 0.2 mg/kg per day. Dosage should be based on ideal dry body weight. The presence of edema or ascites must be considered so that dosage will be based on actual weight unaugmented by these conditions.

The margin of safety in therapy with mechlorethamine HCl is narrow and considerable care must be exercised in the matter of dosage. Repeated examinations of blood are *mandatory* as a guide to subsequent therapy. (See OVERDOSAGE).

Within a few minutes after intravenous injection, mechlorethamine HCl undergoes chemical transformation, combines with reactive compounds, and is no longer present in its active form in the blood stream. Subsequent courses should not be given until the patient has recovered hematologically from the previous course; this is best determined by repeated studies of the peripheral blood elements awaiting their return to normal levels. It is often possible to give repeated courses of mechlorethamine HCl as early as three weeks after treatment.

PREPARATION OF SOLUTION FOR INTRAVENOUS ADMINISTRATION

This drug is highly toxic and both powder and solution must be handled and administered with care. Since mechlorethamine HCl is a powerful vesicant, it is intended primarily for intravenous use, and, in most instances is given by this route. Inhalation of dust or vapors and contact with skin or mucous membranes, especially those of the eyes, must be avoided. Rubber gloves should be worn when handling mechlorethamine HCl. Should accidental eye

DOSAGE AND ADMINISTRATION: *(cont'd)*

contact occur, copious irrigation with water, normal saline or a balanced salt ophthalmic irrigating solution should be instituted immediately, followed by prompt ophthalmological consultation. Should accidental skin contact occur, the affected part must be irrigated immediately with copious amounts of water, for at least 15 minutes, followed by 2 percent sodium thiosulfate solutions. (See also BOXED WARNINGand Special Handling).

Each vial of mechlorethamine HCl contains 10 mg of Mechlorethamine HCl triturated with sodium chloride q.s. 100 mg. In neutral or alkaline aqueous solution it undergoes rapid chemical transformation and is highly unstable. Although solutions prepared according to instructions are acidic and do not decompose as rapidly, they should be prepared immediately before each injection since they will decompose on standing. When reconstituted, mechlorethamine HCl is a clear colorless solution. *Do not use if the solution is discolored or if droplets of water are visible within the vial prior to reconstitution.*

Using a sterile 10 ml syringe, inject 10 ml of Sterile Water for Injection or 10 ml Sodium Chloride Injection into a vial of mechlorethamine HCl. With the needle (syringe attached) still in the rubber stopper, shake the vial several times to dissolve the drug completely. The resultant solution contains 1 mg mechlorethamine HCl per ml.

Parenteral drug products should be inspected visually for particulate matter and discoloration prior to administration whenever solution and container permit.

SPECIAL HANDLING

Due to the drug's toxic and mutagenic properties, appropriate precautions including the use of appropriate safety equipment are recommended for the preparation of mechlorethamine HCl for parenteral administration. The National Institutes of Health presently recommends that the preparation of injectable anti-neoplastic drugs should be performed in a Class II laminar flow biological safety cabinet and that personnel preparing drugs of this class should wear surgical gloves and a closed front surgical-type gown with knit cuffs.[17]

Several other guidelines for proper handling and disposal of anti-cancer drugs have been published and should be considered.[18-22] There is no general agreement that all of the procedures recommended in the guidelines are necessary or appropriate.

Accidental Contact: Should accidental eye contact occur, copious irrigation with water, normal saline or a balanced salt ophthalmic irrigating solution should be instituted immediately, followed by prompt ophthalmological consultation. Should accidental skin contact occur, the affected part must be irrigated immediately with copious amounts of water, for at least 15 minutes, followed by 2 percent sodium thiosulfate solution (See also BOXED WARNING).

TECHNIQUE FOR INTRAVENOUS ADMINISTRATION

Withdraw into the syringe the calculated volume of solution required for a single injection. *Dispose of any remaining solution after neutralization* (See Neutralization of Equipment and Unused Solution). Although the drug may be injected directly into any suitable vein, it is injected preferably into the rubber or plastic tubing of a flowing intravenous infusion set. This reduces the possibility of severe local reactions due to extravasation or high concentration of the drug. Injecting the drug into the tubing rather than adding it to the entire volume of the infusion fluid minimizes a chemical reactions between the drug and the solution. The rate of injection apparently is not critical provided it is completed within a few minutes.

INTRACAVITARY ADMINISTRATION

Nitrogen mustard has been used by intracavitary administration with varying success in certain malignant conditions for the control of pleural,[4-13] peritoneal,[5,6,9,11-16] and pericardial,[5,11-13] effusions caused by malignant cells.

The technic and the dose used by any of these routes varies. Therefore, if mechlorethamine HCl is given by the intracavitary route, the published articles concerning such use should be consulted. *Because of the inherent risks involved, the physician should be experienced in the appropriate injection technics, and be thoroughly aware of the indications, dosages, hazards, and precautions as set forth in the published literature. When using mechlorethamine HCl by the intracavitary routes, the general precautions concerning this agent should be borne in mind.*

As a general guide, reference is made especially to the technics of Weisberger et al.[5,11-13] Intracavitary use is indicated in the presence of pleural, peritoneal, or pericardial effusion due to metastatic tumors. Local therapy with nitrogen mustard is used only when malignant cells are demonstrated in the effusion. Intracavitary injection is not recommended when the accumulated fluid is chylous in nature, since results are likely to be poor.

Paracentesis is first performed with most of the fluid being removed from the pleural or peritoneal cavity. The intracavitary use of mechlorethamine HCl may exert at least some of its effect through production of a chemical poudrage. Therefore, the removal of excess fluid allows the drug to more easily contact the peritoneal and pleural linings. For intrapleural or intrapericardial injection nitrogen mustard is introduced directly through the thoracentesis needle. For intraperitoneal injection it is given through a rubber catheter inserted into the trocar used for paracentesis or through a No. 18 gauge needle inserted at another site. This drug should be injected slowly, with frequent aspiration to insure that a free flow of fluid is present. If fluid cannot be aspirated, pain and necrosis due to injection of solution outside the cavity may occur.[5,1-13] Free flow of fluid also is necessary to prevent injection into a loculated pocket and to insure adequate dissemination of nitrogen mustard.

The usual dose of nitrogen mustard for intracavitary injection is 0.4 mg/kg of body weight, through 0.2 mg/kg (or 10 to 20 mg) has been used by the intrapericardial route[5,11-13] The solution is prepared, as previously described for intravenous injection, by adding 10 ml of Sterile Water for Injection or 10 ml of Sodium Chloride Injection to the vial containing 10 mg of mechlorethamine HCl. (Amounts of diluent of 50 to 100 ml or normal saline have also been used.[4,5]) The position of the patient should be changed every 5 to 10 minutes for an hour after injection to obtain more uniform distribution of the drug throughout the serious cavity. The remaining fluid may be removed from the pleural or peritoneal cavity by paracentesis 24 to 36 hours later. The patient should be followed carefully by clinical and x-ray examination to detect reaccumulation of fluid.

Pain occurs rarely with intrapleural use; it is common with intraperitoneal injections and is often associated with nausea, vomiting, and diarrhea of 2 to 3 days duration. Transient cardiac irregularities may occur with intrapericardial injection. Death, possibly accelerated by nitrogen mustard, has been reported following the use of this agent by the intracavitary route.[9] Although absorption of mechlorethamine HCl when given by the intracavitary route is probably not complete because of its rapid deactivation by body fluids, the systemic effect is unpredictable. The acute side effects such as nausea and vomiting are usually mild. Bone marrow depression is generally milder than when the drug is given intravenously. Care should be taken to avoid use by the intracavitary route when other agents which may suppress bone marrow function are being used systemically.

NEUTRALIZATION OF EQUIPMENT AND UNUSED SOLUTION

To clean rubber gloves, tubing, glassware, etc., after giving mechlorethamine HCl (Mechlorethamine HCl), soak them in an aqueous solution containing equal volumes of sodium thiosulfate (5%) and sodium bicarbonate (5%) for 45 minutes. Excess reagents and reaction products are washed away easily with water. Any unused injection solution should be neutralized by mixing with an equal volume of sodium thiosulfate/sodium bicarbonate solution. Allow the mixture to stand for 45 minutes. Vials that have contained mechlorethamine HCl should be treated in the same way with thiosulfate/bicarbonate solution before disposal.

DOSAGE AND ADMINISTRATION: *(cont'd)*

STORAGE

Store at room temperature. Solutions of mechlorethamine HCl decompose on standing; therefore, solutions of the drug should be prepared immediately before use.

REFERENCES:

1. Calabresi, P.; Parks, R.E., Jr.: Antiproliferative agents and drugs used for immunosuppression, in "The Pharmacological Basis of Therapeutics", L.S. Goodman; A. Gilman (eds.), Ed. 5, New York, Macmillan, 1980, p. 1263. **2.** Kolygin, B.A.: Combination chemotherapy of Hodgkins's disease in children, Cancer Philadelphia 38: 1494-1497, Oct. 1976. **3.** Young, R.C.; DeVita, V.T.: Johnson, R.E.: Hodgkin's Disease in childhood, Blood 42: 163-174, Aug, 1973. **4.** Bass, B.H.: Nitrogen mustard in the palliation of lung cancer, Brit. Med. J. 1:617-620, Feb. 27., 1960. **5.** Bonte, F.J.; Storaasli, J.P.; Weisberger, A.S.: Comparative evaluation of radioactive colloidal gold and nitrogen mustard in the treatment of serious effusions if neoplastic origin., Radiol.67:63-66, July 1956. **6.** Fullerton, C.W.; Reed, P.I.: Nitrogen mustard in treatment of pleural and peritoneal effusions, Can. Med. Ass. J. 79: 190-191, Aug. 1, 1958. **7.** Harris, M.S.: The use of chemotherapy for carcinoma of the lung, J. Int. Coll. Surg. 34 666-673, Nov. 1960. **8.** Hepper, N.G.G.; Carr, D.T.: Intrapleural use of nitrogen mustard in malignant pleural effusion, Minn. Med. 43:374-376, June 1960. **9.** Levison, V.B.: Nitrogen mustard in palliation of malignant effusions, Brit. Med. J. 1: 1143-1145, Apr. 22, 1961. **10.** Taylor, L.: A technique for intrapleural administration of nitrogen mustard compounds, Amer. J. Med. Sci. 233:538-541, May 1957. **11.** Weisberger, A.S.: Direct instillation of nitrogen mustard in the management of malignant effusions, Ann. N.Y. Acd. Sci. 68: 1091-1096, Apr. 24, 1958. **12.** Weisberger, A.S.; Bonte, F.J.; Suhrland, L.G.: Management of malignant serious effusions, Geriat. 11:23-30, Jan. 1956. **13.** Weisberger, A.S.; Levine, B.; Storaasli, J.P.: Use of nitrogen mustard in treatment of serious effusions of neoplastic origin, JAMA 159:1704-1707, Dec. 31 1958. **14.** Brown, F.E.; Wright, H.K.: Hypovolemia following intraperitoneal nitrogen mustard therapy, Surg. Gynecol. Obstet. 121: 528-530, Sept. 1965. **15.** Greenwald, E.S.: Cancer chemotherapy, N.Y. Med. J. 66:2532-2548, Oct. 1, 1966. **16.** Rohn, R.J.; Bond, W.H.: Some indications for the use of chemotherapy in neoplastic disorders, J.Ind. Med. Ass. 50:417-428, Apr. 1957. **17.** National Institutes of Health, Division of Safety, in collaboration with Clinical center pharmacy and nursing staff, and National Cancer Institute; Recommendations for the Safe Handling of Parenteral Antineoplastic Drugs, NIH Publication No. 83-2621. **18.** AMA Council Report: Guidelines for Handling parenteral Antineoplastics, JAMA, March 15, 1985. **19.** National Study Commission on Cytotoxic Exposure - Recommendations for Handling Cytotoxic Agents. Available from Louis P. Jeffrey, Sc. D., Director of Pharmacy Services, Rhode Island Hospital, 593 Eddy Street, Providence Rhode Island 02902. **20.** Clinical Oncological Society of Australia: Guidelines and recommendations for safe handling f antineoplastic agents, Med. J. Australia. 1: 426-428, 1983. **21.** Jones, R.B., et. al: Safe handling of chemotherapeutic agents: A report from the Mount Sinai Medical Center. Ca- A Cancer Journal for Clinicians. Sept/Oct, 258-263, 1983. **22.** American Society of Hospital Pharmacists: Technical assistance bulletin on handling cytotoxic drugs in hospitals, Am. J. Hosp. Pharm. 42: 131-137, 1985.

HOW SUPPLIED - EQUIVALENTS NOT AVAILABLE:

Injection, Dry-Soln - Iart; Intra-Art - 10 mg

20 ml x 4	**$40.41**	**MUSTARGEN, Merck**	**00006-7753-31**

MECLIZINE HYDROCHLORIDE *(001708)*

CATEGORIES: Antiarthritics; Antiemetics; Gastrointestinal Drugs; Motion Sickness; Nausea; Nausea and Vomiting; Vertigo/Motion Sickness/Vomiting; Vomiting; Pregnancy Category B; FDA Approval Pre 1982

BRAND NAMES: *Ancolan*; **Antivert**; *Bonadoxina*; *Bonamina*; *Bonamine* (Germany, Canada, Japan); *Calmonal* (Germany); *Chiclida*; *Dramine*; D-Vert; *Duramesan*; En-Vert; Meclarex; Meclicot; Meclizine Hcl; *Meclozine*; Medivert; Meni-D; *Navicalm*; *Peremesin* (Germany); *Postadoxin* (Germany); *Postafen* (Germany); *Postafene*; Ru-Vert-M; *Sea-Legs*; *Suprimal*; Vertin-32; *Yonyun*
(International brand names outside U.S. in italics)

FORMULARIES: Aetna; BC-BS; CIGNA; FHP; Humana; Kaiser; Medco; Medi-Cal; PruCare; United

DESCRIPTION:

Chemically, Meclizine hydrochloride (abbreviated here as meclizine HCl) is 1-(*p*-chloro-α-phenylbenzyl)-4-(*m*-methylbenzyl) piperazine dihydrochloride monohydrate.

Inert ingredients for the tablets are: dibasic calcium phosphate; magnesium stearate; polyethylene glycol; starch; sucrose. The 12.5 mg tablets also contain: Blue 1. The 25 mg tablets also contain: Yellow 6 Lake; Yellow 10 Lake. The 50 mg tablets also contain: Blue 1 Lake; Yellow 10 Lake.

Inert ingredients for the chewable tablets are: lactose; magnesium stearate; raspberry flavor; Red 40; saccharin sodium; siliceous earth; starch; talc.

CLINICAL PHARMACOLOGY:

Meclizine HCl is an antihistamine which shows marked protective activity against nebulized histamine and lethal doses of intravenously injected histamine in guinea pigs. It has a marked effect in blocking the vasodepressor response to histamine, but only a slight blocking action against acetylcholine. Its activity is relatively weak in inhibiting the spasmogenic action of histamine on isolated guinea pig ileum.

INDICATIONS AND USAGE:

Based on a review of this drug by the National Academy of Sciences-National Research Council and/or other information, FDA has classified the indications as follows:

Effective: Management of nausea and vomiting, and dizziness associated with motion sickness.

Possibly Effective: Management of vertigo associated with diseases affecting the vestibular system.

Final classification of the less than effective indications requires further investigation.

CONTRAINDICATIONS:

Meclizine HCl is contraindicated in individuals who have shown a previous hypersensitivity to it.

WARNINGS:

Since drowsiness may, on occasion, occur with use of this drug, patients should be warned of this possibility and cautioned against driving a car or operating dangerous machinery.

Patients should avoid alcoholic beverages while taking this drug. Due to its potential anticholinergic action, this drug should be used with caution in patients with asthma, glaucoma, or enlargement of the prostate gland.

USAGE IN CHILDREN

Clinical studies establishing safety and effectiveness in children have not been done; therefore, usage is not recommended in children under 12 years of age.

USAGE IN PREGNANCY

Pregnancy Category B: Reproduction studies in rats have shown cleft palates at 25-50 times the human dose. Epidemiological studies in pregnant women, however, do not indicate that meclizine increases the risk of abnormalities when administered during pregnancy. Despite

WARNINGS: *(cont'd)*

the animal findings, it would appear that the possibility of fetal harm is remote. Nevertheless, meclizine, or any other medication, should be used during pregnancy only if clearly necessary.

ADVERSE REACTIONS:

Drowsiness, dry mouth and, on rare occasions, blurred vision have been reported.

DOSAGE AND ADMINISTRATION:

VERTIGO

For the control of vertigo associated with diseases affecting the vestibular system, the recommended dose is 25 to 100 mg daily, in divided dosage, depending upon clinical response.

MOTION SICKNESS

The initial dose of 25 to 50 mg of meclizine HCl should be taken one hour prior to embarkation for protection against motion sickness. Thereafter, the dose may be repeated every 24 hours for the duration of the journey.

HOW SUPPLIED - RATED THERAPEUTICALLY EQUIVALENT:

Tablet, Chewable - Oral - 25 mg

100's	$2.54	Meclizine HCl, H.C.F.A. F F P	99999-1708-01
100's	$2.95	Meclizine Hcl, Major Pharms	00904-2393-60
100's	$3.50	Meclizine Hcl, Consolidated Midland	00223-1164-01
100's	$3.50	Meclizine Hcl, Sidmak Labs	50111-0355-01
100's	$4.17	Meclizine HCl, HL Moore Drug Exch	00839-1401-06
100's	$4.80	Meclizine HCl, Rugby	00536-3990-01
100's	**$50.11**	**ANTIVERT, Roerig Pfizer**	**00662-2120-66**
1000's	$21.00	Meclizine Hcl, Consolidated Midland	00223-1164-02
1000's	$23.40	Meclizine Hcl, Sidmak Labs	50111-0355-03
1000's	$25.40	Meclizine HCl, H.C.F.A. F F P	99999-1708-02
1000's	$27.00	Meclizine Hcl, United Res	00677-0416-10
1000's	$29.17	Meclizine HCl, Rugby	00536-3990-10

Tablet, Uncoated - Oral - 12.5 mg

100's	$2.00	Meclizine Hcl, Harber Pharm	51432-0264-03
100's	$2.66	Meclizine HCl, Camall	00147-0137-10
100's	$2.70	Meclizine HCl, H.C.F.A. F F P	99999-1708-03
100's	$2.75	Meclizine Hcl, Consolidated Midland	00223-1162-01
100's	$3.10	Meclizine Hcl 12.5, Major Pharms	00904-2384-60
100's	$3.70	Meclizine Hcl, Par Pharm	49884-0034-01
100's	$3.78	Meclizine Hcl, Sidmak Labs	50111-0353-01
100's	$3.80	Meclizine Hcl, Goldline Labs	00182-0871-01
100's	$3.95	Meclizine HCl, Geneva Pharms	00781-1345-01
100's	$4.38	Meclizine Hcl, Martec Pharms	52555-0509-01
100's	$4.52	Meclizine Hcl, United Res	00677-0418-01
100's	$4.60	Meclizine Hcl, HL Moore Drug Exch	00839-6009-06
100's	$4.65	Meclizine HCl, Rugby	00536-3986-01
100's	$4.65	Meclizine Hcl, Qualitest Pharms	00603-4319-21
100's	$4.72	Meclizine HCl, Rugby	00536-3985-01
100's	$4.95	Meclizine HCl, Geneva Pharms	00781-1542-01
100's	$5.00	Meclizine Hcl, Aligen Independ	00405-4601-01
100's	$5.06	Meclizine HCl, Schein Pharm (US)	00364-0411-01
100's	$5.84	Meclizine Hcl 12.5, Major Pharms	00904-2384-61
100's	$6.91	Meclizine Hcl, Vangard Labs	00615-1553-13
100's	$7.09	Meclizine Hcl, Medirex	57480-0346-01
100's	$20.80	Meclizine Hcl, Goldline Labs	00182-0871-89
100's	**$31.08**	**ANTIVERT, Roerig Pfizer**	**00662-2100-66**
600's	$108.00	Meclizine Hcl, Medirex	57480-0346-06
1000's	$12.50	Meclicot, C O Truxton	00463-7015-10
1000's	$12.95	Meclizine Hcl, Consolidated Midland	00223-1162-02
1000's	$12.95	Meclizine Hcl, Harber Pharm	51432-0264-06
1000's	$13.25	Meclizine Hcl 12.5, H & H Labs	46703-0005-10
1000's	$17.11	Meclizine HCl, Camall	00147-0137-20
1000's	$18.95	Meclizine Hcl, Major Pharms	00904-2384-80
1000's	$20.64	Meclizine Hcl, Sidmak Labs	50111-0353-03
1000's	$22.01	Meclizine Hcl, United Res	00677-0418-10
1000's	$27.00	Meclizine HCl, H.C.F.A. F F P	99999-1708-04
1000's	$29.80	Meclizine Hcl, Qualitest Pharms	00603-4319-32
1000's	$29.85	Meclizine HCl, Rugby	00536-3986-10
1000's	$30.20	Meclizine HCl, Geneva Pharms	00781-1345-10
1000's	$32.19	Meclizine Hcl, Goldline Labs	00182-0871-10
1000's	$32.19	Meclizine Hcl Tablets 12.5 Mg, Aligen Independ	00405-4601-03
1000's	$32.19	Meclizine Hcl, Par Pharm	49884-0034-10
1000's	$32.19	Meclizine Hcl, Mova Pharms	55370-0810-09
1000's	$32.21	Meclizine HCl, Schein Pharm (US)	00364-0411-02
1000's	$32.80	Meclizine Hcl, Martec Pharms	52555-0509-10
1000's	$34.95	Meclizine Hcl, HL Moore Drug Exch	00839-6009-16
1000's	$36.21	Meclizine HCl, Rugby	00536-3985-10
1000's	$36.25	Meclizine Hcl, Geneva Pharms	00781-1542-10
1000's	**$294.77**	**ANTIVERT, Roerig Pfizer**	**00662-2100-82**

Tablet, Uncoated - Oral - 25 mg

8's	$.20	Meclizine HCl, H.C.F.A. F F P	99999-1708-05
32's	$16.55	VERTIN-32, Alba Pharma	10023-0228-32
100's	$2.54	Meclizine HCl, H.C.F.A. F F P	99999-1708-06
100's	$2.90	Meclizine Hcl 25 Mlt, Harber Pharm	51432-0266-03
100's	$3.05	Meclizine Hcl, Squibb-Mark	57783-6810-01
100's	$3.25	Meclizine Hcl, Consolidated Midland	00223-1163-01
100's	$3.56	Meclizine HCl, Camall	00147-0101-10
100's	$4.60	Meclizine Hcl, Par Pharm	49884-0035-01
100's	$4.80	Meclizine Hcl, Sidmak Labs	50111-0354-01
100's	$4.90	Meclizine Hcl, Goldline Labs	00182-0872-01
100's	$4.90	Meclizine HCl, Geneva Pharms	00781-1375-01
100's	$4.90	Meclizine Hcl, Major Pharms	00904-2350-60
100's	$5.69	Meclizine Hcl, United Res	00677-0419-01
100's	$5.85	Meclizine HCl, Rugby	00536-3988-01
100's	$5.88	Meclizine Hcl, Qualitest Pharms	00603-4320-21
100's	$5.90	Meclizine HCl, Geneva Pharms	00781-1544-01
100's	$5.98	Meclizine Hcl, HL Moore Drug Exch	00839-6010-06
100's	$6.35	Meclizine Hcl, Martec Pharms	52555-0510-01
100's	$6.39	Meclizine Hcl, Major Pharms	00904-2350-61
100's	$7.11	Meclizine Hcl 25, Aligen Independ	00405-4602-01
100's	$7.49	Meclizine HCl, Schein Pharm (US)	00364-0412-01
100's	$7.81	Meclizine Hcl, Vangard Labs	00615-1554-13
100's	$23.91	R U VERT M, Solvay Pharms	00032-7025-01
100's	$24.65	MEDIVERT, Med Tek Pharms	52349-0220-10
100's	$25.65	Meclizine Hcl, Medirex	57480-0347-01
100's	$28.69	MECLIZINE HCL, Amer Preferred	53445-0872-00
100's	$38.00	Meclizine Hcl, Goldline Labs	00182-0872-89
100's	**$49.13**	**ANTIVERT/25, Roerig Pfizer**	**00662-2110-66**
500's	$12.70	Meclizine HCl, H.C.F.A. F F P	99999-1708-07
500's	$40.10	Meclizine Hcl, Camall	00147-0101-05

HOW SUPPLIED - RATED THERAPEUTICALLY EQUIVALENT: *(cont'd)*

600's	$173.40	Meclizine Hcl, Medirex	57480-0347-06
1000's	$17.95	Meclizine Hcl, Consolidated Midland	00223-1163-02
1000's	$18.00	Meclizine Hcl 25 Mlt, Harber Pharm	51432-0266-06
1000's	$18.00	Meclizine Hcl, Squibb-Mark	57783-6810-03
1000's	$24.16	Meclizine HCl, Camall	00147-0101-20
1000's	$25.40	Meclizine HCl, H.C.F.A. F F P	99999-1708-08
1000's	$31.35	Meclizine Hcl, Major Pharms	00904-2350-80
1000's	$33.60	Meclizine Hcl, Sidmak Labs	50111-0354-03
1000's	$37.25	Meclizine HCl, Rugby	00536-3988-10
1000's	$37.48	Meclizine Hcl, Qualitest Pharms	00603-4320-32
1000's	$37.48	Meclizine Hcl, United Res	00677-0419-10
1000's	$39.60	Meclizine Hcl, Martec Pharms	52555-0510-10
1000's	$40.56	Meclizine HCl, Geneva Pharms	00781-1375-10
1000's	$40.89	Meclizine Hcl, Goldline Labs	00182-0872-10
1000's	$40.89	Meclizine Hcl, Aligen Independ	00405-4602-03
1000's	$40.89	Meclizine Hcl, Par Pharm	49884-0035-10
1000's	$40.89	Meclizine Hcl, Mova Pharms	55370-0811-09
1000's	$42.93	Meclizine Hcl, HL Moore Drug Exch	00839-6010-16
1000's	$43.56	Meclizine HCl, Geneva Pharms	00781-1544-10
1000's	$48.56	Meclizine Hcl, Schein Pharm (US)	00364-0412-02
1000's	**$466.34**	**ANTIVERT/25, Roerig Pfizer**	**00662-2110-82**

Tablet, Uncoated - Oral - 50 mg

100's	**$93.35**	**ANTIVERT/50, Roerig Pfizer**	**00662-2140-66**

HOW SUPPLIED - NOT RATED EQUIVALENT:

Capsule - Oral - 30 mg

100's	$15.00	NICO-VERT, Edwards Pharms	00485-0058-01

Tablet, Uncoated - Oral - 32 mg

100's	$54.00	VERTIN-32, Alba Pharma	10023-0228-90

MECLOFENAMATE SODIUM *(001710)*

CATEGORIES: Analgesics; Anti-Inflammatory Agents; Antiarthritics; Antihypertensives; Antipyretics; Arthritis; Central Nervous System Agents; Dysmenorrhea; NSAIDS; Nonsteroidal Anti-Inflammatory; Osteoarthritis; Pain; FDA Approval Pre 1982

BRAND NAMES: *Kyroxan*; **Meclomen**; *Melvon*; *Movens* *(International brand names outside U.S. in italics)*

FORMULARIES: Aetna; BC-BS; FHP; WHO

COST OF THERAPY: $231.11 (Arthritis; Capsule; 50 mg; 4/day; 365 days)

PRIMARY ICD9: 715.99 (Osteoarthritis, Unspecified, Multiple Sites)

DESCRIPTION:

Meclofenamate sodium is N-(2, 6-dichloro-m-tolyl) anthranilic acid, sodium salt, monohydrate. It is an antiinflammatory drug for oral administration. Meclomen capsules contain 50 mg or 100 mg meclofenamic acid as the sodium salt. Also contains lactose, NF; magnesium stearate, NF; silica gel, NF; sodium lauryl sulfate, NF. The capsule shell contains colloidal silicon dioxide, NF; FD&C yellow No. 6, gelatin, NF; sodium lauryl sulfate, NF; titanium dioxide, USP.

It is a white powder with melting point 287° to 291°C, molecular weight 336.15, and water solubility greater than 250 mg/ml.

CLINICAL PHARMACOLOGY:

PHARMACODYNAMICS

Meclofenamate sodium is a nonsteroidal agent which has demonstrated antiinflammatory, analgesic, and antipyretic activity in laboratory animals. The mode of action, like that of other nonsteroidal antiinflammatory agents, is not known. Therapeutic action does not result from pituitary-adrenal stimulation. In animal studies, meclofenamate sodium was found to inhibit prostaglandin synthesis and to compete for binding at the prostaglandin receptor site. *In vitro*, meclofenamate sodium was found to be an inhibitor of human leukocyte 5-lipoxygenase activity. These properties may be responsible for the antiinflammatory action of meclofenamate sodium. There is no evidence that meclofenamate sodium alters the course of the underlying disease.

In several human isotope studies, meclofenamate sodium, at a dosage of 300 mg/day, produced a fecal blood loss of 1 to 2 ml per day, and 2 to 3 ml per day at 400 mg/day. Aspirin, at a dosage of 3.6 g/day, caused a fecal blood loss of 6 ml per day.

In a multiple-dose one-week study in normal human volunteers, meclofenamate sodium had little or no effect on collagen-induced platelet aggregation, platelet count, or bleeding time. In comparison, aspirin suppressed collagen-induced platelet aggregation and increased bleeding time. The concomitant administration of antacids (aluminum and magnesium hydroxides) does not interfere with absorption of meclofenamate sodium.

PHARMACOKINETICS

meclofenamate sodium is rapidly absorbed in man following single and multiple oral doses with peak plasma concentrations occurring in 0.5 to 2 hours. Based on a comparison to a suspension of meclofenamic acid, meclofenamate sodium is completely bioavailable.

The plasma concentrations of meclofenamic acid decline monoexponentially following oral administration. In a study in 10 healthy subjects following a single oral dose the apparent elimination half-life ranged from 0.8 to 5.3 hours. After the administration of meclofenamate sodium for 14 days every 8 hours, the apparent elimination half-life ranged from 0.8 to 2.1 hours with no evidence of accumulation of meclofenamic acid in plasma (see TABLE 1.)

Meclofenamic acid is extensively metabolized to an active metabolite (Metabolite 1; 3-hydroxymethyl metabolite of meclofenamic acid) and at least six other less well characterized minor metabolites. Only this Metabolite l has been shown *in vitro* to inhibit cyclooxygenase activity with approximately one fifth the activity of meclofenamate sodium. Metabolite l (3-hydroxymethyl metabolite of meclofenamic acid) with a mean half-life of approximately 15 hours did accumulate following multiple dosing. After the administration of 100 mg meclofenamate sodium for 14 days every 8 hours, Metabolite l reached a peak plasma concentration of only 1 mcg/ml. By contrast, the peak concentration was 4.8 mcg/ml for the parent compound on both days 1 and 14. Therefore, the accumulation of Metabolite l is probably not clinically significant.

Approximately 70% of the administered dose is excreted by the kidneys with 8%-35% excreted as predominantly conjugated species of meclofenamic acid and Metabolite l (See TABLE 1) Other metabolites, whose excretion rates are unknown, account for the remaining 35%-62% of the dose excreted in the urine. The remainder of the administered dose (approximately 30%) is eliminated in the feces (apparently through biliary excretion). There is insufficient experience to know if meclofenamate sodium or its metabolites accumulate in

CLINICAL PHARMACOLOGY: *(cont'd)*

TABLE 1 SUMMARY OF MECLOFENAMATE SODIUM PHARMACOKINETIC PARAMETERS
Mean (Range) Parameter Value (n = 10)

	Meclofenamic Acid 100 mg[b]	Metabolite l[a]
Cmax mcg/ml[1]	4.8 (1.8-7.2)	1.0 (0.5-1.5)
tmax hr[2]	0.9 (0.5-1.5)	2.4 (0.5-4.0)
Cmin mcg/ml[3]	0.2 (0.5-1.5)	0.4 (0.2-1.1)
Cl/F ml/min[4]	206.0 (126-342)	-
Vd/F liters[5]	23.3 (9.1-43.2)	-
t 1/2 hr[6]	1.3 (0.8-2.1)	15.3[c]
% of Dose in Urine	0.0 -	
Unconjugated		0.5 (0-1.2)
Total	2.7 (0-4.5)	21.6 (7.5-32.6)

[a] 3-Hydroxymethyl metabolite of meclofenamic acid with 20% activity of Meclofenamate sodium *in vitro*
[b] Administered every 8 hours for 14 days
[c] Estimated from mean data
[1] Peak plasma concentration
[2] Time to peak plasma concentration
[3] Trough plasma concentration
[4] Oral clearance
[5] Oral distribution volume
[6] Elimination half-life

patients with compromised renal or hepatic function. Therefore, meclofenamate sodium should be used with caution in these patients (see PRECAUTIONS.) Trace amounts of meclofenamate sodium are excreted in human breast milk.

Meclofenamic acid is greater than 99% bound to plasma proteins over a wide drug concentration range.

Unlike most NSAIDs, which when administered with food have a decrease in rate but not in extent of absorption, meclofenamic acid is decreased in both. Following the administration of meclofenamate sodium capsules one half-hour after a meal, the average extent of bioavailability decreased by 26%, the average peak concentration (Cmax) decreased fourfold and the time to Cmax was delayed by 3 hours.

CLINICAL STUDIES:

Controlled clinical trials comparing meclofenamate sodium with aspirin demonstrated comparable efficacy in rheumatoid arthritis.

The meclofenamate sodium-treated patients had fewer reactions involving the special senses, specifically tinnitus, but more gastrointestinal reactions, specifically diarrhea.

The incidence of patients who discontinued therapy due to adverse reactions was similar for both the meclofenamate sodium and aspirin-treated groups.

The improvement with meclofenamate sodium reported by patients and the reduction of the disease activity as evaluated by both physicians and patients with rheumatoid arthritis are associated with a significant reduction in number of tender joints, severity of tenderness, and duration of morning stiffness.

The improvement reported by patients and as evaluated by physicians in patients treated with meclofenamate sodium for osteoarthritis is associated with a significant reduction in night pain, pain on walking, degree of starting pain, and pain on passive motion. The function of knee joints also improved significantly.

Meclofenamate sodium has been used in combination with gold salts or corticosteroids in patients with rheumatoid arthritis. Studies have demonstrated that meclofenamate sodium contributes to the improvement of patients' conditions while maintained on gold salts or corticosteroids. Data are inadequate to demonstrate that meclofenamate sodium in combination with salicylates produces greater improvement than that achieved with meclofenamate sodium alone.

In controlled clinical trials of patients with mild to moderate pain, meclofenamate sodium 50 mg provided significant pain relief. In these studies of episiotomy and dental pain, meclofenamate sodium 100 mg demonstrated additional benefit in some patients. The onset of analgesic effect was generally within one hour and the duration of action was 4 to 6 hours.

In controlled clinical trials of patients with dysmenorrhea, meclofenamate sodium 100 mg t.i.d. provided significant reduction in the symptoms associated with dysmenorrhea.

In randomized double-blind crossover trials of meclofenamate sodium 100 mg t.i.d. versus placebo in women with heavy menstrual blood loss (MBL), meclofenamate sodium treatment was usually associated with a reduction in menstrual flow.

(Note: For "Scattergram of Menstrual Flow" chart, please refer to original package insert).

In association with this reduction in menstrual blood loss, the duration of menses was decreased by 1 day; tampon/pad usage was decreased by an average of two per day on the 2 days of heaviest flow; and symptoms of dysmenorrhea were significantly reduced.

INDICATIONS AND USAGE:

Meclofenamate sodium is indicated for the relief of mild to moderate pain.

Meclofenamate sodium is also indicated for the treatment of primary dysmenorrhea and for the treatment of idiopathic heavy menstrual blood loss (see CLINICAL PHARMACOLOGY and PRECAUTIONS).

Meclofenamate sodium is also indicated for relief of the signs and symptoms of acute and chronic rheumatoid arthritis and osteoarthritis. As with all nonsteroidal antiinflammatory drugs, selection of meclofenamate sodium requires a careful assessment of the benefit/risk ratio (see WARNINGS, PRECAUTIONS, and ADVERSE REACTIONS).

Meclofenamate sodium is not recommended in children because adequate studies to demonstrate safety and efficacy have not been carried out.

CONTRAINDICATIONS:

Meclofenamate sodium should not be used in patients who have previously exhibited hypersensitivity to it.

Because the potential exists for cross-sensitivity to aspirin or other nonsteroidal antiinflammatory drugs, meclofenamate sodium should not be given to patients in whom these drugs induce symptoms of bronchospasm, allergic rhinitis, or urticaria.

WARNINGS:

RISK OF GI ULCERATION, BLEEDING AND PERFORATION WITH NSAID THERAPY

Serious gastrointestinal toxicity such as bleeding, ulceration, and perforation can occur at any time, with or without warning symptoms, in patients treated chronically with NSAID therapy. Although minor upper gastrointestinal problems, such as dyspepsia, are common, usually developing early in therapy, physicians should remain alert for ulceration and bleeding in patients treated chronically with NSAIDs even in the absence of previous GI tract

WARNINGS: *(cont'd)*

symptoms. In patients observed in clinical trials of several months to 2 years duration, symptomatic upper GI ulcers, gross bleeding, or perforation appear to occur in approximately 1% of patients treated for 3-6 months, and in about 2%-4% of patients treated for one year. Physicians should inform patients about the signs and/or symptoms of serious GI toxicity and what steps to take if they occur.

Studies to date have not identified any subset of patients not at risk of developing peptic ulceration and bleeding. Except for a prior history of serious GI events and other risk factors known to be associated with peptic ulcer disease, such as alcoholism, smoking, etc., no risk factors (*e.g.,* age, sex) have been associated with increased risk. Elderly or debilitated patients seem to tolerate ulceration or bleeding less well than other individuals, and most spontaneous reports of fatal GI events are in this population. Studies to date are inconclusive concerning the relative risk of various NSAIDs in causing such reactions. High doses of any NSAID probably carry a greater risk of these reactions, although controlled clinical trials showing this do not exist in most cases. In considering the use of relatively large doses (within the recommended dosage range), sufficient benefit should be anticipated to offset the potential increased risk of GI toxicity.

PRECAUTIONS:

GENERAL

Patients receiving nonsteroidal antiinflammatory agents, such as meclofenamate sodium, should be evaluated periodically to insure that the drug is still necessary and well tolerated see other PRECAUTIONS, WARNINGSand ADVERSE REACTIONS.

Diarrhea, gastrointestinal irritation and abdominal pain may be associated with meclofenamate sodium therapy. Dosage reduction or temporarily stopping the drug have generally controlled these symptoms (see ADVERSE REACTIONS and DOSAGE AND ADMINISTRATION).

Decreases in hemoglobin and/or hematocrit levels have occurred in approximately 1 of 6 patients, but rarely required discontinuation of meclofenamate sodium therapy. The clinical data revealed no evidence of increased chronic blood loss, bone marrow suppression, or hemolysis to account for the decreases in hemoglobin or hematocrit levels. Patients who are receiving long-term meclofenamate sodium therapy should have hemoglobin and hematocrit values determined if anemia is suspected on clinical grounds.

If a patient develops visual symptoms (see ADVERSE REACTIONS) during meclofenamate sodium therapy, the drug should be discontinued and the patient should have a complete ophthalmologic examination.

When meclofenamate sodium is used in combination with steroid therapy, any reduction in steroid dosage should be gradual to avoid the possible complications of sudden steroid withdrawal.

ELDERLY

Adverse effects are seen more commonly in the elderly; therefore, a lower starting dose and careful follow-up are advised.

EVALUATION OF PATIENTS WITH HEAVY MENSTRUAL BLOOD LOSS

Prior to prescribing meclofenamate sodium for heavy blood flow and primary dysmenorrhea, a thorough risk/benefit assessment should be made that takes into account the results described in the CLINICAL PHARMACOLOGY section. It is recommended that meclofenamate sodium treatment not be prescribed for heavy menstrual flow without establishing its idiopathic nature. Spotting or bleeding between cycles should be evaluated fully and not treated with meclofenamate sodium. Worsening of menstrual blood loss or excessive blood loss failing to respond to meclofenamate sodium should also be evaluated by an appropriate work-up and not treated with meclofenamate sodium.

HEPATIC REACTIONS

As with other nonsteroidal antiinflammatory drugs, borderline elevations of one or more liver tests may occur in some patients. These abnormalities may progress, may remain essentially unchanged, or may be transient with continued therapy. The SGPT (ALT) test is probably the most sensitive indicator of liver dysfunction. Meaningful (three times the upper limit of normal) elevations of SGPT or SGOT (AST) occurred in controlled clinical trials in less than 1% of patients. A patient with symptoms and/or signs suggesting liver dysfunction, or in whom an abnormal liver test has occurred, should be evaluated for evidence of the development of more severe hepatic reaction while on therapy with meclofenamate sodium. Severe hepatic reactions, including jaundice and cases of fatal hepatitis, have been reported with other nonsteroidal antiinflammatory drugs. Although such reactions are rare, if abnormal liver tests persist or worsen, if clinical signs and symptoms consistent with liver disease develop, or if systemic manifestations occur (*e.g.,* eosinophilia, rash), meclofenamate sodium should be discontinued.

RENAL EFFECTS

As with other nonsteroidal antiinflammatory drugs, long-term administration of meclofenamate sodium to animals has resulted in renal papillary necrosis and other abnormal renal pathology. In humans, there have been reports of acute interstitial nephritis with hematuria, proteinuria, and occasionally nephrotic syndrome.

A second form of renal toxicity has been seen in patients with prerenal conditions leading to a reduction in renal blood flow or blood volume, where the renal prostaglandins have a supportive role in the maintenance of renal perfusion. In these patients administration of an NSAID may cause a dose-dependent reduction in prostaglandin formation and may precipitate overt renal decompensation. Patients at greatest risk of this reaction are those with impaired renal function, heart failure, liver dysfunction, those taking diuretics, and the elderly. Discontinuation of NSAID therapy is typically followed by recovery to the pretreatment state.

Since meclofenamate sodium metabolites are eliminated primarily by the kidneys, patients with significantly impaired renal function should be closely monitored; a lower daily dosage should be employed to avoid excessive drug accumulation.

INFORMATION FOR THE PATIENT

Patients should be advised that nausea, vomiting, diarrhea, and abdominal pain have been associated with the use of meclofenamate sodium. The patient should be made aware of a possible drug connection and accordingly should consider discontinuing the drug and contacting his or her physician if any of these conditions are severe.

Women who are taking meclofenamate sodium for heavy menstrual flow should be advised to consult their doctor if they have spotting or bleeding between cycles or worsening of their menstrual blood flow. These symptoms may be signs of the development of a more serious condition that is not appropriately treated with meclofenamate sodium.

Meclofenamate sodium may be taken with meals or milk to control gastrointestinal complaints. Concomitant administration of an antacid (specifically, aluminum and magnesium hydroxides) does not interfere with the absorption of the drug.

Meclofenamate sodium, like other drugs of its class, is not free of side effects. The side effects of these drugs can cause discomfort, and rarely, there are more serious side effects, such as gastrointestinal bleeding, which may result in hospitalization and even fatal outcomes.

PRECAUTIONS: *(cont'd)*

NSAIDs (nonsteroidal antiinflammatory drugs) are often essential agents in the management of arthritis and have a major role in the treatment of pain, but they also may be commonly employed for conditions which are less serious.

Physicians may wish to discuss with their patients the potential risks(see WARNINGS, PRECAUTIONS, and ADVERSE REACTIONS) and likely benefits of NSAID treatment, particularly when the drugs are used for less serious conditions where treatment without NSAIDs may represent an acceptable alternative to both the patient and physician.

LABORATORY TESTS

Patients receiving long-term meclofenamate sodium therapy should have hemoglobin and hematocrit values determined if signs or symptoms of anemia occur.

Low white blood cell counts were rarely observed in clinical trials. These low counts were transient and usually returned to normal while the patient continued on meclofenamate sodium therapy. Persistent leukopenia, granulocytopenia, or thrombocytopenia warrants further clinical evaluation and may require discontinuation of the drug.

When abnormal blood chemistry values are obtained, follow-up studies are indicated.

Elevations of serum transaminase levels and of alkaline phosphatase levels occurred in approximately 4% of patients. An occasional patient had elevations of serum creatinine or BUN levels.

Because serious GI tract ulceration and bleeding can occur without warning symptoms, physicians should follow chronically treated patients for the signs and symptoms of ulceration and bleeding and should inform them of the importance of this follow-up (see Risk of GI Ulceration, Bleeding and Perforation with NSAID Therapy).

CARCINOGENESIS

An 18-month study in rats revealed no evidence of carcinogenicity.

USAGE IN PREGNANCY

Meclofenamate sodium, like aspirin and other nonsteroidal antiinflammatory drugs, causes fetotoxicity, minor skeletal malformations, e.g., supernumerary ribs, and delayed ossification in rodent reproduction trials, but no major teratogenicity. Similarly, it prolongs gestation and interferes with parturition and with normal development of young before weaning. Meclofenamate sodium is not recommended for use during pregnancy, particularly in the 1st and 3rd trimesters based on these animal findings. There are, however, no adequate and well-controlled studies in pregnant women.

USAGE IN NURSING MOTHERS

Trace amounts of meclofenamic acid are excreted in human milk. Because of the possible adverse effects of prostaglandin-inhibiting drugs on neonates, meclofenamate sodium is not recommended for nursing women.

PEDIATRIC USE

Safety and effectiveness in children below the age of 14 have not been established.

DRUG INTERACTIONS:

1. Warfarin: Meclofenamate sodium enhances the effect of warfarin. Therefore, when meclofenamate sodium is given to a patient receiving warfarin, the dosage of warfarin should be reduced to prevent excessive prolongation of the prothrombin time.

2. Aspirin: Concurrent administration of aspirin may lower meclofenamate sodium plasma levels, possible by competing for protein-binding sites. The urinary excretion of meclofenamate sodium is unaffected by aspirin, indicating no change in meclofenamate sodium absorption. Meclofenamate sodium does not affect serum salicylate levels. Greater fecal blood loss results from concomitant administration of both drugs than from either drug alone.

3. Propoxyphene: The concurrent administration of propoxyphene hydrochloride does not affect the bioavailability of meclofenamate sodium.

4. Antacids: Concomitant administration of aluminum and magnesium hydroxides does not interfere with absorption of meclofenamate sodium.

ADVERSE REACTIONS:

INCIDENCE GREATER THAN 1%

The following adverse reactions were observed in clinical trials and included observations from more than 2,700 patients, 594 of whom were treated for one year and 248 for at least 2 years.

Gastrointestinal: The most frequently reported adverse reactions associated with meclofenamate sodium involve the gastrointestinal system.In controlled studies of up to 6 months duration, these disturbances occurred in the following decreasing order of frequency with the approximate incidences in parentheses: diarrhea (10%-33%), nausea with or without vomiting (11%), other gastrointestinal disorders (10%), and abdominal pain.* In long-term uncontrolled studies of up to 4 years duration, one third of the patients had at least one episode of diarrhea some time during meclofenamate sodium therapy.

In approximately 4% of the patients in controlled studies, diarrhea was severe enough to require discontinuation of meclofenamate sodium. The occurrence of diarrhea is dose related, generally subsides with dose reduction, and clears with termination of therapy. The incidence of diarrhea in patients with osteo-arthritis is generally lower than that reported in patients with rheumatoid arthritis.

Other reactions less frequently reported were pyrosis,* flatulence,* anorexia, constipation, stomatitis, and peptic ulcer. The majority of the patients with peptic ulcer had either a history of ulcer disease or were receiving concomitant antiinflammatory drugs, including corticosteroids which are known to produce peptic ulceration.

Cardiovascular: edema

Dermatologic: rash,* urticaria, pruritus

Central Nervous System: headache,* dizziness*

Special Senses: tinnitus

*Incidence between 3% and 9%. Those reactions occurring in 1% to 3% of patients are not marked with an asterisk.

INCIDENCE LESS THAN 1% PROBABLY CAUSALLY RELATED

The following adverse reactions were reported less frequently than 1% during controlled clinical trials and through voluntary reports since marketing. The probability of a causal relationship exists between the drug and these adverse reactions.

Gastrointestinal: bleeding and/or perforation with or without obvious ulcer formation, colitis, cholestatic jaundice

Renal: renal failure

Hematologic: neutropenia, thrombocytopenic purpura, leukopenia, agranulocytosis, hemolytic anemia, eosinophilia, decrease in hemoglobin and/or hematocrit

Dermatologic: erythema multiforme, Stevens-Johnson syndrome, exfoliative dermatitis

Hepatic: alteration of liver function tests

Allergic: lupus and serum sickness-like symptoms

ADVERSE REACTIONS: *(cont'd)*

INCIDENCE LESS THAN 1% CAUSAL RELATIONSHIP UNKNOWN

Other reactions have been reported but under conditions where a causal relationship could not be established. However, in these rarely reported events, that possibility cannot be excluded. Therefore, these observations are listed to alert physicians.

Cardiovascular: palpitations

Central Nervous System: malaise, fatigue, paresthesia, insomnia, depression

Special Senses: blurred vision, taste disturbances, decreased visual acuity, temporary loss of vision, reversible loss of color vision, retinal changes including macular fibrosis, macular and perimacular edema, conjunctivitis, iritis

Renal: nocturia

Gastrointestinal: paralytic ileus

Dermatologic: erythema nodosum, hair loss

OVERDOSAGE:

The following is based on the little information available concerning overdosage with meclofenamate sodium and related compounds. After a massive overdose, CNS stimulation may be manifested by irrational behavior, marked agitation and generalized seizures. Following this phase, renal toxicity (falling urine output, rising creatinine, abnormal urinary cellular elements) may be noted with possible oliguria or anuria and azotemia. A 24-year-old male was anuric for approximately one week after ingesting an overdose of 6-7 grams of meclofenamate sodium. Spontaneous diuresis and recovery subsequently occurred.

Management consists of emptying the stomach by emesis or lavage and instilling an ample dose of activated charcoal into the stomach. There is some evidence that charcoal will actively absorb meclofenamate sodium, but dialysis or hemoperfusion may be less effective because of plasma protein binding. The seizures should be controlled by an appropriate anticonvulsant regimen. Attention should be directed throughout, by careful monitoring, to the preservation of vital functions and fluid-electrolyte balance. Dialysis may be required to correct serious azotemia or electrolyte imbalance.

DOSAGE AND ADMINISTRATION:

USUAL DOSAGE

For Mild to Moderate Pain: the recommended dose is 50 mg every 4 to 6 hours. Doses of 100 mg may be needed in some patients for optimal pain relief (see CLINICAL PHARMACOLOGY). However, the daily dose should not exceed 400 mg (see ADVERSE REACTIONS).

For Excessive Menstrual Blood Loss and Primary Dysmenorrhea: The recommended dose of meclofenamate sodium is 100 mg three times a day, for up to 6 days, starting at the onset of menstrual flow.

For Rheumatoid Arthritis and Osteoarthritis: Including acute exacerbations of chronic disease, the dosage is 200 to 400 mg per day, administered in three or four equal doses.

Therapy should be initiated at the lower dosage, then increased as necessary to improve clinical response. The dosage should be individually adjusted for each patient, depending on the severity of the symptoms and the clinical response. The daily dosage should not exceed 400 mg per day. The smallest dosage of meclofenamate sodium that yields clinical control should be employed.

Although improvement may be seen in some patients in a few days, 2 to 3 weeks of treatment may be required to obtain the optimum therapeutic benefit.

After a satisfactory response has been achieved, the dosage should be adjusted as required. A lower dosage may suffice for long-term administration.

If gastrointestinal complaints occur (see WARNINGS and PRECAUTIONS), meclofenamate sodium may be administered with meals or with milk (see CLINICAL PHARMACOLOGY for a description of food effects). If intolerance occurs, the dosage may need to be reduced. Therapy should be terminated if any severe adverse reactions occur.

Storage: Store at a room temperature below 30°C (86°F). Protect from moisture and light.

HOW SUPPLIED - RATED THERAPEUTICALLY EQUIVALENT:

Capsule, Gelatin - Oral - 50 mg

100's	$15.83	Meclofenamate, H.C.F.A. F F P	99999-1710-01
100's	$22.50	Meclofenamate, US Trading	56126-0414-11
100's	$27.66	Meclofenamate, Bristol Myers Squibb	00003-0622-50
100's	$28.99	Meclofenamate, Lederle Pharm	00005-3480-43
100's	$33.85	Meclofenamate, United Res	00677-1144-01
100's	$33.95	Meclofenamate Sodium, Harber Pharm	51432-0265-03
100's	$34.08	Meclofenamate, Qualitest Pharms	00603-4344-21
100's	$35.50	Meclofenamate, Major Pharms	00904-1413-60
100's	$39.67	Meclofenamate Sodium, Amer Preferred	53445-1270-01
100's	$39.69	Meclofenamate, HL Moore Drug Exch	00839-7274-06
100's	$39.80	Meclofenamate, Schein Pharm (US)	00364-2155-01
100's	$39.95	Meclofenamate, Mylan	00378-2150-01
100's	$43.70	Meclofenamate Sodium, Elkins Sinn	00641-4506-86
100's	**$74.12**	**MECLOMEN, Parke-Davis**	**00071-0268-24**
100's	**$75.92**	**MECLOMEN, Parke-Davis**	**00071-0268-40**
200's	$31.00	Meclofenamate, Raway	00686-0496-20
500's	$36.25	Meclofenamate, Geneva Pharms	00781-2702-01
500's	$79.15	Meclofenamate, H.C.F.A. F F P	99999-1710-02
500's	$98.40	Meclofenamate, Major Pharms	00904-1413-40
500's	$114.90	Meclofenamate, Elkins Sinn	00641-4506-88
500's	$148.60	Meclofenamate, Qualitest Pharms	00603-4344-28
500's	$183.06	Meclofenamate, HL Moore Drug Exch	00839-7274-12
500's	$261.55	Meclofenamate, Mylan	00378-2150-05

Capsule, Gelatin - Oral - 100 mg

100's	$23.93	Meclofenamate, H.C.F.A. F F P	99999-1710-03
100's	$38.30	Meclofenamate, Bristol Myers Squibb	00003-0629-50
100's	$39.00	Meclofenamate, Raway	00686-0497-20
100's	$45.40	Meclofenamate, Qualitest Pharms	00603-4345-21
100's	$45.80	Meclofenamate, United Res	00677-1145-01
100's	$45.90	Meclofenamate, Major Pharms	00904-1414-60
100's	$46.95	Meclofenamate Sodium, Harber Pharm	51432-0263-03
100's	$48.29	Meclofenamate, Geneva Pharms	00781-2703-01
100's	$49.35	Meclofenamate Sodium, Amer Preferred	53445-1271-01
100's	$51.06	Meclofenamate, Bristol Myers Squibb	00003-0692-50
100's	$51.30	Meclofenamate Sodium, Elkins Sinn	00641-4507-86
100's	$52.45	Meclofenamate, Schein Pharm (US)	00364-2156-01
100's	$63.38	Meclofenamate, HL Moore Drug Exch	00839-7275-06
100's	$75.30	Meclofenamate, Parmed Pharms	00349-8638-01
100's	$75.95	Meclofenamate, Mylan	00378-3000-01
100's	**$88.99**	**MECLOMEN, Parke-Davis**	**00071-0269-40**
100's	**$102.62**	**MECLOMEN, Parke-Davis**	**00071-0269-24**
500's	$104.99	Meclofenamate, Balan	00304-1721-05
500's	$119.65	Meclofenamate, H.C.F.A. F F P	99999-1710-04
500's	$132.40	Meclofenamate, Major Pharms	00904-1414-40
500's	$148.50	Meclofenamate, Elkins Sinn	00641-4507-88

HOW SUPPLIED - RATED THERAPEUTICALLY EQUIVALENT: *(cont'd)*

500's	$219.47	Meclofenamate, Qualitest Pharms	00603-4345-28
500's	$230.50	Meclofenamate Sodium, Schein Pharm (US)	00364-2156-05
500's	$261.35	Meclofenamate, HL Moore Drug Exch	00839-7275-12
500's	$261.95	Meclofenamate, Mylan	00378-3000-05
500's	**$440.63**	**MECLOMEN, Parke-Davis**	**00071-0269-30**

MEDROXYPROGESTERONE ACETATE *(001712)*

CATEGORIES: Amenorrhea; Antineoplastics; Cancer; Contraceptives; Endometrial Carcinoma; Hormonal Imbalance; Hormones; Oncologic Drugs; Progesterone; Progestins; Progestogen; Renal Cell Carcinoma; Uterine Bleeding; Osteoporosis*; Sales > $100 Million; FDA Approval Pre 1982; Patent Expiration 1994 Jul; Top 200 Drugs

* Indication not approved by the FDA

BRAND NAMES: Amen; *Aragest*; *Aragest 5*; *Asconale*; *Clinofem* (Germany); *Clinovir*; Curretab; Cycrin; Depo-Provera; Depo-Provera Contraceptive; *Farlutal*; *Gestapuran*; *Hysron*; *Lutoral*; Med-Pro; *Medrone*; *Meprate*; *Perlutex*; *Perlutex Leo*; *Prodasone*; *Progeston*; *Progevera*; **Provera**; *Ralovera*

(International brand names outside U.S. in italics)

FORMULARIES: Aetna; BC-BS; CIGNA; DoD; FHP; Humana; Kaiser; Medco; Medi-Cal; PCS; PruCare; United; WHO

WARNING:

THE USE OF MEDROXYPROGESTERONE ACETATE DURING THE FIRST FOUR MONTHS OF PREGNANCY IS NOT RECOMMENDED.

Progestational agents have been used beginning with the first trimester of pregnancy in an attempt to prevent habitual abortion. There is no adequate evidence that such use is effective when drugs are given during the first four months of pregnancy. Furthermore, in the vast majority of women, the cause of abortion is a defective ovum, which progestational agents could not be expected in influence. In addition, the use of progestational agents, with their uterine relaxant properties, in patients with fertilized defective ova may cause a delay in spontaneous abortion. Therefore, the use of such drugs during the first four months of pregnancy is not recommended.

Several reports suggest an association between intrauterine exposure to progestational drugs in the first trimester of pregnancy and genital abnormalities in male and female fetuses. The risk of hypospadias, 5 to 8 per 1,000 male births in the general population, may be approximately doubled with exposure to these drugs. There are sufficient data to quantify the risk to exposed female fetuses, but insofar as some of these drugs induce mild virilization of the external genitalia of the female fetus, and because of the increased association of hypospadias in the male fetus, it is prudent to avoid the use of these drugs during the first trimester of pregnancy.

If the patient is exposed to medroxyprogesterone acetate during the first four months of pregnancy or if she becomes pregnant while taking this drug, she should be apprised of the potential risks to the fetus.

DESCRIPTION:

Patients should be counseled that this product does not protect against HIV infection (AIDS) and other sexually transmitted diseases.

ORAL TABLETS AND STERILE AQUEOUS SUSPENSION

Oral Tablets: Medroxyprogesterone Acetate Tablets contain medroxyprogesterone acetate, which is a derivative of progesterone. It is a white to off-white, odorless crystalline powder, stable in air, melting between 200 and 210°C. It is freely soluble in chloroform, soluble in acetone and in dioxane, sparingly soluble in alcohol and in methanol, slightly soluble in ether, and insoluble in water.

The chemical name for medroxyprogesterone acetate is Pregn-4-ene-3,20-dione, 17-(acetyloxy)-6-methyl-,(6α)-.

Each Medroxyprogesterone Acetate tablet for oral administration contains 2.5 mg, 5 mg or 10 mg of medroxyprogesterone acetate. Inactive ingredients: calcium stearate, corn starch, lactose, mineral oil, sorbic acid, sucrose, talc. The 2.5 mg tablet contain FD&C Yellow no. 6.

STERILE AQUEOUS SUSPENSION

Medroxyprogesterone Acetate Sterile Aqueous Suspension contains Medroxyprogesterone Acetate which is a derivative of progesterone and is active by the parenteral and oral routes of administration. It is a white to off-white, odorless crystalline powder, stable in air, melting between 200° and 210° C. It is freely soluble in chloroform, soluble in acetone and dioxane, sparingly soluble in ether and insoluble in water.

Medroxyprogesterone Acetate Sterile Aqueous Suspension for intramuscular injection is available in 2 strengths, 100 mg/ml and 400 mg/ml Medroxyprogesterone Acetate.

Each ml of the **100 mg/ml** suspension contains:

Medroxyprogesterone Acetate: 100 mg

Also

Polyethylene Glycol 3350: 27.6 mg

Polysorbate 80: 1.84 mg

Sodium Chloride: 8.3 mg with

Methylparaben: 1.75 mg

Propylparaben: 0.194 mg added as preservatives

Each ml of the **400 mg/ml** suspension contains:

Medroxyprogesterone Acetate: 400 mg

Polyethylene glycol 3350: 20.3 mg

Sodium Sulfate Anhydrous: 11 mg with

Myristyl-Gamma-Picolinium Chloride: 1.69 mg added as a preservative

When necessary, pH was adjusted with sodium hydroxide and/or hydrochloric acid.

CONTRACEPTIVE INJECTION

Depo-Provera Contraceptive Injection contains medroxyprogesterone acetate, a derivative of progesterone, as its active ingredient. Medroxyprogesterone acetate is active by the parenteral and oral routes of administration. It is a white to off-white, odorless crystalline powder that is

DESCRIPTION: *(cont'd)*

stable in air and that melts between 200° C and 210° C. It is freely soluble in chloroform, soluble in acetone and dioxane, sparingly soluble in alcohol and methanol, slightly soluble in ether, and insoluble in water.

The chemical name for medroxyprogesterone acetate is pregn-4-ene-3,20-dione, 17-(acetyloxy)-6-methyl-,(6α)-.

Depo-Provera Contraceptive Injection for intramuscular (IM) injection is available in 150 mg/ml vials each containing 1 ml medroxyprogesterone acetate sterile aqueous suspension.

Each ml contains:

Medroxyprogesterone Acetate: 150 mg
Polyethylene glycol 3350: 28.9 mg
Polysorbate 80: 2.41 mg
Sodium Chloride: 8.68 mg
Methylparaben: 1.37 mg
Propylparaben: 0.150 mg
Water for Injection: qs

When necessary, pH is adjusted with sodium hydroxide and/or hydrochloric acid.

CLINICAL PHARMACOLOGY:

ORAL TABLETS

Medroxyprogesterone acetate, administered orally or parenterally in the recommended doses to women with adequate endogenous estrogen, transforms proliferative into secretory endometrium. Androgenic and anabolic effects have been noted, but the drug is apparently devoid of significant estrogenic activity. While parenterally administered medroxyprogesterone acetate inhibits gonadotropin production, which in turn prevents follicular maturation and ovulation, available data indicate that this does not occur when the usually recommended oral dosage is given as single daily doses.

STERILE AQUEOUS SUSPENSION

Medroxyprogesterone acetate, administered orally or parenterally in the recommended doses to women with adequate endogenous estrogen, transforms proliferative into secretory endometrium.

Medroxyprogesterone Acetate inhibits (in the usual dose range) the secretion of pituitary gonadotropin which in turn, prevents follicular maturation and ovulation.

Because of its prolonged action and the resulting difficulty in predicting the time of withdrawal bleeding following injection, medroxyprogesterone acetate is not recommended in secondary amenorrhea or dysfunctional uterine bleeding. In these conditions oral therapy is recommended.

CONTRACEPTIVE INJECTION

Depo-Provera Contraceptive Injection (medroxyprogesterone acetate), when administered at the recommended dose to women every 3 months, inhibits the secretion of gonadotropins which, in turn, prevents follicular maturation and ovulation and results in endometrial thinning. These actions produce its contraceptive effect.

Following a single 150 mg IM dose of Depo-Provera Contraceptive Injection, medroxyprogesterone acetate concentrations, measured by an extracted radioimmunoassay procedure, increase for approximately 3 weeks to reach peak plasma concentrations of 1 to 7 ng/ml. The levels then decrease exponentially until they become undetectable (<100 pg/ml) between 120 to 200 days following injection. Using an unextracted radioimmunoassay procedure for the assay of medroxyprogesterone acetate in serum, the apparent half-life for medroxyprogesterone acetate following IM administration of Depo-Provera Contraceptive Injection is approximately 50 days.

Women with lower body weights conceive sooner than women with higher body weights after discontinuing Depo-Provera.

The effect of hepatic and/or renal disease on the pharmacokinetics of Depo-Provera Contraceptive Injection is unknown.

INDICATIONS AND USAGE:

ORAL TABLETS

Secondary amenorrhea; abnormal uterine bleeding due to hormonal imbalance in the absence of organic pathology, such as fibroids or uterine cancer.

STERILE AQUEOUS SUSPENSION

Adjunctive therapy and palliative treatment of inoperable, recurrent, and metastatic endometrial or renal carcinoma.

CONTRACEPTIVE INJECTION

Depo-Provera Contraceptive Injection is indicated only for the prevention of pregnancy. It is a long-term injectable contraceptive in women when administered at 3-month intervals. Dosage does not need to be adjusted for body weight.

In five Depo-Provera clinical studies using Depo-Provera, the 12-month failure rate for the group of women treated with Depo-Provera was zero (no pregnancies reported) to 0.7 by Life-Table method. Pregnancy rates with contraceptive measures are typically reported for only the first year of use as shown in TABLE 1. Except for intrauterine devices (IUD), implants, sterilization, and Depo-Provera, the efficacy of these contraceptive measures depends in part on the reliability of use. The effectiveness of Depo-Provera is dependent upon the patient returning every 3 months for reinjection.

CONTRAINDICATIONS:

ORAL TABLETS AND STERILE AQUEOUS SUSPENSION

1. Thrombophlebitis, thromboembolic disorders, cerebral apoplexy or patients with a past history of these conditions.
2. Liver dysfunction or disease.
3. Known or suspected malignancy of breast or genital organs.
4. Undiagnosed vaginal bleeding.
5. Missed abortion.
6. As a diagnostic test for pregnancy.
7. Known sensitivity to medroxyprogesterone acetate (Tablets or suspension).

CONTRACEPTIVE INJECTION

1. Known or suspected pregnancy or as a diagnostic test for pregnancy.
2. Undiagnosed vaginal bleeding.
3. Known or suspected malignancy of the breast.
4. Active thrombophlebitis, or current or past history of thromboembolic disorders, or cerebral vascular disease.
5. Liver dysfunction or disease.
6. Known sensitivity to Depo-Provera (medroxyprogesterone acetate or any of its other ingredients).

TABLE 1 Lowest Expected and Typical Failure Rates* Expressed as Percent of Women Experiencing An Accidental Pregnancy in the first year of Continuous Use

Method	Lowest Expected	Typical
Injectable progestogen		
Depo-Provera	0.3	0.3
Implants		
Norplant (6 capsules)	0.2†	0.2†
Female Sterilization	0.2	0.4
Male Sterilization	0.1	0.15
Pill		3
Combined	0.1	
Progestogen only	0.5	
IUD		3
Progestasert	2	
Copper T 380A	0.8	
Condom	2	12
Diaphragm	6	18
Cap	6	18
Spermicides	3	21
Sponge		
Parous women	9	28
Nulliparous women	6	18
Periodic abstinence	1-9	20
Withdrawal	4	18
No method	85	85

Source: Trussell et al[C-1]
* Lowest expected—when used exactly as directed. Typical—includes those not following directions exactly.
† from Norplant package insert.

WARNINGS:

ORAL TABLETS AND STERILE AQUEOUS SUSPENSION

1. The physician should be alert to the earliest manifestations of thrombotic disorders (thrombophlebitis, cerebrovascular disorders, pulmonary embolism, and retinal thrombosis). Should any of these occur or be suspected, the drug should be discontinued immediately.

2. Long term toxicology studies in the monkey, dog, and rat disclose:

1) Beagle dogs receiving 75 mg/kg and 3 mg/kg every 90 days developed mammary nodules, as did some of the control animals. The nodules appearing in the control animals were intermittent in nature, whereas the nodules in the drug treated animals were larger, more numerous, persistent and there were two high dose animals that developed breast malignancies.

2) Two of the monkeys receiving 150 mg/kg every 90 days developed undifferentiated carcinoma of the uterus. No uterine malignancies were found in monkeys receiving 30 mg/kg, 3 mg/kg, or placebo every 90 days. Transient mammary nodules were found during the study in the control, 3 mg/kg and 30 mg/kg groups, but not in the 150 mg/kg group. At sacrifice, the only nodules extant were in three of the monkeys in the 30 mg/kg group. Upon histopathologic examination these nodules have been determined to be hyperplastic.

3) No uterine or breast abnormalities were revealed in the rat.

The relevance of these findings with respect to human has not been established.

ORAL TABLETS

3. Discontinue medication pending examination if there is sudden partial or complete loss of vision, or if there is a sudden onset of proptosis, diplopia or migraine. If examination reveals papilledema or retinal vascular lesions, medication should be withdrawn.

4. Detectable amounts of progestin have been identified in the milk of mothers receiving the drug. The effect of this on the nursing infant has not been determined.

5. Usage in pregnancy is not recommended (See BOXED WARNING).

STERILE AQUEOUS SUSPENSION

3. The use of medroxyprogesterone acetate Sterile Aqueous Suspension for contraception is investigational since there are unresolved questions relating to its safety for this indication. Therefore, this is not an approved indication.

4. Discontinue medication pending examination if there is sudden partial or complete loss of vision, or if there is a sudden onset or proptosis, diplopia or migraine. If examination reveals papilledema or retinal vascular lesions, medication should be withdrawn.

5. Usage in pregnancy (See BOXED WARNING).

ORAL TABLETS AND STERILE AQUEOUS SUSPENSION

6. Retrospective studies of morbidity and mortality in Great Britain and studies of morbidity in the United States have shown a statistically significant association between thrombophlebitis, pulmonary embolism, and cerebral thrombosis and embolism and the use of oral contraceptives.[1-4] The estimate of the relative risk of thromboembolism in the study by Vessey and Doll[3] was about seven fold, while Sartwell and associates[4] in the United States found a relative risk of 4.4, meaning that the users are several times as likely to undergo thromboembolic disease without evident cause as nonusers. The American study also indicated that the risk did not persist after discontinuation of administration, and that it was not enhanced by long continued administration. The American study was not designed to evaluate a difference between products.

7. Following repeated injections, amenorrhea and infertility may persist for periods of up to 18 months and occasionally longer.

8. The physician should be alert to the earliest manifestations of impaired liver function. Should these occur or be suspected, the drug should be discontinued and the patient's status re-evaluated.

CONTRACEPTIVE INJECTION

1. Bleeding Irregularities: Most women using Depo-Provera Contraceptive Injection experience disruption of menstrual bleeding patterns. Altered menstrual bleeding patterns include irregular or unpredictable bleeding or spotting, or rarely, heavy or continuous bleeding. If abnormal bleeding persists or is severe, appropriate investigation should be instituted to rule out the possibility of organic pathology, and appropriate treatment should be instituted when necessary.

As women continue using Depo-Provera, fewer experience intermenstrual bleeding and more experience amenorrhea. By month 12 amenorrheas was reported by 55% of women, and by month 24 amenorrhea was reported by 68% of women using Depo-Provera.[C-2]

2. Bone Mineral Density Changes: Use of Depo-Provera may be considered among the risk factors for development of osteoporosis. The rate of bone loss is greatest in the early years of use and then subsequently approaches the normal rate of age related fall.

3. Cancer Risks: Long-term case-controlled surveillance of Depo- Provera Contraceptive Injection users found slight or no increased overall risk of breast cancer[C-3] and no overall increased risk of ovarian,[C-4] liver,[C-5] or cervical[C-6] cancer and a prolonged, protective effect of reducing the risk of endometrial[C-7] cancer in the population of users.

WARNINGS: *(cont'd)*

An increased relative risk (RR) of 2.19% (95% C.I. 1.23-3.89)[C-3] of breast cancer has been associated with use of Depo-Provera in women whose first exposure to drug was within the previous 4 years and who were under 35 years of age [C.I. = Confidence Interval]. However, the overall relative risk for ever-users of Depo-Provera was only 1.2% (95% C.I. 0.96 to 1.52).

Note: A RR of 1.0 indicates neither an increased nor a decreased risk of cancer associated with the use of the drug, relative to no use of the drug. In the case of the sub-population with a RR of 2.19, the 95% CI is fairly wide and does not include the value of 1.0, thus inferring an increased risk of breast cancer in the defined subgroup relative to non- users. The value of 2.19 means that women whose first exposure to drug was within the previous 4 years and who are under 35 years of age have 2.19-fold (95% C.I. 1.23 to 3.89-fold) increased risk of breast cancer relative to nonusers. The National Cancer Institute[C-8] reports an average annual incidence rate for breast cancer for US women, all races, age 30 to 34 years of 26.7 per 100,000. A RR of 2.19 thus, increases the possible risk from 26.7 per 58.5 cases per 100,000 women. The attributable risk, thus, is 3.18 per 10,000 women per year.

A statistically insignificant increase in RR estimates of invasive squamous-cell cervical cancer has been associated with use of Depo-Provera in women who were first exposed before the age of 35 years (RR 1.22 to 1.28 and 95% CI 0.93-1.70). The overall, non-significant relative rate of invasive squamous-cell cervical cancer in women who ever used Depo-Provera was estimated to be 1.11 (95% CI 0.96 to 1.29). No trends in risk with duration of use or times since initial or most recent exposure were observed.

4. Thromboembolic Disorders: The physician should be alert to the earliest manifestations of thrombotic disorders (thrombophlebitis, pulmonary embolism, cerebrovascular disorders, and retinal thrombosis). Should any of these occur or be suspected, the drug should not be readministered.

5. Ocular Disorders: Medication should not be readministered pending examination if there is a sudden or partial or complete loss of vision or if there is a sudden onset of proptosis, diplopia, or migraine. If examination reveals papilledema or retinal vascular lesions, medication should not be readministered.

6. Accidental Pregnancies: Infants from accidental pregnancies that occur 1 to 2 months after injection of Depo-Provera Contraceptive Injection may be at an increased risk of low birth weight, which in turn is associated with an increased risk of neonatal death. The attributable risk is low because such pregnancies are uncommon.[C-9-C-10]

A significant increase in incidence of polysyndactyly and chromosomal anomalies was observed among infants of users of Depo-Provera, the former being most pronounced in women under 30 years of age. The unrelated nature of these defects, the lack of confirmation from other studies, the distant preconceptual exposure to Depo-Provera, and the chance effects due to multiple statistical comparisons, make a causal association unlikely.[C-11]

Children exposed to medroxyprogesterone acetate *in utero* and followed to adolescence, showed no evidence of any adverse effects on their health including their physical, intellectual, sexual or social development.

Several reports suggest an association between intrauterine exposure to progestational drugs in the first trimester of pregnancy and genital abnormalities in male and female fetuses. The risk of hypospadia (5 to 8 per 1,000 male births in the general population) may be approximately doubled with exposure to these drugs. There are insufficient data to quantify the risk to exposed female fetuses, but because some of these drugs induce mild virilization of the external genitalia of the female fetus and because of the increased association of hypospadia in the male fetus, it is prudent to avoid use of these drugs during the first trimester of pregnancy.

To ensure that Depo-Provera is not administered inadvertently to a pregnant woman, it is important that the first injection be given only during the first 5 days after the onset of a normal menstrual period within 5 days postpartum if not breast-feeding and if breast-feeding, at the sixth week postpartum (see DOSAGE AND ADMINISTRATION).

7. Ectopic Pregnancy: Health-care providers should be alert to the possibility of an ectopic pregnancy among women using Depo-Provera Contraceptive Injection who become pregnant or complain of severe abdominal pain.

8. Lactation: Detectable amounts of drug have been identified in the milk of mothers receiving Depo-Provera. In nursing mothers treated with Depo-Provera Contraceptive Injection, milk composition, quality, and amount are not adversely affected. Infants exposed to medroxyprogesterone from breast milk have been studied for developmental and behavioral effects through puberty. No adverse effects have been noted.

9. Anaphylaxis and Anaphylactoid Reaction: Anaphylaxis and anaphylactoid reaction have been reported with the use of Depo-Provera. If an anaphylactic reaction occurs appropriate therapy should be instituted. Serious anaphylactic reactions require emergency medical treatment.

PRECAUTIONS:

ORAL TABLETS AND STERILE AQUEOUS SUSPENSION

1. The pretreatment physical examination should include special reference to breast and pelvic organs, as well as Papanicolaou smear.

2. Because progestogens may cause some degree of fluid retention, conditions which might be influenced by this factor, such as epilepsy, migraine, asthma, cardiac or renal dysfunction, require careful observation.

3. In cases of breakthrough bleeding, as in all cases of irregular bleeding per vaginum, nonfunctional causes should be borne in mind. In cases of undiagnosed vaginal bleeding, adequate diagnostic measures are indicated.

4. Patients who have a history of psychic depression should be carefully observed and the drug discontinued if the depression recurs to a serious degree.

5. Any possible influence of prolonged progestin therapy on pituitary, ovarian, adrenal, hepatic or uterine functions awaits further study.

6. A decrease in glucose tolerance has been observed in a small percentage of patients on estrogen-progestin combination drugs. The mechanism of this decrease is obscure. For this reason, diabetic patients should be carefully observed while receiving progestin therapy.

7. The age of the patient constitutes no absolute limiting factor although treatment with progestins may mask the onset of the climacteric.

8. The pathologist should be advised of progestin therapy when relevant specimens are submitted.

9. Because of the occasional occurrence of thrombotic disorders, (thrombophlebitis, pulmonary embolism, retinal thrombosis, and cerebrovascular disorders) in patients taking estrogen-progestin combinations and since the mechanism is obscure, the physician should be alert to the earliest manifestation of these disorders.

10. Studies of the addition of a progestin product to an estrogen replacement regimen for seven or more days of a cycle of estrogen administration have reported a lowered incidence of endometrial hyperplasia. Morphological and biochemical studies of endometrium suggest that 10-13 days of a progestin are needed to provide maximal maturation of the endometrium and to eliminate any hyperplastic changes. Whether this will provide protection from endometrial carcinoma has not been clearly established. There are possible additional risks which may be associated with the inclusion of progestin in estrogen replacement regimen. The potential risks include adverse effects on carbohydrate and lipid metabolism. The dosage used may be important in minimizing these adverse effects.

11. Aminoglutethimide administered concomitantly with medroxyprogesterone acetate may significantly depress the bioavailability of medroxyprogesterone acetate.

Carcinogenesis, Mutagenesis, and Impairment of Fertility: Long-term intramuscular administration of medroxyprogesterone acetate has been shown to produce mammary tumors in beagle dogs (see WARNINGS). There was no evidence of a carcinogenic effect associated with the oral administration of medroxyprogesterone acetate to rats and mice. Medroxyprogesterone acetate was not mutagenic in a battery of *in vitro* or *in vivo* genetic toxicity assays.

Medroxyprogesterone acetate at high doses is an antifertility drug and high doses would be expected to impair fertility until the cessation of treatment.

Information for the Patient: See PATIENT PACKAGE INSERTat end of insert.

CONTRACEPTIVE INJECTION

1. Physical Examination: The pretreatment and annual history and physical examination should include special reference to breast and pelvic organs, as well as a Papanicolaou smear.

2. Fluid Retention: Because progestational drugs may cause some degree of fluid retention, conditions that might be influenced by this condition, such as epilepsy, migraine, asthma, and cardiac or renal dysfunction, require careful observation.

3. Weight Changes: There is a tendency for women to gain weight while on Depo-Provera therapy. From an initial average body weight of 136 lb, women who completed 1 year of therapy with Depo-Provera gained an average of 5.4 lb, Women who completed 2 years of therapy gained an average of 8.1 lb.

Women who completed 4 years gained an average of 13.8 lb. Women who completed 6 years gained an average of 16.5 lb. Two percent of women withdrew from a large-scale clinical trial because of excessive weight gain.

4. Return of Fertility: Depo-Provera Contraceptive Injection has a prolonged contraceptive effect. In a large U.S. study of women who discontinued use of Depo-Provera to become pregnant, data are available for 61% of them. Based on Life-Table analysis of these data, it is expected that 68% of women who do become pregnant may conceive within 12 months, 83% may conceive within 15 months, and 93% may conceive within 18 months from the last injection. The median time to conception for those who do conceive is 10 months following the last injection with a range of 4 to 31 months, and is unrelated to the duration of use. No data are available for 39% of the patients who discontinued Depo-Provera to become pregnant and who were lost to follow-up or changed their mind.

5. CNS Disorders and Convulsions: Patients who have a history of psychic depression should be carefully observed and the drug not be readministered if the depression recurs.

There have been a few reported cases of convulsions in patients who were treated with Depo-Provera Contraceptive Injection. Association with drug use or pre-existing conditions is not clear.

6. Carbohydrate Metabolism: A decrease in glucose tolerance has been observed in some patients on Depo-Provera treatment. The mechanism of this decrease is obscure. For this reason, diabetic patients should be carefully observed while receiving such therapy.

7. Liver Function: If jaundice develops consideration should be given to not re-administering the drug.

8. Protection Against Sexually Transmitted Diseases: Patients should be counseled that this product does not protect against HIV infection (AIDS) and other sexually transmitted diseases.

Laboratory Test Interactions: The pathologist should be advised of progestin therapy when relevant specimens are submitted.

The following laboratory tests may be affected by progestins including Depo-Provera Contraceptive Injection:

a) Plasma and urinary steroid levels are decreased (*e.g.*, progesterone, estradiol, pregnanediol, testosterone, cortisol).

b) Gonadotropin levels are decreased.

c) Sex-hormone binding globulin concentrations are decreased.

d) Protein bound iodine and butanol extractable protein-bound iodine may increase. T_3 uptake values may decrease.

e) Coagulation test values for prothrombin (Factor II), and Factors VII, VIII, IX, and X may increase.

f) Sulfobromophthalein and other liver function test values may be increased.

g) The effects of medroxyprogesterone acetate on lipid metabolism are inconsistent. Both increases and decreases in total cholesterol, triglycerides, low-density lipoprotein (LDL) cholesterol, and high- density lipoprotein (HDL) cholesterol have been observed in studies.

Carcinogenesis: See WARNINGS, section 3.

Pregnancy Category X See WARNINGS, section 8.

Nursing Mothers: See WARNINGS, section 8.

Information for the Patient: See Patient Labeling.

Patient labeling is included with each single dose vial of Depo-Provera Contraceptive Injection to help describe its characteristics to the patient. It is recommended that prospective users be given this labeling and be informed about the risks and benefits associated with the use of Depo-Provera, as compared with other forms of contraception or with no contraception at all. It is recommended that physicians or other health- care providers responsible for those patients advise them at the beginning of treatment that their menstrual cycle may be disrupted and that irregular and unpredictable bleeding or spotting results, and that this usually decreases to the point of amenorrhea as treatment with Depo-Provera continues, without other therapy being required.

DRUG INTERACTIONS:

CONTRACEPTIVE INJECTION

Aminoglutethimide administered concomitantly with the Depo-Provera Contraceptive Injection may significantly depress the serum concentrations of medroxyprogesterone acetate.[C-12] Users of Depo-Provera should be warned of the possibility of decreased efficacy with the use of this or any related drugs.

ADVERSE REACTIONS:

ORAL TABLETS AND STERILE AQUEOUS SUSPENSION

Pregnancy: See BOXED WARNING for possible adverse effects on the fetus.

Breast: Breast tenderness or galactorrhea has been reported rarely.

Skin: Sensitivity reactions consisting of urticaria, pruritus, edema and generalized rash have occurred in an occasional patient. Acne, alopecia and hirsutism have been reported in a few cases.

Thromboembolic Phenomena: Thromboembolic phenomena including thrombophlebitis and pulmonary embolism have been reported.

ADVERSE REACTIONS: *(cont'd)*

The following adverse reactions have been observed in women taking progestins including medroxyprogesterone acetate tablets:

breakthrough bleeding, spotting, change in menstrual flow, amenorrhea, edema, change in weight (increase or decrease), changes in cervical erosion and cervical secretions, cholestatic jaundice, anaphylactoid reactions and anaphylaxis, rash (allergic) with and without pruritus, mental depression, pyrexia, insomnia, nausea, somnolence.

A statistically significant association has been demonstrated between use of estrogen-progestin combination drugs and the following serious adverse reactions: thrombophlebitis; pulmonary embolism and cerebral thrombosis and embolism. For this reason patients on progestin therapy should be carefully observed.

Although available evidence is suggestive of an association, such a relationship has been neither confirmed nor refuted for the following serious adverse reactions:

neuro-ocular lesions, e.g., retinal thrombosis and optic neuritis.

The following adverse reactions have been observed in patients receiving estrogen progestin combination drugs:

rise in blood pressure in susceptible individuals; premenstrual-like syndrome; changes in libido; changes in appetite; cystitis-like syndrome, headache, nervousness; fatigue; backache; hirsutism; loss of scalp hair; erythema multiforme; erythema nodosum; hemorrhagic eruption; itching; dizziness

In view of these observations, patients on progestin therapy should be carefully observed.

The following laboratory results may be altered by the use of estrogen-progestin combination drugs:

Increased sulfobromophthalein retention and other hepatic function tests.

Coagulation Tests: Increase in prothrombin factors VII, VIII, IX and X

Metyrapone test.

Pregnanediol determination.

Thyroid Function: Increase in PBI, and butanol extractable protein bound iodine and decrease in T^3 uptake values.

CONTRACEPTIVE INJECTION

In the largest clinical trial with Depo-Provera Contraceptive Injection, over 3900 women, who were treated for up to 7 years, reported the following adverse reactions, which may or may not be related to the use of Depo-Provera.

The Following Adverse Reactions Were Reported By More Than 5% Of Subjects:

Menstrual irregularities (bleeding or amenorrhea, or both)
Abdominal pain or discomfort Headache
Weight changes
Dizziness
Headache
Asthenia (weakness or fatigue)
Nervousness

Adverse Reactions Reported By 1% To 5% Of Subjects Using Depo-Provera Were:

Decreased libido or anorgasmia
Pelvic Pain
Backache
Breast Pain
Leg Cramps
No hair growth or alopecia
Depression
Bloating
Nausea
Rash
Insomnia
Edema
Leukorrhea
Hot flashes
Acne
Arthralgia
Vaginitis

Events reported by fewer than 1% of subjects included: galactorrhea, melasma, chloasma, convulsions, changes in appetite, gastrointestinal disturbances, jaundice; genitourinary infections, vaginal cysts, dyspareunia, paresthesia, chest pain, pulmonary embolus, allergic reactions, anemia, drowsiness, syncope, dyspnea and asthma, tachycardia, fever, excessive sweating and body odor, dry skin, chills, increased libido, excessive thirst, hoarseness, pain at injection site, blood dyscrasia, rectal bleeding, changes in breast size, breast lumps or nipple bleeding, axillary swelling, breast cancer, prevention of lactation, sensation of pregnancy, lack of return to fertility, paralysis, facial palsy, scleroderma, osteoporosis, uterine hyperplasia, cervical cancer, varicose veins, dysmenorrhea, hirsutism, accidental pregnancy, thrombophlebitis, deep vein thrombosis.

In addition, voluntary reports have been received of anaphylaxis and anaphylactoid reaction with use of Depo-Provera.

DOSAGE AND ADMINISTRATION:

ORAL TABLETS

Secondary Amenorrhea: Medroxyprogesterone acetate tablets may be given in dosages of 5 to 10 mg daily for from 5 to 10 days. A dose for inducing an optimum secretory transformation of an endometrium that has been adequately primed with either endogenous or exogenous estrogen is 10 mg of medroxyprogesterone acetate daily for 10 days. In cases of secondary amenorrhea, therapy may be started at any time. Progestin withdrawal bleeding usually occurs within three to seven days after discontinuing medroxyprogesterone acetate therapy.

Abnormal Uterine Bleeding Due to Hormonal Imbalance in the Absence of Organic Pathology: Beginning on the calculated 16th or 21st day of the menstrual cycle, 5 to 10 mg of medroxyprogesterone acetate may be given daily for from 5 to 10 days. To produce an optimum secretory transformation of an endometrium that has been adequately primed with either endogenous or exogenous estrogen, 10 mg of medroxyprogesterone acetate daily for 10 days beginning on the 16th day of the cycle is suggested. Progestin withdrawal bleeding usually occurs within three to seven days after discontinuing therapy with medroxyprogesterone acetate. Patients with a past history of recurrent episodes of abnormal uterine bleeding may benefit from planned menstrual cycling with medroxyprogesterone acetate.

STERILE AQUEOUS SUSPENSION

This Suspension Is Intended For Intramuscular Administration Only. Endometrial Or Renal Carcinoma: Doses of 400 mg to 1000 mg of medroxyprogesterone acetate Sterile Aqueous Suspension per week are recommended initially. If improvement is noted within a few weeks

DOSAGE AND ADMINISTRATION: *(cont'd)*

or months and the disease appears stabilized, it may be possible to maintain improvement with as little as 400 mg per month. Medroxyprogesterone Acetate is not recommended as primary therapy, but as adjunctive and palliative treatment in advanced inoperable cases including those with recurrent or metastatic disease.

CONTRACEPTIVE INJECTION

The 1-ml vial of Depo-Provera Contraceptive Injection should be vigorously shaken just before use to ensure that the dose being administered represents a uniform suspension.

The recommended dose is 150 mg of Depo-Provera Contraceptive Injection every 3 months administered by deep, IM injection in the gluteal or deltoid muscle. To increase assurance that the patient is not pregnant at the time of the first administration, it is recommended that this injection be given only during the first 5 days after the onset of a normal menstrual period; within 5-days postpartum if not breast-feeding; or, if breast-feeding, at 6 weeks postpartum. If the period between injections is greater than 14 weeks, the physician should determine that the patient is not pregnant before administering the drug.

REFERENCES:

1. Royal College of General Practitioners: Oral contraception and thromboembolic disease. J Coll Gen Pract 13: 267-279, 1967. **2.** Inman WHW, Vessey MP: Investigation of deaths from pulmonary, coronary, and cerebral thrombosis and embolism in women of child-bearing age. Br Med J 2:193-199, 1968. **3.** Vessey MP, Doll R: Investigation of relation between use of oral contraceptives and thromboembolic disease. A further report. Br Med J 2:651-657, 1969. 4. Sartwell PE, Masi AT, Arthes FG, et al: Thromboembolism and oral contraceptives: An epidemiological case-control study. Am J Epidemiol 90:365-380, 1969. **References for Contraceptive Injection (Depo-Provera) C-1.** Trussell J, Hathcer RA, Cates W Jr, Stewart FH, Kost K: A guide to interpreting contraceptive efficacy studies. Obstet Gynecol *76:*558-567, 1990. **C-2.** Schwallie PC, Assenzo JR. Contraceptive use-efficacy study utilizing medroxyprogesterone acetate administered as an intramuscular injection once every 90 days.Fertil Steril. 1973: *24*:331-339. **C-3.** WHO Collaborative Study of Neoplasia and Steroid Contraceptives. Breast cancer and depot-medroxyprogesterone acetate: a multi-national study.Lancet 1991; *338:*833-838. **C-4.** WHO Collaborative study of Neoplasia and Steroid Contraceptives: Depot-medroxyprogesterone acetate (DPMA): and risk of epithelial ovarian cancer. Int J Cancer. 1991; *49:*191-195 **C-5.** WHO Collaborative Study of Neoplasia and Steroid Contraceptives. Depot-medroxyprogesterone acetate (DPMA) and risk of liver cancer. Int J Cancer. 1991;*49:*182-185. **C-6.** WHO Collaborative Study of Neoplasia and Steroid Contraceptives Depot-medroxyprogesterone acetate (DPMA) and risk of invasive squamous-cell cervical cancer. Contraception. 1992;*45*: 299-312. **C-7** WHO Collaborative Study of Neoplasia and Steroid Contraceptives. Depot-medroxyprogesterone acetate (DMPA) and risk of endometrial cancer. Int J Cancer. 1991; *49:*186-190. **C-8** Surveillance, Epidemiology, and End Results: Incidence and Mortality Data, 1973-77, National Cancer Institute Monograph 57, June 1981. (NIH publication No. 81-2330). **C-9** Gray RH, Pardthaisong T:*In Utero* Exposure to steroid contraceptives and survival during infancy. Am J Epidemiol 1991; *134:*804-811. **C-10** Pardthaisong T, Gray RH. *In Utero* exposure to steroid contraceptives and outcome of pregnancy. Am J Epidemiol. 1991;*134*:795-803. **C-11** Pardthaisong T. Gray RH, McDaniel EB, Chandacham A: Steroid Contraceptive use and pregnancy outcome.Teratology. 1988; *38*:51-58. **C-12** Van Deijk WA, Biljham GH, Mellink WAM, and Meulenberg PMM. Influence of aminoglutethimide on plasma levels of medroxyprogesterone acetate: its correlation with serum cortisol. Cancer Treatment Reports 1985; 69:1, 85-90.(Contraceptive Injection: Upjohn, 7/94, 815 461 005, 691412)

PATIENT PACKAGE INSERT:

ORAL TABLETS

Medroxyprogesterone acetate is a progesterone. The information below is that which the U.S. Food and Drug Administration requires be provided for all patients taking progesterones. The information below relates only to the risk to the unborn child associated with use of progesterone during pregnancy. For further information on the use, side effects and other risks associated with this product, ask your doctor.

Warning For Women: Progesterone or progesterone-like drugs have been used to prevent miscarriage in the first few months of pregnancy. No adequate evidence is available to show that they are effective for this purpose. Furthermore, most cases of early miscarriage are due to causes which could not be helped by these drugs.

There is an increased risk of minor birth defects in children whose mothers take this drug during the first 4 months of pregnancy. Several reports suggest an association between mothers who take these drugs in the first trimester of pregnancy and genital abnormalities in male and female babies. The risk to the male baby is the possibility of being born with a condition in which the opening of the penis is on the underside rather than the tip of the penis (hypospadias). Hypospadias occurs in about 5 to 8 per 1,000 male births and is about doubled with exposure to these drugs. There is not enough information to quantify the risk to exposed female fetuses, but enlargement of the clitoris and fusion of the labia may occur, although rarely.

Therefore, since drugs of this type may induce mild masculinization of the external genitalia of the female fetus, as well as hypospadias in the male fetus, it is wise to avoid using the drug during the first trimester of pregnancy.

These drugs have been used as a test for pregnancy but such use is no longer considered safe because of possible damage to a developing baby. Also, more rapid methods for testing for pregnancy are now available.

If you take medroxyprogesterone acetate and later find you were pregnant when you took it, be sure to discuss this with your doctor as soon as possible.

CONTRACEPTIVE INJECTION

Introduction: Every woman who considers using Depo-Provera Contraceptive Injection needs to understand the benefits and risks of this form of birth control and to discuss them with he health-care provider. This leaflet is intended to give you much of the information you will need in order to decide if Depo-Provera is the right choice for you. Your health-care provider will help you compare Depo-Provera with other contraceptive methods and will answer any questions you have after you have read this information.

Depo-Provera is given as an intramuscular injection (a shot) in the buttock or upper arm once every three (3) months. Promptly at the end of the 3-month interval, you will need to return to your health-care provider for your next injection in order to continue your contraceptive protection.

Depo-Provera contains medroxyprogesterone acetate, a chemical similar to (but not the same as) the natural hormone progesterone that is produced by your ovaries during the second half of your menstrual cycle. Depo- Provera acts by preventing your egg cells from ripening. If an egg is not released from the ovaries during your menstrual cycle, it cannot become fertilized by sperm and result in pregnancy. Depo-Provera also causes changes in the lining of your uterus that makes it less likely for pregnancy to occur.

Effectiveness of Depo-Provera Contraceptive Injection: Depo-Provera is over 99% effective, making it one of the most reliable methods of birth control available. This means that the average annual pregnancy rate is less than one for every 100 women who use Depo-Provera. The effectiveness of most contraceptive methods depends in part on how reliably each woman uses the method. The effectiveness of Depo-Provera depends only on the patient returning every three (3) months for her next injection.

The following table (Please refer to TABLE 1 in the INDICATIONS AND USAGE) shows the percent of women who become pregnant while using different kinds of contraceptive methods. It gives both the lowest expected rate of pregnancy (the rate expected in women who use each method exactly as it should be used) and the typical rate of pregnancy (which includes women who became pregnant because they forgot to use their birth control or because they did not follow the directions exactly.

Who Should Not Use Depo-Provera Contraceptive Injection: Certain women should not use Depo-Provera. You should not use Depo-Provera if you have any of these conditions:

if you think you might be pregnant

if you have any vaginal bleeding without a known reason

PATIENT PACKAGE INSERT: *(cont'd)*

if you have had cancer of the breast
if you have had a stroke
if you have or have had blood clots (phlebitis) in your legs
if you have problems with your liver or liver disease
If you are allergic to Depo-Provera (medroxyprogesterone acetate or any of its other ingredients)

Other Things to Consider Before Choosing Depo-Provera Contraceptive Injection: Before your doctor prescribes Depo-Provera, you will have a physical examination. It is important to tell your doctor or health-care provider if you have any of the following:
a family history of cancer of the breast
an abnormal mammogram (breast x-ray), fibrocystic breast disease, breast nodules or lumps, or bleeding from your nipples.
kidney disease
irregular or scanty menstrual periods
high blood pressure
migraine headaches
asthma
epilepsy (convulsions or seizures)
diabetes or a family history of diabetes
a history of depression
if you are taking any prescription or over-the-counter medications

Return of Fertility: Because Depo-Provera is a long-acting birth control method, it takes some time after your last injection for its effect to wear off. Based on results from a large study done in the United States, for women who stop using Depo-Provera in order to become pregnant it is expected that about half of those who become pregnant will do so in about 10 months after their last injection; about two-thirds of those who become pregnant will do so in about 12 months, about 83% of those who become pregnant will do so in about 15 months, and about 93% of those who become pregnant will do so in about 18 months after their last injection. The length of time you use Depo-Provera has no effect on how long it takes you to become pregnant after you stop using it.

RISKS OF USING DEPO-PROVERA CONTRACEPTIVE INJECTION

1. Irregular Menstrual Bleeding: The side effect reported most frequently by women who use Depo-Provera for contraception is a change in their normal menstrual cycle. During the first year of using Depo-Provera, you might have one or more of the following changes:
irregular or unpredictable bleeding or spotting
an increase or decrease in menstrual bleeding, or
no bleeding at all.

Unusually heavy or continuous bleeding, however, is not a usual effect of Depo-Provera and if this happens you should see your health-care provider right away.

With continued use of Depo-Provera, bleeding usually decreased and many women stop having periods completely. In clinical studies of Depo-Provera, 587% of the women studied reported no menstrual bleeding (amenorrhea) after 1 year of use and 68% of the women studied reported no menstrual bleeding after 2 years of use.

The reason that you periods stop is because Depo-Provera causes a resting state in your ovaries. When your ovaries do not release an egg monthly, the regular monthly growth of the lining of your uterus does not occur and, therefore, the bleeding that comes with your normal menstruation does not take place. When you stop using Depo-Provera your menstrual period will usually, in time, return to its normal cycle.

2. Bone Mineral Changes: Use of Depo-Provera may be associated with a decrease in the amount of mineral stored in your bones. This could increase your risk of developing bone fractures. The rate of bone mineral loss is greatest in the early years of Depo-Provera use but, after that, it begins to resemble the normal rate of age-related bone mineral loss.

3. Cancer: Studies of women who have used different forms of contraception found that women who used Depo-Provera for contraception had no increased overall risk of developing cancer of the breast, ovary, uterus, cervix, or liver. However, women under 35 years of age whose first exposure to Depo-Provera was within the previous 4 years may have a slightly increased risk of developing breast cancer similar to that seen with oral contraceptives. You should discuss this with your health-care provider.

4. Accidental Pregnancy: Because Depo-Provera is such an effective contraceptive method, the risk of accidental pregnancy for women who get their shots regularly (every 3 months) is very low. While there have been reports of an increased risk of low birth weight and neonatal infant death or other health problems in infants conceived close to the time of injection, such pregnancies are rare. If you think that you may have become pregnant while using Depo-Provera for contraception, see your health-care provider as soon as possible.

5. Other Risks: Women who use hormone-based contraceptives may have an increased risk of blood clots or stroke. Also, if a contraceptive method fails, there is a possibility that the fertilized egg will begin to develop outside of the uterus (ectopic pregnancy). While these events are rare, you should tell your health-care provider if you have any of the Warning Signals listed in the next section.

Warning Signals: If any of these problems occur following an injection of Depo-Provera, call your health-care provider immediately:
Sharp chest pain, coughing of blood, or sudden shortness of breath (indicating a possible clot in the lung)
Sudden severe headache or vomiting, dizziness or fainting, problems with your eyesight or speech, weakness, or numbness in an arm or leg (indicating a possible stroke)
Severe pain or swelling in the calf (indicating a possible clot in the leg)
Unusually heavy vaginal bleeding
Severe pain or tenderness in the lower abdominal area
Persistent pain, pus, or bleeding at the injection site

SIDE EFFECTS OF DEPO-PROVERA CONTRACEPTIVE INJECTION

1. Weight Gain: You may experience a weight gain while you are using Depo-Provera. About two thirds of the women who used Depo-Provera in the clinical trials reported a weight gain of about 5 pounds during the first year of use. You may continue to gain weight after the first year. Women in one large study who used Depo-Provera for 2 years gained an average total of 8.1 pounds over those 2 years, or approximately 4 pounds per year. Women who continued for 4 years gained an average of 13.8 pounds over those four years, or approximately 3.5 pounds per year. Women who continued for 6 years gained an average total of 16.5 pounds over those 6 years, or approximately 2.75 pounds per year.

2. Other Side Effects: In a clinical study of over 3,900 women who used Depo-Provera for up to 7 years, some women reported the following effects that may or may not have been related to their use of Depo-Provera:
irregular menstrual bleeding
amenorrhea

PATIENT PACKAGE INSERT: *(cont'd)*

headache
nervousness
abdominal cramps
dizziness
weakness or fatigue
decreased sexual desire
leg cramps
nausea
vaginal discharge or irritation
breast swelling and tenderness
bloating
swelling of the hands or feet
backache
depression
insomnia
acne
pelvic pain
no hair growth or excessive hair loss
rash
hot flashes

Other problems were reported by very few of the women in the clinical trials, but some of these could be serious. These include: convulsions, jaundice, urinary tract infections, allergic reactions, fainting, paralysis, osteoporosis, lack of return to fertility, deep vein thrombosis, pulmonary embolus, breast cancer, or cervical cancer. If these or any other problems occur during your use of Depo-Provera, discuss them with your health-care provider.

GENERAL PRECAUTIONS

1. Missed Periods: During the time you are using Depo-Provera for contraception, you may skip a period, or your periods may stop completely. If you have been receiving your Depo-Provera injections regularly every 3 months, then you are probably not pregnant. However, if you think that you may be pregnant, see your health-care provider.

2. Laboratory Test Interactions: If you are scheduled for any laboratory tests, tell your health-care provider that you are using Depo-Provera for contraception. Certain blood tests are effected by hormone such as Depo-Provera.

3. Drug Interactions: Cytadren (aminoglutethimide) is an anti-cancer drug that may significantly decrease the effectiveness of Depo-Provera if the two drugs are given during the same time.

4. Nursing Mothers: Although Depo-Provera can be passed to the nursing infant in the breast milk, no harmful effects have been found in these children. Depo-Provera does not prevent the breasts from producing milk, so it can be used by nursing mothers. However, to minimize the amount of Depo-Provera that is passed to the infant in the first weeks after birth, you should wait until 6 weeks after childbirth before you start using Depo-Provera for contraception.

Administration of Depo-Provera Contraceptive Injection: The recommended dose of Depo-Provera is 150 mg every 3 months given in a single intramuscular injection in the buttock or upper arm. To insure that you are not pregnant at the time of the first injection, it is important that the injection be given only during the first 5 days after the beginning of a normal menstrual period. If used following the delivery of a child, the first Depo-Provera injection should be given within 5 days after childbirth if you are not breast-feeding, or 6 weeks after childbirth if you are breast-feeding. If you wait longer than 3 months between injection, or longer than 6 weeks after childbirth, your health-care provider should determine that you are not pregnant before giving you your Depo-Provera injection.

HOW SUPPLIED - RATED THERAPEUTICALLY EQUIVALENT:

Tablet, Uncoated - Oral - 2.5 mg

30's	**$10.68**	**PROVERA, Pharmacia & Upjohn**	**00009-0064-06**
100's	$29.34	Cycrin, ESI Lederle	59911-5898-01
100's	$29.83	Medroxyprogesterone Acetate, Greenstone	59762-3740-01
100's	**$35.45**	**PROVERA, Pharmacia & Upjohn**	**00009-0064-04**
20000's	**$6559.40**	**PROVERA, Pharmacia & Upjohn**	**00009-0064-12**

Tablet, Uncoated - Oral - 5 mg

30's	**$16.29**	**PROVERA, Pharmacia & Upjohn**	**00009-0286-32**
100's	$44.32	Cycrin, ESI Lederle	59911-5897-01
100's	$45.01	Medroxyprogesterone Acetate, Greenstone	59762-3741-01
100's	**$53.49**	**PROVERA, Pharmacia & Upjohn**	**00009-0286-03**
20000's	**$9896.60**	**PROVERA, Pharmacia & Upjohn**	**00009-0286-42**

Tablet, Uncoated - Oral - 10 mg

30's	**$20.93**	**PROVERA, Pharmacia & Upjohn**	**00009-0050-09**
50's	$11.76	Medroxyprogesterone, Lederle Pharm	00005-3064-18
100's	$46.75	Medroxyprogesterone Acetate, Greenstone	59762-3742-02
100's	$46.75	Cycrin, ESI Lederle	59911-5896-01
100's	**$66.28**	**PROVERA, Pharmacia & Upjohn**	**00009-0050-02**
500's	**$314.99**	**PROVERA, Pharmacia & Upjohn**	**00009-0050-11**

HOW SUPPLIED - NOT RATED EQUIVALENT:

Injection, Susp - Intramuscular - 150 mg/ml

1 ml	$36.90	DEPO-PROVERA CONTRACEPTIVE, Pharmacia & Upjohn	00009-0746-30
1 ml x 25	$922.61	DEPO-PROVERA CONTRACEPTIVE, Pharmacia & Upjohn	00009-0746-35

Injection, Susp - Intramuscular - 400 mg/ml

2.5 ml	$89.37	DEPO-PROVERA, Pharmacia & Upjohn	00009-0626-01
10 ml	$339.32	DEPO-PROVERA, Pharmacia & Upjohn	00009-0626-02

Tablet, Uncoated - Oral - 10 mg

40's	$8.80	Medroxyprogesterone Acetate, Talbert Phcy	44514-0542-25
50's	$7.50	PROGESTONE, Major Pharms	00904-2690-51
50's	$8.40	Medroxyprogesterone, IDE-Interstate	00814-4660-08
50's	$9.75	Medroxyprogesterone, Solvay Pharms	00032-4001-42
50's	$10.11	Medroxyprogesterone, HL Moore Drug Exch	00839-6610-04
50's	$11.90	Medroxyprogesterone Acetate, Intl Labs	00665-4001-42
50's	$12.39	Medroxyprogesterone, Voluntary Hosp	53258-0166-04
50's	$12.40	Medroxyprogesterone, Goldline Labs	00182-1196-19
50's	$12.81	Medroxyprogesterone, Qualitest Pharms	00603-4368-19
50's	$13.10	Medroxyprogesterone, United Res	00677-0803-02
50's	$13.12	Medroxyprogesterone, Rugby	00536-3995-06
50's	$13.73	Medroxyprogesterone, Schein Pharm (US)	00364-0521-50
50's	$13.95	Medroxyprogesterone, Parmed Pharms	00349-2309-50
50's	$14.00	Medroxyprogesterone, Rosemont	00832-0087-26
50's	$14.20	Medroxyprogesterone, Martec Pharms	52555-0463-00

HOW SUPPLIED - NOT RATED EQUIVALENT: *(cont'd)*

50's	$14.82	Medroxyprogesterone Acetate 10, Aligen Independ	00405-4618-50
50's	$17.60	AMEN, Carnrick	00086-0049-05
50's	$25.79	CURRETAB, Solvay Pharms	00032-1007-42
50's	$25.79	Medroxyprogesterone Acetate, Geneva Pharms	00781-1680-50
100's	$11.40	Medroxyprogesterone, Solvay Pharms	00032-4001-06
100's	$13.08	Medroxyprogesterone, HL Moore Drug Exch	00839-6610-06
100's	$16.56	Medroxyprogesterone, US Trading	56126-0480-11
100's	$24.00	Medroxyprogesterone, United Res	00677-0803-01
100's	$25.65	Medroxyprogesterone, Rosemont	00832-0087-00
100's	$26.90	Medroxyprogesterone Acetate, Intl Labs	00665-4001-06
100's	$26.95	Medroxyprogesterone, Parmed Pharms	00349-2309-01
100's	$29.35	AMEN, Carnrick	00086-0049-10
100's	$59.04	Medroxyprogesterone, RID	54807-0550-01
250's	$29.15	Medroxyprogesterone, HL Moore Drug Exch	00839-6610-09
250's	$29.93	Medroxyprogesterone, IDE-Interstate	00814-4660-22
250's	$33.75	PROGESTONE, Major Pharms	00904-2690-70
250's	$35.10	Medroxyprogesterone, Pharmacist Choice	54979-0209-25
250's	$35.25	Medroxyprogesterone, Solvay Pharms	00032-4001-07
250's	$37.50	Medroxyprogesterone, Goldline Labs	00182-1196-02
250's	$42.75	Medroxyprogesterone, Martec Pharms	52555-0463-02
250's	$52.43	Medroxyprogesterone, Rugby	00536-3995-02
250's	$55.00	Medroxyprogesterone, Rosemont	00832-0087-25
250's	$55.11	Medroxyprogesterone, Qualitest Pharms	00603-4368-24
250's	$57.90	Medroxyprogesterone Acetate, Aligen Independ	00405-4618-04
250's	$58.75	Medroxyprogesterone, United Res	00677-0803-03
250's	$58.80	Medroxyprogesterone, Schein Pharm (US)	00364-0521-04
250's	$58.90	Medroxyprogesterone Acetate, Geneva Pharms	00781-1680-25
250's	$59.75	Medroxyprogesterone Acetate, Intl Labs	00665-4001-07
250's	$60.05	Medroxyprogesterone, Parmed Pharms	00349-2309-25
500's	$83.46	Medroxyprogesterone, Parmed Pharms	00349-2309-05
1000's	$224.45	AMEN, Carnrick	00086-0049-90

MEDRYSONE *(001713)*

CATEGORIES: Allergic Reactions; Anti-Inflammatory Agents; Conjunctivitis; EENT Drugs; Episcleritis; Eye, Ear, Nose, & Throat Preparations; Ocular Infections; Ophthalmic Corticosteroids; Ophthalmics; Pregnancy Category C; FDA Approval Pre 1982

BRAND NAMES: *Episona*; **HMS**; *HMS Liquifilm* (Canada); *HMS Liquifilm Ophthalmic Suspension*; *Medricort*; *Medriusar*; *Medrixon* (Mexico); *Medrixon-Ofteno*; *Medrysone Faure* (France); *Ophtocortin* (Germany); *Spectramedryn* (Germany) *(International brand names outside U.S. in italics)*

FORMULARIES: Aetna; Medi-Cal

DESCRIPTION:

HMS(medrysone) 1.0% Liquifilm sterile ophthalmic suspension is a topical anti-inflammatory agent for ophthalmic use.

Chemical Name: 11β-Hydroxy-6α-methylpregna-4-ene-3,20-dione.

CONTAINS:

Medrysone 1.0%

with: Liquifilm (polyvinyl alcohol) 1.4%; benzalkonium chloride 0.004%; edetate disodium; sodium chloride; potassium chloride; sodium phosphate, monobasic; sodium phosphate, dibasic; hydroxypropyl methylcellulose; sodium hydroxide to adjust the pH; and purified water.

CLINICAL PHARMACOLOGY:

HMS (medrysone) is a synthetic corticosteroid with topical anti-inflammatory and anti-allergic activity. Corticosteroids inhibit the inflammatory response to inciting agents of mechanical, chemical or immunological nature of edema, fibrin deposition, capillary dilation and leukocyte migration, capillary proliferation, deposition of collagen and scar formation. Medrysone) has less anti-inflammatory potency than 0.1% dexamethasone. Data from 2 uncontrolled studies[1-2] indicate that in patients with increased intraocular pressure and in those susceptible to a rise in intraocular pressure, there is less effect on pressure with HMS than with dexamethasone or betamethasone.

INDICATIONS AND USAGE:

HMS (medrysone) is indicated for the treatment of allergic conjunctivitis, vernal conjunctivitis, episcleritis, and epinephrine sensitivity.

CONTRAINDICATIONS:

HMS (medrysone) is contraindicated in the following conditions:

Acute superficial herpes simplex

Viral diseases of the conjunctiva and cornea

Ocular tuberculosis

Fungal diseases of the eye

Hypersensitivity to any of the components of the drug.

WARNINGS:

Acte purulent untreated infections of the eye may be masked, enhanced or activated by the presence of corticosteroid medication.

Corneal or scleral perforation occasionally has been reported with prolonged use of topical corticosteroids. In high dosages they have been associated with corneal thinning.

Prolonged use of topical corticosteroids may increase intraocular pressure, with resultant glaucoma, damage to the optic nerve, and defects in visual acuity and fields of vision. However, data from 2 uncontrolled studies[1-2] indicate that in patients with increased intraocular pressure and in those susceptible to a rise in intraocular pressure upon application of topical corticosteroids, there is less effect on pressure with HMS than with dexamethasone or betamethasone.

Prolonged use of topical corticosteroids may rarely be associated with development of posterior subcapsular cataracts.

Systemic absorption and systemic side effects may result with the use of topical corticosteroids.

HMS (medrysone) 1.0% Liquifilm sterile ophthalmic suspension is not recommended for use in iritis and uveitis as its therapeutic effectiveness has not been demonstrated in these conditions.

Corticosteroid medication in the presence of stromal herpes simplex requires great caution; frequent slit-lamp microscopy is suggested.

Prolonged use may aid in the establishment of secondary ocular infections from fungi and viruses liberated from ocular tissue.

PRECAUTIONS:

General: With prolonged use of HMS, the intraocular pressure and the lens should be examined periodically. In persistent corneal ulceration where a corticosteroid has been used, or is in use, fungal infection should be suspected.

Carcinogenesis, Mutagenesis, and Impairment of Fertility: No studies have been conducted in animals r in humans to evaluate the potential of these effects.

Pregnancy Category C: Medrysone has been shown to be embryocidal in rabbits when given in doses 10 and 30 times the human dose. Medrysone was ocularly applied to both eyes of pregnant rabbits 2 drops 4 times per day on day 6 through 18 of gestation. A significant increase in early resorptions was observed in the treated rabbits. There are no adequate or well-controlled studies in pregnant women. Medrysone should be used during pregnancy only if the potential benefit justifies the potential risk to the fetus.

Pediatric Use: Safety and effectiveness in children have not been established.

ADVERSE REACTIONS:

Adverse reactions include occasional transient stinging and burning upon instillation. Increased intraocular pressure, which may be associated with optic nerve damage and defects in the visual fields, and posterior subcapsular cataract formation have been reported rarely with the use of HMS.

OVERDOSAGE:

Overdosage will not ordinarily cause acute problems. If accidentally ingested, drink fluids to dilute.

DOSAGE AND ADMINISTRATION:

Shake well before using. Instill one drop in the conjunctival sac up to every four hours.

Note: Protect from freezing.

REFERENCES:

1. Becker B, Kolker AE. Intraocular pressure response to topical corticosteroids. IN:Leopold IH, ed. Ocular therapy, complications and management. St. Louis:C.V. Mosby, 1967. 2. Spaeth G. Hydroxymethylprogesterone. Arch Ophthalmol 1966; 75:783-787.

HOW SUPPLIED - EQUIVALENTS NOT AVAILABLE:

Suspension - Ophthalmic; Top - 1 %

5 ml	$13.63	HMS STERILE OPHTHALMIC, Allergan-Amer	11980-0074-05
10 ml	$20.93	HMS STERILE OPHTHALMIC, Allergan-Amer	11980-0074-10

MEFENAMIC ACID *(001714)*

CATEGORIES: Analgesics; Anti-Inflammatory Agents; Antipyretics; Central Nervous System Agents; Dysmenorrhea; Menstrual Preparations; NSAIDS; Nonsteroidal Anti-Inflammatory; Pain; Pregnancy Category C; FDA Approval Pre 1982

BRAND NAMES: *Alpain*; *Aprostal*; *Atmose*; *Beafemic*; *Benostan*; *Bonabol* (Japan); *Coslan*; *Drugfenam*; *Dysman* (England); *Dyspen*; *Ecopan*; *Fenal*; *Fenamin*; *Filmefen*; *Johnstal*; *Lysalgo*; *Manic*; *Mefa*; *Mefac*; *Mefalqic*; *Mefeic*; *Mefenal*; *Mefic* (Australia); *Mefix*; *Napan*; *Parkemed* (Germany); *Passton*; *Penadon*; *Pondex*; *Ponsfen*; *Ponstan* (Australia, Asia, England, Canada); *Ponstan (500 mg)*; *Ponstan-500* (Mexico); *Ponstan Forte*; **Ponstel**; *Ponstyl* (France); *Pontal* (Japan); *Potarlon*; *Pynamic*; *Ralgec*; *Youfenam* (Japan); *Zeet*; *Zerrmic*
(International brand names outside U.S. in italics)

FORMULARIES: Aetna

DESCRIPTION:

Ponstel is N-(2,3-xylyl)-anthranilic acid. It is an analgesic agent for oral administration. Ponstel is available in capsules containing 250 mg of mefenamic acid. Each capsule also contains lactose, NF. The capsule shell and/or band contains citric acid, USP; D&C yellow No. 10; FD&C blue No. 1; FD&C red No. 3; FD&C yellow No. 6; gelatin, NF; glycerol monooleate; silicon dioxide, NF; sodium benzoate, NF; sodium lauryl sulfate, NF; titanium dioxide, USP.

It is a white powder with a melting point of 230°-231°C, molecular weight 241.28, and water solubility of 0.004% at pH 7.1.

CLINICAL PHARMACOLOGY:

Ponstel is a nonsteroidal agent with demonstrated antiinflammatory, analgesic, and antipyretic activity in laboratory animals.[1,2] The mode of action is not known. In animal studies, Ponstel was found to inhibit prostaglandin synthesis and to compete for binding at the prostaglandin receptor site.[3]

Pharmacologic studies show Ponstel did not relieve morphine abstinence signs in abstinent, morphine-habituated monkeys.[1]

Following a single 1-gram oral dose, peak plasma levels of 10 mcg/ml occurred in 2 to 4 hours with a half-life of 2 hours. Following multiple doses, plasma levels are proportional to dose with no evidence of drug accumulation. One gram of Ponstel given four times daily produces peak blood levels of 20 mcg/ml by the second day of administration.[4]

Following a single dose, sixty-seven percent of the total dose is excreted in the urine as unchanged drug or as one of two metabolites. Twenty to twenty-five percent of the dose is excreted in the feces during the first three days.[4]

CLINICAL STUDIES:

In controlled, double-blind, clinical trials, Ponstel was evaluated for the treatment of primary spasmodic dysmenorrhea. The parameters used in determining efficacy included pain assessment by both patient and investigator; the need for concurrent analgesic medication; and evaluation of change in frequency and severity of symptoms characteristic of spasmodic dysmenorrhea. Patients received either Ponstel, 500 mg (2 capsules) as an initial dose and 250 mg every 6 hours, or placebo at onset of bleeding or of pain, whichever began first. After three menstrual cycles, patients were crossed over to the alternate treatment for an additional three cycles. Ponstel was significantly superior to placebo in all parameters, and both treatments (drug and placebo) were equally tolerated.

INDICATIONS AND USAGE:

Ponstel is indicated for the relief of moderate pain[5] when therapy will not exceed one week. Ponstel is also indicated for the treatment of primary dysmenorrhea.[5,6]

Studies in children under 14 years of age have been inadequate to evaluate the safety and effectiveness of Ponstel.

CONTRAINDICATIONS:

Ponstel should not be used in patients who have previously exhibited hypersensitivity to it.

Because the potential exists for cross-sensitivity to aspirin or other nonsteroidal antiinflammatory drugs, Ponstel should not be given to patients in whom these drugs induce symptoms of bronchospasm, allergic rhinitis, or urticaria.

Ponstel is contraindicated in patients with active ulceration or chronic inflammation of either the upper or lower gastrointestinal tract.

Ponstel should be avoided in patients with preexisting renal disease.

WARNINGS:

If diarrhea occurs, the dosage should be reduced or temporarily suspended (see ADVERSE REACTIONS and DOSAGE AND ADMINISTRATION). Certain patients who develop diarrhea may be unable to tolerate the drug because of recurrence of the symptoms on subsequent exposure.

Risk of GI Ulceration, Bleeding and Perforation with NSAID Therapy: Serious gastrointestinal toxicity such as bleeding, ulceration, and perforation, can occur at any time, with or without warning symptoms, in patients treated chronically with NSAID therapy. Although minor upper gastrointestinal problems, such as dyspepsia, are common, usually developing early in therapy, physicians should remain alert for ulceration and bleeding in patients treated chronically with NSAIDs even in the absence of previous GI tract symptoms. In patients observed in clinical trials of several months to two years duration, symptomatic upper GI ulcers, gross bleeding or perforation appear to occur in approximately 1% of patients treated for 3-6 months, and in about 2-4% of patients treated for one year. Physicians should inform patients about the signs and/or symptoms of serious GI toxicity and what steps to take if they occur.

Studies to date have not identified any subset of patients not at risk of developing peptic ulceration and bleeding. Except for a prior history of serious GI events and other risk factors known to be associated with peptic ulcer disease, such as alcoholism, smoking, etc., no risk factors (*e.g.,* age, sex) have been associated with increased risk. Elderly or debilitated patients seem to tolerate ulceration or bleeding less well than other individuals and most spontaneous reports of fatal GI events are in this population. Studies to date are inconclusive concerning the relative risk of various NSAIDs in causing such reactions. High doses of any NSAID probably carry a greater risk of these reactions, although controlled clinical trials showing this do not exist in most cases. In considering the use of relatively large doses (within the recommended dosage range), sufficient benefit should be anticipated to offset the potential increased risk of GI toxicity.

PRECAUTIONS:

If rash occurs, administration of the drug should be stopped.

A false-positive reaction for urinary bile, using the diazo tablet test, may result after mefenamic acid administration. If biliuria is suspected, other diagnostic procedures, such as the Harrison spot test, should be performed.

Renal Effects: As with other nonsteroidal antiinflammatory drugs, long-term administration of mefenamic acid to animals has resulted in renal papillary necrosis and other abnormal renal pathology. In humans, there have been reports of acute interstitial nephritis with hematuria, proteinuria and occasionally nephrotic syndrome.

A second form of renal toxicity has been seen in patients with prerenal conditions leading to a reduction in renal blood flow or blood volume, where the renal prostaglandins have a supportive role in the maintenance of renal perfusion. In these patients administration of an NSAID may cause a dose-dependent reduction in prostaglandin formation and may precipitate overt renal decompensation. Patients at greatest risk of this reaction are those with impaired renal function, heart failure, liver dysfunction, those taking diuretics, and the elderly. Discontinuation of NSAID therapy is typically followed by recovery to the pretreatment state.

Since Ponstel is eliminated primarily by the kidneys, the drug should not be administered to patients with significantly impaired renal functions.

As with other nonsteroidal antiinflammatory drugs, borderline elevations of one or more liver tests may occur in some patients. These abnormalities may progress, may remain essentially unchanged, or may be transient with continued therapy. The SGPT (ALT) test is probably the most sensitive indicator of liver dysfunction. Meaningful (3 times the upper limit of normal) elevations of SGPT or SGOT (AST) occurred in controlled clinical trials in less than 1% of patients. A patient with symptoms and/or signs suggesting liver dysfunction, or in whom an abnormal liver test has occurred, should be evaluated for evidence of the development of more severe hepatic reaction while on therapy with Ponstel. Severe hepatic reactions, including jaundice and cases of fatal hepatitis, have been reported with other nonsteroidal antiinflammatory drugs. Although such reactions are rare, if abnormal liver tests persist or worsen, if clinical signs and symptoms consistent with liver disease develop, or if systemic manifestations occur (*e.g.,* eosinophilia, rash, etc.), Ponstel should be discontinued.

Information for the Patient: Patients should be advised that if rash, diarrhea or other digestive problems arise, they should stop the drug and consult their physician.

Patients in whom aspirin or other nonsteroidal antiinflammatory drugs induce symptoms of bronchospasm, allergic rhinitis, or urticaria should be made aware that the potential exists for cross-sensitivity to Ponstel.

The long-term effects, if any, of intermittent Ponstel therapy for dysmenorrhea are not known. Women on such therapy should consult their physician if they should decide to become pregnant.

Ponstel, like other drugs of its class, is not free of side effects. The side effects of these drugs can cause discomfort and, rarely, there are more serious side effects, such as gastrointestinal bleeding, which may result in hospitalization and even fatal outcomes.

NSAIDs (nonsteroidal antiinflammatory drugs) are often essential agents in the management of arthritis and have a major role in the treatment of pain, but they also may be commonly employed for conditions which are less serious.

Physicians may wish to discuss with their patients the potential risks (see WARNINGS, PRECAUTIONS, and ADVERSE REACTIONS) and likely benefits of NSAID treatment, particularly when the drugs are used for less serious conditions where treatment without NSAIDs may represent an acceptable alternative to both the patient and physician.

Laboratory Tests: Because serious GI tract ulceration and bleeding can occur without warning symptoms, physicians should follow chronically treated patients for the signs and symptoms of ulceration and bleeding and should inform them of the importance of this follow-up (see Risk of GI Ulcerations, Bleeding and Perforation with NSAID Therapy.)

Pregnancy Category C Reproduction studies have been performed in rats, rabbits and dogs. Rats given up to 10 times the human dose showed decreased fertility, delay in parturition, and a decreased rate of survival to weaning. Rabbits at 2.5 times the human dose showed an increase in the number of resorptions. There were no fetal anomalies observed in these studies nor in dogs at up to 10 times the human dose.[5]

There are no adequate and well-controlled studies in pregnant women. Because animal reproduction studies are not always predictive of human response, this drug should be used only if clearly needed.

PRECAUTIONS: *(cont'd)*

The use of Ponstel in late pregnancy is not recommended because of the effects on the fetal cardiovascular system of drugs of this class.

Nursing Mothers: Trace amounts of Ponstel may be present in breast milk and transmitted to the nursing infant[7]; thus Ponstel should not be taken by the nursing mother because of the effects on the infant cardiovascular system of drugs of this class.

Use in Children: Safety and effectiveness in children below the age of 14 have not been established.

DRUG INTERACTIONS:

Ponstel may prolong prothrombin time.[5] Therefore, when the drug is administered to patients receiving oral anticoagulant drugs, frequent monitoring of prothrombin time is necessary.

ADVERSE REACTIONS:

Gastrointestinal: The most frequently reported adverse reactions associated with the use of Ponstel involve the gastrointestinal tract. In controlled studies for up to eight months, the following disturbances were reported in decreasing order of frequency: diarrhea (approximately 5% of patients), nausea with or without vomiting, other gastrointestinal symptoms, and abdominal pain.

In certain patients, the diarrhea was of sufficient severity to require discontinuation of medication. The occurrence of the diarrhea is usually dose related, generally subsides on reduction of dosage, and rapidly disappears on termination of therapy.

Other gastrointestinal reactions less frequently reported were anorexia, pyrosis, flatulence, and constipation.

Gastrointestinal ulceration with and without hemorrhage has been reported.

Hematopoietic: Cases of autoimmune hemolytic anemia have been associated with the continuous administration of Ponstel for 12 months or longer. In such cases the Coombs test results are positive with evidence of both accelerated RBC production and RBC destruction. The process is reversible upon termination of Ponstel administration.

Decreases in hematocrit have been noted in 2%-5% of patients and primarily in those who have received prolonged therapy. Leukopenia, eosinophilia, thrombocytopenic purpura, agranulocytosis, pancytopenia, and bone marrow hypoplasia have also been reported on occasion.

Nervous System: Drowsiness, dizziness, nervousness, headache, blurred vision, and insomnia have occurred.

Integumentary: Urticaria, rash, and facial edema have been reported.

Renal: As with other nonsteroidal antiinflammatory agents, renal failure, including papillary necrosis, has been reported. In elderly patients, renal failure has occurred after taking Ponstel for 2-6 weeks. The renal damage may not be completely reversible. Hematuria and dysuria have also been reported with Ponstel.

Other: Eye irritation, ear pain, perspiration, mild hepatic toxicity, and increased need for insulin in a diabetic have been reported. There have been rare reports of palpitation, dyspnea, and reversible loss of color vision.

OVERDOSAGE:

Although doses up to 6000 mg/day have been given, no specific information is available on the management of acute massive overdosage. Should accidental overdosage occur, the stomach should be emptied by inducing emesis or by careful gastric lavage followed by the administration of activated charcoal.[8] Laboratory studies indicate that Ponstel should be adsorbed from the gastrointestinal tract by activated charcoal.[4] Vital functions should be monitored and supported. Because mefenamic acid and its metabolites are firmly bound to plasma proteins, hemodialysis and peritoneal dialysis may be of little value.[4]

DOSAGE AND ADMINISTRATION:

Administration is by the oral route, preferably with food.

The recommended regimen in acute pain for adults and children over 14 years of age is 500 mg as an initial dose followed by 250 mg every six hours as needed, usually not to exceed one week.[5]

For the treatment of primary dysmenorrhea, the recommended dosage is 500 mg as an initial dose followed by 250 mg every 6 hours, starting with the onset of bleeding and associated symptoms. Clinical studies indicate that effective treatment can be initiated with the start of menses and should not be necessary for more than 2 to 3 days.[6]

REFERENCES:

1. Winder CV, et al: Antiinflammatory, antipyretic and antinociceptive properties of N-(2,3-xylyl) anthranilic acid (mefenamic acid). *J Pharmacol Exp Ther* 138: 405-413, 1962. **2.** Wax J, et al: Comparative activities, tolerances and safety of nonsteroidal antiinflammatory agents in rats. *J Pharmacol Exp Ther* 192: 172-178, 1975. **3.** Ferreira SH, Vane JR: Aspirin and prostaglandins, in *The Prostaglandins*, Ramwell PW Ed, Plenum Press, NY, vol. 2, 1974, pp 1-47.4.Glazko AJ: Experimental observations of flufenamic, mefenamic, and meclofenamic acids. Part III. Metabolic disposition, in *Fenamates in Medicine*. A Symposium, London, 1966; *Annals of Physical Medicine*, supplement, pp 23-36, 1967. **5.** Data on file, Medical Affairs Dept, Parke-Davis. **6.** Budoff PW: Use of mefenamic acid in the treatment of primary dysmenorrhea. *JAMA* 241: 2713-2716, 1979. **7.** Buchanan RA, et al: The breast milk excretion of mefenamic acid.*Curr Ther Res* 10:592, 1968. **8.** Corby DG, Decker WJ: Management of acute poisoning with activated charcoal. *Pediatrics* 54:324, 1974.

HOW SUPPLIED - EQUIVALENTS NOT AVAILABLE:

Capsule, Gelatin - Oral - 250 mg

100's	$96.08	PONSTEL, Parke-Davis	00071-0540-24

MEFLOQUINE HYDROCHLORIDE *(001715)*

CATEGORIES: Anti-Infectives; Antimalarial Agents; Antiparasitics; Antiprotozoals; Infections; Malaria; Orphan Drugs; Protozoal Agents; Pregnancy Category C; FDA Class 1A ("Important Therapeutic Advantage"); FDA Approved 1989 May

BRAND NAMES: **Lariam**; *Laricam* (Japan); *Mephaquin*; *Mephaquine* *(International brand names outside U.S. in italics)*

FORMULARIES: BC-BS; PCS; WHO

DESCRIPTION:

Lariam (mefloquine hydrochloride) is an antimalarial agent available as 250-mg tablets of mefloquine hydrochloride (equivalent to 228.0 mg of the free base) for oral administration.

Mefloquine hydrochloride is a 4-quinolinemethanol derivative with the specific chemical name of (R*, S*)-(±)-α-2-piperidinyl-2,8-bis (trifluoromethyl)-4-quinolinemethanol hydrochloride. It is a 2-aryl substituted chemical structural analog of quinine. The drug is a white to almost white crystalline compound, slightly soluble in water.

Mefloquine hydrochloride has a calculated molecular weight of 414.78.

The inactive ingredients are ammonium-calcium alginate, corn starch, crospovidone, lactose, magnesium stearate, microcrystalline cellulose, poloxamer #331 and talc.

CLINICAL PHARMACOLOGY:

Mefloquine is an antimalarial agent which acts as a blood schizonticide. Its exact mechanism of action is not known.

Pharmacokinetic studies of mefloquine in healthy male subjects showed that a significant lag time occurred after drug administration, & the terminal elimination half-life varied widely (13 to 24 days) with a mean of about three weeks. Mefloquine is a mixture of enantiomeric molecules whose rates of release, absorption, transport, action, degradation and elimination may differ. A valid pharmacokinetic model may not exist in such a case.

Additional studies in European subjects showed slightly greater concentrations of drug for longer periods of time. The absorption half-life was 0.36 to 2.0 hours, and the terminal elimination half-life was 15 to 33 days. The primary metabolite was identified and its concentrations were found to surpass the concentrations of mefloquine.

Multiple-dose kinetic studies confirmed the long elimination half-lives previously observed. The mean metabolite to mefloquine ratio measured at steady-state was found to range between 2.3 and 8.6.

The total clearance of the drug, which is essentially all hepatic, is approximately 30 ml/min. The volume of distribution, approximately 20 L/kg, indicates extensive distribution. The drug is highly bound (98%) to plasma proteins and concentrated in blood erythrocytes, the target cells in malaria, at a relatively constant erythrocyte-to-plasma concentration ratio of about 2.

The pharmacokinetics of mefloquine in patients with compromised renal function and compromised hepatic function have not been studied.

In vitro and *in vivo* studies showed no hemolysis associated with glucose-6-phosphate dehydrogenase deficiency. (See ANIMAL PHARMACOLOGY for additional information.)

Microbiology: Strains of *Plasmodium falciparum* resistant to mefloquine have been reported.

INDICATIONS AND USAGE:

Treatment of Acute Malaria Infections: Lariam is indicated for the treatment of mild to moderate acute malaria caused by mefloquine-susceptible strains of *Plasmodium falciparum* (both chloroquine-susceptible and resistant strains) or by *Plasmodium vivax.* There are insufficient clinical data to document the effect of mefloquine in malaria caused by *P. ovale* or *P. malariae.*

Note: Patients with acute *P. vivax* malaria, treated with Lariam, are at high risk of relapse because Lariam does not eliminate exoerythrocytic (hepatic phase) parasites. To avoid relapse, after initial treatment of the acute infection with Lariam, patients should subsequently be treated with an 8-aminoquinoline (*e.g.,* primaquine).

Prevention of Malaria: Lariam is indicated for the prophylaxis of *P. falciparum* and *P. vivax* malaria infections, including prophylaxis of chloroquine-resistant strains of*P. falciparum.*

CONTRAINDICATIONS:

Use of this drug is contraindicated in patients with a known hypersensitivity to mefloquine or related compounds(*e.g.,* quinine).

WARNINGS:

In case of life-threatening, serious or overwhelming malaria infections due to *P. falciparum*, patients should be treated with an intravenous antimalarial drug. Following completion of intravenous treatment, Lariam may be given orally to complete the course of therapy.

Concomitant administration of Lariam and quinine, quinidine or drugs producing beta-adrenergic blockade may produce electrocardiographic abnormalities or cardiac arrest. Concomitant administration of Lariam and quinine or chloroquine may increase the risk of convulsions. (See PRECAUTIONS and DRUG INTERACTIONS).

PRECAUTIONS:

GENERAL

Caution should be exercised with regard to driving, piloting airplanes and operating machines, as dizziness, a disturbed sense of balance neurologic or psychiatric reactions have been reported during the use of Lariam. These effects may occur after therapy is discontinued due to the long half-life of the drug. During prophylactic use, if signs of unexplained anxiety, depression, restlessness or confusion are noticed, these may be considered prodromal to a more serious event. In these cases, the drug must be discontinued. Lariam should be used with caution in patients with psychiatric disturbances because mefloquine use has been associated with emotional disturbances (See ADVERSE REACTIONS.)

This drug has not been administered for longer than 1 year. If the drug is to be administered for a prolonged period, periodic evaluations including liver function tests should be performed. Although retinal abnormalities seen in humans with long-term chloroquine use have not been observed with mefloquine use, long-term feeding of mefloquine to rats resulted in dose-related ocular lesions (retinal degeneration, retinal edema and lenticular opacity at 12.5 mg/kg/day and higher). (see ANIMAL PHARMACOLOGY.) Therefore, periodic ophthalmic examinations are recommended.

Parenteral studies in animals show that mefloquine, a myocardial depressant, possesses 20% of the antifibrillatory action of quinidine and produces 50% of the increase in the PR interval reported with quinine. The effects of mefloquine on the compromised cardiovascular system has not been evaluated. However, transitory and clinically silent ECG alterations have been reported during the use of mefloquine. Alteration included sinus bradycardia, sinus arrhythmia, first degree AV-block, prolongation of the QTc interval and abnormal T waves (see also cardiovascular effects under DRUG INTERACTIONS and ADVERSE REACTIONS). The benefits of Lariam therapy should be weighed against the possibility of adverse effects in patients with cardiac disease.

LABORATORY TESTS

Periodic evaluation of hepatic function should be performed during prolonged prophylaxis.

CARCINOGENESIS, MUTAGENESIS, AND IMPAIRMENT OF FERTILITY

Carcinogenesis: The carcinogenesis potential of mefloquine was studied in rats and mice in 2 year feeding studies at doses up to 30 mg/kg/day. No treatment-related increases in tumor of any type were noted.

Mutagenesis: The mutagenic potential of mefloquine was studied in a variety of assay systems including: Ames test, a host-mediated assay in mice, fluctuation tests and a mouse micronucleus assay. Several of these assays were performed with and without prior metabolic activation. In no instance was evidence obtained for the mutagenicity of mefloquine.

Impairment of Fertility: Fertility studies in rats at doses of 5, 20 and 50 mg/kg/day of mefloquine have demonstrated adverse effects on fertility in the male at the high dose of 50 mg/kg/day, and in the female at doses of 20 and 50 mg/kg/day. Histopathological lesions were noted in the epididymides from male rats at doses of 20 and 50 mg/kg/day. Administration of 250 mg/week of mefloquine (base) in adult males for 22 weeks failed to reveal any deleterious effects on human spermatozoa.

PREGNANCY, TERATOGENIC EFFECTS, PREGNANCY CATEGORY C

Mefloquine has been demonstrated to be teratogenic in rats and mice at a dose of 100 mg/kg/day. In rabbits, a high dose of 160 mg/kg/day was embryotoxic and teratogenic, and a dose of 80 mg/kg/day was teratogenic but not embryotoxic. There are no adequate and well-controlled studies in pregnant women. Mefloquine should be used during pregnancy only if the potential benefit justifies the potential risk to the fetus. Women of childbearing potential who are traveling to areas where malaria is endemic should be warned against becoming pregnant.

NURSING MOTHERS

Mefloquine is excreted in human milk. Based on a study in a few subjects, low concentrations (3% to 4%) of mefloquine were excreted in human milk following a dose equivalent to 250 mg of the free base. Because of the potential for serious adverse reactions in nursing infants from mefloquine, a decision should be made whether to discontinue the drug, taking into account the importance of the drug to the mother.

PEDIATRIC USE

Safety and effectiveness in children have not been established. Two studies of mefloquine in children living in endemic areas for *P. falciparum* were conducted. All children in these studies had at least a low level of parasitemia and 18 to 40% had significant parasitemia with or without mild malaria symptoms. When given 20 to 30 mg/kg of mefloquine as a single dose, all children with fever became afebrile, and 92% of those with significant parasitemia had a satisfactory response to treatment. While incomplete follow-up was obtained in these studies, nausea and vomiting occurred in approximately 10 and 20%, respectively, and dizziness was seen in approximately 40% of children.

DRUG INTERACTIONS:

Drug-drug interactions with Lariam have not been explored in detail. There is one report of cardiopulmonary arrest, with full recovery, in a patient who was taking a beta blocker (propranolol). The effects of mefloquine on the comprised cardiovascular system have not been evaluated. The benefits of Lariam therapy should be weighed against the possibility of adverse effects in patients with cardiac disease.

Lariam should not be used concurrently with quinine or quinidine. If these drugs are to be used in the initial treatment of severe malaria, Lariam administration should be delayed at least 12 hours after the last dose.

Patients taking Lariam while taking valproic acid had loss of seizure control and lower than expected valproic acid blood levels. Therefore, patients concurrently taking antiseizure medication and Lariam should have the blood level of their antiseizure medication monitored and the dosage adjusted appropriately.

In clinical trials the concomitant administration of sulfadoxine and pyrimethamine did not alter the adverse reaction profile.

ADVERSE REACTIONS:

Clinical: At the doses used for treatment of acute malaria infections, the symptoms possibly attributable to drug administration cannot be distinguished from those symptoms usually attributable to the disease itself.

Among subjects who received mefloquine for prophylaxis of malaria, the most frequently observed adverse experience was vomiting (3%). Dizziness, syncope, extrasystoles and other complaints affecting less than 1% were also reported.

Among subjects who received mefloquine for treatment, the most frequently observed adverse experiences included: dizziness, myalgia, nausea, fever, headache, vomiting, chills, diarrhea, skin rash, abdominal pain, fatigue, loss of appetite and tinnitus. Those side effects occurring in less than 1% included bradycardia, hair loss, emotional problems, pruritus, asthenia, transient emotional disturbances and telogen effluvium (loss of resting hair). Seizures have also been reported.

Two serious adverse reactions were cardiopulmonary arrest in one patient shortly after ingesting a single prophylactic dose of mefloquine while concomitantly using propranolol (see WARNINGS and PRECAUTIONS), and encephalopathy of unknown etiology during prophylactic mefloquine administration. The relationship of encephalopathy to drug administration could not be clearly established.

Post Marketing: Post-marketing surveillance indicates that the same adverse experiences are reported during prophylaxis, as well as acute treatment.

The following additional adverse reactions have been reported during post-marketing surveillance: vertigo, visual disturbances and central nervous system disturbances (*e.g.,* psychotic manifestations, hallucinations, confusion, anxiety and depression), Stevens-Johnson Syndrome and erythema multiforma.

Laboratory: The most frequently observed laboratory alterations which could be possibly attributable to drug administration were decreased hematocrit, transient elevation of transaminases, leukopenia and thrombocytopenia. These alterations were observed in patients with acute malaria who received treatment doses of the drug and were attributed to the disease itself.

During prophylactic administration of mefloquine to indigenous populations in malaria-endemic areas, the following occasional alterations in laboratory values were observed: transient elevation of transaminases, leukocytosis or thrombocytopenia.

OVERDOSAGE:

The following procedure is recommended in case of overdosage: Induce vomiting or perform gastric lavage, as appropriate. Monitor cardiac function and neurologic and psychiatric status for at least 24 hours. Provide symptomatic and intensive supportive treatment as reacquired, particularly for cardiovascular disturbances. Treat vomiting or diarrhea with standard fluid therapy.

DOSAGE AND ADMINISTRATION:

(See INDICATIONS AND USAGE)

(a) Treatment of mild to moderate malaria in adults caused by *P. vivax* or mefloquine-susceptible strains of *P. falciparum*-five tablets (1250 mg) mefloquine hydrochloride to be given as a single oral dose. The drug should not be taken on an empty stomach and should be administered with at least 8 oz (240 ml) of water.

If a full treatment course has been administered without clinical cure, alternative treatment should be given. Similarly, if previous prophylaxis with mefloquine has failed, Lariam should not be used for curative treatment.

Note: Patients with acute *P.vivax* malaria, treated with Lariam, are at high risk of relapse because Lariam does not eliminate exoerythrocytic (hepatic phase) parasites. To avoid relapse after initial treatment of the acute infection with Lariam, patients should subsequently be treated with an 8-aminoquinoline (*e.g.,* primaquine).

(b) Malaria prophylaxis-one tablet (250 mg) mefloquine hydrochloride once weekly for four weeks, then one tablet every other week.

Prophylactic drug administration should be begin 1 week prior to departure to an endemic area. Subsequent weekly doses should always be taken on the same day of the week. To reduce the risk of malaria after leaving an endemic area, prophylaxis should be continued for 4 additional weeks. Tablets should not be taken on an empty stomach and should be administered with at least 8 oz (240 ml) of water. It is suggested that the same day of the week be used each time the drug is administered. To avoid development of malaria after return from an endemic area, prophylaxis should be continued for four additional weeks. For

DOSAGE AND ADMINISTRATION: *(cont'd)*

prolonged stays in an endemic area this may be achieved by continuing the recommended dosage schedule, once weekly for four weeks, then once every other week, until the traveler has taken three doses following return to a malaria-free area. Tablets should not be taken on an empty stomach and should be administered with at least 8 oz (240 ml) of water.

ANIMAL PHARMACOLOGY:

Ocular lesions were observed in rats fed mefloquine daily for two years. All surviving rats given 30 mg/kg/day had ocular lesions in both eyes characterized by retinal degeneration, opacity of the lens and retinal edema. Similar but less severe lesions were observed in 80% of female and 22% of male rats fed 12.5 mg/kg/day for two years. At doses of 5 mg/kg/day, only corneal lesions were observed. They occurred in 9% of rats studied.

HOW SUPPLIED:

Lariam is available as scored, white, round tablets, containing 250 mg of mefloquine hydrochloride in unit-dose foil strips in cartons containing 25. Imprint on tablets: LARIAM 250 ROCHE

Tablets should be stored at 15-30°C (59-86°F).

HOW SUPPLIED - EQUIVALENTS NOT AVAILABLE:

Tablet, Uncoated - Oral - 250 mg

25's $172.68 LARIAM, Roche 00004-0172-02

MEGESTROL ACETATE *(001716)*

CATEGORIES: AIDS Related Complex; Anorexia; Antineoplastics; Breast Carcinoma; Cachexia; Endometrial Carcinoma; Hormones; Oncologic Drugs; Weight Loss; Pregnancy Category D; FDA Approval Pre 1982

BRAND NAMES: *Magace*; *Maygace*; **Megace**; *Megestat* (Germany); *Megostat*; *Niagestine*
(International brand names outside U.S. in italics)

FORMULARIES: Aetna; BC-BS; Medi-Cal

WARNING: THE USE OF MEGESTROL ACETATE IS CONTRAINDICATED IN PREGNANCY. Progestational agents have been used beginning with the first trimester of pregnancy in an attempt to prevent habitual abortion. There is no evidence that the use of a high dose progestational agent such as megestrol acetate during any phase of pregnancy is effective for this purpose. Furthermore, in the vast majority of women, the cause of abortion is a defective ovum, which progestational agents could not be expected to influence. In addition, the use of progestational agents, with their uterine- relaxant properties, in patients with fertilized defective ova may cause a delay in spontaneous abortion.

Several reports suggest an association between intrauterine exposure to progestational drugs in the first trimester of pregnancy and genital abnormalities in male and female fetuses. The risk of hypospadias, 5 to 8 per 1,000 male births in the general population, may be approximately doubled with exposure to these drugs. There are insufficient data to quantify the risk to exposed female fetuses. Because of increased genital abnormalities in male and female fetuses induced by some progestational drugs, it is prudent to avoid the use of megestrol acetate during pregnancy.

If the patient is exposed to megestrol acetate during pregnancy or if she becomes pregnant while taking this drug, she should be apprised of the potential risks to the fetus.

DESCRIPTION:

Megestrol acetate is a white, crystalline solid chemically designated as 17α-(acetyloxy)-6-methylpregna-4,6-diene-3,20-dione. Solubility at 37°C in water is 2 mcg per ml, solubility in plasma is 24 mcg per ml. Its molecular weight is 384.51. The empirical formula is $C_{24}H_{32}O_4$.

Tablets: Megestrol acetate, USP is a synthetic, antineoplastic and progestational drug.

Megestrol acetate is supplied as tablets for oral administration containing 20 mg and 40 mg megestrol acetate.

Megace tablets contain the following active ingredients: acacia, calcium phosphate, FD&C Blue No. 1 Aluminum Lake, lactose, magnesium stearate, silicon dioxide colloidal, and starch.

Suspension: Megace (megestrol acetate) Oral Suspension contains megestrol acetate, a synthetic derivative of the naturally occurring steroid hormone, progesterone.

Megace Oral Suspension is supplied as an oral suspension containing 40 mg of micronized megestrol acetate per ml.

Megace Oral Suspension contains the following inactive ingredients: alcohol (max. 0.06% v/v from flavor), citric acid, lemon-lime flavor, polyethylene glycol, polysorbate 80, purified water, sodium benzoate, sodium citrate, sucrose and xanthan gum.

CLINICAL PHARMACOLOGY:

There are several analytical methods used to estimate megestrol acetate plasma concentrations, including gas chromatography-mass fragmentography (GC-MF), high pressure liquid chromatography (HPLC) and radioimmunoassay (RIA). The GC-MF and HPLC methods are specific for megestrol acetate and yield equivalent concentrations. The RIA method reacts to megestrol acetate metabolites and is, therefore, non-specific and indicates higher concentrations than the GC-MF and HPLC methods. The plasma levels by HPLC assay or radioimmunoassay methods are about one-sixth those obtained by the GC method. The plasma levels are dependent not only on the method used, but also on intestinal and hepatic inactivation of the drug, which may be affected by factors such as intestinal tract motility, intestinal bacteria, antibiotics administered, body weight, diet, and liver function.[3,4]

The major route of drug elimination in humans is urine. When radiolabeled megestrol acetate was administered to humans in doses of 4 to 90 mg, the urinary excretion within 10 days ranged from 56.5% to 78.4% (mean 66.4%) and fecal excretion ranged from 7.7% to 30.3% (mean 19.8%). The total recovered radioactivity varied between 83.1% and 94.7% (mean 86.2%). Megestrol acetate metabolites which were identified in urine constituted 5% to 8% of the dose administered and are considered negligible.[5] Respiratory excretion as labeled carbon dioxide and fat storage may have accounted for at least part of the radioactivity not found in the urine and feces.

The relative bioavailability of Megace (megestrol acetate tablets, USP) 40 mg tablets and Megace Oral Suspension has not been evaluated. The effect of food on the bioavailability of Megace Oral Suspension has not been evaluated.

Tablets: While the precise mechanism by which megestrol acetate produces its antineoplastic effects against endometrial carcinoma is unknown at the present time, inhibition of pituitary gonadotropin production and resultant decrease in estrogen secretions may be factors. There is evidence to suggest a local effect as a result of the marked changes brought about by the direct instillation of progestational agents into the endometrial cavity. The antineoplastic action of megestrol acetate on carcinoma of the breast is effected by modifying the action of other steroid hormones and by exerting a direct cytotoxic effect on tumor cells.[1] In metastatic

CLINICAL PHARMACOLOGY: *(cont'd)*

cancer, hormone receptors may be present in some tissues but not others. The receptor mechanism is a cyclic process whereby estrogen produced by the ovaries enters the target cell, forms a complex with cytoplasmic receptor and is transported into the cell nucleus. There it induces gene transcription and leads to the alteration of normal cell functions. Pharmacologic doses of megestrol acetate not only decrease the number of hormone-dependent human breast cancer cells but also is capable of modifying and abolishing the stimulatory effects of estrogen on these cells. It has been suggested[2] that progestins may inhibit in one of two ways: by interfering with either the stability, availability, or turnover of the estrogen receptor complex in its interaction with genes or in conjunction with the progestin receptor complex, by interacting directly with the genome to turn off specific estrogen-responsive genes.

In normal male volunteers (N-23) who received 160 mg of megestrol acetate given as a 40 mg q.i.d. regimen, the oral absorption of megestrol acetate appeared to be variable. Plasma levels were assayed by a high pressure liquid chromatographic (HPLC) procedure. Peak drug levels for the first 40 mg dose ranged from 10 to 56 ng/ml (mean 27.6 ng/ml) and the times to peak concentrations ranged from 1.0-3.0 hours (mean 2.2 hours). Plasma elimination half-life ranged from 13.0 to 104.9 hours (mean 34.2 hours). The steady state plasma concentrations for a 40 mg q.i.d. regimen have not been established.

Suspension: Several investigators have reported on the appetite enhancing property of megestrol acetate and its possible use in cachexia. The precise mechanism by which megestrol acetate produces effects in anorexia and cachexia is unknown at the present time.

Plasma steady state pharmacokinetics of megestrol acetate were evaluated in 10 adults, cachetic male patients with acquired immunodeficiency syndrome (AIDS) and an involuntary weight loss greater than 10% of baseline. Patients received single oral doses of 800 mg/day of Megace Oral Suspension for 21 days. Plasma concentration data obtained on day 21 were evaluated for up to 48 hours past the last dose.

Mean (±1SD) peak plasma concentration (C_{max}) of megestrol acetate was 753 (±539) ng/ml. Mean area under the concentration time- curve (AUC) was 10476 (±7788) ng x hr/ml. Median TMAX value was five hours. Seven of 10 patients gained weight in three weeks.

Additionally, 24 adult, asymptomatic HIV seropositive male subjects were dosed once daily with 750 mg of Megace Oral Suspension. The treatment was administered for 14 days. Mean C_{max} and AUC values 490 (±238) ng/ml and 6779 (±3048) hr x ng/ml respectively. The median TMAX value was three hours. The mean C_{min} value was 202 (±101) ng/ml. The mean % Fl value was 107 (±40).

CLINICAL STUDIES:

SUSPENSION

The clinical efficacy of Megace Oral Suspension was assessed in two clinical trials. One was multicenter, randomized, double-blind, placebo- controlled study comparing megestrol acetate (MA) at doses of 100 mg, 400 mg, and 800 mg per day versus placebo in AIDS patients with anorexia/cachexia and significant weight loss. Of the 270 patients entered on study, 195 met all inclusion/exclusion criteria, had at least two additional post baseline weight measurements over a 12 week period or had one post baseline weight measurement but dropped out for therapeutic failure. The percent of patients gaining five or more pounds at maximum weight gain in 12 study weeks was statistically significantly greater for the 800 mg (64%) and 400 mg (57%) MA-treated groups than for the placebo group (24%). Mean weight increased from baseline to last evaluation in 12 study weeks in the 800 mg MA-treated group by 7.8 pounds, the 400 mg MA group by 4.2 pounds, the 100 mg MA group by 1.9 pounds, and decreased in the placebo group by 1.6 pounds. Mean weight changes at 4, 8, and 12 weeks for patients evaluable for efficacy in the two clinical trials are shown graphically. Changes in body composition during the 12 study weeks as measured by bioelectrical impedance analysis showed increases in non- water body weight in the MA-treated groups (see CLINICAL STUDIES, TABLE 1.) In addition, edema developed or worsened in only 3 patients.

Greater percentages of MA-treated patients, in the 800 mg group (89%) the 400 mg group (68%) and the 100 mg group (72%), than in the placebo- group (50%), showed an improvement in appetite at last evaluation during the 12 study weeks. A statistically significant difference was observed between the 800 mg MA-treated group and the placebo group in the change in caloric intake from baseline to time of maximum weight change. Patients were asked to assess weight change, appetite, appearance, and overall perception of well-being in a 9 question survey. At maximum weight change only the 800 mg MA-treated group gave responses that were statistically significantly more favorable to all questions when compared to the placebo-treated group. A dose response was noted in the survey with positive responses correlating with higher dose for all questions.

The second trial was a multicenter, randomized, double-blind, placebo-controlled study comparing megestrol acetate 800 mg/day versus placebo in AIDS patients with anorexia/cachexia and significant weight loss. Of the 100 patients entered on study, 65 met all inclusion/exclusion criteria, had at least two additional post baseline weight measurements over a 12 week period or had one post baseline weight measurement but dropped out for therapeutic failure. Patients in the 800 mg MA-treated group had a statistically significantly larger increase in mean maximum weight change than patients in the placebo group. From baseline to study week 12, mean weight increased by 11.2 pounds in the MA-treated group and decreased 2.1 pounds in the placebo group. Changes in body composition as measured by bioelectrical impedance analysis showed increases in non-water weight in the MA-treated group (see CLINICAL STUDIES, TABLE 1.) No edema was reported in the MA-treated group. A greater percentage of MA-treated patients (67%) than placebo-treated patients (38%) showed an improvement in appetite at last evaluation during the 12 study weeks; this difference was statistically significant. There were no statistically significant differences between treatment groups in mean caloric change or in daily caloric intake at time to maximum weight change. In the same 9 question survey referenced in the first trial, patients' assessments of weight change, appetite, appearance, and overall perception of well-being showed increases in mean score in MA-treated patients as compared to the placebo group.

In both trials, patients tolerated the drug well and no statistically significant differences were seen between the treatment groups with regard to laboratory abnormalities, new opportunistic infections, lymphocyte counts, T_4 counts, T_8 counts, or skin reactivity tests (See ADVERSE REACTIONS.)

INDICATIONS AND USAGE:

TABLETS

Megestrol acetate is indicated for the palliative treatment of advanced carcinoma of the breast or endometrium (*i.e.,* recurrent, inoperable, or metastatic disease). It should not be used in lieu of currently accepted procedures such as surgery, radiation, or chemotherapy.

SUSPENSION

Megace (megestrol acetate) Oral Suspension is indicated for the treatment of anorexia, cachexia, or an unexplained, significant weight loss in patients with a diagnosis of acquired immunodeficiency syndrome (AIDS).

CONTRAINDICATIONS:

As a diagnostic test for pregnancy. Known or suspected pregnancy.

TABLE 1 Megace (megestrol acetate) Oral Suspension Clinical Efficacy Trials

	Trial 1 Study Accrual Dates 11/88 to 12/90				Trial 2 Study Accrual Dates 5/89 to 4/91	
Megestrol Acetate, mg/day	0	100	400	800	0	800
Entered N	38	82	75	75	48	52
Evaluable N	28	61	53	53	29	36
Mean Change in Weight (lb.) Baseline to to 12 weeks	0.0	2.9	9.3	10.7	-2.1	11.2
% Patients ≥ 5 Pound Gain at Last Evaluation in 12 Wk	21	44	57	64	28	47
Mean Changes in Body Composition*:						
Fat Body Mass (lb.)	0.0	2.2	2.9	5.5	1.5	5.7
Lean Body Mass (lb.)	-1.7	-0.3	1.5	2.5	-1.6	-0.6
Water (liters)	-1.3	-0.3	0.0	0.0	-0.1	-0.1
% Patients With Improved Appetite:						
At Time of Max. Wt. Change	50	72	72	93	48	69
At Last Evaluation in 12 Wk.	50	72	68	89	38	67
Mean Change in Daily Caloric Intake:						
Baseline to Time of Maximum Weight Change	-107	326	308	646	30	464

* Based on Bioelectrical Impedance Analysis Determinations at Last Evaluation in 12 Weeks

WARNINGS:

Megestrol acetate may cause fetal harm when administered to a pregnant woman. For animal data on fetal effects, see PRECAUTIONS, Impairment of Fertility. Fertility and reproduction studies with high doses of megestrol acetate have shown a reversible feminizing effect on some male rat fetuses.[6] There are not adequate and well- controlled studies in pregnant women. If this drug is used during pregnancy, or if the patient becomes pregnant while taking (receiving) this drug, the patient should be apprised of the potential hazard to the fetus. Women of childbearing potential should be advised to avoid becoming pregnant.

Tablets: The use of megestrol acetate in other types of neoplastic disease is not recommended.

Suspension: Megestrol acetate is not intended for prophylactic use to avoid weight loss.

See also PRECAUTIONS, Carcinogenesis, Mutagenesis, and Impairment of Fertility.

PRECAUTIONS:

GENERAL

Tablets: Close surveillance is indicated for any patient treated for recurrent or metastatic cancer. Use with caution in patients with a history of thrombophlebitis.

Suspension: Therapy with Megace Oral Suspension for weight loss should only be instituted after treatable causes of weight loss are sought and addressed. These treatable causes include possible malignancies, systemic infections, gastrointestinal disorders affecting absorption, endocrine disease and renal or psychiatric diseases.

Although the glucocorticoid effects of Megace Oral Suspension in HIV infected individuals have not been evaluated, laboratory evidence of adrenal suppression has been observed which is clinically insignificant.

Effects on HIV viral replication have not been determined.

Use with caution in patients with a history of thromboembolic disease.

INFORMATION FOR THE PATIENT

Patients using megestrol acetate should receive the following instructions.

1. This medication is to be used as directed by the physician.
2. Report any adverse reaction experiences while taking this medication.

Suspension

3. Use contraception while taking this medication if you are a woman capable of becoming pregnant.
4. Notify your physician if you become pregnant while taking this medication.

LABORATORY TESTS:

Tablets: Breast malignancies in which estrogen and/or progesterone receptors are positive are more likely to respond to megestrol acetate.[7,8,9]

CARCINOGENESIS, MUTAGENESIS, AND IMPAIRMENT OF FERTILITY

Tablets

Administration for up to 7 years of megestrol acetate to female dogs is associated with an increased incidence of both benign and malignant tumors of the breast.[10] Comparable studies in rats and studies in monkeys are not associated with an increased incidence of tumors. The relationship of the dog tumors to humans is unknown but should be considered in assessing the benefit-to-risk ratio when prescribing megestrol acetate and in surveillance of patients on therapy.[10,11] Also see WARNINGS.

Suspension

Carcinogenesis: Data on carcinogenesis were obtained from studies conducted in dogs, monkeys and rats treated with megestrol acetate at doses 53.2, 26.6 and 1.3 times *lower* than the proposed dose (13.3 mg/kg/day) for humans. No males were used in the dog and monkey studies. In female beagles, megestrol acetate (0.01, 0.1 or 0.25 mg/kg/day) administered for up to 7 years induced both benign and malignant tumors of the breast. In female monkeys, no tumors were found following 10 years of treatment with 0.01, 0.1 or 0.5 mg/kg/day megestrol acetate. Pituitary tumors were observed in female rats treated with 3.9 or 10 mg/kg/day of megestrol acetate for 2 years. The relationship of these tumors in rats and dogs to humans is unknown but should be considered in assessing the risk-to-benefit ratio when prescribing Megace (megestrol acetate) Oral Suspension and in surveillance of patients on therapy. Also see WARNINGS.

Mutagenesis, Impairment of Fertility: No mutagenesis data are currently available.

Perinatal/postnatal (segment III) toxicity studies were performed in rats at doses (0.05 - 12.5 mg/kg)*less* than that indicated for humans (13.3 mg/kg); in these low dose studies, the reproductive capability of male offspring of megestrol acetate-treated females was impaired. Similar results were obtained in dogs. Pregnant rats treated with megestrol acetate showed a reduction in fetal weight and number of live births, and feminization of male fetuses. No toxicity data are currently available on male reproduction (spermatogenesis).

PREGNANCY CATEGORY X

(See WARNINGS and Impairment of Fertility.) No adequate animal teratology information is available at clinically relevant doses.

PRECAUTIONS: *(cont'd)*

NURSING MOTHERS

Because of the potential for adverse effects on the newborn, nursing should be discontinued if megestrol acetate is required for treatment of cancer.

USE IN HIV INFECTED WOMEN

Suspension: Although megestrol acetate has been used extensively in women for the treatment of endometrial and breast cancers its use in HIV infected women has been limited.

All 10 women in the clinical trials reported breakthrough bleeding.

PEDIATRIC USE

Safety and effectiveness in children have not been established.

ADVERSE REACTIONS:

TABLETS

Weight Gain: Weight gain is a frequent side effect of megestrol acetate.[12,13]This gain has been associated with increased appetite and is not necessarily associated with fluid retention.

Thromboembolic Phenomena: Thromboembolic phenomena including thrombophlebitis and pulmonary embolism have been rarely reported.

Other Adverse Reactions: Nausea and vomiting, edema, breakthrough bleeding, dyspnea, tumor flare, (with or without hypercalcemia), hyperglycemia, glucose intolerance, alopecia, hypertension, carpal tunnel syndrome, and rash.

SUSPENSION

Clinical Adverse Events: Adverse events which occurred in at least 5% of patients in any arm of the two clinical efficacy trials and the open trial are listed by treatment group. All patients listed had at least one post baseline visit during the 12 study weeks. These adverse events should be considered by the physician when prescribing Megace Oral Suspension.

TABLE 2 Adverse Events % of Patients Reporting

	Trial 1 (N=236)				Trial 2 (N=87)		Open Label Trial
Megestrol Acetate mg/day	Placebo 0	100	400	800	Placebo 0	800	1200
No. of Patients	N=34	N=68	N=69	N=65	N=38	N=49	N=176
Diarrhea	15	13	8	15	8	6	10
Impotence	3	4	6	14	0	4	7
Rash	9	9	4	12	3	2	6
Flatulence	9	0	1	9	3	10	6
Hypertension	0	0	0	8	0	0	4
Asthenia	3	2	3	6	8	4	5
Insomnia	0	3	4	6	0	0	1
Nausea	9	4	0	5	3	4	5
Anemia	6	3	3	5	0	0	0
Fever	3	6	4	5	3	2	1
Libido Decreased	3	4	0	5	0	2	1
Dyspepsia	0	0	3	3	5	4	2
Hyperglycemia	3	0	6	3	0	0	3
Headache	6	10	1	3	3	0	3
Pain	6	0	0	2	5	6	4
Vomiting	9	3	0	2	3	6	4
Pneumonia	6	2	0	2	3	0	1
Urinary Freq.	0	0	1	2	5	2	1

Adverse events which occurred in 1% to 3% of all patients enrolled in the two clinical efficacy trials with at least one follow-up visit during the first 12 weeks of the study are listed below by body system. Adverse events occurring less than 1% are not included. There were no significant differences between incidence of these events in patients treated with megestrol acetate and patients treated with placebo.

Body as a Whole: abdominal pain, chest pain, infection, moniliasis and sarcoma

Cardiovascular System: cardiomyopathy and palpitation

Digestive System: constipation, dry mouth, hepatomegaly, increased salivation and oral moniliasis

Hemic and Lymphatic System: leukopenia

Metabolic and Nutritional: LDH increased, edema and peripheral edema

Nervous System: paresthesia, confusion, convulsion, depression, neuropathy, hypesthesia and thinking abnormal

Respiratory System: dyspnea, cough, pharyngitis and lung disorder

Skin and Appendages: alopecia, herpes, pruritus, vesiculobullous rash, sweating and skin disorder

Special Senses: amblyopia

Urogenital System: albuminuria, urinary incontinence, urinary tract infection and gynecomastia

OVERDOSAGE:

No serious unexpected side effects have resulted from studies involving megestrol acetate administered in dosages as high as 1600 mg/day. Oral administration of large, single doses of megestrol acetate (5 grams/kg) did not produce toxic effects in mice.[6] Megestrol acetate has not been tested for dialyzability; however, due to its low solubility it is postulated that this would not be an effective means of treating overdose.

DOSAGE AND ADMINISTRATION:

TABLETS

Breast cancer: 160 mg/day (40 mg q.i.d.)

Endometrial carcinoma: 40-320 mg/day in divided doses

At least 2 months of continuous treatment is considered an adequate period for determining the efficacy of megestrol acetate.

SUSPENSION

The recommended adult initial dosage of Megace Oral Suspension, is 800 mg/day (20 ml/day). Shake container well before using.

In clinical trials evaluating different dose schedules, daily doses of 400 and 800 mg/day were found to be clinically effective.

A plastic dosage cup with 10 ml and 20 ml markings is provided for convenience.

ANIMAL PHARMACOLOGY:

Animal Toxicology: Long-term treatment with Megace may increase the risk of respiratory infections. A trend toward increased frequency of respiratory infections, decreased lymphocyte counts and increased neutrophil counts was observed in a two-year chronic toxicity/carcinogenicity study of megestrol acetate conducted in rats.

HOW SUPPLIED:

Tablets: Megace is supplied as tablets for oral administration containing 20 mg and 40 mg megestrol acetate.

Suspension Megace (megestrol acetate) Oral Suspension is available as a lemon-lime flavored oral suspension containing 40 mg of micronized megestrol acetate per ml. Bottles of 8 fl.oz. (236.6 ml)

STORAGE

Tablets: Store megestrol acetate at room temperature; protect from temperatures above 40°C (104°F).

Suspension: Store Megace Oral Suspension at or below 25°C and dispense in a tight container. Protect from heat.

SPECIAL HANDLING

Tablets and Suspension: There is no threshold limit value established by OSHA, NIOSH, or ACGIH.

Health Hazard Data: Exposure or "overdose" at levels approaching recommended dosing levels could result in side effects described above (see WARNINGS and ADVERSE REACTIONS). Women at risk of pregnancy should avoid such exposure.

REFERENCES:

1. Allegra JC, Kiefer SM: Mechanisms of Action of Progestational Agents, Semin Oncol 12 (Suppl 1): 3, 1985. **2.** DeSombre ER, Kuivanen PC: Progestin Modulation of Estrogen-dependent marker protein synthesis in the endometrium, Semin Oncol 12 (Suppl 1): 6, 1985. **3.** Alexieva-Figusch J, Blankenstein MA, Hop WCJ, *et al:* Treatment of metastatic breast cancer patients with different dosages of megestrol acetate: Dose relations, metabolic and endocrine effects. Eur J Cancer Clin Oncol 20:33-40, 1984. **4.** Gaver RC, Movahhed HS, Farmen RH, Pittman KA: Liquid Chromatographic Procedure for the Quantitative Analysis of Megestrol Acetate in Human Plasma, J Pharm Sci 74:664, 1985. **5.** Cooper JM, Kellie AE: The Metabolism of Megestrol Acetate (17-alpha-acetoxy-6-methylpregna-4, 6-diene-3, 20- dione) in women. Steroids 11:133, 1968. **6.** David A, Edwards K, Fellowes KP, Plummer JM: Anti-ovulatory and other biological properties of Megestrol Acetate, J Reprod Fertil 5:331, 1963. **7.** McGuire WL, Clark GM: The Prognostic Role of Progesterone Receptors in Human Breast Cancer, Semin Oncol 10 (Suppl 4): 2, 1983. **8.** Horwitz KB: The Central Role of Progesterone Receptors and Progestational Agents in the Management and Treatment of Breast Cancer. Semin Oncol 15 (Suppl 1): 14, 1988. **9.** Bonomi P, Johnson P, Anderson K, Wolter J, Bunting N, Strauss A, Roseman D, Shorey W, Econonou S: Primary Hormonal Therapy of Advanced Breast Cancer with Megestrol Acetate: Predictive Value of Estrogen Receptor and Progesterone Receptor Levels. **10.** Nelson LW, Weikel JH Jr., Reno FE: Mammary Nodules in Dogs during Four Year's Treatment with Megestrol Acetate or Chlormadinone Acetate, J Natl Cancer Inst 51: 1303, 1973. **11.** Owen LN, Briggs MH: Contraceptive Steroid Toxicology in the Beagle Dog and its Relevance to Human Carcinogenicity, Curr Med Res Opin 4:309, 1976. **12.** Ansfield FJ, Kallas GJ, Singson JP: Clinical Results with Megestrol Acetate in Patients with Advanced Carcinoma of the Breast. Surg Gynecol Obstet 155: 888, 1982. **13.** Alexieva-Figusch J, van Gilse HA, Hop WCJ, *et al*: Progestin Therapy in Advanced Breast Cancer: Megestrol Acetate - An Evaluation of 160 Treated Cases, Cancer 46:2369, 1980.

HOW SUPPLIED - RATED THERAPEUTICALLY EQUIVALENT:

Tablet, Uncoated - Oral - 20 mg

100's	$41.99	Megestrol, Balan	00304-1882-01
100's	$44.20	Megestrol, Qualitest Pharms	00603-4391-21
100's	$44.63	Megestrol, H.C.F.A. F F P	99999-1716-01
100's	$52.50	Megestrol 20, Major Pharms	00904-3570-60
100's	$60.46	Megestrol, Goldline Labs	00182-1863-01
100's	$61.95	Megestrol, Schein Pharm (US)	00364-2235-01
100's	$62.36	Megestrol Acetate, Par Pharm	49884-0289-01
100's	$62.36	Megestrol, Martec Pharms	52555-0375-01
100's	$64.25	Megestrol, Rugby	00536-4821-01
100's	$64.25	Megestrol, HL Moore Drug Exch	00839-7405-06
100's	$65.30	Megestrol Acetate, Goldline Labs	00182-1863-89
100's	$66.66	Megestrol, Parmed Pharms	00349-8766-01
100's	$66.66	Megestrol Acetate, Aligen Independ	00405-4623-01
100's	**$69.86**	**MEGACE, Mead Johnson**	**00015-0595-01**

Tablet, Uncoated - Oral - 40 mg

100's	$77.93	Megestrol, H.C.F.A. F F P	99999-1716-02
100's	$85.43	Megestrol, United Res	00677-1206-01
100's	$87.40	Megestrol, Major Pharms	00904-3571-60
100's	$91.87	Megestrol, Major Pharms	00904-3571-61
100's	$95.98	Megestrol 40, Balan	00304-1883-01
100's	$99.00	Megestrol, Teva	00093-0674-01
100's	$100.80	Megestrol, Schein Pharm (US)	00364-2234-01
100's	$101.77	Megestrol Acetate, Aligen Independ	00405-4624-01
100's	$102.88	Megestrol, Martec Pharms	52555-0376-01
100's	$104.11	Megestrol, Qualitest Pharms	00603-4392-21
100's	$104.85	Megestrol, Parmed Pharms	00349-8767-01
100's	$105.85	Megestrol Acetate, Goldline Labs	00182-1864-89
100's	$106.00	Megestrol, Goldline Labs	00182-1864-01
100's	$106.37	Megestrol, HL Moore Drug Exch	00839-7406-06
100's	$110.31	Megestrol Acetate, Par Pharm	49884-0290-01
100's	$110.80	Megestrol, Rugby	00536-4822-01
100's	**$124.60**	**MEGACE, Mead Johnson**	**00015-0596-41**
250's	$191.00	Megestrol, Fujisawa USA	00469-5782-50
250's	$192.75	Megestrol, Major Pharms	00904-3571-70
250's	$194.82	Megestrol, H.C.F.A. F F P	99999-1716-03
250's	$240.00	Megestrol, Parmed Pharms	00349-8767-25
250's	$251.75	Megestrol Acetate, Aligen Independ	00405-4624-04
250's	$270.27	Megestrol Acetate, Par Pharm	49884-0290-04
250's	$271.45	Megestrol, Rugby	00536-4822-02
250's	**$305.29**	**MEGACE, Mead Johnson**	**00015-0596-46**
500's	$371.25	Megestrol, Major Pharms	00904-3571-40
500's	$389.65	Megestrol, H.C.F.A. F F P	99999-1716-04
500's	$437.11	Megestrol Acetate, Qualitest Pharms	00603-4392-28
500's	$506.32	Megestrol, HL Moore Drug Exch	00839-7406-12
500's	$529.52	Megestrol Acetate, Par Pharm	49884-0290-05
500's	**$598.14**	**MEGACE, Mead Johnson**	**00015-0596-45**

HOW SUPPLIED - NOT RATED EQUIVALENT:

Suspension - Oral - 40 mg/ml

235.6 ml	**$103.65**	**MEGACE, Mead Johnson**	**00015-0508-42**

MELPHALAN *(001717)*

CATEGORIES: Antineoplastics; Cancer; Chemotherapy; Multiple Myeloma; Myeloma; Nitrogen Mustard Derivatives; Oncologic Drugs; Ovarian Carcinoma; Breast Carcinoma*; Ewing's Sarcoma*; Leukemia*; Melanoma*; Neuroblastoma*; Pregnancy Category D; FDA Approval Pre 1982

* Indication not approved by the FDA

BRAND NAMES: **Alkeran**

FORMULARIES: Aetna; BC-BS; Medi-Cal

COST OF THERAPY: $618.82 (Ovarian Carcinoma; Tablet; 2 mg; 1/day; 365 days)

WARNING:
Melphalan should be administered under the supervision of a qualified physician experienced in the use of cancer chemotherapeutic agents. Severe bone marrow suppression with resulting infection or bleeding may occur. Melphalan is leukemogenic in humans.
Melphalan produces chromosomal aberrations in vitro and in vivo and, therefore, should be considered potentially mutagenic in humans.

DESCRIPTION:

TABLETS AND IV INJECTION

Alkeran (melphalan), also known as L-phenylalanine mustard, phenylalanine mustard, L-PAM, or L-sarcolysin, is a phenylalanine derivative of nitrogen mustard. Alkeran is a bifunctional alkylating agent which is active against selective human neoplastic diseases. It is known chemically as 4-[bis(2-chloroethyl)amino]-*L*-phenylalanine. The molecular formula is $C_{13}H_{18}Cl_2N_2O_2$ and has a molecular weight of 305.20.

Melphalan is the active L-isomer of the compound and was first synthesized in 1953 by Bergel and Stock; the D-isomer, known as medphalan, is less active against certain animal tumors, and the dose needed to produce effects on chromosomes is larger than that required with the L-isomer. The racemic (DL-) form is known as merphalan or sarcolysin.

Melphalan is practically insoluble in water and has a pKa_1 of ~ 2.5.

Alkeran (melphalan) is available in tablet form for oral administration. Each scored tablet contains 2 mg melphalan and the inactive ingredients lactose, magnesium stearate, potato starch, povidone, and sucrose.

Alkeran for injection is supplied as a sterile, non-pyrogenic, freeze-dried powder. Each single-use vial contains melphalan HCl equivalent to 50 mg melphalan and 20 mg povidone. Alkeran for injection is reconstituted using the single diluent provided. Each vial of sterile diluent contains sodium citrate 0.2 g propylene 6.0 ml, ethanol (96%) of 0.52 ml, and Water for Injection to a total of 10 ml. Alkeran for injection is administered intravenously.

CLINICAL PHARMACOLOGY:

Tablets: Melphalan is an alkylating agent of the bischloroethylamine type. As a result, its cytotoxicity appears to be related to the extent of its interstrand cross-linking with DNA, probably by binding at the N^7 position of guanine. Like other bifunctional alkylating agents, it is active against both resting and rapidly dividing tumor cells.

PHARMACOKINETICS

The pharmacokinetics of melphalan after oral administration has been extensively studied in adult patients. Plasma melphalan levels are highly variably after oral dosing, both with respect to the time of the first appearance of melphalan in plasma (range 0 to 336 minutes) and to the peak plasma concentration (range 0.166 to 3.741 mcg/ml) achieved. These results may be due to incomplete intestinal absorption, a variable "first pass" hepatic metabolism, or to rapid hydrolysis. Five patients were studied after both oral and intravenous dosing with 0.6 mg/kg as a single bolus dose by each route. The areas under the plasma concentration-time curves after oral administration averaged 61 ± 26% (± standard deviation; range 25% to 89%) of those following intravenous administration. In 18 patients given a single oral dose of 0.6 mg/kg of melphalan, the terminal plasma half-disappearance time of parent drug was 89.5 ± 50 minutes. The 24-hour urinary excretion of parent drug in these patients was 10 ± 4.5%, suggesting that renal clearance is not a major route of elimination of parent drug.

One study using universally labeled ^{14}C-melphalan, found substantially less radioactivity in the urine of patients given the drug by mouth (30% of administered dose in 9 days) than in the urine of those given it intravenously (35% to 65% in 7 days). Following either oral or intravenous administration, the pattern of label recovery was similar, with the majority being recovered in the first 24 hours. Following oral administration, peak radioactivity occurred in plasma at 2 hours and then disappeared with a half-life of approximately 160 hours. In one patient where parent drug (rather than just radiolabel) was determined, the melphalan half-disappearance time was 67 minutes.

The steady-state volume of distribution of melphalan is 0.5 l/kg. Penetration into cerebrospinal fluid (CSF) is low. The extent of melphalan binding to plasma proteins ranges from 60% to 90% Serum albumin is the major binding protein, while α_1-acid glycoprotein appears to account for about 20% of the plasma protein binding. Approximately 30% of melphalan is (covalently) irreversibly bound to plasma proteins. Interactions with immunoglobulins have been found to be negligible.

Melphalan is eliminated from plasma primarily by chemical hydrolysis to monohydroxy- and dihydroxymelphalan. Aside from these hydrolysis products, no other melphalan metabolites have been observed in humans. Although the contribution of renal elimination to melphalan clearance appears to be low, one pharmacokinetic study showed a significant negative correlation between the elimination rate and constant for melphalan and renal function and a significant negative correlation between renal function and the area under the plasma melphalan concentration/time curve.

IV Injection: Melphalan is an alkylating agent of the bischloroethylamine type. As a result, its cytotoxicity appears to be related to the extent of its interstrand cross-linking with DNA, probably at the N^7 position of guanine. Like other bifunctional alkylating agents, it is active against both resting and rapidly dividing tumor cells.

PHARMACOKINETICS

The pharmacokinetics of melphalan after intravenous administration has been extensively studied in adult patients. Following injection, drug plasma concentrations declined rapidly in a biexponential manner with distribution phase and terminal elimination phase half-lives of approximately 10 and 75 minutes, respectively. Estimates of average total body clearance varied among studies, but typical values of approximately 7 to 9 ml/min/kg (250 to 325 ml/min/m²) were observed. One study has reported that on repeat dosing of 0.5 mg/kg every 6 weeks, the clearance of melphalan decreased from 8.1 ml/min/kg after the first course, to 5.5 ml/min/kg after the third course, but did not decrease appreciably after the third course. Mean (± SD) peak melphalan plasma concentrations in myeloma patients given melphalan intravenously at doses of 10 or 20 mg/m² were 1.2 ± 0.4 and 2.8 ± 1.9 ng/ml, respectively.

The steady-state volume of distribution of melphalan is 0.5 L/kg. Penetration into cerebrospinal fluid (CSF) is low. The extent of melphalan binding to plasma protein ranges from 60 to 90%. Serum albumin is the major binding protein, while α_1-acid glycoprotein appears to account for about 20% of the plasma protein binding. Approximately 30% of the drug is (covalently) irreversibly bound to plasma proteins. Interactions with immunoglobulins have been found to be negligible.

Melphalan is eliminated from plasma primarily through chemical hydrolysis to monohydroxy- and dihydroxymelphalan. Aside from these hydrolysis products, no other melphalan metabolites have been observed in man. Although the contribution of renal elimination to melphalan clearance appears to be low, one study noted an increase in the occurrence of severe leukopenia in patients with elevated BUN after 10 weeks of therapy.

CLINICAL STUDIES:

A randomized trial compared prednisone plus IV melphalan to prednisone plus oral melphalan in the treatment of myeloma. As discussed below, overall response rates at week 22 were comparable; however, because of changes in trial design, conclusions as to the relative activity of the two formulations after week 22 are impossible to make.

Both arms received oral prednisone starting at 0.8 mg/kg/day with tapered over 6 weeks. Melphalan doses in each arm were:

Arm 1: Oral melphalan 0.15 mg/kg/day × 7 followed by 0.05 mg/kg/day when WBC began to rise.

Arm 2: IV melphalan 16 mg/m^2 q 2 weeks × 4 (over 6 weeks) followed by the same dose every 4 weeks.

Doses of melphalan were adjusted according to the criteria found in TABLE 1.

TABLE 1

WBC/mm^3	Platelets	% of full dose
≥ 4000	≥ 100,000	100
≥ 3000	≥ 75,000	75
≥ 2000	≥ 50,000	50
< 2000	< 50,000	0

107 patients were randomized to the oral melphalan arm and 203 patients to the IV melphalan arm. More patients had a poor-risk classification (58% vs. 44%) and high tumor load (51% vs. 34%) on the oral compared to the I.V. arm (p<0.04). Response rates at week 22 are shown in TABLE 2.

TABLE 2

Initial arm	Evaluable patients	Responders n (%)	P
Oral melphalan	100	44 (44%)	P>0.2
IV melphalan	195	74 (38%)	

Because of changes in protocol design after week 22, other efficacy parameters such as response duration and survival cannot be compared.

Severe myelotoxicity (WBC ≤1000 and/or platelets ≤25,000) was more common in the IV melphalan arm (28%) than in the oral melphalan arm (11%).

An association was noted between poor renal function and myelosuppression; consequently, an amendment to the protocol required a 50% reduction in the IV melphalan dose if the BUN was ≥30 mg/dL. The rate of severe leukopenia in the IV arm in the patients with BUN over 30 mg/dl decreased from 50% (8/16) before protocol amendment to 11% (3/28)(P=.01) after the amendment.

Before the dosing amendment, there was a 10% (8/77) incidence of drug-related deaths in the IV arm. After the dosing amendment, this incidence was 3% (3/108). This compares to an overall 1% (1/100) incidence of drug- related death in the oral arm.

INDICATIONS AND USAGE:

Tablets: Melphalan is indicated for the palliative treatment of multiple myeloma and for the palliation of non-resectable epithelial carcinoma of the ovary.

IV Injection: Melphalan HCl for injection is indicated for the palliative treatment of patients with multiple myeloma for whom oral therapy is not appropriate.

CONTRAINDICATIONS:

Tablets and IV Injection: Melphalan should not be used in patients whose disease has demonstrated a prior resistance to this agent. Patients who have demonstrated hypersensitivity to melphalan should not be given the drug.

WARNINGS:

IV INJECTION AND TABLETS

Melphalan should be administered in carefully adjusted dosage by or under the supervision of experienced physicians who are familiar with the drug's actions and the possible complications of its use.

As with other nitrogen mustard drugs, excessive dosage will produce marked bone marrow suppression. Bone marrow suppression is the most significant toxicity associated with melphalan for injection in most patients. Therefore, the following tests should be performed at the start of therapy prior to each subsequent dose of melphalan: platelet count, hemoglobin, white blood cell count and differential. Thrombocytopenia and/or leukopenia are indications to withhold further therapy until the blood cell counts have sufficiently recovered. Frequent blood counts are essential to determine optimal dosage and to avoid toxicity (see PRECAUTIONS, Laboratory Tests). Dose adjustment on the basis of blood counts at the nadir and the day of treatment should be considered.

Hypersensitivity reactions including anaphylaxis have occurred in approximately 2% of patients who received the IV formulation (see ADVERSE REACTIONS). These reactions usually occur after multiple courses of treatment. Treatment is systematic. The infusion should be terminated immediately, followed by the administration of volume expanders, pressor agents, corticosteroids, or antihistamines at the discretion of the physician. If a hypersensitivity reaction occurs, intravenous or oral melphalan should not be readministered since hypersensitivity reactions have also been reported with oral melphalan.

Carcinogenesis: Secondary malignancies, including acute nonlymphocytic leukemia, myeloproliferative syndrome, and carcinoma have been reported in patients with cancer treated with alkylating agents (including melphalan). Some patients also received other chemotherapeutic agents or radiation therapy. Precise quantitation of the risk of acute leukemia, myeloproliferative syndrome, or carcinoma is not possible. Published reports of leukemia in patients who have received melphalan (and other alkylating agents) suggest that the risk of leukemogenesis increases with chronicity of treatment and with cumulative dose. In one study, the 10 year cumulative risk of developing acute leukemia or myeloproliferative syndrome after melphalan therapy was 19.5% for cumulative doses ranging from 730 mg to 9652 mg. In this same study, as well as in an additional study, the 10 year cumulative risk of developing acute leukemia or myeloproliferative syndrome after melphalan therapy was less than 2% for cumulative doses under 600 mg. This does not mean that there is a cumulative dose below which there is no risk of the induction of a second malignancy.

Adequate and well-controlled carcinogenicity studies have not been conducted in animals. However, i.p. administration of melphalan in rats (5.4 to 10.8 mg/m^2) and in mice (2.25 to 4.5 mg/m^2) three times per week for six months followed by 12 months post-dose observation produced peritoneal sarcoma and lung tumors, respectively.

Mutagenesis: Melphalan has been shown to cause chromatid or chromosome damage in humans. Intramuscular administration of melphalan at 6 and 60 mg/m^2 produced structural aberrations of the chromatid and chromosomes in bone marrow cells of Wistar rats.

WARNINGS: *(cont'd)*

Impairment of Fertility: Melphalan causes suppression of ovarian function in pre-menopausal women, resulting in amenorrhea in a significant number of patients. Reversible and irreversible testicular suppression have also been reported.

Pregnancy Category D: Melphalan may cause fetal harm when administered to a pregnant woman. While adequate animal studies have not been conducted with IV melphalan, oral (6 to 18 mg/m^2/day for 10 days) and intraperitoneal (18 mg/m^2/single dose) administration in rats was embryolethal and teratogenic. Malformations resulting from melphalan included alterations of the brain (underdevelopment, deformation, meningocele and encephalocele) and eye (anophthalmia and microphthalmos) reduction of the mandible and tail as well as hepatocele (exomphaly).

There are no adequate and well-controlled studies in pregnant women. If this drug is used during pregnancy, or if the patient becomes pregnant while taking this drug, the patient should be apprised of the potential hazard to the fetus. Women of childbearing potential should be advised to avoid becoming pregnant.

PRECAUTIONS:

GENERAL

Tablets: In all instances where the use of melphalan is considered for chemotherapy, the physician must evaluate the need and usefulness of the drug against the risk of adverse events. Melphalan should be used with extreme caution in patients whose bone marrow reserve may have been compromised by prior irradiation or chemotherapy, or whose marrow function is recovering from previous cytotoxic therapy. If the leukocyte count falls below 3,000/cells/mcg, or the platelet count below 100,000/cells/mcg, melphalan should be discontinued until the peripheral blood cell counts have recovered.

A recommendation as to whether or not dosage reduction should be made routinely in patients with impaired creatinine clearance cannot be made because:

There is considerable inherent patient-to-patient variability in the systemic availability of melphalan in patients with normal renal function.

Only a small amount of the administered dose that appears as parent drug in the urine of patients with normal renal function.

Patients with azotemia should be closely observed, however, in order to make dosage reductions, if required, at the earliest possible time.

IV Injection: In all instances where the use of melphalan for injection is considered for chemotherapy, the physician must evaluate the need and usefulness of the drug against the risk of adverse events. Melphalan should be used with extreme caution in patients whose bone marrow reserve may have been compromised by prior irradiation or chemotherapy or whose marrow function is recovering from previous cytotoxic therapy.

Dose reduction should be considered in patients with renal insufficiency receiving IV melphalan. In one trial, increased bone marrow suppression was observed in patients with BUN levels ≥30 mg/dl. A 50% reduction in the IV melphalan dose decreased the incidence of severe bone marrow suppression in the later portion of the study.

INFORMATION FOR THE PATIENT

Tablets and Injection: Patients should be informed that the major toxicities of melphalan are related to bone marrow suppression,

hypersensitivity reactions, gastrointestinal toxicity, and pulmonary toxicity. The major long-term toxicities are related to infertility and secondary malignancies. Patients should never be allowed to take the drug without close medical supervision and should be advised to consult their physician if they experience skin rash, vasculitis, bleeding, fever, persistent cough, nausea, vomiting, amenorrhea, weight loss, or unusual lumps/masses. Women of childbearing potential should be advised to avoid becoming pregnant.

Laboratory Tests: Periodic complete blood counts with differentials should be performed during the course of treatment with melphalan. At least one determination should be obtained prior to each dose. Patients should be observed closely for consequences of bone marrow suppression, which include severe infections, bleeding, and symptomatic anemia (see WARNINGS.)

Carcinogenesis, Mutagenesis, and Impairment of Fertility: See WARNINGS.

Pregnancy Category D: *Teratogenic Effects:* See WARNINGS.

Nursing Mothers: It is not known whether this drug is excreted in human milk. Melphalan should not be given to nursing mothers.

Pediatric Use: The safety and effectiveness of melphalan in children have not been established.

Geriatric Use: Clinical experience with melphalan has not identified differences in responses between the elderly and younger patients. In general, dose selection for an elderly patient should be cautious, reflecting the greater frequency of decreased hepatic, renal, or cardiac function, and of concomitant disease or other drug therapy.

DRUG INTERACTIONS:

Tablets: There are no known drug/drug interactions with melphalan.

IV Injection: The development of severe renal failure has been reported in patients treated with a single dose of IV melphalan followed by standard oral doses of cyclosporine. Cisplatin may affect melphalan kinetics by inducing renal dysfunction and subsequently altering melphalan clearance. IV melphalan may also reduce the threshold for BCNU lung toxicity. When nalidixic acid IV melphalan are given simultaneously, the incidence of severe hemorrhagic, necrotic enterocolitis has also been reported to increase in pediatric patients.

ADVERSE REACTIONS:

TABLETS AND IV INJECTION

Hematologic Effects: The most common side effect is bone marrow suppression. Although bone marrow suppression frequently occurs, it is usually reversible if melphalan is withdrawn early enough. However, irreversible bone marrow failure has been reported.

Gastrointestinal: Gastrointestinal disturbances such as nausea and vomiting, diarrhea and oral ulceration occur infrequently. Hepatic toxicity, including veno-occlusive bone marrow failure has been reported rarely.

Miscellaneous: Other reported adverse reactions include: pulmonary fibrosis and interstitial pneumonitis, skin hypersensitivity, vasculitis, alopecia, hemolytic anemia. Allergic reactions including rare anaphylaxis, have occurred after multiple courses of treatment.

INJECTION

Hypersensitivity: Acute hypersensitivity reactions including anaphylaxis were reported in 2.4% of 425 patients receiving melphalan for injection for myeloma (see WARNINGS). These reactions were characterized by urticaria, pruritus, edema, and in some patients, tachycardia, bronchospasm, dyspnea, and hypotension. These patients appeared to respond to antihistamine and corticosteroid therapy. If hypersensitivity reaction occurs, IV or oral melphalan should not be readministered since hypersensitivity reactions have also been reported with oral melphalan.

OVERDOSAGE:

Tablets: Overdoses, including doses up to 50 mg/day for 16 days, have been reported. Immediate effects are likely to be vomiting, ulceration of the mouth, diarrhea, and hemorrhage of the gastrointestinal tract. The principal toxic effect is bone marrow suppression. Hematologic parameters should be closely followed for three to six weeks. An uncontrolled study suggests that administration of autologous bone marrow or hematopoietic growth factors (*i.e.,* sargramostim, filgrastim) may shorten the period of pancytopenia. General supportive measures, together with appropriate blood transfusions and antibiotics, should be instituted as deemed necessary by the physician. This drug is not removed from plasma to any significant degree by hemodialysis.[1]

IV Injection: Overdoses resulting in death have been reported. Overdoses, including doses up to 290 mg/m^2, have produced the following symptoms: severe nausea and vomiting, decreased consciousness, convulsions, muscular paralysis and cholinomimetic effects. Severe mucositis, stomatitis, colitis, diarrhea, and hemorrhage of the gastrointestinal tract occur at high doses (>100 mg/m^2). Elevations in liver enzymes and veno-occlusive disease occur infrequently. Significant hyponatremia caused by an associated inappropriate secretion of ADH syndrome has been observed. Nephrotoxicity and adult respiratory distress syndrome have been reported rarely. The principal toxic effect is bone marrow suppression. Hematologic parameters should closely followed for three to six weeks. An uncontrolled study suggests that administration of autologous bone marrow or hematopoietic growth factors (*i.e.,* sargramostim, filgrastim) may shorten the period of pancytopenia. General supportive measures together with appropriate blood transfusions and antibiotics should instituted as deemed necessary by the physician. The drug is not removed from plasma to any significant degree by hemodialysis or hemoperfusion. A pediatric patient survived a 254 mg/m^2 overdose treated with standard supportive care.

DOSAGE AND ADMINISTRATION:

TABLETS

Multiple Myeloma: The usual oral dose is 6 mg (3 tablets) daily. The entire daily dose may be given at one time. The dose is adjusted, as required, on the basis of blood counts done at approximately weekly intervals. After two to three weeks of treatment, the drug should be discontinued for up to four weeks during which time the blood count should be followed carefully. When the white blood cell and platelet counts are rising, a maintenance dose of 2 mg daily may be instituted. Because of the patient-to-patient variation in melphalan plasma levels following oral administration of the drug, several investigators have recommended that the dosage of melphalan be cautiously escalated until some myelosuppression is observed, in order to assure that potentially therapeutic levels of the drug have been reached.

Other dosage regimens have been used by various investigators. Osserman and Takatsuki have used an initial course of 10 mg/day for seven to ten days.[2,3] They report that maximal suppression of the leukocyte and platelet counts occurs within three to five weeks and recovery within four to eight weeks. Continuous maintenance therapy with 2 mg/day is instituted when the white blood cell count is greater that 4,000 cells/µl and the platelet count is greater than 100,000 cells/µl. Dosage is adjusted to between 1 and 3 mg/day depending upon the hematological response. It is desirable to try to maintain a significant degree of bone marrow depression so as to keep the leukocyte count in the range of 3,000 to 3,500 cells/µl.

Hoogstraten *et al* have started treatment with 0.15 mg/kg/day for seven days.[4] This is followed by a rest period of at least 14 days, but it may be as long as five to six weeks. Maintenance therapy is started when the white blood cell and platelet counts are rising. The maintenance dose is 0.05 mg/kg per day or less and is adjusted according to the blood count.

Available evidence suggests that about one third to one half of the patients with multiple myeloma show a favorable response to oral administration of the drug.

One study by Aleutian *et al* has shown that the use of melphalan in combination with prednisone significantly improves the percentage of patients with multiple myeloma who achieve palliation.[5] One regimen has been to administer courses of melphalan at 0.25 mg/kg/day for four consecutive days (or, 0.20 mg/kg/day for five consecutive days) for a total dose of 1 mg/kg per course. These four-to five-day courses are then repeated every four to six weeks if the granulocyte count and the platelet count have returned to normal levels.

It is to be emphasized that response may be very gradual over many months; it is important that repeated courses or continuous therapy be given since improvement may continue slowly over many months, and the maximum benefit may be missed if treatment is abandoned too soon.

In patients with moderate to severe renal impairment, currently available pharmacokinetic data does not justify an absolute recommendation on dosage reduction to those patients, but it may be prudent to use a reduced dose initially.

Epithelial Ovarian Cancer: One commonly employed regimen for the treatment of ovarian carcinoma has been to administer melphalan at a dose of 0.2 mg/kg daily for 5 days as a single course. Courses are repeated every 4 to 5 weeks depending upon hematologic tolerance.[6,7]

Administration for Precautions: Procedures for proper handling and disposal of anticancer drugs should be considered. Several guidelines on this subject have been published[8-14]

There is no general agreement that all of the procedures recommended in the guidelines are necessary or appropriate.

IV INJECTION

The usual intravenous dose is 16 mg/m^2. Dosage reduction of up to 50% should be considered in patients with renal insufficiency (BUN ≥30 mg/dl) (see PRECAUTIONS, General). This drug is administered as a single infusion over 15 to 20 minutes. Melphalan is administered at 2-week intervals for 4 doses, then, after adequate recovery from toxicity, at 4-week intervals. Available evidence suggests about one-third to one- half of the patients with multiple myeloma show a favorable response to the drug. Experience with oral melphalan suggests that repeated courses should be given since improvement may continue slowly over many months, and the maximum benefit may be missed if treatment is abandoned prematurely. Dose adjustment on the basis of blood cell counts at the nadir and day of treatment should be considered.

Administration Precautions: As with other toxic compounds, caution should be exercised in handling and preparing the solutions of melphalan. Skin reactions with accidental exposure may occur. The use of gloves is recommended. If the solution of melphalan contacts the skin or mucosa, immediately wash the skin or mucosa thoroughly with soap and water.

Procedures for proper handling and disposal of anticancer drugs should be considered. Several guidelines have been published. There is no general agreement that all of the procedures recommended in the guidelines are necessary or appropriate.

Parenteral drug products should be visually inspected for particulate matter and discoloration prior to administration whenever solution and container permit. If either occurs, do not use this product.

DOSAGE AND ADMINISTRATION: *(cont'd)*

PREPARATION FOR ADMINISTRATION/STABILITY:

1. Melphalan for injection must be reconstituted by rapidly injecting 10 ml of the supplied diluent directly into the vial of lyophilized powder using a sterile needle (20 gauge or larger needle diameter) and syringe. Immediately shake vial vigorously until a clear solution is obtained. This provides a 5 mg/ml solution of melphalan. Rapid addition of the diluent followed by immediate vigorous shaking is important for proper dissolution.
2. **Immediately** dilute the dose to be administered in 0.9% sodium chloride injection, U.S.P., to a concentration not greater than 0.45 mg/ml.
3. Administer the diluted product over a minimum of 15 minutes.
4. Complete administration within 60 minutes of reconstitution.

The time between constitution/dilution and administration of melphalan should be kept to a minimum because reconstituted and diluted solutions of melphalan are unstable. Over as short a time as 30 minutes a citrate derivative of melphalan has been detected in reconstituted material from the reaction of melphalan with Sterile Diluent for melphalan. Upon further dilution with saline, nearly 1% label strength of melphalan hydrolyzes every 10 minutes.

A precipitate forms if the constituted solution is stored at 5°C. DO NOT REFRIGERATE THE RECONSTITUTED PRODUCT.

REFERENCES:

1. Pallante SL, Fenselau C, Mennel RG, et al. Quantitation by gas chromatography-chemical ionization-mass spectrometry of phenylalanine mustard in plasma of patients. *Cancer Res.* 1980;40:2268-2272. **2.** Osseomucin EF. Therapy of plasma cell myeloma with melphalan (1-phenylalanine mustard). *Proc Am Assoc Cancer Res.* 1963;4:50. Abstract. **3.** Osseomucin EF, Takata K. Plasma cell myeloma: gamma globulin synthesis and structure. A review of biochemical and clinical data, with the description of a newly-recognized and related syndrome, "H-gamma-2-chain" (Franklin's) disease. *Medicin* (Balt). 1963;42:357-384. **4.** Hood B, Sheehe PR, Cuttner J, et al. Melphalan in multiple myeloma. *Blood.* 1967;30:74-83. **5.** Aleutian R, Haut A, Khan AU, et al. Treatment for multiple myeloma: combination chemotherapy with different melphalan dose regimens.*JAMA.* 1969;208:1680-1685. **6.** Smith JP, Rutledge FN: Chemotherapy in advanced ovarian cancer. *Natl Cancer Inst Monogr.*1975;42:141-143. **7.** Young RC, Chabner BA, Hubbard SP, et al. Advanced ovarian adenocarcinoma: a prospective clinical trial of melphalan (L-PAM) versus combination chemotherapy. *N Engl J Med.*1978;299;1261-1266. **8.** Recommendations for the safe handling of parenteral antineoplastic drugs. Washington, DC: Division of Safety, National Institutes of Health; 1983. US Dept of Health and Human Services, Public Health Service publication NIH 83-2621. **9.** AMA Council on Scientific Affairs. Guidelines for handling parenteral antineoplastics. *JAMA.* 1985;253:1590-1591. **10.** National Study Commission on Cytotoxic Exposure. Recommendations for handling cytotoxic agents. 1987. Available from Louis P. Jeffrey, Chairman, National Study Commission on Cytotoxic Exposure. Massachusetts College of Pharmacy and Allied Health Sciences, 179 Longwood Avenue, Boston, Massachusetts, 02115. **11.** Clinical Oncological Society of Australia. Guidelines and recommendations for safe handling of antineoplastic agents. *Med J Australia.* 1983;1:426-428. **12.** Jones RB, Frank R, Mass T. Safe handling of chemotherapeutic agents: a report from the Mount Sinai Medical Center. *CA-A Cancer J for Clin.* 1983;33:258-263. **13.** American Society of Hospital Pharmacists. ASHP technical assistance bulletin on handling cytotoxic and hazardous drugs.*Am J Hosp Pharm.* 1990;47:1033-1049. **14.** Yodaiken RE, Bennett D. OSHA work-practice guidelines for personnel dealing with cytotoxic (antineoplastic) drugs. *Am J Hosp Pharm.*1986;43:1193-1204.

HOW SUPPLIED:

Tablets: Alkeran is supplied as white, scored tablets containing 2 mg melphalan, imprinted with "Alkeran" and "A2A".

Storage: Store at 15° to 25°C (59° to 77°F) in a dry place, protect from light, and dispense in glass.

Injection: Alkeran for injection is supplied in a carton containing one single-use clear glass vial of freeze-dried melphalan hydrochloride equivalent to 50 mg melphalan and one 10 ml clear glass vial of sterile diluent.

Storage: Store at controlled room temperature 15° to 30°C (59° to 86°F) and protect from light.

HOW SUPPLIED - EQUIVALENTS NOT AVAILABLE:

Injection, Solution - Intravenous - 50 mg

1's	$296.99	**ALKERAN, Glaxo Wellcome**	**00173-0130-93**

Tablet, Uncoated - Oral - 2 mg

50's	$84.77	**ALKERAN, Glaxo Wellcome**	**00173-0045-35**

MENADIOL SODIUM DIPHOSPHATE *(001718)*

CATEGORIES: Blood Formation/Coagulation; Celiac Disease; Colitis; Cystic Fibrosis; Enteritis; Hemostatics; Hypoprothrombinemia; Jaundice; Liver Function; Salicylates; Ulcerative Colitis; Vitamin K Activity; Vitamins; Pregnancy Category C; FDA Approval Pre 1982

BRAND NAMES: *Coagen* (Japan); *Kativ* (Japan); *Mena* (Japan); *Synkavit* (England); *Synkavite* (Canada); **Synkayvite**
(International brand names outside U.S. in italics)

FORMULARIES: Aetna; Medi-Cal

DESCRIPTION:

TABLETS

Menadiol sodium diphosphate is a synthetic, water-soluble derivative of menadione (vitamin K_3). Synkayvite is available for oral administration in 5-mg tablets. Each tablet also contains gelatin, lactose, magnesium stearate, corn starch and talc. Chemically, menadiol sodium diphosphate is 2-methyl-1,4-naphthalenediol bis (dihydrogen phosphate) tetrasodium salt, hexahydrate. It is a white to pink hygroscopic powder with a characteristic odor and is very soluble in water and insoluble in alcohol. It has a molecular weight of 530.18.

INJECTION

Menadiol sodium diphosphate injection, a synthetic water-soluble derivative of menadione (vitamin K_3), is a sterile aqueous solution intended for intramuscular, intravenous or subcutaneous administration. Menadiol sodium diphosphate injection is available in the following concentrations:

1-ml Ampuls, 5 mg/ml: each ml contains 5 mg menadiol sodium diphosphate compounded with 2.5 mg sodium metabisulfite, 0.45% phenol as preservative, 0.4% sodium chloride for isotonicity and sodium hydroxide to adjust pH to approximately 8.0.

1-ml Ampuls, 10 mg/ml: each ml contains 10 mg menadiol sodium diphosphate compounded with 2.5 mg sodium metabisulfite, 0.45% phenol as preservative, 0.4% sodium chloride for isotonicity and sodium hydroxide to adjust pH to approximately 8.0.

2-ml Ampuls, 75 mg/2 ml: each 2 ml contains 75 mg menadiol sodium diphosphate compounded with 5 mg sodium metabisulfite, 0.45% phenol as preservative, 0.4% sodium chloride for isotonicity and sodium hydroxide to adjust pH to approximately 8.0.

CLINICAL PHARMACOLOGY:

Menadiol sodium diphosphate is converted *in vivo* to menadione (vitamin K_3). Its potency is approximately one-half that of menadione. Menadiol sodium diphosphate is similar in activity to naturally occurring vitamin K, which is necessary for the synthesis in the liver of blood coagulation factors prothrombin (factor II), proconvertin (factor VII), thromboplastin (factor IX) and Stuart factor (factor X). The prothrombin test is sensitive to the concentra-

CLINICAL PHARMACOLOGY: *(cont'd)*

tions of factors II, VII and X. The mechanism by which vitamin K_1 promotes formation of these clotting factors is not known, but animal data suggest that it acts as an enzyme or catalyst upon a substrate within the liver or combines with an apoenzyme (AE) to form an active enzyme (AE-K) which then is involved in prothrombin synthesis.

Pharmacokinetic data are unavailable because there is no acceptable assay procedure for the determination of menadiol in biological specimens. The physiochemical properties of menadiol sodium diphosphate indicate a negligible potential for absorption problems. The onset and duration of action following oral administration are not known. Vitamin K appears to pass through the placenta.

INDICATIONS AND USAGE:

TABLETS

Menadiol sodium diphosphate tablets are indicated for:

vitamin K deficiency secondary to the administration of antibacterial therapy;

hypoprothrombinemia secondary to obstructive jaundice and biliary fistulas;

hypoprothrombinemia secondary to administration of salicylates.

INJECTION

Menadiol sodium diphosphate injection is indicated for the treatment for hypoprothrombinemia secondary to factors limiting absorption or synthesis of vitamin K, *e.g.*, obstructive jaundice, biliary fistula, sprue, ulcerative colitis, celiac disease, intestinal resection, cystic fibrosis of the pancreas, regional enteritis and antibacterial therapy.

It is also indicated in hypoprothrombinemia secondary to administration of salicylates.

Menadiol sodium diphosphate injection may also be used as a liver function test, although newer functions are available.

CONTRAINDICATIONS:

BOTH FORMS

Vitamin K, or any of its synthetic analogs, should not be administered to the mother *during the last few weeks of pregnancy* as a prophylactic measure against physiologic hypoprothrombinemia or hemorrhagic disease of the newborn.

Menadiol sodium diphosphate is contraindicated in patients with known hypersensitivity to the drug.

WARNINGS:

TABLETS

Menadiol sodium diphosphate and other water-soluble vitamin K analogs are ineffective in the treatment of oral anticoagulant-induced hypoprothrombinemia and should, therefore, not be used in its treatment. Menadiol sodium diphosphate will not counteract the anticoagulant action of heparin.

INJECTION

Menadiol sodium diphosphate injection should not be used in the prophylaxis and treatment of hemorrhagic disease of the newborn because phytonadione is safer than the water-soluble vitamin K analogs.

Menadiol sodium diphosphate and other water-soluble vitamin k analogs are ineffective in the treatment of oral anticoagulant-induced hypoprothrombinemia and, therefore, should not be used in the treatment. Menadiol sodium diphosphate injection contains sodium metabisulfite, a sulfite that may cause allergic-type reactions, including anaphylactic symptoms and life-threatening or less severe asthmatic episodes in certain susceptible people. The overall prevalence of sulfite sensitivity in the general population is unknown and probably low. Sulfite sensitivity is seen more frequently in asthmatic than in non-asthmatic people.

PRECAUTIONS:

General: Temporary resistance to prothrombin-depressing anticoagulants may result, especially when larger doses analogs of menadiol sodium diphosphate are used. If relatively large doses have been employed, it may be necessary when reinstituting anticoagulant therapy to use somewhat larger doses of the prothrombin-depressing anticoagulant or one which has a different mode of action, such as heparin.

Since the liver is the site of metabolic synthesis of prothrombin, hypoprothrombinemia resulting from hepatocellular damage is not corrected by administration of vitamin K. Repeated large doses of vitamin K are not warranted in liver disease if the response to initial use of the vitamin is unsatisfactory (Koller test).

Failure to respond to vitamin K may indicate that a coagulation defect is present or that the condition being treated is unresponsive to vitamin K.

Information for the Patient: To assure safe and effective use of this drug, the following information and instructions should be given to the patient:

1. Take this medication exactly as directed by your doctor. Do not increase or decrease the prescribed dosage, or take it more often, or take it for a longer period of time than instructed.

2. If you miss a dose, take it as soon as possible, and then continue with your normal dosing schedule. Do not take the missed dose if it is almost time for your next dose; continue on your normal schedule and inform your doctor about any doses that you miss. If you have any questions about this, ask your doctor or pharmacist.

3. Inform all doctors and pharmacists that you are taking this medication; other medicines may affect the way this medicine works.

4. Before starting or stopping any other medications, including nonprescription drugs such as aspirin, check with your doctor or pharmacist.

5. A blood test should be performed at regular intervals to determine how this medicine is working. This will help your doctor decide the best dosing schedule for you.

6. Inform your doctor if you are pregnant or become pregnant while using this drug, even though vitamin K has not been shown to cause birth defects or other problems. Also inform your doctor if you are nursing.

Laboratory Tests: The dose, route and frequency of administration and duration of treatment depend on the severity of the prothrombin deficiency and should be regulated by repeated determinations of prothrombin time.

Drug/Laboratory Test Interactions: Menadione has been reported to interfere with the modified Reddy, Jenkins, Thorn procedure for determining urinary 17-hydroxycorticosteroids, producing falsely elevated levels.

Carcinogenesis, Mutagenesis and Impairment of Fertility: Menadiol sodium diphosphate has not undergone adequate animal testing to evaluate carcinogenic potential. The mutagenicity of menadiol sodium diphosphate has not been evaluated in the Ames test. Menadiol sodium diphosphate has not been evaluated for effects on fertility.

Pregnancy Category C: *Teratogenic Effects:* Segment II reproduction studies have not been conducted with menadiol. However, menadione (vitamin K_3) was nonteratogenic in rats at doses of 15 and 150 mg/day. The 150 mg/day dose in rats is approximately 2640 times the maximum human therapeutic dose of 10 mg daily. It is not known whether menadiol sodium diphosphate can cause fetal harm when administered to a pregnant woman or can affect

PRECAUTIONS: *(cont'd)*

reproductive capacity. Menadiol sodium diphosphate should be given to a pregnant woman only if clearly needed. *Nonteratogenic Effects:* Retardation of skeletal ossification and an increase in fetal resorptions have been reported in rats with menadione (vitamin K_3). Menadione and its derivatives have been implicated in producing hemolytic anemia, hyperbilirubinemia and kernicterus in the newborn, especially in premature infants, when administered to the mother prior to delivery or to the newborn. A marked hyperbilirubinemia has been reported in premature infants of mothers given menadione 2 to 112 hours prior to delivery. Menadiol sodium diphosphate given parenterally during labor caused an elevation in prothrombin levels in 16 of 22 infants. (Also see CONTRAINDICATIONS.)

Nursing Mothers: A study has shown that vitamin K is excreted in human milk. This should be considered if it is necessary to administer menadiol sodium diphosphate to a nursing mother.

DRUG INTERACTIONS:

Patients being treated with coumarin and indanedione derivative anticoagulants are extremely sensitive to changes in available vitamin K. Therefore, large doses of menadione or menadiol sodium diphosphate may decrease patient sensitivity to oral anticoagulants, although these vitamin K analogs are ineffective in treating anticoagulant overdosage.

ADVERSE REACTIONS:

Bromsulfalein retention and prolongation of prothrombin time have been reported after maximum doses of vitamin K analogs.

Menadione can induce erythrocyte hemolysis in persons having a genetic deficiency of glucose-6-phosphate dehydrogenase in their red blood cells.

In patients with severe hepatic disease, large doses of menadione may further depress liver function. Paradoxically, the administration of excessive doses of vitamin K or its analogs in an attempt to correct the hypoprothrombinemia associated with severe hepatitis or cirrhosis may actually result in a further depression of the concentration of prothrombin. (Also see PRECAUTIONS, General).

Occasional allergic reactions, such as skin rash and urticaria, have been reported. There have also been minor instances of gastric disturbance.

In infants (particularly premature babies), excessive doses of vitamin K analogs may cause increased bilirubinemia in the first few days of life. This, in turn, may lead to brain damage or even death. Immaturity is apparently an important factor in the appearance of toxic reactions to vitamin K analogs as full-term and larger premature infants demonstrate greater tolerance than smaller premature infants.

OVERDOSAGE:

There are no data on overdosage of menadiol sodium diphosphate in man. The administration of large doses of menadione and its derivatives to animals has resulted in the production of anemia, polycythemia, splenomegaly, renal and hepatic damage and death.

The acute oral toxicity of menadiol sodium diphosphate is as follows: (TABLE 1)

TABLE 1

	$LD_{50} \pm$ S.D.
Mouse	6172 ± 966 mg/kg
Rat	5250 ± 740 mg/kg

The acute intravenous toxicity of menadiol sodium diphosphate is as follows:(TABLE 2)

TABLE 2

	$LD_{50} \pm$ S.D.
Mouse	500 ± 55 mg/kg
Rat	400 ± 65 mg/kg

DOSAGE AND ADMINISTRATION:

TABLETS

The U.S. Recommended Daily Allowances for vitamin K in humans have not been established officially. The adequate daily dietary intake of vitamin K for adults has been estimated to be 70 to 140 mcg. The dietary abundance of vitamin K normally satisfies these requirements.

Following are the usual recommended dosages (TABLE 3):

TABLE 3

For hypoprothrombinemia secondary to obstructive jaundice and biliary fistulas	5 mg daily
For hypoprothrombinemia secondary to the administration of antibacterials or salicylates	5 to 10 mg daily

Store tablets at room temperature (15 to 30°C or 59 to 86°F).

INJECTION

The U.S. Recommended Daily Allowance for vitamin K in humans has not been established officially. The adequate daily dietary intake of vitamin K for adults has been estimated to be 70 to 140 mcg; for infants 10 to 20 mcg; for children and adolescents 15 to 100 mcg. The dietary abundance of vitamin K of normalcy satisfies the requirements except for the neonatal period of 5 to 8 days.

Menadiol sodium diphosphate may be injected subcutaneously, intramuscularly or intravenously. The response after intravenous administration may be more prompt, but more sustained action follows intramuscular or subcutaneous use.

Duration of treatment and frequency of dosage should be governed by blood prothrombin-time determination. In the absence of impaired liver function, a single dose usually corrects hypoprothrombinemia in 8 to 24 hours. Injections should be repeated in 12 hours if tests at this time show no evidence of improvement.

Following are the usual recommended dosages:(TABLE 4)

TABLE 4

	ADULTS	CHILDREN
For treatment of hypoprothrombinemia	5 to 15 mg 1-2 times daily	5 to 10 mg 1-2 times daily
For liver function test	75 mg intravenously	

Parenteral drug products should be inspected visually for particulate matter and discoloration prior to administration, whenever solution and container permit. Menadiol sodium diphosphate injection is incompatible with protein hydrolysate.

DOSAGE AND ADMINISTRATION: *(cont'd)*

Menadiol sodium diphosphate injection need not be refrigerated.

HOW SUPPLIED - EQUIVALENTS NOT AVAILABLE:

Injection, Solution - Intramuscular; - 75 mg/2ml

2 ml x 10 $37.94 SYNKAYVITE, Roche 00004-1925-06

MENINGITIS VACCINE *(001719)*

CATEGORIES: Immunologic; Serums, Toxoids and Vaccines; Vaccines; FDA Pre 1938 Drugs

BRAND NAMES: *FSME-Immun* (Germany); *Mencevax ACWY*; *Menomune*; Menomune-A C Y W-135
(International brand names outside U.S. in italics)

FORMULARIES: WHO

> **WARNING:**
> For special instructions on use of Meningococcal Polysaccharide Vaccine, Groups A, C, Y and W-135 Combined, for Jet Injector Use. (see DOSAGE AND ADMINISTRATION)

DESCRIPTION:

Menomune, Meningococcal Polysaccharide Vaccine Groups, A, C, Y and W-135 Combined, is a freeze-dried preparation of the group-specific polysaccharide antigens from *Neisseria meningitidis*, Group A, Group C, Group Y and Group W-135 for subcutaneous use. The diluent is sterile pyrogen-free distilled water to which thimerosal (mercury derivative) 1: 10,000 is added as a preservative. After reconstitution with diluent as indicated on the label, each 0.5 ml dose contains 50 mcg of "isolated product" from each of Groups A, C, Y and W-135 in isotonic sodium chloride solution preserved with thimerosal (mercury derivative). Each dose of vaccine also contains 2.5 mg to 5 mg of lactose added as a stabilizer.[1] The vaccine when reconstituted is a clear colorless liquid.

THE VACCINE CONFORMS TO W.H.O. REQUIREMENTS.

CLINICAL PHARMACOLOGY:

N. Meningitidis: Causes both endemic and epidemic disease, principally meningitis and meningococcemia. It is the second most common cause of bacterial meningitis in the United States (approximately 20% of all cases), affecting an estimated 3,000-4,000 people each year. The case-fatality rate is approximately 10% for meningococcal meningitis and 20% for meningococcemia, despite therapy with antimicrobial agents, such as penicillin, to which all strains remain highly sensitive.[2]

Within the United States, serogroup B, for which a vaccine is not yet available, accounts for 50%-55% of all cases; serogroup C, for 20%-25%; and serogroup W-135, for 15%. Serogroups Y (10%) and A (1%-2%) account for nearly all remaining cases. Serogroup W-135 has emerged as a major cause of disease only since 1975. While serogroup A causes only a small proportion of endemic disease in the United States, it is the most common cause of epidemics elsewhere.[2]

A study performed using 4 lots of Meningococcal Polysaccharide Vaccine, Groups A, C, Y and W-135 Combined in 150 adults showed at least a 4-fold increase in bactericidal antibodies to all groups in greater than 90 percent of the subjects.[3,4]

A study was conducted in 73 children 2 to 12 years of age. Post- immunization sera were not obtained on four children. Therefore, the seroconversion rates were based on 69 paired samples Seroconversion rates as measured by bactericidal antibody were: Group A - 72 percent, Group C - 58 percent, Group Y - 90 percent and Group W-135 - 82 percent. Seroconversion rates as measured by a 2-fold rise in antibody titers based on Solid Phase Radioimmunoassay were: Group A - 99 percent, Group Y - 97 percent and Group W-135 - 89 percent.[5]

As with any vaccine, vaccination with Meningococcal Polysaccharide Vaccine, Groups A, C, Y and W-135 Combined may not protect 100% of susceptible individuals.

Vaccine Efficacy: Numerous studies have demonstrated the immunogenicity and clinical efficacy of the A and C vaccines. The serogroup A polysaccharide induces antibody in some children as young as 3 months of age, although a response comparable to that seen in adults is not achieved until 4 or 5 years of age; the serogroup C component does not induce a good antibody response before age 18-24 months. The serogroup A vaccine has been shown to have a clinical efficacy of 85%-95% and to be of use in controlling epidemics.[6] A similar level of clinical efficacy has been demonstrated for the serogroup C vaccine, both in American military recruits and in an epidemic. The group Y and W-135 polysaccharides have been shown to be safe and immunogenic in adults and in children over 2 years of age; clinical protection has not been demonstrated directly, but it assumed, based on the production of bactericidal antibody, which for group C has been correlated with clinical protection. The antibody responses to each of the four polysaccharides in the quadrivalent vaccine are serogroup-specific and independent.[2]

Duration of Efficacy: Antibodies against the group A and C polysaccharides decline markedly over the first 3 years following a single dose of vaccine. This antibody decline is more rapid in infants and young children than in adults. Similarly, while vaccine-induced clinical protection probably persists in schoolchildren and adults for at least 3 years, a recent study in Africa has demonstrated a marked decline in the efficacy of the group A vaccine in young children over time. In this study, efficacy declined from greater than 90% to less than 10% over 3 years in those under 4 years of age at the time of vaccination; in older children, efficacy was still 67%, 3 years after vaccination.[2,7]

INDICATIONS AND USAGE:

Meningococcal Polysaccharide Vaccine, Groups A, C, Y and W-135 Combined, is indicated for the following individuals:

1. Persons 2 years of age and above in epidemic or endemic areas as might be determined in a population delineated by neighborhood, school, dormoitory, or the other resonable boundry. The prevalent serogroup in such a situation should match a serogroup in the vaccine.

2. Individuals at particular high-risk to include persons with terminal component complement defiencies and those with anatomic or functional asplenia.

3. Travelers to countries recognized as having hyperendemic or epidemic or epidemic disease such as the part of Sub-Saharan Africa known as the "meningitis belt", which extends from Mauritania in the west to Ethopia in the east.

Vaccinations also should be considered for household or institutional contacts of persons with meningococcal disease as an adjunct to appropriate antibiotic chemoprophlaxis as well as medical and laboratory personnel at risk of exposure to meningococcal disease.

This vaccine will not stimulate protection against infections caused by organisms other than Groups A,C, Y and W-135 meningococci.

CONTRAINDICATIONS:

Immunization should be deferred during the course of any acute illness. Pregnant women should not be immunized since effects of vaccine on the fetus are unknown.

IT IS A CONTRAINDICATIONS TO ADMINISTER MENOMUNE A/C/Y/W-135 TO INDIVIDUALS KNOWN TO BE SENSITIVE TO THIMERSOAL OR AN OTHER COMPONENT OF THE VACCINE.

WARNINGS:

If the vaccine is used in persons receving immunosuppressive therapy, the expected immune response may not be obtained.

PRECAUTIONS:

GENERAL

Epinephrine Injection (1:1000) must be immediately available to combat unexpected anaphylactic or other allergic reactions.

Prior to an injection of any vaccine, all known precautions should be taken to prevent side reactions. This includes a review of the patient's history with respect to possible sensitivity to the vaccine or similar vaccines.

As with any vaccine, vaccination with Meningococcal Polysaccharide Vaccine, Groups A, C, Y and W-135 Combined may not protect 100% of susceptible individuals. Protective antibody levels may be achieved within 10-14 days after vaccination.[2]

Special care should be taken to avoid injecting the vaccine intradermally, intramuscularly, or intravenously since clinical studies have not been done to establish safety and efficacy of the vaccine using these routes of administration.

A seperate, sterile syringe and needle or a sterile disposable unit should be used for each individual patient to prevent transmission of hepatitis and other infections agents from one person to another.

During use it is possible that the nozzle of the Jet Injector Apparatis may become contaminated with blood or serum. In one instance, such contamination has been reported to be associated with transmission to hepatits b disease. Therefore, if blood or serum contamination occurs, the nozzle should be disassembled, cleansed and sterilized before continued use to prevent the possibility of transmission of hepatitis or other infectious agents from one person to another.[8]

PREGNANCY [9]

Pregnancy Category C: Animal reproduction studies have not been conducted with Meningcoccal Polysaccharide Vaccine, Groups A, C, Y and W-135. It is also not known whether Meningococcal Polysaccharide Vaccine, Groups A, C, Y and W-135 can cause fetal harm when administered to a pregnant woman or can affect reproduction capacity.

Experience in Humans: There is no data on the safety of Menomune when administered to a pregnant woman. Therefore, Menomune should not be administered to a pregnant woman, particularly in the first trimester.

Pediatric Use: *THERE ARE NO DATA ON SAFETY AND EFFICACY OF MENOMUNE WHEN ADMINISTERED TO CHILDREN UNDER 2 YEARS OF AGE.*

ADVERSE REACTIONS:

Adverse reactions to meningococcal vaccine are mild and infrequent, consisiting of localized erythema lasting 1-2 days. Up to 2% of young children develop fever transiently after vaccination.[2]

As with the administration of any vaccine, one should expect possible hypersensitivity reactions.

DOSAGE AND ADMINISTRATION:

Parental drug products should be inspected visually for extraneous particulate matter and/or discoloration prior to administration whenever solution and container permit. If these conditions exist, vaccine should not be administered.

Reconstitute the vaccine using only the diluent supplied for this purpose. Draw the volume of diluent shown on the diluent label into a suitable size syringe and inject into the vial containting the vaccine. Shake vial until the vaccine is dissolved. Administer the vaccine subcautaneously.

The immunizing dose is a single injection of 0.5 ml given subcutaneously.

Primary Immunization: For both adults and children, vaccine is administered subcutaneously as a single 0.5 ml dose. The vaccine can be given at the samt time as other immunizations, if needed. Protective antibody levels may be achieved within 10-14 days after vaccination.[2]

Revaccination: Revaccination may be indicated for individuals at high risk of infection, particularly children who were first immunized under 4 years of age; such children should be considered for revaccination after 2 or 3 years if they remain at high risk. The need for revaccination in older children and adults remains unknown.[2]

> **Special instructions for 50 dose Vial of Meningococcal Polysaccharide Vaccine, Groups A, C, Y and W-135 Combined, for Jet Injector Use.**
> **DOSAGE AND ADMINISTRATION:** Parenteral drug products should be inspected visually for extraneous particulate matter and/or discoloration prior to administration whenever solution and container permit. If these conditions exist, vaccine should no tbe administered. Using a suitable syringe and needle and aseptic precautions, transfer the volume of diluent shown on the diluent label into the vial containing the vaccine. Shake vial until the vaccine is dissolved. Administer ONLY with automatic hypodermic jet apparatus. 50 DOSE VIAL NOT TO BE UTILIZED IN NEEDLE AND SYRINGE METHOD OF IMMUNIZATION. If absolutely necessary, syringes and beedles may be used with such containers with caution. However, due to coring of the stopper do NOT insert needle into vial more than 20 times. Discard partially used vial of vaccine. Immunization consists of a single injection of 0.5 ml given subcutaneously. Special care should be taken The immunizing dose is a single injection of 0.5 ml given subcutaneously. Special care should be taken to avoid injecting the vaccine intradermally, intramuscularly, or intravenously by using the deltoid area, since clinical studies have not been done to establish the safety and efficacy of the vaccine using these routes of administration.
> **Caution:** During use it is possible that the nozzle of the Jet Injector Apparatus may become contaminated with blood or serum. In one instance, such contamination has been reported to be associated with the transmission of hepatitis b disease. Therefore, if blood or serum contamination occurs, the nozzle should be disassembled, cleansed and sterilized before continued use to prevent the possibility of transmission of hepatitis or other infectious agents from one person to another.[8]

REFERENCES:

1. Tiesjema RH, et al. Enhanced stability of meningococcal polysaccharide vaccines by using lactose as a menstruum for lyophilization. Bull WHO 55;43-47, 1977. 2. Recommendation of the Immunization Practices Advisory Committee (ACIP). Meningcoccal Vaccines. MMWR 34: 255-259, 1985. 3. Hankins, W.A., et al: Clinical ands serological evaluation of a meningococcal polysaccharide vaccine goups A, C, Y and W-135. proc Soc Exper Biol Med 169: 54-57, 1982. 4. Lepow, M.L., et al: Reactogenicity and immunogenicity of a quadrivalent combined meningcoccal polysaccharide vaccine in children, J. Infect Dis 154: 1033-1036, 1986, 5. Unpublished data available from Connaught Laboratories, Inc., complied 1982. 6. Peltola, H., et al: Clinical efficacy of meningococcus Group A capsular polysaccharide vaccine in children three months to five years of age. N Engl J. Med 297: 686-691, 1977. 7. Reingold, A. L., et al: Age-specific differences in duration of clinical protection after vaccination with meningococcal polysaccharide A vaccine. Lancet. No. 8447: 114-118, 1985. 8. CDC. Hepatitis B associated with jet gun injection - California. MMWR 35: 373-376, 1986. 9. Code of Federal Regulations. 21CFR201.57 (f) (6) (c), 1989.

HOW SUPPLIED:

Vial, 1 Dose, with 0.78 ml vial of diluent.

Vial, 10 Dose, with 6 ml vial of diluent, for administration with needle and syringe (may be used with jet injector although the desired number of doses may not be obtained).

Vial, 50 Dose, with 27.5 ml vial of diluent for JET INJECTOR USE ONLY.

Additional package sizes available on speical order.

Storage: Store freeze-dried vaccine and reconstituted vaccine, when not in use between 2° - 8°C (35° - 45°F). Discard remainder of multidose vials of vaccine within 5 days after reconstitution. The single dose vial should be used within 24 hours of reconstitution.

HOW SUPPLIED - EQUIVALENTS NOT AVAILABLE:

Injection, Lyphl-Soln - Subcutaneous

1's	$52.38	MENOMUNE-A/C/Y/W-135, Connaught Labs	49281-0489-01
10's	$281.31	MENOMUNE A/C/Y/W-135, Connaught Labs	49281-0489-91

MENOTROPINS *(001720)*

CATEGORIES: Anterior Pituitary/Hypothalmic Function; Fertility Agents; Gonadotropins; Hormones; Hypogonadism; In Vitro Fertilization; Infertility; Ovarian Failure; Pituitary Function; Progesterone; Spermatogenesis; Pregnancy Category X; FDA Approval Pre 1982

BRAND NAMES: *HMG*; Humegon; *Menogon 75*; **Pergonal**; *Pergonal 75 75*; *Pergonal 500*
(International brand names outside U.S. in italics)

FORMULARIES: Aetna; BC-BS

DESCRIPTION:

Pergonal (menotropins for injection, USP) is a purified preparation of gonadotropins extracted from the urine of postmenopausal women. Each ampule of Pergonal contains 75 IU or 150 IU of follicle-stimulating hormone (FSH) activity and 75 IU or 150 IU of luteinizing hormone (LH) activity, respectively, plus 10 mg lactose in sterile, lyophilized form. Pergonal is administered by intramuscular injection.

Pergonal is biologically standardized for FSH and LH (ICSH) gonadotropin activities in terms of the Second International Reference Preparation for Human Menopausal Gonadotropins established in September, 1964 by the Expert Committee on Biological Standards of the World Health Organization.

Both FSH and LH are glycoproteins that are acidic and water soluble. Therapeutic class: Infertility.

CLINICAL PHARMACOLOGY:

Women: Pergonal administered for seven to twelve days produces ovarian follicular growth in women who do not have primary ovarian failure. Treatment with Pergonal in most instances results only in follicular growth and maturation. In order to effect ovulation, human chorionic gonadotropin (hCG) must be given following the administration of Pergonal when clinical assessment of the patient indicates that sufficient follicular maturation has occurred.

Men: Pergonal administered concomitantly with human chorionic gonadotropin (hCG) for at least three months induces spermatogenesis in men with primary or secondary pituitary hypofunction who have achieved adequate masculinization with prior hCG therapy.

CLINICAL STUDIES:

Women: The results of the clinical experience and effectiveness of the administration of Pergonal to 1,286 patients in 3,002 courses of therapy are summarized below. The values include patients who were treated with other than the recommended dosage regime. The values for the presently recommended dosage regime are essentially the same (TABLE 1).

TABLE 1

	%
Patients ovulating	75
Patients pregnant	25
Patients aborting	25*
Multiple pregnancies	20†
Twins	15†
Three or more concepti	5†
Fetal abnormalities	1.7†
Hyperstimulation syndrome	1.3

* Based on total pregnancies
† Based on total deliveries

Results by diagnosis group are summarized in TABLE 2 (these values include patients who were treated with other than the present recommended dosage regime):

TABLE 2

	% Pts. Ovul.	% Pts. Preg.	% Abort.	% Multi. Preg.	%Twins	% 3 or More Concepti	% Hyper-stim. Syndr.
Primary Amenorrhea	62	22	14	25	25	0	0
Secondary Amenorrhea	61	28	24	28	18	10	1.9
Secondary Amen. with Galactorrhea	77	42	21	41	31	10	1.2
Polycystic Ovaries	76	26	39	17	17	0	1.1
Anovulatory Cycles	77	24	15	14	9	5	2.0
Miscellaneous	83	20	36	2	2	0	0.1

Men: Clinical results of the treatment of men with primary or secondary hypogonadotropic hypogonadism are as follows:

In the Serono Cooperative study, with an adequate treatment period of 3 to 8 months, 60 of 70 men with primary hypogonadotropic hypogonadism and 8 of 11 men with secondary hypogonadotropic hypogonadism responded with mean increases in their sperm counts from less than 5 to 24 million spermatozoa per milliliter of ejaculate. Forty-one wives of 54 men with primary hypogonadotropic hypogonadism desiring offspring and 7 wives of men with secondary hypogonadotropic hypogonadism conceived. Patients treated with Pergonal and hCG for less than 3 months or with Pergonal alone did not respond to therapy.

A world-wide data search revealed that of 160 recorded pregnancies as the result of use of Pergonal-hCG in men, there were 7 spontaneous abortions, one ectopic pregnancy and 3 congenital anomalies at birth (esophageal atresia in a female infant which was later corrected by surgery, unilateral cryptorchidism, inguinal hernia).

INDICATIONS AND USAGE:

Women: Pergonal and hCG given in a sequential manner are indicated for the induction of ovulation and pregnancy in the anovulatory infertile patient, in whom the cause of anovulation is functional and is not due to primary ovarian failure.

Pergonal and hCG may also be used to stimulate the development of multiple follicles in ovulatory patients participating in an *in vitro* fertilization program.

Men: Pergonal with concomitant hCG is indicated for the stimulation of spermatogenesis in men who have primary or secondary hypogonadotropic hypogonadism.

Pergonal with concomitant hCG has proven effective in inducing spermatogenesis in men with primary hypogonadotropic hypogonadism due to a congenital factor or prepubertal hypophysectomy and in men with secondary hypogonadotropic hypogonadism due to hypophysectomy, craniopharyngioma, cerebral aneurysm or chromophobe adenoma.

Selection of Patients: Women

1. Before treatment with Pergonal is instituted, a thorough gynecologic and endocrinologic evaluation must be performed. Except for those patients enrolled in an *in vitro* fertilization program, this should include a hysterosalpingogram (to rule out uterine and tubal pathology) and documentation of anovulation by means of basal body temperature, serial vaginal smears, examination of cervical mucus, determination of serum (or urine) progesterone, urinary pregnanediol and endometrial biopsy. Patients with tubal pathology should receive Pergonal only if enrolled in an *in vitro* fertilization program.
2. Primary ovarian failure should be excluded by the determination of gonadotropin levels.
3. Careful examination should be made to rule out the presence of an early pregnancy.
4. Patients in late reproductive life have a greater predilection to endometrial carcinoma as well as a higher incidence of anovulatory disorders. Cervical dilation and curettage should always be done for diagnosis before starting. Pergonal therapy in such patients who demonstrate abnormal uterine bleeding or other signs of endometrial abnormalities.
5. Evaluation of the husband's fertility potential should be included in the workup.

Men: Patient selection should be made based on a documented lack of pituitary function. Prior to hormonal therapy, these patients will have low testosterone levels and low or absent gonadotropin levels. Patients with primary hypogonadotropic hypogonadism will have a subnormal development of masculinization, and those with secondary hypogonadotropic hypogonadism will have decreased masculinization.

CONTRAINDICATIONS:

Women: Pergonal is contraindicated in women who have:

1. A high FSH level indicating primary ovarian failure.
2. Uncontrolled thyroid and adrenal dysfunction.
3. An organic intracranial lesion such as a pituitary tumor.
4. The presence of any cause of infertility other than anovulation unless they are candidates for *in vitro* fertilization.
5. Abnormal bleeding of undetermined origin.
6. Ovarian cysts or enlargement not due to polycystic ovary syndrome.
7. Prior hypersensitivity to menotropins.
8. Pergonal is contraindicated in women who are pregnant and may cause fetal harm when administered to a pregnant woman. There are limited human data on the effects of Pergonal when administered during pregnancy.

Men: Pergonal is contraindicated in men who have

1. Normal gonadotropin levels indicating normal pituitary function.
2. Elevated gonadotropin levels indicating primary testicular failure.
3. Infertility disorders other than hypogonadotropic hypogonadism.

WARNINGS:

Pergonal is a drug that should only be used by physicians who are thoroughly familiar with infertility problems. It is a potent gonadotropic substance capable of causing mild to severe adverse reactions in women. Gonadotropin therapy requires a certain time commitment by physicians and supportive health professionals, and its use requires the availability of appropriate monitoring facilities (see PRECAUTIONS, Laboratory Tests). In female patients it must be used with a great deal of care.

Overstimulation of the Ovary During Pergonal Therapy: Ovarian Enlargement: Mild to moderate uncomplicated ovarian enlargement which may be accompanied by abdominal distension and/or abdominal pain occurs in approximately 20% of those treated with Pergonal and hCG, and generally regresses without treatment within two or three weeks.

In order to minimize the hazard associated with the occasional abnormal ovarian enlargement which may occur with Pergonal-hCG therapy, the lowest dose consistent with expectation of good results should be used. Careful monitoring of ovarian response can further minimize the risk of overstimulation.

If the ovaries are abnormally enlarged on the last day of Pergonal therapy, hCG should not be administered in this course of therapy; this will reduce the chances of development of the Ovarian Hyperstimulation Syndrome.

The Ovarian Hyperstimulation Syndrome (OHSS): OHSS is a medical event distinct from uncomplicated ovarian enlargement. OHSS may progress rapidly to become a serious medical event. It is characterized by an apparent dramatic increase in vascular permeability which can result in a rapid accumulation of fluid in the peritoneal cavity, thorax, and potentially, the pericardium. The early warning signs of development of OHSS are severe pelvic pain, nausea, vomiting, and weight gain. The following symptomatology has been seen with cases of OHSS: abdominal pain, abdominal distension, gastrointestinal symptoms, including nausea, vomiting and diarrhea, severe ovarian enlargement, weight gain, dyspnea, and oliguria.

WARNINGS: *(cont'd)*

Clinical evaluation may reveal hypovolemia, hemoconcentration, electrolyte imbalances, ascites, hemoperitoneum, pleural effusions, hydrothorax, acute pulmonary distress, and thromboembolic events (see Pulmonary and Vascular Complications). Transient liver function test abnormalities suggestive of hepatic dysfunction, which may be accompanied by morphologic changes on liver biopsy, have been reported in association with the Ovarian Hyperstimulation Syndrome (OHSS).

OHSS occurs in approximately 0.4% of patients when the recommended dose is administered and in 1.3% of patients when higher than recommended doses are administered. Cases of OHSS are more common, more severe and more protracted if pregnancy occurs. OHSS develops rapidly; therefore patients should be followed for at least two weeks after hCG administration. Most often, OHSS occurs after treatment has been discontinued and reaches its maximum at about seven to ten days following treatment. Usually, OHSS resolves spontaneously with the onset of menses. If there is evidence that OHSS may be developing prior to hCG administration (see PRECAUTIONS, Laboratory Tests, the hCG should be withheld.

If OHSS occurs, treatment should be stopped and the patient hospitalized. Treatment is primarily symptomatic, consisting of bed rest, fluid and electrolyte management, and analgesics if needed. The phenomenon of hemoconcentration associated with fluid loss into the peritoneal cavity, pleural cavity, and the pericardial cavity has been seen to occur and should be thoroughly assessed in the following manner:

1) fluid intake and output
2) weight
3) hematocrit
4) serum and urinary electrolytes
5) urine specific gravity
6) BUN and creatinine
7) abdominal girth

These determinations are to be performed daily or more often if the need arises.

With OHSS there is an increased risk of injury to the ovary. The ascitic, pleural, and pericardial fluid should not be removed unless absolutely necessary to relieve symptoms such as pulmonary distress or cardiac tamponade. Pelvic examination may cause rupture of an ovarian cyst, which may result in hemoperitoneum, and should therefore be avoided. If this does occur, and if bleeding becomes such that surgery is required, the surgical treatment should be designed to control bleeding and to retain as much ovarian tissue as possible. Intercourse should be prohibited in those patients in whom significant ovarian enlargement occurs after ovulation because of the danger of hemoperitoneum resulting from ruptured ovarian cysts.

The management of OHSS may be divided into three phases: the acute, the chronic, and the resolution phases. Because the use of diuretics can accentuate the diminished intravascular volume, diuretics should be avoided except in the late phase of resolution as described below.

Acute Phase: Management during the acute phase should be designed to prevent hemoconcentration due to loss of intravascular volume to the third space and to minimize the risk of thromboembolic phenomena and kidney damage. Treatment is designed to normalize electrolytes while maintaining an acceptable but somewhat reduced intravascular volume. Full correction of the intravascular volume deficit may lead to an unacceptable increase in the amount of third space fluid accumulation. Management includes administration of limited intravenous fluids, electrolytes, and human serum albumin. Monitoring for the development of hyperkalemia is recommended.

Chronic Phase: After stabilizing the patient during the acute phase, excessive fluid accumulation in the third space should be limited by instituting severe potassium, sodium, and fluid restriction.

Resolution Phase: A fall in hematocrit and an increasing urinary output without an increased intake are observed due to the return of third space fluid to the intravascular compartment. Peripheral and or pulmonary edema may result if the kidneys are unable excrete third space fluid as rapidly as it is mobilized. Diuretics may be indicated during the resolution phase if necessary to combat pulmonary edema.

Pulmonary and Vascular Complications: Serious pulmonary conditions (*e.g.,* atelectasis, acute respiratory distress syndrome) have been reported. In addition, thromboembolic events both in association with, and separate from, the Ovarian Hyperstimulation Syndrome have been reported following Pergonal therapy. Intravascular thrombosis and embolism, which may originate in venous or arterial vessels, can result in reduced blood flow to critical organs or the extremities. Sequelae of such events have included venous thrombophlebitis, pulmonary embolism, pulmonary infarction, cerebral vascular occlusion (stroke), and arterial occlusion resulting in loss limb. In rare cases, pulmonary complications and/or thromboembolic events have resulted in death.

Multiple Births: Data from a clinical trial revealed the following results regarding multiple births: Of the pregnancies following therapy with Pergonal and hCG, 80% resulted in single births, 15% in twins, and 5% of the total pregnancies resulted in three or more concepti. The patient and her husband should be advised of the frequency and potential hazards of multiple gestation before starting treatment.

Hypersensitivity/Anaphylactic Reactions: Hypersensitivity/anaphylactic reactions associated with Pergonal administration have been reported in some patients. These reactions presented as generalized urticaria, facial edema, angioneurotic edema, and/or dyspnea suggestive of laryngeal edema. The relationship of these symptoms to uncharacterized urinary proteins is uncertain.

PRECAUTIONS:

GENERAL

Careful attention should be given to diagnosis in the selection of candidates for Pergonal therapy (see INDICATIONS AND USAGE, Selection of Patients.)

INFORMATION FOR THE PATIENT

Prior to therapy with Pergonal, patients should be informed of the duration of treatment and the monitoring of their condition that will be required. Possible adverse reactions (see ADVERSE REACTIONS) and the risk of multiple births should also be discussed.

LABORATORY TESTS

Women: Treatment for Induction of Ovulation

In most instances, treatment with Pergonal results only in follicular growth and maturation. In order to effect ovulation, hCG must be given following the administration of Pergonal when clinical assessment of the patient indicates that sufficient follicular maturation has occurred. This may be directly estimated by measuring serum (or urinary) estrogen levels and sonographic visualization of the ovaries. The combination of both estradiol levels and ultrasonography are useful for monitoring the growth and development of follicles, timing hCG administration, as well as minimizing the risk of the Ovarian Hyperstimulation Syndrome and multiple gestation.

Other clinical parameters which may have potential use for monitoring menotropins therapy include:

PRECAUTIONS: *(cont'd)*

a) Changes in the vaginal cytology
b) Appearance and volume of the cervical mucus
c) Spinnbarkeit
d) Ferning of the cervical mucus

The above clinical indices provide an indirect estimate of the estrogenic effect upon the target organs, and therefore should only be used adjunctively with more direct estimates of follicular development, i.e., serum estradiol and ultrasonography.

The clinical confirmation of ovulation, with the exception of pregnancy, is obtained by direct and indirect indices of progesterone production. The indices most generally used are as follows:

a) A rise in basal body temperature
b) Increase in serum progesterone
c) Menstruation following the shift in basal body temperature

When used in conjunction with indices of progesterone production, sonographic visualization of the ovaries will assist in determining if ovulation has occurred. Sonographic evidence of ovulation may include the following:

a) Fluid in the cul-de-sac
b) Ovarian stigmata
c) Collapsed follicle

Because of the subjectivity of the various tests for the determination of follicular maturation and ovulation, it cannot be overemphasized that the physician should choose tests with which he/she is thoroughly familiar.

Carcinogenesis and Mutagenesis: Long-term toxicity studies in animals have not been performed to evaluate the carcinogenic potential of Pergonal.

Pregnancy Category X See CONTRAINDICATIONS section.

Nursing Mothers: It is not known whether this drug is excreted in human milk. Because many drugs are excreted in human milk, caution should be exercised if Pergonal is administered to a nursing woman.

DRUG INTERACTIONS:

No clinically significant drug/drug or drug/food adverse interactions have been reported during Pergonal therapy.

ADVERSE REACTIONS:

Women: The following adverse reactions, reported during Pergonal therapy, are listed in decreasing order of potential severity:

1. Pulmonary and vascular complications (see WARNINGS)
2. Ovarian Hyperstimulation Syndrome (see WARNINGS)
3. Hemoperitoneum
4. Adnexal torsion (as a complication of ovarian enlargement)
5. Mild to moderate ovarian enlargement
6. Ovarian cysts
7. Abdominal pain
8. Sensitivity of Pergonal (Febrile reactions after the administration of Pergonal have occurred. It is not clear whether or not these were pyrogenic responses or possible allergic reactions. In addition, reports of "flu-like symptoms" including fever, chills, musculoskeletal aches, joint pains, nausea, headache and malaise have also been reported.
9. Gastrointestinal symptoms (nausea, vomiting, diarrhea, abdominal cramps, bloating)
10. Pain, rash, swelling and/or irritation at the site of injection
11. Body rashes
12. Dizziness, tachycardia, dyspnea, tachypnea

The following medical events have been reported subsequent to pregnancies resulting from Pergonal therapy:

1. Ectopic pregnancy
2. Congenital abnormalities

From a study of 287 completed pregnancies following Pergonal-hCG therapy five incidents of birth defects were reported (1.7%). One infant had multiple congenital anomalies consisting of imperforate anus, aplasia of the sigmoid colon, third degree hypospadias, cecovesicle fistula, bifid scrotum, meningocele, bilateral internal tibial torsion, and right metatarsus adductus. Another infant was born with an imperforate anus and possible congenital heart lesions; another had a supernumerary digit; another was born with hypospadias and exstrophy of the bladder; and the fifth child had Down's syndrome. None of the investigators felt that these defects were drug-related. Subsequently one report of an infant death due to hydrocephalus and cardiac anomalies has been received.

Men:

1. Gynecomastia may occur occasionally during Pergonal-hCG therapy. This is a known effect of hCG treatment.
2. Erythrocytosis (hct 50%, hgb 17.8 g%) was recorded in one patient.

DRUG ABUSE AND DEPENDENCE:

There have been no reports of abuse or dependence with Pergonal.

OVERDOSAGE:

Aside from possible ovarian hyperstimulation (see WARNINGS), little is known concerning the consequences of acute overdosage with Pergonal.

DOSAGE AND ADMINISTRATION:

WOMEN:

Dosage: The dose of Pergonal to produce maturation of the follicle must be individualized for each patient. It is recommended that the initial dose to any patient should be 75 IU of FSH/LH per day, **ADMINISTERED INTRAMUSCULARLY,**for seven to twelve days followed by hCG, 5,000 U to 10,000 U, one day after the last dose of Pergonal. Administration of Pergonal should not exceed 12 days in a single course of therapy. The patient should be treated until indices of estrogenic activity, as indicated under PRECAUTIONS above, are equivalent to or greater than those of the normal individual. If serum or urinary estradiol determinations or ultrasonographic visualizations are available, they may be useful as a guide to therapy. If the ovaries are abnormally enlarged on the last day of Pergonal therapy, hCG should not be administered in the last day of Pergonal therapy, hCG should not be administered in this course of therapy; this will reduce the chances of development of the Ovarian Hyperstimulation Syndrome. If there is evidence of ovulation but no pregnancy, repeat this dosage regime for at least two more courses before increasing the dose of Pergonal to 150 IU of FSH/LH per day for seven to twelve days. As before, this dose should be followed by 5,000 U to 10,000 U of hCG one day after the last dose of Pergonal. A Pergonal

DOSAGE AND ADMINISTRATION: *(cont'd)*

dose of 150 IU of FSH/LH per day has proven to be the most effective dose, especially for *in vitro* fertilization. If evidence of ovulation is present, but pregnancy does not ensue, repeat the same dose for two more courses. Doses larger than this are not routinely recommended.

During treatment with both Pergonal and hCG and during a two-week post- treatment period, patients should be examined at least every other day for signs of excessive ovarian stimulation. It is recommended that Pergonal administration be stopped if the ovaries become abnormally enlarged or abdominal pain occurs. Most of the Ovarian Hyperstimulation Syndrome occurs after treatment has been discontinued and reaches its maximum at about seven to ten days post-ovulation. Patients should be followed for at least two weeks after hCG administration.

The couple should be encouraged to have intercourse daily, beginning on the day prior to the administration of hCG until ovulation becomes apparent from the indices employed for the determination of progestational activity. Care should be taken to insure insemination. In the light of the foregoing indices and parameters mentioned, it should become obvious that, unless a physician is willing to devote considerable time to these patients and be familiar with and conduct the necessary laboratory studies, he/she should not use Pergonal.

Administration: Dissolve the contents of one ampule of Pergonal in one to two ml of sterile saline and **ADMINISTER INTRAMUSCULARLY** immediately. Any unused reconstituted material should be discarded. Parenteral drug products should be inspected visually for particulate matter and discoloration prior to administration, whenever solution and container permit.

MEN:

Dosage: Prior to concomitant therapy with Pergonal and hCG, pretreatment with hCG alone (5,000 U three times a week) is required. Treatment should continue for a period sufficient to achieve serum testosterone levels within the normal range and masculinization as judged by the appearance of secondary sex characteristics. Such pretreatment may require four to six months, then the recommended dose of Pergonal is 75 IU FSH/LH **ADMINISTERED INTRAMUSCULARLY,** three times a week and the recommended dose of hCG is 2,000 U twice a week. Therapy should be carried on for a minimum of four more months to insure detecting spermatozoa in the ejaculate, as it takes 74 ± 4 days in the human male for germ cells to reach the spermatozoa stage.

Administration: Dissolve the contents of one ampule of Pergonal in one two ml of sterile saline and **ADMINISTER INTRAMUSCULARLY** immediately. Any unused reconstituted material should be discarded. Parenteral drug products should be inspected visually for particulate matter and discoloration prior to administration, whenever solution and container permit.

If the patient has not responded with evidence of increased spermatogenesis at the end of four months of therapy, treatment may continue with 75 IU FSH/LH three times a week, or the dose can be increased to 150 IU FSH/LH three times a week, with the hCG dose unchanged.

HOW SUPPLIED:

Pergonal is supplied in a sterile lyophilized form as a white to off-white powder or pellet in ampules containing 75 IU or 150 IU FSH/LH activity. The following package combinations are available:

1 ampule 75 IU Pergonal and 1 ampule 2 ml Sodium Chloride Injection (USP).

10 ampules 75 IU Pergonal and 10 ampules 2 ml Sodium Chloride Injection (USP).

100 ampules 75 IU Pergonal and 1 ampule 2 ml Sodium Chloride Injection (USP)

By biological assay, one IU of LH for the Second International Reference Preparation (2nd-IRP) for hMG is biologically equivalent to approximately 1/2 U of hCG.

Lyophilized powder may be stored refrigerated or at a room temperature (3°-25°C/37°-77°F). Protect from light. Use immediately after reconstitution. Discard unused material.

HOW SUPPLIED - RATED THERAPEUTICALLY EQUIVALENT:

Injection, Solution - Intramuscular - 75 unit

1's	$56.65	HUMEGON, Organon	00052-0300-17
1's	**$64.94**	**PERGONAL, Serono Labs**	**44087-0571-07**
5's	$265.20	HUMEGON, Organon	00052-0300-22
10's	**$606.87**	**PERGONAL, Serono Labs**	**44087-5075-03**

Injection, Solution - Intramuscular - 150 unit

1's	$108.77	HUMEGON, Organon	00052-0304-17
1's	**$124.67**	**PERGONAL, Serono Labs**	**44087-5150-01**

MEPENZOLATE BROMIDE *(001726)*

CATEGORIES: Anticholinergic Agents; Antimuscarinics/Antispasmodics; Antispasmodics & Anticholinergics; Autonomic Drugs; Gastrointestinal Drugs; Parasympatholytics; Peptic Ulcer; FDA Approval Pre 1982

BRAND NAMES: **Cantil**; *Trancolon* (Japan)
(International brand names outside U.S. in italics)

FORMULARIES: Medi-Cal

DESCRIPTION:

Cantil tablets for oral administration contain 25 mg mepenzolate bromide USP. The anticholinergic agent mepenzolate bromide USP chemically is 3-[(hydroxydiphenylacetyl)oxy]-1,1-dimethylpiperidinium bromide.

Mepenzolate bromide occurs as a white or light cream-colored powder, which is freely soluble in methanol, slightly soluble in water and chloroform, and practically insoluble in ether.

Each yellow tablet contains 25 mg mepenzolate bromide USP. This tablet also contains inactive ingredients: confectioners' sugar, corn starch, corn syrup solids, FD&C Yellow No. 5 (tartrazine, see PRECAUTIONS), lactose, magnesium stearate and microcrystalline cellulose.

CLINICAL PHARMACOLOGY:

Mepenzolate bromide diminishes gastric acid and pepsin secretion. Mepenzolate bromide also suppresses spontaneous contractions of the colon. Pharmacologically, it is a post-ganglionic parasympathetic inhibitor.

Radiotracer studies in which Cantil-^{14}C was used in animals and humans indicate the absorption following oral administration, as with other quaternary ammonium compounds, is low. Between 3 and 22% of an orally administered dose is excreted in the urine over a 5-day period, with the majority of the radioactivity appearing on Day 1. The remainder appears in the next 5 days in the feces and presumably has not been absorbed.

INDICATIONS AND USAGE:

Mepenzolate bromide is indicated for use as adjunctive therapy in the treatment of peptic ulcer. It has not been shown to be effective in contributing to the healing of peptic ulcer, decreasing the rate of recurrence or preventing complications.

CONTRAINDICATIONS:

1. Glaucoma
2. Obstructive uropathy (for example, bladder neck obstruction due to prostatic hypertrophy)
3. Obstructive disease of the gastrointestinal tract (for example, pyloroduodenal stenosis, achalasia)
4. Paralytic ileus
5. Intestinal atony of the elderly or debilitated patient
6. Unstable cardiovascular status in acute gastrointestinal hemorrhage
7. Toxic megacolon complicating ulcerative colitis
8. Myasthenia gravis
9. Allergic or idiosyncratic reactions to mepenzolate bromide or related compounds

WARNINGS:

In the presence of high environmental temperature, heat prostration (fever and heat stroke due to decreased sweating) can occur with use of mepenzolate bromide.

Diarrhea may be an early symptom of incomplete intestinal obstruction especially in patients with ileostomy or colostomy. In this instance, treatment with this drug would be in appropriate and possibly harmful.

Mepenzolate bromide may produce drowsiness or blurred vision. The patient should be cautioned regarding activities requiring mental alertness such as operating a motor vehicle or other machinery or performing hazardous work while taking this drug.

With overdosage, a curare-like action may occur, i.e. neuromuscular blockade leading to muscular weakness and possible paralysis.

It should be noted that the use of anticholinergic drugs in the treatment of gastric ulcer may produce a delay in gastric emptying time and may complicate such therapy (antral stasis). Psychosis has been reported in sensitive individuals given anticholinergic drugs. CNS signs and symptoms include confusion, disorientation, short-term memory loss, hallucinations, dysarthria, ataxia, coma, euphoria, decreased anxiety, fatigue. These CNS signs and symptoms usually resolve within 12 to 24 hours after discontinuation of the medication.

PRECAUTIONS:

General: Use mepenzolate bromide with caution in the elderly and in all patients with:
1. Autonomic neuropathy
2. Hepatic or renal disease
3. Ulcerative colitis. Large doses may suppress intestinal motility to the point of producing a paralytic ileus and for this reason precipitate or aggravate "toxic megacolon," a serious complication of the disease.
4. Hiatal hernia associated with reflux esophagitis, since anticholinergic drugs may aggravate this condition.
5. Coronary heart disease
6. Congestive heart failure
7. Cardiac arrhythmias
8. Tachycardia
9. Hypertension
10. Prostatic hypertrophy
11. Hyperthyroidism

Investigate any tachycardia before giving anticholinergic (atropine-like) drugs since they may increase the heart rate.

This product contains FD&C Yellow No. 5 (tartrazine), which may cause allergic-type reactions (including bronchial asthma) in certain susceptible individuals. Although the overall incidence of FD&C Yellow No. 5 (tartrazine) sensitivity in the general population is low, it is frequently seen in patients who also have aspirin hypersensitivity.

Information for the Patient: Mepenzolate bromide may produce drowsiness or blurred vision. The patient should be cautioned regarding activities requiring mental alertness, such as operating a motor vehicle or other machinery or performing hazardous work while taking this drug.

Carcinogenesis, Mutagenesis, and Impairment of Fertility: No data are available on long-term potential for carcinogenicity, mutagenicity, or impairment of fertility in animals or humans.

Pregnancy, Teratogenic Effects, Pregnancy Category B: Reproduction studies have been performed in rats and rabbits at doses up to 30 times the human dose (based on 50 kg weight) and have shown no evidence of impaired fertility or harm to the animal fetus. There are, however, no adequate and well controlled studies with mepenzolate bromide in pregnant women. Because animal reproduction studies are not always predictive of human response, mepenzolate bromide should be used during pregnancy only if clearly needed.

Nonteratogenic Effects: No data are available on nonteratogenic effects in the fetus or newborn infant.

Nursing Mothers: It is not known whether mepenzolate bromide is secreted in human milk. Because many drugs are excreted in human milk, caution should be exercised when mepenzolate bromide is administered to a nursing woman.

Pediatric Use Safety and effectiveness in pediatric patients have not been established. Studies in newborn animals (rats) show that younger animals are more sensitive to the toxic effects of mepenzolate bromide than are older animals.

DRUG INTERACTIONS:

The following agents may increase certain actions or side effects of anticholinergic drugs: amantadine, antiarrhythmic agents of class I (*e.g.,* quinidine), antihistamines, antipsychotic agents (*e.g.,* phenothiazines), benzodiazepines, MAO inhibitors, narcotic analgesics (*e.g.,* meperidine), nitrates and other nitrites, sympathomimetic agents, tricyclic antidepressants, and other drugs having anticholinergic activity.

Anticholinergics antagonize the effects of antiglaucoma agents. Anticholinergic drugs in the presence of increased intraocular pressure may be hazardous when taken concurrently with agents such as corticosteroids. (See CONTRAINDICATIONS.)

Anticholinergic agents may affect gastrointestinal absorption of various drugs, such as slowly dissolving dosage forms of digoxin,; increased serum digoxin concentrations may result. Anticholinergic drugs may antagonize the effects of drugs that alter gastrointestinal motility, such as metoclopramide. Because antacids may interfere with the absorption of anticholinergic agents, simultaneous use of these drugs should be avoided. The inhibiting effects of anticholinergic drugs on gastric treat achlorhydria and those used to test gastric secretion.

ADVERSE REACTIONS:

Precise frequency data from controlled clinical studies with mepenzolate bromide are not available.

Gastrointestinal System: vomiting, nausea, constipation, loss of taste, bloated feeling, dry mouth

ADVERSE REACTIONS: *(cont'd)*

Central Nervous System: mental confusion, dizziness, weakness, drowsiness, headache, nervousness.

Ophthalmologic: increased ocular tension, cycloplegia, blurred vision, dilation of the pupil

Dermatologic-Hypersensitivity: anaphylaxis, urticaria

Cardiovascular: tachycardia, palpitations

Genitourinary: urinary retention, urinary hesitancy

Miscellaneous: decreased sweating, drowsiness, insomnia, impotence, suppression of lactation

DRUG ABUSE AND DEPENDENCE:

Tolerance, abuse, or dependence has not been reported with mepenzolate bromide.

OVERDOSAGE:

Signs and Symptoms: The signs and symptoms of overdosage are headache; nausea; vomiting; blurred vision; dilated pupils; hot, dry skin; dizziness; dryness of the mouth; difficulty in swallowing; and CNS stimulation. A curare-like action may occur (*i.e.,* neuromuscular blockade leading to muscular weakness and possible paralysis).

Oral LD_{50}The oral LD_{50} is greater than 750 mg/kg in mice and greater than 1000 mg/kg in rats.

Maximum Human Dose Recorded: The maximum human dose recorded is 375 to 500 mg in a 4-year-old child (no adverse effects reported) and 500 to 750 mg in a 30-year old adult (resulted in death).

Dialysis: It is not known if the drugs is dialyzable.

Treatment: Treatment should consist of gastric lavage, emetics, and activated charcoal. Sedatives (*e.g.,* short-acting barbiturates, benzodiazepines) may be used for management of overt signs of excitement. If indicated, a appropriate parenteral cholinergic agent may be used as an antidote.

DOSAGE AND ADMINISTRATION:

The usual adult dose is 1 or 2 tablets (25 or 50 mg) 4 times a day preferably with meals and at bedtime. Begin with the lower dosage when possible and adjust subsequently according to the patient's response.

Safety and efficacy in children have not been established.

HOW SUPPLIED:

25 mg mepenzolate bromide, compressed yellow tablets debossed MERRELL 37.

Keep tightly closed. Store at room temperature, preferably below 86° F. Protect from excessive heat. Dispense in tight containers with child-resistant closure.

HOW SUPPLIED - EQUIVALENTS NOT AVAILABLE:

Tablet, Uncoated - Oral - 25 mg

100's	$78.90	CANTIL, Hoechst Marion Roussel	00068-0037-01

MEPERIDINE HYDROCHLORIDE *(001727)*

CATEGORIES: Analeptics; Analgesics; Anesthesia; Antipyretics; Central Nervous System Agents; Narcotic Analgesics; Narcotics, Synthetics & Combinations; Opiate Agonists (Controlled); Pain; DEA Class CII; FDA Approval Pre 1982

BRAND NAMES: *Alodan "Gerot"*; *Centralgin*; **Demerol**; *Dolantin* (Germany); *Dolantina*; *Dolantine*; *Dolestine*; *Doloneurin*; *Dolosal* (France); Meperidine Hcl; *Neomochin* (Japan); *Opistan* (Japan); Pethadol; *Pethidine* (England); *Pethidine Injection* (Australia); *Pethidine Roche*; *Pethidine Tablet*; *Petidin*
(International brand names outside U.S. in italics)

FORMULARIES: BC-BS; Medi-Cal; WHO

DESCRIPTION:

Meperidine HCl is ethyl 1-methyl-4-phenylisonipecotate HCl, a white crystalline substance with a melting point of 186°C to 189°C. It is readily soluble in water and has a neutral reaction and a slightly bitter taste. The solution is not decomposed by a short period of boiling.

The syrup is a pleasant-tasting, nonalcoholic, banana-flavored solution containing 50 mg of meperidine HCl, per 5 ml teaspoon (25 drops contain 13 mg of meperidine HCl). The tablets contain 50 mg or 100 mg of the analgesic.

Meperidine HCl injectable is supplied in Carpuject with InterLink and Carpuject Sterile Cartridge-Needle Units, SmartPak Injection Delivery System of 2.5% (25 mg/1 ml), 5% (50 mg/1 ml), 7.5% (75 mg/1 ml), and 10% (100 mg/1 ml). Uni-Amp Unit Dose Pak—ampuls of 5% solution (25 mg/0.5 ml), (50 mg/1 ml), (75 mg/1.5 ml), (100 mg/2 ml), and 10% solution (100 mg/1 ml). Uni-Nest Pak—ampuls of 5% solution (25 mg/0.5 ml), (50 mg/1 ml), (75 mg/1.5), (100 mg/2 ml), and 10% solution (100 mg/1 ml). Multiple-dose vials of 5% and 10% solutions contain metacresol 0.1% as preservative.

The pH of meperidine solutions is adjusted between 3.5 and 6 with sodium hydroxide or hydrochloric acid.

Meperidine HCl, 5 percent solution has a specific gravity of 1.0086 at 20°C and 10 percent solution, a specific gravity of 1.0165 at 20°C.

Inactive Ingredients Tablets: Calcium Sulfate, Dibasic Calcium phosphate, Starch, Stearic Acid, Talc. *Syrup:* Benzoic Acid, Flavor, Liquid Glucose, Purified Water, Saccharin Sodium.

CLINICAL PHARMACOLOGY:

Meperidine HCl is a narcotic analgesic with multiple actions qualitatively similar to those of morphine; the most prominent of these involve the central nervous system and organs composed of smooth muscle. The principal actions of therapeutic value are analgesia and sedation.

There is some evidence which suggests that meperidine may produce less smooth muscle spasm, constipation, and depression of the cough reflex than equianalgesic doses of morphine. Meperidine, in 60 mg to 80 mg parenteral doses, is approximately equivalent in analgesic effect to 10 mg of morphine. The onset of action is lightly more rapid than with morphine, and the duration of action is slightly shorter. Meperidine is significantly less effective by the oral than by the parenteral route, but the exact ratio of oral to parenteral effectiveness is unknown.

INDICATIONS AND USAGE:

For the relief of moderate to severe pain (parenteral and oral forms)

For preoperative medication (parenteral form only)

For support of anesthesia (parenteral form only)

For obstetrical analgesia (parenteral form only)

CONTRAINDICATIONS:

Hypersensitivity of meperidine.

Meperidine is contraindicated in patients who are receiving monoamine oxidase (MAO) inhibitors or those who have recently received such agents. Therapeutic doses of meperidine have occasionally precipitated unpredictable, severe, and occasionally fatal reactions in patients who have received such agents within 14 days. The mechanism of these reactions is unclear, but may be related to a preexisting hyperphenylalaninemia. Some have been characterized by coma, severe respiratory depression, cyanosis, and hypotension, and have resembled the syndrome of acute narcotic overdose. In other reactions the predominant manifestations have been hyperexcitability, convulsions, tachycardia, hyperpyrexia, and hypertension. Although it is not known that other narcotics are free of the risk of such reactions, virtually all of the reported reactions have occurred with meperidine. If a narcotic is needed in such patients, a sensitivity test should be performed in which repeated, small, incremental doses of morphine are administered over the course of several hours while the patient's condition and vital signs are under careful observation. (Intravenous hydrocortisone or prednisolone have been used to treat severe reactions, with the addition of intravenous chlorpromazine in those cases exhibiting hypertension and hyperpyrexia. The usefulness and safety of narcotic antagonists in the treatment of these reactions is unknown.)

Solutions of meperidine and barbiturates are chemically incompatible.

WARNINGS:

Drug Dependence: Meperidine can produce drug dependence of the morphine type and therefore has the potential for being abused. Psychic dependence, physical dependence, and tolerance may develop upon repeated administration of meperidine, and it should be prescribed and administered with the same degree of caution appropriate to the use of morphine. Like other narcotics, meperidine is subject to the provisions of the Federal narcotic laws.

Head Injury and Increased Intracranial Pressure: The respiratory depressant effects of meperidine and its capacity to elevate cerebrospinal fluid pressure may be markedly exaggerated in the presence of head injury, other intracranial lesions, or a preexisting increase in intracranial pressure. Furthermore, narcotics produce adverse reactions which may obscure the clinical course of patients with head injuries. In such patients, meperidine must be used with extreme caution and only if its use is deemed essential.

Intravenous Use: If necessary, meperidine may be given intravenously, but the injection should be given very slowly, preferably in the form of a diluted solution. Rapid intravenous injection of narcotic analgesics, including meperidine, increases the incidence of adverse reactions; severe respiratory depression, apnea, hypotension, peripheral circulatory collapse, and cardiac arrest have occurred. Meperidine should not be administered intravenously in less a narcotic antagonist and the facilities for assisted or controlled respiration are immediately available. When meperidine is given parenterally, especially intravenously, the patient should be lying down.

Asthma and Other Respiratory Conditions: Meperidine should be used with extreme caution in patients having an acute asthmatic attack, patients with chronic obstructive pulmonary disease or cor pulmonale, patients having a substantially decreased respiratory reserve, and patients with preexisting respiratory depression, hypoxia, or hypercapnia. In such patients, even usual therapeutic doses of narcotics may decrease respiratory drive while simultaneously increasing airway resistance to the point of apnea.

Hypotensive Effect: The administration of meperidine may result in severe hypotension in the postoperative patient or any individual whose ability to maintain blood pressure has been compromised by a depleted blood volume or the administration of drugs such as the phenothiazines or certain anesthetics.

Usage in Ambulatory Patients: Meperidine may impair the mental and/or physical abilities required for the performance of potentially hazardous tasks such as driving a car or operating machinery. The patient should be cautioned accordingly.

Meperidine, like other narcotics, may produce orthostatic hypotension in ambulatory patients.

Usage in Pregnancy and Lactation: Meperidine should not be used in pregnant women prior to the labor period, unless in the judgment of the physician the potential benefits outweigh the possible hazards, because safe use in pregnancy prior to labor has not been established relative to possible adverse effects on fetal development.

When used as an obstetrical analgesic, meperidine crosses the placental barrier and can produce depression of respiration and psychophysiologic functions in the newborn. Resuscitation may be required (see OVERDOSAGE).

Meperidine appears in the milk of nursing mothers receiving the drug.

PRECAUTIONS:

As with all intramuscular preparations meperidine intramuscular injection should be injected well within the body of a large muscle.

Supraventricular Tachycardias: Meperidine should be used with caution in patients with atrial flutter and other supraventricular tachycardias because of a possible vagolytic action which may produce a significant increase in the ventricular response rate.

Convulsions: Meperidine may aggravate preexisting convulsions in patients with convulsive disorders. If dosage is escalated substantially above recommended levels because of tolerance development, convulsions may occur in individuals without a history of convulsive disorders.

Acute Abdominal Conditions: The administration of meperidine or other narcotics may obscure the diagnosis of clinical course in patients with acute abdominal conditions.

Special Risk Patients: Meperidine should be given with caution and the initial dose should be reduced in certain patients such as the elderly or debilitated, and those with severe impairment of hepatic or renal function, hypothyroidism, Addison's disease, and prostatic hypertrophy or urethral stricture.

DRUG INTERACTIONS:

Interaction with Other Central Nervous System Depressants: MEPERIDINE SHOULD BE USED WITH GREAT CAUTION AND IN REDUCED DOSAGE IN PATIENTS WHO ARE CONCURRENTLY RECEIVING OTHER NARCOTIC ANALGESICS, GENERAL ANESTHETICS, PHENOTHIAZINES, OTHER TRANQUILIZERS (SEE DOSAGE AND ADMINISTRATION), SEDATIVE-HYPNOTICS (INCLUDING BARBITURATES), TRICYCLIC ANTIDEPRESSANTS AND OTHER CNS DEPRESSANTS (INCLUDING ALCOHOL). RESPIRATORY DEPRESSION, HYPOTENSION, AND PROFOUND SEDATION OR COMA MAY RESULT.

ADVERSE REACTIONS:

The major hazards of meperidine, as with other narcotic analgesics, are respiratory depression and, to a lesser degree, circulatory depression; respiratory arrest, shock, and cardiac arrest have occurred.

ADVERSE REACTIONS: *(cont'd)*

The most frequently observed adverse reactions include lightheadedness, dizziness, sedation, nausea, vomiting, and sweating. These effects seem to be more prominent in ambulatory patients and in those who are not experiencing severe pain. In such individuals, lower dosage are advisable. Some adverse reactions in ambulatory patients may be alleviated if the patients lies down.

Other adverse reactions include:

Nervous System: Euphoria, dysphoria, weakness, headache, agitation, tremor, uncoordinated muscle movements, severe convulsions, transient hallucinations and disorientation, visual disturbances. Inadvertent injection about a nerve trunk may result in sensory-motor paralysis which is usually, though not always, transitory.

Gastrointestinal: Dry mouth, constipation, biliary tract spasm.

Cardiovascular: Flushing of the face, tachycardia, bradycardia, palpitation, hypotension (see WARNINGS), syncope, phlebitis following intravenous injection.

Genitourinary: Urinary retention.

Allergic: Pruritus, urticaria, other skin rashes, wheal and flare over the vein with intravenous injection.

Other: Pain at injection site; local tissue irritation and induration following subcutaneous injection, particularly when repeated; antidiuretic effect.

OVERDOSAGE:

Symptoms: Serious overdosage with meperidine is characterized by respiratory depression (a decrease in respiratory rate and/or tidal volume, Cheyne-Stokes respiration, cyanosis), extreme somnolence progressing to stupor or coma, skeletal muscle flaccidity, cold and clammy skin, and sometimes bradycardia and hypotension. In severe overdosage, particularly by the intravenous route, apnea, circulatory collapse, cardiac arrest, and death may occur.

Treatment: Primary attention should be given to the reestablishment of adequate respiratory exchange through provision of a patent airway and institution of assisted or controlled ventilation. The narcotic antagonist, naloxone HCl, is a specific antidote against respiratory depression which may result from overdosage or unusual sensitivity to narcotics, including meperidine. Therefore, an appropriate dose of this antagonist should be administered, preferably by the intravenous route, simultaneously with efforts at respiratory resuscitation.

An antagonist should not be administered in the absence of clinically significant respiratory or cardiovascular depression.

Oxygen, intravenous fluids, vasopressors, and other supportive measures should be employed as indicated.

In cases of overdosage with meperidine tablets, the stomach should be evacuated by emesis or gastric lavage.

NOTE: In an individual physically dependent on narcotics, the administration of the usual dose of a narcotic antagonist will precipitate an acute withdrawal syndrome. The severity of this syndrome will depend on the degree of physical dependence and the dose of antagonist administered. The use of narcotic antagonists in such individuals should be avoided if possible. If a narcotic antagonist must be used to treat serious respiratory depression in the physically dependent patient, the antagonist should be administered with extreme care and only one-fifth to one-tenth the usual initial dose administered.

DOSAGE AND ADMINISTRATION:

For Relief of Pain Dosage should be adjusted according to the severity of the pain and the response of the patient. While subcutaneous administration is suitable for occasional use, intramuscular administration is preferred when repeated doses are required. If intravenous administration is required, dosage should be decreased and the injection made very slowly, preferably utilizing a diluted solution. Meperidine is less effective orally than on parenteral administration. The dose of meperidine should be proportionately reduced (usually by 25 to 50 percent) when administered concomitantly with phenothiazines and many other tranquilizers since they potentiate the action of meperidine.

Adults: The usual dosage is 50 mg to 150 mg intramuscularly, subcutaneously, or orally, every 3 or 4 hours as necessary.

Children: The usual dosage is 0.5 mg/lb to 0.8 mg/lb intramuscularly, subcutaneously, or orally up to the adult dose, every 3 or 4 hours as necessary.

Each dose of the syrup should be taken in one-half glass of water, since if taken undiluted, it may exert a slight topical anesthetic effect on mucous membranes.

For Preoperative Medication: *Adults:* The usual dosage is 50 mg to 100 mg intramuscularly or subcutaneously, 30 to 90 minutes before the beginning of anesthesia. *Children:* The usual dosage is 0.5 mg/lb to 1 mg/lb intramuscularly or subcutaneously up to the adults does, 30 to 90 minutes before the beginning of anesthesia.

For Support of Anesthesia: Repeated slow intravenous injections of fractional dosages (*e.g.*, 10 mg/ml) or continuous intravenous infusion of a more dilute solution (*e.g.*, 1 mg/ml) should be used. The dose should be titrated to the needs of the patient and will depend on the premedication and type of anesthesia being employed, the characteristics of the particular patient, and the nature and duration of the operative procedure.

For Obstetrical Analgesia: The usual dosage is 50 mg to 100 mg intramuscularly or subcutaneously when pain becomes regular, and may be repeated at 1- to 3-hour intervals.

HOW SUPPLIED - RATED THERAPEUTICALLY EQUIVALENT:

Injection, Solution - Intramuscular; - 10 mg/ml

30 ml	$14.20	MEPERIDINE HCL, Intl Medication	00548-1927-00
30 ml	$14.60	MEPERIDINE HCL, Schein Pharm (US)	00364-3022-56
30 ml x 10	$16.41	Meperidine Hcl, Abbott	00074-6030-04
50 ml x 10	$224.50	MEPERIDINE HCL, Baxter Hlthcare	00338-2691-75

Injection, Solution - Intramuscular; - 25 mg/ml

1 ml x 10	$5.36	Meperidine, Wyeth Labs	00008-0601-02
1 ml x 10	**$5.36**	**DEMEROL, Sanofi Winthrop**	**00024-0324-02**
1 ml x 10	**$8.31**	**DEMEROL, Sanofi Winthrop**	**00024-0324-23**
1 ml x 10	$9.11	Meperidine Hcl, Wyeth Labs	00008-0601-50
1 ml x 10	**$10.15**	**DEMEROL, Sanofi Winthrop**	**00024-0324-42**
1 ml x 25	$9.39	Meperidine Hcl, Elkins Sinn	00641-1120-35
1 ml x 25	$11.05	Meperidine Hcl, Elkins Sinn	00641-0130-25

Injection, Solution - Intramuscular; - 50 mg/ml

0.5 ml x 25	**$12.95**	**DEMEROL UNI-AMP, Sanofi Winthrop**	**00024-0361-04**
0.5 ml x 25	**$12.95**	**DEMEROL UNI-NEST, Sanofi Winthrop**	**00024-0371-04**
1 ml x 10	**$5.87**	**DEMEROL, Sanofi Winthrop**	**00024-0325-02**
1 ml x 10	$5.88	Meperidine, Wyeth Labs	00008-0602-02
1 ml x 10	**$8.81**	**DEMEROL, Sanofi Winthrop**	**00024-0325-33**
1 ml x 10	$9.63	Meperidine Hcl, Wyeth Labs	00008-0602-50
1 ml x 10	**$10.74**	**DEMEROL, Sanofi Winthrop**	**00024-0325-43**
1 ml x 25	$9.96	Meperidine Hcl, Elkins Sinn	00641-1130-35
1 ml x 25	$12.18	Meperidine Hcl, Elkins Sinn	00641-0140-25
1 ml x 25	**$13.15**	**DEMEROL UNI-AMP, Sanofi Winthrop**	**00024-0362-04**
1 ml x 25	**$13.15**	**DEMEROL UNI-NEST, Sanofi Winthrop**	**00024-0372-04**
1.5 ml x 25	**$13.41**	**DEMEROL UNI-AMP, Sanofi Winthrop**	**00024-0363-04**

HOW SUPPLIED - RATED THERAPEUTICALLY EQUIVALENT: *(cont'd)*

1.5 ml x 25	**$13.41**	**DEMEROL UNI-NEST, Sanofi Winthrop**	**00024-0373-04**
2 ml x 25	**$13.69**	**DEMEROL UNI-AMP, Sanofi Winthrop**	**00024-0364-04**
2 ml x 25	**$13.69**	**DEMEROL UNI-NEST, Sanofi Winthrop**	**00024-0374-04**
30 ml	$10.69	Meperidine Hcl, Wyeth Labs	00008-0258-01
30 ml	$15.00	Meperidine Hcl, Steris Labs	00402-0947-30
30 ml	$17.65	Meperidine Hcl, Goldline Labs	00182-9130-66
30 ml	$17.69	Meperidine HCl, Schein Pharm (US)	00364-3026-56
30 ml	**$20.38**	**DEMEROL, Sanofi Winthrop**	**00024-0329-01**
30 ml	$55.97	Meperidine Hcl, Astra USA	00186-1284-01

Injection, Solution - Intramuscular; - 75 mg/ml

1 ml x 10	**$6.34**	**DEMEROL, Sanofi Winthrop**	**00024-0326-02**
1 ml x 10	$6.35	Meperidine, Wyeth Labs	00008-0605-02
1 ml x 10	**$9.25**	**DEMEROL, Sanofi Winthrop**	**00024-0326-33**
1 ml x 10	**$10.88**	**DEMEROL, Sanofi Winthrop**	**00024-0326-44**
1 ml x 25	$10.13	Meperidine Hcl, Elkins Sinn	00641-1140-35
1 ml x 25	$12.98	Meperidine Hcl, Elkins Sinn	00641-0150-25
1 x 10 ml	$10.10	Meperidine HCl, Wyeth Labs	00008-0605-50

Injection, Solution - Intramuscular; - 100 mg/ml

1 ml x 10	**$6.84**	**DEMEROL, Sanofi Winthrop**	**00024-0328-02**
1 ml x 10	$6.85	Meperidine, Wyeth Labs	00008-0613-02
1 ml x 10	**$9.68**	**DEMEROL, Sanofi Winthrop**	**00024-0328-33**
1 ml x 10	$10.60	Meperidine Hcl, Wyeth Labs	00008-0613-50
1 ml x 10	**$11.47**	**DEMEROL, Sanofi Winthrop**	**00024-0328-45**
1 ml x 25	$10.79	Meperidine Hcl, Elkins Sinn	00641-1150-35
1 ml x 25	**$13.69**	**DEMEROL UNI-AMP, Sanofi Winthrop**	**00024-0365-04**
1 ml x 25	**$13.69**	**DEMEROL UNI-NEST, Sanofi Winthrop**	**00024-0375-04**
1 ml x 25	$13.90	Meperidine Hcl, Elkins Sinn	00641-0160-25
20 ml	$12.81	Mepridine Hcl, Steris Labs	00402-0948-20
20 ml	$14.23	Meperidine Hcl, Wyeth Labs	00008-0259-01
20 ml	$17.93	Meperidine HCl, Schein Pharm (US)	00364-3027-55
20 ml	$22.90	Meperidine Hcl, Goldline Labs	00182-9131-65
20 ml	**$26.71**	**DEMEROL, Sanofi Winthrop**	**00024-0331-01**
20 ml	$45.15	Meperidine Hcl, Astra USA	00186-1283-01

Syrup - Oral - 50 mg/5ml

480 ml	**$80.71**	**DEMEROL, Sanofi Winthrop**	**00024-0332-06**
500 ml	$31.87	Meperidine Hcl, Roxane	00054-3545-63

Tablet, Uncoated - Oral - 50 mg

25's	**$13.02**	**DEMEROL, BLISTER PACK HOSPITAL, Sanofi Winthrop**	**00024-0335-02**
100's	$20.15	Meperidine Hcl, Qualitest Pharms	00603-4415-21
100's	$25.50	Meperidine Hcl, Goldline Labs	00182-9140-01
100's	$25.95	Meperidine Hcl, Major Pharms	00904-1977-60
100's	**$71.88**	**DEMEROL, Sanofi Winthrop**	**00024-0335-04**
500's	**$329.12**	**DEMEROL, Sanofi Winthrop**	**00024-0335-06**
1000's	$135.00	PETHADOL, Halsey Drug	00879-0004-10

Tablet, Uncoated - Oral - 100 mg

25's	**$24.63**	**DEMEROL, Sanofi Winthrop**	**00024-0337-02**
100's	$29.19	PETHADOL, Halsey Drug	00879-0005-01
100's	$29.91	Meperidine Hcl, Qualitest Pharms	00603-4416-21
100's	$45.90	Meperidine Hcl, Goldline Labs	00182-9141-01
100's	$53.63	Meperidine Hcl, Rugby	00536-4062-01
100's	**$136.73**	**DEMEROL, Sanofi Winthrop**	**00024-0337-04**
500's	**$643.27**	**DEMEROL, Sanofi Winthrop**	**00024-0337-06**
1000's	$195.50	PETHADOL, Halsey Drug	00879-0005-10

HOW SUPPLIED - NOT RATED EQUIVALENT:

Powder

25 gm	$206.69	Meperidine Hcl, Mallinckrodt	00406-1585-55

MEPERIDINE HYDROCHLORIDE; PROMETHAZINE HYDROCHLORIDE *(001728)*

CATEGORIES: Analeptics; Analgesics; Anesthesia; Antipyretics; Central Nervous System Agents; Narcotics, Synthetics & Combinations; Opiate Agonists (Controlled); Pain; Sedation; Sedatives; DEA Class CII; FDA Approval Pre 1982

BRAND NAMES: **Mepergan**; Meprozine

DESCRIPTION:

FOR COMPLETE PRESCRIBING INFORMATION, REFER TO THE INDIVIDUAL DRUG MONOGRAPHS (MEPERIDINE HYDROCHLORIDE; PROMETHAZINE HYDROCHLORIDE).

INDICATIONS AND USAGE:

CAPSULES

Affords sedation as well as analgesia for moderate pain as seen in postoperative patients, postpartum patients, and in patients with pain associated with malignancies.

INJECTION

As a preanesthetic medication when analgesia and sedation are indicated. As an adjunct to local and general anesthesia.

DOSAGE AND ADMINISTRATION:

CAPSULES

The usual dosage is one capsule every four to six hours as needed for the relief of pain.

INJECTION

Parenteral drug products should be inspected visually for particulate matter and discoloration prior to administration, whenever solution and container permit.

WARNING—BARBITURATES ARE NOT CHEMICALLY COMPATIBLE IN SOLUTION WITH MEPERGAN (MEPERIDINE HYDROCHLORIDE AND PROMETHAZINE HYDROCHLORIDE) AND SHOULD NOT BE MIXED IN THE SAME SYRINGE.

The Tubex Sterile Cartridge-Needle Unit is designed for single-dose use. Vials should be used when required doses are fractions of a milliliter, as indicated below.

Mepergan is usually administered intramuscularly. However, in certain specific situations, the intravenous route may be employed. INADVERTENT INTRA-ARTERIAL INJECTION CAN RESULT IN GANGRENE OF THE AFFECTED EXTREMITY. SUBCUTANEOUS ADMINISTRATION IS CONTRAINDICATED, AS IT MAY RESULT IN TISSUE NECROSIS. INJECTION INTO OR NEAR PERIPHERAL NERVES MAY RESULT IN PERMANENT NEUROLOGICAL DEFICIT.

DOSAGE AND ADMINISTRATION: *(cont'd)*

When used intravenously, the rate should not be greater than 1 ml Mepergan (25 mg of each component) per minute; it is preferable to inject through the tubing of an intravenous infusion set that is known to be functioning satisfactorily.

Adult Dose: 1 to 2 ml (25 to 50 mg of each component) per single injection, which can be repeated every 3 to 4 hours.

Children 12 Years Of Age And Under: 0.5 mg of each component per pound of body weight. The dosage may be repeated every 3 to 4 hours as necessary. For preanesthetic medication the usual adult dose is 2 ml (50 mg of each component) intramuscularly with or without appropriate atropinelike drug. Atropine sulfate, 0.3 to 0.4 mg, or scopolamine hydrobromide, 0.25 to 0.4 mg, in sterile solution may be mixed in the same syringe with Mepergan. Repeat doses of 50 mg or less of both promethazine and meperidine may be administered by either route at 3- to 4-hour intervals, as necessary. As an adjunct to local or general anesthesia, the usual dose is 2 ml (50 mg each of meperidine and promethazine).

HOW SUPPLIED - EQUIVALENTS NOT AVAILABLE:

Capsule, Gelatin - Oral - 50 mg/25 mg

100's	$36.50	Meprozine, Vintage Pharms	00254-4206-28
100's	$36.50	Meperidine/Promethazine, Qualitest Pharms	00603-4424-21
100's	**$56.49**	**MEPERGAN, Wyeth Labs**	**00008-0261-02**

Injection, Solution - Intramuscular; - 25 mg/25 mg

2 ml x 10	**$39.95**	**MEPERGAN, Wyeth Labs**	**00008-0235-50**
10 ml	**$13.75**	**MEPERGAN, Wyeth Labs**	**00008-0234-01**

Injection, Solution - Intramuscular; - 50 mg/50 mg

2 ml x 10	**$36.20**	**MEPERGAN, Wyeth Labs**	**00008-0235-01**

MEPHENTERMINE SULFATE *(001729)*

CATEGORIES: Anesthesia; Autonomic Drugs; Hypotension; Hypotension/Shock; Sympathomimetic Agents; FDA Approval Pre 1982

BRAND NAMES: *Mephentine*; *Wyamine*; **Wyamine Sulfate**
(International brand names outside U.S. in italics)

FORMULARIES: Medi-Cal

DESCRIPTION:

Mephentermine sulfate is a synthetic sympathomimetic drug which is intended for intramuscular or intravenous administration. In addition to the stated quantity of the active ingredient (15 or 30 mg/ml), each ml of the sterile injection solution is buffered to a pH of 5 (pH range of 4 to 6.5) with sodium acetate, and contains not more than 1.8 mg of methylparaben and 0.2 mg of propylparaben.

Mephentermine sulfate occurs as white, usually odorless crystals. It is soluble in water and slightly soluble in alcohol.

The chemical name of mephentermine sulfate is N,α,α-trimethylbenzeneethanamine sulfate (2:1).

CLINICAL PHARMACOLOGY:

Mephentermine sulfate is a sympathomimetic amine that acts indirectly by releasing norepinephrine. Cardiac contraction is enhanced, and cardiac output and systolic and diastolic pressures are usually increased. The pressor response also involves peripheral vasoconstriction. The change in heart rate is variable, depending on the degree of vagal tone; large doses can depress the heart. In some cases the net vascular effect may be vasodilation, which appears not to involve beta-adrenergic receptors. Coronary blood flow is increased, forearm blood flow is reduced, and venous tone is increased. Marked mucosal vasoconstriction can be produced by local application of the drug. CNS effects may occur with large doses of mephentermine. The main effect of therapeutic doses of mephentermine is cardiac stimulation.

Mephentermine is metabolized in the liver by N-demethylation to normephentermine (or phentermine) with subsequent p-hydroxylation to p-hydroxynormephentermine (or p-hydroxyphentermine). The excretion rate of the drug and its metabolites is more rapid in an acidic urine and is only slightly influenced by urine output.

The half-life in humans is reported to be between 17 and 18 hours.

A pressor response occurs almost immediately and persists for 15 to 30 minutes following intravenous injection of therapeutic doses of mephentermine sulfate. Pressor activity occurs within 5 to 15 minutes following intramuscular administration and persists for 1 to 4 hours.

INDICATIONS AND USAGE:

Mephentermine sulfate is indicated in the treatment of hypotension secondary to ganglionic blockade and that occurring with spinal anesthesia.

CONTRAINDICATIONS:

Mephentermine sulfate should not be used in patients with a past history of sensitivity to the drug.

Mephentermine sulfate, like epinephrine and ephedrine, is contraindicated in the treatment of hypotension induced by chlorpromazine, since the sympathomimetic amines will act to potentiate, rather than correct, the hypotension secondary to the adrenolytic effects of chlorpromazine.

Mephentermine sulfate should not be administered in combination with any monoamine-oxidase inhibitor.

WARNINGS:

Persistent hypotension during or after surgery usually indicates hypovolemia and should be treated by replacement of blood volume, rather than with a sympathomimetic such as mephentermine sulfate.

Cyclopropane and halothane are known to sensitize the heart to the arrhythmic action of catecholamines. Serious ventricular arrhythmias may occur in patients under general anesthesia with these agents if sympathomimetic drugs, such as mephentermine, are given to control hypotension.

PRECAUTIONS:

GENERAL

Patients with hyperthyroidism may show an increased responsiveness to vasopressor agents.

Mephentermine sulfate must be used with caution in patients with known cardiovascular diseases and in chronically ill patients, since the drug's action on the cardiovascular system may be profound.

If mephentermine sulfate is to be given to known hypertensives, careful monitoring of the blood pressure is advisable.

PRECAUTIONS: *(cont'd)*

CARCINOGENESIS, MUTAGENESIS, IMPAIRMENT OF FERTILITY

Long-term animal studies have not been performed to evaluate the carcinogenic potential of mephentermine sulfate, nor are there relevant data with regard to mutagenicity or impairment of fertility.

PREGNANCY CATEGORY C

It is not known whether mephentermine sulfate crosses the placental barrier.

Teratogenic Effects: Animal reproduction studies have not been conducted with mephentermine sulfate. It is not known whether mephentermine sulfate can cause fetal harm when administered to a pregnant woman or can affect reproduction capacity. Mephentermine sulfate should be given to a pregnant woman only if clearly needed.

Nonteratogenic Effects: Mephentermine sulfate may increase uterine contractions especially during the third trimester of pregnancy.

LABOR AND DELIVERY

Animal studies indicated that mephentermine sulfate, used during labor, caused a decrease in uterine blood flow. Fetal hypoxia from decreased uterine blood flow secondary to uterine blood flow secondary to uterine vasoconstriction may occur. Transient fetal hypertension (mean arterial blood pressure more than 20% of control) has also been reported with mephentermine sulfate in animal experiments.

NURSING MOTHERS

It is not known whether mephentermine sulfate is excreted in human milk. Because many drugs are excreted in human milk, caution should be exercised when mephentermine sulfate is administered to a nursing woman.

PEDIATRIC USE

Safety and effectiveness of mephentermine sulfate in children have not been established.

DRUG INTERACTIONS:

Administration of mephentermine sulfate to patients who are receiving cyclopropane or halogenated hydrocarbon general anesthetics which increase cardiac irritability may result in serious ventricular arrhythmias. The possibility that digitalis or mercurial diuretics can also sensitize the myocardium to the effects of sympathomimetic drugs should also be considered.

Phenothiazines, including chlorpromazine, may antagonize the pressor effects of mephentermine.

Monoamine-oxidase-inhibitors may potentiate the pressor effects of mephentermine by inhibiting the metabolism of catecholamines.

Drugs such as reserpine and guanethidine, which reduce the quantity of norepinephrine in sympathetic nerve endings, may significantly reduce the pressor response to mephentermine.

ADVERSE REACTIONS:

Adverse reactions to mephentermine sulfate may be especially likely to occur in patients with cardiovascular diseases, hypertension, hyperthyroidism, or other chronic illnesses.

Following the administration of recommended doses of mephentermine sulfate, CNS stimulating effects may result in nervousness and anxiety.

Mephentermine sulfate may produce arrhythmias, including transient extrasystoles, AV block, and hypertension.

OVERDOSAGE:

Effects of overdosage are an extension of the pharmacological activity of mephentermine. In therapy with mephentermine sulfate, cardiac contractility, cardiac output, systolic and diastolic blood pressure are usually raised. The increase in heart rate is variable depending on vagal tone. Large doses may depress the heart. Doses in the range of 3 mg/kg of body weight may alter myocardial conduction by decreasing conduction time and shortening the refractory period. Tachycardia may also be present. Central-nervous-system effects may occur with large doses: hyperexcitability, prolonged wakefulness, weeping, incoherence, convulsions, flushing, tremor, and hallucinations.

Treatment: Therapy of overdosage is symptomatic and supportive. Side effects, in general, disappear rapidly on withdrawal of the drug. Sedation may help to control CNS hyperexcitability. Blood pressure should be followed closely, and cardiac excitability should be monitored by EKG.

Convulsions or cardiac arrhythmias should be treated promptly if they occur. Since arrhythmias produced by mephentermine sulfate may be due to excessive beta-adrenergic stimulation, a beta-blocking agent such as propranolol may be considered.

DOSAGE AND ADMINISTRATION:

Parenteral drug products should be inspected visually for particulate matter and discoloration prior to administration, whenever solution and container permit.

Mephentermine sulfate can be administered intramuscularly without fear of irritation or abnormal tissue reaction. Pressor response is evident 5 to 15 minutes after intramuscular injection and has a duration of 1 to 2 hours. Injection of an undiluted parenteral solution of mephentermine sulfate, containing 30 mg/ml, or a continuous infusion of a solution of mephentermine sulfate, in 5% dextrose in water with a concentration of approximately 1 mg/ml, directly into the vein, is the preferred route for treatment of shock. Intravenous administration of undiluted mephentermine sulfate does not produce vascular irritation and, should extravasation occur, no untoward tissue reaction will develop. Dosage of mephentermine sulfate used in the treatment of shock and hypotension is based on experimental observations that 0.5 mg/kg produces a positive inotropic action, the pharmacologic action of mephentermine sulfate responsible for the pressor effect.

Treatment of hypotension occurring following spinal anesthesia is accomplished by the administration of 30 to 45 mg mephentermine sulfate intravenously in a single injection. Doses of 30 mg may be repeated as necessary to maintain the desired level of blood pressure. An immediate response and maintenance of blood pressure can be accomplished by the continuous intravenous infusion of a 0.1% solution of mephentermine sulfate in 5% dextrose in water (1 mg mephentermine sulfate/ml solution). The rate of flow and duration of this intravenous therapy should be regulated according to the response of the patient.

Treatment of hypotension secondary to spinal anesthesia in the obstetrical patient undergoing Caesarean section, who is known to react more positively to drugs, is accomplished by the administration of an initial dose of 15 mg of mephentermine sulfate intravenously. This dose may be repeated if the response is not adequate.

Prevention of hypotension attendant to spinal anesthesia can be accomplished by the administration of 30 to 45 mg mephentermine sulfate intramuscularly 10 to 20 minutes prior to anesthesia, operation, or termination of the operative procedure.

Preparation Of Intravenous Solution: The 0.1% solution of mephentermine sulfate recommended for continuous intravenous administration can be conveniently prepared in the approximate concentration (0.115%) by adding two 10-ml vials of mephentermine sulfate, 30 mg/ml, to 500 ml of 5% dextrose in water.

Store at room temperature, approximately 25°C (77°F).

HOW SUPPLIED - EQUIVALENTS NOT AVAILABLE:

Injection, Solution - Intramuscular; - 15 mg/ml

2 ml x 25	$64.65	WYAMINE SULFATE, Wyeth Labs	00008-0159-03
10 ml	$10.83	WYAMINE SULFATE, Wyeth Labs	00008-0159-02

Injection, Solution - Intramuscular; - 30 mg/ml

10 ml	$17.18	WYAMINE SULFATE, Wyeth Labs	00008-0224-02

MEPHENYTOIN *(001730)*

CATEGORIES: Anticonvulsants; Central Nervous System Agents; Convulsions; Epilepsy; Hydantoin Anticonvulsants; Neuromuscular; Seizures; Tonic-Clonic Seizures; FDA Approval Pre 1982

BRAND NAMES: *Epilan-Gerot*; *Epilanex* (Germany); **Mesantoin**
(International brand names outside U.S. in italics)

DESCRIPTION:

Mephenytoin is -methyl 5.5-phenyl-ethyl-hydantoin. It may be considered to be the hydantoin homolog of the barbiturate mephobarbital.

Mesantoin Active Ingredient: mephenytoin, USP *Inactive Ingredients:* FD&C Red #3, gelatin, lactose, starch, stearic acid, and sucrose.

CLINICAL PHARMACOLOGY:

Mephenytoin exhibits pharmacologic effects similar to both diphenylhydantoin and the barbiturates in antagonizing experimental seizures in laboratory animals. Mephenytoin produces behavioral and electroencephalographic effects in man which are similar to those produced by barbiturates.

INDICATIONS AND USAGE:

For the control of grand mal, focal, Jacksonian, and psychomotor seizures in those patients who have been refractory to less toxic anticonvulsants.

CONTRAINDICATIONS:

Hypersensitivity to hydantoin products.

WARNINGS:

Mephenytoin should be used only after safer anticonvulsants have been given an adequate trial and have failed.

As with all anticonvulsants, dose reduction must be gradual so as to minimize the risk of precipitating seizures.

Patients should be cautioned about possible additive effects of alcohol and other CNS depressants. Acute alcohol intoxication may increase the anticonvulsant effect due to decreased metabolic breakdown. Chronic alcohol abuse may result in decreased anticonvulsant effect due to enzyme induction.

Usage in Pregnancy: The effects of mephenytoin in human pregnancy and nursing infants are unknown.

Recent reports suggest an association between the use of anticonvulsant drugs by women with epilepsy and an elevated incidence of birth defects in children born to these women. Data are more extensive with respect to diphenylhydantoin and phenobarbital, but these are also the most commonly prescribed anticonvulsants; less systematic or anecdotal reports suggest a possible similar association with the use of all known anticonvulsant drugs.

The reports suggesting an elevated incidence of birth defects in children of drug-treated epileptic women cannot be regarded as adequate to prove a definite cause and effect relationship. There are intrinsic methodologic problems in obtaining adequate data on drug teratogenicity in humans; the possibility also exists that other factors, e.g., genetic factors or the epileptic condition itself, may be more important than drug therapy in leading to birth defects. The great majority of mothers on anticonvulsant medication deliver normal infants. It is important to note that anticonvulsant drugs should not be discontinued in patients in whom the drug is administered to prevent major seizures because of the strong possibility of precipitating status epilepticus with attendant hypoxia and threat to life. In individual cases where the severity and frequency of the seizure disorder are such that the removal of medication does not pose a serious threat to the patient, discontinuation of the drug may be considered prior to and during pregnancy, although it cannot be said with any confidence that even minor seizures do not pose some hazards to the developing embryo or fetus.

The prescribing physician will wish to weigh these considerations in treating or counseling epileptic women of child-bearing potential.

PRECAUTIONS:

The patient taking mephenytoin must be kept under close medical supervision at all times since serious adverse reactions may emerge.

Because the primary site of degradation is the liver, it is recommended that screening tests of liver function precede introduction of the drug.

Some patients may show side reactions as the result of individual sensitivity. These reactions can be broken down into three types respectively according to severity: 1) blood dyscrasias; 2) skin and mucous membrane manifestations; and 3) central effects. The blood, skin and mucous membrane manifestations are the more important since they can be more serious in nature. Since mephenytoin has been reported to produce blood dyscrasias in certain instances, the patient must be instructed that in the event any unusual symptoms develop (*e.g.,* sore throat, fever, mucous membrane bleeding, glandular swelling, cutaneous reaction), he must discontinue the drug and report for examination immediately. It is recommended that blood examinations be made (total white cell count and differential count) during the initial phase of administration. Such tests are best made: a) before starting medication; b) after 2 weeks on a low dosage; c) again after 2 weeks when full dosage is reached; d) thereafter, monthly for a year; e) from then on, every 3 months. If the neutrophils drop to between 2500 and 1600/cu.mm., counts are made every 2 weeks. Stop medication if the count drops to 1600.

ADVERSE REACTIONS:

A number of side effects and toxic reactions have been reported with Mesantoin (mephenytoin) as well as with other hydantoin compounds. Many of these appear to be dose related while others seem to be a manifestation of a hypersensitivity reaction to these drugs.

Blood Dyscrasias: Leukopenia, neutropenia, agranulocytosis, thrombocytopenia and pancytopenia have occurred. Eosinophilia, monocytosis, and leukocytosis have been described. Simple anemia, hemolytic anemia, megaloblastic anemia and aplastic anemia have occurred but are uncommon.

Skin and Mucous Membrane Manifestations: Maculopapular, morbilliform, scarlatiniform, urticarial, purpuric (associated with thrombocytopenia) and non-specific skin rashes have been reported. Exfoliative dermatitis, erythema multiforme (Stevens-Johnson Syndrome), toxic epidermal necrolysis and fatal dermatitides have been described on rare occasions. Skin pigmentation and rashes associated with a lupus erythematosus syndrome have also been reported.

Central Effects: Drowsiness is dose-related and may be reduced by a reduction in dose. Ataxia, diplopia, nystagmus, dysarthria, fatigue, irritability, choreiform movements, depression and tremor have been encountered.

Nervousness, nausea, vomiting, sleeplessness and dizziness may occur during the initial stages of therapy. Generally, these symptoms are transient, often disappearing with continued treatment.

Mental confusion and psychotic disturbances and increased seizures have been reported, but a definite causal relationship with the drug is uncertain.

Miscellaneous: Hepatitis, jaundice and nephrosis have been reported but a definite cause and effect relationship between the drug and these effects has not been established.

Alopecia, weight gain, edema, photophobia, conjunctivitis and gum hyperplasia have been encountered.

Polyarthropathy, pulmonary fibrosis, lupus erythematosus syndrome and lymphadenopathy which simulates Hodgkin's Disease have also been observed.

DOSAGE AND ADMINISTRATION:

Dosage of antiepileptic therapy should be adjusted to the needs of the individual patient. Maintenance dosage is that smallest amount of antiepileptic necessary to suppress seizures completely or reduce their frequency. Optimum dosage is attained by starting with 1/2 or 1 tablet of Mesantoin (mephenytoin) per day during the first week and thereafter increasing the daily dose by 1/2 or 1 tablet at weekly intervals. No dose should be increased until it has been taken for at least 1 week.

The average dose of Mesantoin (mephenytoin) for adults ranges from 2-6 tablets (0.2-0.6 gm.) daily. In some instances it may be necessary to administer as much as 8 tablets or more daily in order to obtain full seizure control. Children usually require from 1-4 tablets (0.1-0.4 gm.) according to nature of seizures and age.

When the physician wishes to replace the anticonvulsant now being employed with Mesantoin (mephenytoin), he should give 1/2-1 tablet of Mesantoin (mephenytoin) daily during the first week and gradually increase the daily dose at weekly intervals while gradually reducing that of the drug being discontinued. The transition can be made smoothly over a period of 3-6 weeks. If seizures are not completely controlled with the dose so attained, the daily dose should then be increased by a one-tablet increment at weekly intervals to the point of maximum effect. If the patient had also been receiving phenobarbital, it is well to continue it until the transition is completed, at which time gradual withdrawal of the phenobarbital may be tried.

HOW SUPPLIED:

Mesantoin Tablets, USP: 100 mg, speckled, pale pink, round, uncoated tablets embossed "78/52" and scored on one side, "S-Sandoz" on the other side. Tablets are scored to permit half-dosage.

Store and Dispense: Below 86°F (30°C); tight container.

HOW SUPPLIED - EQUIVALENTS NOT AVAILABLE:

Tablet, Uncoated - Oral - 100 mg

100's	$28.08	MESANTOIN, Novartis	00078-0052-05

MEPHOBARBITAL *(001731)*

CATEGORIES: Anticonvulsants; Anxiety; Anxiolytics, Sedatives, Hypnotic; Barbiturates; Central Nervous System Agents; Convulsions; Epilepsy; Neuromuscular; Sedatives; Sedatives/Hypnotics; Seizures; Tension; Tonic-Clonic Seizures; Insomnia*; Pregnancy Category D; DEA Class CIV; FDA Pre 1938 Drugs
* Indication not approved by the FDA

BRAND NAMES: **Mebaral**; *Prominal* (England)
(International brand names outside U.S. in italics)

FORMULARIES: Aetna; BC-BS

COST OF THERAPY: $44.90 (Anxiety; Tablet; 32 mg; 3/day; 90 days) vs. Potential Cost of $3,628.44 (Psychoses)

DESCRIPTION:

Mephobarbital, 5-Ethyl-1-methyl-5-phenylbarbituric acid, is a barbiturate with sedative, hypnotic, and anticonvulsant properties. It occurs as a white, nearly odorless, tasteless powder and is slightly soluble in water and in alcohol.

Mebaral is available as tablets for oral administration.

Inactive Ingredients: Lactose, Starch, Stearic Acid, Talc.

CLINICAL PHARMACOLOGY:

Barbiturates are capable of producing all levels of CNS mood alteration from excitation to mild sedation, to hypnosis, and deep coma. Overdosage can produce death. In high enough therapeutic doses, barbiturates induce anesthesia.

Barbiturates depress the sensory cortex, decrease motor activity, alter cerebellar function, and produce drowsiness, sedation, and hypnosis.

Barbiturates are respiratory depressants. The degree of respiratory depression is dependent upon dose. With hypnotic doses, respiratory depression produced by barbiturates is similar to that which occurs during physiologic sleep with slight decrease in blood pressure and heart rate.

Studies in laboratory animals have shown that barbiturates cause reduction in the tone and contractility of the uterus, ureters, and urinary bladder. However, concentrations of the drugs required to produce this effect in humans are not reached with sedative-hypnotic doses.

Barbiturates do not impair normal hepatic function, but have been shown to induce liver microsomal enzymes, thus increasing and/or altering the metabolism of barbiturates and other drugs. See DRUG INTERACTIONS.

Mephobarbital exerts a strong sedative and anticonvulsant action but has a relatively mild hypnotic effect. It reduces the incidence of epileptic seizures in grand mal and petit mal. Mephobarbital usually causes little or no drowsiness or lassitude. Hence, when it is used as a sedative or anticonvulsant, patients usually become more calm, more cheerful, and better adjusted to their surroundings without clouding of mental faculties. Mephobarbital is reported to produce less sedation than does phenobarbital.

CLINICAL PHARMACOLOGY: *(cont'd)*

Barbiturates are weak acids that are absorbed and rapidly distributed to all tissues and fluids with high concentrations in the brain, liver, and kidneys. Lipid solubility of the barbiturates is the dominant factor in their distribution within the body. Barbiturates are bound to plasma and tissue proteins to a varying degree with the degree of binding increasing directly as a function of lipid solubility.

Approximately 50% of an oral dose od mephobarbital is absorbed from the gastrointestinal tract. Therapeutic plasma concentrations for mephobarbital have not been established nor has the half-life been determined. Following oral administration, the onset of action of the drug is 30 to 60 minutes and the duration of action is 10 to 16 hours. The primary route of mephobarbital metabolism is N-demethylation by the microsomal enzymes of the liver to form phenobarbital. Phenobarbital may be excreted in the urine unchanged or further metabolized to *p*- hydroxyphenobarbital and excreted in the urine as glucuronide or sulfate conjugates. About 75% of a single oral dose of mephobarbital is converted to phenobarbital in 24 hours.

Therefore, chronic administration of mephobarbital may lead to an accumulation of phenobarbital (not mephobarbital) in plasma. It has not been determined whether mephobarbital or phenobarbital is the active agent during long-time mephobarbital therapy.

INDICATIONS AND USAGE:

Mephobarbital is indicated for use as a sedative for the relief of anxiety, tension, and apprehension and as an anticonvulsant for the treatment of grand mal and petit mal epilepsy.

CONTRAINDICATIONS:

Hypersensitivity to any barbiturate. Manifest or latent porphyria.

WARNINGS:

Habit Forming: Barbiturates may be habit forming. Tolerance, psychological, and physical dependence may occur with continued use. (See DRUG ABUSE AND DEPENDENCE and CLINICAL PHARMACOLOGY.) Patients who have psychological dependence on barbiturates may increase the dosage or decrease the dosage interval without consulting a physician and may subsequently develop a physical dependence on barbiturates. To minimize the possibility of overdosage or the development of dependence, the prescribing and dispensing of sedative-hypnotic barbiturates should be limited to the amount required for the interval until the next appointment. Abrupt cessation after prolonged use in the dependent person may result in withdrawal symptoms, including delirium, conclusions, and possibly death. Barbiturates should be withdrawn gradually from any patient known to be taking excessive dosage over long periods of time. (See DRUG ABUSE AND DEPENDENCE.)

Acute or Chronic Pain: Caution should be exercised when barbiturates are administered to patients with acute or chronic pain, because paradoxical excitement could be induced or important symptoms could be masked. However, the use of barbiturates as sedatives in the postoperative surgical period and as adjuncts to cancer chemotherapy is well established.

Use in Pregnancy: Barbiturates can cause fetal damage when administered to a pregnant woman. Retrospective, case-controlled studies have suggested a connection between the maternal consumption of barbiturates and a higher than expected incidence of fetal abnormalities. Following oral or parenteral administration, barbiturates readily cross the placental barrier and are distributed throughout fetal tissues with highest concentrations found in the placenta, fetal liver, and brain. Fetal blood levels approach maternal blood levels following parenteral administration.

Withdrawal symptoms occur in infants born to mothers who receive barbiturates throughout the last trimester of pregnancy. (See DRUG ABUSE AND DEPENDENCE.) If this drug is used during pregnancy, or if the patient becomes pregnant while taking this drug, the patient should be apprised of the potential hazard to the fetus.

Synergistic Effects: The concomitant use of alcohol or other CNS depressants may produce additive CNS depressant effects.

PRECAUTIONS:

GENERAL

Barbiturates may be habit forming. Tolerance and psychological and physical dependence may occur with continuing use.(See DRUG ABUSE AND DEPENDENCE.) Barbiturates should be administered with caution, if at all, to patients who are mentally depressed, have suicidal tendencies, or a history of drug abuse.

Elderly or debilitated patients may react to barbiturates with marked excitement, depression, and confusion. In some persons, barbiturates repeatedly produce excitement rather than depression.

In patients with hepatic damage, barbiturates should be administered with caution and initially in reduced doses. Barbiturates should not be administered to patients showing the premonitory signs of hepatic coma.

Status epilepticus may result from the abrupt discontinuation of Mephobarbital, even when administered in small daily doses in the treatment of epilepsy.

Caution and careful adjustment of dosage are required when Mephobarbital is used in patients with impaired renal, cardiac or respiratory function, and in patients with myasthenia gravis and myxedema. The least quantity feasible should be prescribed or dispensed at any one time in order to minimize the possibility of acute or chronic overdosage.

Vitamin D Deficiency: Mephobarbital may increase vitamin D requirements, possibly by increasing vitamin D metabolism via enzyme induction. Rarely, rickets and osteomalacia have been reported following prolonged use of barbiturates.

Vitamin K: Bleeding in the early neonatal period due to coagulation defects may follow exposure to anticonvulsant drugs *in utero*; therefore, vitamin K should be given to the mother before delivery or to the child at birth.

INFORMATION FOR THE PATIENT

Practitioners should give the following information and instructions to patients receiving barbiturates.

1. The use of barbiturates carries with it an associated risk of psychological and/or physical dependence. The patient should he warned against increasing the dose of the drug without consulting a physician.

2. Barbiturates may impair mental and/or physical abilities required for the performance of potentially hazardous tasks (*e.g.,* driving, operating machinery, etc).

3. Alcohol should not be consumed while taking barbiturates. Concurrent use of the barbiturates with other CNS depressants (*e.g.,* alcohol, narcotics, tranquilizers, and antihistamines) may result in additional CNS depressant effects.

LABORATORY TESTS

Prolonged therapy with barbiturates should be accompanied by periodic laboratory evaluation of organ systems, including hematopoietic, renal, and hepatic systems. (See PRECAUTIONS,General and ADVERSE REACTIONS.)

PRECAUTIONS: *(cont'd)*

CARCINOGENESIS, MUTAGENESIS, AND IMPAIRMENT OF FERTILITY

Animal Data: Phenobarbital sodium in carcinogenic in mice and rats after lifetime administration. In mice, it produced benign and malignant liver cell tumors. In rats, benign liver cell tumors were observed very late in life. Phenobarbital is the major metabolite of Mebaral.

Human Data: In a 29-year epidemiological study of 9136 patients who were treated on an anticonvulsant protocol which included phenobarbital, results indicated a higher than normal incidence of hepatic carcinoma. Previously, some of these patients were treated with thorotrast, a drug which is known to produce hepatic carcinomas. Thus, this study did not provide sufficient evidence that phenobarbital sodium is carcinogenic in humans. Phenobarbital is the major metabolite of Mebaral.

A retrospective study of 84 children wit brain tumors matched to 73 normal controls and 78 cancer controls (malignant disease other than brain tumors) suggested an association between exposure to barbiturates prenatally and an increased incidence of brain tumors.

PREGNANCY

Teratogenic Effects: Pregnancy Category D—See WARNINGS—Use in Pregnancy.

Nonteratogenic Effects: Reports of infants suffering from long-term barbiturate exposure *in utero*included the acute withdrawal syndrome of seizures and hyperirritability from birth to a delayed onset on up to 14 days. (See DRUG ABUSE AND DEPENDENCE.)

LABOR AND DELIVERY

Hypnotic doses of these barbiturates do not significantly impair uterine activity during labor. Full anesthetic doses of barbiturates decrease the force and frequency of uterine contractions. Administration of sedative-hypnotic barbiturates to the mother during labor may result in respiratory depression in the newborn. Premature infants are particularly susceptible to the depressant effects of barbiturates. If barbiturates are used during labor and delivery, resuscitation equipment should be available.

Data are currently not available to evaluate the effect of these barbiturates when forceps delivery or other intervention is necessary. Also, data are not available to determine the effect of these barbiturates on the later growth, development, and functional maturation of the child.

NURSING MOTHERS

Caution should be exercised when a barbiturate is administered to a nursing woman since small amounts of barbiturates are excreted in the milk.

DRUG INTERACTIONS:

Most reports of clinically significant drug interactions occurring with the barbiturates have involved phenobarbital. However, the application of these data to other barbiturates appears valid and warrants serial blood level determinations of the relevant drugs when there are multiple therapies.

1. Anticoagulants: Phenobarbital lowers the plasma levels of dicumarol (name previously used: bishydroxycoumarin) and causes a decrease in anticoagulant activity as measured by the prothrombin time. Barbiturates can induce hepatic microsomal enzymes resulting in increased metabolism and decreased anticoagulant response of oral anticoagulants (e.g. warfarin, acenocoumarol, dicumarol, and phenprocoumon). Patients stabilized on anticoagulant therapy may require dosage adjustments if barbiturates are added to or withdrawn from their dosage regimen.

2. Corticosteroids: Barbiturates appear to enhance the metabolism of exogenous corticosteroids probably through the induction of hepatic microsomal enzymes. Patients stabilized on corticosteroid therapy may require dosage adjustments if barbiturates are added to or withdrawn from their dosage regimen.

3. Griseofulvin: Phenobarbital appears to interfere with the absorption of orally administered griseofulvin, thus decreasing its blood level. The effect of the resultant decreased blood levels of griseofulvin on therapeutic response has not been established. However, it would be preferable to avoid concomitant administration of these drugs.

4. Doxycycline: Phenobarbital has been shown to shorten the half-life of doxycycline for as long as 2 weeks after barbiturate therapy is discontinued. This mechanism is probably through the induction of hepatic microsomal enzymes that metabolize the antibiotic. If phenobarbital and doxycycline are administered concurrently, the clinical response to doxycycline should be monitored closely.

5. Phenytoin, Sodium Valproate, Valproic Acid: The effect of barbiturates on the metabolism of phenytoin appears to be variable. Some investigators report an accelerating effect, while others report no effect. Because the effect of barbiturates on the metabolism of phenytoin is not predictable, phenytoin and barbiturate blood levels should be monitored more frequently if these drugs are given concurrently. Sodium valproate and valproic acid appear to decrease barbiturate metabolism; therefore, barbiturate blood levels should be monitored and appropriate dosage adjustments made as indicated.

6. Central Nervous System Depressants: The concomitant use of other central nervous system depressants, including other sedatives or hypnotics, antihistamines, tranquilizers, or alcohol, may produce additive depressant effects.

7. Monoamine Oxidase Inhibitors (MAOI): MAOI prolong the effects of barbiturates probably because metabolism of the barbiturate is inhibited.

8. Estradiol, Estrone, Progesterone, and other Steroidal Hormones: Pretreatment with or concurrent administration of phenobarbital may decrease the effect of estradiol by increasing its metabolism. There have been reports of patients treated with antiepileptic drugs (*e.g.,* phenobarbital) who become pregnant while taking oral contraceptives. An alternate contraceptive method might be suggested to women taking phenobarbital.

ADVERSE REACTIONS:

The following adverse reactions and their incidence were compiled from surveillance of thousands of hospitalized patients. Because such patients may be less aware of certain of the milder adverse effects of barbiturates, the incidence of these reactions may be somewhat higher in fully ambulatory patients.

More than 1 in 100 Patients: The most common adverse reactions estimated to occur at a rate of 1 to 3 patients per 100 is:

Nervous System: Somnolence.

Less than 1 in 100 Patients: Adverse reactions estimated to occur at a rate of less than 1 in 100 patients listed below, grouped by organ system, and by decreasing order of occurrence are:

Nervous System: Agitation, confusion, hyperkinesia, ataxia, CNS depression, nightmares, nervousness, psychiatric disturbance, hallucinations, insomnia, anxiety, dizziness, thinking abnormality.

Respiratory System: Hypoventilation, apnea.

Cardiovascular System: Bradycardia, hypotension, syncope.

Digestive System: Nausea, vomiting, constipation.

Other Reported Reactions: Headache, hypersensitivity reactions (angioedema, skin rashes, exfoliative dermatitis), fever, liver damage, megaloblastic anemia following chronic phenobarbital use.

DRUG ABUSE AND DEPENDENCE:

Mephobarbital is controlled substance in Narcotic Schedule IV. Barbiturates may be habit forming. Tolerance, psychological dependence, and physical dependence may occur especially following prolonged use of high doses of barbiturates. As tolerance to barbiturates develops, the amount needed to maintain the same level of intoxication increase; tolerance to a fatal dosage, however, dose not increase more than two-fold. As this occurs, the margin between an intoxicating dosage and fatal dosage becomes smaller.

Symptoms of acute intoxication with barbiturates include unsteady gait, slurred speech, and sustained nystagmus. Mental signs of chronic intoxication include confusion, poor judgment, irritability, insomnia, and somatic complaints.

Symptoms of barbiturate dependence are similar to those of chronic alcoholism. If an individual appears to be intoxicated with alcohol to a degree that is radically disproportionate to the amount of alcohol in his or her blood the use of barbiturates should be suspected. The lethal dose of barbiturate rate is far less if alcohol is also ingested.

The symptoms of barbiturate withdrawal can be severe and may cause death. Minor withdrawal symptoms may appear 8 to 12 hours after the last dose of barbiturate. These symptoms usually appear in the following order: anxiety, muscle twitching, tremor of hands and fingers, progressive weakness, dizziness, distortion in visual perception, nausea, vomiting, insomnia, and orthostatic hypotension. Major withdrawal symptoms (convulsions and delirium) may occur within 16 hours and last up to 5 days after abrupt cessation of these drugs. Intensity of withdrawal symptoms gradually declines over a period of approximately 15 days. Individuals susceptible to a barbiturate abuse and dependence include alcoholics and opiate abusers, as well as other sedative-hypnotic and amphetamine abusers.

Drug dependence to barbiturates arises from repeated administration of a barbiturate of agent with barbiturate-like effect on a continuous basis, generally in amounts exceeding therapeutic dose levels. The characteristics of drug dependence to barbiturates include: (a) a strong desire or need to continue taking the drug; (b) a tendency to increase the dose; (c) a psychic dependence on the effects of the drug related to subjective and individual appreciation of those effects; and (d) a physical dependence on the effects of the drug requiring its presence for maintenance of homeostasis and resulting in a definite, characteristic, and self-limited abstinence syndrome when the drug is withdrawn.

Treatment of barbiturate dependence consists of cautious and gradual withdrawal of the drug. Barbiturate-dependent patients can be withdrawn by using a number of different withdrawal regimens. In all cases withdrawal takes an extended period of time. One method involves substituting a 30 mg dose of phenobarbital for each 100 mg to 200 mg dose of barbiturate that the patient has been taking. The total daily amount of phenobarbital is then administered in 3 to 4 divided doses, not to exceed to 600 mg daily. Should signs of withdrawal occur on the first day of treatment, a loading dose of 100 mg to 200 mg of phenobarbital may be administered IM in addition to the oral dose. After stabilization on phenobarbital, the total daily dose is decreased by 30 mg a day as long as withdrawal is proceeding smoothly. A modification of this regimen involves initiating treatment at the patient's regular dosage level and decreasing the daily dosage by 10% if tolerated by the patient.

Infants physically dependent on barbiturates may be given phenobarbital 3 mg/kg/day to 10 mg/kg/day. After withdrawal symptoms (hyperactivity, disturbed sleep, tremors, hyperreflexia) are relieved, the dosage of phenobarbital should be gradually decreased and completely withdrawn over a 2-week period.

OVERDOSAGE:

The toxic dose of barbiturates varies considerably. In general, an oral dose of 1 g most barbiturates produces serious poisoning in an adult. Death commonly occurs after 2 g to 10 g of ingested barbiturate. Barbiturate intoxication may be confused with alcoholism, bromide intoxication, and with various neurological disorders.

Acute overdosage with barbiturates is manifested by CNS and respiratory depression which may progress to Cheyne-Stokes respiration, areflexia, constriction of the pupils to a slight degree (though in severe poisoning they may show paralytic dilation), oliguria, tachycardia, hypotension, lowered body temperature, and coma. Typical shock syndrome (apnea, circulatory collapse, respiratory arrest, and death) may occur.

In extreme overdose, all electrical activity in the brain may cease, in which case a "flat" EEG normally equated with clinical death cannot be accepted. This effect is fully reversible unless hypoxic damage occurs. Consideration should be given to the possibility of barbiturate intoxication even in situations that appear to involve trauma.

Complications such as pneumonia, pulmonary edema, cardiac arrhythmias, congestive heart failure, and renal failure may occur. Uremia may increase CNS sensitivity to barbiturates if renal function is impaired. Differential diagnosis should include hypoglycemia, head trauma, cerebrovascular accidents, convulsive states, and diabetic coma.

Treatment of overdosage is mainly supportive and consists of the following:

1. Maintenance of an adequate airway, with assisted respiration and oxygen administration as necessary.

2. Monitoring of vital signs and fluid balance.

3. If the patient is conscious and has not lost the gag reflex, emesis may be induced with ipecac. Care should be taken to prevent pulmonary aspiration of vomitus. After completion of vomiting, 30 g activated charcoal in a glass of water may be administered.

4. If emesis is contraindicated, gastric lavage may be performed with a cuffed endotracheal tube in place with the patient in the face down position. Activated charcoal may be left in the emptied stomach and a saline cathartic administered.

5. Fluid therapy and other standard treatment for shock, if needed.

6. If renal function is normal, forced diuresis may aid in the elimination of the barbiturate. Alkalinization of the urine increases renal excretion of some barbiturates, including mephobarbital (which is metabolized to phenobarbital).

7. Although not recommended as a routine procedure, hemodialysis may be used in severe barbiturate intoxications or if the patient is anuric or in shock.

8. Patient should be rolled from side to side every 30 minutes.

9. Antibiotics should be given if pneumonia is suspected.

10. Appropriate nursing care to prevent hypostatic pneumonia, decubiti aspiration, and other complications of patients with altered states of consciousness.

DOSAGE AND ADMINISTRATION:

Epilepsy: Average dose for adults: 400 mg to 600 mg (6 grains to 9 grains) daily; children under 5 years: 16 mg to 32 mg (1/4 grain to 1/2 grain) three or four times daily; children over 5 years: 32 mg to 64 mg (1/2 grain to 1 grain) three or four times daily. Mephobarbital is best taken at bedtime if seizures generally occur at night, and during the day if attacks are diurnal.

Treatment should be started with a small dose which is gradually increased over four of five days until the optimum dosage is determined. If the patient has been taking some other antiepileptic drug, it should be tapered off as the doses of Mephobarbital are increased, to guard against the temporary marked attacks that may occur when any treatment for epilepsy is changed abruptly. Similarly, when the dose if lowered to a maintenance level or to be discontinued, the amount should be reduced gradually over four of five days.

DOSAGE AND ADMINISTRATION: *(cont'd)*

Special Patient Population: Dosage should be reduced in the elderly or debilitated because these patients may be more sensitive to barbiturates. Dosage should be reduced for patients with impaired renal function or hepatic disease.

Combination with Other Drugs: Mephobarbital may be used in combination with phenobarbital, either in the form of alternating courses or concurrently. When the two drugs are used at the same time, the dose should be about one-half the amount of each used alone. The average daily dose for an adult is from 50 mg to 100 mg (3/4 grain to 1 1/2 grains) of phenobarbital and from 200 mg to 300 mg (3 grains to 4 1/2 grains) of Mephobarbital.

Mephobarbital may also be used with phenytoin sodium; in some cases, combined therapy appears to give better results than either agent used alone, since phenytoin sodium is particularly effective for the psychomotor types of seizure but relatively ineffective for petit mal. When the drugs are employed concurrently, a reduced dose of phenytoin sodium is advisable, but the full dose of Mephobarbital may be given. Satisfactory results have been obtained with an average daily dose of 230 mg (3 1/2 grains) of phenytoin sodium plus about 600 mg (9 grains) of Mephobarbital.

Sedation: *Adults:* 32 mg to 100 mg (1/2 grain to 1 1/2 grains)- -optimum dose, 50 mg (3/4 grain)—three to four times daily. *Children:* 16 mg to 32 mg (1/4 grain to 1/2 grain) three to four times daily.

HOW SUPPLIED:

Tablets: 32 mg (1/2 grain), bottles of 250.
50 mg (3/4 grain), bottles of 250.
100 mg (1 1/2 grains), bottles of 250.

HOW SUPPLIED - EQUIVALENTS NOT AVAILABLE:

Tablet, Uncoated - Oral - 32 mg

250's $41.58 MEBARAL, Sanofi Winthrop 00024-1231-05

Tablet, Uncoated - Oral - 50 mg

250's $59.51 MEBARAL, Sanofi Winthrop 00024-1232-05

Tablet, Uncoated - Oral - 100 mg

250's $79.76 MEBARAL, Sanofi Winthrop 00024-1233-05

MEPIVACAINE HYDROCHLORIDE *(001732)*

CATEGORIES: Analeptics; Anesthesia; Caudal; Dental; Epidural; Local Anesthetics; Pregnancy Category C; FDA Approval Pre 1982

BRAND NAMES: Arestocaine HCl; *Carbocain*; *Carbocain Dental*; *Carbocaina*; **Carbocaine**; *Carbocaine Caudal 1.5%*; *Carbocaine Dental*; Carbocot; *Emcain*; *Isocain* (Canada); Isocaine HCl; *Meaverin* (Germany); Polocaine; *Scandicain* (Germany); *Scandicaine*; *Scandinibsa*; Scandonest Plain; *Tevacaine*
(International brand names outside U.S. in italics)

DESCRIPTION:

THESE SOLUTIONS ARE NOT INTENDED FOR SPINAL ANESTHESIA OR DENTAL USE.

Mepivacaine HCl is 2-Piperidinecarboxamide,*N*-(2,6-dimethylphenyl)-1-methyl-monohydrochloride.

It is a white crystalline odorless power, soluble in water, but very resistant to both acid and alkaline hydrolysis.

Mepivacaine HCl is a local anesthetic available as sterile isotonic solutions in concentrations of 1%, 1.5%, and 2% for injection via local infiltration, peripheral nerve block, and caudal and lumbar epidural blocks.

Mepivacaine HCl is related chemically and pharmacologically to the amide-type local anesthetics. It contains an amide linkage between the aromatic nucleus and the amino group (TABLE 1):

TABLE 1 Composition of Available Solutions*

	1% Single-Dose 30 ml Vial mg/ml	1% Multiple-Dose 50 ml Vial mg/ml	1.5% Single-Dose 30 ml Vial mg/ml	2% Single-Dose 20 ml Vial mg/ml	2% Multiple-Dose 50 ml Vial mg/ml
Mepivacaine HCl	10	10	15	20	20
Sodium chloride	6.6	7	5.6	4.6	5
Potassium chloride	0.3		0.3	0.3	
Calcium chloride	0.33		0.33	0.33	
Methylparaben		1			1

* In Water for Injection.
The pH of the solutions is adjusted between 4.5 and 6.8 with sodium hydroxide or hydrochloric acid.

CLINICAL PHARMACOLOGY:

Local anesthetics block the generation and the conduction of nerve impulses, presumably by increasing the threshold for electrical excitation in the nerve, by slowing the propagation of the nerve impulse and by reducing the rate of rise of the action potential. In general, the progression of anesthesia is related to the diameter, myelination, and conduction velocity of affected nerve fibers. Clinically, the order of loss of nerve function is as follow: pain, temperature, touch, proprioception, and skeletal muscle tone.

Systemic absorption of local produces effects on the cardiovascular and central nervous systems. At blood concentrations achieved with normal therapeutic doses, changes in cardiac conduction, excitability, refractoriness, contractility, and peripheral vascular resistance are minimal. However, toxic blood concentrations depress cardiac conduction and excitability, which may lead to atrioventricular block and ultimately to cardiac arrest. In addition, myocardial contractility is depressed and peripheral vasodilation occurs, leading to decreased cardiac output and arterial blood pressure.

Following systemic absorption, local anesthetics can produce central nervous system stimulation, depression, or both. Apparent central stimulation is manifested as restlessness, tremors, and shivering, progressing to convulsions, followed by depression and coma progressing ultimately to respiratory arrest. However, the local anesthetics have a primary depressant effect on the medulla and on higher centers. The depressed stage may occur without a prior excited stage.

Pharmacokinetics: The rate of systemic absorption of local anesthetics is dependent upon the total dose and concentration of drug administered, the route of administration, the vascularity of the administration site, and the presence or absence of epinephrine in the anesthetic

CLINICAL PHARMACOLOGY: *(cont'd)*

solution. A dilute concentration of epinephrine (1:200,000 or 5 mcg/ml) usually reduces the rate of absorption and plasma concentration of mepivacaine, however, it has been reported that vasoconstrictors do not significantly prolong anesthesia with mepivacaine.

Onset of anesthesia with mepivacaine is rapid, the time of onset for sensory block ranging from about 3 to 20 minutes depending upon such factors as the anesthetic technique, the type of block, the concentration of the solution, and the individual patient. The degree of motor blockade produced is dependent on the concentration of solution. A 0.5% solution will be effective in small superficial nerve blocks while the 1% concentration will block sensory and sympathetic conduction without loss of motor function. The 1.5% solution will provide extensive and often complete motor block and the 2% concentration of mepivacaine will produce complete sensory and motor block of any nerve group.

The duration of anesthesia also varies depending upon the technique and type of block, the concentration, and the individual. Mepivacaine will normally provide anesthesia which is adequate for 2 to 2 1/2 hours of surgery.

Local anesthetics are bound to plasma proteins in varying degrees. Generally, the lower the plasma concentration of drug, the higher the percentage of drug bound to plasma.

Local anesthetic appear to cross the placenta by passive diffusion. The rate and degree of diffusion is governed by the degree of plasma protein binding, the degree of ionization, and the degree of lipid solubility. Fetal/maternal ratios of local anesthetics appear to be inversely related to the degree of plasma protein binding, because only the free, unbound drug is available for placental transfer. Mepivacaine is approximately 75% bound to plasma proteins. The extent of placental transfer is also determined by the degree of ionization and lipid solubility of the drug. Lipid soluble, nonionized drugs readily enter the fetal blood from the maternal circulation.

Depending upon the route of administration, local anesthetics are distributed to some extent to all body tissues, with high concentrations found in highly perfused organs such as the liver, lungs, heart and brain.

Various pharmacokinetic parameters of the local anesthetics can be significantly altered by the presence of hepatic or renal disease, addition of epinephrine, factors affecting urinary pH, renal blood flow, the route of drug administration, and the age of the patient. The half-life of mepivacaine in adults is 1.9 to 3.2 hours and in neonates 8.7 to 9 hours.

Mepivacaine, because of its amide structure, is not detoxified by the circulating plasma esterases. It is rapidly metabolized, with only a small percentage of the anesthetic (5 percent to 10 percent) being excreted unchanged in the urine. The liver is the principal site of metabolism, with over 50% of the administered dose being excreted into the bile as metabolites. Most of the metabolized mepivacaine is probably resorted in the intestine and then excreted into the urine since only a small percentage is found in feces. The principal route of excretion is via the kidney. Most of the anesthetic and its metabolites are eliminated within 30 hours. It has been shown that hydroxylation and N-demethylation, which are detoxification reactions, play important roles in the metabolism of the anesthetic. Three metabolites of mepivacaine have been identified from human adults: two phenols, which are excreted almost exclusively as their glucuronide conjugates, and the N-demethylated compound (2',6'-pipecoloxylidide).

Mepivacaine does not ordinarily produce irritation tissue damage, and does not cause methemoglobinemia when administered in recommended doses and concentration.

INDICATIONS AND USAGE:

Mepivacaine is indicated for production of local or regional analgesia and anesthesia by local infiltration, peripheral nerve block techniques, and central neural techniques including epidural and caudal blocks.

The routes of administration indicated concentration for mepivacaine are (TABLE 2):

TABLE 2

Local infiltration	0.5% (via dilution) or 1%
Peripheral nerve blocks	1% and 2%
Epidural block	1%, 1.5%, 2%
Caudal block	1%, 1.5% 2%

See DOSAGE AND ADMINISTRATION for additional information. Standard textbooks should be consulted to determine the accepted procedures and techniques for the administration of mepivacaine.

CONTRAINDICATIONS:

Mepivacaine is contraindicated in patients with a known hypersensitivity to it or to any local anesthetic agent of the amide-type or to other components of solutions of mepivacaine.

WARNINGS:

LOCAL ANESTHETICS SHOULD ONLY BE EMPLOYED BY CLINICIANS WHO ARE WELL VERSED IN DIAGNOSIS AND MANAGEMENT OF DOSE-RELATED TOXICITY AND OTHER ACUTE EMERGENCIES WHICH MIGHT ARISE FROM THE BLOCK TO BE EMPLOYED, AND THEN ONLY AFTER INSURING THE IMMEDIATE AVAILABILITY OF OXYGEN, OTHER RESUSCITATIVE DRUGS, CARDIOPULMONARY RESUSCITATIVE EQUIPMENT, AND THE PERSONNEL RESOURCE NEEDED FOR PROPER MANAGEMENT OF TOXIC REACTIONS AND RELATED EMERGENCIES. (see also ADVERSE REACTIONSand PRECAUTIONS.) **DELAY IN PROPER MANAGEMENT OF DOSE-RELATED TOXICITY, UNDERVENTILATION FROM ANY CAUSE, AND/OR ALTERED SENSITIVITY MAY LEAD TO THE DEVELOPMENT OF ACIDOSIS, CARDIAC ARREST AND, POSSIBLY, DEATH.**

Local anesthetic solutions containing antimicrobial preservative (*i.e.*, those supplied in multiple dose vials) should not be used for epidural or caudal anesthesia because safety has not been established with regard to intrathecal injection either intentionally or inadvertently, of such preservatives.

It is essential that aspiration for blood or cerebrospinal fluid (where applicable) be done prior to injecting any local anesthetic, both the original dose and all subsequent doses, to avoid intravascular or subarachnoid injection. However, a negative aspiration does not ensure against in intravascular or subarachnoid injection.

Reactions resulting in fatality have occurred on rare occasions with the use of local anesthetics.

Mepivacaine with epinephrine or other vasopressors should not be used concomitantly with ergot-type oxytocic drugs, because a serve persistent hypertension may occur. Likewise, solutions of mepivacaine containing a vasoconstrictor, such as epinephrine, should be used with extreme caution in patients receiving monoamine oxidase inhibitors (MAOI) or antidepressants of the triptyline or imipramine types, because severe prolonged hypertension may result.

Local anesthetic procedures should be used with caution when there is inflammation and/or sepsis in the region of the proposed injection.

Mixing or the prior or intercurrent use of any local anesthetic with mepivacaine cannot be recommended because of insufficient data on the clinical use of such mixtures.

PRECAUTIONS:

General: The safety and effectiveness of local anesthetics depend on proper dosage, correct technique, adequate precautions, and readiness for emergencies. Resuscitative equipment, oxygen, and other resuscitative drug should be available for immediate use. (See WARNINGS and ADVERSE REACTIONS.) During major regional nerve blocks, the patient should have IV fluids running via an indwelling catheter to assure a functioning intravenous pathway. The lowest dosage of local anesthetic that results in effective anesthesia should be used to avoid upon high plasma levels and serious adverse effects. Injections should be made slowly, with frequent aspirations before and during the injection to avoid intravascular inject. Current opinion favors fractional administration with constant attention to the patient, rather than rapid bolus injection. Syringe aspiration should also be performed before and during each supplemental injection in continuous (intermittent catheter techniques. An intravascular injection is still possible even if aspirations for blood are negative).

During the administration of epidural anesthesia, it is recommended that a test dose be administered initially and the effects monitored before the full dose is given. When using a "continuous" catheter technique, test doses should be given prior to both the original and all reinforcing doses, because plastic tubing in the epidural space can migrate into a blood vessel or through the dura. When clinical conditions permit, an effective test dose should contain epinephrine (10 mcg to 15 mcg have been suggested) to serve as a warning of unintended intravascular injection. If injected into a blood vessel, this amount of epinephrine is likely to produce an "epinephrine response" within 45 seconds, consisting of an increase of pulse and blood pressure, circumoral pallor, palpitations, and nervousness in the unsedated patient. The sedated patient may exhibit only a pulse rate increase of 20 or more beats per minute for 15 or more seconds. Therefore, following the test dose, the heart rate should be monitored for a heart rate increase. The test dose should also contain 45 mg to 50 mg of mepivacaine to detect an unintended intrathecal administration. This will be evidenced within a few minutes by sings of spinal block (*e.g.,* decreased sensation of the buttocks, paresis of the legs, or, in the sedated patient, absent knee jerk).

Injection of repeated doses of local anesthetics may cause significant increases in plasma levels with each repeated dose due to slow accumulation of the drug of its metabolites or to slow metabolic degradation. Tolerance to elevated blood levels varies with the status of the patient. Debilitated, elderly patients, and acutely ill patients should be given reduced doses commensurate with their age and physical status. Local anesthetics should also be used with caution in patients with severe disturbances of cardiac rhythm, shock, heart block, or hypotension.

Careful and constant monitoring of cardiovascular and respiratory (adequacy of ventilation) vital signs, and the patient's state of consciousness should be performed after each local anesthetic injection. It should be kept in mind at such times that restlessness, anxiety, incoherent speech, lightheadedness, numbness and tingling of the mouth and lips, metallic taste, tinnitus, dizziness, blurred vision, tremors, twitching, depression, or drowsiness may be early warning signs of central nervous system toxicity.

Local anesthetic solutions containing a vasoconstrictor should be used cautiously and in carefully restricted quantities in areas of the body supplied by end arteries or having otherwise compromised blood supply such as digits, nose, external ear, penis. Patients with hypertensive vascular disease may exhibit exaggerated vasoconstrictor response. Ischemic injury or necrosis may result.

Mepivacaine should be used with caution in patients with known allergies and sensitivities.

Because amide-type local anesthetics such as mepivacaine are metabolized by the liver and excreted by the kidneys, these drugs, especially repeat doses, should be used cautiously in patients with hepatic and renal disease. Patients with severe hepatic disease, because of their inability to metabolize local anesthetics normally, are at a greater risk of developing toxic plasma concentrations. Local anesthetics should also be used with caution in patients with impaired cardiovascular function because they may be less able to compensate for functional changers associated with the prolongation of AV conduction produced by these drugs.

Serious dose-related cardiac arrhythmias may occur if preparations containing a vasoconstrictor such as epinephrine are employed in patients during or following the administration of potent inhalation anesthetics. In deciding whether to use these products concurrently in the same patient, the combined action of both agents upon the myocardium, the concentration and volume of vasoconstrictor used, and the time since injection, when applicable, should be taken into account.

Many drugs used during the conduct of anesthesia are considered potential triggering agents for familial malignant hyperthermia. Because it is not known whether amide-type local anesthetics may trigger this reaction and because the need for supplemental general anesthesia cannot be predicted in advance, it is suggested that a standard protocol for management should be available. Early unexplained signs of tachycardia, tachypnea, labile blood pressure, and metabolic acidosis may precede temperature elevation. Successful outcome is dependent on early diagnosis, prompt discontinuance of the suspect triggering agent(s), and institution of treatment, including oxygen therapy, indicated supportive measures, and dantrolene. (Consult dantrolene sodium intravenous package insert before using.)

Use in Head and Neck Area: Small doses of local anesthetics injected into the head and neck area may produce adverse reactions similar to systemic toxicity seen with unintentional intravascular injections of larger doses. The injection procedures require the utmost care.

Confusion convulsions, respiratory depression, and/or respiratory arrest, and cardiovascular stimulation or depression have been reported. These reactions may be due to intra-arterial injection of the local anesthetic with retrograde flow to the cerebral circulation. Patients receiving these blocks should have their circulation and respiration monitored and be constantly observed. Resuscitative equipment and personnel for treating adverse reactions should be immediately available. Dosage recommendations should not be exceeded.

Information for the Patient: When appropriate, patients should be informed in advance that they may experience temporary loss of sensation and motor activity, usually in the lower half of the body, following proper administration of caudal or epidural anesthesia. Also, when appropriate, the physician should discuss other information including adverse reactions listed in the package insert on mepivacaine.

Carcinogenesis, Mutagenesis, and Impairment of Fertility: Long-term studies in animals of most local anesthetics including mepivacaine to evaluate the carcinogenic potential have not been conducted. Mutagenic potential or the effect of fertility have not been determined. There is no evidence from human data that mepivacaine may be carcinogenic or mutagenic or that it impairs fertility.

Pregnancy Category C: Animal reproduction studies have not been conducted with mepivacaine. There are no adequate and well-controlled studies in pregnant women of the effect of mepivacaine on the developing fetus. Mepivacaine HCl should be used during pregnancy only if the potential benefit justifies the potential risk to the fetus. This does not preclude the use of mepivacaine at term for obstetrical anesthesia or analgesia. (See Labor and Delivery.)

Mepivacaine has been used for obstetrical analgesia by the epidural, caudal, and paracervical routes without evidence of adverse effects on the fetus when no more than the maximum safe dosages are used and strict adherence to technique is followed.

Labor and Delivery: Local anesthetics rapidly cross the placenta, and when used for epidural, paracervical, caudal, or pudendal block anesthesia, can cause varying degrees of maternal, fetal, and neonatal toxicity. (See CLINICAL PHARMACOLOGY, Pharmacokinetics.) The

PRECAUTIONS: *(cont'd)*

incidence and degree of toxicity depend upon the procedure performed, the type and amount of drug used, and the technique of drug administration. Adverse reactions in the parturient, fetus, and neonate involve alterations of the central nervous system, peripheral vascular tone, and cardiac function.

Maternal hypotension has resulted from regional anesthesia. Local anesthetics produce vasodilation by blocking sympathetic nerves. Elevating the patient's legs and positioning her on her left side will help prevent decreases in blood pressure. The fetal heart rate also should be monitored continuously and electronic fetal monitoring is highly advisable.

Epidural, paracervical, caudal, or pudendal anesthesia may alter the forces of parturition through changes in uterine contractility or maternal expulsive efforts. In one study, paracervical block anesthesia was associated with a decrease in the mean duration of first stage labor and facilitation of cervical dilation. Epidural anesthesia has been reported to prolong the second stage of labor by removing the parturient's reflex urge to bear down or by interfering with motor function. The use of obstetrical anesthesia may increase the need for forceps assistance.

The use of some local anesthetics drug products during labor and delivery may be followed by diminished muscle strength and tone for the first day or two of life. The long-term significance of these observations is unknown.

Fetal bradycardia may occur in 20 to 30 percent of patients receiving paracervical block anesthesia with the amide-type local anesthetics and may be associated with fetal acidosis. Fetal heart rate should always be monitored during paracervical anesthesia. Added risk appears to be present in prematurity, postmaturity, toxemia of pregnancy, and fetal distress. The physician should weigh the possible advantages against dangers when considering paracervical block in these conditions. Careful adherence to recommended dosage is of the utmost importance in obstetrical paracervical block. Failure to achieve adequate analgesia with recommended doses should arouse suspicion of intravascular of fetal intracranial injection.

Cases compatible with unintended fetal intracranial injection of local anesthetic solution have been reported following intended paracervical or pudendal block or both. Babies so affected present with unexplained neonatal depression at birth which correlates with high local anesthetic serum levels and usually manifest seizures within six hours. Prompt use of supportive measures combined with forced urinary excretion of the local anesthetic has been used successfully to manage this complication.

Case reports of maternal convulsions and cardiovascular collapse following use of some local anesthetics for paracervical block in early pregnancy (as anesthesia for elective abortion) suggest that systemic absorption under these circumstances may be rapid. The recommended maximum dose of the local anesthetic should not be exceeded. Injection should be made slowly and with frequent aspiration. Allow a five-minute interval between sides.

It is extremely important to avoid aortocaval compression by the gravid uterus during administration of regional block to parturients. To do this, the patient must be maintained in the left lateral decubitus position or a blanket roll or sandbag may be placed beneath the right hip and the gravid uterus displaced to the left.

Nursing Mothers: It is not known whether local anesthetic drugs are excreted in human milk. Because many drugs are excreted in human milk, caution should be exercised when local anesthetics are administered to a nursing woman.

Pediatric Use: Guidelines for the administration of mepivacaine to children are presented in DOSAGE AND ADMINISTRATION.

DRUG INTERACTIONS:

The administration of local anesthetic solution containing epinephrine or norepinephrine to patients receiving monoamine oxidase inhibitors or tricyclic antidepressants may produce severe, prolonged hypertension. Concurrent use of these agents should generally be avoided. In situations when concurrent therapy is necessary, careful patient monitoring is essential.

Concurrent administration of vasopressor drugs and of ergot-type oxytocic drugs may cause severe, persistent hypertension or cerebrovascular accidents.

Phenothiazines and butyrophenones may reduce or reverse the pressor effect of epinephrine.

ADVERSE REACTIONS:

Reactions to mepivacaine are characteristic of those associated with other amide-type local anesthetics. A major cause of adverse reactions to this group of drugs is excessive plasma levels, which may be due to overdosage, inadvertent intravascular injection, or slow metabolic degradation.

Systemic: The most commonly encountered acute adverse experiences which demand immediate countermeasures are related to the central nervous system and the cardiovascular system. These adverse experiences are generally dose related and due to high plasma levels which may result from overdosage, rapid absorption from the injection site, diminished tolerance, or from unintentional intravascular injection of the local anesthetic solution. In addition to systemic dose-related toxicity, unintentional subarachnoid injection of drug during the intended performance of caudal or lumbar epidural block or nerve blocks near the vertebral column (especially in the head and neck region) may result in underventilating or apnea ("Total or High Spinal"). Also, hypotension due to loss of sympathetic tone and respiratory paralysis or underventilation due to cephalad extension of the motor level of anesthesia may occur. This may lead to secondary cardiac arrest if untreated. Factors influencing plasma protein binding, such as acidosis, systemic diseases which alter protein production, or competition of other drugs for protein binding sites, may diminish individual tolerance.

Central Nervous System Reactions: These are characterized by excitation and/or depression. Restlessness, anxiety, dizziness, tinnitus, blurred vision, or tremors may occur, possibly proceeding to convulsions. However, excitement may be transient or absent, with depression being the first manifestation of an adverse reaction. This may quickly be followed by drowsiness merging into unconsciousness and respiratory arrest. Other central nervous system effects may be nausea, vomiting, chills, and constriction of the pupils.

The incidence of convulsions associated with the use of local anesthetics varies with the procedure used and the total dose administered. In a survey of studies of epidural anesthesia, overt toxicity progressing to convulsions occurred in approximately 0.1% of local anesthetic administrations.

Cardiovascular Reactions: High doses or, inadvertent intravascular injection, may lead to high plasma levels and related depression of the myocardium, decreased cardiac output, heart block, hypotension (or sometimes hypertension), bradycardia, ventricular arrhythmias, and possibly cardiac arrest). (See WARNINGS, PRECAUTIONS, and OVERDOSAGE.)

Allergic: Allergic-type reactions rare and may occur as a result of sensitivity to the local anesthetic or to other formulation ingredients, such as the antimicrobial preservative methylparaben, contained in multiple-dose vials. These reactions are characterized by signs such as urticaria, pruritus, erythema, angioneurotic edema (including laryngeal edema), tachycardia, sneezing, nausea, vomiting, dizziness, syncope, excessive sweating, elevated temperature, and possibly, anaphylactoid-like symptomatology (including severe hypotension). Cross sensitivity among members of the amide-type local anesthetic group has been reported. The usefulness of screening for sensitivity has not been definitely established.

ADVERSE REACTIONS: *(cont'd)*

Neurologic: The incidences of adverse neurologic reactions associated with the use of local anesthetics may be related to the total dose of local anesthetic administered and are also dependent upon the particular drug used, the route of administration, and the physical status of the patient. Many of these effects my be related to local anesthetic techniques, with or without a contribution from the drug.

In the practice of caudal or lumbar epidural block, occasional unintentional penetration of the subarachnoid space by the catheter or needle may occur. Subsequent adverse effects may depend partially on the amount of drug administered intrathecally and the physiological and physical effects of a dural puncture. A high spinal is characterized by paralysis of the legs, loss of consciousness, respiratory paralysis, and bradycardia.

Neurologic effects following epidural or caudal anesthesia may include spinal block of varying magnitude (including high or total spinal block); hypotension secondary to spinal block; urinary retention; fecal and urinary incontinence; loss of perineal sensation and sexual function; persistent anesthesia, paresthesia, weakness, paralysis of the lower extremities, and loss of sphincter control all of which may have slow, incomplete, or no recovery; headache; backache; septic meningitis; meningismus; slowing of labor; increased incidence of forceps delivery; cranial nerve palsies due to traction on nerves from loss of cerebrospinal fluid.

Neurologic effects following other procedures or routes of administration may include persistent anesthesia, paresthesia, weakness, paralysis, all of which may have slow, incomplete, or no recovery.

OVERDOSAGE:

Acute emergencies from local anesthetics are generally related to high plasma levels encountered during therapeutic use of local anesthetics or to unintended subarachnoid injection of local anesthetic solution. (See ADVERSE REACTIONS, WARNINGS, and PRECAUTIONS.)

Management of Local Anesthetic Emergencies: The first consideration is prevention, best accomplished by careful and constant monitoring of cardiovascular and respiratory vital signs and the patient's state of consciousness after each local anesthetic injection. At the first sign of change, oxygen should be administered.

The first step in the management of systemic toxic reactions, as well as underventilation or apnea due to unintentional subarachnoid injection of drug solution, consists of immediate attention to the establishment and maintenance of a patent airway and effective assisted or controlled ventilation with 100% oxygen with a delivery system capable of permitting immediate positive airway pressure by mask. This may prevent convulsions if they have not already occurred.

If necessary, use drugs to control the convulsions. A 50 mg to 100 mg bolus IV injection of succinylcholine will paralyze the patient without depressing the central nervous or cardiovascular systems and facilitate ventilation. A bolus IV dose of 5 mg to 10 mg of diazepam or 50 mg to 100 mg of thiopental will permit ventilation and counteract central nervous system stimulation, but these drugs also depress central nervous system, respiratory, and cardiac function, add to postictal depression and may result in apnea. Intravenous barbiturates, anticonvulsant agents, or muscle relaxants should only be administered by those familiar with their use. Immediately after the institution of these ventilatory measures, the adequacy of the circulation should be evaluated. Supportive treatment of circulatory depression may require administration of intravenous fluids, and when appropriate, a vasopressor dictated by the clinical situation (such as ephedrine or epinephrine to enhance myocardial contractile force).

Endotracheal intubation, employing drugs and techniques familiar to the clinician may be indicated after initial administration of oxygen by mask, if difficulty in encountered in the maintenance of a patent airway or if prolonged ventilatory support (assisted or controlled) is indicated.

Recent clinical data from patients experiencing local anesthetic induced convulsions demonstrated rapid development of hypoxia, hypercarbia, and acidosis within a minute of the onset of convulsions. These observations suggest that oxygen consumption and carbon dioxide production are greatly increased during local anesthetic convulsions and emphasize the important of immediate and effective ventilation with oxygen which may avoid cardiac arrest.

If not treated immediately, convulsions with simultaneous hypoxia, hypercarbia, and acidosis, plus myocardial depression from the direct effects of the local anesthetic may result in cardiac arrhythmias, bradycardia, asystole, ventricular fibrillation, or cardiac arrest. Respiratory abnormalities, including apnea, may occur. Underventilation or apnea due to unintentional subarachnoid injection of local anesthetic solution may produce these same signs and also lead to cardiac arrest if ventilatory support is not instituted. If cardiac arrest should occur, standard cardiopulmonary resuscitative measures should be instituted and maintained for a prolonged period if necessary. Recovery has been reported after prolonged resuscitative efforts.

The supine position is dangerous in pregnant women at term because of aortocaval compression by the gravid uterus. Therefore during treatment of systemic toxicity, maternal hypotension, or fetal bradycardia following regional block, the parturient should be maintained in the left lateral decubitus position of possible, or manual displacement of the uterus off the great vessels be accomplished.

The mean seizure dosage or mepivacaine in rhesus monkeys was found to be 18.8 mg/kg with mean arterial plasma concentration of 24.4 mcg/ml. The intravenous and subcutaneous LD_{50} in mice is 23 mg/kg to 35 mg/kg and 280 mg/kg respectively.

DOSAGE AND ADMINISTRATION:

The dose of any local anesthetic administered varies with the anesthetic procedure, the area to be anesthetized, the vascularity of the tissues, the number of neuronal segments to be blocked, the depth of anesthesia and degree of muscle relaxation required, the duration of anesthesia desired, individual tolerance and the physician condition of the patient. The smallest dose and concentration required to produce the desired result should be administered. Dosages of mepivacaine should be reduced for elderly and debilitated patients and patients with cardiac and/or liver disease. The rapid injection of a large volume of local anesthetic solution should be avoided and fractional doses should be used when feasible.

For specific techniques and procedures, refer to standard textbooks.

The recommended single **adult**dose (or the total of series of doses given in one procedure) of mepivacaine for unseated, healthy, normal-sized individuals should not usually exceed 400 mg. The recommended dosage is based on requirements for the average adult and should be reduced for elderly or debilitated patients.

While maximum doses of 7 mg/kg (550 mg) have been administered without adverse effect, these are not recommended, except in exceptional circumstances and under no circumstances should the administration be repeated at intervals of less than 1 1/2 hours. The total dose for any 24-hour period should not exceed 1,000 mg because of a slow accumulation of the anesthetic or its derivatives of slower than normal metabolic degradation or detoxification with repeat administration (See CLINICAL PHARMACOLOGY and PRECAUTIONS).

DOSAGE AND ADMINISTRATION: *(cont'd)*

Children: tolerate the local anesthetic as well as adults. However, the pediatric dose should be ***carefully measured***as a percentage of the total adult dose ***based on weight***, and should not exceed 5 mg/kg to 6 mg/kg (2.5 mg/lb to 3 mg/lb) in children, especially those weighing less than 30 lb. In children ***under 3 years of age or weighing less than 30 lb***concentrations less than 2% (*e.g.,* 0.5% to 1.5%) should be employed.

Unused portions of solutions not containing preservatives, i.e. those supplied in single-dose vials, should be discarded following initial use.

This product should be inspected visually for particulate matter and discoloration prior to administration whenever solution and container permit. Solutions which are discolored or which contain particular matter should not be administered (TABLE 3):

TABLE 3 Recommended Concentrations and Doses of Mepivacaine

Procedure	Concentration	Total Dose ml	Total Dose mg	Comments
Cervical, brachial, intercostal, pudendal nerve block	1%	5-40	50-400	Pudendal block: one half of total dose injected each side.
	2%	5-20	100-400	
Transvaginal block (paracervical plus pudendal)	1%	up to 30 (both sides)	up to 300 (both sides)	One half of total dose injected each side. See PRECAUTIONS.
Paracervical block				
Caudal and epidural block	1% 1.5% 2%	15-30 10-25 10-20	150-300 150-375 200-400	Use only single-dose vials which do not contain a preservative
Infiltration	1%	up to 40	up to 400	An equivalent amount of a 0.5% solution (prepared) by diluting the 1% solution with Sodium Chloride Injection, USP) may be used for large areas.
Therapeutic block (pain management)	1% 2%	1-5 1-5	10-50 20-100	

Unused portions of solutions not containing preservatives should be discarded.

Storage: Store at controlled room temperature between 15 to 30°C (59 to 85°F); brief exposure up to 40°C (104°F) does not adversely affect the product.

HOW SUPPLIED - RATED THERAPEUTICALLY EQUIVALENT:

Injection, Solution - Dental - 2 %

1.8 ml x 20	**$9.96**	**CARBOCAINE W/NEO-COBEFRIN, Cook-Waite Labs**	**00961-0010-04**
1.8 ml x 100	$35.00	POLOCAINE/LEVONORDEFRIN 1:20000, Astra USA	00186-0460-14

Injection, Solution - Dental - 30 mg/ml

1.8 ml x 100	$35.00	POLOCAINE 3%, Astra USA	00186-0440-14

Injection, Solution - Intravenous - 1 %

30 ml	$6.76	POLOCAINE, Astra USA	00186-0412-01
30 ml	**$10.27**	**CARBOCAINE, Sanofi Winthrop**	**00024-0231-01**
30 ml	$10.63	Mepivacaine Hcl, Intl Medication	00548-1102-00
30 ml	$11.44	Mepivacaine Hcl, Intl Medication	00548-1102-02
50 ml	$6.70	Mepivacaine Hcl, Goldline Labs	00182-3053-67
50 ml	$9.58	POLOCAINE, Astra USA	00186-0410-01
50 ml	$10.35	Mepivacaine Hcl, Rugby	00536-5281-80
50 ml	$11.00	Mepivacaine Hcl, Steris Labs	00402-0756-50
50 ml	$12.70	Mepivacaine HCl, Schein Pharm (US)	00364-6770-57
50 ml	**$14.72**	**CARBOCAINE, Sanofi Winthrop**	**00024-0232-01**

Injection, Solution - Intravenous - 1.5 %

30 ml	$9.16	POLOCAINE, Astra USA	00186-0418-01
30 ml	**$14.00**	**CARBOCAINE, Sanofi Winthrop**	**00024-0234-01**

Injection, Solution - Intravenous - 2 %

20 ml	$7.51	POLOCAINE, Astra USA	00186-0422-01
20 ml	**$11.53**	**CARBOCAINE, Sanofi Winthrop**	**00024-0236-01**
50 ml	$5.01	Mepivacaine Hcl, HL Moore Drug Exch	00839-6798-38
50 ml	$11.06	POLOCAINE, Astra USA	00186-0420-01
50 ml	$11.50	Mepivacaine Hcl, Steris Labs	00402-0757-50
50 ml	$13.00	Mepivacaine HCl, Schein Pharm (US)	00364-6771-57
50 ml	**$17.22**	**CARBOCAINE, Sanofi Winthrop**	**00024-0237-01**

MEPROBAMATE *(001734)*

CATEGORIES: Antianxiety Drugs; Anxiety; Anxiolytics, Sedatives, Hypnotic; Central Nervous System Agents; Neuromuscular; Tranquilizers; Skeletal Muscle Hyperactivity*; DEA Class CIV; FDA Approval Pre 1982

* Indication not approved by the FDA

BRAND NAMES: Amosene; *Ansiowas*; *Apo-Meprobamate* (Canada); *Atacin*; *Atraxin* (Japan); *Baprosian*; *Dapaz*; *Disatral*; *Distoncur*; *Epikur*; Equanil; *Harmonin* (Japan); *Medicar*; *Meditran*; *Meposed*; *Meprate* (England); *Meprepose*; Mepriam; *Meprin*; *Mepro*; Meproban-400; *Meprobar*; *Meprodil*; Meprospan; *Miltaun* (Germany); Miltown; Neuramate; *Oasil*; *Oasil-Simes*; *Pertranquil*; *Placidon*; *Praol*; Probate; *Probamyl*; *Procalmadiol*; *Procalmidol*; *Quanil*; *Restenil*; *Sinanin*; *Sycropaz*; *Tensional*; Trancot; *Trankilan*; Tranmep; *Urbilat* (Germany); *Visanon* (Germany)

(International brand names outside U.S. in italics)

FORMULARIES: Aetna; BC-BS; FHP

COST OF THERAPY: $5.04 (Anxiety; Tablet; 400 mg; 3/day; 120 days) vs. Potential Cost of $3,628.44 (Psychoses)

DESCRIPTION:

NOTE: This monograph contains full prescribing information for both meprobamate tablets and Meprospan brand of sustained-release capsules.

Meprobamate is a white powder with a characteristic odor and a bitter taste. It is slightly soluble in water, freely soluble in acetone and alcohol, and sparingly soluble in ether.

TABLETS

Meprobamate tablets contain 200 mg or 400 mg Meprobamate. The inactive ingredients present are lactose, methylcellulose, polacrilin potassium, and stearic acid.

SUSTAINED-RELEASE CAPSULES

Meprospan 400 contains 400 mg meprobamate per capsule.

Other ingredients: corn starch, FD&C Blue #1, FD&C Yellow #6, gelatin, sucrose and other ingredients.

Meprospan 200 contains 200 mg meprobamate per capsule.

Other ingredients: corn starch, FD&C Yellow #6, gelatin, sucrose and other ingredients.

CLINICAL PHARMACOLOGY:

Meprobamate is a carbamate derivative which has been shown (in animal and/or human studies) to have effects at multiple sites in the central nervous system, including the thalamus and limbic system.

INDICATIONS AND USAGE:

Meprobamate is indicated for the management of anxiety disorders or for the short-term relief of the symptoms of anxiety. Anxiety or tension associated with the stress of everyday life usually does not require treatment with an anxiolytic.

The effectiveness of Meprobamate in long-term use, that is, more than 4 months, has not been assessed by systematic clinical studies. The physician should periodically reassess the usefulness of the drug for the individual patient.

CONTRAINDICATIONS:

Acute, intermittent porphyria and allergic or idiosyncratic reactions to Meprobamate or related compounds, such as carisoprodol, mebutamate, tybamate or carbromal.

WARNINGS:

DRUG DEPENDENCE

Physical dependence, psychological dependence, and abuse have occurred. Chronic intoxication from prolonged ingestion of, usually, greater than recommended doses is manifested by ataxia, slurred speech, and vertigo. Therefore, careful supervision of dose and amounts prescribed is advised, as well as avoidance of prolonged administration, especially for alcoholics and other patients with a known propensity for taking excessive quantities of drugs.

Sudden withdrawal of the drug after prolonged and excessive use may precipitate recurrence of preexisting symptoms such as anxiety, anorexia, or insomnia, or withdrawal reactions such as vomiting, ataxia, tremors, muscle twitching, confusional states, hallucinosis, and, rarely, convulsive seizures. Such seizures are more likely to occur in persons with central nervous system damage or preexistent or latent convulsive disorders. Onset of withdrawal symptoms occurs usually within 12 to 48 hours after discontinuation of Meprobamate; symptoms usually cease within the next 12- to 48-hour period.

When excessive dosage has continued for weeks or months, dosage should be reduced gradually over a period of 1 to 2 weeks rather than abruptly stopped. Alternatively, a short-acting barbiturate may be substituted, then gradually withdrawn.

POTENTIALLY HAZARDOUS TASKS

Patients should be warned that Meprobamate may impair the mental or physical abilities required for performance of potentially hazardous tasks, such as driving or operating machinery.

ADDITIVE EFFECTS

Since CNS-suppressant effects of Meprobamate and alcohol or Meprobamate and other psychotropic drugs may be additive, appropriate caution should be exercised with patients who take more than one of these agents simultaneously.

USAGE IN PREGNANCY AND LACTATION

An increased risk of congenital malformations associated with the use of minor tranquilizers (Meprobamate, chlordiazepoxide, and diazepam) during the first trimester of pregnancy has been suggested in several studies. Because use of these drugs is rarely a matter of urgency, their use during this period should almost always be avoided. The possibility that a woman of childbearing potential may be pregnant at the time of institution of therapy should be considered. Patients should be advised that if they become pregnant during therapy or intend to become pregnant they should communicate with their physicians about the desirability of discontinuing the drug.

Meprobamate passes the placental barrier. It is present both in umbilical-cord blood at or near maternal plasma levels and in breast milk of lactating mothers at concentrations two to four times that of maternal plasma. When use of Meprobamate is contemplated in breast-feeding patients, the drug's higher concentrations in breast milk as compared to maternal plasma levels should be considered.

USAGE IN CHILDREN

Meprobamate should not be administered to children under 6 years of age, since there is a lack of documented evidence of safety and effectiveness.

PRECAUTIONS:

The lowest effective dose should be administered, particularly to elderly and/or debilitated patients, in order to preclude oversedation.

Meprobamate is metabolized in the liver and excreted by the kidney; to avoid its excess accumulation caution should be exercised in the administration to patients with compromised liver or kidney function.

Meprobamate occasionally may precipitate seizures in epileptic patients.

The drug should be prescribed cautiously and in small quantities to patients with suicidal tendencies.

ADVERSE REACTIONS:

CENTRAL NERVOUS SYSTEM

Drowsiness, ataxia, dizziness, slurred speech, headache, vertigo, weakness, paresthesias, impairment of visual accommodation, euphoria, overstimulation, paradoxical excitement, fast EEG activity.

ADVERSE REACTIONS: *(cont'd)*

GASTROINTESTINAL

Nausea, vomiting, diarrhea.

CARDIOVASCULAR

Palpitation, tachycardia, various forms of arrhythmia, transient ECG changes, syncope, hypotensive crisis.

ALLERGIC OR IDIOSYNCRATIC

Milder reactions are characterized by an itchy, urticarial, or erythematous maculopapular rash which may be generalized or confined to the groin.

Other reactions have included leukopenia, acute nonthrombocytopenic purpura, petechiae, ecchymoses, eosinophilia, peripheral edema, adenopathy, fever, fixed drug eruption with cross-reaction to carisoprodol, and cross-sensitivity between Meprobamate/mebutamate and Meprobamate/carbromal.

More severe hypersensitivity reactions, rarely reported, include hyperpyrexia, chills, angioneurotic edema, bronchospasm, oliguria, and anuria. Also, anaphylaxis, exfoliative dermatitis, stomatitis, and proctitis. Stevens-Johnson syndrome and bullous dermatitis have occurred.

HEMATOLOGIC (ALSO SEE Allergic or Idiosyncratic)

Agranulocytosis, aplastic anemia have been reported, although no causal relationship has been established, and thrombocytopenic purpura.

OTHER

Exacerbation of porphyric symptoms.

OVERDOSAGE:

Suicidal attempts with Meprobamate have resulted in drowsiness, lethargy, stupor, ataxia, coma, shock, vasomotor and respiratory collapse. Some suicidal attempts have been fatal.

Sustained-Release Capsules: overdosage experience with Meprospan is limited, however:) The following data have been reported in the literature and from other sources. These data are not expected to correlate with each case (considering factors such as individual susceptibility and length of time from ingestion to treatment), but represent the *usual ranges* reported.

Acute Simple Overdose (Meprobamate alone): Death has been reported with ingestion of as little as 12 gm Meprobamate and survival with as much as 40 gm.

BLOOD LEVELS

0.5 to 2.0 mg percent represents the usual blood-level range of Meprobamate after therapeutic doses. The level may occasionally be as high as 3.0 mg percent.

3 to 10 mg percent usually corresponds to findings of mild-to-moderate symptoms of overdosage, such as stupor or light coma.

10 to 20 mg percent usually corresponds to deeper coma, requiring more intensive treatment. Some fatalities occur.

At levels greater than 20 mg percent, more fatalities than survivals can be expected.

Acute Combined Overdose: (Meprobamate With Other Psychotropic Drugs Or Alcohol): Since effects can be additive, a history of ingestion of a low dose of Meprobamate plus any of these compounds (or of a relatively low blood or tissue level) cannot be used as a prognostic indicator.

In cases where excessive doses have been taken, sleep ensues rapidly and blood pressure, pulse, and respiratory rates are reduced to basal levels. Any drug remaining in the stomach should be removed and symptomatic treatment given. Should respiration or blood pressure become compromised, respiratory assistance, central nervous system stimulants, and pressor agents should be administered cautiously as indicated. Diuresis, osmotic (mannitol) diuresis, peritoneal dialysis, and hemodialysis have been used successfully. Careful monitoring of urinary output is necessary, and caution should be taken to avoid overhydration. Relapse and death, after initial recovery, have been attributed to incomplete gastric emptying and delayed absorption.

DOSAGE AND ADMINISTRATION:

TABLETS

Usual adult dose is 1200 to 1600 mg/day in divided doses; doses greater than 2400 mg/day are not recommended. The usual dose for children, ages 6 to 12 years, is 100 to 200 mg, two or three times daily. Meprobamate is not recommended for children under 6 years.

SUSTAINED-RELEASE CAPSULES

The usual adult dosage of Meprospan (meprobamate, sustained-release capsules) is one to two 400 mg capsules in the morning and again at bedtime; doses above 2400 mg daily are not recommended. The usual dosage for children ages six to twelve is one 200 mg capsule in the morning and again at bedtime. Meprobamate is not recommended for children under age six.

Keep tightly closed. Dispense in tight container.

(S.R. Caps, Carter-Wallace, 8/85, IN-072E2-02)

(Tablets, Wyeth Ayerst, 7/87)

HOW SUPPLIED - RATED THERAPEUTICALLY EQUIVALENT:

Tablet, Uncoated - Oral - 200 mg

100's	$1.05	Meprobamate, Anabolic	00722-5435-01
100's	$3.95	Meprobamate, Harber Pharm	51432-0268-03
100's	$3.98	Meprobamate, H.C.F.A. F F P	99999-1734-01
100's	$4.10	Meprobamate, Eon Labs Mfg	00185-0716-01
100's	$4.66	Meprobamate, United Res	00677-0232-01
100's	$4.71	Meprobamate, HL Moore Drug Exch	00839-5070-06
100's	$4.90	Meprobamate, Major Pharms	00904-0044-60
100's	$5.35	Meprobamate, Rugby	00536-4005-01
100's	$5.35	Meprobamate, Qualitest Pharms	00603-4439-21
100's	$5.38	Meprobamate, Aligen Independ	00405-0115-01
100's	$5.63	Meprobamate, IDE-Interstate	00814-4718-14
100's	$6.70	Meprobamate, Schein Pharm (US)	00364-0160-01
100's	$23.80	EQUANIL, Wyeth Labs	00008-0002-03
100's	**$113.12**	**MILTOWN, Wallace Labs**	**00037-1101-01**
1000's	$5.95	Meprobamate, Anabolic	00722-5435-03
1000's	$30.64	Meprobamate, United Res	00677-0232-10
1000's	$30.69	Meprobamate, Rugby	00536-4005-10
1000's	$32.50	Meprobamate, Eon Labs Mfg	00185-0716-10
1000's	$38.04	Meprobamate, Aligen Independ	00405-0115-03
1000's	$39.75	Meprobamate, Schein Pharm (US)	00364-0160-02
1000's	$39.75	Meprobamate, Major Pharms	00904-0044-80
1000's	$39.80	Meprobamate, H.C.F.A. F F P	99999-1734-02

Tablet, Uncoated - Oral - 400 mg

100's	$1.40	Meprobamate, Anabolic	00722-5404-01
100's	$3.20	Blue Cross Neuramate, Halsey Drug	00879-0044-01
100's	$4.50	Meprobamate, Harber Pharm	51432-0270-03
100's	$4.80	Meprobamate, Geneva Pharms	00781-1410-01
100's	$4.80	Meprobamate, H.C.F.A. F F P	99999-1734-03
100's	$5.25	Meprobamate, Eon Labs Mfg	00185-0717-01
100's	$7.00	Meprobamate, Major Pharms	00904-0045-60

HOW SUPPLIED - RATED THERAPEUTICALLY EQUIVALENT: *(cont'd)*

100's	$8.29	Meprobamate, Vangard Labs	00615-0447-13
100's	$8.80	Meprobamate, Goldline Labs	00182-0294-01
100's	$8.80	Meprobamate, United Res	00677-0233-01
100's	$9.00	Meprobamate, Rugby	00536-4006-01
100's	$9.25	Meprobamate, HL Moore Drug Exch	00839-5004-06
100's	$9.35	Meprobamate, Schein Pharm (US)	00364-0161-01
100's	$9.36	Meprobamate, Qualitest Pharms	00603-4440-21
100's	$9.40	Meprobamate, Aligen Independ	00405-0116-01
100's	$29.80	EQUANIL, Wyeth Labs	00008-0001-05
100's	**$138.72**	**MILTOWN, Wallace Labs**	**00037-1001-01**
500's	$24.00	Meprobamate, H.C.F.A. F F P	99999-1734-04
500's	$146.43	EQUANIL, Wyeth Labs	00008-0001-07
500's	**$694.14**	**MILTOWN, Wallace Labs**	**00037-1001-03**
1000's	$7.50	Meprobamate, Anabolic	00722-5404-03
1000's	$12.95	BLUE CROSS NEURAMATE, Halsey Drug	00879-0044-10
1000's	$24.00	Meprobamate White, Calvin Scott	17224-0805-10
1000's	$36.00	TRANCOT, C O Truxton	00463-6177-10
1000's	$44.80	Meprobamate, Eon Labs Mfg	00185-0717-10
1000's	$45.00	Meprobamate, Harber Pharm	51432-0270-06
1000's	$47.95	Meprobamate, Major Pharms	00904-0045-80
1000's	$48.00	Meprobamate, Geneva Pharms	00781-1410-10
1000's	$48.00	Meprobamate, H.C.F.A. F F P	99999-1734-05
1000's	$57.34	Meprobamate, Aligen Independ	00405-0116-03
1000's	$59.25	Meprobamate, Rugby	00536-4006-10
1000's	$59.75	Meprobamate, Parmed Pharms	00349-8830-10
1000's	$59.75	Meprobamate, United Res	00677-0233-10
1000's	$59.80	Meprobamate, Qualitest Pharms	00603-4440-32
1000's	$61.75	Meprobamate, Goldline Labs	00182-0294-10
1000's	$65.11	Meprobamate, Schein Pharm (US)	00364-0161-02
1000's	$66.14	Meprobamate, HL Moore Drug Exch	00839-5004-16
1000's	$89.95	Meproban-400, Quality Res Pharms	52765-1251-00
1000's	**$1361.50**	**MILTOWN, Wallace Labs**	**00037-1001-02**

Tablet, Uncoated - Oral - 600 mg

100's	**$216.12**	**MILTOWN 600, Wallace Labs**	**00037-1601-01**

MERCAPTOPURINE *(001737)*

CATEGORIES: Antimetabolites; Antineoplastics; Cancer; Chemotherapy; Leukemia; Leukemia, Acute Myeloid; Oncologic Drugs; Pregnancy Category D; FDA Approval Pre 1982

BRAND NAMES: *Classen* (Japan); *Ismipur*; *Leukerin* (Japan); *Mercaptopurina*; *Merkaptopurin*; **Purinethol**; *Puri-Nethol* (England, Germany)
(International brand names outside U.S. in italics)

FORMULARIES: Aetna; BC-BS; Medi-Cal; WHO

DESCRIPTION:

CAUTION: Mercaptopurine is a potent drug. It should not be used unless a diagnosis of acute lymphatic leukemia has been adequately established and the responsible physician is knowledgeable in assessing response to chemotherapy.

Purinethol was synthesized and developed by Hitchings, Elion, and associates at the Wellcome Research Laboratories.[1] It is one of a large series of purine analogues which interfere with nucleic acid biosynthesis and has been found active against human leukemias.

Mercaptopurine, known chemically as 1,7-dihydro-6*H*-purine-6-thione monohydrate, is an analogue of the purine bases adenine and hypoxanthine.

Purinethol is available in tablet form for oral administration. Each scored tablet contains 50 mg mercaptopurine and the inactive ingredients corn and potato starch, lactose, magnesium stearate, and stearic acid.

CLINICAL PHARMACOLOGY:

Clinical studies have shown that the absorption of an oral dose of mercaptopurine in man is incomplete and variable, averaging approximately 50% of the administered dose.[2] The factors influencing absorption are unknown. Intravenous administration of an investigational preparation of mercaptopurine revealed a plasma half-disappearance time of 21 minutes in children and 47 minutes in adults. The volume of distribution usually exceeded that of the total body water.[2]

Following the oral administration of ^{35}S-6-mercaptopurine in one subject, a total of 46% of the dose could be accounted for in the urine (as parent drug and metabolites) in the first 24 hours. Metabolites of mercaptopurine were found in urine within the first 2 hours after administration. Radioactivity (in the form of sulfate) could be found in the urine for weeks afterwards.[3]

There is negligible entry of mercaptopurine into cerebrospinal fluid.

Plasma protein binding averages 19% over the concentration range 10 to 50 mcg/ml (a concentration only achieved by intravenous administration of mercaptopurine at doses exceeding 5 to 10 mg/kg).[2]

Monitoring of plasma levels of mercaptopurine during therapy is of questionable value.[3] There is technical difficulty in determining plasma concentrations which are seldom greater than 1 to 2 mcg/ml after a therapeutic oral dose. More significantly, mercaptopurine enters rapidly into the anabolic and catabolic pathways for purines, and the active intracellular metabolites have appreciably longer half-lives than the parent drug. The biochemical effects of a single dose of mercaptopurine are evident long after the parent drug has disappeared from plasma. Because of this rapid metabolism of mercaptopurine to active intracellular derivatives, hemodialysis would not be expected to appreciably reduce toxicity of the drug. There is no known pharmacologic antagonist to the biochemical actions of mercaptopurine *in vivo*.

Mercaptopurine competes with hypoxanthine and guanine for the enzyme hypoxanthine-guanine phosphoribosyltransferase (HGPRTase) and is itself converted to thioinosinic acid (TIMP). This intracellular nucleotide inhibits several reactions involving inosinic acid (IMP), including the conversion of IMP to xanthylic acid (XMP) and the conversion of IMP to adenylic acid (AMP) via adenylosuccinate (SAMP). In addition, 6-methylthioinosinate (MTIMP) is formed by the methylation of TIMP. Both TIMP and MTIMP have been reported to inhibit glutamine-5-phosphoribosylpyrophosphate amidotransferase, the first enzyme unique to the *de novo* pathway for purine ribonucleotide synthesis.[3]

Experiments indicate that radiolabeled mercaptopurine may be recovered from the DNA in the form of deoxythioguanosine.[4] Some mercaptopurine is converted to nucleotide derivatives of 6-thioguanine (6-TG) by the sequential actions of inosinate (IMP) dehydrogenase and xanthylate (XMP) aminase, converting TIMP to thioguanylic acid (TGMP).

Animal tumors that are resistant to mercaptopurine often have lost the ability to convert mercaptopurine to TIMP. However, it is clear that resistance to mercaptopurine may be acquired by other means as well, particularly in human leukemias.

CLINICAL PHARMACOLOGY: *(cont'd)*

It is not known exactly which of any one or more of the biochemical effects of mercaptopurine and its metabolites are directly or predominantly responsible for cell death.[5]

The catabolism of mercaptopurine and its metabolites is complex. In man, after oral administration of ^{35}S-6-mercaptopurine, urine contains intact mercaptopurine, thiouric acid (formed by direct oxidation by xanthine oxidase, probably via 6-mercapto-8-hydroxypurine), and a number of 6-methylated thiopurines. The methylthiopurines yield appreciable amounts of inorganic sulfate.[3] The importance of the metabolism by xanthine oxidase relates to the fact that allopurinol inhibits this enzyme and retards the catabolism of mercaptopurine and its active metabolites. A significant reduction in mercaptopurine dosage is mandatory if a potent xanthine oxidase inhibitor and mercaptopurine are used simultaneously in a patient (see PRECAUTIONS).

INDICATIONS AND USAGE:

Mercaptopurine is indicated for remission induction and maintenance therapy of acute lymphatic leukemia. The response to this agent depends upon the particular subclassification of acute lymphatic leukemia and the age of the patient (child or adult).

Acute Lymphatic (Lymphocytic, Lymphoblastic) Leukemia: Given as a single agent for remission induction, mercaptopurine induces complete remission in approximately 25% of children and 10% of adults. However, reliance upon mercaptopurine alone is not justified for initial remission induction of acute lymphatic leukemia since combination chemotherapy with vincristine, prednisone, and L-asparaginase results in more frequent complete remission induction than with mercaptopurine alone or in combination. The duration of complete remission induced in acute lymphatic leukemia is so brief without the use of maintenance therapy that some form of drug therapy is considered essential. Mercaptopurine, as a single agent, is capable of significantly prolonging complete remission duration; however, combination therapy has produced remission duration longer than that achieved with mercaptopurine alone.

Acute Myelogenous (and Acute Myelomonocytic) Leukemia: As a single agent, mercaptopurine will induce complete remission in approximately 10% of children and adults with acute myelogenous leukemia or its subclassifications. These results are inferior to those achieved with combination chemotherapy employing optimum treatment schedules.

Central Nervous System Leukemia: Mercaptopurine is not effective for prophylaxis or treatment of central nervous system leukemia.

Other Neoplasms: Mercaptopurine is not effective in chronic lymphatic leukemia, the lymphomas (including Hodgkin's Disease), or solid tumors.

CONTRAINDICATIONS:

Mercaptopurine should not be used unless a diagnosis of acute lymphatic leukemia has been adequately established and the responsible physician is knowledgeable in assessing response to chemotherapy.

Mercaptopurine should not be used in patients whose disease has demonstrated prior resistance to this drug. In animals and man, there is usually complete cross-resistance between mercaptopurine and thioguanine.

WARNINGS:

Since drugs used in cancer chemotherapy are potentially hazardous, it is recommended that only physicians experienced with the risks of mercaptopurine and knowledgeable in the natural history of acute leukemias administer this drug.

Bone Marrow Toxicity: The most consistent, dose-related toxicity is bone marrow suppression. This may be manifest by anemia, leukopenia, thrombocytopenia, or any combination of these. Any of these findings may also reflect progression of the underlying disease. Since mercaptopurine may have a delayed effect, it is important to withdraw the medication temporarily at the first sign of an abnormally large fall in any of the formed elements of the blood.

There are rare individuals with an inherited deficiency of the enzyme thiopurine methyltransferase (TPMT) who may be usually sensitive to the myelosuppressive effects of mercaptopurine and prone to developing rapid bone marrow suppression following the initial treatment.[6,7] Substantial dosage reductions may be required to avoid the development of life-threatening bone marrow suppression in these patients. This toxicity may be more profound in patients treated with concomitant allopurinol (see DRUG INTERACTIONS).

Hepatotoxicity: Mercaptopurine is hepatotoxic in animals and man. A small number of deaths have been reported which may have been attributed to hepatic necrosis due to administration of mercaptopurine. Hepatic injury can occur with any dosage, but seems to occur with more frequency when doses of 2.5 mg/kg/day are exceeded. The histologic pattern of mercaptopurine hepatotoxicity includes features of both intrahepatic cholestasis and parenchymal cell necrosis, either of which may predominate. It is not clear how much of the hepatic damage is due to direct toxicity from the drug and how much may be due to a hypersensitivity reaction. In some patients jaundice has cleared following withdrawal of mercaptopurine and reappeared with its reintroduction.[8]

Published reports have cited widely varying incidences of overt hepatotoxicity. In a large series of patients with various neoplastic diseases, mercaptopurine was administered orally in doses ranging from 2.5 mg/kg to 5.0 mg/kg without any evidence of hepatotoxicity. It was noted by the authors that no definite clinical evidence of liver damage could be ascribed to the drug, although an occasional case of serum hepatitis did occur in patients receiving 6-MP who previously had transfusions.[8] In reports of smaller cohorts of adult and pediatric leukemic patients, the incidence of hepatotoxicity ranged from 0 to 6%.[9-11] In an isolated report by Einhorn and Davidsohn, jaundice was observed more frequently (40%), especially when doses exceeded 2.5 mg/kg.[12] Usually, clinically detectable jaundice appears early in the course of treatment (one to two months). However, jaundice has been reported as early as one week and as late as eight years after the start of treatment with mercaptopurine.[13]

Monitoring of serum transaminase levels, alkaline phosphatase, and bilirubin levels may allow early detection of hepatotoxicity. It is advisable to monitor these liver function tests at weekly intervals when first beginning therapy and at monthly intervals thereafter. Liver function tests may be advisable more frequently in patients who are receiving mercaptopurine with other hepatotoxic drugs or with known pre-existing liver disease.

The concomitant administration of mercaptopurine with other hepatotoxic agents requires especially careful clinical and biochemical monitoring of hepatic function. Combination therapy involving mercaptopurine with other drugs not felt to be hepatotoxic should nevertheless be approached with caution. The combination of mercaptopurine with doxorubicin was reported to be hepatotoxic in 10 to 20 patients undergoing remission-induction therapy for leukemia resistant to previous therapy.[14]

The hepatotoxicity has been associated in some cases with anorexia, diarrhea, jaundice, and ascites. Hepatic encephalopathy has occurred.

The onset of clinical jaundice, hepatomegaly, or anorexia with tenderness in the right hypochondrium are immediate indications for withholding mercaptopurine until the exact etiology can be identified. Likewise, any evidence of deterioration in liver function studies, toxic hepatitis, or biliary stasis should prompt discontinuation of the drug and a search for an etiology of the hepatotoxicity.

WARNINGS: *(cont'd)*

Immunosuppression: Mercaptopurine recipients may manifest decreased cellular hypersensitivities and impaired allograft rejection. Induction of immunity to infectious agents or vaccines will be subnormal in these patients; the degree of immunosuppression will depend on antigen dose and temporal relationship to drug. This immunosuppressive effect should be carefully considered with regard to intercurrent infections and risk of subsequent neoplasia.

Pregnancy Category D: Mercaptopurine can cause fetal harm when administered to a pregnant woman. Women receiving mercaptopurine in the first trimester of pregnancy have an increased incidence of abortion; the risk of malformation in offspring surviving first trimester exposure is not accurately known.[15] In a series of twenty-eight women receiving mercaptopurine after the first trimester of pregnancy, three mothers died undelivered, one delivered a stillborn child, and one aborted; there were no cases of macroscopically abnormal fetuses.[16] Since such experience cannot exclude the possibility of fetal damage, mercaptopurine should be used during pregnancy only if the benefit clearly justifies the possible risk to the fetus, and particular caution should be given to the use of mercaptopurine in the first trimester of pregnancy.

There are no adequate and well controlled studies in pregnant women. If this drug is used during pregnancy or if the patient becomes pregnant while taking the drug, the patient should be apprised of the potential hazard to the fetus. Women of childbearing potential should be advised to avoid becoming pregnant.

PRECAUTIONS:

General: The safe and effective use of Purinethol demands a thorough knowledge of the natural history of the condition being treated. After selection of an initial dosage schedule, therapy will frequently need to be modified depending upon the patient's response and manifestations of toxicity.

The most frequent, serious, toxic effect of mercaptopurine is myelosuppression resulting in leukopenia, thrombocytopenia, and anemia.These toxic effects are often unavoidable during the induction phase of adult acute leukemia if remission induction is to be successful. Whether or not these manifestations demand modification or cessation of dosage depends both upon the response of the underlying disease and a careful consideration of supportive facilities (granulocyte and platelet transfusions) which may be available. Life-threatening infections and bleeding have been observed as a consequence of mercaptopurine-induced granulocytopenia and thrombocytopenia. Severe hematologic toxicity may require supportive therapy with platelet transfusions for bleeding, and antibiotics and granulocyte transfusions if sepsis is documented.

If it is not the intent to deliberately induce bone marrow hypoplasia, it is important to discontinue the drug temporarily at the first evidence of an abnormally large fall in white blood cell count, platelet count, or hemoglobin concentration. In many patients with severe depression of the formed elements of the blood due to mercaptopurine, the bone marrow appears hypoplastic on aspiration or biopsy, whereas in other cases it may appear normocellular. The qualitative changes in the erythroid elements toward the megaloblastic series, characteristically seen with the folic acid antagonists and some other antimetabolites, are not seen with this drug.

It is probably advisable to start with smaller dosages in patients with impaired renal function, since the latter might result in slower elimination of the drug and metabolites and a greater cumulative effect.

Information for the Patient: Patients should be informed that the major toxicities of mercaptopurine are related to myelosuppression, hepatotoxicity and gastrointestinal toxicity. Patients should never be allowed to take the drug without medical supervision and should be advised to consult their physician if they experience fever, sore throat, jaundice, nausea, vomiting, signs of local infection, bleeding from any site, or symptoms suggestive of anemia. Women of childbearing potential should be advised to avoid becoming pregnant.

Laboratory Tests: It is recommended that evaluation of the hemoglobin or hematocrit, total white blood cell count and differential count, and quantitative platelet count be obtained weekly while the patient is on mercaptopurine therapy. In cases where the cause of fluctuations in the formed elements in the peripheral blood is obscure, bone marrow examination may be useful for the evaluation of marrow status. The decision to increase, decrease, continue, or discontinue a given dosage of mercaptopurine must be based not only on the absolute hematologic values, but also upon the rapidity with which changes are occurring. In many instances, particularly during the induction phase of acute leukemia, complete blood counts will need to be done more frequently than once weekly in order to evaluate the effect of the therapy.

Carcinogenesis, Mutagenesis, and Impairment of Fertility: Mercaptopurine causes chromosomal aberrations in animals and man and induces dominant-lethal mutations in male mice. In mice, surviving female offspring of mothers who received chronic low doses of mercaptopurine during pregnancy were found sterile or if they became pregnant had smaller litters and more dead fetuses as compared to control animals.[19] Carcinogenic potential exists in man, but the extent of the risk is unknown.

The effect of mercaptopurine on human fertility is unknown for either males or females.

Pregnancy, Teratogenic Effects, Pregnancy Category D: (See WARNINGS.)

Nursing Mothers: It is not known whether this drug is excreted in human milk. Because many drugs are excreted in human milk, and because of the potential for serious adverse reactions in nursing infants from mercaptopurine, a decision should be made whether to discontinue nursing or to discontinue the drug, taking into account the importance of the drug to the mother.

DRUG INTERACTIONS:

Interaction with Allopurinol: When allopurinol and mercaptopurine are administered concomitantly, it is imperative that the dose of mercaptopurine be reduced to one-third to one-quarter of the usual dose. Failure to observe this dosage reduction will result in a delayed catabolism of mercaptopurine and the strong likelihood of inducing severe toxicity.

There is usually complete cross-resistance between Purinethol (mercaptopurine) and thioguanine.

The dosage of mercaptopurine may need to be reduced when this agent is combined with other drugs whose primary or secondary toxicity is myelosuppression. Enhanced marrow suppression has been noted in some patients also receiving trimethoprim-sulfamethoxazole.[17,18]

ADVERSE REACTIONS:

The principal and potentially serious toxic effects of Purinethol are bone marrow toxicity and hepatotoxicity (see WARNINGS).

Hematologic Effects: The most frequent adverse reaction to mercaptopurine is myelosuppression. The induction of complete remission of acute lymphatic leukemia frequently is associated with marrow hypoplasia. Maintenance of remission generally involves multiple drug regimens whose component agents cause myelosuppression. Anemia, leukopenia, and thrombocytopenia are frequently observed. Dosages and schedules are adjusted to prevent life-threatening cytopenias.

ADVERSE REACTIONS: *(cont'd)*

Renal: Hyperuricemia may occur in patients receiving mercaptopurine as a consequence of rapid cell lysis accompanying the antineoplastic effect. Adverse effects can be minimized by increased hydration, urine alkalinization, and the prophylactic administration of a xanthine oxidase inhibitor such as allopurinol. The dosage of mercaptopurine should be reduced to one-third to one-quarter of the usual dose if allopurinol is given concurrently.

Gastrointestinal: Intestinal ulceration has been reported.[20] Nausea, vomiting and anorexia are uncommon during initial administration. Mild diarrhea and sprue-like symptoms have been noted occasionally, but it is difficult at present to attribute these to the medication. Oral lesions are rarely seen, and when they occur they resemble thrush rather than antifolic ulcerations.

An increased risk of pancreatitis may be associated with the investigational use of Purinethol in inflammatory bowel disease.[21-23]

Miscellaneous: While dermatologic reactions can occur as a consequence of disease, the administration of Purinethol has been associated with skin rashes and hyperpigmentation.[24]

Drug fever has been very rarely reported with mercaptopurine. Before attributing fever to mercaptopurine, every attempt should be made to exclude more common causes of pyrexia, such as sepsis, in patients with acute leukemia.

OVERDOSAGE:

Signs and symptoms of overdosage may be immediate such as anorexia, nausea, vomiting and diarrhea; or delayed such as myelosuppression, liver dysfunction and gastroenteritis. Dialysis cannot be expected to clear mercaptopurine. Hemodialysis is thought to be of marginal use due to the rapid intracellular incorporation of mercaptopurine into active metabolites with long persistence. The oral LD_{50} of mercaptopurine was determined to be 480 mg/kg in the mouse and 425 mg/kg in the rat.[25]

There is no known pharmacologic antagonist of mercaptopurine. The drug should be discontinued immediately if unintended toxicity occurs during treatment. If a patient is seen immediately following an accidental overdosage of the drug, it may be useful to induce emesis.

DOSAGE AND ADMINISTRATION:

Induction Therapy: Mercaptopurine is administered orally. The dosage which will be tolerated and be effective varies from patient to patient, and therefore careful titration is necessary to obtain the optimum therapeutic effect without incurring excessive, unintended toxicity. The usual initial dosage for children and adults is 2.5 mg/kg of body weight per day (100 to 200 mg in the average adult and 50 mg in an average 5-year-old child). Children with acute leukemia have tolerated this dose without difficulty in most cases; it may be continued daily for several weeks or more in some patients. If, after four weeks at this dosage, there is no clinical improvement and no definite evidence of leukocyte or platelet depression, the dosage may be increased up to 5 mg/kg daily. A dosage of 2.5 mg/kg per day may result in a rapid fall in leukocyte count within 1 to 2 weeks in some adults with acute lymphatic leukemia and high total leukocyte counts.

The total daily dosage may be given at one time. It is calculated to the nearest multiple of 25 mg. The dosage of mercaptopurine should be reduced to one-third to one-quarter of the usual dose if allopurinol is given concurrently. Because the drug may have a delayed action, it should be discontinued at the first sign of an abnormally large or rapid fall in the leukocyte or platelet count. If subsequently the leukocyte count or platelet count remains constant for two or three days, or rises, treatment may be resumed.

Maintenance Therapy: Once a complete hematologic remission is obtained, maintenance therapy is considered essential. Maintenance doses will vary from patient to patient. A usual daily maintenance dose of mercaptopurine is 1.5 to 2.5 mg/kg/day as a single dose. It is to be emphasized that in children with acute lymphatic leukemia in remission, superior results have been obtained when mercaptopurine has been combined with other agents (most frequently with methotrexate) for remission maintenance. Mercaptopurine should rarely be relied upon as a single agent for the maintenance of remissions induced in acute leukemia.

Procedures for proper handling and disposal of anti-cancer drugs should be considered. Several guidelines on this subject have been published.[26-32]

There is no general agreement that all of the procedures recommended in the guidelines are necessary or appropriate.

REFERENCES:

1. Hitchings GH, Elion GB: The chemistry and biochemistry of purine analogs. *Ann Ny Acad Sci*1954; 60:195-199. **2.** Loo TL, Luce JK, Sullivan MP, et al: Clinical pharmacologic observations on 6-mercaptopurine and 6-methylthiopurine ribonucleoside. *Clin Pharmacol Ther* 1968; 9:180-194. **3.** Elion GB: Biochemistry and pharmacology of purine analogs. *Fed Proc* 1967; 26:898-904. **4.** Scannell JP, Hitchings GH: Thioguanine in deoxyribonucleic acid from tumors of 6-mercaptopurine-treated mice. *Proc Soc Exp Biol Med*1966; 122:627-629. **5.** Paterson ARP, Tidd DM:6-thiopurines, in Sartorelli AC, Johns DG (eds): *Antineoplastic and Immunosuppressive Agents,*Part II. Berlin, Springer-Verlag, 1975, pp 384-403. **6.** Lennard L, Gibson BES, Nicole T. Lilleyman JS. Congenital thiopurine methyltranferase deficiency and 6–mercaptopurine toxicity during treatment for acute lymphoblastic leukemia. *Arch Dis Child.* 1993;69:577–579. **7. 8.** Burchenal JH, Ellison RR, Murphy ML, et al: Clinical studies on 6-mercaptopurine.*Ann N Y Acad Sci* 1954; 60:359-368 **9.** Farber S: Summary of experience with 6-mercaptopurine. *Ann Ny Acad Sci* 1954; 60:412-414. **10.** Fountain JR: Clinical observations of the treatment of leukemia and allied disorders with 6-mercaptopurine. *Ann NY Acad Sci*1954; 60:439-446. **11.** Hyman GA, Gellhorn A, Wolff JA: The therapeutic effect of mercaptopurine in a variety of human neoplastic diseases. *Ann NY Acad Sci* 1954; 60:430-435. **12.**) Einhorn M, Davidsohn I: Hepatotoxicity of mercaptopurine.*JAMA* 1964; 188:802-806. **13.** Schein PS, Winokur SH: Immunosuppressive and cytotoxic chemotherapy: long-term complications.*Ann Intern Med* 1975; 82:84-95. **14.** Stern MH, Minow RA, Casey JH, et al: Hepatotoxicity in patients treated with adriamycin and 6-mercaptopurine for refractory leukemia.*Am J Clin Pathol* 1975; 63:758-759. **15.** Blatt J, Mulvihill JJ, Ziegler JL, et al: Pregnancy outcome following cancer chemotherapy.*Am J Med* 1980; 69:828-832. **16.** Nicholson HO: Cytotoxic drugs in pregnancy. *J Obstet Gynaec Brit Cwlth* 1968; 75:307-312. **17.** Woods WG, Daigle AE, Hutchinson RJ, et al: Myelosuppression associated with co-trimoxazole as a prophylactic antibiotic in the maintenance phase of childhood acute lymphocytic leukemia. *J Pediatr* 1984; 105:639-644. **18.** Rees CA, Lennard L, Lilleyman JS, et al: Disturbance of 6-mercaptopurine metabolism by cotrimoxazole in childhood lymphoblastic leukaemia. *Cancer Chemother Pharmacol*1984; 12:87-89. **19.** Reimers TJ, Sluss PM: 6-mercaptopurine treatment of pregnant mice: effects on second and third generations. *Science*1978; 201:65-67. **20.** Clark PA, Hsia YE, Huntsman RG: Toxic complications of treatment with 6-mercaptopurine. *Br Med J*1960; 1:393-395. **21.** Present DH, Meltzer SJ, Wolke A, et al: Short and long term toxicity to 6-mercaptopurine in the management of inflammatory bowel disease.*Gastroenterology* 1985; 88: 1545. **22.** Bank L, Wright JP: 6-mercaptopurine-related pancreatitis in 2 patients with inflammatory bowel disease, abstract. *Dig Dis Sci* 1984; 29:357-359. **23.** Singleton JW, Law DH, Kelley Jr ML, et al: National Cooperative Crohn's Disease Study: Adverse reactions to study drugs.*Gastroenterology*1979; 77:870-882. **24.** Dreizen S, Bodey GP, Rodriguez V, et al: Cutaneous complications of cancer chemotherapy.*Postgard Med* 1975; 58:150-158. **25.** Unpublished data on file with Glaxo Wellcome Co. **26.** Recommendations for the Safe Handling of Parenteral Antineoplastic Drugs. NIH Publications No. 83-2321. For sale by the Superintendent of Documents, U.S. Government Printing Office, Washington, D.C. 20402. **27.** AMA Council Report. Guidelines for Handling Parenteral Antineoplastics. *JAMA,* March 15, 1985. **28.** National Study Commission on Cytotoxic Exposure - Recommendations for Handling Cytotoxic Agents. Available from Louis P. Jeffrey, Sc.D., Director of Pharmacy Services, Rhode Island Hospital, 593 Eddy Street, Providence, Rhode Island 02902. **29.** Clinical Oncological Society of Australia: Guidelines and recommendations for safe handling of antineoplastic agents. *Med J Australia*1983; 1:426-428. **30.** Jones RB, et al: Safe handling of chemotherapeutic agents: A report from the Mount Sinai Medical Center. *Ca - A Cancer Journal for Clinicians*1983; Sept/Oct:258-263. **31.** American Society of Hospital Pharmacists technical assistance bulletin on handling cytotoxic drugs in hospitals.*AM J Hosp Pharm*1985;42:131-137. **32.** Yodaiken RE, Bennett D. OSHA work-practive guidelines for personel dealing with cytotoxic (antineoplastic) drugs. *Am J Hosp Pharm.* 1986;43:1193–1204.

HOW SUPPLIED:

Pale yellow to buff, scored tablets containing 50 mg mercaptopurine, imprinted with "PURINETHOL" and "04A".

Store at 15-25°C (59-77°F) in a dry place.

HOW SUPPLIED - EQUIVALENTS NOT AVAILABLE:

Tablet, Uncoated - Oral - 50 mg

25's	$61.12	PURINETHOL, Glaxo Wellcome	00173-0807-25
250's	$582.14	PURINETHOL, Glaxo Wellcome	00173-0807-65

MEROPENEM *(003297)*

CATEGORIES: Anti-Infectives; Antibiotics; Antimicrobials; Beta-Lactam Antibiotics; Bacterial Meningitis (Pediatric); Carbapenem Antibiotics; FDA Approved 1996 Jul; Intra-Abdominal Infections; Pregnancy Category B

BRAND NAMES: *Meronem* (England, Germany); *Merrem* (Australia); **Merrem IV**
(International brand names outside U.S. in italics)

PRIMARY ICD9: 136.9 (Unspecified Infections and Parasitic Diseases)

DESCRIPTION:

Meropenem is a sterile, pyrogen-free, synthetic, broad-spectrum, carbapenem antibiotic for intravenous administration. It is (4R, 5S, 6S)-3-[[(3S, 5S)-5-(Dimethylcarbamoyl)-3-pyrrolidinyl]thio]-6-[(1R)-1-hydroxyethyl]-4-methyl-7-oxo-1-azabicyclo[3.2.0]hept-2-ene-2-carboxylic acid trihydrate. Its empirical formula is $C_{17}H_{25}N_3O_5S{\cdot}3H_2O$ with a molecular weight of 437.52.

Meropenem is a white to pale yellow crystalline powder. The solution varies from colorless to yellow depending on the concentration. The pH of freshly constituted solutions is between 7.3 and 8.3. Meropenem is soluble in 5% monobasic potassium phosphate solution, sparingly soluble in water, very slightly soluble in hydrated ethanol, and practically insoluble in acetone or ether.

When constituted as instructed (see DOSAGE AND ADMINISTRATION, PREPARATION OF SOLUTION), each 1 g meropenem vial will deliver 1 g of meropenem and 90.2 mg of sodium as sodium carbonate (3.92 mEq). Each 500 mg meropenem vial will deliver 500 mg meropenem and 45.1 mg of sodium as sodium carbonate (1.96 mEq).

Meropenem in the ADD-Vantage‡ vial is intended for intravenous use only after dilution with the appropriate volume of diluent solution in the Abbott ADD-Vantage diluent container (see DOSAGE AND ADMINISTRATION, Preparation of Solution). Meropenem in the ADD-Vantage vial is available in two strengths. Each 1 g ADD-Vantage vial of meropenem will deliver 90.2 mg of sodium as sodium carbonate (3.92 mEq), and each 500 mg ADD-Vantage vial will deliver 45.1 mg of sodium as sodium carbonate (1.96 mEq).

‡ ADD-Vantage is a registered trademark of Abbott Laboratories Inc.

CLINICAL PHARMACOLOGY:

At the end of a 30-minute intravenous infusion of a single dose of meropenem in normal volunteers, mean peak plasma concentrations are approximately 23 mcg/ml (range 14-26) for the 500 mg dose and the 49 mcg/ml (range 39–58) for the 1 g dose. A 5-minute intravenous bolus injection of meropenem in normal volunteers results in mean peak plasma concentrations of approximately 45 mcg/ml (range 18–65) for the 500 mg dose and 112 mcg/ml (range 83-140) for the 1 g dose.

Following intravenous doses of 500 mg, mean plasma concentrations of meropenem usually decline to approximately 1 mcg/ml at 6 hours after administration.

In subjects with normal renal function, the elimination half-life of meropenem is approximately 1 hour. Approximately 70% of the intravenously administered dose is recovered as unchanged meropenem in the urine over 12 hours, after which little further urinary excretion is detectable. Urinary concentrations of meropenem in excess of 10 mcg/mL are maintained for up to 5 hours after a 500 mg dose. No accumulation of meropenem in plasma or urine was observed with regimens using 500 mg administered every 8 hours or 1 g administered every 6 hours in volunteers with normal renal function.

Plasma protein binding of meropenem is approximately 2%.

There is one metabolite which is microbiologically inactive.

Meropenem penetrates well into most body fluids and tissues including cerebrospinal fluid, achieving concentrations matching or exceeding those required to inhibit most susceptible bacteria. After a single intravenous dose of meropenem, the highest mean concentrations of meropenem were found in tissues and fluids at 1 hour (0.5 to 1.5 hours) after the start of infusion, except where indicated in the tissues and fluids listed in TABLE 1.

TABLE 1 Meropenem Concentrations in Selected Tissues (Highest Concentrations Reported)

Tissue	IV Dose (g)	Number of Samples	Mean [mcg/ml or mcg/(g)]***	Range [mcg/ml or mcg/(g)]
Endometrium	0.5	7	4.2	1.7-10.2
Myometrium	0.5	15	3.8	0.4-8.1
Ovary	0.5	8	2.8	0.8-4.8
Cervix	0.5	2	7.0	5.4-8.5
Fallopian Tube	0.5	9	1.7	0.3-3.4
Skin	0.5	22	3.3	0.5-12.6
Skin	1.0	10	5.3	1.3-16.7
Colon	1.0	2	2.6	2.5-2.7
Bile	1.0	7	14.6 (3 h)	4.0-25.7
Gall Bladder	1.0	1	-	3.9
Interstitial Fluid	1.0	5	26.3	20.9-37.4
Peritoneal Fluid	1.0	9	30.2	7.4-54.6
Lung	1.0	2	4.8 (2 h)	1.4-8.2
Bronchial Mucosa	1.0	7	4.5	1.3-11.1
Muscle	1.0	2	6.1 (2 h)	5.3-6.9
Fascia	1.0	9	8.8	1.5-20
Heart Valves	1.0	7	9.7	6.4-12.1
Myocardium	1.0	10	15.5	5.2-25.5
CSF (Inflamed)	20 mg/kg*	8	1.1 (2 h)	0.2-2.8
	40 mg/kg**	5	3.3 (3 h)	0.9-6.5
CSF (Uninflamed)	1.0	4	0.2 (2 h)	0.1-0.3

* in pediatric patients of age 5 months to 8 years
** in pediatric patients of age 1 month to 15 years
*** at 1 hour unless otherwise noted

The pharmacokinetics of meropenem in pediatric patients 2 years of age or older are essentially similar to those in adults. The elimination half-life for meropenem was approximately 1.5 hours in pediatric patients of age 3 months to 2 years. The pharmacokinetics are linear over the dose range from 10 to 40 mg/kg

Pharmacokinetic studies with meropenem in patients with renal insufficiency have shown that the plasma clearance of meropenem correlates with creatnine clearance. Dosage adjustments are necessary in subjects with renal impairment. (See DOSAGE AND ADMINISTRA-

CLINICAL PHARMACOLOGY: *(cont'd)*

TION, Use in Adults with Renal Impairment.) A pharmacokinetic study with meropenem in elderly patients with renal insufficiency has shown a reduction in plasma clearance of meropenem that correlates with age-associated reduction in creatnine clearance.

Meropenem is hemodialyzable. However, there is no information on the usefulness of hemodialysis to treat overdosage. (See OVERDOSAGE.)

A pharmacokinetic study with meropenem in patients with hepatic impairment has shown no effects of liver disease on the pharmacokinetics of meropenem.

MICROBIOLOGY

The bactericidal activity of meropenem results from the inhibition of cell wall synthesis. Meropenem rapidly penetrates the cell wall of most gram-positive and gram-negative bacteria to reach penicillin-binding-protein (PBP) targets. Its strongest affinities are toward PBPs 2, 3, and 4 of *Escherichia coli* and *Pseudomonas aeruginosa*; and PBPs 1, 2, and 4 of *Staphyloccus aureus*. Bactericidal concentrations (defined as a 3 $\log_{10}$ reduction in cell counts within 12 to 24 hours) are typically 1-2 times the bacteriostatic concentrations or meropenem, with the exception of *Listeria monocytogenes*, against which lethal activity is not observed.

Meropenem has significant stability to hydrolysis by β-lactamases of most categories, both penicillinases and cephalosporinases produced by gram-positive and gram-negative bacteria, with the exception of metallo-β-lactamases. Meropenem should not be used to treat methicillin-resistant staphylococci. Cross resistance is sometimes observed with strains resistant to other carbapenems.

In vitro tests show meropenem to act synergistically with aminoglycoside antibiotics against some isolates of *Pseudomonas aeruginosa*.

Meropenem has been shown to be active against most strains of the following microorganisms, both *in vitro* and in clinical infections (see INDICATIONS AND USAGE).

Gram-Positive Aerobes

Streptococcus pneumoniae (excluding penicillin-resistant strains)
Viridans group streptococci

Note: Penicillin-resistant strains had meropenem MIC_{90}values of 1 or 2 mcg/ml, which is above the 0. 12mcg/ml susceptible breakpoint for this species.

Gram-Negative Aerobes

Escherichia coli
Haemophilus influenzae (β-lactamase and non-β-lactamase-producing)
Klebsiella pneumoniae
Neisseria meningitidis
Pseudomonas aeruginosa

Anaerobes

Bacteroides fragilis
Bacteroides thetaiotaomicron
Peptostreptococcus species

The following *in vitro* data are available, **but their clinical significance is unknown.**

Meropenem exhibits *in vitro* minimum inhibitory concentrations (MICs) of 0.12 mcg/ml against most (≥90%) strains of *Streptococcus pneumoniae*, 0.5 mcg/ml or less against most (≥90%) strains of *Haemophilus influenzae* and 4 mcg/mL or less against most (≥90%) strains of the other microorganisms in the following list; however, the safety and effectiveness of meropenem in treating clinical infections due to these microorganisms have not been established in adequate and well-controlled clinical trials.

Gram-Positive Aerobes

Streptococcus pneumoniae (excluding penicillin-resistant strains)
Viridans group streptococci

Note: Penicillin-resistant strains had meropenem MIC_{90}values of 1 or 2 mcg/ml, which is above the 0.12 mcg/ml susceptible breakpoint for this species.

Gram-Negative Aerobes

Acinetobacter species
Aeromonas hydrophila
Campylobacter jejuni
Citrobacter diversus
Citrobacter freundii
Enterobacter cloacae
Haemophilus influenzae (ampicillin-resistant, non-β-lactamase producing strains [BLNAR strains])
Hafnia alvei
Klebsiella oxytoca
Moraxella catarrhalis (β-lactamase and non-β-lactamase-producing strains)
Morganella morganii
Pasteurella multocida
Proteus mirabilis
Proteus vulgaris
Salmonella species
Serratia marcescens
Shigella species
Yersinia enterocolitica

Anaerobes

Bacteroides distasonis
Bacteroides ovatus
Bacteroides uniformis
Bacteroides ureolyticus
Bacteroides vulgatus
Clostridium difficile
Clostridium perfringens
Eubacterium lentum
Fusobacterium species
Prevotella bivia
Prevotella intermedia
Prevotella melaninogenica
Porphyromonas asacharolytica
Propionbacterium acnes

SUSCEPTIBILITY TESTS

Dilution Techniques: Quantitative methods are used to determine antimicrobial minimal inhibitory concentrations (MICs). These MICs provide estimates of the susceptibility of bacteria to antimicrobial compounds. The MICs should be determined using a standardized procedure. Standardized procedures are based on a dilution method[1] (broth or agar) or equivalent with standardized inoculum concentrations and standardized concentrations of meropenem powder. The MIC values should be interpreted according to the following criteria for indicated aerobic organisms other than *Haemophilus* species and streptococci:

TABLE 2

MIC (mcg/ml)	Interpretation
≤ 4	(S) Susceptible
8	(I) Intermediate
≥ 16	(R) Resistant

Haemophilus Test Media (HTM) and the following interpretive criteria should be used when testing *Haemophilus* species:

TABLE 3

MIC (mcg/ml)	Interpretation
≤ 0.5	(S) Susceptible

The current absence of resistant strains precludes defining any categories other than "Susceptible". Strains yielding results suggestive of a "Nonsusceptible" category should be submitted to a reference laboratory for further testing.

CLINICAL PHARMACOLOGY: *(cont'd)*

The following criteria should be used when testing *Streptococci* and *Streptociccus pneumoniae*:

TABLE 4

MIC (mcg/ml)	Interpretation
≤ 0.12	(S) Susceptible

When testing viridans group streptococci:

TABLE 5

MIC (mcg/ml)	Interpretation
≤ 0.5	(S) Susceptible

The current absence of resistant strains precludes defining any categories other than "Susceptible". Strains yielding results suggestive of a "Nonsusceptible" category should be submitted to a reference laboratory for further testing.

A report of "Susceptible" indicates that the pathogen is likely to be inhibited if the antimicrobial compound in the blood reaches the concentrations usually achievable. A report of "Intermediate" indicates that the result should be considered equivocal, and, if the microorganism is not fully susceptible to alternative, clinically feasible drugs, the test should be repeated. This category implies possible clinical applicability in body sites where the drug is physiologically concentrated or in situations where high dosage of drug can be used. This category also provides a buffer zone which prevents small uncontrolled technical factors from causing major discrepancies in interpretation. A report of "Resistant" indicates that the pathogen in not likely to be inhibited if the antimicrobial compound in the blood reaches the concentrations usually achievable; other therapy should be selected.

Standardized susceptibility test procedures require the use of laboratory control microorganisms to control the technical aspects of the laboratory procedures. Standard meropenem powder should provide the MIC values found in TABLE 6.

TABLE 6

Microorganism	ATCC	MIC (mcg/ml)
Enterococcus faecalis	29212	20.-8.0
Escherichia coli	25922	0.008-0.06
Haemophilus influenzae	49247	0.06-0.25
Pseudomonas aeruginosa	27853	0.25-1.0
Streptococcus pneumoniae	49619	0.06-0.25

Diffusion Techniques: Quantitative methods that require measurement of zone diameters also provide reproducible estimates of the susceptibility of bacteria to antimicrobial compounds. One such standardized procedure[2] requires the use of standardized inoculum concentrations. This procedure uses paper disks impregnated with 10-mcg of meropenem to test the susceptibility of microorganisms to meropenem.

Reports from the laboratory providing results of the standard single-disk susceptibility test with a 10-mcg disk should be interpreted according to the following criteria for indicated aerobic organisms other than *Haemophilus* species and streptococci:

TABLE 7

Zone Diameter (mm)	Interpretation
≥ 16	(S) Susceptible
14-15	(I) Intermediate
≤ 13	(R) Resistant

Haemophilus Test Media and the following criteria should be used when testing *Haemophilus* species:

TABLE 8

Zone Diameter (mm)	Interpretation
≥ 20	(S) Susceptible

The current absence of resistant strains precludes defining any categories other than "Susceptible". Strains yielding results suggestive of a "Nonsusceptible" category should be submitted to a reference laboratory for further testing.

Streptococcus pneumoniae isolates should be tested using 1 mcg/ml oxacillin disk. Isolates with oxacillin zone sizes of ≥20 mm are susceptible (MIC ≤0.06 mcg/ml) to peniclin and can be considered susceptible to meropenem for approved indications, and meropenem need not be tested. A meropenem MIC should be determined on isolates of *S. pneumoniae* with oxacillin zone sizes of ≤19 mm. The disk test does not distinguish penicillin intermediate strains (*i.e.*, MICs = 0.12-1.0 mcg/ml) from strains that are penicillin resistant (*i.e.*, MICs ≥2 mcg/ml). Viridans group streptococci should be tested for meropenem susceptibility using an MIC method. Reliable disk diffusion tests for meropenem do not exist for testing streptococci.

Interpretation should be as stated above for results using dilution techniques. Interpretation involves correlation of the diameter obtained in the disk test with the MIC for meropenem.

As with standardized dilution techniques, diffusion methods require the use of laboratory control microorganisms that are used to control the technical aspects of the laboratory procedures. For the diffusion technique, the 10-mcg meropenem disk should provide the following zone diameters in these laboratory test quality control strains:

TABLE 9

Microorganism	ATCC	Zone Diameter (mm)
Enterococcus faecalis	25922	28-34
Haemophilus influenzae	49247	20-28
Pseudomonas aeruginosa	27853	27-33

Anaerobic Techniques: For anaerobic bacteria, susceptibility to meropenem as MICs can be determined by standardized test methods[3]. The MIC values obtained should be interpreted according to TABLE 10.

TABLE 10

MIC (mcg/ml)	Interpretation
≤ 4	(S) Susceptible
8	(I) Intermediate
≥ 16	(R) Resistant

Interpretation is identical to that stated above for results using dilution techniques.

CLINICAL PHARMACOLOGY: *(cont'd)*

As with other susceptibility techniques, the use of laboratory control microorganisms is required to control the technical aspects of the laboratory standardized procedures. Standardized meropenem powder should provide the MIC values found in TABLE 11.

TABLE 11

Microorganism	ATCC	MIC (mcg/ml)
Bacteroides fragilis	25285	0.06-0.25
Bacteroides thetaiotaomicron	29741	0.125-0.5

CLINICAL STUDIES:

INTRA-ABDOMINAL

One controlled clinical study of complicated intra-abdominal infection was performed in the United States where meropenem was compared to clindamycin/tobramycin. Three controlled clinical studies of complicated intra-abdominal infections were performed in Europe; meropenem was compared to imipenem (two trials) and cefotaxime/metronidazole (one trial).

Using strict evaluablity criteria and microbiologic eradication and clinical cures at follow-up which occurred 7 or more days after completion of therapy, presumptive microbiologic eradication/clinical cure rates and statistical findings were obtained and can be found in TABLE 12.

TABLE 12

Treatment Arm	No. evaluable / No. enrolled (%)	Microbiologic Eradication Rate	Clinical Cure Rate	Outcome
Meropenem	146-516 (28%)	98/146 (67%)	101/146 (69%)	
Imipenem	65/220 (30%)	40/65 (62%)	42/65 (65%)	Meropenem equivalent to control
Cefotaxime/ Metronidazole	26/85 (30%)	22/26 (85%)	22/26 (85%)	Meropenem not equivalent to control
Clindamycin / Tobramycin	50/212 (24%)	38/50 (76%)	38/50 (76%)	Meropenem equivalent to control

The finding that meropenem was not statistically equivalent to cefotaxime/metronidazole may have been due to uneven assignment of more seriously ill patients to the meropenem arm. Currently there is no additional information available to further interpret this observation.

BACTERIAL MENINGITIS

Four hundred forty-six patients (397 pediatric patients ≥3 months to <17 years of age) were enrolled in 4 separate clinical trials and randomized to treatment with meropenem (n=225) at a dose of 40 mg/kg every 8 hours or a comparator drug, *i.e.*, cefotaxime (n=187) or ceftriaxone (n=34), at the approved dosing regimens. A comparable number of patients were found to be clinically evaluable (ranging from 61–68%) and with a similar distribution of pathogens isolated on initial CSF culture.

Patients were defined as clinically not cured if any one of the following three criteria were met:

1. At the 5-7 week post-completion of therapy visit, the patient had any one of the following: moderate to severe motor, behavior or development deficits, hearing loss of >60 decibels in one or both ears, or blindness.

2. During therapy the patient's clinical status necessitated the addition of other antibiotics.

3. Either during or post-therapy, the patient developed a large subdural effusion needing surgical drainage, or a cerebral abscess, or a bacteriologic relapse.

Using the definition, the efficacy rates found in TABLE 13 were obtained per organism. The values represent the number of patients clinically cured/number of clinically evaluable patients, with the percent cure in parentheses.

TABLE 13

Microorganism	Meropenem	Comparator
S. pneumoniae	17/24 (71)	19/30 (63)
H. influenzae (+)	8/10 (80)	6/6 (100)
H. influenzae (-/NT)	44/59 (75)	44/60 (73)
N. meningitidis	30/35 (86)	35/39 (90)
TOTAL (including others)	102/131 (78)	108/140 (77)

(+) β-lactamase producing
(-/NT) non β-lactamase-producing or not tested

Sequelae were the most common reason patients were assessed as clinically not cured.

Five patients were found to be bacteriologically not cured, 3 in the comparator group (1 relapse and 2 patients with cerebral abscesses) and 2 in the meropenem group (1 relapse and 1 with continued growth of *Pseudomonas aeruginosa*).

The adverse events seen were comparable between the two treatment groups both in type and frequency. The meropenem group did have a statistically higher number of patients with transient elevation of liver enzymes. (See ADVERSE REACTIONS.) Rates of seizure activity during therapy were comparable between patients with no CNS abnormalities who received meropenem and those who received comparator agents. In the meropenem IV treated group, 12/15 patients with seizures had late onset seizures (defined as occurring on day 3 or later) versus 7/20 in the comparator arm.

With respect to hearing loss, 263 of the 271 evaluable patients had at least one hearing test performed post-therapy. TABLE 14 shows the degree of hearing loss between the meropenem-treated patients and the comparator-treated patients.

TABLE 14

Degree of Hearing Loss (in one or both ears)	Meropenem (N=128)	Comparator (N=135)
No Loss	61 %	56 %
20 - 40 decibles	20 %	24 %
> 40 - 60 decibles	8 %	7 %
> 60 decibles	9 %	10 %

INDICATIONS AND USAGE:

Meropenem is indicated as single agent therapy for the treatment of the following infections when caused by susceptible strains of the designated microorganisms:

INDICATIONS AND USAGE: *(cont'd)*

Intra-abdominal Infections: Complicated appendicitis and peritonitis caused by viridans group streptococci *Escherichia coli, Klebsiella pneumoniae, Pseudomonas aeruginosa, Bacteroides fragilis, B. thetaiotaomicron*, and *Peptostreptococcus* species.

Bacterial Meningitis (pediatric patients ≥3 months only): Bacterial meningitis caused by *Streptococcus pneumoniae*‡, *Haemophilus influenzae* (β-lactamase and non-β-lacatamase-producing strains), and *Neisseria meningitidis*.

‡ Penicillin-resistant strains have not been studied in clinical trials.

Meropenem has been found to be effective in eliminating concurrent bacteremia in association with bacteria meningitis.

For information regarding use in pediatric patients (3 months of age and older) see Pediatric Use, ADVERSE REACTIONS, and DOSAGE AND ADMINISTRATION sections.

Appropriate cultures should usually be performed before initiating antimicrobial treatment in order to isolate and identify the organisms causing infection and determine their susceptibility to meropenem.

Meropenem is useful as presumptive therapy in the indicated condition (*i.e.*, intra-abdominal infections) prior to the identification of the causative organisms because of its broad spectrum of bactericidal activity.

Antimicrobial therapy should be adjusted, if appropriate, once the results of culture(s) and anti-microbial susceptibility testing are known.

CONTRAINDICATIONS:

Meropenem is contraindicated in patients with known hypersensitivity to any component of this product or to other drugs in the same class or in patients who have demonstrated anaphylactic reactions to β-lactams.

WARNINGS:

SERIOUS AND OCCASIONALLY FATAL HYPERSENSITIVITY (ANAPHYLACTIC) REACTIONS HAVE BEEN REPORTED IN PATIENTS RECEIVING THERAPY WITH β-LACTAMS. THESE REACTIONS ARE MORE LIKELY TO OCCUR IN INDIVIDUALS WITH A HISTORY OF SENSITIVITY TO MULTIPLE ALLERGENS.

THERE HAVE BEEN REPORTS OF INDIVIDUALS WITH A HISTORY OF PENICILLIN HYPERSENSITIVITY WHO HAVE EXPERIENCED SEVERE HYPERSENSITIVITY REACTIONS WHEN TREATED WITH ANOTHER β-LACTAM. BEFORE INITIATING THERAPY WITH MEROPENEM IV, CAREFUL INQUIRY SHOULD BE MADE CONCERNING PREVIOUS HYPERSENSITIVITY REACTIONS TO PENICILLINS, CEPHALOSPORINS, OTHER β-LACTAMS, AND OTHER ALLERGENS. IF AN ALLERGIC REACTION TO MEROPENEM OCCURS, DISCONTINUE THE DRUG IMMEDIATELY. **SERIOUS ANAPHYLACTIC REACTIONS REQUIRE IMMEDIATE EMERGENCY TREATMENT WITH EPINEPHRINE, OXYGEN, INTRAVENOUS STEROIDS, AND AIRWAY MANAGEMENT, INCLUDING INTUBATION. OTHER THERAPY MAY ALSO BE ADMINISTERED AS INDICATED.**

Seizures and other CNS experiences have been reported during treatment with meropenem (see PRECAUTIONS and ADVERSE REACTIONS).

Pseudomembraneous colitis has been reported with nearly all antibacterial agents, including meropenem, and may range in severity from mild to life-threatening. Therefore, it is important to consider this diagnosis in patients who present with diarrhea subsequent to the administration of antibacterial agents.

Treatment with antibacterial agents alters the normal flora of the colon and may permit overgrowth of clostridia. Studies indicate that a toxin produced by *Clostridium difficile* is a primary cause of "antibiotic-associated colitis".

After the diagnosis of pseudomembranous colitis has been established, appropriate therapeutic measures should be initiated. Mild cases of pseudomembranous colitis usually respond to drug discontinuation alone. In moderate-to-severe cases, consideration should be given to management with fluids and electrolytes, protein supplementation, and treatment with an antibacterial drug clinically effective against *Clostridium difficile* colitis.

PRECAUTIONS:

GENERAL

Seizures and other CNS adverse experiences have been reported during treatment with meropenem. These adverse experiences have occurred most commonly in patients with CNS disorders (*e.g.*, brain lesions or history of seizures) or with bacterial meningitis and/or compromised renal function.

During the initial clinical investigations, 2038 immunocompetent adult patients were treated for infections outside the CNS with meropenem (500 mg or 1000 mg every 8 hours). Overall seizures, whether drug related or not, occurred in 0.5% of the meropenem-treated patients. All meropenem-treated patients with seizures had pre-existing contributing factors. Among these are included prior history of seizures or CNS abnormality and concomitant medications with seizure potential. Dosage adjustment is recommended in patients with advanced age and/or reduced renal function. (See DOSAGE AND ADMINISTRATION, Use in Adults with Renal Impairment.)

Close adherence to the recommended dosage regimens is urged, especially in patients with known factors that predispose to convulsive activity. Anticonvulsant therapy should be continued in patients with known seizure disorders. If focal tremors, myoclonus, or seizures occur, patients should be evaluated neurologically, placed on anticonvulsant therapy if not already instituted, and the dosage of meropenem re-examined to determine whether it should be decreased or the antibiotic discontinued.

In patients with renal dysfunction, thrombocytopenia has been observed but no clinical bleeding reported. (See DOSAGE AND ADMINISTRATION, Use in Adults with Renal Impairment.)

There is inadequate information regarding the use of meropenem in patients on hemodialysis.

As with other broad-spectrum antibiotics, prolonged use of meropenem may result in overgrowth of nonsusceptible organisms. Repeated evaluation of the patient is essential. If superinfection does occur during therapy, appropriate measures should be taken.

LABORATORY TESTS

While meropenem possesses the characteristic low toxicity of the β-lactam group of antibiotics, periodic assessment of organ system functions, including renal, hepatic, and hematopoietic, is advisable during prolonged therapy.

CARCINOGENESIS, MUTAGENESIS, IMPAIRMENT OF FERTILITY

Carcinogenesis: Carcinogenesis studies have not been performed.

Mutagenesis: Genetic toxicity studies were performed with meropenem using the bacterial reverse mutation test, the Chinese hamster ovary HGPRT assay, cultured human lymphocytes cytogenic assay, and the mouse micronucleus test. There was no evidence of mutagenic potential found in any of these tests.

PRECAUTIONS: *(cont'd)*

Impairment of Fertility: Reproductive studies were performed with meropenem in rats at doses up to 1000 mg/kg/day, and cynomolgus monkeys at doses up to 360 mg/kg/day (on the basis of AUC comparisons, approximately 1.8 times and 3.7 times, respectively, to the human exposure at the usual dose of 1 g every 8 hours). There was no reproductive toxicity seen.

PREGNANCY CATEGORY B

Reproductive studies have been performed with meropenem in rats at doses of up to 1000 mg/kg/day, and cynomolgus monkeys at doses of up to 360 mg/kg/day (on the basis of AUC comparisons, approximately 1.8 times and 3.7 times, respectively, to the human exposure at the usual dose of 1 g every 8 hours). These studies revealed no evidence of impaired fertility or harm to the fetus due to meropenem, although there were slight changes in fetal body weight at doses of 250 mg/kg/day (on the basis of AUC comparisons, 0.4 times the human exposure at a dose of 1 g every 8 hours) and above in rats. There are, however, no adequate and well-controlled studies in pregnant women. Because animal reproduction studies are not always predictive of human response, this drug should be used in pregnancy only if clearly needed.

PEDIATRIC USE

The safety and effectiveness of meropenem have been established for pediatric patients ≥ 3 months of age. Use of meropenem in pediatric patients with bacterial meningitis is supported by evidence from adequate and well-controlled studies in the pediatric population. Use of meropenem in pediatric patients with intra-abdominal infections is supported by evidence from adequate and well-controlled studies with adults with additional data from pediatric pharmacokinetics studies and controlled clinical trials in pediatric patients. (See CLINICAL PHARMACOLOGY, INDICATIONS AND USAGE, ADVERSE REACTIONS, DOSAGE AND ADMINISTRATION, and CLINICAL STUDIES sections.)

NURSING MOTHERS

It is not known whether this drug is excreted in human milk. Because many drugs are excreted in human milk, caution should be exercised when meropenem is administered to a nursing woman.

DRUG INTERACTIONS:

Probenecid competes with meropenem for active tubular secretion and this inhibits the renal excretion of meropenem. This led to statistically significant increases in the elimination half-life (38%) and in the extent of systemic exposure (56%). Therefore, the coadministration of probenecid with meropenem is not recommended.

Other than probenecid, no specific drug interaction studies were conducted.

ADVERSE REACTIONS:

ADULT PATIENTS

During the initial clinical investigations, 2038 immunocompetent adult patients were treated for infections outside the CNS with meropenem (500 mg or 1000 mg every 8 hours). Deaths in 3 patients were assessed as possibly related to meropenem; 28 (1.4%) patients had meropenem discontinued because of adverse events. Many patients in these trials were severely ill and had multiple background diseases, physiological impairments and were receiving multiple other drug therapies. In the seriously ill patient population, it was not possible to determine the relationship between observed adverse events and therapy with meropenem.

The following adverse reaction frequencies were derived from the clinical trials in the 2038 patients treated with meropenem.

Local Adverse Reactions: Local adverse reactions that were reported, irrespective of the relationship to therapy with meropenem, appear in TABLE 15.

TABLE 15

Inflammation at the injection site	3.0 %
Phlebitis/Thrombophlebitis	1.2 %
Injection site reaction	1.1 %
Pain at the injection site	0.4 %
Edema at the injection site	0.2 %

Systemic Adverse Reactions: Systemic adverse clinical reactions that were reported irrespective of the relationship to meropenem occurring in greater than 1.0 % of the patients were diarrhea (5.0 %), nausea/vomiting (3.9 %), headache (2.8 %), rash (1.7 %), pruritus (1.6 %), apnea (1.2 %), and constipation (1.2 %).

Additional adverse systemic clinical reactions that were reported irrespective of relationship to therapy with meropenem and occurring in less than 1.0 % but greater than 0.1 % of the patients are listed below within each body system in order of decreasing frequency:

Bleeding events [gastrointestinal hemorrhage, melena, epistaxis, and hemoperitoneum] occurred in 0.7 % of meropenem patients.

Body as a Whole: pain, abdominal pain, chest pain, sepsis, shock, fever, abdominal enlargement, back pain, hepatic failure

Cardiovascular: heart failure, heart arrest, tachycardia, hypertension, myocardial infarction, pulmonary embolus, bradycardia, hypotension, syncope

Digestive System: oral moniliasis, anorexia, cholestatic jaundice/jaundice, flatulence, ileus

Hemic/Lymphatic: anemia

Metabolic/Nutritional: peripheral edema, hypoxia

Nervous System: insomnia, agitation/delirium, confusion, dizziness, seizure (See PRECAUTIONS), nervousness, paresthesia, hallucinations, somnolence, anxiety, depression

Respiratory: respiratory disorder, dyspnea

Skin and Appendages: urticaria, sweating

Urogenital System: dysuria, kidney failure

Adverse Laboratory Changes: Adverse laboratory changes that were reported irrespective of relationship to meropenem occurring in greater than 0.2 % of the patients were as follows:

Hepatic: increased SGPT (ALT), SGOT (AST), Alkaline Phosphatase, LDH, and Bilirubin

Hematologic: increased platelets, increased eosinophils, prolonged prothrombin time, prolonged partial thromboplastin time, decreased platelets, positive direct or indirect Coombs test, decreased hemoglobin, decreased hematocrit, decreased WBC, shortened prothrombin time and shortened partial thromboplastin time.

Renal: increased creatinine and increased BUN. *Note:*It is not known if the safety profile of meropenem is changed in patients with varying degrees of renal impairment.

Urinalysis: presence of urine in red blood cells.

PEDIATRIC PATIENTS

Clinical Adverse Reactions: Meropenem was studied in 417 pediatric patients (≥3 months to <13 years of age) with serious bacterial infections at dosages of 10 to 20 mg/kg every 8 hours. The types of clinical adverse events seen in these patients are similar to the adults, with the most common adverse events reported as possibly, probably, or definitely related to meropenem and their rates of occurrence in TABLE 16.

ADVERSE REACTIONS: *(cont'd)*

TABLE 16

Diarrhea	4.3 %
Rash	1.4 %
Vomiting	1.0 %

Meropenem was studied in 198 pediatric patients (≥3 months to <17 years of age) with meningitis at a dosage of 40 mg/kg every 8 hours. The types of clinical adverse events seen in these patients are similar to the adults, with the most common adverse events being reported as possibly, probably, or definitely related to meropenem and their rates of occurrence in TABLE 17.

TABLE 17

Rash (mostly diaper area moniliasis)	3.5 %
Diarrhea	3.5 %
Oral Moniliasis	2.0 %
Glossitis	1.0 %

In the meningitis studies the rates of seizure activity during therapy were comparable between patients with no CNS abnormalities who received meropenem and those who received comparator agent (either cefotaxime or ceftriaxone). In the meropenem IV treated group, 12/15 patients with seizures had late onset seizures (defined as occurring on day 3 or later) versus 7/20 in the comparator arm.

Adverse Laboratory Changes: Laboratory abnormalities seen in the pediatric-aged patients in both the pediatric and the meningitis studies are similar to those reported in adult patients.

There is no experience in pediatric patients with renal impairment.

Post-Marketing Experience: No post-marketing experience is available.

OVERDOSAGE:

In mice and rats, large intravenous doses of meropenem (2200–4000 mg/kg) have been associated with ataxia, dyspnea, convulsions, and mortalities.

Intentional overdosing with meropenem is unlikely, although accidental overdosing might occur if large doses are given to patients with reduced renal function. The largest dose of meropenem administered in clinical trials has been 2 g given intravenously every 8 hours. At this dosage, no adverse pharmacological effects or increased safety risks have been observed.

No specific information is available for the treatment of meropenem overdosage. In the event of an overdose, meropenem should be discontinued and general supportive treatment given until renal elimination takes place. Meropenem and its metabolite are readily dialyzable and effectively removed by hemodialysis; however, no information is available on the use of hemodialysis to treat overdosage.

DOSAGE AND ADMINISTRATION:

Adults: One gram (1 g) by intravenous administration every 8 hours. Meropenem should be given by intravenous infusion, over approximately 15 to 30 minutes or as an intravenous bolus injection (5 to 20 ml) over approximately 3-5 minutes.

Use in Adults with Renal Impairment: Dosage should be reduced in patients with creatinine clearance less than 51 ml/min. (See TABLE 18.)

TABLE 18 Recommended Meropenem Dosage Schedule for Adults With Impaired Renal Function

Creatinine Clearance (ml/min)	Dose (dependent on type of infection)	Dosing Interval
26 - 50	Recommended dose (1000 mg)	Every 12 hours
10 - 25	One-half recommended dose	Every 12 hours
< 10	One-half recommended dose	Every 24 hours

When only serum creatnine is available, the following formula (Cockroft and Gault equation)[4] may be used to estimate creatinine clearance:

Males: Creatinine Clearance (ml/min) = Weight (kg) × (140 - age) ÷ (72 × serum creatinine (mg/dl))

Females: 0.85 × above value

There is inadequate information regarding the use of meropenem in patients on hemodialysis. There is no experience with peritoneal dialysis.

Use in Adults With Hepatic Insufficiency: No dosage adjustment is necessary in patients with impaired hepatic function.

Use in Elderly Patients: No dosage adjustment is required for elderly patients with creatnine clearance values above 50 ml/min.

Use in Pediatric Patients: For pediatric patients from 3 months of age and older, the meropenem dose is 20 or 40 mg/kg every 8 hours (maximum dose is 2 g every 8 hours), depending on the type of infection (intra-abdominal or meningitis). (See TABLE 19.) Pediatric patients weighing over 50 kg should be administered meropenem at a dose of 1 g every 8 hours for intra-abdominal infections and 2 g every 8 hours for meningitis. Meropenem should be given as intravenous infusion over approximately 15 to 30 minutes or as an intravenous bolus injection (5 to 20 mL) over approximately 3-5 minutes.

TABLE 19 Recommended Meropenem Dosage Schedule for Pediatrics With Normal Renal Function

Type of Infection	Dose (mg/kg)	Dosing Interval
Intra-Abdominal	20	Every 8 hours
Meningitis	40	Every 8 hours

There is no experience in pediatric patients with renal impairment.

PREPARATION OF SOLUTION

For Intravenous Bolus Administration: Constitute injection vials (500 mg/20 ml and 1 g/30 ml) with Sterile Water for Injection (See TABLE 20). Shake to dissolve and let stand until clear.

TABLE 20

Vial Size	Amount of Diluent Added (ml)	Approximate Withdrawable Volume (ml)	Approximate Average Concentration (mg/ml)
500 mg/ 20 ml	10	10	50
1 g / 30 ml	20	20	50

DOSAGE AND ADMINISTRATION: *(cont'd)*

For Infusion: Infusion vials (500 mg/100 ml and 1 g/100 ml) may be directly constituted with a compatible infusion fluid. (See Compatibility and Stability.) Alternatively, an injection vial may be constituted, then the resulting solution added to an IV container and further diluted with an appropriate infusion fluid. (See Compatibility and Stability.)

Note: ADD-VANTAGE VIALS ARE NOT TO BE USED IN THIS MANNER.

FOR ADD-VANTAGE VIALS

Add-Vantage vials of meropenem are to be constituted only with Sodium Chloride Injection 0.45 %, Sodium Chloride Injection 0.9 % or Dextrose Injection 5 % in the 50, 100, and 250 mL Abbott ADD-Vantage flexible diluent containers. Meropenem supplied in single-use, ADD-Vantage vials should be prepared as directed:

DIRECTIONS FOR USE OF MEROPENEM IN ADD-VANTAGE VIALS

To open diluent container, peel overwrap from the corner and remove container. Some opacity of the plastic due to moisture absorption during the sterilization process may be observed. This is normal and does not affect the solution quality or safety. The opacity will diminish gradually.

To assemble ADD-Vantage vial and flexible diluent container (use aseptic technique):

1. Remove the protective covers from the top of the vial and the vial port on the diluent container as follows:

a. To remove the breakaway vial cap, swing the pull ring over the top of the vial and pull down far enough to start the opening. Then pull straight up to remove the cap. *Note:* Once the breakaway cap has been removed, do not access vial with syringe.

b. To remove the vial port cover, grasp the tab on the pull ring, pull up to break the three tie strings, then pull back to remove the cover.

2. Screw the vial into the vial port until it will go no further. THE VIAL MUST BE SCREWED IN TIGHTLY TO ASSURE A SEAL. This occurs approximately 1/2 turn (180°) after the first audible click. The clicking sound does not assure a seal; the vial must be turned as far as it will go. *Note:*ONCE VIAL IS SEATED, DO NOT ATTEMPT TO REMOVE.

3. Recheck the vial to assure that it is tight by trying to turn it further in the direction of assembly.

4. Label appropriately.

To Prepare Admixture:

1. Squeeze the bottom of the diluent container gently to inflate the portion of the container surrounding the end of the drug vial.

2. With the other hand, push the drug vial down into the container telescoping the walls of the container. Grasp the inner cap of the vial through the walls of the container.

3. Pull the inner cap from the drug vial. Verify that the rubber stopper has been pulled out and invert the system several times, allowing the drug and diluent to mix.

4. Mix contents thoroughly and use within the specified time.

Preparation For Administration: (Use Aseptic Technique)

1. Confirm the activation and admixture of vial contents.

2. Check for leaks by squeezing container firmly. If leaks are found, discard unit as sterility may be impaired.

3. Close flow control clamp of administration set.

4. Remove cover from outlet port at bottom of container.

5. Insert piercing pin of administration set into port with a twisting motion until the pin is firmly seated. *Note:* See full directions on administration set carton.

6. Lift the free end of the hanger loop on the bottom of the vial, breaking the two tie strings. Bend the loop outward to lock it in the upright position, then suspend container from hanger.

7. Squeeze and release drip chamber to establish proper fluid level in chamber.

8. Open flow control clamp and clear air from set. Close clamp.

9. Attach set to venipuncture device. If device is not indwelling, prime and make venipuncture.

10. Regulate rate of administration with flow control clamp.

WARNING: Do not use flexible container in series connections.

COMPATIBILITY AND STABILITY

Compatibility of meropenem with other drugs has not been established. Meropenem should not be mixed with or physically added to solutions containing other drugs.

Freshly prepared solutions of meropenem should be used whenever possible. However, constituted solutions of meropenem maintain satisfactory potency at controlled room temperature 15°-25°C (59°-77°F) or under refrigeration at 4°C (39°F) as described below. Solutions of intravenous meropenem should not be frozen.

INTRAVENOUS BOLUS ADMINISTRATION

Meropenem injection vials constituted with Sterile Water for Injection for bolus administration (up to 50 mg/ml of meropenem) may be stored for up to 2 hours at controlled room temperature 15°-25°C (59°-77°F) or for up to 12 hours at 4°C (39°F).

INTRAVENOUS INFUSION ADMINISTRATION

Stability in Infusion Vials

Meropenem infusion vials constituted with Sodium Chloride Injection 0.9% (meropenem concentrations ranging from 2.5 to 50 mg/ml) are stable for up to 2 hours at controlled room temperature 15°-25°C (55°-77°F) or for up to 18 hours at 4°C (39°F). Infusion vials of meropenem constituted with Dextrose Injection 5% (meropenem concentrations ranging from 2.5 to 50 mg/ml) are stable for up to 1 hour at controlled room temperature 15°-25°C (59°-77°F) or for up to 8 hours at 4°C (39°F).

Stability in Plastic IV Bags

Solutions prepared for infusion (meropenem concentrations ranging from 1 to 20 mg/ml) may be stored in plastic intravenous bags with diluents as shown in TABLE 21.

Stability in Baxter Minibag Plus

Solutions of meropenem (meropenem concentrations ranging from 2.5 to 20 mg/ml) in Baxter Minibag Plus bags with Sodium Chloride Injection 0.9% may be stored for up to 4 hours at controlled room temperatures 15°-25°C (59°-77°F) or for up to 24 hours at 4°C (39°F). Solutions of meropenem (meropenem concentrations ranging from 2.5 to 20 mg/ml) in Baxter Minibag Plus bags with Dextrose Injection, 0.5% may be stored up to 1 hour at controlled room temperatures 15°-25°C (59°-77°F) for up to 6 hours at 4°C (39°F).

Stability in Plastic Syringes, Tubing, and Intravenous Infusion Sets

Solutions of meropenem (meropenem concentrations ranging from 1 to 20 mg/ml) in Water for Injection of Sodium Chloride Injection 0.9% (for up to 4 hours) or in Dextrose Injection 5.0% (for up to 2 hours) at controlled room temperatures 15°-25°C (59°-77°F) are stable in plastic syringes, plastic tubing, drip chambers, and volume control devices of common intravenous infusion sets.

DOSAGE AND ADMINISTRATION: *(cont'd)*

TABLE 21

	Number of Hours Stable at Controlled Room Temperature 15-25°C (59-77°F)	Number of Hours Stable at 4°C (39°F)
Sodium Chloride Injection 0.9%	4	24
Dextrose Injection 5.0%	1	4
Dextrose Injection 10.0%	1	2
Dextrose and Sodium Chloride Injection 5.0%/0.9%	1	2
Dextrose and Sodium Chloride Injection 5.0%/0.2%	1	4
Potassium Chloride in Dextrose Injection 0.15%/5.0%	1	6
Sodium Bicarbonate in Dextrose Injection 0.02%/5.0%	1	6
Dextrose Injection 5.0% in Normosol-M	1	8
Dextrose Injection 5.0% in Ringers Lactate Injection	1	4
Dextrose and Sodium Chloride Injection 2.5%/0.45%	3	12
Mannitol Injection 2.5%	2	16
Ringers Injection	4	24
Ringers Lactate Injection	4	12
Sodium Lactate Injection 1/6 N	2	24
Sodium Bicarbonate Injection 5.0%	1	4

ADD-Vantage Vials

ADD-Vantage vials diluted in Sodium Chloride Injection 0.45% (meropenem concentrations ranging from 5 to 20 mg/ml) may be stored for up to 6 hours at controlled room temperature 15-25°C (59°-77°F) or for 24 hours at 4°C (39°F). ADD-Vantage vials diluted in Sodium Chloride Injection 0.9% (meropenem concentrations ranging from 1-20 mg/ml) may be stored for up to 4 hours at controlled room temperature 15°-25°C (59°-77°F) or for 24 hours at 4°C (39°F). ADD-Vantage vials diluted with Dextrose Injection 5.0% (meropenem concentrations ranging from 1-20 mg/ml) may be stored for up to one hour at controlled room temperature 15°-25°C (59°-77°F) or for 8 hours at 4°C (39°F).

Note: Parenteral drug products should be inspected visually for particulate matter and discoloration prior to administration, whenever solution and container permit.

REFERENCES:

1. National Committee For Clinical laboratory Standards. Methods for Dilution Antimicrobial Susceptibility Tests for Bacteria that Grow Aerobically —Third Edition. Approved Standard NCCLS Document M7–A3, Vol. 13, No. 25, NCCLS, Villanova, PA, December, 1993. **2.** National Committee for Clinical Laboratory Standards. Performance Standards for Antimicrobial Disk Susceptibility Tests — Fifth Edition. Approved Standard NCCLS Document M2-A5, Vol. 13, No. 24, NCCLS, Villanova, PA. December 1993. **3.** National Committee for Clinical Laboratory Standards. Methods for Antimicrobial Susceptibility Testing of Anaerobic Bacteria —Third Edition. Approved Standard NCCLS Document M11–A3, Vol. 13, No. 26, NCCLS, Villanova, PA. December 1993. **4.** Cockcroft DW, Gault MH. Prediction of creatinine clearance from serum creatinine. Nephron. 1976; 16.31-41.

HOW SUPPLIED:

Merrem IV (meropenem) is supplied in 20 ml and 30 ml injection vials containing sufficient meropenem to deliver 500 mg or 1 g for intravenous administration, respectively. Merrem IV is supplied in 100 ml infusion vials containing sufficient meropenem to deliver 500 mg or 1 g for intravenous administration. The dry powder should be stored at controlled room temperature 20°-25°C (68°-77°F) [see USP].

Merrem IV is also supplied as ADD-Vantage Vials containing sufficient meropenem to deliver 500 mg or 1 g for intravenous administration.

MERSALYL SODIUM; THEOPHYLLINE *(001740)*

CATEGORIES: Diuretics; Electrolytic, Caloric-Water Balance; FDA Approval Pre 1982

BRAND NAMES: Diurette; Mersalo

Prescribing information not available at time of publication.

HOW SUPPLIED - EQUIVALENTS NOT AVAILABLE:

Injection, Solution - Intravenous

30 ml $3.20 MERSALYL-THEOPHYLLINE, Lannett 00527-0130-58

MESALAMINE *(001742)*

CATEGORIES: Anti-Inflammatory Agents; Antipyretics; Central Nervous System Agents; Colitis; Gastrointestinal Drugs; NSAIDS; Nonsteroidal Anti-Inflammatory; Proctitis; Proctosigmoiditis; Salicylates; Ulcerative Colitis; Pregnancy Category B; FDA Approved 1987 Dec

BRAND NAMES: Asacol; *Asacolitin* (Germany); *Claversal* (Germany); *Colitofalk*; *Mesacol*; *Mesasal*; Pentasa; *Pentasa Enema*; *Pentasa SR*; *Pentasa Tab*; **Rowasa**; *Salofalk* (Germany, Canada); *Tidocol*
(International brand names outside U.S. in italics)

FORMULARIES: Aetna; BC-BS; PCS

COST OF THERAPY: $149.71 (Ulcerative Colitis; Tablet; 400 mg; 6/day; 42 days)

DESCRIPTION:

This monograph pertains to the Suspension Enema/Suppositories (Rectal), delayed-release tablet (oral) and controlled release capsule (oral) forms of mesalamine.

Rectal Suspension Enema/Suppositories: The active ingredient is mesalamine, also known as 5-aminosalicylic acid (5-ASA). Chemically, mesalamine is 5-amino-2-hydroxybenzoic acid, and is classified as an anti-inflammatory drug.

The empirical formula is $C_7H_7NO_3$, representing a molecular weight of 153.14.

Each rectal suspension enema is a disposable (60 ml) unit and each unit contains 4 grams of mesalamine. In addition to mesalamine the preparation contains the inactive ingredients potassium metabisulfite, carbomer 934P, edetate disodium, potassium acetate, water and xanthan gum. Sodium benzoate is added as a preservative. The disposable unit consists of an applicator tip protected by a polyethylene cover and lubricated with USP white petrolatum. The unit has a one-way valve to prevent back flow of the dispensed product.

Each suppository contains 500 mg of mesalamine in a base of Hard Fat NF. Each suppository is individually wrapped in foil.

DESCRIPTION: *(cont'd)*

Delayed-Release Tablets: Each delayed-release tablet for oral administration contains 400 mg of mesalamine, an anti-inflammatory drug. The delayed-release tablets are coated with acrylic based resin, Eudragit S (methacrylic acid copolymer B, NF), which dissolves at pH 7 or greater, releasing mesalamine in the terminal ileum and beyond for topical anti-inflammatory action in the colon. Mesalamine has the chemical name 5-amino-2-hydroxybenzoic acid.

It's Molecular Weight is 153.1. It's Molecular Formula is $C_7H_7NO_3$.

Inactive Ingredients: Each tablet contains colloidal silicon dioxide, dibutyl phthalate, edible black ink, iron oxide red, iron oxide yellow, lactose, magnesium stearate, methacrylic acid copolymer B (Eudragit S), polyethylene glycol, povidone, sodium starch glycolate, and talc.

Controlled-Release Capsules: Mesalamine for oral administration is a controlled-release formulation of mesalamine, an aminosalicylate anti-inflammatory agent for gastrointestinal use.

Chemically, mesalamine is 5-amino-2-hydroxybenzoic acid. It has a molecular weight of 153.14.

Each capsule contains 250 mg of mesalamine. It also contains the following inactive ingredients: acetylated monoglyceride, castor oil, colloidal silicon dioxide, ethylcellulose, hydroxypropyl, methylcellulose, starch, stearic acid, sugar, talc, and white wax. The capsule shell contains D&C Yellow #10, FD&C Blue #1, FD&C Green #3, gelatin, titanium dioxide, and other ingredients.

CLINICAL PHARMACOLOGY:

Rectal Suspension Enema/Suppository: Sulfasalazine is split by bacterial action in the colon into sulfapyridine (SP) and mesalamine (5-ASA). It is thought that the mesalamine component is therapeutically active in ulcerative colitis. The usual oral doses of sulfasalazine for active ulcerative colitis in adults is two to four grams per day in divided doses. Four grams of sulfasalazine provide 1.6 g of free mesalamine to the colon. Each mesalamine suspension enema delivers up to 4 g aminosalicylate of mesalamine to the left side of the colon.

Each mesalamine suppository delivers 500 mg of mesalamine to the rectum.

The mechanism of action of mesalamine (and sulfasalazine) is unknown, but appears to be topical rather than systemic. Mucosal production of arachidonic acid (AA) metabolites, both through the cyclooxygenase pathways, i.e. prostanoids, and through the lipoxygenase pathways, i.e. leukotrienes (LTs) and hydroxyeicosatetraenoic acids (HETEs) is increased in patients with chronic inflammatory bowel disease, and it is possible that mesalamine diminishes inflammation by blocking cyclooxygenase and inhibiting prostaglandin (PG) production in the colon.

Preclinical Toxicology: Preclinical studies have shown the kidney to be the major target organ for mesalamine toxicity. Adverse renal function changes were observed in rats after a single 600 mg/kg oral dose, but not after a 200 mg/kg dose. Gross kidney lesions, including papillary necrosis, were observed after a single oral >900 mg/kg dose, and after i.v. doses of >214 mg/kg. Mice responded similarly. In a 13-week oral (gavage) dose study in rats, the high dose of 640 mg/kg/day mesalamine caused deaths, probably due to renal failure, and dose-related renal lesions (papillary necrosis and/or multifocal tubular injury) were seen in most rats given the high dose (males and females) as well as in males receiving lower doses 160 mg/kg/day. Renal lesions were not observed in the 160 mg/kg/day female rats. Minimal tubular epithelial damage was seen in the 40 mg/kg/day males and was reversible. In a six-month oral study in dogs, the no-observable dose level of mesalamine was 40 mg/kg/day and doses of 80 mg/kg/day and higher caused renal pathology similar to that described for the rat.

In a combined 52-week toxicity and 127-week carcinogenicity study in rats, degeneration in kidneys was observed at doses of 100 mg/kg/day and above admixed with diet for 52 weeks, and at 127 weeks increased incidence of kidney degeneration and hyalinization of basement membranes and Bowman's capsules was seen at 100 mg/kg/day and above. In the 12 month eye toxicity study in dogs, Keratoconjunctivitis Sicca (KCS) occurred at oral doses of 40 mg/kg/day and above. The oral preclinical studies were done with a highly bioavailable suspension where absorption throughout the gastrointestinal tract occurred. Although intrarectally administered mesalamine in humans is poorly absorbed, the potential for renal toxicity must be considered (see Pharmacokineticsand PRECAUTIONS).

Delayed-Release Tablets: Mesalamine is thought to be the major therapeutically active part of the sulfasalazine molecule in the treatment of ulcerative colitis. Sulfasalazine is converted to equimolar amounts of sulfapyridine and mesalamine by bacterial action in the colon. The usual oral dose of sulfasalazine for active ulcerative colitis is 3 to 4 grams daily in divided doses, which provides 1.2 to 1.6 grams of mesalamine to the colon.

Controlled-Release Capsules: Sulfasalazine is split by bacterial action in the colon into sulfapyridine (SP) and mesalamine (5- ASA). It is thought that the mesalamine component is therapeutically active in ulcerative colitis. The usual oral dose of sulfasalazine for active ulcerative colitis in adults is 2 to 4 g per day in divided doses. Four grams of sulfasalazine provide 1.6 g of free mesalamine to the colon.

Delayed-Release Tablets and Controlled-Release Capsules: The mechanism of action of mesalamine (and sulfasalazine) is unknown, but appears to be topical rather than systemic. Mucosal production of arachidonic acid (AA) metabolites, both through the cyclooxygenase pathways, i.e., prostanoids, and through the lipoxygenase pathways, i.e., leukotrienes (LTs) and hydroxyeicosatetraenoic acids (HETSs), is increased in patients with chronic inflammatory bowel disease, and it is possible that mesalamine diminishes inflammation by blocking cyclooxygenase and inhibiting prostaglandin (PG) production in the colon.

PHARMACOKINETICS

Rectal Suspension Enema: Mesalamine administered rectally as mesalamine suspension enema is poorly absorbed from the colon and is excreted principally in the feces during subsequent bowel movements. The extent of absorption is dependent upon the retention time of the drug product, and there is considerable individual variation. At steady state, approximately 10 to 30% of the daily 4-gram dose can be recovered in cumulative 24-hour urine collections. Other than the kidney, the organ distribution and other bioavailability characteristics of absorbed mesalamine in man are not known. It is known that the compound undergoes acetylation but whether this process takes place at colonic or systemic sites has not been elucidated.

Whatever the metabolic site, most of the absorbed mesalamine is excreted in the urine as the N-acetyl-5-ASA metabolite. The poor colonic absorption of rectally administered mesalamine is substantiated by the low serum concentration of 5-ASA and N-acetyl-5-ASA seen in ulcerative colitis patients after dosage with mesalamine. Under clinical conditions patients demonstrated plasma levels 10 to 12 hours post mesalamine administration of 2 mcg/ml, about two-thirds of which was the N-acetyl metabolite. While the elimination half-life of mesalamine is short (0.5 to 1.5 h), the acetylated metabolite exhibits a half-life of 5 to 10 hours. In addition, steady state plasma levels demonstrated a lack of accumulation of either free or metabolized drug during repeated daily administrations.

Suppositories: Mesalamine administered in an enema formulation is poorly absorbed from the colon, as shown both by low recovery in urine and by low plasma levels during rectal administration. In plasma and urine, mesalamine occurs largely as its N-acetyl derivative, while the major portion recovered in feces is free mesalamine. The elimination half-life of free mesalamine is 0.5 to 1.5-hr and that of the 5-acetyl metabolite is 5 to 10-hr. Following single doses of mesalamine 500 mg Suppository in normal volunteers, 24-hr urines contained (only) N-acetyl-mesalamine equivalent to 15 to 38% (avg 24%) of the administered dose. This

CLINICAL PHARMACOLOGY: *(cont'd)*

is commensurate with the finding of 3 to 36% (avg. 10%) in urine in a study of mesalamine 4 g rectal suspension in normals. In that study, 40 to 107 (avg. 75%) of the administered dose was recovered in feces. At steady state in ulcerative colitis patients (n=38) being treated with mesalamine rectal suspension, 24-hr urines contained 0 to 41% (avg. 0.37 mcg/ml) of mesalamine equivalent (84% as N-acetyl metabolite). Multiple dose pharmacokinetic studies have not been conducted with mesalamine suppository nor have plasma levels been reported from single dose studies.

Delayed-Release Tablets: Mesalamine tablets are coated with an acrylic-based resin that delays release of mesalamine until it reaches the terminal ileum and beyond. This has been demonstrated in human studies conducted with radiological and serum markers. Approximately 28% of the mesalamine in mesalamine tablets is absorbed after oral ingestion, leaving the remainder available for topical action and excretion in the feces. Absorption of mesalamine is similar in fasted and fed subjects. The absorbed mesalamine is rapidly acetylated in the gut mucosal wall and by the liver. It is excreted mainly by the kidney as N-acetyl-5-amino-salicylic acid.

Mesalamine from orally administered mesalamine tablets appears to be more extensively absorbed than the mesalamine released from sulfasalazine. Maximum plasma levels of mesalamine and N-acetyl-5-aminosalicylic acid following multiple mesalamine doses are about 1.5 to 2 times higher than those following an equivalent dose of mesalamine in the form of sulfasalazine. Combined mesalamine and N-acetyl-5-aminosalicylic acid AUC's and urine dose recoveries following multiple doses of delayed- release tablets are about 1.3 to 1.5 times higher than those following an equivalent dose of mesalamine in the form of sulfasalazine.

The t_{max} for mesalamine and its metabolite, N-acetyl-5-aminosalicylic acid, is usually delayed, reflecting the delayed release, and ranges from 4 to 12 hours. The half-lives elimination ($t1/2_{elm}$) for mesalamine and N-acetyl-5-aminosalicylic acid are usually about 12 hours, but are variable ranging from 2 to 15 hours. There is a large intersubject variability in the plasma concentrations of mesalamine and N-acetyl-5-aminosalicylic acid and in their elimination half-lives following administration of mesalamine tablets.

HUMAN PHARMACOKINETICS AND METABOLISM

Absorption: Controlled-Release Capsules: Mesalamine is an ethylcellulose-coated, controlled-release formulation of mesalamine designed to release therapeutic quantities of mesalamine throughout the gastrointestinal tract. Based on urinary excretion data, 20% to 30% of the mesalamine in mesalamine is absorbed. In contrast, when mesalamine is administered orally as an unformulated 1-g aqueous suspension, mesalamine is approximately 80% absorbed.

Plasma mesalamine concentration peaked at approximately 1 mcg/ml 3 hours following a 1-g mesalamine capsule dose and declined in a biphasic manner. The literature describes a mean terminal half-life of 42 minutes for mesalamine following intravenous administration. Because of the continuous release and absorption of mesalamine from mesalamine throughout the gastrointestinal tract, the true elimination half-life cannot be determined after oral administration. N-acetylmesalamine, the major metabolite of mesalamine, peaked at approximately 3 hours at 1.8 mcg/ml, and its concentration followed a biphasic decline. Pharmacological activities of N-acetylmesalamine are unknown, and other metabolites have not been identified.

Oral mesalamine pharmacokinetics were nonlinear when mesalamine capsules were dosed from 250 mg to 1 g four times daily, with steady-state mesalamine plasma concentrations increasing about nine times, from 0.14 mcg/ml to 1.21 mcg/ml, suggesting saturable first-pass metabolism. N-acetylmesalamine pharmacokinetics were linear.

Elimination: About 130 mg free mesalamine was recovered in the feces following a single 1-g mesalamine dose, which was comparable to the 140 mg of mesalamine recovered from the molar equivalent sulfasalazine tablet dose of 2.5 g. Elimination of free mesalamine and salicylates in feces increased proportionately with a mesalamine dose. N-acetylmesalamine was the primary compound excreted in the urine (19% to 30%) following mesalamine dosing.

CLINICAL STUDIES:

Suppositories: Two double-blind-placebo-controlled multicenter studies were conducted in North America in patients with active ulcerative proctitis. The primary measures of efficacy were the same in both trials. The main difference between the two studies was the dosage regimen: 500 mg three times daily (1.5 g/d) in Study 1 and 500 mg twice daily (1.0 g/d) in Study 2. A total of 173 patients were studied (Study 1, N=79; Study 2, N=94). Patients were evaluated clinically and sigmoidoscopically after three and six weeks of suppository treatment.

Compared to placebo, mesalamine suppository treatment was statistically ($p < .01$) superior in both trials with respect to stool frequency, rectal bleeding, mucosal appearance, disease severity and overall disease activity after both three and six weeks of treatment. Daily diary records indicated significant improvement in rectal bleeding in the first week of therapy while tenesmus and diarrhea improved significantly within two weeks. Investigators rated patients much improved in 84% and 79% with mesalamine in Studies 1 and 2, respectively compared to 41% and 26% with placebo ($p < .001$, $p < .001$).

Normalization of rectal mucosa was achieved by 62% and 60% of mesalamine treated patients in Studies 1 and 2 compared to 25% and 10% of placebo-treated patients ($p < .001$, $p < .001$). The effectiveness of mesalamine suppositories was statistically significant irrespective of sex, extent of proctitis, duration of current episode or duration of disease. Overall the efficacy demonstrated with the twice daily regimen (Study 2) was comparable to that observed with three time daily dosing (Study 1).

EFFICACY

Rectal Suspension Enema: In a placebo-controlled, international, multicenter trial of 153 patients with active distal ulcerative colitis, proctosigmoiditis or proctitis, mesalamine suspension enema reduced the overall disease activity index (DAI) and individual components as follows (TABLE 1):

Differences between mesalamine and placebo were also statistically different in subgroups of patients on concurrent sulfasalazine and in those having an upper disease boundary between 5 and 20 or 20 and 40 cm. Significant differences between mesalamine and placebo were not achieved in those subgroups of patients on concurrent prednisone or with an upper disease boundary between 40 and 50 cm.

Delayed-Release Tablets: Two placebo-controlled studies have demonstrated the efficacy of mesalamine tablets in patients with mildly to moderately active ulcerative colitis. In one randomized, double-blind, multicenter trial of 158 patients. Mesalamine doses of 1.6 g/day and 2.4 g/day were compared to placebo. At the dose of 2.4 g/day, mesalamine tablets reduced the disease activity, with 21 of 43 (49%) mesalamine patients showing improvement in sigmoidoscopic appearance of the bowel compared to 12 of 44 (27%) placebo patients ($p=0.048$). In addition, significantly more patients in the mesalamine 2.4 g/day group showed improvement in rectal bleeding and stool frequency. The 1.6 g/day dose did not produce consistent evidence of effectiveness.

In a second randomized, double-blind, placebo-controlled clinical trial of 6 weeks duration in 87 ulcerative colitis patients, mesalamine tablets, at a dose of 4.8 g/day, gave sigmoidoscopic improvement in 28 of 38 (74%) patients compared to 10 of 38 (26%) placebo patients ($p < 0.001$). Also, more patients in the mesalamine 4.8 g/day group showed improvement in overall symptoms.

CLINICAL STUDIES: *(cont'd)*

TABLE 1 EFFECT OF TREATMENT ON SEVERITY OF DISEASE DATA FROM U.S.-CANADA TRIAL COMBINED RESULTS OF EIGHT CENTERS
Activity Indices, Mean

		n	Baseline	Day 22	End Point	Change Baseline to End-Point†
Overall DAI	Mesalamine	76	7.42	4.05**	3.37***	-55.07%***
	Placebo	77	7.40	6.03	5.83	-21.58%
Stool Frequency	Mesalamine		1.58	1.11*	1.01**	-0.57*
	Placebo		1.92	1.47	1.50	-0.41
Rectal Bleeding	Mesalamine		1.82	0.59***	0.51***	-1.30***
	Placebo		1.73	1.21	1.11	-0.61
Mucosal Inflammation	Mesalamine		2.17	1.22**	0.96***	-1.21**
	Placebo		2.18	1.74	1.61	-0.56
Physician's Assessment of Disease Severity	Mesalamine		1.86	1.13***	0.88***	-0.97***
	Placebo		1.87	1.62	1.55	-0.30

† Percent change for overall DAI only (calculated by taking the average of the change for each individual patient).
* Significant Mesalamine/placebo difference. p < 0.05
** Significant Mesalamine/placebo difference. p < 0.01
*** Significant Mesalamine/placebo difference. p < 0.001
Each parameter has a 4-point scale with a numerical rating: 0=normal, 1=mild, 2=moderate, 3-severe. The four parameters are added together to produce a maximum overall DAI of 12.

The effect of mesalamine on sulfasalazine-induced impairment of male fertility was examined in an open-label study. Nine patients (age <40 years) with chronic ulcerative colitis in clinical remission on sulfasalazine 2-3 g/day were crossed over to an equivalent mesalamine dose (0.8-1.2 g/day) for 3 months. Improvement in sperm count (p <0.02) and morphology (p <0.02) occurred in all cases. Improvement in sperm motility (p 0.001) occurred in 8 of the 9 patients.

Mesalamine Controlled-Release Capsules: In two randomized, double-blind, placebo-controlled, dose-response trials (UC-1 and UC-2) of 625 patients with active mild to moderate ulcerative colitis, mesalamine, at an oral dose of 4 g/day given 1 g four times daily, produced consistent improvement in prospectively identified primary efficacy parameters, PGA, Tx F, and SI as shown in the table below. (TABLE 2)

TABLE 2

Parameter Evaluated	Clinical Trial UC-1 PL (n=90)	Clinical Trial UC-1 Mesalamine 4 g/day (n=95)	Clinical Trial UC-1 Mesalamine 2 g/day (n=97)	Clinical Trial UC-2 PL (n=83)	Clinical Trial UC-2 Mesalamine 4 g/day (n=85)	Clinical Trial UC-2 Mesalamine 2 g/day (n=83)
PGA	36%	59%*	57%*	31%	55%*	41%
Tx F	22%	9%*	18%	31%	9%*	17%*
SI	-2.5	-5.0*	-4.3*	-1.6	-3.8*	-2.6
Remission†	12%	26%*	24%*	12%	27%*	12%

* p < 0.05 vs. placebo.
PGA: (Physician Global Assessment) - proportion of patients with complete or marked improvement.
TxF: Treatment Failure - proportion of patients developing severe or fulminant UC requiring steroid therapy or hospitalization or worsening of the disease at 7 days of therapy, or lack of significant improvement by 14 days of therapy.
SI: Sigmoidscopic Index - an objective measure of disease activity rated by a standard (15-point) scale that includes mucosal vascular pattern, erythema, friability, granularity/ulcerations, and mucopus: improvement over baseline.
†Defined as complete resolution of symptoms plus improvement of endoscopic endpoints. To be considered in remission, patients had a "1" score for one of the endoscopic components (mucosal vascular pattern, erythema, granularity, or friability) and "0" for the others.

INDICATIONS AND USAGE:

Rectal Enema/Suppository: Mesalamine suspension enema is indicated for the treatment of active mild to moderate distal ulcerative colitis, proctosigmoiditis or proctitis.

Mesalamine suppositories are indicated for the treatment of active ulcerative proctitis.

Delayed-Release Tablets and Controlled-Release Capsules: Mesalamine is indicated for the induction of remission and for the treatment of patients with mildly to moderately active ulcerative colitis.

CONTRAINDICATIONS:

Rectal Enema/Suppository: Mesalamine suspension enema is contraindicated for patients known to have hypersensitivity to the drug or any component of this medication.

Mesalamine suppositories are contraindicated for patients known to have hypersensitivity to mesalamine (5-aminosalicylic acid) or to the suppository vehicle [saturated vegetable fatty acid esters (Hard Fat, NF)].

Delayed-Release Tablets and Controlled-Release Capsules: Both of these forms are contraindicated in patients who have demonstrated hypersensitivity to mesalamine, any other components of this medication, or salicylates.

WARNINGS:

Rectal Suspension Enema: Mesalamine suspension enema contains potassium metabisulfite, a sulfite that may cause allergic-type reactions including anaphylactic symptoms and life-threatening or less severe asthmatic episodes in certain susceptible people. The overall prevalence of sulfite sensitivity in the general population is unknown but probably low. Sulfite sensitivity is seen more frequently in asthmatic or in atopic nonasthmatic persons. Epinephrine is the preferred treatment for serious allergic or emergency situations even though epinephrine injection contains sodium or potassium metabisulfite with the above-mentioned potential liabilities. The alternatives to using epinephrine in a life-threatening situation may not be satisfactory. The presence of a sulfite(s) in epinephrine injection should not deter the administration of the drug for treatment of serious allergic or other emergency situations.

Suppositories: None

PRECAUTIONS:

Rectal Suspension Enema/Suppository: Mesalamine has been implicated in the production of an acute intolerance syndrome characterized by cramping, acute abdominal pain and bloody diarrhea, sometimes, fever, headache and a rash; in such cases prompt withdrawal is required. The patients's history of sulfasalazine intolerance, if any, should be re-evaluated. If a rechallenge is performed later in order to validate the hypersensitivity, it should be carried out under close supervision and only if clearly needed, given consideration to reduced dosage.

PRECAUTIONS: *(cont'd)*

In the literature, one patient previously sensitive to sulfasalazine was rechallenged with 400 mg oral mesalamine within eight hours she experienced headache, fever, intensive abdominal colic, profuse diarrhea and was readmitted as an emergency. She responded poorly to steroid therapy and two weeks later a pancolectomy was required.

Rectal Suspension Enema: Although renal abnormalities were not noted in the clinical trials with mesalamine suspension enema, the possibility of increased absorption of mesalamine and concomitant renal tubular damage as noted in the preclinical studies must be kept in mind. Patients on mesalamine suspension enema, especially those on concurrent oral products which liberate mesalamine and those with preexisting renal disease, should be carefully monitored with urinalysis, BUN and creatinine studies.

In a clinical trial most patients who were hypersensitive to sulfasalazine were able to take mesalamine enemas without evidence of any allergic reaction. Nevertheless, caution should be exercised when mesalamine is initially used in patients known to be allergic to sulfasalazine. There patients should be instructed to discontinue therapy if signs of rash or fever become apparent.

While using mesalamine suspension enema some patients have developed pancolitis. However, extension of upper disease boundary and/or flare-ups occurred less often in the mesalamine-treated group than in the placebo-treated group.

Rare instances of pericarditis have been reported with mesalamine containing products including sulfasalazine. Cases of pericarditis have also been reported as manifestations of inflammatory bowel disease. In the cases reported with mesalamine rectal suspension enema there have been positive rechallenges with mesalamine or mesalamine containing products. In one of these cases, however, a second rechallenge with sulfasalazine was negative throughout a 2 month follow-up. Chest pain or dyspnea in patients treated with mesalamine should be investigated with this information in mind. Discontinuation of mesalamine may be warranted in some cases, but rechallenge with mesalamine can be performed under careful clinical observation should the continued therapeutic need for mesalamine be present.

Suppositories: The possibility of increased absorption of mesalamine and concomitant tubular damage as noted in the preclinical studies must be kept in mind. Patients of mesalamine suppositories, especially those on concurrent oral products which liberate mesalamine and those with preexisting renal disease, should be carefully monitored with urinalysis, BUN and creatinine studies.

In a clinical trial most patients who were hypersensitive to sulfasalazine were able to take mesalamine rectally without evidence of any allergic reaction.

Nevertheless, caution should be exercised when mesalamine is initially used in patients known to be allergic to sulfasalazine. These patients should be instructed to discontinue therapy if signs of rash or fever become apparent.

While using mesalamine suppositories a few patients have developed pancolitis. However, extension of upper disease boundary and/or flare-ups occurred less often in the mesalamine-treated group than in the placebo- treated group.

Rare instances of pericarditis have been reported with mesalamine containing products including sulfasalazine. Cases of pericarditis have also been reported as manifestations of inflammatory bowel disease. In the cases reported (with mesalamine enema) there have been positive rechallenges with mesalamine or mesalamine containing products. In one of these cases, however, a second rechallenge with sulfasalazine was negative throughout a 2 month follow-up. Chest pain or dyspnea in patients treated with mesalamine should be investigated with this information in mind. Discontinuation of mesalamine may be warranted in some cases, but rechallenge with mesalamine can be performed under careful observation should the continued therapeutic need for mesalamine be present.

Delayed-Release Tablets: Patients with pyloric stenosis may have prolonged gastric retention of mesalamine which delay release of mesalamine in the colon.

Exacerbation of the symptoms of colitis, thought to have been caused by mesalamine or sulfasalazine has been reported in 3% of patients in controlled clinical trials. This acute reaction, characterized by cramping, abdominal pain, bloody diarrhea, and occasionally by fever, headache, malaise, pruritus, rash, and conjunctivitis, has been reported after the initiation of mesalamine tablets as well as other mesalamine products. Symptoms usually abate when mesalamine tablets are discontinued.

Some patients who have experienced a hypersensitivity reaction to sulfasalazine may have a similar reaction to mesalamine tablets or to other compounds which contain or are converted to mesalamine.

Controlled-Release Tablets: Caution should be exercised if mesalamine is administered to patients with impaired hepatic function.

Mesalamine has been associated with an acute intolerance syndrome that may be difficult to distinguish from a flare of inflammatory bowel disease. Although the exact frequency of occurrence cannot be ascertained, it has occurred in 3% of patients in controlled clinical trials of mesalamine or sulfasalazine. Symptoms include cramping, acute abdominal pain and bloody diarrhea, sometimes fever, headache, and rash. If acute intolerance syndrome is suspected, prompt withdrawal is required. If a rechallenge is performed later in order to validate the hypersensitivity, it should be carried out under close medical supervision at reduced dose and only if clearly needed.

CARCINOGENESIS, MUTAGENESIS, IMPAIRMENT OF FERTILITY

Rectal Suspension Enema and Suppositories: Mesalamine caused no increase in the incidence of neoplastic lesions over controls in a two-year study of Wistar rats fed up to 320 mg/kg/day of mesalamine admixed with diet. Mesalamine is not mutagenic to Salmonella typhimurium tester strains TA98, TA100, TA1535, TA1537, TA1538. There are no reverse mutations in an assay using E. coli strain WP2UVRA. There were no effects in an *in vivo* mouse moicronucleus assay at 600 mg/kg and in an *in vivi* sister chromatid exchange at doses up to 610 mg/kg. No effects on fertility were observed in rats receiving up to 320 mg/kg/day. The oligospermia and infertility in men associated with sulfasalazine have not been reported with mesalamine.

Delayed-Release Tablets Long-term studies in animals have not been performed to evaluate the carcinogenicity potential of mesalamine. Mesalamine was not mutagenic in fluctuation assay in *K. pneumoniae* and Ames assay in *S. typhimurium*. Mesalamine, at oral doses up to 480 mg/kg/day, had no adverse effect on fertility or reproductive performance of male and female rats. The oligospermia and infertility in men associated with sulfasalazine have not been reported with mesalamine delayed-release tablets.

Controlled-Release Capsules Long-term studies of carcinogenic potential of mesalamine in mice and rats are ongoing. No evidence of mutagenicity was observed in an *in vitro* Ames test and in an *in vivo* mouse micronucleus test. No effects on fertility or reproductive performance were observed in male or female rats at doses up to 400 mg/kg/day (2360 mg/M^2). For a 50-kg person (1.3 M^2 body surface area), this represents five times the recommended clinical dose (80 mg/kg/day) on a mg/kg basis and 0.8 times the clinical dose (2960 mg/M^2) on body surface area basis.

Semen abnormalities and infertility in men, which have been reported in association with sulfasalazine, have not been seen with mesalamine capsules during controlled clinical trials.

PRECAUTIONS: *(cont'd)*

PREGNANCY, TERATOGENIC EFFECTS, PREGNANCY CATEGORY B

Rectal Suspension Enema: Teratogenic studies have been performed in rats and rabbits at oral doses up to five and eight times respectively, the maximum recommended human dose, and have revealed no evidence of harm to the embryo or fetus. There are, however, no adequate and well controlled studies in pregnant women for either sulfasalazine or 5-ASA. Because animal reproduction studies are not always predictive of human response, 5-ASA should be used during pregnancy only if clearly needed.

Suppositories: Teratologic studies have been performed in rats and rabbits at oral doses up to ten and sixteen times respectively, the maximum recommended human rectal suppository dose, and have revealed no evidence of harm to the embryo or fetus.

There are, however, no adequate and well-controlled studies in pregnant women. Because animal reproduction studies are not always predictive of human response, this drug should be used during pregnancy only if clearly needed.

Delayed-Release Tablets: Reproduction studies in rats and rabbits at oral doses up to 480 mg/kg/day have revealed no evidence of teratogenic effects or fetal toxicity due to mesalamine. There are, however, no adequate and well-controlled studiies in pregnant women. Because animal production studies are not always predictive of human response, this drug should be used during pregnancy only if clearly needed.

Controlled-Release Capsules: Reproduction studies have been performed in rats at doses up to 1000 mg/kg/day (5900 mg/M^2) and rabbits at doses of 800 mg/kg/day (6856 mg/M^2) and have revealed no evidence of teratogenic effects or harm to the fetus due to mesalamine. There are, however, no adequate and well-controlled studies in pregnant women. Because animal reproduction studies are not always predictive of human response, mesalamine should be used during pregnancy only if clearly needed.

Mesalamine is known to cross the placental barrier.

NURSING MOTHERS

Rectal Suspension Enema and Suppositories: It is not known whether mesalamine or its metabolite(s) are excreted in human milk. As a general rule, nursing should not be undertaken while a patient is on a drug since many drugs are excreted in human milk.

Delayed-Release Tablets: Low concentrations of mesalamine and higher concentrations of its N-acetyl metabolite have been detected in human breast milk. While the clinical significance of this has not been determined, caution should be exercised when mesalamine is administered to a nursing woman.

Controlled-Release Capsules: Minute quantities of mesalamine were distributed to breast milk and amniotic fluid of pregnant women following sulfasalazine therapy. When treated with sulfasalazine at a dose equivalent to 1.25 g/day of mesalamine, 0.02 mcg/ml to 0.08 mcg/ml and trace amounts of mesalamine were measured in amniotic fluid and breast milk, respectively. N-acetylmesalamine, in quantities of 0.07 mcg/ml to 0.77 mcg/ml and 1.13 mcg/ml to 3.44 mcg/ml, was identified in the same fluids, respectively.

Caution should be exercised when mesalamine is administered to a nursing woman.

PEDIATRIC USE

All Forms: Safety and efficacy of mesalamine in pediatric patients have not been established.

RENAL

Delayed-Release Tablets: Renal impairment, including minimal change nephropathy, and acute and chronic interstitial nephritis, has been reported in patients taking mesalamine tablets as well as in patients taking other mesalamine products. In animal studies (rats, dogs), the kidneys is the principal target organ for toxicity. At doses of approximately 750-1000 mg/kg [15-20 times the administered recommended human dose (based on a 50 kg person) on a mg/kg basis and 3-4 times on a mg/m^2 basis], mesalamine causes renal papillary necrosis. **Therefore, caution should be exercised when using mesalamine or other compounds converted to mesalamine or its metabolites in patients with known renal dysfunction or history of renal disease. It is recommended that all patients have an evaluation of renal function prior to initiation of mesalamine tablets and periodically while on mesalamine therapy.**

Controlled-Release Capsules: Caution should be exercised if mesalamine is administered to patients with impaired renal function. Single reports of nephrotic syndrome and interstitial nephritis associated with mesalamine therapy have been described in the foreign literature. There have been rare reports of interstitial nephritis in patients receiving mesalamine. In animal studies, a 13-week oral toxicity study in mice and 13-week and 52-week oral toxicity studies in rats and cynomolgus monkeys have shown the kidney to be the major target organ of mesalamine toxicity. Oral daily doses of 2400 mg/kg in mice and 1150 mg/kg in rats produced renal lesions including granular and hyaline casts, tubular degeneration, tubular dilation, renal infarct, papillary necrosis, tubular necrosis, and interstitial nephritis. In cynomolgus monkeys, oral daily doses of 250 mg/kg or higher produced nephrosis, papillary edema, and interstitial fibrosis. Patients with preexisting renal disease, increased BUN or serum creatinine, or proteinuria should be carefully monitored.

INFORMATION FOR PATIENTS

Delayed-Release Tablets: Patients should be instructed to swallow the mesalamine tablets whole, taking care not to break the outer coating. The outer coating is designed to remain intact to protect the active ingredient and this ensure mesalamine availability for action in the colon. In 2-3% of patients in clinical studies, intact or partially intact tablets have been reported in the stool. If this occurs repeatedly, patients should contact their physician.

DRUG INTERACTIONS:

All Forms: There are no known drug interactions.

ADVERSE REACTIONS:

Rectal Suspension Enema: *Clinical Adverse Experience:* Mesalamine suspension enema is usually well tolerated. Most adverse effects have been mild and transient (TABLE 3).

In addition, the following adverse events have been associated with mesalamine and other mesalamine containing products: nephrotoxicity, pancreatitis, fibrosing, alveolitis and elevated liver enzymes. Cases of pancreatitis and fibrosing alveolitis have been reported as manifestations of inflammatory bowel disease as well.

Hair Loss: Mild hair loss characterized by "more hair in the comb" but no withdrawal from clinical trials has been observed in seven of 815 mesalamine patients but none of the placebo-treated patients. In the literature there are at least six additional patients with mild hair loss who received either mesalamine or sulfasalazine. Retreatment is not always associated with repeated hair loss.

Suppositories: Mesalamine suppository is usually well tolerated. Most adverse effects have been mild and transient. (TABLE 4)

In addition, the following adverse events have been associated with mesalamine and other mesalamine containing products: nephrotoxicity, pancreatitis, fibrosing alveolitis and elevated liver enzymes. Cases of pancreatitis and fibrosing alveolitis have been reported as manifestations of inflammatory bowel disease as well.

Delayed-Release Tablets: Mesalamine tablets have been evaluated in about 1830 inflammatory bowel disease patients (most patients with ulcerative colitis) in controlled and open-label studies. Adverse events seen in clinical trials with mesalamine tablets have generally been mild and reversible. In two short-term (6 weeks) placebo- controlled clinical studies

ADVERSE REACTIONS: *(cont'd)*

TABLE 3 ADVERSE REACTIONS OCCURRING IN MORE THAN 0.1% OF MESALAMINE SUSPENSION ENEMA-TREATED PATIENTS COMPARISON TO PLACEBO)

	MESALAMINE n = 815		PLACEBO n = 128	
SYMPTOM	n	%	n	%
Abdominal Pain/Cramps/Discomfort	66	8.10	10	7.81
Headache	53	6.50	16	12.50
Gas/Flatulence	50	6.13	5	3.91
Nausea	47	5.77	12	9.38
Flu	43	5.28	1	0.78
Tired/Weak/Malaise/Fatigue	28	3.44	8	6.25
Fever	26	3.19	0	0.00
Rash/Spots	23	2.82	4	3.12
Cold/Sore Throat	19	2.33	9	7.03
Diarrhea	17	2.09	5	3.91
Leg/Joint Pain	17	2.09	1	0.78
Dizziness	15	1.84	3	2.34
Bloating	12	1.47	2	1.56
Back Pain	11	1.35	1	0.78
Pain on Insertion of Enema Tip	11	1.35	1	0.78
Hemorrhoids	11	1.35	0	0.00
Itching	10	1.23	1	0.78
Rectal Pain	10	1.23	0	0.00
Constipation	8	0.98	4	3.12
Hair Loss	7	0.86	0	0.00
Peripheral Edema	5	0.61	11	8.59
UT/Urinary Burning	5	0.61	4	3.12
Rectal Pain/Soreness/Burning	5	0.61	3	2.34
Asthenia	1	0.12	4	3.12
Insomnia	1	0.12	3	2.34

TABLE 4 ADVERSE REACTIONS OCCURRING IN MORE THAN 1% OF MESALAMINE SUPPOSITORY TREATED PATIENTS (COMPARISON TO PLACEBO)

	MESALAMINE (N = 168)		PLACEBO (N = 84)	
SYMPTOM	N	%	N	%
Headache	11	6.5	10	11.9
Flatulence	6	3.6	6	7.1
Abdominal Pain	5	3.0	7	8.3
Diarrhea	5	3.0	5	6.0
Dizziness	5	3.0	2	2.4
Rectal Pain	3	1.8	0	0.0
Upper Resp. Infection	3	1.8	2	2.4
Acne	2	1.2	0	0.0
Asthenia	2	1.2	4	4.8
Colitis	2	1.2	0	0.0
Fever	2	1.2	0	0.0
Generalized Edema	2	1.2	1	1.2
Nausea	2	1.2	6	7.1
Rash	2	1.2	0	0.0

involving 245 patients, 155 of whom were randomized to mesalamine tablets, five (3.2%) of the mesalamine patients discontinued mesalamine therapy because of adverse events as compared to two (2.2%) of the placebo patients. Adverse reactions leading to withdrawal from mesalamine tablets included (each in one patient): diarrhea and colitis flare; dizziness, nausea, joint pain, and headache; rash, lethargy and constipation; dry mouth, malaise, lower back discomfort, mild disorientation, mild indigestion and cramping; headache, nausea, malaise, aching, vomiting, muscle cramps, a stuffy head, plugged ears, and fever.

Adverse events occurring at a frequency of 2% or greater in the two short-term, double-blind, placebo-controlled trials mentioned above are listed in TABLE 5. Overall, the incidence of adverse events seen with mesalamine tablets was similar to placebo.

TABLE 5 Frequency (%) of Common Adverse Events Reported inor Placebo in Double-Blind Controlled Studies Ulcerative Colitis Patients Treated with Mesalamine Tablets

	Percent of Patients with Adverse Events	
Event	Placebo (n=87)	Mesalamine tablets (n=152)
Headache	36	35
Abdominal pain	14	18
Eructation	15	16
Pain	8	14
Nausea	15	13
Pharyngitis	9	11
Dizziness	8	8
Asthenia	15	7
Diarrhea	9	7
Back pain	5	7
Fever	8	6
Rash	3	6
Dyspepsia	1	6
Rhinitis	5	5
Arthralgia	3	5
Vomiting	2	5
Constipation	1	5
Hypertonia	3	5
Flatulence	7	3
Flu syndrome	2	3
Chills	2	3
Colitis exacerbation	0	3
Chest pain	2	3
Peripheral edema	2	3
Myalgia	1	3
Pruritus	0	3
Sweating	1	3
Dysmenorrhea	3	3

Of these adverse events, only rash showed a consistently higher frequency with increasing mesalamine dose in these studies. In uncontrolled data, fever, flu syndrome, and headache also seemed dose-related.

In addition, the following adverse reactions were seen in 1-2% of the patients in the controlled studies: malaise, arthritis, increased cough, acne, and conjunctivitis.

ADVERSE REACTIONS: *(cont'd)*

Over 1800 patients have been treated with mesalamine tablets in clinical studies. In addition to the adverse events listed above, the following adverse events also have been reported in controlled clinical studies, open-label studies, or foreign marketing experience. The relationship of the reported events to mesalamine administration is unclear in many cases. Some complaints, including anorexia, joint pains, pyoderma gangrenosum, oral ulcers, and anemia could be part of the clinical presentation of inflammatory bowel disease.

Body as a Whole: Weakness neck pain, abdominal enlargement, facial edema, edema

Cardiovascular: Pericarditis (rare), myocarditis (rare), vasodilation, migraine

Digestive: Anorexia, hepatitis (rare), pancreatitis, gastroenteritis, gastritis, increased appetite, cholecystitis, dry mouth, oral ulcers, perforated peptic ulcer (rare), bloody diarrhea, tenesmus

Hematologic: Agranulocytosis (rare), thrombocytopenia, eosinophilia, leukopenia, anemia, lymphadenopathy

Musculoskeletal: Gout

Nervous: Anxiety, insomnia, depression, somnolence, emotional lability, hyperesthesia, vertigo, nervousness, confusion, paresthesia, tremor, peripheral neuropathy (rare), transverse myelitis (rare), Guillain-Barre syndrome (rare)

Respiratory/Pulmonary: Sinusitis, interstitial pneumonitis, asthma exacerbation

Skin: Alopecia, psoriasis (rare), pyoderma gangrenosum (rare), dry skin, erythema nodosum, urticaria

Special Senses: Ear pain, eye pain, taste perversion, blurred vision, tinnitus

Urogenital: Interstitial nephritis (see also PRECAUTIONS, Renal), minimal change nephropathy (see PRECAUTIONS, Renal), dysuria, urinary urgency, hematuria, epididymitis, menorrhagia

Laboratory Abnormalities: Elevated AST (SGPT) or ALT (SGOT), elevated alkaline phosphatase, elevated serum creatinine and BUN

Hepatitis has been reported to occur rarely with mesalamine tablets. More commonly, asymptomatic elevations of liver enzymes have occurred which usually resolve during continued use or with discontinuation of the drug.

Controlled-Release Capsules: In combined domestic and foreign clinical trials, more than 2100 patients with ulcerative colitis or Crohn's disease received mesalamine therapy. Generally, mesalamine therapy was well tolerated. The most common events (*i.e.*, greater than or equal to 1%) were diarrhea (3.4%), headache (2.0%), nausea (1.8%), abdominal pain (1.7%), dyspepsia (1.6%), vomiting (1.5%), and rash (1.0%).

In two domestic placebo-controlled trials involving over 600 ulcerative colitis patients, adverse events were fewer in mesalamine-treated patients than in the placebo group (mesalamine 14% vs placebo 18%) and were not dose-related. Events occurring at 1% or more are shown in TABLE 6 below. Of these, only nausea and vomiting were more frequent in the mesalamine group. Withdrawal from therapy due to adverse events was more common on placebo than mesalamine (7% vs 4%).

TABLE 6 Adverse Events Occurring in More Than 1% of Either Placebo or Mesalamine Patients in Domestic Placebo-controlled Ulcerative Colitis Trials (Mesalamine Comparison to Placebo)

Event	Mesalamine n=451	Placebo n=173
Diarrhea	16 (3.5%)	13 (7.5%)
Headache	10 (2.2%)	6 (3.5%)
Nausea	14 (3.1%)	—
Abdominal Pain	5 (1.1%)	7 (4.0%)
Melena (Bloody Diarrhea)	4 (0.9%)	6 (3.5%)
Rash	6 (1.3%)	2 (1.2%)
Anorexia	5 (1.1%)	2 (1.2%)
Fever	4 (0.9%)	2 (1.2%)
Rectal Urgency	1 (0.2%)	4 (2.3%)
Nausea and Vomiting	5 (1.1%)	—
Worsening of Ulcerative Colitis	2 (0.4%)	2 (1.2%)
Acne	1 (0.2%)	2 (1.2%)

Clinical laboratory measurements showed no significant abnormal trends for any test, including measurement of hematologic, liver, and kidney function.

The following adverse events, presented by body system, were reported infrequently (*i.e.*, less than 1%) during domestic ulcerative colitis and Crohn's disease trials. In many cases, the relationship to mesalamine has not been established.

Gastrointestinal: abnormal distention, anorexia, constipation, duodenal ulcer, dysphagia, eructation, esophageal ulcer, fecal incontinence, GGTP increase GI bleeding, increased alkaline phosphatase, LDH increase, mouth ulcer, oral moniliases, pancreatitis, rectal bleeding, SGOT increase, SGPT increase, stool abnormalities (color or texture change), thirst

Dermatological: acne, alopecia, dry skin, eczema, erythema nodosum, nail disorder, photosensitivity, pruritus, sweating, urticaria

Nervous System: depression, dizziness, insomnia, somnolence, paresthesia

Cardiovascular: palpitations, pericarditis, vasodilation

Other: albuminuria, amenorrhea, amylase increase, arthralgia, asthenia, breast pain, conjunctivitis, ecchymosis, edema, fever, hematuria, hypomenorrhea, Kawasaki-like syndrome, leg cramps, lichen planus, lipase increase, malaise, menorrhagia, metrorrhagia, myalgia, pulmonary infiltrates, thrombocythemia, thrombocytopenia, urinary frequency

One week after completion of an 8-week ulcerative colitis study, a 72-year old male, with no previous history of pulmonary problems, developed dyspnea. The patient was subsequently diagnosed with interstitial pulmonary fibrosis without eosinophilia by one physician and bronchiolitis obliterans with organizing pneumonitis by a second physician. A causal relationship between this event and mesalamine therapy has not been established.

Published case reports have described infrequent instances of pericarditis, fatal myocarditis, chest pain and T-wave abnormalities, hypersensitivity pneumonitis, pancreatitis, nephrotic syndrome, interstitial nephritis, or hepatitis while receiving mesalamine therapy.

DRUG ABUSE AND DEPENDENCY:

Delayed-Release Tablets: *Abuse:* None reported.

Dependency: Drug dependence has not been reported with chronic administration of mesalamine.

OVERDOSAGE:

Rectal Enema/Suppositories: There have been no documented reports of serious toxicity in man resulting from massive overdosing with mesalamine. Under ordinary circumstances, mesalamine absorption from the colon is limited.

Delayed-Release Tablets: One case of overdosage has been reported. A 3 year-old male ingested 2 grams of mesalamine tablets. He was treated with ipecac and activated charcoal. No adverse events occurred. Oral doses of mesalamine in mice and rats of 5000 mg/kg and 4595 mg/kg, respectively, cause significant lethality.

OVERDOSAGE: *(cont'd)*

Controlled-Release Capsules: Single oral doses of mesalamine up to 5 g/kg in pigs or a single intravenous dose of mesalamine at 920 mg/kg in rats were not lethal.

There is no clinical experience with mesalamine overdosage. Mesalamine is an aminosalicylate, and symptoms of salicylate toxicity may be possible, such as: tinnitus, vertigo, headache, confusion, drowsiness, sweating, hyperventilation, vomiting, and diarrhea. Severe intoxication with salicylates can lead to disruption of electrolyte balance and blood pH, hyperthermia, and dehydration.

Treatment of Overdosage: Since mesalamine is an aminosalicylate, conventional therapy for salicylate toxicity may be beneficial in the event of acute overdosage. This includes prevention of further gastrointestinal tract absorption by emesis and, if necessary, by gastric lavage. Fluid and electrolyte imbalance should be corrected by the administration of appropriate intravenous therapy. Adequate renal function should be maintained.

DOSAGE AND ADMINISTRATION:

Rectal Suspension Enema: The usual dosage of mesalamine suspension enema in 60 ml units is one rectal instillation (4 grams) once a day, preferably at bedtime, and retained for approximately eight hours. While the effect of Mesalamine (mesalamine) may been seen within three to twenty-one days, the usual course of therapy would be from three to six weeks depending on symptoms and sigmoidoscopic findings. Studies available to date have not assessed in mesalamine suspension enema will modify relapse rates after the 6-week short-term treatment.

Patients should be instructed to shake the bottle well to make sure the suspension is homogeneous. The patient should remove the protective sheath from the applicator tip. Holding the bottle at the neck will not cause any of the medication to be discharged. The position most often used is obtained by lying on the left side (to facilitate migration into the sigmoid colon); with the lower leg extended and the upper right leg flexed forward for balance. An alternative is the knee-chest position. The applicator tip should be gently inserted in the rectum pointing toward the umbilicus. A steady squeezing of the bottle will discharge most of the preparation. The preparation should be taken at bedtime with the objective of retaining it all night. Patient instructions are included with every seven units.

Store at controlled room temperature 15°-30°C (59°-86°F).

Suppositories: The usual dosage of mesalamine suppositories 500 mg is one rectal suppository 2 times daily. The suppository should be retained for one to three hours or longer, if possible, to achieve the maximum benefit. While the effect of mesalamine suppositories may be seen within three to twenty-one days, the usual course of therapy would be from three to six weeks depending on symptoms and sigmoidoscopic findings. Studies available to date have not assessed if mesalamine suppositories will modify relapse rates after the six-week short-term treatment.

Store at 19°-26°C (66°-79°F).

Delayed-Release Tablets: The usual dosage in adults is two 400-mg tablets to be taken three times a day for a total daily dose of 2.4 grams for a duration of 6 weeks.

Store at controlled room temperature (59°-86°F or 15°-30°C).

Controlled-Release Capsules: The recommended dosage for the induction of remission and the symptomatic treatment of mildly to moderately active ulcerative colitis is 1 g (4 mesalamine capsules) four times a day for a total daily dose of 4 g. Treatment duration in controlled trials was up to 8 weeks.

Store at controlled room temperature 59-86°F (15-30°C).

REFERENCES:

For a complete listing of references, please refer to the original package insert.

PATIENT PACKAGE INSERT:

Rectal Suspension Enema: *Patient Instructions:*

How to Use this Medication

BEST RESULTS ARE ACHIEVED IF THE BOWEL IS EMPTIED IMMEDIATELY BEFORE THE MEDICATION IS GIVEN

1. Remove the Bottles

a. Remove the bottles from the protective foil pouch by tearing or by using scissors being careful not to squeeze or puncture bottles. Mesalamine rectal suspension is an off-white to tan colored suspension. Once the foil-wrapped unit of seven bottles is opened, all enemas should be used promptly as directed by your physician. **Contents of enemas removed from the foil pouch may darken with time. Slight darkening will not affect potency, however, enemas with dark brown contents should be discarded.**

2. Prepare the Medication for Administration

a. Shake the bottle well to make sure that the medication is thoroughly mixed. *Note:* Mesalamine suspension enema may cause staining of garments, fabrics, painted surfaces, marble, granite, vinyl or other direct contact surfaces.

b. Remove the protective sheath from the applicator tip. Hold the bottle at the neck so as not cause any of the medication to be discharged.

3. Assume the Correct Body Position

a. Best results are obtained by lying on the left side with the left leg extended and the right leg flexed forward for balance.

b. An alternative to lying on the left side is the "knee-chest" position as shown on the original package insert.

4. Administer the Medication

a. Gently insert the lubricated applicator tip into the rectum to prevent damage to the rectal wall, pointed slightly toward the navel.

b. Grasp the bottle firmly, then tilt slightly so that the nozzle is aimed toward the back, squeeze slowly to instill the medication. Steady hand pressure will discharge most of the medication. After administering, withdraw and discard the bottle.

c. Remain in position for at least 30 minutes to allow thorough distribution of the medication internally. Retain the medication all night, if possible.

Suppositories: *Patient Instructions:*

1. Detach one suppository from strip of suppositories.
2. Hold suppository upright and carefully remove the foil wrapper.
3. Avoid excessive handling of suppository, which is designed to melt at body temperature.
4. Insert suppository completely into rectum with gentle pressure, pointed end first.

HOW SUPPLIED - EQUIVALENTS NOT AVAILABLE:

Capsule, Gelatin, Sustained Action - Oral - 250 mg

80's	$27.42	PENTASA, Hoechst Marion Roussel	00088-2010-80
240's	$82.38	PENTASA, Hoechst Marion Roussel	00088-2010-46

Enema - Rectal - 4 gm/60ml

60 ml x 7	**$67.76**	**ROWASA, Solvay Pharms**	**00032-1924-82**

HOW SUPPLIED - EQUIVALENTS NOT AVAILABLE: *(cont'd)*

Suppository - Rectal - 500 mg/supposit

12's	$37.80	ROWASA, Solvay Pharms	00032-1928-46
24's	$71.78	ROWASA, Solvay Pharms	00032-1928-24

Tablet, Enteric Coated - Oral - 400 mg

100's	$59.41	ASACOL, Procter Gamble Pharm	00149-0752-02

MESNA *(001743)*

CATEGORIES: Antineoplastics; Cancer; Detoxifying Agents; Drug Hypersensitivity; Orphan Drugs; Pregnancy Category B; FDA Class 1A ("Important Therapeutic Advantage"); FDA Approved 1988 Dec

BRAND NAMES: *Mesna*; **Mesnex**; *Mexan*; *Uromitexan* (Australia, Europe, Canada) *(International brand names outside U.S. in italics)*

FORMULARIES: BC-BS; Medi-Cal

DESCRIPTION:

Mesnex injection is a detoxifying agent to inhibit the hemorrhagic cystitis induced by ifosfamide (Ifex). The active ingredient mesna is a synthetic sulfhydryl compound designated as sodium-2-mercapto ethanesulfonate with a molecular formula of $C_2H_5NaO_3S_2$ and a molecular weight of 164.18. Its structural formula is as follows: HS-CH_2-CH_2-SO_3-Na.

Mesnex injection is a sterile preservative-free aqueous solution of clear and colorless appearance in clear glass ampules for intravenous administration. Mesnex injection contains 100 mg/ml mesna, 0.25 mg/ml disodium edetate and sodium hydroxide for pH adjustment. The solution has a pH range of 6.5-8.5.

CLINICAL PHARMACOLOGY:

Mesna was developed as a prophylactic agent to prevent the hemorrhagic cystitis induced by ifosfamide.

Analogous to the physiological cysteine-cystine system, following intravenous administration mesna is rapidly oxidized to its only metabolite, mesna disulfide (dimesna). Mesna disulfide remains in the intravascular compartment and is rapidly eliminated by the kidneys.

In the kidney, the mesna disulfide is reduced to the free thiol compound, mesna, which reacts chemically with the urotoxic ifosfamide metabolites (acrolein and 4 hydroxy-ifosfamide) resulting in their detoxification. The first step in the detoxification process is the binding of mesna to 4-hydroxy-ifosfamide forming a non-urotoxic 4-sulfoethylthioifosfamide. Mesna also binds to the double bonds of acrolein and other urotoxic metabolites.

After administration of an 800-mg dose the half-lives of mesna and dimesna in the blood are 0.36 and 1.17 hours, respectively. Approximately 32% and 33% of the administered dose was eliminated in the urine in 24 hours as mesna and dimesna, respectively. The majority of the dose recovered was eliminated within 4 hours. Mesna has a volume of distribution of 0.652 l/kg and a plasma clearance of 1.23 l/kg/hour.

Ifosfamide has been shown to have dose dependent pharmacokinetics in humans. At doses of 2 to 4 g, its terminal elimination half-life is about 7 hours. As a result, in order to maintain adequate levels of mesna in the urinary bladder during the course of elimination of the urotoxic ifosfamide metabolites, repeated doses of mesna are required.

Based of the pharmacokinetic profiles of mesna and ifosfamide as discussed above, mesna was given as bolus doses prior to ifosfamide and at 4 and 8 hours after ifosfamide administration. The hemorrhagic cystitis produced by ifosfamide is dose dependent. At a dose of 1.2 g/m^2 ifosfamide administered daily for 5 days, 16 to 26% of the patients who received conventional uroprophylaxis (high fluid intake, alkalinization if the urine and the administration of diuretics) developed hematuria (>50 rbc/hpf or macrohematuria). In contrast, none of the patients who received mesna together with the dose of ifosfamide developed hematuria. Higher doses of ifosfamide from 2 to 4 g/m^2 administered for three to five days, produced hematuria in 31 to 100% of the patients. When mesna was administered together with these doses of ifosfamide the incidence of hematuria was less than 7%.

INDICATIONS AND USAGE:

Mesna has been shown to be effective as a prophylactic agent in reducing the incidence of ifosfamide induced hemorrhagic cystitis.

CONTRAINDICATIONS:

Mesna is contraindicated in patients known to be hypersensitive to mesna or other thiol compounds.

WARNINGS:

Mesna has been developed as an agent to prevent ifosfamide induced hemorrhagic cystitis. It will not prevent or alleviate an of the other adverse reactions or toxicities associated with ifosfamide therapy.

Mesna does not prevent hemorrhagic cystitis in all patients. Up to 6% of patients treated with mesna have developed hematuria (>50 rbc/hpf or WHO grade 2 and above). As a result, a morning specimen of urine should be examined for the presence of hematuria (red blood cells) each day prior to ifosfamide therapy. If hematuria develops when mesna is given with Ifosfamide according to the recommended dosage schedule, depending on the severity of the hematuria, dosage reductions or discontinuation of ifosfamide therapy may be initiated.

In order to obtain adequate protection, mesna must be administered with each dose of ifosfamide as outlined in the DOSAGE AND ADMINISTRATION section. Mesna is not effective in preventing hematuria due to other pathological conditions such as thrombocytopenia.

PRECAUTIONS:

Laboratory Tests: A false positive test for urinary ketones may arise in patients treated with mesna injection. In this test, a red-violet color develops which, with the addition of glacial acetic acid, will return to violet.

Carcinogenesis, Mutagenesis and Impairment Fertility: No long term animal studies have been performed to evaluate the carcinogenic potential of mesna. The Ames *Salmonella typhimurium* test, mouse micronucleus assay and frequency of sister chromatid exchange and chromosomal aberrations in PHA stimulated lymphocytes in vitro assays revealed no mutagenic activity.

Pregnancy Category C: Reproduction studies in rats and rabbits with oral does up to 1000 mg/kg have revealed no harm to the fetus due to mesna. It is not known whether mesna can cause fetal harm when administered to a pregnant woman or can affect reproductive capacity. Mesna should be given to a pregnant woman only if the benefits clearly outweigh any possible risks.

Teratology studies in rats and rabbits have shown no effects.

PRECAUTIONS: *(cont'd)*

Nursing Mothers: It is not known whether mesna or dimesna are excreted in human milk. Because many drugs are excreted in human milk and because of the potential for adverse reactions in nursing infants, a decision should be made whether to discontinue nursing or discontinue the drug, taking into account the importance of the drug to the mother.

DRUG INTERACTIONS:

In vitro and *in vivo* animal tumor models have shown that mesna does not have any effect on the antitumor efficacy of concomitantly administered cytotoxic agents.

ADVERSE REACTIONS:

Because mesna is used in combination with ifosfamide and other chemotherapeutic agents with documented toxicities, it is difficult to distinguish the adverse reactions which may be due to mesna form those caused by the concomitantly administered cytostatic agents. As a result, the adverse reaction profile of mesna was determined in three Phase I studies (16 subjects) utilizing intravenous and oral administration and two controlled studies in which ifosfamide and mesna were compared to ifosfamide and standard prophylaxis.

In phase I studies in which IV bolus doses of 0.8 to 1.6 g/m^2 mesna administered as single or three repeated doses to a total of 10 patients, a bad taste in the mouth (100%) and soft stools (70%) were reported. At intravenous and oral bolus doses of 2.4 g/m^2 which are approximately 10 times the recommended clinical doses (0.24 g/m^2) headache (50%), fatigue (33%), nausea (33%), diarrhea (83%), limb pain (50%), hypotension (17%) and allergy (17%) have also been reported in the 6 patients who participated in the 6 patients who participated in this study.

In controlled clinical studies, adverse reactions which can be reasonably associated with mesna were vomiting, diarrhea and nausea.

OVERDOSAGE:

There is no known antidote for mesna injection.

DOSAGE AND ADMINISTRATION:

For the prophylaxis of ifosfamide induced hemorrhagic cystitis, mesna may be given on a fractionated dosing schedule of bolus intravenous injections as outlined below (TABLE 1).

Mesna is given as intravenous bolus injections in a dosage equal to 20% of the ifosfamide dosage (w/w) at the time of ifosfamide administration and 4 and 8 hours after each dose of ifosfamide. The total daily dose of mesna is 60% of the ifosfamide dose (TABLE 1).

TABLE 1 Mesna, DOSAGE AND ADMINISTRATION
The recommended dosing schedule is outlined below:

	0 Hours	4 Hours	8 Hours
Ifosfamide	1.2 g/m^2		
Mesna (Mesnex)	240 mg/m^2	240 mg/m^2	240 mg/m^2

In order to maintain adequate protection, this dosing schedule should be repeated on each day that ifosfamide is administered. When the dosage of ifosfamide is adjusted (either increased or decreased), the dose of mesna should be modified accordingly. When exposed to oxygen, mesna is oxidized to the disulfide, dimesna. As a result and unused drug remaining in the ampules after dosing should be discarded and new ampules used for each administration.

Preparation of Intravenous Solutions/Stability: For IV administration the drug can be diluted by adding the contents of a mesna ampule to any of the following fluids obtaining final concentrations of 20 mg mesna/ml fluid:

5% Dextrose Injection, USP

5% Dextrose and Sodium Chloride Injection, USP

0.9% Sodium Chloride Injection, USP

Lactated Ringers's Injection, USP

For example:

One ampule of mesna injection 200 mg/2 ml may be added to 8 ml, or

one ampule of mesna injection 400 mg/ml may be added to 16 ml of any of the solutions listed above to create a final concentration of 20 mg mesna/ml fluid.

Diluted solutions are chemically and physically stable for 24 hours at 25°C (77°F).

It is recommended that solutions of mesna be refrigerated and used within 6 hours.

Mesna is not compatible with cisplatin.

Parenteral drug products should be inspected visually for particulate matter and discoloration prior to administration.

HOW SUPPLIED:

Mesnex (mesna) Injection 100 mg/ml

200 mg Single Dose Ampule, Box of 15 Ampules of 2 ml (*color-ring coding:* turquoise/yellow)

400 mg Single Dose Ampule, Box of 15 Ampules of 4 ml (*color-ring coding:* blue/green)

1 g Single Dose Ampule, Box of 10 Ampules of 10 ml (*color-ring coding:* blue/green) Store at room temperature.

HOW SUPPLIED - EQUIVALENTS NOT AVAILABLE:

Injection, Solution - Intravenous - 1 gm/ampul

10 ml	$740.80	MESNEX, Mead Johnson	00015-3562-41

Injection, Solution - Intravenous - 100 mg/ml

10 ml	$143.06	MESNEX, Mead Johnson	00015-3563-02
10 ml x 10	$1430.64	MESNEX, Mead Johnson	00015-3563-03

Injection, Solution - Intravenous - 200 mg/ampul

2 ml	$222.24	MESNEX, Mead Johnson	00015-3560-41

Injection, Solution - Intravenous - 400 mg/ampul

4 ml	$444.46	MESNEX, Mead Johnson	00015-3561-41

MESORIDAZINE BESYLATE *(001744)*

CATEGORIES: Alcoholism; Antipsychotics/Antimanics; Anxiety; Behavior Problems; Central Nervous System Agents; Depression; Nausea; Nausea and Vomiting; Phenothiazine Tranquilizers; Phenothiazines; Psychotherapeutic Agents; Psychotic Disorders; Schizophrenia; Tension; Tranquilizers; Vomiting; FDA Approval Pre 1982

BRAND NAMES: *Mesorin*; **Serentil**
(International brand names outside U.S. in italics)

FORMULARIES: Aetna; Medi-Cal

COST OF THERAPY: $921.11 (Schizophrenia; Tablet; 50 mg; 3/day; 365 days)

DESCRIPTION:

Serentil, brand of mesoridazine, the besylate salt of a metabolite of thioridazine, is a phenothiazine tranquilizer which is effective in the treatment of schizophrenia, organic brain disorders, alcoholism and psychoneuroses. Mesoridazine is 10-(2(1-methyl-2-piperidyl) ethyl)-2-(methyl-sulfinyl)-phenothiazine (as the besylate).

TABLET, 10 MG FOR ORAL ADMINISTRATION

Active Ingredient: Mesoridazine (as the besylate), 10 mg. *Inactive Ingredients:* Acacia, carnuba wax, colloidal silicon dioxide, FD&C Red No. 40 aluminum lake, lactose, microcrystalline cellulose, povidone, sodium benzoate, starch, stearic acid, sucrose, talc, titanium dioxide, and other ingredients.

TABLET, 25 MG FOR ORAL ADMINISTRATION

Active Ingredient: Mesoridazine (as the besylate), 25 mg. *Inactive Ingredients:* Acacia, carnuba wax, colloidal silicon dioxide, FD&C Red No. 40 aluminum lake, lactose, microcrystalline cellulose, povidone, sodium benzoate, stearic acid, sucrose, talc, titanium dioxide, and other ingredients.

TABLET, 50 MG FOR ORAL ADMINISTRATION

Active Ingredient: Mesoridazine (as the besylate), 50 mg. *Inactive Ingredients:* Acacia, carnuba wax, colloidal silicon dioxide, FD&C Red No. 40 aluminum lake, gelatin, lactose, microcrystalline cellulose, povidone, sodium benzoate, starch, stearic acid, sucrose, talc, titanium dioxide, and other ingredients.

TABLET, 100 MG FOR ORAL ADMINISTRATION

Active Ingredient: Mesoridazine (as the besylate), 100 mg. *Inactive Ingredients:* Acacia, carnuba wax, colloidal silicon dioxide, FD&C Red No. 40 aluminum lake, gelatin, lactose, microcrystalline cellulose, povidone, sodium benzoate, starch, stearic acid, sucrose, talc, titanium dioxide, and other ingredients.

AMPULS, 1 ML FOR INTRAMUSCULAR ADMINISTRATION

Active Ingredient: Mesoridazine (as the besylate), 25 mg. *Inactive Ingredients :* Edetate disodium USP, 0.5 mg; sodium chloride, USP, 7.2 mg; Carbon dioxide gas (bone dry) q.s., water for injection USP, q.s. to 1 ml.

CONCENTRATE FOR ORAL ADMINISTRATION

Active Ingredient: Mesoridazine (as the besylate) 25 mg per ml. *Inactive Ingredients:* Alcohol, 0.61% by volume; citric acid, FD&C Red no. 40; flavors; methylparaben; propylparaben; purified water; sodium citrate; sorbitol.

CLINICAL PHARMACOLOGY:

Based upon animal studies, mesoridazine as with other phenothiazines, acts indirectly on reticular formation, whereby neuronal activity into reticular formation is reduced without affecting its intrinsic ability to activate the cerebral cortex. In addition, the phenothiazines exhibit at least part of their activities, through depression of hypothalamic centers. Neurochemically, the phenothiazines are thought to exert their effects by a central adrenergic blocking action.

INDICATIONS AND USAGE:

In clinical studies mesoridazine has been found useful in the following disease states:

Schizophrenia: Mesoridazine is effective in the treatment of schizophrenia. It substantially reduced the severity of emotional withdrawal, conceptual disorganization, anxiety, tension, hallucinatory behavior, suspiciousness and blunted affect in schizophrenic patients. As with other phenothiazines, patients refractory to previous medication may respond to mesoridazine.

Behavioral Problems in Mental Deficiency and Chronic Brain Syndrome: The effect of mesoridazine, was found to be excellent or good in the management of hyperactivity and uncooperativeness associated with mental deficiency and chronic brain syndrome.

Alcoholism: *Acute and Chronic:* Mesoridazine ameliorates anxiety, tension, depression, nausea and vomiting in both acute and chronic alcoholics without producing hepatic dysfunction or hindering the functional recovery of the impaired liver.

Psychoneurotic Manifestations: Mesoridazine reduces the symptoms of anxiety and tension, prevalent symptoms often associated with neurotic components of many disorders and benefits personality disorders in general.

CONTRAINDICATIONS:

As with other phenothiazines, mesoridazine is contraindicated in severe central nervous system depression or comatose states from any cause. Mesoridazine is contraindicated in individuals who have previously shown hypersensitivity to the drug.

WARNINGS:

Tardive Dyskinesia: Tardive Dyskinesia, a syndrome consisting of potentially irreversible, involuntary, dyskinetic movements may develop in patients treated with neuroleptic (antipsychotic) drugs. Although the prevalence of the syndrome appears to be highest among the elderly, especially elderly women it is impossible to rely upon prevalence estimates to predict, at the inception of neuroleptic treatment, which patients are likely to develop the syndrome. Whether neuroleptic drug products differ in their potential to cause tardive dyskinesia is unknown.

Both the risk of developing the syndrome and the likelihood that it will become irreversible are believed to increase as the duration of treatment and the total cumulative dose of neuroleptic drugs administered to the patient increase. However, the syndrome can develop, although much less commonly, after relatively brief treatment periods at low doses.

There is no known treatment for established cases of tardive dyskinesia, although the syndrome may remit, partially or completely, if neuroleptic treatment is withdrawn, Neuroleptic treatment, itself, however, may suppress (or partially suppress) the signs and symptoms of the syndrome and thereby may possibly mask the underlying disease process. The effect that symptomatic suppression has upon the long-term course of the syndrome is unknown.

Given these considerations, neuroleptics should be prescribed in a manner that is most likely to minimize the occurrence of tardive dyskinesia. Chronic neuroleptic treatment should generally be reserved for patients who suffer from a chronic illness that, 1) is known to respond to neuroleptic drugs, and, 2) for whom alternative, equally effective, but potentially less harmful treatments are *not* available or appropriate. In the patients who do require chronic treatment, the smallest dose and the shortest duration of treatment producing a satisfactory clinical response should be sought. The need for continued treatment should be reassessed periodically.

If signs and symptoms of tardive dyskinesia appear in a patient on neuroleptics, drug discontinuation should be considered. However, some patients may require treatment despite the presence of the syndrome.

(For further information about the description of tardive dyskinesia and its clinical detection, please refer to the sections on PRECAUTIONS, Information for the Patient and ADVERSE REACTIONS.)

WARNINGS: *(cont'd)*

Neuroleptic Malignant Syndrome (NMS): A potentially fatal symptom complex sometimes referred to as Neuroleptic Malignant Syndrome (NMS) has been reported in association with antipsychotic drugs. Clinical manifestations of NMS are hyperreflexia, muscle rigidity, altered mental status and evidence of autonomic instability (irregular pulse or blood pressure, tachycardia, diaphoresis, and cardiac dysrhythmias).

The diagnostic evaluation of patients with this syndrome is complicated. In arriving at a diagnosis, it is important to identify cases where the clinical presentation includes both serious medical illness (*e.g.,* pneumonia, systemic infection etc.) and untreated or inadequately treated extrapyramidal signs and symptoms (EPS). Other important considerations in the differential diagnosis include central anticholinergic toxicity, heat stroke, drug fever and primary central nervous system (CNS) pathology.

The management of NMS should include 1) immediate discontinuation of antipsychotic drugs and other drugs not essential to concurrent therapy, 2) intensive symptomatic treatment and medical monitoring, and 3) treatment of any concomitant serious medical problems for which specific treatments are available. There is no general agreement about specific pharmacological treatment regimens for uncomplicated NMS.

If a patient require antipsychotic drug treatment after recovery from NMS, the potential reintroduction of drug therapy should be carefully considered. The patient should be carefully monitored, since recurrences of NMS have been reported.

Where patients are participating in activities requiring complete mental alertness (*e.g.,* driving) it is advisable to administer the phenothiazines cautiously and to increase the dosage gradually.

Usage in Pregnancy: The safety of this drug in pregnancy has not been established; hence, it should be given only when the anticipated benefits to be derived from treatment exceed the possible risks to mother and fetus.

Usage in Children: The use of mesoridazine in children under 12 years of age is not recommended, because safe conditions for its use have not been established.

Attention should be paid to the fact that phenothiazines are capable of potentiating central nervous system depressants (*e.g.,* anesthetics, opiates, alcohol, etc.) as well as atropine and phosphorus insecticides.

PRECAUTIONS:

While ocular changes have not to date been related to mesoridazine one should be aware that such changes have been seen with other drugs of this class.

Because f possible hypotensive effects, reserve parenteral administration for bedfast patients or for acute ambulatory cases, and keep patient lying down for at least one-half hour after injection.

Leukopenia and/or agranulocytosis have been attributed to phenothiazine therapy. A single case of transient granulocytopenia has been associated with mesoridazine. Since convulsive seizures have been reported, patients receiving anticonvulsant medication should be maintained on that regimen while receiving mesoridazine.

Neuroleptic drugs elevate prolactin levels; the elevation persists during chronic administration. Tissue culture experiments indicate that approximately one-third of human breast cancers are prolactin dependent *in vitro,* a factor of potential importance if the prescription of these drugs is contemplated in a patient with a previously detected breast cancer. Although disturbances such as galactorrhea, amenorrhea, gynecomastia and impotence have been reported, the clinical significance of elevated serum prolactin levels is unknown for most patients.

An increase in mammary neoplasms has been found in rodents after chronic administration of neuroleptic drugs. Neither clinical studies nor epidemiologic studies conducted to date, however, have shown an association between chronic administration of these drugs and mammary tumorigenesis; the available evidence is considered too limited to be conclusive at this time.

Information for the Patient: Given the likelihood that some patients exposed chronically to neuroleptics will develop tardive dyskinesia, it is advised that all patients in whom chronic use is contemplated be given, if possible, full information about this risk.

ADVERSE REACTIONS:

Drowsiness and hypotension were the most prevalent side effects encountered. Side effects tended to reach their maximum level of serenity early with the exception of a few (rigidity and motoric effects) which occurred later in therapy.

With the exceptions of tremor and rigidity, adverse reactions were generally found among those patients who received relatively high doses early in treatment. Clinical data showed no tendency for the investigators to terminate treatment because of side effects.

Mesoridazine had demonstrated remarkably low incidence of adverse reactions when compared with other phenothiazine compounds.

Central Nervous System: Drowsiness, Parkinson's syndrome, dizziness, weakness, tremor, restlessness, ataxia, dystonia, rigidity, slurring, akathisia, motoric reactions (opisthotonos) have been reported.

Autonomic Nervous System: Dry mouth, nausea and vomiting, fainting, stuffy nose, photophobia, constipation and blurred vision have occurred in some instances.

Genitourinary System: Inhibition of ejaculation, impotence, enuresis, incontinence have been reported.

Skin: Itching, rash, hypertrophic papillae of the tongue and angioneurotic edema have been reported.

Cardiovascular System: Hypotension and tachycardia have been reported. EKG changes have occurred in some instances.)

Phenothiazine Derivatives: It should be noted that efficacy, indications, and untoward effects have varied with the different phenothiazines. The physician should be aware that the following have occurred with one or more phenothiazines and should be considered whenever one of these drugs is used.

Autonomic Reactions: Miosis, obstipation, anorexia, paralytic ileus.

Cutaneous Reactions: Erythema, exfoliative dermatitis, contact dermatitis.

Blood, Dyscrasias: Agranulocytosis, leukopenia, eosinophilia, thrombocytopenia, anemia, aplastic anemia, pancytopenia.

Allergic Reactions: Fever, laryngeal edema, angioneurotic edema, asthma.

Hepatotoxicity: Jaundice, biliary stasis.

Cardiovascular Effects: Changes in the terminal portion of the electro cardiogram, including prolongation of the Q-T interval, lowering and inversion of the T wave and appearance of a wave tentatively identified as a bifid T or a U wave, have been observed in some patients receiving the phenothiazine tranquilizers, including mesoridazine. To date, these appear to be due to altered repolarization and not related to myocardial damage. They appear to be reversible. While there is no evidence at present that these changes are in any way precursors of any significant disturbances o cardiac rhythm, it should be noted that sudden and unexpected deaths apparently due to cardiac arrest have occurred in patients previously

ADVERSE REACTIONS: *(cont'd)*

showing characteristic electrocardiographic changes while taking the drug. The use of periodic electrocardiograms has been proposed but would appear to be of questionable value as a predictive device. Hypotension, rarely resulting in cardiac arrest, has been noted.

Extrapyramidal Symptoms: Akathisia, agitation, motor restlessness, dystonic reactions, trismus, torticollis, opisthotonos, oculogyric crises, tremor, muscular rigidity, akinesia.

Tardive Dyskinesia: Chronic use of neuroleptics may be associated with the development of tardive dyskinesia. The salient features of this syndrome are described in the WARNINGS.

The syndrome is characterized by involuntary choreoathetoid movements which variously involve the face tongue, face, mouth, lips, or jaw (*e.g.*, protrusion of the tongue, puffing of cheeks, puckering of the mouth, chewing movements), trunk and extremities. The severity of the syndrome and the degree of impairment produced vary widely.

The syndrome may become clinically recognizable either during treatment, upon dosage reduction, or upon withdrawal of treatment. Movements may decrease in intensity and may disappear altogether if further treatment with neuroleptics is withheld. It is generally believed that reversibility is more likely after short rather than long-term neuroleptic exposure. Consequently, early detection of tardive dyskinesia is important. To increase the likely hood of detecting the syndrome at the earliest possible time, the dosage of Neuroleptic drug should be reduced periodically (if clinically X) and the patient observed for signs of the disorder. This maneuver is critical, for neuroleptic drugs may mask the signs of the syndrome.

Endocrine Disturbances: Menstrual irregularities, altered libido, gynecomastia, lactation, weight gain, edema. False positive pregnancy tests have been reported.

Urinary Disturbances: Retention, incontinence.

Others: Hyperpyrexia. Behavioral effects suggestive of a paradoxical reaction have been reported. These include excitement, bizarre dreams, aggravation of psychoses and toxic confusional states. More recently, a peculiar skin-eye syndrome has been recognized as a side effect following long-term treatment with phenothiazines. This reactions is marked by progressive pigmentation of areas of the skin or conjunctiva and/or accompanied by discoloration of the exposed sclera and cornea described as irregular or stellae in shape have also been reported. Systemic lupus erythematous-like syndrome.

DOSAGE AND ADMINISTRATION:

The dosage of mesoridazine, as in most medications, should be adjusted to the needs of the individual. The lowest effective dosage should always be used. When maximum response is achieved, dosage may be reduced gradually to a maintenance level.

Schizophrenia: For most patients, regardless of severity, a starting dose of 50 mg three times daily is recommended. The usual optimum total daily dose range is 100 - 400 mg per day.

Behavioral Problems in Mental Deficiency and Chronic Brain Syndrome: For most patients a starting dose of 25 mg three times daily is recommended. The usual optimum total daily dose range is 75 - 300 mg per day.

Alcoholism: For most patients the usual starting dose is 25 mg twice daily. The usual optimum total daily dose range is 50 - 200 mg per day.

Psychoneurotic Manifestations: For most patients the usual starting dose is 10 mg three times daily. The usual optimum total daily dose range is 30 - 150 mg per day.

Storage of Concentrate: Below 77°F. Protect from light. Dispense in amber glass bottles only.

The concentrate may be diluted with distilled water, acidified tap water, orange juice or grape juice.

Each dose should be so diluted just prior to administration. Preparation and storage of bulk dilutions is not recommended.

ANIMAL PHARMACOLOGY:

PHARMACOLOGY

Pharmacological studies in laboratory animals have established that mesoridazine has a spectrum of pharmacodynamic action typical of a major tranquilizer. In common with other tranquilizers it inhibits spontaneous motor activity in mice, prolongs thiopental and hexobarbital sleeping time in mice and produces spindles and block of arousal reaction in the EEG of rabbits. It is effective in blocking spinal reflexes in the cat and antagonizes d-amphetamine excitations and toxicity in grouped mice. It shows a moderate adrenergic blocking activity *in vitro* and *in vivo* and antagonizes 5-hydroxytryptamine *in vivo*. Intravenously administered, it lowers the blood pressure of anesthetized dogs. It has a weak antiacetylcholine effect *in vitro*.

The most outstanding activity of mesoridazine is seen in tests developed to investigate antiemotive activity of drugs. Such tests are those in which the rat reacts to acute or chronic stress by increased defecation (emotogenic defecation) or tests in which "emotional mydriasis" is elicited in the mouse by an electric shock. In both of these tests, mesoridazine is effective in reducing emotive reactions. Its ED_{50} in inhibiting emotogenic defecation in the rat is 0.053 mg/kg (subcutaneous administration). Mesoridazine has a potent antiemetic action.

The intravenous ED_{50} against apomorphine-induced emesis in the dog is 0.64 mg/kg. Mesoridazine, in common with other phenothiazines, demonstrates antiarrhythmic activity in anesthetized dogs.

Metabolic studies in the dog and rabbit with tritium labeled mesoridazine demonstrate that the compound is well absorbed from the gastrointestinal tract. The biological half-life of mesoridazine, these studies also suggest that biliary excretion is an important excretion route for mesoridazine and/or its metabolites.

TOXICITY STUDIES

TABLE 1 TOXICITY STUDIES

Acute LD_{50} (mg/kg): Route	Mouse	Rat	Rabbit	Dog
Oral	560 ± 62.5	644 ± 48	MLD = 800	MLD = 800
I.M.	-	509M 584F	405	-
I.V.	26 ± 0.08	-	-	-

Chronic toxicity studies were conducted in rats and dogs. Rats were administered mesoridazine orally seven days per week for a period of seventeen months in doses up to 160 mg/kg per day. Dogs were administered mesoridazine orally seven days per week for a period of thirteen months. The daily dosage of the drug was increased during the period of this test such the "top-dose" group received a daily dose of 120 mg/kg of mesoridazine for the last month of the study.

Untoward effects which occurred upon chronic administration of high dose-levels included:

Rats: Reduction of food intake, slowed weight gain, morphological changes in pituitary-supported endocrine organs, and melanin-like pigment deposition in renal tissues.

Dogs: Emesis, muscle tremors, decreased food intake and death associated with aspiration of oral-gastric contents into the respiratory system. Increased intrauterine resorptions were with mesoridazine in rats at 70 mg/kg and in rabbits at 125 mg/kg but not at 60 and 100 mg/kg, respectively. No drug related teratology was suggested by these reproductive studies.

ANIMAL PHARMACOLOGY: *(cont'd)*

Local irritation from the intramuscular injection of mesoridazine was of the same order of magnitude as with other phenothiazines.

HOW SUPPLIED - EQUIVALENTS NOT AVAILABLE:

Injection, Solution - Intramuscular - 25 mg/ml

1 ml x 20	$89.92	SERENTIL, Boehringer Pharms	00597-0027-02

Liquid - Oral - 25 mg/ml

120 ml	$48.84	SERENTIL, Boehringer Pharms	00597-0025-04

Tablet, Plain Coated - Oral - 10 mg

100's	$55.63	SERENTIL, Boehringer Pharms	00597-0020-01

Tablet, Plain Coated - Oral - 25 mg

100's	$74.58	SERENTIL, Boehringer Pharms	00597-0021-01

Tablet, Plain Coated - Oral - 50 mg

100's	$84.12	SERENTIL, Boehringer Pharms	00597-0022-01

Tablet, Plain Coated - Oral - 100 mg

100's	$103.02	SERENTIL, Boehringer Pharms	00597-0023-01

MESTRANOL; NORETHINDRONE *(001745)*

CATEGORIES: Contraceptives; Hormones; Ovarian Carcinoma; Pregnancy; Progestogen; Progestogen & Estrogen Combinations; Sales > $100 Million; FDA Approval Pre 1982

BRAND NAMES: *Anamai*; Genora; Micronor; Nelova; Norethin; **Norinyl**; *Norinyl-1* (Australia, England, Mexico); *Norinyl-1 28*; *Norinyl-1 28*; *Norinyl 1 50* (Canada); *Norinyl 1 +50*; *Norinyl-28* (Mexico); *Ortho-Novin*; *Ortho-Novin 1 50* (England); Ortho-Novum; *Ortho-Novum 1 50* (Germany, Canada)
(International brand names outside U.S. in italics)

FORMULARIES: Aetna; BC-BS; DoD; Foundation; Medi-Cal; PCS

COST OF THERAPY: $139.56 (Contraceptive; Tablet; 0.05 mg/1 mg; 1/day; 365 days) vs. Potential Cost of $2,351.94 (Pregnancy)

DESCRIPTION:

The chemical name for norethindrone is 17-hydroxy-19-nor-17α-pregn-4-en-20-yn-3-one. The chemical name for mestranol is 3-methoxy-19-nor-17α-pregna-1,3,5(10)-trien-20-yn-17-ol.

Ortho Novum 1/50: Each yellow tablet contains 1 mg of norethindrone and 0.05 mg of mestranol. Inactive ingredients include D&C Yellow No. 10, lactose, magnesium stearate and pregelitanized starch. Each green tablet in the Ortho-Novum 1/50 28 package contains only inert ingredients.

Norethin 1/50: Each white tablet contains 1 mg of norethindrone and 50 mcg of mestranol. Each blue tablet in the Norethin 1/50M-28 package is a placebo containg inert ingredients.

For prescribing information see Ethinyl Estradiol; Norethindrone.

HOW SUPPLIED - RATED THERAPEUTICALLY EQUIVALENT:

Tablet, Uncoated - Oral - 0.05 mg/1 mg

21's	$8.03	Norethindrone W/Mestranol, H.C.F.A. F F P	99999-1745-01
28's	$10.71	Norethindrone W/Mestranol, H.C.F.A. F F P	99999-1745-02
63 (3 x 21)	$52.50	Genora 1/50 21, Rugby	00536-4059-44
126 (6 x 21)	$72.00	Norethin 1/50, Roberts Labs	54092-0072-21
126 (6 x 21)	$90.30	NELOVA 1/50, Warner Chilcott	00047-0942-11
126 (6 x 21)	**$134.79**	**NORINYL 1/50 21, Syntex FP**	**42987-0100-23**
126 (6 x 21)	$138.84	ORTHO-NOVUM 1/50 21, Ortho Pharm	00062-1331-15
168 (6 x 28)	$72.00	Norethin 1/50, Roberts Labs	54092-0072-28
168 (6 x 28)	$90.30	NELOVA 1/50, Warner Chilcott	00047-0947-35
168 (6 x 28)	$105.00	Genora 1/50 28, Rugby	00536-4056-48
168 (6 x 28)	**$134.79**	**NORINYL 1/50 28, Syntex FP**	**42987-0101-24**
168 (6 x 28)	$139.62	ORTHO-NOVUM 1/50 28, Ortho Pharm	00062-1332-15
672 (24 x 28)	**$539.26**	**NORINYL 1/50 28, Syntex FP**	**42987-0101-61**

METAPROTERENOL SULFATE *(001747)*

CATEGORIES: Airway Obstruction; Analgesics; Antiasthmatics/Bronchodilators; Antitussives/Expectorants/Mucolytics; Asthma; Autonomic Drugs; Beta Adrenergic Stimulators; Bronchial Dilators; Bronchitis; Bronchospasm; Emphysema; Gastrointestinal Drugs; Respiratory & Allergy Medications; Sympathomimetic Agents; Sympathomimetics, Beta Agonist; Pregnancy Category C; FDA Approval Pre 1982

BRAND NAMES: *Alotec* (Japan); **Alupent**; *Alutin*; Arm-A-Med; Dey-Dose; Metaprel; *Nonasma*; Prometa
(International brand names outside U.S. in italics)

FORMULARIES: Aetna; BC-BS; CIGNA; FHP; Humana; Kaiser; Medco; Medi-Cal; PruCare; United

COST OF THERAPY: $95.81 (Asthma; Tablet; 20 mg; 3/day; 365 days)

PRIMARY ICD9: 493.90 (Asthma, Unspecified, Without Mention of Status Asthmaticus)

DESCRIPTION:

Metaproterenol sulfate USP 1-(3,5-dihydroxyphenyl)-2-isopropylaminoethanol sulfate, is a white, crystalline, racemic mixture of two optically active isomers. $(C_{11}H_{17}NO_3)_2 \cdot H_2SO_4$ The molecular weight is 520.59

Inhalation Aerosol: Alupent Inhalation Aerosol is a bronchodilator administered by oral inhalation. The metaproterenol sulfate inhalation aerosol containing 75 mg of metaproterenol sulfate as micronized powder is sufficient medication for 100 inhalations. The metaproterenol sulfate inhalation aerosol containing 150 mg of metaproterenol sulfate as micronized powder is sufficient medication for 200 inhalations. Each metered dose delivers through the mouthpiece 0.65 mg of metaproterenol sulfate (each ml contains 15 mg). The inert ingredients are dichlorodifluoromethane, dichlorotetrafluoroethane and trichloromonofluoromethane as propellants, and sorbitan trioleate.

Inhalation Solution: Alupent Inhalation Solution is a bronchodilator administered by oral inhalation via intermittent positive pressure breathing (IPPB) apparatus or nebulizer. It contains metaproterenol sulfate 5% in a pH-adjusted aqueous solution containing benzalkonium chloride and edetate disodium as preservatives.

It differs from isoproterenol hydrochloride by having two hydroxyl groups attached at the meta positions on the benzene ring rather than one at the meta and one at the para position.

DESCRIPTION: *(cont'd)*

Inhalation Solution Unit Dose Vial: Alupent Inhalation solution unit dose vial is a brBonchodilator administered by oral inhalation with the aid of an intermittent positive pressure breathing apparatus (IPPB). It contains metaproterenol sulfate 0.4% or 0.6% in a sterile pH adjusted aqueous solution with edetate disodium and sodium chloride.

It differs from isoproterenol hydrochloride by having two hydroxyl groups attached at the meta positions on the benzene ring rather than one at the meta and one at the para position.

Syrup: Alupent Syrup is an oral bronchodilator. Each teaspoonful (5 ml) of syrup contains 10 mg of metaproterenol sulfate. The inactive ingredients are edetate disodium, FD&C Red No. 40, hydroxyethylcellulose, imitation black cherry flavor, methylparaben, propylparaben, saccharin and sorbitol solution.

Tablets: Alupent in tablet form is an oral bronchodilator. Each tablet contains metaproterenol sulfate 10 mg or 20 mg. The inactive ingredients are colloidal silicon dioxide, corn starch, dibasic calcium phosphate, lactose, magnesium stearate.

CLINICAL PHARMACOLOGY:

INHALATION AEROSOL AND SYRUP

In vitro studies and *in vivo* pharmacologic studies have demonstrated that metaproterenol sulfate has a preferential effect on beta-2 adrenergic receptors compared with isoproterenol. While it is recognized that beta-2 adrenergic receptors are the predominant receptors in the bronchial smooth muscle, recent data indicate that there is a population of beta-2 receptors in the human heart existing in a concentration between 10-50%. The precise function of these, however, is not yet established (see WARNINGS).

INHALATION AEROSOL, INHALATION SOLUTION, SYRUP, AND TABLETS

The pharmacologic effects of beta adrenergic agonist drugs, including metaproterenol sulfate, are at least in part attributable to stimulation through beta adrenergic receptors of intracellular adenyl cyclase, the enzyme which catalyzes the conversion of adenosine triphosphate (ATP) to cyclic-3,5'- adenosine monophosphate (c-AMP). Increased c-AMP levels are associated with relaxation of bronchial smooth muscle and inhibition of release of mediators of immediate hypersensitivity from cells, especially from mast cells.

PHARMACOKINETICS

Inhalation Aerosol: Absorption, biotransformation and excretion studies in humans following administration by inhalation have shown that approximately 3 percent of the actuated dose is absorbed intact through the lungs. The major metabolite, metaproterenol-3-O-sulfate, is produced in the gastrointestinal tract. metaproterenol sulfate is not metabolized by catechol-O methyltransferase nor have glucuronide conjugates been isolated to date.

Inhalation Solution: Absorption, biotransformation and excretion studies following administration by inhalation have not been performed. Following oral administration of tablet and solution, an average of 40% of the drug was excreted as the unchanged drug and its major metabolite, a polar conjugate, metaproterenol-O-sulfate.

Inhalation Solution Unit Dose Vial: Absorption, biotransformation and excretion studies following administration by inhalation have not been performed. Following oral administration in humans, an average of 40% of the drug is absorbed; it is not metabolized by catechol-O-methyltransferase but is excreted primarily as glucuronic acid conjugates.

Syrup and Tablets: Absorption, biotransformation and excretion studies in humans following oral administration have indicated that an average of less than 10% of the drug is absorbed intact; it is not metabolized by catechol-O-methyltransferase nor converted to glucuronide conjugates but is excreted primarily as the polar sulfate conjugate, metaproterenol-3-0-sulfate, formed in the gut.

Inhalation Aerosol: Pulmonary function tests performed concomitantly usually show improvement following aerosol metaproterenol sulfate administration, e.g., an increase in the one-second forced expiratory volume (FEV_1), maximum expiratory flow rate, forced vital capacity, and/or a decrease in airway resistance. The resultant decrease in airway obstruction may relieve the dyspnea associated with bronchospasm.

Tablets: Pulmonary function tests performed after the administration of metaproterenol sulfate usually show improvement, e.g., an increase in the one-second forced expiratory volume (FEV_1), maximum expiratory flow rate, peak expiratory flow rate, forced vital capacity, and/or a decrease in airway resistance. The resultant decrease in airway obstruction may relieve the dyspnea associated with bronchospasm.

Syrup: Pulmonary function has been monitored in controlled single-and multiple-dose studies. The duration of effect of a single dose of metaproterenol sulfate syrup (that is, the period of time during which there is a 15% or greater increase in mean FEV_1) was up to 4 hours.

Inhalation Aerosol: Controlled single- and multiple-dose studies have been performed with pulmonary function monitoring. The duration of effect of a single dose of two to three inhalations of metaproterenol sulfate (that is, the period of time during which there is 20 percent or greater increase in FEV_1) has varied from 1 to 5 hours.

In repetitive-dosing studies (up to q.i.d.) the duration of effect for a similar dose of metaproterenol sulfate has ranged from about 1 to 2.5 hours. Present studies are inadequate to explain the divergence in duration of the FEV_1 effect between single- and repetitive-dosing studies, respectively.

Tablets: In controlled single- and multiple-dose studies in which 319 patients were treated with metaproterenol sulfate tablets (89 patients with 10 mg and 230 patients with 20 mg), a majority (65%) demonstrated improvements in pulmonary function defined as an increase of at least 15% in the one- second forced expiratory volume (FEV_1). For 54% the onset was within 30 minutes. The duration of effect persisted for at least four hours in 51% of those patients who demonstrated a response.

Inhalation Aerosol, Inhalation Solution, Inhalation Solution Unit Dose Vial, Syrup, and Tablets: Recent studies in laboratory animals (minipigs, rodents and dogs) recorded the occurrence of cardiac arrhythmias and sudden death (with histologic evidence of myocardial necrosis) when beta agonists and methylxanthines were administered concurrently. The significance of these findings when applied to humans is currently unknown.

Inhalation Solution and Inhalation Solution Unit Dose Vial: Following controlled single dose studies by an intermittent positive pressure breathing apparatus (IPPB) and by hand bulb nebulizers, significant improvement (15% or greater increase in FEV_1) occurred within 5 to 30 minutes and persisted for periods varying from 2 to 6 hours.

In these studies, the longer duration of effect occurred in the studies in which the drug was administered by IPPB, i.e., 6 hours versus 2 to 3 hours when administered by hand bulb nebulizer. In these studies the doses used were 0.3 ml by IPPB and 10 inhalations by hand bulb nebulizer.

In controlled repetitive dosing studies by IPPB and by hand bulb nebulizer the onset of effect occurred within 5 to 30 minutes and duration ranged from 4 to 6 hours. In these studies the doses used were 0.3 ml b.i.d. or t.i.d. when given by IPPB, and 10 inhalation q.i.d. (no more often than q4h) when given by hand bulb nebulizer. As in the single dose studies, effectiveness was measured as a sustained increase in FEV_1 of 15% or greater. In these repetitive dosing studies there was no apparent difference in duration between the two methods of delivery.

CLINICAL PHARMACOLOGY: *(cont'd)*

Clinical studies were conducted in which the effectiveness of metaproterenol sulfate inhalation solution was evaluated by comparison with that of isoproterenol hydrochloride over periods of two to three months. Both drugs continued to produce significant improvement in pulmonary function throughout this period of treatment.

In two well-controlled studies in children 6-12 years of age with acute exacerbation of asthma, 70% of patients receiving metaproterenol sulfate inhalation solution (0.1 ml-0.2 ml) showed improvement in pulmonary function as demonstrated by a 15% increase in FEV_1 above baseline.

INDICATIONS AND USAGE:

Inhalation Aerosol: Metaproterenol sulfate is indicated as a bronchodilator for bronchial asthma and for reversible bronchospasm which may occur in association with bronchitis and emphysema.

Inhalation Solution: Metaproterenol sulfate inhalation solution is indicated as a bronchodilator in the treatment of asthma and bronchitis or emphysema when a reversible component is present in adults and for the treatment of acute asthmatic attacks in children age 6 years and older.

Inhalation Solution Unit Dose Vial, Syrup, and Tablets: Metaproterenol sulfate inhalation solution, syrup, or tablets is indicated as a bronchodilator for bronchial asthma, and for reversible bronchospasm which may occur in association with bronchitis and emphysema.

CONTRAINDICATIONS:

Use in patients with cardiac arrhythmias associated with tachycardia is contraindicated.

Although rare, immediate hypersensitivity reactions and paradoxical bronchospasm can occur. Therefore, metaproterenol sulfate is contraindicated in patients with a history of hypersensitivity to any of its components.

WARNINGS:

Excessive use of adrenergic aerosols is potentially dangerous. Fatalities have been reported following excessive use of metaproterenol sulfate as with other sympathomimetic inhalation preparations, and the exact cause is unknown. Cardiac arrest was noted in several cases.

Controlled clinical studies and other clinical experience have shown that metaproterenol sulfate, like other beta-adrenergic agonists, can produce a significant cardiovascular effect in some patients, as measured by pulse rate, blood pressure, symptoms, and/or ECG changes.

Paradoxical bronchospasm has been reported after the use of inhaled sympathomimetic drugs and may be life threatening. If it occurs, the preparation should be discontinued immediately and alternative therapy instituted.

Paradoxical bronchoconstriction with repeated excessive administration has been reported with sympathomimetic agents.

metaproterenol sulfate should not be used more often than prescribed. Patients should be advised to contact their physicians in the event that they do not respond to their usual dose of sympathomimetic amine aerosol.

PRECAUTIONS:

GENERAL

Extreme care must be exercised with respect to the administration of additional sympathomimetic agents.

Since metaproterenol is a sympathomimetic amine, it should be used with caution in patients with cardiovascular disorders, including ischemic heart disease, hypertension or cardiac arrhythmias, in patients with hyperthyroidism or diabetes mellitus, and in patients who are unusually responsive to sympathomimetic amines or who have convulsive disorders. Significant changes in systolic and diastolic blood pressure could be expected to occur in some patients after use of any beta adrenergic bronchodilator.

Physicians should recognize that a single dose of nebulized metaproterenol sulfate inhalation solution in the treatment of acute asthma may alleviate symptoms and improve pulmonary function temporarily but fail to completely abort an attack.

INFORMATION FOR THE PATIENT

Extreme care must be exercised with respect to the administration of additional sympathomimetic agents. A sufficient interval of time should elapse prior to administration of another sympathomimetic agent.

Metaproterenol sulfate inhalation solution effects may last up to 6 hours or longer. It should not be used more often than recommended and the patient should not increase the number of inhalations or frequency of use without first consulting the physician. If symptoms of asthma get worse, adverse reactions occur, or the patient does not respond to the usual dose, the patient should be instructed to contact the physician immediately.

A single dose of nebulized metaproterenol sulfate inhalation solution in the treatment of an acute attack of asthma may not completely abort an attack.

Metaproterenol sulfate syrup or tablets should not be used more often than prescribed. If symptoms persist, patients should consult a physician promptly.

CARCINOGENESIS/MUTAGENESIS/IMPAIRMENT OF FERTILITY

Inhalation Aerosol: In an 18-month study in mice, metaproterenol sulfate produced an increase in benign ovarian tumors in females at doses corresponding to 320 and 640 times the maximum recommended dose (based on a 50 kg individual). In a two-year study in rats, a non-significant incidence of benign leiomyomata of the mesovarium was noted at 640 times the maximum recommended dose. The relevance of these findings to man is not known. Mutagenic studies with metaproterenol sulfate have not been conducted. Reproduction studies in rats revealed no evidence of impaired fertility.

Syrup and Tablets: In an 18-month study in mice, metaproterenol sulfate produced a significant increase in benign hepatic adenomas in males and benign ovarian tumors in females at doses corresponding to 31 and 62 times the maximum recommended dose (based on a 50 kg individual). In a two-year study in rats, a non-significant incidence of benign leiomyomata of the mesovarium was noted at 62 times the maximum recommended dose. The relevance of these findings to man is not known. Mutagenicity studies with metaproterenol sulfate have not been conducted. Reproduction studies in rats revealed no evidence of impaired fertility.

CARCINOGENESIS

Inhalation Solution and Inhalation Solution Unit Dose Vial: Long-term studies in mice and rats to evaluate the oral carcinogenic potential of metaproterenol sulfate have not been completed.

Studies of metaproterenol sulfate have not been conducted to determine mutagenic potential or effect on fertility.

PREGNANCY CATEGORY C

Inhalation Aerosol: Metaproterenol sulfate has been shown to be teratogenic and embryotoxic in rabbits when given in doses corresponding to 640 times the maximum recommended dose. These effects included skeletal abnormalities, hydrocephalus and skull bone separation. Results of other studies in rabbits, rats or mice have not revealed any teratogenic, em-

PRECAUTIONS: *(cont'd)*

bryocidal or fetotoxic effects. There are no adequate and well-controlled studies in pregnant women. metaproterenol sulfate should be used during pregnancy only if the potential benefit justifies the potential risk to the fetus.

Inhalation Solution and Inhalation Solution Unit Dose Vial: Metaproterenol sulfate has been shown to be teratogenic and embryocidal in rabbits when given orally in doses 620 times the human inhalation dose; the teratogenic effects included skeletal abnormalities and hydrocephalus with bone separation. Oral reproduction studies in mice, rats and rabbits showed no teratogenic or embryocidal effects at 50 mg/kg, corresponding or/to 310 times the human inhalation dose. There are no adequate and well-controlled studies in pregnant women. metaproterenol sulfate should be used during pregnancy only if the potential benefit justifies the potential risk to the fetus.

Syrup: metaproterenol sulfate has been shown to be teratogenic and embryotoxic in rabbits when given in doses corresponding to 62 times the maximum recommended dose. These effects included skeletal abnormalities, hydrocephalus and skull bone separation. Results of other studies in rabbits, rats or mice have not revealed any teratogenic, embryotoxic or fetotoxic effects. There are no adequate and well-controlled studies in pregnant women. metaproterenol sulfate should be used during pregnancy only if the potential benefit justifies the potential risk to the fetus.

Tablets: Metaproterenol sulfate has been shown to be teratogenic and embryotoxic in rabbits when given orally at doses of 100 mg/kg or 62 times the maximum recommended human oral dose. These effects included skeletal abnormalities, hydrocephalus and skull bone separation.

Embryotoxicity has also been shown in mice when given orally at doses of 50 mg/kg or 31 times the maximum recommended human oral dose. Results of other oral reproduction studies in rats (40 mg/kg) and rabbits (50 mg/kg) have not revealed any teratogenic, embryotoxic or fetotoxic effects. There are no adequate and well-controlled studies in pregnant women. metaproterenol sulfate should be used during pregnancy only if the potential benefit justifies the potential risk to the fetus.

NURSING MOTHERS

It is not known whether metaproterenol sulfate is excreted in human milk; therefore, metaproterenol sulfate should be used during nursing only if the potential benefit justifies the potential risk to the newborn. Because many drugs are excreted in human milk, caution should be exercised when metaproterenol sulfate is administered to a nursing woman.

PEDIATRIC USE

Inhalation Aerosol and Inhalation Solution Unit Dose Vial: Safety and effectiveness in children below the age of 12 have not been established. Studies are currently under way in this age group.

Inhalation Solution: Metaproterenol sulfate inhalation solution may be used in the treatment of acute attacks of asthma in children 6 years and older.

Syrup: Safety and effectiveness in children below the age of 6 have been demonstrated in a limited number of patients. See DOSAGE AND ADMINISTRATIONsection.

Tablets: Metaproterenol sulfate tablets are not recommended for use in children under six years of age because of insufficient clinical data to establish safety and effectiveness.

DRUG INTERACTIONS:

Inhalation Aerosol and Syrup: Other beta adrenergic bronchodilators should not be used concomitantly with metaproterenol sulfate because they may have additive effects. Beta adrenergic agonists should be administered with caution to patients being treated with monoamine oxidase inhibitors or tricyclic antidepressants, since the action of beta adrenergic agonists on the vascular system may be potentiated.

Tablets: Beta adrenergic agonists should be administered with caution to patients being treated with monoamine oxidase inhibitors or tricyclic antidepressants, since the action of beta adrenergic agonists on the vascular system may be potentiated.

ADVERSE REACTIONS:

Adverse reactions are similar to those noted with other sympathomimetic agents.

Inhalation Aerosol: The most frequent adverse reaction to metaproterenol sulfate administered by metered-dose inhaler among 251 patients in 90-day controlled clinical trials was nervousness. This was reported in 6.8% of patients. Less frequent adverse experiences, occurring in 1-4% of patients were headache, dizziness, palpitations, gastrointestinal distress, tremor, throat irritation, nausea, vomiting, cough and asthma exacerbation. Tachycardia occurred in less than 1% of patients.

Inhalation Solution: The following (TABLE 1) summarizes the adverse experiences reported for at least 2% of the 120 patients participating in multiple-dose clinical trials of 60- and 90-day duration.

TABLE 1 Adverse Experiences Occurring In At Least 2% of Patients In 60- and 90-Day Clinical Trials N=120

Adverse Experience	No. of Patients	%
Cough	4	3.3
Headache	4	3.3
Nervousness	17	14.1
Tachycardia	3	2.5
Tremor	3	2.5

The incidence of adverse reactions in children may be somewhat higher. In controlled clinical trials conducted in 160 pediatric patients the incidence of adverse reactions observed at the recommended doses was as follows: tachycardia in 16.6%, tremor 33%, nausea 14% and vomiting 7.7%. The corresponding incidence in placebo-treated patients was: tachycardia 7.6%, tremor 20%, nausea 7.7% and vomiting 2.5%.

In two well-controlled studies in children 6-12 years of age with acute exacerbation of asthma, metaproterenol sulfate inhalation solution was not efficacious in approximately 30% of patients, where efficacy was defined as a 15% increase in FEV_1 above baseline at two or more time points during the one-hour testing period. In 8% of patients there was a decrease in FEV_1 of 10% or more from baseline at two or more time points during the testing period. Insufficient information exists to assess the relationship of drug administration to the decline in pulmonary function observed in these patients, but paradoxical bronchospasm is one possibility.

It is important to recognize that adverse reactions from beta agonist bronchodilator solutions for nebulization may occur with the use of a new container of a product in patients who have previously tolerated that same product without adverse effect. There have been reports that indicate that such patients may subsequently tolerate replacement containers of the same product without adverse effect.

Inhalation Solution Unit Dose Vial: The most frequent adverse reactions to metaproterenol sulfate are nervousness and tachycardia which occur in about 1 in 7 patients, tremor which occurs in about 1 in 20 patients and nausea which occurs in about 1 in 50 patients. Less frequent adverse reactions are hypertension, palpitations, vomiting and bad taste which occur in approximately 1 in 300 patients.

ADVERSE REACTIONS: *(cont'd)*

Syrup: TABLE 2 is a list of adverse experiences derived from 44 clinical trials involving 1,120 patients treated with metaproterenol sulfate syrup.

TABLE 2 Incidence of Adverse Events Occurring in at Least 1% of Patients

Adverse Experience	No. of Patients	% Incidence
Cardiovascular		
Tachycardia	68	6.1
Central Nervous System		
Headache	12	1.1
Nervousness	54	4.8
Gastrointestinal		
Nausea	15	1.3
Musculoskeletal		
Tremor	13	1.6

TABLETS

TABLE 3 is a list of adverse experiences derived from 26 controlled clinical trials with 496 patients treated with metaproterenol sulfate tablets.

TABLE 3 Incidence of Adverse Events Reported Among 496 Patients Treated in 26 Controlled Clinical Trials

Adverse Experience	Number of Patients	Incidence %
Cardiovascular		
Chest Pain	1	.2
Edema	1	.2
Hypertension	2	.4
Palpitations	19	3.8
Tachycardia	85	17.1
Central Nervous System		
Dizziness	12	2.4
Drowsiness	3	.6
Fatigue	7	1.4
Headache	35	7.0
Insomnia	9	1.8
Nervousness	100	20.2
Sensory disturbances	1	.2
Syncope	2	.4
Weakness	1	.2
Dermatological		
Diaphoresis	1	.2
Hives	1	.2
Pruritus	2	.4
Gastrointestinal		
Appetite changes	2	.4
Diarrhea	6	1.2
Gastrointestinal distress	15	3.0
Nausea	18	3.6
Vomiting	4	0.8
Musculoskeletal		
Pain	1	.2
Spasms	1	.2
Tremor	84	16.9
Ophthalmological		
Blurred vision	1	.2
Oro-Otolaryngeal		
Dry mouth/throat	2	.4
Laryngeal changes	1	.2
Bad taste	4	0.8
Respiratory		
Asthma exacerbation	10	2.0
Coughing	1	.2
Other		
Chatty	1	.2
Chills	1	.2
Clonus noted on flexing foot	1	.2
Feverish	2	.4
Flu symptoms	1	.2
Facial and finger puffiness	1	.2

OVERDOSAGE:

The expected symptoms with overdosage are those of excessive beta- stimulation and/or any of the symptoms listed under adverse reactions, e.g., angina, hypertension or hypotension, arrhythmias, nervousness, headache, tremor, dry mouth, palpitation, nausea, dizziness, fatigue, malaise and insomnia.

Treatment consists of discontinuation of metaproterenol sulfate together with appropriate symptomatic therapy or reduction of dosage and/or frequency of administration.

DOSAGE AND ADMINISTRATION:

Inhalation Aerosol: The usual single dose is two to three inhalations. With repetitive dosing, inhalation should usually not be repeated more often than about every three to four hours. Total dosage per day should not exceed 12 inhalations.

Metaproterenol sulfate inhalation aerosol is not recommended for children under 12 years of age.

It is recommended that the physician titrate dosage according to each individual patient's response to therapy.

Store between 59°F (15°C) and 77°F (25°C). Avoid excessive humidity.

Inhalation Solution: The dosage and administration are summarized in the (TABLE 4):

TABLE 4

Population	Method of Administration	Usual Singe Dose	Range	Dilution
Adult	Hand-bulb nebulizer	10 inhalations	5-15 inhalations	No dilution
12 years and older	IPPB or nebulizer	0.3 ml	0.2-0.3 ml	Diluted in approx. 2.5 ml saline solution or other diluent
Pediatric 6-12 years	Nebulizer	0.1 ml	0.1-0.2 ml	Diluted in saline solution to a total volume of 3 ml

DOSAGE AND ADMINISTRATION: *(cont'd)*

Metaproterenol sulfate inhalation solution is administered by oral inhalation via IPPB or nebulizer.

Usually, treatment need not be repeated more often than every four hours to relieve acute attacks of bronchospasm. metaproterenol sulfate inhalation solution may be administered three to four times a day for the treatment of reversible airways disease in adults. A single dose of nebulized metaproterenol sulfate in the treatment of an acute attack of asthma may not completely abort an attack.

As with all medications, the physician should begin therapy with the lowest effective dose and then titrate the dosage according to the individual patient's requirements.

Store between 59°F (15°C) and 77°F (25°C). Protect from light.

Do not use the solution if it is pinkish or darker than slightly yellow or contains the precipitate.

Inhalation Solution Unit Dose Vial: Metaproterenol sulfate inhalation solution unit dose vial is administered by oral inhalation using an IPPB device. The usual adult dose is one vial per nebulization treatment. Each vial of metaproterenol sulfate Inhalation solution 0.4% is equivalent to 0.2 ml metaproterenol sulfate Inhalation solution 5% diluted to 2.5 ml with normal saline; each vial of metaproterenol sulfate inhalation solution 0.6% is equivalent to 0.3 ml metaproterenol sulfate Inhalation solution 5% diluted to 2.5 ml with normal saline.

Usually, treatment need not be repeated more often than every four hours to relieve acute attacks of bronchospasm. As part of a total treatment program in chronic bronchospastic pulmonary diseases, metaproterenol sulfate inhalation solution may be administered three or four times a day.

As with all medications, the physician should begin therapy with the lowest effective dose and then titrate the dosage according to the individual patient's requirements.

metaproterenol sulfate inhalation solution is not recommended for use in children under 12 years of age.

Store between 77°F (25°C). Protect from light.

Do not use the solution if it is pinkish or darker than slightly yellow or contains a precipitate.

Syrup: *Children aged six to nine years or weight under 60 lbs:* one teaspoonful three or four times a day. *Children over nine years or weight over 60 lbs:* two teaspoonfuls three or four times a day. Clinical trial experience in children under the age of six is limited. Of 40 children treated with metaproterenol sulfate syrup for at least one month, daily doses of approximately 1.3 to 2.6 mg/kg were well tolerated. *Adults:* two teaspoonfuls three or four times a day.

It is recommended that the physician titrate the dosage according to each individual patient's response to therapy.

Store between 59°F (15°C) and 86°F (30°C). Protect from light.

Tablets: The usual dose is 20 mg three or four times a day.

Children: Aged six to nine years or weight under 60 lbs.*10 mg:* three or four times a day. Over nine years or weight over 60 lbs. *20 mg:* three or four times a day. Metaproterenol sulfate tablets are not recommended for use in children under six years at this time. (Please refer to the CLINICAL PHARMACOLOGY section for further information on clinical experience with this product.)

It is recommended that the physician titrate dosage according to each individual patient's response to therapy.

Storage for Bottles: Store between 59°F (15°C) and 86°F (30°C). Protect from light.

Storage for Blister Samples: Store between 59°F (15°C) and 77°F (25°C). Protect from light.

HOW SUPPLIED - RATED THERAPEUTICALLY EQUIVALENT:

Aerosol - Inhalation - 650 mcg

10 ml	**$20.02**	**ALUPENT 0.65, Boehringer Pharms**	**00597-0070-17**
14 gm (10 ml)	**$17.92**	**ALUPENT 0.65, Boehringer Pharms**	**00597-0070-18**

Solution - Inhalation - 0.4 %

2.5 ml x 25	$30.75	Metaproterenol Sulfate, Roxane	00054-8613-11
2.5 ml x 25	$30.75	Metaproterenol, Dey Labs	49502-0678-03
2.5 ml x 25	$34.40	Metaproterenol Sulfate, Alpharma	00472-1373-48
2.5 ml x 25	**$41.76**	**ALUPENT, Boehringer Pharms**	**00597-0078-62**
2.5 ml x 100	$68.69	ARM-A-MED, Astra USA	00186-4131-01

Solution - Inhalation - 0.6 %

2.5 ml x 25	$30.75	Metaproterenol Sulfate, Roxane	00054-8614-11
2.5 ml x 25	$30.75	Metaproterenol, Dey Labs	49502-0676-03
2.5 ml x 25	$31.44	Metaproterenolsulfate, HL Moore Drug Exch	00839-7639-07
2.5 ml x 25	$34.40	Metaproterenol Sulfate, Alpharma	00472-1377-48
2.5 ml x 25	**$41.76**	**ALUPENT, Boehringer Pharms**	**00597-0069-62**
2.5 ml x 100	$68.69	ARM-A-MED, Astra USA	00186-4130-01

Solution - Inhalation - 5 %

10 ml	**$14.58**	**ALUPENT, Boehringer Pharms**	**00597-0071-75**
30 ml	$29.25	Metaproterenol Sulfate, Major Pharms	00904-2881-30
30 ml	**$40.15**	**ALUPENT, Boehringer Pharms**	**00597-0071-30**

Syrup - Oral - 10 mg/5ml

480 ml	$6.76	Metaproterenol Sulfate, United Res	00677-1445-33
480 ml	$6.76	Metaproterenol, HL Moore Drug Exch	00839-7442-69
480 ml	$6.76	Metaproterenol, H.C.F.A. F F P	99999-1747-01
480 ml	$13.00	Metaproterenol Sulfate, Morton Grove	60432-0650-16
480 ml	$13.50	Metaproterenol Sulfate, Aligen Independ	00405-3255-16
480 ml	$14.46	METAPREL, Novartis	00078-0211-33
480 ml	$16.04	Metaproterenol, Rugby	00536-1462-85
480 ml	$16.32	Metaproterenol Sulfate, Silarx Pharms	54838-0507-80
480 ml	$16.45	Metaproterenol, Qualitest Pharms	00603-1422-58
480 ml	$17.25	Metaproterenol, Goldline Labs	00182-6080-40
480 ml	$17.25	Metaproterenol Sulfate Syrup 10, Major Pharms	00904-2880-16
480 ml	$17.30	Metaproterenol, Schein Pharm (US)	00364-2417-16
480 ml	$17.90	Metaproterenol Hcl, Copley Pharm	38245-0138-07
480 ml	$23.70	Metaproterenol, Teva	00332-6117-38
480 ml	$23.70	Metaproterenol, Geneva Pharms	00781-6404-16
480 ml	**$33.37**	**ALUPENT, Boehringer Pharms**	**00597-0073-16**

Tablet, Uncoated - Oral - 10 mg

100's	$5.75	Metaproterenol, Raway	00686-2230-09
100's	$7.43	Metaproterenol, Teva	00332-2230-09
100's	$7.43	Metaproterenol, United Res	00677-1253-01
100's	$7.43	Metaproterenol, H.C.F.A. F F P	99999-1747-02
100's	$12.51	Metaproterenol, Qualitest Pharms	00603-4464-21
100's	$15.67	Metaproterenol, Rugby	00536-4437-01
100's	$15.70	Metaproterenol Sulfate, Major Pharms	00904-2878-60
100's	$15.75	Metaproterenol, Goldline Labs	00182-1283-01
100's	$15.75	Metaproterenol, Schein Pharm (US)	00364-2283-01
100's	$15.78	Metaproterenol, HL Moore Drug Exch	00839-7485-06
100's	$16.13	Metaproterenol, Major Pharms	00904-2878-61
100's	$16.42	Metaproterenol Sulfate 10, Aligen Independ	00405-4629-01
100's	$16.49	Metaproterenol Sulfate, Par Pharm	49884-0258-01
100's	**$34.20**	**ALUPENT, Boehringer Pharms**	**00597-0074-01**

Tablet, Uncoated - Oral - 20 mg

100's	$8.75	Metaproterenol, Raway	00686-2232-09
100's	$13.28	Metaproterenol, Teva	00332-2232-09
100's	$13.28	Metaproterenol, United Res	00677-1254-01
100's	$13.28	Metaproterenol, H.C.F.A. F F P	99999-1747-03
100's	$19.35	Metaproterenol, Rugby	00536-4438-01
100's	$19.60	Metaproterenol Sulfate, Major Pharms	00904-2879-60
100's	$19.90	Metaproterenol, Qualitest Pharms	00603-4465-21
100's	$20.93	Metaproterenol, Schein Pharm (US)	00364-2284-01
100's	$20.94	Metaproterenol, Major Pharms	00904-2879-61
100's	$20.99	Metaproterenol, HL Moore Drug Exch	00839-7486-06
100's	$21.00	Metaproternol Sulfate Tablets 20 Mg, Goldline Labs	00182-1284-01
100's	$23.25	Metaproterenol Sulfate, Aligen Independ	00405-4630-01
100's	$23.75	Metaproterenol Sulfate, Par Pharm	49884-0259-01
100's	**$48.59**	**ALUPENT, Boehringer Pharms**	**00597-0072-01**

METARAMINOL BITARTRATE *(001748)*

CATEGORIES: Autonomic Drugs; Brain Damage; Cardiovascular Drugs; Drug Hypersensitivity; Hemorrhage; Hypotension; Hypotension/Shock; Sympathomimetic Agents; Vasopressors; Pregnancy Category C; FDA Approval Pre 1982

BRAND NAMES: **Aramine**; *Levicor*
(International brand names outside U.S. in italics)

FORMULARIES: Medi-Cal

DESCRIPTION:

Metaraminol bitartrate is a potent sympathomimetic amine that increases both systolic and diastolic blood pressure.

Metaraminol bitartrate is (*R*-(*R**,*S**))-α-(1-aminoethyl)-3-hydroxybenzene-methanol(*R*-(*R**,*R**))-2, 3-dihydroxy-butanedioate (1:1) (salt), which is levorotatory. Its empirical formula is $C_9H_{13}NO_2 \cdot C_4H_6O_6$.

Metaraminol bitartrate is a white, crystalline powder with a molecular weight of 317.29, is freely soluble in water, slightly soluble in alcohol, and practically insoluble in chloroform and in ether.

Injection metaraminol bitartrate is a sterile solution.

Each ml Contains: Metaraminol bitartrate equivalent to metaraminol - 10 mg

Inactive ingredients: Sodium chloride - 4.4 mg, Water for Injection q.s. ad - 1 ml, Methylparaben 0.15%, propylparaben 0.02%, and sodium bisulfite 0.2% added as preservatives.

CLINICAL PHARMACOLOGY:

The pressor effect of metaraminol begins in 1 to 2 minutes after intravenous infusion, in about 10 minutes after intramuscular injection, and in 5 to 20 minutes after subcutaneous injection. The effect lasts from about 20 minutes to one hour. Metaraminol has a positive inotropic effect on the heart and a peripheral vasoconstrictor action.

Renal, coronary, and cerebral blood flow are a function of perfusion pressure and regional resistance. In patients with insufficient or failing vasoconstriction, there is additional advantage to the peripheral action of metaraminol, but in most patients with shock, vasoconstriction is adequate and any further increase is unnecessary. Blood flow to vital organs may decrease with metaraminol if regional resistance increases excessively.

The pressor effect of metaraminol is decreased but not reversed by alpha-adrenergic blocking agents. Primary or secondary fall in blood pressure and tachyphylactic response to repeated use are uncommon.

INDICATIONS AND USAGE:

Metaraminol is indicated for prevention and treatment of the acute hypotensive state occurring with spinal anesthesia. It is also indicated as adjunctive treatment of hypotension due to hemorrhage, reactions to medications, surgical complications, and shock associated with brain damage due to trauma or tumor.

CONTRAINDICATIONS:

Use of metaraminol with cyclopropane or halothane anesthesia should be avoided, unless clinical circumstances demand such use.

Hypersensitivity to any component of this product, including sulfites (see WARNINGS).

WARNINGS:

Use of sympathomimetic amines with monoamine oxidase inhibitors or tricyclic antidepressants may result in potentiation of the pressor effect. (See DRUG INTERACTIONS.)

Metaraminol contains sodium bisulfite, a sulfite that may cause allergic-type reactions including anaphylactic symptoms and life-threatening or less severe asthmatic episodes in certain susceptible people. The overall prevalence of sulfite sensitivity in the general population is unknown and probably low. Sulfite sensitivity is seen more frequently in asthmatic than in nonasthmatic people.

PRECAUTIONS:

GENERAL

Caution should be used to avoid excessive blood pressure response. Rapidly induced hypertensive responses have been reported to cause acute pulmonary edema, arrhythmias, cerebral hemorrhage, or cardiac arrest.

Patients with cirrhosis should be treated with caution, with adequate restoration of electrolytes if diuresis ensues. Fatal ventricular arrhythmia was reported in one patient with Laennec's cirrhosis while receiving metaraminol bitartrate. In several instances, ventricular extrasystoles that appeared during infusion of this vasopressor subsided promptly when the rate of infusion was reduced.

With the prolonged action of metaraminol a cumulative effect is possible. If there is an excessive vasopressor response there may be a prolonged elevation of blood pressure even after discontinuation of therapy.

When vasopressor amines are used for long periods, the resulting vasoconstriction may prevent adequate expansion of circulating volume and may cause perpetuation of shock. There is evidence that plasma volume may be reduced in all types of shock, and that the measurement of central venous pressure is useful in assessing the adequacy of the circulating blood volume. Therefore, blood or plasma volume expanders should be used when the principal reason for hypotension or shock is decreased circulating volume.

PRECAUTIONS: *(cont'd)*

Because of its vasoconstrictor effect metaraminol should be given with caution in heart or thyroid disease, hypertension, or diabetes. Sympathomimetic amines may provoke a relapse in patients with a history of malaria.

CARCINOGENESIS, MUTAGENESIS, AND IMPAIRMENT OF FERTILITY

Studies in animals have not been performed to evaluate the mutagenic or carcinogenic potential of metaraminol or its potential to affect fertility.

PREGNANCY CATEGORY C

Animal reproduction studies have not been conducted with metaraminol. It is not known whether metaraminol can cause fetal harm when given to a pregnant woman or can affect reproduction capacity. Metaraminol should be given to a pregnant women only if clearly needed.

NURSING MOTHERS

It is not known whether this drug is secreted in human milk. Because many drugs are secreted in human milk, caution should be exercised when metaraminol is given to a nursing woman.

PEDIATRIC USE

Safety and effectiveness in children have not been established.

DRUG INTERACTIONS:

Metaraminol should be used with caution in digitalized patients, since the combination of digitalis and sympathomimetic amines may cause ectopic arrhythmias.

Monoamine oxidase inhibitors or tricyclic antidepressants may potentiate the action of sympathomimetic amines. Therefore, when initiating pressor therapy in patients receiving these drugs, the initial dose should be small and given with caution. (See WARNINGS.)

ADVERSE REACTIONS:

Sympathomimetic amines, including metaraminol may cause sinus or ventricular tachycardia, or other arrhythmias, especially in patients with myocardial infarction. (See PRECAUTIONS.)

In patients with a history of malaria, these compounds may provoke a relapse.

Abscess formation, tissue necrosis, or sloughing rarely may follow the use of metaraminol. In choosing the site of injection, it is important to avoid those areas recognized as *not* suitable for use of any pressor agent and to discontinue the infusion immediately if infiltration or thrombosis occurs. Although the physician may be forced by the urgent nature of the patient's condition to choose injection sites that are not recognized as suitable, he should, when possible, use the preferred areas of injection. The larger veins of the antecubital fossa or the thigh are preferred to veins in the dorsum of the hand of ankle veins, particularly in patients with peripheral vascular disease, diabetes mellitus, Buerger's disease, or conditions with coexistent hypercoagulability.

OVERDOSAGE:

Overdosage may result in severe hypertension accompanied by headache, constricting sensation in the chest, nausea, vomiting, euphoria, diaphoresis, pulmonary edema, tachycardia, bradycardia, sinus arrhythmia, atrial or ventricular arrhythmia, cerebral hemorrhage, myocardial infarction, cardiac arrest or convulsions.

Should an excessive elevation of blood pressure occur, it may be immediately relieved by a sympatholytic agent, e.g. phentolamine. An appropriate antiarrhythmic agent may also be required.

The Oral LD_{50} in the rat and mouse is 240 mg/kg and 99 mg/kg, respectively.

DOSAGE AND ADMINISTRATION:

metaraminol may be given intramuscularly, subcutaneously, or intravenously, the route depending on the nature and severity of the indication.

Parenteral drug products should be inspected visually for particulate matter and discoloration prior to use, whenever solution and container permit.

Allow at least 10 minutes to elapse before increasing the dose because the maximum effect is not immediately apparent. When the vasopressor is discontinued, observe the patient carefully as the effect of the drug tapers off, so that therapy can be reinitiated promptly if the blood pressure falls too rapidly. The response to vasopressors may be poor in patients with coexistent shock and acidosis. When indicated, established method of shock management should be used, such as blood or fluid replacement.

Intramuscular or Subcutaneous Injection: (for prevention of hypotension see INDICATIONS AND USAGE): The recommended dose is 2 to 10 mg (0.2 to 1 ml). As with other agents given subcutaneously, only the preferred sites of injection, as set forth in standard texts, should be used.

Intravenous Infusion: (for adjunctive treatment of hypotension see INDICATIONS AND USAGE): The recommended dose is 15 to 100 mg (.15 to 10 ml) in 500 ml of Sodium Chloride Injection of 5% Dextrose Injection, adjusting the rate of infusion to maintain the blood pressure at the desired level. Higher concentrations of metaraminol, 150 to 500 mg per 500 ml of infusion fluid, have been used.

If the patient needs more saline or dextrose solution at a rate of flow that would provide an excessive dose of the vasopressor, the recommended volume of infusion fluid (500 ml) should be increased accordingly. Metaraminol may also be added to *less* than 500 ml infusion fluid if a smaller volume desired.

COMPATIBILITY INFORMATION

In addition to Sodium Chloride Injection and Dextrose Injection 5%, the following infusion solutions were found physically and chemically compatible with injection metaraminol when 5 ml injection metaraminol 10 mg/ml (metaraminol equivalent), was added to 5 ml of infusion solution: Ringer's Injection, Lactated Ringer's Injection, Dextran 6% in Saline†, Normosol-R pH 7.4†, a Normosol-M in D5-W†.

When injection metaraminol is mixed with an infusion solution, sterile precautions should be observed. Since infuse solutions generally do not contain preservatives, mixtures should be used within 24 hours.

Direct Intravenous Injection: In severe shock, when time is of great importance this agent should be given by direct intravenous injection. The suggested dose is 0.5 to 5 mg (0.05 to 0.5 ml), followed by an infusion of 15 to 100 mg (1.5 to 10 ml) in 500 ml of infusion fluid described previously.

Vials may be sterilized by autoclave or by immersion in a sterilizing solution.

HOW SUPPLIED:

Injection Aramine 1%, containing metaraminol bitartrate equivalent to 10 mg of metaraminol per ml, is a clear, colorless solution and is supplier as follows:

Storage: Protect from light. Store container in carton until contents have been used. Avoid storage at temperatures below -20°C (-4°F) and above 40°C (104°F)

HOW SUPPLIED - RATED THERAPEUTICALLY EQUIVALENT:

Injection, Solution - Intramuscular; - 10 mg/ml

10 ml	**$11.85**	**ARAMINE, Merck**	**00006-3222-10**
10 ml	$126.38	Metaraminol Bitartrate, Fujisawa USA	00469-9440-90

METAXALONE *(001749)*

CATEGORIES: Autonomic Drugs; Muscle Relaxants; Neuromuscular; Pain; Skeletal Muscle Relaxants; Skeletal Muscle Hyperactivity*; FDA Approval Pre 1982
* Indication not approved by the FDA

BRAND NAMES: **Skelaxin**

DESCRIPTION:

Each pale rose, scored tablet contains: metaxalone, 400 mg.

Skelaxin (metaxalone) has the following chemical name: 5-[(3,4-dimethylphenoxy)methyl]-2-oxazolidinone.

CLINICAL PHARMACOLOGY:

The mechanism of action of metaxalone in humans has not been established, but may be due to general central nervous system depression. It has direct action on the contractile mechanism of striated muscle, the motor end plate or the nerve fiber.

INDICATIONS AND USAGE:

Metaxalone is indicated as an adjunct to rest, physical therapy, and other measures for the relief of discomforts associated with acute, painful musculoskeletal conditions. The mode of action of this drug has not been clearly identified, but may be related to its sedative properties. Metaxalone does not directly relax tense skeletal muscles in man.

CONTRAINDICATIONS:

Metaxalone is contraindicated in individuals who have shown hypersensitivity to the drug. Metaxalone should not be administered to patients with a known tendency to drug induced, hemolytic, or other anemias. It is contraindicated in patients with significantly impaired renal or hepatic function.

PRECAUTIONS:

Elevation in cephalin flocculation tests without concurrent changes in other liver function parameters have been noted. Hence, it is recommended that metaxalone be administered with great care to patients with pre-existing liver damage and that serial liver function studies be performed as required.

False-positive Benedict's tests, due to an unknown reducing substance, have been noted. A glucose-specific test will differentiate findings.

Pregnancy: Reproduction studies have been performed in rats and have revealed no evidence of impaired fertility or harm to the fetus due to metaxalone. Reactions reports from marketing experience have not revealed evidence of fetal injury, but such experience cannot exclude the possibility of infrequent or subtle damage to the human fetus. Safe use of metaxalone has not been established with regard to possible adverse effects upon fetal development. Therefore, metaxalone tablets should not be used in women who are or may become pregnant and particularly during early pregnancy unless in the judgment of the physician the potential benefits outweigh the possible hazards.

Nursing Mothers: It is not known whether this drug is secreted in human milk. As a general rule, nursing should not be undertaken while a patient is on a drug since many drugs are excreted in human milk.

Pediatric Use: Safety and effectiveness in children 12 years of age and below have not been established.

ADVERSE REACTIONS:

The most frequent reactions to metaxalone include nausea, vomiting, gastrointestinal upset, drowsiness, dizziness, headache, and nervousness or "irritability." Other adverse reactions are: hypersensitivity reactions, characterized by a light rash with or without pruritus; leukopenia; hemolytic anemia; jaundice.

OVERDOSAGE:

Gastric lavage and supportive therapy as indicated. (When determining the LD_{50} in rats and mice, progressive sedation, hypnosis and finally respiratory failure were noted as the dosage increased. In dogs, no LD_{50} could be determined as the higher doses produced an emetic action in 15 to 30 minutes). No documented case of major toxicity has been reported.

DOSAGE AND ADMINISTRATION:

The recommended dose for adults and children over 12 years of age is two tablets (800 mg) three to four times a day.

HOW SUPPLIED:

Skelaxin is available as a 400 mg pale rose tablet, inscribed with 8862 on the scored side and "C" on the other.

Store at Controlled Room Temperature, between 15°C and 30°C (59°F and 86°F).

HOW SUPPLIED - EQUIVALENTS NOT AVAILABLE:

Tablet, Uncoated - Oral - 400 mg

100's	**$39.15**	**SKELAXIN, Carnrick**	**00086-0062-10**
500's	**$159.60**	**SKELAXIN, Carnrick**	**00086-0062-50**

METFORMIN HYDROCHLORIDE *(003204)*

CATEGORIES: Antidiabetic Agents; Blood Glucose Regulators; Diabetes; Diabetes Mellitus; Hormones; Hyperglycemia; FDA Class 1P ("Priority Review"); FDA Approved 1994 Dec; Top 200 Drugs; Top 200 Drugs

BRAND NAMES: *Benofomin; Dextin; Diabetmin; Diabex; Diaformin; Diamin; Diaphage; Diformin; Diformin Retard; Fornidd; Geamet; Glucofago; Glucomet; Glucomine; Glucoform; Gluconil;* **Glucophage**; *Glucophage 850; Glucophage Forte* (Mexico); *Glucophage-Mite* (Germany); *Glucophage Retard* (Germany); *Gluformin; Glupermin; Glyciphage; Metforal; Metomin; Miformin; Orabet; Siamformet (International brand names outside U.S. in italics)*

FORMULARIES: PCS

DESCRIPTION:

Metformin hydrochloride is an oral antihyperglycemic drug used in the management of non-insulin-dependent diabetes mellitus (NIDDM). Metformin hydrochloride (N,N-dimethylimidodicarbonimidic diamide hydrochloride) is not chemically or pharmacologically related to the oral sulfonylureas.

Metformin hydrochloride is a white to off-white crystalline compound with a molecular formula of $C_4H_{11}N_5 \cdot HCl$ and a molecular weight of 165.63. Metformin hydrochloride is freely soluble in water and is practically insoluble in acetone, ether and chloroform. The pK_a of metformin is 12.4. The pH of a 1% aqueous solution of metformin hydrochloride is 6.68.

Glucophage tablets contain 500 mg and 850 mg of metformin hydrochloride. In addition, each tablet contains the following inactive ingredients: povidone, magnesium stearate and hydroxypropyl methylcellulose (hypromellose) coating.

CLINICAL PHARMACOLOGY:

Antidiabetic Activity: Metformin HCl is antihyperglycemic agent which improves glucose tolerance in NIDDM subjects, lowering both basal and postprandial plasma glucose. Its pharmacologic mechanisms of action are different from those of sulfonylureas. Metformin HCl decreases hepatic glucose production, decreases intestinal absorption of glucose and improves insulin sensitivity (increases peripheral glucose uptake and utilization). Unlike sulfonylureas. Metformin HCl does not produce hypoglycemia in either diabetic or nondiabetic subjects (except in special circumstances, see PRECAUTIONS) and does not cause hyperinsulinemia. With metformin therapy, insulin secretion remains unchanged while fasting insulin levels and day-long plasma insulin response may actually decrease.

In a double-blind, placebo-controlled, multicenter U.S. clinical trial involving obese NIDDM patients whose hyperglycemia was not adequately controlled with dietary management alone (baseline fasting plasma glucose [FPG] of approximately 240 mg/dl), treatment with metformin HCl (up to 2.55 g/day) for 29 weeks resulted in significant mean net reductions in fasting and postprandial plasma glucose (PPG) and HbA_{1c} of 59 mg/dl, 83 mg/dl, and 1.8%, respectively compared to placebo group (see TABLE 1).

TABLE 1 Metformin HCl vs. Placebo Summary of Mean Changes from Baseline* in Plasma Glucose HbA $_{1C}$ and Body Weight, at Final Visit (29-week study)

	Metformin HCl (n = 141)	Placebo (n = 145)	P-Value
FPG (mg/dl)			
Baseline	241.5	237.7	NS
Change at FINAL VISIT	-53.0	6.3	0.001**
Hemoglobin A_{1C}(%)			
Baseline	8.4	8.2	NS
Change at FINAL VISIT	-1.4	0.4	0.001**
Body Weight (lbs)			
Baseline	201.0	206.0	NS
Change at FINAL VISIT	-1.4	-2.4	NS

* All patients on diet therapy at Baseline
** Statistically significant

Monotherapy with metformin HCl may be effective in patients who have not responded to sulfonylureas or who have only a partial response to sulfonylureas or who have ceased to respond to sulfonylureas. In such patients, if adequate glycemic control is not attained with metformin HCl monotherapy, the combination of metformin HCl and a sulfonylurea may have a synergistic effect, since both agents act to improve glucose tolerance by different but complementary mechanisms.

A 29-week, double-blind, placebo-controlled study of metformin HCl and glyburide alone and in combination, was conducted in obese NIDDM patients who had failed to achieve adequate glycemic control while on maximum doses of glyburide (baseline FPG of approximately 250 mg/dl) (see TABLE 2). Patients randomized to continue on glyburide experienced worsening of glycemic control, with mean increases in FPG, PPG and HbA_{1c} of 14 mg/dl, 3 mg/dl and 0.2%, respectively. In contrast, those randomized to metformin HCl (up to 2.5 g/day) did not experience a deterioration in glycemic control, but rather a slight improvement, with mean reductions in FPG, PPG and Hba_{1c} of 1 mg/dl, 6 mg/dl and 0.4%, respectively. The combination of metformin HCl and glyburide was synergistic in reducing FGP, PPG and HbA_{1c} levels by 63 mg/dl, 65 mg/dl, and 1.7%, respectively. Compared to results of glyburide treatment alone, the net differences with combination treatment were -77 mg/dl, -68 mg/dl and -1.98%, respectively (see TABLE 2).

TABLE 2 Combined Metformin HCl/Glyburide (Comb) vs Glyburide (Glyb) or Metformin HCl (GLU) Monotherapy: Summary of Mean Changes from Baseline* In Plasma Glucose, HbA $_{1c}$ and Body Weight, at Final Visit (29-week study)

	Comb (n=213)	Glyb (n=209)	GLU (n=210)	P-values: Glyb vs Comb	P-values: GLU vs Comb	P-values: GLU vs Glyb
Fasting Plasma Glucose (mg/dl)						
Baseline	250.5	247.5	253.9	NS	NS	NS
Change at FINAL VISIT	-63.5	13.7	-0.9	0.001**	0.001**	0.025**
Hemoglobin A_{1c}(%)						
Baseline	8.8	8.5	8.9	NS	NS	0.007**
Change at FINAL VISIT	-1.7	0.2	-0.4	0.001**	0.001**	0.001**
Body Weight (lbs)						
Baseline	202.2	203.0	204.0	NS	NS	NS
Change at FINAL VISIT	0.9	-0.7	-8.4	0.011**	0.001**	0.001**

* All patients on glyburide, 20 mg/day, at Baseline
** Statistically significant

The magnitude of the decline in fasting blood glucose concentration following the institution of metformin hydrochloride tablets therapy is proportional to the level of fasting hyperglycemia. Non-insulin dependent diabetics with higher fasting glucose concentrations will experience greater declines in plasma glucose and glycosylated hemoglobin.

Metformin HCl has a modest favorable effect on serum lipids, which are often abnormal in NIDDM patients. In clinical studies, particularly when baseline levels were abnormally elevated, metformin HCl, alone or in combination with a sulfonylurea, lowered mean fasting serum triglycerides, total cholesterol and LDL cholesterol levels and had no adverse effects on other lipid levels (see TABLE 3).

In contrast to sulfonylureas body weight of individuals on metformin HCl tends to remain stable or may even decrease somewhat (see TABLE 1 and TABLE 2).

CLINICAL PHARMACOLOGY: *(cont'd)*

TABLE 3 Summary of Mean Percent Reduction of Major Serum Lipid Variables at Final Visit (29-week study)

	Metformin HCl vs. Placebo (%) Change from Baseline		Combined Metformin HCl Glyburide vs. Monotherapy (%) Change from Baseline		
	Metformin HCl (n = 141)	Placebo (n = 145)	Metformin HCl (n = 210)	Metformin HCl/ Glyburide (n = 213)	Glyburide (n = 209)
Total Cholesterol	-5%*	1%	-2%	-4%**	1%
Total Triglycerides	-16%	1%	-3%	-8%**	4%
LDL - Cholesterol	-8%*	1%	-4%	-6%**	3%
HDL - Cholesterol	2%	-1%	5%	3%	1%

* P < 0.05 vs. Placebo
** P < 0.05 vs. Glyburide

In summary, metformin-treated patients showed significant improvement in all parameters of glycemic control (FPG, PPG, and HbA_{1c}), stabilization or decrease in body weight, and a tendency to improvement in the lipid profile, particularly when baseline values are abnormally elevated.

Pharmacokinetics: *Absorption and Bioavailability:* The absolute bioavailability of a 500 mg metformin hydrochloride tablet given under fasting conditions is approximately 50-60%. Studies using single oral doses of metformin tablets of 500 mg and 1500 mg, and 850 mg to 2550 mg, indicate that there is a lack of dose proportionality with increasing doses, which is due to decreased absorption rather than an alteration in elimination. Food decreases the extent and slightly delays the absorption of metformin, as shown by approximately a 40% lower peak concentration and 25% lower AUC in plasma and a 35 minute prolongation of time to peak plasma concentration following administration of a single 850 mg tablet of metformin with food, compared to the same tablet strength administered fasting. The clinical relevance of these decreases is unknown.

Distribution: The apparent volume of distribution (V/F) of metformin following single oral doses of 850 mg averaged 654 ± 358 l. Metformin is negligibly bound to plasma proteins in contrast to sulfonylureas which are more than 90% protein bound. Metformin partitions into erythrocytes, most likely as a function of time. At usual clinical doses and dosing schedules of metformin HCl, steady state plasma concentration of metformin are reached with 24-48 hours and are generally <1 mcg/ml. During controlled clinical trials, maximum metformin plasma levels did not exceed 5 mcg/ml, even at maximum doses.

Metabolism and Elimination: Intravenous single-dose studies in normal subjects demonstrate that metformin is excreted unchanged in the urine and does not undergo hepatic metabolism (no metabolites have been identified in humans) nor biliary excretion. Renal clearance (see TABLE 4) is approximately 3.5 times greater than creatinine clearance which indicates that tubular secretion is the major route of metformin elimination. Following oral administration, approximately 90% of the absorbed drug is eliminated via the renal route within the first 24 hours, with a plasma elimination half-life of approximately 6.2 hours. In blood, the elimination half-life is approximately 17.6 hours, suggesting that the erythrocyte mass may be a compartment of distribution.

Special Populations: *NIDDM Subjects:* In the presence of normal renal function, there are no differences between single or multiple dose pharmacokinetics of metformin between diabetics and nondiabetics (see TABLE 4), nor is there any accumulation of metformin in either group at usual clinical doses.

Renal Insufficiency: In subjects with decreased renal function (based on measured creatinine clearance), the plasma and blood half-life of metformin is prolonged and the renal clearance is decreased in proportion to the decrease in creatinine clearance (see TABLE 4).

Hepatic Insufficiency: No pharmacokinetics studies have been conducted in subjects with hepatic insufficiency.

Geriatrics: Limited data from controlled pharmacokinetic studies of metformin in healthy elderly subjects suggest that total plasma clearance is decreased, the half-life is prolonged and C_{max} is increased, compared to healthy young subjects. From these data, it appears that the change in metformin pharmacokinetics with aging is primarily accounted for by a change in renal function (see TABLE 4).

TABLE 4 Select Mean (± S.D.) Metformin Pharmacokinetics Parameters Following Single or Multiple Oral Doses of Metformin HCl

Subject Groups: Metformin HCl dose[a] (number of subjects)	C_{max}[b] (mcg/ml)	$†_{max}$[2] (hrs)	Renal Clearance (ml/min)
Healthy, nondiabetic adults:			
500 mg SD[d] (24)	1.03 (± 0.33)	2.75 (± 0.81)	600 (± 132)
850 mg SD (74)[e]	1.60 (± 0.38)	2.64 (± 0.82)	552 (± 139)
850 mg t.i.d. for 19 doses[f] (9)	2.01 (± 0.42)	1.79 (± 0.94)	642 (± 173)
Adults with NIDDM:			
850 mg SD (23)	1.48 (± 0.5)	3.32 (± 1.08)	491 (± 138)
850 mg t.i.d. for 19 doses[f] (9)	1.90 (± 0.62)	2.01 (± 1.22)	550 (± 160)
Elderly[g], healthy non-diabetic adults:			
850 mg SD (12)	2.45 (± 0.70)	2.71 (± 1.05)	412 (± 98)
Renal-impaired adults: 850 mg SD			
Mild (CL_{cr}[h] 61-90 ml/min) (5)	1.86 (± 0.52)	3.20 (± 0.45)	384 (± 122)
Moderate (CL_{cr} 31-60 ml/min) (4)	4.12 (± 1.83)	3.75 (± 0.50)	108 (± 57)
Severe (CL_{cr} 10-30 ml/min) (6)	3.93 (± 0.92)	4.01 (± 1.10)	130 (± 90)

[a]-All doses given fasting except the first 18 doses of the multiple dose studies.
[b]-Peak plasma concentration;
[c]-Time to peak plasma concentration;
[d]-SD = single dose;
[e]-Combined results (average means) of five studies mean age 32 years (range 23-59 yrs).
[f]-Kinetic study done following dose 19, given fasting
[g]-Elderly subjects, mean age 71 years (range 65-81 years).
[h]-CL_{cr}= creatinine clearance normalized to body surface area of 1.73 m^2.

Pediatrics: No pharmacokinetic studies have been conducted in pediatric subjects.

Gender: Metformin pharmacokinetic parameters did not differ significantly in diabetic and non-diabetic subjects when analyzed according to gender (males = 19, females = 16). Similarly, in controlled clinical studies in patients with NIDDM, the antihyperglycemic effect of metformin HCl was comparable in males and females.

Race: No studies of metformin pharmacokinetic parameters according to race have been performed. In controlled clinical studies of metformin HCl in patients with NIDDM, the antihyperglycemic effect was comparable in whites (n=249), blacks (n=51) and hispanics (n=24).

INDICATIONS AND USAGE:

Metformin hydrochloride tablets, as monotherapy, is indicated as an adjunct to diet to lower blood glucose in patients with NIDDM whose hyperglycemia cannot be satisfactorily managed on diet alone.

Metformin HCl may used concomitantly with a sulfonylurea when diet and metformin HCl or a sulfonylurea alone do not result in adequate glycemic control.

In initiating treatment for NIDDM, diet should be emphasized as the primary form of treatment. Caloric restriction and weight loss are essential in the obese diabetic patient. Proper dietary management alone may be effective in controlling the blood glucose and symptoms of hyperglycemia. Loss of blood glucose control diet-management alone may be effective in controlling the blood glucose and symptoms of hyperglycemia. Loss of blood glucose control in diet-managed patients may be transient, thus requiring only short-term pharmacologic therapy. The importance of regular physical activity should also be stressed, and cardiovascular risk factors should be identified and corrective measures taken where possible. If this treatment program fails to reduce symptoms and/or blood glucose, the use of metformin HCl alone or metformin HCl plus a sulfonylurea should be considered.

If, after a suitable trial of such treatments, glucose control still has not been achieved, consideration should be given to the use of insulin.

Judgements should be based on regular clinical and laboratory evaluations.

CONTRAINDICATIONS:

Metformin HCl is contraindicated in patients with:

1. Renal disease or renal dysfunction (*e.g.,* as suggested by serum creatinine levels ≥1.5 mg/dl [males], ≥1.4 mg/dl [females] or abnormal creatinine clearance) which may also result from conditions such as cardiovascular collapse (shock), acute myocardial infarction, and septicemia (see WARNINGS and PRECAUTIONS).

2. Metformin HCl should be temporarily withheld in patients undergoing radiologic studies involving parenteral administration of iodinated contrast materials, because use of such products may result in acute alteration of renal function. (See PRECAUTIONS.)

3. Known hypersensitivity to metformin hydrochloride.

4. Acute or chronic metabolic acidosis, including diabetic ketoacidosis, with or without coma. Diabetic ketoacidosis should be treated with insulin.

WARNINGS:

Lactic Acidosis:

Lactic acidosis is a rare, but serious, metabolic complication that can occur due to metformin accumulation during treatment with metformin HCl; when it occurs, it is fatal in approximately 50% cases. Lactic acidosis may also occur in association with a number of pathophysiologic conditions, including diabetes mellitus, and whenever there is significant tissue hypoperfusion and hypoxemia. Lactic acidosis is characterized by elevated blood lactate levels (>5 mmol/l), decreased blood pH, electrolyte disturbances with an increased anion gap, and an increased lactate/pyruvate ratio. When metformin is implicated as the cause of lactic acidosis, metformin plasma levels >mcg/ml are generally found.

The reported incidence of lactic acidosis in patients receiving hydrochloride is very low (approximately 0.03 cases/1,000 patient-years, with approximately 0.015 fatal cases/1,000 patient years). Reported cases have occurred primarily in diabetic patients with significant renal insufficiency, including both intrinsic renal disease and renal hypoperfusion, often in the setting of multiple concomitant medical/surgical problems and multiple concomitant medications. The risk of lactic acidosis increases with the degree of renal dysfunction and the patient's age. The risk of lactic acidosis may, therefore, be significantly decreased by regular monitoring of renal function in patients taking metformin HCl and by use of the minimum effective dose of metformin HCl. In addition, metformin HCl should be promptly withheld in the presence of any condition associated with hypoxemia or dehydration. Because impaired hepatic function may significantly limit the ability to clear lactate, metformin HCl should generally be avoided in patients with clinical or laboratory evidence of hepatic disease. Patients should be cautioned against excessive alcohol intake, either acute or chronic, when taking metformin HCl, since alcohol potentiates the effects of metformin hydrochloride on lactate metabolism. In addition, metformin HCl should be temporarily discontinued prior to any intravascular radiocontrast study and for any surgical procedure (see PRECAUTIONS).

The onset of lactic acidosis often is subtle, and accompanied only by nonspecific symptoms such as malaise, myalgias, respiratory distress, increasing somnolence and nonspecific abdominal distress. There may be associated hypothermia, hypotension and resistant bradyarrhythmias with more marked acidosis. The patient and the patient's physician must be aware of the possible importance of such symptoms and the patient should be instructed to notify the physician immediately if they occur (see PRECAUTIONS). Metformin HCl should be withdrawn until the situation is clarified. Serum electrolytes, ketones, blood glucose and, if indicated, blood pH, lactate levels and even blood metformin levels may be useful. Once a patient is stabilized on any dose level of metformin HCl, gastrointestinal symptoms, which are common during initiation of therapy, are unlikely to be drug related. Later occurrence of gastrointestinal symptoms could be due to lactic acidosis or other serious disease.

Levels of fasting venous plasma lactate above the upper limit of normal but less than 5 mmol/l in patients taking metformin HCl do not necessarily indicate impending lactic acidosis and may be explainable by other mechanisms, such as poorly controlled diabetes or obesity, vigorous physical activity or technical problems in sample handling. (See PRECAUTIONS.)

Lactic acidosis should be suspected in any diabetic patient with metabolic acidosis lacking evidence of ketoacidosis (ketonuria and ketonemia).

Lactic acidosis is a medial emergency that must be treated in a hospital setting. In a patient with lactic acidosis who is taking metformin HCl, the drug should be discontinued immediately and general supportive measures promptly instituted. Because metformin hydro-chloride is dialyzable (with a clearance of up to 170 ml/mn under good hemodynamic conditions), prompt hemodialysis is recommended to correct the acidosis and remove the accumulated metformin. Such management often results in prompt reversal of symptoms and recovery. (See CONTRAINDICATIONS and PRECAUTIONS.)

WARNINGS: *(cont'd)*

SPECIAL WARNING ON INCREASED RISK OF CARDIOVASCULAR MORTALITY: The administration of oral antidiabetic drugs has been reported to be associated with increased cardiovascular mortality as compared to treatment with diet alone or diet plus insulin. This warning is based on the study conducted by the University Group Diabetes program (UGDP), a long-term prospective clinical trial designed to evaluate the effectiveness of glucose-lowering drugs in preventing or delaying vascular complications in patients with non-insulin-dependent diabetes. The study involved 1027 patients who were randomly assigned to one of five treatment groups (*Diabetes*, 19 (Suppl.2):747-830, 1970; *Diabetes*, 24 (Suppl.1):65-184, 1975).

The UGDP reported that patients treated for 5 to 8 years with diet plus a fixed dose of tolbutamide (1.5 g per day) or diet plus a fixed dose of phenformin (100 mg per day), had a rate of cardiovascular mortality approximately 2.5 times that of patients treated with diet alone, resulting in discontinuation of both of these treatments in the UGDP study. Total mortality was increased in both the tolbutamide- and phenformin-treated groups and this increase was statistically significant in the phenformin-treated group. Despite controversy regarding the interpretation of these results, the findings of the UGDP study provide an adequate basis for this warning. The patient should be informed of the potential risks and benefits of metformin HCl and alternative modes of therapy.

Although only one drug in the sulfonylurea category (tolbutamide) and one in the biguanide category (phenformin) were included in this study, it is prudent from a safety standpoint to consider that this warning may also apply to other related oral antidiabetic drugs, in view of the similarities in mode of action and chemical structure among the drugs in each category.

PRECAUTIONS:

GENERAL

Monitoring Renal Function: Metformin HCl is known to be substantially excreted by the kidney and the risk of metformin accumulation and lactic acidosis increases with the degree of impairment of renal function. Thus, patients with serum creatinine levels above the upper limit of normal for their age should not receive metformin HCl. In patients with advanced age, metformin HCl should be carefully titrated to establish the minimum dose for adequate glycemic effect, because aging is associated with reduced renal function. In elderly patients, renal function should be monitored regularly and, generally, metformin HCl should not be titrated to the maximum dose (see DOSAGE AND ADMINISTRATION).

Before initiation of metformin HCl therapy and at least annually thereafter, renal function should be assessed and verified as normal. In patients in whom development of renal dysfunction is anticipated, renal function should be assessed more frequently and metformin HCl discontinued if evidence of renal impairment is present.

Use of Concomitant Medications That May Affect Renal Function Or Metformin Disposition: Concomitant medication(s) that may affect renal function or result in significant hemodynamic change or may interfere with the disposition of metformin HCl, such as cationic drugs that are eliminated by renal tubular secretion (see DRUG INTERACTIONS), should be used with caution.

Radiologic Studies Involving The Use Of Iodinated Contrast Materials (For Example, Intravenous Urogram, Intravenous Cholangiography, Angiography, And Scans With Contrast Materials): Parenteral contrast studies with iodinated materials can lead to acute renal failure and have been associated with lactic acidosis in patients receiving metformin HCl (see CONTRAINDICATIONS). Therefore, in patients in whom any such study is planned, metformin HCl should be withheld for at least 48 hours prior to, and 48 hours subsequent to, the procedure and reinstituted only after renal function has been re-evaluated and found to be normal.

Hypoxic States: Cardiovascular collapse (shock) from whatever cause, acute congestive heart failure, acute myocardial infarction and other conditions characterized by hypoxemia have been associated with lactic acidosis and may also cause prerenal azotemia. When such events occur in patients on metformin HCl therapy, the drug should be promptly discontinued.

Surgical Procedures: Metformin HCl therapy should be temporarily suspended for any surgical procedure (except minor procedures not associated with restricted intake of food and fluids) and should be not restarted until the patient's oral intake has resumed and renal function has been evaluated as normal.

Alcohol Intake: Alcohol is known to potentiate the effect of metformin on lactate metabolism. Patients, therefore, should be warned against excessive alcohol intake, acute or chronic, while receiving metformin HCl.

Impaired Hepatic Function: Since impaired hepatic function has been associated with some cases of lactic acidosis, metformin HCl should generally be avoided in patients with clinical or laboratory evidence of hepatic disease.

Vitamin B_{12} Levels: A decrease to subnormal levels of previously normal serum vitamin B_{12} levels, without clinical manifestations is observed in approximately 7% of patients receiving metformin HCl in controlled clinical trials of 29 weeks duration. Such decrease, possibly due to interference with B_{12} absorption from the B_{12}-intrinsic factor complex, is however, very rarely associated with anemia and appears to be rapidly reversible with discontinuation of metformin HCl or vitamin B_{12}supplementation. Measurement of hematologic parameters on an annual basis is advised in patients on metformin HCl and any apparent abnormalities should be appropriately investigated and managed (see Laboratory Tests).

Certain individuals (those with inadequate vitamin B_{12} or calcium intake or absorption) appear to be predisposed to developing subnormal vitamin B_{12} levels. In these patients, routine serum vitamin B_{12} measurements at two- to three-year intervals may be useful.

Change in Clinical Status Of Previously Controlled Diabetic: A diabetic patient previously well controlled on metformin HCl who develops laboratory abnormalities or clinical illness (especially vague and poorly defined illness) should be evaluated promptly for evidence of ketoacidosis or lactic acidosis. Evaluation should include serum electrolytes and ketones, blood glucose and, if indicated, blood pH, lactate, pyruvate and metformin levels. If acidosis of either form occurs, metformin HCl must be stopped immediately and other appropriate corrective measures initiated (see also WARNINGS).

Hypoglycemia: Hypoglycemia does not occur in patients receiving metformin HCl alone under usual circumstances of use, but could occur when caloric intake is deficient, when strenuous exercise is not compensated by caloric supplementation, or during concomitant use with other glucose-lowering agents (such as sulfonylureas) or ethanol.

Elderly, debilitated or malnourished patients, and those with adrenal or pituitary insufficiency or alcohol intoxication are particularly susceptible to hypoglycemic effects. Hypoglycemia may be difficult to recognize in the elderly, and in people who are taking beta-adrenergic blocking drugs.

Loss of Control of Blood Glucose: When a patient stabilized on any diabetic regimen is exposed to stress such as fever, trauma, infection, or surgery, a temporary loss of glycemic control may occur. At such times, it may necessary to withhold metformin HCl and temporarily administer insulin. metformin HCl may be reinstituted after the acute episode is resolved.

The effectiveness of oral antidiabetic drugs in lowering blood glucose to a targeted level decreases in many patients over a period of time. This phenomenon, which may be due to progression of the underlying disease or to diminished responsiveness to the drug, is known as secondary failure, to distinguish it from primary failure in which the drug is ineffective during initial therapy. Should secondary failure occur with metformin HCl or sulfonylurea

PRECAUTIONS: *(cont'd)*

monotherapy, combined therapy with metformin HCl and sulfonylurea may result in a response. Should secondary failure occur with combined metformin HCl/sulfonylurea therapy, it may be necessary to initiate insulin therapy.

Information for the Patient: Patients should be informed of the potential risks and advantages of metformin HCl and of alternative modes of therapy. They should also be informed about the importance of adherence to dietary instructions, of a regular exercise program, and of regular testing of blood glucose, glycosylated hemoglobin, renal function and hematologic parameters.

The risks of lactic acidosis, its symptoms, and conditions that predispose to its development, as noted in the WARNINGS and PRECAUTIONS secretions should be explained to patients. Patients should be advised to discontinue metformin HCl immediately and to promptly notify their health practitioner if unexplained hyperventilation, myalgia, malaise, unusual somnolence or other nonspecific symptoms occur. Once a patient is stabilized on any dose level of metformin HCl, gastrointestinal symptoms, which are common during initiation of therapy, are unlikely to be drug related. Later occurrence of gastrointestinal symptoms could be due to lactic acidosis or other serious disease.

patients should be counselled against excessive alcohol intake, either acute or chronic, while receiving metformin HCl.

Metformin HCl alone does not usually cause hypoglycemia, although it may occur when metformin HCl is used in conjunction with oral sulfonylureas. When initiating combination therapy, the risks of hypoglycemia, its symptoms and treatment, and conditions that predispose to its development should be explained to patients (see Patient Labeling printed below).

Laboratory Tests: Response to all diabetic therapies should be monitored by periodic measurements of fasting blood glucose and glycosylated hemoglobin levels with a goal of decreasing these levels toward the normal range. During initial dose titration, fasting glucose can be used to determine the therapeutic response. Thereafter, both glucose and glycosylated hemoglobin should be monitored. Measurements of glycosylated hemoglobin may be especially useful for evaluating long-term control (see DOSAGE AND ADMINISTRATION).

Initial and periodic monitoring of hematologic parameters (*e.g.,* hemoglobin/hematocrit and red blood cell indices) and renal function (serum creatinine) should be performed at least on an annual basis. While megaloblastic anemia has rarely been seen with metformin HCl therapy, if this is suspected, vitamin B_{12} deficiency should be excluded.

DRUG INTERACTIONS:

Glyburide: In a single dose interaction study in NIDDM subjects, co-administration of metformin and glyburide did not result in any changes in either-metformin pharmacokinetics or pharmacodynamics. Decrease in glyburide AUC and C_{max} were observed, but were highly variable. The single-dose nature of this study and the lack of correlation between glyburide blood levels and pharmacodynamic effects, makes the clinical significance of this interaction uncertain (see DOSAGE AND ADMINISTRATION, Concomitant Metformin HCl and Oral Sulfonylurea Therapy).

Furosemide: A single-dose, metformin-furosemide drug interaction study in healthy subjects demonstrated that pharmacokinetic parameters of both compounds were affected by co-administration. Furosemide increased the metformin plasma and blood C_{max} by 22% and blood AUC by 15%, without any significant change in metformin renal clearance. When administered with metformin, the C_{max} and AUC of furosemide were 31% and 12% smaller, respectively, than when administered alone, and the terminal half-life was decreased by 32%, without any significant change in furosemide renal clearance. No information is available about the interaction of metformin and furosemide when co-administered chronically.

Nifedipine: A single-dose, metformin-nifedipine drug interaction study in normal healthy volunteers demonstrated that co-administration of nifedipine increased plasma metformin C_{max} and AUC by 20% and 9%, respectively, and increased the amount excreted in the urine. T_{max} and half-life were unaffected. Nifedipine appears to enhance the absorption of metformin. Metformin had minimal effects on nifedipine.

Cationic Drugs: Cationic drugs (*e.g.,* amiloride, digoxin, morphine, procainamide, quinidine, quinidine, ranitidine, triamterene, trimethoprim, and vancomycin) that are eliminated by renal tubular secretion theoretically have the potential for interaction with metformin by competing for common renal tubular transport systems. Such interaction between metformin and oral cimetidine has been observed in normal healthy volunteers in both single- and multiple-dose, metformin-cimetidine drug interaction studies, with a 60% increase in peak metformin plasma and whole blood concentrations and a 40% increase in plasma and whole blood metformin AUC. There was no charge in elimination half-life in the single-dose study. Metformin had no effect on cimetidine pharmacokinetics. Although such interactions remain theoretical (except for cimetidine), careful patient monitoring and dose adjustment of metformin HCl and/or the interfering drug is recommended in patients who are taking cationic medications that are excreted via the proximal renal tubular secretory system.

Other: Certain drugs lend to produce hyperglycemia and may lead to loss of glycemic control. These drugs include thiazide and other diuretics, corticosteroids, phenothiazines, thyroid products, estrogens, oral contraceptives, phenytoin, nicotinic acid, sympathomimetics, calcium channel blocking drugs, and isoniazid. When such drugs are administered to a patient receiving metformin HCl, the patient should be closely observed to maintain adequate glycemic control.

In healthy volunteers, the pharmacokinetics of metformin and propranolol and metformin and ibuprofen were not affected when co-administered in single-dose interaction studies.

Metformin is negligibly bound to plasma proteins and is, therefore, less likely to interact with highly protein-bound drugs such as salicylates, sulfonamides, chloramphenicol, and probenecid, as compared to the sulfonylureas, which are extensively bound to serum proteins.

Carcinogenesis, Mutagenesis, Impairment of Fertility: Long-term carcinogenicity studies have been performed in rats (dosing duration 104 weeks) and mice (dosing duration of 91 weeks) at doses up to and including 900/mg/kg/day and 1500 mg/kg/day, respectively. These doses are both approximately three times the maximum recommended human daily dose on a body surface area basis. No evidence of carcinogenicity with metformin was found in either male or female mice. Similarly, there was no tumorigenic potential observed with metformin in male rats. However, an increased incidence of benign stromal uterine polyps was seen in female rats treated with 900 mg/kg/day.

No evidence of a mutagenic potential of metformin was found in the Ames test (*S. typhimurium*) gene mutation test (mouse lymphoma cells) chromosomal aberrations test (human lymphocytes), or *in-vivo* micronuclei formation test (mouse bone marrow).

Fertility of male or female rats was unaffected by metformin administration at doses as high as 600 mg/kg/day, or approximately two times the maximum recommended human daily dose on a body surface area basis.

Pregnancy, Teratogenic Effects, Pregnancy Category B: Safety in pregnant women has not been established. Metformin was not teratogenic in rats and rabbits at doses up to 600 mg/kg/day, or about two times the maximum recommended human daily dose on a body surface area basis. Determination of fetal concentrations demonstrated a partial placental barrier to metformin. Because animal reproduction studies are not always predictive of human response, any decision to use this drug should be balanced against the benefits and risks.

DRUG INTERACTIONS: *(cont'd)*

Because recent information suggests that abnormal blood glucose levels during pregnancy are associated with a higher incidence of congenital abnormalities, there is a consensus among experts that insulin be used during pregnancy to maintain blood glucose levels as close to normal as possible.

Nursing Mothers: Studies in lactating rats show that metformin is excreted into milk and reaches levels comparable to those in plasma. Similar studies have not been conducted in nursing mothers, but caution should be exercised in such patients, and a decision should be made whether to discontinue nursing or to discontinue the drug, taking into account the importance of the drug to the mother.

Pediatric Use: Safety and effectiveness in children have not been established. Studies in maturity onset diabetes of the young (MODY) have not been conducted.

Geriatric Use: Controlled clinical studies of metformin HCl did not include sufficient numbers of elderly patients to determine whether they respond differently from younger patients, although other reported clinical experience has not identified differences in responses between the elderly and younger patients. Metformin HCl is known to be substantially excreted by the kidney and because the risk of serious adverse reactions to the drug is greater in patients with impaired renal function, it should only be used in patients with normal renal function (see CONTRAINDICATIONS and CLINICAL PHARMACOLOGY, Pharmacokinetics). Because aging is associated with reduced renal function, metformin HCl should be used with caution as age increases. Care should be taken in dose selection and should be based on careful and regular monitoring of renal function. Generally, elderly patients should not be titrated to the maximum dose of metformin HCl (see also DOSAGE AND ADMINISTRATION).

ADVERSE REACTIONS:

Lactic Acidosis: See WARNINGS, PRECAUTIONS and OVERDOSAGE sections.

Gastrointestinal Reactions: Gastrointestinal symptoms (diarrhea, nausea, vomiting, abdominal bloating, flatulence, and anorexia) are the most common reactions to metformin HCl and are approximately 30% more frequent in patients of metformin HCl monotherapy than in placebo-treated patients, particularly during initiation of metformin HCl therapy. These symptoms are generally transient and resolve spontaneously during continued treatment. Occasionally, temporary dose reduction may be useful. In controlled trials, metformin HCl was discontinued due to gastrointestinal reactions in approximately 4% of patients.

Because gastrointestinal symptoms during therapy initiation appear to be dose-related, they may be decreased by gradual dose escalation and by having patients take metformin HCl with meals (see DOSAGE AND ADMINISTRATION).

Because significant diarrhea and/or vomiting may cause dehydration and prerenal azotemia, under such circumstances, metformin HCl should be temporarily discontinued.

For patients who have been stabilized on metformin HCl, nonspecific gastrointestinal symptoms should not be attributed to therapy unless intercurrent illness or lactic acidosis have been excluded.

Special Senses: During initiation if metformin HCl therapy, approximately 3% of patients may complain of an unpleasant or metallic taste, which usually resolves spontaneously.

Dermatologic Reactions: The incidence of rash/dermatitis in controlled clinical trials was comparable to placebo for metformin HCl monotherapy and to sulfonylurea for metformin HCl/sulfonylurea therapy.

Hematologic: (See also PRECAUTIONS.) During controlled clinical trials of 29 weeks duration, approximately 9% of patients on metformin HCl monotherapy and 6% of patients on metformin HCl/sulfonylurea therapy developed asymptomatic subnormal serum vitamin B_{12} levels; serum folic acid levels did not decrease significantly. However, only five cases of megaloblastic anemia have been reported with metformin administration (none during U.S. clinical studies) and no increases incidence of neuropathy has been observed. Therefore, serum B_{12} levels should be appropriately monitored or periodic parenteral B_{12} supplementation considered.

DRUG ABUSE AND DEPENDENCE:

Metformin HCl possesses no pharmacodynamic properties, either primary or secondary, which could be expected to result in abuse as a recreational drug or addiction.

OVERDOSAGE:

Hypoglycemia has not been seen even with ingestion of up to 85 grams of metformin HCl, although lactic acidosis has occurred in such circumstances (see WARNINGS). Metformin is a dialyzable with a clearance of up to 170 ml/min under good hemodynamic conditions. Therefore, hemodialysis may be useful for removal of accumulated drug from patients in whom metformin overdosage is suspected.

DOSAGE AND ADMINISTRATION:

There is no fixed dosage regimen for the management of hyperglycemia in diabetes mellitus with metformin HCl or any other pharmacologic agent. Dosage of metformin HCl must be individualized on the basis of both effectiveness and tolerance, while not exceeding the maximum recommended daily dose of 2550 mg. Metformin HCl should be given in divided doses with meals and should be started at a low dose, with gradual dose escalation, as described below, both to reduce gastrointestinal side effects and to permit identification of the minimum dose required for adequate glycemic control of the patient.

During treatment initiation and dose titration (see USUAL STARTING DOSE), fasting plasma glucose should be used to determine the therapeutic response to metformin HCl and identify the minimum effective dose for the patient. Thereafter, glycosylated hemoglobin should be measured at intervals of approximately three months. **The therapeutic goal should be to decrease both fasting plasma glucose and glycosylated hemoglobin levels to normal or near normal by using the lowest effective dose of metformin HCl, either when used as monotherapy or in combination with sulfonylurea.**

Monitoring blood glucose and glycosylated hemoglobin will also permit detection of primary failure, i.e., inadequate lowering of blood glucose at the maximum recommended dose of medication, and secondary failure, i.e., loss of an adequate blood glucose lowering response after an initial period of effectiveness.

Short-term administration of metformin HCl maybe sufficient during periods of transient loss of control in patients usually well-controlled.

Usual Starting Dose: In general, clinically significant responses are not seen at doses below 1500 mg per day. However, a lower recommended starting dose and gradually increased dosage is advised to minimize gastrointestinal symptoms.

Metformin HCl 500 mg Tablets: The usual starting dose of metformin HCl 500 mg tablets in one tablet b.i.d., given with the morning and evening meals. Dosage increases should be made in increments of one tablet every week, given in divided doses, up to a maximum of 2500 mg per day. Metformin HCl can be administered twice a day up to 2000 mg per day (*e.g.,* 1000 mg b.i.d with morning and evening meals). If a 2500 mg daily dose is required, it may be better tolerated given t.i.d. with meals.

DOSAGE AND ADMINISTRATION: *(cont'd)*

Metformin HCl 850 mg Tablets: The usual starting dose of metformin HCl 850 mg tablets is one tablet daily, given with the morning meal. Dosage increases should be made in increments of one tablet every OTHER week, given in divided doses, up or a maximum of 2550 mg per day. The usual maintenance dose is 850 mg b.i.d. with the morning and evening meals. When necessary, patients may be given 850 mg t.i.d. with meals.

Transfer from Other Antidiabetic Therapy: When transferring patients from standard oral hypoglycemic agents other than chlorpropamide to metformin HCl, no transition period generally is necessary. When transferring patients from chlorpropamide, care should be exercised during the first two weeks because of the prolonged retention of chlorpropamide in the body, leading to overlapping drug effects and possible hypoglycemia.

Concomitant Metformin HCl and Oral Sulfonylurea Therapy: If patients have not responded to four weeks of the maximum dose of metformin HCl monotherapy, consideration should be given to gradual addition of an oral sulfonylurea while continuing metformin HCl at the maximum dose, even if prior primary or secondary failure to a sulfonylurea has occurred. Clinical and pharmacokinetic drug-drug interaction data are currently available only for metformin plus glyburide (glibenclamide). Published clinical information exists for the use of metformin with either chlorpropamide, tolbutamide or glipizide. No published clinical information exists regarding concomitant use of metformin with acetohexamide or tolazamide.

With concomitant metformin HCl and sulfonylurea therapy, the desired control of blood glucose may be obtained by adjusting the dose of each drug. However, attempts should be made to identify the minimum effective dose of each drug to achieve this goal. With concomitant metformin HCl and sulfonylurea therapy, the risk of hypoglycemia associated with sulfonylurea therapy continues and may be increased. Appropriate precautions should be taken.

If patients have not satisfactorily responded to one to three months of concomitant therapy with the maximum dose of metformin HCl and the maximum dose of an oral sulfonylurea, institution of insulin therapy and discontinuation of these oral agents should be considered the maximum dose of an oral sulfonylurea, institution of insulin therapy and discontinuation of these oral agents should be considered.

Specific Patient Populations: Metformin HCl is not recommended for use in pregnancy or for use in children.

The initial and maintenance dosing of metformin HCl should be conservative in patients with advanced age, due to the potential for decreased renal function in this population. Any dosage adjustment should be based on a careful assessment of renal function. Generally, elderly patients should not be titrated to the maximum dose of metformin HCl.

In debilitated or malnourished patients, the dosing should be conservative and based on a careful assessment of renal function.

PATIENT PACKAGE INSERT:

PATIENT INFORMATION ABOUT METFORMIN HCL TABLETS

> **A small number of people who have taken metformin hydrochloride have developed a serious condition called lactic acidosis. Properly functioning kidneys are needed to prevent lactic acidosis. Most people with kidney problems should not take metformin hydrochloride. (See Question Nos. 7 and 11.)**

Q1. WHY DO I NEED TO TAKE METFORMIN HCL?

Your doctor has prescribed metformin hydrochloride to treat your type II diabetes. This is also known as non-insulin-dependent diabetes mellitus (NIDDM).

Q2. WHAT IS TYPE II DIABETES?

People with diabetes are not able to make enough insulin and/or respond normally to the insulin in their body does make. When this happens, sugar (glucose) builds up in the blood. This can lead to serious medical problems including kidney damage, amputations and blindness. Diabetes is also closely linked to heart disease. The main goal of treating diabetes is to lower your blood sugar to a normal level.

Q3. HOW IS TYPE II DIABETES USUALLY CONTROLLED?

High blood sugar can be lowered by diet and exercise, by a number of oral medications and by insulin injections. Before taking metformin hydrochloride you should first try to control your diabetes by exercise and weight loss. Even if you are taking metformin hydrochloride, you should still exercise and follow the diet recommended for your diabetes.

Q4. DOES METFORMIN HYDROCHLORIDE WORK DIFFERENTLY FROM OTHER GLUCOSE-CONTROL MEDICATIONS?

Yes it does. Until metformin hydrochloride was introduced, all the available oral glucose-control medications were from the same chemical group called sulfonylureas. These drugs lower blood sugar primarily by causing more of the body's own insulin to be released. Metformin hydrochloride lowers the amount of sugar in your blood by helping your body respond better to its own insulin. Metformin hydrochloride does not cause your body to produce more insulin. Therefore, metformin hydrochloride rarely causes hypoglycemia (low blood sugar) and doesn't usually cause weight gain.

Q5. WHAT HAPPENS IF MY BLOOD SUGAR IS STILL TOO HIGH?

When blood sugar cannot be lowered enough by either metformin hydrochloride or a sulfonylurea, the two medications may be effective taken together. However, if you are unable to maintain your blood sugar with diet, exercise and glucose-control medication taken orally, then your doctor may prescribe injectable insulin to control your diabetes.

Q6. CAN METFORMIN HCL CAUSE SIDE EFFECTS?

Metformin hydrochloride, like all blood-sugar lowering medications, can cause side effects in some patients. Most of these side effects are minor and will go away after you've taken metformin hydrochloride for a while. However, there are also serious, but rare side effects related to metformin hydrochloride (see PATIENT PACKAGE INSERT, Q8. Are there any serious side effects that Metformin Hydrochloride can cause?).

Q7. WHAT KIND OF SIDE EFFECTS CAN METFORMIN HCL CAUSE?

If side effects occur, they usually occur during the first few weeks of therapy. They are normally minor ones such as diarrhea, nausea and upset stomach. Taking your metformin hydrochloride with meals can help reduce these side effects.

Although these side effects are likely to go away, call your doctor if you have severe discomfort or if these effects last for more than a few weeks. Some patients may need to have their dose lowered or stop taking metformin hydrochloride, either temporarily or permanently. Although these problems occur in up to one-third of patients when they first start taking metformin hydrochloride, you should tell your doctor if the problems come back or start later on during the therapy.

About three out of one hundred people report having a temporary unpleasant or metallic taste when they start taking metformin hydrochloride.

PATIENT PACKAGE INSERT: *(cont'd)*

Q8. ARE THERE ANY SERIOUS SIDE EFFECTS THAT METFORMIN HCL CAN CAUSE?

Metformin hydrochloride rarely causes serious side effects. The most serious side effect that metformin hydrochloride can cause if called lactic acidosis.

Q9. WHAT IS LACTIC ACIDOSIS AND CAN IT HAPPEN TO ME?

Lactic acidosis is caused by a buildup of lactic acid in the blood. Lactic acidosis associated with metformin hydrochloride is rare and has occurred mostly in people whose kidneys were not working normally. Lactic acidosis has been reported in about one in 33,000 patients taking metformin hydrochloride over the course of a year. Although rare, if lactic acidosis does occur, it can be fatal in up to half the cases.

It's also important for your liver to be working normally when you take metformin hydrochloride. Your liver helps remove lactic acid from your bloodstream.

Your doctor will monitor your diabetes and may perform blood tests on you from time to tome to make sure your kidneys and your liver are functioning normally.

There is no evidence that metformin hydrochloride causes harm to the kidneys or liver.

Q10. ARE THERE OTHER RISK FACTORS FOR LACTIC ACIDOSIS?

Your risk of developing lactic acidosis from taking metformin hydrochloride is very low as long as your kidneys and liver are healthy. However, some factors can increase your risk because they can affect kidney and liver function. You should not take metformin hydrochloride if:

You have chronic kidney or liver problems

You drink alcohol excessively (all the time or short-term "binge" drinking)

You are seriously dehydrated (have lost a large amount of body fluids)

You are going to have certain x-ray procedures with injectable contrast agents

You are going to have surgery

You develop a serious condition such as a heart attack, severe infection, or a stroke

Q11. WHAT ARE THE SYMPTOMS OF LACTIC ACIDOSIS?

Some of the symptoms include: feeling very weak, tired or uncomfortable; unusual muscle pain, trouble breathing, unusual or unexpected stomach discomfort, feeling cold, feeling dizzy or lightheaded, or suddenly developing a slow or irregular heartbeat.

If you notice these symptoms, or if your medical condition has suddenly changed, stop taking metformin hydrochloride and call your doctor right away. Lactic acidosis is a medical emergency that must be treated in a hospital.

Q12. WHAT DOES MY DOCTOR NEED TO KNOW TO DECREASE MY RISK OF LACTIC ACIDOSIS?

Tell your doctor if you have an illness that results in severe vomiting, diarrhea and/or fever, or if your intake of fluids is significantly reduced. These situations can lead to severe dehydration, and it may be necessary to stop taking metformin hydrochloride temporarily.

You should let your doctor know if you are going to have any surgery or specialized x-ray procedures that require injection of contrast agents. Metformin hydrochloride therapy will need to be stopped temporarily in such instances.

Q13. CAN I TAKE METFORMIN HYDROCHLORIDE WITH OTHER MEDICATIONS?

Remind your doctor that you are taking metformin hydrochloride when any new drug is prescribed or a change is made in how you take a drug already prescribed. Metformin hydrochloride may interfere with the way some drugs work and some drugs may interfere with the action of metformin hydrochloride.

Q14. WHAT IF I BECOME PREGNANT WHILE TAKING METFORMIN HYDROCHLORIDE?

Tell your doctor if you plan to become pregnant or have become pregnant. As with other oral glucose-control medications, you should not take metformin hydrochloride during pregnancy.

Usually your doctor will prescribe insulin while you are pregnant. As with all medications, you and your doctor should discuss the use of metformin hydrochloride if you are nursing a child.

Q15. ARE THERE OTHER RISKS ASSOCIATED WITH METFORMIN HCL?

There is some evidence that any oral diabetes drug may increase the risk of heart problems. Experts are not sure what the real risk is for heart problems, if any for taking oral diabetes medicine.

Q16. HOW DO I TAKE METFORMIN HCL?

Your doctor will tell you how many metformin hydrochloride tablets to take how often. This should also be printed on the label of your prescription. You will probably be started on a low dose of metformin hydrochloride and your dosage will be increased gradually until your blood sugar is controlled.

Q17. WHERE CAN I GET MORE INFORMATION ABOUT METFORMIN HCL?

This leaflet is a summary of the most important information about metformin HCl. If you have any questions or problems, you should talk to your doctor or other healthcare provider about type II diabetes as well as metformin hydrochloride and its side effects. There is also a leaflet (package insert) written for health professionals that your pharmacist can let you read.

HOW SUPPLIED:

Glucophage is supplied as white, unscored, film-coated, cylindrical, biconvex tablets.

Tablets are debossed with the letters "GL" and either "500" or "850" to indicate strength.

Storage: Store between 15°-30°C (59°-86°F).

HOW SUPPLIED - EQUIVALENTS NOT AVAILABLE:

Tablet, Uncoated - Oral - 500 mg

100's	$46.27	GLUCOPHAGE, Bristol Myers Squibb	00087-6060-05

Tablet, Uncoated - Oral - 850 mg

100's	$78.66	GLUCOPHAGE, Bristol Myers Squibb	00087-6070-05

METHADONE HYDROCHLORIDE *(001753)*

CATEGORIES: Analgesics; Antipyretics; Central Nervous System Agents; Narcotic Addiction; Narcotic Analgesics; Narcotic Detoxification; Narcotics, Synthetics & Combinations; Opiate Agonists (Controlled); Pain; DEA Class CII; FDA Approval Pre 1982

BRAND NAMES: *Adolan*; *Dolmed*; **Dolophine**; Dolophine HCL; *Eptadone*; *L-Polamidon* (Germany); *Mephenon*; *Metadon*; *Metasedin*; Methadone Hcl; Methadose; *Methaforte Linctus*; *Pallidone*; *Physeptone* (England); *Symoron*; *Tussol*; Westadone

(International brand names outside U.S. in italics)

FORMULARIES: Aetna; Medi-Cal

WARNING:
CONDITIONS FOR DISTRIBUTION AND USE OF METHADONE PRODUCTS:
Code of Federal Regulations, Title 21, Sec. 291.505
METHADONE PRODUCTS, WHEN USED FOR THE TREATMENT OF NARCOTIC ADDICTION IN DETOXIFICATION OR MAINTENANCE PROGRAMS, SHALL BE DISPENSED ONLY BY APPROVED HOSPITAL PHARMACIES, APPROVED COMMUNITY PHARMACIES, AND MAINTENANCE PROGRAMS APPROVED BY THE FOOD AND DRUG ADMINISTRATION AND THE DESIGNATED STATE AUTHORITY.
APPROVED MAINTENANCE PROGRAMS SHALL DISPENSE AND USE METHADONE IN ORAL FORM ONLY AND ACCORDING TO THE TREATMENT REQUIREMENTS STIPULATED IN THE FEDERAL METHADONE REGULATIONS (21 CFR 291.505).
FAILURE TO ABIDE BY THE REQUIREMENTS IN THESE REGULATIONS MAY RESULT IN CRIMINAL PROSECUTION, SEIZURE OF THE DRUG SUPPLY, REVOCATION OF THE PROGRAM APPROVAL, AND INJUNCTION PRECLUDING OPERATION OF THE PROGRAM.
A METHADONE PRODUCT, WHEN USED AS AN ANALGESIC, MAY BE DISPENSED IN ANY LICENSED PHARMACY.

DESCRIPTION:

Methadone hydrochloride tablets, USP (3-hepatone, 6-(dimethylamino)-4,4-diphenyl-, hydrochloride) is a white crystalline material that is water soluble. Methadone hydrochloride has the empirical formula $C_{21}H_{27}NO{\cdot}HCl$, and its molecular weight is 345.91.

Each ml contains methadone hydrochloride, 10 mg (0.029 mmol) and sodium chloride of, 0.9%. Sodium hydroxide and/or hydrochloric acid may have been added during manufacture to adjust the pH. The 20-ml vials also contain chlorobutanol (chloroform derivative), 0.5%, as a preservative.

CLINICAL PHARMACOLOGY:

Methadone hydrochloride is a synthetic narcotic analgesic with multiple actions quantitatively similar to those of morphine, the most prominent of which involve the central nervous system & organs composed of smooth muscle. The principal actions of therapeutic value are analgesia and sedation and detoxification or temporary maintenance in narcotic addiction. The methadone abstinence syndrome, although qualitatively similar to that of morphine, differs in that the onset is slower, the course is more prolonged, and the symptoms are less severe.

A parenteral dose of 8 to 10 mg of methadone is approximately equivalent in analgesic effect to 10 mg of morphine. With single-dose administration, the onset and duration of analgesic action of the 2 drugs are similar.

When administered orally, methadone is approximately one-half as potent as when given parenterally. Oral administration results in a delay of the onset, a lowering of the peak, and an increase in the duration of analgesic effect.

INDICATIONS AND USAGE:

For relief of severe pain.

For detoxification treatment of narcotic addiction.

For temporary maintenance treatment of narcotic addiction.

NOTE: If methadone is administered for treatment of heroin dependence for more than 3 weeks, the procedure passes from treatment of the acute withdrawal syndrome (detoxification) to maintenance therapy. Maintenance treatment is permitted to be undertaken only by approved methadone programs. This does not preclude the maintenance treatment of an addict who is hospitalized for medical conditions other than addiction and who requires temporary maintenance during the critical period of his stay or whose enrollment has been verified in a program which has approval for maintenance treatment with methadone.

CONTRAINDICATIONS:

Hypersensitivity to methadone.

WARNINGS:

Methadone hydrochloride, a narcotic, is a Schedule II controlled substance under the Federal Controlled Substances Act. Appropriate security measures should be taken to safeguard stocks of methadone against diversion.

Interaction with Other Central-Nervous-System Depressants: Methadone should be used with caution and in reduced dosage in patients who are concurrently receiving other narcotic analgesics, general anesthetics, phenothiazines, other tranquilizers, sedative-hypnotics, tricyclic antidepressants, and other CNS depressants (including alcohol). Respiratory depression, hypotension, and profound sedation or coma may result.

Anxiety: Since methadone, as used by tolerant subjects as a constant maintenance dosage, is not a tranquilizer, patients who are maintained on this drug will react to life problems and stresses with the same symptoms of anxiety as do other individuals. The physician should not confuse such symptoms with those of narcotic abstinence and should not attempt to treat anxiety by increasing the dosage of methadone. The action of methadone in maintenance treatment is limited to the control of narcotic symptoms and is ineffective for relief of general anxiety.

Head Injury and Increased Intracranial Pressure: The respiratory depressant effects of methadone and its capacity to elevate cerebrospinal-fluid pressure may be markedly exaggerated in the presence of increased intracranial pressure. Furthermore, narcotics produce side effects that may obscure the clinical course of patients with head injuries. In such patients, methadone must be used with caution and only if it is deemed essential.

Asthma and Other Respiratory Conditions: Methadone should be used with caution in patients having an acute asthmatic attack, in those with chronic obstructive pulmonary disease or cor pulmonale, and in individuals with a substantially decreased respiratory reserve, preexisting respiratory depression, hypoxia, or hypercapnia. In such patients, even usual therapeutic doses of narcotics may decrease respiratory drive while simultaneously increasing airway resistance to the point of apnea.

WARNINGS: *(cont'd)*

Hypotensive Effect: The administration of methadone may result in severe hypotension in an individual whose ability to maintain his blood pressure has already been compromised by a depleted blood volume or concurrent administration of such drugs as the phenothiazines or certain anesthetics.

Use in Ambulatory Patients: Methadone may impair the mental and/or physical abilities required for the performance of potentially hazardous tasks, such as driving a car or operating machinery. The patient should be cautioned accordingly.

Methadone, like other narcotics, may produce orthostatic hypotension in ambulatory patients.

Use in Pregnancy: Safe use in pregnancy has not been established in relation to possible adverse effects on fetal development. Therefore, methadone should not be used in pregnant women unless, in the judgment of the physician, the potential benefits outweigh the possible hazards.

Methadone is not recommended for obstetric analgesia because its long duration of action increased the probability of respiratory depression in the newborn.

Usage in Children: Methadone is not recommended for use as an analgesic in children, since documented clinical experience has been insufficient to establish a suitable dosage regiment for the pediatric age group.

PRECAUTIONS:

Special-Risk Patients: Methadone should be given with caution and the initial dose should be reduced in certain patients, such as the elderly or debilitated and those with severe impairment of hepatic or renal function, hypothyroidism, Addison's disease, prostatic hypertrophy, or urethral stricture.

Acute Abdominal Conditions: The administration of methadone or other narcotics may obscure the diagnosis or clinical course in patients with acute abdominal conditions.

DRUG INTERACTIONS:

Pentazocine: Patients who are addicted to heroin or who are on the methadone maintenance program may experience withdrawal symptoms when given pentazocine.

Rifampin: The concurrent administration of rifampin may possibly reduce the blood concentration of methadone to a degree sufficient to produce withdrawal symptoms. The mechanism by which rifampin may decrease blood concentrations of methadone is not fully understood, although enhanced microsomal drug-metabolized enzymes may influence drug disposition.

Monoamine Oxidase (MAO) Inhibitors: Therapeutic doses of meperidine have precipitated severe reactions in patients concurrently receiving monoamine oxidase inhibitors or those who have received such agents within 14 days. Similar reactions thus far have not been reported with methadone; but if the use of methadone is necessary in such patients, a sensitivity test should be performed in which repeated small incremental doses are administered over the course of several hours while the patient's condition and vital signs are under careful observation.

Desipramine: Blood levels of desipramine have increased with concurrent methadone therapy.

ADVERSE REACTIONS:

THE MAJOR HAZARDS OF METHADONE, AS OF OTHER NARCOTIC ANALGESICS, ARE RESPIRATORY DEPRESSION AND, TO A LESSER DEGREE, CIRCULATORY DEPRESSION. RESPIRATORY ARREST, SHOCK, AND CARDIAC ARREST HAVE OCCURRED.

The most frequently observed adverse reactions include lightheadedness, dizziness, sedation, nausea, vomiting, and sweating. These effects seem to be more prominent in ambulatory patients and in those who are not suffering severe pain. In such individuals, lower doses are advisable. Some adverse reactions may be alleviated if the ambulatory patient lies down.

Other adverse reactions include the following:

Central Nervous System: Euphoria, dysphoria, weakness, headache, insomnia, agitation, disorientation, and visual disturbances.

Gastrointestinal: Dry mouth, anorexia, constipation, and biliary tract spasm.

Cardiovascular: Flushing of the face, bradycardia, palpitation, faintness, and syncope.

Genitourinary: Urinary retention or hesitancy, antidiuretic effect, and reduced libido and/or potency.

Allergic: Pruritus, urticaria, other skin rashes, edema, and rarely, hemorrhagic urticaria.

Hematologic: Reversible thrombocytopenia has been described in a narcotics addict with chronic hepatitis.

In addition, pain at injection site; local tissue irritation and induration following subcutaneous injection, particularly when repeated.

DRUG ABUSE AND DEPENDENCE:

METHADONE CAN PRODUCE DRUG DEPENDENCE OF THE MORPHINE TYPE AND, THEREFORE, HAS THE POTENTIAL FOR BEING ABUSED. PSYCHIC DEPENDENCE, PHYSICAL DEPENDENCE, AND TOLERANCE MAY DEVELOP UPON REPEATED ADMINISTRATION OF METHADONE, AND IT SHOULD BE PRESCRIBED AND ADMINISTERED WITH THE SAME DEGREE OF CAUTION APPROPRIATE TO THE USE OF MORPHINE.

OVERDOSAGE:

Signs and Symptoms: Methadone is an opioid and produces effects similar to those of morphine. Symptoms of overdose begin within seconds after intravenous administration and within minutes of nasal, oral, or rectal administration. Prominent symptoms are miosis, respiratory depression, somnolence, coma, cool clammy skin, skeletal muscle flaccidity that may progress to hypotension, apnea, bradycardia and death. Noncardiac pulmonary edema may occur, and monitoring of heart filling pressures may be helpful.

Treatment: To obtain up-to-date information about the treatment of overdose, a good resource is your certified Regional Poison Control Center. Telephone numbers of certified poison control centers are listed in the supplemental section. In managing overdosage, consider the possibility of multiple drug overdoses, interaction among drugs, and usual drug kinetics in your patient.

Initial management of opioid overdose should include the establishment of a secure airway and support of ventilation and perfusion. Naloxone may be given to antagonize opioid effects, but the airway must be secured as vomiting may ensue. **The duration of methadone effect is much longer (36 to 48 hours) than the duration of naloxone effect (1 to 3 hours), and repeated doses (or continuous intravenous infusion) of naloxone may be required.**

If the patient has chronically abused opioids, administration of naloxone may precipitate a withdrawal syndrome that may include yawning, tearing, restlessness, sweating, dilated pupils, piloerection, vomiting, diarrhea, and abdominal cramps. If these symptoms develop, they should abate quickly as the effects of naloxone dissipate.

OVERDOSAGE: *(cont'd)*

If methadone has been taken by mouth, protect the patient's airway and support ventilation and perfusion. Meticulously monitor and maintain, within acceptable limits, the patient's vital signs, blood gases, serum electrolytes, etc. Absorption of drugs from the gastrointestinal tract may be decreased by giving activated charcoal, which, in many cases, is more effective than emesis or lavage; consider charcoal instead of or in addition to gastric emptying. Repeated doses of charcoal over time may hasten elimination of some drugs that have been absorbed. Safeguard the patient's airway when employing gastric emptying or charcoal.

Forced diuresis, peritoneal dialysis, hemodialysis, or charcoal hemoperfusion have not been established as beneficial for an overdose of methadone.

NOTE: IN AN INDIVIDUAL PHYSICALLY DEPENDENT ON NARCOTICS, THE ADMINISTRATION OF THE USUAL DOSE OF A NARCOTIC ANTAGONIST WILL PRECIPITATE AN ACUTE WITHDRAWAL SYNDROME. THE SEVERITY OF THIS SYNDROME WILL DEPEND ON THE DEGREE OF PHYSICAL DEPENDENCE AND THE DOSE OF THE ANTAGONIST ADMINISTERED. THE USE OF A NARCOTIC ANTAGONIST IN SUCH A PERSON SHOULD BE AVOIDED IF POSSIBLE. IF IT MUST BE USED TO TREAT SERIOUS RESPIRATORY DEPRESSION IN THE PHYSICALLY DEPENDENT PATIENT, THE ANTAGONIST SHOULD BE ADMINISTERED WITH EXTREME CARE AND BY TITRATION WITH SMALLER THAN USUAL DOSES OF THE ANTAGONIST.

DOSAGE AND ADMINISTRATION:

For Relief of Pain: Dosage should be adjusted according to the severity of the pain and the response of the patient. Occasionally it may be necessary to exceed the usual dosage recommended in cases of exceptionally severe pain or in those patients who have become tolerant to the analgesic effect of narcotics.

Although subcutaneous administration is suitable for occasional use, intramuscular injection is preferred when repeated doses are required.

The usual adult dosage is 2.5 to 10 mg intramuscularly or subcutaneously every 3 to 4 hours as necessary.

For Detoxification Treatment: THE DRUG SHALL BE ADMINISTERED DAILY UNDER CLOSE SUPERVISION AS FOLLOWS:

A detoxification treatment course shall not exceed 21 days and may not be repeated earlier than 4 weeks after completion of the preceding course.

The oral form of administration is preferred. However, if the patient is unable to ingest oral medication, parenteral administration may be substituted.

In detoxification, the patient may receive methadone when there are significant symptoms of withdrawal. The dosage schedules indicated below are recommended but could be varied in accordance with clinical judgment. Initially,a single oral dose of 15 to 20 mg of methadone will often be sufficient to suppress withdrawal symptoms. Additional methadone may be provided if withdrawal symptoms are not suppressed or if symptoms reappear. When patients are physically dependent on high doses, it may be necessary to exceed these levels. Forty mg/day in single or divided doses will usually constitute an adequate stabilizing dosage level. Stabilization can be continued for 2 to 3 days, and then the amount of methadone normally will be gradually decreased. The rate at which methadone is decreased will be determined separately for each patient. The dose of methadone can be decreased on a daily basis or at 2-day intervals, but the amount of intake shall always be sufficient to keep withdrawal symptoms at a tolerable level. In hospitalized patients, a daily reduction of 20% of the total daily dose may be tolerated and may cause little discomfort. In ambulatory patients, a somewhat slower schedule may be needed. If methadone is administered for more than 3 weeks, the procedure is considered to have progressed from detoxification or treatment of the acute withdrawal syndrome to maintenance treatment, even though the goal and intent may be eventual total withdrawal.

HOW SUPPLIED - RATED THERAPEUTICALLY EQUIVALENT:

Concentrate - Oral - 10 mg/ml

30 ml	$18.51	Methadone Hcl Intensol, Roxane	00054-3553-44
946 ml	$69.99	METHADONE, Roxane	00054-3553-67
960 ml	$42.00	Methadone Hcl, Cherry Flavor, Mallinckrodt	00406-0525-05
960 ml	$85.00	METHADOSE, Mallinckrodt	00406-0527-05

Tablet, Uncoated - Oral - 5 mg

100's	$7.91	METHADOSE, Mallinckrodt	00406-6974-34
100's	$8.04	Methadone Hcl, Roxane	00054-4570-25
100's	**$8.68**	**Dolophine Hcl, Roxane**	**00054-4216-25**
100's	$30.92	Methadone Hcl, Roxane	00054-8553-24

Tablet, Uncoated - Oral - 10 mg

100's	$12.95	Methadose, Mallinckrodt	00406-3454-34
100's	$13.34	Methadone Hcl, Roxane	00054-4571-25
100's	**$14.10**	**Dolophine Hcl, Roxane**	**00054-4217-25**
100's	$35.20	Methadone Hcl, Roxane	00054-8554-24

Tablet, Uncoated - Oral - 40 mg

100's	$32.81	METHADONE HCL, Roxane	00054-4547-25
100's	$35.69	METHADOSE, Mallinckrodt	00406-0540-34
100's	$37.75	METHADONE HCL, Roxane	00054-8547-25

HOW SUPPLIED - NOT RATED EQUIVALENT:

Injection, Solution - Intramuscular; - 10 mg/ml

1 ml x 12	**$23.63**	**DOLOPHINE HCL, Lilly**	**00002-1687-12**
1 ml x 100	**$160.34**	**DOLOPHINE HCL, Lilly**	**00002-1687-02**
20 ml	**$13.85**	**DOLOPHINE HCL, Roxane**	**00054-1218-42**

Powder

50 gm	$380.00	Methadone Hcl, Mallinckrodt	00406-1510-56
100 gm	$760.00	Methadone Hcl, Mallinckrodt	00406-1510-57
500 gm	$3800.00	Methadone Hcl, Mallinckrodt	00406-1510-59

Solution - Oral - 1 mg/ml

500 ml	$27.93	Methadone Hcl, Roxane	00054-3555-63

Solution - Oral - 10 mg/5ml

500 ml	$48.38	Methadone Hcl, Roxane	00054-3556-63

Tablet, Uncoated - Oral - 40 mg

100's	$32.81	METHADONE HCL, Roxane	00054-4538-25

METHAMPHETAMINE HYDROCHLORIDE

(001754)

CATEGORIES: Amphetamines; Anorexients/CNS Stimulants; Appetite Suppressants; Attention Deficit Disorders; Central Nervous System Agents; Obesity; Psychostimulants; Respiratory/Cerebral Stimulant; Stimulants; Sympathomimetic Agents; Weight Loss; Pregnancy Category C; DEA Class CII; FDA Approval Pre 1982

BRAND NAMES: **Desoxyn**; Methampex

FORMULARIES: Aetna

WARNING:
METHAMPHETAMINE HAS A HIGH POTENTIAL FOR ABUSE. IT SHOULD THUS BE TRIED ONLY IN WEIGHT REDUCTION PROGRAMS FOR PATIENTS IN WHOM ALTERNATIVE THERAPY HAS BEEN INEFFECTIVE. ADMINISTRATION OF METHAMPHETAMINE FOR PROLONGED PERIODS OF TIME IN OBESITY MAY LEAD TO DRUG DEPENDENCE AND MUST BE AVOIDED. PARTICULAR ATTENTION SHOULD BE PAID TO THE POSSIBILITY OF SUBJECTS OBTAINING METHAMPHETAMINE FOR NON-THERAPEUTIC USE OR DISTRIBUTION TO OTHERS, AND THE DRUG SHOULD BE PRESCRIBED OR DISPENSED SPARINGLY.

DESCRIPTION:

Methamphetamine hydrochloride chemically known as (S)-N, α-dimethylbenzeneethanamine hydrochloride, is a member of the amphetamine group of sympathomimetic amines.

Methamphetamine HCl is available as gradumet sustained-release tablets containing 5 mg, 10 mg or 15 mg of methamphetamine HCl and as conventional tablets containing 5 mg of methamphetamine HCl, for oral administration. The gradumet is an inert, porous, plastic matrix, which is impregnated with methamphetamine HCl. The drug is leached slowly from the gradumet as it passes through the gastrointestinal tract. The expended matrix is not absorbed and is excreted in the stool.

Desoxyn Inactive Ingredients: *5 mg gradumet tablet:* magnesium stearate, methyl acrylate-methyl methacrylate copolymer, povidone and talc. *10 mg gradumet tablet:* FD&C Yellow No. 6 (sunset yellow), magnesium stearate, methyl acrylate-methyl methacrylate copolymer, povidone and talc. *15 mg gradumet tablet:* FD&C Yellow No. 5 (tartrazine), magnesium stearate, methyl acrylate-methyl methacrylate copolymer, povidone and talc.

CLINICAL PHARMACOLOGY:

Methamphetamine is a sympathomimetic amine with CNS stimulant activity. Peripheral actions include elevation of systolic and diastolic blood pressures and weak bronchodilator and respiratory stimulant action. Drugs of this class used in obesity are commonly known as "anorectics" or "anorexigenics". It has not been established, however, that the action of such drugs in treating obesity is primarily one of appetite suppression. Other central nervous system actions, or metabolic effects, may be involved, for example.

Adult obese subjects instructed in dietary management and treated with "anorectic" drugs, lose more weight on the average than those treated with placebo and diet, as determined in relatively short-term clinical trials.

The magnitude of increased weight loss of drug-treated patients over placebo-treated patients is only a fraction of a pound a week. The rate of weight loss is greatest in the first weeks of therapy for both drug and placebo subjects and tends to decrease in succeeding weeks. The origins of the increased weight loss due to the various possible drug effects are not established. The amount of weight loss associated with the use of an "anorectic" drug varies from trial to trial, and the increased weight loss appears to be related in part to variables other than the drug prescribed, such as the physician-investigator, the population treated, and the diet prescribed. Studies do not permit conclusions as to the relative importance of the drug and non-drug factors on weight loss.

The natural history of obesity is measured in years, whereas the studies cited are restricted to a few weeks duration; thus, the total impact of drug-induced weight loss over that of diet alone must be considered clinically limited.

The mechanism of action involved in producing the beneficial behavioral changes seen in hyperkinetic children receiving methamphetamine is unknown.

In humans, methamphetamine is rapidly absorbed from the gastrointestinal tract. The primary site of metabolism is in the liver by aromatic hydroxylation, N-dealkylation and deamination. At least seven metabolites have been identified in the urine. The biological half-life has been reported in the range of 4 to 5 hours. Excretion occurs primarily in the urine and is dependent on urine pH. Alkaline urine will significantly increase the drug half-life. Approximately 62% of an oral dose is eliminated in the urine within the first 24 hours with about one-third as intact drug and the remainder as metabolites.

INDICATIONS AND USAGE:

Attention Deficit Disorder with Hyperactivity: Methamphetamine HCl is indicated as an integral part of a total treatment program which typically includes other remedial measures (psychological, educational, social) for a stabilizing effect in children over 6 years of age with a behavioral syndrome characterized by the following group of developmentally inappropriate symptoms: moderate to severe distractibility, short attention span, hyperactivity, emotional lability, and impulsivity. The diagnosis of this syndrome should not be made with finality when these symptoms are only of comparatively recent origin. Nonlocalizing (soft) neurological signs, learning disability, and abnormal EEG may or may not be present, and a diagnosis of central nervous system dysfunction may or may not be warranted.

Exogenous Obesity: as a short-term (*i.e.,* a few weeks) adjunct in a regimen of weight reduction based on caloric restriction, for patients in whom obesity is refractory to alternative therapy, e.g. repeated diets, group programs, and other drugs. The limited usefulness of methamphetamine HCl (see CLINICAL PHARMACOLOGY) should be weighed against possible risks inherent in use of the drug, such as those described below.

CONTRAINDICATIONS:

Methamphetamine HCl is contraindicated during or within 14 days following the administration of monoamine oxidase inhibitors; hypertensive crises may result. It is also contraindicated in patients with glaucoma, advanced arteriosclerosis, symptomatic cardiovascular disease, moderate to severe hypertension, hyperthyroidism or known hypersensitivity or idiosyncrasy to sympathomimetic amines. Methamphetamine should not be given to patients who are in an agitated state or who have a history of drug abuse.

WARNINGS:

Tolerance to the anorectic effect usually develops within a few weeks. When this occurs, the recommended dose should not be exceeded in an attempt to increase the effect; rather, the drug should be discontinued (see DRUG ABUSE AND DEPENDENCE.)

Decrements in the predicted growth (*i.e.,* weight gain and/or height) rate have been reported with the long-term use of stimulants in children. Therefore, patients requiring long-term therapy should be carefully monitored.

Usage in Nursing Mothers: Amphetamines are excreted in human milk. Mothers taking amphetamines should be advised to refrain from nursing.

PRECAUTIONS:

GENERAL

Methamphetamine HCl should be used with caution in patients with even mild hypertension.

Methamphetamine should not be used to combat fatigue or to replace rest in normal persons.

Prescribing and dispensing of methamphetamine should be limited to the smallest amount that is feasible at one time in order to minimize the possibility of overdosage.

The 15 mg dosage strength of gradumet tablets contains FD&C Yellow No. 5 (tartrazine) which may cause allergic-type reactions (including bronchial asthma) in certain susceptible individuals. Although the overall incidence of FD&C Yellow No. 5 (tartrazine) sensitivity in the general population is low, it is frequently seen in patients who also have aspirin hypersensitivity.

INFORMATION FOR THE PATIENT

The patient should be informed that methamphetamine may impair the ability to engage in potentially hazardous activities, such as, operating machinery or driving a motor vehicle.

The patient should be cautioned not to increase dosage, except on advice of the physician.

DRUG/LABORATORY TEST INTERACTIONS

Literature reports suggest that amphetamines may be associated with significant elevation of plasma corticosteroids. This should be considered if determination of plasma corticosteroid levels is desired in a person receiving amphetamines.

CARCINOGENESIS, MUTAGENESIS, AND IMPAIRMENT OF FERTILITY

Data are not available on long-term potential for carcinogenicity, mutagenicity, or impairment of fertility.

PREGNANCY CATEGORY C

Teratogenic Effects: Methamphetamine has been shown to have teratogenic and embryocidal effects in mammals given high multiples of the human dose. There are no adequate and well-controlled studies in pregnant women. Methamphetamine HCl should not be used during pregnancy unless the potential benefit justifies the potential risk to the fetus.

Nonteratogenic Effects: Infants born to mothers dependent on amphetamines have an increased risk of premature delivery and low birth weight. Also, these infants may experience symptoms of withdrawal as demonstrated by dysphoria, including agitation and significant lassitude.

NURSING MOTHERS

See WARNINGS.

PEDIATRIC USE

Safety and effectiveness for use as an anorectic agent in children below the age of 12 years have not been established.

Long-term effects of methamphetamine in children have not been established (See WARNINGS.)

Drug treatment is not indicated in all cases of the behavioral syndrome characterized by moderate to severe distractibility, short attention span, hyperactivity, emotional lability and impulsivity. It should be considered only in light of the complete history and evaluation of the child. The decision to prescribe methamphetamine HCl should depend on the physician's assessment of the chronicity and severity of the child's symptoms and their appropriateness for his/her age. Prescription should not depend solely on the presence of one or more of the behavioral characteristics.

When these symptoms are associated with acute stress reactions, treatment with methamphetamine HCl is usually not indicated.

Clinical experience suggests that in psychotic children, administration of methamphetamine HCl may exacerbate symptoms of behavior disturbance and thought disorder.

Amphetamines have been reported to exacerbate motor and phonic tics and Tourette's syndrome. Therefore, clinical evaluation for tics and Tourette's syndrome in children and their families should precede use of stimulant medications.

DRUG INTERACTIONS:

Insulin requirements in diabetes mellitus may be altered in association with the use of methamphetamine and the concomitant dietary regimen.

Guanethidine: Methamphetamine may decrease the hypotensive effect of *guanethidine.*

Monoamine Oxidase Inhibitors: Methamphetamine HCl should not be used concurrently with *monoamine oxidase inhibitors* (see CONTRAINDICATIONS).

Tricyclic Antidepressants: Concurrent administration of *tricyclic antidepressants* and indirect-acting sympathomimetic amines such as the amphetamines, should be closely supervised and dosage carefully adjusted.

Phenothiazines are reported in the literature to antagonize the CNS stimulant action of the amphetamines.

ADVERSE REACTIONS:

The following are adverse reactions in decreasing order of severity within each category that have been reported:

Cardiovascular: Elevation of blood pressure, tachycardia and palpitation.

Central Nervous System: Psychotic episodes have been rarely reported at recommended doses. Dizziness, dysphoria, overstimulation, euphoria, insomnia, tremor, restlessness and headache. Exacerbation of motor and phonic tics and Tourette's syndrome.

Gastrointestinal: Diarrhea, constipation, dryness of mouth, unpleasant taste and other gastrointestinal disturbances.

Hypersensitivity: Urticaria.

Endocrine: Impotence and changes in libido.

Miscellaneous: Suppression of growth has been reported with the long-term use of stimulants in children (see WARNINGS).

DRUG ABUSE AND DEPENDENCE:

Controlled Substance: Methamphetamine HCl is subject to control under DEA schedule II.

Abuse: Methamphetamine HCl has been extensively abused. Tolerance, extreme psychological dependence, and severe social disability have occurred. There are reports of patients who have increased the dosage to many times that recommended. Abrupt cessation following prolonged high dosage administration results in extreme fatigue and mental depression; changes are also noted on the sleep EEG. Manifestations of chronic intoxication with methamphetamine include severe dermatoses, marked insomnia, irritability, hyperactivity, and personality changes. The most severe manifestation of chronic intoxication is psychosis often clinically indistinguishable from schizophrenia.

OVERDOSAGE:

Manifestations of acute overdosage with methamphetamine include restlessness, tremor, hyperreflexia, rapid respiration, confusion, assaultiveness, hallucinations, panic states, hyperpyrexia, and rhabdomyolysis. Fatigue and depression usually follow the central stimulation. Cardiovascular effects include arrhythmias, hypertension or hypotension, and circulatory collapse. Gastrointestinal symptoms include nausea, vomiting, diarrhea, and abdominal cramps. Fatal poisoning usually terminates in convulsions and coma.

Management of acute methamphetamine intoxication is largely symptomatic and includes gastric evacuation and sedation with a barbiturate. Experience with hemodialysis or peritoneal dialysis is inadequate to permit recommendations in this regard.

Acidification of urine increases methamphetamine excretion. Intravenous phentolamine (Regitine) has been suggested for possible acute, severe hypertension, if this complicates methamphetamine overdosage. Usually a gradual drop in blood pressure will result when sufficient sedation has been achieved. Chlorpromazine has been reported to be useful in decreasing CNS stimulation and sympathomimetic effects.

Since the gradumet tablet releases methamphetamine gradually, therapy should be directed at reversing the effects of the ingested drug and at supporting the patient until the symptoms subside. Saline cathartics are useful for hastening the evacuation of the tablets that have not already released medication.

DOSAGE AND ADMINISTRATION:

Methamphetamine HCl is given orally. Methamphetamine should be administered at the lowest effective dosage, and dosage should be individually adjusted. Late evening medication should be avoided because of the resulting insomnia.

ATTENTION DEFICIT DISORDER WITH HYPERACTIVITY

For treatment of children 6 years or older with a behavioral syndrome characterized by moderate to severe distractibility, short attention span, hyperactivity, emotional lability and impulsivity: an initial dose of 5 mg methamphetamine HCl once or twice a day is recommended. Daily dosage may be raised in increments of 5 mg at weekly intervals until an optimum clinical response is achieved. The usual effective dose is 20 to 25 mg daily. The total daily dose may be given as conventional tablets in two divided doses daily or once daily using the gradumet tablet. The gradumet form should not be utilized for initiation of dosage nor until the conventional titrated daily dosage is equal to or greater than the dosage provided in a gradumet tablet.

Where possible, drug administration should be interrupted occasionally to determine if there is a recurrence of behavioral symptoms sufficient to require continued therapy.

For Obesity: one gradumet tablet, 10 or 15 mg, once a day in the morning. Treatment should not exceed a few weeks in duration. Methamphetamine is not recommended for use as an anorectic agent in children under 12 years of age.

Recommended Storage: Store below 86°F (30°C).

HOW SUPPLIED - RATED THERAPEUTICALLY EQUIVALENT:

Tablet, Uncoated - Oral - 5 mg

100's $66.70 DESOXYN, Abbott 00074-3377-04

HOW SUPPLIED - NOT RATED EQUIVALENT:

Tablet, Uncoated, Sustained Action - Oral - 5 mg

100's $179.06 DESOXYN, GRADUMET, Abbott 00074-6941-04

Tablet, Uncoated, Sustained Action - Oral - 10 mg

100's $240.62 DESOXYN, GRADUMET, Abbott 00074-6948-08

Tablet, Uncoated, Sustained Action - Oral - 15 mg

100's $306.96 DESOXYN, GRADUMET, Abbott 00074-6959-07

METHANTHELINE BROMIDE *(001757)*

CATEGORIES: Anticholinergic Agents; Antimuscarinics/Antispasmodics; Autonomic Drugs; Bladder, Neurogenic; Gastrointestinal Drugs; Peptic Ulcer; FDA Approval Pre 1982

BRAND NAMES: **Banthine**; *Vagantin* (Germany)
(International brand names outside U.S. in italics)

FORMULARIES: Medi-Cal

DESCRIPTION:

Banthine oral tablets contain 50 mg of the anticholinergic methantheline bromide, diethyl(2-hydroxyethyl)methylammonium bromide xanthene-9-carboxylate.

Inactive ingredients include acacia, corn starch, FD&C Yellow No. 6, magnesium stearate, sodium sulfate, and talc.

CLINICAL PHARMACOLOGY:

Methantheline bromide inhibits gastrointestinal propulsive motility and diminishes gastric acid secretion. The drug also inhibits the action of acetylcholine at the postganglionic nerve endings of the parasympathetic nervous system.

INDICATIONS AND USAGE:

Methantheline bromide is indicated as adjunctive therapy in the treatment of peptic ulcer. When used for such a condition the effective dose must be titrated to the patients needs.

Methantheline bromide may be used effectively for the treatment of an uninhibited hypertonic neurogenic bladder.

CONTRAINDICATIONS:

Methantheline bromide is contraindicated in patients with:

1. Glaucoma, since mydriasis is to be avoided.

2. Obstructive disease of the gastrointestinal tract (pyloroduodenal stenosis, achalasia, paralytic ileus, etc).

3. Obstructive uropathy (*e.g.,* bladder-neck obstruction due to prostatic hypertrophy).

4. Intestinal atony of elderly or debilitated patients.

5. Severe ulcerative colitis or toxic megacolon complicating ulcerative colitis.

6. Unstable cardiovascular status in acute hemorrhage.

7. Myasthenia gravis.

WARNINGS:

In the presence of a high environmental temperature, heat prostration (fever and heat stroke due to decreased sweating) can occur with the use of methantheline bromide.

Diarrhea may be an early symptom of incomplete intestinal obstruction, especially in patients with ileostomy or colostomy. In this instance treatment with methantheline bromide would be inappropriate and possibly harmful.

With overdosage, a curare-like action may occur, that is, neuromuscular blockade leading to muscular weakness and possible paralysis.

Methantheline bromide may cause increased heart rate and, therefore, should be used with caution in patients with heart disease.

PRECAUTIONS:

General: Methantheline bromide should be used with caution in the elderly and in all patients with autonomic neuropathy, hepatic or renal disease, hyperthyroidism, coronary heart disease, congestive heart failure, cardiac tachyarrhythmias, hypertension, or hiatal hernia associated with reflux esophagitis since anticholinergics may aggravate this condition.

In patients with ulcerative colitis, large doses of methantheline bromide may suppress intestinal motility to the point of producing paralytic ileus and, or for this reason, may precipitate or aggravate toxic megacolon, a serious complication of the disease.

Information for the Patient: Methantheline bromide may produce drowsiness or blurred vision. The patient should be cautioned regarding activities requiring mental alertness, such as operating a motor vehicle or other machinery or performing hazardous work, while taking this drug.

Carcinogenesis, Mutagenesis, and Impairment of Fertility: No long-term fertility, carcinogenicity, or mutagenicity studies have been done with methantheline bromide.

Pregnancy Category C: Animal reproduction studies have not been conducted with methantheline bromide. It is also not known whether methantheline bromide can cause fetal harm when administered to a pregnant woman or can affect reproduction capacity. Methantheline bromidee should be given to a pregnant woman only if clearly needed.

Nursing Mothers: It is not known whether this drug is excreted in human milk. Because many drugs are excreted in human milk, caution should be exercised when methantheline bromide is administered to a nursing woman. Suppression of lactation may occur with anticholinergic drugs.

DRUG INTERACTIONS:

Anticholinergics may delay absorption of other medication given concomitantly.

Excessive cholinergic blockade may occur if methantheline bromide is given concomitantly with belladonna alkaloids, synthetic or semisynthetic anticholinergic agents, narcotic analgesics such as meperidine, Type 1 antiarrhythmic drugs (*e.g.,* disopyramide, procainamide, or quinidine), antihistamines, phenothiazines, tricyclic antidepressants, or other psychoactive drugs. Methantheline bromidee may also potentiate the sedative effect of phenothiazines. Increased intraocular pressure may result from concurrent administration of anticholinergics and corticosteroids.

Concurrent use of methantheline bromide with slow-dissolving tablets of digoxin may cause increased serum digoxin levels. This interaction can be avoided by using only those digoxin tablets that rapidly dissolve by USP standards.

ADVERSE REACTIONS:

Varying degrees of drying of salivary secretions may occur as well as decreased sweating. Ophthalmic side effect include blurred vision, mydriasis, cycloplegia, an increased ocular tension. Other reported adverse reactions include urinary hesitancy and retention, tachycardia, palpitations, loss of the sense of taste, headache, nervousness, mental confusion, drowsiness, weakness, dizziness, insomnia, nausea, vomiting, constipation, bloated feeling, impotence, suppression of lactation, and allergic reactions or drug idiosyncrasies, including anaphylaxis, urticaria, and other dermal manifestations.

OVERDOSAGE:

The symptoms of overdosage with methantheline bromide progress from an intensification of the usual side effects to CNS disturbances (from restlessness and excitement to psychotic behavior), circulatory changes (flushing, fall in blood pressure, circulatory failure), respiratory failure, paralysis, and coma.

Measures to be taken are (1) immediate induction of emesis or lavage of the stomach, (2) injection of physostigmine 0.5 to 2 mg intravenously, repeated as necessary up to a total of 5 mg, and (3) monitoring of vital signs and managing as necessary.

Fever may be treated symptomatically (cooling blanker or alcohol sponging). Excitement of a degree which demands attention may be managed with thiopental sodium 2% solution given slowly intravenously, or diazepam, 5 to 10 mg intravenously or 10 mg intramuscularly. In the event of progression of the curare-like effect to paralysis of the respiratory muscles, mechanical respiration should be instituted and maintained until effective respiratory action returns.

DOSAGE AND ADMINISTRATION:

Peptic ulcer: The usual initial adult dosage is 50 or 100 mg every six hours day and night. The initial dosage recommended applies to the stage of active ulceration; the maintenance dose is approximately half the therapeutic dose.

Uninhibited hypertonic neurogenic bladder: The usual initial dosage is 50 to 100 mg four times daily subsequent adjustment to the patient's requirements.

Pediatrics: Recommended oral dosage for infants and children: *Newborns 0 to 1 months:* 12.5 mg administered twice daily initially and then three times daily; *Infants 1 to 12 months:* 12.5 mg four times daily, gradually increased to 25 mg four times daily; *Children over 1 year:* 12.5 mg to 50 mg four times daily.

HOW SUPPLIED - EQUIVALENTS NOT AVAILABLE:

Tablet, Uncoated - Oral - 50 mg

100's $28.93 BANTHINE, SCS Pharm 00905-1501-31

METHAZOLAMIDE *(001759)*

CATEGORIES: Antiglaucomatous Agents; Carbonic Anhydrase Inhibitors; EENT Drugs; Eye, Ear, Nose, & Throat Preparations; Glaucoma; Intraocular Pressure; Ophthalmics; Pregnancy Category C; FDA Approval Pre 1982

BRAND NAMES: MZM; **Neptazane**

FORMULARIES: Aetna; BC-BS; Medi-Cal; PCS

DESCRIPTION:

Methazolamide, a sulfonamide derivative, is a white crystalline powder, weakly acidic, slightly soluble in water, alcohol and acetone. The chemical name for methazolamide is:*N*-(5-(aminosulfonyl)-3-methyl-1,3,4-thiadiazol-2(3H)-ylidene)-ace tamide.

Molecular formula: $C_5H_8N_4O_3S_2$

Molecular weight: 236.26

Neptazane is available for oral administration as 25 mg and 50 mg tablets containing the following inactive ingredients: Acacia, Alginic Acid, Corn Starch, Dibasic Calcium Phosphate, Gelatin and Magnesium Stearate.

CLINICAL PHARMACOLOGY:

Methazolamide is a potent inhibitor of carbonic anhydrase. Methazolamide is well absorbed from the gastrointestinal tract. Peak plasma concentrations are observed 1 to 2 hours after dosing. In a multiple-dose, pharmacokinetic study, administration of methazolamide 25 mg BID, 50 mg BID and 100 mg BID demonstrated a linear relationship between plasma methazolamide levels and methazolamide dose. Peak plasma concentrations (C_{max}) for the 25 mg, 50 mg and 100 mg BID regimens were 2.5 mcg/ml, 5.1 mcg/ml and 10.7 mcg/ml, respectively. The area under the plasma concentration-time curves (AUC) were 1130 mcg.min/ml, 2571 mcg.min/ml and 5418 mcg.min/ml for the 25 mg, 50 mg and 100 mg dosage regimens, respectively.

Methazolamide is distributed throughout the body including the plasma, cerebrospinal fluid, aqueous humor of the eye, red blood cells, bile and extra-cellular fluid. The mean apparent volume of distribution (V_{area}/F) ranges from 17 to 23 L. Approximately 55% is bound to plasma proteins. The steady-state methazolamide red blood cell: plasma ratio varies with dose and was found to be 27:1, 16:1 and 10:1 following the administration of methazolamide 25 mg BID, 50 mg BID and 100 mg BID, respectively.

The mean steady-state plasma elimination half-life for methazolamide is approximately 14 hours. At steady-state approximately 25% of the dose is recovered unchanged in the urine over the dosing interval. Renal clearance accounts for 20-25% of the total clearance of drug. After repeated BID-TID dosing, methazolamide accumulates to steady state concentration in seven days.

Methazolamide's inhibitory action on carbonic anhydrase decreases the secretion of aqueous humor and results in a decrease in intraocular pressure. The onset of the decrease in intraocular pressure generally occurs within two to four hours, has a peak effect in six to eight hours, and a total duration of ten to eighteen hours.

Methazolamide is sulfonamide derivative; however, it does not have any clinically significant antimicrobial properties. Although methazolamide achieves a high concentration in the cerebrospinal fluid, it is not considered an effective anticonvulsant.

Methazolamide has a weak and transient diuretic effect, therefore use results in an increase in urinary volume, with excretion of sodium, potassium and chloride. The drug should not be used as a diuretic. Inhibition of renal bicarbonate reabsorption produces an alkaline urine. Plasma bicarbonate decreases, and a relative, transient metabolic acidosis may occur due to a disequilibrium in carbon dioxide transport in the red cell. Urinary citrate excretion is decreased by approximately 40% after doses of 100 mg every 8 hours. Uric acid output has been shown to decrease 36% in the first 24 hour period.

INDICATIONS AND USAGE:

Methazolamide is indicated in the treatment of ocular conditions where lowering intraocular pressure is likely to be of therapeutic benefit, such as chronic open-angle glaucoma, secondary glaucoma, and preoperatively in acute-closure glaucoma where lowering the intraocular pressure in desired before surgery.

CONTRAINDICATIONS:

Methazolamide therapy is contraindicated in situations in which sodium and/or potassium serum levels are depressed, in cases of marked kidney or liver disease or dysfunction, in adrenal gland failure, and in hyperchloremic acidosis. In patients with cirrhosis, use may precipitate the development of hepatic encephalopathy.

Long-term administration of methazolamide is contraindicated in patients with angle-closure glaucoma, since organic closure of the angle may occur in spite of lowered intraocular pressure.

WARNINGS:

Fatalities have occurred, although rarely, due to severe reactions to sulfonamides including Stevens-Johnson syndrome, toxic epidermal necrolysis, fulminant hepatic necrosis, agranulocytosis, aplastic anemia, and other blood dyscrasias. Hypersensitivity reactions may recur when a sulfonamide is readministered, irrespective of the route of administration.

If hypersensitivity or other serious reactions occur, the use of this drug should be discontinued.

Caution is advised for patients receiving high-dose aspirin and methazolamide concomitantly, as anorexia, tachypnea, lethargy, coma and death have been reported with concomitant use of high-dose aspirin and carbonic anhydrase inhibitors.

PRECAUTIONS:

General: Potassium excretion is increased initially upon administration of methazolamide and in patients with cirrhosis or hepatic insufficiency could precipitate a hepatic coma.

In patients with pulmonary obstruction or emphysema, where alveolar ventilation may be impaired methazolamide should be used with caution because it may precipitate or aggravate acidosis.

Information for the Patient: Adverse reactions common to all sulfonamide derivatives may occur: anaphylaxis, fever, rash (including erythema multiforme, Stevens-Johnson syndrome, toxic epidermal necrolysis), crystalluria, renal calculus, bone marrow depression, thrombocytopenic purpura, hemolytic anemia, leukopenia, pancytopenia and agranulocytosis. Precaution is advised for early detection of such reactions and the drug should be discontinued and appropriate therapy instituted.

Caution is advised for patients receiving high-dose aspirin and methazolamide concomitantly.

Laboratory Tests: To monitor for hematologic reactions common to all sulfonamides, it is recommended that a baseline CBC and platelet count be obtained on patients prior to initiating methazolamide therapy and at regular intervals during therapy. If significant changes occur, early discontinuance and institution of appropriate therapy are important. Periodic monitoring of serum electrolytes is also recommended.

Carcinogenesis, Mutagenesis, and Impairment of Fertility: Long-term studies in animals to evaluate methazolamide's carcinogenesis potential and its effect on fertility have not been conducted. Methazolamide was not mutagenic in the Ames bacterial test.

Pregnancy, Teratogenic Effects, Pregnancy Category C: Methazolamide has been shown to be teratogenic (skeletal anomalies) in rats when given in doses approximately 40 times the human dose. There are no adequate and well controlled studies in pregnant women. Methazolamide should be used during pregnancy only if the potential benefit justifies the potential risk to the fetus.

PRECAUTIONS: *(cont'd)*

Nursing Mothers: It is not known whether this drug is excreted in human milk. Because many drugs are excreted in human milk and because of the potential for serious adverse reactions in nursing infants from methazolamide, a decision should be made whether to discontinue nursing or to discontinue the drug, taking into account the importance of the drug to the mother.

Pediatric Use: The safety and effectiveness of methazolamide in children have not been established.

DRUG INTERACTIONS:

Methazolamide should be used with caution in patients on steroid therapy because of the potential for developing hypokalemia. Caution is advised for patients receiving high-dose aspirin and methazolamide concomitantly, as anorexia, tachypnea, lethargy, coma and death have been reported with concomitant use of high-dose aspirin and carbonic anhydrase inhibitors (see WARNINGS.)

ADVERSE REACTIONS:

Adverse reactions, occurring most often early in therapy, include, paresthesias, particularly a "tingling" feeling in the extremities; hearing dysfunction or tinnitus; fatigue; malaise; loss of appetite; taste alteration; gastrointestinal disturbances such as nausea, vomiting and diarrhea, polyuria, and occasional instances of drowsiness and confusion.

Metabolic acidosis and electrolyte imbalance may occur.

Transient myopia has been reported. This condition invariably subsides upon diminution or discontinuance of the medication.

Other occasional adverse reactions include urticaria, melena, hematuria, glycosuria, hepatic insufficiency, flaccid paralysis, photosensitivity, convulsions, and rarely, crystalluria and renal calculi. Also see PRECAUTIONS, Information for Patients for possible reactions common to sulfonamide derivatives. Fatalities have occurred although rarely, due to severe reactions to sulfonamides including Stevens-Johnson syndrome, toxic epidermal necrolysis, fulminate hepatic necrosis, agranulocytosis, aplastic anemia, and other blood dyscrasias (see WARNINGS.)

OVERDOSAGE:

No data are available regarding methazolamide overdosage in humans as no cases of acute poisoning with this drug have been reported. Animal data suggest that even a high dose of methazolamide is nontoxic. No specific antidote is known. Treatment should be symptomatic and supportive.

Electrolyte imbalance, development of an acidotic state, and central nervous system effects might be expected to occur. Serum electrolyte levels (particularly potassium) and blood pH levels should be monitored.

Supportive measures may be required to restore electrolyte and pH balance.

DOSAGE AND ADMINISTRATION:

The effective therapeutic dose administered varies from 50 mg to 100 mg 2-3 times daily. The drug may be used concomitantly with miotic and osmotic agents.

Store at Controlled Room Temperature 15°-30°C (59-86°F).

HOW SUPPLIED - RATED THERAPEUTICALLY EQUIVALENT:

Tablet - Oral - 25 mg

100's	$48.25	Methazolamide, Duramed Pharms	51285-0968-02

Tablet - Oral - 50 mg

100's	$72.50	Methazolamide, Duramed Pharms	51285-0969-02

Tablet, Uncoated - Oral - 25 mg

100's	$35.63	Methazolamide, H.C.F.A. F F P	99999-1759-01
100's	$37.14	MZM, Ciba Vision	58768-0106-01
100's	$43.40	Methazolamide, Effcon Labs	55806-0021-03
100's	$43.85	Methazolamide, Lederle Pharm	00005-3519-23
100's	$45.70	Methazolamide, Major Pharms	00904-7781-60
100's	$45.75	Glauctabs, Akorn	17478-0525-01
100's	$47.43	Methazolamide, Qualitest Pharms	00603-4470-21
100's	$47.82	Methazolamide, Schein Pharm (US)	00364-2608-01
100's	$48.00	Methazolamide, Goldline Labs	00182-1075-01
100's	$48.00	Methazolamide, Copley Pharm	38245-0411-10
100's	$49.72	Methazolamide, Geneva Pharms	00781-1072-01
100's	$50.53	Methazolamide, Aligen Independ	00405-4631-01
100's	**$53.13**	**NEPTAZANE, Storz Ophthalm**	**57706-0756-23**

Tablet, Uncoated - Oral - 50 mg

100's	$51.38	Methazolamide, H.C.F.A. F F P	99999-1759-02
100's	$55.43	MZM, Ciba Vision	58768-0116-01
100's	$65.44	Methazolamide, Lederle Pharm	00005-3520-23
100's	$66.58	Methazolamide, Effcon Labs	55806-0020-03
100's	$67.60	Methazolamide, Qualitest Pharms	00603-4471-21
100's	$68.20	Methazolamide, Schein Pharm (US)	00364-2609-01
100's	$68.20	Methazolamide, Major Pharms	00904-7782-60
100's	$69.00	Glauctabs, Akorn	17478-0550-01
100's	$72.00	Methazolamide, Goldline Labs	00182-1076-01
100's	$72.00	Methazolamide, Copley Pharm	38245-0424-10
100's	$72.48	Methazolamide, HL Moore Drug Exch	00839-7835-06
100's	$73.40	Methazolamide, Rugby	00536-5616-01
100's	$74.23	Methazolamide, Geneva Pharms	00781-1071-01
100's	$75.79	Methazolamide, Aligen Independ	00405-4632-01
100's	**$79.30**	**NEPTAZANE, Storz Ophthalm**	**57706-0757-23**

METHENAMINE HIPPURATE *(001761)*

CATEGORIES: Anti-Infectives; Antibacterials; Antimicrobials; Antiseptics, Urinary Tract; Urinary Anti-Infectives; Urinary Antibacterial; Urinary Tract Infections; FDA Approval Pre 1982

BRAND NAMES: *Haiprex*; *Hip-Rex* (Canada); *Hipeksal*; *Hippramine*; *Hippuran*; **Hiprex**; Urex; *Urotractan* (Germany)
(International brand names outside U.S. in italics)

FORMULARIES: Medi-Cal

DESCRIPTION:

Each yellow capsule-shaped tablet contains 1 g methenamine hippurate which is the Hippuric Acid Salt of methenamine (hexamethylene-tetramine). The tablet also contains inactive ingredients: FD&C Yellow No. 5 (tartrazine, see PRECAUTIONS), Magnesium Stearate, Povidone, and Saccharin Sodium.

CLINICAL PHARMACOLOGY:

Microbiology: Methenamine hippurate has antibacterial activity because the methenamine component is hydrolyzed to formaldehyde in acid urine. Hippuric acid, the other component, has some antibacterial activity and also acts to keep the urine acid. The drug is generally active against *E. coli*, enterococci and staphylococci. *Enterobacter aerogenes* is generally resistant. The urine must be kept sufficiently acid for urea-splitting organisms such as *Proteus* and *Pseudomonas* to be inhibited.

Human Pharmacology: Within 1/2 hour after ingestion of a single 1-gram dose of methenamine hippurate, antibacterial activity is demonstrable in the urine. Urine has continuous antibacterial activity when methenamine hippurate is administered at the recommended dosage schedule of 1 gram twice daily. Over 90% of methenamine moiety is excreted in the urine within 24 hours after administration of a single 1-gram dose. Similarly, the hippurate moiety is rapidly absorbed and excreted, and it reaches the urine by both tubular secretion and glomerular filtration. This action may be important in older patients or in those with some degree of renal impairment.

INDICATIONS AND USAGE:

Methenamine hippurate is indicated for prophylactic or suppressive treatment of frequently recurring urinary tract infections when long-term therapy is considered necessary. This drug should only be used after eradication of the infection by other appropriate antimicrobial agents.

CONTRAINDICATIONS:

Methenamine hippurate is contraindicated in patients with renal insufficiency, severe hepatic insufficiency, or severe dehydration. Methenamine preparations should not be given to patients taking sulfonamides because some sulfonamides may form an insoluble precipitate with formaldehyde in the urine.

WARNINGS:

Large doses of methenamine (8 grams daily for 3 to 4 weeks) have caused bladder irritation, painful and frequent micturition, albuminuria, and gross hematuria.

PRECAUTIONS:

1. Care should be taken to maintain an acid pH of the urine, especially when treating infections due to urea-splitting organisms such as *Proteus* and strains of *Pseudomonas*.

2. In a few instances in one study, the serum transaminase levels were slightly elevated during treatment but returned to normal while the patients were still taking methenamine hippurate. Because of this report, it is recommended that liver function studies be performed periodically on patients taking the drug, especially those with liver dysfunction.

3. Use in Pregnancy: In early pregnancy the safe use of methenamine hippurate is not established. In the last trimester, safety is suggested, but not definitely proved. No adverse effects on the fetus were seen in studies in pregnant rats and rabbits.

Methenamine hippurate taken during pregnancy can interfere with laboratory tests of urine estriol (resulting in unmeasurably low values) when acid hydrolysis is used in the laboratory procedure. This interference is due to the presence in the urine of methenamine and/or formaldehyde. Enzymatic hydrolysis, in place of acid hydrolysis, will circumvent this problem.

4. This product contains FD&C Yellow No. 5 (tartrazine), which may cause allergic-type reactions (including bronchial asthma) in certain susceptible individuals. Although the overall incidence of FD&C Yellow No. 5 (tartrazine) sensitivity in the general population is low, it is frequently seen in patients who also have aspirin hypersensitivity.

ADVERSE REACTIONS:

Minor adverse reactions have been reported in less than 3.5% of patients treated. These reactions have included nausea, upset stomach, dysuria, and rash.

DOSAGE AND ADMINISTRATION:

1 tablet (1.0 g) twice daily (morning and night) for adults and children over 12 years of age.

1/2 to 1 tablet (0.5 to 1.0 g) twice daily (morning and night) for children 6 to 12 years of age.

Since the antibacterial activity of methenamine hippurate is greater in acid urine, restriction of alkalinizing foods and medications is desirable. If necessary, as indicated by urinary pH and clinical response, supplemental acidification of the urine should be instituted. The efficacy of therapy should be monitored by repeated urine cultures.

HOW SUPPLIED - RATED THERAPEUTICALLY EQUIVALENT:

Tablet, Uncoated - Oral - 1 gm

100's	$102.60	UREX, 3M Pharms	00089-0371-10
100's	**$105.66**	**HIPREX, Hoechst Marion Roussel**	**00068-0277-61**

METHENAMINE MANDELATE *(001762)*

CATEGORIES: Anti-Infectives; Antibacterials; Antimicrobials; Antiseptics, Urinary Tract; Cystitis; Fever; Pharmaceutical Adjuvants; Pyelonephritis; Urinary Anti-Infectives; Urinary Tract Infections; Pregnancy Category C; FDA Pre 1938 Drugs

BRAND NAMES: *Amigdalin*; *Hexydal*; *Lemandine*; Mandameth; *Mandelamin*; **Mandelamine**; *Mandepiril-S* (Mexico); *Metanamin*; Methenamine; *Reflux*; *Relucin*; *Urocedulamin*
(International brand names outside U.S. in italics)

FORMULARIES: Aetna; Medi-Cal

DESCRIPTION:

Methenamine mandelate USP, a urinary antibacterial agent, is the chemical combination of mandelic acid with methenamine. Methenamine mandelate is available for oral use as film-coated tablets, suspension, and granules.

Each tablet contains 0.5 g or 1 g of methenamine mandelate, USP; and also contains calcium stearate, NF; candelilla wax; colloidal silicon dioxide, NF; croscarmellose sodium, NF; hydroxypropyl methylcellulose; Opaspray brown (0.5 g tablet) or Opaspray purple (1 g tablet); povidone, USP; propylene glycol, USP; and silica gel.

Each teaspoonful of suspension contains 250 mg or 500 mg of methenamine mandelate, USP; and also contains flavors; propylparaben, NF; saccharin sodium, USP; sesame oil, NF and thixcin. The 500 mg per teaspoonful suspension also contains D&C red No. 6 Ba lake.

Each packet of granules contains 1 g of methenamine mandelate, USP; and also contains colloidal silicon dioxide, NF; D&C yellow No. 10; FD&C yellow No. 6 (sunset yellow); flavors; povidone, USP; saccharin sodium, USP; and sucrose, NF.

CLINICAL PHARMACOLOGY: *(cont'd)*

Methenamine mandelate is readily absorbed but remains essentially inactive until it is excreted by the kidney and concentrated in the urine. An acid urine is essential for antibacterial action, with maximum efficacy occurring at pH 5.5 or less. In an acid urine, mandelic acid exerts its antibacterial action and also contributes to the acidification of the urine. Mandelic acid is excreted by both glomerular filtration and tubular excretion. The methenamine component, in an acid urine, is hydrolyzed to ammonia and to the bactericidal agent formaldehyde. There is equally effective antibacterial activity against both gram-positive and gram-negative organisms, since the antibacterial action of mandelic acid and formaldehyde is nonspecific. There are reports that Methenamine mandelate is ineffective in some infections with *Proteus vulgaris* and urea-splitting strains of *Pseudomonas aeruginosa* and *A aerogenes.* Since urea-splitting strains may raise the pH of the urine, particular attention to supplementary acidification is required. However, results in any single case will depend to a large extent on the underlying pathology and the overall management.

INDICATIONS AND USAGE:

Methenamine mandelate is indicated for the suppression or elimination of bacteriuria associated with pyelonephritis, cystitis, and other chronic urinary tract infections; also for infected residual urine sometimes accompanying neurologic diseases. When used as recommended, Methenamine mandelate is particularly suitable for long-term therapy because of its safety and because resistance to the nonspecific bactericidal action of formaldehyde does not develop. Pathogens resistant to other antibacterial agents may respond to Methenamine mandelate because of the nonspecific effect of formaldehyde formed in an acid urine.

Prophylactic use rationale: Urine is a good culture medium for many urinary pathogens. Inoculation by a few organisms (relapse or reinfection) may lead to bacteriuria in susceptible individuals. Thus, the rationale of management in recurring urinary tract infection (bacteriuria) is to change the urine from a growth-supporting to a growth-inhibiting medium. There is a growing body of evidence that long-term administration of Methenamine mandelate can prevent the recurrence of bacteriuria in patients with chronic pyelonephritis.

Therapeutic use rationale: Methenamine mandelate helps to sterilize the urine, and in some situations in which underlying pathologic conditions prevent sterilization by any means, it can help to suppress the bacteriuria. Methenamine mandelate should not be used alone for acute infections with parenchymal involvement causing systemic symptoms such as chills and fever. A thorough diagnostic investigation as a part of the overall management of the urinary tract infection should accompany the use of Methenamine mandelate.

CONTRAINDICATIONS:

Contraindicated in renal insufficiency.

Methenamine mandelate should not be used in patients who have previously exhibited hypersensitivity to it.

PRECAUTIONS:

General: Dysuria may occur (usually at higher than recommended dosage). This can be controlled by reducing the dosage and the acidification. When urine acidification is contraindicated or unattainable (as with some urea-splitting bacteria), the drug is not recommended.

To avoid inducing lipid pneumonia, administer Methenamine mandelate Suspension Forte and Methenamine mandelate Suspension with care to elderly, debilitated or otherwise susceptible patients.

DRUG/LABORATORY TEST INTERACTIONS

Formaldehyde interferes with fluorometric procedures for determination of urinary catecholamines and vanillylmandelic acid (VMA), causing erroneously high results. Formaldehyde also causes falsely decreased urine estriol levels by reacting with estriol when acid hydrolysis techniques are used; estriol determinations which use enzymatic hydrolysis are unaffected by formaldehyde. Formaldehyde causes falsely elevated 17-hydroxycorticosteroid levels when the Porter-Silber method is used and falsely decreased 5-hydroxyindoleacetic acid (5HIAA) levels by inhibiting color development when nitrosonaphthol methods are used.

Pregnancy Category C Animal reproduction studies have not been conducted with Methenamine mandelate. It is also not known whether Methenamine mandelate can cause fetal harm when administered to a pregnant woman or can affect reproduction capacity. Methenamine mandelate should be given to a pregnant woman only if clearly needed.

Since introduction, published reports on the use of Methenamine mandelate in pregnant women have not shown an increased risk of fetal abnormalities from use during pregnancy.

DRUG INTERACTIONS:

Formaldehyde and sulfamethizole form an insoluble precipitate in acid urine; therefore, Methenamine mandelate should not be administered concurrently with sulfamethizole.

ADVERSE REACTIONS:

An occasional patient may experience gastrointestinal disturbance or a generalized skin rash. Microscopic and rarely gross hematuria have been described.

DOSAGE AND ADMINISTRATION:

Directions for using Granules: dissolve contents of packet in 2-4 oz of water immediately before using. Solution formed may remain turbid.

Suspensions: Shake well before using.

The average adult dosage is 4 grams daily given as 1 gram after each meal and at bedtime. Children 6 to 12 should receive half the adult dose and children under 6 years of age should receive 250 mg per 30 lb body weight, four times daily. (See TABLE 1) Since an acid urine is essential for antibacterial activity, with maximum efficacy occurring at pH 5.5 or below, restriction of alkalinizing foods and medication is thus desirable. If testing of urine pH reveals the need, supplemental acidification should be given:

TABLE 1

Adults	Children		Adults	Children
Tablets and Granules			Suspension	
Dosage=1 gram				
1 tablet qid	-	500 mg/5 ml teasp.	2 teaspoonfuls (10 ml) qid	(Ages 6-12) 1 teaspoonful (5 ml) qid
1 packed qid	-			
2 tablets qid	(Aged 6-12) 1 tablet qid		Suspension	
Dosage=0.5 gram				
-	(Ages 6-12) 1 packet qid	250 mg/5 ml teasp.	-	(Age under 6) 1 teasp. (5 ml) per 30 lb body weight qid

Store between 15-30°C (59-86°F).

HOW SUPPLIED - RATED THERAPEUTICALLY EQUIVALENT:

Tablet, Enteric Coated - Oral - 1 gm

100's	$26.50	Methenamine Mandelate, Harber Pharm	51432-0274-03

Tablet, Enteric Coated - Oral - 500 mg

1000's	$147.50	Methenamine Mandelate, Harber Pharm	51432-0272-06

HOW SUPPLIED - NOT RATED EQUIVALENT:

Granules

454 gm	$9.45	Methenamine, Millgood	53118-0524-10
2500 gm	$38.55	Methenamine, Mallinckrodt	00406-5180-05

Suspension - Oral - 250 mg/5ml

480 ml	**$53.88**	**MANDELAMINE, Parke-Davis**	**00071-2173-23**

Suspension - Oral - 500 mg/5ml

480 ml	$37.50	Methenamine Mandelate, Consolidated Midland	00223-6380-00
480 ml	$38.80	Methenamine Mandelate, Goldline Labs	00182-0764-40
480 ml	$48.50	Methenamine Mandelate, Alpharma	00472-0783-16
480 ml	$49.00	Methenamine Mandelate Forte, Schein Pharm (US)	00364-7194-16
480 ml	$55.05	Methenamine Mandelate, Mikart	46672-0621-16
480 ml	**$76.20**	**MANDELAMINE FORTE, Parke-Davis**	**00071-2174-23**

Tablet, Enteric Coated - Oral - 1 gm

100's	$6.95	Methenamine Mandelate, Consolidated Midland	00223-1044-01
100's	$22.53	Methenamine, Aligen Independ	00405-4638-01
100's	$26.10	Methenamine Mandelate, Jerome Stevens	50564-0541-01
100's	$26.12	Methenamine Mandelate, Rugby	00536-4024-01
100's	$26.45	Methenamine Mandelate, Goldline Labs	00182-0187-01
100's	$27.50	Methenamine Mandelate, United Res	00677-0775-01
100's	$27.70	Methenamine Mandelate, Major Pharms	00904-2268-60
100's	**$52.63**	**MANDELAMINE, Parke-Davis**	**00071-0167-24**
250's	$53.20	MANDAMETH, Major Pharms	00904-2268-70
1000's	$49.50	Methenamine Mandelate, Consolidated Midland	00223-1044-02
1000's	$195.00	Methenamine Mandelate, Jerome Stevens	50564-0541-10

Tablet, Enteric Coated - Oral - 500 mg

100's	$5.25	Methenamine Mandelate, Consolidated Midland	00223-1043-01
100's	$14.47	Methenamine, Aligen Independ	00405-4637-01
100's	$15.68	Methenamine Mandelate, Rugby	00536-4022-01
100's	$16.75	Methenamine Mandelate, Goldline Labs	00182-2613-01
100's	$16.75	Methenamine Mandelate, Jerome Stevens	50564-0540-01
100's	$17.60	Methenamine Mandelate, Major Pharms	00904-2267-60
100's	**$32.92**	**MANDELAMINE, Parke-Davis**	**00071-0166-24**
250's	$33.80	MANDAMETH, Major Pharms	00904-2267-70
1000's	$39.50	Methenamine Mandelate, Consolidated Midland	00223-1043-02
1000's	$139.26	Methenamine Mandelate, Rugby	00536-4022-10
1000's	$140.00	Methenamine Mandelate, Jerome Stevens	50564-0540-10

METHENAMINE MANDELATE; SODIUM ACID PHOSPHATE *(001763)*

CATEGORIES: Anti-Infectives; Antibacterials; Antimicrobials; Antiseptics, Urinary Tract; Urinary Anti-Infectives; Urinary Antibacterial; Urinary Tract Infections; Pregnancy Category C; FDA Pre 1938 Drugs

BRAND NAMES: Ty-Methate; Urinary Antiseptic No. 2; Urisedamine; Uritin; Uro-Phosphate; **Uroqid-Acid No. 2**

DESCRIPTION:

Each Uroqid-Acid No. 2 tablet contains methenamine mandelate 500 mg and sodium acid phosphate, monohydrate 500 mg.

CLINICAL PHARMACOLOGY:

Methenamine mandelate is rapidly absorbed and excreted in the urine. Formaldehyde is released by acid hydrolysis from methenamine with bactericidal levels rapidly reached at pH 5.0-5.5. Proportionally less formaldehyde is released as urinary pH approaches 6.0 and insufficient quantities are released above this level for therapeutic response. In acid urine, mandelic acid exerts its antibacterial action and also contributes to the acidification of the urine. Mandelic acid is excreted by both glomerular filtration and tubular excretion. In acid urine, there is equally effective antibacterial activity against both gram-positive and gram-negative organisms, since the antibacterial action of mandelic acid and formaldehyde is nonspecific. With Proteus vulgaris and urea splitting strains of Pseudomonas and Aerobacter, results may be discouraging and particular attention is required in monitoring urinary pH and overall management.

INDICATIONS AND USAGE:

For the suppression or elimination of bacteriuria associated with chronic and recurrent infections of the urinary tract, including pyelitis, pyelonephritis, cystitis, and infected residual urine accompanying neurogenic bladder. When used as recommended, Uroqid-Acid No. 2 is particularly suitable for long-term therapy because of its relative safety and because resistance to the nonspecific bactericidal action of formaldehyde does not develop. Pathogens resistant to other antibacterial agents may respond because of nonspecific effect of formaldehyde formed in an acid urine.

Prophylactic Use Rationale: Urine is a good culture medium for many urinary pathogens. Inoculation by a few organisms (relapse or reinfection) may lead to bacteriuria in susceptible individuals. Thus, the rationale of management in recurring urinary tract infection (bacteriuria) is to change the urine from a growth-supporting to a growth-inhibiting medium. There is a growing body of evidence that long- term administration of methenamine can prevent recurrence of bacteriuria in patients with chronic pyelonephritis.

Therapeutic Use Rationale: Helps to sterilize the urine and, in some situations in which underlying pathological conditions prevent sterilization by any means, can help to suppress bacteriuria. As part of the overall management of the urinary tract infection, a thorough diagnostic evaluation should accompany the use of this product.

CONTRAINDICATIONS:

Uroqid-Acid No. 2 is contraindicated in patients with renal insufficiency, severe hepatic disease, severe dehydration, hyperphosphatemia, and in patients who have exhibited hypersensitivity to any components of this product.

PRECAUTIONS:

General: This product should not be used as the sole therapeutic agent in acute parenchymal infections causing systemic symptoms such as chills and fever.

Uroqid Acid No. 2 contains approximately 83 mg of sodium per tablet and should be used with caution in patients on a sodium-restricted diet.

PRECAUTIONS: *(cont'd)*

Sodium phosphates should be used with caution in the following conditions: cardiac failure; peripheral of pulmonary edema; hypernatremia; hypertension; toxemia of pregnancy; hypoparathyroidism; and acute pancreatitis. High serum phosphate levels increase the incidence of extraskeletal calcification.

Large doses of methenamine (8 grams daily for 3 to 4 weeks) have caused bladder irritation, painful and frequent micturition, albuminuria and gross hematuria. Dysuria may occur, although usually at higher than recommended doses, and can be controlled by reducing the dosage, This product contains a urinary acidifier and can cause metabolic acidosis. Care should be taken to maintain an acidic urinary pH (below 5.5), especially when treating infections due to urea-splitting organisms such as Proteus and strains of Pseudomonas. Drugs and/or foods which produce an alkaline urine should be restricted. Frequent urine pH tests are essential. If acidification of the urine is contraindicated or unattainable, use of this product should be discontinued.

Information for the Patient: To assure an acidic pH, patients should be instructed to restrict or avoid most fruits, milk and milk products, and antacids containing sodium carbonate or bicarbonate.

Laboratory Tests: As with all urinary tract infections, the efficacy of therapy should be monitored by repeated urine cultures. During long-term therapy, careful monitoring of renal function, serum phosphorus and sodium may be required at periodic intervals.

Laboratory Test Interactions: Formaldehyde interferes with fluorometric procedures for determination of urinary catecholamines and vanilmandelic acid (VMA) causing erroneously high results. Formaldehyde also causes falsely decreased urine estriol levels by reacting with estriol when acid hydrolysis techniques are used; estriol determinations which use enzymatic hydrolysis are unaffected by formaldehyde. Formaldehyde causes falsely elevated 17-hydroxycorticosteroid levels when the Porter-Silber method is used and falsely decreased 5-hydroxyindoleacetic acid (5HIAA) levels by inhibiting color development when nitrosonaphthol methods are used.

Carcinogenesis, Mutagenesis, and Impairment of Fertility: Long-term animal studies to evaluate the carcinogenic, mutagenic, or impairment of fertility potential of this product have not been performed.

Pregnancy: Teratogenic Effects, Pregnancy Category C. Animal reproduction studies have not been conducted with Uroqid-Acid No. 2. It is also not known whether Uroqid-Acid No. 2 can cause fetal harm when administered to a pregnant woman or can affect reproductive capacity. Since methenamine is known to cross the placental barrier, Uroqid-Acid No. 2 should be given to a pregnant woman only if clearly needed.

Nursing Mothers: Methenamine is excreted in breast milk. Caution should be exercised when this product is administered to a nursing woman.

DRUG INTERACTIONS:

Formaldehyde and sulfamethizole form an insoluble precipitate in acid urine and increase the risk of crystalluria; therefore, this product should not be used concurrently. Thiazide diuretics, carbonic anhydrase inhibitors, antacids, or urinary alkalinizing agents should not be used concurrently since they may cause the urine to become alkaline and reduce the effectiveness of methenamine by inhibiting its conversion to formaldehyde. Concurrent use of antihypertensives, especially diazoxide, guanethidine, hydralazine, methyldopa, or rauwolfia alkaloids; or corticosteroids, especially mineralocorticoids or corticotropin, with sodium phosphates may result in hypernatremia. Concurrent use of salicylates may lead to increased serum salicylate levels since excretion of salicylates is reduced in acidified urine. Serum salicylate levels should be closely monitored to avoid toxicity.

ADVERSE REACTIONS:

Gastrointestinal disturbances (nausea, stomach upset), generalized skin rash, dysuria, painful or difficult urination may occur occasionally with the use of methenamine preparations. Microscopic and rarely, gross hematuria have also been reported.

Gastrointestinal upset (diarrhea, nausea, stomach pain, and vomiting) may occur with the use of sodium phosphates. Also, bone or joint pain (possible phosphate induced osteomalacia) could occur. The following adverse effects may be observed (primarily from sodium): headaches; dizziness; mental confusion, seizures, weakness or heaviness of legs, unusual tiredness or weakness; muscle cramps; numbness, tingling pain, or weakness of hands or feet; numbness or tingling around lips; fast or irregular heartbeat; shortness of breath or troubled breathing; swelling of feet or lower legs; unusual weight gain; low urine output; unusual thirst.

Directions: Initially, 2 tablets 4 times daily. For maintenance, 2 to 4 tablets daily, in divided doses with a full glass of water.

Dispense in a tight, light resistant container with child-resistant closures.

STORAGE: Keep tightly closed. Store at controlled room temperature 15°-30°C(59°-86°F).

Protect from light.

(Beach Pharmaceuticals, R6/94)

HOW SUPPLIED - EQUIVALENTS NOT AVAILABLE:

Tablet, Coated - Oral - 350 mg/200 mg

100's	$8.95	URINARY ANTISEPTIC NO.2, United Res	00677-1393-01
100's	$18.00	URO PHOSPHATE, ECR Pharms	00095-0031-01
1000's	$99.40	URINARY ANTISEPTIC NO. 2, Eon Labs Mfg	00185-0230-10

Tablet, Coated - Oral - 500 mg/500 mg

100's	$24.00	UROQID ACID NO. 2, Beach Pharms	00486-1114-01

METHICILLIN SODIUM *(001764)*

CATEGORIES: Anti-Infectives; Antibiotics; Antimicrobials; Infections; Penicillins; Staphylococci, Penicillin G Resistant; FDA Approval Pre 1982

BRAND NAMES: *Estafcilina*; *Lucopenin*; *Mechicillin*; **Staphcillin**
(International brand names outside U.S. in italics)

DESCRIPTION:

Methicillin sodium is a semisynthetic antibiotic substance derived from 6-amino-penicillanic acid. It is the sodium salt in a parenteral dosage form. Each gram of methicillin sodium is equivalent to 900 mg methicillin activity and is buffered with 50 mg sodium citrate.

$C_{17}H_{19}N_2NaO_2S°H_2O$ 420.41 (CAS-7246-14-2)

4-Thia-1-azabicyclol(3.2.0)Heptane-2-carboxylic acid, 6((2,6-dimethoxybenzoyl)amino)-3,3-dimethyl-7-oxo-,monosodium salt, monohydrate, (2S-(2α,5α,6β))-.

CLINICAL PHARMACOLOGY:

Microbiology: Penicillinase-resistant penicillins exert a bactericidal action against penicillin-susceptible microorganisms during the state of active multiplication. All penicillins inhibit the biosynthesis of the bacterial cell wall.

CLINICAL PHARMACOLOGY: *(cont'd)*

The drugs in this class are highly resistant to inactivation by staphylococcal penicillinase and are active against penicillinase-producing and nonpenicillinase-producing strains of *Staphylococcus aureus.*

The penicillinase-resistant penicillins are active *in vitro* against a variety of other bacteria.

Susceptibility Testing: Quantitative methods that require measurement of zone diameters or minimal inhibitory concentrations (MICs) give the most precise estimates of antibiotic susceptibility. One such procedure has been recommended for use with discs to test susceptibility to this class of drugs. Interpretations correlate diameters on the disc test with MIC values. A penicillinase-resistant class disc may be used to determine microbial susceptibility to cloxacillin, dicloxacillin, methicillin, nafcillin, and oxacillin. With this procedure, employing a 5 microgram methicillin sodium disc, a report from the laboratory of "susceptible" (zone of at least 14 mm) indicates that the infecting organism is likely to respond to therapy. A report of "resistant" (zone of less than 10 mm) indicates that the infecting organism is not likely to respond to therapy. A report of "intermediate susceptibility" (zone of 10 to 13 mm) suggests that the organism might be susceptible if high doses of the antibiotic are used, or if the infection is confined to tissues and fluids (*e.g.,* urine), in which high antibiotic levels are attained.

In general, all staphylococci should be tested against the penicillin G disc and against the methicillin disc. Routine methods of antibiotic susceptibility testing may fail to detect strains of organisms resistant to the penicillinase-resistant penicillins. For this reason, the use of large inocula and 48-hour incubation periods may be necessary to obtain accurate susceptibility studies with these antibiotics. Bacterial strains which are resistant to one of the penicillinase-resistant penicillins should be considered resistant to all of the drugs in this class.

PHARMACOKINETICS

Methicillin is not acid-resistant and must be administered by intramuscular or intravenous injection. A 1-gram intramuscular dose gives a peak blood level of approximately 12 mcg/ml which drops off to about 1 mcg/ml within a 4-hour period. Methicillin is rapidly excreted unchanged in the urine in individuals with normal kidney function. Impairment in kidney function results in elevated blood levels which may require adjustment of dosage and treatment intervals. Protein binding of methicillin is approximately 40%. The drug penetrates body tissues well, and diffuses readily into pleural, pericardial, and synovial fluids. As with all penicillins, absorption into spinal fluids is poor under normal conditions. However, higher concentrations may be attained in the presence of meningeal inflammation.

INDICATIONS AND USAGE:

The penicillinase-resistant are indicated in the treatment of infections due to penicillinase-producing staphylococci which have demonstrated susceptibility to the drugs. Culture and susceptibility tests should be performed initially to determine the causative organism and their sensitivity to the drug. (See CLINICAL PHARMACOLOGY, Susceptibility Testing.)

The penicillin-resistant penicillins may be used to initiate therapy in suspected cases of resistant staphylococcal infections prior to the availability of laboratory test results. The penicillinase-resistant penicillins should not be used in infections caused by organisms susceptible to penicillin G. If the susceptibility tests indicate that the infection is due to an organism other than a resistant staphylococcus, therapy should not be continued with penicillinase-resistant penicillin.

CONTRAINDICATIONS:

A history of hypersensitivity (anaphylactic) reaction to any penicillin is a contraindication.

WARNINGS:

Serious and occasionally fatal hypersensitivity (anaphylactoid shock with collapse) reactions have occurred in patients receiving penicillin. The incidence of anaphylactoid shock in all penicillin-treated patients is between 0.015 and 0.04 percent. Anaphylactic shock resulting in death has occurred in approximately 0.002 percent of the patients treated. Although anaphylaxis is more frequent following parenteral administration, it has occurred in patients in oral penicillins.

When penicillin therapy is indicated, it should be initiated only after a comprehensive patient drug and allergy history has been obtained. If an allergic reaction occurs, the drug should be discontinued and the patient should receive supportive treatment, e.g., artificial maintenance of ventilation, pressor amines, antihistamines, and corticosteroids. Individuals with a history of penicillin hypersensitivity may also experience allergic reactions when treated with a cephalosporin.

PRECAUTIONS:

General: Penicillinase-resistant penicillins should generally not be administered to patients with a history of sensitivity to any penicillin.

Penicillin should be used with caution in individuals with histories of significant allergies and/or asthma. Whenever allergic reactions occur, penicillin should be withdrawn unless, in the opinion of the physician, the condition being treated is life-threatening and amenable only to penicillin therapy.

The oral route of administration should not be relied upon in patients with severe illness, or with nausea, vomiting, gastric dilation, cardiospasm, or intestinal hypermotility. Occasionally patients will not absorb therapeutic amounts of orally administered penicillin.

The use of antibiotics may result in overgrowth of nonsusceptible organisms. If new infections due to bacteria or fungi occur, the drug should be discontinued and appropriate measures taken.

Laboratory Tests: Bacteriologic studies to determine the causative organisms and their susceptibility to the penicillinase-resistant penicillins should be performed (see CLINICAL PHARMACOLOGY, Microbiology). In the treatment of suspected staphylococcal infections, therapy should be changed to another active agent if culture tests fail to demonstrate the presence of staphylococci.

Periodic assessment of organ system function including renal, hepatic, and hematopoietic should be made during prolonged therapy with penicillinase-resistant penicillins.

Blood cultures, white blood cell, and differential cell counts should be obtained prior to initiation of therapy and at least weekly during therapy with penicillinase-resistant penicillins.

Periodic urinalysis, blood urea nitrogen, and creatinine determinations should be performed during therapy with the penicillinase-resistant penicillins and dosage alterations should be considered if these values become elevated. If any impairment of renal function is suspected or known to exist, a reduction in the total dosage should be considered and blood levels monitored to avoid possible neurotoxic reactions. (See DOSAGE AND ADMINISTRATION.)

SGOT and SGPT values should be obtained periodically during therapy to monitor for possible liver function abnormalities.

Carcinogenesis, Mutagenesis, and Impairment of Fertility: No long-term animal studies have been conducted with these drugs.

Studies on reproduction (nafcillin) in rats and rabbits reveal no fetal or maternal abnormalities before conception and continuously through weaning (one generation).

PRECAUTIONS: *(cont'd)*

Pregnancy Category B: Reproduction studies performed in the mouse, rat, and rabbit have revealed no evidence of impaired fertility or harm to the fetus due the penicillinase-resistant penicillins. Human experience with the penicillins during pregnancy has not shown any positive evidence of adverse effects on the fetus. There are, however, no adequate or well-controlled studies in pregnant women showing conclusively that harmful effects of these drugs on the fetus can be excluded. Because animal reproduction studies are not always predictive of human response, this drug should be administered during pregnancy only if clearly needed.

Nursing Mothers: Penicillins are excreted in breast milk. Caution should be exercised when penicillins are administered to a nursing woman.

Pediatric Use: Because of incompletely developed renal function in newborns, penicillinase-resistant penicillins (especially methicillin) may not be completely excreted, with abnormally high blood levels resulting. Frequent blood levels are advisable in this group with dosage adjustments when necessary. All newborns treated with penicillins should be monitored closely for clinical and laboratory evidence of toxic or adverse effects. (See DOSAGE AND ADMINISTRATION.)

DRUG INTERACTIONS:

Tetracycline, a bacteriostatic antibiotic, may antagonize the bactericidal effect of penicillin and concurrent use of these drugs should be avoided.

ADVERSE REACTIONS:

Body as a Whole: The reported incidence of allergic reactions to penicillin ranges from 0.7 to 10 percent. (See WARNINGS.) Sensitization is usually the result of such treatment but some individuals have had immediate reactions to penicillin when first treatment. In such cases, it is thought that the patients may have had prior exposure to the drug via trace amounts present in milk and vaccines.

Two types of allergic reactions to penicillin are noted clinically, immediate and delayed.

Immediate reactions usually occur within 20 minutes of administration and range in severity from urticaria and pruritus to angioneurotic edema, laryngospasm, bronchospasm, hypotension, vascular collapse, and death. Such immediate anaphylactic reactions are very rare (See WARNINGS) and usually occur after parenteral therapy but have occurred in patients receiving oral therapy. Another type of immediate reaction, an accelerated reaction, may occur between 20 minutes and 48 hours after administration and may include urticaria, pruritus, and fever. Although laryngeal edema, laryngospasm, and hypotension occasionally occur, fatality is uncommon.

Delayed allergic reactions to penicillin therapy usually occur after 48 hours and sometimes as late as 2 to 4 weeks after inhalation of therapy. Manifestations of this type of reaction include serum sickness-like symptoms (*i.e.,* fever, malaise, urticaria, myalgia, arthralgia, abdominal pain) and various skin rashes. Nausea, vomiting, diarrhea, stomatitis, black or hairy tongue, and other symptoms of gastrointestinal irritation may occur, especially during oral penicillin therapy.

Nervous System Reactions: Neurotoxic reactions similar to those observed with penicillin G may occur with large intravenous doses of the penicillinase-resistant penicillins especially in patients with renal insufficiency.

Urogenital Reactions: Renal tubular damage and interstitial nephritis have been associated with the administration of methicillin sodium and infrequently with the administration of nafcillin and oxacillin. Manifestations of this reaction may include rash, fever, eosinophilia, hematuria, proteinuria, and renal insufficiency. Methicillin-induced nephropathy does not appear to be dose-related and is generally reversible upon prompt discontinuation of therapy.

Metabolic Reactions: Agranulocytosis, neutropenia, and bone marrow depression have been associated with the use of methicillin sodium, nafcillin, oxacillin, and cloxacillin. Hepatotoxicity, characterized by fever, nausea, and vomiting associated with abnormal liver function tests, mainly elevated SGOT levels, has been associated with the use of oxacillin and cloxacillin.

DOSAGE AND ADMINISTRATION:

The penicillinase-resistant penicillins are available for oral administration and for intramuscular and intravenous injection. The sodium salts of methicillin, oxacillin, and nafcillin may be administered parenterally and the sodium salts of cloxacillin, dicloxacillin, oxacillin, and nafcillin are available for oral use.

Bacteriologic studies to determine the causative organisms and their sensitivity to the penicillinase-resistant penicillins should always be performed. Duration of therapy varies with the type and severity of infection as well as the overall condition of the patient, therefore, it should be determined by the clinical and bacteriological response of the patient. In severe staphylococcal infections, therapy with penicillinase-resistant penicillins should be continued for at least 14 days. Therapy should be continued for at least 48 hours after the patient has become afebrile, asymptomatic, and cultures are negative. The treatment of endocarditis and osteomyelitis may require a longer term of therapy.

Concurrent administration of the penicillinase-resistant penicillins and probenecid increases and prolongs serum penicillin levels. Probenecid decreases the apparent volume of distribution and slows the rate of excretion by competitively inhibiting renal tubular secretion of penicillin. Penicillin-probenecid therapy is generally limited to those infections where very high serum levels of penicillin are necessary.

Oral preparations of the penicillinase-resistant penicillins should not be used as initial therapy in serious, life-threatening infections. (See PRECAUTIONS, General.) Oral therapy with the penicillinase-resistant penicillins may be used to follow-up the previous use of a parenteral agent as soon as the clinical condition warrants. For intramuscular gluteal injections, care should be taken to avoid sciatic nerve injury. With intravenous administration, particularly in elderly patients, care should be taken because of the possibility of thrombophlebitis.

TABLE 1 Recommended Dosages For Methicillin Sodium

Adults	Infants and Children <40 kg (88 lbs)
1 gram IM every 4 or 6 hours IV every 6 hours	25 mg/kg IM every 6 hours IV not recommended

DIRECTIONS FOR USE

For Intramuscular Use: Use Sterile Water for Injection, USP or Sodium Chloride Injection, USP. Add 1.5 ml to the 1 gram vial, 5.7 ml to the 4 gram vial, and 8.6 ml to the 6 gram vial and withdraw the entire contents. Each 1 ml will contain approximately 500 mg of methicillin sodium. The solutions are stable for 24 hours at room temperature or 4 days under refrigeration.

For Direct Intravenous Use: Further dilute each 1 ml of solution, reconstituted as above, with 25 ml of Sodium Chloride Injection, USP and inject at the rate of 10 ml per minute.

For Administration by Intravenous Drip: Reconstitute as directed above **(For Intramuscular Use)** prior to diluting with Intravenous Solution.

DOSAGE AND ADMINISTRATION: *(cont'd)*

TABLE 2A Stability Periods Of Methicillin Sodium

Concentration mg/ml	Sterile H_2O for Injection	Isotonic Sodium Chloride	M/5 Molar Sodium Lactate Solution
ROOM TEMPERATURE (25°C)			
10-200	24 Hrs	24 hrs	
2-20			8 hrs
10-30			
REFRIGERATION (4°C)			
10-200	7 days	7 days	
10-30			7 days
FROZEN (-15°C)			
19-500	30 days		
20-100		30 days	30 days

TABLE 2B Stability Periods For Methicillin Sodium (Concentration mg/ml In TABLE 2A)

5% Dextrose in H_2O	5% Dextrose in 0.45% NaCl	10% Invert Sugar	Lactated Ringers Solution
ROOM TEMPERATURE (25°C)			
8 Hrs	24 hrs	8 Hrs	8 Hrs
REFRIGERATION (4°C)			
7 days	7 days	7 days	7 days
FROZEN (-15°C)			
30 days	30 days	30 days	30 days

Stability studies on methicillin sodium at concentrations of 2 mg/ml, 10 mg/ml, and 20 mg/ml in various intravenous solutions listed below indicate the drug will lose less than 10% activity at room temperature (70°F) during an 8-hour period.

IV Solution

5% Dextrose in Normal Saline
10% D-Fructose in Water
10% D-Fructose in Normal Saline
Lactated Potassic Saline Injection
5% Plasma Hydrolysate in Water
*10% Invert Sugar in Normal Saline
10% Invert Sugar Plus 0.3% Potassium Chloride in Water
Travert 10% Electrolyte #1
Travert 10% Electrolyte #2
Travert 10% Electrolyte #3

Only those solutions listed above should be used for the intravenous infusion of methicillin sodium. The concentration of the antibiotic should fall within the range specified. The drug concentration and the rate and volume of the infusion should be adjusted so that the total dose of methicillin is administered before the drug loses its stability in the solution in use.

If another agent is used in conjunction with methicillin therapy, **it should not be physically mixed** with methicillin but should be administered separately.

*At a concentration of 2 mg/ml, methicillin sodium is stable for only 4 hours in this solution. Concentrations between 10 mg/ml and 30 mg/ml are stable for 8 hours.

"Piggyback" IV Package: This glass vial contains the labeled quantity of methicillin sodium and is intended for intravenous administration. The diluent and volume are specified on the label of each package.

Pharmacy Bulk Package: This glass vial contains 10 grams methicillin sodium and is designed for use in the pharmacy in preparing IV additives. Add 94 ml Sterile Water for Injection, USP or Sodium Chloride Injection, USP. The resulting solution will contain 100 mg methicillin sodium per ml, which is equivalent to 90 mg per ml methicillin activity.

Following reconstitution in this manner, the resulting solutions are stable for 24 hours at room temperature for 7 days under refrigeration.

CAUTION: NOT TO BE DISPENSED AS A UNIT.

(APOTHECON: 12/90, 796499FF-2)

HOW SUPPLIED - EQUIVALENTS NOT AVAILABLE:

Injection, Dry-Soln - Intramuscular; - 4 gm/vial

4 gm	$20.15	STAPHCILLIN, Mead Johnson	00015-7964-20

Injection, Dry-Soln - Intramuscular; - 900 mg/vial

1 gm	$5.53	STAPHCILLIN, Mead Johnson	00015-7961-20
1 gm	$10.38	STAPHCILLIN, Mead Johnson	00015-7961-28

METHIMAZOLE *(001765)*

CATEGORIES: Antithyroid Agents; Hormones; Hyperthyroidism; Thyroid Preparations; Pregnancy Category D; FDA Approval Pre 1982

BRAND NAMES: *Antitroide-GW*; *Favistan*; *Mercaptizol*; *Mercazole*; *Methimazole*; *Metimazol*; *Strumazol*; **Tapazole**; *Thacapzol*; *Thiamazol* (Germany); *Thycapzol*; *Thyrozol* (Germany); *Tirodril* (Germany); *Unimazole*
(International brand names outside U.S. in italics)

FORMULARIES: Aetna; BC-BS; Medi-Cal; PCS

COST OF THERAPY: $146.18 (Hyperthyroidism; Tablet; 5 mg; 3/day; 365 days)

DESCRIPTION:

Methimazole tablets (1-methylimidazole-2-thiol) is a white crystalline substance that is freely soluble in water. It differs chemically from the drugs of the thiouracil series primarily because it has a 5- instead of a 6-membered ring.

Each tablet contains 5 or 10 mg (43.8 or 87.6 μmol) methimazole, an orally administered antithyroid drug.

Each tablet also contains lactose, magnesium stearate, starch, and talc.

The molecular weight is 114.16, and the empirical formula is $C_4H_6N_2S$.

CLINICAL PHARMACOLOGY:

Methimazole inhibits the synthesis of thyroid hormones and thus is effective in the treatment of hyperthyroidism. The drug does not inactivate existing thyroxine and triiodothyronine that are stored in the thyroid or are circulating in the blood, nor does it interfere with the effectiveness of thyroid hormones given by mouth or by injection.

The actions and use of methimazole are similar to those of propylthiouracil. On a weight basis, the drug is at least 10 times as potent as propylthiouracil, but methimazole may be less consistent in action.

Methimazole is readily absorbed from the gastrointestinal tract. It is metabolized rapidly and requires frequent administration. Methimazole is excreted in the urine.

CLINICAL PHARMACOLOGY: *(cont'd)*

In laboratory animals, various regimens that continuously suppress thyroid function and thereby increase TSH secretion result in thyroid tissue hypertrophy. Under such conditions, the appearance of thyroid and pituitary neoplasms have also been reported. Regimens that have been studied in this regard include antithyroid agents, as well as dietary iodine deficiency, subtotal thyroidectomy, implantation of autonomous thyrotropic hormone-secreting pituitary tumors, and administration of chemical goitrogens.

INDICATIONS AND USAGE:

Tapazole is indicated in the medical treatment of hyperthyroidism. Long-term therapy may lead to remission of the disease. Methimazole may be used to ameliorate hyperthyroidism in preparation for subtotal thyroidectomy or radioactive iodine therapy. Methimazole is also used when thyroidectomy is contraindicated or not advisable.

CONTRAINDICATIONS:

Methimazole is contraindicated in the presence of hypersensitivity to the drug and in nursing mothers because the drug is excreted in milk.

WARNINGS:

Agranulocytosis is potentially a serious side effect of therapy with Methimazole. Patients should be instructed to report to their physicians any symptoms of agranulocytosis, such as fever or sore throat. Leukopenia, thrombocytopenia, and aplastic anemia (pancytopenia) may also occur. The drug should be discontinued in the presence of agranulocytosis, aplastic anemia (pancytopenia), hepatitis, or exfoliative dermatitis. The patient's bone marrow function should be monitored.

Due to the similar hepatic toxicity profiles of Tapazole and propylthiouracil, attention is drawn to the severe hepatic reactions which have occurred with both drugs. There have been rare reports of fulminant hepatitis, hepatic necrosis, encephalopathy, and death. Symptoms suggestive hepatic dysfunction (anorexia, pruritus, right upper quadrant pain, etc.) should prompt evaluation of liver function. Drug treatment should be discontinued promptly in the event of clinically significant evidence of liver abnormality including hepatic transaminase values exceeding 3 times the upper limit of normal.

Methimazole can cause fetal harm when administered to a pregnant woman. Methimazole readily crosses the placental membranes and can induce goiter and even cretinism in the developing fetus. In addition, rare instances of aplasia cutis, as manifested by scalp defects, have occurred in infants born to mothers who received methimazole is used during pregnancy. If methimazole is used during pregnancy, or if the patient becomes pregnant while taking this drug, the patient should be warned of the potential hazard to the fetus.

Since scalp defects have not been reported in offspring of patients treated with propylthiouracil, that agent may be preferable to methimazole in pregnant women requiring treatment with antithyroid drugs.

Postpartum patients receiving methimazole should not nurse their babies.

PRECAUTIONS:

General: Patients who receive methimazole should be under close surveillance and should be cautioned to report immediately any evidence of illness, particularly sore throat, skin eruptions, fever, headache, or general malaise. In such cases, white-blood-cell and differential counts should be made to determine whether agranulocytosis has developed. Particular care should be exercised with patients who are receiving additional drugs known to cause agranulocytosis.

Laboratory Tests: Because methimazole may cause hypoprothrombinemia and bleeding, prothrombin time should be monitored during therapy with the drug, especially before surgical procedures. (See PRECAUTIONS, General).

Periodic monitoring of thyroid function is warranted, and the finding of an elevated TSH warrants a decrease in the dosage of methimazole.

Carcinogenesis, Mutagenesis, and Impairment of Fertility: In a 2 year study, rats were given methimazole at doses of 0.5, 3, and 18 mg/kg/day. These doses were 0.3, 2, and 12 times the 15 mg/day maximum human maintenance dose (when calculated on the basis of surface area). Thyroid hyperplasia, adenoma, and carcinoma developed rats at the two higher doses. The clinical significance of these findings is unclear.

Pregnancy Category D: (See WARNINGS.) methimazole, used judiciously, is an effective drug in hyperthyroidism complicated by pregnancy. In many pregnant women, the thyroid dysfunction diminishes as the pregnancy proceeds; consequently, a reduction in dosage may be possible. In some instances, use of methimazole can be discontinued 2 or 3 weeks before delivery.

Nursing Mothers: The drug appears in human breast milk and its use is contraindicated in nursing mothers (see WARNINGS).

Pediatric Use: See DOSAGE AND ADMINISTRATION.

DRUG INTERACTIONS:

The activity of anticoagulants may be potentiated by anti-vitamin-K activity attributed to methimazole.

ADVERSE REACTIONS:

Major adverse reactions (which occur with much less frequency than the minor adverse reactions) include inhibition of myelopoiesis (agranulocytosis, granulocytopenia, and thrombocytopenia), aplastic anemia, drug fever, a lupuslike syndrome, insulin autoimmune syndrome (which can result in hypoglycemic coma), hepatitis (jaundice may persist for several weeks after discontinuation of the drug), periarteritis, and hypoprothrombinemia. Nephritis occurs very rarely.

Minor adverse reactions include skin rash, urticaria, nausea, vomiting, epigastric distress, arthralgia, paresthesia, loss of taste, abnormal loss of hair, myalgia, headache, pruritus, drowsiness, neuritis, edema, vertigo, skin pigmentation, jaundice, sialadenopathy, and lymphadenopathy.

It should be noted that about 10% of patients with untreated hyperthyroidism have leukopenia (white-blood-cell count of less than 4,000/mm^3), often with relative granulopenia.

OVERDOSAGE:

Signs and Symptoms: Symptoms may include nausea, vomiting, epigastric distress, headache, fever joint pain, pruritus, and edema. Aplastic anemia (pancytopenia) or agranulocytosis may be manifested in hours to days. Less frequent events are hepatitis, nephrotic syndrome, exfoliative dermatitis, neuropathies, and CNS stimulation or depression. Although not well studied, methimazole-induced agranulocytosis is generally associated with doses greater than 40 mg or more in patients older than 40 years of age.

No information is available on the median lethal dose of the drug or the concentration of methimazole in biologic fluids associated with toxicity and/or death.

OVERDOSAGE: *(cont'd)*

Treatment: To obtain up-to-date information about the treatment of overdose, a good resource is your certified Regional Poison Control Center. Telephone numbers of certified poison control centers are listed in *GenRx*. In managing overdosage, consider the possibility of multiple drug overdoses, interaction among drugs, and unusual drug kinetics in your patient.

Protect the patient's airway and support ventilation and perfusion. Meticulously monitor and maintain, within acceptable limits, the patient's vital signs, blood gases, serum electrolytes etc. The patient's bone marrow function should be monitored. Absorption of drugs from the gastrointestinal tract may be decreased by giving activated charcoal, which in many cases, is more effective than emesis or lavage; consider charcoal instead of or in addition to gastric emptying. Repeated doses of charcoal over time may hasten elimination of some drugs that have been absorbed. Safeguard the patient's airway when employing gastric emptying or charcoal.

Forced diuresis, peritoneal dialysis, hemodialysis, or charcoal hemoperfusion have not been established as beneficial for an overdose of methimazole.

DOSAGE AND ADMINISTRATION:

Methimazole is administered orally. It is usually given in 3 equal doses at approximately 8-hour intervals.

Adult: The initial daily dosage is 15 mg for mild hyperthyroidism, 30 to 40 mg for moderately severe hyperthyroidism, and 60 mg for severe hyperthyroidism, divided into 3 doses at 8-hour intervals. The maintenance dosage is 5 to 15 mg daily.

Pediatric: Initially, the daily dosage is 0.4 mg/kg of body weight divided into 3 doses and given at 8-hour intervals. The maintenance dosage is approximately 1/2 of the initial dose.

HOW SUPPLIED:

TapazoleTablets: *5 mg:* white (scored) (No. 1765);*10 mg:* white (scored) (No. 1770).

Store at controlled room temperature, 59° to 86°F (15° to 30°C).

HOW SUPPLIED - EQUIVALENTS NOT AVAILABLE:

Tablet, Uncoated - Oral - 5 mg

100's	**$13.35**	**TAPAZOLE, Lilly**	**00002-1094-02**

Tablet, Uncoated - Oral - 10 mg

100's	**$21.30**	**TAPAZOLE, Lilly**	**00002-1095-02**

METHIONINE *(001766)*

CATEGORIES: Acidifying Agents; Alkalinizing Agents; Antipruritics/Local Anesthetics; Electrolytic, Caloric-Water Balance; Homeostatic & Nutrient; Nutrition, Enteral/Parenteral; Pharmaceutical Adjuvants; Skin/Mucous Membrane Agents; FDA Pre 1938 Drugs

BRAND NAMES: Cotameth; *Methnine*; Odor Scrip; *Oradash*; **Pedameth**; Uranap; *Urosamine*
(International brand names outside U.S. in italics)

FORMULARIES: WHO

Prescribing information not available at time of publication.

HOW SUPPLIED - EQUIVALENTS NOT AVAILABLE:

Capsule, Gelatin - Oral - 200 mg

50's	**$26.74**	**PEDAMETH, Forest Pharms**	**00456-0355-50**
500's	**$218.62**	**PEDAMETH, Forest Pharms**	**00456-0355-02**
1000's	$35.00	Cotameth, C O Truxton	00463-2036-10
1000's	**$140.83**	**PEDAMETH, Forest Pharms**	**00456-1054-00**

Solution - Oral - 75 mg/5ml

480 ml	**$44.52**	**PEDAMETH, Forest Pharms**	**00456-1039-16**

METHIONINE; SODIUM PROPIONATE; UREA *(001767)*

CATEGORIES: Antipruritics/Local Anesthetics; Keratolytic Agents; Skin/Mucous Membrane Agents; Vaginal Preparations; FDA Pre 1938 Drugs

BRAND NAMES: Amino-Cerv

Prescribing information not available at time of publication.

HOW SUPPLIED - EQUIVALENTS NOT AVAILABLE:

Cream - Vaginal

77.96 gm x 12	**$158.39**	**AMINO-CERV, Milex Prod**	**00396-6010-10**
78 gm	**$172.80**	**AMINO-CERV, Milex Prod**	**00396-6010-00**
150 gm	**$15.60**	**AMINO-CERV, Milex Prod**	**00396-6010-30**

METHOCARBAMOL *(001768)*

CATEGORIES: Analgesics; Autonomic Drugs; Muscle Relaxants; Neuromuscular; Pain; Skeletal Muscle Hyperactivity; Skeletal Muscle Relaxants; FDA Approval Pre 1982

BRAND NAMES: *Bolaxin*; Carbacot; *Carbametin* (Japan); *Carxin* (Japan); Delaxin; Forbaxin; *Laxan*; *Lumirelax* (France); Marbaxin-750; Methocarb; *Miolaxin*; *Miowas*; *Myocin*; *Myolax*; *Ortoton* (Germany); *Relaxon*; Ro-Carbamol; **Robaxin**; *Robaxin-750* (England); *Robinax*; Robomol; *Roxin*; *Skedesin*; *Traumacut*; *Tresortil*; *Trolar*
(International brand names outside U.S. in italics)

FORMULARIES: Aetna; BC-BS; DoD; FHP; PCS

DESCRIPTION:

INACTIVE INGREDIENTS: *500 mg Robaxin Tablets:* Corn Starch, FD&C Yellow 6 Aluminum Lake, Hydroxypropyl Cellulose, Hydroxypropyl Methylcellulose, Magnesium Stearate, Polysorbate 20, Povidone, Propylene Glycol, Saccharin Sodium, Sodium Lauryl Sulfate, Sodium Starch Glycolate, Stearic Acid, Titanium Dioxide. *750 mg Robaxin Tablets:* Corn Starch, D&C Yellow 10 Aluminum Lake, FD&C Yellow 6 Aluminum Lake, Hydroxypropyl

DESCRIPTION: *(cont'd)*

Cellulose, Hydroxypropyl Methylcellulose, Magnesium Stearate, Polysorbate 20, Povidone, Propylene Glycol, Saccharin Sodium, Sodium Lauryl Sulfate, Sodium Starch Glycolate, Stearic Acid, Titanium Dioxide.

CLINICAL PHARMACOLOGY:

The mechanism of action of methocarbamol in humans has not been established, but may be due to general central nervous system depression. It has no direct action on the contractile mechanism of striated muscle, the motor end plate or the nerve fiber.

INDICATIONS AND USAGE:

Methocarbamol is indicated as an adjunct to rest, physical therapy, and other measures for the relief of discomforts associated with acute, painful musculoskeletal conditions. The mode of action of this drug has not been clearly identified, but may be related to its sedative properties. Methocarbamol does not directly relax tense skeletal muscles in man.

CONTRAINDICATIONS:

Methocarbamol is contraindicated in patients hypersensitive to any of the ingredients.

WARNINGS:

Since methocarbamol may possess a general central nervous system depressant effect, patients receiving methocarbamol tablets should be cautioned about combined effects with alcohol and other CNS depressants.

Safe use of methocarbamol has not been established with regard to possible adverse effects upon fetal development. Therefore, methocarbamol tablets should not be used in women who are or may become pregnant and particularly during early pregnancy unless in the judgment of the physician the potential benefits outweigh the possible hazards.

PRECAUTIONS:

Safety and effectiveness in children below the age of 12 years have not been established.

It is not known whether this drug is secreted in human milk. As a general rule, nursing should not be undertaken while a patient is on a drug since many drugs are excreted in human milk.

Methocarbamol may cause a color interference in certain screening tests for 5-hydroxyindoleacetic acid (5-HIAA) and vanilmandelic acid (VMA).

ADVERSE REACTIONS:

Lightheadedness, dizziness, drowsiness, nausea, allergic manifestations such as urticaria, pruritus, rash, conjunctivitis with nasal congestion, blurred vision, headache, fever.

DOSAGE AND ADMINISTRATION:

Robaxin 500 mg Adults: initial dosage, 3 tablets q.i.d., maintenance dosage, 2 tablets q.i.d.

Robaxin 750 mg Adults: initial dosage, 2 tablets q.i.d., maintenance dosage, 1 tablet q.4h. or 2 tablets t.i.d.

Six grams a day are recommended for the first 48 to 72 hours of treatment. (For severe conditions 8 grams a day may be administered). Thereafter, the dosage can usually be reduced to approximately 4 grams a day.

Store at controlled room temperature, between 15 and 30°C (59 and 86°F).

HOW SUPPLIED - RATED THERAPEUTICALLY EQUIVALENT:

Injection, Solution - Intramuscular; - 100 mg/ml

10 ml	$3.63	Methocarbamol, HL Moore Drug Exch	00839-6359-30
10 ml	$3.70	Methocarbamol, Steris Labs	00402-0131-10
10 ml	$4.00	Methocarbamol, Consolidated Midland	00223-8150-10
10 ml	$5.18	Methocarbamol, Schein Pharm (US)	00364-6726-54
10 ml	$7.80	Methocarbamol, Rugby	00536-5331-70
10 ml x 5	**$23.63**	**ROBAXIN, AH Robins**	**00031-7409-87**
10 ml x 25	**$106.84**	**ROBAXIN, AH Robins**	**00031-7409-94**

Tablet, Plain Coated - Oral - 500 mg

40's	$2.85	Methocarbamol, Talbert Phcy	44514-0557-25
100's	$6.39	Methocarbamol, Lederle Pharm	00005-3562-23
100's	$6.75	Methocarbamol, H.C.F.A. F F P	99999-1768-01
100's	$7.10	Methocarbamol, West Ward Pharm	00143-1290-01
100's	$8.48	Methocarbamol, Qualitest Pharms	00603-4487-21
100's	$8.50	Methocarbamol, Consolidated Midland	00223-1277-01
100's	$8.68	Methocarbamol, Caremark	00339-5819-12
100's	$8.95	Methocarbamol, United Res	00677-0430-01
100's	$8.95	Methocarbamol 500, Major Pharms	00904-2364-60
100's	$9.00	Methocarbamol, Goldline Labs	00182-0572-01
100's	$9.57	Methocarbamol, Aligen Independ	00405-4635-01
100's	$9.95	Methocarbamol, Raway	00686-0091-20
100's	$10.46	Methocarbamol, HL Moore Drug Exch	00839-5132-06
100's	$11.21	Methocarbamol, Geneva Pharms	00781-1760-01
100's	$11.60	Methocarbamol, Rugby	00536-4026-01
100's	$11.64	Methocarbamol, Schein Pharm (US)	00364-0346-01
100's	$12.00	Methocarbamol, Goldline Labs	00182-0572-89
100's	$13.47	Methocarbamol, Voluntary Hosp	53258-0117-13
100's	$13.77	Methocarbamol 500, Major Pharms	00904-2364-61
100's	$16.50	Methocarbamol, Schein Pharm (US)	00364-0346-90
100's	**$48.55**	**ROBAXIN, AH Robins**	**00031-7429-63**
500's	$29.95	Methocarbamol, Global Source	59618-0555-18
500's	$31.58	Methocarbamol, Lederle Pharm	00005-3562-31
500's	$31.60	Methocarbamol, West Ward Pharm	00143-1290-05
500's	$33.75	Methocarbamol, H.C.F.A. F F P	99999-1768-02
500's	$33.85	Methocarbamol, Aligen Independ	00405-4635-02
500's	$35.50	Methocarbamol, Qualitest Pharms	00603-4487-28
500's	$36.20	Methocarbamol 500, Major Pharms	00904-2364-40
500's	$37.50	Methocarbamol, Consolidated Midland	00223-1277-02
500's	$38.95	Methocarbamol, United Res	00677-0430-05
500's	$39.00	Methocarbomol, Goldline Labs	00182-0572-05
500's	$41.35	Methocarbamol, Geneva Pharms	00781-1760-05
500's	$47.00	Methocarbamol, Schein Pharm (US)	00364-0346-05
500's	$49.61	Methocarbamol, HL Moore Drug Exch	00839-5132-12
500's	$53.50	Methocarbamol, Rugby	00536-4026-05
500's	**$229.11**	**ROBAXIN, AH Robins**	**00031-7429-70**
1000's	$67.50	Methocarbamol, H.C.F.A. F F P	99999-1768-03
1000's	$67.75	Methocarbamol, Rugby	00536-4026-10

Tablet, Plain Coated - Oral - 750 mg

40's	$3.14	Methocarbamol, Talbert Phcy	44514-0558-25
60's	$60.00	METHOCARBAMOL, UDL	51079-0092-98
100's	$7.99	Methocarbamol, Lederle Pharm	00005-3563-23
100's	$8.93	Methocarbamol, H.C.F.A. F F P	99999-1768-04
100's	$9.50	Methocarbamol, West Ward Pharm	00143-1292-01
100's	$10.25	ROBOMOL - 750, Major Pharms	00904-2365-60

HOW SUPPLIED - RATED THERAPEUTICALLY EQUIVALENT: *(cont'd)*

100's	$10.40	Methocarbamol, Qualitest Pharms	00603-4488-21
100's	$10.45	Methocarbamol, Goldline Labs	00182-0573-01
100's	$10.45	Methocarbamol, United Res	00677-0431-01
100's	$10.78	Methocarbamol, Aligen Independ	00405-4636-01
100's	$11.07	Methocarbamol, Caremark	00339-5821-12
100's	$11.85	Methocarbamol 750, Harber Pharm	51432-0278-03
100's	$11.95	Methocarbamol, Consolidated Midland	00223-1278-01
100's	$11.95	Methocarbamol, Raway	00686-0092-20
100's	$12.99	Methocarbamol, Geneva Pharms	00781-1750-01
100's	$13.55	Methocarbamol, Rugby	00536-4027-01
100's	$16.77	Methocarbamol, Voluntary Hosp	53258-0167-13
100's	$17.00	Methocarbamol, Goldline Labs	00182-0573-89
100's	$18.35	Methocarbamol, Schein Pharm (US)	00364-0347-01
100's	$18.56	Methocarbamol, HL Moore Drug Exch	00839-5101-06
100's	$18.68	Methocarbamol, Amer Preferred	53445-0573-01
100's	$21.75	Methocarbamol, Schein Pharm (US)	00364-0347-90
100's	$25.20	Methocarbamol, Geneva Pharms	00781-1750-13
100's	**$69.40**	**ROBAXIN, AH Robins**	**00031-7449-63**
100's	**$71.95**	**ROBAXIN, AH Robins**	**00031-7449-64**
500's	$29.20	Methocarb, H & H Labs	46703-0091-05
500's	$31.95	Methocarbamol 750, H & H Labs	46703-0103-05
500's	$39.52	Methocarbamol, Lederle Pharm	00005-3563-31
500's	$40.25	Methocarbamol, West Ward Pharm	00143-1292-05
500's	$44.65	Methocarbamol, H.C.F.A. F F P	99999-1768-05
500's	$46.75	Methocarbamol, Goldline Labs	00182-0573-05
500's	$47.30	ROBOMOL - 750, Major Pharms	00904-2365-40
500's	$47.35	Methocarbamol, United Res	00677-0431-05
500's	$47.40	Methocarbamol, Qualitest Pharms	00603-4488-28
500's	$49.50	Methocarbamol, Consolidated Midland	00223-1278-05
500's	$49.90	Methocarbamol, Geneva Pharms	00781-1750-05
500's	$50.21	Methocarbamol, Schein Pharm (US)	00364-0347-05
500's	$59.25	Methocarbamol 750, Harber Pharm	51432-0278-05
500's	$62.50	Methocarbamol, Rugby	00536-4027-05
500's	$90.98	Methocarbamol, HL Moore Drug Exch	00839-5101-12
500's	**$326.86**	**ROBAXIN, AH Robins**	**00031-7449-70**
1000's	$18.56	Methocarbamol, HL Moore Drug Exch	00839-5101-16
1000's	$50.30	Methocarbamol, Aligen Independ	00405-4636-02
1000's	$89.30	Methocarbamol, H.C.F.A. F F P	99999-1768-06
1000's	$95.55	Methocarbamol, Rugby	00536-4027-10

METHOHEXITAL SODIUM *(001769)*

CATEGORIES: Analgesics; Anesthesia; Anxiolytics, Sedatives, Hypnotic; Barbiturates; Barbiturate Anesthetics; Central Nervous System Agents; Hypnotics; Injectable Anesthetics; Insomnia; Pregnancy Category B; DEA Class CIV; FDA Approval Pre 1982

BRAND NAMES: *Brietal* (France, England, Canada); *Brietal Sodium*; *Brevimytal* (Germany); *Brevital*; **Brevital Sodium**
(International brand names outside U.S. in italics)

> WARNING:
> This drug should be administered by persons qualified in the use of intravenous anesthetics. Cardiac life support equipment must be immediately available during use of methohexital.

DESCRIPTION:

Methohexital sodium for injection is 2,4,6 (1H,3H,5H)-Pyrimidinetrione, 1-methyl-5-(1-methyl-2-pentynyl)-5-(2-propenyl)-,(±)-, monosodium salt.

Methohexital sodium for injection is a freeze-dried, sterile, nonpyrogenic mixture of methohexital sodium and anhydrous sodium carbonate added as a buffer, which is prepared from an aqueous solution of methohexital, sodium hydroxide, and sodium carbonate. It contains not less than 90% and not more than 110% of the labeled amount of $C_{14}H_{17}N_2NaO_3$. This mixture is ordinarily intended to be reconstituted so as to contain 1% methohexital sodium in Sterile Water for Injection for direct intravenous injection or 0.2% methohexital sodium in 5% dextrose injection (or 0.9% sodium chloride injection) for administration by continuous intravenous drip. The pH of the 1% solution is between 10 and 11; the pH of the 0.2% solution in 5% dextrose is between 9.5 and 10.5.

Methohexital sodium is a rapid, ultrashort-acting barbiturate anesthetic. It occurs as a white, crystalline powder that is freely soluble in water.

CLINICAL PHARMACOLOGY:

Compared with thiamylal and thiopental, methohexital is at least twice as potent on a weight basis, and its duration of action is only about half as long. Although the metabolic fate of methohexital in the body is not clear, the drug does not appear to concentrate in fat depots to the extent that other barbiturate anesthetics do. Thus, cumulative effects are fewer and recovery is more rapid with methohexital than with thiobarbiturates. In experimental animals, the drug cannot be detected in the blood 24 hours after administration.

Methohexital differs chemically from the established barbiturate anesthetics in that it contains no sulfur. Little analgesia is conferred by barbiturates; their use in the presence of pain may result in excitation.

Intravenous administration of methohexital results in rapid uptake by the brain (within 30 seconds) and rapid induction of sleep. With single doses, the rate of redistribution determines duration of pharmacologic effect. Metabolism occurs in the liver through demethylation and oxidation. Side-chain oxidation is the most important biotransformation involved in termination of biologic activity. Excretion occurs via the kidneys through glomerular filtration.

INDICATIONS AND USAGE:

Methohexital sodium can be used as follows:

1. For intravenous induction of anesthesia prior to the use of other general anesthetic agents.

2. For intravenous induction of anesthesia and as an adjunct to subpotent inhalational anesthetic agents (such as nitrous oxide in oxygen) for short surgical procedures; methohexital sodium may be given by infusion or intermittent injection.

3. For use along with other parenteral agents, usually narcotic analgesics, to supplement subpotent inhalational anesthetic agents (such as nitrous oxide in oxygen) for longer surgical procedures.

4. As intravenous anesthesia for short surgical, diagnostic, or therapeutic procedures associated with minimal painful stimuli (see PRECAUTIONS.)

5. As an agent for inducing a hypnotic state.

CONTRAINDICATIONS:

Methohexital sodium is contraindicated in patients in whom general anesthesia is contraindicated, in those with latent or manifest porphyria, or in patients with a known hypersensitivity to barbiturates.

WARNINGS:

(See BOXED WARNING.)

AS WITH ALL POTENT ANESTHETIC AGENTS AND ADJUNCTS, THIS DRUG SHOULD BE ADMINISTERED ONLY BY THOSE TRAINED IN THE ADMINISTRATION OF GENERAL ANESTHESIA, THE MAINTENANCE OF A PATIENT AIRWAY AND VENTILATION, AND THE MANAGEMENT OF CARDIOVASCULAR DEPRESSION ENCOUNTERED DURING ANESTHESIA AND SURGERY.

Because the liver is involved in demethylation and oxidation of methohexital and because barbiturates may enhance preexisting circulatory depression, severe hepatic dysfunction, severe cardiovascular instability, or a shock-like condition may be reason for selecting another induction agent.

Psychomotor seizures may be elicited in susceptible individuals.[1]

Prolonged administration may result in cumulative effects, including extended somnolence, protracted unconsciousness, and respiratory and cardiovascular depression. Respiratory depression in the presence of an impaired airway may lead to hypoxia, cardiac arrest, and death.

The CNS-depressant effect of methohexital sodium may be additive with that of other CNS depressants, including ethyl alcohol and propylene glycol.

Danger Of Intra-Arterial Injection: Unintended intra-arterial injection of barbiturate solutions may be followed by the production of platelet aggregates and thrombosis, starting in arterioles distal to the site of injection. The resulting necrosis may lead to gangrene, which may require amputation. The first sign in conscious patients may be a complaint of fiery burning that roughly follows the distribution path of the injected artery; if noted, the injection should be stopped immediately and the situation reevaluated. Transient blanching may or may not be noted very early; blotchy cyanosis and dark discoloration may then be the first sign in anesthetized patients. There is no established treatment other than prevention. The following should be considered prior to injection:

1. The extent of injury is related to concentration. Concentrations of 1% methohexital will usually suffice; higher concentrations should ordinarily be avoided.

2. Check the infusion to ensure that the catheter is in the lumen of a vein before injection. Injection through a running intravenous infusion may enhance the possibility of detecting arterial placement; however, it should be remembered that the characteristic bright-red color of arterial blood is often altered by contact with drugs. The possibility of aberrant arteries should always be considered.

Postinjury arterial injection of vasodilators and/or arterial infusion of parenteral fluids are generally regarded to be of no value in altering outcome. Animal experiments and published individual case reports concerned with a variety of arteriolar irritants, including barbiturates, suggest that one or more of the following may be of benefit in reducing the area of necrosis:

1. Arterial injection of heparin at the site of injury, followed by systemic anticoagulation.
2. Sympathetic blockade (or brachial plexus blockade in the arm).
3. Intra-arterial glucocorticoid injection at the site of injury, followed by systemic steroids.
4. A recent case report (nonbarbiturate injury) suggests that intra-arterial urokinase may promote fibrinolysis, even if administered late in treatment.

If extravasation is noted during injection of methohexital, the injection should be discontinued until the situation is remedied. Local irritation may result from extravasation; subcutaneous swelling may also serve as a sign of arterial or periarterial placement of the catheter.

PRECAUTIONS:

General: Maintenance of a patient airway and adequacy of ventilation must be ensured during induction and maintenance of anesthesia with methohexital sodium solution. Laryngospasm is common during induction with all barbiturates and may be due to a combination of secretions and accentuated reflexes following induction or may result from painful stimuli during light anesthesia. Transient apnea may be noted during induction, which may impair pulmonary ventilation; the duration of apnea may be longer than that produced by other barbiturate anesthetics. Cardiorespiratory arrest may occur. Intravenous administration of methohexital sodium is often associated with hiccups, coughing, and/or muscle twitching, which may also impair pulmonary ventilation.

Following induction, temporary hypotension and tachycardia may occur.

Recovery from methohexital anesthesia is rapid and smooth. The incidence of postoperative nausea and vomiting is low if the drug is administered to fasting patients. Postanesthetic shivering has occurred in a few instances.

The usual precautions taken with any barbiturate anesthetic pulmonary disease, severe hypertension or hypotension. Myocardial disease, congestive heart failure, severe anemia, or extreme obesity.

Methohexital sodium should be used with extreme caution in patients in status asthmaticus.

Caution should be exercised in debilitated patients or in those with impaired function of respiratory, circulatory, renal, hepatic, or endocrine systems.

Information for the Patient: When appropriate, patients should be instructed as to the hazards of drowsiness that may follow use of methohexital sodium. Outpatients should be released in the company of another individual, and no skilled activities, such as operating machinery or driving a motor vehicle, should be engaged in for 8 to 12 hours.

Laboratory Tests: BSP and liver function studies may be influenced by administration of a single dose of barbiturates.

Carcinogenesis, Mutagenesis, and Impairment of Fertility: Studies of methohexital sodium in animals to evaluate the carcinogenic and mutagenic potential or the effect on fertility have not been conducted. Reproduction studies in animals have revealed no evidence of impaired fertility.[3]

Pregnancy Category B: Reproduction studies have been performed in rabbits and rats at doses up to 4 and 7 times the human dose respectively and have revealed no evidence of impaired fertility or harm to the fetus due to methohexital sodium.[3] There are, however, no adequate and well-controlled studies in pregnant women. Because animal reproduction studies are not always predictive of human response, this drug should be used during pregnancy only if clearly needed.

Labor and Delivery: Methohexital sodium has been used in cesarean section delivery but, because of its solubility and lack of protein binding, it readily and rapidly traverses the placenta.

Nursing Mothers: Caution should be exercised when methohexital sodium is administered to a nursing woman.

Pediatric Use: Safety and effectiveness in children have not been established.

DRUG INTERACTIONS:

Barbiturates may influence the absorption and elimination of other concomitantly used drugs, such as diphenylhydantoin, halothane, anticoagulants, corticosteroids, ethyl alcohol[2], and propylene glycol-containing solutions.

ADVERSE REACTIONS:

Side effects associated with methohexital sodium are extensions of pharmacologic effects and include:

Cardiovascular: Circulatory depression, thrombophlebitis, hypotension, peripheral vascular collapse, and convulsions in association with cardiorespiratory arrest

Respiratory: Respiratory depression (including apnea), cardiorespiratory arrest, laryngospasm, bronchospasm, hiccups, and dyspnea

Neurologic: Skeletal-muscle hyperactivity (twitching), injury to nerves adjacent to injection site, and seizures

Psychiatric: Emergence delirium, restlessness, and anxiety may occur, especially in the presence of postoperative pain

Gastrointestinal: Nausea, emesis, and abdominal pain

Allergic: Erythema, pruritus, and urticaria and cases of anaphylaxis have been reported rarely

Other: Other adverse reactions include pain at injection site, salivation, headache, and rhinitis

DRUG ABUSE AND DEPENDENCE:

Controlled Substance: Methohexital sodium is a Schedule IV drug.

Methohexital sodium may be habit-forming.

OVERDOSAGE:

Signs and Symptoms: The onset of toxicity following an overdose of intravenously administered methohexital will be within seconds of the infusion. If methohexital is administered rectally or is ingested, the onset of toxicity may be delayed. The manifestations of an ultrashort-acting barbiturate in overdose include central nervous system depression, respiratory depression, hypotension, loss of peripheral vascular resistance, and muscular hyperactivity ranging from twitching to convulsive-like movements. Other findings may include convulsions and allergic reactions. Following massive exposure to any barbiturate, pulmonary edema, circulatory collapse with loss of peripheral vascular tone, and cardiac arrest may occur.

Treatment: To obtain up-to-date information about the treatment of overdose, a good resource is your certified Regional Poison Control Center. Telephone numbers of certified poison control centers are listed in the supplemental materials section. In managing overdosage, consider the possibility of multiple drug overdoses, interaction among drugs, and unusual drug kinetics in your patient.

Establish an airway and ensure oxygenation and ventilation. Resuscitative measures should be initiated promptly. For hypotension, intravenous fluids should be administered and the patient's legs raised. If the desirable increase in blood pressure is not obtained, vasopressor and/or inotropic drugs may be used as dictated by the clinical situation.

For convulsions, diazepam intravenously and phenytoin may be required. If the seizures are refractory to diazepam and phenytoin, general anesthesia and paralysis with a neuromuscular blocking agent may be necessary.

Protect the patient's airway and support ventilation and perfusion. Meticulously monitor and maintain, within acceptable limits, the patient's vital signs, blood gases, serum electrolytes, etc. Absorption of drugs from the gastrointestinal tract may be decreased by giving activated charcoal which, in many cases, is more effective than emesis or lavage; consider charcoal instead of or in addition to gastric emptying. Repeated doses of charcoal over time may hasten elimination of some drugs that have been absorbed. Safeguard the patient's airway when employing gastric emptying or charcoal.

DOSAGE AND ADMINISTRATION:

Preanesthetic medication is generally advisable. Methohexital sodium may be used with any of the recognized preanesthetic medications, but the phenothiazines are less satisfactory than the combination of an opiate and a belladonna derivative.

Facilities for assisting respiration and administering oxygen are necessary adjuncts for intravenous anesthesia. Since cardiorespiratory arrest may occur, patients should be observed carefully during and after use of methohexital sodium. Resuscitative equipment (*i.e.,* intubation and cardioversion equipment, oxygen, suction, and a secure intravenous line) and personnel qualified in its use must be immediately available.

Preparation of Solution: FOLLOW DILUTING INSTRUCTIONS EXACTLY.

Diluents: DO NOT USE DILUENTS CONTAINING BACTERIOSTATS.

Sterile Water for Injection is the preferred diluent.

Five percent Dextrose Injection or 0.9% Sodium Chloride Injection may be used. *(Methohexital sodium is not compatible with Lactated Ringer's Injection.)*

Dilution Instruction: For a 1% solution (10 mg/ml), contents of vials should be diluted as follows:

Vial No. 660 (500 mg) add 50 ml of diluent

Vial No. 760 (500 mg) add 50 ml of accompanying diluent

See TABLE 1

TABLE 1

Vial No.	Amount of Diluent to Be Added to the Vial	For 1% Solution Dilute to
663 (2.5 g)	15 ml	250 ml
659 (5 g)	30 ml	500 ml

When the first dilution is made with Vials No. 663 or No. 659, the solution in the vial will be yellow. When further diluted to make a 1% solution, it must be *clear and colorless* or should not be used.

Solutions of methohexital sodium should be freshly prepared and used promptly. Reconstituted solutions of methohexital sodium are chemically stable at room temperature for 24 hours.

For continuous drip anesthesia, prepare a 0.2% solution by adding 500 mg of methohexital sodium to 250 ml of diluent. For this dilution, either 5% glucose solution or isotonic (0.9%) sodium chloride solution is recommended instead of distilled water in order to avoid extreme hypotonicity.

DOSAGE AND ADMINISTRATION: *(cont'd)*

ADMINISTRATION

Methohexital sodium is administered intravenously in a concentration of no higher than 1%. Higher concentrations markedly increase the incidence of muscular movements and irregularities in respiration and blood pressure. Dosage is highly individualized; the drug should be administered only by those completely familiar with its quantitative differences from other barbiturate anesthetics.

Methohexital sodium may be dissolved in Sterile Water for Injection, 5% Dextrose Injection, or Sodium Chloride Injection. For induction of anesthesia, a 1% solution is administered at a rate of about 1 ml/5 seconds. Gaseous anesthetics and/or skeletal-muscle relaxants may be administered concomitantly. The dose required for induction may range from 50 to 120 mg or more but averages about 70 mg. The induction dose usually provides anesthesia for 5 to 7 minutes.

The usual dosage in adults ranges from 1 to 1.5 mg/kg. Data on dosage requirements in children are not available.

Maintenance of anesthesia may be accomplished by intermittent injections of the 1% solution or, more easily, by continuous intravenous drip of a 0.2% solution. Intermittent injections of about 20 to 40 mg (2 to 4 ml of a 1% solution) may be given as required, usually every 4 to 7 minutes. For continuous drip, the average rate of administration is about 3 ml of a 0.2% solution/minute (1 drop/second). The rate of flow must be individualized for each patient. For longer surgical procedures, gradual reduction in the rate of administration is recommended (see WARNINGS.) Other parenteral agents, usually narcotic analgesics, are ordinarily employed along with methohexital sodium during longer procedures.

Parenteral drug products should be inspected visually for particulate matter and discoloration prior to administration, whenever solution and container permit.

COMPATIBILITY INFORMATION

Solutions of methohexital sodium should not be mixed in the same syringe or administered simultaneously during intravenous infusion through the same needle with acid solutions, such as atropine sulfate, Metubine Iodide (Metocurine Iodide Injection, USP, Lilly), and succinylcholine chloride. Alteration of pH may cause free barbituric acid to be precipitated. Solubility of the soluble sodium salts of barbiturates, including methohexital sodium, is maintained only at relatively high (basic) pH.

Because of numerous requests from anesthesiologists for information regarding the chemical compatibility of these mixtures, TABLE 2 contains information obtained from compatibility studies in which a 1% solution of methohexital sodium was mixed with therapeutic amounts of agents whose solutions have a low (acid) pH.

TABLE 2

Active Ingredient	Potency per ml	Vol. Used	Immediate	Physical Change 15 min	30 min	1h
Brevital Sodium	10 mg	10 ml		CONTROL		
Atropine Sulfate	1/150 g	1 ml	None	Haze		
Atropine Sulfate	1/100 g	1 ml	None	Ppt	Ppt	
Succinylcholine chloride	0.5 mg	4 ml	None	None	Haze	
Succinylcholine chloride	1 mg	4 ml	None	None	Haze	
Metocurine Iodide	0.5 mg	4 ml	None	None	Ppt	
Metocurine Iodide	1 mg	4 ml	None	None	Ppt	
Scopolamine hydrobromide	1/120 g	1 ml	None	None	None	Haze
Tubocurarine chloride	3 mg	4 ml	None	Haze		

REFERENCES:

1. Rockoff MA, Goudsuzian NG: Seizures induced by methohexital. *Anesthesiology*1981; 54:333 **2.** Hansten PD: *Drug Interactions*, ed 4 Philadelphia, Lea & Febiger, 1979, p 224. **3.** Gibson WR, et al: Reproduction and teratology studies in rats and rabbits using sodium methohexital, Lilly Toxicology Laboratories, Eli Lilly and Company, Greenfield, Indiana 46140, unpublished manuscript, August 1970.

HOW SUPPLIED:

Storage: Methohexital sodium is stable in Sterile Water for Injection at room temperature 77°F (25°C or below) for at least *6 weeks.* Solutions may be stored and used as long as they remain clear and colorless. Five percent Dextrose Injection or isotonic (0.9%) Sodium Chloride Injection may be used as diluents, but the resulting solutions are not stable for much more than *24 hours.*

The vials may be stored at room temperature 77°F (below 25°C). The expiration period for the vials is 2 years.

HOW SUPPLIED - EQUIVALENTS NOT AVAILABLE:

Injection, Dry-Soln - Intravenous - 2.5 gm/ampul

250 ml x 1	$18.92	BREVITAL SODIUM, Lilly	00002-1449-01
250 ml x 25	$450.38	BREVITAL SODIUM, Lilly	00002-1449-25
250 ml x 25	$517.04	BREVITAL SODIUM, Lilly	00002-1448-25

Injection, Dry-Soln - Intravenous - 5 gm/ampul

5 gm	$44.25	BREVITAL SODIUM, Lilly	00002-1445-01
500 ml x 1	$36.54	BREVITAL SODIUM, Lilly	00002-1447-01
500 ml x 25	$877.10	BREVITAL SODIUM, Lilly	00002-1447-25

Injection, Dry-Soln - Intravenous - 500 mg/ampul

50 ml x 1	$7.61	BREVITAL SODIUM, Lilly	00002-1446-01
50 ml x 1	$11.49	BREVITAL SODIUM, Lilly	00002-1465-01
50 ml x 25	$181.10	BREVITAL SODIUM, Lilly	00002-1446-25

METHOTREXATE SODIUM *(001770)*

CATEGORIES: Anti-Inflammatory Agents; Antineoplastics; Arthritis; Breast Carcinoma; Cancer; Chemotherapy; Choriocarcinoma; Hydatidiform Mole; Immunologic; Immunomodulators; Leukemia; Lung Cancer; Lymphoma; Mycosis Fungoides; NSAIDS; Oncologic Drugs; Orphan Drugs; Osteosarcoma; Psoriasis; Vaccines; FDA Approval Pre 1982

BRAND NAMES: Abitrexate; *Biotrexate*; *Brimexate*; *Canceren*; *Emtexate*; *Emthexat*; *Emthexate*; *Farmitrexat* (Germany); *Farmotrex*; Folex-Pfs; *Lantarel* (Germany); *Ledertrexate* (Australia, France, Mexico); *Maxtrex* (England); *Mexate*; *Metex* (Germany); *Methoblastin* (Australia); Methotrate; *Methotrexate* (Japan); *Methotrexato*; *Metotrexato*; Mexate; *MTX*; *Neotrexate*; **Rheumatrex**; *Texate* (Mexico); *Texate-T* (Mexico); *Tremetex*; *Trexan*; *Trixilem* (Mexico); *Xaken* (Mexico)

(International brand names outside U.S. in italics)

FORMULARIES: Aetna; BC-BS; Medi-Cal; PCS

COST OF THERAPY: $656.74 (Arthritis; Tablet; 2.5 mg; 1/day; 365 days)

PRIMARY ICD9: 715.99 (Osteoarthritis, Unspecified, Multiple Sites)

WARNING:

METHOTREXATE SHOULD BE USED ONLY BY PHYSICIANS WHOSE KNOWLEDGE AND EXPERIENCE INCLUDES THE USE OF ANTIMETABOLITE THERAPY.

THE USE OF METHOTREXATE HIGH DOSE REGIMENTS RECOMMENDED FOR OSTEOSARCOMA REQUIRES METICULOUS CARE (see DOSAGE AND ADMINISTRATION.) HIGH DOSAGE REGIMENS FOR OTHER NEOPLASTIC DISEASES ARE INVESTIGATIONAL AND A THERAPEUTIC ADVANTAGE HAS NOT BEEN ESTABLISHED.

BECAUSE OF THE POSSIBILITY OF SERIOUS TOXIC REACTIONS THE PATIENT SHOULD BE INFORMED BY THE PHYSICIAN OF THE RISKS INVOLVED AND SHOULD BE UNDER A PHYSICIAN'S CONSTANT SUPERVISION.

DEATHS HAVE BEEN REPORTED WITH THE USE OF METHOTREXATE IN THE TREATMENT OF MALIGNANCY, PSORIASES, AND RHEUMATOID ARTHRITIS.

IN THE TREATMENT OF PSORIASIS OR RHEUMATOID ARTHRITIS METHOTREXATE USE SHOULD BE RESTRICTED TO PATIENTS WITH SEVERE, RECALCITRANT, DISABLING DISEASE, WHICH IS NOT ADEQUATELY RESPONSIVE TO OTHER FORMS OF THERAPY, AND ONLY WHEN THE DIAGNOSIS HAS BEEN ESTABLISHED AND AFTER APPROPRIATE CONSULTATION.

1. Methotrexate has been reported to cause fetal death and/or congenital anomalies. Therefore, it is not recommended for women of childbearing potential unless there is clear medical evidence that the benefits can be expected to outweigh the considered risks. Pregnant patients with psoriasis or rheumatoid arthritis should not receive methotrexate. (See CONTRAINDICATIONS.)

2. Periodic monitoring for toxicity, including CBC with differential and platelet counts, and liver and renal function tests is a mandatory part or methotrexate therapy. Periodic liver biopsies may be indicated in some situations. Patients at increased risk for impaired methotrexate elimination (*e.g.*, renal dysfunction, pleural effusion, or ascites) should be monitored more frequently. (See PRECAUTIONS.)

3. Methotrexate causes hepatotoxicity, fibrosis and cirrhosis, but generally only after prolonged use. Acutely, liver enzyme elevations are frequently seen, these are usually transient and asymptomatic, and also do not appear predictive of subsequent hepatic disease. Liver biopsy after sustained use often shows histologic changes, and fibrosis and cirrhosis have been reported; these latter lesions often are not preceded by symptoms or abnormal liver function tests. (See PRECAUTIONS.)

4. Methotrexate-induced lung disease is potentially dangerous lesion, which may occur acutely at any time during therapy and which has been reported at doses as low as 7.5 mg/week. It is not always fully reversible. Pulmonary symptoms (especially a dry, nonproductive cough) may require interruption of treatment and careful investigation.

5. Methotrexate may produce marked bone marrow depression, with resultant anemia, leukopenia, and/or thrombocytopenia.

6. Diarrhea and ulcerative stomatitis require interruption of therapy; otherwise, hemorrhagic enteritis and death from intestinal perforation may occur.

7. Methotrexate therapy in patients with impaired renal function should be undertaken with extreme caution, and at reduced dosages, because renal dysfunction will prolong methotrexate elimination.

8. Unexpected severe (sometimes fatal) marrow suppression concomitant administration of methotrexate (usually in high dosage) along with some nonsteroidal anti-inflammatory drugs (NSAIDs). (See PRECAUTIONS, DRUG INTERACTIONS.)

METHOTREXATE FORMULATIONS AND DILUENTS CONTAINING PRESERVATIVES MUST NOT BE USED FOR INTRATHECAL OR HIGH DOSE METHOTREXATE THERAPY.

DESCRIPTION:

Methotrexate (formerly Amethopterin) is an antimetabolite used in the treatment of certain neoplastic diseases, severe psoriasis, and adult rheumatoid arthritis.

Chemically methotrexate is *N*-(4-(((2,4-diamino-6-pteridinyl) methyl) methylamino)benzoyl)-L -glutamic acid.

Molecular weight: 454.44

Methotrexate Sodium Tablets for oral administration are available in bottles of 100 and in a packaging system designated as the Rheumatrex Methotrexate Sodium Dose Pack for therapy with a weekly dosing schedule of 5 mg, 7.5 mg, 10 mg, 12.5 mg and 15 mg. Methotrexate Sodium Tablets contain an amount of methotrexate sodium equivalent to 2.5 mg of methotrexate and the following inactive ingredients: Lactose, Magnesium Stearate and Pregelatinized Starch. May also contain Corn Starch.

Methotrexate Sodium Injection and for injection products are sterile and non-pyrogenic and may be given by the intramuscular, intravenous, intra-arterial or intrathecal route. (See DOSAGE AND ADMINISTRATION.)However, the preservative formulation contains Benzyl Alcohol and must not be used for intrathecal or high dose therapy.

Methotrexate Sodium Injection, Isotonic Liquid, Preservative Protected is available in 25 mg/ml, 2 ml (50 mg) and 10 ml (250 mg) vials.

Each 25 mg/ml, 2 ml and 10 ml vial contains methotrexate sodium equivalent to 50 mg and 250 mg methotrexate respectively, 0.90% w/v of Benzyl Alcohol as a preservative, and the following inactive ingredients: Sodium Chloride 0.260% w/v and Water for Injection qs ad 100% v. Sodium Hydroxide and, if necessary, Hydrochloric Acid are added to adjust the pH to approximately 8.5.

Methotrexate LPF Sodium (methotrexate sodium injection), Iso-tonic Liquid, Preservative Free, for single use only, is available in 25 mg/ml, 2 ml (50 mg), 4 ml (100 mg), 8 ml (200 mg) and 10 ml (250 mg) vials.

Each 25 mg/ml, 2 ml, 4 ml, 8 ml and 10 ml vial contains methotrexate sodium equivalent to 50 mg, 100 mg, 200 mg and 250 mg methotrexate respectively and the following inactive ingredients: Sodium Chloride 0.490% w/v and Water for Injection qs ad 100% v. Sodium Hydroxide and, if necessary, Hydrochloric Acid are added to adjust the pH to approximately 8.5. The 2 ml, 4 ml, 8 ml and 10 ml solutions contain approximately 0.43 mEq, 0.86 mEq, 1.72 mEq and 2.15 mEq of Sodium per vial, respectively and are isotonic solutions.

DESCRIPTION: *(cont'd)*

Methotrexate Sodium for Injection, Freeze Dried, Preservative Free, Low Sodium, for single use only, is available in 20 mg, 50 mg and 1 g vials.

Each low sodium 20 mg, 50 mg and 1 g vial of cryodesiccated powder contains methotrexate sodium equivalent to 20 mg, 50 mg and 1 g methotrexate respectively. Contains no preservative. Sodium Hydroxide and, if necessary, Hydrochloric Acid are added during manufacture to adjust the pH. The 20 mg vial contains approximately 0.14 mEq of Sodium; the 50 mg vial contains approximately 0.33 mEq of Sodium, and the 1 g vial contains approximately 7 mEq Sodium.

CLINICAL PHARMACOLOGY:

Methotrexate inhibits dihydrofolic acid reductase. Dihydrofolates must be reduced to tetrahydrofolates by this enzyme before they can be utilized as carriers of one-carbon groups in the synthesis of purine nucleotides and thymidylate. Therefore, methotrexate interferes with DNA synthesis, repair, and cellular replication. Actively proliferating tissues such as malignant cells, bone marrow, fetal cells, buccal and intestinal mucosa, and cells of the urinary bladder are in general more sensitive to this effect of methotrexate. When cellular proliferation in malignant tissues is greater than in most normal tissues, methotrexate may impair malignant growth without irreversible damage to normal tissues.

The mechanism of action in rheumatoid arthritis is unknown; it may affect immune function. Two reports describe *in vitro* methotrexate inhibition of DNA precursor uptake by stimulated mononuclear cells, and another describes in animal polyarthritis partial correction by methotrexate of spleen cell hyporesponsiveness and suppressed IL 2 production. Other laboratories, however, have been unable to demonstrate similar effects. Clarification of methotrexate's effect on immune activity and its relation to rheumatoid immunopathogenesis await further studies.

In patients with rheumatoid arthritis, effects of methotrexate on articular swelling and tenderness can be seen as early as 3 to 6 weeks. Although methotrexate clearly ameliorates symptoms of inflammation (pain, swelling, stiffness), there is no evidence that it induces remission of rheumatoid arthritis nor has a beneficial effect been demonstrated on bone erosions and other radiologic changes which result in impaired joint use, functional disability, and deformity.

Most studies of methotrexate in patients with rheumatoid arthritis are relatively short term (3 to 6 months). Limited data from long-term studies indicate that an initial clinical improvement is maintained for at least two years with continued therapy.

In psoriasis, the rate of production of epithelial cells in the skin is greatly increased over normal skin. This differential in proliferation rates is the basis for the use of methotrexate to control the psoriatic process.

Methotrexate in high doses, followed by leucovorin rescue, is used as a part of the treatment of patients with non-metastatic osteosarcoma. The original rationale for high dose methotrexate therapy was based on the concept of selective rescue of normal tissues by leucovorin. More recent evidence suggests that high dose methotrexate may also overcome methotrexate resistance caused by impaired active transport, decreased affinity of dihydrofolic acid reductase for methotrexate, increased levels of dihydrofolic acid reductase resulting from gene amplification, or decreased polyglutamation of methotrexate. The actual mechanism of action is unknown.

Two Pediatric Oncology Group studies (one randomized and one non-randomized) demonstrated a significant improvement in relapse-free survival in patients with non-metastatic osteosarcoma, when high dose methotrexate with leucovorin rescue was used in combination with other chemotherapeutic agents following surgical resection of the primary tumor. These studies were not designed to demonstrate the specific contribution of high dose methotrexate/leucovorin rescue therapy to the efficacy of the combination. However, a contribution can be inferred from the reports of objective responses to this therapy in patients with metastatic osteosarcoma, and from reports of extensive tumor necrosis following preoperative administration of this therapy to patients with non-metastatic osteosarcoma.

PHARMACOKINETICS

Absorption: In adults, oral absorption appears to be dose dependent. Peak serum levels are reached within one to two hours. At doses of 30 mg/m^2 or less, methotrexate is generally well absorbed with a mean bioavailability of about 60%. The absorption of doses greater than 80 mg/m^2 is significantly less, possibly due to a saturation effect.

In leukemic children, oral absorption has been reported to vary widely (23% to 95%). A twenty fold difference between highest and lowest peak levels (C_{max}: 0.11 to 2.3 micromolar after a 20 mg/m^2 dose) has been reported. Significant interindividual variability has also been noted in time to peak concentration (T_{max}: 0.67 to 4 hrs after a 15 mg/m^2 dose) and fraction of dose absorbed. Food has been shown to delay absorption and reduce peak concentration. Methotrexate is generally completely absorbed from parenteral routes of injection. After intramuscular injection, peak serum concentrations occur in 30 to 60 minutes.

Distribution: After intravenous administration, the initial volume of distribution is approximately 0.18 L/kg (18% of body weight) and steady-state volume of distribution is approximately 0.4 to 0.8 L/kg (40% to 80% of body weight). Methotrexate competes with reduced folates for active transport across cell membranes by means of a single carrier-mediated active transport process. At serum concentrations greater than 100 micromolar, passive diffusion becomes a major pathway by which effective intracellular concentrations can be achieved. Methotrexate in serum is approximately 50% protein bound. Laboratory studies demonstrate that it may be displaced from plasma albumin by various compounds including sulfonamides, salicylates, tetracyclines, chloramphenicol, and phenytoin.

Methotrexate does not penetrate the blood-cerebrospinal fluid barrier in therapeutic amounts when given orally or parenterally. High CSF concentrations of the drug may be attained by intrathecal administration.

In dogs, synovial fluid concentrations after oral dosing were higher in inflamed than uninflamed joints. Although salicylates did not interfere with this penetration, prior prednisone treatment reduced penetration into inflamed joints to the level of normal joints.

Metabolism: After absorption, methotrexate undergoes hepatic and intracellular metabolism to polyglutamated forms which can be converted back to methotrexate by hydrolase enzymes. These polyglutamates act as inhibitors of dihydrofolate reductase and thymidylate synthetase. Small amounts of methotrexate polyglutamates may remain in tissues for extended periods. The retention and prolonged drug action of these active metabolites vary among different cells, tissues and tumors. A small amount of metabolism to 7-hydroxymethotrexate may occur at doses commonly prescribed. Accumulation of this metabolite may become significant at the high doses used in osteogenic sarcoma. The aqueous solubility of 7-hydroxymethotrexate is 3 to 5 fold lower than the parent compound. Methotrexate is partially metabolized by intestinal flora after oral administration.

Half-Life: The terminal half-life reported for methotrexate is approximately three to ten hours for patients receiving treatment for psoriasis, or rheumatoid arthritis or low dose antineoplastic therapy (less than 30 mg/m^2). For patients receiving high doses of methotrexate, the terminal half-life is eight to 15 hours.

CLINICAL PHARMACOLOGY: *(cont'd)*

Excretion: Renal excretion is the primary route of elimination and is dependent upon dosage and route of administration. With IV administration, 80% to 90% of the administered dose is excreted unchanged in the urine within 24 hours. There is limited biliary excretion amounting to 10% or less of the administered dose. Enterohepatic recirculation of methotrexate has been proposed.

Renal excretion occurs by glomerular filtration and active tubular secretion. Nonlinear elimination due to saturation of renal tubular reabsorption has been observed in psoriatic patients at doses between 7.5 and 30 mg. Impaired renal function, as well as concurrent use of drugs such as weak organic acids that also undergo tubular secretion, can markedly increase methotrexate serum levels. Excellent correlation has been reported between methotrexate clearance and endogenous creatinine clearance.

Methotrexate clearance rates vary widely and are generally decreased at higher doses. Delayed drug clearance has been identified as one of the major factors responsible for methotrexate toxicity. It has been postulated that the toxicity of methotrexate for normal tissues is more dependent upon the duration of exposure to the drug rather than the peak level achieved. When a patient has delayed drug elimination due to compromised renal function, a third space effusion, or other causes, methotrexate serum concentrations may remain elevated for prolonged periods.

The potential for toxicity from high dose regimens or delayed excretion is reduced by the administration of leucovorin calcium during the final phase of methotrexate plasma elimination. Pharmacokinetic monitoring of methotrexate serum concentrations may help identify those patients at high risk for methotrexate toxicity and aid in proper adjustment of leucovorin dosing. Guidelines for monitoring serum methotrexate levels, and for adjustment of leucovorin dosing to reduce the risk of methotrexate toxicity, are provided in DOSAGE AND ADMINISTRATION.

Methotrexate has been detected in human breast milk. The highest breast milk to plasma concentration ratio reached was 0.08:1.

INDICATIONS AND USAGE:

Neoplastic Diseases: Methotrexate is indicated in the treatment of gestational choriocarcinoma, chorioadenoma destruens and hydatidiform mole.

In acute lymphocytic leukemia, methotrexate is indicated in the prophylaxis of meningeal leukemia and is used in maintenance therapy in combination with other chemotherapeutic agents. Methotrexate is also indicated in the treatment of meningeal leukemia.

Methotrexate is used alone or in combination with other anticancer agents in the treatment of breast cancer, epidermoid cancers of the head and neck, advanced mycosis fungoides, and lung cancer, particularly squamous cell and small cell types. Methotrexate is also used in combination with other chemotherapeutic agents in the treatment of advanced stage non-Hodgkin's lymphomas.

Methotrexate in high doses followed by leucovorin rescue in combination with other chemotherapeutic agents is effective in prolonging relapse-free survival in patients with non-metastatic osteosarcoma who have undergone surgical resection or amputation for the primary tumor.

Psoriasis: Methotrexate is indicated in the symptomatic control of severe, recalcitrant, disabling psoriasis that is not adequately responsive to other forms of therapy, *but only when the diagnosis has been established, as by biopsy and/or after dermatologic consultation.* It is important to ensure that a psoriasis "flare" is not due to an undiagnosed concomitant disease affecting immune responses.

Rheumatoid Arthritis: Methotrexate is indicated in the management of selected adults with severe, active, classical or definite rheumatoid arthritis (ARA criteria) who have had an insufficient therapeutic response to, or are intolerant of, an adequate trial of first line therapy including full dose NSAIDs and usually trial of at least one or more disease modifying antirheumatic drugs.

Aspirin, nonsteroidal anti-inflammatory agents, and/or low dose steroids may be continued, although the possibility of increased toxicity with concomitant use of NSAIDs including salicylates has not been fully explored (see DRUG INTERACTIONS.) Steroids may be reduced gradually in patients who respond to methotrexate. Combined use of methotrexate with gold, penicillamine, hydroxychloroquine, sulfasalazine, or cytotoxic agents, has not been studied and may increase the incidence of adverse effects. Rest and physiotherapy as indicated should be continued.

CONTRAINDICATIONS:

Methotrexate can cause fetal death or teratogenic effects when administered to a pregnant woman. Methotrexate is contraindicated in pregnant patients with psoriasis or rheumatoid arthritis and should be used in the treatment of neoplastic diseases only when the potential benefit outweighs the risk to the fetus. Women of childbearing potential should not be started on methotrexate until pregnancy is excluded and should be fully counseled on the serious risk to the fetus (see PRECAUTIONS) should they become pregnant while undergoing treatment. Pregnancy should be avoided if either partner is receiving methotrexate; during and for a minimum of three months after therapy for male patients, and during and for at least one ovulatory cycle after therapy for female patients. (See BOXED WARNING.)

Because of the potential for serious adverse reactions from methotrexate in breast fed infants, it is contraindicated in nursing mothers.

Patients with psoriasis or rheumatoid arthritis with alcoholism alcoholic liver disease or other chronic lever disease or other chronic liver disease should not receive methotrexate.

Patients with psoriasis or rheumatoid arthritis who have overt or laboratory evidence of immunodeficiency syndromes should not receive methotrexate.

Patients with psoriasis or rheumatoid arthritis who have preexisting blood dyscrasias, such as bone marrow hypoplasia, leukopenia, thrombocytopenia or significant anemia, should not receive methotrexate.

Patients with a known hypersensitivity to methotrexate should not receive the drug.

WARNINGS:

SEE BOXED WARNING.

PRECAUTIONS:

GENERAL

Methotrexate has the potential for serious toxicity. (See BOXED WARNING.) Toxic effects may be related in frequency and severity to dose or frequency of administration but have been seen at all doses. Because they can occur at any time during therapy, it is necessary to follow patients on methotrexate closely. Most adverse reactions are reversible if detected early. When such reactions do occur, the drug should be reduced in dosage or discontinued and appropriate corrective measures should be taken. If necessary, this could include the use of leucovorin calcium (see OVERDOSAGE.) if methotrexate therapy is reinstituted, it should be carried out with caution, with adequate consideration of further need for the drug and with increased alertness as to possible recurrence of toxicity.

PRECAUTIONS: *(cont'd)*

The clinical pharmacology of methotrexate has not been well studied in older individuals. Due to diminished hepatic and renal function as well as decreased folate stores in this population, relatively low doses should be considered, and these patients should be closely monitored for early signs of toxicity.

INFORMATION FOR THE PATIENT

Patients should be informed of the early signs and symptoms of toxicity, of the need to see their physician promptly if they occur, and the need for close follow-up, including periodic laboratory tests to monitor toxicity.

Both the physician and pharmacist should emphasize to the patient that the recommended dose is taken weekly in rheumatoid arthritis and psoriasis, and that mistaken daily use of the recommended dose has led to fatal toxicity. Patients should be encouraged to read the Patient Instructions sheet within the Dose Pack. Prescriptions should not be written or refilled on a PRN basis.

Patients should be informed of the potential benefit and risk in the use of methotrexate. The risk of effects on reproduction should be discussed with both male and female patients taking methotrexate.

LABORATORY TESTS

Patients undergoing methotrexate therapy should be closely monitored so that toxic effects are detected promptly. Baseline assessment should include a complete blood count with differential and platelet counts, hepatic enzymes, renal function tests, and a chest X-ray. During therapy of rheumatoid arthritis and psoriasis, monitoring of these parameters is recommended: hematology at least monthly, and liver and renal function every 1 to 3 months. More frequent monitoring is usually indicated during antineoplastic therapy. *During initial or changing doses,* or during periods of increased risk of elevated methotrexate blood levels (e.g dehydration), more frequent monitoring may also be indicated.

A relationship between abnormal liver function tests and fibrosis or cirrhosis of the liver has not been established. Transient liver function test abnormalities are observed frequently after methotrexate administration and are usually not cause for modification of methotrexate therapy. Persistent liver function test abnormalities just prior to dosing and/or depression of serum albumin may be indicators of serious liver toxicity and require evaluation.

Pulmonary function tests may be useful it methotrexate-induced lung disease is suspected, especially if baseline measurements are available.

CARCINOGENESIS, MUTAGENESIS, AND IMPAIRMENT OF FERTILITY

No controlled human data exist regarding the risk of neoplasia with methotrexate. Methotrexate has been evaluated in a number of animal studies for carcinogenic potential with inconclusive results. Although there is evidence that methotrexate causes chromosomal damage to animal somatic cells and human bone marrow cells, the clinical significance remains uncertain. Assessment of the carcinogenic potential of methotrexate is complicated by conflicting evidence of an increased risk of certain tumors in rheumatoid arthritis. Benefit should be weighed against this potential risk before using methotrexate alone or in combination with other drugs, especially in children or young adults. Methotrexate causes embryotoxicity, abortion, and fetal defects in humans. It has also been reported to cause impairment of fertility, oligospermia and menstrual dysfunction in humans, during and for a short period after cessation of therapy.

PREGNANCY CATEGORY X

Psoriasis and rheumatoid arthritis: Methotrexate is in Pregnancy Category X. See CONTRAINDICATIONS.

NURSING MOTHERS

See CONTRAINDICATIONS.

PEDIATRIC USE

Safety and effectiveness in children have not been established, other than in cancer chemotherapy.

ORGAN SYSTEM TOXICITY

Gastrointestinal: If vomiting, diarrhea, or stomatitis occur, which may result in dehydration, methotrexate should be discontinued until recovery occurs. Methotrexate should be used with extreme caution in the presence of peptic ulcer disease or ulcerative colitis.

Hematologic: Methotrexate can suppress hematopoiesis and cause anemia, leukopenia, and/or thrombocytopenia. In patients with malignancy and preexisting hematopoietic impairment, the drug should be used with caution, if at all. In controlled clinical trials in rheumatoid arthritis (n=128), leukopenia (WBC $<3000/mm^3$) was seen in 2 patients, thrombocytopenia (platelets $<100,000/mm^3$) in 6 patients, and pancytopenia in 2 patients.

In psoriasis and rheumatoid arthritis, methotrexate should be stopped immediately if there is a significant drop in blood counts. In the treatment of neoplastic diseases, methotrexate should be continued only if the potential benefit warrants the risk of severe myelosuppression. Patients with profound granulocytopenia and fever should be evaluated immediately and usually require parenteral broad-spectrum antibiotic therapy.

Hepatic: Methotrexate has the potential for acute (elevated transaminases) and chronic (fibrosis and cirrhosis) hepatotoxicity. Chronic toxicity is potentially fatal; it generally has occurred after prolonged use (generally two years or more) and after a total dose of at least 1.5 grams. In studies in psoriatic patients, hepatotoxicity appeared to be a function of total cumulative dose and appeared to be enhanced by alcoholism, obesity, diabetes and advanced age. An accurate incidence rate has not been determined; the rate of progression and reversibility of lesions is not known. Special caution is indicated in the presence of preexisting liver damage or impaired hepatic function.

Liver function tests, including serum albumin, should be performed periodically prior to dosing but are often normal in the face of developing fibrosis or cirrhosis. These lesions may be detectable only by biopsy.

In psoriasis, the usual recommendation is to obtain a liver biopsy at a total cumulative dose of 1.5 grams. Moderate fibrosis or any cirrhosis normally leads to discontinuation of the drug; mild fibrosis normally suggests a repeat biopsy in 6 months. Milder histologic findings such as fatty change and low grade portal inflammation are relatively common pretherapy. Although these mild changes are usually not a reason to avoid or discontinue methotrexate therapy, the drug should be used with caution.

Clinical experience with liver disease in rheumatoid arthritis is limited, but the same risk factors would be anticipated. Liver function tests are also usually not reliable predictors of histological changes in this population.

When to perform a liver biopsy in rheumatoid arthritis patients has not been established, either in terms of cumulative methotrexate dose or duration of therapy. There is a combined reported experience in 217 rheumatoid arthritis patients with liver biopsies both before and during treatment (after a cumulative dose of at least 1500 mg) and in 714 patients with a biopsy only during treatment. There are 64 (7%) cases of fibrosis and 1 (0.1%) case of cirrhosis. Of the 64 cases of fibrosis, 60 were deemed mild. The reticulin stain is more sensitive for early fibrosis and its use may increase these figures. It is unknown whether even longer use will increase these risks.

Infection or Immunologic States: Methotrexate should be used with extreme caution in the presence of active infection, and is usually contraindicated in patients with over or laboratory evidence of immunodeficiency syndromes. Immunization may be ineffective when given

PRECAUTIONS: *(cont'd)*

during methotrexate therapy. Immunization with live virus vaccines is generally not recommended. There have been reports of disseminated vaccinia infections after smallpox immunization in patients receiving methotrexate therapy. Hypogammaglobulinemia has been reported rarely.

Neurologic: There have been reports of leukoencephalopathy following intravenous administration of methotrexate to patients who have had craniospinal irradiation. Chronic leukoencephalopathy has also been reported in patients with osteosarcoma who received repeated doses of high-dose methotrexate with leucovorin rescue even without cranial irradiation. Discontinuation of methotrexate does not always result in complete recovery.

A transient acute neurologic syndrome has been observed in patients treated with high dosage regimens. Manifestation of this neurologic disorder may include behavioral abnormalities, focal sensorimotor signs and abnormal reflexes. The exact cause is unknown.

After the intrathecal use of methotrexate, the central nervous system toxicity which may occur can be classified as follows: chemical arachnoiditis manifested by such symptoms as headache, back pain, nuchal rigidity, and fever; paresis, usually transient, manifested by paraplegia associated with involvement with one or more spinal nerve roots; leukoencephalopathy manifested by confusion, irritability, somnolence, ataxia, dementia, and occasionally major convulsions.

Pulmonary: Pulmonary symptoms (especially a dry nonproductive cough) or a nonspecific pneumonitis occurring during methotrexate therapy may be indicative of a potentially dangerous lesion and require interruption of treatment and careful investigation. Although clinically variable, the typical patient with methotrexate induced lung disease presents with fever, cough, dyspnea, hypoxemia, and an infiltrate on chest X-ray; infection needs to be excluded. This lesion can occur at all dosages.

Renal: High doses of methotrexate used in the treatment of osteosarcoma may cause renal damage leading to acute renal failure. Nephrotoxicity is due primarily to the precipitation of methotrexate and 7-hydroxymethotrexate in the renal tubules. Close attention to renal function including adequate hydration, urine alkalinization and measurement of serum methotrexate and creatinine levels are essential for safe administration.

OTHER PRECAUTIONS

Methotrexate should be used with extreme caution in the presence of debility.

Methotrexate exits slowly from third space compartments (*e.g.,* pleural effusions or ascites). This results in a prolonged terminal plasma half-life and unexpected toxicity. In patients with significant third space accumulations. It is advisable to evacuate the fluid before treatment and to monitor plasma methotrexate levels.

Lesions of psoriasis may be aggravated by concomitant exposure to ultraviolet radiation. Radiation dermatitis and sunburn may be "recalled" by the use of methotrexate.

DRUG INTERACTIONS:

Nonsteroidal anti-inflammatory drugs should not be administered prior to or concomitantly with the high doses of methotrexate used in the treatment of osteosarcoma. Concomitant administration of some NSAIDs with high dose methotrexate therapy has been reported to elevate and prolong serum methotrexate levels, resulting in deaths from severe hematologic and gastrointestinal toxicity.

Caution should be used when NSAIDs and salicylates are administered concomitantly with lower doses of methotrexate. These drugs have been reported to reduce the tubular secretion of methotrexate in an animal model and may enhance its toxicity.

Despite the potential interactions, studies of methotrexate in patients with rheumatoid arthritis have usually included concurrent use of constant dosage regimens of NSAIDs, without apparent problems. It should be appreciated however, that the doses used in rheumatoid arthritis (7.5 to 15 mg/week) are somewhat lower than those used in psoriasis and that larger doses could lead to unexpected toxicity.

Methotrexate is partially bound to serum albumin, and toxicity may be increased because of displacement by certain drugs, such as salicylates, phenylbutazone, phenytoin, and sulfonamides. Renal tubular transport is also diminished by probenecid; use of methotrexate with this drug should be carefully monitored.

In the treatment of patients with osteosarcoma, caution must be exercised if high-dose methotrexate is administered in combination with a potentially nephrotoxic chemotherapeutic agent (*e.g.,* cisplatin).

Oral antibiotics such as tetracycline, chloramphenicol, and nonabsorbable broad spectrum antibiotics, may decrease intestinal absorption of methotrexate or interfere with the enterohepatic circulation by inhibiting bowel flora and suppressing metabolism of the drug by bacteria.

Vitamin preparations containing folic acid or its derivatives may decrease responses to systemically administered methotrexate. Preliminary animal and human studies have shown that small quantities of intravenously administered leucovorin enter the CSF primarily as 5-methyltetrahydrofolate and, in humans, remain 1 - 3 orders of magnitude lower than the usual methotrexate concentrations following intrathecal administration. However, high doses of leucovorin may reduce the efficacy of intrathecally administered methotrexate.

Folate deficiency states may increase methotrexate toxicity. Trimethoprim/sulfamethoxazole has been reported rarely to increase bone marrow suppression in patients receiving methotrexate, probably by an additive antifolate effect.

ADVERSE REACTIONS:

IN GENERAL, THE INCIDENCE AND SEVERITY OF ACUTE SIDE EFFECTS ARE RELATED TO DOSE AND FREQUENCY OF ADMINISTRATION. THE MOST SERIOUS REACTIONS ARE DISCUSSED ABOVE UNDER ORGAN SYSTEM TOXICITY IN THE PRECAUTIONS SECTION. THAT SECTION SHOULD ALSO BE CONSULTED WHEN LOOKING FOR INFORMATION ABOUT ADVERSE REACTIONS WITH METHOTREXATE.

The most frequently reported adverse reactions include ulcerative stomatitis, leukopenia, nausea, and abdominal distress. Other frequently reported adverse effects are malaise, undue fatigue, chills and fever, dizziness and decreased resistance to infection.

Other adverse reactions that have been reported with methotrexate are listed below by organ system. In the oncology setting, concomitant treatment and the underlying disease make specific attribution of a reaction to methotrexate difficult.

Alimentary System: gingivitis, pharyngitis, stomatitis, anorexia, nausea, vomiting, diarrhea, hematemesis, melena, gastrointestinal ulceration and bleeding, enteritis.

Central Nervous System: headache, drowsiness, blurred vision. Aphasia, hemiparesis, paresis and convulsions have also occurred following administration of methotrexate. **Following low doses, occasional patients have reported transient subtle cognitive dysfunction, mood alteration, or unusual cranial sensations.**

Pulmonary System: interstitial pneumonitis deaths have been reported, and chronic interstitial obstructive pulmonary disease has occasionally occurred.

Skin: erythematous rashes, pruritus, urticaria, photosensitivity, pigmentary changes, alopecia, ecchymosis, telangiectasia, acne, furunculosis.

ADVERSE REACTIONS: *(cont'd)*

Urogenital System: severe nephropathy or renal failure, azotemia, cystitis, hematuria; defective oogenesis or spermatogenesis, transient oligospermia, menstrual dysfunction and vaginal discharge; infertility, abortion, fetal defects.

Other rarer reactions related to or attributed to the use of methotrexate such as opportunistic infection, arthralgia/myalgia, loss of libido/impotence, diabetes, osteoporosis and sudden death. A few cases of anaphylactoid reactions have been reported.

ADVERSE REACTIONS IN DOUBLE-BLIND RHEUMATOID ARTHRITIS STUDIES

The approximate incidences of methotrexate attributed (*i.e.,* placebo rate subtracted) adverse reactions in 12 to 18 week double-blind studies of patients (n=128) with rheumatoid arthritis treated with low-dose oral (7.5 to 15 mg/week) pulse methotrexate, are listed below. Virtually all of these patients were on concomitant nonsteroidal anti-inflammatory drugs and some were also taking low dosages of corticosteroids.

Incidence greater than 10%: Elevated liver function tests 15%, nausea/vomiting 10%.

Incidence 3% to 10%: Stomatitis, thrombocytopenia, (platelet count less than 100,000/mm^3).

Incidence 1% to 3%: Rash/pruritus/dermatitis, diarrhea, alopecia, leukopenia (WBC less than 3000/mm^3), pancytopenia, dizziness.

No pulmonary toxicity was seen in these two trials. Thus, the incidence is probably less than 2.5% (95% C.L.). Hepatic histology was not examined in these short-term studies (see PRECAUTIONS.)

Other less common reactions included decreased hematocrit, headache, upper respiratory infection, anorexia, arthralgias, chest pain, coughing, dysuria, eye discomfort, epistaxis, fever, infection, sweating, tinnitus, and vaginal discharge.

ADVERSE REACTIONS IN PSORIASIS

There are no recent placebo-controlled trials in patients with psoriasis. There are two literature reports (Roenigk, 1969 and Nyfors, 1978) describing large series (n=204, 248) of psoriasis patients treated with methotrexate. Dosage ranged up to 25 mg per week and treatment was administered for up to four years. With the exception of alopecia, photosensitivity, and "burning of skin lesions" (each 3% to 10%), the adverse reaction rates in these reports were very similar to those in the rheumatoid arthritis studies.

OVERDOSAGE:

Leucovorin is indicated to diminish the toxicity and counteract the effect of inadvertently administered overdosages of methotrexate. Leucovorin administration should begin as promptly as possible. As the time interval between methotrexate administration and leucovorin initiation increases, the effectiveness of leucovorin in counteracting toxicity decreases. Monitoring of the serum methotrexate concentration is essential in determining the optimal dose and duration of treatment with leucovorin.

In cases of massive overdosage, hydration and urinary alkalinization may be necessary to prevent the precipitation of methotrexate and/or its metabolites in the renal tubules. Neither hemodialysis nor peritoneal dialysis has been shown to improve methotrexate elimination.

DOSAGE AND ADMINISTRATION:

NEOPLASTIC DISEASES

Oral administration in tablet form is often preferred when low doses are being administered since absorption is rapid and effective serum levels are obtained. Methotrexate sodium injection and for injection may be given by the intramuscular, intravenous, intra-arterial or intrathecal route. However, the preserved formulation contains Benzyl Alcohol and must not be used for intrathecal or high dose therapy. Parenteral drug products should be inspected visually for particulate matter and discoloration prior to administration, whenever solution and container permit.

Choriocarcinoma And Similar Trophoblastic Diseases: Methotrexate is administered orally or intramuscularly in doses of 15 to 30 mg daily for a five-day course. Such courses are usually repeated for 3 to 5 times as required, with rest periods of one or more weeks interposed between courses, until any manifesting toxic symptoms subside. The effectiveness of therapy is ordinarily evaluated by 24 hour quantitative analysis of urinary chorionic gonadotropin (hCG), which should return to normal or less than 50 IU/24 hr usually after the third or fourth course and usually be followed by complete resolution of measurable lesions in 4 to 6 weeks. One to two courses of methotrexate after normalization of hCG is usually recommended. Before each course of the drug careful clinical assessment is essential. Cyclic combination therapy of methotrexate with other antitumor drugs has been reported as being useful.

Since hydatidiform mole may precede choriocarcinoma, prophylactic chemotherapy with methotrexate has been recommended.

Chorioadenoma destruens is considered to be an invasive form of hydatidiform mole. Methotrexate is administered in these disease states in doses similar to those recommended for choriocarcinoma.

Leukemia: Acute lymphoblastic leukemia in children and young adolescents is th most responsive to present day chemotherapy. In young adults and older patients, clinical remission is more difficult to obtain and early relapse is more common.

Methotrexate alone or in combination with steroids was used initially for induction of remission in acute lymphoblastic leukemias. More recently corticosteroid therapy, in combination with other antileukemic drugs or in cyclic combinations with methotrexate included, has appeared to produce rapid and effective remissions. When used for induction, methotrexate in doses of 3.3 mg/m^2 in combination with 60 mg/m^2 of prednisone, given daily, produced remissions in 50% of patients treated, usually within a period of 4 to 6 weeks. Methotrexate in combination with other agents appears to be the drug of choice for securing maintenance of drug - induced remissions. When remission is achieved and supportive care has produced general clinical improvement, maintenance therapy is initiated, as follows: Methotrexate is administered 2 times weekly either by mouth or intramuscularly in total weekly doses of 30 mg/m^2. It has also been given in doses of 2.5 mg/kg intravenously every 14 days. If and when relapse does occur, reinduction of remission can again usually be obtained by repeating the initial induction regimen.

A variety of combination chemotherapy regimens have been used for both induction and maintenance therapy in acute lymphoblastic leukemia. The physician should be familiar with the new advances in antileukemic therapy.

Meningeal Leukemia: In the treatment or prophylaxis of meningeal leukemia, methotrexate must be administered intrathecally. Preservative free methotrexate is diluted to a concentration of 1 mg/ml in an appropriate sterile, preservative free medium such as 0.9% Sodium Chloride Injection, USP.

The cerebrospinal fluid volume is dependent on age and not on body surface area. The CSF is at 40% of the adult volume at birth and reaches the adult volume in several years.

Intrathecal methotrexate administration at a dose of 12 mg/m^2(maximum 15 mg) has been reported to result in low CSF methotrexate concentrations and reduced efficacy in children and high concentrations and neurotoxicity in adults. The following dosage regimen (TABLE 1) is based on age instead of body surface area:

DOSAGE AND ADMINISTRATION: *(cont'd)*

TABLE 1

Age (years)	Dose (mg)
<1	6
1	8
2	10
3 or older	12

in one study in patients under the age of 40, this dosage regimen appeared to result in more consistent CSF methotrexate concentrations and less neurotoxicity. Another study in children with acute lymphocytic leukemia compared this regimen to a dose of 12 mg/m^2 (maximum 15 mg), a significant reduction in the rate of CNS relapse was observed in the group whose dose was based on age.

Because the CSF volume and turnover may decrease with age, a dose reduction may be indicated in elderly patients.

For the treatment of meningeal leukemia, intrathecal methotrexate may be given at intervals of 2 to 5 days. However, administration at intervals of less than 1 week may result in increased subacute toxicity. Methotrexate is administered until the cell count of the cerebrospinal fluid returns to normal. At this point one additional dose is advisable. For prophylaxis against meningeal leukemia, the dosage is the same as for treatment except for the intervals of administration. On this subject, it is advisable for the physician to consult the medical literature.

Untoward side effects may occur with any given intrathecal injection and are commonly neurological in character. Large doses may cause convulsions. Methotrexate given by the intrathecal route appears significantly in the systemic circulation and may cause systemic methotrexate toxicity. Therefore, systemic antileukemic therapy with the drug should be appropriately adjusted, reduced, or discontinued. Focal leukemic involvement of the central nervous system may not respond to intrathecal chemotherapy and is best treated with radiotherapy.

Lymphomas: In Burkitt's tumor, Stages I-II, methotrexate has produced prolonged remissions in some cases. Recommended dosage is 10 to 25 mg/day orally for 4 to 8 days. In Stage III, methotrexate is commonly given concomitantly with other antitumor agents. Treatment in all stages usually consists of several courses of the drug interposed with 7 to 10 day rest periods. Lymphosarcomas in Stage III may respond to combined drug therapy with methotrexate given in doses of 0.625 to 2.5 mg/kg daily.

Mycosis Fungoides: Therapy with methotrexate appears to produce clinical remissions in one half of the cases treated. Dosage is usually 2.5 to 10 mg daily by mouth for weeks or months. Dose levels of drug and adjustment of dose regimen by reduction or cessation of drug are guided by patient response and hematologic monitoring. Methotrexate has also been given intramuscularly in doses of 50 mg once weekly or 25 mg 2 times weekly.

Osteosarcoma: An effective adjuvant chemotherapy regimen requires the administration of several cytotoxic chemotherapeutic agents. In addition to high - dose methotrexate with leucovorin rescue, these agents may include doxorubicin, cisplatin, and the combination of bleomycin, cyclophosphamide and dactinomycin (BCD) in the doses and schedule shown in the table below. The starting dose for high dose methotrexate treatment is 12 grams/m^2. If this dose is not sufficient to produce a peak serum methotrexate concentration of 1,000 micromolar (10^{-3} mol/L) at the end of the methotrexate infusion, the dose may be escalated to 15 grams/m^2 in subsequent treatments. It the patient is vomiting or is unable to tolerate oral medication, leucovorin is given IV or IM at the same dose and schedule (TABLE 2):

TABLE 2

Drug*	Dose*	Treatment Week After Surgery
Methotrexate	12 g/m^2 IV as 4 hour infusion (starting dose)	4,5,6,7,11,12,15,16,29,30,44,45
Leucovorin	15 mg orally every six hours for 10 doses starting at 24 hours after start of methotrexate infusion.	
Doxorubicin† as a single drug	30 mg/m^2/day IV x 3 days	8,17
Doxorubicin†	50 mg/m^2 IV	20,23,33,36
Cisplatin†	100 mg/m^2 IV	20,23,33,36
Bleomycin†	15 units/m^2 IV x 2 days	2,13,26,39,42
Cyclophosphamide† 2,13,26,39,42	600 mg/m^2 IV x 2 days	
Dactinomycin†	0.6 mg/m^2 IV x 2 days	2,13,26,39,42

* Link MP, Goorin AM, Miser AW, et al: The effect of adjuvant chemotherapy on relapse - free survival in patients with osteosarcoma of the extremity. *N Engl J of Med* 1986; 314(No.25): 1600-1606.

† See each respective package insert for full prescribing information.

Dosage modifications may be necessary because of drug induced toxicity. When these higher doses of methotrexate are to be administered, following safety guidelines should be closely observed.

GUIDELINES FOR METHOTREXATE THERAPY WITH LEUCOVORIN RESCUE

1. Administration of methotrexate should be delayed until recovery if:

the WBC count is less than 1500/microliter

the neutrophil count is less than 200/microliter

the platelet count is less than 75,000/microliter

the serum bilirubin level is greater than 1.2 mg/dL

the SGPT level is greater than 450 U

mucositis is present, until there is evidence of healing

persistent pleural effusion is present; this should be drained dry prior to infusion.

2. Adequate renal function must be documented.

a. Serum creatinine must be normal, and creatinine clearance must be greater than 60 ml/min, before initiation of therapy.

b. Serum creatinine must be measured prior to each subsequent course of therapy. If serum creatinine has increased by 50% or more compared to a prior value, the creatinine clearance must be measured and documented to be greater than 60 ml/min (even if the serum creatinine is still with in the normal range).

3. Patients must be well hydrated, and must be treated with sodium bicarbonate for urinary alkalinization.

a. Administer 1,000 ml/m^2 of intravenous fluid over6 hours prior to initiation of the methotrexate infusion. Continue hydration at 125 ml/m^2/hr (3 liters/m^2/day) during the methotrexate infusion, and for 2 days after the infusion has been completed.

DOSAGE AND ADMINISTRATION: *(cont'd)*

b. Alkalinize urine to maintain pH above 7.0 during methotrexate infusion and leucovorin calcium therapy. This can be accomplished by the administration of sodium bicarbonate orally or by incorporation into a separate intravenous solution.

4. Repeat serum creatinine and serum methotrexate 24 hours after starting methotrexate and at least once daily until the methotrexate level is below $5x10^{-8}$ mol/L (0.05 micromolar).

TABLE 3 provides guidelines for leucovorin calcium dosage based upon serum methotrexate levels. See TABLE 3.

5. Patients who experience delayed early methotrexate elimination are likely to develop nonreversible oliguric renal failure. In addition to appropriate leucovorin therapy, these patients require continuing hydration and urinary alkalinization, and close monitoring of fluid and electrolyte status, until the serum methotrexate level has fallen to below 0.05 micromolar and the renal failure has resolved.

6. Some patients will have abnormalities in methotrexate elimination, or abnormalities in renal function following methotrexate administration, which are significant but less severe than the abnormalities described in the table below. These abnormalities may or may not be associated with significant clinical toxicity. If significant clinical toxicity is observed, leucovorin rescue should be extended for an additional 24 hours (total 14 doses over 84 doses over 84 hours) in subsequent courses of therapy. The possibility that the patient is taking other medications which interact with methotrexate (*e.g.,* medications which may interfere with methotrexate binding to serum albumin, or elimination) should always be reconsidered when laboratory abnormalities or clinical toxicities are observed.

TABLE 3 Leucovorin Rescue Schedules Following Treatment With Higher Doses Of Methotrexate

Clinical Situation	Laboratory Findings	Leucovorin Dosage and Duration
Normal Methotrexate Elimination	Serum methotrexate level approximately 10 micromolar at 24 hours after administration, 1 micromolar at 48 hours, and less than 0.2 micromolar at 72 hours.	15 mg PO, IM or IV q 6 hours for 60 hours (10 doses starting at 24 hours after start of methotrexate infusion).
Delayed Late Methotrexate Elimination	Serum methotrexate level remaining above 0.2 micromolar at 72 hours, and more than 0.05 micromolar at 96 hours after administration.	Continue 15 mg PO, IM or IV q six hours, until methotrexate level is less than 0.05 micromolar.
Delayed Early Methotrexate Elimination and/or Evidence of Acute Renal Injury	Serum methotrexate level of 50 micromolar or more at 24 hours, or 5 micromolar or more at 48 hours after administration, OR; a 100% or greater increase in serum creatinine level at 24 hours after methotrexate administration (eg, an increase from 0.5 mg/dL to a level of 1 mg/dL or more).	150 mg IV q three hours, until methotrexate level is less than 1 micromolar; then 15 mg IV q three hours, until methotrexate level is less than 0.05 micromolar.

PSORIASIS AND RHEUMATOID ARTHRITIS

The patient should be fully informed of the risks involved and should be under constant supervision of the physician. (See PRECAUTIONS, Information for the Patient.) Assessment of hematologic, hepatic, renal, and pulmonary function should be made by history. Physical examination, and laboratory tests before beginning, periodically during, and before reinstituting methotrexate therapy (see PRECAUTIONS.) Appropriate steps should be taken to avoid conception during methotrexate therapy. (See PRECAUTIONS and CONTRAINDICATIONS.)

Weekly therapy may be instituted with the Rheumatrex Methotrexate Sodium 2.5 mg Tablet Dose Packs which are designed to provide doses over a range of 5 mg to 15 mg administered as a single weekly dose. The dose packs are not recommended for administration of methotrexate in weekly dose greater than 15 mg. All schedules should be continually tailored to the individual patient. An initial lest dose may be given prior to the regular dosing schedule to detect any extreme sensitivity to adverse effects (see ADVERSE REACTIONS.) Maximal myelosuppression usually occurs in seven to ten days.

Psoriasis: Recommended Starting Dose Schedules

1. Weekly single oral, IM or IV dose schedule: 10 to 25 mg per week until adequate response is achieved.

2. Divided oral dose schedule: 2.5 mg at 12 - hour intervals for three doses.

Dosages in each schedule may be gradually adjusted to achieve optimal clinical response: 30 mg/week should not ordinarily be exceeded.

Once optimal clinical response has been achieved, each dosage schedule should be reduced to the lowest possible amount of drug and to the longest possible rest period. The use of methotrexate may permit the return to conventional topical therapy, which should be encouraged.

Rheumatoid Arthritis: Recommended Starting Dosage Schedules

1. Single oral doses of 7.5 mg once weekly.

2. Divided oral dosages of 2.5 mg at 12 hour intervals for 3 doses given as a course once weekly.

Dosages in each schedule may be adjusted gradually to achieve an optimal response, but not ordinarily to exceed a total weekly dose of 20 mg. Limited experience shows a significant increase in the incidence and severity of serious toxic reactions, especially bone marrow suppression, at doses greater than 20 mg/wk.

Once response has been achieved, each schedule should be reduced, if possible, to the lowest possible effective dose.

Therapeutic response usually begins within 3 to 6 weeks and the patient may continue to improve for another 12 weeks or more.

The optimal duration of therapy is unknown. Limited data available from long-term studies indicate that the initial clinical improvement is maintained for at least two years with continued therapy. When methotrexate is discontinued, the arthritis usually worsens within 3 to 6 weeks.

HANDLING AND DISPOSAL

Procedures for proper handling and disposal of anticancer drugs should be considered. Several guidelines on this subject have been published.[1-6] There is no general agreement that all of the procedures recommended in the guidelines are necessary or appropriate.

RECONSTITUTION OF LOW SODIUM CRYODESICCATED POWDERS

Reconstitute immediately prior to use.

Methotrexate Sodium for Injection should be reconstituted with an appropriate sterile, preservative free medium such as 5% Dextrose Solution, USP, or Sodium Chloride Injection, USP. Reconstitute the 20 and 50 mg vials to a concentration no greater than 25 mg/ml. **The 1 g vial should be reconstituted with 19.4 ml to a concentration of 50 mg/ml.** When high doses of methotrexate are administered by IV infusion, the total dose is diluted in 5% Dextrose Solution.

For intrathecal injection, reconstitute to a concentration of 1 mg/ml with an appropriate sterile, preservative free medium such as Sodium Chloride Injection, USP.

DILUTION INSTRUCTIONS FOR LIQUID METHOTREXATE SODIUM INJECTION PRODUCTS

Methotrexate Sodium Injection, Preservative Protected: If desired, the solution may be further diluted with a compatible medium such as Sodium Chloride Injection, USP. Storage for 24 hours at a temperature of 21 to 25°C results in a product which is within 90% of label potency.

Methotrexate LPF Sodium (methotrexate sodium injection), Isotonic, Preservative Free, for Single Use Only: If desired, the solution may be further diluted immediately prior to use with an appropriate sterile, preservative free medium such as 5% Dextrose Solution, USP or Sodium Chloride Injection, USP.

Storage between 15C (59°F) and 25°C (77°F) is recommended.

Protect From Light.

REFERENCES:

1. Recommendations for the Safe Handling of Parenteral Antineoplastic Drugs. NIH Publications No. 83 - 2621. For sale by the Superintendent of Documents, US Government Printing Office, Washington, DC 20402. **2.** AMA Council Report. Guidelines for Handling Parenteral Antineoplastics. *JAMA,* March 15, 1985. **3.** National Study Commission on Cytotoxic Exposure - Recommendations for Handling Cytotoxic Agents. Available from Louis P. Jeffrey, Sc D, Director of Pharmacy Services, Rhode Island Hospital, 593 Eddy Street, Providence, Rhode Island 02902. **4.** Clinical Oncological Society of Australia: Guidelines and recommendations for safe handling of antineoplastic agents. *Med J Australia* 1983; 1:426-428. **5.** Jones RB, et al. Safe handling of chemotherapeutic agents: A report from the Mount Sinai Medical Center. Ca - *A Cancer Journal for Clinicians* Sept/Oct 1983; 258-263. **6.** American Society of Hospital Pharmacists technical assistance bulletin on handling cytotoxic drugs in hospitals. *Am J Hosp Pharm* 1985; 42:131-137.

HOW SUPPLIED - RATED THERAPEUTICALLY EQUIVALENT:

Injection, Solution - Intramuscular; - 25 mg/ml

2 ml	$14.07	MEXATE-AQ, Mead Johnson	00015-3006-20
2 ml	$136.25	Methotrexate Sodium, Fujisawa USA	00469-2160-10
2 ml x 10	$139.38	METHOTREXATE, Fujisawa USA	00469-1970-10
4 ml	$8.50	Methotrexate Lpf, Lederle Parenterals	00205-5326-18
4 ml	$27.69	MEXATE-AQ, Mead Johnson	00015-3007-20
4 ml x 10	$273.75	METHOTREXATE, Fujisawa USA	00469-1970-20
8 ml	$16.72	Methotrexate Lpf, Lederle Parenterals	00205-5327-30
8 ml x 10	$538.75	METHOTREXATE, Fujisawa USA	00469-1970-30
10 m	$68.06	MEXATE-AQ, Mead Johnson	00015-3008-20
10 ml x 10	$70.19	FOLEX PFS, Pharmacia & Upjohn	00013-2296-91

Injection, Solution - Intramuscular; - 50 mg/vial

2 ml	$4.75	Methotrexate Sodium Parenteral 50, Lederle Parenterals	00205-4556-26
2 ml	$4.75	Methotrexate Lpf, Lederle Parenterals	00205-5325-26
2 ml x 10	$15.20	FOLEX PFS, Pharmacia & Upjohn	00013-2266-91
20 mg	$8.52	MEXATE, Mead Johnson	00015-3050-20
50 mg	$4.75	Methotrexate, Lederle Parenterals	00205-9337-92
50 mg	$13.00	MEXATE, Mead Johnson	00015-3051-20

Injection, Solution - Intramuscular; - 100 mg/vial

4 ml x 10	$30.18	FOLEX PFS, Pharmacia & Upjohn	00013-2276-91
100 mg	$25.64	MEXATE, Mead Johnson	00015-3052-20

Injection, Solution - Intramuscular; - 200 mg/vial

8 ml x 10	$59.10	FOLEX PFS, Pharmacia & Upjohn	00013-2286-91

Tablet - Oral - 2.5 mg

100's	$179.93	Methotrexate Sodium, H.C.F.A. F F P	99999-1770-01

Tablet, Uncoated - Oral - 2.5 mg

8's	$23.00	Methotrexate, Roxane	00054-8550-03
8's	$23.79	Methotrexate, Barr	00555-0572-45
8's	$28.01	METHOTRATE, Lederle Pharm	00005-4507-04
12's	$35.00	Methotrexate, Roxane	00054-8550-05
12's	$35.63	Methotrexate, Barr	00555-0572-46
12's	$41.96	METHOTRATE, Lederle Pharm	00005-4507-05
16's	$49.00	Methotrexate, Roxane	00054-8550-06
16's	$49.53	Methotrexate, Barr	00555-0572-47
16's	$55.99	METHOTRATE, Lederle Pharm	00005-4507-07
20's	$61.00	Methotrexate, Roxane	00054-8550-07
20's	$61.44	Methotrexate, Barr	00555-0572-48
20's	$70.00	METHOTRATE, Lederle Pharm	00005-4507-09
24's	$72.00	Methotrexate, Roxane	00054-8550-10
24's	$73.32	Methotrexate, Barr	00555-0572-49
24's	$83.99	METHOTRATE, Lederle Pharm	00005-4507-91
36's	$106.45	Methotrexate, Major Pharms	00904-1749-73
36's	$112.00	Methotrexate, Aligen Independ	00405-4643-36
36's	$128.95	Methotrexate, Goldline Labs	00182-1539-95
36's	$128.97	Methotrexate, Geneva Pharms	00781-1076-36
36's	$130.05	Methotrexate 2.5 Mg Tablets, Barr	00555-0572-35
36's	$133.88	Methotrexate, Roxane	00054-4550-15
36's	$133.88	Methotrexate, Rugby	00536-3998-36
100's	$269.45	Methotrexate, Qualitest Pharms	00603-4499-21
100's	$282.95	Methotrexate, HL Moore Drug Exch	00839-7905-06
100's	$295.95	Methotrexate 2.5 Mg Tablets, Harber Pharm	51432-0522-03
100's	$298.00	Methotrexate, Aligen Independ	00405-4643-01
100's	$299.95	Methotrexate, Major Pharms	00904-1749-60
100's	$305.16	Methotrexate, Roxane	00054-4550-25
100's	$305.25	Methotrexate 2.5 Mg Tablets, Barr	00555-0572-02
100's	$310.20	Methotrexate, Rugby	00536-3998-01
100's	$314.25	Methotrexate, Geneva Pharms	00781-1076-01
100's	$314.34	Methotrexate 2.5, Goldline Labs	00182-1539-01
100's	$339.50	Methotrexate, Schein Pharm (US)	00364-2499-01
100's	$355.16	Methotrexate, Roxane	00054-8550-25
100's	$363.48	Methotrexate, Mylan	00378-0014-01
100's	$404.09	METHOTRATE, Lederle Pharm	00005-4507-23

HOW SUPPLIED - NOT RATED EQUIVALENT:

Injection, Lyphl-Soln - Intrathecal - 20 mg/vial

20 mg	$2.78	Methotrexate Sodium Parenteral 20, Lederle Parenterals	00205-4654-90

Injection, Solution - Intra-Articular - 2.5 mg/ml

2 ml	$78.75	Methotrexate Sodium, Fujisawa USA	00469-2150-10

Injection, Solution - Intramuscular; - 1 gm/vial

1 gm	$61.44	Methotrexate Sodium Parenteral 1, Lederle Parenterals	00205-4653-02

HOW SUPPLIED - NOT RATED EQUIVALENT: *(cont'd)*

Injection, Solution - Intramuscular; - 25 mg/ml

10 ml x 10	$215.00	Methotrexate Sodium, Voluntary Hosp	53258-2880-03
10 ml x 10	$215.00	Methotrexate Sodium, Voluntary Hosp	53258-2880-30

Injection, Solution - Intramuscular; - 250 mg/vial

10 ml	$20.48	Methotrexate Lpf, Lederle Parenterals	00205-5337-34
10 ml	$20.48	Methotrexate Sodium Parenteral 250, Lederle Parenterals	00205-5338-34
10 ml	$673.13	Methotrexate Sodium, Fujisawa USA	00469-2880-30
250 mg	$63.29	MEXATE, Mead Johnson	00015-3053-20

METHOTRIMEPRAZINE *(001771)*

CATEGORIES: Analgesics; Antipyretics; Anxiety; Anxiolytics, Sedatives, Hypnotic; Central Nervous System Agents; Pain; Phenothiazines; Sedation; FDA Approval Pre 1982

BRAND NAMES: *Hirnamin*; **Levoprome**; *Levozin*; *Methozane*; *Neurocil* (Germany); *Nozinan* (Europe, Canada); *Sinogan*
(International brand names outside U.S. in italics)

DESCRIPTION:

CAUTION: FOLLOWING ADMINISTRATION OF THIS DRUG, ORTHOSTATIC HYPOTENSION, FAINTING, OR DIZZINESS MAY OCCUR. AMBULATION SHOULD BE AVOIDED OR CAREFULLY SUPERVISED FOR AT LEAST SIX HOURS FOLLOWING THE INITIAL DOSE. TOLERANCE TO THIS EFFECT USUALLY DEVELOPS WITH CONTINUED ADMINISTRATION.

Methotrimeprazine is 10H-phenothiazine-10-propanamine, 2-methoxy- N,N, beta-trimethyl-, (—)-. It was formerly called levomepromazine.

It is available as a clear transparent solution of the hydrochloric salt containing 20 mg of methotrimeprazine per ml with benzyl alcohol (0.9% w/v) as a preservative, and with disodium edetate USP (0.065% w/v) and sodium Metabisulfite (0.3% w/v, see WARNINGS) as stabilizers.

It is adjusted to a pH of approximately 4.5 with Sodium Citrate, Citric Acid USP, Anhydrous, and Hydrochloric Acid or Sodium Hydroxide NF. Water for Injection USP q.s. ad 100%.

CLINICAL PHARMACOLOGY:

Methotrimeprazine, a phenothiazine derivative, is a potent central nervous system depressant with sites of action postulated in the thalamus, hypothalamus, reticular and limbic systems, producing supression of sensory impulses, reduction of motor activity, sedation and tranquilization. It raises the pain threshold and produces amnesia. Methotrimeprazine also has antihistamine, anticholinergic and antiadrenalin effects. It is actively metabolized into sulfoxides and glucuronic conjugates and largely excreted into the urine as such. Small amounts of unchanged drug are excreted in the feces and in the urine (1%). Low concentrations of drug occur in the blood serum in man. Elimination into the urine usually continues for several days after intramuscular administration of the drug is discontinued.

Methotrimeprazine produces an analgesic effect in both animals and man comparable to morphine and meperidine. A sedative effect is produced as well. Its use thus far has not been reported to result in signs of addiction, dependence, nor withdrawal symptoms even with large doses or with prolonged administration. Maximum analgesic effect usually occurs within 20-40 minutes after intramuscular injection and is maintained for about 4 hours.

Respiratory depression in the patient or in the newborn during or following preanesthetic or obstetrical use occurs infrequently with Methotrimeprazine. The drug does not appear to affect the cough reflex.

INDICATIONS AND USAGE:

Methotrimeprazine methotrimeprazine is indicated for the relief of pain of moderate to marked degree of severity in nonambulatory patients.

It is indicated for obstetrical analgesia and sedation where respiratory depression is to be avoided.

Methotrimeprazine is indicated as a preanesthetic medication for producing sedation, somnolence and relief of apprehension and anxiety.

CONTRAINDICATIONS:

Methotrimeprazine should not be used:

1. Concurrently with antihypertensive drugs including monoamine oxidase inhibitors.

2. In patients with a history of phenothiazine hypersensitivity.

3. In the presence of overdosage of CNS depressants or comatose states.

4. In the presence of severe myocardial, renal, or hepatic disease.

5. In the presence of clinically significant hypotension.

6. In patients under 12 years of age, since safe and effective use has not been established in children under this age.

WARNINGS:

Methotrimeprazine should be used with caution in women of child-bearing potential and during early pregnancy since its safety for the developing embryo has not been clearly established. A possible antifertility effect has been suggested in that successive generations of animals dosed with this drug have shown a diminution of litter size over the controls. There is no evidence of adverse developmental effect when administered during late pregnancy and labor.

Methotrimeprazine, as with other phenothiazine derivatives, has been found to depress spermatogenesis in experimental animals in doses greatly exceeding the recommended human dose.

Methotrimeprazine exerts additive effects with central nervous system depressant drugs including narcotics, barbiturates, general anesthetics, and certain drugs such as acetylsalicylic acid, meprobamate and reserpine. Consequently, the dosage of methotrimeprazine and of each such drug should be reduced and critically adjusted when used concomitantly or when sequence of use results in overlapping of drug effects.

Contains sodium metabisulfite, a sulfite that may cause allergic-type reactions including anaphylactic symptoms and life-threatening or less severe asthmatic episodes in certain susceptable people. The overall prevalence of sulfite sensitivity in the general population is unknown and probably low. Sulfite sensitivity is seen more frequently in asthmatic than in nonasthmatic people.

PRECAUTIONS:

Methotrimeprazine should be used with caution when given concomitantly with atropine, scopolamine, and succinylcholine in that tachycardia and fall in blood pressure may occur, and undesirable central nervous system effects such as stimulation, delirium, and extrapyramidal symptoms may be aggravated.

Elderly and debilitated patients with heart disease are more sensitive to phenothiazine effects. Therefore, a low initial dose is recommended with adjustment of subsequent doses according to response and tolerance of the patient. The pulse, blood pressure, and general circulatory status should be checked frequently until dosage requirements and responses are stabilized.

Continued administration for more than thirty days has usually been unnecessary and is advised only when narcotic drugs are contraindicated or in terminal illness. When long-term use is anticipated, periodic blood counts and liver function studies are recommended.

Patients should remain in bed or be closely supervised for about 6 hours after each of the first several injections, and not be ambulatory because of the possibility of orthostatic hypotension. Once tolerance to this effect is obtained, tolerance will usually be maintained unless more than several days elapse between subsequent doses. Therapy with vasopressor drugs has been required very rarely. Phenylephrine and methoxamine are suitable vasopressor agents; however, epinephrine should not be used, since a paradoxical decrease in blood pressure may result. Levarterenol should be reserved for hypotension not reversed by other vasopressors.

ADVERSE REACTIONS:

The most important side effects have been those associated with orthostatic hypotension. These effects, which include fainting or syncope, and weakness, usually can be avoided by keeping the patient in a supine position for about 6 hours (occasionally as much as 12 hours) after injection. A drop in blood pressure (usually within the physiological range) often occurs, beginning generally within 10 to 20 minutes following intramuscular injection, and may last 4 to 6 hours (occasionally up to 12 hours). This effect usually diminishes or disappears with continued or intermittent administration. Occasionally, fall in blood pressure may be profound and require immediate restorative measures.

Adverse reactions sometimes encountered include disorientation, dizziness, excessive sedation, weakness, slurring of speech; abdominal discomfort, nausea and vomiting; dry mouth, nasal congestion, difficulties in urination; chills; rarely uterine inertia.

Pain at the site of injection is frequently observed following administration of this drug. Local inflammation and swelling have occurred.

Agranulocytosis and jaundice have been reported following long-term, high- dosage use of this drug. Other adverse effects reported following the use of the phenothiazine family of drugs usually during their administration as psychotherapeutic agents have included:

Blood Dyscrasias: agranulocytosis, pancytopenia, leukopenia, eosinophilia, thrombocytopenia;

Hepatotoxicity: jaundice, biliary stasis;

Extrapyramidal Symptoms: dyskinesia, tilting stance, dystonia, parkinsonism, opisthotonos, hyperreflexia, especially in patients with previous brain damage;

Grand Mal Convulsions ;

Potentiation Of CNS Depressants: opiates, barbiturates, antihistamines, alcohol, analgesics, atropine, phosphorous insecticides, heat; cerebral edema and altered cerebral spinal fluid proteins, reactivation of psychotic processes, catatonia;

Autonomic Reactions: dryness of mouth, constipation cardiac arrest, tachycardia;

Hyperpyrexia ;

Endocrine Disturbances: menstrual and lactation irregularities;

Dermatological Disorder: photosensitivity, itching, erythema, urticaria, pigmentation, rash, exfoliative dermatitis, ocular changes (lenticular and corneal deposits and pigmentary retinopathy);

Hypersensitivity Reactions: angioneurotic, laryngeal, and peripheral edema, anaphylactoid reactions, and asthma.

There is considerable individual variation in type and frequency to these effects and though some are dose-related, many involve individual patient sensitivity. Most of these effects have occurred only on long-term, high-dosage administration and have not necessarily been reported with the recommended analgesic doses of methotrimeprazine.

DOSAGE AND ADMINISTRATION:

ADULT ADMINISTRATION

Methotrimeprazine should be administered by deep intramuscular injection into a large muscle mass. As with other intramuscularly administered drugs, proper injection technique is important to prevent inadvertent injection into a blood vessel, into, or in the region of, a peripheral nerve trunk and to avoid leakage along the needle tract. When multiple injections are used, rotation of the injection sites is advisable. Methotrimeprazine should not be administered subcutaneously as local irritation may occur. Until more experience is obtained, intravenous administration is not recommended.

Methotrimeprazine may be given intramuscularly in the same syringe with either Atropine Sulfate USP or Scopolamine Hydrobromide USP. It should NOT be mixed in the same syringe with other drugs.

The usual adult dose for analgesia is 10 to 20 mg (0.5 to 1.0 ml) administered deeply into a large muscle every 4 to 6 hours as required for pain relief. The dose per injection has varied from 5 to 40 mg (0.25 to 2.0 ml) at intervals of from 1 to 24 hours. A flexible dosage schedule and low initial dose of 10 mg are advisable until individual patient response and tolerance have been determined.

In elderly patients who are more sensitive to phenothiazine effects, an initial dose of 5 to 10 mg (0.25 to 0.5 ml) is suggested. If the patient tolerates the drug, and requires greater pain relief, subsequent doses may be slowly increased.

ANALGESIA FOR ACUTE OR INTRACTABLE PAIN

Initial dose of 10 to 20 mg, with adjustment of subsequent doses, at intervals of 4 to 6 hours as required for relief of pain.

OBSTETRICAL ANALGESIA

During labor, an initial dose of 15 to 20 mg is usually satisfactory. Methotrimeprazine may be repeated in similar or adjusted amounts at intervals as needed for analgesia and sedation.

PREANESTHETIC MEDICATION

The preoperative dose has varied from 2 to 20 mg administered 45 minutes to 3 hours before surgery. A dose of 10 mg is often satisfactory, and 15 to 20 mg, may be used when more sedation is desired. Atropine sulfate USP or Scopolamine Hydrobromide USP may be used concurrently but in lower than usual dosage (See PRECAUTIONS).

POSTOPERATIVE ANALGESIA

In the immediate postoperative period, initial dosage of 2.5 to 7.5 mg is suggested, since residual effects of anesthetic agents and other medications may be additive to the actions of methotrimeprazine. Subsequent doses should be adjusted at intervals of 4 to 6 hours as needed for pain relief. Ambulation must be avoided or carefully supervised(See ADVERSE REACTIONS and PRECAUTIONS).

DOSAGE AND ADMINISTRATION: *(cont'd)*

Store at Controlled Room Temperature 15-30 deg. c (59-86 deg. F).

HOW SUPPLIED - EQUIVALENTS NOT AVAILABLE:

Injection, Solution - Intramuscular - 20 mg/ml

10 ml $181.51 LEVOPROME, Lederle Parenterals 00205-4534-34

METHOXAMINE HYDROCHLORIDE *(001772)*

CATEGORIES: Analeptics; Autonomic Drugs; Cardiovascular Drugs; Central Nervous System Agents; Hypotension; Hypotension/Shock; Respiratory/Cerebral Stimulant; Sympathomimetic Agents; Tachycardia; Vasopressors; Pregnancy Category C; FDA Approval Pre 1982

BRAND NAMES: *Vasoxine*; **Vasoxyl**

(International brand names outside U.S. in italics)

DESCRIPTION:

Methoxamine hydrochloride injection is a sterile solution for intravenous or intramuscular injection, made isotonic with sodium chloride. Each 1 ml ampul contains 20 mg methoxamine hydrochloride. Citric acid anhydrous 0.3% and sodium citrate 0.3% are added as buffers and potassium metabisulfite 0.1% is added as an antioxidant.

Methoxamine hydrochloride is a sympathomimetic amine. It has the empirical formula $C_{11}H_{17}NO_3 \cdot HCl$ and a molecular weight of 247.72. The drug is very soluble in water, soluble in ethanol, but practically insoluble in ether, benzene or chloroform. It is known chemically as α-(1-aminoethyl)-2,5-dimethoxybenzenemethanol hydrochloride.

CLINICAL PHARMACOLOGY:

Methoxamine HCl is an alpha-receptor stimulant which produces a prompt and prolonged rise in blood pressure following parenteral administration. It is especially useful for maintaining blood pressure during operations under spinal anesthesia[1,2,3] and may also be used safely during general anesthesia. Methoxamine HCl does not increase the irritability of the cyclopropane-sensitized heart, making it useful during cyclopropane anesthesia.[4,5] Tachyphylaxis has not been a clinical problem.[1]

The major pharmacological effect of methoxamine HCl is a potent, prolonged pressor action following parenteral administration. Methoxamine HCl differs from most other sympathomimetic amines both in animals[4,6,7] and in man[1,8] by having a predominantly peripheral action and lacking inotropic and chronotropic effects. Methoxamine HCl has less arrhythmogenic potential than other sympathomimetic amines and rarely causes ventricular tachycardia, fibrillation, or increased sinoatrial rate.[4] On occasion, a decrease in rate occurs as blood pressure increases,[1,9,10] apparently caused by a carotid sinus reflex. This bradycardia can be abolished by atropine.[9]

The pressor action appears to be due to peripheral vasoconstriction rather than a centrally mediated effect. Evidence for direct action on blood vessels is provided in part by the observation of intense constriction along the course of a vein into which methoxamine HCl has been injected.[1] methoxamine HCl also increases venous pressure.[8]

Following intravenous administration of methoxamine HCl in dogs[11] and humans,[9,12] the peak pressor effect occurs within 0.5 to 2 minutes. In a group of human surgical patients,[13] the duration of the pressor effect following a single intravenous dose of 2 to 4 mg of methoxamine HCl was 10 to 15 minutes. No clinical pharmacology studies are available concerning the onset and duration of action after administration of recommended intramuscular doses (10 to 15 mg). With administration of 10 to 40 mg methoxamine HCl intramuscularly to patients, however, the peak effect occurs within 15 to 20 minutes, and the duration of action is approximately one and a half hours.[14]

Data from pharmacokinetic studies of methoxamine HCl following either intravenous or intramuscular administration are not available.

INDICATIONS AND USAGE:

Methoxamine HCl is intended for supporting, restoring or maintaining blood pressure during anesthesia (including cyclopropane anesthesia). It can be used to terminate some episodes of supraventricular tachycardia.

CONTRAINDICATIONS:

Methoxamine HCl is contraindicated in patients with severe hypertension, or in patients who are hypersensitive to methoxamine.

WARNINGS:

The use of methoxamine HCl in patients receiving monoamine oxidase inhibitors, tricyclic antidepressants or oxytocic agents such as vasopressin or certain ergot alkaloids may result in potentiation of the pressor effect (see DRUG INTERACTIONS).

Contains potassium metabisulfite, a sulfite that may cause allergic-type reactions including anaphylactic symptoms and life-threatening or less severe asthmatic episodes in certain susceptible people. The overall prevalence of sulfite sensitivity in the general population is unknown and probably low. Sulfite sensitivity is seen more frequently in asthmatic than in nonasthmatic people.

PRECAUTIONS:

GENERAL

Methoxamine HCl, like other vasopressor agents, should be used with caution in patients with hyperthyroidism, bradycardia, partial heart block, myocardial disease, or severe arteriosclerosis. Caution should be exercised to avoid overdosage, preventing undesirable high blood pressure and/or bradycardia. Note: Bradycardia may be abolished with atropine (see OVERDOSAGE). Also, caution should be taken when methoxamine HCl is used closely following the parenteral injection of ergot alkaloids to avoid an excessive rise in blood pressure.

DRUG/LABORATORY TEST INTERACTIONS

Methoxamine HCl may increase plasma cortisol and ACTH levels. Caution should be used when interpreting plasma cortisol and ACTH levels in a patient concurrently receiving methoxamine HCl.[15,16]

CARCINOGENESIS, MUTAGENESIS, AND IMPAIRMENT OF FERTILITY

No long-term animal studies have been performed to evaluate the potential of methoxamine HCl in these areas.

PREGNANCY, TERATOGENIC EFFECTS, PREGNANCY CATEGORY C

Methoxamine HCl has been shown to decrease uterine blood flow, decrease fetal heart rate and adversely affect the fetal acid-base status in pregnant ewes and monkeys at doses comparable to those used in humans. There are no adequate and well-controlled studies in pregnant women. There has been one report of a fetal death; the mother received methoxamine HCl concomitantly with several other drugs. A direct causal relationship to methoxamine HCl was not established. Methoxamine HCl should be used during pregnancy only if the potential benefit justifies the potential risk to the fetus.

PRECAUTIONS: *(cont'd)*

Methoxamine HCl (2.5 mg IV, 1 to 3 times over a 45 min. period) given to 7 pregnant ewes showed a significant deterioration in fetal acid-base status as evidenced by hypoxia, hypercarbia and metabolic acidosis.[17] An inverse relationship between pressor response to methoxamine HCl and uteroplacental blood flow has been shown in 16 pregnant ewes studied at doses ranging from 0.025 mg/kg to 0.2 mg/kg.[18] Uterine blood flow was decreased at all doses, but no significant change in fetal blood gas or acid-base status was demonstrated. Methoxamine HCl administration to 4 fetuses (50 mcg/kg/min for 60 min) and to 4 ewes (25 mcg/kg/min for 30 min) was associated with a decrease in fetal heart rate and uterine blood flow.[19] Nine monkeys studied at an average methoxamine HCl dose of 1.3 mg/kg administered over 57 min showed a decrease in uterine blood flow and a possible association with fetal asphyxia.[20]

LABOR AND DELIVERY

If vasopressor drugs are used to correct hypotension or added to local anesthetic solution during labor and delivery, some oxytocic drugs (vasopressin, ergotamine, ergonovine, methylergonovine) may cause severe persistent hypertension (seeWARNINGS and DRUG INTERACTIONS).

Note: In pregnant animals, methoxamine HCl has been shown to decrease uterine blood flow, possibly resulting in fetal asphyxia. Uterine hypertonus and fetal bradycardia may also be produced. (See ADVERSE REACTIONS and PRECAUTIONS, Pregnancy).

NURSING MOTHERS

It is not known whether this drug is excreted in human milk. Because many drugs are excreted in human milk, caution should be exercised when methoxamine HCl is administered to a nursing woman.

PEDIATRIC USE

Safety and effectiveness in children have not been established.

DRUG INTERACTIONS:

The pressor effect of methoxamine HCl may be markedly potentiated when methoxamine HCl is used in conjunction with monoamine oxidase inhibitors, tricyclic antidepressants, vasopressin or ergot alkaloids such as ergotamine, ergonovine or methylergonovine. Therefore, when initiating pressor therapy in patients receiving these drugs the initial dose should be small and given with caution (see WARNINGS).

ADVERSE REACTIONS:

The following adverse reactions have been observed, but there are insufficient data to support an estimate of their frequency:

Cardiovascular: Excessive blood pressure elevations particularly with high dosage, ventricular ectopic beats

Gastrointestinal: Nausea, vomiting (often projectile)

Central Nervous System: Headache (often severe), anxiety

Integumentary: Sweating, pilomotor response

Genitourinary: Uterine hypertonus, fetal bradycardia (see PRECAUTIONS, Labor and Delivery), urinary urgency.

OVERDOSAGE:

Overdosage of methoxamine HCl may be manifested as an undesirable elevation in blood pressure and/or bradycardia. Should a clinically significant elevation of blood pressure occur that requires treatment, it may be immediately reversed with an alpha-adrenergic blocking agent (*e.g.,* phentolamine). Bradycardia may be abolished by atropine.

DOSAGE AND ADMINISTRATION:

Blood volume depletion should always be corrected before any vasopressor is administered. The usual intravenous dose of methoxamine HCl for emergencies is 3 to 5 mg, injected slowly. Intravenous injection may be supplemented by intramuscular injections to provide a more prolonged effect. The usual intramuscular dose is 10 to 15 mg given shortly before or at the time of administering spinal anesthesia to prevent a fall in blood pressure. The tendency for the blood pressure to fall is greater with higher levels of spinal anesthesia, hence the dosage may be adjusted accordingly; 10 mg may be adequate at lower spinal levels while 15 to 20 mg may be required at high levels of spinal anesthesia. Repeated doses may be given if necessary, but time should be allowed for the previous dose to act (about 15 minutes, see CLINICAL PHARMACOLOGY). For cases of only moderate hypotension, 5 to 10 mg intramuscularly may be adequate.

For purposes of correcting a fall in blood pressure, an intramuscular injection of 10 to 15 mg of methoxamine HCl may be given depending upon the degree of fall. In cases where the systolic pressure falls to 60 mmHg or less, or whenever an emergency exists, an intravenous injection of 3 to 5 mg methoxamine HCl is indicated. This intravenous dose may be accompanied by 10 to 15 mg intramuscularly to provide more prolonged effect.

For termination of episodes of supraventricular tachycardia not responsive to other modes of therapy, the usual dose of methoxamine HCl is 10 mg intravenously, administered by slow push (*i.e.,* 3 to 5 min).

Parenteral drug products should be inspected visually for particulate matter and discoloration prior to administration whenever solution and container permit.

HOW SUPPLIED:

1 ml ampuls, containing 20 mg methoxamine hydrochloride.

Store at 15° to 30°C (59° to 86°F) and protect from light.

REFERENCES:

1. King BD, Dripps RD: The use of methoxamine for maintenance of the circulation during spinal anesthesia. *Surg Gynecol Obstet*1950;90:659-665. **2.** Kistler EM, Ruben JE: Methoxamine in 1 percent procaine as a prophylactic vasopressor in spinal anesthesia.*Arch Surg*1951;62:64-69. **3.** Poe MF: Use of methoxamine hydrochloride as a pressor agent during spinal analgesia.*Anesthesiology* 1952;13:89-93. **4.** Lahti RE, Brill IC, McCawley EL: The effect of methoxamine hydrochloride (Vasoxyl) on cardiac rhythm. *J Pharmacol Exp Ther* 1955;115:268-274. **5.** Stutzman JW, Pettinga FL, Fruggiero EJ: Cardiac effects of methoxamine (β-(2,5-dimethoxy-phenyl)-β-hydroxyisopropylamine HCl) and desoxyephedrine during cyclopropane anesthesia. *J Pharmacol Exp Ther* 1949;97:385-387. **6.** West JW, Faulk AT, Guzman SV: Comparative study of effects of levarterenol and methoxamine in shock associated with acute myocardial ischemia in dogs. *Circ Res*1962;10:712-721. **7.** Goldberg LI, Cotten M, Darby TD, Howell EV: Comparative heart contractile force effects of equipressor doses of several sympathomimetic amines. *J Pharmacol Exp Ther*1953;108:177-185. **8.** Aviado DM, Wnuck AL: Mechanisms for cardiac slowing by methoxamine. *J Pharmacol Exp Ther*1957;119:99-106. **9.** Nathanson MH, Miller H: Clinical observations on a new epinephrin-like compound, methoxamine. *Am J Med Sci*1952;223:270-279. **10.** Stanfield CA, Yu PN: Hemodynamic effects of methoxamine in mitral valve disease. *Circ Res*1960;8:859-864. **11.** Imai S, Shigei T, Hashimoto K: Cardiac actions of methoxamine with special reference to its antagonist action to epinephrine. *Circ Res* 1961;9:552-560. **12.** *The Extra Pharmacopoeia, Martindale*28th Ed., Reynolds, JEF, ed., Pharmaceutical Press (London), pp.19. **13.** Goldberg LI, Bloodwell RD, Braunwald E,*et al.* The direct effects of norepinephrine, epinephrine, and methoxamine on myocardial contractile force in man. *Circ*1960;22:1125-1132. **14.** Data on File, Burroughs Wellcome Co. **15.** Laurian L, Oberman Z. Hoerer E, *et al.*: Low cortisol and growth hormone secretion in response to methoxamine administration in obese subjects. *Isr J Med Sci* 1977;13:477-481. **16.** Nakai Y, Imura H, Yoshimi T, Matsukura S: Adrenergic control mechanism for ACTH secretion in man. *Acta Endocrinol*1973;74:263-270. **17.** Shnider SM, DeLorimier AA, Asling JH, Morishima HO: Vasopressors in obstetrics. II. Fetal hazards of methoxamine administration during obstetric spinal anesthesia. *Am J Obstet Gynecol*1970;106:680-686. **18.** Ralston DH, Shnider SM, DeLorimier AA: Effects of equipotent ephedrine, metaraminol, mephentermine and methoxamine on uterine blood flow in the pregnant ewe.*Anesthesiology*1974;40:354-370. **19.** Oakes GK, Ehrenkranz RA, Walker AM, *et al.*: Effect of α-adrenergic

REFERENCES: *(cont'd)*
agonist and antagonist infusion on the umbilical and uterine circulations of pregnant sheep. *Biol Neonate* 1980;38:229-237. **20.** Eng M, Berges PU, Ueland K, *et al.*:The effects of methoxamine and ephedrine in normotensive pregnant primates.*Anesthesiology* 1971; 35:354-360.

HOW SUPPLIED - EQUIVALENTS NOT AVAILABLE:

Injection, Solution - Intramuscular; - 20 mg/ml

1 ml ampul x 10 $244.22 VASOXYL, Glaxo Wellcome 00173-0957-10

METHOXSALEN *(001773)*

CATEGORIES: Depigmenting/Pigmenting Agents; Dermatologicals; Hypopigmentation; Photosensitizer; Pigmenting Agents; Psoriasis; Skin/Mucous Membrane Agents; Topical; Vitiligo; Pregnancy Category C; FDA Approval Pre 1982

BRAND NAMES: 8-Mop; *Delsoralen*; *Deltasoralen*; *Dermox* (Mexico); *Geroxalen*; Houva-Caps; *Macsoralen*; *Meladinina* (Mexico); *Meladinine* (Germany, France); *Melaoline*; *Methoxsalen*; *Mopsalem*; *Mopsoralen*; **Oxsoralen**; *Oxsoralen Lotion* (Canada); *Oxsoralen Ultra*; *Oxsoralen-Ultra*; *Oxsoralon*; *Oxysoralen*; *Puvasoralen* (England); *Ultra-MOP* (Canada); *UltraMOP Lotion* (Canada)
(International brand names outside U.S. in italics)

FORMULARIES: BC-BS

Methoxsalen with UV radiation should be used only by physicians who have special competence in the diagnosis and treatment of psoriasis and vitiligo and who have special training and experience in photochemotherapy. Psoralen and ultraviolet radiation therapy should be under constant supervision of such a physician. For the treatment of patients with psoriasis, photochemotherapy should be restricted to patients with severe recalcitrant, disabling psoriasis which is not adequately responsive to other forms of therapy, and only when the diagnosis has been supported by biopsy. Because of the possibilities of ocular damage, aging of the skin, and skin cancer (including melanoma), the patient should be fully informed by the physician of the risks inherent in this therapy. When methoxsalen is used in combination with photopheresis, refer to the UVAR System Operator's Manual for specific warnings, cautions, indications, instructions related to photopheresis.

Caution: Oxsoralen-Ultra should not be used interchangeably with regular Oxsoralen. This new dosage form of methoxsalen exhibits significantly greater bioavailability and earlier photo- sensitization onset time than previous methoxsalen dosage forms. Patients should be treated in accordance with the dosimetry specifically recommended for this product. The minimum phototoxic dose (MPD) and phototoxic peak time after drug administration prior to onset of photochemotherapy with this dosage form should be determined.

DESCRIPTION:

Please note the brand names, Oxsoralen-Ultra Capsules, 8-MOP Capsules and Oxsoralen Lotion 1% are used in this monograph where noted.

CAUTION: METHOXSALEN IS A POTENT DRUG. READ ENTIRE BROCHURE BEFORE PRESCRIBING OR DISPENSING THIS MEDICATION.

Oxsoralen (Methoxsalen, 8-Methoxypsoralen) Capsules, 10 mg. Methoxsalen is a naturally occurring photoactive substance found in the seeds of the *Ammi majus* (Umbelliferae) plant. It belongs to a group of compounds known as psoralens, or furocoumarins. The chemical name of methoxsalen is 9-methoxy-7H-furo [3,2-g][1]-benzopyran-7-one.

Topical: WARNING: METHOXSALEN LOTION IS A POTENT DRUG CAPABLE OF PRODUCING SEVERE BURNS IF IMPROPERLY USED. IT SHOULD BE APPLIED ONLY BY A PHYSICIAN UNDER CONTROLLED CONDITIONS FOR LIGHT EXPOSURE AND SUBSEQUENT LIGHT SHIELDING. THIS PREPARATION SHOULD NEVER BE DISPENSED TO A PATIENT.

Each ml of Oxsoralen Lotion contains 10 mg methoxsalen in an inert vehicle containing alcohol (71% v/v), propylene glycol, acetone, and purified water.

CLINICAL PHARMACOLOGY:

The combination treatment regimen of psoralen (P) and ultraviolet radiation of 320-400 nm wavelength commonly referred to as UVA is known by the acronym, PUVA. Skin reactivity to UVA (320-400 nm) radiation is markedly enhanced by the ingestion of methoxsalen.

Methoxsalen is reversibly bound to serum albumin and is also preferentially taken up by epidermal cells. At a dose which is six times larger than that used in humans, it induces mixed function oxidases in the liver of mice. In both mice and man, methoxsalen is rapidly metabolized. Approximately 95% of the drug is excreted as a series of metabolites in the urine within 24 hours. The exact mechanism of action of methoxsalen with the epidermal melanocytes and keratinocytes is not known. The best known biochemical reaction of methoxsalen is with DNA. Methoxsalen, upon photoactivation, conjugates and forms covalent bonds with DNA which leads to the formation of both monofunctional (addition to a single strand of DNA) and bifunctional (crosslinking of psoralen to both strands of DNA) adducts. Reactions with proteins have also been described.

Methoxsalen acts as a photosensitizer. Administration of the drug and subsequent exposure of UVA can lead to cell injury. Orally administered methoxsalen reaches the skin via the blood and UVA penetrates well into the skin. If sufficient cell injury occurs in the skin, an inflammatory reaction occurs. The most obvious manifestation of this reaction is delayed erythema, which may not begin for several hours and peaks at 48-72 hours. The inflammation is followed, over several days to weeks, by repair which is manifested by increased melanization of the epidermis and thickening of the stratum corneum. The mechanisms of therapy are not known. In the treatment of psoriasis, the mechanism is most often assumed to be DNA photodamage and resulting decrease in cell proliferation but other vascular, leukocyte, or cell regulatory mechanisms may also be playing some role. Psoriasis is a hyperproliferative disorder and other agents known to be therapeutic for psoriasis are known to inhibit DNA synthesis.

Oxsoralen-Ultra Capsules: In a well-controlled bioavailability study, Oxsoralen-Ultra capsules reached peak drug levels in the blood of test subjects between 0.5 and 4 hours (Mean = 1.8 hours) as compared to between 1.5 and 6 hours (Mean 3.0 hours) for regular Oxsoralen when administered with 8 ounces of milk. Peak drug levels were 2 to 3 fold greater when the overall extent of drug absorption was approximately two fold greater for Oxsoralen-Ultra as compared to regular Oxsoralen Capsules. Detectable methoxsalen levels were observed up to 12 hours post dose. The drug half-life is approximately 2 hours. Photosensitivity studies demonstrate a shorter time of peak photosensitivity of 1.5 to 2.1 hours vs. 3.9 to 4.25 hours for regular Oxsoralen Capsules. Detectable methoxsalen levels were observed up to 12 hours post dose. The drug half-life is approximately 2 hours. Photosensitivity studies demonstrate a shorter time of peak photosensitivity of 1.5 to 2.1 hours vs. 3.9 to 4.25 hours for regular Oxsoralen capsules. In addition, the mean minimal erythema dose (MED), J/cm^2, for the Oxsoralen-Ultra Capsules is substantially less than that required for regular Oxsoralen Capsules.

8-MOP Capsules: The drug reaches its maximum bioavailability 1 1/2-3 hours after oral administration and may last for up to 8 hours.

INDICATIONS AND USAGE:

Photochemotherapy (methoxsalen with long wave UVA radiation) is indicated for the symptomatic control of severe, recalcitrant, disabling psoriasis not adequately responsive to other forms of therapy and when the diagnosis has been supported by biopsy. Methoxsalen is intended to be administered only in conjunction with a schedule of controlled doses of long wave ultraviolet radiation.

8-MOP Capsules: Photochemotherapy (methoxsalen with long wave ultraviolet radiation) is indicated for the repigmentation of idiopathic vitiligo.

Photopheresis (methoxsalen with long wave ultraviolet radiation of white blood cells) is indicated for use with the UVAR* System in the palliative treatment of the skin manifestations of cutaneous T-cell lymphoma (CTCL) in persons who have not bee responsive to other forms of treatment. WHile this dosage form of methoxsalen has been approved for use in combination with photopheresis, Oxsoralen Ultra Capsules have not been approved for that use.

Topical: As a topical repigmenting agent in vitiligo in conjunction with controlled doses of ultraviolet A (320 - 400 nm) or sunlight.

CONTRAINDICATIONS:

A. Patients exhibiting idiosyncratic reactions to psoralen compounds.

B. Patients possessing a specific history of light sensitive disease states should not initiate methoxsalen therapy except under special circumstances. Diseases associated with photosensitivity include lupus erythematosus, porphyria cutanea tarda, erythropoietic protoporphyria, variegate porphyria, xeroderma pigmentosum, and albinism.

C. Patients with melanoma or possessing a history of melanoma.

D. Patients with invasive squamous cell carcinomas

E. Patients with aphakia, because of the significantly increased risk of retinal damage due to the absence of lenses.

Topical

A. Patients exhibiting idiosyncratic reactions to psoralen compounds or a history of sensitivity reactions to them.

B. Patients exhibiting melanoma or with a history of melanoma.

C. Patients exhibiting invasive skin carcinoma generally.

D. Patients with photosensitivity diseases such as porphyria, acute lupus erythematosus, xeroderma, pigmentosum, etc.

E. Children under 12 since clinical studies to determine the efficacy and safety of treatment in this age group have not been done.

WARNINGS:

ORAL

Skin Burning: Serious burns from either UVA or sunlight (even through window glass) can result if the recommended dosage of the drug and/or exposure schedules are not maintained.

Carcinogenicity

1. Animal Studies: Topical or intraperitoneal methoxsalen has been reported to be a potent photocarcinogen in albino mice and hairless mice. However, methoxsalen given by the oral route to Swiss albino mice suggests this agent exerts a protective effect against ultraviolet carcinogenesis; mice given 8-methoxypsoralen in their diet showed 38% ear tumors 180 days after the start of ultraviolet therapy compared to 62% for controls.

2. Human Studies: A 5.7 year prospective study of 1380 psoriasis patients treated with oral methoxsalen and ultraviolet. A photochemotherapy (PUVA) demonstrated that the risk of cutaneous squamous-cell carcinoma developing at least 22 months following the first PUVA exposure was approximately 12.8 times higher in the high dose patients than in the low dose patients. The substantial dose-dependent increase was observed in patients with neither a prior history of skin cancer nor significant exposure to cutaneous carcinogens. Reduction in PUVA dosage significantly reduces the risk. No substantial dose related increase was noted for basal cell carcinoma according to Stern et al., 1984[14]. Increases appear greatest in patients who have pre-PUVA exposure to 1) prolonged tar and UVB treatment, 2) ionizing radiation, or 3) arsenic.

Roenigk et al., 1980[15], studied 690 patients for up to 4 years and found no increase in the risk of non-melanoma skin cancer, although patients in this cohort has significantly less exposure to PUVA than in the Stern et al. study. After 5 years, two of the 1380 patients in the Stern et al. PUVA study have developed malignant melanoma. In addition, more than 1/5 of the patients in this cohort have developed macular pigmented lesions on the buttocks. While there is no evidence that an increased risk of melanoma exists in PUVA treated patients, these observations indicated the need for continued evaluation of melanoma risk of PUVA treated patients.

In a study in Indian patients treated for 4 years for vitiligo, 12 percent developed keratoses, but not cancer, in the depigmented, vitiliginous areas. Clinically, the keratoses were keratotic papules, actinic keratosis-like macules, nonscaling dome shaped papules, and lichenoid porokeratotic-like papules.

Cataractogenicity

1. Animal Studies: Exposure to large doses of UVA causes cataracts in animals, and this effect is enhanced by the administration of methoxsalen.

2. Human Studies: It has been found that the concentration of methoxsalen in the lens is proportional to the serum level. If the lens is exposed to UVA during the time methoxsalen is present in the lens, photochemical action may lead to irreversible binding of methoxsalen to proteins and the DNA components of the lens. However, if the lens is shielded from UVA, the methoxsalen will diffuse out the lens in a 24 hour period. Patients should be told emphatically to wear UVA absorbing, wrap-around sunglasses for the twenty-four (24) hour period following ingestion of methoxsalen whether exposed to direct or indirect sunlight in the open or through a window glass.

Among patients using proper eye protection, there is no evidence for a significantly increased risk of cataracts in association with PUVA therapy. Thirty-five of 1380 patients have developed cataracts in the five years since their first PUVA treatment. This incidence is comparable to that expected in a population of this size and age distribution. No relationship between PUVA dose and cataract risk in this group has been noted.

Actinic Degeneration: Exposure to sunlight and/or ultraviolet radiation may result in "premature aging" of the skin.

Basal Cell Carcinomas: Patients exhibiting multiple basal cell carcinomas or having a history of basal cell carcinomas should be diligently observed and treated.

Radiation Therapy: Patients having a history of previous x-ray therapy or grenz ray therapy should be diligently observed for signs of carcinoma.

Arsenic Therapy: Patients having a history of previous arsenic therapy should be diligently observed for signs of carcinoma.

Hepatic Diseases: Patients with hepatic insufficiency should be treated with caution since hepatic biotransformation is necessary for drug urinary excretion.

WARNINGS: *(cont'd)*

Cardiac Diseases: Patients with cardiac diseases or others who may be unable to tolerate prolonged standing or exposure to heat stress should not be treated in a vertical UVA chamber.

Total Dosage: The total cumulative dose of UVA that can be given over long periods of time with safety has not yet been established.

Concomitant Therapy: Special care should be exercised in treating patients who are receiving concomitant therapy (either topically or systemically) with known photosensitizing agents such as anthralin, coal tar or coal tar derivatives, griseofulvin, phenothiazines, nalidixic acid, halogenated salicylanilides (bacteriostatic soaps), sulfonamides, tetracyclines, thiazides, and certain organic staining dyes such as methylene blue, toluidine blue, rose bengal, and methyl orange.

TOPICAL

Skin Burns: Serious skin burns either UVA or sunlight (even through window glass) can result if recommended exposure schedule is exceeded and/or protective covering or sunscreens are not used. The blistering of the skin sometimes encountered after UV exposure generally heals without complications or scarring. Suitable covering of the area of application or a topical sunblock should follow the therapeutic UVA exposure.

Carcinogenicity

1. Animal Studies: Topical methoxsalen has been reported to be a potent photocarcinogen in certain strains of mice.

2. Human Studies: None of our clinical investigators reported skin cancer as a complication of topical treatment for vitiligo. However, it is recommended that caution be exercised when the patient is fair-skinned, has a history of prior coal tar UV treatment, or has had ionizing radiation or taken arsenical compounds. Such patients who subsequently have oral psoralen - UVA treatment (PUVA) are at increased risk for developing skin cancer.

Concomitant Therapy: Special care should be exercised in treating patients who are receiving concomitant therapy (either topically or systemically) with known photosensitizing agents such as anthralin, coal tar or coal tar derivatives, griseofulvin, phenothiazines, nalidixic acid, halogenated salicylanilides (bacteriostatic soaps), sulfonamides, tetracyclines, thiazides, and certain organic staining dyes such a methylene blue, toluidine blue, rose bengal, and methyl orange.

PRECAUTIONS:

GENERAL

Oral: Applicable To And Psoriasis Treatment:

1. Before Methoxsalen ingestion, patients must not sunbathe during the 24 hours prior to methoxsalen ingestion and UV exposure. The presence of a sunburn may prevent an accurate evaluation of the patients's response to photochemotherapy.

2.

a. After Methoxsalen ingestion UVA-absorbing wrap-around sunglasses should be worn during daylight for 24 hours after methoxsalen ingestion. The protective eyewear must be designed to prevent entry of stray radiation to the eyes, including that which may enter from the sides of the eyewear. The protective eyewear is used to prevent the irreversible binding of methoxsalen to the proteins and DNA components of the lens. Cataracts form when enough of the binding occurs. Visual discrimination should be permitted by the eyewear for patient well-being and comfort.

b. Patients must avoid sun exposure, even through window glass or cloud cover, for at least 8 hours after methoxsalen ingestion. If sun exposure cannot be avoided, the patient should wear protective devices such as hat and gloves, and/or apply sunscreens which contain ingredients that filter out UVA radiation (*e.g.,* sunscreens containing benzophenone and/or PABA esters which exhibit a sun protective factor equal to or greater than 15). These chemical sunscreens should be applied to all areas that might be exposed to the sun (including lips). Sunscreens should not be applied to areas affected by psoriasis until after the patient has been treated in the UVA chamber.

3.

a. During PUVA therapy, total UVA-absorbing/blocking goggles mechanically designed to give maximal ocular protection must be worn. Failure to do so may increase the risk of cataract formation. A reliable radiometer can be used to verify elimination of UVA transmission through the goggles.

b. Abdominal skin, breasts, genitalia, and other sensitive areas should be protected for approximately 1/3 of the initial exposure time until tanning occurs.

c. Unless affected by disease, male genitalia should be shielded.

4.

a. After combined Methoxsalen/UVA therapy, UVA-absorbing wrap-around sunglasses should be worn during the daylight for 24 hours after combined methoxsalen/UVA therapy.

b. Patients should not sunbathe for 48 hours after therapy. Erythema and/or burning due to photochemotherapy and sunburn due to sun exposure are additive.

Topical: This product should be applied only in small well-defined lesions and preferably on lesions which can be protected by clothing or a sunscreen from subsequent exposure to radiant UVA. If this product is used to treat vitiligo of face or hands, be very emphatic when instructing the patient to keep the treated areas protected from light by the use of protective clothing or sunscreening agents. The area of application may be highly photosensitive for several days and may result in severe burn injury if exposed to additional UV or sunlight.

LABORATORY TESTS

Oral Forms: Patients should have an ophthalmologic examination prior to start of therapy, and thence yearly.

Oxsoralen-Ultra Capsules: Patients should have the following tests prior to the start of therapy and at regular periods thereafter if patients are on extended treatments.

8-MOP Capsules: Patients should have the following tests prior to the start of therapy and should be retested in 6-12 months subsequently. Additional tests at more extended time periods should be conducted as clinically indicated.

a. Complete Blood Count (Hemoglobin or Hematocrit; White Blood Count - if abnormal, a differential count).

b. Anti-nuclear Antibodies.

c. Liver Function Tests

d. Renal Function Tests (Creatinine or Blood Urea Nitrogen).

CARCINOGENESIS

See WARNINGS.

PREGNANCY CATEGORY C

Animal reproduction studies have not been conducted with oral or topical methoxsalen. It is also not known whether methoxsalen can cause fetal harm when administered to a pregnant woman or can affect reproduction capacity. Methoxsalen should be given to a woman only if clearly needed.

PRECAUTIONS: *(cont'd)*

NURSING MOTHERS

8-MOP Capsules: It is not known whether this drug is excreted in human milk. Because many drugs are excreted in human milk, either methoxsalen ingestion or nursing should be discontinued.

Topical: It is not known whether topical methoxsalen is absorbed or excreted in human milk. Caution is advised when topical methoxsalen is used in a nursing mother.

PEDIATRIC USE

Oral: Safety in children has not been established. Potential hazards of long-term therapy include the possibilities of carcinogenicity and cataractogenicity as described in WARNINGSas well as the probability of actinic degeneration which is also described in WARNINGS.

8-MOP Capsules: Safety in children has not been established. Potential hazards of long-term therapy include the possibilities of carcinogenicity and cataractogenicity as described in WARNINGSas well as the probability of actinic degeneration which is also described in WARNINGS.

Topical: Safety and effectiveness in children below the age of 12 years have not been established.

DRUG INTERACTIONS:

See WARNINGS.

ADVERSE REACTIONS:

ORAL

Methoxsalen: The most commonly reported side effect of methoxsalen alone is nausea, which occurs with approximately 10% of all patients. This effect may be minimized or avoided by instructing the patient to take methoxsalen with milk or food, or to divide the dose into two portions, taken approximately one-half hour apart. Other effects include nervousness, insomnia, and depression.

Combined Methoxsalen/UVA Therapy:

1. Pruritus: This adverse reaction occurs with approximately 10% of all patients. In most cases, pruritus can be alleviated with frequent application of bland emollients or other topical agents; severe pruritus may require systemic treatment. If pruritus is unresponsive to these measures, shield pruritic areas from further UVA exposure until the condition resolves. If intractable pruritus is generalized, UVA treatment should be discontinued until the pruritus disappears.

2. Erythema: Mild, transient erythema at 24-48 hours after PUVA therapy is an expected reaction and indicates that a therapeutic interaction between methoxsalen and UVA occurred. Any area showing moderate erythema (greater than Grade 2 - See TABLE 7 for grades of erythema) should be shielded during subsequent UVA exposures until the erythema has resolved. Erythema greater than Grade 2 which appears within 24 hours after UVA treatment may signal a potentially severe burn. Erythema may become progressively worse over the next 24 hours, since the peak erythemal reaction characteristically occurs 48 hours or later after methoxsalen ingestion. The patient should be protected from further UVA exposures and sunlight, and should be monitored closely.

3. Important Differences Between PUVA Erythema and Sunburn: PUVA-induced inflammation differs from sunburn or UVB phototherapy in several ways. The percent transmission of UVB varies between 0% to 34% through skin whereas UVA varies between 1% to 80% transmission; thus UVA is transmitted to a larger percent through the skin. The DNA lesions induced by PUVA are very different from UV-induced thymine dimers and may lead to a DNA crosslink. This DNA lesion may be more problematic to the cell because crosslinks are more lethal and psoralen-DNA photoproducts may be "new" or unfamiliar substrates for DNA repair enzymes. DNA synthesis is also suppressed longer after PUVA. The time course of delayed erythema is different with PUVA and may not involve the usual mediators seen in sunburn. PUVA-induced redness may be just beginning at 24 hours, when UVB erythema has already passed its peak. The erythema dose-response curve is also steeper for PUVA. Compared to equally erythemogenic dose of UVB, the histologic alterations induced by PUVA show more dermal vessel damage and longer duration of epidermal and dermal abnormalities.

4. Other Adverse Reactions: Those reported include edema, dizziness, headache, malaise, depression, hypopigmentation, vesiculation and bullae formation, non-specific rash, herpes simplex, miliaria, urticaria, folliculitis, gastrointestinal disturbances, cutaneous tenderness, leg cramps, hypotension, and extension of psoriasis.

TOPICAL

Systemic adverse reactions have not been reported. The most common adverse reaction is severe burns of the treated area from overexposure to UVA, including sunlight. Treatment must be individualized. Minor blistering of the skin is not a contraindication to further treatment and generally heals without incident. Treatment would be the standard for burn therapy. Since 1953, many studies have demonstrated the safety and effectiveness of topical methoxsalen and UVA for the treatment of vitiligo when used as directed.

OVERDOSAGE:

Oral: In the event of methoxsalen overdosage, induce emesis and keep the patient in the darkened room for at least 24 hours. Emesis is beneficial only within the first 2 to 3 hours after ingestion of methoxsalen, since maximum blood levels are reached by this time.

Topical: This does not apply to topical usage. In the unlikely event that the lotion is ingested, standard procedures for poisoning should be followed, including gastric lavage. Protection from UVA or daylight for hours or days would also be necessary. The patient should be kept in a darkened room.

DOSAGE AND ADMINISTRATION:

OXSORALEN-ULTRA CAPSULES

Caution: Oxsoralen-ultra represents a new dose form of methoxsalen. This new dosage form of methoxsalen exhibits significantly greater bioavailability and earlier photosensitization onset time than previous methoxsalen dosage forms. Each patient should be evaluated by determining the minimum phototoxic dose (MPD) and phototoxic peak time after drug administration prior to onset of photo- photochemotherapy with this dosage form. Human bioavailability studies have indicated the following drug dosage and administration directions are to be used as a guideline only.

8-MOP CAPSULES

Vitiligo Therapy

1. Drug Dosage-Initial Therapy: Two capsules (10 mg each) in one dose taken with milk or in food two to four hours before ultraviolet light exposure.

2. Light Exposure: The exposure time to sunlight should comply with the following guide: (TABLE 1)

Therapy should be on alternate days and never two consecutive days.

DOSAGE AND ADMINISTRATION: *(cont'd)*

TABLE 1

	Basic Skin Color Light	Medium	Dark
Initial Exposure	15 min	20 min	25 min
Second Exposure	20 min	25 min.	30 min.
Third Exposure	25 min.	30 min.	35 min.
Fourth Exposure	30 min.	25 min.	40 min.

Subsequent Exposure: Gradually increase exposure based on erythema and tenderness of the amelanotic skin.

ORAL FORMS

Psoriasis Therapy

1. Drug Dosage-Initial Therapy: The methoxsalen capsules should be taken 1 1/2 to 2 hours before UVA exposure with some food or milk according to the following table (TABLE 2):

TABLE 2

Patient's Weight (kg)	(lbs)	Dose (mg)
< 30	< 65	10
30-50	65-100	20
51-65	101-145	30
66-80	146-175	40
81-90	176-200	50
91-115	201-250	60
> 115	> 250	70

2. Initial Exposure: The initial UVA exposure energy level and corresponding time of exposure is determined by the patient's skin characteristics for sun burning and tanning as follows: (TABLE 3)

TABLE 3

Skin Type		Recommended
I	Always burn, never tan (patients with erythrodermic psoriasis are to be classed as Type I for determination of UVA) dosage.	0.5 J/cm²
II	Always burn, but sometimes tan	1.0 J/cm²
III	Sometime burn, but always tan	1.5 J/cm²
IV	Never burn, always tan	2.0 J/cm²
V*	Moderately pigmented	2.5 J/cm²
VI*	Blacks	3.0 J/cm²

* (Patients with natural pigmentation of these type should be classified into a lower skin type category if the sunburning history so indicates.)

If the MPD is done, start at 1/2 MPD.

Additional drug dosage directions are as follows:

a. Weight Change: In the event that the weight of a patient changes during treatment such that he/she falls into an adjacent weight range/dose category, no change in the dose of methoxsalen is usually required. If, in the physician's opinion, however, a weight change is sufficiently great to modify the drug dose, then an adjustment in the time of exposure to UVA should be made.

b. Dose/Week: The number of doses per week of methoxsalen capsules will be determined by the patient's schedule of UVA exposures. In no case should treatments be given more often than once every other day because the full extent of phototoxic reactions may not be evident until 48 hours after each exposure.

c. Dosage Increase: Dosage may be increased by 10 mg after the fifteenth treatment under the conditions outlined in section PUVA TREATMENT PROTOCOL-CLEARING PHASE;4.b.

UVA Radiation Source Specifications & Information

A. Irradiance Uniformity: The following specifications should be met with the window of the detector held in a vertical plane.

1. Vertical variation: For readings taken at any point along the vertical center axis of the chamber (to within 15 cm from the top and bottom), the lowest reading should not be less than 70 percent of the highest reading.

2. Horizontal variation: Throughout any specific horizontal plane, the lowest reading must be at least 80 percent of the highest reading, excluding the peripheral 3 cm of the patient treatment space.

B. Patient Safety Features: The following safety features should be present:

(1) Protection from electrical hazard: All units should be grounded and conform to applicable electrical codes. The patient or operator should not be able to touch any live electrical parts. There should be ground fault protection.

(2) Protective shielding of lamps: The patient should not be able to come in contact with the bare lamps. In the event of lamp breakage, the patient should not be exposed to broken lamp components.

(3) Hand rails and hand holds: Appropriate supports should be available to the patient.

(4) Patient viewing window: A window which blocks UV should be provided for viewing the patient during treatment.

(5) Door and latches: Patients should be able to open the door from the inside with only slight pressure to the door.

(6) Non-skid floor: The floor should be of a non-skid nature.

(7) Thermoregulation: Sufficient air flow should be provided for patient safely and comfort, limiting temperature within the UVA radiator cabinet to approximately less than 100°F.

(8) Timer: The irradiator should be equipped with an automatic timer which terminates the exposure at the conclusion of a pre-set time interval.

(9) Patient alarm device: An alarm device within the UVA irradiator chamber should be accessible to the patient for emergency activation.

(10) Danger label: The unit should have a label prominently displayed which reads as follows: **DANGER - Ultraviolet radiation - Follow your physicians instructions - Failure to use protective eyewear may result in eye injury.**

C. UVA Exposure Dosimetry Measurements: The maximum radiant exposure or irradiance (within ± 15 percent) of UVA (320-400 nm) delivered to the patient should be determined by using an appropriate radiometer calibrated to be read in Joules/cm² or mW/cm². In the absence of a standard measuring technique approved by the National Bureau of Standards, the system should use a detector corrected to a cosine spatial response. The use and recalibration frequency of such a radiometer for a specific UVA irradiator chamber should be specified by the manufacturer because the UVA dose (exposure) is determined by the design of the irradiator, the number of lamps, and the age of the lamps. If irradiance is measured, the radiometer reading in mW/cm² is used to calculate the exposure time in minutes to deliver the required UVA dose in Joules/cm² to a patient in the UVA irradiator cabinet. The equation is (TABLE 4):

TABLE 4

$$\text{Exposure Time (minutes)} = \frac{\text{Desired UVA Dose (J/cm}^2)}{0.06 \times \text{Irradiance (mW/cm}^2)}$$

Overexposure due to human error should be minimized by using an accurate automatic timing device, which is set by the operator and controlled by energizing and de-energizing the UVA irradiator lamp. The timing device calibration interval should be specified by the manufacturer. Safety systems should be included to minimize the possibility of delivering a UVA exposure which exceeds the prescribed dose, in the event that the timer or radiometer should malfunction.

D. UVA Spectral Output Distribution: The spectral distributions of the lamps should meet the following specifications (TABLE 5):

TABLE 5

Wavelength band (nanometers)	Output[1]
< 310	< 1
310 to 320	1 to 3
320 to 330	4 to 8
330 to 340	11 to 17
340 to 350	18 to 25
350 to 360	19 to 28
360 to 370	15 to 23
370 to 380	8 to 12
380 to 390	3 to 7
390 to 400	1 to 3

[1]As a percentage of total irradiance between 320 and 400 nanometers.

PUVA Treatment Protocol Introduction-Oxsoralen-Ultra Capsules Only

The Oxsoralen-Ultra Capsules reach their maximum bioavailability in 1.5 to 2 hours after ingestion.

On average, the serum level achieved with Oxsoralen-Ultra is twice that obtained with 8-MOP (formerly Oxsoralen) and reach their peak concentration in less than 1/2 the time of the 8-MOP.

As a result the mean MED J/cm² for the Oxsoralen-Ultra Capsules is substantially less than that required for 8-MOP.

Photosensitivity studies demonstrate a shorter time of peak photosensitivity of 1.5 to 2.1 hours vs. 3.9 to 4.25 hours for regular methoxsalen capsules.

A. Initial Exposure: The initial UVA exposures should be conducted according to the guidelines presented previously under DOSAGE AND ADMINISTRATION, B 1 and 2, PSORIASIS THERAPY, Drug dosage-initial Therapy and Exposure).

B. Clearing Phase: Specific recommendations for patient treatment are as follows:

1. Skin Types I, II, and III: Patients with skin types I, II, and III may be treated 2 or 3 times per week. UVA exposure may be held constant or increased by up to 1.0 Joule/cm²at each treatment, according to the patient's response. If erythema occurs, however, do not increase exposure time until erythema resolves. The severity and extent of the patient's erythema may be used to determine whether the next exposure should be shortened, omitted, or maintained at the previous dosage. See ADVERSE REACTIONS for additional information.

2. Skin Types IV, V, and VI: Patients with skin types IV, V and VI may be treated 2 or 3 times per week. UVA exposure may be held constant or increased by up to 1.5 Joules/cm²at each treatment unless erythema occurs. If erythema occurs, follow instructions outlined above in the procedures for patients with skin types I, II, and III.

3. Erythrodermic Psoriasis: Patients with erythrodermic psoriasis should be treated with special attention because pre-existing erythema may obscure observations of possible treatment-related phototoxic erythema. These patients may be treated 2 or 3 times per week, as a Type I patient.

4. Miscellaneous Situations

a. If there is no response after a total of 10 treatments, the exposure of UVA energy may be increased by an additional 0.5-1.0 Joules/cm² above the prior incremental increases for each treatment. (Example: a patient whose exposure dosage is being increased by 1.0 Joule/cm² may now have all subsequent doses increased by 1.5-2.0 Joules/cm².)

b. If there is no response, or only minimal response, after 15 treatments, the dosage of methoxsalen may be increased by 10 mg. (a one-time increase in dosage). This increased dosage may be continued for the remainder of the course of treatment but should not be exceeded.

c. If a patient misses a treatment, the UVA exposure time of the next treatment should not be increased. If more than one treatment is missed, reduce the exposure by 0.5 Joule/cm² for each treatment missed.

d. If the lower extremities are responding as well as the rest of the body and do not show erythema, cover all other body areas and give 25 percent of the present exposure dose as an additional exposure to the lower extremities. This additional exposure to the lower extremities should be terminated if erythema develops on these areas.

e. Non-responsive psoriasis: If a patient's generalized psoriasis is not responding, or if the condition appears to be worsening during treatment, the possibility of a generalized phototoxic reaction should be considered. This may be confirmed by the improvement of the condition following temporary discontinuance of this therapy for two weeks. If no improvement occurs during the interruption of treatment, this patient may be considered a treatment failure.

C. Alternative Exposure Schedule

As an alternative to increasing the UVA exposure at each treatment, the following schedule may be followed: this schedule may reduce the total number of Joules/cm²received by the patient over the entire course of therapy.

1. Incremental increases in UVA exposure for all patients may range from 0.5 to 1.5 Joules/cm²according to the patient's response to therapy.

2. Once Grade 2 clearing (see TABLE 8) has been reached and the patient is progressing adequately, UVA dosage is held constant. This dosage is maintained until Grade 4 clearing is reached.

3. If the rate of clearing significantly decreases, exposure dosage may be increased at each treatment (0.1-1.5 Joules/cm²) until Grade 3 clearing and a satisfactory progress rate is attained. The UVA exposure will be held constant again until Grade 4 clearing is attained. These increases may be used also if the rate of clearing significantly decreases between Grade 3 and Grade 4 response. However, the possibility of a phototoxic reaction should be considered; see Non-responsive Psoriasis, above.

DOSAGE AND ADMINISTRATION: *(cont'd)*

4. In summary, this schedule raises slightly the increments (Joules/cm^2) of UVA dosage, but limits these increases to those periods when the patient is not responding adequately. Otherwise the UVA exposure is held at the lowest effective dose.

D. Maintenance Phase

The goal of maintenance treatment is to keep the patient symptom-free as possible with the least amount of UVA exposure.

1. Schedule of Exposures: When patients have achieved 95 percent clearing or Grade 4 response (TABLE 8), they may be placed on the following maintenance schedules (M_1-M_4), in sequence. It is recommended that each maintenance schedule be adhered to for at least 2 treatments (unless erythema or psoriatic flare occurs, in which case see (2a) and (2b) below).

Maintenance Schedules

M_1 - once/week

M_2 - once/2 weeks

M_3 - once/3 weeks

M_4 - p.r.n. (*i.e.,* for flares)

2. Length Of Exposure: The UVA exposure for the first maintenance treatment of any schedule (except M_4 as noted below) is the same as that of the patient's last treatment under the previous schedule. For skin types I-IV however, it is recommended that the maximum UVA dosage during maintenance treatments not exceed those listed in TABLE 6.

TABLE 6

Skin Type	Joules/cm^2/treatment
I	12
II	14
III	18
IV	22

If the patient develops erythema or new lesions of psoriasis, proceed as follows:

a. Erythema: During maintenance therapy the patients's tan and threshold dose for erythema may gradually decrease. If maintenance treatments produce significant erythema, the exposure to UVA should be decreased by 25 percent until further treatments no longer produce erythema.

b. Psoriasis: If the patient develops new areas of psoriasis during maintenance therapy (but still is classified as having a Grade 4 response), the exposure to UVA may be increased by 0.5-1.5 Joules/cm^2 at each treatment, this is appropriate for all types of patients. These increases are continued until the psoriasis is brought under control and the patient is again clear. The exposure being administered when this clearing is reached should be used for further maintenance treatment.

3. Flares During Maintenance: If the patient flares during maintenance treatment (*i.e.* develops psoriasis on more than 5 percent of the originally involved areas of the body) his maintenance treatment schedule may be changed to the preceding maintenance or clearing schedule. The patient may be kept on his schedule until again 95 percent clear. If the original maintenance treatment schedule is unable to control the psoriasis, the schedule may be changed to a more frequent regimen. If a flare occurs less than 6 weeks after the last treatment, 25 percent of the maximum exposure received during the clearing phase may be used and proceed with the clearing schedule previously followed for this patient (At 95 percent clearing follow regular maintenance until the optimum maintenance schedule is determined for the patient). If more than 6 weeks have elapsed since the last treatment was given, treat patients as if they were beginning therapy insofar as exposure dosages are concerned, since their threshold for erythema may have decreased. (TABLE 7)

TABLE 7 Grades of Erythema

Grade	Erythema Level
0	No erythema
1	Minimally perceptible erythema - faint pink
2	Marked erythema but with no edema
3	Fiery erythema with edema
4	Fiery erythema with edema and blistering

TABLE 8 Response To Therapy

Grade	Criteria	Percent Improvement (compared to original extent of disease
-1	Psoriasis worse	0
0	No change	0
1	Minimal improvement - slightly less scale and/or erythema	5-20
2	Definite improvement - partial flattening of all plaques - less scaling and less erythema	20-50
3	Considerable improvement - nearly complete flattening of all plaques but borders of plaques still palpable	50-95
4	Clearing: complete flattening of plaques including borders; plaques may be outlined by pigmentation	95

TOPICAL

Oxsoralen Lotion is applied to a well-defined areas of vitiligo by the physician and the area is then exposed to a suitable source of UVA. Initial exposure time should be conservative and not exceed that which is predicted to be one-half the minimal erythema dose. Treatment intervals should be required by the erythema response. Treatment intervals should be regulated erythema response; generally once a week is recommended or less often depending on the results. The hands and fingers of the person applying the medication should be protected by gloves or finger cots to avoid photosensitizations and possible burns.

Pigmentation may begin after a few weeks but significant repigmentation may require 6 to 9 months of treatment. Periodic re-treatment may be necessary to retain all of the new pigment. Idiopathic vitiligo is reversible but not equally reversible in every patient. Treatment must be individualized. Repigmentation will vary in completeness, time of onset, and duration. Repigmentation occurs more rapidly in fleshy areas such as face, abdomen, and buttocks and less rapidly over less fleshy areas such as the dorsum of the hands or feet.

HOW SUPPLIED:

Oxsoralen-Ultra Capsules: Oxsoralen-Ultra Capsules, each containing 10 mg of methoxsalen (8-methoxypsoralen) in a soft gelatin capsules.

8-MOP Capsules: 8-MOP Capsules, each containing 10 mg, of methoxsalen (8-methoxalen).

HOW SUPPLIED: *(cont'd)*

Oxsoralen Lotion 1%: Oxsoralen Lotion containing 1% methoxsalen (8-methoxypsoralen). Store at controlled room temperature (15°- 30°C) 59°- 86°F.

HOW SUPPLIED - EQUIVALENTS NOT AVAILABLE:

Capsule, Gelatin - Oral - 10 mg

50's	**$219.69**	**OXSORALEN-ULTRA, ICN Pharms**	**00187-0650-42**
50's	$219.69	8-MOP, ICN Pharms	00187-0651-42

Lotion - Topical - 1 %

30 ml	**$88.75**	**OXSORALEN, ICN Pharms**	**00187-0402-31**

METHSCOPOLAMINE BROMIDE *(001776)*

CATEGORIES: Anticholinergic Agents; Antimuscarinics/Antispasmodics; Autonomic Drugs; Colitis; Constipation; Diarrhea; Diverticulitis; Duodenal Ulcer; Dysmenorrhea; Enteritis; Enterocolitis; Esophagitis; Gastrointestinal Drugs; Hernia; Hyperhidrosis; Irritable Bowel Syndrome; Pancreatitis; Peptic Ulcer; Spasm; Ulcerative Colitis; Migraine*; FDA Approval Pre 1982

* Indication not approved by the FDA

BRAND NAMES: **Pamine**

FORMULARIES: Medi-Cal

DESCRIPTION:

Methscopolamine bromide is an anticholinergic, which occurs as white crystals, or as a white odorless crystalline powder. Methscopolamine bromide melts at about 225° with decomposition. The drug is freely soluble in water, slightly soluble in alcohol, and insoluble in acetone and in chloroform.

The chemical name for methscopolamine bromide is 3-Oxa-9-azoniatricyclo [3.3 1.0^{2,4}]nonane 7-(3-hydroxy-1-oxo-2-phenylpropoxy)-9, 9-dimethyl-, bromide, [7(*S*)-)1α, 2β, 4β, 5α, 7β)]- and the molecular weight is 398.30.

Each Pamine tablet for oral administration contains 2.5 mg of methscopolamine bromide. Inactive ingredients: calcium stearate, cornstarch, lactose, mineral oil, sorbic acid, and sucrose.

CLINICAL PHARMACOLOGY:

Methscopolamine is an anticholinergic agent which possesses most of the pharmacologic actions of that drug class. These include reduction in volume and total acid content of gastric secretion, inhibition of gastrointestinal motility, inhibition of accommodation with resulting blurring vision. Large doses may result in tachycardia.

Pharmacokinetics: Methscopolamine bromide is a quaternary ammonium derivative of scopolamine. As a class, these agents are poorly and unreliably absorbed.[1,2] Total absorption of quaternary ammonium derivatives of the alkaloids in 10-25%. Rate absorption is not available. Quaternary ammonium salts have limited absorption from intact skin, an conjunctival penetration is poor.[1] Little is known of the fate and excretion of most of these agents.[1] Following oral administration, drug effects appear in about one hour and persist for 4 to 6 hours.[2] Methscopolamine bromide has limited ability to cross the blood-brain-barrier,[3,4,5] The drug is excreted primarily in the urine and bile, or as unabsorbed drug in feces.[2] There is no data on the presence of methscopolamine in breast milk; traces of atropine have been found after administration of atropine.[1]

INDICATIONS AND USAGE:

Adjunctive therapy for the treatment of peptic ulcer.

METHOSCOPOLAMINE BROMIDE HAS NOT BEEN SHOWN TO BE EFFECTIVE N CONTRIBUTING TO THE HEALING OF PEPTIC ULCER, DECREASING THE REATE OF RECURRENCE ORT PREVENTING COMPLICATIONS.

CONTRAINDICATIONS:

Glaucoma; obstructive uropathy (*e.g.,* bladder neck obstruction due to prostatic hypertrophy); obstructive disease of the gastrointestinal tract (*e.g.,* pyloroduodenal stenosis, etc.); paralytic ileus; intestinal atony of the elderly or debilitated patient; unstable cardiovascular status in acute hemorrhage; severe ulcerative colitis; toxic megacolon complicating ulcerative colitis; myasthenia gravis.

Pamine is contraindicated in patients who are hypersensitive to it or related drugs.

WARNINGS:

In the presence of high environmental temperature, heat prostration (fever and heat stroke due to decreased sweating) can occur with drug use.

Diarrhea may be an early symptom of incomplete intestinal obstruction, especially in patients with ileostomy or colostomy. In this instance treatment with this drug would inappropriate and possibly harmful.

Methscopolamine bromide may produce drowsiness or blurred vision. The patient should be cautioned regarding activities requiring mental alertness such as operating a motor vehicle of other machinery or performing hazardous work while taking this drug.

With overdosage, a curare-like action may occur, i.e., neuromuscular blockade leading to muscular weakness and possible paralysis.

PRECAUTIONS:

General: Use methscopolamine bromide with caution in the elderly and in all patients with: autonomic neuropathy; hepatic or renal disease; or ulcerative colitis-large doses mat suppress intestinal motility to the point of producing a paralytic ileus and for this reason precipitate or aggravate "toxic megacolon," a serious complication of the disease.

The drug also should be used with caution in patients having hyperthyroidism, coronary heart disease, congestive heart failure, tachyrhythmia, tachycardia, hypertension, or prostatic hypertrophy.

Information for the Patient: See statement under WARNINGS.

Laboratory Tests: Progress of the peptic ulcer under treatment should be followed by upper gastrointestinal contrast radiology or endoscopy to insure healing. Stool tests for occult blood and blood hemoglobin or hematocrit values should be followed to rule out bleeding from the ulcer.

Carcinogenesis, Mutagenesis, and Impairment of Fertility: No long-term studies in animals have been performed to evaluate carcinogenic potential.

Pregnancy, Teratogenic Effects, Pregnancy Category C: Animal reproduction studies have not been conducted with methscopolamine bromide. It also is not known whether methscopolamine bromide can cause fetal harm when administered to a pregnant woman or can affect reproduction capacity. Methscopolamine bromide should be given to a pregnant woman only if clearly needed.

PRECAUTIONS: *(cont'd)*

Nursing Mothers: It is not known whether this drug is excreted in human milk. Because many drugs are excreted in human milk, caution should be exercised when methscopolamine bromide is administered to a nursing woman.

Anticholinergic drugs may suppress lactation.

Pediatric Use: Safety and efficacy in children have not been established.

DRUG INTERACTIONS:

Additive anticholinergic effects may result from concomitant use with antipsychotics, tricyclic antidepressants, and other drugs with anticholinergic effects. Concomitant administration with antacids may interfere with the absorption of methscopolamine bromide.

ADVERSE REACTIONS:

The following adverse reactions have been observed, but there is not enough data to support an estimate of frequency.

Cardiovascular: Tachycardia, palpitation.

Allergic: Severe allergic reaction or drug idiosyncrasies including anaphylaxis.

CNS: Headaches, nervousness, mental confusion, drowsiness, dizziness.

Special Sense: Blurred vision, dilatation of the pupil, cycloplegia, increased ocular tension, loss of taste.

Renal: Urinary hesitancy and retention.

Gastrointestinal: Nausea, vomiting, constipation, bloated feeling.

Dermatologic: Decreased sweating, urticaria and other dermal manifestations.

Miscellaneous: Xerostomia, weakness, insomnia, impotence, suppression of lactation.

OVERDOSAGE:

The symptoms of overdosage with methscopolamine bromide progress from intensification of the usual side effects to CNS disturbances (from restlessness and excitement to psychotic behavior), Circulatory chances (flushing, fall in blood pressure, circulatory failure), respiratory failure, paralysis, and coma.

Measures to be taken are (1) induction of emesis and (2) injection of physostigmine 0.5 to 2 mg intravenously, and repeated as necessary up to a total of 5 mg. Fever may be treated symptomatically)alcohol sponging, ice packs). Excitement of a degree which demands attention may be managed with sodium thiopental 2% solution given slowly intravenously or chloral hydrate (100-200 ml of a 2% solution) by rectal infusion. In the event of progression of the curare-like effect to paralysis of the respiratory muscles, artificial respiration should be instituted and maintained until effective respiratory action returns.

The oral LD_{50} in rats is 1,352 to 2,617 mg/kg.

No data is available on the dialyzability of methscopolamine.

DOSAGE AND ADMINISTRATION:

The average dosage of methscopolamine bromide is 2.5 mg one-half hour before meals and 2.5 to 5 mg at bedtime. A starting dose of 12.5 mg daily will be clinically effective in most patients without the production of appreciable side effects.

Patients whose dosage has been reduced to eliminate or modify side effects often continue to show adequate response both subjectively in relief of symptoms and objectively as measured by antisecretory effects.

If the patient is having severe symptoms which demand prompt relief, the drug maybe started on a daily dosage of 20 mg, administered in doses of 5 mg one-half hour before meals and at bedtime. If very unpleasant side effects develop promptly, the daily dosage should be reduced. If neither symptomatic relief nor side effects appear, the daily dosage may be increased. Some patients have tolerated 30 mg daily with no unpleasant reactions.

The ultimate aim of therapy is to arrive at a dosage which provides maximal clinical effectiveness with a minimum of unpleasant side effects. Many patients report no side effects on a dosage which gives complete relief of symptoms. On the other hand, some patients have reported severe side effects without appreciable symptomatic relief. Such patients must be considered unsuited for this therapy. Usually they have been or will prove to be similarly intolerant to other anticholinergic drugs. If methscopolamine bromide is to be used in a patient who gives a history of such intolerance, it should be started at a low dosage.

REFERENCES:

1. The Pharmacological Basis of Therapeutics,Gilman and Goodman, MacMillan Publ. Co., New York, 6th Ed., 1980. 2. **American Hospital Formulary Service,** American Society of Hospital Pharmacists, Bethesda, Maryland. 3. Domino, E.F., Corasen, G.:Central and Peripheral Effects of Muscarinic Cholinergic Blocking Agents in Man.**Anesthesiology** 28:568-574 (1967). 4. Mogensen, L. and Orinius, E.:Arrhythmic Complications after Parasympathetic Treatment of Bradyarrhythmias in a Coronary Care Unit, **Acta Med. Scand.** 190:495-498 (1971). 5. Neeld, J.B., Jr., et al: Cardiac Rate and Rhythm Changes with Atropine and Methscopolamine, **Clin. Pharmacol. Ther.** 17(3):290-295 (March) 1975.

HOW SUPPLIED:

Pamine Tablets 2.5 mg are available as white, round tablets in the following package size:

Store at controlled room temperature 15°-30°C (59°-86°F).

HOW SUPPLIED - RATED THERAPEUTICALLY EQUIVALENT:

Tablet, Uncoated - Oral - 2.5 mg

100's	$30.80	PAMINE, Bradley Pharms	00482-0061-01

METHSUXIMIDE *(001777)*

CATEGORIES: Anticonvulsants; Central Nervous System Agents; Convulsions; Epilepsy; Neuromuscular; Seizures; Succinimide Anticonvulsants; FDA Approval Pre 1982

BRAND NAMES: **Celontin**; *Petinutin* (Germany)
(International brand names outside U.S. in italics)

FORMULARIES: Aetna; BC-BS; Medi-Cal; PCS

DESCRIPTION:

Methsuximide is an anticonvulsant succinimide, chemically designated as N,2-Dimethyl-2-phenylsuccinimide.

Each Celontin capsule contains 150 mg or 300 mg methsuximide, USP. Also contains starch, NF. The capsule and band contain citric acid, USP; colloidal silicon dioxide, NF; D&C yellow No. 10; FD&C red No. 3; FD&C yellow No. 6 (Sunset Yellow); gelatin, NF; glyceryl monooleate; sodium benzoate, NF; sodium lauryl sulfate, NF. The 150-mg capsule and band also contain FD&C blue No. 1; titanium dioxide, USP. The 300-mg capsule and band also contain polyethylene glycol 200.

CLINICAL PHARMACOLOGY:

Methsuximide suppresses the paroxysmal three cycle per second spike and wave activity associated with lapses of consciousness which is common in absence (petit mal) seizures. The frequency of epileptiform attacks is reduced, apparently by depression of the motor cortex and elevation of the threshold of the central nervous system to convulsive stimuli.

INDICATIONS AND USAGE:

Methsuximide is indicated for the control of absence (petit mal) seizures that are refractory to other drugs.

CONTRAINDICATIONS:

Methsuximide should not be used in patients with a history of hypersensitivity to succinimides.

WARNINGS:

Blood dyscrasias, including some with fatal outcome, have been reported to be associated with the use of succinimides; therefore, periodic blood counts should be performed. Should signs and/or symptoms of infection (*e.g.,* sore throat, fever) develop, blood counts should be considered at that point.

It has been reported that succinimides have produced morphological and functional changes in animal liver. For this reason, methsuximide should be administered with extreme caution to patients with known liver or renal disease. Periodic urinalysis and liver function studies are advised for all patients receiving the drug.

Cases of systemic lupus erythematosus have been reported with the use of succinimides. The physician should be alert to this possibility.

Usage in Pregnancy: Reports suggest an association between the use of anticonvulsant drugs by women with epilepsy and an elevated incidence of birth defects in children born to these women. Data are more extensive with respect to phenytoin and phenobarbital, but these are also the most commonly prescribed anticonvulsants; less systematic or anecdotal reports suggest a possible similar association with the use of all known anticonvulsant drugs.

The reports suggesting an elevated incidence of birth defects in children of drug-treated epileptic women cannot be regarded as adequate to prove a definite cause and effect relationship. There are intrinsic methodologic problems in obtaining adequate data on drug teratogenicity in humans; the possibility also exists that other factors, e.g. genetic factors or the epileptic condition itself, may be more important than drug therapy in leading to birth defects. The great majority of mothers on anticonvulsant medication deliver normal infants. It is important to note that anticonvulsant drugs should not be discontinued in patients in whom the drug is administered to prevent major seizures because of the strong possibility of precipitating status epilepticus with attendant hypoxia and threat to life. In individual cases where the severity and frequency of the seizure disorder are such that the removal of medication does not pose a serious threat to the patient, discontinuation of the drug may be considered prior to and during pregnancy, although it cannot be said with any confidence that even minor seizures do not pose some hazard to the developing embryo or fetus.

The prescribing physician will wish to weigh these considerations in treating or counseling epileptic women of childbearing potential.

PRECAUTIONS:

GENERAL

It is recommended that the physician withdraw the drug slowly on the appearance of unusual depression, aggressiveness, or other behavioral alterations.

As with other anticonvulsants, it is important to proceed slowly when increasing or decreasing dosage, as well as when adding or eliminating other medication. Abrupt withdrawal of anticonvulsant medication may precipitate absence (petit mal) status. Methsuximide, when used alone in mixed types of epilepsy, may increase the frequency of grand mal seizures in some patients.

INFORMATION FOR THE PATIENT

Methsuximide may impair the mental and/or physical abilities required for the performance of potentially hazardous tasks, such as driving a motor vehicle or other such activity requiring alertness, therefore, the patient should be cautioned accordingly.

Patients taking methsuximide should be advised of the importance of adhering strictly to the prescribed dosage regimen.

Patients should be instructed to promptly contact their physician if they develop signs and/or symptoms suggesting an infection (*e.g.,* sore throat, fever).

Advice To The Pharmacist And Patient: Since methsuximide has a relatively low melting temperature (124°F), storage conditions which may promote high temperatures (closed cars, delivery vans, or storage near steam pipes) should be avoided. Do not dispense or use capsules that are not full or in which contents have melted. Effectiveness may be reduced. Protect from excessive heat (104°F).

PREGNANCY

See WARNINGS.

DRUG INTERACTIONS:

Since methsuximide may interact with concurrently administered antiepileptic drugs, periodic serum level determinations of these drugs may be necessary (*e.g.,* methsuximide may increase the plasma concentrations of phenytoin and phenobarbital).

ADVERSE REACTIONS:

Gastrointestinal System: Gastrointestinal symptoms occur frequently and have included nausea or vomiting, anorexia, diarrhea, weight loss, epigastric and abdominal pain, and constipation.

Hemopoietic System: Hemopoietic complications associated with the administration of methsuximide have included eosinophilia, leukopenia, monocytosis and pancytopenia with or without bone marrow suppression.

Nervous System: Neurologic and sensory reactions reported during therapy with methsuximide have included drowsiness, ataxia or dizziness, irritability and nervousness, headache, blurred vision, photophobia, hiccups, and insomnia. Drowsiness, ataxia, and dizziness have been the most frequent side effects noted. Psychologic abnormalities have included confusion, instability, mental slowness, depression, hypochondriacal behavior, and aggressiveness. There have been rare reports of psychosis, suicidal behavior, and auditory hallucinations.

Integumentary System: Dermatologic manifestations which have occurred with the administration of methsuximide have included urticaria, Stevens-Johnson syndrome, and pruritic erythematous rashes.

Cardiovascular: Hyperemia.

Genitourinary System: Proteinuria, microscopic hematuria.

Body as a Whole: Periorbital edema.

OVERDOSAGE:

Acute overdoses may produce nausea, vomiting, and CNS depression including coma with respiratory depression. Methsuximide poisoning may follow a biphasic course. Following an initial comatose state, patients have awakened and then relapsed into a coma within 24 hours. It is believed that an active metabolite of methsuximide, N-desmethylmethsuximide, is responsible for this biphasic profile. It is important to follow plasma levels of N-desmethylmethsuximide in methsuximide poisonings. Levels greater than 40 mcg/ml have caused toxicity and coma has been seen at levels of 150 mcg/ml.

Treatment: Treatment should include emesis (unless the patient is or could rapidly become obtunded, comatose, or convulsing) or gastric lavage, activated charcoal, cathartics and general supportive measures. Charcoal hemoperfusion may be useful in removing the N-desmethyl metabolite of methsuximide. Forced diuresis and exchange transfusions are ineffective.

DOSAGE AND ADMINISTRATION:

Optimum dosage of methsuximide must be determined by trial. A suggested dosage schedule is 300 mg per day for the first week. If required, dosage may be increased thereafter at weekly intervals by 300 mg per day for the three weeks following to a daily dosage of 1.2 g. Because therapeutic effect and tolerance vary among patients, therapy with methsuximide must be individualized according to the response of each patient. Optimal dosage is that amount of methsuximide which is barely sufficient to control seizures so that side effects may be kept to a minimum. The smaller capsule (150 mg) facilitates administration to small children.

Methsuximide may be administered in combination with other anticonvulsants when other forms of epilepsy coexist with absence (petit mal).

Store at controlled room temperature 15-30° C (59-86° F).

Protect from light and moisture.

HOW SUPPLIED - EQUIVALENTS NOT AVAILABLE:

Capsule, Gelatin - Oral - 300 mg

100's	$73.92	CELONTIN, Parke-Davis	00071-0525-24

METHYCLOTHIAZIDE *(001778)*

CATEGORIES: Antihypertensives; Cardiovascular Drugs; Cirrhosis; Congestive Heart Failure; Diuretics; Edema; Electrolytic, Caloric-Water Balance; Glomerulonephritis; Heart Failure; Hypertension; Nephrotic Syndrome; Renal Drugs; Renal Failure; Thiazides; FDA Approval Pre 1982

BRAND NAMES: Aquatensen; **Enduron**; *Enduron-M*; Ethon; *Thiazidil*; *Urimor* *(International brand names outside U.S. in italics)*

FORMULARIES: Aetna; Medi-Cal

DESCRIPTION:

Methyclothiazide is a member of the benzothiadiazine (thiazide) class of drugs. It is an analogue of hydrochlorothiazide and occurs as a white to practically white crystalline powder which is basically odorless. Methyclothiazide is very slightly soluble in water and chloroform, and slightly soluble in alcohol. Chemically, methyclothiazide is represented as 6-chloro-3-(chloromethyl)-3,4-dihydro-2-methyl-2H-1,2,4-benzothiadiazine-7-sulfonamide 1,1-dioxide.

Clinically, methyclothiazide is an oral diuretic-antihypertensive agent. Enduron tablets are available in two dosage strengths containing 2.5 mg and 5 mg of methyclothiazide.

Enduron Inactive Ingredients: *2.5 mg tablets:* corn starch, FD&C Yellow No. 6, lactose, magnesium stearate and talc. *5 mg Tablets:* corn starch, D&C Red No. 36, lactose, magnesium stearate and talc.

CLINICAL PHARMACOLOGY:

The diuretic and saluretic effects of methyclothiazide result from a drug-induced inhibition of the renal tubular reabsorption of electrolytes. The excretion of sodium and chloride is greatly enhanced. Potassium excretion is also enhanced to a variable degree, as it is with the other thiazides. Although urinary excretion of bicarbonate is increased slightly, there is usually no significant change in urinary pH. Methyclothiazide has a per mg natriuretic activity approximately 100 times that of the prototype thiazide, chlorothiazide. At maximal therapeutic dosages, all thiazides are approximately equal in their diuretic/natriuretic effects.

There is significant natriuresis and diuresis within two hours after administration of a single dose of methyclothiazide. These effects reach a peak in about six hours and persist for 24 hours following oral administration of a single dose.

Like other benzothiadiazines, methyclothiazide also has antihypertensive properties, and may be used for this purpose either alone or to enhance the antihypertensive action of other drugs. The mechanism by which the benzothiadiazines, including methyclothiazide, produce a reduction of elevated blood pressure is not known. However, sodium depletion appears to be involved.

Methyclothiazide is rapidly absorbed and slowly eliminated by the kidneys as intact drug but primarily as an inactive metabolite. Additional information on the pharmacokinetics is not known at this time.

INDICATIONS AND USAGE:

Enduron (methyclothiazide) is indicated in the management of hypertension either as the sole therapeutic agent or to enhance the effect of other antihypertensive drugs in the more severe forms of hypertension.

Enduron tablets are indicated as adjunctive therapy in edema associated with congestive heart failure, hepatic cirrhosis, and corticosteroid and estrogen therapy.

Enduron tablets have also been found useful in edema due to various forms of renal dysfunction such as the nephrotic syndrome, acute glomerulonephritis, and chronic renal failure.

Usage in Pregnancy: The routine use of diuretics in an otherwise healthy pregnant woman is inappropriate and exposes mother and fetus to unnecessary hazard. Diuretics do not prevent development of toxemia of pregnancy, and there is no satisfactory evidence that they are useful in the treatment of developed toxemia.

Edema during pregnancy may arise from pathological causes or from the physiological and mechanical consequences of pregnancy. Thiazides are indicated in pregnancy when edema is due to pathologic causes, just as they are in the absence of pregnancy (see PRECAUTIONS, Pregnancy). Dependent edema in pregnancy, resulting from restriction of venous return by the expanded uterus, is properly treated through elevation of the lower extremities and use of support hose; use of diuretics to lower intravascular volume in this case is illogical and unnecessary. There is hypervolemia during normal pregnancy that is harmful to neither the fetus nor the mother (in the absence of cardiovascular disease), but that is associated with edema, including generalized edema, in the majority of pregnant women. If this edema produces discomfort, increased recumbency will often provide relief. In rare instances, this edema may cause extreme discomfort which is not relieved by rest. In these cases, a short course of diuretics may provide relief and may be appropriate.

CONTRAINDICATIONS:

Methyclothiazide is contraindicated in patients with anuria and in patients with a history of hypersensitivity to this compound or other sulfonamide-derived drugs.

WARNINGS:

Methyclothiazide shares with other thiazides the propensity to deplete potassium reserves to an unpredictable degree.

There have been isolated reports that certain nonedematous individuals developed severe fluid and electrolyte derangements after only brief exposure to normal doses of thiazide and non-thiazide diuretics.

Thiazides should be used with caution in patients with renal disease or significant impairment of renal function, since azotemia may be precipitated and cumulative drug effects may occur.

Thiazides should be used with caution in patients with impaired hepatic function or progressive liver disease, since minor alterations of fluid and electrolyte imbalance may precipitate hepatic coma.

Sensitivity reactions may occur in patients with a history of allergy or bronchial asthma.

The possibility of exacerbation or activation of systemic lupus erythematosus has been reported.

Hyperuricemia may occur or frank gout may be precipitated in certain patients receiving thiazide therapy.

PRECAUTIONS:

GENERAL

All patients should be observed for clinical signs of electrolyte imbalances such as dryness of mouth, thirst, weakness, lethargy, drowsiness, restlessness, muscle pains or cramps, muscular fatigue, hypotension, oliguria, tachycardia, and gastrointestinal disturbances such as nausea and vomiting.

Hypokalemia may develop, especially with brisk diuresis, when severe cirrhosis is present, during concomitant use of corticosteroids or ACTH, or after prolonged therapy.

Interference with adequate oral electrolyte intake will also contribute to hypokalemia. Hypokalemia may be avoided or treated by use of potassium supplements or foods with a high potassium content.

Any chloride deficit is generally mild and usually does not require specific treatment except under extraordinary circumstances (as in liver disease or renal disease). Dilutional hyponatremia may occur in edematous patients in hot weather; appropriate therapy is water restriction rather than administration of salt, except in rare instances when the hyponatremia is life threatening. In actual salt depletion, appropriate replacement is the therapy of choice.

Latent diabetes mellitus may become manifest during thiazide administration.

The antihypertensive effects of the drug may be enhanced in the postsympathectomy patient.

If progressive renal impairment becomes evident as indicated by a rising nonprotein nitrogen or blood urea nitrogen, a careful reappraisal of therapy is necessary with consideration given to withholding or discontinuing diuretic therapy.

Thiazides may decrease urinary calcium excretion. Thiazides may cause intermittent and slight elevation of serum calcium in the absence of known disorders of calcium metabolism. Marked hypercalcemia may be evidence of hidden hyperparathyroidism. Thiazides should be discontinued before carrying out tests for parathyroid function.

Thiazides may cause increased concentrations of total serum cholesterol, total triglycerides, and low-density lipoproteins in some patients. Use thiazides with caution in patients with moderate or high cholesterol concentrations and in patients with elevated triglyceride levels.

INFORMATION FOR THE PATIENT

Patients should inform their doctor if they have: 1) had an allergic reaction to methyclothiazide or other diuretics 2) asthma 3) kidney disease 4) liver disease 5) gout 6) systemic lupus erythematosus, or 7) been taking other drugs such as cortisone, digitalis, lithium carbonate, or drugs for diabetes.

The physician should inform patients of possible side effects and caution the patient to report any of the following symptoms of electrolyte imbalance; dryness of the mouth, thirst, weakness, tiredness, drowsiness, restlessness, muscle pains or cramps, nausea, vomiting or increased heart rate.

The physician should advise the patient to take this medication every day as directed. Physicians should also caution patients that drinking alcohol can increase the chance of dizziness.

LABORATORY TESTS

Initial and periodic determinations of serum electrolytes should be performed at appropriate intervals for the purpose of detecting possible electrolyte imbalances such as hyponatremia, hypochloremic alkalosis, and hypokalemia. Serum and urine electrolyte determinations are particularly important when a patient is vomiting excessively or receiving parenteral fluids.

DRUG/LABORATORY TEST INTERACTIONS

Thiazides may decrease serum PBI levels without signs of thyroid disturbance.

Thiazides should be discontinued before carrying out tests for parathyroid function.

CARCINOGENESIS, MUTAGENESIS, AND IMPAIRMENT OF FERTILITY

No data are available concerning the potential for carcinogenicity or mutagenicity in animals or humans. Methyclothiazide did not impair fertility in rats receiving up to 4 mg/kg/day (at least 20 times the maximum recommended human dose of 10 mg, assuming patient weight equal to or greater than 50 kg).

PREGNANCY CATEGORY B

Teratogenic Effects: Reproduction studies performed in rats and rabbits at doses up to 4 mg/kg/day have revealed no evidence of harm to the fetus due to methyclothiazide. There are, however, no adequate and well-controlled studies in pregnant women. Because animal reproduction studies are not always predictive of human response, this drug should be used during pregnancy only if clearly needed.

Nonteratogenic Effects: Thiazides cross the placental barrier and appear in cord blood. The use of thiazides in pregnant women requires that the anticipated benefit be weighed against possible hazards to the fetus. These hazards include fetal or neonatal jaundice, thrombocytopenia and possible other adverse reactions that have occurred in the adult.

NURSING MOTHERS

Thiazides are excreted in breast milk. Because of the potential for serious adverse reactions in nursing infants, a decision should be made whether to discontinue nursing or to discontinue the drug taking into account the importance of the drug to the mother.

PEDIATRIC USE

Safety and effectiveness in children have not been established.

DRUG INTERACTIONS:

Hypokalemia can sensitize or exaggerate the response of the heart to the toxic effects of *digitalis* (*e.g.,* increased ventricular irritability).

Hypokalemia may develop during concomitant use of *steroids* or*ACTH*.

Insulin requirements in diabetic patients may be increased, decreased, or unchanged.

Thiazides may decrease arterial responsiveness to *norepinephrine*. This diminution is not sufficient to preclude effectiveness of the pressor agent for therapeutic use.

Thiazide drugs may increase the responsiveness to *tubocurarine*.

Lithium renal clearance is reduced by thiazides, increasing the risk of lithium toxicity.

Thiazides may add to or potentiate the action of *other antihypertensive drugs*. Potentiation occurs with ganglionic or peripheral adrenergic blocking drugs.

ADVERSE REACTIONS:

Adverse reactions are usually reversible upon reduction of dosage or discontinuation of Enduron tablets. Whenever adverse reactions are moderate or severe, it may be necessary to discontinue the drug.

The following adverse reactions have been observed, but there have not been enough systematic collection of data to support an estimate of their frequency. Consequently the reactions are categorized by organ system and are listed in decreasing order of severity and not frequency.

Body as a Whole: Headache, cramping, weakness.

Cardiovascular System: Orthostatic hypotension (may be potentiated by alcohol, barbiturates, or narcotics).

Digestive System: Pancreatitis, jaundice (intrahepatic cholestatic), sialadenitis, vomiting, diarrhea, nausea, gastric irritation, constipation, anorexia.

Hemic and Lymphatic System: Aplastic anemia, hemolytic anemia, agranulocytosis, leukopenia, thrombocytopenia.

Hypersensitivity Reactions: Anaphylactic reactions, necrotizing angiitis (vasculitis, cutaneous vasculitis), Stevens-Johnson syndrome, respiratory distress including pneumonitis and pulmonary edema, fever, purpura, urticaria, rash, photosensitivity.

Metabolic and Nutritional Disorders: Hyperglycemia, hyperuricemia, electrolyte imbalance (see PRECAUTIONS), hypercalcemia.

Nervous System: Vertigo, dizziness, paresthesias, muscle spasms, restlessness.

Special Senses: Transient blurred vision, xanthopsia.

Urogenital System: Glycosuria.

OVERDOSAGE:

Symptoms of overdosage include electrolyte imbalance and signs of potassium deficiency such as confusion, dizziness, muscular weakness, and gastrointestinal disturbances. General supportive measures including replacement of fluids and electrolytes may be indicated in treatment of overdosage.

DOSAGE AND ADMINISTRATION:

Enduron (methyclothiazide) is administered orally. Therapy should be individualized according to patient response. This therapy should be titrated to gain maximal therapeutic response as well as the minimal dose possible to maintain that therapeutic response.

For edematous conditions: The usual adult dose ranges from 2.5 to 10 mg once daily. Maximum effective single dose is 10 mg; larger single doses do not accomplish greater diuresis, and are not recommended.

For the treatment of hypertension: The usual Adult dose ranges from 2.5 to 5 mg once daily.

If control of blood pressure is not satisfactory after 8 to 12 weeks of therapy with 5 mg once daily, another antihypertensive drug should be added. Increasing the dosage of methyclothiazide will usually not result in further lowering of blood pressure.

Methyclothiazide may be either employed alone for mild to moderate hypertension or concurrently with other hypertensive drugs in the management of more severe forms of hypertension. Combined therapy may provide adequate control of hypertension with lower dosage of the component drugs and fewer or less severe side effects. An enhanced response frequently follows its concurrent administration with Harmonyl (deserpidine) so that dosage of both drugs may be reduced.

When other antihypertensive agents are to be added to the regimen, this should be accomplished gradually. Ganglionic blocking agents should be given at only half the usual dose since their effect is potentiated by pretreatment with Enduron tablets.

Recommended storage: Store below 86°F (30°C).

HOW SUPPLIED - RATED THERAPEUTICALLY EQUIVALENT:

Tablet, Uncoated - Oral - 2.5 mg

100's	$8.00	Methyclothiazide, United Res	00677-0767-01
100's	$8.25	Methyclothiazide, Zenith Labs	00172-2986-60
100's	$8.72	Methyclothiazide, H.C.F.A. F F P	99999-1778-01
100's	$9.70	Methyclothiazide, Geneva Pharms	00781-1803-01
100's	$9.75	Methyclothiazide, Harber Pharm	51432-0289-03
100's	**$41.44**	**ENDURON, Abbott**	**00074-6827-01**
500's	$43.60	Methyclothiazide, H.C.F.A. F F P	99999-1778-02
1000's	$78.38	Methyclothiazide, Zenith Labs	00172-2986-80
1000's	$87.20	Methyclothiazide, H.C.F.A. F F P	99999-1778-03

Tablet, Uncoated - Oral - 5 mg

100's	$5.31	Methyclothiazide, H.C.F.A. F F P	99999-1778-04
100's	$7.45	Methyclothiazide, Aligen Independ	00405-4646-01
100's	$8.50	Methyclothiazide, United Res	00677-0768-01
100's	$8.90	Methyclothiazide, HL Moore Drug Exch	00839-6581-06
100's	$9.98	Methyclothiazide, HL Moore Drug Exch	00839-7938-06
100's	$12.83	Methyclothiazide, Geneva Pharms	00781-1810-01
100's	$12.95	Methyclothiazide, Mylan	00378-0160-01
100's	$19.06	Methyclothiazide, Rugby	00536-4025-01
100's	**$54.83**	**ENDURON, Abbott**	**00074-6812-01**
100's	**$56.61**	**ENDURON, Abbott**	**00074-6812-10**
100's	$114.94	AQUATENSEN, Wallace Labs	00037-0153-92
500's	$26.55	Methyclothiazide, H.C.F.A. F F P	99999-1778-05
500's	$494.81	AQUATENSEN, Wallace Labs	00037-0153-96
1000's	$53.10	Methyclothiazide, H.C.F.A. F F P	99999-1778-06
1000's	$68.00	Methyclothiazide11, United Res	00677-0768-10
1000's	$68.69	Methyclothiazide, Rugby	00536-4041-10
1000's	**$531.82**	**ENDURON, Abbott**	**00074-6812-02**
4500's	$238.95	Methyclothiazide, H.C.F.A. F F P	99999-1778-07
4500's	$4264.52	AQUATENSIN, Wallace Labs	00037-0153-99

METHYCLOTHIAZIDE; RESERPINE *(001780)*

CATEGORIES: Antihypertensives; Cardiovascular Drugs; Diuretics; Hypertension; Renal Drugs; Thiazides; FDA Approval Pre 1982

BRAND NAMES: **Diutensen-R**

DESCRIPTION:

Diutensen-R is a two-component system of active ingredients containing 2.5 mg methyclothiazide and 0.1 mg reserpine per tablet. Diutensen-R thus provides for easier titration of hypersensitive patients than does a three-component system. Diutensen-R tablets are round, white, pink- mottled tablets. NOTE:DIUTENSEN-R previously contained cryptenamine tannate as a third antihypertensive agent.

FOR COMPLETE PRESCRIBING INFORMATION, REFER TO THE INDIVIDUAL DRUG MONOGRAPHS (METHYCLOTHIAZIDE; RESERPINE).

INDICATIONS AND USAGE:

Hypertension.

DOSAGE AND ADMINISTRATION:

As determined by individual titration. The usual adult dosage of Diutensen-R is 1 to 4 tablets a day depending on the individual patient response.

HOW SUPPLIED - EQUIVALENTS NOT AVAILABLE:

Tablet, Uncoated - Oral - 2.5 mg/0.1 mg

100's	**$244.97**	**DIUTENSEN-R, Wallace Labs**	**00037-0274-92**
500's	**$1185.41**	**DIUTENSEN-R, Wallace Labs**	**00037-0274-96**
5000's	**$9793.80**	**Diutensen-R, Wallace Labs**	**00037-0274-99**

METHYLCELLULOSE *(001785)*

CATEGORIES: Autonomic Drugs; Pharmaceutical Adjuvants; Sympathomimetic Agents; FDA Pre 1938 Drugs

BRAND NAMES: *Bulk*; Carbopol 940; *Muciplasma*; Trolamine
(International brand names outside U.S. in italics)

Prescribing information not available at time of publication.

METHYLDOPA *(001787)*

CATEGORIES: Antihypertensives; Cardiovascular Drugs; Central Nervous System Agents; Hypertension; Renal Drugs; Pregnancy Category B; FDA Approval Pre 1982

BRAND NAMES: **Aldomet**; *Aldomet-Forte*; *Aldomet-M*; *Aldometil*; *Aldomin*; *Aldomine*; *Aldopa*; *Alfametildopa*; *Alfametildopa Gen-Far*; *Alphadopa*; *Apo-Methyldopa* (Canada); *Becanta* (Japan); *Densul* (Japan); *Dimal*; *Dopagyt*; *Dopamet* (England, Canada); *Dopasan*; *Dopasian*; *Dopatens*; *Dopegyt*; *Elanpres*; *Emdopa*; *Equibar* (France); *Grospisk* (Japan); *H.G. Metil Dopa*; *Highprepin*; *Hydopa*; *Hypermet*; *Hypolag*; *Hypoten*; *Hy-po-tone*; *L-Domex*; *Lowten* (Mexico); *Medimet*; *Medomet*; *Medopa* (Japan); *Medopal* (Mexico); *Medopren*; *Medoten*; *Meldopa*; *Methopa*; *Metildopa McKesson*; *Methoplain* (Japan); Methyldopate HCl; *Methyldopum*; *Modepres*; *Mopatil* (Mexico); *Novomedopa* (Canada); *Polinal* (Japan); *Presinol* (Germany); *Presinol 500* (Germany); *Presnor*; *Prodop*; *Prodopa*; *Pulsoton* (Mexico); *Scandopa*; *Sembrina*; *Servidopa*; *Siamdopa*; *Sinepress*; *Tensipas*; *Tensodopa*; *Tildopan* (Japan)
(International brand names outside U.S. in italics)

FORMULARIES: Aetna; BC-BS; CIGNA; FHP; Humana; Kaiser; Medco; Medi-Cal; PCS; PruCare; United; WHO

COST OF THERAPY: $49.27 (Hypertension; Tablet; 250 mg; 2/day; 365 days)

PRIMARY ICD9: 401.1 (Essential Hypertension, Benign)

DESCRIPTION:

Methyldopa is an antihypertensive drug.

Methyldopa, the *L*-isomer of alpha-methyldopa, is levo-3-(3, 4-dihydroxyphenyl)-2-methylalanine. Its empirical formula is $C_{10}H_{13}NO_4$, with a molecular weight of 211.22.

Methyldopa is a white to yellowish white, odorless fine powder, and is soluble in water.

Aldomet is supplied as tablets, for oral use, in three strengths: 125 mg, 250 mg, or 500 mg of methyldopa per tablet. Inactive ingredients in the tablets are: calcium disodium edetate, cellulose, citric acid, colloidal silicon dioxide, D&C Yellow 10, ethylcellulose, guar gum, hydroxypropyl methylcellulose, iron oxide, magnesium stearate, propylene glycol, talc, and titanium dioxide.

Aldomet Oral Suspension is supplied as a white to off-white preparation; each 5 ml contains 250 mg of methyldopa and alcohol 1 percent, with benzoic acid 0.1 percent and sodium bisulfite 0.2 percent added as preservatives. Inactive ingredients in the oral suspension are: artificial and natural flavors, cellulose, citric acid, confectioner's sugar, disodium edetate, glycerin, polysorbate, purified water, and sodium carboxymethylcellulose.

Injection Ester HCl (Methyldopate HCl) is an antihypertensive agent for intravenous use. Methyldopate HCl (levo-3-(3, 4-dihydroxyphenyl)-2-methylalanine, ethyl ester hydrochloride) is the ethyl ester of methyldopa, supplied as the HCl salt with a molecular weight of 275.73. Methyldopate HCl is more soluble and stable in solution than methyldopa and is the preferred form for IV use. The empirical formula for methyldopate HCl is $C_{12}H_{16}NO_4 \cdot HCl$.

Injectable Ester HCl is supplied as a sterile solution in 5 ml vials each of which contains Methyldopate HCl (250.0 mg). The inactive ingredients are: citric acid anhydrous (25.0 mg), disodium edetate (2.5 mg), monothioglycerol (10.0 mg), sodium hydroxide to adjust pH. Water for Injection, q.s. to 5 ml, methylparaben 7.5 mg, propylparaben 1 mg, and sodium bisulfite 16 mg added as preservatives.

CLINICAL PHARMACOLOGY:

Methyldopa is an aromatic-amino-acid decarboxylase inhibitor in animals and in man. Although the mechanism of action has yet to be conclusively demonstrated, the antihypertensive effect of methyldopa probably is due to its metabolism to alpha-methylnorepinephrine, which then lowers arterial pressure by stimulation of central inhibitory alpha-adrenergic receptors, false neurotransmission, and/or reduction of plasma renin activity. Methyldopa has been shown to cause a net reduction in the tissue concentration of serotonin, dopamine, norepinephrine, and epinephrine.

CLINICAL PHARMACOLOGY: *(cont'd)*

Only methyldopa, the *L*-isomer of alpha-methyldopa, has the ability to inhibit dopa decarboxylase and to deplete animal tissues of norepinephrine. In man the antihypertensive activity appears to be due solely to the *L*-isomer. About twice the dose of the racemate (*DL*-alpha-methyldopa) is required for equal antihypertensive effect.

Methyldopa has no direct effect on cardiac function and usually does not reduce glomerular filtration rate, renal blood flow, or filtration fraction. Cardiac output usually is maintained without cardiac acceleration. In some patients the heart rate is slowed.

Normal or elevated plasma renin activity may decrease in the course of methyldopa therapy.

Methyldopa reduces both supine and standing blood pressure. Methyldopa usually produces highly effective lowering of the supine pressure with infrequent symptomatic postural hypotension. Exercise hypotension and diurnal blood pressure variations rarely occur.

PHARMACOKINETICS AND METABOLISM

The maximum decrease in blood pressure occurs four to six hours after oral dosage. Once an effective dosage level is attained, a smooth blood pressure response occurs in most patients in 12 to 24 hours. After withdrawal, blood pressure usually returns to pretreatment levels within 24-48 hours.

Methyldopa is extensively metabolized. The known urinary metabolites are: α-methyldopa mono-O-sulfate; 3-0 methyl-α-methyldopa; 3, 4-dihydroxyphenylacetone; α-methyldopamine; 3-0-methyl-α-methyldopamine and their conjugates.

Approximately 70% of the drug which is absorbed is excreted in the urine as methyldopa and its mono-O-sulfate conjugate. The renal clearance is about 130 ml/min in normal subjects and is diminished in renal insufficiency. The plasma half-life of methyldopa is 105 minutes. After oral doses, excretion is essentially complete in 36 hours.

Methyldopa crosses the placental barrier, appears in cord blood, and appears in breast milk.

INDICATIONS AND USAGE:

Tablets And Oral Suspension: Hypertension.

Injection: Hypertension, when parenteral medication is indicated.

The treatment of hypertensive crises may be initiated with injection Methyldopate Ester HCl.

CONTRAINDICATIONS:

Active hepatic disease, such as acute hepatitis and active cirrhosis.

If previous methyldopa therapy has been associated with liver disorders(see WARNINGS.)

Hypersensitivity to any component of these products, including sulfites contained in Oral Suspension Methyldopa and Injection Methyldopate HCl (see WARNINGS.) Methyldopa Tablets do not contain sulfites.

WARNINGS:

It is important to recognize that a positive Coombs test hemolytic anemia, and liver disorders may occur with methyldopa therapy. The rare occurrences of hemolytic anemia of liver disorders could lead to potentially fatal complication unless properly recognized and managed. Read this section carefully to understand these reactions.

With prolonged methyldopa therapy, 10 to 20 percent of patients develop a positive direct Coombs test which usually occurs between 6 and 12 months of methyldopa therapy. Lowest incidence is at daily dosage of 1 g or less. This on rare occasions may be associated with hemolytic anemia, which could lead to potentially fatal complications. One cannot predict which patients with a positive direct Coombs test may develop hemolytic anemia.

Prior existence or development of a positive direct Coombs test is not in itself a contraindication to use of methyldopa. If a positive Coombs test develops during methyldopa therapy, the physician should determine whether hemolytic anemia exists and whether the positive Coombs test may be a problem. For example, in addition to a positive direct Coombs test there is less often a positive indirect Coombs test which may interfere with cross matching of blood.

Before treatment is started, it is desirable to do a blood count (hematocrit, hemoglobin, or red cell count) for a baseline or to establish whether there is anemia. Periodic blood counts should be done during therapy to detect hemolytic anemia. It may be useful to do a direct Coombs test before therapy and at 6 and 12 months after the start of therapy.

If Coombs-positive hemolytic anemia occurs, the cause may be methyldopa and the drug should be discontinued. Usually the anemia remits promptly. If not, corticosteroids may be given and other causes of anemia should be considered. If the hemolytic anemia is related to methyldopa, the drug should not be reinstituted.

When methyldopa causes Coombs positivity alone or with hemolytic anemia, the red cell is usually coated with gamma globulin of the lgG (gamma G) class only. The positive Coombs test may not revert to normal until weeks to months after methyldopa is stopped.

Should the need for transfusion arise in a patient receiving methyldopa, both a direct and an indirect Coombs test should be performed. In the absence of hemolytic anemia, usually only the direct Coombs test will be positive. A positive direct Coombs test alone will not interfere with typing or cross matching. If the indirect Coombs test is also positive, problems may arise in the major cross match and the assistance of a hematologist or transfusion expert will be needed.

Occasionally, fever has occurred within the first 3 weeks of methyldopa therapy, associated in some cases with eosinophilia or abnormalities in one or more liver function tests, such as serum alkaline phosphatase, serum transaminases (SGOT, SGPT), bilirubin, and prothrombin time. Jaundice, with or without fever, may occur with onset usually within the first 2 to 3 months of therapy. In some patients the findings are consistent with those of cholestasis. In others the findings are consistent with hepatitis and hepatocellular injury.

Rarely, fatal hepatic necrosis has been reported after use of methyldopa. These hepatic changes may represent hypersensitivity reactions. Periodic determinations of hepatic function should be done particularly during the first 6 to 12 weeks of therapy or whenever an unexplained fever occurs. If fever, abnormalities in liver function tests, or jaundice appear, stop therapy with methyldopa. If caused by methyldopa, the temperature and abnormalities in liver function characteristically have reverted to normal when the drug was discontinued. Methyldopa should not be reinstituted in such patients.

Rarely, a reversible reduction of the white blood cell count with a primary effect on the granulocytes has been seen. The granulocyte count returned promptly to normal on discontinuance of the drug. Rare cases of granulocytopenia have been reported. In each instance, upon stopping the drug, the white cell count returned to normal. Reversible thrombocytopenia has occurred rarely.

Oral Suspension Methyldopa and Injection Methyldopate HCl (but not Methyldopa Tablets) contain sodium bisulfite, a sulfite that may cause allergic-type reactions including anaphylactic symptoms and life-threatening or less severe asthmatic episodes in certain susceptible people. The overall prevalence of sulfite sensitivity in the general population is unknown and probably low. Sulfite sensitivity is seen more frequently in asthmatic than in nonasthmatic people.

PRECAUTIONS:

GENERAL

Methyldopa should be used with caution in patients with a history of previous liver disease or dysfunction (see WARNINGS.)

Some patients taking methyldopa experience clinical edema or weight gain which may be controlled by use of a diuretic. Methyldopa should not be continued if edema progresses or signs of heart failure appear.

Hypertension has recurred occasionally after dialysis in patients given methyldopa because the drug is removed by this procedure.

Rarely involuntary choreoathetotic movements have been observed during therapy with methyldopa in patients with severe bilateral cerebrovascular disease. Should these movements occur, stop therapy.

LABORATORY TESTS

Blood count, Coombs test, and liver function tests are recommended before initiating therapy and at periodic intervals (see WARNINGS.)

DRUG/LABORATORY TEST INTERACTIONS

Methyldopa may interfere with measurement of: urinary uric acid by the phosphotungstate method, serum creatinine by the alkaline picrate method, and SGOT by colorimetric methods. Interference with spectrophotometric methods for SGOT analysis has not been reported.

Since methyldopa causes fluorescence in urine samples at the same wave lengths as catecholamines, falsely high levels of urinary catecholamines may be reported. This will interfere with the diagnosis of pheochromocytoma. It is important to recognize this phenomenon before a patient with a possible pheochromocytoma is subjected to surgery. Methyldopa does not interfere with measurement of VMA (vanillylmandelic acid), a test for pheochromocytoma, by those methods which convert VMA to vanillin. Methyldopa is not recommended for the treatment of patients with pheochromocytoma. Rarely, when urine is exposed to air after voiding, it may darken because of breakdown of methyldopa or its metabolites.

CARCINOGENESIS, MUTAGENESIS, AND IMPAIRMENT OF FERTILITY

No evidence of a tumorigenic effect was seen when methyldopa was given for two years to mice at doses up to 1800 mg/kg/day or to rats at doses up to 240 mg/kg/day (30 and 4 times the maximum recommended human dose in mice and rats, respectively, when compared on the basis of body weight; 2.5 and 0.6 times the maximum recommended human dose in mice and rats, respectively, when compared on the basis of body surface area; calculations assume a patient weight of 50 kg).

Methyldopa was not mutagenic in the Ames Test and did not increase chromosomal aberration or sister chromatid exchanges in Chinese hamster ovary cells. These *in vitro* studies were carried out both with and without exogenous metabolic activation.

Fertility was unaffected when methyldopa was given to male and female rats at 100 mg/kg/day (1.7 times the maximum daily human dose when compared on the basis of body weight; 0.2 times the maximum daily human dose when compared on the basis of body surface area). Methyldopa decreased sperm count, sperm motility, the number of late spermatids and the male fertility index when given to male rats at 200 and 400 mg/kg/day (3.3 and 6.7 times the maximum daily human dose when compared on the basis of body weight; 0.5 and 1 times the maximum daily human dose when compared on the basis of body surface area).

Long-term studies in animals have not been performed to evaluate the carcinogenic potential of methyldopate hydrochloride; nor have evaluations of this ester's mutagenic potential or potential to affect fertility been carried.

PREGNANCY

Reproduction studies performed with methyldopa at doses up to 1000 mg/kg/day in mice, 200 mg/kg in rabbits and 100 mg/kg in rats revealed no evidence of harm to the fetus. These doses are 16.6 times, 3.3 times and 1.7 times, respectively, the maximum daily human dose when compared on the basis of body weight; 1.4 times, 1.1 times and 0.2 times, respectively, when compared on the basis of body surface area; calculations assume a patient weight of 50 kg. There are, however, no adequate and well-controlled studies in pregnant women in the first trimester of pregnancy. Because animal reproduction studies are not always predictive of human response, Methyldopa should be used during pregnancy only if clearly needed.

Published reports of the use of methyldopa during all trimesters indicate that if this drug is used during pregnancy the possibility of fetal harm appears remote. In five studies, three of which were controlled, involving 332 pregnant hypertensive women, treatment with Methyldopa was associated with an improved fetal outcome. The majority of these women were in the third trimester when methyldopa therapy was begun.

In one study, women who had begun methyldopa treatment between weeks 16 and 20 of pregnancy gave birth to infants whose average head circumference was reduced by a small amount (34.2 ± 1.7 cm vs. 34.6 ± 1.3 cm (mean ± 1 S.D.)). Long-term follow up of 195 (97.5%) of the children born to methyldopa-treated pregnant women (including those who began treatment between weeks 16 and 20) failed to uncover any significant adverse effect on the children. At four years of age, the developmental delay commonly seen in children born to hypertensive mothers was less evident in those whose mothers were treated with methyldopa during pregnancy than those whose mothers were untreated. The children of the treated group scored consistently higher than the children of the untreated group on five major indices of intellectual and motor development. At age seven and one-half developmental scores and intelligence indices showed no significant differences in children of treated or untreated hypertensive women.

Tablets: Pregnancy Category B.

Injection: Pregnancy Category C. Animal reproduction studies have not been conducted with Methyldopate HCl Injection. It is also not known whether Methyldopate HCl Injection can effect reproduction capacity or can cause fetal harm when given to a pregnant woman. Methyldopate HCl should be given to a pregnant woman only if clearly needed.

NURSING MOTHERS

Methyldopa appears in breast milk. Therefore, caution should be exercised when methyldopa is given to a nursing woman.

DRUG INTERACTIONS:

When methyldopa is used with other antihypertensive drugs, potentiation of antihypertensive effect may occur. Patients should be followed carefully to detect side reactions on unusual manifestations of drug idiosyncrasy.

Patients may require reduced doses of anesthetics when on methyldopa. If hypotension does occur during anesthesia, it usually can be controlled by vasopressors. The adrenergic receptors remain sensitive during treatment with methyldopa.

When methyldopa and lithium are given concomitantly the patient should be carefully monitored for symptoms of lithium toxicity. Read the circular for lithium preparations.

ADVERSE REACTIONS:

Sedation, usually transient, may occur during the initial period of therapy or whenever the dose is increased. Headache, asthenia, or weakness may be noted as early and transient symptoms. However, significant adverse effects due to Methyldopa have been infrequent and this agent usually is well tolerated.

ADVERSE REACTIONS: *(cont'd)*

The following adverse reactions have been reported and, within each category, are listed in order of decreasing severity.

Cardiovascular: Aggravation of angina pectoris, congestive heart failure, prolonged carotid sinus hypersensitivity, orthostatic hypotension (decrease daily dosage), edema or weight gain, bradycardia.

Digestive: Pancreatitis, colitis, vomiting, diarrhea, sialadenitis, sore or "black" tongue, nausea, constipation, distension, flatus, dryness of mouth.

Endocrine: Hyperprolactinemia.

Hematologic: Bone marrow depression, leukopenia, granulocytopenia, thrombocytopenia, hemolytic anemia; positive tests for antinuclear antibody, LE cells, and rheumatoid factor, positive Coombs test.

Hepatic: Liver disorders including hepatitis, jaundice, abnormal liver function tests (see WARNINGS.)

Hypersensitivity: Myocarditis, pericarditis, vasculitis, lupus-like syndrome, drug-related fever.

Nervous System / Psychiatric: Parkinsonism, Bell's palsy, decreased mental acuity, involuntary choreoathetotic movements, symptoms of cerebrovascular insufficiency, psychic disturbances including nightmares and reversible mild psychoses or depression, headache, sedation, asthenia or weakness, dizziness, lightheadedness, paresthesias.

Metabolic: Rise in BUN.

Musculoskeletal: Arthralgia, with or without joint swelling; myalgia.

Respiratory: Nasal stuffiness.

Skin: Toxic epidermal necrolysis, rash.

Urogenital: Amenorrhea, breast enlargement, gynecomastia, lactation, impotence, decreased libido.

OVERDOSAGE:

Acute overdosage may produce acute hypotension with other responses attributable to brain and gastrointestinal malfunction (excessive sedation, weakness, bradycardia, dizziness, lightheadedness, constipation, distention, flatus, diarrhea, nausea, vomiting).

In the event of overdosage, symptomatic and supportive measures should be employed. When ingestion is recent, gastric lavage or emesis may reduce absorption. When ingestion has been earlier, infusions may be helpful to promote urinary excretion. Otherwise, management includes special attention to cardiac rate and output, blood volume, electrolyte balance, paralytic ileus, urinary function and cerebral activity.

Sympathomimetic drugs (*e.g.*, levarterenol, epinephrine, Aramine (Metaraminol Bitartrate)) may be indicated. Methyldopa is dialyzable.

The oral LD_{50} of methyldopa is greater than 1.5 g/kg in both the mouse and the rat.

The acute intravenous LD_{50} of Methyldopa Ester HCl in the mouse is 321 mg/kg.

DOSAGE AND ADMINISTRATION:

TABLETS AND ORAL SUSPENSION

Adults

Initiation of Therapy: The usual starting dosage of Methyldopa is 250 mg two or three times a day in the first 48 hours. The daily dosage then may be increased or decreased, preferably at intervals of not less than two days, until an adequate response is achieved. To minimize the sedation, start dosage increases in the evening. By adjustment of dosage, morning hypotension may be prevented without sacrificing control of afternoon blood pressure.

When methyldopa is given to patients on other antihypertensives, the dose of these agents may need to be adjusted to effect a smooth transition. When Methyldopa is given with antihypertensives other than thiazides, the initial dosage of Methyldopa should be limited to 500 mg daily in divided doses; when Methyldopa is added to a thiazide, the dosage of thiazide need not be changed.

Maintenance Therapy: The usual daily dosage of Methyldopa is 500 mg to 2 g in two to four doses. Although occasional patients have responded to higher doses, the maximum recommended daily dosage is 3 g. Once an effective dosage range is attained, a smooth blood pressure response occurs in most patients in 12 to 24 hours. Since methyldopa has a relatively short duration of action, withdrawal is followed by return of hypertension usually within 48 hours. This is not complicated by an overshoot of blood pressure.

Occasionally tolerance may occur, usually between the second and third month of therapy. Adding a diuretic or increasing the dosage of methyldopa frequently will restore effective control of blood pressure. A thiazide may be added at any time during methyldopa therapy and is recommended if therapy has not been started with a thiazide or if effective control of blood pressure cannot be maintained on 2 g of methyldopa daily.

Methyldopa is largely excreted by the kidney and patients with impaired renal function may respond to smaller doses. Syncope in older patients may be related to an increased sensitivity and advanced arteriosclerotic vascular disease. This may be avoided by lower doses.

Children

Initial dosage is based on 10 mg/kg of body weight daily in two to four doses. The daily dosage then is increased or decreased until an adequate response is achieved. The maximum dosage is 65 mg/kg or 3 g daily, whichever is less.

INJECTION

Injection Ester HCl (Methyldopate HCl), when given intravenously in effective doses, causes a decline in blood pressure that may begin in four to six hours and last 10 to 16 hours after injection.

Add the desired dose of Injection Methyldopate HCl to 100 ml of 5% Dextrose Injection USP. Alternatively the desired dose may be given in 5% dextrose in water in a concentration of 100 mg/10 ml. Give this IV infusion slowly over a period of 30 to 60 minutes.

The vial containing Injection Ester HCl (Methyldopate HCl) should be inspected for particulate matter and discoloration before use whenever solution and container permit.

Adults: The usual adult intravenous dosage is 250 to 500 mg at six hour intervals as required. The maximum recommended IV dose is 1 g every six hours.

When control has been obtained, oral therapy with Methyldopa tablets may be substituted for intravenous therapy, starting with the same dosage used for the parenteral route.

Since Methyldopa has a relatively short duration of action, withdrawal is followed by return of hypertension usually within 48 hours. This is not complicated by an overshoot of blood pressure.

Occasionally tolerance may occur, usually between the second and the third month of therapy. Adding a diuretic or increasing the dosage of methyldopa frequently will restore effective control of blood pressure. A thiazide may be added at any time during methyldopa therapy and is recommended if therapy has not been started with a thiazide or if effective control of blood pressure cannot be maintained on 2 g of methyldopa daily.

Methyldopa is largely excreted by the kidney and patients with impaired renal function may respond to smaller doses. Syncope in older patients may be related to an increased sensitivity and advanced arteriosclerotic vascular disease. This may be avoided in lower doses.

DOSAGE AND ADMINISTRATION: *(cont'd)*

Children: The recommended daily dosage is 20 to 40 mg/kg of body weight in divided doses every six hours. The maximum dosage is 65 mg/kg or 3 g daily, whichever is less. When the blood pressure is under control, continue with oral therapy using the tablet form, in the same dosage as the parenteral route.

STORAGE

Store Oral Suspension Methyldopa below 26°C (78°F) in tight, light-resistant container. Protect from freezing.

Store Injection Methyldopate HCl below 30°C (86°F). Protect from freezing.

(Tablets and Oral Suspension: Merck, 12/91, 7398626)

(Injection: Merck, 11/92, 7347135)

HOW SUPPLIED - RATED THERAPEUTICALLY EQUIVALENT:

Injection, Solution - Intravenous - 50 mg/ml

5 ml	$1.98	Methyldopate Hcl, Voluntary Hosp	53258-1950-02
5 ml	$5.30	Methyldopate Hcl, Gensia Labs	00703-1703-01
5 ml	$6.24	Methyldopate Hcl, Am Regent	00517-8905-01
5 ml	$8.06	Methyldopate Hcl, Elkins Sinn	00641-2501-41
5 ml	$8.19	Methyldopate Hcl, Fujisawa USA	00469-1950-20
5 ml	$8.70	Methyldopate Hcl 50, Abbott	00074-3030-01
5 ml	$8.78	Methyldopate 50, Abbott	00074-3405-02
5 ml	**$12.53**	**ALDOMET ESTER HCL, Merck**	**00006-3293-05**
10 ml	$8.58	Methyldopate Hcl, Gensia Labs	00703-1714-01
10 ml	$14.38	Methyldopate Hcl, Fujisawa USA	00469-1950-30
10 ml	$17.36	Methyldopate Hcl, Abbott	00074-3030-02
10 ml	$17.37	Methyldopate Hcl, Abbott	00074-3406-02

Tablet, Plain Coated - Oral - 125 mg

100's	$6.15	Methyldopa, H.C.F.A. F F P	99999-1787-01
100's	$6.75	Methyldopa, US Trading	56126-0374-11
100's	$9.75	Methyldopa, Consolidated Midland	00223-1584-01
100's	$10.67	Methyldopa, Novopharm (US)	55953-0463-40
100's	$10.75	Methyldopa Tablets 125 Mg, Halsey Drug	00879-0606-01
100's	$11.05	Methyldopa, Martec Pharms	52555-0150-01
100's	$11.75	Methyldopa 125, Major Pharms	00904-2399-60
100's	$12.33	Methyldopa, Aligen Independ	00405-4651-01
100's	$12.65	Methyldopa, Sidmak Labs	50111-0475-01
100's	$12.98	Methyldopa, Rugby	00536-4552-01
100's	$13.17	Methyldopa, Novopharm (US)	55953-0463-01
100's	$13.75	Methyldopa, Rugby	00536-5680-01
100's	$14.05	Methyldopa, West Point Pharma	59591-0174-68
100's	$14.05	Methyldopa, Endo Labs	60951-0775-70
100's	$14.84	Methyldopa, HL Moore Drug Exch	00839-7217-06
100's	$14.95	Methyldopa, Harber Pharm	51432-0280-03
100's	**$26.89**	**ALDOMET, Merck**	**00006-0135-68**
500's	$30.75	Methyldopa, H.C.F.A. F F P	99999-1787-02
500's	$53.75	Methyldopa Tablets 125 Mg, Halsey Drug	00879-0606-05
1000's	$61.50	Methyldopa, H.C.F.A. F F P	99999-1787-03
1000's	$87.50	Methyldopa, Consolidated Midland	00223-1584-02

Tablet, Plain Coated - Oral - 250 mg

60's	$13.90	Methyldopa 250, Major Pharms	00904-2400-60
100's	$6.75	Methyldopa, United Res	00677-0973-01
100's	$6.75	Methyldopa, Geneva Pharms	00781-1320-01
100's	$6.75	Methyldopa, Sidmak Labs	50111-0476-01
100's	$6.75	Methyldopa, H.C.F.A. F F P	99999-1787-04
100's	$7.86	Methyldopa, US Trading	56126-0343-11
100's	$12.50	Methyldopa, Consolidated Midland	00223-1585-01
100's	$13.25	Methyldopa, Raway	00686-0200-20
100's	$13.25	Methyldopa, Major Pharms	00904-2410-60
100's	$13.37	Methyldopa, Novopharm (US)	55953-0164-40
100's	$13.37	Methyldopa, Novopharm (US)	55953-0471-40
100's	$13.95	Methyldopa, HL Moore Drug Exch	00839-7778-06
100's	$15.00	Methyldopa, Bristol Myers Squibb	00003-0447-50
100's	$15.40	Methyldopa, Qualitest Pharms	00603-4536-21
100's	$15.65	Methyldopa, Mova Pharms	55370-0815-07
100's	$15.87	Methyldopa, Novopharm (US)	55953-0471-01
100's	$17.90	Methyldopa, West Point Pharma	59591-0152-68
100's	$17.90	Methyldopa, Endo Labs	60951-0776-70
100's	$18.97	Methyldopa, HL Moore Drug Exch	00839-7119-06
100's	$20.95	Methyldopa, Rugby	00536-5681-01
100's	$21.22	Methyldopa, Aligen Independ	00405-4652-01
100's	$22.50	Methyldopa, Zenith Labs	00172-2931-60
100's	$22.50	Methyldopa, Goldline Labs	00182-1732-01
100's	$24.04	Methyldopa, Vangard Labs	00615-2530-13
100's	$25.65	Methyldopa, Medirex	57480-0349-01
100's	$27.95	Methyldopa, Geneva Pharms	00781-1320-13
100's	$28.30	Methyldopa, Goldline Labs	00182-1732-89
100's	$28.37	Methyldopa 250, Major Pharms	00904-2400-61
100's	$29.50	Methydopa, Lederle Pharm	00005-3850-43
100's	$29.70	Methyldopa, Mylan	00378-0611-01
100's	$29.70	Methyldopa, HL Moore Drug Exch	00839-7692-06
100's	$29.70	Methyldopa, Voluntary Hosp	53258-0144-01
100's	$33.21	Methyldopa, Voluntary Hosp	53258-0144-13
100's	**$34.23**	**ALDOMET, Merck**	**00006-0401-68**
500's	$33.75	Methyldopa, H.C.F.A. F F P	99999-1787-06
500's	$81.03	METHYDOPA, Lederle Pharm	00005-3850-31
600's	$162.40	Methyldopa, Medirex	57480-0349-06
1000's	$67.50	Methyldopa, United Res	00677-0973-10
1000's	$67.50	Methyldopa, Geneva Pharms	00781-1320-10
1000's	$67.50	Methyldopa, Novopharm (US)	55953-0471-80
1000's	$67.50	Methyldopa, H.C.F.A. F F P	99999-1787-05
1000's	$92.50	Methyldopa, Consolidated Midland	00223-1585-02
1000's	$99.10	Methyldopa, Major Pharms	00904-2410-80
1000's	$102.50	Methyldopa, Novopharm (US)	55953-0164-80
1000's	$111.10	Methyldopa 250, Major Pharms	00904-2400-80
1000's	$121.43	Methyldopa, HL Moore Drug Exch	00839-7778-16
1000's	$136.11	Methyldopa, Qualitest Pharms	00603-4536-32
1000's	$137.50	Methyldopa, Mova Pharms	55370-0815-09
1000's	$143.00	Methyldopa, Sidmak Labs	50111-0476-03
1000's	$145.56	Methyldopa, Bristol Myers Squibb	00003-0447-75
1000's	$164.35	Methyldopa, West Point Pharma	59591-0152-82
1000's	$164.35	Methyldopa, Endo Labs	60951-0776-90
1000's	$168.00	Methyldopa, Schein Pharm (US)	00364-0707-02
1000's	$168.90	Methyldopa, Aligen Independ	00405-4652-03
1000's	$169.75	Methyldopa, Rugby	00536-5681-10
1000's	$176.06	Methyldopa, Parmed Pharms	00349-8950-10
1000's	$179.54	Methyldopa, HL Moore Drug Exch	00839-7119-16
1000's	$179.95	Methyldopa, Zenith Labs	00172-2931-80
1000's	$179.95	Methyldopa, Goldline Labs	00182-1732-10
1000's	$185.90	Methyldopa, HL Moore Drug Exch	00839-7692-16
1000's	$185.95	Methyldopa, Mylan	00378-0611-10
1000's	$196.86	Methyldopa, Amer Preferred	53445-1785-00

HOW SUPPLIED - RATED THERAPEUTICALLY EQUIVALENT:
(cont'd)

1000's	**$332.28**	**ALDOMET, Merck**	**00006-0401-82**
1200's	**$410.92**	**ALDOMET, 100 X 12, Merck**	**00006-0401-78**

Tablet, Plain Coated - Oral - 500 mg

60's	$21.06	Methyldopa, Voluntary Hosp	53258-0145-60
100's	$12.15	Methyldopa, United Res	00677-0974-01
100's	$12.15	Methyldopa, Geneva Pharms	00781-1322-01
100's	$12.15	Methyldopa, H.C.F.A. F F P	99999-1787-07
100's	$18.68	Methyldopa, US Trading	56126-0344-11
100's	$22.50	Methyldopa, Consolidated Midland	00223-1586-01
100's	$24.00	Methyldopa, Raway	00686-0201-20
100's	$24.24	Methyldopa, Major Pharms	00904-2411-60
100's	$25.08	Methyldopa, Sidmak Labs	50111-0477-01
100's	$25.48	Methyldopa, Novopharm (US)	55953-0165-40
100's	$25.48	Methyldopa, Novopharm (US)	55953-0498-40
100's	$25.95	Methyldopa, HL Moore Drug Exch	00839-7779-06
100's	$26.20	Methyldopa 500, Major Pharms	00904-2401-60
100's	$27.40	Methyldopa, Bristol Myers Squibb	00003-0433-50
100's	$27.98	Methyldopa, Novopharm (US)	55953-0498-01
100's	$27.99	Methyldopa, Caremark	00339-5231-12
100's	$29.70	Methyldopa, Mova Pharms	55370-0816-07
100's	$31.40	Methyldopa, Qualitest Pharms	00603-4537-21
100's	$32.70	Methyldopa, West Point Pharma	59591-0176-68
100's	$32.70	Methyldopa, Endo Labs	60951-0777-70
100's	$35.90	Methyldopa, Zenith Labs	00172-2932-60
100's	$35.90	Methyldopa, Goldline Labs	00182-1733-01
100's	$35.91	Methyldopa, HL Moore Drug Exch	00839-7120-06
100's	$39.04	Methyldopa, Vangard Labs	00615-2531-13
100's	$39.43	Methyldopa, Rugby	00536-5682-01
100's	$44.00	Methyldopa, Schein Pharm (US)	00364-0708-01
100's	$44.30	Methyldopa, Aligen Independ	00405-4653-01
100's	$46.00	Methyldopa, Goldline Labs	00182-1733-89
100's	$46.05	Methyldopa, Geneva Pharms	00781-1322-13
100's	$47.99	Methyldopa, Lederle Pharm	00005-3851-43
100's	$48.25	Methyldopa, Mylan	00378-0421-01
100's	$48.25	Methyldopa, HL Moore Drug Exch	00839-7693-06
100's	$48.32	Methyldopa 500, Major Pharms	00904-2401-61
100's	$58.80	Methyldopa, Voluntary Hosp	53258-0145-01
100's	**$62.53**	**ALDOMET, Merck**	**00006-0516-68**
100's	$64.35	Methyldopa, Voluntary Hosp	53258-0145-13
500's	$60.75	Methyldopa, United Res	00677-0974-05
500's	$60.75	Methyldopa, Geneva Pharms	00781-1322-05
500's	$60.75	Methyldopa, Sidmak Labs	50111-0477-02
500's	$60.75	Methyldopa, Novopharm (US)	55953-0498-70
500's	$60.75	Methyldopa, H.C.F.A. F F P	99999-1787-08
500's	$92.50	Methyldopa, Consolidated Midland	00223-1586-05
500's	$95.90	Methyldopa, Martec Pharms	52555-0152-05
500's	$99.10	Methyldopa, Major Pharms	00904-2411-40
500's	$102.50	Methyldopa, Novopharm (US)	55953-0165-70
500's	$111.10	Methyldopa 500, Major Pharms	00904-2401-40
500's	$121.43	Methyldopa, HL Moore Drug Exch	00839-7779-12
500's	$135.06	Methyldopa, Bristol Myers Squibb	00003-0433-60
500's	$137.88	Methyldopa, Qualitest Pharms	00603-4537-28
500's	$144.85	Methyldopa, West Point Pharma	59591-0176-74
500's	$144.85	Methyldopa, Endo Labs	60951-0777-85
500's	$153.03	Methyldopa, Lederle Pharm	00005-3851-31
500's	$157.40	Methyldopa, Schein Pharm (US)	00364-0708-05
500's	$169.83	Methyldopa, HL Moore Drug Exch	00839-7120-12
500's	$169.83	Methyldopa, HL Moore Drug Exch	00839-7693-12
500's	$170.50	Methyldopa, Parmed Pharms	00349-8951-05
500's	$171.10	Methyldopa, Zenith Labs	00172-2932-70
500's	$171.10	Methyldopa, Goldline Labs	00182-1733-05
500's	$174.50	Methyldopa, Rugby	00536-5682-05
500's	$184.28	Methyldopa, Aligen Independ	00405-4653-02
500's	$186.69	Methyldopa, Amer Preferred	53445-1786-05
500's	$190.85	Methyldopa, Mylan	00378-0421-05
500's	**$308.29**	**ALDOMET, Merck**	**00006-0516-74**
1000's	$121.50	Methyldopa, H.C.F.A. F F P	99999-1787-09
1000's	$264.96	Methyldopa, Lederle Pharm	00005-3851-34

HOW SUPPLIED - NOT RATED EQUIVALENT:
Suspension - Oral - 250 mg/5ml

480 ml	**$60.53**	**ALDOMET, Merck**	**00006-3382-74**

METHYLENE BLUE *(001788)*

CATEGORIES: Antagonists and Antidotes; Antidotes; Antimicrobials; Antiseptics, Urinary Tract; Pharmaceutical Adjuvants; FDA Pre 1938 Drugs

BRAND NAMES: Methylthioninium Chloride; Urolene Blue

FORMULARIES: WHO

Prescribing information not available at time of publication.

HOW SUPPLIED - EQUIVALENTS NOT AVAILABLE:
Injection, Solution - Intravenous - 1 %

1 ml x 10	$44.95	Methylene Blue, Hope Pharms	60267-0400-44
1 ml x 10	$78.13	Methylene Blue, Am Regent	00517-0301-10
1 ml x 10	$80.63	METHYLENE BLUE, Solopak Labs	39769-0287-01
1 ml x 25	$175.00	Methylene Blue, Am Regent	00517-0372-71
1 ml x 25	$400.00	Methylene Blue, Consolidated Midland	00223-8174-01
10 ml x 10	$62.40	Methylene Blue, Hope Pharms	60267-0500-55
10 ml x 10	$101.75	Methylene Blue, Am Regent	00517-0310-10
10 ml x 10	$131.25	METHYLENE BLUE, Solopak Labs	39769-0286-10
10 ml x 25	$293.75	Methylene Blue, Am Regent	00517-0373-71
10 ml x 25	$450.00	Methylene Blue, Consolidated Midland	00223-8175-10
25 x 10 ml	$188.50	Methylene Blue, Pasadena	00418-6521-46

Tablet, Uncoated - Oral - 65 mg

100's	$24.12	UROLENE BLUE, Star Pharms FL	00076-0501-03

METHYLERGONOVINE MALEATE *(001789)*

CATEGORIES: Ergot Preparations; Hormones; Labor and Delivery; Oxytocics; Relaxants/Stimulants, Uterine; Uterine Atony; Uterine Contractions; Pregnancy Category C; FDA Approval Pre 1982

BRAND NAMES: *Demergin*; *Elpan-S* (Japan); *Ergometrine Lek*; *Ergotyl*; *Ingagen-M*; *Methergin* (Europe, Asia, Mexico); **Methergine**; *Mitrotan*; *Utergin*
(International brand names outside U.S. in italics)

FORMULARIES: BC-BS; Medi-Cal; PCS

DESCRIPTION:
methylergonovine maleate is a semi-synthetic ergot alkaloid used for the prevention and control of postpartum hemorrhage.

Methergine is available in sterile ampuls of 1 ml, containing 0.2 mg methylergonovine maleate for intramuscular or intravenous injection and in tablets for oral ingestion containing 0.2 mg methylergonovine maleate.

Methergine Tablets: *Active Ingredient:* methylergonovine maleate USP, 0.2 mg *Inactive Ingredients:* acacia, carnauba wax, D&C Red #7, FD&C Blue #1, lactose, mixed parabens, povidone, sodium benzoate, starch, stearic acid, sucrose, talc, tartaric acid, and titanium dioxide.

Methergine Ampuls: 1 ml, clear, colorless solution *Active Ingredient:* methylergonovine maleate USP, 0.2 mg *Inactive Ingredients:* sodium chloride USP 3 mg, tartaric acid NF 0.25 mg, water for injection USP qs to 1 ml.

Chemically, methylergonovine maleate is designated as ergoline-8-carboxamide, 9,10-didehydro-*N*-(1-(hydroxymethyl)propyl)-6-methyl-, (8β(*S*))-, (*Z*)-2-butenedioate (1:1) (salt).

$C_{20}H_{25}N_3O_2 \cdot C_4H_4O_4$

Molecular weight: 455.51

CLINICAL PHARMACOLOGY:
Methylergonovine maleate acts directly on the smooth muscle of the uterus and increases the tone, rate, and amplitude of rhythmic contractions. Thus, it induces a rapid and sustained tetanic uterotonic effect which shortens the third stage of labor and reduces blood loss. The onset of action after IV administration is immediate; after IM administration, 2-5 minutes, and after oral administration, 5-10 minutes.

Pharmacokinetic studies have utilized radioimmunoassay techniques. After IV injection of 0.2 mg. methylergonovine maleate is rapidly distributed from plasma to peripheral tissues within an alpha-phase half-life of 2-3 minutes or less. The beta-phase elimination half-life is 20-30 minutes or more, but clinical effects continue for about 3 hours.[1,2]

Intramuscular injection of 0.2 mg afforded peak plasma concentrations of over 3 ng/ml at t_{max} of 0.5 hours. After 2 hours, total plasma clearance was 120-240 ml/minute.

After oral administration, bioavailability was reported as 60% with no cumulation after repeated doses. During delivery with parenteral injection, bioavailability increased to 78%.

Excretion is rapid and appears to be partially renal and partially hepatic. Whether the drug is able to penetrate the blood/brain barrier has not been determined.

INDICATIONS AND USAGE:
For routine management after delivery of the placenta; postpartum atony and hemorrhage; subinvolution. Under full obstetric supervision, it may be given in the second stage of labor following delivery of the anterior shoulder.

CONTRAINDICATIONS:
Hypertension; toxemia; pregnancy; and hypersensitivity.

WARNINGS:
This drug should not be administered IV routinely because of the possibility of inducing sudden hypertensive and cerebrovascular accidents. If IV administration is considered essential as a lifesaving measure, methylergonovine maleate should be given slowly over a period of no less than 60 seconds with careful monitoring of blood pressure.

PRECAUTIONS:
GENERAL
Caution should be exercised in the presence of sepsis, obliterative vascular disease, hepatic or renal involvement. Also use with caution during the second stage of labor. The necessity for manual removal of a retained placenta should occur only rarely with proper technique and adequate allowance of time for its spontaneous separation.

CARCINOGENESIS, MUTAGENESIS, AND IMPAIRMENT OF FERTILITY
No long-term studies have been performed in animals to evaluate carcinogenic potential. The effect of the drug on fertility has not been determined.

PREGNANCY CATEGORY C
Animal reproductive studies have not been conducted with methylergonovine maleate. It is also not known whether drug methylergonovine maleate can cause fetal harm or can affect reproductive capacity. Use of methylergonovine maleate is contraindicated during pregnancy. (See INDICATIONS AND USAGE)

LABOR AND DELIVERY
The uterotonic effect of methylergonovine maleate is utilized after delivery to assist involution and decrease hemorrhage, shortening the third stage of labor.

NURSING MOTHERS
Methylergonovine maleate may be administered orally for a maximum of 1 week postpartum to control uterine bleeding. Recommended dosage is 1 tablet (0.2 mg) 3 or 4 times daily. At this dosage level a small quantity of drug appears in mothers' milk. Adverse effects have not been described, but caution should be exercised when methylergonovine maleate is administered to a nursing women.

DRUG INTERACTIONS:
Caution should be exercised when methylergonovine maleate is used concurrently with other vasoconstrictors or ergot alkaloids.

ADVERSE REACTIONS:
The most common adverse reaction is hypertension associated in several cases with seizure and/or headache. Hypotension has also been reported. Nausea and vomiting have occurred occasionally. Rarely observed reactions have included, in order of severity: transient chest pains, dyspnea, hematuria, thrombophlebitis, water intoxication, hallucinations, leg cramps, dizziness, tinnitus, nasal congestion, diarrhea, diaphoresis, palpitation, and foul taste.[3]

DRUG ABUSE AND DEPENDENCE:

Methylergonovine maleate has not been associated with drug abuse or dependence of either a physical or psychological nature.

OVERDOSAGE:

Symptoms of acute overdose may include: nausea, vomiting, abdominal pain, numbness, tingling of the extremities, rise in blood pressure, in severe cases followed by hypotension, respiratory depression, hypothermia, convulsions, and coma.

Because reports of overdosage with methylergonovine maleate are infrequent, the lethal dose in humans has not been established. The oral LD_{50} (in mg/kg) for the mouse is 187, the rat 93, and the rabbit 4.5.[4] Several cases of accidental methylergonovine maleate injection in newborn infants have been reported, and in such cases 0.2 mg represents an overdose of great magnitude. However, recovery occurred in all but one case following a period of respiratory depression, hypothermia, hypertonicity with jerking movements, and, in one case, a single convulsion.

Also, several children 1-3 years of age have accidentally ingested up to 10 tablets (2 mg) with no apparent ill effects. A postpartum patient took 4 tablets at one time in error and reported paresthesias and clamminess as her only symptoms.

Treatment of acute overdosage is symptomatic and includes the usual procedures of:

1. removal of offending drug by inducing emesis, gastric lavage, catharsis, and supportive diuresis.

2. maintenance of adequate pulmonary ventilation, especially if convulsions or coma develop.

3. correction of hypotension with pressor drugs as needed.

4. control of convulsions with standard anti-convulsant agents.

5. control of peripheral vasospasm with warmth to the extremities if needed.[5]

DOSAGE AND ADMINISTRATION:

Parenteral drug products should be inspected visually for particulate matter and discoloration prior to administration.

Intramuscularly: 1 ml, 0.2 mg, after delivery of the anterior shoulder, after delivery of the placenta, or during the puerperium. May be repeated as required, at intervals of 2-4 hours.

Intravenously: Dosage same as intramuscular. (See WARNINGS)

Orally: One tablet, 0.2 mg, 3 or 4 times daily in the puerperium for a maximum of 1 week.

STORE AND DISPENSE

Tablets: Below 77°F; tight, light-resistant container.

Ampuls: Below 77°F; protect from light - administer only if solution is clear and colorless.

REFERENCES:

1. Mantyla, R. and Kants, J.: Clinical Pharmacokinetics of Methylergometrine (Methylergonovine). Int. J. Clin. Pharmacol. Ther. Toxicol. 19(9):386-391, 1981. **2.** Iwamura, S. and Kambegawa, A.: Determinations of Methylergometrine and Dihydroergotoxine in Biological Fluids. J. Pharm. Dyn. 4: 275-281, 1981 **3.** Information on Adverse Reactions supplied by Medical Services Dept., Sandoz Pharmaceuticals, E. Hanover, N.J., based on computerized clinical reports. **4.** Berde, B. and Schild, H.O.: *Ergot Alkaloids and Related Compounds*, Springer-Verlag, New York, 1978, p. 810 **5.** Treatment of Acute Overdosage. Sandoz Dorsey Rx Products. Sandoz Inc., Medical Services Department.

HOW SUPPLIED - EQUIVALENTS NOT AVAILABLE:

Injection, Solution - Intramuscular; - 0.2 mg/ml

20's	$57.24	METHERGINE, Novartis	00078-0053-03
50's	$137.76	METHERGINE, Novartis	00078-0053-04

Tablet, Coated - Oral - 0.2 mg

100's	$51.90	METHERGINE, Novartis	00078-0054-05
100's	$54.36	METHERGINE, Novartis	00078-0054-06
1000's	$505.56	METHERGINE, Novartis	00078-0054-09

METHYLPHENIDATE HYDROCHLORIDE

(001790)

CATEGORIES: Amphetamines; Anorexients/CNS Stimulants; Antidepressants; Antihypertensives; Attention Deficit Disorders; Brain Damage; Central Nervous System Agents; Hyperkinetic Child Syndrome; Methylphenidate; Minimal Cerebral Dysfunction; Narcolepsy; Psychostimulants; Respiratory/Cerebral Stimulant; DEA Class CII; FDA Approval Pre 1982; Top 200 Drugs

BRAND NAMES: *Centedrin*; Methylphenidate Hcl; *Rilatine*; **Ritalin**; Ritalin-SR; *Rubifen*
(International brand names outside U.S. in italics)

FORMULARIES: Aetna; BC-BS; CIGNA; DoD; FHP; Humana; Kaiser; Medco; Medi-Cal; PruCare; United

COST OF THERAPY: $64.36 (Attention Deficit Disorders; Tablet; 10 mg; 2/day; 90 days) vs. Potential Cost of $3,628.44 (Psychoses)

DESCRIPTION:

Methylphenidate hydrochloride USP, abbreviated here as Methylphenidate HCl is a mild central nervous system (CNS) stimulant, available as tablets of 5, 10, and 20 mg for oral administration; Ritalin-SR is available as sustained-release tablets of 20 mg for oral administration. Methylphenidate hydrochloride is methyl α-phenyl-2-piperidineacetate hydrochloride.

Methylphenidate hydrochloride USP is a white, odorless, fine crystalline powder. Its solutions are acid to litmus. It is freely soluble in water and in methanol, soluble in alcohol, and slightly soluble in chloroform and in acetone. Its molecular weight is 269.77.

Inactive Ingredients: Methylphenidate HCl tablets: D&C Yellow No. 10 (5-mg and 20-mg tablets), FD&C Green No. 3 (10-mg tablets), lactose, magnesium stearate, polyethylene glycol, starch (5-mg and 10-mg tablets), sucrose, talc, and tragacanth (20-mg tablets).

Methylphenidate HCl-SR tablets: Cellulose compounds, cetostearyl alcohol, lactose, magnesium stearate, mineral oil, povidone, titanium dioxide, and zein.

CLINICAL PHARMACOLOGY:

Methylphenidate HCl is a mild central nervous system stimulant.

The mode of action in man is not completely understood, but Methylphenidate HCl presumably activates the brain stem arousal system and cortex to produce its stimulant effect.

There is neither specific evidence which clearly establishes the mechanism whereby Methylphenidate HCl produces its mental and behavioral effects in children, nor conclusive evidence regarding how these effects relate to the condition of the central nervous system.

Methylphenidate HCl in the SR tablets is more slowly but as extensively absorbed as in the regular tablets. Relative bioavailability of the SR tablet compared to the Methylphenidate HCl tablet, measured by the urinary excretion of Methylphenidate HCl major metabolite (α-phenyl-2- piperidine acetic acid) was 105% (49-168%) in children and 101% (85-152%) in adults. The time to peak rate in children was 4.7 hours (1.3-8.2 hours) for the SR tablets and 1.9 hours (0.3-4.4 hours) for the tablets. An average of 67% of SR tablet dose was excreted in children as compared to 86% in adults.

INDICATIONS AND USAGE:

ATTENTION DEFICIT DISORDERS, NARCOLEPSY

Attention Deficit Disorders: (previously known as Minimal Brain Dysfunction in Children). Other terms being used to describe the behavioral syndrome below include: Hyperkinetic Child Syndrome, Minimal Brain Damage, Minimal Cerebral Dysfunction, Minor Cerebral Dysfunction.

Methylphenidate HCl is indicated as an integral part of a total treatment program which typically includes other remedial measures (psychological, educational, social) for a stabilizing effect in children with a behavioral syndrome characterized by the following group of developmentally inappropriate symptoms: moderate-to-severe distractibility, short attention span, hyperactivity, emotional lability, and impulsivity. The diagnosis of this syndrome should not be made with finality when these symptoms are only of comparatively recent origin. Nonlocalizing (soft) neurological signs, learning disability, and abnormal EEG may or may not be present, and a diagnosis of central nervous system dysfunction may or may not be warranted.

SPECIAL DIAGNOSTIC CONSIDERATIONS

Specific etiology of this syndrome is unknown, and there is no single diagnostic test. Adequate diagnosis requires the use not only of medical but of special psychological, educational, and social resources.

Characteristics commonly reported include: chronic history of short attention span, distractibility, emotional lability, impulsivity, and moderate-to-severe hyperactivity; minor neurological signs and abnormal EEG. Learning may or may not be impaired. The diagnosis must be based upon a complete history and evaluation of the child and not solely on the presence of one or more of these characteristics.

Drug treatment is not indicated for all children with this syndrome. Stimulants are not intended for use in the child who exhibits symptoms secondary to environmental factors and/or primary psychiatric disorders, including psychosis. Appropriate educational placement is essential and psychosocial intervention is generally necessary. When remedial measures alone are insufficient, the decision to prescribe stimulant medication will depend upon the physician's assessment of the chronicity and severity of the child's symptoms.

CONTRAINDICATIONS:

Marked anxiety, tension, and agitation are contraindications to Methylphenidate HCl, since the drug may aggravate these symptoms. Methylphenidate HCl is contraindicated also in patients known to be hypersensitive to the drug, in patients with glaucoma, and in patients with motor tics or with a family history or diagnosis of Tourette's syndrome.

WARNINGS:

Methylphenidate HCl should not be used in children under six years, since safety and efficacy in this age group have not been established.

Sufficient data on safety and efficacy of long-term use of Methylphenidate HCl in children are not yet available. Although a causal relationship has not been established, suppression of growth (*i.e.*, weight gain, and/or height) has been reported with the long-term use of stimulants in children. Therefore, patients requiring long-term therapy should be carefully monitored.

Methylphenidate HCl should not be used for severe depression of either exogenous or endogenous origin. Clinical experience suggests that in psychotic children, administration of Methylphenidate HCl may exacerbate symptoms of behavior disturbance and thought disorder.

Methylphenidate HCl should not be used for the prevention or treatment of normal fatigue states.

There is some clinical evidence that Methylphenidate HCl may lower the convulsive threshold in patients with prior history of seizures, with prior EEG abnormalities in absence of seizures, and, very rarely, in absence of history of seizures and no prior EEG evidence of seizures. Safe concomitant use of anticonvulsants and Methylphenidate HCl has not been established. In the presence of seizures, the drug should be discontinued.

Use cautiously in patients with hypertension. Blood pressure should be monitored at appropriate intervals in all patients taking Methylphenidate HCl, especially those with hypertension.

Symptoms of visual disturbances have been encountered in rare cases. Difficulties with accommodation and blurring of vision have been reported.

USAGE IN PREGNANCY

Adequate animal reproduction studies to establish safe use of Methylphenidate HCl during pregnancy have not been conducted. Therefore, until more information is available, Methylphenidate HCl should not be prescribed for women of childbearing age unless, in the opinion of the physician, the potential benefits outweigh the possible risks.

PRECAUTIONS:

Patients with an element of agitation may react adversely; discontinue therapy if necessary.

Periodic CBC, differential, and platelet counts are advised during prolonged therapy.

Drug treatment is not indicated in all cases of this behavioral syndrome and should be considered only in light of the complete history and evaluation of the child. The decision to prescribe Methylphenidate HCl should depend on the physician's assessment of the chronicity and severity of the child's symptoms and their appropriateness for his/her age. Prescription should not depend solely on the presence of one or more of the behavioral characteristics.

When these symptoms are associated with acute stress reactions, treatment with Methylphenidate HCl is usually not indicated.

Long-term effects of Methylphenidate HCl in children have not been well established.

DRUG INTERACTIONS:

Methylphenidate HCl may decrease the hypotensive effect of guanethidine. Use cautiously with pressor agents and MAO inhibitors.

Human pharmacologic studies have shown that Methylphenidate HCl may inhibit the metabolism of coumarin anticoagulants, anticonvulsants (phenobarbital, diphenylhydantoin, primidone), phenylbutazone, and tricyclic drugs (imipramine, clomipramine, desipramine). Downward dosage adjustments of these drugs may be required when given concomitantly with Methylphenidate HCl.

ADVERSE REACTIONS:

Nervousness and insomnia are the most common adverse reactions but are usually controlled by reducing dosage and omitting the drug in the afternoon or evening. Other reactions include hypersensitivity (including skin rash, urticaria, fever, arthralgia, exfoliative dermatitis, erythema multiforme with histopathological findings of necrotizing vasculitis, and thrombocytopenic purpura); anorexia; nausea; dizziness; palpitations; headache; dyskinesia; drowsiness; blood pressure and pulse changes, both up and down; tachycardia; angina; cardiac arrhythmia; abdominal pain; weight loss during prolonged therapy. There have been rare reports of Tourette's syndrome. Toxic psychosis has been reported. Although a definite causal relationship has not been established, the following have been reported in patients taking this drug: isolated cases of cerebral arteritis and/or occlusion; leukopenia and/or anemia; transient depressed mood; a few instances of scalp hair loss.

In children, loss of appetite, abdominal pain, weight loss during prolonged therapy, insomnia, and tachycardia may occur more frequently; however, any of the other adverse reactions listed above may also occur.

DRUG ABUSE AND DEPENDENCE:

Methylphenidate HCl should be given cautiously to emotionally unstable patients, such as those with a history of drug dependence or alcoholism, because such patients may increase dosage on their own initiative. Chronically abusive use can lead to marked tolerance and psychic dependence with varying degrees of abnormal behavior. Frank psychotic episodes can occur, especially with parenteral abuse. Careful supervision is required during drug withdrawal, since severe depression as well as the effects of chronic overactivity can be unmasked. Long-term follow-up may be required because of the patient's basic personality disturbances.

OVERDOSAGE:

Signs and symptoms of acute overdosage, resulting principally from overstimulation of the central nervous system and from excessive sympathomimetic effects, may include the following: vomiting, agitation, tremors, hyperreflexia, muscle twitching, convulsions (may be followed by coma), euphoria, confusion, hallucinations, delirium, sweating, flushing, headache, hyperpyrexia, tachycardia, palpitations, cardiac arrhythmias, hypertension, mydriasis, and dryness of mucous membranes.

Treatment consists of appropriate supportive measures. The patient must be protected against self-injury and against external stimuli that would aggravate overstimulation already present. If signs and symptoms are not too severe and the patient is conscious, gastric contents may be evacuated by induction of emesis or gastric lavage. In the presence of severe intoxication, use a carefully titrated dosage of a *short- acting* barbiturate before performing gastric lavage.

Intensive care must be provided to maintain adequate circulation and respiratory exchange; external cooling procedures may be required for hyperpyrexia.

Efficacy of peritoneal dialysis or extracorporeal hemodialysis for Methylphenidate HCl overdosage has not been established.

DOSAGE AND ADMINISTRATION:

Dosage should be individualized according to the needs and responses of the patient.

ADULTS

Tablets: Administer in divided doses 2 or 3 times daily, preferably 30 to 45 minutes before meals. Average dosage is 20 to 30 mg daily. Some patients may require 40 to 60 mg daily. In others, 10 to 15 mg daily will be adequate. Patients who are unable to sleep if medication is taken late in the day should take the last dose before 6 p.m.

SR Tablets: Methylphenidate HCl-SR tablets have a duration of action of approximately 8 hours. Therefore, Methylphenidate HCl-SR tablets may be used in place of Methylphenidate HCl tablets when the 8- hour dosage of Methylphenidate HCl-SR corresponds to the titrated 8-hour dosage of Methylphenidate HCl. Methylphenidate HCl-SR tablets must be swallowed whole and never crushed or chewed.

CHILDREN (6 YEARS AND OVER)

Methylphenidate HCl should be initiated in small doses, with gradual weekly increments. Daily dosage above 60 mg is not recommended.

If improvement is not observed after appropriate dosage adjustment over a one-month period, the drug should be discontinued.

Tablets: Start with 5 mg twice daily (before breakfast and lunch) with gradual increments of 5 to 10 mg weekly.

SR Tablets: Methylphenidate HCl-SR tablets have a duration of action of approximately 8 hours. Therefore, Methylphenidate HCl-SR tablets may be used in place of Methylphenidate HCl tablets when the 8- hour dosage of Methylphenidate HCl-SR corresponds to the titrated 8-hour dosage of Methylphenidate HCl. Methylphenidate HCl-SR tablets must be swallowed whole and never crushed or chewed.

If paradoxical aggravation of symptoms or other adverse effects occur, reduce dosage, or, if necessary, discontinue the drug.

Methylphenidate HCl should be periodically discontinued to assess the child's condition. Improvement may be sustained when the drug is either temporarily or permanently discontinued.

Drug treatment should not and need not be indefinite and usually may be discontinued after puberty.

NOTE: MD Pharm extended release tablets are color-additive free.

PHARMACIST: Dispense in a tight, light resistant container as defined in the USP with a child resistant closure

Store at controlled room temperature 15°–30°C (59°–86°F).

PATIENT INFORMATION:

Methylphenidate is a stimulant used to treat narcolepsy (sudden attacks of uncontrollable sleepiness) and attention deficit hyperactivity disorder. Inform your physician if you are pregnant or nursing. The last dose of this medication should be taken before 6:00 pm, to avoid insomnia. This medication may be taken with or without food. Do not crush or chew sustained release methylphenidate tablets. Methylphenidate may mask the symptoms of tiredness, impair physical coordination; or cause dizziness or drowsiness; use caution while driving or operating hazardous machinery. Notify your physician if you develop very fast or irregular heartbeat, chest tightness or trouble breathing, uncontrolled body movements or seizures. Methylphenidate may be habit forming. Withdrawal symptoms may occur after you stop taking it.

HOW SUPPLIED - RATED THERAPEUTICALLY EQUIVALENT:

Tablet - Oral - 5 mg

100's	$33.29	Methylphenidate Hydrochloride, H.C.F.A. F F P	99999-1790-01

HOW SUPPLIED - RATED THERAPEUTICALLY EQUIVALENT: *(cont'd)*

Tablet - Oral - 10 mg

100's	$46.35	Methylphenidate Hydrochloride, H.C.F.A. F F P	99999-1790-02

Tablet - Oral - 20 mg

100's	$110.25	Methylphenidate Hydrochloride, H.C.F.A. F F P	99999-1790-03

Tablet, Plain Coated, Sustained Action - Oral - 20 mg

100's	$78.73	Methylphenidate Hcl, MD Pharm	43567-0562-07
100's	$78.92	Methylphenidate Hcl, Aligen Independ	00405-0128-01
100's	$79.00	Methylphenidate Hcl, Harber Pharm	51432-0393-03
100's	$80.74	Methylphenidate Hcl, Purepac Pharm	00228-2089-10
100's	$84.55	Methylphenidate, Major Pharms	00904-2773-60
100's	$84.65	Methylphenidate Hcl, Qualitest Pharms	00603-4572-21
100's	$84.75	Methylphenidate Hcl, Parmed Pharms	00349-8834-01
100's	$85.20	Methylphenidate Hcl, Superior	00144-0628-01
100's	$85.49	Methylphenidate Hcl, Schein Pharm (US)	00364-2329-01
100's	$89.93	Methylphenidate Hcl, Goldline Labs	00182-9147-01
100's	$95.64	Methylphenidate HCl, Rugby	00536-4039-01
100's	**$98.41**	**RITALIN-SR, Novartis**	**00083-0016-30**

Tablet, Uncoated - Oral - 5 mg

100's	$25.06	Methylphenidate Hcl, MD Pharm	43567-0531-07
100's	$25.12	Methylphenidate Hcl, Aligen Independ	00405-0125-01
100's	$26.08	Methylphenidate Hcl, Purepac Pharm	00228-2091-10
100's	$28.10	Methylphenidate Hcl, Schein Pharm (US)	00364-0561-01
100's	$28.20	Methylphenidate Hcl, Major Pharms	00904-2768-60
100's	$28.25	Methylphenidate Hcl, Goldline Labs	00182-1173-01
100's	$28.25	Methylphenidate Hcl, Parmed Pharms	00349-8365-01
100's	$28.25	Methylphenidate Hcl, Qualitest Pharms	00603-4569-21
100's	$28.30	Methylphenidate Hcl, Superior	00144-0625-01
100's	$30.44	Methylphenidate HCl, Rugby	00536-4029-01
100's	**$31.32**	**RITALIN, Novartis**	**00083-0007-30**
1000's	$232.74	Methylphenidate Hcl, MD Pharm	43567-0531-12
1000's	$233.33	Methylphenidate Hcl, Aligen Independ	00405-0125-03
1000's	$268.00	Methylphenidate Hcl, Major Pharms	00904-2768-80
1000's	$270.00	Methylphenidate Hcl, Superior	00144-0625-10
1000's	$270.20	Methylphenidate Hcl, Parmed Pharms	00349-8365-10
1000's	$270.30	Methylphenidate Hcl, Qualitest Pharms	00603-4569-32
1000's	$271.32	Methylphenidate Hcl, Schein Pharm (US)	00364-0561-02
1000's	$277.50	Methylphenidate Hcl, Goldline Labs	00182-1173-10
1000's	$289.25	Methylphenidate HCl, Rugby	00536-4029-10

Tablet, Uncoated - Oral - 10 mg

100's	$35.76	Methylphenidate Hcl, Aligen Independ	00405-0126-01
100's	$35.76	Methylphenidate, MD Pharm	43567-0530-07
100's	$35.98	Methylphenidate Hcl, Purepac Pharm	00228-2092-10
100's	$38.55	Methylphenidate Hcl, Schein Pharm (US)	00364-0479-01
100's	$39.00	Methylphenidate Hcl, Superior	00144-0626-01
100's	$39.25	Methylphenidate Hcl, Parmed Pharms	00349-8366-01
100's	$39.50	Methylphenidate Hcl, Qualitest Pharms	00603-4570-21
100's	$39.50	Methylphenidate Hcl, Major Pharms	00904-2769-60
100's	$41.71	Methylphenidate Hcl, Goldline Labs	00182-1066-01
100's	$43.44	Methylphenidate HCl, Rugby	00536-4035-01
100's	**$44.70**	**RITALIN, Novartis**	**00083-0003-30**
1000's	$320.50	Methylphenidate, MD Pharm	43567-0530-12
1000's	$321.31	Methylphenidate Hcl, Aligen Independ	00405-0126-03
1000's	$335.25	Methylphenidate Hcl, Parmed Pharms	00349-8366-10
1000's	$349.00	Methylphenidate Hcl, Rugby	00536-4035-10
1000's	$352.20	Methylphenidate Hcl, Major Pharms	00904-2769-80
1000's	$376.00	Methylphenidate Hcl, Superior	00144-0626-10
1000's	$380.12	Methylphenidate Hcl, Qualitest Pharms	00603-4570-32
1000's	$381.00	Methylphenidate Hcl, Goldline Labs	00182-1066-10
1000's	$391.00	Methylphenidate Hcl, Schein Pharm (US)	00364-0479-02
1000's	$593.63	Methylphenidate HCl, Rugby	00536-4030-10

Tablet, Uncoated - Oral - 20 mg

100's	$49.76	Methylphenidate Hcl, Purepac Pharm	00228-2093-10
100's	$51.44	Methylphenidate Hcl, MD Pharm	43567-0532-07
100's	$52.15	Methylphenidate Hcl, Major Pharms	00904-2770-60
100's	$54.95	Methylphenidate Hcl, Aligen Independ	00405-0127-01
100's	$56.40	Methylphenidate Hcl, Parmed Pharms	00349-8367-01
100's	$56.50	Methylphenidate Hcl, Superior	00144-0627-01
100's	$56.80	Methylphenidate Hcl, Qualitest Pharms	00603-4571-21
100's	$57.00	Methylphenidate Hcl, Goldline Labs	00182-1174-01
100's	$57.12	Methylphenidate Hcl, Schein Pharm (US)	00364-0562-01
100's	$62.49	Methylphenidate HCl, Rugby	00536-4030-01
100's	**$64.30**	**RITALIN, Novartis**	**00083-0034-30**
1000's	$428.40	Methylphenidate Hcl, Major Pharms	00904-2770-80
1000's	$479.04	Methylphenidate Hcl, MD Pharm	43567-0532-12
1000's	$522.03	METHYLPHENIDATE HCL, Aligen Independ	00405-0127-03
1000's	$558.00	Methylphenidate Hcl, Superior	00144-0627-10
1000's	$560.50	Methylphenidate Hcl, Parmed Pharms	00349-8367-10
1000's	$562.50	Methylphenidate Hcl, Goldline Labs	00182-1174-10
1000's	$574.00	Methylphenidate Hcl, Qualitest Pharms	00603-4571-32
1000's	$575.00	Methylphenidate Hcl, Schein Pharm (US)	00364-0562-02

Tablet, extended release - Oral - 20 mg

100's	$110.25	Methylphenidate Hydrochloride, H.C.F.A. F F P	99999-1790-04

METHYLPREDNISOLONE *(001791)*

CATEGORIES: Adrenal Corticosteroids; Adrenal Hyperplasia; Adrenal Insufficiency; Adrenocortical Insufficiency; Airway Obstruction; Allergies; Anabolic Steroids; Anemia; Ankylosing Spondylitis; Anti-Inflammatory Agents; Antiarthritics; Antidiarrhea Agents; Antineoplastics; Arthritis; Aspiration Pneumonitis; Asthma; Atopic Dermatitis; Berylliosis; Bursitis; Cancer; Carditis; Chemotherapy; Choroiditis; Colitis; Conjunctivitis; Corneal Ulcer; Dermatitis; Dermatitis Herpetiformis; Dermatomyositis; Diuresis; Drug Hypersensitivity; Enteritis; Epicondylitis; Erythema Multiforme; Erythroblastopenia; Gastrointestinal Drugs; Glucocorticoids; Gouty Arthritis; Herpes; Herpes Zoster; Hormones; Hypercalcemia; Inflammation; Iridocyclitis; Keratitis; Leukemia; Lupus Erythematosus; Lymphoma; Meningitis; Multiple Sclerosis; Mycosis Fungoides; Nephrotic Syndrome; Neuritis; Ocular Infections; Oncologic Drugs; Ophthalmics; Osteoarthritis; Pain; Pemphigus; Pneumoconiosis; Pneumonitis; Proteinuria; Psoriasis; Purpura; Retinochoroiditis; Rhinitis; Sarcoidosis; Serum Sickness; Spondylitis; Steroids; Synovitis; Synovitis of Osteoarthritis; Tenosynovitis; Thrombocytopenia; Thrombocytopenic Purpura; Thyroiditis; Trichinosis; Tuberculosis; Ulcerative Colitis; Uveitis; FDA Approval Pre 1982

BRAND NAMES: *Esametone*; *Firmacort*; Medlone 21; *Medrate* (Germany); **Medrol**; *Medixon*; *Medrone* (England); Metrocort; *Metypred*; *Reactenol*; *Sieropresol*; *Solomet*; *Summicort*; *Urbason* (Germany); *Urbason Retard* (Germany)
(International brand names outside U.S. in italics)

FORMULARIES: Aetna; BC-BS

COST OF THERAPY: $98.55 (Asthma; Tablet; 4 mg; 1/day; 365 days)

PRIMARY ICD9: 493.90 (Asthma, Unspecified, Without Mention of Status Asthmaticus)

DESCRIPTION:

Methylprednisolone is a glucocorticoid. Glucocorticoids are adrenocortical steroids, both naturally occurring and synthetic, which are readily absorbed from the gastrointestinal tract. Methylprednisolone occurs as a white to practically white, odorless, crystalline powder. It is sparingly soluble in alcohol, in dioxane, and in methanol, slightly soluble in acetone, and in chloroform, and very slightly soluble in ether. It is practically insoluble in water.

The chemical name for methylprednisolone is pregna-1,4-diene-3,20 -dione, 11,17,21-trihydroxy-6-methyl-,(6α, 11β)-and the molecular weight is 374.48.

Each Medrol tablet for oral administration contains 2 mg, 4 mg, 8 mg, 16 mg, 24 mg or 32 mg of methylprednisolone.

Medrol Inactive ingredients: *2 mg:* Calcium Stearate, Corn Starch, Erythrosine Sodium, Lactose, Mineral Oil, Sorbic Acid, Sucrose. *4 and 16 mg:* Calcium Stearate, Corn Starch, Lactose, Mineral Oil, Sorbic Acid, Sucrose, Sucrose. *8 and 32 mg:* Calcium Stearate, Corn Starch, F D & C Yellow No.6, Lactose, Mineral Oil, Sorbic Acid, Sucrose. *24 mg:* Calcium Stearate, Corn Starch, F D & C Yellow No.5, Lactose, Mineral Oil, Sorbic Acid, Sucrose.

CLINICAL PHARMACOLOGY:

Naturally occurring glucocorticoids (hydrocortisone and cortisone), which also have salt-retaining properties, are used as replacement therapy in adrenocortical deficiency states. Their synthetic analogs are primarily used for their potent anti-inflammatory effects in disorders of many organ systems.

Glucocorticoids cause profound and varied metabolic effects. In addition, they modify the body's immune responses to diverse stimuli.

INDICATIONS AND USAGE:

Methylprednisolone is indicated in the following conditions:

Endocrine Disorders: Primary or secondary adrenocortical insufficiency (hydrocortisone or cortisone is the first choice; synthetic analogs may be used in conjunction with mineralocorticoids where applicable; in infancy mineralocorticoid supplementation is of particular importance).

Congenital adrenal hyperplasia

Nonsuppurative thyroiditis

Hypercalcemia associated with cancer

Rheumatic Disorders: As adjunctive therapy for short-term administration (to tide the patient over an acute episode or exacerbation) in:

Rheumatoid arthritis, including juvenile rheumatoid arthritis (selected cases may require low-dose maintenance therapy)
Ankylosing spondylitis
Acute and subacute bursitis
Synovitis of osteoarthritis
Acute nonspecific tenosynovitis
Post-traumatic osteoarthritis
Psoriatic arthritis
Epicondylitis
Acute gouty arthritis

Collagen Diseases: During an exacerbation or as maintenance therapy in selected cases of:

Systemic lupus erythematosus
Systemic dermatomyositis (polymyositis)
Acute rheumatic carditis

Dermatologic Diseases

Bullous dermatitis herpetiformis
Severe erythema multiforme (Stevens-Johnson syndrome)
Severe seborrheic dermatitis
Exfoliative dermatitis
Mycosis fungoides
Pemphigus
Severe psoriasis

Allergic States: Control of severe or incapacitating allergic conditions intractable to adequate trials of conventional treatment:

Seasonal or perennial allergic rhinitis
Drug hypersensitivity reactions
Serum sickness
Contact dermatitis
Bronchial asthma
Atopic dermatitis

Ophthalmic Diseases: Severe acute and chronic allergic and inflammatory processes involving the eye and its adnexa such as:

Allergic corneal marginal ulcers
Herpes zoster ophthalmicus
Anterior segment inflammation
Diffuse posterior uveitis and choroiditis
Sympathetic ophthalmia
Keratitis
Optic neuritis
Iritis and iridocyclitis
Allergic conjunctivitis
Chorioretinitis

Respiratory Diseases

Symptomatic sarcoidosis
Loeffler's syndrome not manageable by other means Fulminating or disseminated pulmonary tuberculosis when used concurrently with appropriate antituberculous chemotherapy
Aspiration pneumonitis
Berylliosis

Hematologic Disorders

Idiopathic thrombocytopenic purpura in adults
Secondary thrombocytopenia in adults
Acquired (autoimmune) hemolytic anemia
Erythroblastopenia (RBC anemia)
Congenital (erythroid) hypoplastic anemia

Neoplastic Diseases: For palliative management of:

Leukemias and lymphomas in adults
Acute leukemia of childhood

Edematous States: To induce a diuresis or remission of proteinuria in the nephrotic syndrome, without uremia, of the idiopathic type or that due to lupus erythematosus.

Gastrointestinal Diseases: To tide the patient over a critical period of the disease in:

Ulcerative colitis
Regional enteritis

Nervous System: Acute exacerbations of multiple sclerosis

Miscellaneous

Tuberculous meningitis with subarachnoid block or impending block when used concurrently with appropriate antituberculous chemotherapy.

Trichinosis with neurologic or myocardial involvement.

CONTRAINDICATIONS:

Systemic fungal infections and known hypersensitivity to components.

WARNINGS:

In patients on corticosteroid therapy subjected to unusual stress, increased dosage of rapidly acting corticosteroids before, during, and after the stressful situation is indicated.

Corticosteroids may mask some signs of infection, and new infections may appear during their use. There may be decreased resistance and inability to localize infection when corticosteroids are used.

Prolonged use of corticosteroids may produce posterior subcapsular cataracts, glaucoma with possible damage to the optic nerves, and may enhance the establishment of secondary ocular infections due to fungi or viruses.

Usage In Pregnancy: Since adequate human reproduction studies have not been done with corticosteroids, the use of these drugs in pregnancy, nursing mothers or women of child-bearing potential requires that the possible benefits of the drug be weighed against the potential hazards to the mother and embryo or fetus. Infants born of mothers who have received substantial doses of corticosteroids during pregnancy, should be carefully observed for signs of hypoadrenalism.

Average and large doses of hydrocortisone or cortisone can cause elevation of blood pressure, salt and water retention, and increased excretion of potassium. These effects are less likely to occur with the synthetic derivatives except when used in large doses. Dietary salt restriction and potassium supplementation may be necessary. All corticosteroids increase calcium excretion.

While on corticosteroid therapy patients should not be vaccinated against smallpox. Other immunization procedures should not be undertaken in patients who are on corticosteroids, especially on high dose, because of possible hazards of neurological complications and a lack of antibody response.

The use of methylprednisolone in active tuberculosis should be restricted to those cases of fulminating or disseminated tuberculosis in which the corticosteroid is used for the management of the disease in conjunction with an appropriate antituberculous regimen.

If corticosteroids are indicated in patients with latent tuberculosis or tuberculin reactivity, close observation is necessary as reactivation of the disease may occur.

During prolonged corticosteroid therapy, these patients should receive chemoprophylaxis.

Children who are on immunosuppressant drugs are more susceptible to infections than healthy children. Chickenpox and measles, for example, can have a more serious or even fatal course in children on immunosuppressant corticosteroids. In such children, or in adults who have not had these diseases, particular care should be taken to avoid exposure. How the dose, route and duration of corticosteroid administration affects the risk of developing a disseminated infection s not known. The contribution of the underlying disease and/or prior corticosteroid treatment to the risk is also not known. If exposed, therapy with varicella zoster immune globulin (VZIG) or pooled intravenous immunoglobin (IVIG), as appropriate, may be indicated. If chickenpox develops, treatment with antiviral agents may be considered.

PRECAUTIONS:

General: Drug-induced secondary adrenocortical insufficiency may be minimized by gradual reduction of dosage. This type of relative insufficiency may persist for months after discontinuation of therapy; therefore, in any situation of stress occurring during that period, hormone therapy should be reinstituted. Since mineralocorticoid secretion may be impaired, salt and/or a mineralocorticoid should be administered concurrently.

There is an enhanced effect of corticosteroids on patients with hypothyroidism and in those with cirrhosis.

Corticosteroids should be used cautiously in patients with ocular herpes simplex because of possible corneal perforation.

The lowest possible dose of corticosteroid should be used to control the condition under treatment, and when reduction in dosage is possible, the reduction should be gradual.

Psychic derangements may appear when corticosteroids are used, ranging from euphoria, insomnia, mood swings, personality changes, and severe depression, to frank psychotic manifestations. Also, existing emotional instability or psychotic tendencies may be aggravated by corticosteroids.

Aspirin should be used cautiously in conjunction with corticosteroids in hypoprothrombinemia.

Steroids should be used with caution in non-specific ulcerative colitis, if there is a probability of impending perforation, abscess or other pyogenic infection; diverticulitis; fresh *intestinal anastomoses*; active or latent peptic ulcer; renal insufficiency; hypertension; osteoporosis; and myasthenia gravis.

Growth and development of infants and children on prolonged corticosteroid therapy should be carefully observed.

Although controlled clinical trials have shown corticosteroids to be effective in speeding the resolution of acute exacerbations of multiple sclerosis, they do not show that corticosteroids affect the ultimate outcome or natural history of the disease. The studies do show that relatively high doses of corticosteroids are necessary to demonstrate a significant effect. (See DOSAGE AND ADMINISTRATION)

Since complications of treatment with glucocorticoids are dependent on the size of the dose and the duration of treatment, a risk/benefit decision must be made in each individual case as to dose and duration of treatment and as to whether daily or intermittent therapy should be used.

The 24 mg tablet contains FD&C Yellow No. 5 (tartrazine) which may cause allergic-type reactions (including bronchial asthma) in certain susceptible individuals. Although the overall incidence of FD&C Yellow No. 5 (tartrazine) sensitivity in the general population is low, it is frequently seen in patients who also have aspirin hypersensitivity.

Convulsions have been reported with concurrent use of methylprednisolone and cyclosporin. Since concurrent use of these agents results in a mutual inhibition of metabolism, it is possible that adverse events associated with the individual use of either drug may be more apt to occur.

Information for the Patient: Patients who are on immunosuppressant doses of corticosteroids should be warned to avoid exposure to chickenpox or measles and, if exposed, to obtain medical advice.

ADVERSE REACTIONS:

Fluid and Electrolyte Disturbances: Sodium retention, Fluid retention, Congestive heart failure in susceptible patients, Potassium loss, Hypokalemic alkalosis, Hypertension.

Musculoskeletal: Muscle weakness, Steroid myopathy, Loss of muscle mass, Osteoporosis, Vertebral compression fractures, Aseptic necrosis of femoral and humeral heads, Pathologic fracture of long bones.

Gastrointestinal: Peptic ulcer with possible perforation and hemorrhage, Pancreatitis, Abdominal distention, Ulcerative esophagitis.

Dermatologic: Impaired wound healing, Thin fragile skin, Petechiae and ecchymoses, Facial erythema, May suppress reactions, Increased sweating to skin tests.

Neurological: Increased intracranial pressure with papilledema (pseudo-tumor cerebri) usually after treatment, Convulsions, Headache, Vertigo.

ADVERSE REACTIONS: *(cont'd)*

Endocrine: Development of Cushingoid state, Suppression of growth in children, Secondary adrenocortical and pituitary unresponsiveness, particularly in times of stress, as in trauma, surgery or illness, Menstrual irregularities, Decreased carbohydrate tolerance, Manifestations of latent diabetes mellitus, Increased requirements of insulin or oral hypoglycemic agents in diabetics.

Ophthalmic: Posterior subcapsular cataracts, Increased intraocular pressure, Glaucoma, Exophthalmos

Metabolic: Negative nitrogen balance due to protein catabolism,

The following additional reactions have been reported following oral as well as parenteral therapy:

Urticaria and other allergic, anaphylactic or hypersensitivity reactions.

DOSAGE AND ADMINISTRATION:

The initial dosage of methylprednisolone may vary from 4 mg to 48 mg of methylprednisolone per day depending on the specific disease entity being treated. In situations of less severity lower doses will generally suffice while in selected patients higher initial doses may be required. The initial dosage should be maintained or adjusted until a satisfactory response is noted. If after a reasonable period of time there is a lack of satisfactory clinical response, Methylprednisolone should be discontinued and the patient transferred to other appropriate therapy.

IT SHOULD BE EMPHASIZED THAT DOSAGE REQUIREMENTS ARE VARIABLE AND MUST BE INDIVIDUALIZED ON THE BASIS OF THE DISEASE UNDER TREATMENT AND THE RESPONSE OF THE PATIENT.

After a favorable response is noted, the proper maintenance dosage should be determined by decreasing the initial drug dosage in small decrements at appropriate time intervals until the lowest dosage which will maintain an adequate clinical response is reached. It should be kept in mind that constant monitoring is needed in regard to drug dosage. Included in the situations which may make dosage adjustments necessary are changes in clinical status secondary to remissions or exacerbations in the disease process, the patient's individual drug responsiveness, and the effect of patient exposure to stressful situations not directly related to the disease entity under treatment; in this latter situation it may be necessary to increase the dosage of Methylprednisolone for a period of time consistent with the patient's condition. If after long-term therapy the drug is to be stopped, it is recommended that it be withdrawn gradually rather than abruptly.

Multiple Sclerosis: In treatment of acute exacerbations of multiple sclerosis daily doses of 200 mg of prednisolone for a week followed by 80 mg every other day for 1 month have been shown to be effective (4 mg of methylprednisolone is equivalent to 5 mg of prednisolone).

ADT (Alternate Day Therapy): Alternate day therapy is a corticosteroid dosing regimen in which twice the usual daily dose of corticoid is administered every other morning. The purpose of this mode of therapy is to provide the patient requiring long-term pharmacologic dose treatment with the beneficial effects of corticoids while minimizing certain undesirable effects, including pituitary-adrenal suppression, the Cushingoid state, corticoid withdrawal symptoms, and growth suppression in children.

The rationale for this treatment schedule is based on two major premises: (a) the anti-inflammatory or therapeutic effect of corticoids persists longer that their physical presence and metabolic effects and (b) administration of the corticosteroid every other morning allows for reestablishment of more nearly normal hypothalamic-pituitary-adrenal (HPA) activity on the off-steroid day.

A brief review of the HPA physiology may be helpful in understanding this rationale. Acting primarily through the hypothalamus a fall in free cortisol stimulates the pituitary gland to produce increasing amounts of corticotropin (ACTH) while a rise in free cortisol inhibits ACTH secretion. Normally the HPA system is characterized by diurnal (circadian) rhythm. Serum levels of ACTH rise from a low point about 10 pm to a peak level about 6 am. Increasing levels of ACTH stimulate adrenal cortical activity resulting in a rise in plasma cortisol with maximal levels occurring between 2 am and 8 am. This rise in cortisol dampens ACTH production and in turn adrenal cortical activity. There is a gradual fall in plasma corticoids during the day with lowest levels occurring about midnight.

The diurnal rhythm of the HPA axis is lost in Cushing's disease, a syndrome of adrenal cortical hyperfunction characterized by obesity with centripetal fat distribution, thinning of the skin with easy bruisability, muscle wasting with weakness, hypertension, latent diabetes, osteoporosis, electrolyte imbalance, etc. The same clinical findings of hyperadrenocorticism may be noted during long-term pharmacologic dose corticoid therapy administered in conventional daily divided doses. It would appear, then, that a disturbance in the diurnal cycle with maintenance of elevated corticoid values during the night may play a significant role in the development of undesirable corticoid effects. Escape from these constantly elevated plasma levels for even short periods of time may be instrumental in protecting against undesirable pharmacologic effects.

During conventional pharmacologic dose corticosteroid therapy, ACTH production is inhibited with subsequent suppression of cortisol production by the adrenal cortex. Recovery time for normal HPA activity is variable depending upon the dose and duration of treatment. During this time the patient is vulnerable to any stressful situation. Although it has been shown that there is considerably less adrenal suppression following a single morning dose of prednisolone (10 mg) as opposed to a quarter of that dose administered every six hours, there is evidence that some suppressive effect on adrenal activity may be carried over into the following day when pharmacologic doses are used. Further, it has been shown that a single dose of certain corticosteroids will produce adrenal cortical suppression for two or more days. Other corticoids, including methylprednisolone, hydrocortisone, prednisone, and prednisolone, are considered to be short acting (producing adrenal cortical suppression for 1 1/4 to 1 1/2 days following a single dose) and thus are recommended for alternate day therapy.

The following should be kept in mind when considering alternate day therapy:

1) Basic principles and indications for corticosteroid therapy should apply. The benefits of ADT should not encourage the indiscriminate use of steroids.

2) ADT is a therapeutic technique primarily designed for patients in whom long-term pharmacologic corticoid therapy is anticipated.

3) In less severe disease processes in which corticoid therapy is indicated, it may be possible to initiate treatment with ADT. More severe disease states usually will require daily divided high dose therapy for initial control of the disease process. The initial suppressive dose level should be continued until satisfactory clinical response is obtained, usually four to ten days in the case of many allergic and collagen diseases. It is important to keep the period of initial suppressive dose as brief as possible particularly when subsequent use of alternate day therapy is intended. Once control has been established, two courses are available: (a) change to ADT and then gradually reduce the amount of corticoid given every other day or (b) following control of the disease process reduce the daily dose of corticoid to the lowest effective level as rapidly as possible and then change over to an alternate day schedule. Theoretically, course (a) may be preferable.

4) Because of the advantages of ADT, it may be desirable to try patients on this form of therapy who have been on daily corticoids for long periods of time (eg, patients with rheumatoid arthritis). Since these patients may already have a suppressed HPA axis, establishing them on ADT may be difficult and not always successful. However, it is recommended that regular attempts be made to change them over. It may be helpful to triple or even quadruple the daily maintenance dose and administer this every other day rather than just doubling the daily dose if difficulty is encountered. Once the patient is again controlled, an attempt should be made to reduce this dose to a minimum.

5) As indicated above, certain corticosteroids, because of their prolonged suppressive effect on adrenal activity, are not recommended for alternate day therapy (*e.g.*, dexamethasone and betamethasone).

6) The maximal activity of the adrenal cortex is between 2 am and 8 am, and it is minimal between 4 pm and midnight. Exogenous corticosteroids suppress adrenocortical activity the least, when given at the time of maximal activity (am).

7) In using ADT it is important, as in all therapeutic situations to individualize and tailor the therapy to each patient. Complete control of symptoms will not be possible in all patients. An explanation of the benefits of ADT will help the patient to understand and tolerate the possible flare-up in symptoms which may occur in the latter part of the off-steroid day. Other symptomatic therapy may be added or increased at this time if needed.

8) In the event of an acute flare-up of the disease process, it may be necessary to return to a full suppressive daily divided corticoid dose for control. Once control is again established alternate day therapy may be reinstituted.

9) Although many of the undesirable features of corticosteroid therapy can be minimized by ADT, as in any therapeutic situation, the physician must carefully weigh the benefit-risk ratio for each patient in whom corticoid therapy is being considered.

Store at controlled room temperature 15 - 30° C (59 - 86° F).

HOW SUPPLIED - RATED THERAPEUTICALLY EQUIVALENT:

Tablet, Uncoated - Oral - 4 mg

21's	$8.00	Methylprednisolone, Rugby	00536-4036-47
21's	$9.20	Methylprednisolone, H.C.F.A. F F P	99999-1791-01
21's	$10.07	Methylprednisolone, Greenstone	59762-3327-01
21's	$10.19	Methylprednisolone, Goldline Labs	00182-1050-03
21's	$10.65	Methylprednisolone, Qualitest Pharms	00603-4593-15
21's	$10.89	Methylprednisolone, Schein Pharm (US)	00364-0467-21
21's	$10.89	Methylprednisolone, United Res	00677-0565-13
21's	$10.90	Methylprednisolone, Rugby	00536-4036-44
21's	$11.00	Methylprednisolone, Duramed Pharms	51285-0301-21
21's	$11.30	Methylprednisolone, Parmed Pharms	00349-8279-21
21's	$11.50	Methyl Prednisolone, Harber Pharm	51432-0282-21
21's	**$11.98**	**MEDROL, Pharmacia & Upjohn**	**00009-0056-04**
21's	$12.02	Methylprednisolone, HL Moore Drug Exch	00839-6224-58
21's	$15.87	Methylprednisolone 4, Aligen Independ	00405-4666-21
21's UD	$10.55	Methylprednisolone, Major Pharms	00904-2175-19
100's	$27.00	Methylprednisolone, Voluntary Hosp	53258-0148-01
100's	$29.87	Methylprednisolone, US Trading	56126-0326-11
100's	$36.28	Methylprednisolone, Voluntary Hosp	53258-0148-13
100's	$43.46	Methylprednisolone, Qualitest Pharms	00603-4593-21
100's	$43.82	Methylprednisolone, H.C.F.A. F F P	99999-1791-02
100's	$48.35	Methylprednisolone, United Res	00677-0565-01
100's	$49.66	Methylprednisolone, Greenstone	59762-3327-02
100's	$50.25	Methylprednisolone, Goldline Labs	00182-1050-01
100's	$50.25	Methylprednisolone, Major Pharms	00904-2175-60
100's	$52.25	Methylprednisolone, Rugby	00536-4036-01
100's	$52.50	Methyl Prednisolone, Harber Pharm	51432-0282-03
100's	$53.26	Methylprednisolone, Schein Pharm (US)	00364-0467-01
100's	$54.00	Methylprednisolone, Duramed Pharms	51285-0301-02
100's	**$59.13**	**MEDROL, Pharmacia & Upjohn**	**00009-0056-02**
100's	**$59.47**	**MEDROL, Pharmacia & Upjohn**	**00009-0056-05**
100's	$59.51	Methylprednisolone, HL Moore Drug Exch	00839-6224-06
100's	$59.95	Methylprednisolone, Parmed Pharms	00349-8279-01
100's	$97.51	Methylprednisolone, Aligen Independ	00405-4666-01
500's	$219.10	Methylprednisolone, H.C.F.A. F F P	99999-1791-03
500's	**$292.51**	**MEDROL, Pharmacia & Upjohn**	**00009-0056-03**

Tablet, Uncoated - Oral - 16 mg

14's	**$17.99**	**MEDROL, Pharmacia & Upjohn**	**00009-0073-02**
50's	$45.90	Methylprednisolone, United Res	00677-1305-02
50's	$52.42	Methylprednisolone, Rugby	00536-4037-06
50's	**$64.14**	**MEDROL, Pharmacia & Upjohn**	**00009-0073-01**

Tablet, Uncoated - Oral - 24 mg

25's	**$37.81**	**MEDROL, Pharmacia & Upjohn**	**00009-0155-01**

Tablet, Uncoated - Oral - 32 mg

25's	**$46.02**	**MEDROL, Pharmacia & Upjohn**	**00009-0176-01**

HOW SUPPLIED - NOT RATED EQUIVALENT:

Tablet, Uncoated - Oral - 2 mg

100's	**$31.26**	**MEDROL, Pharmacia & Upjohn**	**00009-0049-02**

Tablet, Uncoated - Oral - 8 mg

25's	**$20.74**	**MEDROL, Pharmacia & Upjohn**	**00009-0022-01**

METHYLPREDNISOLONE ACETATE *(001792)*

CATEGORIES: Adrenal Corticosteroids; Adrenal Hyperplasia; Adrenal Insufficiency; Adrenocortical Insufficiency; Airway Obstruction; Allergies; Alopecia; Alopecia Areata; Anemia; Ankylosing Spondylitis; Anti-Inflammatory Agents; Antidiarrhea Agents; Antineoplastics; Arthritis; Asthma; Atopic Dermatitis; Berylliosis; Bursitis; Cancer; Carditis; Chemotherapy; Chorioretinitis; Choroiditis; Colitis; Conjunctivitis; Corneal Ulcer; Dermatitis; Dermatitis Herpetiformis; Dermatologicals; Dermatomyositis; Diuresis; Drug Hypersensitivity; Enteritis; Epicondylitis; Erythema Multiforme; Gastrointestinal Drugs; Glucocorticoids; Gouty Arthritis; Granuloma; Granuloma Annulare; Herpes; Herpes Zoster; Hormones; Hypercalcemia; Inflammation; Inflammatory Lesions; Iridocyclitis; Keloids; Keratitis; Laryngeal Edema; Lesions; Leukemia; Lichen Planus; Lichen Simplex Chronicus; Lupus Erythematosus; Lymphoma; Meningitis; Multiple Sclerosis; Mycosis Fungoides; Necrobiosis Lipoidica; Nephrotic Syndrome; Neuritis; Ocular Infections; Ophthalmics; Osteoarthritis; Pemphigus; Pneumoconiosis; Proteinuria; Psoriasis; Retinochoroiditis; Rhinitis; Sarcoidosis; Serum Sickness; Shock; Skin/Mucous Membrane Agents; Spondylitis; Steroids; Synovitis; Synovitis of Osteoarthritis; Tenosynovitis; Thrombocytopenia; Thyroiditis; Transfusion Reactions; Trichinosis; Tuberculosis; Tumors; Ulcerative Colitis; Urticaria; Uveitis; FDA Approval Pre 1982; Top 200 Drugs

BRAND NAMES: Adlone; Deca-Plex; Depapred; Depmedalone; *Depo-Medrate* (Germany); *Depo Medrol*; **Depo-Medrol**; *Depo-Moderin*; Depo-Predate; Depoject; Depopred; Duralone; Edrol-40; *Epizolone-Depot*; *Esametone*; M-Predrol; Mar-Pred; Med-Jec-40; Medipred; Medralone; Medrex; Methylcotolone; Methylone; Methyl-

prednisolone Acetate; Predacorten; Pri-Methylate; Rep-Pred; *Solomet*; *Urbason* (Germany)
(International brand names outside U.S. in italics)

FORMULARIES: BC-BS

DESCRIPTION:

Methylprednisolone Acetate Sterile Aqueous Suspension contains Methylprednisolone Acetate which is the 6-methyl derivative of prednisolone. Methylprednisolone Acetate is a white or practically white, odorless, crystalline powder which melts at about 215° with some decomposition. It is soluble in dioxane, sparingly soluble in acetone, in chloroform, and in methanol, and slightly soluble in ether. It is practically insoluble in water. The chemical name for Methylprednisolone Acetate is pregna-1-4-diene-3,20-dione, 21-(acetyloxy) -11,17-dihydroxy -6 -methyl-(6α,11β)-and the molecular weight is 416.51.

Methylprednisolone Acetate is an anti-inflammatory glucocorticoid, for intramuscular, intrasynovial, soft tissue or intralesional injection. It is available in three strengths: 20 mg/ml; 40 mg/ml; 80 mg/ml.

Each ml of these preparations contains:

Methylprednisolone Acetate: 20 mg, 40 mg, 80 mg

Polyethylene glycol 3350: 29.5 mg, 29.5 mg, 28.2 mg

Polysorbate 80: 1.97 mg, 1.94 mg, 1.88 mg

Monobasic sodium phosphate: 6.9 mg, 6.8 mg, 6.59 mg

Dibasic sodium phosphate USP: 1.44 mg, 1.42 mg, 1.37 mg

Benzyl alcohol: 9.3 mg, 9.16 mg, 8.88 mg added as a preservative

Sodium Chloride was added to adjust tonicity.

When necessary, pH was adjusted with sodium hydroxide and/or hydrochloric acid. The pH of the finished product remains within the USP specified range; i.e., 3.5 to 7.0.

CLINICAL PHARMACOLOGY:

Naturally occurring glucocorticoids (hydrocortisone), which also have salt retaining properties, are used in replacement therapy in adrenocortical deficiency states. Their synthetic analogs are used primarily for their potent anti-inflammatory effects in disorders of many organ systems.

Glucocorticoids cause profound and varied metabolic effects. In addition, they modify the body's immune response to diverse stimuli.

As of November, 1990, the formulation for Methylprednisolone Acetate Sterile Aqueous Suspension was revised. In a bioavailability study with thirty subjects, the new formulation was found to be more bioavailable than the previous formulation. An increase in the extent of Methylprednisolone Acetate absorption was observed for the new formulation as indicated by significantly increased values for area under the serum Methylprednisolone Acetate concentration curve and maximum serum Methylprednisolone Acetate concentration (see TABLE 1). No difference in elimination half-life ($t_{1/2}$calculated from the mean terminal elimination rate) was observed between the two formulations. No medically meaningful differences between the two formulations were seen in relation to vital signs, safety laboratory analyses, formulation effects, local tolerance, or side effects. This increase in absorption is not considered clinically significant (TABLE 1):

TABLE 1

	Previous Formulation	Current Formulation
AUC 0-240 hrs (ng x hr/ml)	1053 (47.3)* (133-2297)**	1286 (39.2) (208-2225)
C_{MAX}(ng/ml)	8.98 (65.9) (0-28.5)	11.8(44.1) (3.37-23.4)
$t_{1/2}$(hr)	139 (46-990)	139 (58-866)

* Coefficient of variation (%)
** Range of values

INDICATIONS AND USAGE:

FOR INTRAMUSCULAR ADMINISTRATION

When oral therapy is not feasible and the strength, dosage form, and route of administration of the drug reasonably lend the preparation to the treatment of the condition, the intramuscular use of Methylprednisolone Acetate Sterile Aqueous Suspension is indicated as follows:

Endocrine Disorders: Primary or secondary adrenocortical insufficiency (hydrocortisone or cortisone is the drug of choice; synthetic analogs may be used in conjunction with mineralocorticoids where applicable; in infancy, mineralocorticoid supplementation is of particular importance)

Acute adrenocortical insufficiency (hydrocortisone or cortisone is the drug of choice; mineralocorticoid supplementation may be necessary, particularly when synthetic analogs are used)

Preoperatively and in the event of serious trauma or illness, in patients with known adrenal insufficiency or when adrenocortical reserve is doubtful:

Congenital adrenal hyperplasia

Hypercalcemia associated with cancer

Nonsuppurative thyroiditis

Rheumatic Disorders: As adjunctive therapy for short-term administration (to tide the patient over an acute episode or exacerbation) in:

Post-traumatic osteoarthritis
Synovitis of osteoarthritis
Rheumatoid arthritis, including juvenile rheumatoid arthritis (selected cases may require low-dose maintenance therapy)
Acute and subacute bursitis
Epicondylitis
Acute nonspecific tenosynovitis
Acute gouty arthritis
Psoriatic arthritis
Ankylosing spondylitis

Collagen Diseases: During an exacerbation or as maintenance therapy in selected cases of:

Systemic lupus erythematosus

Systemic dermatomyositis (polymyositis)

Acute rheumatic carditis

Dermatologic Diseases:

Pemphigus
Severe erythema multiforme (Stevens-Johnson syndrome)
Exfoliative dermatitis
Bullous dermatitis herpetiformis
Severe seborrheic dermatitis
Severe psoriasis
Mycosis fungoides

Allergic States: Control of severe incapacitating allergic conditions intractable to adequate trials of conventional treatment in:

Bronchial asthma
Contact dermatitis
Drug hypersensitivity reactions
Urticarial transfusion reactions

INDICATIONS AND USAGE: *(cont'd)*

Atopic dermatitis
Serum sickness
Seasonal or perennial allergic rhinitis
Acute noninfectious laryngeal edema (epinephrine is the drug of first choice)

Ophthalmic Diseases: Severe acute and chronic allergic and inflammatory processes involving the eye, such as:

Herpes zoster ophthalmicus
Iritis, iridocyclitis
Chorioretinitis
Diffuse posterior uveitis and choroiditis
Optic neuritis
Sympathetic ophthalmia
Anterior segment inflammation
Allergic conjunctivitis
Allergic corneal marginal ulcers
Keratitis

Gastrointestinal Diseases: To tide the patient over a critical period of the disease in:

Ulcerative colitis (systemic therapy)

Regional enteritis(systemic therapy)

Respiratory Diseases

Symptomatic sarcoidosis

Berylliosis

Fulminating or disseminated pulmonary tuberculosis when used concurrently with appropriate antituberculous chemotherapy

Loeffler's syndrome not manageable by other means

Aspiration

Pneumonitis

Hematologic Disorders

Acquired (autoimmune) hemolytic anemia

Secondary thrombocytopenia in adults

Erythroblastopenia (RBC anemia)

Congenital (erythroid) hypoplastic anemia

Neoplastic Diseases: For palliative management of:

Leukemias and lymphomas in adults

Acute leukemia of childhood

Edematous States: To induce diuresis or remission of proteinuria in the nephrotic syndrome, without uremia, of the idiopathic type or that due to lupus erythematosus

Nervous System: Acute exacerbations of multiple sclerosis

Miscellaneous

Tuberculous meningitis with subarachnoid block or impending block when used concurrently with appropriate antituberculous chemotherapy

Trichinosis with neurologic or myocardial involvement

FOR INTRASYNOVIAL OR SOFT TISSUE ADMINISTRATION

Methylprednisolone Acetate is indicated as adjunctive therapy for short-term administration (to tide the patient over an acute episode or exacerbation) in:

Synovitis of osteoarthritis
Rheumatoid arthritis
Acute and subacute bursitis
Acute gouty arthritis
Acute nonspecific tenosynovitis
Post-traumatic osteoarthritis

FOR INTRALESIONAL ADMINISTRATION

Methylprednisolone Acetate is indicated for intralesional use in the following conditions:

Keloids

Localized hypertrophic, infiltrated, inflammatory lesions of:

lichen planus

psoriatic plaques

granuloma annulare

lichen

simplex chronicus (neurodermatitis)

Discoid lupus erythematosus

Necrobiosis lipoidica diabeticorum

Alopecia areata

Methylprednisolone Acetate also may be useful in cystic tumors of an aponeurosis or tendon (ganglia).

CONTRAINDICATIONS:

Methylprednisolone Acetate Sterile Aqueous Suspension is contraindicated for intrathecal administration. Reports of severe medical events have been associated with this route of administration. Methylprednisolone Acetate is contraindicated for use in premature infants because the formulation contains benzyl alcohol. Benzyl alcohol has been reported to be associated with a fatal "gasping syndrome" in premature infants. Methylprednisolone Acetate is also contraindicated in systemic fungal infections and patients with known hypersensitivity to the product and its constituents.

WARNINGS:

This product contains benzyl alcohol which is potentially toxic when administered locally to neural tissue.

Multidose use of Methylprednisolone Acetate Sterile Aqueous Suspension from a single vial requires special care to avoid contamination. Although initially sterile, any multidose use of vials may lead to contamination unless strict aseptic technique is observed. Particular care, such as use of disposable sterile syringes and needles is necessary.

While crystals of adrenal steroids in the dermis suppress inflammatory reactions, their presence may cause disintegration of the cellular elements and physiochemical changes in the ground substance of the connective tissue. The resultant infrequently occurring dermal and/or subdermal changes may form depressions in the skin at the injection site. The degree to which this reaction occurs will vary with the amount of adrenal steroid injected. Regeneration is usually complete within a few months or after all crystals of the adrenal steroid have been absorbed.

In order to minimize the incidence of dermal and subdermal atrophy, care must be exercised not to exceed recommended doses in injections. Multiple small injections into the area of the lesion should be made whenever possible. The technique of intrasynovial and intramuscular injection should include precautions against injection or leakage into the dermis. Injection into the deltoid muscle should be avoided because of a high incidence of subcutaneous atrophy.

It is critical that, during administration of Methylprednisolone Acetate, appropriate technique be used and care taken to assure proper placement of drug.

In patients on corticosteroid therapy subjected to any unusual stress, increased dosage of rapidly acting corticosteroids before, during, and after the stressful situation is indicated.

Corticosteroids may mask some signs of infection, and new infections may appear during their use. There may be decreased resistance and inability to localize infection when corticosteroids are used. Do not use intra-articularly, intrabursally or for intratendinous administration for *local* effect in the presence of acute infection.

WARNINGS: *(cont'd)*

Prolonged use of corticosteroids may produce posterior subcapsular cataracts, glaucoma with possible damage to the optic nerves, and may enhance the establishment of secondary ocular infections due to fungi or viruses.

Usage In Pregnancy: Since adequate human reproduction studies have not been done with corticosteroids, the use of these drugs in pregnancy, nursing mothers, or women of childbearing potential requires that the possible benefits of the drug be weighed against the potential hazards to the mother and embryo or fetus. Infants born of mothers who have received substantial doses of corticosteroids during pregnancy should be carefully observed for signs of hypoadrenalism.

Average and large doses of cortisone or hydrocortisone can cause elevation of blood pressure, salt and water retention, and increased excretion of potassium. These effects are less likely to occur with the synthetic derivatives except when used in large doses. Dietary salt restriction and potassium supplementation may be necessary. All corticosteroids increase calcium excretion.

While on corticosteroid therapy patients should not be vaccinated against smallpox. Other immunization procedures should not be undertaken in patients who are on corticosteroids, especially in high doses, because of possible hazards of neurological complications and lack of antibody response.

The use of Methylprednisolone Acetate in active tuberculosis should be restricted to those cases of fulminating or disseminated tuberculosis in which the corticosteroid is used for the management of the disease in conjunction with appropriate antituberculous regimen.

If corticosteroids are indicated in patients with latent tuberculosis or tuberculin reactivity, close observation is necessary as reactivation of the disease may occur. During prolonged corticosteroid therapy, these patients should receive chemoprophylaxis.

Because rare instances of anaphylactoid reactions have occurred in patients receiving parenteral corticosteroid therapy, appropriate precautionary measures should be taken prior to administration, especially when the patient has a history of allergy to any drug.

Children who are on immunosuppressant drugs are more susceptible to infections than healthy children. Chickenpox and measles, for example, can have a more serious or even fatal course in children on immunosuppressant corticosteroids. In such children, or in adults who have not had these diseases, particular care should be taken to avoid exposure. If exposed, therapy with varicella zoster immune globulin (VZIG) or pooled intravenous immunoglobin (IVIG), as appropriate, may be indicated. If chickenpox develops, treatment with antiviral agents may be considered.

PRECAUTIONS:

GENERAL

Drug-induced secondary adrenocortical insufficiency may be minimized by gradual reduction of dosage. This type of relative insufficiency may persist for months after discontinuation of therapy; therefore, in any situation of stress occurring during that period, hormone therapy should be reinstituted. Since mineralocorticoid secretion may be impaired, salt and/or a mineralocorticoid should be administered concurrently.

When multidose vials are used, special care to prevent contamination of the contents is essential. There is some evidence that benzalkonium chloride is not an adequate antiseptic for sterilizing Methylprednisolone Acetate Sterile Aqueous Suspension multidose vials. A povidone-iodine solution or similar product is recommended to cleanse the vial top prior to aspiration of contents. (See WARNINGS.)

There is an enhanced effect of corticosteroids in patients with hypothyroidism and in those with cirrhosis.

Corticosteroids should be used cautiously in patients with ocular herpes simplex for fear of corneal perforation.

The lowest possible dose of corticosteroid should be used to control the condition under treatment, and when reduction in dosage is possible, the reduction must be gradual.

Psychic derangements may appear when corticosteroids are used, ranging from euphoria, insomnia, mood swings, personality changes, and severe depression to frank psychotic manifestations. Also, existing emotional instability or psychotic tendencies may be aggravated by corticosteroids.

Aspirin should be used cautiously in conjunction with corticosteroids in hypoprothrombinemia.

Steroids should be used with caution in nonspecific ulcerative colitis, if there is a probability of impending perforation, abscess or other pyogenic infection. Caution must also be used in diverticulitis, fresh intestinal anastomoses, active or latent peptic ulcer, renal insufficiency, hypertension, osteoporosis, and myasthenia gravis, when steroids are used as direct or adjunctive therapy.

Growth and development of infants and children on prolonged corticosteroid therapy should be carefully followed.

The following additional precautions apply for parenteral corticosteroids: Intrasynovial injection of a corticosteroid may produce systemic as well as local effects.

Appropriate examination of any joint fluid present is necessary to exclude a septic process.

A marked increase in pain accompanied by local swelling, further restriction of joint motion, fever, and malaise are suggestive of septic arthritis. If this complication occurs and the diagnosis of sepsis is confirmed, appropriate antimicrobial therapy should be instituted.

Local injection of a steroid into a previously infected joint is to be avoided.

Corticosteroids should not be injected into unstable joints.

The slower rate of absorption by intramuscular administration should be recognized.

Although controlled clinical trials have shown corticosteroids to be effective in speeding the resolution of acute exacerbations of multiple sclerosis, they do not show that corticosteroids affect the ultimate outcome or natural history of the disease. The studies do show that relatively high doses of corticosteroids are necessary to demonstrate a significant effect. (See DOSAGE AND ADMINISTRATION.)

Since complications of treatment with glucocorticoids are dependent on the size of the dose and the duration of treatment, a risk/benefit decision must be made in each individual case as to dose and duration of treatment and as to whether daily or intermittent therapy should be used.

Convulsions have been reported with concurrent use of Methylprednisolone Acetate and cyclosporin. Since concurrent use of these agents results in mutual inhibition of metabolism, it is possible that adverse events associated with the individual use of either drug may be more apt to occur.

INFORMATION FOR THE PATIENT

Patients who are on immunosuppressant doses of corticosteroids should be warned to avoid exposure to chickenpox or measles and, if exposed, to obtain medical advice.

ADVERSE REACTIONS:

Adverse reactions are listed in the following table (TABLE 2):

TABLE 2

Fluid and electrolyte disturbances	
Sodium retention	Potassium loss
Fluid retention	Hypokalemic alkalosis
Congestive heart failure in susceptible patients	Hypertension
Musculoskeletal	
Muscle weakness	Vertebral compression fractures
Steroid myopathy	Aseptic necrosis of femoral and humeral heads
Loss of muscle mass	
Osteoporosis	Pathologic fracture of long bones
Gastrointestinal	
Peptic ulcer with possible subsequent perforation and hemorrhage	Abdominal distention
	Ulcerative esophagitis
Pancreatitis	
Dermatologic	
Impaired wound healing	Facial erythema
Thin fragile skin	Increased sweating
Petechiae and ecchymoses	May suppress reactions to skin tests
Neurological	
Convulsions	Vertigo
Increased intracranial pressure with papilledema (pseudotumor cerebri) usually after treatment	Headache
Endocrine	
Menstrual irregularities	Decreased carbohydrate tolerance
Development of Cushingoid state	Manifestations of latent diabetes mellitus
Suppression of growth in children	
Secondary adrenocortical and pituitary unresponsiveness, particularly in times of stress, as in trauma, surgery or illness	Increased requirements for insulin or oral hypoglycemic agents in diabetes
Ophthalmic	
Posterior subcapsular cataracts	Glaucoma
Increased intraocular pressure	Exophthalmos
Metabolic	
Negative nitrogen balance due to protein catabolism	
The following additional adverse reactions are related to parenteral corticosteroid therapy:	
Anaphylactic reaction	Injection site infections following non-sterile administration (seeWARNINGS)
Allergic or hypersensitivity reactions	
Urticaria	
Hyperpigmentation or hypopigmentation	Postinjection flare, following intrasynovial use
Subcutaneous and cutaneous atrophy	
Sterile abscess	Charcot-like arthropathy
Adverse Reactions Reported with the Following Routes of Administration	
Intrathecal/Epidural	
Arachnoiditis	Bowel/bladder dysfunction
Meningitis	Headache
Paraparesis/paraplegia	Seizures
Sensory disturbances	
Intranasal	
Temporary/permanent visual impairment including blindness	Allergic reactions Rhinitis
Ophthalmic	
Temporary/permanent visual impairment including blindness	Infection
	Residue or slough at injection site
Increased intraocular pressure	
Ocular and periocular inflammation including allergic reactions	
Miscellaneous injection sites (scalp, tonsillar fauces, sphenopalatine ganglion)-blindness	

DOSAGE AND ADMINISTRATION:

Because of possible physical incompatibilities, Methylprednisolone Acetate Sterile Aqueous Suspension should not be diluted or mixed with other solutions.

ADMINISTRATION FOR LOCAL EFFECT

Therapy with Methylprednisolone Acetate does not obviate the need for the conventional measures usually employed. Although this method of treatment will ameliorate symptoms, it is in no sense a cure and the hormone has no effect on the cause of the inflammation.

Rheumatoid and Osteoarthritis. The dose for intra-articular administration depends upon the size of the joint and varies with the severity of the condition in the individual patient. In chronic cases, injections may be repeated at intervals ranging from one to five or more weeks depending upon the degree of relief obtained from the initial injection. The doses in the following table (TABLE 3), are given as a general guide:

TABLE 3

Size of Joint	Examples	Range of Dosage
Large	Knees, Ankles, Shoulders	20 to 80 mg
Medium	Elbows, Wrists	10 to 40 mg
Small	Metacarpophalangeal, Interphalangeal, Sternoclavicular, Acromioclavicular	4 to 10 mg

Procedure: It is recommended that the anatomy of the joint involved be reviewed before attempting intra-articular injection. In order to obtain the full anti-inflammatory effect it is important that the injection be made into the synovial space. Employing the same sterile technique as for a lumbar puncture, a sterile 20 to 24 gauge needle (on a dry syringe) is quickly inserted into the synovial cavity. Procaine infiltration is elective. The aspiration of only a few drops of joint fluid proves the joint space has been entered by the needle. *The injection site for each joint is determined by that location where the synovial cavity is most superficial and most free of large vessels and nerves.* With the needle in place, the aspirating syringe is removed and replaced by a second syringe containing the desired amount of Methylprednisolone Acetate. The plunger is then pulled outward slightly to aspirate synovial fluid and to make sure the needle is still in the synovial space. After injection, the joint is moved gently a few times to aid mixing of the synovial fluid and the suspension. The site is covered with a small sterile dressing.

Suitable sites for intra-articular injection are the knee, ankle, wrist, elbow, shoulder, phalangeal, and hip joints. Since difficulty is not infrequently encountered in entering the hip joint, precautions should be taken to avoid any large blood vessels in the area. Joints not suitable

DOSAGE AND ADMINISTRATION: *(cont'd)*

for injection are those that are anatomically inaccessible such as the spinal joints and those like the sacroiliac joints that are devoid of synovial space. Treatment failures are most frequently the result of failure to enter the joint space. Little or no benefit follows injection into surrounding tissue. If failures occur when injections into the synovial spaces are certain, as determined by aspiration of fluid, repeated injections are usually futile. Local therapy does not alter the underlying disease process, and whenever possible comprehensive therapy including physiotherapy and orthopedic correction should be employed.

Following intra-articular steroid therapy, care should be taken to avoid overuse of joints in which symptomatic benefit has been obtained. Negligence in this matter may permit an increase in joint deterioration that will more than offset the beneficial effects of the steroid.

Unstable joints should not be injected. Repeated intra-articular injection may in some cases result in instability of the joint. X-ray follow-up is suggested in selected cases to detect deterioration.

If a local anesthetic is used prior to injection of Methylprednisolone Acetate, the anesthetic package insert should be read carefully and all the precautions observed.

Bursitis: The area around the injection site is prepared in a sterile way and a wheal at the site made with 1 percent procaine hydrochloride solution. A 20 to 24 gauge needle attached to a dry syringe is inserted into the bursa and the fluid aspirated. The needle is left in place and the aspirating syringe changed for a small syringe containing the desired dose. After injection, the needle is withdrawn and a small dressing applied.

Miscellaneous: Ganglion, Tendinitis, Epicondylitis: In the treatment of conditions such as tendinitis or tenosynovitis, care should be taken, following application of a suitable antiseptic to the overlying skin, to inject the suspension into the tendon sheath rather than into the substance of the tendon. The tendon may be readily palpated when placed on a stretch. When treating conditions such as epicondylitis, the area of greatest tenderness should be outlined carefully and the suspension infiltrated into the area. For ganglia of the tendon sheaths, the suspension is injected directly into the cyst. In many cases, a single injection causes a marked decrease in the size of the cystic tumor and may effect disappearance. The usual sterile precautions should be observed, of course, with each injection.

The dose in the treatment of the various conditions of the tendinous or bursal structures listed above varies with the condition being treated and ranges from 4 to 30 mg. In recurrent or chronic conditions, repeated injections may be necessary.

Injections for Local Effect in Dermatologic Conditions: Following cleansing with an appropriate antiseptic such as 70% alcohol, 20 to 60 mg of the suspension is injected into the lesion. It may be necessary to distribute doses ranging from 20 to 40 mg by repeated local injections in the case of large lesions. Care should be taken to avoid injection of sufficient material to cause blanching since this may be followed by a small slough. One to four injections are usually employed, the intervals between injections varying with the type of lesion being treated and the duration of improvement produced by the initial injection.

When multidose vials are used, special care to prevent contamination of the contents is essential. (See WARNINGS.)

ADMINISTRATION FOR SYSTEMIC EFFECT

The intramuscular dosage will vary with the condition being treated. When employed as a temporary substitute for oral therapy, a single injection during each 24-hour period of a dose of the suspension equal to the total daily oral dose of Medrol Tablets (Methylprednisolone Acetate) is usually sufficient. When a prolonged effect is desired, the weekly dose may be calculated by multiplying the daily oral dose by 7 and given as a single intramuscular injection.

Dosage must be individualized according to the severity of the disease and response of the patient. For infants and children, the recommended dosage will have to be reduced, but dosage should be governed by the severity of the condition rather than by strict adherence to the ratio indicated by age or body weight.

Hormone therapy is an adjunct to, and not a replacement for, conventional therapy. Dosage must be decreased or discontinued gradually when the drug has been administered for more than a few days. The severity, prognosis and expected duration of the disease and the reaction of the patient to medication are primary factors in determining dosage. If a period of spontaneous remission occurs in a chronic condition, treatment should be discontinued. Routine laboratory studies, such as urinalysis, two-hour postprandial blood sugar, determination of blood pressure and body weight, and a chest X-ray should be made at regular intervals during prolonged therapy. Upper GI X-rays are desirable in patients with an ulcer history or significant dyspepsia.

In patients with the **adrenogenital syndrome**, single intramuscular injection of 40 mg every two weeks may be adequate. For maintenance of patients with **rheumatoid arthritis**, the weekly intramuscular dose will vary from 40 to 120 mg. The usual dosage for patients with**dermatologic lesions** benefitted by systemic corticoid therapy is 40 to 120 mg of Methylprednisolone Acetate administered intramuscularly at weekly intervals for one to four weeks. In acute severe dermatitis due to poison ivy, relief may result within 8 to 12 hours following intramuscular administration of a single dose of 80 to 120 mg. In chronic contact dermatitis repeated injections at 5 to 10 day intervals may be necessary. In seborrheic dermatitis, a weekly dose of 80 mg may be adequate to control the condition.

Following intramuscular administration of 80 to 120 mg to asthmatic patients, relief may result within 6 to 48 hours and persist for several days to two weeks. Similarly in patients with allergic rhinitis (hay fever) an intramuscular dose may be followed by relief of coryzal symptoms within six hours persisting for several days to three weeks.

If signs of stress are associated with the condition being treated, the dosage of the suspension should be increased. If a rapid hormonal effect of maximum intensity is required, the intravenous administration of highly soluble Methylprednisolone Acetate sodium succinate is indicated.

MULTIPLE SCLEROSIS

In treatment of acute exacerbations of multiple sclerosis daily doses of 200 mg of prednisolone for a week followed by 80 mg every other day for 1 month have been shown to be effective (4 mg of Methylprednisolone Acetate is equivalent to 5 mg of prednisolone).

Store at controlled room temperature 15-30° C (59-86° F)

PATIENT INFORMATION:

Methylprednisolone acetate is a corticosteroid used to treat inflammation, certain types of arthritis, and as replacement therapy when the adrenal cortex gland is not functioning properly. Inform your physician if you are pregnant or nursing. Inform your physician if you have liver or thyroid problems, diabetes, cataracts, or glaucoma. Inform your physician and dentist that you are receiving methylprednisolone. Methylprednisolone should not be discontinued abruptly. Vaccines (including flu shots) may not work well while you are using this medication. Avoid getting methylprednisolone acetate in your eyes, nose, mouth, or on your skin. Methylprednisolone acetate may decrease your immunity, making it easier for you to get an infection. If you are exposed to chickenpox or measles, tell your physician as soon as possible. Notify your physician if you develop unusual weight loss or gain, muscle weakness, black tarry stools, vomiting, puffy face, menstrual irregularities, or unusual tiredness.

HOW SUPPLIED - EQUIVALENTS NOT AVAILABLE:

Injection, Solution - 20 mg/ml

5 ml	**$10.31**	**DEPO-MEDROL, Pharmacia & Upjohn**	**00009-0274-01**
10 ml	$7.50	Methylprednisolone Acetate, Consolidated Midland	00223-8165-10
10 ml	$7.50	Sterile Methylprednisolone Acetate, Schein Pharm (US)	00364-6748-54
10 ml	$7.50	Methylprednisolone Acetate, Steris Labs	00402-0195-10

Injection, Solution - 40 mg/ml

1 ml	$4.66	Methylprednisolone Acetate, Schein Pharm (US)	00364-3064-51
1 ml	**$5.18**	**DEPO-MEDROL, Pharmacia & Upjohn**	**00009-3073-01**
1 ml x 25	$116.50	Methylprednisolone Acetate, Schein Pharm (US)	00364-3064-46
1 ml x 25	**$129.48**	**DEPO-MEDROL, Pharmacia & Upjohn**	**00009-3073-03**
5 ml	$3.65	Methylprednisolone Acetate, Americal Pharm	54945-0570-41
5 ml	$5.85	Methylprednisolone Acetate, Insource	58441-0111-05
5 ml	$6.95	MED-JEC, AF Hauser	52637-0756-05
5 ml	$7.32	Methylprednisolone Acetate, General Inj & Vac	52584-0196-05
5 ml	$7.50	Methylprednisolone Acetate, Consolidated Midland	00223-8166-05
5 ml	$7.75	METHYLCOTOLONE, C O Truxton	00463-1105-05
5 ml	$8.13	ADLONE, UAD Labs	00785-9055-05
5 ml	$8.42	Methylprednisolone Acetate, United Res	00677-1538-20
5 ml	$8.50	Methylprednisolone Acetate, Steris Labs	00402-1069-05
5 ml	$9.90	DEPOPRED, Hyrex Pharms	00314-0840-75
5 ml	$10.26	Methylprednisolone Acetate, Rugby	00536-5380-65
5 ml	$10.50	Methylprednisolone, IDE-Interstate	00814-4780-38
5 ml	$10.67	Methylprednisolone Acetate, HL Moore Drug Exch	00839-7946-25
5 ml	$10.80	Methylprednisolone Acetate, Pasadena	00418-6401-05
5 ml	$11.50	DEP MEDALONE, Forest Pharms	00456-1071-05
5 ml	$12.00	Methylprednisolone Acetate, Goldline Labs	00182-1067-62
5 ml	$12.00	Methylprednisolone Acetate, Goldline Labs	00182-3131-62
5 ml	$12.00	Methylprednisolone Acetate, Schein Pharm (US)	00364-3064-53
5 ml	**$18.82**	**DEPO-MEDROL, Pharmacia & Upjohn**	**00009-0280-02**
5 ml x 25	**$18.82**	**DEPO-MEDROL, Pharmacia & Upjohn**	**00009-0280-32**
10 ml	$6.05	Methylprednisolone Acetate, Americal Pharm	54945-0570-42
10 ml	$10.49	Methylprednisolone Acetate, Balan	00304-1342-56
10 ml	$11.69	Methylprednisolone Acetate, Steris Labs	00402-1069-10
10 ml	$15.05	Methylprednisolone Acteate, HL Moore Drug Exch	00839-7946-30
10 ml	$15.07	Methylprednisolone Acetate, Schein Pharm (US)	00364-3064-54
10 ml	$15.60	Depopred-40, Hyrex Pharms	00314-0842-70
10 ml	$27.10	DEPOJECT-40, Mayrand Pharms	00259-0356-10
10 ml	**$34.24**	**DEPO-MEDROL, Pharmacia & Upjohn**	**00009-0280-03**
10 ml x 25	**$34.24**	**DEPO-MEDROL, Pharmacia & Upjohn**	**00009-0280-33**

Injection, Solution - 80 mg/ml

1 ml	$7.70	Methylprednisolone Acetate, Schein Pharm (US)	00364-3065-51
1 ml	**$8.57**	**DEPO-MEDROL, Pharmacia & Upjohn**	**00009-3475-01**
1 ml x 25	$192.50	Methylprednisolone Acetate, Schein Pharm (US)	00364-3065-46
1 ml x 25	**$214.23**	**DEPO-MEDROL, Pharmacia & Upjohn**	**00009-3475-03**
5 ml	$6.05	Methylprednisolone Acetate, Americal Pharm	54945-0579-41
5 ml	$8.38	Methylprednisolone Acetate, Insource	58441-0112-05
5 ml	$12.00	Methylprednisolone Acetate, Consolidated Midland	00223-8167-05
5 ml	$12.41	Methylprednisolone Acetate, HL Moore Drug Exch	00839-7947-25
5 ml	$12.50	PREDACORTEN 80, Bolan Pharm	44437-0197-05
5 ml	$12.57	Methylprednisolone Acetate, General Inj & Vac	52584-0197-05
5 ml	$12.81	ADLONE, UAD Labs	00785-0956-05
5 ml	$14.42	Methylprednisolone Acetate, HL Moore Drug Exch	00839-6201-25
5 ml	$15.00	METHYLCOTOLONE 80, C O Truxton	00463-1111-05
5 ml	$15.50	Methylprednisolone Acetate, United Res	00677-1539-20
5 ml	$15.60	DEPOPRED, Hyrex Pharms	00314-0841-75
5 ml	$15.66	Sterile Methylprednisolone Acetate, Rugby	00536-5351-65
5 ml	$15.66	Methylprednisolone Acetate, Rugby	00536-5385-65
5 ml	$15.69	Methylprednisolone Acetate, Steris Labs	00402-1070-05
5 ml	$15.70	Methylprednisolone Acetate, Major Pharms	00904-0897-05
5 ml	$15.75	Methylprednisolone Acetate, IDE-Interstate	00814-4782-38
5 ml	$19.20	Methylprednisolone Acetate, Goldline Labs	00182-0332-62
5 ml	$19.20	Methylprednisolone Acetate, Goldline Labs	00182-1068-62
5 ml	$19.20	Methylprednisolone Acetate, Goldline Labs	00182-3132-62
5 ml	$19.20	Methylprednisolone Acetate, Schein Pharm (US)	00364-3065-53
5 ml	$20.00	DEP MEDALONE, Forest Pharms	00456-1072-05
5 ml	$27.10	DEPOJECT-80, Mayrand Pharms	00259-0357-05
5 ml	**$34.24**	**DEPO-MEDROL, Pharmacia & Upjohn**	**00009-0306-02**
5 ml x 25	**$34.24**	**DEPO-MEDROL, Pharmacia & Upjohn**	**00009-0306-10**

METHYLPREDNISOLONE ACETATE; NEOMYCIN SULFATE *(001793)*

CATEGORIES: Adrenal Corticosteroids; Anti-Infectives; Antibiotics; Dermatologicals; Dermatoses; Infections; Skin Infections; Skin/Mucous Membrane Agents; Steroids; FDA Approval Pre 1982

BRAND NAMES: *Neo Moderin*; Neo-Medrol Acetate; *Neo-Medrone* (England)
(International brand names outside U.S. in italics)

DESCRIPTION:

Methylprednisolone is the markedly effective anti-inflammatory corticosteroid synthesized and developed in the Research Laboratories of The Upjohn Company. Clinical studies indicate that topically applied Medrol Acetate Topical (methylprednisolone) is highly active. Neo-Medrol Acetate Topical contains methylprednisolone acetate in a concentration of 0.25% and the broad-spectrum antibiotic, neomycin sulfate, equivalent to 3.5 mg neomycin. Each gram of this preparation contains methylparaben 0.4% and butylparaben 0.3%. The lipid base is composed of saturated and unsaturated free fatty acids; triglycerol and other esters of fatty acids; saturated and unsaturated hydrocarbons; free cholesterol; high-molecular weight alcohol; with water and aromatics. When necessary, pH was adjusted with sulfuric acid.

The synthetic lipid base used in this product was developed in the Research Laboratories of The Upjohn Company and designed to serve as a vehicle for various drugs applied topically to the skin. In composition it is as close as possible to that of the normal skin-lipids. It resembles a cream in appearance but has the feel of an ointment. Clinically it is well tolerated, possessing softening properties without the greasiness of an ointment or the drying effect of cream. Such a base is desirable for replacing the natural lipids of the skin.

CLINICAL PHARMACOLOGY:

Topical steroids are primarily effective because of their anti-inflammatory, antipruritic and vasoconstrictive actions.

Methylprednisolone, one of the most potent corticosteroids, exerts a profound anti-inflammatory action at the tissue level. Studies of anti-inflammatory activity, using the granuloma pouch assay, have shown it to be more potent, on a weight basis, than prednisolone. Similarly a high order of activity has been observed following local application of methylprednisolone. Because of this high order of activity, it is effective topically in the available low concentrations. Prompt control of excessive tissue reaction to allergens, irritants, and trauma may be anticipated following the use of these topical preparations.

CLINICAL PHARMACOLOGY: *(cont'd)*

Methylprednisolone applied locally has been found to be rapidly effective in acute uncomplicated allergic dermatitis. In many instances objective signs of improvement, subsidence of erythema and edema, as well as symptomatic relief occur within a few hours of the first application. With symptomatic relief, further damage to the skin, with subsequent possible infection, is prevented. Following discontinuance of applications no "rebound" activation of lesions has been observed.

Neomycin is an antibacterial substance derived from cultures of the soil organism *Streptomyces fradiae*. It exhibits a wider spectrum of antibacterial activity than does bacitracin, streptomycin, or penicillin and is active against a variety of gram-positive and gram-negative organisms including *staphylococci, Escherichia coli,* and *Hemophilus influenzae*. It is not active against fungi. Neomycin rarely causes resistant strains of microorganisms to develop; in addition, it is unusually nontoxic for human epithelial cells in tissue culture and is nonirritating topically in therapeutic concentrations.

INDICATIONS AND USAGE:

For the treatment of corticosteroid-responsive dermatoses with secondary infection. It has not been demonstrated that this steroid-antibiotic combination provides greater benefit than the steroid component alone after seven days of treatment. (See WARNINGS.)

CONTRAINDICATIONS:

Local application is contraindicated in tuberculosis of the skin, herpes simplex, vaccinia, varicella, and in other cutaneous infections for which an effective antibiotic or chemotherapeutic agent is not available for simultaneous application.

Neo-Medrol Acetate Topical should not be used in individuals with a history of hypersensitivity to any of its components.

WARNINGS:

Because of the potential hazard of nephrotoxicity and ototoxicity, prolonged use of large amounts of this product should be avoided in the treatment of skin infections following extensive burns, trophic ulceration and other conditions where absorption of neomycin is possible.

Because of the concern of nephrotoxicity and ototoxicity associated with neomycin, this combination product should not be used over a wide area or for extended periods of time.

PRECAUTIONS:

This preparation is usually well tolerated. However, neomycin may occasionally induce sensitivity reactions. If signs of irritation or sensitivity should develop, application should be discontinued.

If extensive areas are treated or if the occlusive technique is used, the possibility exists of increased absorption of the corticoid and suitable precautions should be taken.

The safety of the use of topical steroid preparations during pregnancy has not been fully established. Therefore, they should not be used unnecessarily during pregnancy, on extended areas, in large amounts, or for prolonged periods of time.

This product should not be put in the eyes or, if the ear drum is perforated, in the external ear canal.

Note: The prolonged use of antibiotic containing preparations may result in overgrowth of non-susceptible organisms, particularly fungi. If new infections appear during treatment, appropriate therapy should be instituted.

ADVERSE REACTIONS:

When steroid preparations are used for long periods in intertriginous areas or under occlusive dressing, localized atrophy and striae may occur.

Other local adverse reactions associated with topically applied corticoids either with or without occlusive dressings include: burning sensations, itching, irritation, dryness, folliculitis, secondary infection, atrophy of the skin, acneiform eruption and hypopigmentation.

Ototoxicity and nephrotoxicity have been reported following absorption of topically applied neomycin.

According to current medical literature there has been an increase in the prevalence of neomycin hypersensitivity.

DOSAGE AND ADMINISTRATION:

After careful cleansing of the affected skin to minimize the possibility of introducing infection, a small amount is applied and rubbed gently into the involved areas. Application should be made initially one to three times daily. Once control is achieved—usually within a few hours—the frequency of application should be reduced to the minimum necessary to avoid relapses.

HOW SUPPLIED - EQUIVALENTS NOT AVAILABLE:

Cream - Topical - 2.5 mg

30 gm $17.85 NEO-MEDROL ACETATE, Pharmacia & Upjohn 00009-0888-02

METHYLPREDNISOLONE SODIUM SUCCINATE *(001794)*

CATEGORIES: Adrenal Corticosteroids; Adrenal Hyperplasia; Adrenal Insufficiency; Adrenocortical Insufficiency; Airway Obstruction; Allergies; Anemia; Ankylosing Spondylitis; Anti-Inflammatory Agents; Antidiarrhea Agents; Antineoplastics; Arthritis; Asthma; Atopic Dermatitis; Bursitis; Cancer; Carditis; Chemotherapy; Chorioretinitis; Choroiditis; Colitis; Conjunctivitis; Corneal Ulcer; Dermatitis; Dermatitis Herpetiformis; Dermatomyositis; Diuresis; Drug Hypersensitivity; Epicondylitis; Erythema Multiforme; Gastrointestinal Drugs; Glucocorticoids; Gouty Arthritis; Herpes; Herpes Zoster; Hormones; Hypercalcemia; Inflammation; Iridocyclitis; Keratitis; Laryngeal Edema; Leukemia; Lupus Erythematosus; Lymphoma; Meningitis; Multiple Sclerosis; Mycosis Fungoides; Neoplastic Disease; Nephrotic Syndrome; Neuritis; Ocular Infections; Ophthalmics; Osteoarthritis; Pemphigus; Pneumoconiosis; Proteinuria; Psoriasis; Purpura; Retinochoroiditis; Rhinitis; Sarcoidosis; Serum Sickness; Shock; Spondylitis; Steroids; Synovitis; Synovitis of Osteoarthritis; Tenosynovitis; Thrombocytopenia; Thyroiditis; Transfusion Reactions; Trichinosis; Tuberculosis; Ulcerative Colitis; Urticaria; Uveitis; FDA Approval Pre 1982

BRAND NAMES: A-Methapred; *Cryosolona* (Mexico); *Medrate Solubile* (Germany); *Mepsolone*; *Methysol*; *Metypresol*; *Solomet*; *Solu Medrol* (Mexico); **Solu-Medrol**; *Solu-Medrone* (England); *Solu-Moderin*; *Urbason Solubile* (Germany); *Urbason Solubile Forte*; *Urbason Soluble*; *Yumerol*
(International brand names outside U.S. in italics)

DESCRIPTION:

Methylprednisolone Sodium Succinate Sterile Powder contains Methylprednisolone Sodium Succinate as the active ingredient. Methylprednisolone Sodium Succinate, USP, occurs as a white, or nearly white, odorless hygroscopic, amorphous solid. It is very soluble in water and in alcohol; it is insoluble in chloroform and is very slightly soluble in acetone.

The chemical name for Methylprednisolone Sodium Succinate is pregna-1,4-diene-3,20-dione,21-(3-carboxy-1-oxopropoxy)-11,17-dihydroxy-6 -methyl-monosodium salt, (6α, 11β) and the molecular weight is 496.53.

Methylprednisolone Sodium Succinate is so extremely soluble in water that it may be administered in a small volume of diluent and is especially well suited for intravenous use in situations in which high blood levels of methylprednisolone are required rapidly.

Methylprednisolone Sodium Succinate is available in several strengths and packages for intravenous or intramuscular administration.

40 mg ACT-O-VIAL (Upjohn) System (Single-Dose Vial): Each ml (when mixed) contains Methylprednisolone Sodium Succinate equivalent to 40 mg methylprednisolone; also 1.6 mg monobasic sodium phosphate anhydrous; 17.46 mg dibasic sodium phosphate dried; 25 mg lactose hydrous; 8.8 mg benzyl alcohol added as preservative.

125 mg ACT-O-VIAL System (Single-Dose Vial): Each 2 ml (when mixed) contains Methylprednisolone Sodium Succinate equivalent to 125 mg methylprednisolone; also 1.6 mg monobasic sodium phosphate anhydrous; 17.4 mg dibasic sodium phosphate dried; 17.6 mg benzyl alcohol added as preservative.

500 mg Vial: Each 8 ml (when mixed as directed) contains Methylprednisolone Sodium Succinate equivalent to 500 mg methylprednisolone; also 6.4 mg monobasic sodium phosphate anhydrous; 69.6 mg dibasic sodium phosphate dried.

500 mg Vial with Diluent: Each 8 ml (when mixed as directed) contains Methylprednisolone Sodium Succinate equivalent to 500 mg methylprednisolone; also 6.4 mg monobasic sodium phosphate anhydrous; 69.6 mg dibasic sodium phosphate dried; 70.2 mg benzyl alcohol added as preservative.

1 gram Vial: Each 16 ml (when mixed as directed) contains Methylprednisolone Sodium Succinate equivalent to 1 gram methylprednisolone; also 12.8 mg monobasic sodium phosphate anhydrous; 139.2 mg dibasic sodium phosphate dried.

1 gram ACT-O-VIAL System (Single-Dose Vial): Each 8 ml (when mixed) contains Methylprednisolone Sodium Succinate equivalent to 1 gram methylprednisolone; also 12.8 mg monobasic sodium phosphate anhydrous; 139.2 mg dibasic sodium phosphate dried; 66.8 mg benzyl alcohol added as preservative.

2 gram Vial: Each 30.6 ml (when mixed as directed) contains Methylprednisolone Sodium Succinate equivalent to 2 grams methylprednisolone; also 25.6 mg monobasic sodium phosphate anhydrous; 278 mg dibasic sodium phosphate dried.

2 gram Vial with Diluent: Each 30.6 ml (when mixed as directed) contains Methylprednisolone Sodium Succinate equivalent to 2 grams methylprednisolone; also 25.6 mg monobasic sodium phosphate anhydrous; 278 mg dibasic sodium phosphate dried; 273 mg benzyl alcohol added as preservative.

When necessary, the pH of each formula was adjusted with sodium hydroxide so that the pH of the reconstituted solution is within the USP specified range of 7 to 8 and the tonicities are, for the 40 mg per ml solution, 0.50 osmolar; for the 125 mg per 2 ml, 500 mg per 8 ml and 1 gram per 16 ml solutions, 0.40 osmolar; for the 1 gram per 8 ml solution, 0.44 osmolar; for the 2 gram per 30.6 ml solutions, 0.42 osmolar. (Isotonic saline = 0.28 osmolar).

IMPORTANT: Use only the accompanying diluent
or Bacteriostatic Water For Injection with
Benzyl Alcohol when reconstituting Methylprednisolone Sodium Succinate.
Use within 48 hours after mixing.

CLINICAL PHARMACOLOGY:

Methylprednisolone is a potent anti-inflammatory steroid synthesized in the Research Laboratories of The Upjohn Company. It has a greater antiinflammatory potency than prednisolone and even less tendency than prednisolone to induce sodium and water retention.

Methylprednisolone Sodium Succinate has the same metabolic and anti-inflammatory actions as methylprednisolone. When given parenterally and in equimolar quantities, the two compounds are equivalent in biologic activity. The relative potency of Methylprednisolone Sodium Succinate Sterile Powder and hydrocortisone sodium succinate, as indicated by depression of eosinophil count, following intravenous administration, is at least four to one. This is in good agreement with the relative oral potency of methylprednisolone and hydrocortisone.

INDICATIONS AND USAGE:

When oral therapy is not feasible, and the strength, dosage form and route of administration of the drug reasonably lend the preparation to the treatment of the condition, Methylprednisolone Sodium Succinate Sterile Powder is indicated for intravenous or intramuscular use in the following conditions:

Endocrine Disorders: Primary or secondary adrenocortical insufficiency (hydrocortisone or cortisone is the drug of choice; synthetic analogs may be used in conjunction with mineralocorticoids where applicable; in infancy, mineralocorticoid supplementation is of particular importance) Acute adrenocortical insufficiency (hydrocortisone or cortisone is the drug of choice; mineralocorticoid supplementation may be necessary, particularly when synthetic analogs are used).

Preoperatively and in the event of serious trauma or illness, in patients with known adrenal insufficiency or when adrenocortical reserve is doubtful.

Shock unresponsive to conventional therapy if adrenocortical insufficiency exists or is suspected

Congenital adrenal hyperplasia, Nonsuppurative thyroiditis Hypercalcemia associated with cancer.

Rheumatic Disorders: As adjunctive therapy for short-term administration (to tide the patient over an acute episode or exacerbation) in:

Post-traumatic osteoarthritis, Epicondylitis, Synovitis of osteoarthritis, Acute nonspecific tenosynovitis, Rheumatoid arthritis, including juvenile rheumatoid arthritis (select cases may require low-dose maintenance therapy), Acute gouty arthritis, Psoriatic arthritis, Ankylosing spondylitis, Acute and subacute bursitis

Collagen Diseases: During an exacerbation or as maintenance therapy in selected cases of:

Systemic lupus erythematosus, Acute rheumatic carditis, Systemic dermatomyositis (polymyositis)

Dermatologic Diseases: Pemphigus, Bullous dermatitis herpetiformis, Severe erythema multiforme (Stevens-Johnson syndrome), Severe seborrheic dermatitis, Severe psoriasis, Exfoliative dermatitis, Mycosis fungoides

Allergic States: Control of severe or incapacitating allergic conditions intractable to adequate trials of conventional treatment in:

INDICATIONS AND USAGE: *(cont'd)*

Bronchial asthma, Drug hypersensitivity reactions, Contact dermatitis, Urticarial transfusion reactions, Atopic dermatitis, Acute noninfectious laryngeal edema (epinephrine is the drug of first choice), Serum sickness, Seasonal or perennial allergic rhinitis

Ophthalmic Diseases: Severe acute and chronic allergic and inflammatory processes involving the eye, such as:

Herpes zoster ophthalmicus, Sympathetic ophthalmia, Iritis, iridocyclitis, Anterior segment inflammation, Chorioretinitis, Allergic conjunctivitis, Diffuse posterior uveitis and choroiditis, Allergic corneal marginal ulcers, Optic neuritis, Keratitis

Gastrointestinal Diseases: To tide the patient over a critical period of the disease in:

Ulcerative colitis (systemic therapy), Regional enteritis (systemic therapy)

Respiratory Diseases: Symptomatic sarcoidosis, Loeffler's syndrome not manageable by other means, Berylliosis, Aspiration pneumonitis, Fulminating or disseminated pulmonary tuberculosis when used concurrently with appropriate antituberculous chemotherapy

Hematologic Disorders: Acquired (autoimmune) hemolytic anemia, Erythroblastopenia (RBC anemia), Idiopathic thrombocytopenic purpura in adults (IV only; IM administration is contraindicated), Congenital (erythroid) hypoplastic anemia, Secondary thrombocytopenia in adults

Neoplastic Disease: For palliative management of: Leukemias and lymphomas in adults, Acute leukemia of childhood

Edematous States: To induce diuresis or remission of proteinuria in the nephrotic syndrome, without uremia, of the idiopathic type or that due to lupus erythematosus

Nervous System: Acute exacerbations of multiple sclerosis

Miscellaneous: Tuberculous meningitis with subarachnoid block or impending block when used concurrently with appropriate antituberculous chemotherapy

Trichinosis with neurologic or myocardial involvement

CONTRAINDICATIONS:

The use of Methylprednisolone Sodium Succinate Sterile Powder is contraindicated in premature infants because the **40 mg**ACT-O-VIAL, the **125 mg** ACT-O-VIAL, the **1 gram** ACT-O-VIAL system, and the accompanying diluent for the 500 mg and 2 gram vials contain benzyl alcohol. Benzyl alcohol has been reported to be associated with a fatal "Gasping Syndrome" in premature infants. Methylprednisolone Sodium Succinate Sterile Powder is also contraindicated in systemic fungal infections and patients with known hypersensitivity to the product and its constituents.

WARNINGS:

In patients on corticosteroid therapy subjected to any unusual stress, increased dosage of rapidly acting corticosteroids before, during, and after the stressful situation is indicated.

Corticosteroids may mask some signs of infection, and new infections may appear during their use. There may be decreased resistance and inability to localize infection when corticosteroids are used.

A study has failed to establish the efficacy of Methylprednisolone Sodium Succinate in the treatment of sepsis syndrome and septic shock. The study also suggests that treatment of these conditions with Methylprednisolone Sodium Succinate may increase the risk of mortality in certain patients (*i.e.,* patients with elevated serum creatinine levels or patients who develop secondary infections after Methylprednisolone Sodium Succinate).

Prolonged use of corticosteroids may produce posterior subcapsular cataracts, glaucoma with possible damage to the optic nerves, and may enhance the establishment of secondary ocular infections due to fungi or viruses.

Usage in Pregnancy: Since adequate human reproduction studies have not been done with corticosteroids, the use of these drugs in pregnancy, nursing mothers, or women of childbearing potential requires that the possible benefits of the drug be weighed against the potential hazards to the mother and embryo or fetus. Infants born of mothers who have received substantial doses of corticosteroids during pregnancy should be carefully observed for signs of hypoadrenalism.

Average and large doses of cortisone or hydrocortisone can cause elevation of blood pressure, salt and water retention, and increased excretion of potassium. These effects are less likely to occur with the synthetic derivatives except when used in large doses. Dietary salt restriction and potassium supplementation may be necessary. All corticosteroids increase calcium excretion.

While on corticosteroid therapy patients should not be vaccinated against smallpox. Other immunization procedures should not be undertaken in patients who are on corticosteroids, especially on high dose, because of possible hazards of neurological complications and a lack of antibody response.

The use of Methylprednisolone Sodium Succinate Sterile Powder in active tuberculosis should be restricted to those cases of fulminating or disseminated tuberculosis in which the corticosteroid is used for the management of the disease in conjunction with appropriate antituberculous regimen.

If corticosteroids are indicated in patients with latent tuberculosis or tuberculin reactivity, close observation is necessary as reactivation of the disease may occur. During prolonged corticosteroid therapy, these patients should receive chemoprophylaxis.

Because rare instances of anaphylactic (*e.g.,* bronchospasm) reactions have occurred in patients receiving parenteral corticosteroid therapy, appropriate precautionary measures should be taken prior to administration, especially when the patient has a history of allergy to any drug.

There are reports of cardiac arrhythmias and/or circulatory collapse and/or cardiac arrest following the rapid administration of large IV doses of Methylprednisolone Sodium Succinate (greater than 0.5 gram administered over a period of less than 10 minutes). Bradycardia has been reported during or after the administration of large doses of Methylprednisolone Sodium Succinate, and may be unrelated to the speed or duration of infusion.

Children who are on immunosuppressant drugs are more susceptible to infections than healthy children. Chickenpox and measles, for example, can have a more serious or even fatal course in children on immunosuppressant corticosteroids. In such children, or in adults who have not had these diseases, particular care should be taken to avoid exposure. If exposed, therapy with varicella zoster immune globulin (VZIG) or pooled intravenous immunoglobin (IVIG), as appropriate, may be indicated. If chickenpox develops, treatment with antiviral agents may be considered.

PRECAUTIONS:

GENERAL

Drug-induced secondary adrenocortical insufficiency may be minimized by gradual reduction of dosage. This type of relative insufficiency may persist for months after discontinuation of therapy; therefore, in any situation of stress occurring during that period, hormone therapy should be reinstituted. Since mineralocorticoid secretion may be impaired, salt and/or a mineralocorticoid should be administered concurrently.

PRECAUTIONS: *(cont'd)*

There is an enhanced effect of corticosteroids on patients with hypothyroidism and in those with cirrhosis.

Corticosteroids should be used cautiously in patients with ocular herpes simplex because of possible corneal perforation.

The lowest possible dose of corticosteroid should be used to control the condition under treatment, and when reduction in dosage is possible, the reduction should be gradual.

Psychic derangements may appear when corticosteroids are used, ranging from euphoria, insomnia, mood swings, personality changes, and severe depression, to frank psychotic manifestations. Also, existing emotional instability or psychotic tendencies may be aggravated by corticosteroids.

Aspirin should be used cautiously in conjunction with corticosteroids in hypoprothrombinemia.

Steroids should be used with caution in nonspecific ulcerative colitis, if there is a probability of impending perforation, abscess or other pyogenic infection; diverticulitis; fresh intestinal anastomoses; active or latent peptic ulcer; renal insufficiency; hypertension; osteoporosis; and myasthenia gravis.

Growth and development of infants and children on prolonged corticosteroid therapy should be carefully observed.

Although controlled clinical trials have shown corticosteroids to be effective in speeding the resolution of acute exacerbations of multiple sclerosis, they do not show that corticosteroids affect the ultimate outcome or natural history of the disease. The studies do show that relatively high doses of corticosteroids are necessary to demonstrate a significant effect. (See DOSAGE AND ADMINISTRATION.)

Since complications of treatment with glucocorticoids are dependent on the size of the dose and the duration of treatment, a risk/benefit decision must be made in each individual case as to dose and duration of treatment and as to whether daily or intermittent therapy should be used.

Convulsions have been reported with concurrent use of methylprednisolone and cyclosporin. Since concurrent use of these agents results in a mutual inhibition of metabolism, it is possible that adverse events associated with the individual use of either drug may be more apt to occur.

INFORMATION FOR THE PATIENT

Patients who are on immunosuppressant doses of corticosteroids should be warned to avoid exposure to chickenpox or measles and, if exposed, to obtain medical advice.

ADVERSE REACTIONS:

Fluid and Electrolyte Disturbances: Sodium retention, Potassium loss, Fluid retention, Hypokalemic alkalosis, Congestive heart failure in susceptible patients, Hypertension

Musculoskeletal: Muscle weakness, Aseptic necrosis of femoral and humeral heads, Steroid myopathy, Loss of muscle mass, Pathologic fracture of long bones, Severe arthralgia, Osteoporosis, Vertebral compression fractures

Gastrointestinal: Peptic ulcer with possible perforation and hemorrhage, Abdominal distention, Ulcerative esophagitis, Pancreatitis

Dermatologic: Impaired wound healing, Facial erythema, Thin fragile skin, Increased sweating, Petechiae and ecchymoses, May suppress reactions to skin tests

Neurological: Increased intracranial pressure with papilledema (pseudo-tumor cerebri) usually after treatment, convulsions, vertigo, headache

Endocrine: Development of Cushingoid state, Menstrual irregularities, Suppression of growth in children, Decreased carbohydrate tolerance, Secondary adrenocortical and pituitary unresponsiveness, particularly in times of stress, as in trauma, surgery or illness, Manifestations of latent diabetes mellitus, Increased requirements for insulin or oral hypoglycemic agents in diabetes

Ophthalmic: Posterior subcapsular cataracts, Glaucoma, Increased intraocular pressure exophthalmos

Metabolic: Negative nitrogen balance due to protein catabolism

The following *additional* adverse reactions are related to parenteral corticosteroid therapy:

Hyperpigmentation or hypopigmentation

Subcutaneous and cutaneous atrophy

Sterile abscess

Anaphylactic reaction with or without circulatory collapse, cardiac arrest, bronchospasm

Urticaria

Nausea and vomiting

Cardiac arrhythmias; hypotension or hypertension

DOSAGE AND ADMINISTRATION:

When high dose therapy is desired, the recommended dose of Methylprednisolone Sodium Succinate Sterile Powder is 30 mg/kg administered intravenously over at least 30 minutes. This dose may be repeated every 4 to 6 hours for 48 hours.

In general, high dose corticosteroid therapy should be continued only until the patient's condition has stabilized; usually not beyond 48 to 72 hours.

Although adverse effects associated with high dose short-term corticoid therapy are uncommon, peptic ulceration may occur. Prophylactic antacid therapy may be indicated.

In other indications initial dosage will vary from 10 to 40 mg of methylprednisolone depending on the clinical problem being treated. The larger doses may be required for short-term management of severe, acute conditions. The initial dose usually should be given intravenously over a period of several minutes. Subsequent doses may be given intravenously or intramuscularly at intervals dictated by the patient's response and clinical condition. Corticoid therapy is an adjunct to, and not replacement for conventional therapy.

Dosage may be reduced for infants and children but should be governed more by the severity of the condition and response of the patient than by age or size. It should not be less than 0.5 mg per kg every 24 hours.

Dosage must be decreased or discontinued gradually when the drug has been administered for more than a few days. If a period of spontaneous remission occurs in a chronic condition, treatment should be discontinued. Routine laboratory studies, such as urinalysis, two-hour postprandial blood sugar, determination of blood pressure and body weight, and a chest X-ray should be made at regular intervals during prolonged therapy. Upper GI X-rays are desirable in patients with an ulcer history or significant dyspepsia.

Methylprednisolone Sodium Succinate may be administered by intravenous or intramuscular injection or by intravenous infusion, the preferred method for initial emergency use being intravenous injection. To administer by intravenous (or intramuscular) injection, prepare solution as directed. The desired dose may be administered intravenously over a period of several minutes. If desired, the medication may be administered in diluted solutions by adding Water for Injection or other suitable diluent to the **ACT-O-VIAL** and withdrawing the indicated dose.

DOSAGE AND ADMINISTRATION: *(cont'd)*

To prepare solutions for intravenous infusion, first prepare the solution for injection as directed. This solution may then be added to indicated amounts of 5% dextrose in water, isotonic saline solution or 5% dextrose in isotonic saline solution.

MULTIPLE SCLEROSIS

In treatment of acute exacerbations of multiple sclerosis, daily doses of 200 mg of prednisolone for a week followed by 80 mg every other day for 1 month have been shown to be effective (4 mg of methylprednisolone is equivalent to 5 mg of prednisolone).

DIRECTIONS FOR USING THE ACT-O-VIAL SYSTEM

1. Press down on plastic activator to force diluent into the lower compartment.

2. Gently agitate to effect solution.

3. Remove plastic tab covering center of stopper.

4. Sterilize top of stopper with a suitable germicide.

5. Insert needle **squarely through center** of stopper until tip is just visible. Invert vial and withdraw dose.

Storage: Store unreconstituted product at controlled room 15-30° C (59-86° F).

Store solution at controlled room temperature 15-30° (59°-86° F).

Use solution within 48 hours after mixing.

HOW SUPPLIED - RATED THERAPEUTICALLY EQUIVALENT:

Injection, Lyphl-Soln - Intramuscular; - 1 gm/vial

1's	$28.89	Methylprednisolone Sod Succ, Fujisawa USA	00469-1290-60
1's	$30.31	Methylprednisolone Sod Succ, Fujisawa USA	00469-1880-08
1's	$53.50	Methylprednisolone Sod Succ, Elkins Sinn	00641-2508-41
8 ml	$32.21	ACT-O-VIAL SOLU-MEDROL 1, Pharmacia & Upjohn	00009-3389-01
8 ml	$51.67	A-METHAPRED, Abbott	00074-5631-08
1000 mg	$50.68	A-METHAPRED 1000, Abbott	00074-5603-44

Injection, Lyphl-Soln - Intramuscular; - 40 mg/vial

1 ml	**$2.00**	**SOLU-MEDROL 40, Pharmacia & Upjohn**	**00009-0113-12**
1 ml	$2.95	A-METHAPRED, Abbott	00074-5684-01
1's	$2.50	Methylprednisolone Sod Succ, Elkins Sinn	00641-2505-41
1's	$4.00	Methylprednisolone Sod Succ, Consolidated Midland	00223-8160-01
25's	**$50.04**	**SOLU-MEDROL, Pharmacia & Upjohn**	**00009-0113-19**
25's	$67.19	Methylprednisolone Sod Succ, Fujisawa USA	00469-1010-00

Injection, Lyphl-Soln - Intramuscular; - 125 mg/vial

1's	$7.00	Methylprednisolone Sod Succ, Elkins Sinn	00641-2506-41
1's	$12.00	Methylprednisolone Sod Succ, Consolidated Midland	00223-8161-02
1's	$12.50	Methylprednisolone Sod Succ, Consolidated Midland	00223-8160-02
2 ml	**$5.32**	**SOLU-MEDROL, Pharmacia & Upjohn**	**00009-0190-09**
2 ml	$7.79	A-METHAPRED, Abbott	00074-5685-02
25's	$130.00	Methylprednisolone Sod Succin, Fujisawa USA	00469-1020-10
25's	**$132.92**	**SOLU-MEDROL, Pharmacia & Upjohn**	**00009-0190-16**

Injection, Lyphl-Soln - Intramuscular; - 500 mg/vial

1's	$17.03	Methylprednisolone Sod Succ, Fujisawa USA	00469-1280-40
1's	$17.94	Methylprednisolone Sod Succ, Fujisawa USA	00469-1870-70
1's	$30.40	Methylprednisolone Sod Succ, Elkins Sinn	00641-2507-41
4 ml	$20.08	Act-0-Vial Solu-Medrol 500 Mg, Pharmacia & Upjohn	00009-0765-02
4 ml	$30.35	A-METHAPRED, Abbott	00074-5630-04
8 ml	**$20.08**	**SOLU-MEDROL, Pharmacia & Upjohn**	**00009-0887-01**
30's	$37.50	Methylprednisolone Sod Succ, Consolidated Midland	00223-8162-03
500 mg	$29.95	A-METHAPRED 500, Abbott	00074-5601-44

HOW SUPPLIED - NOT RATED EQUIVALENT:

Injection, Solution - Intramuscular; - 2 gm/vial

30 ml	**$54.73**	**SOLU-MEDROL, Pharmacia & Upjohn**	**00009-0796-01**

METHYLTESTOSTERONE *(001795)*

CATEGORIES: Anabolic Steroids; Androgen Deficiency; Androgens; Antiestrogen; Antineoplastics; Breast Carcinoma; Cancer; Cryptorchidism; Delayed Puberty; Hormones; Hypogonadism; Impotence; Oncologic Drugs; Tumors; Breast Engorgement*; Pregnancy Category X; DEA Class CIII; FDA Approval Pre 1982
* Indication not approved by the FDA

BRAND NAMES: **Android**; *Androral*; *Enarmon* (Japan); *Fopou*; *Forton*; *Madiol*; Metandren; Metestone; Oreton Methyl; Primotest; *Testo-B*; *Teston*; *Testotonic "B"*; *Testovis*; Testred; Vigorex; Virilon; *Virormone*
(International brand names outside U.S. in italics)

FORMULARIES: Aetna; BC-BS; FHP; Medi-Cal

DESCRIPTION:

The androgens are steroids that develop and maintain primary and secondary male sex characteristics.

Androgens are derivatives of cyclopentanoperhydrophenanthrene. Endogenous androgens are C-19 steroids with a side chain at C-17, and with two angular methyl groups. Testosterone is the primary endogenous androgen. In their active form, all drugs in the class have a 17-beta hydroxy group. 17-alpha alkylation (methyltestosterone) increases the pharmacologic activity per unit weight compared to testosterone when given orally.

Methyltestosterone, a synthetic derivative of testosterone, is an androgenic preparation given by the oral route in a capsule for. Each capsule contains 10 mg, each tablet contains 10 mg or 25 mg of Methyltestosterone USP. The empirical formula $C_{20}H_{30}O_2$, and a molecular weight of 302.46.

Chemically, Methyltestosterone is 17-β-hydroxy-17-methylandrost-4-en-3-one.

Each Android capsule, for oral administration, contains 10 mg of Methyltestosterone. In addition, each capsule contains the following inactive ingredients: Corn starch NF, Gelatin NF, FD&C Blue #1, FD&C Red #40. 25 mg tablets also contain FD&C Yellow No. 6.

CLINICAL PHARMACOLOGY:

Endogenous androgens are responsible for the normal growth and development of the male sex organs and for the maintenance of secondary sex characteristics. These effects include the growth and maturation of the prostate, seminal vesicles, penis, and scrotum. The development of male hair distribution, such as beard, pubic, chest, and axillary hair; laryngeal enlargement; vocal cord thickening; alterations in body musculature; and fat distribution. Drugs in this class also cause retention of nitrogen, sodium, potassium, and phosphorus, and decreased urinary excretion of calcium. Androgens have been reported to increase protein anabolism and decrease protein catabolism. Nitrogen balance is improved only when there is sufficient intake of calories and protein.

CLINICAL PHARMACOLOGY: *(cont'd)*

Androgens are responsible for the growth spurt of adolescence and for the eventual termination of linear growth, which is brought about by fusion of the epiphyseal growth centers. In children, exogenous androgens accelerate linear growth rates but may cause a disproportionate advancement in bone maturation. Use over long periods may result in fusion of the epiphyseal growth centers and termination of the growth process. Androgens have been reported to stimulate the production of red blood cells by enhancing the production of erythropoietic stimulating factor.

During exogenous administration of androgens, endogenous testosterone release is inhibited through feedback inhibition of pituitary luteinizing hormone (LH). At large doses of exogenous androgens, spermatogenesis may also be suppressed through feedback inhibition of pituitary follicle- stimulating hormone (FSH).

There is a lack of substantial evidence that androgens are effective in fractures, surgery, convalescence, and functional uterine bleeding.

Pharmacokinetics: Testosterone given orally is metabolized by the gut and 44% is cleared by the liver of the first pass. Oral doses as high as 400 mg per day are needed to achieve clinically effective blood levels for full replacement therapy. The synthetic androgen, methyltestosterone is less extensively metabolized by the liver and has a longer half-life. It is more suitable than testosterone for oral administration.

Testosterone in plasma is 98 percent bound to a specific testosterone-estradiol binding globulin, and about 2 percent is free. Generally, the amount of this sex-hormone binding globulin in the plasma will determine the distribution of testosterone between free and bound forms, and the free testosterone concentration will determine its half-life.

About 90 percent of a dose of testosterone is excreted in the urine as glucuronic and sulfuric acid conjugates of testosterone and its metabolites; and 6 percent of a dose is excreted in the feces, mostly in the unconjugated form. Inactivation of testosterone occurs primarily in the liver. Testosterone is metabolized to various 17-keto steroids through two different pathways. There are considerable variations of the half-life of testosterone as reported in the literature, ranging from 10 to 100 minutes.

In many tissues the activity of testosterone appears to depend on reduction to dihydrotestosterone, which binds to cytosol receptor proteins. The steroid-receptor complex is transported to the nucleus where it initials transcription events and cellular changes related to androgen action.

INDICATIONS AND USAGE:

MALES

Androgens are indicated for replacement therapy in conditions associated with a deficiency or absence of endogenous testosterone.

a. Primary hypogonadism (congenital or acquired): testicular failure due to cryptorchidism, bilateral torsions, orchitis, vanishing testis syndrome; or orchidectomy.

b. Hypogonadotropic hypogonadism (congenital or acquired): idiopathic gonadotropin or LHRH deficiency, or pituitary hypothalamic injury from tumors, trauma, or radiation. If the above, conditions occur prior to puberty, androgen replacement therapy will be needed during the adolescent years for development of secondary sexual characteristics. Prolonged androgen treatment will be required to maintain sexual characteristics in these and other males who develop testosterone deficiency after puberty.

c. Androgens may be used to stimulate puberty in carefully selected males with clearly delayed puberty. These patients usually have a familial pattern of delayed puberty that is not secondary to a pathological disorder; puberty is expected to occur spontaneously at a relatively late date. Brief treatment with conservative doses may occasionally be justified in these patients if they do not respond to psychological support. The potential adverse effect on maturation should be discussed with the patient and his parents prior to androgen administration. An x- ray of the hand and wrist to determine bone age should be obtained every 6 months to assess the effect of treatment on the epiphyseal centers (see WARNINGS.)

FEMALES

Androgens may be used secondarily in women with advancing inoperable metastatic (skeletal) mammary cancer who arte 1 to 5 years postmenopausal. Primary goal of therapy in these women include ablation of the ovaries. Other methods of counteracting estrogen activity are adrenalectomy, hypophysectomy, and/or antiestrogen therapy. This treatment has also been used in premenopausal women with breast cancer who have benefitted from oophorectomy and are considered to have a hormone-responsive tumor. Judgment concerning androgen therapy should be made by an oncologist with expertise in this field.

CONTRAINDICATIONS:

Androgens are contraindicated in men with carcinoma of the breast or with known or suspected carcinomas of the prostate, and in women who are or may become pregnant. When administered to pregnant women, androgens cause virilization of the external genitalia of the female fetus. This virilization includes clitoromegaly, abnormal vaginal development, and fusion of genital folds to form a scrotal-like structure. The degree of masculinization is related to the amount of drug given and the age of the fetus, and is most likely to occur in the female fetus when the drugs are given in the first trimester. If the patient becomes pregnant while taking these drugs, she should be apprised of the potential hazard to the fetus.

WARNINGS:

In patients with breast cancer, androgen therapy may cause hypercalcemia by stimulating osteolysis. In this case, the drug should be discontinued.

Prolonged use of high doses of androgens has been associated with the development of peliosis hepatis and hepatic neoplasms including hepatocellular carcinoma (see PRECAUTIONS, Carcinogenesis, Mutagenesis, and Impairment of Fertility). Peliosis hepatis can be a life, threatening or fatal complication

Cholestatic hepatitis and jaundice occur with 17 alpha-alkylandrogens at a relatively low dose. If cholestatic hepatitis with jaundice appears or if liver function tests become abnormal, the androgen should be discontinued and the etiology should be determined. Drug-induced jaundice is reversible when the medication is discontinued.

Geriatric patients treated with androgens may be at an increased risk for the development of prostatic hypertrophy and prostatic carcinoma.

Edema with or without congestive heart failure may be a serious complication in patients with preexisting cardiac, renal, or hepatic disease. In addition to discontinuation of the drug, diuretic therapy may be required.

Gynecomastia frequently develops and occasionally persists in patients being treated for hypogonadism.

Androgen therapy should be used cautiously in healthy males with delayed puberty. The effect on bone maturation should be monitored by assessing bone age of the wrist and hand every 6 months. In children, androgen treatment may accelerate bone maturation without producing compensatory gain in linear growth. This adverse effect may result in compromised adult stature. The younger the child, the greater the risk of compromising final mature height.

WARNINGS: *(cont'd)*

This drug has not been shown to be safe and effective for the enhancement of athletic performance. Because of the potential risk of serious adverse health effects, this drug should not be used for such purpose.

PRECAUTIONS:

GENERAL

Women should be observed for signs of virilization (deepening of the voice, hirsutism, acne, clitoromegaly, and menstrual irregularities). Discontinuation of drug therapy at the time mild virilism becomes evident is necessary to prevent irreversible virilization. Such virilization is usual following androgen use at high doses. A decision may be made by the patient and the physician that some virilization will be tolerated during treatment for breast carcinoma.

INFORMATION FOR THE PATIENT

The physician should instruct patients to report any of the following side effects of androgens:

Adult or Adolescent Males: Too frequent or persistent erection of the penis. Any male adolescent patient receiving androgens for delayed puberty should have bone development checked every six months.

Women: Hoarseness, acne, changes in menstrual periods, or more hair on the face.

All Patients: Any nausea, vomiting, changes in skin color, or ankle swelling.

LABORATORY TESTS

Women with disseminated breast carcinoma should have frequent determinations of urine and serum calcium levels during the coarse of androgen therapy (see WARNINGS.)

1. Because of hematoxicity associated with the use of 17 alpha-alkylated androgens, liver function tests should be obtained periodically.
2. Periodic (every 6 months) X-ray examinations of bone age should be made during treatment of prepubertal males to determine the rate of bone maturation and the effects of androgen therapy on the epiphyseal centers.
3. Hemoglobin and hematocrit should be checked periodically for polycythemia in patients who are receiving high doses of androgens.

Drug/Laboratory Test Interferences: Androgens may decrease levels of thyroxine-binding globulin, resulting in decreased total T4 serum levels and increased resin uptake of T3 and T4. Free thyroid hormone levels remain unchanged, however, and there is no clinical evidence of thyroid dysfunction.

Carcinogenesis, Mutagenesis, and Impairment of Fertility: *Animal Data:* Testosterone has been tested by subcutaneous injection and implantation in mice and rats. The implant induced cervical-uterine tumors in mice, which metastasized in some cases. There is suggestive evidence that injection of testosterone in some strains of female mice increases their susceptibility to hepatoma. Testosterone is also known to decrease the degree of differentiation of chemically induced carcinomas of the liver in rats.

Human Data: There are rare reports of hepatocellular carcinoma in patients receiving long-term therapy with androgens in high doses. Withdrawal of the drugs did not lead to regression of the tumors in all cases.

Geriatric patients treated with androgens may be at an increased risk for the development of prostatic hypertrophy and prostatic carcinoma.

Pregnancy Category X: *Teratogenic Effects:* See CONTRAINDICATIONS.

Nursing Mothers: It is not known whether androgens are excreted in human milk. Because many drugs are excreted in human milk and because of the potential for serious adverse reactions in nursing infants from androgens, a decision should be made whether to discontinue the drug taking into account the importance of the drug to the mother.

Pediatric Use: Androgen therapy should be prescribed very cautiously for use in males with clearly delayed puberty and only by specialists who are aware of the adverse effects on bone maturation. Skeletal maturation must be monitored every 6 months by an X-ray of the hand and wrist (See INDICATIONS AND USAGE and WARNINGS).

DRUG INTERACTIONS:

Anticoagulants: C-17-substituted derivatives of testosterone, such as methandrostenolone, have been reported to decrease the anticoagulant requirements of patients receiving oral anticoagulants. Patients receiving oral anticoagulant therapy require close monitoring, especially when androgen therapy are started or stopped.

Oxyphenbutazone: Concurrent administration of oxyphenbutazone and androgens may result in elevated serum levels of oxyphenbutazone.

Insulin: In diabetic patients, the metabolic effects of androgens may decrease blood glucose levels and insulin requirements.

ADVERSE REACTIONS:

Endocrine and Urogenital:

Female: The most common side effects of androgen therapy are amenorrhea and other menstrual irregularities, inhibition of gonadotropin secretion, and virilization, including deepening of the voice and clitoral enlargement. The latter usually is not reversible after androgens are discontinued. When administrated to a pregnant woman, androgens cause virilization of the external genitalia of the female fetus.

Males: Gynecomastia, and excessive frequency and duration of penile erections may occur. Oligospermia may occur at high dosages (See CLINICAL PHARMACOLOGY.)

Skin and appendages: Hirsutism, male pattern of baldness and acne.

Fluid and Electrolyte Disturbances: Retention of sodium, chloride, water, potassium, calcium, and inorganic phosphates.

Gastrointestinal: Nausea, cholestatic jaundice, alterations in liver function tests, rarely, hepatocellular neoplasms and peliosis hepatis (see WARNINGS.)

Hematologic: Suppression of clotting factors II, V, VII, and X; bleeding in patients on concomitant anticoagulant therapy, and polycythemia.

Nervous System: Increased or decreased libido, headache, anxiety, depression, and generalized paresthesia.

Metabolic: Increased serum cholesterol.

Miscellaneous: Rarely anaphylactoid reactions.

DRUG ABUSE AND DEPENDENCE:

Methyltestosterone capsules and tablets are classified as a schedule III Controlled Substance under the Anabolic Steroids Act of 1990.

OVERDOSAGE:

There have been no reports of acute overdosages with androgens.

DOSAGE AND ADMINISTRATION:

Dosage must be strictly individualized. Methyltestosterone capsules are administered orally. The suggested dosage for androgens varies depending on the age, sex, and diagnosis of the individual patient. Dosage is adjusted according to the patient's response and the appearance of adverse reactions.

Males: In the androgen-deficient male the following guideline for replacement therapy indicates the usual initial dosages:

TABLE 1 Methyltestosterone, DOSAGE AND ADMINISTRATION

Route	Dose	Frequency
Oral	10 - 50 mg	Daily

Various dosage regimens have been used to induce pubertal changes in hypogonadal males; some experts have advocated lower dosages initially, gradually increasing the dose as puberty progresses with or without a decrease to maintenance levels. Other experts emphasize that higher dosages are needed to induce pubertal changes and lower dosages can be used for maintenance after puberty. The chronological and skeletal ages must be taken into consideration both in determining the initial dose and in adjusting the dose.

Doses delayed in puberty generally are in the lower range of that given above, and for a limited duration, for example 4 to 6 months.

Females: Women with metastatic breast carcinoma must be followed closely because androgen therapy occasionally appears to accelerate the disease. Thus, many experts prefer to use the shorter acting androgen preparations rather than those with prolonged activity for treating breast carcinoma, particularly during the early stages of androgen therapy.

TABLE 2 Methyltestosterone, DOSAGE AND ADMINISTRATION: Metastatic Breast Cancer

Route	Dose	Frequency
Oral	50-200 mg	Daily

HOW SUPPLIED:

Android Tablets, 10 mg compressed white, round tablets impressed with the ICN trademark and product identification number 311; bottles of 100.

Android Tablets, 25 mg compressed peach-colored round tablets impressed with the ICN trademark and product identification number 499; bottles of 100.

HOW SUPPLIED - RATED THERAPEUTICALLY EQUIVALENT:

Tablet, Uncoated - Oral - 25 mg

100's	**$325.13**	**ANDROID 25, ICN Pharms**	**00187-0499-06**

HOW SUPPLIED - NOT RATED EQUIVALENT:

Capsule, Gelatin - Oral - 10 mg

10 ml	$26.40	VIRILON, Star Pharms FL	00076-0301-10
100's	$43.20	VIRILON, Star Pharms FL	00076-0301-03
100's	$130.06	TESTRED, ICN Pharms	00187-0901-01
100's	**$130.06**	**ANDROID, ICN Pharms**	**00187-0902-01**
1000's	$402.24	VIRILON, Star Pharms FL	00076-0301-04

Powder

10 gm	$27.20	Methyltestosterone, Paddock Labs	00574-0464-10

Tablet, Sublingual - Oral; Sublingua - 10 mg

100's	$4.95	Methyltestosterone, United Res	00677-0086-01

Tablet, Sublingual - Sublingual - 10 mg

100's	$5.00	Methyltestosterone, Harber Pharm	51432-0284-03

Tablet, Uncoated - Oral - 10 mg

100's	$2.80	Methyltestosterone, Lannett	00527-1078-01
100's	$4.50	Methyltestosterone, United Res	00677-0085-01
100's	$5.00	Methyltestosterone, Harber Pharm	51432-0286-03
100's	$5.50	Methyltestosterone 10, Major Pharms	00904-0807-60
100's	$5.95	Methyltestosterone 10, Major Pharms	00904-0808-60
100's	$10.30	Methyltestosterone 25, Major Pharms	00904-0809-60
100's	**$130.06**	**ORETON METHYL, ICN Pharms**	**00187-0311-01**
100's	**$130.06**	**ANDROID 10, ICN Pharms**	**00187-0311-06**
1000's	$21.48	Methyltestosterone, Lannett	00527-1078-10
1000's	$28.50	Methyltestosterone, Rugby	00536-4634-10

Tablet, Uncoated - Oral - 25 mg

100's	$6.72	Methyltestosterone, Lannett	00527-1140-01
100's	$8.75	Methyltestosterone, Harber Pharm	51432-0288-03
100's	$9.24	Methyltestosterone, United Res	00677-0087-01
1000's	$39.80	Methyltestosterone, Lannett	00527-1140-10

METHYSERGIDE MALEATE *(001797)*

CATEGORIES: Antimigraine/Other Headaches; Autonomic Drugs; Cephalalgia; Ergot Preparations; Headache; Migraine; Pain; Sympatholytic Agents; FDA Approval Pre 1982

BRAND NAMES: *Deseril* (Australia, England); *Desernil* (France); *Deserril*; *Deseryl*; **Sansert**
(International brand names outside U.S. in italics)

FORMULARIES: Aetna; BC-BS

Retroperitoneal Fibrosis, Pleuropulmonary Fibrosis and Fibrotic Thickening of Cardiac Valves May Occur in Patients Receiving Long-term Methysergide Maleate Therapy. Therefore, This Pre- paration Must Be Reserved for Prophylaxis in Patients Whose Vascular Headaches Are Frequent and/or Severe and Uncontrollable and Who Are Under Close Medical Supervision.
(See also WARNINGS)

DESCRIPTION:

Methysergide maleate is a partially synthetic compound structurally related to lysergic acid butanolamide, well-known as methylergonovine in obstetrical practice as an oxytocic agent.

Chemically, methysergide maleate is designated as ergoline-8-carboxamide, 9, 10-didehydro-*N*-[1-(hydroxymethyl)propyl]-1,6- dimethyl-, (8β)-,(*Z*)-2-butenedioate (1:1) (salt).

Methylation in the number 1 position of the ring structure enormously enhances the antagonism to serotonin which is present to a much lesser degree in the partially methylated compound (methylergonovine maleate) as well as profoundly altering other pharmacologic properties.

DESCRIPTION: *(cont'd)*

Sansert Active Ingredient: Methysergide maleate, USP. *Inactive Ingredients:* acacia, carnauba was, colloidal silicon dioxide, FD&C Blue #1, FD&C Yellow #5, gelatin, lactose, malic acid, povidone, sodium benzoate, starch, stearic acid, sucrose, synthetic black iron oxide, talc, and titanium dioxide.

CLINICAL PHARMACOLOGY:

Methysergide maleate has been shown*in vitro* and *in vivo,* to inhibit or block the effects of serotonin, a substance which may be involved in the mechanism of vascular headaches. Serotonin has been variously described as a central neurohumoral agent or chemical mediator, as a "headache substance" acting directly or indirectly to lower pain threshold (others in this category include tyramine; polypeptides, such as bradykinin; histamine; and acetylcholine), as an intrinsic "motor hormone" of the gastrointestinal tract, and as a "hormone" involved in connective tissue reparative processes. Suggestions have been made by investigators as to the mechanism whereby methysergide produces its clinical effects, but this has not been finally established.

INDICATIONS AND USAGE:

For the prevention or reduction of intensity and frequency of vascular headaches in the following kinds of patients:

1. Patients suffering from one or more severe vascular headaches per week.

2. Patients suffering from vascular headaches that are uncontrollable or so severe that preventive therapy is indicated regardless of the frequency of the attack.

CONTRAINDICATIONS:

Pregnancy, peripheral vascular disease, severe arteriosclerosis, severe hypertension, coronary artery disease, phlebitis or cellulitis of the lower limbs, pulmonary disease, collagen diseases or fibrotic processes, impaired liver or renal function, valvular heart disease, debilitated states and serious infections.

WARNINGS:

With long-term, uninterrupted administration, retroperitoneal fibrosis or related conditions — pleuropulmonary fibrosis and cardiovascular disorders with murmurs or vascular bruits have been reported. Patients must be warned to report immediately the following symptoms: cold, numb, and painful hands and feet; leg cramps on walking; any type of girdle, flank, or chest pain, or any associated symptomatology. Should any of these symptoms develop, methysergide should be discontinued. Continuous administration should not exceed 6 months. There must be a drug-free interval of 3-4 weeks after each 6-month course of treatment. The dosage should be reduced gradually during the last 2-3 weeks of each treatment course to avoid "headache rebound."

The drug is not recommended for use in children.

PRECAUTIONS:

All patients receiving methysergide maleate should remain under constant supervision of the physician and be examined regularly for the development of fibrotic or vascular complications (see ADVERSE REACTIONS.)

The manifestations of retroperitoneal fibrosis, pleuropulmonary fibrosis, and vascular shutdown have shown a high incidence of regression once methysergide maleate is withdrawn. These facts should be borne in mind to avoid unnecessary surgical intervention. Cardiac murmurs, which may indicate endocardial fibrosis, have shown varying degrees of regression, with complete disappearance in some and persistence in others.

Methysergide maleate has been specifically designed for the prophylaxis of vascular headache and has no place in the management of the acute attack.

Methysergide maleate tablets contain FD&C Yellow No. 5 (tartrazine) which may cause allergic-type reactions (including bronchial asthma) in certain susceptible individuals. Although the overall incidence of FD&C Yellow No. 5 (tartrazine) sensitivity in the general population is low, it is frequently seen in patients who also have aspirin hypersensitivity.

ADVERSE REACTIONS:

Within the recommended dose levels, the following side effects have been reported:

FIBROTIC COMPLICATIONS

Fibrotic changes have been observed in the retroperitoneal, pleuropulmonary, cardiac, and other tissues, either singly or, very rarely, in combination.

Retroperitoneal Fibrosis: This nonspecific fibrotic process is usually confined to the retroperitoneal connective tissue above the pelvic brim and may present clinically with one or more symptoms such as general malaise, fatigue, weight loss, backache, low grade fever (elevated sedimentation rate), urinary obstruction (girdle or flank pain, dysuria, polyuria, oliguria, elevated BUN), vascular insufficiency of the lower limbs (leg pain, Leriche syndrome, edema of legs, thrombophlebitis). The single most useful diagnostic procedure in suspected cases of retroperitoneal fibrosis is intravenous pyelography. Typical deviation and obstruction of one or both ureters may be observed.

Pleuropulmonary Complications: A similar nonspecific fibrotic process, limited to the pleural and immediately subjacent pulmonary tissues, usually presents clinically with dyspnea, tightness and pain in the chest, pleural friction rubs, and pleural effusion. These findings may be confirmed by chest X-ray.

Cardiac Complications: Nonrheumatic fibrotic thickenings of the aortic root and of the aortic and mitral valves usually present clinically with cardiac murmurs and dyspnea.

Other Fibrotic Complications: Several cases of fibrotic plaques, simulating Peyronie's Disease have been described.

CARDIOVASCULAR COMPLICATIONS

Encroachment of retroperitoneal fibrosis on the aorta, inferior vena cava and their common iliac branches may result in vascular insufficiency of the lower limbs, the presenting features of which are mentioned under Retroperitoneal Fibrosis.

Intrinsic vasoconstriction of large and small arteries, involving one or more vessels, may occur at any stage of therapy. Depending on the vessel involved, this complication may present with chest pain, abdominal pain, or cold, numb, painful extremities with or without paresthesias and diminished or absent pulses. Progression to ischemic tissue damage has rarely been reported. Prompt withdrawal of the drug at the first signs of impaired circulation is recommended (see WARNINGS) to obviate such effects.

Postural hypotension and tachycardia have also been observed.

GASTROINTESTINAL SYMPTOMS

Nausea, vomiting, diarrhea, heartburn, abdominal pain. These effects tend to appear early and can frequently be obviated by gradual introduction of the medication and by administration of the drug with meals. Constipation and elevation of gastric HCl have also been reported.

ADVERSE REACTIONS: *(cont'd)*

CNS SYMPTOMS

Insomnia, drowsiness, mild euphoria, dizziness, ataxia, lightheadedness, hyperesthesia, unworldly feelings (described variously as "dissociation", "hallucinatory experiences", etc.). Some of these symptoms may be associated with vascular headaches, per se, and may, therefore, be unrelated to the drug.

DERMATOLOGICAL MANIFESTATIONS

Facial flush, telangiectasia, and nonspecific rashes have rarely been reported. Increased hair loss may occur, but in many instances the tendency has abated despite continued therapy.

EDEMA

Peripheral edema, and, more rarely, localized brawny edema may occur.

Dependent edema has responded to lowered doses, salt restriction, or diuretics.

WEIGHT GAIN

Weight gain may be a reason to caution patients regarding their caloric intake.

HEMATOLOGICAL MANIFESTATIONS

Neutropenia, eosinophilia.

MISCELLANEOUS

Weakness, arthralgia, myalgia.

DOSAGE AND ADMINISTRATION:

Usual adult dose 4-8 mg daily. Tablets to be given with meals.

Note: There must be a medication-free interval of 3-4 weeks after every 6-month course of treatment (see WARNINGS.)

No pediatric dosage has been established.

If, after a 3-week trial period, efficacy has not been demonstrated, longer administration of methysergide maleate is unlikely to be of benefit.

ANIMAL PHARMACOLOGY:

SEROTONIN ANTAGONISM

Considering structure/effect relationships, it has been demonstrated that methylation of the indole nitrogen in the lysergic acid ring of the alkanolamides fundamentally alters their pharmacologic behavior and is associated with inhibition or blockade of a great variety of serotonin-induced effects:

1. Methysergide maleate is 6 times more active than methylergonovine maleate in antagonizing the effect of serotonin on the rat uterus *in vitro*.*

2. Greater inhibition of the serotonin-induced edema in the rat's paw is revealed by the ED_{50} of 12.9 mcg/kg for methysergide maleate as against 37.4 mcg/kg for methylergonovine maleate.*

3. The more complex effects of serotonin on the cardiovascular system are equally subject to inhibition by methysergide maleate as is evident from the subsequent record of various circulatory parameters in the dog before and after administration of 10 mcg/kg.*

* For illustrated, statistical information, please refer to the manufacturer's current package insert.

TABLE 1 Sansert, Animal Pharmacology and Toxicology

Acute Toxicity	Mice		Rabbits	LD_{50} in mg/kg Rats	
Compound	IV	oral	IV	IV	oral
methysergide maleate	185	581	28	125	2100
methylergonovine maleate	85	187	2.6	23	93

TABLE 2 Sansert, Animal Pharmacology and Toxicology
Rats

Daily Oral Doses mg/kg	No. of Weeks Animals Tested	Mortality
5	50	4/16
20	50	2/16
50	50	2/16
150	17	8/30
450	17	17/30
Control	50	1/16

DOGS

Oral administration of 1, 2, and 5 mg/kg/day of methysergide maleate failed to produce any major signs of toxicity over a period of 6 months.

HOW SUPPLIED:

Sansert: Each tablet contains 2 mg of methysergide maleate, USP. Imprinted "78-58" on one side, "SANDOZ" other side.

HOW SUPPLIED - EQUIVALENTS NOT AVAILABLE:

Tablet, Coated - Oral - 2 mg

100's	$170.82	SANSERT, Novartis	00078-0058-05

METIPRANOLOL HYDROCHLORIDE *(003022)*

CATEGORIES: Beta Adrenergic Blocking Agents; Beta Blockers; Glaucoma; Intraocular Pressure; Ocular Hypertension; Ophthalmics; Pregnancy Category C; FDA Class 1C ("Little or No Therapeutic Advantage"); FDA Approved 1989 Dec

BRAND NAMES: *Beta Ophtiole*; *Betamann* (Germany); *Betanol* (France); *Disorat*; *Glauline*; *Glausyn*; **Optipranolol**; *Ripix*; *Turoptin*
(International brand names outside U.S. in italics)

FORMULARIES: FHP; Medi-Cal; PCS

COST OF THERAPY: (Glaucoma; Solution; 0.3 %; 0.2/day; 365 days)

PRIMARY ICD9: 365.11 (Primary Open-Angle Glaucoma)

DESCRIPTION:

Optipranolol (metipranolol 0.3%) Sterile Ophthalmic Solution contains metipranolol, a nonselective beta-adrenergic receptor blocking agent. Metipranolol is a white, odorless, crystalline powder. The hydrochloride is soluble in water. The molecular weight is 309.38.

The empiric chemical formula of metipranolol is $C_{17}H_{27}NO_4$.

The chemical name of metipranolol is (±)-1-(4-Hydroxy-2, 3, 5-trimethylphenoxy)-3-(isopropylamino)-2-propanol-4-acetate.

DESCRIPTION: *(cont'd)*

Each ml of Optipranolol contains 3 mg of metipranolol. *Inactives:* povidone, glycerol, hydrochloric acid, sodium chloride, edetate disodium, and purified water. Sodium Hydroxide may be added to adjust pH. *Preservative:* Benzalkonium chloride 0.004%.

CLINICAL PHARMACOLOGY:

Metipranolol blocks $beta_1$ and $beta_2$ (non-selective) adrenergic receptors. It does not have significant intrinsic sympathomimetic activity, and has only weak local anesthetic (membrane-stabilizing) and myocardial depressant activity.

Orally administered beta-adrenergic blocking agents reduce cardiac output in both healthy subjects and patients with heart disease. In patients with severe impairment of myocardial function, beta-adrenergic receptor antagonists may inhibit the sympathetic stimulatory effect necessary to maintain adequate cardiac output.

Beta-adrenergic receptor blockade in the bronchi and bronchioles may result in significantly increased airway resistance from unopposed para- sympathetic activity. Such an effect is potentially dangerous in patients with asthma or other bronchospastic conditions (see CONTRAINDICATIONS and WARNINGS).

Metipranolol HCl, when applied topically in the eye, has the action of reducing elevated as well as normal intraocular pressure (IOP), whether or not accompanied by glaucoma. Elevated intraocular pressure is a major risk factor in the pathogenesis of glaucomatous visual field loss. The higher the level of intraocular pressure, the greater the likelihood of glaucomatous visual field loss and optic nerve damage.

The primary mechanism of the ocular hypotensive action of metipranolol is most likely due to a reduction in aqueous humor production. A slight increase in outflow may be an additional mechanism. Metipranolol HCl reduces IOP with little or no effect on pupil size or accommodation.

INDICATIONS AND USAGE:

Metipranolol HCl is indicated in the treatment of ocular conditions where lowering intraocular pressure is likely to be of therapeutic benefit; including patients with ocular hypertension, and patients with chronic open angle glaucoma.

In controlled studies of patients with intraocular pressure greater than 24 mmHg at baseline, metipranolol HCl reduced the average intraocular pressure approximately 20-26%.

The onset of action metipranolol HCl, as measured by a reduction in intraocular pressure, occurs within 30 minutes after a single administration. The maximum effects occurs at about 2 hours. A reduction in intraocular pressure can be demonstrated 24 hours after a single dose. Clinical studies in patients with glaucoma treated for up to two years indicate that an intraocular lowering effect is maintained.

In clinical trials, metipranolol HCl was safety used during concomitant therapy with pilocarpine, epinephrine or acetazolamide.

CONTRAINDICATIONS:

Hypersensitivity to any component of this product.

Metipranolol HCl is contraindicated in patients with bronchial asthma or a history of bronchial asthma, or severe chronic obstructive pulmonary disease; symptomatic sinus bradycardia; greater than a first degree atrioventricular block; cardiogenic shock; or overt cardiac failure.

WARNINGS:

As with other topically applied ophthalmic drugs, this drug may be absorbed systemically. Thus, the same adverse reactions found with systemic administration of beta-adrenergic blocking agents may occur with topical administration. For example, severe respiratory reactions and cardiac reactions, including death due to bronchospasm in patients with asthma, and rarely, death in association with cardiac failure, have been reported following topical application of beta-adrenergic blocking agents(see CONTRAINDICATIONS).

Since metipranolol HCl had a minor effect on heart rate and blood pressure in clinical studies, caution should be observed in treating patients with a history of cardiac failure. Treatment with metipranolol HCl should be discontinued at the first evidence of cardiac failure.

Metipranolol HCl, or other beta-blockers, should not, in general, be administered to patients with chronic obstructive pulmonary disease (*e.g.,* chronic bronchitis, emphysema) of mild or moderate severity (see CONTRAINDICATIONS). However, if the drug is necessary such patients, then it should be administered with caution since it may block bronchodilation produced by endogenous and exogenous catecholamine stimulation of $beta_2$, receptors.

PRECAUTIONS:

General: Because of potential effects of beta-adrenergic receptor blocking agents relative to blood pressure and pulse, these agents should be used with caution in patients with cerebrovascular insufficiency. If signs or symptoms suggesting reduced cerebral blood flow develop following initiation of therapy with metipranolol HCl, alternative therapy should be considered.

Some authorities recommended gradual withdrawal of beta-adrenergic receptor blocking agents in patients undergoing elective surgery. If necessary during surgery, the effects of beta-adrenergic receptor blocking agents may be reversed by sufficient doses of such agonists as isoproterenol, dopamine, dobutamine or levarterenol.

While metipranolol HCl has demonstrated a low potential for systemic effect, it should be used caution in patients with diabetes (especially labile diabetes) because of possible masking of signs and symptoms of acute hypoglycemia.

Beta-adrenergic receptor blocking agents may mask certain signs and symptoms of hyperthyroidism, and their abrupt withdrawal might precipitate a thyroid storm.

Beta-adrenergic blockade has been reported to potentiate muscle weakness consistent with certain myasthenic symptoms (*e.g.,* diplopia, ptosis, and generalized weakness).

Risk of anaphylactic reaction: While taking beta-blockers, patients with a history of severe anaphylactic reaction to a variety of allergens may be more reactive to repeated challenge, either accidental, diagnostic, or therapeutic. Such patients may be unresponsive to the usual doses of epinephrine used to treat allergic reaction.

Ocular: In patients with angle-closure glaucoma, the immediate treatment objective is to re-open the angle by constriction of the pupil with a miotic agent. Metipranolol HCl has little or no effect on the pupil, therefore, when it is used to reduce intraocular pressure in angle-closure glaucoma, it should be used only with concomitant administration of a miotic agent.

Carcinogenesis, Mutagenesis, and Impairment of Fertility: Lifetime studies with metipranolol have been conducted in mice at oral doses of 5, 50, and 100 mg/kg/day and in rats at oral doses of up to 70 mg/kg/day. Metipranolol demonstrated no carcinogenic effect. In the mouse study, female animals receiving the low, but not the intermediate or high dose had an increased number of pulmonary adenomas. The significance of this observation is unknown. In a variety of *in vitro* and *in vivo* bacterial and mammalian cell assays, metipranolol was nonmutagenic.

PRECAUTIONS: *(cont'd)*

Reproduction and fertility studies of metipranolol in rats and mice showed no adverse effect on male fertility at oral doses of to 50 mg/kg/day, and female fertility at oral doses of up to 25 mg/kg/day.

Pregnancy Category C: No drug related effects were reported for the segment II teratology study in fetal rats after administration, during organogenesis, to dams of up to 50 mg/kg/day. Metipranolol HCl has been shown to increase fetal resorption, fetal death, and delayed development when administered orally to rabbits at 50 mg/kg during organogenesis.

There are no adequate and well-controlled studies in pregnant women. Metipranolol HCl should be used during pregnancy only if the potential benefit justifies the potential risk of the fetus.

Nursing Mothers: It is not known whether metipranolol HCl is excreted in human milk. Because many drugs are excreted in human milk, caution should be exercised when metipranolol HCl is administered to nursing women.

Pediatric Use: Safety and effectiveness in children have not been established.

DRUG INTERACTIONS:

Metipranolol HCl should be used with caution in patients who are receiving a beta-adrenergic blocking agent orally, because of the potential for additive effects on systemic beta-blockade.

Close observation of the patient is recommended when a beta-blocker is administered to patients receiving catecholamine-depleting drugs such as reserpine, because of possible additive effects and the production of hypotension and/or bradycardia.

Caution should be used in the coadministration of beta-adrenergic receptor blocking agents, such as metipranolol, and oral or intravenous calcium channel antagonists, because of possible precipitation of left ventricular failure, and hypotension. In patients with impaired cardiac function, who are receiving calcium channel antagonists, coadministration should be avoided.

The concomitant use of beta-adrenergic receptor blocking agents with digitalis and calcium channel antagonists may have additive effects, prolonging atrioventricular conduction time.

Caution should be used in patients using concomitant adrenergic psychotropic drugs.

ADVERSE REACTIONS:

In clinical trials, the use of metipranolol HCl has been associated with transient local discomfort.

Other ocular adverse reactions, such as conjunctivitis, eyelid dermatitis, blepharitis, blurred vision, tearing, browache, abnormal vision, photophobia, and edema have been reported in small numbers of patients, either in U.S. clinical trials or from post-marketing experience in Europe.

Other systemic adverse reactions such as allergic reaction, headache, asthenia, hypertension, myocardial infarct, atrial fibrillation, angina, palpitation bradycardia nausea, rhinitis, dyspnea, epistaxis, bronchitis, coughing, dizziness, anxiety, depression, somnolence, nervousness, arthritis, myalgia, and rash have also been reported in small numbers of patients.

OVERDOSAGE:

No information is available on overdosage metipranolol HCl in humans. The symptoms which might be expected with an overdose of a systemically administered beta-adrenergic receptor blocking agent are bradycardia, hypotension and acute cardiac failure.

DOSAGE AND ADMINISTRATION:

The recommended dose is one drop of metipranolol HCl in the affected eyes twice a day.

In the patients IOP is not at a satisfactory level on this regimen, use of more frequent administration or a large dose of metipranolol HCl is not known to be of benefit. Concomitant therapy to lower intraocular pressure can be instituted.

Store at controlled room temperature 15-30°C (59-86°F).

ANIMAL PHARMACOLOGY:

In rabbits administered metipranolol in one eye at 2 to 4 fold increased concentrations, multi-focal interstitial nephritis was observed in male animals, and lympho-histiocytic and heterophilic interstitial pneumonia was observed female animals. The clinical relevance of these findings is unknown.

For How Supplied Information, Contact Bausch and Lomb (NDA# 19907)

METOCLOPRAMIDE HYDROCHLORIDE

(001798)

CATEGORIES: Acid/Peptic Disorders; Anorexia; Blood Glucose Regulators; Cholinergics; Diabetes; Dyspepsia; GERD; Gastric Emptying; Gastric Stasis; Gastrointestinal Drugs; Gastrointestinal Motility Factor; Intubation; Lesions; Nausea; Nausea and Vomiting; Reflux; Vertigo/Motion Sickness/Vomiting; Pregnancy Category B; FDA Approval Pre 1982

BRAND NAMES: *Ametic*; *Anada*; *Apo-Metoclop* (Canada); *Aputern* (Japan); *Balon*; *Betaclopramide*; *Biwesan*; *Carnotprim Primperan* (Mexico); *Clinamide*; *Clopan*; *Clopamon*; Clopra; *Dibertil*; *Duraclamid* (Germany); *Elitan*; *Emenil*; *Emetal*; *Emex* (Canada); *Emperal*; *Gastronerton* (Germany); *Gastrosil* (Germany); *Gastro-Tablinen* (Germany); *Gastrotrop* (Germany); *Gensil*; *Imperan*; *Macperan*; *Maril*; *Maxeran* (Canada); *Maxeron*; Maxolon; *Meclomid* (Mexico); *Mepra*; *Mepramide*; *Meramide*; *Metagliz*; *Metamide*; Metoclopramide HCl; *Metoclor* (Japan); *Metocobil*; *Metocyl*; *Metolon*; *Metomide*; *Metopram*; *Metramid*; *Mexolon*; Myclopramide; *Mygdalon* (England); *Nausil*; *Neopramiel* (Japan); *Netaf*; *Nilatika*; *Normastin*; Octamide Pfs; *Opram*; *Paspertin* (Germany); *Perinorm*; *Perone*; *Pharmyork*; *Plasil* (Mexico); *Pramin*; *Pramotel* (Mexico); *Primperan* (Europe); *Primperil*; *Prinparl* (Japan); *Priperim*; *Prowel*; *Pulin*; Reclomide; **Reglan**; *Reliveran*; *Setin*; *Terperan* (Japan); *Toast*; *Tomid*; *Ulcofar*; *Vasil*; *Vomitrol*; *Zudaw*
(International brand names outside U.S. in italics)

FORMULARIES: Aetna; BC-BS; CIGNA; FHP; Humana; Kaiser; Medco; Medi-Cal; PCS; PruCare; United; WHO

DESCRIPTION:

For oral administration Reglan 10 mg tablets are white, scored, capsule-shaped tablets engraved Reglan on one side and AHR 10 on the opposite side. *Each tablet contains:* Metoclopramide base 10 mg, (as the monohydrochloride monohydrate) *Inactive Ingredients:* Magnesium Stearate, Mannitol, Microcrystalline Cellulose, Stearic Acid.

DESCRIPTION: *(cont'd)*

Reglan 5 mg Tablets are green, elliptical-shaped tablets engraved Reglan 5 on one side and AHR on the opposite side. *Each tablet contains:* Metoclopramide base 5 mg (as the monohydrochloride monohydrate) *Inactive Ingredients:* Corn Starch, D&C Yellow 10 Lake, FD&C Blue 1 Aluminum Lake, Lactose, Microcrystalline Cellulose, Silicon Dioxide, Stearic Acid.

Reglan Syrup is an orange-colored, palatable, aromatic, sugar-free liquid.*Each 5 ml (1 teaspoonful) contains:* Metoclopramide base 5 mg (as the monohydrochloride monohydrate). *Inactive Ingredients:* Citric Acid, FD&C Yellow 6, Flavors, Glycerin, Methylparaben, Propylparaben, Sorbitol, Water.

For parenteral administration, Metoclopramide Hydrochloride Injection is a clear, colorless, sterile solution with a pH of 4.5-6.5 for intravenous or intramuscular administration.

Contains No Preservative.2 ml and 10 ml **single dose**vials/ampuls; 30 ml **single dose** vial

Each 1 ml contains: Metoclopramide base 5 mg (as the monohydrochloride monohydrate)

Sodium Chloride, USP 8.5 mg, Water for Injection, USP q.s.

pH adjusted, when necessary, with hydrochloric acid and/or sodium hydroxide.

Metoclopramide hydrochloride is a white crystalline, odorless substance, freely soluble in water. Chemically, it is 4-amino-5-chloro-N-[2-(diethylamino)ethyl]-2-methoxy benzamide monohydrochloride monohydrate. Molecular weight: 354.3.

CLINICAL PHARMACOLOGY:

Metoclopramide stimulates motility of the upper gastrointestinal tract without stimulating gastric, biliary, or pancreatic secretions. Its mode of action is unclear. It seems to sensitize tissues to the action of acetylcholine. The effect of metoclopramide on motility is not dependent on intact vagal innervation, but it can be abolished by anticholinergic drugs.

Metoclopramide increases the tone and amplitude of gastric (especially antral) contractions, relaxes the pyloric sphincter and the duodenal bulb, and increases peristalsis of the duodenum and jejunum resulting in accelerated gastric emptying and intestinal transit. It increases the resting tone of the lower esophageal sphincter. It has little, if any effect on the motility of the colon or gallbladder.

In patients with gastroesophageal reflux and low LESP (lower esophageal sphincter pressure), single oral doses of metoclopramide produce dose-related increases in LESP. Effects begin at about 5 mg and increase through 20 mg (the largest dose tested). The increase in LESP from a 5 mg dose lasts about 45 minutes and that of 20 mg lasts between 2 and 3 hours. Increased rate of stomach emptying has been observed with single oral doses of 10 mg.

The antiemetic properties of metoclopramide appear to be a result of its antagonism of central and peripheral dopamine receptors. Dopamine produces nausea and vomiting by stimulation of the medullary chemoreceptor trigger zone (CTZ), and metoclopramide blocks stimulation of the CTZ by agents like l-dopa or apomorphine which are known to increase dopamine levels or to possess dopamine-like effects. Metoclopramide also abolishes the slowing of gastric emptying caused by apomorphine.

Like the phenothiazines and related drugs, which are also dopamine antagonists, metoclopramide produces sedation and may produce extrapyramidal reactions, although these are comparatively rare (see WARNINGS). Metoclopramide inhibits the central and peripheral effects of apomorphine, induces release of prolactin and causes a transient increase in circulating aldosterone levels, which may be associated with transient fluid retention.

The onset of pharmacological action of metoclopramide is 1 to 3 minutes following an intravenous dose, 10 to 15 minutes following intramuscular administration, and 30 to 60 minutes following an oral dose; pharmacological effects persist for 1 to 2 hours.

Pharmacokinetics: Metoclopramide is rapidly and well absorbed. Relative to an intravenous dose of 20 mg, the absolute oral bioavailability of metoclopramide is 80% ± 15.5% as demonstrated in a crossover study of 18 subjects. Peak plasma concentrations occur at about 1-2 hr after a single oral dose. Similar time to peak is observed after individual doses at steady state.

In a single dose study of 12 subjects the area under the drug concentration-time curve increases linearly with doses from 20 to 100 mg. Peak concentrations increase linearly with dose; time to peak concentrations remains the same; whole body clearance is unchanged; and the elimination rate remains the same. The average elimination half-life in individuals with normal renal function is 5-6 hr. Linear kinetic processes adequately describe the absorption and elimination of metoclopramide.

Approximately 85% of the radioactivity of an orally administered dose appears in the urine within 72 hr. Of the 85% eliminated in the urine, about half is present as free or conjugated metoclopramide.

The drug is not extensively bound to plasma proteins (about 30%). The whole body volume of distribution is high (about 3.5 L/kg) which suggests extensive distribution of drug to the tissues.

Renal impairment affects the clearance of metoclopramide. In a study with patients with varying degrees of renal impairment, a reduction in creatinine clearance was correlated with a reduction in plasma clearance, renal clearance, non-renal clearance, and increase in elimination half-life. The kinetios of metoclopramide in the presence of renal impairment remained linear however. The reduction in clearance as a result of renal impairment suggests that adjustment downward of maintenance dosage should be done to avoid drug cumulation.

INDICATIONS AND USAGE:

Symptomatic Gastroesophageal Reflux: Metoclopramide Tablets and Syrup are indicated as short-term (4 to 12 weeks) therapy for adults with symptomatic, documented gastroesophageal reflux who fail to respond to conventional therapy.

The principal effect of metoclopramide is on symptoms of postprandial and daytime heartburn with less observed effect on nocturnal symptoms. If symptoms are confined to particular situations, such as following the evening meal, use of metoclopramide as single doses prior to the provocative situation should be considered, rather than using the drug throughout the day. Healing of esophageal ulcers and erosions has been endoscopically demonstrated at the end of a 12-week trial using doses of 15 mg q.i.d. As there is no documented correlation between symptoms and healing of esophageal lesions, patients with documented lesions should be monitored endoscopically.

Diabetic Gastroparesis (Diabetic Gastric Stasis): Metoclopramide Hydrochloride, USP is indicated for the relief of symptoms associated with acute and recurrent diabetic gastric stasis. The usual manifestations of delayed gastric emptying (*e.g.,* nausea, vomiting, heartburn, persistent fullness after meals and anorexia) appear to respond to Metoclopramide within different time intervals. Significant relief of nausea occurs early and continues to improve over a three-week period. Relief of vomiting and anorexia may precede the relief of abdominal fullness by one week or more.

The Prevention Of Nausea And Vomiting Associated With Emetogenic Cancer Chemotherapy: Metoclopramide HCl Injectable is indicated for the prophylaxis of vomiting associated with emetogenic cancer chemotherapy.

The Prevention Of Postoperative Nausea And Vomiting: Metoclopramide HCl Injectable is indicated for the prophylaxis of postoperative nausea and vomiting in those circumstances where nasogastric suction is undesirable.

INDICATIONS AND USAGE: *(cont'd)*

Small Bowel Intubation: Metoclopramide HCl Injectable may be used to facilitate small bowel intubation in adults and children in whom the tube does not pass the pylorus with conventional maneuvers.

Radiological Examination: Metoclopramide HCl Injectable may be used to stimulate gastric emptying and intestinal transit of barium in cases where delayed emptying interferes with radiological examination of the stomach and/or small intestine.

CONTRAINDICATIONS:

Metoclopramide should not be used whenever stimulation of gastrointestinal motility might be dangerous, e.g., in the presence of gastrointestinal hemorrhage, mechanical obstruction, or perforation.

Metoclopramide is contraindicated in patients with pheochromocytoma because the drug may cause a hypertensive crisis, probably due to release of catecholamines from the tumor. Such hypertensive crises may be controlled by phentolamine.

Metoclopramide is contraindicated in patients with known sensitivity or intolerance to the drug.

Metoclopramide should not be used in epileptics or patients receiving other drugs which are likely to cause extrapyramidal reactions, since the frequency and severity of seizures or extrapyramidal reactions may be increased.

WARNINGS:

Mental depression has occurred in patients with and without prior history of depression. Symptoms have ranged from mild to severe and have included suicidal ideation and suicide. Metoclopramide should be given to patients with a prior history of depression only if the expected benefits outweigh the potential risks.

Extrapyramidal symptoms, manifested primarily as acute dystonic reactions, occur in approximately 1 in 500 patients treated with the usual adult dosages of 30-40 mg/day of metoclopramide. These usually are seen during the first 24-48 hours of treatment with metoclopramide, occur more frequently in children and young adults, and are even more frequent at the higher doses used in prophylaxis of vomiting due to cancer chemotherapy. These symptoms may include involuntary movements of limbs and facial grimacing, torticollis, oculogyric crisis, rhythmic protrusion of tongue, bulbar type of speech, trismus, or dystonic reactions resembling tetanus. Rarely, dystonic reactions may present as stridor and dyspnea, possibly due to laryngospasm. If these symptoms should occur, inject 50 mg Benadryl (diphenhydramine hydrochloride) intramuscularly, and they usually will subside. Cogentin (benztropine mesylate), 1 to 2 mg intramuscularly, may also be used to reverse these reactions.

Parkinsonian-like symptoms have occurred, more commonly within the first 6 months after beginning treatment with metoclopramide, but occasionally after longer periods. These symptoms generally subside within 2-3 months following discontinuance of metoclopramide. Patients with preexisting Parkinson's disease should be given metoclopramide cautiously, if at all, since such patients may experience exacerbation of parkinsonian symptoms when taking metoclopramide.

Tardive Dyskinesia: Tardive dyskinesia, a syndrome consisting of potentially irreversible, involuntary, dyskinetic movements may develop in patients treated with metoclopramide. Although the prevalence of the syndrome appears to be highest among the elderly, especially elderly women, it is impossible to predict which patients are likely to develop the syndrome. Both the risk of developing the syndrome and the likelihood that it will become irreversible are believed to increase with the duration of treatment and the total cumulative dose.

Less commonly, the syndrome can develop after relatively brief treatment periods at low doses; in these cases, symptoms appear more likely to be reversible.

There is no known treatment for established cases of tardive dyskinesia although the syndrome may remit, partially or completely, within several weeks-to-months after metoclopramide is withdrawn. Metoclopramide itself, however, may suppress (or partially suppress) the signs of tardive dyskinesia, thereby masking the underlying disease process. The effect of this symptomatic suppression upon the long-term course of the syndrome is unknown. Therefore, the use of metoclopramide for the symptomatic control of tardive dyskinesia is not recommended.

PRECAUTIONS:

General: In one study in hypertensive patients, intravenously administered metoclopramide was shown to release catecholamines; hence, caution should be exercised when metoclopramide is used in patients with hypertension.

Intravenous injections of undiluted metoclopramide should be made slowly allowing 1 to 2 minutes for 10 mg since a transient but intense feeling of anxiety and restlessness, followed by drowsiness, may occur with rapid administration.

Intravenous administration of Metoclopramide HCl Injectable diluted in a parenteral solution should be made slowly over a period of not less than 15 minutes.

Giving a promotility drug such as metoclopramide theoretically could put increased pressure on suture lines following a gut anastomosis or closure. Although adverse events related to this possibility have not been reported to date, the possibility should be considered and weighed when deciding whether to use metoclopramide or nasogastric suction in the prevention of postoperative nausea and vomiting.

Information for the Patient: Metoclopramide may impair the mental and/or physical abilities required for the performance of hazardous tasks such as operating machinery or driving a motor vehicle. The ambulatory patient should be cautioned accordingly.

Carcinogenesis, Mutagenesis, and Impairment of Fertility: A 77-week study was conducted in rats with oral doses up to about 40 times the maximum recommended human daily dose. Metoclopramide elevates prolactin levels and the elevation persists during chronic administration. Tissue culture experiments indicate that approximately one-third of human breast cancers are prolactin-dependent *in vitro,* a factor of potential importance if the prescription of metoclopramide is contemplated in a patient with previously detected breast cancer. Although disturbances such as galactorrhea, amenorrhea, gynecomastia, and impotence have been reported with prolactin-elevating drugs, the clinical significance of elevated serum prolactin levels is unknown for most patients. An increase in mammary neoplasms has been found in rodents after chronic administration of prolactin-stimulating neuroleptic drugs and metoclopramide. Neither clinical studies nor epidemiologic studies conducted to date, however, have shown an association between chronic administration of these drugs and mammary tumorigenesis; the available evidence is too limited to be conclusive at this time.

An Ames mutagenicity test performed on metoclopramide was negative.

Pregnancy Category B: Reproduction studies performed in rats, mice, and rabbits by the i.v., i.m., s.c. and oral routes at maximum levels ranging from 12 to 250 times the human dose have demonstrated no impairment of fertility or significant harm to the fetus due to metoclopramide. There are, however, no adequate and well-controlled studies in pregnant women. Because animal reproduction studies are not always predictive of human response, this drug should be used during pregnancy only if clearly needed.

Nursing Mothers: Metoclopramide is excreted in human milk. Caution should be exercised when metoclopramide is administered to a nursing mother.

PRECAUTIONS: *(cont'd)*

Pediatric Use: There are insufficient data to support efficacy or make dosage recommendations for metoclopramide in patients less than 18 years of age; therefore, such use is not recommended (see OVERDOSAGE).

DRUG INTERACTIONS:

The effects of metoclopramide on gastrointestinal motility are antagonized by anticholinergic drugs and narcotic analgesics. Additive sedative effects can occur when metoclopramide is given with alcohol, sedatives, hypnotics, narcotics or tranquilizers.

The finding that metoclopramide releases catecholamines in patients with essential hypertension suggests that it should be used cautiously, if at all, in patients receiving monoamine oxidase inhibitors.

Absorption of drugs from the stomach may be diminished (*e.g.,* digoxin) by metoclopramide, whereas the rate and/or extent of absorption of drugs from the small bowel may be increased (*e.g.,* acetaminophen, tetracycline, levodopa, ethanol, cyclosporine).

Gastroparesis (gastric stasis) may be responsible for poor diabetic control in some patients. Exogenously administered insulin may begin to act before food has left the stomach and lead to hypoglycemia. Because the action of metoclopramide will influence the delivery of food to the intestines and thus the rate of absorption, insulin dosage or timing of dosage may require adjustment.

ADVERSE REACTIONS:

In general, the incidence of adverse reactions correlates with the dose and duration of metoclopramide administration. The following reactions have been reported, although in most instances, data do not permit an estimate of frequency:

CNS Effects: Restlessness, drowsiness, fatigue and lassitude occur in approximately 10% of patients receiving the most commonly prescribed dosage of 10 mg q.i.d. (see PRECAUTIONS). Insomnia, headache, confusion, dizziness or mental depression with suicidal ideation (see WARNINGS) occur less frequently. In cancer chemotherapy patients being treated with 1-2 mg/kg per dose, incidence of drowsiness is about 70%. There are isolated reports of convulsive seizures without clear-cut relationship to metoclopramide. Rarely, hallucinations have been reported.

Extrapyramidal Reactions (EPS) . Acute dystonic reactions, the most common type of EPS associated with metoclopramide, occur in approximately 0.2% of patients (1 in 500) treated with 30 to 40 mg of metoclopramide per day. In cancer chemotherapy patients receiving 1-2 mg/kg per dose, the incidence is 2% in patients over the ages of 30-35, and 25% or higher in children and young adults who have not had prophylactic administration of diphenhydramine. Symptoms include involuntary movements of limbs, facial grimacing, torticollis, oculogyric crisis, rhythmic protrusion of tongue, bulbar type of speech, trismus, opisthotonus (tetanus-like reactions) and rarely, stridor and dyspnea possibly due to laryngospasm; ordinarily these symptoms are readily reversed by diphenhydramine (see WARNINGS).

Parkinsonian-like symptoms may include bradykinesia, tremor, cogwheel rigidity, mask-like facies (see WARNINGS).

Tardive dyskinesia most frequently is characterized by involuntary movements of the tongue, face, mouth or jaw, and sometimes by involuntary movements of the trunk and/or extremities; movements may be choreoathetotic in appearance (see WARNINGS).

Motor restlessness (akathisia) may consist of feelings of anxiety, agitation, jitteriness, and insomnia, as well as inability to sit still, pacing, foot-tapping. These symptoms may disappear spontaneously or respond to a reduction in dosage.

Endocrine Disturbances: Galactorrhea, amenorrhea, gynecomastia, impotence secondary to hyperprolactinemia (see PRECAUTIONS). Fluid retention secondary to transient elevation of aldosterone (see CLINICAL PHARMACOLOGY).

Cardiovascular: . Hypotension, hypertension, supraventricular tachycardia, and bradycardia (see CONTRAINDICATIONS and PRECAUTIONS).

Gastrointestinal: Nausea and bowel disturbances, primarily diarrhea.

Hepatic Rarely, cases of hepatotoxicity, characterized by such findings as jaundice and altered liver function tests, when metoclopramide was administered with other drugs with known hepatotoxic potential.

Renal: Urinary frequency and incontinence.

Hematologic: A few cases of neutropenia, leukopenia, or agranulocytosis, generally without clearcut relationship to metoclopramide. Methemoglobinemia, especially with overdosage in neonates (see OVERDOSAGE).

Allergic Reactions: A few cases of rash, urticaria, or bronchospasm, especially in patients with a history of asthma. Rarely, angioneurotic edema, including glossal or laryngeal edema.

Miscellaneous: Visual disturbances. Porphyria. Rare occurrences of neuroleptic malignant syndrome (NMS) have been reported. This potentially fatal syndrome is comprised of the symptom complex of hyperthermia, altered consciousness, muscular rigidity and autonomic dysfunction.

Transient flushing of the face and upper body, without alterations in vital signs, following high doses intravenously.

OVERDOSAGE:

Symptoms of overdosage may include drowsiness, disorientation and extrapyramidal reactions. Anticholinergic or antiparkinson drugs or antihistamines with anticholinergic properties may be helpful in controlling the extrapyramidal reactions. Symptoms are self-limiting and usually disappear within 24 hours.

Hemodialysis removes relatively little metoclopramide, probably because of the small amount of the drug in blood relative to tissues. Similarly, continuous ambulatory peritoneal dialysis does not remove significant amounts of drug. It is unlikely that dosage would need to be adjusted to compensate for losses through dialysis. Dialysis is not likely to be an effective method of drug removal in overdose situations.

Unintentional overdose due to misadministration has been reported in patients between the age ofg 3 months and 7 years with the use of Metoclopramide syrup. While there was no consistent pattern to the reports associated with these overdoses, events included seizures, extrapyramidal reactions, and lethargy.

Methemoglobinemia has occurred in premature and full-term neonates who were given overdoses of metoclopramide (1-4 mg/kg/day orally, intramuscularly or intravenously for 1-3 or more days). Methemoglobinemia has not been reported in neonates treated with 0.5 mg/kg/day in divided doses. Methemoglobinemia can be reversed by the intravenous administration of methylene blue.

DOSAGE AND ADMINISTRATION:

For The Relief Of Symptomatic Gastroesophageal Reflux: Administer from 10 mg to 15 mg Metoclopramide Hydrochloride orally up to q.i.d. 30 minutes before each meal and at bedtime, depending upon symptoms being treated and clinical response (see CLINICAL PHARMACOLOGY and INDICATIONS AND USAGE). If symptoms occur only intermittently or at specific times of the day, use of metoclopramide in single doses up to 20 mg prior to the provoking situation may be preferred rather than continuous treatment. Occasionally, patients (such as elderly patients) who are more sensitive to the therapeutic or adverse effects of metoclopramide will require only 5 mg per dose.

Experience with esophageal erosions and ulcerations is limited, but healing has thus far been documented in one controlled trial using q.i.d. therapy at 15 mg/dose, and this regimen should be used when lesions are present, so long as it is tolerated (see ADVERSE REACTIONS). Because of the poor correlation between symptoms and endoscopic appearance of the esophagus, therapy directed at esophageal lesions is best guided by endoscopic evaluation.

Therapy longer than 12 weeks has not been evaluated and cannot be recommended.

For The Relief Of Symptoms Associated With Diabetic Gastroparesis (Diabetic Gastric Stasis): Administer 10 mg of metoclopramide 30 minutes before each meal and at bedtime for two to eight weeks, depending upon response and the likelihood of continued well-being upon drug discontinuation.

The initial route of administration should be determined by the severity of the presenting symptoms. If only the earliest manifestations of diabetic gastric stasis are present, oral administration of Metoclopramide HCl may be initiated. However, if severe symptoms are present, therapy should begin with Metoclopramide HCl Injectable (IM or IV). Doses of 10 mg may be administered slowly by the intravenous route over a 1-to 2-minute period.

Administration of Metoclopramide HCl Injectable (Metoclopramide Hydrochloride) up to 10 days may be required before symptoms subside, at which time oral administration may be instituted. Since diabetic gastric stasis is frequently recurrent, Metoclopramide HCl therapy should be reinstituted at the earliest manifestation.

For The Prevention Of Nausea And Vomiting Associated With Emetogenic Cancer Chemotherapy: For doses in excess of 10 mg, Metoclopramide HCl Injectable should be diluted in 50 ml of a parenteral solution.

The preferred parenteral solution is Sodium Chloride Injection (normal saline), which when combined with Metoclopramide HCl Injectable, can be stored frozen for up to 4 weeks. Metoclopramide HCl Injectable is degraded when admixed and frozen with Dextrose-5% in Water. Metoclopramide HCl Injectable diluted in Sodium Chloride Injection, Dextrose-5% in Water, Dextrose-5% in 0.45% Sodium Chloride, Ringer's Injection or Lactated Ringer's Injection may be stored up to 48 hours (without freezing) after preparation if protected from light. All dilutions may be stored unprotected from light under normal light conditions up to 24 hours after preparation.

Intravenous infusions should be made slowly over a period of not less than 15 minutes, 30 minutes before beginning cancer chemotherapy and repeated every 2 hours for two doses, then every 3 hours for three doses.

The initial two doses should be 2 mg/kg if highly emetogenic drugs such as cisplatin or dacarbazine are used alone or in combination. For less emetogenic regimens, 1 mg/kg per dose may be adequate.

If extrapyramidal symptoms should occur, inject 50 mg Benadryl (diphenhydramine hydrochloride) intramuscularly, and EPS usually will subside.

For The Prevention Of Postoperative Nausea And Vomiting: Metoclopramide HCl Injectable should be given intramuscularly near the end of surgery. The usual adult dose is 10 mg; however, doses of 20 mg may be used.

To Facilitate Small Bowel Intubation: If the tube has not passed the pylorus with conventional maneuvers in 10 minutes, a single dose (undiluted) may be administered slowly by the intravenous route over a 1-to 2-minute period.

The recommended single dose is: Adults - 10 mg metoclopramide base. Children (6-14 years of age) - 2.5 to 5 mg metoclopramide base; (under 6 years of age) - 0.1 mg/kg metoclopramide base.

To Aid In Radiological Examinations: In patients where delayed gastric emptying interferes with radiological examination of the stomach and/or small intestine, a single dose may be administered slowly by the intravenous route over a 1- to 2-minute period.

For dosage, see intubation above.

Use in Patients with Renal or Hepatic Impairment: Since metoclopramide is excreted principally through the kidneys, in those patients whose creatinine clearance is below 40 ml/min, therapy should be initiated at approximately one-half the recommended dosage. Depending upon clinical efficacy and safety considerations, the dosage may be increased or decreased as appropriate.

See OVERDOSAGE section for information regarding dialysis.

Metoclopramide undergoes minimal hepatic metabolism, except for simple conjugation. Its safe use has been described in patients with advanced liver disease whose renal function was normal.

NOTE: Parenteral drug products should be inspected visually for particulate matter and discoloration prior to administration, whenever solution and container permit.

Admixture Compatibilities. Metoclopramide hydrochloride Injectable is compatible for mixing and injection with the following dosage forms to the extent indicated below:

Physically and Chemically Compatible up to 48 hours. Cimetidine Hydrochloride (SK&F), Mannitol, USP (Abbott), Potassium Acetate, USP (Invenex), Potassium Chloride, USP (ESI), Potassium Phosphate, USP (Invenex).

Physically Compatible up to 48 hours: Ascorbic Acid, USP (Abbott), Benztropine Mesylate, USP (MS&D), Cytarabine, USP (Upjohn), Dexamethasone Sodium Phosphate, USP (ESI, MS&D), Diphenhydramine Hydrochloride, USP (Parke-Davis), Doxorubicin Hydrochloride, USP (Adria), Heparin Sodium, USP (ESI), Hydrocortisone Sodium Phosphate (MS&D), Lidocaine Hydrochloride, USP (ESI), Magnesium Sulfate, USP (ESI) Multi-Vitamin Infusion (must be refrigerated-USV), Vitamin B Complex with Ascorbic Acid. (Roche).

Physically Compatible up to 24 hours (Do not use if precipitation occurs): Aminophylline, USP (ESI), Clindamycin Phosphate, USP (Upjohn), Cyclophosphamide, USP (Mead-Johnson), Insulin, USP (Lilly), Methylprednisolone Sodium Succinate, USP (ESI).

Conditionally Compatible (Use Within one hour after mixing or may be infused directly into the same running IV line): Ampicillin Sodium, USP (Bristol), Calcium Gluconate, USP (ESI), Cisplatin (Bristol), Erythromycin Lactobionate, USP (Abbott), Methotrexate Sodium, USP (Lederle), Penicillin G Potassium, USP (Squibb), Tetracycline Hydrochloride, USP (Lederle).

Incompatible (Do Not Mix). Cephalothin Sodium, USP (Lilly), Chloramphenicol Sodium, USP (Parke-Davis), Sodium Bicarbonate, USP (Abbott).

Store vials and ampuls in carton until used. Do not store open single dose vials or ampuls for later use, as they contain no preservative.

DILUTIONS MAY BE STORED UNPROTECTED FROM LIGHT UNDER NORMAL LIGHT CONDITIONS UP TO 24 HOURS AFTER PREPARATION.

TABLETS, SYRUP AND INJECTABLE SHOULD BE STORED AT CONTROLLED ROOM TEMPERATURE BETWEEN 20œC AND 25œC (68œF AND 86œF).

TABLE 1			
Container	Total contents #	Concentration #	Administration
2 ml single dose vial/ampul	10 mg	5 mg/ml	FOR IV or IM ADMINISTRATION
10 ml single dose vial/ampul	50 mg	5 mg/ml	FOR IV INFUSION ONLY; DILUTE BEFORE USING.
30 ml single dose vial	150 mg	5 mg/ml	FOR IV INFUSION ONLY; DILUTE BEFORE USING
# Metoclopramide base (as the monohydrochloride monohydrate)			

HOW SUPPLIED - RATED THERAPEUTICALLY EQUIVALENT:

Injection, Solution - Intramuscular; - 5 mg/ml

2 ml	$2.93	Metoclopramide, Abbott	00074-1619-01
2 ml	$3.15	Metoclopramide 10, Abbott	00074-1620-01
2 ml	$3.30	Metoclopramide Hcl, Abbott	00074-3413-01
2 ml	$3.75	Metoclopramide Hcl, Abbott	00074-3414-01
2 ml	$58.75	Metoclopramide Hcl Inj 5, Solopak Labs	39769-0066-02
2 ml x 5	**$11.09**	**REGLAN, AH Robins**	**00031-6709-90**
2 ml x 25	$19.00	Metoclopramide Hcl, Voluntary Hosp	53258-3500-01
2 ml x 25	$49.80	Metoclopramide Hcl, Gensia Labs	00703-4502-04
2 ml x 25	**$52.55**	**REGLAN, AH Robins**	**00031-6709-95**
2 ml x 25	$54.06	Metoclopramide Hcl, Fujisawa USA	00469-2170-10
2 ml x 25	$58.75	OCTAMIDE PFS, Pharmacia & Upjohn	00013-6106-95
2 ml x 25	**$58.85**	**REGLAN, AH Robins**	**00031-6709-72**
10 ml x 25	**$227.09**	**REGLAN, AH Robins**	**00031-6709-78**
10 ml x 25	$227.19	OCTAMIDE PFS 50, Pharmacia & Upjohn	00013-6116-95
30 ml x 6	**$153.12**	**REGLAN, AH Robins**	**00031-6709-85**
30 ml x 6	$153.15	OCTAMIDE PFS 150, Pharmacia & Upjohn	00013-6126-70
30 ml x 25	$612.80	OCTAMIDE PFS 150, Pharmacia & Upjohn	00013-6126-95
30 ml x 25	**$613.02**	**REGLAN, AH Robins**	**00031-6709-24**

Syrup - Oral - 5 mg/5ml

1 pt	$8.25	Metoclopramide, Charter Labs	50550-0370-80
10 ml x 10	$69.79	Metoclopramide Hcl, Xactdose	50962-0425-10
10 ml x 100	$57.30	Metoclopramide Syrup 10, Roxane	00054-8563-04
16 oz	$14.75	Metoclopramide, Schein Pharm (US)	00364-2195-16
120 ml	$4.30	Metoclopramide HCl, Silarx Pharms	54838-0508-40
480 ml	$11.97	Metoclopramide HCl, Alpharma	00472-0454-16
480 ml	$12.00	Metoclopramide HCl, Morton Grove	60432-0622-16
480 ml	$12.48	Metoclopramide HCl, Silarx Pharms	54838-0508-80
480 ml	$16.00	Metoclopramide, Teva	00332-6105-38
480 ml	$16.00	Metoclopramide HCl, Liquipharm	54198-0128-16
480 ml	$16.70	Metoclopramide Hcl, Qualitest Pharms	00603-1435-58
480 ml	$17.35	Metoclopramide Hcl, Major Pharms	00904-1073-16
480 ml	$17.75	Metoclopramide Hcl, United Res	00677-1256-33
480 ml	$17.95	Metoclopramide, Goldline Labs	00182-6082-40
480 ml	$18.75	Metoclopramide HCl Syrup, Geneva Pharms	00781-6301-16
480 ml	$22.35	Metoclopramide Hcl, Aligen Independ	00405-3260-16
480 ml	$24.72	Metoclopramide HCl, Rugby	00536-1463-85
480 ml	**$48.39**	**REGLAN, AH Robins**	**00031-6706-25**
500 ml	$19.67	Metoclopramide Hcl, Roxane	00054-3563-63
3840 ml	$92.58	Metoclopramide HCl, Silarx Pharms	54838-0508-00

Tablet, Uncoated - Oral - 5 mg

30's	$4.92	Metoclopramide HCl, H.C.F.A. F F P	99999-1798-01
100's	$5.25	Metoclopramide HCl, US Trading	56126-0408-11
100's	$16.43	Metoclopramide, United Res	00677-1323-01
100's	$16.43	Metoclopramide HCl, H.C.F.A. F F P	99999-1798-02
100's	$19.80	Metoclopramide, Invamed	52189-0227-24
100's	$21.60	Metoclopramide Hcl, ESI Lederle	59911-5814-01
100's	$24.50	Metoclopramide Hcl, Parmed Pharms	00349-8841-01
100's	$24.80	Metoclopramide Hcl, Qualitest Pharms	00603-4616-21
100's	$24.95	Metoclopramide Hcl, Harber Pharm	51432-0781-03
100's	$25.50	Metoclopramide HCl, Teva	00332-2204-09
100's	$27.00	Metoclopramide, Goldline Labs	00182-1898-01
100's	$27.16	Metoclopramide Hcl, Duramed Pharms	51285-0834-02
100's	$27.21	Metoclopramide, Schein Pharm (US)	00364-2549-01
100's	$28.41	Metoclopramide Hcl, Caremark	00339-5232-12
100's	$29.25	Metoclopramide Hcl, Martec Pharms	52555-0523-01
100's	$29.90	Metoclopramide, Major Pharms	00904-1069-60
100's	$31.02	Metoclopramide, Aligen Independ	00405-4671-01
100's	$31.04	Metoclopramide Hcl, HL Moore Drug Exch	00839-7530-06
100's	$31.04	Metoclopramide Hcl, HL Moore Drug Exch	00839-7872-06
100's	$33.20	Metoclopramide, Rugby	00536-4038-01
100's	$40.50	Metoclopramide Hcl, Goldline Labs	00182-1898-89
100's	**$41.46**	**REGLAN, AH Robins**	**00031-6705-63**
100's	$42.53	Metoclopramide Hcl, Vangard Labs	00615-3546-13
100's	**$45.35**	**REGLAN, AH Robins**	**00031-6705-64**
500's	$82.15	Metoclopramide HCl, H.C.F.A. F F P	99999-1798-03
500's	$99.00	Metoclopramide, Invamed	52189-0227-29
500's	$103.93	Metoclopramide Hcl, Qualitest Pharms	00603-4616-28
500's	$124.00	Metoclopramide HCl, Teva	00332-2204-13
500's	$125.25	Metoclopramide, Rugby	00536-4038-05
500's	$125.80	Metoclopramide, Parmed Pharms	00349-8841-05
500's	$130.00	Metoclopramide, Goldline Labs	00182-1898-05
500's	$130.67	Metoclopramide Hcl, HL Moore Drug Exch	00839-7530-12
500's	$130.67	Metoclopramide Hcl, HL Moore Drug Exch	00839-7872-12
500's	$134.55	Metoclopramide, Duramed Pharms	51285-0834-04
500's	$134.80	Metoclopramide, Major Pharms	00904-1069-40
500's	$141.63	Metoclopramide Hcl, Aligen Independ	00405-4671-02
750's	$280.80	Metoclopramide Hcl, Glasgow Pharm	60809-0121-55
750's	$280.80	Metoclopramide Hcl, Glasgow Pharm	60809-0121-72

Tablet, Uncoated - Oral - 10 mg

40's	$39.00	Metoclopramide Hcl, Major Pharms	00904-1070-40
100's	$1.88	Metoclopramide Hcl, United Res	00677-1039-01
100's	$1.88	Metoclopramide HCl, H.C.F.A. F F P	99999-1798-05
100's	$4.35	Metoclopramide HCl, US Trading	56126-0328-11
100's	$6.75	Metoclopramide, Watson Labs	52544-0312-01
100's	$9.45	Metoclopramide, Invamed	52189-0207-24
100's	$9.50	Metoclopramide Hcl, Goldline Labs	00182-1789-01
100's	$9.60	Metoclopramide Hcl, Qualitest Pharms	00603-4617-21
100's	$9.75	Metoclopramide Hcl, Duramed Pharms	51285-0805-02
100's	$15.61	Metoclopramide Hcl, Purepac Pharm	00228-2269-10
100's	$16.51	Metoclopramide Hcl, Caremark	00339-5233-12
100's	$17.21	Metoclopramide Hcl, HL Moore Drug Exch	00839-7127-06
100's	$17.31	Metoclopramide, Rugby	00536-4042-01
100's	$17.35	Metoclopramide Hcl, Major Pharms	00904-1070-60
100's	$17.98	Metoclopramide Hcl, Martec Pharms	52555-0120-01
100's	$19.71	Metoclopramide HCl, Bristol Myers Squibb	00003-0693-50
100's	$19.82	Metoclopramide, Aligen Independ	00405-4672-01
100's	$20.38	Metoclopramide Hcl, ESI Lederle	59911-5815-01

HOW SUPPLIED - RATED THERAPEUTICALLY EQUIVALENT: *(cont'd)*

100's	$21.41	Metoclopramide Hcl, Major Pharms	00904-1070-61
100's	$21.66	Metoclopramide, Teva	00332-2203-09
100's	$22.00	Metoclopramide Hcl, Sidmak Labs	50111-0430-01
100's	$22.90	Metoclopramide HCl, Schein Pharm (US)	00364-0769-01
100's	$25.48	Metoclopramide, Lederle Pharm	00005-4542-23
100's	$25.48	Metoclopramide HCl, Geneva Pharms	00781-1301-01
100's	$27.20	Metoclopramide Hcl, Medirex	57480-0348-01
100's	$27.84	Metoclopramide, Parmed Pharms	00349-8442-01
100's	$29.00	Metoclopramide Hcl, Goldline Labs	00182-1789-89
100's	$29.60	Metoclopramide HCl, Schein Pharm (US)	00364-0769-90
100's	$29.95	Metoclopramide Hcl, Am Generics	58634-0020-01
100's	$31.32	Metoclopramide Hcl, Vangard Labs	00615-2536-13
100's	$31.33	Metoclopramide HCl, Geneva Pharms	00781-1301-13
100's	$38.06	Metoclopramide Hcl, TIE Pharm	55496-5201-09
100's	**$64.79**	**REGLAN, AH Robins**	**00031-6701-63**
100's	**$71.21**	**REGLAN, AH Robins**	**00031-6701-64**
100's	$89.19	Metoclopramide, Aligen Independ	00405-4672-02
500's	$9.40	Metoclopramide Hcl, United Res	00677-1039-05
500's	$9.40	Metoclopramide HCl, H.C.F.A. F F P	99999-1798-04
500's	$27.95	Metoclopramide, Watson Labs	52544-0312-05
500's	$40.86	Metoclopramide Hcl, Qualitest Pharms	00603-4617-28
500's	$41.50	Metoclopramide Hcl, Goldline Labs	00182-1789-05
500's	$41.93	Metoclopramide Hcl, Halsey Drug	00879-0561-05
500's	$72.04	Metoclopramide HCl, Schein Pharm (US)	00364-0769-05
500's	$78.05	Metoclopramide Hcl, Purepac Pharm	00228-2269-50
500's	$84.50	Metoclopramide, Rugby	00536-4042-05
500's	$85.85	Metoclopramide Hcl, Martec Pharms	52555-0120-05
500's	$86.11	Metoclopramide, Parmed Pharms	00349-8442-05
500's	$91.50	Metoclopramide, Invamed	52189-0207-29
500's	$93.48	Metoclopramide HCl, Bristol Myers Squibb	00003-0693-60
500's	$96.68	Metoclopramide Hcl, ESI Lederle	59911-5815-02
500's	$101.84	Metoclopramide, Teva	00332-2203-13
500's	$102.50	Metoclopramide Hcl, Sidmak Labs	50111-0430-02
500's	$104.75	Metoclopramide Hcl, Am Generics	58634-0020-02
500's	$120.85	Metoclopramide, Lederle Pharm	00005-4542-31
500's	$120.85	Metoclopramide HCl, Geneva Pharms	00781-1301-05
500's	**$304.61**	**REGLAN, AH Robins**	**00031-6701-70**
600's	$165.80	Metoclopramide, Medirex	57480-0348-06
1000's	$18.80	Metoclopramide, Teva	00332-2203-15
1000's	$18.80	Metoclopramide, Watson Labs	52544-0312-10
1000's	$18.80	Metoclopramide HCl, H.C.F.A. F F P	99999-1798-06
1000's	$75.47	Metoclopramide Hcl, Halsey Drug	00879-0561-10
1000's	$94.25	Metoclopramide Hcl, Duramed Pharms	51285-0805-05
1000's	$97.27	Metoclopramide HCl, HL Moore Drug Exch	00839-7127-16
1000's	$124.12	Metoclopramide Hcl, Qualitest Pharms	00603-4617-32
1000's	$131.60	Metoclopramide Hcl, Major Pharms	00904-1070-80
1000's	$132.75	Metoclopramide Hcl, Parmed Pharms	00349-8442-10
1000's	$195.50	Metoclopramide HCl, Rugby	00536-4042-10
1000's	$197.00	Metoclopramide Hcl, Sidmak Labs	50111-0430-03
2500's	$181.73	Metoclopramide, Parmed Pharms	00349-8442-52

HOW SUPPLIED - NOT RATED EQUIVALENT:

Concentrate - Oral - 10 mg/ml

30 ml	$19.49	METOCLOPRAMIDE HCL INTENSOL, Roxane	00054-3564-44

Injection, Solution - Intramuscular; - 5 mg/ml

20 ml x 10	$50.00	Metoclopramide Hcl, Jordan Pharms	58196-0226-63

Syrup - Oral - 5 mg/5ml

480 ml	$11.87	Metoclopramide Hcl, HL Moore Drug Exch	00839-7359-69
480 ml	$18.95	Metoclopramide Hcl, Harber Pharm	51432-0627-20

METOCURINE IODIDE *(001799)*

CATEGORIES: Analeptics; Anesthesia; Autonomic Drugs; Convulsions; Curare Derivatives; Muscle Relaxants; Muscles; Neuromuscular Blocking Agents; Non-Depolarizing Muscle Relaxants; Skeletal Muscle Relaxants; Pregnancy Category C; FDA Approval Pre 1982

BRAND NAMES: Metocurine Iodine; **Metubine Iodide**

DESCRIPTION:

THIS DRUG SHOULD BE ADMINISTERED ONLY BY ADEQUATELY TRAINED INDIVIDUALS WHO ARE FAMILIAR WITH ITS ACTIONS, CHARACTERISTICS, AND HAZARDS

Metubine Iodide (Metocurine Iodide Injection, USP, Lilly) is a nondepolarizing muscle relaxant and is presented as a sterile isotonic solution for intravenous injection.

Each ml contains 2 mg metocurine iodide and sodium chloride 0.9% with 0.5% phenol as a preservative. Sodium carbonate and/or hydrochloric acid may have been added during manufacture to adjust the pH in the range of 4 to 4.3.

The empirical formula is: $C_{40}H_{48}I_2N_2O_6$. The molecular weight is 906.64.

CLINICAL PHARMACOLOGY:

Metubine iodide is a methyl analogue of tubocurarine which produces nondepolarizing (competitive) neuromuscular blockade at the myoneural junction. Recent animal studies suggest that metubine iodide does not produce the autonomic ganglionic blockade seen with other nondepolarizing muscle relaxants. Recent clinical findings suggest that metubine iodide reaches the neuromuscular junction more rapidly than does tubocurarine. After intravenous injection, there is rapid onset (1 to 4 minutes) of muscle relaxation with maximum twitch inhibition (96%) in 1.5 to 10 minutes. The maximum effect lasts 35 to 60 minutes. The time of recovery of 50% of control twitch response is in excess of 3 hours.

Following bolus injection of 0.05% mg/kg, the mean terminal half-life of metubine iodide was 3.6 hours (217 minutes). Approximately 50% of the dose was excreted as unchanged drug in the urine over 48 hours, and 2% was excreted unchanged in the bile. Approximately 35% is protein bound, mainly to the beta and gamma globulins.

The use of repeated doses may be accompanied by a cumulative effect. The duration of action and degree of muscle relaxation may be altered by dehydration, body temperature changes, hypocalcemia, excess magnesium, or acid-base imbalance. Concurrently administered general anesthetics, certain antibiotics, and neuromuscular disease may potentiate the neuromuscular blocking action of metubine iodide.

Histamine release with metubine iodide occurs less frequently than with *d*-tubocurarine and is related to dosage and rapidity of administration. Effects on the cardiovascular system (*e.g.*, changes in pulse rate, hypotension) are less than those reported with equipotent doses of *d*-tubocurarine and gallamine.

CLINICAL PHARMACOLOGY: *(cont'd)*

Because the main excretory pathway for metubine iodide is through the kidneys, severe renal disease or conditions associated with poor renal perfusion (shock states) may result in prolonged neuromuscular blockade.

Following intravenous injection in the mother, placental transfer of metubine iodide occurs rapidly, and, after 6 minutes, the fetal plasma concentration is approximately one-tenth the maternal level.

INDICATIONS AND USAGE:

Metubine iodide is indicated as an adjunct to anesthesia to induce skeletal-muscle relaxation. It may be employed to reduce the intensity of muscle contraction in pharmacologically or electrically induced convulsions. It may also be employed to facilitate the management of patients undergoing mechanical ventilation.

CONTRAINDICATIONS:

Metubine iodide is contraindicated in those persons with known hypersensitivity to the drug or to its iodide content.

WARNINGS:

METUBINE IODIDE SHOULD BE ADMINISTERED IN CAREFULLY ADJUSTED DOSES BY OR UNDER THE SUPERVISION OF EXPERIENCED CLINICIANS WHO ARE FAMILIAR WITH THE COMPLICATIONS WHICH MAY OCCUR WITH THE USE OF THIS DRUG. Metubine iodide should not be administered unless facilities for intubation, artificial ventilation, oxygen therapy, and reversal agents are immediately available. The clinician must be prepared to assist or control respiration.

Metubine iodide should be used with extreme caution in patients with myasthenia gravis. In such patients, a peripheral nerve stimulator may be valuable in assessing the effects of administration.

PRECAUTIONS:

General: Metubine iodide should be used with caution in patients with poor renal perfusion or severe renal disease (see CLINICAL PHARMACOLOGY).

Rapid administration of large doses of metubine iodide may produce changes in blood pressure or heart rate or signs of histamine release.

Metubine iodide has no effect on consciousness, pain threshold, or cerebration; therefore, it should be used with adequate anesthesia.

Pregnancy Category C: Intrauterine growth retardation and limb deformities resembling clubfoot were produced by *d*-tubocurarine chloride and succinylcholine chloride when administered to the rat fetus between the 16th and 19th days of gestation or when injected in chick embryos from the 5th to the 15th days of incubation. When *d*-tubocurarine was injected intramuscularly into the interscapular region of the fetuses on the 16th to the 19th day of gestation, the incidence of growth retardation and limb deformity ranged from 21 to 23% and 7 to 8% respectively.

There are no adequate and well-controlled studies of metubine iodide in pregnant women. metubine iodide should be used during pregnancy only if the potential benefit justifies the risk to the fetus.

Labor and Delivery: It is not known whether the use of muscle relaxants during labor or delivery has immediate or delayed adverse effects on the fetus, prolongs the duration of labor, or increases the likelihood that forceps delivery, obstetric intervention, or resuscitation of the newborn will be necessary.

Nursing Mothers: It is not known whether metubine iodide is excreted in human milk. Because many drugs are excreted in human milk, caution should be exercised when metubine iodide is administered to a nursing woman.

Pediatric Use: A clinical study has shown that metubine iodide twice as potent as *d*-tubocurarine in children, but the rate of recovery is the same. There may be slight increase in heart rate, but no change occurs in blood pressure or ECG. Doses calculated on the basis of body weight or body surface area may be applicable when the advantages of nondepolarizing neuromuscular blockade are desired.

DRUG INTERACTIONS:

Synergistic or antagonistic effects may result when depolarizing and nondepolarizing muscle relaxants are administered simultaneously or sequentially.

Parenteral administration of high doses of certain antibiotics may intensify or resemble the neuroblocking action of muscle relaxants. These include neomycin, streptomycin, bacitracin, kanamycin, gentamicin, dihydrostreptomycin, polymyxin B, colistin, sodium colistimethate, and tetracyclines. If muscle relaxants and antibiotics must be administered simultaneously, the patient should be observed closely for any unexpected prolongation of respiratory depression.

Certain general anesthetics have a synergistic action with neuromuscular blocking agents. Diethyl ether, halothane, and isoflurane potentiate the neuromuscular blocking action of other nondepolarizing agents and may be presumed to do so with metubine iodide.

Administration of quinidine shortly after recovery may produce recurrent paralysis.

The effect of diazepam on neuromuscular blockade by metubine iodide is not clear. Until more information is available, patients should be carefully monitored for unexpected drug response and prolongation of action.

The use of magnesium sulfate in preeclamptic patients potentiates the effects of both depolarizing and nondepolarizing muscle relaxants.

ADVERSE REACTIONS:

The most frequently noted adverse reaction is prolongation of the drug's pharmacologic action. Neuromuscular effects may range from skeletal-muscle weakness to a profound relaxation that produces respiration insufficiency or apnea.

Possible adverse reactions include allergic or hypersensitivity reactions to the drug or its iodide content and histamine release when large doses are administered rapidly. Signs of histamine release include erythema, edema, flushing, tachycardia, arterial hypotension, bronchospasm, and circulatory collapse.

Prolonged apnea and respiratory depression have occurred following the use of muscle relaxants. Many physiologic factors, drug interactions, and individual sensitivities may contribute to the development of respiratory paralysis (see CLINICAL PHARMACOLOGY and PRECAUTIONS).

OVERDOSAGE:

An overdose of metubine iodide may result in prolonged apnea, cardiovascular collapse, and sudden release of histamine.

Massive doses of metocurarine are not reversible by the antagonists edrophonium or neostigmine and atropine.

OVERDOSAGE: *(cont'd)*

Overdosage may be avoided by the careful monitoring of response by means of a peripheral nerve stimulator.

The primary treatment for residual neuromuscular blockade with respiratory paralysis or inadequate ventilation is maintenance of the patient's airway and manual or mechanical ventilation.

Accompanying derangements of blood pressure, electrolyte imbalance, or circulating blood volume should be determined and corrected by appropriate fluid and electrolyte therapy.

Residual neuromuscular blockade following surgery may be reversed by the use of anticholinesterase inhibitors such as neostigmine or pyridostigmine bromide and atropine. Prescribing information should be consulted for the appropriate drug selection based on dosage and desired duration of action.

DOSAGE AND ADMINISTRATION:

Metubine iodide should be administered intravenously as a sustained injection over a period of 30 to 60 seconds. INTRAMUSCULAR ADMINISTRATION OF METUBINE IODIDE IS NOT RECOMMENDED. Care must be taken to avoid overdosage. The use of a peripheral nerve stimulator to monitor response will minimize the risk of overdosage. The type of anesthetic used and nature of the surgical procedure will influence the amount of metubine iodide required. Doses of 0.2 to 0.4 mg/kg have been found satisfactory for endotracheal intubation. Relaxation following the initial dose may be expected to be effective for periods of 25 to 90 minutes, with an average of approximately 60 minutes. Supplemental administration may be made as indicated to provide needed surgical relaxation. Supplemental doses average 0.5 to 1 mg. The use of strong anesthetics that potentiate the effect of neuromuscular blocking drugs such as halothane, diethyl ether, isoflurane, or enflurane reduces the requirement for metubine iodide. Incremental doses should be reduced by approximately one-third to one-half.

Recommended Doses for Use During Electroshock Therapy: Doses required for satisfactory relaxation range from 1.75 to 5.5 mg. When the patient is treated for the first time, the drug is administered slowly by the intravenous route as a sustained injection until a head-drop response ensues. After dosage has been established, subsequent injections are completed in 15 to 50 seconds. The average dose ranges from 2 to 3 mg.

Drug Incompatibilities: Metubine iodide is unstable in alkaline solutions. When it is combined with barbiturate solutions, precipitations may occur. Solutions of barbiturates, meperidine, and morphine sulfate should not be administered from the same syringe.

Parenteral drug products should be inspected visually for particulate matter and discoloration prior to administration, whenever solution and container permit.

Store at controlled room temperature 59 to 86°F (15 to 30°C).

Metubine iodide is a clear, colorless solution.

HOW SUPPLIED - EQUIVALENTS NOT AVAILABLE:

Injection, Solution - Intravenous - 2 mg/ml

20 ml $24.18 METUBINE IODIDE, Dista 00777-1421-01

METOLAZONE *(001800)*

CATEGORIES: Antihypertensives; Cardiovascular Drugs; Congestive Heart Failure; Diuretics; Edema; Electrolytic, Caloric-Water Balance; Hypertension; Nephrotic Syndrome; Renal Drugs; Renal Function; Saluretics; Thiazides; Pregnancy Category B; FDA Approval Pre 1982

BRAND NAMES: *Barolyn*; *Diondel*; **Diulo**; *Metenix*; *Metenix 5* (England); Mykrox; *Normelan* (Japan); *Xuret* (England); Zaroxolyn
(International brand names outside U.S. in italics)

FORMULARIES: Aetna; BC-BS; PCS

COST OF THERAPY: $170.85 (Hypertension; Tablet; 2.5 mg; 1/day; 365 days)

PRIMARY ICD9: 401.1 (Essential Hypertension, Benign)

ZAROXOLYN: DO NOT INTERCHANGE ZAROXOLYN TABLETS AND OTHER FORMULATIONS OF METOLAZONE THAT SHARE ITS SLOW AND INCOMPLETE BIOAVAILABILITY AND ARE NOTTHERAPEUTICALLY EQUIVALENT AT THE SAME DOSES TO MYKROX TABLETS, A MORE RAPIDLY AVAILABLE AND COMPLETELY BIOAVAILABLE METOLAZONE PRODUCT. FORMULATIONS BIOEQUIVALENT TO ZAROXOLYN AND FORMULATIONS BIOEQUIVALENT TO MYKROX SHOULD NOT BE INTERCHANGED FOR ONE ANOTHER.

MYKROX: DO NOT INTERCHANGE MYKROX TABLETS ARE A RAPIDLY AVAILABLE FORMULATION OF METOLAZONE FOR ORAL ADMINISTRATION. MYKROX TABLETS AND OTHER FORMULATIONS OF METOLAZONE THAT SHARE ITS MORE RAPID AND COMPLETE BIOAVAILABILITY ARE NOTTHERAPEUTICALLY EQUIVALENT TO ZAROXOLYN TABLETS AND OTHER FORMULATIONS OF METOLAZONE THAT SHARE ITS SLOW AND INCOMPLETE BIOAVAILABILITY. FORMULATIONS BIOEQUIVALENT TO MYKROX AND FORMULATIONS BIOEQUIVALENT TO ZAROXOLYN SHOULD NOT BE INTERCHANGED FOR ONE ANOTHER.

DESCRIPTION:

Zaroxolyn Tablets Zaroxolyn Tablets for oral administration contain 2 1/2, 5, or 10 mg of metolazone, USP, a diuretic/saluretic/antihypertensive drug of the quinazoline class. *Inactive Ingredients:* Magnesium stearate, microcrystalline cellulose and dye: 2 1/2 mg-D&C Red No. 33; 5 mg-FD&C Blue No. 2; 10 mg-D&C Yellow No. 10 and FD&C Yellow No. 6.

Mykrox Tablets: Mykrox Tablets for oral administration contain 1/2 mg of metolazone, USP, a diuretic/saluretic/antihypertensive drug of the quinazoline class. *Inactive Ingredients:* Dibasic calcium phosphate, magnesium stearate, microcrystalline cellulose, pregelatinized starch, sodium starch glycolate.

Metolazone has the molecular formula $C_{16}H_{16}ClN_3O_3S$, the chemical name 7-chloro-1, 2, 3, 4-tetrahydro-2-methyl-3- (2-methylphenyl) -4-oxo-6-quinazolinesulfonamide, and a molecular weight of 365.83.

Metolazone is only sparingly soluble in water, but more soluble in plasma, blood, alkali, and organic solvents.

CLINICAL PHARMACOLOGY:

Metolazone is a quinazoline diuretic, with properties generally similar to the thiazide diuretics. The actions of metolazone result from interference with the renal tubular mechanism of electrolyte reabsorption. Metolazone acts primarily to inhibit sodium reabsorption at the cortical dilution site and to a lesser extent in the proximal convoluted tubule. Sodium and chloride ions are excreted in approximately equivalent amounts. The increased delivery of sodium to the distal tubular exchange site results in increased potassium excretion. Metolazone does not inhibit carbonic anhydrase. A proximal action of metolazone has been

CLINICAL PHARMACOLOGY: *(cont'd)*

shown in humans by increased excretion of phosphate and magnesium ions and by a markedly increased fractional excretion of sodium in patients with severely compromised glomerular filtration. This action has been demonstrated in animals by micropuncture studies.

ZAROXOLYN

When Zaroxolyn Tablets are given, diuresis and saluresis usually begin within one hour and may persist for 24 hours or more. For most patients, the duration of effect can be varied by adjusting the daily dose. High doses may prolong the effect. A single daily dose is recommended. When a desired therapeutic effect has been obtained, it may be possible to reduce dosage to a lower maintenance level.

The diuretic potency of Zaroxolyn at maximum therapeutic dosage is approximately equal to thiazide diuretics. However, unlike thiazides, Zaroxolyn may produce diuresis in patients with glomerular filtration rates below 20 ml/min.

Zaroxolyn and furosemide administered concurrently have produced marked diuresis in some patients where edema or ascites was refractory to treatment with maximum recommended doses of these or other diuretics administered alone. The mechanism of this interaction is unknown (see DRUG INTERACTIONS and WARNINGS).

Maximum blood levels of metolazone are found approximately eight hours after dosing. A small fraction of metolazone is metabolized. Most of the drug is excreted in the unconverted form in the urine.

MYKROX

The antihypertensive mechanism of action of metolazone is not fully understood but is presumed to be related to its saluretic and diuretic properties.

In two double-blind, controlled clinical trials of Mykrox Tablets, the maximum effect on mean blood pressure was achieved within 2 weeks of treatment and showed some evidence of an increased response at 1 mg compared to 1/2 mg. There was no indication of an increased response with 2 mg.

After six weeks of treatment, the mean fall in serum potassium was 0.42 mEq/l at 1/2 mg, 0.66 mEq/l at 1 mg, and 0.7 mEq/l at 2 mg. Serum uric acid increased by 1.1 to 1.4 mg/dl at increasing doses. There were small falls in serum sodium and chloride and a 1.3-2.1 mg/dl increase in BUN at increasing doses.

The rate and extent of absorption of metolazone from Mykrox Tablets were equivalent to those from an oral solution of metolazone. Peak blood levels are obtained within 2 to 4 hours of oral administration with an elimination half-life of approximately 14 hours. Mykrox Tablets have been shown to produce blood levels that are dose proportional between 1/2-2 mg. Steady state blood levels are usually reached in 4-5 days.

In contrast, other formulations of metolazone produce peak blood concentrations approximately 8 hours following oral administration; absorption continues for an additional 12 hours.

INDICATIONS AND USAGE:

ZAROXOLYN

Zaroxolyn is indicated for the treatment of salt and water retention including:

edema accompanying congestive heart failure

edema accompanying renal diseases, including the nephrotic syndrome and states of diminished renal function

Zaroxolyn is also indicated for the treatment of hypertension, alone or in combination with other antihypertensive drugs of a different class. Mykrox Tablets, a more rapidly available form of metolazone, are intended for the treatment of new patients with mild to moderate hypertension. A dose titration is necessary if Mykrox Tablets are to be substituted for Zaroxolyn in the treatment of hypertension.

Usage in Pregnancy: The routine use of diuretics in an otherwise healthy woman is inappropriate and exposes mother and fetus to unnecessary hazard. Diuretics do not prevent development of toxemia of pregnancy, and there is no evidence that they are useful in the treatment of developed toxemia.

Edema during pregnancy may arise from pathologic causes or from the physiologic and mechanical consequences of pregnancy. Zaroxolyn is indicated in pregnancy when edema is due to pathologic causes, just as it is in the absence of pregnancy (see PRECAUTIONS.) Dependent edema in pregnancy resulting from restriction of venous return by the expanded uterus is properly treated through elevation of the lower extremities and use of support hose; use of diuretics to lower intravascular volume in this case is illogical and unnecessary. There is hypervolemia during normal pregnancy which is harmful to neither the fetus nor the mother (in the absence of cardiovascular disease), but which is associated with edema, including generalized edema, in the majority of pregnant women. If this edema produces discomfort, increased recumbency will often provide relief. In rare instances, this edema may cause extreme discomfort which is not relieved by rest. In these cases, a short course of diuretics may be appropriate.

MYKROX

Mykrox Tablets are indicated for the treatment of hypertension, alone or in combination with other antihypertensive drugs of a different class.

MYKROX TABLETS HAVE <u>NOT</u> BEEN EVALUATED FOR THE TREATMENT OF CONGESTIVE HEART FAILURE OR FLUID RETENTION DUE TO RENAL OR HEPATIC DISEASE AND THE CORRECT DOSAGE FOR THESE CONDITIONS AND OTHER EDEMA STATES HAS NOT BEEN ESTABLISHED.

SINCE A SAFE AND EFFECTIVE DIURETIC DOSE HAS NOT BEEN ESTABLISHED, MYKROX TABLETS SHOULD <u>NOT</u> BE USED WHEN DIURESIS IS DESIRED.

Usage in Pregnancy: The routine use of diuretics in an otherwise healthy woman is inappropriate and exposes mother and fetus to unnecessary hazard. Diuretics do not prevent development of toxemia of pregnancy, and there is no evidence that they are useful in the treatment of developed toxemia (see PRECAUTIONS.)

Edema during pregnancy may arise from pathologic causes or from the physiologic and mechanical consequences of pregnancy. Mykrox is not indicated for the treatment of edema in pregnancy. Dependent edema in pregnancy resulting from restriction of venous return by the expanded uterus is properly treated through elevation of the lower extremities and use of support hose; use of diuretics to lower intravascular volume in this case is illogical and unnecessary. There is hypervolemia during normal pregnancy which is harmful to neither the fetus nor the mother (in the absence of cardiovascular disease), but which is associated with edema, including generalized edema, in the majority of pregnant women. If this edema produces discomfort, increased recumbency will often provide relief. In rare instances, this edema may cause extreme discomfort which is not relieved by rest. In these cases, a short course of diuretics may be appropriate.

CONTRAINDICATIONS:

Anuria, hepatic coma or precoma, known allergy or hypersensitivity to metolazone.

WARNINGS:

Rapid Onset Hyponatremia: Rarely, the rapid onset of severe hyponatremia and/or hypokalemia has been reported following initial doses of thiazide and non-thiazide diuretics. When symptoms consistent with severe electrolyte imbalance appear rapidly, drug should be discontinued and supportive measures should be initiated immediately. Parenteral electrolytes may be required. Appropriateness of therapy with this class of drugs should be carefully reevaluated.

Hypokalemia: Hypokalemia may occur with consequent weakness, cramps, and cardiac dysrhythmias. Serum potassium should be determined at regular intervals, and dose reduction, potassium supplementation or addition of a potassium-sparing diuretic instituted whenever indicated. Hypokalemia is a particular hazard in patients who are digitalized or who have or have had a ventricular arrhythmia; dangerous or fatal arrhythmias may be precipitated. Hypokalemia is dose related.

CONCOMITANT THERAPY

Lithium: In general, diuretics should not be given concomitantly with lithium because they reduce its renal clearance and add a high risk of lithium toxicity. Read prescribing information for lithium preparations before use of such concomitant therapy.

Furosemide: Unusually large or prolonged losses of fluids and electrolytes may result when metolazone is administered concomitantly to patients receiving furosemide (see PRECAUTIONSand DRUG INTERACTIONS).

Other Antihypertensive Drugs: When metolazone is used with other antihypertensive drugs, particular care must be taken to avoid excessive reduction of blood pressure, especially during initial therapy.

Cross-Allergy: Cross-allergy, while not reported to date, theoretically may occur when metolazone is given to patients known to be allergic to sulfonamide-derived drugs, thiazides, or quinethazone.

Sensitivity Reactions: Sensitivity reactions (*e.g.*, angioedema, bronchospasm) may occur with or without a history of allergy or bronchial asthma and may occur with the first dose of metolazone.

MYKROX

In controlled clinical trials, 1.5% of patients taking 1/2 mg and 3.1% of patients taking 1 mg of Mykrox daily developed clinical hypokalemia (defined as hypokalemia accompanied by signs or symptoms); 21% of the patients taking 1/2 mg and 30% of the patients taking 1 mg of Mykrox daily developed hypokalemia (defined as a serum potassium concentration below 3.5 mEq/l); in another controlled clinical trial in which the patients started therapy with a serum potassium level greater than 4.0 mEq/l, 8% of patients taking 1/2 mg of Mykrox daily developed hypokalemia (defined as a serum potassium concentration below 3.5 mEq/l).

PRECAUTIONS:

Zaroxolyn: See BOXED WARNING

Mykrox: See BOXED WARNING

GENERAL

Fluid and Electrolytes: All patients receiving therapy with metolazone should have serum electrolyte measurements done at appropriate intervals and be observed for clinical signs of fluid and/or electrolyte imbalance: namely, hyponatremia, hypochloremic alkalosis, and hypokalemia. In patients with severe edema accompanying cardiac failure or renal disease, a low-salt syndrome may be produced, especially with hot weather and a low-salt diet. Serum and urine electrolyte determinations are particularly important when the patient has protracted vomiting, severe diarrhea, or in receiving parenteral fluids. Warning signs of imbalance are: dryness of mouth, thirst, weakness, lethargy, drowsiness, restlessness, muscle pains or cramps, muscle fatigue, hypotension, oliguria, tachycardia, and gastrointestinal disturbances such as nausea and vomiting. Hyponatremia may occur at any time during long term therapy and, on rare occasions, may be life threatening.

The risk of hypokalemia is increased when larger doses are used, when diuresis is rapid, when severe liver disease is present, when corticosteroids are given concomitantly, when oral intake is inadequate or when excess potassium is being lost extrarenally, such as with vomiting or diarrhea.

Thiazide-like diuretics have been shown to increase the urinary excretion of magnesium; this may result in hypomagnesemia.

Glucose Tolerance: Metolazone may raise blood glucose concentrations possibly causing hyperglycemia and glycosuria in patients with diabetes or latent diabetes.

Hyperuricemia: Metolazone regularly causes an increase in serum uric acid and can occasionally precipitate gouty attacks even in patients without a prior history of them.

Azotemia: Azotemia, presumably prerenal azotemia, may be precipitated during the administration of metolazone. If azotemia and oliguria worsen during treatment of patients with severe renal disease, metolazone should be discontinued.

Renal Impairment: Use caution when administering metolazone to patients with severely impaired renal function. As most of the drug is excreted by the renal route, accumulation may occur.

Orthostatic Hypotension: Orthostatic hypotension may occur; this may be potentiated by alcohol, barbiturates, narcotics, or concurrent therapy with other antihypertensive drugs.

Mykrox: In controlled clinical trials, 1.4% of patients treated with Mykrox Tablets (1/2 mg) had orthostatic hypotension; this effect was not reported in the placebo group.

Hypercalcemia: Hypercalcemia may infrequently occur with metolazone, especially in patients taking high doses of vitamin D or with high bone turnover states, and may signify hidden hyperparathyroidism. Metolazone should be discontinued before tests for parathyroid function are performed.

Systemic Lupus Erythematosus: Thiazide diuretics have exacerbated or activated systemic lupus erythematosus and this possibility should be considered with metolazone.

INFORMATION FOR THE PATIENT

Patients should be informed of possible adverse effects, advised to take the medication as directed, and promptly report any possible adverse reactions to the treating physician.

DRUG/LABORATORY TEST INTERACTIONS

None reported.

CARCINOGENESIS, MUTAGENESIS, AND IMPAIRMENT OF FERTILITY

Mice and rats administered metolazone 5 days/week for up to 18 and 24 months, respectively, at daily doses of 2, 10, and 50 mg/kg, exhibited no evidence of a tumorigenic effect of the drug. The small number of animals examined histologically and poor survival in the mice limit the conclusions that can be reached from these studies.

Metolazone was not mutagenic *in vitro* in the Ames Test using Salmonella typhimurium strains TA-97, TA-98, TA-100, TA-102, and TA- 1535.

Reproductive performance has been evaluated in mice and rats. There is no evidence that metolazone possesses the potential for altering reproductive capacity in mice. In a rat study, in which males were treated orally with metolazone at doses of 2, 10, and 50 mg/kg for 127 days prior to mating with untreated females, an increased number of resorption sites was

PRECAUTIONS: *(cont'd)*

observed in dams mated with males from the 50 mg/kg group. In addition, the birth weight of offspring was decreased and the pregnancy rate was reduced in dams mated with males from the 10 and 50 mg/kg groups.

PREGNANCY CATEGORY B

Teratogenic Effects: Reproduction studies performed in mice, rabbits, and rats treated during the appropriate period of gestation at doses up to 50 mg/kg/day have revealed no evidence of harm to the fetus due to metolazone. There are, however, no adequate and well-controlled studies in pregnant women. Because animal reproduction studies are not always predictive of human response, metolazone should be used during pregnancy only if clearly needed. Metolazone crosses the placental barrier and appears in cord blood.

Non-Teratogenic Effects: The use of metolazone in pregnant women requires that the anticipated benefit be weighed against possible hazards to the fetus. These hazards include fetal or neonatal jaundice, thrombocytopenia, and possibly other adverse reactions which have occurred in the adult. It is not known what effect the use of the drug during pregnancy has on the later growth, development, and functional maturation of the child. No such effects have been reported with metolazone.

LABOR AND DELIVERY

Based on clinical studies in which women received metolazone in late pregnancy until the time of delivery, there is no evidence that the drug has any adverse effects on the normal course of labor or delivery.

NURSING MOTHERS

Metolazone appears in breast milk. Because of the potential for serious adverse reactions in nursing infants from metolazone, a decision should be made whether to discontinue nursing or to discontinue the drug, taking into account the importance of the drug to the mother.

PEDIATRIC USE

Safety and effectiveness in children have not been established and such use is not recommended.

DRUG INTERACTIONS:

Diuretics: Furosemide and probably other loop diuretics given concomitantly with metolazone can cause unusually large or prolonged losses of fluid and electrolytes (see WARNINGS).

Other Antihypertensives: When metolazone is used with other antihypertensive drugs, care must be taken, especially during initial therapy. Dosage adjustments of other antihypertensives may be necessary.

Alcohol, Barbiturates, and Narcotics: The hypotensive effects of these drugs may be potentiated by the volume contraction that may be associated with metolazone therapy.

Digitalis Glycosides: Diuretic-induced hypokalemia can increase the sensitivity of the myocardium to digitalis. Serious arrhythmias can result.

Corticosteroids or ACTH: May increase the risk of hypokalemia and increase salt and water retention.

Lithium: Serum lithium levels may increase (see WARNINGS.)

Curariform Drugs: Diuretic-induced hypokalemia may enhance neuromuscular blocking effects of curariform drugs (such as tubocurarine) - the most serious effect would be respiratory depression which could proceed to apnea. Accordingly, it may be advisable to discontinue metolazone three days before elective surgery.

Salicylates and Other Non-Steroidal Anti-Inflammatory Drugs: May decrease the antihypertensive effects of metolazone.

Sympathomimetics: Metolazone may decrease arterial responsiveness to norepinephrine, but this diminution is not sufficient to preclude effectiveness of the pressor agent for therapeutic use.

Insulin and Oral Antidiabetic Agents: See Glucose Tolerance under PRECAUTIONS, General.

Methenamine: Efficacy may be decreased due to urinary alkalizing effect of metolazone.

Anticoagulants: Metolazone, as well as other thiazide-like diuretics, may affect the hypoprothrombinemic response to anticoagulants; dosage adjustments may be necessary.

ADVERSE REACTIONS:

ZAROXOLYN

Zaroxolyn is usually well tolerated, and most reported adverse reactions have been mild and transient. Many Zaroxolyn related adverse reactions represent extensions of its expected pharmacologic activity and can be attributed to either its antihypertensive action or its renal/metabolic actions. The following adverse reactions have been reported. Several are single or comparably rare occurrences. Adverse reactions are listed in decreasing order of severity within body systems.

Cardiovascular: Chest pain/discomfort, orthostatic hypotension, excessive volume depletion, hemoconcentration, venous thrombosis, palpitations.

Central and Peripheral Nervous System: Syncope, neuropathy, vertigo, paresthesias, psychotic depression, impotence, dizziness/lightheadedness, drowsiness, fatigue, weakness, restlessness (sometimes resulting in insomnia), headache

Dermatologic/Hypersensitivity: Necrotizing angitis (cutaneous vasculitis), purpura, dermatitis (photosensitivity), urticaria, and skin rashes

Gastrointestinal: Hepatitis, intrahepatic cholestatic jaundice, pancreatitis, vomiting, nausea, epigastric distress, diarrhea, constipation, anorexia, abdominal bloating

Hematologic: Aplastic/hypoplastic anemia, agranulocytosis, leukopenia.

Metabolic: Hypokalemia, hyponatremia, hyperuricemia, hypochloremia, hypochloremic alkalosis, hyperglycemia, glycosuria, increase in serum urea nitrogen (BUN) or creatinine, hypophosphatemia, hypomagnesemia, hypercalcemia

Musculoskeletal: Joint pain, acute gouty attacks, muscle cramps or spasm.

Other: Transient blurred vision, chills.

In addition, adverse reactions reported with similar antihypertensive-diuretics, but which have not been reported to date for Zaroxolyn include: bitter taste, dry mouth, sialadenitis, xanthopsia, respiratory distress (including pneumonitis), thrombocytopenia, and anaphylactic reactions. These reactions should be considered as possible occurrences with clinical usage of Zaroxolyn.

Whenever adverse reactions are moderate or severe, Zaroxolyn dosage should be reduced or therapy withdrawn.

MYKROX

Adverse experience information is available from more than 14 years of accumulated marketing experience with other formulations of metolazone for which reliable quantitative information is lacking and from controlled clinical trials with Mykrox from which incidences can be calculated.

In controlled clinical trials with Mykrox, adverse experiences resulted in discontinuation of therapy in 6.7-6.8% of patients given 1/2 to 1 mg of Mykrox.

ADVERSE REACTIONS: *(cont'd)*

Adverse experiences occurring in controlled clinical trials with Mykrox with an incidence of >2%, whether or not considered drug-related, are summarized in the following table (TABLE 1).

TABLE 1 Incidence of Adverse Experiences Volunteered or Elicited (by Patient in Percent)*

	Mykrox n = 226†
Dizziness (lightheadedness)	10.2
Headaches	9.3
Muscle Cramps	5.8
Fatigue (malaise, lethargy, lassitude)	4.4
Joint Pain, swelling	3.1
Chest Pain (precordial discomfort)	2.7

* Percent of patients reporting an adverse experience one or more times.
† All doses combined (1/2, 1, and 2 mg).

Some of the adverse effects reported in association with Mykrox also occur frequently in untreated hypertensive patients, such as headache and dizziness, which occurred in 14.8 and 7.4% of patients in a smaller parallel placebo group.

The following adverse effects were reported in less than 2% of the Mykrox treated patients:

Cardiovascular: Cold extremities, edema, orthostatic hypotension, palpitations.

Central and Peripheral Nervous System: Anxiety, depression, dry mouth, impotence, nervousness, neuropathy, weakness, "weird" feeling

Dermatological: Pruritus, rash, skin dryness.

Eyes, Ears, Nose, Throat: Cough, epistaxis, eye itching, sinus congestion, sore throat, tinnitus.

Gastrointestinal: Abdominal discomfort (pain, bloating), bitter taste, constipation, diarrhea, nausea, vomiting.

Genitourinary: Nocturia.

Musculoskeletal: Back Pain.

Other Adverse Experiences: Adverse experiences reported with other marketed metolazone formulations and most thiazide diuretics, for which quantitative data are not available, are listed in decreasing order of severity within body systems. Several are single or rare occurrences.

Cardiovascular: excessive volume depletion, hemoconcentration, venous thrombosis.

Central and Peripheral Nervous System: syncope, paresthesias, drowsiness, restlessness (sometimes resulting in insomnia).

Dermatologic/Hypersensitivity: necrotizing angitis (cutaneous vasculitis), purpura, dermatitis, photosensitivity, urticaria.

Gastrointestinal: hepatitis, intrahepatic cholestatic jaundice, pancreatitis, anorexia.

Hematologic: aplastic (hypoplastic) anemia, agranulocytosis, leukopenia.

Metabolic: hypokalemia (see WARNINGS, Hypokalemia), hyponatremia, hyperuricemia, hypochloremia, hypochloremic alkalosis, hyperglycemia, glycosuria, increase in serum urea nitrogen (BUN) or creatinine, hypophosphatemia, hypomagnesemia, hypercalcemia.

Musculoskeletal: acute gouty attacks.

Other: transient blurred vision, chills.

In addition, rare adverse experiences reported in association with similar antihypertensive-diuretics but not reported to date for metolazone include: sialadenitis, xanthopsia, respiratory distress (including pneumonitis), thrombocytopenia, and anaphylactic reactions. These experiences could occur with clinical use of metolazone.

OVERDOSAGE:

Intentional overdosage has been reported rarely with metolazone and similar diuretic drugs.

Signs and Symptoms: Orthostatic hypotension, dizziness, drowsiness, syncope, electrolyte abnormalities, hemoconcentration and hemodynamic changes due to plasma volume depletion may occur. In some instances depressed respiration may be observed. At high doses, lethargy of varying degree may progress to coma within a few hours. The mechanism of CNS depression with thiazide overdosage is unknown. Also, GI irritation and hypermotility may occur. Temporary elevation of BUN has been reported, especially in patients with impairment of renal function. Serum electrolyte changes and cardiovascular and renal function should be closely monitored.

Treatment: There is no specific antidote available but immediate evacuation of stomach contents is advised. Dialysis is not likely to be effective. Care should be taken when evacuating the gastric contents to prevent aspiration, especially in the stuporous or comatose patient. Supportive measures should be initiated as required to maintain hydration, electrolyte balance, respiration, and cardiovascular and renal function.

DOSAGE AND ADMINISTRATION:

ZAROXOLYN

Effective dosage of Zaroxolyn should be individualized according to indication and patient response. A single daily dose is recommended. Therapy with Zaroxolyn should be titrated to gain an initial therapeutic response and to determine the minimal dose possible to maintain the desired therapeutic response.

Usual Single Daily Dosage Schedules: Suitable initial dosages will usually fall in the ranges given.

Edema of cardiac failure: Zaroxolyn 5 to 20 mg once daily.

Edema of renal disease: Zaroxolyn 5 to 20 mg once daily.

Mild to moderate essential hypertension: Zaroxolyn 2 1/2 to 5 mg once daily.

New patients: Mykrox Tablets (metolazone tablets, USP). If considered desirable to switch patients currently on Zaroxolyn to Mykrox, the dose should be determined by titration starting at one tablet (1/2 mg) once daily and increasing to two tablets (1 mg) once daily if needed.

Treatment of Edematous States: The time interval required for the initial dosage to produce an effect may vary. Diuresis and saluresis usually begin within one hour and persist for 24 hours or longer. When a desired therapeutic effect has been obtained, it may be advisable to reduce the dose if possible. The daily dose depends on the severity of the patient's condition, sodium intake, and responsiveness. A decision to change the daily dose should be based on the results of thorough clinical and laboratory evaluations. If antihypertensive drugs or diuretics are given concurrently with Zaroxolyn, more careful dosage adjustment may be necessary. For patients who tend to experience paroxysmal nocturnal dyspnea, it may be advisable to employ a larger dose to ensure prolongation of diuresis and saluresis for a full 24-hour period.

Treatment of Hypertension: The time interval required for the initial dosage regimen to show effect may vary from three or four days to three to six weeks in the treatment of elevated blood pressure. Doses should be adjusted at appropriate intervals to achieve maximum therapeutic effect.

DOSAGE AND ADMINISTRATION: *(cont'd)*

MYKROX

Therapy should be individualized according to patient response.

For initial treatment of mild to moderate hypertension, the recommended dose is one Mykrox Tablet (1/2 mg) once daily, usually in the morning. If patients are inadequately controlled with one 1/2 mg tablet, the dose can be increased to two Mykrox Tablets (1 mg) once a day. An increase in hypokalemia may occur. Doses larger than 1 mg do not give increased effectiveness.

The same dose titration is necessary if Mykrox Tablets are to be substituted for other dosage forms of metolazone in the treatment of hypertension.

If blood pressure is not adequately controlled with two Mykrox Tablets alone, the dose should not be increased; rather, another antihypertensive agent with a different mechanism of action should be added to therapy with Mykrox tablets.

HOW SUPPLIED:

Zaroxolyn: Zaroxolyn Tablets (metolazone tablets, USP) are shallow biconvex, round tablets, and are available in three strengths:

2 1/2 mg, pink, debossed "Zaroxolyn" on one side, and "2 1/2" on reverse side.

5 mg, blue, debossed "Zaroxolyn" on one side, and "5" on reverse side.

10 mg, yellow, debossed "Zaroxolyn" on one side, and "10" on reverse side.

Mykrox: Mykrox Tablets (metolazone tablets, USP), 1/2 mg are white, flat-faced, round tablets, debossed "Mykrox" on one side, and "1/2" on reverse side.

Storage: Store at room temperature. Dispense in a tight, light-resistant container. Keep out of the reach of children.

HOW SUPPLIED - EQUIVALENTS NOT AVAILABLE:

Tablet, Uncoated - Oral - 0.5 mg

100's	$73.63	MYKROX, Medeva Pharms	53014-0847-71

Tablet, Uncoated - Oral - 2.5 mg

100's	$46.81	ZAROXOLYN, Medeva Pharms	53014-0975-71
100's	$55.64	ZAROXOLYN, Medeva Pharms	53014-0975-72
1000's	$433.64	ZAROXOLYN, Medeva Pharms	53014-0975-90

Tablet, Uncoated - Oral - 5 mg

100's	$53.21	ZAROXOLYN, Medeva Pharms	53014-0850-71
100's	$61.94	ZAROXOLYN, Medeva Pharms	53014-0850-72
1000's	$494.26	ZAROXOLYN, Medeva Pharms	53014-0850-90

Tablet, Uncoated - Oral - 10 mg

100's	$63.68	ZAROXOLYN, Medeva Pharms	53014-0835-71
100's	$71.84	ZAROXOLYN, Medeva Pharms	53014-0835-72
1000's	$591.42	ZAROXOLYN, Medeva Pharms	53014-0835-90

METOPROLOL SUCCINATE *(003115)*

CATEGORIES: Angina; Antianginals; Antiarrhythmic Agents; Beta Adrenergic Blocking Agents; Beta Blockers; Cardiovascular Drugs; Hypertension; Pregnancy Category C; FDA Approved 1992 Jan; Top 200 Drugs; Top 200 Drugs

BRAND NAMES: *Beloc-Zok* (Germany); *Betaloc*; *Betaloc CR*; *Betaloc Zok*; *Betaloc ZOK*; *Betazok*; *Mycol*; *Seloken-Zok* (Mexico); *Selozok*; **Toprol Xl**
(International brand names outside U.S. in italics)

COST OF THERAPY: $162.89 (Hypertension; Tablet; 50 mg; 1/day; 365 days) vs. Potential Cost of $24,027.04 (Coronary Bypass)

PRIMARY ICD9: 401.1 (Essential Hypertension, Benign)

DESCRIPTION:

Toprol-XL, metoprolol succinate, is a beta$_1$-selective (cardioselective) adrenoceptor blocking agent, for oral administration, available as extended release tablets. Toprol-XL has been formulated to provide a controlled and predictable release of metoprolol for once daily administration. The tablets comprise a multiple unit system containing metoprolol succinate in a multitude of controlled release pellets. Each pellet acts as a separate drug delivery unit and is designed to deliver metoprolol continuously over the dosage interval. The tablets contain 47.5 mg, 95 mg and 190 mg of metoprolol succinate equivalent to 50, 100 and 200 mg of metoprolol tartrate, USP, respectively. Its chemical name is (±) 1-(isopropylamino)-3-(p-(2-methoxyethyl) phenoxy)-2-propanol succinate (2:1) (slat).

Metoprolol succinate is a white crystalline powder with a molecular weight of 652.8. It is freely soluble in water; soluble in methanol; sparingly soluble in ethanol; slightly soluble in dichloromethane and 2- propanol; practically insoluble in ethyl-acetate, acetone, diethylether and heptane. Inactive ingredients: Silicone dioxide, Cellulose compounds, Acetyltributyl citrate, Maize starch, Lactose powder, Polyvidone, Magnesium stearate, Polyethylene glycol, Titanium dioxide, Paraffin.

CLINICAL PHARMACOLOGY:

Metoprolol is a beta$_1$-selective (cardioselective) adrenergic receptor blocking agent. This preferential effect is not absolute, however, and at higher plasma concentrations, metoprolol also inhibits beta$_2$-adrenoreceptors, chiefly located in the bronchial and vascular musculature. Metoprolol has no intrinsic sympathomimetic activity, and membrane-stabilizing activity is detectable only at plasma concentrations much greater than required for beta-blockade. Animal and human experiments indicate that metoprolol slows the sinus rate and decreases AV nodal conduction.

Clinical pharmacology studies have confirmed the beta-blocking activity of metoprolol in man, as shown by (1) reduction in heart rate and cardiac output at rest and upon exercise, (2) reduction of systolic blood pressure upon exercise, (3) inhibition of isoproterenol-induced tachycardia, and (4) reduction of reflex orthostatic tachycardia.

The relative beta$_1$-selectivity of metoprolol has been confirmed by the following: (1) In normal subjects, metoprolol is unable to reverse the beta$_2$-mediated vasodilating effects of epinephrine. This contrasts with the effect of nonselective beta-blockers, which completely reverse the vasodilating effects of epinephrine. (2) In asthmatic patients, metoprolol reduces FEV$_1$ and FVC significantly less than a nonselective beta-blocker, propranolol, at equivalent beta$_1$- receptor blocking doses.

In five controlled studies in normal healthy subjects, the same daily doses of Toprol-XL and immediate release metoprolol were compared in terms of the extent and duration of beta$_1$-blockade produced. Both formulations were given in a dose range equivalent to 100-400 mg of immediate release metoprolol per day. In these studies, Toprol-XL was administered once a day and immediate release metoprolol was administered once to four times a day. A sixth controlled study compared the beta$_1$-blocking effects of a 50 mg daily dose of the two formulations. In each study, beta$_1$-blockade was expressed as the percent change from baseline, in exercise heart rate following standardized submaximal exercise tolerance tests at steady state. Toprol- XL administered once a day, and immediate release metoprolol administered once to four times a day, provided comparable total beta$_1$- blockade over 24 hours (area under the beta$_1$-blockade versus time curve) in the dose range 100-400 mg. At a dosage of 50 mg once daily, Toprol-XL produced significantly higher total beta$_1$-blockade over 24 hours than immediate release metoprolol. For Toprol-XL, the percent reduction in exercise heart rate was relatively stable throughout the entire dosage interval and the level of beta$_1$-blockade increased with increasing doses from 50 to 300 mg daily. The effects at peak/trough (*i.e.*, at 24 hours post dosing) were; 14/9, 16/10, 24/14, 27/22 and 27/20% reduction in exercise heart rate for doses of 50, 100, 200, 300 and 400 mg Toprol-XL once a day, respectively. In contrast to Toprol-XL immediate release metoprolol given at a dose of 50-100 mg once a day, produced a significantly larger peak effect on exercise tachycardia, but the effect was not evident at 24 hours. To match the peak to trough ratio obtained with Toprol-XL over the dosing range of 200 to 400 mg, a t.i.d. to q.i.d. divided dosing regimen was required for immediate release metoprolol.

The relationship between plasma metoprolol levels and reduction in exercise heart rate is independent of the pharmaceutical formulation. Using the E_{max} model, the maximal beta$_1$-blocking effect has been estimated to produce a 28.3% reduction in exercise heart rate. Beta$_1$-blocking effects in the range of 30-80% of the maximal effect (corresponding to approximately 8-23% reduction in exercise heart rate) are expected to occur at metoprolol plasma concentrations ranging from 30-540 nmol/L. The concentration-effect curve begins reaching a plateau between 200-300 nmol/L, and higher plasma levels produce little additional beta^1-blocking effect. The relative beta$_1$-selectivity of metoprolol diminishes and blockade of beta$_2$-adrenoceptors increases at higher plasma concentrations.

Although beta-adrenergic receptor blockade is useful in the treatment of angina and hypertension, there are situations in which sympathetic stimulation is vital. In patients with severely damaged hearts, adequate ventricular function may depend on sympathetic drive. In the presence of AV block, beta-blockade may prevent the necessary facilitating effect of sympathetic activity on conduction. Beta$_2$-adrenergic blockade results in passive bronchial constriction by interfering with endogenous adrenergic bronchodilator activity in patients subject to bronchospasm and may also interfere with exogenous bronchodilators in such patients.

HYPERTENSION

The mechanism of the antihypertensive effects of beta-blocking agents has not been elucidated. However, several possible mechanisms have been proposed: (1) competitive antagonism of catecholamines at peripheral (especially cardiac) adrenergic neuron sites, leading to decreased cardiac output; (2) a central effect leading to reduced sympathetic outflow to the periphery; and (3) suppression of renin activity.

In controlled clinical studies, an immediate release dosage form of metoprolol has been shown to be an effective antihypertensive agent when used alone or as concomitant therapy with thiazide-type diuretics at dosages of 100-450 mg daily. Toprol-XL, in dosages of 100 to 400 mg once daily, has been shown to possess comparable β_1-blockade as conventional metoprolol tablets administered two to four times daily. In addition, Toprol-XL administered at a dose of 50 mg once daily has been shown to lower blood pressure 24-hours post-dosing in placebo controlled studies. In controlled, comparative, clinical studies, immediate release metoprolol appeared comparable as an antihypertensive agent to propranolol, methyldopa, and thiazide-type diuretics, and affected both supine and standing blood pressure. Because of variable plasma levels attained with a given dose and lack of consistent relationship of antihypertensive activity to drug plasma concentration, selection of proper dosage requires individual titration.

ANGINA PECTORIS

By blocking catecholamine-induced increases in heart rate, in velocity and extent of myocardial contraction, and in blood pressure, metoprolol reduces the oxygen requirements of the heart at any given level of effort, thus making it useful in the long-term management of angina pectoris. However, in patients with heart failure, beta-adrenergic blockade may increase oxygen requirements by increasing left ventricular fiber length and end-diastolic pressure.

In controlled clinical trials, an immediate release formulation of metoprolol has been shown to be an effective antianginal agent, reducing the number of angina attacks and increasing exercise tolerance. The dosage used in these studies ranged from 100 to 400 mg daily. Toprol-XL, in dosages of 100 to 400 mg once daily, has been shown to possess comparable β_1-blockade as conventional metoprolol tablets administered two to four times daily.

PHARMACOKINETICS

In man, absorption of metoprolol is rapid and complete. Plasma levels following oral administration of conventional metoprolol tablets, however, approximate 50% of levels following intravenous administration, indicating about 50% first-pass metabolism. Metoprolol crosses the blood- brain barrier and has been reported in the CSF in a concentration 78% of the simultaneous plasma concentration.

Plasma levels achieved are highly variable after oral administration. Only a small fraction of the drug (about 12%) is bound to human serum albumin. Elimination is mainly by biotransformation in the liver, and the plasma half-life ranges from approximately 3 to 7 hours. Less than 5% of an oral dose of metoprolol is recovered unchanged in the urine; the rest is excreted by the kidneys as metabolites that appear to have no clinical significance. Following intravenous administration of metoprolol, the urinary recovery of unchanged drug is approximately 10%. The systemic availability and half-life on metoprolol in patients with renal failure do not differ to a clinically significant degree from those in normal subjects. Consequently, no reduction in dosage is usually needed in patients with chronic renal failure.

In comparison to conventional metoprolol, the plasma metoprolol levels following administration of Toprol-XL are characterized by lower peaks, longer time to peak and significantly lower peak to trough variation. The peak plasma levels following once daily administration of Toprol-XL average one-fourth to one-half the peak plasma levels obtained following a corresponding dose of conventional metoprolol, administered once daily or in divided doses. At steady state the average bioavailability of metoprolol following administration of Toprol-XL, across the dosage range of 50 to 400 mg once daily, was 77% relative to the corresponding single or divided doses of conventional metoprolol. Nevertheless, over the 24 hour dosing interval, β_1-blockade is comparable and dose- related (see CLINICAL PHARMACOLOGY.) The bioavailability of metoprolol shows a dose-related, although not directly proportional increase with dose and is not significantly affected by food following Toprol-XL administration.

INDICATIONS AND USAGE:

HYPERTENSION

Toprol-XL tablets are indicated for the treatment of hypertension. They may be used alone or in combination with other antihypertensive agents.

ANGINA PECTORIS

Toprol-XL tablets are indicated in the long-term treatment of angina pectoris.

CONTRAINDICATIONS:

HYPERTENSION AND ANGINA

Toprol-XL is contraindicated in sinus bradycardia, heart block greater than first degree, cardiogenic shock, and overt cardiac failure (see WARNINGS.)

WARNINGS:

HYPERTENSION AND ANGINA

Cardiac Failure: Sympathetic stimulation is a vital component supporting circulatory function in congestive heart failure, and beta-blockade carries the potential hazard of further depressing myocardial contractility and precipitating more severe failure. In hypertensive and angina patients who have congestive heart failure controlled by digitalis and diuretics, Toprol-XL should be administered cautiously. Both digitalis and Toprol-XL slow AV conduction.

In Patients Without a History of Cardiac Failure: Continued depression of the myocardium with beta-blocking agents over a period of time can, in some cases, lead to cardiac failure. At the first sign or symptom of impending cardiac failure, patients should be fully digitalized and/or given a diuretic. The response should be observed closely. If cardiac failure continues, despite adequate digitalization and diuretic therapy, Toprol-XL should be withdrawn.

Ischemic Heart Disease: Following abrupt cessation of therapy with certain beta-blocking agents, exacerbations of angina pectoris and, in some cases, myocardial infarction have occurred. When discontinuing chronically administered Toprol-XL, particularly in patients with ischemic heart disease, the dosage should be gradually reduced over a period of 1-2 weeks and the patient should be carefully monitored. If angina markedly worsens or acute coronary insufficiency develops, Toprol-XL administration should be reinstated promptly, at least temporarily, and other measures appropriate for the management of unstable angina should be taken. Patients should be warned against interruption or discontinuation of therapy without the physician's advice. Because coronary artery disease is common and may be unrecognized, it may be prudent not to discontinue Toprol-XL therapy abruptly even in patients treated only for hypertension.

Bronchospastic Diseases: PATIENTS WITH BRONCHOSPASTIC DISEASES SHOULD, IN GENERAL, NOT RECEIVE BETA-BLOCKERS. Because of its relative $beta_1$-selectivity, however, Toprol-XL may be used with caution in patients with bronchospastic disease who do not respond to, or cannot tolerate, other antihypertensive treatment. Since $beta_1$- selectivity is not absolute, a $beta_2$-stimulating agent should be administered concomitantly, and the lowest possible dose of Toprol-XL should be used (see DOSAGE AND ADMINISTRATION.)

Major Surgery: The necessity or desirability of withdrawing beta-blocking therapy prior to major surgery is controversial; the impaired ability of the heart to respond to reflex adrenergic stimuli may augment the risks of general anesthesia and surgical procedures.

Toprol-XL like other beta-blockers, is a competitive inhibitor of beta-receptor agonists, and its effects can be reversed by administration of such agents, e.g., dobutamine or isoproterenol. However, such patients may be subject to protracted severe hypotension. Difficulty in restarting and maintaining the heart beat has also been reported with beta- blockers.

Diabetes and Hypoglycemia: Toprol-XL should be used with caution in diabetic patients if a beta-blocking agent is required. Beta- blockers may mask tachycardia occurring with hypoglycemia, but other manifestations such as dizziness and sweating may not be significantly affected.

Thyrotoxicosis: Beta-adrenergic blockade may mask certain clinical signs (*e.g.,* tachycardia) of hyperthyroidism. Patients suspected of developing thyrotoxicosis should be managed carefully to avoid abrupt withdrawal of beta-blockade, which might precipitate a thyroid storm.

PRECAUTIONS:

GENERAL

Toprol-XL should be used with caution in patients with impaired hepatic function.

INFORMATION FOR THE PATIENT

Patients should be advised to take Toprol-XL regularly and continuously, as directed, preferably with or immediately following meals. If a dose should be missed, the patient should take only the next scheduled dose (without doubling it). Patients should not discontinue Toprol-XL without consulting the physician.

Patients should be advised (1) to avoid operating automobiles and machinery or engaging in other tasks requiring alertness until the patient's response to therapy with Toprol-XL has been determined; (2) to contact the physician if any difficulty in breathing occurs; (3) to inform the physician or dentist before any type of surgery that he or she is taking Toprol-XL.

LABORATORY TESTS

Clinical laboratory findings may include elevated levels of serum transaminase, alkaline phosphatase, and lactate dehydrogenase.

CARCINOGENESIS, MUTAGENESIS, AND IMPAIRMENT OF FERTILITY

Long-term studies in animals have been conducted to evaluate the carcinogenic potential of metoprolol tartrate. In 2-year studies in rats at three oral dosage levels of up to 800 mg/kg/day, there was no increase in the development of spontaneously occurring benign or malignant neoplasms of any type. The only histologic changes that appeared to be drug related were an increased incidence of generally mild focal accumulation of foamy macrophages in pulmonary alveoli and a slight increase in biliary hyperplasia. In a 21-month study in Swiss albino mice at three oral dosage levels of up to 750 mg/kg/day, benign lung tumors (small adenomas) occurred more frequently in female mice receiving the highest dose than in untreated control animals. There was no increase in malignant or total (benign plus malignant) ling tumors, nor in the overall incidence of tumors or malignant tumors. This 21-month study was repeated in CD-1 mice, and no statistically or biologically significant differences were observed between treated and control mice of either sex for any type of tumor. All mutagenicity tests performed on metoprolol tartrate (a dominant lethal study in mice, chromosome studies in somatic cells, a Salmonella/mammalian-microsome mutagenicity test, and a nucleus anomaly test in somatic interphase nuclei) and metoprolol succinate (a Salmonella/mammalian-microsome mutagenicity test) were negative.

No evidence of impaired fertility due to metoprolol tartrate was observed in a study performed in rats at doses up to 55.5 times the maximum daily human dose of 450 mg.

PREGNANCY CATEGORY C

Metoprolol tartrate has been shown to increase post-implantation loss and decrease neonatal survival in rats at doses up to 55.5 times the maximum daily human dose of 450 mg. Distribution studies in mice confirm exposure of the fetus when metoprolol tartrate is administered to the pregnant animal. These studies have revealed no evidence of impaired fertility or teratogenicity. There are no adequate and well-controlled studies in pregnant women. Because animal reproduction studies are not always predictive of human response, this drug should be used during pregnancy only if clearly needed.

NURSING MOTHERS

Metoprolol is excreted in breast milk in very small quantities. An infant consuming 1 liter of breast milk daily would receive a dose of less than 1 mg of the drug. Caution should be exercised when Toprol-XL is administered to a nursing woman.

PEDIATRIC USE

Safety and effectiveness in children have not been established.

PRECAUTIONS: *(cont'd)*

RISK OF ANAPHYLACTIC REACTIONS

While taking beta-blockers, patients with a history of severe anaphylactic reactions to a variety of allergens may be more reactive to repeated challenge, either accidental, diagnostic or therapeutic. Such patients may be unresponsive to the usual doses of epinephrine used to treat allergic reaction.

DRUG INTERACTIONS:

Catecholamine-depleting drugs (*e.g.,* reserpine) may have an additive effect when given with beta-blocking agents. Patients treated with Toprol-XL plus a catecholamine depletor should therefore be closely observed for evidence of hypotension or marked bradycardia, which may produce vertigo, syncope, or postural hypotension.

ADVERSE REACTIONS:

HYPERTENSION AND ANGINA

Most adverse effects have been mild and transient. The following adverse reactions have been reported for metoprolol tartrate.

Central Nervous System: Tiredness and dizziness have occurred in about 10 of 100 patients. Depression has been reported in about 5 of 100 patients. Mental confusion and short-term memory loss have been reported. Headache, somnolence, nightmares, and insomnia have also been reported.

Cardiovascular: Shortness of breath and bradycardia have occurred in approximately 3 of 100 patients. Cold extremities; arterial insufficiency, usually of the Raynaud type; palpitations; congestive heart failure; peripheral edema; syncope; chest pain; and hypotension have been reported in about 1 of 100 patients (see CONTRAINDICATIONS, WARNINGS, and PRECAUTIONS).

Respiratory: Wheezing (bronchospasm) and dyspnea have been reported in about 1 of 100 patients (see WARNINGS.)

Gastrointestinal: Diarrhea has occurred in about 5 of 100 patients. Nausea, dry mouth, gastric pain, constipation, flatulence, digestive tract disorders and heartburn have been reported in about 1 of 100 patients.

Hypersensitive Reactions: Pruritus or rash have occurred in about 5 of 100 patients. Worsening or psoriasis has also been reported.

Miscellaneous: Peyronie's disease has been reported in fewer than 1 of 100,000 patients. Musculoskeletal pain, blurred vision, decreased libido and tinnitus have also been reported.

There have been rare reports of reversible alopecia, agranulocytosis, and dry eyes. Discontinuation of the drug should be considered if any such reaction is not otherwise explicable. The oculomucocutaneous syndrome associated with the beta-blocker practolol has not been reported with metoprolol.

POTENTIAL ADVERSE REACTIONS

A variety of adverse reactions not listed above have been reported with other beta-adrenergic blocking agents and should be considered potential adverse reactions to Toprol-XL.

Central Nervous System: Reversible mental depression progressing to catatonia; an acute reversible syndrome characterized ny disorientation for time and place, short-term memory loss, emotional lability, slightly clouded sensorium, and decreased performance on neuropsychometrics.

Cardiovascular: Intensification of AV block (see CONTRAINDICATIONS.)

Hematologic: Agranulocytosis, nonthrombocytopenic purpura, thrombocytopenic purpura.

Hypersensitive Reactions: Fever combined with aching and sore throat, laryngospasm, and respiratory distress.

OVERDOSAGE:

ACUTE TOXICITY

No overdosage has been reported with Toprol-XL and no specific overdosage information was obtained with this drug, with the exception of animal toxicology data. However, since Toprol-XL (metoprolol succinate salt) contains the same active moiety, metoprolol, as conventional metoprolol tablets (metoprolol tartrate salt), the recommendations on overdosage for metoprolol conventional tablets are applicable to Toprol-XL.

SIGNS AND SYMPTOMS

Potential signs and symptoms associated with overdosage with metoprolol are bradycardia, hypotension, bronchospasm, and cardiac failure.

TREATMENT

There is no specific antidote.

In general, patients with acute or recent myocardial infarction may be more hemodynamically unstable than other patients and should be treated accordingly. On the basis of the pharmacologic actions of metoprolol tartrate, the following general measures should be employed.

Elimination of the Drug: Gastric lavage should be performed.

Bradycardia: Atropine should be administered. If there is no response to vagal blockade, isoproterenol should be administered cautiously.

Hypotension: A vasopressor should be administered, e.g., levarterenol or dopamine.

Bronchospasm: A $beta_2$-stimulating agent and/or a theophylline derivative should be administered.

Cardiac Failure: A digitalis glycoside and diuretics should be administered. In shock resulting from inadequate cardiac contractility, administration of dobutamine, isoproterenol or glucagon may be considered.

DOSAGE AND ADMINISTRATION:

Toprol-XL is an extended release tablet intended for once-a-day administration. When switching from immediate release metoprolol tablet to Toprol-XL, the same total daily dose of Toprol-XL should be used.

As with immediate release metoprolol, dosages of Toprol-XL should be individualized and titration may be needed in some patients.

Toprol-XL tablets are scored and can be divided; however, the whole or half tablet should be swallowed whole and not chewed or crushed.

HYPERTENSION

The usual initial dosage is 50 to 100 mg daily in a single dose, whether used alone or added to a diuretic. The dosage may be increased at weekly (or longer) intervals until optimum blood pressure reduction is achieved. In general, the maximum effect of any given dosage level will be apparent after 1 week of therapy. Dosages above 400 mg per day have not been studied.

DOSAGE AND ADMINISTRATION: *(cont'd)*

ANGINA PECTORIS

The dosage to Toprol-XL should be individualized. The usual initial dosage is 100 mg daily, given in a single dose. The dosage may be gradually increased at weekly intervals until optimum clinical response has been obtained or there is a pronounced slowing of the heart rate. Dosages above 400 mg per day have not been studied. If treatment is to be discontinued, the dosage should be reduced gradually over a period of 1-2 weeks (see WARNINGS.)

Store at controlled room temperature 15-30°C (59-86°F).

PATIENT INFORMATION:

Metoprolol succinate is used to treat high blood pressure alone or in combination with other medications. This medication can also be used to treat a heart condition called angina. This particular formulation is an extended release product, meaning it can be taken once a day. This medication should be taken as directed, with a meal or right after a meal. The tablets should not be broken or crushed. Do not take a double dose if a dose is missed. This medication should not be stopped abruptly; it should be discontinued slowly over time. If you are taking this medication for high blood pressure, make sure to have your blood pressure checked regularly. If you ever have trouble breathing, call your physician immediately. The most common adverse effects are dizziness and tiredness. It is important to inform all your healthcare providers that you are taking this medication, especially before any surgeries or procedures.

HOW SUPPLIED - EQUIVALENTS NOT AVAILABLE:

Tablet, Coated, Sustained Action - Oral - 50 mg

100's $44.63 TOPROL XL, Astra USA 00186-1090-05

Tablet, Coated, Sustained Action - Oral - 100 mg

100's $67.07 TOPROL XL, Astra USA 00186-1092-05

Tablet, Coated, Sustained Action - Oral - 200 mg

100's $134.14 TOPROL XL, Astra USA 00186-1094-05

METOPROLOL TARTRATE *(001801)*

CATEGORIES: Angina; Antihypertensives; Antianginals; Beta Adrenergic Blocking Agents; Beta Blockers; Cardiovascular Drugs; Hypertension; Myocardial Infarction; Pregnancy Category C; Sales > $500 Million; FDA Approval Pre 1982; Patent Expiration 1993 Dec; Top 200 Drugs

BRAND NAMES: *Apo-Metoprolol* (Canada); *Beloc* (Germany); *Beloc Duriles*; *Beloc Zok*; *Betaloc* (Australia, England, Canada, Japan); *Betaloc CR*; *Betaloc Zok*; *Betalor*; *Betazok*; *Bloxan*; *Cardeloc*; *Cardinol*; *Cardiosel*; *Cardoxone*; *Denex*; *Kenaprol* (Mexico); *Lofarbil*; *Lopresor* (Australia, Germany, England, Canada, Mexico, Japan); *Lopresor Oros*; *Lopresor Retard*; *Lopresor SR* (England); **Lopressor**; *Metolar*; *Metolol*; *Metopress Retard*; *Minax* (Australia); *Mycol*; *Mycol CR*; *Neobloc*; *Prolaken* (Mexico); *Ritmolol* (Mexico); *Selokeen*; *Seloken* (France, Japan, Mexico); *Seloken Retard*; *Seloken Zoc* (Mexico); *Selopral*; *Seloxen*; *Selozok*; *Selo-zok*
(International brand names outside U.S. in italics)

FORMULARIES: Aetna; BC-BS; CIGNA; FHP; Humana; Kaiser; Medco; Medi-Cal; PCS; PruCare; United

COST OF THERAPY: $43.25 (Hypertension; Tablet; 100 mg; 1/day; 365 days)

PRIMARY ICD9: 401.1 (Essential Hypertension, Benign)

DESCRIPTION:

Metoprolol tartrate, is a selective beta$_1$-adrenoreceptor blocking agent, available as 50 - and 100 - mg tablets for oral administration and in 5-ml ampuls for intravenous administration. Each ampul contains a sterile solution of metoprolol tartrate USP, 5 mg and sodium chloride USP, 45 mg. Metoprolol tartrate is (±)-1-(isopropylamino)-3-(*p*-(2-(methoxyethyl) phenoxy)-2-propanol (2:1) *dextro*-tartrate salt.

Metoprolol tartrate is a white, practically odorless, crystalline powder with a molecular weight of 684.82. It is very soluble in water; freely soluble in methylene chloride, in chloroform, and in alcohol; slightly soluble in acetone; and insoluble in ether.

Lopressor Inactive Ingredients: Tablets contain cellulose compounds, colloidal silicon dioxide, D&C Red No. 30 aluminum lake (50-mg tablets), FD&C Blue No. 2 aluminum lake (100-mg tablets), lactose, magnesium stearate, polyethylene glycol, propylene glycol, povidone, sodium starch glycolate, talc, and titanium dioxide.

CLINICAL PHARMACOLOGY:

Metoprolol tartrate is a beta-adrenergic receptor blocking agent. *In vitro* and *in vivo* animal studies have shown that it has a preferential effect on beta$_1$adrenoreceptors, chiefly located in cardiac muscle. This preferential effect is not absolute, however, and at higher doses, metoprolol tartrate also inhibits beta$_2$, adrenoreceptors, chiefly located in the bronchial and vascular musculature.

Clinic pharmacology studies have confirmed the beta-blocking activity of metoprolol in man, as shown by (1) reduction in heart rate and cardiac output at rest and upon exercise, (2) reduction of systolic blood pressure upon exercise, (3) inhibition of isoproterenol-induced tachycardia, and (4) reduction of reflex orthostatic tachycardia.

Relative beta$_1$, selectivity has been confirmed by the following : (1) In normal subjects, metoprolol tartrate is unable to reverse the beta$_2$-mediated vasodilating effects of epinephrine. This contrasts with the effect of nonselective (beta$_1$, plus beta$_2$) beta blockers, which completely reverse the vasodilating effects of epinephrine. (2) In asthmatic patients, metoprolol tartrate reduces FEV_1 and FVC significantly less than a nonselective beta blocker, propranolol, at equivalent beta$_1$-receptor blocking doses.

Metoprolol tartrate has no intrinsic sympathomimetic activity, and membrane-stabilizing activity is detectable only at doses much greater than required for beta blockade. Metoprolol tartrate crosses the blood-brain barrier and has been reported in the CSF in a concentration 78% of the simultaneous plasma concentration. Animal and human experiments indicate that metoprolol tartrate slows the sinus rate and decreases AV nodal conduction.

In controlled clinical studies, metoprolol tartrate has been shown to be an effective antihypertensive agent when used alone or as concomitant therapy with thiazide-type diuretics, at dosages of 100-450 mg daily. In controlled, comparative, clinical studies, metoprolol tartrate has been shown to be as effective an antihypertensive agent as propranolol, methyldopa, and thiazide-type diuretics, and to be equally effective in supine and standing positions.

The mechanism of the antihypertensive effects of beta-blocking agents has not been elucidated. However, several possible mechanisms have been proposed: (1) competitive antagonism of catecholamines at peripheral (especially cardiac) adrenergic neuron sites, leading to decreased cardiac output; (2) a central effect leading to reduced sympathetic outflow to the periphery; and (3) suppression of renin activity.

CLINICAL PHARMACOLOGY: *(cont'd)*

By blocking catecholamine-induced increases in heart rate, in velocity and extent of myocardial contraction, and in blood pressure, metoprolol tartrate reduces the oxygen requirements of the heart at any given level of effort, thus making it useful in the long-term management of angina pectoris. However, in patients with heart failure, beta-adrenergic blockade may increase oxygen requirements by increasing left ventricular fiber length and end-diastolic pressure.

Although beta-adrenergic receptor blockage is useful in the treatment of angina and hypertension, there are situations in which sympathetic stimulation is vital. In patients with severely damaged hearts, adequate ventricular function may depend on sympathetic drive. In the presence of AV block, beta blockade may prevent the necessary facilitating effect of sympathetic activity on conduction. Beta$_2$-adrenergic blockade results in passive bronchial constriction by interfering with endogenous adrenergic blockade results in passive bronchial constriction by interfering with endogenous adrenergic bronchodilator activity in patients subject to bronchospasm and may also interfere with exogenous bronchodilators in such patients.

In controlled clinical trials, metoprolol tartrate, administered two or four times daily, has been shown to be an effective antianginal agent, reducing the number of angina attacks and increasing exercise tolerance. The dosage used in these studies ranged from 100 to 400 mg daily. A controlled, comparative, clinical trial showed that metoprolol tartrate was indistinguishable from propranolol in the treatment of angina pectoris.

In a large (1,395 patients randomized), double-blind, placebo-controlled clinical study, metoprolol tartrate was shown to reduce 3-month mortality by 36% in patients with suspected or definite myocardial infarction.

Patients were randomized and treated as soon as possible after their arrival in the hospital, once their clinical condition had stabilized and their hemodynamic status had been carefully evaluated. Subjects were ineligible if they had hypotension, bradycardia, peripheral signs of shock and/or more than minimal basal rates as signs of congestive heart failure. Initial treatment consisted of intravenous followed by oral administration of metoprolol tartrate or placebo, given in a coronary care or comparable unit. Oral maintenance therapy with metoprolol tartrate or placebo was then continued for 3 months. After this double-blind period, all patients were given metoprolol tartrate and followed up to 1 year.

The median delay from the onset of symptoms to the initiation of therapy was 8 hours in both the metoprolol tartrate and placebo treatment groups. Among patients treated with metoprolol tartrate, there were comparable reductions in 3-month mortality for those treated early (≤8 hours) and those in whom treatment was started later. Significant reductions in the incidence of ventricular fibrillation and in chest paid following initial intravenous therapy were also observed with metoprolol tartrate and were independent of the interval between onset of symptoms and initiation of therapy.

The precise mechanism of action of metoprolol tartrate in patients with suspected or definite myocardial infarction is not known.

In this study, patients treated with metoprolol received the drug both very early (intravenously) and during a subsequent 3-month period, while placebo patients received no beta-blocker treatment for this period. The study thus was able to show a benefit from the overall metoprolol regimen but cannot separate the benefit of very early intravenous treatment from the benefit of later beta-blocker therapy. Nonetheless, because the overall regimen showed a clear beneficial effect on survival without evidence of an early adverse effect on survival, one acceptable dosage regimen is the precise regimen used in the trial. Because the specific benefit of very early treatment remains to be defined however, it is also reasonable to administer the drug orally to patients at a later time as is recommended for certain other beta blockers.

PHARMACOKINETICS

In man, absorption of metoprolol tartrate is rapid and complete. Plasma levels following oral administration, however, approximate 50% of levels following intravenous administration, indicating about 50% first-pass metabolism.

Plasma levels achieved are highly variable after oral administration. Only a small fraction of the drug (about 12%) is bound to human serum albumin. Elimination is mainly by biotransformation in the liver, and the plasma half-life ranges from approximately 3 to 7 hours. Less than 5% of an oral dose of metoprolol tartrate is recovered unchanged in the urine; the rest is excreted by the kidneys as metabolites that appear to have no clinical significance. The systemic availability and half-life of metoprolol tartrate in patients with renal failure do not differ to a clinically significant degree from those in normal subjects. Consequently, no reduction in dosage is usually needed in patients with chronic renal failure.

Significant beta-blocking effect (as measured by reduction of exercise heart rate) occurs within 1 hour after oral administration, and its duration is dose-related. For example, a 50% reduction of the maximum registered effect after single oral doses of 20, 50, and 100 mg occurred at 3.3, 5.0, and 6.4 hours, respectively, in normal subjects. After repeated oral dosages of 100 mg twice daily, a significant reduction in exercise systolic blood pressure was evident at 12 hours.

Following intravenous administration of metoprolol tartrate, the urinary recovery of unchanged drug is approximately 10%. When the drug was infused over a 10-minute period, in normal volunteers, maximum beta blockade was achieved at approximately 20 minutes. Doses of 5 mg and 15 mg yielded a maximal reduction in exercise-induced heart rate of approximately 10% and 15%, respectively. The effect on exercise heart rate decreased linearly with time at the same rate for both doses, and disappeared at approximately 5 hours and 8 hours for the 5-mg and 15-mg doses, respectively.

Equivalent maximal beta-blocking effect is achieved with oral and intravenous doses in the ratio of approximately 2.5:1.

There is a linear relationship between the log of plasma levels and reduction of exercise heart rate. However, antihypertensive activity does not appear to be related to plasma levels. Because of variable plasma levels attained with a given dose and lack of a consistent relationship of antihypertensive activity to dose, selection of proper dosage requires individual titration.

In several studies of patients with acute myocardial infarction, intravenous followed by oral administration of metoprolol tartrate caused a reduction in heart rate, systolic blood pressure, and cardiac output. Stroke volume, diastolic blood pressure, and pulmonary artery end diastolic pressure remained unchanged.

In patients with angina pectoris, plasma concentration measured at 1 hour is linearly related to the oral dose within the range of 50 to 400 mg. Exercise heart rate and systolic blood pressure are reduced in relation to the logarithm of the oral dose of metoprolol. The increase in exercise capacity and the reduction in left ventricular ischemia are also significantly related to the logarithm of the oral dose.

INDICATIONS AND USAGE:

HYPERTENSION

Metoprolol tartrate tablets are indicated for the treatment of hypertension. They may be used alone or in combination with other antihypertensive agents.

ANGINA PECTORIS

Metoprolol tartrate is indicated in the long-term treatment of angina pectoris.

INDICATIONS AND USAGE: *(cont'd)*

MYOCARDIAL INFARCTION

Metoprolol tartrate ampuls and tablets are indicated in the treatment of hemodynamically stable patients with definite or suspected acute myocardial infarction to reduce cardiovascular mortality. Treatment with intravenous metoprolol tartrate can be initiated as soon as the patient's clinical condition allows (see DOSAGE AND ADMINISTRATION, CONTRAINDICATIONS, and WARNINGS). Alternatively, treatment can begin within 3 to 10 days of the acute event (see DOSAGE AND ADMINISTRATION).

CONTRAINDICATIONS:

HYPERTENSION AND ANGINA

Metoprolol tartrate is contraindicated in sinus bradycardia, heart block greater than first degree, cardiogenic shock, and overt cardiac failure (see WARNINGS).

MYOCARDIAL INFARCTION

Metoprolol tartrate is contraindicated in patients with a heart rate $<$ 45 beats/min; second- and third-degree heart block; significant first-degree heart block (P.R. interval $\geq$ 0.24 sec); systolic blood pressure $<$ 100 mmhg; or moderate-to -severe cardiac failure (see WARNINGS).

WARNINGS:

HYPERTENSION AND ANGINA

Cardiac Failure : Sympathetic stimulation is a vital component supporting circulatory function in congestive heart failure, and beta blockade carries the potential hazard of further depressing myocardial contractility and precipitating more severe failure. In hypertensive and angina patients who have congestive heart failure controlled by digitalis and diuretics, metoprolol tartrate should be administered cautiously. Both digitalis and metoprolol tartrate slow AV conduction.

In Patients Without a History of Cardiac Failure: Continued depression of the myocardium with beta-blocking agents over a period of time can, in some cases, lead to cardiac failure. At the first sign or symptom of impending cardiac failure, patients should be fully digitalized and/or given a diuretic. The response should be observed closely. If cardiac failure continues, despite adequate digitalization and diuretic therapy, metoprolol tartrate should be withdrawn.

Ischemic Heart Disease: Following abrupt cessation of therapy with certain beta-blocking agents, exacerbations of angina pectoris and, in some cases, myocardial infarction have occurred. When discontinuing chronically administered metoprolol tartrate, particularly in patients with ischemic heart disease, the dosage should be gradually reduced over a period of 1-2 weeks and the patient should be carefully monitored. If angina markedly worsens or acute coronary insufficiency develops, metoprolol tartrate administration should be reinstated promptly, at least temporarily, and other measures appropriate for the management of unstable angina should be taken. Patients should be warned against interruption or discontinuation of therapy without the physician's advice. Because coronary artery disease is common and may be unrecognized, it may be prudent not to discontinue metoprolol tartrate therapy abruptly even in patients treated only for hypertension.

Bronchospastic Diseases: PATIENTS WITH BRONCHOSPASTIC DISEASES SHOULD, IN GENERAL, NOT RECEIVE BETA BLOCKERS. **Because of its relative $beta_1$ selectivity, however, metoprolol tartrate may be used with caution in patients with bronchospastic disease who do not respond to, or cannot tolerate, other antihypertensive treatment. Since $beta_1$selectivity is not absolute, a $beta_2$-stimulating agent should be administered concomitantly, and the lowest possible dose of metoprolol tartrate should be used. In these circumstances it would be prudent initially to administer metoprolol tartrate in smaller doses three times daily, instead of larger doses two times daily, to avoid the higher plasma levels associated with the longer dosing interval.** (See DOSAGE AND ADMINISTRATION.)

Major Surgery: The necessity or desirability of withdrawing beta-blocking therapy prior to major surgery is controversial; the impaired ability of the heart to respond to reflex adrenergic stimuli may augment the risks of general anesthesia and surgical procedures.

Metoprolol tartrate, like other beta blockers, is a competitive inhibitor of beta-receptor agonists, and its effects can be reversed by administration of such agents, e.g. dobutamine or isoproterenol. However, such patients may be subject to protracted severe hypotension. Difficulty in restarting and maintaining the heart beat has also been reported with beta blockers.

Diabetes and Hypoglycemia: Metoprolol tartrate should be used with caution in diabetic patients if a beta-blocking agent is required. Beta blockers may mask tachycardia occurring with hypoglycemia, but other manifestations such as dizziness and sweating may not be significantly affected.

Thyrotoxicosis: Beta-adrenergic blockade may mask certain clinical signs (*e.g.*, tachycardia) of hyperthyroidism. Patients suspected of developing thyrotoxicosis should be managed carefully to avoid abrupt withdrawal of beta blockade, which might precipitate a thyroid storm.

MYOCARDIAL INFARCTION

Cardiac Failure: Sympathetic stimulation is a vital component supporting circulatory function, and beta blockade carries the potential hazard of depressing myocardial contractility and precipitating or exacerbating minimal cardiac failure.

During treatment with metoprolol tartrate, the hemodynamic status of the patient should be carefully monitored. If heart failure occurs or persists despite appropriate treatment, metoprolol tartrate should be discontinued.

Bradycardia: Metoprolol tartrate produces a decrease in sinus heart rate in most patients; this decrease is greatest among patients with high initial heart rates and least among patients with low initial heart rates. Acute myocardial infarction (particularly inferior infarction) may in itself produce significant lowering of the sinus rate. If the sinus rate decreases to $<$ 40 beats/min, particularly if associated with evidence of lowered cardiac output, atropine (0.25-0.5 mg) should be administered intravenously. If treatment with atropine is not successful, metoprolol tartrate should be discontinued, and cautious administration of isoproterenol or installation of a cardiac pacemaker should be considered.

AV Block: Metoprolol tartrate slows AV conduction and may produce significant first -(P.R interval $\geq$ 0.26 sec), second-, or third-degree heart block. Acute myocardial infarction also produces heart block.

If heart block occurs, metoprolol tartrate should be discontinued and atropine (0.25-0.5 mg) should be administered intravenously. If treatment with atropine is not successful, cautious administration of isoproterenol or installation of a cardiac pacemaker should be considered.

Hypotension: If hypotension (systolic blood pressure $\leq$ 90 mmHg) occurs, metoprolol tartrate should be discontinued, and the hemodynamic status of the patient and the extent of myocardial damage carefully assessed. Invasive monitoring of central venous, pulmonary capillary wedge, and arterial pressures may be required. Appropriate therapy with fluids, positive inotropic agents, balloon counterpulsation, or other treatment modalities should be instituted. If hypotension is associated with sinus bradycardia or AV block, treatment should be directed at reversing these (see above).

WARNINGS: *(cont'd)*

Bronchospastic Disease: PATIENTS WITH BRONCHOSPASTIC DISEASES SHOULD, IN GENERAL, NOT RECEIVE BETA BLOCKERS. Because of its relative $beta_1$ selectivity, metoprolol tartrate may be used with extreme caution in patients with bronchospastic disease. Because it is unknown to what extent $beta_2$ -stimulating agents may exacerbate myocardial ischemia and the extent of infarction, these agents should *not* be used prophylactically. If bronchospasm not related to congestive heart failure occurs, metoprolol tartrate should be discontinued. A theophylline derivative or a $beta_2$agonist may be administered cautiously, depending on the clinical condition of the patient. Both theophylline derivatives and $beta_2$agonists may produce serious cardiac arrhythmias.

PRECAUTIONS:

General: Metoprolol tartrate should be used with caution in patients with impaired hepatic function.

Information for the Patient: Patients should be advised to take metoprolol tartrate regularly and continuously, as directed, with or immediately following meals. If a dose should be missed, the patient should take only the next scheduled dose (without doubling it). Patients should not discontinue metoprolol tartrate without consulting the physician.

Patients should be advised (1) to avoid operating automobiles and machinery or engaging in other tasks requiring alertness until the patient's response to therapy with metoprolol tartrate has been determined; (2) to contact the physician if any difficulty in breathing occurs; (3) to inform the physician or dentist before any type of surgery that he or she is taking metoprolol tartrate.

Laboratory Tests: Clinical laboratory findings may include elevated levels of serum transaminase, alkaline phosphatase, and lactate dehydrogenase.

Carcinogenesis, Mutagenesis, and Impairment of Fertility: Long-term studies in animals have been conducted to evaluate carcinogenic potential. In a 2-year study in rats at three oral dosage levels of up to 800 mg/kg per day, there was no increase in the development of spontaneously occurring benign or malignant neoplasms of any type. The only histologic changes that appeared to be drug related were an increased incidence of generally mild local accumulation of foamy macrophages in pulmonary alveoli and slight increase in biliary hyperplasia. In a 21-month study in Swiss albino mice at three oral dosage levels of up to 750 mg/kg per day, benign lung tumors (small adenomas) occurred more frequently in female mice receiving the highest dose than in untreated control animals. There was no increase in malignant or total (benign plus malignant) lung tumors, nor in the overall incidence of tumors or malignant tumors. This 21-month study was repeated in CD-1 mice, and no statistically or biologically significant differences were observed between treated and control mice of either sex for any type of tumor.

All mutagenicity tests performed (a dominant lethal study in mice, chromosome studies in somatic cells, a Salmonella/mammalian-microsome mutagenicity test, and a nucleus anomaly test in somatic interphase nuclei) were negative.

No evidence of impaired fertility due to metoprolol tartrate was observed in a study performed in rats at doses up to 55.5 times the maximum daily human dose of 450 mg.

Pregnancy Category C: Metoprolol tartrate has been shown to increase postimplantation loss and decrease neonatal survival in rats at doses up to 55.5 times the maximum daily human dose of 450 mg. Distribution studies in mice confirm exposure of the fetus when metoprolol tartrate is administered to the pregnant animal. These studies have revealed no evidence of impaired fertility or teratogenicity. There are no adequate and well-controlled studies in pregnant women. Because animal reproduction studies are not always predictive of human response, this drug should be used during pregnancy only if clearly needed.

Nursing Mothers: Metoprolol tartrate is excreted in breast milk in very small quantity. An infant consuming 1 liter of breast milk daily would receive a dose of less than 1 mg of the drug. Caution should be exercised when metoprolol tartrate is administered to a nursing woman.

Pediatric Use: Safety and effectiveness in children have not been established.

DRUG INTERACTIONS:

Catecholamine-depleting drugs (*e.g.,* reserpine) may have an additive effect when given with beta-blocking agents. Patients treated with metoprolol tartrate plus a catecholamine depletor should therefore be closely observed for evidence of hypotension or marked bradycardia, which may produce vertigo, syncope, or postural hypotension.

Risk of Anaphylactic Reaction . While taking beta-blockers, patients with a history of severe anaphylactic reaction to a variety of allergens may be more reactive to repeated challenge, either accidental, diagnostic, or therapeutic. Such patients may be unresponsive to the usual doses of epinephrine used to treat allergic reaction.

ADVERSE REACTIONS:

HYPERTENSION AND ANGINA

Most adverse effects have been mild and transient.

Central Nervous System: Tiredness and dizziness have occurred in about 10 of 100 patients. Depression has been reported in about 5 of 100 patients. Mental confusion and short-term memory loss have been reported. Headache, nightmares, and insomnia have also been reported.

Cardiovascular: Shortness of breath and bradycardia have occurred in approximately 3 of 100 patients. Cold extremities; arterial insufficiency, usually of the Raynaud type; palpitations; congestive heart failure; peripheral edema; and hypotension have been reported in about 1 of 100 patients. (See CONTRAINDICATIONS, WARNINGS, and PRECAUTIONS.)

Respiratory: Wheezing (bronchospasm) and dyspnea have been reported in about 1 of 100 patients (see WARNINGS).

Gastrointestinal: Diarrhea has occurred in about 5 of 100 patients. Nausea, dry mouth, gastric pain, constipation, flatulence, and heartburn have been reported in about 1 of 100 patients.

Hypersensitive Reactions: Pruritus or rash have occurred in about 5 of 100 patients. Worsening of psoriasis has also been reported.

Miscellaneous: Peyronie's disease has been reported in fewer than 1 of 100,000 patients. Musculoskeletal pain, blurred vision, and tinnitus have also been reported.

There have been rare reports of reversible alopecia, agranulocytosis, and dry eyes. Discontinuation of the drug should be considered if any such reaction is not otherwise explicable.

The oculomucocutaneous syndrome associated with the beta blocker practolol has not been reported with metoprolol tartrate.

MYOCARDIAL INFARCTION

Central Nervous System: Tiredness has been reported in about 1 of 100 patients. Vertigo, sleep disturbances, hallucinations, headache, dizziness, visual disturbances, confusion, and reduced libido have also been reported, but a drug relationship is not clear.

ADVERSE REACTIONS: *(cont'd)*

Cardiovascular: In the randomized comparison of metoprolol tartrate and placebo described in CLINICAL PHARMACOLOGY, the following adverse reactions were reported (TABLE 1):

TABLE 1

	Lopressor	Placebo
Hypotension (Systolic BP <90 mmHg)	27.4%	23.2%
Bradycardia (heart rate <40 beats/min)	15.9%	6.7%
Second-or third-degree heart block	4.7%	4.7%
First-degree heart block (P.R. $\geq$ 0.26 sec)	5.3%	1.9%
Heart failure	27.5%	29.6%

Respiratory: Dyspnea of pulmonary origin has been reported in fewer than 1 of 100 patients.

Gastrointestinal: Nausea and abdominal pain have been reported, but a drug relationship is not clear.

Dermatologic: Rash and worsened psoriasis have been reported, but a drug relationship is not clear.

Miscellaneous: Unstable diabetes and claudication have been reported, but a drug relationship is not clear.

POTENTIAL ADVERSE REACTIONS

A variety of adverse reactions not listed above have been reported with other beta-adrenergic blocking agents and should be considered potential adverse reactions to metoprolol tartrate.

Central Nervous System: Reversible mental depression progressing to catatonia; an acute reversible syndrome characterized by disorientation for time and place, short-term memory loss, emotional lability, slightly clouded sensorium, and decreased performance on neuropsychometrics.

Cardiovascular: Intensification of AV block (see CONTRAINDICATIONS).

Hematologic: Agranulocytosis, nonthrombocytopenic purpura, thrombocytopenic purpura.

Hypersensitive Reactions: Fever combined with aching and sore throat, laryngospasm, and respiratory distress.

OVERDOSAGE:

ACUTE TOXICITY

Several cases of overdosage have been reported, some leading to death. Oral LD_{50}'s (mg/kg): mice, 1158-2460; rats, 3090-4670.

SIGNS AND SYMPTOMS

Potential signs and symptoms associated with overdosage with metoprolol tartrate are bradycardia, hypotension, bronchospasm, and cardiac failure.

TREATMENT

There is no specific antidote.

In general, patients with acute or recent myocardial infarction may be more hemodynamically unstable than other patients and should be treated accordingly (see WARNINGS, Myocardial Infarction).

On the basis of the pharmacologic actions of metoprolol tartrate, the following general measures should be employed:

Elimination of the Drug: Gastric lavage should be performed.

Bradycardia: Atropine should be administered. If there is no response to vagal blockade, isoproterenol should be administered cautiously.

Hypotension: A vasopressor should be administered, e.g. levarterenol or dopamine.

Bronchospasm: A $beta_2$ -stimulating agent and/or a theophylline derivative should be administered.

Cardiac Failure: A digitalis glycoside and diuretic should be administered in shock resulting from inadequate cardiac contractility, administration of dobutamine, isoproterenol, or glucagon may be considered.

DOSAGE AND ADMINISTRATION:

HYPERTENSION

The dosage of metoprolol tartrate should be individualized. Metoprolol tartrate should be taken with or immediately following meals.

The usual initial dosage is 100 mg daily in single or divided doses, whether used alone or added to diuretic. The dosage may be increased at weekly (or longer) intervals until optimum blood pressure reduction is achieved. In general, the maximum effect of any given dosage level will be apparent after 1 week of therapy. The effective dosage range is 100 to 450 mg per day. Dosages above 450 mg per day have not been studied. While once-daily dosing is effective and can maintain a reduction in blood pressure throughout the day, lower doses (especially 100 mg) may not maintain a full effect at the end of the 24-hour period, and larger or more frequent daily doses may be required. This can be evaluated by measuring blood pressure near the end of the dosing interval to determine whether satisfactory control is being maintained throughout the day. $Beta_1$ selectivity diminishes as the dose of metoprolol tartrate is increased.

ANGINA PECTORIS

The dosage of metoprolol tartrate should be individualized. Metoprolol tartrate should be taken with or immediately following meals.

The usual initial dosage is 100 mg daily, given in two divided doses. The dosage may be gradually increased at weekly intervals until optimum clinical response has been obtained or there is pronounced slowing of the heart rate. The effective dosage range is 100 to 400 mg per day. Dosages above 400 mg per day have not been studied. If treatment is to be discontinued, the dosage should be reduced gradually over a period of 1-2 weeks. (See WARNINGS.)

Myocardial Infarction

Early Treatment: During the early phase of definite or suspected acute myocardial infarction, treatment with metoprolol tartrate can be initiated as soon as possible after the patient's arrival in the hospital. Such treatment should be initiated in a coronary care or similar unit immediately after the patient's hemodynamic condition has stabilized.

Treatment in this early phase should begin with the intravenous administration of three bolus injections of 5 mg of metoprolol tartrate each; the injections should be given at approximately 2-minute intervals. During the intravenous administration of metoprolol tartrate, blood pressure, heart rate, and electrocardiogram should be carefully monitored.

In patients who tolerate the full intravenous dose (15 mg), metoprolol tartrate tablets, 50 mg every 6 hours, should be initiated 15 minutes after the last intravenous dose and continued for 48 hours. Thereafter, patients should receive a maintenance dosage of 100 mg twice daily (see Late Treatment).

DOSAGE AND ADMINISTRATION: *(cont'd)*

Patients who appear not to tolerate the full intravenous dose should be started on metoprolol tartrate tablets either 25 mg or 50 mg every 6 hours (depending on the degree of intolerance) 15 minutes after the last intravenous dose or as soon as their clinical condition allows. In patients with severe intolerance, treatment with metoprolol tartrate should be discontinued (see WARNINGS).

Late Treatment: Patients with contraindications to treatment during the early phase of suspected or definite myocardial infarction, patients who appear not to tolerate the full early treatment, and patients in whom the physician wishes to delay therapy for any other reason should be started on metoprolol tartrate tablets, 100 mg twice daily, as soon as their clinical condition allows. Therapy should be continued for at least 3 months. Although the efficacy of metoprolol tartrate beyond 3 months has not been conclusively established, data from studies with other beta blockers suggest that treatment should be continued for 1-3 years.

Note: Parenteral drug products should be inspected visually for particulate matter and discoloration prior to administration, whenever solution and container permit.

Store between 59-86° F (15-30° C). Protect from moisture.

Dispense in tight, light-resistance container (USP).

PATIENT INFORMATION:

Metoprolol is a beta blocker used to treat high blood pressure, angina (chest pain), and decreases the risk of having a repeat heart attack. This medication should be taken even if you feel fine because high blood pressure may not produce physical symptoms. Do not discontinue this medication suddenly without consulting with your physician. Inform your physician if you are pregnant or nursing. Metoprolol should be taken at the same time each day and may be taken with or without food. This medication may cause dizziness, drowsiness, or blurred vision; use caution while driving or operating hazardous machinery. Do not take other medications which may contain alpha-adrenergic stimulants (nasal decongestants, over-the-counter cold preparations) without consulting your physician or pharmacist. Notify your physician if you experience difficulty breathing, slow pulse rate, or swelling of legs or ankles. Metoprolol may alter blood sugar levels or cover up symptoms of very low blood sugar (hypoglycemia) in patients with diabetes.

HOW SUPPLIED - RATED THERAPEUTICALLY EQUIVALENT:

Injection, Solution - Intravenous - 5mg/5ml

3's	**$66.53**	**LOPRESSOR AMPUL 5, Novartis**	**00028-4201-33**
5 ml x 3	$14.67	Metoprolol Tartrate, Schein Pharm (US)	00364-3036-25
5 ml x 12	$54.99	Metoprolol Tartrate, Geneva Pharms	00781-3070-75

Tablet, Coated - Oral - 50 mg

100's	$8.25	Metoprolol Tartrate, H.C.F.A. F F P	99999-1801-01
100's	$10.73	Metoprolol Tartrate, United Res	00677-1482-01
100's	$10.73	Metoprolol Tartrate, Geneva Pharms	00781-1223-01
100's	$41.75	Metoprolol Tartrate, Novopharm (US)	55953-0727-40
100's	$43.00	Metoprolol Tartrate, Goldline Labs	00182-1966-01
100's	$43.00	Metoprolol Tartrate, Goldline Labs	00182-1987-01
100's	$43.50	Metoprolol Tartrate, Major Pharms	00904-7772-60
100's	$43.50	Metoprolol Tartrate, Major Pharms	00904-7820-60
100's	$43.50	Metoprolol Tartrate, Major Pharms	00904-7946-60
100's	$43.53	Metoprolol Tartrate, Apothecon	59772-3692-02
100's	$44.24	Metoprolol Tartrate, Watson Labs	52544-0462-01
100's	$44.51	Metoprolol Tartrate, Qualitest Pharms	00603-4627-21
100's	$45.20	Metoprolol Tartrate, Schein Pharm (US)	00364-2560-01
100's	$45.35	Metoprolol Tartrate, Purepac Pharm	00228-2554-10
100's	$45.35	Metoprolol Tartrate, Mova Pharms	55370-0820-07
100's	$45.90	Metoprolol Tartrate, Mutual Pharm	53489-0366-01
100's	$45.94	Metoprolol Tartrate, Rugby	00536-5604-01
100's	$46.15	Metoprolol Tartrate, Teva	00093-0733-01
100's	$46.80	Metoprolol Tartrate, Geneva Pharms	50752-0308-05
100's	$47.00	Metoprolol Tartrate, Sidmak Labs	50111-0855-01
100's	$47.23	Metoprolol Tartrate, Aligen Independ	00405-5673-01
100's	$47.91	Metoprolol Tartrate, HL Moore Drug Exch	00839-7809-06
100's	$47.91	Metoprolol Tartrate, HL Moore Drug Exch	00839-7841-06
100's	$48.60	Metoprolol Tartrate, Par Pharm	49884-0412-01
100's	$49.00	Metoprolol Tartrate, Vangard Labs	00615-3552-13
100's	$51.15	Metoprolol Tartrate, Geneva Pharms	00781-1371-01
100's	**$52.05**	**LOPRESSOR, Novartis**	**00028-0051-01**
100's	$52.95	Metoprolol Tartrate, Mylan	00378-0032-01
100's	$55.56	Metoprolol Tartrate, Geneva Pharms	00781-1371-13
100's	**$56.54**	**LOPRESSOR, Novartis**	**00028-0051-61**
100's UD	$49.39	Metoprolol Tartrate, Major Pharms	00904-7772-61
500's	$41.25	Metoprolol Tartrate, H.C.F.A. F F P	99999-1801-02
500's	$206.65	Metoprolol Tartrate, Novopharm (US)	55953-0727-70
500's	$226.75	Metoprolol Tartrate, Purepac Pharm	00228-2554-50
500's	$251.55	Metoprolol Tartrate, Mova Pharms	55370-0820-08
1000's	$82.50	Metoprolol Tartrate, H.C.F.A. F F P	99999-1801-03
1000's	$107.30	Metoprolol Tartrate, United Res	00677-1482-10
1000's	$107.30	Metoprolol Tartrate, Geneva Pharms	00781-1223-10
1000's	$413.50	Metoprolol Tartrate, Novopharm (US)	55953-0727-80
1000's	$425.90	Metoprolol Tartrate, Goldline Labs	00182-1987-10
1000's	$429.09	Metoprolol Tartrate, Geneva Pharms	50752-0308-09
1000's	$430.70	Metoprolol Tartrate, Major Pharms	00904-7772-80
1000's	$430.70	Metoprolol Tartrate, Major Pharms	00904-7820-80
1000's	$430.70	Metoprolol Tartrate, Major Pharms	00904-7946-80
1000's	$430.73	Metoprolol Tartrate, Apothecon	59772-3692-05
1000's	$437.83	Metoprolol Tartrate, Watson Labs	52544-0462-10
1000's	$441.50	Metoprolol Tartrate, Goldline Labs	00182-1966-10
1000's	$441.50	Metoprolol Tartrate, Rugby	00536-5604-10
1000's	$445.99	Metoprolol Tartrate, Purepac Pharm	00228-2554-96
1000's	$447.26	Metoprolol Tartrate, Schein Pharm (US)	00364-2560-02
1000's	$448.11	Metoprolol Tartrate, Qualitest Pharms	00603-4627-32
1000's	$454.65	Metoprolol Tartrate, Mutual Pharm	53489-0366-10
1000's	$455.10	Metoprolol Tartrate, Teva	00093-0733-10
1000's	$458.00	Metoprolol Tartrate, Sidmak Labs	50111-0855-03
1000's	$458.00	Metoprolol Tartrate, Sidmak Labs	50111-0855-06
1000's	$458.32	Metoprolol Tartrate, Aligen Independ	00405-5673-03
1000's	$459.80	Metoprolol Tartrate, Par Pharm	49884-0412-10
1000's	$460.62	Metoprolol Tartrate, HL Moore Drug Exch	00839-7809-16
1000's	$460.62	Metoprolol Tartrate, HL Moore Drug Exch	00839-7841-16
1000's	$486.50	Metoprolol Tartrate, Geneva Pharms	00781-1371-10
1000's	$486.73	Metoprolol Tartrate, Mylan	00378-0032-10
1000's	**$515.09**	**LOPRESSOR, Novartis**	**00028-0051-10**
1200's	**$626.83**	**LOPRESSOR, Novartis**	**00028-0051-65**

Tablet, Coated - Oral - 100 mg

60's	$7.11	Metoprolol Tartrate, H.C.F.A. F F P	99999-1801-06
100's	$11.85	Metoprolol Tartrate, H.C.F.A. F F P	99999-1801-04
100's	$15.75	Metoprolol Tartrate, United Res	00677-1483-01
100's	$15.75	Metoprolol Tartrate, Geneva Pharms	00781-1228-01
100's	$62.75	Metoprolol Tartrate, Novopharm (US)	55953-0734-40
100's	$64.60	Metoprolol Tartrate, Goldline Labs	00182-1967-01

HOW SUPPLIED - RATED THERAPEUTICALLY EQUIVALENT: *(cont'd)*

100's	$64.60	Metoprolol Tartrate, Goldline Labs	00182-1988-01
100's	$65.40	Metoprolol Tartrate, Major Pharms	00904-7773-60
100's	$65.40	Metoprolol Tartrate, Major Pharms	00904-7821-60
100's	$65.40	Metoprolol Tartrate, Major Pharms	00904-7947-60
100's	$65.40	Metoprolol Tartrate, Apothecon	59772-3693-02
100's	$65.41	Metoprolol Tartrate, HL Moore Drug Exch	00839-7810-06
100's	$65.41	Metoprolol Tartrate, HL Moore Drug Exch	00839-7842-06
100's	$66.48	Metoprolol Tartrate, Watson Labs	52544-0463-01
100's	$67.41	Metoprolol Tartrate, Purepac Pharm	00228-2555-10
100's	$67.41	Metoprolol Tartrate, Mova Pharms	55370-0821-07
100's	$67.86	Metoprolol Tartrate, Qualitest Pharms	00603-4628-21
100's	$67.91	Metoprolol Tartrate, Schein Pharm (US)	00364-2561-01
100's	$69.00	Metoprolol Tartrate, Mutual Pharm	53489-0367-01
100's	$69.04	Metoprolol Tartrate, Rugby	00536-5605-01
100's	$69.75	Metoprolol Tartrate, Teva	00093-0734-01
100's	$70.13	Metoprolol Tartrate, Vangard Labs	00615-3553-13
100's	$70.30	Metoprolol Tartrate, Geneva Pharms	50752-0309-05
100's	$70.50	Metoprolol Tartrate, Sidmak Labs	50111-0856-01
100's	$70.82	Metoprolol Tartrate, Aligen Independ	00405-4674-01
100's	$71.09	Metoprolol Tartrate, Par Pharm	49884-0413-01
100's	$71.68	Metoprolol Tartrate, Major Pharms	00904-7773-61
100's	$73.99	Metoprolol Tartrate, Geneva Pharms	00781-1372-01
100's	$76.50	Metoprolol Tartrate, Mylan	00378-0047-01
100's	**$78.21**	**LOPRESSOR, Novartis**	**00028-0071-01**
100's	$80.65	Metoprolol Tartrate, Geneva Pharms	00781-1372-13
100's	**$82.07**	**LOPRESSOR, Novartis**	**00028-0071-61**
500's	$59.25	Metoprolol Tartrate, H.C.F.A. F F P	99999-1801-05
500's	$310.60	Metoprolol Tartrate, Novopharm (US)	55953-0734-70
500's	$335.30	Metoprolol Tartrate, Purepac Pharm	00228-2555-50
500's	$335.40	Metoprolol Tartrate, Mova Pharms	55370-0821-08
720's	**$564.00**	**LOPRESSOR, Novartis**	**00028-0071-73**
1000's	$118.50	Metoprolol Tartrate, H.C.F.A. F F P	99999-1801-07
1000's	$157.50	Metoprolol Tartrate, United Res	00677-1483-10
1000's	$157.50	Metoprolol Tartrate, Geneva Pharms	00781-1228-10
1000's	$621.40	Metoprolol Tartrate, Novopharm (US)	55953-0734-80
1000's	$640.00	Metoprolol Tartrate, Goldline Labs	00182-1967-10
1000's	$640.00	Metoprolol Tartrate, Goldline Labs	00182-1988-10
1000's	$645.57	Metoprolol Tartrate, HL Moore Drug Exch	00839-7810-16
1000's	$645.57	Metoprolol Tartrate, HL Moore Drug Exch	00839-7842-16
1000's	$647.25	Metoprolol Tartrate, Major Pharms	00904-7773-80
1000's	$647.25	Metoprolol Tartrate, Major Pharms	00904-7821-80
1000's	$647.25	Metoprolol Tartrate, Major Pharms	00904-7947-80
1000's	$647.30	Metoprolol Tartrate, Apothecon	59772-3693-05
1000's	$657.95	Metoprolol Tartrate, Watson Labs	52544-0463-10
1000's	$663.48	Metoprolol Tartrate, Rugby	00536-5605-10
1000's	$663.55	Metoprolol Tartrate, Teva	00093-0734-10
1000's	$665.54	Metoprolol Tartrate, Purepac Pharm	00228-2555-96
1000's	$665.58	Metoprolol Tartrate, Par Pharm	49884-0413-10
1000's	$668.40	Metoprolol Tartrate, Qualitest Pharms	00603-4628-32
1000's	$672.12	Metoprolol Tartrate, Schein Pharm (US)	00364-2561-02
1000's	$683.20	Metoprolol Tartrate, Mutual Pharm	53489-0367-10
1000's	$688.00	Metoprolol Tartrate, Sidmak Labs	50111-0856-03
1000's	$688.35	Metoprolol Tartrate, Aligen Independ	00405-4674-03
1000's	$699.99	Metoprolol Tartrate, Geneva Pharms	00781-1372-10
1000's	$731.44	Metoprolol Tartrate, Mylan	00378-0047-10
1000's	**$774.06**	**LOPRESSOR, Novartis**	**00028-0071-10**
1200's	**$940.57**	**LOPRESSOR, Novartis**	**00028-0071-65**

METRIZAMIDE *(001802)*

CATEGORIES: Diagnostic Agents; Roentgenography; FDA Approval Pre 1982

BRAND NAMES: Amipaque

Prescribing information not available at time of publication.

HOW SUPPLIED - EQUIVALENTS NOT AVAILABLE:

Injection, Solution - Intravenous - 3.75 gm

1's	$76.56	AMIPAQUE, Nycomed	00407-0044-01

Injection, Solution - Intravenous - 6.75 gm

1's	$127.62	AMIPAQUE, Nycomed	00407-0046-01

METRONIDAZOLE *(001803)*

CATEGORIES: Abdominal Abscess; Amebiasis; Anti-Infectives; Anti-Inflammatory Agents; Antibacterials; Antibiotics; Antidiarrhea Agents; Antifungals; Antimicrobials; Antiparasitics; Antiprotozoals; Bacterial Vaginosis; Bone Infections; Central Nervous System Agents; Dermatologicals; Endocarditis; Endometritis; Gastrointestinal Drugs; Gynecologic Infections; H. Pylori; Hepatic Abscess; Infections; Intra-Abdominal Infections; Joint Infections; Liver Abscess; Local Infections; Lung Abscess; Meningitis; Orphan Drugs; Parasiticidal; Perioperative Prophylaxis; Peritonitis; Pneumonia; Protozoal Agents; Pulmonary Abscess; Respiratory Tract Infections; Rosacea; Septicemia; Sexually Transmitted Diseases; Skin Infections; Skin/Mucous Membrane Agents; Tetracyclines; Topical; Trichomonas; Trichomoniasis; Vaginosis; Peptic Ulcer*; Ulcer*; Pregnancy Category B; FDA Approval Pre 1982
* Indication not approved by the FDA

BRAND NAMES: *Acromona*; *Amibazol*; *Amiyodazol* (Mexico); *Anaerobex*; *Anerobia*; *Apo-Metronidazole* (Canada); *Arcazol*; *Arilin* (Germany); *Ariline*; *Asiazole*; *Asuzol* (Japan); *Camezol*; *Clont* (Germany); *Debetrol*; *Deflamon*; *Elyzol*; *Fladex*; *Flagenase* (Mexico); **Flagyl**; Flagyl 375; *Flasinyl*; *Fossyol* (Germany); *Frotin*; *Fulikan*; *Fuzuzin*; *Klion*; *Medai*; *Melis*; *Metarsal*; Metizol; Metro IV; Metrocream; Metrogel; *Metrogyl*; *Metrolag*; *Metrolex*; *Metronidazole IV* (Australia); *Metronidazol McKesson*; *Metroxyn*; *Metroxyn 500*; *Metrozin*; *Metrozine*; *Metrozole*; Metryl; *Nalox*; *Nida* (Japan); *Nitrozol*; *Norstene*; *Novazole*; *Novonidazole* (Canada); Protostat; *Rozagel* (France); *Rozex* (Australia); *Rozex Gel*; Satric; *Servizol*; *Servizole*; *Supplin*; *Takimetol* (Japan); *Trichex*; *Trichozole*; *Tricowas B*; *Tricowas-B*; *Trikacide*; *Trofonil*; *Vaginyl*; *Vagitrix*; *Vagyl*; *Zadstat* (England)
(International brand names outside U.S. in italics)

FORMULARIES: Aetna; BC-BS; DoD; FHP; Medi-Cal; WHO; PCS

COST OF THERAPY: $0.95 (Baterial Vaginosis; Tablet; 500 mg; 2/day; 7 days)

> WARNING:
> Metronidazole has been shown to be carcinogenic in mice and rats (see PRECAUTIONS.) Unnecessary use of the drug should be avoided. Its use should be reserved for the conditions described in the INDICATIONS AND USAGEsection below.

DESCRIPTION:

Oral: Metronidazole is an oral synthetic antiprotozoal and antibacterial agent, 1-(β-hydroxyethyl)-2-methyl-5-nitroimidazole.

Metronidazole tablets contain 250 mg or 500 mg of metronidazole. Inactive ingredients include cellulose, FD&C Blue No. 2 Lake, hydroxypropyl cellulose, hydroxypropyl methylcellulose, polyethylene glycol, stearic acid, and titanium dioxide.

IV Injection: Metronidazole HCl Sterile IV and Metronidazole Sterile IV, are parenteral dosage forms of the synthetic antibacterial agents 1-(β-hydroxyethyl)-2-methyl-5 - nitroimidazole hydrochloride and 1-(β-hydroxyethyl)-methyl- 5-nitroimidazole, respectively.

Each single-dose vial of lyophilized Metronidazole IV contains sterile, nonpyrogenic Metronidazole HCl, equivalent to 500 mg metronidazole, and 415 mg mannitol.

Each metronidazole IV RTU (Ready-To-Use) 100-ml single-dose plastic container contains a sterile, nonpyrogenic, isotonic, buffered solution of 500 mg metronidazole, 47.6 mg sodium phosphate, 22.9 mg citric acid, and 790 mg sodium chloride in Water for Injection USP. Metronidazole IV RTU has a tonicity of 310 mOsm/L and a pH of 5 to 7. Each container contains 14 mEq of sodium.

The plastic container is fabricated from a specially formulated polyvinyl chloride plastic. Water can permeate from inside the container into the overwrap in amounts insufficient to affect the solution significantly. Solutions in contact with the plastic container can leach out certain of its chemical components in very small amounts within the expiration period, e.g., di 2-ethyhexyl phthalate (DEHP), up to 5 parts per million. However, the safety of the plastic has been confirmed in tests in animal according to USP biological tests for plastic containers as well as by tissue culture toxicity studies.

Topical: Metronidazole Gel contains metronidazole, USP, at a concentration of 7.5 mg per gram (0.75%) in a gelled, purified water solution, containing methyl and propyl parabens, propylene glycol, carbomer 940, and edetate disodium. Metronidazole is classified therapeutically as an antiprotozoal and antibacterial agent. Chemically, metronidazole is named 2-methyl-5- nitro-1*H*-Imidazole-1-ethanol.

CLINICAL PHARMACOLOGY:

Disposition of metronidazole in the body is similar for both oral and intravenous dosage forms, with an average elimination half-life in healthy humans of eight hours.

The major route of elimination of metronidazole and its metabolites is via the urine (60 to 80% of the dose), with fecal excretion accounting for 6 to 15% of the dose. The metabolites that appear in the urine result primarily from side-chain oxidation (1-(β-hydroxyethyl)-2-hydroxymethyl-5-nitroimidazole and 2-methyl-5- nitroimidazole-1-yl-acetic acid) and glucuronide conjugation, with unchanged metronidazole accounting for approximately 20% of the total. Renal clearance of metronidazole is approximately 10 ml/min/1.73m^2.

Metronidazole is the major component appearing in the plasma, with lesser quantities of the 2-hydroxymethyl metabolite also being present. Less than 20% of the circulating metronidazole is bound to plasma proteins. Both the parent compound and the metabolite possess *in vitro* bactericidal activity against most strains of anaerobic bacteria and *in vitro* trichomonacidal activity.

Metronidazole appears in cerebrospinal fluid, saliva, and breast milk in concentrations similar to those found in plasma. Bactericidal concentrations of metronidazole have also been detected in pus from hepatic abscesses.

Following oral administration metronidazole is well absorbed with peak plasma concentrations occurring between one and two hours after administration. Plasma concentrations of metronidazole are proportional to the administered dose. Oral administration of 250 mg, 500 mg, or 2,000 mg produced peak plasma concentrations of 6 mcg/ml, 12 mcg/ml, and 40 mcg/ml, respectively. Studies reveal no significant bioavailability differences between males and females; however, because of weight differences, the resulting plasma levels in males are generally lower.

Decreased renal function dose not alter the single-dose pharmacokinetics of metronidazole. However, plasma clearance of metronidazole is decreased in patients with decreased liver function.

MICROBIOLOGY

*Trichomonas vaginalis, Entamoeba histolytica.*Metronidazole possesses direct trichomonacidal and amebicidal activity against *T. vaginalis* and *E. histolytica.* The *in vitro* minimal inhibitory concentration (MIC) for most strains of these organisms is 1 mcg/ml or less.

Anaerobic Bacteria. Metronidazole is active *in vitro* against most obligate anaerobes, but does not appear to possess any clinically relevant activity against facultative anaerobes or obligate aerobes. Against susceptible organisms, metronidazole is generally bactericidal at concentrations equal to or slightly higher than the minimal inhibitory concentrations. Metronidazole has been shown to have*in vitro* and clinical activity against the following organisms:

Anaerobic gram-negative bacilli, including:

Bacteroides species including the *Bacteroides fragilis* group (*B. fragilis, B. distasonis, B. ovatus, B. thetaiotaomicron, B vulgatus) Fusobacterium* species

Anaerobic gram-positive bacilli, including:

Clostridium species and susceptible strains of *Eubacterium*

Anaerobic gram-positive cocci, including:

Peptococcus species *Peptostreptococcus* species

Susceptibility Testing: Bacteriologic studies should be performed to determine the causative organisms and their susceptibility to metronidazole; however, the rapid, routine susceptibility testing of individual isolates of anaerobic bacteria is not always practical, and therapy may be started while awaiting these results.

Quantitative methods give the most precise estimates of susceptibility to antibacterial drugs. A standardized agar dilution method and a broth microdilution method are recommended.

Control strains are recommended for standardized susceptibility testing. Each time the test is performed, one or more of the following strains should be included: *Clostridium perfringens* ATCC 13124,*Bacteroides fragilis* ATCC 25285, and *Bacteroides thetaiotamicron* ATCC 29741. The mode metronidazole MICs for those three strains are reported to be 0.25, 0.25, and 0.5 mcg/ml, respectively.

A clinical laboratory is considered under acceptable control if the results of the control strains are within one doubling dilution of the mode MICs reported for metronidazole.

A bacterial isolate may be considered susceptible if the MIC value for metronidazole is not more than 16 mcg/ml. An organism is considered resistant if the MIC is greater than 16 mcg/ml. A report of "resistant" from the laboratory indicates that the infecting organism is not likely to respond to therapy.

CLINICAL PHARMACOLOGY: *(cont'd)*

TOPICAL

Bioavailability studies on the administration of 1 gram of metronidazole topical gel to the face, (7.5 mg of metronidazole) of rosacea patients showed a maximum serum concentration of 66 nanograms per milliliter in one patient. This concentration is approximately 100 times less than concentrations afforded by a single 250 mg oral tablet. The serum metronidazole concentrations were below the detectable limits of the assay at the majority of time points in all patients. Three of the patients had no detectable serum concentrations of metronidazole at any time point. The mean dose of gel applied during clinical studies was 600 mg which represents 4.5 mg of metronidazole per application. Therefore, under normal usage levels, the formulation affords minimal serum concentrations of metronidazole.

The mechanisms by which metronidazole topical gel acts in reducing inflammatory lesions of rosacea are unknown, but may include an antibacterial and/or an anti-inflammatory effect.

INDICATIONS AND USAGE:

ORAL TABLETS

Symptomatic Trichomoniasis: Metronidazole is indicated for the treatment of symptomatic trichomoniasis in females and males when the presence of the trichomonad has been confirmed by appropriate laboratory procedures (wet smears and/or cultures).

Asymptomatic Trichomoniasis: Metronidazole is indicated in the treatment of asymptomatic females when the organism is associated with endocervicitis, cervicitis, or cervical erosion. Since there is evidence that presence of the trichomonad can interfere with accurate assessment of abnormal cytological smears, additional smears should be performed after eradication of the parasite.

Treatment of Asymptomatic Consorts: T. vaginalis infection is a venereal disease. Therefore, asymptomatic sexual partners of treated patients should be treated simultaneously if the organism has been found to be present, in the order to prevent reinfection of the partner. The decision as to whether to treat an asymptomatic male partner who has a negative culture or one for whom no culture has been attempted is an individual one. In making this decision, it should be noted that there is evidence that a woman may become reinfected if her consort is not treated. Also, since there can be considerable difficulty in isolating the organism from the asymptomatic male carrier, negative smears and cultures cannot be relied upon in this regard. In any event, the consort should be treated with metronidazole in cases of reinfection.

Amebiasis: Metronidazole is indicated in the treatment of acute intestinal amebiasis (amebic dysentery and amebic liver abscess.

In amebic liver abscess. Metronidazole therapy does not obviate the need for aspiration or drainage of pus.

Anaerobic Bacterial Infections: Metronidazole is indicated in the treatment of serious infections caused by susceptible anaerobic bacteria. Indicated surgical procedures should be performed in conjunction with metronidazole therapy. In a mixed aerobic and anaerobic infection, antibiotics appropriate for the treatment of the aerobic infection should be used in addition to metronidazole.

In the treatment of most serious anaerobic infections, metronidazole IV RTU (metronidazole) is usually administered initially. This may be followed by oral therapy with metronidazole at the discretion of the physician.

Intra-Abdominal Infections, including peritonitis, intra-abdominal abscess, and liver abscess, caused by *Bacteroides* species including the *B. fragilis* group (*B. fragilis, B. distasonis, B. ovatus, B. thetaiotaomicron, B. vulgatus), Clostridium* species,*Eubacterium* species, *Peptococcus* species, and *Peptostreptococcus* species.

Skin and Skin Structure Infections caused by *Bacteroides* species including the *B. fragilis* group, *Clostridium* species,*Peptococcus* species, *Peptostreptococcus* species, and *Fusobacterium* species.

Gynecological Infections, including endometritis, endomyometritis, tubo-ovarian abscess, and postsurgical vaginal cuff infection, caused by*Bacteroides* species including the *B. fragilis* group,*Clostridium* species, *Peptococcus* species, and *Peptostreptococcus* species.

Bacterial Septicemia caused by *Bacteroides* species including the*B. fragilis* group, and *Clostridium* species.

Bone and Joint Infections, as adjunctive therapy, caused by*Bacteroides* species including the *B. fragilis* group.

Central Nervous System (CNS) Infections, including meningitis and brain abscess, caused by *Bacteroides* species including the *B. fragilis* group.

Lower Respiratory Tract Infections, including pneumonia, empyema, and lung abscess, caused by *Bacteroides* species including the *B. fragilis* group.

ENDOCARDITIS caused by *Bacteroides* species including the *B. fragilis* group.

IV INJECTION

Treatment of Anaerobic Infections: Metronidazole IV is indicated in the treatment of serious infections caused by susceptible anaerobic bacteria. Indicated surgical procedures should be performed in conjunction with metronidazole IV therapy. In a mixed aerobic and anaerobic infection, antibiotics appropriate for the treatment of the aerobic infection should be used in addition to metronidazole IV.

Metronidazole IV is effective in *Bacteroides fragilis* infections resistant to clindamycin, chloramphenicol, and penicillin.

Intra—Abdominal Infections, including peritonitis, intra-abdominal abscess, and liver abscess, caused by *Bacteroides* species including the *B. fragilis* group (*B. fragilis, B. distasonis, B. ovatus, B. thetaiotaomicron, B. Vulgatus*), *Clostridium* species, *Eubacterium* species, *Peptococcus* species, and *Peptostreptococcus* species.

Skin and Skin Structure Infections, caused by *Bacteroides* species including the *B. fragilis* group, *Clostridium* species,*Peptococcus* species, *Peptostreptococcus* species, and *Fusobacterium species.*

Gynecological Infections, including endometritis, endomyometritis, tubo- ovarian abscess, and postsurgical vaginal cuff infection, caused by*Bacteroides* species including the *B. fragilis* group,*Clostridium* species, *Peptococcus* species, and *Peptostreptococcus* species.

Bacterial Septicemia, caused by *Bacteroides* species including the*B. fragilis* group, and *Clostridium* species.

Bone and Joint Infection, as adjunctive therapy, caused by*Bacteroides* species including the *B. fragilis* group.

Central Nervous System (CNS) Infections, including meningitis and brain abscess, caused by *Bacteroides* species including the *B. Fragilis* group.

Lower Respiratory Tract Infections, including pneumonia, empyema, and lung abscess, caused by *Bacteroides* species including the *B. Fragilis* group.

Endocarditis, caused by the *Bacteroides* species, including the*B. Fragilis* group.

PROPHYLAXIS

The prophylactic administration of metronidazole IV preoperatively, intraoperatively, and postoperatively may reduce the incidence of postoperative infection in patients undergoing elective colorectal surgery which is classified as contaminated or potentially contaminated.

INDICATIONS AND USAGE: *(cont'd)*

Prophylactic use of metronidazole IV should be discontinued within 12 hours after surgery. If there are signs of infection, specimens for cultures should be obtained for the identification of the causative organism(s) so that appropriate therapy may be given (See DOSAGE AND ADMINISTRATION).

TOPICAL GEL

Metronidazole topical gel is indicated for topical application in the treatment of inflammatory papules, pustules, and erythema of rosacea.

CONTRAINDICATIONS:

IV: Metronidazole is contraindicated in patients with a prior history of hypersensitivity to metronidazole or other nitroimidazole derivatives.

Tablets: Metronidazole is contraindicated in patients with a prior history of hypersensitivity to metronidazole or other nitroimidazole derivatives.

In patients with trichomoniasis, metronidazole is contraindicated during the first trimester of pregnancy. (see WARNINGS.)

Topical Gel: Metronidazole topical gel is contraindicated in individuals with a history of hypersensitivity to metronidazole, parabens, or other ingredients of the formulations.

WARNINGS:

Convulsive Seizures and Peripheral Neuropathy: Convulsive seizures and peripheral neuropathy, the latter characterized mainly by numbness or paresthesia of an extremity, have been reported in patients treated with metronidazole. The appearance of abnormal neurologic signs demands the prompt discontinuation of metronidazole therapy. Metronidazole should be administered with caution to patients with central nervous system diseases.

PRECAUTIONS:

GENERAL

Tablets/IV Injection: Patients with severe hepatic disease metabolize metronidazole slowly, with resultant accumulation of metronidazole and its metabolites in the plasma. Accordingly, for such patients, doses below those usually recommended should be administered cautiously.

Known or previously unrecognized candidiasis may present more prominent symptoms during therapy with metronidazole and requires treatment with a candicidal agent.

Additional Information for IV: Administration of solutions containing sodium ions may result in sodium retention. Care should be taken when administering metronidazole IV RTU to patients receiving corticosteroids or to patients presdisposed to edema.

Metronidazole Topical Gel: Because of the minimal absorption of metronidazole and consequently its insignificant plasma concentration after topical administration, the adverse experiences reported with the oral form of the drug have not been reported with metronidazole topical gel.

Metronidazole Topical Gel has been reported to cause tearing of the eyes. Therefore, contact with the eyes should be avoided. If a reaction suggesting local irritation occurs, patients should be directed to use the medication less frequently, discontinue use temporarily, or discontinue use until further instructions. Metronidazole is a nitroimidazole and should be used with care in patients with evidence of, or history of, blood dyscrasia.

INFORMATION FOR THE PATIENT

Alcoholic beverages should be avoided while taking metronidazole and for at least one day afterward. See DRUG INTERACTIONS.

Topical Gel: This medication is to be used as directed by the physician. It is for external use only. Avoid contact with the eyes.

LABORATORY TESTS

Tablets/IV Injection: Metronidazole is a nitroimidazole and should be used with care in patients with evidence of or history of blood dyscrasia. A mild leukopenia has been observed during its administration; however, no persistent hematologic abnormalities attributable to metronidazole have been observed in clinical studies. Total and differential leukocyte counts are recommended before and after therapy for trichomoniasis and amebiasis, especially if a second course of therapy is necessary, and before and after therapy for anaerobic infection.

DRUG/LABORATORY TEST INTERACTIONS

Tablets/IV Injection: Metronidazole may interfere with certain types of determinations of serum chemistry values, such as aspartate aminotransferase (AST, SGOT), alanine aminotransferase (ALT, SGPT), lactate dehydrogenase (LDH), triglycerides, and hexokinase glucose. Values of zero may be observed. All of the assays in which interference has been reported involve enzymatic coupling of the assay to oxidation-reduction of nicotine adenine dinucleotide ($NAD^+ \leftrightarrow$ NADH). Interference is due to the similarity in absorbance peaks of NADH (340 nm) and metronidazole (322 nm) at pH 7.

CARCINOGENESIS, MUTAGENESIS, AND IMPAIRMENT OF FERTILITY

Tumorigenicity studies in rodents: Metronidazole has shown evidence of carcinogenic activity in a number of studies involving chronic, oral administration in mice and rats.

Prominent among the effects in the mouse was pulmonary tumorigenesis. This has been observed in all six reported studies in that species, including one study in which the animals were dosed on an intermittent schedule (administration during every fourth week only). At very high dose levels (approx. 500 mg/kg/day) there was statistically significant increase in the incidence of malignant liver tumors in males. Also, the published results of one of the mouse studies indicate an increase in the incidence of malignant lymphomas as well as pulmonary neoplasms associated with lifetime feeding of the drug. All these effects are statistically significant.

Several long-term, oral-dosing studies in the rat have been completed. There were statistically significant increase in the incidence of various neoplasms, particularly in mammary and hepatic tumors, among female rats administered metronidazole over those noted in the concurrent female control groups.

Two lifetime tumorigenicity studies in hamsters have been performed and reported to be negative.

Mutagenicity Studies: Although metronidazole has shown mutagenic activity in a number of *in vitro* assay systems, studies in mammals (*in vivo*) have failed to demonstrate a potential for genetic damage.

PREGNANCY, TERATOGENIC EFFECTS, PREGNANCY CATEGORY B

Metronidazole crosses the placental barrier and enters the fetal circulation rapidly. Reproduction studies have been performed in rats at doses up to five times the human dose and have revealed no evidence of impaired fertility or harm to the fetus due to metronidazole. Metronidazole administered intraperitoneally to pregnant mice at approximately the human dose caused fetotoxicity; administered orally to pregnant mice, no fetotoxicity was observed. There are, however, no adequate and well-controlled studies in pregnant women. Because animal reproduction studies are not always predictive of human response, and because metronidazole is a carcinogen in rodents, this drug should be used during pregnancy only if clearly needed (see CONTRAINDICATIONS.)

PRECAUTIONS: *(cont'd)*

Use of metronidazole for trichomoniasis in the second and third trimesters should be restricted to those in whom local palliative treatment has been inadequate to control symptoms.

NURSING MOTHERS

Tablets: Because of the potential for tumorigenicity shown for metronidazole in mouse and rat studies, a decision should be made whether to discontinue nursing or to discontinue the drug, taking into account the importance of the drug to the mother. Metronidazole is secreted in breast milk in concentrations similar to those found in plasma.

Topical Gel: Even though metronidazole topical gel blood levels are significantly lower than those achieved after oral metronidazole, a decision should be made whether to discontinue nursing or to discontinue the drug, taking into account the importance of the drug to the mother.

PEDIATRIC USE

Safety and effectiveness in children have not been established, except for the treatment of amebiasis.

Topical Gel: Safety and effectiveness in children have not been established.

DRUG INTERACTIONS:

TABLETS

Metronidazole has been reported to potentiate the anticoagulant effect of warfarin and other oral coumarin anticoagulants, resulting in a prolongation of prothrombin time. This possible drug interaction should be considered when metronidazole is prescribed for patients on this type of anticoagulant, therapy.

The simultaneous administration of drugs that induce microsomal liver enzymes, such as phenytoin or phenobarbital, may accelerate the elimination of metronidazole, resulting in reduced plasma levels; impaired clearance of phenytoin has also been reported.

The simultaneous administration of drugs that decrease microsomal liver enzyme activity, such as cimetidine, may prolong the half-life and decrease plasma clearance of metronidazole. In patients stabilized on relatively high doses of lithium, short-term metronidazole therapy has been associated with elevation of serum lithium and, in a few cases, signs of lithium toxicity. Serum lithium and serum creatinine levels should be obtained several days after beginning metronidazole to detect any increase that may precede clinical symptoms of lithium intoxication.

Alcoholic beverages should not be consumed during metronidazole therapy and for at least one day afterward because abdominal cramps, nausea, vomiting, headaches, and flushing may occur.

Psychotic reactions have been reported in alcoholic patients who are using metronidazole and disulfiram concurrently. Metronidazole should not be given to patients who have taken disulfiram within the last two weeks.

TOPICAL GEL

Drug interactions are less likely with topical administration but should be kept in mind when metronidazole topical gel is prescribed for patients who are receiving anticoagulant treatment. Oral metronidazole has been reported to potentiate the anticoagulant effect of coumarin and warfarin resulting in a prolongation of prothrombin time.

ADVERSE REACTIONS:

Two serious adverse reactions reported in patients treated with metronidazole have been convulsive seizures and peripheral neuropathy, the latter characterized mainly by numbness or paresthesia of an extremity. Since persistent peripheral neuropathy has been reported in some patients receiving prolonged administration of metronidazole, patients should be specifically warned about these reactions and should be told to stop the drug and report immediately to their physicians if any neurologic symptoms occur.

The most common adverse reactions reported have been referable to the gastrointestinal tract, particularly nausea reported by about 12% of patients, sometimes accompanied by headache, anorexia, and occasionally vomiting; diarrhea; epigastric distress, and abdominal cramping. Constipation has been reported.

The following reactions have also been reported during treatment with metronidazole:

Mouth: A sharp, unpleasant metallic taste is not unusual. Furry tongue, glossitis, and stomatitis have occurred; these may be associated with a sudden overgrowth of *Candida* which may occur during effective therapy.

Hematopoietic: Reversible neutropenia (leukopenia); rarely, reversible thrombocytopenia.

Cardiovascular: Flattening of the T-wave may be seen in electrocardiographic tracings.

Central Nervous System: Convulsive seizures, peripheral neuropathy, dizziness, vertigo, incoordination, ataxia, confusion, irritability, depression, weakness, and insomnia.

Hypersensitivity: Urticaria, erythematous rash, flushing, nasal congestion, dryness of the mouth (or vagina or vulva), and fever.

Renal: Dysuria, cystitis, polyuria, incontinence, and a sense of pelvic pressure. Instances of darkened urine have been reported by approximately one patient in 100,000. Although the pigment which is which is probably responsible for this phenomenon has not been positively identified, it is almost certainly a metabolite of metronidazole and seems to have no clinical significance.

Other: Proliferation of *Candida* in the vagina, dyspareunia, decrease of libido, proctitis, and fleeting joint pains sometimes resembling "serum sickness." If patients receiving metronidazole drink alcoholic beverages, they may experience abdominal distress, nausea, vomiting, flushing, or headache. A modification of the taste of alcoholic beverages has also been reported. Rare cases of pancreatitis, which abated on withdrawal of the drug, have been reported.

Crohn's disease patients are known to have an increased incidence of gastrointestinal and certain extraintestinal cancers. There have been some reports in the medical literature of breast and colon cancer in Crohn,s disease patients who have been treated with metronidazole at high doses for extended periods of time. A cause and effect relationship has not been established. Crohn's disease is not an approved indication for metronidazole.

TOPICAL GEL

Adverse conditions reported include watery (tearing) eyes if the gel is applied too closely to this area, transient redness, and mild dryness, burning and skin irritation. None of the side effects exceeded an incidence of 2% of patients.

OVERDOSAGE:

TABLETS

Single oral doses of metronidazole, up to 15 g, have been reported in suicide attempts and accidental overdoses. Symptoms reported include nausea, vomiting, and ataxia.

Oral metronidazole has been studies as a radiation sensitizer in the treatment of malignant tumors. Neurotoxic effects, including seizures and peripheral neuropathy, have been reported after 5 to 7 days of doses of 6 to 10.4 every other day.

Treatment: There is no specific antidote for metronidazole overdose; therefore, management of the patient should consist of symptomatic and supportive therapy.

OVERDOSAGE: *(cont'd)*

IV INJECTION

Use of dosages of metronidazole HCl IV higher than those recommended has been reported. These include the use of 27 mg/kg three times a day for 20 days, and the use of 75 mg/kg as a single loading dose followed by 7.5 mg/kg maintenance doses. No adverse reactions were reported in either of the two cases.

Single oral doses of metronidazole, up to 15 g, have been reported in suicide attempts and accidental overdoses. Symptoms reported include nausea, vomiting, and ataxia.

Oral metronidazole has been studied as a radiation sensitizer in the treatment of malignant tumors. Neurotoxic effects, including seizures and peripheral neuropathy, have been reported after 5 to 7 days of doses off 6 to 10.4 g every other day.

Treatment: There is no specific antidote for overdose; therefore, management of the patient should consist of symptomatic and supportive therapy.

TOPICAL GEL

There is no human experience with overdosage of metronidazole topical gel. The acute oral toxicity of the metronidazole topical gel formulation was determined to be greater than 5 g/kg (the highest dose given) in albino rats.

DOSAGE AND ADMINISTRATION:

ORAL TABLETS

In elderly patients the pharmacokinetics of metronidazole may be altered and therefore monitoring of serum levels may be necessary to adjust the metronidazole dosage accordingly.

TRICHOMONIASIS

In the Female: *One-day treatment:* two grams of metronidazole, given either as a single dose or in two divided doses of one gram each given in the same day. *Seven-day course of treatment:* 250 mg three times daily for seven consecutive days. There is some indication from controlled comparative studies that cure rates as determined by vaginal smears, signs and symptoms, may be higher after a seven-day course of treatment than after a one-day treatment regimen.

The dosage regimen should be individualized. Single-dose treatment can assure compliance, especially if administered under supervision, in those patients who cannot be relied on to continue the seven-day regimen. A seven-day course of treatment may minimize reinfection of the female long enough to treat sexual contacts. Further, some patients may tolerate one course of therapy better than the other.

Pregnant patients should not be treated during the first trimester with either regimen. If treated during the second or third trimester, the one-day course of therapy should not be used, as it results in higher serum levels which reach the fetal circulation. (See CONTRAINDICATIONS and PRECAUTIONS.)

When repeat courses of the drug are required, it is recommended that an interval of four to six weeks elapse between courses and that the presence of the trichomonad be reconfirmed by appropriate laboratory measures. Total and differential leukocyte counts should be made before and after re-treatment.

In the Male: Treatment should be individualized as for the female.

AMEBIASIS

Adults: *For acute intestinal amebiasis (acute amebic dysentery):* 750 mg orally three times daily for 5 to 10 days. *For amebic liver abscess* : 500 mg or 750 mg orally three times daily for 5 to 10 days.

Children: 36 to 50 mg/kg/24 hours, divided into three doses, orally for 10 days.

ANAEROBIC BACTERIAL INFECTIONS

In the treatment of most serious anaerobic infections, metronidazole HCl IV or metronidazole IV RTU is usually administered initially.

The usual adult *oral* dosage is 7.5 mg/kg every six hours (approx. 500 mg for a 70-kg adult). A maximum of 4 g should not be exceeded during a 24-hours period.

The usual duration of therapy is 7 to 10 days; however, infections of the bone and joint, lower respiratory tract, and endocardium may require longer treatment.

Patients with severe hepatic disease metabolize metronidazole slowly, with resultant accumulation of metronidazole and its metabolites in the plasma. Accordingly, for such patients, doses below those usually recommended should be administered cautiously. Close monitoring of plasma metronidazole levels[2] and toxicity is recommended.

The dose of metronidazole should not be specifically reduced in anuric patients since accumulated metabolites may be rapidly removed by dialysis.

Store below 86°F (30°C) and protect from light.

INTRAVENOUS INJECTION

In elderly patients the pharmacokinetics of metronidazole may be altered and therefore monitoring of serum levels may be necessary to adjust the metronidazole dosage accordingly.

TREATMENT OF ANAEROBIC INFECTIONS

The recommended dosage schedule for *adultsis*:

Loading Dose: 15 mg/kg infused over one hour (approximately 1 g for a 70-kg adult).

Maintenance Dose: 7.5 mg/kg infused over one hour every six hours (approximately 500 mg for a 70-kg adult). The first maintenance dose should be instituted six hours following the initiation of the loading dose.

Parenteral therapy may be changed to oral metronidazole when conditions warrant, based upon the severity of the disease and the response of the patient to metronidazole IV treatment. The usual adult oral dosage is 7.5 mg/kg every six hours.

A maximum of 4 g should not be exceeded during a 24-hour period.

Patients with severe hepatic disease metabolize metronidazole slowly, with resultant accumulation of metronidazole and its metabolites in te plasma. Accordingly, for such patients, doses below those usually recommended should be administered cautiously. Close monitoring of plasma metronidazole levels[1] and toxicity is recommended.

In patients receiving metronidazole in whom gastric secretions are continuously removed by nasogastric aspiration, sufficient metronidazole may be removed in the aspirate to cause a reduction in serum levels.

The dose of metronidazole should not be specifically rescued in anuric patients since accumulated metabolites may be rapidly removed by dialysis.

The usual duration of therapy is 7 to 10 days; however, infections of the bone and joint, lower respiratory tract, and endocardium may require longer treatment.

PROPHYLAXIS

For surgical; prophylactic use, to prevent postoperative infection in contaminated or potentially contaminated colorectal surgery, the recommended dosage schedule for adults is:

a. 15 mg/kg infused over 30 to 60 minutes and completed approximately one hour before surgery; followed by

b. 7.5 mg/kg infused over 30 to 60 minutes at 6 and 12 hours after the initial dose.

DOSAGE AND ADMINISTRATION: *(cont'd)*

It is important that (1) administration of the initial preoperative dose be completed approximately one hour before surgery so that adequate drug levels are present in the serum and tissues at the time of initial incision, and (2) metronidazole IV be administered, if necessary, at 6- hours intervals to maintain effective drug levels. Prophylactic use of metronidazole IV should be limited to the day of surgery only, following the above guidelines.

CAUTION: Metronidazole IV is to be administered by slow intravenous drip infusion only, either as a continuous or intermittent infusion. IV admixtures containing metronidazole and other drugs should be avoided. Additives should not be introduced into the metronidazole IV RTU solution. If used with a primary intravenous fluid system, the primary solution should be discontinued during metronidazole infusion. DO NOT USE EQUIPMENT CONTAINING ALUMINUM (EG, NEEDLES, CANNULAE) THAT WOULD COME IN CONTACT WITH THE DRUG SOLUTION.

METRONIDAZOLE IV

Metronidazole IV cannot be given by direct intravenous injection (IV bolus) because of the low pH (0.5 to 2.0) of the reconstituted product. Metronidazole iv MUST BE FURTHER DILUTED AND NEUTRALIZED FOR IV INFUSION.

Metronidazole IV is prepared for use in two steps:

NOTE: ORDER OF MIXING IS IMPORTANT

A. Reconstitution

B. Dilution in intravenous solution followed by pH neutralization with sodium bicarbonate injection into the dilution.

Reconstitution: To prepare the solution, add 4.4 ml of one of the following diluents and mix thoroughly; Sterile Water for Injection, USP; Bacteriostatic Water for Injection, USP; 0.9% Sodium Chloride Injection, USP; or Bacteriostatic 0.9% Sodium Chloride Injection, USP. The resultant approximate withdrawal volume is 5.0 ml with an approximate concentration of 100 mg/ml.

The pH of the reconstituted product will be in the range will be in the range of 0.5 to 2.0. Reconstituted metronidazole IV is clear, and pale yellow to yellow-green in color.

Dilution in Intravenous Solution: Properly reconstituted metronidazole HCl IV may be added to a glass or plastic IV container not to exceed a concentration of 8 mg/ml. Any of the following intravenous solutions may be used: 0.9% Sodium Chloride Injection, USP; 5% Dextrose Injection, USP; or Lactated Ringer's Injection, USP.

NEUTRALIZATION IS REQUIRED PRIOR TO ADMINISTRATION

The final product should be mixed thoroughly and used within 24 hours.

Neutralization For Intravenous Infusion: Neutralize the intravenous solution containing metronidazole HCl IV with approximately 5 mEq of sodium bicarbonate injection for each 500 mg of metronidazole HCl IV used. Mix thoroughly. The pH of the neutralized intravenous solution will be approximately 6.0 to 7.0. Carbon dioxide gas will be generated with neutralization. It may be necessary to relieve gas pressure within the container.

Note: When the contents of one vial (500 mg) are diluted and neutralized to 100 ml, the resultant concentration is 5 mg/ml. Do not exceed an 8 mg/ml concentration of metronidazole HCl IV in the neutralized intravenous solution, since neutralization will decrease the aqueous solubility and precipitation may occur. DO NOT REFRIGERATE NEUTRALIZED SOLUTION; otherwise, precipitation may occur.

METRONIDAZOLE IV RTU (READY TO USE)

Metronidazole IV RTU is a ready-to-use isotonic solution. **NO DILUTION OR BUFFERING IS REQUIRED**. Do not refrigerate. Each container of metronidazole IV RTU contains 14 mEq of sodium.

Parenteral drug products should be inspected visually for particulate matter and discoloration prior to administration, whenever solution and container permit. Do not use if cloudy or precipitated or if the seal is not intact.

Use sterile equipment. It is recommended that the intravenous administration apparatus be replaced at least once every 24 hours.

Store metronidazole HCl IV, prior to reconstitution, should be stored below 86°F (30°C) and protected from light.

Metronidazole IV RTU should be stored at controlled room temperature, 59° to 86°F (15° to 30°C), and protected from light during storage.

TOPICAL GEL

Apply and rub in a thin film of metronidazole topical solution twice daily, morning and evening, to entire affected areas after washing. Significant therapeutic results should be noticed within three weeks. Clinical studies have demonstrated continuing improvement through nine weeks of therapy.

Area to be treated should be cleansed before application of metronidazole topical gel. Patients may use cosmetics after application of metronidazole topical gel.

REFERENCES:

1. Proposed standard: PSM-11-Proposed Reference Dilution Procedure for Antimicrobic Susceptibility Testing of Anaerobic Bacteria, National Committee for Clinical Laboratory Standards; and Sutter, et al.: Collaborative Evaluation of a Proposed Reference Dilution Method of Susceptibility Testing of Anaerobic Bacteria, Antimicrob. Agents Chemother. *16:*495-502 (Oct.) 1979; and Tally, et al.: *In Vitro*Activity of Thienamycin, Antimicrob. Agents Chemother.*14:*436-438 (Sept.) 1978. **2.** Ralph, E.D., and Kirby, W.M.M.: Bioassay of Metronidazole With Either Anaerobic or Aerobic Incubation, J. Infect. Dis. *132:*587-591 (Nov.) 1975; or Gulaid, et al.: Determination of Metronidazole and Its Major Metabolites in Biological Fluids by High Pressure Liquid Chromatography, Br. J. Clin. Pharmacol. *6:*430-432, 1978.(Tablets: Searle, 7/90, A05709-6; IV Injection: Searle, 7/90, A05034-6; Topicl Gel: Curatek, 10/88, 126297 0789)

HOW SUPPLIED:

Storage and Stability: Reconstituted vials of Metronidazole IV are chemically stable for 96 hours when stored below 86°F (30°C) in room light.

Use diluted and neutralized intravenous solutions containing Metronidazole HCl IV within 24 hours of mixing.

Storage: Store at controlled room temperature.

HOW SUPPLIED - RATED THERAPEUTICALLY EQUIVALENT:

Injection, Solution - Intravenous - 500 mg/100ml

100 ml	$8.88	Metronidazole, Fujisawa USA	00469-1593-00
100 ml	$15.34	Metronidazole, Baxter Hlthcare	00338-1055-48
100 ml	$28.93	Metronidazole, Abbott	00074-7811-24
100 ml	$28.94	Metronidazole In 5% Dextrose, Abbott	00074-7811-37
100 ml	$352.26	Metronidazole, Abbott	00074-1217-11
100 ml x 1	$7.81	Metronidazole Redi-Infusion 500, Elkins Sinn	00641-2337-41
100 ml x 4	$25.73	Metronidazole, Abbott	00074-7811-23
100 ml x 12	$18.88	Metro I.V., McGaw	00264-1939-33
100 ml x 12	$27.68	METRO IV, McGaw	00264-5535-32
100 ml x 24	**$203.88**	**FLAGYL I.V.RTU, SCS Pharm**	**00905-1847-24**
100 ml x 24	$397.34	Metronidazole, Elkins Sinn	00641-7200-97
500 mg x 10	**$167.59**	**FLAGYL I.V., SCS Pharm**	**00905-1804-10**

HOW SUPPLIED - RATED THERAPEUTICALLY EQUIVALENT: *(cont'd)*

Tablet, Plain Coated - Oral - 250 mg

28's	$.92	Metronidazole, H.C.F.A. F F P	99999-1803-01
50's	$1.65	Metronidazole, H.C.F.A. F F P	99999-1803-02
50's	**$67.87**	**FLAGYL, Searle**	**00025-1831-50**
100's	$3.30	Metronidazole, United Res	00677-0690-01
100's	$3.30	Metronidazole, H.C.F.A. F F P	99999-1803-03
100's	$5.52	Metronidazole, US Trading	56126-0095-11
100's	$5.93	Metronidazole, IDE-Interstate	00814-4810-14
100's	$7.11	Metronidazole, Qualitest Pharms	00603-4640-21
100's	$8.75	Metronidazole 250, Major Pharms	00904-1453-60
100's	$10.25	Metronidazole, Raway	00686-0122-20
100's	$10.38	Metronidazole, HL Moore Drug Exch	00839-6415-06
100's	$11.40	Metronidazole, Voluntary Hosp	53258-0146-01
100's	$13.75	Metronidazole, Parmed Pharms	00349-2363-01
100's	$15.00	Metronidazole, Eon Labs Mfg	00185-0551-01
100's	$17.58	Metronidazole, Halsey Drug	00879-0506-01
100's	$18.00	Metronidazole, Voluntary Hosp	53258-0146-13
100's	$18.50	Metronidazole, Teva	00093-0851-01
100's	$18.50	Metronidazole, Zenith Labs	00172-2971-60
100's	$18.50	Metronidazole, Goldline Labs	00182-1330-01
100's	$18.50	Metronidazole, Sidmak Labs	50111-0333-01
100's	$19.10	Metronidazole, Par Pharm	49884-0095-01
100's	$20.00	Metronidazole, Mutual Pharm	53489-0135-01
100's	$20.10	Metronidazole, Geneva Pharms	00781-1742-01
100's	$20.39	Metronidazole, Purepac Pharm	00228-2258-10
100's	$21.45	Metronidazole, Schein Pharm (US)	00364-0595-01
100's	$21.50	Metronidazole, Rugby	00536-4032-01
100's	$21.50	Metronidazole, Martec Pharms	52555-0095-01
100's	$21.82	Metronidazole, Aligen Independ	00405-4677-01
100's	$28.92	Metronidazole 250, Major Pharms	00904-1453-61
100's	$44.70	Metronidazole, Lederle Pharm	00005-3115-23
100's	$45.61	Metronidazole, Bristol Myers Squibb	00003-0488-50
100's	$54.22	Metronidazole, Vangard Labs	00615-1576-13
100's	$55.60	Metronidazole, Medirex	57480-0432-01
100's	$56.10	Metronidazole, Goldline Labs	00182-1330-89
100's	$72.00	Metronidazole, Geneva Pharms	00781-1742-13
100's	$75.30	Metronidazole, Schein Pharm (US)	00364-0595-90
100's	$113.88	PROTOSTAT, Ortho Pharm	00062-1570-01
100's	**$130.58**	**FLAGYL, Searle**	**00025-1831-31**
100's	**$136.09**	**FLAGYL, Searle**	**00025-1831-34**
250's	$8.25	Metronidazole, United Res	00677-0690-03
250's	$8.25	Metronidazole, H.C.F.A. F F P	99999-1803-04
250's	$12.75	Metronidazole, IDE-Interstate	00814-4810-22
250's	$16.15	Metronidazole, Qualitest Pharms	00603-4640-24
250's	$16.95	Metronidazole 250, Major Pharms	00904-1453-70
250's	$25.23	Metronidazole, HL Moore Drug Exch	00839-6415-09
250's	$30.91	Metronidazole, Parmed Pharms	00349-2363-25
250's	$34.75	Metronidazole, Teva	00093-0851-52
250's	$35.00	Metronidazole, Par Pharm	49884-0095-04
250's	$35.50	Metronidazole, Eon Labs Mfg	00185-0551-25
250's	$35.50	Metronidazole, Eon Labs Mfg	00185-0551-52
250's	$35.50	Metronidazole, Mutual Pharm	53489-0135-03
250's	$35.95	Metronidazole, Geneva Pharms	00781-1742-25
250's	$36.00	Metronidazole, Rugby	00536-4032-02
250's	$36.80	Metronidazole, Zenith Labs	00172-2971-65
250's	$36.80	Metronidazole, Goldline Labs	00182-1330-02
250's	$43.41	Metronidazole, Sidmak Labs	50111-0333-06
250's	$43.50	Metronidazole, Aligen Independ	00405-4677-04
250's	$43.60	Metronidazole, Schein Pharm (US)	00364-0595-04
250's	$43.60	Metronidazole, Martec Pharms	52555-0095-02
250's	$104.23	Metronidazole, Lederle Pharm	00005-3115-27
250's	**$308.15**	**FLAGYL, Searle**	**00025-1831-41**
500's	$16.50	Metronidazole, H.C.F.A. F F P	99999-1803-05
500's	$25.65	Metronidazole 250, Major Pharms	00904-1453-40
500's	$34.90	Metronidazole, Qualitest Pharms	00603-4640-28
500's	$52.56	Metronidazole, Halsey Drug	00879-0506-05
500's	$53.00	Metronidazole, Sidmak Labs	50111-0333-02
500's	$53.91	Metronidazole, Parmed Pharms	00349-2363-05
500's	$55.10	Metronidazole, Zenith Labs	00172-2971-70
500's	$55.10	Metronidazole, Goldline Labs	00182-1330-05
500's	$65.75	Metronidazole, Rugby	00536-4032-05
500's	$67.70	Metronidazole, Geneva Pharms	00781-1742-05
500's	$67.75	Metronidazole, Teva	00093-0851-05
500's	$67.90	Metronidazole, Par Pharm	49884-0095-05
500's	$69.90	Metronidazole, Martec Pharms	52555-0095-05
500's	$71.00	Metronidazole, Eon Labs Mfg	00185-0551-05
500's	$147.25	Metronidazole, Amer Preferred	53445-1330-05
500's	$205.15	Metronidazole, Bristol Myers Squibb	00003-0488-60
600's	$120.00	Metronidazole, Medirex	57480-0432-06
1000's	$33.00	Metronidazole, H.C.F.A. F F P	99999-1803-06
1000's	$105.35	Metronidazole, Zenith Labs	00172-2971-80
1000's	$120.00	Metronidazole, Par Pharm	49884-0095-10
2500's	$82.50	Metronidazole, H.C.F.A. F F P	99999-1803-07
2500's	**$2758.03**	**FLAGYL, Searle**	**00025-1831-55**

Tablet, Plain Coated - Oral - 500 mg

50's	$3.41	Metronidazole, H.C.F.A. F F P	99999-1803-08
50's	$8.65	Metronidazole 500, Major Pharms	00904-2694-51
50's	$10.73	Metronidazole, HL Moore Drug Exch	00839-6620-04
50's	$15.19	Metronidazole, Rugby	00536-4019-06
50's	$18.50	Metronidazole, Teva	00093-0852-53
50's	$18.50	Metronidazole, Zenith Labs	00172-3007-48
50's	$18.60	Metronidazole, Schein Pharm (US)	00364-0687-50
50's	$18.75	Metronidazole, Par Pharm	49884-0114-03
50's	$42.39	Metronidazole, Bristol Myers Squibb	00003-0572-40
50's	$103.98	PROTOSTAT, Ortho Pharm	00062-1571-01
50's	**$121.31**	**FLAGYL, Searle**	**00025-1821-50**
100's	$6.83	Metronidazole, United Res	00677-0816-01
100's	$6.83	Metronidazole, H.C.F.A. F F P	99999-1803-09
100's	$12.53	METRINIDAZOLE, IDE-Interstate	00814-4815-14
100's	$18.00	Metronidazole, Raway	00686-0126-20
100's	$21.90	Metronidazole, Voluntary Hosp	53258-0147-01
100's	$26.18	Metronidazole, HL Moore Drug Exch	00839-6620-06
100's	$29.40	Metronidazole, Voluntary Hosp	53258-0147-13
100's	$29.86	Metronidazole, Qualitest Pharms	00603-4641-21
100's	$29.90	Metronidazole, Martec Pharms	52555-0114-01
100's	$29.95	Metronidazole 500, Major Pharms	00904-2694-60
100's	$31.22	Metronidazole, Halsey Drug	00879-0540-01
100's	$31.50	Metronidazole, Mutual Pharm	53489-0136-01
100's	$31.75	Metronidazole, Zenith Labs	00172-3007-60
100's	$31.75	Metronidazole, Goldline Labs	00182-1517-01
100's	$31.75	Metronidazole, Sidmak Labs	50111-0334-01
100's	$31.79	Metronidazole, Geneva Pharms	00781-1747-01

HOW SUPPLIED - RATED THERAPEUTICALLY EQUIVALENT: *(cont'd)*

100's	$31.82	Metronidazole, Aligen Independ	00405-4678-01
100's	$33.15	Metronidazole, Par Pharm	49884-0114-01
100's	$34.75	Metronidazole 500, Eon Labs Mfg	00185-0555-01
100's	$39.96	Metronidazole 500, Major Pharms	00904-2694-61
100's	$46.50	Metronidazole, Rugby	00536-4033-01
100's	$72.39	Metronidazole, Amer Preferred	53445-1517-01
100's	$82.71	Metronidazole, Medirex	57480-0433-01
100's	$83.09	Metronidazole, Bristol Myers Squibb	00003-0572-50
100's	$85.02	Metronidazole, Vangard Labs	00615-1577-13
100's	$90.00	Metronidazole, Harber Pharm	51432-0291-03
100's	$104.95	Metronidazole, Goldline Labs	00182-1517-89
100's	$129.99	Metronidazole, Geneva Pharms	00781-1747-13
100's	$135.15	Metronidazole, Schein Pharm (US)	00364-0687-90
100's	**$237.86**	**FLAGYL, Searle**	**00025-1821-31**
100's	**$244.19**	**FLAGYL, Searle**	**00025-1821-34**
200's	$13.66	Metronidazole, H.C.F.A. F F P	99999-1803-10
200's	$83.70	Metronidazole, Rugby	00536-4033-32
200's	$163.65	Metronidazole, Rugby	00536-4032-32
250's	$17.07	Metronidazole, H.C.F.A. F F P	99999-1803-11
250's	$24.75	Metronidazole, IDE-Interstate	00814-4815-22
250's	$80.38	Metronidazole, Par Pharm	49884-0114-04
500's	$34.15	Metronidazole, H.C.F.A. F F P	99999-1803-12
500's	$35.09	Metronidazole, HL Moore Drug Exch	00839-6620-12
500's	$130.11	Metronidazole, Qualitest Pharms	00603-4641-28
500's	$131.12	Metronidazole, Halsey Drug	00879-0540-05
500's	$132.00	Metronidazole, Sidmak Labs	50111-0334-02
500's	$160.78	Metronidazole, Par Pharm	49884-0114-05
500's	$177.75	Metronidazole, Teva	00093-0852-05
500's	**$1096.84**	**FLAGYL, Searle**	**00025-1821-51**
600's	$257.20	Metronidazole, Medirex	57480-0433-06
1000's	$68.30	Metronidazole, H.C.F.A. F F P	99999-1803-13

HOW SUPPLIED - NOT RATED EQUIVALENT:

Capsule, Gelatin - Oral - 375 mg

50's	**$98.58**	**FLAGYL 375, Searle**	**00025-1942-50**
100's	**$197.76**	**FLAGYL 375, Searle**	**00025-1942-34**

Cream - Topical - 0.75 %

45 gm	$35.00	METROCREAM, Galderma	00299-3836-45

Gel - Topical - 0.75 %

28.4 gm	$23.75	METROGEL, Galderma	00299-3835-28
45 gm	$32.00	METROGEL, Galderma	00299-3835-45

Gel - Vaginal - 0.75 %

70 gm	$25.20	METROGEL-VAGINAL, Curatek Pharms	55326-0200-25

Powder

100 gm	$61.88	Metronidazole, Paddock Labs	00574-0629-01

METYROSINE *(001805)*

CATEGORIES: Autonomic Drugs; Cardiovascular Drugs; Catecholamine Synthesis Inhibitors; Pheochromocytoma; Sympatholytic Agents; Pregnancy Category C; FDA Approval Pre 1982

BRAND NAMES: **Demser**

DESCRIPTION:

Metyrosine is (-)-α-methyl-L-tyrosine.

Metyrosine ((-)-α-methyl-L-tyrosine) (α-MPT) is a white, crystalline compound of molecular weight 195. It is very slightly soluble in water, acetone, and methanol, and insoluble in chloroform and benzene. It is soluble in acidic aqueous solutions. It is also soluble in alkaline aqueous solutions, but is subject to oxidative degradation under these conditions.

Demser is supplied as capsules, for oral administration. Each capsule contains 250 mg metyrosine. Inactive ingredients are colloidal silicon dioxide, gelatin, hydroxypropyl cellulose, magnesium stearate, and titanium dioxide. The capsules may also contain any combination of D&C Red 33, D&C Yellow 10, FD&C Blue 1, and FD&C Blue 2.

CLINICAL PHARMACOLOGY:

Metyrosine inhibits tyrosine hydroxylase, which catalyzes the first transformation. In catecholamine biosynthesis, i.e., the conversion of tyrosine to dihydroxyphenylalanine (DOPA). Because the first step is also the rate-limiting step, blockade of tyrosine hydroxylase activity results in decreased endogenous levels of catecholamines, usually measured as decreased urinary excretion of catecholamines and their metabolites.

In patients with pheochromocytoma, who produce excessive amounts of norepinephrine and epinephrine, administration of one to four grams of metyrosine per day has reduced catecholamine biosynthesis from about 35 to 80 percent as measured by the total excretion of catecholamines and their metabolites (metanephrine and vanillylmandelic acid). The maximum biochemical effect usually occurs within two to three days, and the urinary concentration of catecholamines and their metabolites usually returns to pretreatment levels within three to four days after metyrosine is discontinued. In some patients the total excretion of catecholamines and catecholamine metabolites may be lowered to normal or near normal levels (less than 10 mg/24 hours). In most patients the duration of treatment has been two to eight weeks, but several patients have received metyrosine for periods of one to 10 years.

Most patients with pheochromocytoma treated with metyrosine experience decreased frequency and severity of hypertensive attacks with their associated headache, nausea, sweating, and tachycardia. in patients who respond, blood pressure decreases progressively during the first two days of therapy with metyrosine; after withdrawal, blood pressure usually increases gradually to pretreatment values within two to three days.

Metyrosine is well absorbed from the gastrointestinal tract in animals and in man. From 53 to 88 percent (mean 69 percent) was recovered in the urine as unchanged drug following maintenance oral dosages of 600 to 4000 mg/24 hours in patients with pheochromocytoma or essential hypertension. Less than 1% of the dose was recalled as catechol metabolites.

These metabolites are probably not present in sufficient amounts to contribute to the biochemical effects of metyrosine. The quantities excreted, however, are sufficient to interfere with accurate determination of urinary catecholamines determined by route techniques.

Plasma half-life of metyrosine determined over an 8-hour period after single oral doses was 3.4-3.7 hours in three patients.

For further information refer to: Sjoerdsma, A; Engelman, K: Waldman, T.A.; Cooperman, L.H; Hammond, W.G.: Pheochromocytoma: Current concepts of diagnosis and treatment, Ann. intern. Med. *65*: 1302-1326, Dec. 1966.

INDICATIONS AND USAGE:

Metyrosine is indicated in the treatment of patients with pheochromocytoma for:

1. Preoperative preparation of patients for surgery.

2. Management of patients when surgery is contraindicated

3. Chronic treatment of patients with malignant pheochromocytoma.

Metyrosine is not recommended for the control of essential hypertension.

CONTRAINDICATIONS:

Metyrosine is contraindicated in persons known to be hypersensitive to this compound.

WARNINGS:

MAINTAIN FLUID VOLUME DURING AND AFTER SURGERY

When metyrosine is used preoperatively, alone or especially in combination with alpha-adrenergic blocking drugs, adequate intravascular volume must be maintained intraoperatively (especially after tumor removal) and postoperatively to avoid hypotension and decreased perfusion of vital organs resulting from vasodilatation and expanded volume capacity. Following tumor removal, large volumes of plasma may be needed to maintain blood pressure and central venous pressure within the normal range.

In addition, life-threatening arrhythmias may occur during anesthesia and surgery, and may require treatment with a beta blocker or lidocaine. During surgery, patients should have continuous monitoring of blood pressure and electrocardiogram.

INTRAOPERATIVE EFFECTS

While the preoperative use of metyrosine in patients with pheochromocytoma is thought to decrease intraoperative problems with blood pressure control, metyrosine does not eliminate the danger of hypertensive crises or arrhythmias during manipulation of the tumor, and the alpha-adrenergic blocking drug, phentolamine, may be needed.

INTERACTION WITH ALCOHOL

Metyrosine may add to the sedative effects of alcohol and other CNS depressants, e.g., hypnotics, sedatives, and tranquilizers. (See PRECAUTIONS, Information for the Patient and DRUG INTERACTIONS.)

PRECAUTIONS:

GENERAL

Metyrosine Crystalluria: Crystalluria and urolithiasis have been found in dogs treated with metyrosine at doses similar to those used in humans, and crystalluria has also been observed in a few patients. To minimize the risk of crystalluria, patients should be urged to maintain water intake sufficient to achieve a daily urine volume of 2000 ml or more, particularly when doses greater than 2 g per day are given. Routine examination of the urine should be carried out. Metyrosine will crystallize as needles or rode. If metyrosine crystalluria occurs, fluid intake should be increased further. If crystalluria persists, the dosage should be reduced or the drug discontinued.

Relatively little data regarding long-term use: The total human experience with the drug is quite limited and few patients have been studied long-term. Chronic animal studies have not been carried out. Therefore, suitable laboratory tests should be carried out periodically in patients requiring prolonged use of metyrosine and caution should be observed in patients with impaired hepatic or renal function.

INFORMATION FOR PATIENTS

When receiving metyrosine, patients should be warned about engaging in activities requiring mental alertness and motor coordination, such as driving a motor vehicle or operating machinery metyrosine may have additive side effects with alcohol and other CNS depressants, e.g., hypnotics, sedatives, and tranquilizers.

Patients should be advised to maintain a liberal fluid intake. (See PRECAUTIONS, General.)

LABORATORY TEST INTERFERENCE

Spurious increases in urinary catecholamines may be observed in patients receiving metyrosine due to the presence of metabolites of the drug.

CARCINOGENESIS, MUTAGENESIS, AND IMPAIRMENT OF FERTILITY

Long-term carcinogenic studies in animals and studies on mutagenesis and impairment of fertility have not been performed with metyrosine.

PREGNANCY CATEGORY C

Animal reproduction studies have not been conducted with metyrosine. It is also not known whether metyrosine can cause fetal harm when administered to a pregnant woman or can affect reproduction capacity. Metyrosine should be given to a pregnant woman only if clearly needed.

NURSING MOTHERS

It is not known whether metyrosine is excreted in human milk. Because many drugs are excreted in human mmilk, caution should be exercised when metyrosine is administered to a nursing woman.

PEDIATRIC USE

Safety and effectiveness in children under 12 years of age have not been established.

DRUG INTERACTIONS:

Caution should be observed in administering metyrosine to patients receiving phenothiazines or haloperidol because the extrapyramidal effects of these drugs can be expected to be potentiated by inhibition of catecholamine synthesis.

Concurrent use of metyrosine with alcohol or other CNS depressants can increase their sedative effects. (See WARNINGS and PRECAUTIONS.)

ADVERSE REACTIONS:

CENTRAL NERVOUS SYSTEM

Sedation: The most common adverse reaction to metyrosine is moderate to severe sedation, which has been observed in almost all patients. It occurs at both low and high dosages. Sedative effects begin within the first 24 hours of therapy, are maximal after two to three days and tend to wane during the next few days. Sedation usually is not obvious after one week unless the dosage is increased, but at dosages greater than 2000 mg/day some degree of sedation or fatigue may persist.

In most patients who experience sedation, temporary changes in sleep pattern occur following withdrawal of the drug. Changes consist of insomnia that may last for two or three days and feelings of increased alertness and ambition. Even patients who do not experience sedation while on metyrosine may report symptoms of psychic stimulation when the drug is discontinued.

EXTRAPYRAMIDAL SIGNS

Extrapyramidal signs such as drooling, speech difficulty, and tremor have been reported in approximately 10 percent of patients. These occasionally have been accompanied by trismus and frank parkinsonism.

ADVERSE REACTIONS: *(cont'd)*

ANXIETY AND PSYCHIC DISTURBANCES

Anxiety and psychic disturbances such as depression, hallucinations, disorientation, and confusion may occur. These effects seem to be dose-dependent and may disappear with reduction of dosage.

Diarrhea

Diarrhea occurs in about 10 percent of patients and may be severe. Antidiarrheal agents may be required if continuation of metyrosine is necessary.

Miscellaneous

Infrequently, slight swelling of the breast, galactorrhea, nasal stuffiness, decreased salivation, dry mouth, headache, nausea, vomiting, abdominal pain, and impotence or failure of ejaculation may occur. Crystalluria (see PRECAUTIONS) and transient dysuria and hematuria have been observed in a few patients. Eosinophilia,increased SGOT levels, peripheral edema, and hypersensitivity reactions such as urticaria and pharyngeal edema have been reported rarely.

OVERDOSAGE:

Signs of metyrosine overdosage include those central nervous system effects observed in some patients even at low dosages.

At doses excedding 200 mg/day, some degree of sedation or feeling of fatigue may persist. Doses of 2000-4000 mg/day can result in in anxiety or agitated depression, neuromuscular effects (including fine tremor of the hands, gross tremor of the trunk, tightening of the jaw with trismus), diarrhea, and decreased salivation with dry mouth

Reduction of drug dose or cessation of treatment results in the disappearance of these symptoms.

The acute toxicity of metyrosine was 442 mg/kg and 752 mg/kg in the female mouse and rat respectively.

DOSAGE AND ADMINISTRATION:

The recommended initial dosage of metyrosine for adults and children 12 years of age and older is 250 mg orally four times daily. This may be increased by 250 mg to 500 mg every day to a maximum of 4.0 g/day in divided doses. When used for preoperative preparation, the optimally effective dosage of metyrosine should be given for at least five to seven days.

Optimally effective dosages of metyrosine usually are between 2.0 and 3.0 g/day, and the dose should be titrated by monitoring clinical symptoms and catecholamine excretion. In patients who are hypertensive, dosage should be titrated to achieve normalization of blood pressure and control of clinical symptoms. In patients who are usually normotensive, dosage should be titrated to the amount that will reduce urinary metanephrines and/or vanillylmandelic acid by 50 percent or more.

If patients are not adequately controlled by the use of metyrosine, an alpha-adrenergic blocking agent (phenoxybenzamine) should be added.

Use of metyrosine in children under 12 years of age has been limited and a dosage schedule for this age group cannot be given.

HOW SUPPLIED - EQUIVALENTS NOT AVAILABLE:

Capsule, Gelatin - Oral - 250 mg

100's $142.49 DEMSER, Merck 00006-0690-68

MEXILETINE HYDROCHLORIDE *(001806)*

CATEGORIES: Antiarrhythmic Agents; Arrhythmia; Cardiovascular Drugs; Local Anesthetics; Tachycardia; Pregnancy Category C; FDA Approved 1985 Dec; Patent Expiration 1994 Jun

BRAND NAMES: *Mexihexal* (Germany); *Mexilen*; *Mexitec*; **Mexitil** *(International brand names outside U.S. in italics)*

FORMULARIES: BC-BS; Medi-Cal

COST OF THERAPY: $900.30 (Arrhythmia; Capsule; 200 mg; 3/day; 365 days)

DESCRIPTION:

Mexiletine hydrochloride is an orally active antiarrhythmic agent available as 150 mg, 200 mg and 250 mg capsules. 100 mg of mexiletine hydrochloride is equivalent to 83.31 mg of mexiletine base. It is a white to off-white crystalline powder with slightly bitter taste, freely soluble in water and in alcohol. Mexiletine HCl has a pKa of 9.2.

Chemically, mexiletine HCl is 1-methyl-2-(2, 6-xylyloxy) ethylamine hydrochloride.

Mexitil Capsules contain the following inactive ingredients: colloidal silicon dioxide, corn starch, magnesium stearate, titanium dioxide, gelatin, FD&C Red No. 40, D&C Red No. 28 and FD&C Blue No. 1; the Mexitil 150 mg and 250 mg capsule also contain FD&C yellow No. 10. Mexitil capsules may contain one or more of the following components: sodium lauryl sulfate, sodium propionate, edetate calcium disodium, benzyl alcohol, carboxymethylcellulose sodium, glycerin, butylparaben, propyl paraben, methylparaben, pharmaceutical glaze, ethylene glycol monoethylether, soya lecithin, dimethylpolysiloxane, refined shellac (food grade) and other inactive ingredients.

CLINICAL PHARMACOLOGY:

Mechanism of Action: Mexiletine HCl is a local anesthetic, antiarrhythmic agent, structurally similar to lidocaine, but orally active. In animal studies, mexiletine HCl has been to be effective in the suppression of induced ventricular arrhythmias, including those induced by glycoside toxicity & coronary artery ligation. Mexiletine HCl,like lidocaine, inhibits the inward sodium current, thus reducing the rate of rise of the action potential, Phase O. Mexiletine HCl decreased the effective refractory period (ERP) in Purkinje fibers. The decrease in ERP was of lesser magnitude than the decrease in action potential duration (APD), with a resulting increase in the ERP/APD ratio.

Electrophysiology in Man: Mexiletine is a Class 1B antiarrhythmic compound with electrophysiologic properties in man similar to those of lidocaine, but dissimilar from quinidine, procainamide, and disopyramide.

In patients with normal conduction systems, mexiletine HCl has a minimal effect on cardiac impulse generation and propagation. In clinical trials, no development of second-degree or third-degree AV block was observed. Mexiletine HCl did not prolong ventricular depolarization (QRS duration) or repolarization (QT intervals) as measured by electrocardiography. Theoretically, therefore, mexiletine HCl may be useful in the treatment of ventricular arrhythmias associated with a prolonged QT interval.

In patients with pre-existing conduction defects, depression of the sinus rate, prolongation of sinus nod recovery time, decreased conduction velocity and increased effective refractory period of the intraventricular conduction system have occasionally been observed.

CLINICAL PHARMACOLOGY: *(cont'd)*

The antiarrhythmic effect of mexiletine HCl has been established in controlled comparative trials against placebo, quinidine, procainamide and disopyramide. Mexiletine HCl, at doses of 200-400 mg q8h, produced a significant reduction of ventricular premature beats, paired beats, and episodes of non-sustained ventricular tachycardia compared to placebo and was similar in effectiveness to the active agents. Among all patients entered into the studies, about 30% in each treatment group had a 70% or greater reduction in PVC count and about 40% failed to complete the 3 month studies because of adverse effects. Follow-up of patients from the controlled trials has demonstrated continued effectiveness of mexiletine HCl in long-term use.

Hemodynamics: Hemodynamic studies in a limited number of patients, with normal or abnormal myocardial function, following oral administration of mexiletine HCl, have shown small, usually not statistically significant, decreases in cardiac output and increased in systemic vascular resistance, but no significant negative inotropic effect. Blood pressure and pulse rate remain essentially unchanged. Mild depression of myocardial function, similar to that produced by lidocaine, has occasionally been observed following intravenous mexiletine HCl therapy in patients with cardiac disease.

Pharmacokinetics: Mexiletine HCl is well absorbed (-90%) from the gastrointestinal tract. Unlike lidocaine, its first-pass metabolism is low. Peak blood levels are reached in two to three hours. In normal subjects, the plasma elimination half-life of mexiletine HCl is approximately 10-12 hours. It is 50-60% bound to plasma protein, with a volume of distribution of 5-7 liters/kg. Mexiletine HCl is metabolized in the liver. Approximately 10% is excreted unchanged by the kidney. While urinary pH does not normally have much influence on elimination, marked changes in the urinary pH influence the rate of excretion; acidification accelerates excretion, while alkalinization retards it.

Several metabolites of mexiletine have shown minimal antiarrhythmic activity in animal models. The most active is the minor metabolite N-methylmexiletine, which is less than 20% as potent as mexiletine. The urinary excretion of N-methylmexiletine in man is less than 0.5% Thus the therapeutic activity of mexiletine HCl is due to the parent compound.

Hepatic impairment prolongs the elimination half-life of mexiletine HCl. In eight patients with moderate to severe liver disease, the mean half-life was approximately 25 hours.

Consistent with the limited renal elimination of mexiletine HCl, little change in the half-life has been detected in patients with reduced renal function. In eight patients with creatinine clearance less than 10 ml/min, the mean plasma elimination half-life was 15.7 hours; in seven patients with creatinine clearance between 11-40 ml/min, the mean half-life was 13.4 hours.

The absorption rate of mexiletine HCl is reduced in clinical situations such as acute myocardial infarction in which gastric emptying time is increased. Narcotics, atropine and magnesium-aluminum hydroxide have also been reported to slow the absorption of mexiletine HCl. Metoclopramide has been reported to accelerate absorption.

Mexiletine plasma levels of at least 0.5 mcg/ml are generally required for therapeutic response. An increase in the frequency of central nervous system adverse effects has been observed when plasma levels exceed 2.0 mcg/ml. Thus the therapeutic range is approximately 0.5 to 2.0 mcg/ml. Plasma levels within the therapeutic range can be attained with either three times daily or twice daily dosing but peak to trough differences are greater with the latter regimen, creating the possibility of adverse effects at peak and antiarrhythmic escape at trough. Nevertheless, some patients may be transferred successfully to the twice daily regimen. (See DOSAGE AND ADMINISTRATION.)

INDICATIONS AND USAGE:

Mexiletine HCl is indicated for the treatment of documented ventricular arrhythmias, such as sustained ventricular tachycardia, that, in the judgement of the physicians, are life-threatening. Because of the proarrhythmic effects of mexiletine HCl, its use with lesser arrhythmias is generally not recommended. Treatment of patients with asymptomatic ventricular premature contractions should be avoided.

Initiation of mexiletine HCl treatment, as with other antiarrhythmic agents used to treat life-threatening arrhythmias, should be carried out in the hospital.

Antiarrhythmic drugs have not been shown to enhance survival in patients with ventricular arrhythmias.

CONTRAINDICATIONS:

Mexiletine HCl is contraindicated in the presence of cardiogenic shock or pre-existing second- or third-degree AV block (if no pacemaker is present).

WARNINGS:

Mortality: In the National Heart, Lung and Blood Institute's Cardiac Arrhythmia Suppression Trial (CAST), a long-term, multi-centered, randomized, double-bind study in patients with asymptomatic non-life-threatening ventricular arrhythmias who had had myocardial infarctions more than six days but less than two years previously, and excessive mortality or non-fatal cardiac arrest rate was seen in patients treated with encainide or flecainide (56/730) compared with that seen in patients assigned to matched placebo-treated groups (22/725). The average duration of treatment with encainide or flecainide in this study was ten months.

The applicability of these results to other populations (*e.g.*, those without recent myocardial infarction) or to other antiarrhythmic drugs is uncertain, but at present it is prudent to consider any antiarrhythmic agent to have a significant risk in patients with structural heart disease.

Acute Liver Injury: In postmarketing experience abnormal liver function tests have been reported, some in the first few weeks of therapy with mexiletine HCl. Most of these have been observed in the setting of congestive heart failure or ischemia and their relationship to mexiletine HCl has not been established.

PRECAUTIONS:

General: If a ventricular pacemaker is operative, patients with second or third degree heart block may be treated with mexiletine HCl if continuously monitored. A limited number of patients (45 of 475 in controlled clinical trials) with pre-existing first degree AV block were treated with mexiletine HCl; none of these patients developed second or third degree AV block. Caution should be exercised when it is used in such patients or in patients with pre-existing sinus node dysfunction or intraventricular conduction abnormalities.

Like other antiarrhythmics Mexiletine HCl can cause worsening of arrhythmias. This has been uncommon in patients with less serious arrhythmias (Frequent premature beats or non-sustained ventricular tachycardia; see ADVERSE REACTIONS), but is of greater concern in patients with life-threatening arrhythmias such as sustained ventricular tachycardia. In patients with such arrhythmias subjected to programmed electrical stimulation or to exercise provocation, 10-15% of patients had exacerbation of the arrhythmia, a rate not greater than that of other agents.

Mexiletine HCl should be used with caution in patients with hypotension and severe congestive heart failure because of the potential for aggravating these conditions.

Since mexiletine HCl is metabolized in the liver, and hepatic impairment has been reported to prolong the elimination half-life of mexiletine HCl, patients with liver disease should be followed carefully while receiving mexiletine HCl. The same caution should be observed in patients with hepatic dysfunction secondary to decongestive heart failure.

PRECAUTIONS: *(cont'd)*

Concurrent drug therapy or dietary regimens which may markedly after urinary pH should avoided during mexiletine HCl therapy. The minor fluctuations in urinary pH associated with normal diet do not affect the excretion of mexiletine HCl.

SGOT Elevation and Liver Injury: In three-month controlled trials, elevations of SGOT greater than three times the upper limit of normal occurred in about 1% of both mexiletine-treated and control patients. Approximately 2% of patients in the mexiletine compassionate use program had elevations of SGOT greater than or equal to three times the upper limit of normal. These elevations frequently occurred in association with identifiable clinical events and therapeutic measures such as congestive heart failure, acute myocardial infarction, blood transfusions and other medications. These elevations were often asymptomatic and transient, usually not associated with elevated bilirubin levels and usually did not require discontinuation of therapy. Marked elevations of SGOT (> 1000 U/L) were seen before death in four patients with end-stage cardiac disease (severe congestive heart failure, cardiogenic shock).

Rare instances of severe liver injury, including hepatic necrosis, have been reported in association with mexiletine HCl treatment. It is recommended that patients in whom an abnormal liver test has occurred, or who have signs or symptoms suggesting liver dysfunction, be carefully evaluated. If persistent or worsening elevation of hepatic enzymes is detected, consideration should be given to discontinuing therapy.

Blood Dyscrasias: Among 10,867 patients treated with mexiletine in the compassionate use program, marked leukopenia (neutrophils less than 1000/mm^3) or agranulocytosis were seen in 0.06% and milder depressions of leukocytes were seen in 0.08%, and thrombocytopenia was observed in 0.16%. Many of these patients were seriously ill and receiving concomitant medications with known hematologic adverse effects. Rechallenge with mexiletine in several cases was negative. Marked leukopenia or agranulocytosis did not occur in any patient receiving mexiletine HCl alone; five of the six cases of agranulocytosis were associated with procainamide (sustained release preparations in four) and one with vinblastine. If significant hematologic changes are observed the patient should be carefully evaluated, and, if warranted, mexiletine HCl should be discontinued. Blood counts usually return to normal within one month of discontinuation. (See ADVERSE REACTIONS.)

Convulsions (seizures) did not occur in mexiletine HCl controlled clinical trials. In the compassionate use program, convulsions were reported in about 2 of 1000 patients. Twenty-eight percent of these patients discontinued therapy. Convulsions were reported in patients with and without a prior history of seizures. Mexiletine should be used with caution in patients with known seizure disorder.

CARCINOGENESIS, MUTAGENESIS, AND IMPAIRMENT OF FERTILITY

Studies of carcinogenesis in rats (24 months) and mice (18 months) did not demonstrate any tumorigenic potential. Mexiletine HCl was found to be non-mutagenic in the Ames test. Mexiletine HCl did not impair fertility in the rat.

PREGNANCY, TERATOGENIC EFFECTS, PREGNANCY CATEGORY C

Reproduction studies performed with mexiletine HCl in rats, mice and rabbits at doses up to four times the maximum human oral dose (24 mg/kg in a 50 kg patient) revealed no evidence of teratogenicity or impaired fertility but did show an increase in fetal resorption. There are no adequate and well-controlled studies in pregnant women; this drug should be used in pregnancy only if the potential benefit justifies the potential risk to the fetus.

NURSING MOTHERS

Mexiletine HCl appears in human milk in concentrations similar to those ,observed in plasma. Therefore, if the use of mexiletine HCl is deemed essential, an alternative method of infant feeding should be considered.

PEDIATRIC USE

Safety and effectiveness in children have not been established.

DRUG INTERACTIONS:

In a large compassionate use program mexiletine HCl has been used concurrently with commonly employed antianginal, antihypertensive, and anticoagulant drugs without observed interactions. A variety of antiarrhythmics such as quinidine or propanolol were also added, sometimes with improved control of ventricular ectopy. When phenytoin or other hepatic enzyme inducers such as rifampin and phenobarbital have been taken concurrently with mexiletine HCl, lowered mexiletine HCl plasma levels gave been reported. Monitoring of mexiletine HCl plasma levels is recommended during such concurrent use to avoid ineffective therapy.

In a formal study, benzodiazepine were shown not to effect mexiletine HCl plasma concentration. ECG intervals (PR, QRS, and QT) were not effected by concurrent mexiletine HCl and digoxin, diuretics, or propanolol.

Concurrent administration of cimetidine and mexiletine HCl has been reported to increase, decrease, or leave unchanged mexiletine HCl plasma levels; Therefore patients should be followed carefully during concurrent therapy.

Mexiletine HCl does not alter serum digoxin levels but magnesium-aluminum hydroxide, when used to treat gastrointestinal symptoms due to mexiletine HCl, has been reported to lower serum digoxin levels.

Concurrent use of mexiletine HCl and theophylline may lead to increased plasma theophylline levels. One controlled study in eight normal subjects showed a 72% mean increase (range 35-136%) in plasma theophylline levels. This increase was observed at the first test point which was the second day after starting mexiletine HCl. Theophylline plasma levels returns to pre-mexiletine HCl values within 48 hours after discontinuing mexiletine HCl. If mexiletine HCl and theophylline are to be used concurrently,theophylline blood levels should be monitored, particularly when the mexiletine HCl dose is changed. An appropriate adjustment in the theophylline dose should be considered.

Additionally, in one controlled study in five normal subjects and seven patients, the clearance if caffeine was decreased 50% following the administration of mexiletine HCl.

ADVERSE REACTIONS:

Mexiletine HCl commonly produces reversible gastrointestinal and nervous system adverse reactions but is otherwise well-tolerated. Mexiletine HCl has been evaluated in 483 patients in one-month ad three-month controlled studies and in over 10,000 patients in a large compassionate use program. Dosages in the controlled studies ranged from 600-1200 mg/day: some patients (8%) in the compassionate use program were treated with higher daily doses (1600-3200 mg/day). In the three-month controlled trials comparing mexiletine HCl to quinidine, procainamide and disopyramide, the most frequent adverse reactions were upper gastrointestinal distress (41%), lightheadedness (10.5%), tremor (12.6%) and coordination difficulties (10.2%). Similar frequency and incidence were observed in the one-month placebo-controlled trial. Although these reactions were generally not serious, and were dose-related and reversible with a reduction in dosage, by taking the drug with food or antacid or by therapy discontinuation, they led to therapy discontinuation in 40% of patients in the controlled trials. A tabulation of the adverse events reported in the one-month placebo controlled trial follows (TABLE 1):

A tabulation of adverse reactions occurring in one percent or more of patients in the three-month controlled studies follows (TABLE 2):

ADVERSE REACTIONS: *(cont'd)*

TABLE 1 Mexiletine Hydrochloride, Adverse Reactions
Comparative Incidence (%) of Adverse Events Among Patients Treated with Mexiletine and Placebo in the 4-Week, Double-Blind Crossover Trial

	Mexiletine N = 53	Placebo N = 49
Cardiovascular		
Palpitations	7.5	10.2
Chest Pain	7.5	4.1
Increased Ventricular Arrhythmias/PVC's	1.9	-
Digestive		
Nausea/Vomiting/Heartburn	39.6	6.1
Central Nervous System		
Dizziness/Lightheadedness	26.4	14.3
Tremor	13.2	-
Nervousness	11.3	6.1
Coordination Difficulties	9.4	-
Changes in Sleep Habits	7.5	16.3
Paresthesias/Numbness	3.8	2.0
Weakness	1.9	4.1
Fatigue	1.9	2.0
Tinnitus	1.9	4.1
Confusion/Clouded Sensorium	1.9	2.0
Other		
Headache	7.5	6.1
Blurred Vision/Visual Disturbances	7.5	2.0
Dyspnea	5.7	10.2
Rash	3.8	2.0
Non-specific Edema	3.8	-

TABLE 2 Mexiletine Hydrochloride, Adverse Reactions
Comparative Incidence (%) of Adverse Events Among Patients Treated with Mexiletine or Control Drugs in The 12-week Double-Blind Trials

	Mexiletine N = 430	Quinidine N = 262	Procainamide N = 78	Disopyramide N = 69
Cardiovascular				
Palpitations	4.3	4.6	1.3	5.8
Chest Pain	2.6	3.4	1.3	2.9
Angina/Angina-like Pain	1.7	1.9	2.6	2.9
Increased Ventricular Arrhythmias/PVC's	1.0	2.7	2.7	-
Digestive				
Nausea/Vomiting/Heartburn	39.3	21.4	33.3	14.5
Diarrhea	5.2	33.2	2.6	8.7
Constipation	4.0	-	6.4	11.6
Changes in Appetite	2.6	1.9	-	-
Abdominal Pain/Cramps/Discomfort	1.2	1.5	-	1.4
Central Nervous System				
Dizziness/Lightheadedness	18.9	14.1	14.1	2.9
Tremor	13.2	2.3	3.8	1.4
Coordination Difficulties	9.7	1.1	1.3	-
Changes in Sleep Habits	7.1	2.7	11.5	8.7
Weakness	5.0	5.3	7.7	2.9
Nervousness	5.0	1.9	6.4	5.8
Fatigue	3.8	5.7	5.1	1.4
Speech Difficulties	2.6	0.4	-	-
Confusion/Clouded Sensorium	2.6	-	3.8	-
Paresthesias/Numbness	2.4	2.3	2.6	-
Tinnitus	2.4	1.5	-	-
Depression	2.4	1.1	1.3	1.4
Other				
Blurred Vision/Visual Disturbances	5.7	3.1	5.1	7.2
Headache	5.7	6.9	7.7	4.3
Rash	4.2	3.8	10.3	1.4
Dyspnea/Respiratory	3.3	3.1	5.1	2.9
Dry Mouth	2.8	1.9	5.1	14.5
Arthralgia	1.7	2.3	5.1	1.4
Fever	1.2	3.1	2.6	-

Less than 1%: Syncope, edema, hot flashes, hypertension, short-term memory loss, loss of consciousness, other physiological changes, diaphoresis, urinary hesitancy/retention, malaise, impotence/decreased libido, pharyngitis, congestive heart failure.

An additional group of over 10,000 patients has been treated in a program allowing administration of Mexiletine HCl under compassionate use circumstances. These patients were seriously ill with the large majority on multiple drug therapy. Twenty-four percent of the patients continued in the program for one year or longer. Adverse reactions leading to therapy, discontinuation occurred in 15 percent of patients (usually upper gastrointestinal system or nervous system effects). In general, the more common adverse reactions were similar to those in the controlled trials. Less common adverse events related to mexiletine HCl use include.

Cardiovascular System: Syncope and hypotension, each about 6 in 1000; bradycardia, about 4 in 1000; angina/angina-like pain, about 3 in 1000; edema, atrioventricular block.conduction disturbances and hot flashes, each about 2 in 1000; atrial arrhythmias. hypertension and cardiogenic shock, each about 1 in 1000.

Central Nervous System: Short-term memory loss, about 9 in 1000 patients; hallucinations and other psychological changes, each about 3 in 1000; psychosis and convulsions/seizures, each about 2 in 1000, loss of consciousness, about 6 in 10,000.

Digestive: Dysphagia, about 2 in 1000; peptic ulcer, about 8 in 10,000; upper gastrointestinal bleeding, about 7 in 10,000; esophageal ulceration, about 1 in 10,00. Rare cases of severe hepatitis/acute hepatic necrosis.

Skin: Rare cases of exfoliative dermatitis and Stevens-Johnson Syndrome with Mexiletine HCl treatment have been reported.

Laboratory: Abnormal liver function tests, about 5 in 100 patients, positive ANA and thrombocytopenia, each about 2 in 1000; leukopenia (including neutropenia and agranulocytosis), about 1 in 1000; myelofibrosis, about 2 in 10,000 patients.

Other: Diaphoresis, about 6 in 1000; altered taste, about 5 in 1000; salivary changes, hair loss and impotence/decreased libido, each about 4 in 1000; malaise, about 3 in 100; urinary hesitancy/retention, each about 2 in 1000; hiccups, dry skin, laryngeal and pharyngeal changes and changes in oral mucous membranes, each about 1 in 1000; SLE syndrome about 4 in 10,000.

Hematology: Blood dyscrasias were not seen in the controlled clinical trials but did occur among 10,867 patients treated with mexiletine in the compassionate use program (see PRECAUTIONS).

ADVERSE REACTIONS: *(cont'd)*

Myelofibrosis was reported in two patients in the compassionate use program; one was receiving long-term thiotepa therapy and the other had pretreatment myeloid abnormalities.

In postmarketing experience, there have been isolated, spontaneous reports of pulmonary changes including pulmonary fibrosis during mexiletine HCl therapy with or without other drugs or diseases that are known to produce pulmonary toxicity. A causal relationship to mexiletine HCl therapy has not been established. In addition, there have been isolated reports of exacerbation of congestive heart failure in patients with pre-existing compromised ventricular function.

OVERDOSAGE:

Nine cases of mexiletine HCl overdosage have been reported; two were fatal. In one fatality, 440 mg of the drug was ingested. In the other death, the dose ingested was unknown. There has been a report of non-fatal ingestion of 8000 mg. Symptoms associated with overdosage include nausea, hypotension, sinus bradycardia, paresthesia, seizures, intermittent left bundle branch block and temporary asystole.

There is no specific antidote for mexiletine HCl. Acidification of the urine, which will accelerate the excretion of mexiletine, may be useful. Treatment of overdosage should be supportive, and may include the administration of atropine if hypotension or bradycardia occurs.

DOSAGE AND ADMINISTRATION:

The dosage of mexiletine HCl must be individualized on the basis of response and tolerance, both of which are dose-related. Administration with food or antacid is recommended. Initiate mexiletine HCl therapy with 200 mg every eight hours when rapid control of arrhythmia is not essential. A minimum of two to three days between dose adjustments is recommended. Dose may be adjusted in 50 or 100 mg increments up or down.

As with any antiarrhythmic drug, clinical and electrocardiographic evaluation (including Holter monitoring if necessary for evaluation) are needed to determine whether the desired antiarrhythmic effect has been obtained and to guide titration and dose adjustment.

Satisfactory control can be achieved in most patients by 200 to 300 mg given every eight hours with food or antacid. If satisfactory response had not been achieved at 300 mg q8h, and the patient tolerates mexiletine HCl well, a dose of 400 mg q8h may be tried. As the severity of CNS side effects increases with total daily dose, the dose should not exceed 1200 mg/day.

In general, patients with renal failure will require the usual doses of mexiletine HCl. Patients with severe liver disease, however, may require lower doses and must be monitored closely. Similarly, marked right-sided congestive heart failure can reduce hepatic metabolism and reduce the needed dose. Plasma level may also be affected by certain concomitant drugs (see DRUG INTERACTIONS).

Loading Dose: When rapid control of ventricular arrhythmia is essential, an initial loading dose of 400 mg of mexiletine HCl may be administered, followed by a 200 mg dose in eight hours. Onset of therapeutic effect is usually observed within 30 minutes to two hours.

Q12H Dosage Schedule: Some patients responding to mexiletine HCl may be transferee to a 12-hour dosage schedule to improve convenience and compliance. If adequate suppression is achieved on a mexiletine HCl dose of 300 mg or less every eight hours, the same total daily dose may be given in divided doses every 12 hours while carefully monitoring the degree of suppression of ventricular ectopy. This dose may be adjusted up to a maximum of 450 mg every 12 hours to achieve the desired response.

Transferring to Mexiletine HCl: The following dosage schedule, based on theoretical considerations rather than experimental data, is suggested for transferring patients from other Class I oral antiarrhythmic agents to mexiletine HCl: mexiletine HCl treatment may be initiated with a 200 mg dose, and titrated to response as described above, 6-12 hours after the last dose of quinidine sulfate, 3-6 hours after the last dose of procainamide, 6-12 hours after the last dose of disopyramide or 8-12 hours after the last dose of tocainide.

In patients in whom withdrawal of the previous antiarrhythmic agent is likely to produce life-threatening arrhythmias, hospitalization of the patient is recommended.

When transferring from lidocaine to mexiletine HCl, the lidocaine infusion should be stopped when the first oral dose of mexiletine HCl is administered. The infusion line should be left open until suppression of the arrhythmias appears to be satisfactorily maintained. Consideration should be given to the similarity of the adverse effects of lidocaine and mexiletine HCl and the possibility that they may be additive.

HOW SUPPLIED:

Mexitil is supplied in hard gelatin capsules containing 150 mg, 200 mg, or 250 mg of mexiletine hydrochloride:

Mexitil 150 mg capsules are red and caramel with the marking Bl 66.

Mexitil 200 mg capsules are red with the marking Bl 67.

Mexitil 250 mg capsules are red and aqua green with the marking Bl 68.

Store below 86°F (30°C).

HOW SUPPLIED - RATED THERAPEUTICALLY EQUIVALENT:

Capsule, Gelatin - Oral - 150 mg

100's	$69.05	Mexiletine Hcl, Rugby	00536-5748-01
100's	$69.05	Mexiletine Hcl, HL Moore Drug Exch	00839-8005-06
100's	$69.06	Mexiletine Hcl, Roxane	00054-2616-25
100's	$69.24	Mexiletine Hcl, Novopharm (US)	55953-0739-40
100's	$72.60	Mexiletine Hcl, Roxane	00054-8616-25
100's	$72.60	Mexiletine Hcl, Novopharm (US)	55953-0739-41
100's	**$78.65**	**MEXITIL, Boehringer Pharms**	**00597-0066-01**
100's	**$82.68**	**MEXITIL, Boehringer Pharms**	**00597-0066-61**
500's	$328.89	Mexiletine Hcl, Novopharm (US)	55953-0739-70
1000's	$623.16	Mexiletine Hcl, Novopharm (US)	55953-0739-80

Capsule, Gelatin - Oral - 200 mg

100's	$82.22	Mexiletine Hcl, Novopharm (US)	55953-0740-40
100's	$82.24	Mexiletine Hcl, Roxane	00054-2617-25
100's	$82.24	Mexiletine Hcl, Rugby	00536-5749-01
100's	$82.28	Mexiletine Hcl, HL Moore Drug Exch	00839-8006-06
100's	$86.35	Mexiletine Hcl, Roxane	00054-8617-25
100's	$86.35	Mexiletine Hcl, Novopharm (US)	55953-0740-41
100's	**$93.66**	**MEXITIL, Boehringer Pharms**	**00597-0067-01**
100's	**$98.34**	**MEXITIL, Boehringer Pharms**	**00597-0067-61**
500's	$390.55	Mexiletine Hcl, Novopharm (US)	55953-0740-70
1000's	$739.98	Mexiletine Hcl, Novopharm (US)	55953-0740-80

Capsule, Gelatin - Oral - 250 mg

100's	$95.65	Mexiletine Hcl, HL Moore Drug Exch	00839-8007-06
100's	$95.66	Mexiletine Hcl, Roxane	00054-2618-25
100's	$95.66	Mexiletine Hcl, Novopharm (US)	55953-0741-40
100's	**$108.94**	**MEXITIL, Boehringer Pharms**	**00597-0068-01**

MEZLOCILLIN SODIUM MONOHYDRATEE

(001807)

CATEGORIES: Abdominal Abscess; Anti-Infectives; Antibiotics; Antimicrobials; Broad Spectrum Penicillins; Cellulitis; Cholecystitis; Endometritis; Gonorrhea; Gynecologic Infections; Hepatic Abscess; Intra-Abdominal Infections; Pelvic Inflammatory Disease; Penicillins; Peritonitis; Pulmonary Abscess; Respiratory Tract Infections; Septicemia; Skin Infections; Urinary Tract Infections; Pregnancy Category B; FDA Approval Pre 1982

BRAND NAMES: *Baypen* (France, Germany); **Mezlin**
(International brand names outside U.S. in italics)

DESCRIPTION:

Sterile mezlocillin sodium monohydratee is a semisynthetic broad spectrum penicillin antibiotic for parenteral administration. It is the monohydrate sodium salt of 6-<D-2[3-(methylsulfonyl)-2-OXO- imidazolidine-1-carboxamido]-2-phenyl acetamido> penicillanic acid.

Mezlocillin sodium monohydrate has a molecular weight of 579.6 and contains 42.6 mg (1.85 mEq) of sodium per one gram of mezlocillin activity. The dosage form is supplied as a sterile white to pale yellow crystalline powder, which is freely soluble in water. Each vial contains mezlocillin sodium monohydratee equivalent to 1g, 2g, 3g, or 4g of mezlocillin. When reconstituted, solutions of mezlocillin sodium monohydrate are clear and range from colorless to pale yellow with a pH of 4.5 to 8.0.

CLINICAL PHARMACOLOGY:

Intravenous Administration: In healthy adult volunteers, mean serum levels of mezlocillin 5 minutes after a 5-minute intravenous injection of 1g, 2g or 5g are 100, 253 or 411 mcg/ml, respectively. Serum levels, as noted in TABLE 1, lack dose proportionality.

TABLE 1 Mezlocillin Serum Levels In Adults (mcg/ml) 5 Min IV Injection

DOSE/ 0	5 min	10 min	20 min	30 min	1hr	2hr	3hr	4hr	6hr	8hr
1g 149 (132-185)	100 (64-143)	66 (47-87)	50 (31-87)	40 (22-83)	18 (8-31)	5.3 (3.3-7.7)	2.5 (1.7-3.7)	1.7 (0.7-2.8)	0.5 (0-1.2)	0.1 (0-0.2)
2g 314 (207-362)	253 (161-364)	161 (113-214)	117 (76-174)	82 (55-112)	56 (23-88)	20 (7.5-32)	11 (3.8-16)	4.4 (1.6-8.7)	1.5 (0.5-2.6)	0.5 0.1-1.4)
5g 547 (268-854)	411 (199-597)	357 (246-456)	250 (203-353)	226 (190-333)	131 (104-193)	76 (59-104)	31 (20-40)	13 (6.4--17)	4.6 (2.1--9.4)	1.9 (1.1-3.6)

Fifteen minutes after a 4g intravenous injection (2-5 min), the concentration in serum is 254 mcg/ml. 1 hour and 4 hours later levels are 93 mcg/ml and 9.1 mcg/ml respectively (TABLE 2).

TABLE 2 Mezlocillin Serum Levels In Adults (mcg/ml) 2-5 Min IV Injection

0	15 min	30 min	45 min	1 hr	2 hr	3 hr	4 hr	6 hr
DOSE 4g -	254 (155-400)	163 (99-260)	122 (78-215)	93 (67-133)	47 (22-96)	20 (8-45)	9.1 (6-13)	8.4 (5-17)

After an intravenous infusion (15 min) of 3g, mean levels 15 minutes after dosing are 269 mcg/ml (170-280).

A 30-minute intravenous infusion of 3g produces mean peak concentrations of 263 mcg/ml; 1 hour and 4 hours later the concentrations are 57 mcg/ml and 4.4 mcg/ml respectively (TABLE 3).

TABLE 3 Mezlocillin Serum Levels In Adults (mcg/ml) 30 Min IV Infusion

DOSE	0	5 min	15 min	30 min	45 min	1 hr	2 hr	3 hr	4 hr	6 hr	8 hr
3g	263 (87-489)	170 (6.3-371)	141 (75-301)	109 (56-288)	79 (41-135)	57 (28-100)	26 (14-55)	12 (5.8-26)	4.4 (2.2-6.5)	1.6 (1.0-3.4)	<1

Following intravenous infusion (2 hr.) of a 3g dose of mezlocillin every 4 hours for 7 days, mean peak serum concentrations are higher than 100 mcg/ml, and levels above 50 mcg/ml are maintained throughout dosing.

Intramuscular Administration: Mezlocillin sodium monohydrate is rapidly absorbed after intramuscular injection. In healthy volunteers, the mean peak serum concentration occurs approximately 45 minutes after a single dose of 1g and is about 15 mcg/ml. The oral administration of 1g probenecid before injection produces an increase in mezlocillin serum levels of about 50% After repetitive intramuscular doses of 1g mezlocillin every 6 hours, peak levels in the serum generally range between 35 and 45 mcg/ml. The relationship between the pharmacokinetics of intramuscular and intravenous dosing has not yet been clearly established.

General: As with other penicillins, mezlocillin is excreted primarily by glomerular filtration and tubular secretion. The rate of elimination is dose dependent and related to the degree of renal functional impairment. In patients with normal renal function, approximately 55% of the administered dose is recovered from the urine within the first 6 hours after dosing. Two hours after an intravenous injection of 2g, concentrations of active drug in urine generally exceed 4000 mcg/ml. By 4-6 hours after injection, concentrations usually decline to a range of about 50 to 200 mcg/ml. The serum elimination half-life of mezlocillin after intravenous dosing is approximately 55 minutes.

In patients with reduced renal function, the half-life is only slightly prolonged. Dosage adjustments are usually not necessary except in patients with severe renal impairment. (See DOSAGE AND ADMINISTRATION.) As with other penicillins, mezlocillin is metabolized only slightly, less than 10% of the drug excreted in the urine is in the form of the penicilloate or penilloate. The drug is readily removed from the serum by hemodialysis and, to a lesser extent by peritoneal dialysis.

CLINICAL PHARMACOLOGY: *(cont'd)*

Up to 26% of a dose of mezlocillin is recovered from the bile of patients with normal liver function. Following intravenous doses of 2 to 5g, concentrations of active drug in bile generally range from 500 to 2500 mcg/ml. The biliary excretion of mezlocillin is reduced in patients with common bile duct obstruction.

Mezlocillin is not appreciably absorbed when given orally. Following parenteral administration, the apparent volume of distribution is approximately equal to the extracellular fluid volume. The drug is present in active form in the serum, urine, bile, peritoneal fluid, pleural fluid, bronchial and wound secretions bone and other tissues. As with other penicillins, penetration into the cerebrospinal fluid (CSF) is generally poor, however higher CSF concentrations are obtained in the presence of meningeal inflammation.

Protein binding studies indicate that the degree of mezlocillin binding is low (16-42%) and depends upon testing methods and concentrations of drug studied.

MICROBIOLOGY

Mezlocillin is a bactericidal antibiotic which acts by interfacing with synthesis of cell wall components. It is active against a variety of gram-negative and gram-positive bacteria, including aerobic and anaerobic strains. Mezlocillin is usually active *in vitro* against most strains of the following organisms (TABLE 4).

TABLE 4

Gram-negative bacteria
Escherichia coli Klebsiella species (including *K. pneumoniae*)
Proteus mirabilis Enterobacter species
Proteus vulgaris Shigella species
Morganella morganii (formerly *P. morganii) Pseudomonas aeruginosa* (and other species)
Providencia rettgeri (formerly *P. rettgeri) Haemophilus influenzae*
Providencia stuartii Haemophilus parainfluenzae
Citrobacter species *Neisseria* species
Many strains of*Serratia, Salmonella* and Acinetobacter** are also susceptible.
Gram-positive bacteria *Staphylococcus aureus* (non-penicillinase producing strains);
Beta-hemolytic streptococci (Groups A and B);
Streptococcus pneumoniae (formerly *Diplococcus pneumoniae*);
Streptococcus faecalis (enterococcus)
Anaerobic Organisms *Peptococcus* species;
Peptostreptococcus species;
Clostridium species*; *Bacteroides* species (including *B fragilis* group);
Fusobacterium species*; *Veillonella* species*;
Eubacterium species*

*Mezlocillin has been shown to be active *in vitro* against these organisms, however clinical efficacy has not yet been established. Noteworthy is mezlocillin's broadened spectrum of *in vitro* activity against important pathogenic aerobic gram-negative bacteria, including strains of *Pseudomonas, Klebsiella, Enterobacter, Serratia, Proteus, Escherichia* and *Haemophilus,* as well as *Bacteroides* and other anaerobes, and its excellent inhibitory effect against gram-positive organisms including *Streptococcus faecalis (enterococcus).* It is inactive against penicillinase-producing strains of *Staphylococcus aureus.*

In vitro studies have shown that mezlocillin combined with an aminoglycoside (*e.g.,* gentamicin, tobramycin, amikacin, sisomicin) acts synergistically against strains of *Streptococcus faecalis* and *Pseudomonas aeruginosa.* In some instances, this combination also acts synergistically *in vitro* against other gram-negative bacteria such as *Serratia, Klebsiella* and *Acinetobacter* species.

Mezlocillin is slightly more active when tested at alkaline pH and, as with other penicillins, has reduced activity when tested in vitro with increasing inoculum. The minimum bactericidal concentration (MBC) generally exceeds the minimum inhibitory concentration (MIC) by a factor of 2 or 3. Resistance to mezlocillin in vitro develops slowly (multiple step mutation). Some strains of *Pseudomonas aeruginosa* have developed resistance fairly rapidly. Mezlocillin is not stable in the presence of penicillinase and strains of *Staphylococcus aureus*resistant to penicillin are also resistant to mezlocillin.

Susceptibility Testing

Quantitative methods that require measurement of zone diameters give good estimates of bacterial susceptibility. One such procedure* has been recommended for use with discs to test susceptibility to antimicrobials. When the causative organism is tested by the Kirby-Bauer method of disc susceptibility, a 75 mcg mezlocillin disc should give a zone of 18 mm or greater to indicate susceptibility. Zone sizes of 14 mm or less indicate resistance. Zone sizes of 15 to 17 mm indicate intermediate susceptibility. Susceptible strains of *Haemophilus* and *Neisseria* species give zones of $\geq$ 29 mm, resistant strains $\leq$28 mm. With this procedure a report from the laboratory of "Susceptible" indicates that the infecting organism is likely to respond to therapy. A report of "Resistant" indicates that the infecting organism is not likely to respond to therapy, other therapy should be selected. A report of "Intermediate Susceptibility" suggests that the organism may be susceptible if the infection is confined to tissues and fluids (*e.g.,* urine) in which high antibiotic levels are attained. The mezlocillin disc should be used for testing susceptibility to mezlocillin. In certain conditions, it may be desirable to do additional susceptibility testing by broth or agar dilution techniques. Dilution methods, preferably the agar plate dilution procedure, are most accurate for susceptibility testing of obligate anaerobes. *Enterobacteriaceae, Pseudomonas* species and *Acinetobacter* species are considered susceptible if the MIC of mezlocillin is no greater than 64 mcg/ml and are considered resistant if the MIC is greater than 128 mcg/ml. *Haemophilus* species and *Neisseria* species are considered susceptible if the MIC of mezlocillin is less than or equal to 1 mcg/ml. Mezlocillin standard is available for broth or agar dilution studies

INDICATIONS AND USAGE:

Mezlocillin sodium monohydrate is indicated for the treatment of serious infections caused by susceptible strains of the designated microorganisms in the conditions listed below:

Lower Respiratory Tract Infections including pneumonia and lung abscess caused by *Haemophilus influenzae, Klebsiella* species including *K pneumoniae, Proteus mirabilis. Pseudomonas* species including *P. aeruginosa. E Coli,* and *Bacteroides* species including *B. fragilis.*

Intra-Abdominal Infections including acute cholecystitis, cholangitis, peritonitis, hepatic abscess and intra-abdominal abscess caused by susceptible *E. coli Proteus mirabilis, Klebsiella* species, *Pseudomonas* species, *S. faecalis* (enterococcus).*Bacteroides* species, *Peptococcus* species, and *Peptostreptococcus* species.

Urinary Tract Infections caused by susceptible *E. coli, Proteus mirabilis* the indole positive *Proteus* species,*Morganella morganii; Klebsiella* species, *Enterobacter* species. *Serratia* species, *Pseudomonas* species, *S. faecalis (enterococcus).*

Uncomplicated gonorrhea due to susceptible *Neisseria gonorrhoeae.*

Gynecological Infections including endometritis, pelvic cellulitis, and pelvic inflammatory disease associated with susceptible *Neisseria gonorrhoeae, Peptococcus* species, *Peptostreptococcus* species, *Bacteroides* species, *E. coli, Proteus mirabilis, Klebsiella* species, and *Enterobacter* species

INDICATIONS AND USAGE: *(cont'd)*

Skin And Skin Structure Infections caused by susceptible *S. faecalis* (enterococcus), *E. coli. Proteus mirabilis* the indole positive *Proteus* species. *Proteus vulgaris,* and *Providencia rettgeri, Klebsiella* species, *Enterobacter* species, *Pseudomonas* species,*Peptococcus* species, and *Bacteroides* species.

Septicemia including bacteremia caused by susceptible *E coli, Klebsiella* species, *Enterobacter* species, *Pseudomonas* species, *Bacteroides* species, and *Peptococcus* species.

Mezlocillin has also been shown to be effective for the treatment of infections caused by *Streptococcus* species including Group A*Beta-hemolytic Streptococcus* and *Streptococcus pneumoniae* (formerly *Diplococcus pneumoniae)* however, infections caused by these organisms are ordinarily treated with more narrow spectrum penicillins.

Appropriate culture and susceptibility tests should be performed before treatment in order to isolate and identify organs causing infection and to determine their susceptibility to mezlocillin. Therapy with mezlocillin sodium monohydrate may be initiated before results of these tests are known, once results become available appropriate therapy should be continued.

Mezlocillin's broad spectrum of activity makes it particularly useful for treating mixed infections caused by susceptible strains of both gram negative and gram-positive aerobic or anaerobic bacteria. It is not effective however against infections caused by penicillinase-producing *Staphylococcus aureus.*

In certain severe infections when the causative organisms are unknown, mezlocillin sodium monohydrate may be administered in conjunction with an aminoglycoside or a cephalosporin antibiotic as initial therapy. As soon as results of culture and susceptibility tests become available, antimicrobial therapy should be adjusted if indicated. Culture and sensitivity testing, performed periodically during therapy, will provide information on the therapeutic effect of the antimicrobial and will monitor for the possible emergence of bacterial resistance.

Mezlocillin sodium monohydrate has been used effectively in combination with an aminoglycoside antibiotic for the treatment of life-threatening infections caused by *Pseudomonas aeruginosa.* For the treatment of febrile episodes in immunosuppressed patients with granulocytopenia, mezlocillin sodium monohydrate should be combined with an aminoglycoside or a cephalosporin antibiotic.

Prevention: The administration of mezlocillin sodium monohydrate perioperatively (preoperatively, intraoperatively, and postoperatively) may reduce the incidence of infections in patients undergoing surgical procedures (*e.g.,* vaginal hysterectomy and colorectal surgery) that may be classified as contaminated or potentially contaminated. Effective perioperative use for surgery depends on the time of administration. To achieve effective tissue levels, mezlocillin sodium monohydrate should be given 1/2 hour to 1 1/2 hours before surgery.

In patients undergoing Caesarean section, intraoperative (after clamping the umbilical cord) and postoperative use of mezlocillin sodium monohydrate may reduce the incidence of certain postoperative infections. (See DOSAGE AND ADMINISTRATION.)

For patients undergoing colorectal surgery, preoperative bowel preparation by mechanical cleansing as well as with a non-absorbable antibiotic (e.g, neomycin) is recommended.

If there are signs of infection, specimens for culture should be obtained for identification of the causative organism so that appropriate therapy may be instituted.

CONTRAINDICATIONS:

Mezlocillin sodium monohydrate is contraindicated in patients with a history of hypersensitivity reactions to any of the penicillins.

WARNINGS:

Serious and occasionally fatal hypersensitivity (anaphylactic) reactions have occurred in patients receiving a penicillin. These reactions are more apt to occur in individuals with a history of sensitivity to multiple allergens. There have been reports of individuals with a history of penicillin hypersensitivity reactions who have experienced severe hypersensitivity reactions when treated with a cephalosporin. Before therapy with mezlocillin is instituted careful inquiry should be made to determine whether the patient has had previous hypersensitivity reactions to penicillins, cephalosporins or other drugs. Antibiotics should be used with caution in any patient who has demonstrated some form of allergy, particularly to drugs.

If an allergic reaction occurs during therapy with mezlocillin the drug should be discontinued. SERIOUS ANAPHYLACTOID REACTIONS REQUIRE IMMEDIATE EMERGENCY TREATMENT WITH EPINEPHRINE, OXYGEN, INTRAVENOUS STEROIDS, AND AIRWAY MANAGEMENT, INCLUDING INTUBATION SHOULD ALSO BE PROVIDED AS INDICATED.

PRECAUTIONS:

GENERAL

Although mezlocillin sodium monohydrate shares with other penicillins the low potential for toxicity as with any potent drug, periodic assessment of organ system functions including renal hepatic and hematopoietic is advisable during prolonged therapy. Mezlocillin sodium monohydrate has been reported rarely to cause acute interstitial nephritis.

Bleeding manifestations have occurred in some patients receiving beta-lactam antibiotics. These reactions have been associated with abnormalities of coagulation tests such as clotting time, platelet aggregation and prothrombin time and are more likely to occur in patients with renal impairment. Although mezlocillin sodium monohydrate has rarely been associated with any bleeding abnormalities the possibility of this occurring should be kept in mind particularly in patients with severe renal impairment receiving maximum doses of the drug.

Mezlocillin sodium monohydrate has only rarely been reported to cause hypokalemia however, the possibility of this occurring should also be kept in mind particularly when treating patients with fluid and electrolyte imbalance. Periodic monitoring of serum potassium may be advisable in patients receiving prolonged therapy.

Mezlocillin sodium monohydrate is a monosodium salt containing only 42.6 mg (1.85 mEq) of sodium per gram of mezlocillin. This should be considered when treating patients requiring restricted salt intake.

As with any penicillin, an allergic reaction, including anaphylaxis, may occur during mezlocillin sodium monohydrate administration particularly in a hypersensitive individual.

As with other antibiotics, prolonged use of mezlocillin sodium monohydrate may result in overgrowth of non-susceptible organisms. If this occurs appropriate measures should be taken.

Antimicrobials used in high doses for short periods to treat gonorrhea may mask or delay the symptoms of incubating syphilis. Therefore prior to treatment patients with gonorrhea should also be evaluated for syphilis. Specimens for dark field examination should be obtained from any suspected primary lesion and serologic tests should be performed. Patients treated with mezlocillin sodium monohydrate should under go follow-up serologic tests three months after therapy.

INTERACTIONS WITH DRUGS AND LABORATORY TESTS

As with other penicillins the mixing of mezlocillin with an aminoglycoside in solutions for parenteral administration can result in substantial inactivation of the aminoglycoside.

Probenecid interferes with the renal tubular secretion of mezlocillin, therapy increasing serum concentrations and prolonging serum half-life of the antibiotic.

PRECAUTIONS: *(cont'd)*

High urine concentrations of mezlocillin may produce false positive protein reactions (pseudoproteinuria) with the following methods sulfosalicylic acid and boiling acid test, acetic acid test, biuret reaction and nitric acid test. The bromphenol blue (Multi-stix) reagent strip test has been reported to be reliable.

PREGNANCY: PREGNANCY CATEGORY B

Reproduction studies have been performed in rats and mice at doses up to 2 times the human dose and have revealed no evidence of impaired fertility or harm to the fetus, due to mezlocillin sodium monohydrate. There are however no adequate and well controlled studies in pregnant women. Because animal reproductive studies are not always predictive of human response, this drug should be used during pregnancy only if clearly needed. Mezlocillin crosses the placenta and is found in low concentrations in cord blood and amniotic fluid.

NURSING MOTHERS

Mezlocillin is detected in low concentrations in the milk of nursing mothers, therefore caution should be exercised when mezlocillin sodium monohydrate is administered to a nursing woman.

ADVERSE REACTIONS:

As with other penicillins, the following adverse reactions may occur:

Hypersensitivity Reactions: skin rash, pruritus, urticaria, drug fever, and anaphylactic reactions.

Gastrointestinal Disturbances: abnormal taste sensation, nausea vomiting and diarrhea.

Hemic and Lymphatic Systems: thrombocytopenia, leukopenia, neutropenia, eosinophilia and reduction of hemoglobin or hematocrit.

Abnormalities of Hepatic and Renal Function tTests: elevation of serum aspartate aminotransferase (SGOT), serum alkaline aminotransferase (SGPT), serum alkaline phosphatase, serum bilirubin. Elevation of serum creatinine and/or BUN. Reduction in serum potassium.

Central Nervous System: convulsive seizures or neuromuscular hyperirritability.

Local Reactions: thrombophlebitis with intravenous administration, pain with intramuscular injection.

OVERDOSAGE:

As with other penicillins, mezlocillin sodium monohydrate in overdosage has the potential to cause neuromuscular hyperirritability or convulsive seizures. Hemodialysis if necessary, will aid in removal of the drug from the blood.

DOSAGE AND ADMINISTRATION:

Mezlocillin sodium monohydratee may be administered intravenously or intramuscularly. For serious infections, the intravenous route of administration should be used. Intramuscular doses should not exceed 2g per injection.

The recommended adult dosage for serious infections is 200-300 mg/kg per day given in 4 to 6 divided doses. The usual dose is 3g given every 4 hours (18g/day) or 4g given every 6 hours (16g/day). For life-threatening infections, up to 350 mg/kg per day may be administered but the total daily dosage should ordinarily not exceed 24g (TABLE 5).

TABLE 5 Mezlocillin sodium monohydrate Dosage Guide (Adults)

Condition	Daily Dosage Range	Usual Daily Dosage	Frequency and Route of Administration
Urinary tract infection (uncomplicated)	100 - 125 mg/kg	6-8g	1.5 - 2g every 6 hours IV or IM
Urinary tract infection (complicated)	150 - 200 mg/kg	12g	3g every 6 hours IV
Lower respiratory tract infection			
Intra-abdominal infection			
Gynecological infection	225 - 300 mg/kg	16-18g	4g every 6 hours or 3g every 4 hours IV
Skin & skin structure infection			
Septicemia			

For patients with life-threatening infections, 4g may be administered every 4 hours (24 g/day).

Dosage for any individual patient must take into consideration the site and severity of infection, the susceptibility of the organisms causing infection and the status of the patient's host defense mechanism.

The duration of therapy depends upon the severity of infection. Generally, mezlocillin sodium monohydrate should be continued for at least 2 days after the signs and symptoms of infection have disappeared. The usual duration is 7 to 10 days, however, in difficult and complicated infections, more prolonged therapy may be required. Antibiotic therapy for Group A beta-hemolytic streptococcal infections should be maintained for a least 10 days to reduce the risk of rheumatic fever or glomerulonephritis.

In certain deep-seated infections, involving abscess formation, appropriate surgical drainage should be performed in conjunction with antimicrobial therapy.

For acute, uncomplicated gonococcal urethritis, the usual dose is 1-2g given once intravenously or by intramuscular injection. Probenecid 1g may be given orally at the time of dosing or up to 1/2-hour before. (For full prescribing information, refer to probenecid package insert).

PATIENTS WITH IMPAIRED RENAL FUNCTION

The rate of elimination of mezlocillin is dose dependent and related to the degree of renal function impairment. After an intravenous dose of 3g the serum half-life is approximately 1 hour in patients with creatinine clearances above 60 ml/min, 1.3 hr in those with clearances of 30-59 ml/min, 1.6 hr in those with clearances of 10-29 ml/min and approximately 3.6 hr in patients with clearances of less than 10 ml min. Dosage adjustments of mezlocillin sodium monohydrate are not required in patients with mild impairment of renal function. For patients with a creatinine clearance of ≤30 ml/min (serum creatinine of approximately 3.0 mg% or greater), the following dosage guide, (TABLE 6), may be used.

For life-threatening infections, 3g may be given every 6 hours to patients with creatinine clearances between 10-30 ml/min and 2g every 6 hours to those with clearances less than 10 ml/min.

For patients with serious systemic infection undergoing hemodialysis for renal failure, 3-4g may be administered after each dialysis and then every 12 hours. Patients undergoing peritoneal dialysis may receive 3g every 12 hours.

For patients with renal failure and hepatic insufficiency, measurement of serum levels of mezlocillin will provide additional guidance for adjusting dosage.

DOSAGE AND ADMINISTRATION: *(cont'd)*

TABLE 6 Mezlocillin sodium monohydrate Dosage Guide For Patients With Impaired Renal Function

Creatinine Clearance ml/min	Urinary Tract Infection (Uncomplicated)	Urinary Tract Infection (Complicated)	Serious Systemic Infection
>30	Usual Recommended Dosage		
10-30	1.5g every 8 hours	1.5g every 6 hours	3g every 8 hours
<10	1.5g every 8 hours	1.5g every 8 hours	2g every 8 hours

INTRAVENOUS ADMINISTRATION

Mezlocillin sodium monohydrate may be administered intravenously by intermittent infusion or by direct intravenous injection.

Infusion: Each gram of mezlocillin should be reconstituted by vigorous shaking with at least 10 ml of Sterile Water for Injection, 5% Dextrose Injection or 0.9% Sodium Chloride Injection. The dissolved drug should be further diluted to desired volume (50-100 ml) with an appropriate intravenous solution. (See Compatibility and Stability). The solution of reconstituted drug may then be administered over a period of 30 minutes by direct infusion or through a Y-type intravenous infusion set which may already be in place. If this method or the "piggyback" method of administration is used it is advisable to discontinue temporarily the administration of any other solutions during the infusion of mezlocillin sodium monohydrate.

Injection: The reconstituted solution of mezlocillin sodium monohydrate may also be injected directly into a vein or into intravenous tubing, when administered this way the injection should be given slowly over a period of 3-5 minutes. To minimize venous irritation, the concentration of drug should not exceed 10%.

When mezlocillin sodium monohydrate is given in combination with another antimicrobial, such as an aminoglycoside, each drug should be given separately in accordance with the recommended dosage and routes of administration for each drug.

INTRAMUSCULAR ADMINISTRATION

Each gram of mezlocillin may be reconstituted by vigorous shaking with 3-4 ml of sterile water for injection or with 3-4 ml of 0.5 or 1.0% lidocaine hydrochloride solution (without epinephrine), to yield a final concentration of 250 mg/ml. (For full prescribing information, refer to lidocaine package insert.) Intramuscular doses of mezlocillin sodium monohydrate should not exceed 2g per injection.

As with all intramuscular preparations, mezlocillin sodium monohydrate should be injected well within the body of a relatively large muscle, such as the upper outer quadrant of the buttock (*i.e.,* gluteus maximus) aspiration will help avoid unintentional injection into a blood vessel. Slow injection (12-15 sec) will minimize the discomfort associated with intramuscular administration.

INFANTS AND CHILDREN

Only limited data are available on the safety and effectiveness of mezlocillin sodium monohydrate in the treatment of infants and children with documented serious infection. In the event a child has an infection for which mezlocillin sodium monohydrate may be judged particularly appropriate, the following dosage guide, TABLE 7, may be used.

TABLE 7 Mezlocillin sodium monohydrate Dosage Guide (Newborns)

BODY WEIGHT (gm)	AGE ≤7 DAYS	AGE >7 DAYS
≤2000	75 mg/kg every 12 hours (150 mg/kg/day)	75 mg/kg every 8 hours (225 mg/kg/day)
>2000	75 mg/kg every 12 hours (150 mg/kg/day)	75 mg/kg every 6 hours (300 mg/kg/day)

For infants beyond one month of age and children up to the age of 12 years, 50 mg/kg may be administered every 4 hours (300 mg/kg/day).

The drug may be infused intravenously over 30-minutes or be given by intramuscular injection.

COMPATIBILITY AND STABILITY

Mezlocillin sodium monohydrate at concentrations of 10 mg/ml and 100 mg/ml is stable (loss of potency less than 10%) in the following intravenous solutions for the time periods stated (TABLE 8).

TABLE 8

INTRAVENOUS SOLUTION	STABILITY Controlled Room Temperature	Refrigeration
Sterile Water for Injection, USP	48 hours	7 days
0.9% Sodium Chloride Injection, USP	48 hours	7 days
5% Dextrose Injection, USP	48 hours	7 days
5% Dextrose in 0.225% Sodium Chloride Injection, USP	72 hours	7 days
Lactated Ringer's Injection, USP	72 hours	7 days
5% Dextrose in Electrolyte #75 Injection	72 hours	7 days
5% Dextrose in 0.45% Sodium Chloride Injection, USP	48 hours	48 hours
Ringer's Injection	24 hours	24 hours
10% Dextrose Injection	24 hours	24 hours
5% Fructose Injection	24 hours	24 hours

If precipitation should occur under refrigeration, the product should be warmed to 37°C for 20 minutes in a water bath and shaken well.

*This solution is stable from 10 mg/ml to 50 mg/ml under refrigeration.

Mezlocillin sodium monohydrate at concentrations up to 250 mg/ml is stable for 24 hours at room temperature in the following diluents:

Sterile Water for Injection, USP

0.9% Sodium Chloride Injection, USP

0.5% and 10% Lidocaine Hydrochloride solution (without epinephrine)

Mezlocillin sodium monohydrate is stable for up to 28 days when frozen at -12°C at concentrations up to 100 mg/ml in the following diluents:

Sterile Water for Injection, USP

0.9% Sodium Chloride Injection, USP or 5% Dextrose Injection, USP

HOW SUPPLIED:

Mezlin is a white to pale yellow crystalline powder supplied as listed below:

Mezlin vials and infusion bottles contain mezlocillin sodium equivalent mezlocillin as specified below:

HOW SUPPLIED: *(cont'd)*

Mezlin is also available in ADD-Vantage vials and a Pharmacy Bulk Package.

Unreconstituted Mezlin should be stored at temperatures not exceeding 86°F (30°C). The powder as well as the reconstituted solution of drug may darken slightly, depending upon storage conditions, but potency is not affected.

REFERENCES:

* Bauer, A.W., Kirby, W.M. Sherris, J C., and Turck, M.: Antibiotic Testing by a Standardized Single Disc Method, Am. J. Clin. Pathol., 45.493. 1966. Standardized Disc Susceptibility Test, FEDERAL REGISTER, 39 19182-19184, 1974.

HOW SUPPLIED - EQUIVALENTS NOT AVAILABLE:

Injection, Dry-Soln - Intramuscular; - 1 gm

25 ml	$42.77	MEZLIN 1 GRAM, Bayer	00026-8211-30

Injection, Dry-Soln - Intramuscular; - 2 gm/vial

30 ml	$82.93	MEZLIN 2 GRAM, Bayer	00026-8212-30
100 ml	$89.15	MEZLIN 2 GRAM, Bayer	00026-8212-36

Injection, Dry-Soln - Intramuscular; - 3 gm/vial

20 ml	$125.06	MEZLIN 3 GRAM, Bayer	00026-8213-19
50 ml	$122.47	MEZLIN 3 GRAM, Bayer	00026-8213-35
100 ml	$128.30	MEZLIN 3 GRAM, Bayer	00026-8213-36

Injection, Dry-Soln - Intravenous - 4 gm/vial

20 ml	$158.11	MEZLIN- 4 GRAM, Bayer	00026-8214-19
50 ml	$155.51	MEZLIN- 4 GRAM, Bayer	00026-8214-35
100 ml	$163.28	MEZLIN- 4 GRAM, Bayer	00026-8214-36

Injection, Lyphl-Soln - Intramuscular; - 20 gm/vial

20g x 6	$443.20	MEZLIN, Bayer	00026-8220-31

MICONAZOLE *(001809)*

CATEGORIES: Anti-Infectives; Antibacterials; Antibiotics; Antifungals; Antimicrobials; Candidiasis; Dermatologicals; Fungal Agents; Infections; Meningitis; Skin/Mucous Membrane Agents; Tinea Corporis; Tinea Cruris; Tinea Pedis; Tinea Versicolor; Topical; Sales > $100 Million; FDA Approval Pre 1982

BRAND NAMES: *Acromizol*; *Aflorix*; *Albistat*; *Aloid*; *Andergin*; *Daktarin*; *Deralbine*; *Dermonistat*; *Florid*; *Funcort*; *Fungi-M*; Fungoid; *Gyno-Daktarin*; *Liconar*; *Micatin*; *Miconal*; *Micotef*; *Miracol*; **Monistat**; *Mycorine*; *Mysocort*; *Nazoderm*; *Neomicol*; Ony-Clear Nail; *Zole*
(International brand names outside U.S. in italics)

FORMULARIES: Aetna; BC-BS; Medi-Cal; WHO

COST OF THERAPY: $20.88 (Candidiasis; Suppository; 200 mg; 1/day; 3 days)

DESCRIPTION:

Suppositories: Monistat 3 Vaginal Suppositories are white to off-white suppositories, each containing the antifungal agent, miconazole nitrate, 1-[2,4-Dichloro-β-[(2,4-dichlorobenzyl) oxy]phenethyl]-imidazole mononitrate, 200 mg, in a hydrogenated vegetable oil base. Miconazole nitrate for vaginal use is also available as Monistat 7 Vaginal Cream and Monistat 7 Vaginal Suppositories.

Derm Cream: Monistat-Derm (miconazole nitrate 2%) Cream contains miconazole nitrate 2%, formulated into a water-miscible base consisting of pegoxol 7 stearate, peglicol 5 oleate, mineral oil, benzoic acid, butylated hydroxyanisole and purified water. (Please see above for chemical name).

Intravenous Infusion: Monistat IV (miconazole), 1[2-(2,4 dichlorophenyl)-2-[(2,4-dichlorophenyl)methoxy]ethyl]-1H-imidazole, is a synthetic antifungal agent supplied as a sterile solution for intravenous infusion. Each ml of this solution contains 10 mg of miconazole with 0.115 ml PEG 35 castor oil, 1.0 mg lactic acid USP, 0.5 mg methylparaben, 0.05 mg propylparaben in water for injection. Miconazole IV is a clear, colorless to slightly yellow solution having a pH of 3.7 to 5.7.

CLINICAL PHARMACOLOGY:

Suppositories: Miconazole nitrate exhibits fungicidal activity *in vitro* against species of the genus *Candida*. The pharmacologic mode of action is unknown. Following intravaginal administration of miconazole nitrate, small amounts are absorbed. Administration of a single dose of miconazole nitrate suppositories (100 mg) to healthy subjects resulted in a total recovery from the urine and feces of 0.85% (± 0.43%) of the administered dose.

Animal studies indicate that the drug crossed the placenta and doses above those used in humans result in embryo-and fetotoxicity (80 mg/kg, orally), although this has not been reported in human subjects (See PRECAUTIONS.)

In multi-center clinical trials in 440 women with vulvovaginal candidiasis, the efficacy of treatment with the Monistat 3 Vaginal Suppository for 3 days was compared with treatment for 7 days with Monistat 7 Vaginal Cream. The clinical cure rates (free of microbiological evidence and clinical signs and symptoms of candidiasis at 8-10 days and 30-35 days post-therapy) were numerically lower, although not statistically different, with the 3-Day Suppository when compared with the 7-Day Cream.

Derm Cream: Miconazole nitrate is a synthetic antifungal agent which inhibits the growth of the common dermatophytes,*Trichophyton rubrum*, *Trichophyton mentagrophytes* and *Epidermophyton floccusum*, the yeast-like fungus, *Candida albicans*, and the organism responsible for tinea versicolor (*Malassezia furfur*).

Intravenous Infusion: Monistat IV is rapidly metabolized in the liver and about 14% to 22% of the administered dose is excreted in the urine, mainly as inactive metabolites. The pharmacokinetic profile fits a three compartment open model with the following biologic half life: 0.4, 2.1, and 24.1 hours for each phase respectively. The pharmacokinetic profile of Monistat IV is unaltered in patients with renal insufficiency, including those patients on hemodialysis. The *in vitro* antifungal activity of Monistat IV is very broad. Clinical efficacy has been demonstrated in patients with the following species of fungi: *Coccidioides immitis, Candida albicans, Cryptococcus neoformans, Pseudallescheria boydii (Petriellidium boydii; Allescheria boydii),* and *Paracoccidioides brasiliensis.*

Recommended doses of Monistat IV produce serum concentrations of drug which exceed the *in vitro* minimum inhibitory concentration (MIC) values listed below (TABLE 1):

Doses above 9 mg/kg of Monistat IV produce peak blood levels above 1 mcg/ml in most cases. The drug penetrates into joints.

INDICATIONS AND USAGE:

Suppositories: Monistat 3 Vaginal Suppositories are indicated for the local treatment of vulvovaginal candidiasis (moniliasis). Effectiveness in pregnancy and in diabetic patients has not been established. As Monistat is effective only for candidal vulvovaginitis, the diagnosis

INDICATIONS AND USAGE: *(cont'd)*

TABLE 1 Median Minimal Inhibitory Concentrations of Miconazole in mcg/ml

Clinical Isolates	Median	Range
Coccidioides immitis	0.4	0.1 - 1.6
Candida albicans	0.2	0.1 - 0.8
Cryptococcus neoformans	0.8	0.4 - 1.3
Paracoccidioides brasiliensis	0.24	0.16 - 0.31
Pseudallescheria boydii (Petriellidium boydii)	1.0	0.16 - 10

should be confirmed by KOH smear and/or cultures. Other pathogens commonly associated with vulvovaginitis(*Trichomonas and Haemophilus vaginalis [Gardnerella]*) should be ruled out by appropriate laboratory methods.

Derm Cream: For topical application in the treatment of tinea pedis (athlete's foot), tinea cruris, and tinea corporis caused by*Trichophyton rubrum,* and *Epidermophyton floccosum* in the treatment of cutaneous candidiasis (moniliasis), and in the treatment of tinea versicolor.

Intravenous Infusion: Monistat IV is indicated for the treatment of the following severe systemic fungal infections, based on data derived from open clinical trials: coccidioidomycosis (N=52*), candidiasis (N=151), cryptococcosis (N=13), pseudallescheriosis (petriellidiosis; allescheriosis)(N=12), paracoccidioidomycosis (N=12), and for the treatment of chronic mucocutaneous candidiasis (N=16).

*Represents treatment courses, as some patients were treated more than once.

However, in the treatment of fungal meningitis and *Candida*urinary bladder infections an intravenous infusion alone is inadequate. It must be supplemented with intrathecal administration or bladder irrigation. Appropriate diagnostic procedures should be performed and MIC's should be measured to determine if the organism is susceptible to Monistat.

Monistat IV should only be used to treat severe systemic fungal disease.

CONTRAINDICATIONS:

Suppositories/Intravenous Infusion: Patients known to be hypersensitive to this drug, or its components.

Derm Cream: No known contraindications.

WARNINGS:

Intravenous Infusion: There have been several reports of cardiorespiratory arrest and/or anaphylaxis in patients receiving Monistat IV Excessively rapid administration of the drug may have been responsible in some cases. Rapid injection of undiluted Monistat IV may produce transient tachycardia or dysrhythmia. (See DOSAGE AND ADMINISTRATION.)

Monistat IV should be used only to treat severe systemic fungal diseases.

PRECAUTIONS:

SUPPOSITORIES

General: Discontinue drug if sensitization or irritation is reported during use. The base contained in the suppository formulation may interact with certain latex products, such as the used in vaginal contraceptive diaphragms. Concurrent use is not recommended. Monistat 7 Vaginal Cream may be considered for use under these conditions.

Laboratory Tests: If there is a lack of response to Monistat 3 Vaginal Suppositories, appropriate microbiological studies (standard KOH smear and/or cultures) should be repeated to confirm the diagnosis and rule out other pathogens.

Carcinogenesis, Mutagenesis, Impairment of Fertility: Long-term animal studies to determine carcinogenic potential have not been performed.

Fertility (Reproduction): Oral administration of miconazole nitrate in rats has been reported to produce prolonged gestation. However, this effect was not observed in oral rabbit studies. In addition, signs of fetal and embryo toxicity were reported in rat and rabbit studies, and dystocia was reported in rat studies after oral doses at and above 80 mg per kg. Intravaginal administration did into produce these effects in rats.

Pregnancy: Since imidazoles are absorbed in small amounts from the human vagina, they should not be used in the first trimester of pregnancy unless the physician considers it essential to the welfare of the patient.

Clinical studies, during which miconazole nitrate vaginal cream and suppositories were used for up to 14 days, were reported to include 514 pregnant patients. Follow-up reports available in 471 of these patients reveal no adverse effects or complications attributable to miconazole nitrate therapy in infants born to these women.

Nursing Mothers: It is not known whether miconazole nitrate is excreted in human milk. Because many drugs are excreted in human milk, caution should be exercised when miconazole nitrate is administered to a nursing woman.

DERM CREAM

If a reaction suggesting sensitivity or chemical irritation should occur, use of the medication should be discontinued.

For external use only. Avoid introduction of cream into the eyes.

INTRAVENOUS INFUSION

General: Before a treatment course of Monistat IV is started, the physician should ascertain insofar as possible that the patient is not hypersensitive to the drug product. Monistat IV should be given by intravenous infusion. The treatment should be started under stringent conditions of hospitalization but subsequently may be administered to suitable patients under ambulatory conditions with close clinical monitoring. It is recommended that an initial dose of 200 mg be administered with the physician in attendance. It is also recommended that clinical laboratory monitoring including hemoglobin, hematocrit, electrolytes and lipids be performed.

It should be borne in mind that systemic fungal mycoses may be complications of chronic underlying conditions which in themselves may require appropriate measures.

Since *Pseudoallescheria boydii* is difficult to distinguish histologically from species of *Aspergillus*, it is strongly recommended that cultures be planted.

Pregnancy Category C: Reproduction studies using Monistat IV (miconazole) were performed in rats and rabbits. At intravenous doses of 40 mg/kg in the rat and 20 mg/kg in the rabbit, no evidence of impaired fertility or harm to the fetus appeared. There are no adequate and well- controlled studies using Monistat IV in pregnant women. Monistat IV should be given to a pregnant woman only if clearly needed.

Pediatric Use: The safety of miconazole IV in children under one year has not been extensively studied. However, reports in the literature describe the treatment of 21 neonates for periods ranging from 1 to 56 days at doses ranging from 3 to 50 mg/kg per day in 3 or 4 divided doses. No unanticipated adverse events occurred in children who received these doses. The majority of use was a daily dose in the 15 to 30 mg/kg range. Seven of the eleven evaluable children recovered or improved.

DRUG INTERACTIONS:

Intravenous Infusion: Drugs containing cremophor type vehicles are known to cause electrophoretic abnormalities of the lipoprotein; for example, the values and/or patterns may be altered. These effects are reversible upon discontinuation of treatment but are usually not an indication that treatment should be discontinued.

Interaction with oral and IV anticoagulant drugs, resulting in an enhancement of the anticoagulant effect, may occur. However, this has only been reported with oral (coumarin) administration. In cases of simultaneous treatment with Monistat IV and anticoagulant drugs, the anticoagulant effect should be carefully titrated since reductions of the anticoagulant doses may be indicated.

Interactions between oral miconazole and oral hypoglycemic agents leading to severe hypoglycemia have been reported.

Since concomitant administration of rifampin and ketoconazole (an imidazole) reduces the blood levels of the latter, the concurrent administration of Monistat IV (an imidazole) and rifampin should be avoided.

Ketoconazole (an imidazole) increases the blood level of cyclosporine; therefore there is the possibility of a similar drug interaction involving cyclosporine and Monistat IV (an imidazole). Blood levels of cyclosporine should be monitored if the two drugs must be given concurrently.

Concomitant administration of miconazole with CNS-active drugs such as carbamazepine or phenytoin may alter the metabolism of one or both of the drugs. Therefore, consideration should be given to the advisability of monitoring plasma levels of these drugs. It is not known whether miconazole may affect the metabolism of other CNS-active drugs.

ADVERSE REACTIONS:

Suppositories: During clinical studies with the Monistat 3 Vaginal Suppository (miconazole nitrate, 200 mg) 301 patients were treated. The incidence of vulvovaginal burning, itching or irritation was 2%. Complaints of cramping (2%) and headaches (1.3%) were also reported. Other complaints (hives, skin rash) occurred with less than a 0.5% incidence. The therapy-related dropout rate was 0.3%.

Derm Cream: There have been isolated reports of irritation, burning, maceration, and allergic contact dermatitis with the application of Monistat-Derm.

Intravenous Infusion: Adverse reactions which have been observed with Monistat IV therapy include phlebitis, pruritus, rash, nausea, vomiting, febrile reactions, drowsiness, diarrhea, anorexia and flushes. In the U.S. studies, 29% of 209 patients studied had phlebitis, 21% pruritus, 18% nausea, 10% fever and chills, 9% rash, and 7% emesis. Transient decreases in hematocrit and serum sodium values have been observed following infusion of Monistat IV.

In rare cases, anaphylaxis has occurred.

Thrombocytopenia has also been reported. No serious renal or hepatic toxicity has been reported. If pruritus and skin rashes are severe, discontinuation of treatment may be necessary. Nausea and vomiting can be lessened with antihistaminic or antiemetic drugs given prior to Monistat IV infusion, or by reducing the dose, slowing the rate of infusion, or avoiding administration with foods.

Aggregation of erythrocytes or rouleau formation on blood smears has been reported. Hyperlipemia has occurred in patients and is reported to be due to the vehicle, Cremophor EL (PEG 35 castor oil).

OVERDOSAGE:

Suppositories: Overdosage of miconazole nitrate in humans has not been reported to date. In mice, rats, guinea pigs and dogs, the oral LD 50 values were found to be 578.1, >640, 275.9 and >160 mg/kg, respectively.

DOSAGE AND ADMINISTRATION:

Suppositories: Monistat 3 Vaginal Suppositories: One suppository (miconazole nitrate, 200 mg) is inserted intravaginally once daily at bedtime for three consecutive days. Before prescribing another course of therapy, the diagnosis should be reconfirmed by smears and/or cultures to rule out other pathogens.

Derm Cream: Sufficient Monistat-Derm Cream should be applied to cover affected areas twice daily (morning and evening) in patients with tinea pedis, tinea cruris, tinea corporis, and cutaneous candidiasis, and once daily in patients with tinea versicolor. If Monistat Derm Cream is used in intertriginous areas, it should be applied sparingly and smoothed in well to avoid maceration effects.

Early relief of symptoms (2 to 3 days) is experienced by the majority of patients and clinical improvement may be seen fairly soon after treatment is begun; however *Candida* infections and tinea cruris and corporis should be treated for two weeks and tinea pedis for one month in order to reduce the possibility of recurrence. If a patient shows no clinical improvement after a month of treatment, the diagnosis should be redetermined. Patients with tinea versicolor usually exhibit clinical and mycological clearing after two weeks of treatment.

INTRAVENOUS INFUSION

Dosage

Adults: Doses may vary from 200 to 1200 mg per infusion depending on severity of infection and sensitivity of the organism. The following daily doses, which may be divided over 3 infusions, are recommended (TABLE 2):

TABLE 2

Organism	Dosage Range*	Duration of Successful Therapy (weeks)
Candidiasis	600 to 1800 mg per day	1 to > 20
Cryptococcosis	1200 to 2400 mg per day	3 to > 12
Coccidioidomycosis	1800 to 3600 mg per day	3 to > 20
Pseudoallescheriosis (Petriellidosis; Allescheriosis)	600 to 3000 mg per day	5 to > 20
Paracoccidioidomycosis	200 to 1200 mg per day	2 to > 16

* May be divided over 3 infusions

Repeated courses may be necessitated by relapse or reinfection.

Children: Children under one year: Total daily doses of 15 to 30 mg/kg have been used (See Pediatric Use.).

Children 1 to 12 years: Total daily doses of 20 to 40 mg/kg have generally been adequate. However, a dose of 15 mg/kg body weight per infusion should not be exceeded.

Administration

For daily doses of up to 2400 mg, Monistat IV should be diluted in at least 200 ml of diluent per ampoule and should be administered at a rate of approximately 2 hours per ampoule. For daily doses higher than 2400 mg adjust the rate of infusion and the diluent in terms of patient tolerability (see WARNINGS.)

DOSAGE AND ADMINISTRATION: *(cont'd)*

It is recommended that 0.9% Sodium Chloride Injection be used as the diluent to minimize the possibility of transient hyponatremia following an infusion of Monistat IV. Alternatively, if clinically indicated, 5% Dextrose-Injection may used.

Generally, treatment should be continued until all clinical and laboratory tests no longer indicate that active fungal infection is present. Inadequate periods of treatment may yield poor response an lead to early recurrence of clinical symptoms. The dosing intervals and sites and the duration of treatment vary from patient and depend on the causative organism.

Other Modes of Administration: *Intrathecal:* Administration of the undiluted injectable solution of Monistat IV by the various intrathecal routes (20 mg per dose) is indicated as an adjunct to intravenous treatment in fungal meningitis. Succeeding intrathecal injections may be alternated between lumbar, cervical, and cisternal punctures every 3 to 7 days. *Bladder Instillation:* 200 mg of miconazole in a diluted solution is indicated in the treatment of*Candida* of the urinary bladder.

Suppositories and IV Store at controlled room temperature (15° to 30°C/59° to 86°F).

(IV: Janssen, 3/93, 7614304)

(Suppositories: Ortho Pharmaceuticals, 3/89, 643-10-353-4)

(Derm-Cream: Ortho Pharmaceuticals, 1/92, 631-10-471-9)

HOW SUPPLIED - RATED THERAPEUTICALLY EQUIVALENT:

Suppository - Vaginal - 200 mg

3's	$20.89	Miconazole 3, NMC Labs	23317-0738-03
3's	**$24.36**	**MONISTAT 3, Ortho Pharm**	**00062-5437-01**

HOW SUPPLIED - NOT RATED EQUIVALENT:

Aerosol, Spray - Topical - 2 %

42.5 ml	$16.25	ONY-CLEAR NAIL, Pedinol Pharma	00884-4893-45

Cream - Topical - 2 %

15 gm	$2.01	Miconazole, HL Moore Drug Exch	00839-7715-47
15 gm	**$12.48**	**MONISTAT-DERM, Ortho Pharm**	**00062-5434-02**
30 gm	**$21.00**	**MONISTAT-DERM, Ortho Pharm**	**00062-5434-01**
60 gm	$16.00	Fungoid, Pedinol Pharma	00884-2493-60
85 gm	**$40.74**	**MONISTAT-DERM, Ortho Pharm**	**00062-5434-03**

Injection, Solution - Intrathecal; In - 10 mg/ml

20 ml x 5	**$192.36**	**MONISTAT I.V., Janssen Phar**	**50458-0200-20**

Kit - Topical - 2 %

1's	$13.50	FUNGOID TINCTURE NAIL KIT, Pedinol Pharma	00884-5493-01
1's	$20.25	ONY-CLEAR NAIL TREATMENT, Pedinol Pharma	00884-5593-45

Kit - Topical; Vagina - 200 mg

kit	**$26.52**	**MONISTAT DUAL PAK, Ortho Pharm**	**00062-5429-01**

Package - Topical - 2 mg/0.5 mg

1's	$20.00	FUNGOID & HC, Pedinol Pharma	00884-4193-25

Tampon - Vaginal - 100 mg

5's	**$15.96**	**MONISTAT 5, Ortho Pharm**	**00062-5436-01**

Tincture - Topical - 2 %

29.57 ml	$9.25	FUNGOID, Pedinol Pharma	00884-0293-01
473.12 ml	$92.50	FUNGOID, Pedinol Pharma	00884-0293-16

MIDAZOLAM HYDROCHLORIDE *(001810)*

CATEGORIES: Anesthesia; Angiography; Anxiolytics, Sedatives, Hypnotic; Benzodiazepines; Central Nervous System Agents; General Anesthetics; Injectable Anesthetics; Insomnia; Sedation; Sedatives; Pregnancy Category D; DEA Class CIV; FDA Approved 1985 Dec

BRAND NAMES: *Dormicum* (Europe, Asia); *Hypnovel* (Australia, England, France, Mexico); **Versed**

(International brand names outside U.S. in italics)

Intravenous midazolam HCl has been associated with respiratory depression and respiratory arrest, especially when used for conscious sedation. In some cases, where this was not recognized promptly and treated effectively, death or hypoxic encephalopathy has resulted. Intravenous midazolam HCl should be used only in hospital or ambulatory care settings, including physicians' offices, that provide for continuous monitoring of respiratory and cardiac function. Immediate availability of resuscitative drugs and equipment and personnel trained in their use should be assured. (See WARNINGS.)

The initial intravenous dose for conscious sedation may be as little as 1 mg. but should not exceed 2.5 mg in a normal healthy adult. Lower doses are necessary for older (over 60 years) or debilitated patients and in patients receiving concomitant narcotics or other CNS depressants. The initial dose and all subsequent doses should never be given as a bolus: administer over at least 2 minutes and allow an additional 2 or more minutes to fully evaluate the sedative effect. The use of the 1 mg ml formulation or dilution of the 1 mg/ml or 5 mg ml formulation is recommended to facilitate slower injection. See DOSAGE AND ADMINISTRATION for complete dosing information.

DESCRIPTION:

Midazolam HCl is a water-soluble benzodiazepine available as a sterile parenteral dosage form for intravenous or intramuscular injection. Each ml contains midazolam hydrochloride equivalent to 1 mg or 5 mg midazolam compounded with 0.8% sodium chloride and 0.01% disodium edetate, with 1% benzyl alcohol as preservative: the pH is adjusted to approximately 3 with hydrochloric acid and, if necessary, sodium hydroxide.

Midazolam is a white to light yellow crystalline compound, insoluble in water. The hydrochloride salt of midazolam, which is formed *in situ,* is soluble in aqueous solutions. Chemically, midazolam HCl is 8-chloro-6-(2-fluorophenyl)-1-methyl-4*H*-imidazo(1.5-a)(1.4) benzodiazepine hydrochloride. Midazolam hydrochloride has the empirical formula $C_{18}H_{13}ClFN_3$. Midazolam hydrochloride has a calculated molecular weight of 362.25.

CLINICAL PHARMACOLOGY:

Midazolam HCl is a short-acting benzodiazepine central nervous system depressant.

The effects of midazolam HCl on the CNS are dependent on the dose administered, the route of administration, and the presence or absence of other premedications. Onset time of sedative effects after IM administration was 15 minutes, with peak sedation occurring 30 to 60 minutes following injection. In one study, when tested the following day, 73% of the patients who received midazolam HCl intramuscularly had no recall of memory cards shown 30 minutes following drug administration; 40% had no recall of the memory cards shown 60 minutes following drug administration.

CLINICAL PHARMACOLOGY: *(cont'd)*

Sedation after IV injection was achieved within 3 to 5 minutes; the time of onset is affected by total dose administered and the concurrent administration of narcotic premedication. Seventy-one percent of the patients in the endoscopy studies had no recall of introduction of the endoscope; 82% of the patients had no recall of withdrawal of the endoscope.

When midazolam HCl is given intravenously as an anesthetic induction agent, induction of anesthesia occurs in approximately 1.5 minutes when narcotic premedication has been administered and in 2 to 2.5 minutes without narcotic premedication or with sedative premedication. Some impairment in a test of memory was noted in 90% of the patients studied.

Midazolam HCl, used as directed, does not delay awakening from general anesthesia. Gross tests of recovery after awakening (orientation, ability to stand and walk, suitability for discharge from the recovery room, return to baseline Trieger competency) usually indicate recovery within 2 hours but recovery may take up to 6 hours in some cases. When compared with patients who received thiopental, patients who received midazolam generally recovered at a slightly slower rate.

In patients without intracranial lesions, induction with midazolam HCl is associated with a moderate decrease in cerebrospinal fluid pressure (lumbar puncture measurements), similar to that seen following use of thiopental. Preliminary data in intracranial surgical patients with normal intracranial pressure but decreased compliance (subarachnoid screw measurements); show comparable elevations of intracranial pressure with midazolam HCl and with thiopental during intubation.

Usual intramuscular premedicating doses of midazolam HCl do not depress the ventilatory response to carbon dioxide stimulation to a clinically significant extent. Induction doses of midazolam HCl depress the ventilatory response to carbon dioxide stimulation for 15 minutes or more beyond the duration of ventilatory depression following administration of thiopental. Impairment of ventilatory response to carbon dioxide is more marked in patients with chronic obstructive pulmonary disease (COPD). Sedation with intravenous midazolam HCl does not adversely affect the mechanics of respiration (resistance, static recoil, most lung volume measurements): total lung capacity and peak expiratory flow decrease significantly but static compliance and maximum expiratory flow at 50% of awake total lung capacity (Vmax) increase.

In cardiac hemodynamic studies, induction with midazolam HCl was associated with a slight to moderate decrease in mean arterial pressure, cardiac output, stroke volume and systemic vascular resistance. Slow heart rates (less than 65/minute), particularly in patients taking propranolol for angina, tended to rise slightly; faster heart rates (*e.g.,* 85/minute) tended to slow slightly.

The following preliminary pharmacokinetic data for midazolam have been reported. In normal subjects and healthy patients intravenous midazolam exhibited an elimination half-life of 1.2 to 12.3 hours, a large volume of distribution (0.95 to 6.6 L/kg) and a plasma clearance of 0.15 to 0.77 L/hr/kg. Clinical effects of midazolam HCl do not directly correlate with the blood concentrations of midazolam.

Following intravenous administration, less than 0.03% of the dose is excreted in the urine as intact midazolam. Midazolam is rapidly metabolized to 1-hydroxymethyl midazolam, which is conjugated, with subsequent excretion in the urine. Approximately 45% to 57% of the dose is excreted in the urine as the conjugate of 1-hydroxymethyl midazolam, the major metabolite of midazolam. The half-life of elimination of 1-hydroxymethyl midazolam is similar to the parent compound. The concentration of midazolam is 10- to 30-fold greater than that of 1-hydroxymethyl midazolam after single IV administration.

In a small group of patients (n=11) with congestive heart failure, there appeared to be a 2- to 3-fold increase in the elimination half-life and volume of distribution of midazolam: however, the total body clearance of midazolam appeared to remain unchanged at a single 5-mg intravenous dose. There was no apparent change in the pharmacokinetic profile following the intravenous administration of 5 mg of midazolam to a small group of patients (n=12) with hepatic dysfunction. There was a 1.5- to 2-fold increase in elimination half-life, total body clearance and volume of distribution in a small group of patients (n=15) with chronic renal failure.

In a small group (n=12) of surgical patients, aged 49 to 60 years old, given 0.2 mg kg midazolam intravenously, there appeared to be a small increase in the volume of distribution and elimination half-life with little change in total body clearance compared to an equal number of younger surgical patients (aged 18 to 30).

The mean absolute bioavailability of midazolam following intramuscular administration is greater than 90%. The mean time of maximum midazolam plasma concentrations following intramuscular dosing occurs within 45 minutes postadministration. Peak concentrations of midazolam as well as 1-hydroxymethyl midazolam after intramuscular administration are about one-half of those achieved after equivalent intravenous doses. The pharmacokinetic profile of elimination after intramuscularly administered midazolam is comparable to that observed following intravenous administration of the drug. Dose-linearity relationships have not been adequately defined.

Midazolam is approximately 97% plasma protein-bound in normal subjects and patients with renal failure. In animals, midazolam has been shown to cross the blood-brain barrier. In animals and in humans, midazolam has been shown to cross the placenta and enter into fetal circulation. It is not known whether midazolam is excreted in human milk.

INDICATIONS AND USAGE:

Injectable midazolam HCl is indicated—

intramuscularly for preoperative sedation (induction of sleepiness or drowsiness and relief of apprehension) and to impair memory of perioperative events;

intravenously as an agent for conscious sedation prior to short diagnostic or endoscopic procedures, such as bronchoscopy, gastroscopy, cystoscopy, coronary angiography and cardiac catheterization, either alone or with a narcotic;

intravenously for induction of general anesthesia, before administration of other anesthetic agents. With the use of narcotic premedication, induction of anesthesia can be attained within a relatively narrow dose range and in a short period of time. Intravenous midazolam HCl can also be used as a component of intravenous supplementation of nitrous oxide and oxygen (balanced anesthesia) *for short surgical procedures;* longer procedures have not been studied.

When used intravenously, midazolam HCl is associated with a high incidence of partial or complete impairment of recall for the next several hours. (See CLINICAL PHARMACOLOGY.)

CONTRAINDICATIONS:

Injectable midazolam HCl is contraindicated in patients with a known hypersensitivity to the drug. Benzodiazepines are contraindicated in patients with acute narrow angle glaucoma. Benzodiazepines may be used in patients with open angle glaucoma only if they are receiving appropriate therapy. Measurements of intraocular pressure in patients without eye disease show a moderate lowering following induction with midazolam HCl; patients with glaucoma have not been studied.

CONTRAINDICATIONS: *(cont'd)*

Midazolam HCl is not intended for intrathecal or epidural administration due to the presence of the preservative benzyl alcohol in the dosage form.

WARNINGS:

Midazolam HCl must never be used without individualization of dosage. Prior to the intravenous administration of midazolam HCl in any dose, the immediate availability of oxygen, resuscitative equipment and skilled personnel for the maintenance of a patent airway and support of ventilation should be ensured. Patients should be continuously monitored for early signs of underventilation or apnea, which can lead to hypoxia/cardiac arrest unless effective countermeasures are taken immediately. Vital signs should continue to be monitored during the recovery period. Because intravenous midazolam HCl depresses respiration (see CLINICAL PHARMACOLOGY) and because opioid agonists and other sedatives can add to this depression. midazolam HCl should be administered as an induction agent only by a person trained in general anesthesia and should be used for conscious sedation only in the presence of personnel skilled in early detection of underventilation, maintaining a patent airway and supporting ventilation. **When used for conscious sedation, midazolam HCl should not be administered by rapid or single bolus intravenous administration.**

Serious cardiorespiratory adverse events have occurred. These have included respiratory depression, apnea, respiratory arrest and or cardiac arrest, sometimes resulting in death. There have also been rare reports of hypotensive episodes requiring treatment during or after diagnostic or surgical manipulations in patients who have received midazolam HCl. Hypotension occurred more frequently in the conscious sedation studies in patients premedicated with a narcotic.

Reactions such as agitation, involuntary movements (including tonic/ clonic movements and muscle tremor), hyperactivity and combativeness have been reported. These reactions may be due to inadequate or excessive dosing or improper administration of midazolam HCl; however, consideration should be given to the possibility of cerebral hypoxia or true paradoxical reactions. Should such reactions occur, the response to each dose of midazolam HCl and all other drugs, including local anesthetics, should be evaluated before proceeding.

Concomitant use of barbiturates, alcohol or other central nervous system depressants may increase the risk of underventilation or apnea and may contribute to profound and or prolonged drug effect. Narcotic premedication also depresses the ventilatory response to carbon dioxide stimulation.

Higher risk surgical patients, elderly patients and debilitated patients require lower dosages, whether pre-medicated or not. Patients with chronic obstructive pulmonary disease are unusually sensitive to the respiratory depressant effect of midazolam HCl. Patients with chronic renal failure and patients with congestive heart failure eliminate midazolam more slowly. (See CLINICAL PHARMACOLOGY.) Because elderly patients frequently have inefficient function of one or more organ systems, and because dosage requirements have been shown to decrease with age, reduced initial dosage of midazolam HCl is recommended and the possibility of profound and or prolonged effect should be considered.

Injectable midazolam HCl should not be administered to patients in shock or coma, or in acute alcohol intoxication with depression of vital signs. Particular care should be exercised in the use of intravenous midazolam HCl in patients with uncompensated acute illnesses, such as severe fluid or electrolyte disturbances.

The hazards of intra-arterial injection of midazolam HCl solutions in humans are unknown; therefore, precautions against unintended intra-arterial injection should be taken. Extravasation should also be avoided.

The safety and efficacy of midazolam HCl following non-intravenous and non-intramuscular routes of administration have not been established. Midazolam HCl should only be administered intramuscularly or intravenously.

The decision as to when patients who have received injectable midazolam HCl, particularly on an outpatient basis, may again engage in activities requiring complete mental alertness, operate hazardous machinery or drive a motor vehicle must be individualized. Gross tests of recovery from the effects of midazolam HCl (see CLINICAL PHARMACOLOGY) cannot be relied upon alone to predict reaction time under stress. This drug is never used alone during anesthesia and the contribution of other perioperative drugs and events can vary. It is recommended that no patient operate hazardous machinery or a motor vehicle until the effects of the drug, such as drowsiness, have subsided or until the day after anesthesia and surgery, whichever is longer.

USAGE IN PREGNANCY

An increased risk of congenital malformations associated with the use of benzodiazepine drugs (diazepam and chlordiazepoxide) has been suggested in several studies. If this drug is used during pregnancy, the patient should be apprised of the potential hazard to the fetus.

PRECAUTIONS:

GENERAL

Intravenous doses of midazolam HCl should be decreased for elderly and for debilitated patients. (See WARNINGS and DOSAGE AND ADMINISTRATION). These patients will also probably take longer to recover completely after midazolam HCl administration for the induction of anesthesia.

Midazolam HCl does not protect against the increase in intracranial pressure or against the heart rate rise and or blood pressure rise associated with endotracheal intubation under light general anesthesia.

INFORMATION FOR THE PATIENT

To assure safe and effective use of benzodiazepines, the following information and instructions should be communicated to the patient when appropriate:

1. Inform your physician about any alcohol consumption and medicine you are now taking, including drugs you buy without a prescription. Alcohol has an increased effect when consumed with benzodiazepines: therefore, caution should be exercised regarding simultaneous ingestion of alcohol during benzodiazepine treatment.

2. Inform your physician if you are pregnant or are planning to become pregnant.

3. Inform your physician if you are nursing.

DRUG LABORATORY TEST INTERACTIONS

Midazolam has not been shown to interfere with results obtained in clinical laboratory tests.

CARCINOGENESIS, MUTAGENESIS, AND IMPAIRMENT OF FERTILITY:

Carcinogenesis: Midazolam maleate was administered with diet in mice and rats for two years at dosages of 1.9 and 80 mg/kg/day. In female mice in the highest dose group there was a marked increase in the incidence of hepatic tumors. In high dose male rats there was a small but statistically significant increase in benign thyroid follicular cell tumors. Dosages of 9 mg/kg/day of midazolam maleate (25 times a human dose of 0.35 mg/kg) do not increase the incidence of tumors. The pathogenesis of induction of these tumors is not known. These tumors were found after chronic administration, whereas human use will ordinarily be of single or several doses.

Mutagenesis: Midazolam did not have mutagenic activity in *Salmonella typhimurium* (5 bacterial strains). Chinese hamster lung cells (V79), human lymphocytes, or in the micronucleus test in mice.

PRECAUTIONS: *(cont'd)*

Impairment Of Fertility: A reproduction study in male and female rats did not show any impairment of fertility at dosages up to ten times the human IV dose of 0.35 mg/kg.

PREGNANCY, TERATOGENIC EFFECTS, PREGNANCY CATEGORY D

See WARNINGS.

Segment II teratology studies, performed with midazolam maleate injectable in rabbits and rats at 5 and 10 times the human dose of 0.35 mg/kg, did not show evidence of teratogenicity.

Nonteratogenic effects: Studies in rats showed no adverse effects on reproductive parameters during gestation and lactation. Dosages tested were approximately 10 times the human dose of 0.35 mg/kg.

LABOR AND DELIVERY

In humans, measurable levels of midazolam were found in maternal venous serum, umbilical venous and arterial serum and amniotic fluid, indicating placental transfer of the drug. Following intramuscular administration of 0.05 mg/kg of midazolam, both the venous and the umbilical arterial serum concentrations were lower than maternal concentrations.

The use of injectable midazolam HCl in obstetrics has not been evaluated in clinical studies. Because midazolam is transferred transplacentally and because other benzodiazepines given in the last weeks of pregnancy have resulted in neonatal CNS depression, midazolam HCl is not recommended for obstetrical use.

NURSING MOTHERS

It is not known whether midazolam is excreted in human milk. Because many drugs are excreted in human milk, caution should be exercised when injectable midazolam HCl is administered to a nursing woman.

PEDIATRIC USE

Safety and effectiveness of midazolam HCl in children below the age of 18 years have not been established.

DRUG INTERACTIONS:

The sedative effect of intravenous midazolam HCl is accentuated by premedication, particularly narcotics (*e.g.,* morphine, meperidine and fentanyl) and also secobarbital and Innovar (fentanyl and droperidol). Consequently, the dosage of midazolam HCl should be adjusted according to the type and amount of premedication administered. (See DOSAGE AND ADMINISTRATION.)

A moderate reduction in induction dosage requirements of thiopental (about 15%) has been noted following use of intramuscular midazolam HCl for premedication.

The intravenous administration of midazolam HCl decreases the minimum alveolar concentration (MAC) of halothane required for general anesthesia. This decrease correlates with the dose of midazolam HCl administered.

Although the possibility of minor interactive effects has not been fully studied. Midazolam HCl and pancuronium have been used together in patients without noting clinically significant changes in dosage, onset or duration. Midazolam HCl does not protect against the characteristic circulatory changes noted after administration of succinylcholine or pancuronium and does not protect against the increased intracranial pressure noted following administration of succinylcholine. Midazolam HCl does not cause a clinically significant change in dosage, onset or duration of a single intubating dose of succinylcholine.

No significant adverse interactions with commonly used premedications or drugs used during anesthesia and surgery (including atropine, scopolamine, glycopyrrolate, diazepam, hydroxyzine, d-tubocurarine, succinylcholine and nondepolarizing muscle relaxants) or topical local anesthetics (including lidocaine, dyclonine HCl and Cetacaine) have been observed.

The clearance of midazolam and certain other benzodiazepines may be delayed with the concomitant administration of cimetidine (but not ranitidine). The clinical significance of this interaction is unclear.

ADVERSE REACTIONS:

See WARNINGS concerning serious cardiorespiratory events and possible paradoxical reactions. Fluctuations in vital signs were the most frequently seen findings following parenteral administration of midazolam HCl and included decreased tidal volume and or respiratory rate decrease (23.3% of patients following IV and 10.8% of patients following IM administration) and apnea (15.4% of patients following IV administration), as well as variations in blood pressure and pulse rate.

The following additional adverse reactions were reported after intramuscular administration: headache (1.3%) *Local effects at IM Injection site:* pain (3.7%), induration (0.5%), redness (0.5%), muscle stiffness (0.3%).

The following additional adverse reactions were reported subsequent to intravenous administration: hiccoughs (3.9%), nausea (2.8%), vomiting (2.6%), coughing (1.3%), "oversedation" (1.6%), headache (1.5%), drowsiness (1.2%); *Local effects at the IV site:* tenderness (5.6%), pain during injection (5.0%), redness (2.6%), induration (1.7%), phlebitis (0.4%).

Other adverse experiences, observed mainly following IV injection and occurring at an incidence of less than 1.0%, are as follows:

Respiratory: Laryngospasm, bronchospasm, dyspnea, hyperventilation, wheezing, shallow respirations, airway obstruction, tachypnea.

Cardiovascular: Bigeminy, premature ventricular contractions, vasovagal episode, tachycardia, nodal rhythm.

Gastrointestinal: Acid taste, excessive salivation, retching.

CNS Neuromuscular: Retrograde amnesia, euphoria, confusion, argumentativeness, nervousness, anxiety, grogginess, restlessness, emergence delirium or agitation, prolonged emergence from anesthesia, dreaming during emergence, sleep disturbance, insomnia, nightmares, athetoid movements, ataxia, dizziness, dysphoria, slurred speech, dysphonia, paresthesia.

Special Sense: Blurred vision, diplopia, nystagmus, pinpoint pupils, cyclic movements of eyelids, visual disturbance, difficulty focusing eyes, ears blocked, loss of balance, light-headedness.

Integumentary: Hives, hive-like elevation at injection site, swelling or feeling of burning, warmth or coldness at injection site, rash, pruritus.

Hypersensitivity: Allergic reactions including anaphylactoid reactions, hives, rash, and pruritus.

Miscellaneous: Yawning, lethargy, chills, weakness, toothache, faint feeling, hematoma.

DRUG ABUSE AND DEPENDENCE:

Midazolam is subject to Schedule IV control under the Controlled Substances Act of 1970.

Midazolam was actively self-administered in primate models used to assess the positive reinforcing effects of psychoactive drugs.

Midazolam produced physical dependence of a mild to moderate intensity in cynomolgus monkeys after 5 to 10 weeks of administration. Available data concerning the drug abuse and dependence potential of midazolam suggest that its abuse potential is at least equivalent to that of diazepam.

OVERDOSAGE:

While there is insufficient human data on overdosage with midazolam HCl, the manifestations of midazolam HCl overdosage are expected to be similar to those observed with other benzodiazepines and include sedation, somnolence, confusion, impaired coordination, diminished reflexes, coma and untoward effects on vital signs. No evidence of specific organ toxicity from midazolam HCl overdosage would be expected.

Treatment of Overdosage: Treatment of injectable midazolam HCl overdosage is the same as that followed for overdosage with other benzodiazepines. Respiration, pulse rate and blood pressure should be monitored and general supportive measures should be employed. Attention should be given to the maintenance of a patent airway and support of ventilation. An intravenous infusion should be started. Should hypotension develop, treatment may include intravenous fluid therapy, repositioning, judicious use of vasopressors appropriate to the clinical situation, if indicated, and other appropriate countermeasures. There is no information as to whether peritoneal dialysis, forced diuresis or hemodialysis are of any value in the treatment of midazolam overdosage.

Flumazenil, a specific benzodiazepine-receptor antagonist, is indicated for the complete or partial reversal of the sedative effects of benzodiazepines and may be used in situations when an overdose with a benzodiazepine is known or suspected. Prior to the administration of flumazenil, necessary measures should be instituted to secure airway, ventilation, and intravenous access. Flumazenil is intended as an adjunct to, not as a substitute for proper management of benzodiazepine overdose. Patients treated with flumazenil should be monitored for resedation, respiratory depression and other residual benzodiazepine effects for an appropriate period after treatment. **The prescriber should be aware of a risk of seizure in association with flumazenil treatment, particularly in long-term benzodiazepine users and in cyclic antidepressant overdose.** The complete flumazenil package insert, including CONTRAINDICATIONS, WARNINGS, and PRECAUTIONS, should be consulted prior to use.

DOSAGE AND ADMINISTRATION:

Midazolam HCl is a potent sedative agent which requires slow administration and individualization of dosage. Clinical experience has shown midazolam HCl to be 3 to 4 times as potent per mg as diazepam. BECAUSE SERIOUS AND LIFE-THREATENING CARDIORESPIRATORY ADVERSE EVENTS HAVE BEEN REPORTED, PROVISION FOR MONITORING, DETECTION AND CORRECTION OF THESE REACTIONS MUST BE MADE FOR EVERY PATIENT TO WHOM MIDAZOLAM HCl INJECTION IS ADMINISTERED. REGARDLESS OF AGE OR HEALTH STATUS. Excess doses or rapid or single bolus intravenous administration may result in respiratory depression and/or arrest. (See WARNINGS.)

Reactions such as agitation, involuntary movements, hyperactivity and combativeness have been reported. Should such reactions occur, caution should be exercised before continuing administration of midazolam HCl (See WARNINGS.)

Care should be taken to avoid intra-arterial injection or extravasation.(See WARNINGS.)

Midazolam HCl Injection may be mixed in the same syringe with the following frequently used premedications: morphine sulfate, meperidine, atropine sulfate or scopolamine midazolam HCl Injection is compatible with 5% dextrose in water, 0.9% sodium chloride and lactated Ringer's solution. Both the 1 mg ml and 5 mg ml formulations of midazolam HCl may be diluted with 0.9% sodium chloride or 5% dextrose in water.

Intramuscularly: For preoperative sedation (induction of sleepiness or drowsiness and relief of apprehension) and to impair memory of perioperative events.

For intramuscular use. Midazolam HCl should be injected deep in a large muscle mass.

INTRAVENOUSLY

Conscious Sedation: See INDICATIONS AND USAGE:

Narcotic premedication results in less variability in patient response and a reduction in dosage of midazolam HCl. For peroral procedures, the use of an appropriate topical anesthetic is recommended. For bronchoscopic procedures, the use of narcotic premedication is recommended.

Midazolam HCl 1 mg ml formulation is recommended for conscious sedation, to facilitate slower injection. Both the 1 mg ml and the 5 mg ml formulations may be diluted with 0.9% sodium chloride or 5% dextrose in water.

Induction of Anesthesia: For induction of general anesthesia, before administration of other anesthetic agents.

Injectable midazolam HCl can also be used during maintenance of anesthesia,*for short surgical procedures,* as a component of balanced anesthesia. Effective narcotic premedication is especially recommended in such cases. Long surgical procedures have not been studied.

Usual Adult Dose: The recommended premedication dose of midazolam HCl for good risk (ASA Physical Status I & II) adult patients below the age of 60 years is 0.07 to 0.08 mg/kg IM (approximately 5 mg IM) administered approximately 1 hour before surgery.

The dose must be individualized and reduced when IM midazolam HCl is administered to patients with chronic obstructive pulmonary disease, other higher risk surgical patients, patients 60 or more years of age and patients who have received concomitant narcotics or other CNS depressants (see ADVERSE REACTIONS.) In a study of patients 60 years or older, who did not receive concomitant administration of narcotics, 2 to 3 mg (0.02 to 0.05 mg/kg) of midazolam HCl produced adequate sedation during the preoperative period. The dose of 1 mg IM midazolam HCl may suffice for some older patients if the anticipated intensity and duration of sedation is less critical. As with ant potential respiratory depressant, these patients require observation for signs of cardiorespiratory depression after receiving IM midazolam HCl.

Onset is within 15 minutes, peaking at 30 to 60 minutes. It can be administered concomitantly with atropine sulfate or scopolamine hydrochloride and reduced doses of narcotics.

When used for conscious sedation, dosage must be individualized and titrated. Midazolam HCl should not be administered by rapid or single bolus intravenous administration. Individual response will vary with age, physical status and concomitant medications, but may also vary independent of these factors. (See WARNINGS concerning cardiac/respiratory arrest.)

Healthy adults below the age of 60: Titrate *slowly* to the desired effect, *e.g.,* the initiation of slurred speech. Some patients may respond to as little as 1 mg. No more than 2.5 mg should be given over a period of at least 2 minutes. Wait an additional 2 or more minutes to fully evaluate the sedative effect. If further titration is necessary, continue to titrate, using small increments, to the appropriate level of sedation. Wait an additional 2 or more minutes after each increment to fully evaluate the sedative effect. A total dose greater than 5 mg is not usually necessary to reach the desired endpoint.

If narcotic premedication or other CNS depressants are used, patients will require approximately 30% less midazolam HCl than unpremedicated patients.

Patients age 60 or older, and debilitated or chronically ill patients: Because the danger of underventilation or apnea is greater in elderly patients and those with chronic disease states or decreased pulmonary reserve, and because the peak effect may take longer in these patients, increments should be smaller and the rate of injection slower.

Titrate *slowly* to the desired effect, *e.g.,* the initiation of slurred speech. Some patients may respond to as little as 1 mg. No more than 1.5 mg should be given over a period of no less than 2 minutes. Wait an additional 2 or more minutes to fully evaluate the sedative effect. If

DOSAGE AND ADMINISTRATION: *(cont'd)*

additional titration is necessary. It should be given at a rate of no more than 1 mg over a period of 2 minutes, waiting an additional 2 or more minutes each time to fully evaluate the sedative effect. Total doses greater than 3.5 mg are not usually necessary.

If concomitant CNS depressant premedications are used in these patients, they will require at least 50% less midazolam HCl than healthy young unpremedicated patients.

Maintenance dose: Additional doses to maintain the desired level of sedation may be given in increments of 25% of the dose used to first reach the sedative endpoint, but again only by slow titration, especially in the elderly and chronically ill or debilitated patient. These additional doses should be given *only* after a thorough clinical evaluation clearly indicates the need for additional sedation.

Individual response to the drug is variable, particularly when a narcotic premedication is not used. The dosage should be titrated to the desired effect according to the patient's age and clinical status.

Unpremedicated Patients: In the absence of premedication, an average adult under the age of 55 years will usually require an initial dose of 0.3 to 0.35 mg/kg for induction, administered over 20 to 30 seconds and allowing 2 minutes for effect. If needed to complete induction, increments of approximately 25% of the patient's initial dose may be used, induction may instead be completed with volatile liquid inhalational anesthetics. In resistant cases, up to 0.6 mg/kg total dose may be used for induction, but such larger doses may prolong recovery.

Unpremedicated patients over the age of 55 years usually require less midazolam HCl for induction, an initial dose of 0.3 mg/kg is recommended. Unpremedicated patients with severe systemic disease or other debilitation usually require less midazolam HCl for induction. An initial dose of 0.2 to 0.25 mg/kg will usually suffice. In some cases, as little as 0.15 mg/kg may suffice.

Premedicated Patients: When the patient has received sedative or narcotic premedication, particularly narcotic premedication, the range of recommended doses is 0.15 to 0.35 mg/kg.

In average adults below the age of 55 years, a dose of 0.25 mg/kg, administered over 20 to 30 seconds and allowing 2 minutes for effect will usually suffice.

The initial dose of 0.2 mg/kg is recommended for good risk (ASA I & II) surgical patients over the age of 55 years.

In some patients with severe systemic disease or debilitation, as little as 0.15 mg/kg may suffice.

Narcotic premedication frequently used during clinical trials included fentanyl (1.5 to 2 mcg/kg IV, administered five minutes before induction), morphine (dosage individualized, up to 0.15 mg/kg IM), meperidine (dosage individualized, up to 1 mg/kg IM) and Innovar (0.02 ml/kg IM). Sedative premedications were hydroxyzine pamoate (100 mg orally) and sodium secobarbital (200 mg orally). Except for intravenous fentanyl, administered five minutes before induction, all other premedications should be administered approximately one hour prior to the time anticipated for midazolam HCl induction.

Incremental injections of approximately 25% of the induction dose should be given in response to signs of lightening of anesthesia and repeated as necessary.

Note: Parenteral drug products should be inspected visually for particulate matter and discoloration prior to administration, whenever solution and container permit.

HOW SUPPLIED - EQUIVALENTS NOT AVAILABLE:

Injection, Solution - Intramuscular; - 1 mg/ml

2 ml x 10	$43.37	VERSED STERILE, Roche	00004-1998-06
5 ml x 10	$95.34	VERSED STERILE, Roche	00004-1999-01
10 ml x 10	$170.50	VERSED STERILE, Roche	00004-2000-06

Injection, Solution - Intramuscular; - 5 mg/ml

1 ml x 10	$95.34	VERSED, Roche	00004-1974-01
2 ml x 10	$170.50	VERSED, Roche	00004-1973-01
2 ml x 10	$214.20	VERSED, Roche	00004-1947-01
5 ml x 10	$402.62	VERSED, Roche	00004-1975-01
10 ml x 10	$764.97	VERSED, Roche	00004-1946-01

MIDODRINE HYDROCHLORIDE *(003307)*

CATEGORIES: Alpha Adrenergic Agonists; Hypotension; Orthostatic Hypotension; Postural Hypotension; Pregnancy Category C; FDA Approved 1996 Sep

BRAND NAMES: *Gutron* (France, Germany); *Metligine* (Japan); *Midron*; **ProAmatine**

(International brand names outside U.S. in italics)

WARNING:
Because midodrine HCl can cause marked elevation of supine blood pressure, it should be used in patients whose lives are considerably impaired despite standard clinical care. The indication for use of midodrine HCl in the treatment of symptomatic orthostatic hypotension is based primarily on a change in a surrogate marker of effectiveness, an increase in systolic blood pressure measured one minute after standing, a surrogate marker considered likely to correspond to a clinical benefit. At present, however, clinical benefits of midodrine HCl, principally improved ability to carry out activities of daily living, have not been verified.

DESCRIPTION:

ProAmatine Tablets: *Dosage Form:* 2.5-mg and 5-mg tablets for oral administration. *Active Ingredient:* Midodrine hydrochloride, 2.5 mg or 5 mg. *Inactive Ingredients:* Microcrystalline Cellulose NF, Colloidal Silicone Dioxide NF, Magnesium Stearate NF, Corn Starch NF, Talc USP, FD&C Yellow No. 6 Lake (5-mg tablet).

Pharmacological Classification: Vasopressor/Antihypotensive.

Chemical Names (USAN: Midodrine Hydrochloride): (1) Acetamide, 2-amino-*N* [2-(2,5-dimethoxyphenyl)-2-hydroxyethyl]-monohydrochloride,(±)-; (2) (±)-2-amino-*N*-(β-hydroxy-2,5-dimethoxyphenethyl)acetamide monohydrochloride BAN, INN, JAN: Midodrine.

Molecular Formula: $C_{12}H_{18}N_2O_4HCl$; *Molecular Weight:* 290.7.

Organoleptic Properties: Odorless, white, crystalline powder.

Solubility: *Water:* Soluble. *Methanol:* Sparingly soluble.

pKa: 7.8 (0.3% aqueous solution).

pH: 3.5 to 5.5 (5% aqueous solution).

Melting Range: 200 to 203°C.

CLINICAL PHARMACOLOGY:

Mechanism of Action: Midodrine HCl forms an active metabolite, desglymidodrine, that is an $alpha_1$-agonist, and exerts its actions via activation of the alpha-adrenergic receptors of the arteriolar and venous vasculature, producing an increase in vascular tone and elevation of blood pressure. Desglymidodrine does not stimulate cardiac beta-adrenergic receptors. Desglymidodrine diffuses poorly across the blood-brain barrier, and is therefore not associated with effects on the central nervous system.

Administration of midodrine HCl results in a rise in standing, sitting, and supine systolic and diastolic blood pressure in patients with orthostatic hypotension of various etiologies. Standing systolic blood pressure is elevated by approximately 15 to 30 mmHg at 1 hour after a 10-mg dose of midodrine, with some effect persisting for 2 to 3 hours. Midodrine HCl has no clinically significant effect on standing or supine pulse rates in patients with autonomic failure.

Pharmacokinetics: Midodrine HCl is a prodrug (*i.e.,* the therapeutic effect of orally administered midodrine is due to the major metabolite desglymidodrine, formed by deglycination of midodrine). After oral administration, midodrine HCl is rapidly absorbed. The plasma levels of the prodrug peak after about half an hour, and decline with a half-life of approximately 25 minutes, while the metabolite reaches peak blood concentrations about 1 to 2 hours after a dose of midodrine and has a half-life of about 3 to 4 hours. The absolute bioavailability of midodrine (measured as desglymidodrine) is 93%. The bioavailability of desglymidodrine is not affected by food. Approximately the same amount of desglymidodrine is formed after intravenous and oral administration of midodrine. Neither midodrine nor desglymidodrine is bound to plasma proteins to any significant extent.

Metabolism and Excretion: Thorough metabolic studies have not been conducted, but it appears that deglycination of midodrine to desglymidodrine takes place in many tissues, and both compounds are metabolized in part by the liver. Neither midodrine nor desglymidodrine is a substrate for monoamine oxidase.

Renal elimination of midodrine is insignificant. The renal clearance of desglymidodrine is of the order of 385 ml/minute, most, about 80%, by active renal secretion. The actual mechanism of active secretion has not been studied, but it is possible that it occurs by the base-secreting pathway responsible for the secretion of several other drugs that are base (see also DRUG INTERACTIONS, Potential for Drug Interactions).

CLINICAL STUDIES:

Midodrine has been studied in 3 principal controlled trials, one of 3-weeks duration and 2 of 1 to 2 days duration. All studies were randomized, double-blind and parallel-design trials in patients with orthostatic hypotension of any etiology and supine-to-standing fall of systolic blood pressure of at least 15 mmHg accompanied by at least moderate dizziness/lightheadedness. Patients with pre-existing sustained supine hypertension above 180/110 mmHg were routinely excluded. In a 3-week study in 170 patients, most previously untreated with midodrine, the midodrine-treated patients (10 mg three times daily, with the last dose not later than 6 P.M.) had significantly higher (by about 20 mmHg) 1-minute standing systolic pressure 1 hour after dosing (blood pressures were not measured at other times) for all 3 weeks. After week 1, midodrine-treated patients had small improvements in dizziness/lightheadedness/unsteadiness scores and global evaluations, but these effects were made difficult to interpret by a high early drop-out rate (about 25% vs 5% on placebo). Supine and sitting blood pressure rose 16/8 and 20/10 mmHg, respectively, on average.

In a 2-day study, after open-label midodrine, known midodrine responders received midodrine 10 mg or placebo at 0, 3, and 6 hours. One-minute standing systolic blood pressures were increased 1 hour after each dose by about 15 mmHg and 3 hours after each dose by about 12 mmHg; 3-minute standing pressures were increased also at 1, but not 3, hours after dosing. There were increases in standing time seen intermittently 1 hour after dosing, but not at 3 hours.

In a 1-day, dose-response trial, single doses of 0, 2.5, 10, and 20 mg of midodrine were given to 25 patients. The 10- and 20-mg doses produced increases in standing 1-minute systolic pressure of about 30 mmHg at 1 hour; the increase was sustained in part for 2 hours after 10 mg and 4 hours after 20 mg. Supine systolic pressure was ≥200 mmHg in 22% of patients on 10 mg and 45% of patients on 20 mg; elevated pressures often lasted 6 hours or more.

INDICATIONS AND USAGE:

Midodrine HCl is indicated for the treatment of symptomatic orthostatic hypotension (OH). Because midodrine HCl can cause marked elevation of supine blood pressure (BP>200 mmHg systolic), it should be used in patients whose lives are considerably impaired despite standard clinical care, including non-pharmacologic treatment (such as support stockings), fluid expansion, and lifestyle alterations. The indication is based on midodrine HCl's effect on increases in 1-minute standing systolic blood pressure, a surrogate marker considered likely to correspond to a clinical benefit. At present, however, clinical benefits of midodrine HCl, principally improved ability to perform life activities, have not been established. Further clinical trials are underway to verify and describe the clinical benefits of midodrine HCl.

After initiation of treatment, midodrine HCl should be continued only for patients who report significant symptomatic improvement.

CONTRAINDICATIONS:

Midodrine HCl is contraindicated in patients with severe organic heart disease, acute renal disease, urinary retention, pheochromocytoma or thyrotoxicosis. Midodrine HCl should not be used in patients with persistent and excessive supine hypertension.

WARNINGS:

Supine Hypertension: The most potentially serious adverse reaction associated with midodrine HCl therapy is marked elevation of supine arterial blood pressure (supine hypertension). Systolic pressure of about 200 mmHg were seen overall in about 13.4% of patients given 10 mg of midodrine HCl. Systolic elevations of this degree were most likely to be observed in patients with relatively elevated pretreatment systolic blood pressures (mean 170 mmHg). There is no experience in patients with initial supine systolic pressure above 180 mmHg, as those patients were excluded from the clinical trials. Use of midodrine HCl in such patients is not recommended. Sitting blood pressures were also elevated by midodrine HCl therapy. It is essential to monitor supine and sitting blood pressures in patients maintained on midodrine HCl.

PRECAUTIONS:

General: The potential for supine and sitting hypertension should be evaluated at the beginning of midodrine HCl therapy. Supine hypertension can often be controlled by preventing the patient from becoming fully supine (*i.e.,* sleeping with the head of the bed elevated). The patient should be cautioned to report symptoms of supine hypertension immediately. Symptoms may include cardiac awareness, pounding in the ears, headache, blurred vision, etc. The patient should be advised to discontinue the medication immediately if supine hypertension persists.

Blood pressure should be monitored carefully when midodrine HCl is used concomitantly with other agents that cause vasoconstriction, such as phenylephrine, ephedrine, dihydroergotamine, phenylpropanolamine, or pseudoephedrine.

PRECAUTIONS: *(cont'd)*

A slight slowing of the heart rate may occur after administration of midodrine HCl, primarily due to vagal reflex. Caution should be exercised when midodrine HCl is used concomitantly with cardiac glycosides (such as digitalis), psychopharmacologic agents, beta blockers or other agents that directly or indirectly reduce heart rate. Patients who experience any signs or symptoms suggesting bradycardia (pulse slowing, increased dizziness, syncope, cardiac awareness) should be advised to discontinue midodrine HCl and should be re-evaluated.

Midodrine HCl should be used cautiously in patients with urinary retention problems, as desglymidodrine acts on the alpha-adrenergic receptors of the bladder neck.

Midodrine HCl should be used with caution in orthostatic hypotensive patients who are also diabetic, as well as those with a history of visual problems who are also taking fludrocortisone acetate, which is known to cause an increase in intraocular pressure and glaucoma.

Midodrine HCl use has not been studied in patients with renal impairment. Because desglymidodrine is eliminated via the kidneys, and higher blood levels would be expected in such patients, midodrine HCl should be used with caution in patients with renal impairment, with a starting dose of 2.5 mg (see DOSAGE AND ADMINISTRATION). Renal function should be assessed prior to initial use of midodrine HCl.

Midodrine HCl use has not been studied in patients with hepatic impairment. Midodrine HCl should be used with caution in patients with hepatic impairment, as the liver has a role in the metabolism of midodrine.

Information for the Patient: Patients should be told that certain agents in over-the-counter products, such as cold remedies and diet aids can elevate blood pressure, and therefore, should be used cautiously with midodrine HCl, as they may enhance or potentiate the pressor effects of midodrine HCl (see DRUG INTERACTIONS). Patients should also be made aware of the possibility of supine hypertension. They should also be told to avoid taking their dose if they are to be supine for any length of time (*i.e.,* they should take their last dose of midodrine HCl 3 to 4 hours before bedtime to minimize nighttime supine hypertension.

Laboratory Tests: Since desglymidodrine is eliminated by the kidneys and the liver has a role in its metabolism, evaluation of the patient should include assessment of renal and hepatic function prior to initiating therapy and subsequently, as appropriate.

Carcinogenesis, Mutagenesis, and Impairment of Fertility: Long-term studies have been conducted in rats and mice at dosages of 3 to 4 times the maximum recommended daily human dose on a mg/m^2 basis, with no indication of carcinogenic effects related to midodrine HCl. Studies investigating the mutagenic potential of midodrine HCl revealed no evidence of mutagenicity. Other than the dominant lethal assay in male mice, where no impairment of fertility was observed, there have beer no studies on the effects of midodrine HCl on fertility.

Pregnancy Category C: Midodrine HCl increased the rate of embryo resorption, reduced fetal body weight in rats and rabbits, and decreased fetal survival in rabbits when given in doses 13 (rat) and 7 (rabbit) times the maximum human dose based on body surface area (mg/m^2). There are no adequate and well-controlled studies in pregnant women. Midodrine HCl should be used during pregnancy only if the potential benefit justifies the potential risk to the fetus. No teratogenic effects have been observed in studies in rats and rabbits.

Nursing Mothers: It is not known whether this drug is excreted in human milk. Because many drugs are excreted in human milk, caution should be exercised when midodrine HCl is administered to a nursing woman.

Pediatric Use: Safety and effectiveness in pediatric patients have not been established.

DRUG INTERACTIONS:

When administered concomitantly with midodrine HCl, cardiac glycosides may enhance or precipitate bradycardia, AV block or arrhythmia.

The use of drugs that stimulate alpha-adrenergic receptors (*e.g.,* phenylephrine, pseudoephedrine, ephedrine, phenylpropanolamine or dihydroergotamine) may enhance or potentiate the pressor effects of midodrine HCl. Therefore, caution should be used when midodrine HCl is administered concomitantly with agents that cause vasoconstriction.

Midodrine HCl has been used in patients concomitantly treated with salt-retaining steroid therapy (*i.e.,* fludrocortisone acetate), with or without salt supplementation. The potential for supine hypertension should be carefully monitored in these patients and may be minimized by either reducing the dose of fludrocortisone acetate or decreasing the salt intake prior to initiation of treatment with midodrine HCl. Alpha-adrenergic blocking agents, such as prazosin, terazosin, and doxazosin, can antagonize the effects of midodrine HCl.

Potential for Drug Interactions: It appears possible, although there is no supporting experimental evidence, that the high renal clearance of desglymidodrine (a base) is due to active tubular secretion by the base-secreting system also responsible for the secretion of such drugs as metformin, cimetidine, ranitidine, procainamide, triamterene, flecainide, and quinidine. Thus there may be a potential for drug-drug interactions with these drugs.

ADVERSE REACTIONS:

The most frequent adverse reactions seen in controlled trials were supine and sitting hypertension; paresthesia and pruritus, mainly of the scalp; goosebumps; chills; urinary urge; urinary retention and urinary frequency.

The frequency of these events in a 3-week placebo-controlled trial is shown in TABLE 1.

TABLE 1 Adverse Events

	Placebo n=88		Midodrine n=82	
Event	**# of reports**	**% of patients**	**# of reports**	**% of patients**
Total # of reports	22		77	
Paresthesia*	4	4.5	15	18.3
Piloerection	0	0	11	13.4
Dysuria†	0	0	11	13.4
Pruritis‡	2	2.3	10	12.2
Supine hypertension§	0	0	6	7.3
Chills	0	0	4	4.9
Pain ‖	0	0	4	4.9
Rash	1	1.1	2	2.4

* Includes hyperesthesia and scalp paresthesia.
† Includes dysuria (1), increased urinary frequency (2), impaired urination (1), urinary retention (5), urinary urgency (2).
‡ Includes scalp pruritus.
§ Includes patients who experienced an increase in supine hypertension.
‖ Includes abdominal pain and pain increase.

Less frequent adverse reactions were headache; feeling of pressure/fullness in the head; vasodilation/flushing face; confusion/thinking abnormality; dry mouth; nervousness/anxiety and rash. Other adverse reactions that occurred rarely were visual field defect; dizziness; skin hyperesthesia; insomnia; somnolence; erythema multiforme; canker sore; dry skin; dysuria; impaired urination; asthenia; backache; pyrosis; nausea; gastrointestinal distress; flatulence and leg cramps.

ADVERSE REACTIONS: *(cont'd)*

The most potentially serious adverse reaction associated with midodrine HCl therapy is supine hypertension. The feelings of paresthesia, pruritus, piloerection and chills are pilomotor reactions associated with the action of midodrine on the alpha-adrenergic receptors of the hair follicles. Feelings of urinary urgency, retention and frequency are associated with the action of midodrine on the alpha-receptors of the bladder neck.

OVERDOSAGE:

Symptoms of overdose could include hypertension, piloerection (goosebumps), a sensation of coldness and urinary retention. There are 2 reported cases of overdosage with midodrine HCl, both in young males. One patient ingested midodrine HCl drops, 250 mg, experienced systolic blood pressure of greater than 200 mmHg, was treated with an IV injection of 20 mg of phentolamine, and was discharged the same night without any complaints. The other patient ingested 205 mg of midodrine HCl (41 5-mg tablets), and was found lethargic and unable to talk, unresponsive to voice, but responsive to painful stimuli, hypertensive and bradycardic. Gastric lavage was performed, and the patient recovered fully by the next day without sequelae.

The single doses that would be associated with symptoms of overdosage or would be potentially life-threatening are unknown. The oral LD_{50} is approximately 30 to 50 mg/kg in rats, 675 mg/kg in mice, and 125 to 160 mg/kg in dogs.

Desglymidodrine is dialyzable.

Recommended general treatment, based on the pharmacology of the drug, includes induced emesis and administration of alpha-sympatholytic drugs (*e.g.,* phentolamine).

DOSAGE AND ADMINISTRATION:

The recommended dose of midodrine HCl is 10 mg, 3 times daily. Dosing should take place during the daytime hours when the patient needs to be upright, pursuing the activities of daily life. A suggested dosing schedule of approximately 4-hour intervals is as follows: shortly before or upon rising in the morning, midday, and late afternoon (not later than 6 P.M.). Doses may be given in 3-hour intervals, if required, to control symptoms, but not more frequently. Single doses as high as 20 mg have been given to patients, but severe and persistent systolic supine hypertension occur at a high rate (about 45%) at this dose. In order to reduce the potential for supine hypertension during sleep, midodrine HCl should not be given after the evening meal or less than 4 hours before bedtime. Total daily doses greater than 30 mg have been tolerated by some patients, but their safety and usefulness have not been studied systematically or established. Because of the risk of supine hypertension, midodrine HCl should be continued only in patients who appear to attain symptomatic improvement during initial treatment.

The supine and standing blood pressure should be monitored regularly, and the administration of midodrine HCl should be stopped if supine blood pressure increases excessively.

Because desglymidodrine is excreted renally, dosing in patients with abnormal renal function should be cautious; although this has not been systematically studied, it is recommended that treatment of these patients be initiated using 2.5-mg doses.

Dosing in children has not been adequately studied.

Blood levels of midodrine and desglymidodrine were similar when comparing levels in patients 65 or older vs. younger than 65 and when comparing males vs. females, suggesting dose modifications for these groups are not necessary.

TABLE 2

Suggested dose:	10 mg three times daily; every 3-4 hours	
Suggested dosing schedule:	Dose 1:	Shortly before or upon rising in the morning
	Dose 2:	Midday
	Dose 3:	Late afternoon (not later than 6 PM)

Patients should be told to take their last dose of midorine HCl 3 to 4 hours before bedtime to minimize supine hypertension.

PATIENT INFORMATION:

Midodrine is used for the treatment of abnormally low blood pressure which occurs after standing.

Inform your doctor if you are taking any heart drugs, hormones, or prescription or over the counter cold remedies or diet pills.

Inform your doctor if you are pregnant or if you retain water.

Midodrine may cause high blood pressure; numbness/tingling; itching; goosebumps; chills; urinary retention, urgency or frequency.

May be taken with or without meals. Take at least 3 to 4 hours before bedtime.

HOW SUPPLIED:

ProAmatine is supplied as 2.5-mg and 5-mg tablets for oral administration. The 2.5-mg tablet is white, round, and biplanar, with a bevelled edge, and is scored on one side with "RPC" above and "2.5" below the score, and "003" on the other side. The 5-mg tablet is orange, round, and biplanar, with a bevelled edge, and is scored on one side with "RPC" above and "5" below the score, and "004" on the other side.

Storage: Store from 15 to 25°C (59 to 77°F).

HOW SUPPLIED - EQUIVALENTS NOT AVAILABLE:

Tablet - Oral - 5 mg

100's $140.40 PROAMATINE, Roberts Labs 54092-0004-01

MIFEPRISTONE *(003083)*

CATEGORIES: Abortion; Anti-Progesterone; Contraceptives; FDA Unapproved

BRAND NAMES: **Mifegyne**; RU-486

Prescribing information not available at time of publication.

MIGLITOL *(003310)*

CATEGORIES: Alpha Glucosidase Inhibitors; Antidiabetic Agents; Blood Glucose Regulators; Diabetes; Diabetes Mellitus; FDA Approved 1996 Dec; FDA Class 1S ('Standard Review'); Hormones; Hyperglycemia

BRAND NAMES: **Glyset**

DESCRIPTION:

Miglitol is an oral alpha-glucosidase inhibitor for use in the management of non-insulin dependent diabetes mellitus (NIDDM). Miglitol is a desoxynojirimycin derivative, and is chemically known as 3,4,5-piperidinetriol, 1-(2-hydroxyethyl)-2-(hydroxymethyl)-,[2R-(2α,3β, 4α, 5β)]-. It is a white to pale-yellow powder with a molecular weight of 207.2. Miglitol is soluble in water and has a pK_a of 5.9. Its empirical formula is $C_8H_{17}NO_5$.

Glyset tablets are available as 25 mg, 50 mg, and 100 mg tablets for oral use. The inactive ingredients are starch, microcrystalline cellulose, magnesium stearate, hydroxypropyl methylcellulose, polyethylene glycol, titanium dioxide, polysorbate 80, and iron oxide.

CLINICAL PHARMACOLOGY:

Miglitol is a desoxynojirimycin derivative that delays the digestion of ingested carbohydrates, thereby resulting in a smaller rise in blood glucose concentration following meals. As a consequence of plasma glucose reduction, miglitol reduces levels of glycosylated hemoglobin in patients with Type II (non-insulin-dependent) diabetes mellitus. Systemic nonenzymatic protein glycosylation, as reflected by levels of glycosylated hemoglobin, is a function of average blood glucose concentration over time.

Mechanism of Action: In contrast to sulfonylureas, miglitol does not enhance insulin secretion. The antihyperglycemic action of miglitol results from a reversible inhibition of membrane-bound intestinal α-glucoside hydrolase enzymes. Membrane-bound intestinal α-glucosidases hydrolyze oligosaccharides and disaccharides to glucose and other monosaccharides in the brush border of the small intestine. In diabetic patients, this enzyme inhibition results in delayed glucose absorption and lowering of postprandial hyperglycemia.

Because its mechanism of action is different, the effect of miglitol to enhance glycemic control is additive to that of sulfonylureas when used in combination. In addition, miglitol diminishes the insulinotropic and weight-increasing effects of sulfonylureas.

Miglitol has minor inhibitory activity against lactase and consequently, at the recommended doses, would not be expected to induce lactose intolerance.

PHARMACOKINETICS

Absorption: Absorption of miglitol is saturable at high doses; a dose of 25 mg is completely absorbed, whereas a dose of 100 mg is only 50% to 70% absorbed. For all doses, peak concentrations are reached in 2-3 hours. There is no evidence that systemic absorption of miglitol contributes to its therapeutic effect.

Distribution: The protein binding of miglitol is negligible (<4.0%). Miglitol has a volume of distribution of 0.18 L/kg, consistent with distribution primarily into the extracellular fluid.

Metabolism: Miglitol is not metabolized in man or in any animal species studied. No metabolites have been detected in plasma, urine, or feces, indicating a lack of either systemic or pre-systemic metabolism.

Excretion: Miglitol is eliminated by renal excretion as unchanged drug. Thus, following a 25-mg dose, over 95% of the dose is recovered in the urine within 24 hours. At higher doses, the cumulative recovery of drug from urine is somewhat lower due to the incomplete bioavailability. The elimination half-life from plasma is approximately 2 hours.

Special Populations

Renal Impairment: Because miglitol is excreted primarily by the kidneys, accumulation of miglitol is expected in patients with renal impairment. Patients with creatinine clearance <25 ml/min taking 25 mg 3 times daily exhibited a greater than two-fold increase in miglitol plasma levels as compared to subjects with creatinine clearance >60 ml/min. Dosage adjustment to correct the increased plasma concentrations is not feasible because miglitol acts locally. Little information is available on the safety of miglitol in patients with creatinine clearance <25 ml/min.

Hepatic Impairment: Miglitol pharmacokinetics were not altered in cirrhotic patients relative to healthy control subjects. Since miglitol is not metabolized, no influence of hepatic function on the kinetics of miglitol is expected.

Elderly: The pharmacokinetics of miglitol were studied in elderly and young males (n=8 per group). At a dosage of 100 mg 3 times daily for 3 days, no differences between the two groups were found.

Gender: No significant difference in the pharmacokinetics of miglitol was observed between elderly men and women when body weight was taken into account.

Race: Several pharmacokinetic studies were conducted in Japanese volunteers, with results similar to those observed in Caucasians. A study comparing the pharmacodynamic response to a single 50-mg dose in Black and Caucasian healthy volunteers indicated similar glucose and insulin responses in both populations.

CLINICAL STUDIES:

Clinical Experience in Non-Insulin-Dependent Diabetes Mellitus (NIDDM) Patients on Dietary Treatment Only: Miglitol was evaluated in two US and three non-US controlled, fixed dose, monotherapy studies, in which 735 miglitol-treated patients were evaluated for efficacy analyses. See TABLE 1.

In Study 1, a one-year study in which miglitol was evaluated as monotherapy and also as combination therapy, there was a statistically significantly smaller increase in mean glycosylated hemoglobin (HbA1c) over time in the miglitol 50 mg 3 times daily monotherapy arm compared to placebo. Significant reductions in mean fasting and postprandial plasma glucose levels and in mean postprandial insulin levels were observed in miglitol-treated patients compared with the placebo group.

In Study 2, a 14-week study, there was a significant decrease in HbA1c in patients receiving miglitol 50 mg three times daily or 100 mg 3 times daily compared to placebo. In addition, there were significant reductions in postprandial plasma glucose and postprandial serum insulin levels compared to placebo.

Study 3 was a 6-month, dose-ranging, trial evaluating miglitol at doses from 25 mg 3 times daily to 200 mg 3 times daily. Miglitol produced a greater reduction in HbA1c than placebo at all doses, although the effect was statistically significant only at the 100 mg three times daily and 200 mg 3 times daily doses. In addition, all doses of miglitol produced significant reductions in postprandial plasma glucose and postprandial insulin levels compared to placebo.

Studies 4 and 5 were 6-month studies evaluating 50 and 100 mg 3 times daily, and 100 mg 3 times daily, respectively. As compared to placebo, miglitol produced significant reductions in HbA1c, as well as a significant reduction in postprandial plasma glucose in both studies at the doses employed.

Clinical Experience in NIDDM Patients Receiving Sulfonlyureas: Miglitol was studied as adjunctive therapy to a background of maximal or near-maximal sulfonylurea (SFU) treatment in three large, double blind, randomized studies (two US and one non-US) in which 471 miglitol-treated patients were evaluated for efficacy. See TABLE 2.

Study 6 included patients under treatment with maximal doses of SFU at entry. At the end of this 14-week study, the mean treatment effects on glycosylated hemoglobin (HbA1c) were -0.82% and -0.74% for patients receiving miglitol 50 mg 3 times daily + SFU and miglitol 100 mg 3 times daily + SFU, respectively.

CLINICAL STUDIES: *(cont'd)*

TABLE 1 Miglitol Monotherapy Study Results

Treatment	HbA1c (%) Mean Change from Baseline*	HbA1c (%) Treatment Effect**	1-hour Postprandial Glucose (mg/dl) Mean Change from Baseline	1-hour Postprandial Glucose (mg/dl) Treatment Effect**
1 (US)				
Placebo	+0.71	-	+24	-
Miglitol 50 mg 3× Daily	+0.13	-0.58†	-39	-63†
2 (US)				
Placebo	+0.47	-	+15	-
Miglitol 50 mg 3× Daily	-0.22	-0.69†	-52	-67†
Miglitol 100 mg 3× Daily	-0.28	-0.75†	-59	-74†
3 (US)				
Placebo	+0.18	-	+2	-
Miglitol 25 mg 3× Daily	-0.08	-0.26	-33	-35†
Miglitol 50 mg 3× Daily	-0.22	-0.40	-45	-47†
Miglitol 100 mg 3× Daily	-0.63	-0.81†	-62	-64†
Miglitol 200 mg 3× Daily‡	0.84	-1.02†	-85	-87†
4 (non-US)				
Placebo	+0.01	-	+8	-
Miglitol 50 mg 3× Daily	-0.35	-0.36 †	-20	-28†
Miglitol 100 mg 3 × Daily	-0.57	-0.58†	-25	-33†
5 (non-US)				
Placebo	+0.32	-	+17	-
Miglitol 100 mg 3 × Daily	-0.43	-0.75†	-38	-55†

* Mean baseline ranged from 7.54 to 8.72% in these studies.
** The result of subtracting the placebo group average.
† p≤0.05 ‡ Although the results for the 200 mg 3 times daily are presented for completeness, the maximum recommended dosage of miglitol is 100 mg three times daily.

Study 7 was a one-year study in which miglitol at 25, 50 or 100 mg 3 times daily was added to a maximal dose of glyburide (10 mg twice daily). At the end of this study, the mean treatment effects on HbA1c of miglitol when added to maximum glyburide therapy were -0.30%, -0.62%, and -0.73% with the 25, 50, and 100 mg 3 times daily miglitol dosages, respectively.

In Study 8, the addition of miglitol 100 mg 3 times daily to a background of treatment with glyburide produced an additional mean treatment effect on HbA1c of -0.66%

TABLE 2 Miglitol Plus Sulfonylureas (SFU) Combination Therapy Results

Treatment	HbA1c (%) Mean Change from Baseline*	HbA1c (%) Treatment Effect**	1-hour Postprandial Glucose (mg/dl) Mean Change from Baseline	1-hour Postprandial Glucose (mg/dl) Treatment Effect**
6 (US)				
Placebo + SFU	+0.33	-	-1	-
Miglitol 50 mg t.i.d. + SFU	-0.49	-082†	-69	-68†
Miglitol 100 mg t.i.d. + SFU	-0.41	-0.74†	-73	-72†
7 (US)				
Placebo + SFU	+1.01	-	48	-
Miglitol 25mg t.i.d. + SFU	+0.71	-0.30†	-2	-50†
Miglitol 50 mg t.i.d. + SFU	+0.39	-0.62†	-13	-61†
Miglitol 100 mg 3 × Daily + SFU	+0.28	-0.73†	-33	-81†
8 (non-US)				
Placebo + SFU	+0.16	-	+10	-
Miglitol 100 mg t.i.d. + SFU	-0.50	-0.66†	-36	-46†

* Mean baseline ranged from 8.56 to 9.16 % in these studies.
** The result of subtracting the placebo group average.
† p≤0.05

Dose-Response: Results from controlled, fixed-dose studies of miglitol as monotherapy or as combination treatment with a sulfonylurea were combined to derive a pooled estimate of the difference from placebo in the mean change from baseline in glycosylated hemoglobin (HbA1c) and postprandial plasma glucose.

Because of its mechanism of action, the primary pharmacologic effect of miglitol is manifested as a reduction in postprandial plasma glucose, as shown previously in all of the major clinical trials. Miglitol was statistically different from placebo at all doses in each of the individual studies with respect to effect on mean one-hour postprandial plasma glucose, and there is a dose response from 25 to 100 mg 3 times daily for this efficacy parameter.

INDICATIONS AND USAGE:

Miglitol, as monotherapy, is indicated as an adjunct to diet to improve glycemic control in patients with non-insulin dependent diabetes mellitus (NIDDM) whose hyperglycemia cannot be managed with diet alone. Miglitol may also be used in combination with a sulfonylurea when diet plus either miglitol or a sulfonylurea alone do not result in adequate glycemic control. The effect of miglitol to enhance glycemic control is additive to that of sulfonylureas when used in combination, presumably because its mechanism of action is different.

In initiating treatment for NIDDM, diet should be emphasized as the primary form of treatment. Caloric restriction and weight loss are essential in the obese diabetic patient. Proper dietary management alone may be effective in controlling blood glucose and symptoms of hyperglycemia. The importance of regular physical activity when appropriate should also be stressed. If this treatment program fails to result in adequate glycemic control, the use of miglitol should be considered. The use of miglitol must be viewed by both the physician and patient as a treatment in addition to diet and not as a substitute for diet or as a convenient mechanism for avoiding restraint.

CONTRAINDICATIONS:

Miglitol is contraindicated in patients with:

Diabetic ketoacidosis

Inflammatory bowel disease

Colonic ulceration, or partial intestinal obstruction and in patients predisposed to intestinal obstruction

Chronic intestinal disease associated with marked disorders of digestion or absorption, or with conditions that may deteriorate as a result of increased gas formation in the intestine

Hypersensitivity to the drug or any of its components

PRECAUTIONS:

GENERAL

Hypoglycemia: Because of the mechanism of action, miglitol when administered alone should not cause hypoglycemia in the fasted or postprandial state. Sulfonylurea agents may cause hypoglycemia. Because miglitol given in combination with a sulfonylurea will cause a further lowering of blood glucose, it may increase the hypoglycemic potential of the sulfonylurea, although this was not observed in clinical trials. Oral glucose (dextrose), whose absorption is not delayed by miglitol, should be used instead of sucrose (can sugar) in the treatment of mild-to-moderate hypoglycemia. Sucrose, whose hydrolysis to glucose and fructose is inhibited by miglitol, is unsuitable for the rapid correction of hypoglycemia. Severe hypoglycemia may require the use of either intravenous glucose infusion or glucagon injection.

Loss of Control of Blood Glucose: When diabetic patients are exposed to stress such as fever, trauma, infection, or surgery, a temporary loss of control of blood glucose may occur. At such times, temporary insulin therapy may be necessary.

Renal Impairment: Plasma concentrations of miglitol in renally impaired volunteers were proportionally increased relative to the degree of renal dysfunction. Long-term clinical trials in diabetic patients with significant renal dysfunction (serum creatinine >2.0 mg/dl) have not been conducted. Therefore, treatment of these patients with miglitol is not recommended.

INFORMATION FOR THE PATIENT

The following information should be provided to patients:

Miglitol should be taken orally three times a day at the start (with the first bite) of each main meal. It is important to continue to adhere to dietary instructions, a regular exercise program, and regular testing of urine and/or blood glucose.

Miglitol itself does not cause hypoglycemia even when administered to patients in the fasted state. Sulfonylurea drugs and insulin, however, can lower blood sugar levels enough to cause symptoms or sometimes life-threatening hypoglycemia. Because miglitol given in combination with a sulfonylurea or insulin will cause a further lowering of blood sugar, it may increase the hypoglycemic potential of these agents. The risk of hypoglycemia, its symptoms and treatment, and conditions that predispose to its development should be well understood by patients and responsible family members. Because miglitol prevents the breakdown of table sugar, a source of glucose (dextrose, D-glucose) should be readily available to treat symptoms of low blood sugar when taking miglitol in combination with a sulfonylurea or insulin.

If side effects occur with miglitol, they usually develop during the first few weeks of therapy. They are most commonly mild-to-moderate dose-related gastrointestinal effects, such as flatulence, soft stools, diarrhea, or abdominal discomfort, and they generally diminish in frequency and intensity with time. Discontinuation of drug usually results in rapid resolution of the gastrointestinal symptoms.

LABORATORY TESTS

Therapeutic response to miglitol may be monitored by periodic blood glucose tests. Measurement of glycosylated hemoglobin levels is recommended for the monitoring of long-term glycemic control.

CARCINOGENESIS, MUTAGENESIS, AND IMPAIRMENT OF FERTILITY

Miglitol was administered to mice by the dietary route at doses as high as approximately 500 mg/kg body weight (corresponding to greater than 5 times the exposure in humans based on AUC) for 21 months. In a two-year rat study, miglitol was administered in the diet at exposures comparable to the maximum human exposures based on AUC. There was no evidence of carcinogenicity resulting from dietary treatment with miglitol.

In vitro, miglitol was found to be non-mutagenic in the bacterial mutagenesis (Ames) assay and the eukaryotic forward mutation assay (CHO/HGPRT). Miglitol did not have any clastogenic effects *in vivo* in the mouse micronucleus test. There were no heritable mutations detected in dominant lethal assay.

A combined male and female fertility study in Wistar rats treated orally with miglitol at dose levels of 300 mg/kg body weight (approximately 8 times the maximum human exposure based on body surface area) produced no untoward effect on reproductive performance or capability to reproduce. In addition, survival, growth, development, and fertility of the offspring were not compromised.

PREGNANCY, TERATOGENIC EFFECTS, PREGNANCY CATEGORY B

The safety of miglitol in pregnant women has not been established. Developmental toxicology studies have been performed in rats at doses of 50, 150 and 450 mg/kg, corresponding to levels of approximately 1.5, 4, and 12 times the maximum recommended human exposure based on body surface area. In rabbits, doses of 10, 45, and 200 mg/kg corresponding to levels of approximately 0.5, 3, and 10 times the human exposure were examined. These studies revealed no evidence of fetal malformations attributable to miglitol. Doses of miglitol up to 4 and 3 times the human dose (based on body surface area), for rats and rabbits, respectively, did not reveal evidence of impaired fertility or harm to the fetus. The highest doses tested in these studies, 450 mg/kg in the rat and 200 mg/kg in the rabbit promoted maternal and/or fetal toxicity. Fetotoxicity was indicated by a slight but significant reduction in fetal weight in the rat study and slight reduction in fetal weight, delayed ossification of the fetal skeleton and increase in the percentage of non-viable fetuses in the rabbit study. In the per-postnatal study in rats, the NOAEL (No Observed Adverse Effect Level) was 100 mg/kg (corresponding to approximately four times the exposure to humans, based on the body surface area). An increase in stillborn progeny was noted at the high dose (300 mg/kg) in the rat peri-postnatal study, but not at the high dose (450 mg/kg) in the delivery segment of the rat developmental toxicity study. Otherwise, there was no adverse effect on survival, growth, development, behavior, or fertility in either the rat development toxicity or peri-postnatal studies. There are, however, no adequate and well-controlled studies in pregnant women. Because animal reproduction studies are not always predictive of human response, this drug should be used during pregnancy only if clearly needed.

NURSING MOTHERS

Miglitol has been shown to be excreted in human milk to a very small degree. Total excretion into milk accounted for 0.02% of a 100-mg maternal dose. The estimated exposure to a nursing infant is approximately 0.4% of the maternal dose. Although the levels of miglitol reached in human milk are exceedingly low, it is recommended that miglitol not be administered to a nursing woman.

PEDIATRIC USE

Safety and effectiveness of miglitol in pediatric patients have not been established.

DRUG INTERACTIONS:

Several studies investigated the possible interaction between miglitol and glyburide. In six healthy volunteers given a single dose of 5-mg glyburide on a background of 6 days treatment with miglitol (50 mg 3 times daily for 4 days followed by 100 mg 3 times daily for 2 days) or placebo, the mean C_{max} and AUC values for glyburide were 17% and 25% lower, respectively, when glyburide was given with miglitol. In a study in diabetic patients in which the effects of adding miglitol 100 mg 3 times daily × 7 days or placebo to a background regimen of 3.5 mg glyburide daily were investigated, the mean AUC value for glyburide was 18% lower in the miglitol-treated group, although this difference was not statistically significant. Further information on a potential interaction with glyburide was obtained from one of the large US clinical trials (Study 7) in which patients were dosed with either miglitol or placebo on a background of glyburide 10 mg twice daily. At the 6-month and 1-year clinic visits, patients taking concomitant miglitol 100 mg 3 times daily exhibited mean C_{max} values for glyburide that were 16% and 8% lower, respectively, compared to patients taking glyburide alone. However, these differences were not statistically significant. Thus, although there was a trend toward lower AUC and C_{max} values for glyburide when co-administered with miglitol, no definitive statement regarding a potential interaction can be made based on the foregoing three studies.

The effect of miglitol (100 mg 3 times daily × 7 days) on the pharmacokinetics of a single 1000-mg dose of metformin was investigated in healthy volunteers. Mean AUC and C_{max} values for metformin were 12% to 13% lower when the volunteers were given miglitol as compared with placebo, but this difference was not statistically significant.

In a healthy volunteer study, co-administration of either 50 mg or 100 mg miglitol 3 times daily together with digoxin reduced the average plasma concentrations of digoxin by 19% and 28%, respectively. However, in diabetic patients under treatment with digoxin, plasma digoxin concentrations were not altered by co-administration of miglitol 100 mg 3 times daily × 14 days.

Other healthy volunteer studies have demonstrated that miglitol may significantly reduce the bioavailability or ranitidine and propranolol by 60% and 40%, respectively. No effect of miglitol was observed on the pharmacokinetics or pharmacodynamics of either warfarin or nifedipine.

Intestinal absorbents (*e.g.*, charcoal) and digestive enzyme preparations containing carbohydrate-splitting enzymes (*e.g.*, amylase, pancreatin) may reduce the effect of miglitol and should not be taken concomitantly.

In 12 healthy males, concomitantly administered antacid did not influence the pharmacokinetics or miglitol.

ADVERSE REACTIONS:

Gastrointestinal: Gastrointestinal symptoms are the most common reactions to miglitol. In U.S. placebo-controlled trials, the incidences of abdominal pain, diarrhea, and flatulence were 11.7%, 28.7%, and 41.5%, respectively in 962 patients treated with miglitol 25-100 mg 3 times daily, whereas the corresponding incidences were 4.7%, 10.0%, and 12.0% in 603 placebo-treated patients. The incidence of diarrhea and abdominal pain tended to diminish considerably with continued treatment.

Dermatologic: Skin rash was reported in 4.3% of miglitol-treated patients compared to 2.4% of placebo-treated patients. Rashes were generally transient and most were assessed as unrelated to miglitol by physician-investigators.

Abnormal Laboratory Findings: Low serum iron occurred more often in miglitol-treated patients (9.2%) than in placebo-treated patients (4.2%) but did not persist in the majority of cases and was not associated with reductions in hemoglobin or changes in other hematological indices.

OVERDOSAGE:

Unlike sulfonylureas or insulin, an overdose of miglitol will not result in hypoglycemia. An overdose may result in transient increases in flatulence, diarrhea, and abdominal discomfort. Because of the lack of extra-intestinal effects seen with miglitol, no serious systemic reactions are expected in the event of an overdose.

DOSAGE AND ADMINISTRATION:

There is no fixed dosage regimen for the management of diabetes mellitus with miglitol or any other pharmacologic agent. Dosage of miglitol must be individualized on the basis of both effectiveness and tolerance while not exceeding the maximum recommended dosage of 100 mg 3 times daily. Miglitol should be taken three times daily at the start (with the first bite) of each main meal. Miglitol should be started at 25 mg, and the dosage gradually increased as described below, both to reduce gastrointestinal adverse effects and to permit identification of the minimum dose required for adequate glycemic control of the patient.

During treatment initiation and dose titration, one-hour postprandial plasma glucose may be used to determine the therapeutic response to miglitol and identify the minimum effective dose for the patient. Thereafter, glycosylated hemoglobin should be measured at intervals of approximately three months. The therapeutic goal should be to decrease both postprandial plasma glucose and glycosylated hemoglobin levels to normal or near normal by using the lowest effective dose of miglitol, either a monotherapy or in combination with a sulfonylurea.

Initial Dosage: The recommended starting dose of miglitol is 25 mg, given orally three times daily at the start (with the first bite) of each main meal. However, some patients may benefit by starting at 25 mg once daily to minimize gastrointestinal adverse effects, and gradually increasing the frequency of administration to 3 times daily.

Maintenance Dosage: The usual maintenance dose of miglitol is 50 mg 3 times daily, although some patients may benefit from increasing the dose to 100 mg 3 times daily. In order to allow adaptation to potential gastrointestinal adverse effects, it is recommended that miglitol therapy be initiated at a dosage of 25 mg 3 times daily, the lowest effective dosage, and then gradually titrated upward to allow adaptation. After 4-8 weeks of the 25 mg 3 times daily regimen, the dosage should be increased to 50 mg 3 times daily for approximately three months, following which a glycosylated hemoglobin level should be measured to assess therapeutic response. If, at that time, the glycosylated hemoglobin level is not satisfactory, the dosage may be further increased to 100 mg 3 times daily, the maximum recommended dosage. Pooled data from controlled studies suggest a dose-response for both HbA1c and one-hour postprandial plasma glucose throughout the recommended dosage range. However, no single study has examined the effect on, glycemic control of titrating patient's doses upwards within the same study. If no further reduction in postprandial glucose or glycosylated hemoglobin levels is observed with titration to 100 mg 3 times daily, consideration should be given to lowering the dose. Once an effective and tolerated dosage is established, it should be maintained.

Maximum Dosage: The maximum recommended dosage of miglitol is 100 mg 3 times daily. In one clinical trial, 200 mg 3 times daily gave additional improved glycemic control but increased the incidence of the gastrointestinal symptoms described in ADVERSE REACTIONS.

Patients Receiving Sulfonylureas: Sulfonylurea agents may cause hypoglycemia. There was no increased incidence of hypoglycemia in patients who took miglitol in combination with sulfonylurea agents compared to the incidence of hypoglycemia in patients receiving sulfonylureas alone in any clinical trial. However, miglitol given in combination with a sulfonylurea will cause a further lowering of blood glucose and may increase the risk of hypoglycemia due to the additive effects of the two agents. If hypoglycemia occurs, appropriate adjustments in the dosage of these agents should be made.

PATIENT INFORMATION:

Miglitol is used for the treatment of diabetes.

Do not use this drug if you have a bowel disorder or obstruction, or if you have intestinal disease with digestive or absorption conditions.

This drug is not recommended for patients with kidney disease.

Inform your doctor if you are pregnant or breast-feeding.

PATIENT INFORMATION: *(cont'd)*

When given with other antidiabetic drugs, this medicine may cause severe low-blood sugar. Patients and family members should be aware of the signs of low blood sugar and a source of glucose should always be available.

Miglitol may cause flatulence, soft stools, diarrhea or stomach upset. These symptoms usually lessen in time.

Take 3 times a day at the start (with the first bite) of each main meal. Follow a regular exercise program, dietary control and test for blood/urine glucose.

HOW SUPPLIED:

Glyset is available as 25-mg, 50-mg, and 100-mg light gray, hexagonal-shaped, film-coated tablets. The 25-mg tablet is debossed with the word "GLYSET" on one side and "25" on the other. The 50-mg tablet is debossed with the word "GLYSET" on one side and "50" on the other. The 100-mg tablet is debossed with the word "GLYSET" on one side and "100" on the other.

Storage: Store between 15°-30°C (59°-86°F). For bottles, keep container tightly closed.

MILRINONE LACTATE *(003039)*

CATEGORIES: Cardiotonic Agents; Cardiovascular Drugs; Congestive Heart Failure; Diuretics; Heart Failure; Tachycardia; Vasodilating Agents; FDA Approved 1987 Dec

BRAND NAMES: *Corotrop* (Germany); *Corotrope* (France); **Primacor**
(International brand names outside U.S. in italics)

DESCRIPTION:

Primacor, brand of milrinone lactate injection, is a member of a new class of bipyridine inotropic/vasodilator agents with phosphodiesterase inhibitor activity, distinct from digitalis glycosides or catecholamines. Primacor (milrinone lactate) is designated chemically as 1,6-dihydro-2-methyl-6-oxo-[3,4'-bipyridine]-5-carbonitrile lactate.

Milrinone is an off-white to tan crystalline compound with a molecular weight of 211.2 and an empirical formula of $C_{12}H_9N_3O$. It is slightly soluble in methanol, and very slightly soluble in chloroform and in water. As the lactate salt, it is stable and colorless to pale yellow in solution. Primacor is available as sterile aqueous solutions of the lactate salt of milrinone for injection or infusion intravenously.

Sterile, single-dose vials: Single-dose vials of 10 and 20 ml contain in each ml milrinone lactate equivalent to 1 mg milrinone and 47 mg Dextrose, Anhydrous, USP, in Water for Injection, USP. The pH is adjusted to between 3.2 and 4.0 lactic acid or sodium hydroxide. The total concentration of lactic acid can vary between 0.95 mg/ml and 1.29 mg/ml. These vials require preparation of dilutions prior to administration to patients intravenously.

Pre-Mix Flexible Container: The Flexible Container provides a ready-to-use dilution of milrinone in a volume of 100 ml of 5% Dextrose Injection. Each ml contains milrinone lactate equivalent to 200 mcg milrinone in Water for Injection, USP. The nominal concentration of lactic acid is 0.282 mg/ml. Each ml also contains 49.4 mg Dextrose, Anhydrous, USP. The pH is adjusted to between 3.2 and 4.0 with lactic acid or sodium hydroxide. The flexible plastic container is comprised of polyvinyl chloride with a foil overwrap. Water can permeate the plastic into the overwrap, but the amount is insufficient to significantly affect the pre-mix solution.

CLINICAL PHARMACOLOGY:

Milrinone lactate is a positive inotrope and vasodilator, with little chronotropic activity different in structure and mode of action from either the digitalis glycosides or catecholamines.

Milrinone lactate, at relevant inotropic and vasorelaxant concentrations, is a selective inhibitor of peak III cAMP phosphodiesterase isozyme in cardiac and vascular muscle. This inhibitory action is consistent with cAMP mediated increases in intracellular ionized calcium and contractile force in cardiac muscle, as well as with cAMP dependent contractile protein phosphorylation and relaxation in vascular muscle. Additional experimental evidence also indicates that milrinone lactate is not a beta-adrenergic agonist nor does it inhibit sodium-potassium adenosine triphosphatase activity as do the digitalis glycosides.

Clinical studies in patients with congestive heart failure have shown that milrinone lactate produces dose-related and plasma drug concentration-related increases in the maximum rate of increase of left ventricular pressure. Studies in normal subjects have shown that milrinone lactate produces increases in the slope of the left ventricular pressure-dimension relationship, indicating a direct inotropic effect of the drug. Milrinone lactate also produces dose-related and plasma concentration related increases in forearm blood flow in patients with congestive heart failure, indicating a direct arterial vasodilator activity of the drug.

Both the inotropic and vasodilatory effects have been observed over the therapeutic range of plasma milrinone concentrations of 100 ng/ml to 300 ng/ml.

In addition to increasing myocardial contractility, milrinone lactate improves diastolic function as evidenced by improvements in left ventricular diastolic relaxation.

Pharmacokinetics: Following intravenous injections of 12.5 mcg/kg to 125 mcg/kg to congestive heart failure patients, milrinone lactate had a volume of distribution of 0.38 liters/kg, a mean terminal elimination half-life of 2.3 hours, and a clearance of 0.13 liters/kg/hr. Following intravenous infusions of 0.20 mcg/kg/min to 0.70 mcg/kg/min to congestive heart failure patients, the drug had a volume of distribution of about 0.45 liters/kg, a mean terminal elimination half-life of 2.4 hours and a clearance of 0.14 liters/kg/hr. These pharmacokinetic parameters were not dose-dependent, and the area under the plasma concentration time curve following injections was significantly dose-dependent.

Milrinone lactate has been shown (by equilibrium dialysis) to be approximately 70% bound to human plasma protein.

The primary route of excretion of milrinone lactate in man is via the urine. The major urinary excretion of orally administered milrinone lactate in man are milrinone (83%) and its O-glucuronide metabolite (12%). Elimination in normal subjects via the urine is rapid, with approximately 60% recovered within the first two hours following dosing and approximately 90% recovered within the first eight hours following dosing. The mean renal clearance of milrinone lactate is approximately 0.3 liters/min, indicative of active secretion.

Pharmacodynamics: In patients with depressed myocardial function, milrinone lactate produced a prompt increase in cardiac output and decreases in pulmonary capillary wedge pressure and vascular resistance, without a significant increase in heart rate or myocardial oxygen consumption. These hemodynamic improvements were dose and plasma milrinone concentration related. Hemodynamic improvement during intravenous therapy with milrinone lactate was accompanied by clinical symptomatic improvement, as measured by changes in New York Heart Association classification. The great majority of patients experience improvements in hemodynamic function within 5 to 15 minutes of the initiation of therapy.

CLINICAL PHARMACOLOGY: *(cont'd)*

In studies in congestive heart failure patients, milrinone lactate when administered as a loading injection followed by a maintenance infusion produced significant mean initial increases in cardiac index of 25 percent, 38 percent, and 42 percent at dose regimens of 37.5 mcg/kg/0.375 mcg/kg/min, 50 mcg/kg/0.50 mcg/kg/min, and 75 mcg/kg/0.75 mcg/kg/min, respectively. Over the same range of loading injections and maintenance infusions, pulmonary capillary wedge pressure significantly decreased by 20 percent, 23 percent and 36 percent, respectively, while systemic vascular resistance significantly decreased by 17 percent, 21 percent, and 37 percent. The heart rate was generally unchanged (increases of 3, 3 and 10 percent, respectively). Mean arterial pressure fell by up to 5 percent at the two lower dose regimens, but by 17 percent at the highest dose. Patients evaluated for 48 hours maintained improvements in hemodynamic function, with no evidence of diminished response (tachyphylaxis). A smaller number of patients have received infusions of milrinone lactate for periods of up to 72 hours without evidence of tachyphylaxis.

The duration of therapy should depend upon patient responsiveness. Patients have been maintained on infusions of milrinone lactate for up to 5 days.

Milrinone lactate has a favorable inotropic effect in fully digitized patients without causing signs of glycoside toxicity. Theoretically, in cases of atrial flutter/fibrillation, it is possible that milrinone lactate may increase ventricular response rate because of its slight enhancement of AV node conduction. In these cases, digitalis should be considered prior to the institution of therapy with milrinone lactate.

Improvement in left ventricular function in patients with ischemic heart disease has been observed. The improvement has occurred without inducing symptoms or electrocardiographic signs of myocardial ischemia.

The steady-state plasma milrinone concentrations after approximately 6 to 12 hours of unchanging maintenance infusion of 0.50 mcg/kg/min are approximately 200 ng/ml. Near maximum favorable effects of milrinone lactate on cardiac output and pulmonary capillary wedge pressure are seen at plasma milrinone concentrations in the 150 ng/ml to 250 ng/ml range.

INDICATIONS AND USAGE:

Milrinone lactate is indicated for the short-term intravenous therapy of congestive heart failure. The majority of experience with intravenous milrinone lactate has been in patients receiving digoxin and diuretics.

In some patients injections of milrinone lactate and oral milrinone lactate have been shown to increase ventricular ectopy, including nonsustained ventricular tachycardia. Patients receiving milrinone lactate should be closely monitored during infusion.

CONTRAINDICATIONS:

Milrinone lactate is contraindicated in patients who are hypersensitive to it.

PRECAUTIONS:

General: Milrinone lactate should not be used in patients with severe obstructive aortic or pulmonic valvular disease in lieu of surgical relief of the obstruction. Like other inotropic agents, it may aggravate outflow tract obstruction in hypertrophic subaortic stenosis.

Supraventricular and ventricular arrhythmias have been observed in the high-risk population treated. In some patients, injections of milrinone lactate and oral milrinone lactate have been shown to increase ventricular ectopy, including nonsustained ventricular tachycardia. The potential for arrhythmia, present in congestive heart failure itself, may be increased by many drugs or combinations of drugs. Patients receiving milrinone lactate should be closely monitored during infusion.

Milrinone lactate produces a slight shortening of AV node construction time, indicating a potential for an increased ventricular response rate in patients with atrial flutter/fibrillation which is not controlled with digitalis therapy.

During therapy with milrinone lactate, blood pressure and heart rate should be monitored and the rate of infusion slowed or stopped in patients showing excessive decreases in blood pressure.

If prior vigorous diuretic therapy is suspected to have caused significant decreases in cardiac filling pressure, milrinone lactate should be cautiously administered with monitoring of blood pressure, heart rate, and clinical symptomatology.

Use In Acute Myocardial Infarction: No clinical studies have been conducted in patients in the acute phase of post myocardial infarction. Until further clinical experience with this class of drugs is gained, milrinone lactate is not recommended in these patients.

Laboratory Tests Fluid and Electrolytes: Fluid and electrolyte changes and renal function should be carefully monitored during therapy with milrinone lactate. Improvement in cardiac output with resultant diuresis may necessitate a reduction in the dose of diuretic. Potassium loss due to excessive diuresis may predispose digitalized patients to arrhythmias. Therefore, hypokalemia should be corrected by potassium supplementation in advance of or during use of milrinone lactate.

Carcinogenesis, Mutagenesis, and Impairment of Fertility: Twenty-four months of oral administration of milrinone lactate to mice at doses up to 40 mg/kg/day (about 50 times the human oral therapeutic dose at a 50 kg patient) was unassociated with evidence of carcinogenic potential. Neither was there evidence of carcinogenic potential when milrinone lactate was orally administered to rats at doses up to 5 mg/kg/day (about 6 times the human oral therapeutic dose) for twenty-four months or at 25 mg/kg/day (about 30 times the human oral therapeutic dose) for up to 18 months in males and 20 months in females. Whereas the Chinese Hamster Ovary Chromosome Aberration Assay was positive in the presence of a metabolic activation system, results from the Ames Test, the Mouse Lymphoma Assay, the Micronucleus Test, and the *in vivo* Rat Bone Marrow Metaphase Analysis indicated an absence of mutagenic potential. In reproductive performance studies in rats, milrinone lactate had no effect on male or female fertility at oral doses up to 32 mg/kg/day.

Pregnancy Category C: Oral administration of milrinone lactate to pregnant rats and rabbits during organogenesis produced no evidence of teratogenicity at dose levels up to 40 mg/kg/day and 12 mg/kg/day, respectively. Milrinone lactate did not appear to be teratogenic when administered intravenously to pregnant rats at doses up to 3 mg/kg/day (about 2.5 times the maximum recommended clinical intravenous dose) or pregnant rabbits at doses up to 12 mg/kg/day, although an increased resorption rate was apparent at both 8 mg/kg/day and 12 mg/kg/day (intravenous) in the latter species. There are no adequate and well- controlled studies in pregnant women. Milrinone lactate should be used during pregnancy only if the potential benefit justifies the potential risk to the fetus.

Nursing Mothers: Caution should be exercised when milrinone lactate is administered to nursing women, since it is not known whether it is excreted in human milk.

Pediatric Use: Safety and effectiveness in children have not been established.

Use in Elderly Patients: There are no special dosage recommendations for the elderly patient. Ninety percent of all patients administered milrinone lactate in clinical studies were within the age range of 45 to 70 years, with a mean age of 61 years. Patients in all age groups demonstrated clinically and statistically significant responses. No age-related effects on the incidence of adverse reactions have been observed. Controlled pharmacokinetic studies have not disclosed any age-related effects on the distribution and elimination of milrinone lactate.

DRUG INTERACTIONS:

No untoward clinical manifestations have been observed in limited experience where patients in whom milrinone lactate was used concurrently with the following drugs: digitalis glycosides; lidocaine, quinidine; hydralazine, prazosin; isosorbide dinitrate, nitroglycerin; chlorthalidone, furosemide, hydrochlorothiazide, spironolactone; captopril; heparin, warfarin, diazepam, insulin; and potassium supplements.

Chemical Interactions: There is an immediate chemical interaction which is evidenced by the formulation of a precipitate when furosemide is injected into an intravenous line of an infusion of milrinone lactate. Therefore, furosemide should not be administered in intravenous lines containing milrinone lactate.

ADVERSE REACTIONS:

Cardiovascular Effects: In patients receiving milrinone lactate in Phase II and III clinical trials, ventricular arrhythmias were reported in 12.1%: Ventricular ectopic activity, 8.5%; nonsustained ventricular tachycardia, 2.8%; sustained ventricular tachycardia, 1% and ventricular fibrillation, 0.2% (2 patients experienced more than one type of arrhythmia). Holter recordings demonstrated that in some patients injections of milrinone lactate increased ventricular ectopy, including nonsustained ventricular tachycardia. Life-threatening arrhythmias were infrequent and when present have been associated with certain, underlying factors such as preexisting arrhythmias, metabolic abnormalities (*e.g.,* hypokalemia), abnormal digoxin levels and catheter insertion. Milrinone lactate was not shown to be arrhythmogenic in an electrophysiology study. Supraventricular arrhythmias were reported in 3.8% of the patients receiving milrinone lactate. The incidence of both supraventricular and ventricular arrhythmias has not been related to the dose or plasma milrinone concentration.

Other cardiovascular adverse reactions include hypotension, 2.9% and angina/chest pain, 1.2%

CNS Effects: Headaches, usually mild to moderate in severity, have been reported in 2.9% of patients receiving milrinone lactate.

Other Effects: Other adverse reactions reported, but not definitely related to the administration of milrinone lactate include hypokalemia, 0.6%; tremor, 0.4%; and thrombocytopenia, 0.4%.

OVERDOSAGE:

Doses of milrinone lactate may produce hypotension because of its vasodilator effect. If this occurs, administration of milrinone lactate should be reduced or temporarily discontinued until the patient's condition stabilizes. No specific antidote is known, but general measures for circulatory should be taken.

DOSAGE AND ADMINISTRATION:

Milrinone lactate should be administered with a loading dose followed by a continuous infusion (maintenance dose) according to the following guidelines:

Loading Dose: 50 mcg/kg: Administer slowly over 10 minutes

The table below shows the loading dose in milliliters (ml) of milrinone lactate (1 mg/ml) by patient body weight (kg).

TABLE 1 Loading Dose (ml) Using 1 mg/ml Concentration

Patient Body Weight (kg)										
kg	30	40	50	60	70	80	90	100	110	120
ml	1.5	2.0	2.5	3.0	3.5	4.0	4.5	5.0	5.5	6.0

The loading dose may be given undiluted to a rounded total volume
of 10 or 20 ml (see Maintenance Dose, TABLE 2, for diluents) may simplify the visualization of the injection rate.

TABLE 2 Maintenance Dose

Infusion Rate	Total Daily Dose (24 Hours)	
Minimum 0.375 mcg/kg/min	0.59 mg/kg	Administer as a continuous intravenous infusion
Standard 0.500 mcg/kg/min	0.77 mg/kg	
Maximum 0.750 mcg/kg/min	1.13 mg/kg	

Milrinone lactate drawn from vials should be diluted prior to maintenance dose administration. The diluents that may be used are 0.45% Sodium Chloride Injection USP, 0.9% Sodium Chloride Injection USP, or 5% Dextrose Injection USP. The table below, TABLE 3, shows the volume of diluent in milliliters (ml) that must be added to milrinone lactate vials to achieve concentrations recommended for infusion, 100 mcg/ml, 150 mcg/ml, or 200 mcg/ml, and the resultant total volumes.

TABLE 3

Desired Infusion Concentration mcg/ml	Primacor 1 mg/ml (ml)	Diluent (ml)	Total Volume (ml)
100	10	90	100
100	20	180	200
150	10	56.7	66.7
150	20	113	133
200	10	40	50
200	20	80	100

The infusion rate should be adjusted according to hemodynamic and clinical response. Patients should be closely monitored. in controlled clinical studies, most patients showed an improvement in hemodynamic status as evidenced by increases in cardiac output and reductions in pulmonary capillary wedge pressure.

Note: Dosage Adjustment in Renally Impaired Patients. Dosage may be titrated to the maximum hemodynamic effect and should not exceed 1.13 mg/kg/day. Duration of therapy should depend upon patient responsiveness.

The maintenance dose in ml/hr by patient body weight (kg) may be determined by reference to one of the following three tables, TABLE 4,5 AND 6.

Note: Milrinone lactate supplied in 100 ml Flexible Containers (200 mcg/ml in 5% Dextrose injection) need not be diluted prior to use.

The Flexible Container has a concentration of milrinone equivalent to 200 mcg/ml in 5% Dextrose Injection and is more convenient to use than dilutions prepared from vials. To use the Flexible Container, tear the overwrap at the notch and remove the Pre-Mix solution container. Squeeze the container firmly to check for leaks. Discard the container if leaks are found since the sterility of the product could be affected. Do not add supplementary medication. To prepare the container for administration of milrinone lactate intravenously, use aseptic techniques.

DOSAGE AND ADMINISTRATION: *(cont'd)*

TABLE 4 Milrinone Lactate Infusion Rate (ml/hr) Using 100 mcg/ml Concentration Maintenance Dose

(mcg/kg/min)	Patient Body Weight (kg) 30	40	50	60	70	80	90	100	110	120
0.375	6.8	9.0	11.3	13.5	15.8	18.0	20.3	22.5	24.8	27.0
0.400	7.2	9.6	12.0	14.4	16.8	19.2	21.6	24.0	26.4	28.8
0.500	9.0	12.0	15.0	18.0	21.0	24.0	27.0	30.0	33.0	36.0
0.600	10.8	14.4	18.0	21.6	25.2	28.8	32.4	36.0	39.6	43.2
0.700	12.6	16.8	21.0	25.2	29.4	33.6	37.8	42.0	46.2	50.4
0.750	13.5	18.0	22.5	27.0	31.5	36.0	40.5	45.0	49.5	54.0

TABLE 5 Milrinone Lactate Infusion Rate (ml/hr) Using 150 mcg/ml Concentration Maintenance Dose

(mcg/kg/min)	Patient Body Weight (kg) 30	40	50	60	70	80	90	100	110	120
0.375	4.5	6.0	7.5	9.0	10.5	12.0	13.5	15.0	16.5	18.0
0.400	4.8	6.4	8.0	9.6	11.2	12.8	14.4	16.0	17.6	19.2
0.500	6.0	8.0	10.0	12.0	14.0	16.0	18.0	20.0	22.0	24.0
0.600	7.2	9.6	12.0	14.4	16.8	19.2	21.6	24.0	26.4	28.8
0.700	8.4	11.2	14.0	16.8	19.6	22.4	25.2	28.0	30.8	33.6
0.750	9.0	12.0	15.0	18.0	21.0	24.0	27.0	30.0	33.0	36.0

TABLE 6 Milrinone Lactate Infusion Rate (ml/hr) Using 200 mcg/ml Concentration Maintenance Dose

(mcg/kg/min)	Patient Body Weight (kg) 30	40	50	60	70	80	90	100	110	120
0.375	3.4	4.5	5.6	6.8	7.9	9.0	10.1	11.3	12.4	13.5
0.400	3.6	4.8	6.0	7.2	8.4	9.6	10.8	12.0	13.2	14.4
0.500	4.5	6.0	7.5	9.0	10.5	12.0	13.5	15.0	16.5	18.0
0.600	5.4	7.2	9.0	10.8	12.6	14.4	16.2	18.0	19.8	21.6
0.700	6.3	8.4	10.5	12.6	14.7	16.8	18.9	21.0	23.1	25.2
0.750	6.8	9.0	11.3	13.5	15.8	18.0	20.8	22.5	24.8	27.0

1) The flow control clamp of the administration set closed.

2) The cover of the outlet port at the bottom of the container is removed.

3) Noting the full directions on the administration set carton, the piercing pin of the set is inserted into the port with a twisting motion until it is firmly seated.

4) The container is suspended on the hanger.

5) The drip chamber is squeezed and released to establish the fill level.

6) The flow control clamp is opened to expel air from the set, and then closed.

7) The set is attached to the venipuncture device, primed, and if not indwelling, the venipuncture is performed.

8) The rate of administration is controlled with the flow control clamp. WARNING-DO NOT USE IN SERIES CONNECTIONS.

Intravenous drug products should be inspected visually and should not be used if particulate matter or discoloration is present.

Dosage Adjustment in Renally Impaired Patients: Data obtained from patients with severe renal impairment (creatinine clearance = 0 to 30 ml/min) but without congestive heart failure have demonstrated that the presence of renal impairment significantly increases the terminal elimination half-life of milrinone lactate. Reductions in infusion rate may be necessary in patients with renal impairment. For patients with clinical evidence of renal impairment, the recommended infusion rate can be obtained from the following (TABLE 7).

TABLE 7

Creatinine Clearance (ml/min/1.73 m^2)	Infusion Rate (mcg/kg/min)
5	0.20
10	0.23
20	0.28
30	0.33
40	0.38
50	0.43

ANIMAL PHARMACOLOGY:

Animal Toxicity: Oral and intravenous administration of milrinone lactate to rats and dogs resulted in myocardial degeneration/fibrosis and endocardial hemorrhage, principally affecting the left ventricular papillary muscles. Coronary vascular lesions characterized by periarterial edema and inflammation have been observed in dogs only. The myocardial/endocardial changes are similar to those produced by beta-adrenergic receptor agonists such as isoproterenol, while the vascular changes are similar to those produced by minoxidil and hydralazine. Doses with the recommended clinical dose range (up to 1.13 mg/kg/day) for congestive heart failure patients have not produced significant adverse effects in animals.

HOW SUPPLIED:

Store at controlled room temperature, 15°C to 30°C (59°F-86°F). Avoid freezing.

Exposure of pharmaceutical products to heat should be minimized. Avoid excessive heat. Protect from freezing. It is recommended that the Flexible Containers be stored at room temperature, 25°C (77°F), however, brief exposure up to 40°C (104°F) does not adversely affect the product.

HOW SUPPLIED - EQUIVALENTS NOT AVAILABLE:

Injection, Solution - Intravenous - 1 mg/ml

5 ml x 10	$312.64	PRIMACOR, CARPUJECT, Sanofi Winthrop	00024-1200-05
5 ml x 10	$315.06	PRIMACOR, Sanofi Winthrop	00024-1200-06
10 ml x 10	$595.46	PRIMACOR, Sanofi Winthrop	00024-1200-10
20 ml	$1124.76	PRIMACOR, Sanofi Winthrop	00024-1200-20
100 ml x 10	$1152.00	PRIMACOR, Sanofi Winthrop	00024-1203-01

MINERALS; MULTIVITAMINS *(001816)*

CATEGORIES: EENT Drugs; Electrolyte Solutions; Electrolytic, Caloric-Water Balance; Eye, Ear, Nose, & Throat Preparations; Homeostatic & Nutrient; Mineral Supplements; Nutrition, Enteral/Parenteral; Replacement Solutions; Vitamin B Complex; Vitamins; FDA Pre 1938 Drugs

BRAND NAMES: Amo Endosol Extra; Biotrace; Chromium Trace Element; Conte-Pak-4; M-Trace; M.T.E.; Multe-Pak; Multilyte; Multiple Trace Elements; Multitrace; Neotrace-4; Nonamin; P.T.E.; Pediatrace; Pedte-Pak-4; Pedtrace-4; Pharmalyte; Theracon Forte; Trace Elements; Trace-4; Vitacel; Vitacon Forte

Prescribing information not available at time of publication.

HOW SUPPLIED - RATED THERAPEUTICALLY EQUIVALENT:

Solution - Ophthalmic

515 ml	$61.87	AMO ENDOSOL EXTRA, Allergan	00023-0005-51

HOW SUPPLIED - NOT RATED EQUIVALENT:

Capsule, Gelatin - Oral

100's	$10.00	Therapeutic Vitamin W/Minerals, Contract Pharma	10267-0737-01
100's	$11.00	Vitacon Forte, HL Moore Drug Exch	00839-7508-06
100's	$12.95	Theracon Forte, Goldline Labs	00182-4555-01
100's	$14.00	V-C Forte, Pharmacist Choice	54979-0164-01
100's	$15.48	Vite Con Forte, Jerome Stevens	50564-0542-01
500's	$84.11	Vite Con Forte, Jerome Stevens	50564-0542-05

Injection, Solution - Intravenous

1 ml	$5.73	TRACE-4 MULTIPLE TRACE ELEMENT, Intl Medication	00548-6011-00
1 ml	$58.13	CONTE-PAK-4, Solopak Labs	39769-0057-02
1 ml	$61.25	MTE- 4 CONCENTRATED, Fujisawa USA	00469-9400-00
1 ml	$78.13	MTE-5 CONCENTRATED, Fujisawa USA	00469-2800-00
1 ml x 25	$20.00	Multitrace-4, Am Regent	00517-7201-25
1 ml x 25	$101.75	PEDTRACE-4 PLUS, Fujisawa USA	00469-4410-00
1 ml x 25	$115.73	NEOTRACE-4 PLUS, Fujisawa USA	00469-4420-00
1 ml x 25	$164.06	Multitrace-5, Am Regent	00517-8201-25
1 ml x 25	$164.06	MULTIPLE TRACE ELEMENT, Am Regent	00517-9001-25
2 ml	$121.56	NEOTRACE-4, Fujisawa USA	00469-1410-10
2 ml x 25	$109.38	MTE-4 NEONATAL, Am Regent	00517-0280-25
2 ml x 25	$109.38	Multitrace-4, Am Regent	00517-6202-25
3 ml	$54.69	MULTE-PAK-4, Solopak Labs	39769-0056-05
3 ml	$96.87	PEDTE-PAK-4, Solopak Labs	39769-0058-05
3 ml	$106.88	PEDTRACE-4, Fujisawa USA	00469-1380-03
3 ml	$107.81	PTE-4, Fujisawa USA	00469-8200-03
3 ml	$108.12	PTE-5, Fujisawa USA	00469-1440-03
3 ml	$140.63	MULTE-PAK-5, Solopak Labs	39769-0059-05
3 ml x 25	$31.25	Multitrace-4, Am Regent	00517-9203-25
3 ml x 25	$53.44	M.T.E.-4, Fujisawa USA	00469-8100-31
5 ml	$4.39	TRACE METALS ADDITIVE IN 0.9% SODIUM, Abbott	00074-4592-01
5 ml	$4.52	TRACE ELEMENTS, Abbott	00074-4592-10
5 ml	$6.83	TRACE METALS ADDITIVE, Abbott	00074-4008-01
5 ml	$8.94	Trace Metals, Abbott	00074-4623-15
5 ml x 25	$44.63	M.T.E. 4 PLUS, Fujisawa USA	00469-4390-20
10 ml	$1.89	Chromium Trace Element, McGuff	49072-0125-10
10 ml	$1.89	Manganese Trace Element, McGuff	49072-0477-10
10 ml	$2.59	Selenium Trace Element, McGuff	49072-0625-10
10 ml	$9.68	MULTIPLE TRACE ELEMENT, Am Regent	00517-6010-01
10 ml	$168.44	MULTE-PAK-4, Solopak Labs	39769-0056-10
10 ml	$176.25	MTE-4, Fujisawa USA	00469-8100-30
10 ml	$234.00	MTE-5 CONCENTRATED, Fujisawa USA	00469-2900-30
10 ml	$280.75	M.T.E. -6, Fujisawa USA	00469-3600-30
10 ml	$318.13	MTE-5, Fujisawa USA	00469-1800-30
10 ml	$371.56	M.T.E.-6, Fujisawa USA	00469-2000-30
10 ml	$384.69	PEDTRACE-4, Fujisawa USA	00469-1380-30
10 ml	$390.63	MULTE-PAK-5, Solopak Labs	39769-0059-10
10 ml	$405.00	MTE-4 CONCENTRATED, Fujisawa USA	00469-9800-30
10 ml	$413.44	CONTE-PAK-4, Solopak Labs	39769-0085-10
10 ml	$432.81	M.T.E.-7, Fujisawa USA	00469-1400-30
10 ml x 25	$70.00	MULTIPLE TRACE ELEMENTS, Raway	00686-8010-25
10 ml x 25	$132.81	Multitrace-4, Am Regent	00517-7410-25
10 ml x 25	$132.81	PEDIATRIC MULTIPLE TRACE ELEMENT, Am Regent	00517-8010-25
10 ml x 25	$132.81	Multitrace-5, Am Regent	00517-8510-25
10 ml x 25	$132.81	MULTIPLE TRACE ELEMENT, Am Regent	00517-9010-25
10 ml x 25	$132.81	Trace Elements-4, Am Regent	00517-9310-25
10 ml x 25	$140.63	Multitrace-5, Am Regent	00517-8210-25
10 ml x 25	$141.31	M.T.E. 4 PLUS, Fujisawa USA	00469-4390-30
10 ml x 25	$165.00	MULTIPLE TRACE ELEMENTS, Raway	00686-6010-25
10 ml x 25	$170.00	MULTIPLE TRACE ELEMENTS, Raway	00686-7010-25
10 ml x 25	$310.94	CONCENTRATED MULTIPLE TRACE ELEMENT, Am Regent	00517-7010-25
10 ml x 25	$310.94	Multitrace-4, Am Regent	00517-7210-25
25 ml x 25	$100.00	MULTILYTE-20, Fujisawa USA	00469-0425-25
25 ml x 25	$107.81	MULTILYTE-40, Fujisawa USA	00469-0420-25
30 ml	$371.87	MTE-4, Fujisawa USA	00469-8700-50
30 ml	$396.56	MULTE-PAK-4, Solopak Labs	39769-0084-30
30 ml x 25	$354.02	M.T.E. 4 PLUS, Fujisawa USA	00469-4770-50
50 ml	$46.37	TRACE METALS ADDITIVE IN 0.9% SODIUM, Abbott	00074-4592-50

Solution - Ophthalmic

515 ml x 6	$329.98	B-Salt Forte, Akorn	17478-0930-90

Tablet, Uncoated - Oral

60's	$12.50	Vitacel, Sorter	53879-0200-60

MINERALS; VITAMIN B COMPLEX *(001817)*

CATEGORIES: Blood Formation/Coagulation; Deficiency Anemias; Homeostatic & Nutrient; Multivitamins; Vitamins; FDA Pre 1938 Drugs

BRAND NAMES: May-Vita; Nortonic

Prescribing information not available at time of publication.

HOW SUPPLIED - EQUIVALENTS NOT AVAILABLE:

Elixir - Oral

240 ml	$10.00	Nortonic, Norega Labs	51724-0012-08
480 ml	$16.50	MAY-VITA, Mayrand Pharms	00259-0366-16

MINOCYCLINE HYDROCHLORIDE *(001818)*

CATEGORIES: Acne; Actinomycosis; Amebiasis; Amebicides; Anthrax; Anti-Infectives; Antibiotics; Antimicrobials; Brucellosis; Chancroid; Chlamydia; Cholera; Conjunctivitis; Gonorrhea; Granuloma; Granuloma Inguinale; Infections; Listeriosis; Lyme Disease; Lymphogranuloma; Plague; Pneumonia; Psittacosis; Q Fever; Relapsing Fever; Respiratory Tract Infections; Rickettsial Disease; Rickettsialpox; Rocky Mountain Fever; Sexually Transmitted Diseases; Syphilis; Tetracyclines; Tick Fevers; Trachoma; Tularemia; Typhoid Fever; Typhus; Urethritis; Urinary Tract Infections; Vincent's Infection; Yaws; Pregnancy Category D; Sales > $100 Million; FDA Approval Pre 1982

BRAND NAMES: *Borymycin*; *Cyclimycin*; *Cynomycin*; Dynacin; *Klinomycin* (Germany); *Lederderm*; *Mero*; *Mestacine* (France); *Mino-50*; **Minocin**; *Minocin MR*; *Minoclir 50* (Germany); *Minocyclin 50 Stada* (Germany); *Minogalen* (Germany); *Minoline*; *Minomycin* (Australia, Japan); *Minotab 50*; *Mino-Wolff* (Germany); *Mynocine* (France)

(International brand names outside U.S. in italics)

FORMULARIES: Aetna; BC-BS

COST OF THERAPY: $39.25 (Infections; Capsule; 100 mg; 2/day; 10 days)

PRIMARY ICD9: 136.9 (Unspecified Infections And Parasitic Diseases)

DESCRIPTION:

Minocycline hydrochloride is a semisynthetic derivative of tetracycline, is [4*S*-(4α,4aα,5aα,12aα)]-4,7-bis(dimethylamino)-1,4,4a,5, 5a,6,11,12a- octahydro-3,10,12,12a-tetrahydroxy-1,11-dioxo-2-naphthacenecarboxamide monohydrochloride.

Tablets: Minocin tablets contain minocycline HCl equivalent to 50 or 100 mg minocycline and the following inactive ingredients: FD&C Yellow No. 6, Lactose, Microcrystalline Cellulose, Magnesium Stearate, Povidone, Sodium Lauryl Sulfate, Sodium Starch Glycolate, Sorbitol, Stearic Acid, Titanium Dioxide, Yellow 10 and other ingredients.

Minocin Tablets, 50 mg, containing minocycline HCl equivalent to 50 mg minocycline, are round, convex, orange film-coated tablets engraved with M3 on one side and LL on the other.

Capsules: Minocin pellet-filled capsules for oral administration contain pellets of minocycline HCl equivalent to 50 mg or 100 mg of minocycline in microcrystalline cellulose. The capsule shells contain the following inactive ingredients: Blue 1, Gelatin, Titanium Dioxide and Yellow 10. The 50 mg capsule shells also contain Black and Yellow Iron Oxides.

Intravenous Injection: Each vial, dried by cryodesiccation, contains sterile minocycline HCl equivalent to 100 mg minocycline. When reconstituted with 5 ml of Sterile Water For Injection the pH ranges from 2.0 to 2.8.

CLINICAL PHARMACOLOGY:

ORAL

Microbiology

The tetracyclines are primarily bacteriostatic and are thought to exert their antimicrobial effect by the inhibition of protein synthesis. The tetracyclines, including minocycline HCl, have similar antibacterial spectra of activity against a wide range of gram-negative and gram-positive organisms.

Tablets: Following a single dose of two 100 mg minocycline HCl tablets administered to normal fasting adult volunteers, serum levels ranged from 0.74 to 4.45 mcg/ml in one hour (average 2.24). After 12 hours, they ranged from 0.35 to 2.36 mcg/ml (average 1.25). The serum half-life following a single 200 mg dose ion normal fasting adult volunteers has ranged from 1 to 17 hours.

When minocycline HCl tablets are administered with a meal including milk, the extent of absorption (AUC) is reduced by approximately 33% while the peak serum concentrations are reduced by approximately 32% and delayed by one hour. In previous studies with other dosage forms, the minocycline half-life ranged from 11 to 16 hours in 7 patients with hepatic dysfunction, and from 18 to 69 hours in 5 patients with renal dysfunction. The urinary and fecal recovery of minocycline when administered to 12 normal volunteers is one-half to one-third that of other tetracyclines.

Capsules: Minocycline hydrochloride pellet-filled capsules are rapidly absorbed from the gastrointestinal tract following oral administration. Following a single dose of two 100 mg pellet-filled capsules of minocycline HCl administered to 18 normal fasting adult volunteers, maximum serum concentrations were attained in 1 to 4 hours (average 2.1 hours) and ranged from 2.1 to 5.1 mcg/ml (average 3.5 mcg/ml). The serum half-life in the normal volunteers ranged from 11.1 to 22.1 hours (average 15.5 hours).

When minocycline hydrochloride pellet-filled capsules were given concomitantly with a meal which included dairy products, the extent of absorption of minocycline hydrochloride pellet-filled capsules was not noticeably influenced. The peak plasma concentrations were slightly decreased (11.2%) and delayed by one hour when administered with food, compared to dosing under fasting conditions.

In previous studies with other minocycline dosage forms, the minocycline serum half-life ranged from 11 to 16 hours in 7 patients with hepatic dysfunction, and from 18 to 69 hours in 5 patients with renal dysfunction. The urinary and fecal recovery of minocycline when administered to 12 normal volunteers is one-half to one-third that of other tetracyclines.

Oral: Cross-resistance of these organisms to tetracyclines is common.

While *in vitro* studies have demonstrated the susceptibility of most strains of the following microorganisms, clinical efficacy for infections other than those included in the INDICATIONS AND USAGEsection has not been documented.

Gram-Negative Bacteria: *Bartonella bacilliformis*;*Brucella* species; *Campylobacter fetus*; *Francisella tularensis; Haemophilus ducreyi; Haemophilus influenzae; Listeria monocytogenes; Neisseria gonorrhea;*

Vibrio cholera; *Yersinia pestis.*

Because many strains of the following groups of gram-negative microorganisms have been shown to be resistant to tetracyclines, culture and susceptibility testing are especially recommended:

Acinetobacter species; *Bacteroides* species;*Enterobacter aerogenes;*

Escherichia coli; *Klebsiella* species; *Shigella* species.

Gram-Positive Bacteria: Because many strains of the following groups of gram-positive microorganisms have been shown to be resistant to tetracyclines, culture and susceptibility testing are recommended. Up to 44 percent of strains of *Streptococcus pyogenes* strains have been found to be resistant to tetracycline drugs. Therefore, tetracyclines should not be used for streptococcal disease unless the organism has been demonstrated to be susceptible.

Alpha hemolytic streptococci (viridans group),*Streptococcus pneumoniae*,*Streptococcus pyogenes,*

Other Microorganisms: *Actinomyces* species; *Bacillus anthracis; Balantidium coli; Borrelia recurrentis; Chlamydia psittaci;Chlamydia trachomatis; Clostridium* species;*Entamoeba* species; *Fusobacterium fusiforme;Propionibacterium acnes*; *Treponema pallidum;Treponema pertenue*; *Ureaplasma urealyticum.*

CLINICAL PHARMACOLOGY: *(cont'd)*

Susceptibility Testing

Diffusion Techniques: The use of antibiotic disk susceptibility test methods which measure zone diameter give an accurate estimation of susceptibility of microorganisms to minocycline HCl. One such standard procedure[1] has been recommended for use with disks for testing antimicrobials. Either the 30 mcg tetracycline-class disk or the 30 mcg minocycline disk should be used for the determination of the susceptibility of microorganisms to minocycline.

With this type of procedure a report of "susceptible" from the laboratory indicates that the infecting organism is likely to respond to thereby. A report of "intermediate susceptibility" suggests that the organism would be susceptible if a high dosage is used or if the infection is confined to tissues and fluids (*e.g.,* urine) in which high antibiotic levels are attained. A report of "resistant" indicates that the infecting organism is not likely to respond to therapy. With either the tetracycline-class disk or the minocycline disk, zone sizes of 19 mm or greater indicate susceptibility, zone sizes of 14 mm or less indicate resistance, and zone sizes of 15 to 18 mm indicate intermediate susceptibility.

Standardized procedures require the use of laboratory control laboratory control organisms. The 30 mcg tetracycline disk should give zone diameters between 19 and 28 mm for *Staphylococcus aureus*ATCC 25923 and between 18 and 25 mm for *Escherichia coli* ATCC 25922. The 30 mcg minocycline disk should give zone diameters between 25 and 30 mm for *S. aureus* ATCC 25923 and between 19 and 25 mm for *E. coli*ATCC 25922.

Dilution Techniques: When using the NCCLS agar dilution or broth dilution (including microdilution) method[2] or equivalent, a bacterial isolate may be considered susceptible if the MIC (minimal inhibitory concentration) of minocycline is 4 mcg/ml or less. Organisms are considered resistant if the MIC is 16 mcg/ml or greater. Organisms with an MIC value of less than 16 mcg/ml but greater than 4 mcg/ml are expected to be susceptible if a high dosage is used or if the infection is confined to tissues and fluids (*e.g.,* urine) in which high antibiotic levels are attained.

As with standard dilution methods, dilution procedures require the use of laboratory control organisms. Standard tetracycline powder should give MIC values of 0.25 mcg/ml to 1.0 mcg/ml for *S. aureus* ATCC 25923, and 1.0 mcg/ml to 4.0 mcg/ml for *E. coli* ATCC 25922.

INTRAVENOUS INJECTION

Microbiology

Tube-dilution testing: Microorganisms may be considered susceptible (likely to respond to minocycline therapy) if the minimum inhibitory concentration (MIC) is not more than 4 mcg/ml. Microorganisms may be considered intermediate (harboring partial resistance) if the MIC is 4 to 12.5 mcg/ml and resistant (not likely to respond to minocycline therapy) if the MIC is greater then 12.5 mcg/ml.

Susceptibility Testing: If the Kirby-Bauer method of susceptibility testing (using a 30 mcg tetracycline disc) gives a zone of 18 mm or greater, the bacterial strain is considered to be susceptible to any tetracycline. Minocycline shows moderate *in vitro* activity against certain strains of staphylococci which have been found to be resistant to other tetracyclines. For such strains minocycline susceptibility powder may be used for additional susceptibility testing.

Human Pharmacology: Following a single dose of 200 mg administered intravenously to 10 healthy male volunteers, serum levels ranged from 2.52 to 6.63 mcg/ml (average 4.18), after 12 hours they ranged from 0.82 to 2.64 mcg/ml (average 1.38). In a group of 5 healthy male volunteers serum levels of 1.4 -1.8 mcg/ml were maintained at 12 and 24 hours with doses of 100 mg every 12 hours for three days. When given 200 mg once daily for three days the serum levels had fallen to approximately 1 mcg/ml at 24 hours. The serum half-life following IV doses of 100 mg every 12 hours or 100 mg once daily did not differ significantly and ranged from 15 to 23 hours. The serum half-life following a single 200 mg oral dose in 12 essentially normal volunteers ranged from 11 to 17 hours, in 7 patients with hepatic dysfunction ranged from 11 to 16 hours, and in 5 patients with renal dysfunction from 18 to 69 hours.

Intravenously administered minocycline appears similar to oral doses in excretion. The urinary and fecal recovery of oral minocycline when administered to 12 normal volunteers is one-half to one-third that of other tetracyclines.

INDICATIONS AND USAGE:

ORAL

Minocycline HCl is indicated in the treatment of the following infections due to susceptible strains of the designated microorganisms.

Rocky Mountain spotted fever, typhus fever and the typhus group, Q fever, rickettsialpox and tick fevers caused by rickettsiae.

Respiratory tract infections caused by *Mycoplasma pneumoniae.*

Lymphogranuloma venereum caused by *Chlamydia trachomatis.*

Psittacosis (ornithosis) due to *Chlamydia psittaci.*

Trachoma caused by *Chlamydia trachomatis,* although the infectious agent is not always eliminated, as judged by immunofluorescence. Inclusion conjunctivitis caused by *Chlamydia trachomatis.*

Nongonococcal urethritis and endocervical or rectal infections in adults caused by *Ureaplasma urealyticum* or *Chlamydia trachomatis.*

Relapsing fever due to *Borrelia recurrentis.*

Chancroid caused by *Haemophilus ducreyi.*

Plague due to *Yersinia pestis.*

Tularemia due to *Francisella tularensis.*

Cholera caused by *Vibrio cholerae.*

Campylobacter fetus infections caused by *Campylobacter fetus.*

Brucellosis due to *Brucella* species (in conjunction with streptomycin).

Bartonellosis due to *Bartonella bacilliformis.*

Granuloma inguinale caused by *Calymmatobacterium granulomatis.*

Minocycline is indicated for treatment of infections caused by the following gram-negative microorganisms when bacteriologic testing indicates appropriate susceptibility to the drug:

Escherichia coli; *Enterobacter aerogenes;Shigella* species;

Acinetobacter species.

Respiratory tract infections caused by *Haemophilus influenzae.*

Respiratory tract and urinary tract infections caused by *Klebsiella* species.

Minocycline HCl is indicated for treatment of infections caused by the following gram-positive microorganisms when bacteriologic testing indicates appropriate susceptibility to the drug:

Upper respiratory tract infections caused by *Streptococcus pneumoniae.*

Skin and skin structure infections caused by *Staphylococcus aureus.* (Note: Minocycline is not the drug of choice in the treatment of any type of staphylococcal infection.)

Uncomplicated urethritis in men due to *Neisseria gonorrhoeae* and for the treatment of other gonococcal infections when penicillin is contraindicated.

INDICATIONS AND USAGE: *(cont'd)*

When penicillin is contraindicated, minocycline HCl is an alternative drug in the treatment of the following infections:

Infections in women caused by *Neisseria gonorrhoeae.*

Syphilis caused by *Treponema pallidum.*

Yaws caused by *Treponema pertenue.*

Listeriosis due to *Listeria monocytogenes.*

Anthrax due to *Bacillus anthracis.*

Vincent's infection caused by *Fusobacterium fusiforme.*

Actinomycosis caused by *Actinomyces israelii.*

Infections caused by *Clostridium* species.

In *acute intestinal amebiasis,* minocycline HCl may be a useful adjunct to amebicides.

In severe *acne,* minocycline HCl may be useful adjunctive therapy.

Oral minocycline is indicated in the treatment of asymptomatic carriers of *Neisseria meningitidis* to eliminate meningococci from the nasopharynx. In order to preserve the usefulness of minocycline in the treatment of asymptomatic meningococcal carrier, diagnostic laboratory procedures, including serotyping and susceptibility testing, should be performed to establish the carrier state and the correct treatment. It is recommended that the prophylactic use of minocycline be reserved for situations in which the risk of the meningococcal meningitis is high.

Oral minocycline is not indicated for the treatment of meningococcal infection.

Although no controlled clinical efficacy studies have been conducted, limited clinical data show that oral minocycline HCl has been used successfully in the treatment of infections caused by *Mycobacterium marinum.*

INTRAVENOUS INJECTION

Minocycline HCl is indicated in infections caused by the following microorganisms:

Rickettsiae: (Rocky Mountain spotted fever, typhus fever and the typhus group, Q fever, rickettsialpox, tick fevers).

Mycoplasma pneumoniae (PPLO, Eaton agent).

Agents of psittacosis and ornithosis.

Agents of lymphogranuloma venereum and granuloma inguinale.

The spirochetal agent of relapsing fever *(Borrelia recurrentis).*

The following gram-negative microorganisms:

Haemophilus ducreyi (chancroid); *Yersinia pestis* and *Francisella tularensis,* formerly *Pasteurella pestis* and *Pasteurella tularensis*;

Bartonella bacilliformis; *Bacteroides* species; *Vibrio comma* and *vibrio fetus*; *Brucella* species (in conjunction with streptomycin).

Because many strains of the following groups of microorganisms have been shown to be resistant to tetracyclines, culture and susceptibility testing are recommended.

Minocycline HCl is indicated for treatment of infections caused by the following gram-negative microorganisms, when bacteriologic testing indicates appropriate susceptibility to the drug:

Escherichia coli; *Enterobacter aerogenes* (formerly*Aerobacter aerogenes*); *Shigella* species; *Mima* species and *Herellea* species;

Haemophilus influenzae (respiratory infections);*Klebsiella* species (respiratory and urinary infections).

Minocycline HCl is indicated for treatment of infections caused by the following gram-positive microorganisms when bacteriologic testing indicates appropriate susceptibility to the drug:

Streptococcus species:

Up to 44% of strains of *Streptococcus pyogenes* and 74% of*Streptococcus faecalis* have been found to be resistant to tetracycline drugs. Therefore, tetracyclines should not be used for streptococcal disease unless the organism has been demonstrated to be sensitive.

For upper respiratory infections due to Group A beta-hemolytic streptococci, penicillin is the usual drug of choice, including prophylaxis of rheumatic fever.

Streptococcus pneumoniae,

Staphylococcus aureus, skin and soft tissue infections.

Tetracyclines are not the drugs of choice in the treatment of any type of staphylococcal infection.

When penicillin is contraindicated, tetracyclines are alternative drugs in the treatment of infections due to:

Neisseria gonorrhoeae, and *Neisseria meningitidis;*

Treponema pallidum and *Treponema pertenue* (syphilis and yaws); *Listeria monocytogenes; Clostridium* species;*Bacillus anthracis; Fusobacterium fusiforme* (Vincent's infection); *Actinomyces* species.

In acute intestinal amebiasis, the tetracyclines may be a useful adjunct to amebicides.

Minocycline HCl is indicated in the treatment of trachoma, although the infectious agent is not always eliminated, as judged by immunofluorescence.

Inclusion conjunctivitis may be treated with oral tetracyclines or with a combination of oral and topical agents.

CONTRAINDICATIONS:

This drug is contraindicated in persons who have shown hypersensitivity to any of the tetracyclines.

WARNINGS:

ORAL

MINOCYCLINE HYDROCHLORIDE TABLETS AND PELLET-FILLED CAPSULES, LIKE OTHER TETRACYCLINE-CLASS ANTIBIOTICS, CAN CAUSE FETAL HARM WHEN ADMINISTERED TO A PREGNANT WOMAN. IF ANY TETRACYCLINE IS USED DURING PREGNANCY OR IF THE PATIENT BECOMES PREGNANT WHILE TAKING THESE DRUGS, THE PATIENT SHOULD BE APPRISED OF THE POTENTIAL HAZARD TO THE FETUS. THE USE OF DRUGS OF THE TETRACYCLINE CLASS DURING TOOTH DEVELOPMENT (LAST HALF OF PREGNANCY, INFANCY, AND CHILDHOOD TO THE AGE OF 8 YEARS) MAY CAUSE PERMANENT DISCOLORATION OF THE TEETH (YELLOW-GRAY-BROWN).

This adverse reaction is more common during long-term use of the drug but has been observed following repeated short-term courses. Enamel hypoplasia has also been reported. TETRACYCLINE DRUGS, THEREFORE, SHOULD NOT BE USED IN THIS AGE GROUP UNLESS OTHER DRUGS ARE NOT LIKELY TO BE EFFECTIVE OR ARE CONTRAINDICATED.

WARNINGS: *(cont'd)*

All tetracyclines form a stable calcium complex in any bone forming tissue. A decrease in fibula growth rate has been observed in prematures given oral tetracycline in doses of 25 mg/kg every six hours. This reactions was shown to be reversible when the drug was discontinued.

Results of animal studies indicate that tetracyclines cross the placenta, are found in fetal tissues and can have toxic effects on the developing fetus (often related to retardation of skeletal development). Evidence of embryotoxicity has also been noted in animals treated early in pregnancy.

The anti-anabolic action of the tetracyclines may cause an increase in BUN. While this is not a problem in those with normal renal function, in patients with significantly impaired function, higher serum levels of tetracycline may lead to azotemia, hyperphosphatemia, and acidosis. If renal impairment exists, even usual oral or parenteral doses may lead to excessive systemic accumulation of the drug and possible liver toxicity. Under such conditions, lower than usual total doses are indicated and, if therapy is prolonged, serum level determinations of the drug may be advisable.

Photosensitivity manifested by an exaggerated sunburn reaction has been observed in some individuals taking tetracyclines. This has been reported rarely with minocycline.

Central nervous system side effects including light-headedness, dizziness, or vertigo have been reported. Patients who experience these symptoms should be cautioned about driving vehicles or using hazardous machinery while on minocycline therapy. These symptoms may disappear during therapy and usually disappear rapidly when the drug is discontinued.

INTRAVENOUS INJECTION

In the presence of renal dysfunction, particularly in pregnancy, intravenous tetracycline therapy in daily doses exceeding 2 g has been associated with deaths through liver failure.

When the need for intensive treatment outweighs its potential dangers (mostly during pregnancy or in individuals with known or suspected renal or liver impairment), it is advisable to perform renal and liver function tests before and during therapy. Also tetracycline serum concentrations should be followed.

If renal impairment exists, even unusual oral or parenteral doses may lead to excessive systemic accumulation of the drug and possible liver toxicity. Under such conditions, lower than usual total doses are indicated, and if therapy is prolonged, serum level determinations of the drug may be advisable. This hazard is of particular importance in the parenteral administration of tetracyclines to pregnant or postpartum patients with pyelonephritis. When used under these circumstances, the blood level should not exceed 15 mcg/ml and liver function tests should be made at frequent intervals. Other potentially hepatotoxic drugs should not be used concomitantly.

THE USE OF TETRACYCLINES DURING TOOTH DEVELOPMENT (LAST HALF OF PREGNANCY, INFANCY, AND CHILDHOOD TO THE AGE OF 8 YEARS) MAY CAUSE PERMANENT DISCOLORATION OF THE TEETH (YELLOW-GRAY-BROWN). This adverse reaction is more common during long-term use of the drugs but has been observed following repeated short-term courses. Enamel hypoplasia has also been reported. TETRACYCLINES, THEREFORE, SHOULD NOT BE USED IN THIS AGE GROUP UNLESS OTHER DRUGS ARE NOT LIKELY TO BE EFFECTIVE OR ARE CONTRAINDICATED.

Photosensitivity manifested by an exaggerated sunburn reaction has been observed in some individuals taking tetracyclines. Patients apt to be exposed to direct sunlight or ultraviolet light should be advised that this reaction can occur with tetracycline drugs, and treatment should be discontinued at the first evidence of skin erythema. Studies to date indicate that photosensitivity is rarely reported with minocycline HCl.

The anti-anabolic action of the tetracyclines may cause an increase in BUN. While this is not a problem in those with normal renal function, in patients with significantly impaired function, higher serum levels of tetracycline may lead to azotemia, hyperphosphatemia, and acidosis.

CNS side effects including light-headedness, dizziness or vertigo have been reported. Patients who experience these symptoms may disappear during therapy and usually disappear rapidly when the drug is discontinued.

USAGE IN PREGNANCY

See WARNINGS about use during tooth development.

Results of animal studies indicate that tetracyclines cross the placenta, are found in fetal tissues and can have toxic effects on the developing fetus (often related to retardation of skeletal development). Evidence of embryotoxicity has also been noted in animals treated early in pregnancy.

The safety of minocycline HCl for use during pregnancy has not been established.

USAGE IN NEWBORNS, INFANTS, AND CHILDREN

See above WARNINGS about use during tooth development.

All tetracyclines form a stable calcium complex in any bone forming tissue. A decrease in the fibula growth rate has been observed in prematures given oral tetracycline in doses of 25 mg/kg every six hours. This reaction was shown to be reversible when the drug was discontinued.

Tetracyclines are present in the milk of lactating women who are taking a drug in this class.

PRECAUTIONS:

GENERAL

Oral: As with other antibiotic preparations, use of this drug may result in overgrowth of nonsusceptible organisms, including fungi. If superinfection occurs, the antibiotic should be discontinued and appropriate therapy should be instituted.

Pseudotumor cerebri (benign intracranial hypertension) in adults has been associated with the use of tetracyclines. The usual clinical manifestations are headache and blurred vision. Bulging fontanels have been associated with the use of tetracyclines in infants. While both of these conditions and related symptoms usually resolve soon after discontinuation of the tetracycline, the possibility for permanent sequelae exists.

Incision and drainage or other surgical procedures should be performed in conjunction with antibiotic therapy when indicated.

Intravenous Injection: Pseudotumor cerebri (benign intracranial hypertension) in adults has been associated with the use of tetracyclines. The usual clinical manifestations are headache and blurred vision. Bulging fontanels have been associated with the use of tetracyclines in infants. While both of these conditions and related symptoms usually resolve soon after discontinuation of the tetracycline, the possibility for permanent sequelae exists.

As with other antibiotic preparations, use of this drug may result in overgrowth of non-susceptible organisms, including fungi. If superinfection occurs, the antibiotic should be discontinued and appropriate therapy should be instituted.

In venereal diseases when coexistent syphilis is suspected, darkfield examination should be done before treatment is started and the blood serology repeated monthly for at least four months.

In long-term therapy, periodic laboratory evaluation of organ systems, including hematopoietic, renal and hepatic studies should be performed.

PRECAUTIONS: *(cont'd)*

All infections due to Group A beta-hemolytic streptococci should be treated for at least ten days.

INFORMATION FOR THE PATIENT

Oral: Photosensitivity manifested by an exaggerated sunburn reaction has been observed in some individuals taking tetracyclines. Patients apt to be exposed to direct sunlight or ultraviolet light should be advised that this reaction can occur with tetracycline drugs, and treatment should be discontinued at the first evidence of skin erythema. This reaction has been reported rarely with use of minocycline.

Patients who experience central nervous system symptoms (see WARNINGS) should be cautioned about driving vehicles or using hazardous machinery while on minocycline therapy.

Concurrent use of tetracycline may render oral contraceptives less effective (see DRUG INTERACTIONS.)

Tablets Only: Patients should be informed that minocycline HCl tablets should be taken at least one hour before meals or 2 hours after meals (see DOSAGE AND ADMINISTRATION.)

LABORATORY TESTS

Oral: In venereal diseases when coexistent syphilis is suspected, darkfield examination should be done before treatment is started and the blood serology repeated monthly for at least four months.

In long-term therapy, periodic laboratory evaluation of organ systems, including hematopoietic, renal and hepatic studies should be performed.

DRUG/LABORATORY TEST INTERACTIONS

Oral: False elevations of urinary catecholamine levels may occur due to interference with the fluorescence test.

CARCINOGENESIS, MUTAGENESIS, AND IMPAIRMENT OF FERTILITY

Oral: Dietary administration of minocycline in long term tumorigenicity studies in rats resulted in evidence of thyroid tumor production. Minocycline has also been found to produce thyroid hyperplasia in rats and dogs. In addition, there has been evidence of oncogenic activity in rats in studies with a related antibiotic, oxytetracycline (*i.e.,* adrenal and pituitary tumors). Likewise, although mutagenicity studies of minocycline have not been conducted, positive results in *in vitro* mammalian cell assays (*i.e.,* mouse lymphoma and Chinese hamster lung cells) have been reported for related antibiotics (tetracycline hydrochloride and oxytetracycline). Segment I (fertility and general reproduction) studies have provided evidence that minocycline impairs fertility in male rats.

PREGNANCY CATEGORY D

Oral: Pregnancy Category D (see WARNINGS.)

LABOR AND DELIVERY

Oral: The effect of tetracyclines on labor and delivery is unknown.

NURSING MOTHERS

Oral: Tetracyclines are excreted in milk. Because of the potential for serious adverse reaction in nursing infants from tetracyclines, a decision should be made whether to discontinue the drug, taking into account the importance of the drug to the mother (see WARNINGS.)

PEDIATRIC USE

Oral: See WARNINGS.

DRUG INTERACTIONS:

Because tetracyclines have been shown to depress plasma prothrombin activity, patients who are on anticoagulant therapy may require downward adjustment of their anticoagulant dosage.

Since bacteriostatic drugs may interfere with the bactericidal action of penicillin, it is advisable to avoid giving tetracycline-class drugs in conjunction with penicillin.

Concurrent use of tetracycline may render oral contraceptives less effective.

Oral Only: Absorption of tetracyclines is impaired by antacids containing aluminum, calcium or magnesium and iron-containing preparations.

The concurrent use of tetracycline and methoxyflurane has been reported to result in fatal renal toxicity.

ADVERSE REACTIONS:

Gastrointestinal: Anorexia, nausea, vomiting, diarrhea, glossitis, dysphagia, enterocolitis, pancreatitis, and inflammatory lesions (with monilial overgrowth) in the anogenital region, increases in liver enzymes, and rarely hepatitis have been reported.

These reactions have been caused by both the oral and parenteral administration of tetracyclines.

Skin: Maculopapular erythematous rashes. Exfoliative dermatitis has been reported but is uncommon. Erythema multiforme and rarely Stevens-Johnson syndrome have been reported. Photosensitivity is discussed above (see WARNINGS.) Pigmentation of the skin and mucous membranes has been reported.

Renal Toxicity: Elevations in BUN have been reported and are apparently dose related (see WARNINGS.)

Hypersensitivity Reactions: Urticaria, angioneurotic edema, polyarthralgia, anaphylaxis, anaphylactoid purpura, pericarditis, exacerbation of systemic lupus erythematosus and rarely pulmonary infiltrates with eosinophilia have been reported.

Blood: Hemolytic anemia, thrombocytopenia, neutropenia and eosinophilia have been reported.

Central Nervous System: Bulging fontanels in infants and benign intracranial hypertension (pseudotumor cerebri) in adults (see PRECAUTIONS, General) have been reported. Headache has also been reported.

Other: When given over prolonged periods, tetracyclines have been reported to produce brown-black microscopic discoloration of the thyroid glands. Very rare cases of abnormal thyroid function have been reported.

ORAL ONLY

Due to oral minocycline's virtually complete absorption, side effects to the lower bowel, particularly diarrhea, have been infrequent. The following adverse reactions have been observed in patients receiving tetracyclines.

Rare instances of esophagitis and esophageal ulcerations have been reported in patients taking the tetracycline-class antibiotics in capsule and table form. Most of these patients took the medication immediately before going to bed (see DOSAGE AND ADMINISTRATION.)

Decreased hearing has been rarely reported in patients on minocycline HCl.

Tooth discoloration in children less than 8 years of age (see WARNINGS) and also, rarely, in adults have been reported.

OVERDOSAGE:

In case of overdosage, discontinue medication, treat symptomatically and institute supportive measures.

DOSAGE AND ADMINISTRATION:

ORAL

THE USUAL DOSAGE AND FREQUENCY OF ADMINISTRATION OF MINOCYCLINE DIFFERS FROM THAT OF THE OTHER TETRACYCLINES. EXCEEDING THE RECOMMENDED DOSAGE MAY RESULT IN AN INCREASED INCIDENCE OF SIDE EFFECTS.

Minocycline HCl tablets should be taken at least one hour before meals or 2 hours after meals (see CLINICAL PHARMACOLOGY.)

Minocycline HCl pellet-filled capsules may be taken with or without food(see CLINICAL PHARMACOLOGY.)

Adults: The usual dosage of minocycline HCl tablets and pellet-filled capsules is 200 mg initially followed by 100 mg every 12 hours. Alternatively, if more frequent doses are preferred, two or four 50 mg tablets or pellet-filled capsules may be given initially followed by one 50 mg tablet or pellet-filled capsule four times daily.

For Children Above 8 Years of Age: The usual dosage of minocycline HCl is 4 mg/kg initially followed by 2 mg/kg every 12 hours.

Uncomplicated gonococcal infections other than urethritis and anorectal infections in men: 200 mg initially, followed by 100 mg every 12 hours for a minimum of four days, with post-therapy cultures within 2 to 3 days.

In the treatment of uncomplicated gonococcal urethritis in men, 100 mg every 12 hours for five days is recommended.

For the treatment of syphilis, the usual dosage of minocycline HCl should be administered over a period of 10 to 15 days. Close follow-up, including laboratory tests, is recommended.

In the treatment of meningococcal carrier state, the recommended dosage is 100 mg every 12 hours for five days.

Mycobacterium marinum Infections: Although optimal doses have not been established, 100 mg every 12 hours for 6 to 8 weeks have been used successfully in a limited number of cases.

Uncomplicated urethral, endocervical, or rectal infection in adults caused by *Chlamydia trachomatis* or *Ureaplasma urealyticum*: 100 mg orally, every 12 hours for at least seven days.

Ingestion of adequate amounts of fluids along with capsule and tablet forms of drugs in the tetracycline-class is recommended to reduce the risk of esophageal irritation and ulceration.

In patients with renal impairment (see WARNINGS), the total dosage should be decreased by either reducing the recommended individual doses and/or by extending the time intervals between doses.

Store at Controlled Room Temperature 15-30°C (59-86°F).

Protect from light, moisture and excessive heat.

INTRAVENOUS INJECTION

Note: Rapid administration is to be avoided. Parenteral therapy is indicated only when oral therapy is not adequate or tolerated. Oral therapy should be instituted as soon as possible. If intravenous therapy is given over prolonged periods of time, thrombophlebitis may result.

Adults: Usual adult dose: 200 mg followed by 100 mg every 12 hours and should not exceed 4009 mg in 24 hours. The drug should be initially dissolved and then further diluted to 500-1000 ml with either Sodium Chloride Injection USP, Dextrose Injection USP, Dextrose and Sodium Chloride Injection USP, Ringer's Injection USP, or Lactated Ringer's Injection USP but not in other solutions containing calcium (a precipitate may form).

The reconstituted solutions are stable at room temperature for 24 hours without a significant loss of potency. Any unused portions must be discarded after that period. The final dilution for administration should be administered immediately.

For Children Above Eight Years Of Age: Usual pediatric dose: 4 mg/kg followed by 2 mg/kg every 12 hours.

In Patients With Renal Impairment: (See WARNINGS.)

Total dosage should be decreased by reduction of recommended individual doses and/or by extending time intervals between doses.

Parenteral drug products should be inspected visually for particulate matter and discoloration prior to administration, whenever solution and container permit.

Store at Controlled Room Temperature 15-30°C (59-86°F).

ANIMAL PHARMACOLOGY:

Oral Only: Minocycline HCl has been observed to cause a dark discoloration of the thyroid in experimental animals (rats, minipigs, dogs and monkeys). In the rat, chronic treatment with minocycline HCl has resulted in goiter accompanied by elevated radioactive iodine uptake, and evidence of thyroid tumor production. Minocycline HCl has also been found to produce thyroid hyperplasia in rats and dogs.

REFERENCES:

1. National Committee for Clinical Laboratory Standards, Approved Standard: *Performance Standards for Antimicrobial Disk Susceptibility Tests*, 3rd Edition, Vol. 4(16): M2-A3, Villanova, PA, December 1984. **2.** National Committee for Clinical Laboratory Standards, Approved Standard: *Methods for Dilution Antimicrobial Susceptibility Tests for Bacteria that Grow Aerobically*, 2nd Edition, Vol. 5(22): M7-A, Villanova, PA, December 1985.(Capsules: Lederle, 12/93, 31942-93) (Injection: Lederle, 7/91, 10787-91)

HOW SUPPLIED - RATED THERAPEUTICALLY EQUIVALENT:

Capsule - Oral - 50 mg

100's	$120.50	Minocycline, Duramed Pharms	51285-0991-02

Capsule - Oral - 100 mg

50's	$100.54	Minocycline, Duramed Pharms	51285-0992-50

Capsule, Gelatin - Oral - 50 mg

100's	$49.28	Minocycline HCl, H.C.F.A. F F P	99999-1818-01
100's	$56.93	Minocycline Hcl, United Res	00677-1435-01
100's	$107.99	Minocycline Hcl, HL Moore Drug Exch	00839-7649-06
100's	$110.73	Minocycline Hcl, Harber Pharm	51432-0731-03
100's	$118.00	Minocycline HCl, Schein Pharm (US)	00364-2497-01
100's	$119.86	Minocycline Hcl, Qualitest Pharms	00603-4678-21
100's	$120.00	Minocycline HCl 50, Warner Chilcott	00047-0615-24
100's	$120.00	Minocycline Hcl, Goldline Labs	00182-1102-01
100's	$120.00	Minocycline, Teva	00332-3165-09
100's	$120.00	Minocycline Hcl, Aligen Independ	00405-4680-01
100's	$120.55	Minocycline Hcl, Major Pharms	00904-2413-60
100's	$120.55	Minocycline Hcl, Major Pharms	00904-7682-60
100's	$125.00	Minocycline HCl, Rugby	00536-1482-01
100's	$145.00	Dynacin, Medicis	99207-0497-10
100's	**$163.35**	**MINOCIN, Lederle Pharm**	**00005-5343-23**
250's	$123.20	Minocycline HCl, H.C.F.A. F F P	99999-1818-02
250's	**$407.39**	**MINOCIN, Lederle Pharm**	**00005-5343-27**
500's	$246.40	Minocycline HCl, H.C.F.A. F F P	99999-1818-03
500's	$680.00	Dynacin, Medicis	99207-0497-05
1000's	$492.80	Minocycline HCl, H.C.F.A. F F P	99999-1818-04
1000's	$1051.80	Minocycline Hcl, Warner Chilcott	00047-0615-32

HOW SUPPLIED - RATED THERAPEUTICALLY EQUIVALENT: *(cont'd)*

Capsule, Gelatin - Oral - 100 mg

50's	$90.44	Minocycline Hcl, HL Moore Drug Exch	00839-7650-04
50's	$92.24	Minocycline Hcl, Harber Pharm	51432-0735-05
50's	$97.00	Minocycline HCl, Schein Pharm (US)	00364-2498-50
50's	$97.45	Minocycline Hcl, Major Pharms	00904-7683-51
50's	$98.00	Minocycline Hcl, Goldline Labs	00182-1103-19
50's	$98.00	Minocycline, Teva	00332-3167-07
50's	$98.00	Minocycline Hcl, Qualitest Pharms	00603-4679-19
50's	$98.10	Minocycline Hcl, United Res	00677-1436-02
50's	$98.20	Minocycline Hcl, Aligen Independ	00405-4681-50
50's	$100.05	Minocycline HCl 100, Warner Chilcott	00047-0616-19
50's	$111.25	Minocycline HCl, Rugby	00536-1492-06
50's	$125.00	Dynacin, Medicis	99207-0498-50
50's	**$136.06**	**MINOCIN, Lederle Pharm**	**00005-5344-18**
100's	$196.25	Minocycline Hcl, Major Pharms	00904-2414-61
250's	**$678.61**	**MINOCIN, Lederle Pharm**	**00005-5344-27**
500's	$1045.00	Dynacin, Medicis	99207-0498-05
1000's	$1754.40	Minocycline Hcl, Warner Chilcott	00047-0616-32

HOW SUPPLIED - NOT RATED EQUIVALENT:

Injection, Lyphl-Soln - Intravenous - 100 mg/vial

100 mg	**$32.79**	**MINOCIN, Lederle Parenterals**	**00205-5305-94**

Suspension - Oral - 50 mg/5ml

60 ml	**$30.49**	**MINOCIN, Lederle Pharm**	**00005-5313-56**

MINOXIDIL *(001819)*

CATEGORIES: Alopecia; Antianginals; Antiarrhythmic Agents; Antihypertensives; Baldness; Cardiovascular Drugs; Dermatologicals; Hair Growth Stimulants; Hypertension; Skin/Mucous Membrane Agents; Topical; Vasodilating Agents; Vertigo/Motion Sickness/Vomiting; Pregnancy Category C; Sales > $100 Million; FDA Approval Pre 1982; Patent Expiration 1996 Feb

BRAND NAMES: *Alopexil*; *Alopexy* (France); *Alopexyl* (France); Alostil; *Crecisan*; *Hairex*; *Hairgaine*; *Headway*; *Hebald*; *Kapodin*; *Locion EPC*; Loniten; *Lonnoten*; *Lonolax*; *Lonolox* (Germany); *Lonoten* (France); Minodyl; *Minona*; *Minoxidil Isac*; *Minoximen*; *Mintop*; *Mixidil*; *Modil*; *Multigain*; *Neocapil*; *Neoxidil*; *Pilogan*; *Regaine* (Australia, Europe, Asia, Mexico); *Regrou*; *Regrowth*; **Rogaine**; *Rehair*; *Tiazolin*

(International brand names outside U.S. in italics)

FORMULARIES: Aetna; BC-BS

COST OF THERAPY: $87.60 (Hypertension; Tablet; 2.5 mg; 2/day; 365 days)

PRIMARY ICD9: 401.1 (Essential Hypertension, Benign)

WARNING:
Minoxidil may produce serious adverse effects. It can cause pericardial effusion, occasionally progressing to tamponade, and angina pectoris may be exacerbated. Minoxidil should be reserved for hypertensive patients who do not respond adequately to maximum therapeutic doses of a diuretic and two other antihypertensive agents.
In experimental animals, minoxidil caused several kinds of myocardial lesions as well as other adverse cardiac effects (see Cardiac Lesions in Animals).
Minoxidil must be administered under close supervision, usually concomitantly with therapeutic doses of a beta-adrenergic blocking agent to prevent tachycardia and increased myocardial workload. It must also usually be given with a diuretic, frequently one acting in the ascending limb of the loop of Henle, to prevent serious fluid accusation. Patients with malignant hypertension and those already receiving guanethidine (see WARNINGS) should be hospitalized when minoxidil is first administered so that they can be monitored to avoid too rapid, or large orthostatic, decreases in blood pressure.

DESCRIPTION:

Rogaine Topical Solution: Minoxidil topical solution is a hair growth stimulant. Rogaine contains the active ingredient minoxidil. Minoxidil appears as a white or off-white, odorless crystalline solid that is soluble in water to the extent of approximately 2 mg/ml, is readily soluble in propylene glycol or ethanol, and is almost insoluble in acetone, chloroform or ethyl acetate.

The chemical name for minoxidil is 2,4-pyrimidinediamine, 6-(1-piperidinyl)-, 3-oxide (MW = 209.25).

Rogaine topical solution is available at a concentration of 2% (20 mg minoxidil per milliliter) in a solution of alcohol 60% v/v, propylene glycol, and water.

Loniten Tablets: Loniten tablets contain minoxidil, an antihypertensive peripheral vasodilator. Minoxidil occurs as a white or off-white, odorless, crystalline solid that is soluble in water to the extent of approximately 2 mg/ml, is readily soluble in propylene glycol or ethanol, and is almost insoluble in acetone, chloroform or ethyl acetate. The chemical name for minoxidil is 2,4-pyrimidinediamine, 6-(1-piperidinyl)-, 3-oxide (mw=209.25).

Loniten tablets for oral administration contain either 2.5 mg or 10 mg of minoxidil. Inactive ingredients: cellulose, corn starch, lactose, magnesium stearate, silicon dioxide.

CLINICAL PHARMACOLOGY:

TOPICAL SOLUTION

Pharmacologic Properties and Pharmacokinetics

Minoxidil topical solution stimulates hair growth in individuals with androgenetic alopecia, expressed in males as baldness of the vertex of the scalp and in females as diffuse hair loss or thinning of the frontoparietal areas. The mechanism by which minoxidil stimulates hair growth is not known but like minoxidil some other arterial dilating drugs also stimulate hair growth when given systemically.

Because of its serious side effects oral minoxidil is indicated only for the treatment of hypertension that is symptomatic or associated with target organ damage and is not manageable with maximum therapeutic doses of a diuretic plus two other antihypertensive drugs. It is a direct acting peripheral arterial dilator that reduces blood pressure by decreasing peripheral vascular resistance. Reduction of peripheral arteriolar resistance and the resulting

CLINICAL PHARMACOLOGY: *(cont'd)*

fall in blood pressure trigger sympathetic, vagal inhibitory, and renal homeostatic mechanisms, including increased renin secretion, that lead to increased heart rate and cardiac output and salt and water retention.

The major side effects of oral minoxidil, aside from unwelcome generalized hair growth, result from fluid retention, often profound, and tachycardia, and require that minoxidil be administered in most cases with a beta-blocker or other agent to reduce heart rate and a diuretic, almost always a high ceiling (loop) diuretic. Fluid retention can lead to marked weight gain, local or generalized edema, heart failure, and pleural or pericardial effusion, including cardiac tamponade. Pericarditis has been reported, usually in patients with renal failure or collagen vascular disease, but in some cases these causes of pericarditis do not seem to have been present. The tachycardia and increased cardiac output caused by minoxidil can lead to exacerbation of existing angina or the onset of angina in persons with compromised coronary circulation. It is these serious side effects that have restricted use of oral minoxidil to patients with severe hypertension not controllable with other agents.

In placebo controlled trials involving over 3500 male patients given topical minoxidil for 4 months (longer treatment was given after the placebo group was discontinued) and in over 300 female patients given topical minoxidil for eight months, the typical systemic effects of oral minoxidil (weight gain, edema, tachycardia, fall in blood pressure, and their more serious consequences) were not seen more frequently in patients given topical minoxidil than in those given topical placebo (see ADVERSE REACTIONS). The mean changes from baseline in weight, heart rate, and blood pressure in the treated and placebo groups were similar, and the number of patients experiencing significant changes, such as a blood pressure decrease of 15 mmHg or more diastolic or 30 mmHg or more systolic, a heart rate increase of 15 beats/minute or more, or weight gain of at least 5 pounds, was also similar.

In an effort to explore the potential for systemic effects of topical minoxidil, three concentrations of topical minoxidil (1, 2 and 5%) applied twice daily were compared to low oral doses (2.5 and 5 mg given once daily), and placebo in hypertensive patients (normotensive patients have little or no blood pressure response to minoxidil at dose of 10 mg per day) in a double-blind controlled trial. The 5 mg oral dose had readily detectable effects, a fall in diastolic pressure of about 5 mmHg and an increase in heart rate of 7 beats/minute. No other group had a clear effect, although there was some evidence of a weak and inconsistent effect in the 2.5 mg oral, and possibly the 5% topical, treatments.

The failure to detect evidence of systemic effects during treatment with topical minoxidil reflects the poor absorption of topical minoxidil, which averages about 1.4% (range 0.3 to 4.5%) from normal intact scalp, and was about 2% in the hypertensive patients, whose scalps were shaved.

In a comparison of topical and oral absorption, peak serum levels of unchanged minoxidil after 1 ml b.i.d. of 2% minoxidil solution (the maximum recommended dose) averaged 5.8% (range 1.4% to 12.7%) of the level observed after 2.5 mg b.i.d. oral doses (5 mg is the recommended starting dose of oral minoxidil). Similarly, in the hypertension study, where patients had shaved scalps, mean minoxidil concentrations after 1 ml b.i.d. of 2% topical minoxidil (1.7 ng/ml) were 1/20 the concentrations seen after daily oral doses of 2.5 mg (32.8 ng/ml) or 5 mg (59.2 ng/ml). Blood levels obtained in the large controlled hair growth trials averaged less than 2 ng/ml for the 2% solution. There were, however, occasional values that were higher; about 1% of the patients on 2% minoxidil had serum levels of 5 ng/ml or greater and a few approached 30 ng/ml. It is possible, therefore, that if more than the recommended dose were applied to inflamed skin in an individual with relatively high absorption, blood levels with systemic effects might rarely be obtained. Physicians and patients need to be aware of the possibility.

Serum minoxidil level resulting from administration of minoxidil are governed by the drug's percutaneous absorption rate. Following cessation of topical dosing of minoxidil approximately 95% of systemically absorbed minoxidil is eliminated within four days. The metabolic biotransformation of minoxidil absorbed following administration of minoxidil has not been fully determined.

Minoxidil absorbed following oral administration is metabolized predominantly by conjugation with glucuronic acid at the N-oxide position in the pyrimidine ring but also by conversion to more polar products. Known metabolites exert much less pharmacologic effect than the parent compound. Minoxidil and its metabolites are excreted principally in the urine. Minoxidil does not bind to plasma proteins and its renal clearance corresponds to the glomerular filtration rate. Minoxidil does not enter the central nervous system (CNS) of experimental animals in significant amounts and it does not affect CNS function in man.

Cardiac Lesions in Animals

Minoxidil produces several cardiac lesions in animals. Some are characteristic of agents that cause tachycardia and diastolic hypotension (beta-agonists like isoproterenol, arterial dilators like hydralazine) while others are produced by a narrower range of agents with arterial dilating properties. The significance of these lesions for humans is not clear, as they have not been recognized in patients treated with oral minoxidil at systemically active doses, despite formal review of over 150 autopsies of treated patients.

(a) Papillary muscle/subendocardial necrosis: The most characteristic lesion of minoxidil, seen in rat, dog, and minipig (but not monkeys) is focal necrosis of the papillary muscle and subendocardial areas of the left ventricle. These lesions appear rapidly, within a few days of treatment with doses of 0.5 to 10 mg/kg/day in the dog and minipig, and are not progressive, although they leave residual scars. They are similar to lesions produced by other peripheral arterial dilators, by theobromine, and by beta-adrenergic receptor agonists such as isoproterenol, epinephrine, and albuterol. The lesions are thought to reflect ischemia provoked by increased oxygen demand (tachycardia, increased cardiac output) and relative decrease in coronary flow (decreased diastolic pressure and decreased time in diastole) caused by the vasodilatory effects of these agents coupled with reflex or directly induced tachycardia.

(b) Hemorrhagic lesions: After acute oral minoxidil treatment (0.5 to 10 mg/kg/day) in dogs and minipigs, hemorrhagic lesions are seen in many parts of the heart, mainly in the epicardium, endocardium, and walls of small coronary arteries and arterioles. In minipigs the lesions occur primarily in the left atrium while in dogs they are most prominent in the right atrium, frequently appearing as grossly visible hemorrhagic lesions. With exposure of 1-20 mg/kg/day in the dog for 30 days or longer, there is replacement of myocardial cells by proliferating fibroblasts and angioblasts, hemorrhage and hemosiderin accumulation. These lesions can be produced by topical minoxidil administration that gives systemic absorption of 0.5 to 1 mg/kg/day. Other peripheral dilators, including an experimental agent, nicorandil, and theobromine, have produced similar lesions.

(c) Epicarditis: A less fully studied lesion is focal epicarditis, seen in dogs after 2 days of oral minoxidil. More recently, chronic proliferative epicarditis was observed in dogs treated topically twice a day for 90 days. In a one year oral dog study, serosanguinous pericardial fluid was seen.

(d) Hypertrophy and Dilation: Oral and topical studies in rats, dogs, monkeys (oral only), and rabbits (dermal only) show cardiac hypertrophy and dilation. This is presumed to represent the consequences of prolonged fluid overload; there is preliminary evidence in monkeys that diuretics partly reverse these effects.

Autopsies of over 150 patients who died of various causes after receiving oral minoxidil for hypertension have not revealed the characteristic hemorrhagic (especially atrial) lesions seen in dogs and minipigs. While areas of papillary muscle and subendocardial necrosis were

CLINICAL PHARMACOLOGY: *(cont'd)*

occasionally seen, they occurred in the presence of known pre-existing coronary artery disease and were also seen in patients never exposed to minoxidil in another series using similar, but not identical, autopsy methods.

TABLETS

General Pharmacologic Properties

Minoxidil is an orally effective direct acting peripheral vasodilator that reduces elevated systolic and diastolic blood pressure by decreasing peripheral vascular resistance. Microcirculatory blood flow in animals is enhanced or maintained in all systemic vascular beds. In man, forearm and renal vascular resistance decline; forearm blood flow increases while renal blood flow and glomerular filtration rate are preserved.

Because it causes peripheral vasodilation, minoxidil elicits a number of predictable reactions. Reduction of peripheral arteriolar resistance and the associated fall in blood pressure trigger sympathetic, vagal inhibitory, and renal homeostatic mechanisms, including an increase in renin secretion, that lead to increased cardiac rate and output and salt and water retention. These adverse effects can usually be minimized by concomitant administration of a diuretic and a beta-adrenergic blocking agent or other sympathetic nervous system suppressant.

Minoxidil does not interfere with vasomotor reflexes and therefore does not produce orthostatic hypotension. The drug does not enter the central nervous system in experimental animals in significant amounts, and it does not affect CNS function in man.

Effects on Blood Pressure and Target Organs

The extent and time-course of blood pressure reduction by minoxidil do not correspond closely to its concentration in plasma. After an effective single oral dose, blood pressure usually starts to decline within one-half hour, reaches a minimum between 2 and 3 hours and recovers at an arithmetically linear rate of about 30%/day. The total duration of effect is approximately 75 hours. When minoxidil is administered chronically, once or twice a day, the time required to achieve maximum effect on blood pressure with a given daily dose is inversely related to the size of the dose. Thus, maximum effect is achieved on 10 mg/day within 7 days, on 20 mg/day within 5 days, and on 40 mg/day within 3 days.

The blood pressure response to minoxidil is linearly related to the logarithm of the dose administered. The slope of this log-linear dose-response relationship is proportional to the extent of hypertension and approaches zero at a supine diastolic blood pressure of approximately 85 mm Hg.

When used in severely hypertensive patients resistant to other therapy, frequently with an accompanying diuretic and beta-blocker, minoxidil tablets usually decreased the blood pressure and reversed encephalopathy and retinopathy.

Absorption and Metabolism

Minoxidil is at least 90% absorbed from the GI tract in experimental animals and man. Plasma levels of the parent drug reach maximum within the first hour and decline rapidly thereafter. The average plasma half-life in man is 4.2 hours. Approximately 90% of the administered drug is metabolized, predominantly by conjugation with glucuronic acid at the N-oxide position in the pyrimidine ring, but also by conversion to more polar products. Known metabolites exert much less pharmacologic effect than minoxidil itself; all are excreted principally in the urine. Minoxidil does not bind to plasma proteins, and its renal clearance corresponds to the glomerular filtration rate. In the absence of functional renal tissue, minoxidil and its metabolites can be removed by hemodialysis.

Cardiac Lesions in Animals

Minoxidil produced several types of cardiac lesions in non-primate species:

(a) Dog atrial lesion: Daily oral doses of 0.5 mg/kg for several days to 1 month or longer produced a grossly visible hemorrhagic lesion of the right atrium of the dog. This lesion has not been seen in other species. Microscopic examination showed replacement of myocardial cells by proliferating fibroblasts and angioblasts; phagocytosis; and hemosiderin accumulation in macrophages.

(b) Papillary muscle lesion: Short-term treatment (about 3 days) in several species (dog, rat, minipig) produced necrosis of the papillary muscles, and, in some cases, subendocardial areas of the left ventricle, lesions similar to those produced by other peripheral dilators and by beta-adrenergic receptor agonists such as isoproterenol and epinephrine. These are thought to result from myocardial ischemia resulting from reflex sympathetic or vagal withdrawal-induced tachycardia in combination with hypotension. These lesions were reduced in incidence and severity by beta-adrenergic receptor blockade.

(c) Hemorrhagic lesions: were seen in many parts of the heart, mainly in the epicardium, endocardium, and walls of small coronary arteries and arterioles, after acute minoxidil treatment in dogs, and left atrial hemorrhagic lesions were seen in minipigs.

In addition to these lesions, longer term studies in rats, dogs, and monkeys showed cardiac hypertrophy and (in rats) cardiac dilation. In monkeys, hydrochlorothiazide partly reversed the increased heart weight, suggesting it may be related to fluid overload. In a one-year dog study, serosanguinous pericardial fluid was seen.

Autopsies of 79 patients who dies from various causes and who had received minoxidil did not reveal right atrial or other hemorrhagic pathology of the kind seen in dogs. Instances of necrotic areas in the papillary muscles were seen, but these occurred in the presence of known pre-existing ischemic heart disease and did not appear different from, or more common than, lesions seen in patients never exposed to minoxidil. Studies to date cannot rule out the possibility that minoxidil can be associated with cardiac damage in humans.

CLINICAL STUDIES:

CLINICAL TRIAL EXPERIENCE—MALES

In clinical trails in **males**, three main parameters of efficacy were used: hair counts in a one inch diameter circle on the vertex of the scalp; investigator evaluation of terminal hair regrowth; and patient evaluation of hair regrowth. At the end of four-month placebo-controlled portions of 12 month clinical studies (*i.e.*, baseline to Month 4), minoxidil topical solution (20 mg minoxidil per ml) demonstrated the following efficacy:

Hair Counts: Minoxidil was significantly more effective than placebo in producing hair regrowth as assessed by hair counts. Patients using minoxidil had a mean increase from baseline of 72 non-vellus hairs in the one inch diameter circle compared with a mean increase of 39 non-vellus hairs in patients using the placebo ($P<0.0005$).

Investigator Evaluation: Based on the investigators' evaluation, there was no statistically significant difference in terminal hair regrowth between treatment groups. Eight percent (8%) of the patients using minoxidil demonstrated moderate to dense terminal hair regrowth compared with 4% using the placebo. During the initial four months of treatment, however, very little regrowth of terminal hair can be expected. Although most patients did not demonstrate cosmetically significant regrowth of hair, 26% of the patients showed minimal terminal hair regrowth using minoxidil compared with 16% of those using placebo as assessed by the investigator.

Patient Evaluation: Based on the patients' self evaluation, 26% using minoxidil demonstrated moderate to dense hair regrowth compared with 11% using the placebo ($P<0.0005$).

CLINICAL STUDIES: *(cont'd)*

Patients who continued on minoxidil during the remaining eight months of the 12-month clinical studies (*i.e.*, the non-placebo-controlled portion of the studies) continued to sustain a regrowth response as evaluated by hair counts, investigator evaluation, and patient evaluation.

At the end of the eight month non-placebo-controlled portion of the 12-month clinical studies (*i.e.*, Months 4 to 12), the following results were obtained:

Hair Count: Patients using minoxidil had a mean increase of 112 non-vellus hairs in the same one inch diameter circle as compared to Month 4 (P<0.0005).

Investigator Evaluation: Based on the investigators' evaluation, 39% of the patients achieved moderate to dense terminal hair by Month 12.

Patient Evaluation: Based on the patients assessment, 48% felt they had achieved moderate to dense hair regrowth at Month 12.

Trends in the data suggest that those patients who are younger, who have been balding for a shorter period of time, or who have a smaller area of hair loss may respond better than patients who are older, who have been balding for a longer period of time, or who have a larger area of hair loss.

CLINICAL TRIAL EXPERIENCE—FEMALES

In clinical trials in **females** (age range 18-45 years, 90% who were Caucasian) with Ludwig grade I and II diffuse frontoparietal hair thinning, the main parameters of efficacy were: non-vellus hair counts in a designated 1.0 cm^2 site on the frontoparietal areas of the scalp; investigator evaluation of hair regrowth; and patient evaluation of hair regrowth. Data demonstrate that 44% to 63% (Investigators' evaluation from the international and US multicenter trials, respectively) of women with androgenetic alopecia will have discernible growth of non-vellus hair when treated with minoxidil for 32 weeks versus 29% to 39% for vehicle control treated women.

Two 8-month placebo-controlled studies in females (US multicenter trial and an international multicenter trial) produced the following results:

Hair Counts: Minoxidil was significantly more effective than placebo in producing hair regrowth as assessed by hair counts in both studies. Patients using minoxidil had a mean increase from baseline of 22.7 and 33.2 non-vellus hairs, respectively, in the same 1.0 cm^2 site compared with a mean increase of 11.0 and 19.1 non-vellus hairs, respectively, in patients using placebo (p=0.0004 and p=0.0001, respectively).

Investigator Evaluation: Based on the investigators evaluation 63% (13% moderate and 50% minimal) and 44% (12% moderate and 32% minimal), respectively, of the patients using minoxidil in the two studies achieved hair regrowth at Week-32, compared with 39% (6% moderate and 33% minimal) and 29% (5% moderate and 24% minimal), respectively, of those using placebo (p<0.0005 and p=0.008, respectively).

Patient Evaluation: Based on the patients self evaluation, 59% (19% moderate and 40% minimal) and 55% (1% dense, 24% moderate, and 30% minimal), respectively, of the patients using minoxidil reported hair regrowth at Week-32, compared with 40% (7% moderate and 33% minimal) and 41% (12% moderate and 29% minimal), respectively, of those using placebo (p=0.002 and p=0.013, respectively).

Hair growth was defined as follows:

Investigator Evaluation of Growth:

No visible new hair growth

Minimal growth: Definite growth but no substantial covering of thinning areas

Moderate growth: New growth partially covering thinning areas, less dense than non-thinning areas (readily discernible)

Dense Growth: Full covering of thinning areas; density of hair similar to non-thinning areas

Patient Evaluation of Growth:

No visible hair growth

Minimal hair growth: Barely discernible

Moderate new hair growth: Readily discernible

Dense new hair growth

INDICATIONS AND USAGE:

Topical Solution: Minoxidil topical solution is indicated for the treatment of androgenetic alopecia, expressed in males as baldness of the vertex of the scalp and in females as diffuse hair loss or thinning of the frontoparietal areas. At least four months of twice daily applications of minoxidil are generally required before evidence of hair growth can be expected.

Tablets: Because of the potential for serious adverse effects, minoxidil tablets are indicated only in the treatment of hypertension that is symptomatic or associated with target organ damage and is not manageable with maximum therapeutic doses of a diuretic plus two other antihypertensive drugs. At the present time use in milder degrees of hypertension is not recommended because the benefit-risk relationship in such patients has not been defined.

Minoxidil reduced supine diastolic blood pressure by 20 mm Hg or to 90 mm Hg or less in approximately 75% of patients, most of who had hypertension that could not be controlled by other drugs.

CONTRAINDICATIONS:

Minoxidil is contraindicated in those patients with a history of hypersensitivity to any of the components of the preparation.

Tablets: Minoxidil tablets are contraindicated in pheochromocytoma, because it may stimulate secretion of catecholamines from the tumor through its antihypertensive action.

WARNINGS:

TOPICAL SOLUTION

1. Need for normal scalp: The majority of clinical studies included only healthy patients with normal scalps and no cardiovascular disease. Before starting a patient on minoxidil, the physician should ascertain that the patient has a healthy, normal scalp. Local abrasion or dermatitis may increase absorption and hence increase the risk of side effects.

2. Potential adverse effects: Although extensive use of topical minoxidil has not revealed evidence that enough minoxidil is absorbed to have systemic effects, greater absorption because of misuse or individual variability or unusual sensitivity could lead, at least theoretically, to a systemic effect, and physicians and patients need to be aware of this.

Experience with oral minoxidil has shown the following major cardiovascular effects (the package insert for minoxidil tablets, should be reviewed for details):

salt and water retention, generalized and local edema

pericardial effusion, pericarditis, tamponade

tachycardia

increased frequency of angina or new onset of angina

WARNINGS: *(cont'd)*

If systemic effects were to occur, patients with underlying heart disease, including coronary artery disease and congestive heart failure, would be at particular risk. minoxidil could also have additive effects with other therapy in patients being treated for hypertension.

Patients being considered for minoxidil topical solution should have a history and physical examination. Patients should be advised of the potential risk and a decision should be made by the patient and physician that the benefits outweigh the risks. Patients with a history of underlying heart disease should be aware that adverse effects in them might be especially serious. Patients should be alerted to the possibility of tachycardia and fluid retention and should watch for, and be monitored for, increased heart rate and weight gain or other systemic effects.

TABLETS

Salt and Water Retention: *Congestive Heart Failure:* concomitant use of an adequate diuretic is required—minoxidil tablets must usually be administered concomitantly with a diuretic adequate to prevent fluid retention and possible congestive heart failure; a high ceiling (loop) diuretic is *almost always* required. Body weight should be monitored closely. If minoxidil is used without a diuretic, retention of several hundred milliequivalents of salt and corresponding volumes of water can occur within a few days, leading to increased plasma and interstitial fluid volume and local or generalized edema. Diuretic treatment alone, or in combination with restricted salt intake, will usually minimize fluid retention, although reversible edema did develop in approximately 10% of non-dialysis patients so treated. Ascites has also been reported. Diuretic effectiveness was limited mostly by disease-related impaired renal function. The condition of patients with pre-existing congestive heart failure occasionally deteriorated in association with fluid retention although because of the fall in blood pressure (reduction of afterload), more than twice as many improved than worsened. Rarely, refractory fluid retention may require discontinuation of minoxidil. Provided that the patient is under close medical supervision, it may be possible to resolve refractory salt retention by discontinuing minoxidil for 1 or 2 days and then resuming treatment in conjunction with vigorous diuretic therapy.

Concomitant Treatment to Prevent Tachycardia is Usually Required: Minoxidil increases the heart rate. Angina may worsen or appear for the first time during minoxidil treatment, probably because of the increased oxygen demands associated with increased heart rate and cardiac output. The increase in rate and the occurrence of angina generally can be prevented by the concomitant administration of a beta-adrenergic blocking drug or other sympathetic nervous system suppressant. The ability of beta-adrenergic blocking agents to minimize papillary muscle lesions in animals is further reason to utilize such an agent concomitantly. Round-the-clock effectiveness of the sympathetic suppressant should be ensured.

Pericarditis, Pericardial Effusion, and Tamponade: There have been reports of pericarditis occurring in association with the use of minoxidil. The relationship of this association to renal status is uncertain. Pericardial effusion, occasionally with tamponade, has been observed in about 3% of treated patients not on dialysis, especially those with inadequate or compromised renal function. Although in many cases, the pericardial effusion was associated with a connective tissue disease, the uremic syndrome, congestive heart failure, or marked fluid retention, there have been instances in which these potential causes of effusion were not present. Patients should be observed closely for any suggestion of a pericardial disorder, and echocardiographic studies should be carried out if suspicion arises. More vigorous diuretic therapy, dialysis, pericardiocentesis, or surgery may be required. If the effusion persists, withdrawal of minoxidil should be considered in light of other means of controlling the hypertension and the patient's clinical status.

Interaction with Guanethidine: Although minoxidil does not itself cause orthostatic hypotension, its administration to patients already receiving guanethidine can result in profound orthostatic effects. If at all possible, guanethidine should be discontinued well before minoxidil is begun. Where this is not possible, minoxidil therapy should be started in the hospital and the patient should remain institutionalized until severe orthostatic effects are no longer present or the patient has learned to avoid activities that provoke them.

Hazard of Rapid Control of Blood Pressure: In patients with very severe blood pressure elevation, too rapid control of blood pressure, especially with intravenous agents, can precipitate syncope, cerebrovascular accidents, myocardial infarction and ischemia of special sense organs with resulting decrease or loss of vision or hearing. Patients with compromised circulation or cryoglobulinemia may also suffer ischemic episodes of the affected organs. Although such events have not been unequivocally associated with minoxidil use, total experience is limited at present.

Any patient with malignant hypertension should have initial treatment with minoxidil carried out in a hospital setting, both to assure that blood pressure is falling and to assure that it is not falling more rapidly than intended.

PRECAUTIONS:

TOPICAL SOLUTION

General

Patients treated with minoxidil topical solution should be monitored one month after starting minoxidil and at least every six months thereafter. If systemic effects should occur, discontinue use of minoxidil.

Minoxidil contains an alcohol base which will cause burning and irritation of the eye. In the event of accident contact with sensitive surfaces (eye, abraded skin, and mucous membranes), the area should be bathed with large amounts of cool tap water.

Minoxidil should not be used in conjunction with other topical agents including topical corticosteroids, retinoids, and petrolatum or agents that are known to enhance cutaneous drug absorption.

Minoxidil is for Topical Use Only. Each milliliter of minoxidil contains 20 mg minoxidil. Accidental ingestion of the solution could lead to possible adverse systemic effects (see OVERDOSAGE).

As is the case with other topically applied drugs, decreased integrity of the epidermal barrier caused by inflammation of disease processes in the skin (*e.g.*, excoriations of the scalp, scalp psoriasis, or severe sunburn) may increase percutaneous absorption of minoxidil.

Information for the Patient

A patient information leaflet has been prepared and is included with each package of minoxidil. The text of the leaflet is printed at the end of this insert.

Carcinogenesis, Mutagenesis, and Impairment of Fertility

No evidence of carcinogenicity was detected in rats or rabbits when minoxidil topical solution was applied to the skin for up to one year. Dietary administration of minoxidil to mice for up to 24 months was associated with an increased incidence of malignant lymphomas in females and an increased incidence of hepatic nodules in males. The lymphoma incidence was unrelated to dose level and at all doses was within the range seen in control groups from other studies employing mice from the same colony. The incidence of hepatic nodules was dose dependent, with a significant increase observed at 63 but not at 25 or 10 mg/kg/day. There was no effect of drug on the incidence of malignant tumors of the liver. As with the lymphomas, the incidence of hepatic nodules was within the historical control range for the subject mouse colony. No evidence of carcinogenic potential was obtained from a dietary administration study of minoxidil in rats. However, the rat study involved only 1/3

PRECAUTIONS: *(cont'd)*

the number of animals and half the maximum dosage level evaluated in the mouse experiment, and shorter durations of administration (up to 15 months in males and up to 22 months in females). Minoxidil was not mutagenic in the salmonella (Ames) test, the DNA damage/alkaline elution assay or the rat micronucleus test.

In a study in which male and female rats received one or five times the maximum recommended human oral antihypertensive dose of minoxidil (multiples based on a 50 kg patient) there was a dose-dependent reduction in conception rate.

Pregnancy

Pregnancy Category C. Adequate and well-controlled studies have not been conducted in pregnant woman treated with minoxidil topical solution nor in pregnant women treated with oral minoxidil for hypertension. Oral administration of minoxidil has been associated with evidence of increased fetal resorption in rabbits, but not, rats, when administrated at five times the maximum recommended oral antihypertensive human dose. There was no evidence of teratogenic effects of ORALLY administered minoxidil in rats or rabbits. Subcutaneous administration of minoxidil to pregnant rats at 80 mg/kg/day (approximately 2000 times the maximal systemic human exposure from daily topical administration) was maternally toxic but not teratogenic. Higher subcutaneous doses produced evidence of developmental toxicity. Minoxidil should not be administrated to pregnant woman.

Labor and Delivery

The effects on labor and delivery are unknown.

Nursing Mothers

There has been one report of minoxidil excretion in the breast milk of a woman treated with 5 mg oral minoxidil twice daily for hypertension. Because of the potential for adverse effects in nursing infants from minoxidil absorption, minoxidil should not be administrated to a nursing woman.

Pediatric Use

Safety and effectiveness in patients under 18 years of age have not been established.

Post-Menopausal Use

Efficacy in post-menopausal woman has not been studied.

TABLETS

General

Monitor fluid and electrolyte balance and body weight See WARNINGS, Salt and Water Retention.

Observe patients for signs and symptoms of pericardial effusion: See WARNINGS, Pericarditis, Pericardial Effusion, and Tamponade.

Use after myocardial infarction: Minoxidil tablets have not been used in patients who have had a myocardial infarction within the preceding month. It is possible that a reduction of arterial pressure with minoxidil might further limit blood flow to the myocardium, although this might be compensated by decreased oxygen demand because of lower blood pressure.

Hypersensitivity: Possible hypersensitivity to minoxidil, manifested as a skin rash, has been seen in less than 1% of patients; whether the drug should be discontinued when this occurs depends on treatment alternatives.

Renal failure or dialysis: patients may require smaller doses of minoxidil and should have close medical supervision to prevent exacerbation of renal failure or precipitation of cardiac failure.

Information for the Patient

The patient should be fully aware of the importance of continuing all of his antihypertensive medications and of the nature of symptoms that would suggest fluid overload. A patient brochure has been prepared and is included with each minoxidil package. The text of this brochure is reprinted at the end of the insert.

Laboratory Tests

Those laboratory tests which are abnormal at the time of initiation of minoxidil therapy, such as urinalysis, renal function tests, EKG, chest x-ray, echocardiogram, etc., should be repeated at intervals to ascertain whether improvement or deterioration is occurring under minoxidil therapy. Initially such tests should be performed frequently, e.g., 1-3 month intervals; later as stabilization occurs, at intervals of 6-12 months.

Carcinogenesis, Mutagenesis, and Impairment of Fertility

No evidence of carcinogenicity was detected in rats or rabbits when minoxidil was applied to the skin for up to one year. Dietary administration of minoxidil to mice for up to 24 months was associated with an increased incidence of malignant lymphomas in females and increased incidence of hepatic nodules in males. The lymphoma incidence was unrelated to dose level and at all doses was within the range seen in control groups from other studies employing mice from the same colony. The incidence of hepatic nodules was dose dependent, with a significant increase observed at 63 but not at 25 or 10 mg/kg/day. There was no effect of drug on the incidence of malignant tumors of the liver. As with the lymphomas, the incidence of hepatic nodules was within the historical control range for the subject mouse colony. No evidence of carcinogenic potential was obtained from a dietary administration study of minoxidil in rats. However, the rat study involved only 1/3 the number of animals and half the maximum dosage level evaluated in the mouse experiment, and shorter durations of administration (up to 15 months in males and up to 22 months in females). Minoxidil was not mutagenic in the salmonella (Ames) test; the DNA damage/alkaline elution assay or the rat micronucleus test.

In a study in which male and female rats received one or five times the maximum recommended human oral antihypertensive dose of minoxidil (multiples based on a 50 kg patient) there was a dose-dependent reduction in conception rate.

Pregnancy, Teratogenic Effects, Pregnancy Category C:

Oral administration of minoxidil has been associated with evidence of increased fetal resorption in rabbits, but not rats, when administered at five times the maximum recommended oral antihypertensive human dose. There was no evidence of teratogenic effects in rats and rabbits. Subcutaneous administration of minoxidil to pregnant rats at 80 mg/kg/day was maternally toxic but not teratogenic. Higher subcutaneous doses produced evidence of developmental toxicity. There are no adequate and well controlled studies in pregnant women. Minoxidil should be used during pregnancy only if the potential benefit justifies the potential risk to the fetus.

Labor and Delivery

The effects on labor and delivery are unknown.

Nursing Mothers

There has been one report of minoxidil excretion in the breast milk of a woman treated with 5 mg oral minoxidil twice daily for hypertension. Because of the potential for adverse effects in nursing infants from minoxidil absorption, minoxidil should not be administered to a nursing woman.

Pediatric Use

Use in children has been limited to date, particularly in infants. The recommendations under DOSAGE AND ADMINISTRATION can be considered only a rough guide at present and a careful titration is essential.

PRECAUTIONS: *(cont'd)*

Unapproved Use

Use of minoxidil tablets, in any formulation, to promote hair growth is not an approved indication. While clinical trial with minoxidil topical solution 2% demonstrated that formulation and dosage were safe and effective, the effects of extemporaneous topical formulations and dosages have not been shown to safe or effective. Because systemic absorption of topically applied drug may occur and is dependent on vehicle and/or method of use, extemporaneous topical formulations made from minoxidil should be considered to share in the full range of CONTRAINDICATIONS, WARNINGS, PRECAUTIONS, and ADVERSE REACTIONSlisted here. In addition, skin intolerance to drug and/or vehicle may occur.

DRUG INTERACTIONS:

Topical Solution: There are currently no known drug interactions associated with the use of minoxidil topical solution. Although it has not been clinically demonstrated, there exists the theoretical possibility of absorbed minoxidil potentiating orthostatic hypotension in patients concurrently taking guanethidine.

Tablets: See WARNINGS, Interaction with Guanethidine.

ADVERSE REACTIONS:

TOPICAL SOLUTION

Minoxidil topical solution has been used by 3,857 patients (347 females) enrolled in placebo-controlled trials. The rate of adverse events, grouped by body system, is shown in TABLE 1. Except for dermatologic events, which were more common in the minoxidil group, no individual reaction or body system grouping seemed to be increased in the minoxidil-treated group.

TABLE 1 Medical Event Percent Occurrence By Body System In The Placebo-Control Clinical Trials Involving Minoxidil Topical Solution - All Patients Enrolled

Body System	Minoxidil Soln N=3857 (4-8 months) # PATS.	% OCC.	Placebo N=2717 (4-8 months) # PATS.	% OCC.
Dermatological (irritant dermatitis, allergic contact dermatitis	284	7.36	147	5.41
Respiratory (bronchitis, upper respiratory infection, sinusitis)	276	7.16	233	8.58
Gastrointestinal (diarrhea, nausea, vomiting)	167	4.33	178	6.55
Neurology (headache, dizziness, faintness, light-headedness)	132	3.42	94	3.46
Musculoskeletal (fractures, back pain, tendinitis, aches and pains)	100	2.59	60	2.21
Cardiovascular (edema, chest pain, blood pressure increases/decreases, palpitations, pulse rate increases/decreases)	59	1.53	42	1.55
Allergy (non-specific allergic reactions, hives, allergic rhinitis, facial swelling, and sensitivity)	49	1.27	26	0.96
Metabolic-Nutritional (edema, weight gain)	48	1.24	35	1.29
Special Senses (conjunctivitis, ear infection, vertigo)	45	1.17	33	1.21
Genital Tract (prostatitis, epididymitis, pregnancy, vaginitis, vulvitis, vaginal discharge and itching)	35	0.91	22	0.81
Urinary Tract (urinary tract infections, renal calculi, urethritis)	36	0.93	31	1.14
Endocrine (menstrual changes, breast symptoms)	18	0.47	14	0.52
Psychiatric (anxiety, depression, fatigue)	14	0.36	26	0.96
Hematology (lymphadenopathy, thrombocytopenia, anemia)	12	0.31	15	0.55

Patients have been followed for up to 5 years and there has been no change in incidence or severity of reported reactions.

Additional events reported in postmarketing clinical experience include: eczema, hypertrichosis, local erythema, pruritus, dry skin/scalp flaking, sexual dysfunction, visual disturbances including decreased visual acuity, exacerbation of hair loss, alopecia.

TABLETS

Salt and Water Retention: See WARNINGS, Concomitant Use of Adequate Diuretic is Required. Temporary edema developed in 7% of patients who were not edematous at the start of therapy.

Pericarditis, Pericardial Effusion, and **Tamponade** (see WARNINGS).

Dermatologic: Hypertrichosis-Elongation, thickening, and enhanced pigmentation of fine body hair are seen in about 80% of patients taking minoxidil tablets. This develops within 3 to 6 weeks after starting therapy. It is usually first noticed on the temples, between the eyebrows, between the hairline and the eyebrows, or in the side-burn area of the upper lateral cheek, later extending to the back, arms, legs, and scalp. Upon discontinuation of minoxidil, new hair growth stops, but 1 to 6 months may be required for restoration to pretreatment appearance. No endocrine abnormalities have been found to explain the abnormal hair growth; thus, it is without virilism. Hair growth is especially disturbing to children and women and such patients should be thoroughly informed about this effect before therapy with minoxidil is begun.

Allergic—Rashes have been reported, including rare reports of bullous eruptions, and Stevens-Johnson Syndrome.

Hematologic: Thrombocytopenia and leukopenia (WBC <3000/mm^3) have rarely been reported.

Gastrointestinal: Nausea and/or vomiting has been reported. In clinical trials the incidence of nausea and vomiting associated with the underlying disease has shown a decrease from pretrial levels.

Miscellaneous: Breast tenderness—This developed in less than 1% of patients.

Altered Laboratory Findings: (a) ECG changes—Changes in direction and magnitude of the ECG T-waves occur in approximately 60% of patients treated with minoxidil. In rare instances a large negative amplitude of the T-wave may encroach upon the S-T segment, but the S-T segment is not independently altered. These changes usually disappear with continuance of treatment and revert to the pretreatment state if minoxidil is discontinued. No symptoms have been associated with these changes, nor have there been alterations in blood cell counts or in plasma enzyme concentrations that would suggest myocardial damage. Long-term treatment of patients manifesting such changes has provided no evidence of deteriorating cardiac function. At present the changes appear to be nonspecific and without identifiable clinical significance. (b) Effects of hemodilution—hematocrit, hemoglobin and erythrocyte

ADVERSE REACTIONS: *(cont'd)*

count usually fall about 7% initially and then recover to pretreatment levels. (c) Other—Alkaline phosphatase increased varyingly without other evidence of liver or bone abnormality. Serum creatinine increased an average of 6% and BUN slightly more, but later declined to pretreatment levels.

OVERDOSAGE:

TOPICAL SOLUTION

Increased systemic absorption of minoxidil may potentially occur if more frequent or larger doses of minoxidil (than directed) are used or if minoxidil is applied to large surface areas of the body or areas other than the scalp. There are no known cases of minoxidil overdosage resulting from topical administration of minoxidil.

In a 14-day controlled clinical trial, 1 ml of 3% minoxidil solution was applied eight times daily (six times the recommended dose) to the scalp of 11 normal male volunteers and to the chest of 11 other volunteers. No significant systemic effects were observed in these subjects when compared with a similar number of placebo-treated subjects. All subjects in the study were monitored for vital sign, electrocardiographic, and echocardiographic changes.

In a reported case of accidental ingestion, a 3-year-old male swallowed 1 to 2 ml of a 3% concentration of topical minoxidil solution. After vomiting he was treated in an emergency room. The child was found to be alert and active with no obvious signs of distress. His temperature was 37°C, pulse 152 bpm, respiration 32, and systolic blood pressure 110 by palpation. Cardiovascular, chest, lungs, abdomen, head, skin, and neurological examinations were normal. Blood levels taken indicated a total minoxidil level (glucuronide and unchanged) of 320.6 ng/ml. The child was discharged without sequelae.

Because of the high concentration of minoxidil in minoxidil topical solution, accidental ingestion has the potential of producing systemic effects related to the pharmacologic action of the drug (5 ml of minoxidil topical solution contains 100 mg minoxidil, the maximum adult dose for oral minoxidil administration when used to treat hypertension). Signs and symptoms of minoxidil overdosage would most likely be cardiovascular effects associated with fluid retention and tachycardia. Fluid retention can be managed with appropriate diuretic therapy. Clinically significant tachycardia can be controlled by administration of a beta-adrenergic blocking agent. If encountered, hypotension should be treated by intravenous administration of normal saline. Sympathomimetic drugs, such as norepinephrine and epinephrine, should be avoided because of their excessive cardiac stimulating activity.

Oral LD_{50} in rats has ranged from 1321 to 3492 mg/kg; in mice 2457 to 2648 mg/kg. Minoxidil and its metabolites are hemodialyzable.

TABLETS

There have been only a few instances of deliberate or accidental overdosage with minoxidil tablets. One patient recovered after taking 50 mg of minoxidil together with 500 mg of a barbiturate. When exaggerated hypotension is encountered, it is most likely to occur in association with residual sympathetic nervous system blockade from previous therapy (guanethidine-like effects or alpha-adrenergic blockage), which prevents the usual compensatory maintenance of blood pressure. Intravenous administration of normal saline will help to maintain blood pressure and facilitate urine formation in these patients. Sympathomimetic drugs such as norepinephrine or epinephrine should be avoided because of their excessive cardiac stimulating action. Phenylephrine, angiotensin ii, vasopressin, and dopamine all reverse hypotension due to minoxidil, but should only be used if under-perfusion of vital organ is evident.

Radioimmunoassay can be performed to determine the concentration of minoxidil in the blood. At the maximum adult dose of 100 mg/day, peak blood levels of 1641 ng/ml and 2441 ng/ml were observed two patients, respectively. Due to patient-to-patient variation in blood levels, it is difficult to establish an overdosage warning level. In general, a substantial increase above 2000 ng/ml should be regarded as overdosage, unless the physician is aware that the patient has taken no more than the maximum dose.

Oral LD_{50} in rats has ranged from 1321 to 3492 mg/kg; in mice, 2456 to 2648 mg/kg.

DOSAGE AND ADMINISTRATION:

TOPICAL SOLUTION

Hair and scalp should be dry prior to topical application of minoxidil topical solution. A dose of 1 ml minoxidil topical solution should be applied to the total affected areas of the scalp twice daily. The total daily dosage should not exceed 2 ml. If finger tips are used to facilitate drug applications, hands should be washed afterwards. Twice daily application for four months or longer may be required before evidence of hair regrowth is observed. Onset and degree of hair regrowth may be variable among patients. If hair regrowth is realized, twice daily applications of minoxidil appear necessary for additional or continued hair regrowth. Some anecdotal patient reports indicate that regrown hair and the balding process return to their untreated state three to four months following cessation of the drug.

TABLETS

Patients over 12 years of age: The recommended initial dosage of minoxidil tablets is 5 mg of minoxidil given as a single dose. Daily dosage can be increased to 10, 20 and then to 40 mg in single or divided doses if required for optimum blood pressure control. The effective dosage range is usually 10 to 40 mg per day. The maximum recommended dosage is 100 mg per day.

Patients under 12 years of age: The initial dosage is 0.2 mg/kg minoxidil as a single daily dose. The dosage may be increased in 50 to 100% increments until optimum blood pressure control is achieved. The effective dosage range is usually 0.25 to 1.0 mg/kg/day. The maximum recommended dosage is 50 mg daily (see PRECAUTIONS, Pediatric Use).

Dose frequency: The magnitude of within-day fluctuation of arterial pressure during therapy with minoxidil is directly proportional to the extent of pressure reduction. If supine diastolic pressure has been reduced less than 30 mmHg, the drug need be administered only once a day; if supine diastolic pressure has been reduced more than 30 mm Hg, the daily dosage should be divided into two equal parts.

Frequency of dosage adjustment: Dosage must be titrated carefully according to individual response. Intervals between dosage adjustments normally should be at least 3 days since the full response to given dose is not obtained for at least that amount of time. **Where a more rapid management of hypertension is required, dose adjustments can be made every 6 hours if the patient is carefully monitored.**

Concomitant Therapy: Diuretic and beta-blocker or other sympathetic nervous system suppressant.

Diuretics: Minoxidil must be used in conjunction with a diuretic in conjunction with a diuretic in patients relying on renal function for maintaining salt and water balance. Diuretics have been used at the following dosages when starting therapy with minoxidil: hydrochlorothiazide (50 mg, b.i.d.) or other thiazides at equieffective dosage; chlorthalidone (50 to 100 mg, once daily); furosemide (40 mg, b.i.d). If excessive salt and water retention results in a weight gain of more than 5 pounds, diuretic therapy should be changed to furosemide; if the patient is already taking furosemide, dosage should be increased in accordance with the patient's requirements.

DOSAGE AND ADMINISTRATION: *(cont'd)*

Beta-blocker or other sympathetic nervous system suppressants: When therapy with minoxidil is begun, the dosage of a beta-adrenergic receptor blocking drug should be the equivalent of 80 to 160 mg of propranolol per day in divided doses.

If beta-blockers are contraindicated, methyldopa (250 to 750 mg, b.i.d.) may be used instead. Methyldopa must be given for at least 24 hours before starting therapy with minoxidil because of the delay in the onset of methyldopa's action. Limited clinical experience indicates that clonidine may also be used to prevent tachycardia induced by minoxidil; the usual dosage is 0.1 to 0.2 mg twice daily.

Sympathetic nervous system suppressant may not completely prevent an increase in heart rate due to minoxidil but usually do prevent tachycardia. Typically, patients receiving a beta-blocker prior to initiation of therapy with minoxidil have a bradycardia and can be expected to have an increase in heart rate toward normal when minoxidil is added. When treatment with minoxidil and beta-blocker or other sympathetic nervous system suppressant are begun simultaneously, their opposing cardiac effects usually nullify each other, leading to little change in heart rate.

PATIENT PACKAGE INSERT:

MINOXIDIL TOPICAL SOLUTION

Important Information About minoxidil topical solution (minoxidil 2%)

Your doctor has prescribed minoxidil topical solution for you to use as a hair regrowth stimulant to treat alopecia androgenetica (hair loss). Minoxidil is a prescription medication and therefore should be used only as directed by your doctor.

Please read this booklet thoroughly. It will help you to understand minoxidil topical solution and what to expect from its use. If you have any questions after reading this booklet, or anytime during treatment with minoxidil, you should consult your doctor or ask your pharmacist.

WHAT IS MINOXIDIL?

Minoxidil topical solution, discovered and made by The Upjohn Company, is a standardized topical (for use only on the skin) prescription medication proved effective for the treatment of alopecia androgenetica (hair loss).

Rogaine is a topical solution of minoxidil. Minoxidil in tablet form has been used since 1980 to lower blood pressure. The use of ***minoxidil tablets*** is limited to treatment of patients with severe high blood pressure. When a high enough dosage in tablet form is used to lower blood pressure, certain effects that merit your attention may occur. These effects appear to be dose related (See What are the potential side effects on the heart and circulation when using minoxidil?)

Persons who use minoxidil topical solution have a low level of absorption of minoxidil, much lower than that of persons being treated with ***minoxidil tablets***for high blood pressure. Therefore, the likelihood that a person using minoxidil topical solution will develop the effects associated with ***minoxidil tablets***is very small. In fact, non of these effects has been directly attributed to minoxidil in clinical studies.

Exactly how minoxidil works to stimulate hair growth in some people is not known. Upjohn scientists are doing research in this area.

HOW EFFECTIVE IS MINOXIDIL?

Males: Clinical studies with minoxidil were conducted by physicians in 27 U.S. medical centers involving over 2,300 patients with male pattern baldness involving the top (vertex) of the head. At the end of four months, hair counts showed that on average, the patients using minoxidil topical solution had significantly more hair growth than those who used placebo (a similar solution without the active medication).

Based on the patients' self evaluation at the end of four months, 59% of the patients using minoxidil had minimal to dense hair growth compared with 42% of those using placebo.

By the end of one year, 48% of the people who continued in the study using minoxidil rated their hair growth as moderate or better.

Females: Clinical studies with minoxidil were conducted by physicians in eleven U.S. and ten European medical centers involving over 600 female patients with hair loss. Based on actual hair counts, the women using minoxidil had significantly more hair regrowth at the end of eight months than those who used placebo (a similar solution without the active medication).

Based on the patients' self evaluation, 59% of the U.S. patients using minoxidil reported hair regrowth at Week 32 compared with 40% of those using placebo. Of the 59% reporting hair regrowth, 19% reported moderate and 40% reported minimal hair growth. In the European study, the percentage of patients reporting hair regrowth at Week 32 was 55% among the minoxidil users compared with 41% among the placebo patients. Of the 55% reporting hair regrowth, 1% reported dense, 24% reported moderate and 30% reported minimal hair growth.

In the combined results of the U.S. and European studies, 57% of the women using minoxidil evaluated their hair regrowth as minimal or moderate after 32 weeks compared to 40% of those using placebo.

HOW SOON CAN I EXPECT RESULTS FROM USING MINOXIDIL?

Studies have shown that the response to treatment with minoxidil may vary widely. If you respond to treatment, it usually will take four months or longer before there is evidence of hair growth.

Some patients receiving minoxidil may see faster results than others; others may respond with a slower rate of hair growth. You should not expect visible growth in less than four months.

IF I RESPOND TO MINOXIDIL, WHAT WILL THE HAIR LOOK LIKE?

If you have very little hair and respond to treatment, your first hair growth may be soft, downy, colorless hair that is barely visible. After further treatment the new hair should be the same color and thickness as the other hair on your scalp. If you start with substantial hair, the new hair should be of the same color and thickness as the rest of your hair.

HOW LONG DO I NEED TO USE MINOXIDIL?

Minoxidil is a treatment, not a cure. If you respond to treatment, you will need to continue using minoxidil to maintain or increase hair growth. If you do not begin to show a response to treatment with minoxidil after a reasonable period of time (at least four months or more), your doctor may advise you to discontinue using minoxidil.

WHAT HAPPENS IF I STOP USING MINOXIDIL? WILL I KEEP THE NEW HAIR?

If you stop using minoxidil, you will probably shed the new hair within a few months after stopping treatment.

WHAT IS THE DOSAGE OF MINOXIDIL?

You should apply a 1 ml dose of minoxidil two times a day, once in the morning and once at night. Each bottle should last about 26-30 days. A bottle of minoxidil is 3/4 full. This fill level is intentional so that if the rub-on applicator is used, the tube is not submerged in the solution when the bottle is inverted for dosage administration. The applicators in each package of minoxidil are designed to apply the correct amount of minoxidil with each application. *Please refer to the Instructions for Use.*

PATIENT PACKAGE INSERT: *(cont'd)*

CAN I APPLY MINOXIDIL AND WASH IT OUT AN HOUR LATER?

No. After applying minoxidil it must remain on the scalp for at least 4 hours so that the medication may be absorbed into the scalp. If you prefer, you may wash your hair before applying minoxidil, but the scalp and hair must dry before the application.

SOMETIMES I SEE A RESIDUE ON MY HAIR. IS THIS NORMAL?

In some people, minoxidil will dry in the hair and leave a slight residue. This harmless residue was noted by a small number of patients during the clinical trials for minoxidil. The effectiveness of the product is not altered by the presence of the residue.

WHAT IF I MISS A DOSE OR FORGET TO USE MINOXIDIL?

If you miss one or two daily applications of minoxidil, you should restart your twice-daily application and return to your usual schedule. You should not attempt to make up for missed applications.

CAN I USE MINOXIDIL MORE THAN TWICE A DAY? WILL IT WORK FASTER?

No studies by The Upjohn Company have been carefully conducted to determine the correct amount of minoxidil to use to obtain the most satisfactory results. More frequent applications or use of larger doses (more than 1 ml twice a day) have not been shown to speed up the process of hair growth and may increase the possibility of side effects.

WHAT ARE THE MOST COMMON SIDE EFFECTS REPORTED IN CLINICAL STUDIES WITH MINOXIDIL?

Studies of patients using minoxidil have shown that the most common adverse effects directly attributable to minoxidil topical solution were itching and other skin irritations of the treated area of the scalp.

Other side effects, including light-headedness, dizziness, and headaches were reported by patients using minoxidil or placebo (a similar solution without the active medication). The frequency of these side effects was similar in the minoxidil and placebo groups. For further information about side effects please ask your doctor.

Minoxidil topical solution contains alcohol, which could cause burning or irritation of the eyes, mucous membranes, or sensitive skin areas. If minoxidil accidentally gets into these areas, bathe the area with large amounts of cool tap water. Contact your doctor if irritation persists.

WHAT ARE THE POTENTIAL SIDE EFFECTS ON THE HEART AND CIRCULATION WHEN USING MINOXIDIL?

Although serious side effects have not been attributed to minoxidil in clinical studies, there is a possibility that they could occur because the active ingredient in minoxidil topical solution is the same as in ***minoxidil tablets.***

Minoxidil tablets are used to treat high blood pressure.

Minoxidil tablets lower blood pressure by relaxing the arteries, an effect called vasodilation. Vasodilation leads to retention of fluid an increased heart rate. The following effects have occurred in some patients taking ***minoxidil tablets***for high blood pressure.

1) Increasing heart rate. Some patients have reported that their resting heart rate increased by more than 20 beats per minute.

2) rapid weight gain of more than 5 pounds or swelling (edema) of the face, hands, ankles, or stomach area.

3) Difficulty in breathing, especially when lying down, a result of an increase in body fluids or fluid around the heart.

4) Worsening of, or new onset of, angina pectoris.

When minoxidil topical solution is used on normal skin, very little minoxidil is absorbed and these effects are not expected. If, however, you experience any of the above, discontinue use of minoxidil and consult your doctor. Presumably, such effects would be most likely if greater absorption occurred, e.g., because minoxidil was used on damaged or inflamed skin or in greater than recommended amounts.

In animal studies, minoxidil, in doses higher than would be obtained from topical use in people, has caused important heart structure damage. This kind of damage has not been seen in humans given ***minoxidil tablets***for high blood pressure at effective doses.

WHAT FACTORS MAY INCREASE THE RISK OF SERIOUS SIDE EFFECT WITH MINOXIDIL?

Individuals with known or suspected underlying coronary artery disease or the presence of or predisposition to heart failure would be at particular risk if systemic effects (that is, increased heart rate or fluid retention) of minoxidil were to occur. Physicians, and patients with these kinds of underlying diseases, should be conscious of the potential risk of treatment if they choose minoxidil.

Because absorption of minoxidil may be increased and the risk of side effects may become greater, minoxidil should be applied only to the scalp and should not be used on other parts of the body. You should not use minoxidil if your scalp becomes irritated or is sunburned, and you should not use it along with other topical treatment medication on your scalp.

CAN PEOPLE WITH HIGH BLOOD PRESSURE USE MINOXIDIL?

Individuals with hypertension, including those under treatment with antihypertensive agents, can use minoxidil but should be monitored closely by their doctor. Patients taking guanethidine for high blood pressure should not use minoxidil.

WILL MINOXIDIL CHANGE MY MENSTRUAL CYCLE?

No. Carefully conducted studies have shown that the use of minoxidil will not increase the length of the menstrual cycle (interval between periods) or change the amount of flow or duration of the menstrual period. However, if your menstrual period does not occur at the expected time, you should discontinue the use of minoxidil and consult your doctor as soon as possible.

SHOULD I CONTINUE TO USE MINOXIDIL IF I DESIRE TO BECOME PREGNANT?

If you plan to become pregnant, you should discontinue using minoxidil at least one month before you discontinue your birth control. Adequate and well-controlled studies have not been conducted in pregnant women treated with minoxidil or in pregnant women taking oral minoxidil for the treatment of high blood pressure.

CAN NURSING MOTHERS USE MINOXIDIL?

No. We do not have any data from clinical trials or voluntary reports on minoxidil being reported in the breast milk following use of minoxidil. It should be noted, however, that there has been one report of minoxidil excretion in the breast milk of a woman treated with 5 mg oral minoxidil twice daily for hypertension. Consequently, minoxidil should not be administered to a nursing women.

INSTRUCTIONS FOR USE

Please read this information before using minoxidil topical solution. One ml (or 1 dose) of minoxidil should be applied to the total affected areas of the scalp twice daily. The hair and scalp should be dry before application of minoxidil. Each prescription of minoxidil come with three complimentary, disposable applicators to accommodate your individual preference and needs. You may wish to change the applicator if the condition of your hair changes.

PATIENT PACKAGE INSERT: *(cont'd)*

Each applicator is designed to deliver a measured amount (1 ml, or 1 dose) of solution when used as directed. This amount of minoxidil has been used in extensive clinical studies and determined to be the proper amount for the treatment of alopecia androgenetica (hair loss).

You must understand that twice-daily application for four months or longer may be required before hair regrowth may be observed.

Like all medications, keep minoxidil out of reach of children. In the event of accidental ingestion, contact your doctor. If, after reading this information, you have any questions, consult your doctor or ask your pharmacist.

(Rogaine Topical Solution: Upjohn, 1/94, 813, 264, 012, 691209)

(Loniten Tablets: Upjohn, 12/92, 810 384 415, 691016)

HOW SUPPLIED:

TOPICAL SOLUTION

Minoxidil topical solution is a clear, colorless, to light yellow solution containing 20 mg minoxidil per ml. Store at controlled room temperature 15° to 30° C (59° to 86°F).

HOW SUPPLIED - RATED THERAPEUTICALLY EQUIVALENT:

Tablet, Uncoated - Oral - 2.5 mg

100's	$12.00	Minoxidil, H.C.F.A. F F P	99999-1819-01
100's	$12.15	Minoxidil, United Res	00677-1444-01
100's	$22.01	Minoxidil, Qualitest Pharms	00603-4687-21
100's	$25.50	Minoxidil, Goldline Labs	00182-1602-01
100's	$28.88	Minoxidil, Schein Pharm (US)	00364-2172-01
100's	$33.25	Minoxidil, Rugby	00536-4045-01
100's	$42.40	Minoxidil, Elkins Sinn	00641-4003-86
100's	$43.22	LONITEN, Pharmacia & Upjohn	00009-0121-01
100's	$45.00	Minoxidil, Aligen Independ	00405-4683-01
100's	$45.00	Minoxidil, Par Pharm	49884-0256-01
100's	$45.00	Minoxidil, Martec Pharms	52555-0444-01
100's	$47.25	Minoxidil, HL Moore Drug Exch	00839-7353-06
500's	$60.00	Minoxidil, H.C.F.A. F F P	99999-1819-02
500's	$110.00	Minoxidil, Schein Pharm (US)	00364-2172-05

Tablet, Uncoated - Oral - 10 mg

100's	$15.75	Minoxidil, United Res	00677-1162-01
100's	$15.75	Minoxidil, H.C.F.A. F F P	99999-1819-03
100's	$40.00	Minoxidil, Qualitest Pharms	00603-4688-21
100's	$44.50	Minoxidil 10, Major Pharms	00904-1280-60
100's	$49.45	Minoxidil, Elkins Sinn	00641-4004-86
100's	$53.95	MINOXIDIL, Rugby	00536-4043-01
100's	$54.00	Minoxidil, Goldline Labs	00182-1280-01
100's	$54.00	Minoxidil, Parmed Pharms	00349-8949-01
100's	$54.00	Minoxidil, Aligen Independ	00405-4684-01
100's	$54.00	Minoxidil, Par Pharm	49884-0257-01
100's	$54.50	Minoxidil, Schein Pharm (US)	00364-2173-01
100's	$55.10	Minoxidil, Martec Pharms	52555-0445-01
100's	$56.70	Minoxidil, HL Moore Drug Exch	00839-7342-06
100's	$94.96	LONITEN, Pharmacia & Upjohn	00009-0137-01
100's	$182.80	Minoxidil 10, Major Pharms	00904-1280-40
500's	$199.00	Minoxidil, Parmed Pharms	00349-8949-05
500's	$226.56	Minoxidil, Schein Pharm (US)	00364-2173-05
500's	$238.15	Minoxidil, Elkins Sinn	00641-4004-88
500's	$243.00	Minoxidil, Par Pharm	49884-0257-05
500's	$255.79	Minoxidil, Aligen Independ	00405-4684-02
500's	$470.60	LONITEN, Pharmacia & Upjohn	00009-0137-02

HOW SUPPLIED - NOT RATED EQUIVALENT:

Solution - Topical - 2 %

60 ml	**$60.10**	**ROGAINE, Pharmacia & Upjohn**	**00009-3367-05**
180 ml	**$162.29**	**ROGAINE, Pharmacia & Upjohn**	**00009-3367-19**

MIRTAZAPINE *(003274)*

CATEGORIES: Alpha-2 Receptor Antagonist; Antidepressants; Central Nervous System Agents; Depression; Psychotherapeutic Agents; FDA Approved 1996 Apr

BRAND NAMES: **Remeron**

DESCRIPTION:

Mirtazapine is an antidepressant for oral administration. It has a tetracyclic chemical structure unrelated to selective serotonin reuptake inhibitors, tricyclics or monoamine oxidase inhibitors (MAOI). Mirtazapine belongs to the piperazino-azepine group of compounds. It is designated 1,2,3,4,10,14b-hexahydro-2methylpyrazino [2,1–a] pyrido [2,3–c] benzazepine and has the empirical formula of $C_{17}H_{19}N_3$. Its molecular weight is 265.36.

Mirtazapine is a white to creamy white crystalline powder which is slightly soluble in water.

Remeron is supplied for oral administration as scored film-coated tablets containing 15 or 30 mg of mirtazapine. Each tablet also contains corn starch, hydroxypropyl cellulose, magnesium stearate, colloidal silicon dioxide, lactose and other inactive ingredients.

CLINICAL PHARMACOLOGY:

PHARMACODYNAMICS

The mechanism of action of mirtazapine, as with other antidepressants, is unknown.

Evidence gathered in preclinical studies suggests that mirtazapine enhances central noradrenergic and serotonergic activity. These studies have shown that mirtazapine acts as an antagonist at central presynaptic α_2 adrenergic inhibitory autoreceptors and heteroreceptors, an action that is postulated to result in an increase in central noradrenergic and serotonergic activity.

Mirtazapine is a potent antagonist of $5\text{–}HT_2$and $5\text{–}HT_3$ receptors. Mirtazapine has no significant affinity for the $5\text{–}HT_{1A}$ and $5\text{–}HT_{1B}$ receptors.

Mirtazapine is a potent antagonist histamine (H_1) receptors, a property that may explain its prominent sedative effects.

Mirtazapine is a moderate peripheral α_1 adrenergic antagonist, a property that may explain the occasional orthostatic hypotension reported in association with its use.

Mirtazapine is a moderate antagonist at muscarinic receptors, a property that may explain the relatively low incidence of anticholinergic side effects associated with its use.

PHARMACOKINETICS

Mirtazapine is rapidly and completely absorbed following oral administration and has a half-life of about 20–40 hours. Peak plasma concentrations are reached within about 2 hours following an oral dose. The presence of food in the stomach has a minimal effect on both the rate and extent of absorption and does not require a dosage adjustment.

CLINICAL PHARMACOLOGY: *(cont'd)*

Mirtazapine is extensively metabolized after oral administration. Major pathways of biotransformation are demethylation and hydroxylation followed by glucuronide conjugation. *In vitro* data from human liver microsomes indicate that cytochrome 2D6 and 1A2 are involved in the formulation of the 8–hydroxy metabolite of mirtazapine, whereas cytochrome 3A is considered to be responsible for the formation of the N-desmethyl and N-oxide metabolite. Mirtazapine has an absolute bioavailability of about 50%. It is eliminated predominantly via urine (75%) with 15% in feces. Several unconjugated metabolites possess pharmacological activity but are present in the plasma at very low levels. The (-) enantiomer has an elimination half-life that is approximately twice as long as the (+) enantiomer and therefore achieves plasma levels that are about three times as high as that of the (+) enantiomer.

Plasma levels are linearly related to dose over a dose range of 15 to 80 mg. The mean elimination half-life of mirtazapine after oral administration ranges from approximately 20–40 hours across age and gender subgroups, with females of all ages exhibiting significantly longer elimination half-lives than males (mean half-life of 37 hours for females *vs.* 26 hours for males). Steady state plasma levels of mirtazapine are attained within 5 days, with about 50% accumulation (accumulation ratio = 1.5).

Mirtazapine is approximately 85% bound to plasma proteins over a concentration range of 0.01 to 10 mcg/ml.

Population Subgroups

Liver Disease: Following a single 15 mg oral dose of mirtazapine, the oral clearance of mirtazapine was decreased by approximately 30% in hepatically impaired patients compared to subjects with normal hepatic function. Caution is indicated in administering mirtazapine to patients with compromised hepatic function (see PRECAUTIONS) and DOSAGE AND ADMINISTRATION.

Renal Disease: Following a single 15 mg oral dose of mirtazapine, patients with moderate [glomerular filtration rate (GFR) = 11–39 ml/min/1.73 m^2] and severe [GFR < 10 ml/min/1.73 m^2] renal impairment had reductions in mean oral clearance of mirtazapine of about 30% and 50%, respectively, compared to normal subjects. Caution is indicated in administering mirtazapine to patients with compromised renal function (see PRECAUTIONS) and DOSAGE AND ADMINISTRATION.

Elderly Patients: Following oral administration of mirtazapine 20 mg/day for 7 days to subjects of varying ages (range, 25–74), oral clearance of mirtazapine was reduced in the elderly compared to the younger subjects. The differences were most striking in males, with a 40% lower clearance in elderly males compared to younger males, while the clearance in elderly females was only 10% lower compared to younger females. Caution is indicated in administering mirtazapine to elderly patients (see PRECAUTIONS) and DOSAGE AND ADMINISTRATION.

CLINICAL STUDIES:

CLINICAL TRIALS SHOWING EFFECTIVENESS

The efficacy of mirtazapine as a treatment for depression was established in four placebo-controlled, 6–week trials in adult outpatients meeting DSM-III criteria for major depression. Patients were titrated with mirtazapine from a dose range of 5 mg up to 35 mg/day. Overall, these studies demonstrated mirtazapine to be superior to placebo on at least three of the following four measures: 21–Item Hamilton Depression Rating Scale (HDRS) total score; HDRS Depressed Mood Item; CGI Severity score; and Montgomery and Asberg Depression Rating Scale (MADRS). Superiority of mirtazapine over placebo was also found for certain factors of the HDRS including anxiety/somatization factor and sleep disturbance factor. The mean mirtazapine dose for patients who completed these four studies ranged from 21 to 32 mg/day. A fifth study of similar design utilized a higher dose (up to 50 mg) per day and also showed effectiveness.

Examination of age and gender subsets of the population did not reveal any differential responsiveness on the basis of these subgroups.

INDICATIONS AND USAGE:

Mirtazapine tablets are indicated for the treatment of depression.

The efficacy of mirtazapine in the treatment of depression was established in six week controlled trials of outpatients whose diagnoses corresponded most closely to the Diagnostic and Statistical Manual of Mental Disorders — 3rd edition (DSM-III) category of major depressive disorder (see CLINICAL PHARMACOLOGY.)

A major depressive episode (DSM-IV) implies a prominent and relatively persistent (nearly every day for at least 2 weeks) depressed or dysphoric mood that usually interferes with daily functioning, and includes at least five of the following nine symptoms: depressed mood, loss of interest in usual activities, significant change in weight and/or appetite, insomnia or hypersomnia, psychomotor agitation or retardation, increased fatigue, feelings of guilt or worthlessness, slowed thinking or impaired concentration, suicide attempt or suicidal ideation.

The antidepressant effectiveness of mirtazapine in hospitalized depressed patients has not been adequately studied.

The effectiveness of mirtazapine in long-term use, that is, for more than 6 weeks, has not been systematically evaluated in controlled trials. Therefore, the physician who elects to use mirtazapine for extended periods should periodically evaluate the long-term usefulness of the drug for the individual patient.

CONTRAINDICATIONS:

Mirtazapine tablets are contraindicated in patients with a known hypersensitivity to mirtazapine.

WARNINGS:

AGRANULOCYTOSIS

In premarketing clinical trials, two (one with Sjögren's Syndrome) out of 2796 patients treated with mirtazapine tablets developed agranulocytosis [absolute neutrophil count (ANC) < 500/mm^3 with associated signs and symptoms (*e.g.*, fever, infection, etc.)] and a third patient developed severe neutropenia [ANC < 500/mm^3 without any associated symptoms]. For these three patients, onset of severe neutropenia was detected on days 61, 9, and 14 of treatment, respectively. All three patients recovered after mirtazapine was stopped. These three cases yield a crude incidence of severe neutropenia (with or without associated infection) of approximately 1.1 per thousand patients exposed, with a very wide 95% confidence interval (*i.e.*, 2.2, cases per 10,000 to 3.1 cases per 1000). If a patient develops a sore throat, fever, stomatitis or other signs of infection, along with a low WBC count, treatment with mirtazapine should be discontinued and the patient should be closely monitored.

MAO INHIBITORS

In patients receiving other antidepressants in combination with monoamine oxidase inhibitor (MAOI) and in patients who have recently discontinued an antidepressant drug and then are started on an MAOI, there have been reports of serious, and sometimes fatal, reactions (*e.g.*, including nausea, vomiting, flushing, dizziness, tremor, myoclonus, rigidity, diaphoresis, hyperthermia, autonomic instability with rapid fluctuations of vital signs, seizures, and mental status

WARNINGS: *(cont'd)*

changes ranging from agitation to coma). Although there are no human data pertinent to such an interaction with mirtazapine, it is recommended that mirtazapine not be used in combination with an MAOI, or within 14 days of initiating or discontinuing therapy with an MAOI.

PRECAUTIONS:

GENERAL

Somnolence: In U.S. controlled studies, somnlence was reported in 54% of patients treated with mirtazapine, compared to 18% for placebo and 60% for amitriptyline. In these studies, somnolence resulted in discontinuation for 10.4% of mirtazapine treated patients, compared to 2.2% for placebo. It is unclear whether or not tolerance develops to the somnolent effects of mirtazapine. Because of mirtazapine's potentially significant effects on impairment of performance, patients should be cautioned about engaging in activities requiring alertness until they have been able to assess the drug's effect on their own psychomotor performance (see PRECAUTIONS, Information for the Patient.)

Dizziness: In U.S. controlled studies, dizziness was reported in 7% of patients treated with mirtazapine, compared to 3% for placebo and 14% for amitriptyline. It is unclear whether or not tolerance develops to the dizziness observed in association with the use of mirtazapine.

Increased Appetite/Weight Gain: In U.S. controlled studies, appetite increase was reported in 17% of patients treated with mirtazapine, compared to 2% for placebo and 6% for amitriptyline. In these same trials, weight gain of ≥7% of body weight was reported in 7.5% of patients treated with mirtazapine, compared to 0% for placebo and 5.9% for amitriptyline. In a pool of premarketing U.S. studies, including many patients in long-term, open label treatment, 8% of patients receiving mirtazapine discontinued for weight gain.

Cholesterol/Triglycerides: In U.S. controlled studies, nonfasting cholesterol increases to ≥20% above the upper limits of normal were observed in 15% of patients treated with mirtazapine, compared to 7% for placebo and 8% for amitriptyline. In these same studies, nonfasting triglyceride increases to ≥500 mg/dl were observed in 6% of patients treated with mirtazapine, compared to 3% for placebo and 3% for amitriptyline.

Transaminase Elevations: Clinically significant ALT (SGPT) elevations (≥3 times the upper limit of the normal range) were observed in 2.0% (8/424) of patients exposed to mirtazapine in a pool of short-term U.S. controlled trials, compared to 0.3% (1/328) of placebo patients and 2.0% (3/181) of amitriptyline patients. Most of these patients with ALT increases did not develop signs or symptoms associated with compromised liver function. While some patients were discontinued for the ALT increases, in other cases, the enzyme levels returned to normal despite continued mirtazapine treatment. Mirtazapine should be used with caution in patients with impaired hepatic function (see CLINICAL PHARMACOLOGY, Pharmacokinetics) and DOSAGE AND ADMINISTRATION.

Activation of Mania/Hypomania: Mania/hypomania occurred in approximately 0.2% (3/1,299 patients) of mirtazapine treated patients in U.S. studies. Although the incidence of mania/hypomania was very low during treatment with mirtazapine, it should be used carefully in patients with a history of mania/hypomania.

Seizure: In premarketing clinical trials only one seizure was reported among the 2,796 U.S. and non-U.S. patients treated with mirtazapine. However, no controlled studies have been carried out in patients with a history of seizures. Therefore, care should be exercised when mirtazapine is used in these patients.

Suicide: Suicidal ideation is inherent in depression and may persist until significant remission occurs. As with any patient receiving antidepressants, high-risk patients should be closely supervised during initial drug therapy. Prescriptions of mirtazapine should be written for the smallest quantity consistent with good patient management, in order to reduce the risk of overdose.

Use in Patients with Concomitant Illness: Clinical experience with mirtazapine in patients with concomitant systemic illness is limited. Accordingly, care is advisable in prescribing mirtazapine for patients with diseases or conditions that affect metabolism or hemodynamic responses.

Mirtazapine has not been systemically evaluated or used to any appreciable extent in patients with a recent history of myocardial infarction or other significant heart disease. Mirtazapine was not associated with clinically significant ECG abnormalities in U.S. and non-U.S. placebo controlled trials. Mirtazapine was associated with significant orthostatic hypotension in early clinical pharmacology trials with normal volunteers. Orthostatic hypotension was infrequently observed in clinical trials with depressed patients. Mirtazapine should be used with caution in patients with known cardiovascular or cerebrovascular disease that could be exacerbated by hypotension (history of myocardial infarction, angina, or ischemic stroke) and conditions that would predispose patients to hypotension (dehydration, hypovolemia, and treatment with antihypertensive medication).

Mirtazapine clearance is decreased in patients with moderate [glomerular filtration rate (GFR) = 11–39 ml/min/1.73 m^2] and severe [GFR < 10 ml/min/1.73 m^2] renal impairment, and also in patients with hepatic impairment (see CLINICAL PHARMACOLOGY, Pharmacokinetics.) Caution is indicated in administering mirtazapine to such patients (see DOSAGE AND ADMINISTRATION.)

INFORMATION FOR THE PATIENT

Physicians are advised to discuss the following issues with patients for whom they prescribe mirtazapine:

Agranulocytosis: Patients who are to receive mirtazapine should be warned about the risk of developing agranulocytosis. Patients should be advised to contact their physician if they experience any indication of infection such as fever, chills, sore throat, mucous membrane ulceration or other possible signs of infection. Particular attention should be paid to any flu-like complaints or other symptoms that might suggest infection.

Interference with Cognitive and Motor Performance: Mirtazapine may impair judgement, thinking, and particularly, motor skills, because of its prominent sedative effect. The drowsiness associated with mirtazapine use may impair a patient's ability to drive, use machines or perform tasks that require alertness. Thus, patients should be cautioned about engaging in hazardous activities until they are reasonably certain that mirtazapine therapy does not adversely affect their ability to engage in such activities.

Completing Course of Therapy: While patients may notice improvement with mirtazapine therapy in 1 to 4 weeks, they should be advised to continue therapy as directed.

Concomitant Medication: Patients should be advised to inform their physician if they are taking, or intend to take, any prescription or over-the-counter drugs since there is a potential for mirtazapine to interact with other drugs.

Alcohol: The impairment of cognitive and motor skills produced by mirtazapine has been shown to be additive with those produced by alcohol. Accordingly, patients should be advised to avoid alcohol while taking mirtazapine.

Pregnancy: Patients should be advised to notify their physician if they become pregnant or intend to become pregnant during mirtazapine therapy.

Nursing: Patients should be advised to notify their physician if they are breast-feeding an infant.

LABORATORY TESTS

There are no routine laboratory tests recommended.

PRECAUTIONS: *(cont'd)*

CARCINOGENESIS, MUTAGENESIS, AND IMPAIRMENT OF FERTILITY

Carcinogenesis: Carcinogenicity studies were conducted with mirtazapine given in the diet at doses of 2, 20, and 200 mg/kg/day to mice and 2, 20, and 60 mg/kg/day to rats. The highest doses used are approximately 20 and 12 times the maximum recommended human dose (MRHD of 45 mg/day on a mg/m^2 basis in mice and rats, respectively. There was an increased incidence of hepatocellular adenoma and carcinoma in male mice at the high dose. In rats, there was an increase in hepatocellular adenoma in females at the mid and high doses and in hepatocellular tumors and thyroid follicular adenoma/cystadenoma and carcinoma in males at the high dose. The data suggest that the above effects could possibly be mediated by non-genotoxic mechanisms, the relevance of which to humans is not known.

The doses used in the mouse study may not have been high enough to fully characterize the carcinogenic potential of mirtazapine.

Mutagenesis: Mirtazapine was not mutagenic or clastogenic and did not induce general DNA damage as determined in several genotoxicity tests: Ames test, *in vitro* gene mutation assay in Chinese hamster V 79 cells, *in vitro* sister chromatid exchange assay in cultured rabbit lymphocytes, *in vivo* bone marrow micronucleus test in rats, and unscheduled DNA synthesis assay in HeLa cells.

Impairment of Fertility: In a fertility study in rats, mirtazapine was given at doses up to 100 mg/kg (20 times the maximum recommended human dose (MRHD) on a mg/m^2 basis). Mating and conception were not affected by the drug, but estrous cycling was disrupted at doses that were 3 or more times the MRHD and pre-implantation losses occurred at 20 times the MRHD.

PREGNANCY CATEGORY C

Teratogenic Effects: Reproduction studies in pregnant rats and rabbits at doses up to 100 mg/kg and 40 mg/kg, respectively (20 and 17 times the maximum recommended human dose (MRHD) on a mg/m^2 basis, respectively), have revealed no evidence of teratogenic effects. However, in rats, there was an increase in post-implantation losses in dams treated with mirtazapine. There was an increase in pup deaths during the first 3 days of lactation and a decrease in pup birth weights. The cause of these deaths is not known. These effects occurred at doses that were 20 times the MRHD, but not at 3 times the MRHD, on a mg/m^{2}basis. There are no adequate and well controlled studies in pregnant women. Because animal reproduction studies are not always predictive of human response, this drug should be used during pregnancy only if clearly needed.

NURSING MOTHERS

It is not known whether mirtazapine is excreted in human milk. Because many drugs are excreted in human milk, caution should be exercised when mirtazapine tablets are administered to nursing women.

PEDIATRIC USE

Safety and effectiveness in children have not been established.

GERIATRIC USE

Approximately 190 elderly individuals (≥65 years of age) participated in clinical studies with mirtazapine. No unusual adverse age-related phenomena were identified in this group. Pharmacokinetic studies revealed a decreased clearance in the elderly. Caution is indicated in administering mirtazapine to elderly patients (see CLINICAL PHARMACOLOGY) and DOSAGE AND ADMINISTRATION.

DRUG INTERACTIONS:

As with other drugs, the potential for interaction by a variety of mechanisms (*e.g.,* pharmacodynamic, pharmacokinetic inhibition or enhancement, etc.) is a possibility (see CLINICAL PHARMACOLOGY.)

Drugs Affecting Hepatic Metabolism: The metabolism and pharmacokinetics of mirtazapine may be affected by the induction or inhibition of drug-metabolizing enzymes.

Drugs that are Metabolized by and/or Inhibit Cytochrome P450 Enzymes: Many drugs are metabolized by and/or inhibit various cytochrome P450 enzymes (*e.g.,* 2D6, 1A2, 3A4, etc). *In vitro* studies have shown that mirtazapine is a substrate for several of these enzymes, including 2D6, 1A2, and 3A4. While *in vitro* studies have shown that mirtazapine is not a potent inhibitor of any of these enzymes, an indication that mirtazapine is not likely to have a clinically significant inhibitory effect on the metabolism of other drugs that are substrates for these cytochrome P450 enzymes, the concomitant use of mirtazapine with most other drugs metabolized by these enzymes has not been formally studied. Consequently, it is not possible to make any definitive statements about the risks of coadministration of mirtazapine with such drugs.

Alcohol: Concomitant administration of alcohol (equivalent to 60 g) had a minimal effect on plasma levels of mirtazapine (15 mg) in 6 healthy male subjects. However, the impairment of cognitive and motor skills produced by mirtazapine were shown to be additive with those produced by alcohol. Accordingly, patients should be advised to avoid alcohol while taking mirtazapine.

Diazepam: Concomitant administration of diazepam (15 mg) had a minimal effect on plasma levels of mirtazapine (15 mg) in 12 healthy subjects. However, the impairment of cognitive and motor skills produced by mirtazapine has been shown to be additive with those caused by diazepam. Accordingly, patients should be advised to avoid diazepam and other similar drugs while taking mirtazapine.

ADVERSE REACTIONS:

ASSOCIATED WITH DISCONTINUATION OF TREATMENT

Approximately 16 percent of the 453 patients who received mirtazapine in U.S. 6-week controlled clinical trials discontinued treatment due to an adverse experience, compared to 7 percent of 361 placebo-treated patients in those studies. The most common events (≥1%) associated with discontinuation and considered to be drug related (*i.e.,* those events associated with dropout at a rate at least twice that of placebo) are in TABLE 1.

TABLE 1 COMMON ADVERSE EVENTS ASSOCIATED WITH DISCONTINUATION OF TREATMENT IN 6-WEEK U.S. MIRTAZAPINE TRIALS

	Percentage of Patients Discontinuing with Adverse Event	
Adverse Event	Mirtazapine (n=453)	Placebo (n=361)
Somnolence	10.4%	2.2%
Nausea	1.5%	0%

COMMONLY OBSERVED ADVERSE EVENTS IN U.S. CONTROLLED CLINICAL TRIALS

The most commonly observed adverse events associated with the use of mirtazapine (incidence of 5% or greater) and not observed at an equivalent incidence among placebo-treated patients (mirtazapine incidence at least twice that for placebo) are found in TABLE 2.

ADVERSE REACTIONS: *(cont'd)*

TABLE 2 COMMON TREATMENT-EMERGENT ADVERSE EVENTS ASSOCIATED WITH DISCONTINUATION OF TREATMENT IN 6-WEEK U.S. MIRTAZAPINE TRIALS

	Percentage of Patients Reporting Adverse Event	
Adverse Event	Mirtazapine (n=453)	Placebo (n=361)
Somnolence	54%	18%
Increased Appetite	17%	2%
Weight Gain	12%	2%
Dizziness	7%	3%

ADVERSE EVENTS OCCURRING AT AN INCIDENCE OF 1% OR MORE AMONG MIRTAZAPINE TREATED PATIENTS

TABLE 3 enumerates adverse events that occurred at an incidence of 1% or more, and were frequent than in the placebo group, among mirtazapine-treated patients who participated in short-term U.S. placebo-controlled trials in which patients were dosed in a range of 5 to 60 mg/day. This table shows the percentage of patients in each group who had at least one episode of an event at some time during their treatment. Reported adverse events were classified using a standard COSTART-based dictionary terminology.

The prescriber should be aware that these figures cannot be used to predict the incidence of side effects in the course of usual medical practice where patient characteristics and other factors differ from those which prevailed in the clinical trials. Similarly, the cited frequencies cannot be compared with figures obtained from other investigations involving different treatments, uses and investigators. The cited figures, however, do provide the prescribing physician with some basis for estimating the relative contribution of drug and non-drug factors to the side effect incidence rate in the population studied.

TABLE 3 Incidence Of Adverse Clinical Experiences * (≥ 1%) In Short-Term U.S. Controlled Studies

Body System / Adverse Clinical Experience	Mirtazapine (n=453)	Placebo (n=361)
Body as a Whole		
Asthenia	8%	5%
Flu Syndrome	5%	3%
Back Pain	2%	1%
Digestive System		
Dry Mouth	25%	15%
Increased Appetite	17%	2%
Constipation	13%	7%
Metabolic and Nutritional Disorders		
Weight Gain	12%	2%
Peripheral Edema	2%	1%
Edema	1%	0%
Musculoskeletal System		
Myalgia	2%	1%
Nervous System		
Somnolence	54%	18%
Dizziness	7%	3%
Abnormal Dreams	4%	1%
Thinking Abnormal	3%	1%
Tremor	2%	1%
Confusion	2%	0%
Respiratory System		
Dyspnea	1%	0%
Urogenital System		
Urinary Frequency	2%	1%

*Events reported by at least 1% of patients treated with mirtazapine are included, except the following events which had an incidence on placebo ≥ mirtazapine: headache, infection, pain, chest pain, palpitation, tachycardia, postural hypotension, nausea, dyspepsia, diarrhea, flatulence, insomnia, nervousness, libido decreased, hypertonia, pharyngitis, rhinitis, sweating, amblyopia, tinnitus, taste perversion.

ECG CHANGES

In an analysis of ECGs obtained in U.S. placebo-controlled clinical trial, mirtazapine and placebo-treated patients had a similiar incidence of abnormal changes from baseline at 6–8 weeks of approximately 3%. The abnormalities were generally not considered clinically significant.

OTHER ADVERSE EVENTS OBSERVED DURING THE PREMARKETING EVALUATION OF MIRTAZAPINE

During its premarketing assessment, multiple doses of mirtazapine were administered to 2,796 patients in clinical studies. The conditions and duration of exposure to mirtazapine varied greatly, and included (in overlapping categories) open and double-blind studies, uncontrolled and controlled studies, inpatient and outpatient studies, fixed dose and titration studies. Untoward events associated with its exposure were recorded by clinical investigators using terminology of their own choosing. Consequently, it is not possible to provide a meaningful estimate of the proportion of individuals experiencing adverse events without first grouping similar types of untoward events into a smaller number of standardized event categories.

In the tabulations that follow, reported adverse events were classified using a standard COSTART-based dictionary terminology. The frequencies presented, therefore, represent the proportion of the 2796 patients exposed to multiple doses of mirtazapine who experienced an event of the type cited on at least one occasion while receiving mirtazapine. All reported events are included except those already listed in the previous table, those adverse experiences subsumed under COSTART terms that are either overly general or excessively specific so as to be uninformative, and those events for which a drug cause was very remote.

It is important to emphasize that, although the events reported occurred during treatment with mirtazapine, they were not necessarily caused by it.

Events are further categorized by body system and listed in order of decreasing frequency according to the following definitions: frequent adverse events are those-occurring on one or more occasions in at least 1/100 patients; infrequent adverse events are those occurring in 1/100 to 1/1000 patients; rare events are those occurring in fewer than 1/1000 patients. Only those events not already listed in the previous table appear in this listing. Events of major clinical importance are also described in WARNINGS and PRECAUTIONS.

Body as a Whole: *frequent:*malaise, abdominal pain, abdominal syndrome acute; *infrequent:* chills, fever, face edema, ulcer, photosensitivity reaction, neck rigidity, neck pain, abdomen enlarged; *rare:*cellulitis, chest pain substernal.

Cardiovascular System: *frequent:*hypertension, vasodilatation; *infrequent:*angina pectoris, myocardial infarction, bradycardia, ventricular extrasystoles, syncope, migraine, hypotension; *rare:* atrial arrhythmia, bigeminy, vascular headache, pulmonary embolus, cerebral ischemia, cardiomegaly, phlebitis, left heart failure.

ADVERSE REACTIONS: *(cont'd)*

Digestive System: *frequent:*vomiting, anorexia; *infrequent:*eructation, glossitis, cholecystitis, nausea and vomiting, gum hemorrhage, stomatitis, colitis, liver function tests abnormal; *rare:* tongue discoloration, ulcerative stomatitis, salivary gland enlargement, increased salivation, intestinal obstruction, pancreatitis, aphthous stomatitis, cirrhosis of liver, gastritis, gastroenteritis, oral moniliasis, tongue edema.

Endocrine System: *rare:*goiter, hypothyroidism.

Hemic and Lymphatic System: *rare:*lymphadenopathy, leukopenia, petechia, anemia, thrombocytopenia, lymphocytosis, pancytopenia.

Metabolic and Nutritional Disorders: *frequent:*thirst; *infrequent:*dehydration, weight loss; *rare:* gout, SGOT increased, healing abnormal, acid phosphatase increased, SGPT increased, diabetes mellitus.

Musculoskeletal System: *frequent:*myasthenia, arthralgia; *infrequent:*arthritis, tenosynovitis; *rare:*pathological fracture, osteoporosis fracture, bone pain, myositis, tendon rupture, arthrosis, bursitis.

Nervous system: *frequent:*hypesthesia, apathy, depression, hypokinesia, vertigo, twitching, agitation, anxiety, amnesia, hyperkinesia, paresthesia; *infrequent:*ataxia, delirium, delusions, depersonalization, dyskinesia, extrapyramidal syndrome, libido increased, coordination abnormal, dysarthria, hallucinations, manic reaction, neurosis, dystonia, hostility, reflexes increased, emotional lability, euphoria, paranoid reaction; *rare:*aphasia, nystagmus, akathisia, stupor, dementia, diplopia, drug dependence, paralysis, grand mal convulsion, hypotonia, myoclonus, psychotic depression, withdrawal syndrome.

Respiratory System: *frequent:*cough increased, sinusitis; *infrequent:*epistaxis, bronchitis, asthma, pneumonia; *rare:*asphyxia, laryngitis, pneumothorax, hiccup.

Skin and Appendages: *frequent:*pruritus, rash; *infrequent:*acne exfoliative dermatitis, dry skin, herpes simplex, alopecia; *rare:*urticarial, herpes zoster, skin hypertrophy, seborrhea, skin ulcer.

Special Senses: *infrequent:*eye pain, abnormality of accommodation, conjunctivitis, deafness, keratoconjunctivitis, lacrimation disorder, glaucoma, hyperacusis, ear pain; *rare:*blepharitis, partial transitory deafness, otitis media, taste loss, parosmia.

Urogenital System: *frequent:*urinary tract infection; *infrequent:*kidney calculus, cystitis, dysuria, urinary incontinence, urinary retention, vaginitis, hematuria, breast pain, amenorrhea, dysmenorrhea, leukorrhea, impotence; *rare:*polyuria, urethritis, metrorrhagia, menorrhagia, abnormal ejaculation, breast engorgement, breast enlargement, urinary urgency.

DRUG ABUSE AND DEPENDENCE:

Controlled Substance Class Mirtazapine tablets are not a controlled substance.

Physical and Psychological Dependence Mirtazapine has not been systematically studied in animals or humans for its potential for abuse, tolerance or physical dependence. While clinical trials did not reveal any tendency for any drug-seeking behavior, these observations were not systematic and it is not possible to predict on the basis of this limited experience the extent to which a CNS-active drug will be misused, diverted and/or abused once marketed. Consequently, patients should be evaluated carefully for history of drug abuse, and such patients should be observed closely for signs of mirtazapine misuse or abuse (*e.g.*, development of tolerance, incrementations of dose, drug-seeking behavior).

OVERDOSAGE:

HUMAN EXPERIENCE

There is very limited experience with mirtazapine overdose. In premarketing clinical studies, there were eight reports of mirtazapine overdose alone or in combination with other pharmacological agents The only drug overdose death reported while taking mirtazapine tablets was in combination with amitriptyline and chlorprothixene in a non-U.S clinical study. Based on plasma levels, the mirtazapine dose taken was 30-45 mg, while plasma levels of amitriptyline and chlorprothixene were found to be at toxic levels. All other premarketing overdose cases resulted in full recovery. Signs and symptoms reported in association with overdose included disorientation, drowsiness, impaired memory, and tachycardia. There were no reports of ECG abnormalities, coma or convulsions following overdose with mirtazapine alone.

OVERDOSE MANAGEMENT

Treatment should consist of those general measures employed in the management of overdose with any antidepressant. There are no specific antidotes for mirtazapine. If the patient is unconscious, establish and maintain an airway to ensure adequate oxygenation and ventilation. Gastric evacuation either by the induction of emesis or lavage or both should be considered. Activated charcoal should also be considered in treatment of overdose. Cardiac and vital signs monitoring is recommended along with general symptomatic and supportive measures.

In managing overdosage, consider the possibility of multiple-drug involvement. The physician should consider contacting a poison control center or additional information on the treatment of any overdose.

DOSAGE AND ADMINISTRATION:

INITIAL TREATMENT

The recommended starting dose for mirtazapine is 15 mg/day, administered in a single dose, preferably in the evening prior to sleep. In the controlled clinical trials establishing the antidepressant efficacy of mirtazapine the effective dose range was generally 15-45 mg/day. While the relationship between dose and antidepressant response for mirtazapine has not been adequately explored, patients not responding to the initial 15 mg dose may benefit from dose increases up to a maximum of 45 mg/day. Mirtazapine has an elimination half-life of approximately 20-40 hours; therefore, dose changes should not be made at intervals of less than one to two weeks in order to allow sufficient time for evaluation of the therapeutic response to a given dose.

ELDERLY AND PATIENTS WITH RENAL OR HEPATIC IMPAIRMENT

The clearance of mirtazapine is reduced in elderly patients and in patients with moderate to severe renal or hepatic impairment. Consequently, the prescriber should be aware that plasma mirtazapine levels may be increased in these patient groups, compared to levels observed in younger adults without renal or hepatic impairment (see CLINICAL PHARMACOLOGY, Pharmacokinetics.)

MAINTENANCE/EXTENDED TREATMENT

There is no body of evidence available from controlled trials to indicate how long the depressed patient should be treated with mirtazapine. It is generally agreed, however, that pharmacological treatment for acute episodes of depression should continue for up to six months or longer. Whether the dose of antidepressant needed to induce remission is identical to the dose needed to maintain euthymia is unknown.

SWITCHING PATIENTS TO OR FROM A MONOAMINE OXIDASE INHIBITOR

At least 14 days should elapse between discontinuation of an MAOI and initiation of therapy with mirtazapine. In addition, at least 14 days should be allowed after stopping mirtazapine before starting an MAOI.

PATIENT INFORMATION:

Mirtazapine is used for the treatment of depression.

Contact your physician if you experience signs of infection (fever, chills, sore throat, nose or mouth sores or any flu-like symptoms).

Inform your physician if you are pregnant or are planning to become pregnant or if you are breastfeeding.

May cause drowsiness or tiredness; use caution while driving or operating hazardous machinery.

This drug may interact with many other medications; inform your doctor or pharmacist if you are taking any other medications (including over-the-counter products).

Avoid alcohol while taking this medication.

May cause sleepiness, nausea, increased appetite, weight gain and dizziness.

This medication may be taken with or without food; do not stop taking this medication without consulting your doctor.

HOW SUPPLIED:

Remeron tablets are supplied as: 15 mg tablets - oval, scored, yellow, coated, with "Organon" embossed on one side and "TZ3" on the other side; 30 mg tablets - oval, scored, red-brown, coated, with "Organon" embossed on one side and "TZ5" on the other side in bottles of 30 and unit dose packs, box of 100.

HOW SUPPLIED - EQUIVALENTS NOT AVAILABLE:

Tablets - Oral - 15 mg

30's $59.40 REMERON, Organon 00052-0105-30

MISOPROSTOL *(001820)*

CATEGORIES: Acid/Peptic Disorders; Cytoprotective Agents; Gastric Acid Secretion Inhibitors; Gastric Ulcer; Gastrointestinal Drugs; Prostaglandin Analog; Prostaglandin Anti-Ulcer Drugs; Ulcer; Abortion*; Pregnancy Category X; FDA Approved 1988 Dec; Patent Expiration 1995 Jun

* Indication not approved by the FDA

BRAND NAMES: **Cytotec**; *Symbol*
(International brand names outside U.S. in italics)

FORMULARIES: Aetna; BC-BS; FHP; Medi-Cal; PCS

Misoprostol is contraindicated, because of its abortifacient property, in women who are pregnant. (See PRECAUTIONS.) Patients must be advised of the abortifacient property and warned not to give the drug to others. Misoprostol should not be used in women of childbearing potential unless the patient requires nonsteroidal anti-inflammatory drug (NSAID) therapy and is at high risk of complications from gastric ulcers associated with use of the NSAID, or is at high risk of developing gastric ulceration. In such patients, misoprostol may be prescribed if the patient

is capable of complying with effective contraceptive measures

has received both oral and written warnings of the hazards of misoprostol, the risk of possible contraception failure, and the danger to other women of childbearing potential should the drug be taken by mistake

has had a negative serum pregnancy test within two weeks prior to beginning therapy

will begin misoprostol only on the second or third day of the next normal menstrual period

DESCRIPTION:

Cytotec oral tablets contain either 100 mcg or 200 mcg of misoprostol, a synthetic prostaglandin E_1 analog.

Misoprostol contains approximately equal amounts of the two diastereomers presented below with their enantiomers indicated by (±): and $C_{22}H_{38}O_5$ M.W. = 382.5

(±)methyl 11α,16-dihydroxy-16-methyl-9-oxoprost-13E-en-1-oate.

Misoprostol is a water-soluble, viscous liquid.

Inactive ingredients of Cytotec tablets are hydrogenated castor oil, hydroxypropyl methylcellulose, microcrystalline cellulose, and sodium starch glycolate.

CLINICAL PHARMACOLOGY:

Pharmacokinetics: Misoprostol is extensively absorbed, and undergoes rapid de-esterification to its free acid, which is responsible for its clinical activity and, unlike the parent compound, is detectable in plasma. The alpha side chain undergoes beta oxidation and the beta side chain undergoes omega oxidation followed by reduction of the ketone to give prostaglandin F analogs.

In normal volunteers, misoprostol is rapidly absorbed after oral administration with a T_{max} of misoprostol acid of 12 ± 3 minutes and a terminal half-life of 20-40 minutes.

There is high variability of plasma levels of misoprostol acid between and within studies but mean values after single doses show a linear relationship with dose over the range of 200-400 mcg. No accumulation of misoprostol acid was noted in multiple dose studies; plasma steady state was achieved within two days.

Maximum plasma concentrations of misoprostol acid are diminished when the dose is taken with food and total availability of misoprostol acid is reduced by use of concomitant antacid. Clinical trials were conducted with concomitant antacid, however, so this effect does not appear to be clinically important (TABLE 1):

TABLE 1

Mean ± SD	C_{max}(pg/ml)	AUC(0-4) (pg°hr/ml)	T_{max}(min)
Fasting	811 ± 317	417 ± 135	14 ± 8
With Antacid	689 ± 315	349 ± 108*	20 ± 14
With High Fat Breakfast	303 ± 176*	373 ± 111	64 ± 79*

* Comparisons with fasting results statistically significant, p<0.05.

After oral administration of radiolabeled misoprostol, about 80% of detected radioactivity appears in urine. Pharmacokinetic studies in patients with varying degrees of renal impairment showed an approximate doubling of T 1/2, C_{max}, and AUC compared to normals, but no clear correlation between the degree of impairment and AUC. In subjects over 64 years of age, the AUC for misoprostol acid is increased. No routine dosage adjustment is recommended in older patients or patients with renal impairment, but dosage may need to be reduced if the usual dose is not tolerated.

Misoprostol does not affect the hepatic mixed function oxidase (cytochrome P-450) enzyme systems in animals.

CLINICAL PHARMACOLOGY: *(cont'd)*

Drug interaction studies between misoprostol and several nonsteroidal anti-inflammatory drugs showed no effect on the kinetics of ibuprofen or diclofenac, and a 20% decrease in aspirin AUC, not thought to be clinically significant.

Pharmacokinetic studies also showed a lack of drug interaction with antipyrine and propranolol when these drugs were given with misoprostol. Misoprostol given for one week had no effect on the steady state pharmacokinetics of diazepam when the two drugs were administered two hours apart.

The serum protein binding of misoprostol acid is less than 90% and is concentration-independent in the therapeutic range.

Pharmacodynamics: Misoprostol has both antisecretory (inhibiting gastric acid secretion) and (in animals) mucosal protective properties. NSAIDs inhibit prostaglandin synthesis, and a deficiency of prostaglandins within the gastric mucosa may lead to diminishing bicarbonate and mucus secretion and may contribute to the mucosal damage caused by these agents. Misoprostol can increase bicarbonate and mucus production, but in man this has been shown at doses 200 mcg and above that are also antisecretory. It is therefore not possible to tell whether the ability of misoprostol to prevent gastric ulcer is the result of its antisecretory effect, its mucosal protective effect, or both.

In vitro studies on canine parietal cells using tritiated misoprostol acid as the ligand have led to the identification and characterization of specific prostaglandin receptors. Receptor binding is saturable, reversible, and stereospecific. The sites have a high affinity for misoprostol, for its acid metabolite, and for other E type prostaglandins, but not for F or I prostaglandins and other unrelated compounds, such as histamine or cimetidine. Receptor-site affinity for misoprostol correlates well with an indirect index of antisecretory activity. It is likely that these specific receptors allow misoprostol taken with food to be effective topically, despite the lower serum concentrations attained.

Misoprostol produces a moderate decrease in pepsin concentration during basal conditions, but not during histamine stimulation. It has no significant effect on fasting or postprandial gastrin nor on intrinsic factor output.

Effects on Gastric Acid Secretion: Misoprostol, over the range of 50-200 mcg, inhibits basal and nocturnal gastric acid secretion, and acid secretion in response to a variety of stimuli, including meals, histamine, pentagastrin, and coffee. Activity is apparent 30 minutes after oral administration and persists for at least 3 hours. In general, the effects of 50 mcg were modest and shorter lived, and only the 200-mcg dose had substantial effects on nocturnal secretion or on histamine and meal-stimulated secretion.

Uterine Effects: Misoprostol has been shown to produce uterine contractions that may endanger pregnancy. (See CONTRAINDICATIONSand WARNINGS). In studies in women undergoing elective termination of pregnancy during the first trimester, misoprostol caused partial or complete expulsion of the uterine contents in 11% of the subjects and increased uterine bleeding in 41%.

Other Pharmacologic Effects: Misoprostol does not produce clinically significant effects on serum levels of prolactin, gonadotropins, thyroid-stimulating hormone, growth hormone, thyroxine, cortisol, gastrointestinal hormones (somatostatin, gastrin, vasoactive intestinal polypeptide, and motilin), creatinine, or uric acid. Gastric emptying, immunologic competence, platelet aggregation, pulmonary function, or the cardiovascular system are not modified by recommended doses of misoprostol.

CLINICAL STUDIES:

In a series of small short-term (about one week) placebo-controlled studies in healthy human volunteers, doses of misoprostol were evaluated for their ability to prevent NSAID-induced mucosal injury. Studies of 200 mcg q.i.d. of misoprostol with tolmetin and naproxen, and of 100 and 200 mcg q.i.d. with ibuprofen, all showed reduction of the rate of significant endoscopic injury from about 70-75% on placebo to 10-30% on misoprostol. Doses of 25-200 mcg q.i.d. reduced aspirin-induced mucosal injury and bleeding.

Preventing Gastric Ulcers Caused By Nonsteroidal Anti-Inflammatory Drugs (Nsaids): Two 12-week, randomized, double-blind trials in osteoarthritic patients who had gastrointestinal symptoms but no ulcer on endoscopy while taking an NSAID compared the ability of 200 mcg of misoprostol, 100 mcg of misoprostol, and placebo to prevent gastric ulcer (GU) formation. Patients were approximately equally divided between ibuprofen, piroxicam, and naproxen, and continued this treatment throughout the 12 weeks. The 200-mcg dose caused a marked, statistically significant reduction in gastric ulcers in both studies. The lower dose was somewhat less effective, with a significant result in only one of the studies (TABLE 2):

TABLE 2 Prevention of Gastric Ulcers Induced by Ibuprofen, Piroxicam, or Naproxen(No. of patients with ulcer(s) (%))

Therapy	Therapy Duration 4 Weeks	8 Weeks	12 Weeks	
Study No. 1				
Cytotec 200 mcg q.i.d. (n=74)	1(1.4)	0	0	1(1.4)*
Cytotec 100 mcg q.i.d. (n=77)	3(3.9)	1(1.3)	1(1.3)	5(6.5)*
Placebo (n=76)	11(14.5)	4(5.3)	4(5.3)	19(25.0)
Study No. 2				
Cytotec 200 mcg q.i.d. (n=65)	1(1.5)	1(1.5)	0	2(3.1)*
Cytotec 100 mcg q.i.d. (n=66)	2(3.0)	2(3.0)	1(1.5)	5(7.6)
Placebo (n=62)	6(9.7)	2(3.2)	3(4.8)	11(17.7)
Studies No. 1 & No. 2**				
Cytotec 200 mcg q.i.d. (n=139)	2(1.4)	1(0.7)	0	3(2.2)*
Cytotec 100 mcg q.i.d. (n=143)	5(3.5)	3(2.1)	2(1.4)	10(7.0)*
Placebo (n=138)	17(12.3)	6(4.3)	7(5.1)	30(21.7)

* Statistically significantly different from placebo at the 5% level.
** Combined data from Study No.1 and Study No. 2.

In these trials there were no significant differences between misoprostol and placebo in relief of day or night abdominal pain. No effect of misoprostol in preventing duodenal ulcers was demonstrated, but relatively few duodenal lesions were seen.

In another clinical trial, 239 patients receiving aspirin 650-1300 mg q.i.d. for rheumatoid arthritis who had endoscopic evidence of duodenal and/or gastric inflammation were randomized to misoprostol 200 mcg q.i.d. or placebo for eight weeks while continuing to receive aspirin. The study evaluated the possible interference of misoprostol on the efficacy of aspirin in these patients with rheumatoid arthritis by analyzing joint tenderness, joint swelling, physician's clinical assessment, patient's assessment, change in ARA classification, change in handgrip strength, change in duration of morning stiffness, patient's assessment of pain at rest, movement, interference with daily activity, and ESR. Misoprostol did not interfere with the efficacy of aspirin in these patients with rheumatoid arthritis.

INDICATIONS AND USAGE:

Misoprostol is indicated for the prevention of NSAID (nonsteroidal anti-inflammatory drugs, including aspirin)-induced gastric ulcers in patients at high risk of complications from gastric ulcer, e.g., the elderly and patients with concomitant debilitating disease, as well as patients at high risk of developing gastric ulceration, such as patients with a history of ulcer. Misoprostol has not been shown to prevent duodenal ulcers in patients taking NSAIDs. Misoprostol should be taken for the duration of NSAID therapy. Misoprostol has been shown to prevent gastric ulcers in controlled studies of three months' duration. It had no effect, compared to placebo, on gastrointestinal pain or discomfort associated with NSAID use.

CONTRAINDICATIONS:

See BOXED WARNING.

Misoprostol should not be taken by anyone with a history of allergy to prostaglandins.

WARNINGS:

See BOXED WARNING.

PRECAUTIONS:

INFORMATION FOR THE PATIENT

Misoprostol is contraindicated in women who are pregnant, and should not be used in women of childbearing potential unless the patient requires nonsteroidal anti-inflammatory drug (NSAID) therapy and is at high risk of complications from gastric ulcers associated with the use of the NSAID, or is at high risk of developing gastric ulceration. Women of childbearing potential should be told that they must not be pregnant when misoprostol therapy is initiated, and that they must use an effective contraception method while taking misoprostol.

See BOXED WARNING.

Patients should be advised of the following:

Misoprostol is intended for administration along with nonsteroidal anti-inflammatory drugs (NSAIDs), including aspirin, to decrease the chance of developing an NSAID-induced gastric ulcer.

Misoprostol should be taken only according to the directions given by a physician.

If the patient has questions about or problems with misoprostol, the physician should be contacted promptly.

THE PATIENT SHOULD NOT GIVE MISOPROSTOL TO ANYONE ELSE. Misoprostol has been prescribed for the patient's specific condition, may not be the correct treatment for another person, and may be dangerous to the other person if she were to become pregnant.

The misoprostol package the patient receives from the pharmacist will include a leaflet containing patient information. The patient should read the leaflet before taking misoprostol and each time the prescription is renewed because the leaflet may have been revised.

Keep misoprostol out of the reach of children.

SPECIAL NOTE FOR WOMEN: Misoprostol must not be used by pregnant women. Misoprostol may cause miscarriage. Miscarriages caused by misoprostol may be incomplete, which could lead to potentially dangerous bleeding, hospitalization, surgery, infertility, or maternal or fetal death.

Misoprostol is available only as a unit-of-use package that includes a leaflet containing patient information.

See PATIENT PACKAGE INSERT at the end of this labeling.

CARCINOGENESIS, MUTAGENESIS, AND IMPAIRMENT OF FERTILITY

There was no evidence of an effect of misoprostol on tumor occurrence or incidence in rats receiving daily doses up to 150 times the human dose for 24 months. Similarly, there was no effect of misoprostol on tumor occurrence or incidence in mice receiving daily doses up to 1000 times the human dose for 21 months. The mutagenic potential of misoprostol was tested in several*in vitro* assays, all of which were negative.

Misoprostol, when administered to breeding male and female rats at doses 6.25 times to 625 times the maximum recommended human therapeutic dose, produced dose-related pre- and post-implantation losses and a significant decrease in the number of live pups born at the highest dose. These findings suggest the possibility of a general adverse effect on fertility in males and females.

PREGNANCY CATEGORY X

See BOXED WARNING.

Nonteratogenic Effects: Misoprostol may endanger pregnancy (may cause miscarriage) and thereby cause harm to the fetus when administered to a pregnant woman. misoprostol produces uterine contractions, uterine bleeding, and expulsion of the products of conception. Miscarriages caused by misoprostol may be incomplete. In studies in women undergoing elective termination of pregnancy during the first trimester, misoprostol caused partial or complete expulsion of the products of conception in 11% of the subjects and increased uterine bleeding in 41%. If a woman is or becomes pregnant while taking this drug, the drug should be discontinued and the patient apprised of the potential hazard to the fetus.

Teratogenic Effects: Misoprostol is not fetotoxic or teratogenic in rats and rabbits at doses 625 and 63 times the human dose, respectively.

NURSING MOTHERS

See CONTRAINDICATIONS. It is unlikely that misoprostol is excreted in human milk since it is rapidly metabolized throughout the body. However, it is not known if the active metabolite (misoprostol acid) is excreted in human milk. Therefore, misoprostol should not be administered to nursing mothers because the potential excretion of misoprostol acid could cause significant diarrhea in nursing infants.

PEDIATRIC USE

Safety and effectiveness in children below the age of 18 years have not been established.

DRUG INTERACTIONS:

See CLINICAL PHARMACOLOGY. Misoprostol has not been shown to interfere with the beneficial effects of aspirin on signs and symptoms of rheumatoid arthritis. Misoprostol does not exert clinically significant effects on the absorption, blood levels, and antiplatelet effects of therapeutic doses of aspirin. Misoprostol has no clinically significant effect on the kinetics of diclofenac or ibuprofen.

ADVERSE REACTIONS:

The following have been reported as adverse events in subjects receiving misoprostol:

Gastrointestinal: In subjects receiving misoprostol 400 or 800 mcg daily in clinical trials, the most frequent gastrointestinal adverse events were diarrhea and abdominal pain. The incidence of diarrhea at 800 mcg in controlled trials in patients on NSAIDs ranged from 14-40% and in all studies (over 5,000 patients) averaged 13%. Abdominal pain occurred in 13-20% of patients in NSAID trials and about 7% in all studies, but there was no consistent difference from placebo.

Diarrhea was dose related and usually developed early in the course of therapy (after 13 days), usually was self-limiting (often resolving after 8 days), but sometimes required discontinuation of misoprostol (2% of the patients). Rare instances of profound diarrhea leading to severe dehydration have been reported. Patients with an underlying condition such as inflammatory bowel disease, or those in whom dehydration, were it to occur, would be

ADVERSE REACTIONS: *(cont'd)*

dangerous, should be monitored carefully if misoprostol is prescribed. The incidence of diarrhea can be minimized by administering after meals and at bedtime, and by avoiding coadministration of misoprostol with magnesium-containing antacids.

Gynecological: Women who received misoprostol during clinical trials reported the following gynecological disorders: spotting (0.7%), cramps (0.6%), hypermenorrhea (0.5%), menstrual disorder (0.3%) and dysmenorrhea (0.1%). Postmenopausal vaginal bleeding may be related to misoprostol administration. If it occurs, diagnostic workup should be undertaken to rule out gynecological pathology.

Elderly: There were no significant differences in the safety profile of misoprostol in approximately 500 ulcer patients who were 65 years of age or older compared with younger patients.

Additional adverse events which were reported are categorized as follows:

Incidence Greater Than 1%: In clinical trials, the following adverse reactions were reported by more than 1% of the subjects receiving misoprostol and may be causally related to the drug: nausea (3.2%), flatulence (2.9%), headache (2.4%), dyspepsia (2.0%), vomiting (1.3%), and constipation (1.1%). However, there were no significant differences between the incidences of these events for misoprostol and placebo.

Causal Relationship Unknown: The following adverse events were infrequently reported. Causal relationships between misoprostol and these events have not been established but cannot be excluded:

Body as a Whole: aches/pains, asthenia, fatigue, fever, rigors, weight changes.

Skin: rash, dermatitis, alopecia, pallor, breast pain.

Special Senses: abnormal taste, abnormal vision, conjunctivitis, deafness, tinnitus, earache.

Respiratory: upper respiratory tract infection, bronchitis, bronchospasm, dyspnea, pneumonia, epistaxis.

Cardiovascular: chest pain, edema, diaphoresis, hypotension, hypertension, arrhythmia, phlebitis, increased cardiac enzymes, syncope.

Gastrointestinal: GI bleeding, GI inflammation/infection, rectal disorder, abnormal hepatobiliary function, gingivitis, reflux, dysphagia, amylase increase.

Hypersensitivity: Anaphylaxis

Metabolic: glycosuria, gout, increased nitrogen, increased alkaline phosphatase.

Genitourinary: polyuria, dysuria, hematuria, urinary tract infection.

Nervous System/Psychiatric: anxiety, change in appetite, depression, drowsiness, dizziness, thirst, impotence, loss of libido, sweating increase, neuropathy, neurosis, confusion.

Musculoskeletal: arthralgia, myalgia, muscle cramps, stiffness, back pain.

Blood/Coagulation: anemia, abnormal differential, thrombocytopenia, purpura, ESR increased.

OVERDOSAGE:

The toxic dose of misoprostol in humans has not been determined. Cumulative total daily doses of 1600 mcg have been tolerated, with only symptoms of gastrointestinal discomfort being reported. In animals, the acute toxic effects are diarrhea, gastrointestinal lesions, focal cardiac necrosis, hepatic necrosis, renal tubular necrosis, testicular atrophy, respiratory difficulties, and depression of the central nervous system. Clinical signs that may indicate an overdose are sedation, tremor, convulsions, dyspnea, abdominal pain, diarrhea, fever, palpitations, hypotension, or bradycardia. Symptoms should be treated with supportive therapy. It is not known if misoprostol acid is dialyzable. However, because misoprostol is metabolized like a fatty acid, it is unlikely that dialysis would be appropriate treatment for overdosage.

DOSAGE AND ADMINISTRATION:

The recommended adult oral dose of misoprostol for the prevention of NSAID-induced gastric ulcers is 200 mcg four times daily with food. If this dose cannot be tolerated, a dose of 100 mcg can be used. (See CLINICAL STUDIES.) misoprostol should be taken for the duration of NSAID therapy as prescribed by the physician. Misoprostol should be taken with a meal, and the last dose of the day should be at bedtime.

Dosage for Impaired Renal Function: Adjustment of the dosing schedule in renally impaired patients is not routinely needed, but dosage can be reduced if the 200-mcg dose is not tolerated. (See CLINICAL PHARMACOLOGY.)

ANIMAL PHARMACOLOGY:

Animal Toxicology: A reversible increase in the number of normal surface gastric epithelial cells occurred in the dog, rat, and mouse. No such increase has been observed in humans administered misoprostol for up to one year.

An apparent response of the female mouse to misoprostol in long-term studies at 100 to 1000 times the human dose was hyperostosis, mainly of the medulla of sternebrae. Hyperostosis did not occur in long-term studies in the dog and rat and has not been seen in humans treated with misoprostol.

PATIENT PACKAGE INSERT:

Read this leaflet before taking misoprostol and each time your prescription is renewed, because the leaflet may be changed.

Misoprostol is being prescribed by your doctor to decrease the chance of getting stomach ulcers related to the arthritis/pain medication that you take.

Misoprostol can cause miscarriage, often associated with potentially dangerous bleeding. This may result in hospitalization, surgery, infertility, or death. **Do not take it if you are pregnant and do not become pregnant while taking this medicine.**

If you become pregnant during misoprostol therapy, stop taking misoprostol and contact your physician immediately. Remember that even if you are on a means of birth control it is still possible to become pregnant. Should this occur, stop taking misoprostol and contact your physician immediately.

Misoprostol may cause diarrhea, abdominal cramping, and/or nausea in some people. In most cases these problems develop during the first few weeks of therapy and stop after about a week. You can minimize possible diarrhea by making sure you take misoprostol with food.

Because these side effects are usually mild to moderate and usually go away in a matter of days, most patients can continue to take misoprostol. If you have prolonged difficulty (more than 8 days), or if you have severe diarrhea, cramping and/or nausea, call your doctor.

Take misoprostol only according to the directions given by your physician.

Do not give misoprostol to anyone else. It has been prescribed for your specific condition, may not be the correct treatment for another person, and would be dangerous if the other person were pregnant.

This information sheet does not cover all possible side effects of misoprostol. This patient information leaflet does not address the side effects of your arthritis/pain medication. See your doctor if you have questions.

Keep out of reach of children.

HOW SUPPLIED:

Cytotec 100-mcg tablets are white, round, with SEARLE debossed on one side and 1451 on the other side.

Cytotec 200-mcg tablets are white, hexagonal, with SEARLE debossed above and 1461 debossed below the line on one side and a double stomach debossed on the other side.

Store below 86°F (30°C) in a dry area.

HOW SUPPLIED - EQUIVALENTS NOT AVAILABLE:

Tablet, Uncoated - Oral - 100 mcg

60's	$29.11	CYTOTEC 100 MCG, Searle	00025-1451-60
100's	$50.91	CYTOTEC 100 MCG, Searle	00025-1451-34
120's	$58.20	CYTOTEC 100 MCG, Searle	00025-1451-20

Tablet, Uncoated - Oral - 200 mcg

60's	$42.38	CYTOTEC, Searle	00025-1461-60
100's	$70.63	CYTOTEC, Searle	00025-1461-31
100's	$74.16	CYTOTEC, Searle	00025-1461-34

MITOMYCIN *(001821)*

CATEGORIES: Antineoplastics; Antibiotics; Cancer; Chemotherapy; Cytotoxic Agents; Oncologic Drugs; Stomach Carcinoma; FDA Approval Pre 1982

BRAND NAMES: *Ametycine* (France); *Mitomicina-C*; *Mitomycin* (Germany); *Mitomycin C*; *Mitomycin-C*; *Mitomycin-C Kyowa*; *Mitomycine*; **Mutamycin**
(International brand names outside U.S. in italics)

FORMULARIES: BC-BS; Medi-Cal

Mutamycin should be administered under the supervision of qualified physician experienced in the use of cancer chemotherapeutic agents. Appropriate management of therapy and complications is possible only when adequate diagnostic and treatment facilities are readily available.

Bone marrow suppression, notably thrombocytopenia and leukopenia, which may contribute to overwhelming infections in an already compromised patient, is the most common and severe of the toxic effects of Mutamycin (see WARNINGS and ADVERSE REACTIONS).

Hemolytic Uremic Syndrome (HUS) a serious complication of chemotherapy, consisting primarily of microangiopathic hemolytic anemia, thrombocytopenia, and irreversible renal failure has been reported in patients receiving systemic Mutamycin. The syndrome may occur at any time during systemic therapy with Mutamycin as a single agent or in combination with other cytotoxic drugs, however, most cases occur at doses >/= 60 mg of Mutamycin. Blood product transfusion may exacerbate the symptoms associated with this syndrome.

The incidence of the syndrome has not been defined.

DESCRIPTION:

Mutamycin (also known as mitomycin and/or mitomycin-C) is an antibiotic isolated from the broth of **Streptomyces caespitosus** which has been shown to have antitumor activity. The compound is heat stable, has a high melting point, and is freely soluble in organic solvents.

CLINICAL PHARMACOLOGY:

Mutamycin selectively inhibits the synthesis of deoxyribonucleic and (DNA). The guanine and cytosine content correlates with the degree of Mutamycin-induced cross-linking. At high concentrations of the drug, cellular RNA and protein synthesis are also suppressed.

In humans, Mutamycin is rapidly cleared from the serum after intravenous administration. Time required to reduce the serum concentration by 50% after a 30 mg bolus injection is 17 minutes. After injection of 30 mg, 20 mg, or 10 mg IV, the maximal serum concentrations were 2.4 mcg/ml, 1.7 mcg/ml, and 0.52 mcg/ml, respectively. Clearance is effected primarily by metabolism in the liver, but metabolism occurs in other tissues as well. The rate of clearance is inversely proportional to the maximal serum concentration because, it is thought, of saturation of the degradative pathways.

Approximately 10% of a dose of Mutamycin is excreted unchanged in the urine. Since metabolic pathways are saturated at relatively low doses, the percent of a dose excreted in urine increases with increasing dose. In children, excretion of intravenously administered Mutamycin is similar.

Animal Toxicology - Mutamycin has been found to be carcinogenic in rats and mice. At doses approximating the recommended clinical dose in man, it produces a greater than 100 percent increase in tumor incidence in male Sprague-Dawley rats, and a greater than 50 percent increase in tumor incidence in female Swiss mice.

INDICATIONS AND USAGE:

Mutamycin is not recommended as single-agent, primary therapy. It has been shown to be useful in the therapy of disseminated adenocarcinoma of the stomach or pancreas in proven combinations with other approved chemotherapeutic agents and as palliative treatment when other modalities have failed. Mutamycin is not recommended to replace appropriate surgery and/or radiotherapy.

CONTRAINDICATIONS:

Mutamycin is contraindicated in patients who have demonstrated a hypersensitive or idiosyncratic reaction to it in the past.

Mutamycin is contraindicated in patients with thrombocytopenia, coagulation disorder, or an increase in bleeding tendency due to other causes.

WARNINGS:

Patients being treated with Mutamycin must be observed carefully and frequently during and after therapy.

The use of Mutamycin results in a high incidence of bone marrow suppression, particularly thrombocytopenia and leukopenia. Therefore, the following studies should be obtained repeatedly during therapy and for at least eight weeks following therapy: platelet count, white blood cell count, differential, and hemoglobin. The occurrence of a platelet count below $100{,}000/mm^3$ or a WBC below $4{,}000/mm^3$ or a progressive decline in either is an indication to withhold further therapy until blood counts have recovered above these levels.

Patients should be advised of the potential toxicity of this drug, particularly bone marrow suppression. Deaths have been reported due to septicemia as a result of leukopenia due to the drug.

Patients receiving Mutamycin should be observed for evidence of renal toxicity. Mutamycin should not be given to patients with a serum creatinine greater than 1.7 mg percent.

Usage in Pregnancy - Safe use of Mutamycin in pregnant women has not been established. Teratological changes have been noted in animal studies. The effect of Mutamycin on fertility is unknown.

PRECAUTIONS:

Acute shortness of breath and severe bronchospasm have been reported following the administration of vinca alkaloids in patients who had previously or simultaneously received Mutamycin. The onset of this acute respiratory distress occurred within minutes to hours after the vinca alkaloid injection. The total number of doses for each drug have varied considerably. Bronchodilators, steroids and/or oxygen have produced symptomatic relief.

A few cases of adult respiratory distress syndrome have been reported in patients receiving Mutamycin in combination with other chemotherapy and maintained at FIO_2 concentrations greater than 50% perioperatively. Therefore, caution should be exercised using only enough oxygen to provide adequate arterial saturation since oxygen itself is toxic to the lungs. Careful attention should be paid to fluid balance and overhydration should be avoided.

ADVERSE REACTIONS:

Bone Marrow Toxicity - This was the most common and most serious toxicity, occurring in 605 of 937 patients (64.4%). Thrombocytopenia and/or leukopenia may occur anytime within 8 weeks after onset of therapy with an average time of 4 weeks. Recovery after cessation of therapy was within 10 weeks. About 25% of the leukopenic or thrombocytopenic episodes did not recover. Mutamycin produces cumulative myelosuppression.

Integument and Mucus Membrane Toxicity - This has occurred in approximately 4% of patients treated with Mutamycin. Cellulitis at the injection site has been reported and is occasionally severe. Stomatitis and alopecia also occur frequently. Rashes are rarely reported. The most important dermatological problem with this drug, however, is the necrosis and consequent sloughing of tissue which results if the drug is extravasated during injection. Extravasation may occur with or without an accompanying stinging or burning sensation and even if there is adequate blood return when the injection needle is aspirated. There have been reports of delayed erythema and/or ulceration occurring either at or distant from the injection site, weeks to months after Mutamycin, even when no obvious evidence of extravasation was observed during administration. Skin grafting has been required in some of the cases.

Renal Toxicity - 2% of 1,281 patients demonstrated a statistically significant rise in creatinine. There appeared to be no correlation between total dose administered or duration of therapy and the degree of renal impairment.

Pulmonary Toxicity - This has occurred infrequently but can be severe and may be life threatening. Dyspnea with a nonproductive cough and radiographic evidence of pulmonary infiltrates may be indicative of Mutamycin-induced pulmonary toxicity. If other etiologies are eliminated, Mutamycin therapy should be discontinued. Steroids have been employed as treatment of this toxicity, but the therapeutic value has not been determined. A few cases of adult respiratory distress syndrome have been reported in patients receiving Mutamycin in combination with other chemotherapy and maintained at FIO_2 concentrations greater than 50% perioperatively.

Hemolytic Uremic Syndrome (HUS) - This serious complication of chemotherapy, consisting primarily of microangiopathic hemolytic anemia (hematocrit $\leq$ 25%, thrombocytopenia ($\leq$ 100,000/mm^3), and irreversible renal failure (serum creatinine $\geq$ 1.6 mg/dl) has been reported in patients receiving systemic Mutamycin. Microangiopathic hemolysis with fragmented red blood cells on peripheral blood smears has occurred in 98% of patients with the syndrome. Other less frequent complications of the syndrome may include pulmonary edema (65%), neurologic abnormalities (16%), and hypertension. Exacerbation of the symptoms associated with HUS has been reported in some patients receiving blood product transfusions. A high mortality rate (52%) has been associated with this syndrome.

The syndrome may occur at any time during systemic therapy with Mutamycin as a single agent or in combination with other cytotoxic drugs. Less frequently, HUS has also been reported in patients receiving combinations of cytotoxic drugs not including Mutamycin. Of 83 patients studied, 72 developed the syndrome at total dose exceeding 60 mg of Mutamycin. Consequently, patients receiving $\geq$ 60 mg of Mutamycin should be monitored closely for unexplained anemia with fragmented cells on peripheral blood smear, thrombocytopenia, and decreased renal function.

The incidence of the syndrome has not been defined.

Therapy for the syndrome is investigational.

Cardiac Toxicity -Congestive heart failure, often treated effectively with diuretics and cardiac glycosides, has rarely been reported. Almost all patients who experienced this side effect had received prior doxorubicin therapy.

Acute Side Effects Due to Mutamycin were fever, anorexia, nausea, and vomiting. They occurred in about 14% of 1,281 patients.

Other Undesirable Side Effects that have been reported during Mutamycin therapy have been headache, blurring of vision, confusion, drowsiness syncope, fatigue, edema, thrombophlebitis, hematemesis, diarrhea, and pain. These did not appear to be dose related and were not unequivocally drug related. They may have been due to the primary or metastatic disease processes.

DOSAGE AND ADMINISTRATION:

Mutamycin should be given intravenously only, using care to avoid extravasation of the compound. If extravasation occurs, cellulitis, ulceration, and slough may result.

Each vial contains either mitomycin 5 mg and mannitol 10 mg, mitomycin 20 mg and mannitol 40 mg, or mitomycin 40 mg and mannitol 80 mg. To administer, add Sterile Water for Injection, 10 ml, 40 ml, or 80 ml respectively. Shake to dissolve. If product does not dissolve immediately, allow to stand at room temperature until solution is obtained.

After full hematological recovery (see guide to dosage adjustment) from any previous chemotherapy, the following dosage schedule may be used at 6 to 8 week intervals:

20 mg/m^2 intravenously as a single dose via a functioning intravenous catheter.

Because of cumulative myelosuppression, patients should be fully reevaluated after each course of Mutamycin, and the dose reduced if the patient has experienced any toxicities. Doses greater than 20 mg/m^2 have not been shown to be more effective, and are more toxic than lower doses.

TABLE 1 is suggested as a guide to dosage adjustment:

TABLE 1 Mutamycin, DOSAGE AND ADMINISTRATION Nadir After Prior Dose

Leukocytes/mm^3	Platelets/mm^3	Percentage of Prior Dose to be given
>4000	>100,000	100%
3000-3999	75,000-99,999	100%
2000-2999	25,000-74,999	70%
<2000	<25,000	50%

No repeat dosage should be given until leukocyte count has returned to 4000/mm^3 and platelet count to 100,000/mm^3.

When Mutamycin is used in combination with other myelosuppressive agents, the doses should be adjusted accordingly. If the disease continues to progress after two courses of Mutamycin, the drug should be stopped since chances of response are minimal.

DOSAGE AND ADMINISTRATION: *(cont'd)*

STABILITY

1. Unreconstituted Mutamycin stored at room temperature is stable for the lot life indicated on the package. Avoid excessive heat (over 40°C).

2. Reconstituted with Sterile Water for Injection to a concentration of 0.5 mg per ml, Mutamycin is stable for 14 days refrigerated or 7 days at room temperature.

3. Dilutedin various IV fluids at room temperature, to a concentration of 20 to 40 micrograms per ml (TABLE 2):

TABLE 2 Mutamycin, DOSAGE AND ADMINISTRATION

IV Fluid	Stability
5% Dextrose Injection	3 hours
0.9% Sodium Chloride Injection	12 hours
Sodium Lactate Injection	24 hours

4. The combination of Mutamycin (5 mg to 15 mg) and heparin (1,000 units to 10,000 units) in 30 ml of 0.9% Sodium Chloride Injection is stable for 48 hours at room temperature.

Procedures for proper handling and disposal of anticancer drugs should be considered. Several guidelines on this subject have been published.[1-7]

There is no general agreement that all of the procedures recommended in the guidelines are necessary of appropriate.

REFERENCES:

1 . Recommendations for the Safe Handling of Parenteral Antineoplastic Drugs. NIH Publication No. 83-2621. For sale by the Superintendent of Documents, US Government Printing Office, Washington, DC 20402. **2.** AMA Council Report. Guidelines for Handling Parenteral Antineoplastics, JAMA 1985 March 15. **3.** National Study Commission on Cytotoxic Exposure-Recommendations for Handling Cytotoxic Agents. Available from Louis P. Jeffrey, Sc.D., Chairmen, National Study Commission on Cytotoxic Exposure, Massachusetts College of Pharmacy and Allied Health Sciences, 179 Longwood Avenue, Boston, Massachusetts 02115. **4.** Clinical Oncological Society of Australia. Guidelines and Recommendations for Safe Handling of Antineoplastic Agents. Med J Australia 1983; 1:426-428. **5.** Jones RB, et al: Safe handling of chemotherapeutic agents: A report from the Mount Sinai Medical Center. CA-A Cancer Journal for Clinicians 1983; (Sept/Oct) 258-263. **6.** American Society of Hospital Pharmacists Technical Assistance Bulletin on Handling Cytotoxic Drugs in Hospitals. Am J Hosp Pharm 1985; 42:131-137. **7.** OSHA Work-Practice Guidelines for Personnel Dealing with Cytotoxic (Antineoplastic) Drugs. Am J Hosp Pharm 1986; 43:1193-1204.

HOW SUPPLIED - RATED THERAPEUTICALLY EQUIVALENT:

Injection, Dry-Soln - Intravenous - 5 mg/vial

5 mg $128.77 MUTAMYCIN, Mead Johnson 00015-3001-20

Injection, Dry-Soln - Intravenous - 20 mg

1's $434.87 MUTAMYCIN, Mead Johnson 00015-3002-22

20 mg $434.87 MUTAMYCIN, Mead Johnson 00015-3002-20

HOW SUPPLIED - NOT RATED EQUIVALENT:

Injection, Solution - Intravenous - 40 mg/vial

40 mg $878.63 MUTAMYCIN, Mead Johnson 00015-3059-20

MITOTANE *(001822)*

CATEGORIES: Adrenal Function; Antineoplastics; Cancer; Oncologic Drugs; Pregnancy Category C; FDA Approval Pre 1982

BRAND NAMES: **Lysodren**; *Opeprim* (Japan)
(International brand names outside U.S. in italics)

FORMULARIES: Medi-Cal

Mitotane should be administered under the supervision of a qualified physician experienced in the uses of cancer chemotherapeutic agents. Mitotane should be temporarily discontinued immediately following shock or severe trauma since adrenal suppression is its prime action. Exogenous steroids should be administered in such circumstances, since the depressed adrenal may not immediately start to secret steroids.

DESCRIPTION:

Mitotane is an oral chemotherapeutic agent. It is best known by its trivial name, o,p'-DDD, and is chemically, 1,1-dichloro-2-(0-chlorophenyl)-2-(p-chlorophenyl) ethane.

Mitotane is a white granular solid composed of clear colorless crystals. It is tasteless and has a slight pleasant aromatic odor. It is soluble in ethanol, isoctane and carbon tetrachloride. It has a molecular weight of 320.05.

Inactive ingredients in Lysodren tablets are: avicel, Polyethylene Glycol 4000, silicon dioxide, and starch.

Lysodren is available as 500 mg scored tablets for oral administration.

CLINICAL PHARMACOLOGY:

Mitotane can best be described as an adrenal cytotoxic agent, although it can cause adrenal inhibition, apparently without cellular destruction. Its biochemical mechanism of action is unknown. Data are available to suggest that the drug modifies the peripheral metabolism of steroids as well as directly suppressing the adrenal cortex. The administration of mitotane alters the extra-adrenal metabolism of cortisol in man; leading to a reduction in measurable 17-hydroxy corticosteroids, even though plasma levels of corticosteroids do not fall. The drug apparently causes increased formation of 6-B-hydroxyl cortisol.

Data in adrenal carcinoma patients indicate that about 40% of oral mitotane is absorbed and approximately 10% of administered dose is recovered in the urine as water-soluble metabolite. A variable amount of metabolite (1 to 17%) is excreted in the bile and the balance is apparently stored in the tissues.

Following discontinuation of mitotane, the plasma terminal half life has ranged from 18 to 159 days. In most patients blood levels become undetectable after six to nine weeks. Autopsy data have provided evidence that mitotane is found in most tissues of the body; however, fat tissues are the primary site of storage. Mitotane us converted to a water-soluble metabolite. No unchanged mitotane has been found in urine or bile.

INDICATIONS AND USAGE:

Mitotane is indicated in the treatment of inoperable adrenal cortical carcinoma of both functional and non-functional types.

CONTRAINDICATIONS:

Mitotane should not be given to individuals who have demonstrated a previous hypersensitivity to it.

WARNINGS:

Mitotane should be temporarily discontinued immediately following shock or severe trauma, since adrenal suppression is its prime action. Exogenous steroids should be administered in such circumstances, since the depressed adrenal may not immediately start to secrete steroids.

Mitotane should be administered with care to patients with liver disease other than metastatic lesions from the adrenal cortex, since the metabolism of mitotane may be interfered with and the drug may accumulate.

All possible tumor tissues should be surgically removed from large metastatic masses before mitotane administration is instituted. This is necessary to minimize the possibility of infarction and hemorrhage in the tumor due to a rapid cytotoxic effect of the drug.

Long-term continuous administration f high doses of mitotane may lead to brain damage and impairment of function. Behavioral and neurological assessments should be made at regular intervals when continuous mitotane treatment exceeds two years.

A substantial percentage of the patients treated show signs of adrenal insufficiency. It therefore appears necessary too watch for and institute steroid replacement in those patients. However, some investigators have recommended that steroid replacement therapy be administered concomitantly with mitotane. It has been shown that the metabolism of exogenous steroids is modified and consequently somewhat higher doses than normal replacement therapy may be required.

PRECAUTIONS:

General: Adrenal insufficiency may develop in patients treated with Mitotane, and adrenal steroid replacement should be considered for these patients.

Since sedation, lethargy, vertigo, and other CNS side effect can occur, ambulatory patients should be cautioned about driving, operating machinery, and other hazardous pursuits requiring mental and physical alertness.

Carcinogenesis, Mutagenesis, and Impairment of Fertility: The carcinogenic and mutagenic potential of mitotane are unknown. However, the mechanism of action of this compound suggests that it probably has less carcinogenic potential than other cytotoxic chemotherapeutic drugs.

Pregnancy Category C: Animal reproduction studies have not been conducted with mitotane. It is also not known whether mitotane can cause fetal harm when administered to a pregnant women or can affect reproduction capacity. Mitotane should be given to a pregnant woman only if clearly needed.

Nursing Mothers: It is not known whether this drug is excreted in human milk. Because many drugs are excreted in human milk and because of the potential for adverse reactions in nursing infants from mitotane, a decision should be made whether to discontinue nursing or to discontinue the drug, taking into account the importance of the drug to the mother.

DRUG INTERACTIONS:

Mitotane has been reported to accelerate the metabolism of warfarin by the mechanism of hepatic microsomal enzyme induction, leading to an increase in dosage requirements for warfarin. Therefore, physicians should closely monitor patients for a change in anticoagulant dosage requirements when administering Mitotane to patients on coumarin-type anticoagulants. In addition, mitotane should be given with caution to patients receiving other drugs susceptible to the influence of hepatic enzyme induction.

ADVERSE REACTIONS:

A very high percentage of patients treated with mitotane have shown at least one type off side effects. The main types of adverse reactions consist of the following:

1. Gastrointestinal disturbances, which consist of anorexia, nausea or vomiting, and in some cases diarrhea, occur in about 80% of the patients.

2. Central nervous system side effects occur in 40% of the patients. These consist primarily of depression as manifested by lethargy and somnolence (25%), and dizziness or vertigo (15%).

3. Skin toxicity has been observed in about 15% of the cases. These skin changes consist primarily of transient skin rashes which do not seem to be dose-related. In some instances, this side effect subsided while the patients were maintained on the drug without a change of dose.

Infrequently occurring side effects involve the eye (visual blurring, diplopia, lens opacity, toxic retinopathy); the genitourinary system (hematuria, hemorrhagic cystitis, and albuminuria); cardiovascular system (hypertension, orthostatic hypotension, and flushing); and some miscellaneous effect including generalized aching, hyperpyrexia, and lowered protein bound iodine (PBI).

OVERDOSAGE:

No proven antidotes have been established for mitotane overdosage.

DOSAGE AND ADMINISTRATION:

The recommended treatment schedule is to start the patient at 2 to 6 g of Mitotane per day in divided doses, either three or four times a day. Doses are usually increased incrementally to 9 to 10 g per day. If severe side effects appear, the dose should be reduced until the maximum tolerated dose is achieved. If the patient can tolerate higher doses and improved clinical response appears possible, the dose should be increased until adverse reactions interfere. Experience has shown that the maximum tolerated dose (MTD) will very from 2 to 16 g per day, but has usually been 9 to 10 g per day. The highest doses used in the studies to date were 18 to 19 g per day.

Treatment should be instituted in the hospital until a stable dosage regimen is achieved.

Treatment should be continued as long as clinical benefits are observed. Maintenance of clinical status or slowing of growth of metastatic lesions can be considered clinical benefits if they can clearly be shown to have occurred.

If no clinical benefits are observed after three months at the maximum tolerated dose, the case would generally be considered a clinical failure. However, 10% of the patients who showed a measurable response required more than three months at the MTD. Early diagnosis and prompt institution of treatment improve the probability of a positive clinical response. Clinical effectiveness can be shown by reduction in tumor mass, reduction in pain, weakness or anorexia and reduction of symptoms and signs due to excessive steroid production.

A number of patients have been treated intermittently with treatment being restarted when severe symptoms have reappeared. Patients often do not respond after the third or fourth such course. Experience accumulated to date suggests that continuous treatment with the maximum possible dosage of Mitotane is the best approach.

Procedure for proper handling and disposal of anti-cancer drugs should be considered. Several guideline on this subject have been published.[1-6] There is no general agreement that all of the procedures recommended in the guidelines are necessary or appropriate.

REFERENCES:

1. Recommendations for the Safe Handling or Parenteral Antineoplastic Drugs. NIH Publication No. 83-2621. For sale by the superintendent of Documents, U.S. Government Printing Office, Washington, D.C. 20402 **2.** AMA Council Report. Guidelines for handling Parenteral antineoplastics. JAMA, March 15, 1985. **3.** National Study Commission on Cytotoxic Exposure — Recommendations for Handling Cytotoxic Agents. Available from

REFERENCES: *(cont'd)*

Louis P. Jeffrey, Sc. D., Director of Pharmacy Services, Rhode Island Hospital, 593 Eddy Street, Providence, Rhode Island 02902. **4.** Clinical Oncological Society of Australia: Guidelines and recommendations for Safe Handling of Antineoplastic Agents. Med J. Australia 1:426-428, 1983. **5.** Jones, R.B., et. al. Safe Handling of Chemotherapeutic Agents: A report from the Mount Sinai Medical Center. Ca- A Cancer Journal for Clinicians Sept./Oct. 258-263, 1983. **6.** American Society of Hospital Pharmacists Technical Assistance Bulletin on Handling Cytotoxic Drugs in Hospital. Am. J. Hosp. Pharm. 42:131- 137, 1985.Tablets may be stored at room temperature.

HOW SUPPLIED - EQUIVALENTS NOT AVAILABLE:

Tablet, Enteric Coated - Oral - 500 mg

100's $204.38 LYSODREN, Mead Johnson 00015-3080-60

MITOXANTRONE HYDROCHLORIDE *(001823)*

CATEGORIES: Acute Nonlymphocytic Leukemia; Antimetabolites; Antineoplastics; Breast Carcinoma; Cytotoxic Agents; Leukemia; Oncologic Drugs; Orphan Drugs; Pregnancy Category D; FDA Approved 1987 Dec

BRAND NAMES: *Misostol* (Mexico); *Mitroxone* (Mexico); *Novantone*; *Novantron* (Germany); **Novantrone**; *Oncotron*
(International brand names outside U.S. in italics)

FORMULARIES: BC-BS; Medi-Cal

DESCRIPTION:

Mitoxantrone hydrochloride is a synthetic antineoplastic anthracenedione for intravenous use. Its molecular formula is $C_{22}H_{28}N_4O_6{\cdot}2HCl$ and its molecular weight is 517.41. It is supplied as a concentrate which MUST BE DILUTED PRIOR TO INJECTION. The concentrate is a sterile, non-pyrogenic, dark blue aqueous solution containing mitoxantrone hydrochloride equivalent to 2 mg/ml mitoxantrone free base, with sodium chloride (0.80% w/v), sodium acetate (0.005% w/v), and acetic acid (0.046% w/v) as inactive ingredients. The solution has a pH of 3.0 to 4.5 and contains 0.14 mEq of sodium per ml. The product does not contain preservatives.

1,4-Dihydroxy-5,8 bis((2-((2-hydroxyethyl)amino)ethyl)amino)-9, 10-anthracenedione dihydrochloride

CLINICAL PHARMACOLOGY:

Although its mechanism of action is not fully elucidated, mitoxantrone is a DNA-reactive agent. It has a cytocidal effect on both proliferating and nonproliferating cultured human cells, suggesting lack of cell cycle phase specificity. Pharmacokinetic studies have not been performed in humans receiving multiple daily doses. Pharmacokinetic studies in adult patients following a single intravenous administration of mitoxantrone have demonstrated multi-exponential plasma clearance. Distribution to tissues is rapid and extensive. Distribution to the brain, spinal cord, eye, and spinal fluid in the monkey is low. The apparent steady state volume of distribution exceeds 1000L/m^2. Elimination of drug is slow with an apparent mean terminal plasma half-life of 5.8 days (range 2.3-13.0). The half-life in tissues may be longer.

Multiple intravenous doses in dogs daily for five days resulted in significant accumulation in plasma and tissue. The extent of accumulation was four fold.

Mitoxantrone is 78% bound of plasma proteins in the observed concentration range of 26-455 mg/ml. This binding is independent of concentration and was not affected by the presence of diphenylhydantoin, doxorubicin, methotrexate, prednisone, prednisolone, heparin, or acetylsalicylic acid.

Mitoxantrone is excreted via the renal and hepatobiliary systems. Renal excretion is limited; only 6% - 11% of the dose is recovered in the urine within five days after drug administration. Of the material recovered in the urine, 65% is unchanged drug; the remaining 35% is comprised primarily of two inactive metabolites and their glucuronide conjugates. The metabolites are mono- and dicarboxylic acid derivatives. Hepatobiliary elimination of drug appears to be of greater significance with as much as 25% of the dose recovered in the feces within five days of intravenous dosing. No significant difference in the pharmacokinetics of mitoxantrone was observed in 7 patients with moderately impaired liver function (serum bilirubin 1.3-3.4 mg/dl) as compared with 16 patients without hepatic dysfunction. Results of pharmacokinetic studies on 4 patients with severe hepatic dysfunction (bilirubin greater than 3.4 mg/dl) suggest that these patients have a lower total body clearance and a larger Area under Curve than other patients at a comparable mitoxantrone dose.

In two large randomized multicenter trials, remission induction therapy for ANLL with mitoxantrone 12 mg/m^2 daily for three days as a 10-minute intravenous infusion and cytosine arabinoside 100 mg/m^{2}for seven days given as a continuous 24 hour infusion was compared with daunorubicin 45 mg/m^2 daily by intravenous infusion for three days plus the same dose and schedule of cytosine arabinoside used with mitoxantrone. Patients who had an incomplete antileukemic response received a second induction course in which mitoxantrone or daunorubicin was given for two days and cytosine arabinoside for five days using the same daily dosage schedule. Response rates and median survival information for both the U.S. and international multicenter trials are given in the following table (TABLE 1):

TABLE 1

Trial	% Complete Response(CR)		Median Time to CR (days)		Median Survival Days	
	NOV[1]	DAUN[2]	NOV	DAUN	NOV	DAUN
U.S	63 (62/98)	53 (54/102)	35	42	312	237
Foreign	50 (56/112)	51 (62/123)	36	42	192	230

1 NOV = Novantrone + Cystosine arabinoside
2 DAUN = Daunorubicin + Cystosine arabinoside

In these studies, two consolidation courses were administered to complete responders on each arm. Consolidation therapy consisted of the same drug and daily dosage used for remission induction, but only five days of cytosine arabinoside and two days of mitoxantrone or daunorubicin were given. The first consolidation course was administered 6 weeks after the start of the final induction course if the patient achieved a complete remission. The second consolidation course was generally administered 4 weeks later. Full hematologic recovery was necessary for patients to receive consolidation therapy. For the U.S. trial, median granulocyte nadirs for patients receiving mitoxantrone + cytosine arabinoside for consolidation courses 1 and 2 were 10/mm^3 for both courses, and for those patients receiving daunorubicin + cytosine arabinoside were 170/mm^3 and 260/mm^3, respectively. Median platelet nadirs for patients who received mitoxantrone + cytosine arabinoside for consolidation courses 1 and 2 were 17,000/mm^3 and 14,000/mm^3 respectively, and were 33,000/mm^3 and 22,000/mm^3 in courses 1 and 2 for those patient who received daunorubicin + cytosine arabinoside. The benefit of consolidation therapy in ANLL patients who achieve a complete remission remains controversial. However, in the only well-controlled prospective, randomized multicenter trials

CLINICAL PHARMACOLOGY: *(cont'd)*

with mitoxantrone in ANLL, consolidation therapy was given to all patients who achieved a complete remission. During consolidation in the U.S. study, two myelosuppression related deaths occurred on the mitoxantrone arm and one on the daunorubicin arm. However, in the foreign study there were eight deaths on the mitoxantrone arm during consolidation which were related to the myelosuppression and none on the daunorubicin arm where less myelosuppression occurred.

INDICATIONS AND USAGE:

Mitoxantrone in combination with other approved drug(s) is indicated in the initial therapy of acute nonlymphocytic leukemia (ANLL) in adults. This category includes myelogenous, promyelocytic, monocytic, and erythroid acute leukemias.

CONTRAINDICATIONS:

Mitoxantrone is contraindicated in patients who have demonstrated prior hypersensitivity to it.

WARNINGS:

WHEN MITOXANTRONE IS USED IN DOSES INDICATED FOR THE TREATMENT OF LEUKEMIA, SEVERE MYELOSUPPRESSION WILL OCCUR. THEREFORE, IT IS RECOMMENDED THAT MITOXANTRONE BE ADMINISTERED ONLY BY PHYSICIANS EXPERIENCED IN THE CHEMOTHERAPY OF THIS DISEASE. LABORATORY AND SUPPORTIVE SERVICES MUST BE AVAILABLE FOR HEMATOLOGIC AND CHEMISTRY MONITORING AND ADJUNCTIVE THERAPIES, INCLUDING ANTIBIOTICS: BLOOD AND BLOOD PRODUCTS MUST BE AVAILABLE TO SUPPORT PATIENTS DURING THE EXPECTED PERIOD OF MEDULLARY HYPOPLASIA AND SEVERE MYELOSUPPRESSION. PARTICULAR CARE SHOULD BE GIVEN TO ASSURING FULL HEMATOLOGIC RECOVERY BEFORE UNDERTAKING CONSOLIDATION THERAPY (IF THIS TREATMENT IS USED) AND PATIENTS SHOULD BE MONITORED CLOSELY DURING THIS PHASE.

Patients with preexisting myelosuppression as the result of prior drug therapy should not receive mitoxantrone unless it is felt that the possible benefit from such treatment warrants the risk of further medullary suppression. Because of the possible danger of cardiac effects in patients previously treated with daunorubicin or doxorubicin, the benefit-to-risk ratio of mitoxantrone therapy in such patients should be determined before starting therapy.

The safety of mitoxantrone in patients with hepatic insufficiency is not established. (see CLINICAL PHARMACOLOGY.)

CARDIAC EFFECTS

General: Functional cardiac changes including congestive heart failure and decreases in left ventricular ejection fraction (LVEF) occur with mitoxantrone. Cardiac toxicity may be more common in patients with prior treatment with anthracyclines, prior mediastinal radiotherapy, or with preexisting cardiovascular disease. Such patients should have regular cardiac monitoring of LVEF from the initiation of therapy. In investigational trials of intermittent single doses in other tumor types, patients who received up to the cumulative dose of 140 mg/m^2 had a cumulative 2.6% probability of clinical congestive heart failure. The overall cumulative probability rate of moderate or serious decreases in LVEF at this dose was 13% in comparative trials.

Leukemia: Acute CHF may occasionally occur in patients treated with mitoxantrone for ANLL. In first-line comparative trials of mitoxantrone + cytosine arabinoside vs daunorubicin + cytosine arabinoside in adult patients with previously untreated ANLL, therapy was associated with congestive heart failure in 6.5% of patients on each arm. A causal relationship between drug therapy and cardiac effects is difficult to establish in this setting since myocardial function is frequently depressed by the anemia, fever and infection, and hemorrhage which often accompany the underlying disease.

Pregnancy Category D: Mitoxantrone may cause fetal harm when administered to a pregnant woman. In treated rats, low fetal birth weight and retarded development of the fetal kidney were seen in greater frequency. In rabbits, an increased incidence of premature delivery was observed. Mitoxantrone was not teratogenic in rabbits. There are no adequate and well-controlled studies in pregnant women. If this drug is used during pregnancy, or if the patient becomes pregnant while taking this drug, the patient should be apprised of the potential hazard to the fetus. Women of childbearing potential should be advised to avoid becoming pregnant.

Safety for use by routes other than intravenous administration was not been established.

PRECAUTIONS:

General: Therapy with mitoxantrone should be accompanied by close and frequent monitoring of hematologic and chemical laboratory parameters, as well as frequent patient observation.

Hyperuricemia may occur as a result of rapid lysis of tumor cells by mitoxantrone. Serum uric acid levels should be monitored and hypouricemic therapy instituted prior to the initiation of antileukemic therapy.

Systemic infections should be treated concomitantly with or just prior to commencing therapy with mitoxantrone.

Information for the Patient: Mitoxantrone may impart a blue-green color to the urine for 24 hours after administration, and patients should be advised to expect this during therapy. Bluish discoloration of the sclera may also occur. Patients should be advised of the signs and symptoms of myelosuppression.

Laboratory Tests: Serial complete blood counts and liver function tests are necessary for appropriate dose adjustments. (see DOSAGE AND ADMINISTRATION.)

Carcinogenesis, Mutagenesis: Mitoxantrone can result in chromosomal aberrations in animals and it is mutagenic in bacterial systems. Mitoxantrone caused DNA damage and sister chromatid exchanges *in vitro*.

Pregnancy Category D (see WARNINGS.)

Nursing Mothers: It is not known whether mitoxantrone is excreted in human milk. Because of the potential for serious adverse reactions in infants from mitoxantrone, breast feeding should be discontinued before starting treatment.

Pediatric Use: Safety and effectiveness in children have not been established.

ADVERSE REACTIONS:

Mitoxantrone has been studied in approximately 600 patients with acute nonlymphocytic leukemia. The table below represents the adverse reaction experience in the large U.S. comparative study of mitoxantrone plus cytosine arabinoside vs daunorubicin plus cytosine arabinoside. Experience in the large foreign study was similar. A much wider experience in a variety of other tumor types revealed no additional important reactions other than cardiomyopathy (see WARNINGS.) It should be appreciated that the listed adverse reaction categories include overlapping clinical symptoms related to the same condition e.g. dyspnea, cough and pneumonia. In addition, the listed adverse reactions cannot all necessarily be attributed to chemotherapy as it is often impossible to distinguish effects of the drug and

ADVERSE REACTIONS: *(cont'd)*

effects of the underlying disease. It is clear, however, that the combination of mitoxantrone plus cytosine arabinoside was responsible for nausea and vomiting, alopecia, mucositis/stomatitis, and myelosuppression.

The following table (TABLE 2) summarizes adverse reactions occurring in patients treated with mitoxantrone + cytosine arabinoside in comparison with those who received daunorubicin + cytosine arabinoside for therapy of ANLL in a large multicenter randomized prospective U.S. trial. Adverse reactions are presented as major categories and selected examples of clinically significant subcategories.

TABLE 2

	All Induction (percentage of pts entering induction)		All Consolidation (percentage of pts entering consolidation)	
	NOV N = 102	DAUN N = 102	NOV N = 55	DAUN N = 49
Cardiovascular	26	28	11	24
CHF	5	6	0	0
Arrhythmias	3	3	4	4
Bleeding	37	41	20	6
GI	16	12	2	2
Petechiae/Ecchymoses	7	9	11	2
Gastrointestinal	88	85	58	51
Nausea/Vomiting	72	67	31	31
Diarrhea	47	47	18	8
Abdominal Pain	15	9	9	4
Mucositis/Stomatitis	29	33	18	8
Hepatic	10	11	14	2
Jaundice	3	8	7	0
Infections	66	73	60	43
UTI	7	2	7	2
Pneumonia	9	7	9	0
Sepsis	34	36	31	18
Fungal Infections	15	13	9	6
Renal Failure	8	6	0	2
Fever	78	71	24	18
Alopecia	37	40	22	16
Pulmonary	43	43	24	14
Cough	13	9	9	2
Dyspnea	18	20	6	0
CNS	30	30	34	35
Seizures	4	4	2	8
Headache	10	9	13	8
Eye	7	6	2	4
Conjunctivitis	5	1	0	0

Allergic Reaction: Hypotension, urticaria, dyspnea and rashes have been reported occasionally.

Cutaneous: Phlebitis has been reported infrequently at the site of infusion. There have been rare reports of tissue necrosis following extravasation.

Hematologic: Myelosuppression is rapid in onset and is consistent with the requirement to produce significant marrow hypoplasia in order to achieve a response. The incidences of infection and bleeding seen in the U.S. trial are consistent with those reported for other standard induction regimens.

Gastrointestinal: Nausea and vomiting occurred acutely in most patients, but were generally mild to moderate and could be controlled through the use of antiemetics. Stomatitis/mucositis occurs within one week of therapy.

Cardiovascular: Congestive heart failure, tachycardia, EKG changes including arrhythmias, chest pain and asymptomatic decreases in left ventricular ejection fraction have occurred (see WARNINGS.)

OVERDOSAGE:

There is no known specific antidote for mitoxantrone. Accidental overdoses have been reported. Four patients receiving 140 - 180 mg/m^2as a single bolus injection died as a result of severe leukopenia with infection. Hematologic support and antimicrobial therapy may be required during prolonged periods of medullary hypoplasia.

Although patients with severe renal failure have not been studied, mitoxantrone is extensively tissue bound and it is unlikely that the therapeutic affect or toxicity would be mitigated by peritoneal or hemodialysis.

DOSAGE AND ADMINISTRATION:

(See WARNINGS.)

MITOXANTRONE SOLUTION MUST BE DILUTED PRIOR TO USE. *Combination Initial Therapy for ANLL in Adults:* For induction, the recommended dosage is 12 mg/m^2 of mitoxantrone daily on days 1-3 given as an intravenous infusion, and 100 mg/m^2 of cytosine arabinoside for seven days given as a continuous 24 hours infusion on days 1-7.

Most complete remissions will occur following the initial course of induction therapy. In the event of an incomplete antileukemic response, a second induction course may be given. Mitoxantrone should be given for two days and cytosine arabinoside for five days using the same daily dosage levels.

If severe or life-threatening nonhematologic toxicity is observed during the first induction course, the second induction course should be withheld until toxicity clears.

Consolidation therapy which was used in two large randomized multicenter trials consisted of mitoxantrone 12 mg/m^2 given by intravenous infusion daily for days 1 and 2, and cytosine arabinoside, 100 mg/m^2 for 5 days given as a continuous 24 hour infusion on days 1-5. The first course was given approximately 6 weeks after the final induction course, the second was generally administered 4 weeks after the first. Severe myelosuppression occurred. (See CLINICAL PHARMACOLOGY.)

The dose of mitoxantrone should be diluted to at least 50 ml with either 0.9% Sodium Chloride Injection (USP) or 5% Dextrose Injection (USP). This solution should be introduced slowly into the tubing as a freely running intravenous infusion of 0.9% Sodium Chloride Injection (USP) or 5% Dextrose Injection (USP) over a period of not less than 3 minutes. Unused infusion solutions should be discarded immediately in an appropriate fashion. In the case of multidose use, the remaining portion of the undiluted mitoxantrone concentrate should be stored not longer than 7 days between 15°C (59°F) and 25°C (77°F) or 14 days under refrigeration. If extravasation occurs, the administration should be stopped immediately and restarted in another vein. The nonvesicant properties of mitoxantrone minimized the possibility of severe local reactions following extravasation. However, care should be taken to avoid extravasation at the infusion site and to avoid contact of mitoxantrone with the skin, mucous membranes or eyes.

DOSAGE AND ADMINISTRATION: *(cont'd)*

Skin accidentally exposed to mitoxantrone should be rinsed copiously with warm water and if the eyes are involved, standard irrigation techniques should be used immediately. The use of goggles, gloves, and protective gowns is recommended during preparation and administration of the drug. Spills on equipment and environmental surfaces may be cleaned using an aqueous solution of calcium hypochlorite (5.5 parts calcium hypochlorite in 13 parts by weight of water for each 1 part of mitoxantrone. Absorb the solution with gauze or towels and dispose of these in a safe manner. Appropriate safety equipment such as goggles and gloves should be worn while working with calcium hypochlorite. Mitoxantrone should not be mixed in the same infusion as heparin since a precipitate may form. Because specific compatibility data are not available, it is recommended that mitoxantrone not be mixed in the same infusion with other drugs.

Procedures for proper handling and disposal of anticancer drugs should be considered. Several guidelines on this subject have been published.[1-6] There is no general agreement that all of the procedures recommended in the guidelines are necessary or appropriate.

Mitoxantrone may be further diluted into Dextrose 5% in Water, Normal Saline or Dextrose 5% with Normal Saline and used immediately. DO NOT FREEZE.

Parenteral drug products should be inspected visually for particulate matter and discoloration prior to administration whenever solution and container permit.

Mitoxantrone should be stored between 15°C (59°F) and 25°C (77°F). DO NOT FREEZE.

After the penetration of the stopper, the remaining portion of mitoxantrone may be stored no longer than 7 days between 15°C (59°F) and 25°C (77°F) or 14 days under refrigeration. CONTAINS NO PRESERVATIVE.

REFERENCES:

1. Recommendations for the Safe Handling of Parenteral Antineoplastic Drugs. NIH Publication No. 83-2621. For sale by the Superintendent of Documents, U.S. Government Printing Office, Washington, D.C. 20402. 2. AMA Council Report. Guidelines for Handling Parenteral Antineoplastics.*JAMA*, March 15, 1985. 3. National Study Commission on Cytotoxic Exposure - Recommendations for Handling Cytotoxic Agents. Available from Louis P. Jeffrey, Sc. D., Director of Pharmacy Services, Rhode Island Hospital, 593 Eddy Street, Providence, Rhode Island 02902. 4. Clinical Oncological Society of Australia; Guidelines and recommendations for safe handling of antineoplastic agents. *Med J Australia* 1983; 1:426-428. 5. Jones RB, et al. Safe handling of chemotherapeutic agents: A report from the Mount Sinai Medical Center. *Ca - A Cancer Journal for Clinicians* Sept/Oct 1983; 258-263. 6. American Society of Hospital Pharmacists: Technical assistance bulletin on handling cytotoxic drugs in hospitals. *Am J Hosp Pharm* 1985; 42:131-137.

HOW SUPPLIED - EQUIVALENTS NOT AVAILABLE:

Injection, Solution - Intravenous - 2 mg/ml

10 ml	**$576.03**	**NOVANTRONE, Immunex**	**58406-0640-03**
12.5 ml	**$720.02**	**NOVANTRONE, Immunex**	**58406-0640-05**
15 ml	**$864.04**	**NOVANTRONE, Immunex**	**58406-0640-07**

MIVACURIUM CHLORIDE *(003113)*

CATEGORIES: Anesthesia; Autonomic Drugs; Neuromuscular Blocking Agents; Non-Depolarizing Muscle Relaxants; Short-Acting Neuromuscular Blockers; Skeletal Muscle Relaxants; Tracheal Intubation; Pregnancy Category C; FDA Class 1P ("Priority Review"); FDA Approved 1992 Jan

BRAND NAMES: **Mivacron**

DESCRIPTION:

This drug should be administered only by adequately trained individuals familiar with its actions, characteristics, and hazards.

Mivacurium chloride is a short-acting, nondepolarizing skeletal muscle relaxant for intravenous administration. Mivacurium chloride is (*R*-(*R**,R*-(E)))-2,2'-((1,8-dioxo-4-octene-1,8-diyl)bis(oxy-3,1 -propanediyl))bis(1,2,3,4-tetrahydro-6,7-dimethoxy-2-methyl-1-((3,4,5-trimetho xypheny)methyl) isoquinolinium) dichloride. The molecular formula is $C_{58}H_{80}Cl_2N_2O_{14}$ and the molecular weight is 1100.18.

The partition coefficient of the compound is 0.015 in a 1-octanol/distilled water system at 25°C.

Mivacurium chloride is a mixture of three stereoisomers: (1*R*, 1'*R*, 2*S*, 2'*S*), the trans-trans diester; (1*R*, 1'*R*, 2*R*, 2'*S*), the cis-trans diester; and (1*R*, 1'*R*, 2*R*, 2'*R*), the cis-cis diester. The trans-trans and cis-trans stereoisomers comprise 92% to 96% of mivacurium chloride and their neuromuscular blocking potencies are not significantly different from each other or from mivacurium chloride. The cis-cis diester has been estimated from studies in cats to have one-tenth the neuromuscular blocking potency of the other two stereoisomers.

Mivacurium chloride injection is a sterile, non-pyrogenic solution (pH 3.5 to 5.0) containing mivacurium chloride equivalent to 2 mg/ml mivacurium in Water for injection. Hydrochloric acid may have been added to adjust pH. Mivacurium chloride premixed infusion is a sterile, non-pyrogenic solution (pH 3.5 to 5.0; 260 mOsmol/L-measured) containing mivacurium chloride equivalent to 0.5 mg/ml mivacurium in 5% Dextrose injection USP. Hydrochloric acid may have been added to adjust pH.

CLINICAL PHARMACOLOGY:

Mivacurium chloride (a mixture of three stereoisomers) binds competitively to cholinergic receptors on the motor end-plate to antagonize the action of acetylcholine, resulting in a block of neuromuscular transmission. This action is antagonized by acetylcholinesterase inhibitors, such as neostigmine.

PHARMACODYNAMICS

The time to maximum neuromuscular block is similar for recommended doses of mivacurium chloride and intermediate-acting agents (*e.g.*, atracurium), but longer than for the ultra-short-acting agent, succinylcholine. The clinically effective duration of action of the stereoisomers in mivacurium chloride (a mixture of three stereoisomers) is one-third to one-half that of intermediate-acting agents and 2 to 2.5 times that of succinylcholine.

The average ED_{95} (dose required to produce 95% suppression of the adductor pollicis muscle twitch response to ulnar nerve stimulation) of mivacurium chloride is 0.07 mg/kg (range: 0.06 to 0.09) in adults receiving opioid/nitrous oxide/oxygen anesthesia. The pharmacodynamics of doses of mivacurium chloride $\geq ED_{95}$ administered over 5 to 15 seconds during opioid/nitrous oxide/oxygen anesthesia are summarized in Table 1. The mean time for spontaneous recovery of the twitch response from 25% to 75% of control amplitude is about 6 minutes (range: 3 to 9, n=32) following an initial dose of 0.15 mg/kg mivacurium chloride and 7 to 8 minutes (range: 4 to 24, n=85) following initial doses of 0.20 or 0.25 mg/kg mivacurium chloride.

Volatile anesthetics may decrease the dosing requirement for mivacurium chloride and prolong the duration of action; the magnitude of these effects may be increased as the concentration of the volatile agent is increased. Isoflurane and enflurane (administered with nitrous oxide/oxygen to achieve 1.25 MAC (Minimum Alveolar Concentration)) may decrease the effective dose of mivacurium chloride by as much as 25%, and may prolong the clinically effective duration of action and decrease the average infusion requirement by as much as 35% to 40%. At equivalent MAC values, halothane has little or no effect on the ED_{50} of

CLINICAL PHARMACOLOGY: *(cont'd)*

mivacurium chloride, but may prolong the duration of action and decrease the average infusion requirement by as much as 20% (see CLINICAL PHARMACOLOGY, Individualization of Dosages and DRUG INTERACTIONS).

TABLE 1 Pharmacodynamic Dose Response During Opioid/Nitrous Oxide/Oxygen Anesthesia

Initial Mivacron Dose (mg/kg)	Time to Maximum Block[1] (min)	Time to Spontaneous Recovery[1]: 5% Recovery (min)	25% Recovery[2] (min)	95% Recovery[3] (min)	T_4/T_1 Ratio $\geq$75%[3] (min)	
Adults						
0.07 to 0.10	(n=47)	4.9 (2.0-7.6)	11 (7-19)	13 (8-24)	21 (10-36)	21 (10-36)
0.15	(n=50)	3.3 (1.5-8.8)	13 (6-31)	16 (9-38)	26 (16-41)	26 (15-45)
0.20	(n=50)	2.5 (1.2-6.0)	16 (10-29)	20 (10-36)	31 (15-51)	34 (19-56)
0.25	(n=48)	2.3 (1.0-4.8)	19 (11-29)	23 (14-38)	34 (22-64)	43 (26-75)
Children 2 to 12 Years						
0.11 to 0.12	(n=17)	2.8 (1.2-4.6)	5 (3-9)	7 (4-10)	-	-
0.20	(n=18)	1.9 (1.3-3.3)	7 (3-12)	10 (6-15)	19 (14-26)	16 (12-23)
0.25	(n=9)	1.6 (1.0-2.2)	7 (4-9)	9 (5-12)	-	-

1 Values shown are medians of means from individual studies (range of individual patient values).
2 Clinically effective duration of neuromuscular block.
3 Data available for as few as 40% of adults in specific dose groups and for 22% of children in the 0.20 mg/kg dose group due to administration of reversal agents or additional doses of Mivacron prior to 95% recovery or T_4/T_1 ratio recovery to ≥75%.

Administration of mivacurium chloride over 60 seconds does not alter the time to maximum neuromuscular block or the duration of action. The duration of action of the stereoisomers in mivacurium chloride may be prolonged in patients with reduced plasma cholinesterase (pseudocholinesterase) activity (see PRECAUTIONS, Reduced Plasma Cholinesterase Activity and CLINICAL PHARMACOLOGY, Individualization of Dosages).

Interpatient variability in duration of action occurs with mivacurium chloride as with other neuromuscular blocking agents. However, analysis of data from 224 patients in clinical studies receiving various doses of mivacurium chloride during opioid/nitrous oxide/oxygen anesthesia with a variety of premedicants and varying lengths of surgery indicated that approximately 90% of the patients had clinically effective durations of block within 8 minutes of the median duration predicted from the dose-response data shown in Table 1. Variations in plasma cholinesterase activity, including values within the normal range and values as low as 20% below the lower limit of the normal range, were not associated with clinically significant effects on duration. The variability in duration, however, was greater in patients with plasma cholinesterase activity at or slightly below the lower limit of the normal range.

A dose of 0.15 mg/kg (2 x ED_{95}) mivacurium chloride administered during the induction of thiopental/opioid/nitrous oxide/oxygen anesthesia produced generally good-to-excellent conditions for tracheal intubation in 2.5 minutes. Doses of 0.20 and 0.25 mg/kg (3 and 3.5 x ED_{95}) yielded similar conditions in 2.0 minutes.

Repeated administration of maintenance doses or continuous infusion of mivacurium chloride for up to 2.5 hours is not associated with development of tachyphylaxis or cumulative neuromuscular blocking effects in ASA Physical Status I-II patients. Limited data are available from patients receiving infusions for longer than 2.5 hours. Spontaneous recovery of neuromuscular function after infusion is independent of the duration of infusion and comparable to recovery reported for single doses (TABLE 1).

The neuromuscular block produced by the stereoisomers in mivacurium chloride is readily antagonized by anticholinesterase agents. As seen with other nondepolarizing neuromuscular blocking agents, the more profound the neuromuscular block at the time of reversal, the longer the time and the greater the dose of anticholinesterase agent required for recovery of neuromuscular function.

In children (2 to 12 years), mivacurium chloride has a higher ED_{95}(0.10 mg/kg), faster onset, and shorter duration of action than in adults. The mean time for spontaneous recovery of the twitch response from 25% to 75% of control amplitude is about 5 minutes (n=4) following an initial dose of 0.20 mg/kg mivacurium chloride. Recovery following reversal is faster in children than in adults (TABLE 1).

HEMODYNAMICS

Administration of mivacurium chloride in doses up to and including 0.15 mg/kg (2 x ED_{95}) over 5 to 15 seconds to ASA Physical Status I-II patients during opioid/nitrous oxide/oxygen anesthesia is associated with minimal changes in mean arterial blood pressure (MAP) or heart rate (HR) (TABLE 2).

TABLE 2 Cardiovascular Dose Response During Opioid/Nitrous Oxide/Oxygen Anesthesia

Initial Mivacron Dose (mg/kg)		% of Patients With #>30% Change: MAP Dec	MAP Inc	HR Dec	HR Inc
Adults					
0.07 to 0.10	(n = 49)	0%	2%	0%	0%
0.15	(n = 53)	4%	4%	4%	2%
0.20	(n = 53)	30%	0%	0%	8%
0.25	(n = 44)	39%	2%	0%	14%
Children 2 to 12 years					
0.11 to 0.12	(n = 17)	0%	6%	0%	0%
0.20	(n = 17)	0%	0%	0%	0%
0.25	(n = 8)	13%	0%	0%	0%

Higher doses of ≥0.20 mg/kg (≥3 x ED_{95}) may be associated with transient decreases in MAP and increases in HR in some patients. These decreases in MAP are usually maximal within 1 to 3 minutes following the dose, typically resolve without treatment in an additional 1 to 3 minutes, and are usually associated with increases in plasma histamine concentration. Decreases in MAP can be minimized by administering mivacurium chloride over 30 or 60 seconds (see CLINICAL PHARMACOLOGY, Individualization of Dosages and PRECAUTIONS, General). Analysis of 426 patients in clinical studies receiving initial doses of mivacurium chloride up to and including 0.30 mg/kg (*i.e.*,2 times the recommended intubating dose) during opioid/nitrous oxide/oxygen anesthesia showed that high initial doses and a rapid rate of injection contributed to a greater probability of experiencing a decrease of ≥30% in MAP after mivacurium chloride administration. Obese patients also had a greater

CLINICAL PHARMACOLOGY: *(cont'd)*

probability of experiencing a decrease of ≥30% in MAP when dosed on the basis of actual body weight, thereby receiving a larger dose than if dosed on the basis of ideal body weight (see CLINICAL PHARMACOLOGY, Individualization of Dosages and PRECAUTIONS, General). Children experience minimal changes in MAP or HR after administration of mivacurium chloride doses up to and including 0.20 mg/kg over 5 to 15 seconds, but higher doses (≥0.25 mg/kg) may be associated with transient decreases in MAP (Table 2). Following a dose of 0.15 mg/kg mivacurium chloride administered over 60 seconds, adult patients with significant cardiovascular disease undergoing coronary artery bypass grafting or valve replacement procedures showed no clinically important changes in MAP or HR. Transient decreases in MAP were observed in some patients after doses of 0.20 to 0.25 mg/kg mivacurium chloride administered over 60 seconds. The number of patients in whom these decreases in MAP required treatment was small.

PHARMACOKINETICS

Table 3 describes the results from a study of 9 ASA Physical Status I-II adult patients (31 to 48 years) receiving an infusion of mivacurium chloride at 5 mcg/kg/min for 60 minutes followed by 10 mcg/kg/min for 60 minutes. Mivacurium chloride is a mixture of isomers which do not interconvert *in vivo.* The mivacurium pharmacokinetic parameters presented in Table 3 were determined using a stereospecific assay. The two more potent isomers,*cis-trans* (36% of the mixture) and *trans-trans* (57% of the mixture), have very high clearances that exceed cardiac output reflecting the extensive metabolism by plasma cholinesterase. The volume of distribution is relatively small, reflecting limited tissue distribution secondary to the polarity and large molecular weight of mivacurium. The combination of high metabolic clearance and low distribution volume results in the short elimination half-life of approximately 2 minutes for the two active isomers. The short elimination half-lives and high metabolic clearances of the active isomers are consistent with the short duration of action of mivacurium chloride. The steady-state concentrations of the *cis-trans* and *trans-trans* isomers doubled after the infusion rate was increased from 5 to 10 mcg/kg/min, indicating that their pharmacokinetics are dose-proportional.

TABLE 3 Stereoisomer Pharmacokinetic Parameters [1] of Mivacurium Chloride in ASA Physical Status I-II Adult Patients [2](n=9) During Opioid/Nitrous Oxide/Oxygen Anesthesia

Parameter	*trans-trans* isomer	*cis-trans* isomer
Elimination Half-life $t_{1/2}$, min)	2.3 (1.4-3.6)	2.1 (0.8-4.8)
Volume of Distribution (L/kg)	0.15 (0.06-0.24)	0.27 (0.08-0.56)
Plasma Clearance (ml/min/kg)	53 (32-105)	99 (52-230)

[1]Values shown are mean (range).
[2]Ages 31 to 48 years.

The *cis-cis* isomer (6% of the mixture) has approximately one-tenth the neuromuscular blocking potency of the *trans-trans* and *cis-trans* isomers in cats. In the nine patients shown in Table 3, the volume of distribution of the *cis-cis* isomer averaged 0.31 L/kg (range: 0.18-0.46), the clearance averaged 4.2 ml/min/kg (range: 2.4-5.4), and the half-life averaged 55 minutes (range: 32-102). The neuromuscular blocking potency of the *cis-cis* isomer in humans has not been established; however, modeling of clinical pharmacokinetic-pharmacodynamic data suggests that the *cis-cis* isomer produces minimal (<5%) neuromuscular block during a two-hour infusion. In studies in which infusions of up to 2.5 hours were administered to ASA Physical Status I-II patients, the 25%-75% recovery times were independent of the duration of infusion, suggesting that the *cis-cis* isomer does not contribute significant neuromuscular block during use for up to 2.5 hours. Limited data are available from infusions of longer duration or from patients with compromised elimination capacities (hepatic or renal failure).

METABOLISM AND EXCRETION

Enzymatic hydrolysis by plasma cholinesterase is the primary mechanism for inactivation of mivacurium and yields a quaternary alcohol and a quaternary monoester metabolite. Renal and biliary excretion of unchanged mivacurium are minor elimination pathways; urine and bile are important elimination pathways for the two metabolites. Tests in which these two metabolites were administered to cats and dogs suggest that each metabolite is unlikely to produce clinically significant neuromuscular, autonomic, or cardiovascular effects following administration of mivacurium chloride.

SPECIAL POPULATIONS

The pharmacokinetics of mivacurium isomers has not been studied in the elderly or in patients with renal or hepatic disease using a stereospecific assay. The non-stereospecific, total mivacurium assay used in pharmacokinetic-pharmacodynamic studies in these populations provided preliminary evidence that reduced clearance of one or more isomers is responsible for the longer duration of action of mivacurium chloride seen in patients with end-stage kidney or liver disease. The data did not provide a pharmacokinetic explanation for the 15-20% longer duration of block seen in the elderly. Tables 4 and 5 summarize the pharmacodynamic results in these special populations as compared with young adults (ages 18 to 49 years). No data are available from patients with kidney or liver disease not requiring transplantation.

TABLE 4 Pharmacodynamic Parameters [1] of Mivacurium Chloride In ASA Physical Status I-II Young Adult Patients and Elderly Patients During Isoflurane/Nitrous Oxide/Oxygen Anesthesia

Parameter	Young Adult Patients (18-49 years)		Elderly Patients (68-77 years)
Initial Dose	0.10 mg/kg (n=9)	0.25 mg/kg (n=9)	0.10 mg/kg (n=8)
Maximum Block (%)	98 (83-100)	100 (100-100)	99 (95-100)
Time to Maximum Block (min)	3.2 (2.0-6.0)	1.7 (1.3-2.5)	4.8 (3.0-7.0)
Clinically Effective Duration of Block[2] (min)	17 (9-29)	27 (18-34)	20 (14-28)

[1]Values shown are mean (range).
[2]Time from injection to 25% recovery of the control twitch height.

Renal: The clinically effective duration of action of 0.15 mg/kg mivacurium chloride was about 1.5 times longer in patients with end-stage kidney disease than in healthy patients, presumably due to reduced clearance of one or more isomers.

Hepatic: The clinically effective duration of action of 0.15 mg/kg mivacurium chloride was three times longer in patients with end-stage liver disease than in healthy patients and is likely related to the markedly decreased plasma cholinesterase activity (30% of healthy patient values) which could decrease the clearance of one or more isomers see PRECAUTIONS, Reduced Plasma Cholinesterase Activity.

CLINICAL PHARMACOLOGY: *(cont'd)*

TABLE 5 Pharmacodynamic Parameters [1] of Mivacurium Chloride In ASA Physical Status I-II Patients and In Patients Undergoing Kidney or Liver Transplantation During Isoflurane/Nitrous Oxide/Oxygen Anesthesia

Parameter	Young Adult Patients	Kidney Transplant Patients	Liver Transplant Patients[3]
Initial Dose	0.15 mg/kg (n=8)	0.15 mg/kg (n=9)	0.15 mg/kg (n=8)
Maximum Block (%)	99.8 (98-100)	100 (100-100)	100 (100-100)
Time to Maximum Block (min)	1.9 (0.8-3.5)	2.6 (1.0-4.5)	2.1 (1.0-4.0)
Clinically Effective Duration of Block[2] (min)	19 (12-30)	30 (19-58)	57 (29-80)

[1]Values shown are mean (range).
[2]Time from injection to 25% recovery of the control twitch height.
[3]Liver transplant patients received isoflurane without nitrous oxide.

INDIVIDUALIZATION OF DOSAGES

DOSES OF MIVACURIUM CHLORIDE SHOULD BE INDIVIDUALIZED AND A PERIPHERAL NERVE STIMULATOR SHOULD BE USED TO MEASURE NEUROMUSCULAR FUNCTION DURING MIVACURIUM CHLORIDE ADMINISTRATION IN ORDER TO MONITOR DRUG EFFECT, DETERMINE THE NEED FOR ADDITIONAL DOSES, AND CONFIRM RECOVERY FROM NEUROMUSCULAR BLOCK.

Based on the known actions of mivacurium chloride (a mixture of three stereoisomers) and other neuromuscular blocking agents, these factors should be considered when administering mivacurium chloride.

Renal or Hepatic Impairment: A dose of 0.15 mg/kg mivacurium chloride is recommended for facilitation of tracheal intubation in patients with renal or hepatic impairment. However, the clinically effective duration of block produced by this dose is about 1.5 times longer in patients with end-stage kidney disease and about 3 times longer in patients with end-stage liver disease than in patients with normal renal and hepatic function. Infusion rates should be decreased by as much as 50% in these patients depending on the degree of renal or hepatic impairment see PRECAUTIONS, Renal and Hepatic Disease.

Reduced Plasma Cholinesterase Activity: The possibility of prolonged neuromuscular block following administration of mivacurium chloride must be considered in patients with reduced plasma cholinesterase (pseudocholinesterase) activity. Mivacurium chloride should be used with great caution, if at all, in patients known or suspected of being homozygous for the atypical plasma cholinesterase gene (see WARNINGS.) Doses of 0.03 mg/kg produced complete neuromuscular block for 26 to 128 minutes in three such patients; thus initial doses greater than 0.03 mg/kg are not recommended in homozygous patients. Infusions of mivacurium chloride are not recommended in homozygous patients.

Mivacurium chloride has been used safely in patients heterozygous for the atypical plasma cholinesterase gene and in genotypically normal patients with reduced plasma cholinesterase activity. After recommended intubating doses of mivacurium chloride, the clinically effective duration of block in heterozygous patients may be approximately 10 minutes longer than in patients with normal genotype and normal plasma cholinesterase activity. Lower mivacurium chloride infusion rates are recommended in these patients see PRECAUTIONS, Reduced Plasma Cholinesterase Activity.

Drugs or Conditions Causing Potentiation of or Resistance to Neuromuscular Block: As with other neuromuscular blocking agents, mivacurium chloride may have profound neuromuscular blocking effects in cachectic or debilitated patients, patients with neuromuscular diseases, and patients with carcinomatosis. In these or other patients in whom potentiation of neuromuscular block or difficulty with reversal may be anticipated, the recommended initial dose should be decreased. A test dose of not more than 0.015-0.020 mg/kg, which represents the lower end of the dose-response curve for mivacurium chloride, is recommended in such patients see PRECAUTIONS, General.

The neuromuscular blocking action of the stereoisomers in mivacurium chloride is potentiated by isoflurane or enflurane anesthesia. The recommended initial mivacurium chloride dose of 0.15 mg/kg may be used for intubation prior to the administration of these agents. If mivacurium chloride is first administered after establishment of stable-state isoflurane or enflurane anesthesia (administered with nitrous oxide/oxygen to achieve 1.25 MAC), the initial mivacurium chloride dose should be reduced by as much as 25%, and the infusion rate reduced by as much as 35% to 40%. A greater potentiation of the neuromuscular blocking action of the stereoisomers in mivacurium chloride may be expected with higher concentrations of enflurane or isoflurane. The use of halothane requires no adjustment of the initial dose of mivacurium chloride, but may prolong the duration of action and decrease the average infusion rate by as much as 20% (see DRUG INTERACTIONS.) When mivacurium chloride is administered to patients receiving certain antibiotics, magnesium salts, lithium, local anesthetics, procainamide and quinidine, longer durations of neuromuscular block may be expected and infusion requirements may be lower (see DRUG INTERACTIONS.)

When mivacurium chloride is administered to patients chronically receiving phenytoin or carbamazepine, slightly shorter durations of neuromuscular block may be anticipated and infusion rate requirements may be higher (see DRUG INTERACTIONS.)

Severe acid-base and/or electrolyte abnormalities may potentiate or cause resistance to the neuromuscular blocking action of the stereoisomers in mivacurium chloride. No data are available in such patients and no dosing recommendations can be made see PRECAUTIONS, General.

Burns: While patients with burns are known to develop resistance to nondepolarizing neuromuscular blocking agents, they may also have reduced plasma cholinesterase activity. Consequently, in these patients, a test dose of not more than 0.015-0.020 mg/kg mivacurium chloride is recommended, followed by additional appropriate dosing guided by the use of a neuromuscular block monitor see PRECAUTIONS, General.

Cardiovascular Disease: In patients with clinically significant cardiovascular disease, the initial dose of mivacurium chloride should be 0.15 mg/kg or less, administered over 60 seconds (see CLINICAL PHARMACOLOGY, Hemodynamics and PRECAUTIONS, General).

Obesity: Obese patients (patients weighing ≥30% more than their ideal body weight) dosed on the basis of actual body weight, thereby receiving a larger dose than if dosed on the basis of ideal body weight, had a greater probability of experiencing a decrease of ≥30% in MAP (see CLINICAL PHARMACOLOGY, Hemodynamics and PRECAUTIONS, General). Therefore, in obese patients, the initial dose should be determined using the patient's ideal body weight (IBW), according to the formulae in TABLE 6.

TABLE 6

Men: IBW in kg = [106 + (6 × inches in height above 5 feet)] ÷ 2.2
Women: IBW in kg = [100 + (5 × inches in height above 5 feet)] ÷ 2.2

CLINICAL PHARMACOLOGY: *(cont'd)*

Allergy and Sensitivity: In patients with any history suggestive of a greater sensitivity to the release of histamine or related mediators (*e.g.,* asthma), the initial dose of mivacurium chloride should be 0.15 mg/kg or less, administered over 60 seconds seePRECAUTIONS, General.

INDICATIONS AND USAGE:

Mivacurium chloride is a short-acting neuromuscular blocking agent indicated for inpatients and outpatients, as an adjunct to general anesthesia, to facilitate tracheal intubation and to provide skeletal muscle relaxation during surgery or mechanical ventilation.

CONTRAINDICATIONS:

Mivacurium chloride is contraindicated in patients known to have an allergic hypersensitivity to mivacurium chloride or other benzylisoquinolinium agents, as manifested by reactions such as urticaria or severe respiratory distress or hypotension. Use of mivacurium chloride from multi-dose vials is contraindicated in patients with a known allergy to benzyl alcohol.

WARNINGS:

MIVACURIUM CHLORIDE SHOULD BE ADMINISTERED IN CAREFULLY ADJUSTED DOSAGE BY OR UNDER THE SUPERVISION OF EXPERIENCED CLINICIANS WHO ARE FAMILIAR WITH THE DRUG'S ACTIONS AND THE POSSIBLE COMPLICATIONS OF ITS USE. THE DRUG SHOULD NOT BE ADMINISTERED UNLESS PERSONNEL AND FACILITIES FOR RESUSCITATION AND LIFE SUPPORT (TRACHEAL INTUBATION, ARTIFICIAL VENTILATION, OXYGEN THERAPY), AND AN ANTAGONIST OF MIVACURIUM CHLORIDE ARE IMMEDIATELY AVAILABLE. IT IS RECOMMENDED THAT A PERIPHERAL NERVE STIMULATOR BE USED TO MEASURE NEUROMUSCULAR FUNCTION DURING THE ADMINISTRATION OF MIVACURIUM CHLORIDE IN ORDER TO MONITOR DRUG EFFECT, DETERMINE THE NEED FOR ADDITIONAL DRUG, AND CONFIRM RECOVERY FROM NEUROMUSCULAR BLOCK.

MIVACURIUM CHLORIDE HAS NO KNOWN EFFECT ON CONSCIOUSNESS, PAIN THRESHOLD, OR CEREBRATION. TO AVOID DISTRESS TO THE PATIENT, NEUROMUSCULAR BLOCK SHOULD NOT BE INDUCED BEFORE UNCONSCIOUSNESS.

MIVACURIUM CHLORIDE IS METABOLIZED BY PLASMA CHOLINESTERASE AND SHOULD BE USED WITH GREAT CAUTION, IF AT ALL, IN PATIENTS KNOWN TO BE OR SUSPECTED OF BEING HOMOZYGOUS FOR THE ATYPICAL PLASMA CHOLINESTERASE GENE.

Mivacurium chloride injection and mivacurium chloride premixed infusion are acidic (pH 3.5 to 5.0) and may not be compatible with alkaline solutions having a pH greater than 8.5 (*e.g.,* barbiturate solutions).

PRECAUTIONS:

General: Although mivacurium chloride (a mixture of three stereoisomers) is not a potent histamine releaser, the possibility of substantial histamine release must be considered. Release of histamine is related to the dose and speed of injection.

Caution should be exercised in administering mivacurium chloride to patients with clinically significant cardiovascular disease and patients with any history suggesting a greater sensitivity to the release of histamine or related mediators (*e.g.,* asthma). In such patients, the initial dose of mivacurium chloride should be 0.15 mg/kg or less, administered over 60 seconds; assurance of adequate hydration and careful monitoring of hemodynamic status are important see CLINICAL PHARMACOLOGY, Hemodynamics and CLINICAL PHARMACOLOGY, Individuzation of Dosage.

Obese patients may be more likely to experience clinically significant transient decreases in MAP than non-obese patients when the dose of mivacurium chloride is based on actual rather than ideal body weight. Therefore, in obese patients, the initial dose should be determined using the patient's ideal body weight (see CLINICAL PHARMACOLOGY, Hemodynamics, CLINICAL PHARMACOLOGY, Individualization of Dosages).

Recommended doses of mivacurium chloride have no clinically significant effects on heart rate; therefore, mivacurium chloride will not counteract the bradycardia produced by many anesthetic agents or by vagal stimulation.

Neuromuscular blocking agents may have a profound effect in patients with neuromuscular diseases (*e.g.,* myasthenia gravis and the myasthenic syndrome). In these and other conditions in which prolonged neuromuscular block is a possibility (*e.g.,* carcinomatosis), the use of a peripheral nerve stimulator and a dose of not more than 0.015-0.020 mg/kg mivacurium chloride is recommended to assess the level of neuromuscular block and to monitor dosage requirements (see CLINICAL PHARMACOLOGY, Individualization of Dosages.)

Mivacurium chloride has not been studied in patients with burns. Resistance to nondepolarizing neuromuscular blocking agents may develop in patients with burns, depending upon the time elapsed since the injury and the size of the burn. Patients with burns may have reduced plasma cholinesterase activity which may offset this resistance (see CLINICAL PHARMACOLOGY, Individualization of Dosages.)

Acid-base and/or serum electrolyte abnormalities may potentiate or antagonize the action of neuromuscular blocking agents. The action of neuromuscular blocking agents may be enhanced by magnesium salts administered for the management of toxemia of pregnancy (see CLINICAL PHARMACOLOGY, Individualization of Dosages.)

No data are available to support the use of mivacurium chloride by intramuscular injection.

Renal and Hepatic Disease: The possibility of prolonged neuromuscular block must be considered when mivacurium chloride is used in patients with renal or hepatic disease (see CLINICAL PHARMACOLOGY, Pharmacokinetics.) Most patients with chronic hepatic disease such as hepatitis, liver abscess, and cirrhosis of the liver exhibit a marked reduction in plasma cholinesterase activity. Patients with acute or chronic renal disease may also show a reduction in plasma cholinesterase activity (see CLINICAL PHARMACOLOGY, Individualization of Dosages.)

Reduced Plasma Cholinesterase Activity: The possibility of prolonged neuromuscular block following administration of mivacurium chloride must be considered in patients with reduced plasma cholinesterase (pseudocholinesterase) activity.

Plasma cholinesterase activity may be diminished in the presence of genetic abnormalities of plasma cholinesterase (*e.g.,* patients heterozygous or homozygous for the atypical plasma cholinesterase gene), pregnancy, liver or kidney disease, malignant tumors, infections, burns, anemia, decompensated heart disease, peptic ulcer, or myxedema. Plasma cholinesterase activity may also be diminished by chronic administration of oral contraceptives, glucocorticoids, or certain monoamine oxidase inhibitors and by irreversible inhibitors of plasma cholinesterase (*e.g.,*organophosphate insecticides, echothiophate, and certain antineoplastic drugs).

Mivacurium chloride has been used safely in patients heterozygous for the atypical plasma cholinesterase gene. At doses of 0.10 to 0.20 mg/kg mivacurium chloride, the clinically effective duration of action was 8 to 11 minutes longer in patients heterozygous for the atypical gene than in genotypically normal patients.

PRECAUTIONS: *(cont'd)*

As with succinylcholine, patients homozygous for the atypical plasma cholinesterase gene (1 in 2500 patients) are extremely sensitive to the neuromuscular blocking effect of mivacurium chloride. In three such adult patients, a small dose of 0.03 mg/kg (approximately the ED_{10-20} in genotypically normal patients) produced complete neuromuscular block for 26 to 128 minutes. Once spontaneous recovery had begun, neuromuscular block in these patients was antagonized with conventional doses of neostigmine. One adult patient, who was homozygous for the atypical plasma cholinesterase gene, received a dose of 0.18 mg/kg mivacurium chloride and exhibited complete neuromuscular block for about 4 hours. Response to post-tetanic stimulation was present after 4 hours, all four responses to train-of-four stimulation were present after 6 hours, and the patient was extubated after 8 hours. Reversal was not attempted in this patient.

Malignant Hyperthermia (MH): In a study of MH-susceptible pigs, mivacurium chloride did not trigger MH. Mivacurium chloride has not been studied in MH-susceptible patients. Because MH can develop in the absence of established triggering agents, the clinician should be prepared to recognize and treat MH in any patient undergoing general anesthesia.

Long-Term Use in the Intensive Care Unit (ICU): No data are available on the long-term use of mivacurium chloride in patients undergoing mechanical ventilation in the ICU.

Carcinogenesis, Mutagenesis, Impairment of Fertility: Carcinogenesis and fertility studies have not been performed. Mivacurium chloride was evaluated in a battery of four short-term mutagenicity tests. It was non-mutagenic in the Ames Salmonella assay, the mouse lymphoma assay, the human lymphocyte assay, and the *in vivo* rat bone marrow cytogenetic assay.

Pregnancy, Teratogenic Effects, Pregnancy Category C: Teratology testing in nonventilated pregnant rats and mice treated subcutaneously with maximum subparalyzing doses of mivacurium chloride revealed no maternal or fetal toxicity or teratogenic effects. There are no adequate and well-controlled studies of mivacurium chloride in pregnant women. Because animal studies are not always predictive of human response, and the doses used were subparalyzing, mivacurium chloride should be used during pregnancy only if the potential benefit justifies the potential risk to the fetus.

Labor and Delivery: The use of mivacurium chloride during labor, vaginal delivery, or cesarean section has not been studied in humans and it is not known whether mivacurium chloride administered to the mother has effects on the fetus. Doses of 0.08 and 0.20 mg/kg mivacurium chloride given to female beagles undergoing cesarean section resulted in negligible levels of the stereoisomers in mivacurium chloride in umbilical vessel blood of neonates and no deleterious effects on the puppies.

Nursing Mothers: It is known whether any of the stereoisomers of mivacurium are excreted in human milk. Because many drugs are excreted in human milk, caution should be exercised following administration of mivacurium chloride to a nursing woman.

Pediatric Use: Mivacurium chloride has not been studied in children below the age of 2 years (see CLINICAL PHARMACOLOGY and DOSAGE AND ADMINISTRATION for clinical experience and recommendations for use in children 2 to 12 years of age).

Geriatric Use: Mivacurium chloride was safely administered during clinical trials to 64 elderly (≥65 years) patients, including 31 patients with significant cardiovascular disease (see PRECAUTIONS, General.) The duration of neuromuscular block may be slightly longer in elderly patients than in young adult patients(see CLINICAL PHARMACOLOGY.)

DRUG INTERACTIONS:

Although mivacurium chloride (a mixture of three stereoisomers) has been administered safely following succinylcholine-facilitated tracheal intubation, the interaction between the stereoisomers in mivacurium chloride and succinylcholine has not been systematically studied. Prior administration of succinylcholine can potentiate the neuromuscular blocking effects of nondepolarizing agents. Evidence of spontaneous recovery from succinylcholine should be observed before the administration of mivacurium chloride.

The use of mivacurium chloride before succinylcholine to attenuate some of the side effects of succinylcholine has not been studied.

There are no clinical data on the use of mivacurium chloride with other nondepolarizing neuromuscular blocking agents.

Isoflurane and enflurane (administered with nitrous oxide/oxygen to achieve 1.25 MAC) decrease the ED_{50} of mivacurium chloride by as much as 25% (see CLINICAL PHARMACOLOGY, Pharmacodynamics and CLINICAL PHARMACOLOGY, Individualization of Dosages). These agents may also prolong the clinically effective duration of action and decrease the average infusion requirement of mivacurium chloride by as much as 35% to 40%. A greater potentiation of the neuromuscular blocking effects of the stereoisomers in mivacurium chloride may be expected with higher concentrations of enflurane or isoflurane. Halothane has little or no effect on the ED_{50}, but may prolong the duration of action and decrease the average infusion requirement by as much as 20%.

Other drugs which may enhance the neuromuscular blocking action of nondepolarizing agents such as the stereoisomers in mivacurium chloride include certain antibiotics (*e.g.,* aminoglycosides, tetracyclines, bacitracin, polymyxins, lincomycin, clindamycin, colistin, and sodium colistimethate), magnesium salts, lithium, local anesthetics, procainamide, and quinidine. Drugs that may enhance the neuromuscular blocking effects of mivacurium by a reduction in plasma cholinesterase activity include chronic administration of oral contraceptives, glucocorticoids, or certain monoamine oxidase inhibitors and by irreversible inhibitors of plasma cholinesterase see PRECAUTIONS, Reduced Plasma Cholinesterase Activity.

Resistance to the neuromuscular blocking action of nondepolarizing neuromuscular blocking agents has been demonstrated in patients chronically administered phenytoin or carbamazepine. While the effects of chronic phenytoin or carbamazepine therapy on the action of the stereoisomers in mivacurium chloride are unknown, slightly shorter durations of neuromuscular block may be anticipated and infusion rate requirements may be higher.

ADVERSE REACTIONS:

Observed in Clinical Trials: Mivacurium chloride (a mixture of three stereoisomers) was well tolerated during extensive clinical trials in inpatients and outpatients. Prolonged neuromuscular block, which is an important adverse experience associated with neuromuscular blocking agents as a class, was reported as an adverse experience in 3 of 2074 patients administered mivacurium chloride. The most commonly reported adverse experience following the administration of mivacurium chloride was transient, dose-dependent cutaneous flushing about the face, neck, and/or chest. Flushing was most frequently noted after the initial dose of mivacurium chloride and was reported in about 20% of adult patients who received the recommended dose of 0.15 mg/kg mivacurium chloride over 5 to 15 seconds. When present, flushing typically began within 1 to 2 minutes after the dose of mivacurium chloride and lasted for 3 to 5 minutes. Of 60 patients who experienced flushing after 0.15 mg/kg mivacurium chloride, one patient also experienced mild hypotension that was not treated, and one patient experienced moderate wheezing that was successfully treated.

Overall, hypotension was infrequently reported as an adverse experience in the clinical trials of mivacurium chloride. None of the 397 adults or 63 children who received recommended doses was treated for a decrease in blood pressure associated with administration of mivacurium chloride. Above the recommended dosage range, 1% to 2% of healthy adults

ADVERSE REACTIONS: *(cont'd)*

given ≥0.20 mg/kg over 5 to 15 seconds and 2% to 4% of cardiac surgery patients given ≥0.20 mg/kg over 60 seconds were treated for decreases in blood pressure associated with the administration of mivacurium chloride.

The following adverse experiences were reported in patients administered

Mivacurium chloride (all events judged by investigators during the clinical trials to have a possible causal relationship) (TABLE 7):

TABLE 7

Incidence Greater Than 1%	
Cardiovascular:	Flushing (15%)
Incidence Less Than 1%	
Cardiovascular:	Hypotension, Tachycardia, Bradycardia, Cardiac Arrhythmia, Phlebitis
Respiratory:	Bronchospasm, Wheezing, Hypoxemia
Dermatological:	Rash, Urticaria, Erythema, Injection Site Reaction
Nonspecific:	Prolonged Drug Effect
Neurologic:	Dizziness
Musculoskeletal	Muscle Spasms

OVERDOSAGE:

Overdosage with neuromuscular blocking agents may result in neuromuscular block beyond the time needed for surgery and anesthesia. The primary treatment is maintenance of a patent airway and controlled ventilation until recovery of normal neuromuscular function is assured. Once evidence of recovery from neuromuscular block is observed, further recovery may be facilitated by administration of an anticholinesterase agent (*e.g.* neostigmine, edrophonium) in conjunction with an appropriate anticholinergic agent. (see Antagonism of Neuromuscular Block). Overdosage may increase the risk of hemodynamic side effects, especially decreases in blood pressure. If needed, cardiovascular support may be provided by proper positioning of the patient, fluid administration, and/or vasopressor agent administration.

ANTAGONISM OF NEUROMUSCULAR BLOCK

ANTAGONISTS (SUCH AS NEOSTIGMINE) SHOULD BE ADMINISTERED WHEN COMPLETE NEUROMUSCULAR BLOCK IS EVIDENT OR SUSPECTED. THE USE OF PERIPHERAL NERVE STIMULATOR TO EVALUATE RECOVERY AND ANTAGONISM OF NEUROMUSCULAR BLOCK IS RECOMMENDED.

Administration of 0.030 to 0.064 mg/kg neostigmine or 0.5 mg/kg edrophonium at approximately 10% recovery from neuromuscular block (range: 1 to 15) produced 95% recovery of the muscle twitch response and a T_4T_1 ratio ≥ 75% in about 10 minutes. The times from 25% recovery of the muscle twitch to T_4T_1ratio≥75% following these doses of antagonists averaged about 7 to 9 minutes. In comparison, average times for spontaneous recovery from 25% to T_4T_1 ratio≥75% were 12 to 13 minutes.

Patients administered antagonists should be evaluated for adequate clinical evidence of antagonism, *e.g.,* 5-second head lift and grip strength. Ventilation must be supported until no longer required.

Antagonism may be delayed in the presence of debilitation, carcinomatosis, and the concomitant use of certain broad spectrum antibiotics, or anesthetic agents and other drugs which enhance neuromuscular block or separately cause respiratory depression. (see DRUG INTERACTIONS.) Under such circumstances the management is the same as that of prolonged neuromuscular block (see OVERDOSAGE.)

DOSAGE AND ADMINISTRATION:

MIVACURIUM CHLORIDE SHOULD ONLY BE ADMINISTERED INTRAVENOUSLY.

THE DOSAGE INFORMATION PROVIDED BELOW IS INTENDED AS A GUIDE ONLY. DOSES OF MIVACURIUM CHLORIDE SHOULD BE INDIVIDUALIZED (SEE CLINICAL PHARMACOLOGY, Individualization of Dosages. Factors that may warrant dosage adjustment include but may not be limited to: the presence of significant kidney, liver, or cardiovascular disease, obesity (patients weighing≥30% more than ideal body weight for height), asthma, reduction in plasma cholinesterase activity, and the presence of inhalational anesthetic agents. The use of peripheral nerve stimulator will permit the most advantageous use of mivacurium chloride, minimize the possibility of overdosage or underdosage, and assist in the evaluation of recovery.

ADULTS

Initial Doses: A dose of 0.15 mg/kg mivacurium chloride administered over 5 to 15 seconds is recommended for facilitation of tracheal intubation for most patients. When administered as a component of a thiopental/opioid/nitrous oxide/oxygen induction-intubation technique, 0.15 mg/kg (2 x ED_{95}) mivacurium chloride produces generally good-to-excellent conditions for tracheal intubation in 2.5 minutes. Lower doses of mivacurium chloride may result in a longer time for development of satisfactory intubation conditions. Administration of mivacurium chloride doses above the recommended range (≥0.20 mg/kg) is associated with the development of transient decreases in blood pressure in some patients(see CLINICAL PHARMACOLOGY and ADVERSE REACTIONS).

In patients with clinically significant cardiovascular disease and in patients with any history suggesting a greater sensitivity to the release of histamine or other mediators (*e.g.,* asthma), the dose of mivacurium chloride should be 0.15 mg/kg or less, administered over 60 seconds (see PRECAUTIONS.)

Clinically effective neuromuscular block may be expected to last for 15 to 20 minutes (range: 9 to 38) and spontaneous recovery may be expected to be 95% complete in 25 to 30 minutes (range: 16 to 41) following 0.15 mg/kg mivacurium chloride administered to patients receiving opioid/nitrous oxide/oxygen anesthesia. Maintenance dosing is generally required approximately 15 minutes following an initial dose of 0.15 mg/kg mivacurium chloride during opioid/nitrous oxide/oxygen anesthesia. Maintenance doses of 0.10 mg/kg each provide approximately 15 minutes of additional clinically effective block. For shorter or longer durations of action, smaller or larger maintenance doses may be administered.

The neuromuscular blocking action of mivacurium chloride is potentiated by isoflurane or enflurane anesthesia. The recommended initial mivacurium chloride dose of 0.15 mg/kg may be used to facilitate tracheal intubation prior to the administration of these agents; however, if mivacurium chloride is first administered after establishment of stable-state isoflurane or enflurane anesthesia (administered with nitrous oxide/oxygen to achieve 1.25 MAC), the initial mivacurium chloride dose may be reduced by as much as 25%. Greater reductions in the mivacurium chloride dose may be required with higher concentrations of enflurane or isoflurane. With halothane, which has only a minimal potentiating effect on mivacurium chloride, a smaller dosage reduction may be considered.

Continuous Infusion: Continuous infusion of mivacurium chloride may be used to maintain neuromuscular block. Upon early evidence of spontaneous recovery from an initial dose, an initial infusion rate of 9 to 10 mcg/kg/min is recommended. If continuous infusion is initiated simultaneously with the administration of an initial dose, a lower initial infusion rate should be used (*e.g.,* 4 mcg/kg/min). In either case, the initial infusion rate should be

DOSAGE AND ADMINISTRATION: *(cont'd)*

adjusted according to the response to peripheral nerve stimulation and to clinical criteria. On average, an infusion rate of 6 to 7 mcg/kg/min (range: 1 to 15) may be expected to maintain neuromuscular block within the range of 89% to 99% for extended periods in adults receiving opioid/nitrous oxide/oxygen anesthesia. Reduction of the infusion rate by up to 35% to 40% should be considered when mivacurium chloride is administered during stable-state conditions of isoflurane or enflurane anesthesia (administered with nitrous oxide/oxygen to achieve 1.25 MAC). Greater reductions in the mivacurium chloride infusion rate may be required with greater concentrations of enflurane or isoflurane. With halothane, smaller reductions in infusion rate may be required.

CHILDREN

Initial Doses: Dosage requirements for mivacurium chloride on a mg/kg basis are higher in children than adults. Onset and recovery of neuromuscular block occur more rapidly in children than adults (see CLINICAL PHARMACOLOGY.) The recommended dose of mivacurium chloride for facilitating tracheal intubation in children 2 to 12 years of age is 0.20 mg/kg administered over 5 to 15 seconds. When administered during stable opioid/nitrous oxide/oxygen anesthesia, 0.20 mg/kg of mivacurium chloride produces maximum neuromuscular block in an average of 1.9 minutes (range: 1.3 to 3.3) and clinically effective block for 10 minutes (range: 6 to 15). Maintenance doses are generally required more frequently in children than in adults. Administration of mivacurium chloride doses above the recommended range (>0.20 mg/kg) is associated with transient decreases in MAP in some children see CLINICAL PHARMACOLOGY, Hemodynamics. Mivacurium chloride has not been studied in children below the age of 2 years.

Continuous Infusion: Children require higher mivacurium chloride infusion rates than adults. During opioid/nitrous oxide/oxygen anesthesia the infusion rate required to maintain 89% to 99% neuromuscular block averages 14 mcg/kg/min (range: 5 to 31). The principles for infusion of mivacurium chloride in adults are also applicable to children (See DOSAGE AND ADMINISTRATION, Adults.)

INFUSION RATE TABLES

For adults and children the amount of infusion solution required per hour depends upon the clinical requirements of the patient, the concentration of mivacurium chloride in the infusion solution, and the patient's weight. The contribution of the infusion solution to the fluid requirements of the patient must be considered. Tables 8 and 9 provide guidelines for delivery in ml/hr (equivalent to microdrops/min when 60 microdrops = 1 ml) of mivacurium chloride premixed infusion (0.5 mg/ml) and of mivacurium chloride injection (2 mg/ml).

TABLE 8 Infusion Rates for Maintenance of Neuromuscular Block During Opioid/Nitrous Oxide/Oxygen Anesthesia Using Mivacurium Chloride Premixed Infusion (0.5 mg/ml)

Patient Weight (kg)	Drug Delivery Rate (mcg/kg/min)									
	4	5	6	7	8	10	14	16	18	20
	Infusion Delivery Rate (ml/hr)									
10	5	6	7	8	10	12	17	19	22	24
15	7	9	11	13	14	18	25	29	32	36
20	10	12	15	17	19	24	34	38	43	48
25	12	15	18	21	24	30	42	48	54	60
35	17	21	26	29	34	42	59	67	76	84
50	24	30	36	42	48	60	84	96	108	120
60	29	36	43	50	58	72	101	115	130	144
70	34	42	50	59	67	84	118	134	151	168
80	39	48	58	67	77	96	134	154	173	192
90	44	54	65	76	86	108	151	173	194	216
100	48	60	72	84	96	120	168	192	216	240

TABLE 9 Infusion Rates for Maintenance of Neuromuscular Block During Opioid/Nitrous Oxide/Oxygen Anesthesia Using Mivacurium Chloride Injection (2 mg/ml)

Patient Weight (kg)	Drug Delivery Rate (mcg/kg/min)									
	4	5	6	7	8	10	14	16	18	20
	Infusion Delivery Rate (ml/hr)									
10	1.2	1.5	1.8	2.1	2.4	3.0	4.2	4.8	5.4	6.0
15	1.8	2.3	2.7	3.2	3.6	4.5	6.3	7.2	8.1	9.0
20	2.4	3.0	3.6	4.2	4.8	6.0	8.4	9.6	10.8	12.0
25	3.0	3.8	4.5	5.3	6.0	7.5	10.5	12.0	13.5	15.0
35	4.2	5.3	6.3	7.4	8.4	10.5	14.7	16.8	18.9	21.0
50	6.0	7.5	9.0	10.5	12.0	15.0	21.0	24.0	27.0	30.0
60	7.2	9.0	10.8	12.6	14.4	18.0	25.2	28.8	32.4	36.0
70	8.4	10.5	12.6	14.7	16.8	21.0	29.4	33.6	37.8	42.0
80	9.6	12.0	14.4	16.8	19.2	24.0	33.6	38.4	43.2	48.0
90	10.8	13.5	16.2	18.9	21.6	27.0	37.8	43.2	48.6	54.0
100	12.0	15.0	18.0	21.0	24.0	30.0	42.0	48.0	54.0	60.0

MIVACURIUM CHLORIDE PREMIXED INFUSION IN FLEXIBLE PLASTIC CONTAINERS

The flexible plastic container is fabricated from a specially formulated, nonplasticized, thermoplastic co-polyester (CR3). Water can permeate from inside the container into the overwrap but not in amounts sufficient to affect the solution significantly. Solutions inside the plastic container also can leach out certain of the chemical components in very small amounts before the expiration period is attained. However, the safety of the plastic has been confirmed by tests in animals according to USP biological standards for plastic containers.

Instructions for Use:

1. Tear outer wrap at notch and remove solution container. Check for minute leaks by squeezing container firmly. If leaks are found, discard solution as sterility may be impaired.

2. Close flow control clamp of administration set.

3. Remove cover from outlet port at bottom of container.

4. Insert piercing pin of administration set into port with a twisting motion until the pin is firmly seated.

NOTE: SEE FULL DIRECTIONS ON ADMINISTRATION SET CARTON.

5. Suspend container from hanger.

6. Squeeze and release drip chamber to establish proper fluid level in chamber during infusion.

7. Open flow control clamp to expel air from set. Close clamp.

8. Attach set to intravenous tubing.

9. Regulate rate of administration with flow control clamp.

CAUTION: Additives should not be introduced into this solution. Do not administer unless solution is clear and container is undamaged. Mivacurium chloride premixed infusion is intended for single patient use only. The unused portion of the solution should be discarded.

DOSAGE AND ADMINISTRATION: *(cont'd)*

Warning: Do not use flexible plastic container in series connections.

MIVACURIUM CHLORIDE INJECTION COMPATIBILITY AND ADMIXTURES:

Y-site Administration: Mivacurium chloride injection may not be compatible with alkaline solutions having a pH greater than 8.5 (*e.g.,* barbiturate solutions).

Studies have shown that mivacurium chloride injection is compatible with:

5% dextrose injection USP

0.9% sodium chloride injection USP

5% dextrose and 0.9% sodium chloride injection USP

Lactated Ringer's injection USP

5% Dextrose in Lactated Ringer's injection

Sufentanil citrate injection (Sufenta), diluted as directed

Alfentanil hydrochloride injection (Alfenta), diluted as directed

Fentanyl citrate injection (Sublimaze), diluted as directed

Midazolam hydrochloride injection (Versed), diluted as directed

Droperidol injection (Inapsine), diluted as directed

Compatibility studies with other parenteral products have not been conducted.

Dilution Stability: Mivacurium chloride injection diluted to 0.5 mg mivacurium per ml in 5% Dextrose injection USP, 5% Dextrose and 0.9% Sodium Chloride injection USP, 0.9% Sodium Chloride injection USP, Lactated Ringer's injection USP, or 5% Dextrose in Lactated Ringer's injection is physically and chemically stable when stored in PVC (polyvinyl chloride) bags at 5C to 25C (41F to 77°F) for up to 24 hours. Aseptic techniques should be used to prepare the diluted product. Admixtures of mivacurium chloride should be prepared for single patient use only and used within 24 hours of preparation. The unused portion of diluted mivacurium chloride should be discarded after each case.

NOTE: Parenteral drug products should be inspected visually for particulate matter and discoloration prior to administration whenever solution and container permit. Solutions which are not clear and colorless should not be used.

Storage: Store mivacurium chloride injection at room temperature of 15 to 25°C (59 to 77°F). Avoid exposure to direct ultraviolet light. DO NOT FREEZE.

Recommended storage for mivacurium chloride premixed infusion is room temperature (15 to 25C/59 to 77°F). Avoid excessive heat. Avoid exposure to direct ultraviolet light. Protect from freezing.

HOW SUPPLIED - EQUIVALENTS NOT AVAILABLE:

Injection, Solution - Intravenous - 0.5 mg/ml

50 ml x 24	$392.75	MIVACRON IN DEXTROSE, Glaxo Wellcome	00173-0709-01
100 ml x 24	$691.24	MIVACRON IN DEXTROSE, Glaxo Wellcome	00173-0709-02

Injection, Solution - Intravenous - 2 mg/ml

10 ml x 10	$163.64	MIVACRON, Glaxo Wellcome	00173-0705-95

MOEXIPRIL HYDROCHLORIDE *(003261)*

CATEGORIES: ACE Inhibitors; Angiotensin Converting Enzyme Inhibitors; Antihypertensives; Cardiovascular Drugs; Hypertension; FDA Class 1S ("Standard Review"); FDA Approved 1995 May

BRAND NAMES: Fampress; **Univasc**

FORMULARIES: PCS

WARNING:
USE IN PREGNANCY
When used in pregnancy during the second and third trimesters, ACE inhibitors can cause injury and even death to the developing fetus. When pregnancy is detected, moexipril HCl should be discontinued as soon as possible. See WARNINGS, Fetal/Neonatal Morbidity and Mortality.

DESCRIPTION:

Moexipril HCl has the empirical formula $C_{27}H_{34}N_2O_7$·HCl and a molecular weight of 535.04. It is chemically described as [3S-[2[R*(R*)],3R*]]-2-[2-[[1-(ethoxycarbonyl)-3-phenylpropyl]amino]-1-oxopropyl]-1,2,3,4-tetrahydro- 6,7-dimethoxy-3-isoquinolinecarboxylic acid, monohydrochloride. It is a nonsulfhydryl containing precursor of the active angiotensin-converting enzyme (ACE) inhibitor moexiprilat.

Moexipril hydrochloride is a fine white to off-white powder. It is soluble (about 10% weight-to-volume) in distilled water at room temperature.

Moexipril HCl is supplied as scored, coated tablets containing 7.5 mg and 15 mg of moexipril hydrochloride for oral administration. In addition to the active ingredient, moexipril hydrochloride, the tablet core contains the following inactive ingredients: lactose, magnesium oxide, crospovidone, magnesium stearate and gelatin. The film coating contains hydroxypropyl methylcellulose, hydroxypropyl cellulose, polyethylene glycol 6000, magnesium stearate, titanium dioxide, and ferric oxide.

CLINICAL PHARMACOLOGY:

MECHANISM OF ACTION

Moexipril hydrochloride is a prodrug for moexiprilat, which inhibits ACE in humans and animals. The mechanism through which moexiprilat lowers blood pressure is believed to be primarily inhibition of ACE activity. ACE is a peptidyl dipeptidase that catalyzes the conversion of the inactive decapeptide angiotensin I to the vasoconstrictor substance angiotensin II. Angiotensin II is a potent peripheral vasoconstrictor that also stimulates aldosterone secretion by the adrenal cortex and provides negative feedback on renin secretion. ACE is identical to kininase II, an enzyme that degrades bradykinin, an endothelium-dependent vasodilator. Moexiprilat is about 1000 times as potent as moexipril in inhibiting ACE and kininase II. Inhibition of ACE results in decreased angiotensin II formation, leading to decreased vasoconstriction, increased plasma renin activity, and decreased aldosterone secretion. The latter results in diuresis and natriuresis and a small increase in serum potassium concentration (mean increases of about 0.25 mEq/l were seen when moexipril was used alone, see PRECAUTIONS).

Whether increased levels of bradykinin, a potent vasodepressor peptide, play a role in the therapeutic effects of moexipril remains to be elucidated. Although the principal mechanism of moexipril in blood pressure reduction is believed to be through the renin-angiotensin-aldosterone system, ACE inhibitors have some effect on blood pressure even in apparent low-renin hypertension. As is the case with other ACE inhibitors, however, the antihypertensive effect of moexipril is considerably smaller in black patients, a predominantly low-renin population, than in non-black hypertensive patients.

CLINICAL PHARMACOLOGY: *(cont'd)*

PHARMACOKINETICS AND METABOLISM

Pharmacokinetics: Moexipril's antihypertensive activity is almost entirely due to its deesterified metabolite, moexiprilat. Bioavailability of oral moexipril is about 13% compared to intravenous (IV) moexipril (both measuring the metabolite moexiprilat), and is markedly affected by food, which reduces the peak plasma level (C_{max}) and AUC (see Absorption.) Moexipril should therefore be taken in a fasting state. The time of peak plasma concentration (T_{max}) of moexiprilat is about 1 1/2 hours and elimination half-life ($t_{1/2}$) is estimated at 2 to 9 hours in various studies, the variability reflecting a complex elimination pattern that is not simply exponential. Like all ACE inhibitors, moexiprilat has a prolonged terminal elimination phase, presumably reflecting slow release of drug bound to the ACE. Accumulation of moexiprilat with repeated dosing is minimal about 30%, compatible with a functional elimination $t_{1/2}$of about 12 hours. Over the dose range of 7.5 to 30 mg, pharmacokinetics are approximately dose proportional.

Absorption: Moexipril is incompletely absorbed, with bioavailability as moexiprilat of about 13%. Bioavailability varies with formulation and food intake which reduces C_{max} and AUC by about 70% and 40% respectively after the ingestion of a low-fat breakfast or by 80% and 50% respectively after the ingestion of a high-fat breakfast.

Distribution: The clearance (CL) for moexipril is 441 ml/min and for moexiprilat 232 ml/min with a $t_{1/2}$ of 1.3 and 9.8 hours, respectively. Moexiprilat is about 50% protein bound. The volume of distribution of moexiprilat is about 183 liters.

Metabolism and Excretion: Moexipril is relatively rapidly converted to its active metabolite moexiprilat, but persists longer than some other ACE inhibitor prodrugs, such that its half-life is over one hour and it has a significant AUC. Both moexipril and moexiprilat are converted to diketopiperazine derivatives and unidentified metabolites. After IV administration of moexipril, about 40% of the dose appears in urine as moexiprilat, about 26% as moexipril, with small amounts of the metabolites; about 20% of the IV dose appears in feces, principally as moexiprilat. After oral administration, only about 7% of the dose appears in urine as moexiprilat, about 1% as moexipril, with about 5% as other metabolites. Fifty-two percent of the dose is recovered in feces as moexiprilat and 1% as moexipril.

SPECIAL POPULATIONS

Decreased Renal Function: The effective elimination of $t_{1/2}$ and AUC of both moexipril and moexiprilat are increased with decreasing renal function. There is insufficient information available to characterize this relationship fully, but at creatinine clearances in the range of 10 to 40 ml/min, the $t_{1/2}$ of moexiprilat is increased by a factor of 3 to 4.

Decreased Hepatic Function: In patients with mild to moderate cirrhosis given single 15 mg doses of moexipril, the C_{max} of moexipril was increased by about 50% and the AUC increased by about 120%, while the C_{max} for moexiprilat was decreased by about 50% and the AUC increased by almost 300%.

Elderly Patients: In elderly male subjects (65-80 years old) with clinically normal renal and hepatic function, the AUC and C_{max} of moexiprilat is about 30% greater than those of younger subjects (19-42 years old).

Pharmacokinetic Interactions With Other Drugs: No clinically important pharmacokinetic interactions occurred when moexipril HCl was administered concomitantly with hydrochlorothiazide, digoxin, or cimetidine.

Pharmacodynamics and Clinical Effect: Single and multiple doses of 15 mg or more of moexipril HCl give a sustained inhibition of plasma ACE activity of 80 to 90%, beginning within 2 hours and lasting 24 hours (80%).

In controlled trials, the peak effects of orally administered moexipril increased with the dose administered over a dose range of 7.5 to 60 mg, given once a day. Antihypertensive effects were first detectable about 1 hour after dosing, with a peak effect between 3 and 6 hours after dosing.

Just before (*i.e.,* at trough), the antihypertensive effects were less prominently related to dose and the antihypertensive effect tended to diminish during the 24-hour dosing interval when the drug was administered once a day.

In multiple dose studies in the dose range of 7.5 to 30 mg once a day, moexipril HCl lowered sitting diastolic and systolic blood pressure effects at trough by 3 to 6 mmHg and 4 to 11 mmHg, more than placebo, respectively. There was a tendency toward increased response with higher doses over this range. These effects are typical of ACE inhibitors but, to date, there are no trials of adequate size comparing moexipril with other antihypertensive agents.

The trough diastolic blood pressure effects of moexipril were approximately 3 to 6 mmHg in various studies. Generally, higher doses of moexipril leave a greater fraction of the peak blood pressure effect still present at trough. During dose titration, any decision as to the adequacy of a dosing regimen should be based on trough blood pressure measurements. If diastolic blood pressure control is not adequate at the end of the dosing interval, the dose can be increased or given as a divided (BID) regimen.

During chronic therapy, the antihypertensive effect of any dose of moexipril HCl is generally evident within 2 weeks of treatment, with maximal reduction after 4 weeks. The antihypertensive effects of moexipril HCl have been proven to continue during therapy for up to 24 months.

Moexipril HCl, like other ACE inhibitors, is less effective in decreasing trough blood pressures in blacks than in non-blacks. Placebo-corrected trough group mean diastolic blood pressure effects in blacks in the proposed dose range varied between +1 to -3 mmHg compared with responses in non-blacks of -4 to -6 mmHg.

The effectiveness of moexipril HCl was not significantly influenced by patient age, gender, or weight. Moexipril HCl has been shown to have antihypertensive activity in both pre and postmenopausal women who have participated in placebo-controlled clinical trials.

Formal interaction studies with moexipril have not been carried out with antihypertensive agents other than thiazide diuretics. In these studies, the added effect of moexipril was similar to its effect as monotherapy. In general, ACE inhibitors have less than additive effects with beta- adrenergic blockers, presumably because both work by inhibiting the renin-angiotensin system.

INDICATIONS AND USAGE:

Moexipril HCl is indicated for treatment of patients with hypertension. It may be used alone or in combination with thiazide diuretics.

In using moexipril HCl, consideration should be given to the fact that another ACE inhibitor, captopril, has caused agranulocytosis, particularly in patients with renal impairment or collagen-vascular disease. Available data are insufficient to show that moexipril HCl does not have a similar risk (see WARNINGS.)

In considering use of moexipril HCl, it should be noted that in controlled trials ACE inhibitors have an effect on blood pressure that is less in black patients than in non-blacks. In addition, ACE inhibitors (for which adequate data are available) cause a higher rate of angioedema in black than in non-black patients (see WARNINGS, Angioedema.)

CONTRAINDICATIONS:

Moexipril HCl is contraindicated in patients who are hypersensitive to this product and in patients with a history of angioedema related to previous treatment with an ACE inhibitor.

WARNINGS:

Anaphylactoid and Possibly Related Reactions: Presumably because angiotensin-converting enzyme inhibitors affect the metabolism of eicosanoids and polypeptides, including endogenous bradykinin, patients receiving ACE inhibitors, including moexipril HCl, may be subject to a variety of adverse reactions, some of them serious.

Angioedema: Angioedema involving the face, extremities, lips, tongue, glottis, and/or larynx has been reported in patients treated with ACE inhibitors, including moexipril HCl. Symptoms suggestive of angioedema or facial edema occurred in <0.5% of moexipril-treated patients in placebo-controlled trials. None of the cases were considered life-threatening and all resolved either without treatment or with medication (antihistamines or glucocorticoids). One patient treated with hydrochlorothiazide alone experienced laryngeal edema. No instances of angioedema were reported in placebo-treated patients.

In cases of angioedema, treatment should be promptly discontinued and the patient carefully observed until the swelling disappears. In instances where swelling has been confined to the face and lips, the condition has generally resolved without treatment, although antihistamines have been useful in relieving symptoms.

Angioedema associated with involvement of the tongue, glottis, or larynx, may be fatal due to airway obstruction. Appropriate therapy (*e.g.*, subcutaneous epinephrine solution 1:1000 (0.3 to 0.5 ml) and/or measures to ensure a patent airway) should be promptly provided (see ADVERSE REACTIONS).

Anaphylactoid Reactions During Desensitization: Two patients undergoing desensitizing treatment with hymenoptera venom while receiving ACE inhibitors sustained life-threatening anaphylactoid reactions. In the same patients, these reactions did not occur when ACE inhibitors were temporarily withheld, but they reappeared when the ACE inhibitors were inadvertently readministered.

Anaphylactoid Reactions During Membrane Exposure: Anaphylactoid reactions have been reported in patients dialyzed with high-flux membranes and treated concomitantly with an ACE inhibitor. Anaphylactoid reactions have also been reported in patients undergoing low-density lipoprotein apheresis with dextran sulfate absorption (a procedure dependent upon devices not approved in the United States).

Hypotension: Moexipril HCl can cause symptomatic hypotension, although, as with other ACE inhibitors, this is unusual in uncomplicated hypertensive patients treated with moexipril HCl alone. Symptomatic hypotension was seen in 0.5% of patients given moexipril and led to discontinuation of therapy in about 0.25%. Symptomatic hypotension is most likely to occur in patients who have been salt- and volume-depleted as a result of prolonged diuretic therapy, dietary salt restriction, dialysis, diarrhea, or vomiting. Volume- and salt-depletion should be corrected and, in general, diuretics stopped, before initiating therapy with moexipril HCl (see DRUG INTERACTIONSand ADVERSE REACTIONS).

In patients with congestive heart failure, with or without associated renal insufficiency, ACE inhibitor therapy may cause excessive hypotension, which may be associated with oliguria or progressive azotemia, and rarely, with acute renal failure and death. In these patients, moexipril HCl therapy should be started under close medical supervision, and patients should be followed closely for the first two weeks of treatment and whenever the dose of moexipril or an accompanying diuretic is increased. Care in avoiding hypotension should also be taken in patients with ischemic heart disease, aortic stenosis, or cerebrovascular disease, in whom an excessive decrease in blood pressure could result in a myocardial infarction or a cerebrovascular accident.

If hypotension occurs, the patient should be placed in a supine position and, if necessary, treated with an intravenous infusion of normal saline. Moexipril HCl treatment usually can be continued following restoration of blood pressure and volume.

Neutropenia/Agranulocytosis: Another ACE inhibitor, captopril, has been shown to cause agranulocytosis and bone marrow depression, rarely in patients with uncomplicated hypertension, but more frequently in hypertensive patients with renal impairment, especially if they also have a collagen-vascular disease such as systemic lupus erythematosus or scleroderma. Although there were no instances of severe neutropenia (absolute neutrophil count <500/mm^3) among patients given moexipril HCl, as with other ACE inhibitors, monitoring of white blood cell counts should be considered for patients who have collagen-vascular disease, especially if the disease is associated with impaired renal function. Available data from clinical trials of moexipril HCl are insufficient to show that moexipril HCl does not cause agranulocytosis at rates similar to captopril.

Fetal/Neonatal Morbidity and Mortality: ACE inhibitors can cause fetal and neonatal morbidity and death when administered to pregnant women. Several dozen cases have been reported in the world literature. When pregnancy is detected, ACE inhibitors should be discontinued as soon as possible.

The use of ACE inhibitors during the second and third trimesters of pregnancy has been associated with fetal and neonatal injury, including hypotension, neonatal skull hypoplasia, anuria, reversible or irreversible renal failure, and death. Oligohydramnios has also been reported, presumably resulting from decreased fetal renal function; oligohydramnios in this setting has been associated with fetal limb contractures, craniofacial deformation, and hypoplastic lung development. Prematurity, intrauterine growth retardation, and patent ductus arteriosus have also been reported, although it is not clear whether these were caused by the ACE inhibitor exposure.

Fetal and neonatal morbidity do not appear to have resulted from intrauterine ACE inhibitor exposure limited to the first trimester. Mothers who have used ACE inhibitors only during the first trimester should be informed of this. Nonetheless, when patients become pregnant, physicians should make every effort to discontinue the use of moexipril as soon as possible. Rarely (probably less often than once in every thousand pregnancies), no alternative to ACE inhibitors will be found. In these rare cases, the mothers should be apprised of the potential hazards to their fetuses, and serial ultrasound examinations should be performed to assess the intraamniotic environment.

If oligohydramnios is observed, moexipril should be discontinued unless it is considered life-saving for the mother. Contraction stress (CST), a non-stress test (NST), or biophysical profiling (BPP) may be appropriate, depending upon the week of pregnancy. Patients and physicians should be aware, however, that oligohydramnios may not be detected until after the fetus has sustained irreversible injury.

Infants with histories of *in utero* exposure to ACE inhibitors should be closely observed for hypotension, oliguria, and hyperkalemia. If oliguria occurs, attention should be directed toward support of blood pressure and renal perfusion. Exchange transfusion or peritoneal dialysis may be required as means of reversing hypotension and/or substituting for disordered renal function.

Theoretically, the ACE inhibitor could be removed from the neonatal circulation by exchange transfusion, but no experience with this procedure has been reported.

No embryotoxic, fetotoxic, or teratogenic effects were seen in rats or in rabbits treated with up to 90.9 times and 0.7 times, respectively, the Maximum Recommended Human Dose (MRHD) on a mg/m^{2}basis.

WARNINGS: *(cont'd)*

Hepatic Failure: Rarely, ACE inhibitors have been associated with a syndrome that starts with cholestatic jaundice and progresses to fulminant hepatic necrosis and sometimes death. The mechanism of this syndrome is not understood. Patients receiving ACE inhibitors who develop jaundice or marked elevations of hepatic enzymes should discontinue the ACE inhibitor and receive appropriate medical follow-up.

PRECAUTIONS:

GENERAL

Impaired Renal Function: As a consequence of inhibition of the renin-angiotensin-aldosterone system, changes in renal function may be anticipated in susceptible individuals. There is no clinical experience of moexipril HCl in the treatment of hypertension in patients with renal failure.

Some hypertensive patients with no apparent preexisting renal vascular disease have developed increases in blood urea nitrogen and serum creatinine, usually minor and transient, especially when moexipril HCl has been given concomitantly with a thiazide diuretic. This is more likely to occur in patients with preexisting renal impairment. There may be a need for dose adjustment of moexipril HCl and/or the discontinuation of the thiazide diuretic.

Evaluation Of Hypertensive Patients Should Always Include Assessment Of Renal Function: (see DOSAGE AND ADMINISTRATION.)

Hypertensive Patients With Congestive Heart Failure: In hypertensive patients with severe congestive heart failure, whose renal function may depend on the activity of the renin-angiotensin-aldosterone system, treatment with ACE inhibitors, including moexipril HCl, may be associated with oliguria and/or progressive azotemia and, rarely, acute renal failure and/or death.

Hypertensive Patients With Renal Artery Stenosis: In hypertensive patients with unilateral or bilateral renal artery stenosis, increases in blood urea nitrogen and serum creatinine have been observed in some patients following ACE inhibitor therapy. These increases were almost always reversible upon discontinuation of the ACE inhibitor and/or diuretic therapy. In such patients, renal function should be monitored during the first few weeks of therapy.

Hyperkalemia: In clinical trials, persistent hyperkalemia (serum potassium above 5.4 mEq/l) occurred in approximately 1.3% of hypertensive patients receiving moexipril HCl. Risk factors for the development of hyperkalemia with ACE inhibitors include renal insufficiency, diabetes mellitus, and the concomitant use of potassium-sparing diuretics, potassium supplements, and/or potassium-containing salt substitutes, which should be used cautiously, if at all, with moexipril HCl (see DRUG INTERACTIONS.)

Surgery/Anesthesia: In patients undergoing major surgery or during anesthesia with agents that produce hypotension, moexipril may block the effects of compensatory renin release. If hypotension occurs in this setting and is considered to be due to this mechanism, it can be corrected by volume expansion.

Cough: Presumably due to the inhibition of the degradation of endogenous bradykinin, persistent nonproductive cough has been reported with all ACE inhibitors, always resolving after discontinuation of therapy. ACE inhibitor-induced cough should be considered in the differential diagnosis of cough. In controlled trials with moexipril, cough was present in 6.1% of moexipril patients and 2.2% of patients given placebo.

INFORMATION FOR THE PATIENT

Food: Patients should be advised to take moexipril one hour before meals (see CLINICAL PHARMACOLOGY and DOSAGE AND ADMINISTRATION).

Angioedema: Angioedema, including laryngeal edema, may occur with treatment with ACE inhibitors, usually occurring early in therapy (within the first month). Patients should be so advised and told to report immediately any signs or symptoms suggesting angioedema (swelling of the face, extremities, eyes, lips, tongue, difficulty in breathing) and to take no more moexipril HCl until they have consulted with the prescribing physician.

Symptomatic Hypotension: Patients should be cautioned that lightheadedness can occur with moexipril HCl, especially during the first few days of therapy. If fainting occurs, the patient should stop taking moexipril HCl and consult the prescribing physician.

All patients should be cautioned that excessive perspiration and dehydration may lead to an excessive fall in blood pressure because of reduction in fluid volume. Other causes of volume depletion such as vomiting or diarrhea may also lead to a fall in blood pressure; patients should be advised to consult their physician if they develop these conditions.

Hyperkalemia: Patients should be told not to use potassium supplements or salt substitutes containing potassium without consulting their physician.

Neutropenia: Patients should be told to report promptly any indication of infection (*e.g.*, sore throat, fever) that could be a sign of neutropenia.

Pregnancy: Female patients of childbearing age should be told about the consequences of second- and third-trimester exposure to ACE inhibitors and should also be told that these consequences do not appear to have resulted from intrauterine ACE inhibitor exposure that has been limited to the first trimester. Patients should be asked to report pregnancies to their physicians as soon as possible.

CARCINOGENESIS, MUTAGENESIS, AND IMPAIRMENT OF FERTILITY

No evidence of carcinogenicity was detected on long-term studies in mice and rats at doses up to 14 or 27.3 times the Maximum Recommended Human Dose (MRHD) on a mg/m^2 basis.

No mutagenicity was detected in the Ames test and microbial reverse mutation assay, with and without metabolic activation, or in an *in vivo* nucleus anomaly test. However, increased chromosomal aberration frequency in Chinese hamster ovary cells was detected under metabolic activation conditions at a 20-hour harvest time.

Reproduction studies have been performed in rabbits at oral doses up to 0.7 times the MRHD on a mg/m^2 basis, and in rats up to 90.9 times the MRHD on a mg/m^2 basis. No indication of impaired fertility, reproductive toxicity, or teratogenicity was observed.

PREGNANCY

Pregnancy Categories C (first trimester) and D (second and third trimesters): See WARNINGS, Fetal/Neonatal Morbidity and Mortality.

Nursing Mothers: It is not known whether moexipril HCl is secreted in human milk. Because many drugs are secreted in human milk, caution should be exercised when moexipril HCl is given to a nursing mother.

Geriatric Use: Of the patients who received moexipril HCl in controlled clinical studies, 33% were 65 years of age or older. No overall differences in effectiveness or safety were observed between these patients and younger patients. In elderly patients receiving moexipril HCl, plasma levels of drug are slightly higher and renal clearance is reduced when compared to younger patients, but this did not have detectable consequences.

Pediatric Use: Safety and effectiveness of moexipril HCl in pediatric patients have not been established.

DRUG INTERACTIONS:

Diuretics: Excessive reductions in blood pressure may occur in patients on diuretic therapy when ACE inhibitors are started. The possibility of hypotensive effects with moexipril HCl can be minimized by discontinuing diuretic therapy for several days or cautiously increasing salt intake before initiation of treatment with moexipril HCl. If this is not possible, the starting dose of moexipril should be reduced. (See WARNINGSand DOSAGE AND ADMINISTRATION).

Potassium Supplements and Potassium-Sparing Diuretics: Moexipril HCl can increase serum potassium because it decreases aldosterone secretion. Use of potassium-sparing diuretics (spironolactone, triamterene, amiloride) or potassium supplements concomitantly with ACE inhibitors can increase the risk of hyperkalemia. Therefore, if concomitant use of such agents is indicated, they should be given with caution and the patient's serum potassium should be monitored.

Oral Anticoagulants: Interaction studies with warfarin failed to identify any clinically important effect on the serum concentrations of the anticoagulant or on its anticoagulant effect.

Lithium: Increased serum lithium levels and symptoms of lithium toxicity have been reported in patients receiving ACE inhibitors during therapy with lithium. These drugs should be coadministered with caution, and frequent monitoring of serum lithium levels is recommended. If a diuretic is also used, the risk of lithium toxicity may be increased.

Other Agents: No clinically important pharmacokinetic interactions occurred when moexipril HCl was administered concomitantly with hydrochlorothiazide, digoxin, or cimetidine.

Moexipril HCl has been used in clinical trials concomitantly with calcium-channel-blocking agents, diuretics, H_2 blockers, digoxin, oral hypoglycemic agents, and cholesterol-lowering agents. There was no evidence of clinically important adverse interactions.

ADVERSE REACTIONS:

Moexipril HCl has been evaluated for safety in more than 2500 patients with hypertension; more than 250 of these patients were treated for approximately one year. The overall incidence of reported adverse events was only slightly greater in patients treated with moexipril HCl than patients treated with placebo.

Reported adverse experiences were usually mild and transient, and there were no differences in adverse reaction rates related to gender, race, age, duration of therapy, or total daily dosage within the range of 3.75 mg to 60 mg. Discontinuation of therapy because of adverse experiences was required in 3.4% of patients treated with moexipril HCl and in 1.8% of patients treated with placebo. The most common reasons for discontinuation in patients treated with moexipril HCl were cough (0.7%) and dizziness (0.4%).

All adverse experiences considered at least possibly related to treatment that occurred at any dose in placebo-controlled trials of once-daily dosing in more than 1% of patients treated with moexipril HCl alone and that were at least as frequent in the moexipril HCl group as in the placebo group are shown in the following table (TABLE 1):

TABLE 1 ADVERSE EVENTS IN PLACEBO-CONTROLLED STUDIES

ADVERSE EVENT	MOEXIPRIL HCl (N=674) N (%)	PLACEBO (N=226) N (%)
Cough Increased	41 (6.1)	5 (2.2)
Dizziness	29 (4.3)	5 (2.2)
Diarrhea	21 (3.1)	5 (2.2)
Flu Syndrome	21 (3.1)	0 (0)
Fatigue	16 (2.4)	4 (1.8)
Pharyngitis	12 (1.8)	2 (0.9)
Flushing	11 (1.6)	0 (0)
Rash	11 (1.6)	2 (0.9)
Myalgia	9 (1.3)	0 (0)

Other adverse events occurring in more than 1% of patients on moexipril that were at least as frequent on placebo include: headache, upper respiratory infection, pain, rhinitis, dyspepsia, nausea, peripheral edema, sinusitis, chest pain, and urinary frequency. See WARNINGSand PRECAUTIONS for discussion of anaphylactoid reactions, angioedema, hypotension, neutropenia/agranulocytosis, second and third trimester fetal/neonatal morbidity and mortality, hyperkalemia, and cough.

Other potentially important adverse experiences reported in controlled or uncontrolled clinical trials in less than 1% of moexipril patients or that have been attributed to other ACE inhibitors include the following:

Cardiovascular: Symptomatic hypotension, postural hypotension, or syncope were seen in 9/1750 (0.51%) patients; these reactions led to discontinuation of therapy in controlled trials in 3/1254 (0.24%) patients who had received moexipril HCl monotherapy and in 1/344 (0.3%) patients who had received moexipril HCl with hydrochlorothiazide (see PRECAUTIONS and WARNINGS). Other adverse events included angina/myocardial infarction, palpitations, rhythm disturbances, and cerebrovascular accident.

Renal: Of hypertensive patients with no apparent preexisting renal disease, 1% of patients receiving moexipril HCl alone and 2% of patients receiving moexipril HCl with hydrochlorothiazide experienced increases in serum creatinine to at least 140% of their baseline values (see PRECAUTIONS and DOSAGE AND ADMINISTRATION).

Gastrointestinal: Abdominal pain, constipation, vomiting, appetite/weight change, dry mouth, pancreatitis, hepatitis.

Respiratory: Bronchospasm, dyspnea.

Urogenital: Renal insufficiency, oliguria.

Dermatologic: Apparent hypersensitivity reactions manifested by urticaria, rash, pemphigus, pruritus, photosensitivity.

Neurological and Psychiatric: Drowsiness, sleep disturbances, nervousness, mood changes, anxiety.

Other: Angioedema (see WARNINGS), taste disturbances, tinnitus, sweating, malaise, arthralgia, hemolytic anemia.

CLINICAL LABORATORY TEST FINDINGS

Creatinine and Blood Urea Nitrogen: As with other ACE inhibitors, minor increases in blood urea nitrogen or serum creatinine, reversible upon discontinuation of therapy, were observed in approximately 1% of patients with essential hypertension who were treated with moexipril HCl. Increases are more likely to occur in patients receiving concomitant diuretics and in patients with compromised renal function (see PRECAUTIONS, General.)

Other (causal relationship unknown): Clinically important changes in standard laboratory tests were rarely associated with moexipril HCl administration.

Elevations of liver enzymes and uric acid have been reported. In trials, less than 1% of moexipril-treated patients discontinued moexipril HCl treatment because of laboratory abnormalities. The incidence of abnormal laboratory values with moexipril was similar to that in the placebo-treated group.

OVERDOSAGE:

Human overdoses of moexipril have not been reported. In case reports of overdoses with other ACE inhibitors, hypotension has been the principal adverse effect noted. Single oral doses of 2 g/kg moexipril were associated with significant lethality in mice. Rats, however, tolerated single oral doses of up to 3 g/kg.

No data are available to suggest that physiological maneuvers (*e.g.,* maneuvers to change the pH of the urine) would accelerate elimination of moexipril and its metabolites. The dialyzability of moexipril is not known.

Angiotensin II could presumably serve as a specific antagonist-antidote in the setting of moexipril overdose, but angiotensin II is essentially unavailable outside of research facilities. Because the hypotensive effect of moexipril is achieved through vasodilation and effective hypovolemia, it is reasonable to treat moexipril overdose by infusion of normal saline solution. In addition, renal function and serum potassium should be monitored.

DOSAGE AND ADMINISTRATION:

Hypertension: The recommended initial dose of moexipril HCl in patients not receiving diuretics is 7.5 mg, one hour prior to meals, once daily. Dosage should be adjusted according to blood pressure response. The antihypertensive effect of moexipril HCl may diminish towards the end of the dosing interval. Blood pressure should, therefore, be measured just prior to dosing to determine whether satisfactory blood pressure control is obtained. If control is not adequate, increased dose or divided dosing can be tried. The recommended dose range is 7.5 to 30 mg daily, administered in one or two divided doses one hour before meals. Total daily doses above 60 mg a day have not been studied in hypertensive patients.

In patients who are currently being treated with a diuretic, symptomatic hypotension may occasionally occur following the initial dose of moexipril HCl. The diuretic should, if possible, be discontinued for 2 to 3 days before therapy with moexipril HCl is begun, to reduce the likelihood of hypotension (see WARNINGS). If the patient's blood pressure is not controlled with moexipril HCl alone, diuretic therapy may then be reinstituted. If diuretic therapy cannot be discontinued, an initial dose of 3.75 mg of moexipril HCl should be used with medical supervision until blood pressure has stabilized (see WARNINGSand DRUG INTERACTIONS).

Dosage Adjustment in Renal Impairment: For patients with a creatinine clearance ≤ 40 ml/min/1.73 m^2, an initial dose of 3.75 mg once daily should be given cautiously. Doses may be titrated upward to a maximum daily dose of 15 mg.

HOW SUPPLIED:

Univasc 7.5 mg: Pink colored, biconvex, film-coated and scored with engraved code **707** on the unscored side and **SP** above and **7.5** below the score.

Univasc 15 mg: Salmon colored, biconvex, film-coated and scored with engraved code **715** on the unscored side and **SP** above and **15** below the score.

Store, tightly closed, at controlled room temperature. Protect from excessive moisture.

Dispense in a tight container, if product package is subdivided.

HOW SUPPLIED - EQUIVALENTS NOT AVAILABLE:

Tablet, Uncoated - Oral - 7.5 mg

90's	$35.78	UNIVASC, Schwarz Pharma (US)	00091-3707-09
100's	$39.75	UNIVASC, Schwarz Pharma (US)	00091-3707-01

Tablet, Uncoated - Oral - 15 mg

90's	$35.78	UNIVASC, Schwarz Pharma (US)	00091-3715-09
100's	$39.75	UNIVASC, Schwarz Pharma (US)	00091-3715-01

MOLGRAMOSTIM *(003082)*

CATEGORIES: AIDS Related Complex; Anemia; Bone Marrow Transplantation; Burns; Cytomegalovirus Infections; HIV Infection; Myelodysplastic Syndrome; Neutropenia, Chemotherapy; Platelet Depletion; Retinitis; Recombinant DNA Origin; FDA Unapproved

BRAND NAMES: **Leucomax**; M-Csf; Macrophage-Colony Stimulating Factor

Prescribing information not available at time of publication.

MOLINDONE HYDROCHLORIDE *(001826)*

CATEGORIES: Antipsychotics/Antimanics; Central Nervous System Agents; Neuroleptics; Psychotherapeutic Agents; Psychotic Disorders; Tranquilizers; FDA Approval Pre 1982

BRAND NAMES: **Moban**

FORMULARIES: Medi-Cal

DESCRIPTION:

Molindone hydrochloride is a dihydroindolone compound which is not structurally related to the phenothiazines, the butyrophenones or the thioxanthenes.

Molindone HCl is 3-ethyl-6, 7-dihydro-2-methyl-5-(morpholinomethyl) indol-4(5H)-one hydrochloride. It is a white to off-white crystalline powder, freely soluble in water and alcohol and has a molecular weight of 312.67.

Moban Tablets also contain: *All strengths:* calcium sulfate, lactose, magnesium stearate, microcrystalline, cellulose and povidone. *5 mg:* alginic acid, colloidal silicon dioxide and FD&C Yellow 6. *10 mg:* alginic acid, colloidal silicon dioxide, FD&C Blue 2 and FD&C Red 40. *25 mg:* alginic acid, colloidal silicon dioxide, D&C Yellow 10, FD&C Blue 2, and FD&C Yellow 6. *50 mg:* FD&C Blue 2 and sodium starch glycolate. *100 mg:* FD&C Blue 2, FD&C Yellow 6 and sodium starch glycolate.

Moban Concentrate contains: alcohol, artificial cherry flavor, artificial cover flavor, edetate disodium, glycerin, liquid sugar, methylparaben, propylparaben, sodium metabisulfite, sorbitol solution, and hydrochloric acid reagent grade for pH adjustment.

CLINICAL PHARMACOLOGY:

Molindone hydrochloride has a pharmacological profile in laboratory animals which predominantly resembles that of major tranquilizers causing reduction of spontaneous locomotion and aggressiveness, suppression of a conditioned response and antagonism of the bizarre stereotyped behavior and hyperactivity induced by amphetamines. In addition, molindone HCl antagonizes the depression caused by the tranquilizing agent tetrabenazine.

In human clinical studies tranquilization is achieved in the absence of muscle relaxing or incoordinating effects. Based on EEG studies, molindone HCl exerts its effect on the ascending reticular activating system.

CLINICAL PHARMACOLOGY: *(cont'd)*

Human metabolic studies show molindone HCl to be rapidly absorbed and metabolized when given orally. Unmetabolized drug reached a peak blood level at 1.5 hours. Pharmacological effect from a single oral dose persists for 24-36 hours. There are 36 recognized metabolites with less than 2-3% unmetabolized molindone HCl being excreted in urine and feces.

INDICATIONS AND USAGE:

Molindone HCl is indicated in the management of the manifestations of psychotic disorders. The antipsychotic efficacy of molindone HCl was established in clinical studies which enrolled newly hospitalized and chronically hospitalized, acutely ill, schizophrenic patients as subjects.

CONTRAINDICATIONS:

Molindone hydrochloride is contraindicated in severe central nervous system depression (alcohol, barbiturates, narcotics, etc.) or comatose states, and in patients with known hypersensitivity to the drug.

WARNINGS:

Tardive Dyskinesia: Tardive dyskinesia, a syndrome consisting of potentially irreversible, involuntary, dyskinetic movements, may develop in patients treated with neuroleptic (antipsychotic) drugs. Although the prevalence of the syndrome appears to be highest among the elderly, especially elderly women, it is impossible to rely upon prevalence estimates to predict, at the inception of neuroleptic treatment, which patients are likely to develop the syndrome. Whether neuroleptic drug products differ in their potential to cause tardive dyskinesia is unknown. Both the risk of developing the syndrome and the likelihood that will become irreversible are believed to increase as the duration of treatment and the total cumulative dose of neuroleptic drugs administered to the patient increase. However, the syndrome can develop, although much less commonly, after relatively brief treatment periods at low doses.

There is no known treatment for established cases of tardive dyskinesia, although the syndrome may remit, partially or completely, if neuroleptic treatment is withdrawn. Neuroleptic treatment, itself, however, may suppress (or partially suppress) the signs and symptoms of the syndrome and thereby may possibly mask the underlying disease process. The effect that symptomatic suppression has upon the long-term course of the syndrome is unknown.

Given these considerations, neuroleptics should be prescribed in a manner that is most likely to minimize the occurrence of tardive dyskinesia. Chronic neuroleptic treatment should generally be reserved for patients who suffer from chronic illness that 1) is known to respond to neuroleptic drugs, and 2) for whom alternative, equally effective, but potentially less harmful treatments are *not* available or appropriate. In patients who do require chronic treatment, the smallest dose and the shortest duration of treatment producing a satisfactory clinical response should be sought. The need for continued treatment should be reassessed periodically.

If signs and symptoms of tardive dyskinesia appear in a patient on neuroleptics, drug discontinuation should be considered. However, some patients may require treatment despite the presence of the syndrome.

(For further information about the description of tardive dyskinesia and its clinical detection, please refer to the section on ADVERSE REACTIONS.)

Neuroleptic Malignant Syndrome (NMS): A potentially fatal symptom complex sometimes referred to as Neuroleptic Malignant Syndrome (NMS) has been reported in association with antipsychotic drugs. Clinical manifestations of NMS are hyperpyrexia, muscle rigidity, altered mental status and evidence of autonomic instability (irregular pulse or blood pressure, tachycardia, diaphoresis, and cardiac dysrhythmias).

The diagnostic evaluation of patients with this syndrome is complicated. In arriving at a diagnosis, it is important to identify cases where the clinical presentation includes both serious medical illness (*e.g.,* pneumonia, systemic infection, etc.) and untreated or inadequately treated extrapyramidal signs and symptoms (EPS). Other important considerations in the differential diagnosis include central and anticholinergic toxicity, heat stroke, drug fever and primary central nervous system (CNS) pathology.

The management of NMS should include 1) immediate discontinuation of antipsychotic drugs and other drugs not essential to concurrent therapy, 2) intensive symptomatic treatment and medical monitoring, and 3) treatment of any concomitant serious medical problems for which specific treatments are available. There is no general agreement about specific pharmacological treatment regimens for uncomplicated NMS.

If a patient requires antipsychotic drug treatment after recovery from NMS, the potential reintroduction of drug therapy should be carefully considered. The patient should be carefully monitored, since recurrences or NMS have been reported.

Usage in Pregnancy: Studies in pregnant patients have not been carried out. Reproduction studies have been performed in the following animals (TABLE 1):

TABLE 1

Pregnant Rats oral dose:	
no adverse effect	20 mg/kg/day—2 weeks
no adverse effect	40 mg/kg/day—2 weeks
Pregnant Mice oral dose:	
slight increase resorptions	20 mg/kg/day—10 days
slight increase resorptions	40 mg/kg/day—10 days
Pregnant Rabbits oral dose:	
no adverse effect	5 mg/kg/day—12 days
no adverse effect	10 mg/kg/day—12 days
no adverse effect	20 mg/kg/day—12 days

Animal reproductive studies have not demonstrated a teratogenic potential. The anticipated benefits must be weighed against the unknown risks to the fetus if used in pregnant patients.

Nursing Mothers: Data are not available on the content of molindone HCl in the milk of nursing mothers.

Usage in Children: Use of molindone HCl in children below the age of twelve years is not recommended because safe and effective conditions for its usage have not been established.

Molindone HCl has not been shown effective in the management of behavioral complications in patients with mental retardation.

Sulfites Sensitivity: Molindone HCl Concentrate contains sodium metabisulfite, a sulfite that may cause allergic-type reactions including anaphylactic symptoms and life-threatening or less severe asthmatic episodes in certain susceptible people. The overall prevalence of sulfite sensitivity in the general population is unknown and probably low. Sulfite sensitivity is seen more frequently in asthmatic than in nonasthmatic people.

PRECAUTIONS:

Some patients receiving molindone HCl may note drowsiness initially and they should be advised against activities requiring mental alertness until their response to the drug has been established.

PRECAUTIONS: *(cont'd)*

Increased activity has been noted in patients receiving molindone HCl. Caution should be exercised where increased activity may be harmful.

Molindone HCl does not lower the seizure threshold in experimental animals to the degree noted with more sedating antipsychotic drugs. However, in humans, convulsive seizures have been reported in a few instances.

The physician should be aware that this tablet preparation contains calcium sulfate as an excipient and that calcium ions may interfere with the absorption of preparations containing phenytoin sodium and tetracyclines.

Molindone HCl has an antiemetic effect in animals. A similar effect may occur in humans and may obscure signs of intestinal obstruction or brain tumor.

Neuroleptic drugs elevate prolactin levels; the elevation persists during chronic administration. Tissue culture experiments indicate that approximately one-third of human breast cancers are prolactin dependent*in vitro*, a factor of potential importance if the prescription of these drugs is contemplated in a patient with a previously detected breast cancer. Although disturbances such as galactorrhea, amenorrhea, gynecomastia, and impotence have been reported, the clinical significance of elevated serum prolactin levels is unknown for most patients. An increase in mammary neoplasms has been found in rodents after chronic administration of neuroleptic drugs. Neither clinical studies nor epidemiologic drugs. Neither clinical studies nor epidemiologic studies conducted to date, however, have shown an association between chronic administration of these drugs and mammary tumorigenesis; the available evidence is considered too limited to be conclusive at this time.

DRUG INTERACTIONS:

Potentiation of drugs administered concurrently with molindone HCl has not been reported. Additionally, animal studies have not shown increased toxicity when molindone HCl is given concurrently with representative members of three classes of drugs (*i.e.,* barbiturates, chloral hydrate and antiparkinson drugs).

ADVERSE REACTIONS:

CNS Effects: The most frequently occurring effect is initial drowsiness that generally subsides with continued usage of the drug or lowering of the dose.

Noted less frequently were depression, hyperactivity and euphoria.

Neurological Extrapyramidal Reactions: Extrapyramidal reactions noted below may occur in susceptible individuals and are usually reversible with appropriate management.

Akathisia: Motor restlessness may occur early.

Parkinson Syndrome: Akinesia, characterized by rigidity, immobility and reduction of voluntary movements and tremor, have been observed. Occurrence is less frequent than akathisia.

Dystonic Syndrome: Prolonged abnormal contractions of muscle groups occur infrequently. These symptoms may be managed by the addition of a synthetic antiparkinson agent (other than L-dopa), small doses of sedative drugs, and/or reduction in dosage.

Tardive Dyskinesia: Neuroleptic drugs are known to cause a syndrome of dyskinetic movements commonly referred to as tardive dyskinesia. The movements may appear during treatment or upon withdrawal of treatment and may be either reversible or irreversible (*i.e.,* persistent) upon cessation of further neuroleptic administration.

The syndrome is known to have a variable latency for development and the duration of the latency cannot be determined reliably. It is thus wise to assume that any neuroleptic agent has the capacity to induce the syndrome and act accordingly until sufficient data have been collected to settle the issue definitively for a specific drug product. In the case of neuroleptics known to produce the irreversible syndrome, the following has been observed.

Tardive dyskinesia has appeared in some patients on long-term therapy and has also appeared after drug therapy has been discontinued. The risk appears to be greater in elderly patients on high-dose therapy, especially females. The symptoms are persistent and in some patients appear to be irreversible. The syndrome is characterized by rhythmical involuntary movements of the tongue, face, mouth or jaw (*e.g.,* protrusion of the tongue, puffing of cheeks, puckering of mouth, chewing movements). There may be involuntary movements of extremities.

There is no known effective treatment of tardive dyskinesia; antiparkinsonism agents usually do not alleviate the symptoms of this syndrome. It is suggested that all antipsychotic agents be discontinued if these symptoms appear. Should it be necessary to reinstitute treatment, or increase the dosage of the agent, or switch to a different antipsychotic agent, the syndrome may be masked. It has been reported that fine vermicular movements of the tongue may be an early sign of the syndrome and if the medication is stopped at that time the syndrome may not develop (See WARNINGS.)

Autonomic Nervous System: Occasionally blurring of vision, tachycardia, nausea, dry mouth and salivation have been reported. Urinary retention and constipation may occur particularly if anticholinergic drugs are used to treat extrapyramidal symptoms. One patient being treated with molindone HCl experienced priapism which required surgical intervention, apparently resulting in residual impairment of erectile function.

Laboratory Tests: There have been rare reports of leukopenia and leukocytosis. If such reactions occur, treatment with molindone HCl may continue if clinical symptoms are absent. Alterations of blood glucose, B.U.N., and red blood cells have not been considered clinically significant.

Metabolic and Endocrine Effects: Alteration of thyroid function has not been significant. Amenorrhea has been reported infrequently. Resumption of menses in previously amenorrheic women has been reported. Initially heavy menses may occur. Galactorrhea and gynecomastia have been reported infrequently. Increase in libido has been noted in some patients. Impotence has not been reported. Although both weight gain and weight loss has been in the direction of normal or ideal weight, excessive weight gain has not occurred with molindone HCl.

Hepatic Effects: There have been rare reports of clinically significant alterations in liver function in association with molindone HCl use.

Cardiovascular: Rare, transient, non-specific T wave changes have been reported on E.K.G. Association with a clinical syndrome has not been established. Rarely has significant hypotension been reported.

Ophthalmological: Lens opacities and pigmentary retinopathy have not been reported where patients have received molindone HCl. In some patients, phenothiazine induced lenticular opacities have resolved following discontinuation of the phenothiazine while continuing therapy with molindone HCl.

Skin: Early, non-specific skin rash, probably of allergic origin, has occasionally been reported. Skin pigmentation has not been seen with molindone HCl usage alone.

Molindone HCl has certain pharmacological similarities to other antipsychotic agents. Because adverse reactions are often extensions of the pharmacological activity of a drug, all of the known pharmacological effects associated with other antipsychotic drugs should be kept in mind when molindone HCl is used. Upon abrupt withdrawal after prolonged high dosage an abstinence syndrome has not been noted.

OVERDOSAGE:

Management of Overdose: Symptomatic, supportive therapy should be the rule. Gastric lavage is indicated for the reduction of absorption of molindone HCl which is freely soluble in water.

Since the adsorption of molindone HCl by activated charcoal has not been determined, the use of this antidote must be considered of theoretical value.

Emesis in a comatose patient is contraindicated. Additionally, while the emetic effect of apomorphine is blocked by molindone HCl in animals, this blocking effect has not been determined in humans.

A significant increase in the rate of removal of unmetabolized molindone HCl from the body by forced diuresis, peritoneal or renal dialysis would not be expected. (Only 2% of a single ingested dose of molindone HCl is excreted unmetabolized in the urine.)

However, poor response of the patient may justify use of these procedures.

While the use of laxatives or enemas might be based on general principles, the amount of unmetabolized molindone HCl in feces is less than 1%. Extrapyramidal symptoms have responded to the use of diphenhydramine (Benadryl*), Amantadine HCl (Symmetrel*) and the synthetic anticholinergic antiparkinson agents, (*i.e.,* Artane*, Cogentin*, Akineton*).

DOSAGE AND ADMINISTRATION:

Initial and maintenance doses of molindone HCl should be individualized.

Initial Dosage Schedule: The usual starting dosage is 50-75 mg/day.

Increase to 100 mg/day in 3 or 4 days.

Based on severity of symptomatology, dosage may be titrated up or down depending on individual patient response.

An increase to 225 mg/day may be required in patients with severe symptomatology

Elderly and debilitated patients should be started on lower dosage.

MAINTENANCE DOSAGE SCHEDULE

1. Mild: 5 mg-15 mg three or four times a day.

2. Moderate: 10 mg-25 mg three or four times a day.

3. Severe: 225 mg/day may be required.

HOW SUPPLIED:

As tablets in bottles of 100 with potencies and colors as follows:

5 mg = orange; 10 mg = lavender; 25 mg = light green; 50 mg = blue; 100 mg = tan.

As a concentrate containing 20 mg molindone hydrochloride per ml in 4 oz. (120 ml) bottles.

Store at controlled room temperature (59°-86° F, 15°-30° C). Protect from light.

HOW SUPPLIED - EQUIVALENTS NOT AVAILABLE:

Concentrate - Oral - 20 mg/ml

120 ml	$118.79	MOBAN, Gate Pharms	57844-0920-12

Tablet, Uncoated - Oral - 5 mg

100's	$55.98	MOBAN, Gate Pharms	57844-0914-01

Tablet, Uncoated - Oral - 10 mg

100's	$80.42	MOBAN, Gate Pharms	57844-0915-01

Tablet, Uncoated - Oral - 25 mg

100's	$119.95	MOBAN, Gate Pharms	57844-0916-01

Tablet, Uncoated - Oral - 50 mg

100's	$160.19	MOBAN, Gate Pharms	57844-0917-01

Tablet, Uncoated - Oral - 100 mg

100's	$214.00	MOBAN, Gate Pharms	57844-0918-01

MOLYBDENUM *(001827)*

CATEGORIES: Electrolytic, Caloric-Water Balance; Homeostatic & Nutrient; Mineral Supplements; Replacement Solutions; Vitamins; FDA Pre 1938 Drugs

BRAND NAMES: Ammonium Molybdate; Moly-Pak; Molypen

Prescribing information not available at time of publication.

HOW SUPPLIED - EQUIVALENTS NOT AVAILABLE:

Injection, Solution - Intravenous - 25 mcg/ml

10 ml	$195.31	MOLYPEN, Fujisawa USA	00469-4900-30
10 ml x 25	$157.19	AMMONIUM MOLYBDATE, Am Regent	00517-6610-25

MOMETASONE FUROATE *(001828)*

CATEGORIES: Anti-Inflammatory Agents; Dermatologicals; Dermatoses; Pruritus; Skin/Mucous Membrane Agents; Steroids; Atopic Dermatitis*; Pregnancy Category C; FDA Approved 1987 Apr; Top 200 Drugs
* Indication not approved by the FDA

BRAND NAMES: *Ecural* (Germany); *Elica*; *Elocom* (Canada); Elocon; *Elocon Cream* (Australia); *Elocon Ointment* (Australia); *Elocyn*; *Elomet* (Mexico)
(International brand names outside U.S. in italics)

FORMULARIES: BC-BS; Medi-Cal

DESCRIPTION:

For Dermatologic Use Only

Not for Ophthalmic Use

Elocon products contain mometasone furoate for dermatologic use. Mometasone furoate is a synthetic corticosteroid with anti-inflammatory activity.

Chemically, mometasone furoate is 9α, 21-Dichloro-11β, 17-dihydroxy-16α-methylpregna-1,4-diene-3,20 dione 17-(2-furoate), with the empirical formula $C_{27}H_{30}Cl_2O_6$, and a molecular weight of 521.4.

Mometasone furoate is a white to off-white powder practically insoluble in water, slightly soluble in octanol, and moderately soluble in ethyl alcohol.

Each gram of Elocon Cream 0.1% contains: 1 mg mometasone furoate in a cream base of hexylene glycol, phosphoric acid, propylene glycol stearate, stearyl alcohol and ceteareth-20, titanium dioxide, aluminum starch ocetenylsuccinate, white wax, white petrolatum and purified water.

Each gram of Elocon Ointment 0.1% contains: 1 mg mometasone furoate in an ointment base of hexylene glycol, propylene glycol stearate, white wax, white petrolatum and purified water. May also contain phosphoric acid.

DESCRIPTION: *(cont'd)*

Each gram of Elocon Lotion 0.1% contains: 1 mg of mometasone furoate in a lotion base of isopropyl alcohol (40%), propylene glycol, hydroxypropylcellulose, sodium phosphate and water. May also contain phosphoric acid and sodium hydroxide used to adjust the pH to approximately 4.5.

CLINICAL PHARMACOLOGY:

All Forms: The corticosteroids are a class of compounds comprising steroid hormones secreted by the adrenal cortex and their synthetic analogs. In pharmacologic doses corticosteroids are used primarily for their anti-inflammatory and/or immunosuppressive effects.

Topical corticosteroids, such as mometasone furoate, are effective in the treatment of corticosteroid-responsive dermatoses primarily because of their anti-inflammatory, anti-pruritic, and vasoconstrictive actions. However, while the physiologic, pharmacologic, and clinical effects of the corticosteroids are well known, the exact mechanisms of their actions in each disease are uncertain. Mometasone furoate has been shown to have topical (dermatologic) and systemic pharmacologic and metabolic effects characteristic of this class of drugs.

Pharmacokinetics The extent of percutaneous absorption of topical corticosteroids is determined by many factors including the vehicle, the integrity of the epidermal barrier, and the use of occlusive dressings.(See DOSAGE AND ADMINISTRATION.)Topical corticosteroids can be absorbed from normal intact skin.

Inflammation and/or other disease processes in the skin increase percutaneous absorption. Occlusive dressings substantially increase the percutaneous absorption of topical corticosteroids. (See DOSAGE AND ADMINISTRATION.)

Once absorbed through the skin, topical corticosteroids are handled through pharmacokinetic pathways similar to systemically administered corticosteroids. Corticosteroids are bound to plasma proteins in varying degrees. Corticosteroids are metabolized primarily in the liver and are then excreted by the kidneys. Some of the topical corticosteroids and their metabolites are also excreted into the bile.

Cream The percutaneous absorption of ^{3}H-mometasone furoate was evaluated in rabbits following topical application of both cream (0.1%) and ointment (0.1%) formulations. Approximately 5% of the topically applied dose was systematically absorbed following topical application of the cream and 6% following application of the ointment formulation. Based upon these results it was concluded that mometasone furoate is absorbed to a similar extent following application of either the cream or ointment formulations. Percutaneous absorption studies of ^{3}H-mometasone furoate was also studied in man following topical application of an ointment (0.1%) formulation application of an ointment(0.1%) formulation. Results showed that only about 0.7% of the steroid was systematically absorbed following 8 hours of contact without occlusion. Minimal absorption would be anticipated with the cream formulation.

Cream and Ointment In a study of the effects of mometasone furoate cream on the hypothalamic-pituitary adrenal (HPA) axis, fifteen grams were applied twice daily for seven days to six patients with psoriasis or atopic dermatitis. The cream was applied without occlusion to at least 30% of the body surface. The results suggest that the drug caused a slight lowering of adrenal corticosteroid secretion, although in no case did plasma cortisol levels go below the lower limit of the normal range.

In a study of the effects of mometasone furoate ointment on the hypothalamic-pituitary-adrenal axis, 15 grams were applied twice daily for seven days to six patients with psoriasis or atopic dermatitis. The ointment was applied without occlusion to at least 30% of the body surface. The results suggest that the drug caused a slight lowering of adrenal corticosteroid secretion, although in no case did plasma cortisol levels go below the lower limit of the normal range.

Lotion Mometasone furoate lotion was applied at 15 ml twice daily (30 ml per day) to diseased skin (patients with scalp and body psoriasis) of four patients for seven days, to study its effects on the hypothalamic-pituitary-adrenal (HPA) axis. Plasma cortisol levels for each of the four patients remained well within the normal range and changed little from baseline.

Lotion and Ointment A study using a radio-labelled^{3}H mometasone furoate ointment formulation was performed to measure systemic absorption and excretion. Results showed that approximately 0.7% of the steroid was absorbed during 8 hours of contact, without occlusion, with intact skin of normal volunteers.

INDICATIONS AND USAGE:

Elocon Cream, Ointment and Lotion are indicated for the relief of the inflammatory and pruritic manifestations of corticosteroid-responsive dermatoses.

CONTRAINDICATIONS:

Elocon Cream, Ointment and Lotion are contraindicated in patients who are hypersensitive to mometasone furoate, to other corticosteroids, or to any ingredient in this preparation.

PRECAUTIONS:

General Systemic absorption of potent topical corticosteroids has produced reversible hypothalamic-pituitary-adrenal (HPA) axis suppression, manifestations of Cushing's syndrome, hyperglycemia, and glucosuria in some patients.

Conditions which augment systemic absorption include application of more potent steroids, use over large surface areas, prolonged use, use in areas where the epidermal barrier is disrupted, and the use of occlusive dressings. (See DOSAGE AND ADMINISTRATION.)

Patients receiving a large dose of a potent topical steroid applied to a large surface area or under an occlusive dressing should be evaluated periodically for evidence of HPA axis suppression by using the urinary free cortisol and ACTH stimulation tests. If HPA axis suppression is noted, an attempt should be made to withdraw the drug, to reduce the frequency of application, or to substitute a less potent steroid.

Recovery of HPA axis function is generally prompt and complete upon discontinuation of the drug. Infrequently, signs and symptoms of steroid withdrawal may occur, requiring supplemental systemic corticosteroids.

Children may absorb proportionally larger amounts of topical corticosteroids and thus be more susceptible to systemic toxicity. (See PRECAUTIONS, Pediatric Use.)

If irritation develops, topical corticosteroids should be discontinued and appropriate therapy instituted.

In the presence of dermatological infections, use of an appropriate antifungal or antibacterial agent should be instituted. If a favorable response does not occur promptly, the corticosteroid should be discontinued until the infection has been adequately controlled.

Information for the Patient using topical corticosteroids should receive the following information and instructions. This information is intended to aid in the safe and effective use of this medication. It is not a disclosure of all possible adverse or intended effects.

1. This medication is to be used by the physician. It is for external use only. Avoid contact with the eyes.

2. Patients should be advised not to use this medication for any disorder other than that for which it was prescribed.

3. The treated skin area should not be bandaged or otherwise covered or wrapped as to be occlusive unless directed by the physician. (See DOSAGE AND ADMINISTRATION.)

PRECAUTIONS: *(cont'd)*

4. Patients should report any signs of local adverse reactions.

5. Parents of pediatric patients should be advised not to use tight-fitting diapers or plastic pants on a child being treated in the diaper area, as these garments may constitute occlusive dressing. (See DOSAGE AND ADMINISTRATION.)

Laboratory Tests The following tests may be helpful in evaluating HPA axis suppression:

Urinary free cortisol test

ACTH stimulation test

Carcinogenesis, Mutagenesis, and Impairment of Fertility Long-term animal studies have not been performed to evaluate the carcinogenic potential or the effect on fertility of topical corticosteroids.

Genetic toxicity studies with mometasone furoate, which included the Ames test, mouse lymphoma assay, and a micronucleus test, did not reveal any mutagenic potential.

Pregnancy Category C Corticosteroids are generally teratogenic in laboratory animals when administered systemically at relatively low dosage levels. Corticosteroids have been shown to be teratogenic after dermal application in laboratory animals. There are no adequate and well-controlled studies of teratogenic effects from topically applied corticosteroids in pregnant women. Therefore, topical corticosteroids should be used during pregnancy only if the potential benefit justifies the potential risk to the fetus. Drugs of this class should not be used extensively on pregnant patients in large amounts, or for prolonged periods.

Nursing Mothers It is not known whether topical administration of corticosteroids could result in sufficient systemic absorption to produce detectable quantities in breast milk. Systemically administered corticosteroids are secreted into breast milk in quantities not likely to have a deleterious effect on the infant. Nevertheless, a decision should be made whether to discontinue nursing or to discontinue the drug, taking into account the importance of the drug to the mother.

Pediatric Use *Pediatric patients may demonstrate greater susceptibility to topical corticosteroid-induced HPA axis suppression and Cushing's syndrome than mature patients because of a larger skin surface area to body weight ratio.*

Hypothalamic-pituitary-adrenal (HPA) axis suppression, Cushing's syndrome, and intracranial hypertension have been reported in children receiving topical corticosteroids. Manifestations of adrenal suppression in children include linear growth retardation, delayed weight gain, low plasma cortisol levels, and absence of response to ACTH stimulation. Manifestations of intracranial hypertension include bulging fontanelles, headaches, and bilateral papilledema.

Administration of topical corticosteroids to children should be limited to the least amount compatible with an effective therapeutic regimen. Chronic corticosteroid therapy may interfere with the growth and development of children.

ADVERSE REACTIONS:

The following local adverse reactions were reported with Elocon Cream during clinical studies with 319 patients: burning, 1; pruritus, 1; and signs of skin atrophy, 3.

The following local adverse reactions were reported with Elocon Ointment during clinical studies with 812 patients: burning, 13; pruritus, 8; skin atrophy 8; tingling/stinging, 7; and furunculosis, 3.

The following local adverse reactions were reported with Elocon Lotion during clinical studies with 209 patients: acneform reaction, 2; burning, 4; and itching, 1. In an irritation sensitization study with 156 normal subjects, folliculitis was reported in 4.

The following local adverse reactions have been reported infrequently when other topical dermatologic corticosteroids have been used as recommended. These reactions are listed in an approximate decreasing order of occurrence: burning, itching, irritation, dryness, folliculitis, hypertrichosis, acneiform eruptions, hypopigmentation, perioral dermatitis, allergic contact dermatitis, maceration of the skin, secondary infection, skin atrophy, striae, miliaria.

OVERDOSAGE:

Topically applied corticosteroids can be absorbed in sufficient amounts to produce systemic effects. (See PRECAUTIONS.)

DOSAGE AND ADMINISTRATION:

Lotion Apply a few drops of Elocon Lotion to the affected areas once daily and massage lightly until it disappears. For the most effective and economical use, hold the nozzle of the bottle very close to the affected areas and gently squeeze.

Ointment and Cream Apply a thin film of Elocon Ointment or Cream to the affected skin areas once daily. Do not use occlusive dressings.

PATIENT INFORMATION:

Mometasone is a topical corticosteroid used to treat rashes, skin irritation, and other types of skin problems. Inform your physician if you are pregnant or nursing. This cream is only to be used externally and should not be used in or near the eyes. Gently clean the affected skin before applying the cream. Apply the cream sparingly and rub in gently. Do not apply bandages, dressings, cosmetics or other skin products over the treated area unless directed by your physician. Tight-fitting diapers or plastic pants should not be used on children treated in the diaper area. Avoid applying the cream to the face, genital and rectal areas, armpits, and skin creases for extended lengths of time. Notify your physician if the skin condition being treated gets worse or if irritation, burning, redness, swelling or stinging persists.

HOW SUPPLIED:

Elocon Cream 0.1% is supplied in 15 g and 45 g tubes; boxes of one.

Elocon Ointment 0.1% is supplied in 15 g and 45 g tubes; boxes of one.

Elocon Lotion 0.1% is supplied in 30 ml (275 g) and 60 ml (55 g) bottles; boxes of one

Store Elocon Cream, Ointment, and Lotion between 2 and 30°C (36 and 86°F).

HOW SUPPLIED - EQUIVALENTS NOT AVAILABLE:

Cream - Topical - 0.1 %

15-g	$15.64	ELOCON, Schering	00085-0567-01
45-g	$28.65	ELOCON, Schering	00085-0567-02

Lotion - Topical - 1 mg

30 ml	$16.95	ELOCON, Schering	00085-0854-01
60 ml	$32.35	ELOCON, Schering	00085-0854-02

Ointment - Topical - 0.1 %

15-g	$15.64	ELOCON, Schering	00085-0370-01
45-g	$28.65	ELOCON, Schering	00085-0370-02

MONOBENZONE *(001829)*

CATEGORIES: Depigmenting/Pigmenting Agents; Dermatologicals; Hypopigmentation; Skin Bleaches; Skin/Mucous Membrane Agents; Pregnancy Category C; FDA Approval Pre 1982

BRAND NAMES: **Benoquin**; *Benzoquin*; *Depigman*; *Dermochinona (International brand names outside U.S. in italics)*

DESCRIPTION:

Potent Depigmenting Agent

FOR EXTERNAL USE ONLY

Each gram of Benoquin Cream contains 200 mg of monobenzone, USP, in a water-washable base consisting of purified water, cetyl alcohol, propylene glycol, sodium lauryl sulfate and beeswax.

CLINICAL PHARMACOLOGY:

The mechanism of action of Benoquin is not fully understood. Denton et al.[1] suggested that Benoquin may be converted to hydroquinone, which they found to inhibit the enzymatic oxidation of tyrosine to DOPA.

Iijima and Watanabe[2] suggested a direct action on tyrosinase.

Another suggestion by Denton and his group was that Benoquin acts as an anti-oxidant to prevent SH-group oxidation so that more SH groups are available to inhibit tyrosinase.

The primary role of inflammation in the depigmentation process was studied by Becker and Spencer[3] who suggested that increased cell permeability allows Benoquin to enter the melanocyte to form an antigenic substance which attached to the melanin granule enters the dermis where antibodies are produced, remote positive patch-testing may result.

INDICATIONS AND USAGE:

Monobenzone is indicated for final depigmentation in extensive vitiligo.

Monobenzone is not recommended for freckling, hyperpigmentation due to photosensitization following use of certain perfumes (berlock dermatitis), melasma (chloasma) of pregnancy, and hyperpigmentation following inflammation of the skin. Monobenzone is of no value in the treatment of cafe-au-lait spots, pigmented nevi, malignant melanoma, or pigment resulting from pigments other than melanin including bile, silver, and artificial pigments.

CONTRAINDICATIONS:

Prior history of sensitivity or allergic reaction to this product or any of its ingredients. The safety of topical monobenzone use during pregnancy or in children (12 years and under) has not been established.

WARNINGS:

A. Monobenzone is a potent dipigmenting agent, not a mild cosmetic bleach. Do not use except for final depigmentation in extensive vitiligo.

B. Keep this and all medication out of reach of children. In case of accidental ingestion, call a physician or a poison control center immediately.

PRECAUTIONS:

See WARNINGS

A. Pregnancy Category C: Animal reproduction studies have not been conducted with topical monobenzone. It is also not known whether monobenzone can cause fetal harm when used topically on a pregnant woman or affect reproductive capacity. It is not known to what degree, if any, topical monobenzone is absorbed systemically. Topical monobenzone should be used in pregnant women only when clearly indicated.

B. Nursing Mothers: It is not known whether topical monobenzone is absorbed or excreted in human milk. Caution is advised when topical monobenzone is used by a nursing mother.

C. Pediatric Use: Safety and effectiveness in children below the age of 12 years have not been established.

ADVERSE REACTIONS:

Occasional irritation, a burning sensation, or dermatitis may occur in which case medication should be discontinued and the physician notified immediately.

DOSAGE AND ADMINISTRATION:

Benoquin should be applied to the pigmented area and rubbed in well two or three times daily or as directed by physician. There is no recommended dosage for children under 12 years of age except under the advice and supervision of a physician.

NOTE: Depigmentation is usually observed after one to four months of therapy. If satisfactory results have not been obtained within four months, treatment should be discontinued.

REFERENCES:

1. Denton, C. R.; A.B. Lerner; and T.B. Fitzpatrick: "Inhibition of Melanin Formation by Chemical Agents", **The Journal of Investigative Dermatology**, Vol. 18, No. 2, February, 1952. **2.** Iijima, Susumu and Kazu Watanabe: "Studies on DOPA Reaction: II. Effect of Chemicals on the Reaction", **The Journal of Investigative Dermatology**, Vol. 28, No. 1, January, 1957. **3.** Becker, S.W. and Malcom C. Spencer: "Evaluation of Monobenzone", **The Journal of American Medical Association**, Vol. 180, No. 4, April 28, 1962.

HOW SUPPLIED:

Benoquin Cream should be stored at controlled room temperature (15 - 30°C) 59-86° F.

HOW SUPPLIED - EQUIVALENTS NOT AVAILABLE:

Cream - Topical - 20 %

37.5 gm	$43.06	BENOQUIN, ICN Pharms	00187-0380-34

MONOCHLORACETIC ACID *(001830)*

CATEGORIES: Keratolytic Agents; Skin/Mucous Membrane Agents; FDA Pre 1938 Drugs

BRAND NAMES: Mono-Chlor; Monocete; Verzone

Prescribing information not available at time of publication.

HOW SUPPLIED - EQUIVALENTS NOT AVAILABLE:

Solution - Topical - 80 %

15 ml	$5.95	VERZONE, Dynapedic	10360-1001-01

MORICIZINE HYDROCHLORIDE *(001832)*

CATEGORIES: Antiarrhythmic Agents; Arrhythmia; Cardiovascular Drugs; Tachycardia; Pregnancy Category B; FDA Class 1B ("Modest Therapeutic Advantage"); FDA Approved 1990 Jun

BRAND NAMES: **Ethmozine**

FORMULARIES: Aetna; BC-BS

COST OF THERAPY: $1,061.16 (Arrhythmia; Tablet; 200 mg; 3/day; 365 days)

DESCRIPTION:

Ethmozine (moricizine HCl) is an orally active antiarrhythmic drug available for administration in tablets containing 200 mg, 250 mg and 300 mg of moricizine HCl. The chemical name of moricizine HCl is 10-(3-morpholinopropionyl) phenothiazine-2-carbamic acid ethyl ester HCl.

Moricizine HCl is a white to tan crystalline powder, freely soluble in water and has a pKa of 6.4 (weak base). Ethmozine tablets contain: lactose, microcrystalline cellulose, sodium starch glycolate, magnesium stearate and dyes (FD&C Blue 1, D&C Yellow 10 and FD&C Yellow 6 (200 mg tablet); FD&C Yellow 6 and FD&C Red 40 (250 mg tablet); FD&C Blue 1 (300 mg tablet)).

CLINICAL PHARMACOLOGY:

Mechanism of Action: Moricizine HCl is a Class 1 antiarrhythmic agent with potent local anesthetic activity and myocardial membrane stabilizing effects. Moricizine HCl reduces the fast inward current carried by sodium ions.

In isolated dog Purkinje fibers, moricizine HCl shortens Phase II and III repolarization, resulting in a decreased action potential duration and effective refractory period. A dose-related decrease in the maximum rate of Phase O depolarization (V_{max}) occurs without effect on maximum diastolic potential or action potential amplitude. The sinus node and atrial tissue of the dog are not affected.

Electrophysiology: Electrophysiology studies in patients with ventricular tachycardia have shown that moricizine HCl, at daily doses of 750 mg and 900 mg, prolongs atrioventricular conduction. Both AV nodal conduction time (AH interval) and His-Purkinje conduction time (HV interval) are prolonged by 10-13% and 21-26%, respectively. The PR interval is prolonged by 16-20% and the QRS by 7-18%. Prolongations of 2-5% in the corrected QT interval result from widening of the QRS interval, but there is shortening of the JT interval, indicating an absence of significant effect on ventricular repolarization. Intra-atrial conduction or atrial effective refractory periods are not consistently affected. In patients without sinus node dysfunction, moricizine HCl has minimal effects on sinus cycle length and sinus node recovery time. These effects may be significant in patients with sinus node dysfunction (see PRECAUTIONS, Electrocardiographic Changes/Conduction Abnormalities).

Hemodynamics: In patients with impaired left ventricular function, moricizine HCl has minimal effects on measurements of cardiac performance such as cardiac index, stroke volume index, pulmonary capillary wedge pressure, systemic or pulmonary vascular resistance or ejection fraction, either at rest or during exercise. Moricizine HCl is associated with a small, but consistent increase in resting blood pressure and heart rate. Exercise tolerance in patients with ventricular arrhythmias is unaffected. In patients with a history of congestive heart failure or angina pectoris, exercise duration and rate-pressure product at maximal exercise are unchanged during moricizine HCl administration. Nonetheless, in some cases worsened heart failure in patients with severe underlying heart disease has been attributed to moricizine HCl.

Other Pharmacologic Effects: Although moricizine HCl is chemically related to the neuroleptic phenothiazines, it has no demonstrated central or peripheral dopaminergic activity in animals. Moreover, in patients on chronic moricizine HCl, serum prolactin levels did not increase.

Pharmacokinetics/Pharmacodynamics: The antiarrhythmic and electrophysiologic effects of moricizine HCl are not related in time course or intensity to plasma moricizine concentrations or to the concentrations of any identified metabolite, all of which have short (2-3 hours) half-lives. Following single doses of moricizine HCl, there is a prompt prolongation of the PR interval, which becomes normal within 2 hours, consistent with the rapid fall of plasma moricizine. JT interval shortening, however, peaks at about 6 hours and persists for at least 10 hours. Although an effect on VPD rates is seen within 2 hours after dosing, the full effect is seen after 10-14 hours and persists in full, when therapy is terminated, for more than 10 hours, after which the effect decays slowly, and is still substantial at 24 hours. This suggests either an unidentified, active, long half-life metabolite or a structural or functional "deep compartment" with slow entry from, and release to, the plasma. The following description of parent compound pharmacokinetics is therefore of uncertain relevance to clinical actions.

Following oral administration, moricizine HCl undergoes significant first-past metabolism resulting in an absolute bio-availability of approximately 38%. Peak plasma concentrations of moricizine HCl are usually reached within 0.5-2 hours. Administration 30 minutes after a meal delays the rate of absorption, resulting in lower peak plasma concentrations, but the extent of absorption is not altered. Moricizine HCl plasma levels are proportional to dose over the recommended therapeutic dose range.

The apparent volume of distribution after oral administration is very large ($\geq$ 300 L) and is not significantly related to body weight. Moricizine HCl is approximately 95% bound to human plasma proteins. This binding interaction is independent of moricizine HCl plasma concentration.

Moricizine HCl undergoes extensive biotransformation. Less than 1% of orally administered moricizine HCl is excreted unchanged in the urine. There are at least 26 metabolites, but no single metabolite has been found to represent as much as 1% of the administered dose, and as stated above, antiarrhythmic response has relatively slow onset and offset. Two metabolites are pharmacologically active in at least one animal model: moricizine sulfoxide and phenothiazine-2-carbamic acid ethyl ester sulfoxide. Each of these metabolites represents a small percentage of the administered dose (<0.6%), is present in lower concentrations in the plasma than the parent drug, and has a plasma elimination half-life of approximately three hours.

Moricizine HCl has been shown to induce its own metabolism. Average moricizine HCl plasma concentrations in patients decrease with multiple dosing. This decrease in plasma levels of parent drug does not appear to affect clinical outcome for patients receiving chronic moricizine HCl therapy.

The plasma half-life of moricizine HCl is 1.5-3.5 hours (most values about 2 hours) following single or multiple oral doses in patients with ventricular ectopy. Approximately 56% of the administered dose is excreted in the feces and 39% is excreted in the urine. Some moricizine HCl is also recycled through enterohepatic circulation.

CLINICAL ACTIONS

Moricizine HCl at daily doses of 600-900 mg produces a dose-related reduction in the occurrence of frequent ventricular premature depolarizations (VPDs) and reduces the incidence of nonsustained and sustained ventricular tachycardia (VT). In controlled clinical trials, moricizine HCl has been shown to have antiarrhythmic activity that is generally similar to that of disopyramide, propranolol and quinidine at the doses studied. In controlled and

CLINICAL PHARMACOLOGY: *(cont'd)*

compassionate use programmed electrical stimulation studies (PES), moricizine HCl prevented the induction of sustained ventricular tachycardia in approximately 25% (19/75) of patients. In a post-marketing randomized comparative PES study, moricizine HCl had a response rate of approximately 12% (7/59). Activity of moricizine HCl is maintained during long-term use.

Moricizine HCl is effective in treating ventricular arrhythmias in patients with and without organic heart disease. Moricizine HCl may be effective in patients in whom other antiarrhythmic agents are ineffective, not tolerated and/or contraindicated.

Arrhythmia exacerbation or "rebound" is not noted following discontinuation of moricizine HCl therapy.

INDICATIONS AND USAGE:

Moricizine HCl is indicated for the treatment of documented ventricular arrhythmias, such as sustained ventricular tachycardia, that, in the judgement of the physician are life-threatening. Because of the proarrhythmic effects of moricizine HCl, its use with lesser arrhythmias is generally not recommended. Treatment of patients with asymptomatic ventricular premature contractions should be avoided.

Initiation of moricizine HCl treatment, as with other antiarrhythmic agents used to treat life-threatening arrhythmias, should be carried out in the hospital.

Antiarrhythmic drugs have not been shown to enhance survival in patients with ventricular arrhythmias.

CONTRAINDICATIONS:

Moricizine HCl is contraindicated in patients with pre-existing second- or third-degree AV block and in patients with right bundle branch block when associated with left hemiblock (bifascicular block) unless a pacemaker is present. Moricizine HCl is also contraindicated in the presence of cardiogenic shock or known hypersensitivity to the drug.

WARNINGS:

Mortality moricizine HCl was one of three antiarrhythmic drugs included in the National Heart Lung and Blood Institute's Cardiac Arrhythmia Suppression Trial (CAST I), a long-term multicenter, randomized, double-blind study in patients with asymptomatic non-life-threatening ventricular arrhythmias who had a myocardial infarction more than 6 days, but less than 2 years, previously. An excessive mortality or nonfatal cardiac arrest rate was seen in patients treated with both of the Class IC agents included in the trial, which led to discontinuation of those 2 arms of the trial. The average duration of treatment with these agents was 10 months.

The moricizine HCl and placebo arms of the trial were continued in the NHLBI sponsored CAST II. In this randomized, double-blind trial, patients with asymptomatic non-life-threatening arrhythmias who had a myocardial infarction within 4 to 90 days and left ventricular ejection fraction $\leq$ 0.40 prior to enrollment were evaluated. The average duration of treatment with moricizine HCl in this study was 18 months. The study was discontinued because there was no possibility of demonstrating a benefit toward improved survival with moricizine HCl and because of an evolving adverse trend after long-term treatment.

The applicability of the CAST results to other populations (*e.g.,* those without recent myocardial infarction) is uncertain. Considering the known proarrhythmic properties of moricizine HCl and the lack of evidence of improved survival for any antiarrhythmic drug in patients without life-threatening arrhythmias, the use of moricizine HCl, as well as other antiarrhythmic agents, should be reserved for patients with life-threatening ventricular arrhythmias.

Proarrhythmia: Like other antiarrhythmic drugs, moricizine HCl can provoke new rhythm disturbances or make existing arrhythmias worse. These proarrhythmic effects can range from an increase in the frequency of VPDs to the development of new or more severe ventricular tachycardia, e.g., tachycardia that is more sustained or more resistant to conversion to sinus rhythm, with potentially fatal consequences. It is often not possible to distinguish a proarrhythmic effect from the patient's underlying rhythm disorder, so that the occurrence rates given below must be considered approximations. Note also that drug-induced arrhythmias can generally be identified only when they occur early after starting the drug and when the rhythm can be identified, usually because the patient is being monitored. It is clear from the NIH sponsored CAST (Cardiac Arrhythmia Suppression Trial) that some antiarrhythmic drugs can cause increased sudden death mortality, presumably due to new arrhythmias or asystole that do not appear early after treatment but that represent a sustained increased risk.

Domestic pre-marketing trials included 1072 patients given moricizine HCl; 397 had baseline lethal arrhythmias (sustained VT or VF and non-sustained VT with hemodynamic symptoms) and 576 had potentially lethal arrhythmias (increased VPDs or NSVT in patients with known structural heart disease, active ischemia, congestive heart failure or an LVEF <40% and/or CI <2.0 l/min/m2). In this population there were 40 (3.7%) identified proarrhythmic events, 26 (2.5%) of which were serious, either fatal (6), new hemodynamically significant sustained VT or VF (4), new sustained VT that was not hemodynamically significant (11) or sustained VT that became syncopal/presyncopal when it had not been before (5). Proarrhythmic effects described as incessant ventricular tachycardia were observed in the post-marketing PES study and in post-marketing adverse event reports.

In general, serious proarrhythmic effects in the domestic pre-marketing trials were equally common in patients with more and less severe arrhythmias, 2.5% in the patients with baseline lethal arrhythmias vs. 2.8% in patients with potentially lethal arrhythmias, although the patients with serious effects were more likely to have a history of sustained VT (38% vs. 23%). In post-marketing comparative PES study, patients treated with moricizine HCl (250-300 mg TID) had a proarrhythmia rate of 14% (8/59).

Five of the six fatal proarrhythmic events were in patients with baseline lethal arrhythmias; four had prior cardiac arrests. Rates and severity of proarrhythmic events were similar in patients given 600-900 mg of moricizine HCl per day and those given higher doses. Patients with proarrhythmic events were more likely than the overall population to have coronary artery disease (85% vs. 67%), history of acute myocardial infarction (75% vs. 53%), congestive heart failure (60% vs. 43%), and cardiomegaly (55% vs. 33%). All of the six proarrhythmic deaths were in patients with coronary artery disease; 5/6 each had documented acute myocardial infarction, congestive heart failure, and cardiomegaly.

Electrolyte Disturbances: Hypokalemia, hyperkalemia or hypomagnesemia may alter the effects of Class I antiarrhythmic drugs. Electrolyte imbalances should be corrected before administration of moricizine HCl.

Sick Sinus Syndrome: Moricizine HCl should be used only with extreme caution in patients with sick sinus syndrome, as it may cause sinus bradycardia, sinus pause or sinus arrest.

PRECAUTIONS:

GENERAL

Electrocardiographic Changes/Conduction Abnormalities: Moricizine HCl slows AV nodal and intraventricular conduction, producing dose-related increases in the PR and QRS intervals. In clinical trials, the average increase in the PR interval was 12% and the QRS interval was 14%. Although the QTC interval is increased, this is wholly because of QRS prolongation; the JT interval is shortened, indicating the absence of significant slowing of ventricular repolarization. The degree of lengthening of PR and QRS intervals does not predict efficacy.

PRECAUTIONS: *(cont'd)*

In controlled clinical trials and in open studies, the overall incidence of delayed ventricular conduction, including new bundle branch block pattern, was approximately 9.4%. In patients without baseline conduction abnormalities, the frequency of second-degree AV block was 0.2% and third-degree AV block did not occur. In patients with baseline conduction abnormalities, the frequencies of second-degree AV block and third-degree AV block were 0.9% and 1.4%, respectively.

Moricizine HCl therapy was discontinued in 1.6% of patients due to electrocardiographic changes (0.6% due to sinus pause or asystole, 0.2% to AV block, 0.2% to junctional rhythm, 0.4% to intraventricular conduction delay, and 0.2% to wide QRS and/or PR interval).

In patients with pre-existing conduction abnormalities, moricizine HCl therapy should be initiated cautiously. If second- or third-degree AV block occurs, moricizine HCl therapy should be discontinued unless a ventricular pacemaker is in place. When changing the dose of moricizine HCl or adding concomitant medications which may also affect cardiac conduction, patients should be monitored electrocardiographically.

Hepatic Impairment: Patients with significant liver dysfunction have reduced plasma clearance and an increased half-life of moricizine HCl. Although the precise relationship of moricizine HCl levels to effect is not clear, patients with hepatic disease should be treated with lower doses and closely monitored for excessive pharmacological effects, including effects on ECG intervals, before dosage adjustment. Patients with severe liver disease should be administered moricizine HCl with particular care, if at all. (See DOSAGE AND ADMINISTRATION.)

Renal Impairment: Plasma levels of intact moricizine HCl are unchanged in hemodialysis patients, but a significant portion (39%) of moricizine HCl is metabolized and excreted in the urine. Although no identified active metabolite is known to increase in people with renal failure, metabolites of unrecognized importance could be affected. For this reason, moricizine HCl should be administered cautiously in patients with impaired renal function. Patients with significant renal dysfunction should be started on lower doses and monitored for excessive pharmacologic effects, including ECG intervals, before dosage adjustment. (See DOSAGE AND ADMINISTRATION.)

Congestive Heart Failure: Most patients with congestive heart failure have tolerated the recommended moricizine HCl daily doses without unusual toxicity or change in effect. Pharmacokinetic differences between moricizine HCl patients with and without congestive heart failure were not apparent (see Hepatic Impairment above.) In some cases, worsened heart failure has been attributed to moricizine HCl. Patients with pre-existing heart failure should be monitored carefully when moricizine HCl is initiated.

Effects on Pacemaker Threshold: The effect of moricizine HCl on the sensing and pacing thresholds of artificial pacemakers has not been sufficiently studied. In such patients, pacing parameters must be monitored, if moricizine HCl is used.

CARCINOGENESIS, MUTAGENESIS, AND IMPAIRMENT OF FERTILITY

In a 24-month mouse study in which moricizine HCl was administered in the feed at concentrations calculated to provide doses ranging up to 320 mg/kg/day, ovarian tubular adenomas and granulosa cell tumors were limited in occurrence to moricizine HCl treated animals. Although the findings were of borderline statistical significance, or not statistically significant, historical control data indicate that both of these tumors are uncommon in the strain of mouse studied.

In a 24-month study in which moricizine HCl was administered by gavage to rats at doses of 25, 50 and 100 mg/kg/day, Zymbal's Gland Carcinoma was observed in one mid-dose and two high dose males. This tumor appears to be uncommon in the strain of rat studied. Rats of both sexes showed a dose-related increase in hepatocellular cholangioma (also described as bile ductile cystadenoma or cystic hyperplasia) along with fatty metamorphosis, possibly due to disruption of hepatic choline utilization for phospholipid biosynthesis. The rat is known to be uniquely sensitive to alteration in choline metabolism.

Moricizine HCl was not mutagenic when assayed for genotoxicity in *in vitro* bacterial (Ames test) and mammalian (Chinese hamster ovary/hypoxanthine-guanine phosphoribosyl transferase and sister chromatid exchange) cell systems or in *in vivo* mammalian systems (rat bone cytogenicity and mouse micronucleus).

A general reproduction and fertility study was conducted in rats at dose levels up to 6.7 times the maximum recommended human dose of 900 mg/day (based upon 50 kg human body weight) and revealed no evidence of impaired male or female fertility.

PREGNANCY CATEGORY B

Teratogenic Effects: Teratology studies have been performed with moricizine HCl in rats and in rabbits at doses up to 6.7 and 4.7 times the maximum recommended human daily dose, respectively, and have revealed no evidence of harm to the fetus. There are, however, no adequate and well-controlled studies in pregnant women. Because animal reproduction studies are not always predictive of human response, moricizine HCl should be used during pregnancy only if clearly needed.

Nonteratogenic Effects: In a study in which rats were dosed with moricizine HCl prior to mating, during mating and throughout gestation and lactation, dose levels 3.4 and 6.7 times the maximum recommended human daily dose produced a dose-related decrease in pup and maternal weight gain, possibly related to a larger litter size. In a study in which dosing was begun on Day 15 of gestation, moricizine HCl, at a level 6.7 times the maximum recommended human daily dose, produced a retardation in maternal weight gain but no effect on pup growth.

NURSING MOTHERS

Moricizine HCl is secreted in the milk of laboratory animals and has been reported to be present in human milk. Because of the potential for serious adverse reactions in nursing infants from moricizine HCl, a decision should be made whether to discontinue the drug, taking into account the importance of the drug to the mother.

PEDIATRIC USE

The safety and effectiveness of moricizine HCl in children less than 18 years of age have not been established.

DRUG INTERACTIONS:

No significant changes in serum digoxin levels or pharmacokinetics have been observed in patients or healthy subjects receiving concomitant moricizine HCl therapy. Concomitant use was associated with additive prolongation of the PR interval, but not with a significant increase in the rate of second- or third-degree AV block.

Concomitant administration of cimetidine resulted in a decrease in moricizine HCl clearance of 49% and a 1.4 fold increase in plasma levels in healthy subjects. During clinical trials, no significant changes in the efficacy or tolerance of moricizine HCl have been observed in patients receiving concomitant cimetidine therapy. Patients on cimetidine should have moricizine HCl therapy initiated at relatively low doses, not more than 600 mg/day. Patients should be monitored when concomitant cimetidine therapy is instituted or discontinued or when the moricizine HCl dose is changed.

Concomitant administration of beta blocker therapy did not reveal significant changes in overall electrocardiographic intervals in patients. In one controlled study, moricizine HCl and propranolol administered concomitantly produced a small additive increase in the PR interval.

DRUG INTERACTIONS: *(cont'd)*

Theophylline clearance and plasma half-life were significantly affected by multiple dose moricizine HCl administration when both conventional and sustained release theophylline were given to healthy subjects (clearance increased 44-66% and plasma half-life decreased 19-33%). Plasma theophylline levels should be monitored when concomitant moricizine HCl is initiated or discontinued.

Because of possible additive pharmacologic effects, caution is indicated when moricizine HCl is used with any drug that affects cardiac electrophysiology. Uncontrolled experience in patients indicates no serious adverse interaction during the concomitant use of moricizine HCl and diuretics, vasodilators, antihypertensive drugs, calcium channel blockers, beta-blockers, angiotensin-converting enzyme inhibitors, or warfarin. Plasma warfarin levels, warfarin pharmacokinetics, and prothrombin times were unaffected during multiple dose moricizine HCl administration to young, healthy male subjects in a controlled study. However, there are isolated reports of the need to either increase or decrease warfarin doses after initiation of moricizine HCl. Some patients who were taking warfarin with a stable prothrombin time experienced excessive prolongation of the prothrombin time following the initiation of moricizine HCl. In some cases, liver enzymes also were elevated. Bleeding or bruising may occur. When moricizine HCl is started or stopped in a patient stabilized on warfarin, more frequent prothrombin time monitoring is advisable.

Results from *in vitro* studies do not suggest alterations in moricizine HCl plasma protein binding in the presence of other highly plasma protein bound drugs.

ADVERSE REACTIONS:

The most serious adverse reaction reported for moricizine HCl is proarrhythmia(see WARNINGS.) This occurred in 3.7% of 1072 patients with ventricular arrhythmias who received a wide range of doses under a variety of circumstances.

In addition to discontinuations because of proarrhythmias, in controlled clinical trials and in open studies, adverse reactions led to discontinuation of moricizine HCl in 7% of 1105 patients with ventricular and supraventricular arrhythmias, including 3.2% due to nausea, 1.6% due to ECG abnormalities (principally conduction defects, sinus pause, junctional rhythm, or AV block), 1% due to congestive heart failure, and 0.3-0.4% due to dizziness, anxiety, drug fever, urinary retention, blurred vision, gastrointestinal upset, rash, and laboratory abnormalities.

The most frequently occurring adverse reactions in the 1072 patients (including all adverse experiences whether or not considered moricizine HCl-related by the investigator) were dizziness (15.1%), nausea (9.6%), headache (8.0%), fatigue (5.9%), palpitations (5.8%) and dyspnea (5.7%). Dizziness appears to be related to the size of each dose. In a comparison of 900 mg/day given at 450 mg b.i.d. or 300 mg t.i.d., more than 20% of patients experienced dizziness on the b.i.d. regimen vs. 12% on the t.i.d. regimen.

Adverse reactions reported by less than 5%, but in 2% or greater of the patients were: sustained ventricular tachycardia, hypesthesias, abdominal pain, dyspepsia, vomiting, sweating, cardiac chest pain, asthenia, nervousness, paresthesias, congestive heart failure, musculoskeletal pain, diarrhea, dry mouth, cardiac death, sleep disorders, and blurred vision.

Adverse reactions infrequently reported (in less than 2% of the patients) were:

Cardiovascular: hypotension, hypertension, syncope, supraventricular arrhythmias (including atrial fibrillation/flutter), cardiac arrest, bradycardia, pulmonary embolism, myocardial infarction, vasodilation, cerebrovascular events, thrombophlebitis;

Nervous System: tremor, anxiety, depression, euphoria, confusion, somnolence, agitation, seizure, coma, abnormal gait, hallucinations, nystagmus, diplopia, speech disorder, akathisia, loss of memory, ataxia, abnormal coordination, dyskinesia, vertigo, tinnitus;

Genitourinary: urinary retention or frequency, dysuria, urinary incontinence, kidney pain, impotence, decreased libido;

Respiratory: hyperventilation, apnea, asthma, pharyngitis, cough, sinusitis;

Gastrointestinal: anorexia, bitter taste, dysphagia, flatulence, ileus;

Other: drug fever, hypothermia, temperature intolerance, eye pain, rash, pruritus, dry skin, urticaria, swelling of the lips and tongue, periorbital edema.

During moricizine HCl therapy, two patients developed thrombocytopenia that may have been drug-related. Clinically significant elevations in liver function tests (bilirubin, serum transaminases) and jaundice consistent with hepatitis were rarely reported. Although a cause and effect relationship has not been established, caution is advised in patients who develop unexplained signs of hepatic dysfunction, and consideration should be given to discontinuing therapy.

Three patients developed rechallenge-confirmed drug fever, with one patient experiencing an elevation above 103°F (to 105°F, with rigors). Fevers occurred at about 2 weeks in 2 cases, and after 21 weeks in the third. Fevers resolved within 48 hours of discontinuation of moricizine.

Adverse reactions were generally similar in patients over 65 (n=375) and under 65 (n=697), although discontinuation of therapy for reasons other than proarrhythmia was more common in older patients (13.9% vs. 7.7%). Overall mortality was greater in older patients (9.3% vs. 3.9%), but those were not deaths attributed to treatment and the older patients had more serious underlying heart disease.

TABLE 1 compares the most common (occurrence in more than 2% of the patients) non-cardiac adverse reactions (*i.e.,* drug-related or of unknown relationship) in controlled clinical trials during the first one to two weeks of therapy with moricizine HCl, quinidine, placebo, disopyramide, or propranolol in patients with ventricular arrhythmias.

OVERDOSAGE:

Deaths have occurred after accidental or intentional overdosages of 2,250 and 10,000 mg of moricizine HCl, respectively.

Signs, Symptoms and Laboratory Findings Associated with an Overdosage of Drug: Overdosage with moricizine HCl may produce emesis, lethargy, coma, syncope, hypotension, conduction disturbances, exacerbation of congestive heart failure, myocardial infarction, sinus arrest, arrhythmias (including junctional bradycardia, ventricular tachycardia, ventricular fibrillation and asystole), and respiratory failure.

Lethal Dose in Animals: Oral doses of moricizine HCl of about 200 mg/kg in dogs, 250 mg/kg in monkeys, 420 mg/kg in mice and 905 mg/kg in rats were lethal to about one-half of the animals exposed. Death was usually preceded by tremors, convulsions and respiratory depression.

Recommended General Treatment Procedures: A specific antidote for moricizine HCl has not been identified. In the event of overdosage, treatment should be supportive. Patients should be hospitalized and monitored for cardiac, respiratory and CNS changes. Advanced life support systems, including an intracardiac pacing catheter, should be provided where necessary. Acute overdosage should be treated with appropriate gastric evacuation, and with special care to avoid aspiration. Accidental introduction of moricizine HCl into the lungs of monkeys resulted in rapid arrhythmic death.

TABLE 1 Incidence (%) Of The Most Common Adverse Reactions (Therapy Duration = 1-14 Days)

Adverse Reactions	Moricizine >2% %	No.	Placebo >2% %	No.	Quinidine >2% %	No.	Disopyramide >5% %	No.	Propranolol >5% %	No.
Total No. of Patients	1072		618		110		31		24	
Dizziness	121	11.3	33	5.3	8	7.3	-		2	8.3
Nausea	74	6.9	18	2.9	7	6.4	3	9.7	-	
Headache	62	5.8	27	4.4	-		-		4	16.7
Pain	41	3.8	31	5.0	6	5.5	2	6.5	-	
Dyspnea	41	3.8	22	3.6	-		-		-	
Hypesthesia	40	3.7	-		3	2.7	-		-	
Fatigue	33	3.1	16	2.6	6	5.5	2	6.5	3	12.5
Vomiting	22	2.1	-		-		-		-	
Dry mouth	-		-		-		11	35.5	-	
Nervousness	-		-		-		3	9.7	-	
Blurred Vision	-		-		3	2.7	2	6.5	3	12.5
Diarrhea	-		-		25	22.7	-		-	
Constipation	-		-		-		2	6.5	-	
Somnolence	-		-		-		-		2	8.3
Urinary Retention	-		-		-		4	12.9	-	

DOSAGE AND ADMINISTRATION:

The dosage of moricizine HCl must be individualized on the basis of antiarrhythmic response and tolerance. Clinical, cardiac rhythm monitoring, electrocardiogram intervals, exercise testing, and/or programmed electrical stimulation testing may be used to guide antiarrhythmic response and dosage adjustment. In general, the patients will be at high risk and should be hospitalized for the initiation of therapy (see INDICATIONS AND USAGE.)

The usual adult dosage is between 600 and 900 mg per day, given every 8 hours in three equally divided doses. Within this range, the dosage can be adjusted as tolerated, in increments of 150 mg/day at 3-day intervals, until the desired effect is obtained. Patients with life-threatening arrhythmias who exhibit a beneficial response as judged by objective criteria (Holter monitoring, programmed electrical stimulation, exercise testing, etc.) can be maintained on chronic moricizine HCl therapy. As the antiarrhythmic effect of moricizine HCl persists for more than 12 hours, some patients whose arrhythmias are well-controlled on a Q8H regimen may be given the same total daily dose in a Q12H regimen to increase convenience and help assure compliance. When higher doses are used, patients may experience more dizziness and nausea on the Q12 hour regimen.

Patients with Hepatic Impairment: Patients with hepatic disease should be started at 600 mg/day or lower and monitored closely, including measurement of ECG intervals, before dosage adjustment.

Patients with Renal Impairment: Patients with significant renal dysfunction should be started at 600 mg/day or lower and monitored closely, including measurement of ECG intervals, before dosage adjustment.

Transfer to Moricizine HCl: Recommendations for transferring patients from another antiarrhythmic to moricizine HCl can be given based on theoretical considerations. Previous antiarrhythmic therapy should be withdrawn for 1-2 plasma half-lives before starting moricizine HCl at the recommended dosages. In patients in whom withdrawal of a previous antiarrhythmic is likely to produce life-threatening arrhythmias, hospitalization is recommended (TABLE 2):

TABLE 2

Transferred From	Start Moricizine HCl
Quinidine, Disopyramide	6-12 hours after last dose
Procainamide	3-6 hours after last dose
Encainide, Propafenone,	8-12 hours after last dose
Tocainide, or Mexiletine Flecainide	12-24 hours after last dose

HOW SUPPLIED:

Ethmozine is available as oval, convex, film-coated tablets as follows: 200 mg (light green);

250 mg (light orange)

300 mg (light blue)

Storage: Store at controlled room temperature: 15°-30°C (59°-86°F) in a tightly-closed, light resistant container. Protect from light.

HOW SUPPLIED - EQUIVALENTS NOT AVAILABLE:

Tablet, Coated - Oral - 200 mg

100's $96.91 ETHMOZINE, Roberts Labs 54092-0046-01
100's $96.91 ETHMOZINE, Roberts Labs 54092-0046-52

Tablet, Coated - Oral - 250 mg

100's $115.69 ETHMOZINE, Roberts Labs 54092-0047-01
100's $115.69 ETHMOZINE, Roberts Labs 54092-0047-52

Tablet, Coated - Oral - 300 mg

100's $131.72 ETHMOZINE, Roberts Labs 54092-0048-01
100's $131.72 ETHMOZINE, Roberts Labs 54092-0048-52

MORPHINE SULFATE *(001833)*

CATEGORIES: Analeptics; Analgesics; Anesthesia; Antipyretics; Central Nervous System Agents; Narcotic Analgesics; Narcotics, Synthetics & Combinations; Opiate Agonists (Controlled); Pain; Surgical Post-Operative Pain; Pregnancy Category C; DEA Class CII; FDA Approved 1984 Sep

BRAND NAMES: *Anamorph*; Astramorph-Pf; *Contalgin*; *Continue DR*; *Dolcontin*; *Dolcontin Depottab*; **Duramorph**; *Duromorph* (England); Infumorph; *Kapanol*; *La Morph*; *Longphine SR*; *M-Long* (Germany); *MCR*; *M.I.R.*; *M S Contin* (Canada); MS Contin; *MS-Contin*; MS S; MSIR; *MSP*; *MST*; *MST 10 Mundipharma* (Germany); *MST 30 Mundipharma* (Germany); *MST 60 Mundipharma* (Germany); *MST 100 Mundipharma* (Germany); *MST 200 Mundipharma* (Germany); *MST Continus* (England, Mexico); *MST Continus Retard*; *Morcontin Continus*; *Morficontin*; *Morphine Mixtures*; *Moscontin* (France); *Mundidol Retard*; OMS; *Oramorph* (England); Oramorph SR; RMS; *Ra-Morph*; Roxanol; *Sevredol*; *Statex* (Canada) *(International brand names outside U.S. in italics)*

FORMULARIES: Aetna; BC-BS; FHP; Medi-Cal; WHO; PCS

WARNING:
May be habit forming.

DESCRIPTION:

Morphine sulfate occurs as odorless, white, feathery, silky crystals, cubical masses of crystals, or white crystalline powder. It has a solubility of 1 in 21 parts of water and 1 in 1000 parts of alcohol, but is practically insoluble in chloroform or ether. The octal:water partition coefficient of morphine is 1.42 at physiologic pH and the pK_b is 7.9 for the tertiary nitrogen (mostly ionized at pH 7.4).

The chemical name for morphine sulfate is 7,8-didehydro-4,5α-epoxy-17-methylmorphinan-3,6α-diol sulfate (2:1) (salt), pentahydrate.

The empirical formula is $(C_{17}H_{19}NO_3)_2 \cdot H_2SO_4 \cdot 5H_2O$. Its molecular weight is 758.83

Injection: The injectable form is a sterile solution of morphine sulfate in Water for Injection. Each ml of Morphine Sulfate Injection, USP, contains 15 mg (20 mcgmol) morphine sulfate, with 0.5% chlorobutanol (chloroform derivative) and not more than 0.1% sodium bisulfate.

Oral Solution: Each 5 ml of morphine sulfate immediate release oral solution contains 10 or 20 mg of morphine sulfate.

Oral Solution Concentrate: Each 1 ml of morphine sulfate immediate release oral solution concentrate contains 20 mg of morphine sulfate.

Immediate Release Tablets: Each morphine sulfate immediate release tablet for oral administration contains 15 or 30 mg of morphine sulfate. *Inactive ingredients:* corn starch, lactose, magnesium stearate, and talc.

Immediate Release Capsules: Each morphine sulfate immediate release capsule for oral administration contains 15 or 30 mg of morphine sulfate. *Inactive ingredients:* FD&C Blue No. 1, FD&C Blue No. 2, FD&C Red No. 40, FD&C Yellow No. 6, gelatin, hydroxypropyl methylcellulose, lactose, polyethylene glycol, polysorbate 80, polyvinylpyrrolidone, starch, sucrose, titanium dioxide, and other ingredients. In addition, the 30 mg capsule contains black iron oxide and D&C Red No. 28.

MS Contin Controlled Release Tablets: Each MS Contin controlled release tablet contains either 15, 30, 60, or 100 mg morphine sulfate, USP. *Inactive ingredients:* cetostearyl alcohol, hydroxyethyl cellulose, hydroxypropyl methylcellulose, lactose, magnesium stearate, talc, titanium dioxide and other ingredients and may contain FD&C Blue No.1, FD&C Blue No. 2, FD&C Red No. 40, FD&C Yellow No. 6.

Kadian Controlled Release Capsules: Each Kadian controlled release capsule contains either 20, 50 or 100 mg of morphine sulfate and the following ingredients common to all strengths: hydroxypropyl methylcellulose, ethylcellulose, methacrylic acid copolymer, polyethylene glycol, diethyl phthalate, talc, black ink sw, corn starch and sucrose.

Suppositories: Each Roxanol suppository for rectal administration contains: morphine sulfate: 5, 10, 20, or 30 mg. Each suppository contains morphine sulfate, butylated hydroxyanisole, colloidal silicon dioxide, and hydrogenated suppository base, for rectal administration. Morphine sulfate acts as a narcotic analgesic.

CLINICAL PHARMACOLOGY:

METABOLISM AND PHARMACOKINETICS

Injection

Morphine sulfate is a potent, centrally active analgesic. Other actions include respiratory depression; depression of the cough center; release of antidiuretic hormone; activation of the vomiting center; pupillary constriction; a decrease in gastric, pancreatic, and biliary secretion; a reduction in intestinal motility; an increase in biliary tract pressure; and an increased amplitude of ureteral contractions.

Onset of analgesia following intramuscular or subcutaneous administration occurs within 10 to 30 minutes. The effect persists for 4 to 5 hours.

Approximately 90% of a parenteral dose of morphine appears in the urine within 24 hours as the product of glucuronide conjugation. Most of the remainder is excreted in the bile and eliminated in the feces.

Suppositories

Morphine sulfate given as a rectal suppository can produce analgesic effects and duration similar to that of oral administration at similar dose levels. Analgesic effects are commonly seen 20 to 60 minutes after administration.

Oral Forms

Following oral administration of a given dose of morphine controlled release tablets, the amount ultimately absorbed is essentially the same whether the source is morphine sulfate controlled release or a conventional formulation. Morphine is released from morphine sulfate controlled release somewhat more slowly than from conventional oral preparations. Because of pre-systemic elimination (*i.e.*, metabolism in the gut wall and liver) only about 40% of the administered dose reaches the central compartment.

Morphine is a natural product that is the prototype for the class of natural and synthetic opioid analgesics. Opioids produce a wide spectrum of pharmacologic effects including analgesia, dysphoria, euphoria, somnolence, respiratory depression, diminished gastrointestinal motility, altered circulatory dynamics, histamine release and physical dependence.

Morphine produces both its therapeutic and its adverse effects by interaction with one or more classes of specific opioid receptors located throughout the body. Morphine acts as a pure agonist, binding with and activating opioid receptors at sites in the peri-aqueductal and peri-ventricular grey matter, the ventro-medial medulla and the spinal cord to produce analgesia.

Central Nervous System

The principal actions of therapeutic value of morphine are analgesia, sedation, and alterations of mood. Opioids of this class do not usually eliminate pain, but they do reduce the perception of pain by the central nervous system.

The precise mechanism of analgesic action is unknown. However, specific CNS opiate receptors and endogenous compounds with morphine-like activity have been identified throughout the brain and spinal cord and are likely to play a role in the expression of analgesic effects.

Morphine produces respiratory depression by direct action on brain stem respiratory centers. The mechanism of respiratory depression involves a reduction in the responsiveness of the brain stem respiratory centers to increases in carbon dioxide tension, and to electrical stimulation.

Morphine depresses the cough reflex by direct effect on the cough center in the medulla. Antitussive effects may occur with doses lower than those usually required for analgesia.

Morphine causes miosis, even in total darkness, and little tolerance develops to this effect. Pinpoint pupils are a sign of opioid overdose but are not pathognomonic (*e.g.*, pontine lesions of hemorrhagic or ischemic origins may produce similar findings). Marked mydriasis rather than miosis may be seen due to severe hypoxia in overdose situations.

CLINICAL PHARMACOLOGY: *(cont'd)*

Gastrointestinal Tract and Other Smooth Muscle

Gastric, biliary and pancreatic secretions are decreased by morphine. Morphine causes a reduction in motility associated with an increase in tone in the antrum of the stomach and duodenum. Digestion of food in the small intestine is delayed and propulsive contractions are decreased. Propulsive peristaltic waves in the colon are decreased, while tone is increased to the point of spasm. The end result is constipation. Morphine can cause a marked increase in biliary tract pressure as a result of spasm of the sphincter of Oddi.

Cardiovascular System

Morphine produces peripheral vasodilation which may result in orthostatic hypotension or syncope. Release of histamine can occur and may be induced by morphine and can contribute to opioid-induced hypotension. Manifestations of histamine release and/or peripheral vasodilation may include pruritus, flushing, red eyes and sweating.

Distribution

Once absorbed, morphine is distributed to skeletal muscle, kidneys, liver, intestinal tract, lungs, spleen and brain. The volume of distribution of morphine is approximately 3 to 4 L/kg. Morphine is 30 to 35% reversibly bound to plasma proteins. Although the primary site of action of morphine is in the CNS, only small quantities pass the blood-barrier barrier. Morphine also crosses the placental membranes (see PRECAUTIONS, Pregnancy) and has been found in breast milk (see PRECAUTIONS, Nursing Mothers).

Metabolism

The major pathway of the detoxification of morphine is conjugation, either with D–glucuronic acid in the liver to produce glucuronides or with sulfuric acid to give morphine–3–etheral sulfate. Although a small fraction (less than 5%) of morphine is demethylated, for all practical purposes, virtually all morphine is converted to glucuronide metabolites including morphine–3–glucuronide, M3G (about 50%) and morphine–6–glucuronide, M6G (about 5 to 15%). Studies in healthy subjects and cancer patients have shown that the glucuronide metabolite to morphine mean molar ratios (based on AUC) are similar after both single doses and at steady state for morphine sulfate controlled release capsules, 12 hour tablets and morphine sulfate solution.

M3G has no significant analgesic activity. M6G has shown to have opioid agonist and analgesic activity in humans.

The glucuronide system has a very high capacity and is not easily saturated, even in disease. Therefore, the rate of delivery of morphine to the gut and liver does not influence the total and/or the relative quantities of the various metabolites formed.

The following pharmacokinetic parameters show considerable inter-subject variation but are representative of average values reported in the literature. The volume of distribution (Vd) for morphine is 4 liters per kilogram, and its terminal elimination half-life is approximately 2 to 4 hours.

Following the administration of conventional oral morphine products, approximately fifty percent of the morphine that will reach the central compartment intact reaches it within 30 minutes. Following the administration of an equal amount of morphine sulfate controlled release to normal volunteers, however, this extent of absorption occurs, on average, after 1.5 hours.

Variation in the physical/mechanical properties of a formulation of an oral morphine drug product can affect both its absolute bioavailability and its absorption rate constant (K_a). The basic pharmacokinetic parameters (*e.g.,* volume of distribution [Vd], elimination rate constant [K_e], clearance [Cl]) are fundamental properties of morphine in the organism. However, in chronic use, the possibility that shifts in metabolite to parent drug ratios may occur cannot be excluded.

When immediate release oral morphine is given on a fixed dosing regimen, steady state is achieved in about a day.

For a given dose and dosing interval, the AUC and average blood concentration of morphine at steady state (C_{ss}) will be independent of the specific type of oral formulation administered so long as the formulations have the same absolute bioavailability. The absorption rate of a formulation will, however, affect the maximum (C_{max}) and minimum (C_{min}) blood levels and the times of their occurrence.

While there is no predictable relationship between morphine blood levels and analgesic response, effective analgesia will not occur below some minimum blood level in a given patient. The minimum effective blood level for analgesia will vary among patients, especially among patients who have been previously treated with potent mu (μ) agonist opioids. Similarly, there is no predictable relationship between blood morphine concentration and untoward clinical responses; again, however, higher concentration are more likely to be toxic than lower ones.

Excretion

Approximately 10% of morphine dose is excreted unchanged in the urine. Most of the dose is excreted in the urine as M3G and M6G. A small amount of the glucuronide metabolites is excreted in the bile and there is some minor enterohepatic cycling. Seven to 10% of administered morphine is excreted in the feces.

The mean adult plasma clearance is about 20–30 ml/minute/kg. The effective terminal half-life of morphine after IV administration is reported to be approximately 2.0 hours. Longer plasma sampling in some studies suggests a longer terminal half-life of morphine of about 15 hours.

Controlled Release Capsules

Controlled release capsules contain polymer coated sustained release pellets of morphine sulfate that release morphine significantly more slowly than form morphine sulfate tablets and shorter-acting controlled release oral morphine sulfate preparations. Controlled release capsules activity is primarily due to morphine. One metabolite, morphine–6–glucuronide, has been shown to have analgesic activity, but poorly crosses the blood-brain barrier.

The single-dose pharmacokinetics of Kadian are linear over the dosage range of 30 to 100 mg. The single dose and multiple dose pharmacokinetic parameters of the controlled release capsules in normal volunteers are summarized in TABLE 1.

Immediate and Controlled Release Oral Forms

The elimination of morphine occurs primarily as renal excretion of 3–morphine glucuronide. A small amount of the glucuronide conjugate is excreted in the bile, and there is some minor enterohepatic recycling.

The elimination half-life of morphine is reported to vary between 2 to 4 hours, however, a longer term half-life of about 15 hours has been reported in studies where blood has been sampled up to 48 hours. Thus, steady state is probably achieved on most regimens within a day. Because morphine is primarily metabolized to inactive metabolites, the effects of renal disease on morphine's elimination are not likely to be pronounced. However, as with any drug, caution should be taken to guard against unanticipated accumulation if renal and/or hepatic function is seriously impaired.

Individual differences in the metabolism of morphine suggest that morphine sulfate immediate release oral solutions, tablets and capsules be dosed conservatively according to the dosing initiation and titration recommendations in DOSAGE AND ADMINISTRATION.

CLINICAL PHARMACOLOGY: *(cont'd)*

TABLE 1 Mean Pharmacokinetic Parameters (%coefficient variation) Resulting From a Fasting Single Dose Study in Normal Volunteers and a Multiple Dose Study in Patients with Cancer Pain

Regimen/ Dosage Form	AUC *, † (ng·h/ml)	C_{max} † (ng/ml)	T_{max} (h)	C_{min} † (ng/ml)	Fluctuation‡
Single Dose (n=24)					
Kadian Capsule	271.0 (19.4)	15.6 (24.4)	8.6 (41.1)	na§	na
Controlled Release Tablet	304.3 (19.1)	30.5 (32.1)	2.5 (52.6)	na	na
Morphine Solution	362.4 (42.6)	64.4 (38.2)	0.9 (55.8)	na	na
Multiple Dose (n=24)					
Kadian Capsule q24h	500.9 (38.6)	37.3 (37.7)	10.3 (32.2)	9.9 (52.3)	3.0 (45.5)
Controlled Release Tablet q12h	457.3 (40.2)	36.9 (42.0)	4.4 (53.0)	7.6 (60.3)	4.1 (51.5)

* For single dose AUC=$AUC_{0\text{-}48h}$, for multiple dose AUC=$AUC_{0\text{-}24h}$, at steady state.
† For single dose parameter normalized to 100 mg, for multiple dose parameter normalized to 100 mg per 24 hours.
‡ Steady-state fluctuation in plasma concentrations=C_{max}-C_{min}/C_{min}.
§ Not applicable.

SPECIAL POPULATIONS

Geriatric: The elderly may have increased sensitivity to morphine and may achieve higher and more variable serum levels than younger patients. In adults, the duration of analgesia increases progessively with age, though the degree of analgesia remains unchanged. Morphine sulfate pharmacokinetics have not been investigated in elderly patients (>65 years) although such patients were included in the clinical studies.

Nursing Mothers: Morphine is excreted in the maternal milk, and the milk to plasma morphine AUC ratio is about 2.5:1. The amount of morphine received by the infant depends on the maternal plasma concentration, amount of milk ingested by the infant, and the extent of first pass metabolism.

Pediatric: Infants under 1 month of age have a prolonged elimination half-life and decreased clearance relative to older infants and children. The clearance of morphine and its elimination half-life begin to approach adult values by the second month of life. Children old enough to take capsules should have pharmacokinetic parameters similar to adults, dosed on a per kilogram basis (see PRECAUTIONS, Pediatric Use).

Gender: No meaningful differences between male and female patients were demonstrated in the analysis of the pharmacokinetic data from clinical studies.

Race: Pharmacokinetic differences due to race may exist. Chinese subjects given intravenous morphine in one study had a higher clearance when compared to caucasian subjects (1852 ± 116 ml/min versus 1495 ± 80 ml/min).

Hepatic Failure: The pharmacokinetics of morphine were found to be significantly altered in individuals with alcoholic cirrhosis. The clearance was found to decrease with a corresponding increase in half-life. The M3G and M6G to morphine plasma AUC ratios also decreased in these patients indicating a decrease in metabolic activity.

Renal Insufficiency: The pharmacokinetics of morphine are altered in renal failure patients. AUC is increased and clearance is decreased. The metabolites, M3G and M6G accumulate several fold in renal failure patients compared with healthy subjects.

PHARMACODYNAMICS

The relationship between the blood level of morphine and the analgesic response will depend on the patient's age, state of health, medical condition, and the extent of previous opioid treatment.

A minimum effective concentration (MEC) of morphine for pain relief has been reported as 27.2 ± 14.5 ng/ml (mean ± SD) in cancer patients treated with morphine solution. These results compare with the MEC for plasma morphine reported as 14.7 ± 4.8 ng/ml (mean ± SD) in patients with postoperative pain. The high degree of variation is of clinical significance as it may result in either under-dosing or over-dosing if the dosage is not adjusted to the patient's clinical status and analgesic response (see PRECAUTIONS and DOSAGE AND ADMINISTRATION).

For opioid-tolerant patients the situation is much more complex. Some patients will become rapidly tolerant to the analgesic effects of morphine, and will require high daily oral morphine doses for adequate pain control. Since the development of tolerance to both the therapeutic and adverse effects of opioids is highly individualized, the dose of morphine should be individualized to the patient's condition and should not be based on an arbitrary choice of a dose or blood level to be achieved.

CONTROLLED RELEASE

Absorption: Following the administration of oral morphine solution, approximately 50% of the morphine absorbed reached the systemic circulation within 30 minutes. However, following the administration of an equal amount of morphine sulfate controlled release to healthy volunteers, this occurs, on average, after 8 hours. As with most forms of oral morphine, because of presystemic elimination, only about 20 to 40% of the administered dose reaches the systemic circulation.

Food Effects: While concurrent administration of food slows the rate of absorption of morphine sulfate controlled release, the extent of absorption is not affected and morphine sulfate controlled release can be administered without regard to meals.

Steady State: When morphine sulfate is given on a fixed dosing regimen to patients with chronic pain due to malignancy, steady state is achieved in about two days. At steady state, morphine sulfate controlled release capsules will have significantly lower $C_{max}$and a higher C_{min} than equivalent doses of oral morphine solution and some other controlled release preparations.

When given once-daily (every 24 hours) to 24 patients with malignancy, Kadian (morphine sulfate controlled release capsules) had a similar C_{max} and higher C_{min} at steady state in clinical usage, when compared to twice-daily (every 12 hours) MS Contin (morphine sulfate controlled release tablets), given at an equivalent total daily dosage. Drug-disease interactions are frequently seen in the older and more gravely ill patients, and may result in both altered absorption and reduced clearance as compared to normal volunteers (see PRECAUTIONS, Geriatric,, Hepatic Failure, and, Renal Insufficiency).

Drug-Drug Interactions: The known drug interactions involving morphine are pharmacodynamic, not pharmacokinetic (see DRUG INTERACTIONS).

CLINICAL STUDIES:

Kadian Studies: A total of 177 healthy subjects and 337 patients with cancer pain participated in a total of 15 studies (10 pharmacokinetic and 6 clinical; one study reported both pharmacokinetic and clinical data). Of these individuals, 158 healthy subjects and 268 patients received Kadian. In the controlled clinical studies patients were followed for a

CLINICAL STUDIES: *(cont'd)*

median duration of 7 days and in the open label studies patients were followed for up to 12–24 months. Kadian was compared to oral morphine solution and to either MS Contin or to a 12-hour controlled release morphine tablet bioequivalent to MS Contin using trial designs that followed the clinical and pharmacokinetic performance of each treatment in cancer patients receiving chronic opioid therapy.

In two controlled studies, patients with moderate to severe cancer pain titrated with immediate release morphine (IRM) solution or tablets to a stable total daily dose of morphine for at least three consecutive days, then randomized to Kadian or 12-hour controlled-release morphine for seven days of observation. Kadian given once a day proved similar to the same total dose of morphine given in divided doses in a 12 hour dosage form, with respect to pain relief, use of rescue medication, patient and investigator global assessment, and quality of sleep. Individual patient differences in the pattern of pain control emphasize the need to individualize both dose and dosing interval (see DOSAGE AND ADMINISTRATION).

INDICATIONS AND USAGE:

Injection: Morphine sulfate is a potent analgesic used for the relief of moderate to severe pain. It is also used preoperatively to sedate the patient and allay apprehension, facilitate induction of anesthesia, and reduce anesthetic dosage.

Immediate Release Oral Forms: Morphine sulfate immediate release oral solutions, tablets, capsules are indicated for the relief of moderate to severe pain.

Controlled Release Oral Forms: Morphine sulfate controlled release capsules and tablets are indicated for the management of moderate to severe pain where treatment with an opioid analgesic is indicated for more than a few days (see CLINICAL PHARMACOLOGY and CLINICAL STUDIES).

Morphine sulfate controlled release capsules were developed for use in patients with chronic pain who require repeated dosing with a potent opioid analgesic, and has been tested in patients with pain due to malignant conditions. Morphine sulfate controlled release capsules has not been tested as an analgesic for the treatment of acute pain or in the postoperative setting and is not recommended for such use.

Suppositories: Morphine sulfate suppositories are indicated for the relief of moderate to severe chronic pain, and severe acute pain.

CONTRAINDICATIONS:

Injection: Hypersensitivity to morphine. Because of its stimulating effect on the spinal cord, morphine should not be used in convulsive states, such as those occurring in status epilepticus, tetanus, and strychnine poisoning.

Oral Forms: Morphine sulfate oral products are contraindicated in patients with known hypersensitivity to morphine, morphine salts, or any component of the dose form; in patients with respiratory depression in the absence of resuscitative equipment, and in patients with acute or severe bronchial asthma.

Morphine sulfate oral products are contraindicated in any patient who has or is suspected of having paralytic ileus.

Suppositories: Hypersensitivity to morphine; respiratory insufficiency or depression; severe CNS depression; attack of bronchial asthma; heart failure secondary to chronic lung disease; cardiac arrhythmias; increased intracranial or cerebrospinal fluid pressure; head injuries; brain tumor; acute alcoholism; delirium tremens; convulsive disorders; after biliary tract surgery; suspected surgical abdomen; surgical anastomosis; concomitantly with MAO inhibitors or within 14 days of such treatment.

WARNINGS:

Injection Only: Morphine sulfate injection contains sodium bisulfite, which may cause allergic-type reactions including anaphylactic symptoms and life-threatening or less severe asthmatic episodes in certain susceptible people. The overall prevalence of sulfite sensitivity in the general population is unknown and probably low. Sulfite sensitivity is seen more frequently in asthmatic than in nonasthmatic people.

ALL FORMS

(See also CLINICAL PHARMACOLOGY).

Impaired Respiration: Respiratory depression is the chief hazard of all morphine preparations. Respiratory depression occurs more frequently in elderly and debilitated patients, and those suffering from conditions accompanied by hypoxia, hypercapnia, or upper airway obstruction (when even moderate therapeutic doses may dangerously decrease pulmonary ventilation).

Morphine should be used with extreme caution in patients with chronic obstructive pulmonary disease or cor pulmonale, and in patients having a substantially decreased respiratory reserve (*e.g.* severe kyphoscoliosis), hypoxia, hypercapnia, or pre-existing respiratory depression. In such patients, even usual therapeutic doses of morphine may increase respiratory airway resistance and decrease respiratory drive to the point of apnea.

Head Injury And Increased Intracranial Pressure: The respiratory depressant effects of morphine with carbon dioxide retention and secondary elevation of cerebrospinal fluid pressure may be markedly exaggerated in the presence of head injury, other intracranial lesions, or pre-existing increase in intracranial pressure. Morphine produces effects which may obscure neurologic signs of further increase in pressure in patients with head injuries. Morphine should only be administered under such circumstances when considered essential and then with extreme care.

Hypotensive Effects: All opioid analgesics may cause severe hypotension in an individual whose ability to maintain blood pressure has already been compromised by a depleted blood volume, or a concurrent administration of drugs such as phenothiazines, or general anesthetics. (See DRUG INTERACTIONS). Morphine may produce orthostatic hypotension in ambulatory patients.

Morphine sulfate, like all opioid analgesics, should be administered with caution to patients in circulatory shock, since vasodilation produced by the drug may further reduce cardiac output and blood pressure.

Gastrointestinal Obstruction: Morphine sulfate controlled release capsules should not be given to patients with gastrointestinal obstruction, particularly paralytic ileus, as there is a risk of the product remaining in the stomach for an extended period and the subsequent release of a bolus of morphine when normal gut motility is restored. As with other solid morphine formulations diarrhea may reduce morphine absorption.

Acute Abdominal Conditions: The administration of morphine or other narcotics may obscure the diagnosis or clinical course in patients with acute abdominal conditions.

Special Risk Groups: Morphine sulfate controlled release capsules should be administered with caution, and in reduced dosages in elderly or debilitated patients; patients with severe renal or hepatic insufficiency; patients with Addison's disease; myxedema; hypothyroidism; prostatic hypertrophy or urethral stricture.

Caution should also be exercised in the administration of morphine sulfate to patients with CNS depression, toxic psychosis, acute alcoholism and delirium tremens, and convulsive disorders.

WARNINGS: *(cont'd)*

Morphine sulfate should be used with extreme caution in patients with disorders characterized by hypoxia, since even usual therapeutic doses of narcotics may decrease respiratory drive to the point of apnea while simultaneously increasing airway resistance.

Cordotomy: Patients taking morphine sulfate who are scheduled for cordotomy or other interruption of pain transmission pathways should have morphine sulfate controlled release capsules ceased 24 hours prior to the procedure and the pain controlled by parenteral short-acting opioids. In addition, the post-procedure titration of analgesics for such patients should be individualized to avoid either oversedation or withdrawl syndromes.

Use in Pancreatic/Biliary Tract Disease: Morphine sulfate may cause spasm of the sphincter of Oddi and should be used with caution in patients with biliary tract disease, including acute pancreatitis. Opioids may cause increases in the serum amylase level.

Driving and Operating Machinery: Morphine may impair the mental and/or physical abilities needed to perform potentially hazardous activities such as driving a care or operating machinery. Patients must be cautioned accordingly. Patients should also be warned about the potential combined effects of morphine with other CNS depressants, including other opioids, phenothiazines, sedative/hypnotics and alcohol (see DRUG INTERACTIONS).

PRECAUTIONS:

GENERAL

(See CLINICAL PHARMACOLOGY.)

Injection Only

Supraventricular Tachycardias: Because of a possible vagolytic action that may produce a significant increase in the ventricular response rate, morphine sulfate should be used with caution in patients with atrial flutter and other supraventricular tachycardias.

Convulsions: Morphine sulfate may aggravate preexisting convulsions in patients with convulsive disorders. If dosage is escalated substantially above recommended levels because of tolerance development, convulsions may occur in individuals without a history of convulsive disorders.

Kidney or Liver Dysfunction: Morphine sulfate may have a prolonged duration and cumulative effect in patients with kidney or liver dysfunction.

Oral Forms

(See CLINICAL PHARMACOLOGY.)

Morphine sulfate oral solutions, tablets and capsules are intended for use in patients who require a potent opioid analgesic for analgesic relief of moderate to severe pain.

Selection of patients for treatment with morphine sulfate oral products should be governed by the same principles that apply to the use of morphine and other potent opioid analgesics. Specifically, the increased risks associated with its use in the following populations should be considered: the elderly or debilitated and those with severe impairment of hepatic, pulmonary or renal function; myxedema or hypothyroidism; adrenocortical insufficiency (*e.g.*, Addison's Disease); CNS depression or coma; toxic psychoses; prostatic hypertrophy or urethral stricture; acute alcoholism; delirium tremens; kyphoscoliosis, or inability to swallow.

The administration of morphine, like all opioid analgesics, may obscure the diagnosis or clinical course in patients with acute abdominal conditions.

Morphine may aggravate preexisting convulsions in patients with convulsive disorders.

Morphine should be used with caution in patients about to undergo surgery of the biliary tract, since it may cause spasm of the sphincter of Oddi. Similarly, morphine should be used with caution in patients with acute pancreatitis secondary to biliary tract disease.

Controlled Release Oral Forms

Special Precautions Regarding Morphine Sulfate Controlled Release 200 Tablets: Morphine sulfate controlled release 200 mg tablets are for use only in opioid tolerant patients requiring daily morphine equivalent dosages of 400 mg or more. Care should be taken in its prescription and patients should be instructed against use by individuals other than the patient for whom it was prescribed, as this may have severe medical consequences for that individual.

General: Morphine sulfate controlled release is intended for use in patients who require continuous treatment with a potent opioid analgesic.

The controlled release nature of the formulation allows it to be administered on a more convenient schedule than conventional immediate release oral morphine products (See CLINICAL PHARMACOLOGY). However, morphine sulfate controlled release does not release morphine continuously over the course of a dosing interval. The administration of single doses of morphine sulfate controlled release on a every 12 hour dosing schedule will result in higher peak and lower trough plasma levels than those that occur when an identical daily dose of morphine is administered using conventional oral formulations on a every 4 hour regimen. The clinical significance of greater fluctuations in morphine plasma level has not been systematically evaluated. (See DOSAGE AND ADMINISTRATION.)

As with any potent opioid, it is critical to adjust the dosing regimen for each patient individually, taking into account the patient's prior analgesic treatment experience. Although it is clearly impossible to enumerate every consideration that is important to the selection of the initial dose and dosing interval of morphine sulfate. (See DOSAGE AND ADMINISTRATION.)

INFORMATION FOR THE PATIENT

If clinically advisable, patients receiving morphine sulfate controlled release capsules should be given the following instructions by the physician:

1. While psychological dependence ("addiction") to morphine used in the treatment of pain is very rare, morphine is one of a class of drugs known to be abused and should be handled accordingly.

2. The dose of the drug should not be adjusted without consulting a physician.

3. Morphine may impair mental and/or physical ability required for the performance of potentially hazardous tasks (*e.g.*, driving, operating machinery).

4. Morphine should not be taken with alcohol or other CNS depressants (sleep aids, tranquilizers) because additive effects including CNS depression may occur. A physician should be consulted if other prescription medications are currently being used or are prescribed for future use.

5. For women of childbearing potential who become or are planning to become pregnant, a physician should be consulted regarding analgesics and other drug use.

6. Upon completion of therapy, it may be appropriate to taper morphine dose, rather than abruptly discontinue it.

7. The morphine sulfate controlled release 200 mg tablet is for use only in opioid tolerant patients requiring daily morphine equivalent dosages of 400 mg or more. Special care must be taken to avoid accidental ingestion or the use by individuals (including children) other than the patient for whom it was originally prescribed, as such unsupervised use may have severe, even fatal, consequences.

8. Morphine sulfate controlled release capsules should NOT be opened, chewed, crushed or dissolved. The pellets in the controlled release capsules should NOT be chewed or dissolved.

PRECAUTIONS: *(cont'd)*

9. As with other opioids, patients taking morphine sulfate should be advised that severe constipation could occur and appropriate laxatives, stool softeners and other appropriate treatments should be initiated from the beginning of opioid therapy.

CARCINOGENESIS, MUTAGENESIS, AND IMPAIRMENT OF FERTILITY

Injection and Suppositories: Morphine has no known carcinogenic or mutagenic potential. However, no long-term animal studies are available to support this observation.

Oral Forms: Studies of morphine sulfate in animals to evaluate the drug's carcinogenic and mutagenic potential or the effect on fertility have not been conducted. There are no reports of carcinogenic effects in humans.

In vitro studies have reported that morphine is non-mutagenic in the Ames test with *Salmonella,* and induces chromosomal aberrations in human leukocytes and lethal mutation induction in *Drosophila.* Morphine was found to be mutagenic *in vitro* in human T-cells, increasing the DNA fragmentation. *In vivo,*morphine was mutagenic in the mouse micronucleus test and induced chromosomal aberrations in spermatids and murine lymphocytes.

Chronic opioid abusers (*e.g.* heroin abusers) and their offspring display higher rates of chromosomal damage. However, the rates of chromosomal abnormalities were similar in nonexposed individuals and in heroin users enrolled in long term opioid maintenance programs.

PREGNANCY CATEGORY C

On the basis of the historical use of morphine sulfate during all stages if pregnancy, there is no known risk of fetal abnormality at usual therapeutic dosages. Morphine sulfate should be given to a pregnant woman only if clearly needed.

Teratogenic Effects: Teratogenic effects of morphine have been reported in the animal literature. High parental doses during the second trimester were teratogenic in neurological, soft and skeletal tissue. The abnormalities included encephalopathy and axial skeletal fusions. These doses were often maternally toxic and were 0.3 to 3–fold the maximum recommended human dose (MRHD) on a mg/m^2 basis. The relative contribution of morphine-induced maternal hypoxia and malnutrition, each of which can be teratogenic, has not been clearly defined. Treatment of male rats with approximately 3–fold the MRHD for 10 days prior to mating decreased litter size and viability.

Adequate animal studies on reproduction have not been performed to determine whether morphine affects fertility in males or females. There are no well-controlled studies in women, but marketing experience does not include any evidence of adverse effects on the fetus following routine (short-term) clinical use of morphine sulfate products. Reproductive effects have been observed in mice treated on gestation days 8 and/or 9 with doses ranging from 100 to 500 mg/kg morphine sulfate. Although there is no clearly defined risk, such experience cannot exclude the possibility of infrequent or subtle damage to the human fetus. Morphine sulfate should be used in pregnant women only when clearly needed. See PRECAUTIONS, Labor and Delivery. (Also, see DRUG ABUSE AND DEPENDENCE.)

Nonteratogenic Effects: Morphine given subcutaneously, at non-maternally toxic doses, to rats during the third trimester with approximately 0.15–fold the MRHD caused reversible reductions in brain and spinal cord volume, and testes size and body weight in the offspring, and decreased fertility in female offspring. The offspring of rats and hamsters treated orally or intraperitoneally throughout pregnancy with 0.04– to 0.3–fold the MRHD of morphine have demonstrated delayed growth, motor and sexual maturation and decreased male fertility. Chronic morphine exposure of fetal animals resulted in mild withdrawal, altered reflex and motor skill development, and altered responsivenes to morphine that persisted into adulthood.

There are no well-controlled studies of chronic *in utero* exposure to morphine sulfate in human subjects. However, uncontrolled retrospective studies of human neonates chronically exposed to other opioids *in utero,* demonstrated reduced brain volume which normalized over the first month of life. Infants born to opioid-abusing mothers are more often small for gestational age, have a decreased ventilatory response to CO_2 and increased risk of sudden infant death syndrome.

Infants born from mothers who have been taking morphine chronically may exhibit withdrawal symptoms.

Morphine should only be used during pregnancy if the need for strong opioid analgesia justifies the potential risk to the fetus.

LABOR AND DELIVERY

Morphine sulfate oral products are not recommended for use in women during and immediately prior to labor, where shorter acting analgesics or other analgesic techniques are more appropriate. Occasionally, opioid analgesics may prolong labor through actions which temporarily reduce the strength, duration and frequency of uterine contractions. However, this effect is not consistent and may be offset by an increased rate of cervical dilation which tends to shorten labor.

Morphine readily crosses the placental barrier and should be used with caution in women delivering premature infants since respiratory depression in the neonate may occur. Neonates whose mothers received morphine sulfate during labor should be observed closely for signs of respiratory depression. A specific narcotic antagonist, naloxone, is available for reversal of narcotic-induced respiratory depression in the neonate.

NEONATAL WITHDRAWAL SYNDROME

Chronic maternal use of opiates or opioids during pregnancy coexposes the fetus. The newborn may experience subsequent neonatal withdrawal syndrome (NWS). Manifestations of NWS include irritability, hyperactivity, abnormal sleep pattern, high-pitched cry, tremor, vomiting, diarrhea, weight loss, and failure to gain weight. The onset, duration, and severity of the disorder differ based on such factors as the addictive drug used, time and amount of mother's last dose, and rate of elimination of the drug from the newborn. Approaches to the treatment of this syndrome have included supportive care and, when indicated, drugs such as paragoric or phenobarbital.

NURSING MOTHERS

Low levels of morphine have been detected in human milk. Withdrawal symptoms can occur in breast-feeding infants when maternal administration of morphine sulfate is stopped. Nursing should not be undertaken while a patient is receiving morphine sulfate oral products since morphine may be excreted in the milk. Because of the potential for adverse reactions in nursing infants from morphine sulfate, a decision should be made whether to discontinue nursing or discontinue the drug, taking into account the importance of the drug to the mother.

PEDIATRIC USE

There are studies from the literature reporting the safe and effective use of both immediate and controlled release oral morphine preparations for analgesia in children who were dosed on a per kilogram basis. The safety of morphine sulfate controlled release has not been directly investigated in patients below the age of 18 years and both the dosage form and range of doses available are suitable for the treatment of very small children or those who are not old enough to take capsules safely.

DRUG INTERACTIONS:

CNS Depressants: Morphine should be used with great caution and in reduced dosage in patients who are concurrently receiving other central nervous system (CNS) depressants including sedatives, hypnotics, general anesthetics, antiemetics, phenothiazines, other tranquilizers and alcohol because of the risk of respiratory depression, hypotension and profound sedation or coma. When such combined therapy is contemplated, the initial dose of one or both agents should be reduced by at least 50%.

Opioid analgesics, including morphine sulfate oral products, may enhance the neuromuscular blocking action of skeletal muscle relaxants and produce an increased degree of respiratory depression.
(See WARNINGS.)

Muscle Relaxants: Morphine may enhance the neuromuscular blocking action of skeletal relaxants and produce an increased degree of respiratory depression.

Mixed Agonist/Antagonist Opioid Analgesics: From a theoretical perspective, mixed agonist/antagonist analgesics (*i.e.,* petazocine, nalbupine and butorphanol) should NOT be administered to patients who have received or are receiving a course of therapy with pure opioid agonist analgesic. In these patients, mixed agonist/antagonist analgesics may reduce the analgesic effect and/or may precipitate withdrawal symptoms.

Monoamine Oxidase Inhibitors (MAOIs): MAOIs have been reported to intensify the effects of at least one opioid drug causing anxiety, confusion and significant depression of respiration or coma. We do not recommend the use of morphine sulfate in patients taking MAOIs or within 14 days of stopping such treatment.

Cimetidine: There is an isolated report of confusion and sever respiratory depression when a hemodialysis patient was concurrently administered morphine and cimetidine.

Diuretics: Morphine can reduce the efficacy of diuretics by inducing the release of antidiuretic hormone. Morphine may also lead to acute retention of urine by causing spasm of the sphincter of the bladder, particularly in men with prostatism.

Food: The bioavailability of morphine sulfate controlled release capsules is not significantly affected by food. Capsules should be swallowed whole. The capsules, as well as the pellets contained in the capsules, however, must not be crushed, chewed, or mixed with food due to risk of overdose (see DOSAGE AND ADMINISTRATION and PRECAUTIONS, Information for the Patient).

Generally, the effects of morphine may be potentiated by alkalizing agents and antagonized by acidifying agents. Analgesic effect of morphine is potentiated by chlorpromazine and methocarbamol. CNS depressants such as anesthetics, hypnotics, barbiturates, phenothiazines, chloral hydrate, glutethimide, sedatives, MAO inhibitors (including procarbazine hydrochloride), antihistamines, β-blockers (propranolol), alcohol, furazolidone and other narcotics may enhance the depressant effects of morphine. Morphine may increase anticoagulant activity of coumarin and other anticoagulants.

ADVERSE REACTIONS:

The adverse reactions caused by morphine are essentially the same as those observed with other opioid analgesics. They include the following major hazards: respiratory depression, circulatory depression; respiratory arrest, shock, hypotension and cardiac arrest. (See OVERDOSAGE and WARNINGS.)

MOST FREQUENTLY OBSERVED

Constipation, lightheadedness, dizziness, drowsiness, sedation, nausea, vomiting, sweating, dysphoria and euphoria.

Some of these effects seem to be more prominent in ambulatory patients and in those not experiencing severe pain. Some adverse reactions in ambulatory patients may be alleviated if the patient lies down.

The less severe adverse events seen on initiation of therapy with morphine sulfate are also typical opioid side effects. These events are dose dependent, and their frequency depends on the clinical setting, the patient's level of opioid tolerance, and host factors specific to the individual. They should be expected and managed as a part of opioid analgesia. The most frequent of these include drowsiness, dizziness, constipation and nausea. In many cases, the frequency of these events during initiation of therapy may be minimized by careful individualization of starting dosage, slow titration, and the avoidance of large rapid swings in plasma concentrations of the opioid. Many of these adverse events, will cease or decrease as morphine sulfate therapy is continued and some degree of tolerance is developed, but others may be expected to remain troublesome throughout therapy.

LESS FREQUENTLY OBSERVED REACTIONS

Body as a Whole: Asthenia, accidental injury, fever, pain, chest pain, headache, diaphoresis, chills, flu syndrome, back pain, malaise, withdrawal syndrome

Cardiovascular: Tachycardia, atrial fibrillation, hypotension, hypertension, pallor, facial flushing, palpitations, bradycardia, syncope

Central Nervous System: Confusion, dry mouth, anxiety, abnormal thinking, abnormal dreams, lethargy, depression, tremor, loss of concentration, insomnia, amnesia, paresthesia, agitation, vertigo, foot drop, ataxia, hypethesia, slurred speech, hallucinations, vasodilation, euphoria, apathy, seizures, myoclonus

Endocrine: Hypoatremia due to inappropriate ADH secretion, gynecomastia

Gastrointestinal: Vomiting, anorexia, dysphagia, dyspepsia, diarrhea, abdominal pain, stomach atony disorder, gastro-esophageal reflux, delayed gastric emptying, biliary colic

Hemic and Lymphatic: Anemia, leukopenia, thrombocytopenia

Metabolic and Nutritional: Peripheral edema, hyponatremia, edema

Musculoskeletal: Back pain, bone pain, arthralgia

Respiratory: Hiccup, rhinitis, atelectasis, asthma, hypoxia, dyspnea, respiratory insufficiency, voice alteration, depressed cough reflex, non-cardiogenic pulmonary edema

Skin and Appendages: Rash, decubitis ulcer, pruitis, skin flush

Special Senses: Amblyopia, conjunctivitis, miosis, blurred vision, nystagmus, diplopia

Urogenital: Urinary abnormality, amenorrhea, urinary retention, urinary hesitance, reduced libido, reduced potency, prolonged labor

MANAGEMENT OF EXCESSIVE DROWSINESS

Most patients receiving morphine will experience initial drowsiness. This usually within 3–5 days and is not a cause of concern unless it is excessive, or accompanied by unsteadiness or confusion. Dizziness and unsteadiness may be associated with postural hypotension, particularly in elderly or debilitated patients, and has been associated with syncope and falls in non-tolerant patients started on opiods.

Excessive or persistent sedation should be investigated. Factors to be considered should include: concurrent sedative medications, the presence of hepatic or renal insufficiency, hypoxia or hypercapnia due to exacerbated respiratory failure, intolerance to the dose used (especially in older patients), disease severity and the patient's general condition.

The dosage should be adjusted accordingly to individual needs, but additional care should be used in the selection of initial doses for the elderly patient, the cachectic or gravely ill patient, or in patients not already familiar with opioid analgesic medications to prevent excessive sedation at the onset of treatment.

ADVERSE REACTIONS: *(cont'd)*

MANAGEMENT OF NAUSEA AND VOMITING

Nausea and vomiting is common after single doses of morphine or as an early undesirable effect of chronic opioid therapy. The prescription of a suitable antiemetic should be considered, with the awareness that sedation may result (see DRUG INTERACTIONS). The frequency of nausea and vomiting decreases within a week or so but may persist due to opioid-induced gastric stasis. Metoclopramide is often useful in such patients.

MANAGEMENT OF CONSTIPATION

Virtually all patients suffer from constipation while taking opioids on a chronic basis. Some patients, particularly elderly, debilitated or bedridden patients may become impacted. Tolerance does not usually develop for the constipating effects of opiods. Patients must be cautioned accordingly and laxatives, softeners and other appropriate treatments should be used prophylactically from the beginning of the opioid therapy.

DRUG ABUSE AND DEPENDENCE:

Controlled Substance: Morphine is a Schedule II narcotic.

Morphine can produce drug dependence and therefore, has the potential for being abused. Patients receiving therapeutic dosage regimens of 10 mg every 4 hours for 1 to 2 weeks have exhibited mild withdrawal symptoms. Development of the dependent state is recognizable by an increased tolerance to the analgesic effect and the appearance of purposive phenomena (complaints, pleas, demands, or manipulative actions) shortly before the time of the next scheduled dose. A patient in withdrawal should be treated in a hospital environment. Usually, it is necessary only to provide supportive care with administration of a tranquilizer to suppress anxiety. Severe symptoms of withdrawal may require administration of a replacement narcotic.

Opioid analgesics may cause psychological and physical dependence. (See WARNINGS.) Physical dependence results in withdrawal symptoms in patients who abruptly discontinue the drug or may be precipitated through the administration of drugs with opioid antagonist activity, (*e.g.*, naloxone or mixed agonist/antagonist analgesics) (see OVERDOSAGE).

Physical dependence usually does not occur to a clinically significant degree until after several weeks of continued opioid usage. Tolerance, in which increasingly large doses are required in order to produce the same degree of analgesia, is initially manifested by a shortened duration of analgesic effect, and, subsequently, by decreases in the intensity of analgesia.

In chronic-pain patients and in opioid-tolerant cancer patient, the administration of morphine sulfate should be guided by the degree of tolerance manifested. Physical dependence, per se, is not ordinarily a concern when one is dealing with opioid-tolerant patients whose pain and suffering is associated with an irreversible illness.

If morphine sulfate is abruptly discontinued, abstinence syndrome may occur. The opioid agonist abstinence syndrome is usually mild and is characterized by some or all of the following: restlessness, lacrimation, rhinorrhea, rhinitis, myalgia, abdominal cramping, diarrhea, yawning, perspiration, cutis anserina, restless sleep known as the "yen" and mydriasis during the first 24 hours. These symptoms often increase in severity and over the next 72 hours may be accompanied by increasing irritability, anxiety, weakness, twitching and spasms of muscles; kicking movements; severe backache, abdominal and leg pains; abdominal and muscle cramps; hot and cold flashes; insomnia; nausea, anorexia, vomiting, intestinal spasm, diarrhea; coryza and repetitive sneezing; and increase in body temperature, blood pressure, respiratory rate and heart rate. Because of excessive loss of fluids through sweating, vomiting and diarrhea, there is usually marked weight loss, dehydration, ketosis, and disturbances in acid-base balance. Cardiovascular collapse can occur. Without treatment, most observable symptoms disappear in 5-14 days; however, there appears to be a phase of secondary or chronic abstinence which may last for 2-6 months, characterized by insomnia, irritability, and muscular aches.

If treatment of physical dependence on morphine sulfate oral products is necessary, the patient may be detoxified by gradually reduction of the dosage. Gastrointestinal disturbances or dehydration should be treated accordingly.

Morphine sulfate controlled release has no role in the management of opioid addiction.

Infants born to mothers physically dependent on opioid analgesics may also be physically dependent and exhibit respiratory depression and withdrawal symptoms. (See DRUG ABUSE AND DEPENDENCE.)

OVERDOSAGE:

SIGNS AND SYMPTOMS

Acute overdosage with morphine is manifested by respiratory depression, somnolence progressing to stupor or coma, skeletal muscle flaccidity, cold and clammy skin, constricted pupils, and, sometimes, bradycardia, hypotension and death. Marked mydriasis rather than miosis may be seen due to severe hypoxia in overdose situations.

TREATMENT

In the treatment of overdosage, primary attention should be given to the re-establishment of a patent airway and institution of assisted or controlled ventilation. Gastric contents may need to be emptied to remove unabsorbed drug when a controlled release formula such as morphine sulfate controlled release capsules has been taken. Care should be taken to secure the airway before attempting treatment by gastric emptying or activated charcoal.

The pure opioid antagonists, naloxone or nalmefene, are specific antidotes against respiratory depression which results from opioid overdose. Naloxone (usually 0.4 to 2.0 mg) should be administered intravenously; however, because its duration of action is relatively short, the patient must be carefully monitored until spontaneous respiration is reliably reestablished. If the response to opioid antagonists is suboptimal or not sustained, additional naloxone may be re-administered, as needed, or given by continuous infusion to maintain alertness and respiratory function; however, there is no information available about the cumulative dose of naloxone that may be safely administered.

Opioid antagonists should not be administered in the absence of clinically significant respiratory or circulatory depression secondary to morphine overdose. Such agents should be administered cautiously to persons who are known or suspected to be physically dependent on morphine. In such cases, and abrupt or complete reversal of opioid effects may precipitate an acute abstinence syndrome.

OPIOID TOLERANT INDIVIDUALS

In an individual physically dependent on opioids, administration of the usual dose of the antagonist will precipitate an acute withdrawal syndrome. The severity of the withdrawal syndrome produced will depend on the degree of physical dependence and the dose of the antagonist administered. Use of a narcotic antagonist in such a person should be avoided. If necessary to treat serious respiratory depression in the physically dependent patient the antagonist should be administered with extreme care and by titration with smaller than usual doses of the antagonist.

Supportive measures (including oxygen, vasopressors) should be employed in the management of circulatory shock and pulmonary edema accompanying overdose as indicated. Cardiac arrest or arrhythmias may require cardiac massage or defibrillation.

DOSAGE AND ADMINISTRATION:

INJECTION

Dosage should be adjusted according to the severity of the pain and the response of the patient.

Morphine sulfate injection may be administered subcutaneously, intramuscularly, or intravenously but not intrathecally or epidurally.

For Analgesia

Intravenous Route: *Adults:* 2.5 to 15 mg in 4 to 5 ml of water for injection, injected slowly over a period of 4 to 5 minutes.

Subcutaneous or Intramuscular Route: *Adults:* 10 mg/70 kg of body weight (range, 5 to 20 mg), depending on the cause of the pain and the individual patient; *Children:* (subcutaneous route) 0.1 to 0.2 mg/kg (maximum dose, 15 mg).

For Preanesthetic Medication

The following doses are given 45 to 60 minutes before anesthesia:

Subcutaneous or Intramuscular Route: *Adults:* 10 mg/70 kg of body weight (range, 5 to 20 mg); *Children, 1 Year Of Age And Over:* 0.1 (maximum dose, 10 mg).

Note: Morphine sulfate solutions may darken with age. Do not use if the solution is darker than pale yellow, is discolored in any other way, or contains a precipitate.

Oral Forms: See CLINICAL PHARMACOLOGY, WARNINGS, and PRECAUTIONS.

IMMEDIATE RELEASE ORAL FORMS

Dosage of morphine is a patient-dependent variable, which must be individualized according to patient metabolism, age and disease state, and also response to morphine. Each patient should be maintained at the lowest dosage level that will produce acceptable analgesia. As the patient's well-being improved after successful relief of moderate to severe pain, periodic reduction of dosage and/or extension of dosing interval should be attempted to minimize exposure to morphine.

Usual Adult Oral Dose: 5 to 30 mg every four (4) hours or as directed by physician, administered either as morphine sulfate immediate release oral solutions, morphine sulfate immediate release oral tablets or morphine sulfate immediate release oral capsules. For control of pain in terminal illness, it is recommended that the appropriate dose of morphine sulfate oral products be given on a regularly scheduled basis every four hours at the minimum dose to achieve acceptable analgesia. If converting a patient from another narcotic to morphine sulfate on the basis of standard equivalence tables, a 1 to 3 ratio of parenteral to oral morphine equivalence is suggested. This ratio is conservative and may underestimate the amount of morphine required. If this is the case, the dose of morphine sulfate oral products should be gradually increased to achieve acceptable analgesia and tolerable side effects.

SPRINKLING CONTENTS OF CAPSULE ON FOOD OR LIQUIDS

Morphine sulfate immediate release oral capsules may be carefully opened and the entire beaded contents added to a small amount of cool, soft food, such as applesauce or pudding, or a liquid, such as water or orange juice. The bead-food mixture should be swallowed immediately and not stored for future use.

CONTROLLED RELEASE ORAL TABLETS

> WARNING:
> MORPHINE SULFATE CONTROLLED RELEASE TABLETS ARE TO BE TAKEN WHOLE, AND ARE **NOT TO BE BROKEN, CHEWED OR CRUSHED.**
> **TAKING BROKEN, CHEWED OR CRUSHED MORPHINE SULFATE CONTROLLED RELEASE TABLETS COULD LEAD TO THE RAPID RELEASE AND ABSORPTION OF A POTENTIALLY TOXIC DOSE OF MORPHINE.**

Morphine sulfate controlled release is intended for use in patients who require more than several days continuous treatment with a potent opioid analgesic. The controlled release nature of the formulation allows it to be administered on a more convenient schedule than conventional immediate release oral morphine products. (See CLINICAL PHARMACOLOGY.) However, morphine sulfate controlled release does not release morphine continuously over the course of a dosing interval. The administration of single doses of morphine sulfate controlled release on an every 12 hour dosing schedule will result in higher peak and lower trough plasma levels than those that occur when an identical daily dose of morphine is administered using conventional oral formulations on an every 4 hour regimen. The clinical significance of greater fluctuations in morphine plasma level has not been systematically evaluated.

As with any potent opioid drug product, it is critical to adjust the dosing regimen for each patient individually, taking into account the patient's prior analgesic treatment experience. Although it is clearly impossible to enumerate every consideration that is important to the selection of initial dose and dosing interval of morphine sulfate controlled release, attention should be given to:

1) the daily dose, potency and precise characteristics of the opioid the patient has been taking previously (*e.g.*, whether it is a pure agonist or mixed agonist-antagonist)

2) the reliability of the relative potency estimate used to calculate the dose of morphine needed [N.B. potency estimates may vary with the route of administration]

3) the degree of opioid tolerance, if any

4) the general condition and medical status of the patient,

5) concurrent medication

6) the type and severity of the patient's pain.

The following dosing recommendations, therefore, can only be considered suggested approaches to what is actually a series of clinical decisions in the management of the pain of an individual patient.

Conversion from Conventional Oral Morphine to Morphine Sulfate Controlled Release: A patient's daily morphine requirement is established using immediate release oral morphine (dosing every 4 to 6 hours). The patient is then converted to morphine sulfate controlled release in either of two ways:

1) Kadian or MS Contin: by administering one-half of the patient's 24 hour requirement as morphine sulfate controlled release on an every 12 hour schedule; or,

Note: Kadian should not be given more frequently than every 12 hours.

2) MS Contin Only: by administering one-third of the patient's daily requirement as morphine sulfate controlled release on an every eight hour schedule.

With either method, dose and dosing interval is then adjusted as needed. The MS Contin 15 mg tablet should be used for initial conversion for patients whose total daily requirement is expected to be less than 60 mg. The 30 mg tablet strength is recommended for patients with a daily morphine requirement of 60 to 120 mg. When the total daily dose is expected to be greater than 120 mg, the appropriate combination of tablet strengths should be employed.

Conversion from Parenteral Morphine or Other Opioids (Parenteral or Oral) to Morphine Sulfate Controlled Release: Morphine sulfate controlled release can be administered as the initial oral morphine drug product; in this case, however, particular care must be exercised in

DOSAGE AND ADMINISTRATION: *(cont'd)*

the conversion process. Because of uncertainty about, and intersubject variation in, relative estimates of opioid potency and cross tolerance, initial dosing regimens should be conservative; that is, and underestimation of the 24 hour oral morphine requirement is preferred to an overestimate. To this end, initial individual doses of morphine sulfate controlled release should be estimated conservatively. In patients whose daily morphine requirements are expected to be less than or equal to 120 mg per day, the MS Contin 30 mg tablet strength is recommended for the initial transition period. Once a stable dose regimen is reached, the patient can be converted to the 60 mg or 100 mg tablet strength, or appropriate combination of tablet strengths, if desired.

Estimates of the relative potency of opioids are only approximate and are influenced by route of administration, individual patient differences, and possibly, by an individual's medical condition. Consequently, it is difficult to recommend any fixed rule for converting a patient to morphine sulfate controlled release directly. The following general points should be considered however.

1. Parenteral To Oral Morphine Ratio: Estimates of the oral to parenteral potency of morphine vary. Some authorities suggest that a dose of oral morphine only three times the daily parenteral morphine requirement may be sufficient in chronic use settings.

2. Other Parenteral or Oral Opioids to Oral Morphine: Physicians are advised to refer to published relative potency data, keeping in mind that such ratios are only approximate. In general, it is safest to give half of the estimated daily morphine demand as the initial dose, and to manage inadequate analgesia by supplementation with immediate release morphine. See discussion that follows.

The first dose of morphine sulfate controlled release may be taken with the last dose of any immediate release (short-acting) opioid medication due to the long delay until the peak effect after administration.

Use of Morphine Sulfate Controlled Release as the First Opioid Analgesic: There has been no systematic evaluation of morphine sulfate controlled release as an initial opioid analgesic in the management of pain. Because it may be more difficult to titrate a patient using a controlled release morphine, it is ordinarily advisable to begin treatment using an immediate release formulation.

Individualization Of Dosage

The best use of opioid analgesics in the management of chronic malignant and non-malignant pain is challenging, and is well described in materials published by the World Health Organization and the Agency for Health Care Policy and Research which are available from Zeneca Pharmaceuticals upon request. Morphine sulfate controlled release capsules is a third step drug which is most useful when the patient requires a constant level of opioid analgesia as a "floor" or "platform" from which to manage breakthrough pain. When a patient has reached the point where comfort cannot be provided with a combination of non-opioid medications (NSAIDs and acetaminophen) and intermittent use of moderate or strong opioids, the patient's total opioid therapy should be converted into a 24 hour oral morphine equivalent.

Morphine sulfate controlled release capsules should be started by administering one-half of the estimated total daily oral morphine dose every 12 hours (twice-a-day) or by administering the total daily oral morphine dose every 24 hours (once-a-day). The dose should be titrated no more frequently than every-other-day to allow the patients to stabilize before escalating the dose. If breakthrough pain occurs, the dose may be supplemented with a small dose (less than 20% of the total daily dose) of a short-acting analgesic. Patients who are excessively sedated after a once-a-day dose or who regularly experience inadequate analgesia before the next dose should be switched to twice-a-day dosing.

Patients who do not have a proven tolerance to opioids should be started only on the 20 mg strength, and usually should be increased at a rate not greater than 20 mg every-other-day. Most patients will rapidly develop some degree of tolerance, requiring dosage adjustment until they have achieved their individual best balance between baseline analgesia and opioid side effects such as confusion, sedation and constipation. No guidance can be given as to the recommended maximal dose, especially in patients with chronic pain of malignancy. In such cases the total dose of morphine sulfate controlled release capsules should be advanced until the desired therapeutic endpoint is reached or clinically significant opioid-related adverse reactions intervene.

Considerations in the Adjustment of Dosing Regimens

Whatever the approach, if signs of excessive opioid effects are observed early in a dosing interval, the next dose should be reduced. If this adjustment leads to inadequate analgesia, that is, "breakthrough" pain occurs late in the dosing interval, the dosing interval may be shortened. Alternatively, a supplemental dose of a short-acting analgesic may be given. As experience is gained, adjustments can be made to obtain an appropriate balance between pain relief, opioid side effects, and the convenience of the dosing schedule.

In adjusting dosing requirements, it is recommended that the dosing interval never be extended beyond 12 hours because the administration of very large single doses may lead to acute overdose. (N.B. morphine sulfate controlled release is a controlled release formulation; it does not release morphine continuously over the dosing interval.)

For patients with low daily morphine requirements, the 15 mg tablet should be used.

SPECIAL INSTRUCTIONS FOR MORPHINE SULFATE CONTROLLED RELEASE 200 MG TABLETS

(For use in opioid tolerant patients only.)

The morphine sulfate controlled release 200 mg tablet is for use only in opioid tolerant patients requiring daily morphine equivalent dosages of 400 mg or more. It is recommended that this strength be reserved for patients that have already been titrated to a stable analgesic regimen using lower strengths of morphine sulfate controlled release or other opioid.

CONVERSION FROM KADIAN TO OTHER CONTROLLED RELEASE ORAL MORPHINE FORMULATIONS

Kadian is not bioequivalent to other controlled release morphine preparations. Although for a given dose the same total amount of morphine is available from Kadian as from morphine solution or controlled release morphine tablets, the slow release of morphine from Kadian results in reduced maximum and increased minimum plasma morphine concentrations than with shorter acting morphine products. Conversion from Kadian to the same total daily dose of controlled release morphine preparations may lead to either excessive sedation at peak or inadequate analgesia at trough and close observation and appropriate dosage adjustments are recommended.

CONVERSION FROM MS CONTIN TO PARENTERAL OPIOIDS

When converting a patient from morphine sulfate controlled release to parenteral opioids, it is best to calculate an equivalent parenteral dose, and then initiate treatment at half of this calculated value. For example, to estimate the required 24 hour dose of parenteral morphine for a patient taking Kadian, one would take the 24 hour Kadian dose, divide by and oral to parenteral conversion ration of 3, divide the estimated 24 hour parenteral dose into six divided doses (for a four hour dosing interval), then halve this dose as an initial trial.

DOSAGE AND ADMINISTRATION: *(cont'd)*

For example, to estimate the required parenteral morphine dose for a patient taking 360 mg of Kadian a day, divide the 360 mg daily oral morphine dose by a conversion ration of 1 mg of parenteral morphine for every 3 mg of oral morphine. The estimated 120 mg daily parenteral requirement is then divided into six 20 mg doses, and half of this, or 10 mg, is then given every 4 hours as an initial trial dose.

This approach is likely to require a dosage increase in the first 24 hours for many patients, but is recommended because it is less likely to cause overdose than trying to establish an equivalent dose without titration.

Opioid analgesic agents may not effectively relieve dysesthetic pain, post-herpetic neuralgia, stabbing pains, activity-related pain, and some forms of headache. This does not mean that patients suffering from these types of pain should not be given an adequate trial of opioid analgesics. However, such patients may need to be promptly evaluated for other types of pain therapy.

SUPPOSITORIES

Rectal Administration: Dosage should be adjusted according to the severity of the pain and the response of the patient. Morphine sulfate suppositories are to be administered rectally.

Usual Adult Dose: 10 to 20 mg every 4 hours or as directed by a physician.

Dosage is a patient dependent variable, therefore, increased dosage may be required to achieve adequate analgesia.

For control of severe chronic pain in patients with certain terminal diseases, this drug should be administered on a regularly scheduled basis, every 4 hours, at the lowest dosage level that will achieve adequate analgesia.

Note: Medication may suppress respiration in the elderly, the very ill, and those patients with respiratory problems, therefore lower doses may be required.

Morphine Dosage Reduction: During the first two to three days of effective pain relief, the patient may sleep for many hours. This can be misinterpreted as the effect of excessive analgesic dosing rather than the first sign of relief in a pain exhausted patient. The dose, therefore, should be maintained for at least three days before reduction, if respiratory activity and other vital signs are adequate.

Following successful relief of severe pain, periodic attempts to reduce the narcotic dose should be made. Smaller doses or complete discontinuation of the narcotic analgesic may become feasible due to a physiologic change or the improved mental state of the patient.

SAFETY AND HANDLING

The morphine sulfate controlled release 200 mg tablet strength is for use only in opioid tolerant patients requiring daily morphine equivalent dosages of 400 mg or more. This strength is potentially toxic if accidentally ingested and patients and their families should be instructed to take special care to avoid accidental or intentional ingestion by individuals other than those for whom the medication was originally prescribed.

PATIENT INFORMATION:

This drug is used for moderate to severe pain. Long acting forms of the drug are used for the control of chronic pain due to cancer.

Inform your physician if you are pregnant or taking any medications (including over-the-counter medicine).

Avoid alcohol or other depressants (sleeping pills; tranquilizers).

This drug may cause sleepiness or drowsiness; do not perform potentially hazardous tasks (operating heavy machinery; driving) while taking this drug.

Do not change dosage without checking with your physicians.

Take with or without meals. Do not open, crush or chew the capsule forms of this medication.

May cause nausea, constipation, drowsiness, dizziness or anxiety. Notify you physician or pharmacist if these occur.

HOW SUPPLIED:

MSIR Oral Solution (pleasantly flavored) is dispensed in 10 mg per 5 ml and 20 mg per 5 ml high density, polyethylene plastic, bottles of 120 ml with child-resistant closure.

MSIR Oral Solution Concentrate (unflavored) is dispensed in 20 mg per 1 ml high density, polyethylene plastic, child-resistant closure bottles with child-resistant droppers in 30 ml and 120 mL sizes. Discard opened bottle of oral solution after 90 days. Protect from light.

MSIR Tablets are dispensed as 15 mg round, white scored tablets and 30 mg capsule-shaped, white scored tablets in opaque plastic bottles containing 100 tablets. The 15 mg tablets bear the symbol PF on the scored side and MI 15 on the other side. 30 mg tablets bear the symbol PF on the scored side and MI 30 on the other side.

MSIR Capsules are dispense as 15 mg white opaque capsule body with blue cap in opaque plastic bottles containing 50 capsules. Each capsule bears the symbols PF MSIR 15 and "This End Up".

MS Contin Controlled Release Tablets: The 15 mg tablets are round, blue-colored and bear the symbol PF on one side and M15 on the other side. The 30 mg tablets are round, lavender-colored and bear the symbol PF on one side and M30 on the other side. The 60 mg tablets are round orange-colored and bear the symbol PF on one side and M60 on the other side. The 100 mg tablets are round, gray-colored and bear the symbol PF on one side and M100 on the other side. The 200 mg tablets are capsule-shaped, green-colored and bear the symbol PF on one side and 200 on the other side.

Kadian Sustained Release Capsules: The 20 mg size 4 capsule has a clear cap imprinted KADIAN and clear body imprinted 20 mg. The 50 mg size 2 capsule has a clear cap imprinted KADIAN and clear body imprinted 50 mg. The 100 mg size 0 capsule has a clear cap imprinted KADIAN and clear body imprinted 100 mg.

Roxanol Suppositories: The 5 mg, 10 mg, 20 mg, and 30 mg are supplied in 12 suppository foil packets per carton.

Storage: Store morphine sulfate immediate release oral solutions, tablets, and capsules at controlled room temperature 15° to 30° (59° - 86°F). Dispense in tight, light-resistant container.

HOW SUPPLIED - RATED THERAPEUTICALLY EQUIVALENT:

Injection, Solution - Epidural; Intra - 0.5 mg/ml

2 ml x 10	$76.78	Morphine Sulfate, Preservative Free, Schein Pharm (US)	00364-3015-28
2 ml x 10	$86.95	ASTRAMORPH/PF, Astra USA	00186-1159-03
10 ml	$10.50	Morphine Sulfate, Preservative Free, Schein Pharm (US)	00364-3015-54
10 ml	$62.11	Morphine Sulfate, Abbott	00074-4057-12
10 ml	$68.28	MORPHINE SULFATE, Abbott	00074-3814-12
10 ml x 5	$49.66	ASTRAMORPH/PF, Astra USA	00186-1150-02
10 ml x 5	$53.24	ASTRAMORPH/PF, Astra USA	00186-1152-12
10 ml x 10	**$86.04**	**DURAMORPH, Elkins Sinn**	**00641-1112-33**
30 ml	$15.31	Morphine Sulfate, Abbott	00074-2028-02

HOW SUPPLIED - RATED THERAPEUTICALLY EQUIVALENT: *(cont'd)*

Injection, Solution - Epidural; Intra - 1 mg/ml

2 ml x 10	$82.98	Morphine Sulfate, Preservative Free, Schein Pharm (US)	00364-3016-28
2 ml x 10	$95.81	ASTRAMORPH/PF, Astra USA	00186-1160-03
10 ml	$9.80	Morphine Sulfate, Preservative Free, Schein Pharm (US)	00364-3016-54
10 ml	$15.00	Morphine Sulfate, Intl Medication	00548-3901-00
10 ml	$66.20	Morphine Sulfate, Abbott	00074-4058-12
10 ml	$72.79	MORPHINE SULFATE, Abbott	00074-3815-12
10 ml x 5	$53.04	ASTRAMORPH/PF, Astra USA	00186-1151-02
10 ml x 5	$56.75	ASTRAMORPH/PF, Astra USA	00186-1153-12
10 ml x 10	**$92.19**	**DURAMORPH, Elkins Sinn**	**00641-1114-33**
10 ml x 25	$7.64	Morphine Sulfate, Intl Medication	00548-2901-00
30 ml	$15.00	Morphine Sulfate Inj 1, Intl Medication	00548-1911-00
30 ml	$15.00	Morphine Sulfate, Intl Medication	00548-1931-00
30 ml	$19.74	Morphine Sulfate, Abbott	00074-2029-02
30 ml x 10	$17.09	Morphine Sulfate, Abbott	00074-6023-04
50 ml x 10	$269.50	Morphine Sulfate, Baxter Hlthcare	00338-2689-75
60 ml	$8.94	Morphine Sulfate, Elkins Sinn	00641-2346-41
60 ml	$11.55	Morphine Sulfate, Schein Pharm (US)	00364-2469-58
60 ml	$17.81	Morphine Sulfate, Intl Medication	00548-6548-00
60 ml x 50	$406.23	Morphine Sulfate, Astra USA	00186-1120-81
100 ml	$15.37	MORPHINE SULFATE IN DEXTROSE, Abbott	00074-6062-11
250 ml	$20.52	MORPHINE SULFATE IN DEXTROSE, Abbott	00074-6062-02
500 ml	$27.60	MORPHINE SULFATE IN DEXTROSE, Abbott	00074-6062-03

Injection, Solution - Intramuscular; - 5 mg/ml

1 ml x 25	$15.49	Morphine Sulfate, Elkins Sinn	00641-0168-25

HOW SUPPLIED - NOT RATED EQUIVALENT:

Capsule, Gelatin - Oral - 15 mg

1 ml x 10	$6.81	Morphine Carpuject, Sanofi Winthrop	00024-1257-02
1 ml x 10	$11.06	MORPHINE SULFATE, Sanofi Winthrop	00024-1257-01
50's	$14.45	MSIR, Purdue Frederick	00034-1025-15
60 ml	$13.20	Morphine Sulfate, Schein Pharm (US)	00364-2470-58

Capsule, Gelatin - Oral - 20 mg

60's	$64.79	KADIAN, Zeneca Pharms	00310-0342-60
100's	$107.83	KADIAN, Zeneca Pharms	00310-0342-10
500's	$422.95	KADIAN, Zeneca Pharms	00310-0342-50

Capsule, Gelatin - Oral - 30 mg

50's	$26.97	MSIR, Purdue Frederick	00034-1026-30

Capsule, Gelatin - Oral - 50 mg

60's	$146.39	KADIAN, Zeneca Pharms	00310-0345-60
100's	$230.87	KADIAN, Zeneca Pharms	00310-0345-10

Capsule, Gelatin - Oral - 100 mg

60's	$253.27	KADIAN, Zeneca Pharms	00310-0341-60
100's	$389.83	KADIAN, Zeneca Pharms	00310-0341-10

Capsule,Gelatin - Oral - 50 mg

500's	$999.43	KADIAN, Zeneca Pharms	00310-0345-50

Concentrate - Oral - 100 mg/5ml

120 ml	$70.64	MS/L, Richwood Pharm	58521-0120-58

Injection, Solution - Intramuscular; - 2 mg/ml

1 ml x 10	$7.23	Morphine Sulfate, Wyeth Labs	00008-0649-01
1 ml x 10	$9.82	Morphine Sulfate, Sanofi Winthrop	00024-1257-21
1 ml x 10	$10.98	MORPHINE SULFATE, Wyeth Labs	00008-0649-50
60 ml x 50	$468.75	Morphine Sulfate, Astra USA	00186-1121-81

Injection, Solution - Intramuscular; - 4 mg/ml

1 ml x 10	$7.10	Morphine Carpuject, Sanofi Winthrop	00024-1258-02
1 ml x 10	$7.55	Morphine Sulfate, Wyeth Labs	00008-0653-01
1 ml x 10	$10.19	Morphine Sulfate, Sanofi Winthrop	00024-1258-23
1 ml x 10	$11.06	MORPHINE SULFATE, Sanofi Winthrop	00024-1258-03
1 ml x 10	$11.30	MORPHINE SULFATE, Wyeth Labs	00008-0653-50

Injection, Solution - Intramuscular; - 5 mg/ml

30 ml	$17.50	MORPHINE SULFATE, Intl Medication	00548-1935-00
30 ml x 10	$19.97	Morphine Sulfate, Abbott	00074-6028-04

Injection, Solution - Intramuscular; - 8 mg/ml

1 ml x 10	$7.30	Morphine Carpuject, Sanofi Winthrop	00024-1259-02
1 ml x 10	$7.30	Morphine Carpuject, Sanofi Winthrop	00024-1260-02
1 ml x 10	$7.89	Morphine Sulfate, Wyeth Labs	00008-0655-03
1 ml x 10	$10.62	Morphine Sulfate, Sanofi Winthrop	00024-1260-27
1 ml x 10	$11.06	MORPHINE SULFATE, Sanofi Winthrop	00024-1260-07
1 ml x 10	$11.06	MORPHINE SULFATE, Sanofi Winthrop	00024-2360-07
1 ml x 10	$11.64	MORPHINE SULFATE, Wyeth Labs	00008-0655-50
1 ml x 25	$13.10	Morphine Sulfate, Elkins Sinn	00641-1170-35
1 ml x 25	$15.49	Morphine Sulfate, Elkins Sinn	00641-0170-25
2 ml x 25	$15.00	Morphine Sulfate, Astra USA	00186-1138-13

Injection, Solution - Intramuscular; - 10 mg/ml

1 ml x 10	$7.81	Morphine Carpuject, Sanofi Winthrop	00024-1261-02
1 ml x 10	$8.28	Morphine Sulfate, Wyeth Labs	00008-0656-01
1 ml x 10	$11.06	Morphine Sulfate, Sanofi Winthrop	00024-1261-28
1 ml x 10	$11.06	MORPHINE SULFATE, Sanofi Winthrop	00024-1263-08
1 ml x 10	$12.03	MORPHINE SULFATE, Wyeth Labs	00008-0656-50
1 ml x 25	$13.70	Morphine Sulfate, Elkins Sinn	00641-1180-35
1 ml x 25	$16.09	Morphine Sulfate, Elkins Sinn	00641-0180-25
2 ml x 25	$16.10	Morphine Sulfate, Astra USA	00186-1139-13
3 ml	$13.60	Morphine Sulfate, Abbott	00074-6176-14
6 ml	$16.29	Morphine Sulfate, Abbott	00074-6178-14
10 ml	$85.03	Morphine Sulfate, Abbott	00074-3817-12
10 ml x 1	$11.25	Morphine Sulfate, Elkins Sinn	00641-2343-41
20 ml	$132.60	MORPHINE SULFATE SELECT-A-JET, Intl Medication	00548-6320-00
20 ml	$156.00	INFUMORPH, Elkins Sinn	00641-1131-31

Injection, Solution - Intramuscular; - 15 mg/ml

1 ml x 10	$8.28	Morphine Carpuject, Sanofi Winthrop	00024-1262-02
1 ml x 10	$8.75	Morphine Sulfate, Wyeth Labs	00008-0657-01
1 ml x 10	$11.06	MORPHINE SULFATE, Sanofi Winthrop	00024-1264-10
1 ml x 10	$11.78	Morphine Sulfate, Sanofi Winthrop	00024-1263-20
1 ml x 10	$12.50	Morphine Sulfate, Wyeth Labs	00008-0657-50
1 ml x 25	$14.60	Morphine Sulfate, Elkins Sinn	00641-1190-35
1 ml x 25	$16.99	Morphine Sulfate, Elkins Sinn	00641-0190-25
2 ml x 25	$16.75	Morphine Sulfate, Astra USA	00186-1140-13
20 ml	$10.95	Morphine Sulfate, Harber Pharm	51432-0653-20
20 ml	$13.73	Morphine Sulfate, Schein Pharm (US)	00364-2366-55
20 ml	$13.73	Morphine Sulfate, Steris Labs	00402-0913-20

HOW SUPPLIED - NOT RATED EQUIVALENT: *(cont'd)*

20 ml	$14.50	Morphine Sulfate, Goldline Labs	00182-9139-65
20 ml	$15.47	Morphine Sulfate, Lilly	00002-1637-01
20 ml	$110.56	Morphine Sulfate, Abbott	00074-3819-12
20 ml x 1	$12.38	Morphine Sulfate, Elkins Sinn	00641-2345-41
20 ml x 5	$58.94	Morphine Sulfate, Astra USA	00186-1158-02

Injection, Solution - Intravenous - 0.2 mg/ml

250 ml	$14.87	MORPHINE SULFATE IN DEXTROSE, Abbott	00074-6063-02
500 ml	$16.28	MORPHINE SULFATE IN DEXTROSE, Abbott	00074-6063-03

Injection, Solution - Intravenous - 25 mg/ml

4 ml	$9.44	Morphine Sulfate, Intl Medication	00548-6024-00
4 ml	$9.88	Morphine Sulfate, Intl Medication	00548-6824-00
4 ml	$15.98	Morphine Sulfate, Abbott	00074-6177-14
4 ml	$85.50	MORPHINE SULFATE, Marsam	00209-6859-20
4 ml x 10	$113.25	Morphine Sulfate, Marsam	00209-6855-22
10 ml	$17.71	Morphine Sulfate, Intl Medication	00548-6025-00
10 ml	$18.63	Morphine Sulfate, Intl Medication	00548-6825-00
10 ml	$19.11	Morphine Sulfate, Abbott	00074-6179-14
10 ml	$21.26	MORPHINE SULFATE, King Pharms	60793-0090-10
10 ml	$22.35	MORPHINE SULFATE, Yorpharm	61147-8002-03
10 ml	$132.60	MORPHINE SULFATE SELECT-A-JET, Intl Medication	00548-6325-00
10 ml	$159.25	MORPHINE SULFATE, Marsam	00209-6860-20
10 ml x 10	$212.65	Morphine Sulfate, Marsam	00209-6856-22
20 ml	$17.81	Morphine Sulfate, Astra USA	00186-1135-51
20 ml	$28.63	MORPHINE SULFATE, Intl Medication	00548-7026-00
20 ml	$30.14	Morphine Sulfate, Intl Medication	00548-6026-00
20 ml	$31.63	Morphine Sulfate, Intl Medication	00548-6826-00
20 ml	$35.00	Morphine Sulfate, Schein Pharm (US)	00364-2450-55
20 ml	$36.17	MORPHINE SULFATE, King Pharms	60793-0092-20
20 ml	$36.17	MORPHINE SULFATE, Yorpharm	61147-8002-06
20 ml	$238.85	MORPHINE SULFATE SELECT-A-JET, Intl Medication	00548-6350-00
20 ml	$281.00	INFUMORPH, Elkins Sinn	00641-1132-31
20 ml	$286.75	MORPHINE SULFATE, Marsam	00209-6861-20
20 ml x 10	$361.75	Morphine Sulfate, Marsam	00209-6857-22
40 ml	$64.85	Morphine Sulfate, Intl Medication	00548-6027-00
40 ml	$68.12	Morphine Sulfate, Intl Medication	00548-6827-00
40 ml	$77.82	MORPHINE SULFATE, King Pharms	60793-0093-40
40 ml	$81.75	Morphine Sulfate, Yorpharm	61147-8002-07
40 ml	$539.10	MORPHINE SULFATE, Marsam	00209-6862-20
40 ml x 10	$778.30	Morphine Sulfate, Marsam	00209-6858-22
50 ml	$77.01	MORPHINE SULFATE, Intl Medication	00548-7028-00
50 ml	$85.13	MORPHINE SULFATE, Intl Medication	00548-6038-00
50 ml	$97.28	MORPHINE SULFATE, King Pharms	60793-0094-50
50 ml	$102.19	MORPHINE SULFATE, Yorpharm	61147-8002-05

Injection, Solution - Intravenous - 50 mg/ml

10 ml	$34.14	MORPHINE SULFATE, Intl Medication	00548-6020-00
10 ml	$35.81	MORPHINE SULFATE, Intl Medication	00548-6620-00
10 ml	$42.98	MORPHINE SULFATE, King Pharms	60793-0095-10
10 ml	$42.98	MORPHINE SULFATE, Yorpharm	61147-8003-03
10 ml	$238.85	MORPHINE SULFATE SELECT-A-JET, Intl Medication	00548-6355-00
10 ml	$286.75	MORPHINE SULFATE, Marsam	00209-6867-20
10 ml x 10	$429.90	Morphine Sulfate, Marsam	00209-6863-22
20 ml	$64.88	MORPHINE SULFATE, Intl Medication	00548-7021-00
20 ml	$68.29	MORPHINE SULFATE, Intl Medication	00548-6021-00
20 ml	$71.69	MORPHINE SULFATE, Intl Medication	00548-6621-00
20 ml	$80.00	Morphine Sulfate, Schein Pharm (US)	00364-3067-55
20 ml	$86.03	MORPHINE SULFATE, King Pharms	60793-0091-20
20 ml	$86.03	MORPHINE SULFATE, Yorpharm	61147-8003-06
20 ml x 10	$860.40	Morphine Sulfate, Marsam	00209-6864-22
40 ml	$136.56	MORPHINE SULFATE, Intl Medication	00548-6022-00
40 ml	$143.37	MORPHINE SULFATE, Intl Medication	00548-6622-00
40 ml	$160.00	Morphine Sulfate, Schein Pharm (US)	00364-3067-18
40 ml	$172.05	MORPHINE SULFATE, King Pharms	60793-0096-40
40 ml	$172.05	MORPHINE SULFATE, Yorpharm	61147-8003-07
40 ml x 10	$1720.60	Morphine Sulfate, Marsam	00209-6865-22
50 ml	$162.16	MORPHINE SULFATE, Intl Medication	00548-7023-00
50 ml	$179.24	MORPHINE SULFATE, Intl Medication	00548-6023-00
50 ml	$215.05	MORPHINE SULFATE, King Pharms	60793-0097-50
50 ml	$215.05	MORPHINE SULFATE, Yorpharm	61147-8003-05

Powder

5 gm	$48.50	Morphine Sulfate, Paddock Labs	00574-2006-05
5 gm	$68.13	Morphine Sulfate, Mallinckrodt	00406-1521-53
25 gm	$225.80	Morphine Sulfate, Paddock Labs	00574-2006-25
25 gm	$340.63	Morphine Sulfate, Mallinckrodt	00406-1521-55

Solution - Oral - 10 mg/5ml

5 ml x 40	$24.09	Morphine Sulfate, Roxane	00054-8585-16
100 ml	$8.78	Morphine Sulfate, Roxane	00054-3785-49
120 ml	$8.92	MSIR, Purdue Frederick	00034-0521-02
500 ml	$20.00	Morphine Sulfate Immediate Release, Liquipharm	54198-0144-50
500 ml	$28.15	MSIR, Purdue Frederick	00034-0521-03
500 ml	$28.75	MS/L, Richwood Pharm	58521-0110-50
500 ml	$30.29	Morphine Sulfate, Roxane	00054-3785-63
500 ml	$30.29	MORPHINE SULFATE, Astra USA	00186-1124-95

Solution - Oral - 20 mg/ml

1.5 ml x 25	$28.98	ROXANOL, Roxane	00054-8788-11
30 ml	$16.94	MSIR, Purdue Frederick	00034-0523-01
30 ml	$17.82	OMS, Upsher Smith	00245-0167-31
30 ml	$19.21	MORPHINE SULFATE, Ethex	58177-0886-01
30 ml	$20.16	ROXANOL, Roxane	00054-3751-44
120 ml	$40.00	Morphine Sulfate, Liquipharm	54198-0145-04
120 ml	$63.66	MSIR, Purdue Frederick	00034-0523-02
120 ml	$66.93	OMS, Upsher Smith	00245-0167-04
120 ml	$72.70	MORPHINE SULFATE, Ethex	58177-0886-03
120 ml	$75.69	ROXANOL, Roxane	00054-3751-50
120 ml	$75.69	MORPHINE SULFATE, Astra USA	00186-1123-85
240 ml	$119.16	MORPHINE SULFATE, Ethex	58177-0886-05
240 ml	$127.40	ROXANOL, Roxane	00054-3751-58

Solution - Oral - 20 mg/5ml

2.5 ml x 25	$22.85	RESCUDOSE, Roxane	00054-8789-11
2.5 ml x 25	$23.16	Roxanol, Roxane	00054-8781-11
5 ml x 25	$26.06	Roxanol, Roxane	00054-8785-11
10 ml x 40	$36.31	Morphine Sulfate, Roxane	00054-8586-16
100 ml	$12.50	Morphine Sulfate, Roxane	00054-3786-49
120 ml	$12.22	MSIR, Purdue Frederick	00034-0522-02
500 ml	$48.38	MSIR, Purdue Frederick	00034-0522-03
500 ml	$51.08	Morphine Sulfate, Roxane	00054-3786-63

HOW SUPPLIED - NOT RATED EQUIVALENT: *(cont'd)*

Suppository - Rectal - 5 mg

12's	$9.77	Morphine Sulfate, GW Labs	00713-0193-12
12's	$10.10	Morphine Sulfate, Paddock Labs	00574-7110-12
12's	$12.13	ROXANOL, Roxane	00054-8775-05
12's	$14.35	RMS, Upsher Smith	00245-0160-12
12's UD	$12.21	MS/S, Richwood Pharm	58521-0005-12

Suppository - Rectal - 10 mg

12's	$11.55	Morphine Sulfate 10, GW Labs	00713-0194-12
12's	$11.75	Morphine Sulfate Suppositories 10, Paddock Labs	00574-7112-12
12's	$13.97	ROXANOL, Roxane	00054-8776-05
12's	$16.95	RMS, Upsher Smith	00245-0161-12
12's UD	$15.72	MS/S, Richwood Pharm	58521-0010-12

Suppository - Rectal - 20 mg

12's	$14.05	Morphine Sulfate, GW Labs	00713-0195-12
12's	$14.20	Morphine Sulfate Suppositories 20, Paddock Labs	00574-7114-12
12's	$16.52	ROXANOL, Roxane	00054-8777-05
12's	$20.56	RMS, Upsher Smith	00245-0162-12
12's UD	$19.21	MS/S, Richwood Pharm	58521-0020-12

Suppository - Rectal - 30 mg

12's	$17.85	Morphine Sulfate Suppositories 30, Paddock Labs	00574-7116-12
12's	$19.62	Morphine Sulfate, GW Labs	00713-0196-12
12's	$21.23	ROXANOL, Roxane	00054-8778-05
12's UD	$24.63	MS/S, Richwood Pharm	58521-0030-12
12's UD	$28.71	RMS, Upsher Smith	00245-0163-12

Tablet, Coated, Sustained Action - Oral - 15 mg

25's UD	$21.09	MS CONTIN 15, Purdue Frederick	00034-0514-25
100's	$64.71	Oramorph Sr, Roxane	00054-4790-25
100's	$70.36	Oramorph Sr, Roxane	00054-8790-24
100's	$77.61	MS CONTIN 15, Purdue Frederick	00034-0514-10
500's	$307.42	Oramorph Sr, Roxane	00054-4790-29
500's	$368.68	MS CONTIN 15, Purdue Frederick	00034-0514-90

Tablet, Coated, Sustained Action - Oral - 30 mg

25's	$140.56	ORAMORPH SR, Roxane	00054-8805-24
25's UD	$42.14	MS CONTIN 30, Purdue Frederick	00034-0515-25
50's	$64.71	ORAMORPH SR, Roxane	00054-4805-19
50's	$77.61	MS CONTIN 30, Purdue Frederick	00034-0515-50
100's	$122.98	ORAMORPH SR, Roxane	00054-4805-25
100's	$147.49	MS CONTIN 30, Purdue Frederick	00034-0515-10
250's	$298.17	ORAMORPH SR, Roxane	00054-4805-27
250's	$357.59	MS CONTIN 30, Purdue Frederick	00034-0515-45
500's	$678.37	MS CONTIN 30, Purdue Frederick	00034-0515-90

Tablet, Coated, Sustained Action - Oral - 60 mg

25's	$84.25	MS CONTIN 60, Purdue Frederick	00034-0516-25
25's UD	$70.25	ORAMORPH SR, Roxane	00054-8792-11
100's	$239.97	ORAMORPH SR, Roxane	00054-4792-25
100's	$287.79	MS CONTIN 60, Purdue Frederick	00034-0516-10
500's	$1323.81	MS CONTIN, Purdue Frederick	00034-0516-90

Tablet, Coated, Sustained Action - Oral - 100 mg

25's UD	$110.47	ORAMORPH SR, Roxane	00054-8793-11
25's UD	$131.24	MS CONTIN 100, Purdue Frederick	00034-0517-25
100's	$367.51	ORAMORPH SR, Roxane	00054-4793-25
100's	$436.33	MS CONTIN 100, Purdue Frederick	00034-0517-10
500's	$1777.64	MS CONTIN, Purdue Frederick	00034-0517-90

Tablet, Coated, Sustained Action - Oral - 200 mg

100's	$799.08	MS CONTIN, Purdue Frederick	00034-0513-10
300's	$245.41	MS CONTIN, Purdue Frederick	00034-0513-25

Tablet, Uncoated - Oral - 10 mg

100's	$22.03	Morphine Sulfate, Lilly	00002-2549-02

Tablet, Uncoated - Oral - 15 mg

50's	$8.44	MSIR, Purdue Frederick	00034-0518-15
100's	$16.88	MSIR, Purdue Frederick	00034-0518-10
100's	$17.79	Morphine Sulfate, Roxane	00054-4582-25
100's	$25.36	Morphine Sulfate, Roxane	00054-8582-24
100's	$27.95	Morphine Sulfate, Lilly	00002-2550-02

Tablet, Uncoated - Oral - 30 mg

50's	$14.26	MSIR, Purdue Frederick	00034-0519-30
100's	$28.52	MSIR, Purdue Frederick	00034-0519-10
100's	$30.31	Morphine Sulfate, Roxane	00054-4583-25
100's	$43.05	Morphine Sulfate, Roxane	00054-8583-24
100's	$46.90	Morphine Sulfate, Lilly	00002-2551-02

MORRHUATE SODIUM *(002251)*

CATEGORIES: Cardiovascular Drugs; Sclerosing Agents; Varicose Veins; FDA Pre 1938 Drugs

BRAND NAMES: **Scleromate**; Sodium Morrhuate

DESCRIPTION:

Morrhuate Sodium Injection, U.S.P. is a mixture of the sodium salts of the saturated and unsaturated fatty acids of Cod Liver Oil. Scleromate Morrhuate Sodium Injection, U.S.P. is prepared by the saponification of selected Cod Liver Oils, it is overlaid with filtered Nitrogen to prevent discoloration that occurs on exposure to oxygen. Morrhuate Sodium occurs as a pale-yellowish, granular powder with a slight fishy odor and is soluble in water and in alcohol.

Note: Solid matter may develop a hazy appearance on standing and the injection should not be used if the solid matter does not dissolve completely on warming. The pH of the injection is adjusted to approximately 9.5.

CLINICAL PHARMACOLOGY:

Morrhuate Sodium, when injected into the vein, causes inflammation of the intima and formation of a thrombus. This blood clot occludes of the injected vein and fibrous tissue develops, resulting in the obliteration of the vein.

INDICATIONS AND USAGE:

Morrhuate Sodium Injection is used for the obliteration of primary varicosed veins that consist of simple dilation with competent valves.

Sclerotherapy should not be used in patients with significant valvular or deep vein incompetence. (see PRECAUTIONS)

Although Morrhuate Sodium has been used as a sclerosing agent for the treatment of internal hemorrhoids, there is no substantial evidence that the drug is useful for this purpose.

INDICATIONS AND USAGE: *(cont'd)*

Most patients with symptomatic primary varicosed veins should be treated initially with compression stockings. If this treatment is inadequate, surgery may be required. Sclerosing agents may be useful as a supplement to venous ligation to obliterate residual varicosed veins or in patients who have conditions which increase the risk of surgery. However, many clinicians consider sclerotherapy if not effective may decrease the potential success of later surgery, should this be required.

CONTRAINDICATIONS:

Morrhuate Sodium is contraindicated in patients who have shown a previous hypersensitivity reaction to the drug or to the fatty acids of cod liver oil. Continued administration of the drug is contraindicated when an unusual local reaction at the injection site or a systemic reaction occurs.

Thrombosis induced by Morrhuate Sodium may extend into the deep venous system in patients with significant valvular incompetence, therefore, valvular competency, deep vein patency, and deep vein competency should be determined by angiography and/or by tests such as the Trendelenberg and Perthes before injection of sclerosing agents. The drug is contraindicated for obliterations of superficial veins in patients with persistent occlusion of the deep veins. Morrhuate Sodium is also contraindicated in patients with acute superficial thrombophlebitis; underlying arterial disease; varicosities caused by abdominal and pelvic tumors, uncontrolled diabetes mellitus, thyrotoxicosis, tuberculosis, neoplasms, asthma, sepsis, blood dyscrasias, acute respiratory or skin disease; and in bedridden patients. Treatment with Morrhuate Sodium should be delayed in patients with acute local or systemic infections (including infected ulcers). Extensive therapy with the drug is inadvisable in patients who are severely debilitated or senile.

PRECAUTIONS:

Burning or cramping sensation indicate local reactions. Urticaria may result. Sloughing and necrosis of tissue may occur with extravasation of the drug. Technique development is essential for optimal success in sclerotherapy, therefore the drug should be administered only by a physician familiar with proper injection technique. Drowsiness and headache may occur rarely. Pulmonary embolism has been reported.

Rarely, patients may have, or may develop hypersensitivity to Morrhuate Sodium, characterized by dizziness, weakness, vascular collapse, asthma, respiratory depression, gastrointestinal disturbances (*i.e.,* Nausea, vomiting), and urticaria. Anaphylactic reactions may occur within a few minutes after injection of the drug and are most likely to occur when therapy is reinstituted after an interval of several weeks. Morrhuate Sodium should only be administered when adequate facilities, drugs (*i.e.,* epinephrine, antihistamines, corticosteroids), and personnel are available for the treatment of anaphylactic reactions.

Pregnancy: Safety in use of Morrhuate Sodium during pregnancy has not been established.

DOSAGE AND ADMINISTRATION:

Morrhuate Sodium is administered only by INTRAVENOUS Injection. Care must be taken to avoid extravasation, (see PRECAUTIONS.) Specialized references should be consulted for specific procedures and techniques of administration. When small veins are injected, or the injection solution is cold, or if solid matter has separated in the solution, the ampul or vial should be warmed by immersing in hot water. The solution should become clear on warming; only a clear solution should be used. Because the solution froths easily, a large bore needle should be used to fill the syringe, however, a small bore needle should be used for the injection.

To determine possible sensitivity to the drug, some clinicians recommend injection of 0.25-1 ml of 5% Morrhuate Sodium injection into a varicosity 24 hours before administration of a large dose.

Dosage of Morrhuate Sodium depends on the size and degree of varicosity. The usual adult dose for obliteration of small or medium veins is 50-100 mg (1-2 ml of the 5% injection). For large veins, 150-250 b(3-5 ml of the injection) is used. The drug may be given as multiple injections at one time or in single doses. Therapy may be repeated at 5-7 day intervals, according to the patient's response. Following injection of Morrhuate Sodium, the vein promptly becomes hard and swollen for 2-4 inches, depending on the size and response of the vein. After 24 hours, the vein is hard and slightly tender to the touch (with little or no periphlebitis). The skin around the injection becomes light-bronze; this color usually disappears shortly. An aching sensation and feeling of stiffness usually occur and last approximately 48 hours.

HOW SUPPLIED:

Morrhuate Sodium Injection 5%

NDC-53159-003-01 30 ml Multiple use Vials

Storage: Store below 40 degrees C. (104 degrees F.) preferably in a refrigerator, or between 15-30 degrees C. (59-86 degrees F.)

(Palisades Pharmaceuticals, Inc. 7/85)

HOW SUPPLIED - EQUIVALENTS NOT AVAILABLE:

Injection, Solution - Intravenous - 50 mg/ml

30 ml	$24.95	Morruhate Sodium, Pasadena	00418-5411-30
30 ml	$31.19	Morrhuate Sodium, Am Regent	00517-3065-01
30 ml	**$32.96**	**SCLEROMATE, Palisades Pharms**	**53159-0003-01**
30 ml	$45.88	Sodium Morrhuate, Rugby	00536-7175-75
30 ml	$49.50	SODIUM MORRHUATE, Consolidated Midland	00223-8541-30

MUMPS SKIN TEST ANTIGEN *(001841)*

CATEGORIES: Diagnostic Agents; Mumps; FDA Pre 1938 Drugs

BRAND NAMES: **Msta**

Prescribing information not available at time of publication.

HOW SUPPLIED - EQUIVALENTS NOT AVAILABLE:

Injection, Susp - Intradermal

1 ml x 10	$48.13	MSTA, Connaught Labs	49281-0240-10

MUMPS VIRUS VACCINE LIVE *(001842)*

CATEGORIES: Biologicals; Immunologic; Mumps; Serums, Toxoids and Vaccines; Vaccines; Pregnancy Category C; FDA Pre 1938 Drugs

BRAND NAMES: **Mumpsvax**; *Pariorix*
(International brand names outside U.S. in italics)

DESCRIPTION:

Mumpsvax (Mumps Virus Vaccine Live) is a live virus vaccine for immunization against mumps.

Mumpsvax is a sterile lyophilized preparation of the Jeryl Lynn (B level strain of mumps virus.[1] The virus was adapted to and propagated in cell cultures of chick embryo free of avian leukosis virus and other adventitious agents.

The reconstituted vaccine is for subcutaneous administration. When reconstituted as directed, the dose for injection is 0.5 ml and contains not less than the equivalent of 20,000 $TCID_{50}$ (tissue culture infectious doses) of the U.S. Reference Mumps Virus. Each dose contains approximately 25 mcg of neomycin. The product contains no preservative. Sorbitol and hydrolyzed gelatin are added as stabilizers.

CLINICAL PHARMACOLOGY:

Mumpsvax produces a modified, non-communicable mumps infection in susceptible persons.[2,3] Extensive clinical trials have demonstrated that Mumpsvax is highly immunogenic and well tolerated.[4-17] A single injection of the vaccine has been shown to induce mumps neutralizing antibodies in approximately 97 percent of susceptible children and approximately 93 percent of susceptible adults.[8] The pattern of antibody response closely resembles that observed for natural mumps. Although the antibody level is significantly lower than that following natural infection; it is protective and long lasting.[3] Vaccine-induced antibody levels have been shown to persist for at least 15 years with a rate of decline comparable to that seen in natural infection.[18] If the present pattern continues, it will provide a basis for the expectation that immunity following vaccination will be permanent. However, continued surveillance will be required to demonstrate this point.

INDICATIONS AND USAGE:

Mumpsvax is indicated for immunization against mumps in persons 12 months of age or older. Most adults are likely to have been infected naturally and generally may be considered immune, even if they did not have clinically recognizable disease.[3] A booster is not needed. It is not recommended for infants younger than 12 months because they may retain maternal mumps neutralizing antibodies which may interfere with the immune response.

Evidence indicates that the vaccine will not offer protection when given after exposure to natural mumps.[3] Passively acquired antibody can interfere with the response to live, attenuated-virus vaccines. Therefore, administration of mumps virus vaccine should be deferred until approximately three months after passive immunization.[3]

Individuals planning travel outside the United States, if not immune, can acquire measles, mumps or rubella and import these diseases to the United States. Therefore, prior to International travel, individuals known to be susceptible to one or more of these diseases can receive either a single antigen vaccine (measles, mumps or rubella), or a combined antigen vaccine as appropriate. However, M-M-R*II (Measles, Mumps, and Rubella Virus Vaccine Live) is preferred for persons likely to be susceptible to mumps and rubella; and if single-antigen measles vaccine is not readily available, travelers should receive M-M-R II (Measles, Mumps, and Rubella Virus Vaccine Live) regardless of their immune status to mumps or rubella.[19,20,21]

Revaccination: Children vaccinated when younger than 12 months of age should be revaccinated. Based on available evidence, there is no reason to routinely revaccinate persons who were vaccinated originally when 12 months of age or older. However, persons should be revaccinated if there is evidence to suggest that initial immunization was ineffective.

USE WITH OTHER VACCINES

Routine administration of DTP (diphtheria, tetanus, pertussis) and/or OPV (oral poliovirus vaccine) concomitantly with measles, mumps and rubella vaccines is not recommended because there are insufficient data relating to the simultaneous administration of these antigens. However, the American Academy of Pediatrics has noted that in some circumstances, particularly when the patient may not return, some practitioners prefer to administer all these antigens on a single day. If done, separate sites and syringes should be used for DTP and Mumpsvax.[22]

Mumpsvax should not be given less than one month before or after administration of other virus vaccines.

CONTRAINDICATIONS:

Do not give Mumpsvax to pregnant females; the possible effects of the vaccine on fetal development are unknown at this time. If vaccination of postpubertal females is undertaken, pregnancy should be avoided for three months following vaccination (see PRECAUTIONS, Pregnancy.)

Anaphylactic or anaphylactoid reactions to neomycin (each dose of reconstituted vaccine contains approximately 25 mcg of neomycin).

History of anaphylactic or anaphylactoid reactions to eggs see WARNINGS, HYPERSENSITIVITY TO EGGS.

Any febrile respiratory illness or other active febrile infection.

Active untreated tuberculosis.

Patients receiving immunosuppressive therapy. This contraindication does not apply to patients who are receiving corticosteroids as replacement therapy, e.g., for Addison's disease.

Individuals with blood dyscrasias, leukemia, lymphomas of any type or other malignant neoplasms affecting the bone marrow or lymphatic systems.

Primary and acquired immunodeficiency states, including patients who are immunosuppressed in association with AIDS or other clinical manifestations of infection with human immunodeficiency viruses;[23,24]cellular immune deficiencies; and hypogammaglobulinemic and dysgammaglobulinemic states.

Individuals with a family history of congenital or hereditary immunodeficiency, until the immune competence of the potential vaccine recipient is demonstrated.[25]

WARNINGS:

HYPERSENSITIVITY TO EGGS

Live mumps vaccine is produced in chick embryo cell culture. Persons with a history of anaphylactic, anaphylactoid, or other immediate reactions (*e.g.,* hives, swelling of the mouth and throat, difficulty breathing hypotension, or shock) subsequent to egg ingestion should be vaccinated only with extreme caution. Evidence indicates that persons are not at increased risk if they have egg allergies that are not anaphylactic or anaphylactoid in nature. Such persons may be vaccinated in the usual manner. There is no evidence to indicate that persons with, allergies to chickens or feathers are at increased risk of reaction to the vaccine.[3]

PRECAUTIONS:

GENERAL

Adequate treatment provisions including epinephrine, should be available for immediate use should an anaphylactic or anaphylactoid reaction occur.

PRECAUTIONS: *(cont'd)*

Children and young adults who are known to be infected with human immunodeficiency viruses but without overt clinical manifestations of immunosuppression may be vaccinated; however, the vaccinees should be monitored closely for vaccine-preventable diseases because immunization may be less effective than for uninfected persons.[23,24]

Vaccination should be deferred for at least 3 months following blood or plasma transfusions, or administration of human immune serum globulin.

There are no reports of transmission of live mumps virus from vaccinees to susceptible contacts.

It has been reported that mumps virus vaccine live, may result in a temporary depression of tuberculin skin sensitivity. Therefore, if a tuberculin test is to be done, it should be administered either before or simultaneously with Mumpsvax.[9,26]

As for any vaccine, vaccination with Mumpsvax may not result in seroconversion in 100% of susceptible persons given the vaccine.

PREGNANCY CATEGORY C

Animal reproduction studies have not been conducted with Mumpsvax. It is also not known whether Mumpsvax can cause fetal harm when administered to a pregnant woman or can affect reproduction capacity. Therefore, mumps virus vaccine should not be given to persons known to be pregnant; furthermore, pregnancy should be avoided for three months following vaccination. Although mumps virus is capable of infecting the placenta and fetus, there is no good evidence that it causes congenital malformations in humans. Mumps vaccine virus also has been shown to infect the placenta, but the virus has not been isolated from the fetal tissues from susceptible women who were vaccinated and underwent elective abortions.[3]

NURSING MOTHERS

It is not known whether mumps vaccine virus is secreted in human milk. Therefore, because many drugs are excreted in human milk, caution should be exercised when Mumpsvax is administered to a nursing woman.

ADVERSE REACTIONS:

Burning and/or stinging of short duration at the injection site have been reported.

Anaphylaxis and anaphylactoid reactions have been reported.

Mild fever occurs occasionally. Fever above 103°F (39.4°C) is uncommon.

Mild lymphadenopathy has been reported.

Cough and rhinitis have been reported after vaccination with other mumps-containing vaccines.

Diarrhea has been reported after vaccination with mumps-containing vaccines.

Vasculitis has been reported rarely after vaccination with other mumps-containing vaccines.

Parotitis has been reported to occur in very low incidence, and orchitis rarely, in persons who were vaccinated. In most instances investigated, prior exposure to natural mumps was established. In other instances, whether or not this was due to vaccine or to prior natural mumps exposure or to other causes has not been established.

Reports of purpura and allergic reactions such as wheal and flare at the injection site or urticaria have been extremely rare. Erythema multiforme has also been reported rarely.

Forms of optic neuritis, including retrobulbar neuritis and papillitis may infrequently follow viral infections, and have been reported to occur 1 to 3 weeks following inoculation with some live virus vaccines.

Syncope, particularly at the time of mass vaccination, has been reported.

Very rarely encephalitis, febrile seizures, nerve deafness and other nervous system reactions have occurred in vaccinees. A cause-effect relationship has not been established.

DOSAGE AND ADMINISTRATION:

FOR SUBCUTANEOUS ADMINISTRATION

Do not inject intravenously

The dosage of vaccine is the same for all persons. Inject the total volume (about 0.5 ml) of reconstituted vaccine subcutaneously, preferably into the outer aspect of upper arm. *Do not give immune serum globulin (ISG) concurrently with Mumpsvax.*

During shipment, to insure that there is no loss of potency, the vaccine must be maintained at a temperature of 10°C (50°F) or less.

Before reconstitution, store Mumpsvax at 2 - 8°C (36 - 46°F). *Protect from light.*

CAUTION: A sterile syringe free of preservatives, antiseptics, and detergents should be used for each injection and/or reconstitution of the vaccine because these substances may inactivate the live virus vaccine. A 25 gauge, 5/8" needle is recommended.

To reconstitute, use only the diluent supplied, since it is free of preservatives or other antiviral substances which might inactivate the vaccine.

Single Dose Vial—First withdraw the entire volume of diluent into the syringe to be used for reconstitution. Inject all the diluent in the syringe into the vial of lyophilized vaccine, and agitate to mix thoroughly. Withdraw the entire contents into a syringe and inject the total volume of restored vaccine subcutaneously.

It is important to use a separate sterile syringe and needle for each individual patient to prevent transmission of hepatitis B and other infectious agents from one person to another.

10 Dose Vial (available only to government agencies/institutions)— Withdraw the entire contents (7 ml) of the diluent vial into the sterile syringe to be used for reconstitution, and introduce into the 10 dose vial of lyophilized vaccine. Agitate to ensure thorough mixing. The outer labeling suggests "For Jet Injector or Syringe Use". Use with separate sterile syringes is permitted for containers of 10 doses or less. The vaccine and diluent do not contain preservatives; therefore, the user must recognize the potential contamination hazards and exercise special precautions to protect the sterility and potency of the product. The use of aseptic techniques and proper storage prior to and after restoration of the vaccine and subsequent withdrawal of the individual doses is essential. Use 0.5 ml of the reconstituted vaccine for subcutaneous injection.

It is important to use a separate sterile syringe and needle for each individual patient to prevent transmission of hepatitis B and other infectious agents from one person to another.

50 Dose Vial (available only to government agencies/institutions)— Withdraw the entire contents (30 ml) of the diluent vial into the sterile syringe to be used for reconstitution and introduce into the 50 dose vial of lyophilized vaccine. Agitate to ensure thorough mixing. With full aseptic precautions, attach the vial to the sterilized multidose jet injector apparatus. Use 0.5 ml of the reconstituted vaccine for subcutaneous injection.

Each dose of Mumpsvax contains not less than the equivalent of 20,000 $TCID_{50}$ of the U.S. Reference Mumps Virus.

Parenteral drug products should be inspected visually for particulate matter and discoloration prior to administration. Mumpsvax, when reconstituted, is clear yellow.

DOSAGE AND ADMINISTRATION: *(cont'd)*

STORAGE

It is recommended that the vaccine be used as soon as possible after reconstitution. Protect vaccine from light at all times, since such exposure may inactivate the virus. Store reconstituted vaccine in the vaccine vial in a dark place at 2 - 8°C (36 - 46°F) and discard if not used within 8 hours.

REFERENCES:

1. Buynak, E. B.; Hilleman, M. R.: Live attenuated mumps virus vaccine. 1- Vaccine development, Proc. Soc. Exp. Biol. Med. *123:* 768-775, 1966. **2.** Hilleman, M. R.; Weibel, R. E.; Buynak, E. B.; Stokes, J., Jr.; Whitman, J. E., Jr.: Live, attenuated mumps-virus vaccine.Protective efficacy as measured in a field evaluation, New Engl. J. Med.*276:* 252-258, Feb. 2, 1967 **3.** Recommendation of the Immunization Practices Advisory Committee (ACIP), Mumps Vaccine Morbidity and Mortality Weekly Report*31* (46): 617-620, 625, November 26, 1982. **4.** Burnell, P. A.; Brickman, A.; Steinber, S.: Evaluation of a live attenuated mumps vaccine (Jeryl Lynn), Amer. J. Dis. Child. *118:*435-440, Sept. 1969. **5.** Buynak, E. B.; Hilleman, M. R.; Leagus, M. B.; Whitman, J. E., Jr.; Weibel, R. E.; Stokes, J., Jr.: Jeryl Lynn strain live attenuated mumps virus vaccine. Influence of age, virus dose, lot and gamma globulin administration on response, J. Am. Med. Assoc. *203:* 9-13, Jan. 1, 1968. **6.** Davidson, W. L.; Buynak, E. B.; Leagus, M. B.; Whitman, J. E., Jr.; Hilleman, M. R.: Vaccination of adults with live attenuated mumps virus vaccine, J. Am. Med. Assoc. *201:* 995-998, Sept. 25, 1967. **7.** Furesz, J.; Nagler, F. P.: Vaccination of school children with live mumps virus vaccine, Can. Med. Assoc. J. *102* (11): 1153-1155, May 30, 1970. **8.** Hilleman, M. R.; Buynak, E. B.; Weibel, R. E.; Stokes, J., Jr.: Live, attenuated mumps-virus vaccine, New Engl. J. Med. *278:* 227-232, Feb. 1, 1968. **9.** Horowitz, S. D.; Nagatani, M. S.; Bowen, G. S.; Holloway, A.W.; St. Geme, J. W., Jr.: The acquisition of delayed hypersensitivity following attenuated mumps virus infection, Pediatrics *45* (1): 77-82, Jan. 1970. **10.** Margileth, A. M.; Mella, G. W.; Di Moia, F.: Live mumps virus vaccine: Clinical reactions and serological response in 615 children, Med. Ann. D.C. *37:* 197-201, 1968. **11.** Nickey, L. N.; Huchton, P.; McGee, W. G.: Jeryl Lynn strain live attenuated mumps virus vaccine in a private pediatric practice, South Med. J. *63:* 306-308, March 1970. **12.** Nickey, L. N.; Huchton, P.; McGee, W. G.: Live virus mumps vaccine in pediatrics. Texas Med. *64:* 63-65, Sept. 1968. **13.** Riley, H. D., Jr.; Franco, S. F.; Linares, M. S.; Hughes, J.: Studies of live attenuated mumps virus vaccine, Proc. South. Soc. Ped. Res.*60:* 1351, Dec. 1967 (in Soc. Proc.). **14.** Roth, A.: Immunization with live attenuated mumps virus vaccine in Honolulu. A field trial, Amer. J. Dis. Child. *115:* 459-460, April, 1968. **15.** Stokes, J., Jr.; Weibel, R. E.; Buynak, E. B.; Hilleman, M. R.: Live attenuated mumps virus vaccine. II. Early clinical studies, Pediatrics*39:* 363-371, Mar. 1967. **16.** Sugg, W. C.; Finger, J. A.; Levine, R. H.; Pagano, J. S.: Field evaluation of live virus mumps vaccine, J. Pediatrics *72* (4): 461-466, April, 1968. **17.** Weibel, R. E.; Stokes, J., Jr.; Buynak, E. B.; Whitman, J. E., Jr.; Hilleman, M. R.: Live, attenuated mumps-virus vaccine. 3. Clinical and serologic aspects in a field evaluation, New Engl. J. Med. *276:*245-251, Feb. 2, 1967. **18.** Unpublished data: Files of Merck Sharp & Dohme Research Laboratories. **19.** Recommendations of the Immunization Practices Advisory Committee (ACIP), Measles Prevention, MMWR *36* (26): 409-425, July 10, 1978. **20.** Jong, E. C., The Travel and Tropical Medicine Manual, W. B. Saunders Company, p. 12-16, 1987. **21.** Committee on Immunization Council of Medical Societies, American College of Physicians, Phila., PA, Guide for Adult Immunization, First Edition, 1985. **22.** American Academy of Pediatrics: Report of the Committee on Infectious Disease, Evanston, Ill., p. 17, 1982. **23.** Center for Disease Control: Immunization of Children Infected with Human T-Lymphotropic Virus Type III/Lymphadenopathy-Associated Virus, Annals of Internal Medicine, *106:* 75-78, 1987. **24.** Krasinski, K.; Borkowsky, W.; Krugman, S.: Antibody following measles immunization in children infected with human T-cell lymphotropic virus-type III/lymphadenopathy associated virus (HTLV-III/LAV) (Abstract). In: Program and abstracts of the International Conference on Acquired Immunodeficiency Syndrome, Paris, France, June 29-25, 1986. **25.** Recommendation of the Immunization Practices Advisory Committee (ACIP), General Recommendations on Immunization, Morbidity and Mortality Weekly Report *32* (1): 13, January 14, 1983. **26.** Kupers, T. A.; Petrich, J. M.; Holloway, A. W.; St. Geme, J. W., Jr.: Depression of tuberculin delayed hypersensitivity by live attenuated mumps virus, J. Pediatr. *76:* 716-721, May 1970.

HOW SUPPLIED - EQUIVALENTS NOT AVAILABLE:

Injection, Lyphl-Soln - Subcutaneous - 1 unit/.5ml

0.5 ml	**$12.68**	**MUMPSVAX, Merck**	**00006-4753-00**
0.5 ml x 10	**$113.44**	**MUMPSVAX, Merck**	**00006-4584-00**

MUMPS AND RUBELLA VIRUS VACCINE LIVE *(002195)*

CATEGORIES: Immunologic; Mumps; Rubella; Serums, Toxoids and Vaccines; Vaccines; Pregnancy Category C; FDA Pre 1938 Drugs

BRAND NAMES: **Biavax II**

DESCRIPTION:

Biavax II (Rubella and Mumps Virus Vaccine Live) is a live virus vaccine for immunization against rubella (German measles) and mumps.

Biavax II is a sterile lyophilized preparation of the Wistar RA 27/3 strain of live attenuated rubella virus grown in human diploid cell (WI-38) culture;[1,2] and the Jeryl Lynn (B level) strain of mumps virus grown in cell cultures of chick embryo. The vaccine viruses are the same as those used in the manufacture of Meruvax II (Rubella Virus Vaccine Live) and Mumpsvax (Mumps Virus Vaccine Live). The two viruses are mixed before being lyophilized.

The reconstituted vaccine is for subcutaneous administration. When reconstituted as directed, the dose for injection is 0.5 ml and contains not less than the equivalent of 1,000 $TCID_{50}$ of the U.S. Reference Rubella Virus and 20,000 $TCID_{50}$ of the U.S. Reference Mumps Virus. Each dose contains approximately 25 mcg of neomycin. The product contains no preservative. Sorbitol and hydrolyzed gelatin are added as stabilizers.

CLINICAL PHARMACOLOGY:

Clinical studies of 73 double seronegative children 12 months to 2 years of age demonstrated that Biavax II is highly immunogenic and generally well tolerated. In these studies, a single injection of the vaccine induced rubella hemagglutination-inhibition (HI) antibodies in 100 percent, and mumps neutralizing antibodies in 97 percent of the susceptible children.

The RA 27/3 rubella strain in Biavax II elicits higher immediate postvaccination HI, complement-fixing and neutralizing antibody levels than other strains of rubella vaccine[3-9] and has been shown to induce a broader profile of circulating antibodies including anti-theta and anti-iota precipitating antibodies.[10,11] The RA 27/3 rubella strain immunologically simulates natural infection more closely than other rubella vaccine viruses.[11-13] The increased levels and broader profile of antibodies produced by RA 27/3 strain rubella virus vaccine appear to correlate with greater resistance to subclinical reinfection with the wild virus,[11,13-15] and provide greater confidence for lasting immunity.

Vaccine induced antibody levels following administration of Biavax II have been shown to persist for at least two years without substantial decline.[16] Antibody levels after immunization with Biavax (Rubella and Mumps Virus Vaccine Live), containing the HPV-77 strain of rubella, have persisted for 10.5 years without substantial decline.[17] If the present pattern continues, it will provide a basis for the expectation that immunity following vaccination will be permanent. However, continued surveillance will be required to demonstrate this point.

INDICATIONS AND USAGE:

Biavax II is indicated for simultaneous immunization against rubella and mumps in persons 12 months of age or older. A booster is not needed.

The vaccine is not recommended for infants younger than 12 months because they may retain maternal rubella and mumps neutralizing antibodies which may interfere with the immune response.

Previously unimmunized children of susceptible pregnant women should receive live attenuated rubella vaccine, because an immunized child will be less likely to acquire natural rubella and introduce the virus into the household.

Individuals planning travel outside the United States, if not immune, can acquire measles, mumps or rubella and import these diseases to the United States. Therefore, prior to International travel, individuals known to be susceptible to one or more of these diseases can receive either a single antigen vaccine (measles, mumps, or rubella), or a combined antigen vaccine as appropriate. However, M-M-R* II (Measles, Mumps, and Rubella Virus Vaccine Live) is preferred for persons likely to be susceptible to mumps and rubella; and if a single-antigen measles vaccine is not readily available, travelers should receive M-M-R II (Measles, Mumps, and Rubella Virus Vaccine Live) regardless of their immune status to mumps or rubella.[18,19,20]

NON-PREGNANT ADOLESCENT AND ADULT FEMALES

Immunization of susceptible non-pregnant adolescent and adult females of childbearing age with live attenuated rubella virus vaccine is indicated if certain precautions are observed (see below and PRECAUTIONS). Vaccinating susceptible postpubertal females confers individual protection against subsequently acquiring rubella infection during pregnancy, which in turn prevents infection of the fetus and consequent congenital rubella injury.[21]

Women of childbearing age should be advised not to become pregnant for three months after vaccination and should be informed of the reasons for this precaution.*

It is recommended that rubella susceptibility be determined by serologic testing prior to immunization.** If immune, as evidenced by a specific rubella antibody titer of 1:8 or greater (hemagglutination-inhibition test), vaccination is unnecessary. Congenital malformations do occur in up to seven percent of all live births.[22] Their chance appearance after vaccination could lead to misinterpretation of the cause, particularly if the prior rubella-immune status of vaccinees is unknown.

Postpubertal females should be informed of the frequent occurrence of generally self-limited arthralgia and/or arthritis beginning 2 to 4 weeks after vaccination (see ADVERSE REACTIONS.)

POSTPARTUM WOMEN

It has been found convenient in many instances to vaccinate rubella-susceptible women in the immediate postpartum period. (See Nursing Mothers.)

Revaccination: Children vaccinated when younger than 12 months of age should be revaccinated. Based on available evidence, there is no reason to routinely revaccinate persons who were vaccinated originally when 12 months of age or older. However, persons should be revaccinated if there is evidence to suggest that initial immunization was ineffective.

USE WITH OTHER VACCINES

Routine administration of DTP (diphtheria, tetanus, pertussis) and/or OPV (oral poliovirus vaccine) concomitantly with measles, mumps and rubella vaccines is not recommended because there are insufficient data relating to the simultaneous administration of these antigens. However, the American Academy of Pediatrics has noted that in some circumstances, particularly when the patient may not return, some practitioners prefer to administer all these antigens on a single day. If done, separate sites and syringes should be used for DTP and Biavax II.[23]

Biavax II should not be given less than one month before or after administration of other virus vaccines.

CONTRAINDICATIONS:

Do not give Biavax II to pregnant females; the possible effects of the vaccine on fetal development are unknown at this time. If vaccination of postpubertal females is undertaken, pregnancy should be avoided for three months following vaccination. (See PRECAUTIONS, Pregnancy.)

Anaphylactic or anaphylactoid reactions to neomycin (each dose of reconstituted vaccine contains approximately 25 mcg of neomycin).

History of anaphylactic or anaphylactoid reactions to eggs (see Hypersensitivity To Eggs.)

Any febrile respiratory illness or other active febrile infection.

Active untreated tuberculosis.

Patients receiving immunosuppressive therapy. This contraindication does not apply to patients who are receiving corticosteroids as replacement therapy, e.g., for Addison's disease.

Individuals with blood dyscrasias, leukemia, lymphomas of any type, or other malignant neoplasms affecting the bone marrow or lymphatic systems.

Primary and acquired immunodeficiency states, including patients who are immunosuppressed in association with AIDS or other clinical manifestations of infection with human immunodeficiency viruses;[24,25]cellular immune deficiencies; and hypogammaglobulinemic and dysgammaglobulinemic states.

Individuals with a family history of congenital or hereditary immunodeficiency, until the immune competence of the potential vaccine recipient is demonstrated.[26]

*NOTE: The Immunization Practices Advisory Committee (ACIP) has recommended "In view of the importance of protecting this age group against rubella, reasonable precautions in a rubella immunization program include asking females if they are pregnant, excluding those who say they are, and explaining the theoretical risks to the others."[21]

**NOTE: The Immunization Practices Advisory Committee (ACIP) has stated "When practical, and when reliable laboratory services are available, potential vaccinees of childbearing age can have serologic tests to determine susceptibility to rubella.... However, routinely performing serologic tests for all females of childbearing age to determine susceptibility so that vaccine is given only to proven susceptibles is expensive and has been ineffective in some areas. Accordingly, the ACIP believes that rubella vaccination of a woman who is not known to be pregnant and has no history of vaccination is justifiable without serologic testing."[21]

HYPERSENSITIVITY TO EGGS

Live mumps vaccine is produced in chick embryo cell culture. Persons with a history of anaphylactic, anaphylactoid, or other immediate reactions (*e.g.,* hives, swelling of the mouth and throat, difficulty breathing, hypotension, or shock) subsequent to egg ingestion should not be vaccinated. Evidence indicates that persons are not at increased risk if they have egg allergies that are not anaphylactic or anaphylactoid in nature. Such persons may be vaccinated in the usual manner. There is no evidence to indicate that persons with allergies to chickens or feathers are at increased risk of reaction to the vaccine.[21]

PRECAUTIONS:

GENERAL

Adequate treatment provisions including epinephrine, should be available for immediate use should an anaphylactic or anaphylactoid reaction occur.

Children and young adults who are known to be infected with human immunodeficiency viruses but without overt clinical manifestations of immunosuppression may be vaccinated; however, the vaccinees should be monitored closely for vaccine-preventable diseases because immunization may be less effective than for uninfected persons.[24,25]

Vaccination should be deferred for at least 3 months following blood or plasma transfusions, or administration of human immune serum globulin.

Excretion of small amounts of the live attenuated rubella virus from the nose and throat has occurred in the majority of susceptible individuals 7-28 days after vaccination. There is no confirmed evidence to indicate that such virus is transmitted to susceptible persons who are in contact with the vaccinated individuals. Consequently, transmission through close personal

PRECAUTIONS: *(cont'd)*

contact, while accepted as a theoretical possibility, is not regarded as a significant risk.[21] However, transmission of the rubella vaccine virus to infants via breast milk has been documented (see Nursing Mothers.)

There are no reports of transmission of live attenuated mumps virus from vaccinees to susceptible contacts.

It has been reported that live attenuated rubella and mumps virus vaccines given individually may result in a temporary depression of tuberculin skin sensitivity. Therefore, if a tuberculin test is to be done, it should be administered either before or simultaneously with Biavax II.

As for any vaccine, vaccination with Biavax II may not result in seroconversion in 100% of susceptible persons given the vaccine.

PREGNANCY CATEGORY C

Animal reproduction studies have not been conducted with Biavax II. It is also not known whether Biavax II can cause fetal harm when administered to a pregnant woman or can affect reproduction capacity. Therefore, the vaccine should not be administered to pregnant females; furthermore, pregnancy should be avoided for three months following vaccination (see CONTRAINDICATIONS.)

In counseling women who are inadvertently vaccinated when pregnant or who become pregnant within 3 months of vaccination, the physician should be aware of the following: (1) In a 10 year survey involving over 700 pregnant women who received rubella vaccine within 3 months before or after conception, (of whom 189 received the Wistar RA 27/3 strain) none of the newborns had abnormalities compatible with congenital rubella syndrome;[27] and (2) although mumps virus is capable of infecting the placenta and fetus, there is no good evidence that it causes congenital malformations in humans. Mumps vaccine virus also has been shown to infect the placenta, but the virus has not been isolated from the fetal tissues from susceptible women who were vaccinated and under went elective abortions.[28]

NURSING MOTHERS

It is not known whether mumps vaccine virus is secreted in human milk. Recent studies have shown that lactating postpartum women immunized with live attenuated rubella vaccine may secrete the virus in breast milk and transmit it to breast-fed infants.[29] In the infants with serological evidence of rubella infection, none exhibited severe disease; however, one exhibited mild clinical illness typical of acquired rubella.[30,31] Caution should be exercised when Biavax II is administered to a nursing woman.

ADVERSE REACTIONS:

Burning and/or stinging of short duration at the injection site have been reported.

The adverse clinical reactions associated with the use of Biavax II are those expected to follow administration of the monovalent vaccine given separately. These may include malaise, sore throat, cough rhinitis, headache, dizziness, fever, rash, nausea, vomiting or diarrhea, mild local reactions such as erythema, induration, tenderness and regional lymphadenopathy; parotitis, orchitis, nerve deafness, throm-bocytopenia and purpura; allergic reactions such as wheal and flare at the injection site or urticaria; polyneuritis, and arthralgia and/or arthritis (usually transient and rarely chronic).

Anaphylaxis and anaphylactoid reactions have been reported.

Vasculitis has been reported rarely.

Moderate fever (101 - 102.9°F (38.3 - 39.4°C)) occurs occasionally, and high fever (above 103°F (39.4°C)) occurs less commonly. On rare occasions, children developing fever may exhibit febrile convulsions. Syncope, particularly at the time of mass vaccination, has been reported. Rash occurs infrequently and is usually minimal, but rarely may be generalized. Erythema multiforme has also been reported rarely.

Forms of optic neuritis, including retrobulbar neuritis and papillitis, may infrequently follow viral infections, and have been reported to occur 1 to 3 weeks following inoculation with some live virus vaccines.

Isolated reports of polyneuropathy including Guillain-Barré syndrome have been reported after immunization with rubella-containing vaccines.

Clinical experience with live attenuated rubella and mumps virus vaccines given individually indicates that encephalitis and other nervous system reactions have occurred very rarely. These might occur also with Biavax II.

Arthralgia and/or arthritis (usually transient and rarely chronic), and polyneuritis are features of natural rubella and vary in frequency and severity with age and sex, being greatest in adult females and least in prepubertal children. This type of involvement as well as myalgia and paresthesia have also been reported following administration of Meruvax II (Rubella Virus Vaccine Live).

Chronic arthritis has been associated with natural rubella infection and has been related to persistent virus and/or viral antigen isolated from body tissues. Only rarely have vaccine recipients developed chronic joint symptoms.

Following vaccination in children, reactions in joints are uncommon and generally of brief duration. In women, incidence rates for arthritis and arthralgia are generally higher than those seen in children (children: 0 - 3%; women: 12 - 20%)[32], and the reactions tend to be more marked and of longer duration. Symptoms may persist for a matter of months or on rare occasions for years. In adolescent girls, the reactions appear to be intermediate in incidence between those seen in children and in adult women. Even in older women (35-45 years), these reactions are generally well tolerated and rarely interfere with normal activities.

DOSAGE AND ADMINISTRATION:

FOR SUBCUTANEOUS ADMINISTRATION

Do not inject intravenously.

The dosage of vaccine is the same for all persons. Inject the total volume (about 0.5 ml) of reconstituted vaccine subcutaneously, preferably into the outer aspect of upper arm. *Do not give immune globulin (IG) concurrently with* Biavax II.

During shipment, to insure that there is no loss of potency, the vaccine must be maintained at a temperature of 10°C (50°F) or less.

Before reconstitution, store Biavax II at 2 - 8°C (36 - 46°F). *Protect from light.*

CAUTION: A sterile syringe free of preservatives, antiseptics, and detergents should be used for each injection of the vaccine because these substances may inactivate the live virus vaccine. A 25 gauge, 5/8" needle is recommended.

To reconstitute, use only the diluent supplied, since it is free of preservatives or other antiviral substances which might inactivate the vaccine. First withdraw the entire volume of diluent into the syringe to be used for reconstitution. Inject all the diluent in the syringe into the vial of lyophilized vaccine, and agitate to mix thoroughly. Withdraw the entire contents into a syringe and inject the total volume of restored vaccine subcutaneously.

It is important to use a separate sterile syringe and needle for each individual patient to prevent transmission of hepatitis B virus and other infectious agents from one person to another.

Each dose of Biavax II contains not less than the equivalent of 1,000 $TCID_{50}$ of the U.S. Reference Rubella Virus and 20,000 $TCID_{50}$ of the U.S. Reference Mumps Virus.

DOSAGE AND ADMINISTRATION: *(cont'd)*

Parenteral drug products should be inspected visually for particulate matter and discoloration prior to administration. Biavax II, when reconstituted, is clear yellow.

STORAGE

It is recommended that the vaccine be used as soon as possible after reconstitution. Protect the vaccine from light at all times, since such exposure may inactivate the virus. Store reconstituted vaccine in the vaccine vial in a dark place at 2 - 8°C (36 - 46°F) and discard if not used within eight hours.

REFERENCES:

1) Plotkin, S. A.; Cornfeld, D.; Ingalls, T. H.: Studies of immunization with living rubella virus: Trials in children with a strain cultured from an aborted fetus, Am. J. Dis. Children *110:*381-389, 1965. 2) Plotkin, S. A.; Farquhar, J.; Katz, M.; Ingalls, T. H.: A new attenuated rubella virus grown in human fibroblasts: Evidence for reduced nasopharyngeal excretion, Am. J. Epidemiol. *86:*468-477, 1967. 3) Fogel, A.; Moshkowitz, A.; Rannon, L.; Gerichter, Ch. B.: Comparative trials of RA 27/3 and Cendehill rubella vaccines in adult and adolescent females, Am. J. Epidemiol. *93:* 392-398, 1971. 4) Andzhaparidze, O. G.; Desyatskova, R. G.; Chervonski, G. I.; Pryanichnikova, L. V.: Immunogenicity and reactogenicity of live attenuated rubella virus vaccines, Am. J. Epidemiol. *91:* 527-530, 1970. 5) Freestone, D. S.; Reynolds, G. M.; McKinnon, J. A.; Prydie, J.: Vaccination of schoolgirls against rubella. Assessment of serological status and a comparative trial of Wistar RA 27/3 and Cendehill strain live attenuated rubella vaccines in 13-year-old schoolgirls in Dudley, Br. J. Prev. Soc. Med. *29:* 258-261, 1975. 6) Grillner, L.; Hedstrom, C. E.; Bergstrom, H.; Forssman, L.; Rigner, A.; Lycke, E.: Vaccination against rubella of newly delivered women, Scand. J. Infect. Dis. *5:*237-241, 1973. 7) Grillner, L.: Neutralizing antibodies after rubella vaccination of newly delivered women: a comparison between three vaccines, Scand. J. Infect. Dis. *7:* 169-172, 1975. 8) Wallace, R. B.; Isacson, P.: Comparative trial of HPV-77, DE5 and RA 27/3 live attenuated rubella vaccines, Am. J. Dis. Children *124:* 536-538, 1972. 9) Lalla, M.; Vesikari, T.; Virolainen, M.: Lymphoblast proliferation and humoral antibody response after rubella vaccination, Clin. Exp. Immunol. *15:* 193-202, 1973. 10) LeBouvier, G. L.; Plotkin, S. A.: Precipitin responses to rubella vaccine RA 27/3, J. Infect. Dis. *123:* 220-223, 1971. 11) Horstmann, D. M.: Rubella: the challenge of its control, J. Infect. Dis. *123:* 640-654, 1971. 12) Ogra, P. L.; Kerr-Grant, D.; Umana, G.; Dzierba, J.; Weintraub, D.: Antibody response in serum and nasopharynx after naturally acquired and vaccine induced infection with rubella virus, N. Engl. J. Med.*285:* 1333-1339, 1971. 13) Plotkin, S. A.; Farquhar, J. D.; Ogra, P. L.: Immunologic properties of RA 27/3 rubella virus vaccine, J. Am. Med. Ass. *225:* 585-590, 1973. 14) Liebhaber, H.; Ingalls, T. H.; LeBouvier, G. L.; Horstmann, D. M.: Vaccination with RA 27/3 rubella vaccine. Persistence of immunity and resistance to challenge after two years, Am. J. Dis. Children *123:* 133-136, 1972. 15) Farquhar, J. D.: Follow-up on rubella vaccinations and experience with subclinical reinfection, J. Pediatr. *81:* 460-465, 1972. 16) Weibel, R. E.; Carlson, A. J.; Villarejos, V. M.; Buynak, E. B.; McLean, A. A.; Hilleman, M. R.: Clinical and Laboratory Studies of Combined Live Measles, Mumps, and Rubella Vaccines Using the RA 27/3 Rubella Virus, Proc. Soc. Exp. Biol. Med. *165:* 323-326, 1980. 17) Weibel, R. E.; Buynak, E. B.; McLean, A. A.; Roehm, R. R.; Hilleman, M. R.: Persistence of Antibody in Human Subjects for 7 to 10 years following Administration of Combined Live Attenuated Measles, Mumps, and Rubella Virus Vaccines, Proc. Soc. Exp. Biol. Med. *165:* 260-263, 1980. 18) Recommendations of the Immunization Practices Advisory Committee (ACIP), Measles Prevention, MMWR *36* (26): 409-425, July 10, 1987. 19) Jong, E. C., The Travel and Tropical Medicine Manual, W. B. Saunders Company, p. 12-16, 1987. 20) Committee on Immunization Council of Medical Societies, American College of Physicians, Phila., PA, Guide for Adult Immunization, First Edition, 1985. 21) Recommendation of the Immunization Practices Advisory Committee (ACIP), Morbidity and Mortality Weekly Report *33* (22): 301-310, 315-318, June 8, 1984. 22) McIntosh, R.; Merritt, K. K.; Richards, M. R.; Samuels, M. H; Bellows, M. T.: The incidence of congenital malformations: A study of 5,964 pregnancies, Pediatr. *14:* 505-521, 1954. 23) American Academy of Pediatrics: Report of the Committee on Infectious Disease, Evanston, III., p. 17, 1982. 24) Center for Disease Control: Immunization of Children Infected with Human T-Lymphotropic Virus Type III/Lymphadenopathy-Associated Virus, Annals of Internal Medicine, *106:*75-78, 1987. 25) Krasinski, K.; Borkowsky, W.; Krugman, S.: Antibody following measles immunization in children infected with human T-cell lymphotropic virus-type III/lymphadenopathy associated virus (HTLV-III/LAV) (Abstract). In: Program and abstracts of the International Conference on Acquired Immunodeficiency Syndrome, Paris, France, June 23-25, 1986. 26) Recommendation of the Immunization Practices Advisory Committee (ACIP), General Recommendations on Immunization, Morbidity and Mortality Weekly Report *32* (1): 13, January 14, 1983. 27) Rubella vaccination during pregnancy — United States, 1971-1981, Morbidity and Mortality Weekly Report *31* (35): 477-481, September 10, 1982. 28) Recommendation of the Immunization Practices Advisory Committee (ACIP), Mumps Vaccine Morbidity and Mortality Weekly Report *32* (46): 617-620, 625, November 26, 1982. 29) Losonsky, G. A.; Fishaut, J. M.; Strussenberg, J.; Ogra, P. L.: Effect of immunization against rubella on lactation products. II. Maternal - neonatal interactions. J. Infect. Dis.*145:* 661-666, 1982. 30) Landes, R. D.; Bass, J. W.; Millunchick, E. W.; Oetgen, W. J.: Neonatal rubella following postpartum maternal immunization, J. Pediatr. *97:* 465-467, 1980. 31) Lerman, S. J.: Neonatal rubella following postpartum maternal immunization, J. Pediatr.*98:* 668, 1981. (Letter). 32) Unpublished data from the files of Merck Sharp & Dohme Research Laboratories.

HOW SUPPLIED - EQUIVALENTS NOT AVAILABLE:

Injection, Lyphl-Soln - Subcutaneous - 0.5 ml/vial

0.5 ml	$19.30	BIAVAX II, Merck	00006-4746-00

Injection, Lyphl-Soln - Subcutaneous - 6000 unit

0.5 ml x 10	$169.94	BIAVAX II, Merck	00006-4669-00

MUPIROCIN *(001843)*

CATEGORIES: Anti-Infectives; Antibiotics; Dermatologicals; Impetigo; Local Infections; Skin Infections; Skin/Mucous Membrane Agents; Topical; Pregnancy Category B; FDA Approved 1987 Dec; Top 200 Drugs

BRAND NAMES: **Bactroban**; *Eismycin* (Germany)
(International brand names outside U.S. in italics)

FORMULARIES: Aetna; BC-BS; PCS

DESCRIPTION:

Each gram of Bactroban Ointment 2% contains 20 mg mupirocin in a bland water miscible ointment base consisting of polyethylene glycol 400 and polyethylene glycol 3350 (polyethylene glycol ointment, N.F.). Mupirocin is a naturally occurring antibiotic. The chemical name is (*E*)-(2*S*,3*R*,4*R*,5*S*)-5- [(2*S*,3*S*,4*S*,5*S*)-2,3-Epoxy-5-hydroxy-4-methyl (hexyl) tetrahydro-3,4-dihydroxy-β-methyl-2*H*-pyran-2- crotonic acid, ester with 9-hydroxynonanoic acid.

CLINICAL PHARMACOLOGY:

Mupirocin is produced by fermentation of the organism *Pseudomonas fluorescens.* Mupirocin inhibits bacterial protein synthesis by reversibly and specifically binding to bacterial isoleucyl transfer-RNA synthetase. Due to this mode of action, mupirocin shows no cross resistance with chloramphenicol, erythromycin, fusidic acid, gentamicin, lincomycin, methicillin, neomycin, novobiocin, penicillin, streptomycin, and tetracycline.

Application of ^{14}C-labeled mupirocin ointment to the lower arm of normal male subjects followed by occlusion for 24 hours showed no measurable systemic absorption (<1.1 nanogram mupirocin per milliliter of whole blood). Measurable radioactivity was present in the stratum corneum of these subjects 72 hours after application.

Microbiology: The following bacteria are susceptible to the action of mupirocin *in vitro:* the aerobic isolates of*Staphylococcus aureus* (including methicillin-resistant and β-lactamase producing strains), *Staphylococcus epidermidis, Staphylococcus saprophyticus,* and *Streptococcus pyogenes.*

Only the organisms listed in the INDICATIONS AND USAGE section have been shown to be clinically susceptible to mupirocin.

INDICATIONS AND USAGE:

Bactroban (mupirocin) Ointment is indicated for the topical treatment of impetigo due to: *Staphylococcus aureus,* beta hemolytic Streptococcus*, and *Streptococcus pyogenes.*

*Efficacy for this organism in this organ system was studied in fewer than ten infections.

CONTRAINDICATIONS:

This drug is contraindicated in individuals with a history of sensitivity reactions to any of its components.

WARNINGS:

Bactroban Ointment is not for ophthalmic use.

PRECAUTIONS:

If a reaction suggesting sensitivity or chemical irritation should occur with the use of Bactroban Ointment, treatment should be discontinued and appropriate alternative therapy for the infection instituted. As with other antibacterial products prolonged use may result in overgrowth of nonsusceptible organisms, including fungi.

Bactroban is not formulated for use on mucosal surfaces. Intranasal use has been associated with isolated reports of stinging and drying. Polyethylene glycol can be absorbed from open wounds and damaged skin and is excreted by the kidneys. In common with other polyethylene glycol- based ointments, Bactroban should not be used in conditions where absorption of large quantities of polyethylene glycol is possible, especially if there is evidence of moderate or severe renal impairment.

Pregnancy Category B: Reproduction studies have been performed in rats and rabbits at systemic doses, i.e., orally, subcutaneously, and intramuscularly, up to 100 times the human topical dose and have revealed no evidence of impaired fertility or harm to the fetus due to mupirocin. There are, however, no adequate and well-controlled studies in pregnant women. Because animal studies are not always predictive of human response, this drug should be used during pregnancy only if clearly needed.

Nursing Mothers: It is not known whether Bactroban is present in breast milk. Nursing should be temporarily discontinued while using Bactroban.

ADVERSE REACTIONS:

The following local adverse reactions have been reported in connection with the use of Bactroban Ointment: burning, stinging, or pain in 1.5% of patients; itching in 1% of patients; rash, nausea, erythema, dry skin, tenderness, swelling, contact dermatitis, and increased exudate in less than 1% of patients.

DOSAGE AND ADMINISTRATION:

A small amount of Bactroban Ointment should be applied to the affected area three times daily. The area treated may be covered with a gauze dressing if desired. Patients not showing a clinical response within 3 to 5 days should be re-evaluated.

PATIENT INFORMATION:

Mupirocin is an antibiotic ointment used for the treatment of skin infections. Inform your physician if you are pregnant or nursing. This ointment is only to be used externally and should not be used in or near the eyes. Do not apply this ointment to large open wounds or to burns. Gently clean the affected skin before applying mupirocin. Apply the ointment sparingly and rub in gently. Do not apply cosmetics or other skin products over the treated area unless directed by your physician. Notify your physician if your skin infection does not improve in 3 to 5 days.

HOW SUPPLIED:

Bactroban (mupirocin) Ointment 2% is supplied in 15 gram and 30 gram tubes.

Store between 15° and 30°C (59° and 86°F).

HOW SUPPLIED - EQUIVALENTS NOT AVAILABLE:

Ointment - Topical - 2 %

15 gm x 3	$15.20	BACTROBAN, Beecham	00029-1525-22
30 gm	$28.65	BACTROBAN, Beecham	00029-1525-25

MUROMONAB-CC3 *(001845)*

CATEGORIES: Immunosuppressives; Renal Transplant Allograft Rejection; Renal Transplantation; Pregnancy Category C; Recombinant DNA Origin; FDA Approved 1986 Jun

BRAND NAMES: **Orthoclone OKT-3**

Only physicians experienced in immunosuppressive therapy and management of solid organ transplant patients should use Muromonab-CD3.

Anaphylactic or anaphylactoid reactions may occur following administration of any dose or course of muronmonab-CD3. Serious and occasionally life-threatening systemic, cardiovascular, and central nervous systems reactions have been reported following administration of muronmonab-CD3. These have included: pulmonary edema, especially in patients with volume overload; shock; cardiovascular collapse; cardiac or respiratory arrest; seizures; and coma. Hence, a patient being treated with muronmonab-CD3 must be managed in a facility equipped and staffed for cardiopulmonary resuscitation. (See WARNINGS, Cytokine Release Syndrome, Neuro, Psychiatric Events, Anaphylactic Reactions.)

DESCRIPTION:

Muromonab-CD3 sterile solution is a murine monoclonal antibody to the CD3 antigen of human T cells which functions as an immunosuppressant. It is for intravenous use only. The antibody is a biochemically purified IgG_{2a} immunoglobulin with a heavy chain of approximately 50,000 daltons and a light chain of approximately 25,000 daltons. It is directed to a glycoprotein with a molecular weight of 20,000 in the human T cell surface which is essential for T cell functions. Because it is a monoclonal antibody preparation, muronmonab-CD3 Sterile Solution is a homogeneous, reproducible antibody product with consistent, measurable reactivity to human T cells.

Each 5 ml ampule of Orthoclone Okt-3 Sterile Solution contains 5 mg (1 mg/ml) of muromonab-CD3 in a clear, colorless solution which may contain a few fine translucent protein particles. Each ampule contains a buffered solution (pH 7.0 ± 0.5) of monobasic sodium phosphate (2.25 mg), dibasic sodium phosphate (9.0 mg), sodium chloride (43 mg), and polysorbate 80 (1.0 mg) in water for injection.

The proper name, muromonab-CD3, is derived from the descriptive term murine monoclonal antibody. The CD3 designation identifies the specificity of the antibody as the Cell Differentiation (CD) cluster 3 defined by the First International Workshop on Human Leukocyte Differentiation Antigens.

CLINICAL PHARMACOLOGY:

Muronmonab-CD3 reverses graft injection, most probably by blocking the function of all T cells which play a major role in acute allograft rejection. Muronmonab-CD3 reacts with and blocks the function of a 20,000 dalton molecule (CD3) in the membrane of human T cells that has been associated *in vitro* with the antigen recognition structure of T cells and is essential for signal transduction. In *in vitro* cytolytic assays, muronmonab-CD3 blocks both the generation and function of effector cells. Binding of muronmonab-CD3 to T lymphocytes results in early activation of T cells, which leads to cytokine release, followed by blocking T cell functions. After termination of muronmonab-CD3 therapy, T cell function usually returns to normal within one week.

CLINICAL PHARMACOLOGY: *(cont'd)*

In vivo, muronmonab-CD3 reacts with most peripheral blood cells and T cells in body tissues, but has not been found to react with other hematopoietic elements or other tissues of the body.

A rapid and concomitant decrease in the number of circulating CD2 positive, CD3 positive, CD4 positive, and CD8 positive T cells has observed in patients studied within minutes after the administration of muronmonab-CD3. This decrease in the number of CD3 positive T cells results from the specific interaction between muronmonab-CD3 and the CD3 antigen on the surface of all T lymphocytes. T cell activation results in the release of numerous cytokines/lymphokines, which are felt to be responsible for many of the acute clinical manifestations seen following muronmonab-CD3 administration. (See WARNINGS, Cytokine Release Syndrome, Neuro, Psychiatric Events.)

While CD3 positive cells are not detectable between days two and seven, increasing numbers of circulating CD4 and CD8 positive cells have been observed. The presence of these CD4 and CD8 positive cells has not been shown to affect reversal of rejection. After termination of muromonab-CD3 therapy, CD3 positive cells reappear rapidly and reach pre-treatment levels within a week. In some patients however, increasing numbers of CD3 positive cells have been observed prior to termination of muronmonab-CD3 therapy. This reappearance of CD3 positive cells has been attributed to the development of neutralizing antibodies to muronmonab-CD3, which in turn block its ability to bind to the CD3 antigen or T lymphocytes (see PRECAUTIONS, Sensitization.)

In the initial clinical trials using low doses of prednisone and azathioprine during muronmonab-CD3 therapy for renal allograft rejection, antibodies to muronmonab-CD3 were observed with an incidence of 21% (n=43) for IgM, 86% (n=43) for IgG and 29% (n=35) for IgE. The mean time of appearance of IgG antibodies was 20 ± 2 (mean ± SD) days. Early IgG antibodies appeared towards the end of the second week of treatment in 3% (n=86) of the patients.

Subsequent clinical experience has shown that the dose, duration, and type of immunosuppressive medications used in combination with muronmonab-CD3 may affect both the incidence and magnitude of the host antibody response. Furthermore, immunosuppressive agents used concomitantly with muronmonab-CD3 (*i.e.,* steroids, azathioprine, prednisone, or cyclosporine) have altered the time course of anti-mouse antibody development and the specificity of the antibodies formed (*i.e.,* idiotypic, isotypic, allotypic).

Serum levels of muronmonab-CD3 are measurable using an enzyme-linked immunosorbent assay (ELISA). During the initial clinical trials in renal allograft rejection, in patients treated with 5 mg per day for 14 days, mean serum trough levels of the drug rose over the first three days and then averaged 900 ng/ml on days 3 to 14. Subsequent clinical experience

has demonstrated that circulating serum levels greater than 800 ng/ml of muronmonab-CD3 blocks the function of cytotoxic T cells *in vitro* and *in vivo.* (See PRECAUTIONS, Laboratory Tests.)

Following administration of muronmonab-CD3 *in vivo,* leukocytes have been observed in cerebrospinal and peritoneal fluids. The mechanism for this effect is not completely understood, but probably is related to cytokines altering membrane permeability, rather than an active inflammatory process. (See WARNINGS, Cytokine Release Syndrome, Neuro, Psychiatric Events.)

INDICATIONS AND USAGE:

Muronmonab-CD3 is indicated for the treatment of acute allograft rejection in renal transplant patients.

Muronmonab-CD3 is also indicated for the treatment of steroid-resistant acute allograft rejection in cardiac and hepatic transplant patients.

Acute Renal Rejection: In a controlled randomized clinical trial, muronmonab-CD3 was significantly more effective than conventional high- dose steroid therapy in reversing acute renal allograft rejection of cadaveric renal transplants were treated either with muronmonab-CD3 daily for a mean of 14 days, with concomitant lowering of the dosage of azathioprine and maintenance steroids (62 patients), or with conventional high-dose steroids (60 patients). Muronmonab-CD3 reversed 94% of this rejections compared to a 75% reversal rate obtained with conventional high-dose steroid treatment (p=0.006). The one year Kaplan-Meier (actuarial) estimates of graft survival rates for these patients who had acute rejection were 62% and 45% for muronmonab-CD3 and steroid-treated patients, respectively (p=0.04). At two years the rates were 56% and 42%, respectively (p=0.06).

One- and two-year patient survivals were not significantly different between the two groups, being 85% and 75% for muronmonab-CD3 treated patients and 90% and 85% for steroid-treated patients.

In additional open clinical trials, the observed rate of reversal of acute renal allograft rejection was 92% (n=126) for muronmonab-CD3 therapy. Muronmonab-CD3 was also effective in reversing acute renal allograft rejections in 65% (n=225) of cases where steroids and lymphocyte immune globulin preparations were contraindicated or were not successful (rescue).

Acute Cardiac or Hepatic Allograft Rejection: Muronmonab-CD3 has also been shown to be effective in reversing acute cardiac and hepatic allograft rejection in patients who are unresponsive to high-doses of steroids. Controlled randomized trials have been conducted to evaluate the effectiveness of muronmonab-CD3 compared to conventional therapy as first line treatment for acute cardiac and hepatic allograft rejection.

The raft of reversal in acute cardiac allograft rejection was 90% (n=61) and was 83% for hepatic allograft rejection (n=124) in patients unresponsive to treatment with steroids.

The dosage of other immunosuppressive agents used in conjunction with muronmonab-CD3 should be reduced to the lowest level compatible with an effective therapeutic response. (See WARNINGS; ADVERSE REACTIONS, Infections, Neoplasia; and DOSAGE AND ADMINISTRATION.)

CONTRAINDICATIONS:

Muronmonab-CD3 should not be given to patients who:

are hypersensitive to this or any other product of murine origin;

have anti-mouse antibody titers ≥1:1000;

are in (uncompensated) heart failure or in fluid overload, as evidenced by chest X-ray or a greater than 3 percent weight gain within the week prior to planned muronmonab-CD3 administration;

have a history of seizures, or are predisposed to seizures;

are determined and/or suspected to be pregnant, or who are breast- feeding. (See PRECAUTIONS, Pregnancy, Nursing Mothers.)

WARNINGS:

SEE BOXED WARNING.

Cytokine Release Syndrome: Temporally associated with administration of the first few doses muronmonab-CD3 (particularly, the first two to three doses), most patients have developed an acute clinical syndrome [i.e., Cytokine Release Syndrome (CRS)] that has been attributed to the release of cytokines by activated lymphocytes or monocytes. This clinical syndrome has

WARNINGS: *(cont'd)*

ranged from a more frequently reported mild, self- limited, "flu-like" illness to a less frequently reported severe, life-threatening shock-like reaction, which may include serious cardiovascular and central nervous system manifestations. The syndrome typically begins approximately 30 to 60 minutes after administration of a dose muronmonab-CD3 (but may occur later) and may persist for several hours. The frequency and severity of this symptom complex is usually greatest with the first dose. With each successive dose of muronmonab-CD3, both the frequency and severity of the Cytokine Release Syndrome tends to diminish. Increasing the amount of a dose or resuming treatment after a hiatus may result in a reappearance of the CRS.

Common clinical manifestations of the Cytokine Release Syndrome: may include: high (often spiking, up to 107°F) fever, chills/rigors, headache, tremor, nausea/vomiting, diarrhea, abdominal pain, malaise, muscle/joint aches and pains, and generalized weakness. Less frequently reported adverse experiences include; minor dermatologic reactions (*e.g.*, rash, pruritus, etc.) and a spectrum of often serious, occasionally fatal, cardiorespiratory and neuropsychiatric, adverse experiences. (See WARNINGS, PRECAUTIONS, and ADVERSE REACTIONS, Neuro, Psychiatric Events.)

Cardiorespiratory findings: may include dyspnea, shortness of breath, bronchospasm/wheezing, tachypnea, respiratory arrest/failure/distress, cardiovascular collapse, cardiac arrest, angina/myocardial infarction, chest pain/tightness, tachycardia, hypertension, hemodynamic instability, hypotension including profound shock, heart failure, pulmonary edema (cardiogenic and non-cardiogenic), adult respiratory distress syndrome, hypoxemia, apnea, and arrhythmias. (See BOXED WARNING; PRECAUTIONS; and ADVERSE REACTIONS.)

In the initial renal rejection studies, the most serious post-dose reaction-potentially fatal, severe *pulmonary edema* - occurred in 4.7% of the initial 107 patients. Fluid overload was present before treatment in all of these cases. However, it occurred in 0.0% of the subsequent 311 patients treated with front-dose volume/weight restrictions. In subsequent trials and in post-marketing experience, severe pulmonary edema has occurred in patients who appeared to be euvolemic. The pathogenesis of pulmonary edema may involve all or some of the following: volume overload; increased pulmonary vascular permeability; and/or reduced left ventricular compliance/contractility.

During the first 1 to 3 days of muronmonab-CD3 therapy, some patients have experienced an acute and transient decline in the glomerular filtration rate (GFR) and diminished urine output with a resulting *increase in the level of serum creatinine.* Massive release of cytokines appears to lead to reversible renal functional impairment and/or delayed renal allograft function. Similarly, transient elevations in hepatic transaminases have been reported following administration of the first few doses of muronmonab-CD3.

Patients At Risk: for more serious complications of the Cytokine Release Syndrome may include those with the following conditions: unstable angina; recent myocardial infarction or symptomatic ischemic heart disease; heart failure of any etiology; pulmonary edema of any etiology; any form of chronic obstructive pulmonary disease; intravascular volume overload or depletion of any etiology (*e.g.*, excessive dialysis, recent intensive diuresis, blood loss, etc); cerebrovascular disease; patients with advanced symptomatic vascular disease or neuropathy; a history of seizures; and septic shock. Efforts should be made to correct or stabilize background conditions prior to the initiation of therapy.

Prior to administration of muronmonab-CD3, the patient's volume (fluid) status should be assessed carefully. It is imperative, especially prior to the first few doses, that there be no clinical evidence of volume overload or uncompensated heart failure, including a clear chest x-ray and weight restriction of ≤3% above the patient's minimum weight during the week prior to injection.

Manifestations of the Cytokine Release Syndrome may be prevented or minimized by pretreatment with 8 mg/kg of methylprednisolone (*i.e.,* high-dose steroids), given 1 to 4 hours prior to administration of the first dose of muronmonab-CD3, and closely following recommendations for dosage and treatment duration. (See DOSAGE AND ADMINISTRATION.)

The administration of muronmonab-CD3 should be performed in a facility that is equipped and staffed for cardiopulmonary resuscitation and where a patient can be closely monitored for an appropriate period based on the patient's status.

If any of the more serious presentations of the Cytokine Release Syndrome occur, intensive treatment including oxygen, intravenous fluids, corticosteroids, pressor amines, antihistamines, intubation, etc., may be required.

Anaphylactic Reactions: Serious and occasionally fatal, immediate (usually within 10 minutes) hypersensitivity (anaphylactic) reactions have been reported in patients treated with muronmonab-CD3.**Manifestations of anaphylaxis may appear similar to manifestations of the Cytokine Release Syndrome (described above). It may be impossible to determine the mechanism responsible for any systemic reaction(s).** Reactions attributed to hypersensitivity have been reported less frequently than those attributed to cytokine release. Acute hypersensitivity reactions may be characterized by: cardiovascular collapse, cardiorespiratory arrest, loss of consciousness, hypotension/shock, tachycardia, tingling, angioedema (including laryngeal, pharyngeal, or facial edema), airway obstruction, bronchospasm, dyspena, urticaria, and pruritus.

Serious allergic events, including anaphylactic or anaphylactoid reactions, have been reported to patients re-exposed to muronmonab-CD3 subsequent to their initial course of therapy. Pretreatment with antihistamines and/or steroids may not reliably prevent anaphylaxis in this setting. Possible allergic hazards of retreatment should be weighed against expected therapeutic benefits and alternatives. If retreatment with muronmonab-CD3 is employed, epinephrine and other emergency life-support equipment should be available, and the patient should be monitored closely.

If hypersensitivity is suspected, discontinue the drug immediately, do not resume therapy or re-expose the patient to muronmonab-CD3. Serious acute hypersensitivity reactions may require emergency treatment with 0.3 ml to 0.5 ml aqueous epinephrine (1:1000 dilution) subcutaneously and other resuscitative measures including oxygen, intravenous fluids, antihistamines, corticosteroids, pressor amines, and airway management, as clinically indicated. (See PRECAUTIONS, Cytokine Release Syndrome vs. Anaphylactic Reactions and ADVERSE REACTIONS, Hypersensitivity Reactions.)

Neuro-Psychiatric Events: Seizures, encephalopathy, cerebral edema, aseptic meningitis, and headache have been reported, even following the first dose during therapy with muronmonab-CD3, resulting in part from T cell activation and subsequent systemic-release of cytokines.

Seizures , some accompanied by loss of consciousness or cardiorespiratory arrest, or death, have occurred independently or in conjunction with any of the neurologic syndromes described below. Patients predisposed to seizures may include those with the following conditions: acute tubular necrosis/uremia, fever, infection, a precipitous fall in serum calcium, fluid overload, hypertension, hypoglycemia, history of seizures, and electrolyte imbalances or those who are taking a medication concomitantly that may, by itself, cause seizures.

Between 1987 and 1992, 75 post-marketing reports described seizures, averaging about 12 per year, and including 23 fatalities. More than two-thirds of these reports (53) were of domestic spontaneous origin, and their age and sex distributions were broad. Post-licensure reports generally do not provide sufficient basis for estimation of actual risks (incidence rates for specific adverse events), due to the typically substantial but unknown extent of under-ascertainment of incident events. Nonetheless, the number and regularity of seizure reports with muronmonab-CD3 (muromonab-CD3) indicate that this hazard appears not to be rare. Convulsions should be anticipated clinically with appropriate patient monitoring.

WARNINGS: *(cont'd)*

Manifestations of encephalopathy may include: impaired cognition, confusion, obtundation, altered mental status, auditory/visual hallucinations, psychosis (delirium, paranoia), mood changes (*e.g.*, mania, agitation, combativeness, etc.), diffuse hypotonus, hyperreflexia, myoclonus, tremor, asterixis, involuntary movements, major motor seizures, lethargy/stupor/coma, and diffuse weakness. Approximately one-third of patients with a diagnosis of encephalopathy may have had coexisting aseptic meningitis syndrome.

Cerebral edema: (and other signs of increased vascular permeability *e.g.*, otitis media, nasal and ear stuffiness, etc.) has been seen in patients treated with muronmonab-CD3 and may accompany some of the other neurologic manifestations.

Signs and symptoms of the **aseptic meningitis syndrome** described in association with use of muronmonab-CD3 have included: fever, headache, meningismus (stiff neck), and photophobia. In a post-marketing survey involving 214 renal transplant patients, the incidence of this syndrome was 6%. Fever (89%), headache (44%), neck stiffness (14%), and photophobia (10%) were the most commonly reported symptoms; a combination of these four symptoms occurred in 5% of patients. Diagnosis is confirmed by cerebrospinal fluid (CSF) analysis demonstrating leukocytosis with pleocytosis, elevated protein and normal or decreased glucose, with negative viral, bacterial, and fungal cultures. In any immunosuppressed transplant patient with clinical findings suggesting meningitis, the possibility of infection should be evaluated. Approximately one-third of the patients with a diagnosis of aseptic meningitis had coexisting signs and symptoms of encephalopathy. Most patients with the aseptic meningitis syndrome had a benign course and recovered without any permanent sequelae during therapy or subsequent to its completion or discontinuation.

Headache: is frequently seen after any of the first few doses and may occur in any of the aforementioned neurologic syndromes or by itself.

The following additional neurologic events have each been reported occasionally in post-licensure reports: irreversible blindness, impaired vision, quadri- or paraparesis/plegia, cerebrovascular accident (hemiparesis/plegia), aphasia, transient, ischemic attack, subarachnoid hemorrhage, palsy of the VI cranial nerve, and hearing loss.

Signs or symptoms of encephalopathy, meningitis, seizures, and cerebral edema, with or without headache, have typically been reversible. Headache, aseptic meningitis, seizures, and loss severe forms of encephalopathy resolved in most patients despite continued treatment. However, some events have been irreversible.

Other neurologic events observed in patients treated with muronmonab-CD3 include: post-therapy encephalopathy with or without coexisting metabolic disturbances, post-therapy meningitis, CNS lymphoproliferative disorders and infections. Since these patients usually had both serious and multiple coexisting medical conditions and were also receiving multiple concomitant medications, the association of these events with muronmonab-CD3 treatment in unclear.

Patients who may be at greater risk for CNS adverse experiences: include those with known or suspected CNS disorders (*e.g.*, history of seizure disorder, etc); with cerebrovascular disease (small or large vessel); with conditions having associated neurologic problems (*e.g.*, head trauma, uremia, etc.); with underlying vascular diseases; or who are receiving a medication concomitantly that may, by itself, affect the central nervous system. (See WARNINGS, PRECAUTIONS; ADVERSE REACTIONS, Cytokine Release Syndrome; and DRUG INTERACTIONS.)

Consequences of Immunosuppression: Serious and sometimes fatal infections and neoplasias have been reported in association with immunosuppressive therapies, including those regimens containing muronmonab-CD3.

Infections: Muronmonab-CD3 is usually added to immunosuppressive therapeutic regimens, thereby augmenting the degree immunosuppression. This increase in the total burden of immunosuppression may alter the spectrum of infections observed and increase the risk, the severity, and the potential gravity (morbidity) of infectious complications. During the first month post-transplant, patients are at greatest risk for the following infections: (1) those present prior to transplant, perhaps exacerbated by post-transplant immunosuppression; (2) infection conveyed by the donor organ; and (3) the usual post-operative urinary tract, intravenous line-related, wound, or pulmonary infections due to bacterial pathogens.

Approximately one to six months post-transplant, patients are at risk viral infections [*e.g.*, Cytomegalovirus (CMV), Epstein-Barr Virus (EBV), Herpes simplex virus (HSV), etc.] which produce serious systemic disease and which also increase the overall state of immunosuppression. Clinically significant infections (*e.g.*, pneumonia, sepsis, etc.) may occur with any microorganisms including; *Pneumocystis carinii, Listeria monocytogenes, Aspergillus* species, *Candida* species, *Nocardia asteroides, Legionella,* mycobacteria, gram-negative rods, and gram-positive cocci (staphylococci and streptococci), etc. Opportunistic infections, related to decreased T cell function, are associated with all immunosuppressive modalities employed to treat transplant rejection. Multiple or intensive courses of any anti-T cell antibody preparation, including muronmonab-CD3, which produce profound impairment of cell-mediated immunity, further increase the risk of (opportunistic) infection, especially with the Herpes viruses (HSV, CMV, EBV) and fungi.

Reactivation (1 to 4 months post-transplant) of EBV and CMV has been reported. Infectious syndromes due to CMV have included; fever of unknown origin, pneumonia, viremia, hepatitis, liver/renal dysfunction, gastritis or gastrointestinal ulcerations, pancreatitis, chorioretinitis, leukopenia, and thrombocytopenia. When administration of an antilymphocyte antibody, including muronmonab-CD3, is followed by an immunosuppressive regimen including cyclosporine, there is an increased risk of reactivating CMV and impaired ability to limit its proliferation, resulting in symptomatic and disseminated disease, EBV infection, either primary or reactivated, may play an important role in the development of post-transplant lymphoproliferative disorders. (See WARNINGSand ADVERSE REACTIONS, Neoplasia.)

Anti-Infective prophylaxis may reduce the morbidity associated with certain potential pathogens and should be considered for high-risk patients. Judicious use of immunosuppressive drugs, including type, dosage, and duration, may limit the risk and seriousness of some opportunistic infections. It is also possible to reduce the risk of serious CMV infection by avoiding transplantation of a CMV-seropositive (donor) organ into a seronegative patient.

Neoplasia: As a result of depressed cell-mediated immunity, organ transplant patients have an increased risk of developing malignancies. This risk is evidenced most exclusively by the occurrence of lymphoproliferative disorders (LPD), lymphomas, and skin cancers. In immunosuppressed patients, T cell cytotoxicity is impaired allowing for transformation and proliferation of EBV-Infected B lymphocytes. Transformed B lymphocytes are thought to initiate the oncogenic process that ultimately culminates in the development of most post-transplant lymphoproliferative disorders. (See ADVERSE REACTIONS, Neoplasia.)

Following the initiation of muronmonab-CD3 therapy, patients should be continuously monitored for evidence of LPD, through physical examination and histological evaluation of any suspect lymphoid tissue. Vigilant surveillance is advised, since early detection with subsequent reduction of total immunosuppression may result in regression of some of these lymphoproliferative disorders. Since the potential for the development of LPD is related to the duration and extent (intensity) of total immunosuppression, physicians are advised: to adhere to the recommended dosage and duration of muronmonab-CD3 therapy; to limit the number of courses of muronmonab-CD3 and other anti-T lymphocyte antibody preparations

WARNINGS: *(cont'd)*

administered within a short period of time; and if appropriate, to reduce the dosage(s) of immunosuppressive drugs used concomitantly to the lowest level compatible with an effective therapeutic response. (See DOSAGE AND ADMINISTRATION.)

The long-term risk of neoplastic events in patients being treated with muronmonab-CD3 has been determined.

PRECAUTIONS:

GENERAL

Prior to Treatment with Muronmonab-CD3

Fluid Status: The patient's volume (fluid) status should be assessed carefully. It is imperative, especially prior to the first few doses, that there be no clinical evidence of volume overload or uncompensated heart failure, including a clear chest X-ray and weight restriction of ≤3% above the patient's minimum weight during the week prior to injection.

Fever: If the temperature of the patient exceeds 37.8°C (100°F), it should be lowered by antipyretics before administration of each dose of muronmonab-CD3. The possibility of infection should be evaluated.

Blood Tests: Periodic assessment of organ system functions (renal, hepatic, and hematopoietic) should be performed.

During therapy with muronmonab-CD3: Periodic monitoring to ensure plasma muronmonab-CD3 levels (>800 ng/ml) or T cell clearance (CD3 positive T cells <25 cells/mm^3) is recommended.

Severe Cytokine Release Syndrome Versus Anaphylactic Reactions: It may be very difficult, even impossible, to distinguish between an acute hypersensitivity reaction (*e.g.,* anaphylaxis, angioedema, etc.) and the Cytokine Release Syndrome. Potentially serious signs and symptoms having an immediate onset (usually within 10 minutes) following administration of muronmonab-CD3 are more likely due to acute hypersensitivity; discontinue the drug immediately. If hypersensitivity is suspected, do not resume therapy or re-expose the patient to muronmonab-CD3. Clinical manifestations beginning approximately 30 to 60 minutes (or later) following administration of muronmonab-CD3, are more likely to be cytokine-mediated. (See WARNINGS, Cytokine Release Syndrome, Anaphylactic Reactions.)

Neuro-Psychiatric Events: Since some seizures (and other serious central nervous system events) following muronmonab-CD3 administration have been life-threatening, anti-seizure precautions (*e.g.,* an airway ready to use, if needed) should be taken. (See WARNINGSand ADVERSE REACTIONS, Neuro, Psychiatric Events.)

Infection/Viral-Induced Lymphoproliferative Disorders: Patients must be observed carefully for any signs and symptoms suggesting infection or viral-induced lymphoproliferative disorders (LPD). Anti-infective prophylaxis should be considered for patients at high risk. If infection or viral-induced LPD occur, culture or biopsy as soon as possible, promptly institute appropriate anti-infective therapy, and (if possible) reduce/discontinue immunosuppressive therapy.

When using combinations of immunosuppressive agents, the dose of each agent, including muronmonab-CD3, should be reduced to the lowest level compatible with an effective therapeutic response so as to reduce the potential for and severity of infections and malignant transformations. (SeeWARNINGS, Infections, Neoplasia.)

Low Protein-Binding Filter: Use a low protein-binding 0.2 or 0.22 micrometer (μm) filter to prepare the injections. (See DOSAGE AND ADMINISTRATION instructions.)

Sensitization: Muronmonab-CD3 is a mouse (immunoglobulin) protein that can induce human anti-mouse antibody production) i.e., sensitization) in patients following exposure (see: CLINICAL PHARMACOLOGY). Monitoring for human antibody titers after muronmonab-CD3 therapy is strongly recommended. (See CONTRAINDICATIONS.)

Reduced T cell clearance or impaired ability to maintain adequate muronmonab-CD3 levels provides a basis for adjusting muronmonab-CD3 dosage or for discontinuing therapy. (See WARNINGS, Anaphylactic Reactions ; PRECAUTIONS, Laboratory Tests; ADVERSE REACTIONS, Hypersensitivity Reactions.)

Intravascular Thrombosis: As with other immunosuppressive therapies, arterial or venous thromboses of allografts and other vascular beds (*e.g.,* heart, lungs, brain, bowel, etc.) have been reported in patients treated with muronmonab-CD3. The decision to use muronmonab-CD3 in patients with a history of thrombotic events or underlying vascular disease should take these findings into consideration. Concomitant use of prophylactic anti-thrombotic interventions (*e.g.,* mini-dose heparin, etc.) should be considered. (See ADVERSE REACTIONS.)

INFORMATION FOR THE PATIENT

Patients should be advised:

of the signs and symptoms associated with the Cytokine Release Syndrome, including the potentially serious nature of this symptom complex (*e.g.,* systemic, cardiovascular, neuro-psychiatric events).

to seek medical attention at the first sign of skin rash, urticaria, rapid heartbeat, difficulty in swallowing and breathing, or any swelling that may suggest angioedema or other allergic reaction.

to know how they might react to muronmonab-CD3 before operating an automobile or machinery, or engaging in activities requiring mental alertness and coordination.

of the potential benefits and other risks attendant to the use of muronmonab-CD3. (See BOXED WARNING ; WARNINGS ; PRECAUTIONS ; ADVERSE REACTIONS.)

LABORATORY TESTS

As with many potent drugs, periodic assessment of organ system functions should be performed during treatment with muronmonab-CD3.

The following tests should be monitored prior to and during muronmonab-CD3 therapy:

Renal: BUN, serum creatinine, etc.;

Hepatic: Transaminases, alkaline phosphatase, bilirubin;

Hematopoietic: WBCs and differential, platelet count, etc.;

Chest X-ray within 24 hours before initiating muronmonab-CD3 treatment. *Recommendation: chest X-ray should be free of any evidence of heart failure or fluid overload.*

One of the following immunologic tests should be monitored **during**muronmonab-CD3 therapy:

Plasma muronmonab-CD3 levels (as determined by an ELISA): *target muronmonab-CD3 levels should be ≥800 ng/ml; or*

Quantitative T lymphocyte surface phenotyping (CD3, CD4, CD8); target CD3 positive T cells <25 cells/mm^3.

Testing for human-mouse antibody titers is strongly recommended; *a titer ≥1:1000 is a contraindication for use.* (See CONTRAINDICATIONS and PRECAUTIONS, Sensitization.)

CARCINOGENESIS

Long-term studies have not been performed in laboratory animals to evaluate the carcinogenic potential of muronmonab-CD3. (See WARNINGS and ADVERSE REACTIONS, Neoplasia.)

PRECAUTIONS: *(cont'd)*

PREGNANCY CATEGORY C

Animal reproductive studies have not been conducted with muronmonab-CD3. It is also not known whether muronmonab-CD3 can cause fetal harm when administered to a pregnant woman or can affect reproduction capacity. However, muronmonab-CD3 is an IgG antibody and may cross the human placenta. The effect on the fetus of the release of cytokines and/or immunosuppression after treatment with muronmonab-CD3 is not known. If this drug is used during pregnancy, or the patient should become pregnant while taking this drug, the patient should be apprised of the potential hazard to the fetus. (See CONTRAINDICATIONS, WARNINGS, and ADVERSE REACTIONS.)

NURSING MOTHERS

It is not known whether muronmonab-CD3 is excreted in human milk. Because many drugs are excreted in human milk and because of the potential for serious adverse reactions/oncogenesis shown for muronmonab-CD3 in human studies, a decision should be made to discontinue nursing or to discontinue the drug, taking into account the importance of the drug to the mother. (See CONTRAINDICATIONS.)

PEDIATRIC USE

Safety and effectiveness in children have not been established. No adequately controlled clinical studies have been conducted in children. Published literature[4,10] has reported the use of muronmonab-CD3 in infants/children beginning with a dose of ≤5 mg. Based on immunologic monitoring, the dosage has been adjusted accordingly (see PRECAUTIONS, Laboratory Tests.) Pediatric recipients are reported to be significantly immunosuppressed for a prolonged period of time and therefore, require close monitoring post-therapy for opportunistic infections, particularly varicella (VZV), which poses an infectious complication unique to this population. Gastrointestinal fluid loss secondary to diarrhea and/or vomiting resulting from the Cytokine Release Syndrome may be significant when treating small children and may require parental hydration. It is unknown whether there may be significant long-term sequelae (*e.g.,* neurodevelopmental language difficulties in infants under 1 year of age) related to the occurrence of seizures, high fever, CNS infections, aseptic meningitis, etc., following muronmonab-CD3 treatment. In cases where administration of muronmonab-CD3 would be deemed medically appropriate, more vigilant and frequent monitoring is required for children than in adults. (See BOXED WARNING; WARNINGS; PRECAUTIONS; and ADVERSE REACTIONS.)

DRUG INTERACTIONS:

The following medications are frequently used with muronmonab-CD3 and the information provided below may be helpful in evaluating any adverse events reported in muronmonab-CD3 treated patients.

With *indomethacin*: Encephalopathy and other CNS effects have been reported in patients treated with indomethacin alone and in conjunction with muronmonab-CD3. The mechanism of these effects is unknown.

With *corticosteroids*: Psychosis and infections have been seem in patients treated with corticosteroids alone and in conjunction with muronmonab-CD3.

With *azathioprine*: Infections or malignancies have been reported with azathioprine alone and in conjunction with muronmonab-CD3.

With *cyclosporine*: Seizures, encephalopathy, infections, malignancies and thrombotic events have been reported in patients receiving cyclosporine alone and in conjunction with muronmonab-CD3.

ADVERSE REACTIONS:

Cytokine Release Syndrome: In controlled clinical trials for treatment of acute renal allograft rejection, patients treated with muronmonab-CD3 plus concomitant low-dose immunosuppressive therapy (primarily azathioprine and corticosteroids) were observed to have an increased incidence of adverse experiences during the first two days of treatment, as compared with the group of patients receiving azathioprine and high-dose steroid therapy. During this period the majority of patients experienced pyrexia (90%), of which were 19% were 40.0°C (104°F) or above, and chills (59%). In addition, other adverse experiences occurring in 8% or more of the patients during the first two days of muronmonab-CD3 therapy included: dyspnea (21%), nausea (19%), vomiting (19%), chest pain (14%), diarrhea (14%), tremor (13%), wheezing (13%), headache (11%), tachycardia (10%), rigor (8%), and hypertension (8%). A similar spectrum of clinical manifestations has been observed in open clinical studies and in post-marketing experience involving patients treated with muronmonab-CD3 for rejection following renal, cardiac and hepatic transplantation.

Additional serious and occasionally fatal cardiorespiratory manifestations have been reported following any of the first few doses. (See WARNINGS, Cytokine Release Syndrome and ADVERSE REACTIONS, Cardiovascular, Respiratory.)

In the acute renal allograft rejection trials, potentially fatal pulmonary edema had been reported following the first two doses in less than 2% of the patients treated with muronmonab-CD3. Pulmonary edema was usually associated with fluid overload. However, post-marketing experience revealed that pulmonary edema has occurred in patients who appeared to be euvolemic, presumably as a consequence of cytokine-medicated increased vascular permeability ("leaky capillaries") and/or reduced myocardial contractility/compliance (*i.e.,* left ventricular dysfunction). (See WARNINGS, Cytokine Release Syndrome, and DOSAGE AND ADMINISTRATION.)

Infections: In the controlled randomized renal rejection trial conducted during the pre-cyclosporine era, the most common infections during the first 45 days of muronmonab-CD3 therapy were due to Herpes simplex (27%) and cytomegalovirus (19%). Other severe and life-threatening infections were *Staphylococcus epidermidis* (4.8%),*Pneumocystis carinii* (3.1%), *Legionella* (1.6%),*Cryptococcus* (1.6%), *Serratia* (1.6%) and gram-negative bacteria (1.6%). The incidence of infections was similar in patients treated with muronmonab-CD3 and in patients treated with high-dose steroids.

In clinical trial of acute hepatic rejection refractory to conventional treatment, the most common infections reported in patients treated with muronmonab-CD3 during the first 45 days of the study were cytomegalovirus (15.7% of patients, of which 43% of infections were severe), and Herpes simplex (7.5% patients, of which 10% were severe). Other severe and life-threatening infections were gram-positive infections (9.0% of patients), gram-negative infections (7.5% of patients), viral infections (1.5% of patients), and *Legionella* (0.7% of patients). In another hepatic rejection trial incidence of fungal infections was 34% and infections with the Herpes simplex virus was 31%.

In a clinical trial of acute cardiac rejection refractory to conventional treatment, the most common infections reported in the muronmonab-CD3 group during the first 45 days of the study were Herpes simplex (5% of patients, of which 20% were severe), fungal infections (4% of patients, of which 75% were severe, and cytomegalovirus (3% of patients, of which 33% were severe). No other severe or life-threatening infections were reported during this period.

Clinically significant infections (*e.g.,* pneumonia, sepsis, etc.) due to the following pathogens have been reported:

ADVERSE REACTIONS: *(cont'd)*

Bacterial: *Clostridium* species (including perfringens), *Corynebacterium,* Enteroccus, *Enterobacter aerogenes,Escherichia coli, Klebsiella* species, Nocardia asteroides, *Proteus* species, *Providencia* species, *Pseudomonas aeruginosa, Serratia* species, *Staphylococcus* species, *Streptococcus* species. *Yersinia enterocolitica,* and other gram-negative bacteria.

Fungal: **Aspergillus, Candida,* Cryptococcal, Dermatophytes.

Protozoa: *Pneumocystis carinii, Toxoplasma gondii.*

Viral: Cytomegalovirus* (CMV), Epstein-Barr virus* (EBV), Herpes simplex virus* (HSV), Hepatitis viruses, Varicella virus (VZV).

As a consequence of being a potent immunosuppressive, the incidence and severity of infections with designated(*) pathogens, especially the Herpes family of viruses, may be increased. (See WARNINGS, Infections.)

Neoplasia: In patients treated with muronmonab-CD3, post-transplant lymphoproliferative disorders (LPD) reported have ranged from lymphadenopathy or benign polyclonal B cell hyperplasias to malignant and often fatal monoclonal B cell lymphomas. In post-marketing experience, approximately one-third of the lymphoproliferations reported were benign, and two-thirds were malignant. Classification of these lymphomas has included: B cell, large cell, polyclonal, non-Hodgkin's lymphocytic, T cell, Burkitt's; the majority have not been classified histologically. When malignant lymphomas have been reported, they have appeared to develop soon after transplantation, the majority within the first four months post-treatment. Many of these have been rapidly progressive, widely disseminated at time of diagnosis, and fatal. Carcinomas of the skin have included: basal cell, squamous cell, Kaposi's sarcoma, melanoma, and keratoacanthoma. Other neoplasms infrequently reported include: multiple myeloma, leukemia, carcinoma of the breast, adenocarcinoma, cholangiocarcinoma, and recurrences of pre-existing hepatoma and renal cell carcinoma. (See WARNINGS, Neoplasia.)

Hypersensitivity Reactions: Reported adverse reactions resulting from the formation of antibodies to muronmonab-CD3 have included antigens-antibody (immune complex) mediated syndromes and IgE-mediated reactions. Reported hypersensitivity reactions have ranged from a mild, self-limited rash or pruritus to severe, life-threatening anaphylactic reactions/shock or angioedema (including: swelling of lips, eyelids, laryngeal spasm and airway obstruction with hypoxia). (See WARNINGS, Anaphylactic Reactions.)

Other hypersensitivity reactions have included: ineffectiveness of treatment, serum sickness, arthritis, allergic interstitial nephritis, immune complex deposition resulting in glomerulonephritis, vasculitis, and temporal arteritis, and eosinophilia.

Clinical adverse events occurring trials and post-marketing experience are listed below by body system.

Body as a Whole: fever (including, spiking temperatures as high as 107°F), chills/rigors, flu-like syndrome, fatigue/malaise, generalized weakness, anorexia.

Cardiovascular: cardiac arrest, hypotension/shock, heart failure, cardiovascular collapse, angina/myocardial infarction, tachycardia, bradycardia, hemodynamic instability, hypertension, left ventricular dysfunction, arrhythmias, chest pain/tightness.

Respiratory: respiratory arrest, adult respiratory distress syndrome (ARDS), respiratory failure, pulmonary edema (cardiogenic or noncardiogenic), apnea, dyspnea, bronchospasm, wheezing, shortness of breath, hypoxemia, tachypnea/hyperventilation, abnormal chest sounds, and pneumonia/pneumonitis (bacterial, viral, *P. carinii,* etc.).

Dermatologic: rash, urticaria, pruritus, erythema, flushing, diaphoresis.

Gastrointestinal: diarrhea, nausea/vomiting, abdominal pain, bowel infarction.

Hematopoietic: pancytopenia, aplastic anemia, neutropenia, leukopenia, thrombocytopenia, lymphopenia, leukocytosis, lymphadenopathy; arterial and venous thrombosis of allografts and other vascular beds (*e.g.,* heart, lung, brain, bowel, etc.); disturbances of coagulation.

Hepatobiliary: increases in transaminases (SGOT, SGPT, etc.); hepato/splenomegaly or hepatitis, usually secondary to viral infection or lymphoma.

Neuro-Psychiatric: seizures, lethargy/stupor/coma, encephalopathy, psychotic reactions (delirium), encephalitis, meningitis, cerebral edema, headache, dizziness, tremor, aphasia, quadri- or paraparesis/plegia, obtundation, confusion, altered mental status (*e.g.,* paranoia, etc.), impaired cognition, disorientation, auditory and visual hallucinations, agitation/combativeness, mood changes (*e.g.,* mania, etc.), hypotonus, hyperreflexia, myoclonus, asterixis, involuntary movements, CNS infections, CNS malignancies, cerebrovascular accident, hemiparesis/plegia, transient ischemic attack, subarachnoid hemorrhage.

Musculoskeletal: arthralgia, arthritis, myalgia, stiffness/aches/pains.

Special Senses: blindness, blurred vision, diplopia, hearing loss, otitis media, tinnitus, vertigo, VI cranial nerve palsy, photophobia, conjunctivitis, nasal and ear stuffiness.

Renal: anuria/oliguria; delayed graft function; transient and reversible increases in BUN and serum creatinine; abnormal urinary cytology, including exfoliation of damaged lymphocytes, collecting duct cells and cellular casts.

OVERDOSAGE:

The maximum amount of muronmonab-CD3 that can be safely administered in single or multiple doses has not been determined.

DOSAGE AND ADMINISTRATION:

The recommended dose of muronmonab-CD3 for the treatment of acute renal, steroid-resistant cardiac, or steroid-resistant hepatic allograft rejection is 5 mg per day in a single (**bolus**) intravenous injection for 10 to 14 days. For acute renal rejection, treatment should be begin upon diagnosis. For steroid-resistant cardiac or hepatic allograft rejection, treatment should begin when the treating physician deems a rejection has not been reversed by adequate course of corticosteroid therapy. (See CLINICAL PHARMACOLOGYand PRECAUTIONS, Sensitization, Laboratory Tests.)

For the first few doses, patients should be monitored in a facility equipped and staffed for cardiopulmonary resuscitation with frequent determinations of vital signs. With subsequent doses, the patient should be monitored following muronmonab-CD3 therapy in a facility equipped and staffed for CPR for an appropriate period time of based on the patient's clinical status. Since the Cytokine Release Syndrome may also occur following a treatment hiatus and resumption of therapy, as with the first few doses, exercise vigilant care.

Prior to the administration of any dose of muronmonab-CD3, the patient's temperature should be lowered to <37.8°C (100°F).

Prior to administration of muronmonab-CD3, the patient's volume status should be assessed carefully. It is imperative, especially prior to the first few doses, that there be no clinical evidence of volume overload or uncompensated heart failure, including a clear chest x-ray and weight restriction of ≤3% above the patient's minimum weight during the week prior to injection. (See WARNINGS, Cytokine Release Syndrome, and ADVERSE REACTIONS, Cytokine Release Syndrome.)

Intravenous methylprednisolone sodium succinate 8.0 mg/kg given 1 to 4 hours prior to administering the first dose of muronmonab-CD3 is strongly recommended to decrease the incidence and severity of reactions to the first dose, which have been attributed to the muronmonab-CD3-mediated Cytokine Release Syndrome. Acetaminophen and antihistamines given concomitantly with muronmonab-CD3 may also help to reduce some early reactions. (See WARNINGS, Cytokine Release Syndrome, and ADVERSE REACTIONS, Cytokine Release Syndrome.)

When using concomitant immunosuppressive drugs, the dose of each should be reduced to the lowest level compatible with an effective therapeutic response in order to reduce the potential for malignant transformations and the incidence and/or severity of infections. Maintenance immunosuppression should be resumed approximately three days prior to the cessation of muronmonab-CD3 therapy. (See WARNINGS, Infection, Neoplasia and ADVERSE REACTIONS, Infection, Neoplasia.)

ADMINISTRATION INSTRUCTIONS

1. Prior to administration, parenteral drug products should be inspected visually for particulate matter and discoloration. Because muromonab-CD3 is a protein solution, it may develop a few fine translucent particles which have been shown not affect its potency.

2. No bacteriostatic agent is present in this product; adherence to aseptic technique is advised. Once the ampule is opened, use immediately and discard the unused portion.

3. Prepare muronmonab-CD3 for injection by drawing solution into a syringe through a low protein-binding 0.2 or 0.22 micrometer (μm) filter. Discard filter and attach a new needle for intravenous bolus injection.

4. Since no data is available on compatibility of muronmonab-CD3 with other intravenous substances or additives, other medications/substances should not be added or infused simultaneously through the same intravenous line. If the same intravenous line is used for sequential infusion of several different drugs, the line should be flushed with saline before and after infusion of muronmonab-CD3.

5. Administer muronmonab-CD3 as an intravenous bolus in less than one minute. Do **not** administer by intravenous infusion or in conjunction with other drug solutions.

REFERENCES:

1 . Adair JC, Woodley SL, O'Connell JB, *et al.* Aseptic Meningitis following Cardiac Transplantation: Clinical Characteristics and Relationship to Immunosuppressive Regimen. Neurology 41:249- 252, 1991. **2.** Chatenoud L, Legendre C, Ferran C, *et al.*Corticosteroid Inhibition of the Okt3 - Induced Cytokine-Related Syndrome - Dosage and Kinetics Prerequisites. Transplantation 51:334-338, 1991. **3.** Cockfield SM, Preiksaitis J, Harvey E, Jones C, Herbert D, Keown P, and Halloran PF. Is Sequential Use of ALG and Okt3 in Renal Transplants Associated With an Increased Incidence of Fulminant Post Transplant Lymphoproliferative Disorders? Transplant. Proc.23: 1106-1107, 1991. **4.** Ettenger RB, Marik J. Rosenthal JT, *et al.* Okt3 for Rejection Reversal in Pediatric Renal Transplantation. Clin. Transportation 2:180-184, 1988. **5.** Gaston RS, Deierhoi MH, Patterson T, *et al.* Okt3 First-Dose Reaction: Association with T Cell Subsets and Cytokine Release. Kid. International 39:141-148, 1991. **6.** Goldman M, Abramowicz D, DePauw L, *et al.* Okt3-Induced Cytokine Released Attenuation by High-Dose Methylprednisolone. Lancet2:802-803, 1989. **7.** Ortho Multicenter Transplant Study Group. A Randomized Clinical Trial of Okt3 Monoclonal Antibody for Acute Rejection of Cadaveric Renal Transplants. N. Engl. J. Med 313:337-342, 1985. **8.** Penn I. The Changing Patterns of Posttransplant Malignancies. Transplant Proc. 23: 1101-1103, 1991. **9.** Rubin RH and Tolkoff-Rubin NE. The Impact of Infection on the Outcome of Transplantation. Transplant Proc. 23:2068-2074, 1991. **10.** Schroeder TJ, Ryckman FC, Hurtubise PE, *et al.*Immunological Monitoring during and following Okt3 Therapy in Children. Clin. Transplantation 5:191-196, 1991.

HOW SUPPLIED:

Muronmonab-CD3 is supplied as a sterile solution in packages of 5 ampules. Each 5 ml ampule contains 5 mg of muromonab- CD3.

Storage : Store in a refrigerator at 2° to 8°C (36° to 46°F).

DO NOT FREEZE OR SHAKE.

HOW SUPPLIED - EQUIVALENTS NOT AVAILABLE:

Injection, Solution - Intravenous - 1 mg/ml

5 ml $672.00 ORTHOCLONE OKT-3, Ortho Biotech 59676-0101-01

MYCOPHENOLATE MOFETIL *(003256)*

CATEGORIES: Immunologic; Immunomodulators; Immunosuppressives; Renal Drugs; Renal Transplantation; Transplantation; FDA Class 1P ("Priority Review"); FDA Approved 1995 May

BRAND NAMES: **Cellcept**

Increased susceptibility to infection and the possible development of lymphoma may result from immunosuppression. Only physicians experienced in immunosuppressive therapy and management of renal transplant patients should use mycophenolate mofetil. Patients receiving the drug should be managed in facilities equipped and staffed with adequate laboratory and supportive medical resources. The physician responsible for maintenance therapy should have complete information requisite for the follow-up of the patient.

DESCRIPTION:

Mycophenolate mofetil is the 2-morpholinoethyl ester of mycophenolic acid (MPA), an immunosuppressive agent.

The chemical name for mycophenolate mofetil is 2-morpholinoethyl (E)-6-(1,3-dihydro-4-hydroxy-6-methoxy-7-methyl-3-oxo-5-isobenzofuranyl)-4-methyl-4-hexenoate. It has an empirical formula of $C_{23}H_{31}NO_7$ and a molecular weight of 433.50.

Mycophenolate mofetil is available for oral administration as capsules containing 250 mg of mycophenolate mofetil. Inactive ingredients include croscarmellose sodium, magnesium stearate, povidone (K-90) and pregelatinized starch. The capsule shells contain black iron oxide, FD&C blue #2, gelatin, red iron oxide, silicon dioxide, sodium lauryl sulfate, titanium dioxide, and yellow iron oxide.

Mycophenolate mofetil is a white to off-white crystalline powder. It is slightly soluble in water (43 mcg/ml at pH 7.4); the solubility increases in acidic medium (4.27 mg/ml at pH 3.6) It is freely soluble in acetone, soluble in methanol, and sparingly soluble in ethanol. The apparent partition coefficient in 1-octanol/water (pH 7.4) buffer solution is 238. The pKa values for mycophenolate mofetil are 5.6 for the morpholino group and 8.5 for the phenolic group.

CLINICAL PHARMACOLOGY:

Mechanism of Action: Mycophenolate mofetil has been demonstrated in experimental animal models to prolong the survival of allogeneic transplants (kidney, heart, liver, intestine, limb, small bowel, pancreatic islets, and bone marrow). Mycophenolate mofetil has also been shown to reverse ongoing acute rejection in the canine renal and rat cardiac allograft models. Mycophenolate mofetil also inhibited proliferative arteriopathy in experimental models of aortic and heart allografts in rats, as well as in primate cardiac xenografts. Mycophenolate mofetil was used alone or in combination with other immunosuppressive agents in these studies. Mycophenolate mofetil has been demonstrated to inhibit tumor development and prolong survival in murine tumor transplant models.

Mycophenolate mofetil is rapidly absorbed following oral administration and hydrolyzed to form MPA, which is the active metabolite. MPA is a potent, selective, uncompetitive and reversible inhibitor of inosine monophosphate dehydrogenase (IMPDH), and therefore inhibits the *de novo* pathway of guanosine nucleotide synthesis without incorporation into DNA. Because T- and B-lymphocytes are critically dependent for their proliferation on *de novo* synthesis of purines whereas other cell types can utilize salvage pathways, MPA has potent

CLINICAL PHARMACOLOGY: *(cont'd)*

cytostatic effects on lymphocytes. MPA inhibits proliferative responses of T- and B-lymphocytes to both mitogenic and allospecific stimulation. Addition of guanosine or deoxyguanosine reverses the cytostatic effects of MPA on lymphocytes. MPA also suppresses antibody formation by B-lymphocytes. MPA prevents the glycosylation of lymphocyte and monocyte glycoproteins that are involved in intercellular adhesion to endothelial cells and may inhibit recruitment of leukocytes into sites of inflammation and graft rejection. Mycophenolate mofetil did not inhibit early events in the activation of human peripheral blood mononuclear cells, such as the production of interleukin-1 (IL-1) and interleukin-2 (IL-2), but did not block the coupling of these events to DNA synthesis and proliferation.

Pharmacokinetics: Following oral administration, mycophenolate mofetil undergoes rapid and extensive absorption and complete presystemic metabolism to MPA, the active metabolite. MPA is metabolized to form the phenolic glucuronide of MPA (MPAG) which is not pharmacologically active. Mycophenolate mofetil is not measurable systemically in plasma following oral administration.

Absorption: In 12 healthy volunteers, the mean absolute bioavailability of oral mycophenolate mofetil relative to IV mycophenolate mofetil (based on MPA AUC) was 94%. The area under the plasma-concentration time curve (AUC) for MPA appears to increase in a dose-proportional fashion in renal transplant patients receiving multiple doses of mycophenolate mofetil up to daily doses of 3 g (see TABLE 1on pharmacokinetic parameters in renal transplant patients).

Immediately post-transplant (< 40 days), mean AUC and C_{max} are approximately 50% lower in renal transplant patients than that observed in healthy volunteers or in stable renal transplant patients.

Food (27 g fat, 650 calories) had no effect on the extent of absorption (MPA, AUC) of mycophenolate mofetil when administered at doses of 1.5 g b.i.d. to renal transplant patients. However, MPA C_{max} was decreased by 40% in the presence of food. (See DOSAGE AND ADMINISTRATION.)

Distribution: The mean (± SD) apparent volume of distribution of MPA in twelve healthy volunteers is approximately 3.6 (± 1.5) and 4.0 (± 1.2) l/kg following IV and oral administration, respectively. MPA, at clinically relevant concentrations, is 97% bound to plasma albumin. MPAG is 82% bound to plasma albumin at MPAG concentration ranges that are normally seen in stable renal transplant patients; however, at higher MPAG concentrations (observed in patients with renal impairment or delayed graft function), the binding of MPA may be reduced as a result of competition between MPAG concentrations (observed in patients with renal impairment or delayed graft function), the binding of MPA for protein binding. Mean blood to plasma ratio of radioactivity concentrations was approximately 0.6 indicating that MPA and MPAG do not extensively distribute into the cellular fractions of blood.

In vitro studies to evaluate the effect of other agents on the binding of MPA to human serum albumin (HSA) or plasma proteins showed that salicylate (at 25 mg/dl with HSA) and MPAG (at ≥ 460 mcg/ml with plasma proteins) increased the free fraction of MPA. At concentrations that exceeded what is encountered clinically, cyclosporine, digoxin, naproxen, prednisone, propranolol, tacrolimus, theophylline, tolbutamide, and warfarin did not increase the free fraction of MPA. MPA at concentrations as high as 100 mcg/ml had little effect on the binding of warfarin, digoxin or propranolol, but decreased the binding of theophylline from 53% to 45% and phenytoin from 90% to 87%.

Metabolism: Mycophenolate mofetil undergoes complete presystemic metabolism to MPA, the active metabolite. MPA is metabolized principally by glucuronyl transferase to form the phenolic glucuronide of MPA (MPAG) which is not pharmacologically active. The following metabolites of the 2-hydroxyethyl-morpholino moiety are also recovered in the urine following oral administration of mycophenolate mofetil to healthy subjects: N-(2-carboxymethyl)-morpholine, N-(2-hydroxyethyl)-morpholine, and the N-oxide of N-(2-hydroxyethyl)-morpholine.

Secondary peaks in the plasma MPA concentration-time profile are usually observed 6-12 hours post-dose. The coadministration of cholestyramine (4 g t.i.d.) resulted in approximately a 40% decrease in the MPA AUC (largely as a consequence of lower concentrations in the terminal portion of the profile). These observations suggest that enterohepatic recirculation contributes to MPA plasma concentrations.

Increased plasma concentrations of mycophenolate mofetil metabolites (MPA 50% increase and MPAG about 3-6 fold increase) are observed in patients with renal insufficiency. (See CLINICAL PHARMACOLOGY, Special Populations.)

Excretion: Negligible amount of drug is excreted as MPA (< 1% of dose) in the urine. Orally administered radiolabeled mycophenolate mofetil resulted in complete recovery of the administered dose; with 93% of the administered dose recovered in the urine and 6% recovered in the feces. Most (about 87%) of the administered dose is excreted in the urine as MPAG. MPA and MPAG are usually not removed by hemodialysis. However, at high MPAG plasma concentrations (> 100 mcg/ml), small amounts of MPAG are removed.

Mean (± SD) apparent half-life and plasma clearance of MPA are 17.9 (± 6.5) hours and 193 (± 48) ml/min following oral administration and 16.6 (± 5.8) hours and 177 (± 31) ml/min following IV administration, respectively.

Pharmacokinetics in Healthy Volunteers and Renal Transplant Patients: Shown below are the mean (± SD) pharmacokinetic parameters for MPA following the administration of oral mycophenolate mofetil given as single doses to healthy volunteers and multiple doses to renal transplant patients. As noted below, MPA AUC and C_{max} in early transplant patients (< 40 days post-transplant) are approximately 50% lower as compared to healthy volunteers or to stable renal transplant patients.

TABLE 1 Pharmacokinetic Parameters For Mpa [Mean (± SD)] Following Administration Of Mycophenolate Mofetil To Healthy Volunteers (Single Dose) And Renal Transplant Patient (Multiple Doses)

HealthyVolunteers (no. of subjects)	Dose	T_{max} (h)	C_{max} (mcg/ml)	Total AUC (mcg·h/ml)
(n=129) *(n=117)	1 g	0.80 (± 0.36)	24.5 (± 9.5)	63.9* (± 16.2)
Time After Renal Transplantation (no. of patients)	**Dose**	**T_{max} (h)**	**C_{max} (mcg/ml) (mcg·h/ml)**	**Interdosing Interval AUC_{0-12}**
Early (<40 days) (n=25)	1 g b.i.d.	1.31 (± 0.76)	8.16 (± 4.50)	27.3 (± 10.9)
Early (<40 days) (n=27)	1.5 g b.i.d.	1.21 (± 0.81)	13.5 (± 8.18)	38.4 (± 15.4)
Late (>3 months) (n=23)	1.5 g b.i.d.	0.90 (± 0.24)	24.1 (± 12.1)	65.3 (± 35.4)

SPECIAL POPULATIONS

Shown below are the mean (± SD) pharmacokinetic parameters for MPA following the administration of oral mycophenolate mofetil given as single doses to subjects with renal and hepatic impairment. (TABLE 2)

CLINICAL PHARMACOLOGY: *(cont'd)*

TABLE 2 Pharmacokinetic Parameters For MPA [mean (± SD)] Following Single Doses Of Mycophenolate Mofetil In Chronic Renal And Hepatic Impairment

Renal Impairment (no. of patients)	Dose	T_{max} (h)	C_{max} (mcg/ml)	AUC_{0-96} (mcg·h/ml)
Healthy Volunteers GFR > 80 ml/min/1.73m² (n=6)	1 g	0.75 (± 0.27)	25.3 (± 7.99)	45.0 (± 22.6)
Mild Renal Impairment GFR 50-80 ml/min/1.73m² (n=6)	1 g	0.75 (± 0.27)	26.0 (± 3.82)	59.9 (± 12.9)
Moderate Renal Impairment GFR 25-49 ml/min/1.73m² (n=6)	1 g	0.75 (± 0.27)	19.0 (± 13.2)	52.9 (± 25.5)
Severe Renal Impairment GFR < 25 ml/min/1.73m² (n=7)	1 g	1.00 (± 0.41)	16.3 (± 10.8)	78.6 (± 46.4)
Hepatic Impairment (no. of patients)	**Dose**	**T_{max} (h)**	**C_{max} (mcg/ml)**	**AUC_{0-48} (mcg°h/ml)**
Healthy Volunteers (n=6)	1 g	0.63 (± 0.14)	24.3 (± 5.73)	29.0 (± 5.78)
Alcoholic cirrhosis (n=18)	1 g	0.85 (± 0.58)	22.4 (± 10.1)	29.8 (± 10.7)

Renal Insufficiency: In a single-dose study (6 volunteers per group), plasma MPA AUCs observed in volunteers with severe chronic renal impairment [glomerular filtration rate (GFR) < 25 ml/min/1.73 m²] were about 75% higher relative to those observed in healthy volunteers (GFR > 80 ml/min/1.73 m²). In addition, the single dose plasma MPAG AUC was 3-6 fold higher in volunteers with severe renal impairment than in volunteers with mild renal impairment or healthy volunteers, consistent with the known renal elimination of MPAG. Multiple dosing of mycophenolate mofetil in patients with severe chronic renal impairment has not been studied. No data are available on the safety of long-term exposure to this level of MPAG. (See PRECAUTIONS, Generaland DOSAGE AND ADMINISTRATION.)

In patients with delayed graft function post-transplant, mean MPA AUC_{0-12} was comparable to that seen in post-transplant patients without delayed graft function. Mean plasma MPAG AUC_{0-12} was 2-3 fold higher than in post-transplant patients without delayed graft function. (See PRECAUTIONS, General and DOSAGE AND ADMINISTRATION.)

The pharmacokinetics of mycophenolate mofetil are not altered by hemodialysis. Hemodialysis usually does not remove MPA or MPAG. At high concentrations of MPAG (> 100 mcg/ml), hemodialysis removes only small amounts of MPAG.

Hepatic Insufficiency: In single dose (1 g) study of 18 volunteers with alcoholic cirrhosis and 6 healthy volunteers, hepatic MPA glucuronidation processes appeared to be relatively unaffected by hepatic parenchymal disease when pharmacokinetic parameters of healthy volunteers and alcoholic cirrhosis patients within this study were compared. However, it should be noted that for unexplained reasons, the healthy volunteers in this study had about 50% lower AUC as compared to healthy volunteers in other studies, thus making comparisons between volunteers with alcoholic cirrhosis and healthy volunteers difficult. Effects of hepatic disease on this process probably depend on the particular disease. Hepatic disease with other etiologies may show a different effect.

Pediatrics: Very limited pharmacokinetic data are available for pediatric renal transplant recipients. Data on these patients collected on day 21 post-transplant are presented in the table below. (TABLE 3)

TABLE 3 Pharmacokinetic Parameters For MPA [mean ± (SD)] Following Multiple Oral Doses Of Mycophenolate Mofetil In Pediatric Renal Transplant Patients

Age Range	Dose	T_{max} (h)	C_{max} (mcg/ml)	AUC_{0-12} (mcg·h/ml)
≥ 3 mo to < 6 yr (Mean = 2.75) (n=4)	15 mg/kg b.i.d.	1.25 (± 0.87)	3.70 (± 2.08)	13.6 (± 8.69)
≥ 6 yr to < 12 yr (mean = 9.0) (n=4)	15 mg/kg b.i.d.	0.50 (± 0.00)	13.5 (± 4.48)	23.4 (± 2.84)
≥ 12 yr to 18 yr (Mean = 15.6) (n=5)	15 mg/kg b.i.d.	0.50 (± 0.00)	13.2 (± 6.86)	30.0 (± 8.34)
≥ 12 yr to 18 yr (Mean = 14.0) (n=7)	23 mg/kg b.i.d.	1.14 (± 0.80)	10.6 (± 9.59)	28.3 (± 12.8)

Gender: Data obtained from several studies were pooled to look at any gender related differences in the pharmacokinetics of MPA (data were adjusted to 1 g dose). Mean (± SD) MPA $AUC_{0-12}$for males (n=79) was 32.0 (± 14.5) and for females (n=41) was 36.5 (± 18.8) mcg·h/ml while mean (± SD) MPA C_{max} was 9.96 (± 6.19) in the males and 10.6 (± 5.64) mcg/ml in the females. These differences are not of clinical significance.

Clinical Studies: the safety and efficacy of mycophenolate mofetil in combination with corticosteroids and cyclosporine for the prevention of organ rejection following allogeneic renal transplants were assessed in three randomized, double-blind, multicenter trials.

These studies compared two dose levels of mycophenolate mofetil (1.0 g b.i.d. and 1.5 g b.i.d. with azathioprine (2 studies) or placebo (1 study) when administered in combination with cyclosporine (Sandimmune) and corticosteroids to prevent acute rejection episodes. One study also included antithymocyte globulin (ATGAM) induction therapy. The three studies are described by geographic location of the investigational sites. One study was conducted in the USA at 14 sites, one study was conducted in Europe at 20 sites, and one study was conducted in Europe, Canada, and Australia at a total of 21 sites.

The primary efficacy endpoint was the proportion of patients in each treatment group who experienced treatment failure within the first six months after transplantation (defined as biopsy-proven acute rejection on treatment or the occurrence of death, graft loss or early termination from the study for any reason without prior biopsy-proven rejection). Mycophenolate mofetil, when administered with antithymocyte globulin (ATGAM) induction (one study) and with cyclosporine and corticosteroids (all three studies), was compared to the following three therapeutic regimens: (1) antithymocyte globulin (ATGAM) induction/azathioprine/cyclosporine/corticosteroids, (2) azathioprine/cyclosporine/corticosteroids, and (3) cyclosporine/corticosteroids.

Mycophenolate mofetil, in combination with corticosteroids and cyclosporine reduced (statistically significant at the < 0.05 level) the incidence of treatment failure within the first 6 months following transplantation. The following table (TABLE 4) summarize the results of these studies. These tables show (1) the proportion of patients experiencing treatment failure, (2) the proportion of patients, who experienced biopsy-proven acute rejection on treatment, and (3) early termination, for any reason other than graft loss or death, without a prior biop-

CLINICAL PHARMACOLOGY: *(cont'd)*

sy-proven acute rejection episode. Patients who prematurely discontinued treatment were followed for the occurrence of death or graft loss, and the cumulative incidence of graft loss and patient death are summarized separately. Patients who prematurely discontinued treatment were not followed for the occurrence of acute rejection after termination. More patients discontinued receiving mycophenolate mofetil (without prior biopsy-proven rejection, death or graft loss) than discontinued in the control groups, with the highest rate in the mycophenolate mofetil 3 g/day group. Therefore, the acute rejection rates may be underestimates, particularly in the mycophenolate mofetil 3 g/day group.

TABLE 4A Incidence of Treatment Failure (Biopsy-Proven Rejection of Early Termination for Any Reason)

USA Study (n=499)	CellCept 2 g/day (n=167)	CellCept 3 g/day (n=166)	Azathioprine 1-2 mg/kg/day (n=166)
All treatment failures	31.1%	31.3%	47.6%
Early termination without prior acute rejection*	9.6%	12.7%	6.0%
Biopsy-proven rejection episode on treatment	19.8%	17.5%	38.0%

TABLE 4B

Europe/Canada/ Australia Study (n=503)	CellCept 2 g/day (n=173)	CellCept 3 g/day (n=164)	Azathioprine 100-150 mg/day (n=166)
All treatment failures	38.2%	34.8%	50.0%
Early termination without prior acute rejection*	13.9%	15.2%	10.2%
Biopsy-proven rejection episode on treatment	19.7%	15.9%	35.5%

TABLE 4C

Europe Study (n=491)	CellCept 2 g/day (n=165)	CellCept 3 g/day (n=160)	Placebo (n=166)
All treatment failures	30.3%	38.8%	56.0%
Early termination without prior acute rejection*	11.5%	22.5%	7.2%
Biopsy-proven rejection episode on treatment	17.0%	13.8%	46.4%

* Does not include death and graft loss as reason for early termination

Cumulative incidence of twelve-month graft loss and patient death are presented below. No advantage of mycophenolate mofetil with respect to graft loss and patient death was established. Numerically, patients receiving mycophenolate mofetil 2 g/day and 3 g/day experienced a better outcome than controls in all three studies; patients receiving mycophenolate mofetil 2 g/day experienced a better outcome than mycophenolate mofetil 3 g/day in two of the three studies. Patients in all treatment groups who terminated treatment early were found to have a poor outcome with respect to graft loss and patient death at one year. (TABLE 5)

TABLE 5 Cumulative Incidence of Combined Graft Loss and Patient Death at 12 Mos

Study	CellCept 2 g/day	CellCept 3 g/day	Control (Azathioprine or Placebo)
USA	8.5%	11.5%	12.2%
Europe/ Canada/ Australia	11.7%	11.0%	13.6%
Europe	8.5%	10.0%	11.5%

INDICATIONS AND USAGE:

Mycophenolate mofetil is indicated for the prophylaxis of organ rejection in patients receiving allogenic renal transplants. Mycophenolate mofetil should be used concomitantly with cyclosporine and corticosteroids.

CONTRAINDICATIONS:

Allergic reactions to mycophenolate mofetil have been observed; therefore, mycophenolate mofetil is contraindicated in patients with a hypersensitivity to mycophenolate mofetil, mycophenolic acid or any component of the drug product.

WARNINGS:

(See BOXED WARNING.)

Patients receiving immunosuppressive regimens involving combinations of drugs, including mycophenolate mofetil, as part of an immunosuppressive regimen are at increased risk of developing lymphoma and other malignancies, particularly of the skin. The risk appears to be related to the intensity and duration of immunosuppression rather than to the use of any specific agent. Oversuppression of the immune system can also increase susceptibility to infection. Mycophenolate mofetil has been administered in combination with the following agents in clinical trials: antithymocyte globulin (ATGAM), OKT3 (Orthoclone OKT3), cyclosporine (Sandimmune), and corticosteroids. The efficacy and safety use of mycophenolate mofetil in combination with other immunosuppressive agents have not been determined.

Lymphoproliferative disease or lymphoma developed in patients receiving mycophenolate mofetil with other immunosuppressive agents in approximately 1% of patients in the controlled studies of prevention of rejection. (See ADVERSE REACTIONS.)

Adverse effects on fetal development (including malformations) occurred when pregnant rats and rabbits were dosed during organogenesis. These responses occurred at doses lower than those associated with maternal toxicity, and at doses below the recommended clinical dose. There are no adequate and well-controlled studies in pregnant women. However, mycophenolate mofetil has been shown to have teratogenic effects in animals, it may cause fetal harm when administered to a pregnant woman. Therefore, mycophenolate mofetil should not be used in pregnant women unless the potential benefit justifies the potential risk to the fetus.

Women of childbearing potential should have a negative serum or urine pregnancy test with a sensitivity of at least 50 mIU/ml within 1 week prior to beginning therapy. It is recommended that mycophenolate mofetil therapy should not be initiated by the physician until a report of a negative pregnancy test has been obtained.

WARNINGS: *(cont'd)*

Effective contraception must be used before beginning mycophenolate mofetil therapy, during therapy for 6 weeks following discontinuation of therapy, even where there has been a history of infertility, unless due to hysterectomy. Two reliable forms of contraception must be used simultaneously unless abstinence is the chosen method. If pregnancy does occur during treatment, the physician and patient should discuss the desirability of continuing the pregnancy. (See PRECAUTIONS, Pregnancy and Information for Patients.)

In the three controlled studies for prevention of rejection, similar rates of fatal infections/sepsis (< 2%) occurred in patients while receiving mycophenolate mofetil or control therapy in combination with other immunosuppressive agents. (See ADVERSE REACTIONS.)

Up to 2.0% of patients receiving mycophenolate mofetil for prevention of rejection developed severe neutropenia [absolute neutrophil count (ANC) < 0.5 x 10^3/µl]. (See ADVERSE REACTIONS.) Patients receiving mycophenolate mofetil should be monitored for neutropenia. (See PRECAUTIONS, Laboratory Tests.) The development of neutropenia may be related to mycophenolate mofetil itself, concomitant medications, viral infections, or some combination of these causes. If neutropenia develops (ANC < 1.3 x 10^3/µl dosing with mycophenolate mofetil should be interrupted or the dose reduced, appropriate diagnostic tests performed, and the patient managed appropriately. (See DOSAGE AND ADMINISTRATION.) Neutropenia has been observed most frequently in the period from 31 to 180 days post-transplant in patients treated for prevention of rejection.

PRECAUTIONS:

General: Gastrointestinal tract hemorrhage has been observed in approximately 3% of patients treated with mycophenolate mofetil. Gastrointestinal tract perforations have rarely been observed. Most patients receiving mycophenolate mofetil were also receiving other drugs known to be associated with these complications. Patients with active peptic ulcer disease were excluded from enrollment in studies with mycophenolate mofetil. Because mycophenolate mofetil has been associated with an increased incidence of digestive system adverse events, including infrequent cases of gastrointestinal tract ulceration, hemorrhage, and perforation, mycophenolate mofetil should be administered with caution in patients with active serious digestive system disease.

Subjects with severe chronic renal impairment (GFR < 25 ml/min/1.73 m^2) who have received single doses of mycophenolate mofetil showed higher plasma MPA and MPA AUCs relative to subjects with lesser degrees of renal impairment or normal healthy volunteers. No data are available on the safety of long-term exposure to these levels of MPAG. Doses of mycophenolate mofetil greater than 1 g administered twice a day should be avoided and they should be carefully observed. (See CLINICAL PHARMACOLOGY, Pharmacokinetics and DOSAGE AND ADMINISTRATION.

In patients with delayed graft function post-transplant, mean MPA AUC_{0-12} was comparable, but MPAG AUC_{0-12} was 2-3 fold higher, compared to that seen in post-transplant patients without delayed graft function. In three controlled studies of prevention of rejection, there were 298 of 1,483 patients (20%) with delayed graft function. Although patients with delayed graft function have a higher incidence of certain adverse events (anemia, thrombocytopenia, hyperkalemia) than patients without delayed graft function, these events were not more frequent in patients receiving mycophenolate mofetil than azathioprine or placebo. No dose adjustment is recommended for these patients, however, they should be carefully observed. (See CLINICAL PHARMACOLOGY, Pharmacokinetics and DOSAGE AND ADMINISTRATION.)

It is recommended that mycophenolate mofetil not be administered concomitantly with azathioprine because such concomitant administration has not been studied clinically.

In view of the significant reduction in the AUC of MPA by cholestyramine, caution should be used in the concomitant administration of mycophenolate mofetil with drugs that interfere with enterohepatic recirculation because of the potential to reduce the efficacy of mycophenolate mofetil. (See DRUG INTERACTIONS.)

Information for Patients: Patients should be informed of the need for repeated appropriate laboratory tests while they are receiving mycophenolate mofetil. Patients should be given complete dosage instructions and informed of the increased risk of lymphoproliferative disease and certain other malignancies. Women of childbearing potential should be instructed of the potential risks during pregnancy, and that they should use effective contraception before beginning mycophenolate mofetil therapy, during therapy and for 6 weeks after mycophenolate mofetil has been stopped. (See WARNINGS and PRECAUTIONS, Pregnancy.)

Laboratory Tests: Complete blood counts should be performed weekly during the first month, twice monthly for the second and third months of treatment, then monthly through the first year. (See WARNINGS, ADVERSE REACTIONS, and DOSAGE AND ADMINISTRATION.)

Carcinogenesis, Mutagenesis, Impairment of Fertility: In a 104-week oral carcinogenicity study in mice, mycophenolate mofetil in daily doses up to 180/mg/kg was not tumorigenic. The highest dose tested was 0.5 times the recommended clinical dose (2 g/day) when corrected for differences in body surface area (BSA). In a 104-week oral carcinogenicity study in rats, mycophenolate mofetil in daily doses up to 15 mg/kg was not tumorigenic. The highest dose was 0.08 times the recommended clinical dose when corrected for BSA. While the dosage given to these animals were lower than those given to patients, they were maximal in those species and were considered adequate to evaluate the potential for human risk. (See WARNINGS.)

Mycophenolate mofetil was not genotoxic, with or without metabolic activation, in several assays: the bacterial mutation assay, the yeast mitotic gene conversion assay, the mouse micronucleus aberration assay, or the Chinese hamster ovary cell (CHO) chromosomal aberration assay.

Mycophenolate mofetil had no effect on fertility of male rats at oral doses up to 20 mg/kg/day. This dose represents 0.1 times the recommended clinical dose when corrected for BSA. In a female fertility and reproduction study conducted in rats, oral doses of 4.5 mg/kg/day caused malformations (principally of the head and eyes) in the first—generation offspring in the absence of maternal toxicity. This dose was 0.02 times the recommended clinical dose when corrected for BSA. No effects on fertility or reproductive parameters were evident in the dams or in the subsequent generation.

Pregnancy Category C: In teratology studies in rats and rabbits, fetal resorptions and malformations occurred in rats at 6 mg/kg/day and in rabbits at 90 mg/kg/day, in the absence of maternal toxicity. These levels are equivalent to 0.03-0.92 times the recommended clinical study dose on a BSA basis. In a female fertility and reproduction study conducted in rats, oral doses of 4.5 mg/kg/day caused malformations (principally of the head and eyes) in the first—generation offspring in the absence of maternal toxicity. This dose was 0.02 times the recommended clinical dose when corrected for BSA.

PRECAUTIONS: *(cont'd)*

There are no adequate and well-controlled studies in pregnant women. Mycophenolate mofetil should not be used in pregnant women unless the potential benefit justifies the potential risk to the fetus. Effective contraception must be used before beginning mycophenolate mofetil therapy, during therapy and for 6 weeks after mycophenolate mofetil has been stopped. (See WARNINGS and PRECAUTIONS, Information for Patients.)

Nursing Mothers: Studies in rats treated with mycophenolate mofetil have shown mycophenolic acid to be excreted in milk. It is not known whether this drug is excreted in human milk. Because many drugs are excreted in human milk and because of the potential for serious adverse reactions in nursing infants from mycophenolate mofetil, a decision should be made whether to discontinue nursing or to discontinue the drug, taking into account the importance of the drug to the mother.

Pediatric Patients: Safety and effectiveness in pediatric patients have not been established. Very limited pharmacokinetic data are available in pediatric patients. (See CLINICAL PHARMACOLOGY, Pharmacokinetics.)

DRUG INTERACTIONS:

Drug interaction studies with mycophenolate mofetil have been conducted with acyclovir, antacids, cholestyramine, cyclosporine, ganciclovir, oral contraceptives and trimethoprim/sulfamethoxazole. Drug interaction studies have not been conducted with other drugs that may be commonly administered to renal transplant patients. mycophenolate mofetil has not been administered concomitantly with azathioprine.

Acyclovir: Coadministration of mycophenolate mofetil (1 g) and acyclovir (800 mg) to twelve healthy volunteers resulted in no significant change in MPA AUC and C_{max}. However, MPAG and acyclovir plasma AUCs were increased 10.6% and 21.9%, respectively. Because MPAG plasma concentrations are increased in the presence of renal impairment, as are acyclovir concentrations, the potential exists for the two drugs to compete for tubular secretion further increasing the concentrations of both drugs.

Antacids With Magnesium And Aluminum Hydroxides: Absorption of a single-dose of mycophenolate mofetil (2.0 g) was decreased when administered to ten rheumatoid arthritis patients also taking Maalox TC (10 ml q.i.d.). The C_{max} and AUC_{0-24} for MPA were 33% and 17% lower, respectively, than when mycophenolate mofetil was administered alone under fasting conditions. Mycophenolate mofetil may be administered to patients who are also taking antacids containing magnesium and aluminum hydroxides; however, it is recommended that mycophenolate mofetil and the antacid not be administered simultaneously.

Cholestyramine: Following single-dose administration of 1.5 g mycophenolate mofetil to twelve healthy volunteers pretreated with 4 g t.i.d. of cholestyramine for 4 days, MPA AUC decreased approximately 40%. This decrease is consistent with interruption of enterohepatic recirculation which may be due to binding of recirculating MPAG with cholestyramine in the intestine. mycophenolate mofetil is not recommended to be given with cholestyramine or other agents that may interfere with enterohepatic recirculation.

Cyclosporine: Cyclosporine (Sandimmune) pharmacokinetics (at doses of 275 to 415 mg/day) were unaffected by single and multiple doses of 1.5 g b.i.d. of mycophenolate mofetil in ten stable renal transplant patients. The mean (± SD) AUC_{0-12} and C_{max} of cyclosporine after 14 days of multiple doses of mycophenolate mofetil were 3290 (± 822) ng·h/ml and 753 (± 161) ng/ml, respectively, compared to 3245 (± 1088) ng·h/ml and 700 (± 246) ng/ml, respectively, one week before administration of mycophenolate mofetil. The effect of cyclosporine on mycophenolate mofetil pharmacokinetics could not be evaluated in this study, however, plasma concentrations of MPA were similar to that for healthy volunteers.

Ganciclovir: Following single-dose administration to twelve stable renal transplant patients, no pharmacokinetic interaction was observed between mycophenolate mofetil (1.5 g) and IV ganciclovir (5 mg/kg). Mean (± SD) ganciclovir AUC and C_{max} (n=10) were 54.3 (± 19.0) mcg·h/ml and 11.5 (± 1.8) mcg/ml, respectively after coadministration of the two drugs, compared to 51.0 (± 17.0) mcg°h/ml and 10.6 (± 2.0) mcg/ml, respectively after administration of IV ganciclovir alone. The mean (± SD) AUC and C_{max} of MPA (n=12) after coadministration were 80.9 (± 21.6) mcg°h/ml and 27.8 (± 16.4) mcg·h/ml and 30.9 (± 11.2) mcg/ml, respectively after administration of mycophenolate mofetil alone. Because MPAG plasma concentrations are increased in the presence of renal impairment, as are ganciclovir concentrations, the potential exists for the two drugs to compete for tubular secretion and thus further increases in concentrations of both drugs may occur.

Oral Contraceptives: Following single-dose administration to fifteen healthy women, no pharmacokinetic interaction was observed between mycophenolate mofetil (1.0 g) and two tablets of Ortho-Novum 7/7/7 (1 mg norethindrone [NET] and 35 mcg estradiol ethinyl [EE]). This single-dose study suggests the lack of a gross pharmacokinetic interaction, but cannot exclude the possibility of changes in the pharmacokinetics of the oral contraceptive under long term dosing conditions with mycophenolate mofetil which might adversely affect the efficacy of the oral contraceptive.

Trimethoprim/Sulfamethoxazole : Following single-dose administration of mycophenolate mofetil (1.5 g) to twelve healthy male volunteers on day 8 of a 10 day course of Bactrim DS (trimethoprim 160 mg/sulfamethoxazole 800 mg) administered b.i.d. no effect on the bioavailability of MPA was observed. The mean (± SD) AUC and C_{max} of MPA after concomitant administration were 75.2 (± 19.8) mcg·h/ml and 34.0 (± 6.6) mcg/ml, respectively compared to 79.2 (± 27.9) and 34.2 (± 10.7), respectively after administration of mycophenolate mofetil alone.

Other Interactions: The measured value for renal clearance of MPAG indicates removal occurs by renal tubular secretion as well as glomerular filtration. Consistent with this, coadministration of probenecid, a known inhibitor of tubular secretion, with mycophenolate mofetil in monkeys results in a 3-fold increase in plasma MPAG AUC and a 2-fold increase in plasma MPA AUC. Thus, other drugs known to undergo renal tubular secretion may compete with MPAG and thereby raise plasma concentrations of MPAG or the other drug undergoing tubular secretion.

Drugs that alter the gastrointestinal flora may interact with mycophenolate mofetil by disrupting enterohepatic recirculation. Interference of MPAG hydrolysis may lead to less MPA available for absorption.

ADVERSE REACTIONS:

The principal adverse reactions associated with the administration of mycophenolate mofetil include diarrhea, leukopenia, sepsis and vomiting, and there is evidence of a higher frequency of certain types of infections.

The incidence of adverse events for mycophenolate mofetil was determined in three randomized comparative double-blind trials in prevention of rejection in renal transplant patients. Because of the lower overall reporting of events in the European placebo-controlled, prevention of rejection study, these data were not combined with the other two active controlled prevention trials, but are instead presented separately.

Safety data are summarized below for all patients in the double-blind prevention studies while receiving treatment; approximately 53% of these patients have been treated for more than 1 year. Adverse events that were reported in ≥ 10% of patients in either mycophenolate mofetil treatment group are presented below for the two active-controlled studies combined (USA and Europe/Canada/Australia) and for the one European placebo-controlled study. Opportunistic infections are summarized separately. (TABLE 6)

ADVERSE REACTIONS: *(cont'd)*

TABLE 6A Adverse Events in Prevention of Renal Allograft Rejection USA Study Combined with Europe/Canada/Australia Study

	CellCept 2 g/day (n=336)	CellCept 3 g/day (n=330)	Azathioprine 1-2 mg/kg/day or 100-150 mg/day (n=326
Body as a Whole			
Pain	33.0%	31.2%	32.2%
Abdominal Pain	24.7	27.6	23.0
Fever	21.4	23.3	23.3
Headache	21.4	16.1	21.2
Infection	18.2	20.9	19.9
Sepsis	17.6	19.7	15.6
Asthenia	13.7	16.1	19.9
Chest pain	13.4	13.3	14.7
Back pain	11.6	12.1	14.1
Hemic and Lymphatic			
Anemia	25.6	25.8	23.6
Leukopenia	23.2	34.5	24.8
Thrombocytopenia	10.1	8.2	13.2
Hypochromic anemia	7.4	11.5	9.2
Leukocytosis	7.1	10.9	7.4
Urogenital			
Urinary tract infection	37.2	37.0	33.7
Hematuria	14.0	12.1	11.3
Kidney tubular necrosis	6.3	10.0	5.8
Cardiovascular			
Hypertension	32.4	28.2	32.2
Metabolic and Nutritional			
Peripheral edema	28.6	27.0	28.2
Hypercholesteremia	12.8	8.5	11.3
Hypophosphatemia	12.5	15.8	11.7
Edema	12.2	11.8	13.5
Hypokalemia	10.1	10.0	8.3
Hyperkalemia	8.9	10.3	16.9
Hyperglycemia	8.6	12.4	15.0
Digestive			
Diarrhea	31.0	36.1	20.9
Constipation	22.9	18.5	22.4
Nausea	19.9	23.6	24.5
Dyspepsia	17.6	13.6	13.8
Vomiting	12.5	13.6	9.2
Nausea and vomiting	10.4	9.7	10.7
Oral moniliasis	10.1	12.1	11.3
Respiratory			
Infection	22.0	23.9	19.6
Dyspnea	15.5	17.3	16.6
Cough increased	15.5	13.3	15.0
Pharyngitis	9.5	11.2	8.0
Skin and Appendages			
Acne	10.1	9.7	6.4
Rash	7.7	6.4	10.4
Nervous System			
Tremor	11.0	11.8	12.3
Insomnia	8.9	11.8	10.4
Dizziness	5.7	11.2	11.0

TABLE 6B Europe Study

	Cellcept 2 g/day (n=165)	Cellcept 3 g/day (n=160)	Placebo (n=166)
Body as a Whole			
Sepsis	21.8%	17.5%	13.9%
Infection	12.7	15.6	13.3
Abdominal Pain	12.1	11.9	11.4
Hemic and Lymphatic			
Leukopenia	11.5	16.3	4.2
Urogenital			
Urinary tract infection	45.5	44.4	37.3
Urinary tract disorder	6.7	10.6	4.2
Cardiovascular			
Hypertension	17.6	16.9	19.3
Digestive			
Diarrhea	16.4	18.8	13.9
Respiratory			
Infection	15.8	13.1	9.0
Bronchitis	8.5	11.9	8.4
Pneumonia	3.6	10.6	10.8

The above data demonstrate that in three controlled trials for prevention of rejection, patients receiving 2 g per day of mycophenolate mofetil had an overall better safety profile than did patients receiving 3 g per day of mycophenolate mofetil. Sepsis, which was generally CMV viremia, was slightly more common in patients treated with mycophenolate mofetil, with an incidence of 18-22%, compared to 16% in patients receiving azathioprine and 14% in patients receiving placebo. In the digestive system, diarrhea was most clearly increased in patients receiving mycophenolate mofetil, with an incidence of up to 36%, compared to 21% for patients receiving azathioprine and 14% for patients receiving placebo.

The incidence of malignancies among the 1,483 patients enrolled in controlled trials for the prevention of rejection who were followed for ≥ 1 year was similar to the incidence reported in the literature for renal allograft recipients. There was a slight increase in the incidence of lymphoproliferative disease in the mycophenolate mofetil treatment groups compared to the placebo and azathioprine groups. (See WARNINGS.) The following table (TABLE 7) summarizes the incidence of malignancies observed in the prevention of rejection trials.

Up to 2.0% of patients receiving mycophenolate mofetil for prevention of rejection have developed severe neutropenia [absolute neutrophil count (ANC) < 0.5 x 10^3/µl]. (See WARNINGS, PRECAUTIONS, Laboratory Tests, and DOSAGE AND ADMINISTRATION.)

TABLE 8 shows the incidence of opportunistic infections that occurred in the transplant population in the prevention of rejection trials:

In three controlled studies for prevention of rejection, similar rates of fatal injections/sepsis (< 2%) occurred in patients while receiving mycophenolate mofetil or control therapy in combination with other immunosuppressive agents. (See WARNINGS.)

The following adverse reactions, not mentioned in any of the tables above, were reported with ≥ 3% incidence in patients treated with mycophenolate mofetil:

ADVERSE REACTIONS: *(cont'd)*

TABLE 7 Malignancies Observed in Prevention of Renal Rejection Trials

	CellCept 2 g/day (n=501)	CellCept 3 g/day (n=490)	Placebo 1-2 mg/kg/day or 100-150 mg/day (n=166)	Azathioprine (n=326)
Lymphoma/lymphoproliferative disease	0.6%	1.0%	0.0%	0.3%
Non-melanoma skin carcinoma	4.0	1.6	0.0	2.4
Other malignancy	0.8	1.4	1.8	1.8

TABLE 8A Opportunistic Infections in Prevention of Renal Rejection Trials USA Study Combined with Europe/Canada/Australia Study

	CellCept 2 g/day (n=336)	CellCept 3 g/day (n=330)	Azathioprine 1-2 mg/kg/day or 100-150 mg/day (n=326)
Herpes simplex	16.7%	20.0%	19.0%
CMV			
viremia/syndrome	13.4	12.4	13.8
tissue invasive disease	8.3	11.5	6.1
Herpes zoster	6.0	7.6	5.8
Candida			
fungemia/disseminated	0.6	0.6	0.3
tissue invasive	0.6	0.6	0.3
Aspergillus/Mucor invasive disease	0.3	0.9	0.3
Pneumocystis carinii	0.3	0.0	1.2

TABLE 8B Europe study

	CellCept 2 g/day (n=165)	CellCept 3 g/day (n=160)	Placebo (n=166)
Herpes simplex	15.2%	12.5%	6.0%
CMV			
viremia/syndrome	15.2	15.0	13.3
tissue invasive disease	8.3	11.5	6.1
Herpes zoster	6.7	7.5	2.4
Candida			
fungemia/disseminated	0.0	0.6	0.0
tissue invasive	0.0	0.6	0.0
Pneumocystis carinii	0.0	0.0	2.4

Body As A Whole: abdomen enlarged, accidental injury, chills and fever, cyst, face edema, flu syndrome, hemorrhage, hernia, malaise, pelvic pain

Hemic And Lymphatic: ecchymosis, polycythemia

Urogenital: albuminuria, dysuria, hydronephrosis, impotence, pain, pyelonephritis, urinary frequency, urinary tract disorder

Cardiovascular: angina, pectoris, atrial fibrillation, cardiovascular disorder, hypotension, palpitation, peripheral vascular disorder, postural hypotension, tachycardia, thrombosis, vasodilation

Metabolic And Nutritional: acidosis, alkaline, phosphates increased, creatinine increased, dehydration, gamma glutamyl transpeptidase increased hypercalcemia, hypercalcemia, hypoglycemia, hypoproteinemia, lactic dehydrogenase increased, SGOT increased, SGPT increased, weight gain

Digestive: anorexia, esophagitis, flatulence, gastritis, gastroenteritis, gastrointestinal, hemorrhage, gastrointestinal moniliasis, gingivitis, gum hyperplasia, hepatitis, ileus, infection, liver function tests abnormal, mouth ulceration, rectal disorder

Respiratory: asthma, lung disorder, lung edema, pleural effusion, rhinitis, sinusitis

Skin And Appendages: alopecia, fungal dermatitis, hirsutism, pruritis, skin benign neoplasm, skin disorder, skin hypertrophy, skin ulcer, sweating

Nervous: anxiety, depression, hypertonia, paresthesia, somnolence

Endocrine: diabetes, mellitus, parathyroid disorder

Musculo-Skeletal: arthralgia, joint disorder, leg cramps, myalgia, myasthenia

Special Senses: amblyopia, cataract (not specified), conjunctivitis.

OVERDOSAGE:

There has been no reported experience of overdosage of mycophenolate mofetil in humans. The highest dose administered to renal transplant patients has been 4 g per day. In limited experience with cardiac and hepatic transplant patients, the highest doses used were 4 g or 5 g per day. At doses of 4 g or 5 g per day, there appears to be a higher rate, compared to the use of 3 g per day or less, of gastrointestinal intolerance (nausea, vomiting, and/or diarrhea), and occasional hematologic abnormalities, principally neutropenia, leading to a need to reduce or discontinue dosing.

In acute oral toxicity studies, no deaths occurred in adult mice at doses up to 4000 mg/kg or in adult monkeys at doses up to 1000 mg/kg; these were the highest doses of mycophenolate mofetil tested in these species. These doses represent 11 times the recommended clinical dose when corrected for BSA. In adult rats, deaths occurred after single oral doses of 500 mg/kg of mycophenolate mofetil. The dose represents approximately 3 times the recommended clinical dose when corrected for BSA.

MPA and MPAG are usually not removed by hemodialysis. However, at high MPAG plasma concentrations (> 100 mcg/ml), small amounts of MPAG are removed. By increasing excretion of the drug, MPA can be removed by bile acid sequestrants, such as cholestyramine.

DOSAGE AND ADMINISTRATION:

The initial dose of mycophenolate mofetil should be given within 72 hours following transplantation. A dose of 1.0 g administered twice a day (daily dose of 2 g) is recommended for use in combination with corticosteroids and cyclosporine in renal transplant patients. Although a dose of 1.5 g administered twice daily (daily dose of 3 g) was used in clinical trials and was shown to be safe and effective, no efficacy advantage could be established. Patients receiving 2 g per day of mycophenolate mofetil demonstrated an overall better safety

DOSAGE AND ADMINISTRATION: *(cont'd)*

profile than did patients receiving 3 g per day of mycophenolate mofetil. Food had no effect on MPA AUC, but has been shown to decrease MPA C_{max} by 40%. It is recommended that mycophenolate mofetil be administered on an empty stomach.

Dosage Adjustments: In patients with severe chronic renal impairment (GFR < 25 ml/min/1.73m^2) outside of the immediate post-transplant period, doses of mycophenolate mofetil greater than 1 g administered twice a day should be avoided. These patients should also be carefully observed. No dose adjustments are needed in patients experiencing delayed graft function post-operatively. (See CLINICAL PHARMACOLOGY, Pharmacokinetics and PRECAUTIONS, General.)

If neutropenia develops (ANC < 1.3 x 10^3/µl), dosing with mycophenolate mofetil should be interrupted or the dose reduced, appropriate diagnostic tests performed, and the patient managed appropriately. (See WARNINGS, ADVERSE REACTIONS, and PRECAUTIONS, Laboratory Tests.

Handling and Disposal: Because mycophenolate mofetil has demonstrated teratogenic effects in rats and rabbits, mycophenolate mofetil capsules should not be opened or crushed. Avoid inhalation or direct contact with skin or mucous membranes of the powder contained in mycophenolate mofetil capsules. If such contact occurs, wash thoroughly with soap and water; rinse eyes with plain water.

HOW SUPPLIED:

CellCept capsules are blue/brown, two-piece hard gelatin capsules, printed in black with "CellCept 250" on the blue cap and "Roche" on the brown body.

Storage: Store at 15° to 30° C (59° to 86° F).

HOW SUPPLIED - EQUIVALENTS NOT AVAILABLE:

Capsule, Gelatin - Oral - 250 mg

100's	$187.50	CELLCEPT, Roche	00004-0259-01
500's	$937.50	CELLCEPT, Roche	00004-0259-43

NABUMETONE *(003108)*

CATEGORIES: Analgesics; Antiarthritics; Antipyretics; Arthritis; Central Nervous System Agents; Nonsteroidal Anti-Inflammatory; Osteoarthritis; Pregnancy Category C; FDA Class 1C ("Little or No Therapeutic Advantage"); Sales > $100 Million; FDA Approved 1991 Dec; Top 200 Drugs

BRAND NAMES: *Arthaxan* (Germany); *Arthraxan*; *Consolan*; *Nabuser*; *Prodac*; **Relafen**; *Relif*; *Relifen*; *Relifex* (England, Mexico); *Unimetone*
(International brand names outside U.S. in italics)

FORMULARIES: PCS

COST OF THERAPY: $746.06 (Arthritis; Tablet; 500 mg; 2/day; 365 days)

PRIMARY ICD9: 715.99 (Osteoarthritis, Unspecified, Multiple Sites)

DESCRIPTION:

Nabumetone is a naphthylalkanone designated chemically as 4-(6-methoxy-2-naphthalenyl)-2-butanone.

Nabumetone is a white to off-white crystalline substance with a molecular weight of 228.3. It is nonacidic and practically insoluble in water, but soluble in alcohol and most organic solvents. It has an n-octanol:phosphate buffer partition coefficient of 2400 at pH 7.4.

Tablets for Oral Administration: Each oval-shaped, film-coated tablet contains 500 mg or 750 mg of nabumetone. Inactive ingredients consist of hydroxypropyl methylcellulose, microcrystalline cellulose, polyethylene glycol, polysorbate 80, sodium lauryl sulfate, sodium starch glycolate and titanium dioxide. The 750 mg tablets also contain iron oxides.

CLINICAL PHARMACOLOGY:

Nabumetone is a nonsteroidal anti-inflammatory drug (NSAID) that exhibits anti-inflammatory, analgesic and antipyretic properties in pharmacologic studies. As with other nonsteroidal anti-inflammatory agents, its mode of action is not known. However, the ability to inhibit prostaglandin synthesis may be involved in the anti-inflammatory effect.

The parent compound is a prodrug, which undergoes hepatic biotransformation to the active component, 6-methoxy-2-naphthylacetic acid (6MNA), that is a potent inhibitor of prostaglandin synthesis.

It is acidic and has an n-octanol:phosphate buffer partition coefficient of 0.5 at pH 7.4.

PHARMACOKINETICS

After oral administration, approximately 80% of a radiolabelled dose of nabumetone is found in the urine, indicating that nabumetone is well absorbed from the gastrointestinal tract. Nabumetone itself is not detected in the plasma because, after absorption, it undergoes rapid biotransformation to the principal active metabolite, 6-methoxy-2-naphthylacetic acid (6MNA). Approximately 35% of a 1000 mg oral dose of nabumetone is converted to 6MNA and 50% is converted into unidentified metabolites which are subsequently excreted in the urine. Following oral administration of nabumetone, 6MNA exhibits pharmacokinetic characteristics that generally follow a one-compartment model with first order input and first order elimination.

6MNA is more than 99% bound to plasma proteins. The free fraction is dependent on total concentration of 6MNA and is proportional to dose over the range of 1000 mg to 2000 mg. It is 0.2% to 0.3% at concentrations typically achieved following administration of nabumetone 1000 mg and is approximately 0.6% to 0.8% of the total concentrations at steady state following daily administration of 2000 mg.

Steady-state plasma concentrations of 6MNA are slightly lower than predicted from single-dose data. This may result from the higher fraction of unbound 6MNA which undergoes greater hepatic clearance.

Coadministration of food increases the rate of absorption and subsequent appearance of 6MNA in the plasma but does not affect the extent of conversion of nabumetone into 6MNA. Peak plasma concentrations of 6MNA are increased by approximately one third.

Coadministration with an aluminum-containing antacid had no significant effect on the bioavailability of 6MNA.

6MNA undergoes biotransformation in the liver, producing inactive metabolites that are eliminated as both free metabolites and conjugates. None of the known metabolites of 6MNA has been detected in plasma. Preliminary *in vivo* and *in vitro* studies suggests that unlike other NSAIDs, there is no evidence of enterohepatic recirculation of the active metabolite. Approximately 75% of a radiolabelled dose was recovered in urine in 48 hours. Approximately 80% was recovered in 168 hours. A further 9% appeared in the feces. In the first 48 hours, metabolites consisted of (TABLE 2):

CLINICAL PHARMACOLOGY: *(cont'd)*

TABLE 1 Mean pharmacokinetic parameters of nabumetone active metabolite (6MNA) at steady state following oral administration of 1000 mg or 2000 mg doses of Nabumetone

Abbreviations (units)	Young Adults Mean (±) SD 1000 mg n = 31	Young Adults Mean (±) SD 2000 mg n = 12	Elderly Mean (±) SD 1000 mg n = 27
t_{max} (hours)	3.0(1.0 to 12.0)	2.5(1.0 to 8.0)	4.0(1.0 to 10.0)
$t_{1/2}$ (hours)	22.5 ± 3.7	26.2 ± 3.7	29.8 ± 8.1
Cl_{ss}/F (ml/min)	26.1 ± 17.3	21.0 ± 4.0	18.6 ± 13.4
Vd_{ss}/F (l)	55.4 ± 26.4	53.4 ± 11.3	50.2 ± 25.3

TABLE 2

-nabumetone, unchanged	not detectable
-6-methoxy-2-naphthylacetic acid (6MNA), unchanged	< 1%
-6MNA, conjugated	11%
-6-hydroxy-2-naphthylacetic acid (6HNA), unchanged	5%
-6HNA, conjugated	7%
-4-(6-hydroxy-2-naphthyl)-butan-2-ol, conjugated	9%
-*O*-desmethyl-nabumetone, conjugated	7%
-unidentified minor metabolites	34%
Total % Dose:	73%

Following oral administration of dosages of 1000 mg to 2000 mg to steady state, the mean plasma clearance of 6MNA is 20 to 30 ml/min, and the elimination half-life is approximately 24 hours.

Elderly Patients: Steady-state plasma concentrations in elderly patients were generally higher than in young healthy subjects.(See TABLE 1 for summary of pharmacokinetic parameters.)

Renal Insufficiency: In studies of patients with renal insufficiency, the mean terminal half-life of 6MNA was increased in patients with severe renal dysfunction (creatinine clearance <30 ml/min./1.73m^2). In patients undergoing hemodialysis, steady-state plasma concentrations of the active metabolite were similar to those observed in healthy subjects. Due to extensive protein-binding, 6MNA is not dialyzable.

Hepatic Impairment: Data in patients with severe hepatic impairment are limited. Biotransformation of nabumetone to 6MNA and further metabolism of 6MNA to inactive metabolites is dependent on hepatic function and could be reduced in patients with severe hepatic impairment (history of or biopsy-proven cirrhosis).

SPECIAL STUDIES

Gastrointestinal: Nabumetone was compared to aspirin in inducing gastrointestinal blood loss. Food intake was not monitored. Studies utilizing ^{51}Cr-tagged red blood cells in healthy males showed no difference in fecal blood loss after 3 or 4 weeks' administration of nabumetone 1000 mg or 2000 mg daily when compared to either placebo-treated or nontreated subjects. In contrast, aspirin 3600 mg daily produced an increase in fecal blood loss when compared to the nabumetone-treated, placebo-treated or nontreated subjects. The clinical relevance of the data is unknown.

The following endoscopy trials entered patients who had been previously treated with NSAIDs. These patients had varying baseline scores and different courses of treatment. The trials were not designed to correlate symptoms and endoscopy scores. The clinical relevance of these endoscopy trials, i.e., either G.I. symptoms or serious G.I events, is not known.

Ten endoscopy studies were conducted in 488 patients who had baseline and post-treatment endoscopy. In 5 clinical trials that compared a total of 194 patients on nabumetone 1000 mg daily or naproxen 250 mg or 500 mg twice daily for 3 to 12 weeks. Nabumetone treatment resulted in fewer patients with endoscopically detected lesions (>3 mm). In 2 trials a total of 101 patients on nabumetone 1000 mg or 2000 mg daily or piroxicam 10 mg to 20 mg for 7 to 10 days, there were fewer nabumetone patients with endoscopically detected lesions. In 3 trials of a total of 47 patients on nabumetone 1000 mg daily or indomethacin 100 mg to 150 mg daily for 3 to 4 weeks, the endoscopy scores were higher with indomethacin. Another 12-week trial in a total of 171 patients compared the results of treatment with nabumetone 1000 mg/day to ibuprofen 2400 mg/day and ibuprofen 2400 mg/day plus misoprostol 800 mcg/day. The results showed that patients treated with nabumetone had a lower number of endoscopically detected lesions (>5 mm) than patients treated with ibuprofen alone but comparable to the combination of ibuprofen plus misoprostol. The results did not correlate with abdominal pain.

Other: In 1-week repeat-dose studies in healthy volunteers, nabumetone 1000 mg daily had little effect on collagen-induced platelet aggregation and no effect on bleeding time. In comparison, naproxen 500 mg daily suppressed collagen-induced platelet aggregation and significantly increased bleeding time.

CLINICAL STUDIES:

Osteoarthritis: The use of nabumetone in relieving the signs and symptoms of osteoarthritis was assessed in double-blind controlled trials in which 1,047 patients were treated for 6 weeks to 6 months. In these trials, nabumetone in a dose of 1000 mg/day administered at night was comparable to naproxen 500 mg/day and to aspirin 3600 mg/day.

Rheumatoid Arthritis: The use of nabumetone in relieving the signs and symptoms of rheumatoid arthritis was assessed in double-blind, randomized, controlled trials in which 770 patients were treated for 3 weeks to 6 months. Nabumetone, in a dose of 1000 mg/day administered at night was comparable to naproxen 500 mg/day and to aspirin 3600 mg/day.

In controlled clinical trials of rheumatoid arthritis patients, nabumetone has been used in combination with gold, d-penicillamine and corticosteroids.

Individualization Of Dosing: There is considerable interpatient variation in response to nabumetone. Therapy is usually initiated at a nabumetone dose of 1000 mg daily, then adjusted, if needed, based on clinical response.

In clinical trials with osteoarthritis and rheumatoid arthritis patients, most patients responded to nabumetone in doses of 1000 mg/day administered nightly: total daily dosages up to 2000 mg were used. In open-labelled studies, 1,490 patients were permitted dosage increases and were followed for approximately 1 year (mode). Twenty percent of patients (n=294) were withdrawn for lack of effectiveness during the first year of these open-labelled studies. The following table (TABLE 3) provides patient-exposure to doses used in the U.S. clinical trials:

As with other NSAIDs, the lowest dose should be sought for each patient. Patients weighing under 50 kg may be less likely to require dosages beyond 1000 mg. Therefore, after observing the response to initial therapy, the dose should be adjusted to meet individual patients' requirements.

INDICATIONS AND USAGE:

Nabumetone is indicated for acute and chronic treatment of signs and symptoms of osteoarthritis and rheumatoid arthritis.

TABLE 3 Clinical double-blind and open-labelled trials of Nabumetone in osteoarthritis and rheumatoid arthritis

Nabumetone Dose	Number of Patients		Mean/Mode Duration of Treatment (yrs.)	
	OA	RA	OA	RA
500 mg	17	6	0.4/-	0.2/-
1000 mg	917	701	1.2/1	1.4/1
1500 mg	645	224	2.3/1	1.7/1
2000 mg	15	100	0.6/1	1.3/1

CONTRAINDICATIONS:

Nabumetone is contraindicated in patients who have previously exhibited hypersensitivity to it.

Nabumetone is contraindicated in patients in whom nabumetone, aspirin or other NSAIDs induce asthma, urticaria or other allergic-type reactions. Fatal asthmatic reactions have been reported in such patients receiving NSAIDs.

WARNINGS:

Risk of G.I. Ulceration, Bleeding and Perforation with NSAID Therapy: Serious gastrointestinal toxicity such as bleeding, ulceration and perforation can occur at any time, with or without warning symptoms, in patients treated chronically with NSAID therapy. Although minor upper gastrointestinal problems, such as dyspepsia, are common, usually developing early in therapy, physicians should remain alert for ulceration and bleeding in patients treated chronically with NSAIDs even in the absence of previous G.I. tract symptoms.

In controlled, clinical trials involving 1,677 patients treated with nabumetone (1,140 followed for 1 year and 927 for 2 years), the cumulative incidence of peptic ulcers was 0.3% (95% Cl; 0%, 0.6%) at 3 to 6 months, 0.5% (95% Cl; 0.1%, 0.9%) at 1 year and 0.8% (95% Cl; 0.3%, 1.3%) at 2 years. Physicians should inform patients about the signs and symptoms of serious G.I. toxicity and what steps to take if they occur. In patients with active peptic ulcer, physicians must weigh the benefits of Nabumetone therapy against possible hazards, institute an appropriate ulcer treatment regimen and monitor the patient's progress carefully.

Studies to date have not identified any subset of patients not at risk of developing peptic ulceration and bleeding. Except for a prior history of serious G.I. events and other risk factors known to be associated with peptic ulcer disease, such as alcoholism, smoking, etc., no risk factors (*e.g.,* age, sex) have been associated with increased risk. Elderly or debilitated patients seem to tolerate ulceration or bleeding less well than other individuals and most spontaneous reports of fatal G.I. events are in this population.

High doses of any NSAID probably carry a greater risk of these reactions, although controlled clinical trials showing this do not exist in most cases. In considering the use of relatively large doses (within the recommended dosage range), sufficient benefit should be anticipated to offset the potential increased risk of G.I. toxicity.

PRECAUTIONS:

GENERAL

Renal Effects: As a class, NSAIDs have been associated with renal papillary necrosis and other abnormal renal pathology during long-term administration to animals.

A second form of renal toxicity often associated with NSAIDs is seen in patients with conditions leading to a reduction in renal blood flow or blood volume, where renal prostaglandins have a supportive role in the maintenance of renal perfusion. In these patients, administration of an NSAID results in dose-dependent decrease in prostaglandin synthesis and, secondarily, in a reduction of renal blood flow, which may precipitate overt renal decompensation. Patients at greatest risk of this reaction are those with impaired renal function, heart failure, liver dysfunction, those taking diuretics, and the elderly. Discontinuation of NSAID therapy is typically followed by recovery to the pretreatment state.

Because nabumetone undergoes extensive hepatic metabolism, no adjustment of nabumetone dosage is generally necessary in patients with renal insufficiency. However, as with all NSAIDs, patients with impaired renal function should be monitored more closely than patients with normal renal function (see CLINICAL PHARMACOLOGY, Special Studies.) The oxidized and conjugated metabolites of 6MNA are eliminated primarily by the kidneys. The extent to which these largely inactive metabolites may accumulate in patients with renal failure has not been studied. As with other drugs whose metabolites are excreted by the kidneys, the possibility that adverse reactions (not listed in ADVERSE REACTIONS) may be attributable to these metabolites should be considered.

Hepatic Function: As with other NSAIDs, borderline elevations of one or more liver function tests may occur in up to 15% of patients. These abnormalities may progress, may remain essentially unchanged, or may return to normal with continued therapy. The ALT (SGPT) test is probably the most sensitive indicator of liver dysfunction. Meaningful (3 times the upper limit of normal) elevations of ALT (SGPT) or AST (SGOT) have occurred in controlled clinical trials of Nabumetone in less than 1% of patients. A patient with symptoms and/or signs suggesting liver dysfunction, or in whom an abnormal liver test has occurred, should be evaluated for evidence of the development of a more severe hepatic reaction while on nabumetone therapy. Severe hepatic reactions, including jaundice and fatal hepatitis, have been reported with other NSAIDs. Although such reactions are rare, if abnormal liver tests persist or worsen, if clinical signs and symptoms consistent with liver disease develop, or if systemic manifestations occur (*e.g.,* eosinophilia, rash, etc.), nabumetone should be discontinued. Because nabumetone's biotransformation to 6MNA is dependent upon hepatic function, the biotransformation could be decreased in patients with severe hepatic dysfunction. Therefore, nabumetone should be used with caution in patients with severe hepatic impairment (see Pharmacokinetics, Hepatic Impairment.)

Fluid Retention and Edema: Fluid retention and edema have been observed in some patients taking nabumetone. Therefore, as with other NSAIDs, nabumetone should be used cautiously in patients with a history of congestive heart failure, hypertension or other conditions predisposing to fluid retention.

Photosensitivity: Based on U.V. light photosensitivity testing, nabumetone may be associated with more reactions to sun exposure than might be expected based on skin tanning types.

INFORMATION FOR THE PATIENT

Nabumetone, like other drugs of its class, is not free of side effects. The side effects of these drugs can cause discomfort and, rarely, there are more serious side effects, such as gastrointestinal bleeding, which may result in hospitalization and even fatal outcome.

NSAIDs are often essential agents in the management of arthritis, but they also may be commonly employed for conditions which are less serious. Physicians may wish to discuss with their patients the potential risks(see WARNINGS, PRECAUTIONS, and ADVERSE REACTIONS) and likely benefits of NSAID treatment, particularly when the drugs are used for less serious conditions where treatment without NSAIDs may represent an acceptable alternative to both the patient and the physician.

PRECAUTIONS: *(cont'd)*

LABORATORY TESTS

Because severe G.I. tract ulceration and bleeding can occur without warning symptoms, physicians should follow chronically treated patients for signs and symptoms of ulceration and bleeding, and should inform them of the importance of this follow-up (see WARNINGS, Risk of G.I. Ulceration, Bleeding and Perforation with NSAID Therapy).

CARCINOGENESIS, MUTAGENESIS, AND IMPAIRMENT OF FERTILITY

Carcinogenesis, Mutagenesis: In two-year studies conducted in mice and rats, nabumetone had no statistically significant tumorigenic effect. Nabumetone did not show mutagenetic potential in the Ames test and mouse micronucleus test *in vivo*. However, nabumetone- and 6MNA-treated lymphocytes in culture showed chromosomal aberrations at 80 mcg/ml and higher concentrations (equal to the average human exposure to nabumetone at the maximum recommended dose).

Impairment of Fertility: Nabumetone did not impair fertility of male or female rats treated orally at doses of 320 mg/kg/day (1888 mg/m^2) before mating.

PREGNANCY, TERATOGENIC EFFECTS, PREGNANCY CATEGORY C

Nabumetone did not cause any teratogenic effect in rats given up to 400 mg/kg (2360 mg/m^2) and in rabbits up to 300 mg/kg (3540 mg/m^2) orally. However, increased post-implantation loss was observed in rats at 100 mg/kg (590 mg/m^2) orally and at higher doses (equal to the average human exposure to 6MNA at the maximum recommended human dose). There are no adequate, well-controlled studies in pregnant women. This drug should be used during pregnancy only if clearly needed.

Because of the known effect of prostaglandin-synthesis-inhibiting drugs on the human fetal cardiovascular system (closure of ductus arteriosus), use of Nabumetone during the third trimester of pregnancy is not recommended.

LABOR AND DELIVERY

The effects of nabumetone on labor and delivery in women are not known. As with other drugs known to inhibit prostaglandin synthesis, an increased incidence of dystocia and delayed parturition occurred in rats treated throughout pregnancy.

NURSING MOTHERS

Nabumetone is not recommended for use in nursing mothers because of the possible adverse effects of prostaglandin-synthesis-inhibiting drugs on neonates. It is not known whether nabumetone or its metabolites are excreted in human milk; however, 6MNA is excreted in the milk of lactating rats.

PEDIATRIC USE

Nabumetone is not recommended for use in children because the safety and efficacy in children have not been established.

GERIATRIC USE

Of the 1,677 patients in U.S. clinical studies who were treated with nabumetone, 411 patients (24%) were 65 years of age or older; 22 patients (1%) were 75 years of age or older. No overall differences in efficacy or safety were observed between these older patients and younger ones. Similar results were observed in a 1-year, non-U.S. postmarketing surveillance study of 10,800 nabumetone patients, of whom 4,577 patients (42%) were 65 years of age or older.

DRUG INTERACTIONS:

In vitro studies have shown that, because of its affinity for protein, 6MNA may displace other protein-bound drugs from their binding site. Caution should be exercised when administering nabumetone with warfarin since interactions have been seen with other NSAIDs.

Concomitant administration of an aluminum-containing antacid had no significant effect in the bioavailability of 6MNA. When administered with food or milk, there is more rapid absorption; however, the total amount of 6MNA in the plasma is unchanged (see Pharmacokinetics).

ADVERSE REACTIONS:

Adverse reaction information was derived from blinded-controlled and open-labelled clinical trials and from worldwide marketing experience. In the description below, rates of the more common events (greater than 1%) and many of the less common events (less than 1%) represent results of U.S. clinical studies.

Of the 1,677 patients who received nabumetone during U.S. clinical trials, 1,524 were treated for at least 1 month, 1,327 for at least 3 months, 929 for at least a year and 750 for at least 2 years. Over 300 patients have been treated for 5 years or longer.

The most frequently reported adverse reactions were related to the gastrointestinal tract. They were diarrhea, dyspepsia and abdominal pain.

INCIDENCE ≥1%—PROBABLY CAUSALLY RELATED

Gastrointestinal: Diarrhea (14%), dyspepsia (13%), abdominal pain (12%), constipation*, flatulence*, nausea*, positive stool guaiac*, dry mouth, gastritis, stomatitis, vomiting.

Central Nervous System: Dizziness*, headache*, fatigue, increased sweating, insomnia, nervousness, somnolence.

Dermatologic: Pruritus*, rash*.

Special Senses: Tinnitus*.

Miscellaneous: Edema*.

*Incidence of reported reaction between 3% and 9%. Reactions occurring in 1% to 3% of the patients are unmarked.

INCIDENCE <1%—PROBABLY CAUSALLY RELATEDσ

Gastrointestinal: Anorexia, cholestatic jaundice, duodenal ulcer, dysphagia, gastric ulcer, gastroenteritis, gastrointestinal bleeding, increased appetite, liver function abnormalities, melena.

Central Nervous System: Asthenia, agitation, anxiety, confusion, depression, malaise, paresthesia, tremor, vertigo.

Dermatologic: Bullous eruptions, photosensitivity, urticaria, pseudoporphyria cutanea tarda, *toxic epidermal necrolysis.*

Cardiovascular: Vasculitis.

Metabolic: Weight gain.

Respiratory: Dyspnea, *eosinophilic pneumonia hypersensitivity pneumonitis.*

Genitourinary: Albuminuria, azotemia, *hyperuricemia, interstitial nephritis, nephrotic syndrome, vaginal bleeding.*

Special Senses: Abnormal vision.

Hypersensitivity: *Anaphylactoid reaction, anaphylaxis,* angioneurotic edema.

†Adverse reactions reported only in worldwide postmarketing experience or in the literature, not seen in clinical trials, are considered rarer and are italicized.

INCIDENCE <1%—CAUSAL RELATIONSHIP UNKNOWN†

Gastrointestinal: Bilirubinuria, duodenitis, eructation, gallstones, gingivitis, glossitis, pancreatitis, rectal bleeding.

Central Nervous System: Nightmares.

ADVERSE REACTIONS: *(cont'd)*

Dermatologic: Acne, alopecia, *erythema multiforme, Stevens-Johnson Syndrome.*

Cardiovascular: Angina, arrhythmia, hypertension, myocardial infarction, palpitations, syncope, thrombophlebitis.

Respiratory: Asthma, cough.

Genitourinary: Dysuria, hematuria, impotence, renal stones.

Special Senses: Taste disorder.

Body as a Whole: Fever, chills.

Hematologic/Lymphatic: Anemia, leukopenia, granulocytopenia, thrombocytopenia.

Metabolic/Nutritional: Hyperglycemia, hypokalemia, weight loss.

‡Adverse reactions reported only in worldwide postmarketing experience or in the literature, not seen in clinical trials, are considered rarer and are italicized.

OVERDOSAGE:

Since only one case of nabumetone overdose has been reported, the experience is limited. If acute overdose occurs, it is recommended that the stomach be emptied by vomiting or lavage and general supportive measures be instituted, as necessary. In addition, the use of activated charcoal, up to 60 grams, may effectively reduce nabumetone absorption. Coadministration of nabumetone with charcoal to man has resulted in an 80% decrease in maximum plasma concentrations of the active metabolite.

The one overdose occurred in a 17-year-old female patient who had a history of abdominal pain and was hospitalized for increased abdominal pain following ingestion of 30 nabumetone tablets (15 grams total). Stools were negative for occult blood and there was no fall in serum hemoglobin concentration. The patient had no other symptoms. She was given an H_2-receptor antagonist and discharged from the hospital without sequelae.

DOSAGE AND ADMINISTRATION:

Osteoarthritis and Rheumatoid Arthritis: The recommended starting dose is 1000 mg taken as a single dose with or without food. Some patients may obtain more symptomatic relief from 1500 mg to 2000 mg per day. Nabumetone can be given in either a single or twice-daily dose. Dosages over 2000 mg per day have not been studied. The lowest effective dose should be used for chronic treatment.

PATIENT INFORMATION:

Nabumetone is a non-steroidal anti-inflammatory (NSAID) medication used to relieve pain, treat fever, and decrease inflammation and swelling. It is used commonly to treat osteoarthritis and rheumatoid arthritis. This medication should not be used by those with aspirin allergies producing symptoms of difficult breathing, red itching skin. This class of medications has been associated with ulcer and bleeding in the stomach. This is often relieved by taking the medication with food. Water retention may also occur and you should report any swelling of the feet or difficulty breathing to your physician immediately. This medication can be taken with or without food, however, food often alleviates stomach irritation.

HOW SUPPLIED:

Tablets: Oval-shaped, film-coated: 500 mg-white, imprinted with the product name nabumetone and 500, in bottles of 100 and 500, and in Single Unit Packages of 100 (intended for institutional use only). 750 mg-beige, imprinted with the product name nabumetone and 750, in bottles of 100 and 500, and in Single Unit Packages of 100 (intended for institutional use only).

Store at controlled room temperature (59° to 86°F) in a well-closed container; dispense in light-resistant container.

HOW SUPPLIED - EQUIVALENTS NOT AVAILABLE:

Tablet, Uncoated - Oral - 500 mg

100's	$102.20	RELAFEN, Beecham	00029-4851-20
100's	$102.20	RELAFEN, Beecham	00029-4851-21

Tablet, Uncoated - Oral - 750 mg

100's	$123.15	RELAFEN, Beecham	00029-4852-20

NADOLOL *(001849)*

CATEGORIES: Angina; Antianginals; Antihypertensives; Beta Adrenergic Blocking Agents; Beta Blockers; Cardiovascular Drugs; Hypertension; Pregnancy Category C; Sales > $100 Million; FDA Approval Pre 1982; Patent Expiration 1993 Jan

BRAND NAMES: *Apo-Nadolol*; **Corgard**; *Farmagard*; *Nadic* (Japan); *Solgol* (Germany)
(International brand names outside U.S. in italics)

FORMULARIES: Aetna; BC-BS

COST OF THERAPY: $309.04 (Angina; Tablet; 40 mg; 1/day; 365 days) vs. Potential Cost of $2,683.17 (Angina)

DESCRIPTION:

Nadolol is a synthetic nonselective beta-adrenergic receptor blocking agent designated chemically as 1-(*tert*-butylamino)-3-((5,6,7,8-tetrahydro-*cis*-6,7-dihydroxy-1-naphthyl)oxy)-2-propanol.

Nadolol is a white crystalline powder. It is freely soluble in ethanol, soluble in hydrochloric acid, slightly soluble in water and in chloroform, and very slightly soluble in sodium hydroxide.

Nadolol is available for oral administration as 20 mg, 40 mg, 80 mg, 120 mg, and 160 mg tablets. Inactive ingredients: microcrystalline cellulose, colorant (FD&C Blue No. 2), cornstarch, magnesium stearate, povidone (except 20 mg and 40 mg), and other ingredients.

CLINICAL PHARMACOLOGY:

Nadolol is a nonselective beta-adrenergic receptor blocking agent. Clinical pharmacology studies have demonstrated beta-blocking activity by showing (1) reduction in heart rate and cardiac output at rest and on exercise, (2) reduction of systolic and diastolic blood pressure at rest and on exercise, (3) inhibition of isoproterenol-induced tachycardia, and (4) reduction of reflex orthostatic tachycardia.

Nadolol specifically competes with beta-adrenergic receptor agonists for available beta receptor sites; it inhibits both the beta$_1$ receptors located chiefly in cardiac muscle and the beta$_2$receptors located chiefly in the bronchial and vascular musculature, inhibiting the chronotropic, inotropic, and vasodilator responses to beta-adrenergic stimulation proportionately. Nadolol has no intrinsic sympathomimetic activity and, unlike some other beta-adrenergic blocking agents, nadolol has little direct myocardial depressant activity and does not have an anesthetic-like membrane-stabilizing action. Animal and human studies show that nadolol slows the sinus rate and depresses AV conduction. In dogs, only minimal amounts of

CLINICAL PHARMACOLOGY: *(cont'd)*

nadolol were detected in the brain relative to amounts in blood and other organs and tissues. nadolol has low lipophilicity as determined by octanol/water partition coefficient, a characteristic of certain beta-blocking agents that has been correlated with the limited extent to which these agents cross the blood-brain barrier, their low concentration in the brain, and low incidence of CNS-related side effects.

In controlled clinical studies, nadolol at doses of 40 to 320 mg/day has been shown to decrease both standing and supine blood pressure, the effect persisting for approximately 24 hours after dosing.

The mechanism of the antihypertensive effects of beta-adrenergic receptor blocking agents has not been established; however, factors that may be involved include (1) competitive antagonism of catecholamines at peripheral (non-CNS) adrenergic neuron sites (especially cardiac) leading to decreased cardiac output, (2) a central effect leading to reduced tonic-sympathetic nerve outflow to the periphery, and (3) suppression of renin secretion by blockade of the beta-adrenergic receptors responsible for renin release from the kidneys.

While cardiac output and arterial pressure are reduced by nadolol therapy, renal hemodynamics are stable, with preservation of renal blood flow and glomerular filtration rate.

By blocking catecholamine-induced increases in heart rate, velocity and extent of myocardial contraction, and blood pressure, nadolol generally reduces the oxygen requirements of the heart at any given level of effort, making it useful for many patients in the long-term management of angina pectoris. On the other hand, nadolol can increase oxygen requirements by increasing left ventricular fiber length and end diastolic pressure, particularly in patients with heart failure.

Although beta-adrenergic receptor blockade is useful in treatment of angina and hypertension, there are also situations in which sympathetic stimulation is vital. For example, in patients with severely damaged hearts, adequate ventricular function may depend on sympathetic drive. Beta-adrenergic blockade may worsen AV block by preventing the necessary facilitating effects of sympathetic activity on conduction. Beta$_2$-adrenergic blockade results in passive bronchial constriction by interfering with endogenous adrenergic bronchodilator activity in patients subject to bronchospasm and may also interfere with exogenous bronchodilators in such patients.

Absorption of nadolol after oral dosing is variable, averaging about 30 percent. Peak serum concentrations of nadolol usually occur in three to four hours after oral administration and the presence of food in the gastrointestinal tract does not affect the rate or extent of nadolol absorption. Approximately 30 percent of the nadolol present in serum is reversibly bound to plasma protein.

Unlike many other beta-adrenergic blocking agents, nadolol is not metabolized by the liver and is excreted unchanged, principally by the kidneys.

The half-life of therapeutic doses of nadolol is about 20 to 24 hours, permitting once-daily dosage. Because nadolol is excreted predominantly in the urine, its half-life increases in renal failure (see PRECAUTIONS and DOSAGE AND ADMINISTRATION). Steady-state serum concentrations of nadolol are attained in six to nine days with once-daily dosage in persons with normal renal function. Because of variable absorption and different individual responsiveness, the proper dosage must be determined by titration.

Exacerbation of angina and, in some cases, myocardial infarction and ventricular dysrhythmias have been reported after abrupt discontinuation of therapy with beta-adrenergic blocking agents in patients with coronary artery disease. Abrupt withdrawal of these agents in patients without coronary artery disease has resulted in transient symptoms, including tremulousness, sweating, palpitation, headache, and malaise. Several mechanisms have been proposed to explain these phenomena, among them increased sensitivity to catecholamines because of increased numbers of beta receptors.

INDICATIONS AND USAGE:

Angina Pectoris: Nadolol is indicated for the long-term management of patients with angina pectoris.

Hypertension: Nadolol is indicated in the management of hypertension; it may be used alone or in combination with other antihypertensive agents, especially thiazide-type diuretics.

CONTRAINDICATIONS:

Nadolol is contraindicated in bronchial asthma, sinus bradycardia and greater than first degree conduction block, cardiogenic shock, and overt cardiac failure (see WARNINGS.)

WARNINGS:

Cardiac Failure: Sympathetic stimulation may be a vital component supporting circulatory function in patients with congestive heart failure, and its inhibition by beta-blockade may precipitate more severe failure. Although beta-blockers should be avoided in overt congestive heart failure, if necessary, they can be used with caution in patients with a history of failure who are well-compensated, usually with digitalis and diuretics. Beta-adrenergic blocking agents do not abolish the inotropic action of digitalis on heart muscle.

IN PATIENTS WITHOUT A HISTORY OF HEART FAILURE, continued use of beta-blockers can, in some cases, lead to cardiac failure. Therefore, at the first sign or symptom of heart failure, the patient should be digitalized and/or treated with diuretics, and the response observed closely, or nadolol should be discontinued (gradually, if possible).

Exacerbation of Ischemic Heart Disease Following Abrupt Withdrawal-Hypersensitivity to catecholamines has been observed in patients withdrawn from beta-blocker therapy; exacerbation of angina and, in some cases, myocardial infarction have occurred after abrupt discontinuation of such therapy. When discontinuing chronically administered nadolol, particularly in patients with ischemic heart disease, the dosage should be gradually reduced over a period of one to two weeks and the patient should be carefully monitored. If angina markedly worsens or acute coronary insufficiency develops, nadolol administration should be reinstituted promptly, at least temporarily, and other measures appropriate for the management of unstable angina should be taken. Patients should be warned against interruption or discontinuation of therapy without the physician's advice. Because coronary artery disease is common and may be unrecognized, it may be prudent not to discontinue nadolol therapy abruptly even in patients treated only for hypertension.

Nonallergic Bronchospasm (*e.g.,* chronic bronchitis, emphysema): PATIENTS WITH BRONCHOSPASTIC DISEASES SHOULD IN GENERAL NOT RECEIVE BETA-BLOCKERS. Nadolol should be administered with caution since it may block bronchodilation produced by endogenous or exogenous catecholamine stimulation of beta$_2$ receptors.

Major Surgery: Because beta-blockade impairs the ability of the heart to respond to reflex stimuli and may increase the risks of general anesthesia and surgical procedures, resulting in protracted hypotension or low cardiac output, it has generally been suggested that such therapy should be withdrawn several days prior to surgery. Recognition of the increased

WARNINGS: *(cont'd)*

sensitivity to catecholamines of patients recently withdrawn from beta-blocker therapy, however, has made this recommendation controversial. If possible, beta-blockers should be withdrawn well before surgery takes place. In the event of emergency surgery, the anesthesiologist should be informed that the patient is on beta-blocker therapy. The effects of nadolol can be reversed by administration of beta-receptor agonists such as isoproterenol, dopamine, dobutamine, or levarterenol. Difficulty in restarting and maintaining the heartbeat has also been reported with beta-adrenergic receptor blocking agents.

Diabetes and Hypoglycemia: Beta-adrenergic blockade may prevent the appearance of premonitory signs and symptoms (*e.g.,* tachycardia and blood pressure changes) of acute hypoglycemia. This is especially important with labile diabetics. Beta-blockade also reduces the release of insulin in response to hyperglycemia; therefore, it may be necessary to adjust the dose of antidiabetic drugs.

Thyrotoxicosis: Beta-adrenergic blockade may mask certain clinical signs (*e.g.,* tachycardia) of hyperthyroidism. Patients suspected of developing thyrotoxicosis should be managed carefully to avoid abrupt withdrawal of beta-adrenergic blockade which might precipitate a thyroid storm.

PRECAUTIONS:

Impaired Renal Function: Nadolol should be used with caution in patients with impaired renal function (see DOSAGE AND ADMINISTRATION.)

Information for the Patient: Patients, especially those with evidence of coronary artery insufficiency, should be warned against interruption or discontinuation of nadolol therapy without the physician's advice. Although cardiac failure rarely occurs in properly selected patients, patients being treated with beta-adrenergic blocking agents should be advised to consult the physician at the first sign or symptom of impending failure. The patient should also be advised of a proper course in the event of an inadvertently missed dose.

DRUG INTERACTIONS:

When administered concurrently, the following drugs may interact with beta-adrenergic receptor blocking agents:

Anesthetics, general: exaggeration of the hypotension induced by general anesthetics (see WARNINGS, Major Surgery.)

Antidiabetic drugs (oral agents and insulin): hypoglycemia or hyperglycemia; adjust dosage of antidiabetic drug accordingly (see WARNINGS, Diabetes and Hypoglycemia.)

Catecholamine-depleting drugs (*e.g.,* reserpine): additive effect; monitor closely for evidence of hypotension and/or excessive bradycardia (*e.g.,* vertigo, syncope, postural hypotension).

Response to Treatment for Anaphylactic Reaction While taking beta-blockers, patients with a history of severe anaphylactic reaction to a variety of allergens may be more reactive to repeated challenge, either accidental, diagnostic, or therapeutic. Such patients may be unresponsive to the usual doses of epinephrine used to treat allergic reaction.

Carcinogenesis, Mutagenesis, Impairment of Fertility: In chronic oral toxicologic studies (one to two years) in mice, rats, and dogs, nadolol did not produce any significant toxic effects. In two-year oral carcinogenic studies in rats and mice, nadolol did not produce any neoplastic, preneoplastic, or nonneoplastic pathologic lesions. In fertility and general reproductive performance studies in rats, nadolol caused no adverse effects.

Pregnancy Category C: In animal reproduction studies with nadolol, evidence of embryo and fetotoxicity was found in rabbits, but not in rats or hamsters, at doses 5 to 10 times greater (on a mg/kg basis) than the maximum indicated human dose. No teratogenic potential was observed in any of these species.

There are no adequate and well-controlled studies in pregnant women. Nadolol should be used during pregnancy only if the potential benefit justifies the potential risk to the fetus. Neonates whose mothers are receiving nadolol at parturition have exhibited bradycardia, hypoglycemia, and associated symptoms.

Nursing Mothers: Nadolol is excreted in human milk. Because of the potential for adverse effects in nursing infants, a decision should be made whether to discontinue nursing or to discontinue therapy taking into account the importance of nadolol to the mother.

Pediatric Use: Safety and effectiveness in children have not been established.

ADVERSE REACTIONS:

Most adverse effects have been mild and transient and have rarely required withdrawal of therapy.

Cardiovascular: Bradycardia with heart rates of less than 60 beats per minute occurs commonly, and heart rates below 40 beats per minute and/or symptomatic bradycardia were seen in about 2 of 100 patients. Symptoms of peripheral vascular insufficiency, usually of the Raynaud type, have occurred in approximately 2 to 100 patients. Cardiac failure, hypotension, and rhythm/conduction disturbances have each occurred in about 1 to 100 patients. Single instances of first degree and third degree heart block have been reported; intensification of AV block is a known effect of beta-blockers (see also CONTRAINDICATIONS, WARNINGS, and PRECAUTIONS).

Central Nervous System: Dizziness or fatigue has been reported in approximately 2 of 100 patients; paresthesias, sedation, and change in behavior have each been reported in approximately 6 of 1000 patients.

Respiratory: Bronchospasm has been reported in approximately 1 of 1000 patients (see CONTRAINDICATIONS and WARNINGS.)

Gastrointestinal: Nausea, diarrhea, abdominal discomfort, constipation, vomiting, indigestion, anorexia, bloating, and flatulence have been reported in 1 to 5 of 1000 patients.

Miscellaneous: Each of the following has been reported in 1 to 5 of 1000 patients: rash; pruritus; headache; dry mouth, eyes, or skin; impotence or decreased libido; facial swelling; weight gain; slurred speech; cough; nasal stuffiness; sweating; tinnitus; blurred vision. Reversible alopecia has been reported infrequently.

The following adverse reactions have been reported in patients taking nadolol and/or other beta-adrenergic blocking agents, but no causal relationship to nadolol has been established.

Central Nervous System: Reversible mental depression progressing to catatonia; visual disturbances; hallucinations; an acute reversible syndrome characterized by disorientation for time and place, short-term memory loss, emotional lability with slightly clouded sensorium, and decreased performance on neuropsychometrics.

Gastrointestinal: Mesenteric arterial thrombosis; ischemic colitis; elevated liver enzymes.

Hematologic: Agranulocytosis; thrombocytopenic or nonthrombocytopenic purpura.

Allergic: Fever combined with aching and sore throat; laryngospasm; respiratory distress.

Miscellaneous: Pemphigoid rash; hypertensive reaction in patients with pheochromocytoma; sleep disturbances; Peyronie's disease.

The oculomucocutaneous syndrome associated with the beta-blocker practolol has not been reported with nadolol.

OVERDOSAGE:

Nadolol can be removed from the general circulation by hemodialysis.

In addition to gastric lavage, the following measures should be employed, as appropriate. In determining the duration of corrective therapy, note must be taken of the long duration of the effect of nadolol.

Excessive Bradycardia: Administer atropine (0.25 to 1.0 mg). If there is no response to vagal blockade, administer isoproterenol cautiously.

Cardiac Failure: Administer a digitalis glycoside and diuretic. It has been reported that glucagon may also be useful in this duration.

Hypotension: Administer vasopressors, e.g., epinephrine or levarterenol. (There is evidence that epinephrine may be the drug of choice.)

Bronchospasm: Administer a beta$_2$-stimulating agent and/or a theophylline derivative.

DOSAGE AND ADMINISTRATION:

DOSAGE MUST BE INDIVIDUALIZED. NADOLOL MAY BE ADMINISTERED WITHOUT REGARD TO MEALS.

Angina Pectoris: The usual initial dose is 40 mg nadolol once daily. Dosage may be gradually increased in 40 to 80 mg increments at 3 to 7 day intervals until optimum clinical response is obtained or there is pronounced slowing of the heart rate. The usual maintenance dose is 40 or 80 mg administered once daily. Doses up to 160 or 240 mg administered once daily may be needed.

The usefulness and safety in angina pectoris of dosage exceeding 240 mg per day have not been established. If treatment is to be discontinued, reduce the dosage gradually over a period of one to two weeks (see WARNINGS.)

Hypertension: The usual initial dose is 40 mg nadolol once daily, whether it is used alone or in addition to diuretic therapy. Dosage may be gradually increased in 40 to 80 mg increments until optimum blood pressure reduction is achieved. The usual maintenance dose is 40 to 80 mg administered once daily. Doses up to 240 or 320 mg administered once daily may be needed.

Dosage Adjustment in Renal Failure: Absorbed nadolol is excreted principally by the kidneys and, although nonrenal elimination does occur, dosage adjustments are necessary in patients with renal impairment. The following dose intervals are recommended:

TABLE 1

Creatinine Clearance (ml/min/1.73m^2)	**Dosage Interval (hours)**
>50	24
31-50	24-36
10-30	24-48
<10	40-60

STORAGE

Store at room temperature; avoid excessive heat. Protect from light. Keep bottle tightly closed.

HOW SUPPLIED - RATED THERAPEUTICALLY EQUIVALENT:

Tablet, Uncoated - Oral - 20 mg

100's	$72.40	Nadolol, HL Moore Drug Exch	00839-7869-06
100's	$72.40	Nadolol, Apothecon	59772-2461-01
100's	$73.60	Nadolol, Major Pharms	00904-7816-60
100's	$74.42	Nadolol, Qualitest Pharms	00603-4740-21
100's	$78.18	Nadolol, Apothecon	59772-2461-02
100's	$84.23	Nadolol, UDL	51079-0812-20
100's	$85.50	Nadolol, Mylan	00378-0028-01
100's	**$89.74**	**CORGARD 20, Bristol Myers Squibb**	**00003-0232-50**
100's	**$96.89**	**CORGARD 20, Bristol Myers Squibb**	**00003-0232-51**

Tablet, Uncoated - Oral - 40 mg

100's	$84.67	Nadolol, Qualitest Pharms	00603-4741-21
100's	$84.88	Nadolol, HL Moore Drug Exch	00839-7870-06
100's	$84.88	Nadolol, Apothecon	59772-2462-01
100's	$86.25	Nadolol, Major Pharms	00904-7817-60
100's	$89.10	Nadolol, UDL	51079-0813-20
100's	$91.61	Nadolol, Apothecon	59772-2462-02
100's	$98.84	Nadolol, Mylan	00378-1171-01
100's	**$105.20**	**CORGARD 40, Bristol Myers Squibb**	**00003-0207-50**
100's	**$113.55**	**CORGARD 40, Bristol Myers Squibb**	**00003-0207-53**
1000's	$831.50	Nadolol, Apothecon	59772-2462-03
1000's	$968.25	Nadolol, Mylan	00378-1171-10
1000's	**$1030.55**	**CORGARD 40, Bristol Myers Squibb**	**00003-0207-76**

Tablet, Uncoated - Oral - 80 mg

100's	$116.09	Nadolol, Qualitest Pharms	00603-4742-21
100's	$116.38	Nadolol, HL Moore Drug Exch	00839-7871-06
100's	$116.38	Nadolol, Apothecon	59772-2463-01
100's	$118.30	Nadolol, Major Pharms	00904-7818-60
100's	$120.80	Nadolol, UDL	51079-0814-20
100's	$122.95	Nadolol, Apothecon	59772-2463-02
100's	$135.52	Nadolol, Mylan	00378-1132-01
100's	**$144.24**	**CORGARD 80, Bristol Myers Squibb**	**00003-0241-50**
1000's	$1139.95	Nadolol, Apothecon	59772-2463-03
1000's	$1327.45	Nadolol, Mylan	00378-1132-10
1000's	**$1412.86**	**CORGARD 80, Bristol Myers Squibb**	**00003-0241-76**

Tablet, Uncoated - Oral - 120 mg

100's	$151.68	Nadolol, Apothecon	59772-2464-01
500's	**$188.00**	**CORGARD 120, Bristol Myers Squibb**	**00003-0208-50**
1000's	$1483.50	Nadolol, Apothecon	59772-2464-03
1000's	**$1838.63**	**CORGARD 120, Bristol Myers Squibb**	**00003-0208-76**

Tablet, Uncoated - Oral - 160 mg

100's	$168.70	Nadolol, Apothecon	59772-2465-01
100's	**$209.09**	**CORGARD 160, Bristol Myers Squibb**	**00003-0246-49**

NAFARELIN ACETATE *(001850)*

CATEGORIES: EENT Drugs; Endometriosis; Eye, Ear, Nose, & Throat Preparations; Hormones; Lesions; Lh-Rh Agonist; Pain; Precocious Puberty; Pregnancy Category X; FDA Class 1C ("Little or No Therapeutic Advantage"); FDA Approved 1990 Feb

BRAND NAMES: **Synarel**; *Synarela* (Germany)
(International brand names outside U.S. in italics)

FORMULARIES: Aetna; BC-BS

DESCRIPTION:

NOTE: This monograph contains full prescribing information for two distinct indications of nafarelin acetate:**Endometriosis** and **Central Precocious Puberty**.

Nafarelin acetate nasal solution is intended for administration as a spray to the nasal mucosa. Nafarelin acetate, the active component of nafarelin nasal solution, is a decapeptide with the chemical name: 5-oxo-L-prolyl-L-histidyl-L-tryptophyl-L-seryl-L- tyrosyl-3-(2-naphthyl)-D-alanyl-L-leucyl-L-arginyl-L-prolyl-glycinamide acetate. Nafarelin acetate is a synthetic analog of the naturally occurring gonadotropin-releasing hormone (GnRH).

Nafarelin nasal solution contains nafarelin acetate (2 mg/ml, content expressed as nafarelin base) in a solution of benzalkonium chloride, glacial acetic acid, sodium hydroxide or hydrochloric acid (to adjust pH), sorbitol, and purified water.

After priming the pump unit for nafarelin, each actuation of the unit delivers approximately 100 μL of the spray containing approximately 200 mcg nafarelin base. The contents of one spray bottle are intended to deliver at least 60 sprays.

CLINICAL PHARMACOLOGY:

Nafarelin acetate is a potent agonistic analog of gonadotropin-releasing hormone (GnRH). At the onset of administration, nafarelin stimulates the release of the pituitary gonadotropins, LH and FSH, resulting in a temporary increase of ovarian steroidogenesis. Repeated dosing abolishes the stimulatory effect on the pituitary gland. Twice daily administration leads to decreased secretion of gonadal steroids by about 4 weeks; consequently, tissues and functions that depend on gonadal steroids for their maintenance become quiescent.

Nafarelin acetate is rapidly absorbed into the systemic circulation after intranasal administration. Maximum serum concentrations (measured by RIA) are achieved between 10 and 40 minutes. Following a single dose of 200 mcg base, the observed average peak concentration is 0.6 ng/ml, whereas following a single dose of 400 mcg base, the observed average peak concentration is 1.8 ng/ml. Bioavailability from a 400 mcg dose averaged 2.8%. The average serum half-life of nafarelin following intranasal administration is approximately 3 hours. About 80% of nafarelin acetate is bound to plasma proteins at 4°C. Twice daily intranasal administration of 200 or 400 mcg of nafarelin in 18 healthy women for 22 days did not lead to significant accumulation of the drug. Based on the mean Cmin levels on Days 15 and 22, there appears to be dose proportionally across the two dose levels.

After subcutaneous administration of ^{14}C-nafarelin acetate, 44-55% of the dose was recovered in urine and 18.5-44.2% was recovered in feces. Approximately 3% of the administered dose appears as unchanged nafarelin in urine. The ^{14}C serum half-life of the metabolites was about 85.5 hours. Six metabolites of nafarelin have been identified of which the major metabolite is Tyr-D(2)-Nal-Leu-Arg-Pro-Gly-NH$_2$(5-10). The activity of the metabolites, the metabolism of nafarelin by nasal mucosa, and the pharmacokinetics of the drug in hepatically- and renally-impaired patients have not been determined.

There appeared to be no significant effect of rhinitis, i.e., nasal congestion, on the systemic bioavailability of nafarelin ; however, if the use of a nasal decongestant for rhinitis is necessary during treatment with nafarelin, the decongestant should not be used until at least two hours following dosing of nafarelin.

In controlled clinical studies, nafarelin at doses of 400 and 800 mcg/day for 6 months was shown to be comparable to danazol, 800 mg/day, in relieving the clinical symptoms of endometriosis (pelvic pain, dysmenorrhea, and dyspareunia) and in reducing the size of endometrial implants as determined by laparoscopy. The clinical significance of a decrease in endometriotic lesions is not known at this time and in addition, laparoscopic staging of endometriosis does not necessarily correlate with severity of symptoms.

Nafarelin 400 mcg daily induced amenorrhea in approximately 65%, 80%, and 90% of the patients after 60, 90, and 120 days, respectively. In the first, second, and third post-treatment months, normal menstrual cycles resumed in 4%, 82%, and 100%, respectively, of those patients who did not become pregnant.

At the end of treatment, 60% of patients who received nafarelin, 400 mcg/day, were symptom free, 32% had mild symptoms, 7% had moderate symptoms and 1% had severe symptoms. Of the 60% of patients who had complete relief of symptoms at the end of treatment, 17% had moderate symptoms 6 months after treatment was discontinued, 33% had mild symptoms, 50% remained symptom free, and no patient had severe symptoms.

During the first two months of nafarelin acetate use, some women experience vaginal bleeding of variable duration and intensity. In all likelihood, this bleeding represents estrogen withdrawal bleeding, and is expected to stop spontaneously. If vaginal bleeding continues, the possibility of lack of compliance with the dosing regimen should be considered. If the patient is complying carefully with the regimen, an increase in dose to 400 mcg twice a day should be considered.

There is no evidence that pregnancy rates are enhanced or adversely affected by the use of nafarelin.

INDICATIONS AND USAGE:

ENDOMETRIOSIS

Nafarelin is indicated for management of endometriosis, including pain relief and reduction of endometriotic lesions. Experience with nafarelin for the management of endometriosis has been limited to women 18 years of age and older treated for 6 months.

CENTRAL PRECOCIOUS PUBERTY

Nafarelin is indicated for the treatment of **central precocious puberty (CPP)** (gonadotropin-dependent precocious puberty) in children of both sexes.

The diagnosis of **central precocious puberty (CPP)** is suspected when premature development of secondary sexual characteristics occurs at or before the age of 8 years in girls and 9 years in boys, and is accompanied by significant advancement of bone age and/or a poor adult height prediction. The diagnosis should be confirmed by pubertal gonadal sex steroid levels and a pubertal LH response to stimulation by native GnRH. Pelvic ultrasound assessment in girls usually reveals enlarged uterus and ovaries, the latter often with multiple cystic formations. Magnetic resonance imaging or CT-scanning of the brain is recommended to detect hypothalamic or pituitary tumors, or anatomical changes associated with increased intracranial pressure. Other causes of sexual precocity, such as congenital adrenal hyperplasia, testotoxicosis, testicular tumors and/or other autonomous feminizing or masculinizing disorders must be excluded by proper clinical hormonal and diagnostic imaging examinations.

CONTRAINDICATIONS:

1. Hypersensitivity to GnRH, GnRH agonist analogs or any of the excipients in nafarelin.

2. Undiagnosed abnormal vaginal bleeding.

3. Use in pregnancy or in women who may become pregnant while receiving the drug. Nafarelin may cause fetal harm when administered to a pregnant woman. Major fetal abnormalities were observed in rats, but not in mice or rabbits after administration of nafarelin throughout gestation. There was a dose-related increase in fetal mortality and a decrease in fetal weight in rats (see PRECAUTIONS, Pregnancy. The effects on rat fetal mortality are expected consequences of the alterations in hormonal levels brought about by the drug. If this drug is used during pregnancy or if the patient becomes pregnant while taking this drug, she should be apprised of the potential hazard to the fetus.

CONTRAINDICATIONS: *(cont'd)*

4. Use in women who are breast feeding (see PRECAUTIONS, Nursing Mothers.

WARNINGS:

ENDOMETRIOSIS

Safe use of nafarelin acetate in pregnancy has not been established clinically. Before starting treatment with nafarelin, pregnancy must be excluded.

When used regularly at the recommended dose, nafarelin usually inhibits ovulation and stops menstruation. Contraception is not ensured, however, by taking nafarelin, particularly if patients miss successive doses. Therefore, patients should use nonhormonal methods of contraception. Patients should be advised to see their physician if they believe they may be pregnant. If a patient becomes pregnant during treatment, the drug must be discontinued and the patient must be apprised of the potential risk to the fetus.

CENTRAL PRECOCIOUS PUBERTY

The diagnosis of central precocious puberty (CPP) must be established before treatment is initiated. Regular monitoring of CPP patients is needed to assess both patient response as well as compliance. This is particularly important during the first 6 to 8 weeks of treatment to assure that suppression of pituitary-gonadal function is rapid. Testing may include LH response to GnRH stimulation and circulating gonadal sex steroid levels. Assessment of growth velocity and bone age velocity should begin within 3 to 6 months of treatment initiation.

Some patients may not show suppression of the pituitary-gonadal axis by clinical and/or biochemical parameters. This may be due to lack of compliance with the recommended treatment regimen and may be rectified by recommending that the dosing be done by caregivers. If compliance problems are excluded, the possibility of gonadotropin-independent sexual precocity should be reconsidered and appropriate examinations should be conducted. If compliance problems are excluded and if gonadotropin-independent sexual precocity is not present, the dose of nafarelin may be increased to 1800 mcg/day administered as 600 mcg t.i.d.

PRECAUTIONS:

GENERAL

As with other drugs that stimulate the release of gonadotropins or that induce ovulation, ovarian cysts have been reported to occur in the first two months of therapy with nafarelin acetate. Many, but not all, of these events occurred in patients with polycystic ovarian disease. These cystic enlargements may resolve spontaneously, generally by about four to six weeks of therapy, but in some cases may require discontinuation of drug and/or surgical intervention. The relevance, if any of such events in children is unknown.

INFORMATION FOR THE PATIENT

Endometriosis: An information pamphlet for patients is included with the product. Patients should be aware of the following information:

1. Since menstruation should stop with effective doses of nafarelin acetate, the patient should notify her physician if regular menstruation persists. The cause of vaginal spotting, bleeding or menstruation could be non-compliance with the treatment regimen, or it could be that a higher dose of the drug is required to achieve amenorrhea. The patient should be questioned regarding her compliance. If she is careful and compliant, and menstruation persists to the second month, consideration should be given to doubling the dose of nafarelin. If the patient has missed several doses, she should be counseled on the importance of taking nafarelin regularly as prescribed.

2. Patients should not use nafarelin if they are pregnant, breast feeding, have undiagnosed abnormal vaginal bleeding, or are allergic to any of the ingredients in nafarelin.

3. Safe use of the drug in pregnancy has not been established clinically. Therefore, a nonhormonal method of contraception should be used during treatment. Patients should be advised that if they miss successive doses of nafarelin, breakthrough bleeding or ovulation maybe occur with the potential for conception. If a patient becomes pregnant during treatment, she should discontinue treatment and consult her physician.

4. Those adverse events occurring most frequently in clinical studies with nafarelin are associated with hypoestrogenism; the most frequently reported are hot flashes, headaches, emotional lability, decreased libido, vaginal dryness, acne, myalgia, and reduction in breast size. Estrogen levels returned to normal after treatment was discontinued. Nasal irritation occurred in about 10% of all patients who used intranasal nafarelin.

5. The induced hypoestrogenic state results in a small loss in bone density over the course of treatment, some of which may not be reversible. During one six-month treatment period, this bone loss should not be important. In patients with major risk factors for decreased bone mineral content such as chronic alcohol and/or tobacco use, strong family history of osteoporosis, or chronic use of drugs that can reduce bone mass such as anticonvulsants or corticosteroids, Nafarelin therapy may pose an additional risk. In these patients the risks and benefits must be weighed carefully before therapy with Nafarelin is instituted. Repeated courses of treatment with gonadotropin-releasing hormone analogs are not advisable in patients with major risk factors for loss of bone mineral content.

6. Patients with intercurrent rhinitis should consult their physician for the use of a topical nasal decongestant. If the use of a topical nasal decongestant is required during treatment with nafarelin, the decongestant should not be used until at least 2 hours following dosing with nafarelin.

7. Retreatment cannot be recommended since safety data beyond 6 months are not available.

Central Precocious Puberty (CPP): An information pamphlet for patients is included with the product. Patients and their caregivers should be aware of the following information:

1. Reversibility of the suppressive effects of nafarelin has been demonstrated by the appearance or return of menses, by the return of pubertal gonadotropin and gonadal sex steroid levels, and/or by advancement of secondary sexual development. Semen analysis was normal in the two ejaculated specimens obtained thus far from boys who have been taken off therapy to resume puberty. Fertility has not been documented by pregnancies and the effect of long term use of the drug on fertility is not known.

2. Patients and their caregivers should be adequately counselled to assure full compliance; irregular or incomplete daily doses may result in stimulation of pituitary-gonadal axis.

3. During the first month of treatment with nafarelin, some signs of puberty, e.g., vaginal bleeding or breast enlargement, may occur. This is the expected initial effect of the drug. Such changes should resolve soon after the first month. If such resolution does not occur within the first two months of treatment, this may due to lack of compliance or the presence of gonadotropin independent sexual precocity. If both possibilities are definitively excluded, the dose of nafarelin may be increased to 1800 mcg/day administered as 600 mcg tid.

4. Patients with intercurrent rhinitis should consult their physician for the use of a topical nasal decongestant. If the use of a topical nasal decongestant is required during treatment with nafarelin, the decongestant should not be used until at least 2 hours following dosing with nafarelin.

Sneezing during or immediately after dosing with nafarelin should be avoided, if possible, since this may impair drug absorption.

PRECAUTIONS: *(cont'd)*

DRUG/LABORATORY TEST INTERACTIONS

Endometriosis: Administration of nafarelin in therapeutic doses results in suppression of the pituitary-gonadal system. Normal function is usually restored within 4 to 8 weeks after treatment is discontinued. Therefore, diagnostic tests of pituitary gonadotropic and gonadal functions conducted during treatment and up to 4 to 8 weeks after discontinuation of therapy with nafarelin may be misleading.

CARCINOGENESIS, MUTAGENESIS, AND IMPAIRMENT OF FERTILITY

Carcinogenicity studies of nafarelin were conducted in rats (24 months) at doses up to 100 mcg/kg/day and mice (18 months) at doses up to 500 mcg/kg/day using intramuscular doses (up to 110 times and 560 times the maximum recommended human intranasal dose, respectively). These multiples of the human dose are based on the relative bioavailability of the drug by the two routes of administration. As seen with other GnRH agonists, nafarelin acetate given to laboratory rodents at high doses for prolonged periods induced proliferative responses (hyperplasia and/or neoplasia) of endocrine organs. At 24 months, there was an increase in the incidence of pituitary tumors (adenoma/carcinoma) in high-dose female rats and a dose-related increase in male rats. There was an increase in pancreatic islet cell adenomas in both sexes, and in benign testicular and ovarian tumors in the treated groups. There was a dose-related increase in benign adrenal medullary tumors in treated female rats. In mice, there was a dose-related increase in Harderian gland tumors in males and an increase in pituitary adenomas in high-dose females. No metastases of these tumors were observed. It is known that tumorigenicity in rodents is particularly sensitive to hormonal stimulation.

Mutagenicity studies have been performed with nafarelin acetate using bacterial, yeast, and mammalian systems. These studies provided no evidence of mutagenic potential.

Reproduction studies in male and female rats have shown full reversibility of fertility suppression when drug treatment was discontinued after continuous administration for up to 6 months. The effect of treatment of prepubertal rats on the subsequent reproductive performance of mature animals has not been investigated.

PREGNANCY, TERATOGENIC EFFECTS, PREGNANCY CATEGORY X

See CONTRAINDICATIONS. Intramuscular nafarelin was administered to rats throughout gestation at 0.4, 1.6, and 6.4 mcg/kg/day (about 0.5, 2, and 7 times the maximum recommended human intranasal dose based on the relative bioavailability by the two routes of administration). An increase in major fetal abnormalities was observed in 4/80 fetuses at the highest dose. A similar, repeat study at the same doses in rats and studies in mice and rabbits at doses up to 600 mcg/kg/day and 0.18 mcg/kg/day, respectively, failed to demonstrate an increase in fetal abnormalities after administration throughout gestation. In rats and rabbits, there was a dose-related increase in fetal mortality and a decrease in fetal weight with the highest dose.

NURSING MOTHERS

It is not known whether nafarelin is excreted in human milk. Because many drugs are excreted in human milk, and because the effects of nafarelin on lactation and/or the breast-fed child have not been determined, nafarelin should not be used by nursing mothers.

PEDIATRIC USE

Safety and effectiveness of nafarelin for endometriosis in patients younger than 18 years have not been established.

DRUG INTERACTIONS:

No pharmacokinetic-based drug-drug interaction studies have been conducted with nafarelin. However, because nafarelin acetate is a peptide that is primarily degraded by peptidase and not by cytochrome P-450 enzymes, and the drug is only about 80% bound to plasma proteins at 4°C, drug interactions would not be expected to occur.

ADVERSE REACTIONS:

ENDOMETRIOSIS

As would be expected with a drug which lowers serum estradiol levels, the most frequently reported adverse reactions were those related to hypoestrogenism.

In controlled studies comparing nafarelin (400 mcg/day) and danazol (600 or 800 mg/day), adverse reactions most frequently reported and thought to be drug-related are listed below (for a graphic representation of this data, please consult the original manufacturer's package insert):

Hypoestrogenic: Hot Flashes, Libido Decreased, Vaginal Dryness, Headaches, Emotional Lability, Insomnia

Androgenic: Acne, Myalgia, Breast Size Reduced, Edema, Seborrhea, Weight Gain, Hirsutism, Libido Increased

Local: Nasal Irritation

Miscellaneous: Depression, Weight Loss

In addition, less than 1% of patients experienced paresthesia, palpitations, chloasma, maculopapular rash, eye pain, urticaria, asthenia, lactation, breast engorgement, and arthralgia. In formal clinical trials, immediate hypersensitivity thought to be possibly or probably related to nafarelin occurred in 3 (0.2%) of 1509 healthy subjects or patients.

CHANGES IN BONE DENSITY

After six months of nafarelin treatment, vertebral trabecular bone density and total vertebral bone mass, measured by quantitative computed tomography (QCT), decreased by an average of 8.7% and 4.3%, respectively, compared to pretreatment levels. There was partial recovery of bone density in the post-treatment period; the average trabecular bone density and total bone mass were 4.9% and 3.3% less than the pretreatment levels, respectively. Total vertebral bone mass, measured by dual photon absorptiometry (DPA), decreased by a mean of 5.9% at the end of treatment. Mean total vertebral mass, re-examined by DPA six months after completion of treatment, was 1.4% below pretreatment levels. There was little, if any, decrease in the mineral content in compact bone of the distal radius and second metacarpal. Use of nafarelin for longer than the recommended six months or in the presence of other known risk factors for decreased bone mineral content may cause additional bone loss.

CHANGES IN LABORATORY VALUES DURING TREATMENT

Plasma Enzymes: During clinical trials with nafarelin, regular laboratory monitoring revealed that SGOT and SGPT levels were more than twice the upper limit of normal in only one patient each. There was no other clinical or laboratory evidence of abnormal liver function and levels returned to normal in both patients after treatment was stopped.

Lipids: At enrollment, 9% of the patients in the group taking nafarelin 400 mcg/day group and 2% of the patients in the danazol group had total cholesterol values above 250 mg/dl. These patients also had cholesterol values above 250 mg/dl at the end of treatment.

Of those patients whose pretreatment cholesterol values were below 250 mg/dl, 6% in the group treated with nafarelin and 18% in the danazol group, had post-treatment values above 250 mg/dl.

ADVERSE REACTIONS: *(cont'd)*

The mean (± SEM) pretreatment values for total cholesterol from all patients were 191.8 (4.3) mg/dl in the group treated with nafarelin and 193.1 (4.6) mg/dl in the danazol group. At the end of treatment, the mean values for total cholesterol from all patients were 204.5 (4.8) mg/dl in the Nafarelin group and 207.7 (5.1) mg/dl in the danazol group. These increases from the pretreatment values were statistically significant ($p<0.05$) in both groups.

Triglycerides were increased above the upper limit of 150 mg/dl in 12% of the patients who received nafarelin and in 7% of the patients who received danazol.

At the end of treatment, no patients receiving nafarelin had abnormally low HDL cholesterol fractions (less than 30 mg/dl) compared with 43% of patients receiving danazol. None of the patients receiving nafarelin had abnormally high LDL cholesterol fractions (greater than 190 mg/dl) compared with 15% of those receiving danazol. There was no increase in the LDL/HDL ratio in patients receiving nafarelin, but there was approximately a 2-fold increase in the LDL/HDL ratio in patients receiving danazol.

Other Changes: In comparative studies, the following changes were seen in approximately 10% to 15% of patients. Treatment with nafarelin was associated with elevations of plasma phosphorus and eosinophil counts, and decreases in serum calcium and WBC counts. Danazol therapy was associated with an increase of hematocrit and WBC.

CENTRAL PRECOCIOUS PUBERTY

In clinical trials of 155 pediatric patients, 2.6% reported symptoms suggestive of drug sensitivity, such as shortness of breath, chest pain, urticaria, rash and pruritus.

In these 155 patients treated for an average of 41 months and as long as 80 months (6.7 years), adverse events most frequently reported (>3% of patients) consisted largely of episodes occurring during the first 6 weeks of treatment as a result of the transient stimulatory action of nafarelin upon the pituitary-gonadal axis:

acne (10%)	transient increase in pubic hair (5%)
transient breast enlargement (8%)	body odor (4%)
vaginal bleeding (8%)	seborrhea (3%)
emotional liability (6%)	

Hot flashes, common in adult women treated for endometriosis, occurred in only 3% of treated children and were transient. Other adverse events thought to be drug-related, and occurring in >3% of patients were rhinitis (5%) and white or brownish vaginal discharge (3%). Approximately 3% of patients withdrew from clinical trials due to adverse events.

In one male patient with concomitant congenital adrenal hyperplasia, and who had discontinued treatment 8 months previously to resume puberty, adrenal rest tumors were found in the left testis. Relationship to nafarelin is unlikely.

Regular examinations of the pituitary gland by magnetic resonance imaging (MRI) or computer-assisted tomography (CT) of children during long-term nafarelin therapy as well as during the post-treatment period has occasionally revealed changes in the shape and size of the pituitary gland. These changes include asymmetry and enlargement of the pituitary gland, and a pituitary microadenoma has been suspected in a few children. The relationship of these findings to nafarelin is not known.

OVERDOSAGE:

In experimental animals, a single subcutaneous administration of up to 60 times the recommended human dose (on a mcg/kg basis, not adjusted for bioavailability) had no adverse effects. At present, there is no clinical evidence of adverse effects following overdosage of GnRH analogs.

Based on studies in monkeys, nafarelin is not absorbed after oral administration.

DOSAGE AND ADMINISTRATION:

ENDOMETRIOSIS

For the management of endometriosis, the recommended daily dose of nafarelin is 400 mcg. This is achieved by one spray (200 mcg) into one nostril in the morning and one spray into the other nostril in the evening. Treatment should be started between days 2 and 4 of the menstrual cycle.

In an occasional patient, the 400 mcg daily dose may not produce amenorrhea. For these patients with persistent regular menstruation after 2 months of treatment, the dose of nafarelin may be increased to 800 mcg daily. The 800 mcg dose is administered as one spray into each nostril in the morning (a total of two sprays) and again in the evening.

The recommended duration of administration is six months. Retreatment cannot be recommended since safety data for retreatment are not available. If the symptoms of endometriosis recur after a course of therapy, and further treatment with nafarelin is contemplated, it is recommended that bone density be assessed before retreatment begins to ensure that values are within normal limits.

There appeared to be no significant effect of rhinitis, i.e., nasal congestion, on the systemic bioavailability of nafarelin ; however, if the use of a topical nasal decongestant is necessary during treatment with nafarelin, the decongestant should not be used until at least 2 hours following dosing with nafarelin.

Sneezing during or immediately after dosing with nafarelin should be avoided, if possible, since this may impair drug absorption.

At 400 mcg/day, a bottle of nafarelin provides a 30-day (about 60 sprays) supply. If the daily dose is increased, increase the supply to the patient to ensure uninterrupted treatment for the recommended duration of therapy.

CENTRAL PRECOCIOUS PUBERTY (CPP)

For the treatment of **central precocious puberty (CPP)**, the recommended daily dose of nafarelin is 1600 mcg. The dose can be increased to 1800 mcg daily if adequate suppression cannot be achieved at 1600 mcg/day.

The 1600 mcg dose is achieved by two sprays (400 mcg) into each nostril in the morning (4 sprays) and two sprays into each nostril in the evening (4 sprays), a total of 8 sprays per day. The 1800 mcg dose is achieved by 3 sprays (600 mcg) into alternating nostrils three times a day, a total of 9 sprays per day. The patient's head should be tilted back slightly, and 30 seconds should elapse between sprays.

If the prescribed therapy has been well tolerated by the patient, treatment of CPP with nafarelin should continue until resumption of puberty is desired.

There appeared to be no significant effect of rhinitis, i.e., nasal congestion, on the systemic bioavailability of nafarelin ; however, if the use of a nasal decongestant for rhinitis is necessary during treatment with nafarelin, the decongestant should not be used until at least 2 hours following dosing with nafarelin.

Sneezing during or immediately after dosing with nafarelin should be avoided, if possible, since this may impair drug absorption.

At 1600 mcg/day, a bottle of nafarelin provides about a 7-day supply (about 56 sprays). If the daily dose is increased, increase the supply to the patient to ensure uninterrupted treatment for the duration of therapy.

Store upright at room temperature. Avoid heat above 30°C (86°F). Protect from light. Protect from freezing.

HOW SUPPLIED - EQUIVALENTS NOT AVAILABLE:

Solution - Nasal - 2 mg/ml

10 ml $336.25 SYNAREL NASAL, Syntex Labs 00033-2260-40

NAFCILLIN SODIUM *(001851)*

CATEGORIES: Anti-Infectives; Antibiotics; Antimicrobials; Infections; Penicillins; FDA Approval Pre 1982

BRAND NAMES: Nafcil; Nallpen; **Unipen**; *Vigopen*
(International brand names outside U.S. in italics)

FORMULARIES: BC-BS; Medi-Cal

DESCRIPTION:

Nafcillin sodium for injection is a semisynthetic penicillin derived from the penicillin nucleus, 6-aminopenicillanic acid. Chemically, nafcillin sodium is 6-(2-ethoxy-1-naphthamido)-penicillanic acid monohydrate. It is resistant to inactivation by the enzyme penicillinase (betalactamase).

Each gram of nafcillin is buffered with sodium citrate and contains approximately 2.9 mEq of sodium.

Its molecular formula is $C_{21}H_{21}N_2NaO_5S_1H_2O$ and the molecular weight is 454.47. [CAS-7177-50-6] Monosodium (2*S*,5*R*,6*R*)-6-(2-ethoxy-1-naphthamido)-3,3- dimethyl-7-oxo-4-thia-1-azabicyclo[3.2.0]heptane-2-carboxylate monohydrate.

Nafcillin sodium, equivalent to 500 mg, 1 gram or 2 grams of nafcillin, is a sterile mixture of nafcillin sodium monohydrate and sodium citrate intended for intravenous or intramuscular administration after reconstitution.

CLINICAL PHARMACOLOGY:

PHARMACOKINETICS

In a study of five healthy adults administered a single 500 mg dose of nafcillin by intravenous injection over 7 minutes, the mean plasma concentration of the drug was approximately 30 mcg/ml at 5 minutes after injection. The mean area under the plasma concentration-versus-time curve (AUC) for nafcillin in this study was 18.06 mcg.h/ml.

The serum half-life of nafcillin administered by the intravenous route ranged from 33 to 61 minutes as measured in three separate studies. In contrast to the other penicillinase-resistant penicillins, only about 30% of nafcillin is excreted as unchanged drug in the urine of normal volunteers, and most within the first 6 hours. Nafcillin is primarily eliminated by nonrenal routes, namely hepatic inactivation and excretion in the bile.

Nafcillin binds to serum proteins, mainly albumin. The degree of protein binding reported for nafcillin is 89.9 ± 1.5%. Reported values vary with the method of study and the investigator.

The concurrent administration of probenecid with nafcillin increases and prolongs plasma concentration of nafcillin. Probenecid significantly reduces the total body of nafcillin with renal clearance being decreased to a greater extent than nonrenal clearance.

The penicillinase-resistant penicillins are widely distributed in various body fluids, including bile, pleural, amniotic and synovial fluids. With normal doses insignificant concentrations are found in the aqueous humor of the eye. High nafcillin CSF levels have been obtained in the presence of inflamed meninges.

Renal failure does not appreciably affect the serum half-life of nafcillin; therefore, no modification of the usual nafcillin dosage is necessary in renal failure with or without hemodialysis. Hemodialysis does not accelerate the rate of clearance of nafcillin from the blood.

A study which assessed the effects of cirrhosis and extrahepatic biliary obstruction in man demonstrated that the plasma clearance of nafcillin was significantly decreased in patients with hepatic dysfunction. In these patients with cirrhosis and extrahepatic obstruction, nafcillin excretion in the urine was significantly increased from about 30% to 50% of the administered dose, suggesting that renal disease superimposed on hepatic disease could further decrease nafcillin clearance.

MICROBIOLOGY

Penicillinase-resistant penicillins exert a bactericidal action against penicillin-susceptible microorganisms during the state of active multiplication. All penicillins inhibit the biosynthesis of the bacterial cell wall.

The drugs in this class are highly resistant to inactivation by staphylococcal penicillinase and are active against penicillinase-producing and nonpenicillinase-producing strains of *Staphylococcus aureus.* The penicillinase-resistant penicillins are active *in vitro* against a variety of other bacteria.

SUSCEPTIBILITY TESTS

Diffusion Techniques: Quantitative methods of susceptibility testing that require measurements of zone diameters or minimal inhibitory concentrations (MICs) give the most precise estimates of antibiotic susceptibility. One such procedure has been recommended for use with discs to test susceptibility to this class of drugs. Interpretations correlate diameters on the disc test with MIC values.

A penicillinase-resistant class disc may be used to determine microbial susceptibility to nafcillin.

TABLE 1 shows the interpretation of test results for penicillinase-resistant penicillins using the FDA Standard Disc Test Method (formerly Bauer-Kirby-Sherris-Turck method) of disc bacteriological susceptibility testing for staphylococci with a disc containing 5 mcg of methicillin sodium. With this procedure, a report from a laboratory of "susceptible" indicates that the infecting organism is likely to respond to therapy. A report of "resistant" indicates that the infecting organism is not likely to respond to therapy. A report of "intermediate" susceptibility suggests that the organism might be susceptible if high doses of the antibiotic are used, or if the infection is confined to tissues and fluids (*e.g.*, urine) in which high antibiotic levels are attained.

In general, all staphylococci should be tested against the penicillin G disc and the methicillin disc. Routine methods of antibiotic susceptibility testing may fail to detect strains of organisms resistant to the penicillinase-resistant penicillins. For this reason, the use of large inocula and 48-hour incubation periods may be necessary to obtain accurate susceptibility studies with these antibiotics. Bacterial strains which are resistant to one of the penicillinase-resistant penicillins should be considered resistant to all of the drugs in the class.

TABLE 1 Standardized Disc Test Method Of Bacteriological Susceptibility Testing Using A Class Disc Containing 5mcg Of Methicillin Sodium.

Diameter of Zone indicating "Susceptible":	at least 14 mm
Diameter of Zone indicating "Intermediate":	10-13 mm
Diameter of zone indicating "Resistant":	less than 10 mm

INDICATIONS AND USAGE:

Nafcillin sodium is indicated in the treatment of infections caused by penicillinase-producing staphylococci which have demonstrated susceptibility to the drug. Culture and susceptibility tests should be performed initially to determine the causative organism and its sensitivity to the drug (see CLINICAL PHARMACOLOGY, Susceptibility Tests).

Nafcillin sodium may be used to initiate therapy in suspected cases of resistant staphylococcal infections prior to the availability of laboratory test results. Nafcillin sodium should not be used in infections caused by organisms susceptible to penicillin G. If the susceptibility tests indicate that the infection is due to an organism other than a resistant staphylococcus, therapy should not be continued with nafcillin sodium.

CONTRAINDICATIONS:

A history of a hypersensitivity (anaphylactic) reaction to any penicillin is a contraindication.

WARNINGS:

SERIOUS AND OCCASIONALLY FATAL HYPERSENSITIVITY (anaphylactic) REACTIONS HAVE BEEN REPORTED IN PATIENTS ON PENICILLIN THERAPY. THESE REACTIONS ARE MORE LIKELY TO OCCUR IN INDIVIDUALS WITH A HISTORY OF PENICILLIN HYPERSENSITIVITY AND/OR A HISTORY OF SENSITIVITY TO MULTIPLE ALLERGENS. THERE HAVE BEEN REPORTS OF INDIVIDUALS WITH A HISTORY OF PENICILLIN HYPERSENSITIVITY WHO HAVE EXPERIENCED SEVERE REACTIONS WHEN TREATED WITH CEPHALOSPORINS. BEFORE INITIATING THERAPY WITH NAFCILLIN SODIUM, CAREFUL INQUIRY SHOULD BE MADE CONCERNING PREVIOUS HYPERSENSITIVITY REACTIONS TO PENICILLINS, CEPHALOSPORINS OR OTHER ALLERGENS. IF AN ALLERGIC REACTION OCCURS, NAFCILLIN SODIUM SHOULD BE DISCONTINUED AND APPROPRIATE THERAPY INSTITUTED. **SERIOUS ANAPHYLACTIC REACTIONS REQUIRE IMMEDIATE EMERGENCY TREATMENT WITH EPINEPHRINE, OXYGEN, INTRAVENOUS STEROIDS AND AIRWAY MANAGEMENT, INCLUDING INTUBATION, SHOULD ALSO BE ADMINISTERED AS INDICATED. Pseudomembranous colitis has been reported with nearly all antibacterial agents, including nafcillin, and may range in severity from mild to life-threatening. Therefore, it is important to consider this diagnosis in patients who present with diarrhea subsequent to the administration of antibacterial agents.**

Treatment with antibacterial agents alters the normal flora of the colon and may permit overgrowth of clostridia. Studies indicate that a toxin produced by *Clostridium difficile* is one primary cause of "antibiotic-associated colitis."

After a diagnosis of pseudomembranous colitis has been established, therapeutic measures should be initiated. Mild cases of pseudomembranous colitis usually respond to drug discontinuation alone. In moderate to severe cases, consideration should be given to management with fluids and electrolytes, protein supplementation and treatment with an antibacterial drug clinically effective against *C. difficile* colitis.

PRECAUTIONS:

GENERAL

Nafcillin sodium generally should not be administered to patients with a history of sensitivity to any penicillin.

Penicillin should be used with caution in individuals with histories of significant allergies and/or asthma. Whenever allergic reactions occur, penicillin should be withdrawn unless, in the opinion of the physician, the condition being treated is life-threatening and amenable only to penicillin therapy.

The use of antibiotics may result in overgrowth of nonsusceptible organisms. If new infections due to bacteria or fungi occur, the drug should be discontinued and appropriate measures taken.

The liver/biliary tract is the primary route of nafcillin clearance. Caution should be exercised when patients with concomitant hepatic insufficiency and renal dysfunction are treated with nafcillin. Serum levels should be measured and the dosage adjusted appropriately to avoid possible neurotoxin reactions associated with very high concentrations(see DOSAGE AND ADMINISTRATION.)

LABORATORY TESTS

Bacteriologic studies to determine the causative organisms and their susceptibility to nafcillin should be performed (seeCLINICAL PHARMACOLOGY, Microbiology). In the treatment of suspected staphylococcal infections, therapy should be changed to another active agent if culture tests fail to demonstrate the presence of staphylococci.

Periodic assessment of organ system function including renal, hepatic and hematopoietic should be made during prolonged therapy with nafcillin. White blood cells and differential cell counts should be obtained prior to initiation of therapy and periodically during therapy with nafcillin. Periodic urinalysis, blood urea nitrogen and creatinine determinations should be performed during therapy with nafcillin.

SGOT and SGPT values should be obtained periodically during therapy to monitor for possible liver function abnormalities.

DRUG/LABORATORY TEST INTERACTIONS

Nafcillin in the urine can cause a false-positive urine reaction for protein when the sulfosalicylic acid test is used, but not with the dipstick.

CARCINOGENESIS, MUTAGENESIS, AND IMPAIRMENT OF FERTILITY

No long animal studies have been conducted with nafcillin.

Studies on reproduction in rats and rabbits reveal no fetal or material abnormalities before conception and continuously during weaning (one generation).

PREGNANCY, TERATOGENIC EFFECTS

Pregnancy Category B: Reproduction studies have been performed in the mouse with oral doses up to 20 times the human dose and orally in the rat at doses up to 40 times the human dose and have revealed no evidence of impaired fertility or harm to the rodent fetus due to nafcillin sodium. There are, however, no adequate or well-controlled studies in pregnant women. Because animal reproduction studies are not always predictive of human response, this drug should be used during pregnancy only if clearly needed.

NURSING MOTHERS

Penicillins are excreted in human milk. Caution should be exercised when penicillins are administered to a nursing woman.

PEDIATRIC USE

The liver/biliary tract is the principal route of nafcillin elimination. Because of immature hepatic and renal function in newborns, nafcillin excretion may be impaired with abnormally high serum levels resulting. Serum levels should be monitored and the dosage adjusted appropriately.[1,2] There are no approved neonatal or pediatric dosage regimens for intravenous nafcillin.

DRUG INTERACTIONS:

Tetracycline, a bacteriostatic antibiotic, may antagonize the bactericidal effect of penicillin and concurrent use of these drugs should be avoided. Nafcillin in high dosage regimens, i.e., 2 grams every 4 hours, has been reported to decrease the effects of warfarin. When nafcillin

DRUG INTERACTIONS: *(cont'd)*

and warfarin are used concomitantly, the prothrombin time should be closely monitored and the dose of warfarin adjusted as necessary. This effect may persist for up to 30 days after nafcillin has been discontinued.

Nafcillin when administered concomitantly with cyclosporine has been reported to result in subtherapeutic cyclosporine levels. The nafcillin-cyclosporine interaction was documented in a patient during two separate courses of therapy. When cyclosporine and nafcillin are used concomitantly in organ transplant patients, the cyclosporine levels should be monitored.

ADVERSE REACTIONS:

Body as a Whole: The reported incidence of allergic reactions to penicillin ranges from 0.7% to 10% (see WARNINGS.) Sensitization is usually the result of treatment but some individuals have had immediate reactions to penicillin when first treated. In such cases,it is thought that the patients may have had prior exposure to the drug via trace amounts present in milk or vaccines.

Two types of allergic reactions to penicillins are noted clinically, immediately and delayed.

Immediate reactions usually occur within 20 minutes of administration and range in severity from urticaria and pruritus to angioneurotic edema, laryngospasm, bronchospasm, hypotension, vascular collapse and death. Such immediate anaphylactic reactions are very rare (see WARNINGS) and usually occur after parenteral therapy but have occurred in patients receiving oral therapy. Another type of immediate reaction, an accelerated reaction, may occur between 20 minutes and 48 hours after administration and may include urticaria, pruritus and fever. Although laryngeal edema, laryngospasm and hypotension occasionally occur, fatality is uncommon.

Delayed allergic reactions to penicillin therapy usually occur after 48 hours and sometimes as late as 2 to 4 weeks after initiation of therapy. Manifestations of this type of reaction include serum-sickness-like symptoms (*i.e.,* fever, malaise, urticaria, myalgia, arthralgia, abdominal pain) and various skin rashes. Nausea, vomiting, diarrhea, stomatitis, black or hairy tongue, and other symptoms of gastrointestinal irritation may occur, especially during oral penicillin therapy.

Local Reactions: Pain, swelling and inflammation at the injection site and phlebitis or thrombophlebitis have occurred with intravenous administration of nafcillin (see DOSAGE AND ADMINISTRATION.)

Nervous System Reactions: Neurotoxic reactions similar to those observed with penicillin G could occur with large intravenous doses of nafcillin, especially in patients with concomitant hepatic insufficiency and renal dysfunction (see PRECAUTIONS.)

Urogenital Reactions: Renal tubular damage and interstitial nephritis have been associated infrequently with the administration of nafcillin. Manifestations of this reaction may include rash, fever, eosinophilia, hematuria, proteinuria and renal insufficiency.

Gastrointestinal Reactions: Pseudomembranous colitis has been reported with the use of nafcillin. The onset of pseudomembranous colitis symptoms may occur during or after antibiotic treatment (see WARNINGS.)

Metabolic Reactions: Agranulocytosis, neutropenia and bone marrow depression have been associated with the use of nafcillin.

OVERDOSAGE:

Neurotoxic reactions similar to those observed with penicillin G may arise with intravenous doses of nafcillin especially in patients with concomitant hepatic insufficiency and renal dysfunction (see PRECAUTIONS.)

In the case of overdosage, discontinue nafcillin, treat symptomatically and institute supportive measures are required. Hemodialysis does not increase the rate of clearance of nafcillin from the blood.

DOSAGE AND ADMINISTRATION:

The usual IV dosage for adults is 500 mg every 4 hours. For severe infections, 1 gram every 4 hours is recommended (see TABLE 2.)

Administered slowly over at least 30 to 60 minutes to minimize the risk of vein irritation.

Bacteriologic studies to determine the causative organisms and their sensitivity to nafcillin should always be performed. Duration of therapy varies with the type and severity of infection as well as the overall condition of the patient; therefore, it should be determined by the clinical and bacteriologic responses of the patient. In severe staphylococcal infections, therapy with Nafcillin sodium for Injection should be continued for at least 14 days. Therapy should be continued for at least 48 hours after the patient has become afebrile, asymptomatic and cultures are negative. The treatment of endocarditis and osteomyelitis may require a longer term of therapy.

Concurrent administration of nafcillin and probenecid increases and prolongs serum penicillin levels. Probenecid decreases the apparent volume of distribution and slows the rate of excretion by competitively inhibiting renal tubular secretion of penicillin. Penicillin-probenecid therapy is generally limited to those infections where very high serum levels of penicillin are necessary. For intramuscular gluteal injections, care should be taken to avoid sciatic nerve injury. With intravenous administration, particularly in elderly patients, care should be taken because of the possibility of thrombophlebitis.

Dosage alterations are necessary for patients with renal dysfunction, including those on hemodialysis. Hemodialysis does not accelerate nafcillin clearance from the blood.

For patients with hepatic insufficiency and renal failure, measurement of nafcillin serum levels should be performed and the dosage adjusted accordingly.

Parenteral drug products should be inspected visually for particulate matter and discoloration prior to administration whenever solution and container permit.

Do not add supplementary medication to nafcillin sodium for Injection.

TABLE 2 Recommended Dosages For Nafcillin Sodium

Adult	Infants and Children < 40 kg (88 lbs)	Other Recommendations
500 mg IM every 4-6 Hours IV every 4 hours 1 gram IM or IV every 4 hours (severe infections)	25 mg/kg IM twice daily	Neonates 10 mg/kg IM twice Daily

DIRECTIONS FOR USE

500 mg, 1 gram and 2 gram Standard Vials

For initial reconstitution use Sterile Water for Injection, USP, or Sodium Chloride Injection, USP.

Intramuscular Administration (concentration of 250 mg/ml) (TABLE 3):

DOSAGE AND ADMINISTRATION: *(cont'd)*

TABLE 3

Vial Size	Amount of Diluent to Be Added	Volume After Reconstitution
500 mg	1.7 ml	2 ml
1 gram	3.4 ml	4 ml
2 gram	6.8 ml	8 ml

Add the required amount of Sterile Water for Injection, USP, or Sodium Chloride Injection, Usp, and shake vigorously to reconstitute. As with all intramuscular preparations nafcillin sodium should be injected well within the body of relatively large muscle using techniques and precautions.

After reconstitution, the solution may be frozen (approx. 0°F) and stored for up to 90 days. The thawed solution must be used within 24 hours.

Stability-For IV solution see Stability Period below.

DIRECT INTRAVENOUS ADMINISTRATION (concentration of approximately 16 mg/ml to 87 mg/ml):

Reconstitute the required amount of drug as directed under Intramuscular Administration, withdraw the entire contents, then further dilute with 15 to 30 ml Sodium Chloride Injection, Usp. Administer as slowly as possible to avoid vein irritation.

CONTINUOUS INTRAVENOUS INFUSION

Reconstitute as directed under Intramuscular Administration, withdraw the entire contents, then further dilute with Sodium Chloride Injection, USP, to the desired concentration.

Stability-For IV solution see Stability Period below.

1 gram and 2 gram Piggyback Bottles

Direct Intravenous Administration

Reconstitute as directed under Intramuscular Administration, then further dilute with Sodium Chloride Injection, USP, to the desired concentration. Administer as slowly as possible to avoid vein irritation.

Continuous Intravenous Infusion (concentration of 10 mg/ml to 20 mg/ml):

1 gram Piggyback Bottle: reconstitute with 50 to 100 ml of Sodium Chloride Injection, USP, or 5% Dextrose in Water and shake well.

2 gram Piggyback Bottle: reconstitute with 99 ml of Sodium Chloride Injection, USP, or 5% Dextrose in Water and shake well.

Stability-For IV solutions see Stability Period (TABLE 4) below.

TABLE 4 Stability Period
Intramuscular Solutions/Intravenous Solutions

(concentrations >30 mg/ml to 250 mg/ml)	Room Temperature*	Refrigerated**
Sterile Water for USP Injection,USP	3 days	7 days
Sodium Chloride Injection, USP	3 days	7 days
Intravenous Solutions (concentrations < 30 mg/ml)		
Sodium Chloride Injection, USP	3 days	14 days
5% Dextrose in Water	3 days	14 days

* 21° to 24°C (70° to 75°F)
** 4°C (40°F)

Unused portions of the reconstituted solutions should be discarded after the time periods listed above.

Only those appropriate solutions listed above should be used for the intravenous infusion of nafcillin sodium. The drug concentration, the rate and volume of the infusion should be adjusted so that the dose of nafcillin remains within the stated stability period.

INTRAVENOUS BOLUS INJECTION

Withdraw an appropriate portion of the stock solution containing the recommended dosage and further dilute with 5% Dextrose in Water or Sodium Chloride Injection, USP, to the desired volume. Administer as slowly as possible to avoid vein irritation.

INTRAVENOUS INFUSION

Withdraw the recommended dosage from the stock solution and further dilute with 5% Dextrose in Water or Sodium Chloride Injection, USP, to a concentration ≤30 mg/ml.

Stability/Storage Conditions: The concentrated stock solution (concentration of approx. 100 mg/ml) must be further diluted within 24 hours at room temperature 21° to 24°C (70° to 75°F) or within 72 hours if stored under refrigeration 4°C (40°F).

The diluted solutions (≤30 mg/ml) will remain stable for 72 hours at room temperature 21° to 24°C (70° to 75°F) or 14 days under refrigeration 4°C(40°F). Any unused portion of either solution must be discarded after the time periods listed above.

REFERENCES:

1. Banner W Jr. Gooch WM III, Burckhart G and Korones SB. Pharmacokinetics of nafcillin with low birth rates. Antimicrob Agents Chemother 17:691-694, 1980. 2. O'Connor WJ, Warren GH, Mandala PS, Edrada LS and Rosenman SB. Serum concentrations of nafcillin in newborn infants and children. Antimicrob Agents Chemother 4:188-191, 1964.

HOW SUPPLIED - RATED THERAPEUTICALLY EQUIVALENT:

Injection, Dry-Soln - Intramuscular; - 250 mg/vial

1 gm x 10	**$64.70**	**UNIPEN, Wyeth Labs**	**00008-0751-24**
1 gm x 10	**$65.46**	**UNIPEN, Wyeth Labs**	**00008-0751-16**
2 gm x 10	**$121.95**	**UNIPEN, Wyeth Labs**	**00008-0751-28**
2 gm x 10	**$122.79**	**UNIPEN, Wyeth Labs**	**00008-0751-14**
500 mg x 10	**$32.58**	**UNIPEN, Wyeth Labs**	**00008-0751-08**
500 mg x 10	**$36.33**	**UNIPEN, Wyeth Labs**	**00008-0751-22**

Injection, Dry-Soln - Intravenous - 1 gm/vial

1 gm x 10	$45.40	Nafcillin Sodium, Bristol Myers Squibb	00003-2989-10
1 gm x 10	$63.10	Nafcillin Sodium, Bristol Myers Squibb	00003-2989-20
20 ml x 10	$3.27	NALLPEN, Beecham	00029-6372-22
21 ml x 10	$3.05	NALLPEN ADD-VANTAGE, Beecham	00029-6372-40

Injection, Dry-Soln - Intravenous - 2 gm

2 gm	$6.29	NAFCIL, Mead Johnson	00015-7226-20
2 gm	$6.43	NAFCIL, Mead Johnson	00015-7226-18
2 gm x 10	$87.90	Nafcillin Sodium, Bristol Myers Squibb	00003-2991-10
2 gm x 10	$105.70	Nafcillin Sodium, Bristol Myers Squibb	00003-2991-20
21 ml x 10	$5.60	NALLPEN ADD-VANTAGE, Beecham	00029-6374-40
30 ml x 10	$6.29	NALLPEN, Beecham	00029-6374-27
100 ml x 10	$6.89	NALLPEN, Beecham	00029-6374-21

Injection, Dry-Soln - Intravenous - 10 gm/vial

10 gm	$35.53	NAFCIL, Mead Johnson	00015-7101-28
10 gm x 10	$435.40	Nafcillin Sodium, Bristol Myers Squibb	00003-2993-25
100 ml x 10	$25.95	NALLPEN, Beecham	00029-6376-21

HOW SUPPLIED - RATED THERAPEUTICALLY EQUIVALENT: *(cont'd)*

Injection, Dry-Soln - Intravenous - 500 mg

1 gm	$3.24	NAFCIL, Mead Johnson	00015-7225-20
1 gm	$3.82	NAFCIL, Mead Johnson	00015-7225-18
10 ml x 10	$2.08	NALLPEN, Beecham	00029-6370-25
500 mg	$1.72	NAFCIL, Mead Johnson	00015-7224-20
500 mg x 10	$24.00	Nafcillin Sodium, Bristol Myers Squibb	00003-2987-10

Injection, Solution - Intravenous - 1 gm

1's	$3.62	Nallpen, Beecham	00029-6372-07
1's	$4.50	Nafcillin Sodium, Mead Johnson	00015-7195-28
10's	$31.20	Nafcillin Sodium, Gensia Labs	00703-8218-03
10's	$32.40	Nafcillin Sodium, Gensia Labs	00703-8219-03
20 ml x 10	$40.82	Nafcillin Sodium, Vial, Marsam	00209-6950-22
100 ml x 10	$56.73	Nafcillin Sodium, Piggyback, Marsam	00209-7000-42

Injection, Solution - Intravenous - 2 gm

1's	$6.65	Nallpen, Beecham	00029-6374-07
1's	$9.42	Nafcillin Sodium, Mead Johnson	00015-7196-28
10's	$58.80	Nafcillin Sodium, Gensia Labs	00703-8228-03
10's	$61.20	Nafcillin Sodium, Gensia Labs	00703-8229-03
20 ml x 10	$79.03	Nafcillin Sodium, Vial, Marsam	00209-7100-22
100 ml x 10	$95.04	Nafcillin Sodium, Piggyback, Marsam	00209-7150-42

Injection, Solution - Intravenous - 10 gm

10's	$263.88	Nafcillin Sodium, Gensia Labs	00703-8238-03
100 ml x 10	$391.77	Nafcillin Sodium, Bulk, Marsam	00209-7250-52

Injection, Solution - Intravenous - 500 mg

6 ml x 10	$21.57	Nafcillin Sodium, Vial, Marsam	00209-6900-22
10's	$16.68	Nafcillin Sodium, Gensia Labs	00703-8208-03

HOW SUPPLIED - NOT RATED EQUIVALENT:

Capsule, Gelatin - Oral - 250 mg

100's	**$110.10**	**UNIPEN, Wyeth Labs**	**00008-0057-03**

Injection, Solution - Intravenous - 1 gm

50 ml	$22.21	NALLPEN, Baxter Hlthcare	00338-1017-41

Injection, Solution - Intravenous - 2 gm

100 ml	$31.97	NALLPEN, Baxter Hlthcare	00338-1019-41

NAFTIFINE HYDROCHLORIDE *(001852)*

CATEGORIES: Anti-Infectives; Antifungals; Dermatologicals; Fungal Agents; Infections; Skin/Mucous Membrane Agents; Tinea Corporis; Tinea Cruris; Tinea Pedis; Topical; Pregnancy Category B; FDA Approved 1988 Feb

BRAND NAMES: *Exoderil* (Germany); **Naftin**
(International brand names outside U.S. in italics)

FORMULARIES: BC-BS

COST OF THERAPY: $32.48 (Tinea Pedis; Cream; 1 %; 2/day; 28 days)

DESCRIPTION:

Naftinine HCl cream 1% and gel 1% contains the synthetic, broad-spectrum, antifungal agent naftifine hydrochloride. Naftinine HCl cream 1% and gel 1% are for topical use only.

Chemical Name: (E)-N-Cinnamyl-N-methyl-1-naphthalenemethylamine hydrochloride.

Naftifine hydrochloride has an empirical formula of $C_{21}H_{21}N\text{-}HCl$ and a molecular weight of 323.86.

Active Ingredient: Naftifine hydrochloride 1%.

Naftin Inactive Ingredients: *Cream:* benzyl alcohol, cetyl alcohol, cetyl esters wax, isopropyl myristate, polysorbate 60, purified water, sodium hydroxide, sorbitan monostearate, and stearyl alcohol. Hydrochloric acid may be added to adjust the pH. *Gel:* polysorbate 80, carbomer 934P, diisopropanolamine, edetate disodium, alcohol (52% v/v), and purified water.

CLINICAL PHARMACOLOGY:

Naftifine hydrochloride is a synthetic, allylamine derivative. The following *in vitro* data are available, but their clinical significance is unknown. Naftifine hydrochloride has been shown to exhibit fungicidal activity *in vitro* against a broad spectrum of organisms including *Trichophyton rubrum, Trichophyton mentagrophytes, Trichophyton tonsurans, Epidermophyton floccosum,Microsporum canis, Microsporum audouini,* and *Microsporum gypseum;* and fungistatic activity against *Candida* species, including *Candida albicans.* Naftinine HCl cream 1% and gel 1% have only been shown to be clinically effective against the disease entities listed in the INDICATIONS AND USAGEsection.

Although the exact mechanism of action against fungi is not known, naftifine hydrochloride appears to interfere with sterol biosynthesis by inhibiting the enzyme squalene 2, 3-epoxidase. This inhibition of enzyme activity results in decreased amounts of sterols, especially ergosterol, and a corresponding accumulation of squalene in the cells.

PHARMACOKINETICS

In vitro and *in vivo* bioavailability studies have demonstrated that naftifine penetrates the stratum corneum in sufficient concentration to inhibit the growth of dermatophytes.

Cream: Following a single topical application of 1% naftifine cream to the skin of healthy subjects, systemic absorption of naftifine was approximately 6% of the applied dose. Naftifine and/or its metabolites are excreted via the urine and feces with a half-life of approximately two to three days.

Gel: Following single topical applications of ^{3}H- labeled naftifine gel 1% to the skin of healthy subjects, up to 4.2% of the applied dose was absorbed. Naftifine and/or its metabolites are excreted via the urine and feces with a half-life of approximately two to three days.

INDICATIONS AND USAGE:

Naftinine HCl cream 1% and gel 1% are indicated for the topical application of tinea pedis, tinea cruris and tinea corporis caused by the organisms*Trichophyton rubrum, Trichophyton mentagrophytes, Trichophyton tonsurans** and *Epidermophytonfloccosum.**

*Efficacy for this organism in this organ system was studied in fewer than 10 infections.

CONTRAINDICATIONS:

Naftinine HCl cream 1% and gel 1% are contraindicated in individuals who have shown hypersensitivity to any of its components.

WARNINGS:

Naftinine HCl cream 1% and gel 1% are for topical use only and not for ophthalmic use.

PRECAUTIONS:

General: Naftinine HCl are for external use only. If irritation or sensitivity develops with the use of naftinine HCl cream 1% or gel 1%, treatment should be discontinued and appropriate therapy instituted. Diagnosis of the disease should be confirmed either by direct microscopic examination of a mounting of infected tissue in a solution of potassium hydroxide or by culture on an appropriate medium.

Information for the Patient: The patient should be told to:

1. Avoid the use of occlusive dressings or wrappings unless otherwise directed by the physician.

2. Keep Naftinine HCl cream 1% and gel 1% away from the eyes, nose, mouth and other mucous membranes.

Carcinogenesis, Mutagenesis, and Impairment of Fertility: Long-term studies to evaluate the carcinogenic potential of naftinine HCl cream 1% and gel 1% have not been performed. *In vitro* and animal studies have not demonstrated any mutagenic effect or effect on fertility.

Pregnancy, Teratogenic Effects, Pregnancy Category B Reproduction studies have not been performed in rats and rabbits (via oral administration) at doses 150 times or more the topical human dose and have revealed no evidence of impaired fertility or harm to the fetus due to naftifine. There are, however, no adequate and well-controlled studies in pregnant women. Because animal reproduction studies are not always predictive of human response, the drug should be used during pregnancy only if clearly needed.

Nursing Mothers: It is not known whether this drug is excreted in human milk. Because many drugs are excreted in human milk, caution should be exercised when naftinine HCl cream 1% and gel 1% is administered to a nursing woman.

Pediatric Use: Safety and effectiveness in children have not been established.

ADVERSE REACTIONS:

Cream: During clinical trials with naftin cream 1%, the incidence of adverse reactions was as follows: burning/stinging (6%), dryness (3%), erythema (2%), itching (2%), local irritation (2%).

Gel: During clinical trials with naftinine gel 1%, the incidence of adverse reactions was as follows: burning/stinging (5.0%), itching (1.0%), erythema (0.5%), rash (0.5%), skin tenderness (0.5%).

DOSAGE AND ADMINISTRATION:

Cream: A sufficient quantity of naftinine cream 1% should be gently massaged into the affected and surrounding skin areas once a day. The hands should be washed after application.

If no clinical improvement is seen after four weeks of treatment with naftinine cream 1%, the patient should be re-evaluated.

Note: Store below 30°C (86°F).

Gel: A sufficient quantity of naftinine gel 1% should be gently massaged into the affected and surrounding skin areas twice a day, in the morning and evening. The hands should be washed after application.

If no clinical improvement is seen after four weeks of treatment with naftinine gel 1%, the patient should be re-evaluated.

Note: Store at room temperature.

(Allergan Inc., 5/90, 70104, 9/90, 70147)

HOW SUPPLIED - EQUIVALENTS NOT AVAILABLE:

Cream - Topical - 1 %

15 gm	$13.47	NAFTIN, Allergan	00023-4126-15
30 gm	$22.47	NAFTIN, Allergan	00023-4126-30
60 gm	$34.81	NAFTIN, Allergan	00023-4126-60

Gel - Topical - 1 %

20 gm	$19.05	NAFTIN 1 % GEL, Allergan	00023-4770-20
40 gm	$30.25	NAFTIN 1 % GEL, Allergan	00023-4770-40
60 gm	$35.46	NAFTIN 1 % GEL, Allergan	00023-4770-60

NALBUPHINE HYDROCHLORIDE *(001853)*

CATEGORIES: Analeptics; Analgesics; Anesthesia; Antagonists and Antidotes; Antidotes; Antipyretics; Central Nervous System Agents; Labor; Labor and Delivery; Narcotic Agonist-Antagonist; Narcotics, Synthetics & Combinations; Opiate Partial Agonists; Pain; FDA Approval Pre 1982

BRAND NAMES: **Nubain**; *Nubain SP* (Mexico)
(International brand names outside U.S. in italics)

FORMULARIES: BC-BS

DESCRIPTION:

Nalbuphine Hydrochloride (abbreviated here as nalbuphine HCl) is a synthetic narcotic agonist-antagonist analgesic of the phenanthrene series. It is chemically related to both the widely used narcotic antagonist, naloxone, and the potent narcotic analgesic, oxymorphone.

Nalbuphine HCl is (-)-17-(cyclobutylmethyl)-4,5α-epoxymorphinan-3,6α, 14-triol,HCl. The Molecular weight 393.96.

Nalbuphine HCl Injection is available in two concentrations, 10 mg and 20 mg of nalbuphine HCl per ml. Both strengths contain per ml: 9.4 mg sodium citrate (hydrous) 12.6 mg citric acid (anhydrous), 1 mg sodium metabisulfite, and 1.8 mg methylparaben and 0.2 mg propylparaben as preservatives; pH is adjusted, if necessary, with HCl acid. The 10 mg/ml strength also contains 1 mg sodium chloride per ml.

CLINICAL PHARMACOLOGY:

Nalbuphine HCl is a potent analgesic. Its analgesic potency is essentially equivalent to that of morphine on a milligram basis.

Its onset of action occurs within 2 to 3 minutes after intravenous administration, and in less than 15 minutes following subcutaneous or intramuscular injection. The plasma half-life of nalbuphine is 5 hours and in clinical studies the duration of analgesic activity has been reported to range from 3 to 6 hours.

The narcotic antagonist activity of nalbuphine is one-fourth as potent as nalorphine and 10 times that of pentazocine.

INDICATIONS AND USAGE:

Nalbuphine HCl is indicated for the relief of moderate to severe pain. Nalbuphine HCl can also be used as a supplement to balanced anesthesia, for preoperative and postoperative analgesia, and for obstetrical analgesia during labor and delivery.

CONTRAINDICATIONS:

Nalbuphine HCl Injection should not be administered to patients who are hypersensitive to it.

WARNINGS:

Nalbuphine HCl should be administered as a supplement to general anesthesia only by persons specifically trained in the use of intravenous anesthetics and management of the respiratory effects of potent opioids.

NALOXONE HCL INJECTION, RESUSCITATIVE AND INTUBATION EQUIPMENT AND OXYGEN SHOULD BE READILY AVAILABLE.

Drug Dependence: Nalbuphine HCl has been shown to have a low abuse potential. When compared with drugs which are mixed agonist-antagonists, it has been reported that nalbuphine's potential for abuse would be less than that of codeine and propoxyphene. Psychological and physical dependence and tolerance may follow that abuse or misuse of nalbuphine. Therefore, caution should be observed in prescribing it for emotionally unstable patients, or for individuals with a history of narcotic abuse. Such patients should be closely supervised when long-term therapy is contemplated. Care should be taken to avoid increase in dosage or frequency of administration which in susceptible individuals might result in physical dependence.

Abrupt discontinuation of nalbuphine HCl following prolonged use has been followed by symptoms of narcotic withdrawal, i.e., abdominal cramps, nausea and vomiting, rhinorrhea, lacrimation, restlessness, anxiety, elevated temperature and piloerection.

Use in Ambulatory Patients: Nalbuphine may impair the mental or physical abilities required for the performance of potentially dangerous tasks such as driving a car or operating machinery. Therefore, nalbuphine HCl Injection should be administered with caution to ambulatory patients who should be warned to avoid such hazards.

Use in Emergency Procedures: Maintain patient under observation until recovered from nalbuphine effects that would affect driving or other potentially dangerous tasks.

Usage in Children: Clinical experience to support administration to patients under 18 years is not available at present.

Use in Pregnancy (other than labor): Safe use of nalbuphine HCl in pregnancy has not been established. Although animal reproductive studies have not revealed teratogenic or embryotoxic effects, nalbuphine should only be administered to pregnant women when, in the judgment of the physician, the potential benefits outweigh the possible hazards.

Use During Labor and Delivery: Nalbuphine can produce respiratory depression in the neonate. It should be used with caution in women delivering premature infants.

Head Injury and Increased Intracranial Pressure: The possible respiratory depressant effects and the potential of potent analgesics to elevate cerebrospinal fluid pressure (resulting from vasodilation following CO_2 retention) may be markedly exaggerated in the presence of head injury, intracranial lesions or a pre-existing increase in intracranial pressure. Furthermore, potent analgesics can produce effects which may obscure the clinical course of patients with head injuries. Therefore, nalbuphine HCl Injection should be used in these circumstances only when essential, and then should be administered with extreme caution.

Sulfites Sensitivity: Nalbuphine HCl Injection contains sodium metabisulfite, a sulfite that may cause allergic-type reactions including anaphylactic symptoms and life-threatening or less severe asthmatic episodes in certain susceptible people. The overall prevalence of sulfite sensitivity in the general population is unknown and probably low. Sulfite sensitivity is seen more frequently in asthmatic than in nonasthmatic people.

PRECAUTIONS:

Impaired Respiration: At the usual adult dose of 10 mg/70 kg, nalbuphine HCl causes some respiratory depression approximately equal to that produced by equal doses of morphine. However, in contrast to morphine, respiratory depression is not appreciably increased with higher doses of nalbuphine HCl. Respiratory depression induced by nalbuphine can be reversed by naloxone HCl when indicated. Nalbuphine HCl Injection should be administered with caution at low doses to patients with impaired respiration (*e.g.,* from other medication, uremia, bronchial asthma, severe infection, cyanosis or respiratory obstructions).

Impaired Renal or Hepatic Function: Because nalbuphine is metabolized in the liver and excreted by the kidneys, patients with renal or liver dysfunction may over-react to customary doses. Therefore, in these individuals, nalbuphine HCl Injection should be used with caution and administered in reduced amounts.

Myocardial Infarction: As with all potent analgesics, nalbuphine HCl should be used with caution in patients with myocardial infarction who have nausea or vomiting.

Biliary Tract Surgery: As with all narcotic analgesics, nalbuphine HCl should be used with caution in patients about to undergo surgery of the biliary tract since it may cause spasm of the sphincter of Oddi.

Cardiovascular System: During evaluation of nalbuphine HCl injection in anesthesia, a higher incidence of bradycardia has been reported in patients not administered preoperative atropine.

DRUG INTERACTIONS:

Interaction with Other Central Nervous System Depressants: Although nalbuphine possesses narcotic antagonist activity, there is evidence that in nondependent patients it will not antagonize a narcotic analgesic administered just before, concurrently, or just after an injection of nalbuphine HCl. Therefore, patients receiving at narcotic analgesic, general anesthetics, phenothiazines, or other tranquilizers, sedatives, hypnotics, or other CNS depressants (including alcohol) concomitantly with nalbuphine HCl may exhibit an additive effect. When such combined therapy is contemplated, the dose of one or both agents should be reduced.

ADVERSE REACTIONS:

The most frequent adverse reaction in 1066 patients treated with nalbuphine HCl Injection is sedation 381 (36%).

Less frequent reactions are: sweaty/clammy 99(9%), nausea/vomiting 68(6%), dizziness/vertigo 58(5%), dry mouth 44(4%), and headache 27(3%).

Other adverse reactions which may occur (reported incidence of 1% or less) are:

CNS Effects: Nervousness, depression, restlessness, crying, euphoria, floating, hostility, unusual dreams, confusion, faintness, hallucinations, dysphoria, feeling of heaviness, numbness, tingling, unreality. The incidence of psychotomimetic effects, such as unreality, depersonalization, delusions, dysphoria and hallucinations has been shown to be less than that which occurs with pentazocine.

Cardiovascular: Hypertension, hypotension, bradycardia, tachycardia.

Gastrointestinal: Cramps, dyspepsia, bitter taste.

Respiration: Depression, dyspnea, asthma.

Dermatological: Itching, burning, urticaria.

Miscellaneous: Speech difficulty, urinary urgency, blurred vision, flushing and warmth.

OVERDOSAGE:

Management of Overdosage: The immediate intravenous administration of naloxone HCl is a specific antidote. Oxygen, intravenous fluids, vasopressors and other supportive measures should be used as indicated.

The administration of single doses of 72 mg of nalbuphine HCl subcutaneously to eight normal subjects has been reported to have resulted primarily in symptoms of sleepiness and mild dysphoria.

DOSAGE AND ADMINISTRATION:

The usual recommended adult dose is 10 mg for a 70 kg individual, administered subcutaneously, intramuscularly or intravenously; this dose may be repeated every 3 to 6 hours as necessary. Dosage should be adjusted according to the severity of the pain, physical status of the patient, and other medications which the patient may be receiving. (See Interaction with Other Central Nervous System Depressants under WARNINGS.) In non-tolerant individuals, the recommended single maximum dose is 20 mg, with a maximum total daily dose of 160 mg.

The use of nalbuphine HCl injection as a supplement to balanced anesthesia requires larger doses than those recommended for analgesia. Induction doses of nalbuphine HCl range from 0.3 mg/kg to 3.0 mg/kg intravenously to be administered over a 10 to 15 minute period with maintenance doses of 0.25 mg to 0.50 mg/kg in single intravenous administrations as required. The use of nalbuphine HCl injection may be followed by respiratory depression which can be reversed with the narcotic antagonist naloxone HCl.

Patients Dependent on Narcotics: Patients who have been taking narcotics chronically may experience withdrawal symptoms upon the administration of nalbuphine HCl Injection. If unduly troublesome, narcotic withdrawal symptoms can be controlled by the slow intravenous administration of small increments of morphine, until relief occurs. If the previous analgesic was morphine, meperidine, codeine, or other narcotic with similar duration of activity, one-fourth of the anticipated dose of nalbuphine HCl can be administered initially and the patient observed for signs of withdrawal, i.e., abdominal cramps, nausea and vomiting, lacrimation, rhinorrhea, anxiety, restlessness, elevation of temperature or piloerection. If untoward symptoms do not occur, progressively larger doses may be tried at appropriate intervals until the desired level of analgesia is obtained with nalbuphine HCl.

Parenteral drug products should be inspected visually for particulate matter and discoloration prior to administration whenever solution and container permit.

Store at controlled room temperature 15-30°C(59-86°F).

Protect from light.

HOW SUPPLIED - RATED THERAPEUTICALLY EQUIVALENT:

Injection, Solution - Intramuscular; - 10 mg/ml

1 ml	$4.10	Nalbuphine Hcl, Abbott	00074-1463-01
1 ml	$17.13	Nalbuphine Hcl, Fujisawa USA	00469-2080-00
1 ml x 10	**$10.20**	**NUBAIN, Voluntary Hosp**	**53258-2090-00**
1 ml x 10	**$11.64**	**NUBAIN, Du Pont Merck**	**00590-0395-10**
10 ml	$11.28	Nalbuphine Hcl, Fujisawa USA	00469-2080-30
10 ml	$14.43	Nalbuphine Hcl, HL Moore Drug Exch	00839-7536-30
10 ml	**$22.44**	**NUBAIN, Du Pont Merck**	**00590-0386-01**
10 ml	$26.79	Nalbuphine Hcl, Abbott	00074-1464-01
10 ml x 5	$44.30	Nalbuphine Hcl, Astra USA	00186-1262-12

Injection, Solution - Intramuscular; - 20 mg/ml

1 ml	$5.04	Nalbuphine Hcl, Abbott	00074-1465-01
1 ml	$18.83	Nalbuphine Hcl, Abbott	00074-1466-01
1 ml	$25.38	Nalbuphine Hcl, Fujisawa USA	00469-2090-00
1 ml x 10	**$12.36**	**NUBAIN, Du Pont Merck**	**00590-0398-10**
10 ml	**$11.64**	**Nalbuphine Hcl, Voluntary Hosp**	**53258-2090-03**
10 ml	$18.74	Nalbuphine Hcl, Fujisawa USA	00469-2090-30
10 ml	$19.16	Nalbuphine Hcl, HL Moore Drug Exch	00839-7537-30
10 ml	**$34.92**	**NUBAIN, Du Pont Merck**	**00590-0399-01**
10 ml	$41.44	Nalbuphine Hcl, Abbott	00074-1467-01
10 ml x 5	$50.63	Nalbuphine Hcl, Astra USA	00186-1266-12

NALIDIXIC ACID *(001854)*

CATEGORIES: Anti-Infectives; Antibacterials; Antimicrobials; Antiseptics, Urinary Tract; Quinolones; Urinary Antibacterial; Urinary Tract Infections; FDA Approval Pre 1982

BRAND NAMES: *Acidix* (Mexico); *Anasiron* (Japan); *Betaxina*; *Enexina*; *Faril*; *Gramazine*; *Gramoneg*; *Granexin*; *Mictral*; *Mytacin* (Japan); *Nal-Acid*; *Nalidixin*; *Nalidixio*; *Nalix* (Mexico); *Nalydixine*; *Negacide*; *Negadix*; *Neg-Gram*; **Neggram**; *Negram* (Australia, France, Germany); *Nevigramon*; *Nogram* (Germany); *Notricel*; *Perry*; *Puromylon*; *Urigram*; *Urineg*; *Urodic*; *Youdix* (Japan); *Windol*; *Winlomylon*; *Wintomylon* (Mexico); *Youdix* (Japan)

(International brand names outside U.S. in italics)

FORMULARIES: Aetna; Medi-Cal; WHO

DESCRIPTION:

Nalidixic acid, an oral antibacterial agent, is 1-Ethyl-1, 4-dihydro-7-methyl-4-oxo-1, 8-naphthyridine-3-carboxylic acid. It is a pale yellow, crystalline substance and a very weak organic acid.

Neggram Inactive Ingredients: *Suspension:* Carbomer 934 P, FD&C Red #40, Flavor, Parabens, Purified Water, Saccharin Sodium, Sodium Chloride, Sorbitol Solution. *Caplets:* Hydrogenated Vegetable Oil, Methylcellulose, Microcrystalline Cellulose, Sodium Lauryl Sulfate, Yellow Ferric Oxide.

CLINICAL PHARMACOLOGY:

Nalidix acid has marked antibacterial activity against gram-negative bacteria including *Proteus mirabilis, P. morganii, P. vulgaris,* and *P. rettgeri*; *Escherichia coli*; Enterobacter (Aerobacter), and Klebsiella. Pseudomonas strains are generally resistant to the drug. Nalidix acid is bactericidal and is effective over the entire urinary pH range. Conventional chromosomal resistance to nalidix acid taken in full dosage has been reported to emerge in approximately 2 to 14 percent of patients during treatment; however, bacterial resistance to nalidix acid has not been shown to be transferable via R factor.

PHARMACOLOGY

Following oral administration, nalidix acid is rapidly absorbed from the gastrointestinal tract, partially metabolized in the liver, and rapidly excreted through the kidneys. Unchanged nalidixic acid appears in the urine along with an active metabolite, hydroxynalidixic acid, which has antibacterial activity similar to that of nalidixic acid. Other metabolites include glucuronic acid conjugates of nalidixic acid and hydroxynalidixic acid, and the dicarboxylic acid derivative. The hydroxy metabolite represents 30 percent of the biologically active drug in the blood and 85 percent in the urine. Peak serum levels of active drug average approximately 20 mcg to 40 mcg per ml (90 percent protein bound), one to two hours after administration of a 1 g dose to a fasting normal individual, with a half-live of about 90 minutes. Peak urine levels of active drug average approximately 150 mcg to 200 mcg per ml, three to four hours after administration, with a half-life of about six hours. Approximately four percent of nalidix acid is excreted in the feces. Traces of nalidixic acid were found in blood and urine of an infant whose mother had received the drug during the last trimester of pregnancy.

INDICATIONS AND USAGE:

Nalidix acid is indicated for the treatment of urinary tract infections caused by susceptible gram-negative microorganisms, including the majority of Proteus strains, Klebsiella, Enterobacter (Aerobacter) and *E. coli.* Disc susceptibility testing with 30 mcg disc should be performed prior to administration of the drug, and during treatment if clinical response warrants.

CONTRAINDICATIONS:

Nalidix acid is contraindicated in patients with known hypersensitivity to nalidixic acid and in patients with a history of convulsive disorders.

WARNINGS:

CNS effects including brief convulsions, increased intracranial pressure, and toxic psychosis have been reported rarely. These have occurred in infants and children or in geriatric patients, usually from overdosage or in patients with predisposing factors, and have been completely and rapidly reversible upon discontinuation of the drug. If these reactions occur, nalidix acid should be discontinued and appropriate therapeutic measures instituted; only if rapid disappearance of CNS symptoms does not occur within 48 hours should diagnostic procedures involving risk to the patient be undertaken. (See ADVERSE REACTIONS and OVERDOSAGE.)

PRECAUTIONS:

Blood counts and renal and liver function tests should be performed periodically if treatment is continued for more than two weeks. Nalidix acid should be used with caution in patients with liver disease, epilepsy, or severe cerebral arteriosclerosis. While caution should be used in patients with severe renal failure, therapeutic concentrations of nalidix acid in the urine, without increased toxicity due to drug accumulation in the blood, have been observed in patients on full dosage with creatinine clearances as low as 2 ml/minute to 8 ml/minute.

Patients should be cautioned to avoid under exposure to direct sunlight while receiving nalidix acid. Therapy should be discontinued if photosensitivity occurs.

If bacterial resistance to nalidix acid emerges during treatment, it usually does so within 48 hours, permitting rapid change to another antimicrobial. Therefore, if the clinical response is unsatisfactory or if relapse occurs, cultures and sensitivity tests should be repeated. Underdosage with nalidix acid during initial treatment (with less than 4 g per day for adults) may predispose to emergence of bacterial resistance.(See DOSAGE AND ADMINISTRATION.)

Usage in Prepubertal Children: Recent toxicological studies have shown that nalidixic acid and related drugs can produce erosion of the cartilage in weight-bearing joints and other signs of arthropathy in immature animals of most species tested. No such joint lesions have been reported in man to date. Nevertheless, until the significance of this finding is clarified, care should be exercised when prescribing this product for prepubertal children.

Usage in Pregnancy: Safe use of nalidix acid during the first trimester of pregnancy has not been established. However, the drug has been used during the last two trimesters without producing apparent ill effects in mother or child.

Caution should be used in administering nalidix acid in the days prior to delivery because of the theoretical risk that exposure to maternal nalidixic acid *in utero* may lead to significant blood levels of nalidixic acid in the neonate immediately after birth. Patients using nalidix acid during pregnancy should be advised to discontinue use at the first sign of labor.

DRUG INTERACTIONS:

Nitrofurantoin interferes with the therapeutic action of nalidixic acid.

Cross resistance between nalidix acid and other antimicrobials has been observed only with oxolinic acid.

Nalidixic acid may enhance the effects of oral anticoagulants, warfarin or bishydroxycoumarin, by displacing significant amounts from serum albumin binding sites.

When Benedict's or Fehling's solutions or Clinitest Reagent Tablets are used to test the urine of patients taking nalidix acid, a false-positive reaction for glucose may be obtained, due to the liberation of glucuronic acid from the metabolites excreted. However, a colorimetric test for glucose based on an enzyme reaction (*e.g.,* with Clinistix Reagent Strips or Tes-Tape) does not give a false-positive reaction to the liberated glucuronic acid.

Incorrect values may be obtained for urinary 17-keto and ketogenic steroids in patients receiving nalidix acid, because of an interaction between the drug and the *m*-dinitrobenzene used in the usual assay method. In such cases, the Porter-Silber test for 17-hydroxycorticoids may be used.

ADVERSE REACTIONS:

Reactions reported after oral administration of nalidix acid include *Cns Effects:* drowsiness, weakness, headache, and dizziness and vertigo. Reversible subjective visual disturbances without objective findings have occurred infrequently (generally with each dose during the first few days of treatment). These reactions include overbrightness of lights, change in color perception, difficulty in focusing, decrease in visual acuity, and double vision. They usually disappeared promptly when dosage was reduced or therapy was reduced or therapy was discontinued. Toxic psychosis or brief convulsions have been reported rarely, usually following excessive doses. In general, the convulsions have occurred in patients with predisposing factors such as epilepsy or cerebral arteriosclerosis. In infants and children receiving therapeutic doses of nalidix acid, increased intracranial pressure with bulging anterior fontanel, papilledema, and headache has occasionally been observed. A few cases of 6th cranial nerve palsy have been reported. Although the mechanisms of these reactions are unknown, the signs and symptoms usually disappeared rapidly with no sequelae when treatment was discontinued.*Gastrointestinal:* abdominal pain, nausea, vomiting, and diarrhea. *Allergic:* rash, pruritus, urticaria, angioedema, eosinophilia, arthralgia with joint stiffness and swelling, and rarely, anaphylactoid reaction. Photosensitivity reactions consisting of erythema and bullae on exposed skin surfaces usually resolve completely in 2 weeks to 2 months after nalidix acid is discontinued; however, bullae may continue to appear with successive exposures to sunlight or with mild skin trauma for up to 3 months after discontinuation of drug. (See PRECAUTIONS.) *Other:* rarely, cholestasis, paresthesia, metabolic acidosis, thrombocytopenia, leukopenia, or hemolytic anemia, sometimes associated with glucose-6 phosphate dehydrogenase deficiency.

OVERDOSAGE:

Manifestations: Toxic psychosis, convulsions, increased intracranial pressure, or metabolic acidosis may occur in patients taking more than the recommended dosage. Vomiting, nausea, and lethargy may also occur following overdosage.

Treatment: Reactions are short-lived (two to three hours) because the drug is rapidly excreted. If overdosage is noted early, gastric lavage is indicated. If absorption has occurred, increased fluid administration is advisable and supportive measures such as oxygen and means of artificial respiration should be available. Although anticonvulsant therapy has not been used in the few instances of overdosage reported, it may be indicated in a severe case.

DOSAGE AND ADMINISTRATION:

Adults: The recommended dosage for initial therapy in adults is 1 g administered four times daily for one or two weeks (total daily dose, 4 g). For prolonged therapy, the total daily dose may be reduced to 2 g after the initial treatment period. Underdosage during initial treatment may predispose to emergence of bacterial resistance.

Children: Until further experience is gained, nalidix acid should not be administered to infants younger than three months. Dosage in children 12 years of age and under should be calculated on the basis of body weight. The recommended total daily dosage for initial therapy is 25 mg/lb/day (55 mg/kg/day), administered in four equally divided doses. For prolonged therapy, the total daily dose may be reduced to 15 mg/lb/day (33 mg/kg/day). Nalidix acid suspension or nalidix acid caplets of 250 mg may be used. One 250 mg tablet is equivalent to one teaspoon (5 ml) of the suspension.

ANIMAL PHARMACOLOGY:

Nalidixic acid and related drugs have been shown to cause arthropathy in juvenile animals of most species tested. (See PRECAUTIONS.)

Hydroxynalidixic acid, the principal metabolite of nalidix acid, did not produce any oculotoxic effects at any dosage level in seven species of animals including three primate species. However, oral administration of this metabolite in high doses has been shown to have oculotoxic potential, namely in dogs and cats where it produced retinal degeneration upon prolonged administration leading, in some cases, to blindness.

In experiments with nalidix acid itself, little if any such activity could be elicited in either dogs or cats. Sensitivity to CNS side effects in these species limited the doses of nalidix acid that could be used; this factor, together with a low conversion rate to the hydroxy metabolite in these species, may explain the absence of these effects.

HOW SUPPLIED - RATED THERAPEUTICALLY EQUIVALENT:

Tablet, Uncoated - Oral - 1 gm

100's	$65.45	Nalidixic Acid, Aligen Independ	00405-4692-01
100's	**$190.39**	**NEGGRAM, Sanofi Winthrop**	**00024-1323-04**

Tablet, Uncoated - Oral - 250 mg

56's	**$42.78**	**NEGGRAM, Sanofi Winthrop**	**00024-1321-03**

Tablet, Uncoated - Oral - 500 mg

50's	$29.09	Nalidixic Acid Tablets 500 Mg, Aligen Independ	00405-4691-50
50's	$38.50	Nalidixic Acid, Schein Pharm (US)	00364-2324-50
50's	$40.49	Nalidixic Acid, United Res	00677-1325-02
56's	**$70.65**	**NEGGRAM, Sanofi Winthrop**	**00024-1322-03**
100's	$43.45	Nalidixic Acid Tablets 500 Mg, Aligen Independ	00405-4691-01
100's	$75.50	Nalidixic Acid, Schein Pharm (US)	00364-2324-01
100's	$81.68	Nalidixic Acid, HL Moore Drug Exch	00839-7528-06
500's	**$616.72**	**NEGGRAM, Sanofi Winthrop**	**00024-1322-06**

HOW SUPPLIED - NOT RATED EQUIVALENT:

Suspension - Oral - 250 mg/5ml

480 ml	**$110.01**	**NEGGRAM, Sanofi Winthrop**	**00024-1318-06**

NALMEFENE HYDROCHLORIDE *(003259)*

CATEGORIES: Antagonists and Antidotes; Antidotes; Central Nervous System Agents; Narcotic Antagonists; Opiate Antagonists; FDA Class 1S ("Standard Review"); FDA Approved 1995 Apr

BRAND NAMES: Cervene; **Revex**

DESCRIPTION:

Nalmefene hydrochloride injection, an opioid antagonist, is a 6- methylene analogue of naltrexone.

Molecular Formula: $C_{21}H_{25}NO_3 \cdot HCl$

Molecular Weight: 375.9, CAS # 58895-64-0

Chemical Name: 17-(Cyclopropylmethyl)-4,5α-epoxy-6-methylenemorphinan-3,14-diol, hydrochloride salt.

Nalmefene hydrochloride is a white to off-white crystalline powder which is freely soluble in water up to 130 mg/ml and slightly soluble in chloroform up to 0.13 mg/ml, with a PK_a of 7.6.

Nalmefene HCl is available as a sterile solution for intravenous, intramuscular, and subcutaneous administration in two concentrations, containing 100 mcg or 1.0 mg of nalmefene free base per ml. The 100 mcg/ml concentration contains 110.8 mcg of nalmefene hydrochloride and the 1.0 mg/ml concentration contains 1.108 mg of nalmefene hydrochloride per ml. Both concentrations contain 9.0 mg of sodium chloride per ml and the pH is adjusted to 3.9 with hydrochloric acid.

Concentrations and dosages of nalmefene HCl are expressed as the free base equivalent of nalmefene.

CLINICAL PHARMACOLOGY:

Pharmacodynamics: Nalmefene HCl prevents or reverses the effects of opioids, including respiratory depression, sedation, and hypotension. Pharmacodynamic studies have shown that nalmefene HCl has a longer duration of action than naloxone at fully reversing doses. Nalmefene HCl has no opioid agonist activity.

Nalmefene HCl is not known to produce respiratory depression, psychotomimetic effects, or pupillary constriction. No pharmacological activity was observed when nalmefene HCl was administered in the absence of opioid agonists.

Nalmefene HCl has not been shown to produce tolerance, physical dependence, or abuse potential.

Nalmefene HCl can produce acute withdrawal symptoms in individuals who are opioid dependent.

Pharmacokinetics: Nalmefene exhibited dose proportional pharmacokinetics following intravenous administration of 0.5 mg to 2.0 mg. Pharmacokinetic parameters for nalmefene after a 1 mg intravenous administration in adult male volunteers are listed in TABLE 1.

CLINICAL PHARMACOLOGY: *(cont'd)*

TABLE 1 Mean (CV%) Nalmefene Pharmacokinetic Parameters in Adult Males Following a 1 mg Intravenous Dose

Parameter	Young, N=18	Elderly, N=11
Age	19-32	62-80
C_p at 5 min. (ng/ml)	3.7 (29)	5.8 (38)
V_{dss} (l/kg)	8.6 (19)	8.6 (29)
V_c (l/kg)	3.9 (29)	2.8 (41)
$AUC_{0\text{-}inf}$ (ng-hr/ml)	16.6 (27)	17.3 (14)
Terminal $T_{1/2}$ (hr)	10.8 (48)	9.4 (49)
Cl_{plasma} (l/hr/kg)	0.8 (23)	0.8 (18)

Absorption: Nalmefene was completely bioavailable following intramuscular or subcutaneous administration in 12 male volunteers relative to intravenous nalmefene. The relative bioavailabilities of intramuscular and subcutaneous routes of administration were 101.5% ± 8.1% (Mean ± SD) and 99.7% ± 6.9%, respectively. Nalmefene will be administered primarily as an intravenous bolus, however, nalmefene can be given intramuscularly (IM) or subcutaneously (SC) of venous access cannot be established. While the time to maximum plasma nalmefene concentration was 2.3 ± 1.1 hours following intramuscular and 1.5 ± 1.2 hours following subcutaneous administrations, therapeutic plasma concentrations are likely to be reached within 5-15 minutes after a 1 mg dose in an emergency. Because of the variability in the speed of absorption for IM & SC dosing, and the inability to titrate to effect, great care should be taken if repeated doses must be given by these routes.

Distribution: Following a 1 mg parenteral dose, nalmefene was rapidly distributed. In a study of brain receptor occupancy, a 1 mg dose of nalmefene blocked over 80% of brain opioid receptors within 5 minutes after administration. The apparent volumes of distribution centrally (V_c) and at steady-state (V_{dss}) are 3.9 ± 1.1 l/kg and 8.6 ± 1.7 l/kg, respectively. Ultrafiltration studies of nalmefene have demonstrated that 45% (CV 4.1%) is bound to plasma proteins over a concentration range of 0.1 to 2 mcg/ml. An *in vitro* determination of the distribution of nalmefene in human blood demonstrated that nalmefene distributed 67% (CV 8.7%) into red blood cells and 39% (CV 6.4%) into plasma. The whole blood to plasma ratio was 1.3 (CV 6.6%) over the nominal concentration range in whole blood from 0.376 to 30 ng/ml.

Metabolism: Nalmefene is metabolized by the liver, primarily by glucuronide conjugation, and excreted in the urine. Nalmefene is also metabolized to trace amounts of an N-dealkylated metabolite. Nalmefene glucuronide is inactive and the N-dealkylated metabolite has minimal pharmacological activity. Less than 5% of nalmefene is excreted in the urine unchanged. Seventeen percent (17%) of the nalmefene dose is excreted in the feces. The plasma concentration-time profile in some subjects suggests that nalmefene undergoes enterohepatic recycling.

Elimination: After intravenous administration of 1 mg nalmefene HCl to normal males (ages 19-32), plasma concentrations declined biexponentially with a redistribution and a terminal elimination half-life of 41 ± 34 minutes and 10.8 ± 5.2 hours, respectively. The systemic clearance of nalmefene is 0.8 ± 0.2 l/hr/kg and the renal clearance is 0.08 ± 0.04 l/hr/kg.

SPECIAL POPULATIONS

Elderly: Dose proportionality was observed in nalmefene $AUC_{0\text{-}inf}$ following 0.5 to 2 mg intravenous administration to elderly male subjects. Following a 1 mg intravenous nalmefene dose, there were no significant differences between young (19-32 years) and elderly (62-80 years) adult male subjects with respect to plasma clearance, steady-state volume of distribution, or half-life. There was an apparent age-related decrease in the central volume of distribution (young: 3.9 ± 1.1 l/kg, elderly: 2.8 ± 1.1 l/kg) that resulted in a greater initial nalmefene concentration in the elderly group. While initial nalmefene plasma concentrations were transiently higher in the elderly, it would not be anticipated that this population would require dosing adjustment. No clinical adverse events were noted in the elderly following the 1 mg intravenous nalmefene dose.

Patients with Hepatic Impairment: Subjects with hepatic disease, when compared to matched normal controls, had a 28.3% decrease in plasma clearance of nalmefene (0.56 ± 0.21 l/hr/kg versus 0.78 ± 0.24 l/hr/kg, respectively). Elimination half-life increased from 10.2 ± 2.2 hours to 11.9 ± 2.0 hours in the hepatically impaired. No dosage adjustment is recommended since nalmefene will be administered as an acute course of therapy.

Patients with Renal Impairment: There was a statistically significant 27% decrease in plasma clearance of nalmefene in the end-stage renal disease (ESRD) population during interdialysis (0.57 ± 0.20 l/hr/kg) and a 25% decreased plasma clearance in the ESRD population during intradialysis (0.59 ± 0.18 l/hr/kg) compared to normals (0.79 ± 0.24 l/hr/kg). The elimination half-life was prolonged in ESRD patients from 10.2 ± 2.2 hours in normals to 26.1 ± 9.9 hours. (See DOSAGE AND ADMINISTRATION.)

Gender Differences There has not been sufficient pharmacokinetic study to make a definitive statement as to whether the pharmacokinetics of nalmefene differs between the genders.

CLINICAL STUDIES:

Nalmefene HCl has been administered to reverse the effects of opioids after general anesthesia and in the treatment of overdose. It has also been used to reverse the systemic effects of intrathecal opioids.

Reversal of Postoperative Opioid Depression: Nalmefene HCl (N=326) was studied in 5 controlled trials in patients who had received morphine or fentanyl intraoperatively. The primary efficacy criterion was the reversal of respiratory depression. A positive reversal was defined as both an increase in respiratory rate by 5 breaths per minute and a minimum respiratory rate of 12 breaths per minute. Five minutes after administration, initial single nalmefene HCl doses of 0.1, 0.25, 0.5, or 1.0 mcg/kg had effectively reversed respiratory depression in a dose-dependent manner. Twenty minutes after initial administration, respiratory depression had been effectively reversed in most patients receiving cumulative doses within the recommended range (0.1 to 1.0 mcg/kg). Total doses of nalmefene HCl above 1.0 mcg/kg did not increase the therapeutic response. The postoperative administration of nalmefene HCl at the recommended doses did not prevent the analgesic response to subsequently administered opioids.

Reversal Of The Effect Of Intrathecally Administered Opioids: Intravenous nalmefene HCl at doses 0.5 to 1.0 mcg/kg was administered to 47 patients given intrathecal morphine. One to 2 doses of 0.5 and 1.0 mcg/kg nalmefene HCl reversed respiratory depression in most patients. The administration of nalmefene HCl at the recommended doses did not prevent the analgesic response to subsequently administered opioids.

Management Of Known Or Suspected Opioid Overdose: Nalmefene HCl (N=284) at doses of 0.5 mg to 2.0 mg was studied in 4 trials of patients who were presumed to have taken an opioid overdose. Nalmefene HCl doses of 0.5 mg to 1.0 mg effectively reversed respiratory depression within 2 to 5 minutes in most patients subsequently confirmed to have opioid overdose. A total dose greater than 1.5 mg did not increase the therapeutic response.

INDICATIONS AND USAGE:

Nalmefene HCl is indicated for the complete or partial reversal of opioid drug effects, including respiratory depression, induced by either natural or synthetic opioids.

INDICATIONS AND USAGE: *(cont'd)*

Nalmefene HCl is indicated in the management of known or suspected opioid overdose.

CONTRAINDICATIONS:

Nalmefene HCl is contraindicated in patients with a known hypersensitivity to the product.

WARNINGS:

Use of Nalmefene HCl in Emergencies: Nalmefene HCl, like all drugs in this class, is not the primary treatment for ventilatory failure. In most emergency settings, treatment with nalmefene HCl should follow, not precede, the establishment of a patent airway, ventilatory assistance, administration of oxygen, and establishment of circulatory access.

Risk of Recurrent Respiratory Depression: Accidental overdose with long acting opioids [such as methadone and *levo*-alpha-acetylmethadol (LAAM)] may result in prolonged respiratory depression. Respiratory depression in both the postoperative and overdose setting may be complex and involve the effects of anesthetic agents, neuromuscular blockers, and other drugs. While nalmefene HCl has a longer duration of action than naloxone in fully reversing doses, the physician should be aware that a recurrence of respiratory depression is possible, even after an apparently adequate initial response to nalmefene HCl treatment.

Patients treated with nalmefene HCl should be observed until, in the opinion of the physician, there is no reasonable risk of recurrent respiratory depression.

PRECAUTIONS:

GENERAL

Cardiovascular Risks with Narcotic Antagonists: Pulmonary edema, cardiovascular instability, hypotension, hypertension, ventricular tachycardia, and ventricular fibrillation have been reported in connection with opioid reversal in both postoperative and emergency department settings. In many cases, these effects appear to be the result of abrupt reversal of opioid effects.

Although nalmefene HCl has been used safely in patients with pre-existing cardiac disease, all drugs of this class should be used with caution in patients at high cardiovascular risk or who have received potentially cardiotoxic drugs.(See DOSAGE AND ADMINISTRATION.)

Risk Of Precipitated Withdrawal: Nalmefene HCl, like other opioid antagonists, is known to produce acute withdrawal symptoms and, therefore, should be used with extreme caution in patients with known physical dependence on opioids or following surgery involving high doses of opioids. Imprudent use or excessive doses of opioid antagonists in the postoperative setting has been associated with hypertension, tachycardia, and excessive mortality in patients at high risk for cardiovascular complications. (See PRECAUTIONS.)

Incomplete Reversal Of Buprenorphine: Preclinical studies have shown that nalmefene at doses up to 10 mg/kg (437 times the maximum recommended human dose) produced incomplete reversal of buprenorphine-induced analgesia in animal models. This appears to be a consequence of a high affinity and slow displacement of buprenorphine from the opioid receptors. Hence, nalmefene HCl may not completely reverse buprenorphine-induced respiratory depression.

CARCINOGENESIS, MUTAGENESIS, AND IMPAIRMENT OF FERTILITY

Nalmefene did not have mutagenic activity in the Ames test with five bacterial strains or the mouse lymphoma assay. Clastogenic activity was not observed in the mouse micronucleus test or in the cytogenic bone marrow assay in rats. However, nalmefene did exhibit a weak but significant clastogenic activity in the human lymphocyte metaphase assay in the absence but not in the presence of exogenous metabolic activation. Oral administration of nalmefene up to 1200 $mg/m^2/day$ did not affect fertility, reproductive performance, and offspring survival in rats.

PREGNANCY CATEGORY B

Reproduction studies have been performed in rats (up to 1200 $mg/m^2/day$) and rabbits (up to 2400 $mg/m^2/day$) by oral administration of nalmefene and in rabbits by intravenous administration up to 96 $mg/m^2/day$ (114 times the human dose). There was no evidence of impaired fertility or harm to the fetus. There are, however, no adequate and well-controlled studies in pregnant women. Because animal reproduction studies are not always predictive of human response, this drug should be used during pregnancy only if clearly needed.

NURSING MOTHERS

Nalmefene and its metabolites were secreted into rat milk, reaching concentrations approximately three times those in plasma at one hour and decreasing to about half the corresponding plasma concentrations by 24 hours following bolus administration. As no clinical information is available, caution should be exercised when nalmefene HCl is administered to a nursing woman.

PEDIATRIC USE

Safety and effectiveness of nalmefene HCl in children have not been established.

USE IN NEONATES

The safety and effectiveness of nalmefene HCl in neonates have not been established in clinical studies. In a preclinical study, nalmefene was administered by subcutaneous injection to rat pups at doses up to 205 $mg/m^2/day$ throughout maternal lactation without producing adverse effects. A preclinical study evaluating the irritancy of the dosage form following arterial and venous administration in animals showed no vascular irritancy.

Nalmefene HCl should only be used in the resuscitation of the newborn when, in the opinion of the treating physician, the expected benefits outweigh the risks.

DRUG INTERACTIONS:

Nalmefene HCl has been administered after benzodiazepines, inhalational anesthetics, muscle relaxants, and muscle relaxant antagonists administered in conjunction with general anesthesia. It also has been administered in outpatient settings, both in trials in conscious sedation and in the emergency management of overdose following a wide variety of agents. No deleterious interactions have been observed.

Preclinical studies have shown that both flumazenil and nalmefene can induce seizures in animals. The coadministration of both flumazenil and nalmefene produced fewer seizures than expected in a study in rodents, based on the expected effects of each drug alone. Based on these data, an adverse interaction from the coadministration of the two drugs is not expected, but physicians should remain aware of the potential risk of seizures from agents in these classes.

ADVERSE REACTIONS:

Adverse event information was obtained following administration of nalmefene HCl to 152 normal volunteers and in controlled clinical trials to 1127 patients for the treatment of opioid overdose or for postoperative opioid reversal.

Nalmefene was well tolerated and showed no serious toxicity during experimental administration to healthy individuals, even when given at 15 times the highest recommended dose. In a small number of subjects, at doses exceeding the recommended nalmefene HCl dose, nalmefene produced symptoms suggestive of reversal of endogenous opioids, such as have been reported for other narcotic antagonist drugs. These symptoms (nausea, chills, myalgia, dysphoria, abdominal cramps, and joint pain) were usually transient and occurred at very low frequency.

Such symptoms of precipitated opioid withdrawal at the recommended clinical doses were seen at both postoperative and overdose patients who were later found to have had histories of covert opioid use. Symptoms of precipitated withdrawal were similar to those seen with other opioid antagonists, were transient following the lower doses used in the postoperative setting, and more prolonged following the administration of the larger doses used in the treatment of overdose.

Tachycardia and nausea following the use of nalmefene in the postoperative setting were reported at the same frequencies as for naloxone at equivalent doses. The risk of both these adverse events was low at doses giving partial opioid reversal and increased with increases in dose. Thus, total doses larger than 1.0 mcg/kg in the postoperative setting and 1.5 mg/70 kg in the treatment of overdose are not recommended.

TABLE 2 Relative Frequencies of Common Adverse Reactions With an Incidence Greater Than 1% (all patients, all clinical settings)

Adverse Event	Nalmefene N=1127	Naloxone N=369	Placebo N=77
Nausea	18%	18%	6%
Vomiting	9%	7%	4%
Tachycardia	5%	8%	-
Hypertension	5%	7%	-
Postoperative pain	4%	4%	N/A
Fever	3%	4%	-
Dizziness	3%	4%	1%
Headache	1%	1%	4%
Chills	1%	1%	-
Hypotension	1%	1%	-
Vasodilation	1%	1%	-

INCIDENCE LESS THAN 1%

Cardiovascular: Bradycardia, arrhythmia

Digestive: Diarrhea, dry mouth

Nervous System: Somnolence, depression, agitation, nervousness, tremor, confusion, withdrawal syndrome, myoclonus

Respiratory: Pharyngitis

Skin: Pruritus

Urogenital: Urinary retention

The incidence of adverse events was highest in patients who received more than the recommended dose of nalmefene HCl.

Laboratory findings: Transient increases in CPK were reported as adverse events in 0.5% of the postoperative patients studied. These increases were believed to be related to surgery and not believed to be related to the administration of nalmefene HCl. Increases in AST were reported as adverse events in 0.3% of the patients receiving either nalmefene or naloxone. The clinical significance of this finding is unknown. No cases of hepatitis or hepatic injury due to either nalmefene or naloxone were observed in the clinical trials.

DRUG ABUSE AND DEPENDENCE:

Nalmefene HCl is an opioid antagonist with no agonist activity. It has no demonstrated abuse potential, it is not addictive, and it is not a controlled substance.

OVERDOSAGE:

Intravenous doses of up to 24 mg of nalmefene, administered to healthy volunteers in the absence of opioid agonists, produced no serious adverse reactions, severe signs or symptoms, or clinically significant laboratory abnormalities. As with all opioid antagonists, use in patients physically dependent on opioids can result in precipitated withdrawal reactions that may result in symptoms that require medical attention. Treatment of such cases should be symptomatic and supportive. Administration of large amounts of opioids to patients receiving opioid antagonists in an attempt to overcome a full blockade has resulted in adverse respiratory and circulatory reactions.

DOSAGE AND ADMINISTRATION:

Dosage Forms: IMPORTANT INFORMATION. Nalmefene HCl is supplied in two concentrations which are packaged in ampules of different appearance: an ampul with a blue label containing ONE (1) ml at a concentration suitable for postoperative use (100 mcg/ml) and an ampul with a green label containing TWO (2) ml suitable for the management of overdose (1 mg/ml, 10 times as concentrated, 20 times as much drug). Proper steps should be taken to prevent use of the incorrect dosage form.

General Principles: Nalmefene HCl should be titrated to reverse the undesired effects of opioids. Once adequate reversal has been established, additional administration is not required and may actually be harmful due to unwanted reversal of analgesia or precipitated withdrawal.

Duration of Action: The duration of action of nalmefene HCl is as long as most opioid analgesics. The apparent duration of action of nalmefene HCl will vary, however, depending on the half-life and plasma concentration of the narcotic being reversed, the presence or absence of other drugs affecting the brain or muscles of respiration, and the dose of nalmefene HCl administered. Partially reversing doses of nalmefene HCl (1 mcg/kg) lose their effect as the drug is redistributed through the body, and the effects of these low doses may not last more than 30-60 minutes in the presence of persistent opioid effects. Fully reversing doses (1 mg/70 kg) have been shown to last many hours in both experimental and clinical studies, but may complicate the management of patients who are in pain, at high cardiovascular risk, or who are physically dependent on opioids.

The recommended doses represent a compromise between a desirable controlled reversal and the need for prompt response and adequate duration of action. Using higher dosages or shorter intervals between incremental doses is likely to increase the incidence and severity of symptoms related to acute withdrawal such as nausea, vomiting, elevated blood pressure, and anxiety.

Patients Tolerant To Or Physically Dependent On Opioids Nalmefene HCl may cause acute withdrawal symptoms in individuals who have some degree of tolerance to and dependence on opioids. These patients should be closely observed for symptoms of withdrawal following administration of the initial and subsequent injections of nalmefene HCl. Subsequent doses should be administered with intervals of at least 2-5 minutes between doses to allow the full effect of each incremental dose of nalmefene HCl to be reached.

Recommended Doses for Reversal of Postoperative Opioid Depression Use 100 mcg/ml dosage strength (blue label) and see TABLE 3 for initial doses.

DOSAGE AND ADMINISTRATION: *(cont'd)*

The goal of treatment with nalmefene HCl in the postoperative setting is to achieve reversal of excessive opioid effects without inducing a complete reversal and acute pain. This is best accomplished with an initial dose of 0.25 mcg/kg followed by 0.25 mcg/kg incremental doses at 2-5 minute intervals, stopping as soon as the desired degree of opioid reversal is obtained. A cumulative total dose above 1.0 mcg/kg does not provide additional therapeutic effect.

TABLE 3 Reversal of Postoperative Opioid Depression

Body Weight	ml of Revex 100 mcg/ml Solution
50 kg	0.125
60 kg	0.150
70 kg	0.175
80 kg	0.200
90 kg	0.225
100 kg	0.250

In cases where the patient is known to be at increased cardiovascular risk, it may be desirable to dilute nalmefene HCl 1:1 with saline or sterile water and use smaller initial and incremental doses of 0.1 mcg/kg.

Management of Known or Suspected Opioid Overdose: Use 1.0 mg/ml dosage strength (green label).

The recommended initial dose of nalmefene HCl for non-opioid dependent patients is 0.5 mg/70 kg. If needed, this may be followed by a second dose of 1.0 mg/70 kg, 2- 5 minutes later. If a total dose of 1.5 mg/70 kg has been administered without clinical response, additional nalmefene HCl is unlikely to have an effect. Patients should not be given more nalmefene HCl than is required to restore the respiratory rate to normal, thus minimizing the likelihood of cardiovascular stress and precipitated withdrawal syndrome.

If there is a reasonable suspicion of opioid dependency, a challenge dose of nalmefene HCl 0.1 mg/70 kg should be administered initially. If there is no evidence of withdrawal in 2 minutes, the recommended dosing should be followed.

Nalmefene HCl had no effect in cases where opioids were not responsible for sedation and hypoventilation. Therefore, patients should only be treated with nalmefene HCl when the likelihood of an opioid overdose is high, based on a history of opioid overdose or the clinical presentation of respiratory depression with concurrent pupillary constriction.

Repeated Dosing: Nalmefene HCl is the longest acting of the currently available parenteral opioid antagonists. If recurrence of respiratory depression does occur, the dose should again be titrated to clinical effect using incremental doses to avoid over-reversal.

Hepatic and Renal Disease: Hepatic disease and renal failure substantially reduce the clearance of nalmefene (see Pharmacokinetics.) For single episodes of opioid antagonism, adjustment of nalmefene HCl dosage is not required. However, in patients with renal failure, the incremental doses should be delivered slowly (over 60 seconds) to minimize the hypertension and dizziness reported following the abrupt administration of nalmefene to such patients.

Loss of Intravenous Access: Should intravenous access be lost or not readily obtainable, a pharmacokinetic study has shown that a single dose of nalmefene HCl should be effective within 5-15 minutes after intramuscular or subcutaneous doses of 1.0 mg. (See Pharmacokinetics.)

Safety And Handling: Nalmefene HCl is distributed in sealed ampuls and represents no known risk to health care workers. As with all parenterals, care should be taken to prevent the generation and inhalation of aerosols during preparation and use. Dermal absorption of spilled nalmefene HCl should be prevented by prompt removal of contaminated clothing and rinsing the skin thoroughly with cool water.

Parenteral drug products should be inspected visually for particulate matter and discoloration prior to administration, whenever solution and container permit.

HOW SUPPLIED:

Nalmefene HCl is available in the following presentations:

An ampul containing 1 ml of 100 mcg/ml nalmefene base (Blue Label)

An ampul containing 2 ml of 1 mg/ml nalmefene base (Green Label)

Store at controlled room temperature.

HOW SUPPLIED - EQUIVALENTS NOT AVAILABLE:

Injection, Solution - Intravenous - 1.1 mg/ml

2 ml $43.75 REVEX, Ohmeda Pharm 10019-0311-22

Injection, Solution - Intravenous - 110 mcg/ml

1 ml $3.13 REVEX, Ohmeda Pharm 10019-0315-21

NALOXONE HYDROCHLORIDE *(001855)*

CATEGORIES: Antagonists and Antidotes; Antidotes; Central Nervous System Agents; Diagnostic Agents; Hypotension; Narcotic Antagonists; Opiate Antagonists; Respiratory Depression; Septic Shock; Pregnancy Category B; FDA Approval Pre 1982

BRAND NAMES: *Nalpin*; **Narcan**; *Narcanti* (Germany, Mexico); *Narcotan*; *Zynox* *(International brand names outside U.S. in italics)*

FORMULARIES: WHO

DESCRIPTION:

Naloxone hydrochloride, a narcotic antagonist, is a synthetic congener of oxymorphone. In structure it differs from oxymorphone in that the methyl group on the nitrogen atom is replaced by an allyl group.

The molecular formula is $C_{19}H_{21}NO_4$·HCl.

Naloxone HCl: (-)-17-Allyl-4-5α-epoxy-3, 14 - dihydroxy = morphinan-6-one-hydrochloride

Naloxone hydrochloride occurs as a white to slightly off-white powder, and is soluble in water, in dilute acids, and in strong alkali; slightly soluble in alcohol; practically insoluble in ether and in chloroform.

Naloxone Hydrochloride Injection is available as a sterile solution for intravenous, intramuscular, subcutaneous administration in three concentrations, 0.02 mg, 0.4 mg and 1.0 mg of naloxone hydrochloride per ml. One ml of the 0.02 mg and 0.4 mg strengths contains 8.6 mg of sodium chloride. One ml of the 1.0 mg strength contains 8.35 mg of sodium chloride. One ml of the 0.4 mg and 1.0 mg strengths also contains 2.0 mg of methylparaben and propylparaben as preservatives in a ratio of 9 to 1. pH is adjusted to 3.5 ± 0.5 with hydrochloric acid.

DESCRIPTION: *(cont'd)*

Naloxone HCl injection is also available in a paraben-free formulation in three concentrations; 0.02 mg, 0.4 mg and 1.0 mg of naloxone hydrochloride per ml. One ml of each strength contains 9.0 mg of sodium chloride. Ph is adjusted to 3.5 ± 0.5 with hydrochloric acid.

CLINICAL PHARMACOLOGY:

Naloxone HCl prevents or reverses the effects of opioids including respiratory depression, sedation and hypotension. Also, it can reverse the psychotomimetic and dysphoric effects of agonist-antagonists such as pentazocine.

Naloxone hydrochloride is an essentially pure narcotic antagonist, i.e., it does not possess the "agonistic" or morphine-like properties characteristic of other narcotic antagonists; naloxone hydrochloride does not produce respiratory depression, psychotomimetic effects or pupillary constriction. In the absence of narcotics or agonistic effects of other narcotic antagonists, it exhibits essentially no pharmacologic activity.

Naloxone HCl has not been shown to produce tolerance nor to cause physical or psychological dependence.

In the presence of physical dependence on narcotics, naloxone will produce withdrawal symptoms.

MECHANISM OF ACTION

While the mechanism of action of naloxone is not fully understood, the preponderance of evidence suggests that naloxone antagonizes the opioid effects by competing for the same receptor sites.

When Naloxone Hydrochloride Injection is administered intravenously, the onset of action is generally apparent within two minutes; the onset of action is only slightly less rapid when it is administered subcutaneously or intramuscularly. The duration of action is dependent upon the dose and route of administration of naloxone hydrochloride. Intramuscular administration produces a more prolonged effect than intravenous administration. The requirement for repeat doses of naloxone hydrochloride, however, will also be dependent upon the amount, type and route of administration of the narcotic being antagonized.

Following parenteral administration, naloxone hydrochloride is rapidly distributed in the body. It is metabolized in the liver, primarily by glucuronide conjugation and excreted in urine. In one study, the serum half-life in adults ranged from 30 to 81 minutes (mean 64 ± 12 minutes). In a neonatal study, the mean plasma half-life was observed to be 3.1 ± 0.5 hours.

INDICATIONS AND USAGE:

Naloxone Hydrochloride Injection is indicated for the complete or partial reversal of narcotic depression, including respiratory depression, induced by opioids including natural and synthetic narcotics, propoxyphene, methadone and the narcotic-antagonist analgesics: nalbuphine, pentazocine and butorphanol. Naloxone Hydrochloride Injection is also indicated for the diagnosis of suspected acute opioid overdosage.

CONTRAINDICATIONS:

Naloxone Hydrochloride Injection is contraindicated in patients known to be hypersensitive to it.

WARNINGS:

Naloxone Hydrochloride Injection should be administered cautiously to persons including newborns of mothers who are known or suspected to be physically dependent on opioids. In such cases, an abrupt and complete reversal of narcotic effects may precipitate an acute abstinence syndrome.

The patient who has satisfactorily responded to naloxone should be kept under continued surveillance and repeated doses should be administered, as necessary, since the duration of action of some narcotics may exceed that of naloxone.

Naloxone is not effective against respiratory depression due to non-opioid drugs. Reversal of buprenorpinephrine-induced respiratory depression may be incomplete. If an incomplete response occurs, respirations should be mechanically assisted.

PRECAUTIONS:

In addition to Naloxone Hydrochloride Injection, other resuscitative measures, such as maintenance of a free airway, artificial ventilation, cardiac massage and vasopressor agents should be available and employed, when necessary, to counteract acute narcotic poisoning.

Several instances of hypotension, hypertension, ventricular tachycardia and fibrillation, and pulmonary edema have been reported. These have occurred in postoperative patients most of whom had pre-existing cardiovascular disorders or received other drugs which may have similar adverse cardiovascular effects. Although a direct cause and effect relationship has not been established, Naloxone Hydrochloride Injection should be used with caution in patients with pre-existing cardiac disease or patients who have received potentially cardiotoxic drugs.

CARCINOGENESIS, MUTAGENESIS, AND IMPAIRMENT OF FERTILITY

Carcinogenicity and mutagenicity studies have not been performed with naloxone hydrochloride. Reproductive studies in mice and rats demonstrated no impairment of fertility.

PREGNANCY: PREGNANCY CATEGORY B

Reproduction studies have been performed in mice and rats at doses up to 1,000 times the human dose and have revealed no evidence of impaired fertility or harm to the fetus due to naloxone hydrochloride. There are, however, no adequate and well-controlled studies in pregnant women. Because animal reproduction studies are not always predictive of human response, this drug should be used during pregnancy only if clearly needed.

NURSING MOTHERS

It is not known whether this drug is excreted in human milk. Because many drugs are excreted in human milk, caution should be exercised when Naloxone Hydrochloride Injection is administered to a nursing woman.

ADVERSE REACTIONS:

Abrupt reversal of narcotic depression may result in nausea, vomiting, sweating, tachycardia, increased blood pressure and tremulousness. In postoperative patients, larger than necessary dosage of naloxone hydrochloride may result in significant reversal of analgesia, and in excitement. Hypotension, hypertension, ventricular tachycardia and fibrillation, and pulmonary edema have been associated with the use of naloxone hydrochloride postoperatively (see PRECAUTIONS and DOSAGE AND ADMINISTRATION-USAGE IN ADULTS-Postoperative Narcotic Depression).

OVERDOSAGE:

There is no clinical experience with naloxone hydrochloride overdosage in humans.

OVERDOSAGE: *(cont'd)*

In the mouse and rat, the intravenous LD_{50} is 150 ± 5 mg/kg and 109 ± 4 mg/kg, respectively. In acute subcutaneous toxicity studies in newborn rats, the LD_{50} (95% CL) is 260 (228-296) mg/kg. Subcutaneous injection of 100 mg/kg/day in rats for 3 weeks produced only transient salivation and partial ptosis following injection; no toxic effects were seen at 10 mg/kg/day for 3 weeks.

DOSAGE AND ADMINISTRATION:

Naloxone Hydrochloride Injection may be administered intravenously, intramuscularly, or subcutaneously. The most rapid onset of action is achieved by intravenous administration, and this route is recommended in emergency situations.

Since the duration of action of some narcotics may exceed that of naloxone, the patient should be kept under continued surveillance and repeated doses of naloxone hydrochloride should be administered, as necessary.

INTRAVENOUS INFUSION

Naloxone Hydrochloride Injection may be diluted for intravenous infusion in 0.9% Sodium Chloride Injection or 5% Dextrose Injection. The addition of 2 mg of naloxone hydrochloride in 500 ml of either solution provides a concentration of 0.004 mg/ml. Mixtures should be used within 24 hours. After 24 hours, the remaining unused solution must be discarded. The rate of administration should be titrated in accordance with the patient's response.

Parenteral drug products should be inspected visually for particulate matter and discoloration prior to administration whenever solution and container permit. Naloxone Hydrochloride Injection should not be mixed with preparations containing bisulfite, metabisulfite, long-chain or high molecular weight anions, or any solution having an alkaline pH. No drug or chemical agent should be added to Naloxone Hydrochloride Injection unless its effect on the chemical and physical stability of the solution has first been established.

USAGE IN ADULTS

Narcotic Overdose-Known or Suspected: An initial dose of 0.4 mg to 2 mg of naloxone hydrochloride may be administered intravenously. If the desired degree of counteraction and improvement in respiratory functions is not obtained, it may be repeated at 2 to 3 minute intervals. If no response is observed after 10 mg of naloxone hydrochloride have been administered, the diagnosis of narcotic induced or partial narcotic induced toxicity should be questioned. Intramuscular or subcutaneous administration may be necessary if the intravenous route is not available.

Postoperative Narcotic Depression: For the partial reversal of narcotic depression following the use of narcotics during surgery, smaller doses of naloxone hydrochloride are usually sufficient. The dose of naloxone hydrochloride should be titrated according to the patient's response. For the initial reversal of respiratory depression, Naloxone Hydrochloride Injection should be injected in increments of 0.1 to 0.2 mg intravenously at two- to three-minute intervals to the desired degree of reversal, i.e. adequate ventilation and alertness without significant pain or discomfort. Larger than necessary dosage of naloxone hydrochloride may result in significant reversal of analgesia and increase in blood pressure. Similarly, too rapid reversal may induce nausea, vomiting, sweating or circulatory stress.

Repeat doses of naloxone hydrochloride may be required within one- to two-hour intervals depending upon the amount, type (*i.e.,* short or long acting) and time interval since last administration of narcotic. Supplemental intramuscular doses have been shown to produce a longer lasting effect.

USAGE IN CHILDREN

Narcotic Overdose-Known or Suspected: The usual initial dose in children is 0.01 mg/kg body weight given intravenously. If this dose does not result in the desired degree of clinical improvement, a subsequent dose of 0.1 mg/kg body weight may be administered. If an intravenous route of administration is not available, Naloxone Hydrochloride Injection may be administered intramuscularly or subcutaneously in divided doses. If necessary, Naloxone Hydrochloride Injection can be diluted with Sterile Water for Injection.

Postoperative Narcotic Depression: Follow the recommendations and cautions under **USAGE IN ADULTS-Postoperative Narcotic Depression**. For the initial reversal of respiratory depression, naloxone hydrochloride should be injected in increments of 0.005 mg to 0.01 mg intravenously at two- to three-minute intervals to the desired degree of reversal.

USAGE IN NEONATES

Narcotic Induced Depression: The usual initial dose is 0.01 mg/kg body weight administered IV, IM or Subcutaneously. This dose may be repeated in accordance with adult administration guidelines for postoperative narcotic depression.

When using naloxone hydrochloride injection in neonates, a product containing 0.02 mg/ml should be used.

STORAGE

Protect from light. Store at controlled room temperature 15 - 30°C (59 - 86°F).

(Du Pont, 6108-11/rev.dec.,1990)

HOW SUPPLIED - RATED THERAPEUTICALLY EQUIVALENT:

Injection, Solution - Intramuscular; - 0.02 mg/ml

2 ml	$8.78	Naloxone Hcl Neonatal 0.02, Abbott	00074-1211-01
2 ml	$9.68	Naloxone Hcl Neonatal 0.02, Abbott	00074-1216-01
2 ml x 10	$12.30	Naloxone, Voluntary Hosp	53258-1930-01
2 ml x 10	$14.40	Naloxone, Voluntary Hosp	53258-1920-01
2 ml x 10	$16.88	Naloxone Hcl, Astra USA	00186-1252-13
2 ml x 10	**$18.72**	**NARCAN INJ 0.02, Du Pont Merck**	**00590-0359-10**
2 ml x 10	$29.18	Naloxone HCl, Sanofi Winthrop	00024-1314-27
2 ml x 10	$53.88	Naloxone Hcl, Fujisawa USA	00469-1930-10

Injection, Solution - Intramuscular; - 0.4 mg/ml

1 ml	$8.69	Naloxone Hcl, Intl Medication	00548-1466-00
1 ml	$9.20	Naloxone Hcl 0.4, Abbott	00074-1212-01
1 ml	$10.14	Naloxone Hcl 0.4, Abbott	00074-1215-01
1 ml	$12.90	Naloxone Hcl 0.4, Abbott	00074-1213-01
1 ml	$50.00	Naloxone Hcl Inj 0.4, Solopak Labs	39769-0129-01
1 ml x 10	$9.90	Naloxone, Voluntary Hosp	53258-1910-00
1 ml x 10	$11.88	Naloxone Hcl, Astra USA	00186-1250-13
1 ml x 10	$16.47	Naloxone HCl, Sanofi Winthrop	00024-1313-26
1 ml x 10	**$31.20**	**NARCAN INJ 0.4, Du Pont Merck**	**00590-0358-10**
1 ml x 10	$33.69	Naloxone Hcl, Wyeth Labs	00008-0689-04
1 ml x 10	$52.50	Naloxone 0.4, Elkins Sinn	00641-1451-33
1 ml x 10	$59.75	Naloxone Hcl, Elkins Sinn	00641-0447-23
2 ml	$17.38	Naloxone Hcl, Intl Medication	00548-1467-00
10 ml	**$38.28**	**NARCAN, Du Pont Merck**	**00590-0365-05**
10 ml	$68.14	Naloxone Hcl 0.4, Abbott	00074-1219-01
10 ml x 1	$45.00	Naloxone Hcl, Elkins Sinn	00641-2521-41
10 ml x 5	$24.75	Naloxone Hcl, Astra USA	00186-1254-12

Injection, Solution - Intramuscular; - 1 mg/ml

1 ml x 10	$34.13	Naloxone Hcl, Astra USA	00186-1251-13
2 ml	$21.19	NALOXONE HCL, Intl Medication	00548-1469-00
2 ml	**$45.60**	**NARCAN, Du Pont Merck**	**00590-0377-10**
5 ml x 5	$64.13	Naloxone Hcl, Astra USA	00186-1253-13

HOW SUPPLIED - RATED THERAPEUTICALLY EQUIVALENT: *(cont'd)*

10 ml	**$42.48**	**NARCAN INJ 1, Du Pont Merck**	**00590-0368-05**
10 ml x 5	$153.00	Naloxone Hcl, Astra USA	00186-1255-12

NALOXONE HYDROCHLORIDE; PENTAZOCINE HYDROCHLORIDE *(001856)*

CATEGORIES: Analgesics; Anesthesia; Antipyretics; Central Nervous System Agents; Narcotic Agonist-Antagonist; Narcotics, Synthetics & Combinations; Opiate Partial Agonists; Pain; Pregnancy Category C; DEA Class CIV; FDA Approved 1982 Dec

BRAND NAMES: *Fortalgesic*; *Fortral*; *Fortwin*; *Liticon*; *Peltazon* (Japan); *Pentafen*; *Pentagin* (Japan); *Pentalgina*; *Rafazocine X*; *Sosegen*; *Sosegon* (Japan); *Sosenol*; *Talwin* (Canada); **Talwin Nx**; *Tazcine*
(International brand names outside U.S. in italics)

FORMULARIES: Aetna; BC-BS; FHP

Naloxone with pentazocine is intended for oral use only. Severe, potentially lethal, reactions may result from misuse of naloxone with pentazocine by injection either alone or in combination with other substances. (See DRUG ABUSE AND DEPENDENCE.)

DESCRIPTION:

Naloxone with pentazocine contains pentazocine hydrochloride, USP, equivalent to 50 mg base and is a member of the benzazocine series (also known as the benzomorphan series), and naloxone hydrochloride, USP, equivalent to 0.5 mg base.

Naloxone with pentazocine is an analgesic for oral administration.

Chemically, pentazocine hydrochloride is 1, 2, 3, 4, 5, 6-Hexahydro-6,11 -dimethyl-3-(3-methyl-2-butenyl)-2,6-methano-3-ben-zazocin-8-ol hydrochloride, a white, crystalline substance soluble in acidic aqueous solutions.

Chemically, naloxone hydrochloride is Morphinan-6-one, 4, 5-epoxy-3, 14-dihydroxy-17-(2-propenyl)-, hydrochloride, (5α)-. It is a slightly off-white powder, and is soluble in water and dilute acids.

Talwin Nx Inactive Ingredients: Colloidal Silicon Dioxide, Dibasic Calcium Phosphate, D&C Yellow #10, FD&C Yellow #6, Magnesium Stearate, Microcrystalline Cellulose, Sodium Lauryl Sulfate, Starch.

CLINICAL PHARMACOLOGY:

Pentazocine is a potent analgesic which when administered orally in a 50 mg dose appears equivalent in analgesic effect to 60 mg (1 grain) of codeine. Onset of significant analgesia usually occurs between 15 and 30 minutes after oral administration, and duration of action is usually three hours or longer. Onset and duration of action and the degree of pain relief are related both to dose and the severity of pretreatment pain. Pentazocine weakly antagonizes the analgesic effects of morphine and meperidine; in addition, it produces incomplete reversal of cardiovascular, respiratory, and behavioral depression induced by morphine and meperidine. Pentazocine has about 1/50 the antagonistic activity of nalorphine. It also has sedative activity.

Pentazocine is well absorbed from the gastrointestinal tract. Concentrations in plasma coincide closely with the onset, duration, and intensity of analgesia; peak values occur 1 to 3 hours after oral administration. The half-life in plasma is 2 to 3 hours.

Pentazocine is metabolized in the liver and excreted primarily in the urine. Pentazocine passes into the fetal circulation.

Naloxone when administered orally at 0.5 mg has no pharmacologic activity. Naloxone hydrochloride administered parenterally at the same dose is an effective antagonist to pentazocine and a pure antagonist to narcotic analgesics.

Naloxone with pentazocine is a potent analgesic when administered orally. However, the presence of naloxone in naloxone with pentazocine will prevent the effect of pentazocine if the product is misused by injection.

Studies in animals indicate that the presence of naloxone does not affect pentazocine analgesia when the combination is given orally. If the combination is given by injection the action of pentazocine is neutralized.

INDICATIONS AND USAGE:

Naloxone with pentazocine is intended for oral use only. Severe, potentially lethal, reactions may result from misuse of naloxone with pentazocine by injection either alone or in combination with other substances. (See DRUG ABUSE AND DEPENDENCE.)

Naloxone with pentazocine is indicated for the relief of moderate to severe pain.
Naloxone with pentazocine is indicated for oral use only.

CONTRAINDICATIONS:

Naloxone with pentazocine should not be administered to patients who are hypersensitive to either pentazocine or naloxone.

WARNINGS:

Naloxone with pentazocine is intended for oral use only. Severe, potentially lethal, reactions may result from misuse of naloxone with pentazocine by injection either alone or in combination with other substances. (See DRUG ABUSE AND DEPENDENCE.)

Drug Dependence: Pentazocine can cause a physical and psychological dependence. (See DRUG ABUSE AND DEPENDENCE.)

Head Injury and Increased Intracranial Pressure: As in the case of other potent analgesics, the potential of pentazocine for elevating cerebrospinal fluid pressure may be attributed to CO_2 retention due to the respiratory depressant effects of the drug. These effects may be markedly exaggerated in the presence of head injury, other intracranial lesions, or a preexisting increase in intracranial pressure. Furthermore, pentazocine can produce effects which may obscure the clinical course of patients with head injuries. In such patients. pentazocine must be used with extreme caution and only if its use is deemed essential.

Usage with Alcohol: Due to the potential for increased CNS depressant effects, alcohol should be used with caution in patients who are currently receiving pentazocine.

WARNINGS: *(cont'd)*

Patients Receiving Narcotics: Pentazocine is a mild narcotic antagonist. Some patients previously given narcotics, including methadone for the daily treatment of narcotic dependence, have experienced withdrawal symptoms after receiving pentazocine.

Certain Respiratory Conditions: Although respiratory depression has rarely been reported after oral administration of pentazocine, the drug should be administered with caution to patients with respiratory depression from any cause, severely limited respiratory reserve, severe bronchial asthma, and other obstructive respiratory conditions, or cyanosis.

Acute CNS Manifestations: Patients receiving therapeutic doses of pentazocine have experienced hallucinations (usually visual), disorientation, and confusion which have cleared spontaneously within a period of hours. The mechanism of this reaction is not known. Such patients should be very closely observed and vital signs checked. If the drug is reinstituted, it should be done with caution since these acute CNS manifestations may recur.

PRECAUTIONS:

GENERAL

CNS Effect: Caution should be used when pentazocine is administered to patients prone to seizures; seizures have occurred in a few such patients in association with the use of pentazocine through no cause and effect relationship has been established.

Impaired Renal or Hepatic Function: Decreased metabolism of pentazocine by the liver in extensive liver disease may predispose to accentuation of side effects. Although laboratory tests have not indicated that pentazocine causes or increases renal or hepatic impairment, the drug should be administered with caution to patients with such impairment.

In prescribing pentazocine for long-term use, the physician should take precautions to avoid increases in dose by the patient.

Biliary Surgery: Narcotic drug products are generally considered to elevate biliary tract pressure for varying periods following their administration. Some evidence suggests that pentazocine may differ from other marketed narcotics in this respect (*i.e.,* it causes little or no elevation in biliary tract pressures). The clinical significance of these findings, however, is not yet known.

INFORMATION FOR THE PATIENT

Since sedation, dizziness, and occasional euphoria have been noted, ambulatory patients should be warned not to operate machinery, drive cars, or unnecessarily expose themselves to hazards. Pentazocine may cause physical and psychological dependence when taken alone and may have additive CNS depressant properties when taken in combination with alcohol or other CNS depressants.

Myocardial Infarction: As with all drugs, pentazocine should be used with caution in patients with myocardial infarction who have nausea or vomiting.

CARCINOGENESIS, MUTAGENESIS, AND IMPAIRMENT OF FERTILITY

No long-term studies in animals to test for carcinogenesis have been performed with the components of naloxone with pentazocine.

PREGNANCY CATEGORY C

Animal reproduction studies have not been conducted with naloxone with pentazocine. It is also not known whether naloxone with pentazocine can cause fetal harm when administered to pregnant women or can affect reproduction capacity. Naloxone with pentazocine should be given to pregnant women only if clearly needed. However, animal reproduction studies with pentazocine have not demonstrated teratogenic embryotoxic effects.

LABOR AND DELIVERY

Patients receiving pentazocine during labor have experienced no adverse effects other than those that occur with commonly used analgesics. Naloxone with pentazocine should be used with caution in women delivering premature infants. The effect of naloxone with pentazocine on the mother and fetus, the duration of labor or delivery, the possibility that forceps delivery or other intervention or resuscitation of the newborn may be necessary, or the effect of naloxone with pentazocine on the later growth, development, and functional maturation of the child are unknown at the present time.

NURSING MOTHERS

It is not known whether this drug is excreted in human milk. Because many drugs are excreted in human milk, caution should be exercised when naloxone with pentazocine is administered to a nursing woman.

PEDIATRIC USE

Safety and effectiveness in children below the age of 12 years have not been established.

DRUG INTERACTIONS:

Usage with Alcohol: See WARNINGS.

ADVERSE REACTIONS:

Cardiovascular: Hypotension, tachycardia, syncope.

Respiratory: Rarely, respiratory depression.

Acute CNS Manifestations: Patients receiving therapeutic doses of pentazocine have experienced hallucinations (usually visual), disorientation, and confusion which have cleared spontaneously within a period of hours. The mechanism of this reaction is not known. Such patients should be closely observed and vital signs checked. If the drug is reinstituted it should be done with caution since these acute CNS manifestations may recur.

Other CNS Effects: Dizziness, lightheadedness, hallucinations, sedation, euphoria, headache, confusion, disorientation; infrequently weakness, disturbed dreams, insomnia, syncope, visual blurring and focusing difficulty, depression; and rarely tremor, irritability, excitement, tinnitus.

Autonomic: Sweating; infrequently flushing; and rarely chills.

Gastrointestinal: Nausea, vomiting, constipation, diarrhea, anorexia, rarely abdominal distress.

Allergic: Edema of the face; dermatitis, including pruritus; flushed skin, including plethora; infrequently rash, and rarely urticaria.

Ophthalmic: Visual blurring and focusing difficulty.

Hematologic: Depression of white blood cells (especially granulocytes), which is usually reversible, moderate transient eosinophilia.

Other: Headache, chills, insomnia, weakness, urinary retention, paresthesia.

DRUG ABUSE AND DEPENDENCE:

Controlled Substance: Naloxone with pentazocine is a Schedule IV controlled substance.

There have been some reports of dependence and of withdrawal symptoms with orally administered pentazocine. Patients with a history of drug dependence should be under close supervision while receiving pentazocine orally. There have been rare reports of possible abstinence syndromes in newborns after prolonged use of pentazocine during pregnancy

DRUG ABUSE AND DEPENDENCE: *(cont'd)*

There have been instances of psychological and physical dependence on parenteral pentazocine in patients with a history of drug abuse and rarely, in patients without such a history. Abrupt discontinuance following the extended use of parenteral pentazocine has resulted in withdrawal symptoms.

In prescribing pentazocine for chronic use, the physician should take precautions to avoid increases in dose by the patient.

The amount of naloxone present in naloxone with pentazocine (0.5 mg per tablet) has no action when taken orally and will not interfere with the pharmacologic action of pentazocine. However, this amount of naloxone given by injection has profound antagonistic action to narcotic analgesics.

Severe, even lethal, consequences may result from misuse of tablets by injection either alone or in combination with other substances, such as pulmonary emboli, vascular occlusion, ulceration and abscesses, and withdrawal symptoms in narcotic dependent individuals.

Naloxone with pentazocine contains an opioid antagonist, naloxone (0.5 mg). Naloxone is inactive when administered orally at this dose, and its inclusion in naloxone with pentazocine is intended to curb a form of misuse of oral pentazocine. Parenterally, naloxone is an active narcotic antagonist. Thus, naloxone with pentazocine has a lower potential for parenteral misuse than the previous oral pentazocine formulation Talwin 50 (pentazocine hydrochloride tablets, USP). However, it is still subject to patient misuse and abuse by the oral route.

OVERDOSAGE:

Manifestations: Clinical experience of overdosage with this oral medication has been insufficient to define the signs of this condition.

Treatment: Oxygen, intravenous fluids, vasopressors, and other supportive measures should be employed as indicated. Assisted or controlled ventilation should also be considered. For respiratory depression due to overdosage or unusual sensitivity to pentazocine, parenteral naloxone is a specific and effective antagonist.

DOSAGE AND ADMINISTRATION:

Naloxone with pentazocine is intended for oral use only. Severe, potentially lethal, reactions may result from misuse of naloxone with pentazocine by injection either alone or in combination with other substances. (See DRUG ABUSE AND DEPENDENCE.)

Adults: The usual initial adult dose is 1 tablet every three or four hours. This may be increased to 2 tablets when needed. Total daily dosage should not exceed 12 tablets.

When anti-inflammatory or antipyretic effects are desired in addition to analgesia, aspirin can be administered concomitantly with this product.

Children Under 12 Years of Age: Since clinical experience in children under 12 years of age is limited, administration of this product in this age group is not recommended.

Duration of Therapy: Patients with chronic pain who receive naloxone with pentazocine orally for prolonged periods have only rarely been reported to experience withdrawal symptoms when administration was abruptly discontinued (see WARNINGS). Tolerance to the analgesic effect of pentazocine has also been reported only rarely. However, there is no long-term experience with the oral administration of naloxone with pentazocine.

HOW SUPPLIED:

Talwin Nx Tablets (oblong), yellow, scored, each containing pentazocine hydrochloride equivalent to 50 mg base and naloxone hydrochloride equivalent to 0.5 mg base.

HOW SUPPLIED - EQUIVALENTS NOT AVAILABLE:

Tablet, Uncoated - Oral - 50 mg/0.5 mg

100's	$83.08	TALWIN NX, Sanofi Winthrop	00024-1951-04
250's	$227.92	TALWIN NX, Sanofi Winthrop	00024-1951-24

NALTREXONE HYDROCHLORIDE *(001857)*

CATEGORIES: Alcoholism; Antagonists and Antidotes; Antidotes; Central Nervous System Agents; Narcotic Addiction; Narcotic Antagonists; Opiate Antagonists; Orphan Drugs; Bulimia*; HIV Infection*; Obesity*; Schizophrenia*; Pregnancy Category C; FDA Approved 1984 Nov

* Indication not approved by the FDA

BRAND NAMES: *Antaxone*; *Celupan*; *Nalorex* (France, England); Naltrexone HCl; *Nemexin* (Germany); **Trexan**

(International brand names outside U.S. in italics)

DESCRIPTION:

Naltrexone hydrochloride, an opioid antagonist, is a synthetic congener of oxymorphone with no opioid agonist properties. Naltrexone differs in structure from oxymorphone in that the methyl group on the nitrogen atom is replaced by a cyclopropylmethyl group. Naltrexone HCl is also related to the potent opioid antagonist, naloxone, or n- allylnoroxymorphone (Narcan).

Naltrexone HCl is a white, crystalline compound. The hydrochloride salt is soluble in water to the extent of about 100 mg/cc. Naltrexone HCl is available in scored tablets containing 50 mg of naltrexone HCl.

Naltrexone HCl tablets also contain: alginic acid, FD&C Yellow 6, microcrystalline, cellulose, stearic acid, and sugar.

CLINICAL PHARMACOLOGY:

Pharmacodynamic actions: Naltrexone HCl is a pure opioid antagonist. It markedly attenuates or completely blocks, reversibly, the subjective effects of IV administered opioids.

When co-administered with morphine, on a chronic basis, naltrexone HCl blocks the physical dependence to morphine, heroin and other opioids.

Naltrexone HCl has few, if any, intrinsic actions besides its opioid blocking properties. However, it does produce some pupillary constriction by an unknown mechanism.

The administration of naltrexone HCl is not associated with the development of tolerance or dependence. In subjects physically dependent on opioids, naltrexone HCl will precipitate withdrawal symptomatology.

Clinical studies indicate that 50 mg of naltrexone HCl will block the pharmacologic effects of 25 mg of IV administered heroin for periods as long as 24 hours. Other data suggest that doubling the dose of naltrexone HCl provides blockade for 48 hours, and tripling the dose provides blockade for about 72 hours.

CLINICAL PHARMACOLOGY: *(cont'd)*

Naltrexone HCl blocks the effects of opioids by competitive binding (*i.e.,* analogous to competitive inhibition of enzymes) at opioid receptors. This makes the blockade produced potentially surmountable, but overcoming full naltrexone blockade by administration of very high doses of opiates has resulted in excessive symptoms of histamine release in experimental subjects.

The mechanism of action of naltrexone HCl in alcoholism is not understood; however, involvement of the endogenous opioid system is suggested by preclinical data. Naltrexone HCl, an opioid receptor antagonist, competitively binds to such receptors and may block the effects of endogenous opioids. Opioid antagonists have been shown to reduce alcohol consumption by animals, and naltrexone HCl has been shown to reduce alcohol consumption in clinical studies.

Naltrexone HCl is not aversive therapy and does not cause a disulfiram-like reaction wither as a result of opiate use or ethanol ingestion.

Pharmacokinetics: Naltrexone HCl is a pure opioid receptor antagonist. Although well absorbed orally, naltrexone is subject to significant first pass metabolism with oral bioavailability estimates ranging from 5 to 40%. The activity of naltrexone is believed to be due to both parent and the 6-β-naltrexol metabolite. Both parent drug and metabolites are excreted primarily by the kidney (53% to 79% of the dose), however, urinary excretion of unchanged naltrexone accounts for less than 2% of an oral dose and fecal excretion is a minor elimination pathway. The mean elimination half-life (T-1/2) values for naltrexone and 6-β-naltrexol are 4 hours and 13 hours respectively. Naltrexone and 6-β-naltrexol are dose proportional in terms of AUC and C_{max}over the range of 50 to 200 mg and do not accumulate after 100 mg daily doses.

Absorption: Following oral administration, naltrexone undergoes rapid and nearly complete absorption with approximately 96% of the dose absorbed from the gastrointestinal tract. Peak plasma levels of both naltrexone and 6-β-naltrexol occur within one hour of dosing.

Distribution: The volume of distribution for naltrexone following intravenous administration is estimated to be 1350 liters. *In vitro* tests with human plasma show naltrexone to be 21% bound to plasma proteins over the therapeutic dose range.

Metabolism: The systemic clearance (after intravenous administration) of naltrexone is ~3.5 L/min, which exceeds liver blood flow (~1.2 L/min). This suggests both that naltrexone is a highly extracted drug (>98% metabolized) and that extra-hepatic sites of drug metabolism exist. The major metabolite of naltrexone is 6-β-naltrexol. Two other minor metabolites are 2-hydroxy-3-methoxy-6-β-naltrexol and 2-hydroxy-3-methyl-naltrexone. Naltrexone and its metabolites are also conjugated to form additional metabolic products.

Elimination: The renal clearance for naltrexone ranges from 30-127 ml/min and suggests that renal elimination is primarily by glomerular filtration. In comparison the renal clearance for 6-β-naltrexol ranges from 230-369 ml/min, suggesting an additional renal tubular secretory mechanism. The urinary excretion of unchanged naltrexone accounts for less than 2% of an oral dose; urinary excretion of unchanged and conjugated 6-β-naltrexol accounts for 43% of an oral dose. The pharmacokinetic profile of naltrexone suggests that naltrexone and its metabolites may undergo enterohepatic recycling.

Hepatic and Renal Impairment: Naltrexone appears to have extra- hepatic sites of drug metabolism and its major metabolite undergoes active tubular secretion (see Metabolism. Adequate studies of naltrexone in patients with severe hepatic or renal impairment have not been conducted.

CLINICAL STUDIES:

Alcoholism: The efficacy of naltrexone HCl as an aid to the treatment of alcoholism was tested in placebo-controlled, outpatient, double blind trials. These studies used a dose of naltrexone HCl 50 mg once daily for 12 weeks as an adjunct to social and psychotherapeutic methods when given under conditions that enhanced patients compliance. Patients with psychosis, dementia, and secondary psychiatric diagnoses were excluded from these studies.

In one of these studies, 104 alcohol-dependent patients were randomized to receive either naltrexone HCl 50 mg once daily or placebo. In this study, naltrexone HCl proved superior to placebo in measures of drinking including abstention rates (51% vs. 23%), number of drinking days, and relapse (31% vs. 60%). In a second study with 82 alcohol-dependent patients, the group of patients receiving naltrexone HCl were shown to have lower relapse rates (21% vs. 41%), less alcohol craving, and fewer drinking days compared with patients who received placebo, but these results depended on the specific analysis used.

The clinical use of naltrexone HCl as adjunctive pharmacotherapy for the treatment of alcoholism was also evaluated in a multicenter safety study. This study of 865 individuals with alcoholism included patients with comorbid psychiatric conditions, concomitant medications, polysubstance abuse and HIV disease. Results of this study demonstrated that the side effect profile of naltrexone HCl appears to be similar in both alcoholic and opioid dependent populations, and that serious side effects are uncommon.

In the clinical studies, treatment with naltrexone HCl supported abstinence, prevented relapse and decreased alcohol consumption. In the uncontrolled study, the patterns of abstinence and relapse were similar to those observed in the controlled studies. Naltrexone HCl was not uniformly helpful to all patients, and the expected effect of the drug is a modest improvement in the outcome of conventional treatment.

Treatment of Narcotic Addiction: Naltrexone HCl has been shown to produce complete blockade of the euphoric effects of opioids in both volunteer and addict populations. When administered by means that enforce compliance, it will produce an effective opioid blockade, but has not been shown to affect the use of cocaine or other non-opioid drugs of abuse.

There are no data that demonstrate an unequivocally beneficial effect of naltrexone HCl on rates of recidivism among detoxified, formerly opioid-dependent individuals who self-administer the drug. The failure of the drug in this setting appears to be due to poor medication compliance.

The drug is reported to be of greatest use in good prognosis narcotic addicts who take the drug as part of a comprehensive occupational rehabilitative program, behavioral contract, or other compliance-enhancing protocol. Naltrexone HCl, unlike methadone or LAAM (levo-alpha- acetylmethadol), does not reinforce medication compliance and is expected to have a therapeutic effect only when given under external conditions that support continued use of medication.

Individualization of dosage: DO NOT ATTEMPT TREATMENT WITH NALTREXONE HCL UNLESS, IN THE MEDICAL JUDGEMENT OF THE PRESCRIBING PHYSICIAN, THERE IS NO REASONABLE POSSIBILITY OF OPIOID USE WITHIN THE PAST 7-10 DAYS. IF THERE IS ANY QUESTION OF OCCULT OPIOID DEPENDENCE, PERFORM A NARCAN CHALLENGE TEST.

Treatment of alcoholism: The placebo-controlled studies that demonstrated the efficacy of naltrexone HCl as an adjunctive treatment of alcoholism used a dose regimen of naltrexone HCl 50 mg once daily for up to 12 weeks. Other dose regimens or durations of therapy were not studied in these trials.

CLINICAL STUDIES: *(cont'd)*

Physicians are advised that 5-15% of patients taking naltrexone HCl for alcoholism will complain of non-specific side effects, chiefly gastrointestinal upset. Prescribing physicians have tried using an initial 25 mg dose, splitting the daily dose, and adjusting the time of dosing limited success. No dose or pattern of dosing has been shown to be more effective than any other in reducing these complaints for all patients.

Treatment of Narcotic Dependence: Once the patient has been started on naltrexone HCl, 50 mg once a day will produce adequate clinical blockade of the actions of parenterally administered opioids. As with many non-agonist treatments for addiction, naltrexone HCl is of proven value only when given as part of a comprehensive plan of management that includes some measure to ensure the patient takes the medication.

A flexible approach to a dosing regiment may be employed to enhance compliance. Thus, patients may receive 50 mg of naltrexone HCl every weekday with a 100 mg dose on Saturday or patients may receive 100 mg every other day, or 150 mg every third day. Several of the clinical studies reported in the literature have employed the following dose regimen: 100 mg on Monday, 100 mg on Wednesday, and 150 mg on Friday. This dosing schedule appeared to be acceptable to many naltrexone HCl patients successfully maintaining their opioid-free state.

Experience with the supervised administration of a number of potentially hepatotoxic agents suggests that supervised administration and single doses of naltrexone HCl higher than 50 mg may have an associated increased risk of hepatocellular injury, even though three-times a week dosing has been well tolerated in the addict population and in initial clinical trials in alcoholism. Clinics using this approach should balance the possible risks against the probable benefits and may wish to maintain a higher index of suspicion for drug-associated hepatitis and ensure patients are advised of the need to report non-specific abdominal complaints (see Information for the Patient.)

INDICATIONS AND USAGE:

Naltrexone HCl is indicated in the treatment of alcohol dependence and for the blockade of the effects of exogenously administered opioids.

Naltrexone HCl has not been shown to provide any therapeutic benefit except as part of an appropriate plan of management for the addictions.

CONTRAINDICATIONS:

Naltrexone HCl is contraindicated in:

1) Patients receiving opioid analgesics.

2) Patients currently dependent on opioids.

3) Patients in acute opioid withdrawal (see WARNINGS.)

4) Any individual who has failed the Narcan challenge test or who has a positive urine screen for opioids.

5) Any individual with a history of sensitivity to naltrexone HCl. It is not known if there is any cross-sensitivity with naloxone or the phenanthrene containing opioids.

6) Any individual with acute hepatitis or liver failure.

WARNINGS:

HEPATOTOXICITY

Naltrexone HCl has the capacity to cause dose related hepatocellular injury when given in excessive doses.

Naltrexone HCl is contraindicated in acute hepatitis or liver failure, and its use in patients with active liver disease must be carefully considered in light of its hepatotoxic effects.

The margin of separation between the apparently safe dose of naltrexone HCl and the dose causing hepatic injury appears to be only five-fold or less. Naltrexone HCl does not appear to be hepatoxin at the recommended doses.

Patients should be warned of risk of the risk of hepatic injury and advised to stop the use of naltrexone HCl and seek medical attention if they experience symptoms of acute hepatitis.

Evidence of the hepatotoxic potential of naltrexone HCl is derived primarily from a placebo controlled study in which naltrexone HCl was administered to obese subjects at a dose approximately five-fold that recommended for the blockade of opiate receptors (300 mg per day). In the study, 5 of 26 naltrexone HCl recipients developed elevations or serum transaminase (i.e., peak ALT values ranging from a low of 121 to a high of 532; or 3 to 19 times their baseline values) after three to eight weeks of treatment. Although the patients involved were generally clinically asymptomatic and the transaminase levels of all patients on whom follow-up was obtained returned to (or toward) baseline values in a matter of weeks, the lack of any transaminase elevations of similar magnitude in any of the 24 placebo patients in the same study is persuasive evidence that naltrexone HCl is a direct (*i.e.,* not an idiosyncratic) hepatotoxin.

This conclusion is also supported by evidence from other placebo controlled studies in which exposure to naltrexone HCl at doses above the amount recommended for the treatment of alcoholism or opiate blockade (50 mg/day) consistently produced more numerous and more significant elevations of serum transaminases than did placebo. Transaminase elevations in 3 of 9 patients with Alzheimer's Disease who received naltrexone HCl (at doses up to 300 mg/day) for 5 to 8 weeks in open clinical trial have been reported.

Although no cases of hepatic failure due to naltrexone HCl administration have ever been reported, physicians are advised to consider this as a possible risk of treatment and to use the same care in prescribing naltrexone HCl as they would other drugs with the potential for causing hepatic injury.

Unintended Precipitation of Abstinence: To prevent occurrence of an acute abstinence syndrome, or exacerbation of a pre-existing sub- clinical abstinence syndrome, patients must be opioid-free for a minimum of 7-10 days before starting naltrexone HCl. Since the absence of an opioid drug in the urine is often not sufficient proof that a patient is opioid-free, a Narcan challenge should be employed if the prescribing physician feels there is a risk of precipitating a withdrawal reaction following administration of naltrexone HCl. The Narcan challenge test is described in the DOSAGE AND ADMINISTRATION.

While naltrexone HCl is a potent antagonist with a prolonged pharmacological effect (24 to 72 hours), the blockade produced by naltrexone HCl is surmountable. This is useful in patients who may require analgesia, but poses a potential risk to individuals who attempt, on their own, to overcome the blockade by administering large amounts of exogenous opioids. Indeed, any attempt by the patient to overcome the antagonism by taking opioids is very dangerous and may lead to a fatal overdose. Injury may arise because the plasma concentration of exogenous opioids attained immediately following their acute administration may be sufficient to overcome the competitive receptor blockade.

WARNINGS: *(cont'd)*

As a consequence, the patient may be in immediate danger of suffering life endangering opioid intoxication (*e.g.,* respiratory arrest, circulatory collapse). Also, lesser amounts of exogenous opioids may prove dangerous if they are taken in a manner (*i.e.,* relatively long after the last dose of naltrexone) and in an amount so that they persist in the body longer than effective concentrations of naltrexone and its metabolites. Patients should be told of the serious consequences of trying to overcome the opiate blockade. (See Information for the Patient.)

PRECAUTIONS:

GENERAL

When reversal of naltrexone HCl Blockade is Required: In an emergency situation in patients receiving fully blocking doses of naltrexone HCl, a suggested plan of management is regional analgesia, conscious sedation with a benzodiazepine, use of non-opioid analgesics or general anesthesia.

In a situation requiring opioid analgesia, the amount of opioid required may be greater than usual, and the resulting respiratory depression may be deeper and more prolonged.

A rapidly acting opioid analgesic which minimizes the duration of respiratory depression is preferred. The amounts of analgesic administered should be titrated to the needs of the patient. Non-receptor mediated actions may occur and should be expected (*e.g.,* facial swelling, itching, generalized erythema, or bronchoconstriction) presumably due to histamine release.

Irrespective of the drug chosen to reverse naltrexone HCl blockade, the patient should be monitored closely by appropriately trained personnel in a setting equipped and staffed for cardiopulmonary resuscitation.

When Withdrawal is Accidentally Precipitated With Naltrexone HCl With Naltrexone HCl: Severe opioid withdrawal syndromes precipitated by the accidental ingestion of naltrexone HCl have been reported in opioid-dependent individuals. Symptoms of withdrawal have usually appeared within five minutes of injection of naltrexone HCl and have lasted for up to 48 hours. Mental status changes including confusion, somnolence and visual hallucinations have occurred. Significant fluid losses from vomiting and diarrhea have required IV fluid administration. In all cases patients were closely monitored and therapy with non-opioid medications was tailored to meet individual requirements.

Suicide: The risk of suicide is known to be increased in patients with substance abuse with or without concomitant depression. The risk is not abated by treatment with naltrexone HCl (see ADVERSE REACTIONS.)

INFORMATION FOR THE PATIENT

It is recommended that the prescribing physician relate the following information to patients being treated with naltrexone HCl:

You have been prescribed naltrexone HCl as part of the comprehensive treatment for your alcoholism or drug dependence. You should carry identification to alert medical personnel to the fact that you are taking naltrexone HCl. A naltrexone HCl medication card may be obtained from your physician and can be used for this purpose. Carrying this identification card should help to ensure you that you can obtain adequate treatment in an emergency. If you require medical treatment, be sure to tell the treating physician that you are receiving naltrexone HCl therapy.

You should take naltrexone HCl as directed by your physician. If you attempt to self-administer heroin or any other opiate drug, in small doses, you will not perceive any effect. Most important, however, if you attempt to self-administer large doses of heroin or any other narcotic, you may die or sustain serious injury, including coma.

Naltrexone HCl is well-tolerated in the recommended doses, but may cause liver injury when taken in excess or in people who develop liver disease from other causes. If you develop abdominal pain lasting more than a few days, white bowel movements, dark urine, or yellowing of your eyes, you should stop taking naltrexone HCl immediately and see your doctor as soon as possible.

LABORATORY TESTS

A high index of suspicion for drug-related hepatic injury is critical of the occurrence of liver damage induced by naltrexone HCl is to be detected at the earliest possible time. Evaluations, using appropriate batteries of tests to detect liver injury are recommended at a frequency appropriate to the clinical situation and dose of naltrexone HCl.

Naltrexone HCl does not interfere with thin-layer, gas-liquid, and high pressure liquid chromatographic methods which may be used for the separation and detection of morphine, methadone or quinine in the urine. Naltrexone HCl may or may not interfere with enzymatic methods for the detection of opioids depending on the specificity of the test. Please consult the test manufacturer for specific details.

CARCINOGENESIS, MUTAGENESIS, AND IMPAIRMENT OF FERTILITY:

Carcinogenesis: In a two-year carcinogenicity study in rats, there were small increases in the numbers of mesotheliomas in males, and tumors of vascular origin in both sexes. The number of tumors were within the range seen in historical control groups, except for the vascular tumors in females, where the 4% incidence exceeded the historical maximum of 2%.

Mutagenesis: A total of twenty-two distinct tests were performed using bacterial, mammalian, and tissue culture systems. All tests were negative except for weakly positive findings in the Drosophila recessive lethal assay and non-specific DNA repair tests with *E. coli.* The significance of these findings is undetermined.

Impairment of Fertility: Naltrexone HCl (100 mg/kg, approximately 140 times the human therapeutic dose) caused a significant increase in pseudo-pregnancy in the rat. A decrease in the pregnancy rate of mated female rats also occurred. The relevance of these observations to human fertility is not known.

PREGNANCY CATEGORY C

Naltrexone HCl has been shown to have an embryocidal effect in the rat and rabbit when given in doses approximately 140 times the human therapeutic dose. This effect was demonstrated in rats dosed with naltrexone HCl (100 mg/kg) prior to and throughout gestation, and rabbits treated with 60 mg/kg of naltrexone HCl during the period of organogenesis.

There are no adequate and well-controlled studies in pregnant women. Naltrexone HCl should be used in pregnancy only when the potential benefit justifies the potential risk to the fetus.

LABOR AND DELIVERY

Whether or not naltrexone HCl affects the duration of labor and delivery is unknown.

NURSING MOTHERS

Whether or not naltrexone HCl is excreted in human milk is unknown. Because many drugs are excreted in human milk, caution should be exercised when naltrexone HCl is administered to a nursing mother.

PEDIATRIC USE

The safe use of naltrexone HCl in subjects younger than 18 years old has not been established.

DRUG INTERACTIONS:

Studies to evaluate possible interactions between naltrexone HCl and drugs other than opiates have not been performed. Consequently, caution is advised if the concomitant administration of naltrexone HCl and other drugs is required.

The safety and efficacy of concomitant use of naltrexone HCl and disulfiram is unknown, and the concomitant use of two potentially hepatotoxic medications is not ordinarily recommended unless the probable benefits outweigh the known risks.

Lethargy and somnolence have not been reported following doses of naltrexone HCl and thioridazine.

Patients taking naltrexone HCl may not benefit from opioid containing medicines, such as cough and cold preparations, antidiarrheal preparations, and opioid analgesia must be administered to a patient receiving naltrexone HCl, the amount of opioid required may be greater than usual, and the resulting respiratory depression may be deeper and more prolonged. (see PRECAUTIONS.)

ADVERSE REACTIONS:

During two randomized, double-blind placebo-controlled 12 week trials to evaluate the efficacy of naltrexone HCl as an adjunctive treatment of alcohol dependence, most patients tolerated naltrexone HCl well. In these studies, a total of 93 patients received naltrexone HCl at a dose of 50 mg once daily. Five of these patients discontinued naltrexone HCl because of nausea. No serious adverse events were reported during these two trials.

While extensive clinical studies evaluating the use of naltrexone HCl in detoxified, formerly opioid dependent individuals failed to identify any single, serious untoward risk of naltrexone HCl use, placebo controlled studies employing up to five-fold higher doses of naltrexone HCl (up to 300 mg per day) than that recommended for use in opiate receptor blockade have shown that naltrexone HCl causes hepatocellular injury in a substantial proportion of patients exposed at higher doses (see PRECAUTIONS, Laboratory Tests.

Aside from this finding, and the risk of precipitated opioid withdrawal, available evidence does not incriminate naltrexone HCl, used at any dose, as a cause of any other serious adverse reaction for the patient who is "opioid free." It is critical to recognize that naltrexone HCl can precipitate or exacerbate abstinence signs and symptoms in any individual who is not completely free of exogenous opioids.

Patients with addictive disorders, especially narcotic addiction, are risk for multiple numerous adverse events and abnormal laboratory findings, including liver function abnormalities. Data from both controlled and observational studies suggest that these abnormalities, other than the dose-related hepatotoxicity described above, are not related to the use of naltrexone HCl.

Among opioid free individuals, naltrexone HCl administration at the recommended dose has not been associated with a predictable profile of serious adverse or untoward events. However, as mentioned above, among individuals using opioids, naltrexone HCl may cause serious withdrawal reactions(see CONTRAINDICATIONS, WARNINGS, and DOSAGE AND ADMINISTRATION).

Reported Adverse Events: Naltrexone HCl has not been shown to cause significant increases in complaints in placebo-controlled trials in patients known to be free of opioids for more than 7-10 days. Studies in alcoholic populations and in volunteers in clinical pharmacology studies have suggested that a small fraction of patients may experience an opioid withdrawal-like symptom complex consisting of tearfulness, mild nausea, abdominal cramps, restlessness, bone or joint pain, myalgia, and nasal symptoms. This may represent the unmasking of occult opioid use, or it may represent symptoms attributable to naltrexone. A number of alternative dosing patterns have been recommended to try to reduce the frequency of these complaints (see Individualization of Dosage.)

Alcoholism: In an open label safety study with approximately 570 individuals with alcoholism receiving naltrexone HCl, the following new-onset adverse reactions occurred in 2% or more of the patients: nausea (10%), headache (7%), dizziness (4%), nervousness (4%), fatigue (4%), insomnia (3%), vomiting (3%), anxiety (2%) and somnolence (2%).

Depression (5-7%), suicidal ideation (2%), and attempted suicide (<1%) have been reported in individuals on naltrexone HCl, placebo and in concurrent control groups undergoing treatment for alcoholism. Although no casual relationship with naltrexone HCl is suspected, physicians should be aware that treatment with naltrexone HCl does not reduce the risk of suicide in these patients (see PRECAUTIONS.)

Narcotic Addiction: The following adverse reactions have been reported both at baseline and during the naltrexone HCl clinical trials in narcotic Addiction at an incidence rate of more than 10%:

Difficulty sleeping, anxiety, nervousness, abdominal pain/cramps, nausea and/or vomiting, low energy, joint and muscle pain, and headache.

The incidence was less than 10% for:

Loss of appetite, diarrhea, constipation, increased thirst, increased energy, feeling down, irritability, dizziness, skin rash, delayed ejaculation, decreased potency and chills.

The following events occurred in less than 1% of subjects:

Respiratory: nasal congestion, itching, rhinorrhea, sneezing, sore throat, excess mucus or phlegm, sinus trouble, heavy breathing, hoarseness, cough, shortness of breath.

Cardiovascular: nose bleeds, phlebitis, edema, increased blood pressure, non-specific ECG changes, palpitations, tachycardia.

Gastrointestinal: Excessive gas, hemorrhoids, diarrhea, ulcer.

Musculoskeletal: painful shoulders, legs or knees; tremors, twitching.

Genitourinary: increased frequency of, or discomfort during, urination; increased or decreased sexual interest.

Dermatologic: oily skin, pruritus, acne, athlete's foot, cold sores, alopecia.

Psychiatric: depression, paranoia, fatigue, restlessness, confusion, disorientation, hallucinations, nightmares, bad dreams.

Special Senses: eyes-blurred, burning, light sensitive, swollen, aching, strained; ears "clogged", aching, tinnitus.

General: increased appetite, weight loss, weight gain, yawning, somnolence, fever, dry mouth, head "pounding", inguinal pain, swollen glands, "side" pains, cold feet, "hot spells."

Other: Depression, suicide, attempted suicide and suicidal ideation have been reported in the post-marketing experience with naltrexone HCl used in the treatment of narcotic dependence. No casual relationship has been demonstrated.

Laboratory Tests: With the exception of liver test abnormalities (see WARNINGS, and PRECAUTIONS) results of laboratory tests, like adverse reaction reports have not shown consistent patterns of abnormalities that can be attributed to treatment with naltrexone HCl.

Idiopathic thrombocytopenia purpura was reported in one patient who may have been sensitized to naltrexone HCl in a previous course of treatment with naltrexone HCl. The condition cleared without sequelae after discontinuation of naltrexone HCl and corticosteroid treatment.

DRUG ABUSE AND DEPENDENCE:

Naltrexone HCl is a pure opioid antagonist. It does not lead to physical or psychological dependence. Tolerance to the opioid antagonist effect is not known to occur.

OVERDOSAGE:

There is limited clinical experience with naltrexone HCl overdosage in humans. In one study, subjects who received 800 mg daily naltrexone HCl for up to one week showed no evidence of toxicity.

In acute toxicity studies in the mouse, rat, and dog, cause of death was due to clonic-tonic convulsions and/or respiratory failure.

Treatment: In view of the lack of actual experience in the treatment of naltrexone HCl overdose, patients should be treated symptomatically in a closely supervised environment. Physicians should contact a poison control center for the most up-to-date information.

DOSAGE AND ADMINISTRATION:

IF THERE IS ANY QUESTION OF OCCULT OPIOID DEPENDENCE, PERFORM A NARCAN CHALLENGE TEST AND DO NOT INITIATE NALTREXONE HCL THERAPY UNTIL THE NARCAN CHALLENGE IS NEGATIVE.

Treatment of Alcoholism: A dose of 50 mg once daily is recommended for most patients (see CLINICAL PHARMACOLOGY, Individualization of Dosages).

Naltrexone HCl should be considered as only one of many factors determining the success of treatment of alcoholism. Factors associated with a good outcome in the clinical trials with naltrexone HCl were the type, intensity, and duration of treatment; appropriate management of comorbid conditions; use of community-based support groups; and good medication compliance. To achieve the best possible treatment outcome, appropriate compliance-enhancing techniques should be implemented for all components of the treatment program, especially medication compliance.

Treatment of Narcotic Dependence: Initiate treatment with naltrexone HCl using the following guidelines:

1. Treatment should not be attempted unless the patient has remained opioid-free for at least 7-10 days. Self-reporting of abstinence from opioids in narcotic addicts should be verified by analysis of the patient's urine for absence of opioids. The patient should not be manifesting withdrawal signs or reporting withdrawal symptoms.

2. If there is any question of occult opioid dependence, perform a Narcan challenge test. If signs of opioid withdrawal are still observed following Narcan challenge, treatment with naltrexone HCl should not be attempted. The Narcan challenge can be repeated in 24 hours.

3. Treatment should be initiated carefully, with an initial dose of 25 mg of naltrexone HCl. If no withdrawal signs occur, the patient may be started on 50 mg a day thereafter.

Narcan Challenge Test: The Narcan challenge test should not be performed in a patient showing clinical signs or symptoms of opioid withdrawal, or in a patient whose urine contains opioids. The Narcan challenge test may be administered by either the intravenous or subcutaneous routes.

Intravenous challenge: Following appropriate screening of the patient, 0.8 mg of Narcan should be drawn into a sterile syringe. If the intravenous route of administration is selected, 0.2 mg of Narcan should be injected, and while the needle is still in the patient's vein, the patient should be observed for 30 seconds for evidence of withdrawal signs or symptoms. If there is no evidence of withdrawal, the remaining 0.6 mg of Narcan (naloxone HCl) should be injected, and the patient observed for an additional period of 20 minutes for signs and symptoms of withdrawal.

Subcutaneous challenge: If the subcutaneous route is selected, 0.8 mg should be administered subcutaneously, and the patient observed for signs and symptoms of withdrawal for 20 minutes.

Conditions and technique for observation of patient: During the appropriate period of observation, the patient's vital signs should be monitored and the patient should be monitored for signs of withdrawal. It is also important to question the patient carefully. The signs and symptoms of opioid withdrawal include, but are not limited to, the following:

WITHDRAWAL SIGNS: Stuffiness or running nose, tearing, yawning, sweating, tremor, vomiting or piloerection.

WITHDRAWAL SYMPTOMS: Feeling of temperature change, joint or bone and muscle pain, abdominal cramps, skin crawling, etc.

Interpretation of the Challenge: Warning: the elicitation of the enumerated signs or symptoms indicates a potential risk for the subject, and naltrexone HCl should not be administered. If no signs or symptoms of withdrawal are observed, elicited or reported, NALTREXONE HCL MAY BE ADMINISTERED. If there is any doubt in the observer's mind that the patient is not in an opioid-free state, or is in continuing withdrawal, naltrexone HCl should be withheld for 24 hours and the challenge repeated.

Alternative Dosing Schedules: Once the patient has been started on naltrexone HCl, 50 mg every 24 hours will produce adequate clinical blockade of the actions of parenterally administered opioids (*i.e.,* this dose will block the effects of a 25 mg intravenous heroin challenge). A flexible approach to a dosing regimen may need to be employed in cases of supervised administration. Thus, patients may receive 50 mg of naltrexone HCl every weekday with a 100 mg dose on Saturday, 100 mg every other day, or 150 mg every third day. The degree of blockade produced by naltrexone HCl may be reduced by these extended dosing intervals.

There may be a higher risk of hepatocellular injury with single doses above 50 mg, and use of higher doses and extended dosing intervals should balance the possible risks against the probable benefits (see WARNINGS, and CLINICAL PHARMACOLOGY, Individualization of Dosage).

Patient Compliance: Naltrexone HCl should be considered as only one of many factors determining the success of treatment. To achieve the best possible treatment outcome, appropriate compliance-enhancing techniques should be implemented for all components of the treatment program, including medication compliance.

HOW SUPPLIED:

Naltrexone HCl tablets are available in 50 mg round tablets, scored imprinted with DuPont on one side and NTR on the other. Bottles of 50 tablets.

Protect from light.

(DuPont Merck Pharmaceutical Co., 1/95, 6389-1/Rev.)

HOW SUPPLIED - EQUIVALENTS NOT AVAILABLE:

Tablet, Uncoated - Oral - 50 mg

50's	$227.58	REVIA, Dupont Pharma	00056-0079-50

NANDROLONE DECANOATE *(001858)*

CATEGORIES: Anabolic Steroids; Androgens; Anemia; Blood Formation/Coagulation; Deficiency Anemias; Hormones; Renal Insufficiency; Pregnancy Category X; DEA Class CIII; FDA Approved 1983 Sep

BRAND NAMES: Anabolin La-100; Androlone D; **Deca-Durabolin**; Depo-Nandrolone; Dequibolin-100; Hybolin Decanoate; Kabolin; Nandrobolic L.A.; Nandrolate; Neo-Durabolic; Pri-Andriol La

DESCRIPTION:

Nandrolone decanoate is a sterile solution of nandrolone decanoate, a long acting anabolic agent in sesame oil for intramuscular injection. Each ml contains: 50 mg, 100 mg, or 200 mg nandrolone decanoate in sterile sesame oil. Preservative: 10% benzyl alcohol (50 mg and 100 mg); or 5% (200mg). Chemically it is ESTR-4-en-3-one, 17-((1-oxodecyl) oxy)-,(17β) - 17β - Hydroxyestr-4-en-3-decanoate

CLINICAL PHARMACOLOGY:

Anabolic steroids are synthetic derivatives of testosterone. Certain clinical effects and adverse reactions demonstrate the androgenic properties of this class of drugs. Complete dissociation of anabolic and androgenic effects has not yet been achieved. The actions of anabolic steroids are therefore similar to those of male sex hormones with the possibility of causing serious disturbances of growth and sexual development if given to young children. Anabolic steroids suppress the gonadotropic functions of the pituitary and may exert a direct effect upon the testes.

During exogenous administration of anabolic androgens, endogenous testosterone release is inhibited through inhibition of pituitary luteinizing hormone (LH). At large doses, spermatogenesis may be suppressed through feedback inhibition of pituitary follicle-stimulating hormone (FSH).

Anabolic steroids increase low-density lipoproteins and decrease high-density lipoproteins. These changes revert to normal on discontinuation of treatment.

INDICATIONS AND USAGE:

Nandrolone Decanoate is indicated for the management of the anemia of renal insufficiency and has been shown to increase hemoglobin and red cell mass. Surgically induced anephric patients have been reported to be less responsive.

CONTRAINDICATIONS:

1. Known or suspected carcinoma of the prostate or the male breast.

2. Carcinoma of the breast in females with hypercalcemia (androgenic anabolic steroids may stimulate osteolytic bone resorption).

3. Pregnancy, because of possible masculinization of the female fetus. Androgenic anabolic steroids are known to cause embryotoxicity, fetotoxicity, and masculinization of female animal offspring. Nandrolone Decanoate is contraindicated in women who are or may become pregnant. If this drug is used during pregnancy, or if the patient becomes pregnant while taking this drug, she should be apprised of the potential hazard to the fetus.

4. Nephrosis or nephrotic phase of nephritis.

WARNINGS:

PELIOSIS HEPATIS, A CONDITION IN WHICH LIVER AND SOMETIMES SPLENIC TISSUE IS REPLACED WITH BLOOD-FILLED CYSTS, HAS BEEN REPORTED IN PATIENTS RECEIVING ANDROGENIC ANABOLIC STEROID THERAPY. THESE CYSTS ARE SOMETIMES PRESENT WITH MINIMAL HEPATIC DYSFUNCTION, BUT AT OTHER TIMES THEY HAVE BEEN ASSOCIATED WITH LIVER FAILURE. THEY ARE OFTEN NOT RECOGNIZED UNTIL LIFE-THREATENING LIVER FAILURE OR INTRA-ABDOMINAL HEMORRHAGE DEVELOPS. WITHDRAWAL OF DRUG USUALLY RESULTS IN COMPLETE DISAPPEARANCE OF LESIONS. LIVER CELL TUMORS ARE ALSO REPORTED. MOST OFTEN THESE TUMORS ARE BENIGN AND ANDROGEN-DEPENDENT, BUT FATAL MALIGNANT TUMORS HAVE BEEN REPORTED. WITHDRAWAL OF DRUG OFTEN RESULTS IN REGRESSION OR CESSATION OF PROGRESSION OF THE TUMOR. HOWEVER, HEPATIC TUMORS ASSOCIATED WITH ANDROGENS OR ANABOLIC STEROIDS ARE MUCH MORE VASCULAR THAN OTHER HEPATIC TUMORS AND MAY BE SILENT UNTIL LIFE- THREATENING INTRA-ABDOMINAL HEMORRHAGE DEVELOPS. BLOOD LIPID CHANGES THAT ARE KNOWN TO BE ASSOCIATED WITH INCREASED RISK OF ATHEROSCLEROSIS ARE SEEN IN PATIENTS TREATED WITH ANDROGENS AND ANABOLIC STEROIDS. THESE CHANGES INCLUDE DECREASED HIGH-DENSITY LIPOPROTEIN AND SOMETIMES INCREASED LOW-DENSITY LIPOPROTEIN. THE CHANGES MAY BE VERY MARKED AND COULD HAVE A SERIOUS IMPACT ON THE RISK OF ATHEROSCLEROSIS AND CORONARY ARTERY DISEASE.

Cholestatic hepatitis and jaundice occur with 17-alpha-alkylated androgens at a relatively low dose. If cholestatic hepatitis with jaundice appears or if liver function tests become abnormal, Nandrolone decanoate should be discontinued, and the etiology should be determined. Drug-induced jaundice is reversible when the medication is discontinued.

In patients with breast cancer, anabolic steroid therapy may cause hypercalcemia by stimulating osteolysis. Nandrolone decanoate therapy should be discontinued is hypercalcemia occurs.

Edema with or without congestive heart failure may be a serious complication in patients with preexisting cardiac, renal, or hepatic disease. Concomitant administration of adrenal cortical steroid or ACTH may add to the edema.

In children, androgen therapy may accelerate bone maturation without producing compensatory gain in linear growth. This adverse effect results in compromised adult stature. The younger the child, the greater the risk of compromising final mature height. The effect on bone maturation should be monitored by assessing bone age of the wrist and hand every six months.

Geriatric patients treated with androgenic anabolic steroids may be at an increased risk for the development of prostatic hypertrophy and prostatic carcinoma.

THERE IS NO PERSUASIVE EVIDENCE THAT ATHLETIC PERFORMANCE IS IMPROVED BY USING ANABOLIC STEROIDS.

PRECAUTIONS:

GENERAL

Women should be observed for signs of virilization (deepening of the voice, hirsutism, acne, clitoromegaly). Such virilization is usual following anabolic steroid use in high doses. Discontinuation of drug therapy at time of evidence of mild virilism is necessary to prevent irreversible virilization. Some virilizing changes (facial hair growth, clitoromegaly, deepening of the voice) in women are irreversible even after prompt discontinuance of therapy and are not prevented by the concomitant use of estrogens. Menstrual irregularities may also occur.

Anabolic steroids may cause supression of clotting factors II, V, VII, and X, and an increase in prothrombin time.

Insulin or oral hypoglycemic dosage may need adjustment in diabetic patients who receive anabolic steroids.

INFORMATION FOR THE PATIENT

The physician should instruct patients to report any of the following side effects of androgens:

Adult or Adolescent Males: Too frequent or persistent erections of the penis, appearance of or aggravation of acne.

Females: Hoarseness, acne, changes in menstrual periods, or more hair on the face.

All Patients: Nausea, vomiting, changes in skin color, or ankle swelling.

LABORATORY TESTS

Women with disseminated breast carcinoma should have frequent determination of urine and serum calcium levels during the course of therapy. (See WARNINGS.)

Because of the hepatotoxicity associated with the use of 17-alpha-alkylated androgens, liver function tests should be obtained periodically.

Periodic (every six months) x-ray examinations of bone age should be made during treatment of prepubertal males and females to determine the rate of bone maturation and the effects of androgen therapy on the epiphyseal centers.

Serum lipids and high-density lipoprotein cholesterol determinations should be done periodically as anabolic androgenic steroids have been reported to increase low-density lipoproteins and decrease high-density lipoproteins. Serum cholesterol levels may increase during therapy. Therefore, caution is required when administering these agents to patients with a history of myocardial infarction or coronary artery disease. Serial determinations of serum cholesterol should be made and therapy adjusted accordingly.

Hemoglobin and hematocrit should be checked periodically for polycythemia in patients who are receiving high doses of anabolic steroids.

DRUG/LABORATORY TEST INTERACTIONS

Anabolic steroids may decrease levels of thyroxine-binding globulin, resulting in decreased total T4 serum levels and increased resin uptake of T3 and T4. Free thyroid hormone levels remain unchanged.

Anabolic steroids may cause an increase in prothrombin time.

CARCINOGENESIS, MUTAGENESIS, AND IMPAIRMENT OF FERTILITY

Animal Data: Nandrolone decanoate has not been tested in laboratory animals for carcinogenic or mutagenic effects, or impairment of fertility.

Human Data: Liver cell tumors have been reported in patients receiving long-term therapy with anabolic androgenic steroids in high doses. (See WARNINGS.) Withdrawal of the drugs did not lead to regression of the tumors in all cases.

Geriatric patients treated with anabolic androgenic steroids may be at an increased risk for the development of prostatic hypertrophy and prostate carcinoma.

PREGNANCY, TERATOGENIC EFFECTS, PREGNANCY CATEGORY X

See CONTRAINDICATIONS.

NURSING MOTHERS

It is not known whether anabolic steroids are excreted in human milk. Because of the potential for serious adverse reactions in nursing infants from nandrolone decanoate, a decision should be made whether to discontinue nursing or to discontinue the drug, taking into account the importance of the drug to the mother.

PEDIATRIC USE

Anabolic agents may accelerate epiphyseal maturation more rapidly than linear growth in children, and the effect may continue for six months after the drug has been stopped. Therefore, therapy should be monitored by x-ray studies at six-month intervals in order to avoid the risk of compromising adult height. Anabolic androgenic steroid therapy should be used very cautiously in children and only by specialists who are aware of the effects on bone maturation.

DRUG INTERACTIONS:

Anticoagulants: Anabolic steroids may increase sensitivity to oral anticoagulants. Dosage of the anticoagulant may have to be decreased in order to maintain prothrombin time at the desired therapeutic level. Patients receiving oral anticoagulant therapy require close monitoring, especially when anabolic steroids are started or stopped.

Oral Hypoglycemic Agents: Nandrolone decanoate may inhibit the metabolism of oral hypoglycemic agents.

ADVERSE REACTIONS:

Hepatic: Cholestatic jaundice with, rarely, hepatic necrosis and death. Hepatocellular neoplasms and peliosis hepatis have been reported in association with long-term androgenic anabolic steroid therapy. (See WARNINGS.) Reversible changes in liver function tests also occur, including increased bromsulphalein (BSP) retention, and increases in serum bilirubin, glutamic oxaloacetic transaminase (SGOT), and alkaline phosphatase.

GENITOURINARY SYSTEM: *In Men: Prepubertal:* Phallic enlargement and increased frequency of erections. *Postpubertal:* Inhibition of testicular function, testicular atrophy and oligospermia, impotence, chronic priapism, epididymitis, and bladder irritability. *In Women:* Clitoral enlargement, menstrual irregularities. *In Both Sexes:* Increased or decreased libido.

Central Nervous System: Habituation, excitation, insomnia, depression.

Gastrointestinal: Nausea, vomiting, diarrhea.

Hematologic: Bleeding in patients on concomitant anticoagulant therapy (see DRUG INTERACTIONS).

Breast: Gynecomastia.

Larynx: Deepening of the voice in women.

Hair: Hirsutism and male pattern baldness in women.

Skin: Acne (especially in women and prepubertal boys).

Skeletal: Premature closure of epiphyses in children (see PRECAUTIONS, Pediatric Use).

Fluid and Electrolytes: Edema, retention of serum electrolytes (Sodium, chloride, potassium, phosphate, calcium).

ADVERSE REACTIONS: *(cont'd)*

Metabolic/Endocrine: Decreased glucose tolerance (see PRECAUTIONSand DRUG INTERACTIONS) increased serum levels of low-density lipoproteins and decreased level of high, density lipoproteins, (seePRECAUTIONS, Laboratory Tests) increased creatinine excretion, increased serum levels of creatinine phosphokinase (CPK).

OVERDOSAGE:

There have been no reports of acute overdosage with the anabolics.

DOSAGE AND ADMINISTRATION:

Nandrolone decanoate is intended only for deep intramuscular injection preferably into the gluteal muscle. Dosage should be based on therapeutic response and consideration of the benefit/risk ratio. Duration of therapy will depend on the response of the condition and the appearance of adverse reactions. If possible, therapy should be intermittent.

Nandrolone decanoate should be regarded as adjunctive therapy and adequate quantities of nutrients should be consumed in order to obtain maximal therapeutic effects. When it is used in the treatment of refractory anemias, for example, adequate iron intake is required for a maximal response.

Anemia or Renal Disease: A dose of 50-100 mg per week is recommended for women and 100-200 mg per week for men. Drug therapy should be discontinued if no hematologic improvement is seen within the first six months. When used in the treatment of renal insufficiency, adequate iron intake is required for maximal response. For children from 2 to 13 years of age, the average dose is 25-50 mg every 3 to 4 weeks.

Parenteral drug products should be inspected visually for particulate matter and discoloration prior to administration, whenever solution and container permit.

Store at 15-30°C (59-86°F). Protect from bright light.

HOW SUPPLIED - RATED THERAPEUTICALLY EQUIVALENT:

Injection, Solution - Intramuscular - 50 mg/ml

1 ml x 25	**$131.65**	**DECA-DURABOLIN, Organon**	**00052-0696-71**
2 ml	$5.50	Nandrolone Decanoate, Harber Pharm	51432-0769-02
2 ml	$7.43	Nandrolone Decanoate, Steris Labs	00402-0407-02
2 ml	$9.90	HYBOLIN DECANOATE, Hyrex Pharms	00314-3520-02
2 ml	**$12.30**	**DECA-DURABOLIN, Organon**	**00052-0696-02**
2 ml	$14.05	Nandrolone Decanoate, Goldline Labs	00182-1142-61
2 ml x 10	$109.20	Nandrolone Decanoate, Schein Pharm (US)	00364-6716-47

Injection, Solution - Intramuscular - 100 mg/ml

2 ml	$6.50	Nandrolone Decanoate, Harber Pharm	51432-0771-02
2 ml	$7.43	Nandrolone Decanoate, Steris Labs	00402-0432-02
2 ml	$7.50	Nandrolone Decanoate, Major Pharms	00904-1196-98
2 ml	$11.85	Nandrolone Decanoate, IDE-Interstate	00814-5122-35
2 ml	$12.90	HYBOLIN DECANOATE, Hyrex Pharms	00314-3525-02
2 ml	$14.50	Nandrolone Decanoate, Goldline Labs	00182-1143-61
2 ml	**$21.05**	**DECA-DURABOLIN, Organon**	**00052-0697-02**
2 ml	$208.44	Nandrolone Decanoate, Fujisawa USA	00469-7100-10
2 ml x 10	$113.10	Nandrolone Decanoate, Schein Pharm (US)	00364-6717-47
2 ml x 25	$45.95	Nandrolone Decanoate, Americal Pharm	54945-0525-32
2 ml x 25	**$363.25**	**DECA-DURABOLIN, Organon**	**00052-0697-25**

Injection, Solution - Intramuscular - 200 mg/ml

1 ml	$6.29	Nandrolone Decanoate, Steris Labs	00402-0710-01
1 ml	$6.50	Nandrolone Decanoate, Harber Pharm	51432-0773-01
1 ml	**$20.17**	**DECA-DURABOLIN, Organon**	**00052-0698-01**
1 ml	$208.44	Nandrolone Decanoate, Fujisawa USA	00469-7200-00
1 ml x 25	$241.33	Nandrolone Decanoate, Schein Pharm (US)	00364-2186-46
1 ml x 25	**$382.58**	**DECA-DURABOLIN, Organon**	**00052-0698-25**
1 ml x 25	**$400.75**	**DECA-DURABOLIN, Organon**	**00052-0698-71**

HOW SUPPLIED - NOT RATED EQUIVALENT:

Injection, Solution - Intramuscular - 25 mg/ml

5 ml	$5.00	Nandrolone Phenpropionate, Major Pharms	00904-1207-05

NANDROLONE PHENPROPIONATE *(001859)*

CATEGORIES: Anabolic Steroids; Androgens; Breast Carcinoma; Cancer; Hormones; Pregnancy Category X; DEA Class CIII; FDA Approval Pre 1982

BRAND NAMES: Anabolin; Androlone; *Anadur* (Germany); **Durabolin**; Equibolin-50; *Evabolin*; *Grothic*; Hybolin-Improved; *Metabol*; Nandrobolic; Nandrocot; *Neurabol*; *Noralone*; *Orgabolin*; Protabolin
(International brand names outside U.S. in italics)

DESCRIPTION:

Nandrolone Phenopropionate injection is a sterile solution of nandrolone phenpropionate, a short acting anabolic agent in sesame oil for intramuscular injection. Each ml contains: 25 mg or 50 mg nandrolone phenpropionate in sterile sesame oil. Preservative: 5% benzyl alcohol (25 mg); or 10% (50 mg). Chemically it is Estr-4-en-3-one, 17-(1-oxo-3-phenylpropoxy)-, (17 beta)-

CLINICAL PHARMACOLOGY:

Anabolic steroids are synthetic derivatives of testosterone. Androgens have been reported to increase protein anabolism and decrease protein catabolism. Nitrogen balance is improved with anabolic agents but only when there is sufficient intake of calories and protein. Whether this positive nitrogen balance is of primary benefit in the utilization of protein building dietary substances has not been established.

Certain clinical effects and adverse reactions demonstrate the androgenic properties of this class of drugs. The deletion of the CH3 group from the C-19-position has resulted in reduction of its androgenic properties and retention and enhancement of its anabolic properties.

Thus it is possible to employ doses that provide significant anabolic effects without undesired androgenic effects. Complete dissociation of anabolic and androgenic effects has not been achieved. The actions of anabolic steroids are therefore similar to those of male sex hormones with the possibility of causing serious disturbances of growth and sexual development if given to young children. Anabolic steroids suppress the gonadotropic functions of the pituitary and may exert a direct effect upon the testis.

INDICATIONS AND USAGE:

Effective: For the control of metastatic breast cancer.

CONTRAINDICATIONS:

1. Male patients with carcinoma of the breast or with known or suspected carcinoma of the prostate.

CONTRAINDICATIONS: *(cont'd)*

2. Carcinoma of the breast in some females.
3. Pregnancy because of masculinization of the fetus.
4. Nephrosis or the nephrotic phase of nephritis.

WARNINGS:

1. Anabolic steroids do not enhance athletic ability.
2. Hypercalcemia may develop both spontaneously and as a result of hormonal therapy in women with disseminated breast carcinoma. If it develops while on this agent, the drug should be discontinued.
3. Caution is required in administering these agents to patients with cardiac, renal or hepatic disease. Edema may occur occasionally with or without congestive heart failure. Concomitant administration with adrenal steroids or ACTH may add to the edema.
4. There have been rare reports of hepatocellular neoplasms and peliosis hepatitis in association with long-term androgenic-anabolic steroid therapy. (See PRECAUTIONS, Carcinogenesis, Mutagenesis, and Impairment of Fertility.)
5. Anabolic steroids should be used with caution in patients with benign prostatic hypertrophy.
6. In children, anabolic treatment may accelerate bone maturation without producing compensatory gain in linear growth. This adverse effect may result in compromised adult stature. The younger the child the greater the risk of compromising final mature height. The effect on maturation should be monitored by assessing bone age of the wrist and hand every six months.

PRECAUTIONS:

GENERAL

Women should be observed for signs of virilization (deepening of the voice, hirsutism, acne, clitoromegaly and menstrual irregularities.) Discontinuation of drug therapy at the time of evidence of mild virilism is necessary to prevent irreversible virilization. Such virilization is usual following anabolic use in high doses.

INFORMATION FOR THE PATIENT

The physician should instruct patients to report any of the following side effects of androgenic anabolic steroids:

Women: Hoarseness, acne, changes in menstrual periods, more hair on the face, nausea, vomiting, changes in the skin color or ankle swelling.

LABORATORY TESTS

1. Women with disseminated breast carcinoma should have frequent determination of urine and serum calcium levels during the course of anabolic therapy.
2. Periodic (every 6 months) x-ray examinations of bone age should be made during treatment of children to determine the rate of bone maturation and the effects of anabolic therapy on the epiphyseal centers.
3. Hemoglobin and hematocrit should be checked periodically for polycythemia in patients who are receiving high doses of anabolics.
4. Because of the hepatotoxicity associated with the use of 17-alpha-alkylated anabolic steroids, liver function tests should be obtained periodically.

DRUG/LABORATORY TEST INTERACTIONS

1. Anabolics may decrease levels of the PBI in thyroxine binding capacity and radioactive iodine uptake.
2. Anabolics may cause alterations in the glucose tolerance test and metyrapone test.

CARCINOGENESIS, MUTAGENESIS, IMPAIRMENT OF FERTILITY

Human Data. Long term studies in animals have not been performed to evaluate carcinogenic potential of nandrolone phenpropionate. There are rare reports of hepatocellular carcinoma in patients receiving long-term therapy with anabolics in high doses. Withdrawal of the drugs did not lead to repression of the tumors in all cases. Geriatric patients treated with anabolics may be at an increased risk for the development of prostatic hypertrophy and prostatic carcinoma.

PREGNANCY

Teratogenic Effects. Pregnancy Category X.

(See CONTRAINDICATIONS.)

NURSING MOTHERS

It is not known whether anabolics are excreted in human milk. Because many drugs are excreted in human milk and because of the potential for serious adverse reactions in nursing infants from anabolics, a decision should be made whether to discontinue nursing or to discontinue the drug, taking into account the importance of the drug to the mother.

PEDIATRIC USE

Safety and effectiveness of Nandrolone Phenopropionate in children have not been established.

DRUG INTERACTIONS:

1. Anticoagulants. Anabolic steroids may increase sensitivity to oral anticoagulants. Dosage of the anticoagulant may have to be decreased in order to maintain the prothrombin time at the desired therapeutic level. Patients receiving oral anticoagulant therapy require close monitoring, especially when anabolics are started or stopped.
2. Oxyphenbutazone. Concurrent administration of oxyphenbutazone and androgens may result in elevated serum levels of oxyphenbutazone.
3. Insulin. In diabetic patients the metabolic effects of anabolics may decrease blood glucose and insulin requirements.

ADVERSE REACTIONS:

The following adverse reactions are listed in order of decreasing severity:

1. In Males

a) Prepubertal

1. Phallic enlargement

2. Increased frequency of erections

b) Post-pubertal

1. Inhibition of testicular function and oligospermia

2. Gynecomastia

2. In Females

a) Hirsutism, male pattern baldness, deepening of the voice and clitoral enlargement. These changes are usually irreversible even after prompt discontinuance of therapy and are not prevented by concomitant usage of estrogens,

b) Menstrual irregularities.

3.In Both Sexes

ADVERSE REACTIONS: *(cont'd)*

a) Bleeding of patients on concomitant anticoagulant therapy

b) Premature closure of epiphyses in children

c) Inhibition of gonadotropin secretion

d) Increased or decreased libido

e) Acne (especially in females and prepubertal males)

f) Nausea

g) The electrolytes: retention of sodium, chlorides, water, potassium phosphates and calcium.

h) Increased serum cholesterol

i) Suppression of clotting factors II, V, VII, X

4. There have been rare reports of hepatocellular neoplasm and peliosi hepatitis in association with long-term androgenic-anabolic steroid therapy (See WARNINGS.)

OVERDOSAGE:

There have been no reports of acute overdosage with the anabolics.

DOSAGE AND ADMINISTRATION:

The recommended dosage of Nandrolone Phenpropionate Injection USP in metastatic breast cancer is 50-100 mg/weekly based on therapeutic response, and consideration of the benefit to risk ratio. Duration of therapy will depend on the response of the condition and appearance of adverse reactions. If possible, therapy should be intermittent. Nandrolone is intended only for deep intramuscular injection, into the gluteal muscle preferably.

Store at 15-30°C (59-86°F). Protect from bright light.

HOW SUPPLIED - RATED THERAPEUTICALLY EQUIVALENT:

Injection, Solution - Intramuscular - 25 mg/ml

2 ml	$8.50	HYBOLIN IMPROVED, Hyrex Pharms	00314-3501-02
5 ml	$5.00	Nandrolone Phenpropionate, Fujisawa USA	00469-0603-20
5 ml	$5.95	Nandrolone Phenpropionate, Harber Pharm	51432-0762-05
5 ml	**$16.26**	**DURABOLIN, Organon**	**00052-0691-05**

Injection, Solution - Intramuscular - 50 mg/ml

2 ml	$4.75	Nandrolone Phenpropionate, Harber Pharm	51432-0763-02
2 ml	$4.90	Nandrolone Phenpropionate, Major Pharms	00904-1206-98
2 ml	**$14.79**	**DURABOLIN, Organon**	**00052-0695-02**

NAPHAZOLINE HYDROCHLORIDE *(001860)*

CATEGORIES: Allergies; Antihypertensives; EENT Drugs; Eye, Ear, Nose, & Throat Preparations; Nasal Congestion; Ophthalmic Decongestants; Ophthalmics; Respiratory & Allergy Medications; Topical; Vasoconstrictors; FDA Approval Pre 1982

BRAND NAMES: Ak-Con; Albalon; *Albalon Liquifilm* (Australia); *Albasol*; Allersol; *Clear*; *Clear Eyes* (Australia); *Degest*; I-Naphline; *Imizol*; *Murine*; Muro's Opcon; Nafazair; *Naftazolina*; *Naphacel*; *Naphacel Ofteno* (Mexico); Naphazole; *Naphazolin* (Germany); *Naphcon*; *Naphcon-F*; **Naphcon Forte**; *Nazil*; *Nazil Ofteno* (Mexico); Ocu-Zoline; Opcon; Spectro-Con; Vasocon; *Vistalbalon* (Germany)
(International brand names outside U.S. in italics)

FORMULARIES: Aetna; BC-BS; FHP; Medi-Cal

DESCRIPTION:

Naphazoline HCl is a topical ocular vasoconstrictor prepared as a sterile ophthalmic solution.

ESTABLISHED NAME:

Naphazoline Hydrochloride

CHEMICAL NAME:

1 *H*-Imidazole, 4,5-dihydro-2-(1-naphthalenylmethyl)-,monohydrochloride.

Each ml contains: Active: Naphazoline Hydrochloride 0.1%.

Preservative: Benzalkonium Chloride 0.01%.

Inactive: Boric Acid, Sodium Chloride, Potassium Chloride, Edetate Disodium, Sodium Carbonate and/or Hydrochloric Acid (to adjust pH), Purified Water.

CLINICAL PHARMACOLOGY:

Vasoconstriction through a local adrenergic mechanism on conjunctival blood vessels.

INDICATIONS AND USAGE:

For use as a topical ocular vasoconstrictor.

CONTRAINDICATIONS:

Contraindicated in those persons who have shown hypersensitivity to any component of this preparation.

WARNINGS:

Do not use in presence of narrow angle glaucoma. Patients under therapy with MAO inhibitors may experience a severe hypertensive crisis if given a sympathomimetic drug. Use in infants and children may result in CNS depression leading to coma and marked reduction in body temperature.

PRECAUTIONS:

For topical ophthalmic use only. Use with caution in the presence of hypertension, cardiovascular abnormalities, hyperglycemia, hyperthyroidism, and other medications.

ADVERSE REACTIONS:

Sensitivity reactions may occur.

DOSAGE AND ADMINISTRATION:

Instill one or two drops in the conjunctival sac(s) every three to four hours as needed.

HOW SUPPLIED - RATED THERAPEUTICALLY EQUIVALENT:

Solution - Ophthalmic - 0.1 %

15 ml	$4.72	Naphazoline HCl, H.C.F.A. F F P	99999-1860-01
15 ml	$5.19	Naphazoline HCl, Aligen Independ	00405-6081-15
15 ml	$5.30	Allersol, Ocusoft	54799-0860-15
15 ml	$5.49	Naphazoline, Qualitest Pharms	00603-7178-41
15 ml	$5.95	SPECTRO-CON, Spectrum Scitfc	53268-0344-12
15 ml	$5.99	Naphazoline Hcl, Parmed Pharms	00349-8641-85
15 ml	$6.06	Naphazoline Hcl, HL Moore Drug Exch	00839-6692-31

HOW SUPPLIED - RATED THERAPEUTICALLY EQUIVALENT: *(cont'd)*

15 ml	$6.40	Naphazole, Major Pharms	00904-1906-35
15 ml	$6.45	AK-CON, Akorn	17478-0216-12
15 ml	$6.90	Naphazoline HCl Ophthalmic, Schein Pharm (US)	00364-7421-72
15 ml	$7.05	Naphazoline HCl, Goldline Labs	00182-7032-64
15 ml	$7.15	Naphazoline HCl, Rugby	00536-1702-72
15 ml	$13.16	ALBALON, Allergan-Amer	11980-0154-15
15 ml	$13.80	VASOCON REGULAR, Ciba Vision	00058-2884-15
15 ml	**$14.69**	**NAPHCON FORTE, Alcon-PR**	**00998-0079-15**

HOW SUPPLIED - NOT RATED EQUIVALENT:

Solution - Ophthalmic - 0.1 %

15 ml	$1.50	Nafazair, Raway	00686-0725-06
15 ml	$2.25	Naphazoline Hcl, Logen Pharm	00820-0112-25

NAPHAZOLINE HYDROCHLORIDE; PHENIRAMINE MALEATE *(001861)*

CATEGORIES: Allergies; Antihistamines; DESI Drugs; EENT Drugs; Eye, Ear, Nose, & Throat Preparations; Ocular Infections; Ophthalmic Decongestants; Ophthalmics; Vasoconstrictors; FDA Pre 1938 Drugs

BRAND NAMES: Ak-Con-A; Allersol-A; Muro's Opcon-A; Nafazair A; Naphaz-A; Naphazole-A; Naphazoline-A; *Naphcon A*; **Naphcon-A**; Opcon-A; Spectro-Con-A
(International brand names outside U.S. in italics)

FORMULARIES: Aetna

DESCRIPTION:

Naphazoline Hydrochloride, Pheniramine Maleate is a combination of an antihistamine and a decongestant prepared as a sterile topical ophthalmic solution.

Established name: Naphazoline Hydrochloride

Chemical name: 1 *H*-Imidazole, 4,5-dihydro-2-(1-naphthalenylmethyl)-,monohydrochloride.

Established name: Pheniramine Maleate

Chemical name: *N,N*-Dimethyl-γ-phenyl-2-pyridine-propanamine, (*Z*)-Butenedioic acid.

Each Naphcon-A ml contains: Active: Naphazoline Hydrochloride 0.025%, Pheniramine Maleate 0.3%. Preservative: Benzalkonium Chloride 0.01%. *Inactive:* Boric Acid, Sodium Borate, Edetate Disodium, Sodium Chloride, Sodium Hydroxide and/or Hydrochloric Acid (to adjust pH), and Purified Water.

CLINICAL PHARMACOLOGY:

Naphazoline Hydrochloride, Pheniramine Maleate combines the effects of the antihistamine, pheniramine maleate, and the decongestant, naphazoline.

INDICATIONS AND USAGE:

Based on a review of a related combination of drugs by the National Academy of Sciences — National Research Council and/or other information, FDA has classified the indications as follows: "Possibly" effective: For relief of ocular irritation and/or congestion or for the treatment of allergic or inflammatory ocular conditions. Final classification of the less-than-effective indication requires further investigation.

CONTRAINDICATIONS:

Hypersensitivity to one or more of the components of this preparation.

WARNINGS:

Do not use in the presence of narrow angle glaucoma or in patients predisposed to narrow angle glaucoma. Patients under MAO inhibitors may experience a severe hypertensive crisis if given a sympathomimetic drug such as Naphazoline HCl. Use in infants and children may result in CNS depression leading to coma and marked reduction in body temperature.

PRECAUTIONS:

For topical use only — not for injection. This preparation should be used with caution in elderly patients with severe cardiovascular disease including cardiac arrhythmias; patients with poorly controlled hypertension; patients with diabetes, especially those with a tendency toward diabetic ketoacidosis. To prevent contaminating the dropper tip and solution, care should be taken not to touch the eyelids or surrounding area with the dropper tip of the bottle.

ADVERSE REACTIONS:

The following adverse reactions may occur. Pupillary dilation, increase in intraocular pressure, systemic effects due to absorption (*i.e.,* hypertension, cardiac irregularities, hyperglycemia).

DOSAGE AND ADMINISTRATION:

One or two drops instilled in each eye every 3 or 4 hours or less frequently, as required to relieve symptoms.

Storage: Store at 36 to 80°F. Keep bottle tightly closed when not in use. Protect from light and excessive heat.

HOW SUPPLIED - EQUIVALENTS NOT AVAILABLE:

Solution - Ophthalmic - 0.025 %/0.3 %

15 ml	$3.11	NAPHOPTIC-A SOLUTION, Optopics	52238-0637-15
15 ml	$4.48	Naphazoline Hcl W/Pheniramine, Aligen Independ	00405-6080-15
15 ml	$4.55	Naphazoline/Pheniramine Maleate, Martec Pharms	52555-0175-01
15 ml	$6.88	AK-CON-A, Akorn	17478-0215-12
15 ml	$7.05	Allersol-A Ophthalmic Solution, Ocusoft	54799-0863-15

NAPROXEN *(001864)*

CATEGORIES: Analgesics; Ankylosing Spondylitis; Anti-Inflammatory Agents; Antiarthritics; Antipyretics; Arthritis; Bursitis; Central Nervous System Agents; Dysmenorrhea; Gout; NSAIDS; Nonsteroidal Anti-Inflammatory; Osteoarthritis; Pain; Spondylitis; Migraine*; Pregnancy Category B; Sales > $1 Billion; FDA Approval Pre 1982; Patent Expiration 1993 Dec; Top 200 Drugs
* Indication not approved by the FDA

BRAND NAMES: *Acusprain*; *Anaprox*; *Anax*; *Anexopen*; *Antalgin*; *Apo-Napro-NA* (Canada); *Apo-Naproxen* (Canada); *Apranax* (France, Germany); *Apronax*; *Artagen*; *Arthrisil*; *Artrixen*; *Artroxen*; *Atiflan* (Mexico); *Bipronyl*; *Bonyl*; *Clinosyn*; *Congex*; *Dafloxen* (Mexico); *Danaprox*; *Daprox*; *Diocodal*; *Duk*; *Dysmenalgit* (Germany); EC-Naprosyn; Ec-Naprosyn; *Femex*; *Flanax* (Mexico); *Flanax Forte*; *Flexen*; *Flexin*; *Flexipen*; *Floginax*; *Fuxen* (Mexico); *Genoxen*; *Gibixen*; *Headlon* (Japan); *Inza*; *Laraflex* (England); *Laser*; *Lefaine*; *Leniartil*; *Nafasol*; *Naixan* (Japan); *Nalyxan*; *Napflam*; *Napmel*; *Naposin*; *Napoton*; *Napren*; *Naprium*; *Naprius*; *Naprogesic* (Australia); *Naprontag*; *Naprorex*; **Naprosyn**; *Naprosyn LLE*; *Naprosyn LLE Forte*; *Naprosyne* (France); *Naproxi 250*; *Naproxi 500*; *Naprux*; *Napxen*; *Narma* (Japan); *Narocin*; *Naxen* (Canada, Mexico); *Naxen F*; *Naxid*; *Naxopren*; *Naxyn 250*; *Naxyn 500*; *Noflam*; *Norswel*; *Novonaprox* (Canada); *Nycopren*; *Patxen* (Mexico); *Prafena*; *Prexan*; *Priaxen*; *Primeral*; *Prodexin*; *Pronaxen*; *Proxen* (Germany); *Proxen LE*; *Proxen LLE*; *Rahsen* (Japan); *Rheumaflex*; *Roxen*; *Saritilron* (Japan); *Sinartrin*; *Sinton*; *Soproxen*; *Sutolin*; *Sutony*; *Synflex* (Australia, England); *Tohexen* (Japan); *Traumox*; *U-Ritis*; *Velsay* (Mexico); *Veradol*; *Vinsen*; *Xenar*; *Xenobid*
(International brand names outside U.S. in italics)

FORMULARIES: Aetna; BC-BS; Foundation; Medi-Cal; PCS

COST OF THERAPY: $80.51 (Arthritis; Tablet; 250 mg; 2/day; 365 days)

PRIMARY ICD9: 715.99 (Osteoarthritis, Unspecified, Multiple Sites)

DESCRIPTION:

Naproxen tablets for oral administration each contain 250 mg, 375 mg or 500 mg of naproxen. Naproxen suspension for oral administration contains 125 mg/5 ml of naproxen. Naproxen is a member of the arylacetic acid group of nonsteroidal anti-inflammatory drugs.

The chemical name for naproxen is 2-naphthaleneacetic acid, 5 methoxy- α-methyl-,(+).

Naproxen is an odorless, white to off-white crystalline substance. It is lipid soluble, practically insoluble in water at low pH and freely soluble in water at high pH.

Naproxen suspension for oral administration contains 125 mg/5 ml of naproxen, the active ingredient, in a vehicle of FD&C Yellow #6, fumaric acid, imitation orange flavor, imitation pineapple flavor, magnesium aluminum silicate, methyl paraben, purified water, sodium chloride, sorbitol solution and sucrose.

CLINICAL PHARMACOLOGY:

Naproxen is a nonsteroidal anti-inflammatory drug with analgesic and antipyretic properties. Naproxen sodium, the sodium slat of naproxen, has been developed as an analgesic because it is more rapidly adsorbed. The naproxen anion inhibits prostaglandin synthesis but this its mode of action is unknown.

Naproxen is rapidly and completely absorbed from the gastrointestinal tract. After administration of naproxen, peak plasma levels of naproxen anion are attained in 2 to 4 hours, with steady-state conditions normally achieved after 4-5 doses. The mean biological half-life of the anion in humans is approximately 13 hours, and at therapeutic levels it is greater than 99% albumin bound. Approximately 95% of the dose is excreted in the urine, primarily as naproxen, 6-0-desmethyl naproxen or their conjugates. The rate of excretion has been found to coincide closely with the rate of drug disappearance from the plasma. The drug does not induce metabolizing enzymes.

In children of 5 to 16 years of age with arthritis, plasma naproxen levels following a 5 mg/kg single dose of suspension were found to be similar to those found in normal adults following a 500 mg dose. The terminal half-life appears to be similar in children and adults. Pharmacokinetic studies of naproxen were not performed in children of less than 5 years of age.

The drug was studied in patients with rheumatoid arthritis, osteoarthritis, juvenile arthritis, ankylosing spondylitis, tendinitis and bursitis, and acute gout. It is not a corticosteroid. Improvement in patients treated for rheumatoid arthritis has been demonstrated by a reduction in joint swelling, a reduction in pain, a reduction in direction of morning stiffness, a reduction in disease activity as assesses by both the investigator and the patient, and increased mobility as demonstrated by a reduction in walking time.

In patients with osteoarthritis, the therapeutic action of the drug has been shown by a reduction in joint pain or tenderness, and increase in range of motion in knee joints, increased mobility as demonstrated by a reduction in walking time, and improvement in capacity to perform activities of daily living impaired by the disease.

In clinical studies in patients with rheumatoid arthritis, osteoarthritis, and juvenile arthritis, the drug has been shown to be comparable to aspirin and indomethacin in controlling the aforementioned measures of disease activity, but the frequency and severity if the milder gastrointestinal adverse effects (nausea, dyspepsia, heartburn) and nervous system adverse effects (tinnitus, dizziness, lightheadedness) were less than in both the aspirin- and indomethacin-treated patients. It is not known whether the drug causes less peptic ulceration than aspirin.

In patients with ankylosing spondylitis, the drug has been shown to decrease night pain, morning stiffness and pain at rest. In double-blind studies the drug was shown to be as effective as aspirin, but with fewer side effects.

In patients with acute gout, a favorable response to the drug was shown by significant clearing of inflammatory changes (*e.g.,* decrease in swelling, heat) within 24-48 hours, as well as by relief of pain and tenderness.

This drug may be used safely in combination with gold salts and/or corticosteroids; however, in controlled clinical trials, when added to the regimen of patients receiving corticosteroids it did not appear to cause greater improvement over that seen with corticosteroids alone. Whether the drug could be used in conjunction with partially effective doses of corticosteroids for a "steroid-sparing" effect has not been adequately studied. When added to the regimen of patients receiving gold salts the drug did result in greater improvement. Its use in combination with salicylates is not recommended because data are inadequate to demonstrate that the drug produces greater improvement over that achieved with aspirin alone. Further, there is some evidence that aspirin increases the rate of excretion of the drug.

Generally, improvement due to the drug has not been found to be dependent on age, sex, severity or duration of disease.

In clinical trials in patients with osteoarthritis and rheumatoid arthritis comparing treatments of 750 mg per day with 1,500 mg per day, there were trends toward increased efficacy with the higher dose and a more clear-cut increase in adverse reactions, particularly gastrointestinal reactions severe enough to cause the patient to leave the trial, which approximately doubled.

The drug was studied in patients with mild to moderate pain, and pain relief was obtained within one hour. It is not a narcotic and is not a CNS-acting drug. Controlled double-blind studies have demonstrated the analgesic properties of the drug in, for example, post-operative, post-partum, orthopedic and uterine contraction pain and dysmenorrhea. In dysmenorrheic patients, the drug reduces the level of prostaglandins in the uterus, which correlates with a reduction in the frequency and severity of uterine contractions. Analgesic action has

CLINICAL PHARMACOLOGY: *(cont'd)*

been shown by such measures as a reduction of pain intensity scores, increase in pain relief scores, decrease in numbers of patients requiring additional analgesic medication, and in time for required remedication. The analgesic effect has been found to last for up to 7 hours.

In ^{51}Cr blood loss and gastroscopy studies with normal volunteers, daily administration of 1,000 mg of the drug has been demonstrated to cause statistically significantly less gastric bleeding and erosion than 3,250 mg of aspirin.

INDICATIONS AND USAGE:

Naproxen is indicated for the treatment of rheumatoid arthritis, osteoarthritis, juvenile arthritis, ankylosing spondylitis, tendinitis and bursitis, and acute gout. It is also indicated in the relief of mild to moderate pain, and for the treatment of primary dysmenorrhea.

CONTRAINDICATIONS:

The drug is contraindicated in patients who have had allergic reactions to naproxen. It is also contraindicated in patients in whom aspirin or other nonsteroidal anti-inflammatory/analgesic drugs induce the syndrome of asthma, rhinitis, and nasal polyps. Both types of reactions have the potential of being fatal. Anaphylactoid reactions to naproxen whether of the true allergic type ot the pharmacologic idiosyncratic (e.f., aspirin syndrome) type, usually but not always occur in patients with a known history of such reactions. Therefore, careful questioning of patients for such things as asthma, nasal polyps, urticaria, and hypotension associated with nonsteroidal anti-inflammatory drugs before starting therapy is important. In addition, if such symptoms occur during therapy, treatment should be discontinued.

WARNINGS:

RISK OF GI ULCERATION, BLEEDING AND PERFORATION WITH NSAID THERAPY

Serious gastrointestinal toxicity such as bleeding, ulceration, and perforation, can occur at any time, with or without warning symptoms, in patients treated chronically with NSAID therapy. Although minor upper gastrointestinal problems, such as dyspepsia, are common, usually developing early in therapy, physicians should remain alert for ulceration and bleeding in patients treated chronically with NSAIDs even in the absence of previous GI tract symptoms. In patients observed in clinical trials of several months to two years duration, symptomatic upper GI ulcers, gross bleeding or perforation appear to occur in approximately 1% of patients treated for 3-6 months, and in about 2-4% of patients treated for one year. Physicians should inform patients about the signs and/or symptoms of serious GI toxicity and what steps to take if they occur.

Studies to date have not identified any subset of patients not at risk of developing peptic ulceration and bleeding. Except for a prior history of serious GI events and other risk factors known to be associated with peptic ulcer disease, such as alcoholism, smoking, etc., no risk factors (*e.g.*, age, sex) have been associated with increased risk. Elderly or debilitated patients seem to tolerate ulceration or bleeding less well than other individuals and most spontaneous reports of fatal GI events are in this population. Studies to date are inconclusive concerning the relative risk of various NSAIDs in causing such reactions. High doses of any NSAID probably carry a greater risk of these reactions, although controlled clinical trials showing this do not exist in most cases. In considering the use of relatively large doses (within the recommended dosage range), sufficient benefit should be anticipated to offset the potential increased risk of GI toxicity.

PRECAUTIONS:

GENERAL

NAPROXEN SHOULD NOT BE USED CONCOMITANTLY WITH THE RELATED DRUG *ANAPROX* OR *ANAPROX DS* (NAPROXEN SODIUM) SINCE THEY BOTH CIRCULATE IN PLASMA AS THE NAPROXEN ANION.

Renal Effects: As with other nonsteroidal anti-inflammatory drugs, long-term administration of naproxen to animals has resulted in renal papillary necrosis and other abnormal renal pathology. In humans, there have been reports of acute interstitial nephritis with hematuria, proteinuria, and occasionally nephrotic syndrome.

A second form of renal toxicity has been seen in patients with prerenal conditions leading to a reduction in renal blood flow or blood volume, where the renal prostaglandins have a supportive role in the maintenance of renal perfusion. In these patients, administration of a nonsteroidal anti-inflammatory drug may cause a dose-dependent reduction in prostaglandin formation and may precipitate overt renal decompensation. Patients at greatest risk of this reaction are those with impaired renal function, heart failure, liver dysfunction, those taking diuretics, and the elderly. Discontinuation of nonsteroidal anti-inflammatory therapy is typically followed by recovery to the pretreatment state.

Naproxen and its metabolites are eliminated primarily by the kidneys, therefore, the drug should be used with great caution in patients with significantly impaired renal function and the monitoring of serum creatinine and/or creatinine clearance is advised in these patients. Caution should be used if the drug is given to patients with creatinine clearance of less than 20 ml/minute because accumulation of naproxen metabolites has been seen in patients.

Chronic alcoholic liver disease and probably other forms of cirrhosis reduce the total plasma concentration of naproxen, but the plasma concentration of unbound naproxen is increased. It is prudent to use the lowest effective dose.

One study indicates that, although total plasma concentration of naproxen is unchanged, the unbound plasma fraction of naproxen is increased in the elderly. As with other drugs used in the elderly, it is prudent to use the lowest effective dose.

As with other nonsteroidal anti-inflammatory drugs, borderline elevations of one or more liver tests may occur in up to 15% of patients. These abnormalities may progress, may remain essentially unchanged, or may be transient with continued therapy. The SGPT (ALT) test is probably the most sensitive indicator of liver dysfunction. Meaningful (3 times the upper limit of normal) elevations of SGPT or SGOT (AST) occurred in controlled clinical trials in less than 1% of patients. A patient with symptoms and/or signs suggesting liver dysfunction, or in whom an abnormal liver test has occurred, should be evaluated for evidence of the development of more severe hepatic reaction while on therapy with this drug. Severe hepatic reactions, including jaundice and cases of fatal hepatitis, have been reported with this drug as with other nonsteroidal anti-inflammatory drugs. Although such reactions are rare, if abnormal liver tests persist or worsen, if clinical signs and symptoms consistent with liver disease develop, or if systemic manifestations occur (*e.g.*, eosinophilia, rash, etc.), this drug should be discontinued.

If steroid dosage is reduced or eliminated during therapy, the steroid dosage should be reduced slowly and the patients must be observed closely for any evidence of adverse effects, including adrenal insufficiency and exacerbation of symptoms of arthritis.

Patients with initial hemoglobin values of 10 grams or less who are to receive long-term therapy should have hemoglobin values determined periodically.

Peripheral edema has been observed in some patients. For this reason, the drug should be used with caution in patients with retention, hypertension or heart failure.

Naproxen suspension contains 8 mg/ml of sodium. This should be considered in patients whose overall intake of sodium must be restricted.

PRECAUTIONS: *(cont'd)*

The antipyretic and anti-inflammatory activities of the drug may reduce fever and inflammation, thus diminishing their utility as diagnostic signs in detecting complications of presumed non-infectious, non-inflammatory painful conditions.

Because of adverse eye findings in animal studies with drugs of this class, it is recommended that ophthalmic studies be carried out if any change or disturbance in vision occurs.

INFORMATION FOR THE PATIENT

Naproxen, like other drugs of its class, is not free of side effects. The side effects of these drugs can cause discomfort and, rarely, there are more serious side effects, such as gastrointestinal bleeding, which may result in hospitalization and even fatal outcomes.

NSAIDs (Nonsteroidal Anti-Inflammatory Drugs) are often essential agents in the management of arthritis and have a major role in the treatment of pain, but they also may be commonly employed for conditions which are less serious.

Physicians may wish to discuss with their patients the potential risks (see WARNINGS, PRECAUTIONS, and ADVERSE REACTIONS) and likely benefits of NSAID treatment, particularly when the drugs are used for less serious conditions where treatment without NSAIDs may represent an acceptable alternative to both the patient and physician.

Caution should be exercised by patients whose activities require alertness if they experience drowsiness, dizziness, vertigo or depression during therapy with the drug.

LABORATORY TESTS

Because serious GI tract ulceration and bleeding can occur without warning symptoms, physicians should follow chronically treated patients for the signs and symptoms of ulceration and bleeding and should inform them of the importance of this follow-up (see Risk of GI Ulceration, Bleeding and Perforation with NSAID Therapy.)

DRUG/LABORATORY TEST INTERACTIONS

The drug may decrease platelet aggregation and prolong bleeding time. This effect should be kept in mind when bleeding times are determined.

The administration of the drug may result in increased urinary values for 17-ketogenic steroids because of an interaction between the drug and/or its metabolites with m-dinitrobenzene used in this assay. Although 17 hydroxy-corticosteroid measurements (Porter-Silber test) do not appear to be artifactually altered, it is suggested that therapy with the drug be temporarily discontinued 72 hours before adrenal function tests are performed.

The drug may interfere with some urinary assays of 5-hydroxy indoleacetic acid (5HIAA).

CARCINOGENESIS

A two-year study was performed in rats to evaluate the carcinogenic potential of the drug. No evidence of carcinogenicity was found.

PREGNANCY CATEGORY B

Teratogenic Effects: Reproduction studies have been performed in rats, rabbits, and mice at doses up to 6 times the human dose and have revealed no evidence of impaired fertility or harm to the fetus due to the drug. There are, however, no adequate and well-controlled studies in pregnant women. Because animal reproduction studies are not always predictive of human response, the drug should not be used during pregnancy unless clearly needed. Because of the known effect of drugs of this class on the human fetal cardiovascular system (closure of ductus arteriosus), use during late pregnancy should be avoided.

Non-Teratogenic Effects: As with other drugs known to inhibit prostaglandin synthesis, an increased incidence of dystocia and delayed parturition occurred in rats.

NURSING MOTHERS

The naproxen anion has been found in the milk of lactating women at a concentration of approximately 1% of that found in the plasma. Because of the possible adverse effects of prostaglandin-inhibiting drugs on neonates, use in nursing mothers should be avoided.

PEDIATRIC USE

Safety and effectiveness in children below the age of 2 years have not been established. Pediatric dosing recommendations for juvenile arthritis are based on well-controlled studies (See DOSAGE AND ADMINISTRATION.) There are no adequate effectiveness or dose-response data for other pediatric conditions, but the experience in juvenile arthritis and other use experience have established that single doses of 2.5-5 mg/kg, with a total daily dose not exceeding 15 mg/kg/day, are safe in children over 2 years of age.

DRUG INTERACTIONS:

In vitro studies have shown that naproxen anion, because of its affinity for protein, may displace from their binding sites other drugs which are also albumin-bound. Theoretically, the naproxen anion itself could likewise be displaced. Short-term controlled studies failed to show that taking the drug significantly affects prothrombin times when administered to individuals on coumarin-type anticoagulants. Caution is advised nonetheless, since interactions have been seen with other nonsteroidal agents of this class. Similarly, patients receiving the drug and a hydantoin, sulfonamide or sulfonylurea should be observed for signs of toxicity to these drugs.

The natriuretic effect of the furosemide has been reported to be inhibited by some drugs of this class. Inhibition of renal lithium clearance leading to increases in plasma lithium concentrations has also been reported.

This and other nonsteroidal anti-inflammatory drugs can reduce the antihypertensive effect of propanolol and other beta-blockers.

Probenecid given concurrently increases naproxen anion plasma levels and extends is plasma half-life significantly.

Caution should be used if this drug is administered concomitantly with methotrexate. Naproxen and other nonsteroidal anti-inflammatory drugs have been reported to reduce the tubular secretion of methotrexate in an animal model, possibly enhancing the toxicity of that drug.

ADVERSE REACTIONS:

The following adverse reactions are divided into 3 parts based on frequency and likelihood of causal relationship to naproxen.

INCIDENCE GREATER THAN 1%

Possible Causal Relationship: Adverse reactions reported in controlled clinical trials in 960 patients treated for rheumatoid arthritis or osteoarthritis are listed below. In general, these reactions were reported 2 to 10 times more frequently than they were in studies in the 962 patients treated for mild to moderate pain or for dysmenorrhea.

A clinical study found gastrointestinal reactions to more frequent and more severe in rheumatoid arthritis patients taking 1,500 mg naproxen daily compared to those taking 750 mg daily (See CLINICAL PHARMACOLOGY.)

In controlled clinical trials with about 80 children and in well-monitored open studies with about 400 children with juvenile arthritis, the incidences of rash and prolonged bleeding times were increased, the incidences of gastrointestinal and central nervous system reactions were about the same, and the incidences of other reactions were lower in children than in adults.

ADVERSE REACTIONS: *(cont'd)*

Gastrointestinal: The most frequent complaints reported related to the gastrointestinal tract. They were: constipation*, heartburn*, abdominal pain*, nausea*, dyspepsia, diarrhea, stomatitis.

Central Nervous System: Headache*, dizziness*, drowsiness*, lightheadedness, vertigo.

Dermatologic: Itching (pruritus)*, skin eruption*, ecchymoses*, sweating, purpura.

Special Senses: Tinnitus*, hearing disturbances, visual disturbances.

Cardiovascular: Edema*, dyspnea*, palpitations.

General: Thirst

* Incidence of reported reaction between 3% and 9%. Those reactions occurring in less than 3% of the patients are unmarked.

INCIDENCE LESS THAN 1%

Probable Causal Relationship: The following adverse reactions were reported less frequently than 1% during controlled clinical trial and through voluntary reports since marketing. The probability of a causal relationship exists between the drug and these adverse reactions:

Gastrointestinal: Abnormal liver function tests, gastrointestinal bleeding and/or perforation, hematemesis, jaundice, melena, peptic ulceration with bleeding and/or perforation, vomiting.

Renal: Glomerular nephritis, hematuria, interstitial nephritis, nephrotic syndrome, renal disease, renal failure, renal papillary necrosis.

Hematologic: Eosinophilia, granulocytopenia, leukopenia, thrombocytopenia.

Central Nervous System: Depression, dream abnormalities, inability to concentrate, insomnia, malaise, myalgia and muscle weakness.

Dermatologic: Alopecia, photosensitive dermatitis, skin rashes.

Special Senses: Hearing impairment.

Cardiovascular: Congestive heart failure.

Respiratory: Eosinophilic pneumonitis.

General: Anaphylactoid reactions, menstrual disorders, pyrexia (chills and fever).

Causal Relationship Unknown: Other reactions have been reported in circumstances in which a causal relationship could not be established. However, in these rarely reported events, the possibility cannot be excluded. Therefore, these observations are being listed to serve as alerting information to the physicians:

Hematologic: Aplastic anemia, hemolytic anemia.

Central Nervous System: Aseptic meningitis, cognitive dysfunction.

Dermatologic: Epidermal necrolysis, erythema multiforme, photosensitivity reactions resembling porphyria cutanea tarda and epidermolysis bullosa, Stevens-Johnson syndrome, urticaria.

Gastrointestinal: Non-peptic gastrointestinal ulceration, ulcerative stomatitis.

Cardiovascular: Vasculitis.

General: Angioneurotic edema, hyperglycemia, hypoglycemia.

OVERDOSAGE:

Significant overdosage may be characterized by drowsiness, heartburn, indigestion, nausea or vomiting. A few patients have experienced seizures, but it is not clear whether or not these were drug related. It is not known what dose of the drug would be life threatening. The oral LD_{50} of the drug is 543 mg/kg in rats, 1,234 mg/kg in mice, 4,110 mg/kg in hamsters and greater than 1,000 mg/kg in dogs.

Should a patient ingest a large number of tablets or a large volume of suspension, accidentally or purposefully, the stomach may be emptied and usual supportive measures employed. In animals 0.5 g/kg of activated charcoal was effective in reducing plasma levels of naproxen. Hemodialysis does not decrease the plasma concentration of naproxen because of the high degree of its protein binding.

DOSAGE AND ADMINISTRATION:

A measuring cup marked in 1/2 teaspoon and 2.5 milliliter increments is provided with the suspension. This cup or a teaspoon may be used to measure the appropriate dose.

For Rheumatoid Arthritis, Osteoarthritis, and Ankylosing Spondylitis: The recommended dose of naproxen in adults is 250 mg (10 ml or 2 tsp of suspension), 375 mg (15 ml or 3 tsp), or 500 mg (20 ml or 4 tsp) twice daily (morning and evening). During long-term administration, the dose may be adjusted up or down depending on the clinical response of the patient. A lower daily dose may suffice for long-term administration. The morning and evening doses do not have to be equal in size and the administration of the drug more frequently than twice daily is not necessary. In patients who tolerate lower doses well, the dose may be increased to 1,500 mg per day for limited periods when a higher level of anti-inflammatory/analgesic activity is required. When treating such patients with the 1,500 mg/day dose, the physician should observe sufficient increased clinical benefits to offset the potential increased risk (see CLINICAL PHARMACOLOGY.)

Symptomatic improvement in arthritis usually begins with 2 weeks. However, if improvement is not seen within this period, a trial for an additional 2 weeks should be considered.

For Juvenile Arthritis: The recommended total daily dose of naproxen is approximately 10 mg/kg given in 2 divided doses. One-half of the 250 mg tablet may be used to approximate this dose. The following table may be used as a guide for suspension (TABLE 1):

TABLE 1

Child's Weight	Dose
13 kg (29 lb)	2.5 ml (1/2 tsp) b.i.d.
25 kg (55 lb)	5 ml (1 tsp) b.i.d.
38 kg (84 lb)	7.5 ml (1-1/2 tsp) b.i.d.

For Acute Gout: The recommended starting dose of naproxen is 750 mg (30 ml or 6 tsp), followed by 250 mg (10 ml or 2 tsp) every 8 hours until the attack has subsided.

For Mild to Moderate Pain, Primary Dysmenorrhea and Acute Tendinitis and Bursitis: The recommended starting dose of naproxen is 500 mg (20 ml or 4 tsp), followed by 250 mg (10 ml or 2 tsp) every 6 to 8 hours as required. The total daily dose should not exceed 1,250 mg (50 ml or 10 tsp).

Store naproxen suspension at room temperature; avoid excessive heat, above 40°C (104°F). Dispense in light-resistant container.

Store tablets at room temperature and in well-closed containers; dispense in light-resistant container.

PATIENT INFORMATION:

Naproxen is a non-steroidal anti-inflammatory drug (NSAID) used to treat arthritis, inflammation of the joints, gout, and mild to moderate pain including menstrual cramps. This drug should not be used by those sensitive or allergic to aspirin or who have ever had breathing difficulties, runny nose or itching as a result of taking one of these related medications. Similar to all NSAIDs, including aspirin, naproxen may irritate the stomach.

PATIENT INFORMATION: *(cont'd)*

Stomach irritation can be lessened if naproxen is taken with food. If you have ever had a stomach ulcer and you experience stomach-related problems with this medication, contact your physician. Rarely this drug may cause swelling in the lower legs. If this occurs please contact your physician. Headache, dizziness and drowsiness have also been reported and for this reason, you may want to take the first dose at home. This medicine should be taken as prescribed and should not exceed 1250 mg per day.

HOW SUPPLIED - RATED THERAPEUTICALLY EQUIVALENT:

Suspension - Oral - 125 mg/5ml

15 ml x 25	$50.00	Naproxen, Roxane	00054-8632-11
16's	**$40.87**	**NAPROSYN, Syntex PR**	**18393-0278-20**
20 ml x 25	$66.65	Naproxen, Roxane	00054-8633-11
500 ml	$34.75	Naproxen, Roxane	00054-3630-63

Tablet, Uncoated - Oral - 250 mg

60's	$60.00	NAPROXEN, UDL	51079-0793-98
100's	$11.03	Naproxen, H.C.F.A. F F P	99999-1864-01
100's	$66.10	Naproxen, Roxane	00054-4641-25
100's	$67.05	Naproxen, Qualitest Pharms	00603-4730-21
100's	$67.05	Naproxen, Major Pharms	00904-7745-60
100's	$67.05	Naproxen, West Point Pharma	59591-0253-68
100's	$67.07	Naproxen, Purepac Pharm	00228-2521-10
100's	$67.08	Naproxen, Rugby	00536-5612-01
100's	$67.08	Naproxen, HL Moore Drug Exch	00839-7832-06
100's	$67.08	Naproxen, HL Moore Drug Exch	00839-7881-06
100's	$67.08	Naproxen, Mova Pharms	55370-0139-07
100's	$67.08	Naproxen, Hamilton Pharma	60322-0282-42
100's	$67.10	Naproxen, Mova Pharms	55370-0521-07
100's	$67.10	Naproxen, Novopharm (US)	55953-0517-40
100's	$68.75	Naproxen, Roxane	00054-8641-25
100's	$69.00	Naproxen, Copley Pharm	38245-0146-10
100's	$69.13	Naproxen, Lederle Pharm	00005-3300-43
100's	$71.75	Naproxen, Martec Pharms	52555-0488-01
100's	$71.98	Naproxen, Vangard Labs	00615-3562-13
100's	$72.45	Naproxen, Zenith Labs	00172-4107-60
100's	$72.45	Naproxen, Goldline Labs	00182-1971-01
100's	$72.48	Naproxen, Schein Pharm (US)	00364-2562-01
100's	$72.50	Naproxen, Teva	00093-0147-01
100's	$73.94	Naproxen, Geneva Pharms	00781-1163-01
100's	$73.96	Naproxen, Rugby	00536-4842-01
100's	$74.67	Naproxen, Mylan	00378-0377-01
100's	$75.23	Naproxen, Geneva Pharms	00781-1163-13
100's	$76.22	NAPROXEN, Aligen Independ	00405-4693-01
100's	**$80.54**	**NAPROSYN, Syntex PR**	**18393-0272-42**
500's	$55.15	Naproxen, H.C.F.A. F F P	99999-1864-02
500's	$325.90	Naproxen, Roxane	00054-4641-29
500's	$326.85	Naproxen, Purepac Pharm	00228-2521-50
500's	$326.85	Naproxen, Major Pharms	00904-7745-40
500's	$326.86	Naproxen, Schein Pharm (US)	00364-2562-05
500's	$326.86	Naproxen, Hamilton Pharma	60322-0282-62
500's	$326.90	Naproxen, HL Moore Drug Exch	00839-7832-12
500's	$326.90	Naproxen, HL Moore Drug Exch	00839-7881-12
500's	$326.90	Naproxen, Mova Pharms	55370-0521-08
500's	$326.90	Naproxen, Novopharm (US)	55953-0517-70
500's	$328.42	Naproxen, Aligen Independ	00405-4693-02
500's	$335.00	Naproxen, Copley Pharm	38245-0146-50
500's	$336.83	Naproxen, Lederle Pharm	00005-3300-31
500's	$353.00	Naproxen, Teva	00093-0147-05
500's	$353.00	Naproxen, Zenith Labs	00172-4107-70
500's	$353.00	Naproxen, Goldline Labs	00182-1971-05
500's	$360.40	Naproxen, Geneva Pharms	00781-1163-05
500's	$363.78	Naproxen, Mylan	00378-0377-05
500's	**$392.44**	**NAPROSYN, Syntex PR**	**18393-0272-62**
750's	$518.70	Naproxen, Glasgow Pharm	60809-0117-55
750's	$518.70	Naproxen, Glasgow Pharm	60809-0117-72
1000's	$110.30	Naproxen, H.C.F.A. F F P	99999-1864-03
1000's	$630.54	Naproxen, Purepac Pharm	00228-2521-96
1000's	$630.54	Naproxen, Mova Pharms	55370-0139-09
1000's	$630.54	Naproxen, Hamilton Pharma	60322-0282-66
1000's	$630.60	Naproxen, Novopharm (US)	55953-0517-80
1000's	$649.50	Naproxen, Teva	00093-0147-10
1000's	$649.50	Naproxen, Geneva Pharms	00781-1163-10
1000's	$649.82	Naproxen, HL Moore Drug Exch	00839-7881-16

Tablet, Uncoated - Oral - 375 mg

100's	$15.17	Naproxen, H.C.F.A. F F P	99999-1864-04
100's	$73.12	Naproxen, Zenith Labs	00172-4108-60
100's	$73.12	Naproxen, Goldline Labs	00182-1972-01
100's	$85.40	Naproxen, Roxane	00054-4642-25
100's	$86.20	Naproxen, Qualitest Pharms	00603-4731-21
100's	$86.20	Naproxen, Major Pharms	00904-7746-60
100's	$86.20	Naproxen, West Point Pharma	59591-0254-68
100's	$86.21	Naproxen, Purepac Pharm	00228-2522-10
100's	$86.23	Naproxen, Rugby	00536-5613-01
100's	$86.23	Naproxen, Mova Pharms	55370-0140-07
100's	$86.23	Naproxen, Hamilton Pharma	60322-0283-42
100's	$86.25	Naproxen, HL Moore Drug Exch	00839-7833-06
100's	$86.25	Naproxen, Mova Pharms	55370-0522-07
100's	$86.25	Naproxen, Novopharm (US)	55953-0518-40
100's	$87.92	Naproxen, Aligen Independ	00405-4694-01
100's	$88.00	Naproxen, Roxane	00054-8642-25
100's	$88.81	Naproxen, Lederle Pharm	00005-3301-43
100's	$89.00	Naproxen, Copley Pharm	38245-0443-10
100's	$90.54	Naproxen, Schein Pharm (US)	00364-2563-01
100's	$92.48	Naproxen, Vangard Labs	00615-1504-13
100's	$92.56	Naproxen, Martec Pharms	52555-0489-01
100's	$93.10	Naproxen, Teva	00093-0148-01
100's	$94.99	Naproxen, Geneva Pharms	00781-1164-01
100's	$95.03	Naproxen, Rugby	00536-4843-01
100's	$95.96	Naproxen, Mylan	00378-0555-01
100's	$95.97	Naproxen, Geneva Pharms	00781-1164-13
100's	**$103.52**	**NAPROSYN, Syntex PR**	**18393-0273-42**
500's	$75.85	Naproxen, United Res	00677-1516-05
500's	$75.85	Naproxen, H.C.F.A. F F P	99999-1864-05
500's	$417.20	Naproxen, Roxane	00054-4642-29
500's	$418.15	Naproxen, Qualitest Pharms	00603-4731-28
500's	$418.20	Naproxen, Major Pharms	00904-7746-40
500's	$418.21	Naproxen, Purepac Pharm	00228-2522-50
500's	$418.23	Naproxen, Rugby	00536-5613-05
500's	$418.23	Naproxen, HL Moore Drug Exch	00839-7833-12
500's	$418.23	Naproxen, Hamilton Pharma	60322-0283-62
500's	$418.25	Naproxen, Mova Pharms	55370-0522-08
500's	$418.25	Naproxen, Novopharm (US)	55953-0518-70

HOW SUPPLIED - RATED THERAPEUTICALLY EQUIVALENT: *(cont'd)*

500's	$420.42	Naproxen, Aligen Independ	00405-4694-02
500's	$425.00	Naproxen, Copley Pharm	38245-0443-50
500's	$431.10	Naproxen, Lederle Pharm	00005-3301-31
500's	$438.00	Naproxen, Martec Pharms	52555-0489-05
500's	$439.14	Naproxen, Schein Pharm (US)	00364-2563-05
500's	$451.00	Naproxen, Teva	00093-0148-05
500's	$451.67	Naproxen, Zenith Labs	00172-4108-70
500's	$451.67	Naproxen, Goldline Labs	00182-1972-05
500's	$461.28	Naproxen, Rugby	00536-4843-05
500's	$461.28	Naproxen, Geneva Pharms	00781-1164-05
500's	$465.46	Naproxen, Mylan	00378-0555-05
500's	**$502.14**	**NAPROSYN, Syntex PR**	**18393-0273-62**
750's	$662.98	Naproxen, Glasgow Pharm	60809-0118-55
750's	$662.98	Naproxen, Glasgow Pharm	60809-0118-72
1000's	$151.70	Naproxen, H.C.F.A. F F P	99999-1864-06
1000's	$801.90	Naproxen, HL Moore Drug Exch	00839-7882-16
1000's	$801.91	Naproxen, Purepac Pharm	00228-2522-96
1000's	$801.91	Naproxen, Mova Pharms	55370-0140-09
1000's	$801.91	Naproxen, Hamilton Pharma	60322-0283-66
1000's	$801.95	Naproxen, Novopharm (US)	55953-0518-80
1000's	$807.35	Naproxen, Teva	00093-0148-10
1000's	$807.35	Naproxen, Geneva Pharms	00781-1164-10

Tablet, Uncoated - Oral - 500 mg

100's	$18.23	Naproxen, H.C.F.A. F F P	99999-1864-07
100's	$104.30	Naproxen, Roxane	00054-4643-25
100's	$105.30	Naproxen, Purepac Pharm	00228-2523-10
100's	$105.30	Naproxen, Rugby	00536-5614-01
100's	$105.30	Naproxen, Qualitest Pharms	00603-4732-21
100's	$105.30	Naproxen, HL Moore Drug Exch	00839-7834-06
100's	$105.30	Naproxen, HL Moore Drug Exch	00839-7883-06
100's	$105.30	Naproxen, Major Pharms	00904-7747-60
100's	$105.30	Naproxen, West Point Pharma	59591-0255-68
100's	$105.31	Naproxen, Mova Pharms	55370-0141-07
100's	$105.31	Naproxen, Hamilton Pharma	60322-0287-42
100's	$105.35	Naproxen, Mova Pharms	55370-0524-07
100's	$105.35	Naproxen, Novopharm (US)	55953-0520-40
100's	$107.54	Naproxen, Aligen Independ	00405-4695-01
100's	$108.00	Naproxen, Copley Pharm	38245-0150-10
100's	$108.45	Naproxen, Lederle Pharm	00005-3302-43
100's	$109.00	Naproxen, Roxane	00054-8643-25
100's	$112.35	Naproxen, Martec Pharms	52555-0490-01
100's	$112.36	Naproxen, Schein Pharm (US)	00364-2564-01
100's	$113.70	Naproxen, Teva	00093-0149-01
100's	$113.74	Naproxen, Zenith Labs	00172-4109-60
100's	$113.74	Naproxen, Goldline Labs	00182-1973-01
100's	$115.99	Naproxen, Geneva Pharms	00781-1165-01
100's	$116.04	Naproxen, Rugby	00536-4844-01
100's	$117.22	Naproxen, Mylan	00378-0451-01
100's	$119.23	Naproxen, Geneva Pharms	00781-1165-13
100's	$119.88	Naproxen, Vangard Labs	00615-3563-13
100's	**$126.44**	**NAPROSYN, Syntex PR**	**18393-0277-42**
500's	$91.15	Naproxen, United Res	00677-1517-05
500's	$91.15	Naproxen, H.C.F.A. F F P	99999-1864-08
500's	$509.60	Naproxen, Roxane	00054-4643-29
500's	$510.48	Naproxen, Qualitest Pharms	00603-4732-28
500's	$510.50	Naproxen, Purepac Pharm	00228-2523-50
500's	$510.55	Naproxen, Major Pharms	00904-7747-40
500's	$510.57	Naproxen, Rugby	00536-5614-05
500's	$510.57	Naproxen, HL Moore Drug Exch	00839-7834-12
500's	$510.57	Naproxen, HL Moore Drug Exch	00839-7883-12
500's	$510.57	Naproxen, Mova Pharms	55370-0141-08
500's	$510.57	Naproxen, Hamilton Pharma	60322-0287-62
500's	$510.60	Naproxen, Mova Pharms	55370-0524-08
500's	$510.60	Naproxen, Novopharm (US)	55953-0520-70
500's	$525.00	Naproxen, Copley Pharm	38245-0150-50
500's	$525.18	Naproxen, Aligen Independ	00405-4695-02
500's	$526.19	Naproxen, Lederle Pharm	00005-3302-31
500's	$536.10	Naproxen, Schein Pharm (US)	00364-2564-05
500's	$541.00	Naproxen, Martec Pharms	52555-0490-05
500's	$541.00	Naproxen, Martec Pharms	52555-0499-05
500's	$551.00	Naproxen, Teva	00093-0149-05
500's	$551.40	Naproxen, Zenith Labs	00172-4109-70
500's	$551.40	Naproxen, Goldline Labs	00182-1973-05
500's	$558.24	Naproxen, Mylan	00378-0451-05
500's	$562.99	Naproxen, Geneva Pharms	00781-1165-05
500's	$563.03	Naproxen, Rugby	00536-4844-05
500's	**$613.01**	**NAPROSYN, Syntex PR**	**18393-0277-62**
750's	$813.32	Naproxen, Glasgow Pharm	60809-0119-55
750's	$813.32	Naproxen, Glasgow Pharm	60809-0119-72
1000's	$182.30	Naproxen, H.C.F.A. F F P	99999-1864-09
1000's	$979.35	Naproxen, Purepac Pharm	00228-2523-96
1000's	$979.39	Naproxen, Hamilton Pharma	60322-0287-66
1000's	$979.45	Naproxen, Novopharm (US)	55953-0520-80
1000's	$985.50	Naproxen, Teva	00093-0149-10
1000's	$985.61	Naproxen, Geneva Pharms	00781-1165-10

HOW SUPPLIED - NOT RATED EQUIVALENT:

Tablet, Enteric Coated - Oral - 375 mg

100's	$99.54	EC-NAPROSYN, Syntex PR	18393-0255-42

Tablet, Enteric Coated - Oral - 500 mg

100's	$121.57	EC-NAPROSYN, Syntex PR	18393-0256-42

NAPROXEN SODIUM *(001865)*

CATEGORIES: Analgesics; Ankylosing Spondylitis; Anti-Inflammatory Agents; Antiarthritics; Antipyretics; Arthritis; Bursitis; Central Nervous System Agents; Dysmenorrhea; Gout; NSAIDS; Nonsteroidal Anti-Inflammatory; Osteoarthritis; Pain; Spondylitis; Migraine*; Pregnancy Category B; Sales > $100 Million; FDA Approval Pre 1982; Patent Expiration 1993 Dec
* Indication not approved by the FDA

BRAND NAMES: **Anaprox**; Anaprox DS

FORMULARIES: BC-BS; Foundation

COST OF THERAPY: $107.31 (Arthritis; Tablet; 275 mg; 2/day; 365 days)

PRIMARY ICD9: 715.99 (Osteoarthritis, Unspecified, Multiple Sites)

DESCRIPTION:

Naproxen sodium filmcoated tablets for oral administration each contain 275 mg of naproxen, which is equivalent to 250 mg naproxen with 25 mg (about 1 mEq) sodium. Naproxen sodium filmcoated tablets for oral administration each contain 550 mg of naproxen sodium, which is equivalent to 500 mg naproxen with 50 mg (about 2 mEq) sodium. Naproxen sodium is a member of arylacetic acid group of nonsteroidal anti-inflammatory drugs.

The chemical name of naproxen sodium is 2-naphthaleneacetic acid, 6-methoxy-α-methyl-, sodium salt, (-).

Naproxen sodium is a white to creamy white, crystalline solid, freely soluble in water.

Each naproxen sodium 275 mg tablet contains naproxen sodium, the active ingredient, with lactose, magnesium stearate, and microcrystalline cellulose. The coating suspension may contain hydroxypropyl methylcellulose 2910, Opaspray K-1-4210A, polyethylene glycol 8000 or Opadry YS-1-4215. Each naproxen sodium DS 550 mg tablet contains naproxen sodium, the active ingredient, with magnesium stearate, microcrystalline cellulose, povidone, and talc. The coating suspension may contain hydroxypropyl methylcellulose 2910, Opaspray K-1-4227, polyethylene glycol 8000 or Opadry YS-1-4216.

CLINICAL PHARMACOLOGY:

The sodium salt of naproxen has been developed as an analgesic because it is more rapidly absorbed. Naproxen is a nonsteroidal anti-inflammatory drug with analgesic and antipyretic properties. Naproxen anion inhibits prostaglandin synthesis but beyond this its mode of action is unknown.

Naproxen sodium is rapidly and completely absorbed from the gastrointestinal tract. After administration of naproxen sodium, peak plasma levels of naproxen anion are attained at 1-2 hours with steady-state conditions normally achieved after 4-5 doses. The mean biological half-life of the anion in humans is approximately 13 hours, and at therapeutic levels it is greater than 99% albumin bound. Approximately 95% of the dose is excreted in the urine, primarily as naproxen, 6-0- desmethyl naproxen or their conjugates. The rate of excretion had been found to coincide closely with the rate of drug disappearance from the plasma. The drug does not induce the metabolizing enzymes.

In children of 5 to 16 years of age with arthritis, plasma naproxen levels following a 5 mg/kg single dose of naproxen suspension (see DOSAGE AND ADMINISTRATION) were found to be similar to those found in normal adults following a 500 mg dose. The terminal half-life appears to be similar in children and adults. Pharmacokinetic studies of naproxen were not performed in children less than 5 years of age.

The drug was studied in patients with mild to moderate pain, and pain relief was obtained within 1 hour. It is not a narcotic and is not a CNS-acting drug. Controlled double-blind studies have demonstrated the analgesic properties of the drug in, for example, post-operative, post-partum, orthopedic and uterine contraction pain and dysmenorrhea. In dysmenorrheic patients, the drug reduces the level of prostaglandins in the uterus, which correlates with a reduction in the frequency and severity of uterine contractions. Analgesic action has been shown by such measures as reduction of pain intensity scores, increase in pain relief scores, decrease in numbers of patients requiring additional analgesic medication and delay in time for required remedication. The analgesic effect has been found to last for up to 7 hours.

The drug was studied in patients with rheumatoid arthritis, osteoarthritis, ankylosing spondylitis, tendinitis and bursitis, and acute gout. It is not a corticosteroid. Improvement in patients treated for rheumatoid arthritis has been demonstrated by a reduction in joint swelling, a reduction in pain, a reduction in duration for morning stiffness, a reduction in disease activity as assessed by both the investigator and patient, and by increased mobility as demonstrated by a reduction in walking time.

In patients with osteoarthritis, the therapeutic action of the drug has been shown by a reduction in joint pain or tenderness, an increase in range of motion in knee joints, increased mobility as demonstrated by a reduction in walking time, and improvement in capacity to perform activities of daily living impaired by the disease.

In clinical studies in patients rheumatoid arthritis, osteoarthritis, and juvenile arthritis, the drug has been shown to be comparable to aspirin and indomethacin in controlling the aforementioned measures of disease activity, but the frequency and severity of the milder gastrointestinal adverse effects (nausea, dyspepsia, heartburn) and nervous system adverse effects (tinnitus, dizziness, lightheadedness) were less than in both the aspirin- and indomethacin-treated patients. It is not known whether the drug causes less peptic ulceration than aspirin.

In patients with ankylosing spondylitis, the drug has been shown to decrease night pain, morning stiffness and pain at rest. In double-blind studies the drug was shown to as effective as aspirin, but with fewer side effects.

In patients with acute gout, a favorable response to the drug was shown by significant clearing of inflammatory changes (*e.g.,* decrease in swelling, heat) within 24-48 hours, as well as by relief of pain and tenderness.

The drug may be used in combination with gold salts and/or corticosteroids; however, in controlled clinical trials, when added to the regimen of patients receiving corticosteroids it did not appear to cause greater improvement over that seen with corticosteroids alone. Whether the drug could be used in conjunction with partially effective doses of corticosteroid for a "steroid-sparing" effect has not been adequately studied. When added to the regimen of patients receiving gold salts,the drug did result in greater improvement. Its use in combination with salicylates is not recommended because data are inadequate to demonstrate that the drug produces greater improvement over that achieved with aspirin alone. Further, there is some evidence that aspirin increases the rate of excretion of the drug.

Generally, improvement due to the drug has not been found to be dependent on age, sex, severity or duration of disease.

In clinical trials in patients with osteoarthritis and rheumatoid arthritis comparing treatments of 825 mg per day with 1650 mg per day, there were trends toward increased efficacy with the higher dose and a more clearcut increase in adverse reactions, particularly gastrointestinal reactions severe enough to cause the patient to leave the trial, which approximately doubled.

In ^{51}Cr blood loss and gastroscopy studies with normal volunteers, daily administration of 1100 mg of naproxen sodium has been demonstrated to cause statistically significantly less gastric bleeding and erosion than 3250 mg of aspirin.

INDICATIONS AND USAGE:

Naproxen sodium is indicate in the relief of mild to moderate pain and for the treatment of primary dysmenorrhea.

It is also indicated for the treatment of rheumatoid arthritis, osteoarthritis, juvenile arthritis, ankylosing spondylitis, tendinitis and bursitis and acute gout.

CONTRAINDICATIONS:

The drug is contraindicated in patients who have had allergic reactions to naproxen sodium or to naproxen. It is also contraindicated in patients in whom aspirin or other nonsteroidal anti-inflammatory/analgesic drugs induce the syndrome of asthma, rhinitis, and nasal polyps. Both these types of reactions have the potential of being fatal. Anaphylactoid reactions to naproxen sodium or naproxen, whether of the true allergic type or the pharmacologic idiosyncratic (*e.g.,* aspirin syndrome) type, usually but not always occur in patients with a

CONTRAINDICATIONS: *(cont'd)*

known history of such reactions. Therefore, careful questioning of patients for such things as asthma, nasal polyps, urticaria, and hypotension associated with nonsteroidal anti-inflammatory drugs before starting therapy is important. In addition, if such symptoms occur during therapy, treatment should be discontinued.

WARNINGS:

Risk of GI Ulceration, Bleeding and Perforation with NSAID Therapy: Serious gastrointestinal toxicity such as bleeding, ulceration, and perforation, can occur at any time, with or without warning symptoms, in patients treated chronically with NSAID therapy. Although minor upper gastrointestinal problems, such as dyspepsia, are common, usually developing early in therapy, physicians should remain alert for ulceration and bleeding in patients treated chronically with NSAIDs even in the absence of previous GI tract symptoms. In patients observed in clinical trials of several months to two years' duration, symptomatic upper GI ulcers, gross bleeding or perforation appear to occur in approximately 1% of patients treated for 3-6 months, and in about 2-4% of patients treated for one year. Physicians should inform patients about the signs and/or symptoms of serious toxicity and what steps to take if they occur.

Studies to date have not identified any subset of patients not at risk of developing peptic ulceration and bleeding. Except for a prior history of serious GI events and other risk factors known to be associated with peptic ulcer disease, such as alcoholism, smoking, etc., no risk factors (*e.g.,* age, sex) have been associated with increased risk. Elderly or debilitated patients seem to tolerate ulceration or bleeding less well than other individuals and most spontaneous reports of fatal GI events are in this population. Studies to date are inconclusive concerning the relative risk of various NSAIDs in causing such reactions. High doses of any NSAID probably carry a greater risk of these reactions, although controlled clinical trials showing this do not exist in most cases. In considering the use of relatively large doses (within the recommended dosage range), sufficient benefit should be anticipated to offset the potential increased risk of GI toxicity.

PRECAUTIONS:

GENERAL

NAPROXEN SODIUM SHOULD NOT BE USED CONCOMITANTLY WITH THE RELATED DRUG NAPROXEN SINCE THEY BOTH CIRCULATE IN PLASMA AS THE NAPROXEN ANION.

Renal Effects: As with other nonsteroidal anti-inflammatory drugs, long-term administration of naproxen to animals has resulted in renal papillary necrosis and other abnormal renal pathology. In humans, there have been reports of acute interstitial nephritis with hematuria, proteinuria, and occasionally nephrotic syndrome.

A second form of renal toxicity has been seen in patients with prerenal conditions leading to a reduction in renal blood flow or blood volume, where the renal prostaglandins have a supportive role in the maintenance of renal perfusion. In these patients, administration of a nonsteroidal anti-inflammatory drug may cause a dose-dependent reduction in prostaglandin formation and may precipitate overt renal decompensation. Patients at greatest risk of this reduction are those with impaired renal function, heart failure, liver dysfunction, those taking diuretics, and the elderly. Discontinuation of nonsteroidal anti-inflammatory therapy is typically followed by recovery to the pretreatment state.

Naproxen sodium and its metabolites are eliminated primarily by the kidneys, therefore the drug should be used with great caution in patients with significantly impaired renal function and the monitoring of serum creatinine and/or creatinine clearance is advised in these patients. Caution should be used if the drug is given to patients with creatinine clearance of less than 20 ml/minute because accumulation of naproxen metabolites has been seen in such patients.

Chronic alcoholic liver disease and probably other forms of cirrhosis reduce the total plasma concentration of naproxen, but the plasma concentration of unbound naproxen is increased. Caution is advised when high doses are required and some adjustment of dosage may be required in elderly patients. As with other drugs used in the elderly, it is prudent to use the lowest effective dose.

Studies indicate that although total plasma concentration of naproxen is unchanged, the unbound plasma fraction of naproxen is increased in the elderly. Caution is advised when high doses are required and some adjustment of dosage may be required in elderly patients. As with other drugs used in the elderly, it is prudent to use the lowest effective dose.

As with other nonsteroidal anti-inflammatory drugs, borderline elevations of one or more liver function tests may occur in up to 15% of patients. These abnormalities may progress, may remain essentially unchanged, or may be transient with continued therapy. The SGPT (ALT) test is probably the most sensitive indicator of liver dysfunction. Meaningful (3 times the upper limit of normal) elevations of SGPT or SGOT (AST) occurred in controlled clinical trials in less than 1% of patients. A patient with symptoms and/or signs suggesting liver dysfunction, or in whom an abnormal liver test has occurred, should be evaluated for evidence of the development of more severe hepatic reactions while on therapy with this drug. Severe hepatic reactions, including jaundice and cases of fatal hepatitis, have been reported with this drug as with other nonsteroidal anti-inflammatory drugs. Although such reactions are rare, if abnormal liver tests persist or worsen, if clinical signs and symptoms consistent with liver disease develop, or if systemic manifestations occur (*e.g.,* eosinophilia, rash, etc.), this drug should be discontinued.

If steroid dosage is reduced or eliminated during therapy, the steroid dosage should be reduced slowly and the patients must be observed closely for any evidence of adverse effects, including adrenal insufficiency and exacerbation of symptoms of arthritis.

Patients with initial hemoglobin values of 10 grams or less who are to receive long-term therapy should have hemoglobin values determined periodically.

Peripheral edema has been observed in some patients. Since each naproxen sodium tablet contains approximately 25 mg (about 1 or 2 mEq) of sodium, this should be considered in patients whose overall intake of sodium must be markedly restricted. For these reasons, the drug should be used with caution in patients with fluid retention, hypertension or heart failure.

The antipyretic and anti-inflammatory activities of the drug may reduce fever and inflammation, thus diminishing their utility as diagnostic signs in detecting complications of presumed non-infectious, non-inflammatory painful conditions.

Because of adverse eye findings in animal studies with drugs of this class it is recommended that ophthalmic studies be carried out if any change or disturbance in vision occurs.

INFORMATION FOR THE PATIENT

Naproxen sodium, like other drugs of its class, is not free of side effects. The side effects of these drugs can cause discomfort and, rarely, there are more serious side effects, such as gastrointestinal bleeding, which may result in hospitalization and even fatal outcomes.

NSAIDs (Nonsteroidal Anti-Inflammatory Drugs) are often essential agents in the management of arthritis and have a major role in the treatment of pain, but they also may be commonly employed for conditions which are less serious.

PRECAUTIONS: *(cont'd)*

Physicians may wish to discuss with their patients the potential risks(see WARNINGS, PRECAUTIONS, and ADVERSE REACTIONS) and likely benefits of NSAID treatment, particularly when the drugs are used for less serious conditions where treatment without NSAIDs may represent an acceptable alternative to both the patient and physician.

Caution should be exercised by patients whose activities require alertness if they experience drowsiness, dizziness, vertigo or depression during therapy with the drug.

LABORATORY TESTS

Because serious GI tract ulceration and bleeding can occur without warning symptoms, physicians should follow chronically treated patients for the signs and symptoms of ulceration and bleeding and should inform them of the importance of this follow-up (see Risk of GI Ulcerations, Bleeding and Perforation with NSAID Therapy).

DRUG/LABORATORY TEST INTERACTIONS

The drug may decrease platelet aggregation and prolong bleeding time. This effect should be kept in mind when bleeding times are determined.

The administration of the drug may result in increased urinary values for 17-keratogenic steroids because of an interaction between the drug and/or its metabolites with m-dinitrobenzene used in this assay. Although 17 hydroxy-corticosteroid measurements (Porter-Silber test) do not appear to be artifactually altered, it is suggested that therapy with the drug be temporarily discontinued 72 hours before adrenal function tests are performed.

The drug may interfere with some urinary assays of 5-hydroxy indoleacetic acid (5HIAA).

CARCINOGENESIS

A two-year study was performed in rats to evaluate the carcinogenic potential of the drug. No evidence of carcinogenicity was found.

PREGNANCY CATEGORY B

Teratogenic Effects: Reproduction studies have been performed in rats, rabbits, and mice at doses up to six times the human dose and have revealed no evidence of impaired fertility or harm to the fetus due to the drug. There are, however, no adequate and well- controlled studies in pregnant women. Because animal reproduction studies are not always predictive of human response, the drug should not be used during pregnancy unless clearly needed. Because of the known effect of drugs of this class on the human fetal cardiovascular system (closure of ductus arteriosus), use during late pregnancy should be avoided.

Non-teratogenic Effects: As with other drugs known to inhibit prostaglandin synthesis, an increased incidence of dystocia and delayed parturition occurred in rats.

NURSING MOTHERS

The naproxen anion has been found in the milk of lactating women at a concentration of approximately 1% of that found in the plasma. Because of the possible adverse effects of prostaglandin-inhibiting drugs on neonates, use in nursing mothers should be avoided.

PEDIATRIC USE

Safety and effectiveness in children below the age of 2 years have not been established. Pediatric dosing recommendations for juvenile arthritis are based on well-controlled studies. There are no adequate effectiveness or dose-responsive data for other pediatric conditions, but the experience in juvenile arthritis and other use experience have established that single doses of 2.5-5 mg/kg (as naproxen suspension, see DOSAGE AND ADMINISTRATION), with total daily dose not exceeding 15 mg/kg/day, are safe in children over 2 years of age.

DRUG INTERACTIONS:

In vitro studies have shown that naproxen anion, because if its affinity for protein, may displace from their binding sites other drugs which are also albumin-bound. Theoretically, the naproxen anion itself could likewise be displaced. Short-term controlled studies failed to show that taking the drug significantly affects prothrombin times when administered to individuals on coumarin-type anticoagulants. Caution is advised nonetheless, since interactions have been seen with other nonsteroidal agents of this class. Similarly, patients receiving the drug and a hydantoin, sulfonamide or sulfonylurea should be observed for signs of toxicity to these drugs.

The natriuretic effect of furosemide has been reported to be inhibited by some drugs of this class. Inhibition of renal lithium clearance leading to increases in plasma lithium concentrations has also been reported.

This and other nonsteroidal anti-inflammatory drugs can reduce the antihypertensive effect of propranolol and other beta-blockers.

Probenecid given concurrently increases naproxen anion plasma levels and extends its plasma half-life significantly.

Caution should be used if this drug is administered concomitantly with methotrexate. Naproxen and other nonsteroidal anti-inflammatory drugs have been reported to reduce the tubular secretion of methotrexate in an animal model, possibly enhancing the toxicity of that drug.

ADVERSE REACTIONS:

The following adverse reactions are divided into three parts based on frequency and likelihood o causal relationship to naproxen sodium.

INCIDENCE GREATER THAN 1%

Probable Causal Relationship: Adverse reactions reported in controlled clinical trials in 960 patients treated for rheumatoid arthritis or osteoarthritis are listed below. In general, these reactions were reported 2 to 10 times more frequently than they were in studies in the 962 patients treated for mild to moderate pain or for dysmenorrhea.

A clinical study found gastrointestinal reactions to be more frequent and more severe in rheumatoid arthritis patients taking 1650 mg naproxen sodium daily compared to those taking 825 mg daily (see CLINICAL PHARMACOLOGY.)

In controlled clinical trials with about 80 children and in well monitored open studies with about 400 children with juvenile arthritis, the incidences of rash and prolonged bleeding times were increased, the incidences of gastrointestinal and central nervous system reactions were about the same, and the incidences of other reactions were lower in children than adults.

Gastrointestinal: The most frequent complaints reported related to the gastrointestinal tract. They were: constipation*, heartburn*, abdominal pain*, nausea*, dyspepsia, diarrhea, stomatitis.

Central Nervous System: Headache*, dizziness*, Drowsiness*, lightheadedness, vertigo.

Dermatologic: Itching (pruritus)*,skin eruption*, ecchymoses*, sweating, purpura.

Special Senses: Tinnitus*, hearing disturbances, visual disturbances.

Cardiovascular: Edema*, dyspnea*, palpitations.

General: Thirst.

* Incidence of reported reaction between 3% and 9%. Those reactions occurring in less than 3% of the patients are unmarked.

ADVERSE REACTIONS: *(cont'd)*

INCIDENCE LESS THAN 1%

Probable Causal Relationship: The following adverse reactions were reported less frequently than 1% during controlled clinical trials and through voluntary reports since marketing. The probability of a causal relationship exists between the drug and these adverse reactions.

Gastrointestinal: Abnormal liver function tests, gastrointestinal bleeding, hematemesis, jaundice, melena, peptic ulceration with bleeding and/or perforation, vomiting.

Renal: Glomerular nephritis, hematuria, intestinal nephritis, nephrotic syndrome, renal disease, renal failure, renal papillary necrosis.

Hematologic: Agranulocytosis, eosinophilia, granulocytopenia, leukopenia, thrombocytopenia.

Central Nervous System: Depression, dream abnormalities, inability to concentrate, insomnia, malaise, myalgia and muscle weakness.

Dermatologic: Alopecia, photosensitive dermatitis, skin rashes.

Special Senses: Hearing impairment.

Cardiovascular: Congestive heart failure.

General: Anaphylactoid reactions, menstrual disorders, pyrexia (chills and fever).

Causal Relationship Unknown: Other reactions have been reported in circumstances in which a causal relationship could not be established. However, in these rarely reported events, the possibility cannot be excluded. Therefore these observations are being listed to serve as alerting information to the physicians.

Hematologic: Aplastic anemia, hemolytic anemia.

Dermatologic: Epidermal necrolysis, erythema multiforme, photosensitivity reactions resembling porphyria cutanea tarda and epidermolysis bullosa, Stevens-Johnson syndrome, urticaria.

Gastrointestinal: Non-peptic gastrointestinal ulceration, ulcerative stomatitis.

Cardiovascular: Vasculitis.

General: Angioneurotic edema, hyperglycemia, hypoglycemia.

OVERDOSAGE:

Significant overdosage may be characterized by drowsiness, heartburn, indigestion, nausea or vomiting. Because naproxen sodium may be rapidly absorbed, high and early blood levels should be anticipated. A few patients have experienced seizures, but it is not clear whether or not these were drug related. It is not known what dose of the drug would be life threatening. The oral LD_{50} of the drug is 543 mg/kg in rats, 1234 mg/kg in mice, 4110 mg/kg in hamsters and greater than 1000 mg/kg in dogs.

Should a patient ingest a large number of tablets, accidentally or purposefully, the stomach may be emptied and usual supportive measures employed. In animals 0.5 g/kg of activated charcoal was effective in reducing plasma levels of naproxen. Hemodialysis does not decrease the plasma concentration of naproxen because of the high degree of its protein binding.

DOSAGE AND ADMINISTRATION:

For Mild to Moderate Pain, Primary Dysmenorrhea, and Acute Tendinitis and Bursitis: The recommended starting dose is 550 mg, followed by 275 mg every 6 to 8 hours, as required. The total daily dose should not exceed 5 tablets (1,375 mg).

For Rheumatoid Arthritis, Osteoarthritis, and Ankylosing Spondylitis: The recommended dose in adults is 275 mg or 550 mg twice daily (morning and evening). During long-term administration, the dose may be adjusted up or down depending on the clinical response of the patient. A lower daily dose may suffice for long-term administration. The morning and evening doses do not have to be equal in size and the administration of the drug more frequently than twice daily is not necessary.

In patients who tolerate lower doses well, the dose may be increased to 1650 mg per day for limited periods when a higher level of anti- inflammatory/analgesic activity is required. When treating such patients with the 1650 mg/day dose, the physician should observe sufficient increased clinical benefits to offset the potential increased risk (see CLINICAL PHARMACOLOGY.)

Symptomatic improvement in arthritis usually begins within two weeks. However, if improvement is not seen within this period, a trial for an additional two weeks should be considered.

For Acute Gout: The recommended starting dose is 825 mg, followed by 275 mg every eight hours until the attack has subsided.

For Juvenile Arthritis: The recommended total daily dose is approximately 10 mg/kg given in two divided doses. The 275 mg naproxen sodium tablet is not well suited to this dosage so use of the related drug naproxen as the 250 mg scored tablet or the 125 mg/5 ml suspension is recommended for this indication.

Storage: Store at room temperature in well-closed containers.

HOW SUPPLIED - RATED THERAPEUTICALLY EQUIVALENT:

Tablet, Uncoated - Oral - 275 mg

100's	$14.70	Naproxen Sodium, H.C.F.A. F F P	99999-1865-01
100's	$14.93	Naproxen Sodium, United Res	00677-1513-01
100's	$60.00	Naproxen Sodium, Roxane	00054-4638-25
100's	$60.00	Naproxen Sodium, Roxane	00054-8638-25
100's	$66.85	Naproxen Sodium, Teva	00093-0536-01
100's	$66.85	Naproxen Sodium, Major Pharms	00904-7802-60
100's	$66.86	Naproxen Sodium, Rugby	00536-5606-01
100's	$66.86	Naproxen Sodium, Invamed	52189-0286-24
100's	$66.86	Naproxen Sodium, Hamilton Pharma	60322-0284-42
100's	$66.89	Naproxen Sodium, HL Moore Drug Exch	00839-7889-06
100's	$66.90	Naproxen Sodium, Qualitest Pharms	00603-4733-21
100's	$66.90	Naproxen Sodium, Qualitest Pharms	00603-4753-21
100's	$66.90	Naproxen Sodium, Mova Pharms	55370-0525-07
100's	$66.90	Naproxen Sodium, Novopharm (US)	55953-0531-40
100's	$66.92	Naproxen Sodium, Aligen Independ	00405-4711-01
100's	$67.90	Naproxen Sodium, Martec Pharms	52555-0587-01
100's	$68.65	Naproxen Sodium, Novopharm (US)	55953-0531-41
100's	$68.70	Naproxen Sodium, Vangard Labs	00615-3579-13
100's	$71.50	Naproxen Sodium, Schein Pharm (US)	00364-2553-01
100's	$71.51	Naproxen Sodium, Zenith Labs	00172-4116-60
100's	$71.51	Naproxen Sodium, Goldline Labs	00182-1974-01
100's	$71.51	Naproxen Sodium, Rugby	00536-4841-01
100's	$71.51	Naproxen Sodium, Geneva Pharms	00781-1187-01
100's	$73.70	Naproxen Sodium, Mylan	00378-0537-01
100's	$74.51	Naproxen Sodium, Geneva Pharms	00781-1187-13
100's	**$79.50**	**ANAPROX, Syntex PR**	**18393-0274-42**
500's	$73.50	Naproxen Sodium, H.C.F.A. F F P	99999-1865-02
500's	$300.00	Naproxen Sodium, Roxane	00054-4638-29
500's	$322.70	Naproxen Sodium, Teva	00093-0536-05
500's	$322.70	Naproxen Sodium, Schein Pharm (US)	00364-2553-05
500's	$322.70	Naproxen Sodium, Rugby	00536-5606-05
500's	$322.70	Naproxen Sodium, Major Pharms	00904-7802-40
500's	$322.70	Naproxen Sodium, Invamed	52189-0286-29

HOW SUPPLIED - RATED THERAPEUTICALLY EQUIVALENT: *(cont'd)*

500's	$322.70	Naproxen Sodium, Hamilton Pharma	60322-0284-62
500's	$322.72	Naproxen Sodium, HL Moore Drug Exch	00839-7879-12
500's	$322.72	Naproxen Sodium, HL Moore Drug Exch	00839-7889-12
500's	$322.75	Naproxen Sodium, Mova Pharms	55370-0525-08
500's	$322.75	Naproxen Sodium, Novopharm (US)	55953-0531-70
500's	$324.90	Naproxen Sodium, Aligen Independ	00405-4711-02
500's	$327.60	Naproxen Sodium, Martec Pharms	52555-0587-05
500's	$345.16	Naproxen Sodium, Zenith Labs	00172-4116-70
500's	$345.16	Naproxen Sodium, Goldline Labs	00182-1974-05
500's	$355.70	Naproxen Sodium, Mylan	00378-0537-05
500's	$357.55	Naproxen Sodium, Rugby	00536-4841-05
500's	**$383.72**	**ANAPROX, Syntex PR**	**18393-0274-62**
1000's	$147.00	Naproxen Sodium, H.C.F.A. F F P	99999-1865-03
1000's	$613.25	Naproxen Sodium, Novopharm (US)	55953-0531-80
1000's	$626.00	Naproxen Sodium, Teva	00093-0536-10
1000's	$626.00	Naproxen Sodium, Invamed	52189-0286-30
1000's	$626.04	Naproxen Sodium, Geneva Pharms	00781-1187-10

Tablet, Uncoated - Oral - 550 mg

100's	$24.23	Naproxen Sodium, United Res	00677-1514-01
100's	$24.38	Naproxen Sodium, H.C.F.A. F F P	99999-1865-04
100's	$83.35	Aflaxen, Intl Ethical	11584-0465-01
100's	$90.00	Naproxen Sodium, Roxane	00054-4639-25
100's	$100.00	Naproxen Sodium, Roxane	00054-8639-25
100's	$103.65	Naproxen Sodium, Qualitest Pharms	00603-4734-21
100's	$104.05	Naproxen Sodium, Teva	00093-0537-01
100's	$104.05	Naproxen Sodium, Major Pharms	00904-7803-60
100's	$104.09	Naproxen Sodium, Rugby	00536-5607-01
100's	$104.09	Naproxen Sodium, HL Moore Drug Exch	00839-7890-06
100's	$104.09	Naproxen Sodium, Hamilton Pharma	60322-0286-42
100's	$104.15	Naproxen Sodium, Mova Pharms	55370-0526-07
100's	$104.15	Naproxen Sodium, Novopharm (US)	55953-0533-40
100's	$104.23	Naproxen Sodium, Aligen Independ	00405-4712-01
100's	$104.90	Naproxen Sodium, Invamed	52189-0287-24
100's	$105.45	Naproxen Sodium, Vangard Labs	00615-3580-13
100's	$105.70	Naproxen Sodium, Martec Pharms	52555-0588-01
100's	$105.90	Naproxen Sodium, Novopharm (US)	55953-0533-41
100's	$109.29	Naproxen Sodium, Schein Pharm (US)	00364-2554-01
100's	$111.34	Naproxen Sodium, Zenith Labs	00172-4275-60
100's	$111.34	Naproxen Sodium, Goldline Labs	00182-1975-01
100's	$111.34	Naproxen Sodium, Rugby	00536-4848-01
100's	$111.36	Naproxen Sodium, Geneva Pharms	00781-1188-01
100's	$114.74	Naproxen Sodium, Mylan	00378-0733-01
100's	$116.05	Naproxen Sodium, Geneva Pharms	00781-1188-13
100's	**$123.78**	**ANAPROX DS, Syntex PR**	**18393-0276-42**
500's	$121.15	Naproxen Sodium, United Res	00677-1514-05
500's	$121.90	Naproxen Sodium, H.C.F.A. F F P	99999-1865-05
500's	$450.00	Naproxen Sodium, Roxane	00054-4639-29
500's	$494.37	Naproxen Sodium, Qualitest Pharms	00603-4734-28
500's	$502.55	Naproxen Sodium, Teva	00093-0537-05
500's	$502.55	Naproxen Sodium, Major Pharms	00904-7803-40
500's	$502.56	Naproxen Sodium, Schein Pharm (US)	00364-2554-05
500's	$502.56	Naproxen Sodium, Rugby	00536-5607-05
500's	$502.56	Naproxen Sodium, Invamed	52189-0287-29
500's	$502.56	Naproxen Sodium, Hamilton Pharma	60322-0286-62
500's	$502.59	Naproxen Sodium, HL Moore Drug Exch	00839-7890-12
500's	$502.65	Naproxen Sodium, Mova Pharms	55370-0526-08
500's	$502.65	Naproxen Sodium, Novopharm (US)	55953-0533-70
500's	$505.32	Naproxen Sodium, Aligen Independ	00405-4712-02
500's	$510.20	Naproxen Sodium, Martec Pharms	52555-0588-05
500's	$537.53	Naproxen Sodium, Zenith Labs	00172-4275-70
500's	$537.53	Naproxen Sodium, Goldline Labs	00182-1975-05
500's	$537.53	Naproxen Sodium, Rugby	00536-4848-05
500's	$553.94	Naproxen Sodium, Mylan	00378-0733-05
500's	**$597.59**	**ANAPROX DS, Syntex PR**	**18393-0276-62**
1000's	$243.80	Naproxen Sodium, H.C.F.A. F F P	99999-1865-06
1000's	$955.00	Naproxen Sodium, Novopharm (US)	55953-0533-80
1000's	$974.90	Naproxen Sodium, Teva	00093-0537-10
1000's	$974.90	Naproxen Sodium, Invamed	52189-0287-30
1000's	$974.97	Naproxen Sodium, Geneva Pharms	00781-1188-10

HOW SUPPLIED - NOT RATED EQUIVALENT:

Tablet, Uncoated - Oral - 275 mg

100's	$66.90	Naproxen Sodium, West Point Pharma	59591-0256-68

Tablet, Uncoated - Oral - 550 mg

100's	$104.10	Naproxen Sodium, West Point Pharma	59591-0258-68

NATAMYCIN *(001866)*

CATEGORIES: Anti-Infectives; Antibiotics; Antifungals; Conjunctivitis; EENT Drugs; Eye, Ear, Nose, & Throat Preparations; Keratitis; Ocular Blepharitis; Ocular Infections; Ophthalmics; FDA Approval Pre 1982

BRAND NAMES: **Natacyn**

FORMULARIES: Medi-Cal

DESCRIPTION:

Natamycin 5% Ophthalmic Suspension is a sterile, anti-fungal drug for topical ophthalmic administration.

Established name: Natamycin

Chemical name: Stereoisomer of 22-((3-amino-3,6-dideoxy- β-D-mannopyranosyl)oxy)-1,3,26-trihydroxy-12-methyl-10-oxo-6,11,28-trioxatricyclo(22.3.1.$0^{5,7}$) octacosa-8,14,16,18,20-pentaene-25-carboxylic acid.

Other: pimaricin

Each ml of the suspension contains: Active: natamycin 5% (50 mg/ml). Preservative: benzalkonium chloride 0.02%. Inactive: sodium hydroxide and hydrochloric acid (neutralized to adjust the pH); purified water.

CLINICAL PHARMACOLOGY:

Natamycin is a tetraene polyene antibiotic derived from *Streptomyces natalensis.* It possesses *in vitro* activity against a variety of yeast and filamentous fungi, including *Candida, Aspergillus, Cephalosporium, Fusarium,* and *Penicillium.* The mechanism of action appears to be through binding of the molecule to the sterol moiety of the fungal cell membrane. The polyenesterol complex alters the permeability of the membrane to produce depletion of essential cellular constituents. Although the activity against fungi is dose-related, natamycin is predominantly fungicidal.[9] Natamycin is not effective *in vitro* against gram-positive or gram-

CLINICAL PHARMACOLOGY: *(cont'd)*

negative bacteria. Topical administration appears to produce effective concentrations of natamycin within the corneal stroma, but not in intraocular fluid. Natamycin is not absorbed from the gastrointestinal tract. Systemic absorption should not be expected following topical administration of natamycin 5% ophthalmic suspension. As with other polyene antibiotics, absorption from the gastrointestinal tract is very poor. Studies in rabbits receiving topical natamycin revealed no measurable compound in the aqueous humor or sera but the sensitivity of the measurement was no greater than 2 mg/ml.

INDICATIONS AND USAGE:

Natamycin 5% ophthalmic suspension is indicated for treatment of fungal blepharitis, conjunctivitis, and keratitis caused by susceptible organisms. Natamycin has proven to be the initial drug of choice in *Fusarium solani* keratitis. As in other forms of suppurative keratitis, initial and sustained therapy of fungal keratitis should be determined by the clinical diagnosis, laboratory diagnosis by smear and culture of corneal scrapings, and drug response. Whenever possible, the *in vitro* activity of natamycin against the responsible fungus should be determined. The effectiveness of natamycin as a single agent in fungal endophthalmitis has not been established.

CONTRAINDICATIONS:

Natamycin 5% Ophthalmic Suspension is contraindicated in individuals with a history of hypersensitivity to any of its components.

PRECAUTIONS:

GENERAL

For topical eye use only. NOT FOR INJECTION. Failure of improvement of keratitis following 7-10 days of administration of the drug suggests that the infection may be caused by a microorganism not susceptible to natamycin.

Continuation of therapy should be based on clinical reevaluation and additional laboratory studies.

Adherence of the suspension to areas of epithelial ulceration or retention of the suspension in the fornices occurs regularly. There has only been a limited number of cases in which natamycin has been used, therefore, it is possible that adverse reactions of which we have no knowledge at present may occur. For this reason, patients on this drug should be monitored at least twice weekly. Should suspicion of drug toxicity occur, the drug should be discontinued.

INFORMATION FOR THE PATIENT

Do not touch dropper tip to any surface, as this may contaminate the suspension.

CARCINOGENESIS, MUTAGENESIS, AND IMPAIRMENT OF FERTILITY

There have been no long-term studies done using natamycin in animals to evaluate carcinogenesis, mutagenesis, or impairment of fertility.

PREGNANCY CATEGORY C

Animal reproduction studies have not been conducted with natamycin. It is also not known whether natamycin can cause fetal harm when administered to a pregnant or nursing woman or can affect reproduction capacity. Natamycin 5% ophthalmic suspension should be given to a pregnant woman only if clearly needed.

NURSING MOTHERS

It is not known whether these drugs are excreted in human milk. Because many drugs are excreted in human milk, caution should be exercised when natamycin is administered to a nursing woman.

PEDIATRIC USE

Safety and effectiveness in children have not been established.

ADVERSE REACTIONS:

One case of conjunctival chemosis and hyperemia, thought to be allergic in nature, has been reported.

DOSAGE AND ADMINISTRATION:

SHAKE WELL BEFORE USING. The preferred initial dosage in fungal keratitis is one drop of natamycin 5% ophthalmic suspension instilled in the conjunctival sac at hourly or two-hourly intervals. The frequency of application can be usually be reduced to one drop 6 to 8 times daily after the first 3 to 4 days. Therapy should generally be continued for 14 to 21 days or until there is resolution of active fungal keratitis. In many cases, it may be helpful to reduce the dosage gradually at 4 to 7 day intervals to assure that the replicating organism has been eliminated. Less frequent initial dosage (4 to 6 daily applications) may be sufficient in fungal blepharitis and conjunctivitis.

Storage: May be stored in refrigerator (35-48°F) or at room temperature (46-80°F). *Do not freeze.* Avoid exposure to light and excessive heat. SHAKE WELL BEFORE USING.

REFERENCES:

1. Barckhausen, B.: Die Behandlung der Probleminfektionen das vorderen Augenabschnittes in der Praxis. Landarzt 46:842, 1970. **2.** Cuendet, J. F.; Nouri, A.: Traitement local en ophtalmologie par un nouvel antibiotique fungicide, la "pimaricin." Ophthalmologica 145:297, 1963. **23.** Forster, R. K.; Rebell, G.: "The Diagnosis and Management of Keratomycoses," Arch. Ophth. 93:1134, 1975. **4.** Francois, J.; de Vos, E.: Traitement des mycoses oculaires par la pimaricin. Bull. Soc. beige Ophthal. 131:382, 1962. **5.** Jones, D. B.; Sexton, R.; Rebell, G.: "Mycotic keratitis in South Florida: A Review of Thirty-nine Cases." Transactions ophthal. Soc. U.K. 89:781, 1969. **6.** Jones, D. B.; Forster, R. K.; Rebell, G.: "*Fusarium solani*keratitis treated with Natamycin (pimaricin), 18 consecutive cases." Arch. Ophth. 88:147, 1972. **7.** L'Editeur: Traitment des mycoses oculaires. Presse med. 77:147, 1969. **8.** Vozza, R.; Bagolini, B.: Su di un caso di grave ulcerazione bilaterale delle palpebra de Candida albicans. Bol. Oculist. 43:433, 1964.(Alcon, 2/92, 298904)

HOW SUPPLIED - EQUIVALENTS NOT AVAILABLE:

Suspension - Ophthalmic - 5 %

15 ml $93.75 NATACYN, Alcon 00065-0645-15

NEDOCROMIL SODIUM *(003084)*

CATEGORIES: Airway Obstruction; Anti-Inflammatory Agents; Antiasthmatics/Bronchodilators; Asthma; Respiratory & Allergy Medications; Pregnancy Category B; FDA Class 1S ("Standard Review"); FDA Approved 1992 Dec

BRAND NAMES: *Corotrop* (Germany); *Corotrope* (France); **Primacor**
(International brand names outside U.S. in italics)

PRIMARY ICD9: 493.90 (Asthma, Unspecified, Without Mention of Status Asthmaticus)

DESCRIPTION:

Nedocromil sodium is an inhaled anti-inflammatory agent for the preventive management of asthma. Nedocromil sodium is a pyranoquinoline with the chemical name 4H-Pyrano[3,2-g]quinoline-2,8-dicarboxylic acid, 9-ethyl-6,9-dihydro-4,6-dioxo-10-propyl-, disodium salt, and it has a molecular weight of 415.3. The empirical formula is $C_{19}H_{15}NNa_2O_7$. Nedocromil sodium, a yellow powder, is soluble in water.

Chemical Class: Pyranoquinoline.

Nedocromil sodium inhalation aerosol is a pressurized metered-dose aerosol suspension for oral inhalation containing micronized nedocromil sodium, sorbitan trioleate with dichlorotetrafluoroethane and dichlorodifluoromethane as propellants. Each actuation delivers from the mouthpiece 1.75 mg nedocromil sodium. Each 16.2 g canister provides at least 104 metered inhalations.

CLINICAL PHARMACOLOGY:

Cellular and Animal Studies: Nedocromil sodium has been shown to inhibit the *in vitro* activation of, and mediator release from, a variety of inflammatory cell types associated with asthma, including eosinophils, neutrophils, macrophages, mast cells, monocytes, and platelets. *In vitro* studies on cells obtained by bronchoalveolar lavage from antigen-sensitized macaque monkeys show that nedocromil sodium inhibits the release of mediators including histamine, leukotriene C_4 and prostaglandin D_2. Similar studies with human bronchoalveolar cells showed inhibition of histamine release from the mast cells and beta-glucuronidase release from macrophages.

Nedocromil sodium has been tested in experimental models of asthma using allergic animals and shown to inhibit the development of early and late bronchoconstriction responses to inhaled antigen. The development of airway hyper-responsiveness to nonspecific bronchoconstrictors was also inhibited. Nedocromil sodium reduced antigen-induced increases in airway microvasculature leakage when administered intravenously in a model system.

Pharmacokinetics and Bioavailability: Systemic bioavailability of nedocromil sodium administered as an inhaled aerosol is low. In a single dose study involving 20 healthy subjects who were administered a 3.5 mg dose of nedocromil sodium (2 actuations of 1.75 mg each), the mean AUC was 5.0 ng X hr/ml and the mean Cmax was 1.6 ng/ml attained about 28 minutes after dosing. The mean half life was 3.3 hours. Urinary excretion over 12 hours averaged 3.4% of the administered dose, of which approximately 75% was excreted in the first six hours of dosing.

In a multiple dose study, six healthy volunteers (3 males and 3 females) received a 3.5 mg single dose followed by 3.5 mg four times a day for seven consecutive days. Accumulation of the drug was not observed. Following single and multiple dose inhalations, urinary excretion of nedocromil accounted for 5.6% and 12% of the drug administered, respectively. After intravenous administration, urinary excretion of nedocromil was approximately 70%. The absolute bioavailability of nedocromil was thus 8% (5.6/70) for single and 17% (12/70) for multiple inhaled doses.

Similarly, in a multiple dose study of 12 asthmatic patients, each given a 3.5 mg single dose followed by 3.5 mg four times a day for one month, both single dose and multiple dose inhalation gave a mean high plasma concentration of 2.8 ng/ml between 5 and 90 minutes, mean AUC of 5.6 ng X hr/ml, and a mean terminal half life of 1.5 hours. The mean 24-hour urinary excretion after either single or multiple dose administration represented approximately 5% of the administered dose.

Studies involving very high oral doses of nedocromil (600 mg single dose, and subsequently 200 mg three times a day for seven days), showed an absolute bioavailability of less than 2%. In a radiolabeled (^{14}C) nedocromil study involving two healthy males, urinary excretion accounted for 64% of the dose, fecal excretion for 36%.

Protein Binding: Nedocromil is approximately 89% protein bound to human plasma over a concentration range of 0.5 to 50 mcg/ml. This binding is reversible.

Metabolism: Nedocromil is not metabolized after IV administration and is excreted unchanged.

CLINICAL STUDIES:

Nedocromil sodium has been shown to inhibit acutely the bronchoconstrictor response to several kinds of challenge. Pretreatment with single doses of nedocromil sodium inhibited the bronchoconstriction caused by sulfur dioxide, inhaled neurokinin A, various antigens, exercise, cold air, fog, and adenosine monophosphate.

Nedocromil sodium has no intrinsic bronchodilator, antihistamine, or glucocorticoid activity.

Nedocromil sodium, when delivered by inhalation at the recommended dose, has no known therapeutic systemic activity.

The worldwide clinical trial experience with nedocromil sodium comprises 5352 patients. Studies have been conducted both at twice daily and at four times daily dosage regimens. Evidence from these studies indicates that the four times daily regimen has been more effective than the twice daily regimen. A lower dose (two or three times daily) can be considered in patients under good control on the four times daily regimen (see DOSAGE AND ADMINISTRATION.)

Nedocromil sodium vs. Placebo: The effectiveness of nedocromil sodium given four times daily was examined in a 14 week double-blind, placebo-controlled, parallel group trial in five centers in 120 patients (60/treatment). To be eligible for entry, the asthmatic patients had to be controlled using only sustained-release theophylline (SRT) and beta-agonists. Two weeks after the test therapies were begun the SRT was discontinued and four weeks after that oral beta-agonists were stopped. Beta-agonist metered dose inhalers could still be used after 6 weeks. Efficacy was assessed by symptom scores recorded on diary cards completed on a daily basis by the patients. Each morning the patient recorded nighttime asthma on a 0-2 scale, (0=slept well, no asthma; 1=woke once because of asthma; 2=woke more than once because of asthma). Before bedtime the patients recorded daytime asthma and cough on a 0-5 scale (0=no symptoms or asthma/cough today; 5=asthma/cough symptoms were noticed most of the day and caused a lot of trouble). At the end of the treatment phase, patients and clinicians were asked for their opinions on the effectiveness of the treatment based on a five point scale (1=very effective; 5=made condition worse). The results of these evaluations are shown in TABLE 1; Nedocromil sodium was significantly superior to placebo for all measurements.

The FEV_1 percentage change relative to baseline also favored nedocromil sodium over placebo throughout the study, with an effect seen first at the two week measurement. (For graphic representation of this data, please refer to manufacturer's original package insert).

This study shows that nedocromil sodium improves symptom control and pulmonary function when it is added to a prn inhaled beta-adrenergic bronchodilator regimen and that a beneficial effect could be detected within two weeks.

Nedocromil sodium vs. Cromolyn Sodium vs. Placebo: The effectiveness of nedocromil sodium was compared to cromolyn sodium and placebo in an eight week, double-blind, parallel group, 12 center trial during which medication was given four times daily. Three hundred and six patients were randomized to treatment (103/nedocromil sodium; 104/cromolyn sodium; 99/placebo). All patients were SRT dependent and this drug was stopped prior to starting the test treatment. Efficacy was assessed on the basis of diary card symptom scores and FEV_1. The diary scores were the same as used in the 14 week study except that nighttime

CLINICAL STUDIES: *(cont'd)*

TABLE 1

Variable	Time Period	Tilade Mean	Placebo Mean
Daytime Asthma[1]	Weeks 7-14	1.26	2.08
Nighttime Asthma[2]	Weeks 7-14	0.67	0.96
Cough[1]	Weeks 7-14	0.68	1.49
Patient's Opinion[2]	Week 14	2.27	3.55
Clinician's Opinion[2]	Week 14	2.13	3.48
FEV_1[2] (liters)	Week 2	2.69	2.18
$FEV_1$2 (liters)	Week 6	2.65	2.15
FEV_1[2] (liters)	Week 10	2.55	2.15
FEV_1[2] (liters)	Week 14	2.59	2.10

1 Tilade significantly better than placebo, $p<0.05$
2 Tilade significantly better than placebo, $p<0.01$

symptoms were recorded on a 0-3 scale. The primary efficacy variable was a summary symptom score derived by averaging the scores for daytime asthma, nighttime asthma and cough. The results of the study are shown in TABLE 2.

TABLE 2

Variable	Time Period	Tilade Mean	Placebo Mean	Cromolyn Sodium Mean
Summary Score[1]	Weeks 3-8	1.30	1.76	1.13
Daytime Asthma[1]	Weeks 3-8	1.59	2.05	1.41
Nighttime Asthma[2]	Weeks 3-8	0.91	1.23	0.77
Cough[3]	Weeks 3-8	1.11	1.58	0.93
FEV_1[1]	Weeks 3-8	2.46	2.23	2.56
Patient's Opinion[1]	Week 8	2.54	3.39	2.22
Clinician's Opinion[1]	Week 8	2.60	3.43	2.39

1 Tilade significantly better than Placebo, $p<0.001$
2 Tilade significantly better than Placebo, $p<0.01$, cromolyn sodium significantly better than Tilade, $p<0.05$
3 Tilade significantly better than Placebo, $p<0.05$

This study corroborates the findings of the 14 week study, showing that nedocromil sodium is effective in the management of symptoms and pulmonary function in primary atopic mild to moderate asthmatics. Both active treatments were statistically significantly better than placebo for the primary efficacy variable (summary symptom score); nedocromil sodium and cromolyn sodium were not significantly different for this parameter. A statistically significant difference favoring cromolyn sodium was, however, seen for nighttime asthma and FEV_1.

In laboratory studies, pretreatment with nedocromil sodium before an anticipated challenge can prevent the bronchoconstriction associated with sulfur dioxide, cold air, fog, exercise, allergen challenge, adenosine monophosphate, and neurokinin A. Controlled studies have not been carried out to assess the clinical significance of these findings.

In allergic asthmatics who are well controlled on cromolyn sodium, there is no evidence that the substitution of nedocromil sodium for cromolyn sodium would confer additional benefit to the patient. Efficacy with one agent is not known to be predictive of efficacy with the other.

The presently available data on the relative efficacy of nedocromil sodium and cromolyn sodium are inconclusive.

INDICATIONS AND USAGE:

Nedocromil sodium Inhaler is indicated for maintenance therapy in the management of patients with mild to moderate bronchial asthma. Nedocromil sodium is not indicated for the reversal of acute bronchospasm.

CONTRAINDICATIONS:

Nedocromil sodium inhaler is contraindicated in those patients who have shown hypersensitivity to nedocromil sodium or other ingredients in this preparation.

WARNINGS:

Nedocromil sodium Inhaler is not a bronchodilator and, therefore, should not be used for the reversal of acute bronchospasm, particularly status asthmaticus. Nedocromil sodium should ordinarily be continued during acute exacerbations, unless the patient becomes intolerant to the use of inhaled dosage forms.

As with other inhaled asthma medications, paradoxical bronchospasm, which can be life-threatening, has been reported rarely in postmarketing experience. If it occurs, discontinue treatment with nedocromil sodium immediately and institute alternative therapy.

PRECAUTIONS:

General: If systemic or inhaled steroid therapy is at all reduced, patients must be monitored carefully. Nedocromil sodium has not been shown to be able to substitute for the total dose of steroids.

Information for the Patient: Nedocromil sodium must be taken regularly to achieve benefit, even during symptom-free periods. Because the therapeutic effect depends upon topical application to the lungs, it is essential that patients be properly instructed in the correct method of use (see PATIENT PACKAGE INSERT.) An illustrated leaflet for the patient is included in each nedocromil sodium inhaler pack

Carcinogenesis, Mutagenesis, and Impairment of Fertility: A two-year inhalation chronic/carcinogenicity study of nedocromil sodium in Wistar rats showed no carcinogenic potential. The maximum achievable daily dose of 24 mg/kg corresponded to 86 times the maximum human daily aerosol dose of 0.28 mg/kg (based on eight actuations of 1.75 mg to a 50 kg person). Assuming 5% systemic absorption in man, and comparing calculated exposure to measured exposure in rats, systemic exposure in rats in this study was about 40 times human exposure. A 21-month oral dietary carcinogenicity study of nedocromil sodium performed in B6C3F1 mice with daily doses up to 180 mg/kg showed no carcinogenic potential. Systemic exposure in the mouse, calculated as above for the rats, was about six times that in humans, or about 20 times that in humans based on free drug concentrations in plasma. The exposure of the GI tract in top dose animals corresponded to 643 times the human daily dose since, in man, most of an inhaled dose is subsequently swallowed.

Nedocromil sodium showed no mutagenic potential in the Ames Salmonella/microsome plate assay, mitotic gene conversion in *S. cerevisiae,* mouse lymphoma forward mutation and mouse micronucleus assays.

Reproduction and fertility studies in mice and rats showed no effects on male or female fertility at subcutaneous doses of 100 mg/kg/day.

PRECAUTIONS: *(cont'd)*

Pregnancy Category B: Reproduction studies performed in mice, rats, and rabbits using subcutaneous doses of 100 mg/kg/day, revealed no evidence of impaired fertility or harm to the fetus due to nedocromil sodium. There are, however, no adequate and well-controlled studies in pregnant women. Because animal reproduction studies are not always predictive of human response, this drug should be used during pregnancy only if clearly needed.

Nursing Mothers: It is not known whether this drug is excreted in human milk. Because many drugs are excreted in human milk, caution should be exercised when nedocromil sodium is administered to a nursing woman.

Pediatric Use: Safety and effectiveness in children below the age of 12 years have not been established.

DRUG INTERACTIONS:

Nedocromil sodium has been co-administered with other anti-asthma therapies including inhaled and oral bronchodilators and inhaled corticosteroids. There are no known adverse drug interactions.

ADVERSE REACTIONS:

Nedocromil sodium is generally well tolerated. Adverse event information was derived from 5352 patients receiving nedocromil sodium in controlled and open-label clinical trials of 2-52 weeks in duration. A total of 3538 patients received two inhalations four times a day. An additional 1814 patients received two inhalations twice daily or some other dose regimen. Seventy-three percent of patients were exposed to study drug for eight weeks or longer.

Of the 3538 patients who received two inhalations of nedocromil sodium four times a day, 2042 were in placebo-controlled trials and of these 7% withdrew from the trials due to adverse events, compared to 6% of the 1875 patients who received placebo.

The reasons for withdrawal were generally similar in the nedocromil sodium and placebo-treated groups, except that patients withdrew due to bad taste statistically more frequently on nedocromil sodium than on placebo. Headache reported as severe or very severe was experienced by 1.2 percent of nedocromil sodium patients and 0.9 percent of placebo patients, some with nausea and ill feeling.

The events reported with a frequency of 1% or greater across all placebo-controlled studies are displayed below (TABLE 3) for all patients who received nedocromil sodium or placebo at two inhalations four times daily.

TABLE 3

Adverse Event	% Experiencing AE Tilade (n=2042)	Placebo (n=1875)	% Withdrawing Tilade	Placebo
Special Senses				
Unpleasant Taste*	12.6%	3.6%	2.1%	0.4%
Respiratory System Disorders				
Coughing	7.0	7.2	1.4	1.4
Pharyngitis	5.7	5.0	0.6	0.5
Rhinitis*	4.6	3.0	0.1	0.1
Upper Respiratory Tract Infection*	3.9	2.4	0.1	0.1
Sputum Increased	1.7	1.4	0.1	0.2
Bronchitis	1.2	1.3	0.1	0.1
Dyspnea	2.8	3.8	0.9	1.3
Bronchospasm**	5.4	8.2	1.5	2.3
Gastro-Intestinal Tract				
Nausea*	4.0%	2.1%	1.3%	0.7%
Vomiting*	1.7	0.9	0.2	0.4
Dyspepsia*	1.3	0.6	0.1	0.1
Mouth Dry	1.0	0.9	0.1	0.2
Diarrhea	0.9	0.6	0.1	0.0
Abdominal Pain*	1.2	0.5	0.2	0.1
Central and Peripheral Nervous System				
Dizziness	0.9	1.2	0.1	0.2
Dysphonia	1.0	0.6	0.1	0.1
Body as a Whole				
Headache	6.0	4.7	0.5	0.3
Chest Pain	4.0	3.9	0.9	0.6
Fatigue	1.1	0.7	0.2	0.1
Resistance Mechanism Disorders				
Infection Viral	2.4	3.4	0.1	0.1

* Statistically significant ($p\leq0.05$) higher frequency of events on Tilade.
** Statistically significant ($p\leq0.05$) higher frequency of events on Placebo.
Table includes data from double-blind group comparative studies at four times per day dosing.

Other adverse events present at less than the 1% level of occurrence, but that might be related to nedocromil sodium administration, include rash, arthritis, tremor and a sensation of warmth.

Elevations of SGPT were noted in 3.3% of patients on nedocromil sodium vs. 1.7% on placebo. The average elevation over placebo was 10 I.U. with only two patients increasing by more than 100 I.U. and none becoming ill. The clinical significance of these elevations is unclear.

Rare cases of paradoxical bronchospasm (see WARNINGS) have been reported from post-marketing experience. Isolated cases of pneumonitis with eosinophilia (PIE syndrome) and anaphylaxis have also been reported in which a relationship to drug is undetermined.

OVERDOSAGE:

There is no experience to date with overdose of nedocromil sodium in humans. Animal studies by several routes of administration (inhalation, oral, intravenous, subcutaneous) have demonstrated little potential for significant toxicity in humans from inhalation of high doses of nedocromil sodium. Head shaking/tremor and salivation were observed in beagle dogs following daily inhalation doses of 5 mg/kg and transient hypotension was detected following daily subcutaneous doses of 8 mg/kg. In addition, clonic convulsions were observed in dogs following daily inhalation doses of 20 mg/kg plus subcutaneous doses of 20 mg/kg giving peak plasma levels of 7.6 mcg/ml, some three orders of magnitude greater than peak plasma levels (2.5 ng/ml) of the human daily dose. Specific tests designed to evaluate CNS activity demonstrated no effects due to nedocromil sodium, and nedocromil sodium does not pass the blood brain barrier. Therefore, overdosage is unlikely to result in clinical manifestations requiring more than observation and discontinuation of the drug where appropriate.

DOSAGE AND ADMINISTRATION:

The recommended dosage for symptomatic adults and children (12 years of age and over) is two inhalations four times a day at regular intervals to provide 14 mg of nedocromil sodium per day. Maintenance therapy should be initiated at the same dose. In patients under good control on four times daily dosing (*i.e.,* patients whose only medication need is occasional [not more than twice a week] inhaled or oral beta-agonists, and who have no serious

DOSAGE AND ADMINISTRATION: *(cont'd)*

exacerbations with respiratory infections) a lower dose can be tried. If use of lower doses is attempted, nedocromil sodium should first be reduced to a three times daily regimen (10.5 mg of nedocromil sodium per day) then, after several weeks on continued good control, to twice a day (7 mg of nedocromil sodium per day).

Nedocromil sodium inhaler should be added to the patient's existing treatment regimen (*e.g.,* bronchodilators). When a clinical response to nedocromil sodium Inhaler is evident and if the asthma is under good control, an attempt may be made to decrease concomitant medication usage gradually.

Proper inhalational technique is essential (see PATIENT PACKAGE INSERT.)

Patients should be advised that the optimal effect of nedocromil sodium therapy depends upon its administration at regular intervals, even during symptom-free periods.

PATIENT PACKAGE INSERT:

Metered-Dose Inhaler: The following is one of several acceptable inhalation techniques. If your physician has suggested another method, you should use that method.

(For graphic representation of the following steps, please consult an original copy of the PATIENT PACKAGE INSERT.)

1. To use the nedocromil sodium Inhaler, remove the Mouthpiece Cover and make sure the metal Canister is firmly inserted into the plastic Mouthpiece. **Do not remove the Valve Cover from the metal Cannister.**

2. Shake the Inhaler.

3. Hold the Inhaler away from your mouth, and exhale slowly. **Do not breathe into the Inhaler as moisture could cause it to clog.**

4. Place the Mouthpiece in your mouth and close your lips around it. Tilt your head back, keeping your tongue below the opening of the Inhaler.

5. Press the top of the Canister down firmly at exactly the same time as you begin to inhale. Keep the Canister depressed as you continue to inhale slowly through your mouth until you have taken a full breath. After you have finished your full breath, release the pressure of your finger from the top of the Canister.

6. Remove the Inhaler from your mouth, and **hold your breath** for several seconds before breathing out slowly. This step is very important because it allows the medication to spread throughout your lungs.

7. Repeat Steps 2-6; then replace the Mouthpiece Cover.

8. Keeping the plastic Mouthpiece clean is extremely important to prevent medication build-up and blockage. To clean, simply remove the Canister and Mouthpiece Cover, and wash the Mouthpiece through the top **and** bottom in HOT water. **Never immerse the metal Canister in water.** The Mouthpiece can be washed every day, and should be washed at least twice a week. To dry, shake off excess water and let Mouthpiece air dry in warm place overnight. When the Mouthpiece is completely dry, replace Canister and Mouthpiece Cover.

SUGGESTIONS FOR BEST RESULTS

1. Use the Inhaler every day, as directed by your physician. Do not stop the treatment, or even reduce the dosage during symptom-free periods, without your physician's permission.
2. Before using the Inhaler for the very first time, or the first time in a while, shake the Inhaler and give it one press in the upright position to be sure it's working properly.Note: the Valve Cover should not be removed from the Canister (see Step 1 under Instructions).
3. It is essential that the Canister be pressed at exactly the time as you inhale. It is well worth your time to review this technique with your physician.
4. The dose delivered from the Inhaler can be seen as a fine mist. If you notice this mist escaping from your mouth or nose, you may not be breathing in at the exact moment the Canister is being pressed (see Steps 4 & 5 under Instructions).
5. Keep the Mouthpiece Cover on the Inhaler when not in use so that dirt can't get into it.

Dosage For the treatment of mild to moderate asthma in patients 12 years of age or older, the recommended dosage is two (2) inhalations four times a day at regular intervals. For maintenance therapy, daily dosing frequency will depend upon your physician's assessment of your asthma and may range from four times a day to twice a day at regular intervals.

With regular use, nedocromil sodium will decrease asthma symptoms. However, nedocromil sodium will not relieve the symptoms of an asthma attack once the attack has started.

It is important that you follow your physician's daily dosing instructions — even during symptom-free periods — to achieve optimal benefit from this medication. Please note that nedocromil sodium is **not** a steroid medication.

Benefits which may be achieved from regular use of nedocromil sodium include:

Prevention or reduction of asthma symptoms such as wheezing, chest tightness, cough, and shortness of breath.

Treatment of the bronchial inflammation that causes asthma.

Storage: Store the Inhaler between 2°-30°C (36°-86°F). Do not freeze. Contents under pressure. Do not puncture, incinerate, place near sources of heat, or use with other mouthpieces. Keep out of the reach of children.

Note: The indented statement below is required by the Federal government's Clean Air Act for all products containing or manufactured with chlorofluorocarbons (CFC's).

This product contains CFC-12 and CFC-114, substances which harm the environment by destroying ozone in the upper atmosphere.

Your physician has determined that this product is likely to help your personal health. USE THIS PRODUCT AS DIRECTED, UNLESS INSTRUCTED TO DO OTHERWISE BY YOUR PHYSICIAN. If you have any questions about alternatives, consult with your physician.

For further information about nedocromil sodium, please call our toll-free number: 1-800-2-ASTHMA (1-800-227-8462).

HOW SUPPLIED:

Tilade inhaler is available in 16.2 g canisters providing at least 104 metered inhalations. Available in single and double canister packs. Each pack is supplied with patient instructions and white plastic mouthpiece(s), one per canister, bearing the Tilade logo.

One 16.2 g Canister: (104 Metered Inhalations)

Two 16.2 g Canisters: (2 x 104 Metered Inhalations)

HOW SUPPLIED: *(cont'd)*

Store between 2°-30°C (36°-86°F). Do not freeze. Contents under pressure. Do not puncture, incinerate, place near sources of heat or use with other mouthpieces. Keep out of the reach of children.

Note: The indented statement below is required by the Federal government's Clean Air Act for all products containing or manufactured with chlorofluorocarbons (CFC's).

WARNING: Contains CFC-12 and CFC-114, substances which harm public health and environment by destroying ozone in the upper atmosphere.

A notice similar to the above WARNING has been placed in the "Patient Instructions for Use" portion of this package circular pursuant to EPA regulations.

(Fisons Pharmaceuticals, 10/94, RF302E, 610-1-48)

HOW SUPPLIED - EQUIVALENTS NOT AVAILABLE:

Aerosol - Inhalation - 1.75 mg

16.2 gm	$26.29	TILADE, Fisons	00585-0685-02
32.4 gm	$49.96	TILADE, Fisons	00585-0685-04

NEFAZODONE HYDROCHLORIDE *(003237)*

CATEGORIES: Antidepressants; Central Nervous System Agents; Depression; Depressive Disorder; Psychotherapeutic Agents; Selective Serotonin Reuptake Inhibitors; FDA Class 1S ("Standard Review"); FDA Approved 1994 Dec

BRAND NAMES: **Serzone**

FORMULARIES: Medi-Cal; PCS

COST OF THERAPY: $149.65 (Depression; Tablet; 150 mg; 2/day; 90 days)

PRIMARY ICD9: 311 (Depressive Disorder, Not Elsewhere Classified)

DESCRIPTION:

Nefazodone HCl is an antidepressant for oral administration with a chemical structure unrelated to selective serotonin reuptake inhibitors, tricyclics, tetracyclics, or monoamine oxidase inhibitors (MAOI).

Nefazodone hydrochloride is a synthetically derived phenylpiperazine antidepressant. The chemical name for nefazodone hydrochloride is 2-[3-[4-(3-chlorophenyl)-1-piperazinyl]propyl]-5-ether-2,4-dihydro-4-(2-phenoxyethyl)-3H-1,2,4-triazol-3-one monohydrochloride. The molecular formula is $C_{25}H_{32}ClN_5O_2 \cdot HCl$, which corresponds to a molecular weight of 506.5.

Nefazodone HCl is a nonhygroscopic, white crystalline solid. It is freely soluble in chloroform, soluble in propylene glycol, and slightly soluble in polyethylene glycol and water.

Nefazodone HCl is supplied as hexagonal tablets containing 100 mg, 150 mg, 200 mg, or 250 mg of nefazodone hydrochloride and the following inactive ingredients: microcrystalline cellulose, povidone, sodium starch glycolate, colloidal silicon dioxide, magnesium stearate, and iron oxides (red and/or yellow) as colorants.

CLINICAL PHARMACOLOGY:

Pharmacodynamics: The mechanism of action of nefazodone, as with other antidepressants, is unknown. Preclinical studies have shown that nefazodone inhibits neuronal uptake of serotonin and norepinephrine.

Nefazodone occupies central 5-HT_2 receptors at nanomolar concentrations, and acts as an antagonist at this receptor. Nefazodone was shown to antagonize alpha$_1$-adrenergic receptors, a property which may be associated with postural hypotension. *In vitro* binding studies showed that nefazodone had no significant affinity for the following receptors: alpha$_2$ and beta adrenergic, 5-HT_{1A}, cholinergic, dopaminergic, or benzodiazepine.

Pharmacokinetics: Nefazodone hydrochloride is rapidly and completely absorbed but is subject to extensive metabolism, so that its absolute bioavailability is low, about 20%, and variable. Peak plasma concentrations occur at about one hour and the half-life of nefazodone is 2-4 hours.

Both nefazodone and its pharmacologically similar metabolite, hydroxynefazone, exhibit nonlinear kinetics for both dose and time, with AUC and C_{max} increasing more than proportionally with dose increases and more than expected upon multiple dosing over time, compared to single dosing. For example, in a multiple-dose study involving BID dosing with 50, 100, and 200 mg, the AUC for nefazodone and hydoxynefazodone increased by about 4-fold with an increase in dose from 200 to 400 mg per day; C_{max} increased by about 3-fold with the same dose increase. In a multiple-dose study involving BID dosing with 25, 50, 100, and 150 mg, the accumulation ratios for nefazodone and hydroxynefazodone AUC, after 5 days of BID dosing relative to the first dose, ranged from approximately 3 to 4 at the lower doses (50-100 mg/day) and from 5 to 7 at the higher doses (200-300 mg/day); there were also approximately 2- to 4-fold increases in C_{max} after 5 days of BID dosing relative to the first dose, suggesting extensive and greater than predicted accumulation of nefazodone and its hydroxy metabolite with multiple dosing. Steady-state plasma nefazodone and metabolite concentrations are attained within 4 to 5 days of initiation of BID dosing or upon dose increase or decrease.

Nefazodone is extensively metabolized after oral administration by n-dealkylation and aliphatic and aromatic hydroxylation, and less than 1% of administered nefazodone is excreted unchanged in urine. Attempts to characterize three metabolites identified in plasma, hydroxynefazone (HO-NEF), meta-chlorophenylpiperazine (mCPP), and a triazole-dione metabolite, have been carried out. The AUC (expressed as a multiple of the AUC for nefazodone dosed at 100 mg BID) and elimination half-lives for these three metabolites were as follows:

TABLE 1 AUC Multiples and T1/2 for Three Metabolites of Nefazodone (100 mg BID)

Metabolite	AUC Multiple	T1/2
HO-NEF	0.4	1.5-4 hrs
mCPP	0.07	4-8 hrs
Triazole-dione	4.0	18 hrs

HO-NEF possesses a pharmacological profile qualitatively and quantitatively similar to that of nefazodone. mCPP has some similarities to nefazodone, but also has agonist activity at some serotonergic receptor subtypes. The pharmacological profile of the triazole-dione metabolite has not yet been well characterized. In addition to the above compounds, several other metabolites were present in plasma but have not been tested for pharmacological activity.

After oral administration of radiolabeled nefazodone, the mean half-life of total label ranged between 11 and 24 hours. Approximately 55% of the administered radioactivity was detected in urine and about 20-30% in feces.

Distribution: Nefazodone is widely distributed in body tissues, including the central nervous system (CNS). In humans the volume of distribution of nefazodone ranges from 0.22 to 0.87 L/kg.

CLINICAL PHARMACOLOGY: *(cont'd)*

Protein Binding: At concentrations of 25-2500 ng/ml nefazodone is extensively (>99%) bound to human plasma proteins *in vitro*. While nefazodone did not alter the *in vitro* protein binding of chlorpromazine, desipramine, diazepam, diphenylhydantoin, lidocaine, prazosin, propranolol, verapamil, or warfarin, it is unknown whether or not displacement of either nefazodone or other drugs occurs *in vivo*. There was a 5% decrease in protein binding of haloperidol; this is probably of no clinical significance.

Effect of Food: Food delays the absorption of nefazodone and decreases the bioavailability of nefazodone by approximately 20%.

Renal Disease: In studies involving 29 renally-impaired patients, renal impairment (creatinine clearances ranging from 7 to 60 ml/min/1.73 m^2) had no effect on steady-state nefazodone plasma concentrations.

Liver Disease: In a multiple-dose study of patients with liver cirrhosis, the AUC values for nefazodone and HO-NEF at steady state were approximately 25% greater than those observed in normal volunteers.

Age/Gender Effects: After single doses of 300 mg to younger and older patients, C_{max} and AUC for nefazodone and hydroxynefazodone were up to twice as high in the older patients. With multiple doses, however, differences were much smaller, 10-20%. A similar result was seen for gender, with a higher C_{max} and AUC in women after single doses but no differences after multiple doses.

Treatment with nefazodone HCl should be initiated at half the usual dose in elderly patients, especially women (see DOSAGE AND ADMINISTRATION), but the therapeutic dose range is similar in older and younger patients.

CLINICAL TRIALS SUPPORTING EFFECTIVENESS CLAIM

The efficacy of nefazodone HCl as a treatment for depression was established in two placebo-controlled, short-term trials in outpatients meeting DSM-III or DSM-IIIR criteria for major depression. One was a 6-week dose-titration study comparing nefazodone HCl in dose ranges (up to 300 mg/day and up to 600 mg/day [mean modal dose for this group was about 400 mg/day], on a BID schedule) and placebo. The other was an 8-week dose-titration study comparing nefazodone HCl (up to 600 mg/day; mean modal dose was 375 mg/day), imipramine (up to 300 mg/day), and placebo, all on a BID schedule. Overall these studies demonstrated nefazodone HCl, at doses titrated up to 600 mg/day, to be superior to placebo on at least three of the four following measures: 17-item Hamilton Depression Rating Scale or HDRS (total score), Hamilton Depressed Mood item, CGI severity score, and CGI Improvement score. Significant differences were also found for certain factors of the HDRS (*e.g.,* anxiety factor, sleep disturbance factor, and retardation factor). Two other 6-8 week placebo- and imipramine-controlled studies in depressed outpatients provided additional support for the superiority of nefazodone (titrated up tp 500 or 600 mg/day; mean modal doses of 462 mg/day and 363 mg/day) over placebo.

There were no efficacy studies focusing specifically on the elderly or on men and women separately. Overall, approximately two-thirds of patients in these of patients in these trials were women, and an analysis of the effects of gender on outcome did not suggest any differential responsiveness on the basis of sex. There were too few elderly patients in these trials to reveal possible age-related differences in response.

INDICATIONS AND USAGE:

Nefazodone HCl is indicated for the treatment of depression.

The efficacy of nefazodone HCl in the treatment of depression was established in 6-8 week controlled trials of outpatients whose diagnoses corresponded most closely to the DSM-III or DSM-IIIR category of major depressive disorder (see CLINICAL PHARMACOLOGY.)

A major depressive episode implies a prominent and relatively persistent depressed or dysphoric mood that usually interferes with daily functioning (nearly every day for at least 2 weeks). It must include either depressed mood or loss of interest or pleasure and at least 5 of the following 9 symptoms: depressed mood, loss of interest in usual activities, significant change in weight and/or appetite, insomnia or hypersomnia, psychomotor agitation or retardation, increased fatigue, feelings of guilt or worthlessness, slowed thinking or impaired concentration, a suicide attempt or suicidal ideation.

The antidepressant effectiveness of nefazodone HCl in hospitalized depressed patients has not been adequately studied.

The effectiveness of nefazodone HCl in long-term use, that is, for more than 6 to 8 weeks, has not been systematically evaluated in controlled trials. Therefore, the physician who elects to use nefazodone HCl for extended periods should periodically re-evaluate the long-term usefulness of the drug for the individual patient.

CONTRAINDICATIONS:

Coadministration with terfenadine or astemizole with nefazodone HCl is contraindicated (see WARNINGS and DRUG INTERACTIONS).

Nefazodone HCl is contraindicated in patients with known hypersensitivity to nefazodone or other phenylpiperazine antidepressants.

WARNINGS:

POTENTIAL FOR INTERACTION WITH MONOAMINE OXIDASE INHIBITORS

In patients receiving antidepressants with pharmacological properties similar to nefazodone in combination with a monoamine oxidase inhibitor (MAOI), there have been reports of serious, sometimes fatal, reactions. For a selective serotonin reuptake inhibitor, these reactions have included hyperthermia, rigidity, myoclonus, autonomic instability with possible rapid fluctuations of vital signs, and mental status changes that include extreme agitation progressing to delirium and coma. These reactions have also been reported in patients who have recently discontinued the drug and have been started on a MAOI. Some cases presented with features resembling neuroleptic malignant syndrome. Severe hyperthermia and seizures, sometimes fatal, have been reported in association with the combined use of tricyclic antidepressants and MAOIs. These reactions have also been reported in patients who have recently discontinued these drugs and have been started on an MAOI.

Although the effects of combined use of nefazodone and MAOI have not been evaluated in humans or animals, because nefazodone is an inhibitor of both serotonin and norepinephrine reuptake, it is recommended that nefazodone not be used in combination with an MAOI, or within 14 days of discontinuing treatment with an MAOI. At least 1 week should be allowed after stopping nefazodone before starting an MAOI.

INTERACTION WITH TRIAZOLOBENZODIAZEPINES

Interaction studies of nefazodone with two triazolobenzodiazepines, i.e., triazolam and alprazolam, metabolized by cytochrome $P_{450}IIIA_4$, have revealed substantial and clinically important increases in plasma concentrations of these compounds when administered concomitantly with nefazodone.

TRIAZOLAM

When a single oral 0.25-mg dose of triazolam was coadministered with nefazodone (200 mg BID) at steady state, triazolam half-life and AUC increased 4-fold and peak concentrations increased 1.7-fold. Nefazodone plasma concentrations were unaffected by triazolam.

WARNINGS: *(cont'd)*

Coadministration of nefazodone potentiated the effects of triazolam on psychomotor performance tests. If triazolam is coadministered with nefazodone HCl, a 75% reduction in the initial triazolam dosage is recommended. For many patients, e.g., the elderly, it is recommended that triazolam not be used in combination with nefazodone. No dosage adjustment is required for nefazodone HCl.

ALPRAZOLAM

When alprazolam (1 mg BID) and nefazodone (200 mg BID) were coadministered, steady-state peak concentrations, AUC and half-life values for alprazolam increased by approximately 2-fold. Nefazodone plasma concentrations were unaffected by alprazolam. If alprazolam is coadministered with nefazodone HCl, a 50% reduction in the initial alprazolam dosage is recommended. No dosage adjustment is required for nefazodone HCl.

POTENTIAL TERFENADINE AND ASTEMIZOLE INTERACTIONS

Terfenadine and astemizole are both metabolized by the cytochrome $P_{450}IIIA_4$isozyme,and it has been demonstrated that ketoconazole, erythromycin, and other inhibitors of $IIIA_4$ can block the metabolism of terfenadine and astemizole, resulting in increased plasma concentrations of parent drug. Increased plasma concentrations of terfenadine and astemizole are associated with QT prolongation and with rare cases of serious cardiovascular events, including death, due principally to ventricular tachycardia of the torsades de pointes type. Nefazodone has been shown *in vitro* to be an inhibitor of $IIIA_4$. Consequently, it is recommended that nefazodone not be used in combination with either terfenadine or astemizole (see CONTRAINDICATIONS and PRECAUTIONS).

PRECAUTIONS:

GENERAL

Postural Hypotension: A pooled analysis of the vital signs monitored during placebo-controlled premarketing studies revealed that 5.1% of nefazodone patients compared to 2.5% of placebo patients ($\leq$0.01) met criteria for a potentially important decrease in blood pressure at some time during treatment (systolic blood pressure $\leq$90 mmHg *and* a change from baseline of $\geq$20 mmHg). While there was no difference in the proportion of nefazodone and placebo patients having adverse events characterized as "syncope" (nefazodone, 0.2%; placebo, 0.3%), the rates for adverse events characterized as "postural hypotension" were as follows: nefazodone (2.8%), tricyclic antidepressants (10.9%), SSRI (1.1%), and placebo (0.8%). Thus, the prescriber should be aware that there is some risk of postural hypotension in association with nefazodone use. Nefazodone HCl should be used with caution in patients with known cardiovascular or cerebrovascular disease that could be exacerbated by hypotension (history of myocardial infarction, angina, or ischemic stroke) and conditions that would predispose the patients to hypotension (dehydration, hypovolemia, and treatment with antihypertensive medication).

Activation of Mania/Hypomania: During premarketing testing, hypomania or mania occurred in 0.3% of nefazodone-treated unipolar patients, compared to 0.3% of tricyclic- and 0.4% of placebo-treated patients. In patients classified as bipolar the rate of manic episodes was 1.6% for nefazodone, 5.1% for the combined tricyclic-treated groups, and 0% for placebo-treated patients. Activation of mania/hypomania is a known risk in a small proportion of patients with major affective disorder treated with other marketed antidepressants. As with all antidepressants, nefazodone HCl should be used cautiously in patients with a history of mania.

Suicide: The possibility of a suicide attempt is inherent in depression and may persist until significant remission occurs. Close supervision of high risk patients should accompany initial drug therapy. Prescriptions for nefazodone HCl should be written for the smallest quantity of tablets consistent with good patients management in order to reduce the risk of overdose.

Seizures: During premarketing testing, a recurrence of petit mal seizure was observed in a patient receiving nefazodone who had a history of such seizures. One nonstudy participant took 2000-3000 mg of nefazodone with methocarbamol and alcohol; this person reportedly experienced a convulsion (type not documented).

Priapism: While priapism did not occur during premarketing experience with nefazodone, priapism has been reported with a structurally related drug, trazodone. If patients present with prolonged or inappropriate erections, they should discontinue therapy immediately and consult their physicians. If the condition persists for more than 24 hours, a urologist should be consulted to determine appropriate treatment.

Use in Patients with Concomitant Illness: Nefazodone HCl has not been evaluated or used to any appreciable extent in patients with a recent history of myocardial infarction or unstable heart disease.Patients with these diagnoses were systematically excluded from clinical studies during the product's premarketing testing. Evaluation of electrocardiograms of 1153 patients who received nefazodone in 6- to 8- week, double-blind, placebo-controlled trials did not indicate that nefazodone is associated with the development of clinically important ECG abnormalities. However, sinus bradycardia, defined as heart rate $\leq$50 bpm and a decrease of at least 15 bpm from baseline, was observed in 1.5% of nefazodone-treated patients compared to 0.4% of placebo-treated patients (p $\leq$0.05). Because patients with a recent history of myocardial infarction or unstable heart disease were excluded from clinical trials, such patients should be treated with caution.

In patients with cirrhosis of the liver, the AUC values of nefazodone and HO-NEF were increased by approximately 25%.

INFORMATION FOR THE PATIENT

Physicians are advised to discuss the following issues with patients for whom they prescribe nefazodone HCl:

Time to Response/Continuation: As with all antidepressants, several weeks on treatment may be required to obtain the full antidepressant effect. Once improvement is noted, it is important for patients to continue drug treatment as directed by their physician.

Interference with Cognitive and Motor Performance: Since any psychoactive drug may impair judgement, thinking, or motor skills, patients should be cautioned about operating hazardous machinery, including automobiles, until they are reasonably certain that nefazodone HCl therapy does not adversely affect their ability to engage in such activities.

Pregnancy: Patients should be advised to notify their physician if they become pregnant or intend to become pregnant during therapy.

Nursing: Patients should be advised to notify their physician if they are breast-feeding an infant (see PRECAUTIONS, Nursing Mothers.)

Concomitant Medication: Patients should be advised to inform their physicians if they are taking, or plan to take, any prescription or over-the-counter drugs, since there is a potential for interactions. Significant caution is indicated if nefazodone HCl is to be used in combination with either Halcion or Xanax, and concomitant use with Seldane or Hismanal is contraindicated (see CONTRAINDICATIONS and DRUG INTERACTIONS).

Alcohol: Patients should be advised to avoid alcohol while taking nefazodone HCl.

Allergic Reactions: Patients should be advised to notify their physician if they develop a rash, hives, or a related allergic phenomenon.

LABORATORY TESTS

There are no specific laboratory tests recommended.

PRECAUTIONS: *(cont'd)*

CARCINOGENESIS, MUTAGENESIS, AND IMPAIRMENT OF FERTILITY

Carcinogenesis: There is no evidence of carcinogenicity with nefazodone. The dietary administration of nefazodone to rats and mice for 2 years at daily doses up to 200 mg/kg and 800 mg/kg, respectively, which are approximately 3 and 6 times, respectively, the maximum human daily dose on an mg/m^2 basis, produced no increase in tumors.

Mutagenesis: Nefazodone has been shown to have no genotoxic effects based on the following assays: bacterial mutation assays, a DNA repair assay in cultured rat hepatocytes, a mammalian mutation assay in Chinese hamster ovary cells, an *in vivo* cytogenetics assay in rat bone marrow cells, and a rat dominant lethal study.

Impairment of Fertility A fertility study in rats showed a slight decrease in fertility at 200 mg/kg/day (approximately three times the maximum human daily dose on a mg/m^2 basis) but not at 100 mg/kg/day (approximately 1.5 times the maximum human daily dose on a mg/m^2 basis).

PREGNANCY, TERATOGENIC EFFECTS, PREGNANCY CATEGORY C

Reproduction studies have been performed in pregnant rabbits and rats at daily doses up to 200 and 300 mg/kg, respectively (approximately 6 and 5 times, respectively, the maximum human daily dose on a mg/m^2 basis). No malformations were observed in the offspring as a result of nefazodone treatment. However, increased early pup mortality was seen in rats at a dose approximately five times the maximum human dose, and decreased pup weights were seen at this and lower doses, when dosing began during pregnancy and continued until weaning. The cause of these deaths is not known. The no-effect dose for rat pup mortality was 1.3 times the human dose on a mg/m^2 basis. There are no adequate and well-controlled studies in pregnant women. Nefazodone should be used during pregnancy only if the potential benefit justifies the potential risk to the fetus.

LABOR AND DELIVERY

The effect of nefazodone HCl on labor and delivery in humans is unknown.

NURSING MOTHERS

It is not known whether nefazodone HCl or its metabolites are excreted in human milk. Because many drugs are excreted in human milk, caution should be exercised when nefazodone HCl is administered to a nursing woman.

PEDIATRIC USE

Safety and effectiveness in individuals below 18 years of age have not been established.

GERIATRIC USE

Over 500 elderly (≥65 years) individuals participated in clinical studies with nefazodone. No unusual adverse age-related phenomena were identified in this cohort of elderly patients treated with nefazodone. Due to the increased systemic exposure to nefazodone seen in single dose studies in elderly patients (see CLINICAL PHARMACOLOGY, Pharmacokinetics), treatment should be initiated at half the usual dose, but titration upward should take place over the same range as in younger patients (see DOSAGE AND ADMINISTRATION.) The usual precautions should be observed in elderly patients who have concomitant medical illnesses or who are receiving concomitant drugs.

DRUG INTERACTIONS:

DRUGS HIGHLY BOUND TO PLASMA PROTEIN

Because nefazodone is highly bound to plasma protein (see CLINICAL PHARMACOLOGY, Pharmacokinetics), administration of nefazodone HCl to a patient taking another drug that is highly protein bound may cause increased free concentrations of the other drug, potentially resulting in adverse events. Conversely, adverse effects could result from displacement of nefazodone by highly bound drugs.

CNS ACTIVE DRUGS

Monoamine Oxidase Inhibitors: In patients receiving antidepressants with pharmacological properties similar to nefazodone in combination with a monoamine oxidase inhibitor (MAOI), there have been reports of serious, sometimes fatal, reactions. For a selective serotonin reuptake inhibitor, these reactions have included hyperthermia, rigidity, myoclonus, autonomic instability with possible rapid fluctuations of vital signs, and mental status changes that include extreme agitation progressing to delirium and coma. These reactions have also been reported in patients who have recently discontinued the drug and have been started on a MAOI. Some cases presented with features resembling neuroleptic malignant syndrome. Severe hyperthermia and seizures, sometimes fatal, have been reported in association with the combined use of tricyclic antidepressants and MAOIs. These reactions have also been reported in patients who have recently discontinued these drugs and have been started on an MAOI.

Although the effects of combined use of nefazodone and MAOI have not been evaluated in humans or animals, because nefazodone is an inhibitor of both serotonin and norepinephrine reuptake, it is recommended that nefazodone not be used in combination with an MAOI, or within 14 days of discontinuing treatment with an MAOI. At least 1 week should be allowed after stopping nefazodone before starting an MAOI.

Haloperidol: When a single oral 5-mg dose of haloperidol was coadministered with nefazodone (200 mg BID) at steady state, haloperidol apparent clearance decreased by 35% with no significant increase in peak haloperidol plasma concentrations or time of peak. This change is of unknown clinical significance. Pharmacodynamic effects of haloperidol were generally not altered significantly. There were no changes in the pharmacokinetic parameters for nefazodone. Dosage adjustment of haloperidol may be necessary when coadministered with nefazodone.

Lorazepam: When lorazepam (2 mg BID) and nefazodone (200 mg BID) were coadministered to steady state, there was no change in any pharmacokinetic parameter for either drug compared to each drug administered alone. Therefore, dosage adjustment is not necessary for either drug when coadministered.

Triazolam/Alprazolam: *Triazolam:* When a single oral 0.25-mg dose of triazolam was coadministered with nefazodone (200 mg BID) at steady state, triazolam half-life and AUC increased 4-fold and peak concentrations increased 1.7-fold. Nefazodone plasma concentrations were unaffected by triazolam.

Coadministration of nefazodone potentiated the effects of triazolam on psychomotor performance tests. If triazolam is coadministered with nefazodone HCl, a 75% reduction in the initial triazolam dosage is recommended. For many patients, e.g., the elderly, it is recommended that triazolam not be used in combination with nefazodone. No dosage adjustment is required for nefazodone HCl.

Alprazolam: When alprazolam (1 mg BID) and nefazodone (200 mg BID) were coadministered, steady-state peak concentrations, AUC and half-life values for alprazolam increased by approximately 2-fold. Nefazodone plasma concentrations were unaffected by alprazolam. If alprazolam is coadministered with nefazodone HCl, a 50% reduction in the initial alprazolam dosage is recommended. No dosage adjustment is required for nefazodone HCl.

Alcohol: Although nefazodone did not potentiate the cognitive and psychomotor effects of alcohol in experiments with normal subjects, the concomitant use of nefazodone HCl and alcohol in depressed patients is not advised.

General Anesthetics: Little is known about the potential for interaction between nefazodone and general anesthetics; therefore, prior to elective surgery, nefazodone HCl should be discontinued as long as clinically feasible.

DRUG INTERACTIONS: *(cont'd)*

Other CNS Active Drugs: The use of nefazodone in combination with other CNS-active drugs has not been systematically evaluated. Consequently, caution is advised if concomitant administration of nefazodone HCl and such drugs is required.

Cimetidine: When nefazodone (200 mg BID) and cimetidine (300 mg QD) were coadministered for one week, no change in the steady-state pharmacokinetics of either nefazodone or cimetidine was observed compared to each dosed alone. Therefore, dosage adjustments is not necessary for either drug when coadministered.

CARDIOVASCULAR ACTIVE DRUGS

Digoxin: When nefazodone (200 mg BID) and digoxin (0.2 mg QD) were coadministered for 9 days to healthy male volunteers (n=18) who were phenotyped as $P_{450}IID_6$ extensive metabolizers, C_{max}, C_{min}, and AUC of digoxin were increased by 29%, 27%, and 15%, respectively. Digoxin had no effects on the pharmacokinetics of nefazodone and its active metabolites. Because of the narrow therapeutic index of digoxin, caution should be exercised when nefazodone and digoxin are coadministered; plasma level monitoring for digoxin is recommended.

Propanolol: The coadministration of nefazodone (200 mg BID) and propanolol (40 mg BID) for 5.5 days to healthy male volunteers (n=18), including 3 poor and 15 extensive $P_{450}IID_6$metabolizers, resulted in 30% and 14% reduction in $C_{max}$for the metabolite, 4-hydroxypropranolol. The kinetics of nefazodone, hydroxynefazodone, and triazole-dione were not affected by coadministration of propranolol. However, C_{max} C_{min}, and AUC of m-chlorophenylpiperazine were increased by 23%, 54%, and 28%, respectively. No change in initial dose of either drug is necessary and dose adjustments should be made on the basis of clinical response.

Pharmacokinetics of Nefazodone in "Poor Metabolizers" and Potential Interaction with Drugs that Inhibit and/or are Metabolized by Cytochrome P450 Isozymes

$IIIA_4$ Isozyme: Nefazodone has been shown *in vitro* to be an inhibitor of cytochrome $P_{450}IIIA_4$. This is consistent with the interaction observed between nefazodone and the benzodiazepines triazolam and alprazolam, drugs metabolized by this isozyme. Consequently, caution is indicated in the combined use of nefazodone with any drugs known to be metabolized by the $IIIA_4$ isozyme. In particular, the combined use of nefazodone with either terfenadine or astemizole is contraindicated (see CONTRAINDICATIONS and WARNINGS).

IID_6 Isozyme: A subset (3% to 10%) of the population has reduced activity of the drug-metabolizing enzyme cytochrome $P_{450}II_6$. Such individuals are referred to commonly as "poor metabolizers" of drugs such as debrisoquine, dextromethorphan, and the tricyclic antidepressants. The pharmacokinetics of nefazodone and its major metabolites are not altered in these "poor metabolizers." Plasma concentrations of one major metabolite (mCPP) are increased in this population; th adjustment of nefazodone HCl dosage is not required when administered to "poor metabolizers." Nefazodone and its metabolites have been shown *in vitro* to be extremely weak inhibitors of $P_{450}IID_6$. Thus, it is not likely that nefazodone will decrease the metabolic clearance of drugs metabolized by this isozyme.

IA_2 Isozyme: Nefazodone and its metabolites have been shown*in vitro* not to inhibit cytochrome $P_{450}IA_2$. Thus, metabolic interactions between nefazodone and drugs metabolized by this isozyme are unlikely.

ELECTRO-CONVULSIVE THERAPY (ECT)

There are no clinical studies of the combined use of ECT and nefazodone.

ADVERSE REACTIONS:

ASSOCIATED WITH DISCONTINUATION OF TREATMENT

Approximately 16% of the 3496 patients who received nefazodone HCl in worldwide premarketing clinical trials discontinued treatment due to an adverse experience. The more common (≥1%) events in clinical trials associated with discontinuation and considered to be drug related (*i.e.,* those events associated with dropout at a rate approximately twice or greater for nefazodone HCl compared to placebo) included nausea (3.5%), dizziness (1.9%), insomnia (1.5%), asthenia (1.3%), and agitation (1.2%).

INCIDENCE IN CONTROLLED TRIALS

Commonly Observed Adverse Events in Controlled Clinical Trials: The most commonly observed adverse events associated with the use of nefazodone HCl (incidence of 5% or greater) and not seen at an equivalent incidence among placebo-treated patients (*i.e.,* significantly higher incidence for nefazodone HCl compared to placebo, p≤0.05), derived from the table below, were: somnolence, dry mouth, nausea, dizziness, constipation, asthenia, lightheadedness, blurred vision, confusion, and abnormal vision.

Adverse Events Occurring at an Incidence of 1% or More Among nefazodone HCl-Treated Patients: The table that follows enumerates adverse events that occurred at an incidence of 1% or more, and were more frequent than in the placebo group, among nefazodone HCl-treated patients who participated in short-term (6- to 8-week) placebo-controlled trials in which patients were dosed with nefazodone HCl to ranges of 300 to 600 mg/day. This table shows the percentage of patients in each group who had at least one episode of an event at some time during their treatment. Reported adverse events were classified using a standard COSTART-based Dictionary terminology.

The prescriber should be aware that these figures cannot be used to predict the incidence of side effects in the course of usual medical practice where patient characteristics and other factors differ from those which prevailed in the clinical trials. Similarly, the cited frequencies cannot be compared with figures obtained from other clinical investigations involving different treatments, uses, and investigators. The cited figures, however, do provide the prescribing physician with some basis for estimating the relative contribution of drug and nondrug factors to the side-effect incidence rate in the population studied.

Dose Dependency of Adverse Events: The table that follows (TABLE 3) enumerates adverse events that were more frequent in the nefazodone HCl dose range of 300 to 600 mg/day than in the nefazodone HCl dose range of up to 300 mg/day. This table shows only those adverse events for which there was a statistically significant difference (p ≤0.05 in incidence between the nefazodone HCl dose ranges as well as a difference between the high dose range and placebo.

VITAL SIGN CHANGES

(See PRECAUTIONS, Postural Hypotension)

WEIGHT CHANGES

In a pooled analysis of placebo-controlled premarketing studies, there were no differences between nefazodone and placebo groups in the proportions of patients meeting criteria for potentially important increases or decreases in body weight (a change of ≥7%).

LABORATORY CHANGES

Of the serum chemistry, serum hematology, and urinalysis parameters monitored during placebo-controlled premarketing studies with nefazodone, a pooled analysis revealed a statistical trend between nefazodone and placebo for hematocrit, i.e., 2.8% of nefazodone patients met criteria for a potentially important decrease in hematocrit (≤37% male or ≤32% female) compared to 1.5% of placebo patients (0.05 < ;p ≤0.10). Decreases in hematocrit, presumably dilutional, have been reported with many other drugs that block $alpha_1$-adrenergic receptors. There was no apparent clinical significance of the observed changes in the few patients meeting these criteria.

ADVERSE REACTIONS: *(cont'd)*

TABLE 2 Treatment-Emergent Adverse Experience Incidence in 6- to 8-Week Placebo-Controlled Clinical Trials [1] Nefazodone HCl 300 to 600 mg/day Dose Range

Body System / Preferred Term	Serzone (n=393)	Placebo (n=394)
Body as a Whole		
Headache	36%	33%
Asthenia	11%	5%
Infection	8%	6%
Flu syndrome	3%	2%
Chills	2%	1%
Fever	2%	1%
Neck Rigidity	1%	0
Cardiovascular		
Postural hypotension	4%	1%
Hypotension	2%	1%
Dermatological		
Pruritus	2%	1%
Rash	2%	1%
Gastrointestinal		
Dry Mouth	25%	13%
Nausea	22%	12%
Constipation	14%	8%
Dyspepsia	9%	7%
Diarrhea	8%	7%
Increased appetite	5%	3%
Nausea & Vomiting	2%	1%
Metabolic		
Peripheral edema	3%	2%
Thirst	1%	<1%
Musculoskeletal		
Arthralgia	1%	<1%
Nervous		
Somnolence	25%	14%
Dizziness	17%	5%
Insomnia	11%	9%
Lightheadedness	10%	3%
Confusion	7%	2%
Memory impairment	4%	2%
Paresthesia	4%	2%
Vasodilation[2]	4%	2%
Abnormal Dreams	3%	2%
Concentration decreased	3%	1%
Ataxia	2%	0
Incoordination	2%	1%
Psychomotor retardation	2%	1%
Tremor	2%	1%
Hypertonia	1%	0
Libido decreased	1%	<1%
Respiratory		
Pharyngitis	6%	5%
Cough increased	3%	1%
Special Senses		
Blurred vision	9%	3%
Abnormal vision[3]	7%	1%
Tinnitus	2%	1%
Taste perversion	2%	1%
Visual field defect	1%	0
Urogenital		
Urinary frequency	2%	1%
Urinary tract infection	2%	1%
Urinary retention	2%	1%
Vaginitis[4]	2%	1%
Breast pain[4]	1%	<1%

[1] Events reported by at least 1% of patients treated with Serzone and more frequent than the placebo group are included; incidence is rounded to the nearest 1% (<1% indicates an incidence less than 0.5%). Events for which the Serzone incidence was equal to or less than placebo are not listed in the table, but included the following: abdominal pain, back pain, accidental injury, chest pain, neck pain, palpitation, migraine, sweating, flatulence, vomiting, anorexia, tooth disorder, weight gain, edema, myalgia, cramp, agitation, anxiety, depression, hypesthesia, CNS stimulation, dysphoria, emotional lability, sinusitis, rhinitis, dysmenorrheas[4], dysuria.
[2] Vasodilation—flushing, feeling warm.
[3] Abnormal vision—scotoma, visual trails.
[4] Incidence adjusted for gender.

TABLE 3 Dose Dependency of Adverse Events in Placebo-Controlled Trials [1]

Body System / Preferred Term	Serzone 300-600 mg/day (n=209)	Serzone ≤300 mg/day (n=211)	Placebo (n=212)
Gastrointestinal			
Nausea	23%	14%	12%
Constipation	17%	10%	9%
Somnolence	28%	16%	13%
Dizziness	22%	11%	4%
Confusion	8%	2%	1%
Special Senses			
Abnormal vision	10%	0	2%
Blurred vision	9%	3%	2%
Tinnitus	3%	0	1%

[1] Events for which there was a statistically significant difference ($p \le 0.05$) between the nefazodone dose groups.

ECG CHANGES

Of the ECG parameters monitored during placebo-controlled premarketing studies with nefazodone, a pooled analysis revealed a statistically significant difference between nefazodone and place for sinus bradycardia, i.e., 1.5% of nefazodone patients met criteria for potentially important decrease in heart rate (≤50 bpm and a decrease of ≥15 bpm) compared to 0.4% of placebo patients ($p<0.05$). There was no obvious clinical significance of the observed changes in the few patients meeting these criteria.

OTHER EVENTS OBSERVED DURING THE PREMARKETING EVALUATION OF NEFAZODONE HCL

During its premarketing assessment, multiple doses of nefazodone HCl were administered to 3496 patients in clinical studies, including more than 250 patients treated for at least one year. The conditions and duration of exposure to nefazodone HCl varied greatly, and included (in overlapping categories) open and double-blind studies, uncontrolled and controlled studies, inpatient and outpatient studies, fixed-dose and titration studies. Untoward

ADVERSE REACTIONS: *(cont'd)*

events associated with this exposure were recorded by clinical investigators using terminology of their own choosing. Consequently, it is not possible to provide a meaningful estimate of the proportion of individuals experiencing adverse events without first grouping similar types of untoward events into a smaller number of standardized event categories.

In the tabulations that follow, reported adverse events were classified using a standard COSTART-based Dictionary terminology. The frequencies presented, therefore, represent the proportion of the 3496 patients exposed to multiple doses of nefazodone HCl who experienced an event of the type cited on at least one occasion while receiving nefazodone HCl. All reported events are included except those already listed in the Treatment-Emergent Adverse Experience Incidence Table, those events listed in other safety- related sections of this insert, those adverse experiences listed in other safety-related sections of this insert, those adverse experiences subsumed under COSTART terms that are either overly general or excessively specific as to be uninformative, those events for which a drug cause was very remote, and those events which were not serious and occurred in fewer than two patients.

It is important to emphasize that, although the events reported occurred during treatment with nefazodone HCl, they were not necessarily caused by it.

Events are further categorized by body system and listed in order of decreasing frequency according to the following definitions: frequent adverse events are those occurring on one or more occasions in at least 1/100 patients (only those not already listed in the tabulated results from placebo-controlled trials appear in this listing); infrequent adverse events are those occurring in 1/100 to 1/1000 patients; rare events are those occurring in fewer than 1/1000 patients.

Body as a whole: *Infrequent:* allergic reaction, malaise, photosensitivity reaction, face edema, hangover effect, abdomen enlarged, hernia, pelvic pain, and halitosis. *Rare:* cellulitis.

Cardiovascular system: *Infrequent:* tachycardia, hypertension, syncope, ventricular extrasystoles, and angina pectoris. *Rare:* AV block, congestive heart failure, hemorrhage, pallor, and varicose vein.

Dermatological system: *Infrequent:* dry skin, acne, alopecia, urticaria, maculopapular rash, vesiculobullous rash, and eczema.

Gastrointestinal system: *Frequent:* gastroenteritis.*Infrequent:* eructation, periodontal abscess, abnormal liver function tests, gingivitis, colitis, gastritis, mouth ulceration, stomatitis, esophagitis, peptic ulcer, and rectal hemorrhage.*Rare:* glossitis, hepatitis, dysphagia, gastrointestinal hemorrhage, oral moniliasis, and ulcerative colitis.

Hemic and lymphatic system: *Infrequent:* ecchymosis, anemia, leukopenia, and lymphadenopathy.

Metabolic and nutritional system: *Infrequent:* weight loss, gout, dehydration, lactic dehydrogenase increased, SGOT increased, and SGPT increased. *Rare:* hypercholesteremia and hypoglycemia.

Musculoskeletal system: *Infrequent:* arthritis, tenosynovitis, muscle stiffness, and bursitis. *Rare:* tendinous contracture.

Nervous system: *Infrequent:* vertigo, twitching, depersonalization, hallucinations, suicide attempt, apathy, euphoria, hostility, suicidal thoughts, abnormal gait, thinking abnormal, attention decreased, derealization, neuralgia, paranoid reaction, dysarthria, increased libido, suicide, and myoclonus. *Rare:* hyperkinesia, increased salivation, cerebrovascular accident, hyperesthesia, hypotonia, ptosis, and neuroleptic malignant syndrome.

Respiratory system: *Frequent:* dyspnea and bronchitis.*Infrequent:* asthma, pneumonia, laryngitis, voice alteration, epistaxis, hiccup. *Rare:* hypertension and yawn.

Special senses: *Frequent:* eye pain. *Infrequent:* dry eye, ear pain, abnormality of accommodation, diplopia, conjunctivitis, mydriasis, keratoconjunctivitis, hyperacusis, and photophobia. *Rare:* deafness, glaucoma, night blindness, and taste loss.

Urogenital system: *Frequent:* impotence.[a]*Infrequent:* cystitis, urinary urgency, metrorrhagia[a], amenorrhea[a], polyuria, vaginal hemorrhage[a], breast enlargement[a], menorrhagia[a], urinary incontinence, abnormal ejaculation[a], hematuria, nocturia, and kidney calculus.*Rare:* uterine fibroids enlarged[a], uterine hemorrhage[a], anorgasmia, and oliguria.

[a] Adjusted for gender.

DRUG ABUSE AND DEPENDENCE:

CONTROLLED SUBSTANCE CLASS

Nefazodone HCl is not a controlled substance.

PHYSICAL AND PSYCHOLOGICAL DEPENDENCE

In animal studies, nefazodone did not act as a reinforcer for intravenous self-administration in monkeys trained to self-administer cocaine. suggesting no abuse liability. In a controlled study of abuse liability in human subjects nefazodone showed no potential for abuse.

Nefazodone has not been systematically studied in humans for its potential for tolerance, physical dependence, or withdrawal. While the premarketing clinical experience with nefazodone did not reveal any tendency for a withdrawal syndrome or any drug-seeking behavior, it is not possible to predict on the basis of this limited experience the extent to which a CNS-active drug will be misused, diverted, and/or abused once marketed. Consequently, physicians should carefully evaluate patients for a history of drug abuse and follow such patients closely, observing them for signs of misuse or abuse of nefazodone HCl (*e.g.,* development of tolerance, dose escalation, drug-seeking behavior).

OVERDOSAGE:

HUMAN EXPERIENCE

There is very limited experience with nefazodone overdose. In premarketing clinical studies, there were seven reports of nefazodone overdose alone or in combination with other pharmacological agents. The amount of nefazodone ingested ranged from 1000 mg to 11,200 mg. Commonly reported symptoms from overdose of nefazodone included nausea, vomiting, and somnolence. One nonstudy participant took 2000-3000 mg of nefazodone with methocarbonal and alcohol; this person reportedly experienced a convulsion (type not documented). None of the patients died.

OVERDOSE MANAGEMENT

Overdosage may cause an increase in incidence or severity of any of the reported adverse reactions (see ADVERSE REACTIONS).

There is no specific antidote for nefazodone HCl. Treatment should be symptomatic and supportive in the case of hypotension or excessive sedation. Any patient suspected of having taken an overdose should have the stomach emptied by gastric lavage.

In managing overdosage, consider the possibility of multiple drug involvement/The physician should consider contacting a poison control center on the treatment of any overdose.

DOSAGE AND ADMINISTRATION:

INITIAL TREATMENT

The recommended starting dose for nefazodone HCl is 200 mg/day, administered in two divided doses (BID). In the controlled clinical trials establishing the anti-depressant efficacy of nefazodone HCl, the effective dose range was generally 300 to 600 mg/day. Consequently, most patients, depending on tolerability and the need for further clinical effect, should have

DOSAGE AND ADMINISTRATION: *(cont'd)*

dose increased. Dose increases should occur in increments of 100 mg/day to 200 mg/day, again on a BID schedule, at intervals of no less than 1 week. As with all antidepressants, several weeks on treatment may be required to obtain a full antidepressant response.

DOSAGE FOR ELDERLY OR DEBILITATED PATIENTS

The recommended dose for elderly or debilitated patients is 100 mg/day on a BID schedule. These patients often have reduced nefazodone clearance and/or increased sensitivity to the side effects of CNS-active drugs. It may also be appropriate to modify the rate of subsequent dose titration. As steady-state plasma levels do not change with age, the final target dose based on a careful assessment of the patient's clinical response may be similar in healthy younger and older patients.

MAINTENANCE/CONTINUATION/EXTENDED TREATMENT

There is no body of evidence available from controlled trials to indicate how long the depressed patients should be treated with nefazodone HCl. It is generally agreed, however, that pharmacological treatment for acute episodes of depression should continue for up to six months or longer. Whether the dose of antidepressant needed to induce remission is identical to the dose needed to maintain euthymia is unknown. Although there are no efficacy data that specifically address maintenance antidepressant treatment with nefazodone HCl, the safety of nefazodone in long-term use is supported by data from both double-blind and open-label trials involving more than 250 patients treated for at least one year.

SWITCH PATIENTS TO OR FROM A MONOAMINE OXIDASE INHIBITOR

At least 14 days should elapse between discontinuation of an MAOI and initiation of therapy with nefazodone HCl. In addition, at least 7 days should be allowed after stopping nefazodone HCl before starting an MAOI.

HOW SUPPLIED:

Nefazodone HCl tablets are hexagonal tablets imprinted with BMS and the strength (*i.e.,* 100 mg) on one side and the identification code number on the other. The 100 mg and 150 mg tablets are bisect scored on both tablet faces. The 200 mg and 250 mg tablets are unscored.

Store at room temperature, below 40°C (104°F) and dispense in a tight container.

HOW SUPPLIED - EQUIVALENTS NOT AVAILABLE:

Tablet, Uncoated - Oral - 100 mg

60's	$49.88	SERZONE, Bristol Myers Squibb	00087-0032-31
100's	$83.14	SERZONE, Bristol Myers Squibb	00087-0032-44

Tablet, Uncoated - Oral - 150 mg

60's	$49.88	SERZONE, Bristol Myers Squibb	00087-0039-31
100's	$83.14	SERZONE, Bristol Myers Squibb	00087-0039-01

Tablet, Uncoated - Oral - 200 mg

60's	$49.88	SERZONE, Bristol Myers Squibb	00087-0033-31
100's	$83.14	SERZONE, Bristol Myers Squibb	00087-0033-44

Tablet, Uncoated - Oral - 250 mg

60's	$49.88	SERZONE, Bristol Myers Squibb	00087-0041-31

NELFINAVIR MESYLATE *(003329)*

CATEGORIES: AIDS Related Complex; Anti-Infectives; Antivirals; HIV Infection; Infections; Protease Inhibitors; Viral Agents; FDA Approved 1997 Mar; Pregnancy Category B

BRAND NAMES: Viracept

WARNING:
Nelfinavir mesylate is indicated for the treatment of HIV infection when antiretroviral therapy is warranted. This indication is based on surrogate gate marker changes in patients who received nelfinavir mesylate in combination with nucleoside analogues or alone for up to 24 weeks. At present, there are no results from controlled trials evaluating the effect of therapy with nelfinavir mesylate on clinical progression of HIV infection, such as survival or the incidence of opportunistic infections.

DESCRIPTION:

Nelfinavir mesylate is an inhibitor of the human immunodeficiency virus (HIV) protease.

Viracept Tablets are available for oral administration as a light blue, capsule-shaped tablet in a 250 mg strength (as nelfinavir free base). Each tablet also contains the following inactive ingredients: calcium silicate, crospovidone, magnesium stearate, FD&C blue #2 powder and FD&C blue #2 aluminum lake.

Viracept Oral Powder is available for oral administration in a 50 mg strength (as nelfinavir free base) in bottles. The oral powder also contains the following inactive ingredients; microcrystalline cellulose, maltodextrin, dibasic potassium phosphate, crospovidone, hydroxypropyl methylcellulose, aspartame, sucrose palmitate and natural and artificial flavor.

The chemical name for nelfinavir mesylate is [3S-[2(2S*,3S*),3α,4aβ,8aβ]]-N-(1,1-dimethylethyl)decahydro-2-[2 hydroxy-3-[(3-hydroxy-2-methylbenzoyl)amino]-4-(phenylthio) butyl]-3-isoquinolinecarboxamide mono-methanesulfonate (salt) and the molecular weight is 663.90 (567.79 as the free base).

Nelfinavir mesylate is a white to off-white amorphous, slightly soluble in water at pH ≤4 and freely soluble in methanol, ethanol, isopropanol and propylene glycol.

CLINICAL PHARMACOLOGY:

MICROBIOLOGY

Mechanism of Action: Nelfinavir is an inhibitor of the HIV-1 protease. Inhibition of the viral protease prevents cleavage of the gagpol polyprotein resulting in the production of immature, non-infectious virus.

Antiviral Activity *In Vitro*: The antiviral activity of nelfinavir *in vitro* has been demonstrated in both acute and/or chronic HIV infections in lymphoblastoid cell lines, peripheral blood lymphocytes and monocytes/macrophages. Nelfinavir was found to be active against several laboratory strains of HIV-1 and several clinical isolates of HIV-1 and the HIV-2 strain ROD. The EC_{95} (95% effective concentration) ranged from 7 to 196 nM. In combination with reverse transcriptase inhibitors, nelfinavir demonstrated additive (didanosine or stavudine) to synergistic (zidovudine, lamivudine or zalcitabine). Antiviral activity *in vitro* without enhanced cytotoxicity. Drug combination studies with protease inhibitors (ritonavir, saquinavir or indinavir) showed variable results ranging from antagonistic to synergistic. The clinical relevance of these *in vitro* findings is not known.

Drug Resistance: HIV-1 isolates with reduced susceptibility to nelfinavir have been selected *in vitro.* HIV isolates from selected patients treated with nelfinavir alone or in combination with reverse transcriptase inhibitors were monitored for phenotypic (n=19) and genotypic (n=55) changes in phase I/II trials over a period of 2 to 52 weeks. One or more virus protease mutations at amino acid positions 30, 35, 36, 46, 71, 77 and 88 were detected in >10% of patients with evaluable isoates. Of 19 patients for which both phenotypic and genotypic analyses were performed on clinical isolates, 9 showed reduced susceptibility (5- to 93-fold) to nelfinavir *in vitro.* All 9 patients possessed one or more mutations in the virus protease gene. Amino acid position 30 appeared to be the most frequent mutation site. Phenotypic resistance was defined as a ≥5-fold decrease in viral sensitivity (EC_{95}) *in vitro* compared to baseline. The incidence of the D30N mutation in the virus protease of randomly selected patients receiving nelfinavir monotherapy (n=64) or nelfinavir in combination with zidovudine and lamivudine (n=49) at 12 to 16 weeks of therapy was 56% and 6%, respectively. However, the sample size includes patients with non-amplifiable virus at 12 to 16 weeks of therapy. The clinical relevance of phenotypic and genotypic changes associated with nelfinavir therapy has not been established.

Cross-resistance: HIV isolates obtained from 5 patients during nelfinavir therapy showed a 5- to 93-fold decrease in nelfinavir susceptibility *in vitro* when compared to matched baseline isolates, but did not demonstrate a concordant decrease in susceptibility to indinavir, ritonavir, saquinavir or 141W94, *in vitro.* Conversely, following ritonavir therapy, 6 of 7 clinical isolates with decreased ritonavir susceptibility (8- to 113-fold) *in vitro* compared to baseline also exhibited decreased susceptibility to nelfinavir *in vitro* (5- to 40-fold). An HIV isolate obtained from a patient receiving saquinavir therapy showed decreased susceptibility to saquinavir (7- fold), but did not demonstrate a concordant decrease in susceptibility to nelfinavir *in vitro.* Cross-resistance between nelfinavir and reverse transcriptase inhibitors is unlikely because different enzyme targets are involved. One zidovudine-resistant HIV-1 isolate and one pyridinone-resistant HIV-1 isolate tested *in vitro* retained susceptibility to nelfinavir. Because the potential for HIV cross-resistance between nelfinavir and other protease inhibitors has not been fully explored, it is unknown what effect nelfinavir therapy will have on the activity of coadministered or subsequently administered protease inhibitors.

PHARMACOKINETICS

The pharmacokinetic properties of nelfinavir were evaluated in healthy volunteers and HIV-infected patients; no substantial differences were observed between the two groups.

Absorption: After single and multiple oral doses of 500 to 750 mg (two to three 250 mg tablets) with food, peak nelfinavir plasma concentrations were typically achieved in 2 to 4 hours. After multiple dosing with 750 mg three times daily for 28 days (steady-state), peak plasma concentrations (C_{max}) averaged 3-4 mcg/ml and plasma concentrations prior to the morning dose (trough) were 1-3 mcg/ml (trough sample collection times averaged 11 hours after the previous evening dose). A greater than dose-proportional increase in nelfinavir plasma concentrations was observed after single doses; however, this was not observed after multiple dosing.

Effect of Food on Oral Absorption: Maximum plasma concentrations and area under the plasma concentration-time curve (AUC) were 2- to 3-fold higher under fed conditions compared to fasting. The effect of food on nelfinavir absorption was evaluated in two studies (n=14, total). The meals evaluated contained 517 to 759 Kcal, with 153 to 313 Kcal derived from fat.

Distribution: The apparent volume of distribution following oral administration of nelfinavir was 2-7 L/kg. Nelfinavir in serum is extensively protein-bound (>98%).

Metabolism: Unchanged nelfinavir comprised 82-86% of the total plasma radioactivity after a single oral 750 mg dose of ^{14}C-nelfinavir. *In vitro,* multiple cytochrome P-450 isoforms including CYP3A are responsible for metabolism of nelfinair. One major and several minor oxidative metabolites were found in plasma. The major oxidative metabolite has *in vitro* antiviral activity comparable to the parent drug.

Elimination: The terminal half-life in plasma was typically 3.5 to 5 hours. The majority (87%) of an oral 750 mg dose containing ^{14}C nelfinavir was recovered in the feces; fecal radioactivity consisted of numerous oxidative metabolites (78%) and unchanged nelfinavir (22%). Only 1-2% of the dose was recovered in urine, of which unchanged nelfinavir was the major component.

SPECIAL POPULATIONS

Hepatic or Renal Insufficiency: The pharmacokinetics of nelfinavir have not been studied in patients with hepatic or renal insufficiency; however, less than 2% of nelfinavir is excreted in the urine, so the impact of renal impairment on nelfinavir elimination should be minimal.

Gender and Race: No significant pharmacokinetic differences have been detected between males and females. Pharmacokinetic differences due to race have not been evaluated.

Pediatric: (See PRECAUTIONS, Pediatric Use

CLINICAL STUDIES:

In the clinical studies described below, an experimental branched DNA signal amplification assay was used to estimate the level of circulating HIV RNA in plasma. Using this assay, values below an estimated 1200 copies/ml could not be reliably quantified and were set to 1200 copies/ml in all analyses. The units reported, copies/ml, may not represent actual viral copies on an absolute scale. Consequently HIV RNA results summarized below should not be directly compared to results from other trials utilizing different HIV RNA assays.

Study 511: Nelfinavir Mesylate + Zidovudine + Lamivudine Versus Zidovudine + Lamivudine: Study 511 was double-blind, randomized, placebo controlled trial comparing treatment with zidovudine and lamivudine plus 2 doses of nelfinavir mesylate to zidovudine and lamivudine alone in 297 aniretroviral naive HIV-1 infected patients (median age 35 [range 21 to 63], 89% male and 78% Caucasian). Mean baseline CD_4 cell count was 288 cells/mm^3 and mean baseline plasma HIV RNA was 153,044 copies/ ml (mean of log_{10} baseline plasma HIV RNA was 4.86).

At 24 weeks of therapy, 59, 73 and 30 patients randomized to receive nelfinavir mesylate 500 mg 3 times daily plus zidovudine and lamivudine, nelfinavir mesylate 750 mg 3 times daily plus zidovudine and lamivudine, or zidovudine and lamivudine, respectively, had plasma HIV RNA assigned a value of 1200 copies/ml. The clinical significance of changes in plasma HIV RNA has not been established.

Study 506: Nelfinavir Mesylate + Stavudine Versus Stavudine: Study 506 is an ongoing double blind, randomized, placebo controlled trial comparing treatment with 2 doses of nelfinavir mesylate + stavudine and stavudine monotherapy in 308 HIV-1 infected patients median age 37 [range 21 to 69], 89% male and 75% Caucasian). Sixty-one out of 308 (20%) patients were antiretroviral naive; the remaining patients were experienced (mean duration of antiretroviral therapy 32 months). The mean baseline CD_4 cell count for all patients was 279 cells/mm^3 and the mean baseline plasma HIV RNA was 141,369 copies/ml mean of log_{10} baseline plasma HIV RNA as 4.86). The study allowed for treatment changes in the three study arms based on surrogate marker response or toxicity. By 24 weeks 43, 2 and 4 patients remaining on this study in the stavudine, stavudine plus nelfinavir mesylate 500 mg 3 times daily, and stavudine plus nelfinavir mesylate 750 mg 3 times daily arms, repectively, had altered initial therapy based primarily on their surrogate marker response. For patients receiving stavudine monotherapy, alteration of therapy was primarily the addition of nelfinavir.

At 24 weeks of therapy, 24, 22 and 13 patients randomized to receive nelfinavir mesylate 500 mg 3 times daily plus stavudine, nelfinavir mesylate 70 mg 3 times daily plus stavudine or stavudine alone, respectively, had plasma HIV RNA levels assigned a value of 1200 copies/ ml. The clinical significance of changes in plasma HIV RNA has not been established.

INDICATIONS AND USAGE:

Nelfinavir mesylate is indicated for the treatment of HIV infection when antiretroviral therapy is warranted. This indication is based on surrogate marker changes in patients who received nelfinavir mesylate in combination with nucleoside analogues or alone for up to 24 weeks. At present, there are no results from controlled trials evaluating the effect of therapy with nelfinavir mesylate on clinical progression of HIV infection, such as survival or the incidence of opportunistic infections.

CONTRAINDICATIONS:

Nelfinavir mesylate is contraindicated in patients with clinically significant hypersensitivity to any of its components.

WARNINGS:

Patients with Phenylketonuria: Viracept Oral Powder contains 11.2 mg phenylalanine per gram of powder.

Nelfinavir mesylate should not be administered concurrently with terfenadine, astemizole, cisapride, triazolam or midazolam, because competition for CYP3A by nelfinavir could result in inhibition of the metabolism of these drugs and create the potential for serious and/or life-threatening cardiac arrhythmias or prolonged sedation.

PRECAUTIONS:

GENERAL

Nelfinavir is principally metabolized by the liver. Therefore, caution should be exercised when administering this drug to patients with hepatic impairment.

Resistance/Cross Resistance: Because the potential for HIV cross-resistance between protease inhibitors has not been fully explored, it is unknown what effect nelfinavir therapy will have on the activity of subsequently administered protease inhibitors. (See CLINICAL PHARMACOLOGY, Microbiology).

HEMOPHILIA

There have been reported of increased bleeding, including spontaneous skin hematomas and hemarthrosis, in patients with hemophilia type A and B treated with protease inhibitors. In some patients, additional factor VIII was given. In more than half of the reported cases, treatment with protease inhibitors was continued or reintroduced. A causal relationship has not been established.

INFORMATION FOR THE PATIENT

For optimal absorption, patients should be advised to take nelfinavir mesylate with food. (See CLINICAL PHARMACOLOGY, Pharmacokinetics and DOSAGE AND ADMINISTRATION).

Patients should be informed that nelfinavir mesylate is not a cure for HIV infection and that they may continue to acquire illnesses associated with advanced HIV infection, including opportunistic infections.

Patients should be told that the long-term effects of nelfinavir mesylate are unknown at this time. They should be told that there is currently no data demonstrating that nelfinavir mesylate therapy can reduce the risk of transmitting HIV to others through sexual contact or blood contamination.

Patients should be advised to take nelfinavir mesylate every day as prescribed. Patients should not alter the dose or discontinue therapy without consulting with their doctor. If a dose is missed, patients should take the dose as soon as possible and then return to their normal schedule. However, if a dose is skipped, the patient should not double the next dose.

The most frequent adverse event associated with nelfinavir mesylate is diarrhea, which can usually be controlled with non-prescription drugs, such as loperamide, which slow gastrointestinal motility.

Nelfinavir mesylate may interact with some drugs, therefore, patients should be advised to report to their doctor the use of any other prescription or non-prescription medication.

Patients receiving oral contraceptives should be instructed that alternate or additional contraceptive measures should be used during therapy with nelfinavir mesylate.

CARCINOGENESIS AND MUTAGENESIS

Carcinogenicity studies in animals have not yet been completed. Nelfinavir was not, however, mutagenic or clastogenic in a battery of *in vitro* and *in vivo* tests including microbial mutagenesis (Ames), mouse lymphoma, chromosome aberrations in human lymphocytes, and an *in vivo* rat micronucleus assay.

PREGNANCY CATEGORY B

Comparisons of systemic exposure are based on the steady-state area under the plasma concentration time curve (AUC) observed in humans receiving the recommended therapeutic dose. Nelfinavir produced no effects on either male or female mating and fertility or embryo survival in rat studies at exposures comparable to human therapeutic exposure. There were also no effects on fetal development or maternal toxicity when nelfinavir was administered to pregnant rats at systemic exposures comparable to human exposure. Administration of nelfinavir to pregnant rabbits resulted in no fetal development effects up to a dose at which a slight decrease in maternal body weight was observed; however, even at the highest dose evaluated, systemic exposure in rabbits was significantly lower than human exposure. Additional studies in rats indicated that exposure to nelfinavir in females from mid-pregnancy through lactation had no effect on the survival, growth, and development of the offspring to weaning. Subsequent reproductive performance of these offspring was also not affected by maternal exposure to nelfinavir. However, there are no adequate and well controlled studies in pregnant women. Because animal reproduction studies are not always predictive of human response, nelfinavir mesylate should be used during pregnancy only if clearly needed.

NURSING MOTHERS

The U.S. Public Health Service Centers for Disease Control and Prevention advises HIV-infected women not to breast-feed to avoid postnatal transmission of HIV to a child who may not yet be infected. Studies in lactating rats have demonstrated that nelfinavir is excreted in milk. It is not known whether nelfinavir is excreted in human milk.

PEDIATRIC USE

Nelfinavir was studied in one open-label, uncontrolled trial in 38 pediatric patients ranging in age from 2 to 13 years. In order to achieve plasma concentrations in pediatric patients which approximate those observed in adults, the recommended pediatric dose is 20-30 mg/kg given three times daily, not to exceed 750 mg three times daily. (See DOSAGE AND ADMINISTRATION.)

A similar adverse event profile as seen during the pediatric clinical trial as in adult patients. The evaluation of the antiviral activity of nelfinavir in pediatric patients is ongoing.

The safety, effectiveness and pharmacokinetics of nelfinavir have not been evaluated in pediatric patients below the age of 2 years.

DRUG INTERACTIONS:

The potential ability of nelfinavir to inhibit the major human cytochrome P450 isoforms (CYP3A, CYP2C19, CYP2D6, CYP2C9, CYPlA2 and CYP2E1) has been investigated *in vitro*. Only CYP3A was inhibited at concentrations in the therapeutic range.

DRUG INTERACTIONS: *(cont'd)*

Specific drug interaction studies were formed with nelfinavir and a number of drugs. TABLE 1 and TABLE 2 summarize the effects of coadministration of nelfinavir on the geometric mean AUC and C_{max}.

TABLE 1A Effect of Nelfinair on Coadministered Drug Plasma AUC and C_{max}

Coadministered Dose	Nelfinavir Dose	N
Lamivudine 150 mg Single Dose	750 mg q8h × 7-10 days	11
Stavudine 30-40 mg bid × 56 days	750 mg tid × 56 days	8
Zidovudine 200 mg Single Dose	750 mg q8h × 7-10 days	11
Indinavir 800 mg Single Dose	750 mg q8h × 7 days	6
Ritonavir 500 mg Single Dose	750 m q8h × 5 doses	10
Saquinavir 1200 mg Single Dose	750 mg tid × 4 days	14
Ethinyl estradiol 35 mcg qd × 15 days	750 mg q8h × 7 days	12
Norethindrone 0.4 mg qd × 15 days	760 mg q8h × 7 days	12
Rifabutin 300 mg qd × 8 days	750 mg q8h × 7-8 days	10
Terfenadine 60 mg Single Dose	750 mg q8h × 7 days	12

TABLE 1B Effect of Nelfinair on Coadministered Drug Plasma AUC and C_{max}

Coadministered Drug	AUC (95%Cl)	C_{max}(95%Cl)
Lamivudine 150 mg Single Dose	↑10% (1-20%)	↑31% (5-62%)
Stavudine 30-40 mg bid × 56 days	↔	↔
Zidovudine 200 mg Single Dose	↓35% (28-41%)	↓31% (8-49%)
Indinavir 800 mg Single Dose	↑51% (25-83%)	↔
Ritonavir 500 mg Single Dose	↔	↔
Saquinavir 1200 mg Single Dose	↑392% (271-553%)	↑179% (105-280%)
Ethinyl estradiol 35 mcg qd × 15 days	↓47% (41-63%)	↓28% (14-39%)
Norethindrone 0.4 mg qd × 15 days	↓18% (12-27%)	↔
Rifabutin 300 mg qd × 8 days	↑207% (151-276%)	↑146% (112-186%)
Terfenadine 60 mg Single Dose	Terfenadine plasma concentrations were transiently measurable when coadministered with nelfinavir mesylate*	

* Terfenadine and nelfinavir should not be coadministered

TABLE 2A Effect of Coadministered Drug on Nelfiravir Plasma AUC and C_{max}

Coadministered Drug	Nelfinavir dose	N
Didanosne 200 mg Single Dose	750 mg Single Dose	9
Zidovudine 200 mg + Lamivudine 150 mg Single Dose	750 mg q8h × 7-10 days	11
Indinavir 800 mg q8h × 7 days	750 mg Single Dose	6
Ritonavir 500 mg q8h × 3 doses	750 mg Single Dose	10
Saquinavir 1200 mg tid × 4 days	750 mg Single Dose	14
Ketoconazole 400 mg qd × 7 days	500 mg q8h × 5-6 days	12
Rifabutin 300 mg qd × 8 days	750 mg q8h × 7-8 days	10
Rifampin 600 mg qd × 7 days	750 mg q8h × 5-6 days	12

TABLE 2B Effect of Coadministered Drug on Nelfiravir Plasma AUC and C_{max}

Coadministered Drug	AUC (95%Cl)	C_{max}(95%Cl)
Didanosne 200 mg Single Dose	↔	↔
Zidovudine 200 mg + Lamivudine 150 mg Single Dose	↔	↔
Indinavir 800 mg q8h × 7 days	↑83% (34-150%)	↑31% (13-52%)
Ritonavir 500 mg q8h × 3 doses	↑152% (86-242%)	↑44% (25-67%)
Saquinavir 1200 mg tid × 4 days	↑18% (5-33%)	↔
Ketoconazole 400 mg qd × 7 days	↑35% (21-49%)	↑25% (8-44%)
Rifabutin 300 mg qd × 8 days	↓32% (10-48%)	↓25% (6-38%)
Rifampin 600 mg qd × 7 days	↓82% (77-86%)	↓76% (67-83%)

Nelfinavir is an inhibitor of CYP3A (cytochrome P450 3A). Coadministration of nelfinavir mesylate and drugs primarily metabolized by CYP3A may result in increased plasma concentrations of the other drug that could increase or prolong both its therapeutic and adverse effects. Nelfinavir is metabolized in part by CYP3A. Coadministration of nelfinavir mesylate and drugs that induce CYP3A may decrease nelfinavir plasma concentrations and reduce its therapeutic effect. Coadministration of nelfinavir mesylate and drugs that inhibit CYP3A may increase nelfinavir plasma concentrations.

Based on known metabolic profiles, clinically significant drug interactions are not expected between nelfinavir mesylate and dapsone, trimethoprim/sulfamethoxazole, clarithromycin, azithromycin, erythromycin, itraconazole or fluconazle.

TABLE 3 Drugs That Should Not Be Coadministered With Nelfinavir Mesylate

Drug Class	Drugs Within Class Not to Be Coadministered With Nelfinavir Mesylate
Antihistamines	astemizole, terfenadine
Antimyobacterial agents	rifampin
Benzodiazepines	midazolam, triazolam
GI motility agents	cisapride

TABLE 4 Drugs Which Require A Dose Reduction When Coadministered With Nelfinavir Mesylate

Drug Class	Drugs within Class which Require Dose Reduction
Antimycobacterial agents:	rifabutin

TABLE 5 Other Potentially Clinically Significant Drug Interactions With Nelfinavir Mesylate*

Anticonvulsants: carbamazepine, phenooarbital, phenytoin	May decrease nelfinavir plasma concentrations†
Anti-HIV protease inhibitors: indinavir, ritonavir	May increase nelfinavir plasma concentrations
Oral Contraceptives: ethinyl estradiol, norethindrone	Plasma concentrations may be decreased by nelfinavir mesylate

* This table is not all inclusive
† Nefinavir mesylate may not be effective due to decreased nelfinavir plasma concentrations in patients taking these agents concomitantly.

DRUG INTERACTIONS: *(cont'd)*

ANTIHISTAMINES

Terfenadine: Administration of tefenadine with nelfinavir mesylate resulted in the appearance of unchanged terfenadine in plasma; therefore, nelfinavir mesylate should not be administered concurrently with terfenadine because of the potential for serious and/or life-threatening cardiac arrhythmis. Because a similar interaction is likely, nelfinavir mesylate should also not be administered concurrently with astemizole.

ANTI-HIV PROTEASE INHIBITORS

Indinavir: Coadministration of indinavir with nelfinavir mesylate resulted in an 83% increase in nelfinavir plasma AUC and a 51% increase in indinavir plasma AUC. The safety of this combination has not been established.

Ritonavir: Coadministration of ritonavir with nelfinavir mesylate resulted in a 152% increase in nelfinavir plasma AUC and very little change in ritonavir plasma AUC. The safety of this combination has not been established.

Saquinavir: Coadministration of saquinavir with nelfinavir mesylate resulted in an 18% increase in nelfinavir plasma AUC and a 392% increase in saquinavir plasma AUC. If used in combination, no dose adjustments are needed.

ANTIFUNGAL AGENTS

Ketoconazole: Coadministration of ketoconazole with nelfinavir mesylate resulted in a 35% increase in nelfinavir plasma AUC. This change was not considered clinically significant and no dose adjustment is needed when ketoconazole and nelfinavir mesylate are coadministered.

ANTI-HIV REVERSE TRANSCRIPTASE INHIBITORS

Didanosine: It is recommended that didanosine be administered on an empty stomach; therefore, nelfinavir should be administered (with food) one hour after or more than two hours before didanosine.

Zidovudine: Coadministration of zidovudine and lamivudine with nelfinavir mesylate resulted in a 35% decrease in zidovudine plasma AUC. A dose adjustment is not needed when zidoudine is administered with nelfinavir mesylate.

Little or no change in the pharmacokinetics of either drug was observed when nelfinavir mesylate was coadministered with lamivudine or stavudine.

ANTIMYCOBACTERIAL AGENTS

Rifabutin: Coadministration of rifabutin and nelfinavir mesylate resulted in a 32% decrease in nelfinavir plasma AUC and a 207% increase in rifabutin plasma AUC. It is recommended that the dose of rifabutin be reduced to one-half the usual dose when administered with nelfinavir mesylate.

Rifampin: Coadministration of rifampin and nelfinavir mesylate resulted in an 82% decease in nelfinavir plasma AUC. Nelfinavir mesylate and rifampin should not be coadministered.

ORAL CONTRACEPTIVES

Ethinyl Estradiol And Norethindrone: Coadministration of nelfinavir mesylate with Ovcon-35 resulted in a 47% decrease in ethinyl estradiol and an 18% decease in norethindrone plasma concentrations. Alternate or additional contraceptive measures should be used during therapy with nelfinavir mesylate.

ADVERSE REACTIONS:

The safety of nelfinavir mesylate was studied in over 1500 patients who received drug either alone or in combination with nucleoside analogues (d4T or ZDV/3TC). The majority of adverse events were of mild intensity. The most frequently reported adverse event among patients receiving nelfinavir mesylate was diarrhea, which was generally of mild to moderate intensity.

Drug-related clinical adverse experiences of moderate or severe intensity in ≥2% of patients treated with nelfinavir mesylate coadministered with ZDV plus 3TC (Study 511) or in combination with d4T (Study 506) for up to 24 weeks are presented in TABLE 6A and TABLE 6B.

TABLE 6A Percentage of Patients with Treatment-Emergent* Adverse Events of Moderate or Severe Intensity Reported in ≥2% of Patients

	Study 511 Naive Patients		
Adverse Events	Placebo + ZDV/3TC (n=101)	500 mg tid Nelfinavir Mesylate + ZDV/3TC (n=97)	750 mg tid Nelfinavir Mesylate + ZDV/3TC (n=100)
Body as a Whole			
Abdominal pain	1%	0	0
Asthenia	2%	1%	1%
Digestive System			
Diarrhea	3%	14%	20%
Nausea	4%	3%	7%
Flatulence	0	5%	2%
Skin/Appendages			
Rash	1%	1%	3%

* Includes those adverse events at least possibly related to study drug or of unknown relationship and excludes concurrent HIV conditions.

TABLE 6B Percentage of Patients with Treatment-Emergent* Adverse Events of Moderate or Severe Intensity Reported in ≥2% of Patients

	Study 506 Experienced Patients		
Adverse Events	Placebo + d4T (n=109)	500 mg tid Nelfinavir Mesylate + d4T (n=98)	750 mg tid Nelfinavir Mesylate + d4T (n=101)
Body as a Whole			
Abdominal pain	3%	2%	4%
Asthenia	4%	3%	1%
Digestive System			
Diarrhea	10%	28%	32%
Nausea	1%	3%	2%
Flatulence	4%	8%	3%
Skin/Appendages			
Rash	0	4%	3%

* Includes those adverse events at least possibly related to study drug or of unknown relationship and excludes concurrent HIV conditions.

Adverse events occurring in less than 2% of patients receiving nelfinavir mesylate in all phase II/III clinical trials and considered at least possibly related or of unknown relationship to treatment and of at least moderate severity are listed below.

Body as a Whole: accidental injury, allergic reaction, back pain, fever, headache, malaise, and pain

ADVERSE REACTIONS: *(cont'd)*

Digestive System: anorexia, dyspepsia, epigastric pain, gastrointesinal bleeding, hepatitis, mouth ulceration, pancreatitis and vomiting

Hemic/Lymphatic System: anemia, leukopenia and thrombocytopenia

Metabolic/Nutritional System: increases in alkaline phosphate, amylase creatine phosphokinase, lactic dehydrogenase, SGOT, SGPT and gamma glutamyl transpeptidase; hyperlipemia, hyperuricemia, hypoglycemia, dehydration, and liver function tests abnormal

Musculoskeletal System: arhralgia, arthritis, cramps, myalgia, myasthenia and myopathy

Nervous System: anxiety, depression, dizziness, emotional lability, hyperkinesia, insomnia, migraine, paresthesia, seizures, sleep disorder, somnolence and suicide ideation

Respiratory System: dyspnea, pharyngitis, rhinitis, and sinusitis.

Skin/Appendages: dermatitis, folliculitis, fungal dermatitis, maculopapular rash, pruritus, sweating, and urticaria

Special Senses: acute iritis and eye disorder

Urogenital System: kidney calculus, sexual dysfunction and urine abnormality

LABORATORY ABNORMALITIES

Few patients experienced significant laboratory abnormalities while receiving nelfinavir mesylate. The percentage of patients with marked laboratory abnormalities in Studies 511 and 506 are presented in TABLE 7A and TABLE 7B. Marked laboratory abnormalities are defined as a Grade 3 or 4 abnormality in a patient with a normal baseline value or a Grade 4 abnormality in a patient with a Grade 1 abnormality at baseline.

TABLE 7A Percentage of Patients by Treatment Group With Marked Laboratory Abnormalities* in >2% of Patients

	Study 511 Naive Patients		
Adverse Events	Placebo + ZDV/3TC (n=101)	500 mg tid Nelfinavir Mesylate + ZDV/3TC (n=97)	750 mg tid Nelfinavir Mesylate + ZDV/3TC (n=100)
Hematology			
Hemoglobin	6%	3%	2%
Neutrophils	4%	3%	5%
Lymphocytes	1%	6%	1%
Chemistry			
ALT (SGPT)	6%	1%	1%
AST (SGOT)	4%	1%	0
Creatine Kinase	7%	2%	2%

* Marked laboratory abnormalities are defined as a shift from Grade 0 at baseline to at least Grade 3 or from Grade 1 to Grade 4.

TABLE 7B Percentage of Patients by Treatment Group With Marked Laboratory Abnormalities* in >2% of Patients

	Study 506 Experienced Patients		
Adverse Events	Placebo + d4T (n=109)	500 mg tid Nelfinavir Mesylate + d4T (n=98)	750 mg tid Nelfinavir Mesylate + d4T (n=101)
Hematology			
Hemoglobin	0	0	0
Neutrophils	1%	1%	4%
Lymphocytes	1%	1%	0
Chemistry			
ALT (SGPT)	1%	3%	2%
AST (SGOT)	0	3%	3%
Creatine Kinase	4%	5%	6%

* Marked laboratory abnormalities are defined as a shift from Grade 0 at baseline to at least Grade 3 of from Grade 1 to Grade 4.

OVERDOSAGE:

Human experience of acute overdose with nelfinavir mesylate is limited. There is no specific antidote for overdose with nelfinavir mesylate. If indicated, elimination of unabsorbed drug should be achieved by emesis or gastric lavage. Administration of activated charcoal may also be use to aid removal of unabsorbed drug. Since nelfinavir is highly protein bound, dialysis is unlikely to significantly remove drug from blood.

DOSAGE AND ADMINISTRATION:

Adults: The recommended dose is 750 mg (three 250 mg tablets) three times daily. Nelfinavir mesylate should be taken with a meal or light snack. Antiviral activity is enhanced when nelfinavir mesylate is administered in combination with nucleoside analogues. Therefore, it is recommended at nelfinavir mesylate be used in combination with nucleoside analogues.

Pediatric Patients (2-13 years): The recommended oral dose of nelfinavir mesylate for pediatric patients 2 to 13 years of age is 20-30 mg/kg per dose, three times daily with a meal or a light snack. For children unable to take tablets, nelfinavir mesylate oral powder may be administered. The oral powder may be mixed with a small amount of water, milk, formula, soy formula, soy milk or dietary supplements; once mixed, the entire contents must be consumed in order obtain the full dose. The recommended use period for storage of the product in these media is 6 hours. Acidic food or juice (*e.g.,* orange juice, apple juice or apple sauce) are not recommended to be used in combination with nelfinavir mesylate, because the combination may result in a bitter taste. Nelfinavir mesylate oral powder should not be reconstituted with water in its original container. The recommended pediatric dose of nelfinavir mesylate to be administered three times daily is described in TABLE 8.

TABLE 8 Pediatric Dose to be Administered Three Times Daily

Body Weight		Number of Level 1: : g scoops	tsp.	Number of tablets
7 to < 8.5	15.5 to < 18.5	4	1	-
8.5 to < 10.5	18.5 to < 23	5	1 1/4	-
10.5 < 12	23 to < 26.5	6	1 1/2	-
12 to < 14	26.5 to < 31	7	1 3/4	-
14 to < 16	31 to < 35	8	2	-
16 to < 18	35 to < 39.5	9	2 1/4	-
18 to < 23	39.5 to < 50.5	10	2 1/2	2
≥23	≥50.5	15	3 3/4	3

PATIENT INFORMATION:

Nelfinavir mesylate is used alone or in combination for the treatment of HIV infection. It is not a cure.

PATIENT INFORMATION: *(cont'd)*

Inform your physicians if you are pregnant. Do not breast-feed.

Inform your physician if you are taking any other medication, including over-the-counter medication and birth control pills. An additional method of birth control should be used.

May cause diarrhea, nausea and gas, stomach ache, weakness and rash.

Take exactly as directed. Do not alter or discontinue the dose. If a dose is missed, take as soon as possible then return to your regular schedule. If the dose is skipped, do not double the next dose.

Take this drug with food.

HOW SUPPLIED:

Viracept Tablets, 250 mg are light blue, capsule-shaped tablets engraved with "VIRACEPT" on one side and "250 mg" on the other.

Viracept Oral Powder, 50 mg/g is an off-white powder containing 50 mg (as nelfinavir free base) in each level scoop fill (1 gram).

Nelfinavir mesylate should be stored at 15° to 30°C (59° to 86°F).

HOW SUPPLIED - EQUIVALENTS NOT AVAILABLE:

Powder - Oral - 50 mg

144 g	$49.54	VIRACEPT, Agouron Pharm	63010-0011-90

Tablet - Oral - 250 mg

270's	$464.40	VIRACEPT, Agouron Pharm	63010-0010-27

NEOMYCIN SULFATE *(001868)*

CATEGORIES: Aminoglycosides; Anti-Infectives; Antibiotics; Antimicrobials; Hepatic Coma; Perioperative Prophylaxis; Pharmaceutical Adjuvants; Skin/Mucous Membrane Agents; Topical; Pregnancy Category D; FDA Approval Pre 1982

BRAND NAMES: *Gemicina* (Mexico); Mycifradin; Neo-Rx; *Neomicina*; *Neomycin*; *Neomycine*; *Neomycine Diamant* (France); *Neosulf* (Australia); *Nivemycin* (England); Qrp

(International brand names outside U.S. in italics)

FORMULARIES: BC-BS; Medi-Cal; WHO

> WARNING:
> SYSTEMIC ABSORPTION OF NEOMYCIN OCCURS FOLLOWING ORAL ADMINISTRATION AND TOXIC REACTIONS MAY OCCUR. Patients treated with neomycin should be under close clinical observation because of the potential toxicity associated with their use. NEUROTOXICITY (INCLUDING OTOTOXICITY) AND NEPHROTOXICITY FOLLOWING THE ORAL USE OF NEOMYCIN SULFATE HAVE BEEN REPORTED, EVEN WHEN USED IN RECOMMENDED DOSES. THE POTENTIAL FOR NEPHROTOXICITY, PERMANENT BILATERAL AUDITORY OTOTOXICITY AND SOMETIMES VESTIBULAR TOXICITY IS PRESENT IN PATIENTS WITH NORMAL RENAL FUNCTION WHEN TREATED WITH HIGHER DOSES OF NEOMYCIN AND/OR FOR LONGER PERIODS THAN RECOMMENDED. Serial, vestibular, and audiometric tests, as well as tests of renal function, should be performed (especially in high risk patients). THE RISK OF NEPHROTOXICITY AND OTOTOXICITY IS GREATER IN PATIENTS WITH IMPAIRED RENAL FUNCTION. Ototoxicity is often delayed in onset and patients developing cochlear damage will not have symptoms during therapy to warn them of developing eighth nerve destruction and total or partial deafness may occur long after neomycin has been discontinued.
>
> Neuromuscular blockage and respiratory paralysis have been reported following the oral use of neomycin. The possibility of the occurrence of neuro-muscular blockage and respiratory paralysis should be considered if neomycin is administered, especially to patients receiving anesthetics, neuro-muscular blocking agents such as tubocurarine, succinylcholine, decamethonium, or in patients receiving massive transfusions of citrate anticoagulated blood. If blockage occurs, calcium salts may reverse these phenomena but mechanical respiratory assistance may be necessary.
>
> Concurrent and/or sequential systemic, oral, or topical use of other aminoglycosides including paromomycin and other potentially nephrotoxic and/or neurotoxic drugs such as bacitracin, cisplatin, vancomycin, amphotericin B, polymyxin B, colistin, and viomycin should be avoided because the toxicity may be additive.
>
> Other factors which increase the risk of toxicity are advanced age and dehydration.
>
> The concurrent use of neomycin with potent diuretics such as ethacrynic acid or furosemide should be avoided since certain diuretics by themselves may cause ototoxicity. In addition, when administered intravenously, diuretics may enhance neomycin toxicity by altering the antibiotic concentration in serum and tissue.

DESCRIPTION:

Neomycin sulfate oral solution for oral administration contains neomycin which is an antibiotic obtained from the metabolic products of the actinomycete *Streptomyces fradiae*. Each 5 ml of Neomycin sulfate oral solution contains 125 mg of neomycin sulfate. Inactive ingredients: benzoic acid, FD&C yellow no. 6, flavor, glycerin, methylparaben, propylparaben, sodium phosphate, purified water.

Neomycin B Sulfate: $C_{23}H_{46}N_6O_{13}\cdot 2_{1/2}H_2SO_4$

CLINICAL PHARMACOLOGY:

Neomycin sulfate is poorly absorbed from the normal gastrointestinal tract. The small absorbed fraction is rapidly distributed in the tissues and is excreted by the kidney in keeping with the degree of kidney function. The unabsorbed portion of the drug (approximately 97 percent) is eliminated unchanged in the feces.

Growth of most intestinal bacteria is rapidly suppressed following oral administration of neomycin sulfate, with the suppression persisting for 48-72 hours. Nonpathogenic yeasts and occasionally resistant strains of *Enterobacter aerogenes* (formerly *Aerobacter aerogenes*) replace the intestinal bacteria.

CLINICAL PHARMACOLOGY: *(cont'd)*

As with other aminoglycosides, the amount of systemically absorbed neomycin transferred to the tissues increases cumulatively with each repeated dose administered until a steady state is achieved. The kidney functions as the primary excretory path as well as the tissue binding site with the highest concentration found in the renal cortex. With repeated dosings, progressive accumulation also occurs in the inner ear. Release of tissue bound neomycin occurs slowly over a period of several weeks after dosing has been discontinued.

Protein binding studies have shown that the degree of aminoglycoside protein binding is low and, depending upon the methods used for testing, this may be between 0 and 30 percent.

MICROBIOLOGY

In vitro tests have demonstrated that neomycin is bactericidal and acts by inhibiting the synthesis of protein in susceptible bacterial cells. It is effective primarily against gram-negative bacilli but does have some activity against gram-positive organisms. Neomycin is active*in vitro* against *Escherichia coli* and the*Klebsiella-Enterobacter* group. Neomycin is not active against anaerobic bowel flora.

If susceptibility testing is needed, using a 30 mcg disc, organisms producing zones of 16 mm or greater are considered susceptible. Resistant organisms produce zones of 13 mm or less. Zones greater than 13 mm and less than 16 mm indicate intermediate susceptibility.

INDICATIONS AND USAGE:

HEPATIC COMA (PORTAL-SYSTEMIC ENCEPHALOPATHY)

Neomycin sulfate has been shown to be effective adjunctive therapy in hepatic coma by reduction of the ammonia forming bacteria in the intestinal tract. The subsequent reduction in blood ammonia has resulted in neurologic improvement.

CONTRAINDICATIONS:

Neomycin sulfate oral preparations are contraindicated in the presence of intestinal obstruction and in individuals with a history of hypersensitivity to the drug.

Patients with a history of hypersensitivity or serious toxic reaction to other aminoglycosides may have a cross-sensitivity to neomycin.

Neomycin sulfate oral solution is contraindicated in patients with inflammatory or ulcerative gastrointestinal disease because of the potential for enhanced gastrointestinal absorption of neomycin.

WARNINGS:

(see BOXED WARNING)

Additional manifestations of neurotoxicity may include numbness, skin tingling, muscle twitching, and convulsions.

The risk of hearing loss continues after drug withdrawal.

Aminoglycosides can cause fetal harm when administered to a pregnant woman. Aminoglycoside antibiotics cross the placenta and there have been several reports of total irreversible bilateral congenital deafness in children whose mothers received streptomycin during pregnancy. Although serious side effects to fetus or newborn have not been reported in the treatment of pregnant women with other aminoglycosides, the potential for harm exists. Animal reproduction studies of neomycin have not been conducted. If neomycin is used during pregnancy, or if the patient becomes pregnant while taking this drug, the patient should be apprised of the potential hazard to the fetus.

PRECAUTIONS:

GENERAL

As with other antibiotics, use of oral neomycin may result in overgrowth of nonsusceptible organisms, particularly fungi. If this occurs, appropriate therapy should be instituted.

Neomycin is quickly and almost totally absorbed from body surfaces (except the urinary bladder) after local irrigation and when applied topically in association with surgical procedures. Delayed-onset, irreversible deafness, renal failure, and death due to neuromuscular blockade (regardless of the status of renal function) have been reported following irrigation of both small and large surgical fields with minute quantities of neomycin.

Cross-allergenicity among aminoglycosides has been demonstrated.

Aminoglycosides should be used with caution in patients with muscular disorders such as myasthenia gravis or parkinsonism since these drugs may aggravate muscle weakness because of their potential curare-like effect on the neuromuscular junction.

Small amounts of orally administered neomycin are absorbed through intact intestinal mucosa.

There have been many reports in the literature of nephrotoxicity and/or ototoxicity with the oral use of neomycin. If renal insufficiency develops during oral therapy, consideration should be given to reducing the drug dosage or discontinuing therapy.

An oral neomycin dose of 12 grams per day produces a malabsorption syndrome for a variety of substances including fat, nitrogen, cholesterol, carotene, glucose, xylose, lactose, sodium, calcium, cyanocobalamin and iron.

Orally administered neomycin increases fecal bile acid excretion and reduces intestinal lactase activity.

INFORMATION FOR THE PATIENT

Before administering the drug, patients or members of their families should be informed of possible toxic effects on the eighth nerve. The possibility of acute toxicity increases in premature infants and neonates.

LABORATORY TESTS

Patients with renal insufficiency may develop toxic neomycin blood levels unless doses are properly regulated. If renal insufficiency develops during treatment, the dosage should be reduced or the antibiotic discontinued. To avoid nephrotoxicity and eighth nerve damage associated with high doses and prolonged treatment, the following should be performed prior to and periodically during therapy: urinalysis for increased excretion of protein, decreased specific gravity, casts and cells; renal function tests such as serum creatinine, BUN or creatinine clearance; tests of the vestibulocochlearis nerve (eighth cranial nerve) function.

Serial, vestibular and audiometric tests should be performed (especially in high risk patients). Since elderly patients may have reduced renal function which may not be evident in the results of routine screening tests such as BUN or serum creatinine, a creatinine clearance determination may be more useful.

CARCINOGENESIS, MUTAGENESIS, AND IMPAIRMENT OF FERTILITY

No long-term animal studies have been performed with neomycin sulfate to evaluate carcinogenic or mutagenic potential or impairment of fertility.

PREGNANCY CATEGORY D

(see WARNINGS)

NURSING MOTHERS

It is not know whether neomycin is excreted in human milk but it has been shown to be excreted in cow milk following a single intramuscular injection. Other aminoglycosides have been shown to be excreted in human milk. Because of the potential for serious adverse

PRECAUTIONS: *(cont'd)*

reactions from the aminoglycosides in nursing infants, a decision should be made whether to discontinue nursing or to discontinue the drug, taking into account the importance of the drug to the mother.

PEDIATRIC USE

The safety and efficacy of oral neomycin sulfate in patients less than eighteen years of age have not been established. If treatment of a patient less than eighteen years of age is necessary, neomycin should be used with caution and the period of treatment should not exceed three weeks because of absorption from the gastrointestinal tract.

DRUG INTERACTIONS:

Caution should be taken in concurrent or serial use of other neurotoxic and/or nephrotoxic drugs because of possible enhancement of the nephrotoxicity and/or ototoxicity of neomycin (see BOXED WARNING.)

Caution should also be taken in concurrent or serial use of other aminoglycosides and polymyxins because they may enhance neomycin's nephrotoxicity and/or ototoxicity and potentiate neomycin sulfate's neuromuscular blocking effects.

Oral neomycin inhibits the gastrointestinal absorption of penicillin V, oral vitamin B-12, methotrexate and 5-fluorouracil. The gastrointestinal absorption of digoxin also appears to be inhibited. Therefore, digoxin serum levels should be monitored.

Oral neomycin sulfate may enhance the effect of coumarin in anticoagulants by decreasing vitamin K availability.

ADVERSE REACTIONS:

The most common adverse reactions to oral neomycin sulfate are nausea, vomiting, and diarrhea. The "Malabsorption Syndrome" characterized by increased fecal fat, decreased serum carotene and fall in xylose absorption has been reported with prolonged therapy. Nephrotoxicity, ototoxicity, and neuromuscular blockage have been reported (see BOXED WARNING and PRECAUTIONS).

OVERDOSAGE:

Because of low absorption, it is unlikely that acute overdosage would occur with oral neomycin sulfate. However, prolonged administration could result in sufficient systemic drug levels to produce neurotoxicity, ototoxicity, and/or nephrotoxicity.

Hemodialysis will remove neomycin sulfate from the blood.

DOSAGE AND ADMINISTRATION:

To minimize the risk of toxicity use the lowest possible dose and the shortest possible treatment period to control the condition. Treatment for periods longer than two weeks is not recommended.

HEPATIC COMA

For use as an adjunct in the management of hepatic coma, the recommended dose is 4-12 g per day given in the following regimen:

1. Withdraw protein from diet. Avoid use of diuretic agents.

2. Give supportive therapy including blood products, as indicated.

3. Give Neomycin sulfate oral solution in doses of four to twelve grams of neomycin sulfate per day in divided doses. Treatment should be continued over a period of five to six days during which time protein should be returned incrementally to the diet.

4. If less potentially toxic drugs cannot be used for chronic hepatic insufficiency, neomycin in doses of up to four grams daily may be necessary. The risks for the development of neomycin induced toxicity progressively increase when treatment must be extended to preserve the life of a patient with hepatic encephalopathy who has failed to fully respond. Frequent periodic monitoring of these patients to ascertain the presence of drug toxicity is mandatory (see PRECAUTIONS.) Also, neomycin serum concentrations should be monitored to avoid potentially toxic levels. The benefits to the patient should be weighed against the risks of nephrotoxicity, permanent ototoxicity and neuromuscular blockade following the accumulation of neomycin in the tissues.

STORAGE

Store at controlled room temperature 15-30° C (59-86° F).

(Upjohn, 10/92, 811 947-206, 691015)

HOW SUPPLIED - RATED THERAPEUTICALLY EQUIVALENT:

Powder

10 gm	$5.90	Neomycin Sulfate, Paddock Labs	00574-0440-10
25 gm	$9.56	Neomycin Sulfate, Paddock Labs	00574-0440-25
100 gm	$19.70	Neomycin Sulfate, Paddock Labs	00574-0440-01

Tablet, Uncoated - Oral - 500 mg

100's	$57.05	Neomycin Sulfate, Roxane	00054-8600-25

HOW SUPPLIED - NOT RATED EQUIVALENT:

Ointment - Topical - 0.5 %

30 gm	$2.17	Neomycin Sulfate, Rugby	00536-4805-95
30 gm	$3.50	Neomycin Sulfate, Goldline Labs	00182-5092-34

Solution - Oral - 87.5 mg/5ml

480 ml	$30.12	MYCIFRADIN SULFATE, Pharmacia & Upjohn	00009-0513-02

Tablet, Uncoated - Oral - 500 mg

	$21.85	Neomycin Sulfate, Major Pharms	00904-2703-60
100's	$2.95	Neomycin Sulfate, Geneva Pharms	00781-1400-01
100's	$13.49	Neomycin Sulfate, US Trading	56126-0270-11
100's	$18.16	Neomycin Sulfate, HL Moore Drug Exch	00839-5996-06
100's	$18.48	Neomycin Sulfate, Teva	00332-1177-09
100's	$20.63	Neomycin Sulfate, Rugby	00536-4064-01
100's	$21.70	Neomycin Sulfate, Goldline Labs	00182-0673-01
100's	$23.83	Neomycin Sulfate, United Res	00677-1010-01
100's	$26.27	Neomycin Sulfate, Schein Pharm (US)	00364-2006-01
100's	$36.63	Neomycin Sulfate, Roxane	00054-4600-25

NEOMYCIN SULFATE; POLYMYXIN B SULFATE *(001869)*

CATEGORIES: Aminoglycosides; Anti-Infectives; Antibacterials; Antibiotics; Antimicrobials; Bladder Urine; Burns; Catheter; EENT Drugs; Electrolytic, Caloric-Water Balance; Eye, Ear, Nose, & Throat Preparations; Irrigating Solutions; Ocular Infections; Ophthalmics; Polymyxins; Septicemia; Skin/Mucous Membrane Agents; Urinary Antibacterial; Pregnancy Category D; FDA Approval Pre 1982

BRAND NAMES: Neocin; **Neosporin G.U. Irrigant**; Statrol

FORMULARIES: Medi-Cal

DESCRIPTION:

Note: This monograph contains full prescribing information for the G.U. Irrigant as well as for the Ophthalmic Solution and Ointment.

G.U. IRRIGANT

G.U. Irrigant is a concentrated sterile antibiotic solution to be diluted for urinary bladder irrigation. Each ml contains neomycin sulfate equivalent to 40 mg neomycin base, 200,000 units polymyxin B sulfate and water for injection. The 20-ml multiple dose vial contains, in addition to the above, 1 mg methylparaben (0.1%) added as a preservative.

Neomycin sulfate, an antibiotic of the aminoglycoside group, is the sulfate salt of neomycin B and C produced by *Streptomyces fradiae.* It has a potency equivalent to not less than 600 mcg of neomycin per mg.

Polymyxin B sulfate, a polypeptide antibiotic, is the sulfate salt of polymyxin B_1 and B_2 produced by the growth of*Bacillus polymyxa.* It has the potency of not less than 6,000 polymyxin B units per mg.

OPHTHALMIC SOLUTION AND OINTMENT

This form of this drug is a sterile ophthalmic drug combining two antibacterials in both solution and ointment forms.

Each ml of solution contains: Active: Neomycin Sulfate equivalent to 3.5 mg Neomycin base, Polymyxin B Sulfate 16,250 units. Preservative: Benzalkonium Chloride 0.004%. Vehicle: Hydroxypropyl Methylcellulose 0.5%. Inactive: Boric Acid, Sodium Chloride, Hydrochloric Acid and/or Sodium Hydroxide (to adjust pH), Purified Water.

Each gram of ointment contains: Active: Neomycin Sulfate equivalent to 3.5 mg Neomycin base, polymyxin B Sulfate 10,000 units. Preservatives: Methylparaben 0.05%, Propylparaben 0.01%. Inactive: White Petrolatum, Anhydrous Liquid Lanolin.

CLINICAL PHARMACOLOGY:

G.U. IRRIGANT

After prophylactic irrigation of the intact urinary bladder, neomycin and polymyxin B are absorbed in clinically insignificant quantities. A neomycin serum level of 0.1 mcg/ml was observed in three of the 33 patients receiving the rinse solution. This level is well below that which has been associated with neomycin-induced toxicity.

When used topically, polymyxin B sulfate and neomycin are rarely irritating.

Microbiology: The Neomycin Sulfate/Polymyxin B Sulfate, G.U. Irrigant Sterile solution is bactericidal. The aminoglycosides act by inhibiting normal protein synthesis in susceptible microorganisms. Polymyxins increase the permeability of bacterial cell wall membranes. The solution is active*in vitro* against:

Escherichia coli, Staphylococcus aureus, Haemophilus influenzae, Klebsiella and *Enterobacter* species,*Neisseria* species *Pseudomonas aeruginosa.*

It is not active *in vitro* against *Serratia marcescens* and streptococci.

Bacterial resistance may develop following the use of the antibiotics in the catheter-rinse solution.

OPHTHALMIC SOLUTION AND OINTMENT

The anti-infective components in the combination are included to provide action against specific organisms susceptible to them. Polymyxin B Sulfate is active against gram-negative bacilli including virtually all strains of *Pseudomonas aeruginosa* and most all other strains of*Haemophilus influenzae* species. Neomycin sulfate is active against many strains of both gram-positive and gram-negative organisms including many strains of Proteus.

INDICATIONS AND USAGE:

G.U. Irrigant: Neomycin Sulfate/Polymyxin B Sulfate, G.U. Irrigant is indicated for short-term use (up to 10 days) as a continuous irrigant or rinse in the urinary bladder of abacteriuric patients to prevent bacteriuria and gram-negative rod septicemia associated with the use of indwelling catheters.

Since organisms gain entrance to the bladder by way of, through, and around the catheter, significant bacteriuria is induced by bacterial multiplication in the bladder urine, in the mucoid film often present between catheter and urethra, and in other sites. Urinary tract infection may result from the repeated presence in the urine of large numbers of pathogenic bacteria. The use of closed systems with indwelling catheters has been shown to reduce the risk of infection. A three-way closed catheter system with constant neomycin-polymyxin B bladder rinse is indicated to prevent the development of infection while using indwelling catheters.

If uropathogens are isolated, they should be identified and tested for susceptibility so that appropriate antimicrobial therapy for systemic use can be initiated.

Ophthalmic Solution and Ointment: For the treatment of superficial ocular infections involving the conjunctiva and/or cornea caused by organisms susceptible to Polymyxin B Sulfate and Neomycin Sulfate.

CONTRAINDICATIONS:

G.U. Irrigant: Hypersensitivity to Neomycin, the polymyxins, or any ingredient in the solution is a contraindication to its use. A history of hypersensitivity or serious toxic reaction to an aminoglycoside may also contraindicate the use of any aminoglycoside because of the known cross-sensitivity of patients to drugs of this class.

Ophthalmic Solution and Ointment: Epithelial herpes simplex keratitis (dendritic keratitis), vaccina varicella, and many other viral diseases of the cornea and conjunctiva. Mycobacterial infection of the eye. Fungal diseases of ocular structures. Hypersensitivity to a component of the medication.

WARNINGS:

G.U. IRRIGANT

PROPHYLACTIC BLADDER CARE WITH NEOMYCIN SULFATE/POLYMYXIN B SULFATE, G.U. IRRIGANT STERILE SHOULD NOT BE GIVEN WHERE THERE IS A POSSIBILITY OF SYSTEMIC ABSORPTION. THIS FORM OF THIS DRUG SHOULD NOT BE USED FOR IRRIGATION OTHER THAN FOR THE URINARY BLADDER. Systemic absorption after topical application of neomycin to open wounds, burns, and granulating surfaces is significant and serum concentrations comparable to and often higher than those attained following oral and parenteral therapy have been reported. Absorption of neomycin from the denuded bladder surface has been reported.

However, the likelihood of toxicity following topical irrigation of the intact urinary bladder with Neomycin Sulfate/Polymyxin B Sulfate, G.U. Irrigant Sterile is low since no appreciable amounts of these antibiotics enter the systemic circulation by this route if irrigation does not exceed ten days.

This G.U. irrigant is intended for continuous prophylactic irrigation of the lumen of the intact urinary bladder of patients with indwelling catheters. Patients should be under constant supervision by a physician. Irrigation should be avoided in patients with defects in the bladder mucosa or bladder wall, such as a vesicle rupture, or in association with operative procedures on the bladder wall, because of the risk of toxicity due to systemic absorption

WARNINGS: *(cont'd)*

following diffusion into absorption tissues and spaces. When absorbed, neomycin and polymyxin B are nephrotoxic antibiotics, and the nephrotoxic potentials are additive. In addition, both antibiotics when absorbed, are neurotoxins; neomycin can destroy fibers of the acoustic nerve causing permanent bilateral deafness; neomycin and polymyxin B are additive in their neuromuscular blocking effects, not only in terms of potency and duration but also in terms of characteristics of the blocks produced.

Aminoglycosides, when absorbed, can cause fetal harm when administered to a pregnant woman. Aminoglycoside antibiotics cross the placenta and there have been several reports of total, irreversible, bilateral, congenital deafness in children whose mothers received streptomycin during pregnancy. Although serious side effects have not been reported in the treatment of pregnant women with other aminoglycoside, the potential for harm exists. If Neomycin Sulfate/Polymyxin B Sulfate, G.U. Irrigant Sterile is used during pregnancy, the patient should be apprised of the potential hazard to the fetus (see PRECAUTIONS).

OPHTHALMIC SOLUTION AND OINTMENT

NOT FOR INJECTION INTO THE EYE. Should a sensitivity reaction occur, discontinue use. Ophthalmic ointments may retard corneal wound healing.

PRECAUTIONS:

G.U. IRRIGANT

General: Ototoxicity, nephrotoxicity, and neuromuscular blockade may occur if Neomycin Sulfate/Polymyxin B Sulfate, G.U. Irrigant ingredients are systemically absorbed (see WARNINGS). Absorption of neomycin from the denuded bladder surface has been reported. Patients with impaired renal function, infants, dehydrated patients, elderly patients, and patients receiving high doses of prolonged treatment are especially at risk for the development of toxicity.

Irrigation of the bladder with this irrigant may result in overgrowth of nonsusceptible organisms, including fungi. Appropriate measures should be taken if this occurs. The safety and effectiveness of the preparation for use in the care of patients with recent lower urinary tract surgery have not been established.

Urine specimens should be collected during prophylactic bladder care for urinalysis, culture, and susceptibility testing. Positive cultures suggest the presence of organisms which are resistant to the bladder rinse antibiotics.

Pregnancy, Teratogenic Effects, Pregnancy Category D (See WARNINGS).

OPHTHALMIC SOLUTION AND OINTMENT

The initial prescription and renewal of the medication order beyond 20 ml or 8 g should be made by a physician only after examination of the patient with the aid of magnification such as slit lamp biomicroscopy and, where appropriate, fluorescein staining.

ADVERSE REACTIONS:

G.U. IRRIGANT

Neomycin occasionally causes skin sensitization when applied topically; however, topical application to mucous membranes rarely result in local or systemic hypersensitivity reactions.

Irritation of the urinary bladder mucosa has been reported.

Signs of ototoxicity and nephrotoxicity have been reported following parenteral use of these drugs and following topical use of neomycin (See WARNINGS.)

OPHTHALMIC SOLUTION AND OINTMENT

Adverse reactions have occurred with the anti-infective components. Exact incidence figures are not available since no denominator of treated patients is available.

Reactions occurring most often from the presence of the anti-infective ingredients are allergic sensitizations.

DOSAGE AND ADMINISTRATION:

G.U. IRRIGANT

This preparation is specifically designed for use with "three-way" catheters or with other catheter systems permitting **continuous** irrigation of the urinary bladder. The usual irrigation dose is one 1-ml ampul a day for up to ten days.

Using strict aseptic techniques, the contents of 1-ml ampul of Neomycin Sulfate/Polymyxin B Sulfate, G.U. Irrigant Sterile for irrigation should be added to a 1,000-ml container of isotonic saline solution. This container should then be connected to the inflow of lumen of the "three- way" catheter which has been inserted with full aseptic precautions; use of a sterile lubricant is recommended during insertion into the catheter. The outflow lumen should be connected, via a sterile disposable plastic collection bag. Stringent procedures, such as taping the inflow and outflow junction at the catheter, should be observed when necessary to insure the junctional integrity of the system.

For most patients, the inflow rate of the 1,000-ml saline solution of neomycin and polymyxin B should be adjusted to a slow drip to deliver about 1,000 ml every twenty-four hours. If the patient's urine output exceeds 2 liters per day, it is recommended that the inflow rate be adjusted to deliver 2,000 ml of the solution in a twenty-four hour period.

It is important that the rinse of the bladder be **continuous;** the inflow or rinse should not be interrupted for more than a few minutes.

Preparation of the irrigation solution should be performed with strict aseptic techniques. The prepared solution should be stored at 4°C, and should be used within 48 hours following preparation to reduce the risk of contamination with resistant microorganisms.

Store at 2° to 8°C (36° to 46°F).

OPHTHALMIC SOLUTION AND OINTMENT

Solution: Instill one or two drops in the lower conjunctival sac(s) three or more times daily as required. Ointment: Instill about a half-inch ribbon into the conjunctival sac(s) at night when used adjunctively with the solution.

Not more than 20 ml or 8 mg should be prescribed initially and the prescription should not be refilled without further evaluation as outlined in PRECAUTIONS.

(G.U. Irrigant: Burroughs Wellcome, 3/11/94, 561051)

HOW SUPPLIED - RATED THERAPEUTICALLY EQUIVALENT:

Solution - Irrigation - 40 mg/200,000 u

1 ml ampul x 10	$65.04	NEOSPORIN G U IRRIGANT, Glaxo Wellcome	00173-0748-10
1 ml ampul x 50	$313.45	NEOSPORIN G U IRRIGANT, Glaxo Wellcome	00173-0748-35
1 ml x 25	$76.31	Neomycin-Polymyxin B Sulfates, Schein Pharm (US)	00364-2190-41
1 ml x 25	$76.31	Neomycin & Polymyxin B Sulfates, Steris Labs	00402-0801-81
20 ml	$36.15	Neomycin & Polymyxin B Sulfates, Schein Pharm (US)	00364-2191-55
20 ml	$75.65	NEOSPORIN G U IRRIGANT, Glaxo Wellcome	00173-0748-93

HOW SUPPLIED - NOT RATED EQUIVALENT:

Solution - Ophthalmic - 5 mg/16250 unit

5 ml	$11.25	STATROL, Alcon-PR	00998-0623-05

NEOMYCIN SULFATE; POLYMYXIN B SULFATE; PREDNISOLONE ACETATE *(001870)*

CATEGORIES: Anti-Infectives; Antibiotics; Conjunctivitis; Corneal Inflammation; Corneal Injury; EENT Drugs; Eye, Ear, Nose, & Throat Preparations; Ocular Infections; Ophthalmics; Steroids; Uveitis; FDA Approval Pre 1982

BRAND NAMES: **Poly-Pred**

FORMULARIES: Aetna; Medi-Cal

DESCRIPTION:

LIQUIFILM

Sterile Ophthalmic Suspension

This combination drug sterile ophthalmic suspension is a topical anti-inflammatory/anti-infective combination product for ophthalmic use.

Chemical Name: Prednisolone acetate: 11β, 17, 21-trihydroxypregna-1, 4-dione 21-acetate.

CONTAINS:

Prednisolone acetate (microfine suspension) - 0.5%

neomycin sulfate (equivalent to 0.35% neomycin) - 0.5%

polymyxin B sulfate - 10,000 units/ml

with Liquifilm (polyvinyl alcohol 1.4%); thimerosal (0.001%); polysorbate 80; propylene glycol; sodium acetate; and purified water.

CLINICAL PHARMACOLOGY:

Corticosteroids suppress the inflammatory response to a variety of agents and they probably delay or slow healing. Since corticosteroids may inhibit the body's defense mechanism against infection, a concomitant antimicrobial drug may be used when this inhibition is concerned to be clinically in a particular case.

The anti-infective components in this combination drug are included to provide action against specific organisms susceptible to them. Neomycin sulfate is considered active against a wide range of gram-positive organisms, with effectiveness against many strains of *Proteus, Klebsiella, Staphylococcus aureus, Escherichia coli* and *Haemophilus influenzae.* Polymyxin B Sulfate activity is sharply restricted to gram-negative bacteria, including many strains of *Pseudomonas aeruginosa, Escherichia coli,* and *Haemophilus influenzae.*

When a decision to administer both a corticosteroid and an antimicrobial is made, the administration of such drugs in the combination has the advantage of greater patient is compliance and convenience, with the added assurance that the appropriate dosage of both drugs is administered. When both types of drugs are in the same formulation, compatibility of ingredients is assured and the correct volume of drug is delivered and retained.

The relative potency of corticosteroids depends on the molecular structure, concentration, and release from the vehicle.

INDICATIONS AND USAGE:

A steroid/anti-infective combination is indicated in ocular inflammation when concurrent use of an antimicrobial is judged necessary.

CONTRAINDICATIONS:

Epithelial herpes simplex keratitis (dendritic keratitis), vaccina, varicella, and many other viral diseases of the cornea and conjunctiva. Mycobacterial infection of the eye. Fungal diseases of the ocular structures. Hypersensitivity to component of the medication. Hypersensitivity to the antibiotic component of the medication. (Hypersensitivity to the antibiotic component occurs at a higher rate than for other components).

The use of these combination is always contraindicated after uncomplicated removal of a corneal foreign body.

WARNINGS:

Prolonged use may result in glaucoma with damage to the optic nerve, defects in visual acuity and fields of vision, and posterior subcapsular cataract formation. Prolonged use may suppress the host response and thus increase the hazard of secondary ocular infections. In those diseases causing thinning of the cornea or sclera, perforations have been known to occur with the use of topical steroids. In acute purulent conditions of the eye, steroids may mask infection or enhance existing infection. If these products are used for 10 days or longer, intraocular pressure should be routinely monitored even though it may be difficult in children and uncooperative patients.

Employment of a steroid medication in the treatment of herpes simplex great caution.

PRECAUTIONS:

The initial prescription and renewal of the medication order beyond 20 ml should be made by a physician only after examination of the patient with the aid of magnification, such as slit lamp biomicroscopy and, where appropriate, fluorescein staining.

The possibility of fungal infections of the cornea should be considered after prolonged steroid dosing.

ADVERSE REACTIONS:

Adverse reactions have occurred with steroid/anti-infective combination drugs which can be attributed to the steroid component, the anti-infective component, or the combination. Exact incidence figures are not available since no denomination of treated is available.

Reactions occurring most often from the presence of the anti-infective ingredient are allergic sensitizations. The reactions due to the steroid component in decreasing order of frequency are: elevation of intraocular pressure (IOP) with possible development of glaucoma, and infrequent optic nerve damage; posterior subcapsular cataract formation; and delayed wound healing.

Secondary Infection: The development of secondary infection has occurred after use of combination containing steroids and antimicrobials. Fungal infections of the cornea are particularly prone to develop coincidentally with long-term applications of steroid. The possibility of fungal invasion must be considered in any persistent corneal ulceration where steroid treatment has been used. Secondary bacterial ocular infection following suppression of host responses also occurs.

DOSAGE AND ADMINISTRATION:

To Treat The Eye: 1 or 2 drops every 3 to 4 hours, or more frequently as required. Acute infections may require administration every 30 minutes, with frequency of administration reduced as the infection is brought under control.

To Treat The Lids: Instill 1 or 2 drops in the eye every 3 to 4 hours, close the eye and rub the excess on the lids and lid margins.

Note: Protect from freezing. Shake well before using.

HOW SUPPLIED - EQUIVALENTS NOT AVAILABLE:

Suspension - Ophthalmic; Top - 0.5 %/10000 uni

5 ml	**$16.18**	**POLY-PRED, Allergan**	**00023-0028-05**
10 ml	**$24.99**	**POLY-PRED, Allergan**	**00023-0028-10**

NEOSTIGMINE BROMIDE *(001873)*

CATEGORIES: Autonomic Drugs; Myasthenia Gravis; Neuromuscular; Parasympathomimetic Agents; Pregnancy Category C; FDA Pre 1938 Drugs

BRAND NAMES: **Prostigmin**; *Prostigmina*; *Prostigmine* (Mexico, France); *Stigmine*; *Vagostigmin*; *Vagostin*
(International brand names outside U.S. in italics)

FORMULARIES: Aetna; Medi-Cal; WHO

DESCRIPTION:

Neostigmine bromide, an anticholinesterase agent, is available for oral administration in 15-mg tablets. Each tablet also contains gelatin, lactose, corn starch, stearic acid, sugar and talc.

Chemically, neostigmine bromide is (*m*-hydroxyphenyl)trimethylammonium bromide dimethylcarbamate. It is a white, crystalline, bitter powder, soluble 1:1 in water, with a molecular weight of 303.20.

CLINICAL PHARMACOLOGY:

Neostigmine inhibits the hydrolysis of acetylcholine by competing with acetylcholine for attachment to acetylcholinesterase at sites of cholinergic transmission. It enhances cholinergic action by facilitating the transmission of impulses across neuromuscular junctions. It also has a direct cholinomimetic effect on skeletal muscle and possibly on autonomic ganglion cells and neurons of the central nervous system. Neostigmine undergoes hydrolysis by cholinesterase and is also metabolized by microsomal enzymes in the liver. Protein binding to human serum albumin ranges from 15 to 25 percent.

Neostigmine bromide is poorly absorbed from the gastrointestinal tract following oral administration. As a rule, 15 mg of neostigmine bromide orally is equivalent to 0.5 mg of neostigmine methylsulfate parenterally, due to poor absorption of the tablet from the intestinal tract. In a study in fasting myasthenic patients, the extent of absorption was estimated to be 1 to 2 percent of the ingested 30-mg single oral dose. Peak concentrations in plasma occurred 1 to 2 hours following drug ingestion, with considerable individual variations. The half-life ranged from 42 to 60 minutes with a mean half-life of 52 minutes.

INDICATIONS AND USAGE:

Neostigmine bromide is indicated for the symptomatic treatment of myasthenia gravis. Its greatest usefulness is in prolonged therapy where no difficulty in swallowing is present. In acute myasthenic crisis where difficulty in breathing and swallowing is present, the parenteral form (neostigmine methylsulfate) should be used. The patient can be transferred to the oral form as soon as it can be tolerated.

CONTRAINDICATIONS:

Neostigmine bromide is contraindicated in patients with known hypersensitivity to the drug. Because of the presence of the bromide ion, it should not be used in patients with a previous history of reaction to bromides. It is contraindicated in patients with peritonitis or mechanical obstruction of the intestinal or urinary tract.

WARNINGS:

Neostigmine bromide should be used with caution in patients with epilepsy, bronchial asthma, bradycardia, recent coronary occlusion, vagotonia, hyperthyroidism, cardiac arrhythmias or peptic ulcer. As a rule, 15 mg of neostigmine bromide orally is equivalent to 0.5 mg of neostigmine methylsulfate parenterally, due to poor absorption of the tablet from the intestinal tract. Large doses should be avoided in situations where there might be an increased absorption rate from the intestinal tract. It should be used with caution when co-administered with anticholinergic drugs, in order to avoid reduction of intestinal motility.

PRECAUTIONS:

GENERAL

It is important to differentiate between myasthenic crisis and cholinergic crisis caused by overdosage of neostigmine bromide. Both conditions result in extreme muscle weakness but require radically different treatment. (See OVERDOSAGE.)

CARCINOGENESIS, MUTAGENESIS, AND IMPAIRMENT OF FERTILITY

There have been no studies with neostigmine bromide which would permit an evaluation of its carcinogenic or mutagenic potential. Studies on the effect of neostigmine bromide on fertility and reproduction have not been performed.

PREGNANCY CATEGORY C

Teratogenic Effects: There are no adequate or well-controlled studies of neostigmine bromide in either laboratory animals or in pregnant women. It is not known whether neostigmine bromide can cause fetal harm when administered to a pregnant woman or can affect reproductive capacity. Neostigmine bromide should be given to a pregnant woman only if clearly needed.

Nonteratogenic Effects: Anticholinesterase drugs may cause uterine irritability and induce premature labor when given intravenously to pregnant women near term.

NURSING MOTHERS

It is not known whether neostigmine bromide is excreted in human milk. Because many drugs are excreted in human milk and because of the potential for serious adverse reactions from neostigmine bromide in nursing infants, a decision should be made whether to discontinue nursing or to discontinue the drug, taking into account the importance of the drug to the mother.

PEDIATRIC USE

Safety and effectiveness in children have not been established.

DRUG INTERACTIONS:

Certain antibiotics, especially neomycin, streptomycin and kanamycin, have a mild but definite nondepolarizing blocking action which may accentuate neuromuscular block. These antibiotics should be used in the myasthenic patient only where definitely indicated, and then careful adjustment should be made of adjunctive anticholinesterase dosage.

Local and some general anesthetics, antiarrhythmic agents and other drugs that interfere with neuromuscular transmission should be used cautiously, if at all, in patients with myasthenia gravis; the dose of neostigmine bromide may have to be increased accordingly.

ADVERSE REACTIONS:

Side effects are generally due to an exaggeration of pharmacological effects of which salivation and fasciculation are the most common. Bowel cramps and diarrhea may also occur.

ADVERSE REACTIONS: *(cont'd)*

The following additional adverse reactions have been reported following the use of either neostigmine bromide or neostigmine methylsulfate:

Allergic: Allergic reactions and anaphylaxis.

Neurologic: Dizziness, convulsions, loss of consciousness, drowsiness, headache, dysarthria, miosis and visual changes.

Cardiovascular: Cardiac arrhythmias (including bradycardia, tachycardia, A-V block and nodal rhythm) and nonspecific EKG changes have been reported, as well as cardiac arrest, syncope and hypotension. These have been predominantly noted following the use of the injectable form of neostigmine bromide.

Respiratory: Increased oral, pharyngeal and bronchial secretions, and dyspnea. Respiratory depression, respiratory arrest and bronchospasm have been reported following the use of the injectable form of neostigmine bromide.

Dermatologic: Rash and urticaria.

Gastrointestinal: Nausea, emesis, flatulence and increased peristalsis.

Genitourinary: Urinary frequency.

Musculoskeletal: Muscle cramps and spasms, arthralgia.

Miscellaneous: Diaphoresis, flushing and weakness.

OVERDOSAGE:

Overdosage of neostigmine bromide can cause cholinergic crisis, which is characterized by increasing muscle weakness, and through involvement of the muscles of respiration, may result in death. Myasthenic crisis, due to an increase in the severity of the disease, is also accompanied by extreme muscle weakness and may be difficult to distinguish from cholinergic crisis on a symptomatic basis. However, such differentiation is extremely important because increases in the dose of neostigmine bromide or other drugs in this class, in the presence of cholinergic crisis or of a refractory or "insensitive" state, could have grave consequences. The two types of crises may be differentiated by the use of Tensilon (edrophonium chloride) as well as by clinical judgment.

Treatment of the two conditions differs radically. Whereas the presence of *myasthenic crisis* requires more intensive anticholinesterase therapy, *cholinergic crisis* calls for the prompt withdrawal of all drugs of this type. The immediate use of atropine in cholinergic crisis is also recommended.

Atropine may also be used to abolish or minimize gastrointestinal side effects or other muscarinic reactions; but such use, by masking signs of overdosage, can lead to inadvertent induction of cholinergic crisis.

The LD_{50} of neostigmine methylsulfate in mice is 0.3 $\pm$ 0.02 mg/kg intravenously, 0.54 $\pm$ 0.03 mg/kg subcutaneously, and 0.395 $\pm$ 0.025 mg/kg intramuscularly; in rats the LD_{50} is 0.315 $\pm$ 0.019 mg/kg intravenously, 0.445 $\pm$ 0.032 mg/kg subcutaneously, and 0.423 $\pm$ 0.032 mg/kg intramuscularly.

DOSAGE AND ADMINISTRATION:

The onset of action of neostigmine bromide given orally is slower than when given parenterally, but the duration of action is longer and the intensity of action more uniform. Dosage requirements for optimal results vary from 15 mg to 375 mg per day. In some instances it may be necessary to exceed these dosages, but the possibility of cholinergic crisis must be recognized. The average dose is 10 tablets (150 mg) administered over a 24-hour period. The interval between doses is of paramount importance. The dosage schedule should be adjusted for each patient and changed as the need arises. Frequently, therapy is required day and night. Larger portions of the total daily dose may be given at times when the patient is more prone to fatigue (afternoon, mealtimes, etc.). The patient should be encouraged to keep a daily record of his or her condition to assist the physician in determining an optimal therapeutic regimen.

HOW SUPPLIED - EQUIVALENTS NOT AVAILABLE:

Tablet, Uncoated - Oral - 15 mg

100's	$6.55	Neostigmine Bromide, Lannett	00527-1243-01
100's	**$39.88**	**PROSTIGMIN, ICN Pharms**	**00187-3100-10**

NEOSTIGMINE METHYLSULFATE *(001874)*

CATEGORIES: Analeptics; Antagonists and Antidotes; Autonomic Drugs; Myasthenia Gravis; Parasympathomimetic Agents; Relaxants/Stimulants, Urinary Tract; Urinary Retention; Pregnancy Category C; FDA Pre 1938 Drugs

BRAND NAMES: *Mestastigmin*; *Normastigmin*; *Prostigmin* (England, Germany); *Prostigmin INJ*; **Prostigmin Injectable**; *Prostigmina*; *Prostigmine* (France, Mexico); *Stigmine*; *Tilstigmin*; *Vagostigmin*; *Vagostin*
(International brand names outside U.S. in italics)

FORMULARIES: Aetna; Medi-Cal

DESCRIPTION:

Neostigmine methylsulfate injectable, an anticholinesterase agent, is a sterile aqueous solution intended for intramuscular, intravenous or subcutaneous administration.

Neostigmine methylsulfate Injectable is available in the following concentrations:

Prostigmin Injectable 1:2000 Ampuls: Each ml contains 0.5 mg neostigmine methylsulfate compounded with 0.2% parabens (methyl and propyl) as preservatives and sodium hydroxide to adjust pH to approximately 5.9.

Prostigmin Injectable 1:4000 Ampuls: Each ml contains 0.25 mg neostigmine methylsulfate compounded with 0.2% parabens (methyl and propyl) as preservatives and sodium hydroxide to adjust pH to approximately 5.9.

Prostigmin Injectable 1:1000 Multiple Dose Vials: Each ml contains 1 mg neostigmine methylsulfate compounded with 0.45% phenol as preservative, 0.2 mg sodium acetate, and acetic acid and sodium hydroxide to adjust pH to approximately 5.9.

Prostigmin Injectable 1:2000 Multiple Dose Vials: Each ml contains 0.5 mg neostigmine methylsulfate compounded with 0.45% phenol as preservative, 0.2 mg sodium acetate, and acetic acid and sodium hydroxide to adjust pH to approximately 5.9.

Chemically, neostigmine methylsulfate is (m-hydroxyphenyl) trimethylammonium methylsulfate dimethylcarbamate. It has a molecular weight of 334.39.

CLINICAL PHARMACOLOGY:

Neostigmine inhibits the hydrolysis of acetylcholine by competing with acetylcholine for attachment to acetylcholinesterase at sites of cholinergic transmission. It enhances cholinergic action by facilitating the transmission of impulses across neuromuscular junctions. It also has a direct cholinomimetic effect on skeletal muscle and possibly on autonomic ganglion cells

CLINICAL PHARMACOLOGY: *(cont'd)*

and neurons of the central nervous system. Neostigmine undergoes hydrolysis by cholinesterase and is also metabolized by microsomal enzymes in the liver. Protein binding to human serum albumin ranges from 15 to 25 percent.

Following intramuscular administration, neostigmine is rapidly absorbed and eliminated. In a study of five patients with myasthenia gravis, peak plasma levels were observed at 30 minutes, and the half-life ranged from 51 to 90 minutes. Approximately 80 percent of the drug was eliminated in urine within 24 hours; approximately 50% as the unchanged drug, and 30 percent as metabolites. Following intravenous administration, plasma half-life ranges from 47 to 60 minutes have been reported with a mean half-life of 53 minutes.

The clinical effects of neostigmine usually begin within 20 to 30 minutes after intramuscular injection and last from 2.5 to 4 hours.

INDICATIONS AND USAGE:

Neostigmine methylsulfate is indicated for:

the symptomatic control of myasthenia gravis when oral therapy is impractical.

the prevention and treatment of postoperative distention and urinary retention after mechanical obstruction has been excluded.

reversal of effects of nondepolarizing neuromuscular blocking agents (*e.g.,* tubocurarine, metocurine, gallamine, or pancuronium) after surgery.

CONTRAINDICATIONS:

Neostigmine methylsulfate is contraindicated in patients with known hypersensitivity to the drug. It is also contraindicated in patients with peritonitis or mechanical obstruction of the intestinal or urinary tract.

WARNINGS:

Neostigmine methylsulfate should be used with caution in patients with epilepsy, bronchial asthma, bradycardia, recent coronary occlusion, vagotonia, hyperthyroidism, cardiac arrhythmias or peptic ulcer. When large doses of neostigmine methylsulfate are administered, the prior or simultaneous injection of atropine sulfate may be advisable. Separate syringes should be used for the neostigmine methylsulfate and atropine. Because of the possibility of hypersensitivity in an occasional patient, atropine and antishock medication should always be readily available.

PRECAUTIONS:

GENERAL

It is important to differentiate between myasthenic crisis and cholinergic crisis caused by overdosage of neostigmine methylsulfate. Both conditions result in extreme muscle weakness but require radically different treatment. (See OVERDOSAGE.)

CARCINOGENESIS, MUTAGENESIS AND IMPAIRMENT OF FERTILITY

There have been no studies with neostigmine methylsulfate which would permit an evaluation of its carcinogenic or mutagenic potential. Studies on the effect of neostigmine methylsulfate on fertility and reproduction have not been performed.

PREGNANCY CATEGORY C

Teratogenic Effects: There are no adequate or well-controlled studies of neostigmine methylsulfate in either laboratory animals or in pregnant women. It is not known whether neostigmine methylsulfate can cause fetal harm when administered to a pregnant woman or can affect reproductive capacity. Neostigmine methylsulfate should be given to a pregnant woman only if clearly needed.

Nonteratogenic Effects: Anticholinesterase drugs may cause uterine irritability and induce premature labor when given intravenously to pregnant women near term.

NURSING MOTHERS

It is not known whether neostigmine methylsulfate is excreted in human milk. Because many drugs are excreted in human milk and because of the potential for serious adverse reactions from neostigmine methylsulfate in nursing infants, a decision should be made whether to discontinue nursing or to discontinue the drug, taking into account the importance of the drug to the mother.

PEDIATRIC USE

Safety and effectiveness in children have not been established.

DRUG INTERACTIONS:

Neostigmine methylsulfate does not antagonize, and may in fact prolong, the Phase I block of *depolarizing* muscle relaxants such as succinylcholine or decamethonium. Certain antibiotics, especially neomycin, streptomycin and kanamycin, have a mild but definite nondepolarizing blocking action which may accentuate neuromuscular block. These antibiotics should be used in the myasthenic patient only where definitely indicated, and then careful adjustment should be made of the anticholinesterase dosage. Local and some general anesthetics, antiarrhythmic agents and other drugs that interfere with neuromuscular transmission should be used cautiously, if at all, in patients with myasthenia gravis; the dose of neostigmine methylsulfate may have to be increased accordingly.

ADVERSE REACTIONS:

Side effects are generally due to an exaggeration of pharmacological effects of which salivation and fasciculation are the most common. Bowel cramps and diarrhea may also occur.

The following additional adverse reactions have been reported following the use of either neostigmine bromide or neostigmine methylsulfate.

Allergic: Allergic reactions and anaphylaxis.

Neurologic: Dizziness, convulsions, loss of consciousness, drowsiness, headache, dysarthria, miosis and visual changes.

Cardiovascular: Cardiac arrhythmias (including bradycardia, tachycardia, A-V block and nodal rhythm) and nonspecific EKG changes have been reported, as well as cardiac arrest, syncope and hypotension. These have been predominantly noted following the use of the injectable form of neostigmine methylsulfate.

Respiratory: Increased oral, pharyngeal and bronchial secretions, dyspnea, respiratory depression, respiratory arrest and bronchospasm.

Dermatologic: Rash and urticaria.

Gastrointestinal: Nausea, emesis, flatulence and increased peristalsis.

Genitourinary: Urinary frequency.

Musculoskeletal: Muscle cramps and spasms, arthralgia.

Miscellaneous: Diaphoresis, flushing and weakness.

OVERDOSAGE:

Overdosage of neostigmine methylsulfate can cause cholinergic crisis, which is characterized by increasing muscle weakness, and through involvement of the muscles of respiration, may result in death. Myasthenic crisis, due to an increase in the severity of the disease, is also

OVERDOSAGE: *(cont'd)*

accompanied by extreme muscle weakness and may be difficult to distinguish from cholinergic crisis on a symptomatic basis. However, such differentiation is extremely important because increases in the dose of neostigmine methylsulfate or other drugs in this class, in the presence of cholinergic crisis or of a refractory or "insensitive" state, could have grave consequences. The two types of crises may be differentiated by the use of Tensilon (edrophonium chloride) as well as by clinical judgment.

Treatment of the two conditions differs radically. Whereas the presence of *myasthenic crisis* requires more intensive anticholinesterase therapy, *cholinergic crisis* calls for the prompt withdrawal of all drugs of this type. The immediate use of atropine in cholinergic crisis is also recommended.

Atropine may also be used to abolish or minimize gastrointestinal side effects or other muscarinic reactions; but such use, by masking signs of overdosage, can lead to inadvertent induction of cholinergic crisis.

The LD_{50} of neostigmine methylsulfate in mice is 0.3 ± 0.02 mg/kg intravenously, 0.54 ± 0.03 mg/kg subcutaneously, and 0.395 ± 0.025 mg/kg intramuscularly; in rats the LD_{50} is 0.315 ± 0.019 mg/kg intravenously, 0.445 ± 0.032 mg/kg subcutaneously, and 0.423 ± 0.032 mg/kg intramuscularly.

DOSAGE AND ADMINISTRATION:

Symptomatic Control of Myasthenia Gravis: One ml of the 1:2000 solution (0.5 mg) subcutaneously or intramuscularly. Subsequent doses should be based on the individual patient's response. In most patients, however, oral treatment with neostigmine methylsulfate (neostigmine bromide) tablets, 15 mg each, is adequate for control of symptoms.

Prevention of Postoperative Distention And Urinary Retention: One ml of the 1:4000 solution (0.25 mg) subcutaneously or intramuscularly as soon as possible after operation; repeat every 4 to 6 hours for two or three days.

Treatment of Postoperative Distention: One ml of the 1:2000 solution (0.5 mg) subcutaneously or intramuscularly, as required.

Treatment of Urinary Retention: One ml of the 1:2000 solution (0.5 mg) subcutaneously or intramuscularly. If urination does not occur within an hour, the patient should be catheterized. After the patient has voided, or the bladder has been emptied, continue the 0.5 mg injections every three hours for at least 5 injections.

Reversal of Effects of Nondepolarizing Neuromuscular Blocking Agents: When neostigmine methylsulfate is administered intravenously, it is recommended that atropine sulfate (0.6 to 1.2 mg) also be given intravenously using separate syringes. Some authorities have recommended that the atropine be injected several minutes before the neostigmine methylsulfate rather than concomitantly. The usual dose is 0.5 to 2 mg neostigmine methylsulfate given by *slow* intravenous injection, repeated as required. Only in exceptional cases should the total dose of neostigmine methylsulfate exceed 5 mg. It is recommended that the patient be well ventilated and a patent airway maintained until complete recovery of normal respiration is assured. The optimum time for administration of the drug is during hyperventilation when the carbon dioxide level of the blood is low. It should never be administered in the presence of high concentrations of halothane or cyclopropane. In cardiac cases and severely ill patients, it is advisable to titrate the exact dose of neostigmine methylsulfate required, using a peripheral nerve stimulator device. In the presence of bradycardia, the pulse rate should be increased to about 80/minute with atropine before administering neostigmine methylsulfate.

Parenteral drug products should be inspected visually for particulate matter and discoloration prior to administration, whenever solution and container permit.

HOW SUPPLIED - RATED THERAPEUTICALLY EQUIVALENT:

Injection, Solution - Intramuscular; - 0.5 mg/ml

10 ml x 1	$6.63	Neostigmine Methylsulfate, Vial, Marsam	00209-7750-20

Injection, Solution - Intramuscular; - 1 mg/ml

10 ml x 1	$7.08	Neostigmine Methylsulfate, Vial, Marsam	00209-7800-20

HOW SUPPLIED - NOT RATED EQUIVALENT:

Injection, Solution - Intramuscular; - 0.5 mg/ml

1 ml x 10	$18.25	PROSTIGMIN, ICN Pharms	00187-3101-30
1 ml x 10	$37.20	Neostigmine Methylsulfate, Gensia Labs	00703-2711-03
1 ml x 10	$126.94	PROSTIGMIN 0.5, ICN Pharms	00187-3104-60
10 ml	$4.66	Neostigmine Methylsulfate, Bristol Myers Squibb	00003-2912-12
10 ml	$8.66	Neostigmine Methylsulfate 1:2000 0.5, Abbott	00074-3722-01
10 ml	$9.98	Neostigmine Methylsulfate, Schein Pharm (US)	00364-2368-54
10 ml	$9.98	Neostigmine Methylsulfate, Steris Labs	00402-0916-10
10 ml x 1	$6.56	Neostigmine, Elkins Sinn	00641-2545-41
10 ml x 5	$14.18	Neostigmine Methylsulfate 1:2000, Astra USA	00186-1741-01
10 ml x 10	$50.00	Neostigmine Methylsulfate, Am Regent	00517-0034-10
10 ml x 10	$66.96	Neostigmine Methylsulfate, Gensia Labs	00703-2714-03
10 ml x 10	$67.63	Neostigmine Methylsulfate, Fujisawa USA	00469-3820-30
10 ml x 10	**$117.56**	**PROSTIGMIN, ICN Pharms**	**00187-3100-60**

Injection, Solution - Intramuscular; - 1 mg/ml

unit use vial	$7.01	1.2, Intl Medication	00548-5030-00
10 ml	$4.96	Neostigmine Methylsulfate, Bristol Myers Squibb	00003-2913-10
10 ml	$9.20	Neostigmine Methylsulfate, Schein Pharm (US)	00364-2369-54
10 ml	$9.20	Neostigmine Methylsulfate, Steris Labs	00402-0915-10
10 ml	$11.04	Neostigmine Methylsulfate 1:1000 1, Abbott	00074-3723-01
10 ml	$167.50	PROSTIGMIN, ICN Pharms	00187-3103-50
10 ml x 1	$8.75	Neostigmine Methylsulfate, Elkins Sinn	00641-2540-41
10 ml x 5	$15.49	Neostigmine Methylsulfate 1:1000, Astra USA	00186-1742-01
10 ml x 10	$50.00	Neostigmine Methylsulfate, Am Regent	00517-0033-10
10 ml x 10	$81.72	Neostigmine Methylsulfate, Gensia Labs	00703-2704-03
10 ml x 10	$89.25	Neostigmine Methylsulfate, Fujisawa USA	00469-3830-30

Solution - Intramuscular; - 0.25 mg/ml

1 ml x 10	$14.69	PROSTIGMIN, ICN Pharms	00187-3102-40

NETILMICIN SULFATE *(001875)*

CATEGORIES: Abdominal Abscess; Aminoglycosides; Anti-Infectives; Antibacterials; Antibiotics; Antimicrobials; Infections; Intra-Abdominal Infections; Peritonitis; Respiratory Tract Infections; Sepsis; Septicemia; Skin Infections; Urinary Tract Infections; Pregnancy Category D; Sales > $100 Million; FDA Approved 1983 Feb

BRAND NAMES: *Akocin*; *Certomycin* (Germany); *Netillin* (England); *Netilmicin*; *Netilyn*; *Netrocin*; *Netromicina* (Mexico); *Netromicine* (France); **Netromycin**; *Netromycin IM IV*; *Netromycine*; *Nettacin*; *Zetamicin*
(International brand names outside U.S. in italics)

WARNING:

Patients treated with aminoglycosides should be under close clinical observation because of the potential toxicity associated with the use of these drugs.

Netilmicin has potent neuromuscular blocking potential. Neuromuscular blockade and respiratory paralysis have been reported in animals receiving netilmicin. The possibility of these phenomena occurring in man should be considered if aminoglycosides are administered by any route to patients receiving neuromuscular blocking agents, such as succinylcholine, tubocurarine, or decamethonium, or to patients receiving massive transfusions of citrate-anticoagulated blood. If neuromuscular blockade occurs, calcium salts may lessen it, but mechanical respiratory assistance may also be necessary.

As with other aminoglycosides, netilmicin sulfate injection is potentially nephrotoxic. The risk is greater in patients with impaired renal function, in those who receive high dosage or prolonged therapy, and in the elderly.

Neurotoxicity manifested by ototoxicity, both vestibular and auditory, can occur in patients treated with netilmicin, primarily in those with preexisting renal damage and in patients treated with higher doses and/or for longer periods than recommended. Aminoglycoside-induced ototoxicity is usually irreversible. Other manifestations of aminoglycoside induced neurotoxicity include numbness, skin tingling, muscle twitching, and convulsions.

Renal and eighth cranial nerve functions should be closely monitored, especially in patients with known or suspected impairment of renal function either at onset of therapy or during therapy. Urine should be examined for increased excretion of protein, the presence of cells or casts, and decreased specific gravity. Serum creatinine concentration or blood urea nitrogen should be determined periodically. A more precise measure of glomerular filtration rate is a carefully conducted determination of creatinine clearance rate or, often more practically, an estimate of creatinine clearance based on published nomograms or equations. (See DOSAGE AND ADMINISTRATION.) When feasible it is recommended that serial audiograms be obtained in patients old enough to be tested, particularly in high-risk patients. The dosage of netilmicin should be reduced or administration discontinued if evidence of drug-induced auditory or vestibular toxicity (dizziness, vertigo, tinnitus, nystagmus, or hearing loss) develops during therapy. If evidence of nephrotoxicity occurs, dosage should be adjusted. (See DOSAGE AND ADMINISTRATION, Dosage for Impaired Renal Function. As with the other aminoglycosides, on rare occasions changes in renal and eighth cranial nerve functions may not become manifest until soon after completion of therapy.

Serum concentrations of aminoglycosides should be monitored when feasible to assure adequate levels and to avoid potentially toxic levels. After administration of an appropriate dose of netilmicin, peak serum concentrations occur approximately 30 to 60 minutes after an intramuscular injection or at the end of a one hour intravenous infusion. Dosage should be adjusted so that prolonged peak serum concentrations above 16 mcg/ml are avoided.

When monitoring trough concentrations, dosage should be adjusted so that levels above 4 mcg/ml are avoided. Excessive peak and/or trough serum concentrations of aminoglycosides may increase the risk of renal and eighth cranial nerve toxicity. In the event of overdose or toxic reactions, hemodialysis may aid in removal of netilmicin from the blood, especially if renal function is, or becomes, compromised. Removal of netilmicin by peritoneal dialysis is at a rate considerably less than by hemodialysis.

Concurrent and/or sequential systemic or topical use of other potentially neurotoxic and/or nephrotoxic drugs, such as: cephaloridine, amphotericin B, streptomycin, kanamycin, acyclovir, gentamicin, tobramycin, amikacin, neomycin, vancomycin, bacitracin, polymyxin B, colistin, paromomycin, viomycin, or cisplatin should be avoided. The concurrent use of aminoglycosides with potent diuretics, such as ethacrynic acid or furosemide, should be avoided since certain diuretics by themselves may cause ototoxicity. In addition, when administered intravenously, diuretics may enhance aminoglycoside toxicity by altering the antibiotic concentration in the serum and tissues. Other factors which may increase patient risk of toxicity are advanced age and dehydration.

DESCRIPTION:

Netilmicin sulfate injection contains netilmicin sulfate, USP in clear, sterile aqueous solution with a PH range of 3.5 to 6.0 for intramuscular or intravenous administration. Netilmicin is a semisynthetic, water-soluble antibiotic of the aminoglycoside group, derived from sisomicin. Its chemical name is: *O*-3-Deoxy-4-C -methyl-3-(methylamino)-β-L-arabino-pyranosyl (1→4)-*O*-(2, 6-diamino-2,3,4,6-tetradeoxy-α-D-*glycero*-hex-4-enopyranosyl-(1→6))-2-deoxy-N^3-ethyl-L-streptamine sulfate (2:5) (salt).

Each ml of Netilmicin sulfate injection contains netilmicin sulfate, USP equivalent to 100 mg netilmicin; 10 mg benzyl alcohol as a preservative; 0.1 mg edetate disodium; 2.4 mg sodium metabisulfite; 0.8 mg sodium sulfite; and water for injection, q.s.

CLINICAL PHARMACOLOGY:

Netilmicin is rapidly and completely absorbed after intramuscular injection. Peak serum levels, after intramuscular injection, usually occur within 30 to 60 minutes and levels are measurable for 12 hours. In adult volunteers with normal renal function, peak serum concentration of netilmicin in mcg/ml are usually about 3 to 3.5 times the single intramuscular dose in mg/kg. For example, a dose of 2.0 mg/kg may be expected to result in a peak serum concentration of approximately 7 mcg/ml. At eight or more hours after administration of a dose in the recommended range, serum levels are usually less than 3 mcg/ml. When a single dose of netilmicin is administered by 60-minute intravenous infusion, the peak serum concentrations are similar to those obtained by intramuscular administration. Following a rapid intravenous injection of netilmicin, levels in serum may be transiently 2 to 3 times higher than those of the 60-minute infusion, Netilmicin rapidly distributes to tissues.

The half-life of netilmicin after single doses is usually 2 to 2.5 hours, a half-life which is very similar to that of gentamicin, and is independent of the route of administration. The half-life increases as the dose increases (*e.g.,* 2.2 hours after a 1 mg/kg dose to 3 hours after a 3 mg/kg dose). Approximately 80% of the administered dose is excreted in the urine within 24 hours; the urine netilmicin concentration after a dose often exceeds 100 mcg/ml. There is no evidence or metabolic transformation of netilmicin. The drug is excreted principally by glomerular filtration. Probenecid does not affect renal tubular transport of aminoglycosides. The volume of distribution of netilmicin is approximately 20% of body weight; total body clearance is about 80 ml/min and renal clearance is about 60 ml/min. In multiple-dose studies in volunteers when the drug was administered every 12 hours at doses ranging from 1.0 to 4.0 mg/kg, steady-state levels were obtained by the second day.

The serum levels at steady-state were less than 20% higher than those of the first dose. As with other aminoglycosides, the half-life of netilmicin increases, and its renal clearance decreases with decreasing renal function.

The endogenous creatinine clearance rate and the serum creatinine level have a high correlation with the half-life of netilmicin. Results of these tests can serve as a guide for adjusting dosage in patients with renal impairment.

In patients with marked impairment of renal function, there is a decrease in the concentration of aminoglycosides in urine and in their penetration into defective renal parenchyma. This should be considered when treating patients with urinary tract infections. In one study of adults with renal failure undergoing hemodialysis, netilmicin serum levels were reduced by approximately 63% over an 8-hour dialysis session. Shorter dialysis sessions will remove less drug. No hemodialysis information is available for children. Aminoglycosides are also removed by peritoneal dialysis but at a rate considerably less than by hemodialysis.

Since netilmicin is distributed in extracellular fluid, peak serum concentrations may be lower than usual in patients whose extracellular fluid volume is expanded (*e.g.,* patients with edema or ascites). Serum concentrations of aminoglycosides in febrile patients may be lower than those in afebrile patients given the same dose. When body temperature returns to normal, serum concentrations of the drug may rise. Both febrile and anemic states may be associated with a shorter than usual half-life. (Dosage adjustment is usually not necessary).

In severely burned patients, the half-life of aminoglycosides may be significantly decreased, and serum concentrations resulting from a particular dose may be lower than anticipated.

The elimination half-life of netilmicin in neonates during the first week of life is inversely correlated with body weight, ranging from approximately 8 hours for neonates weighing 1.5 to 2.0 kg to approximately 4.5 hours for 3.0 to 4.0 kg neonates. The elimination half-life of infants and children 6 weeks of age and older is 1.5 to 2.0 hours.

Following parental administration, aminoglycosides can be detected in serum, tissues, and sputum and in pericardial, pleural, synovial, and peritoneal fluids. A variety of methods are available to measure netilmicin concentrations in body fluids; these include microbiologic, enzymatic, and radioimmunoassay techniques. Concentrations in renal cortex may be markedly higher than the usual serum levels.

Minute quantities of aminoglycosides have been detected in the urine for up to 30 days after discontinuing administration. Hepatic secretion is minimal. As with all aminoglycosides, netilmicin diffuses poorly into the subarachnoid space after parenteral administration. Concentrations of netilmicin in cerebrospinal fluid are often low and dependent upon dose and the degree of meningeal inflammation. Netilmicin crosses the placenta and has been detected in cord blood and in the fetus. Studies in nursing mothers indicate that small amounts of the drug are excreted in breast milk. Netilmicin is poorly absorbed from the intact gastrointestinal tract after oral administration. As with other aminoglycosides, the binding of netilmicin to serum proteins is low (0-30%).

Microbiology: Netilmicin is a rapidly acting, broad-spectrum bactericidal antibiotic which appears to act by inhibiting normal protein synthesis in susceptible microorganisms. Netilmicin is active *in vitro* against a wide variety of pathogenic bacteria, primarily gram-negative bacilli and also a few gram-positive organisms including*Citrobacter, Enterobacter, Escherichia coli, Klebsiella,* species,*Proteus mirabilis, Pseudomonas aeruginosa, Salmonella* species,*Shigella* species, and *Staphylococcus* species (penicillin- and methicillin-resistant strains).

Netilmicin is also active *in vitro* against some isolates of*Acinetobacter* and *Neisseria* species, indole-positive*Proteus* species, *Pseudomonas* and *Serratia* species. In addition, netilmicin is active *in vitro* against many strains which have acquired resistance to other aminoglycosides. Such resistance is usually caused by aminoglycoside modifying (inactivating) enzymes. In general, netilmicin is active against organisms which inactivate aminoglycosides by either phosphorylation or adenylylation; it has variable activity against acetylating strains, depending on the specific type. For example, the susceptibility of *Serratia* species producing a combination of adenylylating and acetylating enzymes varies according to the level of acetylating enzyme present. Netilmicin is active *in vitro* against certain strains of gram-negative bacteria resistant to gentamicin and tobramycin: *Citrobacter, Enterobacter* species, *Escherichia coli, Klebsiella, Proteus* (indole-positive), *Pseudomonas, Salmonella,* and *Shigella* species. Netilmicin is active *in vitro* against certain staphylococci resistant to amikacin and tobramycin. Like other aminoglycosides, netilmicin is not active against bacteria with reduced permeability to this class of antibiotics.

Most species of streptococci and anaerobic organisms, such as*Bacteroides* and *Clostridium* species, are resistant to aminoglycosides.

The *in vitro* activity of netilmicin and of other aminoglycosides is affected by media pH, protein content, divalent cation concentration, and inoculum size.

Netilmicin acts synergistically *in vitro*with members of the penicillin class of antibiotics against *Streptococcus faecalis.* It also acts synergistically with those penicillins which are active alone against many strains of *Pseudomonas.* In addition, many, but not all isolates of *Serratia* which are resistant to multiple antibiotics, are inhibited by synergistic combinations of netilmicin with carbenicillin, azlocillin, mezlocillin, cefamandole, cefotaxime, or moxalactam. Tests for antibiotic synergy are necessary.

Susceptibility Testing: Quantitative methods that require measurements of zone diameters give the most precise estimates of antibiotic susceptibility. One such procedure has been recommended for use with discs to test susceptibility to netilmicin. Interpretation involves correlation of the diameters obtained in the disc test with minimal inhibitory concentration (MIC) values for netilmicin.

Reports from the laboratory giving results of the standardized single disc susceptibility test (Bauer, et al. Am J Clin Path 1966; 45:493 and Federal Register 37:20525-20529, 1972), using a 30 mcg netilmicin disc should be interpreted according to the following criteria:

Organisms producing zones of 15 mm or greater, or MIC's of 8.0 mcg or less are considered susceptible, indicating that the tested organism is likely to respond to therapy.

Resistant organisms produce zones of 12 mm or less or MIC's of 16 mcg or greater. A report of "resistant" from the laboratory indicates that the infecting organism is not likely to respond to therapy.

Zones greater than 12 mm and less than 15 mm, or MIC's of greater than 8.0 mcg and less than 16 mcg, indicate intermediate susceptibility. A report of "intermediate" susceptibility suggests that the organism would be susceptible if the infection is confined to tissues and fluids (*e.g.,* urine), in which high antibiotic levels are attained.

Control organisms are recommended for susceptibility testing. Each time the test is performed one or more of the following organisms should be included: *Escherichia coli* ATCC 25922, *Staphylococcus aureus* ATCC 25923, and *Pseudomonas aeruginosa* ATCC 27853. The control organisms should produce zones of inhibition within the following ranges:

Escherichia coli (ATCC 25922) 22-30 mm

CLINICAL PHARMACOLOGY: *(cont'd)*

Staphylococcus aureus (ATCC 25923) 22-31 mm

Pseudomonas aeruginosa (ATCC 27853) 17-23 mm

In certain circumstances, particularly with strains of *Pseudomonas aeruginosa*, it may be desirable to do additional susceptibility testing by the tube or agar dilution method. Netilmicin sulfate powder, a diagnostic reagent, is available for this purpose.

The MIC values of netilmicin for the control strains are the following:

Escherichia coli (ATCC 25922) 0.25-0.5 mcg/ml

Staphylococcus aureus (ATCC 25923) 0.125-0.25 mcg/ml

Pseudomonas aeruginosa (ATCC 27853) 4-8 mcg/ml in media supplemented with calcium and magnesium.

INDICATIONS AND USAGE:

Netilmicin sulfate injection is indicated for the short-term treatment of patients of all ages, including neonates, infants, and children with serious or life-threatening bacterial infections caused by susceptible strains of the designated microorganisms in the diseases listed below:

Complicated Urinary Tract Infections: caused by *Escherichia coli, Klebsiella pneumoniae, Pseudomonas aeruginosa, Enterobacter* species,*Proteus mirabilis, Proteus* species (indole-positive),*Serratia** and *Citrobacter* species, and *Staphylococcus aureus.***

Septicemia: caused by *Escherichia coli, Klebsiella pneumoniae, Pseudomonas aeruginosa, Enterobacter* and *Serratia** species, and *Proteus mirabilis.*

Skin and Skin Structure Infections: caused by *Escherichia coli, Klebsiella pneumoniae, Pseudomonas aeruginosa, Enterobacter* and *Serratia** species, *Proteus mirabilis, Proteus* species (indole-positive), and *Staphylococcus aureus*** (penicillinase- and non-penicillinase-producing strains).

Intra-Abdominal Infections: including peritonitis and intra-abdominal abscess caused by *Escherichia coli, Klebsiella pneumoniae, Pseudomonas aeruginosa, Enterobacter* species, *Proteus mirabilis, Proteus* species (indole-positive), and *Staphylococcus aureus*** (penicillinase- and non-penicillinase-producing strains).

Lower Respiratory Tract Infections: caused by *Escherichia coli, Klebsiella pneumoniae, Pseudomonas aeruginosa, Enterobacter* and *Serratia** species, *Proteus mirabilis, Proteus* species (indole-positive), and *Staphylococcus aureus*** (penicillinase- and non-penicillinase-producing strains).

*See CLINICAL PHARMACOLOGY, Microbiology.

**While not the antibiotic class of first choice, aminoglycosides, including netilmicin, may be considered for the treatment of serious staphylococcal infections when penicillins or other less potentially toxic drugs are contraindicated and bacterial susceptibility tests and clinical judgment indicate their use. They may also be considered in mixed infections caused by susceptible strains of staphylococci and gram-negative organisms.

Aminoglycosides are indicated for those infections for which less potentially toxic antimicrobial agents are ineffective or contraindicated. They are not indicated in the treatment of uncomplicated initial episodes of urinary tract infection unless the causative organisms are resistant to antimicrobial agents having less potential toxicity.

Netilmicin sulfate injection may be considered as initial therapy in suspected or confirmed gram-negative infections, and therapy may be instituted before obtaining results of susceptibility testing. The decision to continue therapy with netilmicin should be based on the results of susceptibility tests, the severity of the infection, and the important additional concepts contained in the "BOXED WARNING above. If the causative organisms are resistant to netilmicin, other appropriate therapy should be instituted.

In serious infections when the causative organisms are unknown, netilmicin may be administered as initial therapy in conjunction with a penicillin-type or cephalosporin-type drug before obtaining results of susceptibility testing. In neonates with suspected sepsis, a penicillin-type drug is also usually indicated as concomitant therapy with netilmicin. If anaerobic organisms are suspected as etiologic agents, other suitable antimicrobial therapy should also be given. Following identification of the organism and its susceptibility, appropriate antibiotic therapy should then be continued.

Netilmicin sulfate injection has been used effectively in combination with carbenicillin or ticarcillin for the treatment of life-threatening infections caused by *Pseudomonas aeruginosa.*

Clinical studies have shown that netilmicin has been effective in the treatment of serious infections caused by some organisms resistant to other aminoglycoside, *i.e.*, gentamicin, tobramycin, and/or amikacin.

Specimens for bacterial culture should be obtained to isolate and identify causative organisms and to determine their susceptibility to netilmicin.

CONTRAINDICATIONS:

Hypersensitivity to netilmicin or to any of the ingredients of the preparation is a contraindication to its use. See WARNINGS if patient is hypersensitive to another aminoglycoside.

WARNINGS:

See BOXED WARNING. If the patient has a history of hypersensitivity or serious toxic reaction to another aminoglycoside, netilmicin should be used very cautiously, if at all, because cross-sensitivity to drugs in this class has been reported.

Aminoglycosides can cause fetal harm when administered to a pregnant woman. Aminoglycoside antibiotics cross the placenta and there have been several reports of total irreversible bilateral congenital deafness in children whose mothers received streptomycin during pregnancy. Although serious side effects to fetus or newborn have not been reported in the treatment of pregnant women with other aminoglycosides, the potential for harm exists. Reproduction studies of netilmicin have been preformed in rats and rabbits using intramuscular and subcutaneous doses approximately 13-15 times the highest adult human dose and have revealed no evidence of impairment of fertility or harm to the fetus. Moreover, there was no evidence of ototoxicity in the offspring of rats treated subcutaneously with netilmicin throughout pregnancy and during the subsequent lactation period. It is not known whether netilmicin sulfate can cause fetal harm when administered to a pregnant woman or can affect reproduction capacity. However, if this drug is used during pregnancy, or if the patient becomes pregnant while taking this drug, the patients should be apprised of the potential hazard to the fetus.

Netilmicin sulfate injection contains sodium metabisulfite and sodium sulfite, which may cause allergic-type reactions including anaphylactic symptoms and life-threatening or less severe asthmatic episodes in certain susceptible people. The overall prevalence of sulfite sensitivity in the general population is unknown and probably low. Sulfite sensitivity is seen more frequently in asthmatic than in nonasthmatic people.

PRECAUTIONS:

GENERAL

Neurotoxic and nephrotoxic antibiotics may be almost completely absorbed from body surfaces (except the urinary bladder) after local irrigation and after topical application during surgical procedures. The potential toxic effects of antibiotics administered in this fashion (neuromuscular blockade, respiratory paralysis, oto- and nephrotoxicity) should be considered. (See BOXED WARNING.

Increased nephrotoxicity has been reported following concomitant administration of aminoglycoside antibiotics with some cephalosporins.

Aminoglycosides should be used with caution in patients with neuromuscular disorders, such as myasthenia gravis, or infant botulism, since these drugs may aggravate muscle weakness because of their potential curare-like effect on the neuromuscular junction.

During or following netilmicin therapy, parasthesias, tetany, positive Chvostek and Trousseau sings, and mental confusion have been described in patients with hypomagnesemia, hypocalcemia, and hypokalemia. When this has occurred in infants, tetany and muscle weakness has been described. Both adults and infants required appropriate corrective electrolyte therapy.

Elderly patients may have reduced renal function which may not be evident in the results of routine screening tests, such as BUN or serum creatinine levels. Determination of creatinine clearance or an estimate based on published nomograms or equations may be more useful. Monitoring of renal function during treatment with netilmicin, as with other aminoglycosides, is particularly important in such patients. A Fanconi-like syndrome, with aminoaciduria and metabolic acidosis, has been reported in some adults and infants being given netilmicin injections.

Patients should be well hydrated during treatment.

Treatment with netilmicin may result in overgrowth of non-susceptible organisms. If this occurs, appropriate therapy is indicated.

LABORATORY TESTS

Tests of Renal Function: Urine should be examined periodically for increased excretion of protein and the presence of cells and casts, keeping in mind the effects of the primary illness on these tests. One or more of the following laboratory measurements should be obtained at the onset of therapy, periodically during therapy, and at, or shortly after the end of therapy:

Creatine clearance rate (either carefully measured or estimated from published nomograms or equations based on the patient's age, sex, body weight, and serum creatinine concentration) (preferred over BUN);

serum creatinine concentration (preferred over BUN);

blood urea nitrogen (BUN).

More frequent testing is desirable if renal function is changing. See also "**PRECAUTIONS, General**" above regarding elderly patients.

Test of Eighth Cranial Nerve Functions: Serial audiometric tests are suggested, particularly when renal function is impaired and/or prolonged aminoglycoside therapy is required; such tests should also be repeated periodically after treatment if there is evidence of a hearing deficit or vestibular abnormality before or during therapy, or when consecutive or concomitant use of other potentially ototoxic drugs is unavoidable.

DRUG/LABORATORY TEST INTERACTIONS

Concomitant cephalosporin therapy may spuriously elevate creatinine determinations.

The inactivation between aminoglycosides and beta-lactam antibiotic described in "**Drug Interactions**" may continue in specimens of body fluids collected for assay, resulting in inaccurate, false low aminoglycoside readings. Such specimens should be properly handled,*i.e.*, assayed promptly, frozen, or treated with beta-lactamase.

CARCINOGENESIS, MUTAGENESIS, AND IMPAIRMENT OF FERTILITY

Life-time carcinogenicity tests have been undertaken in the mouse and rat and no drug-related tumors were observed. Similarly, mutagenesis tests with netilmicin have proven negative, and no impairment in fertility has been observed in the rat.

PREGNANCY CATEGORY D

See WARNINGS.

NURSING MOTHERS

Clinical studies in nursing mothers indicate that small amounts of netilmicin are excreted in breast milk. Because of the potential for serious adverse reactions from aminoglycosides in nursing infants, a decision should be made whether to discontinue nursing or to discontinue the drug, taking into account the importance of the drug to the mother.

PEDIATRIC USE

Aminoglycosides should be used with caution in prematures and neonates because of the renal immaturity of these patients and the resulting prolongation of serum half-life of these drug (also see DOSAGE AND ADMINISTRATION for use in Neonates and Children.)

DRUG INTERACTIONS:

In vitro mixing of an aminoglycoside with beta-lactam-type antibiotics (penicillins or cephalosporins) may result in a significant mutual inactivation. Even when an aminoglycoside and a penicillin-type drug are administered separately by different routes, a reduction in aminoglycoside serum half-life or serum levels has been reported in patients with impaired renal function and in some patients with normal renal function. Usually, such inactivation of the aminoglycoside is clinically significant only in patients with severely impaired renal function. (See also PRECAUTIONS, Drug/Laboratory Test Interactions. See BOXED WARNING regarding concurrent use of potent diuretics, concurrent and/or sequential use of the neurotoxic and/or nephrotoxic antibiotics, and for other essential information. See also PRECAUTIONS, General.

ADVERSE REACTIONS:

Nephrotoxicity: Adverse renal effects due to netilmicin were reported in 7 per 100 patients.

They were demonstrated by a rise in serum creatinine and may have been accompanied by oliguria; the presence of casts, cells or protein in the urine; by rising levels of BUN; or by decreasing creatinine clearance rates. These effects occurred more frequently in the elderly, in patients with a history of renal impairment, and in patients treated for longer periods or with larger doses than recommended. While permanent impairment of renal function may occur following aminoglycoside therapy, observed renal impairment associated with netilmicin was usually mild and reversible after treatment ended while the drug was being excreted.

Neurotoxicity: Adverse effects on both the auditory and vestibular branches of the eighth cranial nerves have been reported.

Audiometric changes associated with netilmicin occurred in approximately 4 per 100 patients. Subjective netilmicin-related hearing loss occurred in about 1 per 250 patients. Vestibular abnormalities related to netilmicin were seen in 1 per 150 patients. Factors which may increase the risk of aminoglycoside-induced ototoxicity include renal impairment (especially if dialysis is required), excessive dosage, dehydration, concomitant administration of ethacrynic acid or furosemide, or previous exposure to other ototoxic drugs.

Peripheral neuropathy or encephalopathy including numbness, skin tingling, muscle twitching, convulsions, and myasthenia gravis-like syndrome have been reported.

ADVERSE REACTIONS: *(cont'd)*

Symptoms include dizziness, vertigo, tinnitus, nystagmus, and hearing loss. Aminoglycoside-induced ototoxicity is usually irreversible. Cochlear damage is usually manifested initially by small changes in audiometric test results at the higher frequencies and may not be associated with subjective hearing loss. Vestibular dysfunction is usually manifested by nystagmus, vertigo, nausea, vomiting, or acute Meniere's syndrome.

The risk of toxic reactions is low in patients with normal renal function who do not receive netilmicin injection at higher doses or for longer periods of time than recommended. Some patients who have had previous neurotoxic reactions to other aminoglycosides have been treated with netilmicin without further neurotoxicity.

Neuromuscular blockade manifested as acute muscular paralysis and apnea can occur following treatment with aminoglycosides. (See BOXED WARNING.

The approximate incidence of other reported adverse reactions to netilmicin injection follows: increased levels of serum transaminase (SGOT or SGPT), alkaline phosphatase, or bilirubin in 15 patients per 1000; rash or itching in 4 or 5 patients per 1000; eosinophilia in 4 patients per 1000; thrombocytosis in 2 patients per 1000; prolonged prothrombin time in 1 patient per 1000.

Fewer than one patient per 1000 was reported to have netilmicin-related anemia, leukopenia, thrombocytopenia, leukemoid reaction, immature circulating white blood cells, hyperkalemia, vomiting, diarrhea, palpitations, hypotension, headache, disorientation, blurred vision, or paresthesias. Local tolerance to intramuscular injection and intravenous infusion of netilmicin is generally excellent, but approximately four patients per 1000 have had severe pain, and similar numbers had induration of hematomas.

OVERDOSAGE:

In the event of overdosage or toxic reaction, netilmicin can be removed from the blood by hemodialysis, and is especially important if renal function is, or becomes, compromised. Although there is no specific information concerning removal of netilmicin by peritoneal dialysis, other aminoglycosides are known to be removed by this method but at a rate considerably less than by hemodialysis.

DOSAGE AND ADMINISTRATION:

Netilmicin injection may be given intramuscularly or intravenously. (See CLINICAL PHARMACOLOGY.) The recommended dosage for both methods of administration is identical.

The patients's pretreatment body weight should be obtained for calculation of correct dosage. The dosage of aminoglycosides in obese patients should be based on an estimate of the lean body mass.

The status of renal function should be estimated by measurement of the serum creatinine concentration or calculation of the endogenous creatinine clearance rate. The blood urea nitrogen (BUN) level is much less reliable for this purpose. Reassessment of renal function should be made periodically during therapy.

In patients with extensive body surface burns, altered pharmacokinetics may result in reduced serum concentrations of aminoglycosides. Measurement of netilmicin serum concentrations is particularly important as a basis for dosage adjustment in such patients.

Duration of Treatment: It is desirable to limit the duration of treatment with aminoglycosides to short-term whenever feasible. The usual duration of treatment of all patients is seven to fourteen days. In complicated infections, a longer course of therapy may be necessary. Although prolonged courses of netilmicin injection have been well tolerated, it is particularly important that patients treated for longer than the usual period be carefully monitored for changes in renal, auditory, and vestibular functions. Dosage should be adjusted if clinically indicated.

Measurement of Serum Concentrations: It is desirable to measure both peak and trough serum concentrations of netilmicin to determine the adequacy and safety of the administered dosage.

When such measurements are feasible, they should be carried out periodically during therapy. Peak serum concentrations are expected to range from 4 to 12 mcg/ml. Dosage should be adjusted to attain the desired peak and trough concentrations and to avoid prolonged peak serum concentrations above 16 mcg/ml. When monitoring trough concentrations (just prior to the next dose), dosage should be adjusted so that levels above 4 mcg/ml are avoided. Inter-patient variation of aminoglycoside serum concentrations occurs in patients with normal or abnormal renal function. Generally, desirable peak and trough concentrations will be in the range of 6-10 and 0.5-2 mcg/ml, respectively.

Determination of the adequacy of a serum level for a particular patient must take into consideration the susceptibility of the causative organism, the severity of the infection, and the status of the patients's host-defense mechanisms.

The dosage recommendations which follow are not intended as rigid schedules, but are provided as guides for initial therapy, or for when the measurement of netilmicin serum levels during therapy is not feasible.

DOSAGE FOR PATIENTS WITH NORMAL RENAL FUNCTION

TABLE 1 shows the recommended dosage of netilmicin injection for patients of various age with normal renal function.

TABLE 1 Dosage Guide For Adults With Normal Renal Function

kg	Patient's Weight* (lb)	For Complicated Urinary Tract Infections, Give 3.0-4.0 mg/kg/day as 1.5-2.0 mg/kg Every 12 Hours mg/dose	For Serious Systemic Infections Give 4.0-6.5 mg/kg/day as 1.3-2.2 mg/kg or 2.0-3.25 mg/kg Every 8 Hours mg/dose	Every 12 Hours mg/dose
40	(88)	60- 80	52- 88	80- 130
45	(99)	68- 90	59- 99	90- 146
50	(110)	75- 100	65- 110	100- 163
55	(121)	83- 110	72- 121	110- 179
60	(132)	90- 120	78- 132	120- 195
65	(143)	98- 130	85- 143	130- 211
70	(154)	105- 140	91- 154	140- 228
75	(165)	113- 150	98- 165	150- 244
80	(176)	120- 160	104- 176	160- 260
85	(187)	128- 170	111- 187	170- 276
90	(198)	135- 180	117- 198	180- 293
95	(209)	143- 190	124- 209	190- 309
100	(220)	150- 200	130- 220	200- 325

* The dosage of aminoglycosides in obese patients should be based on an estimate of the lean body mass.

Although a causal relationship has not been established, administration of injections preserved with benzyl alcohol has been associated with toxicity in neonates. Caution should be used when netilmicin sulfate injection (100 mg/ml) is administered to neonates and children.

Neonates (less than 6 weeks): 4.0 to 6.5 mg/kg/day given as 2.0 to 3.25 mg/kg every 12 hours.

DOSAGE AND ADMINISTRATION: *(cont'd)*

Infants and Children (6 weeks through 12 years): 5.5 to 8.0 mg/kg/day given either as 1.8 to 2.7 mg/kg every 8 hours, or as 2.7 to 4.0 mg/kg every 12 hours.

DOSAGE FOR PATIENTS WITH IMPAIRED RENAL FUNCTION

Dosage must be individualized in patients with impaired renal function to ensure therapeutic levels are attained. There are several methods of doing this; however, dosage adjustment based upon the measurement of serum drug concentrations during treatment is the most accurate.

If netilmicin serum concentrations are not available and renal function is stable, serum creatinine and creatinine clearance values are the most reliable, readily available indicators of the degree of renal impairment for use as a guide for dosage adjustment.

It is also important to recognize that deteriorating renal function may require a greater reduction in dosage than that specified in the guidelines given below for patients with stable renal impairment.

The initial or loading dose is the same as that for a patient with normal renal function. A number of methods are available to adjust the total daily dosage for the degree of renal impairment. Three suggested methods are:

1) Divide the suggested dosage value for patients with normal renal function from Table 1 above by the serum creatinine level to obtain the adjusted size of each dose.

2) If the creatinine clearance rate is known or can be estimated from the serum creatinine levels using the formula given below, the adjusted daily dose of netilmicin may be determined by multiplying the dose given in the Table 1 by:

Patient's Creatinine Clearance Rate % Normal Creatinine Clearance Rate

Creatinine clearance can be estimated from serum creatine levels by the following formula for adult males; multiply by 0.85 for adult females (Nephron, 1976; 16:31-41).

$$C_{cr} = [(140 - Age)(wt.\ Kg)] \div [72 \times S_{cr} (mg/100ml)]$$

The adjusted total daily dose may be administered as one dose at 24-hour intervals, or as 2 or 3 equally divided doses at 12-hour or 8-hour intervals, respectively. Generally, each individual dose should not exceed 3.25 mg/kg. In adults with renal failure who are undergoing hemodialysis, the amount of netilmicin removed from the blood my vary depending upon the dialysis equipment and methods used. (See CLINICAL PHARMACOLOGY.) In adults, a dose of 2.0 mg/kg at the end of each dialysis period is recommended until the results of tests measuring netilmicin serum levels become available. Dosage should then be appropriately adjusted based on these tests.

ALTERNATE DOSING METHOD FOR PATIENTS WITH NORMAL OR IMPAIRED RENAL FUNCTION

An alternate method of determining a dosage regimen (dose and dosing interval) applicable to all ages and all states of renal function (both normal and abnormal) is to employ pharmacokinetic parameters derived from measurements of serum concentrations.

Following the administration of an initial dose of netilmicin and the determination of drug serum concentrations in post-infusion blood samples, the drug's half-life and the patient's elimination rate constant and volume of distribution can be calculated. Desired peak and trough serum levels for a particular patient are then selected by taking into consideration the susceptibility of the causative organism, the severity of infection, and the status of the patient's host-defense mechanisms. The dosage regimen (dose and dosing interval) is then determined using standardized formulae and the appropriate computer program, and the dosage regimen can be adjusted to the nearest practical interval and amount.

ADDITION OF NETILMICIN SULFATE TO VARIOUS INTRAVENOUS PREPARATIONS

In adults, a single dose of netilmicin injection may be diluted in 50 to 200 ml of one of the parenteral solutions listed below (TABLE 2). In infants and children, the volume of diluent should be less according to the fluid requirements of the patient. The solution may be infused over a period of one-half to two hours.

Tested at concentrations of 2.1 to 3.0 mg/ml, netilmicin sulfate has been shown to be stable in the following large volume parenteral solutions for up to 72 hours when stored in glass containers, both when refrigerated and at room temperature. Use after this time period is not recommended.

TABLE 2 Large Volume Parenteral Solutions In Which Netilmicin Sulfate Is Stable

Products/Compositions Tested	Other Trade Names and Manufacturers (Solutions of Same Composition)
Sterile Water for Injection	
0.9% Sodium Chloride Injection alone or with 5% Dextrose	
5% or 10% Dextrose Injection in Water, or 5% Dextrose in Polysal Injection, or 5% Dextrose with Electrolyte #48 or #75	
Ringer's and Lactated Ringer's with 5% Dextrose Injection	
10% Travert with Electrolyte #2 or #3 Injection (Travenol)	Electrolyte #3 (Cooke & Crowley's Solution) with 10% Inverted Sugar Injection (Cutter)
Isolyte E, M, or P with 5% Dextrose Injection	
10% Dextran 40 or 6% Dextran 75 in 5% Dextrose Injection	
Plasma-Lyte 56 or 148 Injection with 5% Dextrose (Travenol)	Normosol-M or R in D5-W (Abbott), Isolyte H or S with 5% Dextrose (McGaw), Polyonic R-148 or M-56 with 5% Dextrose (Cutter)
Plasma-Lyte M Injection 5% Dextrose (Travenol)	Polysal M with 5% Dextrose (Cutter)
Ionosol B in D5-W	
5% Amigen Injection alone or with 5% Dextrose	
Normosol-R	Polyonic R-148 (Cutter), Isolyte S (McGaw), Plasma-Lyte 148 Injection in Water (Travenol)
Polysal (Plain)	
Aminosol 5% Injection	
Fre-Amine II 8.5% Injection	
Plasma-Lyte 148 Injection (approx. pH 7.4) (Travenol)	Normosol-R pH 7.4 (Abbott)
10% Fructose Injection	

Parenteral drug products should be inspected visually for particulate matter and discoloration prior to administration, whenever solution and container permit.

Store between 2 and 30°C (36 and 86°F).

DOSAGE AND ADMINISTRATION: *(cont'd)*

ANIMAL PHARMACOLOGY AND/OR ANIMAL TOXICOLOGY

Netilmicin sulfate, administered by the intravenous and intramuscular routes, has been compared to kanamycin, sisomicin, gentamicin, amikacin, and tobramycin in studies ranging in duration from two weeks to three months. Among the aminoglycosides, netilmicin is one of the more potent neuromuscular-blocking agents; however, in six different species, netilmicin sulfate has proven to be the least nephrotoxic and ototoxic of these aminoglycosides, using morphological as well as functional end points. In the clinical trials nephrotoxicity and ototoxicity occurred at about the same frequency in netilmicin-treated patients as in those treated with other aminoglycosides.

HOW SUPPLIED - EQUIVALENTS NOT AVAILABLE:

Injection, Solution - Intramuscular; - 100mg/ml

1.5 ml x 10	$128.07	NETROMYCIN, Schering	00085-0264-02
15 ml x 5	$405.72	NETROMYCIN, Schering	00085-0264-04

NEVIRAPINE *(003290)*

CATEGORIES: AIDS Related Complex; Antivirals; Dipyridodoazepinone; HIV Infection; Immunomodulators; Non-nucleoside Reverse Transcriptase Inhibitor; Viral Agents; Pregnancy Category C; FDA Approved 1996 Jun

BRAND NAMES: **Viramune**

WARNING:
NEVIRAPINE IS INDICATED FOR USE IN COMBINATION WITH NUCELOSIDE ANALOGUES FOR THE TREATMENT OF HIV-1 INFECTED ADULTS WHO HAVE EXPERIENCED CLINICAL AND/OR IMMUNOLOGIC DETERIORATION. THIS INDICATION IS BASED ON ANALYSIS OF CHANGES IN SURROGATE ENDPOINTS IN STUDIES OF UP TO 48 WEEKS DURATION. AT PRESENT, THERE ARE NO RESULTS FROM CONTROLLED CLINICAL STUDIES EVALUATING THE EFFECT OF NEVIRAPINE WITH NUCLEOSIDE ANALOGUES ON THE CLINICAL PROGRESSION OF HIV-1 INFECTION. SUCH AS THE INCIDENCE OF OPPORTUNISTIC INFECTIONS OR SURVIVAL.
THE DURATION OF BENEFIT FROM ANTIRETROVIRAL THERAPY MAY BE LIMITED. ALTERATION OF ANTIRETROVIRAL THERAPIES SHOULD BE CONSIDERED IF DISEASE PROGRESSION OCCURS WHILE PATIENTS ARE RECEIVING NEVIRAPINE.
RESISTANT VIRUS EMERGES RAPIDLY AND UNIFORMLY WHEN NEVIRAPINE IS ADMINISTERED AS MONOTHERAPY. THEREFORE, NEVIRAPINE SHOULD ALWAYS BE ADMINISTERED IN COMBINATION WITH AT LEAST ONE ADDITIONAL ANTIRETROVIRAL AGENT.
NEVIRAPINE HAS BEEN ASSOCIATED WITH SEVERE RASH, WHICH IN SOME CASES HAVE BEEN LIFE-THREATENING. WHEN SEVERE RASH OCCURS, NEVIRAPINE MUST BE DISCONTINUED.

DESCRIPTION:

Viramune is the brand name for nevirapine (NVP), a non-nucleoside reverse transcriptase inhibitor with activity against Human Immunodeficiency Virus Type 1 (HIV-1). Nevirapine is structurally a member of the dipyridodiazepinone chemical class of compounds.

Viramune is available as tablets for oral administration. Each tablet contains 200 mg of nevirapine and the inactive ingredients microcrystalline cellulose, lactose monohydrate, povidone, sodium starch glycolate, colloidal silicon dioxide and magnesium stearate.

The chemical name of nevirapine is 11-cyclopropyl-5, 11-dihydro-4-methyl-6H-dipyrido[3,2-b:2'.3'-e][1,4]diazepin-6-one. Nevirapine is a white to off-white crystalline powder with the molecular weight of 266.3 and the molecular formula $C_{15}H_{14}N_4O$.

MICROBIOLOGY

Mechanism of Action: Nevirapine is a non-nucleoside reverse transcriptase inhibitor (NNRTI) of HIV-1. Nevirapine binds directly to reverse transcriptase (RT) and blocks the RNA-dependent and DNA-dependent DNA polymerase activities by causing a disruption of the enzyme's catalytic site. The activity of nevirapine does not compete with template or nuceoside triphosphates. HIV-2 RT and eukaryotic DNA polymerases (such as human DNA polymerases α, β, γ, or Δ) are not inhibited by nevirapine.

In Vitro HIV Susceptibility: The relationship between *in vitro*susceptibility of HIV-1 to nevirapine and the inhibition of HIV-1 replication in humans has not been established. The *in vitro* antiviral activity of nevirapine was measured in peripheral blood mononuclear cells, monocyte derived macrophages, and lymphoblastoid cell lines. IC_{50} values (50% inhibitor concentration) ranged from 10-100 nM against laboratory and clinical isolates of HIV-1. In cell culture, nevirapine demonstrated additive to synergistic activity against HIV in drug combination regimens with zidovudine (ZDV), didanosine (ddl), stavudine (d4T), lamivudine (3TC) and saquinavir.

Resistance: HIV isolates with reduced susceptibility (100-250-fold) to nevirapine emerge *in vitro*. Genotypic analysis showed mutations in the HIV RT gene at amino acid positions 181 and/or 106 depending upon the virus strain and cell line employed. Time to emergence of nevirapine resistance in vitro was not altered when selection included nevirapine in combination with several other NNRTIs.

Phenotypic and genotypic changes in HIV-1 isolates from patients treated with either nevirapine (n=24) or nevirapine and ZDV (n=14) were monitored in Phase I/II trials over 1 to ≥12 weeks. After 1 week of nevirapine monotherapy, isolates from 3/3 patients had decreased susceptibility to nevirapine in vitro, one or more of the RT mutations at amino acid positions 103, 106, 108, 181, 188 and 190 were detected in some patients as early as 2 weeks after therapy initiation. By week eight of nevirapine monotherapy, 100% of the patients tested (n=24) had HIV isolates with a > 100-fold decrease in susceptibility to nevirapine *in vitro* compared to baseline, and had one or more of the nevirapine-associated RT resistance mutations; 19 of 24 patients (80%) had isolates with a position 181 mutation regardless of dose. Nevirapine +ZDV combination therapy did not alter the emergence rate of nevirapine-resistant virus or the magnitude of nevirapine resistance *in vitro*; however, a different RT mutation pattern, predominantly distributed amongst amino acid positions 103, 106, 188 and 190, was observed. In patients (6 of 14) whose baseline isolates possessed a wild type RT gene, nevirapine+ZDV combination therapy did not appear to delay emergence of ZDV-resistant RT mutations. The clinical relevance of phenotypic and genotypic changes associated with nevirapine therapy has not been established.

DESCRIPTION: *(cont'd)*

Cross-resistance: Rapid emergence of HIV strains which are cross-resistant to NNRTIs has been observed *in vitro*. Data on cross-resistance between the NNRTI nevirapine and nucleoside analogue RT inhibitors are very limited. In four patients, ZDV-resistant isolates tested *in vitro* retained susceptibility to nevirapine and in six patients, nevirapine-resistant isolates were susceptible to ZDV and ddl. Cross-resistance between nevirapine and HIV protease inhibitors is unlikely because the enzyme targets involved are different.

CLINICAL PHARMACOLOGY:

ABSORPTION AND BIOAVAILABILITY IN ADULTS

Nevirapine is readily absorbed (>90%) after oral administration in healthy volunteers and in adults with HIV-1 infection. Absolute bioavailability in 12 healthy adults following single-dose administration was 93 ± 9% (mean ± SD) for a 50 mg tablet and 91 ± 8% for an oral solution. Peak plasma nevirapine concentrations of 2 ± 0.4 mcg/mL (7.5 μM) were attained by 4 hours following a single 200 mg dose. Following multiple doses, nevirapine peak concentrations appear to increase linearly in the dose range of 200 to 400 mg/day. Steady state trough nevirapine concentrations of 4.5 ± 1.9 mcg/mL (17 ± 7 μM), (n=242) were attained at 400 mg/day.

When nevirapine (200 mg) was administered to 24 healthy adults (12 female, 12 male), with either a high fat breakfast (857 kcal, 50 g fat, 53% of calories from fat) or antacid (Maalox 30 mL), the extent of nevirapine absorption (AUC) was comparable to that observed under fasting conditions. In a separate study in HIV-1 infected patients (n=6), nevirapine steady-state systemic exposure (AUC) was not significantly altered by ddI, which is formulated with an alkaline buffering agent. Nevirapine may be administered with or without food, antacid or ddl.

DISTRIBUTION

Nevirapine is highly lipophilic and is essentially nonionized at physiologic pH. Following intravenous administration to healthy adults, the apparent volume of distribution (Vdss) of nevirapine was 1.21 ± 0.09 L/kg, suggesting that nevirapine is widely distributed in humans. Nevirapine readily crosses the placenta and is found in breast milk. (see PRECAUTIONS: Nursing Mothers). Nevirapine is about 60% bound to plasma proteins in the plasma concentration range of 1–10 mcg/ml. Nevirapine concentrations in human cerebrospinal fluid (n=6) were 45% (± 5%) of the concentrations in plasma: this ratio is approximately equal to the fraction not bound to plasma protein.

METABOLISM/ELIMINATION

In vivo studies in humans and *in vitro* studies with human liver microsomes have shown that nevirapine is extensively biotransformed via cytochrome P450 (oxidative) metabolism to several hydroxylated metabolites. *In vitro* studies with human liver microsomes suggest that oxidative metabolism of nevirapine is medicated primarily by cytochrome P450 isozymes from the CYP3A family, although other isozymes may have a secondary role. In a mass balance/excretion study in eight healthy male volunteers dosed to steady state with nevirapine 200 mg given twice daily followed by a single 50 mg dose of ^{14}C-nevirapine, approximately 91.4 ± 10.5% of the radiolabeled dose was recovered, with urine (81.3 ± 11.1%) representing the primary route of excretion compared to feces (10.1 ± 1.5%). Greater than 80% of the radioactivity in urine was made up of glucuronide conjugates of hydroxylated metabolites. Thus cytochrome P450 metabolism, glucuronide conjugation, and urinary excretion of glucoronidated metabolites represent the primary route of nevirapine biotransformation and elimination in humans. Only a small fraction (<5%) of the radioactivity in urine (representing <3% of the total dose) was made up of parent compound: therefore, renal excretion plays a minor role in elimination of the parent compound.

Nevirapine has been shown to be an inducer of hepatic cytochrome P450 metabolic enzymes. The pharmacokinetics of autoinduction are characterized by an approximately 1.5 to 2 fold increase in the apparent oral clearance of nevirapine as treatment continues from a single dose to two-to-four weeks of dosing with 200–400 mg/day. Autoinduction also results in a corresponding decrease in the terminal phase half-life of nevirapine in plasma from approximately 45 hours (single dose) to approximately 25–30 hours following multiple dosing with 200–400 mg/day.

SPECIAL POPULATIONS

Renal/Hepatic Dysfunction: The pharmacokinetics of nevirapine have not been evaluated in patients with either renal or hepatic dysfunction.

Gender: In one Phase I study in healthy volunteers (15 females, 15 males), the weight-adjusted apparent volume of distribution (Vdss/F) of nevirapine was higher in the female subjects (1.54 L/kg) compared to the males (1.38 L/kg), suggesting that nevirapine was distributed more extensively in the female subjects. However, this difference was offset by a slightly shorter terminal-phase half-life in the females resulting in no significant gender difference in nevirapine oral clearance or plasma concentrations following either single- or multiple-dose administration(s).

Race: An evaluation of nevirapine plasma concentrations (pooled data from several clinical trials) from HIV-1–infected patients (27 Black, 24 Hispanic, 189 Caucasian) revealed no marked difference in nevirapine steady-state trough concentrations (median Cminnss = 4.7 mcg/mL Black, 3.8 mcg/mL Hispanic, 4.3 mcg/mL Caucasian) with long-term nevirapine treatment at 400 mg/day. However, the pharmacokinetics of nevirapine have not been evaluated specifically for the effects of ethnicity.

Age: Nevirapine pharmacokinetics in HIV-1–infected adults do not appear to change with age (range 18–68 years); however, nevirapine has not been extensively evaluated in patients beyond the age of 55 years. Nevirapine is metabolized more rapidly in pediatric patients than in adults. (see PRECAUTIONS: Pediatric Use).

CLINICAL STUDIES:

PATIENTS WITH A PRIOR HISTORY OF NUCLEOSIDE THERAPY

ACTG 241 compared treatment with nevirapine+ZDV+ddl versus ZDV+ddl in 398 HIV-1–infected patients (median age 38 years, 74% Caucasian, 80% male) with CD4+ counts ≤ 350 cells/mm^3 (mean 153 cells/mm^3) and a mean baseline plasma HIV-1 RNA concentration of 4.59 log_{10} copies/mL (38,905 copies/mL), who had received at least 6 months of nucleoside therapy prior to enrollment (median 115 weeks). Treatment doses were nevirapine, 200 mg daily for two weeks, followed by 200 mg twice daily, or placebo: ZDV, 200 mg three times daily; ddl, 200 mg twice daily.

Trial B1 1037 compared treatment with nevirapine+ZDV versus ZDV in 60 HIV-1–infected patients (median age 33 years) 70% Caucasian, 93% male) with CD4+ cell counts between 200 and 500 cells/mm^3(mean 373 cells/mm^3) and a mean baseline plasma HIV-1 RNA concentration of 4.24 log_{10} copies/mL (17,378 copies/mL), who had received between 3 and 24 months of prior ZDV therapy (median 35 weeks). Treatment doses were nevirapine 200 mg daily for 2 weeks, followed by 200 mg twice daily, or placebo: ZDV, 500–600 mg/day.

PATIENTS WITHOUT A HISTORY OF PRIOR ANTIRETROVIRAL THERAPY

B1 Trial 1046 compared treatment with nevirapine+ZDV+ddl versus nevirapine+ZDV versus ZDV+ddl in 151 HIV-1–infected patients (median age 36 years, 94% Caucasian, 93% male) with CD4+ cell counts of 200–600 cells/mm^3 (mean 376 cells/mm^3) and a mean baseline plasma HIV-1 RNA concentration of 4.41 log_{10}copies/ml (25,704 copies/ml). Treatment doses were nevirapine, 200 mg daily for two weeks, followed by 200 mg twice daily, or placebo; ZDV, 200 mg three times daily; ddl, 125 or 200 mg twice daily. Changes in CD4+ cell counts

CLINICAL STUDIES: *(cont'd)*

at 24 weeks: mean levels of CD4+ cell counts in those randomized to nevirapine+ZDV+ddl and ZDV+ddl remained significantly above baseline; however there was no significant difference between these arms. Changes in HIV-1 viral RNA at 24 weeks: there was no significant difference as measured by mean changes in plasma viral RNA between those randomized to nevirapine+ZDV+ddl and ZDV+ddl. However, the proportion of patients whose HIV-1 RNA decreased below the limit of detection (400 copies/mL) was significantly greater for the nevirapine+ZDV+ddl group (27/36 or 75%), when compared to the ZDV+ddl group (18/39 or 46%) or the nevirapine+ZDV group (0/28 or 0%); the clinical significance of this finding is unknown.

INDICATIONS AND USAGE:

Nevirapine in combination with nucleoside analogues is indicated for the treatment of HIV-1 infected adults who have experienced clinical and/or immunologic deterioration. This indication is based on analyses of changes in surrogate endpoints in studies of up to 48 weeks duration. At present, there are no results from controlled clinical trials evaluating the effect of nevirapine with nucleoside analogues on the clinical progression of HIV-1 infection, such as the incidence of opportunistic infections or survival.

The duration of benefit from antiretroviral therapy may be limited. Alteration of antiretroviral therapy should be considered if disease progression occurs while patients are receiving nevirapine.

Resistant virus emerges rapidly and uniformly when nevirapine is administered as monotherapy. Therefore, nevirapine should always be administered in combination with at least one additional antiretroviral agent.

CONTRAINDICATIONS:

Nevirapine is contraindicated in patients with clinically significant hypersensitivity to any of the components contained in the tablet.

WARNINGS:

Severe and life-threatening skin reactions have occurred in patients treated with nevirapine, including Stevens-Johnson syndrome (SJS). Nevirapine must be discontinued in patients developing a severe reash or a rash accompanied by constitutional symptoms such as fever, blistering, oral lesions, conjunctivitis, swelling, muscle or joint aches, or general malaise. (see PRECAUTIONS, Information for the Patient and ADVERSE REACTIONS).

Nevirapine therapy must be initiated with a 14-day lead-in period of 200 mg/day, which has been shown to reduce the frequency of rash. Dose escalation should not occur if rash is observed during this lead-in period until the rash has resolved (see DOSAGE AND ADMINISTRATION.)

PRECAUTIONS:

GENERAL

When administering nevirapine as part of an antiretroviral treatment regimen, the complete product information for each therapeutic component should be consulted before intiation of treatment.

While nevirapine is extensively metabolized by the liver and nevirapine metabolites are extensively eliminated by the kidney, the pharmacokinetics of nevirapine have not been evaluated in patients with either hepatic or renal dysfunction. Therefore, nevirapine should be used with caution in these patient populations.

Abnormal liver function tests have been reported with nevirapine, some in the first few weeks of therapy, including cases of hepatitis. Nevirapine administration should be interrupted in patients experiencing moderate or severe liver function test abnormalities until liver function tests return to baseline values. Nevirapine treatment should be permanently discontinued if liver function abnormalities recur on readministration.

INFORMATION FOR THE PATIENT

Patients should be informed that nevirapine is not a cure for HIV-1 infection, and that they may continue to experience illnesses associated with advanced HIV-1 infection, including opportunistic infections. Treatment with nevirapine has not been shown to reduce the incidence or frequency of such illnesses, and patients should be advised to remain under the care of a physician when using nevirapine.

Patients should be informed that the long-term effects of nevirapine are unknown at this time. They should also be informed that nevirapine therapy has not been shown to reduce the risk of transmission of HIV-1 to others through sexual contact or blood contamination.

Patients should be instructed that the major toxicity of nevirapine is rash and should be advised to promptly notify their physician of any rash. The majority of rashes associated with nevirapine occur within the first 6 weeks of initiation of therapy. Therefore, patients should be monitored carefully for the appearance of rash during this period. Patients should be instructed that dose escalation is not to occur if any rash occurs during the two-week lead-in dosing period, until the rash resolves. Any patient experiencing severe rash or a rash accompanied by constitutional symptoms such as fever, blistering, oral lesions, conjuctivitis, swelling, muscle or joint aches, or general malaise should discontinue medication and consult a physician.

Patients should be informed to take nevirapine every day as prescribed. Patients should not alter the dose without consulting their doctor. If a dose is missed, patients should take the next dose as soon as possible. However, if a dose is skipped, the patient should not double the next dose.

Nevirapine may interact with other drugs; therefore, patients should be advised to report to their doctor the use of any other medications.

Patients should be instructed that oral contraceptives and other hormonal methods of birth control should not be used as a method of contraception in women taking nevirapine.

CARCINOGENESIS, MUTAGENESIS, AND IMPAIRMENT OF FERTILITY

Long-term carcinogenicity studies of nevirapine in animals are currently in progress. In genetic toxicology assays, nevirapine showed no evidence of mutagenic or clastogenic activity in a battery of *in vitro* and *in vivo* assays including microbial assays for gene mutation (Ames: Salmonella strains and *E. coli*), mammalian cell gene mutation assays (CHO/HGPRT), cytogenic assays using a Chinese hamster ovary cell line and a mouse bone marrow micronucleus assay following oral administration. In reproductive toxicology studies, evidence of impaired fertility was seen in female rats at doses providing systemic exposure, based on AUC, approximately equivalent to that provided with the recommended clinical dose of nevirapine.

PREGNANCY CATEGORY C

No observable teratogenicity was detected in reproductive studies performed in pregnant rats and rabbits. In rats, a significant decrease in fetal body weight occurred at doses providing systemic exposure approximately 50% higher, based on AUC, than that seen at the recommended human clinical dose. The maternal and developmental no-observable-effect level dosages in rats and rabbits produced systemic exposures approximately equivalent to or approximately 50% higher, respectively, than those seen at the recommended daily human

PRECAUTIONS: *(cont'd)*

dose, based on AUC. There are no adequate and well-controlled studies in pregnant women. Nevirapine should be used during pregnancy only if the potential benefit justifies the potential risk to the fetus.

NURSING MOTHERS

Preliminary results from an ongoing pharmacokinetic study (ACTG 250) of 10 HIV-1-infected pregnant women who were administered a single oral dose of 100 or 200 mg nevirapine at a median of 5.8 hours before delivery, indicate that nevirapine readily crosses the placenta and is found in breast milk. Consistent with the recommendation by the U.S. Public Health Service Centers for Disease Control and Prevention that HIV-infected mothers not breast-feed their infants to avoid risking postnatal transmission of HIV, mothers should discontinue nursing if they are receiving nevirapine.

PEDIATRIC USE

Safety and effectiveness of nevirapine in pediatric patients have not been established.

Nevirapine has been studied in two open-label, uncontrolled trials (B1 882, B1 892) in 37 HIV-1-infected pediatric patients with a median age of 0.9 years (range: 0.1 to 15 years) who were treated for a median duration of 20.7 months. Seven patients developed rashes while receiving nevirapine. In an ongoing, controlled trial of nevirapine combination therapy in HIV-1-infected pediatric patients (ACTG 245), one of approximately 288 patients treated with nevirapine experienced Stevens-Johnson syndrome.

Because there are no data on multi-dose pharmacokinetics in children, no recommendation on dosing can be made. Based on single-dose pharmacokinetics in 9 HIV-1-infected pediatric patients (age 9 mos. to 14 years) who were administered nevirapine in a suspension formulation, it appears that oral clearance is approximately 2-fold greater in children when compared to adults.

DRUG INTERACTIONS:

No dosage adjustments are required when nevirapine is taken in combination with ZDV, ddl, or ddC. When the ZDV data were pooled from two studies (n=33) in which HIV-1-infected patients received nevirapine 400 mg/day either alone or in combination with 200-300 mg/day ddl or 0.375 to 0.75 mg/day ddC on a background of ZDV therapy, nevirapine produced a non-significant decline of 13% in ZDV AUC and a non-significant increase of 5.8% in ZDV C_{max}. In a subset of patients (n=6) who were administered nevirapine 400 mg/day and ddl on a background of ZDV therapy, nevirapine produced a significant decline of 32% in ZDV AUC and a non-significant decline of 27% in ZDV C_{max}. Paired data suggest that ZDV had no effect on the pharmacokinetics of nevirapine. In one crossover study, nevirapine had no effect on the steady-state pharmacokinetics of either ddl (n=18) or ddC (n=6).

Available data on the potential interactions between nevirapine and other CYP3A substrates are limited and preliminary; therefore, recommendations for dose adjustments cannot be made. (See DRUG INTERACTIONS, Rifampin/Rifabutin for recommendations regarding rifampin, rifabutin, protease inhibitors and oral contraceptives).

In vitro: Studies using human liver microsomes indicated that the formation of nevirapine hydroxylated metabolites was not affected by the presence of dapsone, rifabutin, rifampin, and trimethoprim/sulfamethoxazole. Ketoconazole significantly inhibited the formation of nevirapine hydroxylated metabolites.

In vivo: Monitoring of steady-state nevirapine trough plasma concentrations in patients who received long-term nevirapine treatment in combination with ketoconazole (n=11) revealed no evidence of a significant inhibitory effect on nevirapine metabolism. Steady-state nevirapine trough plasma concentrations were elevated in patients who received cimetidine (+21%, n=11) and macrolides (+12%, n=24), known inhibitors of CYP3A.

Steady-state nevirapine trough concentrations were reduced in patients who received rifabutin (-16%, n=19) and rifampin (-37%, n=3), known inducers of CYP3A. Nevirapine is an inducer of CYP3A, with maximal induction occurring within 2-4 weeks of initiating multiple-dose therapy. Other compounds that are substrates of CYP3A may have decreased plasma concentrations when co-administered with nevirapine. Therefore, careful monitoring of the therapeutic effectiveness of CYP3A-metabolized drugs is recommended when taken in combination with nevirapine (see PRECAUTIONS).

Although clinical studies have not been conducted, induction of CYP3A by nevirapine may result in lower plasma concentrations of other concomitantly administered drugs that are extensively metabolized by CYP3A. Thus, if a patient has been stabilized on a dosage regimen for a drug metabolized by CYP3A, and begins treatment with nevirapine, dose adjustments may be necessary.

Rifampin/Rifabutin: There are insufficient data to assess whether dose adjustments are necessary when nevirapine and rifampin or rifabutin are coadministered. Therefore, these drugs should only be used in combination if clearly indicated and with careful monitoring.

Protease Inhibitors: Nevirapine may decrease plasma concentrations of protease inhibitors. Therefore, until clinical data are available that evaluate the need for dose adjustments, these drugs should not be administered concomitantly with nevirapine.

Oral Contraceptives: There are no clinical data on the effects of nevirapine on the pharmacokinetics of oral contraceptives. Nevirapine may decrease plasma concentrations of oral contraceptives (also other hormonal contraceptives); therefore, these drugs should not be administered concomitantly with nevirapine.

ADVERSE REACTIONS:

The most frequently reported adverse events related to nevirapine therapy were rash, fever, nausea, headache, and abnormal liver function tests.

The major clinical toxicity of nevirapine is rash, with nevirapine-attributable rash occurring in 17% of patients in combination regimens in Phase II/III controlled studies. Thirty-seven percent of patients treated with nevirapine experienced rash compared with 20% of patients treated in control groups of either ZDV+ddl or ZDV alone (TABLES 1Aand 1B). Severe or life-threatening rash occurred in 7.6% of nevirapine-treated patients compared with 1.2% of patients treated in the control groups.

Rashes are usually mild to moderate, maculopapular erythematous cutaneous eruptions, with or without pruritus, located on the trunk, face and extremities. The majority of severe rashes occurred within the first 28 days of treatment: 25% of the patients with severe rashes required hospitalization; and one patient required surgical intervention. All patients recovered. Overall, 7% of patients discontinued nevirapine due to rash.

Table 2 lists treatment-related clinical adverse events that occurred in patients receiving nevirapine in ACTG 241 and in Trials B1 1037 and B1 1011.

Laboratory Abnormalities: TABLE 3 summarizes marked laboratory abnormalities occurring in three controlled studies.

Asymptomatic elevations in GGT levels are more frequent in nevirapine recipients than in controls. Because hepatitis has occasionally been reported in nevirapine-treated patients, monitoring of liver function tests should be considered.

OVERDOSAGE:

There is no known antidote for nevirapine overdosage. No acute toxicities or sequelae were reported for one patient who ingested 800 mg of nevirapine for one day.

OVERDOSAGE: *(cont'd)*

TABLE 1A Percentage of Patients With Rashes in Controlled Trials*

	ACTG 241 †		B1 1037	
	NVP+ZDV +ddl	**ZDV+ddl**	**NVP+ZDV**	**ZDV**
n	197	201	30	30
Rash events of all Grades and all causality	39.6%	23.9%	26.7%	6.7%
Grade 3 or 4 rash events, all causality	8.1%	1.5%	3.3%	0%

* At recommended dose of one 200 mg tablet daily for the first 14 days followed by one 200 mg tablet twice daily
† Trial ACTG 241 was designed to report Grade 3/4 (severe or life-threatening) events: except for several pre-specified events including rash for which all grades are reported.

TABLE 1B Percentage of Patients With Rashes in Controlled Trials*

	B1 1011		COMBINED DATA	
	NVP+ZDV	**ZDV**	**NVP**	**CONTROL**
n	25	24	252	255
Rash events of all Grades and all causality	32.0%	4.2%	37.3%	20.0%
Grade 3 or 4 rash events, all causality	8.0%	0%	7.6%	1.2%

* At recommended dose of one 200 mg tablet daily for the first 14 days followed by one 200 mg tablet twice daily
† Trial ACTG 241 was designed to report Grade 3/4 (severe or life-threatening) events: except for several pre-specified events including rash for which all grades are reported.

TABLE 2 Comparative Incidence of Selected Drug-Related Adverse Events in Controlled Trials

	ACTG 241 Grade 3/4 events		Trial B1 1037 and B1 1011 All severities	
	NVP+ZDV +ddl	**ZDV+ddl**	**NVP+ZDV**	**ZDV alone**
Number of patients	197	201	55	30
Overall incidence of related adverse events	31%	23%	42%	33%
Rash	8	2	20	3
Fever	3	3	11	3
Nausea	5	4	9	3
Headache	3	3	11	0
Diarrhea	2	2	0	0
Abdominal pain	1	2	2	0
Ulcerative stomatitis	0	0	4	0
Peripheral Neuropathy	0	2	0	0
Paraesthesia	1	0	2	0
Myalgia	1	0	2	7
Hepatitis	1	0	4	0

TABLE 3 Percentage of Patients With Marked Laboratory Abnormalities

Data combined for controlled trials ACTG 241, B1 1037 & B1 1011

	Nevirapine n=252	**Control n=255**
Hematology		
Decreases Hg (<8.0 g/dL)	1.2%	2.0%
Decreased platelets (<50,000/mm^3)	0.8	0.8
Decreased neutrophils (<750/mm^3)	11.1	10.2
Blood Chemistry		
Increased ALT (>250 U/L)	3.4	3.5
Increased AST (>250 U/L)	2.0	2.4
Increased CGT (>450 U/L)	2.4	1.2
Increased total bilirubin (>2.5 mg/dL)	0.4	1.2

DOSAGE AND ADMINISTRATION:

The recommended dose for nevirapine is one 200 mg tablet daily for the first 14 days (**this lead-in period should be used because it has been found to lessen the frequency of rash**), followed by one 200 mg tablet twice daily, in combination with nucleoside analogue antiretroviral agents. For concomitantly administered nucleoside therapy, the manufacturer's recommended dosage and monitoring should be followed.

Monitoring of Patients: Clinical chemistry tests, which include liver function tests, should be performed prior to initiating nevirapine therapy and at appropriate intervals during therapy.

Dosage Adjustment: Nevirapine should be discontinued if patients experience severe rash or a rash accompanied by constitutional findings (see WARNINGS). Patients experiencing rash during the 14–day lead-in period of 200 mg/day should not have their nevirapine dose increased until the rash has resolved. (see Information for the Patient)

Nevirapine administration should be interrupted in patients experiencing moderate or severe liver function test abnormalities (excluding GGT), until the liver function test elevations have returned to baseline. Nevirapine may then be restarted at half the previous dose level. Nevirapine should be permanently discontinued if moderate or severe liver function test abnormalities recur. (see PRECAUTIONS)

Patients who interrupt nevirapine dosing for more than 7 days should restart the recommended dosing, using one 200 mg tablet daily for the first 14 days (lead-in) followed by one 200 mg tablet twice daily.

No data are available to recommend a dosage of nevirapine in patients with hepatic dysfunction, renal insufficiency, or undergoing dialysis.

ANIMAL PHARMACOLOGY:

Animal studes have shown that nevirapine is widely distributed to nearly all tissues and readily crosses the blood-brain barrier.

PATIENT INFORMATION:

Nevirapine is used in combination with other AIDS drugs to treat HIV-1–infected adults. Inform your doctor or pharmacist if you are taking any other medications. Inform your doctor if you are pregnant or nursing. This drug may cause severe, life-threatening rash. If

PATIENT INFORMATION: *(cont'd)*

rash occurs or is accompanied by fever, blistering, oral lesions, conjunctivitis, swelling, muscle or joint aches, or general tiredness, stop taking the drug and see your doctor. This drug may interfere with birth control "pills"; use another form of contraception.

Take as directed. Do not alter the dose. If a dose is missed, take the next dose as soon as possible. Do not double-up the next dose. May cause rash, fever, nausea, headache, or diarrhea. Inform your doctor or pharmacist of these occur.

HOW SUPPLIED:

Viramune (nevirapine) Tablets, 200 mg, are white, oval, biconvex tablets, 9.3 mm x 19.1 mm. One side is embossed with "54 193," with a single bisect separating the "54" and "193." The opposite side has a single bisect.

Storage: Store at 15°C-30°C (59°F-86°F). The bottles should be kept tightly closed.

HOW SUPPLIED - EQUIVALENTS NOT AVAILABLE:

Tablet - Oral - 200 mg

100's	$412.80	VIRAMUNE, Roxane	00054-4647-25
100's	$412.80	VIRAMUNE, Roxane	00054-8647-25

NIACIN *(001876)*

CATEGORIES: Cholesterol; Heart Disease; Homeostatic & Nutrient; Hypercholesterolemia; Hyperlipidemia; Hyperlipoproteinemia; Hypolipidemics; Lipotropics; Nutrition, Enteral/Parenteral; Vascular Disorders, Cerebral/Peripheral; Vitamin B Complex; Vitamins; FDA Approval Pre 1982

BRAND NAMES: *Acido Nicotinico*; *Acido Nicotino*; *Akotin*; *Akotin 250*; *Apo-Nicotinic Acid*; *Natinate*; *Nicangin*; *Nicobid*; **Nicolar**; *Niconacid*; Nicotinic Acid; *Nikacid*; Nikotime; *Novoniacin*; *Nyclin* (Japan); *Pepevit* (Mexico); Slo-Niacin; Span Niacin; *Tri-B3* (Canada); *Vitaplex*; Wampocap
(International brand names outside U.S. in italics)

FORMULARIES: Aetna; BC-BS; CIGNA; DoD; FHP; Humana; Kaiser; Medco; Medi-Cal; PCS; PruCare; United

COST OF THERAPY: $49.27 (Hyperlipidemia; Tablet; 500 mg; 6/day; 365 days) vs. Potential Cost of $24,027.04 (Coronary Bypass)

DESCRIPTION:

Niacin or nicotinic acid, a water-soluble B complex vitamin and antihyperlipidemic agent, is 3-pyridinecarboxylic acid. It is a white, crystalline powder, sparingly soluble in water. It has the following structural formula: $C_6H_5NO_2$ with a molecular weight of 123.11.

Each Nicolar tablet, for oral administration, is a scored yellow-colored tablet containing 500 mg of nicotinic acid. In addition, each tablet contains the following inactive ingredients: microcrystalline cellulose, FD&C Yellow No. 5 (tartrazine) (see PRECAUTIONS), magnesium stearate, povidone, and colloidal silica.

CLINICAL PHARMACOLOGY:

The role of low-density lipoprotein (LDL) cholesterol in atherogenesis is supported by pathological observations, clinical studies, and many animal experiments. Observational epidemiological studies have clearly established that high total or LDL (low-density lipoprotein) cholesterol and low HDL (high-density lipoprotein) cholesterol are risk factors for coronary heart disease. The Coronary Drug Project,[1] compared in 1975, was designed to assess the safety and efficacy of nicotinic acid and other lipid-altering drugs in men 30 to 64 years old with a history of myocardial infarction. Over an observation period of five (5) years, nicotinic acid showed a statistically significant benefit in decreasing nonfatal, recurrent myocardial infarctions. The incidence of definite, non-fatal MI was 8.9% for the 1,119 patients randomized to nicotinic acid versus 12.2% for the 2,789 patients who received placebo ($p < 0.004$). Though total mortality was similar in the two groups at five (5) years (24.4% with nicotinic acid versus 25.4% with placebo; p=N.S.), in a fifteen (15) year cumulative follow-up there were 11% (69) fewer deaths in the nicotinic acid group compared to the placebo cohort (52.% versus 58.2%; p=0004).[2]

The Cholesterol-Lowering Atherosclerosis Study (CLAS) was a randomized, placebo-controlled, angiographic trial testing combined colestipol and nicotinic acid therapy in 162 non-smoking males with previous coronary bypass surgery.[3] The primary, per subject cardiac endpoint was global coronary artery change score. After two (2) years, 61% of patients in the placebo cohort showed disease progression by global change score (N=82), compared with only 38.8% of drug-treated subjects (N=80), when both native arteries and grafts were considered ($p < .005$). In a follow- up to this trial in a subgroup of 103 patients treated for four (4) years, again, significantly fewer patients in the drug-treated group demonstrated progression than in the placebo cohort (48% versus 85%, respectively; $p < .0001$).[4]

The Familial Atherosclerosis Treatment Study (FATS) in 146 men ages 62 and younger with apolipoprotein B levels ≥125 mg/dL, established coronary artery disease, and family histories of vascular disease, assessed change in severity of disease in the proximal coronary arteries by quantitative arteriography.[5] Patients were given dietary counselling and randomized to treatment with either conventional therapy with double placebo (or placebo plus colestipol if the LDL-cholesterol was elevated); lovastatin plus colestipol; or nicotinic acid plus colestipol. In the conventional therapy group, 46% of patients had disease progression (and no regression) in at least one of nine proximal coronary segments. In contrast, progression (as the only change) was seen in only 25% in the nicotinic acid plus colestipol group. Though not an original endpoint of the trial, clinical events (death, myocardial infarction, or revascularization for worsening angina) occurred in 10 of 52 patients who received conventional therapy, compared with 2 of 48 who received nicotinic acid plus colestipol.

Nicotinic acid (but not nicotinamide) in gram doses produces an average 10-20% reduction in total and LDL-cholesterol, a 30-70% reduction in triglycerides, and an average 20-35% increase in HDL-cholesterol. The magnitude of individual lipid and lipoprotein responses may be influenced by the severity and type of underlying lipid abnormality. The increase in total HDL is associated with a shift in the distribution of HDL subfractions (as defined by ultra-centrifugation) with an increase in the HDL_2:HDL_3ratio; and an increase in apolipoprotein AI content. The mechanism by which nicotinic acid exerts these effects is not entirely understood, but may involve several actions, including a decrease in esterification of hepatic triglycerides. Nicotinic acid treatment also decreases the serum levels of apolipoprotein B-100 (apo B), the major protein component of the VLDL and LDL fractions, and of lipoprotein, Lp(a), a variant form of LDL independently associated with coronary risk. The effect of nicotinic acid-induced changes in lipids/lipoproteins on cardiovascular morbidity or mortality in individuals without pre-existing coronary disease has not been established.

PHARMACOKINETICS

Following an oral dose, the pharmacokinetic profile of nicotinic acid is characterized by rapid absorption from the gastrointestinal tract and a short plasma elimination half-life. At a 1 gram dose, peak plasma concentrations of 15 to 30 mcg/mL are reached within 30 to 60

CLINICAL PHARMACOLOGY: *(cont'd)*

minutes. Approximately 88% of an oral pharmacologic dose is eliminated by the kidneys as unchanged drug and nicotinuric acid, its primary metabolite. The plasma elimination half-life of nicotinic acid ranges from 20 to 45 minutes.

INDICATIONS AND USAGE:

I. Therapy with lipid-altering agents should be only one component of multiple risk factor intervention in those individuals at significantly increased risk for atherosclerotic vascular disease due to hypercholesterolemia. Nicotinic acid, alone or in combination with a bile-acid binding resin, is indicated as an adjunct to diet for the reduction of elevated total and LDL cholesterol levels in patients with primary hypercholesterolemia (Types IIa and IIb),† when the response to a diet restricted in saturated fat and cholesterol and other nonpharmacologic measures alone has been inadequate (see also the N.C.E.P. treatment guidelines[6]). Prior to initiating therapy with nicotinic acid, secondary causes for hypercholesterolemia (*e.g.,* poorly controlled diabetes mellitus, hypothyroidism, nephrotic syndrome, dysproteinemias, obstructive liver disease, other drug therapy, alcoholism) should be excluded, and a lipid profile performed to measure total cholesterol, HDL-cholesterol, and triglycerides.

II. Nicotinic acid is also indicated as adjunctive therapy for the treatment of adult patients with very high serum triglyceride levels (Types IV and V hyperlipidemia)† who present a risk of pancreatitis and who do not respond adequately to a determined dietary effort to control them. Such patients typically have serum triglyceride levels over 2000 mg/dL and have elevations of VLDL-cholesterol as well as fasting chylomicrons (Type V hyperlipidemia).† Subjects who consistently have total serum or plasma triglycerides below 1000 mg/dL are unlikely to develop pancreatitis. Therapy with nicotinic acid may be considered for those subjects with triglyceride elevations between 1000 and 2000 mg/dL who have a history of pancreatitis or of recurrent abdominal pain typical of pancreatitis. Some Type IV patients with triglycerides under 1000 mg/dL may, through dietary or alcoholic indiscretion, convert to a Type V pattern with massive triglyceride elevations accompanying fasting chylomicronemia, but the influence of nicotinic acid therapy on the risk of pancreatitis in such situations has not been adequately studied. Drug therapy is not indicated for patients with Type I hyperlipoproteinemia, who have elevations of chylomicrons and plasma triglycerides, but who have normal levels of very low density lipoprotein (VLDL). Inspection of plasma refrigerated for 14 hours is helpful in distinguishing Types I, IV, and V hyperlipoproteinemia.[7]

†See Table 1 - Classification of Hyperlipoproteinemias

TABLE 1 Classification of Hyperlipoproteinemias

Type	Lipoproteins elevated	Lipid Elevations major	minor
I (rare)	chylomicrons	TG	↑→C
IIa	LDL	C	-
IIb	LDL, VLDL	C	TG
III (rare)	IDL	C/TG	-
IV	VLDL	TG	↑→C
V (rare)	chylomicrons, VLDL	TG	↑→C

C = cholesterol,
TG = triglycerides,
LDL = low-density lipoprotein,
VLDL = very-low-density lipoprotein,
IDL = intermediate-density lipoprotein.

CONTRAINDICATIONS:

Nicotinic acid is contraindicated in patients with a known hypersensitivity to any component of this medication; significant or unexplained hepatic dysfunction; active peptic ulcer disease; or arterial bleeding.

WARNINGS:

LIVER DYSFUNCTION

Cases of severe hepatic toxicity, including fulminant hepatic necrosis have occurred in patients who have substituted sustained-release (modified-release, timed-release) nicotinic acid products for immediate- release (crystalline) nicotinic acid at equivalent doses.

Liver function tests should be performed on all patients during therapy with nicotinic acid. Serum transaminase levels, including ALT (SGPT), should be monitored before treatment begins, every six weeks to twelve weeks for the first year, and periodically thereafter (*e.g.,* at approximately 6 month intervals). Special attention should be paid to patients who develop elevated serum transaminase levels, and in these patients, measurements should be repeated promptly and then performed more frequently. If the transaminase levels show evidence of progression, particularly if they rise to three times the upper limit of normal and are persistent, the drug should be discontinued. Liver biopsy should be considered if elevation persist beyond discontinuation of the drug.

Nicotinic acid should be used with caution in patients who consume substantial quantities of alcohol and/or have a past history of liver disease. Active liver diseases or unexplained transaminase elevations are contraindication to the use of nicotinic acid.

SKELETAL MUSCLE

Rare cases of rhabdomyolysis have been associated with concomitant administration of lipid-altering doses ($\geq$ 1 g/day) of nicotinic acid and HMG-CoA reductase inhibitors. Physicians contemplating combined therapy with HMG-CoA reductase inhibitors and nicotinic acid should carefully weigh the potential benefits and risks and should carefully monitor patients for any signs and symptoms of muscle pain, tenderness, or weakness, particularly during the initial months of therapy and during any periods of upward dosage titration of either drug. Periodic serum creatine phosphokinase (CPK) and potassium determinations should be considered in such situations, but there is no assurance that such monitoring will prevent the occurrence of severe myopathy.

PRECAUTIONS:

GENERAL

Before instituting therapy with nicotinic acid, an attempt should be made to control hyperlipidemia with appropriate diet, exercise, and weight reduction in obese patients, and to treat other underlying medical problems (see INDICATIONS AND USAGE.)

Patients with a past history of jaundice, hepatobiliary disease, or peptic ulcer should be observed closely during nicotinic acid therapy. Frequent monitoring of liver function tests and blood glucose should be performed to ascertain that the drug is producing no adverse effects on these organ systems. Diabetic patients may experience a dose-related rise in glucose intolerance, the clinical significance of which is unclear. Diabetic or potentially diabetic patients should be observed closely. Adjustment of diet and/or hypoglycemic therapy may be necessary.

PRECAUTIONS: *(cont'd)*

Caution should also be used when nicotinic acid is used in patients with unstable angina or in the acute phase of myocardial infarction, particularly when such patients are also receiving vasoactive drugs such as nitrates, calcium channel blockers, or adrenergic blocking agents.

Elevated uric acid levels have occurred with nicotinic acid therapy, therefore use with caution in patients predisposed to gout.

This product contains FD&C Yellow No. 5 (tartrazine) which may cause allergic-type reactions (including bronchial asthma) in certain susceptible persons. Although the overall incidence of FD&C Yellow No. 5 (tartrazine) sensitivity in the general population is low, it is frequently seen in patients who also have aspirin hypersensitivity.

CARCINOGENESIS, MUTAGENESIS, AND IMPAIRMENT OF FERTILITY

Nicotinic acid administered to mice for a lifetime as a 1% solution in drinking water was not carcinogenic. The mice in this study received approximately 6-8 times a human dose of 3000 milligrams/day as determined on a milligram/square meter basis. Nicotinic acid was negative for mutagenicity in the Ames test. No studies on impairment of fertility have been performed.

PREGNANCY CATEGORY C

Animal reproduction studies have not been conducted with nicotinic acid. It is also not known whether nicotinic acid at doses typically used for lipid disorders can cause fetal harm when administered to pregnant women or whether it can affect reproductive capacity. If a woman receiving nicotinic acid for primary hypercholesterolemia (Types IIa or IIb) becomes pregnant, the drug should be discontinued. If a woman being treated with nicotinic acid for hypertriglyceridemia (Types IV and V) conceives, the benefits and risks of continued drug therapy should be assessed on an individual basis.

NURSING MOTHERS

It is not known whether this drug is excreted in human milk. Because many drugs are excreted in human milk and because of the potential for serious adverse reactions in nursing infants from lipid-altering doses of nicotinic acid, a decision should be made whether to discontinue nursing or to discontinue the drug, taking into account the importance of the drug to the mother.

PEDIATRIC USE

Safety and effectiveness in children and adolescents have not been established.

DRUG INTERACTIONS:

HMG-CoA Reductase Inhibitors: Skeletal Muscle.

Antihypertensive Therapy: Nicotinic acid may potentiate the effects of ganglionic blocking agents and vasoactive drugs resulting in postural hypotension.

Aspirin: Concomitant aspirin may decrease the metabolic clearance of nicotinic acid. The clinical relevance of this finding is unclear.

Other: Concomitant alcohol or hot drinks may increase the side effects of flushing and pruritus and should be avoided at the time of drug ingestion.

ADVERSE REACTIONS:

Cardiovascular: atrial fibrillation and other cardiac arrhythmias; orthostasis; hypotension

Gastrointestinal: dyspepsia; vomiting; diarrhea; peptic ulceration; jaundice; abnormal liver function tests

Skin: mild to severe cutaneous flushing; pruritus; hyperpigmentation; acanthosis nigricans; dry skin

Metabolic: decreased glucose tolerance; hyperuricemia; gout

Eye: toxic amblyopia; cystoid macular edema

Nervous System/Psychiatric: headache

OVERDOSAGE:

Supportive measures should be undertaken in the event of an overdose.

DOSAGE AND ADMINISTRATION:

The usual adult dosage of nicotinic acid is 1 to 2 grams two to three times a day. Doses should be individualized according to the patient's response. Start with one-half tablet (250 mg) as a single daily dose following the evening meal. The frequency of dosing and total daily dose can be increased every four to seven days until the desired LDL- cholesterol and/or triglyceride level is achieved or the first-level therapeutic dose of 1.5 to 2 grams/day is reached. If the patient's hyperlipidemia is not adequately controlled after 2 months at this level, the dosage can then be increased at two to four week intervals to 3 grams/day (1 gram three times per day). In patients with marked lipid abnormalities, a higher dose is occasionally required, but generally should not exceed 6 grams/day.

Flushing of the skin appears frequently and can be minimized by pretreatment with aspirin or non-steroidal anti-inflammatory drugs. Tolerance to this flushing develops rapidly over the course of several weeks. Flushing, pruritus, and gastrointestinal distress are also greatly reduced by slowly increasing the dose of nicotinic acid and avoiding administration on an empty stomach.

Sustained-release (modified-release, timed-release) nicotinic acid preparations should **not** be substituted for equivalent doses of immediate-release (crystalline) nicotinic acid.

HOW SUPPLIED:

Nicolar Tablets (Niacin Tablets, USP) are scored, yellow-colored, oval-shaped 500 mg tablets supplied in bottles containing 100 tablets each.

Dispense in a tight container as defined in the USP. Store at controlled room temperature, 15°-30°C (59°-86°F).

REFERENCES:

1. The Coronary Drug Project Research Group. Clofibrate and Niacin in Coronary Heart Disease. JAMA 1975; 231:360-81. **2.** Canner PL *et al.* Fifteen Year Mortality in Coronary Drug Product Patients: Long-Term Benefit with Niacin. JACC 1986; 8(6):1245-55. **3.** Blankenhorn DH *et al.* Beneficial Effects of Combined Colestipol-Niacin Therapy on Coronary Atherosclerosis and Coronary Venous Bypass Grafts. JAMA1987; 257 (23):3233-40. **4.** Cashin-Hemphill *et al.* Beneficial Effects of Colestipol-Niacin on Coronary Atherosclerosis. JAMA 1990; 264 (23):3013-17. **5.** Brown G *et al.* Regression of Coronary Artery Disease as a Result of Intensive Lipid-Lowering Therapy in Men with High Levels of Apolipoprotein B. NEJM 1990; 323-1289-98. **6.** Report of the National Cholesterol Education Program Expert Panel on Detection, Evaluation, and Treatment of High Blood Cholesterol.Arch. Int. Med. 1988; 148:36-39. **7.** Nikkila EA: Familial lipoprotein lipase deficiency and related disorders of chylomicron metabolism. In Stanbury J.B. *et al.* (eds.): *The Metabolic Basis of Inherited Disease,* 5th ed., McGraw-Hill, 1983, Chap. 30, pp. 622-642.

HOW SUPPLIED - RATED THERAPEUTICALLY EQUIVALENT:

Tablet, Uncoated - Oral - 500 mg

100's	$2.25	Niacin, Harber Pharm	51432-0294-03
100's	$2.96	Niacin, HL Moore Drug Exch	00839-6458-06
100's	$2.99	Niacin, H.C.F.A. F F P	99999-1876-01
100's	$4.34	Niacin, Schein Pharm (US)	00364-1067-01
100's	$5.18	Niacin, IDE-Interstate	00814-5282-14
100's	$5.75	Niacin, Consolidated Midland	00223-1353-01

HOW SUPPLIED - RATED THERAPEUTICALLY EQUIVALENT:
(cont'd)

100's	$15.44	Niacin-Rx, Upsher Smith	00245-0067-11
100's	**$64.40**	**NICOLAR, Rhone-Poulenc Rorer**	**00075-2850-01**
300's	$8.97	Niacin, H.C.F.A. F F P	99999-1876-02
1000's	$13.00	Niacin, Raway	00686-1352-10
1000's	$21.06	Niacin, HL Moore Drug Exch	00839-6458-16
1000's	$23.93	Niacin, IDE-Interstate	00814-5319-30
1000's	$27.50	Niacin, Rugby	00536-4078-10
1000's	$29.90	Niacin, H.C.F.A. F F P	99999-1876-03
1000's	$37.95	Niacin, Consolidated Midland	00223-1353-02

HOW SUPPLIED - NOT RATED EQUIVALENT:

Capsule, Gelatin, Sustained Action - Oral - 125 mg

100's	$3.75	Niacin, United Res	00677-0424-01
100's	$4.95	Niacin, Eon Labs Mfg	00185-0742-01
100's	$5.05	Niacin, Time-Caps Labs	49483-0013-01
100's	$5.10	NIACIN S.R., Major Pharms	00904-0628-60
100's	$5.70	NIACIN S.R., Major Pharms	00904-0629-60
500's	$12.00	Niacin, United Res	00677-0424-05
1000's	$37.41	Niacin, Time-Caps Labs	49483-0013-10
1000's	$42.15	NIACIN S.R., Major Pharms	00904-0629-80
1000's	$47.40	NIACIN S.R., Major Pharms	00904-0628-80
1000's	$47.50	Niacin, Eon Labs Mfg	00185-0742-10

Capsule, Gelatin, Sustained Action - Oral - 250 mg

100's	$4.43	Niacin, IDE-Interstate	00814-5278-14
100's	$4.60	Niacin, United Res	00677-0425-01
100's	$5.75	Niacin, Eon Labs Mfg	00185-0743-01
100's	$5.75	Niacin Td, Qualitest Pharms	00603-4736-21
100's	$5.94	Niacin, Time-Caps Labs	49483-0014-01
250's	$11.45	Niacin, Major Pharms	00904-0629-70
500's	$17.95	Niacin, United Res	00677-0425-05
1000's	$40.11	Niacin Td, Qualitest Pharms	00603-4736-32
1000's	$47.88	Niacin, Time-Caps Labs	49483-0014-10
1000's	$55.00	Niacin, Eon Labs Mfg	00185-0743-10

Capsule, Gelatin, Sustained Action - Oral - 400 mg

100's	$3.63	Niacin T D, HL Moore Drug Exch	00839-6103-06
100's	$4.95	Niacin, Harber Pharm	51432-0343-03
100's	$6.20	Niacin, Major Pharms	00904-0630-60
100's	$6.95	Niacin, Eon Labs Mfg	00185-0744-01
100's	$6.98	Niacin, IDE-Interstate	00814-5280-14
1000's	$67.50	Niacin, Eon Labs Mfg	00185-0744-10

Capsule, Gelatin, Sustained Action - Oral - 500 mg

100's	$7.80	Niacin, Major Pharms	00904-0631-60

Capsule, Gelatin, Sustained Action - Oral - 750 mg

100's	$7.05	Niacin, IDE-Interstate	00814-5284-14

Injection, Solution - Intramuscular; - 100 mg/ml

30 ml	$2.18	Niacin, Lannett	00527-0151-58

NIACINAMIDE *(001880)*

CATEGORIES: Homeostatic & Nutrient; Vitamin B Complex; Vitamins; FDA Pre 1938 Drugs

BRAND NAMES: *Apo-Nicotinamide*; *Bioglan Nicotinamide 250 mg*; *Hipocol* (Mexico); *Nicobion* (France); Nicotinamide; *Nicotivit*; *Nicovital*; *Pepeom Amide*; *Ucemine PP*; *Vitamin B3 Tablets*
(International brand names outside U.S. in italics)

Prescribing information not available at time of publication.

HOW SUPPLIED - EQUIVALENTS NOT AVAILABLE:

Tablet, Uncoated - Oral - 100 mg

100's	$2.40	Niacinamide, Rugby	00536-4068-01

Tablet, Uncoated - Oral - 500 mg

500's	$11.85	Niacinamide, IDE-Interstate	00814-5331-28

NICARDIPINE HYDROCHLORIDE *(001882)*

CATEGORIES: Angina; Antianginals; Antihypertensives; Calcium Channel Blockers; Cardiovascular Drugs; Hypertension; Renal Drugs; Pregnancy Category C; FDA Approved 1988 Dec

BRAND NAMES: *Antagonil* (Germany); *Brodipine*; **Cardene**; Cardene SR; *Cardepine*; *Cardibloc*; *Cardipene*; *Dacarel*; *Dagan*; *Flusemide*; *Lincil*; *Loxen* (France); *Loxen Retard*; *Nerdipine*; *Nicardal*; *Nicarpin*; *Nicodel* (Japan); *Nimicor*; *Perdipina*; *Perdipine* (Japan); *Ranvil*; *Ridene* (Mexico); *Rycarden*; *Rydene*; *Saf Card*; *Vasodin*
(International brand names outside U.S. in italics)

FORMULARIES: Aetna; BC-BS; Foundation; Medi-Cal

COST OF THERAPY: $463.62 (Angina; Capsule; 20 mg; 3/day; 365 days)

DESCRIPTION:

Nicardipine HCl capsules for oral administration each contain 20 mg or 30 mg of nicardipine hydrochloride. Nicardipine HCl is a calcium ion flux inhibitor (slow channel blocker or calcium channel blocker).

Nicardipine hydrochloride is a dihydropyridine structure with the IUPAC (International Union of Pure and Applied Chemistry) chemical name 2- (benzyl-methyl amino)ethyl methyl 1,4-dihydro-2,6-dimethyl-4-(*m*-nitrophenyl)-3,5-pyridinedicarboxylate monohydrochloride.

Nicardipine hydrochloride is a greenish-yellow, odorless, crystalline powder that melts at about 169°C. It is freely soluble in chloroform, methanol, and glacial acetic acid, sparingly soluble in anhydrous ethanol, slightly soluble in n-butanol, water, 0.01 M potassium dihydrogen phosphate, acetone, and dioxane, very slightly soluble in ethyl acetate, and practically insoluble in benzene, ether and hexane. It has a molecular weight of 515.99.

Nicardipine HCl is available in hard gelatin capsules containing 20 mg or 30 mg nicardipine hydrochloride with magnesium stearate and pregelatinized starch as the inactive ingredients. the 20 mg strength is provided in opaque white-white capsules with a brilliant blue band while the 30 mg capsules are opaque light blue-powder blue with a brilliant blue band. The colorants used in the 20 mg capsules are titanium dioxide, D&C Red #7 Calcium Lake and FD&C Blue #1 and the 30 mg capsules use titanium dioxide, FD&C Blue #1, D&C Yellow #10 Aluminum Lake, D&C Red #7 Calcium Lake and FD&C Blue #2.

CLINICAL PHARMACOLOGY:

MECHANISM OF ACTION

Nicardipine HCl is a calcium entry blocker (slow channel blocker or calcium ion antagonist) which inhibits the transmembrane influx of calcium ions into cardiac muscle and smooth muscle without changing serum calcium concentrations. The contractile processes of cardiac muscle and vascular smooth muscle are dependent upon the movement of extracellular calcium ions into these cells through specific ion channels. The effects of nicardipine HCl are more selective to vascular smooth muscle than cardiac muscle. In animal models, nicardipine HCl produces relaxation of coronary vascular smooth muscle at drug levels which cause little or no negative inotropic effect.

PHARMACOKINETICS AND METABOLISM

Nicardipine HCl is completely absorbed following oral doses administered as capsules. Plasma levels are detectable as early as 20 minutes following an oral dose and maximal plasma levels are observed within 30 minutes to two hours (mean T_{max} = 1 hour). While nicardipine HCl is completely absorbed, it is subject to saturable first pass metabolism and the systemic bioavailability is about 35% following a 30 mg oral dose at steady state.

When nicardipine HCl was administered one (1) or three (3) hours after a high fat meal, the mean Cmax and mean AUC were lower (20% to 30%) than when nicardipine HCl was given to fasting subjects. these decreases in plasma observed following a meal may be significant but the clinical trials establishing the efficacy and safety of nicardipine HCl were done in patients without regard to the timing of meals. Thus the results of these trials reflect the effects of meal-induced variability.

The pharmacokinetics of nicardipine HCl are nonlinear due to saturable hepatic first pass metabolism. Following oral administration, increasing doses result in a disproportionate increase in plasma levels. Steady state Cmax values following 20, 30, and 40 mg doses every 8 hours averaged 36, 88, and 133 ng/ml, respectively. Hence, increasing the dose from 20 to 30 mg every 8 hours more than doubled Cmax and increasing the dose from 20 to 40 mg every 8 hours increased Cmax more than 3-fold. A similar disproportionate increase in AUC with dose was observed. Considerable inter-subject variability in plasma levels was also observed.

Post-absorption kinetics of nicardipine HCl are also non-linear, although there is a reproducible terminal plasma half-life that averaged 8.6 hours following 30 and 40 mg doses at steady state (tid). The terminal half-life represents the elimination of less than 5% of the absorbed drug (measured by plasma concentrations). Elimination over the first 8 hours after dosing is much faster with a half-life of 3-4 hours. Steady state plasma levels are achieved after 2 to 3 days of tid dosing (every 8 hours) and are 2-fold higher than after a single dose.

Nicardipine HCl is highly protein bound (>95%) in human plasma over a wide concentration range.

Nicardipine HCl is metabolized extensively by the liver; less than 1% of intact drug is detected in the urine. Following a radioactive oral dose in solution, 60% of the radioactivity was recovered in the urine and 35% in feces. Most of the dose (over 90%) was recovered within 48 hours of dosing. Nicardipine HCl does not induce its own metabolism and does not induce hepatic microsomal enzymes.

The steady-state pharmacokinetics of nicardipine HCl in elderly hypertensive patients (≥65 years) are similar to those obtained in young normal adults. After one week of nicardipine HCl dosing at 20 mg three times a day, the Cmax, Tmax, AUC, terminal plasma half-life, and the extent of protein binding of nicardipine HCl observed in healthy elderly hypertensive patients did not differ significantly from those observed in young normal volunteers.

Nicardipine HCl plasma levels were higher in patients with mild renal impairment (baseline serum creatinine concentration ranged from 1.2 to 5.5 mg/dl) than in normal subjects. After 30 mg nicardipine HCl tid at steady state, Cmax and AUC were approximately 2-fold higher in these patients.

Because nicardipine HCl is extensively metabolized by the liver, the plasma levels of the drug are influenced by changes in hepatic function. Nicardipine HCl plasma levels were higher in patients with severe liver disease (hepatic cirrhosis confirmed by liver biopsy or presence of endoscopically confirmed esophageal varices) than in normal subjects. After 20 mg nicardipine HCl BID at steady state, Cmax and AUC were 1.8 and 4-fold higher, and the terminal half-life was prolonged to 19 hours in these patients.

HEMODYNAMICS

In man, nicardipine HCl produces a significant decrease in systemic vascular resistance. The degree of vasodilation and the resultant hypotensive effects are more prominent in hypertensive patients. In hypertensive patients, nicardipine reduces the blood pressure at rest and during isometric and dynamic exercise. In normotensive patients, a small decrease of about 9 mmHg in systolic and 7 mmHg in diastolic blood pressure may accompany this fall in peripheral resistance. An increase in heart rate may occur in response to the vasodilation and decrease in blood pressure, and in a few patients this heart rate may be pronounced. In clinical studies mean heart rate at time of peak plasma levels was usually increased by 5-10 beats per minute compared to placebo, with the greater increases at higher doses, while there was no difference from placebo at the end of the dosing interval. Hemodynamic studies following intravenous dosing in patients with coronary artery disease and normal or moderately abnormal left ventricular function have shown significant increases in ejection fraction and cardiac output with no significant change, or a small decrease, in left ventricular end-diastolic pressure (LVEDP). Although there is evidence that nicardipine HCl increases coronary blood flow, there is no evidence that this property plays any role in its effectiveness in stable angina. In patients with coronary artery disease, intracoronary administration of nicardipine caused no direct myocardial depression. Nicardipine HCl does, however, have a negative inotropic effect in some patients with severe left ventricular dysfunction and could, in patients with very impaired function, lead to worsened failure.

"Coronary Steal", the detrimental redistribution of coronary blood flow in patients with coronary artery disease (diversion of blood from underperfused areas toward better perfused areas), has not been observed during nicardipine treatment. On the contrary, nicardipine has been shown to improve systolic shortening in normal and hypokinetic segments of myocardial muscle, and radio-nuclide angiography has confirmed that wall motion remained improved during an increase in oxygen demand. Nonetheless, occasional patients have developed increased angina upon receiving nicardipine. Whether this represents steal in those patients, or is the result of increased heart rate and decreased diastolic pressure, is not clear.

In patients with coronary artery disease nicardipine improved L.V. diastolic distensibility during the early filling phase, probably due to a faster rate of myocardial relaxation in previously underperfused areas. There is little or no effect on normal myocardium, suggesting the improvement is mainly by indirect mechanisms such as afterload reduction, and reduced ischemia. Nicardipine has no negative effect on myocardial relaxation at therapeutic doses. The clinical consequences of these properties are as yet undemonstrated.

ELECTROPHYSIOLOGIC EFFECTS

In general, no detrimental effects on the cardiac conduction system were seen with the use of nicardipine HCl.

Nicardipine HCl increased the heart rate when given intravenously during acute electrophysiologic studies, and prolonged the corrected QT interval to a minor degree. The sinus node recovery times and SA conduction times were not affected by the drug. The PA, AH

CLINICAL PHARMACOLOGY: *(cont'd)*

and HV intervals* and the functional and effective refractory periods of the atrium were not prolonged by nicardipine HCl and the relative and effective refractory periods of the His-Purkinje system were slightly shortened after intravenous nicardipine HCl.

* PA = conduction time from high to low right atrium, AH = conduction time from low right atrium to His bundle deflection, or AV nodal conduction time, HV = conduction time through the His bundle and the bundle branch-Purkinje system.

RENAL FUNCTION

There is a transient increase in electrolyte excretion, including sodium. Nicardipine HCl does not cause generalized fluid retention, as measured by weight changes, though 7-8% of patients experience pedal edema..

EFFECTS IN ANGINA PECTORIS

In controlled clinical trials of up to 12 weeks duration in patients with chronic stable angina, nicardipine HCl increased exercise tolerance and reduced nitroglycerin consumption and the frequency of anginal attacks. The antianginal efficacy of nicardipine HCl (20-40 mg) has been demonstrated in four placebo-controlled studies involving 258 patients with chronic stable angina. In exercise tolerance testing, nicardipine HCl significantly increased time to angina, total exercise duration and time to 1 mm ST segment depression. Included among these four studies was a dose-definition in which dose-related improvements in exercise tolerance at one and four hours post-dosing and reduced frequency of anginal attacks were seen at doses of 10, 20 and 30 mg tid. Effectiveness at 10 mg tid was, however, marginal. In a fifth placebo-controlled study, the antianginal efficacy of nicardipine HCl was demonstrated at 8 hours post-dose (trough). The sustained efficacy of nicardipine HCl has been demonstrated over long-term dosing. Blood pressure fell in patients with angina by about 10/8 mmHg at peak blood levels and was little different from placebo at trough blood levels.

EFFECTS IN HYPERTENSION

Nicardipine HCl produced dose-related decreases in both systolic and diastolic blood pressure in clinical trials. The antihypertensive efficacy of nicardipine HCl administered three times daily has been demonstrated in three placebo-controlled studies involving 517 patients with mild to moderate hypertension. The blood pressure responses in the three studies were statistically significant from placebo at peak (1 hour post-dosing) and trough (8 hours post-dosing) although it is apparent that well over half of the antihypertensive effect is lost by the end of the dosing interval. The results from placebo controlled studies of nicardipine HCl given three times daily are shown in the following tables (TABLES 1 and 2).

TABLE 1

SYSTOLIC BP (mmHg)

Dose	Number of Patients	Mean Peak Response	Mean Trough Response	Trough/Peak
20 mg	50	-10.3	-4.9	48%
	52	-17.6	-7.9	45%
30 mg	45	-14.5	-7.2	50%
	44	-14.6	-7.5	51%
40 mg	50	-16.3	-9.5	58%
	38	-15.9	-6.0	38%

TABLE 2

DIASTOLIC BP (mmHg)

Dose	Number of Patients	Mean Peak Response	Mean Trough Response	Trough/Peak
20 mg	50	-10.6	-4.6	43%
	52	- 9.0	-2.9	32%
30 mg	45	-12.8	-4.9	38%
	44	-14.2	-4.3	30%
40 mg	50	-15.4	-5.9	38%
	38	-14.8	-3.7	25%

The responses are shown as differences from the concurrent placebo control group. The large changes between peak and trough effects were not accompanied by observed side effects at peak response times. In a study using 24 hour intra-arterial blood pressure monitoring, the circadian variation in blood pressure remained unaltered, but the systolic and diastolic blood pressures were reduced throughout the whole 24 hours.

When added to beta-blocker therapy, nicardipine HCl further lowers both systolic and diastolic blood pressure.

INDICATIONS AND USAGE:

I. STABLE ANGINA

Nicardipine HCl is indicated for the management of patients with chronic stable angina (effort-associated angina). Nicardipine HCl may be used alone or in combination with beta-blockers.

II. HYPERTENSION

Nicardipine HCl is indicated for the treatment of hypertension. Nicardipine HCl may be used alone or in combination with other anti hypertensive drugs. In administering nicardipine it is important to be aware of the relatively large peak to trough differences in blood pressure effect. (See DOSAGE AND ADMINISTRATION.)

CONTRAINDICATIONS:

Nicardipine HCl is contraindicated in patients with hypersensitivity to the drug.

Because part of the effect of nicardipine HCl is secondary to reduced afterload, the drug is also contraindicated in patients with advanced aortic stenosis. Reduction of diastolic pressure in these patients may worsen rather than improve myocardial oxygen balance.

WARNINGS:

INCREASED ANGINA

About 7% of patients in short-term placebo-controlled angina trials have developed increased frequency, duration or severity of angina on starting nicardipine HCl or at the time of dosage increases, compared with 4% of patients on placebo. Comparisons with beta-blockers also show a greater frequency of increased angina, 4% vs. 1%. The mechanism of this effect has not been established (See ADVERSE REACTIONS.)

USE IN PATIENTS WITH CONGESTIVE HEART FAILURE

Although preliminary hemodynamic studies in patients with congestive heart failure have shown that nicardipine HCl reduced afterload without impairing myocardial contractility, it has a negative inotropic effect *in vitro* and in some patients. Caution should be exercised when using the drug in congestive heart failure patients, particularly in combination with a beta-blocker.

WARNINGS: *(cont'd)*

BETA-BLOCKER WITHDRAWAL

Nicardipine HCl is not a beta blocker and therefore gives no protection against the dangers of abrupt beta-blocker withdrawal; any such withdrawal should be by gradual reduction of the dose of beta-blocker, preferably over 8-10 days.

PRECAUTIONS:

GENERAL

Blood Pressure: Because nicardipine HCl decreases peripheral resistance, careful monitoring of blood pressure during the initial administration and titration of nicardipine HCl is suggested. Nicardipine HCl, like other calcium channel blockers, may occasionally produce symptomatic hypotension. Caution is advised to avoid systemic hypotension when administering the drug to patients who have sustained an acute cerebral infarction or hemorrhage. Because of prominent effects at the time of peak blood levels, initial titration should be performed with measurements of blood pressure at peak effect (1-2 hours after dosing) and just before the next dose.

Use in patients with impaired hepatic function: Since the liver is the major site of biotransformation and since nicardipine HCl is subject to first pass metabolism, the drug should be used with caution in patients having impaired liver function or reduced hepatic blood flow. Patients with severe liver disease developed elevated blood levels (4-fold increase in AUC) and prolonged half-life (19 hours) of nicardipine HCl. (See DOSAGE AND ADMINISTRATION.)

Use in patients with impaired renal function: When nicardipine HCl 20 mg or 30 mg tid was given to hypertensive patients with mild renal impairment, mean plasma concentrations, AUC, and Cmax were approximately 2-fold higher in renally impaired patients than in healthy controls. Doses in these patients must be adjusted. (See CLINICAL PHARMACOLOGY and DOSAGE AND ADMINISTRATION).

CARCINOGENESIS, MUTAGENESIS, AND IMPAIRMENT OF FERTILITY

Rats treated with nicardipine in the diet (at concentrations calculated to provide daily dosage levels of 5, 15 or 45 mg/kg/day) for two years showed a dose-dependent increase in thyroid hyperplasia and neoplasia (follicular adenoma/carcinoma). One and three month studies in the rat have suggested that these results are linked to a nicardipine-induced reduction in plasma thyroxine (T4) levels with a consequent increase in plasma levels of thyroid stimulating hormone (TSH). Chronic elevation of TSH is known to cause hyperstimulation of the thyroid. in rats on an iodine deficient diet, nicardipine administration for one month was associated with thyroid hyperplasia that was prevented by T4 supplementation. Mice treated with nicardipine in the diet (at concentrations calculated to provide daily dosage levels of up to 100 mg/kg/day) for up to 18 months showed no evidence of neoplasia of any tissue and no evidence of thyroid changes. There was no evidence of thyroid pathology in dogs treated with up to 25 mg nicardipine/kg/day for one year and no evidence of effects of nicardipine on thyroid function (plasma T4 and TSH) in man.

There was no evidence of a mutagenic potential of nicardipine in a battery of genotoxicity in tests conducted on microbial indicator organisms, in micronucleus tests in mice and hamsters, or in a sister chromatid exchange study in hamsters.

No impairment of fertility was seen in male or female rats administered nicardipine at oral doses as high as 100 mg/kg/day (50 times the 40 mg tid maximum recommended antianginal or antihypertensive dose in man, assuming a patient weight of 60 kg).

PREGNANCY CATEGORY C

Nicardipine was embryocidal when administered orally to pregnant Japanese White rabbits, during organogenesis, at 150 mg/kg/day (a dose associated with marked body weight gain suppression in the treated doe) but not at 50 mg/kg/day (25 times the maximum recommended antianginal or antihypertensive dose in man). No adverse effects on the fetus were observed when New Zealand albino rabbits were treated, during organogenesis, with up to 100 mg nicardipine/kg/day (a dose associated with significant mortality in the treated doe). In pregnant rats administered nicardipine orally at up to 100 mg/kg/day (50 times the maximum recommended human dose) there was no evidence of embryolethality or teratogenicity. However, dystocia, reduced birth weights, reduced neonatal survival and reduced neonatal weight gain were noted. There are no adequate and well-controlled studies in pregnant women. Nicardipine HCl should be used during pregnancy only if the potential benefit justifies the potential risk to the fetus.

NURSING MOTHERS

Studies in rats have shown significant concentrations of nicardipine HCl in maternal milk following oral administration. For this reason it is recommended that women who wish to breast-feed should not take this drug.

PEDIATRIC USE

Safety and efficacy in patients under the age of 18 have not been established.

GERIATRIC USE

Pharmacokinetic parameters did not differ between elderly hypertensive patients (≥65 years) and healthy controls after one week of nicardipine HCl treatment at 20 mg tid. Plasma nicardipine HCl concentrations in elderly hypertensive patients were similar to plasma concentrations in healthy young adult subjects when nicardipine HCl was administered at doses of 10, 200 and 30 mg tid, suggesting that the pharmacokinetics of nicardipine HCl are similar in young and elderly hypertensive patients. No significant differences in responses to nicardipine HCl have been observed in elderly patients and the general adult population of patients who participated in clinical studies.

DRUG INTERACTIONS:

BETA-BLOCKERS

In controlled clinical studies, adrenergic beta-receptor blockers have been frequently administered concomitantly with nicardipine HCl. The combination is well tolerated.

CIMETIDINE

Cimetidine increases nicardipine HCl plasma levels. Patients receiving the two drugs concomitantly should be carefully monitored.

DIGOXIN

Some calcium blockers may increase the concentration of digitalis preparations in the blood. Nicardipine HCl usually does not alter the plasma levels of digoxin, however, serum digoxin levels should be evaluated after concomitant therapy with nicardipine HCl is initiated.

MAALOX

Co-administration of Maalox TC had no effect on nicardipine HCl absorption.

FENTANYL ANESTHESIA

Severe hypotension has been reported during fentanyl anesthesia with concomitant use of a beta-blocker and a calcium channel blocker. Even though such interactions were not seen during clinical studies with nicardipine HCl, an increased volume of circulating fluids might be required if such an interaction were to occur.

CYCLOSPORINE

Concomitant administration of nicardipine and cyclosporine levels. Plasma concentrations of cyclosporine should therefore be closely monitored, and its dosage reduced accordingly, in patients treated with nicardipine.

DRUG INTERACTIONS: *(cont'd)*

When therapeutic concentrations of *furosemide, propranolol, dipyridamole, warfarin, quinidine,* or *naproxen* were added to human plasma *(in vitro)*, the plasma protein binding of nicardipine HCl was not altered.

ADVERSE REACTIONS:

In multiple-dose U.S. and foreign controlled short-term (up to three months) studies 1910 patients received nicardipine HCl alone or in combination with other drugs. in these studies adverse events were reported spontaneously; adverse experiences were generally not serious but occasionally required dosage adjustment and about 10% of patients left the studies prematurely because of them. Peak responses were not observed to be associated with adverse effects during clinical trials, but physicians should be aware that adverse effects associated with decreases in blood pressure (tachycardia, hypotension, etc.) could occur around the time of the peak effect. Most adverse effects were expected consequences of the vasodilator effects of nicardipine HCl.

ANGINA

The incidence rates of adverse effects in anginal patients were derived from multicenter, controlled clinical trials. Following are the rates of adverse effects for nicardipine HCl (N=520) and placebo (N=310), respectively, that occurred in 0.4% of patients or more. These represent events considered probably drug-related by the investigator (except for certain cardiovascular events which were recorded in a different category). Where the frequency of adverse effects for nicardipine HCl and placebo is similar, causal relationship is uncertain. The only dose-related effects were pedal edema and increased angina.

TABLE 3 Nicardipine Hydrochloride, Adverse Reactions (Incidence of discontinuations shown in parentheses)

Adverse Experience	Cardene (N=520)	Placebo (N=310)
Pedal Edema	7.1 (0)	0.3 (0)
Dizziness	6.9 (1.2)	0.6 (0)
Headache	6.4 (0.6)	2.6 (0)
Asthenia	5.8 (0.4)	2.6 (0)
Flushing	5.6 (3.5)	1.0 (0)
Increased Angina	5.6 (3.5)	4.2 (1.9)
Palpitations	3.3 (0.4)	0.0 (0)
Nausea	1.9 (0)	0.3 (0)
Dyspepsia	1.5 (0.6)	0.6 (0.3)
Dry Mouth	1.4 (0)	0.3 (0)
Somnolence	1.4 (0)	1.0 (0)
Rash	1.2 (0.2)	0.3 (0)
Tachycardia	1.2 (0.2)	0.6 (0)
Myalgia	1.0 (0)	0.0 (0)
Other Edema	1.0 (0)	0.0 (0)
Paresthesia	1.0 (0.2)	0.3 (0)
Sustained Tachycardia	0.8 (0.6)	0.0 (0)
Syncope	0.8 (0.2)	0.0 (0)
Constipation	0.6 (0.2)	0.6 (0)
Dyspnea	0.6 (0)	0.0 (0)
Abnormal ECG	0.6 (0.6)	0.0 (0)
Malaise	0.6 (0)	0.0 (0)
Nervousness	0.6 (0)	0.3 (0)
Tremor	0.6 (0)	0.0 (0)

In addition, adverse events were observed which are not readily distinguishable from the natural history of the atherosclerotic vascular disease in these patients. Adverse events in this category each occurred in <0.4% of patients receiving nicardipine HCl and included myocardial infarction, atrial fibrillation, exertional hypotension, pericarditis, heart block, cerebral ischemia and ventricular tachycardia. it is possible that some of these events were drug-related.

HYPERTENSION

The incidence rates of adverse effects in hypertensive patients were derived from multicenter, controlled clinical trials. Following are the rates of adverse effects for nicardipine HCl (N=1390) and placebo (N=211), respectively, that occurred in 0.4% of patients or more. These represent events considered probably drug-related by the investigator. Where the frequency of adverse effects for nicardipine HCl and placebo is similar, causal relationship is uncertain. The only dose-related effect was pedal edema.

TABLE 4 Nicardipine Hydrochloride, Adverse Reactions (Incidence of discontinuations shown in parentheses)

Adverse Experience	Cardene (N=1390)	Placebo (N=211)
Flushing	9.7 (2.1)	2.8 (0)
Headache	8.2 (2.6)	4.7 (0)
Pedal Edema	8.0 (1.8)	0.9 (0)
Asthenia	4.2 (1.7)	0.5 (0)
Palpitations	4.1 (1.0)	0.0 (0)
Dizziness	4.0 (1.8)	0.0 (0)
Tachycardia	3.4 (1.2)	0.5 (0)
Nausea	2.2 (0.9)	0.9 (0)
Somnolence	1.1 (0.1)	0.0 (0)
Dyspepsia	0.8 (0.3)	0.5 (0)
Insomnia	0.6 (0.1)	0.0 (0)
Malaise	0.6 (0.1)	0.0 (0)
Other Edema	0.6 (0.3)	1.4 (0)
Abnormal Dreams	0.4 (0)	0.0 (0)
Dry mouth	0.4 (0.1)	0.0 (0)
Nocturia	0.4 (0)	0.0 (0)
Rash	0.4 (0.4)	0.0 (0)
Vomiting	0.4 (0.4)	0.0 (0)

RARE EVENTS

The following rare adverse events have been reported in clinical trials or the literature:

Body as a Whole: infection, allergic reaction

Cardiovascular: hypotension, postural hypotension, atypical chest pain, peripheral vascular disorder, ventricular extrasystoles, ventricular tachycardia

Digestive: sore throat, abnormal liver chemistries

Musculoskeletal: arthralgia

Nervous: hot flashes, vertigo, hyperkinesia, impotence, depression, confusion, anxiety

Respiratory: rhinitis, sinusitis

Special Senses: tinnitus, abnormal vision, blurred vision

Urogenital: increased urinary frequency

OVERDOSAGE:

Overdosage with a 600 mg single dose (15 to 30 times normal clinical dose) has been reported. Marked hypotension (blood pressure unobtainable) and bradycardia (heart rate 20 bpm in normal sinus rhythm) occurred, along with drowsiness, confusion and slurred speech. Supportive treatment with a vasopressor resulted in gradual improvement with normal vital signs approximately 9 hours post treatment.

Based on the results obtained in laboratory animals, overdosage may cause systemic hypotension, bradycardia (following initial tachycardia) and progressive atrioventricular conduction block. Reversible hepatic function abnormalities and sporadic focal hepatic necrosis were noted in some animal species receiving very large doses of nicardipine.

For treatment of overdose standard measures (for example, evacuation of gastric contents, elevation of extremities, attention to circulating fluid volume and urine output) including monitoring of cardiac and respiratory functions should be implemented. The patient should be positioned so as to avoid cerebral anoxia. Frequent blood pressure determinations are essential. Vasopressors are clinically indicated for patients exhibiting profound hypotension. Intravenous calcium gluconate may help reverse the effects of calcium entry blockade.

DOSAGE AND ADMINISTRATION:

ANGINA

The dose should be individually titrated for each patient beginning with 20 mg to 40 mg three times daily. Doses in the range of 20-40 mg three times a day have been shown to be effective. At least three days should be allowed before increasing the nicardipine HCl dose to ensure achievement of steady state plasma drug concentrations.

CONCOMITANT USE WITH OTHER ANTIHYPERTENSIVE AGENTS

1. Sublingual NTG may be taken as required to abort acute anginal attacks during nicardipine HCl therapy.

2. Prophylactic Nitrate Therapy - nicardipine HCl may be safely coadministered with short- and long-acting nitrates.

3. Beta-blockers - nicardipine HCl may be safely coadministered with beta-blockers. (See DRUG INTERACTIONS.)

HYPERTENSION

The dose of nicardipine HCl should be individually adjusted according to the blood pressure response beginning with 20 mg three times daily. The effective doses in clinical trials have ranged from 20 mg to 40 mg three times daily. The maximum blood pressure lowering effect occurs approximately 1-2 hours after dosing. **To assess the adequacy of blood pressure response, the blood pressure should be measured at trough (8 hours after dosing). Because of the prominent peak effects of nicardipine, blood pressure should be measured 1-2 hours after dosing, particularly during initiation of therapy.** (See PRECAUTIONS,**Blood Pressure**, INDICATIONS AND USAGE and CLINICAL PHARMACOLOGY, Peak/Trough Effects in Hypertension.) At least three days should be allowed before increasing the nicardipine HCl dose to ensure achievement of steady state plasma drug concentrations.

CONCOMITANT USE WITH OTHER ANTIHYPERTENSIVE AGENTS

1. Diuretics - Nicardipine HCl may be safely coadministered with thiazide diuretics.

2. Beta-blockers - Nicardipine HCl may be safely coadministered with beta-blockers (See DRUG INTERACTIONS.)

SPECIAL PATIENT POPULATIONS

Renal Insufficiency: Although there is no evidence that nicardipine HCl impairs renal function, careful dose titration beginning with 20 mg tid is advised. (See PRECAUTIONS.)

Hepatic Insufficiency: Nicardipine HCl should be administered cautiously in,patients with severely impaired hepatic function. A suggested starting dose of 20 mg twice a day is advised with individual titration based on clinical findings maintaining the twice a day schedule. (See PRECAUTIONS.)

Congestive Heart Failure: Caution is advised when titrating nicardipine HCl dosage in patients with congestive heart failure. (See WARNINGS).

Store bottles at room temperature and dispense in light resistant containers.

Store blister packages at room temperature and protect from excessive humidity and light. To protect from light, product should remain in manufacturer's package until consumed.

HOW SUPPLIED - RATED THERAPEUTICALLY EQUIVALENT:

Capsule - Oral - 20 mg

100's	$42.34	CARDENE 20, Syntex Labs	00033-2437-42
500's	$205.37	CARDENE 20, Syntex Labs	00033-2437-62

Capsule - Oral - 30 mg

100's	$67.32	CARDENE 30, Syntex Labs	00033-2438-42
500's	$326.47	CARDENE 30, Syntex Labs	00033-2438-62

HOW SUPPLIED - NOT RATED EQUIVALENT:

Capsule, Gelatin, Sustained Action - Oral - 30 mg

60's	$39.68	CARDENE SR, Roche	00004-0180-22
200's	$132.26	CARDENE SR, Syntex Labs	00033-2440-60

Capsule, Gelatin, Sustained Action - Oral - 45 mg

60's	$63.02	CARDENE SR, Roche	00004-0181-22
200's	$210.07	CARDENE SR, Roche	00004-0181-91

Capsule, Gelatin, Sustained Action - Oral - 60 mg

60's	$75.47	CARDENE SR, Roche	00004-0182-22
200's	$251.57	CARDENE SR, Syntex Labs	00033-2442-60

Injection, Solution - Intravenous - 25 mg/ampul

10's	$216.36	CARDENE I.V., Wyeth Labs	00008-0812-02

NICOTINE *(003109)*

CATEGORIES: Autonomic Drugs; Central Nervous System Agents; Smoking Cessation; Ulcerative Colitis*; Pregnancy Category D; FDA Class 1C ("Little or No Therapeutic Advantage"); Sales > $100 Million; FDA Approved 1991 Nov
* Indication not approved by the FDA

BRAND NAMES: *Exodus*; Habitrol; *Nicabate*; *Nicabate TTS*; **Nicoderm**; *Nicolan*; *Nicolan Light*; *Nicopatch* (France); *Nicorest* (France); *Nicorette* (Australia, Europe, Canada, Mexico); *Nicostop*; *Nicotinell* (England, Germany, France); *Nicotinell TTS* (Mexico); *Nicotrans*; Nicotrol; *Nikofrenon* (Germany); Prostep; *Stubit*
(International brand names outside U.S. in italics)

FORMULARIES: BC-BS

COST OF THERAPY: $330.50 (Smoking Cessation; Film; 14 mg/24 hr; 1/day; 90 days)

DESCRIPTION:

Nicotine transdermal systems provide systemic delivery of nicotine for 24 hours following its application to intact skin.

Nicotine is a tertiary amine composed of a pyridine and a pyrrolidine ring. It is a colorless to pale yellow, freely water-soluble, strongly alkaline, oily, volatile, hygroscopic liquid obtained from the tobacco plant. Nicotine has a characteristic pungent odor and turns brown on exposure to air or light. Of its two stereoisomers, S(-)-nicotine is the more active and is the more prevalent form in tobacco. The free alkaloid is absorbed rapidly through the skin and respiratory tract.

The Nicoderm system is a multilayered rectangular film containing nicotine as the active agent. For the three doses the composition per unit area is identical. Proceeding from the visible surface toward the surface attached to the skin are (1) an occlusive backing (polyethylene/aluminum/polyester/ethylene-vinyl acetate copolymer); (2) a drug reservoir containing nicotine (in an ethylene-vinyl acetate copolymer matrix); (3) a rate-controlling membrane (polyethylene); (4) a polyisobutylene adhesive; and (5) a protective liner that covers the adhesive layer and must be removed before application to the skin.

Habitrol systems are round, flat, 0.6-mm-thick, multi-layer units containing nicotine as the active agent. Proceeding from the visible surface toward the surface attached to the skin are: (1) a tan-colored aluminized backing film; (2) a pressure sensitive acrylate adhesive; (3) a layer containing a methacrylic acid copolymer solution of nicotine dispersed in a pad of non-woven viscose and cotton; (4) an adhesive layer similar in composition to (2) above; (5) a protective aluminized release liner with overlays the adhesive layer and must be removed prior to use.

The Nicotrol systems are a multilayered, rectangular, thin film laminated units containing nicotine as the active agent. For the treatment and the weaning doses the composition per unit area is identical.

Proceeding from the visible surface toward the surface attached to the skin, there are 3 distinct layers:

1) an outer backing layer composed of a laminated polyester film; 2) a middle layer containing rate - controlling adhesive, a structural nonwoven material and nicotine, and; 3) a disposable liner that protects the system and must be removed prior to use.

Nicotine is the active ingredient; other components of the system are pharmacologically inactive.

NICODERM

The rate of delivery of nicotine to the patient from each system (40 mcg/cm^2-h) is proportional to the surface area. About 73% of the total amount of nicotine remains in the system 24 hours after application. Nicotine transdermal systems are labeled by the dose actually absorbed by the patient. The dose of nicotine absorbed from the nicotine transdermal system represents 68% of the amount released in 24 hours. The other 32% (*e.g.,* 9 mg/day for the 21 mg/day system) volatizes from the edge of the system (TABLE 1).

TABLE 1

Dose Absorbed in 24 Hours (mg/day)	System Area (cm^2)	Total Nicotine Content (mg)
21	22	114
14	15	78
7	7	36

HABITROL

The amount of nicotine delivered to the patient from each system (29 mcg/cm^2-h) is nearly proportional to the surface area. About 60% of the total amount of nicotine remains in the system 24 hours after application. Nicotrol systems are labeled as to the dose actually absorbed by the patient. The dose of nicotine absorbed from a nicotine transdermal system represents 98% of the amount released from the system in 24 hours (TABLE 2).

TABLE 2

Dose Absorbed in 24 hours (mg/day)	System Surface Area (cm^2)	Total Nicotine Content (mg)
21	30	52.5
14	20	35.0
7	10	17.5

NICOTROL

The average amount of nicotine delivered to the patient from each system (31 mcg/cm^2/hr) is approximately proportional to the surface area. About 40% of the total amount of nicotine remains in the system 16 hours after application. Nicotrol systems are labeled with the average amount of nicotine absorbed by the patient over 16 hours. The dose of nicotine absorbed from the nicotine transdermal system represents approximately 95% of the amount released in 16 hours. The remainder of the nicotine is lost via evaporation from the edge (TABLE 3).

TABLE 3

	Dose Absorbed in 16 Hours (mg/day)	System Area (cm^2)	Total Nicotine Content (mg)
Treatment Dose	15	30	24.9
First Weaning Dose	10	20	16.6
Second Weaning Dose	5	10	8.3

CLINICAL PHARMACOLOGY:

PHARMACOLOGIC ACTION

Nicotine, the chief alkaloid in tobacco products, binds stereoselectively to acetylcholine receptors at the autonomic ganglia, in the adrenal medulla, at neuromuscular junctions, and in the brain. Two types of central nervous system effects are believed to be the basis of nicotine's positively reinforcing properties. A stimulating effect, exerted mainly in the cortex via the locus ceruleus, produces increased alertness and cognitive performance. A "reward" effect via the "pleasure system" in the brain is exerted in the limbic system. At low doses the stimulant effects predominate, while at high doses the reward effects predominate. Intermittent intravenous administration of nicotine activates neurohormonal pathways, releasing acetylcholine, norepinephrine, dopamine, serotonin, vasopressin, beta-endorphin, growth hormone, and ACTH.

PHARMACODYNAMICS

The cardiovascular effects of nicotine include peripheral vasoconstriction, tachycardia, and elevated blood pressure. Acute and chronic tolerance to nicotine develops from smoking tobacco or ingesting nicotine preparations. Acute tolerance (a reduction in response for a given dose) develops rapidly (less than 1 hour), but at distinct rates for different physiologic

CLINICAL PHARMACOLOGY: *(cont'd)*

effects (skin temperature, heart rate, subjective effects). Withdrawal symptoms, such as cigarette craving, can be reduced in some individuals by plasma nicotine levels lower than those for smoking.

Withdrawal from nicotine in addicted individuals is characterized by craving, nervousness, restlessness, irritability, mood lability, anxiety, drowsiness, sleep disturbances, impaired concentration, increased appetite, minor somatic complaints (headache, myalgia, constipation, fatigue), and weight gain. Nicotine toxicity is characterized by nausea, abdominal pain, vomiting, diarrhea, diaphoresis, flushing, dizziness, disturbed hearing and vision, confusion, weakness, palpitations, altered respiration, and hypotension.

Nicoderm

The cardiovascular effects of Nicoderm 21 mg/day used continuously for 24 hours and smoking every 30 minutes during waking hours for 5 days were compared. Both regimens elevated heart rate (about 10 beats/min) and blood pressure (about 5 mm Hg) compared with an abstinence period, and these increases were similar between treatments throughout the 24-hour period, including during sleep.

The circadian pattern and release of plasma cortisol following 5 days of treatment with Nicoderm 21 mg/day did not differ from that following 5 days of nicotine abstinence. Urinary excretion of norepinephrine, epinephrine, and dopamine was also similar for Nicoderm 21 mg/day and abstinence.

Habitrol

The cardiovascular effects of habitual 14 mg/day systems used continuously for 24 hours were compared with smoking every hour during waking hours, for 10 days. A small increase in blood pressure was detectable on the first day but not after days. Heart rate was increased by 3-7% and stroke volume decreased by 5-12% on the 10th day of application. Nicotine transdermal treatment had no significant influence on cutaneous blood flow or skin temperature.

Habitrol and Nicotrol

Both smoking and nicotine can increase circulating cortisol and catecholamines, and tolerance does not develop to the catecholamine-releasing effects of nicotine. Changes in the response to a concomitantly administered adrenergic agonist or antagonist should be watched for when nicotine intake is altered during nicotine transdermal therapy and/or smoking cessation (see DRUG INTERACTIONS.)

PHARMACOKINETICS

Nicoderm

Following application of the nicotine transdermal system to the upper body or upper outer arm, approximately 68% of the nicotine released from the system enters the systemic circulation (*e.g.,* 21 mg/day for the highest dose of Nicoderm). The remainder of the nicotine released from the system is lost via evaporation from the edge. All nicotine transdermal systems are labeled by the actual amount of nicotine absorbed by the patient.

The volume of distribution following IV administration of nicotine is approximately 2 to 3 L/kg, and the half-life of nicotine ranges from 1 to 2 hours. The major eliminating organ is the liver, and average plasma clearance is about 1.2 L/min; the kidney and lung also metabolize nicotine. There is no significant skin metabolism of nicotine. More than 20 metabolites of nicotine have been identified, all of which are believed to be less active than the parent compound. The primary metabolite of nicotine in plasma, cotinine, has a half-life of 15 to 20 hours and concentrations that exceed nicotine by 10-fold.

Plasma protein binding of nicotine is $< 5\%$. Therefore, changes in nicotine binding from use of concomitant drugs or alterations of plasma proteins by disease states would not be expected to have significant consequences.

The primary urinary metabolites are cotinine (15% of the dose) and trans-3-hydroxycotinine (45% of the dose). About 10% of nicotine is excreted unchanged in the urine. As much as 30% may be excreted in the urine with high urine flow rates and urine acidification below pH 5.

After nicotine transdermal application, plasma concentrations rise rapidly, plateau within 2 to 4 hours, and then slowly decline until the system is removed; after which they decline more rapidly.

The pharmacokinetic model that best fits the plasma nicotine concentrations from nicotine transdermal systems is an open, two-compartment disposition model with a skin depot through which nicotine enters the central circulation compartment. Nicotine in the adhesive layer is absorbed into and then through the skin, causing the initial rapid rise in plasma concentrations. The nicotine from the reservoir is released slowly through the membrane with a release rate constant approximately 20 times smaller than the skin absorption rate constant, as demonstrated *in vitro* in cadaver skin flux studies and verified by pharmacokinetic trials. Therefore, the slow decline of plasma nicotine concentrations during 4 to 24 hours is determined primarily by the release of nicotine from the system‡.

Following the second daily nicotine transdermal system application, steady-state plasma nicotine concentrations are achieved and are on average 30% higher compared with single-dose applications. Plasma nicotine concentrations are proportional to dose (*i.e.,* linear kinetics are observed) for the three dosages of nicotine transdermal systems. Nicotine kinetics are similar for all sites of application on the upper body and upper outer arm. Plasma nicotine concentrations from Nicoderm 21 mg/day are the same as those from simultaneous use of Nicoderm 14 mg/day and 7 mg/day.

Following removal of the nicotine transdermal system, plasma nicotine concentrations decline in an exponential fashion with an apparent mean half-life of 3 to 4 hours‡ compared with 1 to 2 hours for IV administration, due to continued absorption from the skin depot. Most non-smoking patients will have nondetectable nicotine concentrations in 10 to 12 hours (TABLE 4).

TABLE 4 Steady-State Nicotine Pharmacokinetic Parameters for Nicoderm Systems (Mean, SD, and Range)

	Dose Absorbed (mg/day) 21			14			7		
	Mean	SD	Range	Mean	SD	Range	Mean	SD	Range
C_{max} ng/ml	23	5	13-32	17	3	10-24	8	2	5-12
C_{avg} ng/ml	17	4	10-26	12	3	8-17	6	1	4-10
C_{min} ng/ml	11	3	6-17	7	2	4-11	4	1	3-6
T_{max} h	4	3	1-10	4	3	1-10	4	4	1-18

C_{max}:maximum observed plasma concentration
C_{avg}:average plasma concentration
C_{min}:minimum observed plasma concentration
T_{max}:time of maximum plasma concentration

Half-hourly smoking of cigarettes produces average plasma nicotine concentrations of approximately 44 ng/ml. In comparison, average plasma nicotine concentrations from Nicoderm 21 mg/day are about 17 ng/ml.

CLINICAL PHARMACOLOGY: *(cont'd)*

There are no differences in nicotine kinetics between men and women using nicotine transdermal systems. Linear regression of both AUC and C_{max}vs total body weight shows the expected inverse relationship. Obese men using nicotine transdermal systems had significantly lower AUC and C_{max} values than normal weight men. Men and women having low body weight are expected to have higher AUC and C_{max}values.

Habitrol

The volume of distribution following IV administration of nicotine is approximately 2 to 3 L/kg and the half-life ranges from 1 to 2 hours. The major eliminating organ is the liver, and average plasma clearance is about 1.2 L/min; the kidney and lung also metabolize nicotine. There is no significant skin metabolism of nicotine. More than 20 metabolites of nicotine have been identified, all of which are believed to be less active than the parent compound. The primary metabolite of nicotine in plasma, cotinine, has a half-life of 15-20 hours and concentrations that exceed nicotine by 10-fold.

Plasma protein binding of nicotine is < 5%. Therefore, changes in nicotine binding from use of concomitant drugs or alterations of plasma proteins by disease states would not be expected to have significant consequences.

The primary urinary metabolites are cotinine (15% of the dose) and trans-3-hydroxycotinine (45% of the dose). About 10% of nicotine is excreted unchanged in the urine. As much as 30% may be excreted in the urine with high urine flow rates and urine acidification below pH 5.

The pharmacokinetic model which best fits the plasma nicotine concentrations from nicotine transdermal systems is an open two-compartment disposition model with a skin depot through which nicotine enters the central circulation compartment. The nicotine from the drug matrix is released slowly from the system. Therefore, the decline of plasma nicotine concentrations during the last 12 hours is determined primarily by release of nicotine from the system through the skin.

Following an initial lag time of 1-2 hours, nicotine concentrations increase to a broad peak between 6 and 12 hours and then decrease gradually. Steady state for nicotine is attained within 2 days of initiating nicotine transdermal treatment and average plasma nicotine concentrations are, on average, 25% higher compared to single dose applications. Upon application of a new system and removal of the old system there is, in some patients, a slight and transient (30-60 min) increase in nicotine plasma concentration and its variability. Plasma nicotine concentrations are proportional to dose (i.e. linear kinetics are observed) for the three dosages of nicotine transdermal systems. Nicotine kinetics are similar for all sites of application on the back, abdomen, or side.

Following removal of nicotine transdermal systems, plasma nicotine concentrations decline in an exponential fashion with an apparent mean half-life of 3-4 hours. Most nonsmoking patients will have nondetectable nicotine concentrations in 10 to 12 hours (TABLE 5).

TABLE 5 Steady-State Nicotine Pharmacokinetic Parameters for Habitrol Systems (mean, standard deviation, range)

Parameter (Units)	14 mg/day (N=9) Mean	SD	Range	21 mg/day (N=9) Mean	SD	Range
C_{max} (ng/ml)	12	4	6-16	17	2	13-19
C_{avg} (ng/ml)	9	3	5-12	13	2	9-17
C_{min} (ng/ml)	6	2	3-10	9	2	7-14
T_{max} (hrs)	5	3	0-8	6	3	2-9

C_{max}: maximum observed plasma concentration5
C_{avg}: average plasma concentration
C_{min}: minimum observed plasma concentration
T_{max}: time of maximum plasma concentration

Nicotrol

Following application of the nicotine transdermal system to the upper arm or hip, approximately 95% of the nicotine released from the system enters the systemic circulation. The remainder of the nicotine released from the system is lost via evaporation from the edge. All nicotine transdermal systems are labeled by the average amount of nicotine absorbed by the average patient over 16 hours.

The volume of distribution following IV administration of nicotine is approximately 2 to 3 L/kg and the half-life ranges from 1 to 2 hours. The major eliminating organ is the liver, and average plasma clearance is about 1.2 L/min; the kidney and lung also metabolize nicotine. There is no significant skin metabolism of nicotine. More than 20 metabolites of nicotine have been identified, all of which are believed to be less active than the parent compound. The primary metabolite of nicotine in plasma, cotinine, has a half-life of 15 to 20 hours and concentrations that exceed nicotine by 10-fold.

Plasma protein binding of nicotine is < 5%. Therefore, changes in nicotine binding from use of concomitant drugs or alterations of plasma proteins by disease states would not be expected to have significant effects on nicotine kinetics.

The primary urinary metabolites are cotinine (15% of the dose) and trans-3-hydroxycotinine (45% of the dose). Usually about 10% of nicotine is excreted unchanged in the urine. As much as 30% may be excreted unchanged in the urine with high urine flow rates and acidification below pH 5.

Plasma levels of nicotine obtained with nicotine transdermal systems rise after application, reaching a maximum level after approximately 5-10 hours. The mean peak plasma level of nicotine achieved with the 15 mg/day system is approximately 9-15 ng/ml.

After repeated application nicotine concentrations are not significantly higher than those after a single application. Plasma nicotine concentrations show a slight deviation from dose proportionality for the three nicotine transdermal doses; with increasing system size the increase in concentration is somewhat less than expected. Nicotine kinetics are similar for application on the arm and hip.

Following removal of the nicotine transdermal system after 16 hours of wear, plasma nicotine concentrations decline in an apparently exponential fashion. The half-life after removal was about twice that observed after intravenous infusion, suggesting continued absorption from the skin depot. Patients had nondeductible nicotine concentrations within 10 to 12 hours after removing the system (TABLE 6).

If the 15 mg/day Nicotrol system is left on for 24 hours, as opposed to 16 hours, plasma levels of nicotine decline from a mean of 7.2 to 5.6 ng/ml over the last 8 hours. The smaller systems may be expected to follow a similar pattern at proportionally lower plasma levels.

There are no differences in nicotine kinetics between men and women using nicotine transdermal systems. Linear regression of both AUC and C_{max} vs. total body weight shows the expected inverse relationship. Men and women having low body weight are expected to have higher AUC and C_{max} values.

CLINICAL STUDIES:

NICODERM

The efficacy of nicotine transdermal systems as an aid to smoking cessation was demonstrated in two placebo-controlled, double-blind trials of otherwise healthy patients (n=756) smoking at least one pack of cigarettes per day. The trials consisted of 6 weeks of active

CLINICAL STUDIES: *(cont'd)*

TABLE 6 Steady State Nicotine Pharmacokinetic Parameters for Nicotrol Systems Applied for 16 Hours (Mean ± SD (Range), N = 12)

	Delivery Rate (mg/day) 15* Mean ± SD (Range)	10 Mean ± SD (Range)	5 Mean ± SD (Range)
C_{max} (ng/ml)	13.0 ± 3.1 (7.8 - 17.9)	6.9 ± 2.0 (4.8 - 10.0)	3.5 ± 0.7 (2.7 - 4.7)
C_{avg} 16 (ng/ml)	9.4 ± 2.4 (5.3 - 13.3)	4.9 ± 1.2 (3.0 - 6.8)	2.7 ± 0.5 (2.0 - 3.6)
C_{avg} 24 (ng/ml)	8.7 ± 2.1 (5.2 - 11.8)	4.8 ± 1.0 (3.3 - 6.3)	2.7 ± 0.4 (2.1 - 3.3)
C_{min} (ng/ml)	2.5 ± 0.8 (1.2 - 4.1)	1.4 ± 0.5 (0.5 - 2.4)	0.8 ± 0.3 (0.3 - 1.2)
T_{max} (hrs)	8 ± 3 (4 - 16)	9 ± 4 (6 - 16)	9 ± 4 (3 - 16)

* Data for 15 mg/day system are derived from a different study than the 5 and 10 mg/day systems.
C_{max}: maximum observed plasma concentration
C_{avg}24: average plasma concentration calculated over 24 hrs.
C_{avg}16 : estimated average plasma concentration during the 0 to 16 hour period, calculated as AUC (0-16)/16
C_{min}: minimum observed plasma concentration
T_{max}: time of maximum plasm concentration

-treatment, 6 weeks of weaning off nicotine transdermal systems, and 12 weeks of follow-up on no medication. Quitting was defined as total abstinence from smoking (as determined by patient diary and verified by expired carbon monoxide). The "quit rates" are the proportion of patients enrolled who abstained after week 2.

The two trials in otherwise healthy smokers showed that all nicotine transdermal doses were more effective than placebo, and that treatment with Nicoderm 21 mg/day for 6 weeks provided significantly higher quit rates than the 14 mg/day and placebo treatments at 6 weeks. Data from these two studies are combined in the Quit Rate table. Quit rates were still significantly different after an additional 6-week weaning period and at follow-up 3 months later. All patients were given weekly behavioral supportive care. As shown in the following table, the quit rates on each treatment varied 2- to 3-fold among clinics at 6 weeks (TABLE 7).

TABLE 7 Quit Rates After Week 2 According to Starting Dose (N-756 smokers in 9 clinics)

Nicoderm Delivery Rate (mg/day)	Number of Patients	After 6 weeks Range*	After Weaning Range*	At 6 Months Range*
21	249	32-92%	18-63%	3-50%
14	254	30-61%	15-52%	0-48%
Placebo	253	15-46%	0-38%	0-35%

* Range for 9 centers, number of patients per treatment ranged from 23-34

In a study of smokers with coronary artery disease, 77 patients treated with nicotine transdermal systems (75% on 14 mg/day and 25% on 21 mg/day) had higher quit rates than 78 placebo-treated patients at the end of the 8-week study period (5 weeks of active treatment and 3 weeks of weaning). Nicotine transdermal systems did not affect angina frequency or the appearance of arrhythmias on Holter monitoring in these patients. Symptoms presumed related to nicotine withdrawal and the stress of smoking cessation caused more patients to terminate the study than symptoms thought to be related to nicotine substitution. Seven patients on placebo and one on Nicoderm 14 mg/day dropped out for symptoms probably related to nicotine withdrawal (7 of these 8 patients experienced cardiovascular symptoms), while only two patients dropped out for nicotine-related symptoms (one patient with severe nausea on Nicoderm 14 mg/day and one with nausea and palpitations on Nicoderm 21 mg/day).

Patients who used nicotine transdermal systems in clinical trials had a significant reduction in craving for cigarettes, a major nicotine withdrawal symptom, compared with placebo-treated patients‡. Reduction in craving, as with quit rate, is quite variable. This variability is presumed to be due to inherent differences in patient populations (*e.g.,* patient motivation, concomitant illnesses, number of cigarettes smoked per day, number of years smoking, exposure to other smokers, socioeconomic status) as well as differences among the clinics.

Patients using nicotine transdermal systems dropped out of the trials less frequently than patients receiving placebo. Quit rates for the 56 patients over age 60 were comparable to the quit rates for the 821 patients aged 60 and under.

HABITROL

The efficacy of nicotine transdermal treatment as an aid to smoking cessation was demonstrated in three placebo-controlled, double-blind trials in otherwise healthy patients smoking at least one pack per day (N = 792). In two of the trials nicotine transdermal therapy was combined with concomitant support and in one trial nicotine transdermal was used without concomitant support. In all three trials, patients were treated for 7 weeks (3 weeks of titration and 4 weeks of maintenance) followed by 3 weeks of weaning. Quitting was defined as total abstinence from smoking as measured by patient diary and verified by expired carbon monoxide. The "quit rates" are the proportions of all persons initially enrolled who abstained after week 3.

The two trials in otherwise healthy smokers with concomitant support showed that nicotine transdermal therapy was more effective than placebo after 7 weeks. Quit rates were still significantly different after the additional 3-weeks weaning period. The quit rates varied approximately 2-fold among clinics for each treatment when nicotine transdermal therapy was used with a concomitant support program. Data from these two studies (N=516) are combined in the Quit Rate table. Greater variability and decreased quit rates were demonstrated in both placebo and nicotine transdermal treatment groups when concomitant support was not employed (N=276, see TABLE 8)

TABLE 8 Quit Rates After Weeks 3 by Treatment

Concomitant Support	Treatment	Number of patients	After 7 Weeks (range)	After Weaning (range)
Yes†	Habitrol	260	19-54%	8-43%
	Placebo*	256	9-30%	8-30%
No‡	Habitrol	141	4-28%	4-20%
	Placebo*	135	0-24%	0-22%

* Sub Therapeutic (ST) Placebo systems contained 13% of the nicotine found in the respective-sized active system to allow blinding as to color and odor.
† Two trials with 9 clinics, number of patients per treatment ranged from 22 to 39.
‡ One trial with 5 clinics, number of patients per treatment ranged from 24 to 40.

CLINICAL STUDIES: *(cont'd)*

Patients who used nicotine transdermal treatment in clinical trials had a significant reduction in craving for cigarettes, a major nicotine withdrawal symptom, as compared to placebo-treated patients. Reduction in craving, as with quit rate, is quite variable. This variability is presumed to be due to inherent differences in patient populations, e.g. patient motivation, concomitant illnesses, number of cigarettes smoked per day, number of years smoking, exposure to other smokers, socioeconomic status, etc., as well as differences among the clinics.

Patients using nicotine transdermal systems dropped out of the trials less frequently than did patients receiving placebo. Quit rates for the 32 patients over age 60 were comparable to the quit rates for the 369 patients aged 60 and under.

NICOTROL

The efficacy of nicotine transdermal therapy as an aid to smoking cessation was demonstrated in two single-center, placebo-controlled, double-blind trials in smokers, smoking ≥ 10 cigarettes per day (N = 509), who were healthy or had diseases in their past medical history such as chronic obstructive pulmonary disease, hypertension, or myocardial infarction.

In both clinics nicotine transdermal systems were applied on awakening and removed at bedtime each day. They were used with only limited behavioral support. Patients in both clinics were treated for 12 weeks followed by a 4 to 6 week weaning period. The subjects were followed for 12 months. Quitting was defined as total abstinence from smoking. The "quit rates" are the proportion of all persons initially enrolled who abstained after week 2.

In both clinics nicotine transdermal therapy was more effective than placebo at 6 weeks, 6 months, and 1 year. Data from both are reported in the quit rate table (TABLE 9).

TABLE 9 Quit Rates by Treatment (N = 509 smokers in 2 clinics)*

Treatment Group	Number of Patients	At 6 Weeks	At 6 Months	At 1 year
Nicotrol	258	35-61%	19-35%	12-25%
Placebo	251	7-35%	3-12%	3-9%

* Trials involved 2 clinics; the number of patients per treatment ranged from 107 to 145.

Patients who used nicotine transdermal systems had a significant reduction in craving for cigarettes, a major nicotine withdrawal symptom, compared with placebo-treated patients†. The effect on symptoms, as with quit rate, is quite variable and is presumed to be due to inherent differences in patient populations, e.g. patient motivation, concomitant illness, number of cigarettes smoked per day, number of years smoking, exposure to other smokers, socioeconomic status, etc., as well as differences between the clinics themselves (one Danish, one U.S.).

*Systems worn during waking hours.

Patients using nicotine transdermal systems withdrew from the trials less frequently than did patients receiving placebo. Quit rates for the 79 patients over age 60 were comparable to the quit rates for the 430 patients aged 60 and under.

INDIVIDUALIZATION OF DOSAGE

It is important to make sure that patients read the instructions made available to them and have their questions answered. They should clearly understand the directions for applying and disposing of nicotine transdermal systems. They should be instructed to stop smoking completely when the first system is applied.

The success or failure of smoking cessation depends heavily on the quality, intensity, and frequency of supportive care. Patients are more likely to quit smoking if they are seen frequently and participate in formal smoking cessation programs.

The goal of nicotine transdermal system therapy is complete abstinence. Significant health benefits have not been demonstrated for reduction of smoking. If a patient is unable to stop smoking by the fourth week of therapy, treatment should probably be discontinued. Patients who have not stopped smoking after 4 weeks of nicotine transdermal system therapy are unlikely to quit on that attempt.

Patients who fail to quit on any attempt may benefit from interventions to improve their chances for success on subsequent attempts. These patients should be counselled to determine why they failed and then probably be given a "therapy holiday" before the next attempt. A new quit attempt should be encouraged when the factors that contributed to failure can be eliminated or reduced, and conditions are more favorable.

Based on the clinical trials, a reasonable approach to assisting patients in their attempt to quit smoking is to assign their initial nicotine transdermal system treatment using the recommended dosing schedule (see TABLE 10.) The need for dose adjustment should be assessed during the first 2 weeks. Patients should continue the dose selected with counselling and support over the following month. Those who have successfully stopped smoking during that time should be supported during 4 to 8 weeks of weaning, after which treatment should be terminated.

The symptoms of nicotine withdrawal and excess overlap see ADVERSE REACTIONS and CLINICAL PHARMACOLOGY, Pharmacodynamics. Since patients using nicotine transdermal systems may also smoke intermittently, it may be difficult to determine if patients are experiencing nicotine withdrawal or nicotine excess.

The controlled clinical trials using nicotine transdermal system therapy suggest that abnormal dreams and insomnia are more often symptoms of nicotine excess, while anxiety, somnolence, and depression are more often symptoms of nicotine withdrawal.

Nicoderm and Habitrol

Therapy generally should begin with the Nicoderm 21 mg/day TABLE 10 except if the patient is small (less than 100 pounds), is a light smoker (less than 1/2 pack of cigarettes per day), or has cardiovascular disease (TABLE 10).

TABLE 10

	Dosing Schedule Otherwise Healthy Patients	Other* Patients
Initial/Starting Dose	21 mg/day	14 mg/day
Duration of Treatment	4-8 weeks	4-8 weeks
First Weaning Dose	14 mg/day	7 mg/day
Duration of Treatment	2-4 weeks	2-4 weeks
Second Weaning Dose	7 mg/day	
Duration of Treatment	2-4 weeks	

* Small patient (less than 100 pounds) or light smoker (less than 10 cigarettes/day) or patient with cardiovascular disease

Nicotrol

Therapy should begin with the Nicotrol 15 mg/day dose TABLE 10. If the patient has signs or symptoms suggesting nicotine excess, the 10 mg/day system may be tried (TABLE 11).

TABLE 11 Dosing Schedule

Initial/Starting Dose	15 mg/day
Duration of Treatment	4-12 weeks
First Weaning Dose	10 mg/day
Duration of Treatment	2-4 weeks
Second Weaning Dose	5 mg/day
Duration of Treatment	2-4 weeks

INDICATIONS AND USAGE:

Nicotine transdermal system treatment is indicated as an aid to smoking cessation for the relief of nicotine withdrawal symptoms. Nicotine transdermal system treatment should be used as part of a comprehensive behavioral smoking-cessation program.

The use of Nicoderm and Habitrol systems for longer than 3 months (Nicotrol, 5 months) has not been studied.

CONTRAINDICATIONS:

Use of nicotine transdermal systems is contraindicated in patients with hypersensitivity or allergy to nicotine or to any of the components of the therapeutic system.

WARNINGS:

Nicotine from any source can be toxic and addictive. Smoking causes lung cancer, heart disease, and emphysema and may adversely affect the fetus and the pregnant woman. For any smoker, with or without concomitant disease or pregnancy, the risk of nicotine replacement in a smoking-cessation program should be weighed against the hazard of continued smoking while using nicotine transdermal systems and the likelihood of achieving cessation of smoking without nicotine replacement.

PREGNANCY WARNING

Tobacco smoke, which has been shown to be harmful to the fetus, contains nicotine, hydrogen cyanide, and carbon monoxide. Nicotine has been shown in animal studies to cause fetal harm. It is therefore presumed that nicotine transdermal systems can cause fetal harm when administered to a pregnant woman. The effect of nicotine delivery by nicotine transdermal systems has not been examined in pregnancy (see PRECAUTIONS.)

Therefore pregnant smokers should be encouraged to attempt cessation using educational and behavioral interventions before using pharmacological approaches. If nicotine transdermal systems are used during pregnancy, or if the patient becomes pregnant while using nicotine transdermal systems, the patient should be apprised of the potential hazard to the fetus.

SAFETY NOTE CONCERNING CHILDREN

The amounts of nicotine that are tolerated by adult smokers can produce symptoms of poisoning and could prove fatal if the nicotine transdermal system is applied or ingested by children or pets. Used Nicoderm 21 mg/day systems contain about 73% (83 mg) of their initial drug content (used Habitrol 21 mg/day systems: 60% (32 mg) of initial drug content; used Nicotrol 15 mg/day systems: 40% (10 mg) of initial drug content. Therefore, patients should be cautioned to keep both the used and unused nicotine transdermal systems out of the reach of children and pets.

PRECAUTIONS:

The patient should be urged to stop smoking completely when initiating nicotine transdermal therapy (see DOSAGE AND ADMINISTRATION.) Patients should be informed that if they continue to smoke while using nicotine transdermal systems, they may experience adverse effects due to peak nicotine levels higher than those experienced from smoking alone. If there is a clinically significant increase in cardiovascular or other effects attributable to nicotine, the nicotine transdermal system dose should be reduced or nicotine transdermal system treatment discontinued (see WARNINGS.) Physicians should anticipate that concomitant medications may need dosage adjustment, see DRUG INTERACTIONS.

The use of nicotine transdermal systems beyond 3 months by patients who stop smoking should be discouraged, because the chronic consumption of nicotine by any route can be harmful and addicting.

ALLERGIC REACTIONS

In a 6-week, open-label, dermal irritation and sensitization study of nicotine transdermal systems, 7 of 230 patients exhibited definite erythema at 24 hours after application. Upon rechallenge, 4 patients exhibited mild to moderate contact allergy. Patients with contact sensitization should be cautioned that a serious reaction could occur from exposure to other nicotine-containing products or smoking. In the efficacy trials, erythema following system removal was typically seen in about 14% of patients, some edema in 3%, and dropouts due to skin reactions occurred in 2% of patients.

Patients should be instructed to promptly discontinue the use of nicotine transdermal systems and contact their physicians, if they experience severe or persistent local skin reactions (*e.g.,* severe erythema, pruritus, or edema) at the site of application or a generalized skin reaction (*e.g.,* urticaria, hives, or generalized rash).

Patients using nicotine transdermal therapy concurrently with other transdermal products may exhibit local reactions at both application sites. Reactions were seen in 2 of 7 patients using concomitant Estraderm (estradiol transdermal system) in clinical trials. In such patients, use of one or both systems may have to be discontinued.

SKIN DISEASE

Nicotine transdermal systems are usually well tolerated by patients with normal skin, but may be irritating for patients with some skin disorders (atopic or eczematous dermatitis).

CARDIOVASCULAR OR PERIPHERAL VASCULAR DISEASES

The risks of nicotine replacement in patients with certain cardiovascular and peripheral vascular diseases should be weighed against the benefits of including nicotine replacement in a smoking-cessation program for them. Specifically, patients with coronary heart disease (history of myocardial infarction and/or angina pectoris), serious cardiac arrhythmias, or vasospastic diseases (Buerger's disease, Prinzmetal's variant angina) should be carefully screened and evaluated before nicotine replacement is prescribed.

Tachycardia occurring in association with the use of nicotine transdermal therapy was reported occasionally. If serious cardiovascular symptoms occur with the use of nicotine transdermal therapy, it should be discontinued.

Nicotine transdermal therapy was as well tolerated as placebo in a controlled trial in patients with coronary artery disease (see CLINICAL STUDIES.) One patient on Nicoderm 21 mg/day, two on Nicoderm 14 mg/day, and eight on placebo discontinued treatment due to adverse events.

Nicotine transdermal therapy did not affect angina frequency or the appearance of arrhythmias on Holter monitoring in these patients.

Nicotine transdermal therapy generally should not be used in patients during the immediate post-myocardial infarction period, patients with serious arrhythmias, and patients with severe or worsening angina pectoris.

PRECAUTIONS: *(cont'd)*

RENAL OR HEPATIC INSUFFICIENCY

The pharmacokinetics of nicotine have not been studied in the elderly or in patients with renal or hepatic impairment. However, given that nicotine is extensively metabolized and that its total system clearance is dependent on liver blood flow, some influence of hepatic impairment on drug kinetics (reduced clearance) should be anticipated. Only severe renal impairment would be expected to affect the clearance of nicotine or its metabolites from the circulation CLINICAL PHARMACOLOGY, Pharmacokinetics.

ENDOCRINE DISEASES

Nicotine transdermal therapy should be used with caution in patients with hyperthyroidism, pheochromocytoma, or insulin-dependent diabetes, since nicotine causes the release of catecholamines by the adrenal medulla.

PEPTIC ULCER DISEASE

Nicotine delays healing in peptic ulcer disease; therefore, nicotine transdermal therapy should be used with caution in patients with active peptic ulcers and only when the benefits of including nicotine replacement in a smoking-cessation program outweigh the risks.

ACCELERATED HYPERTENSION

Nicotine therapy constitutes a risk factor for development of malignant hypertension in patients with accelerated hypertension; therefore, nicotine transdermal therapy should be used with caution in these patients and only when the benefits of including nicotine replacement in a smoking-cessation program outweigh the risks.

INFORMATION FOR PATIENT

A patient instruction sheet is included in the package of nicotine transdermal systems dispensed to the patient. The instruction sheet contains important information and instructions on how to properly use and dispose of nicotine transdermal systems. Patients should be encouraged to ask questions of the physician and pharmacist.

Patients must be advised to keep both used and unused systems out of the reach of children and pets.

CARCINOGENESIS, MUTAGENESIS, IMPAIRMENT OF FERTILITY

Nicotine itself does not appear to be a carcinogen in laboratory animals. However, nicotine and its metabolites increased the incidences of tumors in the cheek pouches of hamsters and forestomach of F344 rats, respectively, when given in combination with tumor initiators. One study, which could not be replicated, suggested that cotinine, the primary metabolite of nicotine, may cause lymphoreticular sarcoma in the large intestine in rats.

Nicotine and cotinine were not mutagenic in the Ames *Salmonella* test. Nicotine induced repairable DNA damage in an *E. coli* test system. Nicotine was shown to be genotoxic in a test system using Chinese hamster ovary cells. In rats and rabbits, implantation can be delayed or inhibited by a reduction in DNA synthesis that appears to be caused by nicotine. Studies have shown a decrease in litter size in rats treated with nicotine during gestation.

PREGNANCY CATEGORY D

(See WARNINGS.)

The harmful effects of cigarette smoking on maternal and fetal health are clearly established. These include low birth weight, increased risk of spontaneous abortion, and increased perinatal mortality. The specific effects of nicotine transdermal therapy on fetal development are unknown. Therefore, pregnant smokers should be encouraged to attempt cessation using educational and behavioral interventions before using pharmacological approaches.

Spontaneous abortion during nicotine replacement therapy has been reported; as with smoking, nicotine as a contributing factor cannot be excluded.

Nicotine transdermal therapy should be used during pregnancy only if the likelihood of smoking cessation justifies the potential risk of use of nicotine replacement by the patient who may continue to smoke.

Teratogenicity

Animal Studies: Nicotine was shown to produce skeletal abnormalities in the offspring of mice when given doses toxic to the dams (25 mg/kg IP or SC).

Human Studies: Nicotine teratogenicity has not been studied in humans except as a component of cigarette smoke (each cigarette smoked delivers about 1 mg of nicotine). It has not been possible to conclude whether cigarette smoking is teratogenic to humans.

Other Effects

Animal Studies: A nicotine bolus (up to 2 mg/kg) to pregnant rhesus monkeys caused acidosis, hypercarbia, and hypotension (fetal and maternal concentrations were about 20 times those achieved after smoking 1 cigarette in 5 minutes). Fetal breathing movements were reduced in the fetal lamb after intravenous injection of 0.25 mg/kg nicotine to the ewe (equivalent to smoking 1 cigarette every 20 seconds for 5 minutes). Uterine blood flow was reduced about 30% after infusion of 0.1 mg/kg/min nicotine for 20 minutes to pregnant rhesus monkeys (equivalent to smoking about 6 cigarettes every minute for 20 minutes).

Human Experience: Cigarette smoking during pregnancy is associated with an increased risk of spontaneous abortion, low birth weight infants, and perinatal mortality. Nicotine and carbon monoxide are considered the most likely mediators of these outcomes. The effect of cigarette smoking on fetal cardiovascular parameters has been studied near term. Cigarettes increased fetal aortic blood flow and heart rate and decreased uterine blood flow and fetal breathing movements. Nicotine transdermal therapy has not been studied in pregnant humans.

LABOR AND DELIVERY

The nicotine transdermal system is not recommended to be left on during labor and delivery. The effects of nicotine on a mother or the fetus during labor are unknown.

NURSING MOTHERS

Caution should be exercised when nicotine transdermal therapy is administered to nursing women. The safety of nicotine transdermal therapy in nursing infants has not been examined. Nicotine passes freely into breast milk; the milk to plasma ratio averages 2.9. Nicotine is absorbed orally. An infant has the ability to clear nicotine by hepatic first-pass clearance; however, the efficiency of removal is probably lowest at birth. The nicotine concentrations in milk can be expected to be lower with nicotine transdermal therapy, when used as directed, than with cigarette smoking, as maternal plasma nicotine concentrations are generally reduced with nicotine replacement. The risk of exposure of the infant to nicotine from nicotine transdermal therapy should be weighed against the risks associated with the infant's exposure to nicotine from continued smoking by the mother (passive smoke exposure and contamination of breast milk with other components of tobacco smoke) and from nicotine transdermal therapy alone or in combination with continued smoking.

PEDIATRIC USE

Nicotine transdermal therapy is not recommended for use in children, because the safety and effectiveness of nicotine transdermal therapy in children and adolescents who smoke have not been evaluated.

GERIATRIC USE

Fifty-six patients over the age of 60 participated in clinical trials of nicotine transdermal therapy. Nicotine transdermal therapy appeared to be as effective in this age group as in younger smokers. However, asthenia, various body aches, and dizziness occurred slightly more often in patients over 60 years of age.

DRUG INTERACTIONS:

Smoking cessation, with or without nicotine replacement, may alter the pharmacokinetics of certain concomitant medications.

TABLE 12

May Require a *Decrease* in Dose at Cessation of Smoking	Possible Mechanism
acetaminophen, caffeine, imipramine, oxazepam, pentazocine, propranolol, theophylline	Deinduction of hepatic enzymes on smoking cessation.
insulin	Increase in subcutaneous insulin absorption with smoking cessation.
adrenergic antagonists (*e.g.*, prazosin, labtalol)	Decrease in circulating catecholamines with smoking cessation.

May Require an *Increase* in Dose at Cessation of Smoking	Possible Mechanism
adrenergic agonists (*e.g.*, isoproterenol, phenylephrine)	Decrease in circulating catecholamines with smoking cessation.

ADVERSE REACTIONS:

Assessment of adverse events in the 1,131 patients who participated in controlled clinical trials is complicated by the occurrence of GI and CNS effects of nicotine withdrawal as well as nicotine excess. The actual incidences of both are confounded by concurrent smoking by many of the patients. When reporting adverse events during the trials, the investigators did not attempt to identify the cause of the symptom.

TOPICAL ADVERSE EVENTS

The most common adverse event associated with topical nicotine is a short-lived erythema, pruritus, and/or burning at the application site, which was seen at least once in 47% of patients on the nicotine transdermal system in the clinical trials. Local erythema after system removal was noted at least once in 14% of patients and local edema in 3%. Erythema generally resolved within 24 hours. Cutaneous hypersensitivity (contact sensitization) occurred in 2% of patients on nicotine transdermal systems see PRECAUTIONS, Allergic Reactions.

PROBABLY CAUSALLY RELATED

The following adverse events were reported more frequently in nicotine transdermal-treated patients than in placebo-treated patients or exhibited a dose response in clinical trials.

Digestive system: Diarrhea,* dyspepsia*

Mouth/Tooth disorders: Dry mouth†

Musculoskeletal system: Arthralgia†, myalgia*

Nervous system: Abnormal dreams,* insomnia (23%), nervousness*

Skin and appendages: Sweating†

Frequencies for 21 mg/day system

* Reported in 3% to 9% of patients

† Reported in 1% to 3% of patients

Unmarked if reported in <1% of patients

CAUSAL RELATIONSHIP UNKNOWN

Adverse events reported in nicotine transdermal- and placebo-treated patients at about the same frequency in clinical trials are listed below. The clinical significance of the association between nicotine transdermal systems and these events is unknown, but they are reported as alerting information for the clinician.

Body as a whole: Asthenia,* back pain,* chest pain,† pain*

Digestive system: Abdominal pain,† constipation,* nausea,* vomiting†

Nervous system: Dizziness,* headache (29%), paresthesia

Respiratory system: Cough increased,* pharyngitis,* sinusitis

Skin and appendages: Rash*

Special senses: Taste perversion*

Urogenital system: Dysmenorrhea*

Frequencies for 21 mg/day systems

* Reported in 3% to 9% of patients

Reported in 1% to 3% of patients

Unmarked if reported in <1% of patients

DRUG ABUSE AND DEPENDENCE:

Nicotine transdermal therapy is likely to have a low abuse potential based on differences between it and cigarettes in four characteristics commonly considered important in contributing to abuse: much slower absorption, much smaller fluctuations in blood levels, lower blood levels of nicotine, and less frequent use (*i.e.*, once daily).

Dependence on nicotine polacrilex chewing gum replacement therapy has been reported. Such dependence might also occur from transference to nicotine transdermal systems of tobacco-based nicotine dependence. The use of the system beyond 3 months has not been evaluated and should be discouraged.

To minimize the risk of dependence, patients should be encouraged to withdraw gradually from nicotine transdermal treatment after 4 to 8 weeks of use. Recommended dose reduction is to progressively decrease the dose every 2 to 4 weeks (see DOSAGE AND ADMINISTRATION.)

OVERDOSAGE:

The effects of applying several nicotine transdermal systems simultaneously or swallowing nicotine transdermal systems are unknown (see WARNINGS, Safety Note Concerning Children.)

The oral LD_{50} for nicotine in rodents varies with species but is in excess of 24 mg/kg; death is due to respiratory paralysis. The oral minimum lethal dose of nicotine in dogs is greater than 5 mg/kg. The oral minimum acute lethal dose for nicotine in human adults is reported to be 40 to 60 mg (<1 mg/kg).

Three dogs, each weighing 11 kg, were fed two damaged Nicoderm 14 mg/day systems. Nicotine plasma concentrations of 32 to 79 ng/ml were observed. No ill effects were apparent.

Signs and symptoms of an overdose from a nicotine transdermal system would be expected to be the same as those of acute nicotine poisoning, including pallor, cold sweat, nausea, salivation, vomiting, abdominal pain, diarrhea, headache, dizziness, disturbed hearing and vision, tremor, mental confusion, and weakness. Prostration, hypotension, and respiratory

OVERDOSAGE: *(cont'd)*

failure may ensue with large overdoses. Lethal doses produce convulsions quickly, and death follows as a result of peripheral or central respiratory paralysis or, less frequently, cardiac failure.

OVERDOSE FROM TOPICAL EXPOSURE

The nicotine transdermal system should be removed immediately if the patient shows signs of overdosage, and the patient should seek immediate medical care. The skin surface may be flushed with water and dried. No soap should be used, since it may increase nicotine absorption. Nicotine will continue to be delivered into the bloodstream for several hours see CLINICAL PHARMACOLOGY, Pharmacokinetics after removal of the system because of a depot of nicotine in the skin.

OVERDOSE FROM INGESTION

Persons ingesting nicotine transdermal systems should be referred to a health care facility for management. Due to the possibility of nicotine-induced seizures, activated charcoal should be administered. In unconscious patients with a secure airway, instill activated charcoal via a nasogastric tube. A saline cathartic or sorbitol added to the first dose of activated charcoal may speed gastrointestinal passage of the system. Repeated doses of activated charcoal should be administered as long as the system remains in the gastrointestinal tract since it will continue to release nicotine for many hours.

MANAGEMENT OF NICOTINE POISONING

Other supportive measures include diazepam or barbiturates for seizures, atropine for excessive bronchial secretions or diarrhea, respiratory support for respiratory failure, and vigorous fluid support for hypotension and cardiovascular collapse.

DOSAGE AND ADMINISTRATION:

NICODERM

Patients must desire to stop smoking and should be instructed to *stop smoking immediately* as they begin using nicotine transdermal therapy. The patient should read the patient instruction sheet on nicotine transdermal therapy and be encouraged to ask any questions. Treatment should be initiated with Nicoderm 21 mg/day or 14 mg/day systems, Habitrol 21 mg/day, or Nicotrol 15 mg/day system see CLINICAL STUDIES, Individualization of Dosage.

Once the appropriate dosage is selected the patient should begin 4 to 6 weeks of therapy at that dosage. The patient should stop smoking cigarettes completely during this period. If the patient is unable to stop cigarette smoking within 4 weeks, nicotine transdermal therapy probably should be stopped, since few additional patients in clinical trials were able to quit after this time (TABLE 14).

TABLE 13 Nicoderm and Habitrol — Reccommended Dosing Schedule for Healthy Patients [a] *(see Individualization of Dosage)*

Dose	Duration
Nicoderm 21 mg/day	First 6 Weeks
Nicoderm 14 mg/day	Next 2 Weeks[b]
Nicoderm 7 mg/day	Last 2 Weeks[c]

[a] Start with Nicoderm 14 mg/day for 6 weeks for patients who have cardiovascular disease; weigh less than 100 pounds; smoke less than 1/2 a pack of cigarettes/day. Decrease dose to Nicoderm 7 mg/day for the final 2-4 weeks.
[b] Patients who have successfully abstained from smoking should have their dose of Nicoderm reduced after each 2-4 weeks of treatment until the 7 mg/day dose has been used for 2-4 weeks (see Individualization of Dosage).
[c] The entire course of nicotine substitution and gradual withdrawal should take 8-12 weeks, depending on the size of the initial dose. The use of Nicoderm systems beyond 3 months has not been studied.

TABLE 14 Nicotrol — Recommended Dosing Schedule

Dose	Duration
Nicotrol 15 mg/day	First 12 weeks
Nicotrol 10 mg/day	Next 2 weeks[a]
Nicotrol 5 mg/day	Last 2 weeks[b]

[a] Patients who have successfully abstained from smoking should have their dose of nicotine reduced after each 2-4 weeks of treatment until the Nicotrol 5 mg/day dose has been used for 2-4 weeks.
[b] The entire course of nicotine substitution and gradual withdrawal should take 14-20 weeks. The use of Nicotrol therapy beyond 5 months has not been studied.

The nicotine transdermal system should be applied promptly upon its removal from the protective pouch to prevent evaporative loss of nicotine from the system. Nicotine transdermal systems should be used only when the pouch is intact to assure that the product has not been tampered with.

Nicotine transdermal systems should be applied only once a day to a non-hairy, clean, dry skin site on the upper body or upper outer arm. After 24 hours, the used nicotine transdermal system should be removed and a new system applied to an alternate skin site. Skin sites should not be reused for at least a week. Patients should be cautioned not to continue to use the same system for more than 24 hours.

A Nicotrol system should be applied only once a day to a non-hairy, clean, and dry skin site on the upper arm or the help. Each day a nicotine transdermal systems should be applied upon waking and removed at bedtime.

SAFETY AND HANDLING

The nicotine transdermal system can be a dermal irritant and can cause contact sensitization. Patients should be instructed in the proper use of nicotine transdermal system by using demonstration systems. Although exposure of health care workers to nicotine from nicotine transdermal systems should be minimal, care should be taken to avoid unnecessary contact with active systems. If you do handle active systems, wash with water alone, since soap may increase nicotine absorption. Do not touch your eyes.

DISPOSAL

When the used system is removed from the skin, it should be folded over and placed in the protective pouch that contained the new system. The used system should be immediately disposed of in such a way to prevent its access by children or pets. See patient information for further directions on handling and disposal.

HOW TO STORE

Do not store above 86°F (30°C) because nicotine transdermal systems are sensitive to heat. A slight discoloration of the system is not significant.

Do not store unpouched. Once removed from the protective pouch, nicotine transdermal systems should be applied promptly, since nicotine is volatile and the systems may lose strength.

HOW SUPPLIED - EQUIVALENTS NOT AVAILABLE:

Film, Continuous Release - Percutaneous - 5 mg/16 hr

14's	$49.97	NICOTROL, McNeil Lab	00045-0898-52

Film, Continuous Release - Percutaneous - 7 mg/24 hr

14's	**$49.56**	**NICODERM, Hoechst Marion Roussel**	**00088-0052-61**
30's	$104.37	HABITROL, Novartis	58887-0810-26

Film, Continuous Release - Percutaneous - 10 mg/16 hr

14's	$51.54	NICOTROL, McNeil Lab	00045-0898-53

Film, Continuous Release - Percutaneous - 11 mg/24 hr

7's	$28.35	PROSTEP, Lederle Pharm	00005-2401-90

Film, Continuous Release - Percutaneous - 14 mg/24 hr

14's	**$53.52**	**NICODERM, Hoechst Marion Roussel**	**00088-0051-61**
30's	$110.17	HABITROL, Novartis	58887-0820-26

Film, Continuous Release - Percutaneous - 15 mg/16 hr

14's	$54.17	NICOTROL, McNeil Lab	00045-0898-54

Film, Continuous Release - Percutaneous - 21 mg/24 hr

14's	**$58.32**	**NICODERM, Hoechst Marion Roussel**	**00088-0050-61**
30's	$115.96	HABITROL, Novartis	58887-0830-26

Film, Continuous Release - Percutaneous - 22 mg/24 hr

7's	$30.76	PROSTEP, Lederle Pharm	00005-2402-90

NIFEDIPINE *(001886)*

CATEGORIES: Angina; Antianginals; Antihypertensives; Calcium Channel Blockers; Cardiovascular Drugs; Hypertension; Spasm; Pregnancy Category C; Sales > $1 Billion; FDA Approval Pre 1982; Patent Expiration 1991 Nov; Top 200 Drugs

BRAND NAMES: Adalat; *Adalat 5*; *Adalat 10*; *Adalat 20*; Adalat CC; *Adalat CR*; *Adalat Crono*; *Adalat FT* (Canada); *Adalat GITS*; *Adalat GITS 30*; *Adalat LA* (England); *Adalat Oros* (Australia, Mexico); *Adalat P.A.* (Canada); *Adalat Retard* (England, Germany, Mexico); *Adalate* (France); *Alat*; *Alonix*; *Alonix-S*; *Alpha-Nifedipine Retard*; *Anpine*; *Apo-Nifed* (Canada); *Aprical* (Germany); *Calcibloc*; *Calcigard*; *Calcilat* (England); *Caranta*; *Cardibloc*; *Cardifen*; *Cardiobren* (Japan); *Cardiolat*; *Cardionorm*; *Carvas*; *Citilat*; *Coracten* (England, Germany); *Coral*; *Cordalat*; *Cordipin*; *Corinfar*; *Corotrend* (Germany); *Depin*; *Dignokonstant* (Germany); *Dilcor*; *Duranifin* (Germany); *Ecodipin*; *Ecodipin-E*; *Fedcor*; *Fedcor Retard*; *Fedipin*; *Fenamon*; *Fenamon SR*; *Glopir*; *Hexadilat*; *Lemar* (Japan); *Megalat*; *Myogard*; *Nedipin*; *Nical*; *Nicardia*; *Nifangin*; *Nifdemin*; *Nifebene*; *Nifecard*; *Nifecard Retard*; *Nifecor* (Germany); *Nifedepat* (Germany); *Nifedicor*; *Nifedin*; *Nifedine*; *Nifedipres* (Mexico); *Nifelan*; *Nifelat*; *Nifelat-Q*; *Nificard*; *Nifidine*; *Nifipen*; *Noviken N* (Mexico); *Novo Nifedin* (Canada); *Nyefax*; *Nyefax Retard*; *Orix*; *Osmo-Adalat*; *Pidilat* (Germany); **Procardia**; Procardia XL; *Tibricol*; *Towerat* (Japan); *Vasdalat*; *Vasdalat Retard*; *Zenusin*
(International brand names outside U.S. in italics)

FORMULARIES: Aetna; BC-BS; CIGNA; FHP; Humana; Kaiser; Medco; Medi-Cal; PCS; PruCare; United; WHO

COST OF THERAPY: $96.46 (Angina; Capsule; 10 mg; 3/day; 365 days) vs. Potential Cost of $2,683.17 (Angina)

DESCRIPTION:

Note: This monograph contains full prescribing information for nifedipine capsules and nifedipine extended release tablets.

IMMEDIATE RELEASE CAPSULES AND EXTENDED RELEASE TABLETS

Nifedipine is an antianginal drug belonging to a new class of pharmacological agents, the calcium channel blockers. Nifedipine is 3, 5-pyridinedicarboxylic acid, 1,4-dihydro-2, 6-dimethyl-4-(2-nitrophenyl)-, dimethyl ester, $C_{17}H_{18}N_2O_6$.

Nifedipine is a yellow crystalline substance, practically insoluble in water but soluble in ethanol. It has a molecular weight of 346.3.

CAPSULES

Nifedipine capsules are formulated as soft gelatin capsules for oral administration each containing 10 mg or 20 mg nifedipine.

Inert ingredients in the formulations are: glycerin; peppermint oil; polyethylene glycol; soft gelatin capsules (which contain Yellow 6, and may contain Red Ferric Oxide and other inert ingredients), and water. The 10 mg capsules also contain saccharin sodium.

EXTENDED RELEASE TABLETS

Procardia XL is a trademark for nifedipine GITS. Nifedipine GITS (Gastrointestinal Therapeutic System) Tablet is formulated as a once-a-day controlled-release tablet for oral administration designed to deliver 30, 60, or 90 mg of nifedipine.

Inert ingredients in the formulations are: cellulose acetate; hydroxypropyl cellulose; hydroxypropyl methylcellulose; magnesium stearate; polyethylene glycol; polyethylene oxide; red ferric oxide; sodium chloride; titanium dioxide.

SYSTEM COMPONENTS AND PERFORMANCE

Procardia XL Extended Release Tablet is similar in appearance to a conventional tablet. It consists, however, of a semipermeable membrane surrounding an osmotically active drug core. The core itself is divided into two rounding an osmotically active drug core. The core itself is divided into two layers: an "active" layer containing the drug, and a "push" layer containing pharmacologically inert (but osmotically active) components. As water from the gastrointestinal tract enters the tablet, pressure increases in the osmotic layer and "pushes" against the drug layer, releasing drug through the precision laser-drilled tablet orifice in the active layer.

Procardia XL Extended Release Tablet is designed to provide nifedipine at an approximately constant rate over 24 hours. This controlled rate of drug delivery into the gastrointestinal lumen is independent of pH or gastrointestinal motility. Procardia XL depends for its action on the existence of an osmotic gradient between the contents of the bi-layer core and fluid in the GI tract. Drug delivery is essentially constant as long as the osmotic gradient remains constant, and then gradually falls to zero. Upon swallowing, the biologically inert components of the tablet remain intact during GI transit and are eliminated in the feces as an insoluble shell.

CLINICAL PHARMACOLOGY:

IMMEDIATE RELEASE CAPSULES AND EXTENDED RELEASE TABLETS

Nifedipine is a calcium ion influx inhibitor (slow channel blocker or calcium ion antagonist) and inhibits the transmembrane influx of calcium ions into cardiac muscle and smooth muscle. The contractile processes of cardiac muscle and vascular smooth muscle are depend-

CLINICAL PHARMACOLOGY: *(cont'd)*

ent upon the movement of extracellular calcium ions into these cells through specific ion channels. Nifedipine selectively inhibits calcium ion influx across the cell membrane of cardiac muscle and vascular smooth muscle without changing serum calcium concentrations.

MECHANISM OF ACTION

The precise means by which this inhibition relieves angina has not been fully determined, but includes at least the following two mechanisms:

1) RELAXATION AND PREVENTION OF CORONARY ARTERY SPASM

Nifedipine dilates the main coronary arteries and coronary arterioles, both in normal and ischemic regions, and is a potent inhibitor of coronary artery spasm, whether spontaneous or ergonovine-induced. This property increases myocardial oxygen delivery in patients with coronary artery spasm, and is responsible for the effectiveness of nifedipine in vasospastic (Prinzmetal's or variant) angina. Whether this effect plays any role in classical angina is not clear, but studies of exercise tolerance have not shown an increase in the maximum exercise rate-pressure product, a widely accepted measure of oxygen utilization. This suggests that, in general, relief of spasm or dilation of coronary arteries is not an important factor in classical angina.

2) REDUCTION OF OXYGEN UTILIZATION

Nifedipine regularly reduces arterial pressure at rest and at a given level of exercise by dilating peripheral arterioles and reducing the total peripheral resistance (afterload) against which the heart works. This unloading of the heart reduces myocardial energy consumption and oxygen requirements and probably accounts for the effectiveness of nifedipine in chronic stable angina.

HEMODYNAMICS

Like other slow channel blockers, nifedipine exerts a negative inotropic effect on isolated myocardial tissue. This is rarely, if ever, seen in intact animals or man, probably because of reflex responses to its vasodilating effects. In man, nifedipine causes decreased peripheral vascular resistance and a fall in systolic and diastolic pressure, usually modest (5-10 mmHg systolic), but sometimes larger. In patients with impaired ventricular function, most acute studies have shown some increase in ejection fraction and reduction in left ventricular filling pressure.

IMMEDIATE RELEASE CAPSULES

Pharmacokinetics and Metabolism

Nifedipine is rapidly and fully absorbed after oral administration. The drug is detectable in serum 10 minutes after oral administration, and peak blood levels occur in approximately 30 minutes. Bioavailability is proportional to dose from 10 to 30 mg; half-life does not change significantly with dose. There is little difference in relative bioavailability when nifedipine capsules are given orally and either swallowed whole, bitten and swallowed, or, bitten and held sublingually. However, biting through the capsule prior to swallowing does result in slightly earlier plasma concentrations (27 ng/ml 10 minutes after 10 mg) than if capsules are swallowed intact. It is highly bound by serum proteins. Nifedipine is extensively converted to inactive metabolites and approximately 80 percent of nifedipine and metabolites are eliminated via the kidneys. The half-life of nifedipine in plasma is approximately two hours. There is no information on the effects of renal or hepatic impairment on excretion or metabolism of nifedipine.

There is usually a small increase in heart rate, a reflex response to vasodilation. Measurements of cardiac function in patients with normal ventricular function have generally found a small increase in cardiac index without major effects on ejection fraction, left ventricular end diastolic pressure (LVEDP) or volume (LVEDV).

ELECTROPHYSIOLOGIC EFFECTS

Although like other members of its class, nifedipine decreases sinoatrial node function and atrioventricular conduction in isolated myocardial preparations, such effects have not been seen in studies in intact animals or in man. In formal electrophysiologic studies, predominantly in patients with normal conduction systems, nifedipine has had no tendency to prolong atrioventricular conduction, prolong sinus node recovery time, or slow sinus rate.

EXTENDED RELEASE TABLETS

Procardia XL

Nifedipine is completely absorbed after oral administration. Plasma drug concentrations rise at a gradual, controlled rate after a Procardia XL Extended Release Tablet dose and reach a plateau at approximately six hours after the first dose. For subsequent doses, relatively constant plasma concentrations at the plateau are maintained with minimal fluctuations over the 24 hour dosing interval. About a four-fold higher fluctuation index (ratio of peak to trough plasma concentration) was observed with the conventional immediate release Procardia capsule at t.i.d. dosing than once daily Procardia XL Extended Release Tablet. At steady-state the bioavailability of Procardia XL Extended Release Tablets is 86% relative to Procardia capsules. Administration of the Procardia XL Extended Release Tablets in the presence of food slightly alters the early rate of drug absorption, but does not influence the extent of drug bioavailability. Markedly reduced GI retention time over prolonged periods (*i.e.,* short bowel syndrome), however, may influence the pharmacokinetic profile of the drug which could potentially result in lower plasma concentration. Pharmacokinetics of Procardia XL Extended Release Tablets are linear over the dose range of 30 to 180 mg in that plasma drug concentrations are proportional to dose administered. There was no evidence of dose dumping either in the presence or absence of food for over 150 subjects in pharmacokinetic studies.

Nifedipine is extensively metabolized to highly water-soluble, inactive metabolites accounting for 60 to 80% of the dose excreted in the urine. The elimination half-life of nifedipine is approximately two hours. Only traces (less than 0.1% of the dose) of unchanged form can be detected in the urine. The remainder is excreted in the feces in metabolized form, most likely as a result of biliary excretion. Thus, the pharmacokinetics of nifedipine are not significantly influenced by the degree of renal impairment. Patients in hemodialysis or chronic ambulatory peritoneal dialysis have not reported significantly altered pharmacokinetics of nifedipine. Since hepatic biotransformation is the predominant route for the disposition of nifedipine, the pharmacokinetics may be altered in patients with chronic liver disease. Patients with hepatic impairment (liver cirrhosis) have a longer disposition half-life and higher bioavailability of nifedipine than healthy volunteers. The degree of serum protein binding of nifedipine is high (92-98%). Protein binding may be greatly reduced in patients with renal or hepatic impairments.

Electrophysiologic Effects

Although, like other members of its class, nifedipine causes a slight depression of sinoatrial node function and atrioventricular conduction in isolated myocardial preparations, such effects have not been seen in studies in intact animals or in man. In formal electrophysiologic studies, predominantly in patients with normal conduction systems, nifedipine has had no tendency to prolong atrioventricular conduction or sinus node recovery time, or to slow sinus rate.

CLINICAL PHARMACOLOGY: *(cont'd)*

HEMODYNAMICS

With Procardia XL Extended Release Tablets, these decreases in blood pressure are not accompanied by any significant change in heart rate. Hemodynamic studies in patients with normal ventricular function have generally found a small increase in cardiac index without major effects on ejection fraction, left ventricular end diastolic pressure (LVEDP) or volume (LVEDV).

INDICATIONS AND USAGE:

IMMEDIATE RELEASE CAPSULES AND EXTENDED RELEASE TABLETS

I. Vasospastic Angina

Nifedipine is indicated for the management of vasospastic angina confirmed by any of the following criteria: 1) classical pattern of angina at rest accompanied by ST segment elevation, 2) angina or coronary artery spasm provoked by ergonovine, or 3) angiographically demonstrated coronary artery spasm. In those patients who have had angiography, the presence of significant fixed obstructive disease is not incompatible with the diagnosis of vasospastic angina, provided that the above criteria are satisfied. Nifedipine may also be used where the clinical presentation suggests a possible vasospastic component but where vasospasm has not been confirmed, e.g., where pain has a variable threshold on exertion or in unstable angina where electrocardiographic findings are compatible with intermittent vasospasm, or when angina is refractory to nitrates and/or adequate doses of beta blockers.

II. Chronic Stable Angina

(Classical Effort-Associated Angina)

Nifedipine is indicated for the management of chronic stable angina (effort-associated angina) without evidence of vasospasm in patients who remain symptomatic despite adequate doses of beta blockers and/or organic nitrates or who cannot tolerate those agents.

In chronic stable angina (effort-associated angina) nifedipine has been effective in controlled trials of up to eight weeks duration in reducing angina frequency and increasing exercise tolerance, but confirmation of sustained effectiveness and evaluation of long term safety in these patients are incomplete.

Controlled studies in small numbers of patients suggest concomitant use of nifedipine and beta blocking agents may be beneficial in patients with chronic stable angina, but available information is not sufficient to predict with confidence the effects of concurrent treatment, especially in patients with compromised left ventricular function or cardiac conduction abnormalities. When introducing such concomitant therapy, care must be taken to monitor blood pressure closely since severe hypotension can occur from the combined effects of the drugs. (See WARNINGS.)

EXTENDED RELEASE TABLETS

Procardia XL is also indicated for the treatment of hypertension. It may be used alone or in combination with other antihypertensive agents.

CONTRAINDICATIONS:

Known hypersensitivity reaction to nifedipine.

WARNINGS:

EXCESSIVE HYPOTENSION

Although in most patients, the hypotensive effect of nifedipine is modest and well tolerated, occasional patients have had excessive and poorly tolerated hypotension. These responses have usually occurred during initial titration or at the time of subsequent upward dosage adjustment, and may be more likely in patients on concomitant beta blockers.

Severe hypotension and/or increased fluid volume requirements have been reported in patients receiving nifedipine together with a beta blocking agent who underwent coronary artery bypass surgery using high dose fentanyl anesthesia. The interaction with high dose fentanyl appears to be due to the combination of nifedipine and a beta blocker, but the possibility that it may occur with nifedipine alone, with low doses of fentanyl, in other surgical procedures, or with other narcotic analgesics cannot be ruled out. In nifedipine treated patients where surgery using high dose fentanyl anesthesia is contemplated, the physician should be aware of these potential problems and, if the patient's condition permits, sufficient time (at least 36 hours) should be allowed for nifedipine to be washed out of the body prior to surgery.

INCREASED ANGINA AND/OR MYOCARDIAL INFARCTION

Rarely, patients, particularly those who have severe obstructive coronary artery disease, have developed well documented increased frequency, duration and/or severity of angina or acute myocardial infarction on starting nifedipine or at the time of dosage increase. The mechanism of this effect is not established.

BETA BLOCKER WITHDRAWAL

Patients recently withdrawn from beta blockers may develop a withdrawal syndrome with increased angina, probably related to increased sensitivity to catecholamines. Initiation of nifedipine treatment will not prevent this occurrence and might be expected to exacerbate it by provoking reflex catecholamine release. There have been occasional reports of increased angina in a setting of beta blocker withdrawal and nifedipine initiation. It is important to taper beta blockers if possible, rather than stopping them abruptly before beginning nifedipine.

CONGESTIVE HEART FAILURE

Rarely, patients, usually receiving a beta blocker, have developed heart failure after beginning nifedipine. Patients with tight aortic stenosis may be at greater risk for such an event, as the unloading effect of nifedipine would be expected to be of less benefit to these patients, owing to their fixed impedance to flow across the aortic valve.

PRECAUTIONS:

GENERAL

Hypotension: Because nifedipine decreases peripheral vascular resistance, careful monitoring of blood pressure during the initial administration and titration of nifedipine is suggested. Close observation is especially recommended for patients already taking medications that are known to lower blood pressure. (See WARNINGS.)

Peripheral Edema: Mild to moderate peripheral edema, typically associated with arterial vasodilation and not due to left ventricular dysfunction, occurs in about one in ten patients treated with nifedipine. This edema occurs primarily in the lower extremities and usually responds to diuretic therapy. With patients whose angina is complicated by congestive heart failure, care should be taken to differentiate this peripheral edema from the effects of increasing left ventricular dysfunction.

Extended Release Tablets: As with any other non-deformable material, caution should be used when administering Procardia XL in patients with preexisting severe gastrointestinal narrowing (pathologic or iatrogenic). There have been rare reports of obstructive symptoms in patients with known strictures in association with the ingestion of Procardia XL.

PRECAUTIONS: *(cont'd)*

LABORATORY TESTS

Nifedipine, like other calcium channel blockers, decreases platelet aggregation *in vitro.* Limited clinical studies have demonstrated a moderate but statistically significant decrease in platelet aggregation and increase in bleeding time in some nifedipine patients. This is thought to be a function of inhibition of calcium transport across the platelet membrane. No clinical significance for these findings has been demonstrated.

Positive direct Coombs test with/without hemolytic anemia has been reported.

Although nifedipine has been used safely in patients with renal dysfunction and has been reported to exert a beneficial effect in certain cases, rare, reversible elevations in BUN and serum creatinine have been reported in patients with pre-existing chronic renal insufficiency. The relationship to nifedipine therapy is uncertain in most cases but probable in some.

Immediate Release Capsules: Rare, usually transient, but occasionally significant elevations of enzymes such as alkaline phosphatase, CPK, LDH, SGOT and SGPT have been noted. The relationship to nifedipine therapy is uncertain in most cases, but probable in some. These laboratory abnormalities have rarely been associated with clinical symptoms, however, cholestasis with or without jaundice has been reported. Rare instances of allergic hepatitis have been reported.

Extended Release Tablets: Rare, usually transient, but occasionally significant elevations of enzymes such as alkaline phosphatase, CPK, LDH, SGOT, and SGPT have been noted. The relationship to nifedipine therapy is uncertain in most case, but probable in some. These laboratory abnormalities have rarely been associated with clinical symptoms; however, cholestasis with or without jaundice has been reported. A small (5.4%) increase in mean alkaline phosphatase was noted in patients treated with Procardia XL. This was an isolated finding not associated with clinical symptoms and it rarely resulted in values which fell outside the normal range. Rare instances of allergic hepatitis have been reported. In controlled studies, Procardia XL did not adversely affect serum uric acid, glucose, or cholesterol. Serum potassium was unchanged in patients receiving Procardia XL in the absence of concomitant diuretic therapy, and slightly decreased in patients receiving concomitant diuretics.

INFORMATION FOR THE PATIENT

Extended Release Tablets: Procardia XL Extended Release Tablets should be swallowed whole. Do not chew, divide or crush tablets. Do not be concerned if you occasionally notice in you stool something that looks like a tablet. In Procardia XL, the medication is contained within a nonabsorbable shell that has been specially designed to slowly release the drug for your body to absorb. When this process is completed, the empty tablet is eliminated from your body.

Adalat CC should be taken on an empty stomach. It should not be administered with food.

CARCINOGENESIS, MUTAGENESIS, AND IMPAIRMENT OF FERTILITY

Nifedipine was administered orally to rats for two years and was not shown to be carcinogenic. When given to rats prior to mating, nifedipine caused reduced fertility at a dose approximately 30 times the maximum recommended human dose. *In vivo* mutagenicity studies were negative.

PREGNANCY CATEGORY C

Nifedipine has been shown to be teratogenic in rats when given in doses 30 times the maximum recommended human dose. Nifedipine was embryotoxic (increased fetal resorptions, decreased fetal weight, increased stunted forms, increased fetal deaths, decreased neonatal survival) in rats, mice and rabbits at doses of from 3 to 10 times the maximum recommended human dose. In pregnant monkeys, doses 2/3 and twice the maximum recommended human dose resulted in small placentas and underdeveloped chorionic villi. In rats doses three times maximum human dose and higher caused prolongation of pregnancy. There are no adequate and well controlled studies in pregnant women. Nifedipine should be used during pregnancy only if the potential benefit justifies the potential risk to the fetus.

DRUG INTERACTIONS:

Beta-adrenergic blocking agents: (See INDICATIONS AND USAGEand WARNINGS.)

Experience in over 1400 patients in a non-comparative clinical trial has shown that concomitant administration of nifedipine and beta-blocking agents is usually well tolerated, but there have been occasional literature reports suggesting that the combination may increase the likelihood of congestive heart failure, severe hypotension or exacerbation of angina.

Long acting nitrates: Nifedipine may be safely co-administered with nitrates, but there have been no controlled studies to evaluate the antianginal effectiveness of this combination.

Digitalis: Administration of nifedipine with digoxin increased digoxin levels in nine of twelve normal volunteers. The average increase was 45%. Another investigator found no increase in digoxin levels in thirteen patients with coronary artery disease. In an uncontrolled study of over two hundred patients with congestive heart failure during which digoxin blood levels were not measured, digitalis toxicity was not observed. Since there have been isolated reports of patients with elevated digoxin levels, it is recommended that digoxin levels be monitored when initiating, adjusting, and discontinuing nifedipine to avoid possible over- or under-digitalization.

Coumarin anticoagulants: There have been rare reports of increased prothrombin time in patients taking coumarin anticoagulants to whom nifedipine was administered. However, the relationship to nifedipine therapy is uncertain.

Cimetidine: A study in six healthy volunteers has shown a significant increase in peak nifedipine plasma levels (80%) and area-under-the-curve (74%) after a one week course of cimetidine at 1000 mg per day and nifedipine at 40 mg per day. Ranitidine produced smaller, non-significant increases. The effect may be mediated by the known inhibition of cimetidine on hepatic cytochrome P-450, the enzyme system probably responsible for the first-pass metabolism of nifedipine. If nifedipine therapy is initiated in a patient currently receiving cimetidine, cautious titration is advised.

ADVERSE REACTIONS:

IMMEDIATE RELEASE CAPSULES

In multiple-dose U.S. and foreign controlled studies in which adverse reactions were reported spontaneously, adverse effects were frequent but generally not serious and rarely required discontinuation of therapy or dosage adjustment. Most were expected consequences of the vasodilator effects of nifedipine (TABLE 1):

There is also a large uncontrolled experience in over 2100 patients in the United States. Most of the patients had vasospastic or resistant angina pectoris, and about half had concomitant treatment with beta-adrenergic blocking agents. The most common adverse events were:

Incidence Approximately 10%

Cardiovascular: peripheral edema

Central Nervous System: dizziness or lightheadedness

Gastrointestinal: nausea

Systemic: headache and flushing, weakness

Incidence Approximately 5%

Cardiovascular: transient hypotension

ADVERSE REACTIONS: *(cont'd)*

TABLE 1 Nifedipine, Adverse Reactions

Adverse Effect	Nifedipine (%) (N=226)	Placebo (%) (N=235)
Dizziness, lightheadedness, giddiness	27	15
Flushing, heat sensation	25	8
Headache	23	20
Weakness	12	10
Nausea, heartburn	11	8
Muscle cramps, tremor	8	3
Peripheral edema	7	1
Nervousness, mood changes	7	4
Palpitation	7	5
Dyspnea cough, wheezing	6	3
Nasal congestion, sore throat	6	8

Incidence 2% or Less

Cardiovascular: palpitation

Respiratory: nasal and chest congestion, shortness of breath

Gastrointestinal: diarrhea, constipation, cramps, flatulence

Musculoskeletal: inflammation, joint stiffness, muscle cramps

Central Nervous System: shakiness, nervousness, jitteriness, sleep disturbances, blurred vision, difficulties in balance

Other: dermatitis, pruritus, urticaria, fever, sweating, chills, sexual difficulties.

Incidence Approximately 0.5%

Cardiovascular: syncope. Syncopal episodes did not recur with reduction in the dose of nifedipine or concomitant antianginal medication.

Incidence Less Than 0.5%

Hematologic: thrombocytopenia, anemia, leukopenia, purpura

Gastrointestinal: allergic hepatitis

Oral: gingival hyperplasia

CNS: depression, paranoid syndrome

Special Senses: transient blindness at the peak of plasma level

Other: erythromelalgia, arthritis with ANA (+)

Several of these side effects appear to be dose related. Peripheral edema occurred in about one in 25 patients at doses less than 60 mg per day and in about one patient in eight at 120 mg per day or more. Transient hypotension, generally of mild to moderate severity and seldom requiring discontinuation of therapy, occurred in one of 50 patients at less than 60 mg per day and in one of 20 patients at 120 mg per day or more. Very rarely, introduction of nifedipine therapy was associated with an increase in anginal pain, possibly due to associated hypotension.

In addition, more serious adverse events were observed, not readily distinguishable from the natural history of the disease in these patients. It remains possible, however, that some or many of these events were drug related. Myocardial infarction occurred in about 4% of patients and congestive heart failure or pulmonary edema in about 2%. Ventricular arrhythmias or conduction disturbances each occurred in fewer than 0.5% of patients.

In a subgroup of over 1000 patients receiving nifedipine with concomitant beta blocker therapy, the pattern and incidence of adverse experiences was not different from that of the entire group of nifedipine treated patients (See PRECAUTIONS.)

In a subgroup of approximately 250 patients with a diagnosis of congestive heart failure as well as angina, dizziness or lightheadedness, peripheral edema, headache or flushing each occurred in one in eight patients. Hypotension occurred in about one in 20 patients. Syncope occurred in approximately one patient in 250. Myocardial infarction or symptoms of congestive heart failure each occurred in about one patient in 15. Atrial or ventricular dysrhythmias each occurred in about one patient in 150.

EXTENDED RELEASE TABLETS

Over 1000 patients from both controlled and open trials with Procardia XL Extended Release Tablets in hypertension and angina were included in the evaluation of adverse experiences. All side effects reported during Procardia XL Extended Release Tablet therapy were tabulated independent of their causal relation to medication. The most common side effect reported with Procardia XL was edema which was dose related and ranged in frequency from approximately 10% to about 30% at the highest dose studied (180 mg). Other common adverse experience reported in placebo-controlled trials include (TABLE 2):

TABLE 2

Adverse Effect	Procardia XL (%) (N = 707)	Placebo (%) (N = 266)
Headache	15.8	9.8
Fatigue	5.9	4.1
Dizziness	4.1	4.5
Constipation	3.3	2.3
Nausea	3.3	1.9
Fatigue	5.9	4.1

Of these, only edema and headache were more common in Procardia XL patients than placebo patients.

The following adverse reactions occurred with an incidence of less than 3.0%. With the exception of leg cramps, the incidence of these side effects was similar to that of placebo alone.

Body as a Whole/Systemic: asthenia, flushing, pain

Cardiovascular: palpitations

Central Nervous System: insomnia, nervousness, paresthesia, somnolence

Dermatologic: pruritus, rash

Gastrointestinal: abdominal pain, diarrhea, dry mouth, dyspepsia, flatulence

Musculoskeletal: arthralgia, leg cramps

Respiratory: chest pain (nonspecific), dyspnea

Urogenital: impotence, polyuria

Other adverse reactions were reported sporadically with an incidence of 1.0% or less. These include:

Body as a Whole/System: face edema, fever, hot flashes, malaise, periorbital edema, rigors

Cardiovascular: arrhythmia, hypotension, increased angina, tachycardia, syncope

Central Nervous System: anxiety, ataxia, decreased libido, depression, hypertonia, hypoesthesia, migraine, paroniria, tenor, vertigo

Dermatologic: alopecia, increased sweating, urticaria, purpura

ADVERSE REACTIONS: *(cont'd)*

Gastrointestinal: eructation, gastroesophageal reflux, gum hyperplasia, melena, vomiting, weight increase

Musculoskeletal: back pain, gout, myalgias

Respiratory: coughing, epistaxis, upper respiratory tract infection, respiratory disorder, sinusitis

Special Senses: abnormal lacrimation, abnormal vision, taste perversion, tinnitus

Urogenital/Reproductive: breast pain, dysuria, hematuria, nocturia

Adverse experiences which occurred in less than 1 in 1000 patients cannot be distinguished from concurrent disease states or medications.

The following adverse experiences, reported in less than 1% of patients, occurred under conditions (*e.g.,* open trials, marketing experience) where a causal relationship is uncertain: gastrointestinal irritation, gastrointestinal bleeding.

In multiple-dose U.S. and foreign controlled studies with nifedipine capsules in which adverse reactions were reported spontaneously, adverse effects were frequent but generally not serious and rarely required discontinuation of therapy or dosage adjustment. Most were expected consequences of the vasodilator effects of Procardia (TABLE 3):

TABLE 3

Adverse Effects	Procardia capsules(%) (N=266)	Placebo (%) (N=235)
Dizziness, lightheadedness, giddiness	27	15
Flushing, heat sensation	25	8
Headache	23	20
Weakness	12	10
Nausea, heartburn	11	8
Muscle cramps, tremor	8	3
Peripheral edema	7	1
Nervousness, mood changes	7	4
Palpitation	7	5
Dyspnea, cough, wheezing	6	3
Nasal congestion, sore throat	6	8

There is also a large uncontrolled experience in over 2100 patients in the United States. Most of the patients had vasospastic or resistant angina pectoris, and about half had concomitant treatment with beta-adrenergic blocking agents. The relatively common adverse events were similar in nature to those seen with Procardia XL.

In addition, more serious adverse events were observed, not readily distinguishable from the natural history of the disease in these patients. It remains possible, however, that some or many of these events were drug related. Myocardial infarction occurred in about 4% of patients and congestive heart failure or pulmonary edema in about 2%. Ventricular arrhythmias or conduction disturbances each occurred in fewer than 0.5% of patients.

In a subgroup of over 1000 patients receiving Procardia with concomitant beta blocker therapy, the pattern and incidence of adverse experiences was not different from that of the entire group of Procardia (nifedipine) treated patients (See PRECAUTIONS.)

In a subgroup of approximately 250 patients with a diagnosis of congestive heart failure as well as angina, dizziness or lightheadedness, peripheral edema, headache or flushing each occurred in one in eight patients. Hypotension occurred in about one in 20 patients. Syncope occurred in approximately one patient in 250. Myocardial infarction or symptoms of congestive heart failure each occurred in about one patient in 15. Atrial or ventricular dysrhythmias each occurred in about one patient in 150.

In post-marketing experience, there have been rare reports of exfoliative dermatitis caused by nifedipine.

OVERDOSAGE:

IMMEDIATE RELEASE CAPSULES

Although there is no well documented experience with nifedipine overdosage, available data suggest that gross overdosage could result in excessive peripheral vasodilation with subsequent marked and probably prolonged systemic hypotension. Clinically significant hypotension due to nifedipine overdosage calls for active cardiovascular support including monitoring of cardiac and respiratory function, elevation of extremities, and attention to circulating fluid volume and urine output. A vasoconstrictor (such as norepinephrine) may be helpful in restoring vascular tone and blood pressure, provided that there is no contraindication to its use. Clearance of nifedipine would be expected to be prolonged in patients with impaired liver function. Since nifedipine is highly protein-bound, dialysis is not likely to be of benefit.

EXTENDED RELEASE TABLETS

Experience with nifedipine overdosage is limited. Generally overdosage with nifedipine leading to pronounced hypotension calls for active cardiovascular support including monitoring of cardiovascular and respiratory function, elevation of extremities, judicious use of calcium infusion, pressor agents and fluids. Clearance of nifedipine would be expected to be prolonged in patients with impaired liver function. Since nifedipine is highly protein-bound, dialysis is not likely to be of any benefit.

There has been one reported case of massive overdosage with Procardia XL Extended Release Tablets. The main effects of ingestion of approximately 4800 mg of Procardia XL in a young man attempting suicide as a result of cocaine-induced depression were initial dizziness, palpitations, flushing, and nervousness. Within several hours of ingestion, nausea, vomiting, and generalized edema developed. No significant hypotension was apparent at presentation, 18 hours post-ingestion. Electrolyte abnormalities consisted of a mild, transient elevation of serum creatinine, and modest elevations of LDH and CPK, but normal SGOT. Vital signs remained stable, no electrocardiographic abnormalities were noted and renal function returned to normal within 24 to 48 hours with routine supportive measures alone. No prolonged sequelae were observed.

The effect of a single 900 mg ingestion of Procardia capsules in a depressed anginal patient also on tricyclic antidepressants was loss of consciousness within 30 minutes of ingestion, and profound hypotension, which responded to calcium infusion, pressor agents, and fluid replacement. A variety of ECG abnormalities were seen in this patient with a history of bundle branch block, including sinus bradycardia and varying degrees of AV block. These dictated the prophylactic placement of a temporary ventricular pacemaker, but otherwise resolved spontaneously. Significant hyperglycemia was seen initially in this patient, but plasma glucose levels rapidly normalized without further treatment.

A young hypertensive patient with advanced renal failure ingested 280 mg of Procardia capsules at time, with resulting marked hypotension responding to calcium infusion and fluids. No AV conduction abnormalities, arrhythmias, or pronounced changes in heart rate were noted, nor was there any further deterioration in renal function.

DOSAGE AND ADMINISTRATION:

IMMEDIATE RELEASE CAPSULES

The dosage of nifedipine needed to suppress angina and that can be tolerated by the patient must be established by titration. Excessive doses can result in hypotension.

Therapy should be initiated with the 10 mg capsule. The starting dose is one 10 mg capsule, swallowed whole, 3 times/day. The usual effective dose range is 10-20 mg three times daily. Some patients, especially those with evidence of coronary artery spasm, respond only to higher doses, more frequent administration, or both. In such patients, doses of 20-30 mg three or four times daily may be effective. Doses above 120 mg daily are rarely necessary. More than 180 mg per day is not recommended.

In most cases, nifedipine titration should proceed over a 7-14 day period so that the physician can assess the response to each dose level and monitor the blood pressure before proceeding to higher doses.

If symptoms so warrant, titration may proceed more rapidly provided that the patient is assessed frequently. Based on the patient's physical activity level, attack frequency, and sublingual nitroglycerin consumption, the dose of nifedipine may be increased from 10 mg t.i.d. to 20 mg t.i.d. and then to 30 mg t.i.d. over a three-day period.

In hospitalized patients under close observation, the dose may be increased in 10 mg increments over four- to six-hour periods as required to control pain and arrhythmias due to ischemia. A single dose should rarely exceed 30 mg.

No "rebound effect" has been observed upon discontinuation of nifedipine. However, if discontinuation of nifedipine is necessary, sound clinical practice suggests that the dosage should be decreased gradually with close physician supervision.

CO-ADMINISTRATION WITH OTHER ANTIANGINAL DRUGS

Sublingual nitroglycerin may be taken as required for the control of acute manifestations of angina, particularly during nifedipine titration. See DRUG INTERACTIONS for information on co-administration of nifedipine with beta blockers or long acting nitrates.

EXTENDED RELEASE TABLETS

Dosage must be adjusted according to each patient's needs. Therapy for either hypertension or angina should be initiated with 30 or 60 mg once daily. Procardia XL Extended Release Tablets should be swallowed whole and should not be bitten or divided. In general, titration should proceed over 7-14 day period so that the physician can fully assess the response to each dose level and monitor blood pressure before proceeding to higher doses. Since steady-state plasma levels are achieved on the second day of dosing, if symptoms so warrant, titration may proceed more rapidly provided the patient is assessed frequently. Titration to doses above 120 mg are not recommended.

Angina patients controlled on Procardia capsules alone or in combination with other antianginal medications may be safety switched to Procardia XL Extended Release Tablets at the nearest equivalent total daily dose (e.g. 30 mg t.i.d. of Procardia capsules may be changed to 90 mg once daily of Procardia XL Extended Release Tablets). Subsequent titration to higher or lower doses may be necessary and should be initiated as clinically warranted. Experience with dose greater than 90 mg in patients with angina is limited. Therefore, doses greater than 90 mg should be used with caution and only when clinically warranted.

No "rebound effect" has been observed upon discontinuation of Procardia XL Extended Release Tablets. However, if discontinuation of nifedipine is necessary, sound clinical practice suggests that the dosage should be decreased gradually with close physician supervision.

Care should be taken when dispensing Procardia XL to assure that the extended release dosage form has been prescribed.

CO-ADMINISTRATION WITH OTHER ANTIANGINAL DRUGS

Sublingual nitroglycerin may be taken as required for the control of acute manifestations of angina, particularly during nifedipine titration. See DRUG INTERACTIONS, for information on co-administration of nifedipine with beta blockers or long acting nitrates.

PATIENT INFORMATION:

Nifedipine, known as a calcium channel blocker, is used to treat high blood pressure and some forms of chest pain known as angina. This medication works by relaxing blood vessels and decreasing the pressure on the heart. This can lead to dizziness, headache, lightheadedness, flushing and swelling of the legs. You should report this to your physician because it can often be easily treated with a diuretic (water-pill). This medication is available in an extended-release form allowing for once a day dosing. Some brands must be taken on an empty stomach. Other brands are made in porous capsule which slowly releases the medication. You may notice the empty capsule in your stool. Extended release medications should not be crushed, cut or split because this destroys the slow release mechanism. If you are taking this for high blood pressure, you should have your blood pressure checked regularly to make sure the medication is working.

HOW SUPPLIED:

IMMEDIATE RELEASE CAPSULES

Procardia soft gelatin capsules are supplied in:

Bottles of 100: 10 mg orange #260; 20 mg orange and light brown #261

Bottles of 300: 10 mg orange #260: 20 mg orange and light brown #261

Unit dose packages of 100: 10 mg orange #260; 20 mg orange and light brown #261

The capsules should be protected from light and moisture and stored at controlled room temperature 59° to 77°F (15° to 25°C) in the manufacturer's original container.

EXTENDED RELEASE TABLETS

Procardia XL Extended Release Tablets are supplied as 30 mg, 60 mg and 90 mg round biconvex, rose-pink, film-coated tablets.

Stored below 86°F (30°C)

Protect from moisture and humidity.

HOW SUPPLIED - RATED THERAPEUTICALLY EQUIVALENT:

Capsule, Gelatin - Oral - 10 mg

100's	$8.81	Nifedipine, H.C.F.A. F F P	99999-1886-01
100's	$10.88	Nifedipine, United Res	00677-1398-01
100's	$39.39	Nifedipine, US Trading	56126-0449-11
100's	$39.50	Nifedipine Capsules 10 Mg, Harber Pharm	51432-0345-03
100's	$39.50	Nifedipine, Am Generics	58634-0022-01
100's	$42.20	Nifedipine, Qualitest Pharms	00603-4759-21
100's	$43.05	Nifedipine, HL Moore Drug Exch	00839-7704-06
100's	$43.25	Nifedipine, Major Pharms	00904-7685-60
100's	$43.45	Nifedipine Capsules 10 Mg, Major Pharms	00904-0407-60
100's	$43.45	Nifedipine, Major Pharms	00904-0409-60
100's	$43.45	Nifedipine, Major Pharms	00904-7950-60
100's	$43.75	Nifedipine, Goldline Labs	00182-1547-01
100's	$43.75	Nifedipine, Goldline Labs	00182-1562-01
100's	$43.75	Nifedipine, Schein Pharm (US)	00364-2376-01
100's	$44.05	Nifedipine, Mova Pharms	55370-0156-07
100's	$44.51	Nifedipine, Purepac Pharm	00228-2497-10
100's	$44.51	Nifedipine, Caremark	00339-5717-12

HOW SUPPLIED - RATED THERAPEUTICALLY EQUIVALENT:
(cont'd)

100's	$44.51	Nifedipine, Aligen Independ	00405-4696-01
100's	$44.75	Nifedipine, Rugby	00536-4065-01
100's	$45.86	Nifedipine, Major Pharms	00904-0409-61
100's	$45.93	Nifedipine, Caraco Pharm	57664-0872-08
100's	$45.93	Nifedipine, Caraco Pharm	57664-0972-08
100's	$46.51	ADALAT, Bayer	00026-8811-51
100's	$47.25	Nifedipine, Medirex	57480-0389-01
100's	$48.05	Nifedipine, Geneva Pharms	00781-2504-01
100's	$48.08	Nifedipine, Novopharm (US)	55953-0040-40
100's	$48.08	Nifedipine, Novopharm (US)	55953-0171-40
100's	$48.09	Nifedipine, HL Moore Drug Exch	00839-7564-06
100's	$49.50	Nifedipine, Parmed Pharms	00349-8873-01
100's	$50.40	Nifedipine, Goldline Labs	00182-1547-89
100's	$51.00	Nifedipine, Schein Pharm (US)	00364-2376-90
100's	$51.44	Nifedipine, Novopharm (US)	55953-0040-01
100's	$51.44	Nifedipine, Novopharm (US)	55953-0171-41
100's	$51.83	ADALAT, Bayer	00026-8811-48
100's	**$52.80**	**PROCARDIA, Pfizer Labs**	**00069-2600-66**
100's	$54.43	Nifedipine, Vangard Labs	00615-0360-13
100's	$55.98	Nifedipine, Balan	00304-2294-01
100's	**$58.83**	**PROCARDIA, Pfizer Labs**	**00069-2600-41**
300's	$26.43	Nifedipine, H.C.F.A. F F P	99999-1886-02
300's	$32.64	Nifedipine, United Res	00677-1398-61
300's	$115.50	Nifedipine, Am Generics	58634-0022-02
300's	$118.50	Nifedipine Capsules 10 Mg, Harber Pharm	51432-0345-04
300's	$127.70	Nifedipine, Caraco Pharm	57664-0872-11
300's	$128.25	Nifedipine, Goldline Labs	00182-1547-96
300's	$128.25	Nifedipine, Goldline Labs	00182-1562-96
300's	$128.48	Nifedipine, Mova Pharms	55370-0156-11
300's	$130.40	Nifedipine, HL Moore Drug Exch	00839-7704-13
300's	$130.80	Nifedipine, Rugby	00536-4065-03
300's	$130.88	Nifedipine, Qualitest Pharms	00603-4759-25
300's	$130.95	Nifedipine Capsules 10 Mg, Major Pharms	00904-0407-72
300's	$130.95	Nifedipine, Major Pharms	00904-0409-72
300's	$130.95	Nifedipine, Major Pharms	00904-7685-72
300's	$130.95	Nifedipine, Major Pharms	00904-7950-72
300's	$131.54	Nifedipine, Purepac Pharm	00228-2497-30
300's	$131.54	Nifedipine, Aligen Independ	00405-4696-09
300's	$134.10	Nifedipine, Geneva Pharms	00781-2504-03
300's	$136.70	ADALAT, Bayer	00026-8811-18
300's	$142.31	Nifedipine, Novopharm (US)	55953-0040-60
300's	$142.31	Nifedipine, Novopharm (US)	55953-0171-60
300's	$142.32	Nifedipine, HL Moore Drug Exch	00839-7564-13
300's	$143.88	Nifedipine, Schein Pharm (US)	00364-2376-29
300's	$144.50	Nifedipine, Parmed Pharms	00349-8873-03
300's	**$155.25**	**PROCARDIA, Pfizer Labs**	**00069-2600-72**
600's	$274.60	Nifedipine, Medirex	57480-0389-06
750's	$335.59	Nifedipine, Glasgow Pharm	60809-0300-55
750's	$335.59	Nifedipine, Glasgow Pharm	60809-0300-72
1000's	$88.10	Nifedipine, H.C.F.A. F F P	99999-1886-03
1000's	$402.90	Nifedipine, Caraco Pharm	57664-0872-18
1000's	$404.99	Nifedipine, HL Moore Drug Exch	00839-7564-16
2000's	$176.20	Nifedipine, H.C.F.A. F F P	99999-1886-04
2000's	$690.16	Nifedipine, Novopharm (US)	55953-0171-81
2000's	$724.68	Nifedipine, HL Moore Drug Exch	00839-7564-80

Capsule, Gelatin - Oral - 20 mg

100's	$17.48	Nifedipine, United Res	00677-1399-01
100's	$17.48	Nifedipine, United Res	00677-1434-01
100's	$17.48	Nifedipine, H.C.F.A. F F P	99999-1886-05
100's	$71.00	Nifedipine, Qualitest Pharms	00603-4760-21
100's	$72.00	Nifedipine, Am Generics	58634-0023-01
100's	$77.70	Nifedipine, US Trading	56126-0453-11
100's	$80.00	Nifedipine, Goldline Labs	00182-1548-01
100's	$80.00	Nifedipine, Rugby	00536-4067-01
100's	$80.04	Nifedipine, Purepac Pharm	00228-2530-10
100's	$80.04	Nifedipine, Aligen Independ	00405-4697-01
100's	$80.18	Nifedipine, HL Moore Drug Exch	00839-7565-06
100's	$80.18	Nifedipine, HL Moore Drug Exch	00839-7717-06
100's	$80.50	Nifedipine, Medirex	57480-0390-01
100's	$81.65	Nifedipine, Major Pharms	00904-0408-61
100's	$81.82	Nifedipine, Caremark	00339-5718-12
100's	$82.94	Nifedipine, Caraco Pharm	57664-0873-08
100's	$83.10	Nifedipine, Mova Pharms	55370-0157-07
100's	$83.70	ADALAT, Bayer	00026-8821-51
100's	$84.90	Nifedipine, Major Pharms	00904-0408-60
100's	$84.90	Nifedipine, Major Pharms	00904-7699-60
100's	$84.90	Nifedipine, Major Pharms	00904-7951-60
100's	$86.00	Nifedipine, Goldline Labs	00182-1548-89
100's	$86.50	Nifedipine, Parmed Pharms	00349-8874-01
100's	$86.50	Nifedipine, Schein Pharm (US)	00364-2377-01
100's	$86.50	Nifedipine, Geneva Pharms	00781-2506-01
100's	$90.00	Nifedipine, Schein Pharm (US)	00364-2377-90
100's	$90.00	Nifedipine, Vangard Labs	00615-0359-13
100's	$93.28	ADALAT, Bayer	00026-8821-48
100's	**$95.02**	**PROCARDIA, Pfizer Labs**	**00069-2610-66**
100's	$96.15	Nifedipine, Novopharm (US)	55953-0045-40
100's	$99.52	Nifedipine, Novopharm (US)	55953-0045-01
100's	**$105.91**	**PROCARDIA, Pfizer Labs**	**00069-2610-41**
300's	$52.44	Nifedipine, United Res	00677-1399-61
300's	$52.44	Nifedipine, H.C.F.A. F F P	99999-1886-06
300's	$236.00	Nifedipine, Goldline Labs	00182-1548-96
300's	$236.10	Nifedipine, HL Moore Drug Exch	00839-7565-13
300's	$236.14	Nifedipine, Rugby	00536-4067-03
300's	$236.95	Nifedipine, Am Generics	58634-0023-02
300's	$237.80	Nifedipine, Caraco Pharm	57664-0873-11
300's	$239.85	Nifedipine 20 Mg Capsules, Major Pharms	00904-0408-72
300's	$239.85	Nifedipine, Major Pharms	00904-7951-72
300's	$242.57	Nifedipine, Purepac Pharm	00228-2530-30
300's	$242.57	Nifedipine, Aligen Independ	00405-4697-09
300's	$245.00	Nifedipine, Schein Pharm (US)	00364-2377-29
300's	$245.24	Nifedipine, Mova Pharms	55370-0157-11
300's	$245.50	Nifedipine, Parmed Pharms	00349-8874-03
300's	$246.09	ADALAT, Bayer	00026-8821-18
300's	$249.50	Nifedipine, Harber Pharm	51432-0362-04
300's	**$279.42**	**PROCARDIA, Pfizer Labs**	**00069-2610-72**
300's	$286.54	Nifedipine, Novopharm (US)	55953-0045-60
600's	$442.00	Nifedipine, Medirex	57480-0390-06
750's	$604.20	Nifedipine, Glasgow Pharm	60809-0301-55
750's	$604.20	Nifedipine, Glasgow Pharm	60809-0301-72
1000's	$174.80	Nifedipine, H.C.F.A. F F P	99999-1886-07
1000's	$750.45	Nifedipine, Caraco Pharm	57664-0873-18

HOW SUPPLIED - NOT RATED EQUIVALENT:

Tablet, Coated, Sustained Action - Oral - 30 mg

100's	$90.53	ADALAT CC, Bayer	00026-8841-51
100's	$95.05	ADALAT CC, Bayer	00026-8841-48
100's	**$107.36**	**PROCARDIA XL, Pfizer Labs**	**00069-2650-66**
100's	**$119.61**	**PROCARDIA XL, Pfizer Labs**	**00069-2650-41**
300's	**$315.64**	**PROCARDIA XL, Pfizer Labs**	**00069-2650-72**
5000's	**$5260.66**	**PROCARDIA XL, Pfizer Labs**	**00069-2650-94**

Tablet, Coated, Sustained Action - Oral - 60 mg

100's	$150.59	ADALAT CC, Bayer	00026-8851-51
100's	$164.45	ADALAT CC, Bayer	00026-8851-48
100's	**$185.78**	**PROCARDIA XL, Pfizer Labs**	**00069-2660-66**
100's	**$207.01**	**PROCARDIA XL, Pfizer Labs**	**00069-2660-41**
300's	**$546.18**	**PROCARDIA XL, Pfizer Labs**	**00069-2660-72**
5000's	**$9102.91**	**PROCARDIA XL, Pfizer Labs**	**00069-2660-94**

Tablet, Coated, Sustained Action - Oral - 90 mg

100's	$184.47	ADALAT CC, Bayer	00026-8861-51
100's	$201.44	ADALAT CC, Bayer	00026-8861-48
100's	**$214.35**	**PROCARDIA XL, Pfizer Labs**	**00069-2670-66**
100's	**$238.78**	**PROCARDIA XL, Pfizer Labs**	**00069-2670-41**

NILUTAMIDE *(003247)*

CATEGORIES: Androgen Inhibitors; Antineoplastics; Cancer; Oncologic Drugs; Prostatic Carcinoma; Pregnancy Category C; FDA Approved 1996 Sep

BRAND NAMES: **Nilandron**

DESCRIPTION:

Nilandron tablets contain nilutamide, a nonsteroidal, orally active antiandrogen having the chemical name 5,5-dimethyl 3-[4-nitro3-(trifluoromethyl) phenyl]2,4-imidazolidinedione.

Nilutamide is a microcrystalline, white to practically white powder with a molecular weight of 317.25.

It is freely soluble in ethyl acetate, acetone, chloroform, ethyl alcohol, dichloromethane, and methanol. It is slightly soluble in water [<0.1% W/V at 25°C (77°F)]. It melts between 153°C and 156°C (307.4°F and 312.8°F).

Each Nilandron tablet contains 50 mg nilutamide. Other ingredients in Nilandron tablets are corn starch, lactose, providone, docusate sodium, magnesium stearate, and talc.

CLINICAL PHARMACOLOGY:

MECHANISM OF ACTION

Prostate cancer is known to be androgen sensitive and responds to androgen ablation. In animal studies, nilutamide has demonstrated antiandrogenic activity without other hormonal (estrogen, progesterone, mineralocorticoid, and glucocorticoid) effects. *In vitro*, nilutamide blocks the effects of testosterone at the androgen receptor level. *In vivo*, nilutamide interacts with the androgen receptor and prevents the normal androgenic response.

PHARMACOKINETICS

Absorption: Analysis of blood, urine, and feces samples following a single oral 150 mg dose of [^{14}C]-nilutamide in patients with metastatic prostate cancer showed that the drug is rapidly and completely absorbed and that it yields high and persistent plasma concentrations.

Distribution: After absorption of the drug, there is a detectable distribution phase. There is moderate binding of the drug to plasma proteins and low binding to erythrocytes. The binding is nonsaturable except in the case of alpha-1-glycoprotein, which makes a minor contribution to the total concentration of proteins in the plasma. The results of binding studies do not indicate any effects that would cause nonlinear pharmacokinetics.

Metabolism: The results of a human metabolism study using ^{14}C radiolabelled tablets show that nilutamide is extensively metabolized and less than 2% of the drug is excreted unchanged in urine after 5 days. Five metabolites have been isolated from human urine. Two metabolites display an asymmetric center, due to oxidation of a methyl group, resulting in the formation of D- and L-isomers. One of the metabolites was shown *in vitro*, to possess 25 to 50% of the pharmacological activity of the parent drug, and the D-isomer of the active metabolite showed equal or greater potency compared to the L-isomer. However, the pharmacokinetics and the pharmacodynamics of the metabolites have not been fully investigated.

Elimination: The majority (62%) of orally administered [^{14}C]-nilutamide is eliminated in the urine during the first 120 hours after a single 150 mg dose. Fecal elimination is negligible, ranging from 1.4% to 7% of the dose after 4 to 5 days. Excretion of radioactivity in urine likely continues beyond 5 days. The mean elimination half-life of nilutamide determined in studies in which subject received a single dose of 100-300 mg ranged from 38.0 to 59.1 hours with most values between 41 and 49 hours. The elimination of at least one metabolite is generally longer than that of unchanged nilutamide (59-126 hours). During multiple dosing of 3 x 50 mg twice a day, steady state was reached within 2 to 4 weeks for most patients, and mean steady state $AUC_{0-\infty}$ was 110% higher than the $AUC_{0-\infty}$ obtained from the first dose of 3 x 50 mg. These data and *in vitro* metabolism data suggest that upon multiple dosing metabolic enzyme inhibition may occur for this drug.

CLINICAL STUDIES:

Nilutamide through its antiandrogenic activity can complement surgical castration, which suppresses only testicular androgens. The effects of the combined therapy were studied in patients with previously untreated metastatic prostate cancer.

In a double-blind, randomized, multicenter study that enrolled 457 patients (225 treated with orchiectomy and Nilutamide, 232 treated with orchiectomy and placebo), the Nilutamide group showed a statistically significant benefit in time to progression and time to death. The results are summarized in TABLE 1.

TABLE 1

	Nilutamide	Placebo
Median Survival (Months)	27.3	23.6
Progression-Free Survival (Months)	21.1	14.9
Complete or Partial Regression	41%	24%
Improvement in Bone Pain	54%	37%

INDICATIONS AND USAGE:

Metastatic Prostate Cancer: Nilutamide tablets are indicated for use in combination with surgical castration for the treatment of metastatic prostate cancer (Stage D_2). For maximum benefit, Nilutamide treatment must begin on the same day as or on the day after surgical castration.

CONTRAINDICATIONS:

Nilutamide Tablets are Contraindicated in Patients:

with severe hepatic impairment (baseline hepatic enzymes should be evaluated prior to treatment)

with severe respiratory insufficiency

with hypersensitivity to nilutamide or any component of this preparation.

WARNINGS:

Interstitial Pneumonitis: Interstitial Pneumonitis has been reported in 2% of patients in controlled clinical trials in patients exposed to nilutamide. Patients typically presented with progressive exertional dyspnea, and possibly with cough, chest pain, and fever. X-rays showed interstitial or alveolo- interstitial changes. The suggestive signs of pneumonitis most often occurred within the first three months of nilutamide treatment. A routine chest x-ray should be performed before treatment, and patients should be told to report immediately any dyspnea or aggravation of pre-existing dyspnea.

At the onset of dyspnea or worsening of pre-existing dyspnea at any time during treatment, nilutamide should be interrupted until it can be determined if respiratory symptoms are drug related. A chest x-ray should be obtained, and if there are findings suggestive of interstitial pneumonitis, treatment with nilutamide should be discontinued. The pneumonitis is almost always reversible when treatment is discontinued.

If the chest x-ray appears normal. pulmonary function tests including DL_{CO} (diffusing capability of the lung for carbon monoxide) should be performed. If a significant decrease of DL_{CO} and/or a restrictive pattern is observed on pulmonary function testing, nilutamide treatment should be terminated. In the absence of chest x-ray and pulmonary function test findings consistent with interstitial pneumonitis, treatment with nilutamide can be restarted under close monitoring of pulmonary symptoms.

Because interstitial pneurnonltis was reported in 8 of 47 patients (17%) in a small study performed in Japan, specific caution should be observed in the treatment of Asian patients.

Hepatitis: Hepatitis or marked increases in liver enzymes leading to drug discontinuation occurred in 1% of nilutamide patients in controlled clinical trials;

Serum hepatic enzyme levels should be measured at baseline and at regular intervals (3 months); if transaminases increase over 2-3 times the upper limit of normal, treatment should be discontinued.

Appropriate laboratory testing should be done at the first symptom/sign of liver injury (*e.g.*, jaundice, dark urine, fatigue, abdominal pain, or unexplained gastrointestinal symptoms) and nilutamide treatment must be discontinued immediately if transaminases exceed 3 times the upper limit of normal.

There has been a report of elevated hepatic enzymes followed by death in a 65-year-old patient being treated with nilutamide.

Other: Foreign post marketing surveillance has revealed isolated cases of aplastic anemia in which a causal relationship with nilutamide could not be ascertained.

PRECAUTIONS:

Information for the Patient: Patients should be informed that nilutamide tablets should be started on the day of, or on the day after, surgical castration. They should also be informed that they should not interrupt their dosing of nilutamide or stop taking this medication without consulting their physician. Because of the possibility of interstitial pneumonitis, patients should also be told to report immediately any dyspnea or aggravation of pre-existing dyspnea.

Because of the possibility of hepatitis, patients should be told to consult with their physician should nausea, vomiting, abdominal pain, or jaundice occur.

Because of the possibility of an intolerance to alcohol (facial flushes, malaise, hypotension) following ingestion of nilutamide, it is recommended that intake of alcoholic beverages be avoided by patients who experience this reaction. This effect has been reported in about 5% of patients treated with nilutamide.

In clinical trials 13% to 57% of patients receiving nilutamide reported a delay in adaptation to dark, ranging from seconds to a few minutes, when passing from a lighted area to a dark area. This effect sometimes does not abate as drug treatment is continued. Patients who experience this effect should be cautioned about driving at night or through tunnels. This effect can be alleviated by the wearing of tinted glasses.

Carcinogenesis, Mutagenesis, and Impairment of Fertility: Administration of nilutamide to rats for 18 months at doses of 0, 5, 15, or 45 mg/kg/day produced benign Leydig cell tumors in 35% of the high-dose male rats (AUC exposure in high-dose rats were approximately 1-2 times human AUC exposures with therapeutic doses). The increased incidence of Leydig cell tumors is secondary to elevated luteinizing hormone (LH) concentrations resulting from loss of feedback inhibition at the pituitary. Elevated LH and testosterone concentrations are not observed in castrated men receiving nilutamide. Nilutamide had no effect on the incidence, size, or time of onset of any spontaneous tumor in rats.

Nilutamide displayed no mutagenic effects in a variety of *in vitro* and *in vivo* tests (Ames test, mouse micronucleus test, and two chromosomal aberration tests).

In reproduction studies in rats, nilutamide had no effect on the reproductive function of males and females, and no lethal, teratogenic or growth-suppressive effects on fetuses were found. The maximal dose at which nilutamide did not affect reproductive function in either sex or have an effect on fetuses was estimated to be 45 mg/kg orally (AUC exposures in rats approximately 1-2 times human therapeutic AUC exposures).

Pregnancy Category C: Animal reproduction studies have not been conducted with nilutamide. It is also not known whether nilutamide can cause fetal harm when administered to a pregnant woman or can affect reproductive capacity. Nilutamide should be given to a pregnant woman only if clearly needed.

Pediatric Use: Safety and effectiveness in pediatric patients have not been determined.

DRUG INTERACTIONS:

In vitro, nilutamide has been shown to inhibit the activity of liver cytochrome P-450 isoenzymes and, therefore, may reduce the metabolism of compounds requiring these systems.

Consequently, drugs with a low therapeutic margin, such as vitamin K antagonists, phenytoin and theophylline, could have a delayed elimination and increases in their serum half-life leading to a toxic level. The dosage of these drugs or others with a similar metabolism may need to be modified if they are administered concomitantly with nilutamide. For example, when vitamin K antagonists are administered concomitantly with nilutamide, prothrombin time should be carefully monitored and, if necessary, the dosage of vitamin K antagonists should be reduced.

ADVERSE REACTIONS:

The following adverse experiences were reported during a multicenter clinical trial comparing nilutamide + surgical castration versus placebo + surgical castration. The most frequently reported (greater than 5%) adverse experiences during treatment with nilutamide tablets in combination with surgical castration are listed in TABLE 2. For comparison, adverse experiences seen with surgical castration and placebo are also listed.

TABLE 2

Adverse Experience	Nilutamide + Surgical Castration (N=225) % All	Placebo + Surgical Castration (N=232) % All
Cardiovascular System		
Hypertension	5.3	2.6
Digestive System		
Nausea	9.8	6.0
Constipation	7.1	3.9
Endocrine System		
Hot Flushes	28.4	22.4
Metabolic and Nutritional System		
Increased AST	8.0	3.9
Increased ALT	7.6	4.3
Nervous System		
Dizziness	7.1	3.4
Respiratory System		
Dyspnea	6.2	7.3
Special Senses		
Impaired Adaption to Dark	12.9	1.3
Abnormal Vision	6.7	1.7
Urogenital System		
Urinary Tracy Infection	8.0	9.1

The overall incidence of adverse experiences was 86% (194/225) for the nilutamide group and 81% (188/ 232) for the placebo group. The following adverse experiences were reported during a multicenter clinical trial comparing nilutamide + leuprolide versus placebo + leuprolide. The most frequently reported (greater than 5%) adverse experiences during treatment with nilutamide tablets in combination with leuprolide are listed in TABLE 3. For comparison, adverse experiences seen with leuprolide and placebo are also listed.

TABLE 3

Adverse Experience	Nilutamide + Leuprolide (N=209) % All	Placebo + Leuprolide (N=202) % All
Body as a Whole		
Pain	26.6	27.7
Headache	13.9	10.4
Asthenia	19.1	20.8
Back Pain	11.5	16.8
Abdominal pain	10.0	5.4
Chest pain	7.2	4.5
Flu syndrome	7.2	3.0
Fever	5.3	6.4
Cardiovascular System		
Hypertension	9.1	9.9
Digestive System		
Nausea	23.9	8.4
Constipation	19.6	16.8
Anorexia	11.0	6.4
Dyspepsia	6.7	4.5
Vomiting	5.7	4.0
Endocrine System		
Hot flushes	66.5	59.4
Impotence	11.0	12.9
Libido decreased	11.0	4.5
Hemic and Lymphatic System		
Anemia	7.2	6.4
Metabolic and Nutritional System		
Increased AST	12.9	13.9
Peripheral edema	12.4	17.3
Increased ALT	9.1	8.9
Musculo-Skeletal System		
Bone pain	6.2	5.0
Nervous System		
Insomnia	16.3	15.8
Dizziness	10.0	11.4
Depression	8.6	7.4
Hypesthesia	5.3	2.0
Respiratory System		
Dyspnea	10.5	7.4
Upper respiratory infection	8.1	10.9
Pneumonia	5.3	3.5
Skin and Appendages		
Sweating	6.2	3.0
Body hair loss	5.7	0.5
Dry skin	5.3	2.5
Rash	5.3	4.0
Special Senses		
Impaired adaption to dark	56.9	5.4
Chromatopsia	8.6	0.0
Impaired adaption to light	7.7	1.0
Abnormal Vision	6.2	4.5
Urogenital System		
Testicular atrophy	16.3	12.4
Gynecomastia	10.5	11.9
Urinary tract infection	8.6	21.3
Hematuria	8.1	7.9
Urinary tract disorder	7.2	10.4
Nocturia	6.7	6.4

The overall incidence of adverse experiences is 99.5% (208/209) for the nilutamide group and 98.5% (199/202) for the placebo group. Some frequently occurring adverse experiences, for example hot flushes, impotence, and decreased libido, are known to be associated with low serum androgen levels and known to occur with medical or surgical castration alone. Notable was the higher incidence of visual disturbances (variously described as impaired adaptation to darkness, abnormal vision, and colored vision), which led to treatment discontinuation in 1% to 2% of patients.

ADVERSE REACTIONS: *(cont'd)*

Interstitial pneumonitis occurred in one (<1%) patient receiving nilutamide in combination with surgical castration and in seven patients (3%) receiving nilutamide in combination with leuprolide and one patient receiving placebo in combination with leuprolide. Overall, it has been reported in 2% of patients receiving nilutamide. This included a report of interstitial pneumonitis in 8 of 47 patients (17%) in a small study performed in Japan.

In addition, the following adverse experiences were reported in 2 to 5% of patients treated with nilutamide in combination with leuprolide or orchiectomy.

Body as a Whole: Malaise (2%).

Cardiovascular System: Angina (2%), heart failure (3%), syncope (2%)

Digestive System: Diarrhea (2%), gastrointestinal disorder (2%), gastrointestinal hemorrhage (2%), melena (2%)

Metabolic and Nutritional System: Alcohol Intolerance (5%), edema (2%), weight loss (2%)

Musculoskeletal System: Arthritis (2%).

Nervous System: Dry mouth (2%), nervousness (2%), paresthesia (3%)

Respiratory System Cough increased (2%), interstitial lung disease (2%), lung disorder (4%), rhinitis (2%)

Skin and Appendages: Pruritus (2%).

Special Senses Cataract (2%), photophobia (2%)

Laboratory Values: Haptoglobin increased (2%), leukopenia (3%), alkaline phosphatase increased (3%), BUN increased (2%), creatinine increased (2%), hyperglycemia (4%).

OVERDOSAGE:

One case of massive overdosage has been published. A 79-year-old man attempted suicide by ingesting 13g of nilutamide (*i.e.,* 43 times the maximum recommended dose). Despite immediate gastric lavage and oral administration of activated charcoal, plasma nilutamide levels peaked at 6 times the normal range 2 hours after ingestion. There were no clinical signs or symptoms or changes in parameters such as transaminases or chest x-ray. Maintenance treatment (150 mg/day) was resumed 30 days later.

In repeated-dose tolerance studies, doses of 600 mg/day and 900 mg/day were administered to 9 and 4 patients, respectively. The ingestion of these doses was associated with gastrointestinal disorders, including nausea and vomiting, malaise, headache, and dizziness. In addition, a transient elevation in hepatic enzyme levels was noted in one patient.

Since nilutamide is protein bound, dialysis may not be useful as treatment for overdose. As in the management of overdosage with any drug, it should be borne in mind that multiple agents may have been taken. If vomiting does not occur spontaneously, it should be induced if the patient is alert. General supportive care, including frequent monitoring of the vital signs and close observation of the patient is indicated.

DOSAGE AND ADMINISTRATION:

The recommended dosage is six tablets (50 mg each) once a day for a total daily dose of 300 mg for 30 days followed thereafter by three tablets (50 mg each) once a day for a total daily dosage of 150 mg. Nilutamide tablets can be taken with or without food.

ANIMAL PHARMACOLOGY:

Administration of nilutamide to beagle dogs resulted in drug-related deaths at dose levels that produce AUC exposures in dogs much lower than the AUC exposures of men receiving the therapeutic doses of 150 and 300 mg/day. Nilutamide-induced toxicity in dogs was cumulative with progressively lower doses producing death when given for longer durations. Nilutamide given to dogs at 60 mg/kg/day (1-2 times human AUC exposure) for 1 month produced 100% mortality. Administration of 20 and 30 mg/kg/day nliutamide (½ -1 times human AUC exposure) for 6 months resulted in 20% and 70% mortality in treated dogs. Administration to dogs of 3, 6, and 12 mg/kg/day nilutamide (1/10-1/2 human AUC exposure) for 1 year resulted in 8%, 33%, and 50% mortality, respectively. **A "no-effect level" for nilutamide-induced mortality in dogs was not identified.** Pathology data from the one-year oral toxicity study suggest that the deaths in dogs were secondary to liver toxicity. Marked-to-massive hepatocellular swelling and vacuolization were observed in affected dogs. Liver toxicity in dogs was not consistently associated with elevations of liver enzymes.

Administration of nilutamide to rats at a dose level of 45 mg/kg/day (AUC exposure in rats 1-2 times human therapeutic AUC exposures) for 18 months increased the incidence of lung pathology (granulomatous inflammation and chronic alveolitis).

The hepatic and pulmonary adverse effects observed in nilutamide-treated animals and men are similar to effects observed with another nitroaromatic compound, nitrofurantoin. Nilutamide and nitrofurantoin are both metabolized *in vitro* to nitroanion free-radicals by microsomal NADPH-cytochrome P450 reductase in the lungs and liver of rats and humans.

HOW SUPPLIED:

White, biconvex (with a triangular logo on one face and an internal reference number [168] on the other), cylindrical (about 7 mm in diameter) NILANDRON tablets contain 50 mg of nilutamide

Storage: Store at room temperature between 15°C and 30°C (59°F and 86°F). Protect from light.

NIMODIPINE *(001888)*

CATEGORIES: Aneurysm; Antihypertensives; Calcium Channel Blockers; Cardiovascular Drugs; Hemorrhage; Subarachnoid Hemorrhage; Vasodilating Agents; Hypertension*; Pregnancy Category C; FDA Approved 1988 Dec
* Indication not approved by the FDA

BRAND NAMES: *Admon*; **Nimotop**; *Periplum*; *Vasotop*
(International brand names outside U.S. in italics)

FORMULARIES: Aetna; BC-BS

COST OF THERAPY: $1,325.21 (Subarachnoid Hemorrhage; Capsule; 30 mg; 12/day; 21 days)

DESCRIPTION:

Nimodipine belongs to the class of pharmacological agents known as calcium channel blockers. Nimodipine is isopropyl (2 - methoxyethyl) 1, 4 - dihydro - 2, 6 - dimethyl - 4 - (3 - nitrophenyl) - 3, 5 - pyridine - dicarboxylate. It has a molecular weight of 418.5 and a molecular formula of $C_{21}H_{26}N_2O_7$.

Nimodipine is a yellow crystalline substance, practically insoluble in water.

Nimotop capsules are formulated as soft gelatin capsules for oral administration. Each liquid filled capsule contains 30 mg of nimodipine in a vehicle of glycerin, peppermint oil, purified water and polyethylene glycol 400. The soft gelatin capsule shell contains gelatin, glycerin, purified water and titanium dioxide.

CLINICAL PHARMACOLOGY:

Mechanism of Action: Nimodipine is a calcium channel blocker. The contractile processes of smooth muscle cells are dependent upon calcium ions, which enter these cells during depolarization as slow ionic transmembrane currents. Nimodipine inhibits calcium ion transfer into these cells and thus inhibits contractions of vascular smooth muscle. In animal experiments, nimodipine had a greater effect on cerebral arteries than on arteries elsewhere in the body perhaps because it is highly lipophilic, allowing it to cross the blood-brain barrier; concentrations of nimodipine as high as 12.5 ng/ml have been detected in the cerebrospinal fluid of nimodipine treated subarachnoid hemorrhage (SAH) patients.

Based on animal experiments, it was hoped that nimodipine would prevent cerebral arterial spasm in SAH patients. While the clinical studies described below demonstrate a favorable effect by nimodipine on the severity of neurological deficits caused by cerebral vasospasm following SAH, there is no arteriographic evidence that the drug either prevents or relieves the spasm of these arteries. The actual mechanism of action in humans is, therefore, unknown.

Pharmacokinetics and Metabolism: In man, nimodipine is rapidly absorbed after oral administration, and peak concentrations are generally attained within one hour. The terminal elimination half-life is approximately 8 to 9 hours but earlier elimination rates are much more rapid, equivalent to a half-life of 1-2 hours; a consequence is the need for frequent (every 4 hours) dosing. There were no signs of accumulation when nimodipine was given three times a day for seven days. Nimodipine is over 95% bound to plasma proteins. The binding was concentration independent over the range of 10 ng/ml to 10 mcg/ml. Nimodipine is eliminated almost exclusively in the form of metabolites and less than 1% is recovered in the urine as unchanged drug. Numerous metabolites, all of which are either inactive or considerably less active than the parent compound, have been identified. Because of a high first-pass metabolism, the bioavailability of nimodipine averages 13% after oral administration. The bioavailability is significantly increased in patients with hepatic cirrhosis, with C_{max} approximately double that in normals which necessitates lowering the dose in this group of patients (see DOSAGE AND ADMINISTRATION.) In a study of 24 healthy male volunteers, administration of nimodipine capsules following a standard breakfast resulted in a 68% lower peak plasma concentration and 38% lower bioavailability relative to dosing under fasted conditions.

CLINICAL STUDIES:

Nimodipine has been shown, in 4 randomized, placebo-controlled trials, to reduce the severity of neurological deficits resulting from vasospasm in patients who have had a recent subarachnoid hemorrhage (SAH). The trials used doses ranging from 20-30 mg to 90 mg every 4 hours, with drug given for 21 days in 3 studies, and for at least 18 days in the other. Three of the four trials followed patients for 3-6 months. Three of the trials studied relatively well patients, with all or most patients in Hunt and Hess Grades I-II (essentially free of focal deficits after the initial bleed); the fourth studied much sicker patients, Hunt and Hess Grades III-V. Two studies, one domestic, one French, were similar in design, with relatively unimpaired SAH patients randomized to nimodipine or placebo. In each, a judgment was made as to whether any late-developing deficit was due to spasm or other causes, and the deficits were graded. Both studies showed significantly fewer severe deficits due to spasm in the nimodipine group; the second (French) study showed fewer spasm-related deficits of all severities. No effect was seen on deficits not related to spasm (TABLE 1):

TABLE 1

Study	Dose	Grade*	Patients: Number Analyzed		Any Deficit Due to Spasm	Numbers With Severe Deficit
1.	20-30 mg	I-III	Nimodipine	56	13	1
			Placebo	60	16	8**
2.	60 mg	I-III	Nimodipine	31	4	2
			Placebo	39	11	10**

* Hunt and Hess Grade
** p = 0.03

A Canadian study entered much sicker patients, who had a high rate of death and disability, and used a dose of 90 mg every 4 hours, but was otherwise similar to the first two studies. Analysis of delayed ischemic deficits, many of which result from spasm, showed a significant reduction in spasm-related deficits. Among analyzed patients (72 nimodipine, 82 placebo), there were the following outcomes (TABLE 2):

TABLE 2

	Delayed Ischemic Deficits (DID): Nimodipine n (%)	Delayed Ischemic Deficits (DID): Placebo n (%)	Permanent Deficits: Nimodipine n (%)	Permanent Deficits: Placebo n (%)
DID Spasm Alone	8 (11)*	25 (31)	5 (7)*	22 (27)
DID Spasm Contributing	18 (25)	21 (26)	16 (22)	17 (21)
DID Without Spasm	7 (10)	8 (10)	6 (8)	7 (9)
No DID	39 (54)	28 (34)	45 (63)	36 (44)

* P = 0.001, nimodipine vs placebo

A fourth, large, study was performed in the United Kingdom in SAH patients with all grades of severity (but about 90% were in Grades I-III). Outcomes were not defined as spasm related or not but there was a significant reduction in the overall rate of infarction and severely disabling neurological outcome at 3 months (TABLE 3):

TABLE 3

	Nimodipine	Placebo
Total patients	278	276
Good recovery	199*	169
Moderate disability	24	16
Severe disability	12**	31
Death	43***	60

* p = 0.0444 - good and moderate vs severe and dead
** p = 0.001 - severe disability
*** p = 0.056 - death

A dose-ranging study comparing 30, 60 and 90 mg doses found a generally low rate of spasm-related neurological deficits but no significant relation of response to dose.

The effect of nimodipine on mortality is not yet clear. The large United Kingdom study showed near-significantly improved survival. The two smaller studies (domestic, French) had too few deaths to contribute to this question. The Canadian study, despite showing markedly

CLINICAL STUDIES: *(cont'd)*

decreased spasm-related deficits, showed overall (all patients randomized) greater 90 day mortality, 49/91 (54%) on nimodipine vs 38/97 (39%) on placebo, a significant difference. Most of the deaths appeared, in this very severely ill group (Hunt and Hess Grades III-V), to be consequences of SAH, but a drug effect cannot be ruled out. In this study 90 mg every 4 hours was the dose used, perhaps too high for the very ill population studied. The 90 mg dose is not recommended nor is treatment of Hunt and Hess Grades IV-V patients.

INDICATIONS AND USAGE:

Nimodipine is indicated for the improvement of neurological outcome by reducing the incidence and severity of ischemic deficits in patients with subarachnoid hemorrhage from ruptured congenital aneurysms who are in good neurological condition post-ictus (*e.g.,* Hunt and Hess Grades I-III).

CONTRAINDICATIONS:

None known.

PRECAUTIONS:

GENERAL

Blood Pressure: Nimodipine has the hemodynamic effects expected of a calcium channel blocker, although they are generally not marked. In patients with subarachnoid hemorrhage given nimodipine in clinical studies, about 5% were reported to have had lowering of the blood pressure and about 1% left the study because of this (not all could be attributed to nimodipine). Nevertheless, blood pressure should be carefully monitored during treatment with nimodipine based on its known pharmacology and the known effects of calcium channel blockers.

Hepatic Disease: The metabolism of nimodipine is decreased in patients with impaired hepatic function. Such patients should have their blood pressure and pulse rate monitored closely and should be given a lower dose (see DOSAGE AND ADMINISTRATION.)

Intestinal pseudo-obstruction and ileus have been reported rarely in patients treated with nimodipine. A causal relationship has not been established. The condition has responded to conservative management.

LABORATORY TEST INTERACTIONS

None known.

CARCINOGENESIS, MUTAGENESIS, AND IMPAIRMENT OF FERTILITY

In a two-year study, higher incidences of adenocarcinoma of the uterus and Leydig-cell adenoma of the testes were observed in rats given a diet containing 1800 ppm nimodipine (equivalent to 91 to 121 mg/kg/day nimodipine) than in placebo controls. The differences were not statistically significant, however, and the higher rates were well within historical control range for these tumors in the Wistar strain. Nimodipine was found not to be carcinogenic in a 91-week mouse study but the high dose of 1800 ppm nimodipine-in-feed (546 to 774 mg/kg/day) shortened the life expectancy of the animals. Mutagenicity studies, including the Ames, micronucleus and dominant lethal tests were negative.

Nimodipine did not impair the fertility and general reproductive performance of male and female Wistar rats following oral doses of up to 30 mg/kg/day when administered daily for more than 10 weeks in the males and 3 weeks in the females prior to mating and continued to day 7 of pregnancy. This dose in a rat is about 4 times the equivalent clinical dose of 60 mg q4h in a 50 kg patient.

PREGNANCY CATEGORY C

Nimodipine has been shown to have a teratogenic effect in Himalayan rabbits. Incidences of malformations and stunted fetuses were increased at oral doses of 1 and 10 mg/kg/day administered (by gavage) from day 6 through day 18 of pregnancy but not at 3.0 mg/kg/day in one of two identical rabbit studies. In the second study an increased incidence of stunted fetuses was seen at 1.0 mg/kg/day but not at higher doses. Nimodipine was embryotoxic, causing resorption and stunted growth of fetuses, in Long Evans rats at 100 mg/kg/day administered by gavage from day 6 through day 15 of pregnancy. In two other rat studies, doses of 30 mg/kg/day nimodipine administered by gavage from day 16 of gestation and continued until sacrifice (day 20 of pregnancy or day 21 post partum) were associated with higher incidences of skeletal variation, stunted fetuses and stillbirths but no malformations. There are no adequate and well controlled studies in pregnant women to directly assess the effect on human fetuses. Nimodipine should be used during pregnancy only if the potential benefit justifies the potential risk to the fetus.

NURSING MOTHERS

Nimodipine and/or its metabolites have been shown to appear in rat milk at concentrations much higher than in maternal plasma. It is not known whether the drug is excreted in human milk. Because many drugs are excreted in human milk, nursing mothers are advised not to breast feed their babies when taking the drug.

PEDIATRIC USE

Safety and effectiveness in children have not been established.

DRUG INTERACTIONS:

It is possible that the cardiovascular action of other calcium channel blockers could be enhanced by the addition of nimodipine.

In Europe, nimodipine was observed to occasionally intensify the effect of antihypertensive compounds taken concomitantly by patients suffering from hypertension; this phenomenon was not observed in North American clinical trials.

A study in eight healthy volunteers has shown a 50% increase in mean peak nimodipine plasma concentrations and a 90% increase in mean area under the curve, after a one-week course of cimetidine at 1,000 mg/day and nimodipine at 90 mg/day. This effect may be mediated by the known inhibition of hepatic cytochrome P-450 by cimetidine, which could decrease first-pass metabolism of nimodipine.

ADVERSE REACTIONS:

Adverse experiences were reported by 92 of 823 patients with subarachnoid hemorrhage (11.2%) who were given nimodipine. The most frequently reported adverse experience was decreased blood pressure in 4.4% of these patients. Twenty-nine of 479 (6.1%) placebo treated patients also reported adverse experiences. The events reported with a frequency greater than 1% are displayed TABLE 4A and 4B by dose.

There were no other adverse experiences reported by the patients who were given 0.35 mg/kg q4h, 30 mg q4h or 120 mg q4h. Adverse experiences with an incidence rate of less than 1% in the 60 mg q4h dose group were: hepatitis; itching; gastrointestinal hemorrhage; thrombocytopenia; anemia; palpitations; vomiting; flushing; diaphoresis; wheezing; phenytoin toxicity; lightheadedness; dizziness; rebound vasospasm; jaundice; hypertension; hematoma.

Adverse experiences with an incidence rate less than 1% in the 90 mg q4h dose group were: itching, gastrointestinal hemorrhage; thrombocytopenia; neurological deterioration; vomiting; diaphoresis; congestive heart failure; hyponatremia; decreasing platelet count; disseminated intravascular coagulation; deep vein thrombosis.

ADVERSE REACTIONS: *(cont'd)*

TABLE 4A

Sign/Symptom	Dose q4h Number of Patients (%) Nimodipine 0.35 mg/kg (n=82)	30 mg (n=71)	60 mg (n=494)
Decreased Blood Pressure	1 (1.2)	0	19 (3.8)
Abnormal Liver Function Test	1 (1.2)	0	2 (0.4)
Edema	0	0	2 (0.4)
Diarrhea	0	3 (4.2)	0
Rash	2 (2.4)	0	3 (0.6)
Headache	0	1 (1.4)	6 (1.2)
Gastrointestinal Symptoms	2 (2.4)	0	0
Nausea	1 (1.2)	1 (1.4)	6 (1.2)
Dyspnea	1 (1.2)	0	0
EKG Abnormalities	0	1 (1.4)	0
Tachycardia	0	1 (1.4)	0
Bradycardia	0	0	5 (1.0)
Muscle Pain/Cramp	0	1 (1.4)	1 (0.2)
Acne	0	1 (1.4)	0
Depression	0	1 (1.4)	0

TABLE 4B

Sign/Symptom	Dose q4h Number of Patients (%) Nimodipine 90 mg (n=172)	120 mg (n=4)	Placebo (n=479)
Decreased Blood Pressure	14 (8.1)	2 (50.0)	6 (1.2)
Abnormal Liver Function Test	1 (0.6)	0	7 (1.5)
Edema	2 (1.2)	0	3 (0.6)
Diarrhea	3 (1.7)	0	3 (0.6)
Rash	2 (1.2)	0	3 (0.6)
Headache	0	0	1 (0.2)
Gastrointestinal Symptoms	2 (1.2)	0	0
Nausea	1 (0.6)	0	0
Dyspnea	0	0	0
EKG Abnormalities	1 (0.6)	0	0
Tachycardia	0	0	0
Bradycardia	1 (0.6)	0	0
Muscle Pain/Cramp	1 (0.6)	0	0
Acne	0	0	0
Depression	0	0	0

As can be seen from the table, side effects that appear related to nimodipine use based on increased incidence with higher dose or a higher rate compared to placebo control, included decreased blood pressure, edema and headaches which are known pharmacologic actions of calcium channel blockers. It must be noted, however, that SAH is frequently accompanied by alterations in consciousness which lead to an under reporting of adverse experiences. Patients who received nimodipine in clinical trials for other indications reported flushing (2.1%), headache (4.1%) and fluid retention (0.3%), typical responses to calcium channel blockers. As a calcium channel blocker, nimodipine may have the potential to exacerbate heart failure in susceptible patients or to interfere with A-V conduction, but these events were not observed.

No clinically significant effects on hematologic factors, renal or hepatic function or carbohydrate metabolism have been causally associated with oral nimodipine. Isolated cases of non-fasting elevated serum glucose levels (0.8%), elevated LDH levels (0.4%), decreased platelet counts (0.3%), elevated alkaline phosphatase levels (0.2%) and elevated SGPT levels (0.2%) have been reported rarely.

DRUG ABUSE AND DEPENDENCE:

There have been no reported instances of drug abuse or dependence with nimodipine.

OVERDOSAGE:

There have been no reports of overdosage from the oral administration of nimodipine. Symptoms of overdosage would be expected to be related to cardiovascular effects such as excessive peripheral vasodilation with marked systemic hypotension. Clinically significant hypotension due to nimodipine overdosage may require active cardiovascular support. Norepinephrine or dopamine may be helpful in restoring blood pressure. Since nimodipine is highly protein-bound, dialysis is not likely to be of benefit.

DOSAGE AND ADMINISTRATION:

Nimodipine is given orally in the form of ivory colored, soft gelatin 30 mg capsules for subarachnoid hemorrhage.

The oral dose is 60 mg (two 30 mg capsules) every 4 hours for 21 consecutive days. Oral nimodipine therapy should commence within 96 hours of the subarachnoid hemorrhage.

If the capsule cannot be swallowed, e.g. at the time of surgery, or if the patient is unconscious, a hole should be made in both ends of the capsule with an 18 gauge needle, and the contents of the capsule extracted into a syringe. The contents should then be emptied into the patient's *in situ* naso-gastric tube and washed down the tube with 30 ml of normal saline (0.9%).

Patients with hepatic cirrhosis have substantially reduced clearance and approximately doubled C_{max}. Dosage should be reduced to 30 mg every 4 hours, with close monitoring of blood pressure and heart rate.

HOW SUPPLIED:

Each ivory colored, soft gelatin Nimotop capsule is imprinted with the word Miles and the number 855 and contains 30 mg of nimodipine. The 30 mg capsules are packaged in unit dose foil pouches and supplied in cartons containing 100 capsules. The product is also available in unit dose safety pack foil pouches containing 30 capsules per carton. The capsules should be stored in the manufacturer's original foil package at a controlled room temperature of 59°F to 86°F (15°C to 30°C).

Capsules should be protected from light and freezing.

TABLE 5

	Strength	Capsule Identification
Unit Dose Package of 100:	30 mg	Nimotop
Unit Dose Package of 30:	30 mg	Nimotop

HOW SUPPLIED - EQUIVALENTS NOT AVAILABLE:

Capsule, Elastic - Oral - 30 mg

30's	$165.12	NIMOTOP, Bayer	00026-2855-70
100's	$525.88	NIMOTOP, Bayer	00026-2855-48

NISOLDIPINE *(003246)*

CATEGORIES: Antihypertensives; Calcium Channel Blockers; Cardiovascular Drugs; Hypertension; FDA Class 1S ("Standard Review"); FDA Approved 1995 Feb

BRAND NAMES: *Baymycard* (Germany); **Sular**; *Syscor* (Mexico)
(International brand names outside U.S. in italics)

DESCRIPTION:

Nisoldipine is an extended release tablet dosage form of the dihydropyridine calcium channel blocker nisoldipine. Nisoldipine is 3, 5-pyridinadicarboxylic acid, 1, 4-dihydro-2, 6-dimethyl-4-(2-nitrophenyl)-, methyl, 2-methylpropyl estar, $C_{20}H_{24}N_2O_6$.

Nisoldipine is a yellow crystalline substance, practically insoluble in water but soluble in ethanol. It has a molecular weight of 388.4.

Sular tablets consist of an external coat and an internal core. Both coat and core contain nisoldipine, the coat as a slow release formulation and the core as a fast release formulation. SULAR tablets contain either 10, 20, 30, or 40 mg of nisoldipine for once-a-day oral administration.

Sular Inert ingredients in the formulation are: hydroxypropylcellulose, lactose, corn starch, crospovidone, microcrystalline cellulose, sodium lauryl sulfate, povidone and magnesium stearate. The inert ingredients in the film coating are: hydroxypropylmethylcellulose, polyethylene glycol, ferric oxide, and titanium dioxide.

CLINICAL PHARMACOLOGY:

MECHANISMS OF ACTION

Nisoldipine is a member of the dihydropyridine class of calcium channel antagonists (calcium ion antagonists or slow channel blockers) that inhibit the transmembrane influx of calcium into vascular smooth muscle and cardiac muscle. It reversibly competes with other dihydropyridines for binding to the calcium channel. Because the contratife process of vascular smoothe muscle is dependent upon the movement of extracellular calcium into the muscle through specific ion channels, inhibition of the calcium channel results in dilation of the arterioles. *in vitro* studies show that the effects of nisoldipine on contractile processes are selective, with greater potency on vascular smooth muscle than on cardiac muscle. Although, like other dihydropyridine calcium channel blockers, nisoldipine has negative inotropic effects *in vitro*, studies conducted in intact anesthetized animals have shown that the vasodilating effect occurs at doses lower than those that affect cardiac contractibility.

The effect of nisoldipine on blood pressure is principally a consequence of a dose-related decrease of peripheral vascular resistance. While nisoldipine, like other dihydropyridines, exhibits a mild diuretic effect, most of the antihypertensive activity is attributed to its effect on peripheral vascular resistance.

PHARMACOKINETICS AND METABOLISM

Nisoldipine pharmacokinetics are independent of the dose in the range of 20 to 60 mg, with plasma concentrations proportional to dose. Nisoldipine accumulation during multiple dosing is predictable from a single dose.

Nisoldipine is relatively well absorbed into the systemic circulation with 87% of the radio labeled drug recovered in urine and feces. The absolute bioavailability of nisoldipine is about 5%. Nisoldipine's low bioavailability is due, in part, to pre-systemic metabolism in the gut wall, and this metabolism decreases from the proximal to the distal parts of the intestine. Food with a high fat content has a pronounced effect on the release of nisoldipine from the coat-core formulation and results in a significant increase in peak concentration (C_{max}) by up to 300%. Total exposure, however, is decreased about 25%, presumably because more of the drug is released proximally. This effect appears to be specific for nisoldipine in the controlled release formulation, as a less pronounced food effect was seen with the immediate release tablet. Concomitant intake of a high fat meat with nisoldipine should be avoided.

Maximal plasma concentrations of nisoldipine are reached 6 to 12 hours after dosing. The terminal elimination half-life (reflecting post absorption clearance of nisoldipine) ranges from 7 to 12 hours. $C_{max}$and AUC increase by factors of approximately 1.3 and 1.5, respectively, from first dose to steady state. After oral administration, the concentration of (+) nisoldipine, the active enantiomer, is about 6 times higher than the (-) inactive enantiomer. The plasma protein binding of nisoldipine is very high, with less than 1% unbound over the plasma concentration range of 100 ng/mL to 10 mcg/mL.

Nisoldipine is highly metabolized; 5 major urinary metabolites have been identified. Although 60-80% of an oral dose undergoes urinary excretion, only traces of unchanged nisoldipine are found in urine. The major biotransformation pathway appears to be the hydroxylation of the isobutyl ester. A hydroxylated derivative of the side chain, present in plasma at concentrations approximately equal to the parent compound, appears to be the only active metabolites, and has about 10% of the activity of the parent compound. Cytochrome P_{450} enzymes are believed to play a major role in the metabolism of nisoldipine. The particular isoenzyme system responsible for its metabolism has not been identified, but other dihydropyridines are metabolized by cytochrome P_{450}IIIA4. Nisoldipine should not be administered with grapefruit juice as this has been shown, in a study of 12 subjects, to interfere with nisoldipine metabolism, resulting in a mean increase in C_{max} of about 3-fold (ranging up to about 7-fold) and AUC of almost 2-fold (ranging up to about 5-fold). A similar phenomenon has been seen with several other dihydropyridine calcium channel blockers.

PHARMACODYNAMICS

Hemodynamic Effects: Administration of a single dose of nisoldipine leads to decreased systemic vascular resistance and blood pressure with a transient increase in heart rate. The change in heart rate is greater with immediate release nisoldipine preparations. The effect on blood pressure is directly related to the initial degree of elevation above normal. Chronic administration of nisoldipine results in a sustained decrease in vascular resistance and small increases in stroke index and left ventricular ejection fraction. A study of the immediate release formulation showed no effect of nisoldipine on the renin-angiotensin-aldosterone system or on plasma norepinephrine concentration in normals. Changes in blood pressure in hypertensive patients given nisoldipine were dose related over the range of 10 - 60 mg/day.

Nisoldipine does not appear to have significant negative inotropic activity in intact animals or humans, and did not lead to worsening of clinical heart failure in three small studies of patients with asymptomatic and symptomatic left ventricular dysfunction. There is little information, however, in patients with severe congestive heart failure, and all calcium channel blockers should be used with caution in any patient with heart failure.

Electrophysiologic Effects: Nisoldipine has no clinically important chronotropic effects. Except for mild shortening of sinus cycle, SA conduction time and AH intervals, single oral doses up to 20 mg of immediate release nisoldipine did not significantly change other conduction parameters. Similar electrophysiologic effects were seen with single IV doses, which could be blunted in patients pre-treated with beta-blockers. Dose and plasma level related flattening or inversion of T-waves have been observed in a few small studies. Such reports were concentrated in patients receiving rapidly increased high doses in one study; the phenomenon has not been a cause of safety concern in large clinical trials.

SPECIAL POPULATIONS

Renal dysfunction: Because renal elimination is not an important pathway, bioavaliability and pharmacokinetics of nisoldipine were not significantly different in patients with various degrees of renal impairment. Dosing adjustments in patients with mild to moderate renal impairment are not necessary.

Geriatrics: Elderly patients have been found to have 2 to 3 fold higher plasma concentrations ($C_{max}$and AUC) than young subjects. This should be reflected in more cautious dosing (See DOSAGE AND ADMINISTRATION)

Hepatic Insufficiency: In patients with liver cirrhosis given 10 mg nisoldipine, plasma concentrations of the parent compound were 4 to 5 times higher than those in healthy young subjects. Lower starting and maintenance doses should be used in cirrhotic patients (See DOSAGE AND ADMINISTRATION)

Gender and Race: The effect of gender or race on the pharmacokinetics of nisoldipine has not been investigated.

Disease States: Hypertension does not significantly alter the pharmacokinetics of nisoldipine.

CLINICAL STUDIES:

Clinical Studies in Hypertension The antihypertensive efficacy of nisoldipine was studied in 5 double-blind, placebo-controlled, randomized studies, in which over 600 patients were treated with nisoldipine as monotherapy and about 300 with placebo; 4 of the five studies compared 2 or 3 fixed doses while the fifth allowed titration from 10 - 40 mg. Once daily administration of nisoldipine produced sustained reductions in systolic and diastolic blood pressure at trough, 24 hours post-dose, in these studies, as shown below. Changes in standing blood pressure were similar:

TABLE 1 Mean Supine Trough Systolic And Diastolic Blood Pressure Changes (mm Hg)

Nisoldipine Dose (mg/day)	10 mg	20 mg	30 mg	40 mg	60 mg	10-40 mg titrated
Systolic	6	11	11	14	15	15
Diastolic	3	6	7	7	10	8

In patients receiving atenolol, supine blood pressure reductions with nisoldipine at 20, 40, and 60 mg once daily were 12/6, 19/8, and 22/10 mm Hg, respectively. The sustained antihypertensive effect of nisoldipine was demonstrated by 24 hour blood pressure monitoring and examination of peak and trough effects. The trough/peak ratios ranged from 70 to 100% for diastolic and systolic blood pressure. The mean change in heart rate in these studies was less than one beat per minute. In 4 of the 5 studies, patients received initial doses of 20 - 30 mg nisoldipine without incident (excessive effects on blood pressure or heart rate). The fifth study started patients on lower doses of nisoldipine.

Patient race and gender did not influence the blood pressure lowering effect of nisoldipine. Despite the higher plasma concentration of nisoldipine in the elderly, there was no consistent difference in their blood pressure response except that the 10 mg dose was somewhat more effective than in non-elderly patients. No postural effect on blood pressure was apparent and there was no evidence of tolerance to the antihypertensive effect of nisoldipine in patients treated for up to one year.

INDICATIONS AND USAGE:

Nisoldipine is indicated for the treatment of hypertension. It may be used alone or in combination with other antihypertensive agents.

CONTRAINDICATIONS:

Nisoldipine is contraindicated in patients with known hypersensitivity to dihydropyridine calcium channel blockers.

WARNINGS:

Increased angina and/or myocardial infarction in patients with coronary artery disease: Rarely, patients, particularly those with severe obstructive coronary artery disease, have developed increased frequency, duration and/or severity of angina, or acute myocardial infarction on starting calcium channel blocker therapy or at the time of dosage increase. The mechanism of this effect has not been established. In controlled studies of nisoldipine in patients with angina this was seen about 1.5% of the time in patients given nisoldipine, compared with 0.9% in patients given placebo.

PRECAUTIONS:

GENERAL

Hypotension: Because nisoldipine, like other vasodilators, decreases peripheral vascular resistance, careful monitoring of blood pressure during the initial administration and titration of nisoldipine is recommended. Close observation is especially important for patients already taking medications that are known to lower blood pressure. Although in most patients the hypotensive effect of nisoldipine is modest and well tolerated, occasional patients have had excessive and poorly tolerated hypotension. These responses have usually occurred during initial titration or at the time of subsequent upward dosage adjustment.

Congestive Heart Failure: Although acute hemodynamic studies of nisoldipine in patients with NYHA Class II-IV heart failure have not demonstrated negative inotropic effects, safety of nisoldipine in patients with heart failure has not been established. Caution therefore should be exercised when using nisoldipine in patients with heart failure or compromised ventricular function, particularly in combination with a beta-blocker.

Patients with Hepatic Impairment: Because nisoldipine is extensively metabolized by the liver and, in patients with cirrhosis, it reaches blood concentrations about 5 times those in normals, nisoldipine should be administered cautiously in patients with severe hepatic dysfunction (See DOSAGE AND ADMINISTRATION).

LABORATORY TESTS

Nisoldipine is not known to interfere with the interpretation of laboratory tests.

CARCINOGENESIS, MUTAGENESIS, AND IMPAIRMENT OF FERTILITY

Dietary administration of nisoldipine to male and female rats for up to 24 months (mean doses up to 82 and 111 mg/kg/day, 15 and 19 times the maximum recommended human dose (MRHD) on a mg/m^2 basis, respectively) and female mice for up to 21 months (mean doses of up to 217 mg/kg/day, 20 times the MRHD on a mg/m^2 basis) revealed no evidence of tumorigenic effect of nisoldipine. In male mice receiving a mean dose of 163 mg nisoldipine/kg/day (16 times the MRHD of 60 mg/day on a mg/m^{2}basis), an increased frequency of stomach papilloma, but still within the historical range, was observed. No evidence of stomach neoplasia was observed at lower doses (up to 58 mg/kg/day). Nisoldipine

PRECAUTIONS: *(cont'd)*

was negative when tested in a battery of genotoxicity assays including the Ames test and the CHO/HGRPT assay for mutagenicity and the *in vivo* mouse micronucleus test and *in vitro* CHO cell test for clastogenicity.

When administered to male and female rats at doses of up to 30 mg/kg/day (about 5 times the MRHD on a mg/m^2 basis) nisoldipine had no effect on fertility.

PREGNANCY CATEGORY C

Nisoldipine was neither teratogenic nor fetotoxic at doses that were maternally toxic. Nisoldipine was fetotoxic but not teratogenic in rats and rabbits at doses resulting in maternal toxicity (reduced maternal body weight gain). In pregnant rats, increased fetal resorption (post-implantation loss) was observed at 100 mg/kg/day and decreased fetal weight was observed at both 30 and 100 mg/kg/day. These doses are, respectively, about 5 and 16 times the MRHD when compared on a mg/m^2. In a study in which pregnant rabbits, decreased fetal and placental weights were observed at a dose of 30 mg/kg/day, about 10 times the MRHD when compared on a mg/m^2 basis. In a study in which pregnant monkeys (both treated and control) had high rates of abortion and mortality, the only surviving fetus from a group exposed to a maternal dose of 100 mg nisoldipine/kg/day (about 30 times the MRHD when compared on a mg/m^{2}basis) presented with forelimb and vertebral abnormalities not previously seen in control monkey of the same strain. There are no adequate and well controlled studies in pregnant women. Nisoldipine should be used in pregnancy only if the potential benefit justifies the potential risk to the fetus.

NURSING MOTHERS

It is not known whether nisoldipine is excreted in human milk. Because many drugs are excreted in human milk, a decision should be made to discontinue nursing, or to discontinue nisoldipine, taking into account the importance of the drug to the mother.

DRUG INTERACTIONS:

A 30 to 45% increase in AUC and C_{max} of nisoldipine was observed with concomitant administration of cimetidine 400 mg twice daily. Ranitidine 150 mg twice daily did not interact significantly with nisoldipine (AUC was decreased by 15 - 20%). No pharmacodynamic effects of either H_2 antihistamine were observed.

Pharmacokinetic interactions between nisoldipine and beta-blockers (atenolol, propranolol) were variable and not significant. Propranolol attenuated the heart rate increase following administration of immediate release nisoldipine. The blood pressure effect of nisoldipine tended to be greater in patients on atenolol than in patients on no other antihypertensive therapy.

Quinidine at 648 mg bid decreased the bioavailability (AUC) of nisoldipine by 26%, but not the peak concentration. The immediate release, but not the coat- core formulation of nisoldipine increased plasma quinidine concentrations by about 20%. This interaction was not accompanied by ECG changes and its clinical significance is not known.

No significant interactions were found between nisoldipine and warfarin or digoxin.

ADVERSE REACTIONS:

More than 6000 patients world-wide have received nisoldipine in clinical trials for the treatment of hypertension, either as the immediate release or the nisoldipine extended release formulation. Of about 1,500 patients who received nisoldipine in hypertension studies about 55% were exposed for at least 2 months and about one third were exposed for over 6 months, the great majority at doses of 20 to 60 mg daily.

Nisoldipine is generally well-tolerated. In the U.S. clinical trials of nisoldipine in hypertension, 10.9% of the 921 nisoldipine patients discontinued treatment due to adverse events compared with 2.9% of 280 placebo patients. The frequency discontinuations due to adverse experiences was related to dose, with a 5.4% discontinuation rate at 10 mg daily and a 10.9% discontinuation rate at 60 mg daily.

The most frequently occurring adverse experiences with nisoldipine are those related to its vasodilator properties; these are generally mild and only occasionally lead to patient withdrawal from treatment. The table below, from U.S. placebo-controlled parallel dose response trials of nisoldipine using doses from 10 - 60 mg once daily in patients with hypertension, lists all of the adverse events, regardless of the causal relationship to nisoldipine, which the overall incidence on nisoldipine was both > 1% and greater with nisoldipine than with placebo.

Adverse Event	Nisoldipine (%) (n=663)	Placebo (%) (n=280)
Peripheral Edema	22	10
Headache	22	15
Dizziness	5	4
Pharyngitis	5	4
Vasodilation	4	2
Sinusitis	3	2
Palpitation	3	1
Chest Pain	2	1
Nausea	2	1
Flash	2	1

Only peripheral edema and possibly dizziness appear to be dose related.

Adverse Event	Placebo	Nisoldipine 10mg	20mg	30mg	40 mg	60mg
(Rates in %)	N=280	N=30	N=170	N=105	N=139	N=137
Peripheral Edema	10	7	15	20	27	29
Dizziness	4	7	3	3	4	10

The common adverse events occurred at about the same rate in men as in women, and at a similar rate in patients over age 65 as in those under that age, except that headache was much less common in older patients. Except for peripheral edema and vasodilation, which were more common in whites, adverse event rates were similar in blacks and whites.

The following adverse events occurred in ≤1% of all patients treated for hypertension in U.S. and foreign clinical trials, or with unspecified incidence in other studies. Although a causal relationship of nisoldipine to these events cannot be established, they are listed to alert the physician to a possible relationship with nisoldipine treatment.

Body As A Whole: cellulitis, chills, facial edema, fever, flu syndrome, malaise.

Cardiovascular: atrial fibrillation, cerebrovascular accident, congestive heart failure, first degree AV block, hypertension, hypotension, jugular venous distension, migraine, myocardial infarction, postural hypotension, ventricular extrasystoles, supraventricular tachycardia, syncope, systolic ejection murmur, T wave abnormalities on ECG (flattening, inversion, nonspecific changes), venous insufficiency.

Digestive: abnormal liver function tests, anorexia, colitis, diarrhea, dry mouth, dyspepsia, dysphagia, flatulence, gastritis, gastrointestinal hemorrhage, gingival hyperplasia, glossitis, heptomegaly, increased appetite, melea, mouth ulceration.

ADVERSE REACTIONS: *(cont'd)*

Endocrine: diabetes mellitus, thyroiditis.

Hemic and Lymphatic: anemia, ecchymoses, leukopenia, petechiae.

Metabolic and Nutritional: gout, hypokalemia, increased serum creatinine kinase, increased nonprotein nitrogen, weight gain, weight loss.

Musculoskeletal: arthralgia, arthritis, leg cramps, myalgia, myasthenia, myositis, tenosynovitis.

Nervous: abnormal dreams, abnormal thinking and confusion, amnesia, anxiety, ataxia, cerebral ischemia, decreased libido, depression, hypesthesia, hypertonia, insomnia, nervousness, paresthesia, somnolence, tremor, vertigo.

Respiratory: asthma, dyspnea, and inspiratory wheeze and fine rales, epistaxis, increased cough, laryngitis, pharyngitis, pleural effusion, rhinitis, sinusitis.

Skin and Appendages: acne, alopecia, dry skin, exfoliative dermatitis, fungal dermatitis, herpes simplex, herpes zoster, maculopapular rash, pruritus, pustular rash, skin discoloration, skin ulcer, sweating, urticaria.

Special Senses: abnormal vision, amblyopia, blepharitis, conjunctivitis, ear pain, glaucoma, itchy eyes, keratoconjunctivitis, otitis media, retinal detachment, tinnitus, watery eyes, taste disturbance, temporary unilateral loss of vision, vitreous floater, watery eyes.

Urogenital: dysuria, hematuria, impotence, nocturia, urinary frequency, increased BUN and serum creatinine, vaginal hemorrhage, vaginitis.

In addition to experience with nisoldipine, there is extensive experience with the immediate release formulation of nisoldipine. Adverse events were generally similar to those seen with nisoldipine. Unusual events observed with immediate release nisoldipine but not observed with nisoldipine, were one case each of angioedema and photosensitivity. Spontaneous reports from postmarketing experience with the immediate release formulation of nisoldipine have not revealed any additional adverse events not identified in the above listings.

OVERDOSAGE:

There is no experience with nisoldipine overdosage. Generally, overdosage with other dihydropyridines leading to pronounced hypotension calls for active cardiovascular support including monitoring of cardiovascular support and respiratory function, elevation of extremities. Judicious use of calcium infusion, pressor agents and fluids. Clearance of nisoldipine would be expected to be slowed in patients with impaired liver function. Since nisoldipine is highly protein bound, dialysis is not likely to be of any benefit; however, plasmapheresis may be beneficial.

DOSAGE AND ADMINISTRATION:

The dosage of nisoldipine must be adjusted to each patient's needs. Therapy usually should be initiated with 20 mg orally once daily, then increased by 10 mg per week or longer intervals, to attain adequate control of blood pressure. Usual maintenance dosage is 20 to 40 mg once daily. Blood pressure response increases over the 10 - 60 mg daily dose range but adverse event rates also increase. Doses beyond 60 mg once daily are not recommended. Nisoldipine has been used safely with diuretics, ACE inhibitors, and beta-blocking agents.

Patients over age 65, or patients with impaired liver function are expected to develop higher plasma concentrations of nisoldipine. Their blood pressure should be monitored closely during any dosage adjustment. A starting dose not exceeding 10 mg daily is recommended in these patient groups.

Nisoldipine tablets should be administered orally once daily. Administration with a high fat meal can lead to excessive peak drug concentration and should be avoided. Grapefruit products should be avoided before and after dosing. Nisoldipine is an extended release dosage form and tablets should be swallowed whole, not bitten or divided.

PATIENT INFORMATION:

Nislodipine is used for the treatment of hypertension (high blood pressure). Do not use if you are allergic to calcium channel blockers (*e.g.*, diltiazem hydrochloride). Inform your doctor if you have a history of angina, heart attacks, or liver disease. Also inform your doctor if you are pregnant or nursing. Take one time daily. Nisoldipine is an extended release tablet and should be swallowed whole. Do not chew, crush or break the tablet. Do not take with high fat meal or grapefruit juice. May cause water retention, headache, dizziness, or sore throat.

HOW SUPPLIED:

Sular extended release tablets are supplied as 10 mg, 20 mg, 30 mg, and 40 mg round film coated tablets.

The tablets should be protected from light and moisture and store below 86°F (30°C). Dispense in tight, light-resistant containers.

HOW SUPPLIED - EQUIVALENTS NOT AVAILABLE:

Tablet, Coated - Oral - 10 mg

100's	$82.00	SULAR, Zeneca Pharms	00310-0891-10
100's UD	$82.00	SULAR, Zeneca Pharms	00310-0891-39

Tablet, Coated - Oral - 20 mg

100's	$82.00	SULAR, Zeneca Pharms	00310-0892-10
100's UD	$82.00	SULAR, Zeneca Pharms	00310-0892-39

Tablet, Coated - Oral - 30 mg

100's	$82.00	SULAR, Zeneca Pharms	00310-0893-10
100's UD	$82.00	SULAR, Zeneca Pharms	00310-0893-39

Tablet, Coated - Oral - 40 mg

100's	$82.00	SULAR, Zeneca Pharms	00310-0894-10

NITROFURANTOIN *(001890)*

CATEGORIES: Antibacterials; Anti-Infectives; Antimicrobials; Antiseptics, Urinary Tract; Enterococci Infections; Urinary Anti-Infectives; Urinary Tract Infections; FDA Approval Pre 1982

BRAND NAMES: **Furadantin**; *Furadantin Suspension* (Australia); *Furadantina* (Mexico); *Furadoine* (France); Furalan; Furan; Furanite; Furatoin; *Furobactina*; *Infurin*; Nitrofan; Nitrofuracot; *Urofuran*
(International brand names outside U.S. in italics)

FORMULARIES: Aetna; BC-BS; FHP; Medi-Cal; WHO

DESCRIPTION:

Nitrofurantoin, a synthetic chemical, is a stable, yellow, crystalline compound. Nitrofurantoin is an antibacterial agent for specific urinary tract infections. Nitrofurantoin is available in 50-mg and 100-mg tablets and in 5-mg/ml liquid suspension for oral administration.

1-(((5-nitro-2-furanyl)methylene)amino)-2,4-imidazolidinedione

DESCRIPTION: *(cont'd)*

Furadantin Inactive Ingredients: Nitrofurantoin tablets contain calcium pyrophosphate, magnesium stearate, starch, and sucrose. Nitrofurantoin Oral Suspension contains carboxymethylcellulose sodium, citric acid, flavors, glycerin, magnesium aluminum silicate, methylparaben, propylparaben, purified water, saccharin, sodium citrate, and sorbitol.

CLINICAL PHARMACOLOGY:

Orally administered Nitrofurantoin is readily absorbed and rapidly excreted in urine. Blood concentrations at therapeutic dosage are usually low. It is highly soluble in urine, to which it may impart a brown color. Following a dose regimen of 100 mg q.i.d. for 7 days, average urinary drug recoveries (0-24 hours) on day 1 and day 7 were 42.7% and 43.6%.

Unlike many drugs, the presence of food or agents delaying gastric emptying can increase the bioavailability of Nitrofurantoin, presumably by allowing better dissolution in gastric juices.

Microbiology: Nitrofurantoin, in vitro, is bacteriostatic in low concentrations (5-10 mcg/ml) and is considered bactericidal in higher concentrations. Its mode of action is presumed to be interference with several bacterial enzyme systems. Bacteria develop only a limited resistance to furan derivatives.

While *in vitro* studies have demonstrated the susceptibility of most strains of the following organisms, clinical efficacy for infections other than those included in the INDICATIONS AND USAGE section has not been documented: *Escherichia Coli*, Enterococci (*e.g.,Streptococcus Faecalis*), *Staphylococcus Aureus,Staphylococcus Epidermis.*

NOTE: Some strains of *Enterobacter* species and *Klebsiella* species are resistant to Nitrofurantoin. It is not active against most strains of *Proteus* and *Serratia* species. It has no activity against *Pseudomonas* species.

Antagonism has been demonstrated between nitrofurantoin and both nalidixic acid and oxolinic acid *in vitro.*

Susceptibility Tests: Quantitative methods that require measurement of zone diameters give the most precise estimates of antimicrobial susceptibility. One recommended procedure, (NCCLS, ASM-2)*, uses a disc containing 300 micrograms for testing susceptibility; interpretations correlate zone diameters of this disc test with MIC values for nitrofurantoin. Reports from the laboratory should be interpreted according to the following criteria:

Susceptible organisms produce zones of 17 mm or greater, indicating that the tested organism is likely to respond to therapy.

Organisms of intermediate susceptibility produce zones of 15 to 16 mm, indicating that the tested organism would be susceptible if high dosage is used.

Resistant organisms produce zones of 14 mm or less, indicating that other therapy should be selected.

A bacterial isolate may be considered susceptible if the MIC value for nitrofurantoin is 25 micrograms per ml or less. Organisms are considered resistant if the MIC is 100 micrograms per ml or more.

NOTE: Specimens for culture and susceptibility testing should be obtained prior to and during drug administration.

INDICATIONS AND USAGE:

Nitrofurantoin is specifically indicated for the treatment of urinary tract infections when due to susceptible strains of *E. coli*, enterococci, *S. aureus* (it is not indicated for the treatment or associated renal cortical or perinephric abscesses), and certain susceptible strains of *Klebsiella, Enterobacter,* and *Proteus species.*

CONTRAINDICATIONS:

Anuria, oliguria, or significant impairment of renal function (creatinine clearance under 40 ml per minute) are contraindications. Treatment of this type of patient carries an increased risk of toxicity and is much less effective because of impaired excretion of the drug.

The drug is contraindicated in pregnant patients at term (during labor and delivery) as well as in infants under one month of age because of the possibility of hemolytic anemia in the fetus or in the newborn infant due to immature erythrocyte enzyme systems (glutathione instability).

Nitrofurantoin is also contraindicated in those patients with known hypersensitivity to nitrofurantoin.

WARNINGS:

ACUTE, SUBACUTE OR CHRONIC PULMONARY REACTIONS HAVE BEEN OBSERVED IN PATIENTS TREATED WITH NITROFURANTOIN. IF THESE REACTIONS OCCUR, NITROFURANTOIN SHOULD BE DISCONTINUED AND APPROPRIATE MEASURES TAKEN. REPORTS HAVE CITED PULMONARY REACTIONS AS A CONTRIBUTING CAUSE OF DEATH.

CHRONIC PULMONARY REACTIONS (DIFFUSE INTERSTITIAL PNEUMONITIS OR PULMONARY FIBROSIS, OR BOTH) CAN DEVELOP INSIDIOUSLY. THESE REACTIONS OCCUR RARELY AND GENERALLY IN PATIENTS RECEIVING THERAPY FOR SIX MONTHS OR LONGER. CLOSE MONITORING OF THE PULMONARY CONDITION OF PATIENTS RECEIVING LONG-TERM THERAPY IS WARRANTED AND REQUIRES THAT THE BENEFITS OF THERAPY BE WEIGHED AGAINST POTENTIAL RISKS. (SEE RESPIRATORY REACTIONS.)

Hepatitis, including chronic active hepatitis, occurs rarely. Fatalities have been reported. The onset of chronic active hepatitis may be insidious, and patients receiving long-term therapy should be monitored periodically for changes in liver function. If hepatitis occurs, the drug should be withdrawn immediately and appropriate measures taken.

Peripheral neuropathy, which may become severe or irreversible, has occurred. Fatalities have been reported. Conditions such as renal impairment (creatinine clearance under 40 ml per minute), anemia, diabetes mellitus, electrolyte imbalance, vitamin B deficiency, and debilitating disease may enhance the occurrence of peripheral neuropathy.

Cases of hemolytic anemia of the primaquine sensitivity type have been induced by Nitrofurantoin. Hemolysis appears to be linked to a glucose-6-phosphate dehydrogenase deficiency in the red blood cells of the affected patients. This deficiency is found in 10 percent of Negroes and a small percentage of ethnic groups of Mediterranean and Near-Eastern origin. Hemolysis is an indication for discontinuing Nitrofurantoin; hemolysis ceases when the drug is withdrawn.

PRECAUTIONS:

Carcinogenesis, Mutagenesis: Nitrofurantoin, when fed to female Holtzman rats at levels of 0.3% in a commercial diet for up to 44.5 weeks, was not carcinogenic. Nitrofurantoin was not carcinogenic when female Sprague-Dawley rats were fed a commercial diet with nitrofurantoin levels at 0.1% to 0.187% (total cumulative, 9.25g) for 75 weeks. Further studies of the effects of chronic administration to rodents are in progress.

Results of microbial in vitro tests using *Escherichia Coli,Salmonella Typhimurium,* and *Aspergillus Nidulans* suggest that nitrofurantoin is a weak mutagen. Results of a dominant lethal assay in the mouse were negative.

PRECAUTIONS: *(cont'd)*

Impairment of Fertility: The administration of high doses of nitrofurantoin to rats causes temporary spermatogenic arrest; this is reversible on discontinuing the drug. Doses of 10 mg/kg or greater in healthy human males may, in certain unpredictable instances, produce slight to moderate spermatogenic arrest with a decrease in sperm count.

Pregnancy: The safety of Nitrofurantoin during pregnancy and lactation has not been established. Use of this drug in women of childbearing potential requires that the anticipated benefit be weighed against the possible risks.

Labor and Delivery: See CONTRAINDICATIONS.

Nursing Mothers: Nitrofurantoin has been detected in breast milk, in trace amounts. Caution should be exercised when Nitrofurantoin is administered to a nursing woman, especially if the infant is known or suspected to have a glucose-6-phosphate dehydrogenase deficiency.

Pediatric Use: Contraindicated in infants under one month of age.(See CONTRAINDICATIONS.)

DRUG INTERACTIONS:

Magnesium trisilicate, when administered concomitantly with Nitrofurantoin, reduces both the rate and extent of absorption. The mechanism for this interaction probably is adsorption of drug onto the surface of magnesium trisilicate.

Uricosuric drugs such as probenecid and sulfinpyrazone may inhibit renal tubular secretion of Nitrofurantoin. The resulting increase in serum levels may increase toxicity and the decreased urinary levels could lessen its efficacy as a urinary tract antibacterial.

ADVERSE REACTIONS:

Respiratory: CHRONIC, SUBACUTE, OR ACUTE PULMONARY HYPERSENSITIVITY REACTIONS MAY OCCUR.

CHRONIC PULMONARY REACTIONS OCCUR GENERALLY IN PATIENTS WHO HAVE RECEIVED CONTINUOUS TREATMENT FOR SIX MONTHS OR LONGER. MALAISE, DYSPNEA ON EXERTION, COUGH, AND ALTERED PULMONARY FUNCTION ARE COMMON MANIFESTATIONS WHICH CAN OCCUR INSIDIOUSLY. RADIOLOGIC AND HISTOLOGIC FINDINGS OF DIFFUSE INTERSTITIAL PNEUMONITIS OR FIBROSIS, OR BOTH, ARE ALSO COMMON MANIFESTATIONS OF THE CHRONIC PULMONARY REACTION. FEVER IS RARELY PROMINENT.

THE SEVERITY OF CHRONIC PULMONARY REACTIONS AND THEIR DEGREE OF RESOLUTION APPEAR TO BE RELATED TO THE DURATION OF THERAPY AFTER THE FIRST CLINICAL SIGNS APPEAR. PULMONARY FUNCTION MAY BE IMPAIRED PERMANENTLY, EVEN AFTER CESSATION OF THERAPY. THE RISK IS GREATER WHEN CHRONIC PULMONARY REACTIONS ARE NOT RECOGNIZED EARLY.

In subacute pulmonary reactions, fever and eosinophilia occur less often than in the acute form. Upon cessation of therapy, recovery may require several months. If the symptoms are not recognized as being drug-related and nitrofurantoin therapy is not stopped, the symptoms may become more severe.

Acute pulmonary reactions are commonly manifested by fever, chills, cough, chest pain, dyspnea, pulmonary infiltration with consolidation or pleural effusion on x-ray, and eosinophilia. Acute reactions usually occur within the first week of treatment and are reversible with cessation of therapy. Resolution often is dramatic. (See WARNINGS.)

Gastrointestinal: Hepatitis, including chronic active hepatitis, and cholestatic jaundice occur rarely.

Nausea, emesis, and anorexia occur most often. Abdominal pain and diarrhea are less common gastrointestinal reactions. These dose-related reactions can be minimized by reduction of dosage.

Neurologic: Peripheral neuropathy, which may become severe or irreversible, has occurred. Fatalities have been reported. Conditions such as renal impairment (creatinine clearance under 40 ml per minute), anemia, diabetes mellitus, electrolyte imbalance, vitamin B deficiency, and debilitating diseases may increase the possibility of peripheral neuropathy.

Less frequent reactions, of unknown causal relationship, are nystagmus, vertigo, dizziness, asthenia, headache, and drowsiness.

Dermatologic: Exfoliative dermatitis and erythema multiforme (including Stevens-Johnson Syndrome) have been reported rarely. Transient alopecia also has been reported.

Allergic Reactions: Lupus-like syndrome associated with pulmonary reaction to nitrofurantoin has been reported. Also, angioedema, maculopapular, erythematous or eczematous eruptions, urticaria, rash, and pruritus have occurred. Anaphylaxis, sialoadenitis, pancreatitis, arthralgia, myalgia, drug fever, and chills or chills and fever have been reported.

Hematologic: Agranulocytosis, leukopenia, granulocytopenia, hemolytic anemia, thrombocytopenia, glucose-6-phosphate dehydrogenase deficiency anemia, megaloblastic anemia, and eosinophilia have occurred. Cessation of therapy has returned the blood picture to normal. Aplastic anemia has been reported rarely.

Miscellaneous: As with other antimicrobial agents, superinfections by resistant organisms, e.g., pseudomonas, may occur. However, these are limited to the genitourinary tract because suppression of normal bacterial flora does not occur elsewhere in the body.

OVERDOSAGE:

Occasional incidents of acute overdosage of Nitrofurantoin have not resulted in any specific symptoms other than vomiting. In case vomiting does not occur soon after an excessive dose, induction of emesis is recommended. There is no specific antidote, but a high fluid intake should be maintained to promote urinary excretion of the drug.

DOSAGE AND ADMINISTRATION:

Nitrofurantoin should be given with food to improve drug absorption and, in some patients, tolerance.

Adults: 50-100 mg four times a day - the lower dosage level is recommended for uncomplicated urinary tract infections.

Children: 5-7 mg/kg of body weight per 24 hours, given in four divided doses (contraindicated under one month of age). The following table can be used to calculate an average dose of Nitrofurantoin Oral Suspension (5 mg/ml) for children (one 5-ml teaspoon of Nitrofurantoin oral suspension contains 25 mg of Nitrofurantoin):

TABLE 1

Body Weight: Pounds	Body Weight: Kilograms	No. Teaspoonfuls 4 Times Daily
15 to 26	7 to 11	1/2 (2.5 ml)
27 to 46	12 to 21	1 (5 ml)
47 to 68	22 to 30	1-1/2 (7.5 ml)
69 to 91	31 to 41	2 (10 ml)

DOSAGE AND ADMINISTRATION: *(cont'd)*

Therapy should be continued for one week or for at least 3 days after sterility of the urine is obtained. Continued infection indicates the need for reevaluation.

For long-term suppressive therapy in adults, a reduction of dosage to 50-100 mg at bedtime may be adequate. For long-term suppressive therapy in children, doses as low as 1 mg/kg per 24 hours, given in a single dose or in two divided doses, may be adequate. SEE WARNINGS REGARDING RISKS ASSOCIATED WITH LONG-TERM THERAPY.

Avoid exposure to strong light which may darken the drug. It is stable in storage. It should be dispensed in amber bottles.

HOW SUPPLIED - EQUIVALENTS NOT AVAILABLE:

Suspension - Oral - 25 mg/5ml

60 ml	$20.15	FURADANTIN, Procter Gamble Pharm	00149-0735-15
470 ml	$77.98	FURADANTIN, Procter Gamble Pharm	00149-0735-61

NITROFURANTOIN, MACROCRYSTALLINE

(001891)

CATEGORIES: Anti-Infectives; Antibacterials; Antimicrobials; Antiseptics, Urinary Tract; Infections; Urinary Anti-Infectives; Urinary Antibacterial; Urinary Tract Infections; FDA Approval Pre 1982

BRAND NAMES: *Furadantin Retard*; *Furadantina*; *Furadantina MC*; *Furadantine* (France); *Furadantine-MC*; Macpac; *Macrobid* (England); **Macrodantin**; *Macrodantina* (Mexico); *Macrofuran*; *Macrofurin* (Mexico); Ro-Antoin; *Uro-Tablinen* (Germany); *Uvamin Retard*; *Uvamin-E Retard*
(International brand names outside U.S. in italics)

FORMULARIES: FHP; PCS

COST OF THERAPY: $16.24 (Infections; Capsule; 50 mg; 4/day; 7 days)

PRIMARY ICD9: 136.9 (Unspecified Infections And Parasitic Diseases)

DESCRIPTION:

Macrodantin (nitrofurantoin macrocrystals) is a synthetic chemical of controlled crystal size. It is a stable, yellow, crystalline compound. Macrodantin is an antibacterial agent for specific urinary tract infections. It is available in 25-mg, 50-mg, and 100-mg capsules for oral administration. 1-[[(5-nitro-2-furanyl) methylene]amino]-2, 4- imidazolidinedione.

Macrodantin Inactive Ingredients: Each capsule contains edible black ink, gelatin, lactose, starch, talc, titanium dioxide, and may contain FD&C Yellow No.6 and D&C Yellow No.10.

CLINICAL PHARMACOLOGY:

Macrodantin is a larger crystal form of Furadantin (nitrofurantoin). The absorption of Macrodantin is slower and its excretion somewhat less when compared to Furadantin. Blood concentrations at therapeutic dosage are usually low. It is highly soluble in urine, to which it may impart a brown color.

Following a dose regimen of 100 mg q.i.d. for 7 days, average urinary drug recoveries (0-24 hours) on day 1 and day 7 were 37.9% and 35.0%.

Unlike many drugs, the presence of food or agents delaying gastric emptying can increase the bioavailability of Macrodantin, presumably by allowing better dissolution in gastric juices.

MICROBIOLOGY

Nitrofurantoin is bactericidal in urine at therapeutic doses. The mechanism of the antimicrobial action of nitrofurantoin is unusual among antibacterials. Nitrofurantoin is reduced by bacterial flavoproteins to reactive intermediates which inactivate or alter bacterial ribosomal proteins and other macromolecules. As a result of such inactivations, the vial biochemical processes of protein synthesis, aerobic energy metabolism, DNA synthesis, RNA synthesis, and cell wall synthesis are inhibited. The broad-based nature of this mode of action may explain the lack of acquired bacterial resistance to nitrofurantoin, as the necessary multiple and simultaneous mutations of the target macromolecules would likely be lethal to the bacteria. Development of resistance to nitrofurantoin has not been a significant problem since its introduction in 1953. Cross-resistance with antibiotics and sulfonamides has not been observed, and transferable resistance is, at most, a very rare phenomenon.

Nitrofurantoin, in the form of Macrodantin, has been shown to be active against most strains of the following bacteria both *in vitro* and in clinical infections: (See INDICATIONS AND USAGE.)

Gram-Positive Aerobes *Staphylococcus aureus; Enterococci (e.g., Enterococcus faecalis)*

Gram-Negative Aerobes *Escherichia coli*

NOTE: Some strains of *Enterobacter* species and *Klebsiella* species are resistant to nitrofurantoin.

Nitrofurantoin also demonstrates *in vitro* activity against the following microorganisms, although the clinical significance of these data with respect to treatment with Macrodantin is unknown:

Gram-Positive Aerobes *Coagulase-negative staphylococci (including Staphylococcus epidermidis and Staphylococcus saprophyticus); Streptococcus agalactiae; Group D streptococci; Viridans group streptococci*

Gram-Negative Aerobes *Citrobacter amalonaticus; Citrobacter diversus; Citrobacter freundii; Klebsiella oxytoca; Klebsiella ozaenae*

Nitrofurantoin is not active against most strains of *Proteus* species or *Serratia* species. It has no activity against*Pseudomonas* species.

Antagonism has been demonstrated *in vitro* between nitrofurantoin and quinolone antimicrobial agents. The clinical significance of this finding is unknown.

SUSCEPTIBILITY TESTS

Diffusion Techniques: Quantitative methods that require measurement of zone diameters give the most precise estimate of the susceptibility of bacteria to antimicrobial agents. One such standardized procedure,[1] which has been recommended for use with disks to test susceptibility of organisms to nitrofurantoin, uses the 300-mcg nitrofurantoin disk. Interpretation involves the correlation of the diameter obtained in the disk test with the minimum inhibitory concentration (MIC) for nitrofurantoin.

Reports from the laboratory giving results of the standard single-disk susceptibility test with a 300-mcg nitrofurantoin disk should be interpreted according to the following criteria:

A report of "susceptible" indicates that the pathogen is likely to be inhibited by generally achievable urinary levels. A report of "intermediate" indicates that the result be considered equivocal and, if the organism is not fully susceptible to alternative clinically feasible drugs, the test should be repeated. This category provides a buffer zone which prevents small uncontrolled technical factors from causing major discrepancies in interpretations. A report of "resistant" indicates that achievable concentrations are unlikely to be inhibitory, and other therapy should be selected.

CLINICAL PHARMACOLOGY: *(cont'd)*

TABLE 1

Zone Diameter (mm)	Interpretation
≥17	Susceptible
15-16	Intermediate
≤14	Resistant

Standardized procedures require the use of laboratory control organisms. The 300-mcg nitrofurantoin disk should give the following zone diameters:

TABLE 2

Organism	Zone Diameter (mm)
E. coli ATCC 25922	20-25
S. aureus ATCC 25923	18-22

Dilution Techniques: Use a standardized dilution method[2](broth, agar, microdilution) or equivalent with nitrofurantoin powder. The MIC values obtained should be interpreted according to the following criteria:

TABLE 3

MIC (mcg/ml)	Interpretation
≤32	Susceptible
64	Intermediate
≥128	Resistant

As with standard diffusion techniques, dilution methods require the use of laboratory control organisms. Standard nitrofurantoin powder should provide the following MIC values:

TABLE 4

Organism	MIC (mcg/ml)
E. coli ATCC 25922	4-16
S. aureus ATCC 29213	8-32
E. faecalis ATCC 29212	4-16

INDICATIONS AND USAGE:

Macrodantin is specifically indicated for the treatment of urinary tract infections when due to susceptible strains of *Escherichia coli,* enterococci, *Staphylococcus aureus,* and certain susceptible strains of *Klebsiella* and *Enterobacter* species.

Nitrofurantoin is not indicated for the treatment of pyelonephritis or perinephric abscesses.

Nitrofurantoins lack the broader tissue distribution of other therapeutic agents approved for urinary tract infections. Consequently, many patients who are treated with Macrodantin are predisposed to persistence or reappearance of bacteriuria. Urine specimens for culture and susceptibility testing should be obtained before and after completion of therapy. If persistence or reappearance of bacteriuria occurs after treatment with Macrodantin, other therapeutic agents with broader tissue distribution should be selected. In considering the use of Macrodantin, lower eradication rates should be balanced against the increased potential for systemic toxicity and for the development of antimicrobial resistance when agents with broader tissue distribution are utilized.

CONTRAINDICATIONS:

Anuria, oliguria, or significant impairment of renal function (creatinine clearance under 60 ml per minute or clinically significant elevated serum creatinine) are contraindications. Treatment of this type of patient carries an increased risk of toxicity because of impaired excretion of the drug.

Because of the possibility of hemolytic anemia due to immature erythrocyte enzyme systems (glutathione instability), the drug is contraindicated in pregnant patients at term (38-42 weeks gestation), during labor and delivery, or when the onset of labor is imminent. For the same reason, the drug is contraindicated in neonates under one month of age.

Macrodantin is also contraindicated in those patients with known hypersensitivity to nitrofurantoin.

WARNINGS:

ACUTE, SUBACUTE, OR CHRONIC PULMONARY REACTIONS HAVE BEEN OBSERVED IN PATIENTS TREATED WITH NITROFURANTOIN. IF THESE REACTIONS OCCUR, MACRODANTIN SHOULD BE DISCONTINUED AND APPROPRIATE MEASURES TAKEN. REPORTS HAVE CITED PULMONARY REACTIONS AS A CONTRIBUTING CAUSE OF DEATH.

CHRONIC PULMONARY REACTIONS (DIFFUSE INTERSTITIAL PNEUMONITIS OR PULMONARY FIBROSIS, OR BOTH) CAN DEVELOP INSIDIOUSLY. THESE REACTIONS OCCUR RARELY AND GENERALLY IN PATIENTS RECEIVING THERAPY FOR SIX MONTHS OR LONGER. CLOSE MONITORING OF THE PULMONARY CONDITION OF PATIENTS RECEIVING LONG-TERM THERAPY IS WARRANTED AND REQUIRES THAT THE BENEFITS OF THERAPY BE WEIGHED AGAINST POTENTIAL RISKS. (SEE RESPIRATORY REACTIONS.)

Hepatic reactions, including hepatitis, cholestatic jaundice, chronic active hepatitis, and hepatic necrosis, occur rarely. Fatalities have been reported. The onset of chronic active hepatitis may be insidious, and patients should be monitored periodically for changes in liver function. If hepatitis occurs, the drug should be withdrawn immediately and appropriate measures should be taken.

Peripheral neuropathy (including optic neuritis), which may become severe or irreversible, has occurred. Fatalities have been reported. Conditions such as renal impairment (creatinine clearance under 60 ml per minute or clinically significant elevated serum creatinine), anemia, diabetes mellitus, electrolyte imbalance, vitamin B deficiency, and debilitating disease may enhance the occurrence of peripheral neuropathy. Patients receiving long-term therapy should be monitored periodically for changes in renal function.

Cases of hemolytic anemia of the primaquine-sensitivity type have been induced by nitrofurantoin. Hemolysis appears to be linked to a glucose-6-phosphate dehydrogenase deficiency in the red blood cells of the affected patients. This deficiency is found in 10 percent of Blacks and a small percentage of ethnic groups of Mediterranean and Near-Eastern origin. Hemolysis is an indication for discontinuing Macrodantin; hemolysis ceases when the drug is withdrawn.

PRECAUTIONS:

Information for the Patient: Patients should be advised to take Macrodantin with food to further enhance tolerance and improve drug absorption. Patients should be instructed to complete the full course of therapy; however, they should be advised to contact their physician if any unusual symptoms occur during therapy.

Many patients who cannot tolerate microcrystalline nitrofurantoin are able to take Macrodantin without nausea.

Patients should be advised not to use antacid preparations containing magnesium trisilicate while taking Macrodantin.

Drug/Laboratory Test Interactions: As a result of the presence of nitrofurantoin, a false-positive reaction for glucose in the urine may occur. This has been observed with Benedict's and Fehling's solutions but not with the glucose enzymatic test.

Carcinogenesis, Mutagenesis, and Impairment of Fertility: Nitrofurantoin was not carcinogenic when fed to female Holtzman rats for 44.5 weeks or to female Sprague-Dawley rats for 75 weeks. Two chronic rodent bioassays utilizing male and female Sprague-Dawley rats and two chronic bioassays in Swiss mice and in BDF_1 mice revealed no evidence of carcinogenicity.

Nitrofurantoin presented evidence of carcinogenic activity in female $B6C3F_1$ mice as shown by increased incidences of tubular adenomas, benign mixed tumors, and granulosa cell tumors of the ovary. In male F344/N rats, there were increased incidences of uncommon kidney tubular cell neoplasms, osteosarcomas of the bone, and neoplasms of the subcutaneous tissue. In one study involving subcutaneous administration of 75 mg/kg nitrofurantoin to pregnant female mice, lung papillary adenomas of unknown significance were observed in the F1 generation.

Nitrofurantoin has been shown to induce point mutations in certain strains of *Salmonella typhimurium* and forward mutations in L5178Y mouse lymphoma cells. Nitrofurantoin induced increased numbers of sister chromatid exchanges and chromosomal aberrations in Chinese hamster ovary cells but not in human cells in culture. Results of the sex-linked recessive lethal assay in *Drosophila* were negative after administration of nitrofurantoin by feeding or by injection. Nitrofurantoin did not induce heritable mutation in the rodent models examined.

The significance of the carcinogenicity and mutagenicity findings relative to the therapeutic use of nitrofurantoin in humans is unknown.

The administration of high doses of nitrofurantoin to rats causes temporary spermatogenic arrest; this is reversible on discontinuing the drug. Doses of 10 mg/kg/day or greater in healthy human males may, in certain unpredictable instances, produce a slight to moderate spermatogenic arrest with a decrease in sperm count.

Pregnancy, Teratogenic Effects: Pregnancy Category B. Several reproduction studies have been performed in rabbits and rats at doses up to six times the human dose and have revealed no evidence of impaired fertility or harm to the fetus due to nitrofurantoin. In a single published study conducted in mice at 68 times the human dose (based on mg/kg administered to the dam), growth retardation and a low incidence of minor and common malformations were observed. However, at 25 times the human dose, fetal malformations were not observed; the relevance of these findings to humans is uncertain. There are, however, no adequate and well-controlled studies in pregnant women. Because animal reproduction studies are not always predictive of human response, this drug should be used during pregnancy only if clearly needed.

Non-teratogenic effects: Nitrofurantoin has been shown in one published transplacental carcinogenicity study to induce lung papillary adenomas in the F1 generation mice at doses 19 times the human dose on a mg/kg basis. The relationship of this finding to potential human carcinogenesis is presently unknown. Because of the uncertainty regarding the human implications of these animal data, this drug should be used during pregnancy only if clearly needed.

Labor and Delivery: See CONTRAINDICATIONS.

Nursing Mothers: Nitrofurantoin has been detected in breast milk in trace amounts. Because of the potential for serious adverse reactions from nitrofurantoin in nursing infants under one month of age, a decision should be made whether to discontinue nursing or to discontinue the drug, taking into account the importance of the drug to the mother. (See CONTRAINDICATIONS.)

Pediatric Use: Macrodantin is contraindicated in infants below the age of one month. (See CONTRAINDICATIONS.)

DRUG INTERACTIONS:

Antacids containing magnesium trisilicate, when administered concomitantly with nitrofurantoin, reduce both the rate and extent of absorption. The mechanism for this interaction probably is adsorption of nitrofurantoin onto the surface of magnesium trisilicate.

Uricosuric drugs, such as probenecid and sulfinpyrazone, can inhibit renal tubular secretion of nitrofurantoin. The resulting increase in nitrofurantoin serum levels may increase toxicity, and the decreased urinary levels could lessen its efficacy as a urinary tract antibacterial.

ADVERSE REACTIONS:

Respiratory: CHRONIC, SUBACUTE, OR ACUTE PULMONARY HYPERSENSITIVITY REACTIONS MAY OCCUR.

CHRONIC PULMONARY REACTIONS OCCUR GENERALLY IN PATIENTS WHO HAVE RECEIVED CONTINUOUS TREATMENT FOR SIX MONTHS OR LONGER. MALAISE, DYSPNEA ON EXERTION, COUGH, AND ALTERED PULMONARY FUNCTION ARE COMMON MANIFESTATIONS WHICH CAN OCCUR INSIDIOUSLY. RADIOLOGIC AND HISTOLOGIC FINDINGS OF DIFFUSE INTERSTITIAL PNEUMONITIS OR FIBROSIS, OR BOTH, ARE ALSO COMMON MANIFESTATIONS OF THE CHRONIC PULMONARY REACTION. FEVER IS RARELY PROMINENT.

THE SEVERITY OF CHRONIC PULMONARY REACTIONS AND THEIR DEGREE OF RESOLUTION APPEAR TO BE RELATED TO THE DURATION OF THERAPY AFTER THE FIRST CLINICAL SIGNS APPEAR. PULMONARY FUNCTION MAY BE IMPAIRED PERMANENTLY, EVEN AFTER CESSATION OF THERAPY. THE RISK IS GREATER WHEN CHRONIC PULMONARY REACTIONS ARE NOT RECOGNIZED EARLY.

In subacute pulmonary reactions, fever and eosinophilia occur less often than in the acute form. Upon cessation of therapy, recovery may require several months. If the symptoms are not recognized as being drug-related and nitrofurantoin therapy is not stopped, the symptoms may become more severe.

Acute pulmonary reactions are commonly manifested by fever, chills, cough, chest pain, dyspnea, pulmonary infiltration with consolidation or pleural effusion on x-ray, and eosinophilia. Acute reactions usually occur within the first week of treatment and are reversible with cessation of therapy. Resolution often is dramatic. (See WARNINGS.)

Changes in EKG may occur associated with pulmonary reactions.

Collapse and cyanosis have seldom been reported.

CHRONIC, SUBACUTE, OR ACUTE PULMONARY HYPERSENSITIVITY REACTIONS MAY OCCUR.

ADVERSE REACTIONS: *(cont'd)*

CHRONIC PULMONARY REACTIONS OCCUR GENERALLY IN PATIENTS WHO HAVE RECEIVED CONTINUOUS TREATMENT FOR SIX MONTHS OR LONGER. MALAISE, DYSPNEA ON EXERTION, COUGH, AND ALTERED PULMONARY FUNCTION ARE COMMON MANIFESTATIONS WHICH CAN OCCUR INSIDIOUSLY. RADIOLOGIC AND HISTOLOGIC FINDINGS OF DIFFUSE INTERSTITIAL PNEUMONITIS OR FIBROSIS, OR BOTH, ARE ALSO COMMON MANIFESTATIONS OF THE CHRONIC PULMONARY REACTION. FEVER IS RARELY PROMINENT.

THE SEVERITY OF CHRONIC PULMONARY REACTIONS AND THEIR DEGREE OF RESOLUTION APPEAR TO BE RELATED TO THE DURATION OF THERAPY AFTER THE FIRST CLINICAL SIGNS APPEAR. PULMONARY FUNCTION MAY BE IMPAIRED PERMANENTLY, EVEN AFTER CESSATION OF THERAPY. THE RISK IS GREATER WHEN CHRONIC PULMONARY REACTIONS ARE NOT RECOGNIZED EARLY.

In subacute pulmonary reactions, fever and eosinophilia occur less often than in the acute form. Upon cessation of therapy, recovery may require several months. If the symptoms are not recognized as being drug-related and nitrofurantoin therapy is not stopped, the symptoms may become more severe.

Acute pulmonary reactions are commonly manifested by fever, chills, cough, chest pain, dyspnea, pulmonary infiltration with consolidation or pleural effusion on x-ray, and eosinophilia. Acute reactions usually occur within the first week of treatment and are reversible with cessation of therapy. Resolution often is dramatic. (See WARNINGS.)

Changes in EKG may occur associated with pulmonary reactions.

Collapse and cyanosis have seldom been reported.

Hepatic: Hepatic reactions, including hepatitis, cholestatic jaundice, chronic active hepatitis, and hepatic necrosis, occur rarely.(See WARNINGS.)

Neurologic: Peripheral neuropathy (including optic neuritis), which may become severe or irreversible, has occurred. Fatalities have been reported. Conditions such as renal impairment (creatinine clearance under 60 ml per minute or clinically significant elevated serum creatinine), anemia, diabetes mellitus, electrolyte imbalance, vitamin B deficiency, and debilitating diseases may increase the possibility of peripheral neuropathy. (See WARNINGS.)

Asthenia, vertigo, nystagmus, dizziness, headache, and drowsiness have also been reported with the use of nitrofurantoin.

Benign intracranial hypertension has seldom been reported.

Confusion, depression, euphoria, and psychotic reactions have been reported rarely.

Dermatologic: Exfoliative dermatitis and erythema multiforme (including Stevens-Johnson syndrome) have been reported rarely. Transient alopecia also has been reported.

Allergic: A lupus-like syndrome associated with pulmonary reactions to nitrofurantoin has been reported. Also, angioedema; maculopapular, erythematous, or eczematous eruptions; pruritus; urticaria; anaphylaxis; arthralgia; myalgia; drug fever; and chills have been reported.

Gastrointestinal: Nausea, emesis, and anorexia occur most often. Abdominal pain and diarrhea are less common gastrointestinal reactions. These dose-related reactions can be minimized by reduction of dosage. Sialadenitis and pancreatitis have been reported.

Miscellaneous: As with other antimicrobial agents, superinfections caused by resistant organisms, e.g., *Pseudomonas* species, or *Candida* species, can occur. There are sporadic reports of *Clostridium difficile* superinfections, or pseudomembranous colitis, with the use of nitrofurantoin.

Laboratory Adverse Events: The following laboratory adverse events have been reported with the use of nitrofurantoin: increased AST (SGOT), increased ALT (SGPT), decreased hemoglobin, increased serum phosphorus, eosinophilia, glucose-6-phosphate dehydrogenase deficiency anemia (see WARNINGS), agranulocytosis, leukopenia, granulocytopenia, hemolytic anemia, thrombocytopenia, megaloblastic anemia. In most cases, these hematologic abnormalities resolved following cessation of therapy. Aplastic anemia has been reported rarely.

OVERDOSAGE:

Occasional incidents of acute overdosage of Macrodantin have not resulted in any specific symptoms other than vomiting. Induction of emesis is recommended. There is no specific antidote, but a high fluid intake should be maintained to promote urinary excretion of the drug. It is dialyzable.

DOSAGE AND ADMINISTRATION:

Macrodantin should be given with food to improve drug absorption and, in some patients, tolerance.

Adults: 50-100 mg four times a day—the lower dosage level is recommended for uncomplicated urinary tract infections.

Children: 5-7 mg/kg of body weight per 24 hours, given in four divided doses (contraindicated under one month of age).

Therapy should be continued for one week or for at least 3 days after sterility of the urine is obtained. Continued infection indicates the need for reevaluation.

For long-term suppressive therapy in adults, a reduction of dosage to 50-100 mg at bedtime may be adequate. For long-term suppressive therapy in children, doses as low as 1 mg/kg per 24 hours, given in a single dose or in two divided doses, may be adequate. **SEE WARNINGSSECTION REGARDING RISKS ASSOCIATED WITH LONG-TERM THERAPY.**

REFERENCES:

1. National Committee for Clinical Laboratory Standards. Performance Standards for Antimicrobial Disk Susceptibility Tests - Fourth Edition. Approved Standard NCCLS Document M2-A4, Vol. 10, No. 7, NCCLS, Villanova, PA, 1990. **2.** National Committee for Clinical Laboratory Standards. Methods for Dilution Antimicrobial Susceptibility Tests for Bacteria that Grow Aerobically - Second Edition. Approved Standard NCCLS Document M7-A2, Vol. 10, No. 8, NCCLS, Villanova, PA, 1990.

HOW SUPPLIED:

Macrodantin is available as follows: 25-mg opaque, white capsule imprinted with one black line encircling the capsule and coded "Macrodantin 25 mg" and "0149-0007".*

NDC 0149-0007-05 bottle of 100

50-mg opaque, yellow and white capsule imprinted with two black lines encircling the capsule and coded "Macrodantin 50 mg" and "0149-0008".*

NDC 0149-0008-05 bottle of 100

NDC 0149-0008-66 bottle of 500

NDC 0149-0008-67 bottle of 1000

NDC 0149-0008-77 hospital unit-dose strips in box of 100

100-mg opaque, yellow capsule imprinted with three black lines encircling the capsule and coded "Macrodantin 100 mg" and "0149-0009".*

NDC 0149-0009-05 bottle of 100

NDC 0149-0009-66 bottle of 500

NDC 0149-0009-67 bottle of 1000

HOW SUPPLIED: *(cont'd)*

NDC 0149-0009-77 hospital unit-dose strips in box of 100

* Capsule design, registered trademark of Procter & Gamble Pharmaceuticals.

HOW SUPPLIED - RATED THERAPEUTICALLY EQUIVALENT:

Capsule - Oral - 50 mg

100's	$59.57	Nitrofurantoin, Macrocrystalline, H.C.F.A. F F P	99999-1891-01

Capsule - Oral - 100 mg

100's	$101.22	Nitrofurantoin, Macrocrystalline, H.C.F.A. F F P	99999-1891-02

Capsule, Gelatin - Oral - 25 mg

100's	$41.70	Nitrofurantoin Macrocrystal, Geneva Pharms	00781-2501-01
100's	**$56.46**	**MACRODANTIN, Procter Gamble Pharm**	**00149-0007-05**

Capsule, Gelatin - Oral - 50 mg

100's	$58.00	Nitrofurantoin Macrocrystal, Harber Pharm	51432-0683-03
100's	$58.20	Nitrofurantoin Macrocrystals, Qualitest Pharms	00603-4776-21
100's	$59.57	Nitrofurantoin Macrocrystal, United Res	00677-1224-01
100's	$60.55	Nitrofurantoin Macrocrystals, Martec Pharms	52555-0476-01
100's	$63.25	Nitrofurantoin Macrocrystalline, Warner Chilcott	00047-0788-24
100's	$64.50	Nitrofurantoin Macrocrystal, Goldline Labs	00182-1944-89
100's	$66.10	Nitrofurantoin Macrocrystals, Aligen Independ	00405-4699-01
100's	$66.50	Nitrofurantoin Macro, Rugby	00536-5618-01
100's	$66.75	Nitrofurantoin Macrocrystals, Zenith Labs	00172-2130-60
100's	$66.75	Nitrofurantoin Macrocrystals, Goldline Labs	00182-1944-01
100's	$66.75	Nitrofurantoin (Macrocrystalline), Major Pharms	00904-7721-60
100's	$66.95	Nitrofurantoin Macrocrystal, Geneva Pharms	00781-2502-01
100's	$67.49	Nitrofurantoin, Macro, HL Moore Drug Exch	00839-7518-06
100's	$67.95	Nitrofurantoin Macrocrystal, Geneva Pharms	00781-2502-13
100's	$70.20	Nitrofurantoin Macrocyrstals, Vangard Labs	00615-1308-13
100's	**$74.39**	**MACRODANTIN, Procter Gamble Pharm**	**00149-0008-05**
100's	**$80.57**	**MACRODANTIN, Procter Gamble Pharm**	**00149-0008-77**
500's	$291.00	Nitrofurantoin Macrocrystals, Aligen Independ	00405-4699-02
500's	$307.45	Nitrofurantoin (Macrocrystalline), Major Pharms	00904-7721-40
500's	$318.59	Nitrofurantoin Macrocrystals, Zenith Labs	00172-2130-70
500's	$318.59	Nitrofurantoin Macrocrystals, Goldline Labs	00182-1944-05
500's	$318.59	Nitrofurantoin, Macro, HL Moore Drug Exch	00839-7518-12
500's	$318.60	Nitrofurantoin Macrocrystal, Geneva Pharms	00781-2502-05
500's	**$364.45**	**MACRODANTIN, Procter Gamble Pharm**	**00149-0008-66**
1000's	$558.60	Nitrofurantoin Macrocrystals, Zenith Labs	00172-2130-80
1000's	$617.00	Nitrofurantoin Macrocrystal, Geneva Pharms	00781-2502-10
1000's	**$714.06**	**MACRODANTIN, Procter Gamble Pharm**	**00149-0008-67**

Capsule, Gelatin - Oral - 100 mg

100's	$98.50	Nitrofurantoin Macrocrystals, Qualitest Pharms	00603-4777-21
100's	$98.50	Nitrofurantoin Macrocrystal, Harber Pharm	51432-0741-03
100's	$101.22	Nitrofurantoin Macrocrystals, United Res	00677-1225-01
100's	$102.40	Nitrofurantoin Macrocrystals, Martec Pharms	52555-0477-01
100's	$108.75	Nitrofurantoin Macrocrystals, Zenith Labs	00172-2131-60
100's	$108.75	Nitrofurantoin Macrocrystals, Goldline Labs	00182-1945-01
100's	$108.75	Nitrofurantoin Macrocrystals, Aligen Independ	00405-4700-01
100's	$108.75	Nitrofurantoin (Macrocrystalline), Major Pharms	00904-7722-60
100's	$109.33	Nitrofurantoin Macrocyrstals, Vangard Labs	00615-1309-13
100's	$113.65	Nitrofurantoin Macrocrystal, Geneva Pharms	00781-2503-01
100's	$114.74	Nitrofurantoin, Macro, HL Moore Drug Exch	00839-7519-06
100's	$114.89	Nitrofurantoin Macro, Rugby	00536-5619-01
100's	$116.00	Nitrofurantoin Macrocrystal, Goldline Labs	00182-1945-89
100's	$117.49	Nitrofurantoin Macrocrystal, Geneva Pharms	00781-2503-13
100's	**$126.28**	**MACRODANTIN, Procter Gamble Pharm**	**00149-0009-05**
100's	**$144.96**	**MACRODANTIN, Procter Gamble Pharm**	**00149-0009-77**
500's	$484.00	Nitrofurantoin Macrocrystals, Zenith Labs	00172-2131-70
500's	$542.69	Nitrofurantoin, Macro, HL Moore Drug Exch	00839-7519-12
500's	**$618.76**	**MACRODANTIN, Procter Gamble Pharm**	**00149-0009-66**
1000's	$948.40	Nitrofurantoin Macrocrystals, Zenith Labs	00172-2131-80
1000's	**$1212.31**	**MACRODANTIN, Procter Gamble Pharm**	**00149-0009-67**

NITROFURANTOIN; NITROFURANTOIN, MACROCRYSTALLINE *(003110)*

CATEGORIES: Anti-Infectives; Antibacterials; Cystitis; Infections; Urinary Tract Infections; Pregnancy Category B; FDA Class 1C ("Little or No Therapeutic Advantage"); FDA Approved 1991 Dec; Top 200 Drugs; Top 200 Drugs

BRAND NAMES: **Macrobid**

DESCRIPTION:

FOR COMPLETE PRESCRIBING INFORMATION, REFER TO THE INDIVIDUAL DRUG MONOGRAPHS (NITROFURANTOIN, NITROFURANTOIN, MACROCRYSTALLINE).

INDICATIONS AND USAGE:

This drug combination is indicated only for the treatment of acute uncomplicated urinary tract infections (acute cystitis) caused by susceptible strains of *Escherichia coli* or *Staphylococcus saprophyticus.*

Nitrofurantoin is not indicated for the treatment of pyelonephritis or perinephric abscesses.

Nitrofurantoins lack the broader tissue distribution of other therapeutic agents approved for urinary tract infections. Consequently, many patients who are treated with this drug combination are predisposed to persistence or reappearance of bacteriuria. Urine specimens for culture and susceptibility testing should be obtained before and after completion of therapy. If persistence or reappearance of bacteriuria occurs after treatment with this drug combination, other therapeutic agents with broader tissue distribution should be selected. In considering the use of this drug combination, lower eradication rates should be balanced against the increased potential for systemic toxicity and for the development of antimicrobial resistance when agents with broader tissue distribution are utilized.

DOSAGE AND ADMINISTRATION:

Capsules of this drug combination should be taken with food.

Adults and Children Over 12 Years: One 100-mg capsule every 12 hours for seven days.

PATIENT INFORMATION:

Nitrofurantoin is an antibiotic used to treat urinary tract infections (bladder infections). Improvement in symptoms may be felt within one to two days, however you should continue taking all the medication you have been prescribed. This will fully help cure the infection. This medication should be taken with food to help absorption and decrease the chances of stomach irritation. Do not take antacids within 2 hours of taking this medication. This medication has been reported to cause a false positive test for urine glucose (sugar). In rare instances, respiratory reactions have occurred. Report any unusual side effects to your doctor. If symptoms of bladder infection recur, contact your doctor immediately to receive additional medical attention.

HOW SUPPLIED:

Macrobid is available as 100-mg opaque black and yellow capsules imprinted "Macrobid" on the black portion and "Norwich Eaton" on the yellow portion.

Store at controlled room temperature (59 to 86°F or 15 to 30°C).

HOW SUPPLIED - EQUIVALENTS NOT AVAILABLE:

Capsule, Gelatin - Oral - 100 mg

100's	**$127.91**	**MACROBID, Procter Gamble Pharm**	**00149-0710-01**

NITROFURAZONE *(001892)*

CATEGORIES: Anti-Infectives; Antibacterials; Antibiotics; Burns; Dermatologicals; Local Infections; Skin Grafting; Skin/Mucous Membrane Agents; Topical; Wound Care; Pregnancy Category C; FDA Approval Pre 1982

BRAND NAMES: Actin-N; *Fucorzone*; **Furacin**; *Furacine*; *Furasept*; *Furon*; *Rafuzone* *(International brand names outside U.S. in italics)*

DESCRIPTION:

Chemically: nitrofurazone, 2-((5-nitro-2-furanyl)methylene)hydrazine-carboxamide.

Nitrofurazone soluble dressing is a preparation containing 0.2% nitrofurazone in Solubase (a water-soluble base of polyethylene glycols 3350, 900, and 300).

Nitrofurazone soluble dressing is an antibacterial agent for topical use.

CLINICAL PHARMACOLOGY:

Nitrofurazone soluble dressing is a nitrofuran that is bactericidal for most pathogens commonly causing surface infections, including *Staphylococcus aureus, Streptococcus, Escherichia coli, Clostridium perfringens, Aerobacter aerogenes,* and *Proteus.*

Nitrofurazone soluble dressing inhibits a number of bacterial enzymes, especially those involved in the aerobic and anaerobic degradation of glucose and pyruvate. The activity appears to involve the pyruvate dehydrogenase system as well as citrate synthetase, malate dehydrogenase, glutathione reductase, and pyruvate decarboxylase. Glutathione reductase inhibition may be caused by control of pentose phosphate metabolism. Although nitrofurazone soluble dressing inhibits a variety of enzymes, it is not considered to be a general enzyme inactivator since many enzymes are not inhibited by this compound.

INDICATIONS AND USAGE:

Nitrofurazone soluble dressing is a topical antibacterial agent indicated for adjunctive therapy of patients with second- and third-degree burns when bacterial resistance to other agents is a real or potential problem.

It is also indicated in skin grafting where bacterial contamination may cause graft rejection and/or donor site infection particularly in hospitals with historical resistant-bacteria epidermics.

There is no known evidence of effectiveness of this product in the treatment of minor burns or surface bacterial infections involving wounds, cutaneous ulcers, or the various pyodermas.

CONTRAINDICATIONS:

Known sensitization to any of the components of this preparation is a contraindication for use.

WARNINGS:

Nitrofurazone has been shown to produce mammary tumors when fed at high doses to female Sprague-Dawley rats. The relevance of this to topical use in humans is unknown.

Nitrofurazone soluble dressing should be used with caution in patients with known or suspected renal impairment. The polyethylene glycols in the base can be absorbed through denuded skin and may not be excreted normally by the compromised kidney. This may lead to symptoms of progressive renal impairment such as increased BUN, anion gap, and metabolic acidosis. (NOTE: Nitrofurazone Topical Cream does not contain polyethylene glycols.)

PRECAUTIONS:

GENERAL

Use of topical antimicrobials occasionally allows overgrowth of nonsusceptible organisms including fungi. If this occurs, or if irritation, sensitization or superinfection develops, treatment with nitrofurazone soluble dressing should be discontinued and appropriate therapy instituted.

CARCINOGENESIS, MUTAGENESIS, AND IMPAIRMENT OF FERTILITY

Nitrofurazone has been shown to produce mammary tumors when fed at high doses to female Sprague-Dawley rats. The relevance of this to topical use in humans is unknown. Dietary dosage levels of 60 and 30 mg/kg/day shortened the onset time of the typical mammary gland tumors associated with older female rats. These tumors exhibited the same histological characteristics seen in the spontaneously occurring tumors, and were seen only in the female animals. No mammary tumors were seen in rats treated with nitrofurazone orally in the diet for 1 year at levels of approximately 11 mg/kg/day. Spermatogenic arrest was noted in the male rats in dietary dosage levels of 30 mg/kg/day and above, after one year on test.

PREGNANCY CATEGORY C

Nitrofurazone has been shown to have an embryocidal effect in rabbits when given in oral doses thirty times the human dose. There are no adequate and well controlled studies in pregnant women. Nitrofurazone soluble dressing should be used during pregnancy only if the potential benefit justifies the potential risk to the fetus.

NURSING MOTHERS

It is not known whether this drug is excreted in human milk. Because many drugs are excreted in human milk and because of the potential for tumorigenicity shown for nitrofurazone in animal studies, a decision should be made whether to discontinue nursing or to discontinue the drug, taking into account the importance of the drug to the mother.

PEDIATRIC USE

Safety and effectiveness in children have not been established.

ADVERSE REACTIONS:

Instances of clinical skin reactions have been reported for patients treated with nitrofurazone formulations. Symptoms appear as varying degrees of contact dermatitides such as rash, pruritus, and local edema. Although the exact incidence of such reactions is difficult to determine, historically, a survey of world literature and clinical data indicates an overall incidence of approximately 1%.

Allergic reactions to nitrofurazone soluble dressing should be treated symptomatically.

DOSAGE AND ADMINISTRATION:

Burns: Apply directly to the lesion with a spatula, or first place on gauze, Impregnated gauze may be used. Reapply depending on the preferred dressing technique. Flushing the dressing with sterile saline facilitates its removal.

Preparation of Impregnated Gauze: Sterile gauze strips are placed in a tray and covered with nitrofurazone soluble dressing. Repeat the procedure, adding several layers of gauze for each layer of nitrofurazone soluble dressing. Sprinkling a little sterile water on each layer of dressing will minimize any color change from autoclaving. Cover the tray very loosely and autoclave at 121°C for 30 minutes at 15 to 20 pounds pressure.

To impregnate bandage rolls, place some nitrofurazone soluble dressing in the bottom of a glass jar. Stand rolls on end. Place more nitrofurazone soluble dressing on top. Cover top of jar with aluminum foil. Autoclave at 121°C for 45 minutes at 15 to 20 pounds pressure. Do not store impregnated bandage rolls for more than 24 hours.

Autoclaving more than once is not recommended.

ANIMAL PHARMACOLOGY:

The oral administration of nitrofurazone for 7 days to rats at extremely high dosage levels of 240 mg/kg/day produced severe hepatorenal lesions whereas only renal changes were seen when the dosage level was reduced to 60 mg/kg/day for 60 days.

Dogs treated orally with nitrofurazone for 400 days at levels of 11 mg/kg/day showed no toxic effects related to drug treatment. The single intravenous administration in dogs of 20, 35, or 75 mg/kg nitrofurazone produced clinical signs of lacrimation, salivation, emesis, diarrhea, excitation, weakness, ataxia, and weight loss, whereas 100 mg/kg produced convulsions and death.

There was no evidence of toxicosis in rhesus monkeys treated with doses of nitrofurazone as high as 58 mg/kg/day for 10 weeks and 23 mg/kg/day for 63 weeks.

The peroral LD_{50} of nitrofurazone in mice and rats in 747 and 590 mg/kg respectively.

For bacterial sensitivity tests: Nitrofurazone Sensi-Discs are available from BBL, Division of BioQuest.

HOW SUPPLIED - RATED THERAPEUTICALLY EQUIVALENT:

Ointment - Topical - 0.2 %

20 gm	$.33	Nitrofurazone, H.C.F.A. F F P	99999-1892-01
28 gm	$.46	Nitrofurazone, H.C.F.A. F F P	99999-1892-02
28 gm	**$12.35**	**FURACIN DRESSING, Roberts Labs**	**54092-0310-28**
30 gm	$1.51	Nitrofurazone, Clay Park Labs	45802-0030-03
30 gm	$1.63	Nitrofurazone, H.C.F.A. F F P	99999-1892-03
30 gm	$2.02	BURN, Rugby	00536-1900-95
30 gm	**$19.88**	**FURACIN DRESSING, Roberts Labs**	**54092-0310-56**
56 gm	$3.05	Nitrofurazone, H.C.F.A. F F P	99999-1892-04
454 gm	$6.40	Nitrofurazone, Thames Pharma	49158-0110-16
454 gm	$6.48	Nitrofurazone Soluble Dressing, Clay Park Labs	45802-0030-15
454 gm	$7.58	Nitrofurazone, Rugby	00536-9019-98
454 gm	$7.58	Nitrofurazone, H.C.F.A. F F P	99999-1892-05
454 gm	$24.74	Nitrofurazone, United Res	00677-1085-44
454 gm	**$82.77**	**FURACIN DRESSING, Roberts Labs**	**54092-0310-16**

Solution - Topical - 0.2 %

473 ml	**$66.14**	**FURACIN, Roberts Labs**	**54092-0312-16**
480 ml	$6.48	Nitrofurazone, Clay Park Labs	45802-0031-17
3840 ml	$28.49	Nitrofurazone, Rugby	00536-1510-90
3840 ml	$29.15	Nitrofurazone, Clay Park Labs	45802-0031-18

HOW SUPPLIED - NOT RATED EQUIVALENT:

Cream - Topical - 0.2 %

28 gm	**$17.31**	**FURACIN, Roberts Labs**	**54092-0311-28**

NITROGLYCERIN *(001893)*

CATEGORIES: Analgesics; Anesthesia; Angina; Antianginals; Antihypertensives; Cardiovascular Drugs; Congestive Heart Failure; Coronary Artery Disease; Coronary Vasodilators; Heart Failure; Hypertension; Hypotension; Intubation; Neuromuscular; Nitrates; Pain; Vasodilating Agents; Hypokalemia*; Pregnancy Category C; Sales > $500 Million; FDA Approval Pre 1982; Top 200 Drugs
* Indication not approved by the FDA

BRAND NAMES: *Anginine* (Australia); *Angised*; *Cardinit* (Mexico); *Corditrine* (France); *Coro-Nitro* (Germany); Deponit; *Deponit 5*; *Deponit-5*; *Deponit TTS 5*; *Deponit TTS 10*; *Gilustenon* (Germany); *Glyceryl*; *Lenitral* (France); Mi-Trates; Minitran; *Myovin*; *Natirose*; *Niong Retard*; *Nitradisc* (Germany, Mexico); *Nitradisc Pad*; *Nitradisc TTS*; *Nit-Ret*; *Nitriderm TTS* (France, Germany); Nitro; *Nitro Retard*; *Nitrobaat*; Nitro-Bid; *Nitrobid* (Canada, Japan); *Nitrobid Oint*; Nitrocap T.D.; *Nitrocerin*; Nitrocine; *Nitrocine 5*; *Nitrocontin*; *Nitrocontin Continus* (England); *Nitrocor*; *NitroCor*; Nitrocot; *Nitroderm TTS* (Germany); *Nitroderm TTS Ext*; Nitro-Dur; *Nitro-Dur 5*; *Nitro-Dur 10*; *Nitro Dur TTS*; *Nitrodyl*; *Nitrodyl TTS*; *Nitro-Gesanit Retard* (Germany); *Nitrogard-SR* (Canada); *Nitro-M-Bid*; *Nitro Mack Retard* (Germany); *Nitromack Retard*; *Nitro-Mack Retard*; *Nitromex*; *Nitromint*; *Nitromint Aerosol*; *Nitromint Retard*; Nitro-Par; *Nitropatch*; *Nitroprol*; Nitro-Time; *Nitroderm TTS-5* (Mexico); Nitrodisc; *Nitro-Pflaster* (Germany); Nitrogard; *Nitroglin* (Germany); Nitroglyn; Nitrol; Nitrolin; Nitrolingual; *Nitrolingual Spray* (Australia); *Nitrolong*; Nitronal; Nitrong; *Nitrong Retard*; *Nitrong-SR* (Canada); *Nitropen* (Japan); *Nitroplast*; *Nitropront*; *Nitroprontan*; *Nitrorectal* (Germany); Nitrorex; *Nitro Rorer* (Germany); Nitrospan; Nitrostat; *Nitrovis*; *Nitrozell Retard*; NTS; NTG; *Nysconitrine*; *Percutol*; *Percutol Oint.* (England); *Ratiopharm* (Germany); *Suscard* (England); *Sustac* (England); **Transderm-Nitro**; *Transiderm*; *Transiderm Nitro*; Tridil; *Vasolator* (Japan); *Venitrin*; *Willong*
(International brand names outside U.S. in italics)

FORMULARIES: Aetna; BC-BS; CIGNA; DoD; FHP; Humana; Kaiser; Medco; Medi-Cal; PCS; PruCare; United; WHO

COST OF THERAPY: $70.62 (Angina; Capsule; 6.5 mg; 3/day; 365 days)

DESCRIPTION:

Note: The information in this monograph pertains to the IV form of Nitroglycerin (except where noted otherwise).

IV: FOR INTRAVENOUS USE ONLY: NOT FOR DIRECT INTRAVENOUS INJECTION (MUST BE DILUTED), Nitroglycerin MUST BE DILUTED IN DEXTROSE 5% INJECTION, USP OR SODIUM CHLORIDE (0.9%) INJECTION, USP BEFORE INTRAVENOUS ADMINISTRATION. THE ADMINISTRATION SET USED FOR INFUSION MAY AFFECT THE AMOUNT OF NITROGLYCERIN DELIVERED TO THE PATIENT. (SEE WARNINGS and DOSAGE AND ADMINISTRATIONSECTIONS.)

Caution: SEVERAL PREPARATIONS OF NITROGLYCERIN INJECTION, USP ARE AVAILABLE. THEY DIFFER IN CONCENTRATION AND/OR VOLUME PER VIAL. WHEN SWITCHING FROM ONE PRODUCT TO ANOTHER, ATTENTION MUST BE PAID TO THE DILUTION AND DOSAGE AND ADMINISTRATION INSTRUCTIONS.

Nitroglycerin injection, USP is a clear, practically colorless additive solution for intravenous infusion after dilution. Each milliliter contains 5 mg nitroglycerin and 45 mg propylene glycol.

The solution is sterile, nonpyrogenic, and nonexplosive. Nitroglycerin, an organic nitrate, is a vasodilator. The chemical name for nitroglycerin is 1,2,3 propanetriol trinitrate.

Extended Release Oral Tablets: Each 2.6 mg tablet for oral administration contains 2.6 mg nitroglycerin in extended-release form with light green granules containing corn-starch, D&C Yellow #10 lake and iron oxide. Each 6.5 mg tablet for oral administration contains 6.5 mg nitroglycerin in extended-release form with light orange granules containing cornstarch, D&C Yellow #10 lake, FD&C Yellow #6 lake, iron oxide and povidone.

Sublingual Tablets: This form is manufactured by a process which prevents the migration of nitroglycerin by adding the nonvolatile fixing agent polyethylene glycol 3350. This stabilized formulation has been shown to be more stable and more uniform than conventional molded tablets. Nitroglycerin sublingual tablets contain 0.15 mg (1/400 grain), 0.3 mg (1/200 grain), 0.4 mg (1/150 grain) and 0.6 (1/100 grain) nitroglycerin. Also contains lactose, NF; polyethylene glycol 3350, NF; sucrose, NF.

Ointment: Contains 2% nitroglycerin ointment and lactose in a lanolin and white petrolatum base. Each inch, as squeezed from the tube, contains approximately 15 mg nitroglycerin.

Lingual Aerosol Spray: Nitroglycerin spray is a metered dose aerosol containing nitroglycerin in propellants (dichlorodifluoromethane and dichlorotetrafluoroethane). Each metered dose delivers 0.4 mg of nitroglycerin per spray emission. This product delivers nitroglycerin in the form of spray droplets onto or under the tongue. Inactive ingredients are: caprylic/capric/diglycereryl succinate, ether, flavors.

Transdermal Delivery System: This unit is designed to provide continuous controlled release of nitroglycerin through intact skin. the rate of release is linearly dependent upon the area of the applied system; each cm^2 of applied system delivers approximately 0.02 mg of nitroglycerin per hour. Thus, 3.3, 6.7, 13.3 and 20 cm^2 system delivers approximately 0.1, 0.2. 0.4. and 0.6 mg of nitroglycerin per hour, respectively.

The remainder of nitroglycerin in each system serves as a reservoir and is not delivered in normal use. After 12 hours, for example, each system has delivered about 6% of its original content of nitroglycerin.

This transdermal delivery system contains nitroglycerin in a hypoallergenic, medical grade, acrylic-based polymer adhesive. Each patch is packaged in foil/polymer film laminate.

Prior to use, a protective peel strip is removed from the adhesive surface. Following use, the patch should be discarded in a manner that prevents accidental application or ingestion by children or others.

CLINICAL PHARMACOLOGY:

Relaxation of vascular smooth muscle is the principal pharmacologic action of nitroglycerin. Although venous effects predominate, nitroglycerin produces, in a dose-related manner, dilation of both arterial and venous beds. Dilation of the postcapillary vessels, including large veins, promotes peripheral pooling of blood and decreases venous return to the heart, reducing left ventricular end-diastolic pressure (preload). Arteriolar relaxation reduces systemic vascular resistance and arterial pressure (afterload). Myocardial oxygen consumption or demand (as measured by the pressure-rate product, tension-time index, and stroke-work index) is decreased by both the arterial and venous effects of nitroglycerin, and a more favorable supply-demand ratio can be achieved.

Therapeutic doses of intravenous nitroglycerin reduce systolic, diastolic, and mean arterial blood pressures. Effective coronary perfusion pressure is usually maintained, but can be compromised if blood pressure falls excessively or increased heart rate decreases diastolic filling time.

Elevated central venous and pulmonary capillary wedge pressures, pulmonary vascular resistance, and systemic vascular resistance are also reduced by nitroglycerin therapy. Heart rate is usually slightly increased, presumably a reflex response to the fall in blood pressure. Cardiac index may be increased, decreased, or unchanged. Patients with elevated left ventricular filling pressure and systemic vascular resistance values in conjunction with a depressed cardiac index are likely to experience an improvement in cardiac index. On the other hand, when filling pressures and cardiac index are normal, cardiac index may be slightly reduced by intravenous nitroglycerin.

Nitroglycerin is widely distributed in the body with an apparent volume of distribution of approximately 200 liters in adult male subjects, and is rapidly metabolized to dinitrates and mononitrates, with a short half-life, estimated at one to four minutes. This results in a low plasma concentration after intravenous infusion. At plasma concentrations of between 50 and 500 ng/ml, the binding of nitroglycerin to plasma proteins is approximately 60%, while that of 1,2 dinitroglycerin and 1,3 dinitroglycerin is 60% and 30%, respectively. The activity and half-life of the nitroglycerin metabolites are not well characterized. The mononitrate is not active.

PHARMACOKINETICS

The volume of distribution of nitroglycerin is about 3L/kg, and nitroglycerin is cleared from this volume at extremely rapid rates, with a resulting serum half-life of about 3 minutes. The observed clearance rates (close to 1 L/kg/min) greatly exceed hepatic blood flow; known sites of extrahepatic metabolism include red blood cells and vascular walls.

The first products in the metabolism of nitroglycerin are inorganic nitrate and the 1,2- and 1,3-dinitroglycerols. The dinitrates are less effective vasodilators than nitroglycerin, but they are longer lived in the serum, and their net contribution to the overall effect of chronic nitroglycerin regimes is not known. The dinitrates are further metabolized to (nonvasoactive) mononitrates and, ultimately, to glycerol and carbon dioxide.

To avoid development of tolerance to nitroglycerin, drug-free intervals of 10-12 hours are known to be sufficient; shorter intervals have not been well studied. In one well controlled clinical trial, subjects receiving nitroglycerin appeared to exhibit a rebound or withdrawal effect, so that their exercise tolerance at the end of the daily drug-free interval was *less* than that exhibited by the parallel group receiving placebo.

CLINICAL PHARMACOLOGY: *(cont'd)*

In healthy volunteers, steady-state plasma concentrations of nitroglycerin are reached by about 2 hours after application of a patch and are maintained for the duration of wearing the system (observations have been limited to 24 hours). Upon removal of the patch, the plasma concentration declines with a half-life of about an hour.

CLINICAL STUDIES:

TRANSDERMAL PATCH

Regimens in which nitroglycerin patches were worn for twelve hours daily have been studied in well-controlled trials for up to 4 weeks in duration. Starting about 2 hours after application and continuing until 10-12 hours after application, patches that deliver at least 0.4 mg of nitroglycerin per hour have consistently demonstrated greater antianginal activity than placebo. Lower dose patches have not been well-studied, but in one large, well-controlled trial in which higher-dose patched were also studied, patched delivering 0.2 mg/hr had significantly*less* antianginal activity than placebo.

It is reasonable to believe that the rate of nitroglycerin absorption from patches may vary with the site of application, but this relationship has not been adequately studied.

INDICATIONS AND USAGE:

IV: Nitroglycerin injection, USP is indicated for:

1. Control of blood pressure in perioperative hypertension, i.e., hypertension associated with surgical procedures, especially cardiovascular procedures, such as the hypertension seen during intratracheal intubation, anesthesia, skin incision, sternotomy, cardiac bypass, and in the immediate postsurgical period.

2. Congestive heart failure associated with acute myocardial infarction.

3. Treatment of angina pectoris in patients who have not responded to recommended doses of organic nitrates and/or a beta-blocker.

4. Production of controlled hypotension during surgical procedures.

Extended Release Oral Tablets: Indicated for the prevention of angina pectoris due to coronary artery disease. The onset of action is not sufficiently rapid for this form to be useful in aborting an acute anginal episode.

Sublingual Tablets: Indicated for the prophylaxis, treatment and management of patients with angina pectoris.

Ointment: Indicated for the prevention of angina pectoris due to coronary artery disease. Controlled clinical trials have demonstrated that this form of nitroglycerin is effective in improving exercise tolerance in patients with exertional angina pectoris. Double-blind, placebo-controlled trials have shown significant improvement in exercise time until chest pain for up to six hours after single application of various doses of nitroglycerin ointment (mean doses ranged from 5 to 36 mg) to a 36 square inch area of trunk.

Transdermal Delivery System: This product has been approved by the FDA for the prevention of angina pectoris due to coronary artery disease. The onset of action of transdermal nitroglycerin is not sufficiently rapid for this product to be useful in aborting an acute attack. Tolerance to the anti-anginal effects of nitrates (measured by exercise stress testing) has been shown to be a major factor limiting efficacy when transdermal nitrates are used continuously for longer than 12 hours each day. The development of tolerance can be altered (prevented or attenuated) by use of a noncontinuous (intermittent) dosing schedule with a nitrate-free interval of 10-12 hours.

Controlled clinical trial data suggest that the intermittent use of nitrates is associated with decreased exercise tolerance, on comparison to placebo, during the last part of the nitrate-free interval; the clinical relevance of this observation is unknown, but the possibility of increased frequency of severity of angina during the nitrate-free interval should be considered. Further investigations of the tolerance phenomenon and best regimen are ongoing. A final evaluation of the effectiveness of the product will be announced by the FDA.

CONTRAINDICATIONS:

Nitroglycerin injection, USP should not be administered to individuals with:

1. A known hypersensitivity to nitroglycerin or a known idiosyncratic reaction to organic nitrates.

2. Hypotension or uncorrected hypovolemia, as the use of Nitroglycerin in such states could produce severe hypotension or shock.

3. Increased intracranial pressure (*e.g.,* head trauma or cerebral hemorrhage).

4. Inadequate cerebral circulation.

5. Constrictive pericarditis and pericardial tamponade.

Transdermal Delivery: Allergic reactions to organic nitrates are extremely rare, but they do occur. Nitroglycerin is contraindicated in patients who are allergic to it. Allergy to the adhesives used in nitroglycerin patches have also been reported, and they similarly constitute a contraindication to the use of this product.

WARNINGS:

Nitroglycerin readily migrates into many plastics. To avoid absorption of nitroglycerin into plastic parenteral solution containers, the dilution of nitroglycerin injection, USP should be made only in glass parenteral solution bottles.

Some filters absorb nitroglycerin; they should be avoided.

Forty percent (40%) to eighty percent (80%) of the total amount of nitroglycerin in the final diluted solution for infusion is absorbed by the polyvinyl chloride (PVC) tubing of the intravenous administration sets currently in general use. The higher rates of absorption occur when flow rates are low, nitroglycerin concentrations are high, and tubing is long. Although the rate of loss is highest during the early phase of administration (when flow rates are lowest), the loss is neither constant nor self-limiting; consequently, no simple calculation or correction can be performed to convert the theoretical infusion rate (based on the concentration of the infusion solution) to the actual delivery rate. Because of this problem, Marion Laboratories recommends the use of the least absorptive infusion tubing available (*i.e.,* non-PVC tubing) for infusions of Nitroglycerin IV. DOSING INSTRUCTIONS MUST BE FOLLOWED WITH CARE. IT SHOULD BE NOTED THAT WHEN THE APPROPRIATE INFUSION SETS ARE USED, THE CALCULATED DOSE WILL BE DELIVERED TO THE PATIENT BECAUSE THE LOSS OF NITROGLYCERIN DUE TO ABSORPTION IN STANDARD PVC TUBING WILL BE KEPT TO A MINIMUM. NOTE THAT THE DOSAGES COMMONLY USED IN PUBLISHED STUDIES UTILIZED GENERAL-USE PVC INFUSION SETS, AND RECOMMENDED DOSES BASED ON THIS EXPERIENCE ARE TOO HIGH IF THE LOW ABSORBING INFUSION SETS ARE USED.

A potential safety problem exists with the combined use of some infusion pumps and some non-PVC infusion sets. Because the special tubing required to prevent the absorption of nitroglycerin tends to be less pliable than the conventional PVC tubing normally used with such infusion pumps, the pumps may fail to occlude the infusion sets completely. The results may be excessive flow at low infusion rate settings, causing alarms, or unregulated gravity flow when the infusion pump is stopped; this could lead to over-infusion of nitroglycerin. All

WARNINGS: *(cont'd)*

infusion pumps should be tested with the infusion sets to ensure their ability to deliver nitroglycerin accurately at low flow rates, and to occlude the infusion sets properly when the infusion is stopped.

PRECAUTIONS:

General: Nitroglycerin injection, USP should be used with caution in patients who have severe hepatic or renal disease.

Excessive hypotension, especially for prolonged periods of time, must be avoided because of possible deleterious effects on the brain, heart, liver, and kidney from poor perfusion and the attendant risk of ischemia, thrombosis, and altered function of these organs. Paradoxical bradycardia and increased angina pectoris may accompany nitroglycerin-induced hypotension. Patients with normal or low pulmonary capillary wedge pressure are especially sensitive to the hypotensive effects of Nitroglycerin IV. If pulmonary capillary wedge pressure is being monitored, it will be noted that a fall in wedge pressure precedes the onset of arterial hypotension, and the pulmonary capillary wedge pressure is thus a useful guide to safe titration of the drug.

Nitroglycerin contains alcohol and propylene glycol; safety for intracoronary injection has not been shown.

Carcinogenesis, Mutagenesis, and Impairment of Fertility: No long-term studies in animals were performed to evaluate carcinogenic potential of Nitroglycerin injection, USP.

Pregnancy Category C: Animal reproduction studies have not been conducted with Nitroglycerin. It is also not known whether Nitroglycerin can cause fetal harm when administered to a pregnant woman or can affect reproduction capacity. Nitroglycerin should be given to a pregnant woman only if clearly needed.

Nursing Mothers: It is not known whether nitroglycerin is excreted in human milk. Because many drugs are excreted in human milk, caution should be exercised when Nitroglycerin is administered to a nursing woman.

Pediatric Use: The safety and effectiveness of Nitroglycerin in children have not been established.

ADVERSE REACTIONS:

The most frequent adverse reaction in patients treated with Nitroglycerin is headache, which occurs in approximately 2% of patients. Other adverse reactions occurring in less than 1% of patients are the following: tachycardia, nausea, vomiting, apprehension, restlessness, muscle twitching, retrosternal discomfort, palpitations, dizziness, and abdominal pain.

The following additional adverse reactions have been reported with the oral and/or topical use of nitroglycerin: cutaneous flushing, weakness, and occasionally drug rash or exfoliative dermatitis.

OVERDOSAGE:

Accidental overdosage of Nitroglycerin may result in severe hypotension and reflex tachycardia which can be treated by elevating the legs and decreasing or temporarily terminating the infusion until the patient's condition stabilizes. Since the duration of the hemodynamic effects following Nitroglycerin administration is quite short, additional corrective measures are usually not required. However, if further therapy is indicated, administration of an intravenous alpha-adrenergic agonist (*e.g.,* methoxamine or phenylephrine) should be considered.

DOSAGE AND ADMINISTRATION:

IV

(NOT FOR DIRECT INTRAVENOUS INJECTION)NITROGLYCERIN INJECTION, USP IS A CONCENTRATED, POTENT DRUG WHICH MUST BE DILUTED IN DEXTROSE 5% INJECTION, USP OR SODIUM CHLORIDE (0.9%) INJECTION, USP PRIOR TO ITS INFUSION. NITROGLYCERIN SHOULD NOT BE ADMIXED WITH OTHER DRUGS.

Initial Dilution

Aseptically transfer the desired volume of Nitroglycerin (see TABLE 1)into a glass bottle containing the stated volume of either 5% dextrose injection, USP or 0.9% sodium chloride injection, USP. This yields a final concentration of 100 to 400 mcg/ml (see TABLE 1.) Invert the glass parenteral bottle several times following admixture to assure uniform dilution of nitroglycerin injection.

Maintenance Dilution

It is important to consider the fluid requirements of the patient as well as the expected duration of infusion in selecting the appropriate dilution of Nitroglycerin.

After the initial dosage titration, the concentration of the admixture may be increased, if necessary, to limit fluids given to the patient. The concentration of the infusion solution should not exceed 400 mcg/ml of nitroglycerin.

If the concentration is adjusted, it is imperative to flush or replace the infusion set before a new concentration is utilized. If the set were not flushed, or replaced, it could take minutes to hours, depending upon the flow rate and the dead space of the set, for the new concentration to reach the patient.

TABLE 1A Dilution table

Diluent Volume	Quantity of Nitroglycerin (5 mg/ml)	Approximate Final Concentration
100 ml	10 mg (2 ml)	100 mcg/ml
100 ml	20 mg (4 ml)	200 mcg/ml
100 ml	40 mg (8 ml)	400 mcg/ml
250 ml	25 mg (5 ml)	100 mcg/ml
250 ml	50 mg (10 ml)	200 mcg/ml
250 ml	100 mg (20 ml)	400 mcg/ml
500 ml	50 mg (10 ml)	100 mcg/ml
500 ml	100 mg (20 ml)	200 mcg/ml
500 ml	200 mg (40 ml)	400 mcg/ml

Dosage

Dosage is affected by the type of infusion set used (see WARNINGS.) Although the usual starting adult dose range reported in clinical studies was 25 mcg/min or more, those studies used PVC TUBING. **The use of nonabsorbing tubing will result in the need to use reduced doses.**

When using a nonabsorbing infusion set, initial dosage should be 5 mcg/min delivered through an infusion pump capable of exact and constant delivery of the drug. Subsequent titration must be adjusted to the clinical situation, with dose increments becoming more cautious as partial response is seen. Initial titration should be in 5 mcg/min increments, with increases every three to five minutes until some response is noted. If no response is seen at 20 mcg/min, increments of 10 and later 20 mcg/min can be used. Once a partial blood pressure response is observed, the dose increase should be reduced and the interval between increments should be lengthened. Patients with normal or low left ventricular filling pressure

DOSAGE AND ADMINISTRATION: *(cont'd)*

TABLE 1B Administration Table (60 microdrops = 1 milliliter)

Concentration (mcg/ml)	100	200	400
Dose (mcg/min)	**Flow Rate (microdrops/min = ml/hr)**		
5	3	-	-
10	6	3	-
15	9	-	-
20	12	6	-
30	18	9	-
40	24	12	6
60	36	18	9
80	48	24	12
120	72	36	18
160	96	48	24
240	-	72	36
320	-	96	48
480	-	-	72
640	-	-	96

or pulmonary capillary wedge pressure (*e.g.,* angina patients without other complications) may be hypersensitive to the effects of Nitroglycerin and may respond fully to doses as small as 5 mcg/min. These patients require especially careful titration and monitoring.

There is no fixed optimum dose of Nitroglycerin. Due to variations in the responsiveness of individual patients to the drug, each patient must be titrated to the desired level of hemodynamic function. Therefore, continuous monitoring of physiologic parameters (*e.g.,* blood pressure, heart rate, and pulmonary capillary wedge pressure) MUST BE PERFORMED to achieve the correct dose. Adequate systemic blood pressure and coronary perfusion pressure must be maintained.

Parenteral drug products should be inspected visually for particulate matter and discoloration prior to administration, whenever solution and container permit.

STORE AT CONTROLLED ROOM TEMPERATURE 15-30°C (59-86°F).

PROTECT FROM FREEZING.

EXTENDED RELEASE TABLETS

Careful studies with other formulations of Nitroglycerin have shown that maintenance of continuous 24-hour plasma levels of nitroglycerin results in tolerance (*i.e.,* loss of clinical response). Every dosing regimen should provide a daily nitrate- free interval to avoid the development of this tolerance. The minimum necessary length of such an interval has not yet been defined, but studies with other nitroglycerin formulations have shown that 10-12 hours is sufficient. Large controlled studies with other formulations of nitroglycerin show that no dosing regimen with these tablets should be expected to provide more than about 12 hours of continuous antianginal efficacy per day.

The pharmacokinetics of extended release nitroglycerin tablets, and the clinical effects of multiple-dose regimens, have not been well studied, In clinical trials, the initial regimen of nitroglycerin tablets has been 2.6 to 6.5 mg three times a day, with subsequent upward dose adjustment guided by symptoms and side effects. In one trial, 5 of the 18 subjects were titrated up to a dose of 26 mg four times a day.

STORE AT CONTROLLED ROOM TEMPERATURE BETWEEN 15-30°C (59-86°F).

SUBLINGUAL TABLETS

One tablet should be dissolved under the tongue or in the buccal pouch at the first sign of an acute anginal attack. The dose may be repeated approximately every five minutes until relief is obtained. If the pain persists after a total of three tablets in a fifteen minute period, the physician should be notified. These tablets may be used prophylactically five to ten minutes prior to engaging in activities which might precipitate an acute attack.

STORE AT CONTROLLED ROOM TEMPERATURE BETWEEN 15-30°C (59-86°F).

OINTMENT

When applying the ointment, place the dose-determining applicator supplied with the package printed-side down and squeeze the necessary amount of ointment from the tube onto the applicator. Then place the applicator with the ointment-side down onto the desired area of skin, usually the chest or back. Several studies suggest that absorption of nitroglycerin through the skin varies with the site of the application of the drug. Application of the drug to the skin of the chest is reported to give higher blood levels of nitroglycerin and greater hemodynamic effects than the application of extremities.

The amount of nitroglycerin entering the circulation varies directly with the size of the skin area exposed to the drug and the amount of ointment applied. Although in major clinical trials the dose was often applied to a 6x6-inch (150x150-mm) area of skin, in clinical practice the dose is usually applied to a smaller area. The ointment should be applied in a thin, uniform layer and the dose-to-area ratio kept reasonably constant. For example: 1 inch on a 2x3-inch area; 2 inches on a 3x4-inch area; 3 inches on a 4x5-inch area. When doubling the dose, the surface area over which the ointment is placed should be doubled.

As with all nitrates, clinical studies suggest that clinical response is variable. A suggested starting dose is 1/2 inch (7.5 mg) applied to a 1x3 area every eight hours. Response to treatment should be assessed over the next several days. If angina occurs after ointment has been in place for several hours, the frequency of dosing should be increased (*e.g.,* every six hours). Administer the smallest effective dose three to four times daily, unless clinical response suggests a different regimen. An initiation of therapy or change in dosage, blood pressure (patient standing) should be monitored. Controlled trials have been carried out for up to seven hours after dosing; therefore, it is not known whether the drug is effective in prevention of exertional angina beyond several hours after dosing. The effectiveness of repetitive applications of nitroglycerin ointment for the chronic management of angina pectoris has not been established. Nitroglycerin ointment is not intended for the immediate relief of anginal attacks.

LINGUAL AEROSOL SPRAY

At the onset of an attack, one or two metered doses should be sprayed onto or under the tongue. No more than three metered doses are recommended within a 15-minute period. If the chest pain persists, prompt medical attention is recommended. Nitroglycerin Spray may be used prophylactically five to ten minutes prior to engaging in activities which might precipitate an acute attack.

During application the patient should rest, ideally in the sitting position. The canister should be held vertically with the valve head uppermost and the spray orifice as close to the mouth as possible. The dose should be preferably sprayed onto the tongue by pressing the button firmly and the mouth should be closed immediately after each dose. THE SPRAY SHOULD NOT BE INHALED. Patients should be instructed to familiarize themselves with the position of the spray orifice, which can be identified by the finger rest on top of the valve, in order to facilitate orientation for administration at night.

TRANSDERMAL DELIVERY SYSTEM

The suggested starting dose is between 0.2 mg/hr* and 0.4 mg/hr*. Doses between 0.4 mg/hr* and 0.8 mg/hr* have shown continued effectiveness for 10-12 hours daily for at least one month (the longest period studied) of intermittent administration. Although the minimum nitrate-free interval has not yet been defined, data show that a nitrate-free interval of 10-12 hours is sufficient. Thus, an appropriate dosing schedule for nitroglycerin patches would include a daily patch-on period of 12-14 hours and a patch- off period of 10-12 hours.

Although some well-controlled clinical trials using exercise tolerance testing have shown maintenance of effectiveness when patches are worn continuously, the large majority of such controlled trials have shown the development of tolerance (*i.e.,* complete loss of effect) within the first 24 hours after therapy was initiated. Dose adjustment, even to levels much higher than generally used, did not restore efficacy.

*Release rates for formerly described in terms of drug delivered per 24 hrs. In these terms, the supplied systems would be rated at 2.5 mg/24 hrs. (0.1 mg/hr), 5 mg/24 hrs. (0.2 mg/hr), 10 mg/24 hrs. (0.4 mg/hr), and 15 mg/24 hrs. (0.6 mg/hr.).

STORE AT CONTROLLED ROOM TEMPERATURE BETWEEN 15-30°C (59-86°F). Extremes of temperature and/or humidity should be avoided.

PATIENT INFORMATION:

Nitroglycerin is used to treat chest pain, angina, associated with coronary artery disease. It is available in tablets that are swallowed, tablets that are place under the tongue, a patch, and a paste that is applied to the skin. Nitroglycerin works by dilating blood vessels making it easier for the blood to get to body tissues. Because your body can build up tolerance to this medication, it is not taken continuously as many medications are. It is important to give your body a 10-12 hour drug-free period. The most common side effect is headache. This generally is a mark of effectiveness. Other common side effects include: increased heart rate, nausea, vomiting, apprehension, restlessness, muscle twitching. When using the sublingual tablets - those placed under the tongue - you should feel a burning or tingling. This indicates the drug is effective. You should replace these tablets every six months to ensure they are effective. When using the paste or the patch, make sure to wash your hands after applying the medication to avoid getting the medication into the eyes. You may be asked to remove the patch during the night to provide a drug-free period for your body. When changing from one formulation to another, consult with your pharmacist or physician for proper dosage changes.

HOW SUPPLIED - RATED THERAPEUTICALLY EQUIVALENT:

Film, Continuous Release - Percutaneous - 0.1 mg/hr

30's	$39.18	MINITRAN, 3M Pharms	00089-0301-02

Film, Continuous Release - Percutaneous - 0.2 mg/hr

30's	$39.66	MINITRAN, 3M Pharms	00089-0302-02

Film, Continuous Release - Percutaneous - 0.4 mg/hr

30's	$44.16	MINITRAN, 3M Pharms	00089-0303-02

Film, Continuous Release - Percutaneous - 0.5 mg/hr

30's	**$44.52**	**TRANSDERM-NITRO 0.1, Novartis**	**57267-0902-26**
30's	**$44.52**	**TRANSDERM-NITRO 0.1, Novartis**	**57267-0902-42**
100's	**$148.38**	**TRANSDERM-NITRO 0.1, Novartis**	**57267-0902-30**

Film, Continuous Release - Percutaneous - 0.6 mg/hr

30's	$48.42	MINITRAN, 3M Pharms	00089-0304-02

Film, Continuous Release - Percutaneous - 0.8 mg/hr

30's	**$63.13**	**TRANSDERM-NITRO, Novartis**	**57267-0920-26**
30's	**$63.13**	**TRANSDERM-NITRO, Novartis**	**57267-0920-42**

Film, Continuous Release - Percutaneous - 1 mg/hr

30's	**$45.57**	**TRANSDERM-NITRO 0.2, Novartis**	**57267-0905-26**
30's	**$45.57**	**TRANSDERM-NITRO 0.2, Novartis**	**57267-0905-42**
100's	**$151.87**	**TRANSDERM-NITRO 0.2, Novartis**	**57267-0905-30**

Film, Continuous Release - Percutaneous - 50 mg

30's	**$52.08**	**TRANSDERM-NITRO 0.4, Novartis**	**57267-0910-26**
30's	**$52.08**	**TRANSDERM-NITRO 0.4, Novartis**	**57267-0910-42**
100's	**$173.58**	**TRANSDERM-NITRO 0.4, Novartis**	**57267-0910-30**

Injection, Solution - Intravenous - 0.1 mg/ml

250 ml	$16.01	Nitroglycerin 25, Baxter Hlthcare	00338-1047-02
250 ml	$17.33	NITROGLYCERIN IN D5W, Abbott	00074-1483-02
500 ml	$17.33	NITROGLYCERIN IN D5W, Abbott	00074-1483-03

Injection, Solution - Intravenous - 0.2 mg/ml

250 ml	$16.34	Nitroglycerin 50, Baxter Hlthcare	00338-1049-02
250 ml	$17.33	NITROGLYCERIN IN D5W, Abbott	00074-1482-02

Injection, Solution - Intravenous - 0.4 mg/ml

250 ml	$17.37	Nitroglycerin 100, Baxter Hlthcare	00338-1051-02
250 ml	$19.57	NITROGLYCERIN IN D5W, Abbott	00074-1484-02
500 ml	$24.31	NITROGLYCERIN IN D5W, Abbott	00074-1484-03

Injection, Solution - Intravenous - 5 mg/ml

1 ml	$34.50	NITRO-BID IV, Hoechst Marion Roussel	00088-1800-31
5 ml	$29.43	NITROGLYCERINE, Abbott	00074-4107-01
5 ml	$83.06	NITRO-BID IV, Hoechst Marion Roussel	00088-1800-32
5 ml	$171.88	Nitroglycerin Inj 5, Solopak Labs	39769-0077-05
5 ml x 10	$56.13	Nitroglycerin, Fujisawa USA	00469-4620-20
5 ml x 10	$90.63	Nitroglycerin, Am Regent	00517-4805-10
10 ml	$39.19	Nitroglycerin, Abbott	00074-4104-01
10 ml	$69.13	NITRO-BID IV, Hoechst Marion Roussel	00088-1800-33
10 ml	$375.00	Nitroglycerin Inj 5, Solopak Labs	39769-0077-10
10 ml x 10	$78.75	Nitroglycerin, Fujisawa USA	00469-4620-30
10 ml x 10	$140.63	Nitroglycerin, Am Regent	00517-4810-10
20 ml x 5	$37.50	Nitroglycerin, Voluntary Hosp	53258-1600-04
20 ml x 5	$142.50	Nitroglycerin, Fujisawa USA	00469-1600-40

Injection, Solution - Intravenous - 10 mg/ml

10 ml vial x 10	$90.00	NITROSTAT IV 100, Parke-Davis	00071-4579-45

Kit - Intravenous - 5 mg/ml

1's	$61.73	Nitroglycerin Kit, Abbott	00074-1324-01

HOW SUPPLIED - NOT RATED EQUIVALENT:

Aerosol, Spray - Oral - 0.4 mg/spr

14.49 gm	$24.82	NITROLINGUAL SPRAY, Rhone-Poulenc Rorer	00075-0850-84

Capsule, Gelatin, Sustained Action - Oral - 2.5 mg

60's	$3.44	Nitroglycerin, HL Moore Drug Exch	00839-5146-05
60's	$4.65	Nitroglycerin, Schein Pharm (US)	00364-0174-06
60's	$4.65	Nitroglycerin 2.5, Major Pharms	00904-0643-52
60's	$4.95	Nitroglycerin Slocaps, Eon Labs Mfg	00185-5174-60
60's	$4.95	NITRO-TIME, Time-Caps Labs	49483-0221-06
60's	$5.50	NITRO PAR TD, Parmed Pharms	00349-2102-60
60's	$5.98	Nitroglycerin, Ethex	58177-0004-03
100's	$5.55	Nitroglycerin, Voluntary Hosp	53258-0425-01
100's	$5.58	Nitro-Time, Time-Caps Labs	49483-0221-01
100's	$5.94	Nitroglycerin, Qualitest Pharms	00603-4782-21
100's	$6.00	NITROCOT T.D., C O Truxton	00463-3010-01

HOW SUPPLIED - NOT RATED EQUIVALENT: *(cont'd)*

100's	$6.15	Nitroglycerin, United Res	00677-0485-01
100's	$6.30	Nitroglycerin, Schein Pharm (US)	00364-0174-01
100's	$6.38	Nitroglycerin, Balan	00304-0196-01
100's	$6.50	Nitroglycerin Slocaps, Eon Labs Mfg	00185-5174-01
100's	$6.70	Nitroglycerin 2.5, Major Pharms	00904-0643-60
100's	$6.99	Nitroglycerin, Aligen Independ	00405-4702-01
100's	$8.20	NITROGLYN, Bradley Pharms	00482-1025-01
100's	$8.90	Nitroglycerin Timecap, Goldline Labs	00182-0702-01
100's	$8.90	Nitroglycerin T D, HL Moore Drug Exch	00839-5146-06
100's	$9.10	NITRO PAR TD, Parmed Pharms	00349-2102-01
100's	$9.10	Nitroglycerin, Rugby	00536-4083-01
100's	$9.15	Nitroglycerin, Ethex	58177-0004-04
100's	$10.50	Nitroglycerin, Voluntary Hosp	53258-0425-13
100's	$14.95	Nitroglycerin 2.5, Major Pharms	00904-0643-61
100's	$15.00	Nitroglycerin Timecap, Goldline Labs	00182-0702-89
100's	$16.68	Nitroglycerin, Vangard Labs	00615-0337-13

Capsule, Gelatin, Sustained Action - Oral - 6.5 mg

60's	$4.95	Nitroglycerin 6.5, Major Pharms	00904-0644-52
60's	$5.47	Nitroglycerin, HL Moore Drug Exch	00839-5978-05
60's	$6.42	NITRO-TIME, Time-Caps Labs	49483-0222-06
60's	$6.50	Nitroglycerin Slocaps, Eon Labs Mfg	00185-1235-60
60's	$7.95	NITRO-PAR, Parmed Pharms	00349-2097-60
60's	$8.02	Nitroglycerin, Ethex	58177-0005-03
100's	$6.45	Nitro-Time, Time-Caps Labs	49483-0222-01
100's	$6.61	Nitroglycerin, Qualitest Pharms	00603-4783-21
100's	$6.75	Nitroglycerin, United Res	00677-0486-01
100's	$7.18	Nitroglycerin, Balan	00304-0197-01
100's	$7.35	Nitroglycerin 6.5, Major Pharms	00904-0644-60
100's	$9.44	NITROGLYN, Bradley Pharms	00482-1065-01
100's	$9.55	Nitroglycerin, Schein Pharm (US)	00364-0432-01
100's	$9.56	Nitroglycerin Sustained Release, Lederle Pharm	00005-3292-43
100's	$11.95	NITRO-PAR, Parmed Pharms	00349-2097-01
100's	$12.95	Nitroglycerin Slocaps, Eon Labs Mfg	00185-1235-01
100's	$13.05	Nitroglycerin Timecap, Goldline Labs	00182-0703-01
100's	$13.08	Nitroglycerin T D, HL Moore Drug Exch	00839-5978-06
100's	$13.75	Nitroglycerin, Rugby	00536-4084-01
100's	$13.92	Nitroglycerin, Aligen Independ	00405-4703-01
100's	$13.99	Nitroglycerin, Ethex	58177-0005-04
100's	$17.10	Nitroglycerin Timecap, Goldline Labs	00182-0703-89
100's	$17.45	Nitroglycerin 6.5, Major Pharms	00904-0644-61
100's	$18.71	Nitroglycerin, Vangard Labs	00615-0336-13

Capsule, Gelatin, Sustained Action - Oral - 9 mg

60's	$6.40	Nitroglycerin 9, Major Pharms	00904-0647-52
60's	$7.08	NITRO-TIME, Time-Caps Labs	49483-0223-06
60's	$7.55	Nitroglycerin, HL Moore Drug Exch	00839-6724-05
60's	$9.41	Nitroglycerin, Qualitest Pharms	00603-4784-20
60's	$9.50	Nitroglycerin, Schein Pharm (US)	00364-0664-06
60's	$9.70	NITRO-PAR, Parmed Pharms	00349-8756-60
60's	$9.72	Nitroglycerin, Aligen Independ	00405-4704-31
60's	$9.80	Nitroglycerin, United Res	00677-0967-06
60's	$9.95	Nitroglycerin Slocaps, Eon Labs Mfg	00185-1217-60
60's	$9.99	Nitroglycerin, Goldline Labs	00182-1670-26
60's	$10.95	Nitroglycerin, Rugby	00536-4090-08
60's	$14.96	Nitroglycerin, Ethex	58177-0006-03
100's	$8.25	Nitroglycerin 9, Major Pharms	00904-0647-60
100's	$9.93	Nitro-Time, Time-Caps Labs	49483-0223-01
100's	$13.50	NITRO-PAR, Parmed Pharms	00349-8756-01
100's	$14.90	NITROGLYN, Bradley Pharms	00482-1090-01
100's	$14.95	Nitroglycerin Slocaps, Eon Labs Mfg	00185-1217-01
100's	$15.03	Nitroglycerin, Ethex	58177-0006-04
100's	$16.63	Nitroglycerin S.R., Lederle Pharm	00005-3143-43
100's	$17.95	Nitroglycerin 9, Major Pharms	00904-0647-61
100's	$18.00	Nitroglycerin, Goldline Labs	00182-1670-89

Disk - Percutaneous - 0.2 mg/hr

100's	$173.93	NITRODISC, Roberts Labs	54092-0342-01

Disk - Percutaneous - 0.3 mg/hr

30's	$55.00	NITRODISC, Roberts Labs	54092-0343-30
100's	$183.32	NITRODISC, Roberts Labs	54092-0343-01

Disk - Percutaneous - 0.4 mg/hr

30's	$57.80	NITRODISC, Searle	00025-2068-30

Disk - Percutaneous - 16 mg/pad

30's	$52.18	NITRODISC, Searle	00025-2058-30
100's	$144.94	NITRODISC, Searle	00025-2058-31

Film, Continuous Release - Percutaneous - 0.1 mg/hr

30's	$40.74	NITRO-DUR 2.5, Schering	00085-3305-30
30's	$40.74	NITRO-DUR, Schering	00085-3305-35

Film, Continuous Release - Percutaneous - 0.2 mg/hr

30's	$32.84	Nitroglycerin Transdermal, Rugby	00536-4098-07
30's	$33.06	NITRO TRANSDERM, Goldline Labs	00182-1240-17
30's	$36.60	Nitroglycerin, Qualitest Pharms	00603-4725-16
30's	$37.15	Nitroglycerin, Major Pharms	00904-0652-46
30's	$37.60	Nitroglycerin, HL Moore Drug Exch	00839-7790-19
30's	$39.17	DEPONIT 0.2, Schwarz Pharma (US)	00091-4195-01
30's	$39.17	DEPONIT, Schwarz Pharma (US)	00091-4195-31
30's	$41.35	NITRO-DUR, 5, Schering	00085-3310-30
30's	$41.35	NITRO-DUR, Schering	00085-3310-35
30's	$42.68	Nitroglycerin, Schein Pharm (US)	00364-2501-30
30's	$43.95	TRANSDERMAL-NTG 5, Warner Chilcott	00047-0835-15
30's	$45.95	Nitroglycerin, Mylan	00378-9004-93
90's	$99.65	NITRO-DUR, Schering	00085-3310-09
100's	$130.59	DEPONIT, Schwarz Pharma (US)	00091-4195-11

Film, Continuous Release - Percutaneous - 0.3 mg/hr

30 systems	**$57.39**	**TRANSDERM-NITRO 0.6, Novartis**	**57267-0915-26**
30 systems	**$57.39**	**TRANSDERM-NITRO 0.6, Novartis**	**57267-0915-42**
30's	$45.83	NITRODISC, Searle	00025-2078-30
30's	$46.35	NITRO-DUR, 7.5, Schering	00085-3315-30
30's	$46.35	NITRO-DUR, Schering	00085-3315-35
100's	$2.00	NITRO-DUR, 7.5, Schering	00085-3315-01
100's	$152.77	NITRODISC, Searle	00025-2078-31
100's	**$191.25**	**TRANSDERM-NITRO, Novartis**	**57267-0915-30**

Film, Continuous Release - Percutaneous - 0.4 mg/hr

30 systems	$43.70	DEPONIT, Schwarz Pharma (US)	00091-4196-01
30's	$38.20	Nitroglycerin, Qualitest Pharms	00603-4726-16
30's	$39.33	NITRO-TRANS SYSTEM, Goldline Labs	00182-1267-17
30's	$41.09	Nitroglycerin Transdermal System, Rugby	00536-4111-07
30's	$41.26	Nitroglycerin, HL Moore Drug Exch	00839-7791-19
30's	$43.70	DEPONIT, Schwarz Pharma (US)	00091-4196-31
30's	$44.90	Nitroglycerin, Schein Pharm (US)	00364-2502-30

HOW SUPPLIED - NOT RATED EQUIVALENT: *(cont'd)*

30's	$46.35	NITRO-DUR, 10, Schering	00085-3320-30
30's	$46.35	NITRO-DUR, Schering	00085-3320-35
30's	$46.45	Nitroglycerin, Major Pharms	00904-0653-46
30's	$48.61	TRANSDERMAL-NTG 10, Warner Chilcott	00047-0837-15
30's	$49.95	Nitroglycerin, Mylan	00378-9012-93
90's	$111.71	NITRO-DUR, Schering	00085-3320-09
100's	$145.69	DEPONIT, Schwarz Pharma (US)	00091-4196-11

Film, Continuous Release - Percutaneous - 0.5 mg/hr

30 units	$39.33	Nitroglycerin Transdermal System 0.4, Hercon Labs	49730-0004-30

Film, Continuous Release - Percutaneous - 0.6 mg/hr

30 units	$51.30	Nitroglycerin Transdermal 187.5 mg, Hercon Labs	49730-0002-30
30's	$46.00	Nitroglycerin Transdermal System, Rugby	00536-4112-07
30's	$48.19	Nitroglycerin, Qualitest Pharms	00603-4727-16
30's	$50.26	NITRO-DUR, 15, Schering	00085-3330-30
30's	$50.26	NITRO-DUR, Schering	00085-3330-35
30's	$55.10	NTG, Warner Chilcott	00047-0839-15
30's	$59.25	Nitroglycerin, Major Pharms	00904-0654-46
30's	$59.50	Nitroglycerin, Mylan	00378-9016-93

Film, Continuous Release - Percutaneous - 0.8 mg/hr

30's	$50.26	NITRO-DUR, Schering	00085-0819-30
30's	$50.26	NITRO-DUR, Schering	00085-0819-35

Film, Continuous Release - Percutaneous - 62.5 mg/unit

30 units	$33.06	Nitroglycerin Transdermal System 0.2, Hercon Labs	49730-0001-30

Injection, Conc-Soln - Intravenous - 8 mg/10ml

10 ml	$63.00	NITROSTAT IV 8, Parke-Davis	00071-4572-10

Ointment - Percutaneous - 2 %

1gm x 100	$24.88	NITRO-BID, Hoechst Marion Roussel	00088-1552-49
3 gm x 50	$50.56	NITROL, Savage Labs	00281-5804-48
3 gm x 50	$53.99	NITROL, Savage Labs	00281-5804-59
20 gm	$3.44	NITRO-BID, Hoechst Marion Roussel	00088-1552-20
30 gm	$4.56	Nitroglycerin, Rugby	00536-4820-28
30 gm	$6.95	Nitroglycerin, Fougera	00168-0038-30
30 gm	$8.87	NITROL, Savage Labs	00281-5804-46
60 gm	$6.63	NITRO-BID, Hoechst Marion Roussel	00088-1552-60
60 gm	$6.69	Nitroglycerin, Rugby	00536-4820-25
60 gm	$8.50	Nitroglycerin, Rugby	00536-2558-25
60 gm	$10.40	NITROL, Savage Labs	00281-5804-56
60 gm	$10.62	Nitroglycerin, Fougera	00168-0038-60
60 gm	$16.33	NITROL, Savage Labs	00281-5804-47
60 gm x 6	$56.70	NITROL, Savage Labs	00281-5804-58
100's	$192.62	NITRODISC, Roberts Labs	54092-0344-01

Tablet, Coated, Sustained Action - Oral - 2.6 mg

100's	$29.61	NITRONG, Sanofi Winthrop	00024-1298-10
100's	$30.56	NITRONG, Rhone-Poulenc Rorer	00075-0221-20
100's	$60.35	NITRONG, Rhone Poulenc Rorer	00195-0021-20

Tablet, Coated, Sustained Action - Oral - 6.5 mg

100's	$37.06	NITRONG, Sanofi Winthrop	00024-1299-10
100's	$38.25	NITRONG, Rhone-Poulenc Rorer	00075-0274-20
100's	$43.49	NITRONG, Rhone Poulenc Rorer	00195-0274-20

Tablet, Sublingual - Sublingual - 0.15 mg

100's	$5.46	NITROSTAT, Parke-Davis	00071-0568-24
100's	$11.81	NITROSTAT, Parke-Davis	00071-0568-13

Tablet, Sublingual - Sublingual - 0.3 mg

100's	$6.77	NITROSTAT, Parke-Davis	00071-0569-24

Tablet, Sublingual - Sublingual - 0.4 mg

100's	$6.77	NITROSTAT, Parke-Davis	00071-0570-24
100's	$15.35	NITROSTAT, Parke-Davis	00071-0570-13

Tablet, Sublingual - Sublingual - 0.6 mg

100's	$6.77	NITROSTAT, Parke-Davis	00071-0571-24

Tablet, Uncoated, Sustained Action - Buccal - 1 mg

100's	$37.87	NITROGARD, Forest Pharms	00456-0686-01

Tablet, Uncoated, Sustained Action - Buccal - 2 mg

100's	$40.09	NITROGARD, Forest Pharms	00456-0687-01

Tablet, Uncoated, Sustained Action - Buccal - 3 mg

100's	$43.33	NITROGARD, Forest Pharms	00456-0683-01

NIZATIDINE *(001894)*

CATEGORIES: Acid/Peptic Disorders; Antiulcer Drugs; Duodenal Ulcer; Esophagitis; GERD; Gastric Ulcer; Gastroesophagael Reflux Disease; Gastrointestinal Drugs; Histamine H2 Receptor Antagonists; Ulcer; Dyspepsia*; Gastritis*; Sales > $500 Million; FDA Approved 1988 Apr; Patent Expiration 2002 Dec; Top 200 Drugs
* Indication not approved by the FDA

BRAND NAMES: *Antizid*; **Axid**; *Calmaxid*; *Cronizat*; *Distaxid*; *Gastrax* (Germany); *Naxidine*; *Nizax* (Germany); *Nizaxid* (France); *Panaxid*; *Tazac*; *Zanizal*
(International brand names outside U.S. in italics)

FORMULARIES: Aetna; BC-BS; CIGNA; FHP; Humana; Kaiser; Medco; Medi-Cal; PruCare; United; PCS

COST OF THERAPY: $57.97 (Duodenal Ulcer; Capsule; 300 mg; 1/day; 28 days)

DESCRIPTION:

Axid (Nizatidine, USP) is a histamine H_2-receptor antagonist. Chemically, it is N-[2-[[[2-[(dimethylamino)methyl]-4-thiazolyl] methyl]thio]ethyl]-N'-methyl-2-nitro-1,1-ethenediamine.

Nizatidine has the empirical formula $C_{12}H_{21}N_5O_2S_2$ representing a molecular weight of 331.45. It is an off-white to buff crystalline solid that is soluble in water. Nizatidine has a bitter taste and mild sulfur-like odor. Each Pulvule (capsule) contains for oral administration gelatin, pregelatinized starch, silicone, starch, titanium dioxide, yellow iron oxide, 150 mg (0.45 mmol) or 300 mg (0.91 mmol) of nizatidine, and other inactive ingredients. The 150-mg Pulvule also contains magnesium stearate, and the 300-mg Pulvule also contains carboxymethylcellulose sodium, povidone, red iron oxide, and talc.

CLINICAL PHARMACOLOGY:

Nizatidine is a competitive, reversible inhibitor of histamine at the histamine H_2-receptors, particularly those in the gastric parietal cells.

CLINICAL PHARMACOLOGY: *(cont'd)*

ANTISECRETORY ACTIVITY

Effects on Acid Secretion: Nizatidine significantly inhibited nocturnal gastric acid secretion for up to 12 hours. Nizatidine also significantly inhibited gastric acid secretion stimulated by food, caffeine, betazole, and pentagastrin (TABLE 1).

TABLE 1 Effect of Oral Nizatidine on Gastric Acid Secretion

	Time After Dose (h)	% Inhibition of Gastric Acid Output by Dose (mg) 20-50	75	100	150	300
Nocturnal	Up to 10	57		73		90
Betazole	Up to 3		93		100	99
Pentagastrin	Up to 6		25		64	67
Meal	Up to 4	41	64		98	97
Caffeine	Up to 3		73		85	96

Effects on Other Gastrointestinal Secretions

Pepsin: Oral administration of 75 to 300 mg of nizatidine did not affect pepsin activity in gastric secretions. Total pepsin output was reduced in proportion to the reduced volume of gastric secretions.

Intrinsic Factor: Oral administration of 75 to 300 mg of nizatidine increased betazole-stimulated secretion of intrinsic factor.

Serum Gastrin: Nizatidine had no effect on basal serum gastrin. No rebound of gastrin secretion was observed when food was ingested 12 hours after administration of nizatidine.

Other Pharmacologic Actions:

Hormones: Nizatidine was not shown to affect the serum concentrations of gonadotropins, prolactin, growth hormone, antidiuretic hormone, cortisol, triiodothyronine, thyroxin, testosterone, 5α-dihydrotestosterone, androstenedione, or estradiol.

Nizatidine had no demonstrable antiandrogenic action.

Pharmacokinetics

The absolute oral bioavailability of nizatidine exceeds 70%. Peak plasma concentrations (700 to 1,800 mcg/l for a 150-mg dose and 1,400 to 3,600 mcg/l for a 300-mg dose) occur from 0.5 to 3 hours following the dose. A concentration of 1,000 mcg/l is equivalent to 3 μmol/l; a dose of 300 mg is equivalent to 905 μmoles. Plasma concentrations 12 hours after administration are less than 10 mcg/l. The elimination half-life is 1 to 2 hours, plasma clearance is 40 to 60 l/h, and the volume of distribution is 0.8 to 1.5 l/kg. Because of the short half-life and rapid clearance of nizatidine, accumulation of the drug would not be expected in individuals with normal renal function who take either 300 mg once daily at bedtime or 150 mg twice daily. Nizatidine exhibits dose proportionality over the recommended dose range.

The oral bioavailability of nizatidine is unaffected by concomitant ingestion of propantheline. Antacids consisting of aluminum and magnesium hydroxides with simethicone decrease the absorption of nizatidine by about 10%. With food, the AUC and C_{max} increase by approximately 10%.

In humans, less than 7% of an oral dose is metabolized as N2-monodes-methylnizatidine, an H_2-receptor antagonist, which is the principal metabolite excreted in the urine. Other likely metabolites are the N2-oxide (less than 5% of the dose) and the S-oxide (less than 6% of the dose).

More than 90% of an oral dose of nizatidine is excreted in the urine within 12 hours. About 60% of an oral dose is excreted as unchanged drug. Renal clearance is about 500 ml/min, which indicates excretion by active tubular secretion. Less than 6% of an administered dose is eliminated in the feces.

Moderate to severe renal impairment significantly prolongs the half-life and decreases the clearance of nizatidine. In individuals who are functionally anephric, the half-life is 3.5 to 11 hours, and the plasma clearance is 7 to 14 l/h. To avoid accumulation of the drug in individuals with clinically significant renal impairment, the amount and/or frequency of doses of nizatidine should be reduced in proportion to the severity of dysfunction (see DOSAGE AND ADMINISTRATION.)

Approximately 35% of nizatidine is bound to plasma protein, mainly to α_1-acid glycoprotein. Warfarin, diazepam, acetaminophen, propantheline, phenobarbital, and propranolol did not affect plasma protein binding of nizatidine *in vitro.*

CLINICAL STUDIES:

Active Duodenal Ulcer: In multicenter, double-blind, placebo-controlled studies in the United States, endoscopically diagnosed duodenal ulcers healed more rapidly following administration of nizatidine, 300 mg h.s. or 150 mg b.i.d., than with placebo (TABLE 2). Lower doses, such as 100 mg h.s., had slightly lower effectiveness.

TABLE 2 Healing Response of Ulcers to Nizatidine

	300 mg h.s.		150 mg b.i.d.		Placebo	
	Number Entered	Healed/ Evaluable	Number Entered	Healed/ Evaluable	Number Entered	Healed/ Evaluable
STUDY 1						
Week 2			276	93/265 (35%)*	279	55/260 (21%)
Week 4				198/259 (76%)*		95/243 (39%)
STUDY 2						
Week 2	108	24/103 (23%)*	106	27/101 (27%)*	101	9/93 (10%)
Week 4		65/97 (67%)*		66/97 (68%)*		24/84 (29%)
STUDY 3						
Week 2	92	22/90 (24%)†			98	13/92 (14%)
Week 4		52/85 (61%)*				29/88 (33%)
Week 8		68/83 (82%)*				39/79 (49%)

* P <0.01 as compared with placebo.
† P <0.05 as compared with placebo.

Maintenance of Healed Duodenal Ulcer: Treatment with a reduced dose of nizatidine has been shown to be effective as maintenance therapy following healing of active duodenal ulcers. In multicenter, double-blind, placebo-controlled studies conducted in the United States, 150 mg of nizatidine taken at bedtime resulted in a significantly lower incidence of duodenal ulcer recurrence in patients treated for up to 1 year (TABLE 3).

CLINICAL STUDIES: *(cont'd)*

TABLE 3 Percentage of Ulcers Recurring by 3, 6, and 12 Months in Double-Blind Studies Conducted in the United States

Month	Axid, 150 mg h.s.	Placebo
3	13% (28/208)*	40% (82/204)
6	24% (45/188)*	57% (106/187)
12	34% (57/166)*	64% (112/175)

* P <0.001 as compared with placebo.

Gastroesophageal Reflux Disease (GERD): In 2 multicenter, double-blind, placebo-controlled clinical trials performed in the United States and Canada, nizatidine was more effective than placebo in improving endoscopically diagnosed esophagitis and in healing erosive and ulcerative esophagitis.

In patients with erosive or ulcerative esophagitis, 150 mg b.i.d. of nizatidine given to 88 patients compared with placebo in 98 patients in Study 1 yielded a higher healing rate at 3 weeks (16% vs 7%) and at 6 weeks (32% vs 16%, P<0.05). Of 99 patients on nizatidine and 94 patients on placebo, Study 2 at the same dosage yielded similar results at 6 weeks (21% vs 11%, P<0.05) and at 12 weeks (29% vs 13%,P<0.01).

In addition, relief of associated heartburn was greater in patients treated with nizatidine. Patients treated with nizatidine consumed fewer antacids than did patients treated with placebo.

Active Benign Gastric Ulcer: In a multicenter, double-blind, placebo-controlled study conducted in the United States and Canada, endoscopically diagnosed benign gastric ulcers healed significantly more rapidly following administration of nizatidine than of placebo (TABLE 4).

In a multicenter, double-blind, comparator-controlled study in Europe, healing rates for patients receiving nizatidine (300 mg h.s. or 150 mg b.i.d.) were equivalent to rates for patients receiving a comparator drug, and statistically superior to historical placebo control rates.

TABLE 4

Week	Treatment	Healing Rate	vs. Placebo p-value*
4	Niz 300 mg h.s.	52/153 (34%)	0.342
	Niz 150 mg b.i.d.	65/151 (43%)	0.022
	Placebo	48/151 (32%)	
8	Niz 300 mg h.s.	99/153 (65%)	0.011
	Niz 150 mg b.i.d.	105/151 (70%)	<0.001
	Placebo	78/151 (52%)	

* P-values are one-sided, obtained by Chi-square test, and not adjusted for multiple comparisons.

INDICATIONS AND USAGE:

Nizatidine is indicated for up to 8 weeks for the treatment of active duodenal ulcer. In most patients, the ulcer will heal within 4 weeks.

Nizatidine is indicated for maintenance therapy for duodenal ulcer patients, at a reduced dosage of 150 mg h.s. after healing of an active duodenal ulcer. The consequences of continuous therapy with nizatidine for longer than 1 year are not known.

Nizatidine is indicated for up to 12 weeks for the treatment of endoscopically diagnosed esophagitis, including erosive and ulcerative esophagitis, and associated heartburn due to GERD.

Nizatidine is indicated for up to 8 weeks for the treatment of active benign gastric ulcer. Before initiating therapy, care should be taken to exclude the possibility of malignant gastric ulceration.

CONTRAINDICATIONS:

Nizatidine is contraindicated in patients with known hypersensitivity to the drug. Because cross sensitivity in this class of compounds has been observed, H_2-receptor antagonists, including nizatidine, should not be administered to patients with a history of hypersensitivity to other H_2-receptor antagonists.

PRECAUTIONS:

GENERAL

1. Symptomatic response to nizatidine therapy does not preclude the presence of gastric malignancy.

2. Because nizatidine is excreted primarily by the kidney, dosage should be reduced in patients with moderate to severe renal insufficiency (see DOSAGE AND ADMINISTRATION.)

3. Pharmacokinetic studies in patients with hepatorenal syndrome have not been done. Part of the dose of nizatidine is metabolized in the liver. In patients with normal renal function and uncomplicated hepatic dysfunction, the disposition of nizatidine is similar to that in normal subjects.

Laboratory Tests: False-positive tests for urobilinogen with Multistix may occur during therapy with nizatidine.

Carcinogenesis, Mutagenesis, and Impairment of Fertility: A 2-year oral carcinogenicity study in rats with doses as high as 500 mg/kg/day (about 80 times the recommended daily therapeutic dose) showed no evidence of a carcinogenic effect. There was a dose-related increase in the density of enterochromaffin-like (ECL) cells in the gastric oxyntic mucosa. In a 2-year study in mice, there was no evidence of a carcinogenic effect in male mice; although hyperplastic nodules of the liver were increased in the high-dose males as compared with placebo. Female mice given the high dose of nizatidine (2,000 mg/kg/day, about 330 times the human dose) showed marginally statistically significant increases in hepatic carcinoma and hepatic nodular hyperplasia with no numerical increase seen in any of the other dose groups. The rate of hepatic carcinoma in the high-dose animals was within the historical control limits seen for the strain of mice used. The female mice were given a dose larger than the maximum tolerated dose, as indicated by excessive (30%) weight decrement as compared with concurrent controls and evidence of mild liver injury (transaminase elevations). The occurrence of a marginal finding at high dose only in animals given an excessive and somewhat hepatotoxic dose, with no evidence of a carcinogenic effect in rats, male mice, and female mice (given up to 360 mg/kg/day, about 60 times the human dose), and a negative mutagenicity battery are not considered evidence of a carcinogenic potential for Nizatidine.

Nizatidine was not mutagenic in a battery of tests performed to evaluate its potential genetic toxicity, including bacterial mutation tests, unscheduled DNA synthesis, sister chromatid exchange, mouse lymphoma assay, chromosome aberration tests, and a micronucleus test.

In a 2-generation, perinatal and postnatal fertility study in rats, doses of nizatidine up to 650 mg/kg/day produced no adverse effects on the reproductive performance of parental animals or their progeny.

PRECAUTIONS: *(cont'd)*

Pregnancy, Teratogenic Effects—Pregnancy Category B: Oral reproduction studies in pregnant rats at doses up to 1500 mg/kg/day (9000 mg/m²/day, 40.5 times the recommended human dose based on body surface area) and in pregnant rabbits at doses up to 275 mg/kg/day (3245 mg/m²/day, 14.6 times the recommended human dose based on body surface area) have revealed no evidence of impaired fertility or harm to the fetus due to nizatidine. There are, however, no adequate and well-controlled studies in pregnant women. Because animal reproduction studies are not always predictive of human response, this drug should be used during pregnancy only if clearly needed.

Nursing Mothers: Studies conducted in lactating women have shown that 0.1% of the administered oral dose of nizatidine is secreted in human milk in proportion to plasma concentrations. Because of the growth depression in pups reared by lactating rats treated with nizatidine, a decision should be made whether to discontinue nursing or discontinue the drug, taking into account the importance of the drug to the mother.

Pediatric Use: Safety and effectiveness in children have not been established.

Geriatric Use: Ulcer healing rates in elderly patients are similar to those in younger age groups. The incidence rates of adverse events and laboratory test abnormalities are also similar to those seen in other age groups. Age alone may not be an important factor in the disposition of nizatidine. Elderly patients may have reduced renal function (see DOSAGE AND ADMINISTRATION.)

DRUG INTERACTIONS:

No interactions have been observed between nizatidine and theophylline, chlordiazepoxide, lorazepam, lidocaine, phenytoin, and warfarin. Nizatidine does not inhibit the cytochrome P-450-linked drug-metabolizing enzyme system; therefore, drug interactions mediated by inhibition of hepatic metabolism are not expected to occur. In patients given very high doses (3,900 mg) of aspirin daily, increases in serum salicylate levels were seen when nizatidine, 150 mg b.i.d., was administered concurrently.

ADVERSE REACTIONS:

Worldwide, controlled clinical trials of nizatidine included over 6,000 patients given nizatidine in studies of varying durations. Placebo-controlled trials in the United States and Canada included over 2,600 patients given nizatidine and over 1,700 given placebo. Among the adverse events in these placebo-controlled trials, anemia (0.2% vs 0%) and urticaria (0.5% vs 0.1%) were significantly more common in the nizatidine group.

Incidence in Placebo-Controlled Clinical Trials in the United States and Canada: TABLE 5 lists adverse events that occurred at a frequency of 1% or more among nizatidine-treated patients who participated in placebo-controlled trials. The cited figures provide some basis for estimating the relative contribution of drug and nondrug factors to the side effect incidence rate in the population studied.

TABLE 5 Incidence Of Treatment-Emergent Adverse Events In Placebo-Controlled Clinical Studies In The United States And Canada

	Percentage of Patients Reporting Event	
Body System/Adverse Event*	**Nizatidine (N=2,694)**	**Placebo (N=1,729)**
Body As A Whole		
Headache	16.6	15.6
Abdominal pain	7.5	12.5
Pain	4.2	3.8
Asthenia	3.1	2.9
Back pain	2.4	2.6
Chest pain	2.3	2.1
Infection	1.7	1.1
Fever	1.6	2.3
Surgical procedure	1.4	1.5
Injury, accident	1.2	0.9
Digestive		
Diarrhea	7.2	6.9
Nausea	5.4	7.4
Flatulence	4.9	5.4
Vomiting	3.6	5.6
Dyspepsia	3.6	4.4
Constipation	2.5	3.8
Dry mouth	1.4	1.3
Nausea and vomiting	1.2	1.9
Anorexia	1.2	1.6
Gastrointestinal disorder	1.1	1.2
Tooth disorder	1.0	0.8
Musculoskeletal		
Myalgia	1.7	1.5
Nervous		
Dizziness	4.6	3.8
Insomnia	2.7	3.4
Abnormal dreams	1.9	1.9
Somnolence	1.9	1.6
Anxiety	1.6	1.4
Nervousness	1.1	0.8
Respiratory		
Rhinitis	9.8	9.6
Pharyngitis	3.3	3.1
Sinusitis	2.4	2.1
Cough, increased	2.0	2.0
Skin And Appendages		
Rash	1.9	2.1
Pruritus	1.7	1.3
Special Senses		
Amblyopia	1.0	0.9

* Events reported by at least 1% of nizatidine-treated patients are included.

A variety of less common events were also reported; it was not possible to determine whether these were caused by nizatidine.

Hepatic: Hepatocellular injury, evidenced by elevated liver enzyme tests (SGOT [AST], SGPT [ALT], or alkaline phosphatase), occurred in some patients and was possibly or probably related to nizatidine. In some cases there was marked elevation of SGOT, SGPT enzymes (greater than 500 IU/l) and, in a single instance, SGPT was greater than 2,000 IU/l. The overall rate of occurrences of elevated liver enzymes and elevations to 3 times the upper limit of normal, however, did not significantly differ from the rate of liver enzyme abnormalities in placebo-treated patients. All abnormalities were reversible after discontinuation of nizatidine. Since market introduction, hepatitis and jaundice have been reported. Rare cases of cholestatic or mixed hepatocellular and cholestatic injury with jaundice have been reported with reversal of the abnormalities after discontinuation of nizatidine.

Cardiovascular: In clinical pharmacology studies, short episodes of asymptomatic ventricular tachycardia occurred in 2 individuals administered nizatidine and in 3 untreated subjects.

ADVERSE REACTIONS: *(cont'd)*

CNS: Rare cases of reversible mental confusion have been reported.

Endocrine: Clinical pharmacology studies and controlled clinical trials showed no evidence of antiandrogenic activity due to nizatidine. Impotence and decreased libido were reported with similar frequency by patients who received nizatidine and by those given placebo. Rare reports of gynecomastia occurred.

Hematologic: Anemia was reported significantly more frequently in nizatidine- than in placebo-treated patients. Fatal thrombocytopenia was reported in a patient who was treated with nizatidine and another H_2-receptor antagonist. On previous occasions, this patient had experienced thrombocytopenia while taking other drugs. Rare cases of thrombocytopenic purpura have been reported.

Integumental: Sweating and urticaria were reported significantly more frequently in nizatidine- than in placebo-treated patients. Rash and exfoliative dermatitis were also reported. Vasculitis has been reported rarely.

Hypersensitivity: As with other H_2-receptor antagonists, rare cases of anaphylaxis following administration of nizatidine have been reported. Rare episodes of hypersensitivity reactions (*e.g.*, bronchospasm, laryngeal edema, rash, and eosinophilia) have been reported.

Body as a Whole: Serum sickness-like reactions have occurred rarely in conjunction with nizatidine use.

Genitourinary: Reports of impotence have occurred.

Other: Hyperuricemia unassociated with gout or nephrolithiasis was reported. Eosinophilia, fever, and nausea related to nizatidine administration have been reported.

OVERDOSAGE:

Overdoses of nizatidine have been reported rarely. The following is provided to serve as a guide should such an overdose be encountered.

Signs and Symptoms: There is little clinical experience with overdosage of nizatidine in humans. Test animals that received large doses of nizatidine have exhibited cholinergic-type effects, including lacrimation, salivation, emesis, miosis, and diarrhea. Single oral doses of 800 mg/kg in dogs and of 1,200 mg/kg in monkeys were not lethal. Intravenous median lethal doses in the rat and mouse were 301 mg/kg and 232 mg/kg respectively.

Treatment: To obtain up-to-date information about the treatment of overdose, a good resource is your certified Regional Poison Control Center. Telephone numbers of certified poison control centers are listed at the beginning of *Physicians GenRx*. In managing overdosage, consider the possibility of multiple drug overdoses, interaction among drugs, and unusual drug kinetics in your patient.

If overdosage occurs, use of activated charcoal, emesis, or lavage should be considered along with clinical monitoring and supportive therapy. The ability of hemodialysis to remove nizatidine from the body has not been conclusively demonstrated; however, due to its large volume of distribution, nizatidine is not expected to be efficiently removed from the body by this method.

DOSAGE AND ADMINISTRATION:

Active Duodenal Ulcer: The recommended oral dosage for adults is 300 mg once daily at bedtime. An alternative dosage regimen is 150 mg twice daily.

Maintenance of Healed Duodenal Ulcer: The recommended oral dosage for adults is 150 mg once daily at bedtime.

Gastroesophageal Reflux Disease: The recommended oral dosage in adults for the treatment of erosions, ulcerations, and associated heartburn is 150 mg twice daily.

Active Benign Gastric Ulcer: The recommended oral dosage is 300 mg given either as 150 mg twice daily or 300 mg once daily at bedtime. Prior to treatment, care should be taken to exclude the possibility of malignant gastric ulceration.

Dosage Adjustment for Patients With Moderate to Severe Renal Insufficiency: The dose for patients with renal dysfunction should be reduced (TABLE 6):

TABLE 6 Active Duodenal Ulcer, GERD and Benign Gastric Ulcer

C_{cr}	Dose
20-50 ml/min	150 mg daily
<20 ml/min	150 mg every other day
Maintenance Therapy	
20-50 ml/min	150 mg every other day
<20 ml/min	150 mg every 3 days

Some elderly patients may have creatinine clearances of less than 50 ml/min, and, based on pharmacokinetic data in patients with renal impairment, the dose for such patients should be reduced accordingly. The clinical effects of this dosage reduction in patients with renal failure have not been evaluated.

PATIENT INFORMATION:

Nizatidine is known as a histamine blocker or an H2-receptor blocker. It is used to treat ulcers. Although this drug blocks histamine in the stomach, it cannot be used in place of antihistamine used to treat runny noses and watery eyes. This drug works primarily in the stomach and intestines. In most cases therapy is needed for 4-8 weeks to produce ulcer healing. Some patients may need long term preventative therapy with lower doses taken at bedtime. Nizatidine has no clinically significant drug interactions and few side effects. The most common side effects reported include headache and abdominal pain. This medication must be taken as prescribed for ulcers to heal. You may be asked to follow a certain diet that will not aggravate your ulcer or cause a new one. If you choose to also take antacids, take them two hours before or after taking this medication.

HOW SUPPLIED:

Pulvules: Axid 150 mg (No. 3144) are pale yellow and dark yellow Pulvules with "Lilly 3144" imprinted on one end and "Axid 150 mg" on the other.

Store at controlled room temperature, 59° to 86°F (15° to 30°C).

HOW SUPPLIED - EQUIVALENTS NOT AVAILABLE:

Capsule, Gelatin - Oral - 150 mg

60's	$92.31	AXID, Lilly	00002-3144-60
100's	$158.22	AXID, Lilly	00002-3144-33
620's	$969.65	AXID, Lilly	00002-3144-82

Capsule, Gelatin - Oral - 300 mg

30's	$62.12	AXID, Lilly	00002-3145-85
30's	$89.30	AXID, Lilly	00002-3145-30

NOREPINEPHRINE BITARTRATE *(001898)*

CATEGORIES: Anesthesia; Autonomic Drugs; Cardiac Arrest; Cardiovascular Drugs; Hypotension; Hypotension/Shock; Sympathomimetic Agents; Vasopressors; Pregnancy Category C; FDA Approval Pre 1982

BRAND NAMES: Lavarterenol; **Levophed**

DESCRIPTION:

Norepinephrine (sometimes referred to as *l-arterenol/Levarterenol*or *l-norepinephrine*) is a sympathomimetic amine which differs from epinephrine by the absence of a methyl group on the nitrogen atom.

Norepinephrine Bitartrate is (-)-α-(aminomethyl)-3,4-dihydroxybenzyl alcohol tartrate (1:1) (salt) monohydrate.

Levophed is supplied in sterile aqueous solution in the form of the bitartrate salt to be administered by intravenous infusion following dilution. Norepinephrine is sparingly soluble in water, very slightly soluble in alcohol and ether, and readily soluble in acids. Each ml of Levophed bitartrate injection contains the equivalent of 1 mg base of Levophed, sodium chloride for isotonicity, and not more than 2 mg of sodium metabisulfite as an antioxidant. It has a pH of 3 to 4.5. The air in the ampuls has been displaced by nitrogen gas.

CLINICAL PHARMACOLOGY:

Norepinephrine bitartrate functions as a peripheral vasoconstrictor (alpha-adrenergic action) and as an inotropic stimulator of the heart and dilator of coronary arteries (beta-adrenergic action).

INDICATIONS AND USAGE:

For blood pressure control in certain acute hypotensive states (*e.g.*, pheochromocytomectomy, sympathectomy, poliomyelitis, spinal anesthesia, myocardial infarction, septicemia, blood transfusion, and drug reactions).

As an adjunct in the treatment of cardiac arrest and profound hypotension.

CONTRAINDICATIONS:

Norepinephrine bitartrate should not be given to patients who are hypotensive from blood volume deficits except as an emergency measure to maintain coronary and cerebral artery perfusion until blood volume replacement therapy can be completed. If norepinephrine bitartrate is continuously administered to maintain blood pressure in the absence of blood volume replacement, the following may occur: severe peripheral and visceral vasoconstriction, decreased renal perfusion and urine output, poor systemic blood flow despite "normal" blood pressure, tissue hypoxia, and lactate acidosis.

Norepinephrine bitartrate should also not be given to patients with mesenteric or peripheral vascular thrombosis (because of the risk of increasing ischemia and extending the area of infarction) unless, in the opinion of the attending physician, the administration of norepinephrine bitartrate is necessary as a life-saving procedure.

Cyclopropane and halothane anesthetics increase cardiac autonomic irritability and therefore seem to sensitize the myocardium to the action of intravenously administered epinephrine or norepinephrine. Hence, the use of norepinephrine bitartrate during cyclopropane and halothane anesthesia is generally considered contraindicated because of the risk of producing ventricular tachycardia or fibrillation.

The same type of cardiac arrhythmias may result from the use of norepinephrine bitartrate in patients with profound hypoxia or hypercarbia.

WARNINGS:

Norepinephrine bitartrate should be used with extreme caution in patients receiving monoamine oxidase inhibitors (MAOI) or antidepressants of the triptyline or imipramine types, because severe, prolonged hypertension may result.

Norepinephrine bitartrate injection contains sodium metabisulfite, a sulfite that may cause allergic-type reactions including anaphylactic symptoms and life-threatening or less severe asthmatic episodes in certain susceptible people. The overall prevalence of sulfite sensitivity in the general population is unknown. Sulfite sensitivity is seen more frequently in asthmatic than in nonasthmatic people.

PRECAUTIONS:

GENERAL

Avoid Hypertension: Because of the potency of norepinephrine bitartrate and because of varying response to pressor substances, the possibility always exists that dangerously high blood pressure may be produced with overdoses of this pressor agent. It is desirable, therefore, to record the blood pressure every two minutes from the time administration is started until the desired blood pressure is obtained, then every five minutes if administration is to be continued.

The rate of flow must be watched constantly, and the patient should never be left unattended while receiving norepinephrine bitartrate. Headache may be a symptom of hypertension due to overdosage.

Site of Infusion: Whenever possible, infusions of norepinephrine bitartrate should be given into a large vein, particularly an antecubital vein because, when administered into this vein, the risk of necrosis of the overlying skin from prolonged vasoconstriction is apparently very slight. Some authors have indicated that the femoral vein is also an acceptable route of administration. A catheter tie-in technique should be avoided, if possible, since the obstruction to blood flow around the tubing may cause stasis and increased local concentration of the drug. Occlusive vascular diseases (for example, atherosclerosis, arteriosclerosis, diabetic endarteritis, Buerger's disease) are more likely to occur in the lower than in the upper extremity. Therefore, one should avoid the veins of the leg in elderly patients or in those suffering from such disorders. Gangrene has been reported in a lower extremity when infusions of norepinephrine bitartrate were given in an ankle vein.

Extravasation: The infusion site should be checked frequently for free flow. Care should be taken to avoid extravasation of norepinephrine bitartrate into the tissues, as local necrosis might ensue due to the vasoconstrictive action of the drug. Blanching along the course of the infused vein, sometimes without obvious extravasation, has been attributed to vasa vasorum constriction with increased permeability of the vein wall, permitting some leakage.

This also may progress on rare occasions to superficial slough, particularly during infusion into leg veins in elderly patients or in those suffering from obliterative vascular disease. Hence, if blanching occurs, consideration should be given to the advisability of changing the infusion site at intervals to allow the effects of local vasoconstriction to subside.

IMPORTANT—ANTIDOTE FOR EXTRAVASATION ISCHEMIA:
To prevent sloughing and necrosis in areas in which extravasation has taken place, the area should be infiltrated as soon as possible with 10 ml to 15 ml of saline solution containing from 5 mg to 10 mg of Regitine (brand of phentolamine), an adrenergic blocking agent. A syringe with a

PRECAUTIONS: *(cont'd)*

fine hypodermic needle should be used, with the solution being infiltrated liberally throughout the area, which is easily identified by its cold, hard, and pallid appearance. Sympathetic blockade with phentolamine causes immediate and conspicuous local hyperemic changes if the area is infiltrated within 12 hours. Therefore, phentolamine should be given as soon as possible after the extravasation is noted.

CARCINOGENESIS, MUTAGENESIS, AND IMPAIRMENT OF FERTILITY

Studies have not been performed.

PREGNANCY CATEGORY C

Animal reproduction studies have not been conducted with norepinephrine bitartrate. It is also not known whether norepinephrine bitartrate can cause fetal harm when administered to a pregnant woman or can affect reproduction capacity. Norepinephrine bitartrate should be given to a pregnant woman only if clearly needed.

NURSING MOTHERS

It is not known whether this drug is excreted in human milk. Because many drugs are excreted in human milk, caution should be exercised when norepinephrine bitartrate is administered to a nursing woman.

PEDIATRIC USE

Safety and effectiveness in children has not been established.

DRUG INTERACTIONS:

Cyclopropane and halothane anesthetics increase cardiac automatic irritability and therefore seem to sensitize the myocardium to the action of intravenously administered epinephrine or norepinephrine. Hence, the use of norepinephrine bitartrate during cyclopropane and halothane anesthesia is generally considered contraindicated because of the risk of producing ventricular tachycardia or fibrillation. The same type of cardiac arrhythmias may result from the use of norepinephrine bitartrate in patients with profound hypoxia or hypercarbia.

Norepinephrine bitartrate should be used with extreme caution in patients receiving monoamine oxidase inhibitors (MAOI) or antidepressants of the triptyline or imipramine types, because severe, prolonged hypertension may result.

ADVERSE REACTIONS:

The following reactions can occur:

Body As A Whole: Ischemic injury due to potent vasoconstrictor action tissue hypoxia.

Cardiovascular System: Bradycardia, probably as a reflex result of a rise in blood pressure, arrhythmias.

Nervous System: Anxiety, transient headache.

Respiratory System: Respiratory difficulty.

Skin and Appendages: Extravasation necrosis at injection site.

Prolonged administration of any potent vasopressor may result in plasma volume depletion which should be continuously corrected by appropriate fluid and electrolyte replacement therapy. If plasma volumes are not corrected, hypotension may recur when norepinephrine bitartrate is discontinued, or blood pressure may be maintained at the risk of severe peripheral and visceral vasoconstriction (*e.g.,* decreased renal perfusion) with diminution in blood flow and tissue perfusion with subsequent tissue hypoxia and lactic acidosis and possible ischemic injury. Gangrene of extremities has been rarely reported.

Overdoses or conventional doses in hypersensitive persons (*e.g.,* hyperthyroid patients) cause severe hypertension with violent headache, photophobia, stabbing retrosternal pain, pallor, intense sweating, and vomiting.

OVERDOSAGE:

Overdosage with norepinephrine bitartrate may result in headache, severe hypertension, reflex bradycardia, marked increase in peripheral resistance, and decreased cardiac output. In case of accidental overdosage, as evidenced by excessive blood pressure elevation, discontinue norepinephrine bitartrate until the condition of the patient stabilizes.

DOSAGE AND ADMINISTRATION:

Norepinephrine bitartrate injection is a concentrated, potent drug which must be diluted in dextrose containing solutions prior to infusion. An infusion of norepinephrine bitartrate should be given into a large vein (see PRECAUTIONS.)

Restoration of Blood Pressure in Acute Hypotensive States Blood volume depletion should always be corrected as fully as possible before any vasopressor is administered. When, as an emergency measure, intraaortic pressures must be maintained to prevent cerebral or coronary artery ischemia, norepinephrine bitartrate can be administered before and concurrently with blood volume replacement.

Diluent: Norepinephrine bitartrate should be diluted in 5 percent dextrose injection or 5 percent dextrose and sodium chloride injections. These dextrose containing fluids are protection against significant loss of potency due to oxidation. **Administration in saline solution alone is not recommended.** Whole blood or plasma, if indicated to increase blood volume, should be administered separately (for example, by use of a Y-tube and individual containers if given simultaneously).

Average Dosage: Add a 4 ml ampul (4 mg) of norepinephrine bitartrate to 1,000 ml of a 5 percent dextrose containing solution. Each 1 ml of this dilution contains 4 mcg of the base of norepinephrine bitartrate. Give this solution by intravenous infusion. Insert a plastic intravenous catheter through a suitable bore needle well advanced centrally into the vein and securely fixed with adhesive tape, avoiding, if possible, a catheter tie-in technique as this promotes stasis. An IV drip chamber or other suitable metering device is essential to permit an accurate estimation of the rate of flow in drops per minute. After observing the response to an initial dose of 2 ml to 3 ml (from 8 mcg to 12 mcg of base) per minute, adjust the rate of flow to establish and maintain a low normal blood pressure (usually 80 mm Hg to 100 mm Hg systolic) sufficient to maintain the circulation to vital organs. In previously hypertensive patients, it is recommended that the blood pressure should be raised no higher than 40 mm Hg below the preexisting systolic pressure. The average maintenance dose ranges from 0.5 ml to 1 ml per minute (from 2 mcg to 4 mcg of base).

High Dosage: Great individual variation occurs in the dose required to attain and maintain an adequate blood pressure. In all cases, dosage of norepinephrine bitartrate should be titrated according to the response of the patient. Occasionally much larger or even enormous daily doses (as high as 68 mg base or 17 ampuls) may be necessary if the patient remains hypotensive, but occult blood volume depletion should always be suspected and corrected when present. Central venous pressure monitoring is usually helpful in detecting and treating this situation.

Fluid Intake: The degree of dilution depends on clinical fluid volume requirements. If large volumes of fluid (dextrose) are needed at a flow rate that would involve an excessive dose of the pressor agent per unit of time, a solution more dilute than 4 mcg per ml should be used. On the other hand, when large volumes of fluid are clinically undesirable, a concentration greater than 4 mcg per ml may be necessary.

DOSAGE AND ADMINISTRATION: *(cont'd)*

Duration of Therapy: The infusion should be continued until adequate blood pressure and tissue perfusion are maintained without therapy. Infusions of norepinephrine bitartrate should be reduced gradually, avoiding abrupt withdrawal. In some of the reported cases of vascular collapse due to acute myocardial infarction, treatment was required for up to six days.

Adjunctive Treatment in Cardiac Arrest: Infusions of norepinephrine bitartrate are usually administered intravenously during cardiac resuscitation to restore and maintain an adequate blood pressure after an effective heartbeat and ventilation have been established by other means. [norepinephrine bitartrate's powerful beta-adrenergic stimulating action is also thought to increase the strength and effectiveness of systolic contractions once they occur.]

Average Dosage: To maintain systemic blood pressure during the management of cardiac arrest, norepinephrine bitartrate is used in the same manner as described under Restoration of Blood Pressure in Acute Hypotensive States.

Parenteral drug products should be inspected visually for particulate matter and discoloration prior to use, whenever solution and container permit.

HOW SUPPLIED - EQUIVALENTS NOT AVAILABLE:

Injection, Solution - Intravenous - 0.1 %

4 ml	$15.12	NOREPINEPHRINE BITARTRATE, Abbott	00074-7041-01
4 ml x 10	**$112.80**	**LEVOPHED BITARTRATE, Sanofi Winthrop**	**00024-1123-02**

NOREPINEPHRINE BITARTRATE; PROCAINE HYDROCHLORIDE; PROPOXYCAINE HYDROCHLORIDE *(003120)*

CATEGORIES: Anesthesia; Dental; Injectable Anesthetics; Local Anesthetics; Pregnancy Category C; FDA Approval Pre 1982

BRAND NAMES: **Ravocaine And Novocain W/ Levophed**

DESCRIPTION:

Propoxycaine hydrochloride is 2-(diethylamino)-ethyl 4-amino-2- poxybenzoate monohydrochloride.

It is an odorless white or slightly yellow crystalline solid which is readily soluble in water but incompatible with alkalies.

Procaine hydrochloride is 2-(diethylamino) ethyl *p*-aminobenzoate monohydrochloride.

It is an odorless white crystalline solid which is readily soluble in water but incompatible with alkalies, iodides, and mercurial compounds.

Norepinephrine bitartrate is (-)-α-(aminoethyl)-3,4-dihydroxybenzyl alcohol tartrate (1:1) (salt) monohydrate.

It is a whitish crystalline solid which darkens on exposure to air and light, freely soluble in water (TABLE 1):

TABLE 1 Dental Cartridges May Not Be Autoclaved

Contents:	Per ml	Per cartridge
Propoxycaine hydrochloride	4 mg	7.2 mg
Procaine hydrochloride	20 mg	36 mg
Norepinephrine bitartrate (Equivalent to 0.033 mg Levophed base)	0.067 mg	0.121 mg
Sodium chloride	3.0 mg	5.4 mg
Acetone sodium bisulfite, not more than	2.0 mg	3.6 mg
Water for Injection, q.s. ad pH adjusted between 3.5 and 5.0 with NaOH or HCl.	1.0 ml	1.8 ml

CLINICAL PHARMACOLOGY:

This solution stabilizes the neuronal membrane and prevents the initiation and transmission of nerve impulses, thereby effecting local anesthesia.

The onset of action is usually 2 to 5 minutes and the duration of action is from 2 to 3 hours.

Para-aminobenzoic acid esters are rapidly metabolized through hydrolysis by plasma cholinesterase with some metabolism occurring in the liver.

Norepinephrine bitartrate is a sympathomimetic amine suitable for use as a vasoconstrictor in local anesthetic solutions. It has potent vasoconstrictor action accompanied by decrease in pulse rate.

INDICATIONS AND USAGE:

This solution is indicated for the production of local anesthesia for dental procedures by infiltration injection or nerve block in adults and children.

CONTRAINDICATIONS:

This solution is contraindicated in patients with a known hypersensitivity to local anesthetics of the para-aminobenzoic acid ester group.

This solution should not be used in patients receiving tricyclic antidepressant drugs as 4-to 8-fold potentiation of pressor effect may occur.

WARNINGS:

DENTAL PRACTITIONERS WHO EMPLOY LOCAL ANESTHETICS IN THEIR OFFICES SHOULD BE WELL VERSED IN DIAGNOSIS AND MANAGEMENT OF EMERGENCIES WHICH MIGHT ARISE FROM THEIR USE. RESUSCITATIVE EQUIPMENT, OXYGEN AND OTHER RESUSCITATIVE DRUGS SHOULD BE AVAILABLE FOR IMMEDIATE USE.

Reactions resulting in fatality have occurred on rare occasions with the use of local anesthetics, even in the absence of a history of hypersensitivity.

Solutions which contain a vasoconstrictor should be used with extreme caution for patients whose medical history and physical evaluation suggest the existence of hypertension, arteriosclerotic heart disease, cerebral vascular insufficiency, heart block, thyrotoxicosis, and diabetes, etc.

Contains acetone sodium bisulfite, a sulfite that may cause allergic-type reactions including anaphylactic symptoms and life-threatening or less severe asthmatic episodes in certain susceptible people. The overall prevalence of sulfite sensitivity in the general population is unknown and probably low. Sulfite sensitivity is seen more frequently in asthmatic than in non-asthmatic people.

PRECAUTIONS:

GENERAL

The safety and effectiveness of this solution depend upon proper dosage, correct technique, adequate precautions, and readiness for emergencies. RESUSCITATIVE EQUIPMENT, OXYGEN AND OTHER RESUSCITATIVE DRUGS SHOULD BE AVAILABLE FOR IMMEDIATE USE (see WARNINGS.)

The lowest dose that results in effective anesthesia should be used to avoid high plasma levels and serious undesirable systemic side effects. Repeated administrations may result in accumulation of the anesthetics in plasma.

INJECTIONS SHOULD ALWAYS BE MADE SLOWLY WITH ASPIRATION TO AVOID INTRAVASCULAR INJECTION AND THEREFORE SYSTEMIC REACTION TO BOTH LOCAL ANESTHETIC AND VASOCONSTRICTOR.

Tolerance varies with the status of the patient. Debilitated, elderly patients, acutely ill patients, and children should be given reduced doses commensurate with their weight and physical status.

If sedatives are employed to reduce patient apprehension, use reduced doses, since local anesthetic agents, like sedatives, are central nervous system depressants which in combination may have an additive effect. Young children should be given minimal doses of each agent.

Changes in sensorium such as excitation, disorientation, drowsiness may be early indications of a high blood level of the local anesthetic agents and may occur following inadvertent intravascular administration or rapid absorption.

PEDIATRIC USE

Great care must be exercised in adhering to safe concentrations and dosages for pediatric administration (see DOSAGE AND ADMINISTRATION.)

PREGNANCY CATEGORY C

Animal reproduction studies have not been conducted with this solution. It is also not known whether this solution can cause fetal harm when administered to a pregnant woman or can affect reproduction capacity. This solution should be given to a pregnant woman only if clearly needed.

NURSING MOTHERS

It is not known whether this drug is excreted in human milk. Because many drugs are excreted in human milk, caution should be exercised when this solution is administered to a nursing woman.

Local anesthetic procedures should be used with caution when there is inflammation and/or sepsis in the region of the proposed injection.

This solution should be used with caution in patients with history of hypertension, arteriosclerotic heart disease, cerebral vascular insufficiency, or heart block. Bradycardia may follow administration of this solution.

Mild or even severe headaches may be produced by the systemic action of norepinephrine when the solution is injected too rapidly, and there is rapid absorption from the site of injection.

DRUG INTERACTIONS:

Solutions which contain a vasoconstrictor should also be used with extreme caution in patients receiving drugs known to produce blood pressure alterations (*i.e.,* MAO inhibitors, tricyclic antidepressants, phenothiazines, etc) as either sustained hypertension or hypotension may occur.

Solutions containing a vasoconstrictor should be used cautiously in the presence of diseases which may adversely affect the patient's cardiovascular system. Serious cardiac arrhythmias may occur if preparations containing a vasoconstrictor are employed in patients during or following the administration of potent general anesthetics.

Caution should be used in administering local anesthetics to patients with a history of drug sensitivity or allergy. A thorough history of the patient's prior experience with this and other local anesthetics as well as concomitant or recent drug use should be taken (see CONTRAINDICATIONS). Patients with known sensitivity to the para-aminobenzoic acid ester-type of local anesthetics have not shown cross sensitivity to amide-type drugs.

ADVERSE REACTIONS:

Systemic reactions involving the central nervous system and the cardiovascular system usually result from high plasma levels due to excessive dosage, rapid absorption, or inadvertent intravascular injection.

A small number of reactions may result from hypersensitivity, idiosyncrasy, or diminished tolerance to normal dosage on the part of the patient.

Central nervous system reactions are characterized by excitation and/or depression. Nervousness, dizziness, blurred vision, or tremors may occur followed by drowsiness, convulsions, unconsciousness, and possibly respiratory arrest.

Cardiovascular system reactions may result either from the local anesthetic or from the vasoconstrictor employed, and may include depression of the myocardium, hypotension, profound bradycardia, and cardiac arrest. Cardiovascular reactions may be the result of drugs employed or may result from vasovagal reaction particularly in the sitting position. Early recognition and management of premonitory signs such as sweating, feeling of faintness, changes in heart rate, will avoid resultant cerebral hypoxia which may progress to seizure or cardiovascular catastrophe. Management consists of placing the patient in the recumbent position and administration of oxygen. Should symptoms persist, vasoactive drugs such as ephedrine or methoxamine should be administered intravenously.

Allergic reactions are characterized by cutaneous lesions of delayed onset, or urticaria, edema, and other manifestations of allergy. The detection of sensitivity by skin testing is of limited value. As with other local anesthetics, hypersensitivity, idiosyncrasy, anaphylactoid reactions to this solution have occurred rarely. The reaction may be abrupt and severe, and is not usually dose related.

OVERDOSAGE:

Treatment of a patient with toxic manifestations consists of assuring and maintaining a patent airway and supporting ventilation with oxygen and assisted or controlled ventilation (respiration) as required. This usually will be sufficient in the management of most reactions. Should a convulsion persist despite ventilatory therapy, small increments of anticonvulsive agents may be given intravenously, such as benzodiazepine (*e.g.,* diazepam) or ultra-short acting barbiturates (*e.g.,* pentobarbital or secobarbital). Cardiovascular depression may require circulatory assistance with intravenous fluids and/or vasopressor (*e.g.,* ephedrine) as dictated by the clinical situation. Allergic reactions are rare and may occur as a result of sensitivity to the local anesthetic and are characterized by cutaneous lesions, urticaria, edema, and anaphylactoid type symptomatology. These allergic reactions should be managed by conventional means. The detection of potential sensitivity by skin testing is of limited value.

DOSAGE AND ADMINISTRATION:

As with all local anesthetics, the dose varies and depends upon the area to be anesthetized, vascularity of the tissues, individual tolerance, and the technique of anesthesia. The lowest dose needed to provide effective anesthesia should be administered. For specific techniques and procedures, refer to standard dental manuals and textbooks.

For infiltration and block injections in the upper or lower jaw, the average dose of 1 cartridge will usually suffice.

The 1.8 ml cartridge contains 43.2 mg of the anesthetics (7.2 mg propoxycaine HCl and 36 mg procaine HCl).

Adults: Five cartridges (216 mg of the anesthetics) are usually adequate to effect anesthesia of the entire oral cavity. However, a dose of up to 3 mg per pound of body weight may be administered for one procedure.

Children: Based on a dose of 3 mg per pound of body weight, 5 cartridges maximum, are usually adequate for any procedure.

Using infiltration or regional block anesthesia injections should always be made slowly and with frequent aspiration.

Any unused portion of a cartridge should be discarded.

DISINFECTION OF CARTRIDGES

As in the case of any cartridge, the diaphragm should be disinfected before needle puncture. The diaphragm should be thoroughly swabbed with either pure 91% isopropyl alcohol or 70% ethyl alcohol, USP, just prior to use. Many commercially available alcohol solutions contain ingredients which are injurious to container components, and therefore, should not be used. Cartridges should not be immersed in any solution.

Store at controlled room temperature between 15 and 30°C (59 and 86°F). **Protect from light.**

NORETHINDRONE *(001899)*

CATEGORIES: Amenorrhea; Contraceptives; Endometriosis; Hormonal Imbalance; Hormones; Pregnancy; Progestins; Progestogen; Uterine Bleeding; Pregnancy Category X; FDA Approval Pre 1982

BRAND NAMES: *Dianor*, *Menzol* (England); Micronor; *Micro-Novom*; *Micronovum* (Germany); *Nor-Ethis*; Nor-QD; *Norcolut*; Norethisterone; *Noriday* (England); *Noriday 28*; *Norluten* (France); **Norlutin**; *Primolut N* (Asia, England); *Primolut-N*; *Primulut*; *Shiton*; *Steron*; *Styptin 5*; *Sunolut*; *Utovlan* (England)
(International brand names outside U.S. in italics)

FORMULARIES: Aetna; BC-BS; FHP; Medi-Cal; PCS

WARNING:

THE USE OF NORETHINDRONE DURING THE FIRST FOUR MONTHS OF PREGNANCY IS NOT RECOMMENDED.

Progestational agents have been used beginning with the first trimester of pregnancy in an attempt to prevent habitual abortion. There is no adequate evidence that such use is effective when such drugs are given during the first four months of pregnancy. Furthermore, in the vast majority of women, the cause of abortion is a defective ovum, which progestational agents could not be expected to influence. In addition, the use of progestational agents, with their uterine-relaxant properties, in patients with fertilized defective ova may cause a delay in spontaneous abortion. Therefore, the use of such drugs during the first four months of pregnancy is not recommended.

Several reports suggest an association between intrauterine exposure to progestational drugs in the first trimester of pregnancy and genital abnormalities in male and female fetuses. The risk of hypospadias, 5 to 8 per 1,000 male births in the general population, may be approximately doubled with exposure to these drugs. There are insufficient data to quantify the risk to exposed female fetuses, but insofar as some of these drugs induce mild virilization of the external genitalia of the female fetus, and because of the increased association of hypospadias in the male fetus, it is prudent to avoid the use of these drugs during the first trimester of pregnancy.

If the patient is exposed to norethindrone during the first four months of pregnancy or if she becomes pregnant while taking this drug, she should be apprised of the potential risks to the fetus.

DESCRIPTION:

Norethindrone is the 17 alpha-ethinyl derivative of 19-nortestosterone. It is a progestational agent for oral administration. Each tablet contains 5 mg of norethindrone, USP. Norethindrone also contains: acacia, NF; confectioner's sugar, NF; lactose, NF; magnesium stearate, NF; starch potato, NF; and talc, USP. The chemical name is 17-Hydroxy-19-nor-17 α-pregn-4-en-20-yn-3-one.

Micronor Tablets: *Progestin-Only Oral Contraceptive:* This product is a progestogen oral contraceptive containing the progestational compound norethindrone.Each tablet contains 0.35 mg of norethindrone. Inactive ingredients include D&C Green No. 5, D&C Yellow No. 10, lactose, magnesium stearate, povidone and starch.

CLINICAL PHARMACOLOGY:

Transforms proliferative endometrium into secretory endometrium.

Inhibits (at the usual dose range) the secretion of pituitary gonadotropins, which in turn prevents follicular maturation and ovulation.

May also demonstrate some estrogenic, anabolic or androgenic activity but should not be relied upon.

INDICATIONS AND USAGE:

Norethindrone is indicated in amenorrhea; in abnormal uterine bleeding due to hormonal imbalance in the absence of organic pathology, such as submucous fibroids or uterine cancer; and in endometriosis.

Micronor: For the indication, contraception, see Ethinyl Estradiol; Norethindrone for prescribing information.

CONTRAINDICATIONS:

1. Thrombophlebitis, thromboembolic disorders, cerebral apoplexy or patients with a past history of these conditions
2. Known or suspected carcinoma of the breast
3. Undiagnosed vaginal bleeding

CONTRAINDICATIONS: *(cont'd)*

4. Missed abortion
5. As a diagnostic test for pregnancy

WARNINGS:

Discontinue medication pending examination if there is a sudden partial or complete loss of vision, or if there is sudden onset of proptosis, diplopia or migraine. If examination reveals papilledema or retinal vascular lesions, medication should be withdrawn.

Detectable amounts of progestogens have been identified in the milk of mothers receiving them. The effect of this on the nursing infant has not been determined.

Because of the occasional occurrence of thrombophlebitis and pulmonary embolism in patients taking progestogens, the physician should be alert to the earliest manifestations of the disease.

Masculinization of the female fetus has occurred when progestogens have been used in pregnant women.

Some beagle dogs treated with medroxyprogesterone acetate developed mammary nodules. Although nodules occasionally appeared in control animals they were intermittent in nature, whereas nodules in treated animals were larger and more numerous, and they persisted. There is no general agreement as to whether the nodules are benign or malignant. Their significance with respect to humans has not been established.

PRECAUTIONS:

GENERAL

The pretreatment physical examination should include special reference to breasts and pelvic organs, as well as a Papanicolaou smear.

Because this drug may cause some degree of fluid retention, conditions which might be influenced by this factor, such as epilepsy, migraine, asthma, cardiac or renal dysfunction, require careful observation.

In cases of breakthrough bleeding, as in all cases of irregular bleeding per vaginam, nonfunctional causes should be borne in mind. In cases of undiagnosed vaginal bleeding, adequate diagnostic measures are indicated.

Patients who have a history of psychic depression should be carefully observed and the drug discontinued if the depression recurs to a serious degree.

Any possible influence of prolonged progestogen therapy on pituitary, ovarian, adrenal, hepatic or uterine functions awaits further study.

A decrease in glucose tolerance has been observed in a small percentage of patients on estrogen-progestogen combination drugs. The mechanism of this decrease is obscure. For this reason, diabetic patients should be carefully observed while receiving progestogen therapy.

The age of the patient constitutes no absolute limiting factor although treatment with progestogens may mask the onset of the climacteric.

The pathologist should be advised of progestogen therapy when relevant specimens are submitted.

Steroid hormones are metabolized by the liver; therefore these drugs should be administered with caution in patients with impaired liver function.

CONCOMITANT ESTROGEN USE

Studies of the addition of a progestin product to an estrogen replacement regimen for seven or more days of a cycle of estrogen administration have reported a lowered incidence of endometrial hyperplasia. Morphological and biochemical studies of endometrium suggest that 10 to 13 days of a progestin are needed to provide maximal maturation of the endometrium and to eliminate any hyperplastic changes. Whether this will provide protection from endometrial carcinoma has not been clearly established. There are possible additional risks which may be associated with the inclusion of progestin in estrogen replacement regimens. The potential risks include adverse effects on carbohydrate and lipid metabolism. The dosage used may be important in minimizing these adverse effects.

INFORMATION FOR THE PATIENT

See PATIENT PACKAGE INSERT section.

LABORATORY TESTS

The following laboratory result may be altered by the use of progestogens: Pregnanediol determination.

In addition, the following laboratory results may be altered by the concomitant use of estrogens with progestogens:

1. Hepatic function
2. Coagulation tests; increase in prothrombin, Factors VII, VIII, IX, and X
3. Increase in PBI, BEI and a decrease in T^3 uptake
4. Metyrapone test

CARCINOGENESIS, MUTAGENESIS, AND IMPAIRMENT OF FERTILITY

See WARNINGS.

PREGNANCY CATEGORY X:

See BOXED WARNING.

NURSING MOTHERS

Detectable amounts of progestogens have been identified in the milk of mothers receiving them. Because of the potential for serious adverse reactions in nursing infants from norethindrone, a decision should be made whether to discontinue nursing or to discontinue the drug, taking into account the importance of the drug to the mother.

DRUG INTERACTIONS:

Reduced efficacy and increased incidence of breakthrough bleeding have been associated with concomitant use of rifampin.

ADVERSE REACTIONS:

The following adverse reactions have been observed in women taking progestogens:

breakthrough bleeding	changes in cervical erosion and cervical secretions
spotting	cholestatic jaundice
change in menstrual flow	rash (allergic) with and without pruritus
amenorrhea	melasma or chloasma
edema	mental depression
changes in weight (increase or decrease)	

A statistically significant association has been demonstrated between use of estrogen-progestogen combination drugs and the following serious adverse reactions: thrombophlebitis; pulmonary embolism and cerebral thrombosis and embolism. For this reason patients on progestogen therapy should be carefully observed.

Although available evidence is suggestive of an association, such a relationship has been neither confirmed nor refuted for the following serious adverse reactions:

Neuro-ocular lesions (*e.g.*, retinal thrombosis and optic neuritis.

ADVERSE REACTIONS: *(cont'd)*

The following adverse reactions have been observed in patients receiving estrogen-progestogen combination drugs:

rise in blood pressure in susceptible individuals	fatigue
premenstrual-like syndrome	backache
change in libido	hirsutism
changes in appetite	loss of scalp hair
cystitis-like syndrome	erythema multiforme
headache	erythema nodosum
nervousness	hermorrphagic eruption
dizziness	itching

In view of these observations, patients on progestogen therapy should be carefully observed for their occurrence.

OVERDOSAGE:

Not known.

DOSAGE AND ADMINISTRATION:

Therapy with norethindrone must be adapted to the specific indications and therapeutic response of the individual patient.

This dosage schedule assumes the interval between menses to be 28 days.

Amenorrhea, abnormal uterine bleeding due to hormonal imbalance in the absence of organic pathology: 5 to 20 mg norethindrone starting with the fifth day of the menstrual cycle and ending on the 25th day.

Endometriosis: Initial daily dose of 10 mg norethindrone for two weeks with increments of 5 mg per day of norethindrone every two weeks until 30 mg per day of norethindrone is reached. Therapy may be held at this level for from six to nine months or until annoying breakthrough bleeding demands temporary termination.

REFERENCES:

1. Gal IB, et al: Hormonal pregnancy tests and congenital malformation.*Nature* 216:83, 1967. **2.** Levy EP, et al: Hormone treatment during pregnancy and congenital heart defects. *Lancet* 1:611, 1973. **3.** Nora J, Nora A: Birth defects and oral contraceptives. *Lancet*1:941, 1973. **4.** Janerich DT, et al: Oral contraceptives and congenital limb-reduction defects. *N Engl J Med*291:697, 1974. **5.** Heinonen OP, et al: Cardiovascular birth defects and antenatal exposure to female sex hormones. *N Engl J Med*296:67, 1977.

PATIENT PACKAGE INSERT:

NORETHINDRONE WARNING FOR WOMEN

Progesterone or progesterone-like drugs have been used to prevent miscarriage in the first few months of pregnancy. No adequate evidence is available to show that they are effective for this purpose. Furthermore, most cases of early miscarriage are due to causes which could not be helped by these drugs.

There is an increased risk of minor birth defects in children whose mothers take this drug during the first 4 months of pregnancy. Several reports suggest an association between mothers who take these drugs in the first trimester of pregnancy and genital abnormalities in male and female babies. The risk to the male baby is the possibility of being born with a condition in which the opening of the penis is on the underside rather than the tip of the penis (hypospadias). Hypospadias occurs in about 5 to 8 per 1,000 male births and is about doubled with exposure to these drugs. There is not enough information to quantify the risk to exposed female fetuses, but enlargement of the clitoris and fusion of the labia may occur, although rarely.

Therefore, since drugs of this type may induce mild masculinization of the external genitalia of the female fetus, as well as hypospadias in the male fetus, it is wise to avoid using the drug during the first trimester of pregnancy.

These drugs have been used as a test for pregnancy but such use is no longer considered safe because of possible damage to a developing baby. Also, more rapid methods for testing for pregnancy are now available.

If you take norethindrone and later find you were pregnant when you took it, be sure to discuss this with your doctor as soon as possible.

Storage: Store below 30°C (86°F).

HOW SUPPLIED - EQUIVALENTS NOT AVAILABLE:

Tablet, Uncoated - Oral - 0.35 mg

6 x 42	$164.16	NOR QD, Syntex FP	42987-0107-19
28	$29.22	MICRONOR, Ortho Pharm	00062-1411-01

Tablet, Uncoated - Oral - 5 mg

50's	**$42.88**	**NORLUTIN, Parke-Davis**	**00071-0882-19**

NORETHINDRONE ACETATE *(001900)*

CATEGORIES: Amenorrhea; Endometriosis; Hormonal Imbalance; Hormones; Progestins; Progestogen; Uterine Bleeding; Pregnancy Category X; FDA Approval Pre 1982

BRAND NAMES: Aygestin; *Milligynon*; *Norcolut*; *Nordron*; **Norlutate**; *Norluten-A* (Japan); *Primolut*; *Primolut-Nor* (Germany, Mexico); *Shiton*
(International brand names outside U.S. in italics)

FORMULARIES: Aetna; BC-BS; WHO

WARNING:

THE USE OF NORETHINDRONE ACETATE DURING THE FIRST FOUR MONTHS OF PREGNANCY IS NOT RECOMMENDED.

Progestational agents have been used beginning with the first trimester of pregnancy in an attempt to prevent habitual abortion. There is no adequate evidence that such use is effective when such drugs are given during the first four months of pregnancy. Further-more, in the vast majority of women, the cause of abortion is a defective ovum, which progestational agents could not be expected to influence. In addition, the use of progestational agents, with their uterine relaxant properties, in patients with fertilized defective ova may cause a delay in spontaneous abortion. Therefore, the use of such drugs during the first four months of pregnancy is not recommended.

Several reports suggest an association between intrauterine exposure to progestational drugs in the first trimester of pregnancy and genital abnormalities in male and female fetuses. The risk of hypospadias, 5 to 8 per 1,000 male births in the general population, may be approximately doubled with exposure to these drugs. There are insufficient data to quantify the risk to exposed female fetuses, but insofar as some of these drugs induce mild virilization of the external genitalia of the female fetus, and because of the increased association of hypospadias in the male fetus, it is prudent to avoid the use of these drugs during the first trimester of pregnancy.

If the patient is exposed to Norethindrone Acetate during the first four months of pregnancy or if she becomes pregnant while taking this drug, she should be apprised of the potential risks to the fetus.

DESCRIPTION:

Norethindrone Acetate is the acetic acid ester of norethindrone, which is the 17 alpha-ethinyl derivative of 19-nortestosterone. It is a progestational agent for oral administration. Each tablet contains 5 mg of norethindrone acetate, USP. Norethindrone Acetate also contains: acacia, NF; confectioner's sugar, NF; D&C red No. 30 Al lake; FD&C yellow No. 6 Al lake; lactose, NF; light mineral oil, NF; magnesium stearate, NF; corn starch, NF; and talc, USP. The chemical name is 17-Hydroxy-19-nor-17α-pregn-4-en-20-yn-3-one acetate.

CLINICAL PHARMACOLOGY:

Transforms proliferative endometrium into secretory endometrium. Inhibits (at the usual dose range) the secretion of pituitary gonadotropins, which in turn prevents follicular maturation and ovulation.

May also demonstrate some estrogenic, anabolic or androgenic activity but should not be relied upon.

INDICATIONS AND USAGE:

Norethindrone Acetate is indicated in amenorrhea; in abnormal uterine bleeding due to hormonal imbalance in the absence of organic pathology, such as submucous fibroids or uterine cancer; and in endometriosis.

CONTRAINDICATIONS:

1. Thrombophlebitis, thromboembolic disorders, cerebral apoplexy or patients with a past history of these conditions

2. Known or suspected carcinoma of the breast

3. Undiagnosed vaginal bleeding

4. Missed abortion

5. As a diagnostic test for pregnancy

WARNINGS:

Discontinue medication pending examination if there is a sudden partial or complete loss of vision, or if there is a sudden onset of proptosis, diplopia or migraine. If examination reveals papilledema or retinal vascular lesions, medication should be withdrawn.

Detectable amounts of progestogens have been identified in the milk of mothers receiving them. The effect of this on the nursing infant has not been determined.

Because of the occasional occurrence of thrombophlebitis and pulmonary embolism in patients taking progestogens, the physician should be alert to the earliest manifestations of the disease.

Masculinization of the female fetus has occurred when progestogens have been used in pregnant women.

Some beagle dogs treated with medroxyprogesterone acetate developed mammary nodules. Although nodules occasionally appeared in control animals they were intermittent in nature, whereas nodules in treated animals were larger and more numerous, and they persisted. There is no general agreement as to whether the nodules are benign or malignant. Their significance with respect to humans has not been established.

PRECAUTIONS:

General: The pretreatment physical examination should include special reference to breasts and pelvic organs, as well as a Papanicolaou smear.

Because this drug may cause some degree of fluid retention, conditions which might be influenced by this factor, such as epilepsy, migraine, asthma, cardiac or renal dysfunction, require careful observation.

In cases of breakthrough bleeding, as in all cases of irregular bleeding *per vaginam*, non-functional causes should be borne in mind. In cases of undiagnosed vaginal bleeding, adequate diagnostic measures are indicated.

Patients who have a history of psychic depression should be carefully observed and the drug discontinued if the depression recurs to a serious degree.

Any possible influence of prolonged progestogen therapy on pituitary, ovarian, adrenal, hepatic or uterine functions awaits further study.

A decrease in glucose tolerance has been observed in a small percentage of patients on estrogen-progestogen combination drugs. The mechanism of this decrease is obscure. For this reason, diabetic patients should be carefully observed while receiving progestogen therapy.

The age of the patient constitutes no absolute limiting factor although treatment with progestogens may mask the onset of the climacteric.

The age of the patient constitutes no absolute limiting factor although treatment with progestogens may mask the onset of the climacteric.

The pathologist should be advised of progestogen therapy when relevant specimens are submitted.

Steroid hormones are metabolized in the liver and should be administered with caution in patients with impaired liver function.

Concomitant Estrogen Use: Studies of the addition of a progestin product to an estrogen replacement regimen for seven or more days of a cycle of estrogen administration have reported a lowered incidence of endometrial hyperplasia. Morphological and biochemical studies of endometrium suggest that 10 to 13 days of a progestin are needed to provide maximal maturation of the endometrium and to eliminate any hyperplastic changes. Whether this will provide protection from endometrial carcinoma has not been clearly established. There are possible additional risks which may be associated with the inclusion of progestin in estrogen replacement regimens. The potential risks include adverse effects on carbohydrate and lipid metabolism. The dosage used may be important in minimizing these adverse effects.

Information for the Patient: See PATIENT PACKAGE INSERT.

Laboratory Tests: The following laboratory result may be altered by the use of progestogens: Pregnanediol determination.

In addition, the following laboratory results may be altered by the concomitant use of estrogens with progestogens:

1. Hepatic function

2. Coagulation tests; increase in prothrombin, Factors VII, VIII, IX, and X

3. Increase in PBI, BEI and a decrease in T^3 uptake

PRECAUTIONS: *(cont'd)*

4. Metyrapone test

Carcinogenesis, Mutagenesis, and Impairment of Fertility: See WARNINGS.

Pregnancy Category X: See BOXED WARNING.

Nursing Mothers: Detectable amounts of progestogens have been identified in the milk of mothers receiving them. Because of the potential for serious adverse reactions in nursing infants from Norethindrone Acetate, a decision should be made whether to discontinue nursing or to discontinue the drug, taking into account the importance of the drug to the mother.

DRUG INTERACTIONS:

Reduced efficacy and increased incidence of break-through bleeding have been associated with concomitant use of rifampin.

ADVERSE REACTIONS:

The following adverse reactions have been observed in women taking progestogens:

breakthrough bleeding	changes in cervical erosion and cervical secretions
spotting	cholestatic jaundice
change in menstrual flow	rash (allergic) with and without pruritus
amenorrhea	melasma or chloasma
edema	mental depression
changes in weight (increase or decrease)	

A statistically significant association has been demonstrated between use of estrogen-progestogen combination drugs and the following serious adverse reactions: thrombophlebitis; pulmonary embolism and cerebral thrombosis and embolism. For this reason patients on progestogen therapy should be carefully observed.

Although available evidence is suggestive of an association, such a relationship has been neither confirmed nor refuted for the following serious adverse reactions: neuro-ocular lesions, *e.g.*, retinal thrombosis and optic neuritis.

The following adverse reactions have been observed in patients receiving estrogen-progestogen combination drugs:

rise in blood pressure in susceptible individuals	fatigue
	backache
premenstrual-like syndrome	hirsutism
changes in libido	loss of scalp hair
changes in appetite	erythema multiforme
cystitis-like syndrome	14. erythema nodosum
headache	hemorrhagic eruption
nervousness	itching
dizziness	

In view of these observations, patients on progestogen therapy should be carefully observed for their occurrence.

OVERDOSAGE:

Not known.

DOSAGE AND ADMINISTRATION:

Therapy with Norethindrone Acetate must be adapted to the specific indications and therapeutic response of the individual patient.

This dosage schedule assumes the interval between menses to be 28 days.

Amenorrhea, abnormal uterine bleeding due to hormonal imbalance in the absence of organic pathology: 2.5 to 10 mg Norethindrone Acetate starting with the fifth day of the menstrual cycle and ending on the 25th day.

Endometriosis: Initial daily dose of 5 mg Norethindrone Acetate for two weeks with increments of 2.5 mg per day of Norethindrone Acetate every two weeks until 15 mg per day of Norethindrone Acetate is reached. Therapy may be held at this level for from six to nine months or until annoying breakthrough bleeding demands temporary termination.

REFERENCES:

1. Gal IB, et al: Hormonal pregnancy tests and congenital malformation.*Nature* 216:83, 1967. **2.** Levy EP, et al: Hormone treatment during pregnancy and congenital heart defects. *Lancet* 1:611, 1973. **3.** Nora J, Nora A: Birth defects and oral contraceptives, *Lancet*1:941, 1973. **4.** Janerich DT, et al: Oral contraceptives and congenital limb reduction defects. *N Engl J Med* 291:697, 1974. **5.** Heinonen OP, et al: Cardiovascular birth defects and antenatal exposure to female sex hormones. *N Engl J Med*296:67, 1977.

PATIENT PACKAGE INSERT:

PATIENT LABELING FOR NORETHINDRONE ACETATE WARNING FOR WOMEN

Progesterone or progesterone-like drugs have been used to prevent miscarriage in the first few months of pregnancy. No adequate evidence is available to show that they are effective for this purpose. Furthermore, most cases of early miscarriage are due to causes which could not be helped by these drugs.

There is an increased risk of minor birth defects in children whose mothers take this drug during the first 4 months of pregnancy. Several reports suggest an association between mothers who take these drugs in the first trimester of pregnancy and genital abnormalities in male and female babies. The risk to the male baby is the possibility of being born with a condition in which the opening of the penis is on the underside rather than the tip of the penis (hypospadias). Hypospadias occurs in about 5 to 8 per 1,000 male births and is about doubled with exposure to these drugs. There is not enough information to quantify the risk to exposed female fetuses, but enlargement of the clitoris and fusion of the labia may occur, although rarely.

Therefore, since drugs of this type may induce mild masculinization of the external genitalia of the female fetus, as well as hypospadias in the male fetus, it is wise to avoid using the drug during the first trimester of pregnancy.

These drugs have been used as a test for pregnancy but such use is no longer considered safe because of possible damage to a developing baby. Also, more rapid methods for testing for pregnancy are now available.

If you take Norethindrone Acetate and later find you were pregnant when you took it, be sure to discuss this with your doctor as soon as possible.

Storage - Store below 30°C (86°F).

HOW SUPPLIED - RATED THERAPEUTICALLY EQUIVALENT:

Tablet, Uncoated - Oral - 5 mg

50's	$51.43	AYGESTIN, ESI Lederle	59911-5894-01

NORFLOXACIN *(001901)*

CATEGORIES: Anti-Infectives; Antibacterials; Antibiotics; Antimicrobials; Antiseptics, Urinary Tract; Conjunctivitis; Cystitis; EENT Drugs; Eye, Ear, Nose, & Throat Preparations; Fluoroquinolones; Gonorrhea; Prostatitis; Quinolones; Sexually Transmitted Diseases; Topical; Urinary Antibacterial; Urinary Tract Infections; Pregnancy Category C; Sales > $100 Million; FDA Approved 1986 Oct

BRAND NAMES: *Amicrobin*; *Anquin*; *Apirol*; *Baccidal* (Japan); *Barazan* (Germany); *Biofloxin*; Chibroxin; *Chibroxine* (France); *Chibroxol*; *Floxacin* (Mexico); *Floxenor*; *Fluseminal*; *Foxinon*; *Fulgram*; *Gonorcin*; *Gyrablock*; *Janacin*; *Lexinor* (Asia); *Negaflox*; *Norbactin*; *Norbactin Eye Drops*; *Norflox*; *Norflox Eye*; *Normax Eye Ear Drops*; *Norocin*; *Norofin*; **Noroxin**; *Noroxin Oftalmico* (Mexico); *Noroxine* (France); *Norxacin*; *Noryx*; *Oranor* (Mexico); *Oroflox*; *Orsanac*; *Sofasin*; *Urinox*; *Urisold*; *Urobacid*; *Uroctal*; *Uroflox*; *Uroxacin*; *Utinor* (England); *Xacin*; *Zoroxin*
(International brand names outside U.S. in italics)

FORMULARIES: Aetna; BC-BS; Medi-Cal

COST OF THERAPY: $16.73 (Urinary Infections; Tablet; 400 mg; 2/day; 3 days)

DESCRIPTION:

Noroxin (norfloxacin) is a synthetic, broad spectrum antibacterial agent for oral administration.

Norfloxacin, a fluoroquinolone, is 1-ethyl-6-fluoro-1,4-dihydro- 4-oxo- 7-(1 -piperazinyl)-3-quinolinecarboxylic acid. Its empirical formula is $C_{16}H_{18}FN_3O_3$.

Norfloxacin is a white to pale yellow crystalline powder with a molecular weight of 319.34 and a melting point of about 221°C. It is freely soluble in glacial acetic acid, and very slightly soluble in ethanol, methanol and water.

Tablets: Noroxin is available in 400-mg tablets. Each tablet contains the following inactive ingredients: cellulose, croscarmellose sodium, hydroxypropyl cellulose, hydroxypropyl methylcellulose, iron oxide, magnesium stearate, and titanium dioxide.

Norfloxacin, a fluoroquinolone, differs from non-fluorinated quinolones by having a fluorine atom at the 6 position and a piperazine moiety at the 7 position.

Ophthalmic Solution: Chibroxin (norfloxacin) Ophthalmic Solution is a synthetic broad-spectrum antibacterial agent supplied as a sterile isotonic solution for topical ophthalmic use.

Chibroxin Ophthalmic Solution 0.3% is supplied as a sterile isotonic solution. Each ml contains 3 mg norfloxacin. Inactive ingredients: disodium edetate, sodium acetate, sodium chloride, hydrochloric acid (to adjust pH) and water for injection. Benzalkonium chloride 0.0025% is added as preservative. The pH of Chibroxin is approximately 5.2 and the osmolarity is approximately 285 mOsmol/liter.

Norfloxacin, a fluoroquinolone, differs from quinolones by having a fluorine atom at the 6 position and a piperazine moiety at the 7 position.

CLINICAL PHARMACOLOGY:

TABLETS

In fasting healthy volunteers, at least 30-40% of an oral dose of Noroxin is absorbed. Absorption is rapid following single doses of 200 mg, 400 mg and 800 mg. At the respective doses, mean peak serum and plasma concentrations of 0.8, 1.5 and 2.4 mcg/ml are attained approximately one hour after dosing. The presence of food may decrease absorption. The effective half-life of norfloxacin in serum and plasma is 3-4 hours. Steady-state concentrations of norfloxacin will be attained within two days of dosing.

In healthy elderly volunteers (65-75 years of age with normal renal function for their age), norfloxacin is eliminated more slowly because of their slightly decreased renal function. Drug absorption appears unaffected. However, the effective half-life of norfloxacin in these elderly subjects is 4 hours.

The disposition of norfloxacin in patients with creatinine clearance rates greater than 30 ml/min/1.73m² is similar to that in healthy volunteers. In patients with creatinine clearance rates equal to or less than 30 ml/min/1.73m², the renal elimination of norfloxacin decreases so that the effective serum half-life is 6.5 hours. In these patients, alteration of dosage is necessary (see DOSAGE AND ADMINISTRATION.) Drug absorption appears unaffected by decreasing renal function.

Norfloxacin is eliminated through metabolism, biliary excretion, and renal excretion. After a single 400-mg dose of Noroxin, mean antimicrobial activities equivalent to 278,773, and 82 mcg of norfloxacin/g of feces were obtained at 12, 24, and 48 hours, respectively. Renal excretion occurs by both glomerular filtration and tubular secretion as evidenced by the high rate of renal clearance (approximately 275 ml/min). Within 24 hours of drug administration, 26 to 32% of the administered dose is recovered in the urine as norfloxacin with an additional 5-8% being recovered in the urine as six active metabolites of lesser antimicrobial potency. Only a small percentage (less than 1%) of the dose is recovered thereafter. Fecal recovery accounts for another 30% of the administered dose.

Two to three hours after a single 400-mg dose, urinary concentrations of 200 mcg/ml or more are attained in the urine. In healthy volunteers, mean urinary concentrations of norfloxacin remain above 30 mcg/ml for at least 12 hours following a 400-mg dose. The urinary pH may affect the solubility of norfloxacin. Norfloxacin is least soluble at urinary pH of 7.5 with greater solubility occurring at pHs above and below this value. The serum protein binding of norfloxacin is between 10 and 15%.

The following are mean concentrations of norfloxacin in various fluids and tissues measured 1 to 4 hours post-dose after two 400-mg doses, unless otherwise indicated in TABLE 1

TABLE 1

	Mean Concentrations
Renal Parenchyma	7.3 mcg/g
Prostate	2.5 mcg/g
Seminal Fluid	2.7 mcg/ml
Testicle	1.6 mcg/g
Uterus/Cervix	3.0 mcg/g
Vagina	4.3 mcg/g
Fallopian Tube	1.9 mcg/g
Bile	6.9 mcg/ml (after two 200-mg doses)

Susceptibility Testing

Diffusion Techniques: Quantitative methods that require measurement of zone diameters give the most precise estimate of the susceptibility of bacteria to antimicrobial agents. One such procedure is the National Committee for Clinical Laboratory Standards (NCCLS) approved procedure (M2-A4-Performance Standards for Antimicrobial Disk Susceptibility Tests 1990). This method has been recommended for use with the 10-mcg norfloxacin disk to test susceptibility to norfloxacin. Interpretation involves correlation of the diameters obtained in the disk test with minimum inhibitory concentration (MIC) for norfloxacin. Reports from the

CLINICAL PHARMACOLOGY: *(cont'd)*

laboratory giving results of the standard single-disk susceptibility test with a 10-mcg norfloxacin disk should be interpreted according to the following criteria (these criteria only apply to isolates from urinary tract infections) (TABLE 2)

TABLE 2

Zone diameter (mm)	Interpretation
≥17	(S) Susceptible
13-16	(I) Intermediate
≤12	(R) Resistant

A report of "Susceptible" indicates that the pathogen is likely to be inhibited by generally achievable urine levels. A report of "Intermediate" indicates that the test results be considered equivocal or indeterminate. A report of "Resistant" indicates that achievable concentrations of the antibiotic are unlikely to be inhibitory and other therapy should be selected.

Standardized procedures require the use of laboratory control organisms. The 10-mcg norfloxacin disk should give the following zone diameter (TABLE 3):

TABLE 3

Organism	Zone diameter (mm)
E. coli ATCC 25922	28 - 35
P. aeruginosa ATCC 27853	22 - 29
S. aureus ATCC 25923	17 - 28

Other quinolone antibacterial disks should not be substituted when performing susceptibility tests for norfloxacin because of spectrum differences with norfloxacin. The 10-mcg norfloxacin disk should be used for all *in vitro* testing of isolates using diffusion techniques.

Dilution Techniques: Broth and agar dilution methods, such as those recommended by the NCCLS (M7-A2-Methods for Dilution Antimicrobial Susceptibility Tests for Bacteria that Grow Aerobically 1990), may be used to determine the minimum inhibitory concentration (MIC of norfloxacin. MIC test results should be interpreted according to the following criteria (these criteria only apply to isolates from urinary tract infections) (TABLE 4):

TABLE 4

MIC (mcg/ml)	Interpretation
≤4	(S) Susceptible
8	(I) Intermediate
≥16	(R) Resistant

As with standard diffusion methods, dilution procedures require the use of laboratory control organisms. Standard norfloxacin powder should give the following MIC values (TABLE 5):

TABLE 5

Organism	MIC range (mcg/ml)
E. coli ATCC 25922	0.03-0.12
E. faecalis ATCC 29212	2.0-8.0
P. aeruginosa ATCC 27853	1.0-4.0
S. aureus ATCC 29213	0.05-2.0

TABLETS AND OPHTHALMIC SOLUTION

Microbiology: Norfloxacin has *in vitro* activity against a broad range of gram-positive and gram-negative aerobic bacteria. The fluorine atom at the 6 position provides increased potency against gram-negative organisms, and the piperazine moiety at the 7 position is responsible for antipseudomonal activity.

Norfloxacin inhibits bacterial deoxyribonucleic acid synthesis and is bactericidal. At the molecular level, three specific events are attributed to norfloxacin in *E. coli* cells:

1) inhibition of the ATP-dependent DNA supercoiling reaction catalyzed by DNA gyrase

2) inhibition of the relaxation of supercoiled DNA

3) promotion of double-stranded DNA breakage

Resistance to norfloxacin due to spontaneous mutation *in vitro* is a rare occurrence (range: $10^{-9}$to 10^{-12} cells). Resistant organisms have emerged during therapy with norfloxacin in less than 1% of patients treated. Organisms in which development of resistance is greatest are the following:

PSEUDOMONAS AERUGINOSA

Klebsiella pneumoniae:*Acinetobacter* species *Enterococcus* species: For this reason, when there is a lack of satisfactory clinical response, repeat culture and susceptibility testing should be done. Nalidixic acid-resistant organisms are generally susceptible to norfloxacin *in vitro*; however, these organisms may have higher MICs to norfloxacin than nalidixic acid-susceptible strains. There is generally no cross-resistance between norfloxacin and other classes of antibacterial agents. Therefore, norfloxacin may demonstrate activity against indicated organisms resistant to some other antimicrobial agents including the aminoglycosides, penicillins, cephalosporins, tetracyclines, macrolides, and sulfonamides, including combinations of sulfamethoxazole and trimethoprim. Antagonism has been demonstrated *in vitro* between norfloxacin and nitrofurantoin.

Norfloxacin has been shown to be active against most strains of the following organisms both *in vitro* and in clinical infections (see INDICATIONS AND USAGE.):

Gram-positive aerobes: Enterococcus faecalis, Staphylococcus aureus, Staphylococcus epidermidis, Staphylococcus saprophyticus, Streptococcus agalactiae

Gram-negative aerobes: Citrobacter freundii, Enterobacter aerogenes, Enterobacter cloacae, Escherichia coli, Klebsiella pneumoniae, Neisseria gonorrhoeae, Proteus mirabilis, Proteus vulgaris, Pseudomonas aeruginosa, Serratia marcescens

Norfloxacin has been shown to be active *in vitro* against most strains of the following organisms; however, the clinical significance of these data is unknown.

Gram-Positive Aerobes: Bacillus cereus

Gram-Negative Aerobes: Acinetobacter calcoaceticus, *Aeromonas* species, *Alcaligenes* species, *Campylobacter* species, Citrobacter diversus, Edwardsiella tarda, *Flavobacterium* species, Hafnia alvei, Klebsiella oxytoca, Klebsiella rhinoscleromatis, Morganella morganii, Providencia alcalifaciens, Providencia rettgeri, Providencia stuartii, *Salmonella* species, *Shigella* species, Vibrio cholerae, Vibrio parahemolyticus, Yersinia enterocolitica

Other: Ureaplasma urealyticum

Noroxin is not generally active against obligate anaerobes.

Norfloxacin has not been shown to be active against *Treponema pallidum.* (See WARNINGS.)

CLINICAL STUDIES:

Ophthalmic Solution: Clinical studies were conducted comparing Chibroxin Ophthalmic Solution (n=152) with ophthalmic solutions of tobramycin, gentamicin, and chloramphenicol (n=158) in patients with conjunctivitis and positive bacterial cultures. After seven days of therapy with Chibroxin Ophthalmic Solution, 72 percent of patients were clinically cured. Of those cured, 85 percent had all their pathogens eradicated. Eradication was also achieved in 62 percent (23/37) of patients whose clinical outcome was not completely cured by day seven. These results were similar among all treatment groups.

Another clinical study compared Chibroxin Ophthalmic Solution with placebo in patients with conjunctivitis and positive bacterial cultures. Placebo in this study was the liquid vehicle for Chibroxin Ophthalmic Solution and contained the preservative. After five days of therapy, 64 percent (36/56) of patients on Chibroxin Ophthalmic Solution were clinically cured compared to 50 percent (23/46) of patients receiving placebo. Of those cured, 78 percent had all their pathogens eradicated. Eradication was also achieved in 50 percent (10/20) of patients whose clinical outcome was not completely cured. The response to Chibroxin Ophthalmic Solution was statistically significantly better than the response to placebo.

INDICATIONS AND USAGE:

TABLETS

Noroxin is indicated for the treatment of adults with the following infections caused by susceptible strains of the designated microorganisms:

Urinary Tract Infections: Uncomplicated urinary tract infections (including cystitis) due to *Enterococcus faecalis, Escherichia coli, Klebsiella pneumoniae, Proteus mirabilis, Pseudomonas aeruginosa, Staphylococcus epidermidis, Staphylococcus saprophyticus, Citrobacter freundii*, Enterobacter aerogenes*, Enterobacter cloacae*, Proteus vulgaris*, Staphylococcus aureus*, or Streptococcus agalactiae*.*

Complicated urinary tract infections due to *Enterococcus faecalis, Escherichia coli, Klebsiella pneumoniae, Proteus mirabilis, Pseudomonas aeruginosa,* or *Serratia marcescens*.*

Sexually transmitted diseases (See WARNINGS.): Uncomplicated urethral and cervical gonorrhea due to *Neisseria gonorrhoeae.*

(See DOSAGE AND ADMINISTRATION for appropriate dosing instructions.)

Penicillinase production should have no effect on norfloxacin activity.

Appropriate culture and susceptibility tests should be performed before treatment in order to isolate and identify organisms causing the infection and to determine their susceptibility to norfloxacin. Therapy with norfloxacin may be initiated before results of these tests are known; once results become available, appropriate therapy should be given. Repeat culture and susceptibility testing performed periodically during therapy will provide information not only on the therapeutic effect of the antimicrobial agents but also on the possible emergence of bacterial resistance.

*Efficacy for this organism in this organ system was studied in fewer than 10 infections.

OPHTHALMIC SOLUTION

Chibroxin Ophthalmic Solution is indicated for the treatment of conjunctivitis when caused by susceptible strains of the following bacteria:

*Acinetobacter calcoaceticus**
*Aeromonas hydrophila**
Haemophilus influenzae
*Proteus mirabilis**
*Serratia marcescens**
Staphylococcus aureus
Staphylococcus epidermidis
*Staphylococcus warnerii**
Streptococcus pneumoniae

Appropriate monitoring of bacterial response to topical antibiotic therapy should accompany the use of Chibroxin Ophthalmic Solution.

*Efficacy for this organism was studied in fewer than 10 infections.

CONTRAINDICATIONS:

Tablets and Ophthalmic Solution: Noroxin is contraindicated in patients with a history of hypersensitivity to norfloxacin or the other members of the quinolone group of antibacterial agents, or any other component of these medications.

WARNINGS:

TABLETS

The safety and efficacy of oral norfloxacin in children, adolescents (under the age of 18), pregnant women, and nursing mothers have not been established. (See PRECAUTIONS, Pregnancy, Nursing Mothers and Pediatric Use.) The oral administration of single doses of norfloxacin, 6 times† the recommended human clinical dose (on a mg/kg basis), caused lameness in immature dogs. Histologic examination of the weight-bearing joints of these dogs revealed permanent lesions of the cartilage. Other quinolones also produced erosions of the cartilage in weight-bearing joints and other signs of arthropathy in immature animals of various species. (See ANIMAL PHARMACOLOGY.)

Norfloxacin has not been shown to be effective in the treatment of syphilis. Antimicrobial agents used in high doses for short periods of time to treat gonorrhea may mask or delay the symptoms of incubating syphilis. All patients with gonorrhea should have a serologic test for syphilis at the time of diagnosis. Patients treated with norfloxacin should have a follow-up serologic test for syphilis after three months.

Serious and occasionally fatal hypersensitivity (anaphylactoid or anaphylactic) reactions, some following the first dose, have been reported in patients receiving quinolone therapy. Some reactions were accompanied by cardiovascular collapse, loss of consciousness, tingling, pharyngeal or facial edema, dyspnea, urticaria and itching. Only a few patients had a history of hypersensitivity reactions. If an allergic reaction to norfloxacin occurs, discontinue the drug. Serious acute hypersensitivity reactions may require immediate emergency treatment with epinephrine. Oxygen, intravenous fluids, antihistamines, corticosteroids, pressor amines, and airway management, including intubation, should be administered as indicated.

Convulsions have been reported in patients receiving norfloxacin. Convulsions, increased intracranial pressure, and toxic psychoses have been reported in patients receiving drugs in this class. Quinolones may also cause central nervous system (CNS) stimulation which may lead to tremors, restlessness, lightheadedness, confusion, and hallucinations. If these reactions occur in patients receiving norfloxacin, the drug should be discontinued and appropriate measures instituted.

The effects of norfloxacin on brain function or on the electrical activity of the brain have not been tested. Therefore, until more information becomes available, norfloxacin, like all other quinolones, should be used with caution in patients with known or suspected CNS disorders, such as severe cerebral arteriosclerosis, epilepsy, and other factors which predispose to seizures. (See ADVERSE REACTIONS.)

†Based on a patient weight of 50 kg.

WARNINGS: *(cont'd)*

OPHTHALMIC SOLUTION

Not For Injection Into The Eye: Serious and occasionally fatal hypersensitivity (anaphylactoid or anaphylactic) reactions, some following the first dose, have been reported in patients receiving systemic quinolone therapy. Some reactions were accompanied by cardiovascular collapse, loss of consciousness, tingling, pharyngeal or facial edema, dyspnea, urticaria, and itching. Only a few patients had a history of hypersensitivity reactions. Serious anaphylactoid or anaphylactic reactions require immediate emergency treatment with epinephrine. Oxygen, intravenous steroids and airway management, including intubation, should be administered as indicated.

PRECAUTIONS:

GENERAL

Needle-shaped crystals were found in the urine of some volunteers who received either placebo, 800 mg norfloxacin, or 1600 mg norfloxacin (at or twice the recommended daily dose, respectively) while participating in a double-blind, crossover study comparing single doses of norfloxacin with placebo. While crystalluria is not expected to occur under usual conditions with a dosage regimen of 400 mg b.i.d., as a precaution, the daily recommended dosage should not be exceeded and the patient should drink sufficient fluids to ensure a proper state of hydration and adequate urinary output.

Alteration in dosage regimen is necessary for patients with impaired renal function (see DOSAGE AND ADMINISTRATION.)

Moderate to severe phototoxicity reactions have been observed in patients who are exposed to excessive sunlight while receiving some members of this drug class. Excessive sunlight should be avoided. Therapy should be discontinued if phototoxicity occurs.

Ophthalmic Solution: As with other antibiotic preparations, prolonged use may result in overgrowth of nonsusceptible organisms, including fungi. If superinfection occurs, appropriate measures should be initiated. Whenever clinical judgment dictates, the patient should be examined with the aid of magnification, such as slit lamp biomicroscopy and, where appropriate, fluorescein staining.

INFORMATION FOR THE PATIENT

Tablets: Patients should be advised:

to drink fluids liberally.

that norfloxacin should be taken at least one hour before or at least two hours after a meal.

that multivitamins or other products containing iron or zinc, or antacids should not be taken within the two-hour period before or within the two-hour period after taking norfloxacin. (See DRUG INTERACTIONS)

that norfloxacin can cause dizziness and lightheadedness and, therefore, patients should know how they react to norfloxacin before they operate an automobile or machinery or engage in activities requiring mental alertness and coordination.

that norfloxacin may be associated with hypersensitivity reactions, even following the first dose, and to discontinue the drug at the first sign of a skin rash or other allergic reaction.

to avoid undue exposure to excessive sunlight while receiving norfloxacin and to discontinue therapy if phototoxicity occurs.

that some quinolones may increase the effects of theophylline and/or caffeine. (See DRUG INTERACTIONS.)

Ophthalmic Solution: Patients should be instructed to avoid allowing the tip of the dispensing container to contact the eye or surrounding structures.

Patients should be advised that norfloxacin may be associated with hypersensitivity reactions, even following a single dose, and to discontinue the drug at the first sign of a skin rash or other allergic reaction.

CARCINOGENESIS, MUTAGENESIS, AND IMPAIRMENT OF FERTILITY

No increase in neoplastic changes was observed with norfloxacin as compared to controls in a study in rats, lasting up to 96 weeks at doses 8 - 9 times† the usual human oral dose (on a mg/kg basis).

Norfloxacin was tested for mutagenic activity in a number of *in vivo* and *in vitro* tests. Norfloxacin had no mutagenic effect in the dominant lethal test in mice and did not cause chromosomal aberrations in hamsters or rats at doses 30 - 60 times† the usual human dose (on mg/kg basis). Norfloxacin had no mutagenic activity *in vitro* in the Ames microbial mutagen test, Chinese hamster fibroblasts and V-79 mammalian cell assay. Although norfloxacin was weakly positive in the Rec-assay for DNA repair, all other mutagenic assays were negative including a more sensitive test (V-79).

Norfloxacin did not adversely affect the fertility of male and female mice at oral doses up to 30 times† the usual human dose (on a mg/kg basis).

PREGNANCY, TERATOGENIC EFFECTS, PREGNANCY CATEGORY C

Norfloxacin has been shown to produce embryonic loss in monkeys when given in doses 10 times† the maximum daily total human dose (on a mg/kg basis). At this dose, peak plasma levels obtained in monkeys were approximately 2 times those obtained in humans. There has been no evidence of a teratogenic effect in any of the animal species tested (rat, rabbit, mouse, monkey) at 6 - 50 times† the maximum daily human dose (on a mg/kg basis). There are, however, no adequate and well controlled studies in pregnant women. Norfloxacin should be used during pregnancy only if the potential benefit justifies the potential risk to the fetus.

NURSING MOTHERS

It is not known whether norfloxacin is excreted in human milk.

When a 200-mg dose of Noroxin was administered to nursing mothers, norfloxacin was not detected in human milk. However, because the dose studied was low, because other drugs in this class are secreted in human milk, and because of the potential for serious adverse reactions from norfloxacin in nursing infants, a decision should be made to discontinue nursing or to discontinue the drug, taking into account the importance of the drug to the mother.

PEDIATRIC USE

Tablets: The safety and effectiveness of oral norfloxacin in children and adolescents below the age of 18 years have not been established. Norfloxacin causes arthropathy in juvenile animals of several animal species. (See WARNINGS and ANIMAL PHARMACOLOGY.)

Ophthalmic Solution: Safety and effectiveness in infants below the age of one year have not been established.

Although quinolones including norfloxacin have been shown to cause arthropathy in immature animals after oral administration, topical ocular administration of other quinolones to immature animals has not shown any arthropathy and there is no evidence that the ophthalmic dosage form of those quinolones has any effects on the weight bearing joints.

DRUG INTERACTIONS:

Tablets: Elevated plasma levels of theophylline have been reported with concomitant quinolone use. There have been reports of theophylline-related side effects in patients on concomitant therapy with norfloxacin and theophylline. Therefore, monitoring of theophylline plasma levels should be considered and dosage of theophylline adjusted as required.

DRUG INTERACTIONS: *(cont'd)*

Elevated serum levels of cyclosporine have been reported with concomitant use of cyclosporine with norfloxacin. Therefore cyclosporine serum levels should be monitored and appropriate cyclosporine dosage adjustments made when these drugs are used concomitantly.

Quinolones, including norfloxacin, may enhance the effects of the oral anticoagulant warfarin or its derivatives. When these products are administered concomitantly, prothrombin time or other suitable coagulation tests should be closely monitored.

Diminished urinary excretion of norfloxacin has been reported during the concomitant administration of probenecid and norfloxacin.

The concomitant use of nitrofurantoin is not recommended since nitrofurantoin may antagonize the antibacterial effect of Noroxin in the urinary tract.

Multivitamins, or other products containing iron or zinc, antacids or sucralfate should not be administered concomitantly with, or within 2 hours of, the administration of norfloxacin, because they may interfere with absorption resulting in lower serum and urine levels of norfloxacin.

Some quinolones have also been shown to interfere with the metabolism of caffeine. This may lead to reduced clearance of caffeine and a prolongation of its plasma half-life.

†Based on a patient weight of 50 kg.

Ophthalmic Solution: Specific drug interaction studies have not been conducted with norfloxacin ophthalmic solution. However, the systemic administration of some quinolones has been shown to elevate plasma concentrations of theophylline, interfere with the metabolism of caffeine, and enhance the effects of the oral anticoagulant warfarin and its derivatives. Elevated serum levels of cyclosporine have been reported with concomitant use of cyclosporine with norfloxacin. Therefore, cyclosporine serum levels should be monitored and appropriate cyclosporine dosage adjustments made when these drugs are used concomitantly.

ADVERSE REACTIONS:

URINARY TRACT INFECTIONS

Tablets: In clinical trials involving 1869 patients/subjects, 3.5% reported drug-related adverse experiences. However, the incidence figures below were calculated without reference to drug relationship.

The most common adverse experiences (>1%) were: nausea (4.3%), headache (2.9%), dizziness (1.8%), and fatigue (1.1%).

Additional reactions (0.3%-1%) were: rash, abdominal pain, dyspepsia, somnolence, depression, insomnia, constipation, flatulence, heartburn, dry mouth, diarrhea, fever, vomiting, pruritus, loose stools, back pain and hyperhidrosis.

Less frequent reactions included: erythema, anorexia, bitter taste, and asthenia.

Abnormal laboratory values observed in these patients/subjects were: elevation of ALT (SGPT) (1.6%), decreased WBC and neutrophil count (1.6%), elevation of AST (SGOT) (1.4%), eosinophilia (1.4%), and increased alkaline phosphatase (1.2%). Those occurring less frequently included increased BUN, serum creatinine, and LDH, and decreased hematocrit.

GONORRHEA

In clinical trials involving 228 patients who received a single 800-mg dose, 7.0% of patients reported drug-related adverse experiences. However, the following incidence figures were calculated without reference to drug relationship.

The most common adverse experiences (1%-3.5%) were: dizziness (3.5%), nausea (2.2%), abdominal cramping (1.8%), diarrhea (1.3%), anorexia (1.3%), headache (1.3%), and hyperhidrosis (1.3%).

Additional reactions (0.3%-1%) were: vomiting, constipation, dyspepsia, and tingling of the fingers.

Laboratory adverse changes considered drug-related were reported in 2.2% of patients who received a single 800-mg dose of norfloxacin. These laboratory changes were: decreased hemoglobin and hematocrit (0.9%), decreased platelet count (0.9%), and increased AST (0.4%).

POST MARKETING

The most frequently reported adverse reaction in post-marketing experience is rash.

CNS effects characterized as generalized seizures and myoclonus have been reported with Noroxin. A causal relationship to Noroxin has not been established (see WARNINGS.) Visual disturbances have been reported with drugs in this class.

The following additional adverse reactions have been reported since the drug was marketed:

Hypersensitivity Reactions: Hypersensitivity reactions have been reported including anaphylactoid reactions, angioedema, dyspnea, vasculitis, urticaria, arthritis, arthralgia and myalgia (see WARNINGS.)

Skin: Toxic epidermal necrolysis, Stevens-Johnson syndrome and erythema multiforme, exfoliative dermatitis, pruritus, photosensitivity

Gastrointestinal: Pseudomembranous colitis, hepatitis, jaundice, pancreatitis (rare), stomatitis, anorexia

Renal: Interstitial nephritis, renal failure

Nervous System/Psychiatric: Polyneuropathy including Guillain-Barre Syndrome, ataxia, paresthesia; psychic disturbances including psychotic reactions and confusion

Musculoskeletal: Tendinitis, possible exacerbation of myasthenia gravis

Hematologic: Neutropenia, leukopenia, hemolytic anemia, thrombocytopenia

Special Senses: Transient hearing loss (rare), tinnitus, diplopia

Other adverse events: agranulocytosis, albuminuria, candiduria, crystalluria, cylindruria, dysphagia, elevation of blood glucose, elevation of serum cholesterol, elevation of serum potassium, elevation of serum triglycerides, hematuria, hepatic necrosis, hypoglycemia, nystagmus, postural hypotension, prolongation of prothrombin time, and vaginal candidiasis.

OPHTHALMIC SOLUTION

In clinical trials, the most frequently reported drug-related adverse reaction was local burning or discomfort. Other drug-related adverse reactions were conjunctival hyperemia, chemosis, photophobia and a bitter taste following instillation.

OVERDOSAGE:

TABLETS

No significant lethality was observed in male and female mice and rats at single oral doses up to 4 g/kg.

In the event of acute overdosage, the stomach should be emptied by inducing vomiting or by gastric lavage, and the patient carefully observed and given symptomatic and supportive treatment. Adequate hydration must be maintained.

DOSAGE AND ADMINISTRATION:

TABLETS

Tablets Noroxin should be taken at least one hour before or at least two hours after a meal with a glass of water. Patients receiving Noroxin should be well hydrated (see PRECAUTIONS.)

DOSAGE AND ADMINISTRATION: *(cont'd)*

Normal Renal Function: The recommended daily dose of Noroxin is as described in the following chart (TABLE 6):

TABLE 6

Infection	Description	Unit Dose	Frequency	Duration	Daily Dose
Urinary Tract	Uncomplicated UTI's (cystitis) due to*E. coli, K. pneumoniae,* or *P. mirabilis*	400 mg	q12h	3 days	800 mg
	Uncomplicated UTI's due to other indicated organisms	400 mg	q12h	7-10 days	800 mg
	Complicated UTI's	400 mg	q12h	10-21 days	800 mg
Sexually Transmitted Diseases	Uncomplicated Gonorrhea	800 mg	single dose	1 day	800 mg

Renal Impairment: Noroxin may be used for the treatment of urinary tract infections in patients with renal insufficiency. In patients with a creatinine clearance rate of 30 ml/min/1.73m^2 or less, the recommended dosage is one 400-mg tablet once daily for the duration given above. At this dosage, the urinary concentration exceeds the MICs for most urinary pathogens susceptible to norfloxacin, even when the creatinine clearance is less than 10 ml/min/1.73m^2.

When only the serum creatinine level is available, the following formula (based on sex, weight, and age of the patient) may be used to convert this value into creatinine clearance. The serum creatinine should represent a steady state of renal function.

$$\text{Males:} = [(\text{Weight in kg}) \times (140 - \text{age})] \div [(72) \times \text{Serum Creatnine (mg/ml)}]$$

$$\text{Females} = (0.85) \times (\text{above value})$$

Elderly: Elderly patients being treated for urinary tract infections who have a creatinine clearance of greater than 30 ml/min/1.73m^{2}should receive the dosages recommended under Normal Renal Function.

Elderly patients being treated for urinary tract infections who have a creatinine clearance of 30 ml/min/1.73m^2 or less should receive 400 mg once daily as recommended under Renal Impairment.

OPHTHALMIC SOLUTION

The recommended dose in adults and pediatric patients (one year and older) is one or two drops of Chibroxin Ophthalmic Solution applied topically to the affected eye(s) four times daily for up to seven days. Depending on the severity of the infection, the dosage for the first day of therapy may be one or two drops every two hours during the waking hours.

ANIMAL PHARMACOLOGY:

Tablets: Norfloxacin and related drugs have been shown to cause arthropathy in immature animals of most species tested (see WARNINGS.)

Crystalluria has occurred in laboratory animals tested with norfloxacin. In dogs, needle-shaped drug crystals were seen in the urine at doses of 50 mg/kg/day. In rats, crystals were reported following doses of 200 mg/kg/day.

Embryo lethality and slight maternotoxicity (vomiting and anorexia) were observed in cynomolgus monkeys at doses of 150 mg/kg/day or higher.

Ocular toxicity, seen with some related drugs, was not observed in any norfloxacin-treated animals.

Ophthalmic Solution: The oral administration of single doses of norfloxacin, six times the recommended human oral dose*, caused lameness in immature dogs. Histologic examination of the weight-bearing joints of these dogs revealed permanent lesions of the cartilage. Related drugs also produced erosions of the cartilage in weight-bearing joints and other signs of arthropathy in immature animals of various species.

HOW SUPPLIED:

TABLETS

No. 3522-Tablets Noroxin 400 mg are dark pink, oval shaped, film-coated tablets, coded MSD 705 on one side and Noroxin on the other.

Storage: Tablets Noroxin should be stored in a tightly-closed container. Avoid storage at temperatures above 40°C (104°F).

OPHTHALMIC SOLUTION

Chibroxin Ophthalmic Solution is a clear, colorless to light yellow solution.

No. 3526 — Chibroxin Ophthalmic Solution 0.3% is supplied in a white, opaque, plastic Ocumeter ophthalmic dispenser with a controlled drop tip.

Storage: Store Chibroxin Ophthalmic Solution at room temperature, 15 - 30°C (59 - 86°F). Protect from light.

HOW SUPPLIED - EQUIVALENTS NOT AVAILABLE:

Solution - Ophthalmic - 3 mg/ml

5 ml	$18.04	CHIBROXIN OPHTHALMIC, Merck	00006-3526-03

Tablet, Plain Coated - Oral - 400 mg

20's	**$56.65**	**NOROXIN, Roberts Labs**	**54092-0097-20**
100's	**$278.98**	**NOROXIN, Roberts Labs**	**54092-0097-01**
100's	**$278.98**	**NOROXIN, Roberts Labs**	**54092-0097-52**

NORGESTREL *(001902)*

CATEGORIES: Contraceptives; Hormones; Pregnancy; Progestins; Progestogen; Pregnancy Category X; FDA Approval Pre 1982

BRAND NAMES: *Neogest* (England); **Ovrette**
(International brand names outside U.S. in italics)

FORMULARIES: Aetna; PCS

COST OF THERAPY: $252.29 (Contraceptive; Tablet; 0.075 mg; 1/day; 252 days) vs. Potential Cost of $2,351.94 (Pregnancy)

DESCRIPTION:

Each Ovrette tablet contains 0.075 mg of norgestrel (*dl*-13-beta- ethyl-17-alpha-ethinyl-17-beta-hydroxygon-4-en-3-one). The inactive ingredients present are cellulose, FD&C Yellow 5, lactose, magnesium stearate, and polacrilin potassium.

DESCRIPTION: *(cont'd)*

Each Ovrette tablet contains 0.075 mg of a single active steroid ingredient, norgestrel, a totally synthetic progestogen. The available data suggest that the d(-)enantiomeric form of norgestrel is the biologically active portion. This form amounts to 0.0375 mg per Ovrette tablet.

For prescribing information refer to Ethinyl Estradiol; Norethindrone.

HOW SUPPLIED:

Ovrette tablets (norgestrel tablets are available in containers of 28 yellow, round tablets marked "Wyeth" and "62".

HOW SUPPLIED - EQUIVALENTS NOT AVAILABLE:

Tablet, Uncoated - Oral - 0.075 mg

168 (6 x 28)	**$168.20**	**OVRETTE, Wyeth Labs**	**00008-0062-01**

NORTRIPTYLINE HYDROCHLORIDE *(001903)*

CATEGORIES: Antidepressants; Central Nervous System Agents; Depression; Psychotherapeutic Agents; Tricyclics; Tricyclic Antidepressants; Migraine*; Sales > $100 Million; FDA Approval Pre 1982; Patent Expiration 1992 Nov
* Indication not approved by the FDA

BRAND NAMES: *Allegron* (Australia, England); *Allergron*; *Ateben*; *Aventyl* (England, Canada); Aventyl HCl; *Kareon*; *Lisunim*; *Martimil*; *Noritren* (Japan); *Norline*; *Norpress*; *Nortrilen* (Germany); *Nortrix*; *Nortyline*; *Ortrip*; **Pamelor**; *Paxtibi*; *Sensaval*; *Sensibal*; *Sensival* (Japan); *Vividyl*
(International brand names outside U.S. in italics)

FORMULARIES: Aetna; BC-BS; Foundation; Medi-Cal; PCS

PRIMARY ICD9: 311 (Depressive Disorder, Not Elsewhere Classified)

DESCRIPTION:

Nortriptyline HCl is 1-Propanamine, 3-(10,11-dihydro-*5H*-dibenzo[*a,d*]cyclohepten-5-ylidene)-*N*-methyl-, hydrochloride.

10 mg, 25 mg, 50 mg, and 75 mg Pamelor Capsules: *Active Ingredient:* nortriptyline HCl, USP *Inactive Ingredients:* D&C Yellow #10, FD&C Yellow #6, gelatin, silicone fluid, sodium lauryl sulfate, starch, and titanium dioxide. *May Also Include:* benzyl alcohol, butylparaben, edetate calcium disodium, methylparaben, propylparaben, silicon dioxide, and sodium propionate.

50 mg Capsules: *Inactive Ingredients:* gelatin, silicone fluid, sodium lauryl sulfate, starch, and titanium dioxide. *May Also Include:* benzyl alcohol, butylparaben, edetate calcium disodium, methylparaben, propylparaben, silicon dioxide, sodium bisulfite (capsule shell only), and sodium propionate.

Pamelor Solution: *Active Ingredient:* nortriptyline HCl, USP. *Inactive Ingredients:* alcohol, benzoic acid, flavoring, purified water, and sorbitol.

CLINICAL PHARMACOLOGY:

The mechanism of mood elevation by tricyclic antidepressants is at present unknown. Nortriptyline HCl is not a monoamine oxidase inhibitor. It inhibits the activity of such diverse agents as histamine, 5-hydroxytryptamine, and acetylcholine. It increases the pressor effect of norepinephrine but blocks the pressor response of phenethylamine. Studies suggest that Nortriptyline HCl interferes with the transport, release, and storage of catecholamines. Operant conditioning techniques in rats and pigeons suggest that Nortriptyline HCl has a combination of stimulant and depressant properties.

INDICATIONS AND USAGE:

Nortriptyline HCl is indicated for the relief of symptoms of depression. Endogenous depressions are more likely to be alleviated than are other depressive states.

CONTRAINDICATIONS:

The use of Nortriptyline HCl or other tricyclic antidepressants concurrently with a monoamine oxidase (MAO) inhibitor is contraindicated. Hyperpyretic crises, severe convulsions, and fatalities have occurred when similar tricyclic antidepressants were used in such combinations. It is advisable to have discontinued the MAO inhibitor for at least two weeks before treatment with Nortriptyline HCl is started. Patients hypersensitive to Nortriptyline HCl should not be given the drug.

Cross-sensitivity between Nortriptyline HCl and other dibenzazepines is a possibility.

Nortriptyline HCl is contraindicated during the acute recovery period after myocardial infarction.

WARNINGS:

Patients with cardiovascular disease should be given Nortriptyline HCl only under close supervision because of the tendency of the drug to produce sinus tachycardia and to prolong the conduction time. Myocardial infarction, arrhythmia, and strokes have occurred. The antihypertensive action of guanethidine and similar agents may be blocked. Because of its anticholinergic activity, Nortriptyline HCl should be used with great caution in patients who have glaucoma or a history of urinary retention. Patients with a history of seizures should be followed closely when Nortriptyline HCl is administered, in as much as this drug is known to lower the convulsive threshold. Great care is required if Nortriptyline HCl is given to hyperthyroid patients or to those receiving thyroid medication, since cardiac arrhythmias may develop.

Nortriptyline HCl may impair the mental and/or physical abilities required for the performance of hazardous tasks, such as operating machinery or driving a car; therefore, the patient should be warned accordingly.

Excessive consumption of alcohol in combination with nortriptyline therapy may have a potentiating effect, which may lead to the danger of increased suicidal attempts or overdosage, especially in patients with histories of emotional disturbances or suicidal ideation.

The concomitant administration of quinidine and nortriptyline may result in a significantly longer plasma half-life, higher AUC, and lower clearance of nortriptyline.

Use in Pregnancy: Safe use of Nortriptyline HCl during pregnancy and lactation has not been established; therefore, when the drug is administered to pregnant patients, nursing mothers, or women of childbearing potential, the potential benefits must be weighed against the possible hazards. Animal reproduction studies have yielded inconclusive results.

Usage in Children: This drug is not recommended for use in children, since safety and effectiveness in the pediatric age group have not been established.

PRECAUTIONS:

The use of Nortriptyline HCl in schizophrenic patients may result in an exacerbation of the psychosis or may activate latent schizophrenic symptoms. If the drug is given to overactive or agitated patients, increased anxiety and agitation may occur. In manic-depressive patients, Nortriptyline HCl may cause symptoms of the manic phase to emerge.

Troublesome patient hostility may be aroused by the use of Nortriptyline HCl. Epileptiform seizures may accompany its administration, as is true of other drugs of its class.

When it is essential, the drug may be administered with electroconvulsive therapy, although the hazards may be increased. Discontinue the drug for several days, if possible, prior to elective surgery.

The possibility of a suicidal attempt by a depressed patient remains after the initiation of treatment; in this regard, it is important that the least possible quantity of drug be dispensed at any given time.

Both elevation and lowering of blood sugar levels have been reported.

DRUG INTERACTIONS:

Administration of reserpine during therapy with a tricyclic antidepressant has been shown to produce a "stimulating" effect in some depressed patients.

Close supervision and careful adjustment of the dosage are required when Nortriptyline HCl is used with other anticholinergic drugs and sympathomimetic drugs.

Concurrent administration of cimetidine and tricyclic antidepressants can produce clinically significant increases in the plasma concentrations of the tricyclic antidepressant. The patient should be informed that the response to alcohol may be exaggerated.

A case of significant hypoglycemia has been reported in a type II diabetic patient maintained on chlorpropamide (250 mg/day), after the addition of nortriptyline (125 mg/day).

Drugs Metabolized by P450IID6: The biochemical activity of the drug metabolizing isozyme cytochrome P450IID6 (debrisoquin hydroxylase) is reduced in a subset of the caucasian population (about 7%-10% of caucasians are so called "poor metabolizers"); reliable estimates of the prevalence of reduced P450IID6 isozyme activity among Asian, African and other populations are not yet available. Poor metabolizers have higher than expected plasma concentrations of tricyclic antidepressants (TCAs) when given usual doses. Depending on the fraction of drug metabolized by P450IID6, the increase in plasma concentration may be small, or quite large (8 fold increase in plasma AUC of the TCA).

In addition, certain drugs inhibit the activity of this isozyme and make normal metabolizers resemble poor metabolizers. An individual who is stable on a given dose of TCA may become abruptly toxic when given one of these inhibiting drugs as concomitant therapy. The drugs that inhibit cytochrome P450IID6 include some that are not metabolized by the enzyme (quinidine; cimetidine) and many that are substrates of P450IID6 (many other antidepressants, phenothiazines, and the Type 1C antiarrhythmics propafenone and flecainide). While all the selective serotonin reuptake inhibitors (SSRIs), e.g., fluoxetine, sertraline, and paroxetine, inhibit P450IID6, they may vary in the extent of inhibition. The extent to which SSRI TCA interactions may pose clinical problems will depend on the degree of inhibition and the pharmacokinetics of the SSRI involved. Nevertheless, caution is indicated in the co-administration of TCAs with any of the SSRIs and also in switching from one class to the other. Of particular importance, sufficient time must elapse before initiating TCA treatment in a patient being withdrawn from fluoxetine, given the long half-life of the parent and active metabolite (at lease 5 weeks may be necessary).

Concomitant use of tricyclic antidepressants with drugs that can inhibit cytochrome P450IID6 may require lower doses than usually prescribed for either the tricyclic antidepressant or the other drug. Furthermore, whenever one of these other drugs is withdrawn from co-therapy, an increased dose of tricyclic antidepressant may be required. It is desirable to monitor TCA plasma levels whenever a TCA is going to be co- administered with another drug known to be an inhibitor of P450IID6.

ADVERSE REACTIONS:

Note: Included in the following list are a few adverse reactions that have not been reported with this specific drug. However, the pharmacologic similarities among the tricyclic antidepressant drugs require that each of the reactions be considered when nortriptyline is administered.

Cardiovascular: Hypotension, hypertension, tachycardia, palpitation, myocardial infarction, arrhythmias, heart block, stroke.

Psychiatric: Confusional states (especially in the elderly) with hallucinations, disorientation, delusions; anxiety, restlessness, agitation; insomnia, panic, nightmares; hypomania; exacerbation of psychosis.

Neurologic: Numbness, tingling, paresthesias of extremities; incoordination, ataxia, tremors; peripheral neuropathy; extrapyramidal symptoms; seizures, alteration in EEG patterns; tinnitus.

Anticholinergic: Dry mouth and, rarely, associated sublingual adenitis; blurred vision, disturbance of accommodation, mydriasis; constipation, paralytic ileus; urinary retention, delayed micturition, dilation of the urinary tract.

Allergic: Skin rash, petechiae, urticaria, itching, photosensitization (avoid excessive exposure to sunlight); edema (general or of face and tongue), drug fever, cross-sensitivity with other tricyclic drugs.

Hematologic: Bone marrow depression, including agranulocytosis; eosinophilia; purpura; thrombocytopenia.

Gastrointestinal: Nausea and vomiting, anorexia, epigastric distress, diarrhea, peculiar taste, stomatitis, abdominal cramps, blacktongue.

Endocrine: Gynecomastia in the male, breast enlargement and galactorrhea in the female; increased or decreased libido, impotence; testicular swelling; elevation or depression of blood sugar levels; syndrome of inappropriate ADH (antidiuretic hormone) secretion.

Other: Jaundice (simulating obstructive), altered liver function; weight gain or loss; perspiration; flushing; urinary frequency, nocturia; drowsiness, dizziness, weakness, fatigue; headache; parotid swelling; alopecia.

Withdrawal Symptoms: Though these are not indicative of addiction, abrupt cessation of treatment after prolonged therapy may produce nausea, headache, and malaise.

OVERDOSAGE:

Toxic overdosage may result in confusion, restlessness, agitation, vomiting, hyperpyrexia, muscle rigidity, hyperactive reflexes, tachycardia, ECG evidence of impaired conduction, shock, congestive heart failure, stupor, coma, and CNS stimulation with convulsions followed by respiratory depression. Deaths have occurred following overdosage with drugs of this class.

No specific antidote is known. General supportive measures are indicated, with gastric lavage. Respiratory assistance is apparently the most effective measure when indicated. The use of CNS depressants may worsen the prognosis.

The administration of barbiturates for control of convulsions alleviates an increase in the cardiac work load but should be undertaken with caution to avoid potentiation of respiratory depression.

OVERDOSAGE: *(cont'd)*

Intramuscular paraldehyde or diazepam provides anticonvulsant activity with less respiratory depression than do the barbiturates; diazepam seems to be preferred.

The use of digitalis and/or physostigmine may be considered in case of serious cardiovascular abnormalities or cardiac failure.

The value of dialysis has not been established.

DOSAGE AND ADMINISTRATION:

Nortriptyline HCl is not recommended for children.

Nortriptyline HCl is administered orally in the form of capsules or liquid. Lower than usual dosages are recommended for elderly patients and adolescents. Lower dosages are also recommended for outpatients than for hospitalized patients who will be under close supervision. The physician should initiate dosage at a low level and increase it gradually, noting carefully the clinical response and any evidence of intolerance. Following remission, maintenance medication may be required for a longer period of time at the lowest dose that will maintain remission.

If a patient develops minor side effects, the dosage should be reduced. The drug should be discontinued promptly if adverse effects of a serious nature or allergic manifestations occur.

Usual Adult Dose: 25 mg three or four times daily; dosage should begin at a low level and be increased as required. As an alternate regimen, the total daily dosage may be given once a day. When doses above 100 mg daily are administered, plasma levels of nortriptyline should be monitored and maintained in the optimum range of 50-150 ng/ml. Doses above 150 mg/day are not recommended.

Elderly and Adolescent Patients: 30-50 mg/day, in divided doses, or the total daily dosage may be given once a day.

Capsules: Store and Dispense: Below 86°F (30°C); tight container.

Solution: Store and Dispense: Below 86°F (30°C); tight, light-resistant container.

HOW SUPPLIED - RATED THERAPEUTICALLY EQUIVALENT:

Capsule, Gelatin - Oral - 10 mg

100's	$11.55	Nortriptyline HCl, H.C.F.A. F F P	99999-1903-01
100's	$12.21	Nortriptyline HCl, United Res	00677-1555-01
100's	$35.05	Nortriptyline HCl, Qualitest Pharms	00603-4798-21
100's	$35.41	Nortriptyline HCl, Geneva Pharms	50752-0250-05
100's	$35.89	Nortriptyline Hcl, HL Moore Drug Exch	00839-7798-06
100's	$36.88	Nortriptyline Hcl, Aligen Independ	00405-4705-01
100's	$37.52	Nortriptyline HCl, Rugby	00536-5716-01
100's	$38.15	Nortriptyline HCl, Major Pharms	00904-5029-60
100's	$38.15	Nortriptyline Hcl, Major Pharms	00904-7739-60
100's	$38.15	Nortriptyline Hcl, Major Pharms	00904-7787-60
100's	$38.15	Nortriptyline Hcl, Major Pharms	00904-7795-60
100's	$38.65	Nortriptyline HCl, Teva	00093-0810-01
100's	$38.80	Nortriptyline HCl, Schein Pharm (US)	00364-2508-90
100's	$38.95	Nortriptyline HCl, Geneva Pharms	50752-0250-06
100's	$39.19	Nortriptyline HCl, Schein Pharm (US)	00364-2508-01
100's	$39.65	Nortriptyline HCl, Geneva Pharms	00781-2630-01
100's	$40.65	Nortriptyline HCl, Geneva Pharms	00781-2630-13
100's	$40.96	Nortriptyline HCl, Goldline Labs	00182-1190-01
100's	$42.66	Nortriptyline Hcl, Mylan	00378-1410-01
100's	**$47.40**	**PAMELOR, Novartis**	**00078-0086-05**
100's	**$52.32**	**PAMELOR, Novartis**	**00078-0086-06**
500's	$57.75	Nortriptyline HCl, H.C.F.A. F F P	99999-1903-02
500's	$170.96	Nortriptyline HCl, Schein Pharm (US)	00364-2508-05
500's	$171.00	Nortriptyline HCl, Teva	00093-0810-05
750's	$292.12	Nortriptyline HCl, Glasgow Pharm	60809-0304-55
750's	$292.12	Nortriptyline HCl, Glasgow Pharm	60809-0304-72

Capsule, Gelatin - Oral - 25 mg

100's	$15.90	Nortriptyline HCl, H.C.F.A. F F P	99999-1903-03
100's	$16.83	Nortriptyline HCl, United Res	00677-1556-01
100's	$70.84	Nortriptyline HCl, Geneva Pharms	50752-0251-05
100's	$70.85	Nortriptyline HCl, Qualitest Pharms	00603-4799-21
100's	$71.54	Nortriptyline Hcl, HL Moore Drug Exch	00839-7799-06
100's	$74.38	Nortripyline Hcl, Aligen Independ	00405-4706-01
100's	$74.38	Nortriptyline HCl, Geneva Pharms	50752-0251-06
100's	$74.91	Nortriptyline HCl, Rugby	00536-5717-01
100's	$76.35	Nortriptyline HCl, Major Pharms	00904-5030-60
100's	$76.35	Nortriptyline Hcl, Major Pharms	00904-7740-60
100's	$76.35	Nortriptyline Hcl, Major Pharms	00904-7788-60
100's	$76.35	Nortriptyline Hcl, Major Pharms	00904-7796-60
100's	$77.20	Nortriptyline HCl, Teva	00093-0811-01
100's	$77.51	Nortriptyline HCl, Schein Pharm (US)	00364-2509-90
100's	$79.50	Nortriptyline HCl, Geneva Pharms	00781-2631-01
100's	$80.31	Nortriptyline HCl, Schein Pharm (US)	00364-2509-01
100's	$80.50	Nortriptyline HCl, Geneva Pharms	00781-2631-13
100's	$81.81	Nortriptyline HCl, Goldline Labs	00182-1191-01
100's	$85.15	Nortriptyline Hcl, Mylan	00378-2325-01
100's	**$94.62**	**PAMELOR, Novartis**	**00078-0087-05**
100's	**$99.42**	**PAMELOR, Novartis**	**00078-0087-06**
500's	$79.50	Nortriptyline HCl, H.C.F.A. F F P	99999-1903-04
500's	$346.99	Nortriptyline HCl, Geneva Pharms	50752-0251-08
500's	$364.35	Nortriptyline HCl, HL Moore Drug Exch	00839-7799-12
500's	$374.34	Nortriptyline HCl, Schein Pharm (US)	00364-2509-05
500's	$377.79	Nortriptyline HCl, Geneva Pharms	00781-2631-05
500's	$377.85	Nortriptyline HCl, Teva	00093-0811-05
500's	**$462.90**	**PAMELOR, Novartis**	**00078-0087-08**
750's	$520.48	Nortriptyline HCl, Glasgow Pharm	60809-0305-55
750's	$520.48	Nortriptyline HCl, Glasgow Pharm	60809-0305-72
1000's	$159.00	Nortriptyline HCl, H.C.F.A. F F P	99999-1903-05
1000's	$643.53	Nortriptyline HCl, Schein Pharm (US)	00364-2509-02

Capsule, Gelatin - Oral - 50 mg

100's	$19.43	Nortriptyline HCl, H.C.F.A. F F P	99999-1903-06
100's	$20.57	Nortriptyline Hcl, United Res	00677-1557-01
100's	$124.99	Nortriptyline Hcl, HL Moore Drug Exch	00839-7800-06
100's	$131.65	Nortriptyline Hcl, Qualitest Pharms	00603-4800-21
100's	$133.65	Nortriptyline HCl, Geneva Pharms	50752-0252-05
100's	$136.48	Nortriptyline Hcl, Aligen Independ	00405-4707-01
100's	$137.66	Nortriptyline HCl, Geneva Pharms	50752-0252-06
100's	$145.21	Nortriptyline HCl, Schein Pharm (US)	00364-2510-90
100's	$145.55	Nortriptyline HCl, Teva	00093-0812-01
100's	$149.50	Nortriptyline Hcl, Rugby	00536-5718-01
100's	$149.95	Nortriptyline Hcl, Major Pharms	00904-5031-60
100's	$149.95	Nortriptyline Hcl, Major Pharms	00904-7741-60
100's	$149.95	Nortriptyline Hcl, Major Pharms	00904-7789-60
100's	$149.95	Nortriptyline Hcl, Major Pharms	00904-7797-60
100's	$151.80	Nortriptyline HCl, Schein Pharm (US)	00364-2510-01
100's	$151.95	Nortriptyline HCl, Geneva Pharms	00781-2632-01
100's	$152.95	Nortriptyline HCl, Geneva Pharms	00781-2632-13
100's	$154.24	Nortriptyline Hcl, Goldline Labs	00182-1192-01

HOW SUPPLIED - RATED THERAPEUTICALLY EQUIVALENT: *(cont'd)*

100's	$160.53	Nortriptyline Hcl, Mylan	00378-3250-01
100's	**$178.38**	**PAMELOR, Novartis**	**00078-0078-05**
100's	**$182.94**	**PAMELOR, Novartis**	**00078-0078-06**
500's	$97.15	Nortriptyline HCl, H.C.F.A. F F P	99999-1903-07
500's	$645.18	Nortriptyline HCl, Schein Pharm (US)	00364-2510-05
500's	$645.20	Nortriptyline HCl, Teva	00093-0812-05
640's	**$1039.08**	**PAMELOR, Novartis**	**00078-0078-65**
750's	$1032.45	Nortriptyline Hcl, Glasgow Pharm	60809-0306-55
750's	$1032.45	Nortriptyline Hcl, Glasgow Pharm	60809-0306-72

Capsule, Gelatin - Oral - 75 mg

100's	$24.83	Nortriptyline HCl, H.C.F.A. F F P	99999-1903-08
100's	$26.27	Nortriptyline Hcl, United Res	00677-1558-01
100's	$200.97	Nortriptyline Hcl, Qualitest Pharms	00603-4801-21
100's	$203.79	Nortriptyline HCl, Geneva Pharms	50752-0253-05
100's	$205.32	Nortriptyline Hcl, Aligen Independ	00405-4708-01
100's	$206.48	Nortriptyline HCl, Schein Pharm (US)	00364-2511-90
100's	$209.24	Nortriptyline Hcl, HL Moore Drug Exch	00839-7801-06
100's	$209.90	Nortriptyline HCl, Geneva Pharms	50752-0253-06
100's	$212.50	Nortriptyline Hcl, Major Pharms	00904-5032-60
100's	$212.50	Nortriptyline Hcl, Major Pharms	00904-7742-60
100's	$212.50	Nortriptyline Hcl, Major Pharms	00904-7790-60
100's	$212.50	Nortriptyline Hcl, Major Pharms	00904-7798-60
100's	$221.36	Nortriptyline HCl, Schein Pharm (US)	00364-2511-01
100's	$221.50	Nortriptyline Hcl, Rugby	00536-5719-01
100's	$221.95	Nortriptyline HCl, Teva	00093-0813-01
100's	$221.95	Nortriptyline HCl, Geneva Pharms	00781-2633-01
100's	$235.14	Nortriptyline Hcl, Goldline Labs	00182-1193-01
100's	$244.71	Nortriptyline Hcl, Mylan	00378-4175-01
100's	**$271.92**	**PAMELOR, Novartis**	**00078-0079-05**
500's	$1054.30	Nortriptyline HCl, Teva	00093-0813-05
640's	**$1581.66**	**PAMELOR, Novartis**	**00078-0079-65**
750's	$1574.25	Nortriptyline Hcl, Glasgow Pharm	60809-0307-55
750's	$1574.25	Nortriptyline Hcl, Glasgow Pharm	60809-0307-72

Solution - Oral - 10 mg/5ml

480 ml	$44.00	AVENTYL HCL, Lilly	00002-2468-05
480 ml	**$54.36**	**PAMELOR, Novartis**	**00078-0016-33**

HOW SUPPLIED - NOT RATED EQUIVALENT:

Capsule, Gelatin - Oral - 10 mg

100's	$41.69	AVENTYL HCL, Lilly	00002-0817-02
100's	$46.07	AVENTYL HCL, Lilly	00002-0817-33
500's	$197.66	AVENTYL HCL, Lilly	00002-0817-03

Capsule, Gelatin - Oral - 25 mg

100's	$83.24	AVENTYL HCL, Lilly	00002-0819-02
100's	$87.62	AVENTYL HCL, Lilly	00002-0819-33
500's	$395.55	AVENTYL HCL, Lilly	00002-0819-03

NOVOBIOCIN SODIUM *(001905)*

CATEGORIES: Anti-Infectives; Antibiotics; Antimicrobials; Infections; Urinary Tract Infections; Pregnancy Category C; FDA Approval Pre 1982

BRAND NAMES: Albamycin

> WARNING:
> NOVOBIOCIN SHOULD BE USED ONLY FOR THOSE SERIOUS INFECTIONS WHERE OTHER LESS TOXIC DRUGS ARE INEFFECTIVE OR CONTRAINDICATED.
> NOVOBIOCIN IS ASSOCIATED WITH A HIGH FREQUENCY OF ADVERSE REACTIONS, PRINCIPALLY URTICARIA AND MACULOPAPULAR DERMATITIS. HEPATIC DYSFUNCTION AND BLOOD DYSCRASIAS HAVE OCCURRED LESS FREQUENTLY.
> IN ADDITION, NOVOBIOCIN IS ASSOCIATED WITH THE RAPID AND FREQUENT EMERGENCE OF RESISTANT STRAINS, ESPECIALLY STAPHYLOCOCCI.

DESCRIPTION:

Albamycin Capsules for oral administration contain 250 mg of novobiocin sodium which, in the crystalline state, has a light yellow to white color depending upon the state of subdivision. It is odorless or practically odorless. The sodium salt is freely soluble in water, alcohol, glycerin and propylene glycol. One gram of the calcium salt dissolves in about 250 ml of water, in about 30 ml of alcohol, in about 450 ml of ether and in about 1100 ml of chloroform.

Albamycin Capsules contain the following inactive ingredients: corn starch, edible ink white, erythrosine sodium, FD&C Blue No. 1, gelatin, magnesium stearate, mineral oil, and titanium dioxide.

The chemical name is N-(7-((3-0-(Aminocarbonyl)-5,5-di-C-methyl-4-0-methyl-a-L-lyxopyranosyl)o xy)-4-hydroxy-8-methyl-2-oxo-2H-1-benzopyran-3-yl)-4-hydroxy-3-(3-methyl-2 - butenyl)-benzamide.

CLINICAL PHARMACOLOGY:

Orally administered, novobiocin is rapidly absorbed, producing peak concentrations in the blood within 2 to 3 hours. It diffuses into pleural and ascitic fluid but does not diffuse into the cerebrospinal fluid. Novobiocin is excreted mainly in the bile. Urinary excretion of active drug is low (approximately 3 percent of the dose administered). *In vitro* novobiocin shows activity against *Staphylococcus aureus* and against some strains of *Proteus vulgaris.* It shows no cross resistance with penicillin against resistant strains of *S. aureus;* however, *in vitro* studies indicate that *S. aureus rapidly* develops resistance to novobiocin.

INDICATIONS AND USAGE:

Novobiocin is indicated in the treatment of serious infections due to susceptible strains of *Staphylococcus aureus* when other less toxic antibiotics such as the penicillins, cephalosporins, vancomycin, lincomycin, erythromycin, and the tetracyclines cannot be used. Novobiocin may be useful in the few urinary tract infections caused by proteus species sensitive to novobiocin but resistant to other therapy.

CONTRAINDICATIONS:

Novobiocin is contraindicated in patients with a history of hypersensitivity to this antibiotic.

WARNINGS:

See BOXED WARNING.

Novobiocin has been shown to affect bilirubin metabolism apparently by inhibiting glucuronyl transferase. Therefore, its use should be avoided in newborn and premature infants.

PRECAUTIONS:

General Precautions: Novobiocin possesses a high index of sensitization and appropriate precautions should be taken. If allergic reactions develop during treatment and are not readily controlled by the usual measures, the drug should be discontinued. In the case of development of liver dysfunction, the drug should be stopped. If hematologic studies show evidence of the development of leukopenia or other blood dyscrasias, the drug should be stopped. Should new infections appear during therapy, appropriate measures should be taken and consideration given to discontinuance of novobiocin.

Information for the Patient: Not applicable.

Laboratory Tests: Hepatic and hematologic studies should be made routinely during treatment.

Carcinogenesis, Mutagenesis, and Impairment of Fertility: Animal studies on carcinogenesis, mutagenesis or impairment of fertility have not been performed.

Pregnancy Category C: Animal reproduction studies have not been conducted with novobiocin. It is also not know whether novobiocin can cause fetal harm when administered to a pregnant woman or can affect reproductive capacity. Novobiocin should be given to a pregnant woman only if clearly needed.

Labor and Delivery: Not applicable.

Nursing Mothers: Novobiocin has been reported to appear in human breast milk in the range of 0.34 to 0.54 mg/100 ml. Caution should be exercised when Albamycin Capsules are administered to a nursing woman.

Pediatric Use: See WARNINGS.

DRUG INTERACTIONS:

Novobiocin administration may result in a "pseudojaundice" with yellow discoloration of the skin and plasma. This yellow pigment may interfere with serum bilirubin and icterus index determinations.

Novobiocin may interfere with the hepatic uptake or biliary excretion of sulfobromophthalein in the bromsulphalein (BSP) test.

ADVERSE REACTIONS:

Hypersensitivity Reactions: A relatively high incidence of hypersensitivity reactions has occurred. These have consisted most commonly of skin eruptions, including urticarial, erythematous maculopapular or scarlatiniform rash. Erythema multiforme (Stevens-Johnson Syndrome) has occurred but is rare.

Hematopoietic: Blood dyscrasias including leukopenia, eosinophilia, hemolytic anemia, pancytopenia, agranulocytosis, and thrombocytopenia have occurred.

Hepatic Dysfunction: Liver dysfunction including jaundice, elevation of serum, bilirubin concentration, abnormalities on liver function tests, and impaired bromsulphalein excretion have occurred.

Miscellaneous: Other adverse reactions include nausea and vomiting, loose stools and diarrhea, and intestinal hemorrhage. Alopecia has been reported.

OVERDOSAGE:

Oral LD_{50} in the mouse is 1300 mg/kg.

The dialyzability of novobiocin is not known.

DOSAGE AND ADMINISTRATION:

The recommended dose for adults is 250 mg orally every 6 hours or 500 mg every 12 hours, continued for at least 48 hours after the temperature has returned to normal and all evidence of infection has disappeared. In severe or unusually resistant infections 0.5 g every 6 hours or 1 g every 12 hours may be employed.

The dosage for children on similar schedules is 15 mg per kilogram of body weight per day for moderate acute infections and may be increased to 30 to 45 mg per kilogram of body weight per day for severe infections.

HOW SUPPLIED - EQUIVALENTS NOT AVAILABLE:

Capsule, Gelatin - Oral - 250 mg

100's	$197.35	ALBAMYCIN, Pharmacia & Upjohn	00009-0101-02

NYSTATIN *(001908)*

CATEGORIES: Anti-Infectives; Antiasthmatics/Bronchodilators; Antibacterials; Antibiotics; Antifungals; Antimicrobials; Candidiasis; Central Nervous System Agents; Dermatologicals; Fungal Agents; Gastrointestinal Drugs; Gynecologic Infections; Ocular Infections; Ophthalmics; Otic Preparations; Otologic; Sedatives/Hypnotics; Skin/Mucous Membrane Agents; Topical; Pregnancy Category C; FDA Approval Pre 1982

BRAND NAMES: *Acronistina*; Barstatin; Bio-Statin; *Biofanal* (Germany); Candex; *Candida-Lokalicid* (Germany); *Candio*; *Candio-Hermal* (Germany); *Candistatin*; *Canstat*; *Condio*; *Fongistat*; *Kandistatin*; Korostatin; *Lystin*; *Micostatin* (Mexico); *Moronal* (Germany); *Mycastatin* (Japan); *Mycocide*; **Mycostatin**; *Mycostatine*; *Mycotin*; Mykinac; *Nadostine* (Canada); Nilstat; *Nyaderm* (Canada); Nysert; *Nystacid*; *Nystan* (England); *Nystatin*; Nystex; O-V Statin; *Oranyst*; Pedi-Dry; *Scanytin*; *Statin*; Vagistat
(International brand names outside U.S. in italics)

FORMULARIES: Aetna; BC-BS; DoD; FHP; Medi-Cal; PCS; WHO

DESCRIPTION:

Cream, Topical Powder, and Ointment: Nystatin Cream, Topical Powder, and Ointment are for dermatological use.

Nystatin Cream contains the antifungal antibiotic nystatin at a concentration of 100,000 units per gram in an aqueous, perfumed vanishing cream base containing aluminum hydroxide concentrated wet gel, titanium dioxide, propylene glycol, cetearyl alcohol (and) ceteareth-20, white petrolatum, sorbitol solution, glyceryl monostearate, polyethylene glycol monostearate, sorbic acid and simethicone.

Nystatin Topical Powder provides, in each gram, 100,000 units nystatin dispersed in talc.

Nystatin Ointment provides 100,000 units nystatin per gram in Plastibase (Plasticized Hydrocarbon Gel), a polyethylene and mineral oil gel base.

DESCRIPTION: *(cont'd)*

Oral Suspension (For Extemporaneous Preparation of): This antifungal agent is obtained from *Streptomyces noursei.* It is not known to be a mixture, but the composition has not been completely elucidated. Nystatin A is closely related to amphotericin B. Each is a macrocyclic lactone containing a ketal ring, an all-*trans* polyene system, and a mycosamine (3-amino-3-deoxy-rhamose) moiety.

Nystatin, USP which contains no excipients or preservatives, is a ready-to-use, nonsterile powder for oral administration available in bottles of 150 million, 1 billion and 2 billion units. Each mg contains a minimum of 5000 units.

Oral Suspension and Oral Tablets: Nystatin is an antifungal antibiotic which is both fungistatic and fungicidal *in vitro* against a wide variety of yeasts and yeast-like fungi. It is a polyene antibiotic of undetermined structural formula that is obtained from *Streptomyces noursei.*

Nystatin Oral Suspension is provided for oral administration containing 100,000 units nystatin per ml. Inactive ingredients: alcohol (not > 1% v/v), carboxymethylcellulose sodium, flavors, glycerin, methylparaben, propylparaben, saccharin sodium, sodium phosphate, sucrose (50% w/v), and purified water.

Nystatin Oral Tablets are provided for oral administration as coated tablets containing 500,000 units nystatin. Inactive ingredients: cellulose, colorants (FD&C Blue No. 2 and Yellow No. 6), corn starch, flavor, lactose, magnesium stearate, povidone, stearic acid and other ingredients.

Vaginal Tablets: Nystatin is an antimycotic polyene antibiotic obtained from *Streptomyces noursei.*

Nystatin Vaginal Tablets, USP are available as oval-shaped compressed tablets for intravaginal administration, each containing 100,000 units Nystatin, USP.

Pastilles: Nystatin is a polyene antifungal antibiotic obtained from *Streptomyces noursei.*

Nystatin Pastilles are round, light to dark gold-colored troches designed to dissolve slowly in the mouth. Each pastille provides 200,000 units nystatin. Inactive ingredients: anise oil, cinnamon oil, gelatin, sucrose, and other ingredients.

CLINICAL PHARMACOLOGY:

CREAM, TOPICAL POWDER, AND OINTMENT

Nystatin is an antifungal antibiotic which is both fungistatic and fungicidal *in vitro* against a wide variety of yeasts and yeast-like fungi. It probably acts by binding to sterols in the cell membrane of the fungus with a resultant change in membrane permeability allowing leakage of intracellular components. Nystatin is a polyene antibiotic of undetermined structural formula that is obtained from *Streptomyces noursei,* and is the first well tolerated anti-fungal antibiotic of dependable efficacy for the treatment of cutaneous, oral and intestinal infections caused by *Candida* (Monilia) *albicans* and other Candida species. It exhibits no appreciable activity against bacteria.

Nystatin provides specific therapy for all localized forms of candidiasis. Symptomatic relief is rapid, often occurring within 24 to 72 hours after the initiation of treatment. Cure is effected both clinically and mycologically in most cases of localized candidiasis.

ORAL SUSPENSION (FOR EXTEMPORANEOUS PREPARATION OF), ORAL SUSPENSION, AND ORAL TABLETS

Nystatin probably acts by binding to sterols in the cell membrane of the fungus with a resultant change in membrane permeability allowing leakage of intracellular components. It exhibits no appreciable activity against bacteria or trichomonads.

Following oral administration, nystatin is sparingly absorbed with no detectable blood levels when given in the recommended doses. Most of the orally administered nystatin is passed unchanged in the stool.

VAGINAL TABLETS

Nystatin is both fungistatic and fungicidal *in vitro* against a wide variety of yeasts and yeast-like fungi. Nystatin acts by binding to sterols in the cell membrane of sensitive fungi with a resultant change in membrane permeability allowing leakage of intracellular components. Nystatin exhibits no appreciable activity against bacteria, protozoa, trichomonads or viruses.

Nystatin is not absorbed from intact skin or mucous membranes.

PASTILLES

Nystatin is both fungistatic and fungicidal *in vitro* against a wide variety of yeasts and yeast-like fungi. *Candida albicans* demonstrates no significant resistance to nystatin *in vitro* on repeated subculture in increasing levels of nystatin; other *Candida* species become quite resistant. Generally, resistance does not develop *in vivo.* Nystatin acts by binding to sterols in the cell membrane of susceptible fungi with a resultant change in membrane permeability allowing leakage of intracellular components. Nystatin exhibits no activity against bacteria, protozoa, trichomonads, or viruses.

Pharmacokinetics: Gastrointestinal absorption of nystatin is insignificant. Most orally administered nystatin is passed unchanged in the stool. Significant concentrations of nystatin may appear occasionally in the plasma of patients with renal insufficiency during oral therapy with conventional dosage forms.

Mean nystatin concentrations in excess of those required *in vitro* to inhibit growth of clinically significant *Candida* persisted in saliva for approximately 2 hours after the start of oral dissolution of 2 nystatin pastilles (400,000 units nystatin) administered simultaneously to 12 healthy volunteers.

INDICATIONS AND USAGE:

Cream, Topical Powder, and Ointment: Nystatin topical preparations are indicated in the treatment of cutaneous or mucocutaneous mycotic infections caused by *Candida* (Monilia) *albicans* and other Candida species.

Oral Suspension (For Extemporaneous Preparation of): For the treatment of intestinal and oral cavity infections caused by *Candida (Monilia) albicans.*

Oral Suspension and Pastilles: Nystatin Oral Suspension and Pastilles are indicated for the treatment of candidiasis in the oral cavity.

Oral Tablets: Nystatin Oral Tablets are intended for the treatment of intestinal candidiasis.

Vaginal Tablets: Nystatin Vaginal Tablets, USP are effective for the local treatment of vulvovaginal candidiasis (moniliasis). The diagnosis should be confirmed, prior to therapy, by KOH smears and/or cultures. Other pathogens commonly associated with vulvovaginitis (Trichomonas and *Haemophilus vaginalis*) do not respond to nystatin and should be ruled out by appropriate laboratory methods.

CONTRAINDICATIONS:

Nystatin is contraindicated in patients with a history of hypersensitivity to any of their components.

PRECAUTIONS:

CREAM, TOPICAL POWDER, AND OINTMENT

Should a reaction of hypersensitivity occur the drug should be immediately withdrawn and appropriate measures taken.

PRECAUTIONS: *(cont'd)*

These preparations are not for ophthalmic use.

ORAL SUSPENSION AND ORAL TABLETS

Usage in Pregnancy: No adverse effects or complications have been attributed to nystatin in infants born to women treated with nystatin.

GENERAL

Vaginal Tablets: Discontinue treatment if sensitization or irritation is reported during use.

Pastilles: This medication is not to be used for the treatment of systemic mycoses.

In order to achieve maximum effect from the medication, pastilles must be allowed to dissolve slowly in the mouth; therefore, patients for whom the pastille is prescribed, including children and the elderly, must be competent to utilize the dosage form as intended.

If irritation or hypersensitivity develops with nystatin pastilles, treatment should be discontinued and appropriate therapy instituted.

INFORMATION FOR THE PATIENT

Vaginal Tablets: The patient should be informed of symptoms of sensitization or irritation and told to report them promptly.

The patient should be warned against interruption or discontinuation of medication even during menstruation and even though symptomatic relief may occur within a few days.

The patient should be advised that adjunctive measures such as therapeutic douches are unnecessary and sometimes inadvisable, but cleansing douches may be used by nonpregnant women, if desired, for esthetic purposes.

Pastilles: Patients taking this medication should receive the following information and instructions:

1. Use as directed; the medication is not for any disorder other than for which it was prescribed.

2. Allow the pastille to dissolve slowly in the mouth; **do not chew or swallow the pastille.**

3. The patient should be advised regarding replacement of any missed doses.

4. There should be no interruption or discontinuation of medication until the prescribed course of treatment is completed even though symptomatic relief may occur within a few days.

5. If symptoms of local irritation develop, the physician should be notified promptly.

6. Good oral hygiene, including proper care of dentures, is particularly important for denture wearers.

LABORATORY TESTS

Vaginal Tablets: If there is a lack of response to Nystatin Vaginal Tablets, USP, appropriate microbiological studies should be repeated to confirm the diagnosis and rule out other pathogens before instituting another course of antimycotic therapy (see INDICATIONS AND USAGE.)

Pastilles: If there is a lack of therapeutic response, appropriate microbiological studies (*e.g.,* KOH smears and/or cultures) should be repeated to confirm the diagnosis of candidiasis and rule out other pathogens before instituting another course of therapy.

CARCINOGENESIS, MUTAGENESIS, AND IMPAIRMENT OF FERTILITY

Vaginal Tablets: Long-term studies in animals have not been performed to evaluate carcinogenic potential, mutagenesis, or whether this medication effects fertility in females.

There have been no reports that use of Nystatin Vaginal Tablets by pregnant women increases the risk of fetal abnormalities or affects later growth, development and functional maturation of the child. Nevertheless, because the possibility of harm cannot be ruled out, nystatin vaginal tablets should be used during pregnancy only if the physician considers it essential to the welfare of the patient.

Animal reproduction studies have not been conducted with nystatin vaginal tablets.

Pastilles: Studies have not been performed to evaluate carcinogenic or mutagenic potential, or possible impairment of fertility in males or females.

Animal reproduction studies have not been conducted with nystatin pastilles. It is also not known whether nystatin pastilles can cause fetal harm when administered to a pregnant woman or can affect reproduction capacity. Nystatin pastilles should be dispensed to a pregnant woman only if clearly needed.

PREGNANCY

Pastilles: Pregnancy Category A.

Vaginal Tablets: Pregnancy Category C.

PEDIATRIC USE:

Vaginal Tablets: Safety and effectiveness in children have not been established.

Pastilles: See PRECAUTIONS, General.

ADVERSE REACTIONS:

Cream, Topical Powder, Ointment, and Oral Tablets: Nystatin is virtually nontoxic and nonsensitizing and is well tolerated by all age groups including debilitated infants, even on prolonged administration.

If irritation on topical application should occur, discontinue medication.

Large oral doses have occasionally produced diarrhea, gastrointestinal distress, nausea and vomiting.

Oral Suspension (For Extemporaneous Preparation of), and Oral Suspension: Nystatin is generally well tolerated by all age groups including debilitated infants, even on prolonged administration. Large oral doses have occasionally produced diarrhea, gastrointestinal distress, and possible irritation of the stomach that may result in nausea and vomiting. Rash, including urticaria has been reported rarely. Stevens-Johnson syndrome has been reported very rarely.

Vaginal Tablets: Nystatin is virtually nontoxic and nonsensitizing and is well tolerated by all age groups, even on prolonged administration. Rarely, irritation or sensitization may occur (see PRECAUTIONS.)

Pastilles: Nystatin is generally well-tolerated by all age groups, even during prolonged use. Rarely, oral irritation or sensitization may occur. Nausea has been reported occasionally during therapy.

Large oral doses of nystatin have occasionally produced diarrhea, gastrointestinal distress, nausea and vomiting. Rash, including urticaria has been reported rarely. Stevens-Johnson syndrome has been reported very rarely.

OVERDOSAGE:

Pastilles: Oral doses of nystatin in excess of five million units daily have caused nausea and gastrointestinal upset. There have been no reports of serious toxic effects or superinfections (See CLINICAL PHARMACOLOGY, Pharmacokinetics.)

DOSAGE AND ADMINISTRATION:

CREAM, TOPICAL POWDER, AND OINTMENT

The cream and the ointment should be applied liberally to affected areas twice daily or as indicated until healing is complete. The powder should be applied to candidal lesions two or three times daily until lesions have healed. For fungal infection of the feet caused by Candida species, the powder should be dusted freely on the feet as well as in shoes and socks. The cream is usually preferred to the ointment in candidiasis involving intertriginous areas; very moist lesions, however, are best treated with the topical dusting powder.

The preparations do not stain skin or mucous membranes and they provide a simple, convenient means of treatment.

ORAL SUSPENSION (FOR EXTEMPORANEOUS PREPARATION OF)

Adults and older children: Add 1/8 teaspoonful (approximately 500,000 units) of nystatin, USP to about 1/2 cup of water and stir well. One-eighth teaspoonful of nystatin, USP is equivalent to the recommended dose for adults and children of Nilstat Oral Suspension (4 to 6 ml, or 400,000 to 600,000 units). This powder product contains no preservative and therefore should be used immediately after mixing and should not be stored. It is designed for the extemporaneous preparation of a single dose at a time.

Infections of the oral cavity caused by Candida (Monilia) albicans

Infants: 200,000 units four times daily.

Children and adults: 400,000 to 600,000 units four times daily (one-half dose in each side of mouth).

Note: Limited clinical studies in premature and low-birth weight infants indicate that 100,000 units four times daily is effective.

Local treatment should be continued at least 48 hours after perioral symptoms have disappeared and cultures returned to normal.

It is recommended that the drug be retained in the mouth as long as possible before swallowing.

Intestinal candidiasis (moniliasis)

Usual dosage: 500,000 to 1 million units (approximately 1/8 to 1/4 teaspoonful) three times daily. Treatment should generally be continued for at least 48 hours after clinical cure to prevent relapse.

Store under refrigeration 2-8°C (36-46°F) in tight, light-resistant containers.

Note: The potency of this product cannot be assured for longer than 90 days after the container is first opened.

ORAL SUSPENSION

Infants: 2 ml (200,000 units nystatin) four times daily (1 ml in each side of the mouth).

Note: Limited clinical studies in premature and low birth weight infants indicate that 1 ml four times daily is effective.

Children And Adults: 4-6 ml (400,000 to 600,000 units nystatin) four times daily (one-half of dose in each side of mouth). The preparation should be retained in the mouth as long as possible before swallowing.

Continue treatment for at least 48 hours after perioral symptoms have disappeared and cultures returned to normal.

Storage: Store at room temperature; avoid freezing.

ORAL TABLETS

The usual therapeutic dosage is one to two tablets (500,000 to 1,000,000 units nystatin) three times daily. Treatment should generally be continued for at least 48 hours after clinical cure to prevent relapse.

Storage: Store at room temperature; avoid excessive heat.

VAGINAL TABLETS

The usual dosage is one tablet (100,000 units nystatin) daily for two weeks. The tablets should be deposited high in the vagina by means of the applicator. Instructions for the Patient are enclosed in each package.

Store at controlled room temperature 15-30°C (59-86°F).

PASTILLES

Children and Adults: The recommended dose is one or two pastilles (200,000 or 400,000 units nystatin) four or five times daily for as long as 14 days if necessary. The dosage regimen should be continued for at least 48 hours after disappearance of oral symptoms.

Dosage should be discontinued if symptoms persist after the initial 14 day period of treatment (See PRECAUTIONS, Laboratory Tests.)

Administration: Pastilles must be allowed to dissolve slowly in the mouth, and should not be chewed or swallowed whole.

Storage: Refrigerate between 2° and 8°C (36° and 46°F).

HOW SUPPLIED:

Nilstat Nystatin, USP For Extemporaneous Preparation of Oral Suspension in bottles containing 150 million units, 1 billion units and 2 billion units.

Mycostatin Pastilles, 200,000 units nystatin each, in packages containing 30 pleasant-tasting pastilles.

(Cream, Topical Powder, and Ointment - E.R. Squibb & Sons, Inc. - 2/88, J3-651B) (Oral Suspension (For Extemporaneous Preparation of) - Lederle Laboratories Division - 4/94, 41103-94] (Oral Suspension - E.R. Squibb & Sons, Inc. - 4/92, J3-208L) (Oral Tablets - E.R. Squibb & Sons, Inc. - 12/90, J3-513D) (Vaginal Tablets - Rugby Laboratories, Inc. - 10/89, PO8-375-144) (Pastilles - Bristol Myers Squibb Company - 4/92, P9297-01)

HOW SUPPLIED - RATED THERAPEUTICALLY EQUIVALENT:

Cream - Topical - 100,000 unit/gm

15 gm	$1.45	Nystatin Topical, United Res	00677-0733-40
15 gm	$1.45	Nystatin, H.C.F.A. F F P	99999-1908-01
15 gm	$1.60	Nystatin, Clay Park Labs	45802-0059-35
15 gm	$1.80	Nystatin Topical, Thames Pharma	49158-0149-20
15 gm	$1.88	Nystatin, NMC Labs	23317-0160-15
15 gm	$2.10	Nystatin, Taro Pharms (US)	51672-1289-01
15 gm	$2.12	Nystatin, Geneva Pharms	00781-7005-27
15 gm	$2.15	Nystatin, Teva	00093-0955-15
15 gm	$2.15	Nystatin, HL Moore Drug Exch	00839-7702-47
15 gm	$2.19	Nystatin, Harber Pharm	51432-0766-10
15 gm	$2.20	Nystatin, Qualitest Pharms	00603-7820-74
15 gm	$2.20	Nystatin, Major Pharms	00904-2706-36
15 gm	$2.25	Nystatin, Consolidated Midland	00223-4378-15
15 gm	$2.25	Nystatin Topical, Schein Pharm (US)	00364-7210-72
15 gm	$2.25	Nystatin, IDE-Interstate	00814-5500-93
15 gm	$2.30	Nystatin Topical, Goldline Labs	00182-0982-51
15 gm	$2.30	Nystatin, HL Moore Drug Exch	00839-6130-47
15 gm	$2.59	Nystatin, Fougera	00168-0054-15
15 gm	$3.74	Nystatin, Rugby	00536-4830-20
15 gm	$8.24	NYSTEX, Savage Labs	00281-3208-44
15 gm	**$11.54**	**MYCOSTATIN, Bristol Myers Squibb**	**00003-0579-20**

HOW SUPPLIED - RATED THERAPEUTICALLY EQUIVALENT:

(cont'd)

30 gm	$2.17	Nystatin, H.C.F.A. F F P	99999-1908-02
30 gm	$2.80	Nystatin Topical, Thames Pharma	49158-0149-08
30 gm	$2.87	Nystatin, Qualitest Pharms	00603-7820-78
30 gm	$2.91	Nystatin, United Res	00677-0733-45
30 gm	$2.94	Nystatin, Clay Park Labs	45802-0059-11
30 gm	$3.00	Nystatin, Consolidated Midland	00223-4378-30
30 gm	$3.20	Nystatin, Taro Pharms (US)	51672-1289-02
30 gm	$3.40	Nystatin, Teva	00093-0955-30
30 gm	$3.45	Nystatin Topical, Schein Pharm (US)	00364-7210-56
30 gm	$3.70	Nystatin Topical, Goldline Labs	00182-0982-56
30 gm	$3.75	Nystatin, Geneva Pharms	00781-7005-24
30 gm	$3.75	Nystatin, Major Pharms	00904-2706-31
30 gm	$3.94	Nystatin, Fougera	00168-0054-30
30 gm	$4.25	Nystatin, Rugby	00536-4830-28
30 gm	$4.25	Nystatin, HL Moore Drug Exch	00839-6130-49
30 gm	$4.50	Nystatin, Harber Pharm	51432-0766-11
30 gm	$12.36	NYSTEX, Savage Labs	00281-3208-45
30 gm	**$21.80**	**MYCOSTATIN, Bristol Myers Squibb**	**00003-0579-31**

Ointment - Topical - 100,000 unit/gm

15 gm	$1.45	Nystatin, United Res	00677-1082-40
15 gm	$1.45	Nystatin, H.C.F.A. F F P	99999-1908-03
15 gm	$1.66	Nystatin Topical, Clay Park Labs	45802-0048-35
15 gm	$1.92	Nystatin 100000 Units, NMC Labs	23317-0165-15
15 gm	$2.20	Nystatin, Qualitest Pharms	00603-7821-74
15 gm	$2.23	Nystatin, HL Moore Drug Exch	00839-7128-47
15 gm	$2.25	Nystatin, Consolidated Midland	00223-4379-15
15 gm	$2.30	Nystatin Topical, Goldline Labs	00182-1678-51
15 gm	$2.43	Nystatin Topical, Schein Pharm (US)	00364-7379-72
15 gm	$2.45	Nystatin Topical, Rugby	00536-4781-20
15 gm	$2.46	Nystatin, Major Pharms	00904-2305-36
15 gm	$2.65	Nystatin, Fougera	00168-0007-15
15 gm	$8.24	NYSTEX, Savage Labs	00281-3212-44
15 gm	**$11.54**	**MYCOSTATIN, Bristol Myers Squibb**	**00003-0584-40**
30 gm	$2.91	Nystatin, United Res	00677-1082-45
30 gm	$3.00	Nystatin, Consolidated Midland	00223-4379-30
30 gm	$3.02	Nystatin Topical, Clay Park Labs	45802-0048-11
30 gm	$3.28	Nystatin 100000 Units, NMC Labs	23317-0165-30
30 gm	$3.44	Nystatin, HL Moore Drug Exch	00839-7128-49
30 gm	$3.60	Nystatin, Major Pharms	00904-2305-31
30 gm	$3.60	Nystatin, H.C.F.A. F F P	99999-1908-04
30 gm	$3.70	Nystatin Topical, Goldline Labs	00182-1678-56
30 gm	$3.99	Nystatin, Fougera	00168-0007-30
30 gm	$3.99	Nystatin Topical, Rugby	00536-4781-28
30 gm	$4.50	Nystatin, Harber Pharm	51432-0767-11
30 gm	**$20.86**	**MYCOSTATIN, Bristol Myers Squibb**	**00003-0584-30**

Powder - Oral - 100 %

1's	$48.00	Bio-Statin, Bio-Tech Pharm	53191-0103-03
1's	$60.67	NILSTAT, Lederle Pharm	00005-5421-12
50 mu	$17.50	Nystatin, Paddock Labs	00574-0404-05
150 mu	$43.60	Nystatin, Paddock Labs	00574-0404-15
500 mu	$119.00	Nystatin, Paddock Labs	00574-0404-50
1000 mu	$208.00	Nystatin, Paddock Labs	00574-0404-01
2000 mu	$393.00	Nystatin, Paddock Labs	00574-0404-02
5000 mu	$909.00	Nystatin, Paddock Labs	00574-0404-00

Powder - Topical - 100,000 unit/gm

15 gm	**$22.30**	**MYCOSTATIN, Bristol Myers Squibb**	**00003-0593-20**

Suspension - Oral - 100,000 unit/ml

1 billion units	$374.54	NILSTAT, Lederle Pharm	00005-5421-10
2 billion units	$663.37	NILSTAT, Lederle Pharm	00005-5421-11
5 ml x 40	$43.47	Nystatin, Roxane	00054-8607-16
5 ml x 50	$49.67	Nystatin, Xactdose	50962-0251-05
5 ml x 100	$98.37	Nystatin, Xactdose	50962-0250-05
5 ml x 100	$120.00	Nystatin, Fougera	00168-0037-03
5 ml x 100	**$227.29**	**MYCOSTATIN, Bristol Myers Squibb**	**00003-0588-50**
10 ml x 100	$133.96	Nystatin, Xactdose	50962-0250-10
60 ml	$3.12	Nystatin, United Res	00677-0836-25
60 ml	$3.12	Nystatin, H.C.F.A. F F P	99999-1908-05
60 ml	$4.50	Nystatin, Thames Pharma	49158-0256-48
60 ml	$5.71	Nystatin, Qualitest Pharms	00603-1480-49
60 ml	$5.80	Nystatin, Morton Grove	60432-0537-60
60 ml	$6.25	Nystatin, Alpharma	00472-1320-02
60 ml	$6.49	Nystatin, Goldline Labs	00182-1546-68
60 ml	$6.49	Nystatin, Teva	00332-6109-28
60 ml	$7.36	Nystatin, HL Moore Drug Exch	00839-7703-64
60 ml	$7.50	Nystatin, Major Pharms	00904-2761-03
60 ml	$8.00	Nystatin, Fougera	00168-0037-60
60 ml	$8.08	Nystatin, Roxane	00054-3607-46
60 ml	$8.64	Nystatin, Aligen Independ	00405-3450-56
60 ml	$8.84	Nystatin, HL Moore Drug Exch	00839-6698-64
60 ml	$8.95	Nystatin, Consolidated Midland	00223-6572-60
60 ml	$9.40	Nystatin, Teva	00093-0366-39
60 ml	$9.46	Nystatin, Schein Pharm (US)	00364-2075-58
60 ml	$9.46	Nystatin, Rugby	00536-1220-61
60 ml	$9.46	Nystatin, Geneva Pharms	00781-6105-61
60 ml	$15.72	NILSTAT, Lederle Pharm	00005-5429-18
60 ml	$16.16	NYSTEX, Savage Labs	00281-0037-60
60 ml	**$21.84**	**MYCOSTATIN, Bristol Myers Squibb**	**00003-0588-60**
473 ml	$65.00	Nystatin, Teva	00093-0366-16
480 ml	$24.96	Nystatin, United Res	00677-0836-33
480 ml	$24.96	Nystatin, H.C.F.A. F F P	99999-1908-06
480 ml	$33.85	Nystatin, Morton Grove	60432-0537-16
480 ml	$37.52	Nystatin, Qualitest Pharms	00603-1480-58
480 ml	$40.03	Nystatin, Teva	00332-6109-38
480 ml	$40.03	Nystatin, Alpharma	00472-1320-16
480 ml	$43.45	Nystatin, Goldline Labs	00182-1546-40
480 ml	$44.50	Nystatin, Major Pharms	00904-2761-16
480 ml	$45.00	Nystatin, Harber Pharm	51432-0637-20
480 ml	$51.50	Nystatin, HL Moore Drug Exch	00839-6698-69
480 ml	$52.50	Nystatin, Aligen Independ	00405-3450-16
480 ml	$63.88	Nystatin, Schein Pharm (US)	00364-2075-16
480 ml	$65.00	Nystatin, Consolidated Midland	00223-6572-66
480 ml	$77.11	Nystatin, Rugby	00536-1220-85
480 ml	$77.11	Nystatin, Geneva Pharms	00781-6105-16
480 ml	$101.47	NILSTAT, Lederle Pharm	00005-5429-65
480 ml	**$134.93**	**MYCOSTATIN, Bristol Myers Squibb**	**00003-0588-10**

Tablet - Vaginal - 100,000 unit

15's	$10.96	Nystatin, H.C.F.A. F F P	99999-1908-09
30's	$19.88	Nystatin, H.C.F.A. F F P	99999-1908-10

HOW SUPPLIED - RATED THERAPEUTICALLY EQUIVALENT: *(cont'd)*

Tablet, Plain Coated - Oral - 500,000 unit

10's	$38.95	NILSTAT, Lederle Pharm	00005-5426-60
42 oral & 14 va	$20.19	O-V STATIN, Bristol Myers Squibb	00003-0007-78
100's	$11.93	Nystatin, Geneva Pharms	00781-1305-01
100's	$11.93	Nystatin, H.C.F.A. F F P	99999-1908-07
100's	$12.90	Nystatin, US Trading	56126-0119-11
100's	$15.10	Nystatin, Major Pharms	00904-0672-60
100's	$24.91	Nystatin, HL Moore Drug Exch	00839-6282-06
100's	$25.45	Nystatin, Goldline Labs	00182-1369-01
100's	$25.48	Nystatin, Qualitest Pharms	00603-4830-21
100's	$25.90	Nystatin, United Res	00677-0613-01
100's	$25.90	Nystatin, Mutual Pharm	53489-0400-01
100's	$25.95	Nystatin, Martec Pharms	52555-0119-01
100's	$27.67	Nystatin, Schein Pharm (US)	00364-2051-01
100's	$28.27	Nystatin, Aligen Independ	00405-4714-01
100's	$29.58	Nystatin, Teva	00093-0983-01
100's	$31.95	Nystatin, Eon Labs Mfg	00185-0750-01
100's	$32.00	Nystatin, Parmed Pharms	00349-8710-01
100's	$32.05	Nystatin, Par Pharm	49884-0119-01
100's	$37.36	NILSTAT, Lederle Pharm	00005-5426-23
100's	$44.50	Nystatin, Rugby	00536-4094-01
100's	**$49.69**	**MYCOSTATIN, Bristol Myers Squibb**	**00003-0580-54**
100's	**$55.31**	**MYCOSTATIN, Bristol Myers Squibb**	**00003-0580-53**
500's	$59.65	Nystatin, H.C.F.A. F F P	99999-1908-08
500's	$115.87	Nystatin, Par Pharm	49884-0119-05
1000's	$121.96	Nystatin, Aligen Independ	00405-4714-02

Tablet, Uncoated - Vaginal - 100,000 unit

15's	$4.25	Nystatin, Harber Pharm	51432-0315-07
15's	$8.25	Nystatin Vaginal, Major Pharms	00904-2707-48
15's	$9.85	Nystatin, Sidmak Labs	50111-0375-09
15's	$10.30	Nystatin, Goldline Labs	00182-0981-28
15's	$10.63	Nystatin, Aligen Independ	00405-4719-15
15's	$10.88	Nystatin, Qualitest Pharms	00603-4831-13
15's	$10.95	Nystatin, Rugby	00536-4091-16
15's	$10.96	Nystatin, United Res	00677-1165-39
15's	$12.89	Nystatin, HL Moore Drug Exch	00839-6125-11
30's	$6.65	Nystatin, Harber Pharm	51432-0315-08
30's	$12.78	Nystatin Vaginal, Schein Pharm (US)	00364-7209-30
30's	$14.32	NILSTAT, Lederle Pharm	00005-5428-08
30's	$19.63	Nystatin, Aligen Independ	00405-4719-30
30's	$20.55	Nystatin, Qualitest Pharms	00603-4831-16
30's	$21.40	Nystatin Vaginal, Major Pharms	00904-2707-46
30's	$21.56	Nystatin, Sidmak Labs	50111-0375-10
30's	$23.02	Nystatin, HL Moore Drug Exch	00839-6125-19
50's	**$46.83**	**MYCOSTATIN, Bristol Myers Squibb**	**00003-0457-43**
500's	$78.54	Nystatin, Rugby	00536-4094-05

HOW SUPPLIED - NOT RATED EQUIVALENT:

Capsule, Gelatin - Oral - 1,000,000 unit

100's	$42.00	BIO-STATIN, Bio-Tech Pharm	53191-0192-01

Capsule, Gelatin - Oral - 300,000 unit

100's	$12.95	BIO-STATIN, Bio-Tech Pharm	53191-0098-01

Capsule, Gelatin - Oral - 500,000 unit

100's	$28.80	BIO-STATIN, Bio-Tech Pharm	53191-0009-01

Lozenge - Oral - 200,000 unit

30's	**$30.19**	**MYCOSTATIN PASTILLES, Bristol Myers Squibb**	**00003-0543-20**

Powder - Topical - 100,000 unit/gm

56.7 gm	$12.00	Pedi-Dry, Pedinol Pharma	00884-0394-02

NYSTATIN; TRIAMCINOLONE ACETONIDE

(001909)

CATEGORIES: Anti-Infectives; Antibacterials; Antifungals; Candidiasis; Dermatitis; Dermatologicals; Fungal Agents; Hormones; Pruritus; Skin Infections; Skin/Mucous Membrane Agents; Steroids; Topical; Pregnancy Category C; FDA Approved 1985 May

BRAND NAMES: Dermacomb; Myco Aricidin; Myco Biotic II; Myco II; Myco-Cinolone; Myco-Par; Myco-Triacet II; Mycobiotic II; Mycogen II; **Mycolog II**; Mycomar; Mykacet-II; Mytrex; NCT; NTA; Nyst-Olone II; *Nystadermal*; Tri-Statin II

(International brand names outside U.S. in italics)

FORMULARIES: Aetna; BC-BS; FHP; PCS

DESCRIPTION:

Nystatin/triamcinolone acetonide for dermatologic use contains the antifungal agent nystatin and the synthetic corticosteroid triamcinolone acetonide.

Nystatin is a polyene antimycotic obtained from *Streptomyces noursei*. It is a yellow to light tan powder with a cereal-like odor, very slightly soluble in water, and slightly to sparingly soluble in alcohol.

Triamcinolone acetonide is designated chemically is 9-fluoro- 11β,16α,17,21-tetrahydroxypregna-1,4-diene-3,20-dione cyclic 16,17- acetal with acetone. The white to cream crystalline powder has a slight odor, is practically insoluble in water, and very soluble in alcohol.

Nystatin and Triamcinolone Acetonide Cream is a soft, smooth, cream having a light yellow to buff color. Each gram provides 100,000 units nystatin and 1.0 mg triamcinolone acetonide in an aqueous perfumed vanishing cream base with aluminum hydroxide concentrated wet gel, titanium dioxide, glyceryl monostearate, polyethylene glycol monostearate, simethicone, sorbic acid, propylene glycol, white petrolatum, cetearyl alcohol (and) ceteareth-20, and sorbitol solution.

Nystatin and Triamcinolone Acetonide Ointment provides, in each gram 100,000 units nystatin and triamcinolone acetonide in a protective ointment base, plasticized hydrocarbon gel, a polyethylene and mineral oil gel base.

CLINICAL PHARMACOLOGY:

NYSTATIN

Nystatin exerts its antifungal activity against a variety of pathogenic and nonpathogenic yeasts and fungi by binding to sterols in the cell membrane. The binding process renders the cell membrane incapable of functioning as a selective barrier. Nystatin provides specific anticandidal activity to *Candida* (Monilia) *albicans* and other *Candida* species, but is not active against bacteria, protozoa, trichomonads, or viruses.

Nystatin is not absorbed from intact skin or mucous membranes.

TRIAMCINOLONE ACETONIDE

Triamcinolone acetonide is primarily effective because of its anti-inflammatory, antipruritic and vasoconstrictive actions, characteristic of the topical corticosteroid class of drugs. The pharmacologic effects of the topical corticosteroids are well-known; however, the mechanisms of their dermatologic actions are unclear. Various laboratory methods, including vasoconstrictor assays, are used to compare and predict potencies and/or clinical efficacies of the topical corticosteroids. There is some evidence to suggest that a recognizable correlation exists between vasoconstrictor potency and therapeutic efficacy in man.

Pharmacokinetics: The extent of percutaneous absorption of topical corticosteroids is determined by many factors including the vehicle, the integrity of the epidermal barrier, and the use of occlusive dressings (see DOSAGE AND ADMINISTRATION.)

Topical corticosteroids can be absorbed from normal intact skin. Inflammation and/or other disease processes in the skin increase percutaneous absorption. Occlusive dressings substantially increase the percutaneous absorption of topical (see DOSAGE AND ADMINISTRATION.)

Once absorbed through the skin, topical corticosteroids are handled through pharmacokinetic pathways similar to systemically administered corticosteroids. Corticosteroids are bound to plasma proteins in varying degrees. Corticosteroids are metabolized primarily in the liver and are then excreted by the kidneys. Some of the topical corticosteroids and their metabolites are also excreted into the bile.

NYSTATIN AND TRIAMCINOLONE ACETONIDE

During clinical studies of mild to severe manifestations of cutaneous candidiasis, patients treated with nystatin/triamcinolone acetonide showed a faster and more pronounced clearing of erythema and pruritus than patients treated with nystatin or triamcinolone acetonide alone.

INDICATIONS AND USAGE:

Nystatin/triamcinolone acetonide is indicated for the treatment of cutaneous candidiasis; it has been demonstrated that the nystatin-steroid combination provides greater benefit than the nystatin component alone during the first few days of treatment.

CONTRAINDICATIONS:

This preparation is contraindicated in those patients with a history of hypersensitivity to any of its components.

PRECAUTIONS:

General: Systemic absorption of topical corticosteroids has produced reversible hypothalamic-pituitary-adrenal (HPA) axis suppression, manifestations of Cushing's syndrome, hyperglycemia, and glucosuria in some patients.

Conditions that augment systemic absorption include application of the more potent steroids, use over large surface areas, prolonged use, and the addition of occlusive dressings (see DOSAGE AND ADMINISTRATION.)

Therefore, patients receiving a large dose of any potent topical steroid applied to a large surface area should be evaluated periodically for evidence of HPA axis suppression by using the urinary free cortisol and ACTH stimulation tests, and for impairment of thermal homeostasis. If HPA axis suppression or elevation of the body temperature occurs, an attempt should be made to withdraw the drug, to reduce the frequency of application, or to substitute a less potent steroid.

Recovery of HPA axis function and thermal homeostasis are generally prompt and complete upon discontinuation of the drug. Infrequency, signs and symptoms of steroid withdrawal occur, requiring supplemental systemic corticosteroids.

Children may absorb proportionally larger amounts of topical corticosteroids and thus be more susceptible to systemic toxicity (see PRECAUTIONS, Pediatric Use.)

If irritation or hypersensitivity develops with the combination nystatin and triamcinolone acetonide, treatment should be discontinued and appropriate therapy instituted.

Information for the Patient: Patients using this medication should be receive the following information and instructions:

1. This medication is to be used as directed by the physician. It is for dermatologic use only Avoid contact with the eyes.
2. Patients should be advised not to use this medication for any disorder other than for which it was prescribed.
3. The treated skin area should not be bandaged or otherwise covered or wrapped as to be occluded (see DOSAGE AND ADMINISTRATION.)
4. Patients should report any signs of local adverse reactions.
5. When using this medication in the inguinal area, patients should be advised to apply the cream/ointment sparingly and to wear loosely fitting clothing.
6. Patients of pediatric patient should be advised not to use tight-fitting diapers or plastic pants on a child being treated in the diaper area, as these garments may constitute occlusive dressings.
7. Patients should be advised no preventive measures to avoid reinfection.

Laboratory Tests: If there is a lack of therapeutic response, appropriate microbiological studies (*e.g.*, KOH smears and/or cultures) should be repeated to confirm the diagnosis and rule out other pathogens, before instituting another course of therapy.

A urinary free cortisol test and ACTH stimulation test may be helpful in evaluating hypothalamic-pituitary-adrenal (HPA) axis suppression due to corticosteroid.

Carcinogenesis, Mutagenesis, and Impairment of Fertility: Long-term animal studies have not been performed to evaluate carcinogenic or mutagenic potential, or possible impairment of fertility in males of females.

Pregnancy Category C: There are not teratogenic studies with combined nystatin and triamcinolone acetonide. Corticosteroids are generally teratogenic in laboratory animals when administered systemically at relatively low dosage levels. The more potent corticosteroids have been shown to be teratogenic after dermal application in laboratory animals. Therefore, any topical corticosteroid preparation should be used during pregnancy only if the potential benefit justifies the potential risk to the fetus.

Topical preparations containing corticosteroids should not be used extensively on pregnant patients, in large amounts, or for prolonged periods of time.

PRECAUTIONS: *(cont'd)*

Nursing Mothers: It is not known whether any component of this preparation is excreted in human milk. Because many drugs are excreted in human milk, caution should be exercised during use of this preparation by a nursing woman.

Pediatric Use: In clinical studies of a limited number of pediatric patients ranging in age from two months through 12 years, Nystatin and Triamcinolone Acetonide Cream/Ointment cleared or significantly ameliorated the disease state in most patients.

Pediatric patients may demonstrate greater susceptibility to topical corticosteroid induced hypothalamic-pituitary-adrenal (HPA) axis suppression and Cushing's syndrome than mature patients because of a larger skin surface area to body weight ratio.

HPA axis suppression, Cushing's syndrome, and intracranial hypertension have been reported in children receiving topical corticosteroids. Manifestations of adrenal suppression in children include linear growth retardation, delayed weight gain, low plasma cortisol levels, and absence of response to ACTH stimulation. Manifestations of intracranial hypertension include bulging fontanelles, headaches, and bilateral papilledema.

Administration of topical corticosteroids to children should be limited to the least amount compatible with an effective therapeutic regimen. Chronic corticosteroid therapy may interfere with the growth and development of children.

ADVERSE REACTIONS:

A single case (approximately one percent of patients studied) of acneform eruption occurred with use of combined nystatin and triamcinolone acetonide in clinical studies.

Nystatin is virtually nontoxic and nonsensitizing and is well tolerated by age groups, even during prolonged use. Rarely, irritation may occur.

The following local adverse reactions are reported infrequently with topical corticosteroids (reactions are listed an approximate decreasing order of occurrence): burning, itching, irritation, dryness, folliculitis, hypertrichosis, acneform eruptions, hypopigmentation, perioral dermatitis, allergic contact dermatitis, maceration of the skin, secondary infection, skin atrophy, striae, and miliaria.

OVERDOSAGE:

Topically applied corticosteroids can be absorbed in sufficient amounts to produce systemic effects (see PRECAUTIONS, General); however, acute overdosage and serious adverse effects with dermatologic use are unlikely.

DOSAGE AND ADMINISTRATION:

Nystatin/triamcinolone acetonide is usually applied to the affected areas twice daily in the morning and evening by gently and thoroughly massaging the preparation into the skin. The cream/ointment should be discontinued if symptoms persist after 25 days of therapy (see PRECAUTIONS, Laboratory Tests.)

Nystatin/triamcinolone acetonide should *not* be used with occlusive dressings.

Store at room temperature; avoid freezing.

HOW SUPPLIED - RATED THERAPEUTICALLY EQUIVALENT:

Cream - Topical - 100,000 unit/0.

15 gm	$1.88	Nystatin Triamcinolone, H.C.F.A. F F P	99999-1909-02
30 gm	$3.75	Nystatin Triamcinolone, H.C.F.A. F F P	99999-1909-04
60 gm	$7.50	Nystatin Triamcinolone, H.C.F.A. F F P	99999-1909-05
120 gm	$15.00	Nystatin Triamcinolone, H.C.F.A. F F P	99999-1909-06
120 gm	$15.20	Nystatin W/Triamcinolone, Thames Pharma	49158-0214-12

Cream - Topical - 100,000 unit/1

1.5 gm	$11.49	MYTREX, Savage Labs	00281-0081-08
15 g	$2.05	Nystatin & Triamcinolone Acetonide, Clay Park Labs	45802-0026-35
15 gm	$1.87	N T A, United Res	00677-1063-40
15 gm	$1.90	Nystatin Triamcinolone, Thames Pharma	49158-0214-20
15 gm	$2.40	Nystatin-Triamcinolone, NMC Labs	23317-0150-15
15 gm	$2.40	Nystatin/Triamcinolone, Taro Pharms (US)	51672-1263-01
15 gm	$2.70	MYCOBIOTIC II, HL Moore Drug Exch	00839-7137-47
15 gm	$2.70	MYCO BIOTIC II, HL Moore Drug Exch	00839-7701-47
15 gm	$2.86	N T A, Qualitest Pharms	00603-7810-74
15 gm	$3.00	MYCOGEN II, Goldline Labs	00182-1799-51
15 gm	$3.00	N.G.T., Geneva Pharms	00781-7600-27
15 gm	$3.02	Nyastin & Triamcinolone Acetonide, Schein Pharm (US)	00364-0772-72
15 gm	$3.10	MYCO-TRIACET II, Teva	00093-0232-15
15 gm	$3.25	Myocidin, Major Pharms	00904-2574-36
15 gm	$3.29	TRI-STATIN II, Rugby	00536-4910-20
15 gm	$3.36	Nystatin-Triamcinolone, Fougera	00168-0081-15
15 gm	$4.95	Nystatin W/Triamcinolone, Harber Pharm	51432-0761-10
15 gm	$11.49	MYTREX, Savage Labs	00281-0081-15
15 gm	$14.48	MYCOLOG II, Bristol Myers Squibb	00003-0566-30
30 g	$3.93	Nystatin & Triamcinolone Acetonide, Clay Park Labs	45802-0026-11
30 gm	$3.60	Nystatin Triamcinolone, Thames Pharma	49158-0214-68
30 gm	$3.75	N T A, United Res	00677-1063-45
30 gm	$4.45	N.G.T., Geneva Pharms	00781-7600-03
30 gm	$4.63	N T A, Qualitest Pharms	00603-7810-78
30 gm	$4.71	MYCOBIOTIC II, HL Moore Drug Exch	00839-7137-49
30 gm	$4.71	MYCO BIOTIC II, HL Moore Drug Exch	00839-7701-49
30 gm	$4.75	NYSTATIN-TRIAMCINOLONE ACETONIDE, NMC Labs	23317-0150-30
30 gm	$4.75	Nystatin/Triamcinolone, Taro Pharms (US)	51672-1263-02
30 gm	$4.80	TRI-STATIN II, Rugby	00536-4910-28
30 gm	$4.95	Myocidin, Major Pharms	00904-2574-31
30 gm	$5.10	Nyastin & Triamcinolone Acetonide, Schein Pharm (US)	00364-0772-56
30 gm	$5.30	MYCOGEN II, Goldline Labs	00182-1799-56
30 gm	$5.85	Nystatin-Triamcinolone, Fougera	00168-0081-30
30 gm	$6.15	MYCO-TRIACET II, Teva	00093-0232-30
30 gm	$19.52	MYTREX, Savage Labs	00281-0081-30
30 gm	$24.46	MYCOLOG II, Bristol Myers Squibb	00003-0566-60
60 g	$6.20	Nystatin & Triamcinolone Acetonide, Clay Park Labs	45802-0026-37
60 gm	$5.90	Nystatin Triamcinolone, Thames Pharma	49158-0214-24
60 gm	$7.50	N T A, United Res	00677-1063-43
60 gm	$7.50	Nystatin/Triamcinolone, Taro Pharms (US)	51672-1263-03
60 gm	$7.94	N T A, Qualitest Pharms	00603-7810-88
60 gm	$7.95	N.G.T., Geneva Pharms	00781-7600-35
60 gm	$8.20	Myocidin, Major Pharms	00904-2574-02
60 gm	$8.35	Nyastin & Triamincolone Acetonide, Schein Pharm (US)	00364-0772-58
60 gm	$8.60	Nystatin-Triamcinolone, NMC Labs	23317-0150-60
60 gm	$8.75	TRI-STATIN II, Rugby	00536-4910-25
60 gm	$8.85	MYCOGEN II, Goldline Labs	00182-1799-52
60 gm	$9.67	Nystatin-Triamcinolone, Fougera	00168-0081-60
60 gm	$10.83	MYCO-TRIACET II, Teva	00093-0232-92
60 gm	$11.00	MYCOBIOTIC II, HL Moore Drug Exch	00839-7137-50
60 gm	$11.00	MYCO BIOTIC II, HL Moore Drug Exch	00839-7701-50

HOW SUPPLIED - RATED THERAPEUTICALLY EQUIVALENT: *(cont'd)*

60 gm	$34.02	MYTREX, Savage Labs	00281-0081-60
60 gm	$41.87	MYCOLOG II, Bristol Myers Squibb	00003-0566-65
120 g	$12.94	Nystatin & Triamcinolone Acetonide, Clay Park Labs	45802-0026-52
120 gm	$13.90	Nystatin-Triamcinolone, NMC Labs	23317-0150-04
120 gm	$14.40	Nystatin W/Triamcinolone, Major Pharms	00904-2574-22
120 gm	$15.90	MYCOGEN II, Goldline Labs	00182-1799-57
120 gm	$19.28	Nystatin W/Triamcinolone, Harber Pharm	51432-0761-18
454 gm	$46.00	Nystatin Triamcinolone, Thames Pharma	49158-0214-16
454 gm	$47.02	Nystatin & Triamcinolone Acetonide, Clay Park Labs	45802-0026-05

Ointment - Topical - 100,000 unit/0.

15 gm	$1.73	Nystatin Triamcinolone, H.C.F.A. F F P	99999-1909-08
30 gm	$3.45	Nystatin Triamcinolone, H.C.F.A. F F P	99999-1909-09
60 gm	$6.90	Nystatin Triamcinolone, H.C.F.A. F F P	99999-1909-10

Ointment - Topical - 100,000 unit/1

15 gm	$2.16	Nystatin & Triamcinolone Acetonide, Clay Park Labs	45802-0027-35
15 gm	$2.40	Nystatin-Triamcinolone, NMC Labs	23317-0155-15
15 gm	$2.40	Nystatin/Triamcinolone, Taro Pharms (US)	51672-1272-01
15 gm	$2.77	MYCO-BIOTIC II, HL Moore Drug Exch	00839-7153-47
15 gm	$3.00	MYCOGEN II, Goldline Labs	00182-1800-51
15 gm	$3.00	N T A, Qualitest Pharms	00603-7811-74
15 gm	$3.05	Nyastatin & Triamincolone Acetonide, Schein Pharm (US)	00364-0784-72
15 gm	$3.25	MYOCIDIN, Major Pharms	00904-2699-36
15 gm	$3.35	MYCO-TRIACET II, Teva	00093-0701-15
15 gm	$3.51	Nystatin Triamcinolone, Fougera	00168-0089-15
15 gm	$3.53	TRI-STATIN II, Rugby	00536-4920-20
15 gm	$11.49	MYTREX, Savage Labs	00281-0089-15
15 gm	$14.48	MYCOLOG II, Bristol Myers Squibb	00003-0466-30
30 gm	$3.45	N T A, United Res	00677-1081-45
30 gm	$4.06	Nystatin & Triamcinolone Acetonide, Clay Park Labs	45802-0027-11
30 gm	$4.71	MYCO-BIOTIC II, HL Moore Drug Exch	00839-7153-49
30 gm	$4.75	NYSTATIN-TRIAMCINOLONE ACETONIDE, NMC Labs	23317-0155-30
30 gm	$5.10	N T A, Qualitest Pharms	00603-7811-78
30 gm	$5.30	MYCOGEN II, Goldline Labs	00182-1800-56
30 gm	$5.40	Nyastatin & Triamincolone Acetonide, Schein Pharm (US)	00364-0784-56
30 gm	$5.95	MYCO-TRIACET II, Teva	00093-0701-30
30 gm	$5.95	MYOCIDIN, Major Pharms	00904-2699-31
30 gm	$6.36	Nystatin Triamcinolone, Fougera	00168-0089-30
30 gm	$6.75	TRI-STATIN II, Rugby	00536-4920-28
30 gm	$19.52	MYTREX, Savage Labs	00281-0089-30
30 gm	$24.46	MYCOLOG II, Bristol Myers Squibb	00003-0466-60
60 gm	$6.37	Nystatin & Triamcinolone Acetonide, Clay Park Labs	45802-0027-37
60 gm	$7.50	Nystatin/Triamcinolone, Taro Pharms (US)	51672-1272-03
60 gm	$8.60	Nystatin-Triamcinolone, NMC Labs	23317-0155-60
60 gm	$8.85	MYCOGEN II, Goldline Labs	00182-1800-52
60 gm	$8.96	N T A, Qualitest Pharms	00603-7811-88
60 gm	$10.50	MYOCIDIN, Major Pharms	00904-2699-02
60 gm	$11.00	MYCO-BIOTIC II, HL Moore Drug Exch	00839-7153-50
60 gm	$11.23	Nystatin Triamcinolone, Fougera	00168-0089-60
60 gm	$12.90	TRI-STATIN II, Rugby	00536-4920-25
60 gm	$15.50	Nystatin W/Triamcinolone, Harber Pharm	51432-0765-17
60 gm	$41.87	MYCOLOG II, Bristol Myers Squibb	00003-0466-65
120 gm	$12.94	Nystatin & Triamcinolone Acetonide, Clay Park Labs	45802-0027-52
120 gm	$71.35	MYCOLOG II, Bristol Myers Squibb	00003-0466-50
454 gm	$49.57	Nystatin & Triamcinolone Acetonide, Clay Park Labs	45802-0027-05

OCTREOTIDE ACETATE *(001912)*

CATEGORIES: Acromegaly; Antidiarrhea Agents; Cancer; Tumors; Diarrhea; Hormones; Hypokalemia; Somatostatin-Like Compounds; Tumors; Pregnancy Category B; FDA Approved 1988 Oct

BRAND NAMES: **Sandostatin**; *Sandostatina* (Mexico); *Sandostatine* (France)
(International brand names outside U.S. in italics)

FORMULARIES: Aetna; BC-BS

DESCRIPTION:

Sandostatin (octreotide acetate) Injection, a cyclic octapeptide prepared as a clear sterile solution of octreotide, acetate salt, in buffered sodium chloride for administration by deep subcutaneous (intrafat) or intravenous injection. Octreotide acetate, known chemically as L-Cysteinamide, D-phenylalanyl-L-cysteinyl-L-phenylalanyl-D-tryptophyl-L-lysyl-L-threonyl-N-[2-hydroxy-1-(hydroxymethy l)propyl]-, cyclic (2→7)-disulfide; (R-(R*, R*)) acetate salt, is a long-acting octapeptide with pharmacologic actions mimicking those of the natural hormone somatostatin.

Sandostatin (octreotide acetate) Injection is available as: sterile 1 ml ampuls in 3 strengths, containing 50, 100, or 500 mcg octreotide (as acetate), and sterile 5 ml multi-dose vials in 2 strengths, containing 200 and 1000 mcg/ml of octreotide (as acetate).

Each ampul also contains:

acetic acid, glacial, USP 2.0 mg
sodium acetate trihydrate, USP 2.0 mg
sodium chloride, USP 7.0 mg
water for injection, qs to 1.0 mg

Each ml of the multi-dose vials also contains:

acetic acid, glacial, USP 2.0 mg
sodium acetate trihydrate, USP 2.0 mg
sodium chloride, USP 7.0 mg
phenol, USP 5.0 mg
water for injection, qs to 1.0 mg

Acetic acid and sodium acetate trihydrate are added to provide a buffered solution, pH 4.2 ± 0.3.

The molecular weight of octreotide acetate is 1019.3 (free peptide, $C_{49}H_{66}N_{10}O_{10}S_2$) and its amino acid sequence is:

H-D-Phe-Cys-Phe-D-Trp-Lys-Thr-Cys-Thr-ol,
x CH_3COOH where x = 1.4 to 2.5

CLINICAL PHARMACOLOGY:

Octreotide acetate exerts pharmacological actions similar to the natural hormone somatostatin. It is an even more potent inhibitor of growth hormone, glucagon, and insulin than somatostatin. Like somatostatin, it also suppresses LH response to GnRH, decreases splanchnic blood flow, and inhibits release of serotonin, gastrin, vasoactive intestinal peptide, insulin, glucagon, secretin, motilin, and pancreatic polypeptide.

By virtue of these pharmacological actions, octreotide acetate has been used to treat the symptoms associated with metastatic carcinoid tumors (flushing and diarrhea), and Vasoactive Intestinal Peptide (VIP) secreting adenomas (watery diarrhea).

Octreotide acetate substantially reduces growth hormone and/or IGF-I (somatomedin C) levels in patients with acromegaly.

Single doses of octreotide acetate have been shown to inhibit gallbladder contractility and to decrease bile secretion in normal volunteers. In controlled clinical trials the incidence of gallstone or biliary sludge formation was markedly increased (see WARNINGS.)

Octreotide acetate suppresses secretion of thyroid stimulating hormone (TSH).

Pharmacokinetics: After subcutaneous injection, octreotide is absorbed rapidly and completely from the injection site. Peak concentrations of 5.2 ng/ml (100 mcg dose) were reached 0.4 hours after dosing. Using a specific radioimmunoassay, intravenous and subcutaneous doses were found to be bioequivalent. Peak concentrations and area under the curve values were dose proportional both after subcutaneous or intravenous single doses up to 400 mcg and with multiple doses of 200 mcg t.i.d. (600 mcg/day). Clearance was reduced by about 66% suggesting non- linear kinetics of the drug at daily doses of 600 mcg/day as compared to 150 mcg/day. The relative decrease in clearance with doses above 600 mcg/day is not defined.

In healthy volunteers the distribution of octreotide from plasma was rapid (tα1/2 = 0.2 h), the volume of distribution (Vdss) was estimated to be 13.6 l and the total body clearance was 10 l/hr.

In blood, the distribution into the erythrocytes was found to be negligible and about 65% was bound in the plasma in a concentration- independent manner. Binding was mainly to lipoprotein and, to a lesser extent, to albumin.

The elimination of octreotide from plasma had an apparent half-life of 1.7 hours compared with 1-3 minutes with the natural hormone. the duration of action of octreotide acetate is variable but extends up to 12 hours depending upon the type of tumor. About 32% of the dose is excreted unchanged into the urine. In an elderly population, dose adjustments may be necessary due to a significant increase in the half- life (46%) and a significant decrease in the clearance 926%) of the drug.

In patients with acromegaly, the pharmacokinetics differ somewhat from those in healthy volunteers. A mean peak concentration of 2.8 ng/ml (100 mcg dose) was reached in 0.7 hours under subcutaneous dosing. The volume of distribution (Vdss was estimated to be 21.6 ± 8.5 l and the total body clearance was increased to 18 l/h. The mean percent of the drug bound was 41.2%. The disposition and elimination half-lives were similar to normals.

In patients with severe renal failure requiring dialysis, clearance was reduced to about half that found in normal subjects (from approximately 10 L/h to 4.5 L/h). The effect of hepatic diseases on the disposition of octreotide is unknown.

INDICATIONS AND USAGE:

Acromegaly: Octreotide acetate is indicated to reduce blood levels of growth hormones and IGF-I (somatomedin C) in acromegaly patients who have had inadequate response to or cannot be treated with surgical resection, pituitary irradiation, and bromocriptine mesylate at maximally tolerated doses. The goal is to achieve normalization of growth hormone and IGF-I (somatomedin C) levels (see DOSAGE AND ADMINISTRATION.) In patients with acromegaly. Octreotide acetate reduces growth hormone to within normal ranges in 50% of patients and reduces IGF-I (somatomedin C) to within normal ranges in 50%-60% of patients. Since the effects of pituitary irradiation may not become maximal for several years, adjunctive therapy with octreotide acetate to reduce blood levels of growth hormone and IGF-I (somatomedin C) offers potential benefit before the effects of irradiation are manifested.

Improvement in clinical signs and symptoms or reduction in tumor size or rate of growth were not shown in clinical trials performed with octreotide acetate; these trials were not optimally designed to detect such effects.

Carcinoid Tumors: Octreotide acetate is indicated for the symptomatic treatment of patients with metastatic carcinoid tumors where it suppresses or inhibits the severe diarrhea and flushing episodes associated with the disease.

Octreotide acetate studies were not designed to show an effect on the size, rate of growth or development.

Vasoactive Intestinal Peptide Tumors (VIPomas): Octreotide acetate is indicated for the treatment of the profuse watery diarrhea associated with VIP-secreting tumors. Octreotide acetate studies were not designed to show an effect on the size, rate of growth or development of metastases.

CONTRAINDICATIONS:

Sensitivity to this drug or any of its components.

WARNINGS:

Single doses of octreotide acetate have been shown to inhibit gallbladder contractility and decrease bile secretion in normal volunteers. In clinical trials (primarily patients with acromegaly or psoriasis), the incidence of biliary tract abnormalities was 52% 927% gallstones, 22% sludge without stones, 3% biliary duct dilation). The incidence of stones or sludge in patients who received octreotide acetate for 12 months or longer was 48%. Less than 2% of patients treated with octreotide acetate for 1 month or less developed gallstones. The incidence of gallstones did not appear related to age, sex or dose. like patients without gallbladder abnormalities, the majority of patients developing gallbladder abnormalities on ultrasound had gastrointestinal symptoms. The symptoms were not specific for gallbladder disease. A few patients developed acute cholecystitis, ascending cholangitis, biliary obstruction, cholestatic hepatitis or pancreatitis during octreotide acetate therapy or following its withdrawal. One patient developed ascending cholangitis during octreotide acetate therapy and died.

PRECAUTIONS:

General: Octreotide acetate alters the balance between the counter-regulatory hormones, insulin, glucagon and growth hormone, which may result in hypoglycemia or hyperglycemia. Octreotide acetate also suppresses secretion of thyroid stimulating hormone, which may result in hypothyroidism. Cardiac conduction abnormalities have also occurred during treatment with octreotide acetate. However, the incidence of these adverse events during long-term therapy was determined vigorously only in acromegaly patients who, due to their underlying disease and/or the subsequent treatment they receive are at an increased risk for the development of diabetes mellitus, hypothyroidism, and cardiovascular disease. Although the degree to which these abnormalities are related to octreotide acetate therapy is not clear, new abnormalities of glycemic control, thyroid function and ECG developed during octreotide acetate therapy as described below.

PRECAUTIONS: *(cont'd)*

The hypoglycemia or hyperglycemia which occurs during octreotide acetate therapy is usually mild, but may result in overt diabetes mellitus or necessitate dose changes in insulin or other hypoglycemic agents. Hypoglycemia and hyperglycemia occurred on octreotide acetate in 3% and 15% of acromegalic patients, respectively. Severe hyperglycemia, subsequent pneumonia and death following initiation of octreotide acetate therapy was reported in one patient with no history of hyperglycemia.

In acromegalic patients, 12% developed biochemical hypothyroidism only, 6% developed goiter, and 4% required initiation of thyroid replacement therapy while receiving octreotide acetate. Baseline and periodic assessment of thyroid function (TSH, total and/or free T_4) is recommended during chronic therapy.

In acromegalics, bradycardia (<50 bpm) developed in 21%; conduction abnormalities and arrhythmias each occurred in 9% of patients during octreotide acetate therapy. Other EKG changes observed included QT prolongation, axis shifts, early repolarization, low voltage, R/S transition, and early R wave progression. These ECG changes are not uncommon in acromegalic patients. Dose adjustments in drugs such as beta- blockers that have bradycardia effects may be necessary. In one acromegalic patient with severe congestive heart failure, initiation of octreotide acetate therapy resulted in worsening of CHF with improvement when drug was discontinued. Confirmation of a drug effect was obtained with a positive re-challenge.

Several cases of pancreatitis have been reported in patients receiving octreotide acetate therapy.

Octreotide acetate may alter absorption of dietary fats in some patients.

In patients with severe renal failure requiring dialysis, the half-life of octreotide acetate may be increased, necessitating adjustment of the maintenance dosage.

Depressed vitamin B_{12} levels and abnormal Schilling's tests have been observed in some patients receiving octreotide acetate therapy, and monitoring of vitamin B_{12} levels is recommended during chronic octreotide acetate therapy.

Information for the Patient: Careful instruction in sterile subcutaneous injection technique should be given to the patients and to other persons who may administer octreotide acetate Injection.

Laboratory Tests: Laboratory tests that may be helpful as biochemical markers in determining and following patient response depend on the specific tumor. Based on diagnosis, measurement of the following substances may be useful in monitoring the progress of therapy:

Acromegaly: Growth Hormone, IGF-I (somatomedin C)

Responsiveness to octreotide acetate may be evaluated by determining growth hormone levels at 1-4 hour intervals for 8-12 hours post dose. Alternatively, a single measurement of IGF-I (somatomedin C) level may be made two weeks after drug initiation or dosage change.

Carcinoid: 5-HIAA (urinary 5-hydroxyindole acetic acid), plasma serotonin, plasma Substance P.

VIPoma: VIP (plasma vasoactive intestinal peptide)

Baseline and periodic total and/or free T_4 measurements should be performed during chronic therapy (seePRECAUTIONS, General).

Drug Laboratory Test Interactions: No known interference exists with clinical laboratory tests, including amine or peptide determinations.

Carcinogenesis/Mutagenesis/Impairment of Fertility: Studies in laboratory animals have demonstrated no mutagenic potential of octreotide acetate.

No carcinogenic potential was demonstrated in mice treated subcutaneously for 85-99 weeks at doses up to 2000 mcg/kg/day. In a 116-week subcutaneous study in rats, a 27% and 12% incidence of injection site sarcomas or squamous cell carcinomas was observed in males and females, respectively, at the highest dose level of 1250 mcg/kg/day compared to an incidence of 8%-10% in the vehicle control groups. The increased incidence of injection site tumors was most probably caused by irritation and the high-sensitivity of the rate to repeated subcutaneous injections at the same site. Rotating injection sites would prevent chronic irritation in humans. There have been no reports of injection site tumors in patients treated with octreotide acetate for up to 5 years. There was also a 15% incidence of uterine adenocarcinomas in the 1250 mcg/kg/day females compared to 7% in the saline control females and 0% in the vehicle control females. The presence of endometritis coupled with the absence of corpora lutea, the reduction in mammary fibroadenomas and the presence of uterine dilation suggest that the uterine tumors were associated with estrogen dominance in the aged female rats which does not occur in humans.

Sandostatin (octreotide acetate did not impair fertility in rats at doses up to 1000 mcg/kg/day.

Pregnancy Category B: Reproduction studies have been performed in rats and rabbits at doses up to 30 times the highest human dose and have revealed no evidence of impaired fertility or harm to the fetus due to octreotide acetate. There are, however, no adequate and well-controlled studies in pregnant women. Because animal reproduction studies are not always predictive of human response, this drug should be used during pregnancy only if clearly needed.

Nursing Mothers: It is not known whether this drug is excreted in human milk. Because many drugs are excreted in milk, caution should be exercised when octreotide acetate is administered to a nursing woman.

Pediatric Use: Experience with octreotide acetate in the pediatric population is limited. The youngest patient to receive the drug was 1 month old. Doses of 1-10 mcg/kg body weight were well tolerated in the young patients. A single case of an infant (nesidioblastosis) was complicated by a seizure thought to be independent of octreotide acetate therapy.

DRUG INTERACTIONS:

Octreotide acetate has been associated with alterations in nutrient absorption, so it may have an effect on absorption of orally administered drugs. Concomitant administration of octreotide acetate with cyclosporine may decrease blood levels of cyclosporine and result in transplant rejection.

Patients receiving insulin, oral hypoglycemic agents, beta blockers, calcium channel blockers, or agents to control fluid and electrolyte balance, may require dose adjustments of these therapeutic agents.

ADVERSE REACTIONS:

Gallbladder Abnormalities: Gallbladder abnormalities, especially stones and/or biliary sludge, frequently develop in patients on chronic octreotide acetate therapy (See WARNINGS.)

Cardiac: In acromegalics, sinus bradycardia (<50 bpm) developed in 21% conduction abnormalities and arrhythmias each developed in 9% of patients during octreotide acetate therapy (see PRECAUTIONS, General.

Gastrointestinal: Diarrhea, loose stools, nausea and abdominal discomfort were each seen in 30%-58% of acromegalic patients in US studies although only 2% of the patients discontinued therapy due to these symptoms were seen in 5%-10% of patients with other disorders.

ADVERSE REACTIONS: *(cont'd)*

The frequency of these symptoms was not dose-related, but diarrhea and abdominal discomfort generally resolved more quickly in patients treated with 300 mcg/day than in those treated with 750 mcg/day. Vomiting, flatulence, abnormal stools, distention, and constipation were each seen in less than 10% of patients.

Hypo/Hyperglycemia: Hypoglycemia and hyperglycemia occurred in 3% and 15% of acromegalic patients, respectively, but only in about 1.5% of other patients. Symptoms of hypoglycemia were noted in approximately 2% of patients.

Hypothyroidism: In acromegalics, biochemical hypothyroidism alone occurred in 12% while goiter occurred in 6% during octreotide acetate therapy (see PRECAUTIONS, General.) In patients without acromegaly, hypothyroidism has only been reported in several isolated patients and goiter has not been reported.

Other Adverse Events: Pain on injection was reported in 7.5% and headache in 6%.

OTHER ADVERSE EVENTS 1%-4%

Other events (relationship to drug not established), each observed in 1%-4% of patients, included dizziness, fatigue, weakness, pruritus, joint pain, backache, urinary tract infection, cold symptoms, flu symptoms, injection site hematoma, bruise, edema, flushing, blurred vision, pollakiuria, fat malabsorption, and hair loss.

OTHER ADVERSE EVENTS <1%

Events reported in less than 1% of patients and for which relationship to drug is not established are listed:

Gastrointestinal: hepatitis, jaundice, increase in liver enzymes, GI bleeding, hemorrhoids, appendicitis;

Integumentary: rash, cellulitis, petechiae, urticaria;

Musculoskeletal: arthritis, joint effusion, muscle pain, Raynaud's phenomenon;

Cardiovascular: chest pain, shortness of breath, thrombophlebitis, ischemia, congestive heart failure, hypertension, hypertensive reaction, palpitations, orthostatic BP decrease, tachycardia;

CNS: depression, anxiety, libido decrease, syncope, tremor, seizure, vertigo, Bell's Palsy, paranoia, pituitary apoplexy, increased intraocular pressure;

Respiratory : pneumonia, pulmonary nodule, status asthmaticus;

Endocrine: galactorrhea, hypoadrenalism, diabetes, insipidus, gynecomastia, amenorrhea, polymenorrhea, vaginitis;

Urogenital: nephrolithiasis, hematuria;

Hematologic: anemia, iron deficiency, epistaxis;

Miscellaneous : otitis, allergic reaction, increased CK, visual disturbance.

Evaluation of 20 patients treated for at least 6 months has failed to demonstrate titers of antibodies exceeding background levels. However, antibody titers to octreotide acetate were subsequently reported in three patients and resulted in prolonged duration of drug action in two patients. Anaphylactoid reactions, including anaphylactic sock, have been reported in several patients receiving octreotide acetate.

DRUG ABUSE AND DEPENDENCE:

There are no indication that octreotide acetate has potential for drug abuse or dependence. Octreotide acetate levels in the central nervous system are negligible, even after doses up to 30,000 mcg.

OVERDOSAGE:

No frank overdose has occurred in any patient to date. Intravenous bolus doses of 1 mg (1000 mcg) given to healthy volunteers and of 30 mg (30,000 mcg) IV over 20 minutes and of 120 mg (120,000 mcg) IV over 8 hours to research patients have not resulted in serious ill effects.

Mortality occurred in mice and rats has given 72 mg/kg and 18 mg/kg IV, respectively.

DOSAGE AND ADMINISTRATION:

Octreotide acetate may be administered subcutaneously or intravenously. Subcutaneous injection is the usual route of administration of octreotide acetate for control of symptoms. Pain with subcutaneous administration may be reduced by using the smallest volume that will deliver the desired dose. Multiple subcutaneous injections at the same site within short periods of time should be avoided. Sites should be rotated in a systematic manner.

Parenteral drug products should be inspected visually for particulate matter and discoloration prior to administration. **Do not use if particulates and/or discoloration are observed.** Proper sterile technique should be used in the preparation of parenteral admixtures to minimize the possibility of microbial contamination. **Octreotide acetate is not compatible in Total Parenteral Nutrition (TPN) solutions because of the formation of a glycosyl octreotide conjugate which may decrease the efficacy of the product.**

Octreotide acetate is stable in sterile isotonic saline solutions of dextrose 5% in water for 24 hours. It may be diluted in volumes of 50-200 ml and infused intravenously over 15-30 minutes or administered by IV push over 3 minutes. In emergency situations (*e.g.,* carcinoid crisis) it may be given by rapid bolus.

The initial dosage is 50 mcg, administered twice or three times daily. Upward dose titration is frequently required. Dosage information for patients with specific tumors follows.

Acromegaly: Dosage may be initiated at 50 mcg t.i.d. Beginning with this low dose may permit adaption to adverse gastrointestinal effects for patients who will require higher doses. IGF-I (somatomedin C) levels every 2 weeks can be used to guide titration. Alternatively, multiple growth hormone levels at 0-8 hours after octreotide acetate administration permit more rapid titration of dose. The goal is to achieve growth hormone levels less than 5 ng/ml or IGF-I (somatomedin C) levels less than 1.9 u/ml in males and less than 2.2 u/ml in females. The dose most commonly found to be effective is 100 mcg t.i.d. but some patients require up to 500 mcg t.i.d. for maximum effectiveness. Doses greater than 300 mcg/day seldom result in additional benefit, and if an increase in dose fails to provide additional benefit, the dose should be reduced. IGF-I (somatomedin-C) or growth hormone levels should be reevaluated at 6 month intervals.

Octreotide acetate should be withdrawn yearly for approximately 4 weeks from patients who have received irradiation to assess disease activity. If growth hormone or IGF-I (somatomedin C) levels should be reevaluated at 6 month intervals.

Carcinoid Tumors: The suggested daily dosage of octreotide acetate during the first 2 weeks of therapy ranges from 100-600 mcg/day in 2-4 divided doses (mean daily dosage is 300 mcg). In the clinical studies, the **median** daily maintenance dosage was approximately 450 mcg, but clinical and biochemical benefits were obtained in some patients with as little as 50 mcg, while others required doses up to 1500 mcg/day. However, experience with doses above 750 mcg/day is limited.

VIPomas: Daily dosages of 200-300 mcg in 2-4 divided doses are recommended during the initial 2 weeks of therapy (range 150-750 mcg) to control symptoms of the disease. On an individual basis, dosage may be adjusted to achieve a therapeutic response, but usually doses above 450 mcg/day are not required.

DOSAGE AND ADMINISTRATION: *(cont'd)*

Storage: For prolonged storage, octreotide acetate ampuls and multi-dose vials should be stored in the refrigerator at 2°-8°C (36°-46°F) and protected from light. At room temperature, (20°-30°C or 70°-86°F) The solution can be allowed to come to room temperature prior to administration. Do not warm artificially. After initial use, multiple dose vials should be discarded within 14 days. Ampuls should be opened just prior to administration and the unused portion discarded.

HOW SUPPLIED:

Octreotide acetate Injection is available in 1 ml ampuls and 5 ml multi-dose vials as follows:

Ampuls: 50 mcg/ml octreotide (as acetate); 100 mcg/ml octreotide (as acetate); 500 mcg/ml octreotide (as acetate)

Multi-Dose Vials: 200 mcg/ml octreotide (as acetate); 1000 mcg/ml octreotide (as acetate)

HOW SUPPLIED - EQUIVALENTS NOT AVAILABLE:

Injection, Solution - Intravenous - 0.2 mg/ml

5 ml	$94.20	SANDOSTATIN, Novartis	00078-0183-25

Injection, Solution - Intravenous - 1 mg/ml

5 ml	$463.74	SANDOSTATIN, Novartis	00078-0184-25

Injection, Solution - Subcutaneous - 0.05 mg/ml

1 ml x 50	$236.52	SANDOSTATIN INJ. 0.05, Novartis	00078-0180-04
20 ampules x 1	$95.64	SANDOSTATIN INJ. 0.05, Novartis	00078-0180-03

Injection, Solution - Subcutaneous - 0.1 mg/ml

1 ml x 50	$433.26	SANDOSTATIN, Novartis	00078-0181-04
20 ampules x 1	$175.14	SANDOSTATIN, Novartis	00078-0181-03

Injection, Solution - Subcutaneous - 0.5 mg/ml

1 ml x 50	$1982.52	SANDOSTATIN INJ. 0.5, Novartis	00078-0182-04
20 ampules x 1	$801.12	SANDOSTATIN INJ. 0.5, Novartis	00078-0182-03

OFLOXACIN *(003016)*

CATEGORIES: Antibacterials; Anti-Infectives; Antibiotics; Antimicrobials; Bronchitis; Chlamydia; Chronic Bronchitis; Cystitis; Eye, Ear, Nose, & Throat Preparations; Fluoroquinolones; Gonorrhea; H. Influenzae Pneumonia; Ophthalmics; Pneumonia; Prostatitis; Respiratory Tract Infections; Sexually Transmitted Diseases; Skin Infections; Urethritis; Urinary Antibacterial; Urinary Tract Infections; Tuberculosis*; Pregnancy Category C; FDA Class 1C ("Little or No Therapeutic Advantage"); Sales > $100 Million; FDA Approved 1990 Dec; Top 200 Drugs

* Indication not approved by the FDA

BRAND NAMES: *Akilen*; *Baccidal*; *Bactocin* (Mexico); *Danoflox*; *Effexin*; *Exocine* (France); *Flobacin*; *Floxan*; *Floxil* (Mexico); **Floxin**; *Floxstat* (Mexico); *Inoflox*; *Kinoxacin*; *Loxinter*; *Occidal*; Ocuflox; *Oflocet* (France); *Oflocin*; *Orocin*; *Qinolon*; *Tabrin*; *Taravid*; *Tarivid* (Europe, Japan); *Tarivid Eye Ear*
(International brand names outside U.S. in italics)

FORMULARIES: Aetna; Medi-Cal; PCS

COST OF THERAPY: $43.09 (Urinary Infections; Tablet; 200 mg; 2/day; 7 days)

DESCRIPTION:

TABLETS AND INTRAVENOUS INFUSION

Floxin Tablets and IV are a synthetic broad-spectrum antimicrobial agent for oral or intravenous administration. Chemically, ofloxacin, a fluorinated carboxyquinolone, is the racemate, (±)-9- fluoro-2,3-dihydro-3-methyl-10- (4-methyl-1-piperazinyl)-7-oxo-7H-pyrido[1,2,3-de]-1,4-benzoxazine -6- carboxylic acid. Its empirical formula is $C_{18}H_{20}FN_3O_4$, and its molecular weight is 361.4. Ofloxacin is an off-white to pale yellow crystalline powder. The molecule exists as a zwitterion at the pH conditions in the small intestine. The relative solubility characteristics of ofloxacin at room temperature, as defined by USP nomenclature, indicate that ofloxacin is considered to be *soluble* in aqueous solutions with pH between 2 and 5. It is *sparingly* to *slightly soluble* in aqueous solutions with pH 7 and *freely soluble* in aqueous solutions with pH above 9. Ofloxacin has the potential to form stable coordination compounds with many metal ions. This *in vitro* chelation potential has the following formation order: $Fe^{+3} > Al^{+3} > Cu^{+2} > Ni^{+2} > Pb^{+2} > Zn^{+2} > Mg^{+2} > Ca^{+2} > Ba^{+2}$.

Tablets: Floxin tablets contain the following inactive ingredients: anhydrous lactose, corn starch, hydroxypropyl cellulose, hydroxypropyl methylcellulose, magnesium stearate, polyethylene glycol, polysorbate 80, sodium starch glycolate, titanium dioxide and may also contain synthetic yellow iron oxide.

Intravenous Infusion: Floxin IV IN SINGLE-USE VIALS is a sterile, preservative-free aqueous solution of ofloxacin with pH ranging from 3.5 to 5.5. Floxin IV IN PRE-MIXED BOTTLES and IN PRE-MIXED FLEXIBLE CONTAINERS are sterile, preservative-free aqueous solutions of ofloxacin with pH ranging from 3.8 to 5.8. The color of ofloxacin IV may range from light yellow to amber. This does not adversely affect product potency. Ofloxacin IV IN SINGLE-USE VIALS contains ofloxacin in Water for Injection. Floxin IV IN PRE-MIXED BOTTLES and IN PRE-MIXED FLEXIBLE CONTAINERS are dilute, non-pyrogenic, nearly isotonic pre-mixed solutions that contain ofloxacin in 5% Dextrose (D_5W). Hydrochloric acid and sodium hydroxide may have been added to adjust the pH.

The flexible container is fabricated from a specially formulated non-plasticized, thermoplastic copolyester (CR3). The amount of water that can permeate from the container into the overwrap is insufficient to affect the solution significantly. Solutions in contact with the flexible container can leach out certain of the container's chemical components in very small amounts within the expiration period. The suitability of the container material has been confirmed by tests in animals according to USP biological tests for plastic containers.

OPHTHALMIC SOLUTION

Ofloxacin ophthalmic solution 0.3% is a sterile ophthalmic solution. It is a fluorinated carboxyquinolone anti-infective for topical ophthalmic use.

Chemical Name: (±)-9-Fluoro-2,3-dihydro-3-methyl-10-(4-methyl-1-piperazinyl)-7-oxo-7H-pyrido[1,2,3-de]-1,4 benzoxazine-6-carboxylic acid.

Contains: *Active:* ofloxacin 0.3% (3 mg/ml); *Preservative:* benzalkonium chloride (0.005%); *Inactives:* sodium chloride and purified water. May also contain hydrochloric acid and/or sodium hydroxide to adjust pH.

Ofloxacin ophthalmic solution is unbuffered and formulated with a pH of 6.4 (range - 6.0 to 6.8). It has an osmolality of 300 mOsm/kg. Ofloxacin is a fluorinated 4-quinolone which differs from other fluorinated 4-quinolones in that there is a six member (pyridobenzoxazine) ring from positions 1 to 8 of the basic ring structure.

CLINICAL PHARMACOLOGY:

PHARMACOKINETICS

Tablets: Following oral administration, the bioavailability of ofloxacin in the tablet formulation is approximately 98%. Maximum serum concentrations are achieved one to two hours after an oral dose. Absorption of ofloxacin after single or multiple doses of 200 to 400 mg is predictable, and the amount of drug absorbed increases proportionately with the dose.

Ofloxacin has biphasic elimination. Following multiple oral doses at steady-state administration, the half-lives are approximately 4-5 hours and 20-25 hours. However, the longer half-life represents less than 5% of the total AUC. Accumulation at steady-state can be estimated using a half-life of 9 hours. The total clearance and volume of distribution are approximately similar after single or multiple doses. Elimination is mainly by renal excretion. TABLE 1 shows mean peak serum concentrations in healthy 70-80 kg male volunteers after single oral doses of 200, 300, or 400 mg of ofloxacin or after multiple oral doses of 400 mg.

TABLE 1

Oral Dose	Serum Concentration 2 hours after admin. (mcg/ml)	Area Under the Curve $(AUC_{(0-00)})$(mcg°h/ml)
200 mg single dose	1.5	14.1
300 mg single dose	2.4	21.2
400 mg single dose	2.9	31.4
400 mg steady state	4.6	61.0

Steady-state concentrations were attained after four oral doses and the area under the curve (AUC) was approximately 40% higher than the AUC after single doses. Therefore, after multiple-dose administration of 200 mg and 300 mg doses, peak serum levels of 2.2 mcg/ml and 3.6 mcg/ml, respectively, are predicted at steady-state.

Intravenous Infusion: Following a single intravenous infusion of 200 mg or 400 mg of ofloxacin to normal volunteers, the mean maximum plasma concentrations attained were 2.7 and 4.0 mcg/ml, respectively; the concentrations at 12 hours (h) after dosing were 0.3 and 0.7 mcg/ml, respectively.

Steady-state concentrations were attained after four doses, and the area under the curve (AUC) was approximately 40% higher than the AUC after a single dose. The mean peak and trough plasma steady-state levels attained following intravenous administration of 200 mg of ofloxacin q 12 h for seven days were 2.9 and 0.5 mcg/ml, respectively. Following intravenous doses of 400 mg of ofloxacin q 12 h, the mean peak and trough plasma steady-state levels ranged, in two different studies, from 5.5 to 7.2 mcg/ml and 1.2 to 1.9 mcg/ml, respectively.

Following 7 days of intravenous administration, the elimination half-life of ofloxacin was 6 h (range 5 to 10 h). The total clearance and the volume of distribution were approximately 15 l/h and 120 l, respectively.

Elimination of ofloxacin is primarily by renal excretion. Approximately 65% of a dose is excreted renally within 48 h. Studies indicate that <5% of an administered dose is recovered in the urine as the desmethyl or N- oxide metabolites. Four to eight percent of an ofloxacin dose is excreted in the feces. This indicates a small degree of biliary excretion of ofloxacin.

Tablets and Intravenous Infusion: *In vitro,* approximately 32% of the drug in plasma is protein bound.

The single dose and steady-state plasma profiles of ofloxacin injection were comparable in extent of exposure (AUC) to those of ofloxacin tablets when the injectable and tablet formulations of ofloxacin were administered in equal doses (mg/mg) to the same group of subjects. The mean steady state $AUC_{(0-12)}$ attained after the intravenous administration of 400 mg over 60 min was 43.5 mcg·h/ml; the mean steady state $AUC_{(0-12)}$ attained after the oral administration of 400 mg was 41.2 mcg·h/ml (two one-sided t- test, 90% confidence interval was 103-109).

Between 0 and 6 h following the administration of a single 200 mg oral dose of ofloxacin to 12 healthy volunteers, the average urine ofloxacin concentration was approximately 220 mcg/ml. Between 12 and 24 hours after administration, the average urine ofloxacin level was approximately 34 mcg/ml.

Following oral administration of recommended therapeutic doses, ofloxacin has been detected in blister fluid, cervix, lung tissue, ovary, prostatic fluid, prostatic tissue, skin, and sputum. The mean concentration of ofloxacin in each of these various body fluids and tissues after one or more doses was 0.8 to 1.5 times the concurrent plasma level. Inadequate data are presently available on the distribution or levels of ofloxacin in the cerebrospinal fluid or brain tissue.

Ofloxacin has a pyridobenzoxazine ring that appears to decrease the extent of parent compound metabolism. Between 65% and 80% of an administered oral dose of ofloxacin is excreted unchanged via the kidneys within 48 hours of dosing. Studies indicate that less than 5% of an administered dose is recovered in the urine as the desmethyl or N-oxide metabolites. Four to eight percent of an ofloxacin dose is excreted in the feces. This indicates a small degree of biliary excretion of ofloxacin.

The effect that food has on the absorption of ofloxacin tablets has not been studied.

Following the administration of oral doses of ofloxacin to healthy elderly volunteers (64-74 years of age) with normal renal function, the apparent half-life of ofloxacin was 7 to 8 hours, as compared to approximately 6 hours in younger adults. Drug absorption, however, appears to be unaffected by age.

Clearance of ofloxacin is reduced in patients with impaired renal function (creatinine clearance rate ≤ 50 ml/min), and dosage adjustment is necessary. (See PRECAUTIONS, General and DOSAGE AND ADMINISTRATION).

Ophthalmic Solution: Serum, urine and tear concentrations of ofloxacin were measured in 30 healthy women at various time points during a ten-day course of treatment with ofloxacin ophthalmic solution. The mean serum ofloxacin concentration ranged from 0.4 ng/ml to 1.9 ng/ml. Maximum ofloxacin concentration increased from 1.1 ng/ml on day one to 1.9 ng/ml on day 11 after 4 times daily dosing for 10½ days. Maximum serum ofloxacin concentrations after ten days of topical ophthalmic dosing were more than 1000 times lower than those reported after standard oral doses of ofloxacin.

Tear ofloxacin concentrations ranged from 5.7 to 31 mcg/g during the 40 minute period following the last dose on day 11. Mean tear concentration measured four hours after topical ophthalmic dosing was 9.2 mcg/g.

Corneal tissue concentrations of 4.4 mcg/ml were observed four hours after beginning topical ocular application of two drops of ofloxacin ophthalmic solution every 30 minutes. Ofloxacin was excreted in the urine primarily unmodified.

MICROBIOLOGY

Tablet and IV

Ofloxacin has *in vitro*activity against a broad spectrum of gram-positive and gram-negative aerobic and anaerobic bacteria. Ofloxacin is often bactericidal at concentrations equal to or slightly greater than inhibitory concentrations. Ofloxacin is thought to exert a bactericidal effect on susceptible microorganisms by inhibiting DNA gyrase, an essential enzyme that is a critical catalyst in the duplication, transcription, and repair of bacterial DNA.

CLINICAL PHARMACOLOGY: *(cont'd)*

Cross-resistance has been observed between ofloxacin and other fluoroquinolones. There is generally no cross-resistance between ofloxacin and other classes of antibacterial agents such as beta-lactams or aminoglycosides.

Ofloxacin has been shown to be active against most strains of the following organisms both *in vitro* and in specific clinical infections; (See INDICATIONS AND USAGE).

Many strains of other streptococcal species, *Enterococcus* species, and anaerobes are resistant to ofloxacin.

Ofloxacin has not been shown to be active against *Treponema pallidum.* (See WARNINGS).

Resistance to ofloxacin due to spontaneous mutation *in vitro* is a rare occurrence (range: 10^{-9} to 10^{-11}). To date, emergence of resistance has been relatively uncommon in clinical practice. With the exception of *Pseudomonas aeruginosa* (10%), less than a 4% rate of resistance emergence has been reported for most other species. Although cross-resistance has been observed between ofloxacin and other fluoroquinolones, some organisms resistant to other quinolones may be susceptible to ofloxacin.

Aerobes, Gram-Positive: *Staphylococcus aureus, Staphylococcus epidermidis, Streptococcus pneumoniae.*

Aerobes, Gram-Negative: *Enterobacter cloacae, Haemophilus influenzae, Proteus mirabilis, Pseudomonas aeruginosa, Serratia marcescens**

Anaerobic Species: *Propionibacterium acnes*

*Efficacy for this organism was studied in fewer than 10 infections

The safety and effectiveness of ofloxacin ophthalmic solution in treating ophthalmologic infections due to the following organisms have not been established in adequate and well-controlled clinical trials. Ofloxacin ophthalmic solution has been shown to be active in vitro against most strains of these organisms but the clinical significance in ophthalmologic infections is unknown.

Aerobes, Gram-Positive: *Enterococcus faecalis, Listeria monocytogenes, Staphylococcus capitis, Staphylococcus hominus, Staphylococcus simulans, Streptococcus pyogenes*

Aerobes, Gram-Negative: *Acinetobacter calcoaceticus* var. *anitratus, Acinetobacter calcoaceticus* var. *lwoffii, Citrobacter diversus, Citrobacter freundii, Enterobacter aerogenes, Klebsiella pneumoniae, Moraxella (Branhamella) catarrhalis, Moraxella lacunata, Morganella morganii, Neisseria gonorrhoeae, Pseudomonas acidovorans, Pseudomonas fluorescens, Shigella sonnei*

Other: *Chlamydia trachomatis*

SUSCEPTIBILITY TESTING

Diffusion Techniques: Quantitative methods that require measurement of zone diameters give the most precise estimate of the susceptibility of bacteria to antimicrobial agents. One such standardized procedure[1] that has been recommended for use with disks to test the susceptibility of organisms to ofloxacin uses the 5-mcg ofloxacin disk. Interpretation involves correlation of the diameter obtained in the disk test with the minimum inhibitory concentration (MIC) for ofloxacin.

Reports from the laboratory giving results of the standard single-disk susceptibility test with a 5-mcg ofloxacin disk should be interpreted according to the criteria found in TABLE 2.

TABLE 2

Zone Diameter (mm)	Interpretation
≥ 16	Susceptible
13-15	Intermediate
≤ 12	Resistant

A report of "Susceptible" indicates that the pathogen is likely to be inhibited by generally achievable drug concentrations. A report of "Intermediate" indicates that the result should be considered equivocal, and, if the organism is not fully susceptible to alternative, clinically feasible drugs, the test should be repeated. This category provides a buffer zone that prevents small uncontrolled technical factors from causing major discrepancies in interpretation. A report of "Resistant" indicates that achievable drug concentrations are unlikely to be inhibitory, and other therapy should be selected.

Standardized susceptibility test procedures require the use of laboratory control organisms. The 5-mcg ofloxacin disk should give the zone diameters found in TABLE 3.

TABLE 3

Organism	Zone diameter (mm)
E. coli ATCC 25922	29-33
P. aeruginosa ATCC 27853	17-21
S. aureus ATCC 25923	24-28

Dilution Techniques: Use a standardized dilution method[2](broth, agar, or microdilution) or equivalent with ofloxacin powder. The MIC values obtained should be interpreted according to the criteria found in TABLE 4.

TABLE 4

MIC (mcg/ml)	Interpretation
≤ 2	(S) Susceptible
4	(I) Intermediate
≥ 8	(R) Resistant

As with standard diffusion methods, dilution procedures require the use of laboratory control organisms. Standard ofloxacin powder should give the MIC values found in TABLE 5.

TABLE 5

Organism	MIC Range (mcg/ml)
E. coli ATCC 25922	0.015-0.120
E. faecalis ATCC 29212	1.000-4.000
P. aeruginosa ATCC 27853	1.000-8.000
S. aureus ATCC 25923	0.120-1.000

CLINICAL STUDIES:

OPHTHALMIC SOLUTION

Conjunctivitis: In a randomized, double-masked, multicenter clinical trial, ofloxacin ophthalmic solution was superior to its vehicle after 2 days of treatment in patients with conjunctivitis and positive conjunctival cultures. Clinical outcomes for the trial demonstrated a clinical improvement rate of 86% (54/63) for the ofloxacin treated group versus 72% (48/67) for the placebo treated group after 2 days of therapy. Microbiological outcomes for the same clinical trial demonstrated an eradication rate for causative pathogens of 65% (41/63) for the

CLINICAL STUDIES: *(cont'd)*

ofloxacin treated group versus 25% (17/67) for the vehicle treated group after two days of therapy. Please note that microbiologic eradication does not always correlate with clinical outcome in anti-infective trials.

Corneal Ulcers: In a randomized, double-masked, multi-center clinical trial of 140 subjects with positive cultures, ofloxacin ophthalmic solution treated subjects had an overall clinical success rate (complete reepithelialization and no progression of the infiltrate for two consecutive visits) of 82% (61/74) compared to 80% (53/66) for the fortified antibiotic group, consisting of 1.5% tobramycin and 10% cefazolin solutions. The median time to clinical success was 11 days for the ofloxacin treated group and 10 days for the fortified treatment group.

INDICATIONS AND USAGE:

TABLETS AND INTRAVENOUS INFUSION

Ofloxacin tablets and IV are indicated for the treatment of adults with mild to moderate infections caused by susceptible strains of the designated microorganisms in the infections listed below - when intravenous administration offers a route of administration advantageous to the patient, (*i.e.*, patient cannot tolerate an oral dosage form, etc.).

The safety and effectiveness of the intravenous formulation in treating patients with severe infections have not been established.

NOTE: IN THE ABSENCE OF VOMITING OR OTHER FACTORS INTERFERING WITH THE ABSORPTION OF ORALLY ADMINISTERED DRUG, PATIENTS RECEIVE ESSENTIALLY THE SAME SYSTEMIC ANTIMICROBIAL THERAPY AFTER EQUIVALENT DOSES OF OFLOXACIN ADMINISTERED BY EITHER THE ORAL OR THE INTRAVENOUS ROUTE. THEREFORE, THE INTRAVENOUS FORMULATION DOES NOT PROVIDE A HIGHER DEGREE OF EFFICACY OR MORE POTENT ANTIMICROBIAL ACTIVITY THAN AN EQUIVALENT DOSE OF THE ORAL FORMULATION OF OFLOXACIN.

Lower Respiratory Tract

Acute bacterial exacerbations of chronic bronchitis due to*Haemophilus influenzae* or *Streptococcus pneumoniae.*

Community-acquired Pneumonia due to *Haemophilus influenzae* or *Streptococcus pneumoniae.*

Skin and Skin Structures

Uncomplicated skin and skin structure infections due to*Staphylococcus aureus, Streptococcus pyogenes, or Proteus mirabilis.**

Sexually Transmitted Diseases (See WARNINGS).

Acute, uncomplicated urethral and cervical gonorrhea due to*Neisseria gonorrhoeae.*

Nongonococcal urethritis and cervicitis due to *Chlamydia trachomatis.* **Mixed infections of the urethra and cervix** due to *Chlamydia trachomatis* and *Neisseria gonorrhoeae.*

Urinary Tract

Uncomplicated cystitis due to *Citrobacter diversus,Enterobacter aerogenes, Escherichia coli, Klebsiella pneumoniae, Proteus mirabilis, or Pseudomonas aeruginosa.**

Complicated urinary tract infections due to*Escherichia coli, Klebsiella pneumoniae, Proteus mirabilis, Citrobacter diversus**, or *Pseudomonas aeruginosa.**

Prostate

Prostatitis due to *Escherichia coli.*

* Although treatment of infections due to this organism in this infection demonstrated a clinically acceptable overall outcome, efficacy was demonstrated in fewer than 10 infections.

Appropriate culture and susceptibility tests should be performed before treatment in order to isolate and identify organisms causing the infection and to determine their susceptibility to ofloxacin. Therapy with ofloxacin may be initiated before results of these tests are known; once results become available, appropriate therapy should be continued.

As with other drugs in this class, some strains of *Pseudomonas aeruginosa* may develop resistance fairly rapidly during treatment with ofloxacin. Culture and susceptibility testing performed periodically during therapy will provide information not only on the therapeutic effect of the antimicrobial agent but also on the possible emergence of bacterial resistance.

If anaerobic organisms are suspected of contributing to the infection, appropriate therapy for anaerobic pathogens should be administered.

OPHTHALMIC SOLUTION

Ofloxacin ophthalmic solution is indicated for the treatment of infections caused by susceptible strains of the following bacteria in the conditions listed below:

Conjunctivitis

Gram-positive bacteria: *Staphylococcus aureus, Staphylococcus epidermidis, Streptococcus pneumoniae*

Gram-negative bacteria: Enterobacter cloacae, Haemophilus influenzae, Proteus mirabilis, Pseudomonas aeruginosa

Corneal Ulcers:

Gram-positive bacteria: *Staphylococcus aureus, Staphylococcus epidermidis, Streptococcus pneumoniae*

Gram-negative bacteria: *Pseudomonas aeruginosa, Serratia marcescens**

Anaerobic species: *Propionibacterium acnes*

*Efficacy for this organism was studied in fewer than 10 infections.

CONTRAINDICATIONS:

Ofloxacin is contraindicated in persons with a history of hypersensitivity to ofloxacin, to other quinolones, or to any of the components in this medication.

WARNINGS:

TABLETS AND INTRAVENOUS INFUSION

THE SAFETY AND EFFICACY OF OFLOXACIN IN CHILDREN, ADOLESCENTS (UNDER THE AGE OF 18 YEARS), PREGNANT WOMEN, AND LACTATING WOMEN HAVE NOT BEEN ESTABLISHED. (SEE PEDIATRIC USE, USE IN PREGNANCY, AND NURSING MOTHERS SUBSECTIONS IN PRECAUTIONS).

In the immature rat, the oral administration of ofloxacin at 5 to 16 times the recommended maximum human dose based on mg/kg or 1-3 times based on mg/m^2 increased the incidence and severity of osteochondrosis. The lesions did not regress after 13 weeks of drug withdrawal. Other quinolones also produce similar erosions in the weight- bearing joints and other signs of arthropathy in immature animals of various species. (See ANIMAL PHARMACOLOGY).

Ofloxacin has not been shown to be effective in the treatment of syphilis: Antimicrobial agents used in high doses for short periods of time to treat gonorrhea may mask or delay the symptoms of incubating syphilis. All patients with gonorrhea should have a serologic test for syphilis at the time of diagnosis. Patients treated with ofloxacin should have a follow-up serologic test for syphilis after three months.

WARNINGS: *(cont'd)*

Serious and occasionally fatal hypersensitivity (anaphylactic/anaphylactoid) reactions have been reported in patients receiving therapy with quinolones, including ofloxacin. These reactions often occur following the first dose. Some reactions were accompanied by cardiovascular collapse, hypotension/shock, seizure, loss of consciousness, tingling, angioedema (including tongue, laryngeal, throat or facial edema/swelling, etc.), airway obstruction (including bronchospasm, shortness of breath and acute respiratory distress), dyspnea, urticaria/hives, itching, and other serious skin reactions. A few patients had a history of hypersensitivity reactions. The drug should be discontinued immediately at the first appearance of a skin rash or any other sign of hypersensitivity. Serious acute hypersensitivity reactions may require treatment with epinephrine and other resuscitative measures, including oxygen, intravenous fluids, antihistamines, corticosteroids, pressor amines, and airway management, as clinically indicated. (See PRECAUTIONS and ADVERSE REACTIONS).

Serious and sometimes fatal events of uncertain etiology have been reported in patients receiving therapy with quinolones including, extremely rarely, ofloxacin. These events may be severe and generally occur following the administration of multiple doses. Clinical manifestations may include one or more of the following: fever, rash or severe dermatologic reactions (*e.g.,* toxic epidermal necrolysis, Stevens- Johnson Syndrome, etc.); vasculitis, arthralgia, myalgia, serum sickness; allergic pneumonitis; interstitial nephritis, acute renal insufficiency/failure; hepatitis, jaundice, acute hepatic necrosis/failure; anemia including hemolytic and aplastic, thrombocytopenia, including thrombotic thrombocytopenic purpura, leukopenia, agranulocytosis, pancytopenia, and/or other hematologic abnormalities. The drug should be discontinued immediately at the first appearance of a skin rash or any other sign of hypersensitivity and supportive measures instituted. (See PRECAUTIONS, Information for Patients and ADVERSE REACTIONS).

Convulsions, increased intracranial pressure, and toxic psychosis have been reported in patients receiving quinolones, including ofloxacin. Quinolones, including ofloxacin, may also cause central nervous system stimulation which may lead to: tremors, restlessness/agitation, nervousness/anxiety, lightheadedness, confusion, hallucinations, paranoia and depression, nightmares, insomnia, and rarely suicidal thoughts or acts. These reactions may occur following the first dose. If these reactions occur in patients receiving ofloxacin, the drug should be discontinued and appropriate measures instituted. As with all quinolones, ofloxacin should be used with caution in patients with a known or suspected CNS disorder that may predispose to seizures or lower the seizure threshold (*e.g.,* severe cerebral arteriosclerosis, epilepsy, etc.) or in the presence of other risk factors that may predispose to seizures or lower the seizure threshold (*e.g.,* certain drug therapy, renal dysfunction, etc.). See PRECAUTIONS, General, DRUG INTERACTIONS and ADVERSE REACTIONS.

Pseudomembranous colitis has been reported with nearly all antibacterial agents, including ofloxacin, and may range in severity from mild to life-threatening. Therefore, it is important to consider this diagnosis in patients who present with diarrhea subsequent to the administration of any antibacterial agents.

Treatment with antibacterial agents alters the normal flora of the colon and may permit overgrowth of clostridia. Studies indicate a toxin produced by *Clostridium difficile* is one primary cause of "antibiotic-associated colitis".

After the diagnosis of pseudomembranous colitis has been established, therapeutic measures should be initiated. Mild cases of pseudomembranous colitis usually respond to drug discontinuation alone. In moderate to severe cases, consideration should be given to management with fluids and electrolytes, protein supplementation, and treatment with an antibacterial drug clinically effective against *C. difficile* colitis. (See ADVERSE REACTIONS).

OPHTHALMIC SOLUTION

NOT FOR INJECTION.

Ofloxacin ophthalmic solution should not be injected subconjunctivally, nor should it be introduced directly into the anterior chamber of the eye.

Serious and occasionally fatal hypersensitivity (anaphylactic) reactions, some following the first dose, have been reported in patients receiving systemic quinolones, including ofloxacin. Some reactions were accompanied by cardiovascular collapse, loss of consciousness, angioedema (including laryngeal, pharyngeal or facial edema), airway obstruction, dyspnea, urticaria, and itching. A rare occurrence of Stevens-Johnson syndrome, which progressed to toxic epidermal necrolysis, has been reported in a patient who was receiving topical ophthalmic ofloxacin. If an allergic reaction to ofloxacin occurs, discontinue the drug. Serious acute hypersensitivity reactions may require immediate emergency treatment. Oxygen and airway management, including intubation should be administered as clinically indicated.

PRECAUTIONS:

GENERAL

Intravenous Infusion: Because a rapid or bolus intravenous injection may result in hypotension, **OFLOXACIN INJECTION SHOULD ONLY BE ADMINISTERED BY SLOW INTRAVENOUS INFUSION OVER A PERIOD OF 60 MINUTES.** (See DOSAGE AND ADMINISTRATION).

Tablets and Intravenous Infusion: Adequate hydration of patients receiving ofloxacin should be maintained to prevent the formation of a highly concentrated urine.

Administer ofloxacin with caution in the presence of renal or hepatic insufficiency/impairment. In patients with known or suspected renal or hepatic insufficiency/impairment, careful clinical observation and appropriate laboratory studies should be performed prior to and during therapy since elimination of ofloxacin may be reduced. In patients with impaired renal function (creatinine clearance $\leq$ 50 mg/ml), alteration of the dosage regimen is necessary. (See CLINICAL PHARMACOLOGY and DOSAGE AND ADMINISTRATION).

Moderate to severe phototoxicity reactions have been observed in patients exposed to direct sunlight while receiving some drugs in this class, including ofloxacin. Excessive sunlight should be avoided. Therapy should be discontinued if phototoxicity (*e.g.,* skin eruption, etc.) occurs.

As with all quinolones, ofloxacin should be used with caution in any patient with a known or suspected CNS disorder that may predispose to seizures or lower the seizure threshold (*e.g.,* severe cerebral arteriosclerosis, epilepsy, etc.) or in the presence of other risk factors that may predispose to seizures or lower the seizure threshold (*e.g.,* certain drug therapy, renal dysfunction, etc.). (See WARNINGS and DRUG INTERACTIONS).

As with other quinolones, disturbances of blood glucose, including symptomatic hyper- and hypoglycemia, have been reported, usually in diabetic patients receiving concomitant treatment with an oral hypoglycemic agent (*e.g.,* glyburide/glibenclamide, etc.) or with insulin. In these patients careful monitoring of blood glucose is recommended. If a hypoglycemic reaction occurs in a patient being treated with ofloxacin, discontinue ofloxacin immediately and consult a physician. (See DRUG INTERACTIONSand ADVERSE REACTIONS).

As with any potent drug, periodic assessment of organ system functions, including renal, hepatic, and hematopoietic, is advisable during prolonged therapy. (See WARNINGS and ADVERSE REACTIONS).

Ophthalmic Solution: As with other anti-infectives, prolonged use may result in overgrowth of nonsusceptible organisms, including fungi. If superinfection occurs discontinue use and institute alternative therapy. Whenever clinical judgment dictates, the patient should be

PRECAUTIONS: *(cont'd)*

examined with the aid of magnification, such as slit lamp biomicroscopy and, where appropriate, fluorescein staining. Ofloxacin should be discontinued at the first appearance of a skin rash or any other sign of hypersensitivity reaction.

The systemic administration of quinolones, including ofloxacin, has led to lesions or erosions of the cartilage in weight-bearing joints and other signs of arthropathy in immature animals of various species. Ofloxacin, administered systemically at 10 mg/kg/day in young dogs (equivalent to 110 times the maximum recommended daily *adult ophthalmic* dose) has been associated with these types of effects.

INFORMATION FOR PATIENTS

Tablets and Intravenous Infusion: Patients should be advised:

to drink fluids liberally if able to take fluids by the oral route.

that ofloxacin should not be taken with food.

Tablets and Intravenous Infusion: that ofloxacin may cause neurologic adverse effects (*e.g.*, dizziness, lightheadedness, etc.) and that patients should know how they react to ofloxacin before they operate an automobile or machinery or engage in activities requiring mental alertness and coordination. (See WARNINGS and ADVERSE REACTIONS).

that ofloxacin may be associated with hypersensitivity reactions, even following the first dose, to discontinue the drug at the first sign of a skin rash, hives or other skin reactions, a rapid heartbeat, difficulty in swallowing or breathing, any swelling suggesting angioedema (*e.g.*, swelling of the lips, tongue, face; tightness of the throat, hoarseness, etc.), or any other symptom of an allergic reaction. (See WARNINGS and ADVERSE REACTIONS).

to avoid excessive sunlight or artificial ultraviolet light while receiving ofloxacin and to discontinue therapy if phototoxicity (*e.g.*, skin eruption, etc.) occurs.

that if they are diabetic and are being treated with insulin or an oral hypoglycemic drug, to discontinue ofloxacin immediately if a hypoglycemic reaction occurs and consult a physician. See PRECAUTIONS, General and DRUG INTERACTIONS.

Tablets Only: that mineral supplements, vitamins with iron or minerals, calcium-, aluminum- or magnesium-based antacids or sucralfate should not be taken within the two-hour period before or within the two-hour period after taking ofloxacin. (See DRUG INTERACTIONS).

Ophthalmic Solution: Avoid contaminating the applicator tip with material from the eye, fingers or other source.

Systemic quinolones, including ofloxacin, have been associated with hypersensitivity reactions, even following a single dose. Discontinue use immediately and contact your physician at the first sign of a rash or allergic reaction.

CARCINOGENESIS, MUTAGENESIS, AND IMPAIRMENT OF FERTILITY

Long-term studies to determine the carcinogenic potential of ofloxacin have not been conducted.

Ofloxacin was not mutagenic in the Ames test, *in vitro* and *in vivo* cytogenetic assay, sister chromatid exchange (Chinese Hamster and human cell lines), unscheduled DNA synthesis (UDS) assay using human fibroblasts, the dominant lethal assay, or mouse micronucleus assay. Ofloxacin was positive in the UDS test using rat hepatocyte, and in the mouse lymphoma assay.

In fertility studies in rats, ofloxacin did not affect male or female fertility or morphological or reproductive performance at oral dosing up to 360 mg/kg/day (equivalent to 4000 times the maximum recommended daily ophthalmic dose).

PREGNANCY CATEGORY C

Teratogenic Effects: Ofloxacin has been shown to have an embryocidal effect in rats and in rabbits when given in doses of 810 mg/kg/day (equivalent to 9000 times the maximum recommended daily ophthalmic dose) and 160 mg/kg/day (equivalent to 1800 times the maximum recommended daily ophthalmic dose). These dosages resulted in decreased fetal body weight and increased fetal mortality in rats and rabbits, respectively. Minor fetal skeletal variations were reported in rats receiving doses of 810 mg/kg/day. Ofloxacin has not been shown to be teratogenic at doses as high as 810 mg/kg/day and 160 mg/kg/day when administered to pregnant rats and rabbits, respectively.

Nonteratogenic Effects: Additional studies in rats with doses up to 360 mg/kg/day during late gestation showed no adverse effect on late fetal development, labor, delivery, lactation, neonatal viability, or growth of the newborn.

There are, however, no adequate and well-controlled studies in pregnant women. Ofloxacin should be used during pregnancy only if the potential benefit justifies the potential risk to the fetus.

NURSING MOTHERS

In nursing women a single 200 mg oral dose of ofloxacin resulted in concentrations of ofloxacin in milk that were similar to those found in plasma. It is not known whether ofloxacin is excreted in human milk following topical ophthalmic administration. Because of the potential for serious adverse reactions from ofloxacin in nursing infants, a decision should be made whether to discontinue nursing or to discontinue the drug, taking into account the importance of the drug to the mother.

PEDIATRIC USE

Safety and effectiveness in infants below the age of one year have not been established.

Quinolones, including ofloxacin, have been shown to cause arthropathy in immature animals after oral administration; however, topical ocular administration of ofloxacin to immature animals has not shown any arthropathy. There is no evidence that the ophthalmic dosage form of ofloxacin has any effect on weight bearing joints.

DRUG INTERACTIONS:

TABLETS AND IV

Antacids, Sucralfate, Metal Cations, Multivitamins: *Tablets:* Quinolones form chelates with alkaline earth and transition metal cations. Administration of quinolones with antacids containing calcium, magnesium, or aluminum, with sucralfate, with divalent or trivalent cations such as iron, or with multivitamins containing zinc may substantially interfere with the absorption of quinolones resulting in systemic levels considerably lower than desired. These agents should not be taken within the two-hour period before or within the two-hour period after ofloxacin administration. (See DOSAGE AND ADMINISTRATION). *Intravenous Infusion:* There are no data concerning an interaction of **intravenous** quinolones with **oral** antacids, sucralfate, multi-vitamins, or metal cations. However, no quinolone should be co-administered with any solution containing multivalent cations, *e.g.*, magnesium, through the same intravenous line. (See DOSAGE AND ADMINISTRATION).

Caffeine: Interactions between ofloxacin and caffeine have not been detected.

Cimetidine: Cimetidine has demonstrated interference with the elimination of some quinolones. This interference has resulted in significant increases in half-life and AUC of some quinolones. The potential for interaction between ofloxacin and cimetidine has not been studied.

Cyclosporine: Elevated serum levels of cyclosporine have been reported with concomitant use of cyclosporine with some other quinolones. The potential for interaction between ofloxacin and cyclosporine has not been studied.

DRUG INTERACTIONS: *(cont'd)*

Drugs metabolized by Cytochrome P450 enzymes: Most quinolone antimicrobial drugs inhibit cytochrome P450 enzyme activity. This may result in a prolonged half-life for some drugs that are also metabolized by this system (*e.g.*, cyclosporine, theophylline/methylxanthines, warfarin, etc.) when co-administered with quinolones. The extent of this inhibition varies among different quinolones. (See DRUG INTERACTIONS).

Non-steroidal anti-inflammatory drugs: The concomitant administration of a non-steroidal anti-inflammatory drug, with a quinolone, including ofloxacin, may increase the risk of CNS stimulation and convulsive seizures. (See WARNINGS and PRECAUTIONS, General).

Probenecid: The concomitant use of probenecid with certain other quinolones has been reported to affect renal tubular secretion. The effect of probenecid on the elimination of ofloxacin has not been studied.

Theophylline: Although concurrent administration of some quinolones with theophylline may result in impaired elimination of theophylline, the extent of such impairment varies among different quinolones. Steady-state theophylline levels may increase when ofloxacin and theophylline are administered concurrently. In a pharmacokinetic study involving 15 healthy male subjects, steady-state peak theophylline concentration increased by an average of approximately 9%, and the AUC increased by an average of approximately 13% when oral ofloxacin and theophylline were administered concurrently. In clinical trials with intravenous ofloxacin, theophylline concentrations were determined in 41 patients who were treated with both drugs. In 38 patients, no apparent elevation in the serum theophylline was discernible. Marginal increases above the theophylline therapeutic range were reported in 3 patients; clinical toxicity was, however, not reported in these three patients. Generally, patients receiving theophylline in clinical trials of the intravenous formulation of ofloxacin reported nausea more frequently than those patients not receiving theophylline. As with some other quinolones, concomitant administration of ofloxacin may prolong the half-life of theophylline, elevate serum theophylline levels, and may increase the risk of theophylline-related adverse reactions. Theophylline levels should be closely monitored and theophylline dosage adjustments made, if appropriate, when ofloxacin is co-administered.

Warfarin: Some quinolones have been reported to enhance the effects of the oral anticoagulant warfarin or its derivatives. Therefore, if a quinolone antimicrobial is administered concomitantly with warfarin or its derivatives, the prothrombin time or other suitable coagulation test should be closely monitored.

Antidiabetic agents (*e.g.*, insulin, glyburide/glibenclamide, etc.): Since disturbances of blood glucose, including hyperglycemia and hypoglycemia, have been reported in patients treated concurrently with quinolones and an antidiabetic agent, careful monitoring of blood glucose is recommended when these agents are used concomitantly. (See PRECAUTIONS, General and Information for Patients).

OPHTHALMIC SOLUTION

Specific drug interaction studies have not been conducted with oflaxacin ophthalmic solution. However, the systemic administration of some quinolones has been shown to elevate plasma concentrations of theophylline, interfere with the metabolism of caffeine, and enhance the effects of the oral anticoagulant warfarin and its derivatives, and has been associated with transient elevations in serum creatinine in patients receiving cyclosporine concomitantly.

ADVERSE REACTIONS:

TABLETS AND INTRAVENOUS INFUSION

The following is a compilation of the data for ofloxacin based on clinical experience with both the oral and intravenous formulations. The incidence of drug-related adverse reactions in patients during Phase 2 and 3 clinical trials was 11%. Among patients receiving multiple-dose therapy, 4% discontinued ofloxacin due to adverse experiences.

In clinical trials, the following events were considered likely to be drug-related in patients receiving multiple doses of ofloxacin: nausea 3%, insomnia 3%, headache 1%, dizziness 1%, diarrhea 1%, vomiting 1%, rash 1%, pruritus 1%, external genital pruritus in women 1%, vaginitis 1%, dysgeusia 1%.

In clinical trials, the most frequently reported adverse events, regardless of relationship to drug, were: nausea 10%, headache 9%, insomnia 7%, external genital pruritus in women 6%, dizziness 5%, vaginitis 5%, diarrhea 4%, vomiting 4%.

In clinical trials, the following events, regardless of relationship to drug, occurred in 1 to 3% of patients: Abdominal pain and cramps, chest pain, decreased appetite, dry mouth, dysgeusia, fatigue, flatulence, gastrointestinal distress, nervousness, pharyngitis, pruritus, fever, rash, sleep disorders, somnolence, trunk pain, vaginal discharge, visual disturbances, and constipation.

Additional events, occurring in clinical trials at a rate of less than 1%, regardless of relationship to drug, were:

Body as a whole: asthenia, chills, malaise, extremity pain, pain, epistaxis

Cardiovascular System: cardiac arrest, edema, hypertension, hypotension, palpitations, vasodilation

Gastrointestinal System: dyspepsia

Genital/Reproductive System: burning, irritation, pain and rash of the female genitalia, dysmenorrhea, menorrhagia, metrorrhagia

Musculoskeletal System: arthralgia, myalgia

Nervous System: seizures, anxiety, cognitive change, depression, dream abnormality, euphoria, hallucinations, paresthesia, syncope, vertigo, tremor, confusion

Nutritional/Metabolic: thirst, weight loss

Respiratory System: respiratory arrest, cough, rhinorrhea

Skin/Hypersensitivity: angiodema, diaphoresis, urticaria, vasculitis

Urinary System: dysuria, urinary frequency, urinary retention

The following laboratory abnormalities appeared in $\geq$ 1.0% of patients receiving multiple doses of ofloxacin. It is not known whether these abnormalities were caused by the drug or the underlying conditions being treated.

Hematopoietic: anemia, leukopenia, leukocytosis, neutropenia, neutrophilia, increased band forms, lymphocytopenia, eosinophilia, lymphocytosis, thrombocytopenia, thrombocytosis, elevated ESR

Hepatic: elevated: alkaline phosphatase, AST (SGOT), ALT (SGPT)

Serum chemistry: hyperglycemia, hypoglycemia, elevated creatinine, elevated BUN

Urinary: glucosuria, proteinuria, alkalinuria, hyposthenuria, hematuria, pyuria

Post-Marketing Adverse Events: Additional adverse events, regardless of relationship to drug, reported from worldwide marketing experience with quinolones, including ofloxacin:

Clinical

Cardiovascular System: cerebral thrombosis, pulmonary edema, tachycardia, hypotension/shock, syncope

Endocrine/Metabolic: hyper- or hypoglycemia, especially in diabetic patients on insulin or oral hypoglycemic agents (see PRECAUTIONS, General and DRUG INTERACTIONS).

ADVERSE REACTIONS: *(cont'd)*

Gastrointestinal System: hepatic dysfunction including: hepatic necrosis, jaundice (cholestatic or hepatocellular), hepatitis; instestinal perforation; pseudomembranous colitis, GI hemorrhage; hiccough, painful oral mucosa, pyrosis (see WARNINGS).

Genital/Reproductive System: vaginal candidiasis

Hematopoietic: anemia, including hemolytic and aplastic; hemorrhage, pancytopenia, agranulocytosis, leukopenia, reversible bone marrow depression, thrombocytopenia, thrombotic thrombocytopenic purpura, petechiae, ecchymosis/burning (see WARNINGS).

Musculoskeletal: tendinitis/rupture: weakness

Nervous System: nightmares; suicidal thoughts or acts, disorientation, psychotic reactions, paranoia; phobia, agitation, restlessness, agreesiveness/hostility, manic reaction, emotional lability; peripheral neuropathy, ataxia, incoordination; possible exacerbation of: myasthenia gravis and extrapyramidal disorders; dysphasia, lightheadedness (See WARNINGS and PRECAUTIONS).

Respiratory System: dyspnea, bronchospasm, allergic pneumonitis, stridor (see WARNINGS).

Skin/Hypersensitivity: anaphylactic (-toid) reactions/shock; purpura, serum sickness, erythema multiforme/Stevens-Johnson Syndrome, erythema nodosum, exfoliative dermatitis, hyperpigmentation, toxic epidermal necrolysis, conjunctivitis, photosensitivity, vesiculobullous eruption (see WARNINGS and PRECAUTIONS).

Special Senses: diplopia, nystagmus, blurred vision, disturbances of: taste, smell, hearing and equilibrium, usually reversible following discontinuation.

Urinary System: anuria, polyuria, renal calculi, renal failure, interstitial nephritis, hematuria (see WARNINGS and PRECAUTIONS).

Laboratory

Hematopoietic: prolongation of prothrombin time.

Serum chemistry: acidosis, elevation of: serum triglycerides, serum cholesterol, serum potassium, liver function tests including: GGTP, LDH, bilirubin.

Urinary: albuminuria, candiduria.

In clinical trials using multiple-dose therapy, ophthalmologic abnormalities, including cataracts and multiple punctate lenticular opacities, have been noted in patients undergoing treatment with other quinolones. The relationship of the drugs to these events is not presently established.

CRYSTALLURIA and CYLINDRURIA HAVE BEEN REPORTED with other quinolones.

Intravenous Infusion: Local injection site reactions (phlebitis, swelling, erythema) were reported in approximately 2% of patients treated with the 3.63 mg/ml final infusion concentration of intravenous ofloxacin used in the clinical safety trials. The final infusion concentration of intravenous ofloxacin in the commercially available intravenous preparations is 4.0 mg/ml. To date, individuals administered the 4.0 mg/ml concentration of the intravenous ofloxacin have demonstrated clinically acceptable rates of local injection site reactions. Due to the small difference in concentration, significant differences in local site reactions are unexpected with the 4.0 mg/ml concentration.

OPHTHALMIC SOLUTION

The most frequently reported drug-related adverse reaction was transient ocular burning or discomfort. Other reported reactions include stinging, redness, itching, chemical conjunctivitis/keratitis, periocular/facial edema, foreign body sensation, photophobia, blurred vision, tearing, dryness, and eye pain. Rare reports of dizziness have been received.

OVERDOSAGE:

TABLETS AND INTRAVENOUS INFUSION

Information on overdosage with ofloxacin is limited. One incident of accidental overdosage has been reported. In this case, an adult female received 3 grams of ofloxacin intravenously over 45 minutes. A blood sample obtained 15 minutes after the completion of the infusion revealed an ofloxacin level of 39.4 mcg/ml. In 7 h, the level had fallen to 16.2 mcg/ml, and by 24 h to 2.7 mcg/ml. During the infusion, the patient developed drowsiness, nausea, dizziness, hot and cold flushes, subjective facial swelling and numbness, slurring of speech, and mild to moderate disorientation. All complaints except the dizziness subsided within 1 h after discontinuation of the infusion. The dizziness, most bothersome while standing, resolved in approximately 9 h. Laboratory testing reportedly revealed no clinically significant changes in routine parameters in this patient.

In the event of an acute overdose, the stomach should be emptied. The patient should be observed and appropriate hydration maintained. Ofloxacin is not efficiently removed by hemodialysis or peritoneal dialysis.

DOSAGE AND ADMINISTRATION:

TABLETS

The usual dose of ofloxacin tablets are 200 mg to 400 mg orally every 12 h as described in the dosing chart (TABLE 6). These recommendations apply to patients with normal renal function (*i.e.,* creatinine clearance > 50 ml/min). For patients with altered renal function (*i.e.,* creatinine clearance ≤ 50 ml/min), see the Patients with Impaired Renal Function subsection.

INTRAVENOUS INFUSION

Ofloxacin IV should only be administered by **intravenous** infusion. It is not for intramuscular, intrathecal, intraperitoneal, or subcutaneous administration.

CAUTION: RAPID OR BOLUS INTRAVENOUS INFUSION MUST BE AVOIDED.

Ofloxacin injection should be infused intravenously slowly over a period of not less than 60 minutes. (See PRECAUTIONS).

Single-use vials require dilution prior to administration. (See DOSAGE AND ADMINISTRATION, Preparation for Administration).

The usual dose of ofloxacin injection IV is 200 mg to 400 mg administered by slow infusion over 60 minutes every 12 h as described in the dosing chart (TABLE 6). These recommendations apply to patients with mild to moderate infection and normal renal function (*i.e.,* creatinine clearance > 50 ml/min). For patients with altered renal function (*i.e.,* creatinine clearance ≤ 50 ml/min), see the Patients with Impaired Renal Function subsection.

TABLETS AND INTRAVENOUS INFUSION

TABLETS

Antacids containing calcium, magnesium, or aluminum; sucralfate; divalent or trivalent cations such as iron; or multivitamins containing zinc should not be taken within the two-hour period before, or within the two- hour period after ofloxacin administrations. (See PRECAUTIONS).

TABLETS AND INTRAVENOUS INFUSION

Patients with Impaired Renal Function: Dosage should be adjusted for patients with a creatinine clearance ≤ 50 ml/min.

After a normal initial dose, dosage should be adjusted as follows (TABLE 7):

When only the serum creatinine is known, the formula (TABLE 8) may be used to estimate creatinine clearance.

DOSAGE AND ADMINISTRATION: *(cont'd)*

TABLE 6 Patients with Normal Renal Function

Infection	Description*	Unit Daily Dose	Frequency	Duration	Dose
Lower Respiratory	Exacerbation of Chronic Bronchitis	400 mg	q12h	10 days	800 mg
Tract	Com. Acq. Pneumonia	400 mg	q12h	10 days	800 mg
Skin and Skin	Uncomplicated infections	400 mg	q12h	10 days	800 mg
Structures Sexually Transmitted Diseases	Acute, uncomplicated gonorrhea	400 mg	single dose	1 day	400 mg
	Cervicitis/ urethritis due to *C. trachomatis*	300 mg	q12h	7 days	600 mg
	Cervicitis/ urethritis due to *C. trachomatis* and *N. gonorrhoeae*	300 mg	q12h	7 days	600 mg
Urinary Tract	Cystitis due to *E. coli* or *K. pneumoniae*	200 mg	q12h	3 days	400 mg
	Cystitis due to other approved pathogens	200 mg	q12h	7 days	400 mg
	Complicated UTI's	200 mg	q12h	10 days	400 mg
Prostate	Prostatitis due to *E. coli*	300 mg	q12h	6 wks**	600 mg

* DUE TO THE DESIGNATED PATHOGENS (See INDICATIONS AND USAGE).
** BECAUSE THERE ARE NO SAFETY DATA PRESENTLY AVAILABLE TO SUPPORT THE USE OF THE INTRAVENOUS FORMULATION OF OFLOXACIN FOR MORE THAN 10 DAYS, THERAPY AFTER 10 DAYS SHOULD BE SWITCHED TO THE ORAL TABLET FORMULATION OR OTHER APPROPRIATE THERAPY.

TABLE 7

Creatinine Clearance	Maintenance Dose	Frequency
10-50 ml/min	the usual recommended unit dose	q24h
< 10 ml/min	1/2 the usual recommended unit dose	q24h

TABLE 8 Creatinine clearance (ml/min)

Men: [Weight (kg) × (140-age)] ÷ [72 × serum creatinine (mg/dl)]
Women: 0.85 × the value calculated for men.
The serum creatinine should represent a steady-state of renal function.

Patients with Cirrhosis: The excretion of ofloxacin may be reduced in patients with severe liver function disorders (*e.g.,* cirrhosis with or without ascites). A maximum dose of 400 mg of ofloxacin per day should therefore not be exceeded.

OPHTHALMIC SOLUTION

The recommended dosage regimen for the treatment of **bacterial conjunctivitis** is:

Days 1 and 2: Instill one to two drops every two to four hours in the affected eye(s).

Days 3 through 7: Instill one to two drops four times daily.

The recommended dosage regimen for the treatment of **bacterial corneal ulcer** is:

Days 1 and 2: Instill one to two drops into the affected eye every 30 minutes, while awake. Awaken at approximately four and six hours after retiring and instill one to two drops.

Days 3 through 7 to 9: Instill one to two drops hourly, while awake.

Days 7 to 9 through treatment completion: Instill one to two drops, four times daily.

PREPARATION OF OFLOXACIN INJECTION FOR ADMINISTRATION

Ofloxacin IV in Single-Use Vials: Ofloxacin IV is supplied in single- use vials containing a concentrated ofloxacin solution with the equivalent of 400 mg of ofloxacin in Water for Injection. The 10 ml vials contain 40 mg of ofloxacin/ml and the 20 ml vials contain 20 mg of ofloxacin/ml. **THESE OFLOXACIN IV SINGLE-USE VIALS MUST BE FURTHER DILUTED WITH AN APPROPRIATE SOLUTION PRIOR TO INTRAVENOUS ADMINISTRATION.** (See DOSAGE AND ADMINISTRATION, Compatible Intravenous Solutions). The concentration of the resulting diluted solution should be 4 mg/ml prior to administration.

This parenteral drug product should be inspected visually for discoloration and particulate matter prior to administration.

Since no preservative or bacteriostatic agent is present in this product, aseptic technique must be used in preparation of the final parenteral solution. **Since the vials are for single-use only, any unused portion should be discarded.**

Since only limited data are available on the compatibility of ofloxacin intravenous injection with other intravenous substances, **additives or other medications should not be added to ofloxacin IV in single-use vials or infused simultaneously through the same intravenous line.** If the same intravenous line is used for sequential infusion of several different drugs, the line should be flushed before and after infusion of ofloxacin IV with an infusion solution compatible with ofloxacin IV and with any other drug(s) administrated via this common line.

Prepare the desired dosage of ofloxacin according to TABLE 9.

TABLE 9

Desired Dosage Strength	From 10 ml Vial, Withdraw Volume	From 20 ml Vial, Withdraw Volume	Volume of Diluent	Infusion Time
200 mg	5 ml	10 ml	qs 50 ml	60 min
300 mg	7.5 ml	15 ml	qs 75 ml	60 min
400 mg	10 ml	20 ml	qs 100 ml	60 min

For example, to prepare a 200-mg dose using the 10 ml vial (40 mg/ml), withdraw 5 ml and dilute with a compatible intravenous solution to a total volume of 50 ml.

Compatible Intravenous Solutions: Any of the intravenous solutions listed in TABLE 10 may be used to prepare a 4 mg/ml ofloxacin solution with the appropriate pH values:

DOSAGE AND ADMINISTRATION: *(cont'd)*

TABLE 10

Intravenous Fluids	pH of 4 mg/ml Floxin IV Solution
0.9% Sodium Chloride Injection, USP	4.69
5% Dextrose Injection, USP	4.57
5% Dextrose/0.9% NaCl Injection	4.56
5% Dextrose in Lactated Ringers	4.94
5% Sodium Bicarbonate Injection	7.95
Plasma-Lyte 56/5% Dextrose Injection	5.02
5% Dextrose, 0.45% Sodium Chloride, and 0.15% Potassium Chloride Injection	4.64
Sodium Lactate Injection (M/6)	5.64
Water for Injection	4.66

Ofloxacin IV Pre-Mixed in Single-Use Bottles: Ofloxacin IV is also supplied in 100 ml bottles containing a pre-mixed, ready-to-use ofloxacin solution in D_5W for single-use. **NO FURTHER DILUTION OF THIS PREPARATION IS NECESSARY. Each 100 ml pre-mixed bottle already contains a dilute solution with the equivalent of 400 mg of ofloxacin (4 mg/ml) in 5% Dextrose (D_5W).**

This parenteral drug product should be inspected visually for discoloration and particulate matter prior to administration.

Since no preservative or bacteriostatic agent is present in this product, aseptic technique must be used in preparation of the final parenteral solution. **Since the pre-mixed bottles are for single-use only, any unused portion should be discarded.**

Since only limited data are available on the compatibility of ofloxacin intravenous injection with other intravenous substances, **additives or other medications should not be added to ofloxacin IV in pre-mixed single- use bottles or infused simultaneously through the same intravenous line.** If the same intravenous line is used for sequential infusion of several different drugs, the line should be flushed before and after infusion of ofloxacin IV with an infusion solution compatible with ofloxacin IV and with any other drug(s) administrated via this common line.

Ofloxacin IV Pre-Mixed in Single-Use Flexible Containers: Ofloxacin IV is also supplied in 50 ml and 100 ml flexible containers containing a pre-mixed, ready-to-use ofloxacin solution in D_5W for single-use.**NO FURTHER DILUTION OF THIS PREPARATION IS NECESSARY. Each 50 ml pre- mixed flexible container already contains a dilute solution with the equivalent of 200 mg of ofloxacin (4 mg/ml) in 5% Dextrose (D_5W). Each 100 ml pre-mixed flexible container already contains a dilute solution with the equivalent of 400 mg of ofloxacin (4 mg/ml) in 5% Dextrose (D_5W).**

This parenteral drug product should be inspected visually for discoloration and particulate matter prior to administration.

Since no preservative or bacteriostatic agent is present in this product, aseptic technique must be used in preparation of the final parenteral solution. **Since the pre-mixed flexible containers are for single-use only, any unused portion should be discarded.**

Since only limited data are available on the compatibility of ofloxacin intravenous injection with other intravenous substances, **additives or other medications should not be added to ofloxacin IV in flexible containers or infused simultaneously through the same intravenous line.**If the same intravenous line is used for sequential infusion of several different drugs, the line should be flushed before and after infusion of ofloxacin IV with an infusion solution compatible with ofloxacin IV and with any other drug(s) administrated via this common line.

INSTRUCTIONS FOR THE USE OF OFLOXACIN IV PRE-MIXED IN FLEXIBLE CONTAINERS:

To open:

1. Tear outer wrap at the notch and remove solution container.

2. Check the container for minute leaks by squeezing the inner bag firmly. If leaks are found, or if the seal is not intact, discard the solution, as the sterility may be compromised.

3. Do not use if the solution is cloudy or a precipitate is present.

4. Use sterile equipment.

5. WARNING: Do not use flexible containers in series connections. Such use could result in air embolism due to residual air being drawn from the primary container before administration of the fluid from the secondary container is complete.

Preparation for administration:

1. Close flow control clamp of administration set.

2. Remove cover from port at bottom of container.

3. Insert piercing pin of administration set into port with a twisting motion until the pin is firmly seated. **NOTE: See full directions on administration set carton.**

4. Suspend container from hanger.

5. Squeeze and release drip chamber to establish proper fluid level in chamber during infusion of Ofloxacin IV in Pre-Mixed Flexible Containers.

6. Open flow control clamp to expel air from set. Close clamp.

7. Regulate rate of administration with flow control clamp.

Stability of Ofloxacin IV as Supplied: When stored under recommended conditions, ofloxacin IV, as supplied in 10 ml and 20 ml vials, 100 ml bottles, and 50 ml and 100 ml flexible containers, is stable through the expiration date printed on the label.

Stability of Ofloxacin IV Following Dilution: Ofloxacin IV, when diluted in a compatible intravenous fluid to a concentration between 0.4 mg/ml and 4 mg/ml, is stable for 72 h when stored at or below 75°F or 24°C and for 14 days when stored under refrigeration at 41°F or 5°C in glass bottles or plastic intravenous containers. Solutions that are diluted in a compatible intravenous solution and frozen in glass bottles or plastic intravenous containers are stable for 6 months when stored at -4°F or - 20°C. Once thawed, the solution is stable for up to 14 days, if refrigerated at 36°F to 46°F (2°C to 8°C). **THAW FROZEN SOLUTIONS AT ROOM TEMPERATURE (77°F OR 25°C) OR IN A REFRIGERATOR (46°F OR 8°C). DO NOT FORCE THAW BY MICROWAVE IRRADIATION OR WATER BATH IMMERSION. DO NOT RE-FREEZE AFTER INITIAL THAWING.**

OPHTHALMIC SOLUTION

The recommended dosage regimen for the treatment of **bacterial conjunctivitis** is: *Days 1 and 2* :Instill one to two drops every two to four hours in the affected eye(s). *Days 3 through 7:* Instill one to two drops four times daily.

The recommended dosage regimen for the treatment of **bacterial corneal ulcer** is: *Days 1 and 2:* Instill one to two drops into the affected eye every 30 minutes, while awake. Awaken at approximately four and six hours after retiring and instill one to two drops. *Days 3 through 7 to 9:* Instill one to two drops hourly, while awake. *Days 7 to 9 through treatment completion:* Instill one to two drops, four times daily.

ANIMAL PHARMACOLOGY:

TABLETS AND INTRAVENOUS INFUSION

Ofloxacin, as well as other drugs of the quinolone class, has been shown to cause arthropathies (arthrosis) in immature dogs and rats. In addition, these drugs are associated with an increased incidence of osteochondrosis in rats as compared to the incidence observed in vehicle- treated rats. (See WARNINGS). There is no evidence of arthropathies in fully mature dogs at intravenous doses up to 3 times the recommended maximum human dose (on a mg/m² basis or 5 times based on a mg/kg basis), for a one-week exposure period.

Long-term, high-dose systemic use of other quinolones in experimental animals has caused lenticular opacities; however, this finding was not observed in any animal studies with ofloxacin.

Reduced serum globulin and protein levels were observed in animals treated with other quinolones. In one ofloxacin study, minor decreases in serum globulin and protein levels were noted in female cynomolgus monkeys dosed orally with 40 mg/kg ofloxacin daily for one year. These changes, however, were considered to be within normal limits for monkeys.

Crystalluria and ocular toxicity were not observed in any animals treated with ofloxacin.

REFERENCES:

1. National Committee for Clinical Laboratory Standards,Performance Standards for Antimicrobial Disk Susceptibility Tests— Fourth Edition. Approved Standard NCCLS Document M2-A4, Vol. 10, No. 7, NCCLS, Villanova, PA, 1990. **2.** National Committee for Clinical Laboratory Standards, Methods for Dilution Antimicrobial Susceptibility Tests for Bacteria that Grow Aerobically Second Edition. Approved Standard NCCLS Document M7-A2, Vol. 10, No. 8, NCCLS, Villanova, PA, 1990.

PATIENT INFORMATION:

Oflaxacin is an antibiotic used to treat a variety of infections. It should be used with extreme caution in children and pregnant women. Allergies to this drug have been reports. If you experience a skin rash, hives or difficulty breathing, discontinue the medication and call your physician. Ofloxacin interacts with mineral supplements, vitamins with iron or minerals, calcium-, aluminum- or magnesium-based antacids or sucralfate. Wait at least two hours before taking vitamins or antacids after taking oflaxacin. Ofloxacin should not be taken with food although you are encouraged to drink a lot of fluid. Oflaxacin may cause lightheadedness or dizziness. Take the first dose at home and use caution when operating machinery or driving. Ofloxacin may make your skin more sensitive to the sun. Use appropriate sunscreen and clothing protection while taking this medication. This medication is an antibiotic and should be taken for the full period of time it has been prescribed for. Even if your symptoms improve, continue to take all of the medication.

HOW SUPPLIED:

TABLETS

Floxin tablets are supplied as 200 mg light yellow, 300 mg white, and 400 mg pale gold flim-coated tablets. Each tablet is distinguished by "Floxin" and the appropriate strength. Floxin Tablets are packaged in bottles of 50 tablets (200 mg and 300 mg), 100 tablets (400 mg), and in unit-dose blister strips of 100 tablets.

Floxin Tablets should be stored in well-closed containers. Store below 86°F (30°C).

INTRAVENOUS INFUSION

Single-Use Vials: Floxin (ofloxacin injection) IV is supplied in single-use vials. Each vial contains a concentrated solution with the equivalent of 400 mg of ofloxacin.

Pre-Mixed in Bottles: Floxin (ofloxacin injection) IV pre-mixed in bottles is supplied in 100 ml, single-use, pre-mixed bottles. Each bottle contains a dilute solution with the equivalent of 400 mg of ofloxacin in 5% Dextrose (D_5W).

Pre-Mixed in Flexible Containers: Floxin (ofloxacin injection) IV pre-mixed in flexible containers is supplied as a single-use, pre-mixed solution in 50 ml and 100 ml flexible containers. Each contains a dilute solution with the equivalent of 200 mg or 400 mg of ofloxacin, respectively, in 5% Dextrose (D_5W).

Floxin (ofloxacin injection) IV in single-use vials and pre-mixed in bottles should be stored at controlled room temperature 59°F to 86°F (15°C to 30°C) and protected from light. Floxin IV pre-mixed in flexible containers should be stored at or below 77°F or 25°C; however, brief exposure up to 104°F or 40°C does not adversely affect the product. Avoid excessive heat and protect from freezing and light.

OPHTHALMIC SOLUTION

OCUFLOX 0.3% is supplied sterile in plastic dropper bottles in 1 ml, 5 ml, and 10 ml sizes.

Note: Store at 15-25° C (59-77° F).

HOW SUPPLIED - EQUIVALENTS NOT AVAILABLE:

Injection, Solution - Intravenous - 4 mg/ml

50 ml	$13.80	FLOXIN I.V., Ortho Pharm	00062-1553-01

Injection, Solution - Intravenous - 20 mg/ml

20 ml	$26.40	FLOXIN I.V., Ortho Pharm	00062-1551-01

Injection, Solution - Intravenous - 40 mg/ml

10 ml	$26.40	FLOXIN I.V., Ortho Pharm	00062-1550-01

Solution - Ophthalmic - 0.3 %

5 ml	$18.28	OCUFLOX, Allergan-Amer	11980-0779-05

Tablet, Plain Coated - Oral - 200 mg

50's	$152.86	FLOXIN 200, Ortho Pharm	00062-1540-02
100's	$307.81	FLOXIN 200, Ortho Pharm	00062-1540-05

Tablet, Plain Coated - Oral - 300 mg

50's	$181.92	FLOXIN 300, Ortho Pharm	00062-1541-02
100's	$366.08	FLOXIN 300, Ortho Pharm	00062-1541-05

Tablet, Plain Coated - Oral - 400 mg

100's	$383.71	FLOXIN, Ortho Pharm	00062-1542-01
100's	$386.15	FLOXIN 400, Ortho Pharm	00062-1542-05

OLANZAPINE *(003301)*

CATEGORIES: Antipsychotics/Antimanics; Benzodiazepines; Pregnancy Category C; Psychotic Disorders; Schizophrenia; FDA Approved 1996 Sep

BRAND NAMES: **Zyprexa**

DESCRIPTION:

Olanzapine is an antipsychotic agent that belongs to the thienobenzodiazepine class. The chemical designation is 2-methyl-4-(4-methyl-1-piperazinyl)-l *OH*-thieno[2,3-*b*] [1,5] benzodiazepine. The molecular formula is $C_{17}H_{20}N_4S$, which corresponds to a molecular weight of 312.44.

Olanzapine is a yellow crystalline solid, which is practically insoluble in water.

Olanzapine tablets are intended for oral administration only.

DESCRIPTION: *(cont'd)*

Each Zyprexa tablet contains olanzapine equivalent to 5 mg (16 µmol), 7.5 mg (24 µmol), or 10 mg (32µmol). Inactive ingredients are carnuba wax, color mixture white, crospovidone, FD&C Blue No. 2 Aluminum Lake, hydroxypropyl cellulose, hydroxypropyl methylcellulose, lactose, magnesium stearate, microcrystalline cellulose, and other inactive ingredients.

CLINICAL PHARMACOLOGY:

PHARMACODYNAMICS

Olanzapine is a selective monoaminergic antagonist with high affinity binding to the following receptors: serotonin $5HT_{2A/2C}$ (K_i=4 and 11 nM, respectively), dopamine D_{1-4} (K_i 11- 31 nM), muscarinic M_{1-5} (K_i=1.9-25 nM), histamine H_1 (K_i=7 nM), and adrenergic α_1 receptors (K_i=19 nM). Olanzapine binds weakly to $GABA_A$, BZD, and β adrenergic receptors (K_i>10 µM).

The mechanism of action of olanzapine, as with other antipsychotic drugs, is unknown. However, it has been proposed that this drug's antipsychotic activity is mediated through a combination of dopamine and serotonin type 2 ($5HT_2$) antagonism. Antagonism at receptors other than dopamine and $5HT_2$ with similar receptor affinities may explain some of the other therapeutic and side effects of olanzapine. Olanzapine's antagonism of muscarinic M_{1-5} receptors may explain its anticholinergic effects. Olanzapine's antagonism of histamine H_1 receptors may explain the somnolence observed with this drug. Olanzapine's antagonism of adrenergic α_1 receptors may explain the orthostatic hypotension observed with this drug.

PHARMACOKINETICS

Olanzapine is well absorbed and reaches peak concentrations in approximately 6 hours following an oral dose. It is eliminated extensively by first pass metabolism, with approximately 40% of the dose metabolized before reaching the systemic circulation. Food does not affect the rate or extent of olanzapine absorption.

Olanzapine displays linear kinetics over the clinical dosing range. Its half-life ranges from 21 to 54 hours (5th to 95th percentile; mean of 30 hr), and apparent plasma clearance ranges from 12 to 47 L/hr (5th to 95th percentile; mean of 25 L/hr).

Administration of olanzapine once daily leads to steady-state concentrations in about one week that are approximately twice the concentrations after single doses. Plasma concentrations, half life, and clearance of olanzapine may vary between individuals on the basis of smoking status, gender, and age (see Special Populations).

Olanzapine is extensively distributed throughout the body, with a volume of distribution of approximately 1000 L. It is 93% bound to plasma proteins over the concentration range of 7 to 1100 ng/ml, binding primarily to albumin and α_1-acid glycoprotein.

METABOLISM AND ELIMINATION

Following a single oral dose of ^{14}C labeled olanzapine, 7% of the dose of olanzapine was recovered in the urine as unchanged drug, indicating that olanzapine is highly metabolized. Approximately 57% and 30% of the dose was recovered in the urine and feces, respectively. In the plasma, olanzapine accounted for only 12% of the AUC for total radioactivity, indicating significant exposure to metabolites. After multiple dosing, the major circulating metabolites were the 10-N-glucuronide, present at steady state at 44% of the concentration of olanzapine, and 4'-N-desmethyl olanzapine, present at steady state at 31% of the concentration of olanzapine. Both metabolites lack pharmacological activity at the concentrations observed.

Direct glucuronidation and cytochrome P450 (CYP) mediated oxidation are the primary metabolic pathways for olanzapine. *In vitro* studies suggest that CYPs lA2 and 2D6, and the flavin-containing monooxygenase system are involved in olanzapine oxidation. CYP2D6 mediated oxidation appears to be a minor metabolic pathway *in vivo*, because the clearance of olanzapine is not reduced in subjects who are deficient in this enzyme.

SPECIAL POPULATIONS

Renal Impairment: Because olanzapine is highly metabolized before excretion and only 7% of the drug is excreted unchanged, renal dysfunction alone is unlikely to have a major impact on the pharmacokinetics of olanzapine. The pharmacokinetic characteristics of olanzapine were similar in patients with severe renal impairment and normal subjects, indicating that dosage adjustment based upon the degree of renal impairment is not required. In addition, olanzapine is not removed by dialysis. The effect of renal impairment on metabolite elimination has not been studied.

Hepatic Impairment: Although the presence of hepatic impairment may be expected to reduce the clearance of olanzapine, a study of the effect of impaired liver function in subjects (n=6) with clinically significant (Childs Pugh Classification A and B) cirrhosis revealed little effect on the pharmacokinetics of olanzapine.

Age: In a study involving 24 healthy subjects, the mean elimination half-life of olanzapine was about 1.5 times greater in elderly (>65 years) than in non-elderly subjects (≤65 years). Caution should be used in dosing the elderly, especially if there are other factors that might additively influence drug metabolism and/or pharmacodynamic sensitivity (see DOSAGE AND ADMINISTRATION).

Gender: Clearance of olanzapine is approximately 30% lower in women than in men. There were, however, no apparent differences between men and women in effectiveness or adverse effects. Dosage modifications based on gender should not be needed.

Smoking Status: Olanzapine clearance is about 40% higher in smokers than in nonsmokers, although dosage modifications are not routinely recommended.

Race: No specific pharmacokinetic study was conducted to investigate the effects of race. A cross-study comparison between data obtained in Japan and data obtained in the US suggests that exposure to olanzapine may be about 2-fold greater in the Japanese when equivalent doses are administered. Clinical trial safety and efficacy data, however, did not suggest clinically significant differences among Caucasian patients, patients of African descent, and a third pooled category including Asian and Hispanic patients. Dosage modifications for race are, therefore, not recommended.

Combined Effects: The combined effects of age, smoking, and gender could lead to substantial pharmacokinetic differences in populations. The clearance in young smoking males, for example, may be 3 times higher than that in elderly nonsmoking females. Dosing modification may be necessary in patients who exhibit a combination of factors that may result in slower metabolism of olanzapine (see DOSAGE AND ADMINISTRATION).

CLINICAL STUDIES:

Clinical Efficacy Data: The efficacy of olanzapine in the management of the manifestations of psychotic disorders was established in 2 short-term (6-week) controlled trials of psychotic inpatients who met DSM III-R criteria for schizophrenia. A single haloperidol arm was included as a comparative treatment in one of the two trials, but this trial did not compare these two drugs on the full range of clinically relevant doses for both.

Several instruments were used for assessing psychiatric signs and symptoms in these studies, among them the Brief Psychiatric Rating Scale (BPRS), a multi-item inventory of general psychopathology traditionally used to evaluate the effects of drug treatment in psychosis. The BPRS psychosis cluster (conceptual disorganization, hallucinatory behavior, suspiciousness, and unusual thought content) is considered a particularly useful subset for assessing actively psychotic schizophrenic patients. A second traditional assessment, the Clinical Global Impression (CGI), reflects the impression of a skilled observer, fully familiar with the manifestations

CLINICAL STUDIES: *(cont'd)*

of schizophrenia, about the overall clinical state of the patient. In addition, two more recently developed but less well evaluated scales were employed; these included the 30 item Positive and Negative Symptoms Scale (PANSS), in which is embedded the 18 items of the BPRS, and the Scale for Assessing Negative Symptoms (SANS). The trial summaries below focus on the following outcomes: PANSS total and/or BPRS total; BPRS psychosis cluster; PANSS negative subscale or SANS; and CGI Severity. The results of the trials follow:

(1) In a 6-week, placebo-controlled trial (n=149) involving two fixed olanzapine doses of 1 and 10 mg/day (once daily schedule), olanzapine, at 10 mg/day (but not at 1 mg/day), was superior to placebo on the PANSS total score (also on the extracted BPRS total), on the BPRS psychosis cluster, on the PANSS Negative subscale, and on CGI Severity.

(2) In a 6-week, placebo-controlled trial (n=253) involving 3 fixed dose ranges of olanzapine (5.0 ± 2.5 mg/day, 10.0 ± 2.5 mg/day, and 15.0 ± 2.5 mg/day) on a once daily schedule, the two highest olanzapine dose groups (actual mean doses of 12 and 16 mg/day, respectively) were superior to placebo on BPRS total score, BPRS psychosis cluster, and CGI severity score; the highest olanzapine dose group was superior to placebo on the SANS. There was no clear advantage for the high dose group over the medium dose group.

Examination of population subsets (race and gender) did not reveal any differential responsiveness on the basis of these subgroupings.

INDICATIONS AND USAGE:

Olanzapine is indicated for the management of the manifestations of psychotic disorders.

The antipsychotic efficacy of olanzapine was established in short-term (6-week) controlled trials of schizophrenic inpatients (see CLINICAL STUDIES).

The effectiveness of olanzapine in long-term use, that is, for more than 6 weeks, has not been systematically evaluated in controlled trials. Therefore, the physician who elects to use olanzapine for extended periods should periodically re-evaluate the long-term usefulness of the drug for the individual patient (see DOSAGE AND ADMINISTRATION).

CONTRAINDICATIONS:

Olanzapine is contraindicated in patients with a known hypersensitivity to the product.

WARNINGS:

Neuroleptic Malignant Syndrome (NMS): A potentially fatal symptom complex sometimes referred to as Neuroleptic Malignant Syndrome (NMS) has been reported in association with administration of antipsychotic drugs. Clinical manifestations of NMS are hyperpyrexia, muscle rigidity, altered mental status and evidence of autonomic instability (irregular pulse or blood pressure, tachycardia, diaphoresis and cardiac dysrhythmia). Additional signs may include elevated creatinine phosphokinase, myoglobinuria (rhabdomyolysis), and acute renal failure.

The diagnostic evaluation of patients with this syndrome is complicated. In arriving at a diagnosis, it is important to exclude cases where the clinical presentation includes both serious medical illness (*e.g.,* pneumonia, systemic infection, etc.) and untreated or inadequately treated extrapyramidal signs and symptoms (EPS). Other important considerations in the differential diagnosis include central anticholinergic toxicity, heat stroke, drug fever, and primary central nervous system pathology.

The management of NMS should include: 1) immediate discontinuation of antipsychotic drugs and other drugs not essential to concurrent therapy; 2) intensive symptomatic treatment and medical monitoring; and 3) treatment of any concomitant serious medical problems for which specific treatments are available. There is no general agreement about specific pharmacological treatment regimens for NMS.

If a patient requires antipsychotic drug treatment after recovery from NMS, the potential reintroduction of drug therapy should be carefully considered. The patient should be carefully monitored, since recurrences of NMS have been reported.

Tardive Dyskinesia: A syndrome of potentially irreversible, involuntary, dyskinetic movements may develop in patients treated with antipsychotic drugs. Although the prevalence of the syndrome appears to be highest among the elderly, especially elderly women, it is impossible to rely upon prevalence estimates to predict, at the inception of antipsychotic treatment, which patients are likely to develop the syndrome. Whether antipsychotic drug products differ in their potential to cause tardive dyskinesia is unknown.

The risk of developing tardive dyskinesia and the likelihood that it will become irreversible are believed to increase as the duration of treatment and the total cumulative dose of antipsychotic drugs administered to the patient increase. However, the syndrome can develop, although much less commonly, after relatively brief treatment periods at low doses.

There is no known treatment for established cases of tardive dyskinesia, although the syndrome may remit, partially or completely, if antipsychotic treatment is withdrawn. Antipsychotic treatment, itself, however, may suppress (or partially suppress) the signs and symptoms of the syndrome and thereby may possibly mask the underlying process. The effect that symptomatic suppression has upon the long-term course of the syndrome is unknown.

Given these considerations, olanzapine should be prescribed in a manner that is most likely to minimize the occurrence of tardive dyskinesia. Chronic antipsychotic treatment should generally be reserved for patients (1) who suffer from a chronic illness that is known to respond to antipsychotic drugs, and (2) for whom altemative, equally effective, but potentially less harmful treatments are not available or appropriate. In patients who do require chronic treatment, the smallest dose and the shortest duration of treatment producing a satisfactory clinical response should be sought. The need for continued treatment should be reassessed periodically.

If signs and symptoms of tardive dyskinesia appear in a patient on olanzapine, drug discontinuation should be considered. However, some patients may require treatment with olanzapine despite the presence of the syndrome.

PRECAUTIONS:

GENERAL

Orthostatic Hypotension: Olanzapine may induce orthostatic hypotension associated with dizziness, tachycardia, and in some patients, syncope, especially during the initial dose-titration period, probably reflecting its α_1-adrenergic antagonistic properties. Syncope was reported in 0.6% (15/2500) of olanzapine-treated patients in phase 2-3 studies. The risk of orthostatic hypotension and syncope may be minimized by initiating therapy with 5 mg daily (see DOSAGE AND ADMINISTRATION). A more gradual titration to the target dose should be considered if hypotension occurs. Olanzapine should be used with particular caution in patients with known cardiovascular disease (history of myocardial infarction or ischemia, heart failure, or conduction abnormalities), cerebrovascular disease, and conditions which would predispose patients to hypotension (dehydration, hypovolemia, and treatment with antihypertensive medications).

Seizures: During premarketing testing, seizures occurred in 0.9% (22/2500) of olanzapine treated patients. There were confounding factors that may have contributed to the occurrence of seizures in many of these cases. Olanzapine should be used cautiously in patients with a

PRECAUTIONS: *(cont'd)*

history of seizures or with conditions that potentially lower the seizure threshold (*e.g.,* Alzheimer's dementia). Conditions that lower the seizure threshold may be more prevalent in a population of 65 years or older.

Hyperprolactinemia: As with other drugs that antagonize dopamine D_2 receptors, olanzapine elevates prolactin levels and a modest elevation persists during chronic administration. Tissue culture experiments indicate that approximately one-third of human breast cancers are prolactin dependent *in vitro*, a factor of potential importance if the prescription of these drugs is contemplated in a patient with previously detected breast cancer of this type. Although disturbances such as galactorrhea, amenorrhea, gynecomastia, and impotence have been reported with prolactin-elevating compounds, the clinical significance of elevated serum prolactin levels is unknown for most patients. As is common with compounds which increase prolactin release, an increase in mammary gland neoplasia was observed in the olanzapine carcinogenicity studies conducted in mice and rats (see Carcinogenesis). However, neither clinical studies nor epidemiologic studies have shown an association between chronic administration of this class of drugs and tumorigenesis in humans; the available evidence is considered too limited to be conclusive.

Transaminase Elevations: In placebo-controlled studies, clinically significant ALT (SGPT) elevations (≥3 times the upper limit of the normal range) were observed in 2% (6/243) of patients exposed to olanzapine compared to none (0/115) of the placebo patients. None of these patients experienced jaundice. In two of these patients, liver enzymes decreased toward normal despite continued treatment and in two others, enzymes decreased upon discontinuation of olanzapine. In the remaining two patients, one, seropositive for hepatitis C, had persistent enzyme elevation for four months after discontinuation, and the other had insufficient follow-up to determine if enzymes normalized.

Within the larger premarketing database of about 2400 patients with baseline SGPT ≤90 IU/L, the incidence of SGPT elevation to >200 IU/L was 2% (50/2381). Again, none of these patients experienced jaundice or other symptoms attributable to liver impairment and most had transient changes that tended to normalize while olanzapine treatment was continued.

Among all 2500 patients in clinical trials, about 1% (23/2500) discontinued treatment due to transaminase increases.

Caution should be exercised in patients with signs and symptoms of hepatic impairment, in patients with pre-existing conditions associated with limited hepatic functional reserve, and in patients who are being treated with potentially hepatotoxic drugs. Periodic assessment of transaminases is recommended in patients with significant hepatic disease (see Laboratory Tests).

Potential for Cognitive and Motor Impairment: Somnolence was a commonly reported adverse event associated with olanzapine treatment, occurring at an incidence of 26% in olanzapine patients compared to 15% in placebo patients. This adverse event was also dose related. Somnolence led to discontinuation in 0.4% (9/2500) of patients in the premarketing database.

Since olanzapine has the potential to impair judgment, thinking, or motor skills, patients should be cautioned about operating hazardous machinery, including automobiles, until they are reasonably certain that olanzapine therapy does not affect them adversely.

Body Temperature Regulation: Disruption of the body's ability to reduce core body temperature has been attributed to antipsychotic agents. Appropriate care is advised when prescribing olanzapine for patients who will be experiencing conditions which may contribute to an elevation in core body temperature (*e.g.,* exercising strenuously, exposure to extreme heat, receiving concomitant medication with anticholinergic activity, or being subject to dehydration).

Dysphagia: Esophageal dysmotility and aspiration have been associated with antipsychotic drug use. Two olanzapine-treated patients in a study of olanzapine in Alzheimer's dementia died from aspiration pneumonia. One of these patients had experienced dysphagia prior to the development of aspiration pneumonia. Aspiration pneumonia is a common cause of morbidity and mortality in patients with advanced Alzheimer's dementia. Olanzapine and other antipsychotic drugs should be used cautiously in patients at risk for aspiration pneumonia.

Suicide: The possibility of a suicide attempt is inherent in schizophrenia, and close supervision of high-risk patients should accompany drug therapy. Prescriptions for olanzapine should be written for the smallest quantity of tablets consistent with good patient management, in order to reduce the risk of overdose.

Use in Patients with Concomitant Illness: Clinical experience with olanzapine in patients with certain concomitant systemic illnesses Special Populations, Renal Impairment and Hepatic Impairment is limited.

Olanzapine exhibits *in vitro* muscarinic receptor affinity. In premarketing clinical trials with olanzapine, olanzapine was associated with constipation, dry mouth, and tachycardia, all adverse events possibly related to cholinergic antagonism. Such adverse events were not often the basis for discontinuations from olanzapine, but olanzapine should be used with caution in patients with clinically significant prostatic hypertrophy, narrow angle glaucoma, or a history of paralytic ileus.

Olanzapine has not been evaluated or used to any appreciable extent in patients with a recent history of myocardial infarction or unstable heart disease. Patients with these diagnoses were excluded from premarketing clinical studies. Because of the risk of orthostatic hypotension with olanzapine, caution should be observed in cardiac patients (see PRECAUTIONS, Orthostatic Hypotension).

INFORMATION FOR PATIENTS

Physicians are advised to discuss the following issues with patients for whom they prescribe olanzapine:

Orthostatic Hypotension: Patients should be advised of the risk of orthostatic hypotension, especially during the period of initial dose titration and in association with the use of concomitant drugs that may potentiate the orthostatic effect of olanzapine, (*e.g.,* diazepam or alcohol) (see DRUG INTERACTIONS).

Interference with Cognitive and Motor Performance: Because olanzapine has the potential to impair judgment, thinking, or motor skills, patients should be cautioned about operating hazardous machinery, including automobiles, until they are reasonably certain that olanzapine therapy does not affect them adversely.

Pregnancy: Patients should be advised to notify their physician if they become pregnant or intend to become pregnant during therapy with olanzapine.

Nursing: Patients should be advised not to breast-feed an infant if they are taking olanzapine.

Concomitant Medication: Patients should be advised to inform their physicians if they are taking, or plan to take, any prescription or over-the-counter drugs, since there is a potential for interactions.

Alcohol: Patients should be advised to avoid alcohol while taking olanzapine.

Heat Exposure and Dehydration: Patients should be advised regarding appropriate care in avoiding overheating and dehydration.

LABORATORY TESTS

Periodic assessment of transaminases is recommended in patients with significant hepatic disease (see PRECAUTIONS, Transaminase Elevations).

PRECAUTIONS: *(cont'd)*

CARCINOGENESIS, MUTAGENESIS, IMPAIRMENT OF FERTILITY

Carcinogenesis: Oral carcinogenicity studies were conducted in mice and rats. Olanzapine was administered to mice in two 78-week studies at doses of 3, 10, 30/20 mg/kg/day (equivalent to 0.8-5 times the maximum recommended human daily dose on a mg/m^2 basis) and 0.25, 2, 8 mg/kg/day (equivalent to 0.06-2 times the maximum recommended human daily dose on a mg/m^2 basis). Rats were dosed for 2 years at doses of 0.25, 1, 2.5, 4 mg/kg/day (males) and 0.25, 1, 4, 8 mg/kg/day (females) (equivalent to 0.13-2 and 0.13-4 times the maximum recommended human daily dose on a mg/m^2 basis, respectively). The incidence of liver hemangiomas and hemangiosarcomas was significantly increased in one mouse study in female mice dosed at 8 mg/kg/day (2 times the maximum recommended human daily dose on a mg/m^2 basis). These tumors were not increased in another mouse study in females dosed at 10 or 30/20 mg/l g/day (2-5 times the maximum recommended human daily dose on a mg/m^2 basis); in this study, there was a high incidence of early mortalities in males of the 30/20 mg/kg/day group. The incidence of mammary gland adenomas and adenocarcinomas was significantly increased in female mice dosed at ≥2 mg/kg/day and in female rats dosed at ≥4 mg/kg/day (0.5 and 2 times the maximum recommended human daily dose on a mg/m^2 basis, respectively). Antipsychotic drugs have been shown to chronically elevate prolactin levels in rodents. Serum prolactin levels were not measured during the olanzapine carcinogenicity studies; however, measurements during subchronic toxicity studies showed that olanzapine elevated serum prolactin levels up to 4-fold in rats at the same doses used in the carcinogenicity study. An increase in mammary gland neoplasms has been found in rodents after chronic administration of other antipsychotic drugs and is considered to be prolactin mediated. The relevance for human risk of the finding of prolactin mediated endocrine tumors in rodents is unknown (see PRECAUTIONS, General, Hyperprolactinemia).

Mutagenesis: No evidence of mutagenic potential for olanzapine was found in the Ames reverse mutation test, *in vivo* micronucleus test in mice, the chromosomal aberration test in Chinese hamster ovary cells, unscheduled DNA synthesis test in rat hepatocytes, induction of forward mutation test in mouse lymphoma cells, or *in vivo* sister chromatid exchange test in bone marrow of Chinese hamsters.

Impairment of Fertility: In a fertility and reproductive performance study in rats, male mating performance, but not fertility, was impaired at a dose of 22.4 mg/kg/day and female fertility was decreased at a dose of 3 mg/kg/day (11 and 1.5 times the maximum recommended human daily dose on a mg/m^2 basis, respectively.). Discontinuance of olanzapine treatment reversed the effects on male mating performance. In female rats, the precoital period was increased and the mating index reduced at 5 mg/kg/day (2.5 times the maximum recommended human daily dose on a mg/m^2 basis). Diestrous was prolonged and estrous delayed at 1.1 mg/kg/day (0.6 times the maximum recommended human daily dose on a mg/m^2 basis); therefore olanzapine may produce a delay in ovulation.

PREGNANCY CATEGORY C

In reproduction studies in rats at doses up to 18 mg/kg/day and in rabbits at doses up to 30 mg/kg/day (9 and 30 times the maximum recommended human daily dose on a mg/m^2 basis, respectively) no evidence of teratogenicity was observed. In a rat teratology study, early resorptions and increased numbers of nonviable fetuses were observed at a dose of 18 mg/kg/day (9 times the maximum recommended human daily dose on a mg/m^2 basis). Gestation was prolonged at 10 mg/kg/day (5 times the maximum recommended human daily dose on a mg/m^2 basis). In a rabbit teratology study, fetal toxicity (manifested as increased resorptions and decreased fetal weight) occurred at a maternally toxic dose of 30 mg/kg/day (30 times the maximum recommended human daily dose on a mg/m^2 basis).

Placental transfer of olanzapine occurs in rat pups.

There are no adequate and well-controlled trials with olanzapine in pregnant females. Seven pregnancies were observed during clinical trials with olanzapine, including 2 resulting in normal births, 1 resulting in neonatal death due to a cardiovascular defect, 3 therapeutic abortions, and 1 spontaneous abortion. Because animal reproduction studies are not always predictive of human response, this drug should be used during pregnancy only if the potential benefit justifies the potential risk to the fetus.

LABOR AND DELIVERY

Parturition in rats was not affected by olanzapine. The effect of olanzapine on labor and delivery in humans is unknown.

NURSING MOTHERS

Olanzapine was excreted in milk of treated rats during lactation. It is not known if olanzapine is excreted in human milk. It is recommended that women receiving olanzapine should not breast-feed.

PEDIATRIC USE

Safety and effectiveness in pediatric patients below 18 years of age have not been established.

GERIATRIC USE

Of the 2500 patients in clinical studies with olanzapine, 11% (263) were 65 years of age or over. In general, there was no indication of any different tolerability of olanzapine in the elderly compared to younger adults. Nevertheless, the presence of factors that might decrease pharmacokinetic clearance or increase the pharmacodynamic response to olanzapine should lead to consideration of a lower starting dose (see PRECAUTIONS and DOSAGE AND ADMINISTRATION).

DRUG INTERACTIONS:

The risks of using olanzapine in combination with other drugs have not been extensively evaluated in systematic studies. Given the primary CNS effects of olanzapine, caution should be used when olanzapine is taken in combination with other centrally acting drugs and alcohol.

Because of its potential for inducing hypotension, olanzapine may enhance the effects of certain antihypertensive agents.

Olanzapine may antagonize the effects of levodopa and dopamine agonists.

The Effect of Other Drugs on Olanzapine: Agents that induce CYP1A2 or glucuronyl transferase enzymes, such as omeprazole and rifampin, may cause an increase in olanzapine clearance. Inhibitors of CYPIA2 (*e.g.,* fluvoxamine) could potentially inhibit olanzapine elimination. Because olanzapine is metabolized by multiple enzyme systems, inhibition of a single enzyme may not appreciably decrease olanzapine clearance.

Charcoal: The administration of activated charcoal (1 g) reduced the C_{max} and AUC of olanzapine by about 60%. As peak olanzapine levels are not typically obtained until about 6 hours after dosing, charcoal may be a useful treatment for olanzapine overdose.

Cimetidine and Antacids: Single doses of cimetidine (800 mg) or aluminum- and magnesium-containing antacids did not affect the oral bioavailability of olanzapine.

Carbamazepine: Carbamazepine therapy (200 mg twice daily) causes an approximately 50% increase in the clearance of olanzapine. This increase is likely due to the fact that carbamazepine is a potent inducer of CYPIA2 activity. Higher daily doses of carbamazepine may cause an even greater increase in olanzapine clearance.

Ethanol: Ethanol (45 mg/70 kg single dose) did not have an effect on olanzapine pharmacokinetics.

Warfarin: Warfarin (20 mg single dose) did not affect olanzapine pharmacokinetics.

DRUG INTERACTIONS: *(cont'd)*

Effect of Olanzapine on Other Drugs: *In vitro* studies utilizing human liver microsomes suggest that olanzapine has little potential to inhibit CYPIA2, CYP2C9, CYP2C19, CYP2D6, and CYP3A. Thus, olanzapine is unlikely to cause clinically important drug interactions mediated by these enzymes.

Single doses of olanzapine did not affect the pharmacokinetics of imipramine or its active metabolite desipramine, and warfarin. Multiple doses of olanzapine did not influence the kinetics of diazepam and its active metabolite N-desmethyldiazepam, lithium, ethanol, or biperiden. However, the co-administration of either diazepam or ethanol with olanzapine potentiated the orthostatic hypotension observed with olanzapine. Multiple doses of olanzapine did not affect the pharmacokinetics of theophylline or its metabolites.

ADVERSE REACTIONS:

The premarketing development program for olanzapine included over 3100 patients and/or normal subjects exposed to 1 or more doses of olanzapine. Of these 3100 subjects, 2500 were patients who participated in multiple dose effectiveness trials, and their experience corresponded to approximately 1122 patient-years. The conditions and duration of treatment with olanzapine varied greatly and included (in overlapping categories) open-label and double-blind phases of studies, inpatients and outpatients, fixed-dose and dose-titration studies, and short-term or longer-term exposure. Adverse reactions were assessed by collecting adverse events, results of physical examinations, vital signs, weights, laboratory analytes, ECGs, chest x-rays, and results of ophthalmologic examinations.

Adverse events during exposure were obtained by spontaneous report and recorded by clinical investigators using terminology of their own choosing. Consequently, it is not possible to provide a meaningful estimate of the proportion of individuals experiencing adverse events without first grouping similar types of events into a smaller number of standardized event categories. In the tables and tabulations that follow, standard COSTART dictionary terminology has been used to classify reported adverse events.

The stated frequencies of adverse events represent the proportion of individuals who experienced, at least once, a treatment-emergent adverse event of the type listed. An event was considered treatment emergent if it occurred for the first time or worsened while receiving therapy following baseline evaluation.

ADVERSE FINDINGS OBSERVED IN SHORT-TERM, PLACEBO-CONTROLLED TRIALS

The following findings are based on a pool of two 6-week, placebo-controlled trials in which mean olanzapine doses ranged from 7-16 mg/day.

Adverse Events Associated with Discontinuation of Treatment in Short-Term Placebo-Controlled Trials: Overall, there was no difference in the incidence of discontinuation due to adverse events (5% for olanzapine vs 6% for placebo). However, discontinuations due to increases in SGPT were considered to be drug related (2% for olanzapine vs 0% for placebo) (see PRECAUTIONS).

Adverse Events Occurring at an Incidence of 1% or More Among Olanzapine-Treated Patients in Short-Term, Placebo-Controlled Trials: TABLE 1 enumerates the incidence, rounded to the nearest percent, of treatment-emergent adverse events that occurred during acute therapy (up to 6 weeks) of schizophrenia in 1% or more of patients treated with olanzapine (doses ≥2.5 mg/day) where the incidence in patients treated with olanzapine was greater than the incidence in placebo treated patients.

The prescriber should be aware that the figures in the tables and tabulations cannot be used to predict the incidence of side effects in the course of usual medical practice where patient characteristics and other factors differ from those that prevailed in the clinical trials. Similarly, the cited frequencies cannot be compared with figures obtained from other clinical investigations involving different treatments, uses, and investigators. The cited figures, however, do provide the prescribing physician with some basis for estimating the relative contribution of drug and nondrug factors to the side effect incidence in the population studied.

Commonly Observed Adverse Events in Short-Term, Placebo-Controlled Trials: The most commonly observed adverse events associated with the use of olanzapine (incidence of 5% or greater) and not observed at an equivalent incidence among placebo-treated patients (olanzapine incidence at least twice that for placebo) are in TABLE 2.

Dose Dependency of Adverse Events in Short-Term, Placebo-Controlled Trials: *Extrapyramidal Symptoms:* TABLE 3 enumerates the percentage of patients with treatment-emergent extrapyramidal symptoms as assessed by categorical analyses of formal rating scales during acute therapy in a controlled clinical trial comparing olanzapine at 3 fixed doses with placebo treatment of schizophrenia.

TABLE 4 enumerates the percentage of patients with treatment-emergent extrapyramidal symptoms as assesed by spontaneously reported adverse events during acute therapy in the same controlled clinical trial comparing olanzapine at 3 fixed doses with placebo in the treatment of schizophrenia.

Other Adverse Events: TABLE 5 address dose relatedness for other adverse events using data from a trial involving fixed dosage ranges. It enumerates the percentage of patients with treatment-emergent adverse events for the three fixed-dose range groups and placebo. The data were analyzed using the Cochran-Armitage test, excluding the placebo group, and the table includes only those adverse events for which there was a statistically significant trend.

Vital Sign Changes: Olanzapine is associated with orthostatic hypotension and tachycardia (see PRECAUTIONS).

Weight Gain: In placebo-controlled, 6-week studies, weight gain was reported in 5.6% of olanzapine patients compared to 0.8% of placebo patients. Olanzapine patients gained an average of 2.8 kg, compared to an average 0.4 kg weight loss in placebo patients; 29% of olanzapine patients gained greater than 7% of their baseline weight, compared to 3% of placebo patients. A categorization of patients at baseline on the basis of body mass index (BMI) revealed a significantly greater effect in patients with low BMI compared to normal or overweight patients; nevertheless; weight gain was greater in all 3 olanzapine groups compared to the placebo group. During long-term continuation therapy with olanzapine (238 median days of exposure), 56% of olanzapine patients met the criterion for having gained greater than 7% of their baseline weight. Average weight gain during long-term therapy was 5.4 kg.

Laboratory Changes: An assessment of the premarketing experience for olanzapine revealed an association with asymptomatic increases in SGPT, SGOT, and GGT (see PRECAUTIONS). Olanzapine administration was also associated with increases in serum prolactin (see PRECAUTIONS), with an asymptomatic elevation of the eosinophil in 0.3% of patients, and with an increase in CPK.

Given the concern about neutropenia associated with other psychotropic compounds and the finding of leukopenia associated with the administration of olanzapine in several animal models (see ANIMAL PHARMACOLOGY), careful attention was given to examination of hematologic parameters in premarketing studies with olanzapine. There was no indication of a risk of clinically significant neutropenia associated with olanzapine treatment in the premarketing database for this drug.

ADVERSE REACTIONS: *(cont'd)*

TABLE 1 Treatment-Emergent Adverse Event Incidence in 6-Week Placebo-Controlled Clinical Trials*

Body System/ Adverse Event	Percentage of Patients Reporting Event Olanzapine (N=248)	Placebo (N=118)
Body as a Whole		
Headache	17	15
Fever	5	3
Abdominal Pain	4	2
Back Pain	4	3
Chest Pain	4	2
Neck Rigidity	2	1
Intentional injury	1	0
Cardiovascular System		
Postural hypotension	5	2
Tachycardia	4	1
Hypotension	2	1
Digestive System		
Constipation	9	3
Dry mouth	7	4
Increased appetite	2	1
Metabolic and Nutritional Disorders		
Weight gain	6	1
Peripheral edema	2	0
Lower extremity edema	1	0
Musculoskeletal System		
Joint pain	5	3
Extremity pain (other than joint)	4	3
Twitching	2	1
Nervous System		
Somnolence	26	15
Agitation	23	17
Insomnia	20	19
Nervousness	16	14
Hostility	15	14
Dizziness	11	4
Anxiety	9	8
Personality disorder†	8	4
Akathisia	5	1
Hypertonia	4	3
Tremor	4	3
Amnesia	2	0
Articulation impairment	2	0
Euphoria	2	0
Stuttering	2	0
Respiratory System		
Rhinitis	10	6
Cough increased	5	3
Pharyngitis	5	3
Skin and Appendages		
Vesiculobullous rash	2	1
Special Senses		
Amblyopia	5	4
Blepharitis	2	1
Corneal lesion	1	0
Urogenital System		
Prementrual syndrome‡	2	0

* Events reported by at least 1% of patients treated with olanzapine, except the following events which had an incidence equal to or less than placebo: abnormal dreams, accidental injury, anorexia, apathy, asthenia, cogwheel rigidity, confusion, conjunctivitis, dental pain, diarrhea, depression, dysmenorrhea‡, dyspepsia, ecchymosis, emotional libility, hallucinations, hyperkinesia, hypertension, hypokenesia, joint stiffness, libido increased, myalgia, nausea, paranoid reaction, paresthesia, pruritus, rash, schizophrenic reaction, sweating, thinking abnormal, tooth caries, vaginitis‡, vomiting.
† Personality disorder is the COSTART term for designating non-aggressive objectionable behavior.
‡ Denominator used was for females only (olanzapine, N=41; placebo, N=23).

TABLE 2 Common Treatment-Emergent Adverse Events Associated with the Use of Olanzapine in 6-Week Trials

Adverse Event	Percentage of Patients Reporting Event Olanzapine (N=248)	Placebo (N=118)
Postural hypotension	5	2
Constipation	9	3
Weight gain	6	1
Dizziness	11	4
Personality disorder*	8	4
Akathisia	5	1

* Personality disorder is the COSTART term for designating non-aggressive objectionable behavior.

TABLE 3 Treatment-Emergent Extrapyramidal Symptoms Assessed by Rating Scales Incidence in a Fixed Dosage Range, Placebo-controlled Clinical Trial-Acute Phase*

	Percentage of Patients			
	Placebo	Olanzapine 5 ± 2.5 mg/day	Olanzapine 10 ± 2.5 mg/day	Olanzapine 15 ± 2.5 mg/day
Parkinsonism†	15	14	12	14
Akathisia‡	23	16	19	27

* No statistically significant differences.
† Percentage of patients with a Simpson-Angus Scale total score >3.
‡ Percentage of patients with a Barnes Akathisia Scale global score ≥2.

ECG Changes: Between-group comparisons for pooled placebo-controlled trials revealed no statistically significant olanzapine/placebo differences in the proportions of patients experiencing potentially important changes in ECG parameters, including QT, QTc, and PR intervals. Olanzapine use was associated with a mean increase in heart rate of 2.4 beats per minute compared to no change among placebo patients. This slight tendency to tachycardia may be related to olanzapine's potential for inducing orthostatic changes (see PRECAUTIONS).

OTHER ADVERSE EVENTS OBSERVED DURING THE PREMARKETING EVALUATION OF OLANZAPINE

Following is a list of COSTART terms that reflect treatment-emergent adverse events as defined in the introduction of ADVERSE REACTIONSreported by patients treated with olanzapine at multiple doses ≥1 mg/day during any phase of a trial within the database of

ADVERSE REACTIONS: *(cont'd)*

TABLE 4 Treatment-Emergent Extrapyramidal Symptoms Assessed by Adverse Events Incidence in a Fixed Dosage Range, Placebo-Controlled Clinical Trial-Acute Phase

	Placebo (N=68)	Percentage of Patients Reporting Event Olanzapine 5 ± 2.5 mg/day (N=65)	Olanzapine 10 ± 2.5 mg/day (N=64)	Olanzapine 15 ± 2.5 mg/day (N=69)
Dystonic events†	1	3	2	3
Parkinsonism events‡	10	8	14	20
Akathisia events§	1	5	11*	10*
Dyskinetic events ‖	4	0	2	1
Residual events¶	1	2	5	1
Any extrapyramidal event	16	15	25	32*

* Statistically significantly different from placebo.
† Patients with the following COSTART terms were counted in this category: dystonia, generalized spasm, neck rigidity, oculoyric crisis, opisthontonos, torticollis.
‡ Patients with the following COSTART terms were counted in this category: akinesia, cogwheel rigidity, extrapyramidal syndrome, hypertonia, hypokinesia, masked facies, tremor.
§ Patients with the following COSTART terms were counted in this category: akathisia, hyperkinesia.
‖ Patients with the following COSTART terms were counted in this category: buccoglossal syndrome, choreoathetosis, dyskinesia, tardive dyskinesia.
¶ Patients with the following COSTART terms were counted in this category: movement disorder, myoclonus, twitching.

TABLE 5 Treatment-Emergent Adverse Events for the Three Fixed-Dose Range Groups and Placebo

Adverse Event	Placebo (N=68)	Percentage of Patients Reporting Event Olanzapine 5 ± 2.5 mg/day (N=65)	Olanzapine 10 ± 2.5 mg/day (N=64)	Olanzapine 15 ± 2.5 mg/day (N=69)
Asthenia	15	8	9	20
Dry mouth	4	3	5	13
Nausea	9	0	2	9
Somnolence	16	20	30	39
Tremor	3	0	5	7

2500 patients. All reported events are included except those already listed in TABLE 1 or elsewhere in labeling, those events for which a drug cause was remote, those event terms which were so general as to be uninformative, and events reported only once and which did not have a substantial probability of being acutely life-threatening. It is important to emphasize that, although the events reported occurred during treatment with olanzapine, they were not necessarily caused by it.

Events are further categorized by body system and listed in order of decreasing frequency according to the following definitions: frequent adverse events are those occurring in at least 1/100 patients (only those not already listed in the tabulated results from placebo-controlled trials appear in this listing); infrequent adverse events are those occurring in 1/100 to 1/1000 patients; rare events are those occurring in fewer than 1/1000 patients.

Body as a Whole: *Frequent:* flu syndrome and suicide attempt; *Infrequent:*chills, chills and fever, face edema, hangover effect, malaise, moniliasis, neck pain, pelvic pain, and photosensitivity reaction; *Rare:*abdomen enlarged and sudden death.

Cardiovascular System: *Infrequent:*cerebrovascular accident, hemorrhage, migraine, palpitation, vasodilatation, and ventricular extrasystoles; *Rare:*heart arrest.

Digestive System: *Frequent:* increased salivation, nausea and vomiting, and thirst; *Infrequent:* aphthous stomatitis, dysphagia, eructation, esophagitis, fecal incontinence, flatulence, gastritis, gastroenteritis, gingivitis, glossitis, hepatitis, melena, mouth ulceration, oral moniliasis, periodontal abscess, rectal hemorrhage, stomatitis, and tongue edema; *Rare:*enteritis, esophageal ulcer, and tongue discoloration.

Endocrine System: *Infrequent:*diabetes mellitus and goiter; *Rare:* diabetic acidosis.

Hemic and Lymphatic System: *Infrequent:*cyanosis, leukocytosis, lymphadenopathy, and thrombocythemia.

Metabolic and Nutritional Disorders: *Frequent:*weight loss; *Infrequent:*alkaline phosphatase increased, bilirubinemia, dehydration, hyperglycemia, hyperkalemia, hyperuricemia, hypoglycemia, hypokalemia, hyponatremia, ketosis, and water intoxication;*Rare:*hypercholesteremia and hyperlipemia.

Musculoskeletal System: *Infrequent:*arthritis, back and hip pain, bursitis, leg cramps, myasthenia, and rheumatoid arthritis; *Rare:*bone pain and myopathy.

Nervous System: *Frequent:* tardive dyskinesia; *Infrequent:*abnormal gait, alcohol misuse, antisocial reaction, ataxia, CNS stimulation, coma, delirium, depersonalization, hypesthesia, hypotonia, incoordination, libido decreased, obsessive compulsive symptoms, phobias, somatization, stimulant misuse, stupor, vertigo, and withdrawal syndrome; *Rare:*facial paralysis, neuralgia, nystagmus, and subarachnoid hemorrhage.

Respiratory System: *Frequent:* dyspnea; *Infrequent:*apnea, asthma, epistaxis, hemoptysis, hyperventilation, and voice alteration; *Rare:*laryngitis.

Skin and Appendages: *Infrequent:*alopecia, contact dermatitis, dry skin, eczema hirsutism, seborrhea, skin ulcer, and urticaria; *Rare:*maculopapular rash and skin discoloration.

Special Senses: *Infrequent:* cataract, deafness, diplopia, dry eyes, ear pain, eye hemorrhage, eye inflammation, eye pain, ocular muscle abnormality, taste perversion, and tinnitus; *Rare:* abnormality of accommodation, glaucoma, keratoconjunctivitis, macular hypopigmentation, mydriasis, and pigment deposits lens.

Urogenital System: *Frequent:* hematuria, metrorrhagia*, urinary incontinence, and urinary tract infection;*Infrequent:*abnormal ejaculation*, amenorrhea*, breast pain, cystitis, decreased menstruation*, dysuria, increased menstruation*, female lactation, impotence*, menorrhagia*, polyuria, pyuria, urinary retention, urinary frequency, urination impaired, and uterine fibroids enlarged*; *Rare:* albuminuria.

*Adjusted for gender.

DRUG ABUSE AND DEPENDENCE:

Controlled Substance Class: Olanzapine is not a controlled substance.

Physical and Psychological Dependence: In studies prospectively designed to assess abuse and dependence potential, olanzapine was shown to have acute depressive CNS effects but little or no potential of abuse or physical dependence in rats administered oral doses up to 15 times the maximum daily human dose (20 mg) and rhesus monkeys administered oral doses up to 8 times the maximum daily human dose on a mg/m² basis.

DRUG ABUSE AND DEPENDENCE: *(cont'd)*

Olanzapine has not been systematically studied in humans for its potential for abuse, tolerance, or physical dependence. While the clinical trials did not reveal any tendency for any drug-seeking behavior, these observations were not systematic, and it is not possible to predict on the basis of this limited experience the extent to which a CNS-active drug will be misused, diverted, and/or abused once marketed. Consequently, patients should be evaluated carefully for a history of drug abuse, and such patients should be observed closely for signs of misuse or abuse of olanzapine (*e.g.*, development of tolerance, increases in dose, drug-seeking behavior).

OVERDOSAGE:

Human Experience: In premarketing trials involving more than 3100 patients and/or normal subjects, accidental or intentional acute overdosage of olanzapine was identified in 67 patients. In the patient taking the largest identified amount, 300 mg, the only symptoms reported were drowsiness and slurred speech. In the limited number of patients who were evaluated in hospitals, including the patient taking 300 mg, there were no observations indicating an adverse change in laboratory analytes or ECG. Vital signs were usually within normal limits following overdoses.

Overdosage Management: The possibility of multiple drug involvement should be considered. In case of acute overdosage, establish and maintain an airway and ensure adequate oxygenation and ventilation. Gastric lavage (after intubation, if patient is unconscious) and administration of activated charcoal together with a laxative should be considered. The possibility of obtundation, seizures, or dystonic reaction of the head and neck following overdose may create a risk of aspiration with induced emesis. Cardiovascular monitoring should commence immediately and should include continuous electrocardiographic monitoring to detect possible arrhythmias.

There is no specific antidote to olanzapine. Therefore, appropriate supportive measures should be initiated. Hypotension and circulatory collapse should be treated with appropriate measures such as intravenous fluids and/or sympathomimetic agents. (Do not use epinephrine, dopamine, or other sympathomimetics with beta-agonist activity, since beta stimulation may worsen hypotension in the setting of olanzapine-induced alpha blockade.) Close medical supervision and monitoring should continue until the patient recovers.

DOSAGE AND ADMINISTRATION:

Usual Dose: Olanzapine should be administered on a once-a-day schedule without regard to meals, generally beginning with 5 to 10 mg initially, with a target dose of 10 mg/day within several days. Further dosage adjustments, if indicated, should generally occur at intervals of not less than 1 week, since steady state for olanzapine would not be achieved for approximately 1 week in the typical patient. When dosage adjustments are necessary, dose increments/decrements of 5 mg daily are recommended.

Antipsychotic efficacy was demonstrated in a dose range of 10 to 15 mg/day in the clinical trials. However, doses above 10 mg/day were not demonstrated to be more efficacious than the 10 mg/day dose. An increase to a dose greater than target dose of 10 mg/day (*i.e.*, to a dose of 15 mg/day or greater) is recommended only after clinical assessment. The safety of doses above 20 mg/day has not been evaluated in clinical trials.

Dosing in Special Populations: The recommended starting dose is 5 mg in patients who are debilitated, who have a predisposition to hypotensive reactions, who otherwise exhibit a combination of factors that may result in slower metabolism of olanzapine (*e.g.*, nonsmoking female patients ≥ 65 years of age), or who may be more pharmacodynamically sensitive to olanzapine (see CLINICAL PHARMACOLOGY; also see PRECAUTIONS, Use in Patients with Concomitant Illness and DRUG INTERACTIONS). When indicated, dose escalation should be performed with caution in these patients.

Maintenance Treatment: While there is no body of evidence available to answer the question of how long the patient treated with olanzapine should remain on it, the effectivenss of maintenance treatment is well established for many other antipsychotic drugs. It is recommended that responding patients be continued on olanzapine, but at the lowest dose needed to maintain remission. Patients should be periodically reassessed to determine the need for mainentance treatment.

ANIMAL PHARMACOLOGY:

In animal studies with olanzapine, the peincipal hematologic findings were reversible peripheral cytopenias in individual dogs dosed at 10 mg/kg (17 times the maximum recommended human daily dose on a mg/m² basis), dose-related decreased in lymphocytes and neutrophils in mice, and lymphopenia in rats. A few dogs treated with 10 mg/kg developed reversible neutropenia and/or reversible hemolytic anemia between 1 and 10 months of treatment. Dose-related decreases in lymphocytes and neutrophils were seen in mice given doses of 10 mg/kg (equal to 2 times the maximum recommended human daily dose on a mg/m² basis) in studies 3 months' duration. Nonspecific lymphopenia, consistent with decreased body weight gain, occurred in rats receiving 22.5 mg/kg (11 times the maximum recommended human daily dose on a mg/m² basis) for 6 to 12 months. No evidence of bone marrow cytotoxicity was found in any of the species examined. Bone marrows were normocellular or hypercellular, indicating that the reductions in circulating blood cells were probably due to peripheral (non-marrow) factors.

HOW SUPPLIED:

Zyprexa tablets are white, round, film-coated, and imprinted in blue ink with LILLY and the tablet number: 5 mg imprinted with "4115", 7.5 mg imprinted with "4116", 10 mg imprinted with "4117".

Store at controlled room temperature, 20° to 25°C (68° to 77°F). The USP defines controlled room temperature as a temperature maintained thermostatically that encompasses the usual and customary working environment of 20° to 25°C (68° to 77°F); that results in a mean kinetic temperature calculated to be not more than 25°C; and that allows for excursions between 15° and 30°C (59° and 86°F) that are experienced in pharmacies, hospitals, and warehouses.

Protect from light and moisture.

HOW SUPPLIED - EQUIVALENTS NOT AVAILABLE:

Tablet - Oral - 5 mg

100's $524.40 ZYPREXA, Lilly 00002-4115-33

Tablet - Oral - 7.5 mg

100's $524.40 ZYPREXA, Lilly 00002-4116-33

Tablet - Oral - 10 mg

100's $774.00 ZYPREXA, Lilly 00002-4117-33

OLOPATADINE HYDROCHLORIDE *(003317)*

CATEGORIES: Allergies; Antihistamines; Conjunctivitis; EENT Drugs; Eye, Ear, Nose, & Throat Preparations; FDA Approved 1996 Dec; Ophthalmics; Respiratory & Allergy Medications

BRAND NAMES: **Patanol**

DESCRIPTION:

Olopatadine HCl ophthalmic solution 0.1% is a sterile ophthalmic solution containing olopatadine, a relatively selective H_1-receptor antagonist and inhibitor of histamine release from the mast cell for topical administration to the eyes. Olopatadine HCl is a white, crystalline, water-soluble powder with a molecular weight of 373.88. The chemical name is 11-[(Z)-3-(Dimethylamino)propylidene]-6-11-dihydrodibenz[b,e] oxepin-2-acetic acid hydrochloride.

Each ml of olopatadine HCl ophthalmic solution 0.1% contains: *Active:* 1.11 olopatadine hydrochloride equivalent to 1 mg olopatadine. *Preservative:* benzalkonium chloride 0.01%. *Inactives:* dibasic sodium phosphate; sodium chloride; hydrochloric acid/sodium hydroxide (adjust pH); and purified water.

CLINICAL PHARMACOLOGY:

Olopatadine is an inhibitor of the release of histamine from the mast cell and a relatively selective histamine H_1-antagonist that inhibits the *in vivo* and *in vitro* type 1 immediate hypersensitivity reaction. Olopatadine is devoid of effects on alpha-adrenergic, dopamine, muscarinic type 1 and 2, and seratonin receptors. Following topical ocular administration in man, olopatadine was shown to have low systemic exposure. Two studies in normal volunteers (totaling 24 subjects) dosed bilaterally with olopatadine 0.15% ophthalmic solution once every 12 hours for 2 weeks demonstrated plasma concentrations to be generally below the quantitation limit of the assay (<0.5 ng/ml). Samples in which olopatadine was quantifiable were typically found within 2 hours of dosing and ranged from 0.5 to 1.3 ng/ml. The half-life in plasma was approximately 3 hours, and ellimination was predominantly through renal excretion. Approximately 60-70% of the dose was recovered in the urine as parent drug. Two metabolites, the mono-desmethyl and the N-oxide, were detected at low concentrations in the urine. Results from conjunctival antigen challenge studies demonstrated that olopatadine HCl ophthalmic solution 0.1%, when subjects were challenged with antigen both initially and up to 8 hours after dosing, was significantly more effective than its vehicle in preventing ocular itching associated with allergic conjunctivitis.

INDICATIONS AND USAGE:

Olopatadine HCl ophthalmic solution 0.1% is indicated for the temporary prevention of itching of the eye due to allergic conjunctivitis.

CONTRAINDICATIONS:

Hypersensitivity to any component of this product.

WARNINGS:

For topical use only. Not for injection. Patients should be instructed not to instill olopatadine HCl ophthalmic solution 0.1% while wearing contact lenses.

PRECAUTIONS:

Information for the Patient: To prevent contaminating the dropper tip and solution, care should be taken not to touch the eyelids or surrounding areas with the dropper tip of the bottle. Keep bottle tightly closed when not in use.

Carcinogenesis, Mutagenesis, and Impairment of Fertility: Olopatadine administered orally was not carcinogenic in mice and rats in doses up to 500 mg/kg/day and 200 mg/kg/day, respectively. Based on a 40 µl drop size, these doses were 78,125 and 31,250 times higher than the maximum recommended ocular human dose (MROHD). No mutagenic potential was observed when olopatadine was tested in an *in vitro* bacterial reverse mutation (Ames) test, an *in vitro* mammalian chromosome aberration assay or an *in vivo* mouse micronucleus test. Olopatadine administered to male and female rats at oral doses of 62,500 times MROHD level resulted in a slight decrease in the fertility index and reduced implantation rate; no effects on reproductive function were observed at doses of 7,800 times the maximum recommended ocular human use level.

Pregnancy: Pregnancy Category C: Olopatadine was found not to be teratogenic in rats and rabbits. However, rats treated at 600 mg/kg/day, or 93,750 times the MROHD and rabbits treated at 400 mg/kg/day, or 62,500 times the MROHD, during organogenesis showed a decrease in live fetuses. There are, however no adequated and well controlled studies in pregnant women. Because animal studies are not always predictive of human responses, this drug should be used in pregnant women only if the potential benefit to the mother justifies the potential risk to the embryo or fetus.

Nursing Mothers: Olopatadine has been identified in the milk of nursing rats following oral administration. It is not known whether topical ocular administration could result in sufficient systemic absorption to produce detectable quantities in the human breast milk. Nevertheless, caution should be exercised when olopatadine HCl ophthalmic solution 0.1% is administered to a nursing mother.

Pediatric Use: Safety and effectiveness in pediatric patients below the age of 3 years have not been established.

ADVERSE REACTIONS:

Headaches were reported at an incidence of 7%. The following additional ocular and nonocular adverse reactions were reported at an incidence of less than 5%:

Ocular: Burning or stinging, dry eye, foreign body sensation, hyperemia, keratitis, lid edema, and pruritis.

Nonocular: Asthenia, cold syndrome, pharyngitis, rhinitis, sinusitis, and taste perversion.

DOSAGE AND ADMINISTRATION:

The recommended dose is one to two drops in each affected eye two times per day at an interval of 6 to 8 hours.

PATIENT INFORMATION:

Olopatadine is used for prevention of itching of the eye due to allergic conjunctivitis.

Inform physician if you are pregnant or nursing.

Do not instill while wearing contact lenses.

May cause headache, burning or stinging, dry eye, foreign body sensation, redness or inflammation of the eyes, lid swelling and itching, general weakness, cold syndrome, sore throat, rhinitis, sinusitis and tast disturbance.

Instill twice daily at 6 to 8 hour intervals.

HOW SUPPLIED:

Olopatadine HCl ophthalmic solution 0.1% is supplied in 5 ml plastic DROP-TAINER dispensers.

Storage: Store at 39° F to 86° F (4° C to 30° C).

OLSALAZINE SODIUM *(003017)*

CATEGORIES: Anti-Inflammatory Agents; Antipyretics; Central Nervous System Agents; Colitis; Gastrointestinal Drugs; Nonsteroidal Anti-Inflammatory; Ulcerative Colitis; Pregnancy Category C; FDA Class 1B ("Modest Therapeutic Advantage"); FDA Approved 1990 Jul

BRAND NAMES: **Dipentum**

FORMULARIES: Aetna; BC-BS

COST OF THERAPY: $903.44 (Ulcerative Colitis; Capsule; 250 mg; 4/day; 365 days)

DESCRIPTION:

The active ingredient in Dipentum (olsalazine sodium) Capsules is a sodium salt of a salicylate, disodium 3, 3'-azobis (6-hydroxybenzoate) a compound that is effectively bioconverted to 5-aminosalicylic acid (5-ASA), which has anti-inflammatory activity in ulcerative colitis. Its empirical formula is $C_{14}H_8N_2Na_2O_6$ with a molecular weight of 346.21.

Olsalazine sodium is a yellow crystalline powder which melts with decomposition at 240°C. It is the sodium salt of a weak acid, soluble in water and DMSO, and practically insoluble in ethanol, chloroform and ether. Olsalazine sodium has acceptable stability under acidic or basic conditions.

Dipentum is supplied in hard gelatin capsules for oral administration. The inert ingredient in each 250 mg capsule of olsalazine sodium is magnesium stearate. The capsule shell has the following inactive ingredients: black iron oxide, caramel, gelatin, and titanium dioxide.

CLINICAL PHARMACOLOGY:

After oral administration, olsalazine has limited systemic bioavailability. Based on oral and intravenous dosing studies, approximately 2.4% of a single 1.0 g oral dose is absorbed. Less than 1% of olsalazine is recovered in the urine. The remaining 98- 99% of an oral dose will reach the colon where each molecule is rapidly converted into two molecules of 5-aminosalicylic acid (5- ASA) by colonic bacteria and the low prevailing redox potential found in this environment. The liberated 5-ASA is absorbed slowly resulting in very high local concentrations in the colon.

The conversion of olsalazine to mesalamine (5-ASA) in the colon is similar to that of sulfasalazine, which is converted into sulfapyridine and mesalamine. It is thought that the mesalamine component is therapeutically active in ulcerative colitis (A.K. Azad-Kahn et al, *LANCET*, 2: 892-895, 1977). The usual dose of sulfasalazine for maintenance of remission in patients with ulcerative colitis is 2 grams daily, which would provide approximately 0.8 gram of mesalamine to the colon. More than 0.9 gram of mesalamine would usually be made available in the colon from 1 gram of olsalazine.

The mechanism of action of mesalamine (and sulfasalazine) is unknown, but appears to be topical rather than systemic. Mucosal production of arachidonic acid (AA) metabolites, both through the cyclooxygenase pathways, i.e., prostanoids, and through the lipoxygenase pathways, i.e., leukotrienes (LTs) and hydroxyeicosatetraenoic acids (HETEs) is increased in patients with chronic inflammatory bowel disease, and it is possible that mesalamine diminishes inflammation by blocking cyclooxygenase and inhibiting prostaglandin (PG) production in the colon.

Pharmacokinetics: The pharmacokinetics of olsalazine are similar in both healthy volunteers and in patients with ulcerative colitis. Maximum serum concentrations of olsalazine appear after approximately 1 hour, and even after a 1.0 g single dose are low, e.g., 1.6 - 6.2 umol/l. Olsalazine, has a very short serum half-life, approximately 0.9 hours. Olsalazine is more than 99% bound to plasma proteins. It does not interfere with protein binding of warfarin. The urinary recovery of olsalazine is below 1%. Total recovery of oral 14C-labeled olsalazine in animals and humans ranges from 90 to 97%.

Approximately 0.1% of an oral dose of olsalazine is metabolized in the liver to olsalazine-O-sulfate (olsalazine-S). Olsalazine-S, in contrast to olsalazine has a half-life of 7 days. Olsalazine-S accumulates to steady state within 2-3 weeks. Patients on daily doses of 1.0 g olsalazine for 2-4 years show a stable plasma concentration of olsalazine-S (3.3-12.4 umol/l). Olsalazine-S, is more than 99% bound to plasma proteins. Its long half-life is mainly due to slow dissociation from the protein binding site. Less than 1% of both olsalazine and olsalazine-S appears undissociated in plasma.

5-aminosalicylic acid (5-ASA): Serum concentration of 5-ASA are detected after 4-8 hours. The peak levels of 5-ASA after an oral dose of 1.0 g olsalazine are low, i.e., 0-4.3 umol/l. Of the total 5-ASA found in the urine, more than 90% is in the form of N-acetyl- 5-ASA (Ac-5-ASA). Only small amounts of 5-ASA are detected.

N-acetyl-5-ASA (Ac-5-ASA), the major metabolite of 5-ASA found in plasma and urine, is acetylated (deactivated) in at least two sites, the colonic epithelium and the liver. Ac-5-ASA is found in the serum, with peak values of 1.7-8.7 µmol/l after a single 1.0 g dose. Approximately 20% of the total 5-ASA is recovered in the urine, where it is found almost exclusively as Ac-5-ASA. The remaining 5-ASA is partially acetylated and is excreted in the feces. From fecal dialysis, the concentration of 5-ASA in the colon following olsalazine has been calculated to be 18-49 mmol/l.

No accumulation of 5-ASA or Ac-5-ASA in plasma has been detected. 5-ASA and Ac-5-ASA are 74 and 81%, respectively, bound to plasma proteins.

Animal Toxicology: Preclinical subacute and chronic toxicity studies in rats have shown the kidney to be the major target organ of olsalazine toxicity. At an oral daily dose of 400 mg/kg or higher, olsalazine treatment produced nephritis and tubular necrosis in a 4-week study; interstitial nephritis and tubular calcinosis in a 6-month study, and renal fibrosis, mineralization and transitional cell hyperplasia in a 1 year study.

CLINICAL STUDIES:

Two controlled studies have demonstrated the efficacy of olsalazine as maintenance therapy in patients with ulcerative colitis. In the first, ulcerative colitis patients in remission were randomized to olsalazine 500 mg B.I.D. or placebo, and relapse rates for a six month period of time were compared. For the 52 patients randomized to olsalazine, 12 relapses occurred, while for the 49 placebo patients, 22 relapses occurred. This difference in relapse rates was significant (p<.02).

In the second study, 164 ulcerative colitis patients in remission were randomized to olsalazine 500 mg B.I.D. or sulfasalazine 1 gram B.I.D., and relapse rates were compared after six months. The relapse rate for olsalazine was 19.5% while that for sulfasalazine was 12.2%, a non-significant difference.

INDICATIONS AND USAGE:

Olsalazine is indicated for the maintenance of remission of ulcerative colitis in patients who are intolerant of sulfasalazine.

CONTRAINDICATIONS:

Hypersensitivity to salicylates.

PRECAUTIONS:

General: Overall, approximately 17% of subjects receiving olsalazine in clinical studies reported diarrhea sometime during therapy. This diarrhea resulted in withdrawal of treatment in 6% of patients. This diarrhea appears to be dose related, although it may be difficult to distinguish from the underlying symptoms of the disease.

Exacerbation of the symptoms of colitis thought to have been caused by mesalamine or sulfasalazine has been noted.

Although renal abnormalities were not reported in clinical trials with olsalazine, there have been rare reports from post-marketing experience(see ADVERSE REACTIONS.) Therefore, the possibility of renal tubular damage due to absorbed mesalamine or its n-acetylated metabolite, as noted in the ANIMAL TOXICOLOGY section must be kept in mind, particularly for patients with pre-existing renal disease. In these patients, monitoring with urinalysis, BUN and creatinine determinations is advised.

Information for the Patient: Patients should be instructed to take olsalazine with food. The drug should be taken in evenly divided doses. Patients should be informed that about 17% of subjects receiving olsalazine during clinical studies reported diarrhea some time during therapy. If diarrhea occurs, patients should contact their physician.

Drug/Laboratory Test Interactions: None known.

Carcinogenesis, Mutagenesis, and Impairment of Fertility: In a two year oral rat carcinogenicity study, olsalazine was tested in male and female Wistar rats at daily doses of 200, 400 and 800 mg/kg/day (approximately 10 to 40 times the human maintenance dose, based on a patient weight of 50 kg and a human dose of 1 g). Urinary bladder transitional cell carcinomas were found in three male rats (6%, p=0.022, exact trend test) receiving 40 times the human dose and were not found in untreated male controls. In the same study, urinary bladder transitional cell carcinoma and papilloma occurred in 2 untreated control female rats (2%). No such tumors were found in any of the female rats treated at doses up to 40 times the human dose.

In an eighteen month oral mouse carcinogenicity study, olsalazine was tested in male and female CD-1 mice at daily doses of 500, 1000 and 2000 mg/kg/day (approximately 25 to 100 times the human maintenance dose). Liver hemangiosarcomata were found in two male mice (4%) receiving olsalazine at 100 times the human dose, while no such tumor occurred in the other treated male mice groups or any of the treated female mice. The observed incidence of this tumor is within the 4% incidence in historical controls.

Olsalazine was not mutagenic in *in vitro*Ames tests, mouse lymphoma cell mutation assays, human lymphocyte chromosomal aberration tests and the*in vivo* rat bone marrow cell chromosomal aberration test.

Olsalazine in a dose range of 100 to 400 mg/kg/day (approximately 5 to 20 times the human maintenance dose) did not influence the fertility of male or female rats. The oligospermia and infertility in men associated with sulfasalazine have not been reported with olsalazine.

Pregnancy, Teratogenic Effects, Pregnancy Category C: Olsalazine has been shown to produce fetal developmental toxicity as indicated by reduced fetal weights, retarded ossifications and immaturity of the fetal visceral organs when given during organogenesis to pregnant rats in doses 5 to 20 times the human dose (100 to 400 mg/kg). There are no adequate and well-controlled studies in pregnant women. Olsalazine should be used during pregnancy only if the potential benefit justifies the potential risk to the fetus.

Nursing Mothers: Oral administration of olsalazine to lactating rats in doses 5 to 20 times the human dose produced growth retardation in their pups. It is not known whether this drug is excreted in human milk. Because many drugs are excreted in human milk, caution should be exercised when olsalazine is administered to a nursing woman.

Pediatric Use: Safety and effectiveness in a pediatric population have not been established.

DRUG INTERACTIONS:

Increased prothrombin time in patients taking concomitant warfarin has been reported.

ADVERSE REACTIONS:

Olsalazine has been evaluated in ulcerative colitis patients in remission as well as those with acute disease. Both sulfasalazine- tolerant and intolerant patients have been studied in controlled clinical trials. Overall, 10.4% of patients discontinued olsalazine because of an adverse experience compared with 6.7% of placebo patients. The most commonly reported adverse reactions leading to treatment withdrawal were diarrhea or loose stools (olsalazine 5.9%; placebo 4.8%), abdominal pain and rash or itching (slightly more than 1% of patients receiving olsalazine). Other adverse reactions to olsalazine leading to withdrawal occurred in fewer than 1% of patients (TABLE 1).

TABLE 1 Adverse Reactions Resulting in Withdrawal From Controlled Studies

	Total	
	Olsalazine (N=441)	Placebo (N=208)
Diarrhea/Loose Stools	26 (5.9%)	10 (4.8%)
Nausea	3	2
Abdominal Pain	5 (1.1%)	0
Rash/Itching	5 (1.1%)	0
Headache	3	0
Heartburn	2	0
Rectal Bleeding	1	0
Insomnia	1	0
Dizziness	1	0
Anorexia	1	0
Light Headedness	1	0
Depression	1	0
Miscellaneous	4 (0.9%)	3 (1.4%)
Total Number of Patients Withdrawn	46 (10.4%)	14 (6.7%)

For those controlled studies, the comparative incidences of adverse reactions reported in 1% or more patients treated with olsalazine or placebo are provided in TABLE 2.

Over 2,500 patients have been treated with olsalazine in various controlled and uncontrolled clinical studies. In these as well as in the post- marketing experience, olsalazine was administered mainly to patients intolerant to sulfasalazine. There have been rare reports of the following adverse effects in patients receiving olsalazine. These were often difficult to distinguish from possible symptoms of the underlying disease or from the effects of prior and/or concomitant therapy. A casual relationship to the drug has not been demonstrated for some of these reactions.

ADVERSE REACTIONS: *(cont'd)*

TABLE 2 Comparative Incidence (%) Of Adverse Effects Reported By One Percent Or More Of Ulcerative Colitis Patients Treated With Olsalazine Or Placebo In Double Blind Controlled Studies

Adverse Event	Olsalazine (N = 441) %	Placebo (N = 208) %
Digestive System		
Diarrhea	11.1	6.7
Abdominal Pain/Cramps	10.1	7.2
Nausea	5.0	3.9
Dyspepsia	4.0	4.3
Bloating	1.5	1.4
Anorexia	1.3	1.9
Vomiting	1.0	-
Stomatitis	1.0	-
Increased Blood in Stool	-	3.4
CNS/Psychiatric		
Headache	5.0	4.8
Fatigue/Drowsiness/Lethargy	1.8	2.9
Depression	1.5	-
Vertigo/Dizziness	1.0	-
Insomnia	-	2.4
Skin		
Rash	2.3	1.4
Itching	1.3	-
Musculoskeletal		
Arthralgia/Joint Pain	4.0	2.9
Miscellaneous		
Upper Respiratory Infection	1.5	-

Digestive: Pancreatitis, diarrhea with dehydration, increased blood in stool, rectal bleeding, flare in symptoms, rectal discomfort, epigastric discomfort, flatulence.

Rare cases of granulomatous hepatitis and nonspecific, reactive hepatitis have been reported in patients receiving olsalazine. Additionally, a patient developed mild cholestatic hepatitis during treatment with sulfasalazine and experienced the same symptoms two weeks later after the treatment was changed to olsalazine. Withdrawal of olsalazine led to complete recovery in these cases.

Neurologic: Paresthesia, tremors, insomnia, mood swings, irritability, fever, chills, rigors.

Dermatologic: Erythema nodosum, photosensitivity, erythema, hot flashes, alopecia.

Musculoskeletal: Muscle cramps.

Cardiovascular/Pulmonary: Pericarditis, second degree heart block, interstitial pulmonary disease, hypertension, orthostatic hypotension, peripheral edema, chest pains, tachycardia, palpitations, bronchospasm, shortness of breath.

A patient who developed thyroid disease 9 days after starting Dipentum was given propranolol and radioactive iodine and subsequently developed shortness of breath and nausea. The patient died 5 days later with signs and symptoms of acute diffuse myocarditis.

Genitourinary: Frequency, dysuria, hematuria, proteinuria, nephrotic syndrome, interstitial nephritis, impotence, menorrhagia.

Hematologic: Leukopenia, neutropenia, lymphopenia, eosinophilia, thrombocytopenia, anemia, hemolytic anemia, reticulocytosis.

Laboratory: ALT (SGPT) or AST (SGOT) elevated beyond the normal range.

Special Senses: Tinnitus, dry mouth, dry eyes, watery eyes, blurred vision.

DRUG ABUSE AND DEPENDENCE:

Abuse: None reported.

Dependence: Drug dependence has not been reported with chronic administration of olsalazine.

OVERDOSAGE:

No overdosage has been reported in humans. Maximum single oral doses of 5 g/kg in mice and rats and 2 g/kg in dogs were not lethal. Symptoms of acute toxicity were decreased motor activity and diarrhea in all species tested and in addition, vomiting in dogs.

DOSAGE AND ADMINISTRATION:

The usual dosage in adults for maintenance of remission is 1.0 g/day in two divided doses.

HOW SUPPLIED:

Beige colored capsules, containing 250 mg olsalazine sodium imprinted with "Dipentum 250 mg" on the capsule shell. Packaged in bottles of 100.

Storage: Controlled Room Temperature (15-30°C/59-86°F)

HOW SUPPLIED - EQUIVALENTS NOT AVAILABLE:

Capsule, Gelatin - Oral - 250 mg

100's $61.88 DIPENTUM, Pharmacia & Upjohn 00013-0105-01

OMEPRAZOLE *(001916)*

CATEGORIES: Antiulcer Drugs; Duodenal Ulcer; Endocrine Adenomas; Esophagitis; GERD; Gastric Acid Secretion Inhibitors; Gastroesophagael Reflux Disease; Gastrointestinal Drugs; Hypersecretory Conditions; Mastocytosis; Proton Pump Inhibitors; Reflux; Ulcer; Zollinger-Ellison Syndrome; Pregnancy Category C; Sales > $1 Billion; FDA Approved 1989 Sep; Top 200 Drugs

BRAND NAMES: *Antra* (Germany); *Audazol*; *Desec*; *Dudencer*; *Epirazole*; *Gastroloc* (Germany); *Gibancer*; *Inhibitron* (Mexico); *Inhipump*; *Logastric*; *Lomac*; Losec; *Miracid*; *Mopral* (France); *Nilsec*; *Ocid*; *Omed*; *Omezol*; *Omid*; *Omizac*; *Omisec*; *OMP*; *OMZ*; *Ortanol*; *Ozoken* (Mexico); *Parizac*; *Peptilcer*; *Prazidec* (Mexico); **Prilosec**; *Ramezol*; *Result*; *Ulsen* (Mexico); *Zefxon*
(International brand names outside U.S. in italics)

FORMULARIES: BC-BS; Medi-Cal; PCS

COST OF THERAPY: $101.64 (Duodenal Ulcer; Capsule; 20 mg; 1/day; 28 days)

DESCRIPTION:

The active ingredient in Prilosec Delayed-Release Capsules is a substituted benzimidazole, 5-methoxy-2-[[(4-methoxy-3, 5-dimethyl-2-pyridinyl) methyl] sulfinyl]-1*H*-benzimidazole, a compound that inhibits gastric acid secretion. Its empirical formula is $C_{17}H_{19}N_3O_3S$, with a molecular weight of 345.42.

DESCRIPTION: *(cont'd)*

Omeprazole is a white to off-white crystalline powder which melts with decomposition at about 155°C. It is a weak base, freely soluble in ethanol and methanol, and slightly soluble in acetone and isopropanol and very slightly soluble in water. The stability of omeprazole is a function of pH; it is rapidly degraded in acid media, but has acceptable stability under alkaline conditions.

Prilosec is supplied as delayed-release capsules for oral administration. Each delayed-release capsule contains either 10 mg or 20 mg of omeprazole in the form of enteric-coated granules with the following inactive ingredients: cellulose, disodium hydrogen phosphate, hydroxypropyl cellulose, hydroxypropyl methylcellulose, lactose, mannitol, sodium lauryl sulfate and other ingredients. The capsule shells have the following inactive ingredients: gelatin-NF, FD&C Blue #1, FD&C Red #40, D&C Red #28, titanium dioxide, synthetic black iron oxide, isopropanol, butyl alcohol, FD&C Blue #2, D&C Red #7 Calcium Lake, and, in addition, the 10 mg capsule shell also contains D&C Yellow #10.

CLINICAL PHARMACOLOGY:

PHARMACOKINETICS AND METABOLISM

Omeprazole delayed-release capsules contain an enteric-coated granule formulation of omeprazole (because omeprazole is acid-labile), so that absorption of omeprazole begins only after the granules leave the stomach. Absorption is rapid, with peak plasma levels of omeprazole occurring within 0.5 to 3.5 hours. Peak plasma concentrations of omeprazole and AUC are approximately proportional to doses up to 40 mg, but because of a saturable first-pass effect, a greater than linear response in peak plasma concentration and AUC occurs with doses greater than 40 mg. Absolute bioavailability (compared to intravenous administration) is about 30-40% at doses of 20-40 mg, due in large part to presystemic metabolism. In healthy subjects the plasma half-life is 0.5 to 1 hour, and the total body clearance is 500-600 ml/min. Protein binding is approximately 95%.

The bioavailability of omeprazole increases slightly upon repeated administration of omeprazole delayed-release capsules.

Following single dose oral administration of a buffered solution of omeprazole, little if any unchanged drug was excreted in urine. The majority of the dose (about 77%) was eliminated in urine as at least six metabolites. Two were identified as hydroxyomeprazole and the corresponding carboxylic acid. The remainder of the dose was recoverable in feces. This implies a significant biliary excretion of the metabolites of omeprazole. Three metabolites have been identified in plasma—the sulfide and sulfone derivatives of omeprazole, and hydroxyomeprazole. These metabolites have very little or no antisecretory activity.

In patients with chronic hepatic disease, the bioavailability increased to approximately 100% compared to an IV dose, reflecting decreased first-pass effect, and the plasma half-life of the drug increased to nearly 3 hours compared to the half-life in normals of 0.5-1 hour. Plasma clearance averaged 70 ml/min, compared to a value of 500-600 ml/min in normal subjects.

In patients with chronic renal impairment, whose creatinine clearance ranged between 10 and 62 ml/min/1.73 m^2, the disposition of omeprazole was very similar to that in healthy volunteers, although there was a slight increase in bioavailability. Because urinary excretion is a primary route of excretion of omeprazole metabolites, their elimination slowed in proportion to the decreased creatinine clearance.

The elimination rate of omeprazole was somewhat decreased in the elderly, and bioavailability was increased. Omeprazole was 76% bioavailable when a single 40 mg oral dose of omeprazole (buffered solution) was administered to healthy elderly volunteers, versus 58% in young volunteers given the same dose. Nearly 70% of the dose was recovered in urine as metabolites of omeprazole and no unchanged drug was detected. The plasma clearance of omeprazole was 250 ml/min (about half that of young volunteers) and its plasma half-life averaged one hour, about twice that of young healthy volunteers.

In pharmacokinetic studies of single 20 mg omeprazole doses, an increase in AUC of approximately four-fold was noted in Asian subjects compared to Caucasians.

Dose adjustment, particularly where maintenance of healing of erosive esophagitis is indicated, for the hepatically impaired and Asian subjects should be considered.

PHARMACOKINETICS: COMBINATION THERAPY WITH CLARITHROMYCIN

Omeprazole 40 mg daily was given in combination with clarithromycin 500 mg every 8 hours to healthy adult male subjects. The steady state plasma concentrations of omeprazole were increased (C_{max}, AUC_{0-24}, and $T_{1/2}$ increases of 30%, 89% and 34% respectively) by the concomitant administration of clarithromycin. The observed increases in omeprazole plasma concentration were associated with the following pharmacological effects. The mean 24-hour gastric pH value was 5.2 when omeprazole was administered alone and 5.7 when coadministered with clarithromycin.

The plasma levels of clarithromycin and 14-hydroxy-clarithromycin were increased by the concomitant administration of omeprazole. For clarithromycin, the mean C_{max} was 10% greater, the mean C_{min} was 27% greater, and the mean $AUC_{0-8}$was 15% greater when clarithromycin was administered with omeprazole than when clarithromycin was administered alone. Similar results were seen for 14-hydroxy-clarithromycin, the mean C_{max} was 45% greater, the mean C_{min} was 57% greater, and the mean $AUC_{0-8}$was 45% greater. Clarithromycin concentrations in the gastric tissue and mucus were also increased by concomitant administration of omeprazole.

TABLE 1 Clarithromycin Tissue Concentrations 2 hours after Dose [1]

Tissue	Clarithromycin	Clarithromycin + Omeprazole
Antrum	10.48 ± 2.01 (n=5)	19.96 ± 4.71 (n=5)
Fundus	20.81 ± 7.64 (n=5)	24.25 ± 6.37 (n=5)
Mucus	4.15 ± 7.74 (n=4)	39.29 ± 32.79 (n=4)

[1]Mean ± SD (mcg/g)

For more information on clarithromycin pharmacokinetics and microbiology, consult the Clarithromycin monograph, Clinical Pharmacology section.

PHARMACODYNAMICS

Mechanism of Action: Omeprazole belongs to a new class of antisecretory compounds, the substituted benzimidazoles, that do not exhibit anticholinergic or H_2 histamine antagonistic properties, but that suppress gastric acid secretion by specific inhibition of the H^+/K^+ ATPase enzyme system at the secretory surface of the gastric parietal cell. Because this enzyme system is regarded as the acid (proton) pump within the gastric mucosa, omeprazole has been characterized as a gastric acid-pump inhibitor, in that it blocks the final step of acid production. This effect is dose-related and leads to inhibition of both basal and stimulated acid secretion irrespective of the stimulus. Animal studies indicate that after rapid disappearance from plasma, omeprazole can be found within the gastric mucosa for a day or more.

Antisecretory Activity: After oral administration, the onset of the antisecretory effect of omeprazole occurs within one hour, with the maximum effect occurring within two hours. Inhibition of secretion is about 50% of maximum at 24 hours and the duration of inhibition lasts up to 72 hours. The antisecretory effect thus lasts far longer than would be expected from the very short (less than one hour) plasma half-life, apparently due to prolonged binding

CLINICAL PHARMACOLOGY: *(cont'd)*

to the parietal H^+/K^+ ATPase enzyme. When the drug is discontinued, secretory activity returns gradually, over 3 to 5 days. The inhibitory effect of omeprazole on acid secretion increases with repeated once-daily dosing, reaching a plateau after four days.

Results from numerous studies of the antisecretory effect of multiple doses of 20 mg and 40 mg of omeprazole in normal volunteers and patients are in TABLE 2. The "max" value represents determinations at a time of maximum effect (2-6 hours after dosing), while "min" values are those 24 hours after the last dose of omeprazole.

TABLE 2 Range of Mean Values from Multiple Studies of the Mean Antisecretory Effects of Omeprazole After Multiple Daily Dosing

Parameter	Omeprazole 20 mg		Omeprazole 40 mg	
	Max	Min	Max	Min
% Decrease in Basal Acid Output	78*	58-80	94*	80-93
% Decrease in Peak Acid Output	79*	50-59	88*	62-68
% Decrease in 24-hr. Intragastric Acidity		80-97		92-94

* Single Studies

Single daily oral doses of omeprazole ranging from a dose of 10 mg to 40 mg have produced 100% inhibition of 24-hour intragastric acidity in some patients.

Enterochromaffin-like (ECL) Cell Effects: In 24-month carcinogenicity studies in rats, a dose-related significant increase in gastric carcinoid tumors and ECL cell hyperplasia was observed in both male and female animals (see PRECAUTIONS, Carcinogenesis, Mutagenesis, Impairment of Fertility). Hypergastrinemia secondary to prolonged and sustained hypochlorhydria has been postulated to be the mechanism by which ECL cell hyperplasia and gastric carcinoid tumors develop. Omeprazole may also affect other cells in the gastrointestinal tract (*e.g.,* G cells), either directly or by inducing sustained hypochlorhydria, but this possibility has not been extensively studied.

Human gastric biopsy specimens from about 200 patients treated continuously with omeprazole for an average of over 12 months have not detected ECL cell effects of omeprazole similar to those seen in rats. Longer term data are needed to rule out the possibility of an increased risk for the development of gastric tumors in patients receiving long-term therapy with omeprazole.

Serum Gastrin Effects: In studies involving more than 200 patients, serum gastrin levels increased during the first 1 to 2 weeks of once-daily administration of therapeutic doses of omeprazole in parallel with inhibition of acid secretion. No further increase in serum gastrin occurred with continued treatment. In comparison with histamine H_2-receptor antagonists, the median increases produced by 20 mg doses of omeprazole were higher (1.3 to 3.6 fold vs. 1.1 to 1.8 fold increase). Gastrin values returned to pretreatment levels, usually within 1 to 2 weeks after discontinuation of therapy.

Other Effects: Systemic effects of omeprazole in the CNS, cardiovascular and respiratory systems have not been found to date. Omeprazole, given in oral doses of 30 or 40 mg for 2 to 4 weeks, had no effect on thyroid function, carbohydrate metabolism, or circulating levels of parathyroid hormone, cortisol, estradiol, testosterone, prolactin, cholecystokinin or secretin.

No effect on gastric emptying of the solid and liquid components of a test meal was demonstrated after a single dose of omeprazole 90 mg. In healthy subjects, a single IV dose of omeprazole (0.35 mg/kg) had no effect on intrinsic factor secretion. No systematic dose-dependent effect has been observed on basal or stimulated pepsin output in humans.

However, when intragastric pH is maintained at 4.0 or above, basal pepsin output is low, and pepsin activity is decreased.

As do other agents that elevate intragastric pH, omeprazole administered for 14 days in healthy subjects produced a significant increase in the intragastric concentrations of viable bacteria. The pattern of the bacterial species was unchanged from that commonly found in saliva. All changes resolved within three days of stopping treatment.

CLINICAL STUDIES:

Duodenal Ulcer Disease: *Active Duodenal Ulcer:* In a multicenter, double-blind, placebo-controlled study of 147 patients with endoscopically documented duodenal ulcer, the percentage of patients healed (per protocol) at 2 and 4 weeks was significantly higher with omeprazole 20 mg once a day than with placebo ($p \leq 0.01$) (Table 3).

TABLE 3 Treatment of Active Duodenal Ulcer % of Patients Healed

	Omeprazole 20 mg a.m. (n = 99)	Placebo a.m. (n = 48)
Week 2	*41	13
Week 4	*75	27

* ($p \leq 0.01$)

Complete daytime and nighttime pain relief occurred significantly faster ($p \leq 0.01$) in patients treated with omeprazole 20 mg than in patients treated with placebo. At the end of the study, significantly more patients who had received omeprazole had complete relief of daytime pain ($p \leq 0.05$) and nighttime pain ($p \leq 0.01$).

In a multicenter, double-blind study of 293 patients with endoscopically documented duodenal ulcer, the percentage of patients healed (per protocol) at 4 weeks was significantly higher with omeprazole 20 mg once a day than with ranitidine 150 mg b.i.d. ($p < 0.01$) (Table 4).

TABLE 4 Treatment of Active Duodenal Ulcer % of Patients Healed

	Omeprazole 20 mg a.m. (n = 145)	Ranitidine 150 mg b.i.d. (n = 148)
Week 2	42	34
Week 4	*82	63

* ($p < 0.01$)

Healing occurred significantly faster in patients treated with omeprazole than in those treated with ranitidine 150 mg b.i.d. ($p < 0.01$).

In a foreign multinational randomized, double-blind study of 105 patients with endoscopically documented duodenal ulcer, 20 mg and 40 mg of omeprazole were compared to 150 mg b.i.d. of ranitidine at 2, 4 and 8 weeks. At 2 and 4 weeks both doses of omeprazole were statistically superior (per protocol) to ranitidine, but 40 mg was not superior to 20 mg of omeprazole, and at 8 weeks there was no significant difference between any of the active drugs (Table 5).

CLINICAL STUDIES: *(cont'd)*

TABLE 5 Treatment of Active Duodenal Ulcer % of Patients Healed

	Prilosec 20 mg (n = 34)	Prilosec 40 mg (n = 36)	Ranitidine 150 mg b.i.d. (n = 35)
Week 2	*83	*83	53
Week 4	*97	*100	82
Week 8	100	100	94

* ($p \le 0.01$)

Duodenal Ulcer Recurrence: Four randomized double blind clinical studies with *H. pylori* infection and active duodenal ulcer disease compared omeprazole plus clarithromycin to omeprazole. Two of these studies, one in the U.S., the other in the U.S. and Canada, included a clarithromycin alone arm. The dose regimen in the two multicenter U.S. studies (n=498) was omeprazole 40 mg q.d. plus clarithromycin 500 mg t.i.d. for 14 days followed by omeprazole 20 mg q.d. for 14 days; omeprazole 40 mg q.d. for 14 days followed by omeprazole 20 mg q.d. for 14 days; clarithromycin 500 mg t.i.d. for 14 days. Two foreign studies (n=369) compared omeprazole and clarithromycin to omeprazole, and did not include a clarithromycin alone arm. The dose regimen was the same as that used in the U.S. studies except for one study (M92–812b) where omeprazole 40 mg q.d. was used throughout the 28 day treatment period. Endpoints studied were: eradication of *H. pylori*, duodenal ulcer healing and recurrence. *H. pylori* status was determined by histology and another bacteriological test. For a given patient, *H. pylori* was considered eradicated if at least one of these tests was negative, and none was positive.

The combination of omeprazole and clarithromycin was effective in eradicating *H. pylori*.

TABLE 6 H. pylori Eradication Rates % of Patients Cured† [95% Confidence Inverval]

U.S. Studies	Omeprazole + Clarithromycin	Omeprazole	Clarithromycin
Study M93-067	*74 [61, 85] (n=58)	0 [0, 6] (n=55)	34 [20, 50] (n=44)
Study M93-100	*64 [51, 76] (n=64)	0 [0, 6] (n=62)	38 [24, 53] (n=48)
Non U.S. Studies			
Study M92-812b	*83 [72, 91] (n=69)	1 [0, 7] (n=75)	N/A
Study M93-058	*74 [64-83] (n=93)	4 [1, 10] (n=96)	N/A

† Evaluable patients with confirmed duodenal ulcer and *H. pylori* infection at baseline who are healed at week 4, and for whom results were available for the 4-6 week post-treatment visit are included in this analysis
* ($p \le 0.01$) versus omeprazole or clarithromycin

Ulcer healing was not significantly different when clarithromycin was added to omeprazole therapy compared to omeprazole therapy alone.

The combination of omeprazole and clarithromycin was effective in eradicating *H. pylori* and reduced duodenal ulcer recurrence.

TABLE 7 Duodenal Ulcer Recurrence Rates by *H. pylori* Eradication Status % of Patients with Ulcer Recurrence

	H. pylori eradicated#	*H. pylori* not eradicated#
U.S. Studies†		
6 months post-treatment		
Study M93-067	*35 (n=49	60 (n=88)
Study M93-100	*8 (n=53)	60 (n=106)
Non U.S. Studies$^{\Delta}$		
6 months post-treatment		
Study M92-812b	*5 (n=43)	46 (n=78)
Study M93-058	*6 (n=53)	43 (n=107)
12 months post-treatment		
Study M92-812b	*5 (n=39)	68 (n=71)

H. pylori eradication status assessed at same timepoint as ulcer recurrence
† Combined results for omeprazole + clarithromycin, omeprazole, and clarithromycin treatment arms
$^{\Delta}$Combined results for omeprazole + clarithromycin and omeprazole treatment arms
* ($p \le 0.01$) versus proportion with duodenal ulcer recurrence who were not *H. pylori* eradicated

Gastric Ulcer: In a U.S. multicenter, double-blind, study of omeprazole 40 mg once a day, 20 mg once a day, and placebo in 520 patients with endoscopically diagnosed gastric ulcer, the following results were obtained.

TABLE 8 Treatment of Gastric Ulcer; % of Patients Healed; All Patients Treated

	Omeprazole 20 mg q.d. (n=202)	Omeprazole 40 mg q.d. (n=214)	Placebo (n=104)
Week 4	47.5**	55.6**	30.8
Week 8	74.8**	82.7**,+	48.1

** ($p < 0.01$) omeprazole 40 mg or 20 mg versus placebo
+($p < 0.05$) omeprazole 40 mg versus 20 mg

For the stratified groups of patients with ulcer size less than or equal to 1 cm, no difference in healing rates between 40 mg and 20 mg was detected at either 4 or 8 weeks. For patients with ulcer size greater than 1 cm, 40 mg was significantly more effective than 20 mg at 8 weeks.

In a foreign, multinational, double-blind study of 602 patients with endoscopically diagnosed gastric ulcer, omeprazole 40 mg once a day, 20 mg once a day, and ranitidine 150 mg twice a day were evaluated.

TABLE 9 Treatment of Gastric Ulcer; % of Patients Healed (All Patients Treated)

	Omeprazole 20 mg q.d. (n=200)	Omeprazole 40 mg q.d. (n=187)	Ranitidine 150 mg b.i.d. (n=199)
Week 4	63.5	78.1**,++	56.3
Week 8	81.5	91.4**,++	78.4

** ($P<0.01$) omeprazole 40 mg versus ranitidine
++($p<0.01$) omeprazole 40 mg versus 20 mg

Gastroesophageal Reflux Disease (GERD): *Symptomatic GERD:* A placebo controlled study was conducted in Scandinavia to compare the efficacy of omperazole 20 mg or 10 mg once daily for up to 4 weeks in the treatment of heartburn and other symptoms in GERD patients without erosive esophagitis. Results are shown in TABLE 10.

CLINICAL STUDIES: *(cont'd)*

TABLE 10

	% Successful Symptomatic Outcome‡ Omeprazole 20 mg a.m.	Omeprazole 10 mg a.m.	Placebo a.m.
All patients	46*,† (n=205)	31 † (n=199)	13 (n=105)
Patients with confirmed GERD	56*,† (n=115)	36† (n=109)	14 (n=59)

‡ Defined as complete resolution of heartburn
* ($p<0.005$) versus 10 mg
† ($p<0.005$) versus placebo

Erosive Esophagitis: In a U.S. multicenter double-blind placebo controlled study of 20 mg or 40 mg of omeprazole delayed-release capsules in patients with symptoms of GERD and endoscopically diagnosed erosive esophagitis of grade 2 or above, the percentage healing rates (per protocol) are shown in TABLE 11.

TABLE 11

Week	20 mg Omeprazole (n = 83)	40 mg Omeprazole (n = 87)	Placebo (n = 43)
4	39**	45**	7
8	74**	75**	14

** ($p<0.01$) omeprazole versus placebo.

In this study, the 40 mg dose was not superior to the 20 mg dose of omeprazole in the percentage healing rate. Other controlled clinical trials have also shown that omeprazole is effective in severe GERD. In comparisons with histamine H_2-receptor antagonists in patients with erosive esophagitis, grade 2 or above, omeprazole in a dose of 20 mg was significantly more effective than the active controls. Complete daytime and nighttime heartburn relief occurred significantly faster ($p<0.01$) in patients treated with omeprazole than in those taking placebo or histamine H_2-receptor antagonists.

In this and five other controlled GERD studies, significantly more patients taking 20 mg omeprazole (84%) reported complete relief of GERD symptoms than patients receiving placebo (12%).

Long Term Maintenance Treatment of Erosive Esophagitis: In a U.S. double-blind, randomized, multicenter, placebo controlled study, two dose regimens of omeprazole were studied in patients with endoscopically confirmed healed esophagitis. Results to determine maintenance of healing of erosive esophagitis are shown below (Table 12).

TABLE 12 Life Table Analysis

	Omeprazole 20 mg q.d. (n = 138)	Omeprazole 20 mg 3 days per week (n = 137)	Placebo (n = 131)
Percent in endoscopic remission at 6 months	*70	34	11

* ($p<0.01$) Omeprazole 20 mg q.d. versus omeprazole 20 mg 3 consecutive days per week or placebo.

In an international multicenter double-blind study, omeprazole 20 mg daily and 10 mg daily were compared to ranitidine 150 mg twice daily in patients with endoscopically confirmed healed esophagitis. The table (Table 13) below provides the results of this study for maintenance of healing of erosive esophagitis.

TABLE 13 Life Table Analysis

	Omeprazole 20 mg q.d. (n = 131)	Omeprazole 10 mg q.d. (n = 133)	Ranitidine 150 mg b.i.d. (n = 128)
Percent in endoscopic remission at 12 months	*77	‡58	46

* ($p=0.01$) Omeprazole 20 mg q.d. versus omeprazole 10 mg q.d. or Ranitidine.
‡ ($p=0.03$) Omeprazole 10 mg q.d. versus Ranitidine.

In patients who initially had grades 3 or 4 erosive esophagitis, for maintenance after healing 20 mg daily of omeprazole was effective, while 10 mg did not demonstrate effectiveness.

Pathological Hypersecretory Conditions: In open studies of 136 patients with pathological hypersecretory conditions, such as Zollinger-Ellison (ZE) syndrome with or without multiple endocrine adenomas, omeprazole delayed-release capsules significantly inhibited gastric acid secretion and controlled associated symptoms of diarrhea, anorexia, and pain. Doses ranging from 20 mg every other day to 360 mg per day maintained basal acid secretion below 10 mEq/hr in patients without prior gastric surgery, and below 5 mEq/hr in patients with prior gastric surgery.

Initial doses were titrated to the individual patient need, and adjustments were necessary with time in some patients (see DOSAGE AND ADMINISTRATION.) Omeprazole was well tolerated at these high dose levels for prolonged periods (>5 years in some patients). In most ZE patients, serum gastrin levels were not modified by omeprazole. However, in some patients serum gastrin increased to levels greater than those present prior to initiation of omeprazole therapy. At least 11 patients with ZE syndrome on long-term treatment with omeprazole developed gastric carcinoids. These findings are believed to be a manifestation of the underlying condition, which is known to be associated with such tumors, rather than the result of the administration of omeprazole. (See ADVERSE REACTIONS.)

INDICATIONS AND USAGE:

DUODENAL ULCER

Omeprazole delayed-release capsules are indicated for short-term treatment of active duodenal ulcer. Most patients heal within four weeks. Some patients may require an additional four weeks of therapy.

Omeprazole delayed-release capsules, in combination with clarithromycin, are also indicated for the treatment of patients with *H. pylori* infection and active duodenal ulcer to eradicated *H. pylori*. Eradication of *H. pylori* has been shown to reduce the risk of duodenal ulcer recurrence (see CLINICAL STUDIES and DOSAGE AND ADMINISTRATION).

In patients who fail therapy, susceptibility testing should be done. If resistance to clarithromycin is demonstrated or susceptibility testing is not possible, alternative antimicrobial therapy should be instituted. (See the Clarithromycin monograph, **Microbiology** section.)

INDICATIONS AND USAGE: *(cont'd)*

GASTRIC ULCER

Omeprazole delayed-release capsules are indicated for the short-term treatment (4–8 weeks) of active benign gastric ulcer. (See CLINICAL STUDIES.)

TREATMENT OF GASTROESOPHAGEAL REFLUX DISEASE (GERD)

Symptomatic GERD: Omeprazole delayed-release capsules are indicated for the treatment of heartburn and other symptoms associated with GERD.

Erosive Esophagitis: Omeprazole delayed-release capsules are indicated for the short-term treatment (4-8 weeks) of erosive esophagitis which has been diagnosed by endoscopy (See CLINICAL STUDIES.)

The efficacy of omeprazole used for longer than 8 weeks in these patients has not been established. In the rare instance of a patient not responding to 8 weeks of treatment, it may be helpful to give up to an additional 4 weeks of treatment. If there is recurrence of erosive esophagitis or GERD symptoms (*e.g.,* heartburn), additional 4-8 week courses of omeprazole may be considered

Maintenance of Healing of Erosive Esophagitis: Omeprazole delayed-release capsules are indicated to maintain healing of erosive esophagitis.

Controlled studies do not extend beyond 12 months.

Pathological Hypersecretory Conditions: Omeprazole delayed-release capsules are indicated for the long-term treatment of pathological hypersecretory conditions (*e.g.,* Zollinger-Ellison syndrome, multiple endocrine adenomas and systemic mastocytosis).

CONTRAINDICATIONS:

Omeprazole delayed-release capsules are contraindicated in patients with known hypersensitivity to any component of the formulation.

PRECAUTIONS:

General: Symptomatic response to therapy with omeprazole does not preclude the presence of gastric malignancy.

Atrophic gastritis has been noted occasionally in gastric corpus biopsies from patients treated long-term with omeprazole.

Information for Patients: Omeprazole delayed-release capsules should be taken before eating. Patients should be cautioned that the omeprazole delayed-release capsule should not be opened, chewed or crushed, and should be swallowed whole.

Carcinogenesis, Mutagenesis, Impairment of Fertility: In two 24-month carcinogenicity studies in rats, omeprazole at daily doses of 1.7, 3.4, 13.8, 44.0 and 140.8 mg/kg/day (approximately 4 to 352 times the human dose, based on a patient weight of 50 kg and a human dose of 20 mg) produced gastric ECL cell carcinoids in a dose-related manner in both male and female rats; the incidence of this effect was markedly higher in female rats, which had higher blood levels of omeprazole. Gastric carcinoids seldom occur in the untreated rat. In addition, ECL cell hyperplasia was present in all treated groups of both sexes. In one of these studies, female rats were treated with 13.8 mg omeprazole/kg/day (approximately 35 times the human dose) for one year, then followed for an additional year without the drug. No carcinoids were seen in these rats. An increased incidence of treatment-related ECL cell hyperplasia was observed at the end of one year (94% treated vs 10% controls). By the second year the difference between treated and control rats was much smaller (46% vs 26%) but still showed more hyperplasia in the treated group. An unusual primary malignant tumor in the stomach was seen in one rat (2%). No similar tumor was seen in male or female rats treated for two years. For this strain of rat no similar tumor has been noted historically, but a finding involving only one tumor is difficult to interpret. A 78-week mouse carcinogenicity study of omeprazole did not show increased tumor occurrence, but the study was not conclusive.

Omeprazole was not mutagenic in an *in vitro* Ames *Salmonella typhimurium* assay, an *in vitro* mouse lymphoma cell assay and an *in vivo* rat liver DNA damage assay. A mouse micronucleus test at 625 and 6250 times the human dose gave a borderline result, as did an*in vivo* bone marrow chromosome aberration test. A second mouse micronucleus study at 2000 times the human dose, but with different (suboptimal) sampling times, was negative.

In a rat fertility and general reproductive performance test, omeprazole in a dose range of 13.8 to 138.0 mg/kg/day (approximately 35 to 345 times the human dose) was not toxic or deleterious to the reproductive performance of parental animals.

Pregnancy Category C: Teratology studies conducted in pregnant rats at doses up to 138 mg/kg/day (approximately 345 times the human dose) and in pregnant rabbits at doses up to 69 mg/kg/day (approximately 172 times the human dose) did not disclose any evidence for a teratogenic potential of omeprazole.

In rabbits, omeprazole in a dose range of 6.9 to 69.1 mg/kg/day (approximately 17 to 172 times the human dose) produced dose-related increases in embryo-lethality, fetal resorptions and pregnancy disruptions. In rats, dose-related embryo/fetal toxicity and postnatal developmental toxicity were observed in offspring resulting from parents treated with omeprazole 13.8 to 138.0 mg/kg/day (approximately 35 to 345 times the human dose). There are no adequate or well-controlled studies in pregnant women. Sporadic reports have been received of congenital abnormalities occurring in infants born to women who have received omeprazole during pregnancy. Omeprazole should be used during pregnancy only if the potential benefit justifies the potential risk to the fetus.

Nursing Mothers: It is not known whether omeprazole is excreted in human milk. In rats, omeprazole administration during late gestation and lactation at doses of 13.8 to 138 mg/kg/day (35 to 345 times the human dose) resulted in decreased weight gain in pups. Because many drugs are excreted in human milk, because of the potential for serious adverse reactions in nursing infants from omeprazole, and because of the potential for tumorigenicity shown for omeprazole in rat carcinogenicity studies, a decision should be made whether to discontinue nursing or to discontinue the drug, taking into account the importance of the drug to the mother.

Pediatric Use: Safety and effectiveness in children have not been established.

DRUG INTERACTIONS:

Omeprazole can prolong the elimination of diazepam, warfarin and phenytoin, drugs that are metabolized by oxidation in the liver. Although in normal subjects no interaction with theophylline or propranolol was found, there have been clinical reports of interaction with other drugs metabolized via the cytochrome P-450 system (*e.g.,* cyclosporine, disulfiram, benzodiazepines). Patients should be monitored to determine if it is necessary to adjust the dosage of these drugs when taken concomitantly with omeprazole.

Because of its profound and long lasting inhibition of gastric acid secretion, it is theoretically possible that omeprazole may interfere with absorption of drugs where gastric pH is an important determinant of their bioavailability (*e.g.,* ketoconazole, ampicillin esters, and iron salts). In the clinical trials, antacids were used concomitantly with the administration of omeprazole.

ADVERSE REACTIONS:

Omeprazole delayed-release capsules were generally well tolerated during domestic and international clinical trials in 3096 patients.

ADVERSE REACTIONS: *(cont'd)*

In the U.S. clinical trial population of 465 patients (including duodenal ulcer, Zollinger-Ellison syndrome and resistant ulcer patients), the following adverse experiences were reported to occur in 1% or more of patients on therapy with omeprazole. Numbers in parentheses indicate percentages of the adverse experiences considered by investigators as possibly, probably or definitely related to the drug (Table 14):

TABLE 14

	Omeprazole (n=465)	Placebo (n=64)	Ranitidine (n=195)
Headache	6.9 (2.4)	6.3	7.7 (2.6)
Diarrhea	3.0 (1.9)	3.1 (1.6)	2.1 (0.5)
Abdominal Pain	2.4 (0.4)	3.1	2.1
Nausea	2.2 (0.9)	3.1	4.1 (0.5)
URI	1.9	1.6	2.6
Dizziness	1.5 (0.6)	0.0	2.6 (1.0)
Vomiting	1.5 (0.4)	4.7	1.5 (0.5)
Rash	1.5 (1.1)	0.0	0.0
Constipation	1.1 (0.9)	0.0	0.0
Cough	1.1	0.0	1.5
Asthenia	1.1 (0.2)	1.6 (1.6)	1.5 (1.0)
Back Pain	1.1	0.0	0.5

The following adverse reactions which occurred in 1% or more of omeprazole-treated patients have been reported in international double- blind, and open-label, clinical trials in which 2,631 patients and subjects received omeprazole (Table 15).

TABLE 15 Incidence of Adverse Experiences ≥ 1%, Causal Relationship Not Assessed

	Omeprazole (n=2631)	Placebo (n=120)
Body As A Whole, Site Unspecified		
Abdominal Pain	5.2	3.3
Asthenia	1.3	0.8
Digestive System		
Constipation	1.5	0.8
Diarrhea	3.7	2.5
Flatulence	2.7	5.8
Nausea	4.0	6.7
Vomiting	3.2	10.0
Acid regurgitation	1.9	3.3
Nervous System/Psychiatric		
Headache	2.9	2.5

Additional adverse experiences occurring in < 1% of patients or subjects in domestic and/or international trials, or occurring since the drug was marketed, are shown below within each body system. In many instances, the relationship to omeprazole was unclear.

Body As a Whole: Fever, pain, fatigue, malaise, abdominal swelling

Cardiovascular: Chest pain or angina, tachycardia, bradycardia, palpitation, elevated blood pressure, peripheral edema

Gastrointestinal: Pancreatitis (some fatal), anorexia, irritable colon, flatulence, fecal discoloration, esophageal candidiasis, mucosal atrophy of the tongue, dry mouth. During treatment with omeprazole, gastric fundic gland polyps have been noted rarely. These polyps are benign and appear to be reversible when treatment is discontinued. Gastro-duodenal carcinoids have been reported in patients with ZE syndrome on long-term treatment with omeprazole. This finding is believed to be a manifestation of the underlying condition, which is known to be associated with such tumors.

Hepatic: Mild and, rarely, marked elevations of liver function tests [ALT (SGPT), AST (SGOT), γ-glutamyl transpeptidase, alkaline phosphatase, and bilirubin (jaundice)]. In rare instances, overt liver disease has occurred, including hepatocellular, cholestatic, or mixed hepatitis, liver necrosis (some fatal), hepatic failure (some fatal), and hepatic encephalopathy.

Metabolic/Nutritional: Hypoglycemia, weight gain

Musculoskeletal: Muscle cramps, myalgia, muscle weakness, joint pain, leg pain

Nervous System/Psychiatric: Psychic disturbances including depression, aggression, hallucinations, confusion, insomnia, nervousness, tremors, apathy, somnolence, anxiety, dream abnormalities; vertigo; paresthesia; hemifacial dysesthesia

Respiratory: Epistaxis, pharyngeal pain

Skin: Rash and, very rarely, cases of severe generalized skin reactions including toxic epidermal necrolysis (TEN; some fatal), Stevens-Johnson syndrome, and erythema multiforme (some severe); skin inflammation, urticaria, angioedema, pruritus, alopecia, dry skin, hyperhidrosis

Special Senses: Tinnitus, taste perversion

Urogenital: Interstitial nephritis (some with positive rechallenge), urinary tract infection, microscopic pyuria, urinary frequency, elevated serum creatinine, proteinuria, hematuria, glycosuria, testicular pain, gynecomastia

Hematologic: Rare instances of pancytopenia, agranulocytosis (some fatal), thrombocytopenia, neutropenia, anemia, leucocytosis, and hemolytic anemia have been reported.

The incidence of clinical adverse experiences in patients greater than 65 years of age was similar to that in patients 65 years of age or less.

OVERDOSAGE:

There is no experience to date with deliberate overdosage. Dosages of up to 360 mg/day have been well tolerated. No specific antidote is known. Omeprazole is extensively protein bound and is, therefore, not readily dialyzable. In the event of overdosage, treatment should be symptomatic and supportive.

Lethal doses of omeprazole after single oral administration are about 1500 mg/kg in mice and greater than 4000 mg/kg in rats, and about 100 mg/kg in mice and greater than 40 mg/kg in rats given single intravenous injections. Animals given these doses showed sedation, ptosis, convulsions, and decreased activity, body temperature, and respiratory rate and increased depth of respiration.

DOSAGE AND ADMINISTRATION:

Duodenal Ulcer: The recommended adult oral dose is 40 mg once daily for 4-8 weeks. (See CLINICAL STUDIES and INDICATIONS AND USAGE.)

Gastroesophageal Reflux Disease (GERD): The recommended adult oral dose for the treatment of patients with symptomatic GERD and no esophageal lesions is 20 mg daily for up to 4 weeks. The recommended adult oral dose for the treatment of patients with erosive esophagitis and accompanying symptoms due to GERD is 20 mg daily for 4 to 8 weeks (see INDICATIONS AND USAGE.)

Maintenance of Healing of Erosive Esophagitis: The recommended adult oral dose is 20 mg daily. (See CLINICAL STUDIES.)

DOSAGE AND ADMINISTRATION: *(cont'd)*

Pathological Hypersecretory Conditions: The dosage of omeprazole in patients with pathological hypersecretory conditions varies with the individual patient. The recommended adult oral starting dose is 60 mg once a day. Doses should be adjusted to individual patient needs and should continue for as long as clinically indicated. Doses up to 120 mg t.i.d. have been administered. Daily dosages of greater than 80 mg should be administered in divided doses. Some patients with Zollinger- Ellison syndrome have been treated continuously with omeprazole for more than 5 years.

No dosage adjustment is necessary for patients with renal impairment, hepatic dysfunction or for the elderly.

Omeprazole delayed-release capsules should be taken before eating. In the clinical trials, antacids were used concomitantly with omeprazole.

Patients should be cautioned that the omeprazole delayed-release capsule should not be opened, chewed or crushed, and should be swallowed whole.

PATIENT INFORMATION:

Omeprazole is used to treat ulcers and acid reflux. Generally 4 to 8 weeks of therapy are needed. If symptoms persist, contact your physician for additional evaluation. Very few side effects were reported with this medication. Most commonly reported side effects include: headache, diarrhea and abdominal pain. Omeprazole is available in a delayed-release capsule and it should be taken whole, not crushed or broken. The capsules should be taken before meals. It is ok to take this medication with antacids.

HOW SUPPLIED:

No. 3426: Prilosec Delayed-Release Capsules, 10 mg: are opaque, hard gelatin, apricot and amethyst colored capsules, coded 606 on cap and Prilosec 10 on the body.

No. 3440: Prilosec Delayed-Release Capsules, 20 mg: are opaque, hard gelatin, amethyst colored capsules, coded 742 on cap and Prilosec 20 on body.

Storage: Store Prilosec Delayed-Release Capsules in a tight container protected from light and moisture. Store between 15°C and 30°C (59°F and 86°F).

HOW SUPPLIED - EQUIVALENTS NOT AVAILABLE:

Capsule, Gelatin, Sustained Action - Oral - 10 mg

30's	$97.56	PRILOSEC, Astra Merck	61113-0606-31
100's	$325.20	PRILOSEC, Astra Merck	61113-0606-28
100's	$325.20	PRILOSEC, Astra Merck	61113-0606-68

Capsule, Gelatin, Sustained Action - Oral - 20 mg

30's	$108.90	PRILOSEC, Astra Merck	61113-0742-31
100's	$363.01	PRILOSEC, Astra Merck	61113-0742-28
1000's	$3630.12	PRILOSEC, Astra Merck	61113-0742-82

ONDANSETRON HYDROCHLORIDE *(003031)*

CATEGORIES: Antiemetics; Cancer; Central Nervous System Agents; Chemotherapy; 5-HT3 Receptor Antagonist; Gastrointestinal Drugs; Nausea; Nausea and Vomiting; Serotonin Antagonists; Vomiting; Dementia*; Schizophrenia*; Pregnancy Category B; FDA Class 1B ("Modest Therapeutic Advantage"); Sales > $500 Million; FDA Approved 1991 Jan

* Indication not approved by the FDA

BRAND NAMES: *Emeset; Oncoden;* **Zofran**; *Zofron*
(International brand names outside U.S. in italics)

FORMULARIES: Kaiser; Medi-Cal; PCS

COST OF THERAPY: $117.73 (Nausea; Tablet; 8 mg; 3/day; 2 days)

DESCRIPTION:

The active ingredient in Zofran Injection and Zofran Injection Premixed is ondansetron hydrochloride (HCl), and the active ingredient in Zofran Tablets is ondansetron HCl as the dihydrate, the racemic form of ondansetron and a selective blocking agent of the serotonin 5-HT_3 receptor type. Chemically it is (±) 1, 2, 3, 9-tetrahydro-9-methyl-3- [(2-methyl-1H-imidazol-1-yl) methyl] -4H-carbazol-4-one, monohydrochloride, dihydrate.

The empirical formula is $C_{18}H_{19}N_3O{\cdot}HCl{\cdot}2H_2O$, representing a molecular weight of 365.9.

Ondansetron HCl and ondansetron HCl dihydrate are a white to off-white powder that is soluble in water and normal saline.

Sterile Injection for Intravenous Administration: Each 1 ml of aqueous solution in the 2-ml single-dose vial contains 2 mg of ondansetron as the hydrochloride dihydrate; 9.0 mg of sodium chloride, USP; and 0.5 mg of citric acid monohydrate, USP and 0.25 mg of sodium citrate dihydrate, USP as buffers in Water for Injection, USP.

Each 1 ml of aqueous solution in the 20-ml multidose vial contains 2 mg of ondansetron as the hydrochloride dihydrate; 8.3 mg of sodium chloride, USP; 0.5 mg of citric acid monohydrate, USP and 0.25 mg of sodium citrate dihydrate, USP as buffers; and 1.2 mg of methylparaben, NF and 0.15 mg of propylparaben, NF as preservatives in Water for Injection, USP.

Ondansetron injection is a clear, colorless, nonpyrogenic, sterile solution for intravenous (IV) injection. The pH of the injection solution is 3.3 to 4.0.

Sterile, Premixed Solution for Intravenous Administration in Single-dose, Flexible Plastic Containers: Each 50 ml contains ondansetron 32 mg (as the hydrochloride dihydrate); dextrose 2500 mg; and citric acid 26 mg and sodium citrate 11.5 mg as buffers in Water for Injection, USP. It contains no preservatives. The osmolarity of this solution is 270 mOsm/l (approx.), and the pH is 3.0 to 4.0.

The flexible plastic container is fabricated from a specially formulated, nonplasticized, thermoplastic co-polyester (CR3). Water can permeate from inside the container into the overwrap but not in amounts sufficient to affect the solution significantly. Solutions inside the container also can leach out certain of the chemical components in very small amounts before the expiration period is attained. However, the safety of the plastic has been confirmed by tests in animals according to USP biological standards for plastic containers.

Zofran Tablets: Each 4-mg Zofran Tablet for oral administration contains ondansetron HCl dihydrate equivalent to 4 mg of ondansetron. Each 8-mg Zofran Tablet for oral administration contains ondansetron HCl dihydrate equivalent to 8 mg of ondansetron. Each tablet also contains the inactive ingredients lactose, microcrystalline cellulose, pregelatinized starch, hydroxypropyl methylcellulose, magnesium stearate, titanium dioxide, iron oxide yellow (8-mg tablet only), and sodium benzoate (4-mg tablet only).

CLINICAL PHARMACOLOGY:

PHARMACODYNAMICS

Ondansetron is a selective 5-HT_3 receptor antagonist. While ondansetron's mechanism of action has not been fully characterized, it is not a dopamine-receptor antagonist. Serotonin receptors of the 5-HT_3 type are present both peripherally on vagal nerve terminals and centrally in the chemoreceptor trigger zone of the area postrema. It is not certain whether ondansetron's antiemetic action in chemotherapy-induced emesis is mediated centrally, peripherally, or in both sites. However, cytotoxic chemotherapy appears to be associated with release of serotonin from the enterochromaffin cells of the small intestine. In humans, urinary 5-HIAA (5-hydroxyindoleacetic acid) excretion increases after cisplatin administration in parallel with the onset of emesis. The released serotonin may stimulate the vagal afferents through the 5-HT_3receptors and initiate the vomiting reflex.

In animals, the emetic response to cisplatin can be prevented by pretreatment with an inhibitor of serotonin synthesis, bilateral abdominal vagotomy and greater splanchnic nerve section, or pretreatment with a serotonin 5-HT_3 receptor antagonist.

In normal volunteers, single IV doses of 0.15 mg/kg of ondansetron had no effect on esophageal motility, gastric motility, lower esophageal sphincter pressure, or small intestinal transit time. In another IV study in six normal male volunteers, a 16-mg dose infused over 5 minutes showed no effect of the drug on cardiac output, heart rate, stroke volume, blood pressure, or electrocardiogram (ECG). Multiday administration of ondansetron has been shown to slow colonic transit in normal volunteers. Ondansetron has no effect on plasma prolactin concentrations.

Intravenous ondansetron does not alter the respiratory depressant effects produced by alfentanil or the degree of neuromuscular blockade produced by atracurium. Interactions with general or local anesthetics have not been studied.

PHARMACOKINETICS

Injection

Ondansetron is extensively metabolized in humans, with approximately 5% of a radiolabeled dose recovered as the parent compound from the urine. The primary metabolic pathway is hydroxylation on the indole ring followed by glucuronide or sulfate conjugation.

In normal volunteers, the mean pharmacokinetic data in TABLE 1 have been determined following a single 0.15-mg/kg IV dose.

TABLE 1 Pharmacokinetics in Normal Volunteers

Age-group	n	Peak Plasma Concentration (ng/ml)	Mean Elimination Half-life (h)	Plasma Clearance (l/h/kg)
19-40	11	102	3.5	0.381
61-74	12	106	4.7	0.319
≥ 75	11	170	5.5	0.262

From a single-dose infusion study, patients with severe hepatic impairment showed a fivefold and those with mild-to-moderate liver impairment a twofold reduction in mean plasma clearance, with increases in the mean apparent volume of distribution of less than twofold, as compared to normals. The mean half-life of 3.6 hours in normals increased to 9.2 hours in patients with mild-to-moderate hepatic impairment and was prolonged to 20.6 hours in patients with severe hepatic insufficiency.

A reduction in clearance and increase in elimination half-life are seen in patients over 75 years old. In clinical trials with patients with cancer, there was neither a difference in safety nor efficacy between patients over 65 years of age and those under 65 years of age; there was an insufficient number of patients over 75 years of age to permit conclusions in that age-group. No adjustment in dosage is recommended in the elderly.

In adult cancer patients, the mean elimination half-life was 4.0 hours, and there was no difference in the multidose pharmacokinetics over a 4-day period. In a study of 21 pediatric cancer patients (aged 4 to 18 years) who received three IV doses of 0.15 mg/kg of ondansetron at 4-hour intervals, patients older than 15 years of age exhibited ondansetron pharmacokinetic parameters similar to those of adults. Patients aged 4 to 12 years generally showed higher clearance and somewhat larger volume of distribution than adults. Most pediatric patients younger than 15 years of age with cancer had a shorter (2.4 hours) ondansetron plasma half-life than patients older than 15 years of age. It is not known whether these differences in ondansetron plasma half-life may result in differences in efficacy between adults and some young children (see CLINICAL STUDIES, Pediatric Studies.)

In a study of 21 pediatric patients (aged 3 to 12 years) who were undergoing surgery requiring anesthesia for a duration of 45 minutes to 2 hours, a single IV dose of ondansetron, 2 mg (3 to 7 years) or 4 mg (8 to 12 years), was administered immediately prior to anesthesia induction. Mean weight-normalized clearance and volume of distribution values in these pediatric patients were similar to those previously reported for young adults. Mean terminal half-life was slightly reduced in pediatric patients (range, 2.5 to 3 hours) in comparison with adults (range, 3 to 3.5 hours).

In normal volunteers (19 to 39 years old, n=23), the peak plasma concentration was 264 ng/ml following a single 32-mg dose administered as a 15-minute IV infusion. The mean elimination half-life was 4.1 hours. Systemic exposure to 32 mg of ondansetron was not proportional to dose as measured by comparing dose-normalized AUC values to an 8-mg dose. This is consistent with a small decrease in systemic clearance with increasing plasma concentrations.

Plasma protein binding of ondansetron as measured *in vitro* was 70% to 76%, with binding constant over the pharmacologic concentration range (10 to 500 ng/ml). Circulating drug also distributes into erythrocytes.

A positive lymphoblast transformation test to ondansetron has been reported, which suggests immunologic sensitivity to ondansetron.

Tablets

Ondansetron is extensively metabolized in humans, with approximately 5% of a radiolabeled dose recovered from the urine as the parent compound. The primary metabolic pathway is hydroxylation on the indole ring followed by subsequent glucuronide or sulfate conjugation. Although some nonconjugated metabolites have pharmacologic activity, these are not found in plasma concentrations likely to significantly contribute to the biological activity of ondansetron.

Oral ondansetron is well absorbed and undergoes limited first-pass metabolism. Following the administration of a single 8-mg ondansetron tablet to healthy, young, male volunteers and from pooled studies, the time to peak plasma ondansetron concentration is approximately 1.7 hours, the terminal elimination half-life is approximately 3 hours, and bioavailability is approximately 56%. Gender differences were shown in the disposition of ondansetron given as a single dose. The extent and rate of ondansetron's absorption is greater in women than men. Slower clearance in women, a smaller apparent volume of distribution (adjusted for weight) and higher absolute bioavailability resulted in higher plasma ondansetron levels. These higher plasma levels may in part be explained by differences in body weight between men and women. It is not known whether these gender-related differences were clinically important. More detailed pharmacokinetic information is contained in TABLE 2 taken from one study.

CLINICAL PHARMACOLOGY: *(cont'd)*

TABLE 2 Pharmacokinetics in Normal Volunteers: Single 8-mg Oral Dose

Age-group (years)	Mean Weight (kg)	n	Peak Plasma Concentration (ng/ml)	Time of Peak Plasma Concentration (h)	Mean Elimination Half-life (h)	Systemic Plasma Clearance l/h/kg	Absolute Bioavailability
18-40 M	69.0	6	26.2	2.0	3.1	0.403	0.483
F	62.7	5	42.7	1.7	3.5	0.354	0.663
61-74 M	77.5	6	24.1	2.1	4.1	0.384	0.585
F	60.2	6	52.4	1.9	4.9	0.255	0.643
≥ 75 M	78.0	5	37.0	2.2	4.5	0.277	0.619
F	67.6	6	46.1	2.1	6.2	0.249	0.747

Both AUC and C_{max} more than double on increasing the tablet dose from 8 to 16 mg (123% and 118%, respectively). This may result from saturation of first-pass metabolism leading to greater oral bioavailability at 16 mg than 8 mg.

The administration of oral ondansetron with food increases significantly (about 17%) the extent of absorption of ondansetron. The peak plasma concentration and time to peak plasma concentration are not significantly affected. This change in the extent of absorption is not believed to be of any clinical relevance.

There was no significant effect of antacid administration on the pharmacokinetics of orally administered ondansetron.

Because ondansetron undergoes extensive metabolism, the modest reduction in clearance in the over 75 age-group was not unexpected. However, since there was a difference in neither safety nor efficacy between patients over 65 years of age and those under 65 years of age, no adjustment in dosage is required in the elderly.

Plasma protein binding of ondansetron as measured *in vitro* was 70% to 76% over the concentration range of 10 to 500 ng/ml. Circulating drug also distributes into erythrocytes.

CLINICAL STUDIES:

INJECTION

Chemotherapy-Induced Nausea and Vomiting

In a double-blind study of three different dosing regimens of ondansetron injection, 0.015 mg/kg, 0.15 mg/kg, and 0.30 mg/kg, each given three times during the course of cancer chemotherapy, the 0.15-mg/kg dosing regimen was more effective than the 0.015-mg/kg dosing regimen. The 0.30-mg/kg dosing regimen was not shown to be more effective than the 0.15-mg/kg dosing regimen.

Cisplatin-Based Chemotherapy: In a double-blind study in 28 patients, ondansetron injection (three 0.15-mg/kg doses) was significantly more effective than placebo in preventing nausea and vomiting induced by cisplatin-based chemotherapy. Treatment response is in TABLE 3.

TABLE 3 Prevention of Chemotherapy-Induced Nausea and Emesis in Single-Day Cisplatin Therapy*

	Ondansetron Injection	Placebo	P Value†
Number of patients	14	14	
Treatment response			
0 Emetic episodes	2 (14%)	0 (0%)	
1-2 Emetic episodes	8 (57%)	0 (0%)	
3-5 Emetic episodes	2 (14%)	1 (7%)	
More than 5 emetic episodes/rescued	2 (14%)	13 (93%)	0.001
Median number of emetic episodes	1.5	Undefined‡	
Median time to first emetic episode (h)	11.6	2.8	0.001
Median nausea scores (0-100) §	3	59	0.034
Global satisfaction with control of nausea and vomiting (0-100)‖	96	10.5	0.009

* Chemotherapy was high dose (100 and 120 mg/m²; Ondansetron Injection n=6, placebo n=5) or moderate dose (50 and 80 mg/m²; Ondansetron Injection n=8, placebo n=9). Other chemotherapeutic agents included fluorouracil, doxorubicin, and cyclophosphamide. There was no difference between treatments in the types of chemotherapy that would account for differences in response.
† Efficacy based on "all patients treated" analysis.
‡ Median undefined since at least 50% of the patients were rescued or had more than five emetic episodes.
§ Visual analog scale assessment of nausea: 0=no nausea, 100=nausea as bad as it can be.
‖ Visual analog scale assessment of satisfaction: 0=not at all satisfied, 100=totally satisfied.

Ondansetron was compared with metoclopramide in a single-blind trial in 307 patients receiving cisplatin ≥ 100 mg/m² with or without other chemotherapeutic agents. Patients received the first dose of ondansetron or metoclopramide 30 minutes before cisplatin. Two additional ondansetron doses were administered 4 and 8 hours later, or five additional metoclopramide doses were administered 2, 4, 7, 10, and 13 hours later. Cisplatin was administered over a period of 3 hours or less. Episodes of vomiting and retching were tabulated over the period of 24 hours after cisplatin. The results of this study are summarized in TABLE 4.

Forty-one of the ondansetron patients were over 65 years of age. The complete response rate (zero emetic episodes) was 41% in this group compared with 40% in those 65 years old or younger.

In a stratified, randomized, double-blind, parallel group, multicenter study, a single 32-mg dose of ondansetron was compared with three 0.15-mg/kg doses in patients receiving cisplatin doses of either 50 to 70 mg/m² or ≥ 100 mg/m². Patients received the first ondansetron dose 30 minutes before cisplatin. Two additional ondansetron doses were administered 4 and 8 hours later to the group receiving three 0.15-mg/kg doses. In both strata, significantly fewer patients on the single 32-mg dose than those receiving the three-dose regimen failed (TABLE 5).

Cyclophosphamide-Based Chemotherapy: In a double-blind, placebo-controlled study of ondansetron injection (three 0.15-mg/kg doses) in 20 patients receiving cyclophosphamide (500-600 mg/m²) chemotherapy, ondansetron injection was significantly more effective than placebo in preventing nausea and vomiting. The results are summarized in TABLE 6.

Re-treatment: In uncontrolled trials, 127 patients receiving cisplatin (median dose, 100 mg/m²) and ondansetron who had two or fewer emetic episodes were re-treated with ondansetron and chemotherapy, mainly cisplatin, for a total of 269 re-treatment courses (median, 2; range, 1 to 10). No emetic episodes occurred in 160 (59%), and two or fewer emetic episodes occurred in 217 (81%) retreatment courses.

Pediatric Studies: Four open-label, noncomparative (one US, three foreign) trials have been performed with 209 pediatric cancer patients aged 4 to 18 years given a variety of cisplatin or noncisplatin regimens. In the three foreign trials, the initial ondansetron injection dose ranged from 0.04 to 0.87 mg/kg for a total dose of 2.16 to 12 mg. This was followed by the oral administration of ondansetron ranging from 4 to 24 mg daily for 3 days. In the US trial, ondansetron was administered intravenously (only) in three doses of 0.15 mg/kg each for a total daily dose of 7.2 to 39 mg. In these studies, 58% of the 196 evaluable patients had a complete response (no emetic episodes) on day 1. Thus, prevention of emesis in these children was essentially the same as for patients older than 18 years of age. Overall, ondansetron injection was well tolerated in these pediatric patients.

CLINICAL STUDIES: *(cont'd)*

TABLE 4 Prevention of Emesis Induced by Cisplatin (≥ 100 mg/m ²) Single-Day Therapy*

	Ondansetron Injection	Metoclopramide	P Value
Dose	0.15 mg/kg × 3	2 mg/kg × 6	
Number of patients in efficacy population	136	138	
Treatment response			
0 Emetic episodes	54 (40%)	41 (30%)	
1-2 Emetic episodes	34 (25%)	30 (22%)	
3-5 Emetic episodes	19 (14%)	18 (13%)	
More than 5 emetic episodes/rescued	29 (21%)	49 (36%)	
Comparison of treatments with respect to 0 Emetic episodes	54/136	41/138	0.083
More than 5 emetic episodes/rescued	29/136	49/138	0.009
Median number of emetic episodes	1	2	0.005
Median time to first emetic episode (h)	20.5	4.3	<0.001
Global satisfaction with control of nausea and vomiting (0-100)†	85	63	0.001
Acute dystonic reactions	0	8	0.005
Akathisia	0	10	0.002

* In addition to cisplatin, 68% of patients received other chemotherapeutic agents, including cyclophosphamide, etoposide, and fluorouracil. There was no difference between treatments in the types of chemotherapy that would account for differences in response.
† Visual analog scale assessment: 0=not at all satisfied, 100=totally satisfied.

TABLE 5 Prevention of Chemotherapy-Induced Nausea and Emesis in Single-Dose Therapy

	Ondansetron Dose 0.15 mg/kg x 3	Ondansetron Dose 32 mg x 1	P Value
High-dose cisplatin (≥100 mg/m²)			
Number of patients	100	102	
Treatment response			
0 Emetic episodes	41 (41%)	49 (48%)	0.315
1-2 Emetic episodes	19 (19%)	25 (25%)	
3-5 Emetic episodes	4 (4%)	8 (8%)	
More than 5 emetic episodes/rescued	36 (36%)	20 (20%)	0.009
Median time to first emetic episode (h)	21.7	23	0.173
Median nausea scores (0-100)*	28	13	0.004
Medium-dose cisplatin (50-70 mg/m²)			
Number of Patients	101	93	
Treatment response			
0 Emetic episodes	62 (61%)	68 (73%)	0.083
1-2 Emetic episodes	11 (11%)	14 (15%)	
3-5 Emetic episodes	6 (6%)	3 (3%)	
More than 5 emetic episodes/rescued	22 (22%)	8 (9%)	0.011
Median time to first emetic episode (h)	Undefined†	Undefined	0.084
Median nausea scores (0-100)*	9	3	0.131

* Visual analog scale assessment: 0=no nausea, 100=nausea as bad as it can be.
† Median undefined since at least 50% of patients did not have any emetic episodes.

TABLE 6 Prevention of Chemotherapy-Induced Nausea and Emesis in Single-Day Cyclophosphamide Therapy*

	Ondansetron Injection	Placebo	P Value†
Number of Patients	10	10	
Treatment response			
0 Emetic episodes	7 (70%)	0 (0%)	0.001
1-2 Emetic episodes	0 (0%)	2 (20%)	
3-5 Emetic episodes	2 (20%)	4 (40%)	
More than 5 emetic episodes/rescued	1 (10%)	4 (40%)	0.131
Median number of emetic episodes	0	4	0.008
Median time to first emetic episode (h)	Undefined‡	8.79	
Median nausea scores (0-100) §	0	60	0.001
Global satisfaction with control of nausea and vomiting (0-100) ‖	100	52	0.008

* Chemotherapy consisted of cyclophosphamide in all patients, plus other agents, including fluorouracil, doxorubicin, methotrexate, and vincristine. There was no difference between treatments in the type of chemotherapy that would account for differences in response.
† Efficacy based on "all patients treated" analysis.
‡ Median undefined since at least 50% of patients did not have any emetic episodes.
§ Visual analog scale assessment of nausea: 0=no nausea, 100=nausea as bad as it can be.
‖ Visual analog scale assessment of satisfaction: 0=not at all, satisfied, 100=totally satisfied.

Postoperative Nausea and Vomiting

Prevention of Postoperative Nausea and Vomiting: Adult surgical patients who received ondansetron immediately before the induction of general balanced anesthesia (barbiturate: thiopental, methohexital or thiamylal; opioid: alfentanil or fentanyl; nitrous oxide; neuromuscular blockade: succinylcholine/curare and/or vecuronium or atracurium; and supplemental isoflurane) were evaluated in two double-blind US studies involving 554 patients. Ondansetron injection (4 mg) IV given over 2 to 5 minutes was significantly more effective than placebo. The results of these studies are summarized below in TABLE 7.

CLINICAL STUDIES: *(cont'd)*

TABLE 7 Prevention of Postoperative Nausea and Vomiting

	Ondansetron 4 mg IV	Placebo	P value
Study 1			
Emetic episodes:			
Number of patients	136	139	
Treatment response over 24-hour postoperative period			
0 Emetic episodes	103 (76%)	64 (46%)	< 0.001
1 Emetic episodes	13 (10%)	17 (12%)	
More than 1 emetic episode/rescued	20 (15%)	58 (42%)	
Nausea assessments:			
Number of patients	134	136	
No nausea over 24-hr postoperative period	56 (42%)	39 (29%)	
Study 2			
Emetic episodes:			
Number of patients	136	143	
Treatment response over 24-hr postoperative period			
0 Emetic episodes	85 (63%)	63 (44%)	0.002
1 Emetic episode	16 (12%)	29 (20%)	
More than 1 emetic episodes/rescued	35 (26%)	51 (36%)	
Nausea assessments:			
Number of patients	125	133	
No nausea over 24-hr postoperative period	48 (38%)	42 (32%)	

The study populations in all trials thus far consisted of mainly women undergoing laparoscopic procedures. While some men were included in some trials with similar results, clearance of the drug is more rapid in men and sufficient numbers of men have not been clinically studied to be certain that efficacy and safety have been established. Few patients undergoing major abdominal surgery have been studied.

Pediatric Studies: Three double-blind, placebo-controlled studies have been performed (one US, two foreign) in 1409 male and female patients (2 to 12 years of age) undergoing general anesthesia with nitrous oxide. The surgical procedures included tonsillectomy with or without adenoidectomy, strabismus surgery, herniorrhaphy, and orchidopexy. Patients were randomized to either single IV doses of ondansetron (0.1 mg/kg for children weighing 40 kg or less, a single 4 mg dose for children weighing more than 40 kg) or placebo. Study drug was administered over at least 30 seconds, immediately prior to or following anesthesia induction. Ondansetron was significantly more effective than placebo in preventing nausea and vomiting. The results of these studies are summarized in TABLE 8.

TABLE 8 Prevention of Further Postoperative Nausea and Vomiting

Treatment Response Over 24 Hours	Ondansetron n (%)	Placebo n (%)	P value
Study 1			
Number of patients	205	210	
0 Emetic episodes	140 (68%)	82 (39%)	≤0.001
Failure*	65 (32%)	128 (61%)	
Study 2			
Number of patients	112	110	
0 Emetic episodes	68 (61%)	38 (35%)	≤0.001
Failure*	44 (39%)	72 (65%)	
Study 3			
Number of patients	206	206	
0 Emetic episodes	123 (60%)	96 (47%)	≤0.01
Failure*	83 (40%)	110 (53%)	
Nausea assessments†:			
Number of patients	185	191	
None	119 (64%)	99 (52%)	≤0.01

* Failure was one or more emetic epsiodes, rescued, or withdrawn.
† Nausea measured as none, mild or severe.

Prevention of Further Postoperative Nausea and Vomiting: Adult surgical patients receiving general balanced anesthesia (barbiturate: thiopental, methohexital or thiamylal; opioid: alfentanil or fentanyl; nitrous oxide; neuromuscular blockade: succinylcholine/curare and/or vecuronium or atracurium; and supplemental isoflurane) who received no prophylactic antiemetics and who experienced nausea and/or vomiting within 2 hours postoperatively were evaluated in two double-blind US studies involving 441 patients. Patients who experienced an episode of postoperative nausea and/or vomiting were given ondansetron injection (4 mg) IV over 2 to 5 minutes, and this was significantly more effective than placebo. The results of these studies are summarized in TABLE 9.

The study populations in all trials thus far consisted of mainly women undergoing laparoscopic procedures. While some men were included in some trials with similar results, clearance of the drug is more rapid in men and sufficient numbers of men have not been clinically studied to be certain that efficacy and safety have been established. Few patients undergoing major abdominal surgery have been studied.

Pediatric Studies: One double-blind, placebo-controlled US study was performed in 351 male and female outpatients (2 to 12 years of age) who received general anesthesia with nitrous oxide and no prophylactic antiemetics. Surgical procedures were unrestricted. Patients who experienced two or more emetic episodes within 2 hours following discontinuation of nitrous oxide were randomized to a single IV dose of ondansetron (0.1 mg/kg for children weighing 40 kg or less, a single 4 mg dose for children weighing more than 40 kg) or placebo administered over at least 30 seconds. Ondansetron was significantly more effective than placebo in preventing further episodes of nausea and vomiting. The results of these studies are summarized in TABLE 10.

TABLETS

Chemotherapy-Induced Nausea and Vomiting

In one double-blind US study in 67 patients, ondansetron tablets were significantly more effective than placebo in preventing vomiting induced by cyclophosphamide-based chemotherapy containing doxorubicin. Treatment response is based on the total number of emetic episodes over the 3-day study period. The results of this study is summarized in TABLE 11.

In one double-blind US study in 336 patients, ondansetron tablets 8 mg administered twice a day were as effective as ondansetron tablets 8 mg administered three times a day in preventing nausea and vomiting induced by cyclophosphamide-based chemotherapy containing either methotrexate or doxorubicin. Treatment response is based on the total number of emetic episodes over the 3-day study period. The results of this study are summarized in TABLE 12.

CLINICAL STUDIES: *(cont'd)*

TABLE 9 Prevention of Further Postoperative Nausea and Vomiting

	Ondansetron 4 mg IV	Placebo	P value
Study 1			
Emetic episodes: Number of patients	104	117	
Treatment response 24 hrs after study drug			
0 Emetic episodes	49 (47%)	19 (16%)	<0.001
1 Emetic episode	12 (12%)	9 (8%)	
More than 1 emetic episode/rescued	43 (41%)	89 (76%)	
Median time to first emetic episode (min)*	55.0	43.0	
Nausea assessments:			
Number of patients	98	102	
Mean nausea score over 24-hr postoperative period†	1.7	3.1	
Study 2			
Emetic episodes:			
Number of patients	112	108	
Treatment response 24 hrs after study drug			
0 Emetic episodes	49 (44%)	28 (26%)	0.006
1 Emetic episode	14 (13%)	3 (3%)	
More than 1 emetic episode/rescued	49 (44%)	77 (71%)	
Median time to first emetic episode (min)*	60.5	34.0	
Nausea assessments:			
Number of patients	105	85	
Mean nausea score over 24-hr postoperative period†	1.9	2.9	

* After administration of study drug.
† Nausea measured on a scale of 0-10 with 0=no nausea, 10=nausea as bad as it can be.

TABLE 10 Prevention of Further Postoperative Nausea and Vomiting

Treatment Response Over 24 Hours	Ondansetron n (%)	Placebo n (%)	P value
Study 1			
Number of patients	180	171	
0 Emetic episodes	96 (53%)	29 (17%)	≤0.001
Failure*	84(47%)	142 (83%)	

* Failure was one or more emetic epsiodes, rescued, or withdrawn.

TABLE 11 Emetic Episodes: Treatment Response

	Ondansetron 8 mg b.i.d. Oral*	Placebo	P value
Number of patients	33	34	
Treatment response			
0 Emetic episodes	20 (61%)	2 (6%)	<0.001
1-2 Emetic episodes	6 (18%)	8 (24%)	
More than 2 emetic episodes/withdrawn	7 (21%)	24 (71%)	<0.001
Median number of emetic episodes	0.0	Undefined†	
Median time to first emetic episode (h)	Undefined‡	6.5	

* The first dose was administered 30 minutes before the start of emetogenic chemotherapy, with a subsequent dose 8 hours after the first dose. An 8-mg tablet was administered twice a day for 2 days after completion of chemotherapy.
† Median undefined since at least 50% of the patients were withdrawn or had more than two emetic episodes.
‡ Median undefined since at least 50% of patients did not have any emetic episodes.

TABLE 12 Emetic Episodes: Treatment Response

	Ondansetron 8 mg b.i.d. Oral*	Ondansetron 8 mg t.i.d Oral†
Number of patients	165	171
Treatment response		
0 Emetic episodes	101 (61%)	99 (58%)
1-2 Emetic episodes	16 (10%)	17 (10%)
More than 2 emetic episodes/withdrawn	48 (29%)	55 (32%)
Median number of emetic episodes	0.0	0.0
Median time to first emetic episode (h)	Undefined‡	Undefined‡
Median nausea scores (0-100) §	6	6

* The first dose was administered 30 minutes before the start of emetogenic chemotherapy, with a subsequent dose 8 hours after the first dose. An 8-mg tablet was administered twice a day for 2 days after completion of chemotherapy.
† The first dose was administered 30 minutes before the start of emetogenic chemotherapy, with subsequent doses 4 and 8 hours after the first dose. An 8-mg tablet was administered three times a day for 2 days after completion of chemotherapy.
‡ Median undefined since at least 50% of patients did not have any emetic episodes.
§ Visual analog scale assessment: 0=no nausea, 100=nausea as bad as it can be.

Re-treatment: In uncontrolled trials, 148 patients receiving cyclophosphamide-based chemotherapy were re-treated with 8 mg 3 times a day of oral ondansetron during subsequent chemotherapy for a total of 396 re-treatment courses. No emetic episodes occurred in 314 (79%) of the retreatment courses, and only one to two emetic episodes occurred in 43 (11%) of the retreatment courses.

Pediatric Studies: Three open-label, uncontrolled, foreign trials have been performed with 182 patients 4 to 18 years old with cancer who were given a variety of cisplatin or noncisplatin regimens. In these foreign trials, the initial dose of ondansetron injection ranged from 0.04 to 0.87 mg/kg for a total dose of 2.16 to 12 mg. This was followed by the oral administration of ondansetron ranging from 4 to 24 mg daily for 3 days. In these studies, 58% of the 170 evaluable patients had a complete response (no emetic episodes) on day 1. Two studies showed the response rates for patients less than 12 years of age who received 4 mg of ondansetron three times a day to be similar to those in patients 12 to 18 years of age who

CLINICAL STUDIES: *(cont'd)*

received 8 mg of ondansetron three times daily. Thus, prevention of emesis in these children was essentially the same as for patients older than 18 years of age. Overall, ondansetron tablets were well tolerated in these pediatric patients.

Elderly Patients: One hundred thirty-seven (137) patients 65 years of age or older have received oral ondansetron. Prevention of emesis was similar to that in patients younger than 65 years of age and adverse reactions were not seen in increased frequency.

Radiation-Induced Nausea and Vomiting: Total Body Irradiation

In a randomized, double-blind study in 20 patients, ondansetron tablets (8 mg given 1.5 hours before each fraction of radiotherapy for 4 days) were significantly more effective than placebo in preventing vomiting induced by total body irradiation. Total body irradiation consisted of 11 fractions (120 cGy per fraction) over 4 days for a total of 1320 cGy. Patients received three fractions for 3 days, than two fractions on day 4.

Single High-Dose Fraction Radiotherapy: Ondansetron was significantly more effective than metoclopramide with respect to complete control of emesis (0 emetic episodes) in a double-blind trial in 105 patients receiving single high-dose radiotherapy (800 to 1000 cGy) over an anterior or posterior field size of $\geq$80 cm^2 to the abdomen. Patients received the first dose of ondansetron (8 mg) or metoclopramide (10 mg) 1 to 2 hours before radiotherapy. If radiotherapy was given in the morning, two additional doses of study treatment were given (one tablet late afternoon and one tablet before bedtime). If radiotherapy was given in the afternoon, patients took only one further tablet that day before bedtime. Patients continued the oral medication on a t.i.d basis for 3 days.

Daily Fractionated Radiotherapy: Ondansetron was significantly more effective than prochlorperazine with respect to complete control of emesis (0 emetic episodes) in a double-blind trial in 135 patients receiving a 1- to 4-week course of fractionated radiotherapy (180 cGy doses) over a field size of $\geq$100 cm^2 to the abdomen. Patients received the first dose of ondansetron (8 mg) or prochlorperazine (10 mg) 1 to 2 hours before the patient received the first daily radiotherapy fraction, with two subsequent doses on a 3 times a day basis. Patients continued the oral medication on a 3 times a day basis on each day of radiotherapy.

Postoperative Nausea and Vomiting: Surgical patients who received ondansetron 1 hour before the induction of general balanced anesthesia (barbiturate: thiopental, methohexital or thiamylal; opioid: alfentanil, sufentanil, morphine, or fentanyl; nitrous oxide; neuromuscular blockade: succinylcholine/curare or gallamine and/or vecuronium, pancuronium, or atracurium; and supplemental isoflurane or enflurane) were evaluated in two double-blind studies (one US, one foreign) involving 865 patients. Ondansetron tablets (16 mg) were significantly more effective than placebo in preventing postoperative nausea and vomiting.

The study populations in all trials thus far consisted of women undergoing inpatient surgical procedures. No studies have been performed in males. No controlled clinical study comparing ondansetron tablets to ondansetron injection has been performed.

INDICATIONS AND USAGE:

Injection

1. Prevention of nausea and vomiting associated with initial and repeat courses of emetogenic cancer chemotherapy, including high-dose cisplatin. Efficacy of the 32-mg single dose beyond 24 hours in these patients has not yet been established.

2. Prevention of postoperative nausea and/or vomiting. As with other antiemetics, routine prophylaxis is not recommended for patients in whom there is little expectation that nausea and/or vomiting will occur postoperatively. In patients where nausea and/or vomiting must be avoided postoperatively, ondansetron injection is recommended even where the incidence of postoperative nausea and/or vomiting is low. For patients who have nausea and/or vomiting postoperatively, ondansetron injection may be given to prevent further episodes (see CLINICAL STUDIES.)

Tablets

1. Prevention of nausea and vomiting associated with initial and repeat courses of moderately emetogenic cancer chemotherapy.

2. Prevention of nausea and vomiting associated with radiotherapy in patients receiving either total body irradiation, single high-dose fraction to the abdomen, or daily fractions to the abdomen.

3. Prevention of postoperative nausea and/or vomiting. As with other antiemetics, routine prophylaxis is not recommended for patients in whom there is little expectation that nausea and/or vomiting will occur postoperatively. In patients where nausea and/or vomiting must be avoided postoperatively, ondansetron tablets are recommended even where the incidence of postoperative nausea and/or vomiting is low.

CONTRAINDICATIONS:

Ondansetron is contraindicated for patients known to have hypersensitivity to the drug.

WARNINGS:

Hypersensitivity reactions have been reported in patients who have exhibited hypersensitivity to other selective 5–HT_3 receptor antagonists.

PRECAUTIONS:

Ondansetron is not a drug that stimulates gastric or intestinal peristalsis. It should not be used instead of nasogastric suction. The use of ondansetron in patients following abdominal surgery or in patients with chemotherapy-induced nausea and vomiting may mask a progressive ileus and/or gastric distension.

Carcinogenesis, Mutagenesis, Impairment of Fertility: Carcinogenic effects were not seen in 2-year studies in rats and mice with oral ondansetron doses up to 10 and 30 mg/kg per day, respectively. Ondansetron was not mutagenic in standard tests for mutagenicity. Oral administration of ondansetron up to 15 mg/kg per day did not affect fertility or general reproductive performance of male and female rats.

Pregnancy, Teratogenic Effects, Pregnancy Category B: Reproduction studies have been performed in pregnant rats and rabbits at IV doses up to 4 mg/kg per day and at daily oral doses up to 15 and 30 mg/kg per day, respectively, and have revealed no evidence of impaired fertility or harm to the fetus due to ondansetron. There are, however, no adequate and well-controlled studies in pregnant women. Because animal reproduction studies are not always predictive of human response, this drug should be used during pregnancy only if clearly needed.

Nursing Mothers: Ondansetron is excreted in the breast milk of rats. It is not known whether ondansetron is excreted in human milk. Because many drugs are excreted in human milk, caution should be exercised when ondansetron is administered to a nursing woman.

Pediatric Use: Little information is available about dosage in children 2 years of age or younger (injection) or children 4 years of age or younger (tablet) (see DOSAGE AND ADMINISTRATION, Pediatric Use.)

Use in Elderly Patients: Dosage adjustment is not needed in patients over the age of 65 (see CLINICAL PHARMACOLOGY.) Prevention of nausea and vomiting in elderly patients was no different than in younger age-groups.

DRUG INTERACTIONS:

Ondansetron does not itself appear to induce or inhibit the cytochrome P-450 drug-metabolizing enzyme system of the liver. Because ondansetron is metabolized by hepatic cytochrome P-450 drug-metabolizing enzymes, inducers or inhibitors of these enzymes may change the clearance and, hence, the half-life of ondansetron. On the basis of available data, no dosage adjustment is recommended for patients on these drugs. Tumor response to chemotherapy in the P 388 mouse leukemia model is not affected by ondansetron. In humans, carmustine, etoposide, and cisplatin do not affect the pharmacokinetics of ondansetron.

Use in Surgical Patients: The coadministration of ondansetron had no effect on the pharmacokinetics and pharmacodynamics of temazepam.

ADVERSE REACTIONS:

INJECTION

Chemotherapy-Induced Nausea and Vomiting: The following adverse events have been reported in individuals receiving ondansetron at a dosage of three 0.15-mg/kg doses or as a single 32-mg dose in clinical trials. These patients were receiving concomitant chemotherapy, primarily cisplatin, and IV fluids. Most were receiving a diuretic (TABLE 13).

TABLE 13 Principal Adverse Events in Comparative Trials

Number of Patients With Event	Ondansetron Injection 0.15 mg/kg x 3 n=419	Ondansetron Injection 32 mg x 1 n=220	Metoclopramide n=156	Placebo n=34
Diarrhea	16%	8%	44%	18%
Headache	17%	25%	7%	15%
Fever	8%	7%	5%	3%
Akathisia	0%	0%	6%	0%
Acute dystonic reactions*	0%	0%	5%	0%

* See Central Nervous System below.

The following have been reported during controlled clinical trials or in the routine management of patients. The percentage figures are based on clinical trial experience.

Gastrointestinal: Constipation has been reported in 11% of chemotherapy patients receiving multiday ondansetron.

Hepatic: In comparative trials in cisplatin chemotherapy patients with normal baseline values of aspartate transaminase (AST) and alanine transaminase (ALT), these enzymes have been reported to exceed twice the upper limit of normal in approximately 5% of patients. The increases were transient and did not appear to be related to dose or duration of therapy. On repeat exposure, similar transient elevations in transaminase values occurred in some courses, but symptomatic hepatic disease did not occur.

There have been reports of liver failure and death in patients with cancer receiving concurrent medications including potentially hepatotoxic cytotoxic chemotherapy and antibiotics. The etiology of the liver failure is unclear.

Integumentary: Rash has occurred in approximately 1% of patients receiving ondansetron.

Central Nervous System: There have been rare reports consistent with, but not diagnostic of, extrapyramidal reactions in patients receiving ondansetron.

Cardiovascular: Rare instances of tachycardia, angina (chest pain), bradycardia, hypotension, syncope, and electrocardiographic alterations, including second degree heart block. In many cases the relationship to ondansetron injection was unclear.

Special Senses: Transient blurred vision, in some cases associated with abnormalities of accommodation, and transient dizziness during or shortly after IV infusion.

Local Reactions: Pain, redness, and burning at site of injection.

Other: Rare cases of hypokalemia and grand mal seizures have been reported. The relationship to ondansetron injection was unclear. Rare cases of hypersensitivity reactions, sometimes severe (*e.g.*, anaphylaxis, bronchospasm, shortness of breath, hypotension, shock, angioedema, urticaria), have also been reported.

Postoperative Nausea and Vomiting: The following adverse events have been reported in $\geq$2% of people receiving ondansetron at a dosage of 4 mg IV over 2 to 5 minutes in clinical trials. Rates of these events were not significantly different in the ondansetron and placebo groups. These patients were receiving multiple concomitant perioperative and postoperative medications (TABLE 14).

TABLE 14

	Ondansetron Injection 4 mg IV n=547 patients	Placebo n=547 patients
Headache	92 (17%)	77 (14%)
Dizziness	67 (12%)	88 (16%)
Musculoskeletal pain	57 (10%)	59 (11%)
Drowsiness/sedation	44 (8%)	37 (7%)
Shivers	38 (7%)	39 (7%)
Malaise/fatigue	25 (5%)	30 (5%)
Injection site reaction	21 (4%)	18 (3%)
Urinary retention	17 (3%)	15 (3%)
Postoperative CO_2-related pain*	12 (2%)	16 (3%)
Chest pain (unspecified)	12 (2%)	15 (3%)
Anxiety/agitation	11 (2%)	16 (3%)
Dysuria	11 (2%)	9 (2%)
Hypotension	10 (2%)	12 (2%)
Fever	10 (2%)	6 (1%)
Cold sensation	9 (2%)	8 (1%)
Pruritus	9 (2%)	3 (<1%)
Paresthesia	9 (2%)	2 (<1%)

* Sites of pain included abdomen, stomach, joints, rib cage, shoulder.

Pediatric Use: The following were the most commonly reported adverse events in pediatric patients receiving ondansetron (0.1 mg/kg for children weighing 40 kg or less, a single 4 mg dose for children weighing more than 40 kg) adminstered intravenously over at least 30 seconds. Rates of these events were not significantly different in the ondasteron and placebo groups. These patients were receiving multiple concomitant perioperative and postoperative medications.

TABLETS

Chemotherapy-Induced Nausea and Vomiting: The following adverse events have been reported in adults receiving either 8 mg of ondansetron two to three times a day for 3 days or placebo in four trials. These patients were receiving concurrent chemotherapy, primarily cyclophosphamide-based regimens (TABLE 16).

Central Nervous System: There have been rare reports consistent with, but not diagnostic of, extrapyramidal reactions in patients receiving ondansetron.

ADVERSE REACTIONS: *(cont'd)*

TABLE 15 Frequency of Adverse Events From Controlled Studies

Adverse Event	Ondansetron n=755 Patients	Placebo n=731 Patients
Wound problem	80 (11%)	86 (12%)
Anxiety/agitation	49 (6%)	47 (6%)
Headache	44 (6%)	43 (6%)
Drowsiness/sedation	41 (5%)	56 (8%)
Pyrexia	32(4%)	41 (6%)

TABLE 16 Principal Adverse Events in US Trials: 3 Days of Oral Therapy

Event	Ondansetron 8 mg b.i.d. n=242	Ondansetron 8 mg t.i.d n=415	Placebo n=262
Headache	58 (24%)	113 (27%)	34 (13%)
Malaise/fatigue	32 (13%)	37 (9%)	6 (2%)
Constipation	22 (9%)	26 (6%)	1 (<1%)
Diarrhea	15 (6%)	16 (4%)	10 (4%)
Dizziness	13 (5%)	18 (4%)	12 (5%)
Abdominal pain	3 (1%)	13 (3%)	1 (<1%)
Xerostomia	5 (2%)	6 (1%)	1 (<1%)
Weakness	0 (0%)	7 (2%)	1 (<1%)

Hepatic: In 723 patients receiving cyclophosphamide-based chemotherapy in US clinical trials, AST and/or ALT values have been reported to exceed twice the upper limit of normal in approximately 1% to 2% of patients receiving oral ondansetron. The increases were transient and did not appear to be related to dose or duration of therapy. On repeat exposure, similar transient elevations in transaminase values occurred in some courses, but symptomatic hepatic disease did not occur. The role of cancer chemotherapy in these biochemical changes cannot be clearly determined.

There have been reports of liver failure and death in patients with cancer receiving concurrent medications including potentially hepatotoxic cytotoxic chemotherapy and antibiotics. The etiology of the liver failure is unclear.

Integumentary: Rash has occurred in approximately 1% of patients receiving ondansetron.

Other: Rare cases of anaphylaxis, bronchospasm, tachycardia, angina (chest pain), hypokalemia, electrocardiographic alterations, vascular occlusive events, and grand mal seizures have been reported. Except for bronchospasm and anaphylaxis, the relationship to ondansetron was unclear.

Radiation-Induced Nausea and Vomiting: The adverse events reported in patients receiving ondansetron and concurrent radiotherapy were similar to those reported in patients receiving ondansetron and concurrent chemotherapy. The most frequently reported adverse events were headache, constipation, and diarrhea.

Postoperative Nausea and Vomiting: The following adverse events have been reported in ≥5% of patients receiving ondansetron at a dosage of 16 mg orally in clinical trials. With the exception of headache, rates of these events were not significantly different in the ondansetron and placebo groups. These patients were receiving multiple concomitant perioperative and postoperative medications (TABLE 17).

TABLE 17 Frequency of Adverse Events From Controlled Studies

Adverse Event	Ondansetron 16 mg (n=550)	Placebo (n=531)
Wound problem	152 (28%)	162 (31%)
Drowsiness/sedation	112 (20%)	122 (23%)
Headache	49 (9%)	27 (5%)
Hypoxia	49 (9%)	35 (7%)
Pyrexia	45 (8%)	34 (6%)
Dizziness	36 (7%)	34 (6%)
Gynecological disorder	36 (7%)	33 (6%)
Anxiety/agitation	33 (6%)	29 (5%)
Bradycardia	32 (6%)	30 (6%)
Shiver (s)	28 (5%)	30 (6%)
Urinary rentention	28 (5%)	18 (3%)
Hypotension	27 (5%)	32 (6%)
Pruritus	27 (5%)	20 (4%)

DRUG ABUSE AND DEPENDENCE:

Animal studies have shown that ondansetron is not discriminated as a benzodiazepine nor does it substitute for benzodiazepines in direct addiction studies.

OVERDOSAGE:

There is no specific antidote for ondansetron overdose. Patients should be managed with appropriate supportive therapy. Individual intravenous doses as large as 145 mg and total daily intravenous doses (three doses) as large as 252 mg have been inadvertently administered without significant adverse events. These doses are more than 10 times the recommended daily dose.

Hypotension (and faintness) occurred in a patient that took 48 mg of oral ondansetron. The events resolved completely.

"Sudden blindness" (amaurosis) of 2 to 3 minutes' duration plus severe constipation occurred in one patient that was administered 72 mg of ondansetron intravenously as a single dose. Following infusion of 32 mg over only a 4-minute period, a vasovagal episode with transient second degree heart block was observed. In all instances, the events resolved completely.

DOSAGE AND ADMINISTRATION:

INJECTION

Prevention of Chemotherapy-Induced Nausea and Vomiting

The recommended IV dosage of ondansetron is a single 32-mg dose or three 0.15-mg/kg doses. A single 32-mg dose is infused over 15 minutes beginning 30 minutes before the start of emetogenic chemotherapy. The recommended infusion rate should not be exceeded (see OVERDOSAGE.) With the three-dose (0.15-mg/kg) regimen, the first dose is infused over 15 minutes beginning 30 minutes before the start of emetogenic chemotherapy. Subsequent doses (0.15 mg/kg) are administered 4 and 8 hours after the first dose of ondansetron injection.

Ondansetron injection should not be mixed with solutions for which physical and chemical compatibility have not been established. In particular, this applies to alkaline solutions as a precipitate may form.

Vial: DILUTE BEFORE USE. Ondansetron injection should be diluted in 50 ml of 5% dextrose injection or 0.9% sodium chloride injection before administration.

DOSAGE AND ADMINISTRATION: *(cont'd)*

Flexible Plastic Container: Ondansetron injection premixed, 32 mg in 5% dextrose, 50 ml **REQUIRES NO DILUTION.**

Pediatric Use: DILUTE BEFORE USE. On the basis of the limited available information (see CLINICAL STUDIES, Pediatric Studies and CLINICAL PHARMACOLOGY, Pharmacokinetics), the dosage in children 4 to 18 years of age should be three 0.15-mg/kg doses (see above). Little information is available about dosage in children 2 years of age or younger.

Use in the Elderly: The dosage recommendation is the same as for the general population.

Ondansetron Injection Premixed in Flexible Plastic Containers: Instructions for Use: *To Open:* Tear outer wrap at notch and remove solution container. Check for minute leaks by squeezing container firmly. If leaks are found, discard unit as sterility may be impaired.

Preparation for Administration: Use aseptic technique.

1. Close flow control clamp of administration set.

2. Remove cover from outlet port at bottom of container.

3. Insert piercing pin of administration set into port with a twisting motion until the pin is firmly seated. NOTE: See full directions on administration set carton.

4. Suspend container from hanger.

5. Squeeze and release drip chamber to establish proper fluid level in chamber during infusion of ondansetron injection premixed.

6. Open flow control clamp to expel air from set. Close clamp.

7. Attach set to venipuncture device. If device is not indwelling, prime and make venipuncture.

8. Perform venipuncture.

9. Regulate rate of administration with flow control clamp.

Caution: Ondansetron injection premixed in flexible plastic containers is to be administered by IV drip infusion only. Ondansetron injection premixed should not be mixed with solutions for which physical and chemical compatibility have not been established. In particular, this applies to alkaline solutions as a precipitate may form. If used with a primary IV fluid system, the primary solution should be discontinued during ondansetron injection premixed infusion.

Do not administer unless solution is clear and container is undamaged.

Warning: Do not use flexible container in series connections.

Prevention of Postoperative Nausea and/or Vomiting

The recommended IV dosage of ondansetron is 4 mg administered intravenously in not less than 30 seconds, preferably over 2 to 5 minutes, immediately before induction of anesthesia, or postoperatively if the patient experiences nausea and/or vomiting occurring shortly after surgery.

Vial: Ondansetron injection **REQUIRES NO DILUTION.**

Repeat dosing for patients who continue to experience nausea and/or vomiting postoperatively has not been studied. While recommended as a fixed dose for patients weighing more than 40 kg, few patients above 80 kg have been studied.

Pediatric Use: The recommended IV dosage of ondansetron for pediatric patients 2 to 12 years of age is 0.1 mg/kg for children weighing 40 kg or less, or a single 4 mg dose for children weighing more than 40 kg. The rate of administration should not be less than 30 seconds, preferably over 2 to 5 minutes. Little information is available about dosage in children younger than 2 years of age.

Use in the Elderly: NO DILUTION NECESSARY. The dosage recommendation is the same as for the general population.

Dosage Adjustment for Patients With Impaired Renal Function: No specific studies have been conducted in patients with renal insufficiency.

Dosage Adjustment for Patients With Impaired Hepatic Function: In patients with severe hepatic impairment according to Child-Pugh[1] criteria, a single maximal daily dose of 8 mg to be infused over 15 minutes beginning 30 minutes before the start of the emetogenic chemotherapy is recommended. There is no experience beyond first-day administration of ondansetron.

Stability: Ondansetron injection is stable at room temperature under normal lighting conditions for 48 hours after dilution with the following IV fluids: 0.9% sodium chloride injection, 5% dextrose injection, 5% dextrose and 0.9% sodium chloride injection, 5% dextrose and 0.45% sodium chloride injection, and 3% sodium chloride injection.

Although ondansetron injection is chemically and physically stable when diluted as recommended, sterile precautions should be observed because diluents generally do not contain preservative. After dilution, do not use beyond 24 hours.

Note: Parenteral drug products should be inspected visually for particulate matter and discoloration before administration whenever solution and container permit.

Precaution: Occasionally, ondansetron precipitates at the stopper/vial interface in vials stored upright. Potency and safety are not affected. If a precipitate is observed, resolubilize by shaking the vial vigorously.

TABLETS

Prevention of Nausea and Vomiting Associated With Moderately Emetogenic Cancer Chemotherapy

The recommended oral dosage of ondansetron tablets is one 8-mg tablet given twice a day. The first dose should be administered 30 minutes before the start of emetogenic chemotherapy, with a subsequent dose 8 hours after the first dose. One 8-mg ondansetron tablet should be administered twice a day (every 12 hours) for 1 to 2 days after completion of chemotherapy.

Pediatric Use: For patients 12 years of age and older, the dosage is the same as for adults. For patients 4 through 11 years of age, the dosage is one 4-mg tablet given three times a day. The first dose should be administered 30 minutes before the start of emetogenic chemotherapy, with subsequent doses 4 and 8 hours after the first dose. One 4-mg ondansetron tablet should be administered three times a day (every 8 hours) for 1 to 2 days after completion of chemotherapy.

Use in the Elderly: The dosage is the same as for the general population.

Prevention of Nausea and Vomiting Associated With Radiotherapy, Either Total Body Irradiation, or Single High-Dose Fraction or Daily Fractions to the Abdomen

The recommended oral dosage of ondansetron tablets is one 8-mg tablet given three times a day.

For total body irradiation, an 8-mg dose should be administered 1 to 2 hours before each fraction of radiotherapy administered each day.

For single high-dose fraction radiotherapy to the abdomen, an 8-mg dose should be administered 1 to 2 hours before radiotherapy, with subsequent doses every 8 hours after the first dose for 1 to 2 days after completion of radiotherapy.

For daily fractionated radiotherapy to the abdomen, an 8-mg dose should be administered 1 to 2 hours before radiotherapy, with subsequent doses every 8 hours after the first dose for each day radiotherapy is given.

DOSAGE AND ADMINISTRATION: *(cont'd)*

Pediatric Use: There is no experience with the use of ondansetron tablets in the prevention of radiation-induced nausea and vomiting in children.

Use in the Elderly: The dosage recommendation is the same as for the general population.

Postoperative Nausea and Vomiting

The recommended oral dosage is 16 mg given as a single dose (2 8-mg tablets) 1 hour before induction of anesthesia.

Pediatric Use: There is no experience with the use of ondansetron tablets in the prevention of postoperative nausea and vomiting in children.

Use in the Elderly: The dosage is the same as for the general population.

Dosage Adjustment for Patients With Impaired Renal Function

No specific studies have been conducted in patients with renal insufficiency.

Dosage Adjustment for Patients With Impaired Hepatic Function

In patients with severe hepatic insufficiency, clearance is reduced, apparent volume of distribution is increased with a resultant increase in plasma half-life, and bioavailability approaches 100%. In such patients, a total daily dose of 8 mg should not be exceeded.

HOW SUPPLIED:

Zofran Tablets, *4 mg:* (Ondansetron HCl dihydrate equivalent to 4 mg of ondansetron), are white, oval, film-coated tablets engraved with "Zofran" on one side and "4" on the other. *8 mg:* (Ondansetron HCl dihydrate equivalent to 8 mg of ondansetron), are yellow, oval, film-coated tablets engraved with "Zofran" on one side and "8" on the other.

Store between 2° and 30°C (36° and 86°F). Protect from light.

REFERENCES:

1. Pugh RNH, Murray-Lyon IM, Dawson JL, Pietroni MC, Williams R. Transection of the oesophagus for bleeding oesophageal varices. *Brit J Surg.* 1973;60:646-649.

HOW SUPPLIED - EQUIVALENTS NOT AVAILABLE:

Injection, Solution - Intravenous - 2 mg/ml

2 ml x 5	$122.26	ZOFRAN, Glaxo Wellcome	00173-0442-02
20 ml	$244.43	ZOFRAN, Glaxo Wellcome	00173-0442-00

Injection, Solution - Intravenous - 32 mg/50 ml

50 ml	$1238.44	ZOFRAN, Glaxo Wellcome	00173-0461-00

Tablet, Coated - Oral - 4 mg

3's	$35.32	ZOFRAN, Glaxo Wellcome	00173-0446-04
30's	$346.30	ZOFRAN, Glaxo Wellcome	00173-0446-00
100's	$1177.87	ZOFRAN, Glaxo Wellcome	00173-0446-02

Tablet, Coated - Oral - 8 mg

3's	$58.86	ZOFRAN, Glaxo Wellcome	00173-0447-04
30's	$576.90	ZOFRAN, Glaxo Wellcome	00173-0447-00
100's	$1962.23	ZOFRAN, Glaxo Wellcome	00173-0447-02

OPIUM *(001917)*

CATEGORIES: Antidiarrhea Agents; Antipyretics; Central Nervous System Agents; Gastrointestinal Drugs; Opiate Agonists (Controlled); Opium Preparations; DEA Class CII; FDA Pre 1938 Drugs

BRAND NAMES: Pantopon; Paregoric

FORMULARIES: Medi-Cal

Prescribing information not available at time of publication.

HOW SUPPLIED - EQUIVALENTS NOT AVAILABLE:

Liquid - Oral - 4 mg/ml

480 ml	$4.80	PAREGORIC, Lannett	00527-0766-27
3840 ml	$24.88	PAREGORIC, Lannett	00527-0766-28

Tincture - Oral - 10 %

4 oz	$42.10	Opium, Lilly	00002-2606-58
16 oz	$152.50	Opium, Lilly	00002-2606-05

OPIUM ALKALOIDS *(001918)*

CATEGORIES: Analgesics; Antipyretics; Central Nervous System Agents; Hypnotics; Narcotics, Synthetics & Combinations; Opiate Agonists (Controlled); Opium Preparations; Pain; Sedatives; Pregnancy Category C; DEA Class CII; FDA Pre 1938 Drugs

BRAND NAMES: **Pantopon**

DESCRIPTION:

Hydrochlorides of opium alkaloids, a narcotic analgesic, is a sterile injectable preparation for intramuscular and subcutaneous administration. It contains all the alkaloids of opium in a highly purified form free from inert matter and in approximately the same proportions as they occur in nature.

Hydrochlorides of opium alkaloids is a yellowish-gray powder which is freely soluble in water. The approximate composition of Pantopon is as follows: anhydrous morphine — 50 percent, and bases of secondary opium alkaloids — 29.9 to 34.2 percent. One part of Pantopon is equivalent to five parts of opium, U.S.P.

One ml of Pantopon contains 20 mg hydrochlorides of opium alkaloids compounded with 6% alcohol, 136 mg glycerin, 0.2% parabens (methyl and propyl) as preservatives, and either acetic acid, sodium hydroxide, or both, as necessary to adjust pH to approximately 3.3.

CLINICAL PHARMACOLOGY:

The action of Pantopon is essentially that of opium. Pantopon, therefore, exhibits not only the action of morphine but also the actions of codeine, papaverine and other alkaloids present in opium. The other alkaloids in opium alkaloids enhance the sedative and analgesic effects of morphine and tend to minimize its undesirable side effects. Pharmacokinetic data on opium alkaloids are not available; however, data are available on morphine, the major component of opium alkaloids.

Morphine acts as an agonist interacting with stereo-specific receptors in the brain and other tissues; the receptor sites are distributed throughout the CNS and are present in highest concentrations in the limbic system, thalamus, striatum, hypothalamus, midbrain and spinal cord. Morphine is well absorbed after subcutaneous and intramuscular administration. When therapeutic concentrations of morphine are present in plasma, approximately one-third of the drug is protein bound. Unbound morphine accumulates in parenchyma tissues (such as lung, liver, kidney and spleen) and skeletal muscle; however, 24 hours following the last dose, concentrations of the drug in these tissues are quite low.

The half-life of morphine in plasma is about 2.5 to 3 hours in young adults; in older patients, the half-life may be more prolonged. The major metabolic pathway for the drug is conjugation with glucuronic acid and the major route of elimination is through glomerular filtration. Ninety percent of the total excretion takes place during the first 24 hours after administration, although traces of the drug are detectable in the urine for well over 48 hours. About 7 to 10% of administered morphine eventually appears in the feces.

INDICATIONS AND USAGE:

Opium alkaloids is indicated in conditions in which the analgesic, sedative-hypnotic or narcotic effect of an opiate is needed. It is recommended for the relief of severe pain in place of morphine.

CONTRAINDICATIONS:

Opium alkaloids is contraindicated in patients with a known hypersensitivity to this drug or to other opiates.

WARNINGS:

Drug Dependence: *Opium alkaloids may be habit forming.* Opium alkaloids can produce drug dependence of the morphine type and has the potential for being abused. Psychological and physical dependence and tolerance may develop upon repeated administration of opium alkaloids; it should be prescribed and administered with the same degree of caution appropriate to the use of morphine.

Intravenous Use: Opium alkaloids should not be administered intravenously. Rapid intravenous injection of narcotic analgesics increases the incidence of adverse reactions; severe respiratory depression, apnea, hypotension, peripheral circulatory collapse and cardiac arrest have occurred.

Interaction with Other Central Nervous System Depressants: Opium alkaloids should be used with great caution and in reduced dosage in patients who are concurrently receiving other narcotic analgesics, general anesthetics, tranquilizers (including phenothiazines), sedative-hypnotics (including barbiturates), tricyclic antidepressants, MAO inhibitors and other CNS depressants, including alcohol. Respiratory depression, hypotension and profound sedation or coma may result.

Hypotensive Effects: The administration of opium alkaloids may result in severe hypotension in the postoperative patient or in any individual whose ability to maintain blood pressure has been compromised by a depleted blood volume or by the administration of drugs, such as phenothiazines or certain anesthetics.

Head Injury: The respiratory depressant effects of opium alkaloids may be markedly exaggerated in the presence of head injury or other intracranial lesions. Furthermore, narcotics produce adverse reactions which may obscure the clinical course of patients with head injuries. In such patients opium alkaloids must be used with extreme caution and only if its use is deemed essential.

Asthma and Other Respiratory Conditions: Opium alkaloids should be used with extreme caution in patients with bronchial asthma, chronic obstructive pulmonary disease or *cor pulmonale*. Similarly, it should be used with extreme caution in patients having a decreased respiratory reserve or with pre-existing respiratory depression, hypoxia or hypercapnia. In such patients, usual therapeutic doses of narcotics may decrease respiratory drive while simultaneously increasing airway resistance to the point of apnea.

PRECAUTIONS:

General: The administration of opium alkaloids or other narcotics may obscure the diagnosis or clinical course in patients with acute abdominal conditions. Opium alkaloids should be administered with caution and the initial dose should be reduced in patients who are elderly or debilitated and in those patients with severe impairment of hepatic or renal function, hypothyroidism, Addison's disease, toxic psychosis, and prostatic hypertrophy or urethral stricture.

Information for Patients: *In the unlikely event that opium alkaloids would be administered to ambulatory patients,* they should be cautioned that opium alkaloids may impair the mental and/or physical abilities required for the performance of potentially hazardous tasks such as driving a car or operating machinery.

Carcinogenesis, Mutagenesis, Impairment Of Fertility: There have been no studies performed with opium alkaloids to permit an evaluation of its carcinogenic or mutagenic potential. Studies have not been performed to determine the effect of opium alkaloids on fertility and reproduction.

Pregnancy, Teratogenic Effects, Pregnancy Category C: Animal studies have demonstrated the teratogenicity of morphine, the major component of opium alkaloids, in rats, mice and hamsters.

There are no adequate or well-controlled studies of opium alkaloids in either laboratory animals or in pregnant women. It is also not known whether opium alkaloids can cause fetal harm when administered to a pregnant woman or if it can affect reproductive capacity. Opium alkaloids should be used during pregnancy only if the potential benefit justifies the potential risk to the fetus.

Nursing Mothers: It has been reported that morphine is excreted in human milk in microgram amounts. Because of the potential for serious adverse reactions from opium alkaloids in nursing infants, a decision should be made whether to discontinue nursing or to discontinue the drug, taking into account the importance of the drug to the mother.

Pediatric Use: Safety and effectiveness in children have not been established.

DRUG INTERACTIONS:

See WARNINGS.

ADVERSE REACTIONS:

Note: Included in this listing are adverse reactions which have not been reported with this specific drug; however, the pharmacologic similarities among the narcotics require that each of the reactions be considered with opium alkaloids administration.

Neurologic: Respiratory depression and arrest, pinpoint pupils, visual disturbances, coma, sedation, dizziness, headache, tremors, uncoordinated muscle movements. Inadvertent injection in close proximity to a nerve may result in a sensory-motor paralysis which is usually, though not always, transitory.

Psychiatric: Delirium, euphoria, dysphoria, weakness, agitation, hallucinations.

Cardiovascular: Hypotension, collapse, tachycardia, bradycardia, palpitation.

Dermatologic: Rash, urticaria (local and generalized), pruritus.

Gastrointestinal: Nausea, emesis, constipation, dry mouth, biliary tract spasm.

Genitourinary: Urinary retention.

Miscellaneous: Diaphoresis, flushing, pain at the site of injection, anaphylactoid reactions.

DRUG ABUSE AND DEPENDENCE:

Opium alkaloids is subject to Schedule II control under the Federal Controlled Substances Act of 1970. This drug can produce drug dependence of the morphine type and, therefore, has the potential for being abused. Psychological and physical dependence and tolerance may develop upon repeated administration of opium alkaloids, and consequently the same precautions should be taken in administering the drug as with morphine. A narcotic order is required.

OVERDOSAGE:

Serious overdosage with opium alkaloids is characterized by respiratory depression (a decrease in respiratory rate and/or tidal volume, Cheyne-Stokes respiration, cyanosis), extreme somnolence progressing to stupor or coma, skeletal muscle flaccidity, cold and clammy skin, and sometimes bradycardia and hypotension. In severe overdosage, apnea, circulatory collapse, cardiac arrest and death may occur. The triad of coma, pinpoint pupils and depressed respiration strongly suggests opioid poisoning.

Primary attention should be given to the reestablishment of adequate respiratory exchange through provision of a patent airway and through the institution of assisted or controlled ventilation. The narcotic antagonist, naloxone hydrochloride (Narcan), is a specific antidote against respiratory depression resulting from narcotic overdosage or unusual sensitivity to narcotics. An appropriate dose of this antagonist should be administered, preferably by the intravenous route, simultaneously with efforts at respiratory resuscitation.

An antagonist should not be administered in the absence of clinically significant respiratory or cardiovascular depression.

Oxygen, intravenous fluids, vasopressors and other supportive measures should be employed if needed.

NOTE: The administration of the usual dose of a narcotic antagonist will precipitate an acute withdrawal syndrome in patients physically dependent on narcotics. The severity of this syndrome will depend on the degree of physical dependence and the dose of the antagonist administered. The use of narcotic antagonists in such patients should be avoided if possible. If a narcotic antagonist must be used in physically dependent patients to treat serious respiratory depression, the antagonist should be administered with extreme care using only one-fifth to one-tenth the usual initial dose.

The intravenous LD_{50} of opium alkaloids in mice is 96 to 99 mg/kg.

DOSAGE AND ADMINISTRATION:

One-third grain (20 mg) of Pantopon with a morphine content of 1/6 grain (10 mg) is therapeutically equivalent to and is usually administered where 1/4 grain (15 mg) of morphine is indicated.

Usual Adult Dosage: 5 to 20 mg (1/12 to 1/3 grain) approximately every 4 to 5 hours according to the individual needs and severity of pain. Administer only by intramuscular or subcutaneous injection.

Parenteral drug products should be inspected visually for particulate matter and discoloration prior to administration, whenever solution and container permit.

For How Supplied Information, Contact Roche (NDA# NULL)

ORPHENADRINE CITRATE *(001920)*

CATEGORIES: Analgesics; Anticholinergic Agents; Antiparkinson Agents; Autonomic Drugs; Neuromuscular; Pain; Skeletal Muscle Hyperactivity; Skeletal Muscle Relaxants; Pregnancy Category C; FDA Approval Pre 1982

BRAND NAMES: Banflex; *Biorfen* (England); *Biorphen* (England); *Distalene*; *Disipal* (Canada); Flexoject; Flexon; Flexor; Marflex; Mio-Rel; Myolin; Myophen; Myotrol; Neocyten; Noradex; **Norflex**; O'Flex; *Opheryl*; Orflagen; Orfro; Orphenate; *Prolongatum*; Qualaflex; Tega-Flex
(International brand names outside U.S. in italics)

FORMULARIES: Aetna

DESCRIPTION:

Orphenadrine citrate is the citrate salt of orphenadrine (2-dimethylaminoethyl 2-methylbenzhydryl ether citrate). It occurs as a white, crystalline powder having a bitter taste. It is practically odorless; sparingly soluble in water, slightly soluble in alcohol.

Each Orphenadrine Citrate Tablet contains 100 mg orphenadrine citrate. Orphenadrine Citrate Tablets also contain: calcium stearate, ethylcellulose, and lactose. Orphenadrine Citrate Injection contains 60 mg of orphenadrine citrate in aqueous solution in each ampul. Orphenadrine Citrate Injection also contains: sodium bisulfite NF, 2.0 mg; sodium chloride USP, 5.8 mg; sodium hydroxide, to adjust pH; and water for injection USP, q.s. to 2 ml.

CLINICAL PHARMACOLOGY:

The mode of therapeutic action has not been clearly identified, but may be related to its analgesic properties. Orphenadrine citrate also possesses anti-cholinergic actions.

INDICATIONS AND USAGE:

Orphenadrine citrate is indicated as an adjunct to rest, physical therapy, and other measures for the relief of discomfort associated with acute painful musculoskeletal conditions. The mode of action of the drug has not been clearly identified, but may be related to its analgesic properties. Orphenadrine citrate does not directly relax tense skeletal muscles in man.

CONTRAINDICATIONS:

Contraindicated in patients with glaucoma, pyloric or duodenal obstruction, stenosing peptic ulcers, prostatic hypertrophy or obstruction of the bladder neck, cardio-spasm (megaesophagus) and myasthenia gravis.

Contraindicated in patients who have demonstrated a previous hypersensitivity to the drug.

WARNINGS:

Some patients may experience transient episodes of light-headedness, dizziness or syncope. Orphenadrine Citrate may impair the ability of the patient to engage in potentially hazardous activities such as operating machinery or driving a motor vehicle; ambulatory patients should therefore be cautioned accordingly.

Orphenadrine Citrate Injection contains sodium bisulfite, a sulfite that may cause allergic-type reactions including anaphylactic symptoms and life-threatening or less severe asthmatic episodes in certain susceptible people. The overall prevalence of sulfite sensitivity in the general population is unknown and probably low. Sulfite sensitivity is seen more frequently in asthmatic than nonasthmatic people.

WARNINGS: *(cont'd)*

Pregnancy Category C: Pregnancy category C. Animal reproduction studies have not been conducted with Orphenadrine Citrate. It is also not known whether Orphenadrine Citrate can cause fetal harm when administered to a pregnant woman or can affect reproduction capacity. Orphenadrine Citrate should be given to a pregnant woman only if clearly needed.

Usage in Children: Safety and effectiveness in children have not been established; therefore, this drug is not recommended for use in the pediatric age group.

PRECAUTIONS:

Confusion, anxiety and tremors have been reported in few patients receiving propoxyphene and orphenadrine concomitantly. As these symptoms may be simply due to an additive effect, reduction to dosage and/or discontinuation of one or both agents is recommended in such cases.

Orphenadrine citrate should be used with caution in patients with tachycardia, cardiac decompensation, coronary insufficiency, cardiac arrhythmias.

Safety of continuous long-term therapy with orphenadrine has not been established. Therefore, if orphenadrine is prescribed for prolonged use, periodic monitoring of blood, urine and liver function values is recommended.

ADVERSE REACTIONS:

Adverse reactions of orphenadrine are mainly due to the mild anti-cholinergic action of orphenadrine, and are usually associated with higher dosage. Dryness of the mouth is usually the first adverse effect to appear. When the daily dose is increased, possible adverse effects include: tachycardia, palpitation, urinary hesitancy or retention, blurred vision, dilation of pupils, increased ocular tension, weakness, nausea, vomiting, headache, dizziness, constipation, drowsiness, hypersensitivity reactions, pruritus, hallucinations, agitation, tremor, gastric irritation, and rarely urticaria and other dermatoses. Infrequently, an elderly patient may experience some degree of mental confusion. These adverse reactions can usually be eliminated by reduction in dosage. Very rare cases of aplastic anemia associated with the use of orphenadrine tablets have been reported. No causal relationship has been established.

Rare instances of anaphylactic reaction have been reported associated with the intramuscular injection of Orphenadrine Citrate Injection.

DOSAGE AND ADMINISTRATION:

Tablets: *Adults:* Two tablets per day; one in the morning and one in the evening.

Injection: *Adults:* One 2 ml ampul (60 mg) intravenously or intramuscularly; may be repeated every 12 hours. Relief may be maintained by 1 Orphenadrine Citrate tablet twice daily.

Store at controlled room temperature, 15-30°C (59-86°F).

HOW SUPPLIED - RATED THERAPEUTICALLY EQUIVALENT:

Injection, Solution - Intramuscular; - 30 mg/ml

2 ml x 5	$29.90	MIO-REL, Intl Ethical	11584-1016-05
2 ml x 6	**$57.78**	**NORFLEX, 3M Pharms**	**00089-0540-06**
2 ml x 25	$85.00	Orphenadrine Citrate, Schein Pharm (US)	00364-2182-42
2 ml x 25	$85.00	Orphenadrine Citrate, Steris Labs	00402-0354-82
2 ml x 25	$91.65	MYOPHEN, Teral Labs	51234-0514-02
2 ml x 25	$142.50	MIO-REL, Intl Ethical	11584-1016-02
10 ml	$6.25	Orphenadrine Citrate, Major Pharms	00904-0858-10
10 ml	$7.50	Orfro, C O Truxton	00463-1092-10
10 ml	$8.00	Orphenadrine Citrate, Consolidated Midland	00223-8200-10
10 ml	$8.00	Orphenadrine Citrate, Consolidated Midland	00223-8201-10
10 ml	$8.80	Orphenadrine Citrate, Steris Labs	00402-0129-10
10 ml	$11.90	Orphenadrine Citrate, Schein Pharm (US)	00364-6747-54
10 ml	$12.00	BANFLEX, Forest Pharms	00456-1092-10
10 ml	$12.00	MYOPHEN, Alba Pharma	10023-0190-10
10 ml	$21.50	Flexor Injectable 30 Mg/Ml, Deliz	58238-0301-10
10 ml	$22.65	FLEXOJECT, Mayrand Pharms	00259-0322-10

HOW SUPPLIED - NOT RATED EQUIVALENT:

Tablet, Plain Coated, Sustained Action - Oral - 100 mg

100's	**$126.54**	**NORFLEX, 3M Pharms**	**00089-0221-16**
100's	**$149.94**	**NORFLEX, 3M Pharms**	**00089-0221-10**
500's	**$712.02**	**NORFLEX, 3M Pharms**	**00089-0221-50**

OXACILLIN SODIUM *(001923)*

CATEGORIES: Anti-Infectives; Antibacterials; Antibiotics; Antimicrobials; Infections; Penicillins; Pregnancy Category B; FDA Approval Pre 1982

BRAND NAMES: Bactocill; *Bristopen* (France); Prostaphlin; *Stapenor* (Germany); Staphaloxin
(International brand names outside U.S. in italics)

FORMULARIES: Aetna

DESCRIPTION:

CAPSULES AND ORAL SOLUTION

Oxacillin sodium is an antibacterial agent of the isoxazolyl penicillin series. It is a penicillinase-resistant, acid resistant, semi-synthetic penicillin suitable for oral administration. Oxacillin sodium is available for administration as an oral solution and capsules.

Inactive ingredient in oxacillin sodium capsules: Lactose, Magnesium Stearate and FD&C Yellow No.6.

Inactive ingredients in oxacillin sodium oral solution are: FD&C Red No. 40, natural & artificial flavorings, potassium alginate, sodium benzoate, sodium citrate, sodium saccharin, and sucrose.

INJECTION

Oxacillin Sodium For Injection, USP, is a semisynthetic antibiotic substance derived from 6-amino-penicillanic acid. It is the sodium salt in a parenteral dosage form. Each gram of Oxacillin Sodium contains approximately 2.5 mEq of sodium and is buffered with 20 mg dibasic sodium phosphate.

CAPSULES, ORAL SOLUTION, AND INJECTION

$C_{19}H_{18}N_3NaO_5S \cdot H_2O$ 441.43 (CAS 7240-38-2)

4-Thia-1-azabicyclo(3.2.0)heptane-2-carboxylic acid, 3,3 dimethyl-6-(((5-methyl-3-phenyl-4-isoxazolyl)carbonyl) amino)-7-oxo-monosodium salt, monohydrate, (2S-(2α,5α,6β)).

CLINICAL PHARMACOLOGY:

MICROBIOLOGY

Penicillinase-resistant penicillins exert a bactericidal action against penicillin-susceptible microorganisms during the state of active multiplication. All penicillins inhibit the biosynthesis of the bacterial cell wall.

CLINICAL PHARMACOLOGY: *(cont'd)*

The drugs in this class are highly resistant to inactivation by staphylococcal penicillinase and are active against penicillinase producing and non-penicillinase producing strains of *staphylococcus aureus.*

The penicillinase-resistant penicillins are active *in vitro* against a variety of other bacteria.

SUSCEPTIBILITY TESTING

Quantitative methods of susceptibility testing that require measurement of zone diameters or minimal inhibitory concentrations (MICs) give the most precise estimates of antibiotic susceptibility. One such procedure has been recommended for use with discs to test susceptibility to this class of drugs. Interpretations correlate diameters on the disc test with MIC values. A penicillinase-resistant class disk may be used to determine microbial susceptibility to cloxacillin, dicloxacillin, methicillin, nafcillin, and oxacillin. With this procedure, employing a 5 microgram methicillin sodium disc, a report from the laboratory of "susceptible" (zone of at least 14 mm) indicates that the infecting organism is likely to respond to therapy. A report of "resistant" (zone of less than 10 mm) indicates that the infecting organism is not likely to respond to therapy. A report of "intermediate susceptibility" (zone of 10 to 13 mm) suggests that the organism might be susceptible if high doses of the antibiotic are used, or if the infection is confined to tissues and fluids (*e.g.,* urine), in which high antibiotic levels are attained.

In general, all staphylococci should be tested against the penicillin G disc and against the methicillin disc. Routine methods of antibiotic susceptibility testing may fail to detect strains of organisms resistant to the penicillinase-resistant penicillins. For this reason, the use of large inocula and the 48-hour incubation periods may be necessary to obtain accurate susceptibility studies with these antibiotics. Bacterial strains which are resistant to one of the penicillinase-resistant penicillins should be considered resistant to all of the drugs in the class.

PHARMACOKINETICS

Capsules and Oral Solution: Oxacillin sodium is resistant to destruction by acid. Absorption of oxacillin sodium after oral administration is rapid but incomplete. A single 250-mg oral dose gives a 1-hour peak serum level of 1.65 mcg/ml. A-500 mg dose peaks at about 2.6 mcg/ml. Peak serum levels with the oral solution occur somewhat earlier, about one-half hour after dosing. A single dose of 250-mg oral solution gives a peak serum level of 1.9 mcg/ml; of 500-mg 4.8 mcg/ml.

Once absorbed, oxacillin sodium binds to serum protein, mainly albumin. The degree of protein binding reported varies with the method of study and the investigator, but generally has been found to be $94.2 \pm 2.1\%$. Oral absorption of oxacillin is delayed when the drug is administered after meals.

Oxacillin sodium, with normal doses, has insignificant concentrations in the cerebrospinal and ascitic fluids. It is found in therapeutic concentrations in the pleural, bile, and amniotic fluids. Oxacillin is rapidly excreted as unchanged drug in the urine by glomerular filtration and active tubular secretion.

Injection: Oxacillin Sodium, with normal doses, has significant concentrations in the cerebrospinal and ascitic fluids. It is found in therapeutic concentrations in the pleural, bile, and amniotic fluids. Oxacillin is rapidly excreted as unchanged drug in the urine by glomerular filtration and active tubular secretion.

Oxacillin Sodium binds to serum protein, mainly albumin. The degree of protein binding reported varies with the method of study and the investigator, but generally has been found to be $94.2 \pm 2.1\%$.

Intramuscular injections give peak serum levels 30 minutes after injection. A 250 mg dose gives a level of 5.3 mcg/ml while a 500 mg dose peaks at 10.9 mcg/ml. Intravenous injection gives a peak about 5 minutes after the injection is completed. Slow IV dosing with 500 mg gives a 5 minute peak of 43 mcg/ml with a half-life of 20 to 30 minutes.

INDICATIONS AND USAGE:

The penicillinase-resistant penicillins are indicated in the treatment of infections caused by penicillinase-producing staphylococci which have demonstrated susceptibility to the drugs. Culture and susceptibility tests should be performed initially to determine the causative organisms and their sensitivity to the drug (see CLINICAL PHARMACOLOGY, Susceptibility Testing.)

The penicillinase-resistant penicillins may be used to initiate therapy in suspected cases of resistant staphylococcal infections prior to the availability of laboratory test results. The penicillinase-resistant penicillins should not be used in infections caused by organisms susceptible to penicillin G. If the susceptibility tests indicate that the infection is due to an organism other than a resistant staphylococcus, therapy should not be continued with a penicillinase-resistant penicillin.

CONTRAINDICATIONS:

A history of hypersensitivity (anaphylactic) reaction to any penicillin is a contraindication.

WARNINGS:

Serious and occasionally fatal hypersensitivity (anaphylactic shock with collapse) reactions have occurred in patients receiving penicillin. The incidence of anaphylactic shock in all penicillin-treated patients is between 0.015 and 0.04 percent. Anaphylactic shock resulting in death has occurred in approximately 0.002 percent of the patients treated. Although anaphylaxis is more frequent following a parenteral administration, it has occurred in patients receiving oral penicillins.

When penicillin therapy is indicated, it should be initiated only after a comprehensive patient drug and allergy history has been obtained. If an allergic reaction occurs, the drug should be discontinued and the patient should receive supportive treatment, e.g., artificial maintenance of ventilation, pressor amines, antihistamines, and corticosteroids. Individuals with a history of penicillin hypersensitivity may also experience allergic reactions when treated with a cephalosporin.

PRECAUTIONS:

General: Penicillinase-resistant penicillins should generally not be administered to patients with a history of sensitivity to any penicillin.

Penicillin should be used with caution in individuals with histories of significant allergies and/or asthma. Whenever allergic reactions occur, penicillin should be withdrawn unless, in the opinion of the physician, the condition being treated is life-threatening and amenable only to penicillin therapy.

The oral route of administration should not be relied upon in patients with severe illness, or with nausea, vomiting, gastric dilation, cardiospasm, or intestinal hypermotility. Occasionally patients will not absorb therapeutic amounts of orally administered penicillin.

The use of antibiotics may result in overgrowth of nonsusceptible organisms. If new infections due to bacteria or fungi occur, the drug should be discontinued and appropriate measures taken.

Information for the Patient (Oral Administration): *Capsules and Oral Solution:*Patients receiving penicillins should be given the following information and instructions by the physician:

PRECAUTIONS: *(cont'd)*

1. Patients should be told that penicillin is an antibacterial agent which will work with the body's natural defenses to control certain types of infections. They should be told that the drug should not be taken if they have had an allergic reaction to any form of penicillin previously, and to inform the physician of any allergies or previous allergic reactions to any drugs they may have had (see WARNINGS.)

2. Patients who have previously experienced an anaphylactic to penicillin should be instructed to wear a medical identification tag or bracelet.

3. Because most antibacterial agents taken by mouth are best absorbed on an empty stomach, patients should be directed, unless circumstances warrant otherwise, to take penicillin one hour before meals or two hours after eating (see CLINICAL PHARMACOLOGY, Pharmacokinetics.)

4. Patients should be told to take the entire course of therapy prescribed, even if fever and other symptoms have stopped (see PRECAUTIONS, General.)

5. If any of the following reactions occur, stop taking your prescription and notify the physician: shortness of breath, wheezing, skin rash, mouth irritation, black tongue, sore throat, nausea, vomiting, diarrhea, fever, swollen joints, or any unusual bleeding or bruising (see ADVERSE REACTIONS.)

6. Do not take any additional medications without physician approval, including non-prescription drugs such as antacids, laxatives, or vitamins.

7. Discard any liquid forms of penicillin after 7 days if stored at room temperature or after 14 days if refrigerated.

Laboratory Tests: Bacteriologic studies to determine the causative organisms and their susceptibility to the penicillinase-resistant penicillins should be performed (see CLINICAL PHARMACOLOGY, Microbiology.) In the treatment of suspected staphylococcal infections, therapy should be changed to another active agent if culture tests fail to demonstrate the presence of staphylococci.

Periodic assessment of organ system function including renal, hepatic, and hematopoietic should be made during prolonged therapy with the penicillinase-resistant penicillins.

Blood cultures, white blood cell, and differential cell counts should be obtained prior to initiation of therapy and at least weekly during therapy with penicillinase-resistant penicillins.

Periodic urinalysis, blood urea in nitrogen; and creatinine determinations should be performed during therapy with the penicillinase-resistant penicillins and dosage alterations should be considered if these values become elevated. If any impairment of renal function is suspected or known to exist, a reduction in the total dosage should be considered and blood levels monitored to avoid possible neurotoxic reactions (See DOSAGE AND ADMINISTRATION.)

SGOT and SGPT values should be obtained periodically during therapy to monitor for possible liver function abnormalities.

Carcinogenesis, Mutagenesis, and Impairment of Fertility: No long-term animal studies have been conducted with these drugs.

Studies on reproduction (nafcillin) in rats and rabbits reveal no fetal or maternal abnormalities before conception and continuously through weaning (one generation).

Pregnancy Category B: Reproduction studies performed in the mouse, rat, and rabbit have revealed no evidence of impaired fertility or harm to the fetus due to the penicillinase-resistant penicillins. Human experience with the penicillins during pregnancy has not shown any positive evidence of adverse effects on the fetus. There are, however, no adequate or well-controlled studies in pregnant women showing conclusively that harmful effects of these drugs on the fetus can be excluded. Because animal reproduction studies are not always predictive of human response, this drug should be used during pregnancy only if clearly needed.

Nursing Mothers: Penicillins are excreted in breast milk. Caution should be exercised when penicillins are administered to a nursing woman.

Pediatric Use: Because of incompletely developed renal function in newborns, penicillinase-resistant penicillins (especially methicillin) may not be completely excreted, with abnormally high blood levels resulting. Frequent blood levels are advisable in this group with dosage adjustments when necessary. All newborns treated with penicillins should be monitored closely for clinical and laboratory evidence of toxic or adverse effects (see DOSAGE AND ADMINISTRATION.)

DRUG INTERACTIONS:

Tetracycline, a bacteriostatic antibiotic, may antagonize the bactericidal effect of penicillin and concurrent use of these drugs should be avoided.

ADVERSE REACTIONS:

Body as a Whole: The reported incidence of allergic reactions to penicillins ranges from 0.7 to 10 percent (see WARNINGS.) Sensitization is usually the result of treatment but some individuals have had immediate reactions to penicillin when first treated. In such cases, it is thought that the patients may have had prior exposure to the drug via trace amounts present in milk and vaccines.

Two types of allergic reactions to penicillin are noted clinically,

immediate and delayed.

Immediate reactions usually occur within 20 minutes of administration and range in severity from urticaria and pruritus to angioneurotic edema, laryngospasm, bronchospasm, hypotension, vascular collapse, and death. Such immediate anaphylactic reactions are very rare (see WARNINGS) and usually occur after parenteral therapy but have occurred in patients receiving oral therapy. Another type of immediate reaction, an accelerated reaction, may occur between 20 minutes and 48 hours after administration and may include urticaria, pruritus, and fever. Although laryngeal edema, laryngospasm, and hypotension occasionally occur, fatality is uncommon.

Delayed allergic reactions to penicillin therapy usually occur after 48 hours and sometimes as late as 2 to 4 weeks after initiation of therapy. Manifestations of this type of reaction include serum sickness-like symptoms (*i.e.,* fever, malaise, urticaria, myalgia, arthralgia, abdominal pain) and various skin rashes. Nausea, vomiting, diarrhea, stomatitis, black or "hairy" tongue, and other symptoms of gastrointestinal irritation may occur, especially during oral penicillin therapy.

Nervous System Reactions: Neurotoxic reactions similar to those observed with penicillin G may occur with large intravenous doses of the penicillinase-resistant penicillins especially in patients with renal insufficiency.

Urogenital Reactions: Renal tubular damage and interstitial nephritis have been associated with the administration of methicillin sodium and infrequently with the administration of nafcillin and oxacillin. Manifestations of this reaction may include rash, fever, eosinophilia, hematuria, proteinuria, and renal insufficiency. Methicillin-induced nephropathy does not appear to be dose-related and is generally reversible upon prompt discontinuation of therapy.

Gastrointestinal Reactions: Pseudomembranous colitis has been reported with the use of Oxacillin Sodium (and other broad spectrum antibiotics); therefore, it is important to consider its diagnosis in patients who develop diarrhea in association with antibiotic use.

ADVERSE REACTIONS: *(cont'd)*

Treatment with broad spectrum antibiotic alters normal flora of the colon and may permit overgrowth of clostridia. Studies indicate a toxin produced by *Clostridium difficile* is one primary cause of antibiotic-associated colitis. Cholestyramine and colestipol resins have been shown to bind the toxin *in vitro*.

Mild cases of colitis may respond to drug discontinuance alone.

Moderate to severe cases should be managed with fluid, electrolyte and protein supplementation as indicated.

When the colitis is not relieved by drug discontinuance or when it is severe, oral vancomycin is the treatment of choice for antibiotic-associated pseudomembranous colitis produced by c. difficile. Other causes of colitis should also be considered.

Metabolic Reactions: Agranulocytosis, neutropenia, and bone marrow depression have been associated with the use of methicillin sodium, nafcillin, oxacillin, and cloxacillin. Hepatotoxicity, characterized by fever, nausea, and vomiting associated with abnormal liver function tests, mainly elevated SGOT levels, has been associated with the use of oxacillin and cloxacillin.

DOSAGE AND ADMINISTRATION:

The penicillinase-resistant penicillins are available for oral administration and for intramuscular and intravenous injection. The sodium salts of methicillin, oxacillin, and nafcillin may be administered parenterally and the sodium salts of cloxacillin, dicloxacillin, oxacillin, and nafcillin are available for oral use.

Bacteriologic studies to determine the causative organisms and their sensitivity to the penicillinase-resistant penicillins should always be performed. Duration of therapy varies with the type and severity of infection as well as the overall condition of the patient, therefore, it should be determined by the clinical and bacteriological response of the patient. In severe staphylococcal infections, therapy with penicillinase-resistant penicillins should be continued for at least 14 days. Therapy should be continued for at least 48 hours after the patient has become afebrile, asymptomatic, and cultures are negative. The treatment of endocarditis and osteomyelitis may require a longer term of therapy.

Concurrent administration of the penicillinase-resistant penicillins and probenecid increases and prolongs serum penicillin levels. Probenecid decreases the apparent volume of distribution and slows the rate of excretion by competitively inhibiting renal tubular secretion of penicillin. Penicillin-probenecid therapy is generally limited to those infections where very high serum levels of penicillin are necessary.

Oral preparations of the penicillinase-resistant penicillins should not be used as initial therapy in serious, life-threatening infections. Oral therapy with the penicillinase-resistant penicillins may be used to follow-up the previous use of a parenteral agent as soon as the clinical condition warrants. For intramuscular gluteal injections, care should be taken to avoid sciatic nerve injury. With intravenous administration, particularly in elderly patients, care should be taken because of the possibility of thrombophlebitis. (See TABLE 1.)

DIRECTIONS FOR DISPENSING ORAL SOLUTION

Prepare these formulations at the time of dispensing. For ease in preparation, add water to the bottle in two portions and shake well after each addition. Add the total amount of water as directed on the package being dispensed. The reconstituted formulation is stable or 3 days at room temperature or 14 days under refrigeration.

TABLE 1 Recommended For Oxacillin Sodium For Injection, Usp

Adults	Infants and Children 40 kg (88 lbs)	Other Recommendations
250-500 mg IM or IV every 4-6 hours (mild to moderate infections)	50 mg/kg/day IM or IV in equally divided doses every 6 hours (mild to moderate infections)	
1 gram IM or IV every 4-6 hours severe infections)	100 mg/kg/day IM or IV in equally divided doses every 4-6 hours (severe infections)	Premature and neonates 25 mg/kg/day IM or IV

DIRECTIONS FOR USE

For Intramuscular Use: Use Sterile Water for Injection USP. Add 1.4 ml to the 250 mg vial, 2.7 ml to the 500 mg vial, 5.7 ml to the 1 gram vial, 11.5 ml to the 2 gram vial, and 23 ml to the 4 gram vial. Shake well until a clear solution is obtained. After constitution, vials will contain 250 mg of active drug per 1.5 ml of solution. The constituted solution is stable for 3 days at 70°F or for one week under refrigeration (40°F).

For Direct Intravenous Use: Use Sterile Water for Injection USP or Sodium Chloride Injection, USP. Add 5 ml to the 250 mg and 500 mg vials; 10 ml to the 1 gram vial; 20 ml to the 2 gram vial; and 40 ml to the 4 gram vial. Withdraw the entire contents and administer slowly over a period of approximately 10 minutes.

For Administration by Intravenous Drip: Constitute as directed above (For Direct Intravenous Use) prior to diluting with Intravenous Solution.

TABLE 2A Stability Periods For Oxacillin Sodium For Injection, Usp

Concentration mg/ml	Sterile Water for Injection	Isotonic Sodium Chloride	M/6 Molar Sodium Lactate Solution	%5 Dextrose in Water
Room Temperature (25°C)				
10 - 100	4 days	4 days		
10 - 30			24 hours	
0.5 - 2				6 hours
Refrigeration (4°C)				
10 - 100	7 days	7 days		
10 - 30			4 days	4 days
Frozen (-15°C)				
50 - 100	30 days			
250/1.5 ml	30 days			
100		30 days		
10 - 100			30 days	30 days

Table 2B lists the stability periods of additional solutions with oxacillin sodium added.

Stability studies on oxacillin sodium at concentrations of 0.5 mg/ml and 2 mg/ml in various intravenous solutions listed below indicate the drug will lose less than 10% activity at room temperature (70°F) during a 6 hour period.

IV Solution

5% Dextrose in Normal Saline	10% Invert Sugar Plus 0.3% Potassium Chloride in Water
10% D-Fructose in Water	Travert 10% Electrolyte #1
10% D-Fructose in Normal Saline	Travert 10% Electrolyte #2
Lactated Potassic Saline Injection	Travert 10% Electrolyte #3
10% Invert Sugar in Normal Saline	

DOSAGE AND ADMINISTRATION: *(cont'd)*

TABLE 2B Stability Periods In Oxacillin Sodium For Injection, Usp

Concentration mg/ml	5% Dextrose in 0.45% NaCl	10% Invert Sugar	Lactated Ringer's Solution
Room Temperature (25°C)			
10 - 30	24 hours		
0.5 - 2		6 hours	6 hours
Refrigeration (4°C)			
10 - 30	4 days	4 days	4 days
Frozen (-15°C)			
10 - 100	30 days	30 days	30 days

Only those solutions listed above should be used for the intravenous infusion of oxacillin sodium. The concentration of the antibiotic should fall within the range specified. The drug concentration and the rate and volume of the infusion should be adjusted so that the total dose of oxacillin is administered before the drug loses its stability in the solution in use.

If another agent is used in conjunction with oxacillin therapy, it should not be physically mixed with oxacillin but should be administered separately.

"Piggyback" IV Package: This glass vial contains the labeled quantity and is intended for intravenous administration. The diluent and volume are specified on the label of each package.

Discard solution after 24 hours at room temperature.

Pharmacy Bulk Package: This glass vial contains 10 grams oxacillin sodium and is designed for use in the pharmacy in preparing IV additives. Add 93 ml sterile water for injection USP or sodium chloride injection USP. The resulting solution will contain 100 mg oxacillin sodium per ml.

Following reconstitution in this manner, the resulting solutions are stable for 4 days at room temperature or 7 days under refrigeration.

CAUTION: NOT TO BE DISPENSED AS A UNIT.

Storage: Store sterile powder at controlled room temperature 15-30° C (59-86° F).

(Capsules and Oral Solution: Apothecon, 1/89)

(Injection: SmithKline Beecham, 1/92, BT:L2)

HOW SUPPLIED - RATED THERAPEUTICALLY EQUIVALENT:

Capsule, Gelatin - Oral - 250 mg

100's	$21.75	Oxacillin, Teva	00332-3115-09
100's	$21.75	Oxacillin Sodium, United Res	00677-0932-01
100's	$21.75	Oxacillin Sodium, H.C.F.A. F F P	99999-1923-01
100's	$22.00	Oxacillin Sodium, Raway	00686-0162-20
100's	$28.40	Oxacillin Sodium, HL Moore Drug Exch	00839-6412-06
100's	$28.71	Oxacillin Sodium, Qualitest Pharms	00603-4927-21
100's	$28.75	Oxacillin Sodium, Major Pharms	00904-2709-60
100's	$28.88	Oxacillin Sodium, Rugby	00536-1150-01
100's	$29.00	Oxacillin Sodium, Goldline Labs	00182-1340-01
100's	$29.90	Oxacillin Sodium, Aligen Independ	00405-4726-01
100's	$30.08	Oxacillin Sodium, Schein Pharm (US)	00364-2059-01
100's	$30.50	BACTOCILL, Beecham	00029-6010-30
100's	$75.96	PROSTAPHLIN, Mead Johnson	00015-7977-66

Capsule, Gelatin - Oral - 500 mg

100's	$32.60	Oxacillin Sodium, Raway	00686-0163-20
100's	$41.93	Oxacillin, Teva	00332-3117-09
100's	$41.93	Oxacillin Sodium, United Res	00677-0933-01
100's	$41.93	Oxacillin Sodium, H.C.F.A. F F P	99999-1923-02
100's	$53.20	Oxacillin Sodium, Major Pharms	00904-2710-60
100's	$53.45	Oxacillin Sodium, HL Moore Drug Exch	00839-6413-06
100's	$54.45	Oxacillin Sodium, Qualitest Pharms	00603-4928-21
100's	$55.29	Oxacillin Sodium, Aligen Independ	00405-4727-01
100's	$55.42	Oxacillin Sodium, Schein Pharm (US)	00364-2060-01
100's	$56.45	Oxacillin Sodium, Goldline Labs	00182-1341-01
100's	$56.85	BACTOCILL, Beecham	00029-6015-30
100's	$57.05	Oxacillin Sodium, Rugby	00536-1160-01

Injection, Dry-Soln - Intramuscular; - 1 gm/vial

1 gm	$3.82	PROSTAPHLIN, Mead Johnson	00015-7981-20
1 gm	$3.95	PROSTAPHLIN, Mead Johnson	00015-7981-18
1 gm	$5.15	PROSTAPHLIN, Mead Johnson	00015-7981-28
1 gm x 10	$61.80	Oxacillin Sodium, Bristol Myers Squibb	00003-2712-10
1 gm x 10	$83.30	Oxacillin Sodium, Bristol Myers Squibb	00003-2712-20
1's	$4.04	Bactocill, Beecham	00029-6025-07
1's	$11.50	PROSTAPHLIN, Mead Johnson	00015-7981-89
10's	$39.48	Oxacillin Sodium, Gensia Labs	00703-8318-03
10's	$41.88	Oxacillin Sodium, Gensia Labs	00703-8319-03
20 ml x 10	$55.57	Oxacillin Sodium, Vial, Marsam	00209-8000-22
20ml x 10	$3.68	BACTOCILL, Beecham	00029-6025-22
21 ml x 10	$3.40	BACTOCILL ADD-VANTAGE, Beecham	00029-6025-40
100 ml x 10	$74.89	Oxacillin Sodium, Piggyback, Marsam	00209-8050-42

Injection, Dry-Soln - Intramuscular; - 2 gm/vial

1's	$6.29	Bactocill, Beecham	00029-6028-07
2 gm	$7.33	PROSTAPHLIN, Mead Johnson	00015-7970-20
2 gm	$7.47	PROSTAPHLIN, Mead Johnson	00015-7970-18
2 gm	$8.67	PROSTAPHLIN, Mead Johnson	00015-7970-28
2 gm x 10	$118.80	Oxacillin Sodium, Bristol Myers Squibb	00003-2713-10
2 gm x 10	$140.50	Oxacillin Sodium, Bristol Myers Squibb	00003-2713-20
10's	$76.68	Oxacillin Sodium, Gensia Labs	00703-8328-03
10's	$78.00	Oxacillin Sodium, Gensia Labs	00703-8329-03
20 ml x 10	$106.83	Oxacillin Sodium, Vial, Marsam	00209-8100-22
21 ml x 10	$5.30	BACTOCILL ADD-VANTAGE, Beecham	00029-6028-40
30 ml x 10	$5.94	BACTOCILL, Beecham	00029-6028-27
100 ml x 10	$7.42	BACTOCILL, Beecham	00029-6028-21
100 ml x 10	$126.36	Oxacillin Sodium, Piggyback, Marsam	00209-8150-42

Injection, Dry-Soln - Intramuscular; - 4 gm

1's	$41.13	PROSTAPHLIN, Mead Johnson	00015-7300-99
50 ml x 10	$11.10	BACTOCILL, Beecham	00029-6030-26

Injection, Dry-Soln - Intramuscular; - 10 gm/vial

10 gm	$47.16	PROSTAPHLIN, Mead Johnson	00015-7103-28
10 gm x 10	$594.60	Oxacillin Sodium, Bristol Myers Squibb	00003-2715-25
10's	$351.48	Oxacillin Sodium, Gensia Labs	00703-8338-03
100 ml x 10	$28.20	BACTOCILL, Beecham	00029-6032-21
100 ml x 10	$535.05	Oxacillin Sodium, Bulk, Marsam	00209-8300-52

Injection, Dry-Soln - Intramuscular; - 500 mg/vial

6 ml x 10	$28.48	Oxacillin Sodium, Vial, Marsam	00209-7950-22
10 ml x 10	$2.43	BACTOCILL, Beecham	00029-6020-25

HOW SUPPLIED - RATED THERAPEUTICALLY EQUIVALENT: *(cont'd)*

10's	$20.40	Oxacillin Sodium, Gensia Labs	00703-8308-03
500 mg	$1.96	PROSTAPHLIN, Mead Johnson	00015-7979-20
500 mg x 10	$31.70	Oxacillin Sodium, Bristol Myers Squibb	00003-2711-10

Powder, Reconstitution - Oral - 250 mg/5ml

100 ml	$4.69	Oxacillin Sodium, Rugby	00536-1170-82
100 ml	$5.25	Oxacillin, Teva	00332-4157-32
100 ml	$5.25	Oxacillin Sodium, H.C.F.A. F F P	99999-1923-03
100 ml	$5.60	Oxacillin Sodium, Major Pharms	00904-1519-04
100 ml	$5.80	Oxacillin Sodium, Goldline Labs	00182-7069-70
100 ml	$5.95	Oxacillin Sodium, Qualitest Pharms	00603-6584-64
100 ml	$14.58	PROSTAPHLIN, Mead Johnson	00015-7985-40

HOW SUPPLIED - NOT RATED EQUIVALENT:

Injection, Dry-Soln - Intramuscular; - 1 gm/vial

50 ml	$22.21	Bactocill 1 Gm Injection, Baxter Hlthcare	00338-1013-41

Injection, Dry-Soln - Intramuscular; - 2 gm/vial

50 ml	$31.97	Bactocill 2 Gm Injection, Baxter Hlthcare	00338-1015-41

OXAMNIQUINE *(001924)*

CATEGORIES: Anthelmintics; Anti-Infectives; Antiparasitics; Helminths; Parasiticidal; Trematodes; Pregnancy Category C; FDA Approval Pre 1982

BRAND NAMES: **Vansil**

FORMULARIES: WHO

DESCRIPTION:

Oxamniquine is a tetrahydroquinoline derivative for the oral treatment of Schistosoma Mansoni infections. It is 1,2,3,4,-tetrahydro-2-(((1-methylethyl) amino)methyl)-7-nitro-6-quinolinemethanol.

Oxamniquine is a yellow-orange crystalline solid which is sparingly soluble in water, but soluble in methanol, acetone, and chloroform.

Oxamniquine capsules contain 250 mg of oxamniquine.

CLINICAL PHARMACOLOGY:

Oxamniquine is well absorbed when administered orally. Human plasma concentrations reach a peak at 1 to 1.5 hours after oral administration of therapeutic doses, with a plasma half-life of 1 to 2.5 hours. It is extensively metabolized to inactive acidic metabolites which are largely excreted in the urine.

Male schistosomes are more susceptible than females, but after treatment with oxamniquine the residual female schistosomes cease to lay eggs thus losing the parasitological aspect of their pathological significance. Animal studies with immature S. Mansoni infections have demonstrated oxamniquine to be highly active in the immediate post-infection phase. Oxamniquine significantly reduces the egg load of S. Mansoni.

INDICATIONS AND USAGE:

Oxamniquine is indicated for all stages of S. Mansoni infection, including the acute phase & the chronic phase with hepatosplenic involvement.

CONTRAINDICATIONS:

At present, there are no known contraindications to the administration of oxamniquine.

WARNINGS:

In rare instances epileptiform convulsions have been observed within the first few hours after ingestion of oxamniquine. When a convulsion occurred, it was mostly in a patient with a previous history of a convulsive condition.

Oxamniquine should be used with care in such individuals and they should remain under medical supervision with facilities available to treat a convulsion should it occur.

PRECAUTIONS:

Pregnancy Category C: Oxamniquine has been shown to have an embryocidal effect in rabbits and mice when given in doses 10 times the human dose.

There are no adequate and well controlled studies in pregnant women. Oxamniquine should be used during pregnancy only if the potential benefit justifies the potential risk to the fetus.

Nursing Mothers: It is not known whether this drug is excreted in human milk.

Because many drugs are excreted in human milk, caution should be exercised when oxamniquine is administered to a nursing mother.

ADVERSE REACTIONS:

Oxamniquine is generally well tolerated and toleration is improved if the doses are given after food. Transitory dizziness/drowsiness occurred in approximately one-third of the patients assessed. Other effects observed to a lesser degree are headache, nausea, vomiting, abdominal pain and anorexia. Urticaria has also been reported. In rare instances epileptiform convulsions have been observed (see WARNINGS).

Minor and transient abnormalities in laboratory data have been observed after treatment with oxamniquine which were not considered to be drug-related and were of no clinical significance.

They included rare instances of mild to moderate liver enzyme elevations but there was no evidence of hepatotoxicity even in patients with severe hepatosplenic involvement. There was evidence, however, of liver abnormalities in animals with the female rat being uniquely sensitive to relatively low doses.

DOSAGE AND ADMINISTRATION:

Adults: The recommended doage is 12 to 15 mg per kilogram of body weight given as a single oral dose in patients with Western Hemisphere strains of S.

Mansoni. The recommended capsule dosage according to body weight is as follows:

Body Weight (kg)	No. of Capsules (250 mg)
30- 40	2
41- 60	3
61- 80	4
81-100	5

DOSAGE AND ADMINISTRATION: *(cont'd)*

Children: The recommended dosage for children under 30 kg in weight is 20 mg/kg of body weight given in two divided doses of 10 mg/kg in one day with an interval of 2 to 8 hours between doses. Toleration is improved if the doses are given after food.

HOW SUPPLIED - EQUIVALENTS NOT AVAILABLE:

Capsule, Gelatin - Oral - 250 mg

24's	$106.79	VANSIL, Pfizer Labs	00069-6410-24

OXANDROLONE *(001925)*

CATEGORIES: Anabolic Steroids; Androgens; Hormones; Infections; Osteoporosis; Pain; Steroids; Weight Gain; Pregnancy Category X; DEA Class CIII

BRAND NAMES: *Lonavar* (Japan); **Oxandrin**; *Vasorome* (Japan)
(International brand names outside U.S. in italics)

COST OF THERAPY: $2,737.50 (Osteoporosis; Tablet; 2.5 mg; 2/day; 365 days) vs. Potential Cost of $8,326.27 (Back Procedures)

DESCRIPTION:

Oxandrin oral tablets contain 2.5 mg of the anabolic steroid oxandrolone. Oxandrolone is 17β-hydroxy-17α-methyl-2-oxa-5α-androstan-3-one.

Inactive ingredients include corn starch, lactose, magnesium stearate, and hydroxypropyl methylcellulose.

CLINICAL PHARMACOLOGY:

Anabolic steroids are synthetic derivatives of testosterone. Certain clinical effects & adverse reactions demonstrate the androgenic properties of this class of drugs. Complete dissociation of anabolic and androgenic effects has not been achieved.

The actions of anabolic steroids are therefore similar to those of male sex hormones with the possibility of causing serious disturbances of growth and sexual development if given to young children. Anabolic steroids suppress the gonadotropic functions of the pituitary and may exert a direct effect upon the testes.

During exogenous administration of anabolic androgens, endogenous testosterone release is inhibited through inhibition of pituitary luteinizing hormone (LH). At large doses, spermatogenesis may be suppressed through feedback inhibition of pituitary follicle-stimulating hormone (FSH).

Anabolic steroids have been reported to increase low-density lipoproteins and decrease high-density lipoproteins. These levels revert to normal on discontinuation of treatment.

INDICATIONS AND USAGE:

Oxandrin is indicated as adjunctive therapy to promote weight gain after weight loss following extensive surgery, chronic infections, or severe trauma, and in some patients who without definite pathophysiologic reasons fail to gain or to maintain normal weight, to offset the protein catabolism associated with prolonged administration of corticosteroids, and for the relief of the bone pain frequently accompanying osteoporosis. (See DOSAGE AND ADMINISTRATION.)

CONTRAINDICATIONS:

1. Known or suspected carcinoma of the prostate or the male breast.

2. Carcinoma of the breast in females with hypercalcemia (androgenic anabolic steroids may stimulate osteolytic bone resorption).

3. Pregnancy, because of the possible masculinization of the fetus. Oxandrolone has been shown to cause embryotoxicity, fetotoxicity, infertility, and masculinization of female animal offspring when given in doses 9 times the human dose.

4. Nephrosis or nephrotic phase of nephritis.

5. Hypercalcemia.

WARNINGS:

PELIOSIS HEPATITIS, A CONDITION IN WHICH LIVER AND SOMETIMES SPLENIC TISSUE IS REPLACED WITH BLOOD-FILLED CYSTS, HAS BEEN REPORTED IN PATIENTS RECEIVING ANDROGENIC ANABOLIC STEROID THERAPY. THESE CYSTS ARE SOMETIMES PRESENT WITH MINIMAL HEPATIC DYSFUNCTION, BUT AT OTHER TIMES THEY HAVE BEEN ASSOCIATED WITH LIVER FAILURE. THEY ARE OFTEN RECOGNIZED UNTIL LIFE-THREATENING LIVER FAILURE OR INTRA-ARTERIAL HEMORRHAGE DEVELOPS. WITHDRAWAL OF DRUG USUALLY RESULTS IN COMPLETE DISAPPEARANCE OF LESIONS.

LIVER CELL TUMORS ARE ALSO REPORTED. MOST OFTEN THESE TUMORS ARE BENIGN AND ANDROGEN-DEPENDENT, BUT FATAL MALIGNANT TUMORS HAVE BEEN REPORTED. WITHDRAWAL OF DRUG OFTEN RESULTS IN REGRESSION OR CESSATION OF PROGRESSION OF THE TUMOR. HOWEVER, HEPATIC TUMORS ASSOCIATED WITH ANDROGENS OR ANABOLIC STEROIDS ARE MUCH MORE VASCULAR THAN OTHER HEPATIC TUMORS AND MAY BE SILENT UNTIL LIFE- THREATENING INTRA-ABDOMINAL HEMORRHAGE DEVELOPS, BLOOD LIPID THAT ARE KNOWN TO BE ASSOCIATED WITH INCREASED RISK OF ATHEROSCLEROSIS ARE SEEN IN PATIENTS TREATED WITH ANDROGENS OR ANABOLIC STEROIDS. THESE CHANGES INCLUDE DECREASED HIGH-DENSITY LIPOPROTEINS AND SOMETIMES INCREASED LOW-DENSITY LIPOPROTEINS. THE CHANGES MAY BE VERY MARKED AND COULD HAVE A SERIOUS IMPACT ON THE RISK OF ATHEROSCLEROSIS AND CORONARY ARTERY DISEASE.

Cholestatic hepatitis and jaundice may occur with 17-alpha-alkylated androgens at a relatively low dose. If cholestatic hepatitis with jaundice appears or if liver function tests become abnormal, oxandrolone should be discontinued and the etiology should be determined. Drug-induced jaundice is reversible when the medication is discontinued.

In patients with breast cancer, anabolic steroid therapy may cause hypercalcemia by stimulating osteolysis. Oxandrolone therapy should be discontinued if hypercalcemia occurs.

WARNINGS: *(cont'd)*

Edema with or without congestive heart failure may be a serious complication in patients with preexisting cardiac, renal, or hepatic disease. Concomitant administration of adrenal cortical steroids or ACTH may increase the edema.

In children, androgen therapy may accelerate bone maturation without producing compensatory gain in linear growth. This adverse effect results in compromised adult height. The younger the child, the greater the risk of compromising final mature height. The effect on maturation should be monitored by assessing bone age of the left wrist and hand every six months. (See PRECAUTIONS, Laboratory Tests.)

Geriatric patients treated with androgenic anabolic steroids may be at an increased risk for the development of prostatic hypertrophy and prostatic carcinoma.

ANABOLIC STEROIDS HAVE NOT BEEN SHOWN TO ENHANCE ATHLETIC ABILITY.

PRECAUTIONS:

GENERAL

Women should be observed for signs of virilization (deepening of the voice, hirsutism, acne, clitoromegaly). Discontinuation of drug therapy at the time of evidence of mild virilism is necessary to prevent irreversible virilization. Some virilizing changes in women are irreversible even after prompt discontinuance of therapy and are not prevented by concomitant use of estrogens. Menstrual irregularities may also occur.

Anabolic steroids may cause suppression of clotting factors II, V, VII, and X, and an increase in prothrombin time.

INFORMATION FOR THE PATIENT

The physician should instruct patients to report any of the following side effects of androgens:

Males: Too frequent or persistent erections of the penis, appearance or aggravation of acne.

Females: Hoarseness, acne, changes in menstrual periods, or more facial hair.

All patients: Nausea, vomiting, changes in skin color, or ankle swelling.

LABORATORY TESTS

Women with disseminated breast carcinoma should have frequent determination of urine and serum calcium levels during the course of therapy (see WARNINGS).

Because of the hepatotoxicity associated with the use of 17-alpha-alkylated androgens, liver function tests should be obtained periodically.

Periodic (every 6 months) x-ray examinations of bone age should be made during treatment of children to determine the rate of bone maturation and the effects of androgen therapy on the epiphyseal centers.

Serum lipids and high-density lipoprotein cholesterol determinations should be done periodically as androgenic anabolic steroids have been reported to increase low-density lipoproteins and decrease high-density lipoproteins. Serum cholesterol levels may increase during therapy. Therefore, caution is required when administering these agents to patients with a history of myocardial infarction or coronary artery disease. Serial determinations of serum cholesterol should be made and therapy adjusted accordingly.

Hemoglobin and hematocrit should be checked periodically for polycythemia in patients who are receiving high doses of anabolic steroids.

DRUG/LABORATORY TEST INTERACTIONS

Anabolic steroids may decrease levels of thyroxine-binding globulin, resulting in decreased total T_4 serum levels and increased resin uptake of T_3 and T_4. Free thyroid hormone levels remain unchanged. In addition, a decrease in PBI and radioactive iodine uptake may occur.

CARCINOGENESIS, MUTAGENESIS, AND IMPAIRMENT OF FERTILITY

Animal data: Oxandrolone has not been tested in laboratory animals for carcinogenic or mutagenic effects. In two-year chronic oral rat studies, a dose related reduction of spermatogenesis and decreased organ weights (tests, prostate, seminal vesicles, ovaries, uterus, adrenals, and pituitary) were shown.

Human data: Liver cell tumors have been reported in patients receiving long-term therapy with androgenic anabolic steroids in high doses (see WARNINGS). Withdrawal of the drugs did not lead to regression of the tumors in all cases.

Geriatric patients treated with androgenic anabolic steroids may be at an increased risk for the development of prostatic hypertrophy and prostatic carcinoma.

PREGNANCY CATEGORY X

Teratogenic effects: See CONTRAINDICATIONS.

NURSING MOTHERS

It is not known whether anabolic steroids are excreted in human milk. Because of the potential for serious adverse reactions in nursing infants from oxandrolone, a decision should be made whether to discontinue nursing or to discontinue the drug, taking into account the importance of the drug to the mother.

PEDIATRIC USE

Anabolic agents may accelerate epiphyseal maturation more rapidly than linear growth in children and the effect may continue for six months after the drug has been stopped. Therefore, therapy should be monitored by x-ray studies at six-months intervals in order to avoid the risk of compromising adult height. Androgenic anabolic steroid therapy should be used very cautiously in children and only by specialists who are aware of the effect on bone maturation. (See WARNINGS.)

DRUG INTERACTIONS:

Anticoagulants: Anabolic steroids may increase sensitivity to oral anticoagulants. Dosage of the anticoagulant may have to be decreased in order to maintain desired prothrombin time. Patients receiving oral anticoagulant therapy require close monitoring, especially when anabolic steroids are started or stopped.

Oral hypoglycemic agents: Oxandrolone may inhibit the metabolism of oral hypoglycemic agents.

Adrenal steroids or ACTH: In patients with edema, concomitant administration with adrenal cortical steroids or ACT may increase the edema.

ADVERSE REACTIONS:

The following adverse reactions have been associated with use of anabolic steroids:

Hepatic: Cholestatic jaundice with, rarely, hepatic necrosis and death. Hepatocellular neoplasms and peliosis hepatitis with long term therapy (see WARNINGS). Reversible changes in liver function tests also occur including increased bromsulfophthalein (BSP) retention, and increases in serum bilirubin, aspartate aminotransferase (AST, SGOT), and alkaline phosphatase.

In Males: *Prepubertal:* Phallic enlargement and increased frequency or persistence of erections. *Postpubertal:* Inhibition of testicular function, testicular atrophy and oligospermia, impotence, chronic priapism, epididymitis, and bladder irritability.

In Females: Clitoral enlargement, menstrual irregularities.

ADVERSE REACTIONS: *(cont'd)*

CNS: Excitation, insomnia, depression, and changes in libido.

Gastrointestinal: Nausea, vomiting, diarrhea.

Hematologic: Bleeding in patients on concomitant anticoagulant therapy.

Breast: Gynecomastia.

Larynx: Deepening of the voice in females.

Hair: Hirsutism and male pattern baldness in females.

Skin: Acne (especially in females and prepubertal males).

Skeletal: Premature closure of epiphyses in children (see PRECAUTIONS, Pediatric Use).

Fluid and electrolytes: edema, retention of serum electrolytes (sodium chloride, potassium, phosphate, calcium).

Metabolic/Endocrine: Decreased glucose tolerance (see PRECAUTIONS), increased serum levels of low-density lipoproteins and decreased level of high-density lipoproteins (see PRECAUTIONS, Laboratory Tests), increased creatinine excretion, increased serum levels of creatinine phosphokinase (CPK). Masculinization of the fetus. Inhibition of gonadotropin secretion.

DRUG ABUSE AND DEPENDENCE:

Oxandrolone is classified as a controlled substance under the Anabolic Steroids Control Act of 1990 and has been assigned to Schedule III (non-narcotic).

OVERDOSAGE:

No symptoms or signs associated with overdosage have been reported. It is possible that sodium and water retention may occur..

The oral LD_{50} of oxandrolone in mice and dogs is greater then 5,000 mg/kg. No specific antidote is known, but gastric lavage may be used.

DOSAGE AND ADMINISTRATION:

Therapy with anabolic steroids is adjunctive to and not a replacement for conventional therapy. The duration of therapy with oxandrolone will depend on the response of the patient and the possible appearance of adverse reactions. Therapy should be intermittent.

Adults: The *usual adult*dosage of Oxandrin is one 2.5 mg tablet two to four times daily. However, the response of individuals to anabolic steroids varies, and a daily dosage of as little as 2.5 mg or as much as 20 mg may be required to achieve the desired response. A course of therapy of two to four weeks is usually adequate. This may be repeated from intermittently as indicated.

Children: For children the total *daily* dosage of oxandrolone is $\leq$ 0.1 mg per kilogram body weight or $\leq$ 0.045 mg per pound of body weight. This may be repeated intermittently as indicated.

HOW SUPPLIED:

Oxandrin 2.5-mg tablets are oval, white, and scored with BTG on one side and "11" on each side of the scoreline on the other side.

HOW SUPPLIED - EQUIVALENTS NOT AVAILABLE:

Tablet, Uncoated - Oral - 2.5 mg

100's $375.00 OXANDRIN, BTG Pharms 54396-0111-11

OXAPROZIN *(003140)*

CATEGORIES: Analgesics; Anti-Inflammatory Agents; Antiarthritics; Arthritis; Central Nervous System Agents; NSAIDS; Nonsteroidal Anti-Inflammatory; Osteoarthritis; Pain; FDA Class 1S ("Standard Review"); Sales > $100 Million; FDA Approved 1992 Oct; Patent Expiration 1997 Oct; Top 200 Drugs

BRAND NAMES: **Daypro**; *Deflam*; *Duraprox*
(International brand names outside U.S. in italics)

DESCRIPTION:

Daypro (oxaprozin) is a nonsteroidal anti-inflammatory drug (NSAID), chemically designated as 4,5-diphenyl-2-oxazole-propionic acid.

The empirical formula for oxaprozin is $C_{18}H_{15}NO_3$, and the molecular weight is 293. Oxaprozin is a white to off-white powder with a slight odor and a melting point of 162°C to 163°C. It is slightly soluble in alcohol and insoluble in water, with an octanol/water partition coefficient of 4.8 and physiologic pH (7.4). The pK_a in water is 4.3.

Daypro oral caplets contain 600 mg of oxaprozin.

Inactive ingredients in Daypro oral caplets are microcrystalline cellulose, hydroxypropyl methylcellulose, methylcellulose, magnesium stearate, polacrilin potassium, starch, polyethylene glycol, titanium dioxide.

CLINICAL PHARMACOLOGY:

Oxaprozin is a nonsteroidal anti-inflammatory drug (NSAID) that has been shown to have anti-inflammatory, analgesic, and antipyretic properties in animal models. As with other nonsteroidal anti-inflammatory agents, all of the modes of action of oxaprozin are not fully established. Oxaprozin is an inhibitor of several steps along the arachidonic acid pathway of prostaglandin synthesis, and one of its modes of action is presumed to be due to the inhibition of prostaglandin synthesis at the site of inflammation.

Pharmacodynamics: Acute analgesic effects are demonstrable in humans after a single 1200 mg dose of oxaprozin, but anti-inflammatory effects are not reliably achieved after a single dose. Because of the long half-life of oxaprozin, it takes several days of dosing to reach steady state (see Pharmacokinetics.)

Pharmacokinetics: The pharmacokinetics of oxaprozin have been evaluated in approximately 400 individuals which have included patients with rheumatoid arthritis, osteoarthritis, healthy elderly volunteers, and patients with cardiac, renal, and hepatic disease.

Oxaprozin demonstrates high oral bioavailability (95%), with peak plasma concentrations occurring between 3 and 5 hours after dosing. Food may reduce the rate of absorption of oxaprozin, but the extent of absorption is unchanged. Antacids have no effect on the rate or extent of oxaprozin absorption.

As is true for most NSAIDs, approximately 99.9% of the oxaprozin present in plasma is bound to albumin. The fraction of the drug present in the tissues across the therapeutic dosage range ranges between 40% and 60% of the total drug in the body and is proportional to dose, since the tissue sites are not saturated with the usual clinical doses.

(A graph showing "the amount of oxaprozin in the plasma and in the tissue as a function of dose and the concentration of the free drug" is available in the original manufacturer's package insert.)

CLINICAL PHARMACOLOGY: *(cont'd)*

Unbound oxaprozin is the pharmacologically active component; it is able to distribute into tissues and to be cleared from the body. The average unbound concentration is a function of the tissue-bound and plasma-bound drug, and it increases proportionally with dose.

As the amount of oxaprozin in the tissues increases at higher dose, the plasma concentration of oxaprozin is limited by saturation of plasma protein binding. In addition, the increase in free (unbound) oxaprozin results in an increase in clearance. Both of these contribute to the total plasma concentration of oxaprozin increasing less than proportionately with dose.

Oxaprozin kinetics were modeled using a two-compartment model with first-order absorption and protein binding that becomes saturable in the clinical dosage range. As the dose is increased from 600 to 1200 mg daily, the steady state clearance of total oxaprozin increases from 0.25 to 0.34 l/hr, the steady state apparent volume of distribution increases from 10 to 12.5 l, and the accumulation of half-life decreases from 25 to 21 hours. The terminal elimination half-life is approximately twice as long as the accumulation half-life because of the increased binding and decreased clearance at lower concentrations. Steady state concentrations in clinical usage are achieved in 4 to 7 days.

Plasma levels of total oxaprozin (free and bound drug) in studies of patients taking 600 to 1200 mg/day for several months ranged from 98 to 230 mcg/ml, corresponding to estimated levels of free drug ranging from about 0.10 to 0.40 mcg/ml.

Oxaprozin is primarily metabolized in the liver, by both microsomal oxidation (65%) and glucuronic acid conjugation (35%). A small amount (<5%) of active phenolic metabolites is produced, but the contribution to overall activity is minimal. All conjugated metabolites are inactive.

Biliary excretion of unchanged oxaprozin is a minor elimination pathway, and enteropathic recycling of oxaprozin is insignificant. The glucuronide metabolites can be recovered from the urine (65%) and feces (35%), while unchanged oxaprozin is poorly excreted.

Renal dysfunction appears to alter oxaprozin binding and to reduce unbound clearance and unbound volume of distribution; dosage reductions should be made (See PRECAUTIONS, General.)

Age, gender, and well-compensated cardiac failure do not affect the plasma protein binding or the pharmacokinetics of oxaprozin.

Like other NSAIDs exhibiting a degree of protein binding and had a primarily metabolic route of elimination, oxaprozin had the potential for drug-drug interactions (see DRUG INTERACTIONS.)

CLINICAL STUDIES:

Rheumatoid Arthritis: Daypro was evaluated for managing the signs and symptoms of rheumatoid arthritis in placebo and active controlled clinical trials in a total of 646 patients. Daypro was given in single or divided daily doses of 600 to 1800 mg/day and was found to be comparable to 2600 to 3900 mg/day of aspirin. At these doses there was a trend (over all trials) for oxaprozin to be more effective and cause fewer gastrointestinal side effects than aspirin.

Daypro was given as a once-a-day dose of 1200 mg in most of the clinical trials, but larger doses (up to 26 mg/kg or 1800 mg/day) were used in selected patients. In some patients, Daypro may be better tolerated in divided doses. Due to its long half-life, several days of Daypro therapy were needed for the drug to reach its full effect (See Individualization Of Dosage.)

Osteoarthritis: Daypro was evaluated for the management of the signs and symptoms of osteoarthritis in a total of 616 patients in active controlled clinical trials against aspirin (N=464), piroxicam (N=102), and other NSAIDs. Daypro was given both in variable (600 to 1200 mg/day) and in fixed (1200 mg/day) dosing schedules in either single or divided doses. In these trials, oxaprozin was found to be comparable to 2600 to 3200 mg/day doses of aspirin or 20 mg/day doses of piroxicam. Oxaprozin was effective both in once daily and in divided dosing schedules. In controlled clinical trials several days of oxaprozin therapy were needed for the drug to reach its full effects (see Individualization Of Dosage).

INDIVIDUALIZATION OF DOSAGE

Daypro, like other NSAIDs, shows considerable inter-individual differences in both pharmacokinetics and clinical response (pharmacodynamics). Therefore, the dosage for each patient should be individualized according to the patient's response to therapy.

The usual starting dose for most normal weight patients with rheumatoid arthritis is 1200 mg, once a day.

The usual starting dose for normal weight patients with mild to moderate osteoarthritis is 600 mg, once a day.

In cases where a quick onset of action is important, the pharmacokinetics of oxaprozin allow therapy to be started with a <u>one-time</u> loading dose of 1200 to 1800 mg (not to exceed 26 mg/kg).

Doses larger than 1200 mg/day should be reserved for patients who weigh more than 50 kg, have normal renal and hepatic function, are at low risk of peptic ulcer, and whose severity of disease justifies maximal therapy. Physicians should ensure that patients are tolerating doses in the 600 to 1200 mg/day range without gastroenterologic, renal hepatic, or dermatologic adverse effects before advancing to the larger doses.

The maximum recommended total daily dosage is 1800 mg in divided doses.

Most patients will tolerate once-a-day dosing with Daypro, although divided doses may be tried in patients unable to tolerate single doses. As with all drugs of this class, the frequency and severity of adverse events will depend on the dose of the drug, the age and physical condition of the patient, any concurrent medical diagnoses, individual vulnerability, and the duration of therapy. In clinical trials of oxaprozin, no clear dose-response relationship was seen for serious adverse effects, but physicians are cautioned that the reported safety data were developed in patients who had successfully taken lower doses of Daypro before being advanced above 1200 mg/day.

Experience with other NSAIDs has shown that starting therapy with maximal doses in patients at increased risk due to renal or hepatic disease, low body weight, advanced age, a known ulcer diathesis, or known sensitivity to NSAID effects is likely to increase the frequency of adverse events and is not recommended (see PRECAUTIONS.)

INDICATIONS AND USAGE:

Daypro is indicated for acute and long-term use in the management of the signs and symptoms of osteoarthritis and rheumatoid arthritis.

CONTRAINDICATIONS:

Daypro should not be used in patients with previously demonstrated hypersensitivity to oxaprozin or any of its components or in individuals with the complete or partial syndrome of nasal polyps, angioedema, and bronchospastic reactivity to aspirin or other nonsteroidal anti- inflammatory drugs (NSAIDs).

Severe and occasionally fatal asthmatic and anaphylactic reactions have been reported in patients receiving NSAIDs, and there have been rare reports of anaphylaxis in patients taking oxaprozin.

WARNINGS:

Risk Of Gastrointestinal (Gi) Ulceration, Bleeding, And Perforation With Nonsteroidal Anti-Inflammatory Drug Therapy: Serious gastrointestinal toxicity, such as bleeding, ulceration, and perforation, can occur at any time, with or without warning symptoms, in patients treated with NSAIDs. Although minor upper gastrointestinal problems, such as dyspepsia, are common, and usually develop early in therapy, physicians should remain alert for ulceration and bleeding in patients treated chronically NSAIDs, even in the absence of previous GI tract symptoms. In patients observed in clinical trials for several months to 2 years, symptomatic upper GI ulcers, gross bleeding, or perforation appear to occur in approximately 1% of patients treated for 3 to 6 months, and in about 2% to 4% of patients treated for 1 year. Physicians should inform patients about the signs and symptoms of serious GI toxicity and what steps to take if they occur.

Patients at risk for developing peptic ulceration and bleeding are those with a prior history of serious GI events, alcoholism, smoking, or other factors known to be associated with peptic ulcer disease. Elderly or debilitated patients seem to tolerate ulceration or bleeding less well than other individuals, and most spontaneous reports of fatal GI events are in these populations. Studies to date are inconclusive concerning the relative risk of various nonsteroidal anti-inflammatory drugs (NSAIDs) in causing such reactions. High doses of any NSAID probably carry a greater risk of these reactions, and substantial benefit should be anticipated to patients prior to prescribing maximal doses of Daypro.

PRECAUTIONS:

GENERAL

Hepatic Effects: As with other nonsteroidal anti- inflammatory drugs, borderline elevations of one or more liver tests may occur in up to 15% of patients. These abnormalities may progress, remain essentially unchanged, or resolve with continued therapy. The SGPT (ALT) test is probably the most sensitive indicator of liver dysfunction. Meaningful (3 times the upper limit of normal) elevations of SGOT (AST) occurred in controlled clinical trials of Daypro (oxaprozin) in just under 1% of patients. A patient with symptoms and/or signs suggesting liver dysfunction or in whom an abnormal liver test has occurred should be evaluated for evidence of the development of more severe hepatic reaction while on therapy with this drug. Severe hepatic reactions including jaundice have been reported with Daypro, and there may be a risk of fatal hepatitis with oxaprozin, such as those seen with other NSAIDs. Although such reactions are rare, if abnormal liver tests persist or worsen, clinical signs and symptoms consistent with liver disease develop, or systemic manifestations occur (eosinophilia, rash, fever), Daypro should be discontinued.

Well-compensated hepatic cirrhosis does not appear to alter the disposition of unbound oxaprozin, so dosage adjustment is not necessary. However, the primary route of elimination of oxaprozin is hepatic metabolism, so caution should be observed in patients with severe hepatic dysfunction.

Renal Effects: Acute interstitial nephritis, hematuria, and proteinuria have been reported with Daypro as with some other NSAIDs. Long-term administration of some nonsteroidal anti-inflammatory drugs to animals has resulted in renal papillary necrosis and other abnormal renal pathology. This was not observed with oxaprozin, but the clinical significance of this difference is unknown.

A second form of renal toxicity has been seen in patients with preexisting conditions leading to a reduction in renal blood flow, where the renal prostaglandins have a supportive role in the maintenance of renal perfusion. In these patients administration of a nonsteroidal anti-inflammatory drug may cause a dose-dependent reduction in prostaglandin formation and may precipitate overt renal decompensation. Patients at the greatest risk of this reaction are those with previously impaired renal function, heart failure, or liver dysfunction, those taking diuretics, and the elderly. Discontinuation of nonsteroidal anti-inflammatory drug therapy is often followed by recovery to the pretreatment state. Those patients at high risk should have renal function monitored if they have signs or symptoms that may be consistent with mild azotemia, such as malaise, fatigue, or loss of appetite. As with all NSAID therapy, patients may occasionally develop some elevation of serum creatinine and BUN levels without any signs or symptoms.

The pharmacokinetic of oxaprozin may be significantly altered in patients with renal insufficiency or in patients who are undergoing hemodialysis. Such patients should be started on doses of 600 mg/day, with cautious dosage increases if the desired effect is not obtained. Oxaprozin is not dialyzed because of its high degree of protein binding.

Like other NSAIDs, Daypro may worsen fluid retention by the kidneys in patients with uncompensated cardiac failure due to its effect on prostaglandins. It should be used with caution in patients with a history of hypertension, cardiac decompensation, in patients on chronic diuretic therapy, or in those with other conditions predisposing to fluid retention.

Photosensitivity: Oxaprozin has been associated with rash and/or mild photosensitivity in dermatologic testing. An increased incidence of rash on sun-exposed skin was seen in some patients in the clinical trials.

Recommended Laboratory Testing: Because serious GI tract ulceration and bleeding can occur without warning symptoms, physicians should follow chronically treated patients for signs and symptoms of ulceration and bleeding and should inform them of the importance of follow-up (see WARNINGS.)

Anemia may occur in patients receiving oxaprozin or other NSAIDs. This may be due to fluid retention, gastrointestinal blood loss, or an incompletely described effect upon erythrogenesis. Patients on long-term treatment with Daypro should have their hemoglobin or hemocrit values determined at appropriate intervals as determined by the clinical situation.

Oxaprozin, like other NSAIDs, can affect platelet aggregation and prolong bleeding time. Daypro should be used with caution in patients with underlying hemostatic defects or in those who are undergoing surgical procedures where a high degree of hemostasis is needed.

INFORMATION FOR THE PATIENT

Daypro, like other drugs of its class, nonsteroidal anti-inflammatory drugs (NSAIDs), is not free of side effects. The side effects of these drugs can cause discomfort and, rarely, serious side effects, such as gastrointestinal bleeding, which may result in hospitalization and even fatal outcomes.

NSAIDS are often essential agents in the management of arthritis, but they may also be commonly employed for conditions that are less serious.

Physicians may wish to discuss with their patients the potential risks (see WARNINGS, PRECAUTIONS, and ADVERSE REACTIONS) and likely benefits of Daypro treatment, particularly in less-serious conditions where treatment without Daypro may represent an acceptable alternative to both the patient and the physician.

Patients receiving Daypro may benefit from physician instruction in the symptoms of the more common or serious gastrointestinal, renal, hepatic, hematologic, and dermatologic adverse effects.

LABORATORY TEST INTERACTIONS

False positive urine drug screening tests for benzodiazepines have been reported in patients taking Daypro. This is due to cross-reactivity. Confirmatory testing is recommended when such screening test results are positive.

PRECAUTIONS: *(cont'd)*

CARCINOGENESIS, MUTAGENESIS, AND IMPAIRMENT OF FERTILITY

In oncogenicity studies, oxaprozin administration for 2 years was associated with the exacerbation of liver neoplasms (hepatic adenomas and carcinomas) in male CD mice, but not in females CD mice or rats. The significance of this species-specific finding to man is unknown.

Oxaprozin did not display mutagenic potential. Results from the Ames test, forward mutation in yeast and chinese hamster ovary (CHO) cells, DNA repair testing in CHO cells, micronucleus testing in mouse bone marrow, chromosomal aberration testing in human lymphocytes, and cell transformation testing in mouse fibroblast all showed no evidence of genetic toxicity or cell-transforming ability.

Oxaprozin administration was not associated with impairment of fertility in male and female rats at oral doses up to 200 mg/kg/day (1180 mg/m^2); the usual human dose is 17 mg/kg/day (629 mg/m^2). However, testicular degeneration was observed in beagle dogs treated with 37.5 to 150 mg/kg/day (750 to 3000 mg/m^2) of oxaprozin for 6 months, or 37.5 mg/kg/day for 42 days, a finding not confirmed in other species. The clinical relevance of this finding is not known.

PREGNANCY, TERATOGENIC EFFECTS, PREGNANCY CATEGORY C

There are no adequate and well-controlled studies in pregnant women. Teratology studies with oxaprozin were performed in mice, rats, and rabbits. In mice and rats, no drug-related developmental abnormalities were observed at 50 to 200 mg/kg/day of oxaprozin (225 to 900 mg/m^2). However, in rabbits, infrequent malformed fetuses were observed in dams treated with 7.5 to 30 mg/kg/day of oxaprozin (the usual human dosage range). Oxaprozin should be used during pregnancy only if the potential benefits justify the potential risks to the fetus.

LABOR AND DELIVERY

The effect of oxaprozin in pregnant women is unknown. NSAIDs are known to delay parturition, to accelerate closure of the fetal ductus arteriosus, and to be associated with dystocia. Oxaprozin is known to have caused decreases in pup survival in rat studies. Accordingly, the use of oxaprozin during late pregnancy should be avoided.

NURSING MOTHERS

Studies of oxaprozin excretion in human milk have not been conducted; however, oxaprozin was found in the milk of lactating rats. Since the effects of oxaprozin on infants are not known, caution should be exercised if oxaprozin is administered to nursing women.

PEDIATRIC USE

Safety and effectiveness of Daypro in children have not been established.

GERIATRIC USE

No adjustment of the dose of Daypro is necessary in the elderly for *pharmacokinetic* reasons, although many elderly may need to receive a reduced dose because of low body weight or disorders associated with aging. No significant differences in the pharmacokinetic profile for oxaprozin were seen in studies in the healthy elderly.

Although selected elderly patients in controlled clinical trials tolerated Daypro as well as younger patients, caution should be exercised in treating the elderly, and extra care should be taken when choosing a dose. As with any NSAID, the elderly are likely to tolerate adverse reactions less well than younger patients.

DRUG INTERACTIONS:

Aspirin: Concomitant administration of Daypro and aspirin is not recommended because oxaprozin displaces salicylates from plasma protein binding sites to a much greater extent than salicylates displace oxaprozin. Coadministration would be expected to increase the risk of salicylate toxicity.

Oral Anticoagulants: The anticoagulant effects of warfarin were not affected by the coadministration of 1200 mg/day of Daypro. Nevertheless, caution should be exercised when adding any drug that affects platelet function to the regimen of patients receiving oral anticoagulants.

H_2-receptor antagonists: The total body clearance of oxaprozin was reduced by 20% in subjects who concurrently received therapeutic doses of cimetidine or ranitidine; no other pharmacokinetic parameter was affected. A change of clearance of this magnitude lies within the range of normal variation and is unlikely to produce a clinically detectable difference in the outcome of therapy.

Beta-blockers: Subjects receiving 1200 mg Daypro qd with 100 mg metoprolol bid exhibited statistically significant but transient increases in sitting and standing blood pressures after 14 days. Therefore, as with all NSAIDs, routine blood pressure monitoring should be considered in these patients when starting Daypro therapy.

Other drugs: The coadministration of oxaprozin and antacids, acetaminophen, or conjugated estrogens resulted in no statistically significant changes in pharmacokinetic parameters in single- and/or multiple-dose studies. The interaction of oxaprozin with lithium and cardiac glycosides has not been studied.

ADVERSE REACTIONS:

Adverse reaction data were derived from patients who received Daypro in multidose, controlled, and open-label clinical trials, and from foreign marketing experience. Rates for events occurring in more than 1% of patients, and for most of the less common events, are based on 2253 patients who took 1200 to 1800 mg Daypro per day in clinical trials. Of these, 1721 were treated for at least 1 month, 971 for at least 3 months, and 366 for more than 1 year. Rates for the rarer events and for events reported from foreign marketing experience are difficult to estimate accurately and are only listed as less than 1%.

The adverse event rates below refer to the incidence in the first month of use. Most of the events were seen by this time for common adverse reactions. However, the cumulative incidence can be expected to rise with continued therapy, and some events, such as gastrointestinal bleeding (see WARNINGS), seem to occur at a constant or possibly increasing rate over time.

The most frequently reported adverse reactions were related to the gastrointestinal tract. They were nausea (8%) and dyspepsia (8%).

INCIDENCE GREATER THAN 1%

In clinical trials the following adverse reactions occurred at an incidence greater than 1% and are probably related to treatment. Reactions occurring in 3% to 9% of patients treated with Daypro are indicated by an asterisk (*); those reactions occurring in less than 3% of patients are unmarked.

Digestive system: abdominal pain/distress, anorexia, constipation*, diarrhea*, dyspepsia*, flatulence, nausea*, vomiting.

Nervous system: CNS inhibition (depression, sedation, somnolence, or confusion), disturbance of sleep.

Skin and appendages: rash*.

Special senses: tinnitus.

Urogenital system: dysuria or frequency.

ADVERSE REACTIONS: *(cont'd)*

INCIDENCE LESS THAN 1%

Probable causal relationship: The following adverse reactions were reported in clinical trials at an incidence of less than 1% or were reported from foreign experience. Those reactions reported only from foreign marketing experience are in *italics*. The probability of causal relationship exists between the drug and these adverse reactions.

Body as a whole: anaphylaxis.

Cardiovascular system: edema, blood pressure changes.

Digestive system: peptic ulceration and/or GI bleeding (see WARNINGS), liver function abnormalities including hepatitis (see PRECAUTIONS), stomatitis, hemorrhoidal or rectal bleeding.

Hematologic system: anemia, thrombocytopenia, leukopenia, ecchymoses.

Metabolic system: weight gain, weight loss.

Nervous system: weakness, malaise.

Respiratory system: symptoms of upper respiratory tract infection.

Skin: pruritus, urticaria, photosensitivity, *exfoliative dermatitis, erythema multiforme, Stevens-Johnson syndrome, toxic epidermal necrolysis (Lyell's syndrome).*

Special senses: blurred vision, conjunctivitis.

Urogenital: *acute interstitial nephritis*, hematuria, renal insufficiency, decreased menstrual flow.

Causal relationship unknown: The following adverse reactions occurred at an incidence of less than 1% in clinical trials, or were suggested from marketing experience, under circumstances where a causal relationship could not be definitely established. They are listed as alerting information for the physician.

Cardiovascular system: palpitations.

Digestive system: alteration in taste.

Respiratory system: sinusitis, pulmonary infections.

Skin and appendages: alopecia.

Special Senses: hearing decrease.

Urogenital system: increase in menstrual flow.

DRUG ABUSE AND DEPENDENCE:

Daypro is a non-narcotic drug. Usually reliable animal studies have indicated that Daypro has no known addiction potential in humans.

OVERDOSAGE:

No patient experienced either an accidental or intentional overdosage of Daypro in the clinical trials of the drug. Symptoms following acute overdosage with other NSAIDs are usually limited to lethargy, drowsiness, nausea, vomiting, and epigastric pain and are generally reversible with supportive care. Gastrointestinal bleeding and coma have occurred following NSAID overdose. Hypertension, acute renal failure, and respiratory depression are rare.

Patients should be managed by symptomatic and supportive care following and NSAID overdose. There are no specific antidotes. Gut decontamination may be indicated in patients seen within 4 hours of ingestion with symptoms or following a large overdose (5 to 10 times the usual dose). This should be accomplished via emesis and/or activated charcoal (60 to 100 g in adults, 1 to 2 g/kg in children) with an osmotic cathartic. Forced diuresis, alkalization of the urine, or hemoperfusion would probably not be useful due to the high degree of protein binding of oxaprozin.

DOSAGE AND ADMINISTRATION:

Rheumatoid Arthritis: The usual daily dose of Daypro in the management of the signs and symptoms of rheumatoid arthritis is 1200 mg (two 600 mg caplets) once a day. Both smaller and larger doses may be required in individual patients (see Individualization Of Dosage.)

Osteoarthritis: The usual daily dose of Daypro for the management of the signs and symptoms of moderate to severe osteoarthritis is 1200 mg (two 600 mg caplets) once a day. For patients of low body weight or with milder disease, an initial dosage of one 600 mg caplet once a day may be appropriate (see Individualization Of Dosage.)

Regardless of the indication, the dosage should be individualized to the lowest effective dose of Daypro to minimize adverse effects, and the maximum recommended total daily dose is 1800 mg (or 26 mg/kg, whichever is lower) in divided doses.

Safety And Handling: Daypro is supplied as a solid dosage form in closed containers, it is not known to produce contact dermatitis, and poses no known risk to healthcare workers. It may be disposed of in accordance with applicable local regulations governing the disposal of pharmaceuticals.

PATIENT INFORMATION:

Oxaprozin is a nonsteroidal anti-inflammatory agent used to treat the signs and symptoms of osteoarthritis and rheumatoid arthritis. Oxaprozin decreases pain and inflammation. If you are sensitive to aspirin or other nonsteroidal anti-inflammatory agents, you may be sensitive to oxaprozin. This drug, and others related to it, can cause ulcers in those with a history of ulcers or those sensitive to these drugs. Oxaprozin may cause sensitivity to light. Use appropriate skin protection (clothing or sunscreen) when in the sun. Nausea and heartburn are the most commonly reported effects. These can be minimized by taking the medication with food.

HOW SUPPLIED:

Daypro 600-mg caplets are white, capsule-shaped, scored, film-coated, with DAYPRO debossed on one side and 1381 on the other side.

Keep bottles tightly closed and store below 86°F (30°C). Disclose in a tight, light-resistant container with a child resistant closure. Protect the unit dose from light.

HOW SUPPLIED - EQUIVALENTS NOT AVAILABLE:

Tablet, Uncoated - Oral - 600 mg

100's	$121.17	DAYPRO, Searle	00025-1381-31
100's	$124.81	DAYPRO, Searle	00025-1381-34

OXAZEPAM *(001926)*

CATEGORIES: Alcohol Withdrawal; Alcoholism; Analgesics; Antianxiety Drugs; Anxiety; Anxiolytics, Sedatives, Hypnotic; Benzodiazepines; Central Nervous System Agents; Tension; Tranquilizers; Insomnia*; DEA Class CIV; FDA Approval Pre 1982

* Indication not approved by the FDA

BRAND NAMES: *Adumbran* (Germany); *Alepam* (Australia); *Alopam*; *Anxiolit*; *Anxiolit Retard*; *Apo-Oxazepam* (Canada); *Azutranquil* (Germany); *Benzotran*; *Durazepam* (Germany); *Enidrel*; *Hilong* (Japan); *Medopam*; *Murelax* (Australia); *Nesontil*; *Noctazepam* (Germany); *Novoxapam* (Canada); *Opamox*; *Oxaline*; *Oxa-Puren* (Germany); *Oxepam*; *Ox-Pam*; *Praxiten* (Germany); *Primizum* (Japan); *Propax* (Japan); *Proxam*; *Psiquiwas*; *Purata*; *Quilibrex*; **Serax**; *Serepax* (Australia); *Seresta* (France); *Sigacalm* (Germany); *Sobile*; *Sobril*; *Vaben*; *Wakazepam* (Japan); *Wakezepam*; *Zapex* (Canada)
(International brand names outside U.S. in italics)

FORMULARIES: Aetna; BC-BS

COST OF THERAPY: $20.26 (Anxiety; Capsule; 10 mg; 3/day; 120 days)

DESCRIPTION:

Oxazepam is the first of a chemically new series of compounds, the 3-hydroxybenzodiazepinones. A new therapeutic agent providing versatility and flexibility in control of common emotional disturbances, this product exerts prompt action in a wide variety of disorders associated with anxiety, tension, agitation, and irritability, and anxiety associated with depression. In tolerance and toxicity studies on several animal species, this product reveals significantly greater safety factors than related compounds (chlordiazepoxide and diazepam) and manifests a wide separation of effective doses and doses inducing side effects.

Oxazepam capsules contain 10 mg, 15 mg, or 30 mg oxazepam.

The inactive ingredients present in Serax are gelatin, lactose, titanium dioxide, and other ingredients. Each dosage strength also contains the following: 10 mg—D&C Red 22, D&C Red 28, and FD&C Blue 1; 15 mg—FD&C Red 40 and FD&C Yellow 6; 30 mg—D&C Red 28, FD&C Red 40, and FD&C Blue 1.

Oxazepam tablets contain 15 mg oxazepam. The inactive ingredients present in Serax are FD&C Yellow 5, lactose, magnesium stearate, methylcellulose, and polacrilin potassium.

Oxazepam is 7 chloro-1,3-dihydro-3-hydroxy-5-phenyl-2*H*-1,4-benzodiazepin-2-one. A white crystalline powder with a molecular weight of 286.7.

CLINICAL PHARMACOLOGY:

Pharmacokinetic testing in twelve volunteers demonstrated that when given as a single 30 mg dose, the capsule, tablet, and suspension were equivalent in extent of absorption. For the capsule and tablet, peak plasma levels averaged 450 ng/ml and were observed to occur about 3 hours after dosing. The mean elimination half-life for oxazepam was approximately 8.2 hours (range 5.7 to 10.9 hours).

This product has a single, major inactive metabolite in man, a glucuronide excreted in the urine.

ANIMAL PHARMACOLOGY AND TOXICOLOGY

In mice, Oxazepam exerts an anticonvulsant (anti-Metrazol) activity at 50-percent-effective doses of about 0.6 mg/kg orally. (Such anticonvulsant activity of benzodiazepines correlates with their tranquilizing properties.) To produce ataxia (rotabar test) and sedation (abolition of spontaneous motor activity), the 50-percent-effective doses of this product are greater than 5 mg/kg orally. Thus, about ten times the therapeutic (anticonvulsant) dose must be given before ataxia ensues, indicating a wide separation of effective doses and doses inducing side effects.

In evaluation of antianxiety activity of compounds, conflict behavioral tests in rats differentiate continuous response for food in the presence of anxiety-provoking stress (shock) from drug-induced motor incoordination. This product shows significant separation of doses required to relieve anxiety and doses producing sedation or ataxia. Ataxia-producing doses exceed those of related CNS-acting drugs.

Acute oral LD_{50} in mice is greater than 5000 mg/kg, compared to 800 mg/kg for a related compound (chlordiazepoxide).

Subacute toxicity studies in dogs for four weeks at 480 mg/kg daily showed no specific changes; at 960 mg/kg two out of eight died with evidence of circulatory collapse. This wide margin of safety is significant compared to chlordiazepoxide HCl, which showed nonspecific changes in six dogs at 80 mg/kg. On chlordiazepoxide, two out of six died with evidence of circulatory collapse at 127 mg/kg, and six out of six died at 200 mg/kg daily. Chronic toxicity studies of Oxazepam in dogs at 120 mg/kg/day for 52 weeks produced no toxic manifestation.

Fatty metamorphosis of the liver has been noted in six-week toxicity studies in rats given this product at 0.5% of the diet. Such accumulations of fat are considered reversible, as there is no liver necrosis or fibrosis.

Breeding studies in rats through two successive litters did not produce fetal abnormality.

Oxazepam has not been adequately evaluated for mutagenic activity.

In a carcinogenicity study, Oxazepam was administered with diet to rats for two years. Male rats receiving 30 times the maximum human dose showed a statistical increase, when compared to controls, in benign thyroid follicular cell tumors, testicular interstitial cell adenomas, and prostatic adenomas. An earlier published study reported that mice fed dietary dosages of 35 or 100 times the human daily dose of Oxazepam for 9 months developed a dose-related increase in liver adenomas.[1] In an independent analysis of some of the microscopic slides from this mouse study several of these tumors were classified as liver carcinomas. At this time, there is no evidence that clinical use of Oxazepam is associated with tumors.

INDICATIONS AND USAGE:

Oxazepam is indicated for the management of anxiety disorders or for the short-term relief of the symptoms of anxiety. Anxiety or tension associated with the stress of everyday life usually does not require treatment with an anxiolytic.

Anxiety associated with depression is also responsive to Oxazepam therapy.

This product has been found particularly useful in the management of anxiety, tension, agitation, and irritability in older patients.

Alcoholics with acute tremulousness, inebriation, or with anxiety associated with alcohol withdrawal are responsive to therapy.

The effectiveness of Oxazepam in long-term use, that is, more than 4 months, has not been assessed by systematic clinical studies. The physician should periodically reassess the usefulness of the drug for the individual patient.

CONTRAINDICATIONS:

History of previous hypersensitivity reaction to Oxazepam. Oxazepam is not indicated in psychoses.

WARNINGS:

As with other CNS-acting drugs, patients should be cautioned against driving automobiles or operating dangerous machinery until it is known that they do not become drowsy or dizzy on Oxazepam therapy.

WARNINGS: *(cont'd)*

Patients should be warned that the effects of alcohol or other CNS-depressant drugs may be additive to those of Oxazepam, possibly requiring adjustment of dosage or elimination of such agents.

Physical And Psychological Dependence: Withdrawal symptoms, similar in character to those noted with barbiturates and alcohol (convulsions, tremor, abdominal and muscle cramps, vomiting, and sweating), have occurred following abrupt discontinuance of Oxazepam. The more severe withdrawal symptoms have usually been limited to those patients who received excessive doses over an extended period of time. Generally milder withdrawal symptoms (*e.g.,* dysphoria and insomnia) have been reported following abrupt discontinuance of benzodiazepines taken continuously at therapeutic levels for several months. Consequently, after extended therapy, abrupt discontinuation should generally be avoided and a gradual dosage-tapering schedule followed. Addiction-prone individuals (such as drug addicts or alcoholics) should be under careful surveillance when receiving Oxazepam or other psychotropic agents because of the predisposition of such patients to habituation and dependence.

Use In Pregnancy: An increased risk of congenital malformations associated with the use of minor tranquilizers (chlordiazepoxide, diazepam, and meprobamate) during the first trimester of pregnancy has been suggested in several studies. Oxazepam, a benzodiazepine derivative, has not been studied adequately to determine whether it, too, may be associated with an increased risk of fetal abnormality. Because use of these drugs is rarely a matter of urgency, their use during this period should almost always be avoided. The possibility that a woman of childbearing potential may be pregnant at the time of institution of therapy should be considered. Patients should be advised that if they become pregnant during therapy or intend to become pregnant they should communicate with their physician about the desirability of discontinuing the drug.

PRECAUTIONS:

Although hypotension has occurred only rarely, Oxazepam should be administered with caution to patients in whom a drop in blood pressure might lead to cardiac complications. This is particularly true in the elderly patient.

Oxazepam 15 mg tablets, *but none of the other available dosage forms of this product,* contain FD&C Yellow 5 (tartrazine) which may cause allergic-type reactions (including bronchial asthma) in certain susceptible individuals. Although the overall incidence of FD&C Yellow 5 (tartrazine) sensitivity in the general population is low, it is frequently seen in patients who also have aspirin hypersensitivity.

Information for the Patient: To assure the safe and effective use of Oxazepam, patients should be informed that, since benzodiazepines may produce psychological and physical dependence, it is advisable that they consult with their physician before either increasing the dose or abruptly discontinuing this drug.

ADVERSE REACTIONS:

The necessity for discontinuation of therapy due to undesirable effects has been rare. Transient, mild drowsiness is commonly seen in the first few days of therapy. If it persists, the dosage should be reduced. In few instances, dizziness, vertigo, headache, and rarely syncope have occurred either alone or together with drowsiness. Mild paradoxical reactions, i.e., excitement, stimulation of affect, have been reported in psychiatric patients; these reactions may be secondary to relief of anxiety and usually appear in the first two weeks of therapy.

Other side effects occurring during Oxazepam therapy include rare instances of minor diffuse skin rashes—morbilliform, urticarial, and maculopapular—nausea, lethargy, edema, slurred speech, tremor, and altered libido. Such side effects have been infrequent and are generally controlled with reduction of dosage.

Although rare, leukopenia and hepatic dysfunction including jaundice have been reported during therapy. Periodic blood counts and liver-function tests are advisable.

Ataxia with Oxazepam has been reported in rare instances and does not appear to be specifically related to dose or age.

Although the following side reactions have not as yet been reported with Oxazepam, they have occurred with related compounds (chlordiazepoxide and diazepam): paradoxical excitation with severe rage reactions, hallucinations, menstrual irregularities, change in EEG pattern, blood dyscrasias including agranulocytosis, blurred vision, diplopia, incontinence, stupor, disorientation, fever, and euphoria.

Transient amnesia or memory impairment has been reported in association with the use of benzodiazepines.

DOSAGE AND ADMINISTRATION:

Because of the flexibility of this product and the range of emotional disturbances responsive to it, dosage should be individualized for maximum beneficial effects (TABLE 1):

TABLE 1

Usual Dose	
Mild-to-moderate anxiety, with associated tension, irritability, agitation, or related symptoms of functional origin or secondary to organic disease.	10 to 15 mg, 3 or 4 times daily
Severe anxiety syndromes, agitation, or anxiety associated with depression.	15 to 30 mg, 3 or 4 times daily
Older patients with anxiety, tension, irritability, and agitation.	Initial dosage: 10 mg, 3 times daily. If necessary, increase cautiously to 15 mg, 3 or 4 times daily.
Alcoholics with acute inebriation, tremulousness, or anxiety on withdrawal.	15 to 30 mg, 3 or 4 times daily.

This product is not indicated in children under 6 years of age. Absolute dosage for children 6 to 12 years of age is not established.

HOW SUPPLIED:

Serax (oxazepam) Capsules and Tablets are available in the following dosage strengths:

10 mg,white and pink capsule banded with Wyeth logo and marked "SERAX", "10", and "51".

15 mg, white and red capsule banded with Wyeth logo and marked "SERAX", "15", and "6".

30 mg, white and maroon capsule banded with Wyeth logo and marked "SERAX", "30", and "52".

15 mg, yellow, five-sided tablet with a raised "S" and a "15" on one side and "WYETH" and "317" on reverse side.

Store at room temperature, approx. 25° C (77° F).

Keep tightly closed.

Dispense in tight container.

REFERENCES:

1. FOX, K.A.; LAHCEN, R.B.: Liver-cell Adenomas and Peliosis Hepatis in Mice Associated with Oxazepam. Res. Commun. Chem. Pathol. Pharmacol. *8*:481-488, 1974.

HOW SUPPLIED - RATED THERAPEUTICALLY EQUIVALENT:

Capsule, Gelatin - Oral - 10 mg

25's	$1.40	Oxazepam, H.C.F.A. F F P	99999-1926-01
100's	$5.63	Oxazepam, H.C.F.A. F F P	99999-1926-02
100's	$6.03	Oxazepam, United Res	00677-1181-01
100's	$21.13	Oxazepam, Bristol Myers Squibb	00003-0574-50
100's	$22.20	Oxazepam, Qualitest Pharms	00603-4950-21
100's	$23.25	Oxazepam, Rugby	00536-4879-01
100's	$23.34	Oxazepam, HL Moore Drug Exch	00839-7501-06
100's	$23.39	Oxazepam, Purepac Pharm	00228-2067-10
100's	$24.92	Oxazepam, Caremark	00339-4023-12
100's	$25.94	Oxazepam, Aligen Independ	00405-0132-01
100's	$26.00	Oxazepam, Zenith Labs	00172-4804-60
100's	$26.00	Oxazepam, Goldline Labs	00182-1230-01
100's	$26.00	Oxazepam, Parmed Pharms	00349-8865-01
100's	$26.10	Oxazepam, Major Pharms	00904-1890-60
100's	$26.25	Oxazepam, Martec Pharms	52555-0233-01
100's	$27.16	Oxazepam, Vangard Labs	00615-0409-13
100's	$28.50	Oxazepam, Geneva Pharms	00781-2809-01
100's	$28.51	Oxazepam, Warner Chilcott	00047-0690-24
100's	$28.51	Oxazepam, Schein Pharm (US)	00364-2154-01
100's	**$55.20**	**SERAX, Wyeth Labs**	**00008-0051-07**
100's	**$70.48**	**SERAX, Wyeth Labs**	**00008-0051-02**
500's	$28.15	Oxazepam, H.C.F.A. F F P	99999-1926-03
500's	$65.70	Oxazepam, Elkins Sinn	00641-4508-88
500's	$73.10	Oxazepam, Major Pharms	00904-1890-40
500's	$101.59	Oxazepam, Purepac Pharm	00228-2067-50
500's	$111.15	Oxazepam, Zenith Labs	00172-4804-70
500's	$117.00	Oxazepam, Aligen Independ	00405-0132-02
500's	**$331.73**	**SERAX, Wyeth Labs**	**00008-0051-03**

Capsule, Gelatin - Oral - 15 mg

25's	$1.76	Oxazepam, H.C.F.A. F F P	99999-1926-04
100's	$7.05	Oxazepam, H.C.F.A. F F P	99999-1926-05
100's	$7.50	Oxazepam, United Res	00677-1182-01
100's	$27.40	Oxazepam, Bristol Myers Squibb	00003-0599-50
100's	$29.46	Oxazepam, Purepac Pharm	00228-2069-10
100's	$30.86	Oxazepam, Vangard Labs	00615-0410-13
100's	$32.00	Oxazepam, Zenith Labs	00172-4805-60
100's	$32.00	Oxazepam, Goldline Labs	00182-1231-01
100's	$32.10	Oxazepam, Martec Pharms	52555-0234-01
100's	$32.18	Oxazepam, Caremark	00339-4025-12
100's	$32.70	Oxazepam, Aligen Independ	00405-0133-01
100's	$33.51	Oxazepam, Qualitest Pharms	00603-4951-21
100's	$33.90	Oxazepam, Major Pharms	00904-1891-60
100's	$34.16	Oxazepam, HL Moore Drug Exch	00839-7502-06
100's	$34.28	Oxazepam, Rugby	00536-4877-01
100's	$36.33	Oxazepam, Warner Chilcott	00047-0665-24
100's	$36.33	Oxazepam, Parmed Pharms	00349-8866-01
100's	$36.33	Oxazepam, Geneva Pharms	00781-2810-01
100's	$36.75	Oxazepam, Schein Pharm (US)	00364-2152-01
100's	**$69.11**	**SERAX, Wyeth Labs**	**00008-0006-10**
100's	**$88.59**	**SERAX, Wyeth Labs**	**00008-0006-02**
500's	$35.25	Oxazepam, H.C.F.A. F F P	99999-1926-06
500's	$85.45	Oxazepam, Elkins Sinn	00641-4509-88
500's	$130.75	Oxazepam, Bristol Myers Squibb	00003-0599-60
500's	$139.79	Oxazepam, Purepac Pharm	00228-2069-50
500's	$146.90	Oxazepam, Zenith Labs	00172-4805-70
500's	$146.90	Oxazepam, Major Pharms	00904-1891-40
500's	$147.50	Oxazepam, Aligen Independ	00405-0133-02
500's	$159.69	Oxazepam, HL Moore Drug Exch	00839-7502-12
500's	$164.10	Oxazepam, Rugby	00536-4877-05
500's	$178.99	Oxazepam, Geneva Pharms	00781-2810-05
500's	$179.00	Oxazepam, Parmed Pharms	00349-8866-05
500's	**$422.60**	**SERAX, Wyeth Labs**	**00008-0006-04**

Capsule, Gelatin - Oral - 30 mg

25's	$2.28	Oxazepam, H.C.F.A. F F P	99999-1926-07
100's	$9.15	Oxazepam, H.C.F.A. F F P	99999-1926-08
100's	$9.75	Oxazepam, United Res	00677-1183-01
100's	$39.85	Oxazepam, Major Pharms	00904-1982-60
100's	$41.17	Oxazepam, Purepac Pharm	00228-2073-10
100's	$41.25	Oxazepam, Zenith Labs	00172-4806-60
100's	$41.25	Oxazepam, Goldline Labs	00182-1232-01
100's	$41.35	Oxazepam, Bristol Myers Squibb	00003-0159-50
100's	$42.05	Oxazepam, Martec Pharms	52555-0235-01
100's	$42.14	Oxazepam, Caremark	00339-4027-12
100's	$42.78	Oxazepam, HL Moore Drug Exch	00839-7503-06
100's	$43.11	Oxazepam, Qualitest Pharms	00603-4952-21
100's	$43.42	Oxazepam, Aligen Independ	00405-0134-01
100's	$43.56	Oxazepam, Rugby	00536-4878-01
100's	$43.90	Oxazepam, Major Pharms	00904-1892-60
100's	$47.05	Oxazepam, Vangard Labs	00615-0411-13
100's	$48.99	Oxazepam, Geneva Pharms	00781-2811-01
100's	$49.00	Oxazepam, Warner Chilcott	00047-0667-24
100's	$49.00	Oxazepam, Parmed Pharms	00349-8867-01
100's	$49.01	Oxazepam, Schein Pharm (US)	00364-2153-01
100's	**$98.65**	**SERAX, Wyeth Labs**	**00008-0052-09**
100's	**$128.14**	**SERAX, Wyeth Labs**	**00008-0052-02**
500's	$45.75	Oxazepam, H.C.F.A. F F P	99999-1926-09
500's	$130.60	Oxazepam, Elkins Sinn	00641-4510-88
500's	$189.20	Oxazepam, Major Pharms	00904-1982-40
500's	$195.94	Oxazepam, Zenith Labs	00172-4806-70
500's	$205.83	Oxazepam, Purepac Pharm	00228-2073-50
500's	**$621.10**	**SERAX, Wyeth Labs**	**00008-0052-04**

Tablet, Uncoated - Oral - 15 mg

100's	$26.45	Oxazepam 15, Major Pharms	00904-1894-60
100's	**$88.59**	**SERAX, Wyeth Labs**	**00008-0317-01**

OXICONAZOLE NITRATE *(001927)*

CATEGORIES: Anti-Infectives; Antifungals; Dermatologicals; Fungal Agents; Infections; Skin Infections; Skin/Mucous Membrane Agents; Tinea Corporis; Tinea Cruris; Tinea Pedis; Topical; Pregnancy Category B; FDA Approved 1988 Dec

BRAND NAMES: *Myfungar* (Germany, Mexico); *Oceral*; *Oceral GB* (Germany); **Oxistat**
(International brand names outside U.S. in italics)

FORMULARIES: Aetna; BC-BS; Medi-Cal

DESCRIPTION:

Potency expressed as oxiconazole.

For Topical Dermatologic Use Only - Not for Ophthalmic or Intravaginal Use.

Oxistat Cream and lotion formulations contain the antifungal active compound oxiconazole nitrate.

Chemically, oxiconazole nitrate is 2',4'-dichloro-2-imidazol-1-ylacetophenone (*Z*)-[0-(2,4-dichlorobenzyl) oxime], mononitrate, with the empirical formula:
$C_{18}H_{13}CL_4N_3{\cdot}HNO_3$, and
a molecular weight of 492.15.

Oxiconazole nitrate is a nearly white crystalline powder, soluble in methanol; sparingly soluble in ethanol, chloroform, and acetone; and very slightly soluble in water.

Oxistat Cream contains 10 mg/g of oxiconazole as oxiconazole nitrate in a white to off-white, opaque cream base of purified water USP, white petrolatum USP, stearyl alcohol NF, propylene glycol USP, polysorbate 60 NF, cetyl alcohol NF, and benzoic acid USP 0.2% as a preservative.

Oxistat Lotion contains 10 mg of oxiconazole/g of lotion in white to off- white, opaque lotion base of purified water USP, white petrolatum USP, stearyl alcohol NF, propylene glycol USP, polysorbate 60 NF, cetyl alcohol NF, and benzoic acid USP 0.2% as a preservative.

CLINICAL PHARMACOLOGY:

Five hours after application of 2.5 mg/cm² of oxiconazole nitrate cream onto human skin, the concentration of oxiconazole nitrate was demonstrated to be 16.2 µmol in the epidermis, 3.64 µmol in the upper corium, and 1.29 µmol in the deeper corium. Systemic absorption of oxiconazole nitrate appears to be low. Less than 0.3% of the applied dose of oxiconazole nitrate was recovered in the urine of volunteer subjects up to 5 days after application of the cream formulation.

Neither *in vitro* or *in vivo* studies have been conducted to establish relative activity between the lotion and cream formulations.

Microbiology: Oxiconazole nitrate is an imidazole derivative whose antifungal activity is derived primarily from the inhibition or ergosterol biosynthesis, which is critical for cellular membrane integrity. It has *in vitro* activity against a wide range of pathogenic fungi.

Oxiconazole has been shown to be active against most strains of the following organisms both *in vitro* and in clinical infections at indicated body sites: (See INDICATIONS AND USAGE.)

Epidermophyton floccosum
Trichophyton mentagrophytes
Trichophyton rubrum

The following *in vitro* data are available;*however, their clinical significance is unknown.* Oxiconazole exhibits satisfactory *in vitro*MIC's against most strains of the following organisms; however, the safety and efficacy of oxiconazole in treating clinical infections due to these organisms have not been established in adequate and well-controlled clinical trials:

Candida albicans
Malassezia Furfur
Microsporum audouini
Microsporum canis
Microsporum gypseum
Trichophyton tonsurans
Trichophyton violaceum

CLINICAL STUDIES:

Tinea Pedis Studies: The following definitions were applied to the clinical and microbiological outcomes in patients enrolled in the clinical trials that form the basis for the approvals of Oxistat Lotion and Oxistat Cream.

THERE ARE NO HEAD-TO-HEAD COMPARISON TRIALS OF THE OXISTAT CREAM AND LOTION FORMULATIONS IN THE TREATMENT OF TINEA PEDIS.

Definitions

1. Clinical Improvement: Greater than 50% improvement in the clinically signs and symptoms above the baseline assessment.

2. Clinical Cure: Greater than 90% improvement in the clinical signs and symptoms above the baseline assessment.

3. Mycological Cure: No evidence (culture and KOH preparation) of the baseline (original) pathogen in a specimen from the affected area taken at the 2-week post-treatment visit.

4. Overall Cure: Both a clinical cure (see above) and a microbiologic eradication (see above) at the 2-week post-treatment visit.

Lotion Formulation: The clinical trial for the lotion formulation line extension involved 332 evaluable patients with clinically and microbiologically established tinea pedis. Of these evaluable patients, 64% were diagnosed with hyperkeratotic plantar tinea pedis and 28% with interdigital tinea pedis. Seventy-seven had disease secondary to infection with *T. rubrum*, 18% had disease secondary to infection with *T. Mentagrophytes*, and 4% had disease secondary to infection with *E. floccosum*.

The results of this clinical trial at the 2-week post-treatment follow-up visit are shown in TABLE 1.

TABLE 1

Patient Outcome Category	**Oxistat Lotion b.i.d.**	**Oxistat Lotion q.d.**	**Vehicle**
Clinical Improvement	82%	80%	50%
Clinical Cure	52%	43%	18%
Mycological Cure	67%	64%	28%
Overall Cure	41%	34%	10%

In this study, the improvement and cure rates of the b.i.d.- and q.d.-treated groups did not differ significantly (95% confidence interval) from each other bit were statistically (95% confidence interval) superior to the vehicle-treated group.

Cream Formulation: The two pivotal trials for the cream formulation involved 281 evaluable patients (total from both trials) with clinically and microbiologically established tinea pedis.

The combined results of these two clinical trials at the 2-week post-treatment follow-up visit are shown in TABLE 2.

All the improvement and cure rates of the b.i.d.- and q.d.- treated groups did not differ significantly (95% confidence interval) from each other but were statistically (95% confidence interval) superior to the vehicle-treated group.

TABLE 2			
Patient Outcome Category	Oxistat Cream b.i.d	q.d.	Vehicle
Clinical Improvement	84%	83%	49%
Mycological Cure	77%	79%	33%
Overall Cure	52%	43%	14%

INDICATIONS AND USAGE:

Oxistat Cream and Lotion are indicated for the topical treatment of the following dermal infections: tinea pedis, tinea cruris, and tinea corporis due to *Trichophyton rubrum, Trichophyton mentagrophytes,* or *Epidermophyton floccosum.* (See DOSAGE AND ADMINISTRATION and CLINICAL STUDIES.)

CONTRAINDICATIONS:

Oxistat Cream and Lotion are contraindicated in individuals who have shown hypersensitivity to any of their components.

WARNINGS:

Oxistat Cream and Lotion is not for ophthalmic or intravaginal use.

PRECAUTIONS:

General: If a reaction suggesting sensitivity or chemical irritation should occur with the use of Oxistat Cream or Lotion, treatment should be discontinued and appropriate therapy instituted. Oxistat Cream and Lotion are for external dermal use only. Avoid introduction of Oxistat Cream or Lotion into the eyes or vagina.

Carcinogenesis, Mutagenesis, and Impairment of Fertility: Although no long-term studies in animals have been performed to evaluate carcinogenic potential, no evidence of mutagenic effect was found in two mutation assays (Ames test and Chinese hamster V79 *in vitro* cell mutation assay) or in two cytogenetic assays (human peripheral blood lymphocyte *in vitro* chromosome aberration assay and *in vivo* micronucleus assay in mice).

Reproductive studies revealed no impairment of fertility in rats at oral doses of 3 mg/kg per day in females (one time the human dose based on mg/m^2) and 15 mg/kg per day in males (four times the human dose based on mg/m^2). However, at doses above this level, the following effects were observed: a reduction in the fertility parameters of males and females, a reduction in the number of sperm in vaginal smears, extended estrous cycle, and a decrease in mating frequency.

Pregnancy, Teratogenic Effects, Pregnancy Category B: Reproduction studies have been performed in rabbits, rats, and mice at oral doses up to 100, 150, and 200 mg/kg per day (57, 40, and 27 times the human dose based on mg/m^2), respectively, and revealed no evidence of harm to the fetus due to oxiconazole nitrate. There are, however, no adequate and well-controlled studies in pregnant women. Because animal reproduction studies are not always predictive of human response, this drug should be used during pregnancy only if clearly needed.

Nursing Mothers: Since oxiconazole is excreted in human milk, caution should be exercised when the drug is administered to a nursing woman.

ADVERSE REACTIONS:

(Numbers in this section include patients treated both once daily and twice daily combined)

During clinical trials, 41 (4.3%) of 955 patients treated with oxiconazole nitrate 1% cream, reported adverse reactions thought to be related to drug therapy. These reactions included pruritus (1.6%), burning (1.4%), irritation and allergic contact dermatitis (0.4% each), folliculitis (0.3%), erythema (0.2%); and papules, fissuring, maceration, rash, stinging, and nodules (0.1% each).

In a controlled, multicenter clinical trial, 7 (2.6%) of 269 patients treated with oxiconazole nitrate lotion, 1%, reported adverse reactions thought to be related to drug therapy. These reactions included burning and stinging (0.7% each) and pruritus, scaling, tingling, pain, and dyshidrotic eczema (0.4% each).

OVERDOSAGE:

When a 5% oxiconazole cream was applied at a rate of 1 g/kg to approximately 10% of body surface area of a group of 40 male and female rats for 35 days, 3 deaths and severe dermal inflammation were reported.

DOSAGE AND ADMINISTRATION:

Oxistat Cream or Lotion should be applied to cover affected and immediately surrounding areas once to twice daily in patients with tinea pedis, tinea corporis, or tinea cruris. Tinea corporis and tinea cruris should be treated for 2 weeks and tinea pedis for 1 month to reduce the possibility of recurrence. If a patient shows no clinical improvement after the treatment period, the diagnosis should be reviewed.

HOW SUPPLIED:

Store between 15° and 30°C (59° and 86°F).

HOW SUPPLIED - EQUIVALENTS NOT AVAILABLE:

Cream - Topical - 1 %

15 gm	**$14.38**	**OXISAT, Glaxo Wellcome**	**00173-0423-00**
30 gm	**$24.00**	**OXISTAT, Glaxo Wellcome**	**00173-0423-01**
60 gm	**$35.41**	**OXISTAT, Glaxo Wellcome**	**00173-0423-04**

Lotion - Topical - 1 %

30 ml	**$24.00**	**OXISTAT, Glaxo Wellcome**	**00173-0448-01**

OXTRIPHYLLINE *(001929)*

CATEGORIES: Airway Obstruction; Antiasthmatics/Bronchodilators; Asthma; Bronchial Dilators; Bronchitis; Bronchospasm; Chronic Bronchitis; Emphysema; Respiratory & Allergy Medications; Respiratory Muscle Relaxant; Smooth Muscle Relaxants; Xanthine Derivatives; Pregnancy Category C; FDA Approval Pre 1982

BRAND NAMES: *Apo Oxtriphyllin* (Canada); *Brondecon*; *Brondecon-PD*; *Cholecyl*; **Choledyl**; *Choledyl Pediatrico*; *Choledyl Retard*; Cholegyl; *Euspirax* (Germany); *Euspirax Forte* (Germany); *Euspirax Retard* (Germany); *Theocolin* (Japan)
(International brand names outside U.S. in italics)

FORMULARIES: Medi-Cal

COST OF THERAPY: $316.12 (Asthma; Tablet; 200 mg; 3/day; 365 days)

PRIMARY ICD9: 493.90 (Asthma, Unspecified, Without Mention of Status Asthmaticus)

DESCRIPTION:

Note: The information in this monograph pertains to Oxtriphylline delayed-release and sustained-action tablets.

Oxtriphylline delayed-release tablets contain oxtriphylline which is the choline salt of theophylline. Theophylline is a bronchodilator structurally classified as a xanthine derivative. It occurs as a white, odorless, crystalline powder having a bitter taste. Theophylline anhydrous has the chemical name 1*H*-Purine-2, 6-dione, 3,7-dihydro-1,3-dimethyl-.

The molecular formula is $C_{12}H_{21}N_5O_3$. The molecular weight is 283.33.

Oxtriphylline tablets are available as enteric, sugar-coated tablets intended for oral administration, containing 100 mg or 200 mg oxtriphylline (64 mg and 127 mg of theophylline anhydrous, respectively). Each tablet also contains acacia, NF; precipitated calcium carbonate, USP; tribasic calcium phosphate, NF; carnauba wax; confectioner's sugar, NF; gelatin, NF; kaolin, USP; magnesium stearate, NF; pharmaceutical glaze; starch, NF; sucrose, NF; talc, USP; titanium dioxide, USP; tragacanth, NF; and white wax, NF. The 100-mg tablet also contains D&C red No. 7 Lake and FD&C yellow No. 6 Lake. The 200-mg tablet also contains D&C yellow No. 10.

Each film-coated Oxtriphylline sustained-action tablet contains 400 mg or 600 mg Oxtriphylline (equivalent to 254 mg or 383 mg anhydrous theophylline, respectively). Each tablet also contains: candelilla wax; confectioner's sugar, NF; magnesium stearate, NF; Opaseal pharmaceutical sealant; talc, USP; and other ingredients. The 400-mg tablet also contains Opaspray pink and triethyl citrate. The 600-mg tablet also contains Opaspray tan.

Each sustained-action tablet contains Oxtriphylline in a tablet matrix specially designed for the prolonged release of the drug in the gastrointestinal tract. Following the release of the drug, the expended wax tablet matrix, which is not absorbed, may be detected in the stool.

CLINICAL PHARMACOLOGY:

Theophylline directly relaxes the smooth muscle of the bronchial airways and pulmonary blood vessels, thus acting mainly as a bronchodilator and smooth muscle relaxant. It has also been demonstrated that aminophylline has a potent effect on diaphragmatic contractility in normal persons and may then be capable of reducing fatigability and thereby improve contractility in patients with chronic obstructive airways disease. The exact mode of action remains unsettled. Although theophylline does cause inhibition of phosphodiesterase with a resultant increase in intracellular cyclic AMP, other agents similarly inhibit the enzyme producing a rise of cyclic AMP but are unassociated with any demonstrable bronchodilation. Other mechanisms proposed include an effect on translocation of intracellular calcium; prostaglandin antagonism; stimulation of catecholamines endogenously; inhibition of cyclic guanosine monophosphate metabolism and adenosine receptor antagonism. None of these mechanisms has been proved, however.

In vitro, theophylline has been shown to act synergistically with beta agonists, and there are now available data which do demonstrate an additive effect in vivo with combined use.

PHARMACOKINETICS

The half-life of theophylline is influenced by a number of known variables. It may be prolonged in chronic alcoholics, particularly those with liver disease (cirrhosis or alcoholic liver disease), in patients with congestive heart failure, and in those patients taking certain other drugs (see DRUG INTERACTIONS.) Newborns and neonates have extremely slow clearance rates compared to older infants and children, i.e., those over 1 year. Older children have rapid clearance rates while most nonsmoking adults have clearance rates between these two extremes. In premature neonates, the decreased clearance is related to oxidative pathways that have yet to be established (TABLE 1):

TABLE 1 Theophylline Elimination Characteristics	Half-Life (in hours)	
	Range	Mean
Children	1-9	3.7
Adults	3-15	7.7

In cigarette smokers (1-2 packs/day) the mean half-life is 4-5 hours, much shorter than in nonsmokers. The increase in clearance associated with smoking is presumably due to stimulation of the hepatic metabolic pathway by components of cigarette smoke. The duration of this effect after cessation of smoking is unknown but may require 6 months to 2 years before the rate approaches that of the nonsmoker.

Additional information for sustained-action tablets: Film coated tablets are less irritating to the gastric mucosa than aminophylline.

Oxtriphylline sustained-action tablets have been formulated to provide therapeutic serum levels when administered every 12 hours and minimize the peaks and valleys of serum levels commonly found with shorter acting theophylline products.

The sustained action characteristic of Oxtriphylline sustained-action has been demonstrated in studies in human subjects. Single and multiple dose studies have shown equivalent steady-state theophylline plasma levels of sustained-action tablets given every 12 hours when compared with an equal total daily dose of (the nonsustained action) Oxtriphylline elixir given every six hours.

INDICATIONS AND USAGE:

Oxtriphylline is indicated for relief and/or prevention of symptoms from asthma and reversible bronchospasm associated with chronic bronchitis and emphysema.

CONTRAINDICATIONS:

Oxtriphylline is contraindicated in individuals who have shown hypersensitivity to its components. It is also contraindicated in patients with active peptic ulcer disease, and in individuals with underlying seizure disorders (unless receiving appropriate anticonvulsant medication).

WARNINGS:

Serum levels above 20 mcg/ml are rarely found after appropriate administration of the recommended doses. However, in individuals in whom theophylline plasma clearance is reduced *for any reason*, even conventional doses may result in increased serum levels and potential toxicity. Reduced theophylline clearance has been documented in the following readily identifiable groups: 1) patients with impaired liver function; 2) patients over 55 years of age, particularly males and those with chronic lung disease; 3) those with cardiac failure from any cause; 4) patients with sustained high fever; 5) neonates and infants under 1 year of age; and 6) those patients taking certain drugs (see DRUG INTERACTIONS). Frequently, such patients have markedly prolonged theophylline serum levels following discontinuation of the drug.

Reduction of dosage and laboratory monitoring is especially appropriate in the above individuals.

Serious side effects such as ventricular arrhythmias, convulsions or even death may appear as the first sign of toxicity without any previous warning. Less serious signs of theophylline toxicity (*i.e.,* nausea and restlessness) may occur frequently when initiating therapy, but are usually transient; when such signs are persistent during maintenance therapy, they are often

WARNINGS: *(cont'd)*

associated with serum concentrations above 20 mcg/ml. Stated differently; *serious toxicity is not reliably preceded by less severe side effects.* A serum concentration measurement is the only reliable method of predicting potentially life-threatening toxicity.

Many patients who require theophylline exhibit tachycardia due to their underlying disease process so that the cause/effect relationship to elevated serum theophylline concentrations may not be appreciated.

Theophylline products may cause dysrhythmia and/or worsen preexisting arrhythmias and any significant change in rate and/or rhythm warrants monitoring and further investigation.

Studies in laboratory animals (minipigs, rodents, and dogs) recorded the occurrence of cardiac arrhythmias and sudden death (with histologic evidence of myocardial necrosis) when beta-agonists and methylxanthines were administered concurrently. The significance of these findings when applied to humans is currently unknown.

PRECAUTIONS:

GENERAL

On the average, theophylline half-life is shorter in cigarette and marijuana smokers than in nonsmokers, but smokers can have half-lives as long as nonsmokers. Theophylline should not be administered concurrently with other xanthines. Use with caution in patients with hypoxemia, hypertension, or those with history of peptic ulcer. Theophylline may occasionally act as a local irritant to the GI tract although gastrointestinal symptoms are more commonly centrally mediated and associated with serum drug concentrations over 20 mcg/ml.

Information for the Patient: Tablets should not be chewed, or crushed or dissolved.

The importance of taking only the prescribed dose and time interval between doses should be reinforced.

LABORATORY TESTS

Serum levels should be monitored periodically to determine the theophylline level associated with observed clinical response and as the method of predicting toxicity. For such measurements, the serum sample should be obtained at the time of peak concentration, 1 to 2 hours after administration for immediate release products. It is important that the patient will not have missed or taken additional doses during the previous 48 hours and that dosing intervals will have been reasonably equally spaced. DOSAGE ADJUSTMENT BASED ON SERUM THEOPHYLLINE MEASUREMENTS WHEN THESE INSTRUCTIONS HAVE NOT BEEN FOLLOWED MAY RESULT IN RECOMMENDATIONS THAT PRESENT RISK OF TOXICITY TO THE PATIENT.

DRUG-LABORATORY TEST INTERACTIONS

Currently available analytical methods, including high pressure liquid chromatography and immunoassay techniques, for measuring serum theophylline levels are specific. Metabolites and other drugs generally do not affect the results. Other new analytic methods are also now in use. The physician should be aware of the laboratory method used and whether other drugs will interfere with the assay for theophylline.

CARCINOGENESIS, MUTAGENESIS, AND IMPAIRMENT OF FERTILITY

Long-term carcinogenicity studies have not been performed with theophylline.

Chromosome-breaking activity was detected in human cell cultures at concentrations of theophylline up to 50 times the therapeutic serum concentration in humans. Theophylline was not mutagenic in the dominant lethal assay in male mice given theophylline intraperitoneally in doses up to 30 times the maximum daily oral dose.

Studies to determine the effect on fertility have not been performed with theophylline.

PREGNANCY

Category C - Animal reproduction studies have not been conducted with oxtriphylline. It is not known whether theophylline can cause fetal harm when administered to a pregnant woman or can affect reproduction capacity. Oxtriphylline should be given to a pregnant woman only if clearly needed.

NURSING MOTHERS

Theophylline is distributed into breast milk and may cause irritability or other signs of toxicity in nursing infants. Because of the potential for serious adverse reactions in nursing infants from theophylline, a decision should be made whether to discontinue nursing or to discontinue the drug, taking into account the importance of the drug to the mother.

PEDIATRIC USE

Sufficient numbers of infants under the age of 1 year have not been studied in clinical trials to support use in this age group; however, there is evidence recorded that the use of dosage recommendations for older infants and young children (16 mg/kg/24 hours) may result in the development of toxic serum levels. Such findings very probably reflect differences in the metabolic handling of the drug related to absent or undeveloped enzyme systems. Consequently, the use of the drug in this age group should carefully consider the associated benefits and risks. If used, the maintenance dose must be conservative and in accord with the following guidelines:

INITIAL THEOPHYLLINE MAINTENANCE DOSAGE

Premature Infants:

Up to 24 days postnatal age -1 mg/kg q 12h

Beyond 24 days postnatal age -1.5 mg/kg q 12h

Infants 6 to 52 Weeks:

((0.2 X age in weeks)+5)X kg body wt=24 hour dose in mg.

Up to 26 weeks, divide into q 8h dosing intervals.

From 26-52 weeks, divide into q 6h dosing intervals.

Final dosage should be guided by serum concentration after a steady state no further accumulation of drug) has been achieved.

DRUG INTERACTIONS:

Toxic synergism with ephedrine has been documented and may occur with other sympathomimetic bronchodilators. In addition, the following drug interactions have been demonstrated (TABLE 2):

TABLE 2

Theopylline with	
Allopurinol (high-dose)	Increased serum theophylline levels
Cimetidine	Increased serum theophylline levels
Erythromycin, Troleandomycin	Increased serum theophylline levels
Lithium Carbonate	Increased renal excretion of lithium
Oral Contraceptives	Increased serum theophylline levels
Phenytoin	Decreased theophylline and phenytoin serum levels
Rifampin	Decreased serum theophylline levels

ADVERSE REACTIONS:

The following adverse reactions have been observed, but there has not been enough systematic collection of data to support an estimate of their frequency. The most consistent adverse reactions are usually due to overdosage.

1. Gastrointestinal: nausea, vomiting, epigastric pain, hematemesis, diarrhea.

2. Central nervous system: headaches, irritability, restlessness, insomnia, reflex hyperexcitability, muscle twitching, clonic and tonic generalized convulsions.

3. Cardiovascular: palpitation, tachycardia, extrasystoles, flushing, hypotension, circulatory failure, ventricular arrhythmias.

4. Respiratory: tachypnea.

5. Renal: potentiation of diuresis.

6. Others: alopecia, hyperglycemia, inappropriate ADH syndrome, rash.

OVERDOSAGE:

MANAGEMENT

It is suggested that the management principles (consistent with the clinical status of the patient when first seen) outlined below be instituted and that simultaneous contact with a Regional Poison Control Center be established. In this way both updated information and individualization regarding required therapy may be provided.

When potential oral overdose is established and seizure has not occurred:

a. If patient is alert and seen within the early hours after ingestion, induction of emesis may be of value. Gastric lavage has been demonstrated to be of no value in influencing outcome in patients who present more than 1 hour after ingestion.

b. Administer a cathartic. Sorbitol solution is reported to be of value.

c. Administer repeated doses of activated charcoal and monitor theophylline serum levels.

d. Prophylactic administration of phenobarbital has been shown to increase the seizure threshold in laboratory animals, and administration of this drug can be considered.

If patient presents with a seizure:

a. Establish an airway.

b. Administer oxygen.

c. Treat the seizure with intravenous diazepam, 0.1 to 0.3 mg/kg up to 10 mg. If seizures cannot be controlled, the use of general anesthesia should be considered.

d. Monitor vital signs, maintain blood pressure and provide adequate hydration.

If postseizure coma is present:

a. Maintain airway and oxygenation.

b. If a result of oral medication, follow above recommendations to prevent absorption of the drug, but intubation and lavage will have to be performed instead of inducing emesis, and the cathartic and charcoal will need to be introduced via large bore gastric lavage tube.

c. Continue to provide full supportive care and adequate hydration until the drug is metabolized. In general, drug metabolism is sufficiently rapid so as not to warrant dialysis. If repeated oral activated charcoal is ineffective (as noted by stable or rising serum levels), charcoal hemoperfusion may be indicated.

DOSAGE AND ADMINISTRATION:

Tablets should not be chewed, or crushed or dissolved.

Effective use of theophylline (*i.e.,* the concentration of drug in the serum associated with optimal benefit and minimal risk of toxicity) is considered to occur when the theophylline concentration is maintained from 10 to 20 mcg/ml. The early studies from which these levels were derived were carried out in patients immediately or shortly after recovery from acute exacerbations of their disease (some hospitalized with status asthmaticus).

Although the 20 mcg/ml level remains appropriate as a critical value (above which toxicity is more likely to occur) for safety purposes, additional data are now available which indicate that the serum theophylline concentrations required to produce maximum physiologic benefit may, in fact, fluctuate with the degree of bronchospasm present and are variable. Therefore, the physician should individualize the range appropriate to the patient's requirements, based on both symptomatic response and improvement in pulmonary function. It should be stressed that serum theophylline concentrations maintained at the upper level of the 10 to 20 mcg/ml range may be associated with potential toxicity when factors known to reduce theophylline clearance are operative. (See WARNINGS.)

If it is not possible to obtain serum level determinations, restriction of the daily dose (in otherwise healthy adults) to not greater than 13 mg/kg/day (of anhydrous theophylline), to a maximum of 900 mg, in divided doses will result in relatively few patients exceeding serum levels of 20 mcg/ml and the resultant greater risk of toxicity.

Caution should be exercised for younger children who cannot complain of minor side effects. Older adults, those with cor pulmonale, congestive heart failure, and/or liver disease may have unusually low dosage requirements and thus may experience toxicity at the maximal dosage recommended below.

Theophylline does not distribute into fatty tissue. Dosage should be calculated on the basis of lean (ideal) body weight where mg/kg doses are presented.

FREQUENCY OF DOSING

When immediate release products with rapid absorption are used, dosing to maintain serum levels generally requires administration every 6 hours. This is particularly true in children, but dosing intervals up to 8 hours may be satisfactory in adults since they eliminate the drug at a slower rate. Some children and adults requiring higher than average doses (those having rapid rates of clearance, e.g., half-lives of under 6 hours) may benefit and be more effectively controlled during chronic therapy when given products with sustained-release characteristics since these provide longer dosing intervals and/or less fluctuation in serum concentration between dosing.

Dosage guidelines are approximations only, and the wide range of theophylline clearance between individuals (particularly those with concomitant disease) makes indiscriminate usage hazardous.

DOSAGE GUIDELINES

The following dosage information relates to initiation and titration of daily dosage requirements utilizing a nonsustained action form of Oxtriphylline (*e.g.,* Oxtriphylline Tabs, Elixir).

Acute Symptoms of Bronchospasm Requiring Rapid Attainment of Theophylline Serum Levels for Bronchodilation.

NOTE: Status asthmaticus should be considered a medical emergency and is defined as that degree of bronchospasm which is not rapidly responsive to usual doses of conventional bronchodilators. Optimal therapy for such patients frequently requires both *additional medication,* parenterally administered, and *close monitoring,* preferably in an intensive care setting.

Patients not currently receiving theophylline products (TABLE 3):

Patients currently receiving theophylline products:

Determine, where possible, the time, amount, dosage form, and route of administration of the last dose the patient received.

DOSAGE AND ADMINISTRATION: *(cont'd)*

TABLE 3 Oxtriphylline Dosage

	Oral Loading	Maintenance
Children age 1 to 9 years	7.8 mg/kg *(5 mg/kg)	6.2 mg/kg q 6 hours *(4 mg/kg q 6 hours)
Children age 9 to 16 years and smokers	7.8 mg/kg *(5 mg/kg)	4.7 mg/kg q 6 hours *(3 mg/kg q 6 hours)
Otherwise healthy nonsmoking adults	7.8 mg/kg *(5 mg/kg)	4.7 mg/kg q 8 hours *(3 mg/kg q 8 hours)
Older patients and patients with cor pulmonale	7.8 mg/kg *(5 mg/kg)	3.1 mg/kg q 8 hours *(2 mg/kg q 8 hours)
Patients with congestive heart failure	7.8 mg/kg *(5 mg/kg)	1.6-3.1 mg/kg q 12 hours *(1-2 mg/kg q 12 hours)

* Anhydrous theophylline included in ().

The loading dose for theophylline will be based on the principle that each 0.8 mg/kg oxtriphylline (equivalent to 0.5 mg/kg of theophylline) administered as a loading dose will result in a 1 mcg/ml increase in serum theophylline concentration. Ideally, the loading dose should be deferred if a serum theophylline concentration can be obtained rapidly.

If this is not possible, the clinician must exercise judgment in selecting a dose based on the potential for benefit and risk. When there is sufficient respiratory distress to warrant a small risk, then 4 mg/kg of oxtriphylline (equivalent to 2.5 mg/kg of theophylline) administered in rapidly absorbed form is likely to increase the serum concentration by approximately 5 mcg/ml. If the patient is not experiencing theophylline toxicity, this is unlikely to result in dangerous adverse effects.

Subsequent to the decision regarding use of a loading dose for this group of patients, the maintenance dosage recommendations are the same as those described above.

Chronic Therapy

Theophylline is a treatment for the management of reversible bronchospasm (asthma, chronic bronchitis and emphysema) to prevent symptoms and maintain patent airways. A dosage form which allows small incremental doses is desirable for initiating therapy. A liquid preparation should be considered for children to permit both greater ease of and more accurate dosage adjustment. Slow clinical titration is generally preferred to assure acceptance and safety of the medication, and to allow the patient to develop tolerance to transient caffeine-like side effects.

Initial Dose: 25 mg*/kg/24 hours or 625 mg/24 hours (whichever is less) of oxtriphylline in divided doses at 6- or 8-hour intervals.

*25 mg oxtriphylline = 16 mg anhydrous theophylline.

Increasing Dose: The above dosage may be increased in approximately 25-percent increments at 3-day intervals as long as the drug is tolerated; until clinical response is satisfactory or the maximum dose as indicated in section III (below) is reached. The serum concentration may be checked at these intervals, but at a minimum, should be determined at the end of this adjustment period.

It is important that no patient be maintained on any dosage that is not tolerated. When instructing patients to increase dosage according to the schedule above, they should be told not to take a subsequent dose if apparent side effects occur and to resume therapy at a lower dose once adverse effects have disappeared.

Maximum Dose of Oxtriphylline Where the Serum Concentration Is Not Measured

DO NOT ATTEMPT TO MAINTAIN ANY DOSE THAT IS NOT TOLERATED.

Not to exceed the following: (or 1400 mg **(900 mg) whichever is less; TABLE 4:)

TABLE 4

Age 1-9 years	37.5 mg/kg/day	**(24 mg/kg/day)
Age 9-12 years	31 mg/kg/day	**(20 mg/kg/day)
Age 12-16 years	28 mg/kg/day	**(18 mg/kg/day)
Age 16 years and older	20 mg/kg/day	**(13 mg/kg/day)

** Anhydrous theophylline indicated in ().

Measurement of Serum Theophylline Concentrations During Chronic Therapy

If the above maximum doses are to be maintained or exceeded, serum theophylline measurement is essential (see PRECAUTIONS, Laboratory Testsfor guidance).

Final Adjustment of Dosage

Dosage adjustment after serum theophylline measurement (TABLE 5):

TABLE 5

If serum theophylline is:		Directions:
Within desired range		Maintain dosage if tolerated.
Too high	20 to 25 mcg/ml	Decrease doses by about 10% and recheck serum level after 3 days.
	25 to 30 mcg/ml	Skip the next dose and decrease subsequent doses by about 25%. Recheck serum level after 3 days.
	over 30 mcg/ml	Skip next 2 doses and decrease subsequent doses by 50%. Recheck serum level after 3 days.
Too low		Increase dosage by 25% at 3 day intervals until either the desired serum concentration and/or clinical response in achieved. The total daily dose may need to be administered at more frequent intervals if symptoms occur repeatedly at the end of a dosing interval.

The serum concentration may be rechecked at appropriate intervals, but at least at the end of any adjustment period. When the patient's condition is otherwise clinically stable and none of the recognized factors which alter elimination are present, measurement of serum levels need be repeated only every 6 to 12 months.

Additional Dosing Information For The Sustained-Action Tablets: Therapy should be initiated and daily dosage requirements established utilizing a non-sustained action form of Oxtriphylline.

If the total daily maintenance dosage requirement of the Oxtriphylline nonsustained preparation is established at approximately 1200 mg, Oxtriphylline sustained-action 600 mg tablets, one every 12 hours, may be substituted to provide smoother steady-state theophylline levels

DOSAGE AND ADMINISTRATION: *(cont'd)*

and the convenience of bid-dosage. Similarly, if the total daily maintenance dosage is established at approximately 800 mg, Oxtriphylline sustained-action 400 mg, one every 12 hours may be substituted.

Store at controlled room temperature 15-30°C (59-86°F).

HOW SUPPLIED - EQUIVALENTS NOT AVAILABLE:

Tablet, Coated, Sustained Action - Oral - 400 mg

100's $35.89 CHOLEDYL SA, Parke-Davis 00071-0214-24

Tablet, Coated, Sustained Action - Oral - 600 mg

100's $43.06 CHOLEDYL SA, Parke-Davis 00071-0221-24

Tablet, Enteric Coated - Oral - 200 mg

100's $28.87 CHOLEDYL, Parke-Davis 00071-0211-24

OXYBUTYNIN CHLORIDE *(001930)*

CATEGORIES: Antipsychotics/Antimanics; Antispasmodics; Bladder, Neurogenic; Central Nervous System Agents; Dysuria; Genitourinary Muscle Relaxant; Relaxants/Stimulants, Urinary Tract; Smooth Muscle Relaxants; Urinary Incontinence; Vertigo/Motion Sickness/Vomiting; Pregnancy Category B; FDA Approval Pre 1982

BRAND NAMES: *Cystrin* (England); **Ditropan**; *Dridase* (Germany); *Novitropan*; *Oxyban*; *Novitropan*; *Tropax*
(International brand names outside U.S. in italics)

FORMULARIES: Aetna; BC-BS; DoD; FHP; PCS

DESCRIPTION:

Each scored biconvex, engraved blue tablet contains 5 mg of oxybutynin chloride. Each 5 ml of syrup contains 5 mg of oxybutynin chloride. Chemically, oxybutynin chloride is d.l (racemic) 4-diethylamino-2-butynyl phenylcyclo-hexylglycolate hydrochloride. The empirical formula of oxybutynin chloride is $C_{22}H_{31}NO_3 \cdot HCl$.

Oxybutynin chloride is a white crystalline solid with a molecular weight of 393.9. It is readily soluble in water and acids, but relatively insoluble in alkalis.

Oxybutynin chloride tablets Also contains: calcium stearate, FD&C Blue #1 Lake, lactose, and microcrystalline cellulose.

Oxybutynin chloride syrup Also contains: citric acid, FD&C Green #3, glycerin, methylparaben, flavor, sodium citrate, sorbitol, sucrose, and water. Oxybutynin chloride tablets and Syrup are for oral administration.

Therapeutic Category: Antispasmodic, anticholinergic.

CLINICAL PHARMACOLOGY:

Oxybutynin chloride exerts direct antispasmodic effect on smooth muscle and inhibits the muscarinic action of acetylcholine on smooth muscle. Oxybutynin chloride exhibits only one fifth of the anticholinergic activity of atropine on the rabbit detrusor muscle, but four to ten times the antispasmodic activity. No blocking effects occur at skeletal neuromuscular junctions or autonomic ganglia (antinicotinic effects).

Oxybutynin chloride relaxes bladder smooth muscle. In patients with conditions characterized by involuntary bladder contractions, cystometric studies have demonstrated that oxybutynin chloride increases bladder (vesical) capacity, diminishes the frequency of uninhibited contractions of the detrusor muscle, and delays the initial desire to void. Oxybutynin chloride thus decreases urgency and the frequency of both incontinent episodes and voluntary urination.

Oxybutynin chloride was well tolerated in patients administered the drug in controlled studies of 30 days' duration and in uncontrolled studies in which some of the patients received the drug for 2 years. Pharmacokinetic information is not currently available.

INDICATIONS AND USAGE:

Oxybutynin chloride is indicated for the relief of symptoms of bladder instability associated with voiding in patients with uninhibited neurogenic or reflex neurogenic bladder (*i.e.,* urgency, frequency, urinary leakage, urge incontinence, dysuria).

CONTRAINDICATIONS:

Oxybutynin chloride is contraindicated in patients with untreated angle closure glaucoma and in patients with untreated narrow anterior chamber angles since anticholinergic drugs may aggravate these conditions.

It is also contraindicated in partial or complete obstruction of the gastrointestinal tract, paralytic ileus, intestinal atony of the elderly or debilitated patient, megacolon, toxic megacolon complicating ulcerative colitis, severe colitis, and myasthenia gravis. It is contraindicated in patients with obstructive uropathy and in patients with unstable cardiovascular status in acute hemorrhage.

Oxybutynin chloride is contraindicated in patients who have demonstrated hypersensitivity to the product.

WARNINGS:

Oxybutynin chloride, when administered in the presence of high environmental temperature, can cause heat prostration (fever and heat stroke due to decreased sweating).

Diarrhea may be an early symptom of incomplete intestinal obstruction, especially in patients with ileostomy or colostomy. In this instance treatment with oxybutynin chloride would be inappropriate and possibly harmful.

Oxybutynin chloride may produce drowsiness or blurred vision. The patient should be cautioned regarding activities requiring mental alertness such as operating a motor vehicle or other machinery or performing hazardous work while taking this drug.

Alcohol or other sedative drugs may enhance the drowsiness caused by oxybutynin chloride.

PRECAUTIONS:

Oxybutynin chloride should be used with caution in the elderly and in all patients with autonomic neuropathy, hepatic or renal disease. Oxybutynin chloride may aggravate the symptoms of hyperthyroidism, coronary heart disease, congestive heart failure, cardiac arrhythmias, hiatal hernia, tachycardia, hypertension, and prostatic hypertrophy. Administration of oxybutynin chloride to patients with ulcerative colitis may suppress intestinal motility to the point of producing a paralytic ileus and precipitate or aggravate toxic megacolon, a serious complication of the disease.

Carcinogenesis, Mutagenesis, and Impairment of Fertility: A 24-month study in rats at dosages up to approximately 400 times the recommended human dosage showed no evidence of carcinogenicity.

PRECAUTIONS: *(cont'd)*

Oxybutynin chloride showed no increase of mutagenic activity when tested in *Schizosaccharomyces pompholiciformis. Saccharomyces cerevisiae* and *Salmonella typhimurium* test systems. Reproduction studies in the hamster, rabbit, rat, and mouse have shown no definite evidence of impaired fertility.

Pregnancy Category B: Reproduction studies in the hamster, rabbit, rat, and mouse have shown no definite evidence of impaired fertility or harm to the animal fetus. The safety of oxybutynin chloride administered to women who are or who may become pregnant has not been established. Therefore, oxybutynin chloride should not be given to pregnant women unless, in the judgment of the physician, the probable clinical benefits outweigh the possible hazards.

Nursing Mothers: It is not known whether this drug is excreted in human milk. Because many drugs are excreted in human milk, caution should be exercised when oxybutynin chloride is administered to a nursing woman.

Pediatric Use: The safety and efficacy of oxybutynin chloride administration have been demonstrated for children 5 years of age and older (see DOSAGE AND ADMINISTRATION.) However, as there is insufficient clinical data for children under age 5, oxybutynin chloride is not recommended for this age group.

ADVERSE REACTIONS:

Following administration of Oxybutynin chloride, the symptoms that can be associated with the use of other anticholinergic drugs may occur.

Cardiovascular: Palpitations, tachycardia, vasodilation

Dermatologic: Decreased sweating, rash

Gastrointestinal/Genitourinary: Constipation, decreased gastrointestinal motility, dry mouth, nausea, urinary hesitance and retention

Nervous System: Asthenia, dizziness, drowsiness, hallucinations, insomnia, restlessness

Ophthalmic: Amblyopia, cycloplegia, decreased lacrimation, mydriasis

Other: Impotence, suppression of lactation

OVERDOSAGE:

The symptoms of overdosage with oxybutynin chloride may be any of those seen with other anticholinergic agents. Symptoms may include signs of central nervous system excitation (*e.g.,* restlessness, tremor, irritability, convulsions, delirium, hallucinations), flushing, fever, nausea, vomiting, tachycardia, hypotension or hypertension, respiratory failure, paralysis, and coma.

In the event of an overdose or exaggerated response, treatment should be symptomatic and supportive. Maintain respiration and induce emesis or perform gastric lavage (emesis is contraindicated in precomatose, convulsive, or psychotic state). Activated charcoal may be administered as well as a cathartic. Physostigmine may be considered to reverse symptoms of anticholinergic intoxication. Hyperpyrexia may be treated symptomatically with ice bags or other cold applications and alcohol sponges.

DOSAGE AND ADMINISTRATION:

TABLETS

Adults: The usual dose is one 5-mg tablet two to three times a day. The maximum recommended dose is one 5-mg tablet four times a day.

Pediatric patients over 5 years of age: The usual dose is one 5-mg tablet two times a day. The maximum recommended dose is one 5-mg tablet three times a day.

SYRUP

Adults: The usual dose is one teaspoon (5 mg/5 ml) syrup two to three times a day. The maximum recommended dose is one teaspoon (5 mg/5 ml) syrup four times a day.

Pediatric patients over 5 years of age: The usual dose is one teaspoon (5 mg/5 ml) two times a day. The maximum recommended dose is one teaspoon (5 mg/5 ml) three times a day.

Store at controlled room temperature (59-86°F).

HOW SUPPLIED - RATED THERAPEUTICALLY EQUIVALENT:

Syrup - Oral - 5 mg/5ml

480 ml	**$49.38**	**DITROPAN, Hoechst Marion Roussel**	**00088-1373-18**

Tablet, Uncoated - Oral - 5 mg

100's	$17.84	Oxybutynin, United Res	00677-1255-01
100's	$17.84	Oxybutynin, H.C.F.A. F F P	99999-1930-01
100's	$19.31	Oxybutynin, US Trading	56126-0404-11
100's	$28.15	Oxybutynin, Qualitest Pharms	00603-4975-21
100's	$28.25	Oxybutynin, Medirex	57480-0434-01
100's	$30.00	Oxybutynin Chloride 5 Mg Tablets, Major Pharms	00904-2821-60
100's	$32.00	Oxybutinin, Raway	00686-0628-20
100's	$36.00	Oxybutynin, Schein Pharm (US)	00364-2310-01
100's	$36.50	Oxybutynin, Goldline Labs	00182-1289-01
100's	$36.50	Oxybutynin, Parmed Pharms	00349-8827-01
100's	$36.95	Oxybutynin, Martec Pharms	52555-0105-01
100's	$38.59	Oxybutynin, Sidmak Labs	50111-0456-01
100's	$38.60	Oxybutynin Chloride, Rugby	00536-5672-01
100's	$38.60	Oxybutynin, Geneva Pharms	00781-1629-01
100's	$38.60	Oxybutynin, HL Moore Drug Exch	00839-7504-06
100's	$38.68	Oxybutynin Chloride Tablets 5 Mg, Aligen Independ	00405-4735-01
100's	$38.79	Oxybutynin, Major Pharms	00904-2821-61
100's	$39.99	Oxybutynin Chloride, Geneva Pharms	00781-1629-13
100's	$42.25	Oxybutynin, Goldline Labs	00182-1289-89
100's	$44.36	Oxybutynin, Vangard Labs	00615-3512-13
100's	**$45.56**	**DITROPAN, Hoechst Marion Roussel**	**00088-1375-47**
100's	**$49.75**	**DITROPAN, Hoechst Marion Roussel**	**00088-1375-49**
500's	$89.20	Oxybutynin Chloride, United Res	00677-1255-05
500's	$89.20	Oxybutynin, H.C.F.A. F F P	99999-1930-02
500's	$139.00	Oxybutynin, Parmed Pharms	00349-8827-05
500's	$151.20	Oxybutynin, Sidmak Labs	50111-0456-02
500's	$180.00	Oxybutynin, Goldline Labs	00182-1289-05
500's	$183.35	Oxybutynin Chloride, Rugby	00536-5672-05
600's	$169.60	Oxybutynin, Medirex	57480-0434-06
750's	$317.70	Oxybutynin Chloride, Glasgow Pharm	60809-0116-55
750's	$317.70	Oxybutynin Chloride, Glasgow Pharm	60809-0116-72
1000's	$178.40	Oxybutynin, H.C.F.A. F F P	99999-1930-03
1000's	$200.80	Oxybutynin, Elkins Sinn	00641-4020-89
1000's	$202.45	Oxybutynin Chloride, Major Pharms	00904-2821-80
1000's	$250.95	Oxybutynin, Parmed Pharms	00349-8827-10
1000's	$279.41	Oxybutynin, Qualitest Pharms	00603-4975-32
1000's	$286.50	Oxybutynin Chloride, Martec Pharms	52555-0105-10
1000's	$299.25	Oxybutynin, Sidmak Labs	50111-0456-03
1000's	$300.00	Oxybutynin Chloride, Aligen Independ	00405-4735-03
1000's	$322.91	Oxybutynin, HL Moore Drug Exch	00839-7504-16
1000's	**$444.06**	**DITROPAN, Hoechst Marion Roussel**	**00088-1375-58**

OXYCODONE HYDROCHLORIDE *(001932)*

CATEGORIES: Analgesics; Antipyretics; Central Nervous System Agents; Narcotic Analgesics; Narcotics, Synthetics & Combinations; Opiate Agonists (Controlled); Pain; DEA Class CII; FDA Pre 1938 Drugs

BRAND NAMES: *Endone*; **Roxicodone**; *Supeudol* (Canada)
(International brand names outside U.S. in italics)

DESCRIPTION:

Each tablet contains: Oxycodone Hydrochloride - 5 mg (WARNING: May be habit forming)

Each 5 ml Oral Solution contains: Oxycodone Hydrochloride - 5 mg (WARNING: May be habit forming)

Each ml Intensol contains: Oxycodone Hydrochloride - 20 mg (WARNING: May be habit forming)

Roxicodone Inactive ingredients: The tablet contains microcrystalline cellulose and stearic acid. The oral solution contains alcohol, FD&C Red No. 40, flavoring, glycol, sorbitol, water, and other ingredients.

Oxycodone is a 14-hydroxydihydrocodeinone, a white odorless, crystalline powder which is derived from the opium alkaloid, thebaine.

CLINICAL PHARMACOLOGY:

The analgesic ingredient, oxycodone, is a semi-synthetic narcotic with multiple actions qualitatively similar to those of morphine; the most prominent of these involve the central nervous system and organs composed of smooth muscle. The principal actions of therapeutic value of oxycodone are analgesia and sedation.

Oxycodone is similar to codeine and methadone in that it retains at least one half of its analgesic activity when administered orally.

INDICATIONS AND USAGE:

For the relief of moderate to moderately severe pain.

CONTRAINDICATIONS:

Hypersensitivity to oxycodone

WARNINGS:

Usage in ambulatory patients: Oxycodone may impair the mental and/or physical abilities required for the performance of potentially hazardous tasks such as driving a car or operating machinery. The patient using this drug should be cautioned accordingly.

Interaction with other central nervous system: Patients receiving other narcotic analgesics, general anesthesia, phenothiazines, other tranquilizers, sedative-hypnotics or other CNS depressants (including alcohol) concomitantly with oxycodone HCl may exhibit an additive CNS depression. When such combined therapy is contemplated, the dose of one or both agents should be reduced.

Usage in Pregnancy: Safe use in pregnancy has not been established relative to possible adverse effects on fetal development. Therefore, this drug should not be used in pregnant women unless, in the judgment of the physician, the potential benefits outweigh the possible hazards.

Usage in children: This drug should not be administered to children.

PRECAUTIONS:

Head injury and increased intracranial pressure: The respiratory depressant effects on narcotics and their capacity to elevate cerebrospinal fluid pressure may be markedly exaggerated in the presence of head injury, other intracranial legions or a pre-existing increase in intracranial pressure. Furthermore, narcotics produce adverse reactions which may obscure the clinical course of patients with head injuries.

Acute abdominal conditions : The administration of this drug or other narcotics may obscure the diagnosis or clinical course in patients with acute abdominal conditions.

Special risk patients: This drug should be given with caution to certain patients such as the elderly, or debilitated, and those with severe impairments of hepatic or renal function, hypothyroidism, Addison's disease and prostatic hypertrophy or urethral stricture.

DRUG INTERACTIONS:

The CNS depressant effects of oxycodone HCl may be additive with that of other CNS depressants. See WARNINGS.

ADVERSE REACTIONS:

The most frequently observed adverse reactions include light headedness, dizziness, sedation, nausea, and vomiting. These effects seem to be more prominent in ambulatory than in nonambulatory patients, and some of these adverse reactions may be alleviated if the patient lies down.

Other adverse reactions include euphoria, dysphoria, constipation, skin rash and pruritus.

DRUG ABUSE AND DEPENDENCE:

Drug Dependence: Oxycodone can produce drug dependence of the morphine type, and therefore, has the potential for being abused. Psychic dependence, physical dependence and tolerance may develop upon repeated administration of this drug, and it should be prescribed and administered with the same degree of caution appropriate to the use of other narcotic containing medications. Like other narcotic-containing medications, this drug is subject to the Federal Controlled Substance Act.

OVERDOSAGE:

Signs and Symptoms: Serious overdosage of oxycodone HCl is characterized by respiratory depression (a decrease in respiratory rate and/or tidal volume, Cheyne-Stokes respiration, cyanosis), extreme somnolence, progressing to stupor or coma skeletal muscle flaccidity, cold and clammy skin, and sometimes bradycardia and hypotension. In serious overdosage, apnea, circulatory collapse, cardiac arrest, and death may occur.

Treatment: Primary attention should be given to the reestablishment of adequate respiratory exchange through provision of a patent airway and the institution of assisted or controlled ventilation. The narcotic antagonist naloxone is a specific antidote against respiratory depression which may result from overdosage or unusual sensitivity to narcotics, including oxycodone. Therefore, an appropriate dose: 0.4 mg should be administered, preferably by the IV route, simultaneously with efforts at respiration resuscitation. Since the duration of action of oxycodone may exceed that of the antagonist, the patient should be kept under continued surveillance and repeated doses of the antagonist should be administered as needed to maintain adequate respiration.

An antagonist should not be administered in the absence of clinically significant respiratory or cardiovascular depression.

OVERDOSAGE: *(cont'd)*

Oxygen, IV fluids, vasopressors and other supportive measures should be employed as indicated. Gastric emptying may be useful in removing unabsorbed drug.

DOSAGE AND ADMINISTRATION:

Dosage should be adjusted to the severity of the pain and the response of the patient. It may occasionally be necessary to exceed the usual recommended dosage in cases of more severe pain or in those patients who have become more tolerant to the analgesic effects of narcotics. This drug is given orally. The usual adult dose is 5 mg every 6 hours as needed for pain.

HOW SUPPLIED - EQUIVALENTS NOT AVAILABLE:

Solution - Oral - 5 mg/5ml

5 ml x 40	**$54.21**	**ROXICODONE, Roxane**	**00054-8782-16**
500 ml	$40.44	Oxycodone Hcl, Roxane	00054-3682-63

Solution - Oral - 20 mg/ml

30 ml	$39.38	OXYCODONE HCL, Roxane	00054-3683-44

Tablet, Uncoated - Oral - 5 mg

100's	**$30.14**	**ROXICODONE, Roxane**	**00054-4657-25**
100's	**$41.25**	**ROXICODONE, Roxane**	**00054-8657-24**

OXYMETHOLONE *(001934)*

CATEGORIES: Anabolic Steroids; Androgens; Anemia; Hormones; Iron Deficiency; Myelofibrosis; Pyridoxine Deficiency; Steroids; Pregnancy Category X; DEA Class CIII; FDA Approval Pre 1982

BRAND NAMES: *Anadrol* (Japan); **Anadrol-50**; *Anapolon* (England); *Anapolon 50* (Australia, Canada); *Daricon*; *Manir* (France); *Synasteron*; *Zenalosyn*
(International brand names outside U.S. in italics)

DESCRIPTION:

Anadrol (oxymetholone) tablets for oral administration each contain 50 mg of the steroid oxymetholone, a potent anabolic and androgenic drug.

The chemical name for oxymetholone is 17β-hydroxy-2-(hydroxymethylene)-17-methyl-5α-androstan-3-one.

Inactive ingredients-lactose, magnesium stearate, povidone, starch.

CLINICAL PHARMACOLOGY:

Anabolic steroids are synthetic derivatives of testosterone. Nitrogen balance is improved with anabolic agents but only when there is sufficient intake of calories & protein. Whether this positive nitrogen balance is of primary benefit in the utilization of protein-building dietary substances has not been established. Oxymetholone enhances the production and urinary excretion of erythropoietin in patients with anemias due to bone marrow failure and often stimulates erythropoiesis in anemias due to deficient red cell production.

Certain clinical effects and adverse reactions demonstrate the androgenic properties of this class of drugs. Complete dissociation of anabolic and androgenic effects has not been achieved. The actions of anabolic steroids are therefore similar to those of male sex hormones with the possibility of causing serious disturbances of growth and sexual development if given to young children. They suppress the gonadotropic functions of the pituitary and may exert a direct effect upon the testes.

INDICATIONS AND USAGE:

Anadrol-50 is indicated in the treatment of anemias caused by deficient red cell production. Acquired aplastic anemia, congenital aplastic anemia, myelofibrosis and the hypoplastic anemias due to the administration of myelotoxic drugs often respond.

Anadrol-50 should not replace other supportive measures such as transfusion, correction of iron, folic acid, vitamin B_{12} or pyridoxine deficiency, antibacterial therapy and the appropriate use of corticosteroids.

CONTRAINDICATIONS:

1. Carcinoma of the prostate or breast in male patients.

2. Carcinoma of the breast in females with hypercalcemia; androgenic anabolic steroids may stimulate osteolytic resorption of bones.

3. Oxymetholone can cause fetal harm when administered to pregnant women. It is contraindicated in women who are or may become pregnant. If the patient becomes pregnant while taking the drug, she should be apprised of the potential hazard to the fetus.

4. Nephrosis or the nephrotic phase of nephritis.

5. Hypersensitivity to the drug.

6. Severe hepatic dysfunction.

WARNINGS:

The following conditions have been reported in patients receiving androgenic anabolic steroids as a general class of drugs:

Peliosis hepatis, a condition in which liver and sometimes splenic tissue is replaced with blood-filled cysts, has been reported in patients receiving androgenic anabolic steroid therapy. These cysts are sometimes present with minimal hepatic dysfunction, but at other times they have been associated with liver failure. They are often not recognized until life-threatening liver failure or intra-abdominal hemorrhage develops. Withdrawal of drug usually results in complete disappearance of lesions.

Liver cell tumors are also reported. Most often these tumors are benign and androgen-dependent but fatal malignant tumors have been reported. Withdrawal of drug often results in regression or cessation of progression of the tumor. However, hepatic tumors associated with androgens or anabolic steroids are much more vascular than other hepatic tumors and may be silent until life-threatening intra-abdominal hemorrhage develops.

Blood lipid changes that are known to be associated with increased risk of atherosclerosis are seen in patients treated with androgens and anabolic steroids. These changes include high density lipoprotein and sometimes increased low density lipoprotein. The changes may be very marked and could have a serious impact on the risk of atherosclerosis and coronary artery disease.

Cholestatic hepatitis and jaundice occur with 17-alpha-alkylated androgens at relatively low doses. Clinical jaundice may be painless, with or without pruritus. It may also be associated with acute hepatic enlargement and right upper-quadrant pain, which has been mistaken for

WARNINGS: *(cont'd)*

acute (surgical) obstruction of the bile duct. Drug-induced jaundice is usually reversible when the medication is discontinued. Continued therapy has been associated with hepatic coma and death. Because of the hepatotoxicity associated with oxymetholone administration, periodic liver function tests are recommended.

In patients with breast cancer, anabolic steroid therapy may cause hypercalcemia by stimulating osteolysis. In this case, the drug should be discontinued.

Edema with or without congestive heart failure may be a serious complication in patients with pre-existing cardiac, renal or hepatic disease. Concomitant administration with adrenal steroids or ACTH may add to the edema. This is generally controllable with appropriate diuretic and/or digitalis therapy.

Geriatric male patients treated with androgenic anabolic steroids may be at an increased risk for the development of prostate hypertrophy and prostatic carcinoma.

Anabolic steroids have not been shown to enhance athletic ability.

PRECAUTIONS:

GENERAL

Women should be observed for signs of virilization (deepening of the voice, hirsutism, acne, and clitoromegaly). To prevent irreversible change, drug therapy must be discontinued when mild virilism is first detected. Such virilization is usual following androgenic anabolic steroid use at high doses. Some virilizing changes in women are irreversible even after prompt discontinuance of therapy and are not prevented by concomitant use of estrogens. Menstrual irregularities, including amenorrhea, may also occur.

The insulin or oral hypoglycemic dosage may need adjustment in diabetic patients who receive anabolic steroids.

Anabolic steroids may cause suppression of clotting factors II, V, VII and X, and an increase in prothrombin time.

INFORMATION FOR THE PATIENT

The physician should instruct patients to report any of the following side effects of androgens.

Adult or Adolescent Males: Too frequent or persistent erections of the penis, appearance or aggravation of acne.

Women: Hoarseness, acne, changes in menstrual periods, or more hair on the face.

All Patients: Any nausea, vomiting, changes in skin color or ankle swelling.

LABORATORY TESTS

Women with disseminated breast carcinoma should have frequent determination of urine and serum calcium levels during the course of androgenic anabolic steroid therapy (see WARNINGS.)

Because of the hepatotoxicity associated with the use of 17-alpha-alkylated androgens, liver function tests should be obtained periodically.

Periodic (every 6 months) x-ray examinations of bone age should be made during treatment of prepubertal patients to determine the rate of bone maturation and the effects of androgenic anabolic steroid therapy on the epiphyseal centers.

Anabolic steroids have been reported to lower the level of high-density lipoproteins and raise the level of low-density lipoproteins. These changes usually revert to normal on discontinuation of treatment. Increased low-density lipoproteins and decreased high-density lipoproteins are considered cardiovascular risk factors. Serum lipids and high-density lipoprotein cholesterol should be determined periodically.

Hemoglobin and hematocrit should be checked periodically for polycythemia in patients who are receiving high doses of anabolics.

Because iron deficiency anemia has been observed in some patients treated with oxymetholone, periodic determination of the serum iron and iron binding capacity is recommended. If iron deficiency is detected, it should be appropriately treated with supplementary iron.

Oxymetholone has been shown to decrease 17-ketosteroid excretion.

DRUG/LABORATORY TEST INTERFERENCES

Therapy with androgenic anabolic steroids may decrease levels of thyroxine-binding globulin resulting in decreased total T_4 serum levels and increased resin uptake of T_3 and T_4. Free thyroid hormone levels remain unchanged and there is no clinical evidence of thyroid dysfunction. Altered tests usually persist for 2-3 weeks after stopping anabolic therapy.

Anabolic steroids may cause an increase in prothrombin time.

Anabolic steroids have been shown to alter fasting blood sugar and glucose tolerance tests.

CARCINOGENESIS, MUTAGENESIS, AND IMPAIRMENT OF FERTILITY

Animal data: Testosterone has been tested by subcutaneous injection and implantation in mice and rats. The implant induced cervical-uterine tumors in mice, which metastasized in some cases. There is suggestive evidence that injection of testosterone into some strains of female mice increases their susceptibility to hepatoma. Testosterone is also known to increase the number of tumors and decrease the degree of differentiation of chemically induced carcinomas of the liver in rats.

Human data: There are rare reports of hepatocellular carcinoma in patients receiving long-term therapy with anabolics in high doses. Withdrawal of the drugs did not lead to regression of the tumors in all cases.

Geriatric patients treated with androgens may be at an increased risk of developing prostatic hypertrophy and prostatic carcinoma although conclusive evidence to support this concept is lacking.

This compound has not been tested for mutagenic potential. However, as noted above, carcinogenic effects likely occur through a hormonal mechanism rather than by a direct chemical interaction mechanism.

Impairment of fertility was not tested directly in animal species. However, as noted below under ADVERSE REACTIONS, oligospermia in males and amenorrhea in females are potential adverse effects of treatment with Anadrol tablets. Therefore, impairment of fertility is a possible outcome of treatment with Anadrol.

PREGNANCY CATEGORY X

See CONTRAINDICATIONS.

NURSING MOTHERS

It is not known whether anabolics are excreted in human milk. Because of the potential for serious adverse reactions in nursed infants from anabolics, women who take oxymetholone should not nurse.

PEDIATRIC USE

Anabolic/androgenic steroids should be used very cautiously in children and only by specialists who are aware of their effects on bone maturation.

Anabolic agents may accelerate epiphyseal maturation more rapidly than linear growth in children, and the effect may continue for 6 months after the drug has been stopped. Therefore, therapy should be monitored by x-ray studies at 6-month intervals in order to avoid the risk of compromising the adult height.

DRUG INTERACTIONS:

Anabolic steroids may increase sensitivity to anticoagulants; therefore dosage of an anticoagulant may have to be decreased in order to maintain the prothrombin time at the desired therapeutic level.

ADVERSE REACTIONS:

Hepatic: Cholestatic jaundice with, rarely, hepatic necrosis and death. Hepatocellular neoplasms an peliosis hepatis have been reported in association with long-term androgenic anabolic steroid therapy (see WARNINGS.)

CNS:

Excitation, insomnia.

Gastrointestinal: Nausea, vomiting, diarrhea.

Hematologic: Bleeding in patients on concomitant anticoagulant therapy, iron-deficiency anemia.

Leukemia has been observed in patients with aplastic anemia treated with oxymetholone. The role, if any, of oxymetholone is unclear because malignant transformation has been seen in blood dyscrasias and leukemia has been reported in patients with aplastic anemia who have not been treated with oxymetholone.

Breast: Gynecomastia.

Larynx: Deepening of the voice in women.

Hair: Hirsutism and male-pattern baldness in women, male-pattern of hair loss in postpubertal males.

Skin: Acne (especially in women and prepubertal boys).

Skeletal: Premature closure of epiphyses in children (see PRECAUTIONS, Pediatric Use), muscle cramps.

Body as a Whole: Chills.

Fluid and Electrolytes: Edema, retention of serum electrolytes (sodium, chloride, potassium, phosphate, calcium).

Metabolic/Endocrine: Decreased glucose tolerance (see PRECAUTIONS), increased serum levels of low-density lipoproteins and decreased levels of high-density lipoproteins (see PRECAUTIONS, Laboratory Tests), increased creatine and creatinine excretion, increased serum levels of creatinine phosphokinase (CPK). Reversible changes in liver function tests also occur including increased bromsulphalein (BSP) retention and increases in serum bilirubin, glutamic oxaloacetic transaminase (SGOT), and alkaline phosphatase.

Genitourinary System: *In Men: Prepubertal:* Phallic enlargement and increased frequency of erections. *Postpubertal:* Inhibition of testicular function, testicular atrophy and oligospermia, impotence, chronic priapism, epididymitis, bladder irritability, and decrease in seminal volume. *In Women:* Clitoral enlargement, menstrual irregularities. *In both sexes:* Increased or decreased libido.

DRUG ABUSE AND DEPENDENCE:

CONTROLLED SUBSTANCE: Anadrol-50 is considered to be a controlled substance and is listed in Schedule III.

OVERDOSAGE:

There have been no reports of acute overdosage with anabolics.

DOSAGE AND ADMINISTRATION:

The recommended daily dose in children and adults is 1-5 mg/kg body weight per day. The usual effective dose is 1-2 mg/kg/day but higher doses may be required and the dose should be individualized. Response is not often immediate and a minimum trial of three to six months should be given. Following remission, some patients may be maintained without the drug; others may be maintained on an established lower daily dosage. A continued maintenance dose is usually necessary in patients with congenital aplastic anemia.

HOW SUPPLIED - EQUIVALENTS NOT AVAILABLE:

Tablet, Uncoated - Oral - 50 mg

100's	$88.06	ANADROL-50, Syntex Labs	00033-2902-42

OXYMORPHONE HYDROCHLORIDE *(001935)*

CATEGORIES: Analgesics; Anesthesia; Antipyretics; Anxiety; Central Nervous System Agents; Edema; Labor and Delivery; Narcotic Analgesics; Narcotics, Synthetics & Combinations; Opiate Agonists (Controlled); Pain; Pulmonary Edema; DEA Class CII; FDA Approval Pre 1982

BRAND NAMES: **Numorphan**

FORMULARIES: Medi-Cal

DESCRIPTION:

Oxymorphone hydrochloride is a semi-synthetic narcotic substitute for morphine, is a potent analgesic.

Oxymorphone hydrochloride occurs as a white or slightly off-white, odorless powder, sparingly soluble in alcohol and ether, but freely soluble in water.

Numorphan Injection is available in two concentrations, 1 mg and 1.5 mg of oxymorphone hydrochloride per ml. Both strengths contain sodium chloride 0.8%; with methylparaben 0.18%, propylparaben 0.02% and sodium dithionite 0.1%, as preservatives. pH is adjusted with sodium hydroxide.

CLINICAL PHARMACOLOGY:

Oxymorphone hydrochloride is a potent narcotic analgesic. Administered parenterally, 1 mg of oxymorphone hydrochloride is approximately equivalent in analgesic activity to 10 mg of morphine sulfate.

The onset of action is rapid; initial effects are usually perceived within 5 to 10 minutes. Its duration of action is approximately 3 to 6 hours.

Oxymorphone hydrochloride produces mild sedation and causes little depression of the cough reflex. These properties make it particularly useful in postoperative patients.

INDICATIONS AND USAGE:

Oxymorphone hydrochloride is indicated for the relief of moderate to severe pain. This drug is also indicated parenterally for preoperative medication, for support of anesthesia, for obstetrical analgesia, and for relief of anxiety in patients with dyspnea associated with acute left ventricular failure and pulmonary edema.

CONTRAINDICATIONS:

Oxymorphone hydrochloride in children under 12 years of age has not been established. This drug should not be used in patients known to be hypersensitive to morphine analogs.

WARNINGS:

May be habit forming: As with other narcotic drugs, tolerance and addiction may develop. The addicting potential of the drug appears to be about the same as for morphine.

Like other narcotic-containing medications, oxymorphone hydrochloride is subject to the Federal Controlled Substances Act.

Sulfites Sensitivity: Oxymorphone hydrochloride contains sodium dithionite, a sulfite that may cause allergic-type reactions including anaphylactic symptoms and life-threatening or less severe asthmatic episodes in certain susceptible people. The overall prevalence of sulfite sensitivity in the general population is unknown and probably low. Sulfite sensitivity is seen more frequently in asthmatic than in nonasthmatic people.

PRECAUTIONS:

The same care and caution should be taken when administering oxymorphone hydrochloride as when other potent analgesics are used. It should be borne in mind that some respiratory depression may occur as with all potent narcotics especially when other analgesic and/or anesthetic drugs with depressant action have been given shortly before administration of oxymorphone hydrochloride.

The respiratory depressant effects of narcotics and their capacity to elevate cerebrospinal fluid pressure may be markedly exaggerated in the presence of head injury, other intracranial lesions or a pre-existing increase in intracranial pressure.

Furthermore, narcotics produce adverse reactions which may obscure the clinical course of patients with head injuries.

As with other analgesics, caution must also be exercised in elderly and debilitated patients and in patients who are known to be sensitive to central nervous system depressants, such as those with cardiovascular, pulmonary, or hepatic disease, in hypothyroidism (myxedema), acute alcoholism, delirium tremens, convulsive disorders, bronchial asthma and kyphoscoliosis. Debilitated and elderly patients and those with severe liver diseases should receive smaller doses of oxymorphone hydrochloride.

DRUG INTERACTIONS:

Interactions with other central nervous system depressants: Patients receiving other narcotic analgesics, general anesthetics, phenothiazines, other tranquilizers, sedatives, hypnotics or other CNS depressants (including alcohol) concomitantly with oxymorphone hydrochloride may exhibit an additive CNS depression. When such combined therapy is contemplated, the dose of one or both agents should be reduced.

Safe use in pregnancy has not been established (relative to possible adverse effects on fetal development). As with other analgesics, the use of oxymorphone hydrochloride in pregnancy, in nursing mothers, or in women of child-bearing potential requires that the possible benefits of the drug be weighted against the possible hazards to the mother and child.

ADVERSE REACTIONS:

As with all potent narcotic analgesics, possible side effects include drowsiness, nausea, vomiting, miosis, itching, dysphoria, light-headedness, and headache. Respiratory depression may occur with oxymorphone as with other narcotics.

OVERDOSAGE:

Signs and Symptoms: Serious overdosage with oxymorphone hydrochloride is characterized by respiratory depression, (a decrease in respiratory rate and/or tidal volume, Cheyne-Stokes respiration, cyanosis), extreme somnolence progressing to stupor or coma, skeletal muscle flaccidity, cold and clammy skin, and sometimes bradycardia and hypotension. In severe overdosage, apnea, circulatory collapse, cardiac arrest and death may occur.

Treatment: Primary attention should be given to the reestablishment of adequate respiratory exchange through provision of a patent airway and the institution of assisted or controlled ventilation. The narcotic antagonist naloxone hydrochloride (Narcan) is a specific antidote against respiratory depression which may result from overdosage or unusual sensitivity to narcotics including oxymorphone. Therefore, an appropriate dose of naloxone hydrochloride should be administered (usual initial adult dose 0.4 mg-2 mg) preferably by the intravenous route and simultaneously with efforts at respiratory resuscitation. Since the duration of action of oxymorphone may exceed that of the antagonist, the patient should be kept under continued surveillance and repeated doses of the antagonist should be administered as needed to maintain adequate respiration.

Oxygen, intravenous fluids, vasopressors and other supportive measures should be employed as indicated.

DOSAGE AND ADMINISTRATION:

Usual Adult Dosage of Oxymorphone Hydrochloride Injection: Subcutaneous or Intramuscular administration: Initially 1 mg to 1.5 mg, repeated every 4 to 6 hours as needed. Intravenous: 0.5 mg initially. In nondebilitated patients the dose can be cautiously increased until satisfactory pain relief is obtained. For analgesia during labor 0.5 mg to 1 mg intramuscularly is recommended.

HOW SUPPLIED - EQUIVALENTS NOT AVAILABLE:

Injection, Solution - Intramuscular; - 1 mg/ml

1 ml x 10	$37.25	NUMORPHAN, Du Pont Merck	00590-0370-10

Injection, Solution - Intramuscular; - 1.5 mg/ml

1 ml x 10	$48.75	NUMORPHAN, Du Pont Merck	00590-0373-10
10 ml	$47.50	NUMORPHAN, Du Pont Merck	00590-0374-01

Suppository - Rectal - 5 mg

6's	$30.56	NUMORPHAN, Du Pont Merck	00590-0761-06

OXYPHENBUTAZONE *(001936)*

CATEGORIES: Antiarthritics; Antigout; Antipyretics; Central Nervous System Agents; Nonsteroidal Anti-Inflammatory; Pain; FDA Pre 1938 Drugs

BRAND NAMES: *Mefaril*; *Omnizona*; *Oxifen*; *Phlogont* (Germany); *Reducin*; *Sioril*; *Sponderil*; *Tanderil*

(International brand names outside U.S. in italics)

Prescribing information not available at time of publication.

HOW SUPPLIED - RATED THERAPEUTICALLY EQUIVALENT:

Tablet, Plain Coated - Oral - 100 mg

100's	$23.00	Oxyphenbutazone Usp 100, Harber Pharm	51432-0321-03

OXYQUINOLINE *(001940)*

CATEGORIES: Anti-Infectives; Local Infections; Skin/Mucous Membrane Agents

BRAND NAMES: Oxychinol

Prescribing information not available at time of publication.

HOW SUPPLIED - EQUIVALENTS NOT AVAILABLE:

Tablet, Uncoated - Oral - 64.8 mg

100's $12.60 OXYCHINOL, Ferndale Labs 00496-0269-02

OXYTETRACYCLINE HYDROCHLORIDE *(001942)*

CATEGORIES: Acne; Amebiasis; Amebicides; Anti-Infectives; Antibiotics; Antimicrobials; Conjunctivitis; Granuloma; Granuloma Inguinale; Infections; Lymphogranuloma; Parasiticidal; Pneumonia; Polymyxins; Psittacosis; Q Fever; Relapsing Fever; Rheumatic Fever; Rickettsial Disease; Rickettsialpox; Rocky Mountain Fever; Skin/Mucous Membrane Agents; Syphilis; Tetracyclines; Topical; Trachoma; Typhoid Fever; Typhus; Urinary Tract Infections; Vincent's Infection; Yaws; Lyme Disease*; FDA Approval Pre 1982

* Indication not approved by the FDA

BRAND NAMES: *Acu-Oxytet*; *Aknin*; *BTH-S 250 Broncho-Tetra-Holz* (Germany); *Chemotrex 500*; *Clinmycin*; *Corsamycin*; *Cotet*; E.P. Mycin; *Geomicina*; *Intermycin*; *Leydoxycline*; *Macocyn* (Germany); *Olinmycin*; *Oxacycle*; *Oxitet*; *Oxitetraciclina Gen-Far*; *Oxy*; *Oxy-Dumocyclin*; Oxy-Kesso-Tetra; *Oxycin*; *Oxycyclin*; *Oxylag*; *Rorap*; *Servicyclin*; *Terramicina*; **Terramycin**; *Terramycine*; Tija; Uri-Tet

(International brand names outside U.S. in italics)

FORMULARIES: Aetna; Medi-Cal

DESCRIPTION:

(Note: This monograph pertains to oxytetracycline HCL capsules and the IM solution—which contains 2% lidocaine).

Oxytetracycline is a product of the metabolism of *Streptomyces rimosus* and is one of the family of tetracycline antibiotics.

Oxytetracycline diffuses readily through the placenta into the fetal circulation, into the pleural fluid and, under some circumstances, into the cerebrospinal fluid. It appears to be concentrated in the hepatic system and excreted in the bile, so that it appears in the feces, as well as in the urine, in a biologically active form.

Inert ingredients in the capsule formulation are: glucosamine hydrochloride; hard gelatin capsules (which may contain Red 3, Yellow 10 and other inert ingredients); magnesium stearate; sodium lauryl sulfate; starch.

The composition of Terramycin IM solution (2% lidocaine) is shown in TABLE 1:

TABLE 1 Composition contents per ml (m/v)

Ingredient	2 ml Single Dose Ampules 100 mg/2 ml	2 ml Single Dose Ampules 250 mg 2 ml	10 ml Vial Multidose 50 mg/ml (10 ml (5 x 2 ml Doses))
oxytetracycline	50 mg	125 mg	50 mg
lidocaine	2.0%	2.0%	2.0%
magnesium chloride hexahydrate	2.5%	6.0%	2.5%
sodium formaldehyde sulfoxylate	0.5%	0.5%	0.3%
α-monothioglycerol	—	—	1.0%
monoethanolamine	appr. 1.7%	appr. 4.2%	appr. 2.6%
citric acid	—	—	1.0%
propyl gallate	—	—	0.02%
propyl glycol	75.2%	67.0%	74.1%
water	18.8%	16.8%	18.5%

CLINICAL PHARMACOLOGY:

Oxytetracycline is primarily bacteriostatic and is thought to exert its antimicrobial effect by the inhibition of protein synthesis. Oxytetracycline is active against a wide range of gram-negative and gram- positive organisms.

The drugs in the tetracycline class have closely similar antimicrobial spectra, and cross resistance among them is common. Microorganisms may be considered susceptible if the M.I.C. (minimum inhibitory concentration) is not more than 4.0 mcg/ml and intermediate if the M.I.C. is 4.0 to 12.5 mcg/ml.

Susceptibility plate testing: A tetracycline disc may be used to determine microbial susceptibility to drugs in the tetracycline class. If the Kirby-Bauer method of disc susceptibility testing is used, a 30 mcg tetracycline disc should give a zone of at least 19 mm when tested against a tetracycline-susceptible bacterial strain.

Tetracyclines are readily absorbed and are bound to plasma proteins in varying degree. They are concentrated by the liver in the bile, and excreted in the urine and feces at high concentrations and in a biologically active form.

INDICATIONS AND USAGE:

Oxytetracycline is indicated in infections caused by the following microorganisms:

Rickettsiae (Rocky Mountain spotted fever, typhus fever and the typhus group, Q fever, rickettsialpox, and tick fevers).

Mycoplasma pneumoniae (PPLO, Eaton Agent).

Agents of psittacosis and ornithosis.

Agents of lymphogranuloma venereum and granuloma inguinale.

The spirochetal agent of relapsing fever (*Borrelia recurrentis*).

The following gram-negative microorganisms:

Haemophilus ducreyi (chancroid).

Pasteurella pestis, and *Pasteurella tularensis.*

Bartonella bacilliformis.

Bacteroides species.

Vibrio comma and *Vibrio fetus.*

Brucella species (in conjunction with streptomycin).

Because many strains of the following groups of microorganisms have been shown to be resistant to tetracyclines, culture and susceptibility testing are recommended.

INDICATIONS AND USAGE: *(cont'd)*

Oxytetracycline is indicated for treatment of infections caused by the following gram-negative microorganisms, when bacteriologic testing indicates appropriate susceptibility to the drug:

Escherichia coli.

Enterobacter aerogenes (formerly Aerobacter aerogenes).

Shigella species.

Mima species and *Herellea* species,

Haemophilus influenzae (respiratory infections).

Klebsiella species (respiratory and urinary infections).

Oxytetracycline is indicated for treatment of infections caused by the following gram-positive microorganisms when bacteriologic testing indicates appropriate susceptibility to the drug:

Streptococcus species:

Up to 44 percent of strains of *Streptococcus pyogenes* and 74 percent of *Streptococcus faecalis* have been found to be resistant to tetracycline drugs. Therefore, tetracyclines should not be used for streptococcal disease unless the organism has been demonstrated to be sensitive.

For upper respiratory infections due to Group A beta-hemolytic streptococci, penicillin is the usual drug of choice, including prophylaxis of rheumatic fever.

Diplococcus pneumoniae,

Staphylococcus aureus, skin and soft-tissue infections. Oxytetracycline is not the drug of choice in the treatment of any type of staphylococcal infections.

When penicillin is contraindicated, tetracyclines are alternative drugs in the treatment of infections due to:

Neisseria gonorrhoeae,

Treponema pallidum and *Treponema pertenue* (syphilis and yaws).

Listeria monocytogenes.

Clostridium species.

Bacillus anthracis.

Fusobacterium fusiforme (Vincent's infection).

Actinomyces species.

In acute intestinal amebiasis, the tetracyclines may be a useful adjunct to amebicides.

Tetracyclines are indicated in the treatment of trachoma, although the infectious agent is not always eliminated, as judged by immunofluorescence.

Inclusion conjunctivitis may be treated with oral tetracyclines or with a combination of oral and topical agents.

CONTRAINDICATIONS:

This drug is contraindicated in persons who have shown hypersensitivity to any of the tetracyclines.

WARNINGS:

THE USE OF DRUGS OF THE TETRACYCLINE CLASS DURING TOOTH DEVELOPMENT (LAST HALF OF PREGNANCY, INFANCY, AND CHILDHOOD TO THE AGE OF 8 YEARS) MAY CAUSE PERMANENT DISCOLORATION OF THE TEETH (YELLOW-GRAY-BROWN). This adverse reaction is more common during long term use of the drugs but has been observed following repeated short term courses. Enamel hypoplasia has also been reported. *TETRACYCLINE DRUGS, THEREFORE, SHOULD NOT BE USED IN THIS AGE GROUP UNLESS OTHER DRUGS ARE NOT LIKELY TO BE EFFECTIVE OR ARE CONTRAINDICATED.*

If renal impairment exists, even usual oral or parenteral doses may lead to excessive systemic accumulation of the drug and possible liver toxicity. Under such conditions, lower than usual total doses are indicated and, if therapy is prolonged, serum level determinations of the drug may be advisable.

Photosensitivity manifested by an exaggerated sunburn reaction has been observed in some individuals taking tetracyclines. Patients apt to be exposed to direct sunlight or ultraviolet light should be advised that this reaction can occur with tetracycline drugs, and treatment should be discontinued at the first evidence of skin erythema.

The antianabolic action of the tetracyclines may cause an increase in BUN. While this is not a problem in those with normal renal function, in patients with significantly impaired function, higher serum levels of tetracycline may lead to azotemia, hyperphosphatemia, and acidosis.

Usage In Pregnancy: See above WARNINGS about use during tooth development.

Results of animal studies indicate that tetracyclines cross the placenta, are found in fetal tissues and can have toxic effects on the developing fetus (often related to retardation of skeletal development). Evidence of embryotoxicity has also been noted in animals treated early in pregnancy.

Usage In Newborns, Infants, And Children. See above WARNINGS about use during tooth development.

All tetracyclines form a stable calcium complex in any bone forming tissue. A decrease in the fibula growth rate has been observed in prematures given oral tetracycline in doses of 25 mg/kg every 6 hours. This reaction was shown to be reversible when the drug was discontinued.

Tetracyclines are present in the milk of lactating women who are taking a drug in this class.

Additional Information For IM Solution: This hazard of renal impairment is of particular importance in the parenteral administration of tetracyclines to pregnant or postpartum patients with pyelonephritis. When used under these circumstances, the blood level should not exceed 15 mcg/ml and liver function tests should be made at frequent intervals. Other potentially hepatoxic drugs should not be prescribed concomitantly.

(In the presence of renal dysfunction, particularly in pregnancy, IV tetracycline therapy in daily doses exceeding 2 grams has been associated with deaths due to liver failure).

This product contains sodium formaldehyde sulfoxylate which serves as an antioxidant. Upon oxidation, this compound can form a potential sulfiting agent. Sulfiting agents may cause allergic-type reactions including anaphylactic symptoms and life-threatening or less severe asthmatic episodes in certain susceptible people. The overall-prevalence of sulfite sensitivity in the general population is unknown and probably low. Sulfite sensitivity is seen more frequently in asthmatic than in nonasthmatic people.

PRECAUTIONS:

As with other antibiotic preparations, use of this drug may result in overgrowth of nonsusceptible organisms, including fungi. If superinfection occurs, the antibiotic should be discontinued and appropriate therapy instituted.

In venereal diseases when coexistent syphilis is suspected, a dark field examination should be done before treatment is started and the blood serology repeated monthly for at least 4 months.

PRECAUTIONS: *(cont'd)*

Because tetracyclines have been shown to depress plasma prothrombin activity, patients who are on anticoagulant therapy may require downward adjustment of their anticoagulant dosage.

In long term therapy, periodic laboratory evaluation of organ systems, including hematopoietic, renal and hepatic studies should be performed.

All infections due to Group A beta-hemolytic streptococci should be treated for at least 10 days.

Since bacteriostatic drugs may interfere with the bactericidal action of penicillin, it is advisable to avoid giving tetracycline in conjunction with penicillin.

Additional information for IM solution (2% lidocaine): As with all intramuscular preparations, Terramycin (oxytetracycline) intramuscular solution should be injected well within the body of a relatively large muscle.

Adults: The preferred site is the upper outer quadrant of the buttock (*i.e.*, glutenous maximus), or the mid-lateral thigh.

Children: It is recommended that intramuscular injections be given preferably in the mid-lateral muscles of the thigh. In infants and small children the periphery of the upper outer quadrant of the gluteal region should be used only when necessary, such as in burn patients, in order to minimize the possibility of damage to the sciatic nerve.

The deltoid area should be used only if well developed such as in certain adults and older children and then only with caution to avoid radial nerve injury. Intramuscular injections should not be made into the lower and mid-thirds of the upper arm. As with all other intramuscular injection, aspiration is necessary to help avoid inadvertent injection into a blood vessel.

ADVERSE REACTIONS:

Gastrointestinal: anorexia, nausea, vomiting, diarrhea, glossitis, dysphagia, enterocolitis, and inflammatory lesions (with monilial overgrowth) in the anogenital region. These reactions have been caused by both the oral and parenteral administration of tetracyclines. Rare instances of esophagitis and esophageal ulcerations have been reported in patients receiving capsule and tablet forms of drugs in the tetracycline class. Most of these patients took medications immediately before going to bed. (See DOSAGE AND ADMINISTRATION.)

Skin: maculopapular and erythematous rashes. Exfoliative dermatitis has been reported but is uncommon. Photosensitivity is discussed above. (See WARNINGS.)

Renal toxicity: Rise in BUN has been reported and is apparently dose related. (See WARNINGS.)

Hypersensitivity reactions: urticaria, angioneurotic edema, anaphylaxis, anaphylactoid purpura, pericarditis and exacerbation of systemic lupus erythematosus.

Bulging fontanels in infants and benign intracranial hypertension in adults have been reported in individuals receiving full therapeutic dosages. These conditions disappeared rapidly when the drug was discontinued.

Blood: Hemolytic anemia, thrombocytopenia, neutropenia and eosinophilia have been reported.

When given over prolonged periods, tetracyclines have been reported to produce brown-black microscopic discoloration of thyroid glands. No abnormalities of thyroid function studies are known to occur.

Local irritation may be present after intramuscular injection. The injection should be deep, with care taken not to injure the sciatic nerve nor inject intravascularly.

DOSAGE AND ADMINISTRATION:

CAPSULES

Adults: Usual daily dose, 1-2 g divided in four equal doses, depending on the severity of the infection.

For children above eight years of age: Usual daily dose, 10-20 mg per pound (25-50 mg/kg) of body weight divided in four equal doses.

Therapy should be continued for at least 24-48 hours after symptoms and fever have subsided.

For treatment of brucellosis, 500 mg oxytetracycline four times daily for 3 weeks should be accompanied by streptomycin, 1 gram intramuscularly twice daily the first week, and once daily the second week.

For treatment of uncomplicated gonorrhea, when penicillin is contraindicated, tetracycline may be used for the treatment of both males and females in the following divided dosage schedule: 1.5 grams initially followed by 0.5 gram q.i.d. for a total of 9.0 grams.

For treatment of syphilis, a total of 30-40 grams in equally divided doses over a period of 10-15 days should be given. Close follow-up, including laboratory tests, is recommended.

Administration of adequate amounts of fluid along with capsule and tablet forms of drugs in the tetracycline class is recommended to wash down the drugs and reduce the risk of esophageal irritation and ulceration. (See ADVERSE REACTIONS.)

Concomitant therapy: Antacids containing aluminum, calcium, or magnesium impair absorption and should not be given to patients taking oral tetracyclines.

Food and some dairy products also interfere with absorption. Oral forms of tetracyclines should be given 1 hour before or 2 hours after meals. Pediatric oral dosage forms should not be given with milk formulas and should be given at least 1 hour prior to feeding.

In patients with renal impairment (See WARNINGS.) Total dosage should be decreased by reduction of recommended individual doses and/or by extending time intervals between doses.

In the treatment of streptococcal infections, a therapeutic dose of oxytetracycline should be administered for at least 10 days.

INTRAMUSCULAR ADMINISTRATION

Adults: The usual daily dose is 250 mg administered once every 24 hours or 300 mg given in divided doses at 8 to 12 hour intervals.

For children above eight years of age: 15-25 mg/kg of body weight up to a maximum of 250 mg per single daily injection. Dosage may be divided and given at 8-12 hour intervals.

Intramuscular therapy should be reserved for situations in which oral therapy is not feasable.

The intramuscular administration of oxytetracycline produces lower blood levels than oral administration in the recommended dosages. Patients placed on intramuscular oxytetracycline should be changed to the oral dosage form as soon as possible. If rapid, high blood pressure levels are needed, oxytetracycline should be administered intravenously.

In patients with renal impairment: (See WARNINGS.) Total dosage should be decreased by reduction of recommended individual doses and/or by extending time intervals between doses.

(Intramuscular Solution: Roerig, 3/87, 70-1051-00-2)

HOW SUPPLIED - RATED THERAPEUTICALLY EQUIVALENT:

Capsule, Gelatin - Oral - 250 mg

100's	$16.58	Oxytetracycline Hcl, Rugby	00536-4101-01
100's	**$68.07**	**TERRAMYCIN, Pfizer Labs**	**00069-0730-66**
1000's	$86.10	Oxytetracycline Hcl, Rugby	00536-4101-10

OXYTETRACYCLINE HYDROCHLORIDE; PHENAZOPYRIDINE HYDROCHLORIDE; SULFAMETHIZOLE *(001943)*

CATEGORIES: Anti-Infectives; Antibacterials; Antibiotics; Antimicrobials; Cystitis; Infections; Prostatitis; Pyelitis; Pyelonephritis; Sulfonamides; Tetracyclines; Urinary Tract Infections; Urethritis; FDA Pre 1938 Drugs

BRAND NAMES: **Urobiotic-250**; *Urobiotic*; *Urobiotico*
(International brand names outside U.S. in italics)

DESCRIPTION:

Each capsule contains Oxytetracycline hydrochloride equivalent to: 250 mg oxytetracycline; Sulfamethizole: 250 mg; Phenazopyridine hydrochloride: 50 mg

Inert ingredients in the Urobiotic-250 formulation are: hard gelatin capsules (which may contain Green 3, Yellow 6, Yellow 10 and other inert ingredients); magnesium stearate; sodium lauryl sulfate; starch.

CLINICAL PHARMACOLOGY:

Urobiotic-250 is a product designed for use specifically in urinary tract infections.

Terramycin (oxytetracycline HCl) is a widely used antibiotic with clinically proved activity against gram-positive and gram-negative bacteria, rickettsiae, spirochetes, large viruses, and certain protozoa. Terramycin is well tolerated and well absorbed after oral administration. It diffuses readily through the placenta and is present in the fetal circulation. It diffuses into the pleural fluid, and under some circumstances, into the cerebrospinal fluid. Oxytetracycline HCl appears to be concentrated in the hepatic system and is excreted in the bile. It is excreted in the urine and in the feces, in high concentrations, in a biologically active form.

Sulfamethizole is a chemotherapeutic agent active against a number of important gram-positive and gram-negative bacteria. This sulfonamide is well absorbed, has a low degree of acetylation, and is extremely soluble. Because of these features and its rapid renal excretion, sulfamethizole has a low order of toxicity and provides prompt and high concentrations of the active drug in the urinary tract.

Phenazopyridine is an orally absorbed agent which produces prompt and effective local analgesia and relief of urinary symptoms by virtue of its rapid excretion in the urinary tract. These effects are confined to the genitourinary system and are not accompanied by generalized sedation or narcosis.

INDICATIONS AND USAGE:

Based on a review of this drug by the National Academy of Sciences-National Research Council and/or other information, FDA has classified the indications as follows:

"Lacking substantial evidence of effectiveness as a fixed combination":

Urobiotic-250 is indicated in the therapy of a number of genitourinary infections caused by susceptible organisms. These infections include the following: pyelonephritis, pyelitis, ureteritis, cystitis, prostatitis, and urethritis.

Since both Terramycin and sulfamethizole provide effective levels in blood, tissue, and urine, Urobiotic-250 provides a multiple antimicrobial approach at the site of infection. Both antibacterial components are active against the most common urinary pathogens, including Escherichia coli, Pseudomonas aeruginosa, Aerobacter aerogenes, Streptococcus faecalis, Streptococcus hemolyticus, and Micrococcus pyogenes. Urobiotic-250 is particularly useful in the treatment of infections caused by bacteria more sensitive to the combination than to either component alone. The combination is also of value in those cases with mixed infections, and in those instances where the causative organism is unknown pending laboratory isolation.

Final classification of the less than effective indications requires further investigation. Clinical studies to substantiate the efficacy of Urobiotic-250 are ongoing. Completion of these ongoing studies will provide data for final classification of these indications.

CONTRAINDICATIONS:

This drug is contraindicated in individuals who have shown hypersensitivity to any of its components.

This drug, because of the sulfonamide component, should not be used in patients with a history of sulfonamide sensitivities, and in pregnant females at term.

WARNINGS:

If renal impairment exists, even usual oral or parenteral doses may lead to excessive systemic accumulation of the drug and possible liver toxicity. Under such conditions, lower than usual doses are indicated and if therapy is prolonged, tetracycline serum level determinations may be advisable.

Oxytetracycline HCl, which is one of the ingredients of Urobiotic-250, may form a stable calcium complex in any bone-forming tissue with no serious harmful effects reported thus far in humans. However, use of oxytetracycline during tooth development (last trimester of pregnancy, neonatal period and early childhood) may cause discoloration of the teeth (yellow-grey-brownish). This effect occurs mostly during long term use of the drug but it also has been observed in usual short treatment courses.

Because of its sulfonamide content, this drug should be used only after critical appraisal in patients with liver damage, renal damage, urinary obstruction, or blood dyscrasias. Deaths have been reported from hypersensitivity reactions, agranulocytosis, aplastic anemia, and other blood dyscrasias associated with sulfonamide administration. When used intermittently, or for a prolonged period, blood counts and liver and kidney function tests should be performed.

Certain hypersensitive individuals may develop a photodynamic reaction precipitated by exposure to direct sunlight during the use of this drug. This reaction is usually of the photoallergic type which may also be produced by other tetracycline derivatives. Individuals

WARNINGS: *(cont'd)*

with a history of photosensitivity reactions should be instructed to avoid exposure to direct sunlight while under treatment with this or other tetracycline drugs, and treatment should be discontinued at first evidence of skin discomfort.

NOTE: Reactions of a photoallergic nature are exceedingly rare with Terramycin (oxytetracycline HCl). Phototoxic reactions are not believed to occur with Terramycin.

PRECAUTIONS:

As with all antibiotic preparations, use of this drug may result in overgrowth of nonsusceptible organisms, including fungi. If superinfection occurs, the antibiotic should be discontinued and appropriate specific therapy should be instituted. This drug should be used with caution in persons having histories of significant allergies and/or asthma.

ADVERSE REACTIONS:

Glossitis, stomatitis, proctitis, nausea, diarrhea, vaginitis, and dermatitis, as well as reactions of an allergic nature, may occur during oxytetracycline HCl therapy, but are rare. If adverse reactions, individual idiosyncrasy, or allergy occur, discontinue medication. Rare instances of esophagitis and esophageal ulcerations have been reported in patients receiving capsule forms of drugs in the tetracycline class. Most of these patients took medications immediately before going to bed. (See DOSAGE AND ADMINISTRATION.)

With oxytetracycline therapy bulging fontanels in infants and benign intracranial hypertension in adults have been reported in individuals receiving full therapeutic dosages. These conditions disappeared rapidly when the drug was discontinued.

As in all sulfonamide therapy, the following reactions may occur: nausea, vomiting, diarrhea, hepatitis, pancreatitis, blood dyscrasias, neuropathy, drug fever, skin rash, injection of the conjunctiva and sclera, petechiae, purpura, hematuria and crystalluria. The dosage should be decreased or the drug withdrawn, depending upon the severity of the reaction.

DOSAGE AND ADMINISTRATION:

Urobiotic-250 is recommended in adults only. A dose of 1 capsule four times daily is suggested. In refractory cases 2 capsules four times a day may be used.

Therapy should be continued for a minimum of seven days or until bacteriologic cure in acute urinary tract infections.

Administration of adequate amounts of fluid along with capsule forms of drugs in the tetracycline class is recommended to wash down the drugs and reduce the risk of esophageal irritation and ulceration. (See ADVERSE REACTIONS.)

To aid absorption of the drug, it should be given at least one hour before or two hours after eating. Aluminum hydroxide gel given with antibiotics has been shown to decrease their absorption and is contraindicated.

HOW SUPPLIED - EQUIVALENTS NOT AVAILABLE:

Capsule, Gelatin - Oral - 250 mg/50 mg/25

50's	$65.34	UROBIOTIC, Roerig	00049-0920-50

OXYTETRACYCLINE HYDROCHLORIDE; POLYMYXIN B SULFATE *(001944)*

CATEGORIES: Anti-Infectives; Antibiotics; Conjunctivitis; EENT Drugs; Eye, Ear, Nose, & Throat Preparations; Infections; Ocular Infections; Ophthalmics; Tetracyclines; FDA Approval Pre 1982

BRAND NAMES: Aktetra; *Oxymycin*; *Poxytrin*; *Terramicina con Polimixina* (Mexico); *Terramycin* (Germany); *Terramycin Eye*; *Terramycin Ophthalmic Ointment*; **Terramycin W Polymyxin**; *Terramycin with Polmyxin B*; *Terramycine*
(International brand names outside U.S. in italics)

DESCRIPTION:

Each gram of sterile ointment contains oxytetracycline HCl equivalent to 5 mg oxytetracycline, 10,000 units of polymyxin B sulfate, white petrolatum, and liquid petrolatum.

CLINICAL PHARMACOLOGY:

Terramycin is a widely used antibiotic with clinically proved activity against gram-positive and gram-negative bacteria, rickettsiae, spirochetes, large viruses, and certain protozoa.

Polymyxin B Sulfate, one of a group of related antibiotics derived from*Bacillus polymyxa*, is rapidly bactericidal. This action is exclusively against gram-negative organisms. It is particularly effective against *Pseudomonas aeruginosa (B. pyocyaneus),* and Koch-Weeks bacillus, frequently found in local infections of the eye.

There is thus made available a particularly effective antimicrobial combination of the broad-spectrum antibiotic Terramycin as well as polymyxin B sulfate against primarily causative or secondarily infecting organisms.

INDICATIONS AND USAGE:

The sterile preparation, Terramycin with Polymyxin B Sulfate Ophthalmic Ointment, is indicated for the treatment of superficial ocular infections involving the conjunctiva and/or cornea caused by Terramycin with Polymyxin B Sulfate-susceptible organisms.

It may be administered topically alone, or as an adjunct to systemic therapy.

It is effective in infections caused by susceptible strains of staphylococci, streptococci, pneumococci, *Hemophilus influenzae, Pseudomonas aeruginosa,* Koch-Weeks bacillus, and *Proteus.*

CONTRAINDICATIONS:

This drug is contraindicated in individuals who have shown hypersensitivity to any of its components.

PRECAUTIONS:

As with all antibiotic preparations, use of this drug may result in overgrowth of nonsusceptible organisms, including fungi. If superinfection occurs, the antibiotic should be discontinued and appropriate specific therapy should be instituted.

ADVERSE REACTIONS:

Terramycin with Polymyxin B Sulfate Ophthalmic Ointment is well tolerated by the epithelial membranes and other tissues of the eye. Allergic or inflammatory reactions due to individual hypersensitivity are rare.

DOSAGE AND ADMINISTRATION:

Approximately 1/2 inch of the ointment is squeezed from the tube onto the lower lid of the affected eye two to four times daily.

DOSAGE AND ADMINISTRATION: *(cont'd)*

The patient should be instructed to avoid contamination of the lip of the tube when applying the ointment.

HOW SUPPLIED - EQUIVALENTS NOT AVAILABLE:

Ointment - Ophthalmic - 1/8 oz

1's	$7.17	TERRAMYCIN W/POLYMYCIN B SULFATE, Roerig	00049-0801-08
3.5 gm	$10.50	Aktetra, Akorn	17478-0230-35

OXYTOCIN *(001945)*

CATEGORIES: Abortion; Diabetes; Galactokinetic; Hemorrhage; Hormones; Labor; Labor and Delivery; Lactation; Oxytocics; Pregnancy; Relaxants/Stimulants, Uterine; Uterine Contractions; FDA Approval Pre 1982

BRAND NAMES: *Orasthin* (Germany); *Orasthin INJ*; *Oxytocin S INJ*; *Oxiton INJ*; *Partocon INJ*; **Pitocin**; *Pitocin INJ*; *Piton S*; *Piton S INJ*; *Synthetic Oxytocin INJ*; Syntocinon; *Syntocinon INJ* (Australia, Germany, England, France); *Syntocinon Spray*; *Utron INJ*
(International brand names outside U.S. in italics)

FORMULARIES: Aetna; BC-BS; WHO

DESCRIPTION:

Note: This monograph contains complete prescribing information for the Injection as well as the Nasal Spray forms of Oxytocin.

Injection: Pitocin (oxytocin injection, USP) is a sterile, clear, colorless solution of synthetic oxytocin, for intravenous infusion or intramuscular injection. Pitocin is a nonapeptide found in pituitary extracts from mammals. It is standardized to contain 10 units of oxytocic hormone/ml and contains 0.5% Chloretone (chlorobutanol, a chloroform derivative) as a preservative, with the pH adjusted with acetic acid. The hormone is prepared synthetically to avoid possible concentration with vasopressin (ADH) and other small polypeptides with biologic activity. Pitocin has the empirical formula $C_{43}H_{6651}O_{12}S_2$ (molecular weight 1007.19).

Nasal Spray: Each ml contains 40 USP Units (International Units) Oxytocin and the following: chlorobutanol, NF max, 0.05%; citric acid, USP; dried sodium phosphate, USP, glycerin, USP; methylparaben, NF; propylparaben, NF; purified water, USP; sodium chloride, USP; sorbitol solution, USP.

Oxytocin is one of the polypeptide hormones of the pituitary gland. The pharmacologic and clinical properties of Oxytocin nasal solution, USP (nasal spray) are identical with the oxytocic and galactokinetic principle of the natural hormone.

Synthetic Oxytocin has the formula $C_{43}H_{66}N_{12}0_{12}S_2$, with a molecular weight of 1007.19

Since Oxytocin, a polypeptide, is subject to inactivation by the proteolytic enzymes of the alimentary tract, it is **not absorbed from the gastrointestinal tract**.

CLINICAL PHARMACOLOGY:

INJECTION

Uterine motility depends on the formation of the contractile protein actomyosin under the influence of the Ca^{2+} -dependent phosphorylating enzyme myosin light-chain kinase. Oxytocin promotes contractions by increasing the intracellular Ca^{2+}. Oxytocin has specific receptors in the myometrium and the receptor concentration increases greatly during pregnancy, reaching a maximum in early labor at term. The response to a given dose of oxytocin is very individualized and depends on the sensitivity of the uterus, which is determined by the oxytocin receptor concentration. However, the physician should be aware of the fact that oxytocin even in its pure form has inherent pressor and antidiuretic properties which may become manifest when large doses are administered. These properties are though to be due to the fact that oxytocin and vasopressin differ in regard to only two of the eight amino acids (see PRECAUTIONS.)

Oxytocin is distributed throughout the extracellular fluid. Small amounts of the drug probably reach the fetal circulation. Oxytocin has a plasma half-life of about 1 to 6 minutes which is decreased in late pregnancy and during lactation. Following intravenous administration of oxytocin, uterine response occurs almost immediately and subsides within 1 hour. Following intramuscular injection of the drug, uterine response occurs within 3 to 5 minutes and persists for 2 to 3 hours. Its rapid removal from plasma is accomplished largely by the kidney and the liver. Only small amounts are excreted in urine unchanged.

NASAL SPRAY

Oxytocin nasal spray acts specifically on the myoepithelial elements surrounding the alveoli of the breast, and making up the walls of the lactiferous ducts, causing their smooth muscle fibers to contract and thus force milk into the large ducts of the sinuses where it is more readily available to the baby. Oxytocin does not possess galactopoietic properties and its use is intended only for the purpose of milk ejection.

Pharmacokinetics: Oxytocin nasal solution (nasal spray) is promptly absorbed by the nasal mucosa to enter the systemic circulation. Intranasal application of the spray preparation, however, is a practical and effective method of administration. Half-life is extremely short - less than 10 minutes - and Oxytocin is then rapidly removed from the plasma by the kidney, liver, and lactating mammary gland. The enzyme oxytocinase is believed to be elaborated by placental and uterine tissues. This enzyme inactivates the hormone by cleavage of the cysteine- tyrosine peptide bond. Excretion is mainly urinary following inactivation of metabolites.[2]

INDICATIONS AND USAGE:

INJECTION

> IMPORTANT NOTICE
> **Elective induction of labor is defined as the initiation of labor in a pregnant individual who has no medical indications for induction. Since the available data are inadequate to evaluate the benefits-to-risks considerations. Pitocin is not indicated for elective induction of labor.**

Antepartum: Pitocin is indicated for the initiation or improvement of uterine contractions, where this is desirable and considered suitable for reasons of fetal or maternal concern, in order to achieve vaginal delivery. It is indicated for (1) induction of labor in patients with a medical indication for initiation of labor, such as Rh problems, maternal diabetes, preeclampsia at or near term, when delivery is in the best interest of mother and fetus or when membranes are prematurely ruptured and delivery is indicated; (2) stimulation or reinforcement of labor, as in selected cases of uterine inertia; (3) as adjunctive therapy in the management of incomplete or inevitable abortion. In the first trimester, curettage is generally considered primary therapy. In second trimester abortion, oxytocin infusion will often be successful in emptying the uterus. Other means of therapy, however, may be required in such cases.

INDICATIONS AND USAGE: *(cont'd)*

Postpartum: Pitocin is indicated to produce uterine contractions during the third stage of labor and to control postpartum bleeding or hemorrhage.

Nasal Spray: Oxytocin nasal solution (nasal spray) is indicated to assist the initial postpartum milk ejection from the breasts once milk formulation has commenced.

CONTRAINDICATIONS:

Injection: Antepartum use of Pitocin is contraindicated in any of the following circumstances:

1. Where there is significant cephalopelvic disproportion;

2. In unfavorable fetal positions or presentations, such as transverse lies, which are undeliverable without conversion prior to delivery;

3. In obstetrical emergencies where the benefit-to-risk ratio for either the fetus or the mother favors surgical intervention;

4. In fetal distress where delivery is not imminent;

5. Where adequate uterine activity fails to achieve satisfactory progress;

6. Where the uterus is already hyperactive or hypertonic;

7. In cases where vaginal delivery is contraindicated, such as invasive cervical carcinoma, active herpes genitalis, total placenta previa, vase previa, and cord presentation or prolapse of the cord;

8. In patients with hypersensitivity to the drug.

Nasal Spray: Pregnancy and hypersensitivity are the only known contraindications.

WARNINGS:

Injection: Pitocin, when given for induction of labor on augmentation of uterine activity, should be administered only by the intravenous route and with adequate medical supervision in a hospital.

PRECAUTIONS:

GENERAL

Injection

1. All patients receiving intravenous oxytocin must be under continuous observation by trained personnel who have a thorough knowledge of the drug and qualified to identify complications. A physician qualified to manage any complications should be immediately available. Electric fetal monitoring provides the best means for early detection of overdosage (see OVERDOSAGE.) However, it must be born in mind that only intrauterine pressure recording can accurately measure the intrauterine pressure during contractions. A fetal scalp electrode provides a more dependable recording of the fetal heart rate than any external monitoring system.

2. When properly administered, oxytocin should stimulate uterine contractions similar to those seen in normal labor. Overstimulation of the uterus by improper administration can be hazardous to both mother and fetus. Even with proper administration and adequate supervision, hypertonic contractions can occur in patients whose uteri are hypersensitive to oxytocin. This fact must be considered by the physician in exercising his judgement regarding patient selection.

3. Except in unusual circumstances, oxytocin should not be administered in the following conditions: fetal distress, partial placenta, previa, prematurity, borderline cephalopelvic disproportion, and major surgery on the cervix or uterus including cesarean section, overdistention of the uterus, grand multiparity, or past history of uterine sepsis or of traumatic delivery. Because of the variability of the combinations of factors which may be present in the conditions listed above, the definition of "unusual circumstances" must be left to the judgment of the physician. The decision can only be made by carefully weighing the potential benefits which oxytocin can provide in a given case against rare but definite potential for the drug to produce hypertonicity or tetanic spasm.

4. Maternal deaths due to hypertensive episodes, subarachnoid hemorrhage, rupture of the uterus, fetal deaths due to various cases have been reported associated with the use of parenteral oxytocic drugs for induction of labor or the augmentation in the first and second stages of labor

5. Oxytocin has been shown to have an intrinsic antidiuretic effect, acting to increase water reabsorption from the glomerular filtrate. Consideration should, therefore, be given to the possibility of water intoxication, particularly when oxytocin is administered continuously by infusion and the patient is receiving fluids by mouth.

6. When oxytocin is used for induction or reinforcement of already existent labor, patients should be carefully selected. Pelvic adequacy must be considered and maternal and fetal conditions evaluated before the drug.

CARCINOGENESIS, MUTAGENESIS, AND IMPAIRMENT OF FERTILITY

There are no animal or human studies on the carcinogenicity and mutagenicity of this drug, nor is there any information on its effect on fertility.

PREGNANCY

Injection

Teratogenic Effects: Animal reproduction studies have not been conducted with oxytocin. There are no known indications for use in the first trimester of pregnancy other than in relation to spontaneous or induced abortion. Based on the wide experience with this drug and its chemical structure and pharmacological properties, it would not be expected to present a risk of fetal abnormalities when used as indicated.

Nonteratogenic Effects: See ADVERSE REACTIONS in the fetus or infant.

Nasal Spray

Pregnancy Category X (see CONTRAINDICATIONS) Oxytocin nasal solution, USP (nasal spray) is contraindicated during pregnancy since it may provoke a uterotonic effect to precipitate contractions and abortions. Its proper use is during the first week postpartum, as needed.

LABOR AND DELIVERY

See INDICATIONS AND USAGE.

Nasal Spray: No particular information regarding any special care to be exercised by the practitioner for safe and effective use of the drug is known at this time.

INFORMATION FOR THE PATIENT

The squeeze bottle should be held in an upright position when administering the drug to the nose and the patient should be in an sitting position rather than lying down. If preferred, the solution can be instilled in drop form by inverting the squeeze bottle and exerting very gentle pressure on its walls.

NURSING MOTHERS

While harmful effects on the newborn have not been reported, it should be noted that Oxytocin nasal solution, USP (nasal spray) is intended to be used only for **initial** milk propulsion and ejection during the first week postpartum, and not for continued use. Caution shall be exercised when Oxytocin nasal solution, USP (nasal spray) is administered to a nursing mother since Oxytocin is known to be excreted in human milk.

DRUG INTERACTIONS:

Injection: Severe hypertension has been reported when oxytocin was given three to four hours following prophylactic administration of a vasoconstrictor in conjunction with caudal block anesthesia. Cyclopropane anesthesia may modify oxytocin's cardiovascular effects, so as to produce unexpected results such as hypotension. Maternal sinus bradycardia with abnormal atrioventricular rhythms has also been noted when oxytocin was used concomitantly with cyclopropane anesthesia.

ADVERSE REACTIONS:

Injection: The following adverse reactions have been reported in the mother Anaphylactic reaction, Nausea, Postpartum hemorrhage, Vomiting, Cardiac arrhythmia, Premature ventricular contractions, Fatal afibrinogenemia, Pelvic hematoma.

Excessive dosage or hypersensitivity to the drug may result in uterine hypertonicity, spasm, tetanic contraction, or rupture of the uterus.

The possibility of increased blood loss and afibrinogenemia should be kept in mind when administering the drug.

Severe water intoxication with convulsions and coma has occurred, associated with a slow oxytocin infusion over a 24-hour period. Maternal death due to oxytocin-induced water intoxication has been reported.

The following adverse reactions have been reported in the fetus or infant: Due to induced uterine motility: Bradycardia, Premature ventricular contractions and other arrhythmias, Permanent CNS or brain damage, Fetal death. Due to use of oxytocin in the mother: Low Apgar scores at five minutes, Neonatal jaundice, Neonatal retinal hemorrhage.

Nasal Spray: Lack of efficacy has been the most frequent adverse effect (seven cases), followed by nasal irritation and/or rhinorrhea, uterine bleeding, excessive uterine contractions, and lacrimation.

One case each of seizure and "psychotic state" are the most severe reactions reported. No other reactions have been described.[3]

DRUG ABUSE AND DEPENDENCE:

Nasal Spray: These problems have not been encountered with Oxytocin nasal solution, USP (nasal spray). This may be due to the fact that synthetic Oxytocin acts like the natural posterior pituitary hormone. Also, its clinical use is limited to the first week following delivery, to assist in initial milk letdown.

OVERDOSAGE:

Injection: Overdosage with oxytocin depends essentially on uterine hyperactivity whether or not due to hypersensitivity to this agent. Hyperstimulation with strong (hypertonic) or prolonged (tetanic) contractions, or a resting tone of 15 to 20 mmH_2O or more between contractions can lead to tumultuous labor, uterine rupture, cervical and vaginal lacerations, postpartum hemorrhage, uteroplacental hypoperfusion, and variable deceleration of fetal heart, fetal hypoxia, hypercapnia, or death. Water intoxication with convulsions, which is caused by the inherent antidiuretic effect of oxytocin, is a serious complication that may occur if large doses (40 to 50 milliunits/minute) are infused for long periods. Management consists of immediate discontinuation of oxytocin and symptomatic and supportive therapy.

Nasal Spray: No case of overdosage with Oxytocin nasal solution, USP (nasal spray) has been reported since the preparation became commercially available in 1961. It is theoretically possible for the very large doses to be self-administered depending on the topical tolerance of the nasal mucosa. With such massive use, painful uterine contractions could be induced, although these effects persist for only about 15 minutes.[4] Also, an antidiuretic effect could occur resulting in water intoxification. Should this ensue, diuresis should be forced with appropriate agents such as furosemide.[5]

DOSAGE AND ADMINISTRATION:

INJECTION

Parenteral drug products should be inspected visually for particulate matter and discoloration prior to administration whenever solution and container permit.

The dosage of oxytocin is determined by uterine response. The following dosage information is based upon the various regimens and indications in general use.

Induction or Stimulation of Labor

Intravenous infusion (drip method) is the only acceptable method of parenteral administration of Pitocin for the induction or stimulation of labor. Accurate control of the rate of infusion flow is essential and is best accomplished by an infusion pump. It is convenient to piggyback the Pitocin infusion on a physiologic electrolyte solution, permitting the Pitocin infusion to be stopped abruptly without interrupting the electrolyte infusion. This is done in the following way.

Preparation

a. The standard solution for infusion of Pitocin is prepared by adding the contents of one 1-ml ampoule containing 10 units of oxytocin to 1000 ml of 0.9% aqueous sodium chloride or Ringer's lactate. The combined solution containing 10 milliunits (mU) of oxytocin/ml is rotated in the infusion bottle for thorough mixing. The same concentration can be obtained by mixing the contents of one 0.5 ml ampoule, containing 5 units of oxytocin, with 500 ml of electrolyte solution.

b. Establish the infusion with a separate bottle of physiologic electrolyte solution not containing Pitocin.

c. Attach (piggyback) the Pitocin-containing bottle with the infusion pump to the infusion line as close to the infusion site as possible.

Administration: The initial dose should be 0-5-1 mU/min (equal to 3-6 ml of the dilute oxytocin solution per hour). At 30-60 minute intervals the dose should be gradually increased in the increments desired frequency of contractions has been reached and labor has progressed to 5-6 cm dilation, the dose may be reduced by similar increments.

Studies of the concentrations of oxytocin in the maternal plasma during Pitocin infusion have shown that infusion rates up to 6 mU/min give the same oxytocin levels that are found in spontaneous labor. At term, higher infusion rates should be given with great care, and rates exceeding 9-10 mU/min are rarely required. Before term, when the sensitivity of the uterus is lower because of a lower concentration of oxytocin receptors, a higher infusion rate may be required.

Monitoring

a. Electronically monitor the uterine activity and the fetal heart rate throughout the infusion of Pitocin. Attention should be given to tonus, amplitude and frequency of contractions and to the fetal heart rate in relation to uterine contractions. If uterine contractions become too powerful, the infusion can be abruptly stopped and oxytocic stimulation of the uterine musculature will soon wane. (see PRECAUTIONS.)

b. Discontinue the infusion of Pitocin immediately in the event of uterine and hyperactivity and/or fetal distress. Administer oxygen to the mother, who preferably should be put in a lateral position. The condition of mother and fetus should immediately be evaluated by the responsible physician and appropriate steps taken.

DOSAGE AND ADMINISTRATION: *(cont'd)*

Control of Postpartum Uterine Bleeding

Intravenous infusion (drip method): If the patient has an intravenous infusion running, 10 to 40 units of oxytocin may be added tot he bottle, depending on the amount of electrolyte or dextrose solution remaining (maximum 40 units to 1000 ml). Adjust the infusion rate to sustain uterine concentration and control uterine atony.

Intramuscular Administration: (One ml) Ten (10) units of Pitocin can be given after the delivery of the placenta.

Treatment of Incomplete, Inevitable or Elective Abortion

Intravenous infusion of 10 units of Pitocin added to 500 ml of a physiologic saline solution or 5% dextrose in-water solution may help the uterus contract after a suction or sharp curettage for an incomplete, inevitable or elective abortion.

Subsequent to intra-amniotic injection of hypertonic saline, professionals, urea, etc, for midtrimester elective abortion, the injection-to-abortion time may be shortened by infusion of Pitocin at the rate of 10 to 20 milliunits (20 to 40 drops) per minute. The total dose should not exceed 30 units in a 12-hour period due to the risk of water intoxication.

NASAL SPRAY

One spray into one or both nostrils two to three minutes before nursing or pumping of breasts.

REFERENCES:

Nasal Spray 1. U.S.P. XXI, p. 777, **2.** Goodman and Gilman: The Pharmacological Basis of Therapeutics. Sixth Ed., 937-8. **3.** Data collected by the Medical Services Department, Sandoz Pharmaceuticals Corporation. **4.** Boglin, N.E.: The use of intranasal oxytocin for the induction of labor. Zbl. Gynak. **85**:193-199 (Feb 9) 1963. **5.** Sandoz Overdosage Manual, 1984, Syntocinon Injection. **Injection** : **1.** Seitchik J, Castillo M: Oxytocin augmentation of dysfunctional labor. I. Clinical Data. *Am J Obstet Gynecol*1982; 144:889-905. **2.** Seitchik j, Castillo M: Oxytocin augmentation of dysfunctional labor. II. Multuparous patients.*Am J Obstet Gynecol* 1983; 145:777-780. **3.** Fuchs A, Goeschen K, Husslein P, et al: Oxytocin and the initiation of human parturition. III. Plasma concentrations of oxytocin and 13, 14-dihydro-15-keto-prostaglandin $F_2\alpha$ in spontaneous and oxytocin-induced labor at term. *Am J Obstet Gynecol* 1983; 145:497-502. **4.** Seitchik J, Amico J, et al: Oxytocin augmentation of dysfunctional labor. IV. Oxytocin pharmacokinetics. *Am J Obstet Gynecol* 1984; 150:225- 228. **5.** American College of Obstetricians and Gynecologists: ACOG Technical Bulletin Number 110-November 1987: Induction and augmentation of labor.

HOW SUPPLIED:

Injection: Store between 15° and 25°C (59° and 77°F).

Nasal Spray: : Store below 77°; DO NOT FREEZE.

(Injection, Parke-Davis, 5/94, 4160G069)

(Nasal Spray, Sandoz, 7/88, St-ZZ13)

HOW SUPPLIED - RATED THERAPEUTICALLY EQUIVALENT:

Injection, Solution - Intramuscular; - 10 unit/ml

1 ml	**$9.49**	**PITOCIN, Parke-Davis**	**00071-4160-03**
1 ml	**$18.30**	**PITOCIN, Parke-Davis**	**00071-4160-40**
1 ml x 25	$24.38	Oxytocin, Fujisawa USA	00469-0012-06
10 ml	**$6.13**	**PITOCIN, Parke-Davis**	**00071-4160-10**
10 ml x 25	**$23.74**	**PITOCIN, Parke-Davis**	**00071-4160-45**
10 ml x 25	$64.00	Oxytocin, Voluntary Hosp	53258-0012-02
10 ml x 25	$118.13	Oxytocin, Fujisawa USA	00469-0012-25
50's	$141.78	SYNTOCINON, Novartis	00078-0060-04

PACLITAXEL *(003073)*

CATEGORIES: Antineoplastics; Breast Carcinoma; Chemotherapy; Oncologic Drugs; Ovarian Carcinoma; Lung Cancer*; Melanoma*; FDA Class 1P ("Priority Review"); Sales > $500 Million; FDA Approved 1992 Dec

* Indication not approved by the FDA

BRAND NAMES: BMY-45622; **Taxol**

FORMULARIES: Medi-Cal

COST OF THERAPY: $3,200.13 (Ovarian Carcinoma; Injection; 30 mg/5ml; 0.25/day; 365 days)

WARNING:

Paclitaxel for injection voncentrate should be administered under the supervision of a physician experienced in the use of cancer chemotherapeutic agents. Appropriate management of complications is possible only when adequate diagnostic and treatment facilities are readily available.

Severe hypersensitivity reactions characterized by dyspnea and hypotension requiring treatment, angioedema, and generalized urticaria have occurred in 2% of patients receiving paclitaxel. One of these reactions was fatal in a patient treated without premedication in a Phase I study. Patients receiving paclitaxel should be pretreated with corticosteroids, diphenhydramine, and H2 antagonists to prevent these reactions. (See DOSAGE AND ADMINISTRATION.) Patients who experience severe hypersensitivity reactions to paclitaxel should not be rechallenged with the drug.

Paclitaxel therapy should not be given to patients with baseline neutrophil counts of less than 1,500 cells/mm3. In order to monitor the occurrence of bone marrow suppression, primarily neutropenia, which may be severe and result in infection, it is recommended that frequent peripheral blood cell counts be performed on all patients receiving paclitaxel.

DESCRIPTION:

Taxol for Injection Concentrate is a clear colorless to slightly yellow viscous solution. It is supplied as a nonaqueous solution intended for dilution with a suitable parenteral fluid prior to intravenous infusion. Taxol is available in 30 mg (5 ml) single-dose vials. Each ml of sterile nonpyrogenic solution contains 6 mg paclitaxel, 527 mg Cremophor EL (polyoxyethylated castor oil) and 49.7% (v/v) dehydrated alcohol, USP.

Paclitaxel is a natural product with antitumor activity. The chemical name for paclitaxel is 5β,20-Epoxy-1,2α,4,7β,10β,13α-hexahydroxytax-11-en-9-one 4,10-diacetate 2-benzoate 13-ester with *(2R,3S)*-*N*-benzoyl-3-phenylisoserine.

Paclitaxel is a white to off-white crystalline powder with the empirical formula $C_{47}H_{51}NO_{14}$ and a molecular weight of 853.9. It is highly lipophilic, insoluble in water, and melts at around 216-217°C.

CLINICAL PHARMACOLOGY:

Paclitaxel is a novel antimicrotubule agent that promotes the assembly of microtubules from tubulin dimers and stabilizes microtubules by preventing depolymerization. This stability results in the inhibition of the normal dynamic reorganization of the microtubule network that is essential for vital interphase and mitotic cellular functions. In addition, paclitaxel induces abnormal arrays or "bundles" of microtubules throughout the cell cycle and multiple asters of microtubules during mitosis.

Following intravenous administration of paclitaxel, paclitaxel plasma concentrations declined in a biphasic manner. The initial rapid decline represents distribution to the peripheral compartment and elimination of the drug. The later phase is due, in part, to a relatively slow efflux of paclitaxel from the peripheral compartment.

Pharmacokinetic parameters of paclitaxel following 3- and 24-hour infusions of paclitaxel at dose levels of 135 and 175 mg/m²were determined in a Phase 3 randomized study in ovarian cancer patients and are summarized in the following table (TABLE 1):

TABLE 1 Summary of Non-Compartment Pharmacokinetic Parameters Mean (% Coefficient of Variation) Values by Single-Dose and Infusion

Dose (mg/m^2)	Infusion Duration (h)	N (patients)	C_{max} (ng/ml)	AUC (0-∞) (ng-h/ml)	T-HALF (h)	CL_T ($l/h/m^2$)
135	24	2	195	6300	52.7	21.7
175	24	4	365(33)	7993(29)	15.7(56)	23.8(35)
135	3	7	2170(21)	7952(23)	13.1(45)	17.7(20)
175	3	5	3650(30)	15007(27)	20.2(85)	12.2(25)

C_{max} - Maximum plasma concentration
AUC(0-∞) - Area under the plasma concentration-time curve from time 0 to infinity
CL_T - Total body clearance

It appeared that with the 24-hour infusion of paclitaxel, a 30% increase in dose (135 mg/m^2 versus 175 mg/m^2) increased the C_{max} by 87% whereas the $AUC(0\text{-}_{00})$ remained proportional. However, with a 3-hour infusion, for a 30% increase in dose, the $C_{max}$and $AUC(0\text{-}_{00})$ were increased by 68% and 89%, respectively. The mean apparent volume of distribution in steady state, with the 24-hour infusion of paclitaxel ranged from 227 to 688 l/m^2, indicating extensive extravascular distribution and/or tissue binding of paclitaxel.

The pharmacokinetics of paclitaxel were also evaluated in adult cancer patients who received single doses of 15-135 mg/m^2given be 1- hour infusions (n=15, 30-275 mg/m^2given by 6-hour infusions (n=36), and 200-275 mg/m^2given by 24-hour infusions (n=54) in Phase 1 & 2 studies. Values for total body clearance and volume of distribution were consistent with the findings in the Phase 3 study.

In vitro studies of binding to human serum proteins, using paclitaxel concentrations ranging from 0.1 to 50 mcg/ml, indicate that between 89-98% of drug is bound; the presence of cimetidine, ranitidine, dexamethasone, or diphenhydramine did not affect protein binding of paclitaxel.

The disposition of paclitaxel has not been fully elucidated in humans. After intravenous administration of 15-275 mg/m^2doses of paclitaxel as 1, 6, or 24-hour infusions, mean (SD) values for cumulative urinary recovery of unchanged drug ranged from 1.3% (0.5%) to 12.6% (16.2%)) of the dose, indicating extensive non-renal clearance. Paclitaxel has been demonstrated to be metabolized in the liver in animals and there is evidence suggesting hepatic metabolism in humans. High paclitaxel concentrations have been reported in the bile of patients treated with paclitaxel. The effect of renal or hepatic dysfunction on the disposition of paclitaxel has not been investigated.

Possible interactions of paclitaxel with concomitantly administered medications have not been formally investigated.

CLINICAL STUDIES:

Ovarian Carcinoma: Data from five Phase 1 & 2 clinical studies (189 patients), a multicenter, randomized Phase 3 study (407 patients) as well as an interim analysis of data from more than 300 patients enrolled in a treatment referral center program were used in support of the use of paclitaxel for injection concentrate in patients who have failed initial or subsequent chemotherapy for metastatic carcinoma of the ovary. Two of the Phase 2 studies (92 patients) utilized an initial dose of 135 to 170 mg/m^2 in most patients (>90%) administered over 24 hours by continuous infusion. Response rates in these two studies were 22% (95% CI = 11-37%) and 30% (95% CI = 18-46%) with a total of six complete and 18 partial responses in 92 patients. The median duration of overall response in these two studies measured from the first day of treatment was 7.2 months (range: 3.5-15.8 months) and 7.5 months (range: 5.3-17.4 months), respectively. The median survival was 8.1 months (range: 0.2- 36.7 months) and 15.9 months (range: 1.8-34.5+ months).

The Phase 3 study had a bifactorial design and compared the efficacy and safety of paclitaxel, administered at two different doses (135 or 175 mg/m^2) and schedules (3- or 24-hour infusion). The overall response rate for the 407 patients was 16.2% (95% CI = 12.8-20.2%), with 6 complete and 60 partial responses. Duration of response, measured from the first day of treatment was 8.3 months (range: 3.2-21.6 months). Median time to progression was 3.7 months (range: 0.1+-25.1+ months). Median survival was 11.5 months (range: 0.2-26.3+ months).

Response rates, median survival and median time to progression for the 4 arms are given in the following table (TABLE 2). The arms are listed by dose and schedule ($mg{\cdot}m^2$/hours). Comparisons between study arms should be done with caution in view of the bifactorial study design and small sample sizes per arm.

TABLE 2 Key Efficacy Parameters in the Phase 3 Ovarian Carcinoma Study

	175/3 (n=96)	175/24 (n=106)	135/3 (n=99)	135/24 (n=106)
•**Response**				
-rate (percent)	14.6	21.7	15.2	13.2
-95% Confidence Interval	(8.5-23.6)	(14.5-31.0)	(9.0-24.1)	(7.7-21.5)
•**Time to Progression**				
-median (months)	4.4	4.2	3.4	2.8
-95% Confidence Interval	(3.0-5.6)	(3.5-5.1)	(2.8-4.2)	(1.9-4.0)
•**Survival**				
-median (months)	11.5	11.8	13.1	10.7
-95% Confidence Interval	(8.4-14.4)	(8.9-14.6)	(9.1-14.6)	(8.1-13.6)

Analyses were performed as planned by the study protocol, by comparing the two doses (135 or 175 mg/m^2) irrespective of the schedule (3 or 24 hours) and the two schedules irrespective of dose.

Patients receiving the 175 mg/m^2 dose achieved a higher response rate than those receiving the 135 mg/m^2 dose: 18% vs. 14% (p=0.28). No difference in response rate was detected when comparing the 3-hour with the 24-hour infusion: 15% vs. 17% (p=0.50). Patients receiving the 175 mg/m^2 dose of paclitaxel had a longer time to progression than those receiving the 135

CLINICAL STUDIES: *(cont'd)*

mg/m²dose: median 4.2 vs. 3.1 months (p=0.03). Time to progression was longer for patients receiving the 3-hour vs. the 24-hour infusion: 4.0 months vs. 3.7 months (p=0.08). No difference in survival according to dose or schedule was observed.

Paclitaxel remained active in patients who had developed resistance to platinum-containing therapy (defined as tumor progression while on, or tumor relapse within 6 months from completion of, platinum-containing regimens) with response rates of 14% in the Phase 3 study and 31% in the Phase 1 & 2 clinical studies.

The adverse event profile in the Phase 3 study was consistent with that seen for a pooled analysis performed on 812 patients treated in ten clinical studies (see ADVERSE REACTIONS.) For the 403 patients who received paclitaxel in the Phase 3 study, the following table (TABLE 3) shows the incidence of some key adverse events by treatment arm. The arms are listed by dose and schedule (mg/m²/hours).

TABLE 3 Frequency of Key Adverse Events in the Phase 3 Ovarian Carcinoma Study

		Percent of Patients 175/3 (n=95)	175/24 (n=105)	135/3 (n=98)	135/24 (n=105)
•Bone Marrow					
Neutropenia	< 2,000/mm³	78	98	78	98
	< 500/mm³	27	75	14	67
Thrombocytopenia	< 100,000/mm²	4	18	8	6
	< 50,000/mm³	1	7	2	1
Anemia	< 11 g/dl	84	90	68	88
	< 8 g/dl	11	12	6	10
Infections		26	29	20	18
•Hypersensitivity Reaction*					
All		41	45	38	45
Severe		2	0	2	1
•Peripheral Neuropathy					
Any symptoms		63	60	55	42
Severe symptoms		1	2	0	0
•Mucositis					
Any symptoms		17	35	21	25
Severe symptoms		0	3	0	2

* All patients received premedication

Myelosuppression was dose and schedule related, with the schedule effect being more prominent. The development of severe hypersensitivity reactions (HSRs) was rare: 1% of the patients and 0.2% of the courses overall. There was no apparent dose or schedule effect seen for the HSRs. Additionally, peripheral neuropathy was clearly dose-related, but schedule did not appear to affect the incidence.

The results of the randomized study support the use of paclitaxel at doses of 135 to 175 mg/m² administered by a 3-hour infusion. The same doses administered by 24-hour infusion were more toxic:the bifactorial study design and small sample size per arm preclude definitive conclusions regarding relative efficacy between the 4 arms of the study.

Breast Carcinoma: Data from 83 patients accrued in three phase 2 open label studies and from 471 patients enrolled in a phase 3 randomized study were available to support the use of paclitaxel in patients with metastatic breast carcinoma.

Phase 2 open-label studies: Two studies were conducted in 53 patients previously treated with a maximum of one prior chemotherapeutic regimen. Paclitaxel was administered in these 2 trials as a 24-hour infusion at initial doses of 250 mg/m² (with G-CSF support) or 200 mg/m². The response rates were 57% (95% Cl: 37-75%) and 52% (95% Cl: 32-72%), respectively. The third phase 2 study evaluated quality of life changes and was conducted in extensively pretreated patients who had failed anthracycline therapy and who had received a minimum of 2 chemotherapy regimens for the treatment of metastatic disease. The dose of paclitaxel was 200 mg/m² as a 24-hour infusion with G-CSF support. Nine of 30 patients analyzed achieved a partial response, for a response rate of 30% (95% Cl: 15-50%).

Phase 3 randomized study: This multicenter trial was conducted in patients previously treated with one or two regimens of chemotherapy. Patients were randomized to receive paclitaxel at a dose of either 175 mg/m² or 135 mg/m² given as a 3-hour infusion. In the 471 patients enrolled, 60% had symptomatic disease with impaired performance status at study entry, and 73% had visceral metastases. These patients had failed prior chemotherapy either in the adjuvant setting (30%), the metastatic setting (39%), or both (31%). Sixty-seven percent of the patients had been previously exposed to anthracyclines and 23% of them had disease considered resistant to this class of agents.

The overall response rate for the 454 evaluable patients was 26% (95% Cl: 22-30%), with 17 complete and 99 partial responses. The median duration of response, measured from the first day of treatment, was 8.1 months (range: 3.4-18.1+ months). Overall for the 471 patients, the median time to progression was 3.5 months (range: 0.03-17.1 months). Median survival was 11.7 months (range: 0-18.9 months).

Response rates, median survival and median time to progression for the 2 arms are given in the following table (TABLE 4). The arms are listed by dose and schedule (mg·m²/hours).

TABLE 4 Key Efficacy Parameters in the Phase 3 Breast Carcinoma Study

	175/3 (n=235)	135/3 (n=236)
•Response		
rate (percent)	28	22
95% Confidence Interval	(22-34)	(17-27)
•Time to Progression		
median (months)	4.2	3.0
95% Confidence Interval	(3.2-4.6)	(2.5-3.8)
•Survival		
median (months)	11.7	10.5
95% Confidence Interval	(10.0-13.8)	(9.0-12.8)

For the 458 patients who received paclitaxel for injection concentrate in the Phase 3 study, the following table (TABLE 5) shows the incidence of some key adverse events by treatment arm (each arm was administered by a 3-hour infusion).

Myelosuppression and peripheral neuropathy were dose related. There was one severe hypersensitivity reaction (HSR) observed at the dose of 135 mg/m².

INDICATIONS AND USAGE:

Paclitaxel is indicated, after failure of first-line or subsequent chemotherapy for the treatment of metastatic carcinoma of the ovary.

Paclitaxel is indicated for the treatment of breast cancer after failure of combination chemotherapy for metastatic disease or relapse within 6 months of adjuvant chemotherapy. Prior therapy should have included an anthracycline unless clinically contraindicated.

TABLE 5 Frequency of Key Adverse Events in the Phase 3 Breast Carcinoma Study

		Percent of Patients 175 mg/m² (n=229)	135 mg/m² (n=229)
•Bone Marrow			
Neutropenia*	< 2,000/mm³	90	81
	< 500/mm³	28	19
Thrombocytopenia*	< 100,000/mm³	11	7
	< 50,000/mm³	3	2
Anemia*	< 11 g/dl	55	47
	< 8 g/dl	4	2
Infections		23	15
Febrile Neutropenia		2	2
•Hypersensitivity Reaction**			
All		36	31
Severe		0	<1
•Peripheral Neuropathy			
Any symptoms		70	46
Severe symptoms		7	3
•Mucositis			
Any symptoms		23	17
Severe symptoms		3	<1

* Based on worst course analysis
** All patients received premedication

CONTRAINDICATIONS:

Paclitaxel is contraindicated in patients who have a history of hypersensitivity reactions to paclitaxel, or other drugs formulated in Cremophor EL (polyoxyethylated castor oil).

Paclitaxel should not be used in patients with baseline neutropenia of < 1,500 cells/mm³.

WARNINGS:

Patients should be pretreated with corticosteroids (such as dexamethasone), diphenhydramine and H_2 antagonists (such as cimetidine or ranitidine) before receiving paclitaxel. (See DOSAGE AND ADMINISTRATION.) Severe hypersensitivity reactions characterized by dyspnea and hypotension requiring treatment, angioedema, and generalized urticaria have occurred in 2% of patients receiving paclitaxel. These reactions are probably histamine-mediated. One of these reactions was fatal in a patient with pulmonary metastases who was a participant in a Phase I trial. This patient received no premedication; the first course of paclitaxel, which was uneventful, was administered at 190 mg/m²infused over three hours. Within a few minutes from the beginning of a second course of paclitaxel, the patient developed severe hypotension and died. Patients who experience severe hypersensitivity reactions to paclitaxel should not be rechallenged with the drug.

Bone marrow suppression (primarily neutropenia) is dose-dependent and is the dose-limiting toxicity. Neutrophil nadirs occurred at a median of 11 days. Paclitaxel should not be administered to patients with baseline neutrophil counts of less than 1,500 cells/mm³. Frequent monitoring of blood counts should be instituted during paclitaxel treatment. Patients should not be re-treated with subsequent cycles of paclitaxel until neutrophils recover to a level > 1,500 cells/mm³ and platelets recover to a level > 100,000 cells/mm³.

Severe conduction abnormalities have been documented in < 1% of patients during paclitaxel therapy and in some cases requiring pacemaker placement. If patients develop significant conduction abnormalities during paclitaxel infusion, appropriate therapy should be administered and continuous cardiac monitoring should be performed during subsequent therapy with paclitaxel.

Paclitaxel may cause fetal harm when administered to a pregnant woman. Paclitaxel has been shown to be embryo- and feto-toxic in rats and rabbits and to decrease fertility in rats. In these studies, paclitaxel was shown to result in abortions, decreased corpora lutea, a decrease in implantations and live fetuses, and increased resorptions and embryo-fetal deaths. No gross external, soft tissue or skeletal alterations occurred. There are no studies in pregnant women. If paclitaxel is used during pregnancy, or if the patient becomes pregnant while receiving this drug, the patient should be apprised of the potential hazard. Women of childbearing potential should be advised to avoid becoming pregnant during therapy with paclitaxel.

PRECAUTIONS:

GENERAL

Contact of the undiluted concentrate with plasticized polyvinyl chloride (PVC) equipment or devices used to prepare solutions for infusion is not recommended. In order to minimize patient exposure to the plasticizer DEHP [di-(2-ethylhexyl)phthalate], which may be leached from PVC infusion bags or sets, diluted paclitaxel solutions should preferably be stored in bottles (glass, polypropylene) or plastic bags (polypropylene, polyolefin) and administered through polyethylene-lined administration sets.

Paclitaxel should be administered through an in-line filter with a microporous membrane not greater than 0.22 microns. Use of filter devices such as IVEX-2 filters which incorporate short inlet and outlet PVC-coated tubing has not resulted in significant leaching of DEHP.

Hematology: Paclitaxel for injection concentrate therapy should not be administered to patients with baseline neutrophil counts of less than 1,500 cells/mm³. In order to monitor the occurrence of myelotoxicity, it is recommended that frequent peripheral blood cell counts be performed on all patients receiving paclitaxel. Patients should not be re-treated with subsequent cycles of paclitaxel until neutrophils recover to a level > 1,500 cells/mm³ and platelets recover to a level > 100,000 cells/mm³. In the case of severe neutropenia (<500 cells/mm³ for seven days or more) during a course of paclitaxel therapy, a 20% reduction in dose for subsequent courses of therapy is recommended.

Hypersensitivity Reactions: Patients with a history of severe hypersensitivity reactions to products containing Cremophor EL (*e.g.,* cyclosporin for injection concentrate and teniposide for injection concentrate) should not be treated with paclitaxel. In order to avoid the occurrence of severe hypersensitivity reactions, all patients treated with paclitaxel should be premedicated with corticosteroids (such as dexamethasone), diphenhydramine and H_2 antagonists (such as cimetidine or ranitidine). Minor symptoms such as flushing, skin reactions, dyspnea, hypotension or tachycardia do not require interruption of therapy. However, severe reactions, such as hypotension requiring treatment, dyspnea requiring bronchodilators, angioedema or generalized urticaria require immediate discontinuation of paclitaxel and aggressive symptomatic therapy. Patients who have developed severe hypersensitivity reactions should not be rechallenged with paclitaxel.

Cardiovascular: Hypotension and bradycardia have been observed during administration of paclitaxel, but generally do not require treatment. Frequent vital sign monitoring, particularly during the first hour of paclitaxel infusion, is recommended. Continuous cardiac monitoring is not required except for patients with serious conduction abnormalities. (See WARNINGS.)

Nervous System: Although, the occurrence of peripheral neuropathy is frequent, the development of severe symptomatology is unusual and requires a dose reduction of 20% for all subsequent courses of paclitaxel.

PRECAUTIONS: *(cont'd)*

Hepatic: There is no evidence that the toxicity of paclitaxel is enhanced in patients with elevated liver enzymes, but no data are available for patients with severe baseline cholestasis. However, evidence suggests that the liver plays an important role in the metabolism of paclitaxel. As a result, since there are no data available from patients with severe liver disease, caution should be exercised when administering paclitaxel to patients with severe hepatic impairment.

CARCINOGENESIS, MUTAGENESIS, AND IMPAIRMENT OF FERTILITY

The carcinogenic potential of paclitaxel has not been studied. Paclitaxel has been shown to be mutagenic *in vitro* (chromosome aberrations in human lymphocytes) and *in vivo* (micronucleus test in mice) mammalian test systems, however, it did not induce mutagenicity in the Ames test or the CHO/HGPRT gene mutation assay. Paclitaxel at an IV dose of 1 mg/kg (6 mg/m^2) produced low fertility and fetal toxicity in rats. Paclitaxel has also been shown to be maternal and embryo-fetal toxic in rabbits receiving the drug at an IV dose of 3 mg/kg (33 mg/m^2) during organogenesis. (See WARNINGS.)

PREGNANCY CATEGORY D

(See WARNINGS.)

NURSING MOTHERS

It is not known whether the drug is excreted in human milk. Because many drugs are excreted in human milk and because of the potential for serious adverse reactions in nursing infants, it is recommended that nursing be discontinued when receiving paclitaxel therapy.

PEDIATRIC USE

The safety and effectiveness of paclitaxel in children have not been established.

DRUG INTERACTIONS:

In a Phase I trial[1] using escalating doses of paclitaxel (110-200 mg/m^2) and cisplatin (50 or 75 mg/m^2) given as sequential infusions, myelosuppression was more profound when paclitaxel was given after cisplatin that with the alternate sequence (*i.e.,* paclitaxel before cisplatin). Pharmacokinetic data from these patients demonstrated a decrease in paclitaxel clearance of approximately 33% when paclitaxel was administered following cisplatin.

Based on *in vitro* data, there is the possibility of an inhibition of paclitaxel metabolism in patients treated with ketoconazole. As a result, caution should be exercised when treating patients with paclitaxel when they are receiving ketoconazole as concomitant therapy.

ADVERSE REACTIONS:

Data in the following table (TABLE 6) are based on the experience of 812 patients (493 with ovarian carcinoma and 319 with breast carcinoma) enrolled in 10 studies. Two hundred and seventy-five patients were treated in 8 Phase 2 studies with paclitaxel doses ranging from 135 to 300 mg/m^{2}administered over 24 hours (in 4 of these studies, G-CSF was administered as hematopoietic support). Three hundred and one patients were treated in the randomized Phase 3 ovarian carcinoma study which compared two doses (135 or 175 mg/m^2) and two schedules (3 or 24 hours) of paclitaxel. Two hundred and thirty-six patients with breast carcinoma received paclitaxel (135 or 175 mg/m^2) administered over 3 hours in a controlled study.

TABLE 6 Summary of Adverse Events in 812 Patients Receiving Paclitaxel

		% Incidence
•Bone Marrow		
Neutropenia	< 2,000/mm^3	90
	< 500/mm^3	52
Leukopenia	< 4,000/mm^3	90
	< 1,000/mm^3	17
Thrombocytopenia	< 100,000/mm^3	20
	< 50,000/mm^3	7
Anemia	< 11 g/dl	78
	< 8 g/dl	16
Infections		30
Bleeding		14
Red Cell Transfusions		25
Platelet Transfusions		2
•Hypersensitivity Reaction*		
All		41
Severe		2
•Cardiovascular		
Vital Sign Changes**		
Bradycardia (N=537)		3
Hypotension (N=532)		12
Significant Cardiovascular Events		1
•Abnormal ECG		
All Pts		23
Pts with normal baseline (N=559)		14
•Peripheral Neuropathy		
Any symptoms		60
Severe symptoms		3
•Myalgia/Arthralgia		
Any symptoms		60
Severe symptoms		8
•Gastrointestinal		
Nausea and vomiting		52
Diarrhea		38
Mucositis		31
•Alopecia		87
•Hepatic (Pts with normal baseline and on study data)		
Bilirubin elevations (N=765)		7
Alkaline phosphatase elevations (N=575)		22
AST (SGOT) elevations (N=591)		19
•Injection Site Reaction		13

* All patients received premedication
** During the first 3-hours of infusion

None of the observed toxicities were clearly influenced by age.

The following data relate to the overall safety database of 812 patients treated in clinical studies. In addition, rare events have been reported from the postmarketing experience or from other clinical studies. The frequency and severity of adverse events are generally similar between patients receiving paclitaxel for the treatment of ovarian or breast carcinoma. The frequency and severity of key adverse events for the Phase 3 ovarian and breast carcinoma studies are presented in tabular form by treatment are in CLINICAL STUDIES

Hematologic: Bone marrow suppression was the major dose-limiting toxicity of paclitaxel. Neutropenia, the most important hematologic toxicity, was dose and schedule dependent and generally rapidly reversible. Among patients treated in the Phase 3 ovarian study with a 3-hour infusion, neutrophil counts decline below 500 cells/mm^3 in 13% of the patients treated with a dose of 135 mg/m^2 compared to 27% at a dose of 175 mg/m^2 (p=0.05). In the same

ADVERSE REACTIONS: *(cont'd)*

study, severe neutropenia (<500 cells/mm^3) was more frequent with the 24-hour than with the 3-hour infusion; infusion duration had a greater impact on myelosuppression than dose. Neutropenia did not appear to increase with cumulative exposure and did not appear to be more frequent nor more severe for patients previously treated with radiation therapy.

Fever was frequent (12% of all treatment courses). Infectious episodes occurred in 30% of all patients and 9% of all courses; these episodes were fatal in 1% of all patients, and included sepsis, pneumonia and peritonitis. In the Phase 3 ovarian study, infectious episodes were reported in 19% of the patients given either 135 or 175 mg/m^{2}dose by a 3 hour infusion. Urinary tract infections and upper respiratory tract infections were the most frequently reported infectious complications.

Thrombocytopenia was uncommon, and almost never severe (<50,000 cells/mm^3). Twenty percent of the patients experienced a drop in their platelet count below 100,000 cells/mm^3 at least once while on treatment; 7% had a platelet count <50,000 cells/mm^3 at the time of their worst nadir. Among the 812 patients, bleeding episodes were reported in 4% of all courses and by 14% of all patients but most of the hemorrhagic episodes were localized and the frequency of these events was unrelated to the paclitaxel for injection concentrate dose and schedule. In the Phase 3 ovarian study, bleeding episodes were reported in 10% of the patients receiving either the 135 or 175 mg/m^2 dose given by a 3-hour infusion; no patients treated with the 3-hour infusion received platelet transfusions.

Anemia (Hb <11 g/dl) was observed in 78% of all patients and was severe (Hb <8 g/dl) in 16% of the cases. No consistent relationship between dose or schedule and frequency of anemia was observed. Among all patients with normal baseline hemoglobin, 69% became anemic on study but only 7% had severe anemia. Red cell transfusions were required in 25% of all patients and in 12% of those with normal baseline hemoglobin levels.

Hypersensitivity Reactions (HSRs): All patients received premedication prior to paclitaxel (See WARNINGS and PRECAUTIONS, Hypersensitivity Reactions). The frequency and severity of HSRs were not affected by the dose or schedule of paclitaxel administration. In the Phase 3 ovarian study the 3-hour infusion was not associated with a greater increase in HSRs when compared to the 24-hour infusion. Hypersensitivity reactions were observed in 20% of all courses and in 41% of all patients. These reactions were severe in less than 2% of the patients and 1% of the courses. No severe reactions were observed after course 3 and severe symptoms occurred generally within the first hour of paclitaxel infusion. The most frequent symptoms observed during these severe reactions were dyspnea, flushing, chest pain and tachycardia.

The minor hypersensitivity reactions consisted mostly of flushing (28%), rash (12%), hypotension (4%), dyspnea (2%), tachycardia (2%) and hypertension (1%). The frequency of hypersensitivity reactions remained relativity stable during the entire treatment period.

Cardiovascular: Hypotension, during the first 3-hours of infusion, occurred in 12% of all patients and 3% of all courses administered. Bradycardia, during the first 3-hours of infusion, occurred in 3% of all patients and 1% of all courses. In Phase 3 ovarian study, neither dose nor schedule had an effect on the frequency of hypotension and bradycardia. These vital sign changes most often caused no symptoms and required neither specific therapy nor treatment discontinuation. The frequency of hypotension and bradycardia were not influenced by prior anthracycline therapy.

Significant cardiovascular events possibly related to paclitaxel occurred in approximately 1% of all patients. These events included syncope, rhythm abnormalities, hypertension and venous thrombosis. One of the patients with syncope treated with paclitaxel at 175 mg/m^2 over 24-hours had progressive hypotension and died. The arrhythmias included asymptomatic ventricular tachycardia, bigeminy and complete AV block requiring pacemaker placement.

Electrocardiogram (ECG) abnormalities were common among patients at baseline. ECG abnormalities on study did not usually result in symptoms, were not dose-limiting, and required no intervention. ECG abnormalities were noted in 23% of all patients. Among patients with a normal ECG prior to study entry, 14% of all patients developed an abnormal tracing while on study. The most frequently reported ECG modifications were non- specific repolarization abnormalities, sinus bradycardia, sinus tachycardia and premature beats. Among patients with normal ECG at baseline, prior therapy with anthracylines did not influence the frequency of ECG abnormalities.

Neurologic: The frequency and severity of neurologic manifestations were dose-dependent, but were not influenced by infusion duration. Peripheral neuropathy was observed in 60% of all patients (3% severe) and in 52% (2% severe) of the patients without pre-existing neuropathy.

The frequency of peripheral neuropathy increased with cumulative dose. Neurologic symptoms were observed in 27% of the patients after the first course of treatment and 34-51% from 2 to 10.

Peripheral neuropathy was the cause of paclitaxel discontinuation in 1% of all patients. Sensory symptoms have usually improved or resolved within several months of paclitaxel discontinuation. The incidence of neurologic symptoms did not increase in the subset of patients previously treated with cisplatin. Pre-existing neuropathies resulting from prior therapies are not a contraindication for paclitaxel therapy.

Other than peripheral neuropathy, serious neurologic events following paclitaxel administration have been rare (<1%) and have included grand mal seizures, syncope, ataxia and neuroencephalopathy.

Rare reports of autonomic neuropathy resulting in paralytic ileus have been received as part of the continuing surveillance of paclitaxel safety.

Arthralgia/Myalgia: There was no consistent relationship between dose or schedule of paclitaxel and the frequency or severity of arthralgia/myalgia. Sixty percent of all patients treated experienced arthralgia/myalgia; 8% experienced severe symptoms. The symptoms were usually transient, occurred two or three days after paclitaxel administration, and resolved within a few days. The frequency and severity of musculoskeletal symptoms remained unchanged throughout the treatment period.

Hepatic: No relationship was observed between liver function abnormalities and either dose or schedule of paclitaxel administration. Among patients with normal baseline liver function 7%, 22% and 19% had elevations in bilirubin, alkaline phosphatase and AST (SGOT), respectively. Prolonged exposure to paclitaxel was not associated with cumulative hepatic toxicity.

Rare reports of hepatic necrosis and hepatic encephalopathy leading to death have been received as part of the continuing surveillance of paclitaxel safety.

Gastrointestinal (GI): Nausea/vomiting, diarrhea and mucositis were reported by 52%, 38% and 31% of all patients, respectively. These manifestations were usually mild to moderate. Mucositis was schedule dependent and occurred more frequently with the 24-hour than with the 3- hour infusion.

Rare reports of intestinal obstruction, intestinal perforation and ischemic colitis have been received as part of the continuing surveillance of paclitaxel safety.

ADVERSE REACTIONS: *(cont'd)*

Injection Site Reaction: Injection site reactions, including reactions secondary to extravasation, were usually mild and consisted of erythema, tenderness, skin discoloration, or swelling at the injection site. These reactions have been observed more frequently with 24-hour infusion than with 3-hour infusion. A specific treatment for extravasation reactions is unknown at this time.

Rare reports of more severe events such as phlebitis and cellulitis have been received as part of the continuing surveillance of paclitaxel safety.

Other Clinical Events: Alopecia was observed in almost all (87%) of the patients. Transient skin changes due to paclitaxel related hypersensitivity reactions have been observed, but no other skin toxicities were significantly associated with paclitaxel administration. Nail changes (changes in pigmentation or discoloration of nail bed) were uncommon (2%). Edema was reported in 21% of all patients (17% of those without baseline edema); only 1% had severe edema and none of these patients required treatment discontinuation. Edema was most commonly focal and disease-related. Edema was observed in 5% of all courses for patients with normal baseline and did not increase with time on study.

Rare reports of skin abnormalities related to radiation recall have been received as part of the continuing surveillance of paclitaxel safety.

OVERDOSAGE:

There is no known antidote for paclitaxel for injection concentrate overdosage. The primary anticipated complications of overdosage would consist of bone marrow suppression, peripheral neurotoxicity and mucositis.

DOSAGE AND ADMINISTRATION:

Note: Contact of the undiluted concentrate with plasticized PVC equipment or devices used to prepare solutions for infusion is not recommended. In order to minimize patient exposure to the plasticizer DEHP [di-(2- ethylhexyl)phthalate], which may be leached from PVC infusion bags or sets, diluted paclitaxel solutions should be stored in bottles (glass, propylene) or plastic bags (polypropylene, polyolefin) and administered through polyethylene-lined administration sets.

All patients should be premedicated prior to paclitaxel administration in order to prevent severe hypersensitivity reactions. Such premedication may consist of dexamethasone 20 mg PO administered approximately 12 and 6 hours before paclitaxel, diphenhydramine (or its equivalent) 50 mg IV 30 to 60 minutes prior to paclitaxel, and cimetidine (300 mg) or ranitidine (50 mg) IV 30 to 60 minutes before paclitaxel.

In patients with carcinoma of the ovary, paclitaxel has been used at several doses and schedules; however, the optimal regimen is not yet clear (see CLINICAL PHARMACOLOGY.) In patients previously treated with chemotherapy for ovarian cancer, the recommended regimen is paclitaxel 135 mg/m^2 or 175 mg/m^{2}administered intravenously over three hours every three weeks.

For patients with carcinoma of the breast, paclitaxel at a dose of 175 mg/m^2 administered intravenously over 3 hours every three weeks has been shown to be effective after failure of chemotherapy for metastatic disease or relapse within 6 months of adjuvant chemotherapy.

Courses of paclitaxel should not be repeated until the neutrophil count is at least 1,500 cells/mm^3 and the platelet count is at least 100,000 cells/mm^3. Patients who experience severe neutropenia (neutrophil <500 cells/mm^{3}for a week or longer) or severe peripheral neuropathy during paclitaxel therapy should have dosage reduced by 20% for subsequent courses of paclitaxel. The incidence of neurotoxicity and the severity of neutropenia increase with dose.

Preparation and Administration Precautions: Paclitaxel is a cytotoxic anticancer drug and, as with other potentially toxic compounds, caution should be exercised in handling paclitaxel. The use of gloves is recommended. If paclitaxel solution contacts the skin, wash the skin immediately and thoroughly with soap and water. If paclitaxel contacts mucous membranes, the membranes should be flushed thoroughly with water.

Preparation for Intravenous Administration: Paclitaxel for Injection Concentrate must be diluted prior to infusion. Paclitaxel should be diluted in 0.9% Sodium Chloride Injection, USP, 5% Dextrose Injection, USP, 5% Dextrose and 0.9% Sodium Chloride Injection, USP or 5% Dextrose in Ringer's Injection to a final concentration of 0.3 to 1.2 mg/ml. The solutions are physically and chemically stable for up to 27 hours at ambient temperature (approximately 25°C) and room lighting conditions. Parenteral drug products should be inspected visually for particulate matter and discoloration prior to administration whenever solution and container permit.

Upon preparation, solutions may show haziness, which is attributed to the formulation vehicle. No significant losses in potency have been noted following simulated delivery of the solution through IV tubing containing an in-line (0.22 micron) filter.

Data collected for the presence of the extractable plasticizer DEHP [di- (2-ethylhexyl) phthalate] show that levels increase with time and concentration when dilutions are prepared in PVC containers. Consequently, the use of plasticized PVC containers and administration sets is not recommended. Paclitaxel solutions should be prepared and stored in glass, polypropylene, or polyolefin containers. Non-PVC containing administration sets, such as those which are polyethylene-lined, should be used.

Paclitaxel should be administered through an in-line filter with a microporous membrane not greater than 0.22 microns. Use of filter devices such as IVEX-2 filters which incorporate short inlet and outlet PVC-coated tubing has not resulted in significant leaching of DEHP.

Stability: Unopened vials of paclitaxel are stable until the date indicated on the package when stored under refrigeration, 2°- 8°C (36°-46°F), in the original package. Freezing does not adversely affect the product. Upon refrigeration components in the paclitaxel vial may precipitate, but will redissolve upon reaching room temperature with little or no agitation. There is no impact on product quality under these circumstances. If the solution remains cloudy or if an insoluble precipitate is noted, the vial should be discarded. Solutions for infusion prepared as recommended are stable at ambient temperature (approximately 25°C) and lighting conditions for up to 27 hours.

HOW SUPPLIED:

Storage: Store the vials in original cartons under refrigeration, 2°-8°C (36°-46°F). Retain in the original package to protect from light.

Handling and Disposal: Procedures for proper handling and disposal of anticancer drugs should be considered. Several guidelines on this subject have been published.[2-6] There is no general agreement that all of the procedures recommended in the guidelines are necessary or appropriate.

REFERENCES:

1. Rowinsky EK, et al: Sequences of paclitaxel and Cisplatin: A Phase I and Pharmacologic Study. J Clin Oncol 1991: 9(9):1692-1703. **2.** Recommendations for the Safe Handling of Parenteral Antineoplastic Drugs. NIH Publication No. 83-2621. For sale by the Superintendent of Documents, US Government Printing Office, Washington, DC 20402. **3.** AMA Council Report. Guidelines for Handling Parenteral Antineoplastics. JAMA 1985; 253 (11): 1590-1592. **4.** National Study Commission on Cytotoxic Exposure - Recommendations for Handling Cytotoxic Agents. Available from Louis P. Jeffrey, ScD, Chairman, National Study Commission on Cytotoxic Exposure. Massachusetts College of Pharmacy and Allied Health Sciences, 179 Longwood Avenue, Boston, Massachusetts, 02115. **5.** Clinical Oncological Society of Australia. Guidelines and Recommendations for Safe Handling of Antineoplastic Agents. Med J Australia 1983; 1:426-428. **6.** Jones RB, et al: Safe Handling of Chemotherapeutic Agents: A Report from the Mount Sinai Medical Center. Ca-A Cancer Journal for Clinicians

REFERENCES: *(cont'd)*

1983; (Sept/Oct) 258-263. **7.** American Society of Hospital Pharmacists Technical Assistance Bulletin on Handling Cytotoxic and Hazardous Drugs. Am J Hosp Pharm 1990; 47:1033-1049. **8.** OSHA Work-Practice Guidelines for Personnel Dealing with Cytotoxic (Antineoplastic) Drugs. Am J Hosp Pharm 1986; 43:1193-1204.

HOW SUPPLIED - EQUIVALENTS NOT AVAILABLE:

Injection, Solution - Intravenous - 30 mg/5ml

5 ml $175.35 TAXOL, Mead Johnson 00015-3475-27

PAMIDRONATE DISODIUM *(003067)*

CATEGORIES: Biphosphonates; Bone Metabolism Regulators; Bone Resorption Inhibitors; Calcium Metabolism; Hypercalcemia Of Malignancy; Hypercalcemic Agents; Oncologic Drugs; Osteolytic Bone Metastases of Breast Cancer; Osteolytic Lesions of Multiple Myeloma; Paget's Disease; Tumors; Osteoporosis*; Pregnancy Category C; FDA Class 1B ("Modest Therapeutic Advantage"); FDA Approved 1991 Oct

* Indication not approved by the FDA

BRAND NAMES: **Aredia**

DESCRIPTION:

Aredia, pamidronate disodium, (APD), is a bone-resorption inhibitor available in 30-mg, 60-mg, or 90-mg vials for intravenous administration. Each 30-mg, 60-mg, and 90-mg vial contains, respectively, 30 mg, 60 mg, and 90 mg of sterile, lyophilized pamidronate disodium and 470 mg, 400 mg, and 375 mg of mannitol, USP. The pH of a 1% solution of pamidronate disodium in distilled water is approximately 8.3. Aredia, a member of the group of chemical compounds known as bisphosphonates, is an analog of pyrophosphate. Pamidronate disodium is designated chemically as phosphonic acid (3-amino-1-hydroxypropylidene) bis-, disodium salt, pentahydrate, (APD).

Pamidronate disodium is a white-to-practically-white powder. It is soluble in water and in 2N sodium hydroxide, sparingly soluble in 0.1N hydrochloric acid and in 0.1N acetic acid, and practically insoluble in organic solvents. Its molecular formula is $C_3H_9NO_7P_2NA_2{\cdot}5H_20$ and its molecular weight is 369.1.

Inactive Ingredients: Mannitol, USP, and phosphoric acid (for adjustment to pH 6.5 prior to lyophilization).

CLINICAL PHARMACOLOGY:

The principal pharmacologic action of pamidronate disodium is inhibition of bone resorption. Although the mechanism of antiresorptive action is not completely understood, several factors are thought to contribute to this action. Pamidronate disodium absorbs to calcium phosphate (hydroxyapatite) crystals in bone and may directly block dissolution of this mineral component of bone. *In vitro* studies also suggest that inhibition of osteoclast activity contributes to inhibition of bone resorption. In animal studies, at doses recommended for the treatment of hypercalcemia, pamidronate disodium inhibits bone resorption apparently without inhibiting bone formation and mineralization. Of relevance to the treatment of hypercalcemia of malignancy is the finding that pamidronate disodium inhibits the accelerated bone resorption that results from osteoclast hyperactivity induced by various tumors in animal studies.

PHARMACOKINETICS

Cancer patients (n=24) who had minimal or no bony involvement were given an intravenous infusion of 30, 60, or 90 mg of pamidronate disodium over 4 hours and 90 mg of pamidronate over 24 hours (TABLE 1).

TABLE 1 Mean (SD, CV%) Pamidronate Pharmacokinetic Parameters in Cancer Patients (n=6 for each group)

Dose (infusion rate)	Maximum Concentration (mcg/ml)	Percent of dose excreted in urine	Total Clearance (ml/min)	Renal Clearance (ml/min)
30 mg (4 hrs)	0.73 (0.14, 19.1%)	43.9 (14.0, 31.9%)	136 (44, 32.4%)	58 (27, 46.5%)
60 mg (4 hrs)	1.44 (0.57, 39.6%)	47.4 (47.4%, 54.4%)	88 (56, 63.6%)	42 (28, 66.7%)
90 mg (4 hrs)	2.61 (0.74, 28.3%)	45.3 (25.8, 56.9%)	103 (37, 35.9%)	44 (16, 36.4%)
90 mg (24 hrs)	1.38 (1.97, 142.7%)	47.5 (10.2, 21.5%)	101 (58, 57.4%)	52 (42, 80.8%)

Distribution: The mean ± SD body retention of pamidronate was calculated to be 54 ± 16% of the dose over 120 hours.

Metabolism: Pamidronate is not metabolized and is exclusively eliminated by renal excretion.

Excretion: After administration of 30, 60, and 90 mg of pamidronate disodium over 4 hours, and 90 mg of pamidronate disodium over 24 hours, an overall mean ± SD of 46 ± 16% of the drug was excreted unchanged in the urine within 120 hours. Cumulative urinary excretion was linearly related to dose. The mean ± SD elimination half-life is 28 ± 7 hours. Mean ± SD total and renal clearances of pamidronate were 107 ± 50 ml/min and 49 ± 28 ml/min, respectively. The rate of elimination from bone has not been determined.

Special Populations

There are no data available on the effects of age, gender, or race on the pharmacokinetics of pamidronate.

Pediatric: Pamidronate is not labeled for use in the pediatric population.

Renal Insufficiency: The pharmacokinetics of pamidronate were studied in cancer patients (n=19) with normal and varying degrees of renal impairment. Each patient received a single 90 mg dose of pamidronate disodium infused over 4 hours. The renal clearance of pamidronate in patients was found to closely correlate with creatinine clearance. A trend toward a lower percentage of drug excreted unchanged in urine was observed in renally impaired patients. Adverse experiences noted were not found to be related to changes in renal clearance of pamidronate. Given the recommended dose, 90 mg infused over 4 hours, excessive accumulation of pamidronate in renally impaired patients is not anticipated if pamidronate is administered on a monthly basis.

Hepatic Insufficiency: There are no human pharmacokinetic data for pamidronate disodium in patients who have hepatic insufficiency.

Drug-Drug Interactions: There are no human pharmacokinetic data for drug interactions with pamidronate disodium.

After intravenous administration of radiolabeled pamidronate in rats, approximately 50%-60% of the compound was rapidly absorbed by bone and slowly eliminated from the body by the kidneys. In rats given 10 mg/kg bolus injections of radiolabeled pamidronate disodium, approximately 30% of the compound was found in the liver shortly after administration and was then redistributed to bone or eliminated by the kidneys over 24-48 hours. Studies in rats injected with radiolabeled pamidronate disodium showed that the compound was rapidly

CLINICAL PHARMACOLOGY: *(cont'd)*

cleared from the circulation and taken up mainly by bones, liver, spleen, teeth, and tracheal cartilage. Radioactivity was eliminated from most soft tissues within 1-4 days; was detectable in liver and spleen for 1 and 3 months, respectively; and remained high in bones, trachea, and teeth for 6 months after dosing. Bone uptake occurred preferentially in areas of high bone turnover. The terminal phase of elimination half-life in bone was estimated to be approximately 300 days.

PHARMACODYNAMICS

Serum phosphate levels have been noted to decrease after administration of pamidronate disodium, presumably because of decreased release of phosphate from bone and increased renal excretion as parathyroid hormone levels, which are usually suppressed in hypercalcemia associated with malignancy, return toward normal. Phosphate therapy was administered in 30% of the patients in response to a decrease in serum phosphate levels. Phosphate levels usually returned toward normal within 7-10 days.

Urinary calcium/creatinine and urinary hydroxyproline/creatinine ratios decrease and usually return to within or below normal after treatment with pamidronate disodium. These changes occur within the first week after treatment, as do decreases in serum calcium levels, and are consistent with an antiresorptive pharmacologic action.

HYPERCALCEMIA OF MALIGNANCY

Osteoclastic hyperactivity resulting in excessive bone resorption is the underlying pathophysiologic derangement in metastatic bone disease and hypercalcemia of malignancy. Excessive release of calcium into the blood as bone is resorbed results in polyuria and gastrointestinal disturbances, with progressive dehydration and decreasing glomerular filtration rate. This, in turn, results in increased renal resorption of calcium, setting up a cycle of worsening systemic hypercalcemia. Correction of excessive bone resorption and adequate fluid administration to correct volume deficits are therefore essential to the management of hypercalcemia.

Most cases of hypercalcemia associated with malignancy occur in patients who have breast cancer; squamous-cell tumors of the lung or head and neck; renal-cell carcinoma; and certain hematologic malignancies, such as multiple myeloma and some types of lymphomas. A few less-common malignancies, including vasoactive intestinal-peptide-producing tumors and cholangiocarcinoma, have a high incidence of hypercalcemia as a metabolic complication. Patients who have hypercalcemia of malignancy can generally be divided into two groups, according to the pathophysiologic mechanism involved.

In humoral hypercalcemia, osteoclasts are activated and bone resorption is stimulated by factors such as parathyroid-hormone-related protein, which are elaborated by the tumor and circulate systemically. Humoral hypercalcemia usually occurs in squamous-cell malignancies of the lung or head and neck or in genitourinary tumors such as renal-cell carcinoma or ovarian cancer. Skeletal metastases may be absent or minimal in these patients.

Extensive invasion of bone by tumor cells can also result in hypercalcemia due to local tumor products that stimulate bone resorption by osteoclasts. Tumors commonly associated with locally mediated hypercalcemia include breast cancer and multiple myeloma.

Total serum calcium levels in patients who have hypercalcemia of malignancy may not reflect the severity of hypercalcemia, since concomitant hypoalbuminemia is commonly present. Ideally, ionized calcium levels should be used to diagnose and follow hypercalcemic conditions; however, these are not commonly or rapidly available in many clinical situations. Therefore, adjustment of the total serum calcium value for differences in albumin levels is often used in place of measurement of ionized calcium; several nomograms are in use for this type of calculation (See DOSAGE AND ADMINISTRATION.)

PAGET'S DISEASE

Paget's disease of bone (osteitis deformans) is an idiopathic disease characterized by chronic, focal areas of bone destruction complicated by concurrent excessive bone repair, affecting one or more bones. These changes result in thickened but weakened bones that may fracture or bend under stress. Signs and symptoms may be bone pain, deformity, fractures, neurological disorders resulting from cranial and spinal nerve entrapment and from spinal cord and brain stem compression, increased cardiac output to the involved bone, increased serum alkaline phosphatase levels (reflecting increased bone formation) and/or urine hydroxyproline excretion (reflecting increased bone resorption).

OSTEOLYTIC BONE METASTASES OF BREAST CANCER AND OSTEOLYTIC LESIONS OF MULTIPLE MYELOMA

Osteolytic bone metastases commonly occur in patients with multiple myeloma or breast cancer. These cancers demonstrate a phenomenon known as osteotropism, meaning they possess an extraordinary affinity for bone. The distribution of osteolytic bone metastases in these cancers is predominantly in the axial skeleton, particularly in the spine, pelvis, and ribs, rather than the appendicular skeleton, although lesions in the proximal femur and humerus are not uncommon. This distribution is similar to the red bone marrow in which slow blood flow possibly assists attachment of metastatic cells. The surface-to-volume ratio of trabecular bone is much higher than cortical bone, and therefore disease processes tend to occur more floridly in trabecular bone than at sites of cortical tissue.

These bone changes can result in patients having evidence of osteolytic skeletal destruction leading to severe bone pain that requires either radiation therapy or narcotic analgesics (or both) for symptomatic relief. These changes also cause pathologic fractures of bone in both the axial and appendicular skeleton. Axial skeletal fractures of the vertebral bodies may lead to spinal cord compression or vertebral body collapse with significant neurologic complications. Also patients may experience episode(s) of hypercalcemia.

CLINICAL STUDIES:

HYPERCALCEMIA OF MALIGNANCY

In one double-blind clinical trial, 52 patients who had hypercalcemia of malignancy were enrolled to receive 30 mg, 60 mg, or 90 mg of pamidronate disodium as a single 24-hour intravenous infusion if their corrected serum calcium levels were 12.0 mg/dl after 48 hours of saline hydration.

The mean baseline-corrected serum calcium for the 30 mg, 60 mg and 90 mg groups were 13.8 mg/dl, 13.8 mg/dl and 13.3 mg/dl, respectively.

The majority of patients (64%) had decreases in albumin-corrected serum calcium levels by 24 hours after initiation of treatment. Mean-corrected serum calcium levels at days 2-7 after initiation of treatment with pamidronate disodium were significantly reduced from baseline in all three dosage groups. As a result, by 7 days after initiation of treatment with pamidronate disodium, 40%, 61%, and 100% of the patients receiving 30 mg, 60 mg, and 90 mg of pamidronate disodium, respectively, had normal corrected serum calcium levels. Many patients (33%-53%) in the 60-mg and 90-mg dosage groups continued to have normal-corrected serum calcium levels, or a partial response (15% decrease of corrected serum calcium from baseline), at day 14.

In a second double-blind, controlled clinical trial, 65 cancer patients who had corrected serum calcium levels of 12.0 mg/dl after at least 24 hours of saline hydration were randomized to receive either 60 mg of pamidronate disodium as a single 24-hour intravenous infusion or 7.5 mg/kg of Didronel (etidronate disodium) as a 2-hour intravenous infusion daily for 3 days. Thirty patients were randomized to receive pamidronate disodium and 35 to receive Didronel.

CLINICAL STUDIES: *(cont'd)*

The mean baseline-corrected serum calcium for the pamidronate disodium 60 mg and Didronel groups were 14.6 mg/dl and 13.8 mg/dl, respectively.

By day 7, 70% of the patients in the pamidronate disodium group and 41% of the patients in the Didronel group had normal-corrected serum calcium levels ($P<0.05$). When partial responders (≥15% decrease of serum calcium from baseline) were also included, the response rates were 97% for the pamidronate disodium group and 65% for the Didronel group ($P<0.01$). Mean corrected serum calcium for the pamidronate disodium and Didronel groups decreased from baseline values to 10.4 and 11.2 mg/dl, respectively, on day 7. At day 14, 43% of patients in the pamidronate disodium group and 18% of patients in the Didronel group still had normal-corrected serum calcium levels, or maintenance of a partial response. For responders in the pamidronate disodium and Didronel groups, the median duration of response was similar (7 and 5 days, respectively). The time course of effect on corrected serum calcium is summarized in TABLE 2.

TABLE 2 Change in Corrected Serum Calcium by Time from Initiation of Treatment

Time (hr)	Mean Change from Baseline in Corrected Serum Calcium (mg/dl) Pamidronate Disodium	Didronel	P-Value[1]
Baseline	14.6	13.8	
24	-0.3	-0.5	
48	-1.5	-1.1	
72	-2.6	-2.0	
96	-3.5	-2.0	<0.01
168	-4.1	-2.5	<0.01

[1]Comparison between treatment groups

In a third multicenter, randomized, parallel double-blind trial, a group of 69 cancer patients with hypercalcemia was enrolled to receive 60 mg of pamidronate disodium as a 4- or 24-hour infusion, which was compared to a saline treatment group. Patients who had a corrected serum calcium level of 12.0 mg/dl after 24 hours of saline hydration were eligible for this trial.

The mean baseline-corrected serum calcium levels for pamidronate disodium 60-mg 4-hour infusion, pamidronate disodium 60-mg 24-hour infusion, and saline infusion were 14.2 mg/dl, 13.7 mg/dl, and 13.7 mg/dl, respectively.

By day 7 after initiation of treatment, 78%, 61%, and 22% of the patients had normal-corrected serum calcium levels for the 60-mg 4-hour infusion, 60-mg 24-hour infusion, and saline infusion, respectively. At day 14, 39% of the patients in the pamidronate disodium 60-mg 4-hour infusion group and 26% of the patients in the pamidronate disodium 60-mg 24-hour infusion group had normal-corrected serum calcium levels or maintenance of a partial response.

For responders, the median duration of complete responses was 4 days and 6.5 days for pamidronate disodium 60-mg 4-hour infusion and pamidronate disodium 60-mg 24-hour infusion, respectively.

In all three trials, patients treated with pamidronate disodium had similar response rates in the presence or absence of bone metastases. Concomitant administration of furosemide did not affect response rates.

Thirty-two patients who had recurrent or refractory hypercalcemia of malignancy were given a second course of 60 mg of pamidronate disodium over a 4- or 24-hour period. Of these, 41% showed a complete response and 16% showed a partial response to the retreatment, and these responders had about a 3-mg/dl fall in mean-corrected serum calcium levels 7 days after retreatment.

Unlike pamidronate disodium 60 mg, the drug has not been investigated in a controlled clinical trial employing a 90-mg dose infused over a 4-hour period.

PAGET'S DISEASE

In one, double-blind, clinical trial, 64 patients with moderate to severe Paget's disease of bone were enrolled to receive 5 mg, 15 mg, or 30 mg of pamidronate disodium as a single 4-hour infusion on 3 consecutive days, for total doses of 15 mg, 45 mg, and 90 mg of pamidronate disodium.

The mean baseline serum alkaline phosphatase levels were 1409 U/L, 983 U/L, and 1085 U/L, and the mean baseline urine hydroxyproline/creatinine ratios were 0.25, 0.19, and 0.19 for the 15-mg, 45-mg, and 90-mg groups, respectively.

The effects of pamidronate disodium on serum alkaline phosphatase (SAP) and urine hydroxyproline/creatinine ratios (UOHP/C) are summarized in TABLE 3.

TABLE 3 Percent of Patients With Significant % Decreases in SAP and UOHP/C

% Decrease	SAP 15 mg	SAP 45 mg	SAP 90 mg	UOHP/C 15 mg	UOHP/C 45 mg	UOHP/C 90 mg
50	26	33	60	15	47	72
30	40	65	83	35	57	85

The medium maximum percent decreases from baseline in serum alkaline phosphatase and urine hydroxyproline/creatinine ratios were 25%, 41%, and 57%, and 25%, 47%, and 61% for the 15-mg, 45-mg, and 90-mg groups, respectively. The median time to response (50% decrease) for serum alkaline phosphatase was approximately 1 month for the 90-mg group, and the response duration ranged from 1 to 372 days.

No statistically significant differences between treatment groups, or statistically significant changes from baseline were observed for the bone pain response, mobility, and global evaluation in the 45-mg and 90-mg groups. Improvement in radiologic lesions occurred in some patients in the 90-mg group.

Twenty-five patients who had Paget's disease were retreated with 90 mg of pamidronate disodium. Of these, 44% had a 50% decrease in serum alkaline phosphatase from baseline after treatment, and 39% had a 50% decrease in urine hydroxyproline/creatinine ratio from baseline after treatment.

OSTEOLYTIC LESIONS OF MULTIPLE MYELOMA

In a double-blind, randomized, placebo-controlled trial, 392 patients with advanced multiple myeloma were enrolled to receive pamidronate disodium or placebo in addition to their underlying antimyeloma therapy to determine the effect of pamidronate disodium on the occurrence of skeletal-related events (SRE's). SRE's were defined as episodes of pathologic fractures, radiation therapy to bone, surgery to bone, and spinal cord compression. Patients received either 90 mg of pamidronate disodium or placebo as a monthly 4-hour intravenous infusion for 9 months. Of the 392 patients, 377 were evaluable for efficacy (196 pamidronate disodium, 181 placebo). The proportion of patients developing any SRE was significantly smaller in the pamidronate disodium group (24% vs 41%, $P<0.001$), and the mean skeletal morbidity rate (#SRE/year) was significantly smaller for pamidronate patients than for placebo patients (mean: 1.1 vs.2.1, P,.02). The times to the first SRE occurrence, pathological fracture, and radiation to bone were significantly longer in the pamidronate disodium group

CLINICAL STUDIES: *(cont'd)*

(P=.001,.006 and.046, respectively). Moreover, fewer pamidronate disodium patients suffered any pathologic fracture (17% vs 30%, P=.004) or needed radiation to bone (14% vs 22%, P=.049).

In addition, decreases in pain scores from baseline occurred at the last measurement for those pamidronate disodium patients with pain at baseline (P=.026) but not in the placebo group. At the last measurement, a worsening from baseline was observed in the placebo group for the Spitzer quality of life variable (P<0.001) and ECOG performance status (P<.011) while there was no significant deterioration from baseline in these parameters observed in pamidronate disodium-treated patients.*

After 21 months, the proportion of patients experiencing any skeletal event remained significantly smaller in the pamidronate disodium group than the placebo group (P=.015). In addition, the mean skeletal morbidity rate (#SRE/year) was 1.3 vs 2.2 for pamidronate disodium patients vs placebo patients (P=.008), and time to first SRE was significantly longer in the pamidronate disodium group compared to placebo (P=.016). Fewer pamidronate disodium patients suffered vertebral pathologic fractures (16% vs 27%, P=.005). Survival of all patients was not different between treatment groups.

OSTEOLYTIC BONE METASTASES OF BREAST CANCER

Two double-blind, randomized, placebo-controlled trials compared the safety and efficacy of 90 mg of pamidronate disodium infused over 2 hours every 3 to 4 weeks for 12 months to that of placebo in preventing SREs in breast cancer patients with osteolytic bone metastases who had one or more predominantly lytic metastases of at least 1 cm in diameter: one in patients being treated with antineoplastic chemotherapy and the second in patients being treated with hormonal antineoplastic therapy at trial entry.

382 patients receiving chemotherapy were randomized, 185 to pamidronate disodium and 197 to placebo. 372 patients receiving hormonal therapy were randomized, 182 to pamidronate disodium and 190 to placebo. All but three patients were evaluable for efficacy. The efficacy results on SREs are shown in TABLES 4 and 5.

TABLE 4 Breast Cancer Patients Receiving Chemotherapy

	Any SRE		Radiation‡	
N	A 185	P 195	A 185	P 195
Skeletal Morbidity Rate (#SRE/year) Mean	2.1	3.3	0.6	1.1
P-Value	<.01		<.01	
Proportion of patients having an SRE	43%	56%	19%	33%
P-Value	<.01		<.01	
Median Time to SRE (months)	13.1	7.0	NR**	NR**
P-Value	<.01		<.01	

‡ Radiation to bone was a secondary endpoint.

** NR=Not Reached.

TABLE 5 Breast Cancer Patients Receiving Hormonal Therapy

	Any SRE		Radiation†	
N	A 182	P 189	A 182	P 189
Skeletal Morbidity Rate (#SRE/year) Mean	2.4	3.5	0.6	1.1
P-Value	.05		<.01	
Proportion of patients having an SRE	47%	55%	21%	33%
P-Value	.11		.01	
Median Time to SRE (months)	10.9	7.4	NR**	NR**
P-Value	.16		<.01	

† Radiation to bone was a secondary endpoint.

** NR=Not Reached.

Bone lesion response was radiographically assessed at baseline and at 3, 6, and 12 months. The complete + partial response rate was 33% in pamidronate disodium patients and 18% in placebo patients treated with chemotherapy (P=.001). No difference was seen between pamidronate disodium and placebo in hormonally-treated patients.

Pain and analgesic scores, ECOG performance status and Spitzer quality of life index were measured at baseline and periodically during the trials. The changes from baseline to the last measurement carried forward are shown in TABLES 6A and 6B.

TABLE 6A Mean Change ([Dgr]) from Baseline‡ at Last Measurement

	Breast Cancer Patients Receiving Chemotherapy				
	Pamidronate Disodium		Placebo		
	N	Mean [Dgr]	N	Mean [Dgr]	A vs P P-Value*
Pain Score	175	+0.3	183	+1.1	<.05
Analgesic Score	175	+0.3	183	+0.9	.05
ECOG PS	178	+0.6	186	+0.8	.03
Spitzer QOL	177	-1.2	185	-1.6	.11

‡ Decreases in pain, analgesic scores and ECOG PS, and increases in Spitzer QOL indicate an improvement from baseline.

* The statistical significance of analyses of these secondary endpoints of pain, quality of life, and performance status in all three trials may be overestimated since numerous analyses were performed.

TABLE 6B Mean Change ([Dgr]) from Baseline‡ at Last Measurement

	Breast Cancer Patients Receiving Hormonal Therapy				
	Pamidronate Disodium		Placebo		
	N	Mean [Dgr]	N	Mean [Dgr]	A vs P P-Value*
Pain Score	173	-0.3	179	+0.8	<.01
Analgesic Score	173	+0.4	179	+1.5	<.01
ECOG PS	175	+0.5	182	+0.6	.23
Spitzer QOL	173	-0.9	181	-1.4	.07

‡ Decreases in pain, analgesic scores and ECOG PS, and increases in Spitzer QOL indicate an improvement from baseline.

* The statistical significance of analyses of these secondary endpoints of pain, quality of life, and performance status in all three trials may be overestimated since numerous analyses were performed.

INDICATIONS AND USAGE:

Hypercalcemia of Malignancy: Pamidronate disodium, in conjunction with adequate hydration, is indicated for the treatment of moderate or severe hypercalcemia associated with malignancy, with or without bone metastases. Patients who have either epidermoid or non-epidermoid tumors respond to treatment with pamidronate disodium. Vigorous saline hydration, an integral part of hypercalcemia therapy, should be initiated promptly and an attempt should be made to restore the urine output to about 2 L/day throughout treatment. Mild or asymptomatic hypercalcemia may be treated with conservative measures (*i.e.*, saline hydration, with or without loop diuretics). Patients should be hydrated adequately throughout the treatment, but overhydration, especially in those patients who have cardiac failure, must be avoided. Diuretic therapy should not be employed prior to correction of hypovolemia. The safety and efficacy of pamidronate disodium in the treatment of hypercalcemia associated with hyperparathyroidism or with other non-tumor-related conditions has not been established.

Paget's Disease: Pamidronate disodium is indicated for the treatment of patients with moderate to severe Paget's disease of bone. The effectiveness of pamidronate disodium was demonstrated primarily in patients with serum alkaline phosphatase 3 times the upper limit of normal. Pamidronate disodium therapy in patients with Paget's disease has been effective in reducing serum alkaline phosphatase and urinary hydroxyproline levels by 50% in at least 50% of patients, and by 30% in at least 80% of patients. Pamidronate disodium therapy has also been effective in reducing these biochemical markers in patients with Paget's disease who failed to respond, or no longer responded to other treatments.

Osteolytic Bone Metastases of Breast Cancer and Osteolytic Lesions of Multiple Myeloma: Pamidronate disodium is indicated, in conjunction with standard antineoplastic therapy, for the treatment of osteolytic bone metastases of breast cancer and osteolytic lesions of multiple myeloma. The pamidronate disodium treatment effect appeared to be smaller in the study of breast cancer patients receiving hormonal therapy than in the study of those receiving chemotherapy (see CLINICAL STUDIES, Osteolytic Bone Metastases of Breast Cancer and Osteolytic Lesions of Multiple Myeloma.

CONTRAINDICATIONS:

Pamidronate disodium is contraindicated in patients with clinically significant hypersensitivity to pamidronate disodium or other bisphosphonates.

WARNINGS:

In both rats and dogs, nephropathy has been associated with intravenous (bolus and infusion) administration of pamidronate disodium.

Two 7-day intravenous infusion studies were conducted in the dog wherein pamidronate disodium was given for 1, 4, or 24 hours at doses of 1-20 mg/kg for up to 7 days. In the first study, the compound was well tolerated at 3 mg/kg (1.7 x highest recommended human dose [HRHD] for a single intravenous infusion) when administered for 4 or 24 hours, but renal findings such as elevated BUN and creatinine levels and renal tubular necrosis occurred when 3 mg/kg was infused for 1 hour and at doses of 10 mg/kg. In the second study, slight renal tubular necrosis was observed in 1 male at 1 mg/kg when infused for 4 hours. Additional findings included elevated BUN levels in several treated animals and renal tubular dilation and/or inflammation at 1 mg/kg after each infusion time.

Pamidronate disodium was given to rats at doses of 2, 6, and 20 mg/kg and to dogs at doses of 2, 4, 6, and 20 mg/kg as a 1-hour infusion, once a week, for 3 months followed by a 1-month recovery period. In rats, nephrotoxicity was observed at 6 mg/kg and included increased BUN and creatinine levels and tubular degeneration and necrosis. These findings were still present at 20 mg/kg at the end of the recovery period. In dogs, moribundity/death and renal toxicity occurred at 20 mg/kg as did kidney findings of elevated BUN and creatinine levels at 6 mg/kg and renal tubular degeneration at 4 mg/kg. The kidney changes were partially reversible at 6 mg/kg. In both studies, the dose level that produced no adverse renal effects was considered to be 2 mg/kg (1.1 x HRHD for a single intravenous infusion).

Patients who receive an intravenous infusion of pamidronate disodium should have periodic evaluations of standard laboratory and clinical parameters of renal function.

Studies conducted in young rats have reported the disruption of dental dentine formation following single- and multi-dose administration of bisphosphonates. The clinical significance of these findings is unknown.

PRECAUTIONS:

General: Standard hypercalcemia-related metabolic parameters, such as serum levels of calcium, phosphate, magnesium, and potassium, should be carefully monitored following initiation of therapy with pamidronate disodium. Cases of asymptomatic hypophosphatemia (12%), hypokalemia (7%), hypomagnesemia (11%), and hypocalcemia (5-12%), were reported in pamidronate disodium-treated patients. Rare cases of symptomatic hypocalcemia (including tetany) have been reported in association with pamidronate disodium therapy. If hypocalcemia occurs, short-term calcium therapy may be necessary. In Paget's disease of bone, 17% of patients treated with 90 mg of pamidronate disodium showed serum calcium levels below 8 mg/dl.

Pamidronate disodium has not been tested in patients who have class Dc renal impairment (creatinine >5.0 mg/dl), and in few multiple myeloma patients with serum creatinine 3.0 mg/dl (See CLINICAL PHARMACOLOGY, Pharmacokinetics) Clinical judgement should determine whether the potential benefit outweighs the potential risk in such patients.

Laboratory Tests: Serum calcium, electrolytes, phosphate, magnesium and creatinine, and CBC differential, and hematocrit/hemoglobin must be closely monitored in patients treated with pamidronate disodium. Patients who have preexisting anemia, leukopenia, or thrombocytopenia should be monitored carefully in the first 2 weeks following treatment.

Carcinogenesis, Mutagenesis, Impairment of Fertility: In a 104-week carcinogenicity study (daily oral administration) in rats, there was a positive dose response relationship for benign adrenal pheochromocytoma in males ($p<0.00001$). Although this condition was also observed in females, the incidence was not statistically significant. When the dose calculations were adjusted to account for the limited oral bioavailability of pamidronate disodium in rats, the

PRECAUTIONS: *(cont'd)*

lowest daily dose associated with adrenal pheochromocytoma was similar to the intended clinical dose. Adrenal pheochromocytoma was also observed in low numbers in the control animals and is considered a relatively common spontaneous neoplasm in the rat. Pamidronate disodium (daily oral administration) was not carcinogenic in an 80-week study in mice.

Pamidronate disodium was nonmutagenic in six mutagenicity assays: Ames test,*Salmonella* and *Escherichia*/liver-microsome test, nucleus-anomaly test, sister-chromatid-exchange study, point-mutation test, and micronucleus test in the rat.

In rats, decreased fertility occurred in first-generation offspring of parents who had received 150 mg/kg of pamidronate disodium orally; however, this occurred only when animals were mated with members of the same dose group. Pamidronate disodium has not been administered intravenously in such a study.

Pregnancy Category C: There are no adequate and well-controlled studies in pregnant women.

Bolus intravenous studies conducted in rats and rabbits determined that pamidronate disodium produces maternal toxicity and embryo/fetal effects when given during organogenesis at doses of 0.6 to 8.3 times the highest recommended human dose for a single intravenous infusion. As it has been shown that pamidronate disodium can cross the placenta in rats and has produced marked maternal and nonteratogenic embryo/fetal effects in rats and rabbits, it should not be given to women during pregnancy.

Nursing Mothers: It is not known whether pamidronate disodium is excreted in human milk. Because many drugs are excreted in human milk, caution should be exercised when pamidronate disodium is administered to a nursing woman.

Pediatric Use: Safety and effectiveness of pamidronate disodium in children have not been established.

DRUG INTERACTIONS:

Concomitant administration of a loop diuretic had no effect on the calcium-lowering action of pamidronate disodium.

ADVERSE REACTIONS:

Hypercalcemia of Malignancy: Transient mild elevation of temperature by at least 1°C was noted 24 to 48 hours after administration of pamidronate disodium in 34% of patients in clinical trials. In the saline trial, 18% of patients had a temperature elevation of at least 1°C 24 to 48 hours after treatment.

Drug-related local soft-tissue symptoms (redness, swelling or induration and pain on palpitation) at the site of catheter insertion were most common (18%) in patients treated with 90 mg of pamidronate disodium. When all on-therapy events are considered, that rate rises to 41%. Symptomatic treatment resulted in rapid resolution in all patients.

Rare cases of uveitis, iritis, and episcleritis have been reported, including one case of scleritis, and one case of uveitis upon separate rechallanges.

Four of 128 patients (3%) who received pamidronate disodium during the three U.S. controlled hypercalcemia clinical studies were reported to have had seizures, 2 of whom had preexisting seizure disorders. None of the seizures were considered to be drug-related by the investigators. However, a possible relationship between the drug and the occurrence of seizures cannot be ruled out. It should be noted that in the saline arm 1 patient (4%) had a seizure.

At least 15% of patients treated with pamidronate disodium for hypercalcemia of malignancy also experienced the following adverse events during a clinical trial:

General: Fluid overload, generalized pain.

Cardiovascular: Hypertension.

Gastrointestinal: Abdominal pain, anorexia, constipation, nausea, vomiting.

Genitourinary: Urinary tract infection.

Musculoskeletal: Bone pain.

Laboratory abnormality: Anemia, hypokalemia, hypomagnesemia, hypophosphatemia.

Many of these adverse experiences may have been related to the underlying disease state.

TABLE 7 lists the adverse experiences considered to be treatment-related during comparative, controlled U.S. trials.

Paget's Disease: Transient mild elevation of temperature >1°C above pretreatment baseline was noted within 48 hours after completion of treatment in 21% of the patients treated with 90 mg of pamidronate disodium in clinical trials.

Drug-related musculoskeletal pain and nervous system symptoms (dizziness, headache, paresthesia, increased sweating) were more common in patients with Paget's disease with 90 mg of pamidronate disodium than in patients with hypercalcemia of malignancy treated with the same dose.

Adverse experiences considered to be related to trial drug, which occurred in at least 5% of patients with Paget's disease treated with 90 mg of pamidronate disodium in two U.S. clinical trials, were fever, nausea, back pain, and bone pain.

At least 10% of all pamidronate disodium-treated patients with Paget's disease also experienced the following adverse experiences during clinical trials:

Cardiovascular: Hypertension

Musculoskeletal: Arthrosis, bone pain

Nervous system: Headache

Most of these adverse experiences may have been related to the underlying disease state.

Osteolytic Bone Metastases of Breast Cancer and Osteolytic Lesions of Multiple Myeloma: The most commonly reported (>15%) adverse experiences occurred with similar frequencies in the pamidronate disodium and placebo treatment groups, and most of these adverse experiences may have been related to the underlying disease state or antimyeloma therapy.

Toxicities commonly associated with chemotherapy, including cytopenia, infection, nausea and vomiting, and cachexia, were not more frequent or severe in pamidronate disodium patients than in placebo patients, although viral infection, herpes zoster, and anorexia all occurred more frequently in the pamidronate disodium arm of the study. Mineral and electrolyte disturbances, including hypocalcemia, were reported rarely and in similar percentages of pamidronate disodium-treated patients compared with those in the placebo group. The reported frequencies of hypocalcemia, hypokalemia, hypophosphatemia, and hypomagnesemia for pamidronate disodium treated patients were 3.0%, 8.7%, 1.6% and 3.8%, respectively, and for placebo-treated patients were 1.2%, 10.6%, 1.7% and 4.2%, respectively. In previous hypercalcemia of malignancy trials, patients treated with pamidronate disodium (60 or 90 mg over 24 hours) developed electrolyte abnormalities more frequently (see ADVERSE REACTIONS, Hypercalcemia of Malignancy.

Arthralgias and myalgias were reported slightly more frequently in the pamidronate disodium group than in the placebo group (11.5% and 22.6% vs 8.0% and 16.9%, respectively).

In multiple myeloma patients, there were five pamidronate disodium-related serious and unexpected adverse experiences. Four of these were reported during the 12-month extension of the multiple myeloma trial. Three of the reports were of worsening renal function developing in patients with progressive multiple myeloma or multiple myeloma-associated

ADVERSE REACTIONS: *(cont'd)*

TABLE 7 Treatment-Related Adverse Experiences Reported in Three U.S. Controlled Clinical Trials

	Percent of Patients				
	Pamidronate Disodium		Didronel		Saline
	60 mg over 4 hr	60 mg over 24 hr	90 mg over 24 hr	7.5 mg/kg x 3 days	
	n=23	n=73	n=17	n=35	n=23
General					
Edema	0	1	0	0	0
Fatigue	0	0	12	0	0
Fever	26	19	18	9	0
Fluid overload	0	0	0	6	0
Infusion-site reaction	0	4	18	0	0
Moniliasis	0	0	6	0	0
Rigors	0	0	0	0	4
Gastrointestinal					
Abdominal pain	0	1	0	0	0
Anorexia	4	1	12	0	0
Constipation	4	0	6	3	0
Diarrhea	0	1	0	0	0
Dyspepsia	4	0	0	0	0
Nausea	4	0	18	6	0
Stomatitis	0	1	0	3	0
Vomiting	4	0	0	0	0
Respiratory					
Dyspnea	0	0	0	3	0
Rales	0	0	6	0	0
Rhinitis	0	0	6	0	0
Upper respiratory infection	0	3	0	0	0
CNS					
Anxiety	0	0	0	0	4
Convulsions	0	0	0	3	0
Insomnia	0	1	0	0	0
Nervousness	0	0	0	0	4
Psychosis	4	0	0	0	0
Somnolence	0	1	6	0	0
Taste Perversion	0	0	0	3	0
Cardiovascular					
Atrial fibrillation	0	0	6	0	4
Atrial flutter	0	1	0	0	0
Cardiac failure	0	1	0	0	0
Hypertension	0	0	6	0	4
Syncope	0	0	6	0	0
Tachycardia	0	0	6	0	4
Endocrine					
Hypothyroidism	0	0	6	0	0
Hemic and Lymphatic					
Anemia	0	0	6	0	0
Leukopenia	4	0	0	0	0
Neutropenia	0	1	0	0	0
Thrombocytopenia	0	1	0	0	0
Musculoskeletal					
Myalgia	0	1	0	0	0
Urogenital					
Uremia	4	0	0	0	0
Laboratory Abnormalities					
Hypocalcemia	0	1	12	0	0
Hypokalemia	4	4	18	0	0
Hypomagnesemia	4	10	12	3	4
Hypophosphatemia	0	9	18	3	0
Abnormal liver function	0	0	0	3	0

amyloidosis. The fourth report was the adult respiratory distress syndrome developing in a patient recovering from pneumonia and acute gangrenous cholecystitis. One pamidronate disodium-treated patient experienced allergic reactions (of moderate severity) characterized by swollen and itchy eyes, runny nose, and scratchy throat within 24 hours after the sixth infusion.

In the breast cancer trials, there were four pamidronate disodium-related adverse experiences, all moderate in severity, that caused a patient to discontinue participation in the trial. One was due to interstitial pneumonitis, another to malaise and dyspnea. One pamidronate patient discontinued the trial due to a symptomatic hypocalcemia. Another pamidronate disodium patient discontinued due to severe bone pain after each infusion, which the investigator felt was trial-drug-related.

OVERDOSAGE:

There have been several cases of drug maladministration of intravenous pamidronate disodium in hypercalcemia patients with total doses of 225 mg to 300 mg given over 2 1/2 to 4 days. All of these patients survived, but they experienced hypocalcemia that required intravenous and/or oral administration of calcium.

In addition, one obese woman (95 kg) who was treated with 285 mg of pamidronate disodium/day for 3 days, experienced high fever (39.5°C), hypotension (from 170/90 mmHg to 90/60 mmHg), and transient taste perversion, noted about 6 hours after the first infusion. The fever and hypotension were rapidly corrected with steroids.

If overdosage occurs, symptomatic hypocalcemia could also result; such patients should be treated with short-term intravenous calcium.

DOSAGE AND ADMINISTRATION:

Hypercalcemia of Malignancy: Consideration should be given to the severity of as well as the symptoms of hypercalcemia. Vigorous saline hydration alone may be sufficient for treating mild, asymptomatic hypercalcemia. Overhydration should be avoided in patients who have potential for cardiac failure. In hypercalcemia associated with hematologic malignancies, the use of glucocorticoid therapy may be helpful.

Moderate Hypercalcemia: The recommended dose of pamidronate disodium in moderate hypercalcemia (corrected serum calcium* of approximately 12-13.5 mg/dl) is 60 to 90 mg. The 60-mg dose is given as an initial, SINGLE-DOSE, intravenous infusion over at least 4 hours. The 90-mg dose must be given by an initial, SINGLE-DOSE, intravenous infusion over 24 hours.

Severe Hypercalcemia: The recommended dose of pamidronate disodium in severe hypercalcemia (corrected serum calcium* >13.5 mg/dl) is 90 mg. The 90-mg dose must be given by an initial, SINGLE-DOSE, intravenous infusion over 24 hours.

DOSAGE AND ADMINISTRATION: *(cont'd)*

TABLE 8 Commonly Reported Adverse Experiences in Three U.S. Controlled Clinical Trials

	Pamidronate Disodium 90 mg over 2 hr N=367 %	Pamidronate Disodium 90 mg over 4 hr N=205 %	All Pamidronate Disodium 90 mg N=572 %	Placebo N=573 %
General				
Asthenia	16.6	16.1	16.4	15.4
Fatigue	29.7	31.7	30.4	35.5
Fever	33.5	39.0	35.5	30.5
Metastases	21.3	1.0	14.0	13.6
Digestive System				
Anorexia	22.9	17.1	20.8	18.0
Constipation	27.2	28.3	27.6	30.9
Diarrhea	22.9	26.8	24.3	26.2
Dyspepsia	11.4	17.6	13.6	12.4
Nausea	55.6	35.6	48.4	46.4
Pain, Abdominal	16.1	19.5	17.3	14.0
Vomiting	39.0	16.6	30.9	28.1
Hemic and Lymphatic				
Anemia	28.1	47.8	35.1	32.6
Granulocytopenia	14.7	20.5	16.8	17.3
Thrombocytopenia	7.9	16.6	11.0	13.1
Musculoskeletal System				
Myalgia	21.0	25.4	22.6	16.9
Skeletal Pain	58.6	61.0	59.4	69.1
CNS				
Headache	23.7	24.4	24.0	19.7
Insomnia	18.8	17.1	18.2	17.3
Respiratory System				
Coughing	18.3	26.3	21.2	18.8
Dyspnea	24.0	22.0	23.3	18.7
Upper Respiratory Infection	12.8	32.2	19.8	20.9
Urogenital System				
Urinary Tract Infection	13.9	15.6	14.5	10.8

*Albumin-corrected serum calcium (CCa, mg/dl) = serum calcium, mg/dl + 0.8 (4.0-serum albumin, g/dl).

Retreatment: A limited number of patients have received more than one treatment with pamidronate disodium for hypercalcemia. Retreatment with pamidronate disodium, in patients who show complete or partial response initially, may be carried out if serum calcium does not return to normal or remain normal after initial treatment. **It is recommended that a minimum of 7 days elapse before retreatment, to allow for full response to the initial dose.** The dose and manner of retreatment is identical to that of the initial therapy.

Paget's Disease: The recommended dose of pamidronate disodium in patients with moderate to severe Paget's disease of bone is 30 mg daily, administered as a 4-hour infusion on 3 consecutive days for a total dose of 90 mg.

Retreatment: A limited number of patients with Paget's disease have received more than one treatment of pamidronate disodium in clinical trials. When clinically indicated, patients should be retreated at the dose of initial therapy.

Osteolytic Bone Lesions of Multiple Myeloma: The recommended dose of pamidronate disodium in patients with osteolytic bone lesions of multiple myeloma is 90 mg administered as a 4-hour infusion given on a monthly basis.

Patients with marked Bence-Jones proteinuria and dehydration should receive adequate hydration prior to pamidronate disodium infusion.

Limited information is available on the use of pamidronate disodium in multiple myeloma patients with a serum creatinine ≥3.0 mg/dl.

The optimal duration of therapy is not yet known (see CLINICAL STUDIES.)

Osteolytic Bone Metastases of Breast Cancer: The recommended dose of pamidronate disodium in patients with osteolytic bone metastases is 90 mg administered over a 2-hour infusion given every 3-4 weeks.

Pamidronate disodium has been frequently used with doxorubicin, fluorouracil, cyclophosphamide, methotrexate, mitoxantrone, vinblastine, dexamethasone, prednisone, melphalan, vincristine, megesterol, and tamoxifen. It has been given less frequently with etoposide, cisplatin, cytabrine, paclitaxel, and aminoglutethimide.

PREPARATION OF SOLUTION:

Reconstitution: Pamidronate disodium is reconstituted by adding 10 ml of Sterile Water for Injection, USP, to each vial, resulting in a solution of 30 mg/10 ml, 60 mg/10 ml, or 90 mg/10 ml. The pH of the reconstituted solution is 6.0-7.4. The drug should be completely dissolved before the solution is withdrawn.

Hypercalcemia of Malignancy: The daily dose must be administered as an intravenous infusion over at least 4 hours for the 60 mg dose, and over 24 hours for the 90 mg dose. The recommended dose should be diluted in 1000 ml of sterile 0.45% or 0.9% Sodium Chloride, USP, or 5% Dextrose Injection, USP. This infusion is stable for up to 24 hours at room temperature.

Paget's Disease: The recommended dose of 30 mg should be diluted in 500 ml of sterile 0.45% or 0.9% Sodium Chloride, USP, or 5% Dextrose Injection, USP, and administered over a 4-hour period for 3 consecutive days.

Osteolytic Bone Metastases of Breast Cancer: The recommended dose of 90 mg should be diluted in 250 mL of sterile 0.45% or 0.9% Sodium Chloride, USP, or 5% dextrose injection, USP, and administered over a 2 hour period, every 3-4 weeks.

Osteolytic Bone Lesions of Multiple Myeloma: The recommended dose of 90 mg should be diluted in 500 ml of sterile 0.45% or 0.9% Sodium Chloride, USP, or 5% Dextrose Injection, USP, and administered over a 4-hour period on a monthly basis.

Pamidronate disodium must not be mixed with calcium-containing infusion solutions, such as Ringer's solution and should be given.

Note: Parenteral drug products should be inspected visually for particulate matter and discoloration prior to administration, whenever solution and container permit.

HOW SUPPLIED:

30 mg: each vial contains 30 mg of sterile, lyophilized pamidronate disodium and 470 mg of mannitol, USP.

HOW SUPPLIED: *(cont'd)*

60 mg: each vial contains 60 mg of sterile, lyophilized pamidronate disodium and 400 mg of mannitol, USP.

90 mg: each vial contains 90 mg of sterile, lyophilized pamidronate disodium and 375 mg of mannitol, USP.

Pamidronate disodium reconstituted with Sterile Water for Injection may be stored under refrigeration at 36° - 46°F (2°- 8°C) for up to 24 hours.

Storage: Do not store above 86°F (30°C).

HOW SUPPLIED - EQUIVALENTS NOT AVAILABLE:

Injection, Solution - Intravenous - 30 mg

4's $708.95 AREDIA, Novartis 00083-2601-04

Injection, Solution - Intravenous - 60 mg

1's $354.47 AREDIA, Novartis 00083-2606-01

Injection, Solution - Intravenous - 90 mg

1's $531.71 AREDIA, Novartis 00083-2609-01

PANCREATIN *(001948)*

CATEGORIES: Cystic Fibrosis; Digestants; Enzymes & Digestants; Gastrointestinal Drugs; Pregnancy Category C; FDA Pre 1938 Drugs

BRAND NAMES: *Bioglan Panazyme*; Creon; *Creon Forte*; **Donnazyme**; Entozyme; *Festal*; *Festal-N*; *Kreon* (Germany); *Kreon 25000*; *Ozym* (Germany); *Pancrex*; *Pancrex V*; *Pancrex V Forte*; *Pankreatin* (Germany); *Pankreo-N*; *Pankreon* (Germany); *Pankrotanon*; *Panpur-N* (Germany); *Viokase*
(International brand names outside U.S. in italics)

FORMULARIES: Aetna

Prescribing information not available at time of publication.

HOW SUPPLIED - EQUIVALENTS NOT AVAILABLE:

Tablet, Uncoated - Oral - 500 mg

100's $33.48 DONNAZYME, AH Robins 00031-4650-63

PANCRELIPASE *(001949)*

CATEGORIES: Abdominal Distention; Cystic Fibrosis; Diarrhea; Digestants; Enzymes & Digestants; Flatulence; Gastrointestinal Drugs; Pancreatic Enzymes; Pancreatitis; Steatorrhea; FDA Pre 1938 Drugs

BRAND NAMES: *Alipase* (France); Amylase; Amylase Lipase Protease; *Combizym*; *Combizym Compositum*; *Cotazym* (Canada); *Cotazym-65 B* (Canada); *Cotazym ECS*; **Cotazym-S**; *Cotazym-S Forte*; Creon; Creon 5; Encron 10; Encron-10; Entolase; Enzymase 16; Festalan; Ilozyme; *Krebsilasi*; Ku-Zyme Hp; Lipase; Panase; Pancote; Pancrease; *Pancrease HL* (England); *Pancrease MT 4* (Canada); *Pancrease MT 10* (Canada); *Pancrease MT 16* (Canada); Pancreatic Enzyme; Pancreatin 10; Pancrelipase 10000; Pancrelipase Mt 16; Pancrelipase Mt-16; *Pancrex*; Pancron 10; *Panga*; *Pankrease*; Panokase; *Panzytrat*; *Prolipase*; Promylin; Protease; Protilase; Protilase Mt 16; Ultrase; Ultrase Mt; Vio-Moore; *Vitazyme*; Zymase
(International brand names outside U.S. in italics)

FORMULARIES: Aetna; BC-BS; FHP; Humana; Kaiser; Medi-Cal; PCS

DESCRIPTION:

(Note: This monograph pertains to the Enteric Coated Microspheres, and the Enteric Coated Microtablets, or MT.)

MICROSPHERES

Pancrease pancrelipase capsules are a white, dye-free, orally administered capsule containing enteric coated microspheres of porcine pancreatic enzyme concentrate, predominately steapsin (pancreatic lipase), amylase and protease. Each capsule contains no less than:

Lipase 4,000 U.S.P. Units
Amylase 20,000 U.S.P. Units
Protease 25,000 U.S.P. Units

Inactive ingredients include cellulose acetate phthalate, diethyl phthalate, gelatin, povidone, sodium starch glycollate, corn starch, sugar, talc and titanium dioxide.

MICROTABLETS

Pancrease MT pancrelipase capsules are orally administered capsules containing enteric coated microtablets of porcine pancreatic enzyme concentrate, predominately steapsin (pancreatic lipase), amylase and protease.

Each Pancrease MT 4 capsule contains:
Lipase 4,000 U.S.P. Units
Amylase 12,000 U.S.P. Units
Protease 12,000 U.S.P. Units

Each Pancrease MT 10 capsule contains:
Lipase 10,000 U.S.P. Units
Amylase 30,000 U.S.P. Units
Protease 30,000 U.S.P. Units

Each Pancrease MT 16 capsule contains:
Lipase 16,000 U.S.P. Units
Amylase 48,000 U.S.P. Units
Protease 48,000 U.S.P. Units

Each Pancrease MT 25 capsule contains:
Lipase 25,000 U.S.P. Units
Amylase 75,000 U.S.P. Units
Protease 75,000 U.S.P. Units

Inactive ingredients include: benzyl alcohol, cellulose, crospovidone, gelatin, iron oxide, magnesium stearate, methacrylic acid, copolymer, methylparaben, polydimethylsiloxane, propylparaben, sodium laurel sulfate, silicon dioxide, talc, titanium dioxide, triethylcitrate, wax and other trace ingredients.

CLINICAL PHARMACOLOGY:

Pancrease pancrelipase capsules resist gastric inactivation and deliver predictable, high levels of biologically active enzymes into the duodenum. The enzymes catalyze the hydrolysis of fats into glycerol and fatty acids, protein into proteoses and derived substances, and starch into dextrins and sugars. Pancrease capsules are effective in controlling steatorrhea and its consequences at low daily dosage levels.

INDICATIONS AND USAGE:

PANCREASE PANCRELIPASE CAPSULES ARE INDICATED FOR PATIENTS WITH EXOCRINE PANCREATIC ENZYME DEFICIENCY AS IN BUT NOT LIMITED TO:

cystic fibrosis

chronic pancreatitis

post-pancreatectomy

post-gastrointestinal bypass surgery (*e.g.,* Billroth II gastroenterostomy)

ductal obstruction from neoplasm (*e.g.,* of the pancreas or common bile duct).

CONTRAINDICATIONS:

PANCREASE PANCRELIPASE CAPSULES ARE CONTRAINDICATED IN PATIENTS KNOWN TO BE HYPERSENSITIVE TO PORK PROTEIN.

(PANCREASE MT CAPSULES ARE CONTRAINDICATED IN PATIENTS WITH ACUTE PANCREATITIS OR WITH ACUTE EXACERBATIONS OF CHRONIC PANCREATIC DISEASES).

WARNINGS:

SHOULD HYPERSENSITIVITY OCCUR, DISCONTINUE MEDICATION AND TREAT SYMPTOMATICALLY.

PRECAUTIONS:

MICROSPHERES

TO PROTECT ENTERIC COATING, MICROSPHERES SHOULD NOT BE CRUSHED OR CHEWED. Where swallowing of capsules is difficult, they may be opened and the microspheres shaken onto a small quantity of a soft food (*e.g.,* applesauce, gelatin, etc.), which does not require chewing, and swallowed immediately. Contact of the microspheres with foods having a pH greater than 5.5 can dissolve the protective enteric shell.

Pregnancy Category C: Diethyl phthalate, an enteric coating component of pancrease pancrelipase capsules has been shown with high intraperitoneal dosing to be teratogenic in rats. However, when this coating was administered orally to rats up to 100 times the human dose, no teratogenic or embryocidal effects were observed. There were no adequate and well-controlled studies in pregnant women. Pancrease capsules should be used in pregnancy only if the potential benefit justifies the potential risk to the fetus.

MICROTABLETS (MT)

TO PROTECT ENTERIC COATING, MICROSPHERES SHOULD NOT BE CRUSHED OR CHEWED. Where swallowing of capsules is difficult, they may be opened and the microtablets shaken onto a small quantity of a soft food (*e.g.,* applesauce, gelatin, etc.), which does not require chewing, and swallowed immediately. Contact of the microspheres with foods having a pH greater than 6.0 can dissolve the protective enteric shell.

Pregnancy Category C: Animal reproduction studies have not been conducted with pancrease MT pancrelipase capsules. It is not known whether this drug can cause fetal harm when administered to a pregnant woman or can effect reproduction capacity. Pancrease MT should be given to a pregnant woman only if clearly needed.

ADVERSE REACTIONS:

THE MOST FREQUENTLY REPORTED ADVERSE REACTIONS TO PANCREASE PANCRELIPASE ARE GASTROINTESTINAL IN NATURE. LESS FREQUENTLY, ALLERGIC-TYPE REACTIONS HAVE ALSO BEEN OBSERVED. EXTREMELY HIGH DOSES OF EXOGENOUS PANCREATIC ENZYMES HAVE BEEN ASSOCIATED WITH HYPERURICOSURIA AND HYPERURICEMIA.

DOSAGE AND ADMINISTRATION:

MICROSPHERES

Usual dosage: One or two capsules during each meal and one capsule with snacks. Occasionally a third capsule with meals may be required depending upon individual requirements for control of steatorrhea.

MICROTABLETS (MT)

Dosage should be adjusted according to the severity of the exocrine pancreatic enzyme deficiency. The number of capsules or capsule strength given with meals and/or snacks should be estimated by assessing which dose minimizes steatorrhea and maintains good nutritional status.

In some patients with pancreatic enzyme deficiency, satisfactory responses have been achieved with dosages (expressed in U.S.P. units of lipase) similar to the ones stated below. However, dosages should be adjusted according to the response of the patient.

Children 7 to 12 years: 4,000 to 12,000 units (more if necessary) with each meal and with snacks.

Children 1 to 6 years: 4,000 to 8,000 units with each meal and 4,000 units with snacks.

Children under 1 year: Dosage for children under 6 months of age has not yet been established. Children 6 months to 1 year have responded to 2,000 units of lipase per meal.

The assessment of the end points in children is aided by charting growth curves.

Adults: 4,000 to 25,000 units (more if necessary) with each meal and with snacks.

Keep bottle tightly closed. Store at controlled room temperature (15 - 30°C, 59-86°), in a dry place. Do not refrigerate.

HOW SUPPLIED - EQUIVALENTS NOT AVAILABLE:

Capsule, Enteric Coated - Oral - 12000 unit/4000

100's	$16.90	Pancote, Econolab	55053-0400-01
100's	$19.65	ENTOLASE, AH Robins	00031-5025-63
100's	$25.30	Panase, Qualitest Pharms	00603-5021-21
100's	$25.40	Pancrelipase, Alphagen Labs	59743-0025-01
100's	$25.84	PANCREASE MT 4, McNeil Lab	00045-0341-60
100's	$26.75	PANCOTE, Econolab	55053-0323-01
100's	$28.24	PROTILASE, Rugby	00536-4929-01
100's	$58.10	ULTRASE MT 12, Scandipharm	58914-0002-10
100's	$87.16	ULTRASE MT 18, Scandipharm	58914-0018-10
100's	$96.34	ULTRASE MT 20, Scandipharm	58914-0004-10
250's	$52.45	Pancrelipase, Major Pharms	00904-3470-70
250's	$58.00	Panase, Qualitest Pharms	00603-5021-24
250's	$58.10	Pancrelipase, Alphagen Labs	59743-0025-25
250's	$60.00	PANCOTE, Econolab	55053-0323-02

HOW SUPPLIED - EQUIVALENTS NOT AVAILABLE: *(cont'd)*

500's	$93.25	ENTOLASE, AH Robins	00031-5025-70
500's	$460.15	ULTRASE MT 20, Scandipharm	58914-0004-50

Capsule, Enteric Coated - Oral - 20000 unit/4000

100's	$23.54	PANCRELIPASE, Geneva Pharms	00781-2219-01
100's	$25.27	ULTRASE, Scandipharm	58914-0045-10
100's	$27.00	COTAZYM - S, Organon	00052-0388-91
100's	$28.15	Amylase/Lipase/Protease, Aligen Independ	00405-4481-01
100's	$29.50	PANCREATIC ENZYME, Goldline Labs	00182-1554-01
100's	$29.94	PANCRELIPASE, United Res	00677-1322-01
100's	$31.69	CREON 5, Solvay Pharms	00032-1205-01
100's	$32.80	PANCREASE, McNeil Lab	00045-0095-60
100's	$35.25	Pancron 10, Pecos	59879-0505-01
100's	$38.14	Pancrelipase 10000, United Res	00677-1576-01
100's	$47.62	CREON 10, Solvay Pharms	00032-1210-01
100's	$91.12	CREON 20, Solvay Pharms	00032-1220-01
100's	$129.17	PANCREASE MT 20, McNeil Lab	00045-0346-60
250's	$40.49	PANCRELIPASE, HL Moore Drug Exch	00839-7526-09
250's	$56.07	PANCRELIPASE, Geneva Pharms	00781-2219-25
250's	$78.12	PANCREASE, McNeil Lab	00045-0095-69
250's	$78.74	CREON 5, Solvay Pharms	00032-1205-07
250's	$116.67	CREON 10, Solvay Pharms	00032-1210-07
250's	$223.25	CREON 20, Solvay Pharms	00032-1220-07
500's	$127.05	COTAZYM - S, Organon	00052-0388-95

Capsule, Enteric Coated - Oral - 30000 unit/1000

100's	$56.16	ZYMASE, Organon	00052-0393-91
100's	$64.58	PANCREASE MT 10, McNeil Lab	00045-0342-60
100's	$93.33	Protilase Mt 16, Rugby	00536-5711-01
100's	$99.50	Pancrelipase Mt-16, Pecos	59879-0122-01

Capsule, Enteric Coated - Oral - 75000 unit/2500

100's	$89.95	Pancrelipase Mt 16, Goldline Labs	00182-1999-01
100's	$90.15	Pancrelipase Mt 16, United Res	00677-1543-01
100's	$103.70	PANCREASE MT 25, McNeil Lab	00045-0343-60

Capsule, Gelatin - Oral - 30000 unit/8000

100's	$19.95	COTAZYM, Organon	00052-0381-91
100's	$35.87	KU-ZYME HP, Schwarz Pharma (US)	00091-3525-01
500's	$94.48	COTAZYM, Organon	00052-0381-95

Capsule, Gelatin, Sustained Action - Oral - 6000 unit

100's	$28.98	ULTRASE MT 6, Scandipharm	58914-0001-10

Powder - Oral - 70000 unit/1680

4 oz	$60.41	VIOKASE, AH Robins	00031-9115-12
8 oz	$102.85	VIOKASE, AH Robins	00031-9115-25

Tablet, Uncoated - Oral - 30000 unit/8000

100's	$12.81	VIO-MOORE, HL Moore Drug Exch	00839-7618-06
100's	$15.70	Panokase, Major Pharms	00904-3472-60
100's	$16.58	PANOKASE, Rugby	00536-4395-01
100's	$17.00	Pancrelipase, Goldline Labs	00182-1741-01
100's	$17.22	PANOKASE, Econolab	55053-0320-01
100's	$18.13	Amylase/Lipase/Protease, Aligen Independ	00405-4482-01
100's	$24.83	VIOKASE, AH Robins	00031-9111-63
250's	$119.04	ILOZYME, Savage Labs	00281-2001-19
500's	$71.50	Panokase, Major Pharms	00904-3472-40
500's	$77.55	PANOKASE, Econolab	55053-0320-05
500's	$111.74	VIOKASE, AH Robins	00031-9111-70

PANCURONIUM BROMIDE *(001950)*

CATEGORIES: Analeptics; Anesthesia; Autonomic Drugs; Endotracheal Intubation; Muscle Relaxants; Non-Depolarizing Muscle Relaxants; Neuromuscular Blocking Agents; Skeletal Muscle Relaxants; Pregnancy Category C; FDA Approval Pre 1982

BRAND NAMES: *Bromurex* (Mexico); *Curon-B*; *Midblock*; *Panconium*; *Panslan*; *Pavulon* (Asia, Europe, Canada); **Pavulon**
(International brand names outside U.S. in italics)

> **WARNING:**
> This drug should be administered by adequately trained individuals familiar with its actions, characteristics, and hazards.

DESCRIPTION:

Pancuronium injection is a nondepolarizing neuromuscular blocking agent chemically designated as the aminosteroid 2 beta, 16 beta - dipiperidino-5 alpha-androstane-3 alpha, 17-beta diol diacetate dimethobromide.

Pancuronium is supplied as a sterile, nonpyrogenic solution for injection. Each ml contains 1 mg or 2 mg pancuronium bromide, 2 mg sodium acetate and 1% benzyl alcohol as preservative. The solution is adjusted to isotonicity with sodium chloride and to a pH of 4 with acetic acid and/or sodium hydroxide; water is used as the solvent.

CLINICAL PHARMACOLOGY:

Pancuronium is a nondepolarizing neuromuscular blocking agent processing all of the characteristic pharmacological actions of this class of drugs (curariform). It acts by competing for cholinergic receptors at the motor end-plate. The antagonism to acetylcholine is inhibited and neuromuscular block is reversed by anticholinesterase agents such as pyridostigmine, neostigmine, and edrophonium. Pancuronium is approximately 1/3 less potent than vecuronium and approximately 5 times as potent as d-tubocurarine; the duration of neuromuscular blockage produced by pancuronium is longer than that of vecuronium at initially equipotent doses.

The ED95 (dose required to produce 95% suppression of muscle twitch response) is approximately 0.05 mg/kg under balanced anesthesia and 0.03 mg/kg under halothane anesthesia. These doses produce effective skeletal muscle relaxation (as judged by time from maximum effect to 25% recovery of control twitch height) for approximately 22 minutes; the duration from injection to 90% recovery of control twitch height is approximately 65 minutes. The intubating dose of 0.1 mg/kg (balanced anesthesia) will effectively abolish twitch response within approximately 4 minutes; time from injection to 25% recovery from this dose is approximately 100 minutes.

Supplemental doses to maintain muscle relaxation slightly increase the magnitude of block and significantly increase the duration of block. The use of a peripheral nerve stimulator is of benefit in assessing the degree of neuromuscular blockade.

The most characteristic circulatory effects of pancuronium, studied under halothane anesthesia, are a moderate rise in heart rate, mean arterial pressure and cardiac output; systemic vascular resistance is not changed significantly and central venous pressure may fall slightly.

CLINICAL PHARMACOLOGY: *(cont'd)*

The heart rate is inversely related to the rate immediately before administration of pancuronium, is blocked by prior administration of atropine, and appears unrelated to the concentration of halothane or dose of pancuronium.

Data on histamine assays and available clinical experience indicate that hypersensitivity reactions such as bronchospasm, flushing, redness, hypotension, tachycardia, and other reactions commonly associated with histamine release are rare. (See ADVERSE REACTIONS.)

Pharmacokinetics: The elimination half-life of pancuronium has been reported to range between 89-161 minutes. The volume of distribution ranges from 241-280 ml/kg and plasma clearance is approximately 1.1-1.90 ml/minute/kg. Approximately 40% of the total dose of pancuronium has been recovered in urine as unchanged pancuronium and its metabolites while approximately 11% has been recovered in bile. As much as 25% of an injected dose may be recovered as 3-hydroxy metabolite, which is half as potent a blocking agent as pancuronium. Less than 5% of the injected dose is recovered as 17-hydroxy metabolite and 3,17-dihydroxy metabolite, which have been judged to be approximately 50 times less potent that pancuronium. Pancuronium exhibits strong binding to gamma globulin and moderate binding to albumin. Approximately 13% is unbound to plasma protein. In patients with cirrhosis the volume of distribution is increased by approximately 50%, the plasma clearance is decreased by approximately 22% and the elimination half-life is doubled. Similar results were noted in patients with biliary obstruction, except that plasma clearance was less than half the normal rate. The initial total dose to achieve adequate relaxation may thus be high in patients with hepatic and/or biliary tract dysfunction, while the duration of action is greater than usual.

The elimination half-life is doubled and the plasma clearance is reduced by approximately 60% in patients with renal failure. The volume of distribution is variable, and in some cases elevated. The rate of recovery of neuromuscular blockade, as determined by peripheral nerve stimulation is variable and sometimes very much slower than normal.

INDICATIONS AND USAGE:

Pancuronium injection is indicated as an adjunct to general anesthesia, to facilitate tracheal intubation and to provide skeletal muscle relaxation during surgery or mechanical ventilation.

CONTRAINDICATIONS:

Pancuronium is contraindicated in patients known to be hypersensitive to the drug.

WARNINGS:

PANCURONIUM SHOULD BE ADMINISTERED IN CAREFULLY ADJUSTED DOSES BY OR UNDER THE SUPERVISION OF EXPERIENCED CLINICIANS WHO ARE FAMILIAR WITH ITS ACTIONS AND THE POSSIBLE COMPLICATIONS THAT MIGHT OCCUR FOLLOWING ITS USE. THE DRUG SHOULD NOT BE ADMINISTERED UNLESS FACILITIES FOR INTUBATION, ARTIFICIAL RESPIRATION, OXYGEN THERAPY, AND REVERSAL AGENTS ARE IMMEDIATELY AVAILABLE. THE CLINICIAN MUST BE PREPARED TO ASSIST OR CONTROL RESPIRATION.

In patients who are known to have myasthenia gravis or the myasthenic (Eaton-Lambert) syndrome, small doses of pancuronium may have profound effects. In such patients, a peripheral nerve stimulator and use of a small test dose may be of value in monitoring the response to administration of muscle relaxants.

PRECAUTIONS:

USE OF A PERIPHERAL NERVE STIMULATOR WILL USUALLY BE OF VALUE FOR MONITORING OF NEUROMUSCULAR BLOCKING EFFECT, AVOIDING OVERDOSAGE AND ASSISTING IN EVALUATION OF RECOVERY.

General: Although pancuronium has been used successfully in many patients with pre-existing pulmonary, hepatic, or renal disease, caution should be exercised in these situations.

Renal Failure: A major portion of pancuronium, as well as an active metabolite, are recovered in urine. The elimination of half-life is doubled and the plasma clearance is reduced in patients with renal failure; at the same time, the rate of recovery of neuromuscular blockade is variable and sometimes very much slower than normal (See Pharmacokinetics.) This information should be taken into consideration if pancuronium is selected, for other reasons, to be used in a patient with renal failure.

Altered Circulation Time: Conditions associated with slower circulation time in cardiovascular disease, old age, edematous states resulting in increased volume of distribution may contribute to a delay in onset time; therefore dosage should not be increased.

Hepatic and/or Biliary Tract Disease: The doubled elimination half-life and reduced plasma clearance determined in patients with hepatic and/or biliary tract disease, as well as limited data showing that recovery time is prolonged an average of 65% in patients with biliary tract obstruction, suggests that prolongation of neuromuscular blockage may occur. At the same time, these conditions are characterized by an approximately 50% increase in volume of distribution of pancuronium, suggesting that the total initial dose to achieve adequate relaxation may in some cases be high. The possibility of slower onset, higher total dosage and prolongation of neuromuscular blockade must be taken into consideration when pancuronium is used in these patients (See also Pharmacokinetics).

Long Term Use in I.C.U.: In the intensive care unit, in rare cases, long-term use of neuromuscular blocking drugs to facilitate mechanical ventilation may be associated with prolonged paralysis and/or skeletal muscle weakness, that may be first noted during attempts to wean such patients from the ventilator. Typically, such patients receive other drugs such as broad spectrum antibiotics, narcotics and/or steroids and may have electrolyte imbalance and diseases which lead to electrolyte imbalance, hypoxic episodes of varying duration, acid-base imbalance and extreme debilitation, any of which may enhance the actions of a neuromuscular blocking agent. Additionally, patients immobilized for extended periods frequently develop symptoms consistent with disuse muscle atrophy. Therefore, when there is a need for long- term mechanical ventilation, the benefits-to-risk ratio of neuromuscular blockade must be considered.

Continuous infusion or intermittent bolus dosing to support mechanical ventilation, has not been studied sufficiently to support dosage recommendations.

UNDER THE ABOVE CONDITIONS, APPROPRIATE MONITORING, SUCH AS USE OF A PERIPHERAL NERVE STIMULATOR, TO ASSESS THE DEGREE OF NEUROMUSCULAR BLOCKADE, MAY PRECLUDE INADVERTENT EXCESS DOSING.

SEVERE OBESITY OR NEUROMUSCULAR DISEASE: Patients with severe obesity or neuromuscular disease may pose airway and/or ventilatory problems requiring special care before, during and after the use of neuromuscular blocking agents such as pancuronium.

C.N.S.: Pancuronium has no known effect on consciousness, the pain threshold or cerebration. Administration should be accompanied by adequate anesthesia or sedation.

Drug/Laboratory Test Interactions: None known.

Carcinogenesis, Mutagenesis, and Impairment of Fertility: Long-term studies in animals have not been performed to evaluate carcinogenic or mutagenic potential or impairment of fertility.

PRECAUTIONS: *(cont'd)*

Pregnancy Category C: Animal reproduction studies have not been performed. It is not known whether pancuronium can cause fetal harm when administered to a pregnant woman or can affect reproduction capacity. Pancuronium should be given to a pregnant woman only if the administering clinician decides that the benefits outweigh the risks.

Pancuronium may be used in operative obstetrics (Cesarean section), but reversal of pancuronium may be unsatisfactory in patients receiving magnesium sulfate for toxemia of pregnancy, because magnesium salts enhance neuromuscular blockade. Dosage should usually be reduced as indicated, in such cases. It is also recommended that the interval between use of pancuronium and delivery be reasonably short to avoid clinically significant placental transfer.

Pediatric Use: Dose response studies in children indicate that, with the exception of neonates, dosage requirements are the same as for adults. Neonates are especially sensitive to non-depolarizing neuromuscular blocking agents, such as pancuronium during the first month of life. It is recommended that a test dose of 0.02 mg/kg be given first in this group to measure responsiveness.

The prolonged use of pancuronium for the management of neonates undergoing mechanical ventilation has been associated in rare cases with severe skeletal muscle weakness that may first be noted during attempts to wean such patients from the ventilator; such patients usually receive other drugs such as antibiotics which may enhance neuromuscular blockade. Microscopic changes consistent with disuse atrophy have been noted at autopsy. Although a cause-and-effect relationship has not been established, the benefits-to-risk ratio must be considered when there is a need for neuromuscular blockade to facilitate long-term mechanical ventilation of neonates.

Rare cases of unexplained, clinically significant methemoglobinemia have been reported in premature neonates undergoing emergency anesthesia and surgery which included combined use of pancuronium, fentanyl and atropine. A direct cause-and-effect relationship between the combined use of these drugs and the reported cases of methemoglobinemia has not been established.

DRUG INTERACTIONS:

Prior administration of succinylcholine may enhance the neuromuscular blocking effect of pancuronium and increase its duration of action. If succinylcholine is used before pancuronium the administration of pancuronium should be delayed until the patient starts recovering from succinylcholine-induced neuromuscular blockade.

If a small dose of pancuronium is given at least 3 minutes prior to the administration of succinylcholine, in order to reduce the incidence and intensity of succinylcholine-induced fasiculations, this dose may induce a degree of neuromuscular block sufficient to cause respiratory depression in some patients.

Other nondepolarizing neuromuscular blocking agents (vecuronium, atracurium, d-tubocurarine, metocurine, and gallamine) behave in a clinically similar fashion to pancuronium. The combinations of pancuronium-metocurine and pancuronium-d-tubocurarine are significantly more potent than the additive effects of each of the individual drugs given alone, however, the duration of blockade of these combinations is not prolonged. There are insufficient data to support concomitant use of pancuronium and the other three above mentioned muscle relaxants in the same patients.

Inhalational Anesthetics: Use of volatile inhalational anesthetics such as enflurane, isoflurane, and halothane with pancuronium will enhance neuromuscular blockade. Potentiation is most prominent with use of enflurane and isoflurane.

With the above agents, the intubating dose of pancuronium may be the same as with balanced anesthesia unless the inhalational anesthetic has been administered for a sufficient time at a sufficient dose to have reached clinical equilibrium. The relatively long duration of action of pancuronium should be taken into consideration when the drug is selected for intubation in these circumstances.

Clinical experience and animal experiments suggest that pancuronium should be given with caution to patients receiving chronic tricyclic antidepressant therapy who are anesthetized with halothane because severe ventricular arrhythmias may result from this combination. The severity of the arrhythmias appear in part related to the dose of pancuronium.

Antibiotics: Parenteral/intraperitoneal administration of high doses of certain antibiotics may intensify or produce neuromuscular block on their own. The following antibiotics have been associated with various degrees of paralysis: aminoglycosides (such as neomycin, streptomycin, kanamycin, gentamicin, and dihydrostreptomycin); tetracyclines; bacitracin; polymyxin B; colistin; and sodium colistimethate. If these or other newly introduced antibiotics are used preoperatively or in conjunction with pancuronium, unexpected prolongation of neuromuscular block should be considered a possibility.

Other: Experience concerning injection of quinidine during recovery from use of other muscle relaxants suggests that recurrent paralysis may occur. This possibility must also be considered for pancuronium injection.

Electrolyte imbalance and diseases which lead to electrolyte imbalance, such as adrenal cortical insufficiency, have been shown to alter neuromuscular blockade. Depending on the nature of the imbalance, either enhancement or inhibition may be expected. Magnesium salts, administered for the management of toxemia or pregnancy, may enhance the neuromuscular blockade.

ADVERSE REACTIONS:

Neuromuscular: The most frequent adverse reaction to non-depolarizing blocking agents as a class consists of an extension of drug's pharmacological action beyond the time period needed. This may vary from skeletal muscle weakness to profound and prolonged skeletal muscle paralysis resulting in respiratory insufficiency or apnea. (See PRECAUTIONS, Pediatric Use.)

Inadequate reversal of the neuromuscular blockade is possible with pancuronium as with all curariform drugs. These adverse experiences are managed by manual or mechanical ventilation until recovery is judged adequate.

Prolonged paralysis and/or skeletal muscle weakness have been reported after long-term use to support mechanical ventilation in the intensive care unit.

Cardiovascular: See discussion of circulatory effects in CLINICAL PHARMACOLOGY.

Gastrointestinal: Salivation is sometimes noted during very light anesthesia, especially if no anticholinergic premedication is used.

Skin: An occasional transient rash is noted accompanying the use of pancuronium.

Other: Although histamine release is not a characteristic action of pancuronium, rare hypersensitivity reactions such as bronchospasm, flushing, redness, hypotension, tachycardia and other reactions possibly mediated by histamine release have been reported.

OVERDOSAGE:

The possibility of iatrogenic overdosage can be minimized by carefully monitoring the muscle twitch response to peripheral nerve stimulation.

OVERDOSAGE: *(cont'd)*

Excessive doses of pancuronium produces enhanced pharmacological effects. Residual neuromuscular blockade beyond the time period needed may occur with pancuronium as with other neuromuscular blockers. This may be manifested by skeletal muscle weakness, decreased respiratory reserve, low tidal volume, or apnea. A peripheral nerve stimulator may be used to assess the degree of residual neuromuscular blockade and help to differentiate residual neuromuscular blockade from other causes of decreased respiratory reserve.

Pyridostigmine bromide injection, neostigmine, or edrophonium, in conjunction with atropine or glycopyrrolate, will usually antagonize the skeletal muscle relaxant action of pancuronium. Satisfactory reversal can be judged by adequacy of skeletal muscle tone and by adequacy of respiration. A peripheral nerve stimulator may also be used to monitor restoration of twitch response.

Failure of prompt reversal (within 30 minutes) may occur in the presence of extreme debilitation, carcinomatosis, and with concomitant use of certain broad spectrum antibiotics, or anesthetic agents and other drugs which enhance neuromuscular blockade or cause respiratory depression of their own. Under such circumstances, the management is the same as that of prolonged neuromuscular blockade. Ventilation must be supported by artificial means until the patients has resumed control of his respiration. Prior to the use of reversal agents, reference should be made to the specific package insert of the reversal agent.

DOSAGE AND ADMINISTRATION:

Pancuronium injection is for intravenous use only. This drug should be administered by or under the supervision of experienced clinicians familiar with the use of neuromuscular blocking agents. DOSAGE MUST BE INDIVIDUALIZED IN EACH CASE. The dosage information which follows is derived from studies based upon units of drug per unit of body weight and is intended to serve as a guide only. Since potent inhalational anesthetics or prior use of succinylcholine may enhance the intensity and duration of pancuronium (See DRUG INTERACTIONS), the lower end of the recommended initial dosage range may suffice when pancuronium is first used after intubation with succinylcholine and/or after maintenance doses of volatile liquid inhalational anesthetics are started. To obtain maximum clinical benefits of pancuronium and to minimize the possibility of overdosage, the monitoring of muscle twitch response to a peripheral nerve stimulator is advised.

In adults under balance anesthesia the initial intravenous dosage range is 0.04 to 0.1 mg/kg. Later incremental doses starting at 0.01 mg/kg may be used. These increments slightly increase the magnitude of the blockade and significantly increase the duration of blockade, because a significant number of myoneural junctions are still blocked when there is clinical need for more drug.

If pancuronium is used to provide skeletal muscle relaxation for endotracheal intubation, a bolus dose of 0.06 to 0.1 mg/kg are recommended. Conditions satisfactory for intubation are usually present within 2 to 3 minutes. (See PRECAUTIONS.)

Dosage in Children: Dose response studies in children indicate that, with the exception of neonates, dosage requirements are the same as for adults. Neonates are especially sensitive to nondepolarizing neuromuscular blocking agents, such as pancuronium during the first month of life. It is recommended that a test dose of 0.02 mg/kg be given first in this group to measure responsiveness.

Cesarean Section: The dosage to provide relaxation for intubation and operation is the same as for general surgical procedures. The dosage to provide relaxation, following usage of succinylcholine for intubation (See DRUG INTERACTIONS), is the same as for general surgical procedures.

Compatibility: Pancuronium is compatible in solution with:

0.9% sodium chloride injection

5% dextrose and sodium chloride injection

5% dextrose injection

Lactated Ringer's injection

Parenteral drug products should be inspected visually for particulate matter and discoloration prior to administration, whenever solution and container permit.

When mixed with the above solutions in glass or plastic containers, pancuronium will remain stable in solution for 48 hours with no alteration in potency or pH; no decomposition is observed and there is no absorption to either the glass or plastic container.

Storage: Both concentrations of pancuronium will maintain full clinical potency for six months if kept at a room temperature of 18-22°C. (65 to 72°F); or for 2 years when refrigerated at 2-8°C. (36 to 46°F).

HOW SUPPLIED - RATED THERAPEUTICALLY EQUIVALENT:

Injection, Solution - Intravenous - 1 mg/ml

10 ml	$21.19	Pancuronium Bromide, Abbott	00074-4646-01
10 ml x 5	$63.75	Pancuronium Bromide, Astra USA	00186-1322-12
10 ml x 10	$133.08	Pancuronium Bromide 1, Gensia Labs	00703-2804-03
10 ml x 25	$350.00	Pancuronium Bromide, Elkins Sinn	00641-2547-45
10 ml x 25	**$353.20**	**PAVULON, Organon**	**00052-0443-25**

Injection, Solution - Intravenous - 2 mg/ml

2 ml	$15.95	Pancuronium Bromide 2, Abbott	00074-4645-01
2 ml	$58.81	Pancuronium Bromide, Astra USA	00186-1333-23
2 ml x 10	$48.00	Pancuronium Bromide, Astra USA	00186-1334-03
2 ml x 10	$49.06	Pancuronium Bromide, Astra USA	00186-1336-23
2 ml x 10	$54.00	Pancuronium Bromide, Astra USA	00186-1331-13
2 ml x 25	$141.30	Pancuronium Bromide, Gensia Labs	00703-2812-04
2 ml x 25	**$151.60**	**PAVULON, Organon**	**00052-0444-26**
2 ml x 25	$156.25	PANCURONIUM BROMIDE, Elkins Sinn	00641-0469-25
5 ml	$39.79	Pancuronium Bromide 2, Abbott	00074-4645-02
5 ml x 10	$112.50	Pancuronium Bromide, Astra USA	00186-0692-01
5 ml x 10	$112.50	Pancuronium Bromide, Astra USA	00186-1335-03
5 ml x 10	$125.63	Pancuronium Bromide, Astra USA	00186-1332-13
5 ml x 10	$133.88	Pancuronium Bromide, Astra USA	00186-0676-01
5 ml x 25	$311.40	Pancuronium Bromide 2, Gensia Labs	00703-2823-04
5 ml x 25	$324.25	Pancuronium Bromide, Elkins Sinn	00641-2546-25
5 ml x 25	$331.25	Pancuronium Bromide, Elkins Sinn	00641-1476-35
5 ml x 25	**$334.90**	**PAVULON, Organon**	**00052-0444-25**
5 ml x 25	$337.81	Pancuronium Bromide, Elkins Sinn	00641-2546-45

PAPAIN; UREA *(001952)*

CATEGORIES: Burns; Decubitus Ulcer; Deodorants; Dermatologicals; Enzymes; Enzymes & Digestants; Fibrinolytic & Proteolytic; Furunculosis; Lesions; Mucous Membrane Agents; Skin/Mucous Membrane Agents; Varicose Veins; Wound Care; FDA Pre 1938 Drugs

BRAND NAMES: **Panafil**; Panafil-White

DESCRIPTION:

Panafil Ointment is an enzymatic debriding healing ointment which contains standardized Papain 10%, Urea U.S.P. 10% and Chlorophyllin Copper Complex 0.5% in a hydrophilic base. Inactive ingredients are: While Petrolatum, U.S.P.; Propylene Glycol, U.S.P; Stearyl Alcohol, N.F.; Sorbitan Monostearate, N.F.; Polyoxyl 40 Stearate, N.F.; Boric Acid, N.F.; Sodium Borate, N.F.; Chlorobutanol (Anhydrous), N.F. as a preservative.

Panafil-White ointment is an enzymatic debriding ointment containing standardized Papain (10,000 Rystan Units of enzyme activity per gm of ointment) and Urea USP 10% in a hydrophilic base. One Rystan Unit is that quantity which under specified conditions will clot 10 microliters of milk substrate in 1 minute at 40°C. Inactive ingredients are Purified Water, USP; Propylene Glycol, USP; White Petrolatum, USP; Stearyl Alcohol, NF; Sorbitan Monostearate, NF; Polyoxyl 40 Stearate, NF; Boric Acid, NF; Sodium Borate, NF; Chlorobutanol (Anhydrous), NF as a preservative.

CLINICAL PHARMACOLOGY:

Papain, the proteolytic enzyme derived from the fruit of carica papaya, is a potent digestant of nonviable protein matter, but is harmless to viable tissue. It has the unique advantage of being active over a wide pH range, 3 to 1 2. Despite its recognized value as a digestive agent, papain is relatively ineffective when used alone as a debriding agent, primarily because it requires the presence of activators to exert its digestive function.

In Panafil Ointment, urea is combined with papain to provide two supplementary chemical actions: 1) to expose by solvent action the activators of papain (sulfhydryl groups) which are always present, but not necessarily accessible, in the nonviable tissue or debris of lesions, and 2) to denature the nonviable protein matter in lesions and thereby render it more susceptible to enzymatic digestion. In pharmacologic studies involving digestion of beef powder, Miller[1] showed that the combination of papain and urea produced twice as much digestion as papain alone.

Chlorophyllin Copper Complex adds healing action to the cleansing action of the proteolytic papain-urea combination. The basic wound-healing properties of Chlorophyllin Copper Complex are promotion of healthy granulations, control of local inflammation and reduction of wound odors.[2] Specifically, Chlorophyllin Copper Complex inhibits the hemagglutinating and inflammatory properties of protein degradation products in the wounds, including the products of enzymatic digestion thus providing an additional protective factor.[1,3] The incorporation of Chlorophyllin Copper Complex in Panafil Ointment permits its continuous use for as long as desired to help produce and then maintain a clean wound base and to promote healing.

INDICATIONS AND USAGE:

Panafil Ointment is suggested for treatment of acute and chronic lesions such as varicose, diabetic and decubitus ulcers, burns, postoperative wounds, pilonidal cyst wounds, carbuncles and miscellaneous traumatic or infected wounds.

Panafil Ointment is applied continuously throughout treatment of these conditions (1) for enzymatic debridement of necrotic tissue and liquefaction of fibrinous, purulent debris, (2) to keep the wound clean, and simultaneously (3) to promote normal healing.

CONTRAINDICATIONS:

None known.

PRECAUTIONS:

See DOSAGE AND ADMINISTRATION.

Not to be used in eyes.

ADVERSE REACTIONS:

Panafil Ointment is generally well tolerated and nonirritating. A small percentage of patients may experience a transient "burning" sensation on application of the ointment. Occasionally, the profuse exudate resulting from enzymatic digestion may cause irritation. In such cases, more frequent changes of dressings until exudate diminishes will alleviate discomfort.

DOSAGE AND ADMINISTRATION:

Apply Panafil Ointment directly to lesion and cover with appropriate dressing. When practicable, daily or twice daily changes of dressings are preferred. Longer intervals between redressings (two or three days) have proved satisfactory and Panafil Ointment may be applied under pressure dressings. At each redressing, the lesion should be irrigated with isotonic saline solution or other mild cleansing solution (except hydrogen peroxide solution, which may inactivate the papain) to remove any accumulation of liquefied necrotic material.

NOTE: Papain may also be inactivated by the salts of heavy metals (lead, silver, mercury, etc.) Contact with medications containing these metals should be avoided.

REFERENCES: 1.-3. Data on file. (Rystan Company Inc.)

HOW SUPPLIED - EQUIVALENTS NOT AVAILABLE:

Ointment - Topical - 10 %/10 %

30 gm	**$28.13**	**PANAFIL-WHITE, Rystan**	**00263-5148-01**
30 gm	**$28.19**	**PANAFIL, Rystan**	**00263-5145-01**
454 gm	**$186.37**	**PANAFIL, Rystan**	**00263-5145-16**

Powder

120 gm	$14.00	Papain, Millgood	53118-0621-04

PAPAVERINE HYDROCHLORIDE *(001953)*

CATEGORIES: Arrhythmia; Cardiovascular Drugs; Impotence*; Ischemia; Myocardial Ischemia; Nasal Congestion*; Peripheral Vasodilators; Spasm; Vascular Disorders, Cerebral/Peripheral; Vasodilating Agents; FDA Pre 1938 Drugs
* Indication not approved by the FDA

BRAND NAMES: *Angioverin '100'* (Mexico); Cerespan; Delapav; Genabid; Marpap; *Optenyl* (Germany); *Pameion*; Papacon; *Papaverine 60*; Papaverine Hcl; *Papaverini*; Para-Time; **Pavabid**; Pavacels; Pavacot; Pavagen; Pavased; Pavaspan; Pavasule; Pavatab-200; Pavatym; Paverine Spancap; Paverolan; Vasal
(International brand names outside U.S. in italics)

FORMULARIES: Aetna

COST OF THERAPY: $48.54 (Arrhythmia; Capsule; 150 mg; 2/day; 365 days) vs. Potential Cost of $3,462.83 (Arrhythmia)

DESCRIPTION:

NOTE: This monograph contains complete prescribing information for the Capsule and Injection forms of Papaverine Injection.

DESCRIPTION: *(cont'd)*

CAPSULES

Each capsulet contains Papaverine HCl 150 mg. Also contains calcium stearate, starch, stearic acid, sucrose, talc, and other ingredients.

INJECTION

This product is to be used by used by or under the direction of a physician.

Each ampoule or vial contains a sufficient amount to permit withdrawal and administration of the volume specified on the label.

Papaverine Hydrochloride (HCl) is the hydrochloride of an alkaloid obtained from opium or prepared synthetically. It belongs to the benzylisoquinoline group of alkaloids. It does not contain a phenanthrene group as do morphine and codeine.

Papaverine hydrochloride is 6,7-dimethoxy-1-veratrylisoquinoline hydrochloride and contains, on the dried basis, not less than 98.5% of $C_{20}H_{21}NO_4 \cdot HCl$. The molecular weight is 375.85.

Papaverine HCl occurs as white crystals or white crystalline powder. 1g dissolves in about 30 ml of water and in 120 ml of alcohol. It is soluble in chloroform and practically insoluble in ether.

Papaverine HCl Injection is a clear, colorless to pale-yellow solution.

Papaverine HCl, for parenteral administration, is a smooth-muscle relaxant that is available in ampoules or vials containing 30 mg/ml (88.4 μmol/l) of papaverine base. Each ampoule or vial also contains edetate disodium, 0.005%. Sodium hydroxide may have been added during manufacture to adjust the pH.

CLINICAL PHARMACOLOGY:

CAPSULES

The main actions of papaverine are exerted on cardiac and smooth muscle. Like quinidine, papaverine acts directly on the heart muscle to depress conduction and prolong the refractory period. Papaverine relaxes various smooth muscles. This relaxation may be prominent if spasm exists. The muscle cell is not paralyzed by papaverine, and still responds to drugs and other stimuli causing contraction. The antispasmodic effect is a direct one, and unrelated to muscle innervation. Papaverine is practically devoid of effects on the central nervous system.

Papaverine relaxes the smooth musculature of the larger blood vessels, especially coronary, systemic peripheral, and pulmonary arteries. Perhaps by its direct vasodilating action on cerebral blood vessels, papaverine increases cerebral blood flow and decreases cerebral vascular resistance in normal subjects; oxygen consumption is unaltered. These effects may explain the benefit reported from the drug in cerebral vascular encephalopathy.

The direct actions of papaverine on the heart to depress conduction and irritability and to prolong the refractory period of the myocardium provide the basis for its clinical trial in abrogating atrial and ventricular premature systoles and ominous ventricular arrhythmias. The coronary vasodilator action could be an additional factor of therapeutic value when such rhythms are secondary to insufficiency or occlusion of the coronary arteries.

In patients with acute coronary thrombosis, the occurrence of ventricular rhythms is serious and requires measures designed to decrease myocardial irritability. Papaverine may have advantages over quinidine, used for a similar purpose, in that it may be given in an emergency by the intravenous route, does not depress myocardial contraction or cause cinchonism, and produces coronary vasodilation.

INJECTION

The most characteristic effect of papaverine is relaxation of the tonus of all smooth muscle, especially when it has been spasmodically contracted. Papaverine HCl apparently acts directly on the muscle itself. This relaxation is noted in the *vascular system* and *bronchial musculature* and in the *gastrointestinal, biliary,* and *urinary tracts.*

The main actions of papaverine are exerted on cardiac and smooth muscle. Papaverine relaxes various smooth muscles, especially those of larger arteries; this relaxation may be prominent if spasm exists. The antispasmodic effect is a direct one and unrelated to muscle innervation, and the muscle still responds to drugs and other stimuli causing contraction. Papaverine has minimal actions on the central nervous system, although very large doses tend to produce some sedation and sleepiness in some patients. In certain circumstances, mild respiratory stimulation can be observed, but this is therapeutically inconsequential. Papaverine stimulates respiration by acting on carotid and aortic body chemoreceptors.

INDICATIONS AND USAGE:

CAPSULES

For the relief of cerebral and peripheral ischemia associated with arterial spasm and myocardial ischemia complicated by arrhythmias.

INJECTION

Papaverine is recommended in various conditions accompanied by spasm of smooth muscle, such as *vascular spasm* associated with acute myocardial infarction (coronary occlusion), angina pectoris, peripheral and pulmonary embolism, peripheral vascular disease in which there is a vasospastic element, or certain cerebral angiospastic states; and *visceral spasm*, as in ureteral, biliary, or gastrointestinal colic.

CONTRAINDICATIONS:

INJECTION

Intravenous injection of papaverine is contraindicated in the presence of complete atrioventricular heart block. When conduction is depressed, the drug may produce transient ectopic rhythms of ventricular origin, either premature beats or paroxysmal tachycardia.

Papaverine hydrochloride is not indicated for the treatment of impotence by intracorporeal injection. The intracorporeal injection of papaverine hydrochloride has been reported to have resulted in persistent priapism requiring medical and surgical intervention.

PRECAUTIONS:

GENERAL

Capsules: Use with caution in patients with glaucoma. Hepatic hypersensitivity has been reported with gastrointestinal symptoms, jaundice, eosinophilia, and altered liver function tests. Discontinue medication if these occur.

Injection: Papaverine Hydrochloride Injection should not be added to Lactated Ringer's Injection, because precipitation would result.

Papaverine HCl should be used with caution in patients with glaucoma. The medication should be discontinued if hepatic hypersensitivity with gastrointestinal symptoms, jaundice, or eosinophilia becomes evident or if liver function test vales become altered.

USAGE IN PREGNANCY

Pregnancy Category C: No teratogenic effects were observed in rats when papaverine hydrochloride was administered subcutaneously as a single agent. It is not known whether papaverine can cause fetal harm when administered to a pregnant woman or can affect reproduction capacity. Papaverine hydrochloride should be given to a pregnant woman only if clearly needed.

PRECAUTIONS: *(cont'd)*

NURSING MOTHERS

It is not known whether this drug is excreted in human milk. Because many drugs are excreted in human milk, caution should be exercised when papaverine HCl is administered to a nursing woman.

USAGE IN CHILDREN

Safety and effectiveness in children have not been established.

ADVERSE REACTIONS:

CAPSULES

Although occurring rarely, the reported side effects of papaverine include nausea, abdominal distress, anorexia, constipation, malaise, drowsiness, vertigo, sweating, headache, diarrhea, and skin rash.

INJECTION

The following side effect have been reported: general discomfort, nausea, abdominal discomfort, anorexia, constipation or diarrhea, skin rash, malaise, vertigo, headache, intensive flushing of the face, perspiration, increase in the depth of respiration, increase in heart rate, a slight rise in blood pressure, and excessive sedation.

DRUG ABUSE AND DEPENDENCE:

Drug dependence resulting from the abuse of many of the selective depressants, including papaverine HCl, has been reported.

OVERDOSAGE:

SIGNS AND SYMPTOMS

Injection: The symptoms of toxicity from papaverine HCl often result from vasomotor instability and include nausea, vomiting, weakness, central nervous system depression, nystagmus, diplopia, diaphoresis, flushing, dizziness, and sinus tachycardia. In large overdoses, papaverine is a potent inhibitor of cellular respiration and a weak calcium antagonist. Following an oral overdose of 15 g, metabolic acidosis with hyperventilation, hyperglycemia, and hypokalemia have been reported. No information on toxic serum concentrations is available.

Following intravenous overdosing in animals, seizures, tachyarrhythmias, and ventricular fibrillation have been reported. The oral median lethal dose in rats is 360 mg/kg.

TREATMENT

To obtain up-to-date information about the treatment of overdose, a good resource is your certified Regional Poison Control Center. Telephone numbers of certified regional poison control centers are listed in *Physicians GenR$_X$*. In managing overdosage, consider the possibility of multiple drug overdoses, interaction among drugs, and unusual drug kinetics in your patient.

Protect the patient's airway and support ventilation and perfusion. Meticulously monitor vital signs, blood gases, blood chemistry values, and other variables.

If convulsions occur, consider diazepam, phenytoin or phenobarbital. If the seizures are refractory, general anesthesia with thiopental or halothane and paralysis with a neuromuscular blocking agent may be necessary.

For hypotension, consider intravenous fluids, elevation of the legs, and an inotropic vasopressor, such as dopamine or levarterenol. Theoretically, calcium gluconate may be helpful in treating some of the toxic cardiovascular effects of papaverine: monitor the ECG and plasma calcium concentrations.

Forced diuresis, peritoneal dialysis, hemodialysis, or charcoal hemoperfusion have not been established as beneficial for an overdose of papaverine hydrochloride.

DOSAGE AND ADMINISTRATION:

CAPSULES

One capsule every 12 hours. In difficult cases administration may be increased to one capsule every 8 hours or two capsules every 12 hours.

INJECTION

Papaverine hydrochloride may be administered intravenously or intramuscularly. The intravenous route is recommended when an immediate effect is desired, but the drug *must be injected slowly* over the course of 1 or 2 minutes to avoid uncomfortable or alarming side effects.

Parenteral administration of papaverine hydrochloride in doses of 1 to 4 ml is repeated every 3 hours as indicated. In the treatment of cardiac extrasystoles, 2 doses may be given 10 minutes apart.

(Capsules: Marion Merrell Dow)

(Injection: Lilly, 90/10, PA 0343 AMP)

HOW SUPPLIED - EQUIVALENTS NOT AVAILABLE:

Capsule, Gelatin, Sustained Action - Oral - 150 mg

100's	$6.65	Papaverine Hcl, Qualitest Pharms	00603-5043-21
100's	$6.75	PAPACON, Consolidated Midland	00223-1358-01
100's	$7.37	Papaverine Hcl, Eon Labs Mfg	00185-5156-01
100's	$7.75	Papaverine Hcl, Sidmak Labs	50111-0318-01
100's	$7.90	GENABID, Goldline Labs	00182-0181-01
100's	$7.95	Papaverine Hcl 150, Major Pharms	00904-2180-60
100's	$8.09	PAVAGEN, Rugby	00536-4124-01
100's	$8.32	Papaverine, United Res	00677-0171-01
100's	$8.37	Papaverine Hcl, HL Moore Drug Exch	00839-1441-06
100's	$8.52	Para-Time, Time-Caps Labs	49483-0019-01
100's	$8.62	Papaverine Hcl, Aligen Independ	00405-4757-01
100's	$8.88	Papaverine HCl, Schein Pharm (US)	00364-0181-01
100's	$9.00	PAVACOT T.D., C O Truxton	00463-3011-01
100's	$9.95	Papaverine HCl, Geneva Pharms	00781-2000-01
100's	$12.93	Papaverine Hcl 150, Major Pharms	00904-2180-61
100's	**$27.81**	**PAVABID PLATEAU, Hoechst Marion Roussel**	**00088-1555-47**
500's	$34.58	PAVAGEN, Rugby	00536-4124-05
1000's	$49.50	Papaverine Hcl, Consolidated Midland	00223-1358-03
1000's	$58.15	Papaverine Hcl, Sidmak Labs	50111-0318-03
1000's	$60.25	Papaverine Hcl 150, Major Pharms	00904-2180-80
1000's	$60.69	Papaverine, United Res	00677-0171-10
1000's	$60.74	Papaverine Hcl, HL Moore Drug Exch	00839-1441-16
1000's	$63.37	Papaverine Hcl, Qualitest Pharms	00603-5043-32
1000's	$63.50	GENABID, Goldline Labs	00182-0181-10
1000's	$65.72	Papaverine Hcl, Aligen Independ	00405-4757-03
1000's	$65.84	PAVAGEN, Rugby	00536-4124-10
1000's	$65.95	Papaverine HCl, Geneva Pharms	00781-2000-10
1000's	$66.73	Papaverine Hcl, Eon Labs Mfg	00185-5156-10
1000's	$76.38	Para-Time, Time-Caps Labs	49483-0019-10
1000's	$79.80	PAVACOT T.D., C O Truxton	00463-3011-10

HOW SUPPLIED - EQUIVALENTS NOT AVAILABLE: *(cont'd)*

Injection, Solution - Intramuscular; - 30 mg/ml

2 ml	$3.50	Papaverine Hcl, Am Regent	00517-4002-05
2 ml	$8.72	PAPAVERINE HCL, King Pharms	60793-0015-02
2 ml	$9.00	PAPAVERINE HCL, Yorpharm	61147-8009-01
2 ml x 12	$18.08	Papaverine Hcl, Lilly	00002-1664-12
2 ml x 100	$120.01	Papaverine Hcl, Lilly	00002-1664-02
10 ml	$16.88	Papaverine Hcl, Am Regent	00517-4010-01
10 ml	$33.48	PAPAVERINE HCL, Yorpharm	61147-8009-03
10 ml	$37.37	PAPAVERINE HCL, King Pharms	60793-0015-10

Tablet, Uncoated - Oral - 100 mg

100's	$11.76	PAPAVERINE HCL, Lilly	00002-2055-02

Tablet, Uncoated - Oral - 300 mg

100's	$7.95	PAVATINE, Major Pharms	00904-2179-60

PARALDEHYDE *(001957)*

CATEGORIES: Anticonvulsants; Anxiolytics, Sedatives, Hypnotic; Central Nervous System Agents; Neuromuscular; Sedatives/Hypnotics; DEA Class CIV; FDA Pre 1938 Drugs

BRAND NAMES: Paral

Prescribing information not available at time of publication.

HOW SUPPLIED - EQUIVALENTS NOT AVAILABLE:

Injection, Solution - Intramuscular; - 100 %

5 ml x 25	$175.00	Paraldehyde, Consolidated Midland	00223-8240-05
30 ml	$212.16	PARAL, Forest Pharms	00456-0762-30

PARAMETHADIONE *(001958)*

CATEGORIES: Anticonvulsants; Central Nervous System Agents; Convulsions; Epilepsy; Neuromuscular; Oxazolidinedione Anticonvulsant; Seizures; Pregnancy Category D; FDA Approval Pre 1982

BRAND NAMES: **Paradione**

BECAUSE OF ITS POTENTIAL TO PRODUCE FETAL MALFORMATIONS AND SERIOUS SIDE EFFECTS, PARAMETHADIONE SHOULD ONLY BE UTILIZED WHEN OTHER LESS TOXIC DRUGS HAVE BEEN FOUND INEFFECTIVE IN CONTROLLING ABSENCE (PETIT MAL) SEIZURES.

DESCRIPTION:

Paramethadione is an antiepileptic agent. An oxazolidinedione compound, it is chemically identified as 5-Ethyl- 3, 5- dimethyl-2,4-oxazolidinedione.

Paradione is a synthetic, oily, slightly water-soluble liquid. It is supplied in capsule form for oral use only. The capsules are available in two dosage strengths. One strength contains 150 mg the other 300 mg of paramethadione per capsule.

Inactive Ingredients: *150 mg capsule:* FD&C Yellow No. 6, gelatin, glycerin, methylparaben, olive oil ethyl ester and propylparaben. *300 mg capsule:* FD&C Blue No. 1, FD&C Yellow No. 5 (tartrazine), FD&C Yellow No. 6, gelatin, glycerin, methylparaben, olive oil ethyl ester and propylparaben.

CLINICAL PHARMACOLOGY:

Paramethadione has been shown to prevent pentylenetetrazol-induced & thujone-induced seizures in experimental animals; the drug has a less marked effect on seizures induced by picrotoxin, procaine, cocaine, or strychnine. Unlike the hydantoins and antiepileptic barbiturates, paramethadione does not modify the maximal seizure pattern in patients undergoing electroconvulsive therapy. Paramethadione has a sedative effect that may increase to the point of ataxia when excessive doses are used. A toxic dose of the drug in animals (approximately 1 g/kg) produced sleep, unconsciousness, and respiratory depression.

Paramethadione is rapidly absorbed from the gastrointestinal tract. It is demethylated by liver microsomes to an active N-demethylated metabolite, and is excreted slowly in this form by the kidney; almost no unmetabolized paramethadione is excreted.

INDICATIONS AND USAGE:

Paramethadione is indicated for the control of absence (petit mal) seizures that are refractory to treatment with other drugs.

CONTRAINDICATIONS:

Paramethadione is contraindicated in patients with a known hypersensitivity to the drug.

WARNINGS:

Paramethadione may cause serious side effects. Strict medical supervision of the patient is mandatory, especially during the initial year of therapy.

USAGE DURING PREGNANCY

THERE ARE MULTIPLE REPORTS IN THE CLINICAL LITERATURE WHICH INDICATE THAT THE USE OF ANTIEPILEPTIC DRUGS DURING PREGNANCY RESULTS IN AN INCREASED INCIDENCE OF BIRTH DEFECTS IN THE OFFSPRING. DATA ARE MORE EXTENSIVE WITH RESPECT TO TRIMETHADIONE, PARAMETHADIONE, PHENYTOIN AND PHENOBARBITAL THAN WITH OTHER ANTIEPILEPTIC DRUGS.

THEREFORE, ANTIEPILEPTIC DRUGS SUCH AS PARAMETHADIONE SHOULD BE ADMINISTERED TO WOMEN OF CHILDBEARING POTENTIAL ONLY IF THEY ARE CLEARLY SHOWN TO BE ESSENTIAL IN THE MANAGEMENT OF THEIR SEIZURES. EFFECTIVE MEANS OF CONTRACEPTION SHOULD ACCOMPANY THE USE OF PARAMETHADIONE IN SUCH PATIENTS. IF A PATIENT BECOMES PREGNANT WHILE TAKING PARAMETHADIONE, TERMINATION OF THE PREGNANCY SHOULD BE CONSIDERED. A PATIENT WHO REQUIRES THERAPY WITH PARAMETHADIONE AND WHO WISHES TO BECOME PREGNANT SHOULD BE ADVISED OF THE RISKS.

REPORTS HAVE SUGGESTED THAT THE MATERNAL INGESTION OF ANTIEPILEPTIC DRUGS, PARTICULARLY BARBITURATES, IS ASSOCIATED WITH A NEONATAL COAGULATION DEFECT THAT MAY CAUSE BLEEDING DURING THE EARLY (USUALLY WITHIN 24 HOURS OF BIRTH) NEONATAL PERIOD. THE POSSIBILITY OF THE OCCURRENCE OF THIS DEFECT WITH THE USE OF PARAMETHADIONE SHOULD BE KEPT IN MIND. THE DEFECT IS CHARACTERIZED BY DECREASED LEVELS OF VITAMIN K-DEPENDENT CLOTTING FACTORS, AND PROLONGATION OF EITHER THE PROTHROMBIN TIME OR THE PARTIAL

WARNINGS: *(cont'd)*

THROMBOPLASTIN TIME, OR BOTH. IT HAS BEEN SUGGESTED THAT PROPHYLACTIC VITAMIN K BE GIVEN TO THE MOTHER ONE MONTH PRIOR TO, AND DURING DELIVERY, AND TO THE INFANT, INTRAVENOUSLY, IMMEDIATELY AFTER BIRTH.

PRECAUTIONS:

General: Abrupt discontinuation of paramethadione may precipitate absence (petit mal) status. Paramethadione should always be withdrawn gradually unless serious adverse effects dictate otherwise. In the latter case, another antiepileptic may be substituted to protect the patient.

Paramethadione should be withdrawn promptly if skin rash appears, because of the grave possibility of the occurrence of exfoliative dermatitis or severe forms of erythema multiforme. Even a minor acneiform or morbilliform rash should be allowed to clear completely before treatment with paramethadione is resumed; reinstitute therapy cautiously.

Paramethadione should ordinarily not be used in patients with severe blood dyscrasias.

Hepatitis has been associated rarely with the use of oxazolidinediones. Jaundice or other signs of liver dysfunction are an indication for withdrawal of paramethadione. Paramethadione should ordinarily not be used in patients with severe hepatic impairment.

Fatal nephrosis has been reported with the use of oxazolidinediones. Persistent or increasing albuminuria, or the development of any other significant renal abnormality, is an indication for withdrawal of the drug. Paramethadione should ordinarily not be used in patients with severe renal dysfunction.

Hemeralopia has occurred with the use of oxazolidinedione compounds; this appears to be an effect of the drugs on the neural layers of the retina, and usually can be reversed by a reduction in dosage. Scotomata are an indication for withdrawal of the drug. Caution should be observed when treating patients who have diseases of the retina or optic nerve.

Manifestations of systemic lupus erythematosus have been associated with the use of the oxazolidinediones, as they have with the use of certain other antiepileptics. Lymphadenopathies simulating malignant lymphoma have also occurred. Lupus-like manifestations or lymph node enlargement are indications for withdrawal of paramethadione. Signs and symptoms may disappear after discontinuation of therapy, and specific treatment may be unnecessary.

A myasthenia gravis-like syndrome has been associated with the chronic use of the oxazolidinediones. Symptoms suggestive of this condition are indications for withdrawal of paramethadione.

The 300 mg capsule of Paradione contains FD&C Yellow No. 5 (tartrazine) which may cause allergic-type reactions (including bronchial asthma) in certain susceptible individuals. Although the overall incidence of FD&C Yellow No. 5 (tartrazine) sensitivity in the general population is low, it is frequently seen in patients who also have aspirin hypersensitivity.

Information for Patients: Patients should be advised to report immediately such signs and symptoms, as sore throat, fever, malaise, easy-bruising, petechiae, or epistaxis, or others that may be indicative of an infection or bleeding tendency.

Laboratory Tests: A complete blood count should be done prior to initiating therapy with paramethadione, and at monthly intervals thereafter. A marked depression of the blood count is an indication for withdrawal of the drug. If no abnormality appears within 12 months, the interval between blood counts may be extended. A moderate degree of neutropenia with or without a corresponding drop in the leukocyte count is not uncommon. Therapy need not be withdrawn unless the neutrophil count is 2500 or less; more frequent blood examinations should be done when the count is less than 3,000. Other blood dyscrasias, including leukopenia, eosinophilia, thrombocytopenia, pancytopenia, agranulocytosis, hypoplastic anemia, and fatal aplastic anemia, have occurred with the use of oxazolidinediones.

Liver function tests should be done prior to initiating therapy with paramethadione and at monthly intervals thereafter.

A urinalysis should be done prior to initiating therapy with paramethadione and at monthly intervals thereafter.

Carcinogenesis: No data are available on long-term potential for carcinogenicity in animals or humans.

Pregnancy Category D: See WARNINGS section.

Nursing Mothers: It is not known whether this drug is excreted in human milk. Because many drugs are excreted in human milk and because of the potential for serious adverse reactions in nursing infants from paramethadione, a decision should be made whether to discontinue nursing or to discontinue the drug, taking into account the importance of the drug to the mother.

DRUG INTERACTIONS:

Drugs known to cause toxic effects similar to those of the oxazolidinediones should be avoided or used only with extreme caution during therapy with paramethadione.

ADVERSE REACTIONS:

The following side effects in decreasing order of severity, have been associated with the use of oxazolidinedione compounds. Although not all of them have been reported with the use of paramethadione, the possibility of their occurrence should be kept in mind when the drug is prescribed.

Renal: Fatal nephrosis has occurred. Albuminuria.

Hematologic: Fatal aplastic anemia, hypoplastic anemia, pancytopenia, agranulocytosis, leukopenia, neutropenia, thrombocytopenia, eosinophilia, retinal and petechial hemorrhages, vaginal bleeding, epistaxis, and bleeding gums.

Hepatic: Hepatitis has been reported rarely.

Dermatologic: Acneiform or morbilliform skin rash that may progress to severe forms of erythema multiforme or to exfoliative dermatitis. Hair loss.

CNS/Neurologic: A myasthenia gravis-like syndrome has been reported. Precipitation of tonic-clonic (grand mal) seizures, vertigo, personality changes, increased irritability, drowsiness, headache, paresthesias, fatigue, malaise, and insomnia.

Drowsiness usually subsides with continued therapy. If it persists, a reduction in dosage is indicated.

Ophthalmologic: Diplopia, hemeralopia, and photophobia.

Cardiovascular: Changes in blood pressure.

Gastrointestinal: Vomiting, abdominal pain, gastric distress, nausea, anorexia, weight loss, and hiccups.

Other: Lupus erythematosus, and lymphadenopathies simulating malignant lymphoma, have been reported.

Pruritus associated with lymphadenopathy and hepatosplenomegaly has occurred in hypersensitive individuals.

OVERDOSAGE:

Symptoms of acute paramethadione overdosage include drowsiness, nausea, dizziness, ataxia, visual disturbances. Coma may follow massive overdosage.

Gastric evacuation, either by induced emesis, or by lavage, or both, should be done immediately. General supportive care, including frequent monitoring of the vital signs and close observation of the patient, are required.

It has been reported that alkalinization of the urine may be expected to increase the excretion of the N-demethylated metabolite of paramethadione.

A blood count and a careful evaluation of hepatic and renal function should be done following recovery.

DOSAGE AND ADMINISTRATION:

Paramethadione is administered orally.

Usual Adult Dosage: 0.9 - 2.4 g daily in 3 or 4 equally divided doses (*i.e.,* 300 - 600 mg 3 or 4 times daily).

Initially, give 0.9 g daily; increase this dose by 300 mg at weekly intervals until therapeutic results are seen or until toxic symptoms appear.

Maintenance dosage should be the least amount of drug required to maintain control.

Children's Dosage: Usually 0.3-0.9 g daily in 3 or 4 equally divided doses.

Recommended Storage: 59 - 86°F (15 - 30°C).

HOW SUPPLIED - EQUIVALENTS NOT AVAILABLE:

Capsule, Elastic - Oral - 150 mg

100's	$42.67	PARADIONE, Abbott	00074-3976-01

PAREGORIC *(001960)*

CATEGORIES: Analgesics; Antidiarrhea Agents; Gastrointestinal Drugs; Pain; DEA Class CIII; FDA Pre 1938 Drugs

FORMULARIES: Aetna; Medi-Cal

Prescribing information not available at time of publication.

HOW SUPPLIED - EQUIVALENTS NOT AVAILABLE:

Liquid - Oral - 0.35 mg/ml

480 ml	$3.12	Paregoric, Purepac Pharm	00228-2020-16
480 ml	$7.30	Paregoric, HR Cenci	00556-0257-16
480 ml	$7.30	Paregoric, Harber Pharm	51432-0642-20
480 ml	$8.03	Paregoric, Alpharma	00472-0802-16
480 ml	$8.05	Paregoric, United Res	00677-0634-33
480 ml	$8.05	Paregoric, HL Moore Drug Exch	00839-7075-69
480 ml	$8.95	Paregoric, Major Pharms	00904-0802-16
480 ml	$9.12	Paregoric, Morton Grove	60432-0457-16
480 ml	$9.15	Paregoric, Qualitest Pharms	00603-1494-58
480 ml	$9.25	Paregoric, Geneva Pharms	00781-6130-16
480 ml	$9.68	Paregoric, IDE-Interstate	00814-5790-82
480 ml	$10.57	Paregoric, Aligen Independ	00405-0145-16
480 ml	$11.30	Paregoric, Goldline Labs	00182-0757-40
3840 ml	$35.87	Paregoric, HR Cenci	00556-0257-28

Solution - Oral - 0.4 %/0.4 %/0.4

480 ml	$9.00	Paregoric, Halsey Drug	00879-0035-16
3840 ml	$35.94	Paregoric, Halsey Drug	00879-0035-28

Tincture - Oral - 0.35 mg/ml

1 pt	$9.13	Paregoric, Rugby	00536-1501-85

PAROMOMYCIN SULFATE *(001962)*

CATEGORIES: Amebiasis; Amebicides; Aminoglycosides; Anti-Infectives; Antimicrobials; Antiprotozoals; Hepatic Coma; Parasiticidal; FDA Approval Pre 1982

BRAND NAMES: *Gabbroral*; *Humagel* (France); **Humatin**
(International brand names outside U.S. in italics)

FORMULARIES: Medi-Cal

DESCRIPTION:

Humatin is a broad spectrum antibiotic produced by *Streptomyces rimosus* var. *paromomycinus.* It is a white, amorphous, stable, water-soluble product supplied as capsules containing the equivalent of 250 mg paromomycin.

The capsule contains D&C yellow No. 10; FD&C blue No. 1; FD&C red No. 3; FD&C yellow No. 6; gelatin, NF; and titanium dioxide, USP.

CLINICAL PHARMACOLOGY:

The *in vitro* and *in vivo* antibacterial action of paromomycin closely parallels that of neomycin. It is poorly absorbed after oral administration, with almost 100% of the drug recoverable in the stool.

INDICATIONS AND USAGE:

Humatin is indicated for intestinal amebiasis—acute and chronic (NOTE-It is not effective in extraintestinal amebiasis); management of hepatic coma—as adjunctive therapy.

CONTRAINDICATIONS:

Paromomycin sulfate is contraindicated in individuals with a history of previous hypersensitivity reactions to it. It is also contraindicated in intestinal obstruction.

PRECAUTIONS:

The use of this antibiotic, as with other antibiotics, may result in an overgrowth of nonsusceptible organisms, including fungi. Constant observation of the patient is essential. If new infections caused by nonsusceptible organisms appear during therapy, appropriate measures should be taken.

The drug should be used with caution in individuals with ulcerative lesions of the bowel to avoid renal toxicity through inadvertent absorption.

ADVERSE REACTIONS:

Nausea, abdominal cramps, and diarrhea have been reported in patients on doses over 3 g daily.

DOSAGE AND ADMINISTRATION:

INTESTINAL AMEBIASIS

Adults and Children: Usual dose-25 to 35 mg/kg body weight daily, administered in three doses with meals, for five to ten days.

MANAGEMENT OF HEPATIC COMA

Adults: Usual dose-4 g daily in divided doses, given at regular intervals for five to six days.

HOW SUPPLIED - EQUIVALENTS NOT AVAILABLE:

Capsule, Gelatin - Oral - 250 mg

16's	$27.61	HUMATIN, Parke-Davis	00071-0529-09
100's	$197.88	HUMATIN, Parke-Davis	00071-0529-24

PAROXETINE HYDROCHLORIDE *(003130)*

CATEGORIES: Antidepressants; Central Nervous System Agents; Depression; Depressive Disorder; Fatigue; Psychotherapeutic Agents; Selective Serotonin Reuptake Inhibitors; Panic Disorder*; Pregnancy Category B; FDA Class 1S ("Standard Review"); Sales > $500 Million; FDA Approved 1992 Dec; Top 200 Drugs
* Indication not approved by the FDA

BRAND NAMES: Aropax; *Aropax 20* (Australia); **Paxil**; Seroxat
(International brand names outside U.S. in italics)

FORMULARIES: BC-BS; Medi-Cal; PCS

COST OF THERAPY: $170.91 (Depression; Tablet; 20 mg; 1/day; 90 days) vs. Potential Cost of $2,456.15 (Depression)

PRIMARY ICD9: 311 (Depressive Disorder, Not Elsewhere Classified)

DESCRIPTION:

Paxil (paroxetine hydrochloride) is an orally administered antidepressant with a chemical structure unrelated to other selective serotonin reuptake inhibitors or to tricyclic, tetracyclic or other available antidepressants agents. It is the hydrochloride salt of a phenylpiperidine compound identified chemically as (-)-*trans*-4*R*-(4'-fluorophenyl)-3*S*-[(3',4'-methylenedioxyphenoxy) methyl] piperidine hydrochloride hemihydrate and has the empirical formula of $C_{19}H_{20}FNO_3{\cdot}HCl{\cdot}1/2H_2O$. The molecular weight is 374.8 (329.4 as free base).

Paroxetine hydrochloride is an odorless, off-white powder, having a melting point range of 120 to 138°C and a solubility of 5.4 mg/ml in water.

Each film-coated tablet contains paroxetine hydrochloride equivalent to paroxetine as follows: 20 mg-pink (scored); 30 mg-blue. Inactive ingredients consist of dibasic calcium phosphate dihydrate, hydroxypropyl methylcellulose, magnesium stearate, polyethylene glycols, polysorbate 80, sodium starch glycolate, titanium dioxide and one or more of the following: D&C Red No. 30, FD&C Blue No. 2.

CLINICAL PHARMACOLOGY:

Pharmacodynamics: The antidepressant action of paroxetine is presumed to be linked to potentiation of serotonergic activity in the central nervous system resulting from inhibition of neuronal reuptake of serotonin (5-hydroxy-tryptamine, 5-HT). Studies at clinically relevant doses in humans have demonstrated that paroxetine blocks the uptake of serotonin into human platelets. *In vitro* studies in animals also suggest that paroxetine is a potent and highly selective inhibitor of neuronal serotonin reuptake and has only very weak effects on norepinephrine and dopamine neuronal reuptake. *In vitro*radioligand binding studies indicate that paroxetine has little affinity for muscarinic alpha$_1$-, alpha$_2$-, beta-adrenergic-, dopamine (D_2)-, 5-HT_1-, 5-HT_2,- and histamine (H_1)-receptors; antagonism of muscarinic, histaminergic, and alpha$_1$-adrenergic receptors has been associated with various anticholinergic, sedative and cardiovascular effects for other psychotropic drugs.

Because the relative potencies of paroxetine's major metabolites are at most 1/50 of the parent compound, they are essentially inactive.

Pharmacokinetics: Paroxetine hydrochloride is completely absorbed after oral dosing of a solution of the hydrochloride salt. In a study in which normal male subjects (n=15) received 30 mg tablets daily for 30 days, steady-state paroxetine concentrations were achieved by approximately 10 days for most subjects, although it might take substantially longer in an occasional patient. At steady state, mean values of C_{max}, T_{max}, C_{min}, and $T_{1/2}$were 61.7 ng/ml (CV 45%), 5.2 hr. (CV (10%), 30.7 ng/ml (CV 67%) and 21.0 hr. (CV 32%), respectively. The steady-state C_{max} and C_{min} values were about 6 and 14 times what would be predicted from a single-dose studies. Steady-state drug exposure based on AUC_{0-24} was about 8 times greater than would have been predicted from single-dose data in these subjects. The excess accumulation is a consequence of the fact that one of the enzymes that metabolizes paroxetine is readily saturable.

In steady-state dose proportionality studies involving elderly and nonelderly patients, at doses of 20 to 40 mg daily for the elderly and 20 to 50 mg daily for the nonelderly, some nonlinearity was observed in both populations, again reflecting a saturable metabolic pathway. In comparison to C_{min} values after 20 mg daily, values after 40 mg were only about 2 to 3 times greater than doubled.

Paroxetine is extensively metabolized after oral administration. The principal metabolites are polar and conjugated products of oxidation and methylation, which are readily cleared. Conjugates with gluconic acid and sulfate predominate, and major metabolites have been isolated and identified. Data indicate that the metabolites have no more than 1/50 the potency of the parent compound at inhibiting serotonin uptake. The metabolism of paroxetine is accomplished in part by cytochrome $P_{450}IID_6$. Saturation of this enzyme at clinical doses appears to account for the nonlinearity of paroxetine kinetics with increasing dose and increasing duration of treatment. The role of this enzyme in paroxetine metabolism also suggests potential drug-drug interactions (see PRECAUTIONS.)

Approximately 64% of a 30 mg oral solution dose of paroxetine was excreted in the urine with 2% as the parent and 62% as metabolites over a 10-day post-dosing period. About 36% was excreted in the feces (probably via the bile), mostly as metabolites and less than 1% as the parent compound over the 10-day post-dosing period.

Distribution: Paroxetine distributes throughout the body, including the CNS, with only 1% remaining in the plasma.

Protein Binding: Approximately 95% and 93% of paroxetine is bound to plasma protein at 100 ng/ml and 400 ng/ml, respectively. Under clinical conditions, paroxetine concentrations would normally be less than 400 ng/ml. Paroxetine does not alter the *in vitro*protein binding of phenytoin or warfarin.

Renal and Liver Disease: Increased plasma concentrations of paroxetine occur in subjects with renal and hepatic impairment. The mean plasma concentrations in patients with creatinine clearance below 30 ml/min was approximately 4 times greater than seen in normal volunteers. Patients with creatinine clearance of 30 to 60 ml/min and patients with hepatic functional impairment had about a 2-fold increase in plasma concentrations (AUC, C_{max}).

CLINICAL PHARMACOLOGY: *(cont'd)*

The initial dosage should therefore be reduced in patients with severe renal or hepatic impairment, and upward titration, if necessary, should be at increased intervals (see DOSAGE AND ADMINISTRATION.)

Elderly Patients: In a multiple-dose study in the elderly at daily paroxetine doses of 20, 30 and 40 mg, C_{min}concentrations were about 70% to 80% greater than the respective C_{min}concentrations in nonelderly subjects. Therefore the initial dosage in the elderly should be reduced. (See DOSAGE AND ADMINISTRATION.)

CLINICAL STUDIES:

Depression: The efficacy of paroxetine hydrochloride as a treatment for depression has been established in 6 placebo-controlled studies of patients with depression (ages 18 to 73). In these studies paroxetine hydrochloride was shown to be significantly more effective than placebo in treating depression by at least 2 of the following measures: Hamilton Depression Rating Scale (HDRS), the Hamilton depressed mood item, and the Clinical Global Impression (CGI)—Severity of illness. Paroxetine hydrochloride was significantly better than placebo in improvement of the HDRS sub-factor scores, including the depressed mood item, sleep disturbance factor and anxiety factor.

A study of depressed outpatients who had responded to paroxetine hydrochloride (HDRS total score <8) during an initial 8-week open-treatment phase and were then randomized to continuation on paroxetine hydrochloride or placebo for 1 year demonstrated a significantly lower relapse rate for patients taking paroxetine hydrochloride (15%) compared to those on placebo (39%). Effectiveness was similar for male and female patients.

Obsessive Compulsive Disorder: The effectiveness of paroxetine hydrochloride in the treatment of obsessive compulsive disorder (OCD) was demonstrated in two 12–week multicenter placebo-controlled studies of adult outpatients (Studies 1 and 2). Patients in all studies had moderate to severe OCD (DSM-IIIR) with mean baseline ratings on the Yale Brown Obsessive Compulsive Scale (YBOCS) total score ranging from 23 to 26. Study 1, a dose-range finding study where patients were treated with fixed doses of 20, 40 or 60 mg of paroxetine/day demonstrated that daily doses of paroxetine 40 and 60 mg are effective in the treatment of OCD. Patients receiving doses of 40 and 60 mg paroxetine experienced a mean reduction of approximately 6 and 7 points respectively on the YBOCS total score which was significantly greater than the approximate 4 point reduction at 20 mg and a 3 point reduction in the placebo-treated patients. Study 2 was a flexible dose study comparing paroxetine (20 to 60 mg daily) with clomipramine (25 to 250 mg daily). In this study, patients receiving paroxetine experienced a mean reduction of approximately 7 points on the YBOCS total score which was significantly greater than the mean reduction of approximately 4 points in the placebo-treated patients.

The following table provides the outcome classification by treatment group on Global Improvement items of the Clinical Global Impressions (CGI) scale for Study 1.

TABLE 1 Outcome Classification (%) on CGI-Global Improvement Item for Completers in Study 1

Outcome Classification	Placebo (N=74)	Paroxetine HCl 20 mg (N=75)	Paroxetine HCl 40 mg (N=66)	Paroxetine HCl 60 mg (N=66)
Worse	14%	7%	7%	3%
No Change	44%	35%	22%	19%
Minimally Improved	24%	33%	29%	34%
Much Improved	11%	18%	22%	24%
Very Much Improved	7%	7%	20%	20%

Subgroup analyses did not indicate that there were any differences in treatment outcomes as a function of age or gender.

The long-term maintenance effects of paroxetein hydrochloride in OCD were demonstrated in a long-term extension to Study 1. Patients who were responders on paroxetine during the 3–month double-blind phase and a 6–month extension on open-label paroxetine (20 to 60 mg/day) were randomized to either paroxetine or placebo in a 6–month double-blind relapse prevention phase. Patients randomized to paroxetine were significantly less likely to relapse than comparably treated patients who were randomized to placebo.

Panic Disorder: The effectiveness of paroxetine hydrochloride in the treatment of panic disorder was demonstrated in three 10 to 12 week multicenter, placebo-controlled studies of adult outpatients (Studies 1–3). Patients in all studies had panic disorder (DSM-IIIR), with or without agoraphobia. In these studies, paroxetine hydrochloride was shown to be significantly more effective than placebo in treating panic disorder by at least 2 out of 3 measures of panic attack frequency and on the Clinical Global Impression Severity of Illness score.

Study 1 was a 10–week dose-range finding study: patients were treated with fixed paroxetine doses of 10, 20, or 40 mg/day or placebo. A significant difference from placebo was observed only for the 40 mg/day group. At endpoint, 76% of patients receiving paroxetine 40 mg/day were free of panic attacks, compared to 44% of placebo-treated patients.

Study 2 was a 12–week flexible-dose study comparing paroxetine (10 to 60 mg daily) and placebo. At endpoint, 51% of paroxetine patients were free of panic attacks compared to 32% of placebo-treated patients.

Study 3 was a 12–week flexible-dose study comparing paroxetine (10 to 60 mg daily) to placebo in patients concurrently receiving standardized cognitive behavioral therapy. At endpoint, 33% of the paroxetine-treated patients showed a reduction to 0 or 1 panic attacks compared to 14% of placebo patients.

In both Studies 2 and 3, the mean paroxetine dose for completers at endpoint was approximately 40 mg/day of paroxetine.

In both Studies 2 and 3, the mean paroxetine dose for completers at endpoint was approximately 40 mg/day of paroxetine.

Long-term maintenance effects of paroxetine hydrochloride in panic disorder were demonstrated in an extension to Study 1. Patients who were responders during the 10–week double-blid phase and during a 3–month double-blind extension phase were randomized to either paroxetine (10, 20, or 40 mg/day) or placebo in a 3–month double-blind relapse prevention phase. Patients randomized to paroxetine were significantly less likely to relapse than comparably treated patients who were randomized to placebo.

Subgroup analyses did not indicate that there were any differences in treatment outcomes as a function of age or gender.

INDICATIONS AND USAGE:

DEPRESSION

Paroxetine hydrochloride is indicated for the treatment of depression.

The efficacy of paroxetein hydrochloride in the treatment of a major depressive episode was established in 6-week controlled trials of outpatients whose diagnoses corresponded most closely to the DSM-III category of major depressive disorder (See CLINICAL PHARMACOLOGY.)

INDICATIONS AND USAGE: *(cont'd)*

A major depressive episode implies a prominent and relatively persistent depressed or dysphoric mood that usually interferes with daily functioning (nearly every day for at least 2 weeks); it should include at least 4 of the following 8 symptoms: change in appetite, change in sleep, psychomotor agitation or retardation, loss of interest in usual activities or decrease in sex drive, increased fatigue, feelings of guilt or worthlessness, slowed thinking or impaired concentration, and a suicide attempt or suicidal ideation.

The antidepressant action of paroxetine hydrochloride in hospitalized depressed patients has not been adequately studied.

The efficacy of paroxetine hydrochloride in maintaining an antidepressant response for up to 1 year was demonstrated in a placebo-controlled trial (see CLINICAL PHARMACOLOGY.)

Nevertheless, the physician who elects to use paroxetine hydrochloride for extended periods should periodically re-evaluate for long-term usefulness of the drug for the individual patient.

OBSESSIVE COMPULSIVE DISORDER

Paroxetine hydrochloride is indicated for the treatment of obsessions and compulsions in patients with obsessive compulsive disorder (OCD) as defined in the DSM-IV. The obsessions or compulsions cause marked distress, are time-consuming, or significantly interfere with social or occupational functioning.

The efficacy of paroxetine hydrochloride was established in two 12 week trials with obsessive compulsive outpatients whoe diagnoses corresponded most closely to the DSM-IIIR category of obsessive compulsive disorder (see CLINICAL STUDIES.)

Obsessive compulsive disorder is characterized by recurrent and persistent ideas, thoughts, impulses or images (obsessions) that are egodystonic and/or repetitive, purposeful and intentional behaviors (compulsions) that are recognized by the person as excessive or unreasonable.

Long-term maintenance of efficacy was demonstrated in a 6–month relapse prevention trial. In this trial, patients assigned to paroxetine showed a lower relapse rate compared to patients on placebo (see CLINICAL PHARMACOLOGY.) Nevertheless, the physicians who elects to use paroxetine hydrochloride for extended periods should periodically reevaluate the long-term usefulness of the drug for the individual patient (see DOSAGE AND ADMINISTRATION.)

PANIC DISORDER

Paroxetine hydrochloride is indicated for the treatment of panic disorder, with or without agoraphobia, as defined in DSM-IV. Panic disorder is characterized by the occurrence of unexpected panic attacks and associated concern about having additional attacks, worry about the implications or consequences of the attacks, and/or a significant change in behavior related to the attacks.

The efficacy of paroxetine hydrochloride was established in three 10 to 12 week trials in panic disorder patients whose diagnoses corresponded to the DSM-IIIR category of panic disorder (see CLINICAL STUDIES.)

Panic disorder (DSM-IV) is characterized by recurrent unexpected panic attacks (*i.e.*, a discrete period of intense fear or discomfort in which four (or more) of the following symptoms develop abruptly and reach a peak within 10 minutes: [(1) palpitations; (2) sweating; (3) trembling or shaking; (4) sensations of shortness of breath or smothering; (5) feeling of choking; (6) chest pain or discomfort; (7) nausea or abdominal distress; (8) feeling dizzy, unsteady, lightheaded, or faint; (9) derealization (feelings of unreality) or depersonalization (being detached from oneself); (10) fear of losing control; (11) fear of dying; (12) paresthesias (numbness or tingling sensations); (13) chills or hot flashes.])

Long-term maintenance of efficacy was demonstrated in a 3–month relapse prevention trial. In this trial, patients with panic disorder assigned to paroxetine demonstrated a lower relapse rate compared to patients on placebo (see CLINICAL PHARMACOLOGY.) Nevertheless, the physician who prescribes paroxetine hydrochloride for extended periods should periodically reevaluate the long-term usefulness of the drug for the individual patient.

CONTRAINDICATIONS:

Concomitant use in patients taking monoamine oxidase inhibitors (MAOIs) is contraindicated (see WARNINGS.)

WARNINGS:

POTENTIAL FOR INTERACTION WITH MONOAMINE OXIDASE INHIBITORS.

In patients receiving another serotonin reuptake inhibitor drug in combination with a monoamine oxidase inhibitor (MAOI), there have been reports of serious, sometimes fatal, reactions including hyperthermia, rigidity, myoclonus, autonomic instability with possible rapid fluctuations of vital signs, and mental status changes that include extreme agitation progressing to delirium and coma. These reactions have also been reported in patients who have recently discontinued that drug and have been started on a MAOI. Some cases presented with features resembling neuroleptic malignant syndrome. While there are no human data showing such an interaction with paroxetine, limited animal data on the effects of combined use of paroxetine and MAOIs suggest that these drugs may act synergistically to elevate blood pressure and evoke behavioral excitation. Therefore, it is recommended that paroxetine hydrochloride not be used in combination with a MAOI, or within 14 days of discontinuing treatment with a MAOI. At least 2 weeks should be allowed after stopping paroxetine before starting a MAOI.

PRECAUTIONS:

GENERAL

Activation of Mania/Hypomania: During premarketing testing, hypomania or mania occurred in approximately 1.0% of paroxetine-treated unipolar patients compared to 1.1% of active-control and 0.3% of placebo-treated unipolar patients. In a subset of patients classified as bipolar, the rate of manic episodes was 2.2% for paroxetine and 11.6% for the combined active-control groups. As with all antidepressants, paroxetine should be used cautiously in patients with a history of mania.

Seizures: During premarketing testing, seizures occurred in 0.1% of paroxetine-treated patients, a rate similar to that associated with other antidepressants. Paroxetine should be used cautiously in patients with a history of seizures. It should be discontinued in any patient who develops seizures.

Suicide: The possibility of a suicide attempt is inherent in depression and may persist until significant remission occurs. Close supervision of high-risk patients should accompany initial drug therapy. Prescriptions for paroxetine should be written for the smallest quantity of tablets consistent with good patient management, in order to reduce the risk of overdose.

Hyponatremia: Several cases of hyponatremia have been reported. The hyponatremia appeared to be reversible when paroxetine was discontinued. The majority of these occurrences have been in elderly individuals, some in patients taking diuretics or who were otherwise volume depleted.

Abnormal Bleeding: There have been several reports of abnormal bleeding (mostly ecchymosis and purpural) associated with paroxetine treatment, including a report of impaired platelet aggregation. While a causal relationship to paroxetine is unclear, impaired platelet aggregation may result from platelet serotonin depletion and contribute to such occurrences.

PRECAUTIONS: *(cont'd)*

Use in Patients with Concomitant Illness: Clinical experience with paroxetine hydrochloride in patients with certain concomitant systemic illness is limited. Caution is advisable in using paroxetine hydrochloride in patients with diseases or conditions that could affect metabolism or hemodynamic responses.

Paroxetine hydrochloride has not been evaluated or used to any appreciable extent in patients with a recent history of myocardial infarction or unstable heart disease. Patients with these diagnoses were excluded from clinical studies during the product's premarket testing. Evaluations of electrocardiograms of 682 patients who received paroxetein hydrochloride in double-blind, placebo-controlled trials, however, did not indicate that paroxetine hydrochloride is associated with the development of significant ECG abnormalities. Similarly, paroxetine hydrochloride does not cause any clinically important changes in heart rate or blood pressure.

Increased plasma concentrations of paroxetine occur in patients with severe renal impairment (creatinine clearance <30 ml/min.) or severe hepatic impairment. A lower starting dose should be used in such patients (see DOSAGE AND ADMINISTRATION.)

INFORMATION FOR PATIENTS

Physicians are advised to discuss the following issues with patients for whom they prescribe paroxetine hydrochloride.

Interference with Cognitive and Motor Performance: Any psychoactive drug may impair judgment, thinking or motor skills. Although in controlled studies paroxetine hydrochloride has not been shown to impair psychomotor performance, patients should be cautioned about operating hazardous machinery, including automobiles, until they are reasonably certain that paroxetine hydrochloride therapy does not affect their ability to engage in such activities.

Contemplating Course of Therapy: While patients may notice improvement with paroxetine hydrochloride therapy in 1 to 4 weeks, they should be advised to continue therapy as directed.

Concomitant Medication: Patients should be advised to inform their physician if they are taking, or plan to take, any prescription or over-the-counter drugs, since there is a potential for interactions.

Alcohol: Although paroxetine hydrochloride has not been shown to increase the impairment of mental and motor skills caused by alcohol, patients should be advised to avoid alcohol while taking paroxetine hydrochloride.

Pregnancy: Patients should be advised to notify their physician if they become pregnant or intend to become pregnant during therapy.

Nursing: Patients should be advised to notify their physician if they are breast-feeding an infant. See PRECAUTIONS, Nursing Mothers.

Laboratory Tests There are no specific laboratory tests recommended.

CARCINOGENESIS, MUTAGENESIS, IMPAIRMENT OF FERTILITY

Carcinogenesis: Two-year carcinogenicity studies were conducted in mice and rats given paroxetine in the diet at 1, 5, and 25 mg/kg/day (mice) and 1, 5 and 20 mg/kg/day (rats). The maximum doses in these studies were approximately 25 (mouse) and 20 (rat) times the maximum dose recommended for human use on a mg/kg basis or 2.5 (mouse) and 5.8 (rat) times the maximum recommended human dose on a mg/m^2 basis. There was a significantly greater number of male rats in the high-dose group with reticulum cell sarcomas (1/100, 0/50, 0/50 and 4/50 for control, low-, middle- and high-dose groups, respectively) and a significantly increased linear trend across dose groups for the occurrence of lymphoreticular tumors in male rats. Female rats were not affected. Although there was a dose-related increase in the number of tumors in mice, there was no drug-related increase in the number of mice with tumors. The relevance of these findings to humans is unknown.

Mutagenesis: Paroxetine produced no genotoxic effects in a battery of 5 *in vitro* and 2 *in vivo* assays that included the following: bacterial mutation assay, mouse lymphoma mutation assay, unscheduled DNA synthesis assay, and tests for cytogenetic aberrations *in vivo*in mouse bone marrow and *in vitro* in human lymphocytes and in a dominant lethal test in rats.

Impairment of Fertility: Serotonergic compounds are known to affect reproductive function in animals. Impaired reproductive function (*i.e.,* reduced pregnancy rate, increased pre- and post- implantation losses, decreased viability of pups) was found in reproduction studies in rats at doses of paroxetine which were 15 or more times the highest recommended human dose on a mg/kg basis, or 4.4 times on a mg/m^{2}basis. Irreversible lesions occurred in the reproductive tract of male rats after dosing in toxicity studies for 2 to 52 weeks. These lesions, which consisted of vacuolation of epididymal tubular epithelium and atrophic changes in the seminiferous tubules of the testes with arrested spermatogenesis occurred at doses which were 25 times the highest recommended human dose on a mg/kg basis of 7.3 times on a mg/m^2 basis.

Pregnancy, Teratogenic Effects, Pregnancy Category C: Reproduction studies performed at doses up to 50 mg/kg/day in rats and 6 mg/kg/day in rabbits administered during organogenesis. These doses are equivalent to 9.7 (rat) and 2.2 (rabbit) times the maximum recommended human dose (MRHD) for depression (50 mg) and 8.1 (rat) and 1.9 (rabbit) times the MRHD for OCD, on a mg/m^2 basis. These studies have revealed no evidence of teratogenic effects. However, in rats, there was an increase in pup deaths during the first 4 days of lactation when dosing occurred during the last trimester of gestation and continued throughout lactation. This effect occurred at a dose of 1 mg/kg/day or 0.19 times (mg/m^2) the MRHD for depression and at 0.16 times (mg/m^2) the MRHD for OCD. The no-effect dose for rat pup mortality was not determined. The cause of these deaths is not known. There are no adequate and well-controlled studies in pregnant women. Because animal reporduction studies are not always predictive of human response, this drug should be used during pregnancy only if the potential benefit justifies the potential risk to the fetus.

Labor and Delivery: The effect of paroxetine on labor and delivery in humans is unknown.

Nursing Mothers: Like many other drugs, paroxetine is secreted in human milk, and caution should be exercised when paroxetine hydrochloride is administered to a nursing woman.

Usage in Children: Safety and effectiveness in children have not been established.

Geriatric Use: In worldwide paroxetine hydrochloride clinical trials, 17% of paroxetine hydrochloride- treated patients (approximately 700) were 65 years of age or older. Pharmacokinetic studies revealed a decreased clearance in the elderly, and a lower starting dose is recommended; there were, however, no overall differences in the adverse event profile between elderly and younger patients, and effectiveness was similar in younger and older patients. (See CLINICAL PHARMACOLOGY and DOSAGE AND ADMINISTRATION.)

DRUG INTERACTIONS:

Tryptophan: As with other serotonin reuptake inhibitors, an interaction between paroxetine and tryptophan may occur when they are co-administered. Adverse experiences, consisting primarily of headache, nausea, sweating and dizziness, have been reported when tryptophan was administered to patients taking paroxetine hydrochloride. Consequently, concomitant use of paroxetine hydrochloride with tryptophan is not recommended.

Monoamine Oxidase Inhibitors: (See CONTRAINDICATIONS) and WARNINGS.

Warfarin: Preliminary data suggest that there may be a pharmacodynamic interaction (that causes an increased bleeding diathesis in the face of unaltered prothrombin time) between paroxetine and warfarin. Since there is little clinical experience, the concomitant administration of paroxetine hydrochloride and warfarin should be undertaken with caution.

Drugs Affecting Hepatic Metabolism: The metabolism and pharmacokinetics of paroxetine may be affected by the induction or inhibition of drug-metabolizing enzymes.

Cimetidine: Cimetidine inhibits many cytochrome P_{450} (oxidative) enzymes. In a study where paroxetine hydrochloride (30 mg q.d.) was dosed orally for 4 weeks, steady-state plasma concentrations of paroxetine were increased by approximately 50% during co-administration with oral cimetidine (300 mg t.i.d.) for the final week. Therefore, when these drugs are administered concurrently, dosage adjustment of paroxetine hydrochloride after the 20 mg starting dose should be guided by clinical effect. The effect of paroxetine on cimetidine's pharmacokinetics was not studied.

Phenobarbital: Phenobarbital induces many cytochrome P_{450}(oxidative) enzymes. When a single oral 30 mg dose of paroxetine hydrochloride was administered at phenobarbital steady state (100 mg q.d. for 14 days), paroxetine AUC and $T_{1/2}$were reduced (by an average of 25% and 38%, respectively) compared to paroxetine administered alone. The effect of paroxetine on phenobarbital pharmacokinetics was not studied. Since paroxetine hydrochloride exhibits nonlinear pharmacokinetics, the results of this study may not address the case where the 2 drugs are both being chronically dosed. No initial paroxetine hydrochloride dosage adjustment is considered necessary when co- administered with phenobarbital; any subsequent adjustment should be guided by clinical effect.

Phenytoin: When a single oral 30 mg dose of paroxetine hydrochloride was administered at phenytoin steady state (300 mg q.d. for 14 days), paroxetine AUC and $T_{1/2}$ were reduced (by an average of 50% and 35%, respectively) compared to paroxetine hydrochloride administered alone. In a separate study, when a single oral 300 mg dose of phenytoin was administered at paroxetine steady state (30 mg q.d. for 14 days), phenytoin AUC was slightly reduced (12% on average) compared to phenytoin administered alone. Since both drugs exhibit nonlinear pharmacokinetics, the above studies may not address the case where the 2 drugs are both being chronically dosed. No initial dosage adjustments are considered necessary when these drugs are co- administered; any subsequent adjustments should be guided by clinical effect.

Drug Metabolized by Cytochrome $P_{450}IID_6$: Concomitant use of with drugs metabolized by cytochrome $P_{450}IID_6$ has not been formally studied but may require lower doses than usually prescribed for either paroxetine hydrochloride or the other drug. Many drugs, including most antidepressants (paroxetine, other SSRIs and many tricyclics), are metabolized by the cytochrome P_{450} isozyme $P_{450}IID_6$. In most patients (>90%), this $P_{450}IID_6$ isozyme is saturated early during paroxetine hydrochloride dosing. Like other agents that are metabolized by $P_{450}IID_6$, paroxetine may significantly inhibit the activity of this isozyme.

Therefore, co-administration of paroxetine hydrochloride with other drugs that are metabolized by this isozyme, including certain antidepressants (*e.g.,* nortriptyline, amitriptyline, imipramine, desipramine and fluoxetine), phenothiazines (*e.g.,* thioridazine) and Type 1C antiarrhythmics (*e.g.,* propafenone, flecainide and encainide), or that inhibit this enzyme (*e.g.,* quinidine), should be approached with caution.

At steady state, when the $P_{450}IID_6$ pathway is essentially saturated, paroxetine clearance is governed by alternative P_{450} isozymes which, unlike $P_{450}IID_6$, show no evidence of saturation. (see PRECAUTIONS, Tricyclic Antidepressants.

Drugs Metabolized by Cytochrome $P_{450}IIIA_4$: An *in vivo* interaction study involving the co-administration under steady-state conditions of paroxetine and terfenadine, a substrate for cytochrome $P_{450}IIIA_4$, revealed no effect of paroxetine or terfenadine pharmacokinetics. In addition, *in vitro* studies have shown ketoconazole, a potent inhibitor of $P_{450}IIIA_4$ activity, to be at least 100 times more potent than paroxetine as an inhibitor of the metabolism of several substrates for this enzyme, including terfenadine, astemizole, cisapride, triazolam, and cyclosporin. Based on the assumption that the relationship between paroxetine's *in vitro* K and its lack of effect on terfenadine's *in vivo* clearance predicts its effect on other $IIIA_4$ substrates, paroxetine's extent of inhibition of $IIIA_4$ activity is not likely to be of clinical significance.

Tricyclic Antidepressants (TCA): Caution is indicated in the co-administration of tricyclic antidepressants (TCAs) with paroxetine hydrochloride, because paroxetine may inhibit TCA metabolism. Plasma TCA concentrations may need to be monitored, and the dose of TCA may need to be reduced, if a TCA is co-administered with paroxetine hydrochloride (see PRECAUTIONS: Drugs Metabolized by Cytochrome $P_{450}IID_5$

Drugs Highly Bound to Plasma Protein: Because paroxetine is highly bound to plasma protein, administration of paroxetine hydrochloride to a patient taking another drug that is highly protein bound may cause increased free concentrations of the other drug, potentially resulting in adverse events. Conversely, adverse effects could result from displacement of paroxetine by other highly bound drugs.

Alcohol: Although paroxetine hydrochloride does not increase the impairment of mental and motor skills caused by alcohol, patients should be advised to avoid alcohol while taking paroxetine hydrochloride.

Lithium: A multiple-dose study has shown that there is no pharmacokinetic interaction between paroxetine hydrochloride and lithium carbonate. However, since there is little clinical experience, the concurrent administration of paroxetine and lithium should be undertaken with caution.

Digoxin: The steady-state pharmacokinetics of paroxetine was not altered when administered with digoxin at steady state. Mean digoxin AUC at steady state decreased by 15% in the presence of paroxetine. Since there is little clinical experience, the concurrent administration of paroxetine and digoxin should be undertaken with caution.

Diazepam: Under steady-state conditions, diazepam does not appear to affect paroxetine kinetics. The effects of paroxetine on diazepam were not evaluated.

DRUG INTERACTIONS: *(cont'd)*

Procyclidine: Daily oral dosing of paroxetine hydrochloride (30 mg q.d.) increased steady-state AUC_{0-24}, C_{Max} and C_{min} values of procyclidine (5 mg oral q.d.) by 35%, 37%, and 67%, respectively, compared to procyclidine alone at steady state. If anticholinergic effects are seen, the dose of procyclidine should be reduced.

Beta-Blockers: In a study where propranolol (80 mg b.i.d.) was dosed orally for 18 days, the established steady-state plasma concentrations of propranolol were unaltered during co-administration with paroxetine hydrochloride (30 mg q.d.) for the final 10 days. The effects of propranolol on paroxetine have not been evaluated. See ADVERSE REACTIONS, Postmarketing Reports.

Theophylline: Reports of elevated theophylline levels associated with paroxetine hydrochloride treatment have been reported. While this interaction has not been formally studied, it is recommended that theophylline levels be monitored when these drugs are concurrently administered.

Electroconvulsive Therapy (ECT): There are no clinical studies of the combined use of ECT and paroxetine hydrochloride.

ADVERSE REACTIONS:

Associated with Discontinuation of Treatment Twenty-one percent (881/4,126) of paroxetine hydrochloride patients in worldwide clinical trials discontinued treatment due to an adverse event. The most common events (≥1%) associated with discontinuation and considered to be drug related (*i.e.,* those events associated with dropout at a rate approximately twice or greater for paroxetine compared to placebo) included (TABLE 1):

TABLE 1

CNS	
Somnolence	2.3%
Insomnia	1.9%
Agitation	1.3%
Tremor	1.3%
Anxiety	1.1%
Gastrointestinal	
Nausea	3.4%
Diarrhea	1.0%
Dry mouth	1.0%
Vomiting	1.0%
Other	
Asthenia	1.7%
Abnormal ejaculation	1.6%
Sweating	1.1%

COMMONLY OBSERVED ADVERSE EVENTS

Depression: The most commonly observed adverse events associated with the use of paroxetine (incidence of 5% or greater and incidence for paroxetine hydrochloride at least twice that for placebo, derived from Table 2 below) were: asthenia, sweating, nausea, decreased appetite, somnolence, dizziness, insomnia, tremor, nervousness, ejaculatory disturbance and other male genital disorders.

Obsessive Compulsive Disorder: The most commonly observed adverse events associated with the use of paroxetine (incidence of 5% or greater and incidence for paroxetine hydrochloride at least twice that of placebo, derived from Table 3 below) were: nausea, dry mouth, decreased appetite, constipation, dizziness, somnolence, tremor, sweating, impotence and abnormal ejaculation.

Panic Disorder: The most commonly observed adverse events associated with the use of paroxetine (incidence of 5% or greater and incidence for paroxetine hydrochloride at least twice that for placebo, derived from Table 3 below) were: asthenia, sweating, decreased appetite, libido decreased, tremor, abnormal ejaculation, female genital disorders and impotence.

INCIDENCE IN CONTROLLED CLINICAL TRIALS

Depression: Table 2 enumerates adverse events that occurred at an incidence of 1% or more among paroxetine-treated patients who participated in short-term (6-week) placebo-controlled trials in which patients were dosed in a range of 20 to 50 mg/day. Reported adverse events were classified using a standard COSTART-based Dictionary terminology.

The prescriber should be aware that these figures cannot be used to predict the incidence of side effects in the course of usual medical practice where patient characteristics and other factors differ from those which prevailed in the clinical trials. Similarly, the cited frequencies cannot be compared with figures obtained from other clinical investigations involving different treatments, uses and investigators. The cited figures, however, do provide the prescribing physician with some basis for estimating the relative contribution of drug and nondrug factors to the side effect incidence rate in the population studied (TABLE 2):

TABLE 2A Treatment-Emergent Adverse Experience Incidence in Placebo-Controlled Clinical Trials[1]

Body System	Preferred Term	Paroxetine HCl (n=421)	Placebo (n=421)
Body as a Whole	Headache	17.6%	17.3%
	Asthenia	15.0%	5.9%
	Abdominal Pain	3.1%	4.0%
	Fever	1.7%	1.7%
	Chest Pain	1.4%	2.1%
	Trauma	1.4%	0.5%
	Back Pain	1.2%	2.4%
Cardiovascular	Palpitation	2.9%	1.4%
	Vasodilation	2.6%	0.7%
	Postural Hypotension	1.2%	0.5%
Dermatologic	Sweating	11.2%	2.4%
	Rash	1.7%	0.7%
Gastrointestinal	Nausea	25.7%	9.3%
	Dry Mouth	18.1%	12.1%
	Constipation	13.8%	8.6%
	Diarrhea	11.6%	7.6%
	Decreased Appetite	6.4%	1.9%
	Flatulence	4.0%	1.7%
	Vomiting	2.4%	1.7%
	Oropharynx Disorder[2]	2.1%	0.0%
	Dyspepsia	1.9%	1.0%
	Increased Appetite	1.4%	0.5%

ADVERSE REACTIONS: *(cont'd)*

TABLE 2B

Body System & Preferred Term	Paroxetine HCl (n=421)	Placebo (n=421)
Musculoskeletal		
Myopathy	2.4%	1.4%
Myalgia	1.7%	0.7%
Myasthenia	1.4%	0.2%
Nervous System		
Somnolence	23.3%	9.0%
Dizziness	13.3%	5.5%
Insomnia	13.3%	6.2%
Tremor	8.3%	1.9%
Nervousness	5.2%	2.6%
Anxiety	5.0%	2.9%
Paresthesia	3.8%	1.7%
Libido Decreased	3.3%	0.0%
Agitation	2.1%	1.9%
Drugged Feeling	1.7%	0.7%
Myoclonus	1.4%	0.7%
CNS Stimulation	1.2%	3.6%
Confusion	1.2%	0.2%
Respiration		
Respiratory Disorder[3]	5.9%	6.4%
Yawn	3.8%	0.0%
Pharyngitis	2.1%	2.9%
Special Senses		
Blurred Vision	3.6%	1.4%
Taste Perversion	2.4%	0.2%
Urogenital System		
Ejaculatory Disturbance[4,5]	12.9%	0.0%
Other Male Genital Disorders[4,6]	10.0%	0.0%
Urinary Frequency	3.1%	0.7%
Urination Disorder[7]	2.9%	0.2%
Female Genital Disorders[4-8]	1.8%	0.0%

1 Events reported by at least 1% of patients treated with Paxil (paroxetine hydrochloride) are included.
2 Includes mostly "lump in throat" and "tightness in throat."
3 Includes mostly "cold symptoms" or "URI."
4 Percentage corrected for gender.
5 Mostly "ejaculatory delay."
6 Includes "anorgasmia", "erectile difficulties," "delayed ejaculation/orgasm," and "sexual dysfunction," and "impotence."
7 Includes mostly "difficulty with micturition" and "urinary hesitancy."
8 Includes mostly "anorgasmia" and "difficulty reaching climax/orgasm."

TABLE 3A Treatment Emergent Adverse Experience Incidence in Placebo-Controlled Clinical Trials for Obsessive Compulsive Disorder[1]

Body System	Preferred Term	Paroxetine HCl (n=542)	Placebo (n=285)
Body As A Whole	Asthenia	22%	14%
	Abdominal Pain		
	Chest Pain	3%	2%
	Back Pain	-	-
	Chills	2%	1%
Cardiovascular	Vasodilation	4%	1%
	Palpitation	2%	0%
Dermatologic	Sweating	9%	3%
	Rash	3%	2%
Gastrointestinal	Nausea	23%	10%
	Dry Mouth	18%	9%
	Constipation	16%	6%
	Diarrhea	10%	10%
	Decreased Appetite	9%	3%
	Increased Appetite	4%	3%

TABLE 3B Obsessive Compulsive Disorder

Body System & Preferred Term	Paroxetine HCl (n=542)	Placebo (n=285)
Nervous System		
Insomnia	24%	13%
Somnolence	24%	7%
Dizziness	12%	6%
Tremor	11%	1%
Nervousness	9%	8%
Libido Decreased	7%	4%
Agitation	-	-
Anxiety	-	-
Abnormal Dreams	4%	1%
Concentration Impaired	3%	2%
Depersonalization	3%	0%
Myoclonus	3%	0%
Amnesia	2%	1%
Respiratory System		
Rhinitis	-	-
Special Senses		
Abnormal Vision	4%	2%
Taste Perversion	2%	0%
Urogenital System		
Abnormal Ejaculation[2]	23%	1%
Female Genital Disorder[2]	3%	0%
Impotence[2]	8%	1%
Urinary Frequency	3%	1%
Urinary Impaired	3%	0%
Urinary Tract Infection	2%	1%

Obsessive Compulsive Disorder and Panic Disorder: Tables 3A and 3B enumerate adverse events that occurred at a frequency of 2% or more among OCD patients on paroxetine hydrochloride who participated in placebo-controlled trials of 12-weeks duration in which patients were dosed in a range of 20 to 60 mg/day or among patients with panic disorder on paroxetine hydrochloride who participated in placebo-controlled trials of 10 to 12 weeks duration in which patients were dosed in a range of 10 to 60 mg/day.

ADVERSE REACTIONS: *(cont'd)*

TABLE 3C Treatment Emergent Adverse Experience Incidence in Placebo-Controlled Clinical Trials for Panic Disorder[1]

Body System	Preferred Term	Paroxetine HCl (n=489)	Placebo (n=324)
Body As A Whole	Asthenia	14%	5%
	Abdominal Pain	4%	3%
	Chest Pain	-	-
	Back Pain	3%	2%
	Chills	2%	1%
Cardiovascular	Vasodilation	-	-
	Palpitation	-	-
Dermatologic	Sweating	14%	6%
	Rash	-	-
Gastrointestinal	Nausea	23%	17%
	Dry Mouth	18%	11%
	Constipation	8%	5%
	Diarrhea	12%	7%
	Decreased Appetite	7%	3%
	Increased Appetite	2%	1%

TABLE 3D Panic Disorder

Body System & Preferred Term	Paroxetine HCl (n=489)	Placebo (n=324)
Nervous System		
Insomnia	18%	10%
Somnolence	19%	11%
Dizziness	14%	10%
Tremor	9%	1%
Nervousness	-	-
Libido Decreased	9%	1%
Agitation	5%	4%
Anxiety	5%	4%
Abnormal Dreams	-	-
Concentration Impaired	-	-
Depersonalization	-	-
Myoclonus	3%	2%
Amnesia	-	-
Respiratory System		
Rhinitis	3%	0%
Special Senses		
Abnormal Vision	-	-
Taste Perversion	-	-
Urogenital System		
Abnormal Ejaculation[2]	21%	1%
Female Genital Disorder[2]	9%	1%
Impotence[2]	5%	0%
Urinary Frequency	2%	0%
Urinary Impaired	-	-
Urinary Tract Infection	2%	1%

1. Events reported by at least 2% of OCD or panic disorder paroxetine hydrochloride-treated patients are included, except the following events which had an incidence on placebo ≥ paroxetine hydrochloride. [OCD]: abdominal pain, agitation, anxiety, back pain, cough increased, depression, headache, hyperkinesia, infection, paresthesia, pharyngitis, respiratory disorder, rhinitis and sinusitis [panic disorder]: abnormal dreams, abnormal vision, chest pain, cough increased, depersonalization, depressions, dysmenorrhea, dyspepsia, flu syndrome, headache, infection, myalgia, nervousness, palpitation, paresthesia, pharyngitis, rash, respiratory disorder, sinusitis, taste perversion, trauma, urination impaired and vasodilation.
2. Percentage corrected for gender.

Dose Dependency of Adverse Events: A comparison of adverse event rates in a fixed-dose study comparing paroxetine hydrochloride 10, 20, 30 and 40 mg/day with placebo revealed a clear dose dependency for some of the more common adverse events associated with paroxetine hydrochloride use, as shown in the following table (TABLE 4):

TABLE 4 Treatment-Emergent Adverse Experience Incidence in a Dose-Comparison Trial*

Body System/ Preferred Term	Placebo n=51	Paxil 10 mg n=102	20 mg n=104	30 mg n=101	40 mg n=102
Body As A Whole					
Asthenia	0.0%	2.9%	10.6%	13.9%	12.7%
Dermatology					
Sweating	2.0%	1.0%	6.7%	8.9%	11.8%
Gastrointestinal					
Constipation	5.9%	4.9%	7.7%	9.9%	12.7%
Decreased Appetite	2.0%	2.0%	5.8%	4.0%	4.9%
Diarrhea	7.8%	9.8%	19.2%	7.9%	14.7%
Dry Mouth	2.0%	10.8%	18.3%	15.8%	20.6%
Nausea	13.7%	14.7%	26.9%	34.7%	36.3%
Nervous System					
Anxiety	0.0%	2.0%	5.8%	5.9%	5.9%
Dizziness	3.9%	6.9%	6.7%	8.9%	12.7%
Nervousness	0.0%	5.9%	5.8%	4.0%	2.9%
Paresthesia	0.0%	2.9%	1.0%	5.0%	5.9%
Somnolence	7.8%	12.7%	18.3%	20.8%	21.6%
Tremor	0.0%	0.0%	7.7%	7.9%	14.7%
Special Senses					
Blurred Vision	2.0%	2.9%	2.9%	2.0%	7.8%
Urogenital System					
Abnormal Ejaculation	0.0%	5.8%	6.5%	10.6%	13.0%
Impotence	0.0%	1.9%	4.3%	6.4%	1.9%
Male Genital Disorders	0.0%	3.8%	8.7%	6.4%	3.7%

* Rule for including adverse events in table: incidence at least 5% for one of paroxetine groups and ≥ twice the placebo incidence for at least one paroxetine group.

In a fixed-dose study comparing placebo and paroxetine hydrochloride 20, 40 and 60 mg in the treatment of OCD, there was no clear relationship between adverse events and the dose of paroxetine hydrochloride to which patients were assigned. No new adverse events were observed in hte paroxetine hydrochloride 60 mg dose group compared to any of the other treatment groups.

In a fixed-dose study comparing placebo and paroxetine hydrochloride 10, 20 and 40 mg in the treatment of panic disorder, there was no clear relationship between adverse events and the dose of paroxetine hydrochloride to which patients were assigned, except for asthenia, dry

ADVERSE REACTIONS: *(cont'd)*

mouth, anxiety, libido decreased, tremor and abnormal ejaculation. In flexible dose studies, no new adverse events were observed in patients receiving paroxetine hydrochloride 60 mg compared to any of the other treatment groups.

Adaptation to Certain Adverse Events: Over a 4- to 6-week period, there was evidence of adaptation to some adverse events with continued therapy (*e.g.,* nausea and dizziness), but less to other effects (*e.g.,* dry mouth, somnolence and asthenia).

Weight and Vital Sign Changes: Significant weight loss may be an undesirable result of treatment with paroxetine for some patients but, on average, patients in controlled trials had minimal (about 1 pound) weight loss vs. smaller changes on placebo and active control. No significant changes in vital signs (systolic and diastolic blood pressure, pulse and temperature) were observed in patients treated with paroxetine in controlled clinical trials.

ECG Changes: In an analysis of ECGs obtained in 682 patients treated with paroxetine and 415 patients treated with placebo in controlled clinical trials, no clinically significant changes were seen in the ECGs of either group.

Liver Function Tests: In placebo-controlled clinical trials, patients treated with paroxetine exhibited abnormal values on liver function tests at no greater rate than that seen in placebo-treated patients. In particular, the paroxetine-vs.-placebo comparison for alkaline phosphatase was 0% vs. 0%. SGOT 0.3% vs. 0.3%, SGPT 1% vs. 0.3% and bilirubin 0% vs. 0.8%.

Other Events Observed During the Premarketing Evaluation of Paroxetine Hydrochloride: During its premarketing assessment, multiple doses of paroxetine were administered to 4,126 patients in phase 2 and 3 studies. The conditions and duration of exposure to paroxetine varied greatly and included (in overlapping categories) open and double-blind studies, uncontrolled and controlled studies, inpatient and outpatient studies, and fixed-dose and titration studies. Untoward events associated with this exposure were recorded by clinical investigators using terminology of their own choosing. Consequently, it is not possible to provide a meaningful estimate of the proportion of individuals experiencing adverse events without first grouping similar types of untoward events into a smaller number of standardized event categories.

In the tabulations that follow, reported adverse events were classified using a standard COSTART-based Dictionary terminology. The frequencies presented, therefore, represent the proportion of the 4,126 patients exposed to multiple doses of paroxetine hydrochloride who experienced an event of the type cited on at least one occasion while receiving paroxetine. All reported events are included except those already listed in TABLE 2, those reported in terms so general as to be uninformative and those events where a drug cause was remote. It is important to emphasize that although the events reported occurred during treatment with paroxetine, they were not necessarily caused by it.

Events are further categorized by body system and listed in order of decreasing frequency according to the following definitions: frequent adverse events are those occurring on one or more occasions in at least 1/100 patients (only those not already listed in the tabulated results from placebo-controlled trials appear in this listing); infrequent adverse events are those occurring in 1/100 to 1/1000 patients; rare events are those occurring in fewer than 1/1000 patients. Events of major clinical importance are also described in the PRECAUTIONS section.

Body as a Whole: *frequent:* chills, malaise; *infrequent:* allergic reaction, carcinoma, face edema, moniliasis, neck pain; *rare:*abscess, adrenergic syndrome, cellulitis, neck rigidity, pelvic pain, peritonitis, ulcer.

Cardiovascular System: *frequent:* hypertension, syncope, tachycardia; *infrequent:*bradycardia, conduction abnormalities, electrocardiogram abnormal, hypotension, migraine, peripheral vascular disorder; *rare:*angina pectoris, arrhythmia, atrial fibrillation, bundle branch block, cerebral ischemia, cerebrovascular accident, congestive heart failure, low cardiac output, myocardial infarct, myocardial ischemia, pallor, phlebitis, pulmonary embolus, supraventricular extrasystoles, thrombosis, varicose vein, vascular headache, ventricular extrasystoles.

Digestive System: *infrequent:*bruxism, dysphagia, eructation, glossitis, increased salivation, liver function tests abnormal, mouth ulceration, rectal hemorrhage; *rare:*aphthous stomatitis, bloody diarrhea, bulimia, colitis, duodenitis, esophagitis, fecal impactions, fecal incontinence, gastritis, gastroenteritis, gingivitis, hematemesis, hepatitis, ileus, jaundice, melena, peptic ulcer, salivary gland enlargement, stomach ulcer, stomatitis, tongue edema, tooth caries.

Endocrine System: *rare:*diabetes mellitus, hyperthyroidism, hypothyroidism, thyroiditis.

Hemic and Lymphatic Systems: *infrequent:* anemia, leukopenia, lymphadenopathy, purpura; *rare:* abnormal erythrocytes, eosinophilia, leukocytosis, lymphedema, abnormal lymphocytes, lymphocytosis, microcytic anemia, monocytosis, normocytic anemia.

Metabolic and Nutritional: *frequent:* edema, weight gain, weight loss; *infrequent:*hyperglycemia, peripheral edema, thirst; *rare:*alkaline phosphatase increased, bilirubinemia, dehydration, gout, hypercholesteremia, hypocalcemia, hypoglycemia, hypokalemia, hyponatremia, SGOT increased, SGPT increased.

Musculoskeletal System: *infrequent:* arthralgia, arthritis; *rare:* arthrosis, bursitis, myositis, osteoporosis, tetany.

Nervous System: *frequent:*amnesia, CNS stimulation, concentration impaired, depression, emotional lability, vertigo; *infrequent:* abnormal thinking, akinesia, alcohol abuse, ataxia, convulsion, depersonalization, hallucinations, hyperkinesia, hypertonia, incoordination, lack of emotion, manic reaction, paranoid reaction; *rare:*abnormal electroencephalogram, abnormal gait, antisocial reaction, choreoathetosis, delirium, delusions, diplopia, drug dependence, dysarthria, dyskinesia, dystonia, euphoria, fasciculations, grand mal convulsion, hostility, hyperalgesia, hypokinesia, hysteria, libido increased, manic-depressive reaction, meningitis, myelitis, neuralgia, neuropathy, nystagmus, paralysis, psychosis, psychotic depression, reflexes increased, stupor, withdrawal syndrome.

Respiratory System: *frequent:* cough increased, rhinitis; *infrequent:* asthma, bronchitis, dyspnea, epistaxis, hyperventilation, pneumonia, respiratory flu, sinusitis; *rare:*carcinoma of lung, hiccups, lung fibrosis, sputum increased.

Skin and Appendages: *frequent:* pruritus; *infrequent:*acne, alopecia, dry skin, ecchymosis, eczema, furunculosis, urticaria; *rare:* angioedema, contact dermatitis, erythema nodosum, maculopapular rash, photosensitivity, skin discoloration, skin melanoma.

Special Senses: *infrequent:*abnormality of accommodation, ear pain, eye pain, mydriasis, otitis media, taste loss, tinnitus; *rare:*amblyopia, cataract, conjunctivitis, corneal ulcer, exophthalmos, eye hemorrhage, glaucoma, hyperacusis, otitis externa, photophobia.

Urogenital System: *infrequent:*abortion, amenorrhea, breast pain, cystitis, dysmenorrhea, dysuria, menorrhagia, nocturia, polyuria, urethritis, urinary incontinence, urinary retention, urinary urgency, vaginitis; *rare:* breast atrophy, breast carcinoma, breast neoplasm, female lactation, hematuria, kidney calculus, kidney function abnormal, kidney pain, mastitis, nephritis, oliguria, prostatic carcinoma, vaginal moniliasis.

ADVERSE REACTIONS: *(cont'd)*

Postmarketing Reports: Voluntary reports of adverse events in patients taking paroxetine that have been received since market introduction and not listed above that may have no causal relationship with the drug include elevated liver function tests (the most severe case was a death due to liver necrosis, and one other case involved grossly elevated transaminases associated with severe liver dysfunction), toxic epidermal necrolysis, priapism, thrombocytopenia, syndrome of inappropriate ADH secretion, symptoms suggestive of prolactinemia and galactorrhea, neuroleptic malignant syndrome-like events; extrapyramidal symptoms which have included dystonia, akathisia, bradykinesia, cogwheel rigidity, hypertonia, oculogyric crisis which has been associated with concomitant use of pimozide, tremor and trismus; and serotonin syndrome, associated in some cases with concomitant use of serotonergic drugs and with drugs which may have impaired paroxetine metabolism (symptoms have included agitation, confusion, diaphoresis, hallucinations, hyperreflexia, myoclonus, shivering, tachycardia and tremor). There have been spontaneous reports that abrupt discontinuation may lead to symptoms such as dizziness, sensory disturbances, agitation or anxiety, nausea and sweating; these events are generally self-limiting.

DRUG ABUSE AND DEPENDENCE:

Controlled Substance Class: Paroxetine is not a controlled substance.

Physical and Psychologic Dependence: Paroxetine has not been systematically studied in animals or humans for its potential for abuse, tolerance or physical dependence. While the clinical trials did not reveal any tendency for any drug-seeking behavior, these observations were not systematic and it is not possible to predict on the basis of this limited experience the extent to which a CNS-active drug will be misused, diverted and/or abused once marketed. Consequently, patients should be evaluated carefully for history of drug abuse, and such patients should be observed closely for signs of paroxetine misuse or abuse (*e.g.*, development of tolerance, incrementations of dose, drug-seeking behavior).

OVERDOSAGE:

Human Experience: No deaths were reported following acute overdose with paroxetine alone or in combination with other drugs and/or alcohol (18 cases, with doses up to 850 mg) during premarketing clinical trials. Signs and symptoms of overdose with paroxetine included: nausea, vomiting, drowsiness, sinus tachycardia and dilated pupils. There were no reports of ECG abnormalities, coma or convulsions following overdosage with paroxetine alone.

Overdosage Management: Treatment should consist of those general measures employed in the management of overdosage with any antidepressant. There are no specific antidotes for paroxetine. Establish and maintain an airway; ensure adequate oxygenation and ventilation. Gastric evacuation either by the induction of emesis or lavage or both should be performed. In most cases, following evacuation, 20 to 30 grams of activated charcoal may be administered every 4 to 6 hours during the first 24 to 48 hours after ingestion. An ECG should be taken and monitoring of cardiac function instituted if there is any evidence of abnormality. Supportive care with frequent monitoring of vital signs and careful observation is indicated. Due to the large volume of distribution of paroxetine, forced diuresis, dialysis, hemoperfusion and exchange transfusion are unlikely to be of benefit.

A specific caution involves patients taking or recently having taken paroxetine who might ingest by accident or intent excessive quantities of a tricyclic antidepressant. In such a case, accumulation of the parent tricyclic and its active metabolite may increase the possibility of clinically significant sequelae and extend the time needed for close medical observation.

In managing overdosage, consider the possibility of multiple-drug involvement. The physician should consider contacting a poison control center for additional information on the treatment of any overdose. Telephone numbers for certified poison control centers are listed in *Physicians GenRx*.

DOSAGE AND ADMINISTRATION:

DEPRESSION

Depression Usual Initial Dosage: Paroxetine should be administered as a single daily dose, usually in the morning. The recommended initial dose is 20 mg/day. Patients were dosed in a range of 20 to 50 mg/day in the clinical trials demonstrating the antidepressant effectiveness of paroxetine hydrochloride. As with all antidepressants, the full antidepressant effect may be delayed. Some patients not responding to a 20 mg dose may benefit from dose increases, in 10 mg/day increments, up to a maximum of 50 mg/day. Dose changes should occur at intervals of at least 1 week.

Maintenance Therapy: There is no body of evidence available to answer the question of how long the patient treated with paroxetine hydrochloride should remain on it. It is generally agreed that acute episodes of depression require several months or longer of sustained pharmacologic therapy. Whether the dose of an antidepressant needed to induce remission is identical to the dose needed to maintain and/or sustain euthymia is unknown.

Systematic evaluation of the efficacy of paroxetine hydrochloride has shown that efficacy is maintained for periods of up to 1 year with doses that averaged about 30 mg.

OBSESSIVE COMPULSIVE DISORDER

Usual Initial Dosage: Paroxetine should be administered as a single daily dose, usually in the morning. The recommended dose of paroxetine hydrochloride in the treatment of OCD is 40 mg daily. Patients should be started on 20 mg/day and the dose can be increased in 10 mg/day increments. Dose changes should occur at intervals of at least 1 week. Patients were dosed in a range of 20 to 60 mg/day in the clinical trials demonstrating the effectiveness of paroxetine hydrochloride in the treatment of OCD. The maximum dosage should not exceed 60 mg/day.

Maintenance Therapy: Long-term maintenance of efficacy was demonstrated in a 6–month relapse prevention trial. In this trial, patients with OCD assigned to paroxetine demonstrated a lower relapse rate compared to patients on placebo (see CLINICAL PHARMACOLOGY.) OCD is a chronic condition, and it is reasonable to consider continuation for a responding patient. Dosage adjustments should be made to maintain the patient on the lowest effective dosage, and patients should be periodically reassessed to determine the need for continued treatment.

PANIC DISORDER

Usual Initial Dosage: Paroxetine should be administered as a single daily dose, usually in the morning. The target dose of paroxetine hydrochloride in the treatment of panic disorder is 40 mg/day. Patients should be started on 10 mg/day. Dose changes should occur in 10 mg/week increments and at intervals of at least 1 week. Patients were dosed in a range of 10 to 60 mg/day in the clinical trials demonstrating the effectiveness of paroxetine hydrochloride. The maximum dosage should not exceed 60 mg/day.

DOSAGE AND ADMINISTRATION: *(cont'd)*

Maintenance Therapy: Long-term maintenance of efficacy was demonstrated in a 3–month relapse prevention trial. In this trial, patients with panic disorder assigned to paroxetine demonstrated a lower relapse rate compared to patients on placebo (see CLINICAL PHARMACOLOGY.) Panic disorder is a chronic condition, and it is reasonable to consider continuation for a responding patient. Dosage adjustments should be made to maintain the patient on the lowest effective dosage, and patients should be periodically reassessed to determine the need for continued treatment.

Dosage for Elderly or Debilitated, and Patients with Severe Renal or Hepatic Impairment: The recommended initial dose is 10 mg/day for elderly patients, debilitated patients, and/or patients with severe renal or hepatic impairment. Increases may be made if indicated. Dosage should not exceed 40 mg/day.

Switching Patients to or from a Monoamine Oxidase Inhibitor: At least 14 days should elapse between discontinuation of a MAOI and initiation of paroxetine hydrochloride therapy. Similarly, at least 14 days should be allowed after stopping paroxetine hydrochloride before starting an MAOI.

PATIENT INFORMATION:

Paroxetine HCl is used to treat depression, panic disorder and obsessive-compulsive disorders. Paroxetine HCl should not be taken if you are currently taking monoamine oxidase inhibitors. If you have been prescribed a monoamine oxidase inhibitor by another physician please call them for advice. Any drug which affects the central nervous system can cause drowsiness or lethargy. This drug has rarely been associated with this effect but caution is warranted while driving or operating machinery. Avoid drinking alcohol. Please consult with your physician or pharmacist whenever you are using another medication, especially over-the-counter medications since there may be interactions. Paroxetine is generally taken once a day, in the morning. It may take 4 or more weeks before improvement is symptoms is seen. You are encouraged to continue therapy until advised by your physician to stop.

HOW SUPPLIED:

Paxil is supplied as film-coated, modified-oval tablets.

Storage: Store at controlled room temperature (15° to 30°C; 59° to 86°F).

HOW SUPPLIED - EQUIVALENTS NOT AVAILABLE:

Tablet, Film-Coated - Oral - 10 mg

10 mg x 30	**$56.80**	**PAXIL, Beecham**	**00029-3210-13**

Tablet, Film-Coated - Oral - 40 mg

40 mg x 30	$64.44	PAXIL, Beecham	00029-3213-13

Tablet, Uncoated - Oral - 20 mg

30's	**$57.00**	**PAXIL, Beecham**	**00029-3211-13**
100's	**$189.90**	**PAXIL, Beecham**	**00029-3211-20**
100's	**$193.80**	**PAXIL, Beecham**	**00029-3211-21**

Tablet, Uncoated - Oral - 30 mg

30's	**$58.65**	**PAXIL, Beecham**	**00029-3212-13**

PEGADEMASE BOVINE *(003024)*

CATEGORIES: Adenosine Deanimase Deficiency; Antibiotics; Immunodeficiency Disease; Orphan Drugs; Severe Combined Immunodeficiency; Pregnancy Category C; FDA Class 1A ("Important Therapeutic Advantage"); FDA Approved 1990 Mar

BRAND NAMES: **Adagen**; PEG-ADA

DESCRIPTION:

Pegademase bovine injection is a modified enzyme used for enzyme replacement therapy for the treatment of severe combined immunodeficiency disease (SCID) associated with a deficiency of adenosine deaminase.

Pegademase bovine injection is supplied in an isotonic, pyrogen free, sterile solution, pH 7.2-7.4, for intramuscular injection only. The solution is clear and colorless. It is supplied in 1.5 ml single-dose vials.

The chemical name for pegademase bovine injection is (monomethoxypolyethylene glycol succinimidyl)$_{11-17}$-adenosine deaminase. It is a conjugate of numerous strands of monomethoxypolyethylene glycol (PEG), molecular weight 5,000, covalently attached to the enzyme adenosine deaminase (ADA). ADA (adenosine deaminase EC 3.5.4.4) used in the manufacture of pegademase bovine injection is derived from bovine intestine.

The structural formula of pegademase bovine injection is:

$[CH_3\text{-}(OCH_2CH_2)x\text{-}O\text{-}C\text{-}CH_2CH_2\text{-}C\text{-}NH]y$-adenosine deaminase

x = 114 oxyethylene groups per PEG strand.

y = 11-17 primary amino groups of lysine onto which succinyl PEG is attached.

Each milliliter of pegademase bovine injection contains: Pegademase bovine: 250 units*; Monobasic sodium phosphate, USP: 1.20 mg; Dibasic sodium phosphate, USP: 5.58 mg; Sodium Chloride, USP: 8.50 mg; Water for injection, USP: q.s. to 1.0 ml

*One unit of activity is defined as the amount of ADA that converts 1 μM of adenosine to inosine per minute at 25°C and pH 7.3.

CLINICAL PHARMACOLOGY:

Severe Combined Immunodeficiency Disease Associated with ADA Deficiency: Severe combined immunodeficiency disease (SCID) associated with a deficiency of ADA is a rare, inherited, and often fatal disease. In the absence of the ADA enzyme, the purine substrates adenosine and 2'-deoxyadenosine accumulate, causing metabolic abnormalities that are directly toxic to lymphocytes.

The immune deficiency can be cured by bone marrow transplantation. When a suitable bone marrow donor is unavailable or when bone marrow transplantation fails, non-selective replacement of the ADA enzyme has been provided by periodic irradiated red blood cell transfusions. However, transmission of viral infections and iron overload are serious risks associated with irradiated red blood cell transfusions, and relatively few ADA deficient patients have benefited from chronic transfusion therapy.

CLINICAL PHARMACOLOGY: *(cont'd)*

Pegademase bovine injection provides specific and direct replacement of the deficient enzyme, but will not benefit patients with immunodeficiency due to other causes.

In patients with ADA deficiency, rigorous adherence to a schedule of pegademase bovine injection administration can eliminate the toxic metabolites of ADA deficiency and result in improved immune function. It is imperative that treatment with pegademase bovine injection be carefully monitored by measurement of the level of ADA activity in plasma. Monitoring of the level of deoxyadenosine triphosphate (dATP) in erythrocytes is also helpful in determining that the dose of pegademase bovine injection is adequate.

Mechanism of Action: Pegademase bovine injection provides specific replacement of the deficient enzyme.

In the absence of the enzyme ADA, the purine substrates adenosine, 2'-deoxyadenosine and their metabolites are toxic to lymphocytes. The direct action of pegademase bovine injection is the correction of these metabolic abnormalities. Improvement in immune function and diminished frequency of opportunistic infections compared with the natural history of combined immunodeficiency due to ADA deficiency only occurs after metabolic abnormalities are corrected. There is a lag between the correction of the metabolic abnormalities and improved immune function. This period of time is variable, and has been reported to be from a few weeks to as long as 6 months. In contrast to the natural history of combined immunodeficiency disease due to ADA deficiency, a trend toward diminished frequency of opportunistic infections and fewer complications of infections has occurred in patients receiving pegademase bovine injection.

Pharmacokinetics: The pharmacokinetics and biochemical effects of pegademase bovine injection have been studied in six children ranging in age from 6 weeks to 12 years with SCID associated with ADA deficiency.

After the intramuscular injection of pegademase bovine injection, peak plasma levels of ADA activity were reached 2 to 3 days following administration. The plasma elimination half-life of ADA following the administration of pegademase bovine injection was variable, even for the same child. The range was 3 to >6 days. Following weekly injections of pegademase bovine injection at 15 U/kg, the average trough level of ADA activity in plasma was between 20 and 25 μmol/hr/ml.

Biochemical Effects: The changes in red blood cell deoxyadenosine nucleotide (dATP) and S-adenosylhomocysteine hydrolase (SAHase) have been evaluated. In patients with ADA deficiency, inadequate elimination of 2'-deoxyadenosine caused a marked elevation in dATP and a decrease in SAHase level in red blood cells. Prior to treatment with pegademase bovine injection, the levels of dATP in the red blood cells ranged from 0.056 to 0.899 μmol/ml of erythrocytes. After 2 months of maintenance treatment with pegademase bovine injection, the levels decreased to 0.007 to 0.015 μmol/ml. The normal value of dATP is below 0.001 μmol/ml. In the same period of time, the levels of SAHase increased from the pretreatment range of 0.09 to 0.22 nmol/hr/mg protein to a range of 2.37 to 5.16 nmol/hr/mg protein. The normal value for SAHase is 4.18 ± 1.9 nmol/hr/mg protein.

The optimal dosage and schedule of administration of pegademase bovine injection should be established for each patient, based on monitoring of plasma ADA activity levels (trough levels before maintenance injection), biochemical markers of ADA deficiency (primarily red cell dATP content), and parameters of immune function. Since improvement in immune function follows correction of metabolic abnormalities, maintenance dosage in individual patients should be aimed at achieving the following biochemical goals: 1) maintain plasma ADA activity (trough levels) in the range of 15-35 μmol/hr/ml (assayed at 37°C); and 2) decline in erythrocyte dATP to ≤0.005-0.015 μmol/ml packed erythrocytes, or ≤1% of the total erythrocyte adenine nucleotide (ATP + dATP) content, with a normal ATP level, as measured in a pre-injection sample.

In vitro immunologic data (lymphocyte response to mitogens and lymphocyte surface antigens) were obtained, but their clinical significance is unknown. Prior to treatment with pegademase bovine injection, immune status was significantly below normal, as indicated by <10% of normal mitogen responses and circulating mononuclear cells bearing T-cell surface antigens. These parameters improved, though not always to normal, within 2 to 6 months of therapy.

INDICATIONS AND USAGE:

Pegademase bovine injection is indicated for enzyme replacement therapy for adenosine deaminase (ADA) deficiency in patients with severe combined immunodeficiency disease (SCID) who are not suitable candidates for—or who have failed—bone marrow transplantation. Pegademase bovine injection is recommended for use in infants from birth or in children of any age at the time of diagnosis. Pegademase bovine injection is not intended as a replacement for HLA identical bone marrow transplant therapy. Pegademase bovine injection is also not intended to replace continued close medical supervision and the initiation of appropriate diagnostic tests and therapy (*e.g.,* antibiotics, nutrition, oxygen, gammaglobulin) as indicated for intercurrent illnesses.

CONTRAINDICATIONS:

There is no evidence to support the safety and efficacy of pegademase bovine injection as preparatory or support therapy for bone marrow transplantation. Since pegademase bovine injection is administered by intramuscular injection, it should be used with caution in patients with thrombocytopenia and should not be used if thrombocytopenia is severe.

PRECAUTIONS:

Warnings: At present, testing prior to distribution may not assure the initial and continuing potency of each new lot of pegademase bovine injection. Any laboratory or clinical indication of a decrease in potency of pegademase bovine injection should be reported immediately by telephone to the manufacturer (Telephone number is located in the SUPPLIER PROFILES SECTION of Physicians GenRx).

General: There have been no reports of hypersensitivity reactions in patients who have been treated with pegademase bovine injection.

One of 12 patients showed an enhanced rate of clearance of plasma ADA activity after 5 months of therapy at 15 U/kg/week. Enhanced clearance was correlated with the appearance of an antibody that directly inhibited both unmodified ADA and pegademase bovine injection. Subsequently, the patient was treated with twice weekly intramuscular injections at an increased dose of 20 U/kg, or a total weekly dose of 40 U/kg. No adverse effects were observed at the higher dose and effective levels of plasma ADA were restored. After 4 months, the patient returned to a weekly dosage schedule of 20 U/kg and effective plasma levels have been maintained.

Appropriate care to protect immune deficient patients should be maintained until improvement in immune function has been documented. The degree of immune function improvement may vary from patient to patient and, therefore, each patient will require appropriate care consistent with immunologic status.

Laboratory Tests: The treatment of SCID associated with ADA deficiency with pegademase bovine injection should be monitored by measuring plasma ADA activity and red blood cell dATP levels.

PRECAUTIONS: *(cont'd)*

Plasma ADA activity and red cell dATP should be determined prior to treatment. Once treatment with pegademase bovine injection has been initiated, a desirable range of plasma ADA activity (trough level before maintenance injection) should be 15-35 μmol/hr/ml. This minimum trough level will ensure that plasma ADA activity from injection to injection is maintained above the level of total erythrocyte ADA activity in the blood of normal individuals.

Plasma ADA activity (pre-injection) should be determined every 1-2 weeks during the first 8-12 weeks of treatment in order to establish an effective dose of pegademase bovine injection. After two months of maintenance treatment with pegademase bovine injection, red cell dATP levels should decrease to a range of ≤0.005 to 0.015 μmol/ml. The normal value of dATP is below 0.001 μmol/ml. Once the level of dATP has fallen adequately, it should be measured 2-4 times a year during the remainder of the first year and 2-3 times a year thereafter, assuming no interruption in therapy.

Between 3 and 9 months, plasma ADA should be determined twice a month, then monthly until after 18-24 months of treatment with pegademase bovine injection.

Patients who have successfully been maintained on therapy for two years should continue to have plasma ADA measured every 2-4 months and red cell dATP measured twice yearly. More frequent monitoring would be necessary if therapy were interrupted or if an enhanced rate of clearance of plasma ADA activity develops.

Once effective ADA plasma levels have been established, should a patient's plasma ADA activity level fall below 10 μmol/hr/ml (which cannot be attributed to improper dosing, sample handling or antibody development) then all patients receiving this lot of pegademase bovine injection will be required to have a blood sample for plasma ADA determination taken prior to their next injection of pegademase bovine injection. The index patient will require re-testing for determination of plasma ADA activity prior to his/her next injection of pegademase bovine injection. If this value, as well as the value from one of the other patients from a different site, is less than 10 μmol/hr/ml then the lot in use will be recalled and replaced with a new clinical lot by the manufacturer.

Immune function, including the ability to produce antibodies, generally improves after 2-6 months of therapy, and matures over a longer period. Compared with the natural history of combined immunodeficiency disease due to ADA deficiency, a trend toward diminished frequency of opportunistic infections and fewer complications of infections has occurred in patients receiving pegademase bovine injection. However, the lag between the correction of the metabolic abnormalities and improved immune function with a trend toward diminished frequency of infections and complications of infection is variable, and has ranged from a few weeks to approximately 6 months. Improvement in the general clinical status of the patient may be gradual (as evidenced by improvement in various clinical parameters) but should be apparent by the end of the first year of therapy.

Antibody to pegademase bovine injection may develop in patients and may result in more rapid clearance of pegademase bovine injection. Antibody to pegademase bovine injection should be suspected if a persistent fall in pre-injection levels of plasma ADA to <10 μmol/hr/ml occurs. If other causes for a decline in plasma ADA levels can be ruled out [such as improper storage of pegademase bovine injection vials (freezing or prolonged storage at temperatures above 8°C), or improper handling of plasma samples (*e.g.,* repeated freezing and thawing during transport to laboratory)], then a specific assay for antibody to ADA and pegademase bovine injection (ELISA, enzyme inhibition) should be performed.

In patients undergoing treatment with pegademase bovine injection, a decline in immune function, with increased risk of opportunistic infections and complications of infection, will result from failure to maintain adequate levels of plasma ADA activity [whether due to the development of antibody to pegademase bovine injection, to improper calculation of pegademase bovine injection dosage, to interruption of treatment or to improper storage of pegademase bovine injection with subsequent loss of activity]. If a persistent decline in plasma ADA activity occurs, immune function and clinical status should be monitored closely and precautions should be taken to minimize the risk of infection. If antibody to ADA or pegademase bovine injection is found to be the cause of a persistent fall in plasma ADA activity, then adjustment in the dosage of pegademase bovine injection and other measures may be taken to induce tolerance and restore adequate ADA activity.

Carcinogenesis, Mutagenesis, and Impairment of Fertility: Long-term carcinogenic studies in animals have not been performed with pegademase bovine injection nor have studies been performed on impairment of fertility.

Pegademase bovine injection did not exhibit a mutagenic effect when tested against *Salmonella typhimurium* strains in the Ames assay.

Pregnancy Category C: Animal reproduction studies have not been conducted with pegademase bovine injection. It is also not known whether pegademase bovine injection can cause fetal harm when administered to a pregnant woman or can affect reproduction capacity. Pegademase bovine injection should be given to a pregnant woman only if clearly needed.

Nursing Mothers: It is not known whether pegademase bovine injection is excreted in human milk. Because many drugs are excreted in human milk, caution should be exercised when pegademase bovine injection is administered to a nursing woman.

DRUG INTERACTIONS:

There are no known drug interactions with pegademase bovine injection. However, Vidarabine is a substrate for ADA and 2'-deoxycoformycin is a potent inhibitor of ADA. Thus, the activities of these drugs and pegademase bovine injection could be substantially altered if they are used in combination with one another.

ADVERSE REACTIONS:

Clinical experience with pegademase bovine injection has been limited. The following adverse reactions have been reported: headache in one patient and pain at the injection site in two patients.

OVERDOSAGE:

There is no documented experience with pegademase bovine injection overdosage. An intraperitoneal dose of 50,000 U/kg of pegademase bovine injection in mice resulted in weight loss up to 9%.

DOSAGE AND ADMINISTRATION:

Before prescribing pegademase bovine injection the physician should be thoroughly familiar with the details of this prescribing information. For further information concerning the essential monitoring of pegademase bovine injection therapy, the prescribing physician should contact the manufacturer (address and phone number are located in the SUPPLIER PROFILE SECTION of Physicians GenRx).

Pegademase bovine injection is recommended for use in infants from birth or in children of any age at the time of diagnosis.

Parenteral drug products should be inspected visually for particulate matter and discoloration prior to administration, whenever solution and container permits.

DOSAGE AND ADMINISTRATION: *(cont'd)*

Pegademase bovine injection should not be diluted nor mixed with any other drug prior to administration. Pegademase bovine injection should be administered every 7 days as an intramuscular injection. The dosage of pegademase bovine injection should be individualized. The recommended dosing schedule is 10 U/kg for the first dose, 15 U/kg for the second dose, and 20 U/kg for the third dose. The usual maintenance dose is 20 U/kg per week. Further increases of 5 U/kg/week may be necessary, but a maximum single dose of 30 U/kg should not be exceeded. Plasma levels of ADA more than twice the upper limit of 35 μmol/hr/ml have occurred on occasion in several patients, and have been maintained for several weeks in one patient who received twice weekly injections (20 U/kg per dose) of pegademase bovine injection. No adverse effects have been observed at these higher levels; there is no evidence that maintaining pre-injection plasma ADA above 35 μmol/hr/ml produces any additional clinical benefits.

Dose proportionality has not been established and patients should be closely monitored when the dosage is increased. Pegademase bovine injection is not recommended for intravenous administration.

The optimal dosage and schedule of administration should be established for each patient based on monitoring of plasma ADA activity levels (trough levels before maintenance injection) and biochemical markers of ADA deficiency (primarily red cell dATP content). Since improvement in immune function follows correction of metabolic abnormalities, maintenance dosage in individual patients should be aimed at achieving the following biochemical goals: 1) maintain plasma ADA activity (trough levels before maintenance injection) in the range of 15-35 μmol/hr/ml (assayed at 37°C); and 2) decline in erythrocyte dATP to ≤0.005-0.015 μmol/ml packed erythrocytes, or ≤1% of the total erythrocyte adenine nucleotide (ATP + dATP) content, with a normal ATP level, as measured in a pre-injection sample. In addition, continued monitoring of immune function and clinical status is essential in any patient with a primary immunodeficiency disease and should be continued in patients undergoing treatment with pegademase bovine injection.

Refrigerate. Store between + 2°C and + 8°C (36°F and 46°F). DO NOT FREEZE. Adagen (pegademase bovine) Injection should not be stored at room temperature. This product should not be used if there are any indications that it may have been frozen.

REFERENCES:

1. Hershfield MS, Buckley RH, Greenberg ML, et al. Treatment of adenosine deaminase deficiency with polyethylene glycol-modified adenosine deaminase. N Engl J Med 1987; 316:589-96. **2.** Levy Y, Hershfield MS, Fernandez-Mejia C, Polmar ST, Scudiery D, Berger M, Sorensen RU. Adenosine deaminase deficiency with late onset of recurrent infections: response to treatment with polyethylene glycol-modified adenosine deaminase. J Pediatr 1988; 113:312-17. **3.** Kredich NM, Hershfield MS. Immunodeficiency diseases caused by adenosine deaminase deficiency and purine nucleoside phosphorylase deficiency. 6th ed. In: Scriver CR, Beaudet AL, Sly WS, Valle D, eds. The metabolic basis of inherited disease. New York: McGraw Hill, 1989; 1045-75. **4.** Hirschhorn R. Inherited enzyme deficiencies and immunodeficiency: adenosine deaminase (ADA) and purine nucleoside phosphorylase (PNP) deficiencies. Clin Immunol Immunopathol 1986; 40:157-65. **5.** Hirschhorn R, Roegner-Maniscalco V, Kuritsky L, Rosen FS. Bone marrow transplantation only partially restores purine metabolites to normal adenosine deaminase-deficient patients. J. Clin Invest 1981; 68:1387-93. **6.** Polmar AH, Stern RC, Schwartz AL, Wetzler EM, Chase PA, Hirschhorn R. Enzyme replacement therapy for adenosine deaminase deficiency and severe combined immunodeficiency. N Engl J Med 1976; 295:1337-43. **7.** Rubinstein A, Hirschhorn R, Sicklick M, Murphy RA. In vivo and in vitro effects of thymosin and adenosine deaminase on adenosine-deaminase-deficient lymphocytes. N Engl J Med 1979; 300:387-92. **8.** Hirschhorn R, Papageorgiou PS, Kesarwala HH, Taft LT. Amelioration of neurologic abnormalities after "enzyme replacement" in adenosine deaminase deficiency. N Engl J Med 1980; 303:377-80. **9.** Hirschhorn R, Ratech H, Rubinstein A, et al. Increased excretion of modified adenine nucleosides by children with adenosine deaminase deficiency. Pediatr Res 1982; 16:362-9. **10.** Polmar SH. Enzyme replacement and other biochemical approaches to the therapy of adenosine deaminase deficiency. In: Elliott K, Whelan J, eds. Enzyme defects and immune dysfunction. Amsterdam: Excerpta Medica, 1979; 213-30.

HOW SUPPLIED:

Adagen (pegademase bovine) injection is a clear, colorless solution for intramuscular injection. Each vial contains 250 units/ml and is supplied as a 1.5 ml single-use vial, in boxes of 4 vials.

HOW SUPPLIED - EQUIVALENTS NOT AVAILABLE:

Injection, Solution - Intramuscular - 250 unit/ml

1.5 ml $2200.00 ADAGEN, Enzon 57665-0001-01

PEGASPARGASE *(003199)*

CATEGORIES: Acute Lymphoblastic Leukemia; Antineoplastics; Chemotherapy; Leukemia; Oncologic Drugs; Orphan Drugs; FDA Approved 1994 Feb

BRAND NAMES: **Oncaspar**; L-Asparaginase

FORMULARIES: Medi-Cal

DESCRIPTION:

Oncaspar, the ENZON trademark for pegaspargase, is a modified version of the enzyme L-asparaginase. It is an oncolytic agent used in combination chemotherapy for the treatment of patients with acute lymphoblastic leukemia who are hypersensitive to native forms of L-asparaginase (as described in CLINICAL PHARMACOLOGY).

The generic name for Oncaspar is pegaspargase. The chemical name is monomethoxypolyethylene glycol succinimidyl L-asparaginase. L- asparaginase is modified by covalently conjugating units of monomethoxypolyethylene glycol (PEG), molecular weight of 5,000, to the enzyme, forming the active ingredient PEG-L-asparaginase. The L- asparaginase (L-asparagine amidohydrolase, type EC-2, EC 3.5.1.1) used in the manufacture of Oncaspar is derived from *Escherichia coli.* ENZON purchases the enzyme L-asparaginase in bulk from Merck, Sharp and Dohme, Division of Merck & Co., Inc., West Point, PA 19486, U.S. License Number 2. Merck & Co., Inc. supplies bulk L-asparaginase as a licensed intermediate for further manufacture by ENZON into PEG-L-asparaginase. Merck & Co., Inc. can only assume responsibility for the bulk intermediate supplied to ENZON.

Oncaspar is supplied as an isotonic sterile solution in phosphate buffered saline, pH 7.3, for intramuscular or intravenous administration only. The solution is clear, colorless and contains no preservatives. It is supplied in 5mL single-dose vials.

Oncaspar activity is expressed in International Units (IU) according to the recommendation of the International Union of Biochemistry. One IU of L-asparaginase is defined as that amount of enzyme required to generate 1 μmol of ammonia per minute at pH 7.3 and 37°C.

Each milliliter of Oncaspar contains:

PEG-L-asparaginase: 750 IU ± 20%

Monobasic sodium phosphate, USP: 1.20 mg ± 5%

Dibasic sodium phosphate, USP: 5.58 mg ± 5%

Sodium chloride, USP: 8.50 mg ± 5%

Water for injection, USP: qs to 1.0 mL

The specific activity of Oncaspar is at least 85 IU per milligram protein.

CLINICAL PHARMACOLOGY:

Leukemic cells are unable to synthesize asparagine due to a lack of asparagine synthetase and are dependent on an exogenous source of asparagine for survival. Rapid depletion of asparagine which results from treatment with the enzyme L-asparaginase, kills the leukemic cells. Normal cells, however, are less affected by the rapid depletion due to their ability to synthesize asparagine. This is an approach to therapy based on a specific metabolic defect in some leukemic cells which do not produce asparagine synthetase.[1]

In a study in predominately L-asparaginase naive adult patients with leukemia and lymphoma, initial plasma levels of L-asparaginase following intravenous administration were determined. Plasma half-life did not appear to be influenced by dose levels, and it could not be correlated with age, sex, surface area, renal or hepatic function, diagnosis or extent of disease. Apparent volume of distribution was equal to estimated plasma volume. L-asparaginase was measurable for at least 15 days following the initial treatment with pegaspargase. The enzyme could not be detected in the urine.[2]

In a study of newly diagnosed pediatric patients with acute lymphoblastic leukemia (ALL) who received either a single intramuscular injection of pegaspargase (2,500 IU/m^2), *E. coli* L-asparaginase (25,000 IU/m^2), or *Erwinia* L-asparaginase (25,000 IU/m^2) the plasma half-lives for the three forms of L-asparaginase were:[3]

TABLE 1

PLASMA HALF-LIVES OF THREE FORMS OF L-ASPARAGINASE

TREATMENT GROUP	NO. OF PATIENTS	MEAN (DAYS)	STANDARD DEVIATION
ONCASPAR	10	5.73	3.24
E. Coli L-asparaginase	17	1.24	0.17
Erwinia L-asparaginase	10	0.65	0.13

In this same study of newly diagnosed pediatric ALL patients, the *in vivo* early leukemic cell kill after a single intramuscular injection of native *E. coli* L-asparaginase (25,000 IU/m^2),*Erwinia* L-asparaginase (25,000 IU/m^2), and pegaspargase (25,000 IU/m^2) during a five day "investigational window" was studied.[4] Bone marrow aspirates were taken before and five days after a single dose of one of the three different forms of L- asparaginase. Rhodamine-124 (RH-123), a selectively incorporated fluorescent mitochondrial dye, was used in an *in vitro* assay on the bone marrow aspirates to ascertain cell viability. The percent reduction of viable lymphoblasts at day five for each group is presented in the following table:[4]

TABLE 2

RHODAMINE-123 (*IN VIVO* CELL KILL)

TREATMENT GROUP	NO. OF PATIENTS	PERCENT REDUCTION OF VIABLE LYMPHOBLASTS AT DAY 5 MEAN ± S.D.
ONCASPAR	21	55.7 ± 10.2
E. Coli L-asparaginase	28	57.8 ± 10.1
Erwinia L-asparaginase	19	57.9 ± 13.8

In three pharmacokinetic studies, 37 relapsed ALL patients received pegaspargase at 2,500 IU/m^2 every two weeks. The plasma half-life of pegaspargase was 3.24 ± 1.83 days in nine patients who were previously hypersensitive to native L-asparaginase and 5.69 ± 3.25 days in 28 non-hypersensitive patients. The area under the curve was 9.50 ± 3.95 IU/mL/day in the previously hypersensitive patients, and 9.83 ± 5.94 IU/mL/day in the non-hypersensitive patients.

HYPERSENSITIVITY REACTIONS

Hypersensitivity reactions to *E. coli*L-asparaginase have been reported in the literature in 3% to 73% of patients.[1] Patients in pegaspargase clinical studies were considered to be previously hypersensitive if they experienced a systemic rash, urticaria, bronchospasm, laryngeal edema, or hypotension following administration of any form of native L- asparaginase. Patients were also considered to be previously hypersensitive if they experienced local erythema, urticaria, or swelling, greater than two centimeters, for at least ten minutes following administration of any form of native L-asparaginase. The National Cancer Institute Common Toxicity Criteria (CTC) were used to classify the severity of the hypersensitivity reactions. These are: grade 1 — transient rash (mild); grade 2— mild bronchospasm (moderate); grade 3 — moderate bronchospasm and/or serum sickness (severe); grade 4 — hypotension and/or anaphylaxis (life-threatening). Additionally, most transient local urticaria were considered grade 2 hypersensitivity reactions, while most sustained urticaria distant from the injection site were considered grade 3 hypersensitivity reactions. In general, the moderate to life-threatening hypersensitivity reactions were considered dose-limiting; that is, they required L-asparaginase treatment to be discontinued.

In separate studies, pegaspargase was administered intravenously to 48 patients and intramuscularly to 126 patients. The incidence of hypersensitivity reactions when pegaspargase was administered intramuscularly was 30% in patients who were previously hypersensitive to native L- asparaginase and 11% in non-hypersensitive patients (p-value of 0.007). The incidence of hypersensitivity reactions when pegaspargase was administered intravenously was 60% in patients who were previously hypersensitive to native L-asparaginase and 12% in non-hypersensitive patients. Since only five previously hypersensitive patients received pegaspargase intravenously, no meaningful analysis of the incidence of hypersensitivity reactions was possible between either the previously hypersensitive and non-hypersensitive patients, or between the intravenous and intramuscular routes of administration.

The overall incidence of hypersensitivity reactions in 174 patients who received pegaspargase in five clinical studies is shown in the table below:

TABLE 3

INCIDENCE OF ONCASPAR HYPERSENSITIVITY REACTIONS

		CTC Grade of Hypersensitivity Reaction				
PATIENT STATUS	N	1	2	3	4	TOTAL
Previously Hypersensitive Patients	62	7	8	4	1	20 (32%)
Non-Hypersensitive Patients	112	5	4	1	1	11 (10%)
Total Patients	174	12	12	5	2	31 (18%)

The probability of a previously hypersensitive or non-hypersensitive patient completing 8 doses of pegaspargase therapy without developing a dose-limiting hypersensitivity reaction was 77% and 95%, respectively.

All of the 62 hypersensitive patients treated with pegaspargase in five clinical studies had previously hypersensitivity reactions to one or more of the native forms of L-asparaginase. Of the 35 patients who had previous hypersensitivity reactions to *E. Coli* L-asparaginase only, 5

CLINICAL PHARMACOLOGY: *(cont'd)*

(14%) had pegaspargase dose-limiting hypersensitivity reactions. Of the 27 patients who had hypersensitivity reactions to both *E. coli* and *Erwinia* L-asparaginase, 7 (26%) had pegaspargase dose- limiting hypersensitivity reactions. The overall incidence of dose- limiting hypersensitivity reactions in 174 patients treated with pegaspargase was 9% (19% in 62 hypersensitive and 3% in 112 non-hypersensitive patients). Of the total of 9% dose-limiting hypersensitivity reactions, 1% were anaphylactic (CTC grade 4) and the other 8% were ≤ CTC grade 3.

CLINICAL ACTIVITY

Pegaspargase was evaluated as part of combination therapy in four open label studies comprising 42 multiply-relapsed, previously hypersensitive acute leukemia patients [39 (93%) with ALL] at a dose of 2,000 or 2,500 IU/m^2 administered intramuscularly or intravenously every 14 days during induction combination chemotherapy. The reinduction response rate was 50% (36% complete remissions and 14% partial remissions), with a 95% confidence interval of 35% to 65%. This response rate is comparable to that reported in the literature for relapsed patients treated with native L-asparaginase as part of combination chemotherapy.[1]

Pegaspargase was also shown to have some activity as a single agent in multiply-relapsed hypersensitive ALL patients, the majority of whom were pediatric. Treatment with pegaspargase resulted in three responses (one complete remission and two partial remissions) in nine previously hypersensitive patients who would not have been able to receive any further L-asparaginase treatment.

Pegaspargase was also studied in non-hypersensitive, relapsed ALL patients who were randomized to receive two doses of pegaspargase at 2,500 IU/m^2 every 14 days or twelve doses of *E. coli* L- asparaginase at 10,000 IU/m^{2}three times a week during a 28 induction combination chemotherapy regimen (which included vincristine and prednisone). Although the enrollment in this study was too small to be conclusive, the data showed that for 20 patients there was no significant difference between the overall response rates of 60% and 50%, respectively, or the complete remission rates of 50% and 50%, respectively.

Pegaspargase was administered during maintenance therapy regimens to 33 previously hypersensitive patients. The average number of doses received during maintenance therapy was 5.8 (range of 1 to 24) and the average duration of maintenance therapy was 126 (range of 1 to 513) days for this patient population.

INDICATIONS AND USAGE:

Pegaspargase is indicated for patients with acute lymphoblastic leukemia who require L-asparaginase in their treatment regimen, but have developed hypersensitivity to the native forms of L-asparaginase (see CLINICAL PHARMACOLOGY.) Pegaspargase, like native L-asparaginase, is generally used in combination with other chemotherapeutic agents, such as vincristine, methotrexate, cytarabine, daunorubicin, and doxorubicin.[1,3] Use of pegaspargase as a single agent should only be undertaken when multi-agent chemotherapy is judged to be inappropriate for the patient.

CONTRAINDICATIONS:

Pegaspargase is contraindicated in patients with pancreatitis or a history of pancreatitis. Pegaspargase is contraindicated in patients who have had significant hemorrhagic events associated with prior L-asparaginase therapy. Pegaspargase is also contraindicated in patients who have had previous serious allergic reactions, such as generalized urticaria, bronchospasm, laryngeal edema, hypotension, or other unacceptable adverse reactions to pegaspargase.

WARNINGS:

It is recommended that pegaspargase be given under the supervision of an individual who is qualified by training and experience to administer cancer chemotherapeutic agents.

Especially in patients with known hypersensitivity to the other forms of L-asparaginase, hypersensitivity reactions to pegaspargase, including life-threatening anaphylaxis, may occur during therapy. As a routine precaution, patients should be kept under observation for one hour with resuscitation equipment and other agents necessary to treat anaphylaxis (epinephrine, oxygen, intravenous steroids, etc.) available.

PRECAUTIONS:

GENERAL

This drug may be a contact irritant, and the solution must be handled and administered with care. Gloves are recommended. Inhalation of vapors and contact with skin or mucous membranes, especially those of the eyes, must be avoided. In case of contact, wash with copious amounts of water for at least 15 minutes. Anaphylactic reactions require the immediate use of epinephrine, oxygen, intravenous steroids, and antihistamines. Patients taking pegaspargase are at higher than usual risk for bleeding problems, especially with simultaneous use of other drugs that have anticoagulant properties, such as aspirin, and non-steroidal anti-inflammatories (see DRUG INTERACTIONS.) Pegaspargase may have immunosuppressive activity. Therefore, it is possible that use of the drug in patients may predispose the patient to infection. Severe hepatic and central nervous system toxicity following multi-agent chemotherapy that includes pegaspargase may occur. Caution appears warranted when treating patients with pegaspargase given in combination with hepatotoxic agents, particularly when liver dysfunction is present.

Patients undergoing pegaspargase therapy must be carefully monitored and the therapeutic regimen adjusted according to response and toxicity. Physicians using a given treatment regimen incorporating pegaspargase should be thoroughly familiar with its benefits and risks.

INFORMATION FOR THE PATIENT

Patients should be informed of the possibility of hypersensitivity reactions, including immediate anaphylaxis, to pegaspargase. Patients taking pegaspargase are at higher than usual risk for bleeding problems. Patients should be instructed that the simultaneous use of pegaspargase with other drugs that may increase the risk of bleeding should be avoided (see DRUG INTERACTIONS.) Pegaspargase may affect the ability of the liver to function normally in some patients. Therapy with pegaspargase may increase the toxicity of other medications (see DRUG INTERACTIONS.) Pegaspargase may have immunosuppressive activity. Therefore, it is possible that use of the drug in patients may predispose the patient to infection. Patients should notify their physicians of any adverse reactions that occur.

LABORATORY TESTS

A fall in circulating lymphoblasts is often noted after initiating therapy. This may be accompanied by a marked rise in serum uric acid. As a guide to the effects of therapy, the patient's peripheral blood count and bone marrow should be monitored.

Frequent serum amylase determinations should be obtained to detect early evidence of pancreatitis (see CONTRAINDICATIONS). Blood sugar should be monitored during therapy with pegaspargase because hyperglycemia may occur. When using pegaspargase in conjunction with hepatotoxic chemotherapy, patients should be monitored for liver dysfunction. Pegaspargase may affect a number of plasma proteins; therefore, monitoring of fibrinogen, PT, and PTT may be indicated.

PRECAUTIONS: *(cont'd)*

CARCINOGENESIS, MUTAGENESIS, AND IMPAIRMENT OF FERTILITY

Long-term carcinogenic studies in animals have not been performed with pegaspargase nor have studies been performed on impairment of fertility. Pegaspargase did no exhibit a mutagenic effect when tested against *Salmonella typhimurium* strains in the Ames assay.

PREGNANCY CATEGORY C

Animal reproduction studies have not been conducted with pegaspargase. It is also not known whether pegaspargase can cause fetal harm when administered to a pregnant woman or can affect reproduction capacity. Pegaspargase should be given to a pregnant woman only if clearly needed.

NURSING MOTHERS

It is not known whether pegaspargase is excreted in human milk. Because many drugs are excreted in human milk and because of the potential for serious adverse reactions due to pegaspargase in nursing infants, a decision should be made to discontinue nursing or discontinue the drug, taking into account the importance of the drug to the mother.

DRUG INTERACTIONS:

Unfavorable interactions of L-asparaginase with some antitumor agents have been demonstrated.[1] It is recommended, therefore, that pegaspargase be used in combination regimens only by physicians familiar with the benefits and risks of a given regimen. Depletion of serum proteins by pegaspargase may increase the toxicity of other drugs which are protein bound. Additionally, during the period of its inhibition of protein synthesis and cell replication, pegaspargase may interfere with the action of drugs such as methotrexate, which require cell replication for their lethal effects. Pegaspargase may interfere with the enzymatic detoxification of other drugs, particularly in the liver. Physicians using a given treatment regimen should be thoroughly familiar with its benefits and risks.

Imbalances in coagulation factors have been noted with the use of pegaspargase predisposing to bleeding and/or thrombosis. Caution should be used when administering any concurrent anticoagulant therapy, such as coumadin, heparin, dipyridamole, aspirin, or nonsteroidal anti-inflammatories.

ADVERSE REACTIONS:

Adverse reactions have been reported in adults and pediatric patients. Overall, the adult patients treated with pegaspargase had a somewhat higher incidence of known L-asparaginase toxicities, except for hypersensitivity reactions, than the pediatric patients treated with pegaspargase.

Excluding hypersensitivity reactions, the most frequently occurring known L-asparaginase related toxicities and adverse experiences reported for the 174 patients in clinical studies were chemical hepatotoxicities and coagulopathies, the majority of which did not result in any significant clinical events. The incidence of significant clinical events included clinical pancreatitis (1%), hyperglycemia requiring insulin therapy (3%), and thrombosis (4%).

The following adverse reactions related to pegaspargase were reported for 174 patients in five clinical studies.

The adverse reactions reported most frequently (greater than 5%) were allergic reactions (which may have included rash, erythema, edema, pain, fever, chills, urticaria, dyspnea, or bronchospasm), SGPT increase, nausea and/or vomiting, fever, and malaise.

The adverse reactions reported occasionally (greater than 1% but less than 5%) were anaphylactic reactions, dyspnea, injection site hypersensitivity, lip edema, rash, urticaria, abdominal pain, chills, pain in the extremities, hypotension, tachycardia, thrombosis, anorexia, diarrhea, jaundice, abnormal liver function test, decreased anticoagulant effect, disseminated intravascular coagulation, decreased fibrinogen, hemolytic anemia, leukopenia, pancytopenia, thrombocytopenia, increased thromboplastin, injection site pain, injection site reaction, bilirubinemia, hyperglycemia, hyperuricemia, hypoglycemia, hypoproteinemia, peripheral edema, increased SGOT, arthralgia, myalgia, convulsion, headache, night sweats, and paresthesia.

The adverse reactions reported rarely (less than 1%) were bronchospasm, petechial rash, face edema, lesional edema, sepsis, septic shock, chest pain, endocarditis, hypertension, constipation, flatulence, gastrointestinal pain, hepatomegaly, increased appetite, liver fatty deposits, coagulation disorder, increased coagulation time, decreased platelet count, purpura, increased amylase, edema, excessive thirst, hyperammonemia, hyponatremia, weight loss, bone pain, joint disorder, confusion, dizziness, emotional lability, somnolence, increased cough, epistaxis, upper respiratory infection, erythema simplex, pruritus, hematuria, increased urinary frequency, and abnormal kidney function.

The following pegaspargase related adverse reactions have been observed in patients with hematologic malignancies, primarily acute lymphoblastic leukemia (approximately 75%), non-Hodgkins lymphoma (approximately 13%), acute myelogenous leukemia (approximately 3%), and a variety of solid tumors (approximately 9%):

Hypersensitivity Reactions: a variety of hypersensitivity reactions have occurred. These reactions may be acute or delayed, and include acute anaphylaxis, bronchospasm, dyspnea, urticaria, arthralgia, erythema, induration, edema, pain, tenderness, hives, swelling, lip edema, chills, fever, and skin rashes (see WARNINGS AND CONTRAINDICATIONS.)

Pancreatic Function: pancreatitis, sometimes fulminant and fatal, has occurred. Increased serum amylase and lipase have also occurred.

Liver Function: a variety of liver function abnormalities have been observed, including elevations of SGOT, SGPT, and bilirubin (direct and indirect). Jaundice, ascites, and hypoalbuminemia, which may be associated with peripheral edema, have been observed. These abnormalities usually are reversible on discontinuance of therapy, and some reversal may occur during the course of therapy. Fatty changes in the liver and liver failure have occurred.

Hematologic: hypofibrinogenemia, prolonged prothrombin times, prolonged partial thromboplastin times, and decreased antithrombin III have been observed. Superficial and deep venous thrombosis, sagittal sinus thrombosis, venous catheter thrombosis, and atrial thrombosis have occurred. Leukopenia, agranulocytosis, pancytopenia, thrombocytopenia, disseminated intravascular coagulation, severe hemolytic anemia, and anemia have been observed. Clinical hemorrhage, which may be fatal; easy bruisability, and ecchymosis have also been observed.

Metabolic: mild to severe hyperglycemia has been observed in low incidence, and usually responds to discontinuation of pegaspargase and the judicious use of intravenous fluid and insulin. Hypoglycemia, increased thirst and hyponatremia, uric acid nephropathy, hyperuricemia, hypoproteinemia, and peripheral edema have also been observed. Hypoalbuminemia, proteinuria, weight loss, and metabolic acidosis have occurred. Therapy with pegaspargase is associated with an increase in blood ammonia during the conversion of L-asparagine to aspartic acid by the enzyme.

Neurologic: status epilepticus and temporal lobe seizures, somnolence, coma, malaise, mental status changes, dizziness, emotional lability, headache, lip numbness, finger paresthesia, mood changes, night sweats, and a Parkinson-like syndrome have occurred. Mild to severe confusion, disorientation, and paresthesia have also occurred. These side effects usually have reversed spontaneously after treatment was stopped.

ADVERSE REACTIONS: *(cont'd)*

Renal: increased BUN, increased creatinine, increased urinary frequency, hematuria due to thrombopenia, severe hemorrhagic cystitis, renal dysfunction, and renal failure have been observed.

Cardiovascular: chest pain, subacute bacterial endocarditis, hypertension, severe hypotension, and tachycardia have occurred.

Digestive: anorexia, constipation, decreased appetite, diarrhea, indigestion, flatulence, gas, gastrointestinal pain, mucositis, hepatomegaly, elevated gamma-glutamyltranspeptidase, increased appetite, mouth tenderness, severe colitis, and nausea and/or vomiting have been observed.

Musculoskeletal: diffuse and local musculoskeletal pain, arthralgia, joint stiffness, and cramps have occurred.

Respiratory: cough, epistaxis, severe bronchospasm, and upper respiratory infection have been observed.

Skin/Appendages: itching, alopecia, fever blister, purpura, hand whiteness and fungal changes, nail whiteness and ridging, erythema simplex, jaundice, and petechial rash have occurred.

General: localized edema, injection site reactions (including pain, swelling, or redness), malaise, infection, sepsis, fatigue, and septic shock may occur.

OVERDOSAGE:

Three patients received 10,000 IU/m^2 of pegaspargase as an intravenous infusion. One patient experienced a slight increase in liver enzymes. A second patient developed a rash ten minutes after the start of the infusion, which was controlled with the administration of an antihistamine and by slowing down the infusion rate. A third patient did not experience any adverse reactions.

DOSAGE AND ADMINISTRATION:

As a component of selected multiple agent regimens, the recommended dose of pegaspargase is 2,500 IU/m^2 every 14 days by either the intramuscular or intravenous route of administration.

The preferred route of administration, however, is the intramuscular route because of the lower incidence of hepatotoxicity, coagulopathy, and gastrointestinal and renal disorders compared to the intravenous route of administration.

The safety and effectiveness of pegaspargase have been established in patients with known previous hypersensitivity to L-aparaginase whose ages ranged from 1 to 21 years old. The recommended dose of pegaspargase for children with a body surface area $\geq$ 0.6 m^2 is 2,500 IU/m^2 administered every 14 days. The recommended dose of pegaspargase for children with a body surface area < 0.6 m^{2}is 82.5 IU/kg administered every 14 days.

Do not administer pegaspargase if there is any indication that the drug has been frozen. Although there may not be an apparent change in the appearance of the drug, pegaspargase's activity is destroyed after freezing.

When administering pegaspargase intramuscularly, the volume at a single injection site should be limited to 2 mL. If the volume to be administered is greater than 2 mL, multiple injection sites should be used.

When administered intravenously, pegaspargase should be given over a period of 1 to 2 hours in 100 mL of sodium chloride or dextrose injection 5%, through an infusion that is already running.

Anaphylactic reactions require the immediate use of antihistamines, epinephrine, oxygen, and intravenous steroids.

Use pegaspargase as the sole induction agent should be undertaken only in an unusual situation when a combined regimen, which uses other chemotherapeutic agents such as vincristine, methotrexate, cytarabine, daunorubicin, or doxorubicin is inappropriate because of toxicity or other specific patient-related factors, or in patients refractory to other therapy. When pegaspargase is to be used as the sole induction agent, the recommended dosage regimen is also 2,500 IU/m^2 every 14 days.

When a remission is obtained, appropriate maintenance therapy may be instituted. pegaspargase may be used as part of a maintenance regimen.

Parenteral drug products should be inspected visually for particulate matter, cloudiness or discoloration prior to administration, whenever solution and container permit.

HOW SUPPLIED:

DOSAGE FORM

Oncaspar: Use only one dose per vial; do not re-enter the vial. Discard unused portions. Do not save unused drug for later administration.

Sterile solution for injection in ready to use single-use vials. Preservative free.

QUANTITY PER INDIVIDUAL CONTAINER

5 mL per vial containing 750 IU/mL Oncaspar in a clear, colorless, phosphate buffered saline solution, pH 7.3. Each vial contains 3.750 IU of Oncaspar.

HANDLING AND STORAGE

Avoid excessive agitation. DO NOT SHAKE.

Keep refrigerated at + 2°C to + 8°C (36°F to 46°F).

Do not use if cloudy or if precipitate is present.

Do not use if stored at room temperature for more than 48 hours.

DO NOT FREEZE. Do not use product if it is known to have been frozen. Freezing destroys activity, which cannot be detected visually.

U.S. Patent 4,179,337 and pat. pending

ENZON, Inc., 40 Kingsbridge Road, Piscataway, NJ 08854-3998 USA

REFERENCES:

1. Capizzi, RL and Holcenberg, JS. Asparaginase. IN: Holland and Frei (eds). *Cancer Med* third edition, Lea and Febiger, Phila. PA, 1993. **2.** Ho, DH, et al. Clinical pharmacology of polyethylene glycol-Lasparaginase. *Drug Metab Dispos* 14 (3): 349-352, 1986. **3.** Asselin, BL, et al. Comparative Pharmacokinetic Studies of Three L-asparaginase Preparations. *J Clin Oncology* (11):1780- 1786, 1993. **4.** Data on File at ENZON. **5.** Clavell, LA, et al. Four-agent induction and intensive asparaginase therapy for treatment of childhood acute lymphoblastic leukemia. *N Engl J Med*315(11):657-663. 1986.(Rhone-Poulenc Rorer, 03/94, ON63J394(10-50)A)

HOW SUPPLIED - EQUIVALENTS NOT AVAILABLE:

Injection, Solution - Intravenous - 750 unit/ml

5 ml $1225.00 ONCASPAR, Rhone-Poulenc Rorer 00075-0640-05

PEMOLINE *(001963)*

CATEGORIES: Anorexients/CNS Stimulants; Attention Deficit Disorders; Central Nervous System Agents; Psychostimulants; Respiratory/Cerebral Stimulant; Stimulants; Narcolepsy*; Pregnancy Category B; DEA Class CIV; FDA Approval Pre 1982

* Indication not approved by the FDA

BRAND NAMES: *Betanamin* (Japan); **Cylert**; *Tradon* (Germany)
(International brand names outside U.S. in italics)

FORMULARIES: Aetna; BC-BS; FHP; Medi-Cal; PCS

DESCRIPTION:

Pemoline is a central nervous system stimulant. Pemoline is structurally dissimilar to the amphetamines and methylphenidate.

It is an oxazolidine compound and is chemically identified as 2-amino-5-phenyl-2-oxazolin-4-one.

Pemoline is a white, tasteless, odorless powder, relatively insoluble (less than 1 mg/ml) in water, chloroform, ether, acetone, and benzene; its solubility in 95% ethyl alcohol is 2.2 mg/ml.

Cylert is supplied as tablets containing 18.75 mg, 37.5 mg or 75 mg of pemoline for oral administration. Cylert is also available as chewable tablets containing 37.5 mg of pemoline.

Cylert Inactive Ingredients: *18.75 mg tablet:* corn starch, gelatin, lactose, magnesium hydroxide, polyethylene glycol and talc. *37.5 mg tablet:* corn starch, FD&C Yellow No. 6, gelatin, lactose, magnesium hydroxide, polyethylene glycol and talc. *37.5 mg chewable tablet:* corn starch, FD&C Yellow No. 6, magnesium hydroxide, magnesium stearate, mannitol, polyethylene glycol, povidone, talc and artificial flavor. *75 mg tablet:* corn starch, gelatin, iron oxide, lactose, magnesium hydroxide, polyethylene glycol and talc.

CLINICAL PHARMACOLOGY:

Pemoline has a pharmacological activity similar to that of other known central nervous system stimulants; however, it has minimal sympathomimetic effects. Although studies indicate that pemoline may act in animals through dopaminergic mechanisms, the exact mechanism and site of action of the drug in man is not known.

There is neither specific evidence which clearly establishes the mechanism whereby pemoline produces its mental and behavioral effects in children, nor conclusive evidence regarding how these effects relate to the condition of the central nervous system.

Pemoline is rapidly absorbed from the gastrointestinal tract. Approximately 50% is bound to plasma proteins. The serum half-life of pemoline is approximately 12 hours. Peak serum levels of the drug occur within 2 to 4 hours after ingestion of a single dose. Multiple dose studies in adults at several dose levels indicate that steady state is reached in approximately 2 to 3 days. In animals given radiolabeled pemoline, the drug was widely and uniformly distributed throughout the tissues, including the brain.

Pemoline is metabolized by the liver. Metabolites of pemoline include pemoline conjugate, pemoline dione, mandelic acid, and unidentified polar compounds. Pemoline is excreted primarily by the kidneys with approximately 50% excreted unchanged and only minor fractions present as metabolites.

Pemoline has a gradual onset of action. Using the recommended schedule of dosage titration, significant clinical benefit may not be evident until the third or fourth week of drug administration.

INDICATIONS AND USAGE:

Pemoline is indicated in Attention Deficit Disorder (ADD) with hyperactivity as an integral part of a total treatment program which typically includes other remedial measures (psychological, educational, social) for a stabilizing effect in children with a behavioral syndrome characterized by the following group of developmentally inappropriate symptoms: moderate to severe distractibility, short attention span, hyperactivity, emotional lability, and impulsivity. The diagnosis of this syndrome should not be made with finality when these symptoms are only of comparatively recent origin. Nonlocalizing (soft) neurological signs, learning disability, and abnormal EEG may or may not be present, and a diagnosis of central nervous system dysfunction may or may not be warranted.

CONTRAINDICATIONS:

Pemoline is contraindicated in patients with known hypersensitivity or idiosyncrasy to the drug. Pemoline should not be administered to patients with impaired hepatic function. (See ADVERSE REACTIONS.)

WARNINGS:

Decrements in the predicted growth (*i.e.,* weight gain and/or height) rate have been reported with the long-term use of stimulants in children. Therefore, patients requiring long-term therapy should be carefully monitored.

PRECAUTIONS:

GENERAL

Clinical experience suggests that in psychotic children, administration of pemoline may exacerbate symptoms of behavior disturbance and thought disorder.

Pemoline should be administered with caution to patients with significantly impaired renal function.

LABORATORY TESTS

Liver function tests should be performed prior to and periodically during therapy with pemoline. The drug should be discontinued if abnormalities are revealed and confirmed by follow-up tests. (See "ADVERSE REACTIONS" section regarding reports of abnormal liver function tests, hepatitis and jaundice.)

CARCINOGENESIS, MUTAGENESIS, AND IMPAIRMENT OF FERTILITY

Carcinogenesis: Long-term studies have been conducted in rats with doses as high as 150 mg/kg/day for eighteen months. There was no significant difference in the incidence of any neoplasm between treated and control animals.

Mutagenesis: Data are not available concerning long-term effects on mutagenicity in animals or humans.

Impairment of Fertility: The results of studies in which rats were given 18.75 and 37.5 mg/kg/day indicated that pemoline did not affect fertility in males or females at those doses.

PREGNANCY CATEGORY B

Teratogenic Effects: Reproduction studies have been performed in rats and rabbits at doses of 18.75 and 37.5 mg/kg/day and have revealed no evidence of impaired fertility or harm to the fetus. There are, however, no adequate and well-controlled studies in pregnant women. Because animal reproduction studies are not always predictive of human response, this drug should be used during pregnancy only if clearly needed.

PRECAUTIONS: *(cont'd)*

Nonteratogenic Effects: Studies in rats have shown an increased incidence of stillbirths and cannibalization when pemoline was administered at a dose of 37.5 mg/kg/day. Postnatal survival of offspring was reduced at doses of 18.75 and 37.5 mg/kg/day.

NURSING MOTHERS

It is not known whether this drug is excreted in human milk. Because many drugs are excreted in human milk, caution should be exercised when pemoline is administered to a nursing woman.

PEDIATRIC USE

Safety and effectiveness in children below the age of 6 years have not been established.

Long-term effects of pemoline in children have not been established (See WARNINGS.)

CNS stimulants, including pemoline, have been reported to precipitate motor and phonic tics and Tourette's syndrome. Therefore, clinical evaluation for tics and Tourette's syndrome in children and their families should precede use of stimulant medications.

Drug treatment is not indicated in all cases of ADD with hyperactivity and should be considered only in light of complete history and evaluation of the child. The decision to prescribe pemoline (pemoline) should depend on the physician's assessment of the chronicity and severity of the child's symptoms and their appropriateness for his/her age. Prescription should not depend solely on the presence of one or more of the behavioral characteristics.

DRUG INTERACTIONS:

The interaction of pemoline with other drugs has not been studied in humans. Patients who are receiving pemoline concurrently with other drugs, especially drugs with CNS activity, should be monitored carefully.

Decreased seizure threshold has been reported in patients receiving pemoline concomitantly with *antiepileptic medications.*

ADVERSE REACTIONS:

The following are adverse reactions in decreasing order of severity within each category associated with pemoline:

Hepatic: There have been reports of hepatic dysfunction including elevated liver enzymes, hepatitis and jaundice in patients taking pemoline. The occurrence of elevated liver enzymes is not rare and these reactions appear to be reversible upon drug discontinuance. Most patients with elevated liver enzymes were asymptomatic. Although no causal relationship has been established, there have been rare reports of hepatic related fatalities involving patients taking pemoline.

Hematopoietic: There have been isolated reports of aplastic anemia.

Central Nervous System: The following CNS effects have been reported with the use of pemoline: convulsive seizures; literature reports indicate that pemoline may precipitate attacks of Gilles de la Tourette syndrome; hallucinations; dyskinetic movements of the tongue, lips, face and extremities; abnormal oculomotor function including nystagmus and oculogyric crisis; mild depression; dizziness; increased irritability; headache; and drowsiness.

Insomnia is the most frequently reported side effect of pemoline; it usually occurs early in therapy prior to an optimum therapeutic response. In the majority of cases it is transient in nature or responds to a reduction in dosage.

Gastrointestinal: Anorexia and weight loss may occur during the first weeks of therapy. In the majority of cases it is transient in nature; weight gain usually resumes within three to six months.

Nausea and stomach ache have also been reported.

Genitourinary: A case of elevated acid phosphatase in association with prostatic enlargement has been reported in a 63 year old male who was treated with pemoline for sleepiness. The acid phosphatase normalized with discontinuation of pemoline and was again elevated with rechallenge.

Miscellaneous: Suppression of growth has been reported with the long-term use of stimulants in children. (See WARNINGS.) Skin rash has been reported with pemoline.

Mild adverse reactions appearing early during the course of treatment with pemoline often remit with continuing therapy. If adverse reactions are of a significant or protracted nature, dosage should be reduced or the drug discontinued.

DRUG ABUSE AND DEPENDENCE:

Controlled Substance: Pemoline is subject to control under DEA schedule IV.

Abuse: Pemoline failed to demonstrate a potential for self-administration in primates. However, the pharmacologic similarity of pemoline to other psychostimulants with known dependence liability suggests that psychological and/or physical dependence might also occur with pemoline. There have been isolated reports of transient psychotic symptoms occurring in adults following the long-term misuse of excessive oral doses of pemoline. Pemoline should be given with caution to emotionally unstable patients who may increase the dosage on their own initiative.

OVERDOSAGE:

Signs and symptoms of acute overdosage, resulting principally from overstimulation of the central nervous system and from excessive sympathomimetic effects, may include the following: vomiting, agitation, tremors, hyperreflexia, muscle twitching, convulsions (may be followed by coma), euphoria, confusion, hallucinations, delirium, sweating, flushing, headache, hyperpyrexia, tachycardia, hypertension and mydriasis. Treatment consists of appropriate supportive measures. The patient must be protected against self-injury and against external stimuli that would aggravate over-stimulation already present. If signs and symptoms are not too severe and the patient is conscious, gastric contents may be evacuated. Chlorpromazine has been reported in the literature to be useful in decreasing CNS stimulation and sympathomimetic effects.

Efficacy of peritoneal dialysis or extracorporeal hemodialysis for pemoline overdosage has not been established.

DOSAGE AND ADMINISTRATION:

Pemoline is administered as a single oral dose each morning. The recommended starting dose is 37.5 mg/day. This daily dose should be gradually increased by 18.75 mg at one week intervals until the desired clinical response is obtained. The effective daily dose for most patients will range from 56.25 to 75 mg. The maximum recommended daily dose of pemoline is 112.5 mg.

Clinical improvement with pemoline is gradual. Using the recommended schedule of dosage titration, significant benefit may not be evident until the third or fourth week of drug administration.

Where possible, drug administration should be interrupted occasionally to determine if there is a recurrence of behavioral symptoms sufficient to require continued therapy.

HOW SUPPLIED - EQUIVALENTS NOT AVAILABLE:

Tablet, Chewable - Oral - 37.5 mg

100's $128.97 CYLERT, Abbott **00074-6088-13**

Tablet, Uncoated - Oral - 18.75 mg

100's $75.28 CYLERT, Abbott **00074-6025-13**

Tablet, Uncoated - Oral - 37.5 mg

100's $118.31 CYLERT, Abbott **00074-6057-13**

Tablet, Uncoated - Oral - 75 mg

100's $204.31 CYLERT, Abbott **00074-6073-13**

PENBUTOLOL SULFATE *(001964)*

CATEGORIES: Antihypertensives; Beta Adrenergic Blocking Agents; Beta Blockers; Cardiovascular Drugs; Hypertension; Pregnancy Category C; FDA Approved 1989 Jan

BRAND NAMES: *Betapresin* (Mexico); *Betapressin* (Germany, Japan); **Levatol** *(International brand names outside U.S. in italics)*

FORMULARIES: Medi-Cal

COST OF THERAPY: $362.37 (Hypertension; Tablet; 20 mg; 1/day; 365 days)

PRIMARY ICD9: 401.1 (Essential Hypertension, Benign)

DESCRIPTION:

Levatol (penbutolol sulfate) is a synthetic β-receptor antagonist for oral administration. The chemical name of penbutolol sulfate is (S)-1-tert-Butylamino-3-(o-cyclopentylphenoxy)-2-propanol sulfate. It is provided as the levorotatory isomer.

The empirical formula for penbutolol sulfate is:

$C_{36}H_{60}N_2O_8S$.

Its molecular weight is 680.94. A dose of 20 mg is equivalent to 29.4 μmol.

Penbutolol is a white, odorless, crystalline powder. Penbutolol sulfate is available as tablets for oral administration. Each tablet contains 20 mg of penbutolol sulfate. It also contains corn starch, D & C Yellow No. 10, lactose, magnesium stearate, povidone, silicon dioxide, talc, titanium dioxide, and other inactive ingredients.

CLINICAL PHARMACOLOGY:

Penbutolol is a β-1, β-2 (nonselective) adrenergic receptor antagonist. Experimental studies showed a dose-dependent increase in heart rate in reserpinized (norepinephrine-depleted) rats given penbutolol intravenously at doses of 0.25 to 1.0 mg/kg, suggesting that penbutolol has some intrinsic sympathomimetic activity. In human studies, however, heart rate decreases have been similar to those seen with propranolol.

Penbutolol antagonizes the heart rate effects of exercise and infused isoproterenol. The β-blocking potency of penbutolol is approximately 4 times that of propranolol. An oral dose of less than 10 mg will reduce exercise-induced tachycardia to one-half its usual level; maximum antagonism follows doses of 10 to 20 mg. The peak effect is between 1.5 and 3 hours after oral administration. The duration of effect exceeds 20 hours during a once-daily dosing regimen. During chronic administration of penbutolol, the duration of antihypertensive effects permits a once-daily dosage schedule.

Acute hemodynamic effects of penbutolol have been studied following single intravenous doses between 0.1 and 4 mg. The cardiovascular responses included significant reductions in heart rate, left ventricular maximum dP/dt, cardiac output, stroke volume index, stroke work, and stroke work index. Systolic pressure and mean arterial pressure were reduced, and total peripheral resistance was increased.

Chronic administration of penbutolol to hypertensive patients results in the hemodynamic pattern typical of β-adrenergic blocking drugs: a reduction in cardiac index, heart rate, systolic and diastolic blood pressures, and the product of heart rate and mean arterial pressure both at rest and with all levels of exercise, without significant change in total peripheral resistance. Penbutolol causes a reduction in left ventricular contractility. Penbutolol decreases glomerular filtration rate, but not significantly.

Clinical trial doses of 10 to 80 mg per day in single daily doses have reduced supine and standing systolic and diastolic blood pressures. In most studies, effects were small, generally a change in blood pressure 5 to 8/3 to 5 mm Hg greater than seen with a placebo measured 24 hours after dosing. It is not clear whether this relatively small effect reflects a characteristic of penbutolol or the particular population studied (the population had relatively mild hypertension but did not appear unusual in other respects). In a direct comparison of penbutolol with adequate doses of twice daily propranolol, no difference in blood pressure effect was seen. In a comparison of placebo and 10-, 20-, and 40-mg single daily doses of penbutolol, no significant dose-related difference was seen in response to active drug at 6 weeks, but, compared to the 10-mg dose, the two larger doses showed greater effects at 2 and 4 weeks and reached their maximum effect at 2 weeks. In several studies, dose, increases from 40 to 80 mg were without additional effect on blood pressure. Response rates to penbutolol are unaffected by sex or age but are greater in caucasians than blacks.

Penbutolol decreases plasma renin activity in normal subjects and in patients with essential and renovascular hypertension. The mechanisms of the antihypertensive actions of β-receptor antagonists have not been established. However, factors that may be involved are: (1) competitive antagonism of catecholamines at peripheral adrenergic receptor sites (especially cardiac) that leads to decreased cardiac output; (2) a central-nervous-system (CNS) action that results in a decrease in tonic sympathetic neural outflow to the periphery; and (3) a reduction of renin secretion through blockade of β-receptors involved in release of renin from the kidneys.

Penbutolol dose dependently increases the RR and QT intervals. There is no influence on the PR, QRS, or QT_c (corrected) intervals.

Pharmacokinetics: Following oral administration, penbutolol is rapidly and completely absorbed. Peak plasma concentrations of penbutolol occur between 2 and 3 hours after oral administration and are proportional to single and multiple doses between 10 and 40 mg once a day. The average plasma elimination half-life of penbutolol is approximately 5 hours in normal subjects. There is no significant difference in the plasma half-life of penbutolol in healthy elderly persons or patients on renal dialysis. Twelve to 24 hours after oral administration of doses up to 120 mg, plasma concentrations of parent drug are 0% to 10% of the peak level. No accumulation of penbutolol is observed in hypertensive patients after 8 days of therapy at doses of 40 mg daily or 20 mg twice a day. Penbutolol is approximately 80% to 98% bound to plasma proteins.

The metabolism of penbutolol in humans involves conjugation and oxidation. The metabolites are excreted principally in the urine. When radiolabeled penbutolol was administered to humans, approximately 90% of the radioactivity was excreted in the urine. Approximately 1/6 of the dose of penbutolol was recovered as penbutolol conjugate, while the remaining fraction was not identified. Conjugated penbutolol has a plasma elimination half-life of approximately

CLINICAL PHARMACOLOGY: *(cont'd)*

20 hours in healthy persons, 25 hours in healthy elderly persons, and 100 hours in patients on renal dialysis. Thus, accumulation of penbutolol conjugate may be expected upon multiple-dosing in renal insufficiency. An oxidative metabolite of penbutolol, 4-hydroxy penbutolol, has been identified in small quantities in plasma and urine. It is 1/8 to 1/15 times as active as the parent compound in blocking isoproterenol-induced β-adrenergic receptor responses in isolated guinea-pig trachea and is 1/8 to 1 times as potent in anesthetized dogs.

INDICATIONS AND USAGE:

Penbutolol sulfate is indicated in the treatment of mild to moderate arterial hypertension. It may be used alone or in combination with other antihypertensive agents, especially thiazide-type diuretics.

CONTRAINDICATIONS:

Penbutolol sulfate is contraindicated in patients with cardiogenic shock, sinus bradycardia, second and third degree atrioventricular conduction block, bronchial asthma, and those with known hypersensitivity to this product (see WARNINGS).

WARNINGS:

Cardiac Failure: Sympathetic stimulation may be essential for supporting circulatory function in patients with heart failure, and its inhibition by β-adrenergic receptor blockade may precipitate more severe failure. Although β-blockers should be avoided in overt congestive heart failure, penbutolol sulfate can, if necessary, by used with caution in patients with a history of cardiac failure who are well compensated, on treatment with vasodilators, digitalis and/or diuretics. Both digitalis and penbutolol slow AV conduction. Beta-adrenergic receptor antagonists do not inhibit the inotropic action of digitalis on heart muscle. If cardiac failure persists, treatment with penbutolol sulfate should be discontinued.

Patients Without History of Cardiac Failure: Continued depression of the myocardium with β-blocking agents over a period of time can, in some cases, lead to cardiac failure. At the first evidence of heart failure, patients receiving penbutolol sulfate should be given appropriate treatment, and the response should be closely observed. If cardiac failure continues despite adequate intervention with appropriate drugs, penbutolol sulfate should be withdrawn (gradually, if possible).

Exacerbation of Ischemic Heart Disease Following Abrupt Withdrawal: Hypersensitivity to catecholamines has been observed in patients who were withdrawn from therapy with β-blocking agents; exacerbation of angina and, in some cases, myocardial infarction have occurred after abrupt discontinuation of such therapy. When discontinuing penbutolol sulfate, particularly in patients with ischemic heart disease the dosage should be reduced gradually over a period of 1 to 2 weeks and the patient should be monitored carefully. If angina becomes more pronounced or acute coronary insufficiency develops, administration of penbutolol sulfate should be reinstated promptly, at least on a temporary basis, and appropriate measures should be taken for the management of unstable angina. Patients should be warned against interruption or discontinuation of therapy without the physician's advice. Because coronary artery disease is common and may not be recognized, it may not be prudent to discontinue penbutolol sulfate abruptly, even in patients who are being treated only for hypertension.

Nonallergic Bronchospasm (*e.g.,* chronic bronchitis, emphysema): Penbutolol sulfate is contraindicated in bronchial asthma. In general, patients with bronchospastic diseases should not receive β-blockers. Penbutolol sulfate should be administered with caution because it may block bronchodilation produced by endogenous catecholamine stimulation of β-2 receptors.

Anesthesia and Major Surgery: The necessity, or desirability, of withdrawal of a β-blocking therapy prior to major surgery is controversial. Beta-adrenergic receptor blockade impairs the ability of the heart to respond to β-adrenergically mediated reflex stimuli. Although this might be of benefit in preventing arrhythmic response, the risk of excessive myocardial depression during general anesthesia may be enhanced and difficulty in restarting and maintaining the heart beat has been reported with β-blockers. If treatment is continued, particular care should be taken when using anesthetic agents that depress the myocardium, such as ether, cyclopropane, and trichloroethylene, and it is prudent to use the lowest possible dose of penbutolol sulfate. Penbutolol sulfate like other β-blockers, is a competitive inhibitor of β-receptor agonists, and its effect on the heart can be reversed by cautious administration of such agents (*e.g.,* dobutamine or isoproterenol *see* Overdose). Manifestations of excessive vagal tone (*e.g.,* profound bradycardia, hypotension) may be corrected with atropine 1 to 3 mg IV in divided doses.

Diabetes Mellitus and Hypoglycemia: Beta-adrenergic receptor blockade may prevent the appearance of signs and symptoms of acute hypoglycemia, such as tachycardia and blood pressure changes. This is especially important in patients with labile diabetes. Beta-blockade also reduces the release of insulin in response to hyperglycemia; therefore, it may be necessary to adjust the dose of hypoglycemic drugs. Beta-adrenergic blockade may also impair the homeostatic response to hypoglycemia; in that event, the spontaneous recovery from hypoglycemia may be delayed during treatment with β-adrenergic receptor antagonists.

Thyrotoxicosis: Beta-adrenergic blockade may mask certain clinical signs (*e.g.,* tachycardia) of hyperthyroidism. Patients suspected of developing thyrotoxicosis should be managed carefully to avoid abrupt withdrawal of β-adrenergic receptor blockers that might precipitate a thyroid storm.

PRECAUTIONS:

Information for Patients: Patients, especially those with evidence of coronary artery insufficiency, should be warned against interruption or discontinuation of penbutolol sulfate without the physician's advice. Although cardiac failure rarely occurs in properly selected patients, those being treated with β-adrenergic receptor antagonists should be advised of the symptoms of heart failure and to report such symptoms immediately, should they develop.

Risk of Anaphylactic Reactions: While taking β-blockers, patients with a history of severe anaphylactic reactions ot a variety of allergens may be more reactive to repeated challenge, either accidental, diagnostic, or therapeutic. Such patients may be unresponsive to the usual doses of epinephrine used to treat allergic reactions.

Carcinogenesis, Mutagenesis, and Impairment of Fertility: There was no evidence of carcinogenicity observed in a 21-month study in mice of 2-year study in rats. Mice were given penbutolol in the diet for 18 months at doses up to 395 mg/kg/day (about 500 times the maximum recommended dose of 40 mg in a 50 kg person). Rats were given 141 mg/kg/day for the same length of time. Mice were observed for 3 months and rats for 5.5 to 7 months after termination of treatment before necropsy was performed.

No evidence of mutagenic activity of penbutolol was seen in the *Salmonella* mutagenicity test (Ames test), in point mutation induction test (*Saccharomyces*), and the micronucleus test.

Penbutolol had not adverse effects on fertility or general reproduction performance in mice and rats at oral doses up to 172 mg/kg/day.

Pregnancy, Teratogenic Effects, Pregnancy Category C: Teratology studies in rats and rabbits revealed no teratogenic effects related to treatment with penbutolol at oral doses up to 200 mg/kg/day (250 times the maximum recommended human dose). In rabbits, a slight increase in the intrauterine fetal mortality and a reduced 24-hour offspring survival rats were observed

PRECAUTIONS: *(cont'd)*

in the groups treated with 125 mg/kg/day (156 times the maximum recommended dose) but not in the groups treated with 0.2 and 5 mg (0.25 to 6 times the maximum recommended dose).

There are no adequate and well-controlled studies in pregnant women. Penbutolol sulfate should be used during pregnancy only if the potential benefit justifies the potential risk to the fetus.

Nonteratogenic Effects: In a perinatal and postnatal study in rats, the pup body weight and pup survival rate were reduced at the highest dose level of 160 mg/kg/day (200 times the maximum recommended dose).

Nursing Mothers: It is not known whether penbutolol sulfate is excreted in human milk. Because many drugs are excreted in human milk, caution should be exercised when penbutolol sulfate is administered to a nursing woman.

Usage in Children: Safety and effectiveness of penbutolol sulfate in children have not been established.

DRUG INTERACTIONS:

Penbutolol sulfate has been used in combination with hydrochlorothiazide in at least 100 patients without unexpected adverse reactions.

In one study, the combination of penbutolol and alcohol increased the number of errors in the eye-hand psychomotor function test.

Penbutolol increases the volume of distribution of lidocaine in normal subjects. This could results in a requirement for higher loading doses of lidocaine.

Cimetidine has no effect on the clearance of penbutolol. The major metabolite of penbutolol is a glucuronide, and it has been shown that cimetidine does not inhibit glucuronidation.

Synergistic hypotensive effects, bradycardia, and arrhythmias have been reported in some patients receiving β-adrenergic blocking agents when an oral calcium antagonist was added to the treatment regimen.

Generally, penbutolol sulfate should not be used in patients receiving catecholamine-depleting drugs.

ADVERSE REACTIONS:

Penbutolol sulfate is usually well tolerated in properly selected patients. Most adverse effects observed during clinical trials have been mild and reversible.

Table 1 lists the adverse reactions reported from 4 controlled studies conducted in the United States involving once-a-day administration of penbutolol sulfate (at doses ranging from 10 to 120 mg) as monotherapy or in combination with hydrochlorothiazide. Penbutolol sulfate doses above 40 mg/day are not, however, recommended. The tablet includes only those events where the prevalence rate in the penbutolol sulfate group was at least 1.5%, or where the reaction is of particular interest.

Over a dose range 10 to 40 mg, once a day fatigue, nausea, and sexual impotence occurred at a greater frequency as the dose was increased (TABLE 1).

TABLE 1 ADVERSE REACTIONS DURING CONTROLLED US STUDIES

Body System Experience	Penbutolol (N=628)	Placebo (N=212)	Propranolol (N=266)
Body as a Whole	%	%	%
Asthenia	1.6	0.9	4.9
Pain, chest	2.4	2.8	2.3
Pain, limb	2.4	1.4	1.5
Digestive System			
Diarrhea	3.3	1.9	2.6
Nausea	4.3	0.9	2.3
Dyspepsia	2.7	1.4	5.3
Nervous System			
Dizziness	4.9	2.4	4.2
Fatigue	4.4	1.9	2.6
Headache	7.8	6.1	7.5
Insomnia	1.9	0.9	2.6
Respiratory System			
Cough	2.1	0.5	1.1
Dyspnea	2.1	1.4	3.4
Upper respiratory	2.5	3.3	4.9
Skin and Appendages			
Sweating, excessive	1.6	0.5	2.3
Urogenital System			
Impotence, sexual	0.5	0.0	0.8

In a double-blind clinical trial comparing penbutolol sulfate (40 mg and greater once a day) and propranolol (40 mg or more twice a day), heart rates of less than 60 beats/min were recorded at least once in 25% of the patient in the group receiving penbutolol sulfate and in 37% of the patients in the propranolol group. Corresponding figures for heat rates of less than 50 beats/min were 1.2% of 6% respectively. No symptoms associated with bradycardia were reported.

Discontinuations of penbutolol sulfate because of adverse reactions have ranged between 2.4% and 6.9% of patients in double-blind, parallel, controlled groups that were given placebo. The frequency and severity of adverse reactions have not increased during long-term administration of penbutolol sulfate. The prevalence of adverse reactions reported from 4 controlled clinical trials (referred to in TABLE 1) as reasons for discontinuations of therapy by ≥ 0.5% of the penbutolol sulfate groups is listed in TABLE 2.

TABLE 2 DISCONTINUATIONS DURING CONTROLLED US STUDIES

Body System Experience	Penbutolol (N=628)	Placebo (N=212)	Propranolol (N=266)
Body as a Whole	%	%	%
Asthenia	0.6	0.0	0.4
Pain, chest	0.6	1.4	0.4
Digestive System			
Nausea	0.8	0.0	0.8
Nervous System			
Depression	0.6	0.5	0.8
Dizziness	0.6	0.0	0.4
Fatigue	0.5	0.5	0.0
Headache	0.6	0.5	0.4

Potential Adverse Effects: In addition, certain adverse effects not listed above have been reported with other β-blocking agents and should also be considered as potential adverse effects of penbutolol sulfate.

ADVERSE REACTIONS: *(cont'd)*

Central Nervous System: Reversible mental depression progressing to catatonia (an acute syndrome characterized by disorientation for time and place), short-term memory loss, emotional lability, slightly clouded sensorium, and decreased performance (neuropsychometrics).

Cardiovascular: Intensification of AV block (see CONTRAINDICATIONS).

Allergic: Erythematous rash, fever combined with aching and sore throat, laryngospasm, and respiratory distress.

Hematologic: Agranulocytosis, nonthrombocytopenic and thrombocytopenic purpura.

Gastrointestinal: Mesenteric arterial thrombosis and ischemic colitis.

Miscellaneous: Reversible alopecia and Peyronie's disease. The oculomucocutaneous syndrome associated with the β-blocker practolol has not been reported with penbutolol sulfate during investigational use and extensive foreign clinical experience.

OVERDOSAGE:

There is not actual experience with penbutolol sulfate overdose. The signs and symptoms that would be expected with overdosage of β-adrenergic receptor antagonists are symptomatic bradycardia, hypotension, bronchospasm and acute cardiac failure. In addition to discontinuation of penbutolol sulfate, gastric emptying, and close observation of the patient, the following measures might be considered as appropriate:

Excessive Bradycardia: Administer atropine sulfate to induce vagal blockade. If bradycardia persists, intravenous isoproterenol hydrochloride may be administered cautiously; larger than usual doses may be needed. In refractor cases, the use of transvenous cardiac pacemaker may be necessary.

Hypotension: Sympathomimetic drug therapy, such as dopamine, dobutamine, or levarterenol, may be considered if hypotension persists despite correction of bradycardia. In refractor cases, administration of glucagon hydrochloride has been reported to be useful.

Bronchospasm: A β-2-agonist or isoproterenol hydrochloride may be administered. Additional therapy with aminophylline may be considered.

Acute Cardiac Failure: Institute conventional therapy immediately. Intravenous administration of dobutamine and glucagon hydrochloride has been reported to be useful.

Heart Block (Second or Third Degree): Isoproterenol hydrochloride or a transvenous cardiac pacemaker may be used.

DOSAGE AND ADMINISTRATION:

The usual starting and maintenance dose of penbutolol sulfate, used alone in combination with other antihypertensive agents, such as thiazide-type diuretics, is 20 mg given once daily.

Doses of 40 mg and 80 mg have been well tolerated but have not been shown to give a greater antihypertensive effect. The full effect of a 20- or 40-mg dose is seen by the end of 2 weeks. A dose of 10 mg also lowers blood pressure, but the full effect is not seen for 4 to 6 weeks.

Store at controlled room temperature 15°-30°C (59°-86°F).

Keep tightly closed and protect from light.

ANIMAL PHARMACOLOGY:

Studies in rats indicated that the combination of penbutolol, triamterene, and hydrochlorothiazide (up to 40, 50 and 25 mg/kg respectively) increased the incidence and severity of renal tubular dilation and regeneration when compared to that in rats treated only with triamterene and hydrochlorothiazide. Dogs administered the same doses of triamterene and hydrochlorothiazide alone and in combination with penbutolol had an increase in serum alkaline phosphatase and serum alanine transferase, but there were no gross or microscopic abnormalities observed. No significant toxicologic findings were observed in rats and dogs treated with a combination of penbutolol and hydrochlorothiazide.

HOW SUPPLIED - EQUIVALENTS NOT AVAILABLE:

Tablet, Uncoated - Oral - 20 mg

100's $99.28 LEVATOL, Schwarz Pharma (US) 00091-4500-15

PENCICLOVIR *(003304)*

CATEGORIES: Anti-Infectives; Antimicrobials; Antivirals; Dermatologicals; FDA Approved 1996 Sep; Fever Blisters; Herpes Simplex; Lesions; Pregnancy Category B; Topical; Viral Agents

BRAND NAMES: **Denavir**; *Vectavir* (Germany)
(International brand names outside U.S. in italics)

DESCRIPTION:

Penciclovir is an antiviral agent active against herpes viruses. Denavir is available for topical administration as a 1% white cream. Each gram of Denavir contains 10 mg of penciclovir and the following inactive ingredients: cetomacrogol 1000 BP, cetostearyl alcohol, mineral oil, propylene glycol, purified water and white petrolatum.

Chemically, penciclovir is known as 9-[4-hydroxy-3-(hydroxymethyl) butyl]guanine. Its molecular formula is $C_{10}H_{15}N_5O_3$; its molecular weight is 253.26. It is a synthetic acyclic guanine derivative.

Penciclovir is a white to pale yellow solid. At 20°C it has a solubility of 0.2 mg/ml in methanol, 1.3 mg/ml in propylene, and 1.7 mg/ml in water. In aqueous buffer (pH 2) the solubility is 10.0 mg/ml. Penciclovir is not hygrpscopic. Its partition coefficient in n-octanol/water at pH 7.5 is 0.024 (logP = -1.62).

CLINICAL PHARMACOLOGY:

MICROBIOLOGY

Mechanism of Antiviral Activity: The antiviral compound penciclovir has *in vitro* inhibitory activity against herpes simplex virus types 1 (HSV-1) and 2 (HSV-2). In cells infected with HSV-1 or HSV-2, viral thymidine kinase phosphorylates penciclovir to a monophosphate form which, in turn, is converted to penciclovir triphosphate by cellular kinases. *In vitro* studies demonstrate that penciclovir triphosphate inhibits HSV polymerase competitively with deoxyguanosine triphosphate. Consequently, herpes viral DNA synthesis and, therefore, replication are selectively inhibited.

Antiviral Activity *In Vitro* and *In Vivo*: In cell culture studies, penciclovir has antiviral activity against HSV-1 and HSV-2. Sensitivity test results, expressed as the concentration of the drug required to inhibit growth of the virus by 50% (IC_{50}) or 99% (IC_{99}) in cell culture, vary depending upon a number of factors, including the assay protocols. See TABLE 1

Drug Resistance: Penciclovir-resistant mutants of HSV can result from qualitative changes in viral thymidine kinase or DNA polymerase. The most commonly encountered acyclovir-resistant mutants that are deficient in viral thymidine kinase are also resistant to penciclovir.

CLINICAL PHARMACOLOGY: *(cont'd)*

TABLE 1

Method of Assay	Virus Type	Cell Type	IC_{50} (mcg/ml)	IC_{99} (mcg/ml)
Plaque Reduction	HSV-1 (c.i.)	MRC-5	0.2-0.6	
	HSV-1 (c.i.)	WISH	0.04-0.5	
	HSV-2 (c.i.)	MRC-5	0.9-2.1	
	HSV-2 (c.i.)	WISH	0.1-0.8	
Virus Yield Reduction	HSV-1 (c.i.)	MRC-5		0.4-0.5
	HSV-2 (c.i.)	MRC-5		0.6-0.7
DNA Synthesis Inhibition	HSV-1 (SC16)	MRC-5	0.04	
	HSV-2 (MS)	MRC-5	0.05	

(c.i.) Clinical isolates. The latent state of any herpes virus not known to respond to any antiviral therapy.

PHARMACOKINETICS

Measurable penciclovir concentration were not detected in plasma or urine of healthy male volunteers (n=12) following single or repeat application of the 1% cream at a dose of 180 mg penciclovir daily (approximately 67 times the estimated usual clinical dose).

Pediatric Patients: The systemic absorption of penciclovir following topical administration has not been evaluated in patients <18 years of age.

CLINICAL STUDIES:

Penciclovir was studied in two double-blind, placebo (vehicle)-controlled trials for the treatment of recurrent herpes labialis in which otherwise healthy adults were randomized to either penciclovir or placebo. Therapy was to be initiated by the subjects within one hour of noticing signs or symptoms and continued for 4 days, with application of study medication every 2 hours while awake. In both studies, the mean duration of lesions was approximately one-half day shorter in the subjects treated with penciclovir (N=1,516) as compared to subjects treated with placebo (N=1,541) (approximately 4 days versus 5 days, respectively). The mean duration of lesion pain was also approximately one-half-day shorter in the penciclovir group compared to the placebo group.

INDICATIONS AND USAGE:

Penciclovir cream is indicated for the treatment of recurrent herpes labialis (cold sores) in adults.

CONTRAINDICATIONS:

Penciclovir is contraindicated in patients with known hypersensitivity to the product or any of its components.

PRECAUTIONS:

GENERAL

Penciclovir should only be used on herpes labialis on the lips and face. Because no data are available, application to human mucous membranes is not recommended. Particular care should be taken to avoid application in or near the eyes since it may cause irritation. The effect of penciclovir has not been established in immunocompromised patients.

CARCINOGENESIS, MUTAGENESIS, AND IMPAIRMENT OF FERTILITY

In clinical trials, systemic drug exposure following the topical administration of penciclovir cream was negligible, as the penciclovir content of all plasma and urine samples was below the limit of assay detection (0.1 mcg/ml and 10 mcg/ml, respectively). However, for the purpose of inter-species dose comparisons presented in the following sections, an assumption of 100% absorption of penciclovir from the topically applied product has been used. Based on use of the maximal recommended topical dose of penciclovir of 0.05 mg/kg/day and an assumption of 100% absorption, the maximum theoretical plasma AUC_{0-24} hours for penciclovir is approximately 0.129 mcg·h/ml.

Carcinogenesis: Two-year carcinogenicity studies were conducted with famciclovir (the oral pro-drug of penciclovir) in rats and mice. An increase in the incidence of mammary adenocarcinoma (a common tumor in female rats in the strain used) was seen in female rats receiving 600 mg/kg/day) (approximately 395 times the maximum theoretical human exposure to penciclovir following application of the topical product, based on area under the plasma concentration curve comparison [24 hour AUC]). No increases in tumor incidence were seen among male rats treated at doses up to 240 mg/kg/day (approximately 190 times the maximum theoretical human AUC for penciclovir), or in male and female mice at doses up to 600 mg/kg/day (approximately 100 times the maximum theoretical human AUC for penciclovir).

Mutagenesis: When tested *in vitro*, penciclovir did not cause an increase in gene mutation in the Ames assay using multiple strains of *S. typhimurium* or *E. coli* (at up to 20,000 mcg/plate), nor did it cause an increase in unscheduled DNA repair in mammalian HeLa S3 cells(at up to 5,000 mcg/ml). However, an increase in clastogenic responses was seen with penciclovir in the L5178Y mouse lymphoma cell assay at doses ≥1000 mcg/ml) and, in human lymphocytes incubated *in vitro* at doses ≥250 mcg/ml. When tested *in vivo*, penciclovir caused an increase in micronuclei in mouse bone marrow following the intravenous administration of doses ≥500 mg/kg (≥810 times the maximum human dose, based on body surface area conversion.)

Impairment of Fertility: Testicular toxicity was observed in multiple animal species (rats and dogs) following repeated intravenous administration of penciclovir (160 mg/kg/day and 100 mg/kg/day, respectively, approximately 1155 and 3255 times the maximum theoretical human AUC). Testicular changes seen in both species included atrophy of the seminiferous tubules and reductions in epididymal sperm counts and/or an increased incidence of sperm with abnormal morphology or reduced motility. Adverse testicular effects were related to an increasing dose or duration of exposure to penciclovir. No adverse testicular or reproductive effects (fertility and reproductive function) were observed in rats after 10 to 13 weeks dosing at 80 mg/kg/day, or testicular effects in dogs after 13 weeks dosing at 30 mg/kg/day (575 and 845 times the maximum theoretical human AUC, respectively). Intravenously administered penciclovir had no effect on fertility or reproductive performance in female rats at doses of up to 80 mg/kg/day (260 times the maximum human dose [BSA]).

There was no evidence of any clinically significant effects on sperm count, motility or morphology in 2 placebo-controlled clinical trails of famciclovir [the oral prodrug of penciclovir], 250 mg twice daily; n=66) in immunocompetent men with recurrent genital herpes, when dosing and follow-up were maintained for 18 weeks and 8 weeks, respectively (approximately 2 and 1 spermatogenic cycles in the human).

PREGNANCY, TERATOGENIC EFFECTS, PREGNANCY CATEGORY B

No adverse effects on the course and outcome of pregnancy or on fetal development were noted in rats and rabbits following the intravenous administration of penciclovir at doses of 80 and 60 mg/kg/day, respectively (estimated human equivalent doses of 13 and 18 mg/kg/day for the rat and rabbit, respectively, based on body surface area conversion; the body surface area doses being 260 and 355 times the maximum recommended dose following

PRECAUTIONS: *(cont'd)*

topical application of the penciclovir cream. There are, however, no adequate and well-controlled studies in pregnant women. Because animal reproduction studies are not always predictive of human response, penciclovir should be used during pregnancy only if clearly needed.

NURSING MOTHERS

There is no information on whether penciclovir is excreted in human milk after topical administration. However, following oral administration of famciclovir (the oral prodrug of penciclovir) to lactating rats, penciclovir was excreted in breast milk at concentrations higher than those seen in the plasma. Therefore, a decision should be made whether to discontinue the drug, taking into account the importance of the drug to the mother. There are no data on the safety of penciclovir in newborns.

PEDIATRIC USE

Safety and effectiveness in pediatric patients have not been established.

GERIATRIC USE

In 74 patients ≥65 years of age, the adverse events profile was comparable to that observed in younger patients.

ADVERSE REACTIONS:

In two double-blind, placebo-controlled trials, 1516 patients were treated with penciclovir cream and 1541 with placebo. The most frequently reported adverse event was headache, which occurred in 5.3% of the patients treated with penciclovir and 5.8% of the placebo-treated patients. The rates of reported local adverse reactions are shown in TABLE 2. One or more local adverse reactions were reported by 2.7% of the patients treated with penciclovir and 3.9% of the placebo-treated patients.

TABLE 2 Local Adverse Reactions Reported in Phase III Trials

	Penciclovir n=1516 %	Placebo n=1541 %
Application site reaction	1.3	1.8
Hypesthesia/ Local anesthesia	0.9	1.4
Taste perversion	0.2	0.3
Pruritus	0.0	0.3
Pain	0.0	0.1
Rash (erythematous)	0.1	0.1
Allergic reaction	0.0	0.1

Two studies, enrolling 108 healthy subjects, were conducted to evaluate the dermal tolerance of 5% penciclovir cream (a 5-fold higher concentration than the commercial formulation) compared to vehicle using repeated occluded patch testing methodology. The 5% penciclovir cream induced mild erythema in approximately one-half of the subjects exposed, an irritancy profile similar to the vehicle control in terms of severity and proportion of subjects with a response. No evidence of sensitization was observed.

OVERDOSAGE:

Since penciclovir is poorly absorbed following oral administration, adverse reactions related to penciclovir ingestion are unlikely. There is no information on overdose.

DOSAGE AND ADMINISTRATION:

Penciclovir should be applied every 2 hours during waking hours for a period of 4 days. Treatment should be started as early as possible (*i.e.,* during the prodrome or when lesions appear).

PATIENT INFORMATION:

Penciclovir is used for the treatment of herpes simplex virus of the lips and face. Do not use on mucous membranes.

Inform your doctor if you are pregnant or nursing.

Apply every 2 hours during waking hours. Begin treatment as soon as lesions appear.

May cause headaches and local redness/ irritation.

HOW SUPPLIED:

Denavir is supplied in a 2 gram tube containing 10 mg of penciclovir per gram.

Store at or below 30°C (86°F). Do not freeze.

PENICILLAMINE *(001965)*

CATEGORIES: Antagonists and Antidotes; Antiarthritics; Arthritis; Chelating Agents; Cystinuria; Heavy Metal Antagonists; Renal Drugs; Wilson's Disease; FDA Approval Pre 1982

BRAND NAMES: *Artamin*; *Atamir*; *Cupripen*; **Cuprimine**; Depen; *Distamine* (England); *D-Penamine* (Australia); *Kelatin*; *Kelatine*; *Mercaptyl*; *Metalcaptase* (Japan); *Penicillamine*; *Pendramine* (England); *Sufortanon*
(International brand names outside U.S. in italics)

FORMULARIES: Aetna; BC-BS; PCS; WHO

WARNING:
Physicians planning to use penicillamine should thoroughly familiarize themselves with its toxicity, special dosage considerations, and therapeutic benefits. Penicillamine should never be used casually. Each patient should remain constantly under the close supervision of the physician. Patients should be warned to report promptly any symptoms suggesting toxicity.

DESCRIPTION:

Penicillamine is a chelating agent used in the treatment of Wilson's disease. It is also used to reduce cystine excretion in cystinuria and to treat patients with severe, active rheumatoid arthritis unresponsive to conventional therapy (see INDICATIONS AND USAGE.) It is 3-mercapto-D-valine. It is a white or practically white, crystalline powder, freely soluble in water, slightly soluble in alcohol, and insoluble in ether, acetone, benzene, and carbon tetrachloride. Although its configuration is D, it is levorotatory as usually measured (TABLE 1):

The empirical formula is $C_5H_{11}NO_2S$, giving it a molecular weight of 149.21.

It reacts readily with formaldehyde or acetone to form a thiazolidine-carboxylic acid.

DESCRIPTION: *(cont'd)*

TABLE 1

$[\alpha]^{25°}_{D} = -62.5° \pm 2°$ (c = 1, 1N NaOH),
calculated on a dried basis.

Capsules Cuprimine (Penicillamine) for oral administration contain either 125 mg or 250 mg of penicillamine. Each capsule contains the following inactive ingredients: D & C Yellow 10, gelatin, lactose, magnesium stearate, and titanium dioxide. The 125 mg capsule also contains iron oxide.

CLINICAL PHARMACOLOGY:

Penicillamine is a chelating agent recommended for the removal of excess copper in patients with Wilson's disease. From *in vitro* studies which indicate that one atom of copper combines with two molecules of penicillamine, it would appear that one gram of penicillamine should be followed by the excretion of about 200 milligrams of copper; however, the actual amount excreted is about one percent of this.

Penicillamine also reduces excess cystine excretion in cystinuria. This is done, at least in part, by disulfide interchange between penicillamine and cystine, resulting in formation of penicillamine-cysteine disulfide, a substance that is much more soluble than cystine and is excreted readily.

Penicillamine interferes with the formation of cross-links between tropocollagen molecules and cleaves them when newly formed.

The mechanism of action of penicillamine in rheumatoid arthritis is unknown although it appears to suppress disease activity. Unlike cytotoxic immunosuppressants, penicillamine markedly lowers IgM rheumatoid factor but produces no significant depression in absolute levels of serum immunoglobulins. Also unlike cytotoxic immunosuppressants which act on both, penicillamine *in vitro* depresses T-cell activity but not B-cell activity.

In vitro, penicillamine dissociates macroglobulins (rheumatoid factor) although the relationship of the activity to its effect in rheumatoid arthritis is not known.

In rheumatoid arthritis, the onset of therapeutic response to penicillamine may not be seen for two or three months. In those patients who respond, however, the first evidence of suppression of symptoms such as pain, tenderness, and swelling is generally apparent within three months. The optimum duration of therapy has not been determined. If remissions occur, they may last from months to years, but usually require continued treatment (see DOSAGE AND ADMINISTRATION.)

In all patients receiving penicillamine, it is important that penicillamine be given on an empty stomach, at least one hour before meals or two hours after meals, and at least one hour apart from any other drug, food, or milk. This permits maximum absorption and reduces the likelihood of inactivation by metal binding in the gastrointestinal tract.

Methodology for determining the bioavailability of penicillamine is not available; however, penicillamine is known to be a very soluble substance.

INDICATIONS AND USAGE:

Penicillamine is indicated in the treatment of Wilson's disease, cystinuria, and in patients with severe, active rheumatoid arthritis who have failed to respond to an adequate trial of conventional therapy. Available evidence suggests that penicillamine is not of value in ankylosing spondylitis.

Wilson's Disease: Wilson's disease (hepatolenticular degeneration) results from the interaction of an inherited defect and an abnormality in copper metabolism. The metabolic defect, which is the consequence of the autosomal inheritance of one abnormal gene from each parent, manifests itself in a greater positive copper balance than normal. As a result, copper is deposited in several organs and appears eventually to produce pathologic effects most prominently seen in the brain, where degeneration is widespread; in the liver, where fatty infiltration, inflammation, and hepatocellular damage progress to postnecrotic cirrhosis; in the kidney, where tubular and glomerular dysfunction results; and in the eye, where characteristic corneal copper deposits are known as Kayser-Fleischer rings.

Two types of patients require treatment for Wilson's disease: (1) the symptomatic, and (2) the asymptomatic in whom it can be assumed the disease will develop in the future if the patient is not treated.

Diagnosis, suspected on the basis of family or individual history, physical examination, or a low serum concentration of ceruloplasmin*, is confirmed by the demonstration of Kayser-Fleischer rings or, particularly in the asymptomatic patient, by the quantitative demonstration in a liver biopsy specimen of a concentration of copper in excess of 250 mcg/g dry weight.

Treatment has two objectives:

(1) to minimize dietary intake and absorption of copper.

(2) to promote excretion of copper deposited in tissues.

The first objective is attained by a daily diet that contains no more than one or two milligrams of copper. Such a diet should exclude, most importantly, chocolate, nuts, shellfish, mushrooms, liver, molasses, broccoli, and cereals enriched with copper, and be composed to as great an extent as possible of foods with a low copper content. Distilled or demineralized water should be used if the patient's drinking water contains more than 0.1 mg of copper per liter.

For the second objective, a copper chelating agent is used.

In symptomatic patients this treatment usually produces marked neurologic improvement, fading of Kayser-Fleischer rings, and gradual amelioration of hepatic dysfunction and psychic disturbances.

Clinical experience to date suggests that life is prolonged with the above regimen.

Noticeable improvement may not occur for one to three months. Occasionally, neurologic symptoms become worse during initiation of therapy with penicillamine. Despite this, the drug should not be discontinued permanently, although temporary interruption may result in clinical improvement of the neurological symptoms but it carries an increased risk of developing a sensitivity reaction upon resumption of therapy (see WARNINGS.)

Treatment of asymptomatic patients has been carried out for over ten years. Symptoms and signs of the disease appear to be prevented indefinitely if daily treatment with penicillamine can be continued.

Cystinuria: Cystinuria is characterized by excessive urinary excretion of the dibasic amino acids, arginine, lysine, ornithine, and cystine, and the mixed disulfide of cysteine and homocysteine. The metabolic defect that leads to cystinuria is inherited as an autosomal, recessive trait. Metabolism of the affected amino acids is influenced by at least two abnormal factors: (1) defective gastrointestinal absorption and (2) renal tubular dysfunction.

Arginine, lysine, ornithine, and cysteine are soluble substances, readily excreted. There is no apparent pathology connected with their excretion in excessive quantities.

Cystine, however, is so slightly soluble at the usual range of urinary pH that it is not excreted readily, and so crystallizes and forms stones in the urinary tract. Stone formation is the only known pathology in cystinuria.

INDICATIONS AND USAGE: *(cont'd)*

Normal daily output of cystine is 40 to 80 mg. In cystinuria, output is greatly increased and may exceed 1 g/day. At 500 to 600 mg/day, stone formation is almost certain. When it is more than 300 mg/day, treatment is indicated.

Conventional treatment is directed at keeping urinary cystine diluted enough to prevent stone formation, keeping the urine alkaline enough to dissolve as much cystine as possible, and minimizing cystine production by a diet low in methionine (the major dietary precursor of cystine). Patients must drink enough fluid to keep urine specific gravity below 1.010, take enough alkali to keep urinary pH at 7.5 to 8, and maintain a diet low in methionine. This diet is not recommended in growing children and probably is contraindicated in pregnancy because of its low protein content (see PRECAUTIONS.)

When these measures are inadequate to control recurrent stone formation, penicillamine may be used as additional therapy. When patients refuse to adhere to conventional treatment, penicillamine may be a useful substitute. It is capable of keeping cystine excretion to near normal values, thereby hindering stone formation and the serious consequences of pyelonephritis and impaired renal function that develop in some patients.

Bartter and colleagues depict the process by which penicillamine interacts with cystine to form penicillamine-cysteine mixed disulfide as:

CSSC + PS' ⇊ CS' + CSSP

PSSP + CS' ⇊ PS' + CSSP

CSSC + PSSP ∫ 2 CSSP

CSSC = Cystine

CS' = deprotonated cysteine

PSSP = penicillamine

PS' = deprotonated penicillamine sulfhydryl

CSSP = penicillamine-cysteine mixed disulfide

In this process, it is assumed that the deprotonated form of penicillamine, PS', is the active factor in bringing about the disulfide interchange.

Rheumatoid Arthritis: Because penicillamine can cause severe adverse reactions, its use in rheumatoid arthritis should be restricted to patients who have severe, active disease and who have failed to respond to an adequate trial of conventional therapy. Even then, benefit-to-risk ratio should be carefully considered. Other measures, such as rest, physiotherapy, salicylates, and corticosteroids should be used, when indicated, in conjunction with penicillamine (see PRECAUTIONS.)

*For quantitative test for serum ceruloplasmin see: Morell, A. G.; Windsor, J.; Sternlieb, I.; Scheinberg, I. H.: Measurement of the concentration of ceruloplasmin in serum by determination of its oxidase activity, in "Laboratory Diagnosis of Liver Disease", F. W. Sunderman;F. W. Sunderman, Jr. (eds.), St. Louis, Warren H. Green, Inc., 1968, pp. 193-195.

CONTRAINDICATIONS:

Except for the treatment of Wilson's disease or certain cases of cystinuria, use of penicillamine during pregnancy is contraindicated (see WARNINGS.)

Although breast milk studies have not been reported in animals or humans, mothers on therapy with penicillamine should not nurse their infants.

Patients with a history of penicillamine-related aplastic anemia or agranulocytosis should not be restarted on penicillamine (see WARNINGS) and ADVERSE REACTIONS.

Because of its potential for causing renal damage, penicillamine should not be administered to rheumatoid arthritis patients with a history or other evidence of renal insufficiency.

WARNINGS:

The use of penicillamine has been associated with fatalities due to certain diseases such as aplastic anemia, agranulocytosis, thrombocytopenia, Good-pasture's syndrome, and myasthenia gravis.

Because of the potential for serious hematological and renal adverse reactions to occur at any time, routine urinalysis, white and differential blood cell count, hemoglobin determination, and direct platelet count must be done every two weeks for at least the first six months of penicillamine therapy and monthly thereafter. Patients should be instructed to report promptly the development of signs and symptoms of granulocytopenia and/or thrombocytopenia such as fever, sore throat, chills, bruising or bleeding. The above laboratory studies should then be promptly repeated.

Leukopenia and thrombocytopenia have been reported to occur in up to five percent of patients during penicillamine therapy. Leukopenia is of the granulocytic series and may or may not be associated with an increase in eosinophils. A confirmed reduction in, WBC below 3500/mm^{3}mandates discontinuance of penicillamine therapy. Thrombocytopenia may be on an idiosyncratic basis, with decreased or absent megakaryocytes in the marrow, when it is part of an aplastic anemia. In other cases the thrombocytopenia is presumably on an immune basis since the number of megakaryocytes in the marrow has been reported to be normal or sometimes increased. The development of a platelet count below 100,000/mm^3, even in the absence of clinical bleeding, requires at least temporary cessation of penicillamine therapy. A progressive fall in either platelet count or WBC in three successive determinations, even though values are still within the normal range, likewise requires at least temporary cessation.

Proteinuria and/or hematuria may develop during therapy and may be warning signs of membranous glomerulopathy which can progress to a nephrotic syndrome. Close observation of these patients is essential. In some patients the proteinuria disappears with continued therapy; in others, penicillamine must be discontinued. When a patient develops proteinuria or hematuria the physician must ascertain whether it is a sign of drug-induced glomerulopathy or is unrelated to penicillamine.

Rheumatoid arthritis patients who develop moderate degrees of proteinuria may be continued cautiously on penicillamine therapy, provided that quantitative 24-hour urinary protein determinations are obtained at intervals of one to two weeks. Penicillamine dosage should not be increased under these circumstances. Proteinuria which exceeds 1 g/24 hours, or proteinuria which progressively increasing, requires either discontinuance of the drug or a reduction in the dosage. In some patients, proteinuria has been reported to clear following reduction in dosage.

In rheumatoid arthritis patients penicillamine should be discontinued if unexplained gross hematuria or persistent microscopic hematuria develops.

In patients with Wilson's disease or cystinuria the risks of continued penicillamine therapy in patients manifesting potentially serious urinary abnormalities must be weighed against the expected therapeutic benefits.

When penicillamine is used in cystinuria, an annual x-ray for renal stones is advised. Cystine stones form rapidly, sometimes in six months.

Up to one year or more may be required for any urinary abnormalities to disappear after penicillamine has been discontinued.

Because of rare reports of intrahepatic cholestasis and toxic hepatitis, liver function tests are recommended every six months for the duration of therapy.

WARNINGS: *(cont'd)*

Goodpasture's syndrome has occurred rarely. The development of abnormal urinary findings associated with hemoptysis and pulmonary infiltrates on x-ray requires immediate cessation of penicillamine.

Obliterative bronchiolitis has been reported rarely. The patient should be cautioned to report immediately pulmonary symptoms such as exertion, dyspnea, unexplained cough or wheezing. Pulmonary function studies should be considered at that time.

Myasthenic syndrome sometimes progressing to myasthenia gravis has been reported. Ptosis and diplopia, with weakness of the extraocular muscles are often early signs of myasthenia. In the majority of cases, symptoms of myasthenia have receded after withdrawal of penicillamine.

Most of the various forms of pemphigus have occurred during treatment with penicillamine. Pemphigus vulgaris and pemphigus foliaceus are reported most frequently, usually as a late complication of therapy. The seborrhea-like characteristics of pemphigus foliaceus may obscure an early diagnosis. When pemphigus is suspected, penicillamine should be discontinued. Treatment has consisted of high doses of corticosteroids alone or, in some cases, concomitantly with an immunosuppressant. Treatment may be required for only a few weeks or months, but may need to be continued for more than a year.

Once instituted for Wilson's disease or cystinuria, treatment with penicillamine should, as a rule, be continued on a daily basis. Interruptions for even a few days have been followed by sensitivity reactions after reinstitution of therapy.

Use in Pregnancy: Penicillamine has been shown to be teratogenic in rats when given in doses 6 times higher than the highest dose recommended for human use. Skeletal defects, cleft palates and fetal toxicity (resorptions) has been reported.

There are no controlled studies on the use of penicillamine in pregnant women. Although normal outcomes have been reported, characteristic congenital cutis laxa and associated birth defects have been reported in infants born of mothers who received therapy with penicillamine during pregnancy. Penicillamine should be used in women of childbearing potential only when the expected benefits outweigh the possible hazards. Women on therapy with penicillamine who are of childbearing potential should be apprised of this risk advised to report promptly any missed menstrual periods or other indications of possible pregnancy, and followed closely for early recognition of pregnancy.

Wilson's Disease: Reported experience* shows that continued treatment with penicillamine throughout pregnancy protects the mother against relapse of the Wilson's disease, and that discontinuation of penicillamine has deleterious effects on the mother.

If penicillamine is administered during pregnancy to patients with Wilson disease, it is recommended that the daily dosage be limited to 1 g. If cesarean section is planned, the daily dosage should be limited to 250 mg during the last six weeks of pregnancy and postoperatively until wound healing is complete.

Cystinuria: If possible, penicillamine should not be given during pregnancy to women with cystinuria (see CONTRAINDICATIONS.) There are reports of women with cystinuria on therapy with penicillamine who gave birth to infants with generalized connective tissue defects who died following abdominal surgery. If stones continue to form in these patients, the benefits of therapy to the mother must be evaluated against the risk to the fetus.

Rheumatoid Arthritis: Penicillamine should not be administered to rheumatoid arthritis patients who are pregnant (see CONTRAINDICATIONS) and should be discontinued promptly in patients in whom pregnancy is suspected or diagnosed.

There is a report that a woman with rheumatoid arthritis treated with less than one gram a day of penicillamine during pregnancy gave birth (cesarean delivery) to an infant with growth retardation, flattened face with broad nasal bridge, low set ears, short neck with loose skin folds, and unusually lax body skin.

PRECAUTIONS:

Some patients may experience drug fever, a marked febrile response tp penicillamine, usually in the second to third week following initiation of therapy. Drug fever may sometimes be accompanied by a macular cutaneous eruption.

In the case of drug fever in patients with Wilson's disease or cystinuria penicillamine should be temporarily discontinued until the reaction subsides. Then penicillamine should be reinstituted with a small dose that is gradually increased until the desired dosage is attained. Systemic steroid therapy may be necessary, and is usually helpful, in such patients in whom toxic reactions develop a second or third time.

In the case of drug fever in rheumatoid arthritis patients, because other treatments are available, penicillamine should be discontinued and another therapeutic alternative tried since experience indicates that the febrile reaction will recur in a very high percentage of patients upon readministration of penicillamine.

The skin and mucous membranes should be observed for allergic reactions. Early and late rashes have occurred. Early rash occurs during the first few months of treatment and is more common. It is usually a generalized pruritic, erythematous, maculopapular or morbilliform rash and resembles the allergic rash seen with other drugs. Early rash usually disappears within days after stopping penicillamine and seldom recurs when the drug is restarted at a lower dosage. Pruritus and early rash may often be controlled by the concomitant administration of antihistamines. Less commonly, a late rash may be seen, usually after six months or more of treatment, and requires discontinuation of penicillamine. It is usually on the trunk, is accompanied by intense pruritus, and is usually unresponsive to topical corticosteroid therapy. Late rash may take weeks to disappear after penicillamine is stopped and usually recurs if the drug is restarted.

The appearance of a drug eruption accompanied by fever, arthralgia, lymphadenopathy or other allergic manifestations usually requires discontinuation of penicillamine.

Certain patients will develop a positive antinuclear antibody (ANA) test and some of these may show a lupus erythematosus-like syndrome similar to drug-induced lupus associated with other drugs. The lupus erythematosus-like syndrome is not associated with hypocomplementemia and may be present without nephropathy. The development of a positive ANA test does not mandate discontinuance of the drug; however, the physician should be alerted to the possibility that a lupus erythematosus-like syndrome may develop in the future.

Some patients may develop oral ulcerations which in some cases have the appearance of aphthous stomatitis. The stomatitis usually recurs on rechallenge but often clears on a lower dosage. Although rare, cheilosis, glossitis and gingivostomatitis have also been reported. These oral lesions are frequently dose-related and may preclude further increase in penicillamine dosage or require discontinuation of the drug.

Hypogeusia (a blunting or diminution in taste perception) has occurred in some patients. This may last two to three months or more and may develop into a total loss of taste; however, it is usually self-limited despite continued penicillamine treatment. Such taste impairment is rare in patients with Wilson's disease.

Penicillamine should not be used in patients who are receiving concurrently gold therapy, antimalarial or cytotoxic drugs, oxyphenbutazone or phenylbutazone because these drugs are also associated with similar serious hematologic and renal adverse reactions. Patients who have had gold salt therapy discontinued due to a major toxic reaction may be at greater risk of serious adverse reactions with penicillamine but not necessarily of the same type.

PRECAUTIONS: *(cont'd)*

Patients who are allergic to penicillin may theoretically have cross-sensitivity to penicillamine. The possibility of reactions from contamination of penicillamine by trace amounts of penicillin has been eliminated now that penicillamine is being produced synthetically rather than as a degradation product of penicillin.

Because of their dietary restrictions, patients with Wilson's disease and cystinuria should be given 25 mg/day of pyridoxine during therapy, since penicillamine increases the requirement for this vitamin. Patients also may receive benefit from a multivitamin preparation, although there is no evidence that deficiency of any vitamin other than pyridoxine is associated with penicillamine. In Wilson's disease, multivitamin preparations must be copper-free.

Rheumatoid arthritis patients whose nutrition is impaired should also be given a daily supplement of pyridoxine. Mineral supplements should not be given, since they may block the response to penicillamine.

Iron deficiency may develop, especially in children and in menstruating women. In Wilson's disease, this may be a result of adding the effects of the low copper diet, which is probably also low in iron, and the penicillamine to the effects of blood loss or growth. In cystinuria, a low methionine diet may contribute to iron deficiency, since it is necessarily low in protein. If necessary, iron may be given in short courses, but a period of two hours should elapse between administration of penicillamine and iron, since orally administered iron has been shown to reduce the effects of penicillamine.

Penicillamine causes an increase in the amount of soluble collagen. In the rat this results in inhibition of normal healing and also a decrease in tensile strength of intact skin. In man this may be the cause of increased skin friability at sites especially subject to pressure or trauma, such as shoulders, elbows, knees, toes, and buttocks. Extravasations of blood may occur and may appear as pupuric areas, with external bleeding if the skin is broken, or as vesicles containing dark blood. Neither type is progressive. There is no apparent association with bleeding elsewhere in the body and no associated coagulation defect has been found. Therapy with penicillamine may be continued in the presence of these lesions. They may not recur if dosage is reduced. Other reported effects probably due to the action of penicillamine on collagen are excessive wrinkling of the skin and development of small, white papules at venipuncture and surgical sites.

The effects of penicillamine on collagen and elastin make it advisable to consider a reduction in dosage to 250 mg/day, when surgery is contemplated. Reinstitution of full therapy should be delayed until wound healing is complete.

Carcinogenesis: Long-term animal carcinogenicity studies have not been done with penicillamine. There is a report that five of ten autoimmune disease-prone NZB hybrid mice developed lymphocytic leukemia after 6 months' intraperitoneal treatment with a dose of 400 mg/kg penicillamine 5 days per week.

Nursing Mothers: See CONTRAINDICATIONS.

Usage in Children: The efficacy of penicillamine in juvenile rheumatoid arthritis has not been established.

*Scheinberg, I.H.; Sternlieb, I.: N. Engl. J. Med. *293*:1300-1302, Dec. 18, 1975

ADVERSE REACTIONS:

Penicillamine is a drug with a high incidence of untoward reactions, some of which are potentially fatal. Therefore, it is mandatory that patients receiving penicillamine therapy remain under close medical supervision throughout the period of drug administration (see WARNINGS) and PRECAUTIONS.

Reported incidences (%) for the most commonly occurring adverse reactions in rheumatoid arthritis patients are noted, based on 17 representative clinical trials reported in the literature (1270 patients).

Allergic: Generalized pruritus, early and late rashes (5%), pemphigus (see WARNINGS), and drug eruptions which may be accompanied by fever, arthralgia, or lymphadenopathy have occurred (see WARNINGS and PRECAUTIONS). Some patients may show a lupus erythematosus-like syndrome similar to drug-induced lupus produced by other pharmacological agents (see PRECAUTIONS.)

Urticaria and exfoliative dermatitis have occurred.

Thyroiditis has been reported; hypoglycemia in association with anti-insulin antibodies has been reported. These reactions are extremely rare.

Some patients may develop a migratory polyarthralgia, often with objective synovitis (see DOSAGE AND ADMINISTRATION.)

Gastrointestinal: Anorexia, epigastric pain, nausea, vomiting, or occasional diarrhea may occur (17%).

Isolated cases of reactivated peptic ulcer have occurred, as have hepatic dysfunction and pancreatitis. Intrahepatic cholestasis and toxic hepatitis have been reported rarely. There have been a few reports of increased serum alkaline phosphatase, lactic dehydrogenase, and positive cephalin flocculation and thymol turbidity tests.

Some patients may report a blunting, diminution, or total loss of taste perception (12%); or may develop oral ulcerations. Although rare, cheilosis, glossitis, and gingivostomatitis have been reported (see PRECAUTIONS.)

Gastrointestinal side effects are usually reversible following cessation of therapy.

Hematological: Penicillamine can cause bone marrow depression (see WARNINGS.) Leukopenia (2%) and thrombocytopenia (4%) have occurred. Fatalities have been reported as a result of thrombocytopenia, agranulocytosis, aplastic anemia, and sideroblastic anemia.

Thrombotic thrombocytopenic purpura, hemolytic anemia, red cell aplasia, monocytosis, leukocytosis, eosinophilia, and thrombocytosis have also been reported.

Renal: Patients on penicillamine therapy may develop proteinuria (6%) and/or hematuria which, in some, may progress to the development of the nephrotic syndrome as a result of an immune complex membranous glomerulopathy (see WARNINGS.)

Central Nervous System: Tinnitus, optic neuritis and peripheral sensory and motor neuropathies (including polyradiculoneuropathy, i.e., Guillain-Barre syndrome) have been reported. Muscular weakness may or may not occur with the peripheral neuropathies. Visual and psychic disturbances have been reported.

Neuromuscular: Myasthenia gravis (see WARNINGS.)

Other: Adverse reactions that have been reported rarely include thrombophlebitis; hyperpyrexia (see PRECAUTIONS); falling hair or alopecia; lichen planus; polymyositis; dermatomyositis; mammary hyperplasia; elastosis perforans serpiginosa; toxic epidermal necrolysis; anetoderma (cutaneous macular atrophy); and Goodpasture's syndrome, a severe and ultimately fatal glomerulonephritis associated with intra-alveolar hemorrhage (see WARNINGS.) Fatal renal vasculitis has also been reported. Allergic alveolitis, obliterative bronchiolitis, interstitial pneumonitis and pulmonary fibrosis have been reported in patients with severe rheumatoid arthritis, some of whom were receiving penicillamine. Bronchial asthma also has been reported.

Increased skin friability, excessive wrinkling of skin, and development of small white papules at venipuncture and surgical sites have been reported (see PRECAUTIONS.)

The chelating action of the drug may cause increased excretion of other heavy metals such as zinc, mercury and lead.

ADVERSE REACTIONS: *(cont'd)*

There have been reports associating penicillamine with leukemia. However, circumstances involved in these reports are such that a cause and effect relationship to the drug has not been established.

DOSAGE AND ADMINISTRATION:

In all patients receiving penicillamine, it is important that penicillamine be given on an empty stomach, at least one hour before meals or two hours after meals, and at least one hour apart from any other drug, food, or milk. Because penicillamine increases the requirement for pyridoxine, patients may require a daily supplement of pyridoxine (see PRECAUTIONS.)

Wilson's Disease: Optimal dosage can be determined by measurement of urinary copper excretion and the determination of free copper in the serum. The urine must be collected in copper-free glassware, and should be quantitatively analyzed for copper before and soon after initiation of therapy with penicillamine.

Determination of 24-hour urinary copper excretion is of greatest value in the first week of therapy with penicillamine. In the absence of any drug reaction, a dose between 0.75 and 1.5 g that results in an initial 24-hour cupriuresis of over 2 mg should be continued for about three months, by which time the most reliable method of monitoring maintenance treatment is the determination of free copper in the serum. This equals the difference between quantitatively determined total copper and ceruloplasmin-copper. Adequately treated patients will usually have less than 10 mcg free copper/dl of serum. It is seldom necessary to exceed a dosage of 2 g/day. If the patient is intolerant to therapy with penicillamine, alternative treatment is trientine hydrochloride.

In patients who cannot tolerate as much as 1 g/day initially, initiating dosage with 250 mg/day, and increasing gradually to the requisite amount, gives closer control of the effects of the drug and may help to reduce the incidence of adverse reactions.

Cystinuria: It is recommended that penicillamine be used along with conventional therapy. By reducing urinary cystine, it decreases crystalluria and stone formation. In some instances, it has been reported to decrease the size of, and even to dissolve, stones already formed.

The usual dosage of penicillamine in the treatment of cystinuria is 2 g/day for adults, with a range of 1 to 4 g/day. For children, dosage can be based on 30 mg/kg/day. The total daily amount should be divided into four doses. If four equal doses are not feasible, give the larger portion at bedtime. If adverse reactions necessitate a reduction in dosage, it is important to retain the bedtime dose.

Initiating dosage with 250 mg/day, and increasing gradually to the requisite amount, gives closer control of the effects of the drug and may help to reduce the incidence of adverse reactions.

In addition to taking penicillamine, patients should drink copiously. It is especially important to drink about a pint of fluid at bedtime and another pint once during the night when urine is more concentrated and more acid than during the day. The greater the fluid intake, the lower the required dosage of penicillamine.

Dosage must be individualized to an amount that limits cystine excretion to 100-200 mg/day in those with no history of stones, and below 100 mg/day in those who have had stone formation and/or pain. Thus, in determining dosage, the inherent tubular defect, the patient's size, age, and rate of growth, and his diet and water intake all must be taken into consideration.

The standard nitroprusside cyanide test has been reported useful as a qualitative measure of the effective dose*: Add 2 ml of freshly prepared 5 percent sodium cyanide to 5 ml of a 24-hour aliquot of protein-free urine and let stand ten minutes. Add 5 drops of freshly prepared 5 percent sodium nitroprusside and mix. Cystine will turn the mixture magenta. If the result is negative, it can be assumed that cystine excretion is less than 100 mg/g creatinine.

Although penicillamine is rarely excreted unchanged, it also will turn the mixture magenta. If there is any question as to which substance is causing the reaction, a ferric chloride test can be done to eliminate doubt: Add 3 percent ferric chloride dropwise to the urine. Penicillamine will turn the urine an immediate and quickly fading blue. Cystine will not produce any change in appearance.

Rheumatoid Arthritis: The principal rule of treatment with penicillamine in rheumatoid arthritis is patience. The onset of therapeutic response is typically delayed. Two or three months may be required before the first evidence of a clinical response is noted (see CLINICAL PHARMACOLOGY.)

When treatment with penicillamine has been interrupted because of adverse reactions or other reasons, the drug should be reintroduced cautiously by starting with a lower dosage and increasing slowly.

Initial Therapy: The currently recommended dosage regimen in rheumatoid arthritis begins with a single daily dose of 125 mg or 250 mg which is thereafter increased at one to three month intervals, by 125 mg or 250 mg/day, as patient response and tolerance indicate. If a satisfactory remission of symptoms is achieved, the dose associated with the remission should be continued (see Maintenance Therapy.) If there is no improvement and there are no signs of potentially serious toxicity after two to three months of treatment with doses of 500-750 mg/day, increases of 250 mg/day at two to three month intervals may be continued until a satisfactory remission occurs (see Maintenance Therapy) or signs of toxicity develop (see WARNINGS and PRECAUTIONS). If there is no discernible improvement after three to four months of treatment with 1000 to 1500 mg of penicillamine/day, it may be assumed the patient will not respond and penicillamine should be discontinued.

Maintenance Therapy: The maintenance dosage of penicillamine must be individualized, and may require adjustment during the course of treatment. Many patients respond satisfactorily to a dosage within the 500-750 mg/day range. Some need less.

Changes in maintenance dosage levels may not be reflected clinically or in the erythrocyte sedimentation rate for two to three months after each dosage adjustment.

Some patients will subsequently require an increase in the maintenance dosage to achieve maximal disease suppression. In those patients who do respond, but who evidence incomplete suppression of their disease after the first six to nine months of treatment, the daily dosage of penicillamine may be increased by 125 mg or 250 mg/day at three-month intervals. It is unusual in current practice to employ a dosage in excess of 1 g/day, but up to 1.5 g/day has sometimes been required.

Management of Exacerbations: During the course of treatment some patients may experience an exacerbation of disease activity following an initial good response. These may be self-limited and can subside within twelve weeks. They are usually controlled by the addition of non-steroidal anti-inflammatory drugs, and only if the patient has demonstrated a true "escape" phenomenon (as evidenced by failure of the flare to subside within this time period) should an increase in the maintenance dose ordinarily be considered.

In the rheumatoid patient, migratory polyarthralgia due to penicillamine is extremely difficult to differentiate from an exacerbation of the rheumatoid arthritis. Discontinuance or a substantial reduction in dosage of penicillamine for up to several weeks will usually determine which of these processes is responsible for the arthralgia.

DOSAGE AND ADMINISTRATION: *(cont'd)*

Duration of Therapy: The optimum duration of therapy with penicillamine in rheumatoid arthritis has not been determined. If the patient has been in remission for six months or more, a gradual, stepwise dosage reduction in decrements of 125 mg or 250 mg/day at approximately three month intervals may be attempted.

Concomitant Drug Therapy: Penicillamine should not be used in patients who are receiving gold therapy, antimalarial or cytotoxic drugs, oxyphenbutazone, or phenylbutazone (see PRECAUTIONS.) Other measures, such as salicylates, other non-steroidal anti-inflammatory drugs, or systemic corticosteroids, may be continued when penicillamine is initiated. After improvement commences, analgesic and anti-inflammatory drugs may be slowly discontinued as symptoms permit. Steroid withdrawal must be done gradually, and many months of treatment with penicillamine may be required before steroids can be completely eliminated.

Dosage Frequency: Based on clinical experience dosages up to 500 mg/day can be given as a single daily dose. Dosages in excess of 500 mg/day should be administered in divided doses.

Storage: Keep container tightly closed.

REFERENCES:

* Lotz, M.; Potts, J. T. and Bartter, F. C.: Brit. Med. J. *2*:521, Aug. 28, 1965 (in Medical Memoranda).

HOW SUPPLIED - EQUIVALENTS NOT AVAILABLE:

Capsule, Gelatin - Oral - 125 mg

100's $64.88 **CUPRIMINE, Merck** **00006-0672-68**

Capsule, Gelatin - Oral - 250 mg

100's $92.63 **CUPRIMINE, Merck** **00006-0602-68**

Tablet, Coated - Oral - 250 mg

100's $148.24 DEPEN TITRATABLE, Wallace Labs 00037-4401-01

PENICILLIN G BENZATHINE *(001966)*

CATEGORIES: Anti-Infectives; Antibiotics; Antimicrobials; Bejel; Chorea; Glomerulonephritis; Infections; Penicillins; Pinta; Respiratory Tract Infections; Rheumatic Fever; Sexually Transmitted Diseases; Yaws; Lyme Disease*; Otitis Media*; Pregnancy Category B; FDA Approval Pre 1982
* Indication not approved by the FDA

BRAND NAMES: *Benzadar*; *Benzanil Simple* (Mexico); Benzathine Benzylpenicillin; *Benzetacil*; *Benzetacil A.P.* (Mexico); *Benzetacil L.A.*; *Benzetacil L-A*; *Benzilfan* (Mexico); **Bicillin L-A**; *Bicillin LA 1.2*; *Bicillin LA 2.4*; *Cepacilina*; *Diaminocillina*; *Durabiotic*; *Extencilline* (France); *Lentopenil* (Mexico); *Lutecilina 1.200*; *Mycin*; *Penadur*; *Penadur L.A.*; *Penadur L-A*; *Penadur LA*; *Pencom*; *Penadur - LA*; *Penidural*; *Penidure LA 6*; *Penidure LA 12*; *Penidure LA 24*; *Penilente*; *Penilente - LA*; Permapen; *Retarcilina*; *Retarpen*; *Wycillina A P*
(International brand names outside U.S. in italics)

FORMULARIES: BC-BS; WHO

DESCRIPTION:

Sterile Penicillin G Benzathine suspension, is prepared by the reaction of dibenzylethylene diamine with two molecules of Penicillin G. It is chemically designated as 3,3-dimethyl-7-oxo-6-(2-phenylacetamido)-4-thia- 1-azabicyclo (3.2.0)heptane-2-carboxylic acid compound with *N,N'*- dibenzylethylenediamine (2:1), tetrahydrate.

It is available for deep intramuscular injection. It contains sterile Penicillin G Benzathine in aqueous suspension with sodium citrate buffer and, as w/v, approximately 0.5% lecithin, 0.6% carboxymethylcellulose, 0.6% povidone, 0.1% methylparaben, and 0.01% propylparaben. It occurs as a white, crystalline powder and is very slightly soluble in water and sparingly soluble in alcohol.

Sterile Penicillin G Benzathine suspension in the multiple-dose vial formulation is viscous and opaque. It contains the equivalent of 300,000 units per ml of Penicillin G as the benzathine salt. Read CONTRAINDICATIONS, WARNINGS, PRECAUTIONS, and DOSAGE AND ADMINISTRATION prior to use.

CLINICAL PHARMACOLOGY:

GENERAL

Penicillin G Benzathine has an extremely low solubility and, thus, the drug is slowly released from intramuscular injection sites. The drug is hydrolyzed to Penicillin G. This combination of hydrolysis and slow absorption results in blood serum levels much lower but much more prolonged than other parenteral Penicillins.

Intramuscular administration of 300,000 units of Penicillin G Benzathine in adults results in blood levels of 0.03 to 0.05 units per ml, which are maintained for 4 to 5 days. Similar blood levels may persist for 10 days following administration of 600,000 units and for 14 days following administration of 1,200,000 units. Blood concentrations of 0.003 units per ml may still be detectable 4 weeks following administration of 1,200,000 units.

Approximately 60% of Penicillin G is bound to serum protein. The drug is distributed throughout the body tissues in widely varying amounts. Highest levels are found in the kidneys with lesser amounts in the liver, skin, and intestines. Penicillin G penetrates into all other tissues and the spinal fluid to a lesser degree. With normal kidney function, the drug is excreted rapidly by tubular excretion. In neonates and young infants and in individuals with impaired kidney function, excretion is considerably delayed.

MICROBIOLOGY

Penicillin G exerts a bactericidal action against penicillin-susceptible microorganisms during the stage of active multiplication. It acts through the inhibition of biosynthesis of cell-wall mucopeptide. It is not active against the penicillinase-producing bacteria, which include many strains of staphylococci.

The following *in-vitro* data are available, but their clinical significance is unknown. Penicillin G exerts high *in-vitro* activity against staphylococci (except penicillinase-producing strains), streptococci (Groups A, C, G, H, L, and M), and pneumococci. Other organisms susceptible to Penicillin G are *Neisseria gonorrhoeae, Corynebacterium diphtheriae, Bacillus anthracis,* Clostridia species,*Actinomyces bovis, Streptobacillus moniliformis, Listeria monocytogenes,* and *Leptospira* species. *Treponema pallidum* is extremely susceptible to the bactericidal action of Penicillin G.

Susceptibility Test: If the Kirby-Bauer method of disc susceptibility is used, a 20-unit penicillin disc should give a zone greater than 28 mm when tested against a penicillin-susceptible bacterial strain.

INDICATIONS AND USAGE:

Intramuscular Penicillin G Benzathine is indicated in the treatment of infections due to Penicillin-G-sensitive microorganisms that are susceptible to the low and very prolonged serum levels common to this particular dosage form. Therapy should be guided by bacteriological studies (including sensitivity tests) and by clinical response.

INDICATIONS AND USAGE: *(cont'd)*

The following infections will usually respond to adequate dosage of intramuscular Penicillin G Benzathine:

Mild-to-moderate infections of the upper-respiratory tract due to susceptible streptococci.

Venereal Infections: Syphilis, yaws, bejel, and pinta.

Medical Conditions in which Penicillin G Benzathine Therapy is Indicated as Prophylaxis:

Rheumatic Fever and/or Chorea: Prophylaxis with Penicillin G Benzathine has proven effective in preventing recurrence of these conditions. It has also been used as follow-up prophylactic therapy for rheumatic heart disease and acute glomerulonephritis.

CONTRAINDICATIONS:

A history of a previous hypersensitivity reaction to any of the penicillins is a contraindication.

Do not inject into or near an artery or nerve.

WARNINGS:

Penicillin G Benzathine should only be prescribed for the indications listed in this insert.

Serious and occasionally fatal hypersensitivity (anaphylactoid) reactions have been reported in patients receiving penicillin. Although anaphylaxis is more frequent following parenteral administration, it has occurred in patients on oral penicillins. These reactions are more apt to occur in individuals with a history of sensitivity to multiple allergens.

There are reports of patients with a history of penicillin hypersensitivity reactions who experienced severe hypersensitivity reactions when treated with a cephalosporin. Before therapy with a penicillin, careful inquiry should be made about previous hypersensitivity reactions to penicillins, cephalosporins, and other allergens. If an allergic reaction occurs, the drug should be discontinued and appropriate therapy should be instituted. Serious anaphylactoid reactions require immediate emergency treatment with epinephrine. Oxygen, intravenous steroids, airway management, including intubation, should also be administered as indicated.

Inadvertent intravascular administration, including inadvertent direct intraarterial injection or injection immediately adjacent to arteries, of Sterile Penicillin G Benzathine suspension and other penicillin preparations has resulted in severe neurovascular damage, including transverse myelitis with permanent paralysis, gangrene requiring amputation of digits and more proximal portions of extremities, and necrosis and sloughing at and surrounding the injection site. Such severe effects have been reported following injections into the buttock, thigh, and deltoid areas. Other serious complications of suspected intravascular administration which have been reported include immediate pallor, mottling, or cyanosis of the extremity both distal and proximal to the injection site, followed by bleb formation; severe edema requiring anterior and/or posterior compartment fasciotomy in the lower extremity. The above-described severe effects and complications have most often occurred in infants and small children. Prompt consultation with an appropriate specialist is indicated if any evidence of compromise of the blood supply occurs at, proximal to, or distal to the site of injection.[1-9] See CONTRAINDICATIONS, PRECAUTIONS and DOSAGE AND ADMINISTRATION.

Quadriceps femoris fibrosis and atrophy have been reported following repeated intramuscular injections of penicillin preparations into the anterolateral thigh.

Injection into or near a nerve may result in permanent neurological damage.

PRECAUTIONS:

General: Penicillin should be used with caution in individuals with histories of significant allergies and/or asthma.

Care should be taken to avoid intravenous or intraarterial administration, or injection into or near major peripheral nerves or blood vessels, since such injection may produce neurovascular damage. See CONTRAINDICATIONS, WARNINGS and DOSAGE AND ADMINISTRATION.

Prolonged use of antibiotics may promote the overgrowth of nonsusceptible organisms, including fungi. Should superinfection occur, appropriate measures should be taken.

Laboratory Tests: In streptococcal infections, therapy must be sufficient to eliminate the organism; otherwise, the sequelae of streptococcal disease may occur. Cultures should be taken following completion of treatment to determine whether streptococci have been eradicated.

Pregnancy Category B: Reproduction studies performed in the mouse, rat, and rabbit have revealed no evidence of impaired fertility or harm to the fetus due to Penicillin G. Human experience with the penicillins during pregnancy has not shown any positive evidence of adverse effects on the fetus. There are, however, no adequate and well-controlled studies in pregnant women showing conclusively that harmful effects of these drugs on the fetus can be excluded. Because animal reproduction studies are not always predictive of human response, this drug should be used during pregnancy only if clearly needed.

Nursing Mothers: Soluble Penicillin G is excreted in breast milk. Caution should be exercised when Penicillin G Benzathine is administered to a nursing woman.

Carcinogenesis, Mutagenesis, Impairment Of Fertility: No long-term animal studies have been conducted with this drug.

Pediatric Use: See INDICATIONS AND USAGE and DOSAGE AND ADMINISTRATION."

DRUG INTERACTIONS:

Tetracycline, a bacteriostatic antibiotic, may antagonize the bactericidal effect of penicillin, and concurrent use of these drugs should be avoided.

Concurrent administration of penicillin and probenecid increases and prolongs serum penicillin levels by decreasing the apparent volume of distribution and slowing the rate of excretion by competitively inhibiting renal tubular secretion of penicillin.

ADVERSE REACTIONS:

As with other penicillins, untoward reactions of the sensitivity phenomena are likely to occur, particularly in individuals who have previously demonstrated hypersensitivity to penicillins or in those with a history of allergy, asthma, hay fever, or urticaria.

As with other treatments for syphilis, the Jarisch-Herxheimer reaction has been reported.

The following have been reported with parenteral penicillin G:

General: Hypersensitivity reactions including the following: skin eruptions (maculopapular to exfoliative dermatitis), urticaria, laryngeal edema, fever, eosinophilia; other serum-sicknesslike reactions (including chills, fever, edema, arthralgia, and prostration); anaphylaxis. Note: Urticaria, other skin rashes, and serum-sicknesslike reactions may be controlled with antihistamines and, if necessary, systemic corticosteroids.

Whenever such reactions occur, Penicillin G should be discontinued unless, in the opinion of the physician, the condition being treated is life-threatening and amenable only to therapy with Penicillin G. Serious anaphylactic reactions require the immediate use of epinephrine, oxygen, and intravenous steroids.

Hematologic: Hemolytic anemia, leukopenia, thrombocytopenia.

Neurologic: Neuropathy.

ADVERSE REACTIONS: *(cont'd)*

Urogenital: Nephropathy.

OVERDOSAGE:

Penicillin in overdosage has the potential to cause neuromuscular hyperirritability or convulsive seizures.

DOSAGE AND ADMINISTRATION:

STREPTOCOCCAL (GROUP A) UPPER RESPIRATORY INFECTIONS (FOR EXAMPLE, PHARYNGITIS)

Adults: a single injection of 1,200,000 units;

Older Children: a single injection of 900,000 units;

Infants and Children (under 60 lbs.): 300,000 to 600,000 units.

SYPHILIS

Primary, secondary, and latent: 2,400,000 units (1 dose).

Late (tertiary and neurosyphilis): 2,400,000 units at 7-day intervals for three doses.

Congenital: *under 2 years of age:* 50,000 units/kg/body weight; *ages 2 to 12 years:* adjust dosage based on adult dosage schedule.

YAWS, BEJEL, AND PINTA

1,200,000 units (1 injection).

PROPHYLAXIS—FOR RHEUMATIC FEVER AND GLOMERULONEPHRITIS

Following an acute attack, Penicillin G Benzathine (parenteral) may be given in doses of 1,200,000 units once a month or 600,000 units every 2 weeks.

Administer by DEEP INTRAMUSCULAR INJECTION in the upper, outer quadrant of the buttock. In infants and small children, the midlateral aspect of the thigh may be preferable. When doses are repeated, vary the injection site.

After selection of the proper site and insertion of the needle into the selected muscle, aspirate by pulling back on the plunger. While maintaining negative pressure for 2 to 3 seconds, carefully observe the barrel of the syringe immediately proximal to the needle hub for appearance of blood or any discoloration. Blood or "typical blood color" may *not* be seen if a blood vessel has been entered—only a mixture of blood and Sterile Penicillin G Benzathine suspension. The appearance of any discoloration is reason to withdraw the needle and discard the syringe. If it is elected to inject at another site, a new syringe and needle should be used. If no blood or discoloration appears, inject the contents of the syringe slowly. Discontinue delivery of the dose if the subject complains of severe immediate pain at the injection site or if in infants and young children symptoms or signs occur suggesting onset of severe pain.

Because of the high concentration of suspended material in this product, the needle may be blocked if the injection is not made at a slow, steady rate.

Parenteral drug products should be inspected visually for particulate matter and discoloration prior to administration whenever solution and container permit.

Store in a refrigerator.

CDC GUIDELINES FOR TREATMENT OF SEXUALLY TRANSMITTED DISEASES

Syphilis:[1] Early syphilis - Primary, secondary or latent syphilis of $<$ 1 year's duration: 2.4 million units IM in single dose.

Syphilis of $>$ 1 year's duration, gummas and cardiovascular syphilis - Latent, cardiovascular or late benign syphilis: 2.4 million units once weekly for 3 weeks.

Neurosyphilis: Aqueous penicillin G, 12 to 24 million units/day IV (2 to 4 million units every 4 hours) for 10 to 14 days. Many recommend benzathine penicillin G, 2.4 million units IM weekly for 3 doses following completion of this regimen; or aqueous procaine penicillin G, 2.4 million units/day IM *plus* probenecid 500 mg orally 4 times daily, both for 10 to 14 days. Many recommend benzathine penicillin G, 2.4 million units IM weekly for 3 doses following completion of this regimen.

1 CDC 1989 Sexually Transmitted Diseases Treatment Guidelines. Morbidity and Mortality Weekly Report 1989 Sept. 1;38(No. S-8):1–43.

REFERENCES:

1. SHAW, E.: Transverse myelitis from injection of penicillin. *Am. J. Dis. Child., 111:*548, 1966. **2.** KNOWLES, J.: Accidental intraarterial injection of penicillin. *Am. J. Dis. Child., 111:*552, 1966. **3.** DARBY, C. et al: Ischemia following an intragluteal injection of benzathine-procaine penicillin G mixture in a one-year-old boy. *Clin. Pediatrics, 12:*485, 1973. **4.** BROWN, L. & NELSON, A.: Postinfectious intravascular thrombosis with gangrene. *Arch. Surg., 94:*652, 1967. **5.** BORENSTINE, J.: Transverse myelitis and penicillin (Correspondence).*Am. J. Dis. Child., 112:*166, 1966. **6.** ATKINSON, J.: Transverse myelopathy secondary to penicillin injection.*J. Pediatrics, 75:*867, 1969. **7.** TALBERT, J. et al: Gangrene of the foot following intramuscular injection in the lateral thigh: A case report with recommendations for prevention. *J. Pediatrics, 70:*110, 1967. **8.** FISHER, T.: Medicolegal affairs. *Canad. Med. Assoc. J., 112:*395, 1975. **9.** SCHANZER, H. et al: Accidental intraarterial injection of penicillin G. *JAMA, 242:* 1289, 1979.

HOW SUPPLIED - EQUIVALENTS NOT AVAILABLE:

Injection, Susp - Intramuscular - 300,000 unit/ml

10 ml	$22.28	BICILLIN LA, Wyeth Labs	00008-0163-01

Injection, Susp - Intramuscular - 600,000 unit/ml

1 ml x 10	$75.66	BICILLIN LA, Wyeth Labs	00008-0021-08
2 ml disposable	$50.10	PERMAPEN ISOJECT AQUEOUS, Roerig	00049-0210-35
2 ml x 10	$131.03	BICILLIN LA, Wyeth Labs	00008-0021-07
4 ml x 10	$268.50	BICILLIN LA, Wyeth Labs	00008-0021-12

PENICILLIN G BENZATHINE; PENICILLIN G PROCAINE *(001967)*

CATEGORIES: Anti-Infectives; Antibiotics; Antimicrobials; Arthritis; Bacteremia; Chorea; Erysipelas; Glomerulonephritis; Infections; Meningitis; Otitis Media; Penicillins; Pericarditis; Peritonitis; Pinta; Pneumonia; Respiratory Tract Infections; Rheumatic Fever; Scarlet Fever; Streptococcal Infection; FDA Approval Pre 1982

BRAND NAMES: **Bicillin C-R**

DESCRIPTION:

Bicillin C-R (Penicillin G Benzathine and Penicillin G Procaine suspension), contains equal amounts of the benzathine and Procaine salts of Penicillin G. It is available for deep intramuscular injection.

Penicillin G Benzathine is prepared by the reaction of dibenzylethylene diamine with two molecules of Penicillin G. It is chemically designated as 3,3-dimethyl-7-oxo-6-(2-phenylacetamido)-4-thia-1-azabicyclo(3.2.0) heptane-2-carboxylic acid compound with *N,N'*-dibenzylethylenediamine (2:1), tetrahydrate. It occurs as a white, crystalline powder and is very slightly soluble in water and sparingly soluble in alcohol.

Penicillin G Procaine, 3,3-dimethyl-7-oxo-6-(2-phenylacetamido)-4-thia-1-azabicyclo (3.2.0) heptane-2-carboxylic acid 2-(diethylamino)ethyl p- aminobenzoate compound (1:1) monohydrate, is an equimolar salt of procaine and Penicillin G. It occurs as white crystals or a white, microcrystalline powder and is slightly soluble in water.

DESCRIPTION: *(cont'd)*

Bicillin C-R (Penicillin G Benzathine and Penicillin G Procaine suspension) contains in each ml the equivalent of 150,000 units of Penicillin G as the Benzathine salt and 150,000 units of Penicillin G as the procaine salt in a stabilized aqueous suspension with sodium citrate buffer; and as w/v, approximately 0.5% lecithin, 0.55% carboxymethylcellulose, 0.55% povidone, 0.1% methylparaben, and 0.01% propylparaben.

Bicillin C-R suspension in the multiple-dose-vial formulation is viscous and opaque. Read CONTRAINDICATIONS, WARNINGS, PRECAUTIONS and DOSAGE AND ADMINISTRATION prior to use.

CLINICAL PHARMACOLOGY:

GENERAL

Penicillin G Benzathine and Penicillin G Procaine have a low solubility and, thus, the drugs are slowly released from intramuscular injection sites. The drugs are hydrolyzed to Penicillin G. This combination of hydrolysis and slow absorption results in blood serum levels much lower but more prolonged than other parenteral penicillins.

Intramuscular administration of 600,000 units of Bicillin C-R in adults usually produces peak blood levels of 1.0 to 1.3 units per ml within 3 hours; this level falls to an average concentration of 0.32 units per ml at 12 hours, 0.19 units per ml at 24 hours, and 0.03 units per ml at seven days.

Intramuscular administration of 1,200,000 units of Bicillin C-R in adults usually produces peak blood level of 2.1 to 2.6 units per ml within 3 hours; this level falls to an average concentration of 0.75 units per ml at 12 hours, 0.28 units per ml at 24 hours, and 0.04 units per ml at seven days.

Approximately 60% of Penicillin G is bound to serum protein. The drug is distributed throughout the body tissues in widely varying amounts. Highest levels are found in the kidneys with lesser amounts in the liver, skin, and intestines. Penicillin G penetrates into all other tissues and the spinal fluid to a lesser degree. With normal kidney function, the drug is excreted rapidly by tubular excretion. In neonates and young infants and in individuals with impaired kidney function, excretion is considerably delayed.

MICROBIOLOGY

Penicillin G exerts a bactericidal action against penicillin-susceptible microorganisms during the stage of active multiplication. It acts through the inhibition of biosynthesis of cell-wall mucopeptide. It is not active against the penicillinase-producing bacteria, which include many strains of staphylococci. The following *in-vitro* data are available, but their clinical significance is unknown. Penicillin G exerts high *in-vitro* activity against staphylococci (except penicillinase-producing strains), streptococci (Groups A, C, G, H, L, and M), and pneumococci. Other organisms susceptible to Penicillin G are *Neisseria gonorrhoeae, Corynebacterium diphtheriae, Bacillus anthracis,* Clostridia species, *Actinomyces bovis, Streptobacillus moniliformis, Listeria monocytogenes,* and Leptospira species. *Treponema pallidum* is extremely susceptible to the bactericidal action of Penicillin G.

Susceptibility Test: If the Kirby-Bauer method of disc susceptibility is used, a 10-unit penicillin disc should give a zone greater than 28 mm when tested against a penicillin-sensitive bacterial strain.

INDICATIONS AND USAGE:

This drug is indicated in the treatment of moderately severe infections due to penicillin-G-susceptible microorganisms that are susceptible to serum levels common to this particular dosage form. Therapy should be guided by bacteriological studies (including susceptibility testing) and by clinical response.

Bicillin C-R is indicated in the treatment of the following in children of all ages:

Moderately severe to severe infections of the upper-respiratory tract, scarlet fever, erysipelas, and skin and soft-tissue infections due to susceptible streptococci.

Note: Streptococci in Groups A, C, G, H, L, and M are very sensitive to Penicillin G. Other groups, including Group D (enterococci), are resistant. Penicillin G sodium or potassium is recommended for streptococcal infections with bacteremia.

Moderately severe pneumonia and otitis media due to susceptible pneumococci.

Note: Severe pneumonia, empyema, bacteremia, pericarditis, meningitis, peritonitis, and arthritis of pneumococcal etiology are better treated with Penicillin G sodium or potassium during the acute stage.

When high, sustained serum levels are required, Penicillin G sodium or potassium, either IM or IV, should be used. This drug should not be used in the treatment of venereal diseases, including syphilis, gonorrhea, yaws, bejel, and pinta.

CONTRAINDICATIONS:

A previous hypersensitivity reaction to any penicillin or to procaine is a contraindication.

Do not inject into or near an artery or nerve.

WARNINGS:

The combination of Penicillin G Benzathine and Penicillin G Procaine should only be prescribed for the indications listed in this insert.

Serious and occasionally fatal hypersensitivity (anaphylactoid) reactions have been reported in patients receiving penicillin. Although anaphylaxis is more frequent following parenteral administration, it has occurred in patients on oral penicillins. These reactions are more apt to occur in individuals with a history of sensitivity to multiple allergens.

There are reports of patients with a history of penicillin hypersensitivity reactions who experienced severe hypersensitivity reactions when treated with a cephalosporin. Before therapy with a penicillin, careful inquiry should be made about previous hypersensitivity reactions to penicillins, cephalosporins, and other allergens. If an allergic reaction occurs, the drug should be discontinued and appropriate therapy should be instituted. Serious anaphylactoid reactions require immediate emergency treatment with epinephrine. Oxygen, intravenous steroids, airway management, including intubation, should also be administered as indicated.

Inadvertent intravascular administration, including inadvertent direct intraarterial injection or injection immediately adjacent to arteries, of Bicillin C-R and other penicillin preparations has resulted in severe neurovascular damage, including transverse myelitis with permanent paralysis, gangrene requiring amputation of digits and more proximal portions of extremities, and necrosis and sloughing at and surrounding the injection site. Such severe effects have been reported following injections into the buttock, thigh, and deltoid areas. Other serious complications of suspected intravascular administration which have been reported include immediate pallor, mottling, or cyanosis of the extremity both distal and proximal to the injection site, followed by bleb formation; severe edema requiring anterior and/or posterior compartment fasciotomy in the lower extremity. The above-described severe effects and complications have most often occurred in infants and small children. Prompt consultation with an appropriate specialist is indicated if any evidence of compromise of the blood supply occurs at, proximal to, or distal to the site of injection.[1-9] See CONTRAINDICATIONS, PRECAUTIONS and DOSAGE AND ADMINISTRATION.

Quadriceps femoris fibrosis and atrophy have been reported following repeated intramuscular injections of penicillin preparations into the anterolateral thigh.

WARNINGS: *(cont'd)*

Injection into or near a nerve may result in permanent, neurological damage.

PRECAUTIONS:

General: Penicillin should be used with caution in individuals with histories of significant allergies and/or asthma.

Care should be taken to avoid intravenous or intraarterial administration, or injection into or near major peripheral nerves or blood vessels, since such injections may produce neurovascular damage. See CONTRAINDICATIONS, WARNINGS and DOSAGE AND ADMINISTRATION

A small percentage of patients are sensitive to procaine. If there is a history of sensitivity, make the usual test: Inject intradermally 0.1 ml of a 1 to 2 percent procaine solution. Development of an erythema, wheal, flare, or eruption indicates procaine sensitivity. Sensitivity should be treated by the usual methods, including barbiturates, and procaine penicillin preparations should not be used. Antihistaminics appear beneficial in treatment of procaine reactions.

The use of antibiotics may result in overgrowth of nonsusceptible organisms. Constant observation of the patient is essential. If new infections due to bacteria or fungi appear during therapy, the drug should be discontinued and appropriate measures taken.

Whenever allergic reactions occur, penicillin should be withdrawn unless, in the opinion of the physician, the condition being treated is life-threatening and amenable only to penicillin therapy.

In prolonged therapy with penicillin, and particularly with high-dosage schedules, periodic evaluation of the renal and hematopoietic systems is recommended.

Laboratory Tests: In streptococcal infections, therapy must be sufficient to eliminate the organism; otherwise, the sequelae of streptococcal disease may occur. Cultures should be taken following completion of treatment to determine whether streptococci have been eradicated.

Pregnancy Category B: Reproduction studies performed in the mouse, rat, and rabbit have revealed no evidence of impaired fertility or harm to the fetus due to Penicillin G. Human experience with the penicillins during pregnancy has not shown any positive evidence of adverse effects on the fetus. There are, however, no adequate and well-controlled studies in pregnant women showing conclusively that harmful effects of these drugs on the fetus can be excluded. Because animal reproduction studies are not always predictive of human response, this drug should be used during pregnancy only if clearly needed.

Nursing Mothers: Soluble Penicillin G is excreted in breast milk. Caution should be exercised when Penicillin G Benzathine and Penicillin G Procaine are administered to a nursing woman.

Carcinogenesis, Mutagenesis, Impairment Of Fertility: No long-term animal studies have been conducted with these drugs.

Pediatric Use: See INDICATIONS AND USAGE and DOSAGE AND ADMINISTRATION.

DRUG INTERACTIONS:

Tetracycline, a bacteriostatic antibiotic, may antagonize the bactericidal effect of penicillin, and concurrent use of these drugs should be avoided.

Concurrent administration of penicillin and probenecid increases and prolongs serum penicillin levels by decreasing the apparent volume of distribution and slowing the rate of excretion by competitively inhibiting renal tubular secretion of penicillin.

ADVERSE REACTIONS:

As with other penicillins, untoward reactions of the sensitivity phenomena are likely to occur, particularly in individuals who have previously demonstrated hypersensitivity to penicillins or in those with a history of allergy, asthma, hay fever, or urticaria.

The following have been reported with parenteral Penicillin G:

General: Hypersensitivity reactions including the following: skin eruptions (maculopapular to exfoliative dermatitis), urticaria, laryngeal edema, fever, eosinophilia; other serum-sicknesslike reactions (including chills, fever, edema, arthralgia, and prostration); anaphylaxis. Note: Urticaria, other skin rashes, and serum-sicknesslike reactions may be controlled with antihistamines and, if necessary, systemic corticosteroids. Whenever such reactions occur, Penicillin G should be discontinued unless, in the opinion of the physician, the condition being treated is life-threatening and amenable only to therapy with Penicillin G. Serious anaphylactic reactions require the immediate use of epinephrine, oxygen, and intravenous steroids.

Hematologic: Hemolytic anemia, leukopenia, thrombocytopenia.

Neurologic: Neuropathy.

Urogenital: Nephropathy.

OVERDOSAGE:

Penicillin in overdosage has the potential to cause neuromuscular hyperirritability or convulsive seizures.

DOSAGE AND ADMINISTRATION:

Shake multiple-dose vial vigorously before withdrawing the desired dose.

Administer by DEEP INTRAMUSCULAR INJECTION in the upper, outer quadrant of the buttock. In infants and small children, the midlateral aspect of the thigh may be preferable. When doses are repeated, vary the injection site.

After selection of the proper site and insertion of the needle into the selected muscle, aspirate by pulling back on the plunger. While maintaining negative pressure for 2 to 3 seconds, carefully observe the neck of the syringe immediately proximal to the needle hub for appearance of blood or any discoloration. Blood or "typical blood color" may *not* be seen if a blood vessel has been entered—only a mixture of blood and Bicillin C-R. The appearance of any discoloration is reason to withdraw the needle and discard the syringe. If it is elected to inject at another site, a new syringe and needle should be used. If no blood or discoloration appears, inject the contents of the syringe slowly. Discontinue delivery of the dose if the subject complains of severe immediate pain at the injection site or if in infants and young children symptoms or signs occur suggesting onset of severe pain.

Because of the high concentration of suspended material in this product, the needle may be blocked if the injection is not made at a slow, steady rate.

STREPTOCOCCAL INFECTIONS GROUP A

Infections of the upper-respiratory tract, skin and soft-tissue infections, scarlet fever, and erysipelas.

The following doses are recommended:

Adults and children over 60 lbs. in weight: 2,400,000 units.

Children from 30 to 60 lbs.: 900,000 units to 1,200,000 units.

Infants and children under 30 lbs.: 600,000 units.

DOSAGE AND ADMINISTRATION: *(cont'd)*

Note: Treatment with the recommended dosage is usually given at a single session using multiple IM sites when indicated. An alternative dosage schedule may be used, giving one-half (1/2) the total dose on day 1 and one-half (1/2) on day 3. This will also insure the penicillinemia required over a 10-day period; however, this alternate schedule should be used only when the physician can be assured of the patient's cooperation.

PNEUMOCOCCAL INFECTIONS (EXCEPT PNEUMOCOCCAL MENINGITIS)

600,000 units in children and 1,200,000 units in adults, repeated every 2 or 3 days until the temperature is normal for 48 hours. Other forms of penicillin may be necessary for severe cases.

Parenteral drug products should be inspected visually for particulate matter and discoloration prior to administration whenever solution and container permit.

Store in a refrigerator.

REFERENCES:

1. SHAW, E.: Transverse myelitis from injection of penicillin. *Am. J. Dis. Child., 111*:548, 1966. **2.** KNOWLES, J.: Accidental intraarterial injection of penicillin. *Am. J. Dis. Child., 111*:552, 1966. **3.** DARBY, C. et al: Ischemia following an intragluteal injection of benzathine-procaine penicillin G mixture in a one-year-old boy. *Clin. Pediatrics, 12*:485, 1973. **4.** BROWN, L. & NELSON, A.: Postinfectious intravascular thrombosis with gangrene. *Arch. Surg., 94*:652, 1967. **5.** BORENSTINE, J.: Transverse myelitis and penicillin (Correspondence).*Am. J. Dis. Child., 112*:166, 1966. **6.** ATKINSON, J.: Transverse myelopathy secondary to penicillin injection.*J. Pediatrics, 75*:867, 1969. **7.** TALBERT, J. et al: Gangrene of the foot following intramuscular injection in the lateral thigh: A case report with recommendations for prevention. *J. Pediatrics, 70*:110, 1967. **8.** FISHER, T.: Medicolegal affairs. *Canad. Med. Assoc. J., 112*:395, 1975. **9.** SCHANZER, H. et al: Accidental intraarterial injection of penicillin G. *JAMA, 242*:1289, 1979.

HOW SUPPLIED - EQUIVALENTS NOT AVAILABLE:

Injection, Susp - Intramuscular - 150000 unit/150

10 ml	$15.06	BICILLIN CR, Wyeth Labs	00008-0176-01

Injection, Susp - Intramuscular - 300000 unit/300

1 ml x 10	**$53.21**	**BICILLIN C-R, Wyeth Labs**	**00008-0026-17**
2 ml x 10	**$104.48**	**BICILLIN C-R, Wyeth Labs**	**00008-0026-16**
4 ml x 10	**$223.74**	**BICILLIN C-R, Wyeth Labs**	**00008-0026-22**

Injection, Susp - Intramuscular - 900000 unit/300

2 ml x 10	$108.71	BICILLIN CR 900/300, Wyeth Labs	00008-0079-01

PENICILLIN G POTASSIUM *(001968)*

CATEGORIES: Anti-Infectives; Antibacterials; Antibiotics; Antimicrobials; Arthritis; Chorea; Dental; Endocarditis; Enterococci Infections; Erysipelas; Gingivitis; Infections; Meningitis; Otitis Media; Penicillins; Pharyngitis; Pneumococcal Infections; Respiratory Tract Infections; Rheumatic Fever; Scarlet Fever; Septicemia; Skin Infections; Streptococcal Infection; Vincent's Infection; Pregnancy Category B; FDA Approval Pre 1982

BRAND NAMES: Aoracillin B; *Cristapen*; *K-Cillin*; *Megacillin* (Canada); *Novopen-G* (Canada); Orpeneed; Pen-G; **Pentids**; Pfizerpen; Truxcillin
(International brand names outside U.S. in italics)

FORMULARIES: Aetna; Medi-Cal

DESCRIPTION:

TABLETS

Active: Penicillin G Potassium USP

Inactive: Calcium Carbonate USP, Povidone USP, Magnesium Stearate NF, Sodium Starch Glycolate NF, Sodium Lauryl Sulfate NF, and other trace inactive ingredients (NO sulfiting agents).

Penicillin G Potassium is provided is oral dosage form as white compressed tablets buffered with calcium carbonate.

INJECTION

Buffered penicillin G potassium for Injection is a sterile, pyrogen-free powder for reconstitution. Buffered penicillin G potassium for injection is an antibacterial agent for IM, continuous drip, intrapleural or other local infusion, and intrathecal administration.

Each million units contains approximately 6.8 milligrams of sodium (0.3 mEq) and 65.6 mg of potassium (1.68 mEq).

Chemically, this drug is monopotassium 3,3-dimethyl-7-oxo-6-(2-phenylacetamido)-4-thia-l'azabicyclo (3.2.0) heptane-2-carboxylate. It has a molecular weight of 372.48.

Penicillin G potassium is a colorless or white crystal, or a white crystalline powder which is odorless, or practically so, and moderately hygroscopic. Penicillin G potassium is very soluble in water. The pH of the reconstituted product is between 6.0-8.5.

CLINICAL PHARMACOLOGY:

Penicillin G exerts a bactericidal action against penicillin-sensitive micro-organisms during the stage of active multiplication. It acts through the inhibition of biosynthesis of cell wall mucopeptide. It is not active against the penicillinase producing bacteria, which include many strains of staphylococci. Penicillin G exerts high *in vitro* activity against the nonpenicillinase producing bacteria, which include many strains of staphylococci. Penicillin G exerts high *in vitro* activity against staphylococci (except penicillinase-producing strains), streptococci (groups A, C, G, H, L, and M) and pneumococci. Other organisms, sensitive to penicillin G are *Neisseria gonorrhoeae*, *Corynebacterium diphtheriae*, *Bacillus anthracis*, Clostridia,*Actinomycesbovis*, *Streptobacillus moniliformis*, *Listeria monocytogenes*, and Leptospira. *Treponema palladium*is extremely sensitive to the bactericidal action of penicillin G. Some species of gram negative bacilli are sensitive to moderate to high concentrations of the drug obtained with intravenous administration. These include most strains of *Escherichia coli*, all strains of *Proteus mirabilis*, Salmonella and Shigella and some strains of *Aerobacter aerogenes* and *Alcaligenes faecalis*.

TABLETS

Oral preparations of penicillin G are only slightly affected by normal gastric acidity (pH of 2-3.5); however a pH below 2.0 may partially or totally inactivate penicillin G. Oral penicillin G is absorbed in the upper small intestine, chiefly the duodenum; however, based on serum level and urinary excretion data only approximately 30% of the dose is absorbed. For this reason 4-5 times the dose of oral penicillin G must be given to obtain a blood level comparable to that obtained with parenteral penicillin G. Since gastric acidity, stomach emptying time and other factors affecting may vary considerably, serum levels may be appreciably reduced to non-therapeutic levels in certain individuals.

Approximately 60% of penicillin G is bound to serum protein. The drug is distributed throughout the body tissues in widely varying amounts. Highest levels are found in the kidneys with lesser amounts in the liver, skin and intestines. Penicillin G penetrates into all other tissues to a lesser degree with very limited amounts found in the cerebrospinal fluid. With normal kidney function the drug is excreted rapidly by tubular excretion. In neonates

CLINICAL PHARMACOLOGY: *(cont'd)*

and young infants and in individuals with impaired kidney function, excretion is considerably delayed. Approximately 20% of a dose of oral penicillin G is excreted in the urine under normal circumstances.

INJECTION

Aqueous penicillin G is rapidly absorbed following both intramuscular and subcutaneous injection. Initial blood levels following parenteral administration are high but not transient. Penicillins bind to serum proteins, mainly albumin. Therapeutic levels of the penicillins are easily achieved under normal circumstances in extracellular fluid and most other body tissues. Penicillins are distributed in varying degrees into pleural, pericardial, peritoneal, ascitic, synovial, and interstitial fluids. Penicillins are excreted in breast milk. Penetration into the cerebrospinal fluid, eyes, and prostate is poor. Penicillins are rapidly excreted in the urine by glomerular filtration and active tubular secretion, primarily as unchanged drug. Approximately 60 percent of the total dose of 300,000 units is excreted in the urine within this 5 hour period. For this reason high and frequent doses are required to maintain the elevated serum levels desirable in treating certain severe infections in individuals with normal kidney function. In neonates and young infants, and in individuals with impaired kidney function, excretion is considerably delayed.

Penicillin acts synergistically with gentamicin or tobramycin against many strains of enterococci.

Susceptibility Testing: Penicillin G Susceptibility Powder or 10 units penicillin G Susceptibility Discs may be used to determine microbial susceptibility to penicillin G using one of the following standard methods recommended by the National Committee for Laboratory Standards:

M2-M3, "Performance Standards for Antimicrobial Disk Susceptibility Tests"

M7-A, "Methods for Dilution Antimicrobial Susceptibility Tests for Bacteria that Grow Aerobically"

M11-A, "Reference Agar Dilution Procedure for Antimicrobial Susceptibility Testing of Anaerobic Bacteria"

M17-P, "Alternative Methods for Antimicrobial Susceptibility Testing of Anaerobic Bacteria"

Tests should be interpreted by the following criteria (TABLES 1 & 2):

TABLE 1 Zone Diameter, Nearest Whole mm

	Susceptible	Moderately Susceptible	Resistant
Staphylococci	≥29	-	≤28
N. gonorrhoeae	≥20	-	≤19
Enterococci	-	≥15	≤14
Non-enterococcal streptococci and *L. monocytogenes*	≥28	20-27	≤19

TABLE 2 Approximate MIC Correlates

	Susceptible	Resistant
Staphylococci	≤0.1 mcg/ml	β-lactamase
N. gonorrhoeae	≤0.1 mcg/ml	β-lactamase
Enterococci	-	≥16 mcg/ml
Non-enterococcal streptococci and *L. monocytogenes*	≤0.12 mcg/ml	≥ 4 mcg/ml

Interpretations of susceptible, intermediate, and resistant correlate zone size diameters with MIC values. A laboratory report of "susceptible" indicates that the suspected causative microorganism most likely will respond to therapy with penicillin G. A laboratory test of "resistant" indicates that the infecting microorganism most likely will not respond to therapy. A laboratory report of "moderately susceptible" indicates that the microorganism is most likely susceptible if a high dose of penicillin G is used, or if the infection is such that high levels of penicillin G may be attained, as in urine. A report of "intermediate" using the disk diffusion method may be considered an equivocal result, and dilution tests may be indicated.

Control organisms are recommended for susceptibility testing. Each time the test is performed the following organisms should be included. The range for zones of inhibition is shown below:

Control Organism: (ATCC 25923)

Zone of Inhibition Range: 27-35

INDICATIONS AND USAGE:

TABLETS

Oral penicillin G is indicated in the treatment of mild to moderately severe infections due to penicillin G sensitive micro-organisms that are sensitive to the low serum levels common to this particular dosage form. Therapy should be guided by bacteriological studies (including sensitivity tests) and by clinical response.

NOTE: Severe pneumonia, empyema, bacteremia, pericarditis, meningitis, and arthritis should not be treated with oral penicillin during the acute stage.

Indicated surgical procedures should be performed.

The following infections will usually respond to adequate dosage of oral penicillin G.

1. Streptococcal Infections: (Group A) (without bacteremia). Mild to moderate infections of the upper respiratory tract, skin and soft tissue infections, scarlet fever, and mild very erysipelas.

NOTE: Streptococci in groups A, C, H, G, L and M are very sensitive to penicillin G. Other groups, including group D (enterococcus) are resistant.

2. Pneumococcal Infections: Mild to moderately severe infections of the respiratory tract.

3. Staphylococcal Infections: Penicillin G sensitive. Mild infections of the skin and soft tissues.

NOTE: Reports indicate an increasing number of strains of staphylococci resistant to penicillin G, emphasizing the need for culture and sensitivity studies in treating suspected staphylococcal infections.

4. Fusospirochetosis: (Vincent's gingivitis and pharyngitis) - Mild to moderately severe infection of the oropharynx usually respond with oral penicillin G.

NOTE: Necessary dental care should be accomplished in infections involving the gum tissue.

5. Medical Conditions in Which Oral Penicillin G Therapy is Indicated as Prophylaxis:

(a) **For the prevention of recurrence following rheumatic fever and/or chorea.** Prophylaxis with oral penicillin G on a continuing basis has proven effective in preventing recurrence of these conditions.

(b) Prevention of bacteremia following tooth extraction.

NOTE: Oral penicillin G should not be used as adjunctive prophylaxis for genito-urinary instrumentation or surgery, lower intestinal tract surgery, sigmoidoscopy and childbirth.

INDICATIONS AND USAGE: *(cont'd)*

(c) "Oral penicillin G is not recommended for short-term prevention of bacterial endocarditis in patients with valvular heart disease undergoing dental or surgical procedures."

INJECTION

Aqueous penicillin G (parenteral) is indicated in the therapy of severe infections caused by penicillin G susceptible microorganisms when rapid and high penicillin levels are required in the conditions listed below. Therapy should be guided by bacteriological studies (including susceptibility tests) and by clinical response.

The following infections will usually respond to adequate dosage of aqueous penicillin G (parenteral):

NOTE: Streptococci in groups A, C, H, G, L, and M are very sensitive to penicillin G. Some group D organisms are sensitive to the high serum levels obtained with aqueous penicillin G.

Aqueous penicillin G (parenteral) is the penicillin dosage form of choice for bacteremia, empyema, severe pneumonia, pericarditis, endocarditis, meningitis, and other severe infections caused by sensitive trains of the gram-positive species listed above.

Pneumococcal Infections: *Staphylococcal infections* penicillin G sensitive.

Other Infections: Anthrax, Actinomycosis, Clostridial infections (including tetanus), Diphtheria (to prevent carrier state), Erysipeloid *(Erysipelothrix insidiosa)* endocarditis,

Fusospirochetal Infections: Severe infections of the oropharynx (Vincent's), lower respiratory tract and genital area due to *Fusobacterium fusiformisans* spirochetes.

Gram-Negative Bacillary Infections (Bacteremias): *(E. coli, A. aerogenes, A. faecalis,* Salmonella, Shigella and *P. mirabilis),* Listeria infections *(Listeria monocytogenes),* Meningitis and endocarditis, Pasteurella infections *(Pasteurella multocida),* Bacteremia and meningitis, Ratbite fever *(Spirillum minus* or *Streptobacillus moniliformis),* Gonorrheal endocarditis and arthritis *(N. gonorrhoeae),* Syphilis *(t. pallidum)* including congenital syphilis, Meningococcic meningitis.

Although no controlled clinical efficacy studies have been conducted, aqueous crystalline penicillin G for injection and penicillin G procaine suspension have been suggested by the American Heart Association and the American Dental Association for use as part of a combined parenteral-oral regimen for prophylaxis against bacterial endocarditis in patients with congenital heart disease or rheumatic, or other acquired valvular heart disease when they undergo dental procedures and surgical procedures of the upper respiratory tract.[1] Since it may happen that *alpha* hemolytic streptococci relatively resistant to penicillin may be found when patients are receiving continuous oral penicillin for secondary prevention of rheumatic fever, prophylactic agents other than penicillin may be chosen for these patients and prescribed in addition to their continuous rheumatic fever prophylactic regimen.

NOTE: When selecting antibiotics for the prevention of bacterial endocarditis the physician or dentist should read the full joint statement of the American Heart Association and the American Dental Association.[1]

CONTRAINDICATIONS:

A previous hypersensitivity reaction to any penicillin is a contraindication.

WARNINGS:

Serious and occasionally fatal hypersensitivity (anaphylactoid) reactions have been reported in patients on penicillin therapy. Although anaphylaxis is more frequent following parenteral therapy, it has occurred in patients on oral penicillins. These reactions are more apt to occur in individuals with history of sensitivity to multiple allergens.

There have been well documented reports of individuals with a history of penicillin hypersensitivity reactions who have experienced severe hypersensitivity reactions when treated with a cephalosporin. Before therapy with a penicillin, careful inquiry should be made concerning previous hypersensitivity reactions to penicillin, cephalosporins, and other allergens.

TABLETS

If an allergic reaction occurs, the drug should be discontinued and the patient treated with the usual agents e.g., pressor amines, antihistamines and corticosteroids.

INJECTION

If an allergic reaction occurs, the drug should be discontinued and the appropriate therapy instituted. Serious anaphylactoid reactions require immediate emergency treatment with epinephrine. Oxygen, intravenous steroids, and airway management including intubation, should also be administered as indicated.

PRECAUTIONS:

Penicillin should be used with caution in individuals with histories of significant allergies and/or asthma.

The oral route of administration should not be relied upon in patients with severe illness, or with nausea, vomiting gastric dilatation, cardiospasm or intestinal hypermotility.

Occasional patients will not absorb therapeutic amounts of orally administered penicillin.

In streptococcal infections, therapy must be sufficient to eliminate that organism (10 days minimum); otherwise the sequelae or streptococcal disease may occur. Culture should be taken following completion of treatment to determine whether streptococci have been eradicated.

TABLETS

Prolonged use of antibiotics may promote the overgrowth of nonsusceptible organisms, including fungi. Should superinfection occur, appropriate measures should be taken.

INJECTION

Intramuscular Therapy: Care should be taken to avoid intravenous or accidental intraarterial administration, or injection into or near major peripheral nerves or blood vessels, since such injections may produce neurovascular damage. Particular care should be taken with IV administration because of the possibility of thrombophlebitis.

The use of antibiotics may result in overgrowth of nonsusceptible organisms. Constant observation of the patient is essential. If new infections due to bacteria or fungi appear during therapy, the drug should be discontinued and appropriate measures taken. Whenever allergic reactions occur, penicillin should be withdrawn unless, in the opinion of the physician, the condition being treated is life threatening and amenable only to penicillin therapy.

Aqueous penicillin G by the intravenous route in high doses (above 10 million units), should be administered slowly because of the adverse effects of electrolyte imbalance from either the potassium or sodium content of the penicillin. Potassium penicillin G contains 1.7 mEg potassium and 0.3 mEq sodium per million units. The patient's renal, cardiac, and vascular status should be evaluated and if impairment of function is suspected or known to exist a reduction in the total dosage should be evaluated and if impairment of function is suspected or known to exist a reduction in the total dosage should be considered. Frequent evaluation of electrolyte balance, renal and hematopoietic function is recommended during therapy when high doses of intravenous aqueous penicillin G are used.

Laboratory Tests: In prolonged therapy with penicillin, periodic evaluation of the renal, hepatic, and hematopoietic systems is recommended foe organ system dysfunction. This is particularly important in prematures, neonates and other infants, and when high doses are used.

PRECAUTIONS: *(cont'd)*

Positive Coomb's tests have been reported after large intravenous doses.

Monitor serum potassium and implement corrective measures when necessary.

When treating gonococcal infections in which primary and secondary syphilis are suspected, proper diagnostic procedures, including dark field examinations, should be done before receiving penicillin and monthly serological tests made for at least four months. All cases of penicillin treated syphilis should receive clinical and serological examinations every six months for two to three years.

In suspected staphylococcal infections, proper laboratory studies, including susceptibility tests, should be performed.

In streptococcal infections, cultures should be taken following completion of treatment to determine whether streptococci have been eradicated. Therapy must be sufficient to eliminate the organism (a minimum of 10 days); otherwise the sequelae of streptococcal disease (*e.g.*, endocarditis, rheumatic fever) may occur.

Carcinogenesis, Mutagenesis, and Impairment of Fertility: No information on long-term studies are available on the carcinogenesis, mutagenesis, ot the impairment of fertility with the use of penicillins.

Pregnancy, Teratogenic Effects, Pregnancy Category B: Reproduction studies performed in the mouse, rat, and rabbit have revealed no evidence of impaired fertility or harm to the fetus due to penicillin G. Human experience with the penicillins during pregnancy has not shown any positive evidence of adverse effects on the fetus. There are, however, no adequate and well controlled studies in pregnant women showing conclusively that harmful effects of these drugs on the fetus can be excluded. Because animal reproduction studies are not always predictive of human response, this drug should be used during pregnancy only if clearly needed.

Nursing Mothers: Penicillins are excreted in human milk. Caution should be exercised wen penicillin G is administered to a nursing woman.

Pediatric Use: Penicillins are excreted largely unchanged by the kidney. Because of incompletely developed renal function in infants, the rate of elimination will be slow. Use caution in administering to newborns and evaluate organ system function frequently.

DRUG INTERACTIONS:

Concurrent administration of bacteriostatic antibiotics (*e.g.*, erythromycin, tetracycline) may diminish the bactericidal effects of penicillins by slowing the rate of bacterial growth. Bactericidal agents work most effective against the immature cell wall of rapidly proliferating microorganisms. This has been demonstrated *in vitro*; however, the clinical significance of this interaction is not well documented. There are few clinical situations in which the concurrent use of "static" and "cidal" antibiotics are indicated. However, in selected circumstances in which such therapy is appropriate, using adequate doses of antibacterial agents and beginning penicillin therapy first, should minimize the potential for interaction.

Penicillin blood levels may be prolonged by concurrent administration of probenecid which blocks the renal tubular secretion of penicillins.

Displacement of penicillin from plasma protein binding sites will elevate the level of free penicillin in the serum.

ADVERSE REACTIONS:

TABLETS

Although the incidence of reactions to oral penicillin has been reported with much less frequency than following parenteral therapy, it should be remembered that all degrees of hypersensitivity including fatal anaphylaxis, have been reported with oral penicillin.

The most common reactions to oral penicillin are nausea, vomiting, epigastric distress, diarrhea, and black hairy tongue. The hypersensitivity reactions reported are skin eruptions (maculo-papular to exfoliative dermatitis), urticaria and other serum sickness reactions, laryngeal edema and anaphylaxis. Fever and eosinophilia may frequently be the only reaction observed. Hemolytic anemia, leukopenia, thrombocytopenia, neuropathy, and nephropathy are infrequent reactions and usually associated with high doses of parenteral penicillin.

INJECTION

Penicillin is a substance of low toxicity but does have a significant index of sensitization. The following hypersensitivity reactions have been reported: skin rashes ranging from maculopapular eruptions to exfoliative dermatitis; urticaria; and reactions resembling serum sickness, including chills, fever, edema, arthralgia and prostration. Severe and occasionally fatal anaphylaxis has occurred (see WARNINGS).

Hemolytic anemia, leucopenia, thrombocytopenia, nephropathy, and neuropathy are rarely observed adverse reactions and are usually associated with high intravenous dosage. Patients given continuous intravenous therapy with penicillin G potassium in high dosage (10 million to 100 million units daily) may suffer severe or even fatal potassium poisoning, particularly if renal insufficiency is present. Hyperreflexia, convulsions, and coma may be indicative of this syndrome.

Cardiac arrhythmias and cardiac arrest may also occur. (High dosage of penicillin G sodium may result in congestive heart failure due to high sodium intake.)

The Jarisch-Herxheimer reaction has been reported in patients treated for syphilis.

OVERDOSAGE:

INJECTION

Neurological adverse reactions, including convulsions, may occur with the attainment of high CSF levels of beta-lactams. In case of overdosage, discontinue medication, treat symptomatically, and institute supportive measures as required.

Penicillin G potassium is hemodialzyable.

DOSAGE AND ADMINISTRATION:

TABLETS

The dosage of penicillin G (oral) should be determined according to the sensitivity of the causative micro-organism and the severity of infection, and adjusted to the clinical response of the patient.

Oral penicillin G should be given at least 1 hour before or 2 hours after meals. The usual dosage recommendation for adults and children 12 years and over is as follows:

Streptococcal Infections: Mild to moderately severe-of the upper respiratory tract and including scarlet fever and mild erysipelas.

200,000-250,000 units q. 6-8 hours for 10 days for mild infections.

400,000-5000,000 units q. 8 hours for 10 days for moderately severe infections.

800,000 units may be given q. 12 hours.

Pneumococcal Infections: Mild to moderately severe-of the respiratory tract, including otitis media.

400,000-5000,000 units q. 6 hours until the patient has been afebrile for at least 2 days.

Staphylococcal Infections: Mild infections of skin and soft tissue (culture and sensitivity tests should be performed).

DOSAGE AND ADMINISTRATION: *(cont'd)*

200,000-5000,000 units q. 6-8 hours until infection is cured.

Fusospirochetosis (Vincent's Infection): of the oropharynx: Mild to moderately severe infections.

400,000-500,000 units q. 6-8 hours.

For the prevention of recurrence following rheumatic fever and/or chorea:

200,000-250,000 units twice daily on a continuing basis.

NOTE: Therapy for children 12 years of age is calculated on the basis of body weight. For infants and small children the suggested dose is 25,000 to 90,000 units per kg per day in 3 to 6 divided doses.

Storage: Store at 15-30°C (59-86°F).

Dispense in a tight, child-resistant container.

INJECTION

Severe Infections due to Susceptible Strains of Streptococci, Pneumococci and Staphylococci: bacteremia, pneumonia, endocarditis, pericarditis, empyema, meningitis, and other severe infections-a minimum of 5 million units daily.

Syphilis: Aqueous Penicillin G may be used in the treatment of acquired and congenital syphilis, but because of necessity of frequent dosage, hospitalization is recommended. Dosage and duration of therapy will be determined by age of patient and stage of the disease.

Gonorrheal Endocarditis: a minimum of 5 million units daily.

Meningococcic Meningitis: 1-2 million units by the IM route every 2 hours, or continuous IV drip of 20-30 million units daily.

Actinomycosis: 1-6 million units/day for cervicofacial cases; 10- 20 million units daily for thoracic and abdominal disease.

Clostridial Infections: 20 million units/day; penicillin is adjunctive therapy to antitoxin

Fusospirochetal Infections: severe infections of oropharynx, lower respiratory tract, and genital area—5-10 million units/day.

Rat-bite Fever (Spirillum Minus or Streptobacillus Moniliformis): 12-15 million units/day for 3-4 weeks.

LISTERIA INFECTIONS (LISTERIA MONOCYTOGENES)

Neonates: 500,000 to 1 million units/day

Adults with Meningitis: 15-20 million units/day for 2 weeks

Adults with Endocarditis: 15-20 million units/day for 4 weeks.

PASTEURELLA INFECTIONS (PASTEURELLA MULTOCIDA)

Bacteremia and meningitis—4-6 million units/day for 2 weeks.

ERYSIPELOID (ERYSIPELOTHRIX INSIDIOSA)

Endocarditis: 20-20 million units/day for 4-6 weeks.

Gram-Negative Bacillary Infections (E. Coli, Enterobacter Aerogens, A Faecalis: Salmonella, Shigella and *Proteus mirabilis).*

Bacteremia: 20-80 units day.

Diphtheria: (carrier state); 300,000-400,000 units of penicillin/day in divided doses for 10-12 days.

Anthrax: A minimum of 5 million units of penicillin/day in divided doses until cure is effected.

For prophylaxis against bacterial endocarditis (American Heart Association, 1977. Prevention of bacterial endocarditis. Circulation.**56** :139A-143A) in patients with congenital heart disease or rheumatic or other acquired valvular heart disease, when undergoing dental procedures or surgical procedures of the upper respiratory tract, use a combined parenteral-oral regimen. One million units of aqueous crystalline-penicillin G (30,000 units/kg in children) intramuscularly, mixed with 600,000 units of procaine penicillin G (600,000 units for children) should be given one-half to one hour before the procedure. Oral penicillin V (phenoxymethyl penicillin), 500 mg for adults or 250 mg for children less than 60 lb, should be given every 6 hours for 8 doses. Doses for children should not exceed recommendations for adults for a single dose or for a 24 hour period.

RECONSTITUTION

The following table, (TABLE 3), shows the amount of solvent required for solutions of various concentrations:

TABLE 3

Approx. Desired Concentrations (units/ml)	Approx. Volume (ml) 1,000,000 units	Solvent Vial of 5,000,000	Infusion Only 20,000,000 units
50,000	20.0	—	—
100,000	10.0	—	—
250,000	4.0	18.2	75.0
500,000	1.8	8.2	33.0
750,000	—	4.8	—
1,000,000	—	3.2	11.5

When the required volume of solvent is greater than the capacity of the vial, the penicillin can be dissolved by first injecting only a potion of the solvent into the vial, then withdrawing the resultant solution and combining it with thr remainder of the solvent in a larger sterile container.

Buffered penicillin G potassium for Injection is highly water soluble. It may be dissolved in small amounts of Water for Injection, or Sterile Isotonic Sodium Chloride Solution for parenteral use. All solutions should be stored in a refrigerator. When refrigerated, penicillin solutions may be stored for seven days without significant loss of potency.

Penicillin G potassium for Injection may be given intramuscularly or by continuous drip for dosages of 500,000, 1,000,000, or 5,000,000 units. It is also suitable for intrapleural, intraarticulare, and other local instillations.

THE 20,000,000 UNIT DOSAGE MAY BE ADMINISTERED BY INTRAVENOUS INFUSION ONLY.

(1) Intramuscular Injection: Keep total volume of injection small. The IM route is the preferred route of administration. Solutions containing up to 100,000 units of penicillin per ml of diluent may be used with a minimum of discomfort. Greater concentrations of penicillin G per ml is physically possible and may be employed where therapy demands. When larger doses are required, it may be advisable to administer aqueous solutions of penicillin by means of continuous IV drip.

(2) Continuous Intravenous Drip: Determine the volume of fluid and rate of its administration required by the patient in a 24 hour period in the usual manner of fluid therapy, and add the appropriate daily dosage of penicillin to this fluid. For example, if an adult patient requires 2 liters of fluid in 24 hours and a daily dosage of 10 million units of penicillin, add 5 million units to 1 liter and adjust the rate of flow so the liter will be infused in 12 hours.

(3) Intrapleural or Other Local Infusions: If fluid is aspirated, give infusion in a volume equal to 1/4 or 1/2 the amount of fluid aspirated, otherwise, prepare as for intramuscular injection.

DOSAGE AND ADMINISTRATION: *(cont'd)*

(4) Intrathecal Use: The intrathecal use of penicillin in meningitis must be highly individualized. It should be employed only with full consideration of the possible irritating effects of penicillin when used by this route. The preferred route of therapy in bacterial meningitides is intravenous, supplemented by intravenous injection.

Parenteral drug products should be inspected visually for particulate matter and discoloration prior to administration, whenever solution and container permit.

Sterile solution may be left in the refrigerator for one week without significant loss of potency.

CDC GUIDELINES FOR TREATMENT OF SEXUALLY TRANSMITTED DISEASES

Syphilis:[1] *Neurosyphilis:* 12 to 24 million units/day IV (2 to 4 million units every 4 hours) for 10 to 14 days. Many recommend benzathine penicillin G 2.4 million units IM weekly for 3 weeks following the completion of this regimen.

Congenital Syphilis: *Symptomatic or Asymptomatic Infants: Newborns:* 50,000 units/kgday IV every 8 to 12 hours for 10 to 14 days. If >1 day of therapy is missed, restart the entire course. *Infants (after newborn period):* 50,000 units/kg every 4 to 6 hours for 10 to 14 days.

Gonococcal Infections:[1] *Infants With Disseminated Gonococcal Infection Or Gonococcal Ophthalmia (Hospitalization Recommended):* If the gonococcal isolate is proven to be susceptible to penicillin: 100,000 units/kg/day in 2 equal doses (4 equal doses per day for infants >1 week old). Increase the dose to 150,000 units/kg/day for meningitis.

[1] CDC 1989 Sexually Transmitted Diseases Treatment Guidelines. *Morbidity and Mortality Weekly Report* 1989 Sept. 1;38 (No. S-8):1–43.

HOW SUPPLIED - RATED THERAPEUTICALLY EQUIVALENT:

Injection, Solution - Intravenous - 1,000,000 unit/

10 ml x 10	$13.25	Penicillin G Potassium, Bristol Myers Squibb	00003-0634-41
20 ml x 10	$14.56	Penicillin G Potassium, Vial, Marsam	00209-8570-22
100's	$192.34	Penicillin G Potassium, Lilly	00002-1406-02

Injection, Solution - Intravenous - 5,000,000 unit/

5mmu x 10	$29.00	PFIZERPEN, Roerig	00049-0520-83
30 ml x 10	$27.38	Penicillin G Potassium, Bristol Myers Squibb	00003-0673-71
50 ml x 10	$40.00	Penicillin G Potassium, Vial, Marsam	00209-8574-22

Injection, Solution - Intravenous - 10,000,000 unit

10 vial	$66.63	Penicillin G Potassium, Bristol Myers Squibb	00003-0734-11
50 ml x 10	$70.00	Penicillin G Potassium, Vial, Marsam	00209-8578-22

Injection, Solution - Intravenous - 20,000,000 unit

1 ml x 10	$75.75	Penicillin G Potassium, Bristol Myers Squibb	00003-0735-31
20mmu x 1	$8.49	PFIZERPEN, Roerig	00049-0530-28
20mmu x 10	$86.87	PFIZERPEN, Roerig	00049-0530-83
100 ml x 10	$110.85	Penicillin G Potassium, Vial, Marsam	00209-8580-22

Powder, Reconstitution - Oral - 400,000 unit/5m

100 ml	**$2.46**	**PENTIDS 400, Bristol Myers Squibb**	**00003-0743-39**
200 ml	**$4.17**	**PENTIDS 400, Bristol Myers Squibb**	**00003-0743-54**

Tablet, Uncoated - Oral - 200,000 unit

100's	**$7.70**	**PENTIDS, Bristol Myers Squibb**	**00003-0164-50**

Tablet, Uncoated - Oral - 250,000 unit

100's	$6.95	Potassium Penicillin G Buffered, United Res	00677-0097-01
100's	$8.27	Potassium Penicillin G, Geneva Pharms	00781-1615-01
100's	$8.78	Penicillin G Potassium, HL Moore Drug Exch	00839-5142-06

Tablet, Uncoated - Oral - 400,000 unit

100's	$7.50	Penicillin G Potassium, Aligen Independ	00405-4774-01
100's	$10.73	Penicillin G Potassium, Rugby	00536-1000-01
100's	$11.62	Potassium Penicillin G, Geneva Pharms	00781-1985-01
100's	**$12.39**	**PENTIDS '400', Bristol Myers Squibb**	**00003-0165-50**

Tablet, Uncoated - Oral - 800,000 unit

100's	**$18.59**	**PENTIDS '800', Bristol Myers Squibb**	**00003-0168-50**

HOW SUPPLIED - NOT RATED EQUIVALENT:

Injection, Solution - Intravenous - 1,000,000 unit/

50 ml	$12.99	Penicillin G Potassium, Baxter Hlthcare	00338-1021-41

Injection, Solution - Intravenous - 2,000,000 unit/

50 ml	$13.52	Penicillin G Potassium, Baxter Hlthcare	00338-1023-41

Injection, Solution - Intravenous - 3,000,000 unit/

50 ml	$14.03	Penicillin G Potassium, Baxter Hlthcare	00338-1025-41

Powder, Reconstitution - Oral - 200,000 unit/5m

100 ml	**$1.90**	**PENTIDS, Bristol Myers Squibb**	**00003-0746-38**

PENICILLIN G PROCAINE *(001969)*

CATEGORIES: Anthrax; Anti-Infectives; Antibiotics; Antimicrobials; Arthritis; Bacteremia; Bejel; Dental; Endocarditis; Enterococci Infections; Erysipelas; Erysipeloid; Fever; Gingivitis; Gonorrhea; Heart Disease; Infections; Meningitis; Middle Ear Infections; Otitis Media; Penicillins; Pericarditis; Perioperative Prophylaxis; Peritonitis; Pharyngitis; Pinta; Pneumococcal Infections; Pneumonia; Respiratory Tract Infections; Rheumatic Fever; Scarlet Fever; Septicemia; Skin Infections; Streptococcal Infection; Syphilis; Vincent's Infection; Yaws; Pregnancy Category B; FDA Approval Pre 1982

BRAND NAMES: *Aquicilina;* Crysticillin AS; Duracillin AS; *Farmaproina; Fradicilina 600; Novocillin; PAM;* **Pfizerpen AS**; *Procapen; Procillin;* Provaine Pencillin; Wycillin

(International brand names outside U.S. in italics)

FORMULARIES: BC-BS; Medi-Cal; WHO

DESCRIPTION:

Penicillin G procaine is a highly potent antibacterial agent effective against a wide variety of pathogenic organisms. It is an equimolecular compound of procaine and penicillin G in aqueous suspension for intramuscular administration.

Penicillin G procaine is supplied in 10 ml vials (3,000,000 units).

Chemically, Penicillin G procaine is: 3,3-Dimethyl-7-oxo-6-(2-phenylacetamido)-4-thia-1-azabicyclo (3.2.0) heptane-2-carboxylic acid compound with 2-(diethylamino) ethyl-*p*-aminobenzoate (1:1) monohydrate.

It has a molecular weight of 588.72.

Penicillin G procaine is a white, fine crystal, or a white, very fine microcrystalline powder. Penicillin G procaine is odorless or practically so and 1 gram is soluble in 250 ml water. The pH of the aqueous suspension is between 5.0-7.5.

CLINICAL PHARMACOLOGY:

Penicillin G procaine is an equimolecular compound of procaine and penicillin G administered intramuscularly as a suspension. It dissolves slowly at the site of injection, giving a plateau type of blood level at about 4 hours, which falls slowly over a period of the next 15-20 hours.

Approximately 60% of penicillin G is bound to serum protein. The drug is distributed throughout the body tissues in widely varying amounts. Highest levels are found in the kidneys with lesser amounts in the liver, skin, and intestines. Penicillin G penetrates into all other tissues to a lesser degree with a very small level found in the cerebrospinal fluid. With normal kidney function the drug is excreted rapidly by tubular excretion. In neonates and young infants, and in individuals with impaired kidney function, excretion is considerably delayed. Approximately 60%-90% of a dose of parenteral penicillin G is excreted in the urine within 24-36 hours. Penicillin G crosses the placental barrier and is found in the amniotic fluid and cord serum.

MICROBIOLOGY

Penicillin G exerts a bactericidal action against penicillin-susceptible microorganisms during the stage of active multiplication. It acts through the inhibition of biosynthesis of cell wall mucopeptide. It is not active against the penicillinase-producing bacteria, which include many strains of staphylococci. While *in vitro* studies have demonstrated the susceptibility of most strains of the following organisms, clinical efficacy for infections other than those included in INDICATIONS AND USAGE has not been documented. Penicillin G exerts high *in vitro* activity against staphylococci (except penicillinase-producing strains), streptococci (groups A, C, G, H, L, and M), and pneumococci. Other organisms sensitive to penicillin G are *N. gonorrhoeae, Corynebacterium diphtheriae, Bacillus anthracis,* Clostridia, *Actinomyces bovis, Streptobacillus moniliformis, Listeria monocytogenes,* and Leptospira. *Treponema pallidum* is extremely sensitive to the bactericidal action of penicillin G.

Penicillin acts synergistically with gentamicin or tobramycin against many strains of enterococci.

Susceptibility Testing: Penicillin G Susceptibility Powder or 10 units Penicillin G Susceptibility Discs may be used to determine microbial susceptibility to penicillin G using one of the following standard methods recommended by the National Committee for Laboratory Standards:

M2-A3, "Performance Standards for Antimicrobial Disk Susceptibility Tests"

M7-A, "Methods for Dilution Antimicrobial Susceptibility Tests for Bacteria that Grow Aerobically"

M11-A, "Reference Agar Dilution Procedure for Antimicrobial Susceptibility Testing of Anaerobic Bacteria"

M17-P, "Alternative Methods for Antimicrobial susceptibility Testing of Anaerobic Bacteria"

Tests should be interpreted by the following criteria (TABLE 1):

TABLE 1

Zone Diameter, nearest whole mm

	Susceptible	**Moderately Susceptible**	**Resistant**
Staphylococci	≥29	-	≤28
N. gonorrhoeae	≥20	-	≤19
Enterococci	-	≥15	≤14
Non-enterococcal streptococci and*L. monocytogenes*	≥28	20-27	≤19

Approximate MIC Correlates

	Susceptible	**Resistant**
Staphylococci	≤0.1 mcg/ml	β-lactamase
N. gonorrhoeae	≤0.1 mcg/ml	β-lactamase
Enterococci	-	≥16 mcg/ml
Non-enterococcal streptococci and*L. monocytogenes*	≤0.12 mcg/ml	≥4 mcg/ml

Interpretations of susceptible, intermediate, and resistant correlate zone size diameters with MIC values. A laboratory report of "susceptible" indicates that the suspected causative microorganism most likely will respond to therapy with penicillin G. A laboratory report of "resistant" indicates that the infecting microorganism most likely will not respond to therapy. A laboratory report of "moderately susceptible" indicates that the microorganism is most likely susceptible if a high dosage of penicillin G is used, or if the infection is such that high levels of penicillin G may be attained as in urine. A report of "intermediate" using the disk diffusion method may be considered an equivocal result, and dilution tests may be indicated.

Control organisms are recommended for susceptibility testing. Each time the test is performed the following organisms should be included. The range for zones of inhibition is shown below (TABLE 2):

TABLE 2

Control Organism	**Zone of Inhibition Range**
Staphylococcus aureus (ATCC 25923)	27-35

INDICATIONS AND USAGE:

Penicillin G procaine is indicated in the treatment of moderately severe infections in both adults and children due to penicillin G-susceptible microorganisms that are susceptible to the low and persistent serum levels common to this particular dosage form in the indications listed below. Therapy should be guided by bacteriological studies (including susceptibility tests) and by clinical response.

NOTE: When high sustained serum levels are required, aqueous penicillin G either IM or IV should be used.

The following infections will usually respond to adequate dosages of intramuscular penicillin G procaine.

Streptococcal Infections Group A (Without Bacteremia): Moderately severe to severe infections of the upper respiratory tract (including middle ear infections - otitis media), skin and soft tissue infections, scarlet fever, and erysipelas.

NOTE: Streptococci in groups A, C, H, G, L, and M are very sensitive to penicillin G. Other groups, including group D (enterococcus) are resistant. Aqueous penicillin is recommended for streptococcal infections with bacteremia.

Pneumococcal Infections: Moderately severe infections of the respiratory tract (including middle ear infections-otitis media).

INDICATIONS AND USAGE: *(cont'd)*

NOTE: Severe pneumonia, empyema, bacteremia, pericarditis, meningitis, peritonitis, and purulent or septic arthritis of pneumococcal etiology are better treated with aqueous penicillin G during the acute stage.

Staphylococcal Infections: Penicillin G-sensitive. Moderately severe infections of the skin and soft tissues.

NOTE: Reports indicate an increasing number of strains of staphylococci resistant to penicillin G emphasizing the need for culture and sensitivity studies in treating suspected staphylococcal infections.

Indicated surgical procedures should be performed.

Fusospirochetosis (Vincent's Gingivitis And Pharyngitis): Moderately severe infections of the oropharynx respond to therapy with penicillin G procaine.

NOTE: Necessary dental care should be accomplished in infections involving the gum tissue.

Treponema pallidum: (syphilis); all stages.

N. gonorrhoeae;: acute and chronic (without bacteremia).

Yaws, Bejel, Pinta: *C. diphtheriae*-penicillin G procaine as an adjunct to antitoxin for prevention of the carrier stage.

Anthrax: *Streptobacillus moniliformis* and *Spirillum minus* infections (rat bite fever).

Erysipeloid: Subacute bacterial endocarditis (group A streptococcus) only in extremely sensitive infections.

Prophylaxis Against Bacterial Endocarditis: Although no controlled clinical efficacy studies have been conducted, aqueous crystalline penicillin G for injection and penicillin G procaine suspension have been suggested by the American Heart Association and the American Dental Association for use as part of a combined parenteral-oral regimen for prophylaxis against bacterial endocarditis in patients with congenital heart disease or rheumatic, or other acquired valvular heart disease when they undergo dental procedures and surgical procedures of the upper respiratory tract.[1] Since it may happen that *alpha* hemolytic streptococci relatively resistant to penicillin may be found when patients are receiving continuous oral penicillin for secondary prevention of rheumatic fever, prophylactic agents other than penicillin may be chosen for these patients and prescribed in addition to their continuous rheumatic fever prophylactic regimen.

NOTE: When selecting antibiotics for the prevention of bacterial endocarditis the physician or dentist should read the full joint statement of the American Heart Association and the American Dental Association.[1]

CONTRAINDICATIONS:

A previous hypersensitivity reaction to any penicillin or procaine is a contraindication.

WARNINGS:

Serious and occasionally fatal hypersensitivity (anaphylactoid) reactions have been reported in patients on penicillin therapy. These reactions are more likely to occur in individuals with a history of penicillin hypersensitivity and/or a history of sensitivity to multiple allergens. There have been reports of individuals with a history of penicillin hypersensitivity who have experienced severe reactions when treated with cephalosporins. Before initiating therapy with any penicillin, careful inquiry should be made concerning previous hypersensitivity reactions to penicillin, cephalosporins, or other allergens. If an allergic reaction occurs, the drug should be discontinued and the appropriate therapy instituted. Serious anaphylactoid reactions require immediate emergency treatment with epinephrine. Oxygen, intravenous steroids, and airway management-including intubation, should be administered as indicated.

Immediate toxic reactions to procaine may occur in some individuals, particularly when a large single dose is administered in the treatment of gonorrhea (4.8 million units). These reactions may be manifested by mental disturbances including anxiety, confusion, agitation, depression, weakness, seizures, hallucinations, combativeness, and expressed "fear of impending death." The reactions noted in carefully controlled studies occurred in approximately one in 500 patients treated for gonorrhea. Reactions are transient, lasting from 15-30 minutes.

PRECAUTIONS:

General: Penicillin should be used with caution in individuals with histories of significant allergies and/or asthma.

Intramuscular Therapy: Care should be taken to avoid intravenous or accidental intraarterial administration, or injection into or near major peripheral nerves or blood vessels, since such injections may produce neurovascular damage.

As with all intramuscular preparations, Penicillin G procaine should be injected well within the body of a relatively large muscle. *Adults:* The preferred site is the upper outer quadrant of the buttock (*i.e.,* gluteus maximus), or the mid-lateral thigh. *Children:* It is recommended that intramuscular injections be given preferably in the mid-lateral muscles of the thigh. In infants and small children the periphery of the upper outer quadrant of the gluteal region should only be used when necessary, such as in burn patients, in order to minimize the possibility of damage to the sciatic nerve.

The deltoid area should be used only if well developed, such as in certain adults and older children, and then only with caution to avoid radial nerve injury. Intramuscular injections should not be made into the lower and mid-third of the upper arm. As with all intramuscular injections, aspiration is necessary to help avoid inadvertent injection into a blood vessel.

In streptococcal infections, therapy must be sufficient to eliminate the organism (10 days minimum), otherwise the sequelae of streptococcal disease may occur. Cultures should be taken following completion of treatment to determine whether streptococci have been eradicated.

The use of antibiotics may result in overgrowth of nonsusceptible organisms. Constant observation of the patient is essential. If new infections due to bacteria or fungi appear during therapy, the drug should be discontinued and appropriate measures taken. whenever allergic reactions occur, penicillin should be withdrawn unless, in the opinion of the physician, the condition being treated is life threatening and amenable only to penicillin therapy.

A small percentage of patients are sensitive to procaine. If there is a history of sensitivity make the usual test: Inject intradermally 0.1 ml of a 1 to 2 percent solution. Development of an erythema, wheal, flare, or eruption indicates procaine sensitivity. Sensitivity should be treated by the usual methods, including barbiturates, and penicillin G procaine preparations should not be used. Antihistamines appear beneficial in treatment of procaine reactions.

Laboratory Tests: In prolonged therapy with penicillin, periodic evaluation of the renal, hepatic, and hematopoietic systems is recommended. This is particularly important in prematures, neonates and other infants, and when high doses are used.

When treating gonococcal infections in which primary or secondary syphilis may be suspected, proper diagnostic procedures, including dark field examinations, should be done. In all cases in which concomitant syphilis is suspected, monthly serological tests should be made for at least four months. All cases of penicillin treated syphilis should receive clinical and serological examinations every six months for two to three years.

In suspected staphylococcal infections, proper laboratory studies, including susceptibility tests, should be performed.

PRECAUTIONS: *(cont'd)*

In streptococcal infections, cultures should be taken following completion of treatment to determine whether streptococci have been eradicated.

Carcinogenesis, Mutagenesis, and Impairment of Fertility: No information or long-term studies are available on the carcinogenesis, mutagenesis, or the impairment of fertility with the use of penicillin.

Pregnancy, Teratogenic Effects, Pregnancy Category B: Reproduction studies performed in the mouse, rat, and rabbit have revealed no evidence of impaired fertility or harm to the fetus due to penicillin G. Human experience with the penicillins during pregnancy has not shown any positive evidence of adverse effects on the fetus. There are, however, no adequate and well controlled studies in pregnant women showing conclusively that harmful effects of these drugs on the fetus can be excluded. Because animal reproduction studies are not always predictive of human response, this drug should be used during pregnancy only if clearly needed.

Nursing Mothers: Penicillin G procaine has been reported in milk. Caution should be exercised when penicillin G is administered to a nursing woman.

Pediatric Use: Penicillins are excreted largely unchanged by the kidney. Because of incompletely developed renal function in infants, the rate of elimination will be slow. Use caution in administering to newborns and evaluate organ system function frequently.

DRUG INTERACTIONS:

Concurrent administration of bacteriostatic antibiotics (*e.g.,* erythromycin, tetracycline) may diminish the bactericidal effects of penicillins by slowing the rate of bacterial growth. Bactericidal agents work most effectively against the immature cell wall of rapidly proliferating microorganisms. This has been demonstrated *in vitro;* however, the clinical significance of this interaction is not well documented. There are few clinical situations in which the concurrent use of "static" and "cidal" antibiotics are indicated. However, in selected circumstances in which such therapy is appropriate, using adequate doses of antibacterial agents and beginning penicillin therapy first, should minimize the potential for interaction.

Penicillin blood levels may be prolonged by concurrent administration of probenecid which blocks the renal tubular secretion of penicillins.

Displacement of penicillins from plasma protein binding sites will elevate the level of free penicillin in the serum.

ADVERSE REACTIONS:

Penicillin is a substance of low toxicity, but does possess a significant index of sensitization. The following hypersensitivity reactions associated with use of penicillin have been reported: skin rashes, ranging from maculopapular eruptions to exfoliative dermatitis; urticaria; serum sickness-like reactions, including chills, fever, edema, arthralgia, and prostration. Severe and often fatal anaphylaxis has been reported (see WARNINGS). As with other treatments for syphilis, the Jarisch-Herxheimer reaction has been reported.

Procaine toxicity manifestations have been reported (see WARNINGS). Procaine hypersensitivity reactions have not been reported with this drug.

OVERDOSAGE:

In case of overdosage, discontinue medication, treat symptomatically, and institute supportive measures as required.

Convulsions have been reported in individuals receiving 4.8 million units.

Penicillin is hemodialyzable.

DOSAGE AND ADMINISTRATION:

Pediatric Dosage Schedule: In children under 3 months of age, the absorption of aqueous penicillin G produces such high and sustained levels that penicillin G procaine dosage forms offer no advantages and are usually unnecessary.

In children under 12 years of age, dosage should be adjusted in accordance with the age and weight of the child, and the severity of the infection.

Under 2 years of age, the dose may be divided between the two buttocks if necessary.

Penicillin G procaine (aqueous) is for intramuscular injection only.

RECOMMENDED DOSAGE FOR PENICILLIN G PROCAINE AQUEOUS

Pneumonia: (pneumococcal), moderately severe (uncomplicated): 600,000-1,000,000 units daily.

Streptococcal Infections: (group A), moderately severe to severe tonsillitis, erysipelas, scarlet fever, upper respiratory tract, skin and soft tissue: 600,000-1,000,000 units daily for a minimum of 10 days.

Staphylococcal Infections: moderately severe to severe: 600,000-1,000,000 units daily.

Bacterial Endocarditis: (group A streptococci), only in extremely sensitive infections: 600,000-1,000,000 units daily.

For prophylaxis against bacterial endocarditis[1] in patients with congenital heart disease or rheumatic or other acquired valvular heart disease, when undergoing dental procedures or surgical procedures of the upper respiratory tract, use a combined parenteral-oral regimen. One million units of aqueous crystalline penicillin G (30,000 units/kg in children) intramuscularly, mixed with 600,000 units penicillin G (600,000 units for children) should be given one-half to one hour before the procedure. Oral penicillin V (phenoxymethyl penicillin), 500 mg for adults or 250 mg for children less than 60 lb, should be given every six hours for 8 doses. Doses for children should not exceed recommendations for adults for a single dose or for a 24 hour period.

Syphilis: Primary, secondary and latent with a negative spinal fluid in adults and children over 12 years of age: 600,000 units daily for 8 days, total 4,800,000 units.

Late (Tertiary Neurosyphilis And Latent Syphilis): with positive spinal fluid examination or no spinal fluid examination): 600,000 units daily for 10-15 days, total 6-9 million units.

Congenital Syphilis: (early and late) 50,000 units/kg per day for a minimum of 10 days.

Yaws, Bejel, and Pinta: Treatment as syphilis in corresponding stage of disease.

Gonorrheal Infections: (uncomplicated) Men or women-4.8 million units intramuscularly divided into at least two doses and injected at different sites at one visit, together with 1 gram of oral probenecid, preferably given at least 30 minutes prior to the injection.

NOTE: Gonorrheal endocarditis should be treated intensively with aqueous penicillin G.

Diphtheria Adjunctive Therapy With Antitoxin: 300,000-600,000 units daily.

Diphtheria Carrier State: 300,000 units daily for 10 days.

Anthrax Cutaneous: 600,000-1,000,000 units/day.

Vincent's Infection (Fusospirochetosis): 600,000-1,000,000 units/day.

Erysipeloid: 600,000-1,000,000 units/day.

Streptobacillus moniliformis and *Spirillum minus* (rat Bite Fever): 600,000-1,000,000 units/day.

Parenteral drug products should be inspected visually for particulate matter and discoloration prior to administration, whenever solution and container permit.

DOSAGE AND ADMINISTRATION: *(cont'd)*

The product should be stored between 2°-8°C (36°-46°F).

CDC GUIDELINES FOR TREATMENT OF SEXUALLY TRANSMITTED DISEASES

Neurosyphilis:[1] (as An Alternative To The Recommended Regimen Of Penicillin G Aqueous) 2 to 4 million units/day plus probenecid 500 mg orally 4 times daily, both for 10 to 14 days; many recommend benzathine penicillin G 2.4 million units weekly for 3 doses following the completion of this regimen.

Congenital Syphilis:[1] Symptomatic and asymptomatic infants: 50,000 units/kg/day (administered once IM) for 10 to 14 days.

[1] CDC 1989 Sexually Transmitted Diseases Treatment Guidelines. *Morbidity and Mortality Weekly Report* 1989 Sept. 1; 38 (No. S-8):1–43.

REFERENCES:

1. American Heart Association, 1977. Prevention of Bacterial Endocarditis. Circulation **56**:139A-143A.

HOW SUPPLIED - RATED THERAPEUTICALLY EQUIVALENT:

Injection, Solution - Intramuscular - 600,000 unit/ml

1 ml x 10	$28.96	WYCILLIN, Wyeth Labs	00008-0018-10
2 ml x 10	$48.21	WYCILLIN, Wyeth Labs	00008-0018-08
4 ml x 10	$102.69	WYCILLIN, Wyeth Labs	00008-0018-12
12 ml x 10	$35.90	CRYSTICILLIN 600 A.S., Bristol Myers Squibb	00003-0309-51

HOW SUPPLIED - NOT RATED EQUIVALENT:

Injection, Susp - Intramuscular - 300,000 unit/ml

10 ml x 10	$18.34	CRYSTICILLIN 300 A.S., Bristol Myers Squibb	00003-0299-51

PENICILLIN G PROCAINE; PROBENECID

(001970)

CATEGORIES: Anti-Infectives; Antibiotics; Antimicrobials; Gonorrhea; Infections; Penicillins; Pharyngitis; Sexually Transmitted Diseases; Urethritis; FDA Pre 1938 Drugs

BRAND NAMES: Wycillin & Probenecid

DESCRIPTION:

Disposable Syringe and Tablets

Wycillin is for deep IM injection only.

The Wycillin disposable syringe is designed to provide a stable aqueous suspension of sterile penicillin G procaine; ready for immediate use. This eliminates the necessity for addition of any diluent, required for the usual dry formulation of injectable penicillin.

Each syringe, 2,400,000 units (4 ml size), contains penicillin G procaine in a stabilized aqueous suspension with sodium citrate buffer; and as w/v, approximately 0.5% lecithin, 0.5% carboxymethylcellulose, 0.5% povidone, 0.1% methylparaben, and 0.01% propylparaben.

Wycillin must be stored in a refrigerator. Keep from freezing. This will prevent deterioration and assure that no significant loss of potency occurs within the expiration date.

Probenecid is a uricosuric and renal tubular-blocking agent. Probenecid tablets contain 0.5 gram probenecid. The inactive ingredients present are calcium stearate, D&C Yellow 10, gelatin, hydroxypropyl methylcellulose, iron oxide, magnesium carbonate, polyethylene glycol, starch, talc, and titanium dioxide.

Wycillin suspension in the disposable syringe formulation is viscous and opaque. Read "Contraindications," "Warnings," "Precautions," and DOSAGE AND ADMINISTRATION sections prior to use.

CLINICAL PHARMACOLOGY:

Penicillin G exerts a bactericidal action against penicillin-sensitive microorganisms during the stage of active multiplication. It acts through the inhibition of biosynthesis of cell-wall mucopeptide. It is not active against the penicillinase-producing bacteria, which include many strains of staphylococci. *Neisseria gonorrhoeae* are included among the various organisms which are sensitive to penicillin G. Penicillin G procaine is an equimolecular salt of procaine and penicillin G, administered intramuscularly as a suspension. It dissolves slowly at the site of injection, giving a plateau type of blood level at about 4 hours which falls slowly over a period of the next 15 to 20 hours. Approximately 60% to 90% of a dose of penicillin G is excreted in the urine within 24 to 36 hours.

Approximately 60% of penicillin G is bound to serum protein. The drug is distributed throughout the body tissues in widely varying amounts, with highest levels found in the kidneys and lesser amounts in the liver, skin, and intestines. Penicillin G penetrates into all other tissues to a lesser degree, with a very small level found in the cerebrospinal fluid. With normal kidney function, the drug is excreted rapidly by tubular excretion. In neonates and young infants and in individuals with impaired kidney function, excretion is considerably delayed.

Probenecid inhibits the tubular reabsorption of urate, thus increasing the urinary excretion of uric acid and decreasing serum uric acid levels. It also inhibits the tubular excretion of penicillin and usually increases penicillin plasma levels, regardless of the route by which the antibiotic is given. A 2-fold to 4-fold elevation has been demonstrated for various penicillins. Probenecid does not influence plasma concentrations of salicylates, nor the excretion of streptomycin, chloramphenicol, chlortetracycline, oxytetracycline, or neomycin.

INDICATIONS AND USAGE:

Wycillin and Probenecid is indicated for the single-dose treatment of uncomplicated (without bacteremia) urethral, cervical, rectal, or pharyngeal infections caused by *Neisseria gonorrhoeae* (gonorrhea) in men and women.

Susceptibility studies should be performed when recurrent infections or resistant strains are encountered. Urethritis and the presence of gram-negative diplococci in urethral smears are strong presumptive evidence of gonorrhea. Culture or fluorescent antibody studies will confirm the diagnosis. Therapy may be instituted prior to obtaining results of susceptibility testing.

CONTRAINDICATIONS:

A history of a previous hypersensitivity reaction to any of the penicillins or to Probenecid is a contraindication.

Probenecid is not recommended in persons with known blood dyscrasias or uric acid kidney stones or during an acute attack of gout. It is not recommended in conjunction with penicillin G procaine suspension in the presence of known renal impairment.

Do not inject into or near an artery or nerve.

WARNINGS:

PENICILLIN G PROCAINE

Serious and occasionally fatal hypersensitivity (anaphylactoid) reactions have been reported in patients on penicillin therapy. Serious anaphylactoid reactions require immediate emergency treatment with epinephrine. Oxygen and intravenous corticosteroids should also be administered as indicated. Although anaphylaxis is more frequent following parenteral therapy, it has occurred in patients on oral penicillins. These reactions are more apt to occur in individuals with a history of sensitivity to multiple allergens.

There have been well-documented reports of individuals with a history of penicillin-hypersensitivity reactions who have experienced severe hypersensitivity reactions when treated with a cephalosporin. Before therapy with a penicillin, careful inquiry should be made concerning previous hypersensitivity reactions to penicillins, cephalosporins, and other allergens. If an allergic reaction occurs, the drug should be discontinued and the patient treated with the usual agents, e.g., pressor amines, antihistamines, and corticosteroids.

Immediate toxic reactions to procaine may occur in some individuals, particularly when a large single dose is administered in the treatment of gonorrhea (4.8 million units). These reactions may be manifested by mental disturbances, including anxiety, confusion, agitation, depression, weakness, seizures, hallucinations, combativeness, and expressed "fear of impending death." The reactions noted in carefully controlled studies occurred in approximately one in 500 patients treated for gonorrhea. Reactions are transient, lasting from 15 to 30 minutes.

Inadvertent intravascular administration, including inadvertent direct intra-arterial injection or injection immediately adjacent to arteries, of Wycillin and other penicillin preparations has resulted in severe neurovascular damage, including transverse myelitis with permanent paralysis, gangrene requiring amputation of digits and more proximal portions of extremities, and necrosis and sloughing at and surrounding the injection site. Such severe effects have been reported following injections into the buttock, thigh, and deltoid areas. Other serious complications of suspected intravascular administration which have been reported include immediate pallor, mottling, or cyanosis of the extremity, both distal and proximal to the injection site, followed by bleb formation; severe edema requiring anterior and/or posterior compartment fasciotomy in the lower extremity. The above-described severe effects and complications have most often occurred in infants and small children. Prompt consultation with an appropriate specialist is indicated if any evidence of compromise of the blood supply occurs at, proximal to, or distal to the site of injection.[1-9] See "Contraindications," "Precautions," and DOSAGE AND ADMINISTRATION sections.

Quadriceps femoris fibrosis and atrophy have been reported following repeated intramuscular injections of penicillin preparations into the anterolateral thigh.

Injection into or near a nerve may result in permanent neurological damage.

PROBENECID

Exacerbation of gout following therapy with Probenecid may occur; in such cases colchicine therapy is advisable.

In patients on Probenecid, the use of salicylates in either small or large doses is not recommended because it antagonizes the uricosuric action of Probenecid. Patients on Probenecid who require a mild analgesic agent should receive acetaminophen rather than salicylates, even in small doses.

USAGE IN PREGNANCY

The safety of these drugs for use in pregnancy has not been established.

PRECAUTIONS:

PENICILLIN G PROCAINE

When treating gonococcal infections in which primary or secondary syphilis may be suspected, proper diagnostic procedures, including dark-field examinations, should be done. In all cases in which concomitant syphilis is suspected, monthly serological tests should be made for at least four months. Patients with gonorrhea, who also have syphilis, should be given additional appropriate parenteral penicillin treatment.

Penicillin should be used with caution in individuals with histories of significant allergies and/or asthma. When administering Wycillin, care should be taken to avoid intravenous or intra-arterial administration, or injection into or near major peripheral nerves or blood vessels, since such injections may produce neurovascular damage. See CONTRAINDICATIONS, WARNINGS and DOSAGE AND ADMINISTRATION sections.

A small percentage of patients are sensitive to procaine. If there is a history of sensitivity, make the usual test: Inject intradermally 0.1 ml of a 1- to 2-percent procaine solution. Development of an erythema, wheal, flare, or eruption indicates procaine sensitivity. Sensitivity should be treated by the usual methods, including barbiturates, and procaine penicillin preparations should not be used. Antihistaminics appear beneficial in treatment of procaine reactions.

PROBENECID

Use Probenecid with caution in patients with a history of peptic ulcer. A reducing substance may appear in the urine of patients receiving Probenecid. Although this disappears with discontinuance of therapy, a false diagnosis of glycosuria may be made because of a false-positive Benedict's test.

ADVERSE REACTIONS:

WYCILLIN

Penicillin is a substance of low toxicity but does possess a significant index of sensitization. The following hypersensitivity reactions associated with use of penicillin have been reported: skin rashes, ranging from maculopapular eruptions to exfoliative dermatitis; urticaria; serum-sicknesslike reactions, including chills, fever, edema, arthralgia, and prostration. Severe and often fatal anaphylaxis has been reported (see WARNINGS). As with other treatments for syphilis, the Jarisch-Herxheimer reactions has been reported.

Procaine toxicity manifestations have been reported (see WARNINGS). Although procaine hypersensitivity reactions have not been reported with this drug, there are patients who are sensitive to procaine (see PRECAUTIONS).

PROBENECID

The following are the principal adverse reactions which have been reported as associated with the use of Probenecid, generally with more prolonged or repeated administration: hypersensitivity reactions (including anaphylaxis), nephrotic syndrome, hepatic necrosis, aplastic anemia; also other anemias, including hemolytic anemia related to genetic deficiency of glucose-6-phosphate dehydrogenase.

DOSAGE AND ADMINISTRATION:

Parenteral drug products should be inspected visually for particulate matter and discoloration prior to administration, whenever solution and container permit.

Penicillin G procaine (aqueous) is for intramuscular injection only. Administer by DEEP INTRAMUSCULAR INJECTION in the upper, outer quadrant of the buttock. When doses are repeated, vary the injection site.

The Wyeth disposable syringe for this product incorporates several features that are designed to facilitate its use.

DOSAGE AND ADMINISTRATION: *(cont'd)*

A single small indentation, or "dot," has been punched into the metal ring that surrounds the neck of the syringe near the base of the needle. It is important that this "dot" be placed in a position so that it can be easily visualized by the operator following the intramuscular insertion of the syringe needle.

After selection of the proper site and insertion of the needle into the selected muscle, aspirate by pulling back on the plunger. While maintaining negative pressure for 2 to 3 seconds, carefully observe the barrel of the syringe immediately proximal to the location of the "dot" for appearance of blood or any discoloration. Blood or "typical blood color" may *not* be seen if a blood vessel has been entered— only a mixture of blood and Wycillin. The appearance of any discoloration is reason to withdraw the needle and discard the syringe. If it is elected to inject at another site, a new syringe should be used. If no blood or discoloration appears, inject the contents of the syringe slowly. Discontinue delivery of the dose if the subject complains of severe immediate pain at the injection site or if in infants and young children symptoms or signs occur suggesting onset of severe pain.

Although some isolates of *Neisseria gonorrhoeae* have decreased susceptibility to penicillin, this inherent resistance is relative, not absolute, and penicillin in large doses remains the drug of choice for these strains. Strains producing penicillinase, however, are resistant to penicillin G, and a drug other than penicillin G should be used.

GONORRHEAL INFECTIONS (UNCOMPLICATED) MEN OR WOMEN

Aqueous penicillin G procaine, 4.8 million units intramuscularly, divided into at least two doses and injected at different sites at one visit, together with 1 gram (2 tablets, 0.5 gram each) of Probenecid orally, given just before the injections. Physicians are cautioned to use no less than the recommended dosages.

NOTE: Treatment of severe complications of gonorrhea should be individualized, using large amounts of short-acting penicillin. Gonorrheal endocarditis should be treated intensively with aqueous penicillin G. Prophylactic or epidemiologic treatment for gonorrhea (male and female) is accomplished with the same treatment schedules as for the uncomplicated gonorrhea.

RETREATMENT

The National Center for Disease Control, Venereal Disease Branch, U.S. Department of Health, Education and Welfare, Atlanta, Georgia, recommends:

Test of cure procedures at approximately 7 to 14 days after therapy. In the male, a gram-stained smear is adequate if positive; otherwise, a culture specimen should be obtained from the anterior urethra. In the female, culture specimens should be obtained from both the endocervical and anal canal sites.

Retreatment in the male is indicated if the urethral discharge persists for three or more days following initial therapy and the smear or culture remains positive. Follow-up treatment consists of 4,800,000 units of aqueous penicillin G procaine, intramuscular, divided in two injection sites at a single visit.

In uncomplicated gonorrhea in the female, retreatment is indicated if follow-up cervical or rectal cultures remain positive for *N. gonorrhoeae*. Follow-up treatment consists of 4,800,000 units of aqueous penicillin G procaine daily on two successive days.

SYPHILIS

All gonorrhea patients should have a serologic test for syphilis at the time of diagnosis. Patients with gonorrhea who also have syphilis should be given additional treatment appropriate to the stage of syphilis.

Store in a refrigerator—Keep from freezing.

REFERENCES:

1. SHAW, E.: Transverse myelitis from injection of penicillin. *Am. J. Dis. Child., 111*:548, 1966. 2. KNOWLES, J.: Accidental intra-arterial injection of penicillin.*Am. J. Dis. Child., 111*: 552, 1966. 3. DARBY, C. et al: Ischemia following an intragluteal injection of benzathine-procaine penicillin G mixture in a one-year-old boy. *Clin. Pediatrics, 12*:485, 1973. 4. BROWN, L. & NELSON, A.: Postinfectious intravascular thrombosis with gangrene. *Arch. Surg., 94*:652, 1967. 5. BORENSTINE, J.: Transverse myelitis and penicillin (Correspondence).*Am. J. Dis. Child., 112*: 166, 1966. 6. ATKINSON, J.: Transverse myelopathy secondary to penicillin injection.*J. Pediatrics, 75*: 867, 1969. 7. TALBERT, J. et al: Gangrene of the foot following intramuscular injection in the lateral thigh: A case report with recommendations for prevention. *J. Pediatrics, 70*:110, 1967. 8. FISHER, T.: Medicolegal affairs. *Canad. Med. Assoc. J., 112*:395, 1975. 9. SCHANZER, H. et al: Accidental intra-arterial injection of penicillin G. *JAMA, 242*:1289, 1979.

HOW SUPPLIED - EQUIVALENTS NOT AVAILABLE:

Kit - Intramuscular; - 2400000 unit/0.

1 kit $20.85 WYCILLIN, Wyeth Labs   00008-2517-01

PENICILLIN G SODIUM *(003040)*

CATEGORIES: Actinomycosis; Anthrax; Anti-Infectives; Antibiotics; Arthritis; Bacteremia; Dental; Diphtheria; Endocarditis; Erysipeloid; Fever; Genitourinary Tract Infections; Gingivitis; Heart Disease; Meningitis; Penicillins; Pericarditis; Perioperative Prophylaxis; Pharyngitis; Pneumococcal Infections; Pneumonia; Rat-Bite Fever; Respiratory Tract Infections; Rheumatic Fever; Streptococcal Infection; Syphilis; Tetanus; Vincent's Infection; FDA Approval Pre 1982

DESCRIPTION:

Penicillin G Sodium for Injection is crystalline penicillin G sodium as a sterile powder. The preparation contains approximately 28 mg citrate buffer (composed of sodium citrate and not more than 0.92 mg citric acid) and 2.0 mEq sodium per million units of penicillin.

CLINICAL PHARMACOLOGY:

Penicillin G is bactericidal against penicillin-susceptible microorganisms during the stage of active multiplication. It acts by inhibiting biosynthesis of cell-wall mucopeptide. It is not active against the penicillinase-producing bacteria, which include many strains of staphylococci. Penicillin G is highly active in vitro against staphylococci (except penicillinase-producing strains), streptococci (groups A, C, G, H, L, and M) and pneumococci. Other organisms susceptible in vitro to penicillin G are Neisseria gonorrhoea, Corynebacterium diphtheriae, Bacillus anthracis, Clostridia, Actinomyces bovis, Streptobacillus moniliformis, Listeria monocytogenes, and Leptospira; Treponema pallidum is extremely susceptible. Some species of gram-negative bacilli are susceptible to moderate to high concentrations of penicillin G obtained with intravenous administration. These include most strains of Escherichia coli; all strains of Proteus mirabilis, Salmonella, and Shigella; and some strains of Enterobacter aerogenes (formerly Aerobacter aerogenes) and Alcaligenes faecalis.

Susceptibility plate testing: If the Kirby-Bauer method of disc susceptibility is used, a 10 u penicillin disc should give a zone greater than 28 mm when tested against a penicillin-susceptible bacterial strain.

Aqueous penicillin G is rapidly absorbed following both intramuscular and subcutaneous injection. Approximately 60 percent of the total dose of 300,000 u is excreted in the urine within this five-hour period. Therefore, high and frequent doses are required to maintain the elevated serum levels desirable in treating certain severe infections in individuals with normal kidney function. In neonates and young infants and in individuals with impaired kidney function, excretion is considerably delayed.

INDICATIONS AND USAGE:

Penicillin G Sodium for Injection is indicated in the treatment of severe infections caused by penicillin G-susceptible microorganisms when rapid and high penicillinemia is required. Therapy should be guided by bacteriological studies, including susceptibility tests, and by clinical response.

The following infections will usually respond to adequate dosage:

Streptococcal Infections: *Note:* Streptococci in groups A, C, G, H, L, and M are very susceptible to penicillin G. Some group D organisms are susceptible to the high serum levels obtained with aqueous penicillin G. Aqueous penicillin G sodium is the penicillin dosage form of choice for bacteremia, empyema, severe pneumonia, pericarditis, endocarditis, meningitis, and other severe infections caused by susceptible strains of the gram-positive species listed above.

Pneumococcal infections; staphylococcal infections;penicillin g-susceptible; anthrax; actinomycosis; clostridial infections (including tetanus); diphtheria (to prevent the carrier state); erysipeloid endocarditis (erysipelothrix insidiosa); vincent's gingivitis and pharyngitis (fusospirochetosis); severe infections of the oropharynx (Note: necessary dental care should be accomplished in infections involving gum tissue.) and lower respiratory tract and genital area infections due to f. fusiformisans spirochetes; gram-negative bacillary infections (bacteremias) - (E. coli, E. aerogenes, A. faecalis, Salmonella, Shigella and P. mirabilis); listeria infections (l. monocytogenes); meningitis and endocarditis; pasteurella infections (P. multocida): Bacteremia and meningitis; rat-bite fever (S.minus or S. moniliformis); gonorrheal endocarditis and arthritis (N. gonorrhoea); syphilis (T. pallidum) including congenital syphilis; meningococcic meningitis.

Prevention Of Bacterial Endocarditis (Patients Unable To Take Oral Antibiotics): Although no controlled clinical efficacy studies have been conducted, aqueous crystalline penicillin G for injection (EXCEPT penicillin G procaine suspension) has been suggested by the American Heart Association and the American Dental Association for prophylaxis against bacterial endocarditis in patients with congenital heart disease or rheumatic or other acquired valvular heart disease when they undergo dental procedures and surgical procedures of the upper respiratory tract. Since it may happen that ALPHA hemolytic streptococci relatively resistant to penicillin may be found when patients are receiving continuous oral penicillin for secondary prevention of rheumatic fever, prophylactic agents other than penicillin may be chosen for these patients and prescribed in addition to their continuous rheumatic fever prophylactic regimen. NOTE: WHEN SELECTING ANTIBIOTICS FOR THE PREVENTION OF BACTERIAL ENDOCARDITIS THE PHYSICIAN OR DENTIST SHOULD READ THE FULL JOINT STATEMENT OF THE AMERICAN HEART ASSOCIATION AND THE AMERICAN DENTAL ASSOCIATION.

CONTRAINDICATIONS:

Contraindicated in patients with a history of hypersensitivity to any penicillin.

WARNINGS:

Serious and occasional fatal hypersensitivity (anaphylactoid) reactions have been reported in patients on penicillin therapy. Although anaphylaxis is more frequent following parenteral administration, it has occurred in patients on oral penicillins. These reactions are more apt to occur in individuals with a history of sensitivity to multiple allergens.

There have been well-documented reports of individuals with a history of penicillin hypersensitivity who have experienced severe hypersensitivity reactions when treated with cephalosporins. Before therapy with a penicillin, careful inquiry should be made concerning previous hypersensitivity reactions to penicillins, cephalosporins, and other allergens. If an allergic reaction occurs, the drug should be discontinued and the patient treated with the usual agents, e.g., pressor amines, antihistamines, and corticosteroids. Serious anaphylactoid reactions are not controlled by antihistamines alone, and require such emergency measures as the immediate use of epinephrine, aminophylline, oxygen, and intravenous corticosteroids.

PRECAUTIONS:

Penicillin should be used with caution in individuals with histories of significant allergies and/or asthma.

In prolonged therapy with penicillin and particularly with high dosage schedules, periodic evaluation of the renal and hematopoietic systems is recommended.

In streptococcal infections, therapy must be sufficient to eliminate the organism (10 days minimum); otherwise the sequelae of streptococcal disease may occur. Cultures should be taken following the completion of treatment to determine whether streptococci have been eradicated.

In high doses (above 10 million u), intravenous aqueous penicillin G sodium should be administered slowly because of the adverse effects of electrolyte imbalance from the sodium content of the penicillin. The patient's renal, cardiac and vascular status should be evaluated and if impairment of function is suspected or known to exist, a reduction int he total dosage should be considered. Frequent evaluation of electrolyte balance, and renal and hematopoietic function is recommended during therapy when high doses of intravenous aqueous penicillin G sodium are used.

Prolonged use of antibiotics may promote overgrowth of nonsusceptible organisms, including fungi. Should superinfection occur, appropriate measures should be taken. Indwelling intravenous catheters encourage superinfection and should be avoided whenever possible.

Therapy of susceptible infections should be accompanied by any indicated surgical procedures. In suspected staphylococcal infections, proper laboratory studies, including susceptibility tests, should be performed.

When treating gonococcal infections in which primary or secondary syphilis may be suspected, proper diagnostic procedures, including darkfield examinations, should be done. In all cases in which concomitant syphilis is suspected, monthly serological tests should be made for at least four months. All cases of penicillin treated syphilis should receive clinical and serological examinations every six months for at least two or three years.

Any entry into the container to effect solution of the powder or withdrawal of contents must be accomplished with strict aseptic technique and sterile equipment.

ADVERSE REACTIONS:

Penicillin is a substance of low toxicity but does possess a significant index of sensitization.

The hypersensitivity reactions reported are skin rashes ranging from maculopapular eruptions to exfoliative dermatitis; urticaria; and serum sickness-like reactions including chills, fever, edema, arthralgia, and prostration. Severe and occasionally fatal anaphylaxis has occurred (see WARNINGS).

Hemolytic anemia, leukopenia, thrombocytopenia, neuropathy, and nephropathy are rarely observed adverse reactions and are usually associated with high intravenous dosage. Urticaria, other skin rashes, and serum sickness-like reactions may be controlled by antihistamines and, if necessary, corticosteroids. When ever such reactions occur, penicillin should be discontinued unless, in the opinion of the physician, the condition being treated is life-threatening and amenable only to penicillin therapy. High dosage of penicillin G sodium may result in congestive heart failure due to high sodium intake.

The Jarisch-Herxheimer reaction has been reported in patients treated for syphilis.

DOSAGE AND ADMINISTRATION:

Penicillin G Sodium for Injection may be given intramuscularly or by continuous intravenous drip.

The usual dosage recommendation is as follows:

Severe Infections Due To Susceptible Strains Of Streptococci, Pneumococci, And Staphylococci; Bacteremia, Pneumonia, Endocarditis, Pericarditis, Empyema, Meningitis And Other Severe Infections: a minimum of 5 million u daily. *Anthrax:* a minimum of 5 million u/day in divided doses until cure is effected; *Actinomycosis:* 1 to 6 million u/day for cervicofacial cases; 10 to 20 million u/day for thoracic and abdominal disease; *Clostridial Infections (As Adjunctive Therapy To Antitoxin):* 20 million u/day; *Diphtheria:* Adjunctive therapy to antitoxin for prevention of the carrier state: 300,000 to 400,000 u/day in divided doses for 10 to 12 days; *Erysipeloid: Endocarditis:* 2 to 20 million u/day for four to six weeks; *Fusospirochetal Infections (Fusospirochetosis):* severe infections of the oropharynx, lower respiratory tract and genital areas: 5 to 10 million u/day; *Gram-Negative Bacillary Infections:* (E. coli, E. aerogenes, A. faecalis, Salmonella, Shigella, and P. mirabilis); Bacteremia: 20 to 80 million u/day; *Listeria Infections (L. Monocytogenes): Neonates:* 500,000 to 1 million u/day; *Adults With Meningitis:* 15 to 20 million u/day for two weeks; *Adults With Endocarditis:* 15 to 20 million u/day for four weeks; *Pasteurella Infections (P.Multocida): Bacteremia And Meningitis:* 4 to 6 million u/day for two weeks; *Rat-Bite Fever (S. Minus Or S. Moniliformis):* 12 to 15 million u/day for three to four weeks.

Gonorrheal Endocarditis And Arthritis: A minimum of 5 million u daily.

Syphilis: Aqueous penicillin G sodium may be used in the treatment of acquired and congenital syphilis but, because of the necessity of frequent dosage, hospitalization is recommended. Dosage and duration of therapy is determined by the age of the patient and the stage of the disease.

Meningococcic Meningitis: 1 to 2 million u IM every two hours or continuous IV drip of 20 to 30 million u/day.

PREVENTION OF BACTERIAL ENDOCARDITIS (Patients unable to take oral antibiotics) - For prophylaxis against bacterial endocarditis in patients with congenital heart disease or rheumatic or other acquired valvular heart disease when undergoing dental procedures or surgical procedures of the upper respiratory tract, administer 2 million u (50,000 u/kg for children) aqueous penicillin G, EXCEPT penicillin G procaine suspension, intravenously or intramuscularly 30 to 60 minutes before the procedure and 1 million u (25,000 u/kg for children) six hours later. Doses for children should not exceed recommendations for adults for a single dose or for a 24-hour period.

Preparation Of Solutions: Solutions of penicillin should be prepared as follows: Loosen powder. Hold vial horizontally and rotate it while slowly directing the stream of diluent against the wall of the vial. Shake vial vigorously after all the diluent has been added. Depending on the route of administration, use Sterile Water for Injection USP, isotonic Sodium Chloride Injection USP, or Dextrose Injection USP.

NOTE: Penicillins are rapidly inactivated in the presence of carbohydrate solutions at alkaline pH.

Reconstitute with 23 ml, 18ml, 8 ml, or 3 ml diluent to provide concentrations of 200,000 u, 250,000 u, 500,000 u, or 1,000,000 u per ml, respectively.

Storage: The dry powder is relatively stable and may be stored at room temperature without significant loss of potency. Sterile solutions may be kept in the refrigerator one week without significant loss of potency. Solutions prepared for intravenous infusion are stable at room temperature for at least 24 hours.

HOW SUPPLIED - EQUIVALENTS NOT AVAILABLE:

Injection, Dry-Soln - Intramuscular; - 5,000,000 unit/

10's	$66.00	Penicillin G Sodium, Bristol Myers Squibb	00003-0668-05
50 ml x 10	$67.50	Penicillin G Sodium, Vial, Marsam	00209-8586-22

PENICILLIN V POTASSIUM *(001971)*

CATEGORIES: Anti-Infectives; Antibacterials; Antibiotics; Antimicrobials; Chorea; Dental; Endocarditis; Erysipelas; Gingivitis; Heart Disease; Infections; Otitis Media; Penicillins; Perioperative Prophylaxis; Pharyngitis; Renal Drugs; Respiratory Tract Infections; Rheumatic Fever; Scarlet Fever; Skin Infections; Streptococcal Infection; Vincent's Infection; Pregnancy Category B; Sales > $100 Million; FDA Approval Pre 1982; Top 200 Drugs

BRAND NAMES: *Abbocillin VK*; *Acipen*; *Anapenil* (Mexico); *Antibiocin* (Germany); *Apsin VK*; *Apo-Pen-VK* (Canada); *Arcasin* (Germany); *Asillin*; *Beapen*; Beepen-Vk; Betapen-Vk; *Calciopen*; Caropen-Vk; *Cilacil*; *Cilicaine*; *Cilicaine VK*; *Cliacil*; *Compocillin*; *Compocillin VK*; *Copen*; *Crystapen V*; *Darocillin*; *Deltacillin*; *Distaquaine V-K* (England); *DuraPenicillin* (Germany); *Eropen*; *Fenocin*; *Fenospen*; *Fenoxcillin*; *Fenoxypen*; *Interpen*; *Isocillin* (Germany); *Ispenoral*; *Kaypen*; *Kavepenin*; *L.P.V.*; Lanacillin Vk; Ledercillin Vk; *Len V.K.*; *Medoxypen*; *Megacillin*; *Megacillin Oral* (Germany); *Microcillin-VK*; *Micropen-VK*; *Milcopen*; *Monocillin-E*; *Nadopen-V* (Canada); *Newcillin* (Japan); *Novo-VK*; *Novopen*; *Novopen-VK* (Canada); Ora-Vk; *Oracilina*; *Oracillin VK*; *Oracilline*; Orpeneed Vk; *Orpenic*; *Ospen* (France); *Ospen 250*; *Ospen-KV*; *PVF K* (Canada); *PVK*; *P.V.O.*; *Pen-V*; *Pen V*; Pen-Vee K; *Pen Vee K*; *Penadur-VK Mega*; Penapar-Vk; Penicillin-Vk; *Penoral*; *Penoxilin*; *Pentabs*; *Pentacillin*; *Pentid*; *Pentranex*; *Pen-Vi-K* (Mexico); *Penvisil*; Pfizerpen-Vk; Phenoxymethylpenicillin; *Primcillin*; *Rafapen V-K*; Robicillin VK; *Rocilin*; Ropen Vk; *Roscopenin*; *Servipen-V*; *Stabilin V-K*; *Stabillin V-K*; Suspen; *Trepopen*; *Trepopen VK*; Uticillin Vk; *V-Cil-K*; **V-Cillin K**; *V-Kal-K* (Japan); *V-Penicillin Kalium* (Japan); *Vamosyn*; Veetids; *Vepicombin*; Win-Cillin Vk

(International brand names outside U.S. in italics)

FORMULARIES: Aetna; BC-BS; CIGNA; DoD; FHP; Foundation; Humana; Kaiser; Medco; Medi-Cal; PruCare; United; WHO

COST OF THERAPY: $3.27 (Pharyngitis; Tablet; 500 mg; 4/day; 10 days) vs. Potential Cost of $7,048.46 (Respiratory Infections)

DESCRIPTION:

Penicillin V potassium, USP is the potassium salt of penicillin V, USP. This chemically improved form combines acid stability with immediate solubility and rapid absorption. It is designated 4-thia-1-azabicyclo[3.2.0]-heptane-2-carboxylic acid, 3,3 -dimethyl-7-oxo-6-[(phenoxyacetyl)amino]-, monopotassium salt, [2S-(2α,5α,6β)]-. The empirical formula is $C_{16}H_{17}KN_2O_5S$, and the molecular weight is 388.48.

Each tablet contains penicillin V potassium equivalent to 250 mg (400,000 units) or 500 mg (800,000 units) penicillin V. The tablets also contain lactose, magnesium stearate, povidone, starch, stearic acid, and other inactive ingredients.

DESCRIPTION: *(cont'd)*

After being mixed as directed, each 5 ml of the oral solution will contain penicillin V potassium equivalent to 250 mg (400,000 units) penicillin V. The suspension also contains citric acid, F D & C Red No. 40, flavors, saccharin, sodium citrate, and sucrose.

The potassium content of the tablets and oral solution is listed below (TABLE 1).

TABLE 1

Size	Potassium (mEq)	Potassium (mg)
TABLETS		
250 mg (400,000 units)	0.72	28.06
500 mg (800,000 units)	1.44	56.12
ORAL SOLUTION		
250 mg (400,000 units) 5 ml	0.72	28.06

CLINICAL PHARMACOLOGY:

Penicillin V potassium is bactericidal against penicillin-susceptible microorganisms during the stage of active multiplication. It produces its effect by inhibiting biosynthesis of cell-wall mucopeptide. It is not active against the penicillinase-producing bacteria, which include many strains of staphylococci. The drug exerts high *in vitro* activity against staphylococci (except penicillinase-producing strains), streptococci (groups A, C, G, H, L, and M), and pneumococci. Other organisms susceptible *in vitro* to penicillin V are*Corynebacterium diphtheriae, Bacillus anthracis,* clostridia,*Actinomyces bovis, Streptobacillus moniliformis, Listeria monocytogenes, Leptospira,* and *Neisseria gonorrhoeae.Treponema pallidium* is extremely susceptible.

Penicillin V potassium has the distinct advantage over penicillin G in being resistant to inactivation by gastric acid. It may be given with meals; however, blood levels are slightly higher when the drug is given on an empty stomach. Average blood levels are 2 to 5 times higher than those following the same dose of oral penicillin G and also show much less individual variation.

Once absorbed, about 80% of penicillin V potassium is bound to serum protein. Tissue levels are highest in the kidneys, and lesser amounts appear in the liver, skin, and intestines. Small concentrations are found in all other body tissues and the cerebrospinal fluid. The drug is excreted as rapidly as it is absorbed in individuals with normal kidney function; however, recovery of the drug from the urine indicates that only about 25% of the dose given is absorbed. In neonates, young infants, and individuals with impaired kidney function, excretion is considerably delayed.

INDICATIONS AND USAGE:

Penicillin V potassium is indicated in the treatment of mild to moderately severe infections due to microorganisms whose susceptibility to penicillin G is within the range of serum levels common to this particular dosage form. Therapy should be guided by bacteriologic studies (including susceptibility tests) and by clinical response.

NOTE: Severe pneumonia, empyema, bacteremia, pericarditis, meningitis, and arthritis should not be treated with penicillin V during the acute stage.

Indicated surgical procedures should be performed.

The following infections will usually respond to adequate dosage of penicillin V:

Streptococcal Infections (without bacteremia): Mild to moderate infections of the upper respiratory tract, scarlet fever, and mild erysipelas.

NOTE: Streptococci groups A, C, G, H, L, and M are very susceptible to penicillin. Other groups, including group D (enterococcus), are resistant.

Pneumococcal Infections: Mild to moderately severe infections of the respiratory tract.

Staphylococcal Infections Susceptible to Penicillin G: Mild infections of the skin and soft tissues.

NOTE: Reports indicate an increasing number of strains of staphylococci resistant to penicillin G, which emphasizes the need for culture and susceptibility studies in treating suspected staphylococcal infections.

Fusospirochetosis (Vincent's Gingivitis and Pharyngitis): Mild to moderately severe infections of the oropharynx usually respond to therapy with oral penicillin.

NOTE: Necessary dental care should be accomplished in infections involving the gum tissue.

Medical Conditions in Which Oral Penicillin Therapy Is Indicated as Prophylaxis: To prevent recurrence following rheumatic fever and/or chorea. Prophylaxis with oral penicillin on a continuing basis has proved effective in preventing recurrence of these conditions.

Although no controlled clinical efficacy studies have been conducted, penicillin V has been suggested by the American Heart Association and the American Dental Association for use as an oral regimen for prophylaxis against bacterial endocarditis in patients with congenital heart disease or rheumatic or other acquired valvular heart disease when they undergo dental procedures and surgical procedures of the respiratory tract.[1]

Since α-hemolytic streptococci relatively resistant to penicillin may be found when patients are receiving continuous oral penicillin for secondary prevention of rheumatic fever, prophylactic agents other than penicillin may be chosen for these patients and prescribed in addition to their continuous prophylactic regimen for rheumatic fever.

Oral penicillin should not be used as adjunctive prophylaxis for genitourinary instrumentation or surgery, lower intestinal tract surgery, sigmoidoscopy, and childbirth.

NOTE: When selecting antibiotics for the prevention of bacterial endocarditis, the physician or dentist should read the full joint statement of the American Heart Association and the American Dental Association.[1]

CONTRAINDICATIONS:

A previous hypersensitivity reaction to any penicillin is a contraindication.

WARNINGS:

SERIOUS AND OCCASIONALLY FATAL HYPERSENSITIVITY (ANAPHYLACTIC) REACTIONS HAVE BEEN REPORTED IN PATIENTS RECEIVING PENICILLIN THERAPY. THESE REACTIONS ARE MORE LIKELY TO OCCUR IN INDIVIDUALS WITH A HISTORY OF PENICILLIN HYPERSENSITIVITY AND/OR A HISTORY OF SENSITIVITY TO MULTIPLE ALLERGENS. THERE HAVE BEEN REPORTS OF INDIVIDUALS WITH A HISTORY OF PENICILLIN HYPERSENSITIVITY WHO HAVE EXPERIENCED SEVERE REACTIONS WHEN TREATED WITH CEPHALOSPORINS. BEFORE INITIATING THERAPY WITH PENICILLIN V POTASSIUM, CAREFUL INQUIRY SHOULD BE MADE CONCERNING PREVIOUS HYPERSENSITIVITY REACTIONS TO PENICILLINS, CEPHALOSPORINS, OR OTHER ALLERGENS. IF AN ALLERGIC REACTION OCCURS, PENICILLIN V POTASSIUM SHOULD BE DISCONTINUED AND APPROPRIATE THERAPY INSTITUTED. **SERIOUS ANAPHYLACTIC REACTIONS REQUIRE IMMEDIATE EMERGENCY TREATMENT WITH EPINEPHRINE. OXYGEN, INTRAVENOUS STEROIDS, AND AIRWAY MANAGEMENT, INCLUDING INTUBATION, SHOULD ALSO BE ADMINISTRATED AS INDICATED.**

WARNINGS: *(cont'd)*

Pseudomembranous colitis has been reported with nearly all antibacterial agents including penicillins, and may range in severity from mild to life-threatening. Therefore, it is important to consider this diagnosis in patients who present with diarrhea subsequent to the administration of antibacterial agents.

Treatment with antibacterial agents alters the normal flora of the colon and may permit overgrowth of clostridia. Studies indicate that a toxin produced by *Clostridium difficile* is one primary cause of "antibiotic-associated colitis."

After the diagnosis of pseudomembranous colitis has been established, therapeutic measures should be initiated. Mild cases of pseudomembranous colitis usually respond to drug discontinuation alone. In moderate to severe cases, consideration should be given to management with fluids and electrolytes, protein supplementation, and treatment with an antibacterial drug clinically effective against *C. difficile* colitis.

PRECAUTIONS:

Penicillin should be used with caution in individuals with histories of significant allergies and/or asthma.

The oral route of administration should not be relied upon in patients with severe illness or with nausea, vomiting, gastric dilatation, cardiospasm, or intestinal hypermotility.

Occasional patients will not absorb therapeutic amounts of orally administered penicillin.

In streptococcal infections, therapy must be sufficient to eliminate the organism (a minimum of 10 days); otherwise, the sequelae of streptococcal disease may occur. Cultures should be taken following completion of treatment to determine whether streptococci have been eradicated.

Prolonged use of antibiotics may promote the overgrowth of nonsusceptible organisms, including fungi. If superinfection occurs, appropriate measures should be taken.

ADVERSE REACTIONS:

Although reactions have been reported much less frequently after oral than after parenteral penicillin therapy, it should be remembered that all degrees of hypersensitivity, including fatal anaphylaxis, have been observed with oral penicillin.

The most common reactions to oral penicillin are nausea, vomiting, epigastric distress, diarrhea, and black, hairy tongue. The hypersensitivity reactions noted are skin eruptions (ranging from maculopapular to exfoliative dermatitis); urticaria; reactions resembling serum sickness, including chills, fever, edema, arthralgia, and prostration; laryngeal edema; and anaphylaxis. Fever and eosinophilia may frequently be the only reactions observed. Hemolytic anemia, leukopenia, thrombocytopenia, neuropathy, and nephropathy are infrequent reactions and are usually associated with high doses of parenteral penicillin.

OVERDOSAGE:

Signs and Symptoms: Symptoms of large oral overdose of penicillin may cause nausea, vomiting, stomach pain, diarrhea, and, in rare cases, major motor seizures. If other symptoms are present, consideration must also be given to the possibility of an allergic reaction or symptoms secondary to a concurrent medication or other underlying disease state, especially in adults.

Treatment: To obtain up-to-date information about the treatment of overdose, a good resource is your certified Regional Poison Control Center. Telephone numbers of certified poison control centers are listed in *Physicians GenRx*. In managing overdosage, consider the possibility of multiple drug overdoses, interaction among drugs, and unusual drug kinetics in your patient.

Ensure adequate ventilation and protect the patient's airway while attempting to limit drug absorption. In oral overdosage, consideration must be given to emesis or lavage to evacuate the stomach, and administration of activated charcoal by mouth or via lavage tube with a cathartic such as sorbitol may hasten drug elimination. Penicillin may be removed by hemodialysis. No specific antidote is known to be effective.

DOSAGE AND ADMINISTRATION:

The dosage of penicillin V potassium should be determined according to the susceptibility of the causative microorganism and the severity of infection and should be adjusted to the clinical response of the patient.

The usual dosage recommendations for adults and children 12 years and over are as follows:

Streptococcal Infections: Mild to moderately severe infections of the upper respiratory tract, including scarlet fever and mild erysipelas: 200,000 to 500,000 units every 6 to 8 hours for 10 days.

Pneumococcal Infections: Mild to moderately severe infections of the respiratory tract, including otitis media: 400,000 to 500,000 units every 6 hours until the patient has been afebrile for at least 2 days.

Staphylococcal Infections: Mild infections of skin and soft tissue (culture and susceptibility tests should be performed): 400,000 to 500,000 units every 6 to 8 hours.

Fusospirochetosis (Vincent's Infection) of the Oropharynx: Mild to moderately severe infections: 400,000 to 500,000 units every 6 to 8 hours.

Prophylaxis in the Following Conditions: To prevent recurrence following rheumatic fever and/or chorea: 200,000 to 250,000 units twice daily on a continuing basis.

For prophylaxis against bacterial endocarditis[1] in patients with congenital heart disease or rheumatic or other acquired valvular heart disease when undergoing dental procedures or surgical procedures of the upper respiratory tract, 1 of 2 regimens may be selected:

(1) For the oral regimen, the usual adult dosage is 2 g of penicillin V (1 g for children less than 30 kg) 1 hour before the procedure and then 1 g (500 mg for children less than 30 kg) 6 hours later.

(2) For patients unable to take oral antibiotics, 2,000,000 units of aqueous penicillin G (50,000 units/kg for children) IV or IM may be substituted 30 to 60 minutes before the procedure and 1,000,000 units (25,000 units/kg for children) 6 hours later.

For patients with prosthetic valves and for those at highest risk for endocarditis, ampicillin, 1 to 2 g (50 mg/kg for children), plus gentamicin, 1.5 mg/kg (2 mg/kg for children), IM or IV, may be given one- half hour prior to the procedure, followed by 1 g of oral penicillin V 6 hours later. Alternatively, the parenteral regimen should be repeated once every 8 hours later.

Children's antibiotic dosages should not exceed the maximum adult doses.

NOTE: Therapy for children under 12 years of age is calculated on the basis of body weight. For infants and small children, the suggested daily dose is 25,000 to 90,000 units (15 to 50 mg)/kg in 3 to 6 divided doses.

After being mixed, the solution should be stored in a refrigerator. It may be kept for 14 days without significant loss of potency. Shake well before using. Keep tightly closed.

Tablets should be stored at controlled room temperature, 59° to 86°F (15° to 30°C).

REFERENCES:

1. Dajani AS, Bisno AL, et al: Prevention of bacterial endocarditis. Recommendations by the American Heart Association. *JAMA*, 1990;264:2919.

PATIENT INFORMATION:

Penicillin V potassium is an antibiotic used to treat a variety of infections, most notably strep throat. This drug is also used to prevent infections (bacterial endocarditis) in patients with congenital heart disease or rheumatic or other acquired valvular heart disease. Penicillin is taken before dental procedures and surgical procedures in these patients. This drug should not be used by those with allergies to penicillin and you should consult with your pharmacist or physician if you are allergic to penicillin before taking this medication. The most common side effects from penicillin include: nausea, vomiting, epigastric distress, and diarrhea. Because this medication is used to treat infections, it should be taken as prescribed. Even if your symptoms are better, the entire supply of medication should be taken to ensure the infection is cured. Liquid forms of penicillin must be refrigerated and shaken before administered.

HOW SUPPLIED - RATED THERAPEUTICALLY EQUIVALENT:

Powder, Reconstitution - Oral - 125 mg/5ml

100 ml	$1.21	BETAPEN-VK, Mead Johnson	00015-7506-59
100 ml	$1.27	Penicillin V Potassium, Harber Pharm	51432-0695-14
100 ml	$1.65	Penicillin VK, H.C.F.A. F F P	99999-1971-01
100 ml	$1.72	Penicillin V Potassium, Harber Pharm	51432-0696-14
100 ml	$1.74	VEETIDS 125, Bristol Myers Squibb	00003-0681-44
100 ml	$1.74	Penicillin V, HL Moore Drug Exch	00839-5189-73
100 ml	$1.81	PEN-VEE K, Wyeth Labs	00008-0004-06
100 ml	$1.86	LEDERCILLIN VK, Lederle Pharm	00005-3874-46
100 ml	$2.04	Penicillin V, United Res	00677-0109-27
100 ml	$2.16	PENICILLIN-VK, Goldline Labs	00182-0276-70
100 ml	$2.16	Penicillin VK, Teva	00332-4125-32
100 ml	$2.16	Penicillin V Potassium, Major Pharms	00904-4001-04
100 ml	$2.25	Penicillin V, Rugby	00536-2540-82
100 ml	$2.28	Penicillin VK, Qualitest Pharms	00603-6605-64
100 ml	$2.38	Penicillin VK, Warner Chilcott	00047-2449-17
100 ml	$2.51	Penicillin-Vk, Aligen Independ	00405-3500-60
100 ml x 6	$2.00	BEEPEN-VK, Beecham	00029-6165-23
150 ml	$2.40	LEDERCILLIN VK, Lederle Pharm	00005-3874-49
150 ml	$2.47	Penicillin VK, H.C.F.A. F F P	99999-1971-02
150 ml	**$3.84**	**V-CILLIN K, Lilly**	**00002-2307-68**
200 ml	$2.05	Penicillin V Potassium, Harber Pharm	51432-0695-16
200 ml	$2.24	Penicillin VK, H.C.F.A. F F P	99999-1971-03
200 ml	$2.36	Penicillin V Potassium, HL Moore Drug Exch	00839-5189-78
200 ml	$2.50	BETAPEN-VK, Mead Johnson	00015-7506-70
200 ml	$2.92	Penicillin V Potassium, Harber Pharm	51432-0696-16
200 ml	$2.99	VEETIDS 125, Bristol Myers Squibb	00003-0681-54
200 ml	$3.03	Penicillin V, United Res	00677-0109-29
200 ml	$3.08	LEDERCILLIN VK, Lederle Pharm	00005-3874-60
200 ml	$3.14	PEN-VEE K, Wyeth Labs	00008-0004-07
200 ml	$3.25	Penicillin V, Rugby	00536-2540-84
200 ml	$3.34	PENICILLIN-VK, Goldline Labs	00182-0276-73
200 ml	$3.34	Penicillin VK, Teva	00332-4125-36
200 ml	$3.34	Penicillin VK, Qualitest Pharms	00603-6605-68
200 ml	$3.34	Penicillin V Potassium, Major Pharms	00904-4001-08
200 ml	$3.47	Penicillin VK, Warner Chilcott	00047-2449-20
200 ml	$3.92	Penicillin-Vk, Aligen Independ	00405-3500-70
200 ml	**$4.24**	**V-CILLIN K, Lilly**	**00002-2307-89**
200 ml x 6	$3.05	BEEPEN-VK, Beecham	00029-6165-24

Powder, Reconstitution - Oral - 250 mg/5ml

100 ml	$1.67	BETAPEN-VK, Mead Johnson	00015-7507-59
100 ml	$1.88	Penicillin VK, H.C.F.A. F F P	99999-1971-04
100 ml	$2.11	LEDERCILLIN VK, Lederle Pharm	00005-3875-46
100 ml	$2.21	Penicillin V, HL Moore Drug Exch	00839-5190-73
100 ml	$2.25	VEETIDS 250, Bristol Myers Squibb	00003-0682-44
100 ml	$2.50	Penicillin VK, United Res	00677-0110-27
100 ml	$2.73	Pen Vee K, Wyeth Labs	00008-0036-04
100 ml	$2.89	Penicillin VK, Schein Pharm (US)	00364-2024-61
100 ml	$2.95	Penicillin VK, Teva	00332-4127-32
100 ml	$2.95	PENICILLIN-VK, Rugby	00536-2560-82
100 ml	$2.95	Penicillin V Potassium, Major Pharms	00904-4004-04
100 ml	$3.03	Penicillin-Vk, Aligen Independ	00405-3525-60
100 ml	$3.08	Penicillin VK, Qualitest Pharms	00603-6606-64
100 ml	$3.24	BETAPEN-VK, Mead Johnson	00015-7507-40
100 ml	$3.24	Penicillin VK, Warner Chilcott	00047-2506-17
100 ml	**$4.46**	**V-CILLIN K, Lilly**	**00002-2316-48**
100 ml	$5.07	PENICILLIN-VK, Goldline Labs	00182-0308-73
100 ml x 6	$2.60	BEEPEN-VK, Beecham	00029-6170-23
150 ml	$2.82	Penicillin VK, H.C.F.A. F F P	99999-1971-06
150 ml	$3.06	LEDERCILLIN VK, Lederle Pharm	00005-3875-49
150 ml	$3.79	PEN VEE K, Wyeth Labs	00008-0036-03
150 ml	**$6.72**	**V-CILLIN K, Lilly**	**00002-2316-68**
200 ml	$2.95	PENICILLIN-VK, Goldline Labs	00182-0308-70
200 ml	$3.08	Penicillin VK, H.C.F.A. F F P	99999-1971-05
200 ml	$3.36	BETAPEN-VK, Mead Johnson	00015-7507-70
200 ml	$3.42	Penicillin V, HL Moore Drug Exch	00839-5190-78
200 ml	$3.79	VEETIDS 250, Bristol Myers Squibb	00003-0682-54
200 ml	$4.04	LEDERCILLIN VK, Lederle Pharm	00005-3875-60
200 ml	$4.06	Pen Vee K, Wyeth Labs	00008-0036-05
200 ml	$4.30	Penicillin VK, United Res	00677-0110-29
200 ml	$4.31	Penicillin VK, Purepac Pharm	00228-2328-83
200 ml	$4.65	PENICILLIN-VK, Rugby	00536-2560-84
200 ml	$5.07	Penicillin VK, Teva	00332-4127-36
200 ml	$5.07	Penicillin VK, Qualitest Pharms	00603-6606-68
200 ml	$5.07	Penicillin V Potassium, Major Pharms	00904-4004-08
200 ml	$5.10	Penicillin VK, Schein Pharm (US)	00364-2024-63
200 ml	$5.30	BETAPEN-VK, Mead Johnson	00015-7507-64
200 ml	$5.31	Penicillin VK, Warner Chilcott	00047-2506-20
200 ml	$5.42	Penicillin-Vk, Aligen Independ	00405-3525-70
200 ml	**$7.65**	**V-CILLIN K, Lilly**	**00002-2316-89**
200 ml x 6	$4.35	BEEPEN-VK, Beecham	00029-6170-24

Tablet, Uncoated - Oral - 125 mg

100's	**$10.86**	**V-CILLIN K, Lilly**	**00002-0327-02**

Tablet, Uncoated - Oral - 250 mg

40's	$2.08	Penicillin VK, H.C.F.A. F F P	99999-1971-07
40's	$36.63	LEDERCILLIN VK, Lederle Pharm	00005-3865-61
100's	$4.17	Penicillin V Potassium, Harber Pharm	51432-0332-03
100's	$4.68	BETAPEN-VK, Mead Johnson	00015-7508-64
100's	$5.22	Penicillin VK, Geneva Pharms	00781-1205-01
100's	$5.22	Penicillin VK, H.C.F.A. F F P	99999-1971-08
100's	$5.25	Penicillin V Potassium, IDE-Interstate	00814-5863-14
100's	$5.25	Penicillin V Potassium, IDE-Interstate	00814-5866-14
100's	$5.34	Penicillin VK, Teva	00332-1171-09
100's	$5.34	Penicillin VK, Teva	00332-1172-09
100's	$5.50	Penicillin V K, Major Pharms	00904-2450-60
100's	$6.00	PEN-V, Goldline Labs	00182-0869-01
100's	$6.07	Penicillin V Oval, Schein Pharm (US)	00364-2021-01

HOW SUPPLIED - RATED THERAPEUTICALLY EQUIVALENT: *(cont'd)*

100's	$6.49	LEDERCILLIN VK, Lederle Pharm	00005-3865-23
100's	$7.13	VEETIDS, Bristol Myers Squibb	00003-0115-50
100's	$7.20	Penicillin-VK, Aligen Independ	00405-4762-01
100's	$7.20	Penicillin-Vk, Aligen Independ	00405-4768-01
100's	$7.31	Penicillin VK, United Res	00677-0107-01
100's	$7.31	Penicillin VK, United Res	00677-0411-01
100's	$7.36	Penicillin VK, HL Moore Drug Exch	00839-5187-06
100's	$7.36	Penicillin VK, HL Moore Drug Exch	00839-5188-06
100's	$7.41	Penicillin VK, Purepac Pharm	00228-2324-10
100's	$7.65	Penicillin V, Rugby	00536-2520-01
100's	$7.65	Penicillin V, Rugby	00536-2527-01
100's	$8.12	Penicillin VK 250, Warner Chilcott	00047-0648-24
100's	$12.24	PEN-VEE K, Wyeth Labs	00008-0059-02
100's	$13.34	PEN-VEE K, Wyeth Labs	00008-0059-10
100's	**$21.46**	**V-CILLIN K, Lilly**	**00002-0329-02**
100's	$41.70	Penicillin V Potassium, Harber Pharm	51432-0332-06
500's	$26.10	Penicillin VK, H.C.F.A. F F P	99999-1971-09
500's	$48.13	PEN-VEE K, Wyeth Labs	00008-0059-04
500's	**$101.27**	**V-CILLIN K, Lilly**	**00002-0329-03**
1000's	$30.00	Truxcillin-Vk 250 Mg Tablets, C O Truxton	00463-5017-10
1000's	$42.38	Penicillin V Potassium, IDE-Interstate	00814-5866-30
1000's	$42.79	Penicillin VK, Teva	00332-1171-15
1000's	$42.79	Penicillin VK, Teva	00332-1172-15
1000's	$43.00	Penicillin V K, Major Pharms	00904-2450-80
1000's	$45.90	PENICILLIN-V, Goldline Labs	00182-0116-10
1000's	$45.90	PEN-V, Goldline Labs	00182-0869-10
1000's	$47.20	BETAPEN-VK, Mead Johnson	00015-7508-85
1000's	$51.47	Penicillin-Vk Tablets 250 Mg, Aligen Independ	00405-4762-03
1000's	$51.47	Penicillin-Vk, Aligen Independ	00405-4768-03
1000's	$52.20	Penicillin VK, H.C.F.A. F F P	99999-1971-10
1000's	$53.45	Penicillin VK, HL Moore Drug Exch	00839-5187-16
1000's	$53.45	Penicillin VK, HL Moore Drug Exch	00839-5188-16
1000's	$56.51	Penicillin V Oval, Schein Pharm (US)	00364-2021-02
1000's	$57.12	Penicillin VK, Qualitest Pharms	00603-5067-32
1000's	$57.25	Penicillin V, Rugby	00536-2520-10
1000's	$57.25	Penicillin V, Rugby	00536-2527-10
1000's	$58.75	Penicillin VK, United Res	00677-0107-10
1000's	$59.40	Penicillin VK, Geneva Pharms	00781-1205-10
1000's	$59.47	Penicillin VK 250, Warner Chilcott	00047-0648-32
1000's	$59.50	Penicillin V Potassium, Mylan	00378-0111-10
1000's	$59.50	Penicillin V Potassium, Mylan	00378-0195-10
1000's	$59.70	BEEPEN-VK, Beecham	00029-6150-33
1000's	$59.83	VEETIDS, Bristol Myers Squibb	00003-0115-75
1000's	$60.07	LEDERCILLIN VK, Lederle Pharm	00005-3865-34

Tablet, Uncoated - Oral - 500 mg

40's	$3.27	Penicillin VK, H.C.F.A. F F P	99999-1971-11
100's	$8.18	Penicillin VK, H.C.F.A. F F P	99999-1971-12
100's	$8.86	BETAPEN-VK, Mead Johnson	00015-7509-64
100's	$9.24	Penicillin VK, Teva	00332-1173-09
100's	$9.24	Penicillin VK, Teva	00332-1174-09
100's	$9.51	ROBICILLIN VK, AH Robins	00031-8227-63
100's	$9.75	Penicillin V Potassium, IDE-Interstate	00814-5870-14
100's	$9.75	Penicillin V Potassium, IDE-Interstate	00814-5871-14
100's	$9.90	Penicillin V Potassium, Major Pharms	00904-2451-60
100's	$11.40	PENICILLIN-V, Goldline Labs	00182-0115-01
100's	$11.40	PEN-V, Goldline Labs	00182-1537-01
100's	$11.68	Penicillin VK, HL Moore Drug Exch	00839-1766-06
100's	$11.68	Penicillin VK, HL Moore Drug Exch	00839-6393-06
100's	$12.25	Penicillin-VK, Aligen Independ	00405-4763-01
100's	$12.25	Penicillin-Vk, Aligen Independ	00405-4769-01
100's	$12.32	Penicillin VK, Purepac Pharm	00228-2330-10
100's	$12.38	Penicillin VK, United Res	00677-0108-01
100's	$12.38	Penicillin VK, United Res	00677-0576-01
100's	$12.81	LEDERCILLIN VK, Lederle Pharm	00005-3866-23
100's	$12.99	Penicillin VK Oval, Schein Pharm (US)	00364-2058-01
100's	$13.20	Penicillin V, Rugby	00536-2530-01
100's	$13.20	Penicillin VK Oval, Rugby	00536-2537-01
100's	$13.55	VEETIDS, Bristol Myers Squibb	00003-0116-50
100's	$14.91	Penicillin VK, Warner Chilcott	00047-0673-24
100's	$15.30	Penicillin VK, Geneva Pharms	00781-1655-01
100's	$15.33	Penicillin VK, Qualitest Pharms	00603-5068-21
100's	$15.35	Penicillin V Potassium, Mylan	00378-0112-01
100's	$15.35	Penicillin V Potassium, Mylan	00378-0198-01
100's	$23.01	Pen Vee K, Wyeth Labs	00008-0390-01
100's	$26.13	PEN VEE K, Wyeth Labs	00008-0390-04
100's	**$40.60**	**V-CILLIN K, Lilly**	**00002-0346-02**
100's	$87.95	Penicillin VK, United Res	00677-0108-10
300's	$59.52	Penicillin VK, Warner Chilcott	00047-0673-30
500's	$40.90	Penicillin VK, H.C.F.A. F F P	99999-1971-14
500's	$44.44	BETAPEN-VK, Mead Johnson	00015-7509-81
500's	$61.25	BEEPEN-VK, Beecham	00029-6160-32
500's	$62.44	LEDERCILLIN VK, Lederle Pharm	00005-3866-31
500's	**$190.07**	**V-CILLIN K, Lilly**	**00002-0346-03**
1000's	$67.76	Penicillin VK, HL Moore Drug Exch	00839-1766-16
1000's	$81.00	Penicillin V Potassium, Major Pharms	00904-2452-80
1000's	$81.80	Penicillin VK, H.C.F.A. F F P	99999-1971-13
1000's	$84.54	Penicillin VK, Teva	00332-1173-15
1000's	$84.54	Penicillin VK, Teva	00332-1174-15
1000's	$84.54	Penicillin V K, Major Pharms	00904-2451-80
1000's	$85.95	Penicillin V, Rugby	00536-2530-10
1000's	$85.95	Penicillin VK Oval, Rugby	00536-2537-10
1000's	$87.95	Penicillin V Potassium, United Res	00677-0576-10
1000's	$88.00	PENICILLIN-V, Goldline Labs	00182-0115-10
1000's	$88.00	PEN-V, Goldline Labs	00182-1537-10
1000's	$89.93	Penicillin VK Oval, Schein Pharm (US)	00364-2058-02
1000's	$89.93	Penicillin V Potassium, IDE-Interstate	00814-5870-30
1000's	$89.93	Penicillin VK, IDE-Interstate	00814-5871-30
1000's	$96.82	VEETIDS, Bristol Myers Squibb	00003-0116-75
1000's	$97.50	Penicillin V Potassium, Mylan	00378-0112-10
1000's	$97.50	Penicillin V Potassium, Mylan	00378-0198-10
1000's	$99.47	Penicillin-Vk, Aligen Independ	00405-4769-03
1000's	$103.37	Penicillin-VK, Aligen Independ	00405-4763-03

PENTAERYTHRITOL TETRANITRATE *(001972)*

CATEGORIES: Angina; Antianginals; Cardiovascular Drugs; Central Nervous System Agents; DESI Drugs; Nitrates; Vasodilating Agents; FDA Pre 1938 Drugs

BRAND NAMES: *Dilcoran*; *Dilcoran 80* (Germany); *Dilcoran Retard*; Duotrate; *Maxicardyl*; *Mycardol* (England); *Nitrodex* (France); P.E.T.N.; *Pectolex* (Japan); Pentet; Pentol; Pentylan; **Peritrate**; *Peritrate Forte* (Canada); *Peritrate L.P.*; *Peritrate Retard*; *Peritrate SA* (Canada); *Peritrate Sincroni*; Perphenazine; Tetraneed
(International brand names outside U.S. in italics)

FORMULARIES: Medi-Cal

DESCRIPTION:

Pentaerythritol tetranitrate is a nitric acid ester of a tetrahydric alcohol (pentaerythritol).

Pentaerythritol Acetate 10 mg and 20 mg contain alginic acid, NF; D&C yellow No. 10; FD&C blue No. 1; gelatin, NF; lactose, NF; methylcellulose, USP; propylparaben, NF; corn starch, NF; stearic acid, NF; and may also contain magnesium stearate, NF. Pentaerythritol Acetate 40 mg contains D&C yellow No. 10 Al lake; D&C red No. 30 Al lake; lactose, NF; povidone, USP; silicon dioxide, NF; corn starch, NF; stearic acid, NF; and confectioner's sugar, NF.

CLINICAL PHARMACOLOGY:

The exact cause of angina pectoris (that is, the pain associated with coronary artery disease) remains obscure despite the numerous and often conflicting hypotheses concerning its pathophysiology. Therapy at the present time, therefore, remains essentially empirical. Customarily, clinical improvement has been measured by: reduction in (1) number, intensity and duration of angina pectoris attacks and (2) necessity for glyceryl trinitrate intake for prevention or relief of anginal attacks, Pentaerythritol Acetate has been reported in clinical usage to reduce in number and severity the incidence of angina pectoris attacks, with concomitant reduction in glyceryl trinitrate intake.

In the evaluation of Pentaerythritol Acetate in angina pectoris, clinical improvement has been customarily measured subjectively by: reduction in number and severity of attacks and necessity for glyceryl trinitrate intake for prevention or abortion of anginal attacks. Individual patterns of angina pectoris differ widely as does the symptomatic response to antianginal agents such as pentaerythritol tetranitrate. The published literature contains both favorable and unfavorable clinical reports. In conjunction with total management of the patient with angina pectoris, Pentaerythritol Acetate has been accepted as safe for prolonged administration and widely regarded as useful.

INDICATIONS AND USAGE:

INDICATIONS AND USAGE:
Based on a review of this drug by the National Academy of Sciences—National Research Council and/or other information, FDA has classified the indications as follows:
"Possibly" effective: Pentaerythritol Acetate is indicated for the relief of angina pectoris (pain associated with coronary artery disease). It is not intended to abort the acute anginal episode but is widely regarded as useful in the prophylactic treatment of angina pectoris.
Final classification of the less-than-effective indications requires further investigation.

CONTRAINDICATIONS:

Pentaerythritol Acetate is contraindicated in patients who have a history of sensitivity to the drug.

WARNINGS:

Data supporting the use of Pentaerythritol Acetate during the early days of the acute phase of myocardial infarction (the period during which clinical and laboratory findings are unstable) are insufficient to establish safety.

This drug can act as a physiological antagonist to norepinephrine, acetylcholine, histamine, and many other agents.

PRECAUTIONS:

Should be used with caution in patients who have glaucoma. Tolerance to this drug and cross-tolerance to other nitrites and nitrates may occur.

ADVERSE REACTIONS:

Side effects reported to date have been predominantly related to rash (which requires discontinuation of medication) and headache and gastrointestinal distress, which are usually mild and transient with continuation of medication. In some cases severe persistent headaches may occur.

In addition, the following adverse reactions to nitrates such as pentaerythritol tetranitrate have been reported in the literature:

(a) Cutaneous vasodilatation with flushing.

(b) Transient episodes of dizziness and weakness, as well as other signs of cerebral ischemia associated with postural hypotension, may occasionally develop.

(c) An occasional individual exhibits marked sensitivity to the hypotensive effects of nitrite, and severe responses (nausea, vomiting, weakness, restlessness, pallor, perspiration and collapse) can occur, even with the usual therapeutic doses. Alcohol may enhance this effect.

DOSAGE AND ADMINISTRATION:

Pentaerythritol Acetate may be administered in individualized doses up to 160 mg a day. Dosage can be initiated at one 10 mg or 20 mg tablet q.i.d. and titrated upward to 40 mg (two 20 mg tablets or one 40 mg tablet) q.i.d. one-half hour before or one hour after meals and at bedtime. Tablets can be chewed or swallowed whole.

Store at controlled room temperature 15-30°C (59-86°F).

ANIMAL PHARMACOLOGY:

In a series of carefully designed studies in pigs, Pentaerythritol Acetate was administered for 48 hours before an artificially induced occlusion of a major coronary artery and for seven days thereafter. The pigs were sacrificed at various intervals for periods up to six weeks. The result showed a significantly larger number of survivors in the drug-treated group. Damage to myocardial tissue in the drug-treated survivors was less extensive than in the untreated group. Studies in dogs subjected to oligemic shock through progressive bleeding have demonstrated

ANIMAL PHARMACOLOGY: *(cont'd)*

that Pentaerythritol Acetate is vasoactive at the postarteriolar level, producing increased blood flow and better tissue perfusion. These animal experiments cannot be translated to the drug's actions in humans.

HOW SUPPLIED - EQUIVALENTS NOT AVAILABLE:

Tablet, Uncoated - Oral - 10 mg

100's	**$16.02**	**PERITRATE, Parke-Davis**	**00071-0013-24**
250's	$13.45	Pentaerythritol Tetranitrate 10, Major Pharms	00904-2147-70
500's	$10.40	PENTYLAN, Lannett	00527-1202-05
1000's	$18.00	PENTYLAN, Lannett	00527-1202-10
1000's	$29.90	Pentaerythritol Tetranitrate 10, Major Pharms	00904-2147-80

Tablet, Uncoated - Oral - 20 mg

100's	$3.20	PENTYLAN, Lannett	00527-1208-01
100's	**$21.18**	**PERITRATE, Parke-Davis**	**00071-0001-24**
250's	$17.25	Pentaerythritol Tetranitrate 20, Major Pharms	00904-2165-70
500's	$13.20	PENTYLAN, Lannett	00527-1208-05
1000's	$24.00	PENTYLAN, Lannett	00527-1208-10
1000's	$37.40	Pentaerythritol Tetranitrate 20, Major Pharms	00904-2165-80

Tablet, Uncoated - Oral - 40 mg

100's	**$37.81**	**PERITRATE, Parke-Davis**	**00071-0008-24**

Tablet, Uncoated, Sustained Action - Oral - 80 mg

100's	**$51.29**	**PERITRATE SA, Parke-Davis**	**00071-0004-24**

PENTAMIDINE ISETHIONATE *(001975)*

CATEGORIES: AIDS Related Complex; Anti-Infectives; Antiprotozoals; HIV Infection; Orphan Drugs; Parasiticidal; Pneumocystis Carinii Pneumonia; Protozoal Agents; Kaposi's Sarcoma*; Pregnancy Category C; FDA Approved 1984 Oct
* Indication not approved by the FDA

BRAND NAMES: Nebupent; *Pentacarinat* (Australia, Europe, Mexico, Canada); **Pentam 300**
(International brand names outside U.S. in italics)

FORMULARIES: Aetna; BC-BS; Medi-Cal; WHO

DESCRIPTION:

INHALATION SOLUTION

NebuPent (Pentamidine Isethionate), an anti-protozoal agent, is a sterile and nonpyrogenic lyophilized product. After reconstitution with Sterile Water for Injection, USP, NebuPent is administered by inhalation via the Respirgard II nebulizer [Marquest, Englewood, CO]. (see DOSAGE AND ADMINISTRATION.)

INJECTION

Pentam 300 (sterile pentamidine isethionate),

an anti-protozoal agent, is a nonpyrogenic lyophilized product. After reconstitution, it should be administered by intramuscular or intravenous (IM or IV) routes. (See DOSAGE AND ADMINISTRATION.)

Pentamidine isethionate is a white crystalline powder soluble in water and glycerin and insoluble in ether, acetone, and chloroform. It is chemically designated as 4,4'-diamidino-diphenoxypentane di- (β-hydroxyethanesulfonate) with the following empirical formula: $C_{23}H_{36}N_4O_{10}S_2$ with a molecular weight of 592.68.

Each vial contains: Pentamidine isethionate - 300 mg

CLINICAL PHARMACOLOGY:

MICROBIOLOGY

Inhalation Solution and Injection: Pentamidine isethionate, an aromatic diamidine, is known to have activity against *Pneumocystis carinii.* The mode of action is not fully understood. *In vitro* studies with mammalian tissues and the protozoan *Crithidia oncopelti* indicate that the drug interferes with nuclear metabolism producing inhibition of the synthesis of DNA, RNA, phospholipids and proteins.

PHARMACOKINETICS

Inhalation Solution: In 5 AIDS patients with suspected *Pneumocystis carinii* pneumonia (PCP), the mean concentrations of pentamidine determined 18 to 24 hours after inhalation therapy were 23.2 ng/ml (range 5.1 to 43.0 ng/ml) in bronchoalveolar lavage fluid and 705 ng/ml (range, 140 to 1336 ng/ml) in sediment after administration of a 300 mg single dose via the Respirgard II nebulizer. In 3 AIDS patients with suspected PCP, the mean concentrations of pentamidine determined 18 to 24 hours after a 4 mg/kg intravenous dose were 2.6 ng/ml (range 1.5 to 4.0 ng/ml) in bronchoalveolar lavage fluid and 9.3 ng/ml (range, 6.9 to 12.8 ng/ml) in sediment. In the patients who received aerosolized pentamidine, the peak plasma levels of pentamidine were at or below the lower limit of detection of the assay (2.3 ng/ml).

Following a single 2-hour intravenous infusion of 4 mg/kg of pentamidine isethionate to 6 AIDS patients, the mean plasma Cmax, T 1/2 and clearance were 612 ± 371 ng/ml, 6.4 ± 1.3 hr and 248 ± 91 l/hr respectively. In another study of aerosolized pentamidine in 13 AIDS patients with acute PCP who received 4 mg/kg/day administered via the Ultra Vent jet nebulizer, peak plasma levels of pentamidine averaged 18.8 ± 11.9 ng/ml after the first dose. During the next 14 days of repeated dosing, the highest observed Cmax averaged 20.5 ± 21.2 ng/ml. In a third study, following daily administration of 600 mg of inhaled pentamidine isethionate with the Respirgard II nebulizer for 21 days in 11 patients with acute PCP, mean plasma levels measured shortly after the 21st dose averaged 11.8 ± 10.0 ng/ml. Plasma concentrations after aerosol administration are substantially lower than those observed after a comparable intravenous dose. The extent of pentamidine accumulation and distribution following chronic inhalation therapy are not known.

In rats, intravenous administration of a 5 mg/kg dose resulted in concentrations of pentamidine in the liver and kidney that were 87.5 and 62.3-fold higher, respectively, than levels in those organs following 5 mg/kg administered as an aerosol.

No pharmacokinetic data are available following aerosol administration of pentamidine in humans with impaired hepatic or renal function.

Injection: Little is known about the drug's pharmacokinetics. Preliminary studies have shown that in seven patients treated with daily IM doses of pentamidine at 4 mg/kg for 10 to 12 days, plasma concentrations were between 0.3 and 0.5 mcg/ml. The levels did not appreciably change with time after injection or from day to day. Higher plasma levels were encountered in patients with an elevated BUN. The patients continued to excrete decreasing amounts of pentamidine in urine up to six to eight weeks after cessation of the treatment.

CLINICAL PHARMACOLOGY: *(cont'd)*

Tissue distribution has been studied in mice given a single intraperitoneal injection of pentamidine at 10 mg/kg. The concentration in the kidneys was the highest followed by that in the liver. In mice, pentamidine was excreted unchanged, primarily via the kidneys with some elimination in the feces. The ratio of amounts excreted in the urine and feces (4:1) was constant over the period of study.

INDICATIONS AND USAGE:

INHALATION SOLUTION

NebuPent is indicated for the prevention of *Pneumocystis carinii*pneumonia (PCP) in high-risk, HIV-infected patients defined by one or both of the following criteria:

i. a history of one or more episodes of PCP

ii. a peripheral CD4+ (T4 helper/inducer) lymphocyte count less than or equal to 200/mm^3.

These indications are based on the results of an 18-month randomized, dose-response trial in high risk HIV-infected patients and on existing epidemiological data from natural history studies.

The patient population of the controlled trial consisted of 408 patients, 237 of whom had a history of one or more episodes of PCP. The remaining patients without a history of PCP included 55 patients with Kaposi's sarcoma and 116 patients with other AIDS diagnoses, ARC or asymptomatic HIV infection. Patients were randomly assigned to receive NebuPent via the Respirgard II nebulizer at one of the following three doses: 30 mg every two weeks (n=135), 150 mg every two weeks (n=134) or 300 mg every four weeks (n=139). The results of the trial demonstrated a significant protective effect ($p<0.01$) against PCP with the 300 mg every four week dosage regimen compared to the 30 mg every two week dosage regimen. The 300 mg dose regimen reduced the risk of developing PCP by 50 to 70% compared to the 30 mg regimen. A total of 293 patients (72% of all patients) also received zidovudine at sometime during the trial.

The analysis of the data demonstrated the efficacy of the 300 mg dose even after adjusting for the effect of zidovudine.

The results of the trial further demonstrate that the dose and frequency of dosing are important to the efficacy of NebuPent prophylaxis in that multiple analyses consistently demonstrated a trend toward greater efficacy with 300 mg every four weeks as compared to 150 mg every two weeks.

No dose-response was observed for reduction in overall mortality; however, mortality from PCP was low in all three dosage groups.

INJECTION

Pentam 300 (sterile pentamidine isethionate) is indicated for the treatment of pneumonia due to *Pneumocystis carinii.*

CONTRAINDICATIONS:

INHALATION SOLUTION

NebuPent is contraindicated in patients with a history of an anaphylactic reaction to inhaled or parenteral pentamidine isethionate.

INJECTION

Once the diagnosis of *Pneumocystis carinii* pneumonia has been firmly established, there are no absolute contraindications to the use of pentamidine isethionate.

WARNINGS:

INHALATION SOLUTION

The potential for development of acute PCP still exists in patients receiving NebuPent prophylaxis. Therefore, any patient with symptoms suggestive of the presence of a pulmonary infection, including but not limited to dyspnea, fever or cough, should receive a thorough medical evaluation and appropriate diagnostic tests for possible acute PCP as well as for other opportunistic and non-opportunistic pathogens. The use of NebuPent may alter the clinical and radiographic features of PCP and could result in an atypical presentation, including but not limited to mild disease or focal infection.

Prior to initiating NebuPent prophylaxis, symptomatic patients should be evaluated appropriately to exclude the presence of PCP. The recommended dose of NebuPent for the prevention of PCP is insufficient to treat acute PCP.

INJECTION

Fatalities due to severe hypotension, hypoglycemia, acute pancreatitis and cardiac arrhythmias have been reported in patients treated with pentamidine isethionate, both by the IM and IV routes. Severe hypotension may result after a single dose (see PRECAUTIONS.) The administration of the drug should, therefore, be limited to the patients in whom*Pneumocystis carinii* has been demonstrated. Patients should be closely monitored for the development of serious adverse reactions (see PRECAUTIONS and ADVERSE REACTIONS).

PRECAUTIONS:

INHALATION SOLUTION

IMPORTANT: DO NOT MIX THE NEBUPENT SOLUTION WITH ANY OTHER DRUGS. DO NOT USE THE RESPIRGARD II NEBULIZER TO ADMINISTER A BRONCHODILATOR. (See DOSAGE AND ADMINISTRATION.)

PULMONARY

Inhalation of NebuPent may induce bronchospasm or cough. This has been noted particularly in some patients who have a history of smoking or asthma. In clinical trials, cough and bronchospasm were the most frequently reported adverse experiences associated with NebuPent administration (38% and 15%, respectively of patients receiving the 300 mg dose); however less than 1% of the doses were interrupted or terminated due to these effects. For the majority of patients, cough and bronchospasm were controlled by administration of an aerosolized bronchodilator (only 1% of patients withdrew from the study due to treatment-associated cough or bronchospasm). In patients who experience bronchospasm or cough, administration of an inhaled bronchodilator prior to giving each NebuPent dose may minimize recurrence of the symptoms.

GENERAL

Inhalation Solution: The extent and consequence of pentamidine accumulation following chronic inhalation therapy are not known. As a result, patients receiving NebuPent should be closely monitored for the development of serious adverse reactions that have occurred in patients receiving parenteral pentamidine, including hypotension, hypoglycemia, hyperglycemia, hypocalcemia, anemia, thrombocytopenia, leukopenia, hepatic or renal dysfunction, ventricular tachycardia, pancreatitis and Stevens-Johnson syndrome.

Extrapulmonary infection with *P. carinii* has been reported infrequently. Most, but not all, of the cases have been reported in patients who have a history of PCP. The presence of extrapulmonary pneumocystosis should be considered when evaluating patients with unexplained signs and symptoms.

Cases of acute pancreatitis have been reported in patients receiving aerosolized pentamidine. NebuPent should be discontinued if signs or symptoms of acute pancreatitis develop.

PRECAUTIONS: *(cont'd)*

Injection: Pentamidine isethionate should be used with caution in patients with hypertension, hypotension, hypoglycemia, hyperglycemia, hypocalcemia, leukopenia, thrombocytopenia, anemia, and hepatic or renal dysfunction.

Patients may develop sudden, severe hypotension after a single dose of pentamidine isethionate, whether given IV or IM. Therefore, patients receiving the drug should be lying down and the blood pressure should be monitored closely during administration of the drug and several times thereafter until the blood pressure is stable. Equipment for emergency resuscitation should be readily available. If pentamidine isethionate is administered IV, it should be infused over a period of 60 minutes.

Pentamidine isethionate-induced hypoglycemia has been associated with pancreatic islet cell necrosis and inappropriately high plasma insulin concentrations. Hyperglycemia and diabetes mellitus, with or without preceding hypoglycemia, have also occurred, sometimes several months after therapy with pentamidine isethionate. Therefore, blood glucose levels should be monitored daily during therapy with pentamidine isethionate, and several times thereafter.

LABORATORY TESTS

The following tests should be carried out before, during and after therapy:

a) Daily blood urea nitrogen and serum creatinine determinations.

b) b) Daily blood glucose determinations.

c) Complete blood count and platelet count.

d) Liver function test, including bilirubin, alkaline phosphatase, AST (SGOT), and ALT (SGPT).

e) Serum calcium determinations.

f) Electrocardiograms at regular intervals.

CARCINOGENESIS, MUTAGENESIS, AND IMPAIRMENT OF FERTILITY

No studies have been conducted to evaluate the potential of pentamidine isethionate as a carcinogen, mutagen, or cause of impaired fertility.

PREGNANCY CATEGORY C

Animal reproduction studies have not been conducted with pentamidine isethionate. It is also not known whether pentamidine isethionate can cause fetal harm when administered to a pregnant woman or can affect reproduction capacity. Pentamidine isethionate should be given to a pregnant woman only if clearly needed. Pentamidine isethionate should not be given to a pregnant woman unless the potential benefits are judged to outweigh the unknown risk.

NURSING MOTHERS

Inhalation Solution: It is not known whether NebuPent is excreted in human milk. Because of the potential for serious adverse reactions in nursing infants from NebuPent, a decision should be made whether to discontinue nursing or to discontinue the drug, taking into account the importance of the drug to the mother. Because many drugs are excreted in human milk, NebuPent should not be given to a nursing mother unless the potential benefits are judged to outweigh the unknown risk.

PEDIATRIC USE

Inhalation Solution: The safety and effectiveness of NebuPent in children have not been established.

DRUG INTERACTIONS:

Inhalation Solution: While specific studies on drug interactions with NebuPent have not been conducted, the majority of patients in clinical trials received concomitant medications, including zidovudine, with no reported interactions.

ADVERSE REACTIONS:

INHALATION SOLUTION

The most frequent adverse effects attributable to NebuPent administration are cough and bronchospasm (reported by 38% and 15%, respectively, of patients receiving 300 mg every four weeks).

The most frequently reported adverse experiences in the controlled clinical trials in which 607 patients were treated with NebuPent (139 patients at 300 mg every four weeks, 232 at 150 mg every two weeks, 101 at 100 mg every two weeks and 135 at 30 mg every two weeks) using the Respirgard II nebulizer were as follows:

53-72%: fatigue, bad (metallic) taste, shortness of breath and decreased appetite; 31-47%: dizziness and rash; 10-23%: nausea, pharyngitis, chest pain or congestion, night sweats, chills and vomiting.

In nearly all cases neither the relationship to treatment or underlying disease nor the severity of adverse experiences was recorded.

Other less frequently occurring adverse experiences (reported by greater than 1% and up to 5% of patients in two clinical trials) were pneumothorax, diarrhea, headache, anemia (generally associated with zidovudine use), myalgia, abdominal pain and edema.

From a total experience with 1130 patients adverse events reported with a frequency of 1% or less were as follows. No causal relationship to treatment has been established for these adverse events.

General: Allergic reaction and extrapulmonary pneumocystosis.

Cardiovascular: Tachycardia, hypotension, hypertension, palpitations, syncope, cerebrovascular accident, vasodilation and vasculitis.

Metabolic: Hypoglycemia, hyperglycemia, and hypocalcemia.

Gastrointestinal: Gingivitis, dyspepsia, oral ulcer/abscess, gastritis, gastric ulcer, hypersalivation, dry mouth, splenomegaly, melena, hematochezia, esophagitis, colitis, and pancreatitis.

Hematological: Pancytopenia, neutropenia, eosinophilia and thrombocytopenia.

Hepatorenal: Hepatitis, hepatomegaly, hepatic dysfunction, renal failure, flank pain and nephritis.

Musculoskeletal: Arthralgia.

Neurological: Tremors, confusion, anxiety, memory loss, seizure, neuropathy, paresthesia, insomnia, hypesthesia, drowsiness, emotional lability, vertigo, paranoia, neuralgia, hallucination, depression and unsteady gait.

Respiratory: Rhinitis, laryngitis, laryngospasm, hyperventilation, hemoptysis, gagging, eosinophilic or interstitial pneumonitis, pleuritis, cyanosis, tachypnea, and rales.

Skin: Pruritus, erythema, dry skin, desquamation and urticaria.

Special Senses: Eye discomfort, conjunctivitis, blurred vision, blepharitis and loss of taste and smell.

Urogenital: Incontinence.

Reproductive: Miscarriage.

INJECTION

CAUTION: Fatalities due to severe hypotension, hypoglycemia, acute pancreatitis and cardiac arrhythmias have been reported in patients treated with pentamidine isethionate, both by the IM and IV routes. The administration of the drug should, therefore, be limited to the patients in whom *Pneumocystis carinii* has been demonstrated.

ADVERSE REACTIONS: *(cont'd)*

Of 424 patients treated with pentamidine isethionate, 244 (57.5%) developed some adverse reaction. Most of the patients had the acquired immunodeficiency syndrome (AIDS). In the following (TABLE 1), "Severe" refers to life-threatening reactions or reactions that required immediate corrective measures and led to discontinuation of pentamidine isethionate.

TABLE 1

Adverse Reactions	Number	%
Severe		
Leukopenia (<1000/mm³)	12	2.8
Hypoglycemia (<25 mg/dl)	10	2.4
Thrombocytopenia (<20,000/mm³)	7	1.7
Hypotension (<60 mm Hg systolic)	4	0.9
Acute renal failure		
(serum creatinine >6 mg/dl)	2	0.5
Hypocalcemia	1	0.2
Stevens-Johnson syndrome	1	0.2
Ventricular tachycardia	1	0.2
Total number of patients with severe effects*	37	8.7
Moderate		
Elevated serum creatinine		
(2.4 to 6.0 mg/dl)	98	23.1
Sterile abscess, pain, or induration at the site of IM injection	47	11.1
Elevated liver function tests	37	8.7
Leukopenia	32	7.5
Nausea, anorexia	25	5.9
Hypotension	17	4.0
Fever	15	3.5
Hypoglycemia	15	3.5
Rash	14	3.3
Bad taste in mouth	7	1.7
Confusion/hallucinations	7	1.7
Anemia	5	1.2
Neuralgia	4	0.9
Thrombocytopenia	4	0.9
Hyperkalemia	3	0.7
Phlebitis	3	0.7
Dizziness (without hypotension)	2	0.5
Other moderate adverse reactions**	5	1.2
Total number of patients with moderate adverse reactions*	207	48.8

* Patients total may not equal sum of reactions, since some patients had more than one reaction.

** Each of the following moderate adverse reactions was reported in one patient: Hypocalcemia, abnormal ST segment of electrocardiogram, bronchospasm, diarrhea, and hyperglycemia.

OVERDOSAGE:

INHALATION SOLUTION

Overdosage has not been reported with NebuPent. The symptoms and signs of overdosage are not known.

A serious overdosage, to the point of producing systemic drug levels similar to those following parenteral administration, would have the potential of producing similar types of serious systemic toxicity. (See PRECAUTIONS.)

Available clinical pharmacology data (see CLINICAL PHARMACOLOGY) suggest that a dose up to 40 times the recommended NebuPent dosage would be required to produce systemic levels similar to a single 4 mg/kg intravenous dose.

DOSAGE AND ADMINISTRATION:

INHALATION SOLUTION

IMPORTANT: NEBUPENT MUST BE DISSOLVED ONLY IN STERILE WATER FOR INJECTION, USP. DO NOT USE SALINE SOLUTION FOR RECONSTITUTION BECAUSE THE DRUG WILL PRECIPITATE. DO NOT MIX THE NEBUPENT SOLUTION WITH ANY OTHER DRUGS. DO NOT USE THE RESPIRGARD II NEBULIZER TO ADMINISTER A BRONCHODILATOR.

RECONSTITUTION

The contents of one vial (300 mg) must be dissolved in 6 mL Sterile Water for Injection, USP. Place the entire reconstituted contents of the vial into the Respirgard II nebulizer reservoir for administration.

DOSAGE

The recommended adult dosage of NebuPent for the prevention of*Pneumocystis carinii* pneumonia is 300 mg once every four weeks administered via the Respirgard II nebulizer.

The dose should be delivered until the nebulizer chamber is empty (approximately 30 to 45 minutes). The flow rate should be 5 to 7 liters per minute from a 40 to 50 pounds per square inch (PSI) air or oxygen source. Alternatively, a 40 to 50 PSI air compressor can be used with flow limited by setting the flowmeter at 5 to 7 liters per minute or by setting the pressure at 22 to 25 PSI. Low pressure (less than 20 PSI) compressors should not be used.

STABILITY

Freshly prepared solutions for aerosol use are recommended. After reconstitution with sterile water, the NebuPent solution is stable for 48 hours in the original vial at room temperature if protected from light.

Store the dry product at controlled room temperature 15° - 30°C (59° - 86°F).

Protect the dry product and the reconstituted solution from light.

INJECTION

Pentamidine isethionate should be administered IM or IV only. The recommended regimen for adults and children is 4 mg/kg once a day for 14 days. The benefits and risks of therapy with pentamidine isethionate for more than 14 days are not well defined.

INTRAMUSCULAR INJECTION

The contents of one vial (300 mg) should be dissolved in 3 ml of Sterile Water for Injection, USP. The calculated daily dose should then be withdrawn and administered by deep IM injection.

INTRAVENOUS INJECTION

The contents of one vial should first be dissolved in 3 to 5 ml of Sterile Water for Injection, USP, or 5% Dextrose Injection, USP. The calculated dose of pentamidine isethionate should then be withdrawn and diluted further in 50 to 250 ml of 5% Dextrose Injection, USP. **The diluted IV solutions containing pentamidine isethionate should be infused over a period of 60 minutes.**

DOSAGE AND ADMINISTRATION: *(cont'd)*

Aseptic technique should be employed in preparation of all solutions. Parenteral drug products should be inspected visually for particulate matter and discoloration prior to administration.

Stability: Intravenous infusion solutions of pentamidine isethionate at 1 mg and 2.5 mg/ml prepared in 5% Dextrose Injection, USP are stable at room temperature for up to 24 hours.

Store the dry product at controlled room temperature 15° - 30°C (59° - 86°F). Protect the dry product and reconstituted solution from light.

Discard unused portions.

(Fujisawa Pharmaceutical Company, Inhalation Solution, 2/91, 45474A)

(Fujisawa Pharmaceutical Company, Injection, 11/92, 45485B)

HOW SUPPLIED - RATED THERAPEUTICALLY EQUIVALENT:

Injection, Solution - Intravenous - 300 mg

1's	$113.54	Pentamidine Isethionate, Abbott	00074-4548-01
1's	$113.54	Pentamidine Isethionate, Abbott	00074-4548-49
5's	$468.00	Pentacarinat, Centeon	00053-1000-05
10's	$987.50	PENTAM, Fujisawa Pharm (US)	57317-0211-03

HOW SUPPLIED - NOT RATED EQUIVALENT:

Aerosol - Inhalation - 300 mg

1's	$98.75	NEBUPENT, Fujisawa Pharm (US)	57317-0210-06

PENTAZOCINE LACTATE *(001977)*

CATEGORIES: Analgesics; Anesthesia; Antipyretics; Central Nervous System Agents; Narcotic Agonist-Antagonist; Narcotics, Synthetics & Combinations; Opiate Partial Agonists; Pain; DEA Class CIV; FDA Approval Pre 1982; Patent Expiration 1995 Aug

BRAND NAMES: *Fortral* (Australia, France); *Fortwin*; *Liticon*; *Ospronim*; *Pentafen*; *Pentawin*; *Sosegon*; *Susevin*; **Talwin**

(International brand names outside U.S. in italics)

DESCRIPTION:

Pentazocine lactate injection is a member of the benzozocine series (also known as the benzomorphan series). Chemically, pentazocine lactate is 1,2,3,4,5,6-hexahydro -6, 11-dimethyl-3-(3-methyl-2-butenyl) -2,6-methano-3-benzazocin-8-ol lactate, a white, crystalline substance soluble in acidic aqueous solutions.

CLINICAL PHARMACOLOGY:

Pentazocine lactate is a potent analgesic and 30 mg is usually as effective an analgesic as morphine 10 mg or meperidine 75 mg to 100 mg; however, a few studies suggest the pentazocine lactate to morphine ratio may range from 20 mg to 40 mg pentazocine lactate to 10 mg morphine. The duration of analgesia may sometimes be less than that of morphine. Analgesia usually occurs within 15 to 20 minutes after intramuscular or subcutaneous injection and within 2 to 3 minutes after intravenous injection. Pentazocine lactate weakly antagonizes the analgesic effects of morphine, meperidine, and phenazocine; in addition, it produces incomplete reversal of cardiovascular, respiratory, and behavioral depression induced by morphine and meperidine. Pentazocine lactate has about 1/50 the antagonistic activity of nalorphine. It also has sedative activity.

INDICATIONS AND USAGE:

For the relief of moderate to severe pain. Pentazocine lactate may also be used for preoperative or preanesthetic medication and as a supplement to surgical anesthesia.

CONTRAINDICATIONS:

Pentazocine lactate should not be administered to patients who are hypersensitive to it.

WARNINGS:

Drug Dependence: *Special care should be exercised in prescribing pentazocine for emotionally unstable patients and for those with a history of drug misuse. Such patients should be closely supervised when greater than 4 or 5 days of therapy is contemplated. There have been instances of psychological and physical dependence on pentazocine lactate in patients with such a history and, rarely, in patients without such a history. Extended use of parenteral pentazocine lactate may lead to physical or psychological dependence in some patients. When pentazocine lactate is abruptly discontinued, withdrawal symptoms such as abdominal cramps, elevated temperature, rhinorrhea, restlessness, anxiety, and lacrimation may occur. However, even when these have occurred, discontinuance has been accomplished with minimal difficulty. In the rare patient in whom more than minor difficulty has been encountered, reinstitution of parenteral pentazocine lactate with gradual withdrawal has ameliorated the patient's symptoms. Substituting methadone or other narcotics for pentazocine lactate in the treatment of the pentazocine abstinence syndrome should be avoided. There have been rare reports of possible abstinence syndromes in newborns after prolonged use of pentazocine lactate during pregnancy.*

In prescribing parenteral pentazocine lactate for chronic use, particularly if the drug is to be self-administered, the physician should be precautions to avoid increases in dose and frequency of injection by the patient.

Just as with all medication, the oral form of pentazocine lactate is preferable for chronic administration.

Tissue Damage of Injection Sites: Severe sclerosis of the skin, subcutaneous tissues, and underlying muscle have occurred of the injection sites of patients who have received multiple doses of pentazocine lactate. Constant rotation of injection sites is, therefore, essential. In addition, animal studies have demonstrated that pentazocine lactate is tolerated less well subcutaneously than intramuscularly. (See DOSAGE AND ADMINISTRATION.)

Head Injury and Increased Intracranial Pressure: As in the case of other potent analgesics, the potential of pentazocine lactate injection for elevating cerebrospinal fluid pressure may be attributed to CO_2retention due to the respiratory depressant effects of the drug. These effects may be markedly exaggerated in the presence of head injury, other intracranial lesions, or a preexisting increase in intracranial pressure. Furthermore, pentazocine lactate can produce effects which may obscure the clinical course of patients with head injuries. In such patients, pentazocine lactate must be used with extreme caution and only if its use is deemed essential.

Usage in Pregnancy: Safe use of pentazocine lactate during pregnancy (other than labor) has not been established. Animal reproduction studies have not demonstrated teratogenic or embryotoxic effects. However, pentazocine lactate should not be administered to pregnant patients (other than labor) only when, in the judgment of the physician, the potential benefits outweigh the possible hazards. Patients receiving pentazocine lactate during labor have experienced no adverse effects other than those that occur with commonly used analgesics. Pentazocine lactate should be used with caution in women delivering premature infants.

WARNINGS: *(cont'd)*

Acute CNS Manifestations: Patients receiving therapeutic doses of pentazocine have experienced hallucinations (usually visual), disorientation, and confusion which have cleared spontaneously within a period of hours. The mechanism of this reaction is not known. Such patients should be closely observed and vital signs checked. If the drug is reinstituted, it should be done with caution since these acute CNS manifestations may recur.

Dur to the potential for increased CNS depressant effects, alcohol should be used with caution in patients who are currently receiving pentazocine.

Usage in Children: Because clinical experience in children under twelve years of age is limited, the use of pentazocine lactate in this age group is not recommended.

Ambulatory Patients: Since sedation, dizziness, and occasional euphoria have been noted, ambulatory patients should be warned not to operate machinery, drive cars, or unnecessarily expose themselves to hazards.

Myocardial Infarction: Caution should be exercised in the intravenous use of pentazocine for patients with acute myocardial infarction accompanied by hypertension or left ventricular failure. Data suggest that intravenous administration of pentazocine increases systemic and pulmonary arterial pressure and systemic vascular resistance in patients with acute myocardial infarction.

NOTE: Acetone sodium bisulfite, a sulfite that may cause allergic-type reactions including anaphylactic symptoms and life-threatening or less severe asthmatic episodes in certain susceptible people, is contained in both Carpuject Sterile Cartridge-Needle Unit and multiple-dose vials. The overall prevalence of sulfite sensitivity in the general population in unknown and probably low. Sulfite sensitivity is seen more frequently in asthmatic than in nonasthmatic people.

The ampuls in the Uni-Amp Pak and the Uni-Nest Pak do not contain acetone sodium bisulfite.

PRECAUTIONS:

Certain Respiratory Conditions: The possibility that pentazocine lactate may cause respiratory depression should be considered in treatment of patients with bronchial asthma. pentazocine lactate should be administered only with caution and in low dosage to patients with respiratory depression (*e.g.,* from other medication, uremia, or severe infection), severely limited respiratory reserve, obstructive respiratory conditions, or cyanosis.

Impaired Renal or Hepatic Function: Although laboratory tests have not indicated that pentazocine lactate causes or increase renal or hepatic impairment, the drug should be administered with caution to patients with such impairment. Extensive liver disease appears to predispose to greater side effects (*e.g.,* marked apprehension, anxiety, dizziness, sleepiness) from the usual clinical dose, and may be the result of decreased metabolism of the drug by the liver.

Biliary Surgery: Narcotic drug products are generally considered to elevate biliary tract pressure for varying periods following their administration. Some evidence suggests that pentazocine may differ from other marketed narcotics in this respect (*i.e.,* it causes little or no elevation in biliary tract pressures). The clinical significance of these findings, however, is not yet known.

Patients Receiving Narcotics: Pentazocine lactate is a mild narcotic antagonist. Some patients previously given narcotics, including methadone for the daily treatment of narcotic dependence, have experienced withdrawal symptoms after receiving pentazocine lactate.

CNS Effect: Caution should be used when pentazocine lactate is administered to patients prone to seizures; seizures have occurred in a few such patients in association with the use of pentazocine lactate although no cause and effect relationship has been established.

Use in Anesthesia: Concomitant use of CNS depressants with parenteral pentazocine lactate may produce additive CNS depression. Adequate equipment and facilities should be available to identify and treat systemic emergencies should they occur.

ADVERSE REACTIONS:

The most commonly occurring reactions are: nausea, dizziness or lightheadedness, vomiting, euphoria.

Dermatologic Reactions: Soft tissue induration, nodules, and cutaneous depression can occur at injection sites. Ulceration (sloughing) and severe sclerosis of the skin and subcutaneous tissues (and, rarely underlying muscle) have been reported after multiple doses. Other reported dermatologic reactions include diaphoresis, sting on injection, flushed skin including plethora, dermatitis including pruritus.

Infrequently Occurring Reactions Are: *Respiratory:* respiratory depression, dyspnea, transient apnea in a small number of newborn infants whose mothers received pentazocine lactate during labor; *Cardiovascular:* circulatory depression, shock, hypertension; *CNS effects:* dizziness, lightheadedness, hallucinations, sedation, euphoria, headache, confusion, disorientation; infrequently weakness, disturbed dreams, insomnia, syncope, visual blurring and focusing difficulty, depression; and rarely tremor, irritability, excitement, tinnitus.*Gastrointestinal:* constipation, dry mouth; *Other:* urinary retention, headache, paresthesia, alterations in rate or strength of uterine contractions during labor.

Rarely Reported Reactions Include: *Neuromuscular And Psychiatric:* muscle tremor, insomnia, disorientation, hallucinations;*Gastrointestinal:* taste alteration, diarrhea and cramps;*Ophthalmic:* blurred vision, nystagmus, diplopia, miosis;*Hematologic:* depression of white bloods cells (especially granulocytes), which is usually reversible, moderate transient eosinophilia; *Other:* tachycardia, weakness or faintness, chills, allergic reactions including edema of the face, toxic epidermal necrolysis.

See Acute CNS Manifestations and Drug Dependence under WARNINGS.

OVERDOSAGE:

Manifestations: Clinical experience with pentazocine lactate overdosage has been insufficient to define the signs of this condition.

Treatment: Oxygen, intravenous fluids, vasopressors, and other supportive measures should be employed as indicated. Assisted or controlled ventilation should also be considered. For respiratory depression due to overdosage or unusual sensitivity to pentazocine lactate, parenteral naloxone is a specific and effective antagonist.

DOSAGE AND ADMINISTRATION:

Adults, Excluding Patients in Labor: The recommended single parenteral dose is 30 mg by intramuscular, subcutaneous, or intravenous route. This may be repeated every 3 to 4 hours. Doses in excess of 30 mg intravenously or 60 mg intramuscularly or subcutaneously are not recommended. Total daily dosage should not exceed 360 mg.

The subcutaneous route of administration should be used only when necessary because of possible severe tissue damage at injection sites (see WARNINGS). When frequent injections are needed, the drug should be administered intramuscularly. In addition, constant rotation of injection sites (*e.g.,* the upper outer quadrants of the buttocks, mid-lateral aspects of the thighs, and the deltoid areas) is essential.

DOSAGE AND ADMINISTRATION: *(cont'd)*

Patients in Labor: A single, intramuscular 30 mg dose has been most commonly administered. An intravenous 20 mg dose has given adequate pain relief to some patients in labor when contractions become regular, and this dose may be given two or three times of two-to three-four intervals, as needed.

Children Under 12 Years of Age: Since clinical experience in children under twelve years of age is limited, the use of pentazocine lactate in this age group is not recommended.

Caution: Pentazocine lactate should not be mixed in the same syringe with soluble barbiturates because precipitation will occur.

HOW SUPPLIED - EQUIVALENTS NOT AVAILABLE:

Injection, Solution - Intravenous - 30 mg/ml

1 ml x 10	$19.52	TALWIN, Sanofi Winthrop	00024-1917-02
1 ml x 25	$98.72	TALWIN, Sanofi Winthrop	00024-1924-04
1 ml x 25	$98.72	TALWIN, Sanofi Winthrop	00024-1924-14
1.5 ml x 10	$21.91	TALWIN, Sanofi Winthrop	00024-1918-02
1.5 ml x 25	$113.51	TALWIN, Sanofi Winthrop	00024-1925-04
2 ml x 10	$25.33	TALWIN, Sanofi Winthrop	00024-1919-02
2 ml x 25	$133.52	TALWIN, Sanofi Winthrop	00024-1926-04
2 ml x 25	$133.52	TALWIN, Sanofi Winthrop	00024-1926-14
10 ml	$31.49	TALWIN, Sanofi Winthrop	00024-1916-01

PENTOBARBITAL SODIUM *(001978)*

CATEGORIES: Analeptics; Anesthesia; Anticonvulsants; Anxiolytics, Sedatives, Hypnotic; Barbiturates; Central Nervous System Agents; Hypnotics; Insomnia; Neuromuscular; Sedatives; Sedatives/Hypnotics; Convulsions*; Epilepticus*; Pregnancy Category D; DEA Class CII; DEA Class CIII; FDA Approval Pre 1982
* Indication not approved by the FDA

BRAND NAMES: *Carbrital*; *Embutal*; *Medinox Mono* (Germany); *Mintal* (Japan); Nembutal; *Novopentobarb* (Canada); *Pentobarbitone*; *Prodormol*; Sodium Pentobarbital; *Sombutol*
(International brand names outside U.S. in italics)

FORMULARIES: Medi-Cal

COST OF THERAPY: $3.65 (Insomnia; Capsule; 100 mg; 1/day; 7 days)

DESCRIPTION:

WARNING-MAY BE HABIT FORMING The barbiturates are nonselective central nervous system depressants which are primarily used as sedative hypnotics. The barbiturates and their sodium salts are subject to control under the Federal Controlled Substances Act (See DRUG ABUSE AND DEPENDENCE.)

Barbiturates and substituted pyrimidine derivatives in which the basic structure common to these drugs is barbituric acid, a substance which has no central nervous system (CNS) activity. CNS activity is obtained by substituting alkenyl, or aryl groups on the pyrimidine ring. Pentobarbital sodium) is chemically represented by sodium 5-ethyl-5-(1-methylbutyl) barbiturate.

Capsules, Suppositories, and Injection: The sodium salt of pentobarbital occurs as a white, slightly bitter powder which is freely soluble in water and alcohol but practically insoluble in benzene and ether.

Capsules: Pentobarbital sodium capsules for oral administration contain either 50 mg or 100 mg of pentobarbital sodium.

Elixir: Pentobarbital elixir for oral use contains 18.2 mg pentobarbital (equivalent to 20 mg pentobarbital sodium) per 5 ml.

Suppositories: Each rectal suppository contains either 30 mg, 60 mg, 120 mg, or 200 mg of pentobarbital sodium.

Solution: Pentobarbital sodium injection is a sterile solution for intravenous or intramuscular injection. Each ml contains pentobarbital sodium 50 mg, in a vehicle of propylene glycol, 40%, alcohol, 10% and water for injection, to volume. The pH is adjusted to approximately 9.5 with hydrochloric acid and/or sodium hydroxide.

CLINICAL PHARMACOLOGY:

Barbiturates are capable of producing all levels of CNS mood alteration from excitation to mild sedation, to hypnosis, and deep coma. Overdosage can produce death. In high enough therapeutic doses, barbiturates induce anesthesia.

Barbiturates depress the sensory cortex, decrease motor activity, alter cerebellar function, and produce drowsiness, sedation, and hypnosis.

Barbiturate-induced sleep differs from physiological sleep. Sleep laboratory studies have demonstrated that barbiturates reduce the amount of time spent in the rapid eye movement (REM) phase of sleep or dreaming stage. Also, Stages III and IV sleep are decreased. Following abrupt cessation of barbiturates used regularly, patients may experience markedly increased dreaming, nightmares, and/or insomnia. Therefore, withdrawal of a single therapeutic dose over 5 or 6 days has been recommended to lessen the REM rebound and disturbed sleep which contribute to drug withdrawal syndrome (for example, decrease the dose from 3 to 2 doses a day for 1 week).

In studies, secobarbital sodium and pentobarbital sodium have been found to lose most of their effectiveness for both inducing and maintaining sleep by the end of 2 weeks of continued drug administration at fixed doses. The short-, intermediate-, and, to a lesser degree, long-acting barbiturates have been widely prescribed for treating insomnia. Although the clinical literature abounds with claims that the short-acting barbiturates are superior for producing sleep while the intermediate-acting compounds are more effective in maintaining sleep, controlled studies have failed to demonstrate these differential effects. Therefore, as sleep medications, the barbiturates are of limited value beyond short-term use.

Barbiturates have little analgesic action at subanesthetic doses. Rather, in subanesthetic doses these drugs may increase the reaction to painful stimuli. All barbiturates exhibit anticonvulsant activity in anesthetic doses. However, of the drugs in this class, only phenobarbital, mephobarbital, and metharbital have been clinically demonstrated to be effective as oral anticonvulsants in subhypnotic doses.

Barbiturates are respiratory depressants. The degree of respiratory depression is dependent upon dose. With hypnotic doses, respiratory depression produced by barbiturates is similar to that which occurs during physiologic sleep with slight decrease in blood pressure and heart rate.

Studies in laboratory animals have shown that barbiturates cause reduction in the tone and contractility of the uterus, ureters, and urinary bladder. However, concentrations of the drugs required to produce this effect in humans are not reached with sedative-hypnotic doses.

Barbiturates do not impair normal hepatic function, but have been shown to induce liver microsomal enzymes, thus increasing and/or altering the metabolism of barbiturates and other drugs. (See DRUG INTERACTIONS.)

CLINICAL PHARMACOLOGY: *(cont'd)*

PHARMACOKINETICS

Barbiturates are absorbed in varying degrees following oral, rectal, or parenteral administration. The salts are more rapidly absorbed than are the acids. The rate of absorption is increased if the sodium salt is ingested as a dilute solution or taken on an empty stomach.

The onset of action for oral or rectal administration varies from 20 to 60 minutes. For IM administration, the onset of action is slightly faster. Following IV administration, the onset of action ranges from almost immediately for pentobarbital sodium to 5 minutes for phenobarbital sodium. Maximal CNS depression may not occur until 15 minutes or more after IV administration for phenobarbital sodium.

Duration of action, which is related to the rate at which the barbiturates are redistributed throughout the body, varies among persons and in the same person from time to time.

No studies have demonstrated that the different routes of administration are equivalent with respect to bioavailability.

Barbiturates are weak acids that are absorbed and rapidly distributed to all tissues and fluids with high concentrations in the brain, liver, and kidneys. Lipid solubility of the barbiturates is the dominant factor in their distribution within the body. The more lipid soluble the barbiturate, the more rapidly it penetrates all tissues of the body. Barbiturates are bound to plasma and tissue proteins to a varying degree of binding increasing directly as function of lipid solubility.

Phenobarbital has the lowest lipid solubility, lowest plasma binding, lowest brain protein binding, the longest delay in onset of activity, and the longest duration of action. At the opposite extreme is secobarbital which has the highest lipid solubility, plasma protein binding, brain protein binding, the shortest delay in onset of activity, and the shortest duration of action. Butabarbital is classified as an intermediate barbiturate.

The plasma half-life for pentobarbital in adults is 15 to 50 hours and appears to be dose dependent.

Barbiturates are metabolized primarily by the hepatic microsomal enzyme system, and the metabolic products are excreted in the urine, and less commonly, in the feces. Approximately 25 to 50 percent of a dose of aprobarbital or phenobarbital is eliminated unchanged in the urine, whereas the amount of other barbiturates excreted unchanged in the urine is negligible. The excretion of unmetabolized barbiturate is one feature that distinguishes the long-acting category from those belonging to other categories which are almost entirely metabolized. The inactive metabolites of the barbiturates are excreted as conjugates of glucuronic acid.

CAPSULES AND ELIXIR

In TABLE 1, the barbiturates are classified according to their duration of action. This classification should not be used to predict the exact duration of effect, but the grouping of drugs should be used as a guide in the selection of barbiturates.

TABLE 1 Classification, Onset, and Duration of Action of Commonly used Barbiturates Taken Orally

Classification	Onset of action	Duration of action
Long-acting Phenobarbital.	1 hour or longer	10 to 12 hours
Intermediate Amobarbital Butabarbital.	3/4 to 1 hour	6 to 8 hours
Short-acting Pentobarbital Secobarbital.	10 to 15 minutes	3 to 4 hours

INDICATIONS AND USAGE:

CAPSULES, ELIXIR, AND INJECTION

Oral

a. Sedatives.

b. Hypnotics, for the short-term treatment of insomnia, since they appear to lose their effectiveness for sleep induction and sleep maintenance after 2 weeks (See CLINICAL PHARMACOLOGY.)

c. Preanesthetics.

SUPPOSITORIES

Barbiturates administered rectally are absorbed from the colon and are used when oral or parenteral administration may be undesirable.

Rectal

1. Sedative.

2. Hypnotic, for the short-term treatment of insomnia, since they appear to lose their effectiveness for sleep induction and sleep maintenance after 2 weeks (See CLINICAL PHARMACOLOGY).

INJECTION

Parenteral

a. Sedatives.

b. Hypnotics, for the short-term treatment of insomnia, since they appear to lose their effectiveness for sleep induction and sleep maintenance after 2 weeks (See CLINICAL PHARMACOLOGY).

c. Preanesthetics.

d. Anticonvulsant, in anesthetic doses, in the emergency control of certain acute convulsive episodes, e.g., those associated with status epilepticus, cholera, eclampsia, meningitis, tetanus, and toxic reactions to strychnine or local anesthetics.

CONTRAINDICATIONS:

Barbiturates are contraindicated in patients with known barbiturate sensitivity. Barbiturates are also contraindicated in patients with a history of manifest or latent porphyria.

WARNINGS:

1. Habit Forming: Barbiturates may be habit forming. Tolerance, psychological and physical dependence may occur with continued use. (See DRUG ABUSE AND DEPENDENCE and Pharmacokinetics). Patients who have psychological dependence on barbiturates may increase the dosage or decrease the dosage interval without consulting a physician and may subsequently develop a physical dependence on barbiturates. To minimize the possibility of overdosage or the development of dependence, the prescribing and dispensing of sedative-hypnotic barbiturates should be limited to the amount required for the interval until the next appointment. Abrupt cessation after prolonged use in the dependent person may result in withdrawal symptoms, including delirium, convulsions, and possibly death. Barbiturates should be withdrawn gradually from any patient known to be taking excessive dosage over long periods of time. (See DRUG ABUSE AND DEPENDENCE).

2. Acute or Chronic Pain: Caution should be exercised when barbiturates are administered to patients with acute or chronic pain, because paradoxical excitement could be induced or important symptoms could be masked. However, the use of barbiturates as sedatives in the postoperative surgical period and as adjuncts to cancer chemotherapy is well established.

WARNINGS: *(cont'd)*

3. Use in Pregnancy: Barbiturates can cause fetal damage when administered to a pregnant women. Retrospective, case-controlled studies have suggested a connection of barbiturates and a higher than expected incidence of fetal abnormalities. Following oral or parenteral administration, barbiturates readily cross the placental barrier and are distributed throughout fetal tissues with highest concentrations found in the placenta, fetal liver, and brain. It is presumed that this effect will also be seen following rectal administration.

4. Synergistic Effects: The concomitant use of alcohol or other CNS depressants may produce additive CNS depressant effects.

Withdrawal symptoms occur in infants born to mothers who receive barbiturates throughout the last trimester of pregnancy. (See DRUG ABUSE AND DEPENDENCE.) If this drug is used during pregnancy, or if the patient becomes pregnant while taking this drug, the patient should be apprised of the potential hazard to the fetus.

INJECTION

IV aAdministration: Too rapid administration may cause respiratory depression, apnea, laryngospasm or vasodilation with fall in blood pressure.

Fetal blood levels approach maternal blood levels following parenteral administration.

PRECAUTIONS:

GENERAL

Barbiturates may be habit forming. Tolerance and psychological and physical dependence may occur with continuing use. (See DRUG ABUSE AND DEPENDENCE) Barbiturates should be administered with caution, if at all, to patients who are mentally depressed, have suicidal tendencies, or a history of drug abuse.

Elderly or debilitated patients may react to barbiturates with marked excitement, depression, and confusion. In some persons, barbiturates repeatedly produce excitement rather than depression.

In patients with hepatic damage, barbiturates should be administered with caution and initially in reduced doses. Barbiturates should not be administered to patients showing the premonitory signs of hepatic coma.

The 100 mg dosage strength of pentobarbital sodium capsules contains FD&C Yellow No. 5 (tartrazine) which may cause allergic-type reactions (including bronchial asthma) in certain susceptible individuals. Although the overall incidence of FD&C Yellow No. 5 (tartrazine) sensitivity in the general population is low, it is frequently seen in patients who also have aspirin hypersensitivity.

Parenteral solutions of barbiturates are highly alkaline. Therefore, extreme care should be taken to avoid perivascular extravasation or intra-arterial injection. Extravascular injection may cause local tissue damage with subsequent necrosis; consequences of intra-arterial injection may vary from transient pain to gangrene of the limb. Any complaint of pain in the limb warrants stopping the injection.

Capsules: The 100 mg dosage strength of pentobarbital sodium capsules contains FD&C Yellow No. 5 (tartrazine) which may cause allergic-type reactions (including bronchial asthma) in certain susceptible individuals. Although the overall incidence of FD&C Yellow No. 5 (tartrazine) sensitivity in the general population is low, it is frequently seen in patients who also have aspirin hypersensitivity.

INFORMATION FOR THE PATIENT

Practitioners should give the following information and instructions to patients receiving barbiturates.

1. The use of barbiturates carries with it an associated risk of psychological and/or physical dependence. The patients should be warned against increasing the dose of the drug without consulting a physician.

2. Barbiturates may impair mental and/or physical abilities required for the performance of potentially hazardous tasks (*e.g.,* driving, operating machinery, etc.).

3. Alcohol should not be consumed while taking barbiturates with other CNS depressants (*e.g.,* alcohol, narcotics, tranquilizers, and antihistamines) may result in additional CNS depressant effects.

LABORATORY TESTS

Prolonged therapy with barbiturates should be accompanied by periodic laboratory evaluation of organ systems, including hematopoietic, renal, and hepatic systems. (See PRECAUTIONS, General and ADVERSE REACTIONS.)

CARCINOGENESIS

1. Animal Data: Phenobarbital sodium is carcinogenic in mice and rats after lifetime administration. In mice, it produced benign and malignant liver cell tumors. In rats, benign liver cell tumors were observed very late in life.

2. Human Data: In a 29-year epidemiological study of 9,136 patients who were treated on an anticonvulsant protocol that included phenobarbital, results indicated a higher than normal incidence of hepatic carcinoma. Previously some of these patients were treated with thorotrast, a drug that is known to produce hepatic carcinomas. Thus, this study did not provide sufficient evidence that phenobarbital sodium is carcinogenic in humans.

Data from one retrospective study of 235 children in which the types of barbiturates are not identified suggested an association between exposure to barbiturates prenatally and an increased incidence of brain tumor. (Gold, E., et al., "Increased Risk of Brain Tumors in Children Exposed to Barbiturates," Journal of National Cancer Institute, 61: 1031-1034, 1978).

PREGNANCY

1. Pregnancy, Teratogenic Effects, Pregnancy Category D: See WARNINGS, Use in Pregnancy.

2. Nonteratogenic Effects: Reports of infants suffering from long-term barbiturate exposure in utero included the acute withdrawal syndrome of seizures and hyperirritability from birth to a delayed onset of up to 14 days. (See DRUG ABUSE AND DEPENDENCE).

LABOR AND DELIVERY

Hypnotic doses of these barbiturates do not appear to significantly impair uterine a activity during labor. Full anesthetic doses of barbiturates decrease the force and frequency of uterine contractions. Administration of sedative-hypnotic barbiturates to the mother during labor may result in respiratory depression in the newborn. Premature infants are particularly susceptible to the depressant effects of barbiturates. If barbiturates are used during labor and delivery, resuscitation equipment should be available.

Data are currently not available to evaluate the effect of these barbiturates when forceps delivery or other intervention is necessary. Also, data are not available to determine the effect of these barbiturates on the later growth, development, and functional maturation of the child.

NURSING MOTHERS

Caution should be exercised when a barbiturate is administered to a nursing woman since small amounts of barbiturates are excreted in the milk.

DRUG INTERACTIONS:

Most reports of clinically significant drug interactions occurring with the barbiturates have involved phenobarbital. However, the application of these data to other barbiturates appears valid and warrants serial blood level determinations of the relevant drugs when there are multiple therapies.

1. Anticoagulants: Phenobarbital lowers the plasma levels of dicumarol (name previously used: bishydroxycoumarin) and causes a decrease in anticoagulant activity as measured by the prothrombin time. Barbiturates can induce hepatic microsomal enzymes resulting in increased metabolism and decreased anticoagulant response of oral anticoagulants (*e.g.,* warfarin, acenocoumarol, dicumarol and phenprocoumon). Patients stabilized on anticoagulant therapy may require dosage adjustments if barbiturates are added to or withdrawn from their dosage regimen.

2. Corticosteroids: Barbiturates appear to enhance the metabolism of exogenous corticosteroids probably through the induction of hepatic microsomal enzymes. Patients stabilized on corticosteroid therapy may require dosage adjustments if barbiturates are added to or withdrawn from their dosage regimen.

3. Griseofulvin: Phenobarbital appears to interfere with the absorption of orally administered griseofulvin, thus decreasing its blood level. The effect of the resultant decreased blood levels of griseofulvin on therapeutic response has not been established. However, it would be preferable to avoid concomitant administration of these drugs.

4. Doxycycline: Phenobarbital has been shown to shorten the half-life of doxycycline for as long as 2 weeks after barbiturate therapy is discontinued.

This mechanism is probably through the induction of hepatic microsomal enzymes that metabolize the antibiotic. If phenobarbital and doxycycline are administered concurrently, the clinical response to doxycycline should be monitored closely.

5. Phenytoin, Sodium Valproate, Valproic Acid: The effect of barbiturates on the metabolism of phenytoin appears to be variable. Some investigators report an accelerating effect, while others report no effect. Because the effect of barbiturates on the metabolism of phenytoin is not predictable, phenytoin and barbiturate blood levels should be monitored more frequently if these drugs are given concurrently. Sodium valproate and valproic acid appear to decrease barbiturate metabolism; therefore, barbiturate blood levels should be monitored and appropriate dosage adjustments made as indicated.

6. Central Nervous System Depressants: The concomitant use of other central nervous system depressants, including other sedatives or hypnotics, antihistamines, tranquilizers, or alcohol, may produce additive depressant effects.

7. Monoamine Oxidase Inhibitors (MAOI): MAOI prolong the effects of barbiturates probably because metabolism of the barbiturate is inhibited.

8. Estradiol, Estrone, Progesterone And Other Steroidal Hormones: Pretreatment with or concurrent administration of phenobarbital may decrease the effect of estradiol by increasing its metabolism. There have been reports of patients treated with antiepileptic drugs (*e.g.,* phenobarbital) who became pregnant while taking oral contraceptives. An alternate contraceptive method might be suggested to women taking phenobarbital.

ADVERSE REACTIONS:

The following adverse reactions and their incidence were compiled from surveillance of thousands of hospitalized patients. Because such patients may be less aware of certain of the milder adverse effects of barbiturates, the incidence of these reactions may be somewhat higher in fully ambulatory patients.

More Than 1 In 100 Patients: The most common adverse reaction estimated to occur at a rate of 1 to 3 patients per 100 is: *Nervous System:* Somnolence.

Less Than 1 In 100 Patients: Adverse reactions estimated to occur at a rate of less than 1 in 100 patients listed below, grouped by organ system, and by decreasing order of occurrence are:

Nervous System: Agitation, confusion, hyperkinesia, ataxia, CNS depression, nightmares, nervousness, psychiatric disturbance, hallucinations, insomnia, anxiety, dizziness, thinking abnormality.

Respiratory System: Hypoventilation, apnea.

Cardiovascular System: Bradycardia, hypotension, syncope.

Digestive System: Nausea, vomiting, constipation.

Other Reported Reactions: Headache, injection site reactions, hypersensitivity reactions (angioedema, skin rashes, exfoliative dermatitis), fever, liver damage, megaloblastic anemia following chronic phenobarbital use.

DRUG ABUSE AND DEPENDENCE:

Capsules, Elixir, and Injection: Pentobarbital sodium capsules and elixir are subject to control by the Federal Controlled Substances Act under DEA schedule II.

Suppositories: Pentobarbital sodium suppositories are subject to control by the Federal Controlled Substances Act under DEA schedule III.

CAPSULES, ELIXIR, SUPPOSITORIES, AND INJECTION

Barbiturates may be habit forming. Tolerance, psychological dependence, and physical dependence may occur especially following prolonged use of high doses of barbiturates. Daily administration in excess of 400 milligrams (mg) of pentobarbital or secobarbital for approximately 90 days is likely to produce some degree of physical dependence. A dosage of from 600 to 800 mg taken for at least 35 days is sufficient to produce withdrawal seizures. The average daily dose for the barbiturate addict is usually about 1.5 grams. As tolerance to barbiturates develops, the amount needed to maintain the same level of intoxication increases; tolerance to a fatal dosage, however, does not increase more than two-fold. As this occurs, the margin between an intoxicating dosage and fatal dosage becomes smaller.

Symptoms of acute intoxication with barbiturates include unsteady gait, slurred speech, and sustained nystagmus. Mental signs of chronic intoxication include confusion, poor judgment, irritability, insomnia, and somatic complaints.

Symptoms of barbiturate dependence are similar to those of chronic alcoholism. If an individual appears to be intoxicated with alcohol to a degree that is radically disproportionate to the amount of alcohol in his or her blood the use of barbiturates should be suspected. The lethal dose of a barbiturate is far less if alcohol is also ingested.

The symptoms of barbiturate withdrawal can be severe and may cause death. Minor withdrawal symptoms may appear 8 to 12 hours after the last dose of a barbiturate. These symptoms usually appear in the following order: anxiety, muscle twitching, tremor of hands and fingers, progressive weakness, dizziness, distortion in visual perception, nausea, vomiting, insomnia, and orthostatic hypotension. Major withdrawal symptoms (convulsions and delirium) may occur within 16 hours and last up to 5 days after abrupt cessation of these drugs. Intensity of withdrawal symptoms gradually declines over a period of approximately 15 days. Individuals susceptible to barbiturate abuse and dependence include alcoholics and opiate abusers, as well as other sedative-hypnotic and amphetamine abusers.

Drug dependence to barbiturates arises from repeated administration of a barbiturate or agent with barbiturate-like effect on a continuous basis, generally in amounts exceeding therapeutic dose levels. The characteristics of drug dependence to barbiturates include: (a) a

DRUG ABUSE AND DEPENDENCE: *(cont'd)*

strong desire or need to continue taking the drug; (b) a tendency to increase the dose; (c) a psychic dependence on the effects of the drug related to subjective and individual appreciation of those effects; and (d) a physical dependence on the effects of the drug requiring its presence for maintenance of homeostasis and resulting in a definite, characteristic, and self-limited abstinence syndrome when the drug is withdrawn.

Treatment of barbiturate dependence consists of cautious and gradual withdrawal of the drug. Barbiturate-dependent patients can be withdrawn by using a number of different withdrawal regimens. In all cases withdrawal takes an extended period of time. One method involves substituting a 30 mg dose of phenobarbital for each 100 to 200 mg dose of barbiturate that the patient has been taking. The total daily amount of phenobarbital is then administered in 3 to 4 divided doses, not to exceed 600 mg daily. Should signs of withdrawal occur on the first day of treatment, a loading dose of 100 to 200 mg of phenobarbital may be administered IM in addition to the oral dose. After stabilization on phenobarbital, the total daily dose is decreased by 30 mg a day as long as withdrawal is proceeding smoothly. A modification of this regimen involves initiating treatment at the patient's regular dosage level and decreasing the daily dosage by 10 percent if tolerated by the patient.

Infants physically dependent on barbiturates may be given phenobarbital 3 to 10 mg/kg/day. After withdrawal symptoms (hyperactivity, disturbed sleep, tremors, hyperreflexia) are relieved, the dosage of phenobarbital should be gradually decreased and completely withdrawn over a 2-week period.

OVERDOSAGE:

CAPSULES, ELIXIR AND SUPPOSITORIES

The toxic dose of barbiturates varies considerably. In general, an oral dose of 1 gram of most barbiturates produces serious poisoning in an adult. Death commonly occurs after 2 to 10 grams of ingested barbiturate. Barbiturate intoxication may be confused with alcoholism, bromide intoxication, and with various neurological disorders.

Acute overdosage with barbiturates is manifested by CNS and respiratory depression which may progress to Cheyne-Stokes respiration, areflexia, constriction of the pupils to a slight degree (though in severe poisoning they may show paralytic dilation), oliguria, tachycardia, hypotension, lowered body temperature, and coma. Typical shock syndrome (apnea, circulatory collapse, respiratory arrest, and death) may occur.

In extreme overdose, all electrical activity in the brain may cease, in which case a "flat" EEG normally equated with clinical death cannot be accepted. This effect is fully reversible unless hypoxic damage occurs. Consideration should be given to the possibility of barbiturate intoxication even in situations that appear to involve trauma.

Complications such as pneumonia, pulmonary edema, cardiac arrhythmias, congestive heart failure, and renal failure may occur. Uremia may increase CNS sensitivity to barbiturates. Differential diagnosis should include hypoglycemia, head trauma, cerebrovascular accidents, convulsive states, and diabetic coma. Blood levels from acute overdosage for some barbiturates are listed in TABLE 2.

TABLE 2 Concentration of Barbiturate in the Blood Versus Degree of CNS Depression — Blood barbiturate level in ppm (mcg/ml)

	Degree of depression in nontolerant persons*				
Onset/duration	**1**	**2**	**3**	**4**	**5**
Pentobarbital					
Fast/short	≤2	0.5 to 3	10 to 15	12 to 25	15 to 40
Secobarbital					
Fast/short	≤2	0.5 to 5	10 to 15	15 to 25	15 to 40
Amobarbital					
Intermediate/intermediate	≤3	2 to 10	30 to 40	30 to 60	40 to 80
Butabarbital					
Intermediate/intermediate	≤5	3 to 25	40 to 60	50 to 80	60 to 100
Phenobarbital					
Slow/long	≤10	5 to 40	50 to 80	70 to 120	100 to 200

* Categories of degree of depression in nontolerant persons:

1. Under the influence and appreciably impaired for purposes of driving a motor vehicle or performing tasks requiring alertness and unimpaired judgment and reaction time.

2. Sedated, therapeutic range, calm, relaxed, and easily aroused.

3. Comatose, difficult to arouse, significant depression of respiration.

4. Compatible with death in aged or ill persons or in presence of obstructed airway, other toxic agents, or exposure to cold.

5. Usual lethal level, the upper end of the range includes those whoreceived some supportive treatment.

Treatment of overdosage is mainly supportive and consists of the following:

1. Maintenance of an adequate airway, with assisted respiration and oxygen administration as necessary.

2. Monitoring of vital signs and fluid balance.

3. If the patient is conscious and has not lost the gag reflex, emesis may be induced with ipecac. Care should be taken to prevent pulmonary aspiration of vomitus. After completion of vomiting, 30 grams activated charcoal in a glass of water may be administered.

4. If emesis is contraindicated, gastric lavage may be performed with a cuffed endotracheal tube in place with the patient in the face down position. Activated charcoal may be left in the emptied stomach and a saline cathartic administered.

5. Fluid therapy and the standard treatment for shock, if needed.

6. If renal function is normal, forced diuresis may aid in the elimination of the barbiturate. Alkalinization of the urine increases renal excretion of some barbiturates, especially phenobarbital, also aprobarbital, and mephobarbital (which is metabolized to phenobarbital).

7. Although not recommended as a routine procedure, hemodialysis may be used in severe barbiturate intoxications or if the patient is anuric or in shock.

8. Patient should be rolled from side to side every 30 minutes.

9. Antibiotics should be given if pneumonia is suspected.

10. Appropriate nursing care to prevent hypostatic pneumonia, decubiti, aspiration, and other complications of patients with altered states of consciousness.

DOSAGE AND ADMINISTRATION:

CAPSULES

Adults: The usual hypnotic dose consists of 100 mg at bedtime.

Children: The preoperative dose is 2 to 6 mg/kg/24 hours (maximum 100 mg), depending on age, weight, and the desired degree of sedation.

The proper hypnotic dose for children must be judged on the basis of individual age and weight.

DOSAGE AND ADMINISTRATION: *(cont'd)*

Dosages of barbiturates must be individualized with full knowledge of their particular characteristics and recommended rate of administration. Factors of consideration are the patient's age, weight, and condition.

Special Patient Population: Dosage should be reduced in the elderly or debilitated because these patients may be more sensitive to barbiturates. Dosage should be reduced for patients with impaired renal function or hepatic disease.

Recommended storage: Store below 86°F (30°C).

ELIXIR

Adults: Daytime sedation can ordinarily be provided by one 5-ml teaspoonful of the elixir taken 3 or 4 times per day.

The usual hypnotic dose consists of the equivalent to 100 mg pentobarbital sodium provided by 5 teaspoonfuls pentobarbital elixir.

Children: Daytime sedation can be provided by 2 to 6 mg/kg/24 hours, depending on age, weight, and the desired degree of sedation.

The proper hypnotic dose for children must be judged on the basis of individual age and weight.

Dosages of barbiturates must be individualized with full knowledge of their particular characteristics and recommended rate of administration. Factors of consideration are the patient's age, weight and condition.

Special Patient Population: Dosage should be reduced in the elderly or debilitated because these patients may be more sensitive to barbiturates. Dosage should be reduced for patients with impaired renal function or hepatic disease.

Recommended Storage: Store below 86°F (30°C). Avoid freezing.

Dispense in a USP tight, light-resistant, glass container.

SUPPOSITORIES

Typical hypnotic doses for adults and children are given below. These are intended only as a guide, and administration should be adjusted to the individual needs of each patient. For sedation, in children 5-14 years and in adults, reduce dose appropriately.

Adults (average To Above Average Weight): one 120 mg or one 200 mg suppository.

Children: *12-14 years (80-110 lbs.):* one 60 mg or one 120 mg suppository *5-12 years (40-80 lbs.):* one 60 mg suppository *1-4 years (20-40 lbs.):* one 30 mg or one 60 mg suppository *2 months-1 year (10-20 lbs.):* one 30 mg suppository.

Suppositories should not be divided.

Dosages of barbiturates must be individualized with full knowledge of their particular characteristics and recommended rate of administration. Factors of consideration are the patient's age, weight, and condition.

Special Patient Population: Dosage should be reduced in the elderly or debilitated because these patients more sensitive to barbiturates. Dosage should be reduced for patients with impaired renal function or hepatic disease.

Store in a refrigerator (36-46°F).

INJECTION

Dosages of barbiturates must be individualized with full knowledge of their particular characteristics and recommended rate of administration. Factors of consideration are the patient's age, weight, and condition. Parenteral routes should be used only when oral administration is impossible or impractical.

Intramuscular Administration: IM injection of the sodium salts of barbiturates should be made deeply into a large muscle, and a volume of 5 ml should not be exceeded at any one site because of possible tissue irritation. After IM injection of a hypnotic dose, the patient's vital signs should be monitored. The usual adult dosage of pentobarbital sodium solution is 150 to 200 mg as a single IM injection; the recommended pediatric dosage ranges from 2 to 6 mg/kg as a single IM injection not to exceed 100 mg.

Intravenous Administration: Pentobarbital sodium solution should not be admixed with any other medication or solution. IV injection is restricted to conditions in which other routes are not feasible, either because the patient is unconscious (as in cerebral hemorrhage, eclampsia, or status epilepticus), or because the patient resists (as in delirium), or because prompt action is imperative. Slow IV injection is essential, and patients should be carefully observed during administration. This requires that blood pressure, respiration, and cardiac function be maintained, vital signs be recorded, and equipment for resuscitation and artificial ventilation be available. The rate of IV injection should not exceed 50 mg/min for pentobarbital sodium.

There is no average intravenous dose of pentobarbital sodium solution that can be relied on to produce similar effects in different patients. The possibility of overdose and respiratory depression is remote when the drug is injected slowly in fractional doses.

A commonly used initial dose for the 70 kg adult is 100 mg. Proportional reduction in dosage should be made for pediatric or debilitated patients. At least one minute is necessary to determine the full effect of intravenous pentobarbital. If necessary, additional small increments of the drug may be given up to a total of from 200 to 500 mg for normal adults.

Anticonvulsant Use: In convulsive states, dosage of pentobarbital sodium solution should be kept to a minimum to avoid compounding the depression which may follow convulsions. The injection must be made slowly with due regard to the time required for the drug to penetrate the blood-brain barrier.

Special Patient Population: Dosage should be reduced in the elderly or debilitated because these patients may be more sensitive to barbiturates. Dosage should be reduced for patients with impaired renal function or hepatic disease.

Inspection: Parenteral drug products should be inspected visually for particulate matter and discoloration prior to administration, whenever solution containers permit. Solutions for injection showing evidence of precipitation should not be used.

Exposure of pharmaceutical products to heat should be minimized. Avoid excessive heat. Protect from freezing. It is recommended that the product be stored at room temperature 86°F (30°C); however, brief exposure up to 104°F (40°C) does not adversely affect the product.

HOW SUPPLIED - RATED THERAPEUTICALLY EQUIVALENT:

Capsule, Gelatin - Oral - 50 mg

100's	$33.31	NEMBUTAL SODIUM, Abbott	00074-3150-11

Capsule, Gelatin - Oral - 100 mg

100's	$52.16	NEMBUTAL SODIUM, Abbott	00074-3114-01
100's	$53.94	NEMBUTAL SODIUM, Abbott	00074-3114-21
500's	$252.95	NEMBUTAL SODIUM, Abbott	00074-3114-02

Injection, Solution - Intramuscular; - 50 mg/ml

2 ml	$25.89	PENTOBARBITAL SODIUM, Wyeth Labs	00008-0303-50
2 ml x 10	$22.14	Sodium Pentobarbital, Wyeth Labs	00008-0303-02
2 ml x 25	$58.45	NEMBUTAL SODIUM, Abbott	00074-6899-04
20 ml	$11.58	NEMBUTAL SODIUM, Abbott	00074-3778-04
50 ml	$21.58	NEMBUTAL SODIUM, Abbott	00074-3778-05

HOW SUPPLIED - NOT RATED EQUIVALENT:

Elixir - Oral - 20 mg/5ml
480 ml $64.74 NEMBUTAL, Abbott 00074-3142-01

Suppository - Rectal - 30 mg
12's $41.46 NEMBUTAL SODIUM, Abbott 00074-3272-01

Suppository - Rectal - 60 mg
12's $48.65 NEMBUTAL SODIUM, Abbott 00074-3148-01

Suppository - Rectal - 120 mg
12's $54.24 NEMBUTAL SODIUM, Abbott 00074-3145-01

Suppository - Rectal - 200 mg
12's $66.69 NEMBUTAL SODIUM, Abbott 00074-3164-01

PENTOSAN POLYSULFATE SODIUM *(003306)*

CATEGORIES: Anticoagulants; Bladder Pain; Cystitis; Interstitial Cystitis; Low Molecular Weight Heparin; Pregnancy Category B; FDA Approved 1996 Sep

BRAND NAMES: **Elmiron**

DESCRIPTION:

Pentosan polysulfate sodium is a semi-synthetically produced heparin-like macromolecular carbohydrate derivative which chemically and structurally resembles glycosaminoglycans. It is a white odorless powder, slightly hygroscopic and soluble in water to 50% at pH 6. It has a molecular weight of 4000 to 6000 Dalton.

Elmiron (Pentosan polysulfate sodium) is supplied in white opaque hard gelatin capsules containing 100 mg pentosan polysulfate sodium, microcrystalline cellulose, and magnesium stearate. It is formulated for oral use.

CLINICAL PHARMACOLOGY:

General: Pentosan polysulfate sodium is a low molecular weight heparin-like compound. It has anticoagulant and fibrinolytic effects. The mechanism of action of pentosan polysulfate sodium in interstitial cystitis is not known.

PHARMACOKINETICS

Absorption: In preliminary clinical studies with different doses of radio labeled pentosan polysulfate sodium, absorption was approximately 3% of the administered dose (n=3).

Distribution: Preclinical studies with parenterally administered radio labeled pentosan polysulfate sodium showed distribution to the uroepithelium of the genitourinary tract with lesser amounts found in the liver, spleen, lung, skin, periosteum, and bone marrow. Erythrocyte penetration is low in animals.

Metabolism: Preliminary literature studies of metabolism in 5 healthy volunteers with radio labeled drug suggest that 68% of the dose, at about 1 hour after IV administration, undergoes partial desulfation in the liver and spleen. In another study of 3 healthy volunteers, partial depolymerization occurs in the kidney. Both the desulfation and depolymerization can be saturated with continued dosing.

Excretion: In preliminary clinical studies in 8 healthy male volunteers, the elimination half-life or pentosan polysulfate sodium had a mean value at 24 hours after IV injection of 40 mg. The elimination half-life in urine following orally administered radio labeled pentosan polysulfate sodium was determined to be 4.8 hours for the unchanged drug.

In preliminary human studies in 3 healthy male volunteers, after single doses of radio labeled drug, urinary excretion averaged 3.5% of the administered dose. After multiple doses of pentosan polysulfate sodium, urine excretion of radioactivity averaged 11% of the administered dose.

Further analysis of the urinary fraction obtained after repeated dosing showed that about 3% of the dose may be unchanged pentosan polysulfate sodium.

Special Populations: Dose adjustments in geriatric patients and in patients with hepatic or renal impairment were not studied.

PHARMACODYNAMICS

The mechanism by which pentosan polysulfate sodium achieves its effects in patients is unknown. In preliminary clinical models, pentosan polysulfate sodium adhered to the bladder wall mucosal membrane. The drug may act as a buffer to control cell permeability preventing irritating solutes in the urine from reaching the cells.

Food Effects: The effect of food on absorption of pentosan polysulfate sodium in not known. In clinical trials, pentosan polysulfate sodium was administered with water 1 hour before or 2 hours after meals.

CLINICAL STUDIES:

Pentosan polysulfate sodium was evaluated in two clinical trials for the relief of pain in patients with chronic interstitial cystitis (IC). All patients met the NIH definition of IC based upon the results of cystoscopy, cytology, and biopsy. One blinded, randomized, placebo controlled study evaluated 151 patients (145 women, 5 men, 1 unknown) with a mean age of 44 years (range 18 to 81). Approximately equal numbers of patients received either placebo or pentosan polysulfate sodium 100 mg three times a day for 3 months. Clinical improvement in bladder pain was based upon the patient's own assessment. In this study, 28/74 (38%) of patients who received pentosan polysulfate sodium and 13/74 (18%) of patients who received placebo, showed greater than 50% improvement in bladder pain (p=0.005).

A second clinical trial, the physician's usage study was a prospectively designed retrospective analysis of 2499 patients who received pentosan polysulfate sodium 300 mg a day without blinding. Of the 2499 patients, 2220 were women, 254 were men, and 25 were of unknown sex. The patients had a mean age of 47 years and 23% were over 60 years of age. By 3 months, 1307 (52%) of the patients had dropped out or were ineligible for analysis, overall, 1192 (48%) received pentosan polysulfate sodium for 3 months; 892 (36%) received pentosan polysulfate sodium for 6 months; and 598 (24%) received pentosan polysulfate sodium for one year.

Patients had unblinded evaluations every 3 months for the patient's rating of overall change in pain in comparison to baseline and for the difference calculated in "pain/discomfort" scores. At baseline, pain/discomfort scores for the original 2499 patients were severe or unbearable in 60%, moderate in 33%, and mild or none in 7% of patients. The extent of the patients' pain improvement is shown in TABLE 1.

At 3 months, 722/2499 (29%) of the patients originally in the study had pain scores that improved by one or two categories. By 6 months, in the 892 patients who continued taking pentosan polysulfate sodium, an additional 116/2499 (5%) of patients had improved pain scores. After 6 months, the percent of patients who reported the first onset of pain relief was less than 1.5% of patients who originally entered in the study (see TABLE 2.)

INDICATIONS AND USAGE:

Pentosan polysulfate sodium is indicated for the relief of bladder pain or discomfort associated with interstitial cystitis.

TABLE 1 Pain Scores in Reference to Baseline in Open Label Physician's Usage Study (N=2499) [1]

Efficacy Parameter	3 Months[2]	6 Months[3]
Patient Rating of Overall Change in Pain (Recollection of difference between current pain and baseline pain)[3]	N=1161 Median=3 Mean =3.44 Cl: (3.37, 3.51)	N=724, Median=4 Mean=3.91 Cl: (3.83, 3.99)
Change in Pain/ Discomfort Score (Calculated difference in scores at the time point and baseline)[4]	N=1440 Median =1 Mean=0.51 Cl: (0.45, 0.57)	N=904 Median=1 Mean=0.66 Cl: (0.61, 0.71)

1 Trial not designed to detect onset of pain relief.
2 Cl = 95% confidence interval
3 6-point scale; 1=worse, 2=no better, 3=slightly improved, 4=moderately improved, 5=greatly improved, 6=symptom gone
4 3-point scale; 1=none or mild, 2=moderate, 3=severe or unbearable

TABLE 2 Number (%) of Patients with New Relief of Pain/Discomfort [1] in the Open Label Physician's Usage Study (N=2499)

	At 3 Months[2] (n=1192)	At 5 Months[3] (n=892)
Considering only the patients who continued treatment	722/1192 (61%)	116/892 (13%)
Considering all the patients originally enrolled in the study	722/2499 (29%)	116/2499 (5%)

1 First-time improvement in pain/discomfort score by 1 or 2 categories.
2 Number (%) of patients with improvement of pain/discomfort scores at 3 months when compared to baseline.
3 Number (%) of patients without pain/discomfort improvement at 3 months who had improvement at 6 months.

CONTRAINDICATIONS:

Pentosan polysulfate sodium is contraindicated in patients with unknown hypersensitivity to the drug, structurally related compounds, or excipients.

WARNINGS:

None.

PRECAUTIONS:

GENERAL

Pentosan polysulfate sodium is a weak anticoagulant (1/15 the activity of heparin). Bleeding complications of ecchymosis, epistaxis, and gum hemorrhage have been reported (see ADVERSE REACTIONS.) Patients undergoing invasive procedures or having signs/symptoms of underlying coagulopathy or other increased risk of bleeding (due to other therapies such as coumarin anticoagulants, heparin, t-PA, streptokinase, or high dose aspirin) should be evaluated for hemorrhage. Patients with diseases such as aneurysms, thrombocytopenia, hemophilia, gastrointestinal ulcerations, polyps, or diverticula should be carefully evaluated before starting pentosan polysulfate sodium.

A similar product that was given subcutaneously, sublingually, or intramuscularly (and not initially metabolized by the liver) is associated with delayed immunoallergic thrombocytopenia with symptoms of thrombosis and hemorrhage. Caution should be exercised when using pentosan polysulfate sodium in patients who have a history of heparin-induced thrombocytopenia.

Hepatic Insufficiency: Pentosan polysulfate sodium is desulfated by both the liver and the spleen. The extent to which hepatic insufficiency or splenic disorders may increase the bioavailability of the parent or active metabolites of pentosan polysulfate sodium is not known. Caution should be exercised when using pentosan polysulfate sodium in these patients.

Mildly (<2.5 × normal) elevated transaminase, alkaline phosphatase, gamma-glutmyl transpeptidase, and lactic dehydrogenase occurred in 1.2% of patients. The increases usually appeared 3 to 12 months after the start of pentosan polysulfate sodium therapy, and were not associated with jaundice or other clinical signs or symptoms. These abnormalities are usually transient, may remain essentially unchanged, or may rarely progress with continued use. Increases in PTT and PT (<1 for both) or thrombocytopenia (0.2%) were noted.

Alopecia is associated with pentosan polysulfate and with heparin products. In clinical trials of pentosan polysulfate sodium, alopecia could begin within the first 4 weeks of treatment. Ninety-seven percent (97%) of the cases of alopecia reported were alopecia areata, limited to a single area on the scalp.

Information for the Patient: Patients should take the drug as prescribed, in the dosage prescribed, and no more frequently than prescribed. Patients should be reminded that pentosan polysulfate sodium has a weak anticoagulant effect. This effect may increase bleeding times.

Laboratory Test Findings: Pentosan polysulfate sodium did not affect prothrombin time (PT) or partial prothrombin time (PTT) up to 1200 mg per day in 24 healthy male subjects treated for eight days. Pentosan polysulfate sodium also inhibits the generation of factor Xa in plasma and inhibits thrombin-induced platelet aggregation in human platelet rich plasma *ex vivo*. (See PRECAUTIONS, Hepatic Insufficiency.)

Carcinogenesis, Mutagenesis, and Impairment of Fertility: Long term studies in animals have not been performed to evaluate the carcinogenic potential of pentosan polysulfate sodium. Pentosan polysulfate sodium was not clastogenic or mutagenic when tested in the mouse micronucleus test or the Ames test (*S. typhimurium*). The effect of pentosan polysulfate sodium on spermatogenesis has not been investigated.

Pregnancy Category B: Reproduction studies have been performed in mice and rats with intravenous daily doses of 15 mg/kg and in rabbits with 7.5 mg/kg. These doses are 0.42 and 0.14 times the daily oral human doses of pentosan polysulfate sodium when normalized to body surface area. These studies did not reveal evidence of impaired fertility or harm to the fetus from pentosan polysulfate sodium. Direct *in vitro* bathing of cultured mouse embryos with pentosan polysulfate sodium (PPS) at a concentration of 1 mg/ml may cause reversible limb bud abnormalities. Adequate and well controlled studies have not been performed in pregnant women. Because animal studies are not always predictive of human response, this drug should be used in pregnancy only if clearly needed.

Nursing Mothers: It is not known whether this drug is excreted in human milk. Because many drugs are excreted in human milk, caution should be exercised when pentosan polysulfate sodium is administered to a nursing woman.

Pediatric Use: Safety and effectiveness in pediatric patients below the age of 16 years have not been established.

DRUG INTERACTIONS:

Drug – drug interactions not studied.

ADVERSE REACTIONS:

Pentosan polysulfate sodium was evaluated in clinical trials in a total of 2627 patients (2343 women, 262 men, 22 unknown) with a mean age of 47 [range 18 to 88 with 581 (22%) over 60 years of age]. Of the 2627 patients, 128 patients were in a 3 month trial and the remaining 2499 patients were in a long term unblinded trial.

Deaths occurred in 6/2627 (0.2%) patients who received the drug over a period of 3 to 75 months. The deaths appear to be related to other concurrent illnesses or procedures, except in one patient for whom the cause was not known.

Serious adverse events occurred in 33/2627 (1.3%) patients. Two patients had severe abdominal pain or diarrhea and dehydration that required hospitalization. Because there was not a control group of patients with interstitial cystitis who were concurrently evaluated, it is difficult to determine which events are associated with pentosan polysulfate sodium and which events are associated with concurrent illness, medicine, or other factors.

TABLE 3 Adverse Experience in Placebo-Controlled Clinical Trials of Pentosan Polysulfate Sodium 100 mg Three Times a Day for 3 Months

Body System/ Adverse Experience		Pentosan Polysulfate Sodium (n=128)	Placebo (n=130)
CNS	Overall Number of Patients*	3	5
	Insomnia	1	0
	Headache	1	3
	Severe Emotional Lability/Depression	2	1
	Nystagmus/Dizziness	1	1
	Hyperkinesia	1	1
GI	Overall Number of Patients	7	7
	Nausea	3	3
	Diarrhea	3	6
	Dyspepsia	1	0
	Jaundice	0	1
	Vomiting	0	2
Skin / Allergic	Overall Number of Patients	2	4
	Rash	0	2
	Pruritus	0	2
	Lacrimation	1	1
	Rhinitis	1	1
	Increased Sweating	1	0
Other	Overall Number of Patients	1	3
	Amenorrhea	0	1
	Arthralgia	0	1
	Vaginitis	1	1
Total Events		17	27
Total Number of Patients Reporting Adverse Events		13	19

* Within a body system, the individual events do not sum to equal overall number of patients because a patient may have more than one event.

The adverse events described below were reported in an unblinded clinical trial of 2499 interstitial cystitis patients treated with pentosan polysulfate sodium. Of the original 2499 patients, 1192 (48%) received pentosan polysulfate sodium for 3 months; 892 (36%) received pentosan polysulfate sodium for 6 months; and 598 (24%) received pentosan polysulfate sodium for one year, 355 (14%) received pentosan polysulfate sodium for 2 years, and 145 (6%) received pentosan polysulfate sodium for 4 years.

Frequency (1 to 4%)

Alopecia (4%)
Diarrhea (4%)
Nausea (4%)
Headache (3%)
Rash (3%)
Dyspepsia (2%)
Abdominal Pain (2%)
Liver Function Abnormalities (1%)
Dizziness (1%)

Frequency (≤1%)

Digestive: Vomiting, mouth ulcer, colitis, esophagitis, gastritus, flatulence, constipation, anorexia, gum hemorrhage.

Hematologic: Anemia, ecchymosis, increased prothrombin time, increased partial prothromboplastin time, leukopenia, thrombocytopenia.

Hypersensitive Reactions: Allergic reaction, photosensitivity.

Respiratory System: Pharyngitis, rhinitis, epistaxis, dyspnea.

Skin and Appendages: Pruritis, urticaria.

Special Senses: Conjunctivitis, tinnitus, optic neuritis, amblyopia, retinal hemorrhage.

OVERDOSAGE:

Overdosage has not been reported. Based upon the pharmacodynamics of the drug, toxicity is likely to be reflected as anticoagulation, bleeding, thrombocytopenia, liver function abnormalities, and gastric distress. (See CLINICAL PHARMACOLOGY) and PRECAUTIONS. In the event of acute overdosage, the patient should be given gastric lavage if possible, carefully observed and given symptomatic and supportive treatment.

DOSAGE AND ADMINISTRATION:

The recommended dose of pentosan polysulfate sodium is 300 mg/day taken as one 100 mg capsule orally three times daily. The capsules should be taken with water at least 1 hour before meals or 2 hours after meals.

Patients receiving pentosan polysulfate sodium should be reassessed after 3 months. If improvement has not occurred and if limiting adverse events are not present, pentosan polysulfate sodium may be continued for another 3 months. The clinical value and risks of continued treatment in patients whose pain has not improved by 6 months is not known.

PATIENT INFORMATION:

Pentosan polysulfate sodium is used for the treatment of bladder pain and discomfort due to interstitial cystitis.

Inform your doctor if you are pregnant or nursing.

Inform your doctor if you have liver disease or if you ever had bleeding or hemorrhaging.

Inform your doctor if you have hemophilia, ulcers, clotting problems, or are taking aspirin, warfarin, or any anticlotting medications.

May cause alopecia (localized hair loss), diarrhea, nausea, headache, rash, or stomach upset. Inform your doctor or pharmacist if these occur.

Take with water at least 1 hour before or 2 hours after meals.

HOW SUPPLIED:

Elmiron is supplied in white opaque hard gelatin capsules imprinted "BNP7600" containing 100 mg pentosan polysulfate sodium.

Storage: Store at controlled room temperature 15° to 30°C (59° to 86°F).

HOW SUPPLIED - EQUIVALENTS NOT AVAILABLE:

Capsule - Oral - 100 mg

100's $156.25 ELMIRON, Baker Norton Pharms 00575-7600-01

PENTOSTATIN *(003065)*

CATEGORIES: Adenosine Deaminase Inhibitor; Antineoplastics; Hairy Cell Leukemia; Leukemia; Oncologic Drugs; Orphan Drugs; Pregnancy Category D; FDA Class 1A ("Important Therapeutic Advantage"); FDA Approved 1991 Oct

BRAND NAMES: **Nipent**

FORMULARIES: Medi-Cal

WARNING:
Pentostatin for Injection should be administered under the supervision of a physician qualified and experienced in the use of cancer chemotherapeutic agents. The use of higher doses than those specified (see DOSAGE AND ADMINISTRATION) is not recommended. Dose- limiting severe renal, liver, pulmonary, and CNS toxicities occurred in Phase 1 studies that used pentostatin at higher doses (20-50 mg/m^{2}in divided doses over 5 days) than recommended.
In a clinical investigation in patients with refractory chronic lymphocytic leukemia using pentostatin at the recommended dose in combination with fludarabine phosphate, 4 of 6 patients entered in the study had severe or fatal pulmonary toxicity. The use of pentostatin in combination with fludarabine phosphate is not recommended.

DESCRIPTION:

Nipent (pentostatin for injection) is supplied as a sterile, apyrogenic, lyophilized powder in single-dose vials for intravenous administration. Each vial contains 10 mg of pentostatin and 50 mg of mannitol USP. The pH of the final product is maintained between 7.0 and 8.5 by addition of sodium hydroxide or hydrochloric acid.

Pentostatin, also known as 2'-deoxycoformycin (DCF), is a potent inhibitor of the enzyme adenosine deaminase and is isolated from fermentation cultures of *Streptomyces antibioticus*. Pentostatin is known chemically as (R)-3-(2-deoxy-β-D-*erythro*-pentofuranosyl)-3,6,7,8-tetrahydroimidazo(4,5-d)(1,3)diazepin-8-ol with a molecular formula of $C_{11}H_{16}N_4O_4$ and a molecular weight of 268.27.

Pentostatin is a white to off-white solid, freely soluble in distilled water.

CLINICAL PHARMACOLOGY:

MECHANISM OF ACTION

Pentostatin is a potent transition state inhibitor of the enzyme adenosine deaminase (ADA). The greatest activity of ADA is found in cells of the lymphoid system with T-cells having higher activity than B-cells and T-cell malignancies higher ADA activity than B-cell malignancies. Pentostatin inhibition of ADA, particularly in the presence of adenosine or deoxyadenosine, leads to cytotoxicity, and this is believed to be due to elevated intracellular levels of dATP which can block DNA synthesis through inhibition of ribonucleotide reductase. Pentostatin can also inhibit RNA synthesis as well as cause increased DNA damage. In addition to elevated dATP, these mechanisms may contribute to the overall cytotoxic effect of pentostatin. The precise mechanism of pentostatin's antitumor effect, however, in hairy cell leukemia is not known.

PHARMACOKINETICS/DRUG METABOLISM

A tissue distribution and whole-body autoradiography study in the rat revealed that radioactivity concentrations were highest in the kidneys with very little central nervous system penetration.

In man, following a single dose of 4 mg/m^{2}of pentostatin infused over 5 minutes, the distribution half-life was 11 minutes, the mean terminal half-life was 5.7 hours, the mean plasma clearance was 68 ml/min/m^2, and approximately 90% of the dose was excreted in the urine as unchanged pentostatin and/or metabolites as measured by adenosine deaminase inhibitory activity. The plasma protein binding of pentostatin is low, approximately 4%.

A positive correlation was observed between pentostatin clearance and creatinine clearance (CrCl) in patients with creatinine clearance values ranging from 60 ml/min to 130 ml/min.[1] Pentostatin half-life in patients with renal impairment (CrCl<50 ml/min, n=2) was 18 hours, which was much longer than that observed in patients with normal renal function (CrCl>60 ml/min, n=14), about 6 hours.

CLINICAL STUDIES:

One hundred thirty-three patients with hairy cell leukemia previously treated with alpha-interferon were treated with pentostatin in five clinical studies. Forty-four of these patients were established to be refractory to alpha-interferon and were evaluable for response to pentostatin. The majority of these patients were treated during studies conducted at the M.D. Anderson Hospital and by the Cancer and Leukemia Group B (CALGB). At M.D. Anderson pentostatin was administered at a dose of 4 mg/m^{2}every other week for 3 months and responding patients received 3 additional months. CALGB patients received 4 mg/m^2 of pentostatin every other week for 3 months and responding patients were treated monthly for up to 9 additional months. A complete response required clearing of the peripheral blood and bone marrow of hairy cells, normalization of organomegaly and lymphadenopathy, and recovery of the hemoglobin to at least 12 g/dl, platelet count to at least 100,000/mm^3, and granulocyte count to at least 1500/mm^3. A partial response required that the percentage of hairy cells in the blood and bone marrow decrease by more than 50%, enlarged organs and lymph nodes had to decrease by more than 50%, and hematologic parameters had to meet the same criteria as for a complete response. For those patients who were clearly refractory to alpha-interferon, the complete response rate was 58% and the partial response rate was 28% giving a total response rate (complete plus partial responses) of 86%. The median time to achieve a response was 4.7 months with a range of 2.9 to 24.1 months. Occasionally a complete response has occurred after discontinuation of treatment. The duration of response ranged from 1.4 months to 35.1+ months in the CALGB study (median >7.7 months) and from 1.3+ months to 31.2+ months for the M.D. Anderson study (median >15.2 months). The median duration of follow-up ranged from 3.9 months in the CALGB study to 19.3 months in the M.D. Anderson study. Only 4 of 20 and 2 of 13 responding patients had relapsed, respectively.

CLINICAL STUDIES: *(cont'd)*

Responding patients with abnormal peripheral blood counts at the start of therapy showed increases in their hemoglobin, granulocyte count, and platelet count in response to treatment with pentostatin.

INDICATIONS AND USAGE:

Pentostatin is indicated as single agent treatment for adult patients with alpha-interferon-refractory hairy cell leukemia (HCL). Alpha-interferon-refractory disease is defined as progressive disease after a minimum of 3 months of alpha-interferon treatment or no response after a minimum of 6 months of alpha-interferon treatment.

CONTRAINDICATIONS:

Pentostatin is contraindicated in patients who have demonstrated hypersensitivity to pentostatin.

WARNINGS:

See BOXED WARNING.

Patients with hairy cell leukemia may experience myelosuppression primarily during the first few courses of treatment. Patients with infections prior to pentostatin treatment have in some cases developed worsening of their condition leading to death, whereas others have achieved complete response. Patients with infection should be treated only when the potential benefit of treatment justifies the potential risk to the patient. Efforts should be made to control the infection before treatment is initiated or resumed.

In patients with progressive hairy cell leukemia, the initial courses of pentostatin treatment were associated with worsening of neutropenia. Therefore, frequent monitoring of complete blood counts during this time is necessary. If severe neutropenia continues beyond the initial cycles, patients should be evaluated for disease status, including a bone marrow examination.

Elevations in liver function tests occurred during treatment with pentostatin and were generally reversible.

Renal toxicity was observed at higher doses in early studies; however, in patients treated at the recommended dose, elevations in serum creatinine were usually minor and reversible. There were some patients who began treatment with normal renal function who had evidence of mild to moderate toxicity at a final assessment. (See DOSAGE AND ADMINISTRATION.)

Rashes, occasionally severe, were commonly reported and may worsen with continued treatment. Withholding of treatment may be required. (See DOSAGE AND ADMINISTRATION.)

PREGNANCY CATEGORY D

Pentostatin can cause fetal harm when administered to a pregnant woman. Pentostatin was administered intravenously at doses of 0, 0.01, 0.1, or 0.75 mg/kg/day (0, 0.06, 0.6, and 4.5 mg/m^2) to pregnant rats on days 6 through 15 of gestation. Drug-related maternal toxicity occurred at doses of 0.1 and 0.75 mg/kg/day (0.6 and 4.5 mg/m^2). Teratogenic effects were observed at 0.75 mg/kg/day (4.5 mg/m^2) manifested by increased incidence of various skeletal malformations. In a dose range-finding study, pentostatin was administered intravenously to rats at doses of 0, 0.05, 0.1, 0.5, 0.75, or 1 mg/kg/day (0, 0.3, 0.6, 3, 4.5, 6 mg/m^2) on days 6 through 15 of gestation. Fetal malformations that were observed were an omphalocele at 0.05 mg/kg (0.3 mg/m^2), gastroschisis at 0.75 mg/kg and 1 mg/kg (4.5 and 6 mg/m^2), and a flexure defect of the hindlimbs at 0.75 mg/kg (4.5 mg/m^2). Pentostatin was also shown to be teratogenic in mice when administered as a single 2 mg/kg (6 mg/m^2) intraperitoneal injection on day 7 of gestation. Pentostatin was not teratogenic in rabbits when administered intravenously on days 6 through 18 of gestation at doses of 0, 0.005, 0.01, or 0.02 mg/kg/day (0, 0.015, 0.03, or 0.06 mg/m^2); however maternal toxicity, abortions, early deliveries, and deaths occurred in all drug-treated groups. There are no adequate and well-controlled studies in pregnant women. If pentostatin is used during pregnancy, or if the patient becomes pregnant while taking (receiving) this drug, the patient should be apprised of the potential hazard to the fetus. Women of childbearing potential receiving pentostatin should be advised to avoid becoming pregnant.

PRECAUTIONS:

GENERAL

Therapy with pentostatin requires regular patient observation and monitoring of hematologic parameters and blood chemistry values. If severe adverse reactions occur, the drug should be withheld (see DOSAGE AND ADMINISTRATION), and appropriate corrective measures should be taken according to the clinical judgment of the physician.

Pentostatin treatment should be withheld or discontinued in patients showing evidence of nervous system toxicity.

INFORMATION FOR THE PATIENT

Patients should be advised of the signs and symptoms of adverse events associated with pentostatin therapy. (See ADVERSE REACTIONS.)

LABORATORY TESTS

Prior to initiating therapy with pentostatin, renal function should be assessed with a serum creatinine and/or a creatinine clearance assay.(See CLINICAL PHARMACOLOGY and DOSAGE AND ADMINISTRATION.) Complete blood counts and serum creatinine should be performed before each dose of pentostatin and at other appropriate periods during therapy (see DOSAGE AND ADMINISTRATION.) Severe neutropenia has been observed following the early courses of treatment with pentostatin and therefore frequent monitoring of complete blood counts is recommended during this time. If hematologic parameters do not improve with subsequent courses, patients should be evaluated for disease status, including a bone marrow examination. Periodic monitoring of the peripheral blood for hairy cells should be performed to assess the response to treatment.

In addition, bone marrow aspirates and biopsies may be required at 2 to 3 month intervals to assess the response to treatment.

CARCINOGENESIS, MUTAGENESIS, AND IMPAIRMENT OF FERTILITY

Carcinogenesis: No animal carcinogenicity studies have been conducted with pentostatin.

Mutagenesis: Pentostatin was nonmutagenic when tested in*Salmonella typhimurium* strains TA-98, TA-1535, TA-1537, and TA-1538. When tested with strain TA-100, a repeatable statistically significant response trend was observed with and without metabolic activation. The response was 2.1 to 2.2 fold higher than the background at 10 mg/plate, the maximum possible drug concentration. Formulated pentostatin was clastogenic in the in vivo mouse bone marrow micronucleus assay at 20, 120, and 240 mg/kg. Pentostatin was not mutagenic to V79 Chinese hamster lung cells at the HGPRT locus exposed 3 hours to concentrations of 1 to 3 mg/ml, with or without metabolic activation. Pentostatin did not significantly increase chromosomal aberrations in V79 Chinese hamster lung cells exposed 3 hours to 1 to 3 mg/ml in the presence or absence of metabolic activation.

Impairment of Fertility: No fertility studies have been conducted in animals; however, in a 5-day intravenous toxicity study in dogs, mild seminiferous tubular degeneration was observed with doses of 1 and 4 mg/kg. The possible adverse effects on fertility in humans have not been determined.

PRECAUTIONS: *(cont'd)*

PREGNANCY

Pregnancy Category D: (See WARNINGS)

NURSING MOTHERS

It is not known whether pentostatin is excreted in human milk. Because many drugs are excreted in human milk, and because of the potential for serious adverse reactions in nursing infants from pentostatin, a decision should be made whether to discontinue nursing or discontinue the drug, taking into account the importance of pentostatin to the mother.

PEDIATRIC USE

Safety and effectiveness in children or adolescents have not been established.

DRUG INTERACTIONS:

Allopurinol and pentostatin are both associated with skin rashes. Based on clinical studies in 25 refractory patients who received both pentostatin and allopurinol, the combined use of pentostatin and allopurinol did not appear to produce a higher incidence of skin rashes than observed with pentostatin alone. There has been a report of one patient who received both drugs and experienced a hypersensitivity vasculitis that resulted in death. It was unclear whether this adverse event and subsequent death resulted from the drug combination.

Biochemical studies have demonstrated that pentostatin enhances the effects of vidarabine, a purine nucleoside with antiviral activity. The combined use of vidarabine and pentostatin may result in an increase in adverse reactions associated with each drug. The therapeutic benefit of the drug combination has not been established.

The combined use of pentostatin and fludarabine phosphate is not recommended because it may be associated with an increased risk of fatal pulmonary toxicity (see WARNINGS.)

ADVERSE REACTIONS:

The following adverse events were reported during clinical studies with pentostatin in patients with hairy cell leukemia who were refractory to alpha-interferon therapy. Most patients experienced an adverse event. The drug association of these adverse events in particular cases is uncertain as they may be associated with the disease itself (*e.g.,* fever, infection, anemia), but other events, such as the gastrointestinal symptoms, hematologic suppression, rashes, and abnormal liver function tests, can in many cases be attributed to the drug. Most adverse events that were assessed for severity were either mild (52% of reports) or moderate (26% of reports) and diminished in frequency with continued therapy. Eleven percent of patients withdrew from treatment due to an adverse event.

The following table (TABLE 1) lists adverse events that occurred in at least 21 (11%) of 197 alpha-interferon-refractory patients with hairy cell leukemia:

TABLE 1

Adverse Event*	Number (%) of Patients (N = 197)
Leukopenia	118(60)
Nausea and Vomiting	104(53)
Fever	83(42)
Infection	70(36)
Anemia	68(35)
Thrombocytopenia	64(32)
Fatigue	57(29)
Rash	52(26)
Nausea	43(22)
Pain	40(20)
Hepatic Disorder/Elevated Liver Function Tests	38(19)
Skin Disorder	34(17)
Increased Cough	33(17)
Upper Respiratory Infection	31(16)
Anorexia	32(16)
Genitourinary Disorder	30(15)
Diarrhea	29(15)
Headache	25(13)
Lung Disorder	24(12)
Allergic Reaction	22(11)
Chills	22(11)
Myalgia	22(11)
Neurologic Disorder, CNS	21(11)

* Occurring in at least 11% of patients

Adverse events that occurred in 3% to 10% of alpha-interferon-refractory patients are as follows. The drug relatedness of many of these adverse events is uncertain.

Body as a Whole: Death, sepsis, chest pain, abdominal pain, back pain, flu syndrome, asthenia, malaise, and neoplasm

Cardiovascular System: Arrhythmia, abnormal electrocardiogram, thrombophlebitis, and hemorrhage

Digestive System: Constipation, flatulence, and stomatitis

Hemic and Lymphatic System: Ecchymosis, lymphadenopathy, and petechia

Metabolic and Nutritional System: Weight loss, peripheral edema, increased lactate dehydrogenase (LDH)

Musculoskeletal System: Arthralgia

Nervous System: Anxiety, confusion, depression, dizziness, insomnia, nervousness, paresthesia, somnolence, and abnormal thinking

Respiratory System: Bronchitis, dyspnea, epistaxis, lung edema, pneumonia, pharyngitis, rhinitis, and sinusitis

Skin and Appendages: Eczema, dry skin, herpes simplex, herpes zoster, maculopapular rash, pruritus, seborrhea, skin discoloration, sweating, and vesiculobullous rash

Special Senses: Abnormal vision, conjunctivitis, ear pain, and eye pain

Urogenital System: Hematuria and dysuria, increased BUN, and increased creatinine

The remaining adverse events occurred in less than 3% of patients; their relationship to pentostatin is uncertain: *Body as a Whole:* abscess, enlarged abdomen, ascites, cellulitis, cyst, face edema, fibrosis, granuloma, hernia, injection-site hemorrhage, injection-site inflammation, moniliasis, neck rigidity, pelvic pain, photosensitivity reaction, anaphylactoid reaction, immune system disorder, mucous membrane disorder, neck pain; *Cardiovascular System:* aortic stenosis, arterial anomaly, cardiomegaly, congestive heart failure, flushing, cardiac arrest, hypertension, myocardial infarct, palpitation, shock, and varicose vein; *Digestive System:* colitis, dysphagia, eructation, gastritis, gastrointestinal hemorrhage, gum hemorrhage, hepatitis, hepatomegaly, intestinal obstruction, jaundice, leukoplakia, melena, periodontal abscess, proctitis, abnormal stools, dyspepsia, esophagitis, gingivitis, hepatic failure, mouth disorder; *Hemic and Lymphatic System:* abnormal erythrocytes, leucocytosis, pancytopenia, purpura, splenomegaly, eosinophilia, hematologic disorder, hemolysis, lymphoma-like reaction, thrombocythemia; *Metabolic and Nutritional System:* acidosis, increased creatine phos-

ADVERSE REACTIONS: *(cont'd)*

phokinase, dehydration, diabetes mellitus, increased gamma globulins, gout, abnormal healing, hypocholesterolemia, weight gain, hyponatremia; *Musculoskeletal System:* arthritis, bone pain, osteomyelitis, pathological fracture;*Nervous System:* agitation, amnesia, apathy, ataxia, central nervous system depression, coma, convulsion, abnormal dreams, depersonalization, emotional lability, facial paralysis, abnormal gait, hyperesthesia, hypesthesia, hypertonia, incoordination, decreased libido, neuropathy, postural dizziness, decreased reflexes, stupor, tremor, vertigo; *Respiratory System:* asthma, atelectasis, hemoptysis, hyperventilation, hypoventilation, laryngitis, larynx edema, lung fibrosis, pleural effusion, pneumothorax, pulmonary embolus, increased sputum; *Skin and Appendages:* acne, alopecia, contact dermatitis, exfoliative dermatitis, fungal dermatitis, psoriasis, benign skin neoplasm, subcutaneous nodule, skin hypertrophy, urticaria; *Special Senses:* blepharitis, cataract, deafness, diplopia, exophthalmos, lacrimation disorder, optic neuritis, otitis media, parosmia, retinal detachment, taste perversion, tinnitus; *Urogenital System:* albuminuria, fibrocystic breast, glycosuria, gynecomastia, hydronephrosis, kidney failure, oliguria, polyuria, pyuria, toxic nephropathy, urinary frequency, urinary retention, urinary tract infection, urinary urgency, impaired urination, urolithiasis, and vaginitis.

One patient with hairy cell leukemia treated with pentostatin during another clinical study developed unilateral uveitis with vision loss.

OVERDOSAGE:

No specific antidote for pentostatin overdose is known. Pentostatin administered at higher doses (20-50 mg/m^2 in divided doses over 5 days) than recommended was associated with deaths due to severe renal, hepatic, pulmonary, and CNS toxicity. In case of overdose, management would include general supportive measures through any period of toxicity that occurs.

DOSAGE AND ADMINISTRATION:

It is recommended that patients receive hydration with 500 to 1,000 ml of 5% Dextrose in 0.5 Normal Saline or equivalent before pentostatin administration. An additional 500 ml of 5% Dextrose or equivalent should be administered after pentostatin is given.

The recommended dosage of pentostatin for the treatment of alpha-interferon-refractory hairy cell leukemia is 4 mg/m^2 every other week. Pentostatin may be administered intravenously by bolus injection or diluted in a larger volume and given over 20 to 30 minutes. See Preparation Of Intravenous Solution.

Higher doses are not recommended.

No extravasation injuries were reported in clinical studies.

The optimal duration of treatment has not been determined. In the absence of major toxicity and with observed continuing improvement, the patient should be treated until a complete response has been achieved. Although not established as required, the administration of two additional doses has been recommended following the achievement of a complete response.

All patients receiving pentostatin at 6 months should be assessed for response to treatment. If the patient has not achieved a complete or partial response, treatment with pentostatin should be discontinued.

If the patient has achieved a partial response, pentostatin treatment should be continued in an effort to achieve a complete response. At any time thereafter that a complete response is achieved, two additional doses of pentostatin are recommended. Pentostatin treatment should then be stopped. If the best response to treatment at the end of 12 months is a partial response, it is recommended that treatment with pentostatin be stopped.

Withholding or discontinuation of individual doses may be needed when severe adverse reactions occur. Drug treatment should be withheld in patients with severe rash, and withheld or discontinued in patients showing evidence of nervous system toxicity.

Pentostatin treatment should be withheld in patients with active infection occurring during the treatment but may be resumed when the infection is controlled.

Patients who have elevated serum creatinine should have their dose withheld and a creatinine clearance determined. There are insufficient data to recommend a starting or a subsequent dose for patients with impaired renal function (creatinine clearance <60 ml/min).

Patients with impaired renal function should be treated only when the potential benefit justifies the potential risk. Two patients with impaired renal function (creatinine clearances 50 to 60 ml/min) achieved complete response without unusual adverse events when treated with 2 mg/m^2.

No dosage reduction is recommended at the start of therapy with pentostatin in patients with anemia, neutropenia, or thrombocytopenia. In addition, dosage reductions are not recommended during treatment in patients with anemia and thrombocytopenia if patients can be otherwise supported hematologically. Pentostatin should be temporarily withheld if the absolute neutrophil count falls during treatment below 200 cells/mm^3 in a patient who had an initial neutrophil count greater than 500 cells/mm^{3}and may be resumed when the count returns to predose levels.

PREPARATION OF INTRAVENOUS SOLUTION

1. Procedures for proper handling and disposal of anticancer drugs should be followed. Several guidelines on this subject have been published.[2-7] There is no general agreement that all of the procedures recommended in the guidelines are necessary or appropriate. Spills and wastes should be treated with a 5% sodium hypochlorite solution prior to disposal.

2. Protective clothing including polyethylene gloves must be worn.

3. Transfer 5 ml of Sterile Water for Injection USP to the vial containing pentostatin and mix thoroughly to obtain complete dissolution of a solution yielding 2 mg/ml. Parenteral drug products should be inspected visually for particulate matter and discoloration prior to administration.

4. Pentostatin may be given intravenously by bolus injection or diluted in a larger volume (25 to 50 ml) with 5% Dextrose Injection USP or 0.9% Sodium Chloride Injection USP. Dilution of the entire contents of a reconstituted vial with 25 ml or 50 ml provides a pentostatin concentration of 0.33 mg/ml or 0.18 mg/ml respectively for the diluted solutions.

5. Pentostatin solution when diluted for infusion with 5% Dextrose Injection USP or 0.9% Sodium Chloride Injection USP does not interact with PVC infusion containers or administration sets at concentrations of 0.18 mg/ml to 0.33 mg/ml.

STABILITY

Pentostatin vials are stable at refrigerated storage temperature 2 to 8°C (36 to 46°F) for the period stated on the package. Vials reconstituted or reconstituted and further diluted as directed may be stored at room temperature and ambient light but should be used within 8 hours because Nipent contains no preservatives.

Storage: Store pentostatin vials under refrigerated storage conditions 2 to 8°C (36 to 46°F).

REFERENCES:

1. Malspeis L, et. al. Clinical Pharmacokinetics of 2'-Deoxycoformycin. Cancer Treatment Symposia 2:7-15, 1984. 2. Recommendations for the safe handling of parenteral antineoplastic drugs. NIH publication 83-2621. For sale by the Superintendent of Documents, US Government Printing Office, Washington, DC 20402. 3. AMA council report. Guidelines for handling parenteral antineoplastics. JAMA 253:590-2, 1985. 4. National Study Commission on Cytotoxic Exposure—Recommendations for handling cytotoxic agents. Director of Pharmacy Services, Rhode Island Hospital, 593 Eddy Street, Providence, RI 02902. 5. Clinical Oncological Society of Australia: Guidelines and recommendations for safe handling of antineoplastic agents. Med J Australia 1:426-8,

REFERENCES: *(cont'd)*

1983. 6. Jones RB, et. al. Safe handling of chemotherapeutic agents: A report from the Mount Sinai Medical Center. CA: A Cancer Journal for Clinicians 33:258-63, 1983. 7. American Society of Hospital Pharmacists technical assistance bulletin on handling cytotoxic and hazardous drugs. Am J Hosp Pharm 47:1033-49, 1990.

HOW SUPPLIED - EQUIVALENTS NOT AVAILABLE:

Injection, Solution - Intravenous - 10 mg

1's $1440.00 NIPENT, Parke-Davis 00071-4243-01

PENTOXIFYLLINE *(001980)*

CATEGORIES: Arterial Disease; Cardiovascular Drugs; Claudication; Hemorrheologic Agents; Vascular Disease; Vascular Disorders, Cerebral/Peripheral; Vasodilating Agents; Pregnancy Category C; Sales > $100 Million; FDA Approved 1984 Aug; Patent Expiration 1994 Aug; Top 200 Drugs

BRAND NAMES: *Artal*; *Azupentat* (Germany); *Ceretal*; *Ebisanin*; *Elorgan*; *Erytral*; *Flexital*; *Harine*; *Hemovas*; *Oxopurin 400 SR*; *Penlol*; *Pentoxi*; *Peridane* (Mexico); *Pexal*; *Sipental*; *Tarontal*; *Techlon*; *Torental* (France); **Trental**
(International brand names outside U.S. in italics)

FORMULARIES: Aetna; BC-BS; Medi-Cal; WellPoint

DESCRIPTION:

Trental (pentoxifylline) tablets for oral administration contain 400 mg of the active drug and the following inactive ingredients: benzyl alcohol NF, D&C Red No. 27 Aluminum Lake or FD&C Red No. 3, hydroxypropyl methylcellulose USP, magnesium stearate NF, polyethylene glycol NF, povidone USP, talc USP, titanium dioxide USP, and other ingredients in a controlled-release formulation. Trental is a tri-substituted xanthine derivative designated chemically as 1-(5-oxohexyl)-3, 7-dimethylxanthine that, unlike theophylline, is a hemorrheologic agent, i.e., an agent that affects blood viscosity. Pentoxifylline is soluble in water and ethanol, and sparingly soluble in toluene. The CAS Registry Number is 6493-05-6.

CLINICAL PHARMACOLOGY:

MODE OF ACTION

Pentoxifylline and its metabolites improve the flow properties of blood by decreasing its viscosity. In patients with chronic peripheral arterial disease, this increases blood flow to the affected microcirculation and enhances tissue oxygenation. The precise mode of action of pentoxifylline and the sequence of events leading to clinical improvement are still to be defined. Pentoxifylline administration has been shown to produce dose related hemorrheologic effects, lowering blood viscosity, and improving erythrocyte flexibility. Leukocyte properties of hemorrheologic importance have been modified in animal and *in vitro* human studies. Pentoxifylline has been shown to increase leukocyte deformability and to inhibit neutrophil adhesion and activation. Tissue oxygen levels have been shown to be significantly increased by therapeutic doses of pentoxifylline in patients with peripheral arterial disease.

PHARMACOKINETICS AND METABOLISM

After oral administration in aqueous solution pentoxifylline is almost completely absorbed. It undergoes a first-pass effect and the various metabolites appear in plasma very soon after dosing. Peak plasma levels of the parent compound and its metabolites are reached within 1 hour. The major metabolites are Metabolite I (1-[5-hydroxyhexyl]-3,7-dimethylxanthine) and Metabolite V (1-[3- carboxypropyl] -3, 7-dimethylxanthine), and plasma levels of these metabolites are 5 and 8 times greater, respectively, than pentoxifylline.

Following oral administration of aqueous solutions containing 100 to 400 mg of pentoxifylline, the pharmacokinetics of the parent compound and Metabolite I are dose-related and not proportional (non-linear), with half-life and area under the blood-level time curve (AUC) increasing with dose. The elimination kinetics of Metabolite V are not dose-dependent. The apparent plasma half-life of pentoxifylline varies from 0.4 to 0.8 hours and the apparent plasma half-lives of its metabolites vary from 1 to 1.6 hours. There is no evidence of accumulation or enzyme induction (Cytochrome P_{450}) following multiple oral doses.

Excretion is almost totally urinary; the main biotransformation product is Metabolite V. Essentially no parent drug is found in the urine. Despite large variations in plasma levels of parent compound and its metabolites, the urinary recovery of Metabolite V is consistent and shows dose proportionality. Less than 4% of the administered dose is recovered in feces. Food intake shortly before dosing delays absorption of an immediate-release dosage form but does not affect total absorption. The pharmacokinetics and metabolism of Trental (pentoxifylline) have not been studied in patients with renal and/or hepatic dysfunction, but AUC was increased and elimination rate decreased in an older population (60-68 years) compared to younger individuals (22-30 years).

After administration of the 400 mg controlled-release Trental tablet, plasma levels of the parent compound and its metabolites reach their maximum within 2 to 4 hours and remain constant over an extended period of time. The controlled release of pentoxifylline from the tablet eliminates peaks and troughs in plasma levels for improved gastrointestinal tolerance.

INDICATIONS AND USAGE:

Trental is indicated for the treatment of patients with intermittent claudication on the basis of chronic occlusive arterial disease of the limbs. Trental can improve function and symptoms but is not intended to replace more definitive therapy, such as surgical bypass, or removal of arterial obstructions when treating peripheral vascular disease.

CONTRAINDICATIONS:

Trental should not be used in patients with recent cerebral and/or retinal hemorrhage or in patients who have previously exhibited intolerance to this product or methylxanthines such as caffeine, theophylline, and theobromine.

PRECAUTIONS:

General: Patients with chronic occlusive arterial disease of the limbs frequently show other manifestations of arteriosclerotic disease. Trental has been used safely for treatment of peripheral arterial disease in patients with concurrent coronary artery and cerebrovascular diseases, but there have been occasional reports of angina, hypotension, and arrhythmia. Controlled trials do not show that Trental causes such adverse effects more often than placebo, but, as it is a methylxanthine derivative, it is possible some individuals will experience such responses. Patients on Warfarin should have more frequent monitoring of prothrombin times, while patients with other risk factors complicated by hemorrhage (*e.g.*, recent surgery, peptic ulceration, cerebral and/or retinal bleeding) should have periodic examinations for bleeding including hematocrit and/or hemoglobin.

Carcinogenesis, Mutagenesis and Impairment of Fertility: Long-term studies of the carcinogenic potential of pentoxifylline were conducted in mice and rats by dietary administration of the drug at doses up to approximately 19 times (450 mg/kg) the maximum recommended human daily dose (MRHD) of 24 mg/kg for 18 months in mice and 18 months in rats with an additional 6 months without drug exposure in the latter. No carcinogenic potential for pentoxifylline was noted in the mouse study. In the rat study, there was a

PRECAUTIONS: *(cont'd)*

statistically significant increase in benign mammary fibroadenomas in females in the high dose group (19 x MRHD). The relevance of this finding to human use is uncertain since this was only a marginal statistically significant increase for a tumor that is common in aged rats. Pentoxifylline was devoid of mutagenic activity in various strains of *Salmonella* (Ames test) when tested in the presence and absence of metabolic activation.

Pregnancy: Category C. Teratogenic studies have been performed in rats and rabbits at oral doses up to about 25 and 10 times the maximum recommended human daily dose (MRHD) of 24 mg/kg, respectively. No evidence of fetal malformation was observed. Increased resorption was seen in rats at 25 times MRHD. There are, however, no adequate and well controlled studies in pregnant women. Because animal reproduction studies are not always predictive of human response, Trental should be used during pregnancy only if clearly needed.

Nursing Mothers: Pentoxifylline and its metabolites are excreted in human milk. Because of the potential for tumorigenicity shown for pentoxifylline in rats, a decision should be made whether to discontinue nursing or discontinue the drug, taking into account the importance of the drug to the mother.

Pediatric Use: Safety and effectiveness in pediatric patients have not been established.

DRUG INTERACTIONS:

Although a causal relationship has not been established, there have been reports of bleeding and/or prolonged prothrombin time in patients treated with Trental with and without anticoagulants or platelet aggregation inhibitors. Patients on Warfarin should have more frequent monitoring of prothrombin times, while patients with other risk factors complicated by hemorrhage (*e.g.*, recent surgery, peptic ulceration) should have periodic examinations for bleeding including hematocrit and/or hemoglobin. Concomitant administration of Trental and theophylline-containing drugs leads to increased theophylline levels and theophylline toxicity in some individuals. Such patients should be closely monitored for signs of toxicity and have their theophylline dosage adjusted as necessary. Trental has been used concurrently with antihypertensive drugs, beta blockers, digitalis, diuretics, antidiabetic agents, and antiarrhythmics, without observed problems. Small decreases in blood pressure have been observed in some patients treated with Trental; periodic systemic blood pressure monitoring is recommended for patients receiving concomitant antihypertensive therapy. If indicated, dosage of the antihypertensive agents should be reduced.

ADVERSE REACTIONS:

Clinical trials were conducted using either controlled-release Trental (pentoxifylline) tablets for up to 60 weeks or immediate-release Trental capsules for up to 24 weeks. Dosage ranges in the tablet studies were 400 mg bid to tid and in the capsule studies, 200-400 mg tid.

The table (TABLE 1) summarizes the incidence (in percent) of adverse reactions considered drug related, as well as the numbers of patients who received controlled-release Trental tablets, immediate-release Trental capsules, or the corresponding placebos. The incidence of adverse reactions was higher in the capsule studies (where dose related increases were seen in digestive and nervous system side effects) than in the tablet studies. Studies with the capsule include domestic experience, whereas studies with the controlled-release tablets were conducted outside the U.S. The table (TABLE 1) indicates that in the tablet studies few patients discontinued because of adverse effects.

TABLE 1 INCIDENCE (%) OF SIDE EFFECTS

	Controlled-Release Immediate-Release Tablets Commercially Available		Immediate-Release Capsules Used only for Controlled Clinical Trials	
	Trental	**Placebo**	**Trental**	**Placebo**
(Numbers of Patients at Risk)	(321)	(128)	(177)	(138)
Discontinued for Side Effect	3.1	0	9.6	7.2
CARDIOVASCULAR SYSTEM				
Angina/Chest Pain	0.3	-	1.1	2.2
Arrhythmia/Palpitation	-	-	1.7	0.7
Flushing	-	-	2.3	0.7
DIGESTIVE SYSTEM				
Abdominal Discomfort	-	-	4.0	1.4
Belching/Flatus/Bloating	0.6	-	9.0	3.6
Diarrhea	-	-	3.4	2.9
Dyspepsia	2.8	4.7	9.6	2.9
Nausea	2.2	0.8	28.8	8.7
Vomiting	1.2	-	4.5	0.7
NERVOUS SYSTEM				
Agitation/Nervousness	-	-	1.7	0.7
Dizziness	1.9	3.1	11.9	4.3
Drowsiness	-	-	1.1	5.8
Headache	1.2	1.6	6.2	5.8
Insomnia	-	-	2.3	2.2
Tremor	0.3	0.8	-	-
Blurred Vision	-	-	2.3	1.4

Trental has been marketed in Europe and elsewhere since 1972. In addition to the above symptoms, the following have been reported spontaneously since marketing or occurred in other clinical trials with an incidence of less than 1%; the causal relationship was uncertain:

Cardiovascular: dyspnea, edema, hypotension.

Digestive: anorexia, cholecystitis, constipation, dry mouth/thirst.

Nervous: anxiety, confusion, depression, seizures.

Respiratory: epistaxis, flu-like symptoms, laryngitis, nasal congestion.

Skin and Appendages: brittle fingernails, pruritus, rash, urticaria, angioedema.

Special Senses: blurred vision, conjunctivitis, earache, scotoma.

Miscellaneous: bad taste, excessive salivation, leukopenia, malaise, sore throat/swollen neck glands, weight change.

A few rare events have been reported spontaneously worldwide since marketing in 1972. Although they occurred under circumstances in which a causal relationship with pentoxifylline could not be established, they are listed to serve as information for physicians: "Cardiovascular— angina, arrhythmia, tachycardia, anaphylactoid reactions." Digestive—hepatitis, jaundice, increased liver enzymes; and Hemic and Lymphatic—decreased serum fibrinogen, pancytopenia, aplastic anemia, leukemia, purpura, thrombocytopenia."

OVERDOSAGE:

Overdosage with Trental (pentoxifylline) has been reported in pediatric patients and adults. Symptoms appear to be dose related. A report from a poison control center on 44 patients taking overdoses of enteric-coated pentoxifylline tablets noted that symptoms usually occurred 4-5 hours after ingestion and lasted about 12 hours. The highest amount ingested was 80 mg/kg; flushing, hypotension, convulsions, somnolence, loss of consciousness, fever, and agitation occurred. All patients recovered.

In addition to symptomatic treatment and gastric lavage, special attention must be given to supporting respiration, maintaining systemic blood pressure, and controlling convulsions. Activated charcoal has been used to adsorb pentoxifylline in patients who have overdosed.

DOSAGE AND ADMINISTRATION:

The usual dosage of Trental in controlled-release tablet form is one tablet (400 mg) three times a day with meals.

While the effect of Trental may be seen within 2 to 4 weeks, it is recommended that treatment be continued for at least 8 weeks. Efficacy has been demonstrated in double-blind clinical studies of 6 months duration.

Digestive and central nervous system side effects are dose related. If patients develop these side effects it is recommended that the dosage be lowered to one tablet twice a day (800 mg/day). If side effects persist at this lower dosage, the administration of Trental should be discontinued.

PATIENT INFORMATION:

Pentoxifylline is used to treat a condition known as intermittent claudication which is where blood vessels in the arms or legs are somewhat blocked. This drug works by making blood cells more flexible making it easier for them to squeeze through small openings in the vessels. This drug doesn't directly improve the situation but does relieve symptoms such as pain in the extremities. Those intolerant of caffeine, theophylline or theobromine may be suited to take this drug. The most common side effects reported with pentoxifylline include nausea, dizziness, heartburn and belching. These side effects are related to the dose and decreasing the dose decreases the side effects. Improvement in symptoms may not be seen for 8 weeks. Therapy should be continued and re-assessed regularly.

HOW SUPPLIED:

Trental is available for oral administration as 400 mg pink film-coated oblong tablets imprinted Trental.

Store at controlled room temperature (59 to 86°F).

Dispense in well-closed, light-resistant containers.

Protect blisters from light.

HOW SUPPLIED - EQUIVALENTS NOT AVAILABLE:

Tablet, Coated, Sustained Action - Oral - 400 mg

100's	$56.55	TRENTAL, Hoechst Marion Roussel	00039-0078-10
100's	$59.04	TRENTAL, Hoechst Marion Roussel	00039-0078-11
5000's	$2827.50	TRENTAL, Hoechst Marion Roussel	00039-0078-80

PERGOLIDE MESYLATE *(001986)*

CATEGORIES: Anticholinergic Agents; Antiparkinson Agents; Autonomic Drugs; Dopamine Receptor Agonists; Extrapyramidal Movement Disorders; Neuromuscular; Parkinsonism; Pregnancy Category B; FDA Approved 1988 Dec

BRAND NAMES: *Celance* (England); *Parkotil* (Germany); *Pergolide*; **Permax**
(International brand names outside U.S. in italics)

FORMULARIES: Aetna; Medi-Cal; PCS

COST OF THERAPY: $559.54 (Parkinsonism; Tablet; 0.05 mg; 3/day; 365 days)

DESCRIPTION:

Pergolide Mesylate is an ergot derivative dopamine receptor agonist at both D_1 and D_2 receptor sites. Pergolide mesylate is chemically designated as 8β-[(Methylthio)methyl]-6-propylergoline monomethanesulfonate.

The formula weight of the base is 314.5; 1 mg of base corresponds to 3.18 μmol.

Pergolide Mesylate is provided for oral administration in tablets containing 0.05 mg (0.159 μmol), 0.25 mg (0.795 μmol), or 1 mg (3.18 μmol) pergolide as the base. The tablets also contain croscarmellose sodium, iron oxide, lactose, magnesium stearate, and povidone. The 0.05-mg tablet also contains methionine, and the 0.25-mg tablet also contains F D & C Blue No. 2.

CLINICAL PHARMACOLOGY:

Pharmacodynamic Information: Pergolide mesylate is a potent dopamine receptor agonist. Pergolide is 10 to 1,000 times more potent than bromocriptine on a milligram per milligram basis in various *in vitro* and *in vivo* test systems. Pergolide mesylate inhibits the secretion of prolactin in humans; it causes a transient rise in serum concentrations of growth hormone and a decrease in serum concentrations of luteinizing hormone. In Parkinson's disease, pergolide mesylate is believed to exert its therapeutic effect by directly stimulating postsynaptic dopamine receptors in the nigrostriatal system.

Pharmacokinetic Information (Absorption, Distribution, Metabolism, and Elimination): Information on oral systemic bioavailability of pergolide mesylate is unavailable because of the lack of a sufficiently sensitive assay to detect the drug after the administration of a single dose. However, following oral administration of ^{14}C radiolabeled pergolide mesylate, approximately 55% of the administered radioactivity can be recovered from the urine and 5% from expired CO_2, suggesting that a significant fraction is absorbed. Nothing can be concluded about the extent of presystemic clearance, if any.

Data on postabsorption distribution of pergolide are unavailable.

At least 10 metabolites have been detected, including N-despropylpergolide, pergolide sulfoxide, and pergolide sulfone. Pergolide sulfoxide and pergolide sulfone are dopamine agonists in animals. The other detected metabolites have not been identified and it is not known whether any other metabolites are active pharmacologically.

The major route of excretion is the kidney.

Pergolide is approximately 90% bound to plasma proteins. This extent of protein binding may be important to consider when pergolide mesylate is coadministered with other drugs known to affect protein binding.

INDICATIONS AND USAGE:

Pergolide Mesylate is indicated as adjunctive treatment to levodopa/carbidopa in the management of the signs and symptoms of Parkinson's disease.

Evidence to support the efficacy of pergolide mesylate as an antiparkinsonian adjunct was obtained in a multicenter study enrolling 376 patients with mild to moderate Parkinson's disease who were intolerant to *l*-dopa/carbidopa as manifested by moderate to severe dyskinesia and/or on-off phenomena. On average, the patients evaluated had been on *l*-dopa/

INDICATIONS AND USAGE: *(cont'd)*

carbidopa for 3.9 years (range, 2 days to 16.8 years). The administration of pergolide mesylate permitted a 5% to 30% reduction in the daily dose of *l*-dopa. On average, these patients treated with pergolide mesylate maintained an equivalent or better clinical status than they exhibited at baseline.

CONTRAINDICATIONS:

Pergolide mesylate is contraindicated in patients who are hypersensitive to this drug or other ergot derivatives.

WARNINGS:

Symptomatic Hypotension: In clinical trials, approximately 10% of patients taking pergolide mesylate with *l*-dopa versus 7% taking placebo with *l*-dopa experienced symptomatic orthostatic and/or sustained hypotension, especially during initial treatment. With gradual dosage titration, tolerance to the hypotension usually develops. It is therefore important to warn patients of the risk, to begin therapy with low doses, and to increase the dosage in carefully adjusted increments over a period of 3 to 4 weeks (see DOSAGE AND ADMINISTRATION).

Hallucinosis: In controlled trials, pergolide mesylate with *l*-dopa caused hallucinosis in about 14% of patients as opposed to 3% taking placebo with *l*-dopa. This was of sufficient severity to cause discontinuation of treatment in about 3% of those enrolled; tolerance to this untoward effect was not observed.

Fatalities: In the placebo-controlled trial, 2 of 187 patients treated with placebo died as compared with 1 of 189 patients treated with pergolide mesylate. Of the 2,299 patients treated with pergolide mesylate in premarketing studies evaluated as of October 1988, 143 died while on the drug or shortly after discontinuing it. Because the patient population under evaluation was elderly, ill, and at high risk for death, it seems unlikely that pergolide mesylate played any role in these deaths, but the possibility that pergolide shortens survival of patients cannot be excluded with absolute certainty.

In particular, a case-by-case review of the clinical course of the patients who died failed to disclose any unique set of signs, symptoms, or laboratory results that would suggest that treatment with pergolide caused their deaths. Sixty-eight percent (68%) of the patients who died were 65 years of age or older. No death (other than a suicide) occurred within the first month of treatment; most of the patients who died had been on pergolide for years. A relative frequency of the causes of death by organ system are: Pulmonary failure/Pneumonia, 35%; Cardiovascular, 30%; Cancer, 11%; Unknown, 8.4%; Infection, 3.5%; Extrapyramidal syndrome, 3.5%; Stroke, 2.1%; Dysphagia, 2.1%; Injury, 1.4%; Suicide, 1.4%; Dehydration, 0.7%; Glomerulonephritis, 0.7%.

PRECAUTIONS:

General: Caution should be exercised when administering pergolide mesylate to patients prone to cardiac dysrhythmias.

In a study comparing pergolide mesylate and placebo, patients taking pergolide mesylate were found to have significantly more episodes of atrial premature contractions (APCs) and sinus tachycardia.

The use of pergolide mesylate in patients on *l*-dopa may cause and/or exacerbate preexisting states of confusion and hallucinations (see WARNINGS) and preexisting dyskinesia. Also, the abrupt discontinuation of pergolide mesylate in patients receiving it chronically as an adjunct to *l*-dopa may precipitate the onset of hallucinations and confusion; these may occur within a span of several days. Discontinuation of pergolide should be undertaken gradually whenever possible, even if the patient is to remain on *l*-dopa.

A symptom complex resembling the neuroleptic malignant syndrome (NMS) (characterized by elevated temperature, muscular rigidity, altered consciousness, and autonomic instability), with no other obvious etiology, has been reported in association with rapid dose reduction, withdrawal of, or changes in antiparkinsonian therapy, including pergolide.

Information for the Patient: Patients and their families should be informed of the common adverse consequences of the use of pergolide mesylate (see ADVERSE REACTIONS) and the risk of hypotension (see WARNINGS).

Patients should be advised to notify their physician if they become pregnant or intend to become pregnant during therapy.

Patients should be advised to notify their physician if they are breast feeding an infant.

Laboratory Tests: No specific laboratory tests are deemed essential for the management of patients on Pergolide Mesylate. Periodic routine evaluation of all patients, however, is appropriate.

Carcinogenesis, Mutagenesis, and Impairment of Fertility: A 2-year carcinogenicity study was conducted in mice using dietary levels of pergolide mesylate equivalent to oral doses of 0.6, 3.7, and 36.4 mg/kg/day in males and 0.6, 4.4, and 40.8 mg/kg/day in females. A 2-year study in rats was conducted using dietary levels equivalent to oral doses of 0.04, 0.18, and 0.88 mg/kg/day in males and 0.05, 0.28, and 1.42 mg/kg/day in females. The highest doses tested in the mice and rats were approximately 340 and 12 times the maximum human oral dose administered in controlled clinical trials (6 mg/day equivalent to 0.12 mg/kg/day).

A low incidence of uterine neoplasms occurred in both rats and mice. Endometrial adenomas and carcinomas were observed in rats. Endometrial sarcomas were observed in mice. The occurrence of these neoplasms is probably attributable to the high estrogen/progesterone ratio that would occur in rodents as a result of the prolactin-inhibiting action of pergolide mesylate. The endocrine mechanisms believed to be involved in the rodents are not present in humans. However, even though there is no known correlation between uterine malignancies occurring in pergolide-treated rodents and human risk, there are no human data to substantiate this conclusion.

Pergolide mesylate was evaluated for mutagenic potential in a battery of tests that included an Ames bacterial mutation assay, a DNA repair assay in cultured rat hepatocytes, an *in vitro* mammalian cell- point-mutation assay in cultured L5178Y cells, and a determination of chromosome alteration in bone marrow cells of Chinese hamsters. A weak mutagenic response was noted in the mammalian cell-point-mutation assay only after metabolic activation with rat liver microsomes. No mutagenic effects were obtained in the 2 other *in vitro* assays and in the *in vivo* assay. The relevance of these findings in humans is unknown.

A fertility study in male and female mice showed that fertility was maintained at 0.6 and 1.7 mg/kg/day but decreased at 5.6 mg/kg/day. Prolactin has been reported to be involved in stimulating and maintaining progesterone levels required for implantation in mice and, therefore, the impaired fertility at the high dose may have occurred because of depressed prolactin levels.

Pregnancy Category B: Reproduction studies were conducted in mice at doses of 5, 16, and 45 mg/kg/day and in rabbits at doses of 2, 6, and 16 mg/kg/day. The highest doses tested in mice and rabbits were 375 and 133 times the 6 mg/day maximum human dose administered in controlled clinical trials. In these studies, there was no evidence of harm to the fetus due to pergolide mesylate.

There are, however, no adequate and well-controlled studies in pregnant women. Among women who received pergolide mesylate for endocrine disorders in premarketing studies, there were 33 pregnancies that resulted in healthy babies and 6 pregnancies that resulted in

PRECAUTIONS: *(cont'd)*

congenital abnormalities (3 major, 3 minor); a causal relationship has not been established. Because human data are limited and because animal reproduction studies are not always predictive of human response, this drug should be used during pregnancy only if clearly needed.

Nursing Mothers: It is not known whether this drug is excreted in human milk. The pharmacologic action of pergolide mesylate suggests that it may interfere with lactation. Because many drugs are excreted in human milk and because of the potential for serious adverse reactions to pergolide mesylate in nursing infants, a decision should be made whether to discontinue nursing or to discontinue the drug, taking into account the importance of the drug to the mother.

Pediatric Use: Safety and effectiveness in children have not been established.

DRUG INTERACTIONS:

Dopamine antagonists, such as the neuroleptics (phenothiazines, butyrophenones, thioxanthenes) or metoclopramide, ordinarily should not be administered concurrently with Pergolide Mesylate (a dopamine agonist); these agents may diminish the effectiveness of Pergolide Mesylate.

Because pergolide mesylate is approximately 90% bound to plasma proteins, caution should be exercised if pergolide mesylate is coadministered with other drugs known to affect protein binding.

ADVERSE REACTIONS:

Commonly Observed: In premarketing clinical trials, the most commonly observed adverse events associated with use of pergolide mesylate which were not seen at an equivalent incidence among placebo-treated patients were: nervous system complaints, including dyskinesia, hallucinations, somnolence, insomnia; digestive complaints, including nausea, constipation, diarrhea, dyspepsia; and respiratory system complaints, including rhinitis.

Associated With Discontinuation of Treatment: Twenty-seven percent (27%) of approximately 1,200 patients receiving pergolide mesylate for treatment of Parkinson's disease in premarketing clinical trials in the US and Canada discontinued treatment due to adverse events. The events most commonly causing discontinuation were related to the nervous system (15.5%), primarily hallucinations (7.8%) and confusion (1.8%).

Fatalities: See WARNINGS.

Incidence in Controlled Clinical Trials: The table that follows, (TABLE 1), enumerates adverse events that occurred at a frequency of 1% or more among patients taking pergolide mesylate who participated in the premarketing controlled clinical trials comparing pergolide mesylate with placebo. In a double-blind, controlled study of 6 months' duration, patients with Parkinson's disease were continued on*l*-dopa/carbidopa and were randomly assigned to receive either pergolide mesylate or placebo as additional therapy.

The prescriber should be aware that these figures cannot be used to predict the incidence of side effects in the course of usual medical practice where patient characteristics and other factors differ from those which prevailed in the clinical trials. Similarly, the cited frequencies cannot be compared with figures obtained from other clinical investigations involving different treatments, uses, and investigators. The cited figures, however, do provide the prescribing physician with some basis for estimating the relative contribution of drug and nondrug factors to the side-effect incidence rate in the population studied.

Events Observed During the Premarketing Evaluation of Pergolide Mesylate: This section reports event frequencies evaluated as of October 1988 for adverse events occurring in a group of approximately 1,800 patients who took multiple doses of pergolide mesylate. The conditions and duration of exposure to pergolide mesylate varied greatly, involving well-controlled studies as well as experience in open and uncontrolled clinical settings. In the absence of appropriate controls in some of the studies, a casual relationship between these events and treatments with pergolide mesylate cannot be determined.

The following enumeration by organ system describes events in terms of their relative frequency of reporting in the data base. Events of major clinical importance are also described in the WARNINGS and PRECAUTIONS sections.

The following definitions of frequency are used: frequent adverse events are defined as those occurring in at least 1/100 patients; infrequent adverse events are those occurring in 1/100 to 1/1,000 patients; rare events are those occurring in fewer than 1/1,000 patients.

Body as a Whole

Frequent: headache, asthenia, accidental injury, pain, abdominal pain, chest pain, back pain, flu syndrome, neck pain, fever

Infrequent: facial edema, chills, enlarged abdomen, malaise, neoplasm, hernia, pelvic pain, sepsis, cellulitis, moniliasis, abscess, jaw pain, hypothermia

Rare: acute abdominal syndrome, LE syndrome

Cardiovascular System

Frequent: postural hypotension, syncope, hypertension, palpitations, vasodilatations, congestive heart failure

Infrequent: myocardial infarction, tachycardia, heart arrest, abnormal electrocardiogram, angina pectoris, thrombophlebitis, bradycardia, ventricular extrasystoles, cerebrovascular accident, ventricular tachycardia, cerebral ischemia, atrial fibrillation, varicose vein, pulmonary embolus, AV block, shock

Rare: vasculitis, pulmonary hypertension, pericarditis, migraine, heart block, cerebral hemorrhage

Digestive System

Frequent: nausea, vomiting, dyspepsia, diarrhea, constipation, dry mouth, dysphagia

Infrequent: flatulence, abnormal liver function tests, increased appetite, salivary gland enlargement, thirst, gastroenteritis, gastritis, periodontal abscess, intestinal obstruction, nausea and vomiting, gingivitis, esophagitis, cholelithiasis, tooth carries, hepatitis, stomach ulcer, melena, hepatomegaly, hematemesis, eructation

Rare: sialadenitis, peptic ulcer, pancreatitis, jaundice, glossitis, fecal incontinence, duodenitis, colitis, cholecystitis, aphthous stomatitis, esophageal ulcer

Endocrine System

Infrequent: hypothyroidism, adenoma, diabetes mellitus, ADH inappropriate

Rare: Endocrine disorder, thyroid adenoma

Hemic and Lymphatic System

Frequent: anemia

Infrequent: leukopenia, lymphadenopathy, leukocytosis, thrombocytopenia, petechia, megaloblastic anemia, cyanosis

Rare: purpura, lymphocytosis, eosinophilia, thrombocythemia, acute lymphoblastic leukemia, polycythemia, splenomegaly

Metabolic and Nutritional System

Frequent: peripheral edema, weight loss, weight gain;

Infrequent: dehydration, hypokalemia, hypoglycemia, iron deficiency anemia, hyperglycemia, gout, hypercholesteremia

ADVERSE REACTIONS: *(cont'd)*

TABLE 1 Incidence of Treatment-Emergent Adverse Experiences in the Placebo-Controlled Clinical Trial Percentage of Patients Reporting Events

Body System/Adverse Event*	Pergolide Mesylate N = 189	Placebo N = 187
BODY AS A WHOLE		
Pain	7.0	2.1
Abdominal pain	5.8	2.1
Injury, accident	5.8	7.0
Headache	5.3	6.4
Asthenia	4.2	4.8
Chest pain	3.7	2.1
Flu syndrome	3.2	2.1
Neck pain	2.7	1.6
Back pain	1.6	2.1
Surgical procedure	1.6	<1
Chills	1.1	0
Face edema	1.1	0
Infection	1.1	0
CARDIOVASCULAR		
Postural hypotension	9.0	7.0
Vasodilatation	3.2	<1
Palpitation	2.1	<1
Hypotension	2.1	<1
Syncope	2.1	1.1
Hypertension	1.6	1.1
Arrhythmia	1.1	<1
Myocardial infarction	1.1	<1
DIGESTIVE		
Nausea	24.3	12.8
Constipation	10.6	5.9
Diarrhea	6.4	2.7
Dyspepsia	6.4	2.1
Anorexia	4.8	2.7
Dry mouth	3.7	<1
Vomiting	2.7	1.6
HEMIC AND LYMPHATIC		
Anemia	1.1	<1
METABOLIC AND NUTRITIONAL		
Peripheral edema	7.4	4.3
Edema	1.6	0
Weight gain	1.6	0
MUSCULOSKELETAL		
Arthralgia	1.6	2.1
Bursitis	1.6	<1
Myalgia	1.1	<1
Twitching	1.1	0
NERVOUS SYSTEM		
Dyskinesia	62.4	24.6
Dizziness	19.1	13.9
Hallucinations	13.8	3.2
Dystonia	11.6	8.0
Confusion	11.1	9.6
Somnolence	10.1	3.7
Insomnia	7.9	3.2
Anxiety	6.4	4.3
Tremor	4.2	7.5
Depression	3.2	5.4
Abnormal dreams	2.7	4.3
Personality disorder	2.1	<1
Psychosis	2.1	0
Abnormal gait	1.6	1.6
Akathisia	1.6	0
Extrapyramidal syndrome	1.6	1.1
Incoordination	1.6	<1
Paresthesia	1.6	3.2
Akinesia	1.1	1.1
Hypertonia	1.1	0
Neuralgia	1.1	<1
Speech disorder	1.1	1.6
RESPIRATORY SYSTEM		
Rhinitis	12.2	5.4
Dyspnea	4.8	1.1
Epistaxis	1.6	<1
Hiccup	1.1	0
SKIN AND APPENDAGES		
Rash	3.2	2.1
Sweating	2.1	2.7
SPECIAL SENSES		
Abnormal vision	5.8	5.4
Diplopia	2.1	0
Taste perversion	1.6	0
Eye disorder	1.1	0
UROGENITAL SYSTEM		
Urinary frequency	2.7	6.4
Urinary tract infection	2.7	3.7
Hematuria	1.1	<1

* Events reported by at least 1% of patients receiving pergolide mesylate are included.

Rare: electrolyte imbalance, cachexia, acidosis, hyperuricemia

Musculoskeletal System

Frequent: twitching, myalgia, arthralgia

Infrequent: bone pain, tenosynovitis, myositis, bone sarcoma, arthritis

Rare: osteoporosis, muscle atrophy, osteomyelitis

Nervous System

Frequent: dyskinesia, dizziness, hallucinations, confusion, somnolence, insomnia, dystonia, paresthesia, depression, anxiety, tremor, akinesia, extrapyramidal syndrome, abnormal gait, abnormal dreams, incoordination, psychosis, personality disorder, nervousness, choreoathetosis, amnesia, paranoid reaction, abnormal thinking

Infrequent: akathisia, neuropathy, neuralgia, hypertonia, delusions, convulsion, libido increased, euphoria, emotional lability, libido decreased, vertigo, myoclonus, coma, apathy, paralysis, neurosis, hyperkinesia, ataxia, acute brain syndrome, torticollis, meningitis, manic reaction, hypokinesia, hostility, agitation, hypotonia

Rare: stupor, neuritis, intracranial hypertension, hemiplegia, facial paralysis, brain edema, myelitis, hallucinations and confusion after abrupt discontinuation

Respiratory System

Frequent: rhinitis, dyspnea, pneumonia, pharyngitis, cough increased

ADVERSE REACTIONS: *(cont'd)*

Infrequent: epistaxis, hiccup, sinusitis, bronchitis, voice alteration, hemoptysis, asthma, lung edema, pleural effusion, laryngitis, emphysema, apnea, hyperventilation

Rare: pneumothorax, lung fibrosis, larynx edema, hypoxia, hypoventilation, hemothorax, carcinoma of lung

Skin and Appendages System

Frequent: sweating, rash

Infrequent: skin discoloration, pruritus, acne, skin ulcer, alopecia, dry skin, skin carcinoma, seborrhea, hirsutism, herpes simplex, eczema, fungal dermatitis, herpes zoster

Rare: vesiculobullous rash, subcutaneous nodule, skin nodule, skin benign neoplasm, lichenoid dermatitis

Special Senses System

Frequent: abnormal vision, diplopia

Infrequent: otitis media, conjunctivitis, tinnitus, deafness, taste perversion, ear pain, eye pain, glaucoma, eye hemorrhage, photophobia, visual field defect

Rare: blindness, cataract, retinal detachment, retinal vascular disorder

Urogenital System

Frequent: urinary tract infection, urinary frequency, urinary incontinence, hematuria, dysmenorrhea

Infrequent: dysuria, breast pain, menorrhagia, impotence, cystitis, urinary retention, abortion, vaginal hemorrhage, vaginitis, priapism, kidney calculus, fibrocystic breast, lactation, uterine hemorrhage, urolithiasis, salpingitis, pyuria, metrorrhagia, menopause, kidney failure, breast carcinoma, cervical carcinoma

Rare: amenorrhea, bladder carcinoma, breast engorgement, epididymitis, hypogonadism, leukorrhea, nephrosis, pyelonephritis, urethral pain, uricaciduria, withdrawal bleeding.

Postintroduction Reports

Voluntary reports of adverse events temporally associated with pergolide that have been received since market introduction and which may have no causal relationship with the drug, include the following: neuroleptic malignant syndrome.

OVERDOSAGE:

There is no clinical experience with massive overdosage. The largest overdose involved a young hospitalized adult patient who was not being treated with pergolide mesylate but who intentionally took 60 mg of the drug. He experienced vomiting, hypotension, and agitation. Another patient receiving a daily dosage of 7 mg of pergolide mesylate unintentionally took 19 mg/day for 3 days, after which his vital signs were normal but he experienced severe hallucinations. Within 36 hours of resumption of the prescribed dosage level, the hallucinations stopped. One patient unintentionally took 14 mg/day for 23 days instead of her prescribed 1.4 mg/day dosage. She experienced severe involuntary movements and tingling in her arms and legs. Another patient who inadvertently received 7 mg instead of the prescribed 0.7 mg experienced palpitations, hypotension, and ventricular extrasystoles. The highest total daily dose (prescribed for several patients with refractory Parkinson's disease) has exceeded 30 mg.

Symptoms: Animal studies indicate that the manifestations of overdosage in man might include nausea, vomiting, convulsions, decreased blood pressure, and CNS stimulation. The oral median lethal doses in mice and rats were 54 and 15 mg/kg respectively.

Treatment: To obtain up-to-date information about the treatment of overdose, a good resource is your certified Regional Poison Control Center. Telephone numbers of certified poison control centers are listed in the beginning of *Physicians GenRx*. In managing overdosage, consider the possibility of multiple drug overdoses, interaction among drugs, and unusual drug kinetics in your patient.

Management of overdosage may require supportive measures to maintain arterial blood pressure. Cardiac function should be monitored; an antiarrhythmic agent may be necessary. If signs of CNS stimulation are present, a phenothiazine or other butyrophenone neuroleptic agent may be indicated; the efficacy of such drugs in reversing the effects of overdose has not been assessed.

Protect the patient's airway and support ventilation and perfusion. Meticulously monitor and maintain, within acceptable limits, the patient's vital signs, blood gases, serum electrolytes, etc. Absorption of drugs from the gastrointestinal tract may be decreased by giving activated charcoal, which, in many cases, is more effective than emesis or lavage; consider charcoal instead of or in addition to gastric emptying. Repeated doses of charcoal over time may hasten elimination of some drugs that have been absorbed. Safeguard the patient's airway when employing gastric emptying or charcoal.

There is no experience with dialysis or hemoperfusion, and these procedures are unlikely to be of benefit.

DOSAGE AND ADMINISTRATION:

Administration of Pergolide Mesylate should be initiated with a daily dosage of 0.05 mg for the first 2 days. The dosage should then be gradually increased by 0.1 or 0.15 mg/day every third day over the next 12 days of therapy. The dosage may then be increased by 0.25 mg/day every third day until an optimal therapeutic dosage is achieved.

Pergolide Mesylate is usually administered in divided doses 3 times per day. During dosage titration, the dosage of concurrent *l*-dopa/carbidopa may be cautiously decreased.

In clinical studies, the mean therapeutic daily dosage of Pergolide Mesylate was 3 mg/day. The average concurrent daily dosage of *l*-dopa/carbidopa (expressed as *l*-dopa) was approximately 650 mg/day. The efficacy of Pergolide Mesylate at doses above 5 mg/day has not been systematically evaluated.

HOW SUPPLIED:

Tablets (Scored): 0.05 mg, ivory, 0.25 mg, green, 1 mg, pink

Store at controlled room temperature, 59° to 86°F (15° to 30°C).

HOW SUPPLIED - EQUIVALENTS NOT AVAILABLE:

Tablet, Uncoated - Oral - 0.05 mg

30's	$15.33	PERMAX, Athena	59075-0615-30

Tablet, Uncoated - Oral - 0.25 mg

100's	$106.20	PERMAX, Athena	59075-0625-10

Tablet, Uncoated - Oral - 1 mg

100's	$352.60	PERMAX, Athena	59075-0630-10

PERINDOPRIL ERBUMINE *(003191)*

CATEGORIES: ACE Inhibitors; Angiotensin Converting Enzyme Inhibitors; Antihypertensives; Cardiovascular Drugs; Hypertension; Pregnancy Category D; FDA Class 1S ("Standard Review"); FDA Approved 1993 Dec

BRAND NAMES: **Aceon**; *Acertil*; *Coversum* (Germany); *Coversyl* (Australia, France, England); *Prexum*
(International brand names outside U.S. in italics)

Prescribing information not available at time of publication.

PERMETHRIN *(001987)*

CATEGORIES: Anti-Infectives; Antiparasitics; Arthropods; Dermatologicals; Lice; Ovicide; Parasiticidal; Pediculicides; Scabicides/Pediculicides; Skin/Mucous Membrane Agents; Topical; Pregnancy Category B; FDA Approved 1986 Mar

BRAND NAMES: Elimite; *Lyclear* (England); *Lyclear Dermal Cream*; *Lyclear Scabies Cream*; **Nix**; *Nix Cream*; *Nix Creme Rinse* (Canada); *Nix Dermal Cream* (Canada); *Nok*; *Novo-Herklin 2000* (Mexico); *Quellada Creme Rinse*; *Quellada Head Lice Treatment*; *Scabmite*; *Zehu-Ze*
(International brand names outside U.S. in italics)

FORMULARIES: Medi-Cal; PCS; WHO

DESCRIPTION:

Nix (Permethrin) 1% Creme Rinse is a topical pediculicide and ovicide for the treatment of infestation with *Pediculus humanus* var. *capitis* (the head louse) and its nits (eggs). The product is a creme rinse, each gram containing Permethrin 10 mg (1%). Inactive ingredients are: stearalkonium chloride, hydrolyzed animal protein, cetyl alcohol, polyoxyethylene 10 cetyl ether, hydroxyethylcellulose, balsam canada, fragrance, citric acid, propylene glycol and FD&C Yellow No. 6. Also contains isopropyl alcohol 200 mg (20%) and added as preservatives, methylparaben 2 mg (0.2%), propylparaben 0.8 mg (0.08%) and imidazolidinyl urea 2 mg (0.2%).

Permethrin is a mixture of the *cis* and *trans* isomers of the synthetic pyrethroid (+-)-3-phenoxybenzyl 3-(2,2-dichlorovinyl)-2,2-dimethylcyclopropanecarboxylate (*cis trans*/25:75). It is a yellow to light orange-brown low melting solid or viscous liquid. The molecular weight is 391.29.

CLINICAL PHARMACOLOGY:

Permethrin is a synthetic pyrethroid, active against lice, ticks, mites, and fleas. It acts on the nerve cell membrane to disrupt the sodium channel current by which the polarization of the membrane is regulated. Delayed repolarization and paralysis of the pests are the consequences of this disturbance.

Permethrin is rapidly metabolized by ester hydrolysis to inactive metabolites which are excreted primarily in the urine. Although the amount of permethrin absorbed after a single application of the 1% Creme Rinse has not been determined precisely, preliminary data suggest it is less than 2% of the amount applied. Residual persistence of Nix is detectable on the hair for at least 10 days following a single application.

PEDICULICIDAL/OVICIDAL ACTIVITIES:

In vitro data indicate that permethrin has pediculicidal and ovicidal activity against *Pediculus humanus var. capitis*. The high cure rate (97-99%) of Nix in patients with head lice demonstrated at 14 days following a single application is attributable to a combination of its pediculicidal and ovicidal activities and its residual persistence on the hair which may also prevent reinfestation.

INDICATIONS AND USAGE:

Nix is indicated for the single-application treatment of infestation with *Pediculus humanus var. capitis* (the head louse) and its nits (eggs). Retreatment for recurrences is required in less than 1% of patients since the ovicidal activity may be supplemented by residual persistence in the hair. If live lice are observed after at least seven days following the initial application, a second application can be given.

CONTRAINDICATIONS:

Nix is contraindicated in patients with known hypersensitivity to any of its components, to any synthetic pyrethroid or pyrethrin, or to chrysanthemums.

WARNINGS:

If hypersensitivity to Nix occurs, discontinue use.

PRECAUTIONS:

GENERAL:

Head lice infestation is often accompanied by pruritus, erythema, and edema. Treatment with Nix may temporarily exacerbate these conditions.

INFORMATION FOR THE PATIENT:

Patients with head lice should be advised that itching, redness, or swelling of the scalp may occur after application of Nix. If irritation persists, they should consult their physician. Nix is not irritation to the eyes; however, patients should be advised to avoid contact with eyes during application and to flush with water immediately if Nix gets in the eyes. In order to prevent accidental ingestion by children, the remaining contents of Nix should be discarded after use.

Combing of nits following treatment with Nix is not necessary for effective treatment. However, patients may do so for cosmetic or other reasons. The nits are easily combed from the hair treated with Nix after drying.

CARCINOGENESIS, MUTAGENESIS, AND IMPAIRMENT OF FERTILITY:

Six carcinogenicity bioassays were evaluated with permethrin, three each in rats and mice. No tumorigenicity was seen in the rat studies. However, species-specific increases in pulmonary adenomas, a common benign tumor of mice of high spontaneous background incidence, were seen in the three mouse studies. In one of these studies there was an increased incidence of pulmonary alveolar-cell carcinomas and benign liver adenomas only in female mice when permethrin was given in their food at a concentration of 5000 ppm. Mutagenicity assays, which give useful correlative data for interpreting results from carcinogenicity bioassays in rodents, were negative. Permethrin showed no evidence of mutagenic potential in a battery of *in vitro* and *in vivo* genetic toxicity studies.

Permethrin did not have any adverse effect on reproductive function at a dose of 180 mg/kg/day orally in a three-generation rat study.

PRECAUTIONS: *(cont'd)*

PREGNANCY:

Teratogenic Effects: Pregnancy Category B: Reproduction studies have been performed in mice, rats, and rabbits (200-400 mg/kg/day orally) and have revealed no evidence of impaired fertility or harm to the fetus due to permethrin. There are, however, no adequate and well-controlled studies in pregnant women. Because animal reproduction studies are not always predictive of human response, this drug should be used during pregnancy only if clearly needed.

NURSING MOTHERS:

It is not known whether this drug is excreted in human milk. Because many drugs are excreted in human milk and because of the evidence for tumorigenic potential of permethrin in animal studies, consideration should be given to discontinuing nursing temporarily or withholding the drug while the mother is nursing.

PEDIATRIC USE:

Nix is safe and effective in children two years of age and older. Safety and effectiveness in children less than two years of age have not been established.

ADVERSE REACTIONS:

The most frequent adverse reaction to Nix is pruritus. This is usually a consequence of head lice infestation itself, but may be temporarily aggravated following treatment with Nix, 5.9% of patients in clinical studies experienced mild temporary itching; 3.4% experienced mild transient burning/stinging, tingling, numbness, or scalp discomfort; and 2.1% experienced mild transient erythema, edema, or rash of the scalp.

OVERDOSAGE:

No instance of accidental ingestion of Nix has been reported. If ingested, gastric lavage and general supportive measures should be employed.

DOSAGE AND ADMINISTRATION:

Adults and Children: Nix is intended for use after the hair has been washed with shampoo, rinsed with water and towel dried. Apply a sufficient volume of Nix to saturate the hair and scalp. Nix should remain on the hair for 10 minutes before being rinsed off with water. A single treatment is sufficient to eliminate head lice infestation. Combing of nits is not required for therapeutic efficacy, but may be done for cosmetic or other reasons.

SHAKE WELL BEFORE USING.

Store at 15-25°C (59-77°F).

HOW SUPPLIED - EQUIVALENTS NOT AVAILABLE:

Cream - Topical - 5 %

60 gm	$17.09	ELIMITE, Allergan	00023-7915-60

PERPHENAZINE *(001988)*

CATEGORIES: Antidepressants; Antipsychotics/Antimanics; Central Nervous System Agents; Nausea; Phenothiazine Tranquilizers; Psychotherapeutic Agents; Psychotic Disorders; Tranquilizers; Vertigo/Motion Sickness/Vomiting; Vomiting; FDA Approval Pre 1982

BRAND NAMES: *APO-Perphenazine* (Canada); *Decentan* (Germany); *Fentazin* (England); *F-Mon* (Japan); *Leptopsique* (Mexico); *Peratsin*; *Pernamed*; *Perphenan*; *Pernazine*; *Perzine-P*; *PMS Perphenazine* (Canada); *Porazine*; *Trilifan*; *Trilifan Retard* (France); **Trilafon**; *Trilafon Concentrate* (Canada); *Triomin*
(International brand names outside U.S. in italics)

FORMULARIES: Aetna; BC-BS; Medi-Cal

COST OF THERAPY: $110.78 (Psychotic Disorders; Tablet; 4 mg; 3/day; 90 days)

DESCRIPTION:

Perphenazine products contain perphenazine, USP (4-[3-(2-chlorophenothiazin-10-yl)propyl]-1-piperazineethanol), a piperazinyl phenothiazine having the chemical formula, $C_{21}H_{26}ClN_3OS$. They are available as Tablets, 2, 4, 8, and 16 mg; Concentrate, 16 mg perphenazine per 5 ml and alcohol less than 0.1%; and Injection, perphenazine 5 mg per 1 ml.

The inactive ingredients for Perphenazine Tablets, 2, 4, 8, and 16 mg, include: acacia, black iron oxide, butylparaben, calcium phosphate, calcium sulfate, carnauba wax, corn starch, gelatin, lactose, magnesium stearate, potato starch, sugar, titanium dioxide, white wax and other ingredients. May also contain talc.

The inactive ingredients for Perphenazine Concentrate include: alcohol, citric acid, flavors, menthol, sodium phosphate, sorbitol, sugar, and water.

The inactive ingredients for Perphenazine Injection include: citric acid, sodium bisulfite, sodium hydroxide, and water.

CLINICAL PHARMACOLOGY:

Perphenazine has actions at all levels of the central nervous system, particularly the hypothalamus. However, the site and mechanism of action of therapeutic effect are not known.

INDICATIONS AND USAGE:

Perphenazine is indicated for use in the management of the manifestations of psychotic disorders; and for the control of severe nausea and vomiting in adults.

Perphenazine has not been shown effective for the management of behavioral complications in patients with mental retardation.

CONTRAINDICATIONS:

Perphenazine products are contraindicated in comatose or greatly obtunded patients and in patients receiving large doses of central nervous system depressants (barbiturates, alcohol, narcotics, analgesics, or antihistamines); in the presence of existing blood dyscrasias, bone marrow depression, or liver damage; and in patients who have shown hypersensitivity to Perphenazine products, their components, or related compounds.

Perphenazine products are also contraindicated in patients with suspected or established subcortical brain damage, with or without hypothalamic damage, since a hyperthermic reaction with temperatures in excess of 104°F may occur in such patients, sometimes not until 14 to 16 hours after drug administration. Total body ice-packing is recommended for such a reaction; antipyretics may also be useful.

WARNINGS:

Tardive dyskinesia, a syndrome consisting of potentially irreversible, involuntary, dyskinetic movements, may develop in patients treated with neuroleptic (antipsychotic) drugs. Although the prevalence of the syndrome appears to be highest among the elderly, especially elderly

WARNINGS: *(cont'd)*

women, it is impossible to rely upon prevalence estimates to predict, at the inception of neuroleptic treatment, which patients are likely to develop the syndrome. Whether neuroleptic drug products differ in their potential to cause tardive dyskinesia is unknown.

Both the risk of developing the syndrome and the likelihood that it will become irreversible are believed to increase as the duration of treatment and the total cumulative dose of neuroleptic drugs administered to the patient increase. However, the syndrome can develop, although much less commonly, after relatively brief treatment periods at low doses.

There is no known treatment for established cases of tardive dyskinesia, although the syndrome may remit, partially or completely, if neuroleptic treatment is withdrawn. Neuroleptic treatment itself, however, may suppress (or partially suppress) the signs and symptoms of the syndrome, and thereby may possibly mask the underlying disease process. The effect that symptomatic suppression has upon the long-term course of the syndrome is unknown.

Given these considerations, neuroleptics should be prescribed in a manner that is most likely to minimize the occurrence of tardive dyskinesia. Chronic neuroleptic treatment should generally be reserved for patients who suffer from a chronic illness that, 1) is known to respond to neuroleptic drugs, and, 2) for whom alternative, equally effective, but potentially less harmful treatments are not available or appropriate. In patients who do require chronic treatment, the smallest dose and the shortest duration of treatment producing a satisfactory clinical response should be sought. The need for continued treatment should be reassessed periodically.

If signs and symptoms of tardive dyskinesia appear in a patient on neuroleptics, drug discontinuation should be considered. However, some patients may require treatment despite the presence of the syndrome.

(For further information about the description of tardive dyskinesia and its clinical detection, please refer to Information for Patients and ADVERSE REACTIONS.)

Perphenazine Injection contains sodium bisulfite, a sulfite that may cause allergic-type reactions including anaphylactic symptoms and life-threatening or less severe asthmatic episodes in certain susceptible people. The overall prevalence of sulfite sensitivity is seen more frequently in asthmatic than in nonasthmatic people.

Neuroleptic Malignant Syndrome (NMS) A potentially fatal symptom complex, sometimes referred to as Neuroleptic Malignant Syndrome (NMS), has been reported in association with antipsychotic drugs. Clinical manifestations of NMS are hyperpyrexia, muscle rigidity, altered mental status and evidence of autonomic instability (irregular pulse or blood pressure, tachycardia, diaphoresis, and cardiac dysrhythmias).

The diagnostic evaluation of patients with this syndrome is complicated. In arriving at a diagnosis, it is important to identify cases where the clinical presentation includes both serious medical illness (*e.g.,* pneumonia, systemic infection, etc.) and untreated or inadequately treated extrapyramidal signs and symptoms (EPS). Other important considerations in the differential diagnosis include central anticholinergic toxicity, heat stroke, drug fever and primary central nervous system (CNS) pathology.

The management of NMS should include 1) immediate discontinuation of antipsychotic drugs and other drugs not essential to concurrent therapy, 2) intensive symptomatic treatment and medical monitoring, and 3) treatment of any concomitant serious medical problems for which specific treatments are available. There is no general agreement about specific pharmacological treatment regimens for uncomplicated NMS.

If a patient requires antipsychotic drug treatment after recovery from NMS, the reintroduction of drug therapy should be carefully considered. The patient should be carefully monitored, since recurrences of NMS have been reported.

If hypotension develops, epinephrine should not be administered since its action is blocked and partially reversed by perphenazine. If a vasopressor is needed, norepinephrine may be used. Severe, acute hypotension has occurred with the use of phenothiazines and is particularly likely to occur in patients with mitral insufficiency or pheochromocytoma. Rebound hypertension may occur in pheochromocytoma patients.

Perphenazine products can lower the convulsive threshold in susceptible individuals; they should be used with caution in alcohol withdrawal and in patients with convulsive disorders. If the patient is being treated with an anticonvulsant agent, increased dosage of that agent may be required when Perphenazine products are used concomitantly.

Perphenazine products should be used with caution in patients with psychic depression.

Perphenazine may impair the mental and/or physical abilities required for the performance of hazardous tasks such as driving a car or operating machinery; therefore, the patient should be warned accordingly.

Perphenazine products are not recommended for children under 12 years of age.

Usage in Pregnancy: Safe use of Perphenazine during pregnancy and lactation has not been established; therefore, in administering the drug to pregnant patients, nursing mothers, or women who may become pregnant, the possible benefits must be weighed against the possible hazards to mother and child.

PRECAUTIONS:

The possibility of suicide in depressed patients remains during treatment and until significant remission occurs. This type of patient should not have access to large quantities of this drug.

As with all phenothiazine compounds, perphenazine should not be used indiscriminately. Caution should be observed in giving it to patients who have previously exhibited severe adverse reactions to other phenothiazines. Some of the untoward actions of perphenazine tend to appear more frequently when high doses are used. However, as with other phenothiazine compounds, patients receiving Perphenazine products in any dosage should be kept under close supervision.

Neuroleptic drugs elevate prolactin levels; the elevation persists during chronic administration. Tissue culture experiments indicate that approximately one-third of human breast cancers are prolactin dependent *in vitro,* a factor of potential importance if the prescription of these drugs is contemplated in a patient with a previously detected breast cancer. Although disturbances such as galactorrhea, amenorrhea, gynecomastia, and impotence have been reported, the clinical significance of elevated serum prolactin levels is unknown for most patients. An increase in mammary neoplasms has been found in rodents after chronic administration of neuroleptic drugs. Neither clinical studies nor epidemiologic studies conducted to date, however, have shown an association between chronic administration of these drugs and mammary tumorigenesis; the available evidence is considered too limited to be conclusive at this time.

The antiemetic effect of perphenazine may obscure signs of toxicity due to overdosage of other drugs, or render more difficult the diagnosis of disorders such as brain tumors or intestinal obstruction.

A significant, not otherwise explained, rise in body temperature may suggest individual intolerance to perphenazine, in which case it should be discontinued.

Patients on large doses of a phenothiazine drug who are undergoing surgery should be watched carefully for possible hypotensive phenomena. Moreover, reduced amounts of anesthetics or central nervous system depressants may be necessary.

PRECAUTIONS: *(cont'd)*

Since phenothiazines and central nervous system depressants (opiates, analgesics, antihistamines, barbiturates) can potentiate each other, less than the usual dosage of the added drug is recommended and caution is advised when they are administered concomitantly.

Use with caution in patients who are receiving atropine or related drugs because of additive anticholinergic effects and also in patients who will be exposed to extreme heat or phosphorus insecticides.

The use of alcohol should be avoided, since additive effects and hypotension may occur. Patients should be cautioned that their response to alcohol may be increased while they are being treated with Perphenazine products. The risk of suicide and the danger of overdose may be increased in patients who use alcohol excessively due to its potentiation of the drug's effect.

Blood counts and hepatic and renal functions should be checked periodically. The appearance of signs of blood dyscrasias requires the discontinuance of the drug and institution of appropriate therapy. If abnormalities in hepatic tests occur, phenothiazine treatment should be discontinued. Renal function in patients on long-term therapy should be monitored; if blood urea nitrogen (BUN) becomes abnormal, treatment with the drug should be discontinued.

The use of phenothiazine derivatives in patients with diminished renal function should be undertaken with caution.

Use with caution in patients suffering from respiratory impairment due to acute pulmonary infections, or in chronic respiratory disorders such as severe asthma or emphysema.

In general, phenothiazines, including perphenazine, do not produce psychic dependence. Gastritis, nausea and vomiting, dizziness, and tremulousness have been reported following abrupt cessation of high-dose therapy. Reports suggest that these symptoms can be reduced by continuing concomitant antiparkinson agents for several weeks after the phenothiazine is withdrawn.

The possibility of liver damage, corneal and lenticular deposits, and irreversible dyskinesias should be kept in mind when patients are on long-term therapy.

Because photosensitivity has been reported, undue exposure to the sun should be avoided during phenothiazine treatment.

Information for the Patient: This information is intended to aid in the safe and effective use of this medication. It is not a disclosure of all possible adverse or intended effects.

Given the likelihood that a substantial proportion of patients exposed chronically to neuroleptics will develop tardive dyskinesia, it is advised that all patients in whom chronic use is contemplated be given, if possible, full information about this risk. The decision to inform patients and/or their guardians must obviously take into account the clinical circumstances and the competency of the patient to understand the information provided.

ADVERSE REACTIONS:

Not all of the following adverse reactions have been reported with this specific drug; however, pharmacological similarities among various phenothiazine derivatives require that each be considered. With the piperazine group (of which perphenazine is an example), the extrapyramidal symptoms are more common, and others (*e.g.,* sedative effects, jaundice, and blood dyscrasias) are less frequently seen.

CNS Effects: *Extrapyramidal reactions:* opisthotonus, trismus, torticollis, retrocollis, aching and numbness of the limbs, motor restlessness, oculogyric crisis, hyperreflexia, dystonia, including protrusion, discoloration, aching and rounding of the tongue, tonic spasm of the masticatory muscles, tight feeling in the throat, slurred speech, dysphagia, akathisia, dyskinesia, parkinsonism, and ataxia. Their incidence and severity usually increase with an increase in dosage, but there is considerable individual variation in the tendency to develop such symptoms. Extrapyramidal symptoms can usually be controlled by the concomitant use of effective antiparkinsonian drugs, such as benztropine mesylate, and/or by reduction in dosage. In some instances, however, these extrapyramidal reactions may persist after discontinuation of treatment with perphenazine.

Persistent Tardive Dyskinesia: As with all antipsychotic agents, tardive dyskinesia may appear in some patients on long-term therapy or may appear after drug therapy has been discontinued. Although the risk appears to be greater in elderly patients on high-dose therapy, especially females, it may occur in either sex and in children. The symptoms are persistent and in some patients appear to be irreversible. The syndrome is characterized by rhythmical, involuntary movements of the tongue, face, mouth or jaw (*e.g.,* protrusion of tongue, puffing of cheeks, puckering of mouth, chewing movements). Sometimes these may be accompanied by involuntary movements of the extremities. There is no known effective treatment for tardive dyskinesia; antiparkinsonism agents usually do not alleviate the symptoms of this syndrome. It is suggested that all antipsychotic agents be discontinued if these symptoms appear. Should it be necessary to reinstitute treatment, or increase the dosage of the agent, or switch to a different antipsychotic agent, the syndrome may be masked. It has been reported that fine, vermicular movements of the tongue may be an early sign of the syndrome, and if the medication is stopped at that time the syndrome may not develop.

Other CNS Effects: Include cerebral edema; abnormality of cerebrospinal fluid proteins; convulsive seizures, particularly in patients with EEG abnormalities or a history of such disorders; and headaches.

Neuroleptic malignant syndrome has been reported in patients treated with neuroleptic drugs (see WARNINGS for further information.)

Drowsiness may occur, particularly during the first or second week, after which it generally disappears. If troublesome, lower the dosage. Hypnotic effects appear to be minimal, especially in patients who are permitted to remain active.

Adverse behavioral effects include paradoxical exacerbation of psychotic symptoms, catatonic-like states, paranoid reactions, lethargy, paradoxical excitement, restlessness, hyperactivity, nocturnal confusion, bizarre dreams, and insomnia.

Hyperreflexia has been reported in the newborn when a phenothiazine was used during pregnancy.

Autonomic Effects: dry mouth or salivation, nausea, vomiting, diarrhea, anorexia, constipation, obstipation, fecal impaction, urinary retention, frequency or incontinence, bladder paralysis, polyuria, nasal congestion, pallor, myosis, mydriasis, blurred vision, glaucoma, perspiration, hypertension, hypotension, and change in pulse rate occasionally may occur. Significant autonomic effects have been infrequent in patients receiving less than 24 mg perphenazine daily.

Adynamic ileus occasionally occurs with phenothiazine therapy and if severe can result in complications and death. It is of particular concern in psychiatric patients, who may fail to seek treatment of the condition.

Allergic Effects: urticaria, erythema, eczema, exfoliative dermatitis, pruritus, photosensitivity, asthma, fever, anaphylactoid reactions, laryngeal edema, and angioneurotic edema; contact dermatitis in nursing personnel administering the drug; and in extremely rare instances, individual idiosyncrasy or hypersensitivity to phenothiazines has resulted in cerebral edema, circulatory collapse, and death.

ADVERSE REACTIONS: *(cont'd)*

Endocrine Effects: lactation, galactorrhea, moderate breast enlargement in females and gynecomastia in males on large doses, disturbances in the menstrual cycle, amenorrhea, changes in libido, inhibition of ejaculation, syndrome of inappropriate ADH (antidiuretic hormone) secretion, false positive pregnancy tests, hyperglycemia, hypoglycemia, glycosuria.

Cardiovascular Effects: postural hypotension, tachycardia (especially with sudden marked increase in dosage), bradycardia, cardiac arrest, faintness, and dizziness. Occasionally the hypotensive effect may produce a shock-like condition. ECG changes, nonspecific (quinidine-like effect) usually reversible, have been observed in some patients receiving phenothiazine tranquilizers.

Sudden death has occasionally been reported in patients who have received phenothiazines. In some cases the death was apparently due to cardiac arrest; in others, the cause appeared to be asphyxia due to failure of the cough reflex. In some patients, the cause could not be determined nor could it be established that the death was due to the phenothiazine.

Hematological Effects: agranulocytosis, eosinophilia, leukopenia, hemolytic anemia, thrombocytopenic purpura, and pancytopenia. Most cases of agranulocytosis have occurred between the fourth and tenth weeks of therapy. Patients should be watched closely, especially during that period, for the sudden appearance of sore throat or signs of infection. If white blood cell and differential cell counts show significant cellular depression, discontinue the drug and start appropriate therapy. However, a slightly lowered white count is not in itself an indication to discontinue the drug.

Other Effects: Special considerations in long-term therapy include pigmentation of the skin, occurring chiefly in the exposed areas; ocular changes consisting of deposition of fine particulate matter in the cornea and lens, progressing in more severe cases to star-shaped lenticular opacities; epithelial keratopathies; and pigmentary retinopathy. Also noted: peripheral edema, reversed epinephrine effect, increase in PBI not attributable to an increase in thyroxine, parotid swelling (rare), hyperpyrexia, systemic lupus erythematosus-like syndrome, increases in appetite and weight, polyphagia, photophobia, and muscle weakness.

Liver damage (biliary stasis) may occur. Jaundice may occur, usually between the second and fourth weeks of treatment, and is regarded as a hypersensitivity reaction. Incidence is low. The clinical picture resembles infectious hepatitis but with laboratory features of obstructive jaundice. It is usually reversible; however, chronic jaundice has been reported.

Side effects with intramuscular Perphenazine Injection have been infrequent and transient. Dizziness or significant hypotension after treatment with Perphenazine Injection is a rare occurrence.

OVERDOSAGE:

In the event of overdosage, emergency treatment should be started immediately. All patients suspected of having taken an overdose should be hospitalized as soon as possible.

Manifestations: Overdosage of perphenazine primarily involves the extrapyramidal mechanism and produces the same side effects described under ADVERSE REACTIONS, but to a more marked degree. It is usually evidenced by stupor or coma; children may have convulsive seizures.

Treatment: Treatment is symptomatic and supportive. There is no specific antidote. The patient should be induced to vomit even if emesis has occurred spontaneously. Pharmacologic vomiting by the administration of ipecac syrup is a preferred method. It should be noted that ipecac has a central mode of action in addition to its local gastric irritant properties, and the central mode of action may be blocked by the antiemetic effect of Perphenazine products. Vomiting should not be induced in patients with impaired consciousness. The action of ipecac is facilitated by physical activity and by the administration of 8 to 12 fluid ounces of water. If emesis does not occur within 15 minutes, the dose of ipecac should be repeated. Precautions against aspiration must be taken, especially in infants and children. Following emesis, any drug remaining in the stomach may be adsorbed by activated charcoal administered as a slurry with water. If vomiting is unsuccessful or contraindicated, gastric lavage should be performed. Isotonic and one-half isotonic saline are the lavage solutions of choice. Saline cathartics, such as milk of magnesia, draw water into the bowel by osmosis and therefore, may be valuable for their action in rapid dilution of bowel content.

Standard measures (oxygen, intravenous fluids, corticosteroids) should be used to manage circulatory shock or metabolic acidosis. An open airway and adequate fluid intake should be maintained. Body temperature should be regulated. Hypothermia is expected, but severe hyperthermia may occur and must be treated vigorously. (See CONTRAINDICATIONS.)

An electrocardiogram should be taken and close monitoring of cardiac function instituted if there is any sign of abnormality. Cardiac arrhythmias may be treated with neostigmine, pyridostigmine, or propranolol. Digitalis should be considered for cardiac failure. Close monitoring of cardiac function is advisable for not less than five days. Vasopressors such as norepinephrine may be used to treat hypotension, but epinephrine should NOT be used.

Anticonvulsants (an inhalation anesthetic, diazepam, or paraldehyde) are recommended for control of convulsions, since perphenazine increases the central nervous system depressant action, but not the anticonvulsant action of barbiturates.

If acute parkinson-like symptoms result from perphenazine intoxication, benztropine mesylate or diphenhydramine may be administered.

Central nervous system depression may be treated with nonconvulsant doses of CNS stimulants. Avoid stimulants that may cause convulsions (*e.g.*, picrotoxin and pentylenetetrazol).

Signs of arousal may not occur for 48 hours.

Dialysis is of no value because of low plasma concentrations of the drug.

Since overdosage is often deliberate, patients may attempt suicide by other means during the recovery phase. Deaths by deliberate or accidental overdosage have occurred with this class of drugs.

DOSAGE AND ADMINISTRATION:

Dosage must be individualized and adjusted according to the severity of the condition and the response obtained. As with all potent drugs, the best dose is the lowest dose that will produce the desired clinical effect. Since extrapyramidal symptoms increase in frequency and severity with increased dosage, it is important to employ the lowest effective dose. These symptoms have disappeared upon reduction of dosage, withdrawal of the drug, or administration of an antiparkinsonian agent.

Prolonged administration of doses exceeding 24 mg daily should be reserved for hospitalized patients or patients under continued observation for early detection and management of adverse reactions. An antiparkinsonian agent, such as trihexyphenidyl hydrochloride or benztropine mesylate, is valuable in controlling drug-induced extrapyramidal symptoms.

PERPHENAZINE TABLETS

Suggested dosages for Tablets for various conditions follow:

Moderately Disturbed Nonhospitalized Psychotic Patients: Tablets 4 to 8 mg t.i.d. initially; reduce as soon as possible to minimum effective dosage.

Hospitalized Psychotic Patients: Tablets 8 to 16 mg b.i.d. to q.i.d.; avoid dosages in excess of 64 mg daily.

Severe Nausea And Vomiting In Adults: Tablets 8 to 16 mg daily in divided doses; 24 mg occasionally may be necessary; early dosage reduction is desirable.

DOSAGE AND ADMINISTRATION: *(cont'd)*

PERPHENAZINE INJECTION

Intramuscular Administration: The injection is used when rapid effect and prompt control of acute or intractable conditions is required or when oral administration is not feasible. Perphenazine Injection, administered by deep intramuscular injection, is well tolerated. The injection should be given with the patient seated or recumbent, and the patient should be observed for a short period after administration.

Therapeutic effect is usually evidenced in 10 minutes and is maximal in 1 to 2 hours. The average duration of effective action is 6 hours, occasionally 12 to 24 hours.

Pediatric dosage has not yet been established. Children over 12 years may receive the lowest limit of adult dosage.

The usual initial dose is 5 mg (1 ml). This may be repeated every 6 hours. Ordinarily, the total daily dosage should not exceed 15 mg in ambulatory patients or 30 mg in hospitalized patients. When required for satisfactory control of symptoms in severe conditions, an initial 10-mg intramuscular dose may be given. Patients should be placed on oral therapy as soon as practicable. Generally, this may be achieved within 24 hours. In some instances, however, patients have been maintained on injectable therapy for several months. It has been established that Perphenazine Injection is more potent than Perphenazine Tablets. Therefore, equal or higher dosage should be used when the patient is transferred to oral therapy after receiving the injection.

Psychotic Conditions: While 5 mg of the Injection has a definite tranquilizing effect, it may be necessary to use 10-mg doses to initiate therapy in severely agitated states. Most patients will be controlled and amenable to oral therapy within a maximum of 24 to 48 hours. Acute conditions (hysteria, panic reaction) often respond well to a single dose, whereas in chronic conditions, several injections may be required. When transferring patients to oral therapy, it is suggested that increased dosage be employed to maintain adequate clinical control. This should be followed by gradual reduction to the minimal maintenance dose which is effective.

Severe Nausea And Vomiting In Adults: To obtain rapid control of vomiting, administer 5 mg (1 ml); in rare instances it may be necessary to increase the dose to 10 mg; in general, higher doses should be given only to hospitalized patients.

INTRAVENOUS ADMINISTRATION

The intravenous administration of Perphenazine Injection is seldom required. This route of administration should be used with particular caution and care, and only when absolutely necessary to control severe vomiting, intractable hiccoughs, or acute conditions, such as violent retching during surgery. Its use should be limited to recumbent hospitalized adults in doses not exceeding 5 mg. When employed in this manner, intravenous injection ordinarily should be given as a diluted solution by either fractional injection or a slow drip infusion. In the surgical patient, slow infusion of not more than 5 mg is preferred. When administered in divided doses, Perphenazine Injection should be diluted to 0.5 mg/ml (1 ml mixed with 9 ml of physiologic saline solution), and not more than 1 mg per injection given at not less than one- to two-minute intervals. Intravenous injection should be discontinued as soon as symptoms are controlled and should not exceed 5 mg. The possibility of hypotensive and extrapyramidal side effects should be considered and appropriate means for management kept available. Blood pressure and pulse should be monitored continuously during intravenous administration. Pharmacologic and clinical studies indicate that intravenous administration of norepinephrine should be useful in alleviating the hypotensive effect.

Perphenazine Concentrate: In hospitalized psychotic patients, the usual dosage range is 8 to 16 mg b.i.d. to q.i.d., depending on the severity of symptoms and individual response. Although a number of investigators have employed higher dosage, a total daily dose of more than 64 mg ordinarily is not required. The Concentrate should be diluted only with water, saline, Seven-Up, homogenized milk, carbonated orange drink, and pineapple, apricot, prune, orange, V-8, tomato, and grapefruit juices. Perphenazine Concentrate should not be mixed with beverages containing caffeine (coffee, cola), tannics (tea), or pectinates (apple juice), since physical incompatibility may result. Suggested dilution is approximately two fluid ounces of diluent for each 5 ml (16 mg) teaspoonful of Perphenazine Concentrate. For convenience in measuring smaller doses, a graduated dropper marked to measure 8 mg or 4 mg is supplied with each bottle.

Tablets: Store between 2° and 25°C (36° and 77°F).

Concentrate: Protect from light. Store between 2° and 30°C (36° and 86°F). Shake well before using. Store in carton until completely used.

Injection: Protect from light. Store in carton until completely used.

HOW SUPPLIED - RATED THERAPEUTICALLY EQUIVALENT:

Tablet, Coated - Oral - 2 mg

100's	$29.93	Perphenazine, H.C.F.A. F F P	99999-1988-01
100's	$31.43	Perphenazine, United Res	00677-1385-01
100's	$39.60	Perphenazine, Major Pharms	00904-1872-61
100's	$40.50	Perphenazine, Harber Pharm	51432-0804-03
100's	$40.55	Perphenazine, Qualitest Pharms	00603-5090-21
100's	$40.80	Perphenazine, Warrick Pharms	59930-1600-01
100's	$40.90	Perphenazine, Major Pharms	00904-1872-60
100's	$42.53	Perphenazine, Schein Pharm (US)	00364-2623-01
100's	$42.86	Perphenazine, HL Moore Drug Exch	00839-7423-06
100's	$44.25	Perphenazine, Teva	00093-0789-01
100's	$44.30	Perphenazine, Parmed Pharms	00349-8773-01
100's	$45.50	Perphenazine, Zenith Labs	00172-3667-60
100's	$45.50	Perphenazine, Goldline Labs	00182-1865-01
100's	$45.50	Perphenazine, Martec Pharms	52555-0569-01
100's	$45.51	Perphenazine, Geneva Pharms	00781-1046-01
100's	$46.00	Perphenazine, Rugby	00536-4131-01
100's	$53.89	Perphenazine, Geneva Pharms	00781-1046-13
100's	**$63.90**	**TRILAFON, Schering**	**00085-0705-04**
500's	$149.65	Perphenazine, H.C.F.A. F F P	99999-1988-02
500's	$168.28	Perphenazine, HL Moore Drug Exch	00839-7423-12
500's	$178.15	Perphenazine, Major Pharms	00904-1872-40
500's	$190.80	Perphenazine, Zenith Labs	00172-3667-70
500's	$202.50	Perphenazine, Harber Pharm	51432-0804-05

Tablet, Coated - Oral - 4 mg

100's	$41.03	Perphenazine, H.C.F.A. F F P	99999-1988-03
100's	$41.93	Perphenazine, United Res	00677-1386-01
100's	$54.70	Perphenazine, Qualitest Pharms	00603-5091-21
100's	$54.85	Perphenazine, Major Pharms	00904-1873-60
100's	$55.22	Perphenazine, Aligen Independ	00405-4780-01
100's	$55.49	Perphenazine, Harber Pharm	51432-0806-03
100's	$55.50	Perphenazine, Warrick Pharms	59930-1603-01
100's	$56.81	Perphenazine, Major Pharms	00904-1873-61
100's	$57.75	Perphenazine, Schein Pharm (US)	00364-2624-01
100's	$58.25	Perphenazine, HL Moore Drug Exch	00839-7424-06
100's	$60.65	Perphenazine, Parmed Pharms	00349-8774-01
100's	$60.75	Perphenazine, Teva	00093-0790-01
100's	$64.90	Perphenazine, Zenith Labs	00172-3668-60
100's	$64.90	Perphenazine, Goldline Labs	00182-1866-01
100's	$64.90	Perphenazine, Martec Pharms	52555-0570-01
100's	$64.91	Perphenazine, Geneva Pharms	00781-1047-01

HOW SUPPLIED - RATED THERAPEUTICALLY EQUIVALENT:
(cont'd)

100's	$65.00	Perphenazine, Rugby	00536-4132-01
100's	$74.65	Perphenazine, Geneva Pharms	00781-1047-13
100's	**$87.42**	**TRILAFON, Schering**	**00085-0940-05**
500's	$205.15	Perphenazine, H.C.F.A. F F P	99999-1988-04
500's	$233.87	Perphenazine, HL Moore Drug Exch	00839-7424-12
500's	$239.25	Perphenazine, Major Pharms	00904-1873-40
500's	$264.85	Perphenazine, Zenith Labs	00172-3668-70
500's	$264.85	Perphenazine, Goldline Labs	00182-1866-05
500's	$265.05	Perphenazine, Harber Pharm	51432-0806-05

Tablet, Coated - Oral - 8 mg

100's	$49.65	Perphenazine, H.C.F.A. F F P	99999-1988-05
100's	$50.25	Perphenazine, United Res	00677-1388-01
100's	$64.95	Perphenazine, Qualitest Pharms	00603-5092-21
100's	$65.60	Perphenazine, Major Pharms	00904-1874-60
100's	$67.27	Perphenazine, Harber Pharm	51432-0808-03
100's	$67.30	Perphenazine, Aligen Independ	00405-4781-01
100's	$67.45	Perphenazine, Warrick Pharms	59930-1605-01
100's	$68.56	Perphenazine, Major Pharms	00904-1874-61
100's	$70.19	Perphenazine, HL Moore Drug Exch	00839-7425-06
100's	$70.87	Perphenazine, Schein Pharm (US)	00364-2625-01
100's	$73.60	Perphenazine, Parmed Pharms	00349-8775-01
100's	$75.85	Perphenazine, Teva	00093-0791-01
100's	$77.85	Perphenazine, Zenith Labs	00172-3669-60
100's	$77.85	Perphenazine, Goldline Labs	00182-1867-01
100's	$77.85	Perphenazine, Martec Pharms	52555-0571-01
100's	$77.86	Perphenzaine, Geneva Pharms	00781-1048-01
100's	$78.00	Perphenazine, Rugby	00536-4133-01
100's	$98.00	Perphenazine, Geneva Pharms	00781-1048-13
100's	**$106.08**	**TRILAFON, Schering**	**00085-0313-05**
250's	$124.12	Perphenazine, H.C.F.A. F F P	99999-1988-06
500's	$248.25	Perphenazine, H.C.F.A. F F P	99999-1988-07
500's	$278.10	Perphenazine, Major Pharms	00904-1874-40
500's	$286.50	Perphenazine, HL Moore Drug Exch	00839-7425-12
500's	$319.00	Perphenazine, Zenith Labs	00172-3669-70
500's	$319.00	Perphenazine, Goldline Labs	00182-1867-05

Tablet, Coated - Oral - 16 mg

100's	$67.13	Perphenazine, H.C.F.A. F F P	99999-1988-08
100's	$80.78	Perphenazine, United Res	00677-1389-01
100's	$89.25	Perphenazine, Major Pharms	00904-1875-60
100's	$90.65	Perphenazine, Warrick Pharms	59930-1610-01
100's	$90.67	Perphenazine, Harber Pharm	51432-0809-03
100's	$90.82	Perphenazine Tablets 16 Mg, Aligen Independ	00405-4782-01
100's	$94.50	Perphenazine, Schein Pharm (US)	00364-2626-01
100's	$95.18	Perphenazine, HL Moore Drug Exch	00839-7426-06
100's	$98.55	Perphenazine, Teva	00093-0792-01
100's	$107.55	Perphenazine, Zenith Labs	00172-3670-60
100's	$107.55	Perphenazine, Goldline Labs	00182-1868-01
100's	$107.55	Perphenazine, Martec Pharms	52555-0572-01
100's	$107.56	Perphenazine, Geneva Pharms	00781-1049-01
100's	$108.00	Perphenazine, Rugby	00536-4134-01
100's	$114.10	Perphenazine, Geneva Pharms	00781-1049-13
100's	**$142.73**	**TRILAFON, Schering**	**00085-0077-05**
500's	$335.65	Perphenazine, H.C.F.A. F F P	99999-1988-09
500's	$411.75	Perphenazine, Major Pharms	00904-1875-40
500's	$435.00	Perphenazine, Zenith Labs	00172-3670-70

HOW SUPPLIED - NOT RATED EQUIVALENT:

Injection, Solution - Intramuscular; - 5 mg/ml

1 ml x 100	**$541.64**	**TRILAFON, Schering**	**00085-0012-04**

Liquid - Oral - 16 mg/5ml

120 ml	**$36.40**	**TRILAFON CONCENTRATE, Schering**	**00085-0363-02**

PHENACEMIDE *(001993)*

CATEGORIES: Anticonvulsants; Central Nervous System Agents; Convulsions; Epilepsy; Hydantoin Anticonvulsants; Neuromuscular; Seizures; Pregnancy Category D; FDA Approval Pre 1982

BRAND NAMES: *Phenuron* (Japan); **Phenurone**
(International brand names outside U.S. in italics)

DESCRIPTION:

Phenacemide is a valuable antiepileptic drug for use in selected patients with epilepsy. Since therapy with Phenurone involves certain risks, *physicians should thoroughly familiarize themselves with the undesirable side effects which may occur and the precautions to be observed.* Phenacemide is a substituted acetyl urea derivative. Chemically phenacemide is identified as N-(aminocarbonyl)-benzeneacetamide.

Phenurone tablets contain 500 mg phenacemide for oral administration. *Inactive Ingredients:* Corn starch, lactose and talc.

CLINICAL PHARMACOLOGY:

In experimental animals, phenacemide in doses well below those causing neurological signs, elevates the threshold for minimal electroshock convulsions and abolished the tonic phase of maximal electroshock seizures. The drug prevents or modifies seizures induced by pentylenetetrazol or other convulsants. In comparative tests, phenacemide was found to be equal or more effective than other commonly used antiepileptics against complex partial (psychomotor) seizures which were induced in mice by low frequency stimulation of the cerebral cortex. Studies in mice have shown that phenacemide exerts a synergistic antiepileptic effect with mephenytoin, phenobarbital, or trimethadione.

Given orally to laboratory animals, phenacemide has a low acute toxicity. In mice, slight ataxia appears at 400 mg/kg and light sleep occurs at 800 mg/kg. In high doses the drug causes marked ataxia and coma, the fatal dose being in the range of 3 to 5 g/kg for mice, rats and cats.

Phenacemide is metabolized by the liver, however, further definition of human pharmacokinetics has not been determined.

INDICATIONS AND USAGE:

Phenacemide is indicated for the control of severe epilepsy, particularly mixed forms of complex partial (psychomotor) seizures, refractory to other drugs.

CONTRAINDICATIONS:

Phenacemide should not be administered unless other available antiepileptics have been found to be ineffective in satisfactorily controlling seizures.

WARNINGS:

Phenacemide can produce serious side effects as well as direct organ toxicity. As a consequence its use entails the assumption of certain risks which must be weighed against the benefit to the patient.*Ordinarily phenacemide should not be administered unless other available antiepileptics have been found to be ineffective in controlling seizures.*

Death attributable to liver damage during therapy with phenacemide has been reported. Phenacemide should be used with caution in patients with a history of previous liver dysfunction. If jaundice or other signs of hepatitis appear, the drug should be discontinued.

Aplastic anemia has occurred in association with phenacemide therapy, and death from this condition has been reported. Phenacemide should ordinarily not be used in patients with severe blood dyscrasias. Marked depression of the blood count is an indication for withdrawal of the drug.

USAGE DURING PREGNANCY

Phenacemide can cause fetal harm when administered to a pregnant women. There are multiple reports in the clinical literature which indicate that the use of antiepileptic drugs during pregnancy results in an increased incidence of birth defects in the offspring. Reports have also suggested that the maternal ingestion of antiepileptic drugs, particularly barbiturates, is associated with a neonatal coagulation defect that may cause bleeding during the early (usually within 24 hours of birth) neonatal period. The possibility of the occurrence of this defect with the use of phenacemide should be kept in mind. The defect is characterized by decreased levels of vitamin K-dependent clotting factors, and prolongation of either the prothrombin time or the partial thromboplastin time, or both. It has been suggested that vitamin K be given prophylactically to the mother one month prior to and during delivery, and to the infant, intravenously, immediately after birth. If this drug is used during pregnancy, or if the patient becomes pregnant while taking this drug, the patient should be apprised of the potential hazard to the fetus.

PRECAUTIONS:

General: Extreme caution must be exercised in treating patients who previously have shown personality disorders. It may be advisable to hospitalize such patients during the first week of treatment. Personality changes, including attempts at suicide and the occurrence of psychoses requiring hospitalization, have been reported during therapy with phenacemide. Severe or exacerbated personality changes are an indication for withdrawal of the drug.

Phenacemide should be used with caution in patients with a history of previous liver dysfunction.

Phenacemide should be administered with caution to patients with a history of allergy, particularly in association with the administration of other antiepileptics. The drug should be discontinued at the first sign of a skin rash or other allergic manifestation.

Information for Patients: The patient and his family should be aware of the possibility of personality changes so the family can watch for changes in the behavior of the patient such as decreased interest in surrounding, depression, or aggressiveness.

The patient should be told to report immediately any symptoms indicative of a developing blood dyscrasia such as malaise, sore throat, or fever.

Laboratory Tests: Liver function tests should be performed before and during therapy. Death attributable to liver damage during therapy with phenacemide has been reported. If jaundice or other signs of hepatitis appear, the drug should be discontinued.

Complete blood counts should be made before instituting phenacemide, and at monthly intervals thereafter. If no abnormality appears within 12 months, the interval between blood counts may be extended. Blood changes have been reported with leukopenia (leukocyte count of 4,000 or less per cubic millimeter of blood) as the most commonly observed effect. However, aplastic anemia has occurred in association with phenacemide therapy, and death from this condition has been reported. *The total number of each cellular element per cubic millimeter is a better index of possible blood dyscrasia than the percentage of cells.* Marked depression of the blood count is an indication for withdrawal of the drug.

Similarly, as nephritis has occasionally occurred in patients on phenacemide, the urine should be examined at regular intervals. Abnormal urinary findings are an indication for discontinuance of therapy.

Carcinogenesis: No data are available on long-term potential for carcinogenicity in animals or humans.

Pregnancy Category D: See WARNINGS section.

Nursing Mothers: It is not known whether this drug is excreted in human milk. Because many drugs are excreted in human milk and because of the potential for serious adverse reactions in nursing infants from phenacemide, a decision should be made whether to discontinue nursing or to discontinue the drug, taking into account the importance of the drug to the mother.

Pediatric Use: Safety and effectiveness in children below the age of 5 years have not been established.

DRUG INTERACTIONS:

Extreme caution is essential if phenacemide is administered with any other antiepileptic which is known to cause similar toxic effects.

Considerable caution should be exercised if phenacemide is administered concurrently with Peganone (ethotoin) since paranoid symptoms have been reported during therapy with this combination.

ADVERSE REACTIONS:

The following adverse effects associated with phenacemide are listed by decreasing order of frequency based on data from one large clinical study.[1]

Psychiatric: Psychic changes (17 in 100 patients).

Gastrointestinal: Gastrointestinal disturbances (8 in 100 patients), including anorexia (5 in 100 patients) and weight loss (less than 1 in 100 patients).

Dermatologic: Skin rash (5 in 100 patients). Stevens-Johnson Syndrome with epidermal necrolysis has been reported in one non-fatal case.

CNS: Drowsiness (4 in 100 patients), headache (2 in 100 patients), insomnia (1 in 100 patients), dizziness and paresthesias (less than 1 in 100 patients).

Hematopoietic: Blood dyscrasias (primarily leukopenia), including fatal aplastic anemia (2 in 100 patients).

Hepatic: Hepatitis, including fatalities (2 in 100 patients).

Renal: Abnormal urinary findings, including a rise in serum creatine[2], and nephritis (1 in 100 patients or less).

Other: Fatigue, fever, muscle pain and palpitation (less than 1 in 100 patients).

OVERDOSAGE:

Symptoms of acute overdosage include excitement or mania, followed by drowsiness, ataxia and coma. In one case of acute overdosage, dizziness was followed by coma which lasted nearly 24 hours. Treatment should be started by inducing emesis; gastric lavage may be

OVERDOSAGE: *(cont'd)*

considered as an alternative or adjunct. General supportive measures will be necessary. A careful evaluation of liver and kidney function, mental state, and the blood-forming organs should be made following recovery.

DOSAGE AND ADMINISTRATION:

Phenacemide is administered orally.

Since phenacemide may produce serious toxic effects, it is strongly recommended that the dosage be held to the minimum amount necessary to achieve an adequate therapeutic effect.

For adults the usual starting dose is 1.5 g daily, administered in three divided doses of 500 mg each. After the first week, if seizures are not controlled and the drug is well tolerated, an additional 500 mg tablet may be taken upon arising. In the third week, if necessary, the dosage may be further increased by another 500 mg at bedtime. Satisfactory results have been noted in some patients on an initial dose of 250 mg three times per day. The effective total daily dose for adults usually ranges from 2 to 3 g, although some patients have required as much as 5 g daily.

For the pediatric patient from 5 to 10 years of age, approximately one-half the adults dose is recommended. It should be given at the same intervals as for adults.

Phenacemide may be administered alone or in conjunction with other antiepileptics. However, extreme caution must be exercised if other antiepileptics cause toxic effects similar to phenacemide.

When phenacemide is to replace other antiepileptic medication, the latter should be withdrawn gradually as the dosage of phenacemide is increased to maintain seizure control.

HOW SUPPLIED:

Phenurone, grooved, white, 500 mg tablets are supplied in bottles of 100.

REFERENCES:

1. Tyler, M. W., King, E. Q.: Phenacemide in Treatment of Epilepsy. JAMA 147: 17-21 (1951). 2. Richards, R.K., Bjornsson, T. D., Waterbury, L. D.: Rise in Serum and Urine Creatinine After Phenacemide. Clin. Pharmacol. Ther. 23: 430-437 (1978).

HOW SUPPLIED - EQUIVALENTS NOT AVAILABLE:

Tablet, Uncoated - Oral - 500 mg

100's	**$52.86**	**PHENURONE, Abbott**	**00074-3971-05**

PHENAZOPYRIDINE HYDROCHLORIDE

(001995)

CATEGORIES: Analgesics; Antibacterials; Antimicrobials; Antipruritics/Local Anesthetics; Antiseptics, Urinary Tract; Phenazopyridine; Skin/Mucous Membrane Agents; Urinary Tract Infections; Pregnancy Category B; FDA Pre 1938 Drugs

BRAND NAMES: *Anazo*; *Azodine*; Azo-Standard; Eridium; Geridium; *Phenazo* (Canada); Phenazodine; *Phendiridine*; *Pirimir* (Mexico); Pyridiate; **Pyridium**; *Pyronium*; Ro-Pyridine; *Sedural*; Urodine; Urodol; *Urogesic*; *Urohman* (Japan); *Uropydine*; *Uroprin*; *Uropyridin* (Japan); Viridium
(International brand names outside U.S. in italics)

FORMULARIES: Aetna; BC-BS; CIGNA; DoD; FHP; Humana; Kaiser; Medco; Medi-Cal; PCS; PruCare; United

DESCRIPTION:

Phenazopyridine hydrochloride (abbreviated here as Phenazopyridine HCl) is chemically designated 2.6-Pyridinediamine, 3-(phenylazo), monohydrochloride. It is a urinary tract analgesic agent for oral administration. Phenazopyridine HCl tablets contain 100 mg or 200 mg Phenazopyridine HCl. Also contains carnauba wax, NF; corn starch, NF; D and C red No. 7; FD and C blue No. 2; FD and C yellow No. 6; gelatin, NF; lactose, NF; magnesium stearate, NF; methylcellulose, USP; sodium starch glycolate, NF; sucrose, NF; titanium dioxide, USP; white wax, NF.

CLINICAL PHARMACOLOGY:

Phenazopyridine HCl is excreted in the urine where it exerts a topical analgesic effect on the mucosa of the urinary tract. This action helps to relieve pain, burning, urgency and frequency. The precise mechanism of action is not known.

The pharmacokinetic properties of Phenazopyridine HCl have not been determined. Phenazopyridine is rapidly excreted by the kidneys, with as much as 65% of an oral dose being excreted unchanged in the urine.

INDICATIONS AND USAGE:

Phenazopyridine HCl is indicated for the symptomatic relief of pain, burning, urgency, frequency, and other discomforts arising from irritation of the lower urinary tract mucosa caused by infection, trauma, surgery, endoscopic procedures, or the passage of sounds or catheters. The use of Phenazopyridine HCl for relief of symptoms should not delay definitive diagnosis and treatment of causative conditions. Because it provides only symptomatic relief, prompt appropriate treatment of the cause of pain must be instituted and Phenazopyridine HCl should be discontinued when symptoms are controlled.

The analgesic action may reduce or eliminate the need for systemic analgesics or narcotics. It is, however, compatible with antibacterial therapy and can help to relieve pain and discomfort during the interval before antibacterial therapy controls the infection. Treatment of a urinary tract infection with Phenazopyridine HCl should not exceed 2 days because there is a lack of evidence that the combined administration of Phenazopyridine HCl and an antibacterial provides greater benefit than administration of the antibacterial alone after 2 days. (See DOSAGE AND ADMINISTRATION.)

CONTRAINDICATIONS:

Phenazopyridine HCl should not be used in patients who have previously exhibited hypersensitivity to it. The use of Phenazopyridine HCl is contraindicated in patients with renal insufficiency.

PRECAUTIONS:

GENERAL:

A yellowish tinge of the skin or sclera may indicate accumulation due to impaired renal excretion and the need to discontinue therapy.

The decline in renal function associated with advanced age should be kept in mind.

INFORMATION FOR THE PATIENT:

Phenazopyridine HCl produces an orange to red color in the urine and may stain fabric. Staining of contact lenses has been reported.

PRECAUTIONS: *(cont'd)*

LABORATORY TEST INTERACTIONS:

Due to its properties as an azo dye, Phenazopyridine HCl may interfere with urinalysis based on spectrometry or color reactions.

CARCINOGENESIS, MUTAGENESIS, AND IMPAIRMENT OF FERTILITY:

Long-term administration of Phenazopyridine HCl has induced neoplasia in rats (large intestine) and mice (liver). Although no association between Phenazopyridine HCl and human neoplasia has been reported, adequate epidemiological studies along these lines have not been conducted.

PREGNANCY CATEGORY B:

Reproduction studies have been performed in rats at doses up to 50 mg/kg/day and have revealed no evidence of impaired fertility or harm to the fetus due to Phenazopyridine HCl. There are, however, no adequate and well controlled studies in pregnant women. Because animal reproduction studies are not always predictive of human response, this drug should be used during pregnancy only if clearly needed.

NURSING MOTHERS:

No information is available on the appearance of Phenazopyridine HCl or its metabolites in human milk.

ADVERSE REACTIONS:

Headache, rash, pruritus and occasional gastrointestinal disturbance. An anaphylactoid-like reaction has been described. Methemoglobinemia, hemolytic anemia, renal and hepatic toxicity have been reported, usually at overdosage levels (see OVERDOSAGE.)

OVERDOSAGE:

Exceeding the recommended dose in patients with good renal function or administering the usual dose to patients with impaired renal function (common in elderly patients) may lead to increased serum levels and toxic reactions. Methemoglobinemia generally follows a massive, acute overdose. Methylene blue, 1 to 2 mg/kg body weight intravenously or ascorbic acid 100 to 200 mg given orally should cause prompt reduction of the methemoglobinemia and disappearance of the cyanosis which is an aid in diagnosis. Oxidative Heinz body hemolytic anemia may also occur, and "bite cells" (degmacytes) may be present in a chronic overdosage situation. Red blood cell G-6-PD deficiency may predispose to hemolysis. Renal and hepatic impairment and occasional failure, usually due to hypersensitivity, may also occur.

DOSAGE AND ADMINISTRATION:

100-mg tablets: Adult dosage is two tablets 3 times a day after meals. 200-mg tablets: Adult dosage is one tablet 3 times a day after meals.

When used concomitantly with an antibacterial agent for the treatment of a urinary tract infection, the administration of Phenazopyridine HCl should not exceed 2 days.

Store at controlled room temperature 15°-30°C (59°-86°F).

HOW SUPPLIED - EQUIVALENTS NOT AVAILABLE:

Tablet, Coated - Oral - 100 mg

30's	$4.35	Phenazopyridine Hcl, Manufac Chems	00148-9125-03
30's	$4.40	Phenazopyridine Hcl, Manufac Chems	00148-9130-03
100's	$5.50	PHENYLAZO-DIAMINO-PYRIDINE HCL, Consolidated Midland	00223-1442-01
100's	$5.80	Phenazopyridine Hcl, Manufac Chems	00148-9125-01
100's	$5.85	Phenazopyridine Hcl, Manufac Chems	00148-9130-01
100's	$6.08	Phenazopyridine Hcl, US Trading	56126-0278-11
100's	$9.60	Phenazopyridine Hcl, Voluntary Hosp	53258-0168-13
100's	$10.24	Phenazopyridine Hcl, United Res	00677-0575-01
100's	$10.25	Phenazopyridine Hcl, Major Pharms	00904-0191-60
100's	$10.25	Phenazopyridine Hcl, Major Pharms	00904-7922-60
100's	$10.50	GERIDIUM, Goldline Labs	00182-0138-01
100's	$10.50	Phenazopyridine Hcl, Vintage Pharms	00254-4971-28
100's	$10.50	Phenazopyridine Hcl, Qualitest Pharms	00603-5141-21
100's	$10.50	Phenazopyridine HCl, Geneva Pharms	00781-1510-01
100's	$10.59	Phenazopyridine Hcl, Parmed Pharms	00349-8741-01
100's	$10.61	PHENAZPYRIDINE HCL, Schein Pharm (US)	00364-0286-01
100's	$11.25	PYRIDIATE, Rugby	00536-4388-01
100's	$12.25	Phenazopyridine Hcl, Alpharma	00472-0196-10
100's	$14.25	UROGESIC, Edwards Pharms	00485-0046-01
100's	$16.95	Phenazopyridine Hcl, Parmed Pharms	00349-8975-01
100's	$29.95	Phenazopyridine HCl, HL Moore Drug Exch	00839-1503-06
100's	$30.95	Phenazopyridine Hcl, Alphagen Labs	59743-0013-01
100's	$43.60	PHENAZOPYRIDINE HCL, Aligen Independ	00405-4792-01
100's	**$44.78**	**PYRIDIUM, Parke-Davis**	**00071-0180-40**
100's	**$52.76**	**PYRIDIUM, Parke-Davis**	**00071-0180-24**
1000's	$27.50	PHENYLAZO-DIAMINO-PYRIDINE HCL, Consolidated Midland	00223-1442-02
1000's	$36.00	Phenazopyridine Hcl, Manufac Chems	00148-9130-02
1000's	$57.50	Pyridiate, Harber Pharm	51432-0402-06
1000's	$73.35	Phenazopyridine Hcl, Major Pharms	00904-0191-80
1000's	$73.35	Phenazopyridine Hcl, Major Pharms	00904-7922-80
1000's	$79.63	Phenazopyridine Hcl, Vintage Pharms	00254-4971-38
1000's	$79.63	Phenazopyridine Hcl, Qualitest Pharms	00603-5141-32
1000's	$89.90	PYRIDIATE, Rugby	00536-4388-10
1000's	$94.00	GERIDIUM, Goldline Labs	00182-0138-10
1000's	$269.95	Phenazopyridine HCl, HL Moore Drug Exch	00839-1503-16
1000's	$283.50	Phenazopyridine Hcl, Alphagen Labs	59743-0013-10
1000's	**$417.08**	**PYRIDIUM, Parke-Davis**	**00071-0180-32**

Tablet, Coated - Oral - 200 mg

30's	$4.80	Phenazopyridine Hcl, Manufac Chems	00148-9135-03
30's	$8.50	Urodol, Dayton Labs	52041-0042-09
30's	$8.50	Urodol, Dayton Labs	52041-0042-13
100's	$6.55	Phenazopyridine Hcl, Manufac Chems	00148-9135-01
100's	$6.59	Phenazopyridine Hcl, US Trading	56126-0279-11
100's	$7.50	Phenazopyridine Hcl, Consolidated Midland	00223-1443-01
100's	$12.00	Phenazopyridine Hcl, Voluntary Hosp	53258-0169-13
100's	$13.70	Phenazopyridine, Parmed Pharms	00349-8742-01
100's	$18.90	Phenazopyridine Hcl, Major Pharms	00904-0192-60
100's	$18.90	Phenazopyridine Hcl, Major Pharms	00904-7923-60
100's	$19.35	Phenazopyridine, United Res	00677-0804-01
100's	$19.95	Phenazopyridine HCl, Geneva Pharms	00781-1512-01
100's	$22.00	GERIDIUM, Goldline Labs	00182-0904-01
100's	$22.48	Phenazopyridine Hcl, Alpharma	00472-0197-10
100's	$23.13	Phenazopyridine Hcl, Vintage Pharms	00254-4972-28
100's	$23.13	Phenazopyridine Hcl, Qualitest Pharms	00603-5142-21
100's	$23.95	PYRIDATE NO.2, Rugby	00536-4392-01
100's	$25.00	Urodol, Dayton Labs	52041-0042-15
100's	$25.69	PHENAZOPYRIDINE HCL, Schein Pharm (US)	00364-0321-01
100's	$29.95	PHENAZOPYRIDINE HCL, Parmed Pharms	00349-8976-01
100's	$59.10	Phenazopyridine Hcl, Alphagen Labs	59743-0014-01
100's	$59.95	Phenazopyridine, HL Moore Drug Exch	00839-1556-06

HOW SUPPLIED - EQUIVALENTS NOT AVAILABLE: *(cont'd)*

100's	$84.01	PHENAZOPYRIDINE HCL, Aligen Independ	00405-4793-01
100's	**$91.70**	**PYRIDIUM, Parke-Davis**	**00071-0181-40**
100's	**$101.69**	**PYRIDIUM, Parke-Davis**	**00071-0181-24**
500's	$92.40	Phenazopyridine Hcl, Vintage Pharms	00254-4972-38
1000's	$34.50	Phenazopyridine Hcl, Consolidated Midland	00223-1443-02
1000's	$42.00	Phenazopyridine, Parmed Pharms	00349-8742-10
1000's	$53.85	Phenazopyridine Hcl, Manufac Chems	00148-9135-02
1000's	$65.00	Pyridiate, Harber Pharm	51432-0404-06
1000's	$92.40	Phenazopyridine Hcl, Qualitest Pharms	00603-5142-32
1000's	$98.97	PYRIDATE NO.2, Rugby	00536-4392-10
1000's	$101.55	Phenazopyridine Hcl, Major Pharms	00904-0192-80
1000's	$101.55	Phenazopyridine Hcl, Major Pharms	00904-7923-80
1000's	$489.95	Phenazopyridine, HL Moore Drug Exch	00839-1556-16
1000's	$546.11	Phenazopyridine Hcl, Alphagen Labs	59743-0014-10
1000's	**$765.78**	**PYRIDIUM, Parke-Davis**	**00071-0181-32**

PHENAZOPYRIDINE HYDROCHLORIDE; SULFISOXAZOLE *(001997)*

CATEGORIES: Anti-Infectives; Antibacterials; Antimicrobials; Pain; Phenazopyridine; Sulfonamides; Urinary Tract Infections; Pregnancy Category C; FDA Approved 1990 Aug

BRAND NAMES: **Azo-Gantrisin**; Azo-Sulfisoxazole; Azo-Truxazole; Sul-Azo

DESCRIPTION:

Sulfisoxazole, an antibacterial sulfonamide, is*N*'-(3,4-dimethyl-5-isoxazolyl) sulfanilamide. It is a white to slightly yellowish, odorless, slightly bitter, crystalline powder which is soluble in alcohol and very slightly soluble in water. Sulfisoxazole has an empirical formula of $C_{11}H_{13}N_3O_3S$, and a molecular weight of 267.30.

Phenazopyridine hydrochloride, a local urinary analgesic, is 2,6-diamino-3-(phenylazo) pyridine monohydrochloride. It is a light or dark red to dark violet, odorless, slightly bitter, crystalline powder with an empirical formula of $C_{11}H_{11}N_5$·HCl, and a molecular weight of 249.70.

FOR COMPLETE PRESCRIBING INFORMATION REFER TO THE INDIVIDUAL DRUG MONOGRAPHS (PHENAZOPYRIDINE HYDROCHLORIDE; SULFISOXAZOLE).

INDICATIONS AND USAGE:

Azo Gantrisin is indicated for the initial treatment of uncomplicated urinary tract infections caused by susceptible strains of the following microorganisms: *Escherichia coli, Klebsiella species, Enterobacter species, Proteus mirabilis, Proteus vulgaris* and *Staphylococcus aureus* when relief of symptoms of pain, burning or urgency is needed during the first 2 days of therapy. There is a lack of evidence that the combination of sulfisoxazole and phenazopyridine hydrochloride provides greater benefit than sulfisoxazole alone after 2 days. Therefore, treatment with Azo Gantrisin should not exceed 2 days, and the remaining therapeutic course should be completed with sulfisoxazole alone. (See DOSAGE AND ADMINISTRATION.)

The frequency of resistant organisms limits the usefulness of sulfonamides as sole therapy in the treatment of urinary tract infections.

Important Note: *In vitro* susceptibility tests for sulfonamides are not always reliable. When the patient is already taking sulfonamides, follow-up cultures should have aminobenzoic acid added to the culture media.

DOSAGE AND ADMINISTRATION:

The recommended dosage in adults is 4 tablets initially, followed by 2 tablets four times daily for up to two days. **Treatment with Azo Gantrisin should not exceed 2 days.** A full course of therapy for an uncomplicated urinary tract infection should be completed with sulfisoxazole alone.

HOW SUPPLIED:

Each red, film-coated Azo Gantrisin tablet contains 500 mg sulfisoxazole and 50 mg phenazopyridine HCl. Imprint on tablets: AZO GANTRISIN ROCHE.

HOW SUPPLIED - EQUIVALENTS NOT AVAILABLE:

Tablet, Coated - Oral - 50 mg/500 mg

100's	$9.75	Azo Sulfisoxazole, Manufac Chems	00148-9410-01
100's	$9.75	Azosulfisoxazole, Pharmacist Choice	54979-0143-01
100's	$10.62	Azo-Sulfisoxazole, Qualitest Pharms	00603-2385-21
500's	$156.56	AZO GANTRISIN, Roche	00004-0012-14
1000's	$84.80	Azo Sulfisoxazole, Manufac Chems	00148-9410-02

PHENDIMETRAZINE TARTRATE *(001998)*

CATEGORIES: Amphetamines; Anorexients/CNS Stimulants; Appetite Suppressants; Central Nervous System Agents; Methylphenidate; Obesity; Psychostimulants; Respiratory/Cerebral Stimulant; Weight Loss; DEA Class CIII; DEA Class CIV; FDA Approval Pre 1982

BRAND NAMES: Adipost; Adphen; Alphazine; Anorex; Appecon; Bontril; Cam-Metrazine; Dital; Dyrexan-O.D.; Melfiat; Metra; Neocurb; Obalan; Obe-Del; *Obesan-X*; Obezine; P.D.M.; Panrexin; Parzine; Phen 35; Phenazine; Phendiet; Phendimetrazine Bitartrate; Phenzene; **Plegine**; Prelu-2; Pt 105; Qrp-105; Rapdone; Rexigen Forte; Slyn-Ll; Sprx; Stabec-105; Statobex; Tega-Nil; Trimstat; Trimtabs; Wehless; Weightrol; X-Trozine
(International brand names outside U.S. in italics)

FORMULARIES: Aetna

DESCRIPTION:

Chemical Name: (+)-3,4-Dimethyl-2-phenylmorpholine Tartrate.

Phendimetrazine tartrate is the dextro isomer of Phendimetrazine tartrate. Phendimetrazine tartrate is a white, odorless powder with a bitter taste. It is soluble in water, methanol, and ethanol.

Plegine contains these inactive ingredients: D&C Yellow No. 10, FD&C Yellow No. 6, Lactose, NF, Magnesium Stearate, NF, Polyethylene Glycol 8000, NF.

CLINICAL PHARMACOLOGY:

Phendimetrazine tartrate is a phenylalkylamine sympathomimetic with pharmacologic activity similar to the prototype drugs of this class used in obesity, the amphetamines. Actions include central nervous system (CNS) stimulation and elevation of blood pressure. Tachyphylaxis and tolerance have been demonstrated with all drugs of this class in which these phenomena have been looked for.

Drugs of this class used in obesity are commonly known as "anorectics" or "anorexigenics." It has not been established, however, that the action of such drugs in treating obesity is primarily one of appetite suppression. Other CNS actions, or metabolic effects, may be involved.

Adult obese subjects instructed in dietary management and treated with "anorectic" drugs, lose more weight on the average than those treated with placebo and diet, as determined in relatively short-term clinical trials.

The magnitude of increased weight loss of drug-treated patients over placebo-treated patients is only a fraction of a pound a week. The rate of weight loss is greatest in the first weeks of therapy for both drug and placebo subjects and tends to decrease in succeeding weeks. The possible origins of the increased weight loss due to the various drug effects are not established. The amount of weight loss associated with use of an "anorectic" drug varies from trial to trial, and the increased weight loss appears to be related, in part, to variables other than the drug prescribed, such as the physician-investigator, the population treated, and the diet prescribed. Studies do not permit conclusions as to the relative importance of the drug and non-drug factors on weight loss.

The natural history of obesity is measured in years, whereas the studies cited are restricted to a few weeks' duration; thus, the total impact of drug-induced weight loss over that of diet alone must be considered clinically limited.

INDICATIONS AND USAGE:

Phendimetrazine tartrate is indicated in the management of exogenous obesity as a short-term adjunct (a few weeks) in a regimen of weight reduction based on caloric restriction. The limited usefulness of agents of this class should be measured against possible risk factors inherent in their use (see CLINICAL PHARMACOLOGY).

CONTRAINDICATIONS:

Known hypersensitivity or idiosyncratic reactions to sympathomimetics.

Advanced arteriosclerosis, symptomatic cardiovascular disease, moderate and severe hypertension, hyperthyroidism, glaucoma.

Highly nervous or agitated patients.

Patients with a history of drug abuse.

Patients taking other CNS stimulants, including monamine oxidase inhibitors.

WARNINGS:

Drug Dependence: Phendimetrazine tartrate is related chemically and pharmacologically to the amphetamines. Amphetamines and related stimulant drugs have been abused extensively, and the possibility of phendimetrazine tartrate abuse should be kept in mind when evaluating the desirability of including a drug as part of a weight reduction program. Abuse of amphetamines and related drugs may be associated with intense psychological dependence and severe social dysfunction. There are reports of patients who have increased the dosage to many times that recommended. Abrupt cessation following prolonged high-dosage administration results in extreme fatigue and mental depression; changes are also noted on the sleep EEG. Manifestations of chronic intoxication with anorectic drugs include severe dermatoses, marked insomnia, irritability, hyperactivity, and personality changes. The most severe manifestation of chronic intoxication is psychosis, often indistinguishable clinically from schizophrenia.

Tolerance to the anorectic effect of phendimetrazine tartrate develops within a few weeks. When this occurs, its use should be discontinued; the maximum recommended dose should not be exceeded.

Use of phendimetrazine tartrate within 14 days following the administration of monamine oxidase inhibitors may result in a hypertensive crisis.

Abrupt cessation of administration following prolonged high dosage results in extreme fatigue and depression. Because of the effect on the central nervous system phendimetrazine tartrate may impair the patient's ability to engage in potentially hazardous activities such as operating machinery or driving a motor vehicle; the patient should therefore be cautioned accordingly.

Usage in Pregnancy: Safe use in pregnancy has not been established. Until more information is available, phendimetrazine tartrate should not be taken by women who are, or may become, pregnant unless, in the opinion of the physician, the potential benefits outweigh the possible hazards.

Usage in Children: Phendimetrazine tartrate is not recommended for use in children under 12 years of age.

PRECAUTIONS:

Caution is to be exercised in prescribing phendimetrazine tartrate for patients with even mild hypertension.

Insulin requirements in diabetes mellitus may be altered in association with the use of phendimetrazine tartrate and the concomitant dietary regimen.

Phendimetrazine tartrate may decrease the hypotensive effect of guanethidine.

The least amount feasible should be prescribed or dispensed at one time in order to minimize the possibility of overdosage.

ADVERSE REACTIONS:

Central Nervous System: Over-stimulation, restlessness, insomnia, agitation, flushing, tremor, sweating, dizziness, headache, psychotic states, blurring of vision.

Cardiovascular: Palpitation, tachycardia, elevated blood pressure.

Gastrointestinal: Mouth dryness, nausea, diarrhea, constipation, stomach pain.

Genitourinary: Urinary frequency, dysuria, changes in libido.

OVERDOSAGE:

Acute overdosage of phendimetrazine tartrate may manifest itself by the following signs and symptoms: unusual restlessness, confusion, belligerence, hallucinations, and panic states. Fatigue and depression usually follow the central stimulation. Cardiovascular effects include arrhythmias, hypertension or hypotension, and circulatory collapse. Gastrointestinal symptoms include nausea, vomiting, diarrhea, and abdominal cramps. Poisoning may result in convulsions, coma, and death.

The management of overdosage is largely symptomatic. It includes sedation with a barbiturate. If hypertension is marked, the use of a nitrate or rapid-acting alpha receptor-blocking agent should be considered. Experience with hemodialysis or peritoneal dialysis is inadequate to permit recommendations for its use.

DOSAGE AND ADMINISTRATION:

Usual Adult Dosage: 1 tablet (35 mg) bid or tid, one hour before meals.

Dosage should be individualized to obtain an adequate response with the lowest effective dosage. In some cases, 1/2 tablet per dose may be adequate; dosage should not exceed 2 tablets tid.

HOW SUPPLIED - RATED THERAPEUTICALLY EQUIVALENT:

Capsule, Gelatin - Oral - 35 mg

1000's	$19.00	Phenzene Capsules 35 Mg, Calvin Scott	17224-0630-10
1000's	$31.00	PHENZENE, Calvin Scott	17224-0624-10
1000's	$31.00	PHENZENE, Calvin Scott	17224-0627-10
1000's	$31.00	PHENZENE 35, Calvin Scott	17224-0650-10
1000's	$45.00	Phendiet, C O Truxton	00463-2043-10
1000's	$53.00	Phendimetrazine Tartrate, Rexar	00478-5466-10
1000's	$53.00	Phendimetrazine Tartrate, Rexar	00478-5472-10
1000's	$53.00	Phendimetrazine Tartrate, Rexar	00478-5473-10

Tablet, Uncoated - Oral - 35 mg

100's	$4.25	NEOCURB, Pasadena	00418-6591-41
100's	$5.00	Phendimetrazine Tartrate, Camall	00147-0103-10
100's	$5.00	Phendimetrazine Tartrate, Camall	00147-0105-10
100's	$5.00	CAM METRAZINE, Camall	00147-0106-10
100's	$5.00	Cam-Metrazine, Camall	00147-0132-10
100's	$5.00	Phendimetrazine Tartrate, Camall	00147-0135-10
100's	$5.00	Phendimetrazine Tartrate, Camall	00147-0165-10
100's	$5.00	Phendimetrazine Tartrate, Camall	00147-0166-10
100's	$5.00	Phendimetrazine, United Res	00677-0399-01
100's	$5.10	Phendimetrazine, Eon Labs Mfg	00185-4057-01
100's	$7.50	Phendimetrazine Tartrate, United Res	00677-1499-01
100's	$7.50	Phendimetrazine Tartrate, H.C.F.A. F F P	99999-1998-01
100's	$8.50	Phendimetrazine Tartrate, Rexar	00478-5460-01
100's	$8.98	CAM-METRAZINE, Camall	00147-0107-10
100's	$10.85	BONTRIL PDM, Carnrick	00086-0048-10
100's	$15.71	STATOBEX, Teva	00093-0071-01
100's	**$69.81**	**PLEGINE, Ayerst**	**00046-0755-81**
1000's	$15.75	Phenzene, Calvin Scott	17224-0601-10
1000's	$16.75	PHENZENE, Calvin Scott	17224-0604-10
1000's	$16.75	PHENZENE, Calvin Scott	17224-0620-10
1000's	$16.75	Phenzene, Calvin Scott	17224-6021-10
1000's	$16.75	Phenzene, Calvin Scott	17224-6031-10
1000's	$17.47	Rapdone, Macnary	55982-0001-01
1000's	$18.25	Phen 35, H & H Labs	46703-0034-10
1000's	$19.00	Phenzene, Calvin Scott	17224-0600-10
1000's	$21.40	Phendimetrazine Tartrate, Eon Labs Mfg	00185-4057-10
1000's	$21.40	Phendimetrazine Tartrate, Eon Labs Mfg	00185-4095-10
1000's	$23.05	Phendimetrazine Tartrate, Eon Labs Mfg	00185-4055-10
1000's	$23.75	Phendimetrazine, United Res	00677-0399-10
1000's	$25.25	Phendimetrazine, Rosemont	00832-0202-10
1000's	**$26.80**	**PLEGINE, Major Pharms**	**00904-4270-80**
1000's	$29.85	Phendimetrazine, IDE-Interstate	00814-6035-30
1000's	$30.00	Weightrol, Vortech Pharms	00298-1879-11
1000's	$39.65	Phendimetrazine Tartrate, Rugby	00536-5617-10
1000's	$39.90	Phendimetrazine Tartrate, Hyrex Pharms	00314-0135-20
1000's	$45.62	CAM METRAZINE, Camall	00147-0103-20
1000's	$45.62	CAM METRAZINE, Camall	00147-0105-20
1000's	$45.62	CAM METRAZINE, Camall	00147-0106-20
1000's	$45.62	CAM-METRAZINE, Camall	00147-0107-20
1000's	$47.91	Phendimetrazine, HL Moore Drug Exch	00839-5108-16
1000's	$47.91	Phendimetrazine, HL Moore Drug Exch	00839-5955-16
1000's	$47.91	Phendimetrazine, Pink, HL Moore Drug Exch	00839-5956-16
1000's	$48.10	Phendimetrazine Tartrate, Camall	00147-0165-20
1000's	$48.10	Phendimetrazine Tartrate, Camall	00147-0166-20
1000's	$48.65	Phendimetrazine Yellow, Rugby	00536-4160-10
1000's	$50.30	Phendimetrazine Tartrate, Rexar	00478-5457-10
1000's	$50.30	Phendimetrazine Tartrate, Rexar	00478-5458-10
1000's	$50.30	Phendimetrazine Tartrate, Rexar	00478-5459-10
1000's	$50.30	Phendimatrazine Tartrate, Rexar	00478-5460-10
1000's	$55.12	Cam-Metrazine, Camall	00147-0132-20
1000's	$55.12	Phendimetrazine - Speckled, Camall	00147-0135-20
1000's	$63.75	BONTRIL PDM, Carnrick	00086-0048-90
1000's	$75.00	Phendimetrazine Tartrate, United Res	00677-1499-10
1000's	$75.00	Phendimetrazine Tartrate, H.C.F.A. F F P	99999-1998-02
1000's	$110.30	STATOBEX, Teva	00093-0071-10
5000's	$176.50	CAM-METRAZINE, Camall	00147-0107-30
5000's	$200.10	Phendimetrazine Tartrate, Camall	00147-0103-30
5000's	$200.10	Phendimetrazine Tartrate, Camall	00147-0105-30
5000's	$200.10	Phendimetrazine Tartrate, Camall	00147-0106-30
5000's	$216.00	Phendimetrazine Tartrate, Rexar	00478-5460-50
5000's	$244.00	Phendimatrazine Tartrate, Rexar	00478-5458-50
5000's	$375.00	Phendimetrazine Tartrate, H.C.F.A. F F P	99999-1998-03

HOW SUPPLIED - NOT RATED EQUIVALENT:

Capsule, Gelatin, Sustained Action - Oral - 105 mg

100's	$19.71	Phendimetrazine Tartrate, Rexar	00478-5462-01
100's	$24.75	BONTRIL SLOW RELEASE, Carnrick	00086-0047-10
100's	$29.88	APPECON, Lunsco	10892-0117-10
100's	$98.96	PRELU-2, Boehringer Pharms	00597-0064-01
250's	$44.35	Phendimetrazine Tartrate, Rexar	00478-5462-02
500's	$73.92	Phendimetrazine Tartrate, Rexar	00478-5462-05
1000's	$75.00	PHENZENE BROWN/CLEAR, Calvin Scott	17224-0640-10
1000's	$123.20	Phendimetrazine Tartrate, Rexar	00478-5462-10
1000's	$126.00	Phendiet-105, C O Truxton	00463-3029-10
1000's	$130.00	Phendimetrazine Tartrate, Hyrex Pharms	00314-5462-10
1000's	$350.00	Qrp-105, Quality Res Pharms	52765-2201-00

PHENELZINE SULFATE *(001999)*

CATEGORIES: Antidepressants; Anxiety; Central Nervous System Agents; Depression; MAO Inhibitors; Monoamine Oxidase Inhibitors; Psychotherapeutic Agents; Cocaine Addiction*; FDA Approval Pre 1982

* Indication not approved by the FDA

BRAND NAMES: *Nardelzine*; **Nardil**

(International brand names outside U.S. in italics)

FORMULARIES: Aetna; BC-BS

COST OF THERAPY: $108.64 (Depression; Tablet; 15 mg; 3/day; 90 days)

PRIMARY ICD9: 311 (Depressive Disorder, Not Elsewhere Classified)

DESCRIPTION:

Phenelzine Sulfate is a potent inhibitor of monoamine oxidase (MAO). Chemically, it is a hydrazine derivative.

Each tablet contains phenelzine sulfate equivalent to 15 mg of phenelzine base. Also contains: acacia, NF; calcium carbonate; carnauba wax, NF; corn starch, NF; FD and C yellow No. 6; gelatin, NF; kaolin, USP; magnesium stearate, NF; mannitol, USP; pharmaceutical glaze, NF; povidone, USP; sucrose, NF; talc, USP; white wax, NF; white wheat flour.

CLINICAL PHARMACOLOGY:

Monoamine oxidase is a complex enzyme system, widely distributed throughout the body. Drugs that inhibit monoamine oxidase in the laboratory are associated with a number of clinical effects. Thus, it is unknown whether MAO inhibition *per se*, other pharmacologic actions, or an interaction of both, is responsible for the clinical effects observed. Therefore, the physician should become familiar with all the effects produced by drugs of this class.

INDICATIONS AND USAGE:

Phenelzine Sulfate has been found to be effective in depressed patients clinically characterized as "atypical," "nonendogenous," or "neurotic." These patients often have mixed anxiety and depression and phobic or hypochondriacal features. There is less conclusive evidence of its usefulness with severely depressed patients with endogenous features.

Phenelzine Sulfate should rarely be the first antidepressant drug used. Rather, it is more suitable for use with patients who have failed to respond to the drugs more commonly used for these conditions.

CONTRAINDICATIONS:

Phenelzine Sulfate is contraindicated in patients with known sensitivity to the drug, pheochromocytoma, congestive heart failure, a history of liver disease, or abnormal liver function tests.

The potentiation of sympathomimetic substances and related compounds by MAO inhibitors may result in hypertensive crises (see WARNINGS). Therefore, patients being treated with Phenelzine Sulfate should not take **sympathomimetic drugs** (including amphetamines, cocaine, methylphenidate, dopamine, epinephrine and norepinephrine) or related compounds (including methyldopa, L-dopa, L-tryptophan, L-tyrosine, and phenylalanine). Hypertensive crises during Phenelzine Sulfate therapy may also be caused by the ingestion of foods with a high concentration of tyramine or dopamine. Therefore, patients being treated with Phenelzine Sulfate should avoid high protein food that has undergone protein breakdown by aging, fermentation, pickling, smoking, or bacterial contamination; patients should also avoid cheeses (especially aged varieties), pickled herring, beer, wine, liver, yeast extract (including brewer's yeast in large quantities), dry sausage (including Genoa salami, hard salami, pepperoni, and Lebanon bologna), pods of broad beans (fava beans), and yogurt. Excessive amounts of caffeine and chocolate may also cause hypertensive reactions.

WARNINGS:

Important

The most serious reactions to Phenelzine Sulfate involve changes in blood pressure.

Hypertensive Crises: The most important reaction associated with Phenelzine Sulfate administration is the occurrence of hypertensive crises, which have sometimes been fatal.

These crises are characterized by some or all of the following symptoms: occipital headache which may radiate frontally, palpitation, neck stiffness or soreness, nausea, vomiting, sweating (sometimes with fever and sometimes with cold, clammy skin), dilated pupils, and photophobia. Either tachycardia or bradycardia may be present and can be associated with constricting chest pain.

Note: Intracranial bleeding has been reported in association with the increase in blood pressure.

BLOOD PRESSURE SHOULD BE OBSERVED FREQUENTLY TO DETECT EVIDENCE OF ANY PRESSOR RESPONSE IN ALL PATIENTS RECEIVING PHENELZINE SULFATE. THERAPY SHOULD BE DISCONTINUED IMMEDIATELY UPON THE OCCURRENCE OF PALPITATION OR FREQUENT HEADACHES DURING THERAPY.

RECOMMENDED TREATMENT IN HYPERTENSIVE CRISIS: If a hypertensive crisis occurs, Phenelzine Sulfate should be discontinued immediately and therapy to lower blood pressure should be instituted immediately. On the basis of present evidence, phentolamine is recommended. (The dosage reported for phentolamine is 5 mg intravenously.) Care should be taken to administer this drug slowly in order to avoid producing an excessive hypotensive effect. Fever should be managed by means of external cooling.

Warning to the patient: All patients should be warned that the following foods, beverages and medications must be avoided while taking Phenelzine Sulfate, and for two weeks after discontinuing use.

FOODS AND BEVERAGES TO AVOID

Meat and Fish: Pickled herring, Liver, Dry sausage (including Genoa salami, hard salami, pepperoni, and Lebanon bologna)

Vegetables: Broad bean pods (fava bean pods)

Dairy Products: Cheese (cottage cheese and cream cheese are allowed), Yogurt

Beverages: Beer and wine, Alcohol-free and reduced-alcohol beer and wine products.

Miscellaneous: Yeast extract (including brewer's yeast in large quantities), Excessive amounts of chocolate and caffeine.

Also, any spoiled or improperly refrigerated, handled or stored protein-rich foods such as meats, fish, and dairy products, including foods that may have undergone protein changes by aging, pickling, fermentation, or smoking to improve flavor should be avoided.

OTC MEDICATIONS TO AVOID

Cold and cough preparations (including those containing dextromethorphan)
Nasal decongestants (tablets, drops or spray)
Hay-fever medications
Sinus medications
Asthma inhalant medications
Antiappetite medicines
Weight-reducing preparations
"Pep" pills
L-tryptophan containing preparations

Also, certain prescription drugs should be avoided. Therefore, patients under the care of another physician or dentist should inform him/her that they are taking Phenelzine Sulfate.

WARNINGS: *(cont'd)*

Patients should be warned that the use of the above foods, beverages or medications may cause a reaction characterized by headache and other serious symptoms due to a rise in blood pressure, with the exception of dextromethorphan which may cause reactions similar to those seen with meperidine.

Patients should be instructed to report promptly the occurrence of headache or other unusual symptoms.

Use in Pregnancy: The safe use of Phenelzine Sulfate during pregnancy or lactation has not been established. The potential benefit of this drug, if used during pregnancy, lactation or in women of childbearing age, should be weighed against the possible hazard to the mother or fetus.

Doses of Phenelzine Sulfate in pregnant mice well exceeding the maximum recommended human dose have caused a significant decrease in the number of viable offspring per mouse. In addition, the growth of young dogs and rats has been retarded by doses exceeding the maximum human dose.

Use in Children: Phenelzine Sulfate is not recommended for patients under 16 years of age, since there are no controlled studies of safety in this age group.

Phenelzine Sulfate, as with other hydrazine derivatives, has been reported to induce pulmonary and vascular tumors in an uncontrolled lifetime study in mice.

PRECAUTIONS:

In depressed patients, the possibility of suicide should always be considered and adequate precautions taken. It is recommended that careful observations of patients undergoing Phenelzine Sulfate treatment be maintained until control of depression is achieved. If necessary, additional measures (ECT, hospitalization, etc) should be instituted.

All patients undergoing treatment with Phenelzine Sulfate should be closely followed for symptoms of postural hypotension. Hypotensive side effects have occurred in hypertensive as well as normal and hypotensive patients. Blood pressure usually returns to pretreatment levels rapidly when the drug is discontinued or the dosage is reduced.

Because the effect of Phenelzine Sulfate on the convulsive threshold may be variable, adequate precautions should be taken when treating epileptic patients.

Of the more severe side effects that have been reported with any consistency, hypomania has been the most common. This reaction has been largely limited to patients in whom disorders characterized by hyperkinetic symptoms coexist with, but are obscured by, depressive affect; hypomania usually appeared as depression improved. If agitation is present, it may be increased with Phenelzine Sulfate. Hypomania and agitation have also been reported at higher than recommended doses or following long-term therapy.

Phenelzine Sulfate may cause excessive stimulation in schizophrenic patients; in manic-depressive states it may result in a swing from a depressive to a manic phase.

MAO inhibitors, including Phenelzine Sulfate, potentiate hexobarbital hypnosis in animals. Therefore, barbiturates should be given at a reduced dose with Phenelzine Sulfate.

MAO inhibitors inhibit the destruction of serotonin and norepinephrine, which are believed to be released from tissue stores by rauwolfia alkaloids. Accordingly, caution should be exercised when rauwolfia is used concomitantly with an MAO inhibitor, including Phenelzine Sulfate.

There is conflicting evidence as to whether or not MAO inhibitors affect glucose metabolism or potentiate hypoglycemic agents. This should be kept in mind if Phenelzine Sulfate is administered to diabetics.

DRUG INTERACTIONS:

Phenelzine Sulfate should not be used in combination with dextromethorphan or with CNS depressants such as alcohol and certain narcotics. Excitation, seizures, delirium, hyperpyrexia, circulatory collapse, coma, and death have been reported in patients receiving MAOI therapy who have been given a single dose of meperidine. Phenelzine Sulfate should not be administered together with or in rapid succession to other MAO inhibitors because HYPERTENSIVE CRISES and convulsive seizures, fever, marked sweating, excitation, delirium, tremor, coma, and circulatory collapse may occur (TABLE 1).

TABLE 1 List of MAO Inhibitors

Generic Name	Trademark
pargyline hydrochloride	Eutonyl (Abbott Laboratories)
pargyline hydrochloride and methyclothiazide	Eutron (Abbott Laboratories)
furazolidone	Furoxone (Eaton Laboratories)
isocarboxazid	Marplan (Roche)
procarbazine	Matulane (Roche)
tranylcypromine	Parnate (Smith Kline & French Laboratories)

Phenelzine Sulfate should also not be used in combination with buspirone HCl, since several cases of elevated blood pressure have been reported in patients taking MAO inhibitors who were then given buspirone HCl. At least 10 days should elapse between the discontinuation of Phenelzine Sulfate and the institution of another antidepressant or buspirone HCl, or the discontinuation of another MAO inhibitor and the institution of Phenelzine Sulfate.

There have been reports of serious reactions (including hyperthermia, rigidity, myoclonic movements and death) when fluoxetine has been combined with an MAO inhibitor. Therefore, Phenelzine Sulfate should not be used in combination with fluoxetine. Allow at least five weeks between discontinuation of fluoxetine and initiation of Phenelzine Sulfate and at least 10 days between discontinuation of Phenelzine Sulfate and initiation of fluoxetine.

Patients taking Phenelzine Sulfate should not undergo elective surgery requiring general anesthesia. Also they should not be given cocaine or local anesthesia containing sympathomimetic vasoconstrictors. The possible combined hypotensive effects of Phenelzine Sulfate and spinal anesthesia should be kept in mind. Phenelzine Sulfate should be discontinued at least 10 days prior to elective surgery.

Concomitant Use with Dibenzazepine Derivative Drugs

If the decision is made to administer Phenelzine Sulfate concurrently with other antidepressant drugs, or within less than 10 days after discontinuation of antidepressant therapy, the patient should be cautioned by the physician regarding the possibility of adverse drug interaction (TABLE 2).

Phenelzine Sulfate should be used with caution in combination with antihypertensive drugs, including thiazide diuretics and β-blockers, since exaggerated hypotensive effects may result. MAO inhibitors including Phenelzine Sulfate, are contraindicated in patients receiving guanethidine.

TABLE 2 Phenelzine Sulfate, Drug Interactions

Generic Name	Trademark
nortriptyline hydrochloride	Aventyl (Eli Lilly & Co)
amitriptyline hydrochloride	Elavil (Merck Sharp & Dohme)
amitriptyline hydrochloride	Endep (Roche)
perphenazine and amitriptyline hydrochloride	Etrafon (Schering Corporation)
perphenazine and amitriptyline hydrochloride	Triavil (Merck Sharp & Dohme)
clomipramine hydrochloride	Anafranil (CIBA-Geigy)
desipramine hydrochloride	Norpramin (Merrell-National)
desipramine hydrochloride	Pertofrane (USV)
imipramine hydrochloride	Tofranil (Geigy)
doxepin	Adapin (Pennwalt)
doxepin	Sinequan (Pfizer)
carbamazepine	Tegretol (Geigy)
cyclobenzaprine HCl	Flexeril (Merck Sharp & Dohme)
amoxapine	Asendin (Lederle)
maprotiline HCl	Ludiomil (CIBA)
trimipramine maleate	Surmontil (Wyeth)
protriptyline HCl	Vivactil (Merck Sharp & Dohme)

ADVERSE REACTIONS:

Phenelzine Sulfate is a potent inhibitor of monoamine oxidase. Because this enzyme is widely distributed throughout the body, diverse pharmacologic effects can be expected to occur. When they occur, such effects tend to be mild or moderate in severity (see below), often subside as treatment continues, and can be minimized by adjusting dosage; rarely is it necessary to institute counteracting measures or to discontinue Phenelzine Sulfate.

Common Side Effects Include:

Nervous System: Dizziness, headache, drowsiness, sleep disturbances (including insomnia and hypersomnia), fatigue, weakness, tremors, twitching, myoclonic movements, hyperreflexia.

Gastrointestinal: Constipation, dry mouth, gastrointestinal disturbances, elevated serum transaminases (without accompanying signs and symptoms).

Metabolic: Weight gain.

Cardiovascular: Postural hypotension, edema.

Genitourinary: Sexual disturbances, i.e., anorgasmia and ejaculatory disturbances.

Less Common Mild To Moderate Side Effects (Some Of Which Have Been Reported In A Single Patient Or By A Single Physician) Include:

Nervous System: Jitteriness, palilalia, euphoria, nystagmus, paresthesias.

Genitourinary: Urinary retention.

Metabolic: Hypernatremia.

Dermatologic: Skin rash, sweating.

Special senses: Blurred vision, glaucoma.

Although Reported Less Frequently, And Sometimes Only Once, Additional Severe Side Effects Include:

Nervous System: Ataxia, shock-like coma, toxic delirium, manic reaction, convulsions, acute anxiety reaction, precipitation of schizophrenia, transient respiratory and cardiovascular depression following ECT.

Gastrointestinal: To date, fatal progressive necrotizing hepatocellular damage has been reported in very few patients. Reversible jaundice.

Hematologic: Leukopenia.

Metabolic: Hypermetabolic syndrome (which may include, but is not limited to, hyperpyrexia, tachycardia, tachypnea, muscular rigidity, elevated CK levels, metabolic acidosis, hypoxia, coma and may resemble an overdose).

Respiratory: Edema of the glottis.

Withdrawal may be associated with nausea, vomiting and malaise.

An uncommon withdrawal syndrome following abrupt withdrawal of Phenelzine Sulfate has been infrequently reported. Signs and symptoms of this syndrome generally commence 24 to 72 hours after drug discontinuation and may range from vivid nightmares with agitation to frank psychosis and convulsions. This syndrome generally responds to reinstitution of low-dose Phenelzine Sulfate therapy followed by cautious downward titration and discontinuation.

OVERDOSAGE:

Note: For management of *hypertensive crises* see WARNINGS.

Accidental or intentional overdosage may be more common in patients who are depressed. It should be remembered that multiple drugs and/or alcohol may have been ingested.

Depending on the amount of overdosage with Phenelzine Sulfate, a varying and mixed clinical picture may develop, involving signs and symptoms of central nervous system and cardiovascular stimulation and/or depression. Signs and symptoms may be absent or minimal during the initial 12-hour period following ingestion and may develop slowly thereafter, reaching a maximum in 24-48 hours. Death has been reported following overdosage. Therefore, immediate hospitalization, with continuous patient observation and monitoring throughout this period, is essential.

Signs and symptoms of overdosage may include, alone or in combination, any of the following: drowsiness, dizziness, faintness, irritability, hyperactivity, agitation, severe headache, hallucinations, trismus, opisthotonus, rigidity, convulsions, and coma; rapid and irregular pulse, hypertension, hypotension and vascular collapse; precordial pain, respiratory depression and failure, hyperpyrexia, diaphoresis, and cool, clammy skin.

Intensive symptomatic and supportive treatment may be required. Induction of emesis or gastric lavage with instillation of charcoal slurry may be helpful in early poisoning, provided the airway has been protected against aspiration. Signs and symptoms of central nervous system stimulation, including convulsions, should be treated with diazepam, given slowly intravenously. Phenothiazine derivatives and central nervous system stimulants should be avoided. Hypotension and vascular collapse should be treated with intravenous fluids and, if necessary, blood pressure titration with an intravenous infusion of dilute pressor agent. It should be noted that adrenergic agents may produce a markedly increased pressor response.

Respiration should be supported by appropriate measures, including management of the airway, use of supplemental oxygen, and mechanical ventilatory assistance, as required.

Body temperature should be monitored closely. Intensive management of hyperpyrexia may be required. Maintenance of fluid and electrolyte balance is essential.

There are no data on the lethal dose in man. The pathophysiologic effects of massive overdosage may persist for several days, since the drug acts by inhibiting physiologic enzyme systems. With symptomatic and supportive measures, recovery from *mild* overdosage may be expected within 3 to 4 days.

OVERDOSAGE: *(cont'd)*

Hemodialysis, peritoneal dialysis, and charcoal hemoperfusion may be of value in massive overdosage, but sufficient data are not available to recommend their routine use in these cases.

Toxic blood levels of phenelzine have not been established, and assay methods are not practical for clinical or toxicological use.

DOSAGE AND ADMINISTRATION:

Initial Dose: The usual starting dose of Phenelzine Sulfate is one tablet (15 mg) three times a day.

Early Phase Treatment: Dosage should be increased to at least 60 mg per day at a fairly rapid pace consistent with patient tolerance. It may be necessary to increase dosage up to 90 mg per day to obtain sufficient MAO inhibition. Many patients do not show a clinical response until treatment at 60 mg has been continued for at least 4 weeks.

Maintenance Dose: After maximum benefit from Phenelzine Sulfate is achieved, dosage should be reduced slowly over several weeks. Maintenance dose may be as low as 1 tablet, 15 mg, a day or every other day, and should be continued for as long as is required.

Store between 15-30°C (59-86°F).

HOW SUPPLIED - EQUIVALENTS NOT AVAILABLE:

Tablet, Sugar Coated - Oral - 15 mg

100's	**$40.24**	**NARDIL 15, Parke-Davis**	**00071-0270-24**

PHENIRAMINE; PHENYLPROPANOLAMINE; PYRILAMINE *(002002)*

CATEGORIES: Allergies; Antihistamines; Antitussives/Expectorants/Mucolytics; Autonomic Drugs; Common Cold; Cough Preparations; Decongestants; Nasal Congestion; Respiratory & Allergy Medications; Sympathomimetic Agents; FDA Pre 1938 Drugs

BRAND NAMES: Chem-Hist; Cophene-X; Delhistine D; Liqui-Minic; Maxihist-D; Metahistine D; Multihist-D; Multihistamine-D Pediatric; Poly-D; Poly-Histine-D; Polyhistamine; Polyhistamine Ppa; Rolatuss; Tri-P; Triamill; **Triaminic**; Trihist-D; *Triominic*; Triphenyl; Tussanil; Uni Multi Hist D Pediatric; Uni-Multihist D
(International brand names outside U.S. in italics)

Prescribing information not available at time of publication.

HOW SUPPLIED - EQUIVALENTS NOT AVAILABLE:

Capsule, Gelatin, Sustained Action - Oral - 8 mg/25 mg/8 mg

100's	$39.95	Multihistamine-D Pediatric, Pecos	59879-0506-01
100's	$40.95	Uni Multi Hist D Pediatric, United Res	00677-1575-01
100's	$55.80	POLY-HISTINE-D PED CAPS, Bock Pharma	00563-1658-01

Capsule, Gelatin, Sustained Action - Oral - 16 mg/50 mg/16

30's	$10.26	POLY-HISTINE-D, Bock Pharma	00563-1656-30
100's	$45.48	Poly-D, Qualitest Pharms	00603-5230-21
100's	$52.45	Delhistine D, HL Moore Drug Exch	00839-8017-06
100's	$54.62	Uni-Multihist D, United Res	00677-1550-01
100's	$55.71	Multihist-D, Highland Pkging	55782-0130-01
100's	$59.50	Polyhistamine, Pecos	59879-0117-01
100's	$59.95	Polyhistamine Ppa, Goldline Labs	00182-2612-01
100's	$59.97	Delhistine D, Rugby	00536-5729-01
100's	$80.21	POLY-HISTINE-D, Bock Pharma	00563-1656-01

Elixir - Oral - 4 mg/12.5 mg/4

120 ml	$5.24	Poly-Histine-D Elixir, Bock Pharma	00563-1662-04

Elixir - Oral

15 ml	$6.29	Tri-P, Cypress Pharm	60258-0448-15
15 ml	$6.95	Phenylprop/Pyrilamine/Pheniram, Aligen Independ	00405-3530-61
15 ml	$10.33	Liqui-Minic, Liquipharm	54198-0139-15
473 ml	$17.10	Liqui-Histine D, Liquipharm	54198-0157-16
473 ml	$18.96	Polytine D, Am Generics	58634-0010-01
473 ml	$19.95	Metahistine D, Econolab	55053-0830-16
480 ml	$16.40	Poly-D, Alphagen Labs	59743-0007-16
480 ml	$18.89	Metahistine D, HL Moore Drug Exch	00839-7846-69
480 ml	$18.91	Poly-D, Qualitest Pharms	00603-1528-58
480 ml	$19.04	Uni-Multihist D, United Res	00677-1489-33
480 ml	$19.50	Trihist-D, Cypress Pharm	60258-0226-16
480 ml	$19.81	Kg-Hist D, King Pharms	60793-0034-16
480 ml	$24.03	Trihist-D, Aligen Independ	00405-3878-16

Liquid - Oral - 4 mg/12.5 mg/4

480 ml	$28.53	POLY-HISTINE-D, Bock Pharma	00563-1662-16

Syrup - Oral - 10 mg/20 mg/10

15 ml	**$11.08**	**TRIAMINIC, Novartis**	**00043-0506-15**

Tablet, Coated, Sustained Action - Oral - 25 mg/50 mg/25

100's	**$41.35**	**TRIAMINIC TR, Novartis**	**00043-0020-51**
250's	**$66.77**	**TRIAMINIC TR, Novartis**	**00043-0020-52**

PHENIRAMINE; PHENYLTOLOXAMINE; PYRILAMINE *(002003)*

CATEGORIES: Allergies; Antihistamines; Common Cold; Respiratory & Allergy Medications; FDA Pre 1938 Drugs

BRAND NAMES: Delhistine D; Liqui-Histine; Poly-D; **Poly-Histine**

Prescribing information not available at time of publication.

HOW SUPPLIED - EQUIVALENTS NOT AVAILABLE:

Elixir - Oral - 4 mg/4 mg/4 mg

473 ml	$16.40	Poly-D, Alphagen Labs	59743-0107-16
473 ml	$17.00	Liqui-Histine, Liquipharm	54198-0156-16
480 ml	$19.71	Delhistine D, Rugby	00536-2702-85
480 ml	**$28.53**	**POLY-HISTINE, Bock Pharma**	**00563-1647-16**

PHENOBARBITAL *(002005)*

CATEGORIES: Anesthesia; Anticonvulsants; Anxiolytics, Sedatives, Hypnotic; Barbiturates; Central Nervous System Agents; Cholera; Convulsions; Drug Hypersensitivity; Epilepsy; Epilepticus; Hypnotics; Insomnia; Local Anesthetics; Meningitis; Neuromuscular; Sedatives; Sedatives/Hypnotics; Seizures; Status Epilepticus; Tetanus; Tonic-Clonic Seizures; Pregnancy Category D; DEA Class CIV; FDA Pre 1938 Drugs

BRAND NAMES: *Andral*; *Atrofen*; *Barbilettae*; *Barbiphenyl*; Barbita; *Dormiral*; *Fenemal*; *Fenemal NM Pharma*; *Fenobarb*; *Fenobarbital*; *Gardenal* (France); *Gardenale*; *Lethyl*; *Linasen* (Japan); *Luminal* (Germany); Luminal Sodium; *Luminale*; *Luminaleren*; *Luminaletas*; *Luminaletten* (Germany); *Luminalettes*; *Phenaemal* (Germany); *Phenaemaletten* (Germany); *Phenobal* (Japan); Phenobarbital Sodium; *Phenobarbitone* (Australia); *Phenotal*; *Sedofen*; Solfoton
(International brand names outside U.S. in italics)

FORMULARIES: Aetna; BC-BS; CIGNA; DoD; FHP; Humana; Kaiser; Medco; Medi-Cal; PCS; PruCare; United; WHO

COST OF THERAPY: $0.23 (Insomnia; Tablet; 100 mg; 1/day; 7 days)

DESCRIPTION:

The barbiturates are nonselective central nervous system (CNS) depressants which are primarily used as sedative hypnotics and are also anticonvulsants in subhypnotic doses. The barbiturates and their sodium salts are subject to control under the Federal Controlled Substances Act.

Barbiturates are substituted pyrimidine derivatives in which the basic structure common to these drugs is barbituric acid, a substance which has no CNS activity. CNS activity is obtained by substituting alkyl, alkenyl, or aryl groups on the pyrimidine ring. Phenobarbital is 5- ethyl-t-phenylbarbituric acid and has the empirical formula $C_{12}H_{12}N_2O_3$. Its molecular weight is 232.24.

Tablets: The tablets from Eli Lilly contain 15 mg (0.064 mmol), 30 mg (0.129 mmol), 60 mg (0.258 mmol), or 100 mg (0.431 mmol) phenobarbital. The tablets also contain cornstarch, lactose, magnesium, stearate, and talc.

Phenobarbital occurs as white, odorless, glistening, small crystals or as white, crystalline powder. It is very slightly soluble in water and is soluble in alcohol.

Injectable: Do not use if solution is discolored or contains a precipitate.

The sodium salt of phenobarbital is available as a sterile parenteral solution. It occurs as a white, slightly bitter powder or crystals; it is very soluble in alcohol, and practically insoluble in ether or chloroform.

In the TUBEX and TUBEX BLUE POINTE (Wyeth) Sterile Cartridge Units each milliliter contains 30, 60, or 130 mg phenobarbital sodium in a special vehicle containing 10% alcohol and approximately 75% propylene glycol; when required during manufacture, the pH is adjusted with hydrochloric acid.

Phenobarbital is designated chemically as 5-ethyl-5-phenylbarbiturate.

CLINICAL PHARMACOLOGY:

Barbiturates are capable of producing all levels of CNS mood alteration from excitation to mild sedation, to hypnosis, and deep coma. Overdosage can produce death. In high enough therapeutic doses, barbiturates induce anesthesia.

Barbiturates depress the sensory cortex, decrease motor activity, alter cerebellar function, and produce drowsiness, sedation, and hypnosis.

Barbiturate-induced sleep differs from physiological sleep. Sleep laboratory studies have demonstrated that barbiturates reduce the amount of time spent in the rapid-eye-movement (REM) phase of sleep or dreaming stage. Also, Stages III and IV sleep are decreased. Following abrupt cessation of barbiturates used regularly, patients may experience markedly increased dreaming, nightmares, and/or insomnia. Therefore, withdrawal of a single therapeutic dose over 5 or 6 days has been recommended to lessen the REM rebound and disturbed sleep which contribute to drug-withdrawal syndrome (for example, decrease the dose from 3 to 2 doses a day for 1 week).

The short, intermediate and, to a lesser degree, long-acting barbiturates have been widely prescribed for treating insomnia. Although the clinical literature abounds with claims that the short-acting barbiturates are superior for producing sleep while the intermediate- acting compounds are more effective in maintaining sleep, controlled studies have failed to demonstrate these differential effects. Therefore, as sleep medications, the barbiturates are of limited value beyond short-term use.

Barbiturates have little analgesic action at subanesthetic doses. Rather, in subanesthetic doses these drugs may increase the reaction to painful stimuli. All barbiturates exhibit anticonvulsant activity in anesthetic doses. However, of the drugs in this class, only phenobarbital, mephobarbital, and metharbital are effective as oral anticonvulsants in subhypnotic doses.

Barbiturates are respiratory depressants. The degree of respiratory depression is dependent upon dose. With hypnotic doses, respiratory depression produced by barbiturates is similar to that which occurs during physiologic sleep with slight decrease in blood pressure and heart rate.

Studies in laboratory animals have shown that barbiturates cause reduction in the tone and contractility of the uterus, ureters, and urinary bladder. However, concentrations of the drugs required to produce this effect in humans are not reached with sedative-hypnotic doses.

Barbiturates do not impair normal hepatic function, but have been shown to induce liver microsomal enzymes, thus increasing and/or altering the metabolism of barbiturates and other drugs. (See DRUG INTERACTIONS.)

PHARMACOKINETICS

Barbiturates are absorbed in varying degrees following oral, rectal, or parenteral administration. The salts are more rapidly absorbed than are the acids. The rate of absorption is increased if the sodium salt is ingested as a dilute solution or taken on an empty stomach.

Duration of action, which is related to the rate at which the barbiturates are redistributed throughout the body, varies among persons and in the same person from time to time.

Phenobarbital is classified as a long-acting barbiturate when taken orally. Its onset of action is 1 hour or longer, and its duration of action ranges from 10 to 12 hours.

No studies have demonstrated that the different routes of administration are equivalent with respect to bioavailability.

Barbiturates are weak acids that are absorbed and rapidly distributed to all tissues and fluids with high concentrations in the brain, liver, and kidneys. Lipid solubility of the barbiturates is the dominant factor in their distribution within the body. The more lipid soluble the barbiturate, the more rapidly it penetrates all tissues of the body. Barbiturates are bound to plasma and tissue proteins to a varying degree, with the degree of binding increasing directly as a function of lipid solubility.

Phenobarbital has the lowest lipid solubility, lowest plasma binding, lowest brain-protein binding, the longest delay in onset of activity, and the longest duration of action.

CLINICAL PHARMACOLOGY: *(cont'd)*

Phenobarbital plasma half-life values in adults range from 53 to 118 hours (mean 79 hours) and 60 to 180 hours (mean 110 hours) in children and newborns (age 48 hours or less).

Barbiturates are metabolized primarily by the hepatic microsomal enzyme system, and the metabolic products are excreted in the urine, and less commonly, in the feces. Approximately 25 to 50 percent of a dose of phenobarbital is eliminated unchanged in the urine, whereas the amount of other barbiturates excreted unchanged in the urine is negligible. The excretion of unmetabolized barbiturate is one feature that distinguishes the long-acting category from those belonging to other categories which are almost entirely metabolized. The inactive metabolites of the barbiturates are excreted as conjugates of glucuronic acid.

Additional Information For Injection: Following IV administration, the onset of action is 5 minutes for phenobarbital sodium. Maximal CNS depression may not occur until 15 minutes or more after IV administration. The onset of action of IM administration of barbiturates is slightly faster than the oral route. The onset of action of the oral route varies between 20 and 60 minutes.

INDICATIONS AND USAGE:

Sedative

Hypnotic, for the short-term treatment of insomnia, since barbiturates appear to lose their effectiveness for sleep induction and sleep maintenance after 2 weeks (see CLINICAL PHARMACOLOGY).

Preanesthetic

Tablets: *Anticonvulsant:* For the treatment of generalized and partial seizures.

Injection: For the treatment of generalized tonic-clonic and cortical focal seizures. And, in the emergency control of certain acute convulsive episodes, *e.g.,* those associated with status epilepticus, cholera, eclampsia, meningitis, tetanus, and toxic reactions to strychnine or local anesthetics. Phenobarbital sodium may be administered IM or IV as an anticonvulsant for emergency use. When administered IV, it may require 15 or more minutes before reaching peak concentrations in the brain. Therefore, injecting phenobarbital sodium until the convulsions stop may cause the brain level to exceed that required to control the convulsions and lead to severe barbiturate- induced depression.

CONTRAINDICATIONS:

Barbiturates are contraindicated in patients with known barbiturate sensitivity. Barbiturates are also contraindicated in patients with a history of manifest or latent porphyria or marked impairment of liver function, or with severe respiratory disease where dyspnea or obstruction is evident. Large doses are contraindicated in nephritic subjects. Barbiturates should not be administered to persons with known previous addiction to the sedative/hypnotic group, since ordinary doses may be ineffectual and may contribute to further addiction.

Intra-arterial administration is contraindicated. Its consequences vary from transient pain to gangrene. Subcutaneous administration produces tissue irritation, ranging from tenderness and redness to necrosis, and it not recommended. (See DOSAGE AND ADMINISTRATION, Treatment of Adverse Effects Due to Inadvertent Error in Administration.)

WARNINGS:

Habit-Forming: Barbiturates may be habit-forming. Tolerance, psychological and physical dependence may occur with continued use. (See DRUG ABUSE AND DEPENDENCE and CLINICAL PHARMACOLOGY,Pharmacokinetics. Patients who have psychological dependence on barbiturates may increase the dosage or decrease the dosage interval without consulting a physician and may subsequently develop a physical dependence on barbiturates. To minimize the possibility of overdosage or the development of dependence, the prescribing and dispensing of sedative-hypnotic barbiturates should be limited to the amount required for the interval until the next appointment. Abrupt cessation after prolonged use in the dependent person may result in withdrawal symptoms, including delirium, convulsions, and possibly death. Barbiturates should be withdrawn gradually from any patient known to be taking excessive dosage over long periods of time (see DRUG ABUSE AND DEPENDENCE).

IV Administration: Too-rapid administration may cause respiratory depression, apnea, laryngospasm, or vasodilation with fall in blood pressure.

Acute Or Chronic Pain: Caution should be exercised when barbiturates are administered to patients with acute or chronic pain, because paradoxical excitement could be induced or important symptoms could be masked. However, the use of barbiturates as sedatives in the postoperative surgical period and as adjuncts to cancer chemotherapy is well established.

Use In Pregnancy: Barbiturates can cause fetal damage when administered to a pregnant woman. Retrospective, case-controlled studies have suggested a connection between the maternal consumption of barbiturates and a higher than expected incidence of fetal abnormalities. Following oral or parenteral administration, barbiturates readily cross the placental barrier and are distributed throughout fetal tissues, with highest concentration found in the placenta, fetal liver, and brain. Fetal blood levels approach maternal blood levels following parenteral administration.

Withdrawal symptoms occur in infants born to mothers who receive barbiturates throughout the last trimester of pregnancy. (See DRUG ABUSE AND DEPENDENCE.) If phenobarbital is used during pregnancy, or if the patient becomes pregnant while taking this drug, the patient should be apprised of the potential hazard to the fetus.

Synergistic Effects: The concomitant use of alcohol or other CNS depressants may produce additive CNS depressant effects.

PRECAUTIONS:

GENERAL

Barbiturates may be habit-forming. Tolerance and psychological and physical dependence may occur with continuing use. (See DRUG ABUSE AND DEPENDENCE.) Barbiturates should be administered with caution, if at all, to patients who are mentally depressed, have suicidal tendencies, or a history of drug abuse.

Elderly or debilitated patients may react to barbiturates with marked excitement, depression, and confusion. In some persons, barbiturates repeatedly produce excitement rather than depression.

In patients with hepatic damage, barbiturates should be administered with caution and initially in reduced doses. Barbiturates should not be administered to patients showing the premonitory signs of hepatic coma.

Untoward reactions may occur in the presence of fever, hyperthyroidism, diabetes mellitus, and severe anemia.

Intramuscular injection should be confined to a total volume of 5 ml and made in a large muscle in order to avoid possible tissue irritation.

Parenteral solutions of barbiturates are highly alkaline. Therefore, extreme care should be taken to avoid perivascular extravasation or intra-arterial injection.

Extravascular injection may cause local tissue damage with subsequent necrosis; consequences of intra-arterial injection may vary from transient pain to gangrene of the limb. Any complaint of pain in the limb warrants stopping the injection.

PRECAUTIONS: *(cont'd)*

INFORMATION FOR THE PATIENT

Practitioners should give the following information and instructions to patients receiving barbiturates:

The use of barbiturates carries with it an associated risk of psychological and/or physical dependence. The patient should be warned against increasing the dose of the drug without consulting a physician.

Barbiturates may impair mental and/or physical abilities required for the performance of potentially hazardous tasks (*e.g.,* driving, operating machinery, etc.).

Alcohol should not be consumed while taking barbiturates. Concurrent use of the barbiturates with other CNS depressants (*e.g.,* alcohol, narcotics, tranquilizers, and antihistamines) may result in additional CNS depressant effects.

LABORATORY TESTS

Prolonged therapy with barbiturates should be accompanied by periodic laboratory evaluation of organ systems, including hematopoietic, renal, and hepatic systems. (See PRECAUTIONS, General and ADVERSE REACTIONS).

CARCINOGENESIS, MUTAGENESIS, AND IMPAIRMENT OF FERTILITY

Animal Data: Phenobarbital sodium is carcinogenic in mice and rats after lifetime administration. In mice, it produced benign and malignant liver-cell tumors. In rats, benign liver-cell tumors were observed very late in life.

Human Data: In a 29-year epidemiological study of 9,136 patients who were treated on an anticonvulsant protocol which included phenobarbital, results indicated a higher than normal incidence of hepatic carcinoma. Previously, some of these patients were treated with thorotrast, a drug which is known to produce hepatic carcinomas. Thus, this study did not provide sufficient evidence that phenobarbital sodium is carcinogenic in humans.

A retrospective study of 84 children with brain tumors matched to 73 normal controls and 78 cancer controls (malignant disease other than brain tumors) suggested an association between exposure to barbiturates prenatally and an increased incidence of brain tumors.

PREGNANCY CATEGORY D

Teratogenic Effects: See WARNINGS, Use in Pregnancy.

Nonteratogenic Effects: Reports of infants suffering from long- term barbiturate exposure *in utero* included the acute withdrawal syndrome of seizures and hyperirritability from birth to a delayed onset of up to 14 days. (See DRUG ABUSE AND DEPENDENCE.)

LABOR AND DELIVERY

Hypnotic doses of these barbiturates do not appear to significantly impair uterine activity during labor. Full anesthetic doses of barbiturates decrease the force and frequency of uterine contractions. Administration of sedative-hypnotic barbiturates to the mother during labor may result in respiratory depression in the newborn. Premature infants are particularly susceptible to the depressant effects of barbiturates. If barbiturates are used during labor and delivery, resuscitation equipment should be available.

Data are currently not available to evaluate the effect of these barbiturates when forceps delivery or other intervention is necessary. Also, data are not available to determine the effect of these barbiturates on the later growth, development, and functional maturation of the child.

NURSING MOTHERS

Caution should be exercised when a barbiturate is administered to a nursing woman, since small amounts of barbiturates are excreted in the milk.

DRUG INTERACTIONS:

Anticoagulants: Phenobarbital lowers the plasma levels of dicumarol (name previously used: bishydroxycoumarin) and causes a decrease in anticoagulant activity as measured by the prothrombin time. Barbiturates can induce hepatic microsomal enzymes, resulting in increased metabolism and decreased anticoagulant response of oral anticoagulants (*e.g.,* warfarin, acenocoumarol, dicumarol, and phenprocoumon). Patients stabilized on anticoagulant therapy may require dosage adjustments if barbiturates are added to or withdrawn from their dosage regimen.

Corticosteroids: Barbiturates appear to enhance the metabolism of exogenous corticosteroids, probably through the induction of hepatic microsomal enzymes. Patients stabilized on corticosteroid therapy may require dosage adjustments if barbiturates are added to or withdrawn from their dosage regimen.

Griseofulvin: Phenobarbital appears to interfere with the absorption of orally administered griseofulvin, thus decreasing its blood level. The effect of the resultant decreased blood levels of griseofulvin on therapeutic response has not been established. However, it would be preferable to avoid concomitant administration of these drugs.

Doxycycline: Phenobarbital has been shown to shorten the half- life of doxycycline for as long as 2 weeks after barbiturate therapy is discontinued.

This mechanism is probably through the induction of hepatic microsomal enzymes that metabolize the antibiotic. If phenobarbital and doxycycline are administered concurrently, the clinical response to doxycycline should be monitored closely.

Phenytoin, Sodium Valproate, Valproic Acid: The effect of barbiturates on the metabolism of phenytoin appears to be variable. Some investigators report an accelerating effect, while others report no effect. Because the effect of barbiturates on the metabolism of phenytoin is not predictable, phenytoin and barbiturate blood levels should be monitored more frequently if these drugs are given concurrently. Sodium valproate and valproic acid appear to decrease barbiturate metabolism; therefore, barbiturate blood levels should be monitored and appropriate dosage adjustments made as indicated.

Central Nervous System Depressants: The concomitant use of other central nervous system depressants, including other sedatives or hypnotics, antihistamines, tranquilizers, or alcohol, may produce additive depressant effects.

Monoamine Oxidase Inhibitors (MAOI): MAOI prolong the effects of barbiturates, probably because metabolism of the barbiturate is inhibited.

Estradiol, Estrone, Progesterone, and Other Steroidal Hormones: Pretreatment with or concurrent administration of phenobarbital may decrease the effect of estradiol by increasing its metabolism. There have been reports of patients treated with antiepileptic drugs (*e.g.,* phenobarbital) who became pregnant while taking oral contraceptives. An alternate contraceptive method might be suggested to women taking phenobarbital.

ADVERSE REACTIONS:

The following adverse reactions and their incidence were compiled from surveillance of thousands of hospitalized patients. Because such patients may be less aware of certain of the milder adverse effects of barbiturates, the incidence of these reactions may be somewhat higher in fully ambulatory patients.

More Than 1 In 100 Patients: The most common adverse reaction estimated to occur at a rate of 1 to 3 patients per 100 is: *Nervous System:* Somnolence.

Less Than 1 In 100 Patients: Adverse reactions estimated to occur at a rate of less than 1 in 100 patients listed below, grouped by organ system, and by decreasing order of occurrence are: *Nervous System:* Agitation, confusion, hyperkinesia, ataxia, CNS depression, nightmares,

ADVERSE REACTIONS: *(cont'd)*

nervousness, psychiatric disturbance, hallucinations, insomnia, anxiety, dizziness, thinking abnormality. *Respiratory System:* Hypoventilation, apnea. *Cardiovascular System:* Bradycardia, hypotension, syncope. *Digestive System:* Nausea, vomiting, constipation. *Other Reported Reactions:* Headache, injection-site reactions, hypersensitivity reactions (angioedema, skin rashes, exfoliative dermatitis), fever, liver damage, megaloblastic anemia following chronic phenobarbital use.

DRUG ABUSE AND DEPENDENCE:

Barbiturates may be habit-forming. Tolerance, psychological dependence, and physical dependence may occur, especially following prolonged use of high doses of barbiturates. As tolerance to barbiturates develops, the amount needed to maintain the same level of intoxication increases; tolerance to a fatal dosage, however, does not increase more than two-fold. As this occurs, the margin between an intoxicating dosage and fatal dosage becomes smaller.

Symptoms of acute intoxication with barbiturates include unsteady gait, slurred speech, and sustained nystagmus. Mental signs of chronic intoxication include confusion, poor judgement, irritability, insomnia, and somatic complaints.

Symptoms of barbiturate dependence are similar to those of chronic alcoholism. If an individual appears to be intoxicated with alcohol to a degree that is radically disproportionate to the amount of alcohol in his or her blood, the use of barbiturates should be suspected. The lethal dose of a barbiturate is far less if alcohol is also ingested.

The symptoms of barbiturate withdrawal can be severe and may cause death. Minor withdrawal symptoms may appear 8 to 12 hours after the last dose of a barbiturate. These symptoms usually appear in the following order: anxiety, muscle twitching, tremor of hands and fingers, progressive weakness, dizziness, distortion in visual perception, nausea, vomiting, insomnia, and orthostatic hypotension. Major withdrawal symptoms (convulsions and delirium) may occur within 16 hours and last up to 5 days after abrupt cessation of these drugs. Intensity of withdrawal symptoms gradually declines over a period of approximately 15 days. Individuals susceptible to barbiturate abuse and dependence include alcoholics and opiate abusers, as well as other sedative- hypnotic and amphetamine abusers.

Drug dependence to barbiturates arises from repeated administration of a barbiturate or agent with barbiturate-like effect on a continuous basis, generally in amounts exceeding therapeutic dose levels. The characteristics of drug dependence to barbiturates include: **(a)** a strong desire or need to continue taking the drug; **(b)** a tendency to increase the dose; **(c)** a psychic dependence on the effects of the drug related to subjective and individual appreciation of these effects; and **(d)** a physical dependence on the effects of the drug requiring its presence for maintenance of homeostasis and resulting in a definite, characteristic, and self-limited abstinence syndrome when the drug is withdrawn.

Treatment of barbiturate dependence consists of cautious and gradual withdrawal of the drug. If withdrawal symptoms appear, dosage is maintained at that level or increased slightly until symptoms disappear.

The total daily dose of phenobarbital may normally be decreased by 10 percent if tolerated by the patient. Severely dependent individuals may generally be withdrawn over a period of two to three weeks.

Infants physically dependent on barbiturates may be given phenobarbital, 3 to 10 mg/kg/day. After withdrawal symptoms (hyperactivity, disturbed sleep, tremors, hyperreflexia) are relieved, the dosage of phenobarbital should be gradually decreased and completely withdrawn over a 2-week period.

OVERDOSAGE:

The toxic dose of barbiturates varies considerably. In general, an oral dose of 1 gram of most barbiturates produces serious poisoning in an adult. Death commonly occurs after 2 to 10 grams of ingested barbiturate. Barbiturate intoxication may be confused with alcoholism, bromide intoxication, and with various neurological disorders.

Acute overdosage with barbiturates is manifested by CNS and respiratory depression which may progress to Cheyne-Stokes respiration, areflexia, constriction of the pupils to a slight degree (though in severe poisoning they may show paralytic dilation), oliguria, tachycardia, hypotension, lowered body temperature, and coma. Typical shock syndrome (apnea, circulatory collapse, respiratory arrest, and death) may occur.

In extreme overdose, all electrical activity in the brain may cease, in which case a "flat" EEG, normally equated with clinical death, cannot be accepted. This effect is fully reversible unless hypoxic damage occurs. Consideration should be given to the possibility of barbiturate intoxication even in situations that appear to involve trauma.

Complications such as pneumonia, pulmonary edema, cardiac arrhythmias, congestive heart failure, and renal failure may occur. Uremia may increase CNS sensitivity to barbiturates if renal function is impaired. Differential diagnosis should include hypoglycemia, head trauma, cerebrovascular accidents, convulsive states, and diabetic coma.

Blood levels from acute overdosage, causing CNS depression, for phenobarbital range from 5 ppm (mcg/ml) to 200 ppm (mcg/ml).

Treatment of overdosage is mainly supportive and consists of the following:

1. Maintenance of an adequate airway, with assisted respiration and oxygen administration as necessary.

2. Monitoring of vital signs and fluid balance.

3. Fluid therapy and other standard treatment for shock, if needed.

4. If renal function is normal, forced diuresis may aid in the elimination of the barbiturate. Alkalinization of the urine increases renal excretion of some barbiturates, especially phenobarbital, also aprobarbital, and mephobarbital (which is metabolized to phenobarbital).

5. Although not recommended as a routine procedure, hemodialysis may be used in severe barbiturate intoxications or if the patient is anuric or in shock.

6. Patient should be rolled from side to side every 30 minutes.

7. Antibiotics should be given if pneumonia is suspected.

8. Appropriate nursing care to prevent hypostatic pneumonia, decubiti, aspiration, and other complications of patients with altered states of consciousness.

DOSAGE AND ADMINISTRATION:

Dosages of barbiturates must be individualized with full knowledge of their particular characteristics and recommended rate of administration. Factors of consideration are the patient's age, weight, and condition.

TABLETS

Sedation: For sedation, the drug may be administered in single doses of 30 to 120 mg repeated at intervals; frequency will be determined by the patient's response. It is generally considered that no more than 400 mg of phenobarbital should be administered during a 24-hour period.

Adults: *Daytime Sedation:* 30 to 120 mg daily in 2 to 3 divided doses. *Oral Hypnotic:* 100 to 200 mg.

DOSAGE AND ADMINISTRATION: *(cont'd)*

Anticonvulsant Use: Clinical laboratory reference values should be used to determine the therapeutic anticonvulsant level of phenobarbital in the serum. To achieve the blood levels considered therapeutic in children, higher per-kilogram dosages are generally necessary for phenobarbital and most other anticonvulsants. In children and infants, phenobarbital at a loading dose of 15 to 20 mg/kg produces blood levels of about 20 mcg/ml shortly after administration

Phenobarbital has been used in the treatment and prophylaxis of febrile seizures. However, it has not been established that prevention of febrile seizures influences the subsequent development of epilepsy.

Adults: 60 to 200 mg/day.

Children: 3 to 6 mg/kg/day.

Special Patient Populations: Dosage should be reduced in the elderly or debilitated because these patients may be more sensitive to barbiturates. Dosage should be reduced for patients with impaired renal function or hepatic disease.

INJECTION

Suggested doses of phenobarbital sodium for specific indications:

Pediatric Dosage: Recommended by the American Academy of Pediatrics (Intended as a guide)

Preoperative Sedation: 1 to 3 mg/kg IM or IV

Anticonvulsion: 4 to 6 mg/kg/day for 7 to 10 days to blood level of 10 to 15 mcg/ml or 10 to 15 mg/kg/day IM or IV

Status Epilepticus: 15 to 20 mg/kg over 10 to 15 minutes IV

Adult Dosage: (Intended as a Guide)

Daytime Sedation: 30 to 120 mg daily in 2 to 3 divided doses IM or IV

Bedtime Hypnosis: 100 to 320 mg IM or IV

Preoperative Sedation: IM only; 100 to 200 mg 60 to 90 minutes before surgery

Acute Convulsions: 200 to 320 mg IM or IV, repeated in 6 hours as necessary.

Parenteral routes should be used only when oral administration is impossible or impractical.

The TUBEX BLUE POINTE Sterile Cartridge Unit (Wyeth) is suitable for substances to be administered intravenously only. It is intended for use with injection sets specifically manufactured as "needle-less" injection systems. TUBEX BLUE POINTE (Wyeth) is compatible with Abbott's Life- Shield pre-pierced reseal injection site, Baxter's InterLink Injection Site, and B. Braun Medical's SafSite Reflux Valve. Consult manufacturer's recommendations regarding "Directions for USe" of the "needle-less" system. It is also intended for admixture with, and convenient administration of, various medicaments when using Drug Vial Adapters for "needle-less" injection systems.

The TUBEX Sterile Cartridge-Needle Unit (Wyeth) is suitable for substances to be administered intravenously or intramuscularly.

IM injection of the sodium salts of barbiturates should be made deeply into a large muscle, and a volume of 5 ml should not be exceeded at any one site because of possible tissue irritation. After IM injection of a hypnotic dose, the patient's vital signs should be monitored.

IV injection is restricted to conditions in which other routes are not feasible, either because the patient is unconscious (as in cerebral hemorrhage, eclampsia, or status epilepticus), or because the patient resists (as in delirium), or because prompt action is imperative. Slow IV injection is essential, and patients should be carefully observed during administration. This requires that blood pressure, respiration, and cardiac function be maintained, vital signs be recorded, and equipment for resuscitation and ventilation be available. The rate of IV injection for adults should not exceed 60 mg/mn for phenobarbital sodium.

Any vein may be used, but preference should be given to a larger vein (to minimize the risk of irritation with the possibility of resultant thrombosis). Avoid administration into varicose veins, because circulation there is retarded. Inadvertent injection into or adjacent to an artery has resulted in gangrene requiring amputation of an extremity or a portion thereof. Careful technique, including aspiration, is necessary to avoid inadvertent intra-arterial injection.

Treatment of Adverse Effects due to Inadvertent Error in Administration: Extravasation into subcutaneous tissues causes tissue irritation. This may vary from slight tenderness and redness to necrosis. Recommended treatment includes the application of moist heat and the injection of 0.05% procaine solution into the affected area.

Intra-arterial injection of any barbiturate must be avoided. The accidental intra-arterial injection of a small amount of the solution may cause spasm and severe pain along the course of the artery. The injection should be terminated if the patient complains of pain or if other indications of accidental intra-arterial injection occur, such as a white hand with cyanosed skin or patches of discolored skin and delayed onset of hypnosis.

The consequences of intra-arterial injection of phenobarbital can vary from transient pain to gangrene. It is not possible to formulate strict rules for management of such accidents. The following procedures have been suggested: 1) release of the tourniquet or restrictive garments to permit dilution of injected drug, 2) relief of arterial spasm by injecting 10 ml of a 1% procaine solution into the artery and, if considered necessary, brachial plexus block, 3) prevention of thrombosis by early anticoagulant therapy, and 4) supportive treatment.

Anticonvulsant Use: A therapeutic anticonvulsant level of phenobarbital in the serum is 10 to 25 mcg/ml. To achieve the blood levels considered therapeutic in children, higher per-kilogram dosages are generally necessary for phenobarbital and higher per-kilogram dosages are generally necessary for phenobarbital and most other anticonvulsants. In children and infants, phenobarbital at loading doses of 15 to 20 mg/kg produces blood levels of about 20 mcg/ml shortly after administration.

In status epilepticus, it is imperative to achieve therapeutic blood levels of a barbiturate (or other anticonvulsants) as rapidly as possible. When administered intravenously, phenobarbital sodium may require 15 minutes or more to attain peak concentrations in the brain. If phenobarbital sodium is injected continuously until the convulsions stop, the brain concentration would continue to rise and could eventually exceed that required to control the seizures. A barbiturate-induced depression may occur along with a postictal depression once the seizures are controlled, therefore, it is important to use the minimal amount required, and to wait for the anticonvulsant effect to develop before administering a second dose.

Phenobarbital has been used in the treatment and prophylaxis of febrile seizures. However, it has not been established that prevention of febrile seizures influences the subsequent development of epilepsy.

Special Patient Population: Dosage should be reduced in the elderly or debilitated because these patients may be more sensitive to barbiturates. Dosage should be reduced for patients with impaired renal function or hepatic disease.

Inspection: Parenteral drug products should be inspected visually for particulate matter and discoloration prior to administration, whenever solution and container permit. Solutions for injection showing evidence of precipitation should not be used.

Storage: *Tablets:* Keep tightly closed. Store at controlled room temperature, 59° to 86°F (15° to 30°C). *Injection:* Store at room temperature, approximately 25°C (77°F)

(TABLETS: Eli Lilly and Company, 10/30/91)

(INJECTION: Wyeth Laboratories, 3/22/94)

HOW SUPPLIED - EQUIVALENTS NOT AVAILABLE:

Capsule, Gelatin - Oral - 16 mg

100's	$12.00	SOLFOTON, ECR Pharms	00095-0025-01

Elixir - Oral - 20 mg/5ml

5 ml x 100	$45.77	Phenobarbital, Roxane	00054-8704-04
7.5 ml x 100	$47.99	Phenobarbital, Roxane	00054-8701-04
480 ml	$4.00	Phenobarbital, Century Pharms	00436-0585-16
480 ml	$4.40	Phenobarbital, Purepac Pharm	00228-2024-16
480 ml	$4.50	Phenobarbital, Harber Pharm	51432-0644-20
480 ml	$4.50	Phenobarbital, Liquipharm	54198-0130-16
480 ml	$5.00	Phenobarbital, Schein Pharm (US)	00364-7046-16
480 ml	$5.00	Phenobarbital, HR Cenci	00556-0112-16
480 ml	$5.10	Phenobarbital, Halsey Drug	00879-0049-16
480 ml	$5.13	Phenobarbital, Alpharma	00472-1015-16
480 ml	$5.25	Phenobarbital, Major Pharms	00904-1015-16
480 ml	$5.31	Phenobarbital, Qualitest Pharms	00603-1508-58
480 ml	$5.50	Phenobarbital, Morton Grove	60432-0026-16
480 ml	$5.52	Phenobarbital, HL Moore Drug Exch	00839-5398-69
480 ml	$5.77	Phenobarbital, Aligen Independ	00405-0155-16
480 ml	$5.80	Phenobarbital, Goldline Labs	00182-0314-40
480 ml	$5.95	Phenobarbital, United Res	00677-0805-33
480 ml	$6.53	Phenobarbital, Rugby	00536-1590-85
480 ml	$11.13	Phenobarbital, Lilly	00002-2438-05
960 ml	$6.25	Phenobarbital, Century Pharms	00436-0585-32
3785 ml	$35.83	Phenobarbital, Goldline Labs	00182-0314-41
3840 ml	$22.27	Phenobarbital, Liquipharm	54198-0130-28
3840 ml	$25.00	Phenobarbital, Century Pharms	00436-0585-28
3840 ml	$25.69	Phenobarbital, Rugby	00536-1590-90
3840 ml	$29.07	Phenobarbital, Morton Grove	60432-0026-28
3840 ml	$29.22	Phenobarbital, Major Pharms	00904-1015-28
3840 ml	$29.91	Phenobarbital, Harber Pharm	51432-0644-21
3840 ml	$30.99	Phenobarbital, HR Cenci	00556-0112-28
3840 ml	$31.53	Phenobarbital, Halsey Drug	00879-0049-28
3840 ml	$31.57	Phenobarbital, Alpharma	00472-1015-28
3840 ml	$48.65	Phenobarbital, Lilly	00002-2438-06

Injection, Solution - Intramuscular; - 30 mg/ml

1 ml x 10	$21.20	Phenobarbital Sodium, Wyeth Labs	00008-0499-01
1 ml x 10	$24.95	PHENOBARBITAL SODIUM, Wyeth Labs	00008-0499-50

Injection, Solution - Intramuscular; - 60 mg/ml

1 ml x 10	$23.66	SODIUM PHENOBARBITAL, Wyeth Labs	00008-0747-01
1 ml x 10	$27.41	PHENOBARBITAL SODIUM, Wyeth Labs	00008-0747-50
1 ml x 25	$23.16	PHENOBARBITAL SODIUM, Elkins Sinn	00641-0476-25

Injection, Solution - Intramuscular; - 130 mg/ml

1 ml x 10	$26.00	SODIUM PHENOBARBITAL, Wyeth Labs	00008-0304-01
1 ml x 10	$29.75	PHENOBARBITAL SODIUM, Wyeth Labs	00008-0304-50
1 ml x 25	$27.60	PHENOBARBITAL SODIUM, Elkins Sinn	00641-0477-25
1 ml x 100	$318.16	LUMINAL SODIUM, Sanofi Winthrop	00024-1171-06

Powder

125 gm	$13.81	PHENOBARBITAL, Mallinckrodt	00406-6588-01
125 gm	$21.38	PHENOBARBITAL SODIUM, Mallinckrodt	00406-6593-01
500 gm	$76.74	PHENOBARBITAL SODIUM, Mallinckrodt	00406-6593-03

Tablet, Uncoated - Oral - 15 mg

10 tab x 10	$5.92	Phenobarbital, Roxane	00054-8703-25
100's	$3.00	Phenobarbital, Lilly	00002-1031-02
100's	$4.65	Phenobarbital, Medirex	57480-0504-01
100's	$4.86	Phenobarbital, Major Pharms	00904-3815-61
100's	$7.80	SOLFOTON, ECR Pharms	00095-0023-01
600's	$44.20	Phenobarbital, Medirex	57480-0504-06
1000's	$5.73	Phenobarbital, West Ward Pharm	00143-1445-10
1000's	$7.24	Phenobarbital, Aligen Independ	00405-0148-03
1000's	$7.25	Phenobarbital, C O Truxton	00463-6160-10
1000's	$7.88	Phenobarbital, Vintage Pharms	00254-5011-38
1000's	$7.99	Phenobarbital, Purepac Pharm	00228-2026-96
1000's	$8.20	Phenobarbital, United Res	00677-0236-10
1000's	$8.49	Phenobarbital, Geneva Pharms	00781-1091-10
1000's	$8.75	Phenobarbital, Harber Pharm	51432-0342-06
1000's	$8.85	Phenobarbital, Rugby	00536-4170-10
1000's	$9.40	Phenobarbital, Qualitest Pharms	00603-5165-32
1000's	$9.66	Phenobarbital, Eon Labs Mfg	00185-0015-10
1000's	$9.95	Phenobarbital, Parmed Pharms	00349-8868-10
1000's	$10.90	Phenobarbital, Major Pharms	00904-3815-80
1000's	$15.51	Phenobarbital, HL Moore Drug Exch	00839-1478-16

Tablet, Uncoated - Oral - 30 mg

10 tab x 10	$6.95	Phenobarbital, Roxane	00054-8705-25
10 x 25	$18.85	Phenobarbital, Wyeth Labs	00008-0268-04
100's	$3.07	Phenobarbital, Lilly	00002-1032-02
100's	$4.43	Phenobarbital, Lilly	00002-1032-33
100's	$4.55	Phenobarbital, Vangard Labs	00615-0421-47
100's	$5.53	Phenobarbital, Medirex	57480-0505-01
600's	$46.20	Phenobarbital, Medirex	57480-0505-06
750's	$32.06	Phenobarbital, Glasgow Pharm	60809-0507-55
750's	$32.06	Phenobarbital, Glasgow Pharm	60809-0507-72
1000's	$6.95	Phenobarb, Calvin Scott	17224-0803-10
1000's	$7.21	Phenobarbital, West Ward Pharm	00143-1450-10
1000's	$8.10	Phenobarbital, C O Truxton	00463-6145-10
1000's	$8.53	Phenobarbital, Vintage Pharms	00254-5012-38
1000's	$8.80	Phenobarbital, Major Pharms	00904-3827-80
1000's	$9.12	Phenobarbital, Aligen Independ	00405-0149-03
1000's	$9.95	Phenobarbital, Harber Pharm	51432-0344-06
1000's	$10.68	Phenobarbital, United Res	00677-0237-10
1000's	$10.73	Phenobarbital, Rugby	00536-4224-10
1000's	$10.80	Phenobarbital, Eon Labs Mfg	00185-0030-10
1000's	$10.98	Phenobarbital, Parmed Pharms	00349-8869-10
1000's	$11.15	Phenobarbital, Qualitest Pharms	00603-5166-32
1000's	$11.80	Phenobarbital, Purepac Pharm	00228-2028-96
1000's	$11.95	Phenobarbital, Major Pharms	00904-3816-80
1000's	$13.75	Phenobarbital, Goldline Labs	00182-0292-10
1000's	$13.75	Phenobarbital, Geneva Pharms	00781-1110-10
1000's	$15.22	Phenobarbital, Lilly	00002-1032-04
1000's	$17.94	Phenobarbital, HL Moore Drug Exch	00839-1484-16

Tablet, Uncoated - Oral - 60 mg

10 tab x 10	$7.27	Phenobarbital, Roxane	00054-8708-25
100's	$2.66	Phenobarbital, Vintage Pharms	00254-5013-28
100's	$2.98	Phenobarbital, Qualitest Pharms	00603-5167-21
100's	$4.54	Phenobarbital, Lilly	00002-1037-02
100's	$5.70	Phenobarbital, Vangard Labs	00615-0418-27
250's	$20.20	Phenobarbital, Wyeth Labs	00008-0320-04
1000's	$11.42	Phenobarbital, Vintage Pharms	00254-5013-38
1000's	$13.45	Phenobarbital, United Res	00677-0762-10

HOW SUPPLIED - EQUIVALENTS NOT AVAILABLE: *(cont'd)*

1000's	$15.70	Phenobarbital, Qualitest Pharms	00603-5167-32
1000's	$18.90	Phenobarbital, Goldline Labs	00182-0590-10
1000's	$24.21	Phenobarbital, Lilly	00002-1037-04
1000's	$30.38	Phenobarbital, HL Moore Drug Exch	00839-6257-16

Tablet, Uncoated - Oral - 100 mg

10 tab x 10	$7.45	Phenobarbital, Roxane	00054-8707-25
100's	$3.31	Phenobarbital, Vintage Pharms	00254-5014-28
100's	$3.98	Phenobarbital, Qualitest Pharms	00603-5168-21
100's	$5.75	Phenobarbital, Lilly	00002-1033-02
1000's	$18.50	Phenobarbital, United Res	00677-0238-10
1000's	$18.65	Phenobarbital, Harber Pharm	51432-0346-06
1000's	$19.40	Phenobarbital, Major Pharms	00904-2066-80
1000's	$19.50	Phenobarbital, C O Truxton	00463-6152-10
1000's	$37.73	Phenobarbital, HL Moore Drug Exch	00839-5154-16

PHENOBARBITAL; PHENYTOIN *(002007)*

CATEGORIES: Anticonvulsants; Antiepileptics; Barbiturates; Central Nervous System Agents; Convulsions; Epilepsy; Hydantoin Anticonvulsants; Neuromuscular; Seizures; Tonic-Clonic Seizures; Sales > $100 Million; FDA Pre 1938 Drugs

BRAND NAMES: **Dilantin With Phenobarbital**

FORMULARIES: BC-BS; Medi-Cal

DESCRIPTION:

Dilantin (phenytoin sodium) is related to the barbiturates in chemical structure, but has a five-membered ring. The chemical name is sodium 5,5-diphenyl-2,4-imidazolidinedione.

FOR COMPLETE PRESCRIBING INFORMATION REFER TO THE INDIVIDUAL DRUG MONOGRAPHS (PHENOBARBITAL; PHENYTOIN).

INDICATIONS AND USAGE:

Dilantin with Phenobarbital is indicated for the control of generalized tonic-clonic (grand mal) and complex partial (psychomotor, temporal lobe) seizures, only in those patients who require both drugs for seizure control and who previously have had their daily anticonvulsant requirements determined by the administration of the two drugs separately. Combinations should not be used to initiate anticonvulsant therapy and are provided as a convenience for epileptic patients.

Phenytoin serum level determinations may be necessary for optimal dosage adjustments.

DOSAGE AND ADMINISTRATION:

Serum concentrations should be monitored and care should be taken when switching a patient from the sodium salt to the free acid form.

Dilantin Kapseals, Dilantin Parenteral, and Dilantin with Phenobarbital are formulated with the sodium salt of phenytoin. The free acid form of phenytoin is used in Dilantin-30 Pediatric and Dilantin-125 Suspensions and Dilantin Infatabs. Because there is approximately an 8% increase in drug content with the free acid form over that of the sodium salt, dosage adjustments and serum level monitoring may be necessary when switching from a product formulated with the free acid to a product formulated with the sodium salt and vice versa.

The combination of Dilantin with Phenobarbital Kapseals is provided as a convenience for epileptic patients who require both drugs for seizure control. Anticonvulsant therapy should be initiated with either phenytoin or phenobarbital and, if indicated, the other drug can then be added. If the total daily doses of the two drugs used separately are within those given below, the combination of Dilantin with Phenobarbital Kapseals can then be substituted in equivalent amounts. When plasma level determinations are necessary for optimal dosage adjustments, the clinically effective level of Dilantin is usually 10 to 20 mcg/ml and for phenobarbital 10 to 30 mcg/ml in adults. Serum blood level determinations are especially helpful when possible drug interactions are suspected.

If either the phenytoin or phenobarbital dosage requires adjustment, this should be done by switching the patient to separate phenytoin and phenobarbital dosage forms in order to enable subsequent dosage adjustment of either or both drugs.

The recommended starting phenobarbital dose for children is 2 to 3 mg/kg/day in two or three equally divided doses.

The recommended starting Dilantin dose for children is 5 mg/kg/day in two or three equally divided doses.

Adult Dosage: *For maintenance:* Usually three or four capsules daily. An increase to six capsules daily may be made, if necessary.

Pediatric Dosage: *For maintenance:* Individualized to a maximum of 300 mg Dilantin daily.

Protect from moisture and light.

Storage: Store below 30°C (86°F).

HOW SUPPLIED - RATED THERAPEUTICALLY EQUIVALENT:

Capsule, Gelatin - Oral - 32 mg/100 mg

100's	**$25.50**	**DILANTIN WITH PHENOBARBITAL, Parke-Davis**	**00071-0531-24**

HOW SUPPLIED - NOT RATED EQUIVALENT:

Capsule, Gelatin - Oral - 16 mg/100 mg

100's	**$23.84**	**DILANTIN WITH PHENOBARBITAL 15, Parke-Davis**	**00071-0375-24**

PHENOL *(002009)*

CATEGORIES: Anti-Infectives; Local Infections; Skin/Mucous Membrane Agents; FDA Pre 1938 Drugs

FORMULARIES: WHO

Prescribing information not available at time of publication.

HOW SUPPLIED - EQUIVALENTS NOT AVAILABLE:

Crystals

2500 gm	$46.55	Phenol U.S.P. Crystals, Mallinckrodt	00406-0605-05

Liquid

480 ml	$55.74	Phenol, Paddock Labs	00574-0640-16

PHENOXYBENZAMINE HYDROCHLORIDE

(002013)

CATEGORIES: Antihypertensives; Autonomic Drugs; Cardiovascular Drugs; Hypertension; Pheochromocytoma; Sympatholytic Agents; Vasodilating Agents; Pregnancy Category C; FDA Approval Pre 1982

BRAND NAMES: *Dibenyline* (Australia, England); **Dibenzyline**; *Dibenzyran* (Germany)
(International brand names outside U.S. in italics)

FORMULARIES: Aetna; BC-BS

DESCRIPTION:

Each Dibenzyline capsule, with red cap and red body, is imprinted SKF and E33 and contains phenoxybenzamine hydrochloride, 10 mg. Inactive ingredients consist of benzyl alcohol, cetylpyridinium chloride, D&C Red No. 33, FD&C Red No. 3, FD&C Yellow No. 6, gelatin, lactose, sodium lauryl sulfate and trace amounts of other inactive ingredients.

Dibenzyline is N-(2-Chloroethyl)-N-(1-methyl-2-phenoxyet hyl)benzylamine hydrochloride.

Phenoxybenzamine hydrochloride is a colorless, crystalline powder with a molecular weight of 340.3 which melts between 136° and 141°C. It is soluble in water, alcohol and chloroform; insoluble in ether.

CLINICAL PHARMACOLOGY:

Dibenzyline (phenoxybenzamine hydrochloride) is a long-acting, adrenergic, *alpha*-receptor blocking agent which can produce and maintain "chemical sympathectomy" by oral administration. It increases blood flow to the skin, mucosa and abdominal viscera, and lowers both supine and erect blood pressures. It has no effect on the parasympathetic system.

Twenty to 30 percent of orally administered phenoxybenzamine appears to be absorbed in the active form.[1]

The half-life of orally administered phenoxybenzamine hydrochloride is not known; however, the half-life of intravenously administered drug is approximately 24 hours. Demonstrable effects with intravenous administration persist for at least three to four days, and the effects of daily administration are cumulative for nearly a week.[1]

INDICATIONS AND USAGE:

Pheochromocytoma, to control episodes of hypertension and sweating. If tachycardia is excessive, if may be necessary to use a beta-blocking agent concomitantly.

CONTRAINDICATIONS:

Conditions where a fall in blood pressure may be undesirable.

WARNINGS:

Dibenzyline-induced *alpha*-adrenergic blockade leaves *beta*-adrenergic receptors unopposed. Compounds that stimulate both types of receptors may therefore produce an exaggerated hypotensive response and tachycardia.

PRECAUTIONS:

GENERAL

Administer with caution in patients with marked cerebral or coronary arteriosclerosis or renal damage. Adrenergic blocking effect may aggravate symptoms of respiratory infections.

CARCINOGENESIS, MUTAGENESIS, AND IMPAIRMENT OF FERTILITY

Phenoxybenzamine hydrochloride has shown in vitro mutagenic activity in the Ames test and in the mouse lymphoma assay; It has not shown mutagenic activity in the micronucleus test in mice. In rats and mice repeated intraperitoneal administration of phenoxybenzamine hydrochloride resulted in peritoneal sarcomas. Chronic oral dosing in rats has produced malignant tumors in the gastrointestinal tract. The majority of these tumors were found in the nonglandular stomach of the rats.

In chronic oral studies in rats, ulcerative and/or erosive gastritis of the glandular stomach occurred which was probably drug related.

PREGNANCY, TERATOGENIC EFFECTS, PREGNANCY CATEGORY C

Adequate reproductive studies have not been performed with Dibenzyline (phenoxybenzamine hydrochloride). It is also not known whether Dibenzyline can cause fetal harm when administered to a pregnant woman. Dibenzyline should be given to a pregnant woman only if clearly needed.

NURSING MOTHERS

It is not known whether this drug is excreted in human milk. Because many drugs are excreted in human milk, and because of the potential for serious adverse reactions from phenoxybenzamine hydrochloride, a decision should be made whether to discontinue nursing or to discontinue the drug, taking into account the importance of the drug to the mother.

PEDIATRIC USE

Safety and effectiveness in children have not been established.

DRUG INTERACTIONS:

Dibenzyline (phenoxybenzamine hydrochloride) may interact[2] with compounds that stimulate both *alpha*- and *beta*-adrenergic receptors (*i.e.*, epinephrine) to produce an exaggerated hypotensive response and tachycardia. (See WARNINGS.)

Dibenzyline blocks hyperthermia production by levarterenol, and blocks hypothermia production by reserpine.

ADVERSE REACTIONS:

The following adverse reactions have been observed, but there are insufficient data to support an estimate of their frequency.

Autonomic Nervous System*: Postural hypotension, tachycardia, inhibition of ejaculation, nasal congestion, miosis.

Miscellaneous: Gastrointestinal irritation, drowsiness, fatigue.

*These so-called "side effects" are actually evidence of adrenergic blockade and vary according to the degree of blockade.

OVERDOSAGE:

Signs and Symptoms: These are largely the result of block of the sympathetic nervous system and of the circulating epinephrine. They may include postural hypotension resulting in dizziness or fainting: tachycardia, particularly postural; vomiting; lethargy; shock.

Treatment: When symptoms and signs of overdosage exist, discontinue the drug. Treatment of circulatory failure, if present, is a prime consideration. In cases of mild overdosage, recumbent position with legs elevated usually restores cerebral circulation. In the more severe cases, the usual measures to combat shock should be instituted. Usual pressor agents are not effective. Epinephrine is contraindicated because it stimulates both *alpha* and *beta* receptors; since *alpha* receptors are blocked, the net effect of epinephrine administration is vasodilation and a further drop in blood pressure (epinephrine reversal).

The patient may have to be kept flat for 24 hours more in the case of overdose, as the effect of drug is prolonged. Leg bandages and an abdomen binder may shorten the period of disability.

IV infusion of levarterenol bitartrate may be used to combat severe hypotensive reactions, because it stimulates *alpha* receptors primarily. Although Dibenzyline (phenoxybenzamine hydrochloride) is an *alpha* adrenergic blocking agent, a sufficient dose of levarterenol bitartrate will overcome this effect.

The oral LD_{50} for phenoxybenzamine hydrochloride approximately 2000 mg/kg in rats and approximately 500 mg/kg in guinea pigs.

DOSAGE AND ADMINISTRATION:

The dosage should be adjusted to fit the needs of each patient. Small initial doses should be *slowly* increased until the desired effect is obtained or the side effect from blockade become troublesome. *After each increase, the patient should be observed on that level before instituting another increase.* The dosage should be carried to a point where symptomatic relief and/or objective improvement are obtained, but not so high that the side effects from blockade become troublesome.

Initially, 10 mg of Dibenzyline (phenoxybenzamine hydrochloride) twice a day. Dosage should be increased every other day, usually to 20 to 40 mg two to three times a day, until an optimal dosage is obtained as judged by blood pressure control.

REFERENCES:

1 .Weiner, N.: Drugs That Inhibit Adrenergic Nerves and Block Adrenergic Receptors, in Goodman A. and Gilman, A., *The Pharmacological Basis of Therapeutics* , ed. 6, New York, Macmillan Publishing Co., 1980, p. 179; p. 182. 2. Martin, E.W.: Drug Interactions Index *1978/1979* Philadelphia, J.B. Lippincott Co., 1978, pp 209-210

HOW SUPPLIED - EQUIVALENTS NOT AVAILABLE:

Capsule, Gelatin - Oral - 10 mg

100's $62.40 DIBENZYLINE, SKB Pharms 00007-3533-20

PHENSUXIMIDE *(002015)*

CATEGORIES: Anticonvulsants; Antiepileptics; Central Nervous System Agents; Epilepsy; Neuromuscular; Seizures; Succinimide Anticonvulsants; FDA Approval Pre 1982

BRAND NAMES: **Milontin**

FORMULARIES: BC-BS; Medi-Cal

DESCRIPTION:

Milontin (phensuximide) is an anticonvulsant succinimide, chemically designated as N-Methyl-2-phenylsuccinimide.

Each Milontin capsule contains 500 mg phensuximide, USP. The capsule and band contain citric acid, USP; colloidal silicon dioxide, NF; D&C yellow No. 10; FD&C red No. 3; FD&C yellow No. 6; gelatin, NF; glyceryl monooleate; polyethylene glycol 200; sodium benzoate, NF; sodium lauryl sulfate, NF.

CLINICAL PHARMACOLOGY:

Phensuximide suppresses the paroxysmal three cycle per second spike and wave activity associated with lapses of consciousness which is common in absence (petit mal) seizures. The frequency of epileptiform attacks is reduced, apparently by depression of the motor cortex and elevation of the threshold of the central nervous system to convulsive stimuli.

INDICATIONS AND USAGE:

Milontin is indicated for the control of absence (petit mal) seizures.

CONTRAINDICATIONS:

Phensuximide should not be used in patients with a history of hypersensitivity to succinimides.

WARNINGS:

Blood dyscrasias, including some with fatal outcome, have been reported to be associated with the use of succinimides; therefore, periodic blood counts should be performed. Should signs and/or symptoms of infection (*e.g.,* sore throat, fever) develop, blood counts should be considered at that point.

It has been reported that succinimides have produced morphological and functional changes in animal liver. For this reason, phensuximide should be administered with extreme caution to patients with known liver or renal disease. Periodic urinalysis and liver function studies are advised for all patients receiving the drug.

Cases of systemic lupus erythematosus have been reported with the use of succinimides. The physician should be alert to this possibility.

USAGE IN PREGNANCY:

Reports suggest an association between the use of anticonvulsant drugs by women with epilepsy and an elevated incidence of birth defects in children born to these women. Data are more extensive with respect to phenytoin and phenobarbital, but these are also the most commonly prescribed anticonvulsants; less systematic or anecdotal reports suggest a possible similar association with the use of all known anticonvulsant drugs.

The reports suggesting an elevated incidence of birth defects in children of drug-treated epileptic women cannot be regarded as adequate to prove a definite cause and effect relationship. There are intrinsic methodologic problems in obtaining adequate data on drug teratogenicity in humans; the possibility also exists that other factors, e.g., genetic factors or the epileptic condition itself, may be more important than drug therapy in leading to birth defects. The great majority of mothers on anticonvulsant medication deliver normal infants. It is important to note that anticonvulsant drugs should not be discontinued in patients in whom the drug is administered to prevent major seizures because of the strong possibility of precipitating status epilepticus with attendant hypoxia and threat to life. In individual cases where the severity and frequency of the seizure disorder are such that the removal of medication does not pose a serious threat to the patient, discontinuation of the drug may be considered prior to and during pregnancy, although it cannot be said with any confidence that even minor seizures do not pose some hazard to the developing embryo or fetus.

The prescribing physician will wish to weigh these considerations in treating or counseling epileptic women of childbearing potential.

PRECAUTIONS:

GENERAL:

Phensuximide, when used alone in mixed types of epilepsy, may increase the frequency of grand mal seizures in some patients.

As with other anticonvulsants, it is important to proceed slowly when increasing or decreasing dosage, as well as when adding or eliminating other medication. Abrupt withdrawal of anticonvulsant medication may precipitate absence (petit mal) status.

INFORMATION FOR THE PATIENT:

Phensuximide may impair the mental and/or physical abilities required for the performance of potentially hazardous tasks, such as driving a motor vehicle or other such activity requiring alertness, therefore, the patient should be cautioned accordingly.

Patients taking phensuximide should be advised of the importance of adhering strictly to the prescribed regimen.

Patients should be instructed to promptly contact their physician if they develop signs and/or symptoms suggesting an infection (*e.g.,* sore throat, fever).

PREGNANCY:

See WARNINGS.

DRUG INTERACTIONS:

Since Milontin (phensuximide), as a member of the succinimide class, may interact with concurrently administered antiepileptic drugs, periodic serum level determinations of these drugs may be necessary.

ADVERSE REACTIONS:

Gastrointestinal System: Gastrointestinal symptoms such as nausea, vomiting, and anorexia occur frequently, but may be the result of overdosage.

Nervous System: Neurologic and sensory reactions reported during therapy with phensuximide have included drowsiness, dizziness, ataxia, headache, dreamlike state, and lethargy. Side effects such as drowsiness and dizziness may be relieved by a reduction in total dosage.

Integumentary System: Dermatologic manifestations reported to be associated with the administration of phensuximide have included pruritus, skin eruptions, erythema multiforme, Stevens-Johnson syndrome, erythematous rashes, and alopecia.

Genitourinary System: Genitourinary complications which have been reported include urinary frequency, renal damage, and hematuria.

Hemopoietic System: Hemopoietic complications associated with the administration of phensuximide include granulocytopenia, transient leukopenia, and pancytopenia with or without bone marrow suppression.

Musculoskeletal System: Muscular weakness.

OVERDOSAGE:

Acute overdoses may produce nausea, vomiting, and CNS depression including coma with respiratory depression.

TREATMENT:

Treatment should include emesis (unless the patient is, or could rapidly become, obtunded, comatose, or convulsing) or gastric lavage, activated charcoal, cathartics and general supportive measures. Forced diuresis and exchange transfusions are ineffective.

DOSAGE AND ADMINISTRATION:

Milontin is administered by the oral route in doses of 0.5 to 1 g two or three times daily. As with other anticonvulsant medication, the dosage should be adjusted to suit individual requirements. The total dosage, irrespective of age, may therefore vary between 1 and 3 g per day, the average being 1.5 g.

Milontin may be administered in combination with other anticonvulsants when other forms of epilepsy coexist with absence (petit mal).

Store at controlled room temperature 15-30°C (59-86°F). Protect from moisture.

HOW SUPPLIED - EQUIVALENTS NOT AVAILABLE:

Capsule, Gelatin - Oral - 0.5 gm

100's $72.23 MILONTIN, Parke-Davis 00071-0393-24

PHENTERMINE HYDROCHLORIDE *(002016)*

CATEGORIES: Amphetamines; Anorexients/CNS Stimulants; Appetite Suppressants; Central Nervous System Agents; Obesity; Psychostimulants; Respiratory/Cerebral Stimulant; Weight Loss; DEA Class CIV; FDA Approval Pre 1982; Top 200 Drugs

BRAND NAMES: Adipex-P; Anoxine-Am; Atti-Plex P; *Behapront*; Curban; Dapex-37.5; **Fastin**; Fastophen; *Minobese-Forte*; Obe-Mar; Obe-Nix; Obephen; Obermine; Obestin-30; Oby-Cap; Oby-Trim; Ona-Mast; *Panbesy*; *Panbesyl*; *Panbesyl Nyscaps*; Panshape M; Phentercot; Phentride; Phentrol; Pro-Fast; *Redusa*; Supramine; T-Diet; Tara-30; Teramin; Termene; Tora; *Umine*; Umi-Pex 30; Zantryl

(International brand names outside U.S. in italics)

DESCRIPTION:

Each phentermine hydrochloride capsule contains phentermine hydrochloride, 30 mg (equivalent to 24 mg Phentermine).

Phentermine Hydrochloride is a white crystalline powder, very soluble in water and alcohol. Chemically, the product is phenyl-tertiary-butylamine hydrochloride. *Inactive Ingredients:* F D & C Blue 1, Methylcellulose, Polyethylene Glycol, Starch, Titanium Dioxide, Sucrose and Invert Sugar. The branding ink used on the gelatin capsules contains: Ethyl Alcohol, F D & C Blue 1 Aluminum Lake, Isopropyl Alcohol, n-Butyl Alcohol, Propylene Glycol, Pharmaceutical Shellac (modified) or Refined Shellac (Food Grade).

CLINICAL PHARMACOLOGY:

Phentermine hydrochloride is a sympathomimetic amine with pharmacologic activity similar to the prototype drugs of this class used in obesity, the amphetamines. Actions include central nervous system stimulation and elevation of blood pressure. Tachyphylaxis and tolerance have been demonstrated with all drugs of this class in which these phenomena have been looked for.

Drugs of this class used in obesity are commonly known as "anorectics" or "anorexigenics." It has not been established that the action of such drugs in treating obesity is primarily one of appetite suppression. Other central nervous system actions, or metabolic effects may be involved, for example.

Adult obese subjects instructed in dietary management and treated with "anorectic" drugs, lose more weight on the average than those treated with placebo and diet, as determined in relatively short-term clinical trials.

CLINICAL PHARMACOLOGY: *(cont'd)*

The magnitude of increased weight loss of drug-treated patients over placebo-treated patients is only a fraction of a pound a week. The rate of weight loss is greatest in the first weeks of therapy for both drug and placebo subjects and tends to decrease in succeeding weeks. The possible origins of the increased weight loss due to the various drug effects are not established. The amount of weight loss associated with the use of an "anorectic" drug varies from trial to trial, and the increased weight loss appears to be related in part to variables other than the drugs prescribed, such as the physician-investigator, the population treated, and the diet prescribed. Studies do not permit conclusions as to the relative importance of the drug and non-drug factors on weight loss.

The natural history of obesity is measured in years, whereas the studies cited are restricted to a few weeks duration; thus, the total impact of drug-induced weight loss over that of diet alone must be considered clinically limited.

INDICATIONS AND USAGE:

Phentermine hydrochloride is indicated in the management of exogenous obesity as a short term (a few weeks) adjunct in a regimen of weight reduction based on caloric restriction. The limited usefulness of agents of this class (see CLINICAL PHARMACOLOGY) should be measured against possible risk factors inherent in their use such as those described below.

CONTRAINDICATIONS:

Advanced arteriosclerosis, symptomatic cardiovascular disease, moderate to severe hypertension, hyperthyroidism, known hypersensitivity, or idiosyncrasy to the sympathomimetic amines, glaucoma.

Agitated states.

Patients with a history of drug abuse.

During or within 14 days following the administration of monoamine oxidase inhibitors (hypertensive crises may result).

WARNINGS:

Tolerance to the anorectic effect usually develops within a few weeks. When this occurs, the recommended dose should not be exceeded in an attempt to increase the effect; rather, the drug should be discontinued.

Phentermine hydrochloride may impair the ability of the patient to engage in potentially hazardous activities such as operating machinery or driving a motor vehicle; the patient should therefore be cautioned accordingly.

Drug Dependence: Phentermine hydrochloride is related chemically and pharmacologically to the amphetamines. Amphetamines and related stimulant drugs have been extensively abused, and the possibility of abuse of phentermine hydrochloride should be kept in mind when evaluating the desirability of including a drug as part of a weight reduction program. Abuse of amphetamines and related drugs may be associated with intense psychological dependence and severe social dysfunction. There are reports of patients who have increased the dosage to many times that recommended. Abrupt cessation following prolonged high dosage administration results in extreme fatigue and mental depression; changes are also noted on the sleep EEG. Manifestations of chronic intoxication with anorectic drugs include severe dermatoses, marked insomnia, irritability, hyperactivity, and personality changes. The most severe manifestation of chronic intoxications is psychosis, often clinically indistinguishable from schizophrenia.

Usage in Pregnancy: Safe use in pregnancy has not been established. Use of phentermine hydrochloride by women who are or who may become pregnant, and those in the first trimester of pregnancy, requires that the potential benefit be weighed against the possible hazard to mother and infant.

Usage in Children: Phentermine hydrochloride is not recommended for use in children under 12 years of age.

PRECAUTIONS:

Caution is to be exercised in prescribing phentermine hydrochloride for patients with even mild hypertension.

Insulin requirements in diabetes mellitus may be altered in association with the use of phentermine hydrochloride and the concomitant dietary regimen.

Phentermine hydrochloride may decrease the hypotensive effect of guanethidine.

The least amount feasible should be prescribed or dispensed at one time in order to minimize the possibility of overdosage.

DRUG INTERACTIONS:

Concomitant use of alcohol with phentermine hydrochloride may result in an adverse drug interaction.

ADVERSE REACTIONS:

Cardiovascular: Palpitation, tachycardia, elevation of blood pressure.

Central Nervous System: Overstimulation, restlessness, dizziness, insomnia, euphoria, dysphoria, tremor, headache; rarely psychotic episodes at recommended doses.

Gastrointestinal: Dryness of the mouth, unpleasant taste, diarrhea, constipation, other gastrointestinal disturbances.

Allergic: Urticaria.

Endocrine: Impotence, changes in libido.

OVERDOSAGE:

Manifestations of acute overdosage with phentermine include restlessness, tremor, hyperreflexia, rapid respiration, confusion, assaultiveness, hallucinations, panic states. Fatigue and depression usually follow the central stimulation. Cardiovascular effects include arrhythmias, hypertension or hypotension, and circulatory collapse. Gastrointestinal symptoms include nausea, vomiting, diarrhea, and abdominal cramps. Fatal poisoning usually terminates in convulsions and coma.

Management of acute phentermine intoxication is largely symptomatic and includes lavage and sedation with a barbiturate. Experience with hemodialysis or peritoneal dialysis is inadequate to permit recommendations in this regard. Acidification of the urine increases phentermine excretion. Intravenous phentolamine (REGITINE) has been suggested for possible acute, severe hypertension, if this complicates phentermine overdosage.

DOSAGE AND ADMINISTRATION:

Exogenous Obesity: One capsule at approximately 2 hours after breakfast for appetite control. Late evening medication should be avoided because of the possibility of resulting insomnia.

Administration of one capsule (30 mg) daily has been found to be adequate in depression of the appetite for twelve to fourteen hours.

Phentermine hydrochloride is not recommended for use in children under 12 years of age.

PATIENT INFORMATION:

Phentermine HCl is used to produce weight loss. It should only be used for a few weeks because long term use has not been adequately studied. Those with advanced heart disease, high blood pressure, thyroid problems, or glaucoma should use this drug only on the advice of a physician. Alcohol should be avoided. The most common adverse reactions include increased heart rate, palpitations, restlessness, dizziness, insomnia, euphoria, dysphoria, tremor, and headache. This medication should be taken early in the day to best control appetite. Taking this medication late in the day can interfere with sleep patterns. This medication is most effective when used in combination with behavior modification and dietary control.

HOW SUPPLIED - RATED THERAPEUTICALLY EQUIVALENT:

Capsule, Gelatin - Oral - 15 mg

100's	$3.91	Phentermine Hydrochloride, Eon Labs Mfg	00185-0644-01
1000's	$25.32	Phentermine Hcl, Eon Labs Mfg	00185-0644-10

Capsule, Gelatin - Oral - 30 mg

100's	$4.43	Phentermine HCl, H.C.F.A. F F P	99999-2016-01
100's	$4.50	Phentermine Hcl, Genetco	00302-5030-01
100's	$4.55	Phentermine Hcl, Eon Labs Mfg	00185-0647-01
100's	$5.25	CURBAN, Pasadena	00418-0198-30
100's	$5.78	Phentermine Hcl, Genetco	00302-5031-01
100's	$5.95	Phentermine Hcl, Eon Labs Mfg	00185-5000-01
100's	$6.15	Phentermine Hcl, Major Pharms	00904-3921-60
100's	$6.30	Phentermine Hcl, IDE-Interstate	00814-6077-14
100's	$6.30	Phentermine Hcl, IDE-Interstate	00814-6078-14
100's	$6.63	Phentermine Hcl, Qualitest Pharms	00603-5190-21
100's	$8.38	Phentermine Hcl, United Res	00677-0460-01
100's	$8.54	Phentermine Hcl, Rosemont	00832-0204-00
100's	$8.80	Phentermine Hcl, Goldline Labs	00182-1026-01
100's	$8.98	OBY-CAP, Richwood Pharm	58521-0333-01
100's	$9.90	PHENTAMINE, Major Pharms	00904-0614-60
100's	$10.05	Phentermine Hcl, Aligen Independ	00405-4796-01
100's	$10.05	Phentermine HCl 30 Mg, Geneva Pharms	00781-2415-01
100's	$13.24	Phentermine Hcl, Camall	00147-0199-10
100's	$18.00	Phentermine HCl, Rugby	00536-4235-01
100's	$18.00	Phentermine HCl, Rugby	00536-4236-01
100's	$18.00	Phentermine HCl, Rugby	00536-4271-01
100's	$19.75	Phentermine HCl, Camall	00147-0198-10
100's	$19.75	Phentermine HCl, Camall	00147-0201-10
100's	$19.75	Phentermine HCl, Camall	00147-0202-10
100's	$20.95	Phentermine Hcl, Harber Pharm	51432-0348-03
100's	$80.00	ZANTRYL, Ion	11808-0555-01
100's	**$98.90**	**FASTIN, Beecham**	**00029-2205-30**
150's	**$107.45**	**FASTIN, Beecham**	**00029-2205-31**
450's	$19.93	Phentermine HCl, H.C.F.A. F F P	99999-2016-03
450's	**$430.45**	**FASTIN, Beecham**	**00029-2205-39**
500's	$22.15	Phentermine HCl, H.C.F.A. F F P	99999-2016-04
500's	$35.98	OBY-CAP, Richwood Pharm	58521-0333-05
1000's	$6.95	Phentermine Hcl, Rexar	00478-5469-01
1000's	$24.00	Phentermine Yellow, Calvin Scott	17224-0608-10
1000's	$24.00	Phentermine Red/Yellow, Calvin Scott	17224-0612-10
1000's	$24.00	Termene, Calvin Scott	17224-0613-10
1000's	$24.00	Termene, Calvin Scott	17224-0619-10
1000's	$25.25	Phentermine Hcl, Eon Labs Mfg	00185-0635-10
1000's	$25.25	Phentermine Hcl, Eon Labs Mfg	00185-0640-10
1000's	$31.88	Phentermine Hcl, Eon Labs Mfg	00185-0647-10
1000's	$32.95	Phentermine Blue/Clear, Calvin Scott	17224-0609-10
1000's	$38.50	Phentermine Hcl, Rexar	00478-5465-10
1000's	$38.50	Phentermine Hcl, Rexar	00478-5468-10
1000's	$38.50	Phentermine Hcl, Rexar	00478-5469-10
1000's	$38.50	Phentermine Hcl, Rexar	00478-5474-10
1000's	$38.90	Phentermine Hcl, Hyrex Pharms	00314-0206-10
1000's	$39.30	Phentermine Hcl, Major Pharms	00904-3921-80
1000's	$39.95	FASTOPHEN, AF Hauser	52637-0030-10
1000's	$40.94	Phentermine Hcl, Qualitest Pharms	00603-5190-32
1000's	$41.63	Phentermine Hcl, IDE-Interstate	00814-6078-30
1000's	$43.84	Phentermine Hcl, Aligen Independ	00405-4796-03
1000's	$43.84	Phentermine Hcl, Rosemont	00832-0204-10
1000's	$44.30	Phentermine HCl, H.C.F.A. F F P	99999-2016-02
1000's	$48.75	PHENTAMINE, Major Pharms	00904-0614-80
1000's	$49.50	Phentermine Hcl, United Res	00677-0460-10
1000's	$49.95	Phentermine Hcl, Eon Labs Mfg	00185-5000-10
1000's	$49.95	Phentrol 2, Vortech Pharms	00298-3925-11
1000's	$58.20	Phentermine Hcl, Goldline Labs	00182-1026-10
1000's	$79.95	Tara-30 No.1, Quality Res Pharms	52765-2204-00
1000's	$93.69	Phentermine HCl, HL Moore Drug Exch	00839-5099-16
1000's	$93.69	Phentermine HCl, HL Moore Drug Exch	00839-6298-16
1000's	$124.45	Phentermine HCl, Camall	00147-0198-20
1000's	$124.45	Phentermine HCl, Camall	00147-0201-20
1000's	$124.45	Phentermine HCl, Camall	00147-0202-20
1000's	$126.00	Phentermine Hcl, Camall	00147-0199-20
1000's	$126.00	Phentermine HCl, Camall	00147-0200-20
1000's	$126.00	Phentermine HCl, Camall	00147-0233-20
1000's	$126.00	Phentermine HCl, Camall	00147-0240-20
1000's	$129.95	Phentermine HCl, Rugby	00536-4235-10
1000's	$129.95	Phentermine HCl, Rugby	00536-4236-10
1000's	$129.95	Phentermine HCl, Rugby	00536-4271-10

Capsule, Gelatin - Oral - 37.5 mg

100's	$14.03	Phentermine HCl, H.C.F.A. F F P	99999-2016-05
100's	$27.75	Phentermine HCl, Camall	00147-0231-10
100's	$27.75	Phentermine HCl, Camall	00147-0234-10
100's	$27.75	Phentermine HCl, Camall	00147-0235-10
100's	$39.80	PRO-FAST SR, Am Pharms	58605-0503-01
100's	$76.20	OBENIX, Abana Pharms	12463-0217-01
100's	$104.26	ADIPEX-P, Gate Pharms	57844-0019-01
500's	$55.31	Phentermine Hcl, Camall	00147-0231-05
500's	$55.31	Phentermine Hcl, Camall	00147-0234-05
500's	$55.31	Phentermine Hcl, Camall	00147-0235-05
500's	$70.15	Phentermine HCl, H.C.F.A. F F P	99999-2016-06
1000's	$29.95	Supramine, Calvin Scott	17224-0632-10
1000's	$29.95	Supramine, Calvin Scott	17224-0633-10
1000's	$29.95	Supramine, Calvin Scott	17224-0634-10
1000's	$29.95	Supramine, Calvin Scott	17224-0635-10
1000's	$29.95	Supramine, Calvin Scott	17224-0637-10
1000's	$29.95	Supramine, Calvin Scott	17224-0638-10
1000's	$92.50	Phentermine Hcl, Camall	00147-0250-20
1000's	$140.30	Phentermine HCl, H.C.F.A. F F P	99999-2016-07
1000's	$174.50	Phentermine HCl, Camall	00147-0231-20
1000's	$174.50	Phentermine HCl, Camall	00147-0234-20
1000's	$174.50	Phentermine HCl, Camall	00147-0235-20
1000's	$174.50	Phentermine HCl, Camall	00147-0251-20
1000's	$174.50	Phentermine HCl, Camall	00147-0253-20

HOW SUPPLIED - RATED THERAPEUTICALLY EQUIVALENT: *(cont'd)*

1000's	$174.50	Phentermine HCl, Camall	00147-0254-20
1000's	$175.00	Atti-Plex P, Quality Res Pharms	52765-2101-00

Tablet, Uncoated - Oral - 8 mg

100's	$28.42	PRO-FAST SA, Am Pharms	58605-0504-01
1000's	$22.50	Phentermine Hcl, Goldline Labs	00182-0204-10
1000's	$55.50	Phentermine, Rugby	00536-4288-10
1000's	$69.82	Phentermine HCl, Camall	00147-0102-20
1000's	$69.82	Phentermine HCl, Camall	00147-0136-20

Tablet, Uncoated - Oral - 37.5 mg

100's	$7.43	Phentermine Hcl, United Res	00677-0829-01
100's	$11.28	Phentermine Hcl, Qualitest Pharms	00603-5191-21
100's	$11.40	Phentermine Hcl, Goldline Labs	00182-0205-01
100's	$12.08	Phentermine Hcl, Rugby	00536-4237-01
100's	$12.08	Phentermine HCl, H.C.F.A. F F P	99999-2016-08
100's	$31.50	Phentermine HCl, Camall	00147-0232-10
100's	$31.50	Phentermine HCl, Camall	00147-0248-10
100's	$102.43	ADIPEX-P, Gate Pharms	57844-0009-01
400's	$48.32	Phentermine HCl, H.C.F.A. F F P	99999-2016-09
400's	$389.32	ADIPEX-P, Gate Pharms	57844-0009-26
500's	$60.40	Phentermine HCl, H.C.F.A. F F P	99999-2016-10
1000's	$62.90	Phentermine Hcl, Goldline Labs	00182-0205-10
1000's	$120.80	Phentermine HCl, H.C.F.A. F F P	99999-2016-11
1000's	$212.82	Phentermine HCl, Camall	00147-0232-20
1000's	$212.82	Phentermine HCl, Camall	00147-0248-20
1000's	$225.00	Phentermine HCl, Rugby	00536-4237-10
1000's	$838.19	ADIPEX-P, Gate Pharms	57844-0009-10

HOW SUPPLIED - NOT RATED EQUIVALENT:

Capsule, Gelatin - Oral - 18.75 mg

100's	$21.50	Phentermine HCl, Camall	00147-0249-10
100's	$35.00	Pro-Fast Hs, Am Pharms	58605-0508-01
1000's	$20.00	Termene Capsules 18.75 Mg, Calvin Scott	17224-0677-10
1000's	$102.90	Phentermine HCl, Camall	00147-0249-20

PHENTERMINE RESIN COMPLEX *(003123)*

CATEGORIES: Amphetamines; Anorexients/CNS Stimulants; Appetite Suppresants; Central Nervous System Agents; Obesity; Psychostimulants; Respiratory/Cerebral Stimulant; Weight Loss; DEA Class CIV; FDA Approval Pre 1982

BRAND NAMES: *Adipex*; *Adipex Retard*; *Adipomin*; *Diminex* (Mexico); *Duromine* (Australia, England); **Ionamin**; *Ionamin Forte*; *Ionamine*; *Mirapront*; *Novirasin* *(International brand names outside U.S. in italics)*

DESCRIPTION:

Phentermine Resin Complex '15' and Phentermine Resin Complex '30' contain 15 mg and 30 mg respectively of phentermine as the cationic exchange resin complex. Phentermine is α, α-dimethyl phenethylamine (phenyl-tertiary-butylamine).

Inactive Ingredients: D&C Yellow No. 10, dibasic calcium phosphate, FD&C Yellow No. 6, gelatin, iron oxides (15 mg capsules only), lactose, magnesium stearate, titanium dioxide.

CLINICAL PHARMACOLOGY:

Phentermine Resin Complex is a sympathomimetic amine with pharmacologic activity similar to the prototype drug of this class used in obesity, amphetamine (d- and d *l*-amphetamine). Actions include central nervous system stimulation and elevation of blood pressure. Tachyphylaxis and tolerance have been demonstrated with all drugs of this class in which these phenomena have been looked for.

Drugs of this class used in obesity are commonly known as "anorectics" or "anorexigenics." It has not been established, however, that the action of such drugs in treating obesity is primarily one of appetite suppression. Other central nervous system actions, or metabolic effects may be involved.

Adult obese subjects instructed in dietary management and treated with "anorectic" drugs, lose more weight on the average than those treated with placebo and diet, as determined in relatively short-term clinical trials.

The magnitude of increased weight loss of drug-treated patients over placebo-treated patients is only a fraction of a pound a week. The rate of weight loss is greatest in the first weeks of therapy for both drug and placebo subjects and tends to decrease in succeeding weeks. The possible origins of the increased weight loss due to the various drug effects are not established. The amount of weight loss associated with the use of an "anorectic" drug varies from trial to trial, and the increased weight loss appears to be related in part to variables other than the drugs prescribed, such as the physician-investigator, the population treated, and the diet prescribed. Studies do not permit conclusions as to the relative importance of the drug and non-drug factors on weight loss.

The natural history of obesity is measured in years, whereas the studies cited are restricted to a few weeks' or months' duration; thus, the total impact of drug-induced weight loss over that of diet alone must be considered clinically limited.

The bioavailability of Phentermine Resin Complex has been studied in humans in which blood levels of phentermine were measured by a gas chromatography method. Blood levels obtained with the 15 mg and 30 mg resin complex formulations indicated slower absorption with a reduced but prolonged peak concentration and without a significant difference in prolongation of blood levels when compared with the same doses of phentermine hydrochloride. The clinical significance of these differences is not known. In clinical trials establishing the efficacy of Phentermine Resin Complex, a single daily dose produced an effect comparable to that produced by other regimens of "anorectic" drug therapy.

INDICATIONS AND USAGE:

Phentermine Resin Complex is indicated in the management of exogenous obesity as a short-term (a few weeks) adjunct in a regimen of weight reduction based on caloric restriction. The limited usefulness of agents of this class(see CLINICAL PHARMACOLOGY) should be measured against possible risk factors inherent in their use such as those described below.

CONTRAINDICATIONS:

Advanced arteriosclerosis, symptomatic cardiovascular disease, moderate to severe hypertension, hyperthyroidism, known hypersensitivity, or idiosyncrasy to the sympathomimetic amines, glaucoma.

Agitated states.

Patients with a history of drug abuse.

During or within 14 days following the administration of monoamine oxidase inhibitors (hypertensive crises may result).

WARNINGS:

If tolerance to the "anorectic" effect develops, the recommended dose should not be exceeded in an attempt to increase the effect: rather, the drug should be discontinued.

Phentermine Resin Complex may impair the ability of the patient to engage in potentially hazardous activities such as operating machinery or driving a motor vehicle; the patient should therefore be cautioned accordingly.

When using CNS active agents, consideration must always be given to the possibility of adverse interactions with alcohol.

PRECAUTIONS:

Caution is to be exercised in prescribing Phentermine Resin Complex for patients with even mild hypertension. Insulin requirements in diabetes mellitus may be altered in association with the use of Phentermine Resin Complex and the concomitant dietary regimen.

Phentermine Resin Complex may decrease the hypotensive effect of adrenergic neuron blocking drugs.

The least amount feasible should be prescribed or dispensed at one time in order to minimize the possibility of overdosage.

Usage in Pregnancy: Safe use in pregnancy has not been established. Use of Phentermine Resin Complex by women who are or may become pregnant requires that the potential benefit be weighed against the possible hazard to mother and infant.

Usage in Children: Phentermine Resin Complex is not recommended for use in children under 12 years of age.

DRUG INTERACTIONS:

When using CNS active agents, consideration must always be given to the possibility of adverse interactions with alcohol.

ADVERSE REACTIONS:

Cardiovascular: Palpitation, tachycardia, elevation of blood pressure.

Central Nervous System: Overstimulation, restlessness, dizziness, insomnia, euphoria, dysphoria, tremor, headache; rarely psychotic episodes at recommended doses with some drugs in this class.

Gastrointestinal: Dryness of the mouth, unpleasant taste, diarrhea, constipation, other gastrointestinal disturbances.

Allergic: Urticaria.

Endocrine: Impotence, changes in libido.

DRUG ABUSE AND DEPENDENCE:

Phentermine Resin Complex is related chemically and pharmacologically to amphetamine (d- and d *l*-amphetamine) and other stimulant drugs that have been extensively abused. The possibility of abuse of Phentermine Resin Complex should be kept in mind when evaluating the desirability of including a drug as part of a weight reduction program. Abuse of amphetamine (d- and d *l*-amphetamine) and related drugs may be associated with intense psychological dependence and severe social dysfunction. There are reports of patients who have increased the dosage of some of these drugs to many times that recommended. Abrupt cessation following prolonged high dosage administration results in extreme fatigue and mental depression; changes are also noted on the sleep EEG. Manifestations of chronic intoxication with anorectic drugs include severe dermatoses, marked insomnia, irritability, hyperactivity, and personality changes. The most severe manifestation of chronic intoxications is psychosis, often clinically indistinguishable from schizophrenia.

OVERDOSAGE:

Manifestations of acute overdosage may include restlessness, tremor, hyperreflexia, rapid respiration, confusion, assaultiveness, hallucinations, panic states.

Fatigue and depression usually follow the central stimulation.

Cardiovascular effects include arrhythmias, hypertension, or hypotension and circulatory collapse. Gastrointestinal symptoms include nausea, vomiting, diarrhea, and abdominal cramps. Overdosage of pharmacologically similar compounds has resulted in fatal poisoning, usually terminating in convulsions and coma.

Management of acute Phentermine Resin Complex intoxication is largely symptomatic and includes lavage and sedation with a barbiturate. Experience with hemodialysis or peritoneal dialysis is inadequate to permit recommendation in this regard. Intravenous phentolamine (Regitine) has been suggested on pharmacologic grounds for possible acute, severe hypertension, if this complicates overdosage.

DOSAGE AND ADMINISTRATION:

One capsule daily, before breakfast or 10-14 hours before retiring. For individuals exhibiting greater drug responsiveness, Phentermine Resin Complex '15' will usually suffice. Phentermine Resin Complex '30' is recommended for less responsive patients. Phentermine Resin Complex is not recommended for use in children under 12 years of age.

Phentermine Resin Complex capsules should be swallowed whole.

HOW SUPPLIED:

Ionamin Capsules (phentermine resin) are available in two strengths:

15 mg, yellow/grey capsules, imprinted with "Ionamin 15."

Bottle of 100's

Bottle of 400's

30 mg, yellow/yellow capsules, imprinted with "Ionamin 30."

Bottle of 100's

Bottle of 400's

Dispense in a tight container. Store at room temperature. Keep out of the reach of children.

HOW SUPPLIED - EQUIVALENTS NOT AVAILABLE:

Capsule, Gelatin, Sustained Action - Oral - 15 mg

100's	$106.25	IONAMIN, Medeva Pharms	53014-0903-71
400's	$389.91	IONAMIN, Medeva Pharms	53014-0903-84

Capsule, Gelatin, Sustained Action - Oral - 30 mg

100's	$121.76	IONAMIN, Medeva Pharms	53014-0904-71
400's	$446.36	IONAMIN, Medeva Pharms	53014-0904-84

PHENTOLAMINE MESYLATE *(002017)*

CATEGORIES: Antihypertensives; Autonomic Drugs; Diagnostic Agents; Hypertension; Necrosis; Pheochromocytoma Test; Sympatholytic Agents; Impotence*; Pregnancy Category C; FDA Approval Pre 1982

* Indication not approved by the FDA

BRAND NAMES: *Regitin* (Germany); **Regitine**; *Rogitene* (Canada); *Rogitine* (England)

(International brand names outside U.S. in italics)

DESCRIPTION:

Phentolamine Mesylate USP, is an antihypertensive, available in vials for intravenous and intramuscular administration. Each vial contains phentolamine mesylate USP, 5 mg, and mannitol USP, 25 mg, in sterile, lyophilized form.

Phentolamine mesylate is 4,5-dihydro-2-(N-(*m*-hydroxyphenyl)-N-(*p*-methylphenyl)amin omethyl)-1*H*-imidazole 1:1 methanesulfonate.

Phentolamine mesylate USP is a white or off-white, odorless crystalline powder with a molecular weight of 377.46. Its solutions are acid to litmus. It is freely soluble in water and in alcohol, and slightly soluble in chloroform. It melts at about 178°C.

CLINICAL PHARMACOLOGY:

Phentolamine Mesylate produces an alpha-adrenergic block of relatively short duration. It also has direct, but less marked, positive inotropic and chronotropic effects on cardiac muscle and vasodilator effects on vascular smooth muscle.

Phentolamine Mesylate has a half-life in the blood of 19 minutes following intravenous administration. Approximately 13% of a single intravenous dose appears in the urine as unchanged drug.

INDICATIONS AND USAGE:

Phentolamine Mesylate is indicated for the prevention or control of hypertensive episodes that may occur in a patient with pheochromocytoma as a result of stress or manipulation during preoperative preparation and surgical excision.

Phentolamine Mesylate is indicated for the prevention of treatment of dermal necrosis and sloughing following intravenous administration or extravasation of norepinephrine.

Phentolamine Mesylate is also indicated for the diagnosis of pheochromocytoma by the Phentolamine Mesylate blocking test.

CONTRAINDICATIONS:

Myocardial infarction, history of myocardial infarction, coronary insufficiency, angina, or other evidence suggestive of coronary artery disease; hypersensitivity to phentolamine or related compounds.

WARNINGS:

Myocardial infarction, cerebrovascular spasm, and cerebrovascular occlusion have been reported to occur following the administration of Phentolamine Mesylate, usually in association with marked hypotensive episodes.

For screening tests in patients with hypertension, the generally available urinary assay of catecholamines or other biochemical assays have largely replaced the Phentolamine Mesylate and other pharmacological tests for reasons of accuracy and safety. None of the chemical or pharmacological tests is infallible in the diagnosis of pheochromocytoma. The Phentolamine Mesylate blocking test is not the procedure of choice and should be reserved for cases in which additional confirmatory evidence is necessary and the relative risks involved in conducting the test have been considered.

PRECAUTIONS:

GENERAL

Tachycardia and cardiac arrhythmias may occur with the use of Phentolamine Mesylate or other alpha-adrenergic blocking agents. When possible, administration of cardiac glycosides should be deferred until cardiac rhythm returns to normal.

CARCINOGENESIS, MUTAGENESIS, AND IMPAIRMENT OF FERTILITY

Long-term carcinogenicity studies, mutagenicity studies, and fertility studies have not been conducted with Phentolamine Mesylate.

PREGNANCY CATEGORY C

Administration of Phentolamine Mesylate to pregnant rats and mice at oral doses 24-30 times the usual daily human dose (based on a 60-kg human) resulted in slightly decreased growth and slight skeletal immaturity of the fetuses. Immaturity was manifested by increased incidence of incomplete or unossified calcanei and phalangeal nuclei of the hind limb and of incompletely ossified sternebrae. At oral doses 60 times the usual daily human dose (based on a 60-kg human), a slightly lower rate of implantation was found in the rat. Phentolamine Mesylate did not affect embryonic or fetal development in the rabbit at oral doses 20 times the usual daily human dose (based on a 60-kg human). No teratogenic or embryotoxic effects were observed in the rat, mouse, or rabbit studies.

There are no adequate and well-controlled studies in pregnant women. Phentolamine Mesylate should be used during pregnancy only if the potential benefit justifies the potential risk to the fetus.

NURSING MOTHERS

It is not known whether this drug is excreted in human milk. Because many drugs are excreted in human milk and because of the potential for serious adverse reactions in nursing infants from Phentolamine Mesylate, a decision should be made whether to discontinue nursing or to discontinue the drug, taking into account the importance of the drug to the mother.

PEDIATRIC USE

See DOSAGE AND ADMINISTRATION.

DRUG INTERACTIONS:

See DOSAGE AND ADMINISTRATION, Diagnosis of pheochromocytoma, Preparation.

ADVERSE REACTIONS:

Acute and prolonged hypotensive episodes, tachycardia, and cardiac arrhythmias have been reported. In addition, weakness, dizziness, flushing, orthostatic hypotension, nasal stuffiness, nausea, vomiting, and diarrhea may occur.

OVERDOSAGE:

ACUTE TOXICITY

No deaths due to acute poisoning with Phentolamine Mesylate have been reported.

Oral LD_{50}'s (mg/kg): mice, 1000; rats, 1250.

SIGNS AND SYMPTOMS

Overdosage with Phentolamine Mesylate is characterized chiefly by cardiovascular disturbances, such as arrhythmias, tachycardia, hypotension, and possibly headache, sweating, pupillary contraction, visual disturbances; nausea, vomiting diarrhea; hypoglycemia.

OVERDOSAGE: *(cont'd)*

TREATMENT

There is no specific antidote.

A decrease in blood pressure to dangerous levels or other evidence of shock like conditions should be treated vigorously and promptly. The patient's legs should be kept raised and a plasma expander should be administered. If necessary, intravenous infusion of norepinephrine, titrated to maintain blood pressure at the normotensive level, and all available supportive measures should be included. Epinephrine should not be used, since it may cause a paradoxical reduction in blood pressure.

DOSAGE AND ADMINISTRATION:

The reconstituted solution should be used upon preparation and should not be stored.

Note: Parenteral drug products should be inspected visually for particulate matter and discoloration prior to administration, whenever solution and container permit.

PREVENTION OR CONTROL OF HYPERTENSIVE EPISODES IN THE PATIENT WITH PHEOCHROMOCYTOMA.

For preoperative reduction of elevated blood pressure, 5 mg of Phentolamine Mesylate (1 mg for children) is injected intravenously or intramuscularly 1 or 2 hours before surgery, and repeated if necessary.

During surgery, Phentolamine Mesylate (5 mg for adults, 1 mg for children) is administered intravenously as indicated, to help prevent or control paroxysms of hypertension, tachycardia, respiratory depression, convulsions, or other effects of epinephrine intoxication. (Postoperatively norepinephrine may be given to control the hypotension that commonly follows complete removal of a pheochromocytoma.)

PREVENTION OR TREATMENT OF DERMAL NECROSIS AND SLOUGHING FOLLOWING INTRAVENOUS ADMINISTRATION OR EXTRAVASATION OF NOREPINEPHRINE.

For Prevention: 10 mg of Phentolamine Mesylate is added to each liter of solution containing norepinephrine. The pressor effect of norepinephrine is not affected.

For Treatment: 5-10 mg of Phentolamine Mesylate in 10 ml of saline is injected into the area of extravasation within 12 hours.

DIAGNOSIS OF PHEOCHROMOCYTOMA - PHENTOLAMINE MESYLATE BLOCKING TEST.

The test is most reliable in detecting pheochromocytoma in patients with sustained hypertension and least reliable in those with paroxysmal hypertension. False-positive tests may occur in patients with hypertension without pheochromocytoma.

Intravenous

Preparation

The CONTRAINDICATIONS and WARNINGS, and PRECAUTIONS sections should be reviewed. Sedatives, analgesics, and all other medications except those that might be deemed essential (such as digitalis and insulin) are withheld for at least 24 hours, and preferably 48-72 hours, prior to the test. Antihypertensive drugs are withheld until blood pressure returns to the untreated, hypertensive level. This test is not performed on a patient who is normotensive.

Procedure

The patient is kept at rest in the supine position throughout the test, preferably in a quiet, darkened room. Injection of Phentolamine Mesylate is delayed until blood pressure is stabilized, as evidenced by blood pressure readings taken every 10 minutes for at least 30 minutes.

Five milligrams of Phentolamine Mesylate is dissolved in 1 ml of Sterile Water for Injection. The dose for adults is 5 mg; for children, 1 mg.

The syringe needle is inserted into the vein, and injection is delayed until pressor response to venipuncture has subsided.

Phentolamine Mesylate is injected rapidly. Blood pressure is recorded immediately after injection, at 30-second intervals for the first 3 minutes, and at 60-second intervals for the next 7 minutes.

Interpretation

A positive response, suggestive of pheochromocytoma, is indicated when the blood pressure is reduced more than 35 mmHg systolic and 25 mmHg diastolic. A typical positive response is a reduction in pressure of 60 mmHg systolic and 25 mmHg diastolic. Usually, maximal effect is evident within 2 minutes after injection. A return to preinjection pressure commonly occurs within 15-30 minutes but may occur more rapidly.

If blood pressure decreases to a dangerous level, the patient should be treated as outlined under OVERDOSAGE.

A positive response should always be confirmed by other diagnostic procedures, preferably by measurement of urinary catecholamines or their metabolites.

A negative response is indicated when the blood pressure is elevated, unchanged, or reduced less than 35 mmHg systolic and 25 mmHg diastolic after injection of Phentolamine Mesylate. A negative response to this test does not exclude the diagnosis of pheochromocytoma especially in patients with paroxysmal hypertension in whom the incidence of false-negative responses is high.

Intramuscular

If the intramuscular test for pheochromocytoma is preferred, preparation is the same as for the intravenous test. Five milligrams of Phentolamine Mesylate is then dissolved in 1 ml of Sterile Water of Injection. The dose for adults is 5 mg intramuscularly; for children 3 mg. Blood pressure is recorded every 5 minutes for 30-45 minutes following injection. A positive response is indicated when the blood pressure is reduced 35 mmHg systolic and 25 mmHg diastolic, or more, within 20 minutes following injection.

Store between 59 and 86°F.

HOW SUPPLIED - EQUIVALENTS NOT AVAILABLE:

Injection, Conc, W/Buf - Intramuscular; - 5 mg

2 vial	$58.53	REGITINE MESYLATE LYOPHILIZED, Novartis	00083-6830-02

PHENYLBUTAZONE *(002019)*

CATEGORIES: Analgesics; Ankylosing Spondylitis; Anti-Inflammatory Agents; Antiarthritics; Antigout; Antipyretics; Arthritis; Central Nervous System Agents; Gouty Arthritis; NSAIDS; Nonsteroidal Anti-Inflammatory; Pain; Spondylitis; Pregnancy Category C; FDA Approval Pre 1982

BRAND NAMES: *Apo-Phenylbutazone* (Canada); Azolid; *Baliomel* (Japan); *Basireuma*; *Bumzolidina*; *Butacote* (England); *Butadion*; *Butapirazol*; Butatab; **Butazolidin**; *Butazolidina* (Mexico); *Butazolidine* (France); Butazone-100; *Butrex*; *Exrheudon N* (Germany); *Fenilblan*; *Fenilbutazona*; *Fenilbutazona Gen-Far*; *Fenilbutazona McKesson*; *Fenilbutazona MK*; *Fenibutol*; *Ipirheumax*; *Ircodin* (Japan); *Irgapan*; *Irgapyrin* (Japan); *Redalin*; *Reumuzol*; *Zolandin*
(International brand names outside U.S. in italics)

COST OF THERAPY: $174.65 (Arthritis; Capsule; 100 mg; 3/day; 365 days)

PRIMARY ICD9: 715.99 (Osteoarthritis, Unspecified, Multiple Sites)

WARNING:

Because of the increased risk of agranulocytosis and aplastic anemia (see ADVERSE REACTIONS), Phenylbutazone is not recommended as initial therapy for any of its indications. It should be used only after other nonsteroidal anti-inflammatory drugs have been tried and found unsatisfactory. Phenylbutazone cannot be considered a simple analgesic and should never be administered casually. If it is used, the following caution should be observed:

Therapy should not be initiated until a careful detailed history is taken and complete physical and laboratory examinations, including an examination of red cells, white cells and platelets, have been made. These examinations should be repeated if any signs or symptoms suggesting blood dyscrasia appear.

Patients should be told to discontinue use of the drug and report to the physician immediately any sign of:

Fever, sore throat, or lesions in the mouth (symptoms of blood dyscrasia)

Dyspepsia, epigastric pain; symptoms of anemia; unusual bleeding or bruising; black or tarry stools, or other evidence of intestinal ulceration;

Skin rashes

Significant weight gain or edema

The risk of aplastic anemia is greater in women, in the elderly of both sexes, and with chronic therapy, but even short-term exposure of healthy young persons can result in fetal aplastic anemia.

A trial period of 1 week of therapy is considered adequate to determine the therapeutic effect of the drug. In the absence of a favorable response, therapy should be discontinued.

In patients 60 years and over, the drug should be restricted to short-term treatment periods only - if possible, 1 week maximum.

If long-term treatment is necessary, the lowest possible effective dose should be used, and patients should be adequately warned (see Information for the Patient) and closely monitored.

DESCRIPTION:

Phenylbutazone is closely related chemically and pharmacologically, including effects, to the pyrazole compounds aminopyrine and antipyrine.

Phenylbutazone is 4-Butyl-1,2-diphenyl-3,5-pyrazolidinedione, with a molecular weight of 308.38.

It is very slightly soluble in water; freely soluble in acetone and in ether, soluble in alcohol.

Phenylbutazone is available as capsules and tablets containing 100 mg of phenylbutazone.

This product contains the following inactive ingredients: Colloidal Silicon Dioxide, NF, D&C Yellow No. 10 (Capsules only), FD&C Blue #2 Lake (Tablets only), FD&C Yellow No. 6 Aluminum Lake (Tablets only), Gelatin NF (Capsules only), Hydroxypropyl Methylcellulose (Tablets only), Microcrystalline Cellulose NF, Polyethylene Glycol NF, (Tablets only), Polysorbate 80 NF (Tablets only), Pregelatinized Starch NF, Propylene Glycol USP (Tablets only), Sodium Starch Glycolate NF, Starch NF (Corn), Steric Acid NF, and Titanium Dioxide USP.

CLINICAL PHARMACOLOGY:

Phenylbutazone is a nonsalicylate, nonsteroidal, anti-inflammatory drug. It has anti-inflammatory, anti-pyretic, analgesic and mild uricosuric properties that produce symptomatic relief but do not alter the disease process.

The exact mechanism of the anti-inflammatory effects of phenylbutazone has not been elucidated, but clinical pharmacology studies have shown that phenylbutazone inhibits certain factors believed to be involved in the inflammatory process. These processes are (1) prostaglandin synthesis; (2) leukocyte migration; (3) release and activity of lysosomal enzymes.

PHARMACOKINETICS

Phenylbutazone is rapidly absorbed after oral administration and distributed partially into an extravascular compartment, with about one third remaining in plasma. About 98% of the drug in plasma is bound to albumin.

After administration of single 100-, 300-, and 600-mg doses, the mean elimination half-life is approximately 77 (54-99) hours (n=6). There is a linear relationship between dose and area-under-the-curve.

After the administration of phenylbutazone, a peak plasma concentration is attained within approximately 1-4 hours.

Elimination half-lives corresponding to the apparent elimination rate constant in each subject do not differ greatly for the first and last doses administered.

The pharmacokinetics of single doses of phenylbutazone can be described by a two-component open model. Steady-state plasma concentrations of phenylbutazone are about four times higher than the peak concentration after the first single dose.

Steady-state plasma concentrations of the major, active metabolite, oxyphenylbutazone, are about 50% of those of phenylbutazone. Less than 2% of the dose appears in the urine as oxyphenbutazone.

At steady-state, 61% of ^{14}C-labelled phenylbutazone can be recovered from the urine and 27% from the feces. However, only about 1% of total urinary radioactivity is eliminated in the urine as unchanged drug. The sum of nonconjugated urinary metabolites (oxyphenbutazone, γ-hydroxyphenylbutazone, p, γ-dihydroxyphenylbutazone) and phenylbutazone itself amount to only about 10%. About 40% of the drug (total urinary radioactivity) is excreted in the urine as the C-4 glucuronide of phenylbutazone and an additional 12% is the C-4 glucuronide of γ-hydroxyphenylbutazone.

INDICATIONS AND USAGE:

Phenylbutazone is indicated for the relief of symptoms associated with the following conditions, but only after other therapeutic measures, including other nonsteroidal, anti-inflammatory drugs, have been tried and found unsatisfactory: active ankylosing spondylitis, acute gouty arthritis, active rheumatoid arthritis, and acute attacks of degenerative joint disease of the hips and knees.

CONTRAINDICATIONS:

Phenylbutazone is contraindicated in patients with hypersensitivity to phenylbutazone or oxyphenbutazone, and in patients who have a bronchospastic reaction to aspirin or other nonsteroidal anti- inflammatory drugs.

WARNINGS:

Hematologic: Phenylbutazone can cause aplastic anemia and agranulocytosis (see ADVERSE REACTIONS.) If patients develop any signs or symptoms suggesting a blood cell dyscrasia, then an examination of red cells, white cells, and platelets should be performed. If there is any significant change in the total leukocyte count, relative decrease in granulocytes, appearance of immature forms, or fall in hematocrit or platelet count, treatment with this drug should be discontinued immediately and a complete hematologic investigation should be made. Hematologic toxicity may occur shortly after initiation of therapy or after prolonged treatment; it may develop abruptly or gradually and may become apparent days or weeks after cessation of therapy. It is manifested by the appearance of anemia, leukopenia, thrombocytopenia, or clinically significant hemorrhage diathesis.

Gastrointestinal: Risk of GI Ulceration, Bleeding and Perforation with NSAID Therapy: Serious gastrointestinal toxicity such as bleeding, ulceration, and perforation, can occur at any time, with or without warning symptoms, in patients treated chronically with NSAID therapy. Although minor upper gastrointestinal problems such as dyspepsia, are common, usually developing early in therapy, physicians should remain alert for ulceration and bleeding in patients treated chronically with NSAIDs even in the absence of previous GI tract symptoms. In patients observed in clinical trials of several months to two years duration, symptomatic upper GI ulcers, gross bleeding or perforation appear to occur in approximately 1% of patients treated for 3-6 months, and in about 2-4% of the patients treated for one year. Physicians should inform patients about the signs and/or symptoms of serious GI toxicity and what steps to take if they occur.

Studies to date have not identified any subset of patients not at risk of developing peptic ulceration and bleeding. Except for a prior history of serious GI events and other risk factors known to be associated with peptic ulcer disease, such as alcoholism, smoking, etc., no risk factors (*e.g.,* age, sex) have been associated with increased risk. Elderly or debilitated patients seem to tolerate ulceration or bleeding less well than other individuals and most spontaneous reports of fatal GI events are in this population. Studies to date are inconclusive concerning the relative risk of various NSAIDs in causing such reactions. High doses of any NSAID probably carry a greater risk of these reactions, although controlled clinical trials showing this do not exist in most cases. In considering the use of relatively large doses (within the recommended dosage range), sufficient benefit should be anticipated to offset the potential increased risk of GI toxicity.

Hepatic: As with other nonsteroidal anti-inflammatory drugs, borderline elevations of values measured by one or more liver tests may occur in up to 15% of patients. These abnormalities may progress, may remain essentially unchanged, or may be transient with continued therapy. The SGPT (ALT) test is probably the most sensitive indicator of liver dysfunction. Meaningful elevations (three times the upper limit of normal) of SGPT or SGOT (AST) have occurred in controlled clinical trials in less than 1% of patients. A patient with symptoms and/or signs suggesting liver dysfunction, or in whom abnormal liver test results have occurred, should be evaluated for evidence of the development of more severe hepatic reactions while on therapy with phenylbutazone. Severe hepatic reactions, including jaundice and cases of fatal hepatitis, have been reported with phenylbutazone as with other nonsteroidal anti- inflammatory drugs. Although such reactions are rare, if abnormal liver tests persist or worsen, if clinical signs and symptoms consistent with liver disease develop or if systemic manifestations (eosinophilia, rash, etc.) occur, therapy with phenylbutazone should be discontinued.

Respiratory: Like other drugs that inhibit prostaglandin synthetase activity, such as aspirin and sulfinpyrazone, phenylbutazone may precipitate acute episodes of asthmatic attacks in patients with asthma (see CONTRAINDICATIONS.)

PRECAUTIONS:

General: Because serious adverse reactions or aggravation of existing medical problems can occur and have been reported, phenylbutazone should be used with caution in patients with incipient cardiac failure; blood dyscrasias; pancreatitis; parotitis; stomatitis; polymyalgia rheumatica; temporal arteritis; severe renal, cardiac and hepatic disease; and in patients with a history of peptic ulcer disease or with symptoms of gastrointestinal inflammation or active ulceration, inflammatory bowel disease of Crohn's disease.

Renal Effects: As with other nonsteroidal anti-inflammatory drugs, long-term administration of phenylbutazone to animals has resulted in renal papillary necrosis and other abnormal renal pathology. In humans, there have been reports of acute interstitial nephritis with hematuria, proteinuria, and occasionally nephrotic syndrome.

A second form of renal toxicity has been seen in patients with prerenal conditions leading to a reduction in renal blood flow or blood volume, where the renal prostaglandins have a supportive role in the maintenance of renal perfusion. In these patients administration of NSAID may cause a dose-dependent reduction on prostaglandin formation and may precipitate overt renal decompensation. Patients at greatest risk of this reaction are those with impaired renal function, heart failure, liver dysfunction, those taking diuretics, and the elderly. Discontinuation of NSAID therapy is typically followed by recovery to the pretreatment statement.

Patients with significantly impaired renal function should be closely monitored: a lower daily dose should be anticipated to avoid excessive drug accumulation.

Patients reporting visual disturbances while receiving the drug should discontinue treatment and have an ophthalmologic examination, because ophthalmic adverse reactions have been reported (see ADVERSE REACTIONS, Special Senses.)

Phenylbutazone increases sodium retention. As with other non-steroidal anti-inflammatory drugs, phenylbutazone should be used with caution in patients with whom fluid retention would aggravate an underlying condition such as severe cardiac or renal disease.

From age 40 on, the possibility of adverse reactions increases, and therefore phenylbutazone should be used with commensurately greater care in these patients.

Information for the Patient: Phenylbutazone, like other drugs of its class, is not free of side effects. The side effects of these drugs can cause discomfort and, rarely, there are more serious side effects, such as blood disorders and gastrointestinal bleeding, which may result in hospitalization and even fatal outcomes. Patients should be told to discontinue use of the drug and report lesions in the mouth (symptoms of blood dyscrasia); dyspepsia, epigastric pain, symptoms of anemia; unusual bleeding of bruising; black or tarry stools, or other evidence of intestinal ulceration; skin rashes; or significant weight gain or edema. Patients should also be warned not to exceed the recommended dosage, since this may lead to toxic effects.

Physicians should discuss with their patients the potential risks (see WARNINGS, PRECAUTIONS, and ADVERSE REACTIONS) and likely benefits of phenylbutazone treatment.

Laboratory Tests: Therapy should not be initiated until a careful detailed history is taken and complete physical and laboratory examinations, including an examination of red cells, white cells, and platelets, have been made. These examinations should also be made if any signs of symptoms appear suggesting depression of the formed blood elements.

PRECAUTIONS: *(cont'd)*

Because serious GI tract ulceration and bleeding can occur without symptoms, physicians should follow chronically treated patients for the signs and symptoms of ulceration and bleeding and inform them of the importance of this follow-up (see WARNINGS, Gastrointestinal.)

Drug/Laboratory Test Interactions: Phenylbutazone reduces iodine uptake by the thyroid and may interfere with laboratory tests of thyroid function. (Thyroid hyperplasia, goiters, and hypothyroidism have also been reported; see ADVERSE REACTIONS.)

Carcinogenesis, Mutagenesis, and Impairment of Fertility: Long-term carcinogenicity studies in animals have not been performed with phenylbutazone.

An increased incidence of chromosome anomalies has been reported in cultured leukocyte cells from patients receiving therapeutic doses of phenylbutazone. In other similar studies in humans and horses, results were inconclusive or negative. In Chinese-hamster fibroblast cells in vitro, chromosome aberrations were inducted at a concentration of phenylbutazone exceeding 20 times the human plasma levels of 43 mg/L. In mice, Chinese hamsters, and rats given up to 33 times the maximum daily human dose of phenylbutazone, no evidence of mutagenic activity or adverse effects on fertility was found. Phenylbutazone was not mutagenic in bacteria or fungi.

Pregnancy Category C: Reproduction studies in rats and rabbits given phenylbutazone in oral doses up to 16 times the maximum daily human dose have revealed no evidence of teratogenicity due to phenylbutazone. However, slightly reduced litter sizes were observed after oral or subcutaneous administration of phenylbutazone to pregnant rats or rabbits; an increase in stillbirths and reduced survival of offspring were observed after oral administration of 3.5 times the maximum daily human dose of phenylbutazone to rats during late pregnancy and lactation.

There are no adequate and well-controlled studies in pregnant women. However, phenylbutazone may appear in cord blood. Phenylbutazone should be used during pregnancy only if the potential benefit justifies the potential risk to the fetus.

Nursing Mothers: Phenylbutazone is excreted in breast milk in small quantity. Because of the potential for serious adverse reactions in nursing infants from phenylbutazone, a decision should be made whether to discontinue nursing or to discontinue use of the drug, taking into account the importance of the drug to the mother.

Pediatric Use: Safety and effectiveness in children 14 years of age or younger have not been established.

DRUG INTERACTIONS:

See CONTRAINDICATIONS.

Phenylbutazone competitively displaces other drugs, *e.g.,* other anti-inflammatory agents, oral anti-coagulants, oral antidiabetics, sulfonamides, sodium valproate and phenytoin, from serum-binding sites. The activity, duration of effect, and toxicity of the displaced drugs may thus be increased. Phenylbutazone accentuates the prothrombin depression produced by coumarin-type anti-coagulants. When administered alone, phenylbutazone does not affect prothrombin activity.

Phenylbutazone may induce the hepatic microsomal metabolism of dicoumarol, amidopyrine, digitoxin, hexobarbital, and cortisone. Conversely, it may inhibit the metabolism of phenytoin. Concomitant administration of phenylbutazone and phenytoin may result in increased serum levels of phenytoin which could lead to increased phenytoin toxicity.

Inducers of hepatic microsomal enzymes, e.g., barbiturates, promethazine, chlorpheniramine, rifampin, and corticosteroids (prednisone), may decrease the half-life of Phenylbutazone.

The effects of methotrexate, insulin, antidiabetic and sulfonamide drugs may be potentiated by phenylbutazone. Phenylbutazone increases the serum concentration of lithium by increasing tubular reabsorption, and it reduces the renal clearance of sulfonylureas. Methylphenidate is reported to prolong the half-life of phenylbutazone and to increase the serum level of oxyphenbutazone. Cholestyramine reduces the enteral absorption of phenylbutazone.

ADVERSE REACTIONS:

Aplastic anemia and agranulocytosis are the most serious adverse reactions that have been reported with the use of phenylbutazone. An incidence of 2.2 deaths from aplastic anemia and agranulocytosis per 100,000 exposures to phenylbutazone was reported by Inman, in a review of all deaths in England and Wales from October 1974 through September 1975 in which aplastic anemia or agranulocytosis was considered a primary or contributing case of death. The study found an increased risk with long- term use and use in elderly patients, especially women, with a rate of 6.5 deaths per 100,000 elderly women (over age 65). These data, while generated under conditions of use which differ from those presently recommended in the United Stages, indicate the need for careful consideration in any contemplated long-term use or use in the elderly.

The following adverse reactions have been reported with phenylbutazone and oxyphenbutazone:

Incidence Greater Than 1%

Gastrointestinal: (see WARNINGS) Abdominal discomfort and distress (3- 9%); nausea; dyspepsia, including indigestion and heartburn.

Dermatologic: Rash

Cardiovascular/Fluid and Electrolyte: Edema, water retention (3-9%).

Incidence Less Than 1%: (Causal Relationship Probable)

Hematologic: (see WARNINGS) Aplastic anemia; agranulocytosis; bone marrow depression; thrombocytopenia; pancytopenia; leukopenia; anemia; hemolytic anemia.

Gastrointestinal: (see WARNINGS) Vomiting; abdominal distention with flatulence; constipation; diarrhea; esophagitis; gastritis; salivary gland enlargement; stomatitis, sometimes with ulceration; ulceration and perforation of the intestinal tract, including acute and reactivated peptic ulcer; exacerbation of inflammatory bowel disease of Crohn's disease; anemia due to occult gastrointestinal bleeding; hepatitis.

Hypersensitive Reactions: Urticaria; anaphylactic shock; arthralgia; fever; vasculitis; Lyell's syndrome; serum sickness; Stevens-Johnson syndrome; activation of systemic lupus erythematosus; aggravation of temporal arteritis.

Dermatologic: Pruritus; erythema nodosum; erythema multiforme; nonthrombocytopenic purpura.

Cardiovascular/Fluid and Electrolyte: Sodium and chloride retention; fluid retention and plasma dilution; congestive heart failure; metabolic acidosis; respiratory alkalosis; hypertension; pericarditis; interstitial myocarditis.

Renal: Hematuria; proteinuria; ureteral obstruction with uric acid crystals; anuria; glomerulonephritis; acute tubular necrosis; cortical necrosis; renal stones; nephrotic syndrome; impaired renal function an renal failure; interstitial nephritis.

Central Nervous System: Headache; drowsiness; agitation; confusional states and lethargy; tremors; numbness; weakness.

Endocrine-Metabolic: Hyperglycemia.

Special Senses, Otic: hearing loss; tinnitus.

Incidence Less Than 1%: (Causal Relationship Unknown)

ADVERSE REACTIONS: *(cont'd)*

Hematologic: Leukemia. (There have been reports associating phenylbutazone with leukemia. However, the circumstances involved in these reports are such that a causal relationship to the drug has not been clearly established.

Special Senses, Ocular: (see PRECAUTIONS, General) Blurred vision; optic neuritis; toxic amblyopia; scotomata; retinal detachment; retinal hemorrhage; oculomotor palsy.

Endocrine-Metabolic: Thyroid hyperplasia; goiters associated with hyperthyroidism and hypothyroidism (see PRECAUTIONS, Drug/Laboratory Test Interactions ; pancreatitis.

OVERDOSAGE:

Acute Toxicity: The lowest known lethal doses are 14 g (45 year old man) and 2 g (3 year old child). The highest known doses that have been survived are 40 g (20 year old man) and 5 g (3 year old boy). Oral LD_{50}'s (mg/kg): mice, 650; rats, 364; guinea pigs, 1220.

SIGNS AND SYMPTOMS

The first signs and symptoms, referable chiefly to the stomach and the nervous system, appear 1 to hours after ingestion of the overdosage in children and somewhat later in adults.

The signs and symptoms of phenylbutazone poisoning can be summarized as follows:

Mild poisoning

Nausea, abdominal pain, drowsiness

Severe Poisoning

Early Onset: Upper abdominal pain, nausea, vomiting, hematemesis, diarrhea, restlessness, dizziness, agitation, hallucinations, psychosis, coma, convulsions (more prevent in children) hyperpyrexia, electrolyte disturbances, hyperventilation, alkalosis or acidosis, respiratory arrest, hypotension, hypertension, cyanosis.

Late Onset (2-7 Days): Acute renal failure, edema, hematuria, oliguria, abnormal laboratory test results, jaundice, electrocardiographic abnormalities, cardiac arrest, blood dyscrasias (anemia, thrombocytopenia, leukopenia, leukocytosis, hypoprothrombinemia).

Abnormalities evident on laboratory tests after overdosage may include respiratory or metabolic acidosis, impaired hepatic or renal function, and abnormalities of formed blood elements.

Treatment: There is no specific antidote.

In the alert patients, the stomach should be emptied promptly by induced emesis followed by lavage. In the obtunded patient the airway should be secured with a cuffed endotracheal tube before lavage; emesis should not be induced. Adequate respiratory exchange should be maintained; respiratory stimulants should be used. Shock should be treated with appropriate supportive measures. Seizures should be controlled with intravenous diazepam or short-acting barbiturates. Hemoperfusion has been used as an adjunct of supportive therapy in cases with poor prognosis.

DOSAGE AND ADMINISTRATION:

Phenylbutazone should be used at the smallest effective dosage that provides rapid relief of severe symptoms. If a favorable symptomatic response to treatment is not obtained after 1 week, use of the drug should be discontinued as soon as possible.

In elderly patients (60 years and over), every effort should be made to discontinue therapy on, or as soon as possible after, the seventh day, because of the increased risk of severe or fatal toxic reactions in this age group.

The drug should be taken with milk or with meals so that the possibility of gastric upset will be minimized.

In selecting the appropriate dosage, the physician should consider the patient's age, weight, general health, and any other factors that may influence the patient's response to the drug.

RHEUMATOID ARTHRITIS, ANKYLOSING SPONDYLITIS, AND ACUTE ATTACKS OF DEGENERATIVE JOINT DISEASE

Initial Dosage: The initial daily dosage in adult patients is 300-600 mg in three to four divided doses. Maximum therapeutic response is usually obtained with a total dose of 400 mg. A trial period of 1 week of therapy is considered adequate to adequate to determine the therapeutic effect of the drug; in the absence of a favorable response, therapy should be discontinued.

Maintenance Dosage: When improvement is obtained, the dosage should be promptly decreased to the minimum effective level necessary to maintain relief and not exceed 400 mg daily, because of the possibility of cumulative toxicity. A satisfactory clinical response may be obtained with daily doses as low as 100-200 mg.

Acute Gouty Arthritis: Satisfactory results may be obtained after an initial dose of 400 mg every 4 hours. The articular inflammation usually subsides within 4 days. Treatment should not be continued longer than 1 week.

Storage: Store at controlled room temperature 15 - 30° (59 - 86°F).

HOW SUPPLIED - RATED THERAPEUTICALLY EQUIVALENT:

Capsule, Gelatin - Oral - 100 mg

100's	$15.95	Phenylbutazone, Harber Pharm	51432-0350-03
1000's	$114.88	Phenylbutazone, Rugby	00536-4305-10

Tablet, Uncoated - Oral - 100 mg

100's	$19.80	Phenylbutazone, United Res	00677-0649-01

PHENYLEPHRINE HYDROCHLORIDE *(002020)*

CATEGORIES: Allergies; Analeptics; Anesthesia; Autonomic Drugs; Cardiovascular Drugs; Cough Preparations; Cycloplegics/Mydriatics; Decongestants; EENT Drugs; Eye, Ear, Nose, & Throat Preparations; Hypotension; Hypotension/Shock; Mydriasis; Mydriatics; Nasal Congestion; Ophthalmics; Refraction; Renal Drugs; Respiratory & Allergy Medications; Sympathomimetic Agents; Tachycardia; Uveitis; Vasoconstrictors; Vasopressors; Pregnancy Category C; FDA Pre 1938 Drugs

BRAND NAMES: Ah-Chew D; Ak-Dilate; Dilatair; *Drosin*; *Efrin*; *Efrin-10*; *Efrisel*; *Fenilefrina*; I-Phrine; *Isopto Frin* (Australia); *Metaoxedrin*; *Minims*; *Minims Phenylephrine Hydrochloride* (England); *Minims Phenylephrine HCL 10%*; Murocoll-2; Mydfrin; *Nefrin-Ofteno*; *Neosynephrine*; **Neo-Synephrine**; *Neo-Synephrine Ophthalmic Viscous 10%*; Neofrin; *Neosynephrine*; *Neosynephrine 10% Chibret* (France); *Neosynephrine Faure 10%* (France); Ocu-Phrin; *Oftan-Metaoksedrin*; *Optistin*; *Phenylephrine*; Phenylephrine Hcl; *Prefrin*; *Pupiletto Forte*; *Pupiletto-Forte*; Ricobid-D; Spectro-Dilate; Spectro-Nephrine; Storz-Fen; *Vistafrin*; *Vistosan* (Germany) *(International brand names outside U.S. in italics)*

FORMULARIES: Aetna; BC-BS; FHP; Medi-Cal; PCS

WARNING:
PHYSICIANS SHOULD THOROUGHLY FAMILIARIZE THEMSELVES WITH THE COMPLETE CONTENTS OF THIS INSERT BEFORE PRESCRIBING PHENYLEPHRINE HYDROCHLORIDE.

DESCRIPTION:

(Note: This monograph contains information on the 2.5% ophthalmic solution, the 10% ophthalmic solution, and the 1% injection). Phenylephrine HCl is a sterile topical ophthalmic solution.

Established Name: Phenylephrine Hydrochloride

Chemical Name (2.5%, 10%, and Injection): Benzenemethanol, 3-hydroxy-α-((methylamino) methyl)-, hydrochloride (*S*)-.

Each ml Contains: *Active:* Phenylephrine HCl 2.5%. *Preservative:* Benzalkonium Chloride 0.01%. *Inactive:* Boric Acid, Sodium Bisulfite, Edetate Disodium, Sodium Hydroxide and/or Hydrochloric Acid (to adjust pH), Purified Water.

CLINICAL PHARMACOLOGY:

2.5% / 10% Solution: Phenylephrine HCl 2.5% is an alpha receptor sympathetic agonist used in local ocular disorders because of its vasoconstrictor and mydriatic action. It exhibits rapid and moderately prolonged action, and it produces little rebound vasodilatation. Systemic side effects are uncommon.

The action of different concentrations of ophthalmic solutions of Phenylephrine HCl 2.5% is shown in TABLE 1.

TABLE 1 Phenylephrine HCl, Clinical Pharmacology

Strength of solution	Mydriasis Maximal (min)	Mydriasis Recovery Time (hrs)	Paralysis of accommodation
2.5	15-60	3	trace
10	10-60	6	slight

1% Injection: Phenylephrine HCl provides vasoconstriction that lasts longer than that of epinephrine and ephedrine. Responses are more sustained than those to epinephrine, lasting 20 minutes after intravenous and as long as 50 minutes after subcutaneous injection. It's action on the heart contrasts sharply with that of epinephrine and ephedrine, in that it slows the heart rate and increases the stroke output, producing no disturbance in the rhythm of the pulse.

Phenylephrine is a powerful postsynaptic alpha-receptor stimulant with little effect on the beta receptors of the heart. In therapeutic doses it produces little if any stimulation of either spinal cord or cerebrum. a singular advantage of this drug is the fact that repeated injections produce comparable effects.

The predominant actions of Phenylephrine are on the cardiovascular system. Parenteral administration causes a rise in systolic and diastolic pressures in man and other species. Accompanying the pressure response to Phenylephrine is a marked reflex bradycardia that can be blocked by atropine; after atropine, large doses of the drug increase the heart rate only slightly. In man, cardiac output is slightly decreased and peripheral resistance is considerably increased. Circulation time is slightly prolonged, and venous pressure is slightly increased; venous constriction is not marked. Most vascular beds are constricted; renal splanchnic, cutaneous, and limb blood flows are reduced but coronary blood blow is increased. Pulmonary vessels are constricted, and pulmonary arterial pressure is raised.

The drug is a powerful vasoconstrictor, with properties very similar to those of norepinephrine but almost completely lacking the chronotropic and inotropic actions on the heart. Cardiac irregularities are seen only very rarely even with large doses.

INDICATIONS AND USAGE:

2.5% / 10% Solution: Phenylephrine HCl is recommended as a vasoconstrictor, decongestant, and mydriatic in a variety of ophthalmic conditions and procedures. Some of its uses are for pupillary dilatation in uveitis (to prevent or aid in the disruption of posterior synechia formation), for many ophthalmic surgical procedures and for refraction without cycloplegia. Phenylephrine HCl 2.5% may also be used for funduscopy, and other diagnostic procedures.

1% Injection: Phenylephrine HCl 1% Injection is intended for the maintenance of an adequate level of blood pressure during spinal and inhalation anesthesia and for the treatment of vascular failure in shock, shocklike states, and drug-induced hypotension, or hypersensitivity. It is also employed to overcome paroxysmal superventricular tachycardia, to prolong spinal anesthesia, and as a vasoconstrictor in regional analgesia.

CONTRAINDICATIONS:

Ophthalmic solutions, (both strengths), of phenylephrine HCl are contraindicated in patients with anatomically narrow angles or narrow angle glaucoma. Phenylephrine HCl may be contraindicated in some low birth weight infants and some elderly adults with severe arteriosclerotic cardiovascular or cerebrovascular disease. Phenylephrine HCl may be contraindicated during intraocular operative procedures when the corneal epithelial barrier has been disturbed. This preparation is also contraindicated in persons with a known sensitivity to phenylephrine HCl or any of its components.

Additional information for the 10% Solution: Contraindicated in infants and in patients with aneurysms.

1% Injection: Phenylephrine HCl Injection should not be used with patients with severe hypertension, ventricular tachycardia, or in patients who are hypersensitive to it.

WARNINGS:

10% Solution: There have been reports associating the use of Phenylephrine HCl 10% ophthalmic solutions with the development of serious cardiovascular reactions, including ventricular arrhythmias and myocardial infarctions. These episodes, some ending fatally, have usually occurred in elderly patients with preexisting cardiovascular diseases.

1% Injection: If used in conjunction with oxytocic drugs, the pressure effect of sympathomimetic pressor amines is potentiated (see The obstetrician should be warned that some oxytocic drugs may cause severe persistent hypertension and that even a rupture of a cerebral blood vessel may occur during the postpartum period.

Contains sodium metabisulfite, a sulfite that may cause allergic-type reactions including anaphylactic symptoms and life-threatening or less severe asthmatic episodes in certain susceptible people. The overall prevalence of sulfite sensitivity in the general population is unknown and probably low. Sulfite sensitivity is seen more frequently in asthmatic than in nonasthmatic people.

PRECAUTIONS:

Both Solution Strengths: Ordinarily, any mydriatic, including phenylephrine HCl, is contraindicated in patients with glaucoma, since it may occasionally raise intraocular pressure. However, when temporary dilatation of the pupil may free adhesions, this advantage may temporarily outweigh the danger from coincident dilatation of the pupil. Rebound miosis has been reported in older persons one day after receiving phenylephrine HCl ophthalmic solutions, and reinstillation of the drug may produce less mydriasis than previously. This may be of clinical importance in dilating the pupils of older subjects prior to retinal detachment or cataract surgery. The lacrimal sac should be compressed by digital pressure for one minute after instillation to avoid excessive systemic absorption.

Due to a strong action of the drug on the dilator muscle, older individuals may also develop transient pigment floaters in the aqueous humor 40 to 45 minutes following the administration of phenylephrine HCl ophthalmic solution. The appearance may be similar to anterior uveitis or to a microscopic hyphema. To prevent pain, a drop of suitable topical anesthetic may be applied before using. Prolonged exposure to air or strong light may cause oxidation and discoloration. Do not use if solution is brown or contains a precipitate.

Additional information for the 10% solution: A significant elevation in blood pressure is rare but has been reported following conjunctival instillation of recommended doses of Phenylephrine HCl 10%. Caution, therefore, should be exercised in administering the 10% solutions to children of low body weight, the elderly, and patients with insulin-dependent diabetes, hypertension, hyperthyroidism, generalized arteriosclerosis, or cardiovascular disease. The posttreatment blood pressure of these patients, and any patients who develop symptoms, should be carefully monitored.

To prevent pain, a drop of suitable topical anesthetic may be applied before using the 10 percent ophthalmic solution.

It has ben reported that the concomitant use of Phenylephrine HCl 10% ophthalmic solutions and systemic beta blockers has caused acute hypertension and, in one case, the rupture of a congenital cerebral aneurysm. This drug may potentiate the cardiovascular depressant effects of potent inhalation anesthetic agents.

1% Injection: Should be employed only with extreme caution in elderly patients or in patients with hyperthyroidism, bradycardia, partial heart block, myocardial disease, or severe arteriosclerosis.

Vasopressors, particularly metaraminol, may cause serious cardiac arrhythmias during halothane anesthesia and therefore should be used only with great caution or not at all.

The pressor effect of sympathomimetic pressor amines is markedly potentiated in patients receiving MAO inhibitors. Therefore, when initiating pressor therapy in these patients, the initial dose should be small and used with due caution. The pressor response of adrenergic agents may also be potentiated by tricyclic antidepressants.

Carcinogenesis, Mutagenesis, and Impairment of Fertility: No long- term animal studies have been done to evaluate the potential of Phenylephrine HCl Injection in these areas.

Pregnancy Category C: Animal reproduction studies have not been conducted with this drug. It is also not known whether Phenylephrine HCl Injection can cause fetal harm when administered to a pregnant woman or can affect reproduction capacity. This drug should be given to a pregnant women only if clearly needed.

Labor and Delivery: If vasopressor drugs are either used to correct hypotension or added to the local anesthetic solution, the obstetrician should be cautioned that some oxytocic drugs may cause severe persistent hypertension and that a rupture of a cerebral blood vessel may occur during the postpartum period (see WARNINGS.)

Nursing Mothers: It is not known whether this drug is excreted in human milk. Because many are excreted in human milk, caution should be exercised when Phenylephrine HCl Injection is administered to a nursing woman.

Pediatric Use: To combat hypotension during special anesthesia in children, a dose of 0.5 mg to 1 mg per 25 pounds body weight, administered subcutaneously or IM, is recommended.

DRUG INTERACTIONS:

2.5% Solution: Not for intraocular use. As with other adrenergic drugs, when it is administered simultaneously with, or up to 21-days after, administration of monoamine oxidase (MAO) inhibitors, careful supervision and adjustment of dosages are required since exaggerated adrenergic effects may result. The pressor response of adrenergic agents may also be potentiated by tricyclic antidepressants. Systemic side effects are more common in patients taking beta adrenergic blocking agents such as propranolol.

ADVERSE REACTIONS:

(Pertains only to the injection)

Headache, reflex bradycardia, excitability, restlessness, and rarely arrhythmias.

OVERDOSAGE:

(Pertains only to the injection)

Overdosage may induce ventricular extrasystoles and short paroxysms of ventricular tachycardia, a sensation of fullness in the head and tingling of the extremities.

Should an excessive elevation of blood pressure occur, it may be immediately relieved by an α-adrenergic blocking agent, eg, phentolamine. The oral LD_{50} in the rat is 350 mg/kg, in the mouse 120 mg/kg

DOSAGE AND ADMINISTRATION:

2.5% Solution - Vasoconstriction and Pupil Dilatation: Phenylephrine HCl 2.5% is especially useful when rapid and powerful dilatation of the pupil without cycloplegia and reduction of congestion in the capillary bed are desired. A drop of a suitable topical anesthetic may be applied, followed in a few minutes by 1 drop of the on the upper limbus. The anesthetic prevents stinging and consequent dilution of the solution by lacrimation. It may occasionally be necessary to repeat the instillation after one hour, again preceded by the use of the topical anesthetic.

UVEITIS

Posterior Synechia: Phenylephrine HCl 2.5% may be used in patients with uveitis when synechiae are present or may develop. The formation of synechia may be prevented by the use of this ophthalmic solution and atropine or other cycloplegics to produce wide dilatation of the pupil. For recently formed posterior synechiae one drop of may be applied to the upper surface of the cornea and be repeated as necessary, not to exceed three times. Treatment may be continued the following day, if necessary. Atropine sulfate and the application of hot compresses should also be used if indicated.

MYDRIATICS/CYCLOPLEGICS

Glaucoma: Phenylephrine HCl 2.5% may be used with miotics in patients with open angle glaucoma. It reduces the difficulties experienced by the patient because of the small field produced by miosis, and still it permits and often supports the effect of the miotic in lowering the intraocular pressure in open angle glaucoma. Hence, there may be marked improvement in visual acuity after using Phenylephrine HCl 2.5% in conjunction with miotic drugs.

DOSAGE AND ADMINISTRATION: *(cont'd)*

Surgery: When a short-acting mydriatic is needed for wide dilatation of the pupil before intraocular surgery, Phenylephrine HCl 2.5% (or the 10%) may be applied topically from 30 to 60 minutes before the operation.

Refraction: Phenylephrine HCl 2.5% may be used effectively to increase mydriasis with homatropine hydrobromide, cyclopentolate hydrochloride, tropicamide hydrochloride and atropine sulfate.

For Adults: One drop of the preferred cycloplegic is placed in each eye, followed in 5 minutes by one drop of Phenylephrine HCl 2.5%.

Since adequate cycloplegia is achieved at different time intervals after the instillation of the necessary number of drops, different cycloplegics will require different waiting periods to achieve adequate cycloplegia.

For Children: For a "one application method," Phenylephrine HCl 2.5% may be combined with one of the preferred rapid acting cycloplegics to produce adequate cycloplegia.

Ophthalmoscopic Examination: One drop of Phenylephrine HCl 2.5% is placed in each eye. Sufficient mydriasis to permit examination is produced in 15 to 30 minutes. Dilatation lasts from one to three hours.

Diagnostic Procedures: Provocative Test for Angle Closure Glaucoma: Phenylephrine HCl 2.5% may be used cautiously as a provocative test when interval narrow angle closure glaucoma is suspected. Intraocular tension and gonioscopy are performed prior to and after dilatation of the pupil with phenylephrine HCl. A "significant" intraocular pressure (IOP) rise combined with gonioscopic evidence of angle closure indicates an anterior segment anatomy capable of angle closure. A negative test does not rule this out. This pharmacologically induced angle closure glaucoma may not simulate real life conditions and other causes for transient elevations of IOP should be excluded.

Retinoscopy (Shadow Test): When dilatation of the pupil without cycloplegic action is desired for retinoscopy, may be used.

NOTE: Heavily pigmented irides may require larger doses in all of the above procedures.

Blanching Test: One or two drops of Phenylephrine HCl 2.5% should be applied to the injected eye. After five minutes, examine for perilimbal blanching. If blanching occurs, the congestion is superficial and probably does not indicate iridocyclitis.

10% Solution - Vasoconstriction and Pupil Dilatation: (same as 2.5%, please see above)

Uveitis: Posterior Synechiae: (also see 2.5%, above). Phenylephrine HCl 10% ophthalmic solution may be used in patients with uveitis when synechiae are present or may develop. The formation of synechiae may be prevented by the use of the 10% solution and atropine to produce wide dilation of the pupil. It should be emphasized, however, that the vasoconstrictor effect of this drug may be antagonistic to the increase of local blood flow in uveal infection.

To free recently formed posterior synechiae, 1 drop of the 10 percent ophthalmic solution may be applied to the upper surface of the cornea. On the following day, treatment may be continued if necessary. In the interim, hot compresses should be applied for five or ten minutes three times a day, with 1 drop of a 1 or 2 percent solution of atropine sulfate before and after each series of compresses.

Glaucoma: In certain patients with glaucoma, temporary reduction of intraocular tension may be attained by producing vasoconstriction of the intraocular vessels; this may be accompanied by placing 1 drop of the 10 % solution on the upper surface of the cornea. This treatment may be repeated as often as necessary.

Storage (2.5 and 10% Solutions): Store at 36 to 80°F. Protect from light and excessive heat.

1% Injection: Generally injected subcutaneously, intramuscularly, slowly intravenously, or in dilute solution as a continuous IV infusion. In patients with paroxysmal superventricular tachycardia and, if indicated, in case of emergency, Phenylephrine HCl is administered directly intravenously. The dose should be adjusted according to the pressure response. Dosage calculations are shown in TABLE 2.

TABLE 2 Phenylephrine, DOSAGE AND ADMINISTRATION
Dosage Calculations

Dose Required	Use Phenylephrine HCl 1%
10 mg	1 ml
5 mg	0.5 ml
1 mg	0.1 ml

For convenience in intermittent IV administration, dilute 1 ml Phenylephrine HCl 1% with 9 ml Sterile Water for Injection, USP, to yield 0.1% Phenylephrine HCl (TABLE 3).

TABLE 3 Phenylephrine HCl, DOSAGE AND ADMINISTRATION

Dose Required	Use Diluted Phenylephrine HCl (0.1%)
0.1 mg	0.1 ml
0.2 mg	0.2 ml
0.5 mg	0.5 ml

Mild or Moderate Hypotension: *Subcutaneously or Intramuscularly:* Usual dose, from 1 mg to 10 mg. Initial dose should not exceed 5 mg. *Intravenously:* Usual dose, 0.2 mg. Range, from 0.1 mg to 0.5 mg. Initial dose should not exceed 0.5 mg.

Injections should not be repeated more often than every 10 to 15 minutes. A 5 mg IM dose should raise blood pressure for one to two hours. A 0.5 mg IV dose should elevate the pressure for about 15 minutes.

SEVERE HYPOTENSION AND SHOCK - INCLUDING DRUG-RELATED HYPOTENSION

Blood volume depletion should always be corrected as fully as possible before any vasopressor is administered. When, as an emergency measure, intra-aortic pressures must be maintained to prevent cerebral or coronary artery ischemia, Phenylephrine HCl can be administered before and concurrently with blood volume replacement.

Hypotension and occasionally severe shock may result from overdosage or idiosyncracy following the administration of certain drugs, especially adrenergic and ganglionic blocking agents, rauwolfia and veratrum alkaloids, and phenothiazine tranquilizers. patients who receive a phenothiazine derivative as preoperative medication are especially susceptible to these reactions. As an adjunct in the management of such episodes, Phenylephrine HCl 1% is a suitable agent for restoring blood pressure.

Higher initial and maintenance doses of Phenylephrine HCl are required in patients with persistent or untreated severe hypotension or shock. Hypotension produced by powerful peripheral adrenergic blocking agents, chlorpromazine, or pheochromocytometoctomy may also require more intensive therapy.

Continuous Infusion: Add 10 mg of the drug (1 ml of 1 percent solution) to 500 ml of Dextrose Injection, USP, or Sodium Chloride Injection, USP (providing a 1:50,000 solution). To raise the blood pressure rapidly, start to infusion at about 100 mcg to 180 mcg per minute (based on 20 drops per ml this would be 100 to 180 drops per minute). When the blood pressure is stabilized (at a low normal level for the individual), a maintenance rate of

DOSAGE AND ADMINISTRATION: *(cont'd)*

40 mcg to 60 mcg per minute usually suffices (based on 20 drops per ml this would be 40 mcg to 60 mcg per minute). If the drop size of the infusion system varies from the 20 drops per ml, the dose must be adjusted accordingly.

If a prompt initial pressor response is not obtained, additional increments of Phenylephrine HCl (10 mg or more) are added to the infusion bottle. The rate of flow is then adjusted until the desired blood pressure level is obtained. (In some cases, a more potent vasopressor such as norepinephrine biurate, may be required). Hypertension should be avoided. The blood pressure should be checked frequently. Headache and/or bradycardia may indicate hypertension. Arrhythmias are rare.

SPINAL ANESTHESIA-HYPOTENSION

Routine parenteral use of Phenylephrine HCl has been recommended for the prophylaxis and treatment of hypotension during spinal anesthesia. It is best administered subcutaneously or intramuscularly three to four minutes before injection of the spinal anesthetic. The total requirement for high anesthetic levels is usually 3 mg, and for the lower levels, 2 mg. For hypotensive emergencies during spinal anesthesia, this drug may be given IV, using an initial dose of 0.2 mg. Any subsequent dose should not exceed the previous dose by more than 0.1 mg to 0.2 mg and no more than 0.5 mg should be administered in a single dose. To combat hypotension during spinal anesthesia in children, a dose of 0.5 mg to 1 mg per 25 pounds body weight, administered subcutaneously or IM, is recommended.

PROLONGATION OF SPINAL ANESTHESIA

The addition of 2 mg to 5 mg of Phenylephrine HCl to the anesthetic solution increases the duration of motor block by as much as approximately 50% without any increase in the incidence of complications such as nausea, vomiting, or blood pressure disturbances.

VASOCONSTRICTOR FOR REGIONAL ANALGESIA

Concentrations about 10 times those employed when epinephrine is used as a vasoconstrictor are recommended. The optimum strength is 1:20,000 (made by adding 1 mg of Phenylephrine HCl to every 20 ml of local anesthetic solution). Some pressor responses can be expected when 2 mg or more are injected.

PAROXYSMAL SUPERVENTRICULAR TACHYCARDIA

Rapid IV Injection (within 20 to 30 seconds) is recommended; the initial dose should not exceed 0.5 mg, and subsequent doses, which are determined by the initial blood pressure response, should not exceed the preceding dose by more than 0.1 mg to 0.2 mg and should never exceed 1 mg.

Protect from light if removed from carton or dispensing bin.

HOW SUPPLIED - EQUIVALENTS NOT AVAILABLE:

Injection, Solution - Intramuscular; - 10 mg/ml

1 ml x 25	$50.70	Phenylephrine Hcl, Gensia Labs	00703-1631-04
1 ml x 25	$78.13	Phenylephrine Hcl, Am Regent	00517-0299-25
1 ml x 25	$80.00	Phenylephrine Hcl, Schein Pharm (US)	00364-2426-46
1 ml x 25	**$192.95**	**NEO-SYNEPHRINE, Sanofi Winthrop**	**00024-1342-04**
1 ml x 50	**$113.56**	**NEO-SYNEPHRINE, Sanofi Winthrop**	**00024-1340-02**
5 ml x 25	$390.63	PHENYLEPHRINE HCL, Am Regent	00517-0405-25
25's	$76.88	Phenylephrine Hcl, Elkins Sinn	00641-0482-25

Solution - Nasal - 0.25 %

480 ml	$2.82	Phenylephrine Hcl, Rugby	00536-1620-85

Solution - Ophthalmic - 2.5 %

2 ml	$2.25	Phenylephrine Hcl, Apotex	60505-7512-01
2 ml	$2.75	PHENOPTIC, Optopics	52238-0718-02
2 ml	$3.44	AK-DILATE, Akorn	17478-0200-20
2 ml	$3.70	Neofrin, Ocusoft	54799-0530-02
3 ml	$5.94	MYDFRIN, Alcon	00065-0342-03
5 ml	$2.30	Phenylephrine Hcl, Apotex	60505-7512-02
5 ml	$4.00	PHENOPTIC, Optopics	52238-0718-05
5 ml	$11.56	MYDFRIN, Alcon-PR	00998-0342-05
15 ml	$2.50	Phenylephrine Hcl, Apotex	60505-7512-05
15 ml	$4.75	Phenylephrine Hcl, Rugby	00536-2410-72
15 ml	$5.40	PHENOPTIC, Optopics	52238-0718-15
15 ml	$5.55	NEOFRIN 2.5% OPTHALMIC, Ocusoft	54799-0530-15
15 ml	$5.94	AK-DILATE, Akorn	17478-0200-12
15 ml	$6.02	Phenylephrine Hcl, Steris Labs	00402-0798-15
15 ml	$7.83	Phenylephrine HCl, Schein Pharm (US)	00364-7376-72
15 ml	**$20.01**	**NEO-SYNEPHRINE, Sanofi Winthrop**	**00024-1358-01**

Solution - Ophthalmic - 10 %

1 ml x 12	$25.80	Phenylephrine HCl, Ciba Vision	00058-0780-12
2 ml	$4.69	AK-DILATE, Akorn	17478-0205-20
5 ml	$5.55	Neofrin Ophthalmic Solution 10%, Ocusoft	54799-0531-05
5 ml	$5.60	Phenylephrine Hcl, Steris Labs	00402-0799-05
5 ml	$6.25	AK-DILATE, Akorn	17478-0205-10
5 ml	$7.78	Phenylephrine Hydrochloride Ophthalmic S, Schein Pharm (US)	00364-2370-53
5 ml	**$18.56**	**NEO-SYNEPHRINE VISCOUS, Sanofi Winthrop**	**00024-1362-01**
5 ml	**$19.13**	**NEO-SYNEPHRINE, Sanofi Winthrop**	**00024-1359-01**

Suspension - Oral - 1 mg/ml

118.3 ml	$22.00	RICOBID-D, Teral Labs	51234-0156-04

Tablet, Chewable - Oral - 10 mg

100's	$36.25	AH-CHEW D, WE Pharm	59196-0007-01

PHENYLEPHRINE HYDROCHLORIDE; PHENYLPROPANOLAMINE; PSEUDOEPHEDRINE *(002024)*

CATEGORIES: Autonomic Drugs; Common Cold; Cough Preparations; Respiratory & Allergy Medications; Sympathomimetic Agents; FDA Pre 1938 Drugs

BRAND NAMES: No-Hist; No-Hist-S

Prescribing information not available at time of publication.

HOW SUPPLIED - EQUIVALENTS NOT AVAILABLE:

Capsule, Gelatin - Oral

100's	$18.00	NO-HIST, Dunhall Pharms	00217-0415-01

PHENYLEPHRINE HYDROCHLORIDE; PROMETHAZINE HYDROCHLORIDE *(002021)*

CATEGORIES: Allergies; Anesthesia; Antihistamines; Antitussives/Expectorants/Mucolytics; Common Cold; Cough Preparations; Decongestants; Expectorants; Influenza; Nasal Congestion; Respiratory & Allergy Medications; Rhinitis; Pregnancy Category C; FDA Approved 1984 Apr

BRAND NAMES: Phen-Tuss A.D.; **Phenergan Vc**; Pherazine Vc; Promethazine Vc

FORMULARIES: BC-BS; Medi-Cal

DESCRIPTION:

FOR COMPLETE PRESCRIBING INFORMATION REFER TO THE INDIVIDUAL DRUG MONOGRAPHS (PHENYLEPHRINE HYDROCHLORIDE; PROMETHAZINE HYDROCHLORIDE).

INDICATIONS AND USAGE:

Phenylephrine HCl and Promethazine HCl is indicated for the temporary relief of upper respiratory symptoms, including nasal congestion, associated with allergy or the common cold.

DOSAGE AND ADMINISTRATION:

The recommended adult dose is one teaspoon (5 ml) every 4 to 6 hours, not to exceed 30.0 ml in 24 hours. For children 6 years to under 12 years of age, the dose is one-half to one teaspoon (2.5 to 5.0 ml) repeated at 4- to 6-hour intervals, not to exceed 30.0 ml in 24 hours. For children 2 years to under 6 years of age, the dose is one-quarter to one-half teaspoon (1.25 to 2.5 ml) every 4 to 6 hours.

Phenylephrine HCl and Promethazine HCl is not recommended for children under 2 years of age.

Keep bottles tightly closed and store at room temperature between 15 and 25°C (59 and 77°F).

HOW SUPPLIED - RATED THERAPEUTICALLY EQUIVALENT:

Syrup - Oral - 5 mg/6.25 mg/5m

118 ml	$2.80	PHENAMETH VC PLAIN, Major Pharms	00904-1512-00
120 ml	$0.94	Promethazine Vc, H.C.F.A. F F P	99999-2021-01
120 ml	$2.00	Promethazine Vc, HR Cenci	00556-0346-04
120 ml	$2.20	Promethazine Vc, Morton Grove	60432-0605-04
120 ml	$2.38	Prometh Vc Plain, Alpharma	00472-1628-04
120 ml	$2.38	Promethazine Vc, Qualitest Pharms	00603-1582-54
120 ml	$2.50	Promethazine Vc Plain, Rugby	00536-1785-97
120 ml	$2.63	Promethazine Vc Plain, HL Moore Drug Exch	00839-7060-65
120 ml	$2.85	PHERAZINE VC SYRUP, Halsey Drug	00879-0514-04
120 ml x 24	**$132.05**	**PHENERGAN VC, Wyeth Labs**	**00008-0551-02**
240 ml	$1.87	Promethazine Vc, H.C.F.A. F F P	99999-2021-03
473 ml	$15.00	PHEN-TUSS A.D., Bergmar Pharm	58173-0033-16
480 ml	$1.94	Promethazine Vc Plain, United Res	00677-0964-33
480 ml	$3.74	Promethazine Vc, H.C.F.A. F F P	99999-2021-02
480 ml	$5.20	Promethazine Vc, HR Cenci	00556-0346-16
480 ml	$6.90	Promethazine Vc, Qualitest Pharms	00603-1582-58
480 ml	$7.33	Promethazine Vc Plain, HL Moore Drug Exch	00839-7060-69
480 ml	$8.50	Prometh Vc Plain, Goldline Labs	00182-1711-40
480 ml	$8.55	Promethazine Vc Plain, Rugby	00536-1785-85
480 ml	$8.70	Promethazine Vc, Morton Grove	60432-0605-16
480 ml	$9.00	Prometh VC Plain Syrup, Schein Pharm (US)	00364-0860-16
480 ml	$9.90	Promethazine VC Plain, Major Pharms	00904-1512-16
480 ml	$10.50	PHERAZINE VC SYRUP, Halsey Drug	00879-0514-16
480 ml	$11.30	Prometh Vc Plain, Alpharma	00472-1628-16
480 ml	$11.30	Promethazine Vc Plain, Geneva Pharms	00781-6635-16
480 ml	**$19.86**	**PHENERGAN VC, Wyeth Labs**	**00008-0551-03**
3785 ml	$41.24	PHENAMETH VC PLAIN, Major Pharms	00904-1512-28
3840 ml	$29.95	Promethazine Vc, H.C.F.A. F F P	99999-2021-04
3840 ml	$31.20	Promethazine Vc Plain, Rugby	00536-1785-90
3840 ml	$31.37	Promethazine Vc, HR Cenci	00556-0346-28
3840 ml	$31.49	Prometh Vc Plain, Goldline Labs	00182-1711-41
3840 ml	$36.39	Prometh Vc Plain, Alpharma	00472-1628-28
3840 ml	$36.75	PHERAZINE VC SYRUP, Halsey Drug	00879-0514-28
3840 ml	$65.86	Promethazine Vc Plain, HL Moore Drug Exch	00839-7060-70
4000 ml	$31.20	Promethazine Vc, H.C.F.A. F F P	99999-2021-05

HOW SUPPLIED - NOT RATED EQUIVALENT:

Syrup - Oral - 5 mg/6.25 mg/5m

120 ml	$1.65	Promethazine Vc, Major Pharms	00904-1512-20
120 ml	$1.95	Promethazine Vc, Harber Pharm	51432-0663-18
120 ml	$2.57	Promethazine Vc, Aligen Independ	00405-3625-76
120 ml	$2.75	Promethazine Vc, Consolidated Midland	00223-6346-01
480 ml	$4.90	Promethazine Vc, Harber Pharm	51432-0663-20
480 ml	$5.50	Promethazine Vc, Consolidated Midland	00223-6346-02
480 ml	$5.64	Promethazine Vc, Aligen Independ	00405-3625-16
480 ml	$6.00	Promethazine Vc, ESI Lederle	59911-5820-03
3840 ml	$22.46	Promethazine Vc, Harber Pharm	51432-0663-21
3840 ml	$32.49	Promethazine Vc, Consolidated Midland	00223-6346-03

PHENYLEPHRINE HYDROCHLORIDE; SULFACETAMIDE SODIUM *(002023)*

CATEGORIES: Anti-Infectives; Antibacterials; Conjunctivitis; Corneal Ulcer; EENT Drugs; Eye, Ear, Nose, & Throat Preparations; Infections; Ocular Infections; Ophthalmic Decongestants; Sulfonamides; Trachoma; Pregnancy Category C; FDA Pre 1938 Drugs

BRAND NAMES: **Vasosulf**

DESCRIPTION:

Sulfacetamide sodium-phenylephrine hydrochloride ophthalmic solution is a sterile solution for ophthalmic administration having the following composition: *Sulfacetamide Sodium* 150 mg/ml; (bacteriostatic antibacterial) *Phenylephrine Hydrochloride* 1.25 mg/ml (sympathomimetic);

In a solution of mono and dibasic sodium phosphate, sodium thiosulfate, poloxamer 188 and purified water, preserved with methylparaben and propylparaben. Hydrochloric acid added to adjust pH when necessary.

The chemical name for sulfacetamide sodium is Acetamide, N-((4-aminophenyl)sulfonyl)-, monosodium salt, monohydrate.

The chemical name for phenylephrine hydrochloride is Benzenemethanol, 3-hydroxy-alpha-(methylamino)-methyl)-, hydrochloride (R)-.

CLINICAL PHARMACOLOGY:

Sulfacetamide sodium exerts a bacteriostatic effect against a wide range of gram-positive and gram-negative microorganisms by restricting through competition with p-aminobenzoic acid, the synthesis of folic acid which bacteria require for growth. Phenylephrine hydrochloride is an alpha sympathetic receptor agonist producing vasoconstriction.

INDICATIONS AND USAGE:

Sulfacetamide Na-Phenylephrine Hcl ophthalmic solution is indicated for the treatment of conjunctivitis, corneal ulcer, and other superficial ocular infections due to susceptible microorganisms, and an adjunctive in systemic sulfonamide therapy of trachoma.

CONTRAINDICATIONS:

Contraindicated in persons hypersensitive to one or more of the components of this preparation.

PRECAUTIONS:

The solutions are incompatible with silver preparations. Local anesthetics related to p-aminobenzoic acid may antagonize the action of the sulfonamides. Bacteria initially sensitive to sulfonamides may acquire resistance to the drug.

Nonsusceptible organisms, including fungi, may proliferate with the use of this preparation.

Sulfonamides are inactivated by the p-aminobenzoic acid present in purulent exudates.

If signs of hypersensitivity or other untoward reactions occur, discontinue use of the preparation.

To prevent contaminating the dropper tip and solution, care should be taken not to touch the eye-lids or surrounding area with the dropper tip of the bottle. Keep bottle tightly closed when not in use and protect from light. Do not use if the solution has darkened or contains a precipitate.

For topical use only.

Carcinogenesis, Mutagenesis, and Impairment of Fertility: There have been no long-term studies done using sulfacetamide and/or phenylephrine in animals to evaluate carcinogenic potential.

Pregnancy Category C Animal reproduction studies have not been conducted with sulfacetamide and/or phenylephrine. It is also not known whether sulfacetamide and/or phenylephrine can cause fetal harm when administered to a pregnant woman or can affect reproduction capacity. Sulfacetamide and/or phenylephrine should be given to a pregnant woman only if clearly needed.

Nursing Mothers: It is not known whether these drugs are excreted in human milk. Because many drugs are excreted in human milk, caution should be exercised when sulfacetamide and/or phenylephrine is administered to a nursing woman.

Pediatric Use: Safety and effectiveness in children have not been established.

ADVERSE REACTIONS:

Headache or browache, blurred vision, local irritation, burning, transient stinging, transient epithelial keratitis, and reactive hyperemia. Sensitization reactions to sulfacetamide sodium may occur, although rarely.

Reactions occurring most often from the presence of the anti-infective ingredient are allergic sensitizations. Although hypersensitivity reactions to sulfacetamide sodium are rare, instances of Stevens-Johnson syndrome, systemic lupus erythematosus (in one case producing a fatal outcome), exfoliative dermatitis, toxic epidermal necrolysis, and photosensitivity have been reported following the use of sulfonamide preparations.

DOSAGE AND ADMINISTRATION:

Instill one or two drops into lower conjunctival sac every two or three hours during the day, less often at night.

HOW SUPPLIED - EQUIVALENTS NOT AVAILABLE:

Solution - Ophthalmic - 1.25 mg/150 mg

5 ml	**$9.30**	**VASOSULF OPHTHALMIC, Ciba Vision**	**00058-2883-05**
15 ml	**$12.54**	**VASOSULF OPHTHALMIC, Ciba Vision**	**00058-2883-15**

PHENYLPROPANOLAMINE HYDROCHLORIDE *(002027)*

CATEGORIES: Allergies; Anorexients/CNS Stimulants; Autonomic Drugs; Central Nervous System Agents; Nasal Congestion; Respiratory & Allergy Medications; Respiratory/Cerebral Stimulant; Sympathomimetic Agents; FDA Pre 1938 Drugs

BRAND NAMES: *Acutrim*; *Dexatrim*; *Disudrin*; *Fansia*; *Fugoa N*; Kleer; *Kontexin Retard*; *Monydrin*; *Monydrin Depottab*; *Pinru*; Propan; *Restaslim*;' Rhindecon; *Rinexin*; *Rinexin Depottab* ; *Slimfit*; *Slimomin*
(International brand names outside U.S. in italics)

Prescribing information not available at time of publication.

HOW SUPPLIED - EQUIVALENTS NOT AVAILABLE:

Capsule, Gelatin, Sustained Action - Oral - 75 mg

1000's	$28.00	Propan, C O Truxton	00463-3033-10

PHENYTOIN *(002029)*

CATEGORIES: Anticonvulsants; Antiepileptics; Central Nervous System Agents; Convulsions; Epilepsy; Hydantoin Anticonvulsants; Neuromuscular; Seizures; Tonic-Clonic Seizures; Sales > $100 Million; FDA Approval Pre 1982; Top 200 Drugs

BRAND NAMES: *Aladdin*; *Aleviatin*; *Antisacer*; *Cumatil*; *Dantoin*; *Decatona*; **Dilantin Infatabs**; Dilantin Injection; Dilantin Suspension; *Dintoina*; *Ditoin*; *Ditomed*; *Epamin*; *Epanutin*; *Epilantin-E*; *Eptoin*; *Fenantoin*; *Fenytoin*; *Hidantoina*; *Hydantin*; *Hydantol*; *Lehydan*; *Neosidantoina*; *Phenilep*; *Pyoredol*; *Zentropil*
(International brand names outside U.S. in italics)

FORMULARIES: Aetna; BC-BS; CIGNA; DoD; FHP; Humana; Kaiser; Medco; Medi-Cal; PCS; PruCare; United; WHO

DESCRIPTION:

(Note: This monograph pertains to the tablets, the pediatric oral suspension, and the injection.)

Phenytoin is an antiepileptic drug.

DESCRIPTION: *(cont'd)*

Phenytoin is related to the barbiturates in chemical structure, but has a five-membered ring. The chemical name is 5,5-diphenyl-2,4-imidazolidinedione.

Each Phenytoin Infatab, for oral administration, contains 50 mg phenytoin, USP. Also contains: D&C yellow No. 10, Al lake; FD&C yellow No. 6, Al lake; flavor; saccharin sodium, USP; sucrose, NF; talc, USP; and other ingredients.

Each teaspoonful of suspension contains 30 mg or 125 mg of phenytoin, USP with a maximum alcohol content not greater than 0.6 percent. Also contains carboxymethylcellulose sodium, USP; citric acid, anhydrous, USP; flavors; glycerin, USP; magnesium aluminum silicate, NF; polysorbate 40 NF; purified water, USP; sodium benzoate, NF; sucrose, NF; vanillin, NF. The 30 mg per teaspoonful suspension also contains D&C red No.33; FD&C red No. 40. The 125 mg per teaspoonful suspension also contains FD&C yellow No. 6.

Phenytoin sodium injection, USP is a sterile solution for IM or slow IV use, containing in each ml phenytoin sodium 50 mg, propylene glycol 0.4 ml and alcohol 0.1 ml in Water for Injection, ph 10.0-12.3; sodium hydroxide added, if needed, for pH adjustment.

Important Note: The parenteral form of this drug must be administered slowly. In adults, do not exceed 50 mg per minute intravenously. In neonates, the drug should be administered at a rate not exceeding 1-3 mg/kg/min.

CLINICAL PHARMACOLOGY:

Phenytoin is an antiepileptic drug which can be useful in the treatment of epilepsy. The primary site of action appears to be the motor cortex where spread of seizure activity is inhibited. Possibly by promoting sodium efflux from neurons, phenytoin tends to stabilize the threshold against hyperexcitability caused by excessive stimulation or environmental changes capable of reducing membrane sodium gradient. This includes the reduction of posttetanic potentiation at synapses. Loss of posttetanic potentiation prevents cortical seizure foci from detonating adjacent cortical areas. Phenytoin reduces the maximal activity of brain stem centers responsible for the tonic phase of tonic-clonic (grand mal) seizures.

Clinical studies using Phenytoin Infatabs have shown an average plasma half-life of 14 hours with a range of 7 to 29 hours. Steady-state therapeutic levels are achieved at least 7 to 10 days (5-7 half-lives) after initiation of therapy with recommended doses of 300 mg/day. The plasma half-life in man after oral administration of the pediatric suspension phenytoin averages 22 hours, with a range of 7 to 42 hours. Steady-state therapeutic levels are achieved at least 7 to 10 days (5-7 half-lives) after initiation of therapy with recommended doses of 300 mg/day.

When serum level determinations are necessary, they should be obtained at least 5-7 half-lives after treatment initiation, dosage change, or addition or subtraction of another drug to the regimen so that equilibrium or steady-state will have been achieved. Trough levels provide information about clinically effective serum level range and confirm patient compliance and are obtained just prior to the patient's next scheduled dose. Peak levels indicate an individual's threshold for emergence of dose-related side effects and are obtained at the time of expected peak concentration. For Phenytoin Infatabs peak levels occur 1 1/2-3 hours after administration.

Optimum control without clinical signs of toxicity occurs more often with serum levels between 10 and 20 mcg/ml, although some mild cases of tonic-clonic (grand mal) epilepsy may be controlled with lower serum levels of phenytoin.

In most patients maintained at a steady dosage, stable phenytoin serum levels are achieved. There may be wide interpatient variability in phenytoin serum levels with equivalent dosages. Patients with unusually low levels may be noncompliant or hypermetabolizers of phenytoin. Unusually high levels result from liver disease, congenital enzyme deficiency or drug interactions which result in metabolic interference. The patient with large variations in phenytoin plasma levels, despite standard doses, presents a difficult clinical problem. Serum level determinations in such patients may be particularly helpful. As phenytoin is highly protein bound, free phenytoin levels may be altered in patients whose protein binding characteristics differ from normal.

Most of the drug is excreted in the bile as inactive metabolites which are then reabsorbed from the intestinal tract and excreted in the urine. Urinary excretion of phenytoin and its metabolites occurs partly with glomerular filtration but, more importantly, by tubular secretion. Because phenytoin is hydroxylated in the liver by an enzyme system which is saturable at high plasma levels small incremental doses may increase the half-life and produce very substantial increases in serum levels, when these are in the upper range. The steady-state level may be disproportionately increased, with resultant intoxication, from an increase in dosage of 10% or more.

Clinical studies show that chewed and unchewed Phenytoin Infatabs are bioequivalent, yield approximately equivalent plasma levels, and are more rapidly absorbed than 100-mg Phenytoin Kapseals.

Additional Information For The Injection: The plasma half-life in man after IV administration ranges from 10 to 15 hours. Optimum control without clinical signs of toxicity occurs most often with serum levels between 10 and 20 mcg/ml.

A fall in plasma levels may occur when patients are changed from oral to IM administration. The drop is caused by slower absorption, as compared to oral administration, due to poor water solubility of phenytoin. IV administration is the preferred route for producing therapeutic serum levels.

There are occasions when IM administration may be required, i.e. postoperatively, in comatose patients, for GI upsets. During these periods, a sufficient dose must be administered intramuscularly to maintain the plasma level within the therapeutic range. Where oral dosage is resumed following IM usage, the oral dose should be properly adjusted to compensate for the slow continuing IM absorption to avoid toxic syndromes.

Patients stabilized on a daily oral regimen of phenytoin experience a drop in peak blood levels to 50-60 percent of stable levels if crossed over to an equal dose administered intramuscularly. However, the IM depot of poorly soluble material is eventually absorbed, as determined by urinary excretion of 5-(p-hydroxyphenyl)-5-phenylhydantoin (HPPH), the principal metabolite, as well as the total amount of drug eventually appearing in the blood.

A short-term (one week) study indicates that patients do not experience the expected drop in blood levels when crossed over to the IM route if the phenytoin IM dose is increased by 50% over the previously established oral dose. To avoid drug cumulation due to absorption from the muscle depots, it is recommended that for the first week back on oral phenytoin, the dose will be reduced to half of the original oral dose (one-third of the IM dose). Experience for periods greater than one week is lacking and blood level monitoring is recommended. For administration of phenytoin in patients who cannot take oral medication for periods greater than a week, gastric intubation may be considered.

INDICATIONS AND USAGE:

Phenytoin Infatabs are indicated for the control of generalized tonic-clonic (grand mal) and complex partial (psychomotor, temporal lobe) seizures and prevention and treatment of seizures occurring during or following neurosurgery. Phenytoin serum level determinations may be necessary for optimal dosage adjustments (see DOSAGE AND ADMINISTRATION and CLINICAL PHARMACOLOGY).

CONTRAINDICATIONS:

Phenytoin is contraindicated in those patients who are hypersensitive to phenytoin or other hydantoins.

Additional Information For The Injection: Because of its effect on ventricular automaticity, phenytoin is contraindicated in sinus bradycardia, sino-atrial block, second and third degree A-V block, and patients with Adams-Stokes syndrome.

WARNINGS:

Abrupt withdrawal of phenytoin in epileptic patients may precipitate status epilepticus. When, in the judgment of the clinician, the need for dosage reduction, discontinuation, or substitution of alternative antiepileptic medication arises, this should be done gradually. However, in the event of an allergic or hypersensitivity reaction, rapid substitution of alternative therapy may be necessary. In this case, alternative therapy should be an anti-epileptic drug not belonging to the hydantoin chemical class.

There have been a number of reports suggesting a relationship between phenytoin and the development of lymphadenopathy (local or generalized) including benign lymph node hyperplasia, pseudolymphoma, lymphoma, and Hodgkin's disease. Although a cause and effect relationship has not been established, the occurrence of lymphadenopathy indicates the need to differentiate such a condition from other types of lymph node pathology. Lymph node involvement may occur with or without symptoms and signs resembling serum sickness, e.g. fever, rash and liver involvement. In all cases of lymphadenopathy, follow-up observation for an extended period is indicated and every effort should be made to achieve seizure control using alternative antiepileptic drugs.

Acute alcoholic intake may increase phenytoin serum levels while chronic alcoholic use may decrease serum levels.

In view of isolated reports associating phenytoin with exacerbation of porphyria, caution should be exercised in using this medication in patients suffering from this disease.

USE IN PREGNANCY

A number of reports suggest an association between the use of antiepileptic drugs by women with epilepsy and a higher incidence of birth defects in children born to these women. Data are more extensive with respect to phenytoin and phenobarbital, but these are also the most commonly prescribed antiepileptic drugs; less systematic or anecdotal reports suggest a possible similar association with the use of all known antiepileptic drugs.

The reports suggesting a higher incidence of birth defects in children of drug-treated epileptic women cannot be regarded as adequate to prove a definite cause and effect relationship. There are intrinsic methodologic problems in obtaining adequate data on drug teratogenicity in humans; genetic factors or the epileptic condition itself may be more important than drug therapy in leading to birth defects. The great majority of mothers on antiepileptic medication deliver normal infants. It is important to note that antiepileptic drugs should not be discontinued in patients in whom the drug is administered to prevent major seizures, because of the strong possibility of precipitating status epilepticus with attendant hypoxia and threat to life. In individual cases where the severity and frequency of the seizure disorder are such that the removal of medication does not pose a serious threat to the patient, discontinuation of the drug may be considered prior to and during pregnancy, although it cannot be said with any confidence that even minor seizures do not pose some hazard to the developing embryo or fetus. The prescribing physician will wish to weigh these considerations in treating or counseling epileptic women of childbearing potential.

In addition to the reports of increased incidence of congenital malformations, such as cleft lip/palate and heart malformations, in children of women receiving phenytoin and other antiepileptic drugs, there have more recently been reports of a fetal hydantoin syndrome. This consists of prenatal growth deficiency, microcephaly and mental deficiency in children born to mothers who have received phenytoin, barbiturates, alcohol, or trimethadione. However, these features are all interrelated and are frequently associated with intrauterine growth retardation from other causes.

There have been isolated reports of malignancies, including neuroblastoma, in children whose mothers received phenytoin during pregnancy.

An increase in seizure frequency during pregnancy occurs in a high proportion of patients, because of altered phenytoin absorption or metabolism. Periodic measurement of serum phenytoin levels is particularly valuable in the management of a pregnant epileptic patient as a guide to an appropriate adjustment of dosage. However, postpartum restoration of the original dosage will probably be indicated.

Neonatal coagulation defects have been reported within the first 24 hours in babies born to epileptic mothers receiving phenobarbital and/or phenytoin. Vitamin K has been shown to prevent or correct this defect and has been recommended to be given to the mother before delivery and to the neonate after birth.

Additional Information For The Injection: IV administration should not exceed 50 mg per minute. In neonates, the drug should be administered at a rate not exceeding 1-3 mg/kg/min.

Severe cardiotoxic reactions and fatalities have been reported with atrial and ventricular conduction depression and ventricular fibrillation. Severe complications are most commonly encountered in elderly or gravely ill patients.

Hypotension usually occurs when the drug is administered rapidly by the IV route.

PRECAUTIONS:

GENERAL

The liver is the chief site of biotransformation of phenytoin; patients with impaired liver function, elderly patients, or those who are gravely ill may show early signs of toxicity.

A small percentage of individuals who have been treated with phenytoin have been shown to metabolize the drug slowly. Slow metabolism may be due to limited enzyme availability and lack of induction; it appears to be genetically determined.

Phenytoin should be discontinued if a skin rash appears (see WARNINGS regarding drug discontinuation). If the rash is exfoliative, purpuric, or bullous or if lupus erythematosus, Stevens-Johnson syndrome, or toxic epidermal necrolysis is suspected, use of this drug should not be resumed and alternative therapy should be considered. (See ADVERSE REACTIONS.) If the rash is of a milder type (measles-like or scarlatiniform), therapy may be resumed after the rash has completely disappeared. If the rash recurs upon reinstitution of therapy, further phenytoin medication is contraindicated.

Phenytoin and other hydantoins are contraindicated in patients who have experienced phenytoin hypersensitivity. Additionally, caution should be exercised if using structurally similar (*e.g.*, barbiturates, succinimides, oxazolidinediones and other related compounds) in these same patients.

Hyperglycemia, resulting from the drug's inhibitory effects on insulin release, has been reported. Phenytoin may also raise the serum glucose level in diabetic patients.

Osteomalacia has been associated with phenytoin therapy and is considered to be due to phenytoin's interference with Vitamin D metabolism.

Phenytoin is not indicated for seizures due to hypoglycemic or other metabolic causes. Appropriate diagnostic procedures should be performed as indicated.

Phenytoin is not effective for absence (petit mal) seizures. If tonic-clonic (grand mal) and absence (petit mal) seizures are present, combined drug therapy is needed.

PRECAUTIONS: *(cont'd)*

Serum levels of phenytoin sustained above the optimal range may produce confusional states referred to as "delirium," "psychosis," or "encephalopathy," or rarely irreversible cerebellar dysfunction. Accordingly, at the first sign of acute toxicity, plasma levels are recommended. Dose reduction of phenytoin therapy is indicated if plasma levels are excessive; if symptoms persist, termination is recommended. (See WARNINGS.)

INFORMATION FOR THE PATIENT

Patients taking phenytoin should be advised of the importance of adhering strictly to the prescribed dosage regimen, and of informing the physician of any clinical condition in which it is not possible to take the drug orally as prescribed, e.g. surgery, etc.

Patients should also be cautioned on the use of other drugs or alcoholic beverages without first seeking the physician's advice.

Patients should be instructed to call their physician if skin rash develops.

The importance of good dental hygiene should be stressed in order to minimize the development of gingival hyperplasia and its complications.

LABORATORY TESTS

Phenytoin serum level determinations may be necessary to achieve optimal dosage adjustments.

DRUG/LABORATORY TEST INTERACTIONS

Phenytoin may cause decreased serum levels of protein-bound iodine (PBI). It may also produce lower than normal values for dexamethasone or metyrapone tests. Phenytoin may cause increased serum levels of glucose, alkaline phosphatase, and gamma glutamyl transpeptidase (GGT).

CARCINOGENESIS

See WARNINGS section for information on carcinogenesis.

PREGNANCY

See WARNINGS section.

NURSING MOTHERS

Infant breast-feeding is not recommended for women taking this drug because phenytoin appears to be secreted in low concentrations in human milk.

Additional Information For The Injection: The addition of Phenytoin sodium injection, USP to IV infusion is not recommended due to lack of solubility and resultant precipitation.

Each injection of Phenytoin sodium should be followed by an injection of sterile saline through the same needle or IV catheter to avoid venous irritation due to the alkalinity of the solution. Continuous infusion should be avoided. Soft tissue irritation and inflammation has occurred at the site of injection with and without extravasation of intravenous phenytoin. Soft tissue irritation varying from slight tenderness to extensive necrosis and sloughing has been noted. Subcutaneous or perivascular injection should be avoided.

DRUG INTERACTIONS:

There are many drugs which may increase or decrease phenytoin levels or which phenytoin may affect. Serum level determinations for phenytoin are especially helpful when possible drug interactions are suspected. The most commonly occurring drug interactions are listed below:

1. Drugs which may increase phenytoin serum levels include: acute alcohol intake, amiodarone, chloramphenicol, chlordiazepoxide, diazepam, dicumarol, disulfiram, estrogens, H_2-antagonists, halothane, isoniazid, methylphenidate, phenothiazines, phenylbutazone, salicylates, succinimides, sulfonamides, tolbutamide, trazodone.

2. Drugs which may decrease phenytoin serum levels include: carbamazepine, chronic alcohol abuse, reserpine, and sucralfate. Moban brand of Molindone Hydrochloride contains calcium ions which interfere with the absorption of phenytoin. Ingestion times of phenytoin and antacid preparations containing calcium should be staggered in patients with low serum phenytoin levels to prevent absorption problems.

3. Drugs which may either increase or decrease phenytoin serum levels include: phenobarbital, sodium valproate, and valproic acid. Similarly, the effect of phenytoin on phenobarbital, valproic acid and sodium valproate serum levels is unpredictable.

4. Although not a true drug interaction, tricyclic antidepressants may precipitate seizures in susceptible patients and phenytoin dosage may need to be adjusted.

5. Drugs whose efficacy is impaired by phenytoin include: corticosteroids, coumarin anticoagulants, digitoxin, doxycycline, estrogens, furosemide, oral contraceptives, quinidine, rifampin, theophylline, vitamin D.

ADVERSE REACTIONS:

Central Nervous System:

The most common manifestations encountered with phenytoin therapy are referable to this system and are usually dose-related. These include nystagmus, ataxia, slurred speech, decreased coordination and mental confusion. Dizziness, insomnia, transient nervousness, motor twitchings, and headache have also been observed.

There have also been rare reports of phenytoin induced dyskinesias, including chorea, dystonia, tremor and asterixis, similar to those induced by phenothiazine and other neuroleptic drugs.

A predominantly sensory peripheral polyneuropathy has been observed in patients receiving long-term phenytoin therapy.

Gastrointestinal System:

Nausea, vomiting, constipation, toxic hepatitis and liver damage.

Integumentary System: Dermatological manifestations sometimes accompanied by fever have included scarlatiniform or morbilliform rashes. A morbilliform rash (measles-like) is the most common; other types of dermatitis are seen more rarely. Other more serious forms which may be fatal have included bullous, exfoliative or purpuric dermatitis, lupus erythematosus, Stevens-Johnson syndrome, and toxic epidermal necrolysis (see PRECAUTIONS.)

Hemopoietic System: Hemopoietic complications, some fatal, have occasionally been reported in association with administration of phenytoin. These have included thrombocytopenia, leukopenia, granulocytopenia, agranulocytosis, and pancytopenia with or without bone marrow suppression. While macrocytosis and megaloblastic anemia have occurred, these conditions usually respond to folic acid therapy. Lymphadenopathy including benign lymph node hyperplasia, pseudolymphoma, lymphoma, and Hodgkin's disease have been reported (see WARNINGS).

CONNECTIVE TISSUE SYSTEM

Coarsening of the facial features, enlargement of the lips, gingival hyperplasia, hypertrichosis and Peyronie's disease.

Cardiovascular: Periarteritis nodosa.

IMMUNOLOGIC

Hypersensitivity syndrome (which may include, but is not limited to, symptoms such as arthralgias, eosinophilia, fever, liver dysfunction, lymphadenopathy or rash), systemic lupus erythematosus, and immunoglobulin abnormalities.

ADVERSE REACTIONS: *(cont'd)*

Additional Information For The Injection: The most notable signs of toxicity associated with the IV use of this drug are cardiovascular collapse and/or central nervous system depression. Hypotension does occur when the drug is administered rapidly by the IV route. The *rate* of administration is very important; it should not exceed 50 mg per minute in adults, and 1-3 mg/kg/min in neonates. At this rate, toxicity should be minimized. Severe cardiotoxic reactions and fatalities have been reported with atrial and ventricular conduction depression and ventricular fibrillation. Severe complications are most commonly encountered in elderly or gravely ill patients.

Local irritation, inflammation, tenderness, necrosis and sloughing have been reported with or without the extravasation of IV phenytoin.

Systemic lupus erythematous, periarteris nodosa, toxic hepatitis, liver damage and immunoglobulin abnormalities may occur.

OVERDOSAGE:

The lethal dose in children is not known. The lethal dose in adults is estimated to be 2 to 5 grams. The initial symptoms are nystagmus, ataxia, and dysarthria. Other signs are tremor, hyperreflexia, lethargy, slurred speech, nausea, vomiting. The patient may become comatose and hypotensive. Death is due to respiratory and circulatory depression.

There are marked variations among individuals with respect to phenytoin plasma levels where toxicity may occur. Nystagmus on lateral gaze usually appears at 20 mcg/ml, ataxia at 30 mcg/ml, dysarthria and lethargy appear when the plasma concentration is over 40 mcg/ml, but as high a concentration as 50 mcg/ml has been reported without evidence of toxicity. As much as 25 times the therapeutic dose has been taken to result in a serum concentration over 100 mcg/ml with complete recovery.

TREATMENT

Treatment is nonspecific since there is no known antidote.

The adequacy of the respiratory and circulatory systems should be carefully observed and appropriate supportive measures employed. Hemodialysis can be considered since phenytoin is not completely bound to plasma proteins. Total exchange transfusion has been used in the treatment of severe intoxication in children.

In acute overdosage the possibility of other CNS depressants, including alcohol, should be borne in mind.

DOSAGE AND ADMINISTRATION:

Infatabs: When given in equal doses, Phenytoin Infatabs yield higher plasma levels than Phenytoin Kapseals. For this reason serum concentrations should be monitored and care should be taken when switching a patient from the sodium salt to the free acid form.

Phenytoin Kapseals, Phenytoin Parenteral, and Phenytoin with Phenobarbital are formulated with the sodium salt of phenytoin. The free acid form of phenytoin is used in Phenytoin-30 Pediatric and Phenytoin-125 Suspensions and Phenytoin Infatabs. Because there is approximately an 8% increase in drug content with the free acid form over that of the sodium salt, dosage adjustments and serum level monitoring may be necessary when switching from a product formulated with the free acid to a product formulated with the sodium salt and vice versa.

GENERAL

Not for once a day dosing.

Dosage should be individualized to provide maximum benefit. In some cases, serum blood level determinations may be necessary for optimal dosage adjustments-the clinically effective serum level is usually 10-20 mcg/ml. With recommended dosage, a period of seven to ten days may be required to achieve steady-state blood levels with phenytoin and changes in dosage (increase or decrease) should not be carried out at intervals shorter than seven to ten days.

Phenytoin Infatabs can be either chewed thoroughly before being swallowed or swallowed whole.

ADULT DOSAGE

Patients who have received no previous treatment may be started on two Infatabs three times daily, and the dose is then adjusted to suit individual requirements. For most adults, the satisfactory maintenance dosage will be six to eight Infatabs daily; an increase to twelve Infatabs daily may be made, if necessary.

PEDIATRIC DOSAGE

Initially, 5 mg/kg/day in two or three equally divided doses, with subsequent dosage individualized to a maximum of 300 mg daily. A recommended daily maintenance dosage is usually 4 to 8 mg/kg. Children over 6 years old may require the minimum adult dose (300 mg/day). If the daily dosage cannot be divided equally, the larger dose should be given before retiring.

Phenytoin Infatabs: Store at controlled room temperature 15-30°C (59°-86°F). Protect from moisture.

Phenytoin supplied in other forms: Store below 30°C (86°F).

Pediatric Oral Suspension: Dosage should be individualized to provide maximum benefit. In some cases, serum blood level determinations may be necessary for optimal dosage adjustments-the clinically effective serum level is usually 10-20 mcg/ml. With recommended dosage, a period of seven to ten days may be required to achieve steady-state blood levels with phenytoin and changes in dosage (increase or decrease) should not be carried out at intervals shorter than seven to ten days.

Adult Dosage: Patients who have received no previous treatment may be started on one teaspoonful (5 ml) of Phenytoin-125 suspension three times daily, and the dosage may then be adjusted to suit individual requirements. An increase to five teaspoonfuls daily may be made, if necessary.

Pediatric Dose: Initially, 5 mg/kg/day in two or three equally divided doses, with subsequent dosage individualized to a maximum of 300 mg daily. A recommended daily maintenance dosage is usually 4 to 8 mg/kg. Children over 6 years may require the minimum adult dose (300 mg/day).

Injection: The addition of Phenytoin Sodium Injection, USP to IV infusion is not recommended due to lack of solubility and resultant precipitation.

Not to exceed 50 mg per minute, intravenously in adults, and not exceeding 1-3 mg/kg/min in neonates. There is a relatively small margin between full therapeutic effect and minimally toxic doses of this drug.

The solution is suitable for use as long as it remains free of haziness and precipitate. Upon refrigeration or freezing, a precipitate might form; this will dissolve again after the solution is allowed to stand at room temperature. The product is still suitable for use. Only a c lear solution should be used. A faint yellow coloration may develop; however,this has no effect on the potency of the solution.

In the treatment of status epilepticus, the IV route is preferred because of the delay in absorption of phenytoin when administered intramuscularly.

Serum concentrations should be monitored and care should be taken when switching a patient from the sodium salt to the free acid form.

DOSAGE AND ADMINISTRATION: *(cont'd)*

STATUS EPILEPTICUS

In adults, a loading dose of 10 to 15 mg/kg should be administered slowly intravenously, at a rate not exceeding 50 mg per minute (this will require approximately 20 minutes in a 70 kg patient). The loading dose should be followed by maintenance doses of 100 mg orally or intravenously every 6-8 hours.

Recent work in neonates and children has shown that absorption pH phenytoin is unreliable after oral administration, but a loading dose of 15-20 mg/kg pH phenytoin intravenously will usually produce plasma concentrations of phenytoin within the generally accepted therapeutic range (10-20 mcg/ml). The drug should be injected slowly intravenously at a rate not exceeding 1-3 mg/kg/min.

Phenytoin Sodium Injection, USP should be injected *slowly* and directly into a large vein through a large-gauge needle or IV catheter. Each injection of IV phenytoin should be followed by an injection of sterile saline through the same needle or catheter to avoid local venous irritation due to the alkalinity of the solution. Continuous infusion should be avoided; the addition of phenytoin sodium injection, USP to IV infusion fluids is not recommended because of the likelihood of precipitation.

Continuous monitoring of the electrocardiogram and blood pressure is essential. The patient should be observed for signs of respiratory depression. Determination of phenytoin plasma levels is advised when using phenytoin in the management of status epilepticus and in the subsequent establishment of maintenance dosage.

Other measures, including concomitant administration of an IV benzodiazepine such as diazepam, or an IV short acting barbiturate, will usually be necessary for rapid control of seizures because of the required slow rate of administration of phenytoin.

If administration of Phenytoin Sodium Injection, USP does not terminate seizures, the use of other anticonvulsants, IV barbiturates, general anesthesia and other appropriate measures should be considered.

IM administration should not be used in the treatment of status epilepticus because the attainment of peak plasma levels may require up to 24 hours.

NEUROSURGERY

Prophylactic dosage-100 to 200 mg (2 to 4 ml) intramuscularly at approximately 4 hour intervals during surgery and continued during the postoperative period. When IM administration is required for a patient previously stabilized orally, compensating dosage adjustments are necessary to maintain therapeutic plasma levels. An IM dose 50% greater than the oral dose is necessary to maintain these levels. When returned to oral administration, the dose should be reduced by 50% of the original dose for one week to prevent excessive plasma levels due to sustained release from intramuscular tissue sites.

If the patient requires more than a week of IM phenytoin, alternative routes should be explored, such as gastric intubation. For time periods less than one week, the patient shifted back from IM administration should receive one half the original dose for the same period of time the patient received IM phenytoin. Monitoring plasma levels would help prevent a fall into the sub-therapeutic range. Serum blood level determinations are especially helpful when possible drug interactions are suspected.

Parenteral drug products should be inspected visually for particulate matter and discoloration prior to administration, whenever solution and container permit.

Store at controlled room temperature 15-30°C (59-86°F).

PATIENT INFORMATION:

Phenytoin is used to treat seizure disorders. This drug should not be used by some patients with specific heart diseases. This medication must be monitored very closely and therefore you will have blood drawn periodically to determine how much drug is in your blood. The medication works best when the level of medication in the blood is kept constant. When blood levels get too low, a seizure may result. When blood levels get too high, side effects occur. Blood levels should normally be between 10 to 20 micrograms per milliliter. It may take several dose adjustment to find the right dose for you. It is very important then to take the medication exactly as prescribed. This is also one medication where changing between brands is not recommended. Alcoholic beverages should be avoided. This medication has many side effects and you should discuss all medicines with your doctor or pharmacist. If you develop a rash call your doctor or pharmacist immediately. You may be instructed on the importance of oral hygiene. This drug, with long term use, can cause gum growth. Other common side effects include: eye movements, loss of coordination, confusion and slurred speech. Report any of these side effects to your doctor or pharmacist immediately.

HOW SUPPLIED - RATED THERAPEUTICALLY EQUIVALENT:

Injection, Solution - Intramuscular; - 50 mg/ml

2 ml	$2.43	Phenytoin Sodium 50, Abbott	00074-1317-01
2 ml	$78.13	Phenytoin Sodium, Solopak Labs	39769-0034-02
2 ml x 10	$12.94	Phenytoin Sodium, Sanofi Winthrop	00024-1549-01
2 ml x 10	$49.32	DILANTIN, Parke-Davis	00071-4488-41
2 ml x 25	$25.00	Phenytoin Sodium, Elkins Sinn	00641-1465-35
2 ml x 25	$36.00	DILANTIN, Parke-Davis	00071-4488-45
2 ml x 25	$40.00	Phenytoin Sodium Injection, Elkins Sinn	00641-0493-25
5 ml	$2.85	Phenytoin Sodium 50, Abbott	00074-1317-02
5 ml	$5.49	Phenytoin Sodium Kit, Abbott	00074-1185-01
5 ml	$84.38	Phenytoin Sodium, Solopak Labs	39769-0034-05
5 ml x 10	$20.71	Phenytoin Sodium, Sanofi Winthrop	00024-1549-05
5 ml x 25	$15.00	Phenytoin Sodium, Voluntary Hosp	53258-1615-02
5 ml x 25	$42.00	DILANTIN, Parke-Davis	00071-4475-45
5 ml x 25	$47.50	Phenytoin Sodium, Elkins Sinn	00641-2555-45
5 ml x 25	$51.46	Phenytoin Sodium, Sanofi Winthrop	00024-1549-25

Suspension - Oral - 125 mg/5ml

4 ml x 50	$54.04	Phenytoin, Xactdose	50962-0228-04
4 ml x 50	$69.56	Phenytoin, UDL	51079-0674-10
4 ml x 100	$107.00	Phenytoin, Xactdose	50962-0225-04
12 ml x 100	$248.41	Phenytoin, Xactdose	50962-0225-12
240 ml	$29.66	DILANTIN-125, Parke-Davis	00071-2214-20

HOW SUPPLIED - NOT RATED EQUIVALENT:

Tablet, Chewable - Oral - 50 mg

10 x 10	**$29.00**	**DILANTIN INFATABS, Parke-Davis**	**00071-0007-40**
100's	**$20.45**	**DILANTIN INFATABS, Parke-Davis**	**00071-0007-24**

PHENYTOIN SODIUM CAPSULES *(002030)*

CATEGORIES: Anticonvulsants; Antiepileptics; Central Nervous System Agents; Central Pain Syndromes; Convulsions; Epilepsy; Hydantoin Anticonvulsants; Neuromuscular; Seizures; Tonic-Clonic Seizures; Sales > $100 Million; FDA Approval Pre 1982

BRAND NAMES: *Aleviatin* (Japan); *Antisacer*; *Cumatil*; *Difhydan*; *Di-hydan* (France); **Dilantin**; Dilantin Kapseals; *Dintoina*; *Diphantoine*; *Diphantoine-Z*; Diphen; Diphentoin; Diphenylan Sodium; *Ditoin*; *Ditomed*; Dyatoin; *Epamin*; *Epanutin* (England, Germany); *Epilan-D*; *Epilantin*; *Epileptin*; *Epsolin*; *Eptoin*; *Fenatoin NM*; *Fenidantoin S 100* (Mexico); *Fenitron* (Mexico); *Fenytoin* (Germany); *Hidanil*; *Hydantin*; *Hydantol* (Japan); *Lehydan*; *Neosidantoina*; *Nuctane* (Mexico); *Phenhydan* (Germany); *Phenilep*; *Phenytoin KP*; Phenytex; Prompt Phenytoin Sodium; *Pyoredol* (France); *Zentropil* (Germany)
(International brand names outside U.S. in italics)

FORMULARIES: Aetna; BC-BS; CIGNA; DoD; FHP; Humana; Kaiser; Medco; Medi-Cal; PCS; PruCare; United

COST OF THERAPY: $74.46 (Epilepsy; Capsule; 100 mg; 3/day; 365 days)

DESCRIPTION:

Phenytoin sodium is an antiepileptic drug. Phenytoin sodium is related to the barbiturates in chemical structure, but has a five-membered ring. The chemical name is sodium 5, 5-diphenyl-2, 4-imidazolidinedione.

Each Phenytoin Sodium Capsules USP—contains 30 mg or 100 mg phenytoin sodium, USP. Also contains lactose, NF; sucrose, NF; talc, USP; and other ingredients. The capsule shell and band contain colloidal silicon dioxide, NF; FD&C red No. 3; gelatin, NF; glyceryl monooleate; sodium lauryl sulfate, NF. The Phenytoin Sodium Capsules 30-mg capsule shell and band also contain citric acid, USP; FD&C blue No. 1; sodium benzoate, NF; titanium dioxide, USP. The Phenytoin Sodium Capsules 100-mg capsule shell and band also contain FD&C yellow No. 6; hydrogen peroxide 3%; polyethylene glycol 200. Product in vivo performance is characterized by a slow and extended rate of absorption with peak blood concentrations expected in 4 to 12 hours as contrasted to *Prompt Phenytoin Sodium Capsules,* USP with a rapid rate of absorption with peak blood concentration expected in 1 1/2 to 3 hours.

CLINICAL PHARMACOLOGY:

Phenytoin is an antiepileptic drug which can be useful in the treatment of epilepsy. The primary site of action appears to be the *motor cortex* where spread of seizure activity is inhibited. Possibly by promoting sodium efflux from neurons, phenytoin tends to*stabilize* the threshold against hyperexcitability caused by excessive stimulation or environmental changes capable of reducing membrane sodium gradient. This includes the reduction of posttetanic potentiation at synapses. Loss of posttetanic potentiation prevents cortical seizure foci from detonating adjacent cortical areas. Phenytoin reduces the maximal activity of brain stem centers responsible for the tonic phase of tonic-clonic (grand mal) seizures.

The plasma half-life in man after oral administration of phenytoin averages 22 hours, with a range of 7 to 42 hours. Steady-state therapeutic levels are achieved at least 7 to 10 days (5-7 half-lives) after initiation of therapy with recommended doses of 300 mg/day.

When serum level determinations are necessary, they should be obtained at least 5-7 half-lives after treatment initiation, dosage change, or addition or subtraction of another drug to the regimen so that equilibrium or steady-state will have been achieved. Trough levels provide information about clinically effective serum level range and confirm patient compliance and are obtained just prior to the patient's next scheduled dose. Peak levels indicate an individual's threshold for emergence of dose-related side effects and are obtained at the time of expected peak concentration. For Phenytoin Sodium Capsules Kapseals peak serum levels occur 4-12 hours after administration.

Optimum control without clinical signs of toxicity occurs more often with serum levels between 10 and 20 mcg/ml, although some mild cases of tonic-clonic (grand mal) epilepsy may be controlled with lower serum levels of phenytoin.

In most patients maintained at a steady dosage, stable phenytoin serum levels are achieved. There may be wide interpatient variability in phenytoin serum levels with equivalent dosages. Patients with unusually low levels may be noncompliant or hypermetabolizers of phenytoin. Unusually high levels result from liver disease, congenital enzyme deficiency or drug interactions which result in metabolic interference. The patient with large variations in phenytoin plasma levels, despite standard doses, presents a difficult clinical problem. Serum level determinations in such patients may be particularly helpful. As phenytoin is highly protein bound, free phenytoin levels may be altered in patients whose protein binding characteristics differ from normal.

Most of the drug is excreted in the bile as inactive metabolites which are then reabsorbed from the intestinal tract and excreted in the urine. Urinary excretion of phenytoin and its metabolites occurs partly with glomerular filtration but, more importantly, by tubular secretion. Because phenytoin is hydroxylated in the liver by an enzyme system which is saturable at high plasma levels, small incremental doses may increase the half-life and produce very substantial increases in serum levels, when these are in the upper range. The steady-state level may be disproportionately increased, with resultant intoxication, from an increase in dosage of 10% or more.

INDICATIONS AND USAGE:

Phenytoin Sodium Capsules is indicated for the control of generalized tonic-clonic (grand mal) and complex partial (psychomotor, temporal lobe) seizures and prevention and treatment of seizures occurring during or following neurosurgery.

Phenytoin serum level determinations may be necessary for optimal dosage adjustments (see DOSAGE AND ADMINISTRATION and CLINICAL PHARMACOLOGY).

CONTRAINDICATIONS:

Phenytoin is contraindicated in those patients who are hypersensitive to phenytoin or other hydantoins.

WARNINGS:

Abrupt withdrawal of phenytoin in epileptic patients may precipitate status epilepticus. When, in the judgment of the clinician, the need for dosage reduction, discontinuation, or substitution of alternative antiepileptic medication arises, this should be done gradually. However, in the event of an allergic or hypersensitivity reaction, rapid substitution of alternative therapy may be necessary. In this case, alternative therapy should be an antiepileptic drug not belonging to the hydantoin chemical class.

There have been a number of reports suggesting a relationship between phenytoin and the development of lymphadenopathy (local or generalized) including benign lymph node hyperplasia, pseudolymphoma, lymphoma, and Hodgkin's Disease. Although a cause and effect relationship has not been established, the occurrence of lymphadenopathy indicates the need to differentiate such a condition from other types of lymph node pathology. Lymph node involvement may occur with or without symptoms and signs resembling serum sickness, e.g., fever, rash and liver involvement.

In all cases of lymphadenopathy, follow-up observation for an extended period is indicated and every effort should be made to achieve seizure control using alternative antiepileptic drugs.

WARNINGS: *(cont'd)*

Acute alcoholic intake may increase phenytoin serum levels while chronic alcoholic use may decrease serum levels.

In view of isolated reports associating phenytoin with exacerbation of porphyria, caution should be exercised in using this medication in patients suffering from this disease.

USE IN PREGNANCY

A number of reports suggests an association between the use of antiepileptic drugs by women with epilepsy and a higher incidence of birth defects in children born to these women. Data are more extensive with respect to phenytoin and phenobarbital, but these are also the most commonly prescribed antiepileptic drugs; less systematic or anecdotal reports suggest a possible similar association with the use of all known antiepileptic drugs.

The reports suggesting a higher incidence of birth defects in children of drug-treated epileptic women cannot be regarded as adequate to prove a definite cause and effect relationship. There are intrinsic methodologic problems in obtaining adequate data on drug teratogenicity in humans; genetic factors or the epileptic condition itself may be more important than drug therapy in leading to birth defects. The great majority of mothers on antiepileptic medication deliver normal infants. It is important to note that antiepileptic drugs should not be discontinued in patients in whom the drug is administered to prevent major seizures, because of the strong possibility of precipitating status epilepticus with attendant hypoxia and threat to life. In individual cases where the severity and frequency of the seizure disorder are such that the removal of medication does not pose a serious threat to the patient, discontinuation of the drug may be considered prior to and during pregnancy, although it cannot be said with any confidence that even minor seizures do not pose some hazard to the developing embryo or fetus. The prescribing physician will wish to weigh these considerations in treating or counseling epileptic women of childbearing potential.

In addition to the reports of increased incidence of congenital malformation, such as cleft lip/palate and heart malformations, in children of women receiving phenytoin and other antiepileptic drugs, there have more recently been reports of a fetal hydantoin syndrome. This consists of prenatal growth deficiency, microcephaly and mental deficiency in children born to mothers who have received phenytoin, barbiturates, alcohol, or trimethadione. However, these features are all inter-related and are frequently associated with intrauterine growth retardation from other causes.

There have been isolated reports of malignancies, including neuroblastoma, in children whose mothers received phenytoin during pregnancy.

An increase in seizure frequency during pregnancy occurs in a high proportion of patients, because of altered phenytoin absorption or metabolism. Periodic measurement of serum phenytoin levels is particularly valuable in the management of a pregnant epileptic patient as a guide to an appropriate adjustment of dosage. However, postpartum restoration of the original dosage will probably be indicated.

Neonatal coagulation defects have been reported within the first 24 hours in babies born to epileptic mothers receiving phenobarbital and/or phenytoin. Vitamin K has been shown to prevent or correct this defect and has been recommended to be given to the mother before delivery and to the neonate after birth.

PRECAUTIONS:

GENERAL

The liver is the chief site of biotransformation of phenytoin; patients with impaired liver function, elderly patients, or those who are gravely ill may show early signs of toxicity.

A small percentage of individuals who have been treated with phenytoin has been shown to metabolize the drug slowly. Slow metabolism may be due to limited enzyme availability and lack of induction; it appears to be genetically determined.

Phenytoin should be discontinued if a skin rash appears (see WARNINGS regarding drug discontinuation). If the rash is exfoliative, purpuric, or bullous or if lupus erythematosus, Stevens-Johnson syndrome, or toxic epidermal necrolysis is suspected, use of this drug should not be resumed and alternative therapy should be considered. (See ADVERSE REACTIONS.) If the rash is of a milder type (measles-like or scarlatiniform), therapy may be resumed after the rash has completely disappeared. If the rash recurs upon reinstitution of therapy, further phenytoin medication is contraindicated.

Phenytoin and other hydantoins are contraindicated in patients who have experienced phenytoin hypersensitivity. Additionally, caution should be exercised if using structurally similar compounds (*e.g.,* barbiturates, succinimides, oxazolidinediones and other related compounds) in these same patients.

Hyperglycemia, resulting from the drug's inhibitory effects on insulin release, has been reported. Phenytoin may also raise the serum glucose level in diabetic patients.

Osteomalacia has been associated with phenytoin therapy and is considered to be due to phenytoin's interference with Vitamin D metabolism.

Phenytoin is not indicated for seizures due to hypoglycemic or other metabolic causes. Appropriate diagnostic procedures should be performed as indicated.

Phenytoin is not effective for absence (petit mal) seizures. If tonic-clonic (grand mal) and absence (petit mal) seizures are present, combined drug therapy is needed.

Serum levels of phenytoin sustained above the optimal range may produce confusional states referred to as "delirium," "psychosis," or "encephalopathy," or rarely irreversible cerebellar dysfunction. Accordingly, at the first sign of acute toxicity, plasma levels are recommended. Dose reduction of phenytoin therapy is indicated if plasma levels are excessive; if symptoms persist, termination is recommended. (See WARNINGS.)

INFORMATION FOR THE PATIENT

Patients taking phenytoin should be advised of the importance of adhering strictly to the prescribed dosage regimen, and of informing the physician of any clinical condition in which it is not possible to take the drug orally as prescribed, e.g., surgery, etc.

Patients should also be cautioned on the use of other drugs or alcoholic beverages without first seeking the physician's advice.

Patients should be instructed to call their physician if skin rash develops.

The importance of good dental hygiene should be stressed in order to minimize the development of gingival hyperplasia and its complications.

Do not use capsules which are discolored.

Laboratory Tests: Phenytoin serum level determinations may be necessary to achieve optimal dosage adjustments.

Drug/Laboratory Test Interactions: Phenytoin may cause decreased serum levels of protein-bound iodine (PBI). It may also produce lower than normal values for dexamethasone or metyrapone tests. Phenytoin may cause increased serum levels of glucose, alkaline phosphatase, and gamma glutamyl transpeptidase (GGT).

Carcinogenesis: See WARNINGS for information on carcinogenesis.

Pregnancy: See WARNINGS.

Nursing Mothers: Infant breast-feeding is not recommended for women taking this drug because phenytoin appears to be secreted in low concentrations in human milk.

DRUG INTERACTIONS:

There are many drugs which may increase or decrease phenytoin levels or which phenytoin may affect. Serum level determinations for phenytoin are especially helpful when possible drug interactions are suspected. The most commonly occurring drug interactions are listed.

1. Drugs which may increase phenytoin serum levels include: acute alcohol intake, amiodarone, chloramphenicol, chlordiazepoxide, diazepam, dicumarol, disulfiram, estrogens, H_2-antagonists, halothane, isoniazid, methylphenidate, phenothiazines, phenylbutazone, salicylates, succinimides, sulfonamides, tolbutamide, trazodone.

2. Drugs which may decrease phenytoin levels include: carbamazepine, chronic alcohol abuse, reserpine, and sucralfate. Moban brand of molindone hydrochloride contains calcium ions which interfere with the absorption of phenytoin. Ingestion times of phenytoin and antacid preparations containing calcium should be staggered in patients with low serum phenytoin levels to prevent absorption problems.

3. Drugs which may either increase or decrease phenytoin serum levels include: phenobarbital, sodium valproate, and valproic acid. Similarly, the effect of phenytoin on phenobarbital, valproic acid and sodium valproate serum levels is unpredictable.

4. Although not a true drug interaction, tricyclic antidepressants may precipitate seizures in susceptible patients and phenytoin dosage may need to be adjusted.

5. Drugs whose efficacy is impaired by phenytoin include: corticosteroids, coumarin anticoagulants, digitoxin, doxycycline, estrogens, furosemide, oral contraceptives, quinidine, rifampin, theophylline, vitamin D.

ADVERSE REACTIONS:

Central Nervous System: The most common manifestations encountered with phenytoin therapy are referable to this system and are usually dose-related. These include nystagmus, ataxia, slurred speech, decreased coordination and mental confusion. Dizziness, insomnia, transient nervousness, motor twitchings, and headaches have also been observed. There have also been rare reports of phenytoin induced dyskinesias, including chorea, dystonia, tremor and asterixis, similar to those induced by phenothiazine and other neuroleptic drugs.

A predominantly sensory peripheral polyneuropathy has been observed in patients receiving long-term phenytoin therapy.

Gastrointestinal System: Nausea, vomiting, constipation, toxic hepatitis and liver damage.

Integumentary System: Dermatological manifestations sometimes accompanied by fever have included scarlatiniform or morbilliform rashes. A morbilliform rash (measles-like) is the most common; other types of dermatitis are seen more rarely. Other more serious forms which may be fatal have included bullous, exfoliative or purpuric dermatitis, lupus erythematosus, Stevens-Johnson syndrome, and toxic epidermal necrolysis (see PRECAUTIONS).

Hemopoietic System: Hemopoietic complications, some fatal, have occasionally been reported in association with administration of phenytoin. These have included thrombocytopenia, leukopenia, granulocytopenia, agranulocytosis, and pancytopenia with or without bone marrow suppression. While macrocytosis and megaloblastic anemia have occurred, these conditions usually respond to folic acid therapy. Lymphadenopathy including benign lymph node hyperplasia, pseudolymphoma, lymphoma, and Hodgkin's Disease have been reported (see WARNINGS).

Connective Tissue System: Coarsening of the facial features, enlargement of the lips, gingival hyperplasia, hypertrichosis and Peyronie's Disease.

Cardiovascular: Periarteritis nodosa.

Immunologic: Hypersensitivity syndrome (which may include, but is not limited to, symptoms such as arthralgias, eosinophilia, fever, liver dysfunction, lymphadenopathy or rash), systemic lupus erythematosus, and immunoglobulin abnormalities.

OVERDOSAGE:

The lethal dose in children is not known. The lethal dose in adults is estimated to be 2 to 5 grams. The initial symptoms are nystagmus, ataxia, and dysarthria. Other signs are tremor, hyperreflexia, lethargy, slurred speech, nausea, vomiting. The patient may become comatose and hypotensive. Death is due to respiratory and circulatory depression.

There are marked variations among individuals with respect to phenytoin plasma levels where toxicity may occur. Nystagmus, on lateral gaze, usually appears at 20 mcg/ml, ataxia at 30 mcg/ml, dysarthria and lethargy appear when the plasma concentration is over 40 mcg/ml, but as high a concentration as 50 mcg/ml has been reported without evidence of toxicity. As much as 25 times the therapeutic dose has been taken to result in a serum concentration over 100 mcg/ml with complete recovery.

TREATMENT

Treatment is nonspecific since there is not known antidote.

The adequacy of the respiratory and circulatory systems should be carefully observed and appropriate supportive measures employed. Hemodialysis can be considered since phenytoin is not completely bound to plasma proteins. Total exchange transfusion has been used in the treatment of severe intoxication in children.

In acute overdosage the possibility of other CNS depressants, including alcohol, should be borne in mind.

DOSAGE AND ADMINISTRATION:

Serum concentrations should be monitored in changing from Extended Phenytoin Sodium Capsules, USP to Prompt Phenytoin Sodium Capsules, USP, and from the sodium salt to the free acid form.

Phenytoin Sodium Capsules, Phenytoin Sodium Capsules Parenteral, and Phenytoin Sodium Capsules with Phenobarbital are formulated with the sodium salt of phenytoin. The free acid form of phenytoin is used in Phenytoin Sodium Capsules-30 Pediatric and Phenytoin Sodium Capsules-125 Suspensions and Phenytoin Sodium Capsules Infatabs. Because there is approximately an 8% increase in drug content with the free acid form over that of the sodium salt, dosage adjustments and serum level monitoring may be necessary when switching from a product formulated with the free acid to a product formulated with the sodium salt and vice versa.

GENERAL

Dosage should be individualized to provide maximum benefit. In some cases, serum blood level determinations may be necessary for optimal dosage adjustments—the clinically effective serum level is usually 10-20 mcg/ml. With recommended dosage, a period of seven to ten days may be required to achieve steady-state blood levels with phenytoin and changes in dosage (increase or decrease) should not be carried out at intervals shorter than seven to ten days.

ADULT DOSAGE

Divided Daily Dosage: Patients who have received no previous treatment may be started on one 100-mg Extended Phenytoin Sodium Capsule three times daily and the dosage then adjusted to suit individual requirements. For most adults, the satisfactory maintenance dosage will be one capsule three to four times a day. An increase up to two capsules three times a day may be made, if necessary.

DOSAGE AND ADMINISTRATION: *(cont'd)*

Once-A-Day Dosage: In adults, if seizure control is established with divided doses of three 100-mg Phenytoin Sodium Capsules capsules daily, once-a-day dosage with 300 mg of extended phenytoin sodium capsules may be considered. Studies comparing divided doses of 300 mg with a single daily dose of this quantity indicated absorption, peak plasma levels, biologic half-life, difference between peak and minimum values, and urinary recovery were equivalent. Once-a-day dosage offers a convenience to the individual patient or to nursing personnel for institutionalized patients and is intended to be used only for patients requiring this amount of drug daily. A major problem in motivating noncompliant patients may also be lessened when the patient can take this drug once a day. However, patients should be cautioned not to miss a dose, inadvertently.

Only extended phenytoin sodium capsules are recommended for once-a-day dosing. Inherent differences in dissolution characteristics and resultant absorption rates of phenytoin due to different manufacturing procedures and/or dosage forms preclude such recommendation for other phenytoin products. When a change in the dosage form or brand is prescribed, careful monitoring of phenytoin serum levels should be carried out.

Loading Dose: Some authorities have advocated use of an oral loading dose of phenytoin in adults who require rapid steady-state serum levels and where intravenous administration is not desirable. This dosing regimen should be reserved for patients in a clinic or hospital setting where phenytoin serum levels can be closely monitored. Patients with a history of renal or liver disease should not receive the oral loading regimen.

Initially, one gram of phenytoin capsules is divided into 3 doses (400 mg, 300 mg, 300 mg) and administered at two-hourly intervals. Normal maintenance dosage is then instituted 24 hours after the loading dose, with frequent serum level determinations.

PEDIATRIC DOSAGE

Initially, 5 mg/kg/day in two or three equally divided doses, with subsequent dosage individualized to a maximum of 300 mg daily. A recommended daily maintenance dosage is usually 4 to 8 mg/kg. Children over 6 years old may require the minimum adult dose (300 mg/day).

Store below 30°C (86°F). Protect from light and moisture.

HOW SUPPLIED:

Kapseal 362, transparent #3 capsule with an orange band—Dilantin 100 mg
Kapseal 365, transparent #4 capsule with a pink band—Dilantin 30 mg

HOW SUPPLIED - EQUIVALENTS NOT AVAILABLE:

Capsule, Gelatin - Oral - 30 mg

100's	**$19.72**	**DILANTIN, Parke-Davis**	**00071-0365-24**

Capsule, Gelatin - Oral - 100 mg

10 x 10	**$23.96**	**DILANTIN, Parke-Davis**	**00071-0362-40**
100's	$6.80	Prompt Phenytoin Sodium, Zenith Labs	00172-2057-60
100's	**$21.72**	**DILANTIN, Parke-Davis**	**00071-0362-24**
1000's	$49.50	DI-PHEN, C O Truxton	00463-2007-10
1000's	$61.90	Phenytoin Sodium, Major Pharms	00904-2057-80
1000's	$63.20	Prompt Phenytoin Sodium, Zenith Labs	00172-2057-80
1000's	$63.20	PROMPT PHENYTOIN SODIUM 100, Goldline Labs	00182-0197-10
1000's	**$217.20**	**DILANTIN, Parke-Davis**	**00071-0362-32**

PHYSOSTIGMINE *(003153)*

CATEGORIES: Acetylcholine Protector; Alzheimer's Disease; Anticholinergic Agents; Central Nervous System Agents; Dementia; Neuromuscular; FDA Unapproved

BRAND NAMES: **Synapton**

Prescribing information not available at time of publication.

PHYSOSTIGMINE SALICYLATE *(002032)*

CATEGORIES: Anticholinergic Drug Inhibitors; Anticholinesterase; Antidotes; Autonomic Drugs; EENT Drugs; Eye, Ear, Nose, & Throat Preparations; Glaucoma; Miotics; Ophthalmics; Parasympathomimetic Agents; FDA Pre 1938 Drugs

BRAND NAMES: Antilirium; Eserine Salicylate; **Isopto Eserine**

FORMULARIES: Medi-Cal

Prescribing information not available at time of publication.

HOW SUPPLIED - EQUIVALENTS NOT AVAILABLE:

Injection, Solution - Intramuscular; - 1 mg/ml

2 ml x 10	$73.25	Physostigmine Salicylate, Hope Pharms	60267-0600-66
2 ml x 12	$111.16	ANTILIRIUM, Forest Pharms	00456-1037-12

Solution - Ophthalmic - 0.25 %

15 ml	**$11.87**	**ISOPTO ESERINE 1/4 %, Alcon-PR**	**00998-0261-15**

Solution - Ophthalmic - 0.5 %

15 ml	**$12.50**	**ISOPTO ESERINE, Alcon**	**00065-0262-15**
15 ml	**$12.50**	**ISOPTO ESERINE 1/2 %, Alcon-PR**	**00998-0262-15**

PHYSOSTIGMINE SULFATE *(002033)*

CATEGORIES: Autonomic Drugs; EENT Drugs; Eye, Ear, Nose, & Throat Preparations; Glaucoma; Miotics; Ophthalmics; Parasympathomimetic Agents; FDA Pre 1938 Drugs

BRAND NAMES: **Eserine Sulfate**

Prescribing information not available at time of publication.

HOW SUPPLIED - EQUIVALENTS NOT AVAILABLE:

Ointment - Ophthalmic - 0.25 %

3.5 gm	**$2.85**	**Eserine Sulfate, Consolidated Midland**	**00223-4122-03**
3.5 gm	$6.25	Physostigmine Sulfate, Fougera	00168-0068-38

PHYSOSTIGMINE; PILOCARPINE *(002034)*

CATEGORIES: EENT Drugs; Eye, Ear, Nose, & Throat Preparations; Glaucoma; Miotics; Ophthalmics; FDA Pre 1938 Drugs

BRAND NAMES: **Isopto P-Es**

Prescribing information not available at time of publication.

HOW SUPPLIED - EQUIVALENTS NOT AVAILABLE:

Solution - Ophthalmic - 0.25 %/2 %

15 ml	$15.00	ISOPTO P-ES, Alcon-PR	00998-0233-15

PHYTONADIONE *(002035)*

CATEGORIES: Anticoagulant Antagonists; Blood Formation/Coagulation; Hemorrhagic Disease; Hemostatics; Hypoprothrombinemia; Jaundice; Prothrombin Deficiency; Vitamin K Activity; Vitamins; Pregnancy Category C; FDA Approval Pre 1982

BRAND NAMES: Aquamephyton; *Kaywan*; **Konakion**; *Konakion 10 mg*; *Konakion (10 mg)* (England, Germany, Mexico); Mephyton; Phytomenadione; *Vitak* (Japan); Vitamin K1 Roche

(International brand names outside U.S. in italics)

FORMULARIES: Aetna; BC-BS; FHP; Medi-Cal; WHO

DESCRIPTION:

Phytonadione is a vitamin which is a clear, yellow to amber, viscous, and nearly odorless liquid. It is insoluble in water, soluble in chloroform and slightly soluble in ethanol. It has a molecular weight of 450.70.

Phytonadione is 2-methyl-3-phytyl-1, 4-naphthoquinone. Its empirical formula is $C_{31}H_{46}O_2$.

TABLETS

Mephyton (Phytonadione, MSD) tablets containing 5 mg of phytonadione are yellow, compressed tablets, scored on one side. Inactive ingredients are acacia, calcium phosphate, colloidal silicon dioxide, lactose, magnesium stearate, starch, and talc.

INJECTION

Konakion (phytonadione/Roche) injection, a prothrombogenic vitamin, is an essentially clear, light yellow, sterile, aqueous dispersion of vitamin K_1. It is intended for intramuscular administration only. Konakion injection is available in the following concentrations:

0.5 ml Ampuls: Each 0.5 ml contains 1 mg phytonadione (vitamin K_1) compounded with 10 mg polysorbate 80, 0.45% phenol as preservative, 10.4 mg propylene glycol, 0.17 mg sodium acetate and 0.00002 ml glacial acetic acid.

1 ml Ampuls: Each ml contains 10 mg phytonadione (vitamin K_1) compounded with 40 mg polysorbate 80, 20.7 mg propylene glycol, 0.8 mg sodium acetate and 0.00006 ml glacial acetic acid.

Phytonadione is a fat-soluble naphthoquinone derivative which is identical to naturally occurring vitamin K_1. Chemically, phytonadione is 1,4-naphthalenedione, 2 methyl-3-(3,7,11,15-tetra-methyl-2-hexadecenyl)-(R-(R*,R*-(E))). It is a clear, yellow to amber, very viscous liquid and in insoluble in water and slightly soluble in alcohol.

CLINICAL PHARMACOLOGY:

Phytonadione tablets possess the same type and degree of activity as does naturally-occurring vitamin K, which is necessary for the production via the liver of active prothrombin (factor II), proconvertin (factor VII), plasma thromboplastin component (factor IX), and Stuart factor (factor X). The prothrombin test is sensitive to the levels of three of these four factors—II, VII, and X. Vitamin K is an essential cofactor for a microsomal enzyme that catalyzes the post-translational carboxylation of multiple, specific, peptide-bound glutamic acid residues in inactive hepatic precursors of factors II, VII, IX, and X. The resulting gamma-carboxyglutamic acid residues convert the precursors into active coagulation factors that are subsequently secreted by liver cells into the blood.

Oral phytonadione is adequately absorbed from the gastrointestinal tract only if bile salts are present. After absorption, phytonadione is initially concentrated in the liver, but the concentration declines rapidly. Very little vitamin K accumulates in tissues. Little is known about the metabolic fate of vitamin K. Almost no free unmetabolized vitamin K appears in bile or urine.

In normal animals and humans, phytonadione is virtually devoid of pharmacodynamic activity. However, in animals and humans deficient in vitamin K, the pharmacological action of vitamin K is related to its normal physiological function; that is, to promote the hepatic biosynthesis of vitamin K-dependent clotting factors.

Mephyton tablets generally exert their effect within 6 to 10 hours.

Following intramuscular injection, phytonadione is readily absorbed, almost entirely by way of the lymph. After absorption, phytonadione is initially concentrated in the liver, but the concentration declines rapidly.

Following intravenous administration of titrated vitamin K_1, the half-life of elimination of tritiated vitamin K_1, the half-life of elimination of phytonadione ranged from two to four hours. The lipid-soluble radioactivity in the plasma, which is assumed to represent the injected phytonadione, was rapidly cleared and resembles the clearance of orally administered phytonadione.

The action of aqueous dispersion when administered parenterally is generally detectable within an hour or two, and hemorrhage is usually controlled within three to six hours. A normal prothrombin level may often be obtained in 12 to 14 hours.

INDICATIONS AND USAGE:

Phytonadione is indicated in the following coagulation disorders which are due to faulty formation of factors II, VII, IX and X when caused by vitamin K deficiency or interference with vitamin K activity.

Phytonadione is indicated in:

anticoagulant-induced prothrombin deficiency caused by coumarin or indanedione derivatives;

hypoprothrombinemia secondary to antibacterial therapy;

hypoprothrombinemia secondary to administration of salicylates;

hypoprothrombinemia secondary to obstructive jaundice or biliary fistulas but only if bile salts are administered concurrently, since otherwise the oral vitamin K will not be absorbed.

INDICATIONS AND USAGE: *(cont'd)*

ADDITIONAL INDICATION FOR INJECTION

prophylaxis and therapy of hemorrhagic disease of the newborn.

In the prophylaxis and treatment of hemorrhagic disease of the newborn, phytonadione injection (Konakion) has demonstrated a greater margin of safety than that of the water-soluble vitamin K analogs.

CONTRAINDICATIONS:

Hypersensitivity to any component of this medication.

WARNINGS:

An immediate coagulant effect should not be expected after administration of phytonadione.

Konakion does not directly counteract the effects of oral anticoagulants, but it promotes the synthesis of prothrombin by the liver, usually within two hours. Fresh plasma or blood transfusions may be required for severe blood loss or lack of response to vitamin K.

Phytonadione will not counteract the anticoagulant action of heparin.

When vitamin K_1 is used to correct excessive anticoagulant-induced hypoprothrombinemia, anticoagulant therapy still being indicated, the patient is again faced with the clotting hazards existing prior to starting the anticoagulant therapy. Phytonadione is not a clotting agent, but overzealous therapy with vitamin K_1 may restore conditions which originally permitted thromboembolic phenomena. Dosage should be kept as low as possible, and prothrombin time should be checked regularly as clinical conditions indicate.

Repeated large doses of vitamin K are not warranted in liver disease if the response to initial use of the vitamin is unsatisfactory. Failure to respond to vitamin K may indicate a congenital coagulation defect or that the condition being treated is unresponsive to vitamin K.

PRECAUTIONS:

GENERAL

Temporary resistance to prothrombin-depressing anticoagulants may result, especially when larger doses of phytonadione are used. If relatively large doses have been employed, it may be necessary when reinstituting anticoagulant therapy to use somewhat larger doses of the prothrombin-depressing anticoagulant, or to use one which acts on a different principle, such as heparin sodium.

Since the liver is the site of metabolic synthesis of prothrombin, hypoprothrombinemia resulting from hepatocellular damage is not corrected by administration of vitamin K. Repeated large doses of vitamin K are not warranted in liver disease if the response to initial use of the vitamin is unsatisfactory (Koller test).

Failure to respond to vitamin K may indicate that a coagulation defect is present or that the condition being treated is unresponsive to vitamin K.

LABORATORY TESTS

Prothrombin time should be checked regularly as clinical conditions indicate.

CARCINOGENESIS, MUTAGENESIS, AND IMPAIRMENT OF FERTILITY

Studies of carcinogenicity or impairment of fertility have not been performed with phytonadione. Phytonadione at concentrations up to 2000 mcg/plate with or without metabolic activation, was negative in the Ames microbial mutagen test.

PREGNANCY CATEGORY C

Animal reproduction studies have not been conducted with phytonadione. It is also not known whether phytonadione can cause fetal harm when administered to a pregnant woman or can affect reproduction capacity. Phytonadione should be given to a pregnant woman only if clearly needed.

Nonteratogenic effects: Retardation of skeletal ossification has been reported in mice with vitamin K_2 (menaquinone).

PEDIATRIC USE

Safety and effectiveness in children have not been established with phytonadione. Hemolysis, jaundice, and hyperbilirubinemia in newborns, particularly in premature infants, have been reported with vitamin K.

Therefore, the recommended dose should not be exceeded (See ADVERSE REACTIONS and DOSAGE AND ADMINISTRATION).

NURSING MOTHERS

A study has shown that vitamin K is excreted in human milk. This should be considered if it is necessary to administer phytonadione to a nursing mother.

DRUG INTERACTIONS:

Because vitamin K_1 is a pharmacologic antagonist to coumarin and indanedione derivatives, patients being treated with these anticoagulants should not receive phytonadione except for the treatment of excessive hypoprothrombinemia.

ADVERSE REACTIONS:

Transient "flushing sensations" and "peculiar" sensations of taste have been observed with parenteral phytonadione, as well as rare instances of dizziness, rapid and weak pulse, profuse sweating, brief hypotension, dyspnea, and cyanosis.

Although phytonadione has a greater margin of safety than the water-soluble vitamin K analogs, hyperbilirubinemia has been reported in the newborn, particularly in prematures when used at 5 to 10 times the recommended dosage. This effect, with the possibility of attendant kernicterus, should be considered if such dosages are deemed necessary.

In patients with sever hepatic disease, large doses of phytonadione may further depress liver function. Paradoxically, the administration of excessive doses of vitamin K or its analogs in an attempt to correct hypoprothrombinemia associated with severe hepatitis or cirrhosis may actually result in a further depression of the concentration of prothrombin (also see PRECAUTIONS, General).

INJECTION

Allergic Reactions: The possibility of allergic reactions, including an anaphylactoid reaction, should be kept in mind.

Miscellaneous: Pain, swelling and tenderness at the injection site have occurred rarely

OVERDOSAGE:

The intravenous and oral $LD_{50}s$ in the mouse are approximately 1.17 g/kg and greater than 24.18 g/kg, respectively.

If anticoagulation is needed following overdosage of phytonadione, heparin may be used.

DOSAGE AND ADMINISTRATION:

PHYTONADIONE TABLETS

See TABLE 1.

DOSAGE AND ADMINISTRATION: *(cont'd)*

TABLE 1 Phytonadione Tablets
Summary of Dosage Guidelines (See text for details)

Adults	Initial Dosage
Anticoagulant - Induced Prothrombin Deficiency (caused by coumarin or indanedione derivatives)	2.5 mg - 10 mg or up to 25 mg (rarely 50 mg)
Hypoprothrombinemia due to other causes (Antibiotics; Salicylates or other drugs; Factors limiting absorption or synthesis)	2.5 mg - 25 mg or more (rarely up to 50 mg)

Anticoagulant-Induced Prothrombin Deficiency in Adults

To correct excessively prolonged prothrombin times caused by oral anticoagulant therapy—2.5 to 10 mg or up to 25 mg initially is recommended. In rare instances 50 mg may be required. Frequency and amount of subsequent doses should be determined by prothrombin time response or clinical condition. (See WARNINGS.) If, in 12 to 48 hours after oral administration, the prothrombin time has not been shortened satisfactorily, the dose should be repeated.

Hypoprothrombinemia Due to Other Causes in Adults

If possible, discontinuation or reduction of the dosage of drugs interfering with coagulation mechanisms (such as salicylates, antibiotics) is suggested as an alternative to administering concurrent Mephyton. The severity of the coagulation disorder should determine whether the immediate administration of Myphyton is required in addition to discontinuation or reduction of interfering drugs.

A dosage of 2.5 to 25 mg or more (rarely up to 50 mg) is recommended, the amount and route of administration depending upon the severity of the condition and response obtained.

The oral route should be avoided when the clinical disorder would prevent proper absorption. Bile salts must be given with the tablets when the endogenous supply of bile to the gastrointestinal tract is deficient.

Storage: Protect from light.

PHYTONADIONE INJECTION

The U.S. Recommended Daily allowances for vitamin K in humans have not been established officially. The adequate daily dietary intake of vitamin K for adults has been estimated to be 70 to 140 mcg; for infants 10 to 20 mcg; for children and adolescents 15 to 100 mcg. The dietary abundance of vitamin K normally satisfies these requirements except for the neonatal period of 5 to 8 days.

Prevention and Therapy of Neonatal Hemorrhage Due to Vitamin K Deficiency: Vitamin K_1 0.5 to 1.0 mg should be administered intramuscularly to the infant immediately after delivery. This may be repeated after two to three weeks if the mother has received anticoagulant, anticonvulsant, antituberculous or recent antibiotic therapy during her pregnancy. These mothers may be given 1.0 to 5.0 mg of vitamin K_1 intramuscularly 12 to 24 hours before delivery. Due to inefficient placental transport, however, this should not be considered a substitute for the prophylactic administration if vitamin K_1 to the infant immediately after delivery.

For the treatment of severe, life-threatening hemorrhage, administration of blood or blood products such as fresh frozen plasma, in addition to parenteral vitamin K_1, may be needed (see WARNINGS).

When the expected clinical response is not observed, additional coagulation studies should be carried out to more clearly define the cause of the bleeding.

Because of the possibility that breast-fed infants who develop diarrhea may have decreased bacterial synthesis, as well as insufficient dietary intake of vitamin K, the American Academy of Pediatrics recommends that breast-fed infants who develop diarrhea that persists for longer than a few days should be given an additional injection of vitamin K_1(1.0 mg).

Therapy of Hypoprothrombinemia Induced by Anticoagulant Therapy (except Heparin) in Adults: Vitamin K_1 should be administered intramuscularly at the dose of 5 to 10 mg initially; up to 20 mg if necessary.

In the presence of severe or active bleeding, transfusion of blood or fresh frozen plasma may be required (see WARNINGS).

Therapy of Hypoprothrombinemia Due to Other Causes in Adults (TABLE 2):

TABLE 2 Phytonadione

Antibacterial therapy:	5 to 20 mg intramuscularly.
Other drugs (*e.g.*, salicylates):	2 to 20 mg intramuscularly.
Factors limiting synthesis or absorption of vitamin K:	2 to 20 mg intramuscularly.

In older children and adults, injection of phytonadione should be in the upper outer quadrant of the buttocks. In infants and young children, the anterolateral aspect of the thighs or the deltoid region is preferred so that danger of sciatic nerve injury is avoided.

It is recommended that phytonadione be injected by itself, since phytonadione injection has been reported to be incompatible with many drugs in admixtures.

Parenteral drug products should be inspected visually for particulate matter and discoloration prior to administration, whenever solution and container permit. Slight opalescence may occur with phytonadione ampuls, but this does not affect the safety or potency of the product.

Phytonadione is stable in air, but it is photosensitive, decomposing with loss of potency on exposure to light. Therefore it should be stored in a dark place and protected from light at all times. Phytonadione injection need not be refrigerated.

STORE AT ROOM TEMPERATURE (15 to 30°C; 59 to 86°F). DO NOT FREEZE. PROTECT FROM LIGHT AT ALL TIMES.

(Tablets: Merck, 3/91, 7469513)

HOW SUPPLIED - EQUIVALENTS NOT AVAILABLE:

Injection, Emulsion - Intramuscular; - 1 mg/0.5ml

0.5 ml	$2.36	VITAMIN K1, Abbott	00074-9157-01
0.5 ml	$5.00	Phytonadione, Intl Medication	00548-1140-00
0.5 ml x 25	$57.98	AQUAMEPHYTON, Merck	00006-7784-33

Injection, Emulsion - Intramuscular; - 10 mg/ml

1 ml	$4.75	VITAMIN K1, Abbott	00074-9158-01
1 ml x 6	$28.37	AQUAMEPHYTON, Merck	00006-7780-64
1 ml x 25	$113.15	AQUAMEPHYTON, Merck	00006-7780-66
2.5 ml	$11.91	AQUAMEPHYTON, Merck	00006-7782-30
5 ml	$23.64	AQUAMEPHYTON, Merck	00006-7782-03

Tablet, Uncoated - Oral - 5 mg

100's	$52.20	MEPHYTON, Merck	00006-0043-68

PILOCARPINE *(003122)*

CATEGORIES: Antiglaucomatous Agents; EENT Drugs; Eye, Ear, Nose, & Throat Preparations; Glaucoma; Intraocular Pressure; Miotics; Mydriasis; Ocular Hypertension; Ophthalmics; Parasympathomimetic Agents; Pregnancy Category C; FDA Approved 1984 Oct

BRAND NAMES: *Ocusert Pilo-20* (Canada, England); *Ocusert Pilo-40* (Canada, England); *Ocusert Pilocarpine* (England); *Pilocarpol* (Germany); *Pilomin* *(International brand names outside U.S. in italics)*

FORMULARIES: Medi-Cal; WHO

DESCRIPTION:

Ocusert pilocarpine system is an elliptically shaped unit designed for continuous release of pilocarpine following placement in the cul-de-sac of the eye. Clinical evaluation in appropriate patients has demonstrated therapeutic efficacy of the system in the eye for one week. Two strengths are available, Pilo-20 and Pilo-40.

Pilocarpine systems contain a core reservoir consisting of pilocarpine and alginic acid. Pilocarpine is designated chemically as 2(3H)-Furanone, 3-ethyldihydro-4((1-methyl-1H-imidazol-5-yl) methyl)-, (3S-cis)-.

The core is surrounded by a hydrophobic ethylene/vinyl acetate (EVA) copolymer membrane which controls the diffusion of pilocarpine from the Pilocarpine system into the eye. The Pilo-40 membrane contains di(2-ethylhexyl) phthalate, which increases the rate of diffusion of pilocarpine across the EVA membrane. Of the total content of pilocarpine in the Pilo-20 or Pilo-40 system (5 mg or 11 mg, respectively), a portion serves as the thermodynamic diffusional energy source to release the drug and remains in the unit at the end of the week's use. The alginic acid component of the core is not released from the system. The readily visible white margin around the system contains titanium dioxide. The Pilo-20 system is 5.7 x 13.4 mm on its axes and 0.3 mm thick; the Pilo-40 system is 5.5 x 13 mm on its axes and 0.5 mm thick.

Release Rate Concept: With the Pilocarpine system form of therapy, the particular strength is described by the rated release, the mean release rate of drug from the system over seven days, in micrograms per hour. To cover the range of drug therapy needed to control the increased intraocular pressure associated with the glaucomas, two rated releases of pilocarpine from the Pilocarpine system are available, 20 and 40 micrograms per hour, for one week.

During the first few hours of the seven day time course, the release rate is higher than that prevailing over the remainder of the one-week period. The system releases drug at three times the rated value in the first hours and drops to the rated value in approximately six hours. A total of 0.3 mg to 0.7 mg pilocarpine (Pilo-20 or Pilo-40, respectively) is released during this initial six-hour period (one drop of 2% pilocarpine ophthalmic solution contains 1 mg pilocarpine). During the remainder of the seven day period the release rate is within ±20% of the rated value.

CLINICAL PHARMACOLOGY:

Pilocarpine is released from the Pilocarpine system as soon as it is placed in contact with the conjunctival surfaces. Pilocarpine is a direct acting parasympathomimetic drug which produces pupillary constriction, stimulates the ciliary muscle, and increases aqueous humor outflow facility. Because of its action on ciliary muscle, pilocarpine induces transient myopia, generally more pronounced in younger patients. In association with the increase in outflow facility, there is a decrease in intraocular pressure.

Preclinical Results: The levels of ^{14}C-pilocarpine in the ocular tissues of rabbits following Pilocarpine system and eyedrop administration have been determined. The Pilocarpine system produces constant low pilocarpine levels in the ciliary body and iris. Following ^{14}C-pilocarpine eyedrop treatment, the initial levels of pilocarpine in the cornea, aqueous humor, ciliary body and iris are 3 to 5 times higher than the corresponding levels with the Pilocarpine system, declining over the next six hours to approximately the tissue concentrations maintained by the Pilocarpine system. In contrast, in the conjunctiva, lens, and vitreous the ^{14}C-pilocarpine concentrations remain consistently high from eyedrops and do not return to the constant low levels maintained by the Pilocarpine system. Pilocarpine does not accumulate in ocular tissues during Pilocarpine system use. These studies in rabbits have not been done in humans.

Clinical Results: The ocular hypotensive effect of both the Pilo-20 and Pilo-40 systems is fully developed within 1 1/2 to 2 hours after placement in the cul-de-sac. A satisfactory ocular hypotensive response is maintained around-the-clock. Intraocular pressure reduction for an entire week is achieved with the Pilocarpine system from either 3.4 mg or 6.7 mg pilocarpine (20 or 40 mcg/hour times 24 hours/day times 7 days, respectively), as compared with 28 mg administered as a 2% ophthalmic solution four times a day.

During the first several hours after insertion of a pilocarpine system into the conjunctival cul-de-sac, induced myopia may occur. In contrast to the fluctuating and high levels of induced myopia typical of pilocarpine administration by eyedrop, the amount of induced myopia with Pilocarpine systems decreases after the first several hours to a low baseline level, approximately 0.5 diopters or less, which persists for the therapeutic life of the Pilocarpine system. Pilocarpine-induced miosis approximately parallels the induced myopia.

Of the 302 patients who used the Pilocarpine system in clinical studies for more than two weeks, 229 (75%) preferred it to previously used pilocarpine eyedrops. This percentage increased with further wearing experience.

INDICATIONS AND USAGE:

Pilocarpine system is indicated for control of elevated intraocular pressure in pilocarpine responsive patients. Clinical studies have demonstrated Pilocarpine system efficacy in certain glaucomatous patients.

The patient should be instructed on the use of the Pilocarpine system and should read the package insert instructions for use. The patient should demonstrate to the ophthalmologist his ability to place, adjust and remove the units.

Concurrent Therapy: Pilocarpine systems have been used concomitantly with various ophthalmic medications. The release rate of pilocarpine from the Pilocarpine system is not influenced by carbonic anhydrase inhibitors, epinephrine or timolol ophthalmic solutions, fluorescein, or anesthetic, antibiotic, or antiinflammatory steroid ophthalmic solutions. Systemic reactions consistent with an increased rate of absorption from the eye of an autonomic drug, such as epinephrine, have been observed. The occurrence of mild bulbar conjunctival edema, which is frequently present with epinephrine ophthalmic solutions, is not influenced by the pilocarpine system.

CONTRAINDICATIONS:

Pilocarpine system is contraindicated where pupillary constriction is undesirable, such as for glaucomas associated with acute inflammatory disease of the anterior segment of the eye, and glaucomas occurring or persisting after extracapsular cataract extraction where posterior synechiae may occur.

WARNINGS:

Patients with acute infectious conjunctivitis or keratitis should be given special consideration and evaluation prior to the use of the pilocarpine system.

Damaged or deformed systems should not be placed or retained in the eye. Systems believed to be associated with an unexpected increase in drug action should be removed and replaced with a new system.

PRECAUTIONS:

GENERAL

Pilocarpine system safety in retinal detachment patients and in patients with filtration blebs has not been established. The conjunctival erythema and edema associated with epinephrine ophthalmic solutions are not substantially altered by concomitant pilocarpine system therapy. The use of pilocarpine drops should be considered when intense miosis in desired in certain ocular conditions.

CARCINOGENESIS, MUTAGENESIS, AND IMPAIRMENT OF FERTILITY

No long-term carcinogenicity and reproduction studies in animals have been conducted with the Pilocarpine system.

PREGNANCY CATEGORY C

Although the use of the pilocarpine system has not been reported to have adverse effect on pregnancy, the safety of its use in pregnant women has not been absolutely established. While systemic absorption of pilocarpine from the Pilocarpine system is highly unlikely, pregnant women should use it only if clearly needed.

NURSING MOTHERS

It is not known whether pilocarpine is excreted in human milk. Because many drugs are excreted in human milk, caution should be exercised when the Pilocarpine system is used by a nursing woman.

PEDIATRIC USE

Safety and effectiveness in children have not been established.

DRUG INTERACTIONS:

Although ophthalmic solutions have been used effectively in conjunction with the Pilocarpine system, systemic reactions consistent with an increased rate of absorption from the eye of an autonomic drug, such as epinephrine, have been observed. In rare instances, reactions of this type can be severe.

ADVERSE REACTIONS:

Ciliary spasm is encountered with pilocarpine usage but is not a contraindication to continued therapy unless the induced myopia is debilitating to the patient. Irritation from pilocarpine has been infrequently encountered and may require cessation of therapy depending on the judgment of the physician. True allergic reactions are uncommon but require discontinuation of therapy should they occur. Corneal abrasion and visual impairment have been reported with use of the Pilocarpine System.

Although withdrawal of the peripheral iris from the anterior chamber angle by miosis may reduce the tendency for narrow angle closure, miotics can occasionally precipitate angle closure by increasing the resistance to aqueous flow from posterior to anterior chamber. Miotic agents may also cause retinal detachment; thus, care should be exercised with all miotic therapy especially in young myopic patients.

Some patients may notice signs of conjunctival irritation, including mild erythema with or without a slight increase in mucous secretion when they first use pilocarpine systems. These symptoms tend to lessen or disappear after the first week of therapy. In rare instances a sudden increase in pilocarpine effects has been reported during system use.

DOSAGE AND ADMINISTRATION:

Initiation of Therapy: A patient whose intraocular pressure has been controlled by 1% or 2% pilocarpine eyedrop solution has a higher probability of pressure control with the Pilo-20 system than a patient who has used a higher strength pilocarpine solution and might require Pilo-40 therapy. However, there is no direct correlation between the Pilocarpine system (Pilo-20 and Pilo-40) and the strength of pilocarpine eyedrop solutions required to achieve a given level of pressure lowering. The Pilocarpine system reduces the amount of drug necessary to achieve adequate medical control; therefore, therapy may be started with the Pilocarpine-20 system irrespective of the strength of pilocarpine solution the patient previously required. Because of the patient's age, family history, and disease status or progression, however, the ophthalmologist may elect to begin therapy with the Pilo-40. The patient should then return during the first week of therapy for evaluation of his intraocular pressure, and as often thereafter as the ophthalmologist deems necessary.

If the pressure is satisfactorily reduced with the Pilocarpine-20 system the patient should continue its use, replacing each unit every 7 days. If the physician desires intraocular pressure reduction greater than that achieved by the Pilo-20 system, the patient should be transferred to the Pilo-40 system. If necessary, an epinephrine ophthalmic solution of a carbonic anhydrase inhibitor may be used concurrently with Pilocarpine system.

After a satisfactory therapeutic regimen has been established with the Pilocarpinecarpine system, the frequency of follow-up should be determined by the ophthalmologist according to the status of the patient's disease process.

Placement and Removal of the Pilocarpine System: The Pilocarpine system is readily placed in the eye by the patient, according to patient instructions provided in the package. The instructions also describe procedures for removal of the system. It is strongly recommended that the patient's ability to manage the placement and removal of the system be reviewed at the first patient visit after initiation of therapy.

Since the pilocarpine-induced myopia from the Pilocarpine systems may occur during the first several hours of therapy (average of 1.4 diopters in a group of young subjects), the patient should be advised to place the system into the conjunctival cul-de-sac at bedtime. By morning the induced myopia is at a stable level (about 0.5 diopters or less in young subjects).

Sanitary Handling: Patients should be instructed to wash their hands thoroughly with soap and water before touching or manipulating the Pilocarpine system. In the event a displaced unit contacts unclean surfaces, rinsing with cool tap water before replacing is advisable. Obviously bacteriologically contaminated units should be discarded and replaced with a fresh unit.

Pilocarpine System Retention in the Eye: During the initial adaptation period, the Pilocarpine unit may slip out of the conjunctival cul-de-sac onto the cheek. The patient is usually aware of such movement and can replace the unit without difficulty.

In those patients in whom retention of the Pilocarpine unit is a problem, superior cul-de-sac placement is often more desirable. The Pilocarpine unit can be manipulated from the lower to the upper conjunctival cul-de-sac by a gentle digital massage through the lid, a technique readily learned by the patient. If possible the unit should be moved before sleep to the upper conjunctival cul-de-sac for best retention. Should the unit slip out of the conjunctival cul-de-sac during sleep, its ocular hypotensive effect following loss continues for a period of time comparable to that following instillation of eyedrops. The patient should be instructed to check for the presence of the Pilocarpine unit before retiring at night and upon arising.

DOSAGE AND ADMINISTRATION: *(cont'd)*

STORAGE AND HANDLING

Store under refrigeration (36° - 46°F).

(91/04)

HOW SUPPLIED - EQUIVALENTS NOT AVAILABLE:

Insert - Ophthalmic - 20 mcg/hr

8's	$34.20	OCUSERT PILO, Alza	17314-4064-03

Insert - Ophthalmic - 40 mcg/hr

8's	$34.20	OCUSERT PILO, Alza	17314-4086-03

PILOCARPINE HYDROCHLORIDE *(002036)*

CATEGORIES: Antiglaucomatous Agents; Chemotherapy; Conjunctivitis; Corneal Ulcer; EENT Drugs; Eye, Ear, Nose, & Throat Preparations; Glaucoma; Hyperosmotic Agents; Intraocular Pressure; Miotics; Mydriasis; Ocular Hypertension; Ophthalmics; Parasympathomimetic Agents; Xerostomia; FDA Approved 1984 Oct

BRAND NAMES: Adsorbocarpine; Akarpine; *Asthenopin*; *Cendo Carpine*; *Glaucocarpine*; I-Pilopine; *Isopto Carpina*; Isopto Carpine; *Isopto Pilocarpine* (France); *Liocarpina*; *Miocarpine* (Canada); *O.P.D.*; Ocu-Carpine; *Oftan-Pilocarpin* ; *P.V. Carpine Liquifilm Ophthalimic Solution* (Australia); *Pil Ofteno* (Mexico); *Pilo Grin* (Mexico); *Pilocarpin*; *Pilogel* (Germany); *Pilogel HS*; Pilokair; *Pilokarpin Isopto* ; *Pilomann*; **Pilopine HS**; *Pilopt Eye Drops* (Australia); Pilosol; Pilostat; *Pilotonina*; Salagen; *Sanpilo*; *Sno Pilo* (England); Spectro-Pilo; *Spersacarpin* (Germany); *Spersacarpine*; Storzine; *Vistacarpin* (Germany); *Ximex Opticar*
(International brand names outside U.S. in italics)

FORMULARIES: Aetna; BC-BS; CIGNA; DoD; FHP; Humana; Kaiser; Medco; Medi-Cal; PCS; PruCare; United

PRIMARY ICD9: 365.11 (Primary Open-Angle Glaucoma)

DESCRIPTION:

Established name: Pilocarpine Hydrochloride

Pilocarpine, with a chemical name of 2(*3H*)-Furanone, 3-ethyldihydro-4-[(1-methyl-1*H*-imidazol-5-yl)-methyl]-, monohydrochloride, (*3S-cis*), has a molecular weight of 244.72.

OPHTHALMIC GEL

Pilocarpine hydrochloride 4% gel is a sterile topical ophthalmic aqueous gel which contains more than 90% water and employs CARBOPOL 940, a synthetic high molecular weight crosslinked polymer of acrylic acid to impart a high viscosity. The active ingredient, pilocarpine hydrochloride, is a cholinergic.

Pilocarpine HCl HS Gel Each Gram Contains: *Active:* Pilocarpine hydrochloride 4% (40 mg). *Preservative:* Benzalkonium chloride 0.008%. *Inactive:* Carbopol 940, edetate disodium, hydrochloric Aacid and/or sodium hydroxide (to adjust pH) and purified water.

TABLETS

Pilocarpine hydrochloride is a cholinergic agonist for oral use. Pilocarpine hydrochloride is a hygroscopic, odorless, bitter tasting white crystal or powder which is soluble in water and alcohol and virtually insoluble in most non-polar solvents.

Each Salagen Tablet for oral administration contains 5 mg of pilocarpine hydrochloride. Inactive ingredients in the tablet, the tablet's film coating, polishing, and branding are: carnauba wax, hydroxypropyl methylcellulose, iron oxide, microcrystalline cellulose, stearic acid, titanium dioxide and other ingredients.

OPHTHALMIC SOLUTION

Pilocarpine hydrochloride ophthalmic solution is a sterile solution for ophthalmic administration having the following composition:

Plastic Squeeze Bottle: 5, 10, 20, 30, 40, or 60 mg/ml of pilocarpine hydrochloride... (cholinergic/parasympathomimetric) in a buffered solution of boric acid, potassium chloride, hydroxypropylmethyl cellulose, sodium carbonate, edetate disodium and purified water, preserved with benzalkonium chloride.

Dropperettes Applicator: 10, 20, or 40 mg/ml of pilocarpine hydrochloride (cholinergic/parasympathomimetric) is an isotonic, buffered solution of boric acid, potassium chloride and purified water, preserved with benzalkonium chloride.

CLINICAL PHARMACOLOGY:

OPHTHALMIC

Pilocarpine is a direct acting cholinergic parasympathomimetic agent which acts through direct stimulation of muscarinic neuro receptors and smooth muscle such as the iris and secretory glands. Pilocarpine produces miosis through contraction of the iris sphincter causing increased tension on the scleral spur and opening of the trabecular meshwork spaces to facilitate outflow of aqueous humor. Outflow resistance is thereby reduced, lowering intraocular pressure.

TABLETS

Pharmacodynamics: Pilocarpine is a cholinergic parasympathomimetic agent exerting a broad spectrum of pharmacologic effects with predominant muscarinic action. Pilocarpine, in appropriate dosage, can increase secretion by the exocrine glands. The sweat, salivary, lacrimal, gastric, pancreatic, and intestinal glands and the mucous cells of the respiratory tract may be stimulated. When applied topically to the eye as a single dose it causes miosis, spasm of accommodation, and may cause a transitory rise in intraocular pressure followed by a more persistent fall. Dose-related smooth muscle stimulation of the intestinal tract may cause increased tone, increased motility, spasm, and tenesmus. Bronchial smooth muscle tone may increase. The tone and motility of urinary tract, gallbladder, and biliary duct smooth muscle may be enhanced. Pilocarpine may have paradoxical effects on the cardiovascular system. The expected effect of a muscarinic agonist is vasosuppression, but administration of pilocarpine may produce hypotension after a brief episode of hypotension. Bradycardia and tachycardia have both been reported with use of pilocarpine.

In a study in 12 healthy male volunteers there was a dose-related increase in unstimulated salivary flow following single 5 and 10 mg oral doses of pilocarpine hydrochloride. The stimulatory effect was time-related with an onset at 20 minutes and peak at 1 hour with a duration of 3 to 5 hours.(See CLINICAL PHARMACOLOGY,Pharmacokinetics.)

In a 12 week randomized, double-blind, placebo-controlled study in 207 patients (placebo, N=65; 5 mg, N=73; 10 mg, N=69), increases from baseline (means 0.072 and 0.112 ml/min, ranges -0.690 to 0.728 and -0.380 to 1.689) of whole saliva flow for the 5 mg (63%) and 10 mg (90%) tablet, respectively, were seen 1 hour after the first dose of pilocarpine hydrochloride. Increases in unstimulated parotid flow were seen following the first dose (means 0.025 and 0.046 ml/min, ranges 0 to 0.414 and -0.070 to 1.002 ml/min for the 5 and 10 mg dose, respectively). In this study, no correlation existed between the amount of increase in salivary flow and the degree of symptomatic relief. (see CLINICAL STUDIES.)

CLINICAL PHARMACOLOGY: *(cont'd)*

Pharmacokinetics: In a multiple-dose pharmacokinetic study in male volunteers following 2 days of 5 or 10 mg of oral pilocarpine hydrochloride tablets given at 8 a.m., noontime, and 6 p.m., the mean elimination half-life was 0.76 hours for the 5 mg dose and 1.35 for the 10 mg dose. T_{max} values were 1.25 hours and 0.85 hours. C_{max} values were 15 ng/ml and 41 ng/ml. The AUC trapezoidal values were 33h (ng/ml) and 108 h)ng/ml), respectively, for the 5 and 10 mg doses following the last 6 hour dose.

Pharmacokinetics in elderly male volunteers (n=11) were comparable to those in younger men. I five healthy elderly female volunteers, the mean C_{max} and AUC were approximately twice that of elderly males and young normal volunteers.

When taken with a high fat meal by 12 healthy volunteers, there was a decrease in the rate of absorption of pilocarpine from pilocarpine hydrochloride. Mean $T_{max's}$ were 1.47 and 0.87 hours, respectively.

Limited information is available about the metabolism and elimination of pilocarpine in humans. Inactivation of pilocarpine is thought to occur at neuronal synapses and probably in plasma. Pilocarpine and its minimally active or inactive degradation products, including pilocarpic acid, are excreted in the urine.

CLINICAL STUDIES:

A 12 week randomized, double-blind, placebo- controlled study in 207 patients (142 men, 65 women) was conducted in patients whose mean age was 58.5 years with a range of 19 to 77; the racial distribution was Caucasian 95%, Black 4%, and other 1%. In this population, a statistically significant improvement in mouth dryness occurred in the 5 and 10 mg Salagen Tablet treated patients compared to placebo treated patients. The 5 and 10 mg treated patients could not be distinguished. (See CLINICAL STUDIES, Pharmacodynamics.)

Another 12 week, double-blind, randomized placebo-controlled study was conducted in 162 patients whose mean age was 57.8 years with a range of 27 to 80; the racial distribution was Caucasian 88%, Black 10%, and other 2%. The effects of placebo were compared to 2.5 mg three times a day of pilocarpine hydrochloride for 4 weeks followed by titration to 5 mg three times a day and 10 mg three times a day. Lowering of the dose was necessary because of adverse events in 3 of 67 patients treated with 5 mg of pilocarpine hydrochloride and in 7 of 66 patients treated with 10 mg of pilocarpine hydrochloride. After 4 weeks of treatment, 2.5 mg of pilocarpine hydrochloride three times a day was comparable to placebo in relieving dryness. In patients treated with 5 mg and 10 mg of pilocarpine hydrochloride, the greatest improvement in dryness was noted in patients with no measurable salivary flow at baseline.

In both studies, some patients noted improvement in the global assessment of their xerostomia, speaking without liquids, and a reduced need for supplemental oral comfort agents.

In the two placebo-controlled clinical trials, the most common adverse events related to drug, and increasing in rate as dose increases, were sweating, nausea, rhinitis, chills, flushing, urinary frequency, dizziness, and asthenia. The most common adverse experience causing withdrawal from treatment was sweating (5 mg=<1%; 10 mg=12%).

INDICATIONS AND USAGE:

OPHTHALMIC GEL

Pilocarpine hydrochloride is a miotic (parasympathomimetic) used to control intraocular pressure. It may be used in combination with other miotics, beta blockers, carbonic anhydrase inhibitors, sympathomimetics or hyperosmotic agents.

OPHTHALMIC SOLUTION

Pilocarpine hydrochloride ophthalmic solution is indicated for the treatment of primary open-angle glaucoma and also to lower intraocular pressure prior to surgery for acute angle-closure glaucoma. It may be used in combination with other miotics, beta adrenergic blocking agents, carbonic anhydrase inhibitors, hyperosmotic agents, or ephinephrine.

TABLETS

Pilocarpine hydrochloride are indicated for the treatment of symptoms of xerostomia from salivary gland hypofunction caused by radiotherapy for cancer of the head and neck.

CONTRAINDICATIONS:

OPHTHALMIC

Miotics are contraindicated where constriction is undesirable such as in acute iritis; and in those persons showing hypersensitivity to any of their components.

TABLETS

Tablets are contraindicated in patients with uncontrolled asthma, known hypersensitivity to pilocarpine, and when miosis is undesirable, (*e.g.,* in acute iritis and in narrow-angle (angle closure) glaucoma).

WARNINGS:

OPHTHALMIC GEL

For topical use only.

TABLETS

Cardiovascular Disease: Patients with significant cardiovascular disease may be unable to compensate for transient changes in hemodynamics or rhythm induced by pilocarpine. Pulmonary edema has been reported as a complication of pilocarpine toxicity from high ocular doses given for acute angle closure glaucoma. Pilocarpine should be administered with caution in and under close medical supervision of patients with cardiovascular disease.

Ocular: Careful examination of the fundus should be carried out prior to initiating therapy with pilocarpine. An association of ocular pilocarpine use and retinal detachment in patients with preexisting retinal disease has been reported. The systemic blood level that is associated with this finding is not known.

Ocular formulations of pilocarpine have been reported to cause visual blurring which may result in decreased visual acuity, especially at night and in patients with central lens changes, and to cause impairment of depth perception. Caution should be advised while driving at night or performing hazardous activities in reduced lighting.

Pulmonary Disease: Pilocarpine has been reported to increase airway resistance, bronchial smooth muscle tone, and bronchial secretions. Pilocarpine hydrochloride should be administered with caution to and under close medical supervision in patients with controlled asthma, chronic bronchitis, or chronic obstructive pulmonary disease.

PRECAUTIONS:

OPHTHALMIC

The miosis usually causes difficulty in dark adaptation. Patient should be advised to exercise caution in night driving and other hazardous occupations in poor illumination.

Solution: Not for internal use. To prevent contaminating the dropper tip and solution, care should be taken not to touch the eyelids or surroundings areas with the dropper tip of the bottle.

PRECAUTIONS: *(cont'd)*

TABLETS

General: Pilocarpine toxicity is characterized by an exaggeration of its parasympathomimetic effects. These may include: headache, visual disturbance, lacrimation, sweating, respiratory distress, gastrointestinal spasm, nausea, vomiting, diarrhea, atrioventricular block, tachycardia, bradycardia, hypotension, hypertension, shock, mental confusion, cardiac arrythmia, and tremors.

The dose-related cardiovascular pharmacologic effects of pilocarpine include hypotension, hypertension, bradycardia, and tachycardia.

Pilocarpine should be administered with caution to patients with known or suspected cholelithiasis or biliary tract disease. Contractions of the gallbladder or biliary smooth muscle could precipitate complications including cholecystitis, cholangitis, and biliary obstruction.

Pilocarpine may increase ureteral smooth muscle tone and could theoretically precipitate renal colic (or "ureteral reflux"), particularly in patients with nephrolithiasis.

Cholinergic agonists may have dose-related central nervous system effects. This should be considered when treating patients with underlying cognitive or psychiatric disturbances.

Renal Insufficiency: The pharmacokinetics of orally administered pilocarpine in patients with renal and V) disease is not known.

Information for the Patient: Patients should be informed that pilocarpine may cause visual disturbances, especially at night, that could impair their ability to drive safely.

If a patient sweats excessively while taking pilocarpine hydrochloride and cannot drink enough liquid, the patients should consult a physician. Dehydration may develop.

Carcinogenesis, Mutagenesis, Impairment of Fertility: No definitive long term animal studies have evaluated the carcinogenic potential of pilocarpine hydrochloride.

No evidence that pilocarpine hydrochloride has the potential to cause genetic toxicity was obtained in a series of studies that included: 1) bacterial assays (Salmonella and E. coli) for reverse gene mutations; 2) an *in vitro* chromosome aberration in a Chinese hamster ovary cell line; 3) an *in vivo* chromosome aberration assay (micronucleus test) in mice; and 4) a primary DNA damage assay (unscheduled DNA synthesis) in rat hepatocyte primary cultures. In a published report, male rats who received pilocarpine at a dosage of 39 mg/kg/day (approximately 11 times the maximum recommended dose for a 60 kg human based on body surface area [mg/m^2] estimates) exhibited morphologic evidence of reduced spermatogenesis. The possibility that pilocarpine may impair male fertility in humans cannot be excluded.The effects of pilocarpine on male and female fertility in humans have not been systematically studied.

Pregnancy Category C: Pilocarpine hydrochloride was associated with a reduction in the mean fetal body weight and an increase in the incidence of skeletal variations when given to pregnant rats at a dosage of 90 mg/kg/day (approximately 26 times the maximum recommended dose for a 60 kg human based upon body surface area [mg/m^2] estimates). These effects may have been secondary to maternal toxicity. There are no adequate and well-controlled studies in pregnant women. pilocarpine hydrochloride should be used during pregnancy only if the potential benefit justifies the potential risk to the fetus.

Nursing Mothers: It is not known whether this drug is excreted in human milk. Because many drugs are excreted in human milk and because of the potential for serious adverse reactions in nursing infants from pilocarpine hydrochloride, a decision should be made whether to discontinue nursing or to discontinue the drug, taking into account the importance of the drug to the mother.

Pediatrics: Safety and effectiveness of this drug in children have not been established.

Geriatric Use: In the placebo-controlled clinical trials (see CLINICAL STUDIES) the mean age of patients was approximately 58 years (range 19 to 80). Of these patients, 97/369 (61/217 receiving pilocarpine) were over the age of 65 years. In the healthy volunteer studies, 15/150 subjects were over the age of 65 years. In both study populations, the adverse events reported by those over 65 years and those 65 years and younger were comparable. Of the 15 elderly volunteers (5 women, 10 men), the 5 women had higher $C_{max's}$and AUC's than the men. (See CLINICAL PHARMACOLOGY, Pharmacokinetics.)

OPHTHALMIC

Carcinogenesis, Mutagenesis, and Impairment of Fertility: There have been no long term studies done using pilocarpine in animals to evaluate carcinogenic potential.

Pregnancy Category C: Animal reproduction studies have not been conducted with pilocarpine. It is also not know whether pilocarpine an cause fetal harm when administered to a pregnant woman or can affect reproduction capacity. Pilocarpine should be given to pregnant women only if clearly needed.

Nursing Mothers: It is not known whether this drug is excreted in human milk. Because many drugs are excreted in human milk caution should be exercised when pilocarpine is administered to a nursing woman.

DRUG INTERACTIONS:

Tablets

Pilocarpine should be administered with caution to patients taking beta adrenergic antagonists because of the possibility of conduction disturbances. Drugs with parasympathomimetic effects administered concurrently with pilocarpine would be expected to result in additive pharmacologic effects. Pilocarpine might antagonize the anticholinergic effects of drugs used concomitantly. These effects should be considered when anticholinergic properties may be contributing to the therapeutic effect of concomitant medication (*e.g.,* atropine, inhaled ipratropium).

ADVERSE REACTIONS:

OPHTHALMIC GEL

Pilocarpine HCl gel is usually well tolerated. In a controlled clinical study in 78 glaucomatous patients treated for 30 days, there were no significant differences in the type or severity of adverse effects associated with the instillation of pilocarpine gel at bedtime or the four daily instillations of pilocarpine 4% drops. The following adverse experiences associated with pilocarpine therapy have been reported: lacrimation, burning or discomfort, temporal or periorbital headache, ciliary spasm, conjunctival vascular congestion, superficial keratitis and induced myopia. Ocular reactions usually occur during initiation of therapy and often will not persist with continued therapy. Reduced visual acuity in poor illumination is frequently experienced by older individuals and in those with lens opacity. A subtle corneal granularity was observed in about 10% of patients treated with pilocarpine gel. In a control patient group treated with other therapies including pilocarpine drops, timolol, or epinephrine, the incidence was the same as reported among the individuals treated with pilocarpine gel. In both groups, the corneal granularity was asymptomatic and visual acuity was not affected. Rare cases of retinal detachment have been reported during treatment with miotic agents; thus care should be exercised with all miotic therapy, especially in young myopic patients. Lens opacity may occur with prolonged use of pilocarpine.

OPHTHALMIC SOLUTION

Ocular: Ciliary spasm, conjunctival vascular congestion, temporal or supraorbital headache, lacrimation, and induced myopia may occur. This is especially true for younger individuals who have recently started administration. Reduced visual acuity in poor illumination is

ADVERSE REACTIONS: *(cont'd)*

frequently experienced with older individuals and individuals with lens opacity. Miotic agents may also cause **retinal detachment**; thus, care should be exercised with all miotic therapy especially in young miotic patients. Lens opacity may occur with prolonged use of pilocarpine.

Systemic: Systemic reactions following topical administration, although extremely rare, have included hypertension, tachycardia, bronchiolar spasm, pulmonary edema, salivation, sweating, nausea, vomiting, and diarrhea.

TABLETS

In controlled studies, 217 patients received pilocarpine, of whom 68% were men and 32% were women. Race distribution was 91% Caucasian, 8% Black, and 1% of other origin. Mean age was approximately 58 years. The majority of patients were between 50 and 64 years (51%), 33% were 65 years and older and 16% were younger than 50 years of age.

The most frequent adverse experiences associated with pilocarpine hydrochloride were a consequence of the expected pharmacologic effects of pilocarpine.

TABLE 1

Adverse Event	Placebo t.i.d. n=152	5 mg t.i.d. n=141	10 mg t.i.d. n=121
Sweating	9%	29%	68%
Nausea	4	6	15
Rhinitis	7	5	14
Chills	<1	3	14
Flushing	3	8	13
Urinary Frequency	7	9	12
Dizziness	4	5	12
Asthenia	3	6	12

In addition, the following adverse events (≥1% incidence) were reported at doses of 5 and 10 mg in the controlled clinical trials:

TABLE 2

Adverse Event	Placebo t.i.d. n=152	Pilocarpine HCl t.i.d. n=212
Headache	8%	11%
Dyspepsia	5	7
Lacrimation	8	6
Diarrhea	5	6
Edema	4	5
Abdominal Pain	4	4
Amblyopia	2	4
Vomiting	1	4
Pharyngitis	8	3
Hypertension	1	3
Conjunctivitis	4	2
Tachycardia	1	2
Epistaxis	1	2
Tremor	0	2
Dysphagia	<1	2
Voice Alteration	0	2
Rash	4	1
Taste Perversion	2	1
Sinusitis	2	1
Abnormal Vision	1	1
Myalgias	1	1
Pruritus	<1	1

THE FOLLOWING EVENTS WERE REPORTED RARELY IN TREATED PATIENTS (<1%): Causal relation is unknown.

Body as a whole: body odor, hypothermia, mucous membrane abnormality

Cardiovascular: bradycardia, ECG abnormality, palpitations, syncope

Digestive: anorexia, increased appetite, esophagitis, gastrointestinal disorder, tongue disorder

Hematologic: leukopenia, lymphadenopathy

Nervous: anxiety, confusion, depression, abnormal dreams, hyperkinesia, hypesthesia, nervousness, paresthesias, speech disorder, twitching

Respiratory: increased sputum, stridor, yawning

Skin: seborrhea

Special Senses: deafness, eye pain, glaucoma

Urogenital: dysuria, metrorrhagia, urinary impairment

In long-term treatment were two patients with underlying cardiovascular disease of whom one experienced a myocardial infarct and another an episode of syncope. The association with drug in uncertain.

The following adverse experiences have been reported rarely with ocular pilocarpine: malignant glaucoma, macular hole, shock, middle ear disturbance, A-V block, depression, delusion, eyelid twitching, visual hallucination, confusion, agitation, dermatitis, ciliary congestion, and iris cysts.

OVERDOSAGE:

OPHTHALMIC

Systemic reactions following topical administration are extremely rare.

TABLETS

Management Of Overdosage: Pilocarpine fatal overdosage resulting from poisoning has been reported in the scientific literature at doses presumed to be greater than 100 mg in two hospitalized patients. 100 mg of pilocarpine is considered potentially fatal. Overdosage should be treated with atropine titration (0.5 mg to 1.0 mg given subcutaneously or intravenously) and supportive measures to maintain respiration and circulation. Epinephrine (0.3 mg to 1.0 mg, subcutaneously or intramuscularly) may also be of value in the presence of severe cardiovascular depression or bronchoconstriction. It is not known if pilocarpine is dialyzable.

DOSAGE AND ADMINISTRATION:

OPHTHALMIC GEL

Apply a one-half inch ribbon in the lower conjunctival sac of the affected eye(s) once a day at bedtime. Under selected conditions, more frequent instillations may be indicated.

Store in a refrigerator (36°F-46°F) until dispensed to patient. Do not freeze. Patient may store at room temperature and should discard any unused portion after eight weeks.

DOSAGE AND ADMINISTRATION: *(cont'd)*

OPHTHALMIC SOLUTION

The initial dose is one or two drops. This may be repeated up to six times daily. The frequency of instillation and concentration of pilocarpine ophthalmic solution are determined by the severity of the glaucoma and miotic response of the patient.

During acute phases, the miotic must be instilled into the unaffected eye to prevent an attack of angle-closure glaucoma.

TABLETS

The recommended oral dose of pilocarpine hydrochloride for the initiation of treatment is 5 mg three times a day. Titration up to 10 mg three times a day may be considered for patients who have not responded adequately and who can tolerate lower doses. the incidence of the most common adverse events increases with dose. The lowest dose that is tolerated and effective should be used for maintenance.

HOW SUPPLIED:

Tablets: Salagen Tablets, 5 mg, are white, film coated, round tablets, coded MGI 705. Each tablet contains 5 mg pilocarpine hydrochloride.

Store at Controlled Room Temperature 15°-30°C (59°-86°F).

HOW SUPPLIED - EQUIVALENTS NOT AVAILABLE:

Crystals

3.5 gm	$44.86	Pilocarpine Hcl, Mallinckrodt	00406-6656-30
30 gm	$274.02	Pilocarpine Hcl, Mallinckrodt	00406-6656-34
125 gm	$1065.94	Pilocarpine Hcl, Mallinckrodt	00406-6656-01

Gel - Ophthalmic - 4 %

3.5 gm	**$23.13**	**PILOPINE HS, Alcon**	**00065-0215-35**
5 gm	**$21.25**	**Pilocarpine Hs Gel, Alcon**	**00065-0215-05**

Solution - Ophthalmic - 0.25 %

15 ml	$12.81	ISOPTO CARPINE, Alcon-PR	00998-0201-15

Solution - Ophthalmic - 0.5 %

15 ml	$2.34	Pilocarpine Hcl, Apotex	60505-7486-05
15 ml	$4.28	Pilocarpine Hcl, Caremark	00339-5963-52
15 ml	$4.31	Pilocarpine HCl, HL Moore Drug Exch	00839-6076-31
15 ml	$4.50	Pilocarpine Hcl, Martec Pharms	52555-0995-01
15 ml	$4.50	Pilocarpine Hcl, Adv Remedies	57685-0020-15
15 ml	$4.67	Pilocarpine Hcl Sterile Opthalmic S, Steris Labs	00402-0860-15
15 ml	$4.70	Pilosol, Ocusoft	54799-0521-15
15 ml	$4.82	Pilocarpine, Schein Pharm (US)	00364-2350-72
15 ml	$4.82	Pilocarpine HCl, Rugby	00536-2495-72
15 ml	$10.44	PILOCAR OPHTHALMIC, Ciba Vision	00058-2514-15
15 ml	$12.81	ISOPTO CARPINE, Alcon-PR	00998-0202-15
15 ml x 2	$15.96	PILOCAR OPHTHALMIC, Ciba Vision	00058-2514-34
30 ml	$14.69	ISOPTO CARPINE, Alcon-PR	00998-0202-30

Solution - Ophthalmic - 1 %

1 ml x 12	$25.80	PILOCAR OPHTHALMIC, Ciba Vision	00058-0781-12
2 ml x 12	$51.00	Pilocarpine Hcl, Alcon	00065-0728-12
15 ml	$2.55	Pilocarpine Hcl, Apotex	60505-7487-05
15 ml	$4.93	Pilocarpine Hcl, HL Moore Drug Exch	00839-5517-31
15 ml	$4.95	Pilocarpine Hcl, Consolidated Midland	00223-6700-15
15 ml	$4.95	Pilosol, Ocusoft	54799-0522-15
15 ml	$5.11	Pilocarpine Hcl, Qualitest Pharms	00603-7247-41
15 ml	$5.15	Pilocarpine Hcl, Martec Pharms	52555-0996-01
15 ml	$5.25	Pilocarpine Hcl, Goldline Labs	00182-0301-64
15 ml	$5.26	Pilocarpine Hcl, Caremark	00339-5965-52
15 ml	$5.30	Pilocarpine, United Res	00677-0910-30
15 ml	$5.30	Pilocarpine Hcl, Major Pharms	00904-2714-35
15 ml	$5.60	Pilocarpine Hcl, Aligen Independ	00405-6120-15
15 ml	$5.95	Pilocarpine HCl, Rugby	00536-2500-72
15 ml	$6.10	Pilocarpine Hcl, Steris Labs	00402-0863-15
15 ml	$6.49	Pilocarpine HCl, Fougera	00168-0173-15
15 ml	$6.56	AKARPINE, Akorn	17478-0223-12
15 ml	$7.95	Pilocarpine, Schein Pharm (US)	00364-7131-72
15 ml	$8.00	Pilocarpine Hcl, Geneva Pharms	00781-7040-85
15 ml	$10.74	PILOCAR OPHTHALMIC, Ciba Vision	00058-2515-15
15 ml	$12.81	ISOPTO CARPINE, Alcon-PR	00998-0203-15
15 ml	$12.81	ADSORBOCARPINE, Alcon-PR	00998-0212-15
15 ml x 2	$16.50	PILOCAR OPHTHALMIC, Ciba Vision	00058-2515-34
30 ml	$8.18	Pilocarpine, Rugby	00536-2500-96
30 ml	$8.30	Pilocarpine Hcl, Goldline Labs	00182-0301-66
30 ml	$8.91	Pilocarpine Hcl, Qualitest Pharms	00603-7247-42
30 ml	$9.22	Pilocarpine Hcl, Aligen Independ	00405-6120-22
30 ml	$9.90	Pilocarpine, Major Pharms	00904-2714-30
30 ml	$19.69	ISOPTO CARPINE, Alcon-PR	00998-0203-30

Solution - Ophthalmic - 2 %

1 ml x 12	$25.80	PILOCAR OPHTHALMIC, Ciba Vision	00058-0782-12
2 ml	$51.00	Pilocarpine Hcl, Alcon	00065-0752-12
15 ml	$3.10	Pilocarpine Hcl, Apotex	60505-7488-05
15 ml	$5.30	Pilosol, Ocusoft	54799-0523-15
15 ml	$6.00	Pilokair, Raway	00686-0681-06
15 ml	$6.50	Pilocarpine Hcl, Qualitest Pharms	00603-7249-41
15 ml	$6.56	AKARPINE, Akorn	17478-0224-12
15 ml	$6.71	Pilocarpine Hcl, Aligen Independ	00405-6121-15
15 ml	$6.76	Pilocarpine Hcl, Caremark	00339-5967-52
15 ml	$6.90	Pilocarpine Hydrochloride, United Res	00677-0911-30
15 ml	$6.90	Pilocarpine Hcl, Martec Pharms	52555-0997-01
15 ml	$6.95	Pilocarpine Hcl, HL Moore Drug Exch	00839-5518-31
15 ml	$6.95	Pilocarpine Hcl, Major Pharms	00904-2715-35
15 ml	$7.05	Pilocarpine Hcl, Goldline Labs	00182-0303-64
15 ml	$7.50	Pilocarpine Hcl, Consolidated Midland	00223-6701-15
15 ml	$7.59	Pilocarpine Hcl, Steris Labs	00402-0864-15
15 ml	$7.94	Pilocarpine HCl, Fougera	00168-0174-15
15 ml	$10.03	Pilocarpine, Schein Pharm (US)	00364-7132-72
15 ml	$10.03	Pilocarpine HCl, Rugby	00536-2521-72
15 ml	$10.10	Pilocarpine HCl, Geneva Pharms	00781-7042-85
15 ml	$10.74	PILOCAR OPHTHALMIC, Ciba Vision	00058-2516-15
15 ml	$13.13	ISOPTO CARPINE, Alcon-PR	00998-0204-15
15 ml	$13.13	ADSORBOCARPINE, Alcon-PR	00998-0213-15
15 ml x 2	$16.62	PILOCAR OPHTHALMIC, Ciba Vision	00058-2516-34
30 ml	$11.65	Pilocarpine Hcl, Goldline Labs	00182-0303-66
30 ml	$11.72	Pilocarpine, Rugby	00536-2521-96
30 ml	$11.90	Pilocarpine, Major Pharms	00904-2715-30
30 ml	$12.08	Pilocarpine Hcl, Qualitest Pharms	00603-7249-42
30 ml	$13.43	Pilocarpine Hcl, Aligen Independ	00405-6121-22
30 ml	$19.69	ISOPTO CARPINE, Alcon-PR	00998-0204-30

Solution - Ophthalmic - 3 %

15 ml	$3.33	Pilocarpine Hcl, Apotex	60505-7489-05
15 ml	$6.74	Pilocarpine Hcl, Qualitest Pharms	00603-7251-41

HOW SUPPLIED - EQUIVALENTS NOT AVAILABLE: *(cont'd)*

15 ml	$6.75	Pilocarpine Hcl, Major Pharms	00904-2716-35
15 ml	$7.20	Pilocarpine Hcl, Martec Pharms	52555-0998-01
15 ml	$7.40	Pilocarpine Hcl, Caremark	00339-5969-52
15 ml	$7.50	Pilocarpine Hcl, Goldline Labs	00182-0304-64
15 ml	$7.90	Pilocarpine, Schein Pharm (US)	00364-7133-72
15 ml	$7.90	Pilocarpine Hcl Sterile Ophthalmic, Steris Labs	00402-0865-15
15 ml	$8.13	Pilocarpine Hcl, Aligen Independ	00405-6122-15
15 ml	$11.52	PILOCAR OPHTHALMIC, Ciba Vision	00058-2517-15
15 ml	$14.06	ISOPTO CARPINE, Alcon-PR	00998-0205-15
15 ml x 2	$18.48	PILOCAR OPHTHALMIC, Ciba Vision	00058-2517-34
30 ml	$21.56	ISOPTO CARPINE, Alcon-PR	00998-0205-30

Solution - Ophthalmic - 4 %

1 ml x 12	$25.80	PILOCAR OPHTHALMIC, Ciba Vision	00058-0783-12
2 ml	$51.00	Pilocarpine Hcl, Alcon	00065-0756-12
15 ml	$3.60	Pilocarpine Hcl, Apotex	60505-7490-05
15 ml	$6.55	Pilosol, Ocusoft	54799-0524-15
15 ml	$7.04	Pilocarpine Hcl, Qualitest Pharms	00603-7253-41
15 ml	$7.49	Pilocarpine Hcl, HL Moore Drug Exch	00839-5520-31
15 ml	$7.51	Pilocarpine Hcl, Caremark	00339-5971-52
15 ml	$7.60	Pilocarpine Hcl, United Res	00677-0912-30
15 ml	$7.83	Pilocarpine Hcl, Steris Labs	00402-0866-15
15 ml	$7.88	Pilocarpine Hcl, Aligen Independ	00405-6123-15
15 ml	$7.90	Pilocarpine Hydrochloride, Martec Pharms	52555-0999-01
15 ml	$7.95	Pilocarpine Hcl, Goldline Labs	00182-0305-64
15 ml	$7.95	Pilocarpine Hcl, Major Pharms	00904-2717-35
15 ml	$8.16	AKARPINE, Akorn	17478-0226-12
15 ml	$8.22	Pilocarpine, Schein Pharm (US)	00364-7134-72
15 ml	$8.69	Pilocarpine HCl, Fougera	00168-0175-15
15 ml	$11.15	Pilocarpine HCl, Rugby	00536-2561-72
15 ml	$11.15	Pilocarpine Hcl, Geneva Pharms	00781-7044-85
15 ml	$11.52	PILOCAR OPHTHALMIC, Ciba Vision	00058-2518-15
15 ml	$14.06	ISOPTO CARPINE, Alcon-PR	00998-0206-15
15 ml	$14.06	ADSORBOCARPINE, Alcon-PR	00998-0214-15
15 ml x 2	$18.60	PILOCAR OPHTHALMIC, Ciba Vision	00058-2518-34
30 ml	$12.37	Pilocarpine, Rugby	00536-2561-96
30 ml	$12.50	Pilocarpine Hcl, Goldline Labs	00182-0305-66
30 ml	$12.60	Pilocarpine Hcl, United Res	00677-0912-62
30 ml	$13.30	Pilocarpine Hcl, Qualitest Pharms	00603-7253-42
30 ml	$14.21	Pilocarpine Hcl, Aligen Independ	00405-6123-22
30 ml	$14.30	Pilocarpine, Major Pharms	00904-2717-30
30 ml	$21.56	ISOPTO CARPINE, Alcon-PR	00998-0206-30

Solution - Ophthalmic - 5 %

15 ml	$5.01	Pilocarpine Hcl, Aligen Independ	00405-6119-15
15 ml	$11.87	ISOPTO CARPINE, Alcon-PR	00998-0207-15

Solution - Ophthalmic - 6 %

15 ml	$8.15	Pilocarpine Hcl, Geneva Pharms	00781-6555-85
15 ml	$8.91	Pilocarpine Hcl, Apotex	60505-7491-05
15 ml	$10.15	Pilocarpine Hcl, HL Moore Drug Exch	00839-5521-31
15 ml	$10.91	Pilocarpine Hcl, Qualitest Pharms	00603-7257-41
15 ml	$11.52	Pilocarpine Hcl Serile Ophthalmic S, Steris Labs	00402-0861-15
15 ml	$11.63	Pilocarpine Hcl, Caremark	00339-5973-52
15 ml	$12.10	Pilocarpine, Schein Pharm (US)	00364-7135-72
15 ml	$12.46	Pilocarpine Hcl, Aligen Independ	00405-6124-15
15 ml	$12.48	PILOCAR, Ciba Vision	00058-2519-15
15 ml	$12.69	Pilocarpine HCl, Fougera	00168-0176-15
15 ml	$13.13	Pilocarpine HCl, Rugby	00536-2580-72
15 ml	$15.62	ISOPTO CARPINE, Alcon-PR	00998-0208-15
30 ml	$20.70	PILOCAR, Ciba Vision	00058-2519-34
30 ml	$23.44	ISOPTO CARPINE, Alcon-PR	00998-0208-30

Solution - Ophthalmic - 8 %

15 ml	$17.50	ISOPTO CARPINE, Alcon-PR	00998-0209-15

Solution - Ophthalmic - 10 %

15 ml	$20.00	ISOPTO CARPINE, Alcon-PR	00998-0211-15

Tablet, Coated - Oral - 5 mg

100's	$107.40	SALAGEN, MGI Pharma	58063-0705-10

PILOCARPINE NITRATE *(002037)*

CATEGORIES: Antiglaucomatous Agents; Compliance Aids; EENT Drugs; Eye, Ear, Nose, & Throat Preparations; Glaucoma; Intraocular Pressure; Miotics; Mydriasis; Ocular Hypertension; Ophthalmics; Parasympathomimetic Agents; Pregnancy Category C; FDA Pre 1938 Drugs

BRAND NAMES: *Carpo-Miotic*; *Chibro-Pilocarpin* (Germany); *Chibro-Pilocarpine*; *Minims Pilocarpine* (Australia); *Minims Pilocarpine Nitrate* (England); *Minims Pilocarpinenitraat*; *P.V. Carpine* ; *P.V. Carpine Liquifilm* (Canada); **Pilagan**; *Pilo* (France); *Pilocar*, *Pilocarpine Nitrate*; *Pilopos* (Germany); *PV Carpine*
(International brand names outside U.S. in italics)

FORMULARIES: Aetna

COST OF THERAPY: $97.13 (Glaucoma; Solution; 1 %; 0.4/day; 365 days)

PRIMARY ICD9: 365.11 (Primary Open-Angle Glaucoma)

DESCRIPTION:

Pilocarpine Nitrate Liquifilm sterile ophthalmic solution is a topical parasympathomimetic agent for ophthalmic use.

Chemical Name: 2(3*H*)-Furanone, 3-ethyldihydro-4-((1-methyl-1*H*-imadazol- 5-yl)methyl)-,(3S-*cis*)-, mononitrate.

Contains: Pilocarpine nitrate - 1%, 2%, 4% with Liquifilm (polyvinyl alcohol) 1.4%; chlorobutanol (chloral derivative) 0.5% as a preservative; sodium acetate; sodium chloride; citric acid; menthol; camphor; phenol; eucalyptol; and purified water.

CLINICAL PHARMACOLOGY:

Pilocarpine Nitrate is a direct acting parasympathomimetic drug which duplicates the muscarinic effects of acetylcholine, but has no nicotinic effects. Pilocarpine stimulates secretory glands and smooth muscles and has no effect on striated muscles. Pilocarpine is effective in the treatment of glaucoma by improving the facility of outflow and by decreasing aqueous secretion.

INDICATIONS AND USAGE:

Pilocarpine Nitrate Liquifilm is indicated for:

1. The control of intraocular pressure in glaucoma.

INDICATIONS AND USAGE: *(cont'd)*

2. Emergency relief of mydriasis in an acutely glaucomatous situation.

3. To reverse mydriasis caused by cycloplegic agents.

CONTRAINDICATIONS:

Pilocarpine Nitrate Liquifilm is contraindicated in persons showing hypersensitivity to any of its ingredients.

WARNINGS:

Pilocarpine is readily absorbed systemically through the conjunctiva. Excessive application (instillation) may elicit systemic toxicity symptoms in some individuals.

PRECAUTIONS:

General Pilocarpine has been reported to elicit retinal detachment in individuals with pre-existing retinal disease or predisposed to retinal tears. Fundus examination is advised for all patients prior to initiation of pilocarpine therapy.

Carcinogenesis, Mutagenesis, and Impairment of Fertility No studies have been conducted in animals or in humans to elevate the potential of these effects.

Pregnancy Category C Animal reproduction studies have not been conducted with pilocarpine. It is also not known whether pilocarpine can cause fetal harm when administered to a pregnant woman or can affect reproduction capacity. Pilocarpine should be given to a pregnant woman only if clearly needed.

PEDIATRIC USE Safety and effectiveness in children has not been established.

ADVERSE REACTIONS:

Adverse reactions associated with topical pilocarpine therapy include: visual blurring due to miosis and accommodative spasm, poor dark adaptation caused by the failure of the pupil in reduced illumination, and conjunctival hyperemia.

Miotics have been reported to cause lens opacities in susceptible individuals after prolonged use.

Systemic reactions following topical use of pilocarpine are rare.

OVERDOSAGE:

Should accidental overdosage in the eye(s) occur, flush with water or normal saline. If accidentally ingested, induce emesis or perform gastric lavage. Observe patients for signs of pilocarpine toxicity. i.e., salivation, lacrimation, sweating, nausea, vomiting and diarrhea. If these occur, therapy with anticholinergics (atropine) may be necessary. Bronchial constriction may be a problem in asthmatic patients.

DOSAGE AND ADMINISTRATION:

1. For glaucoma, the recommended dosage is 1 to 2 drops two or four times a day of the selected concentration; patient response may be variable.

2. To aid in emergency miosis, 1 to 2 drops of one of the higher concentrations should be used.

3. The dosage and strength required to reverse mydriasis depends on the cycloplegic used.

Note: Shake well before use. Protect from freezing. Keep out of reach of children.

(Allergan, PR7248 30-12J)

HOW SUPPLIED - EQUIVALENTS NOT AVAILABLE:

Powder

30 gm	$307.82	Pilocarpine Nitrate, Mallinckrodt	00406-6662-03

Solution - Ophthalmic - 1 %

15 ml	**$9.98**	**PILAGAN OPHTHALMIC, Allergan-Amer**	**11980-0879-45**

Solution - Ophthalmic - 2 %

15 ml	**$10.35**	**PILAGAN OPHTHALMIC, Allergan-Amer**	**11980-0878-45**

Solution - Ophthalmic - 4 %

15 ml	**$10.74**	**PILAGAN, Allergan-Amer**	**11980-0877-45**

PIMOZIDE *(002038)*

CATEGORIES: Central Nervous System Agents; Psychotherapeutic Agents; Tics; Tourette Syndrome; Tranquilizers; Pregnancy Category C; FDA Approved 1984 Jul

BRAND NAMES: *Frenal (1mg, 4 mg)*; *Neurap*; **Orap**; *Orap (1 mg)*; *Orap (4 mg)*; *Orap Forte (4 mg)*; *Pimodac*
(International brand names outside U.S. in italics)

DESCRIPTION:

Pimozide is an orally active antipsychotic agent of the diphenylbutylpiperidine series. The structural formula of pimozide, 1-[1- [4,4- bis(4-fluorophenyl) -butyl]-4- piperidinyl] -1,3-dihydro-2*H*-benzimidazol-2-one.

The solubility of pimozide in water is less than 0.01 mg/ml; it is slightly soluble in most organic solvents.

Each white Pimozide tablet contains 2 mg of pimozide and the following inactive ingredients: calcium stearate, cellulose, lactose and corn starch.

CLINICAL PHARMACOLOGY:

Pharmacodynamic Actions: Pimozide is an orally active antipsychotic drug product which shares with other antipsychotics the ability to blockade dopaminergic receptors on neurons in the central nervous system. Although its exact mode of action has not been established, the ability of pimozide to suppress motor and phonic tics in Tourette's Disorder is thought to be a function of its dopaminergic blocking activity. However, receptor blockade is often accompanied by a series of secondary alterations in central dopamine metabolism and function which may contribute to both pimozide's therapeutic and untoward effects. In addition, pimozide, in common with other antipsychotic drugs, has various effects on other central nervous system receptor systems which are not fully characterized.

Metabolism and Pharmacokinetics: More than 50% of a dose of pimozide is absorbed after oral administration. Based on the pharmacokinetic and metabolic profile, pimozide appears to undergo significant first pass metabolism. Peak serum levels occur generally six to eight hours (range 4-12 hours) after dosing. Pimozide is extensively metabolized, primarily by N-dealkylation in the liver. Two major metabolites have been identified, 1-(4-piperidyl)-2-benzimidazolinone and 4,4-bis(4-fluorophenyl) butyric acid. The antipsychotic activity of these metabolites is undetermined. The major route of elimination of pimozide and its metabolites is through the kidney.

CLINICAL PHARMACOLOGY: *(cont'd)*

The mean serum elimination half-life of pimozide in schizophrenic patients was approximately 55 hours. There was a 13-fold interindividual difference in the area under the serum pimozide level-time curve and an equivalent degree of variation in peak serum levels among patients studied. The significance of this is unclear since there are few correlations between plasma levels and clinical findings.

Effects of food, disease or concomitant medication upon the absorption, distribution, metabolism and elimination of pimozide are not known.

INDICATIONS AND USAGE:

Pimozide is indicated for the suppression of motor and phonic tics in patients with Tourette's Disorder who have failed to respond satisfactorily to standard treatment. Pimozide is not intended as a treatment of first choice nor is it intended for the treatment for tics that are merely annoying or cosmetically troublesome. Pimozide should be reserved for use in Tourette's Disorder patients whose development and/or daily life function is severely compromised by the presence of motor and phonic tics.

Evidence supporting approval of Pimozide for use in Tourette's Disorder was obtained in two controlled clinical investigations which enrolled patients between the ages of 8 and 53 years. Most subjects in the two trials were 12 or older.

CONTRAINDICATIONS:

1. Pimozide is contraindicated in the treatment of simple tics or tics other than those associated with Tourette's Disorder.

2. Pimozide should not be used in patients taking drugs that may, themselves, cause motor and phonic tics (*e.g.,* pemoline, methylphenidate and amphetamines) until such patients have been withdrawn from these drugs to determine whether or not the drugs, rather than Tourette's Disorder, are responsible for the tics.

3. Because Pimozide prolongs the QT interval of the electrocardiogram it is contraindicated in patients with congenital long QT syndrome, patients with a history of cardiac arrhythmias, or patients taking other drugs which prolong the QT interval of the electrocardiogram (see DRUG INTERACTIONS.)

4. Pimozide is contraindicated in patients with severe toxic central nervous system depression or comatose states from any cause.

5. Pimozide is contraindicated in patients with hypersensitivity to it. As it is not known whether cross-sensitivity exists among the antipsychotics, Pimozide should be used with appropriate caution in patients who have demonstrated hypersensitivity to other antipsychotic drugs.

WARNINGS:

The use of Pimozide in the treatment of Tourette's Disorder involves different risk/benefit considerations than when antipsychotic drugs are used to treat other conditions. Consequently, a decision to use Pimozide should take into consideration the following (see also PRECAUTIONS, Information for the Patient).

Tardive Dyskinesia: A syndrome consisting of potentially irreversible, involuntary, dyskinetic movements may develop in patients treated with antipsychotic drugs. Although the prevalence of the syndrome appears to be highest among the elderly, especially elderly women, it is impossible to rely upon prevalence estimates to predict, at the inception of antipsychotic treatment, which patients are likely to develop the syndrome. Whether antipsychotic drug products differ in their potential to cause tardive dyskinesia is unknown.

Both the risk of developing tardive dyskinesia and the likelihood that it will become irreversible are believed to increase as the duration of treatment and the total cumulative dose of antipsychotic drugs administered to the patient increase. However, the syndrome can develop, although much less commonly, after relatively brief treatment periods at low doses.

There is no known treatment for established cases of tardive dyskinesia, although the syndrome may remit, partially or completely, if antipsychotic treatment is withdrawn. Antipsychotic treatment, itself, however, may suppress (or partially suppress) the signs and symptoms of the syndrome and thereby possibly mask the underlying process. The effect that symptomatic suppression has upon the long-term course of the syndrome is unknown.

Given these considerations, antipsychotic drugs should be prescribed is a manner that is most likely to minimize the occurrence of tardive dyskinesia. Chronic antipsychotic treatment should generally be reserved for patients who suffer from a chronic illness that, 1) is known to respond to antipsychotic drugs, and, 2) for whom alternative, equally effective, but potentially less harmful treatments are not available or appropriate. In patients who do require chronic treatment, the smallest dose and the shortest duration of treatment producing a satisfactory clinical response should be sought. The need for continued treatment should be reassessed periodically.

If signs and symptoms of tardive dyskinesia appear in a patient on antipsychotics, drug discontinuation should be considered. However, some patients may require treatment despite the presence of the syndrome.

(For further information about the description of tardive dyskinesia and its clinical detection, please refer to ADVERSE REACTIONS and PRECAUTIONS- Information for Patients.)

Neuroleptic Malignant Syndrome (NMS): A potentially fatal syndrome complex sometimes referred to as Neuroleptic Malignant Syndrome (NMS) has been reported in association with antipsychotic drugs. Clinical manifestations of NMS are hyperpyrexia, muscle rigidity, altered mental status (including catatonic signs) and evidence of autonomic instability (irregular pulse or blood pressure, tachycardia, diaphoresis, and cardiac dysrhythmias). Additional signs may include elevated creatinine phosphokinase, myoglobinuria (rhabdomyolysis) and acute renal failure.

The diagnostic evaluation of patients with this syndrome is complicated. In arriving at a diagnosis, it is important to identify cases where the clinical presentation includes both serious medical illness (*e.g.,* pneumonia, systemic infection, etc.) and untreated or inadequately treated extrapyramidal signs and symptoms (EPS). Other important considerations in the differential diagnosis include central anticholinergic toxicity, heat stroke, drug fever and primary central nervous system (CNS) pathology.

The management of NMS should include 1) immediate discontinuation of antipsychotic drugs and other drugs not essential to concurrent therapy, 2) intensive symptomatic treatment and medical monitoring, and 3) treatment of any concomitant serious medical problems for which specific treatments are available. There is no general agreement about specific pharmacological treatment regimens for uncomplicated NMS.

If a patient requires antipsychotic drug treatment after recovery from NMS, the potential reintroduction of drug therapy should be carefully considered. The patient should be carefully monitored, since recurrences of NMS have been reported.

Hyperpyrexia, not associated with the above symptom complex, has been reported with other antipsychotic drugs.

Other: Sudden, unexpected deaths have occurred in experimental studies of conditions other than Tourette's Disorder. These deaths occurred while patients were receiving dosages in the range of 1 mg per kg. One possible mechanisms for such deaths is prolongations of the QT interval predisposing patients to ventricular arrhythmia. An electrocardiogram should be performed before Pimozide treatment is initiated and periodically thereafter, especially during the period of dose adjustment.

Pimozide may have a tumorigenic potential. Based on studies conducted in mice, it is known that Pimozide can produce a dose related increase in pituitary tumors. The full significance of this finding is not known, but should be taken into consideration in the physician's and patient's decisions to use this drug product. This finding should be given special consideration when the patient is young and chronic use of Pimozide is anticipated. (See PRECAUTIONS, Carcinogenesis, Mutagenesis, and Impairment of Fertility.)

PRECAUTIONS:

General: Pimozide may impair the mental and/or physical abilities required for the performance of potentially hazardous tasks, such as driving a car or operating machinery, especially during the first few days of therapy.

Pimozide produces anticholinergic side effects and should be used with caution in individuals whose conditions may be aggravated by anticholinergic activity.

Pimozide should be administered cautiously to patients with impairment of liver or kidney function, because it is metabolized by the liver and excreted by the kidneys.

Antipsychotics should be administered with caution to patients receiving anticonvulsant medication, with a history of seizures, or with EEG abnormalities, because they may lower the convulsive threshold. If indicated, adequate anticonvulsant therapy should be maintained concomitantly.

Information for the Patient: Treatment with Pimozide exposes the patient to serious risks. A decision to use Pimozide chronically in Tourette's Disorder is one that deserves full consideration by the patient (or patient's family) as well as by the treating physician. Because the goal of treatment is symptomatic improvement, the patient's view of the need for treatment and assessment of response are critical in evaluating the impact of therapy and weighing its benefits against the risks. Since the physician is the primary source of information about the use of a drug in any disease it is recommended that the following information be discussed with patients and/or their families.

Pimozide is intended only for use in patients with Tourette's Disorder whose symptoms are severe and who cannot tolerate, or who do not respond to Haldol (haloperidol).

Given the likelihood that a proportion of patients exposed chronically to antipsychotics will develop tardive dyskinesia, it is advised that all patients in whom chronic use is contemplated be given, if possible, full information about this risk. The decision to inform patients and/or their guardians must obviously take into account the clinical circumstances and the competency of the patient to understand the information provided.

There is limited information available on the use of Pimozide in children under 12 years of age.

The information available on Pimozide from foreign marketing experience and from U.S. clinical trials indicate that Pimozide has a side effect profile similar to that of other antipsychotic drugs. Patients should be informed that all types of side effects associated with the use of antipsychotics may be associated with the use of Pimozide.

In addition, sudden unexpected deaths have occurred in patients taking high doses of Pimozide for conditions other than Tourette's Disorder. These deaths may have been the result of an effect of Pimozide upon the heart. Therefore, patients should be instructed not to exceed the prescribed dose of Pimozide and they should realize the need for the initial ECG and for follow-up ECGs during treatment.

Also, pimozide, at a dose about 15 times that given humans, caused an increase in the number of benign tumors of the pituitary gland in female mice. It is not possible to say how important this is. Similar tumors were not seen in rats given pimozide, nor at lower doses in mice, which is reassuring. However, any such finding must be considered to suggest a possible risk of long term use of the drug.

Laboratory Tests: An ECG should be done at baseline and periodically thereafter throughout the period of dose adjustment. Any indication of prolongation of the QT_c interval beyond an absolute limit of 0.47 seconds (children) or 0.52 seconds (adults), or more than 25% above the patient's original baseline should be considered a basis for stopping further dose increase (see CONTRAINDICATIONS) and considering a lower dose.

Since hypokalemia has been associated with ventricular arrhythmias, potassium insufficiency, secondary to diuretics, diarrhea, or other cause, should be corrected before Pimozide therapy is initiated and normal potassium maintained during therapy.

Carcinogenesis, Mutagenesis, and Impairment of Fertility: Carcinogenicity studies were conducted in mice and rats. In mice, Pimozide causes a dose-related increase in pituitary and mammary tumors.

When mice were treated for up to 18 months with pimozide, pituitary gland changes developed in females only. These changes were characterized as hyperplasia at doses approximating the human dose and adenoma at doses about fifteen times the maximum recommended human dose on a mg per kg basis. The mechanism for the induction of pituitary tumors in mice is not known.

Mammary gland tumors in female mice were also increased, but these tumors are expected in rodents treated with antipsychotic drugs which elevate prolactin levels. Chronic administration of an antipsychotic also causes elevated prolactin levels in humans. Tissue culture experiments indicate that approximately one-third of human breast cancers are prolactin-dependent *in vitro,* a factor of potential importance if the prescription of these drugs is contemplated in a patient with a previously detected breast cancer. Although disturbances such as galactorrhea, amenorrhea, gynecomastia, and impotence have been reported with antipsychotic drugs, the clinical significance of elevated serum prolactin levels is unknown for most patients. Neither clinical studies nor epidemiologic studies conducted to date have shown an association between chronic administration of these drugs and mammary tumorigenesis. The available evidence, however, is considered too limited to be conclusive at this time.

In a 24 month carcinogenicity study in rats, animals received up to 50 times the maximum recommended human dose. No increased incidence of overall tumors or tumors at any site was observed in either sex. Because of the limited number of animals surviving this study, the meaning of these results is unclear.

Pimozide did not have mutagenic activity in the Ames test with four bacterial test strains, in the mouse dominant lethal test or in the micronucleus test in rats.

Reproduction studies in animals were not adequate to assess all aspects of fertility. Nevertheless, female rats administered Pimozide had prolonged estrus cycles, an effect also produced by other antipsychotic drugs.

Pregnancy Category C: Reproduction studies performed in rats and rabbits at oral doses up to 8 times the maximum human dose did not reveal evidence of teratogenicity. In the rat, however, this multiple of the human dose resulted in decreased pregnancies and in the retarded development of fetuses. These effects are thought to be due to an inhibition or delay in implantation which is also observed in rodents administered other antipsychotic drugs. In the rabbit, maternal toxicity, mortality, decreased weight gain, and embryotoxicity including

PRECAUTIONS: *(cont'd)*

increased resorptions were dose related. Because animal reproduction studies are not always predictive of human response, pimozide should be given to a pregnant woman only if the potential benefits to treatment clearly outweigh the potential risks.

Labor and Delivery: This drug has no recognized use in labor or delivery.

Nursing Mothers: It is not known whether pimozide is excreted in human milk. Because many drugs are excreted in human milk and because of the potential for tumorigenicity and unknown cardiovascular effects in the infant, a decision should be made whether to discontinue nursing or to discontinue the drug, taking into account the importance of the drug to the mother.

Pediatric Use: Although Tourette's Disorder most often has its onset between the ages of 2 and 15 years, information on the use and efficacy of Pimozide in patients less than 12 years of age is limited.

A 24 week open label study in 36 children between the age of 2 and 12 demonstrated that pimozide has a similiar safety profile in this age group as in older patients and there were no safety findings that would preclude its use in this age group.

Because its use and safety have not been evaluated in other childhood disorders, Pimozide is not recommended for use in any condition other than Tourette's Disorder.

DRUG INTERACTIONS:

Because Pimozide prolongs the QT interval of the electrocardiogram, an additive effect on QT interval would be anticipated if administered with other drugs such as phenothiazines, tricyclic antidepressants or antiarrhythmic agents, which prolong the QT interval. Such concomitant administration should not be undertaken (see CONTRAINDICATIONS.)

Pimozide may be capable of potentiating CNS depressants, including analgesics, sedatives, anxiolytics, and alcohol.

ADVERSE REACTIONS:

GENERAL

Extrapyramidal Reactions: Neuromuscular (extrapyramidal) reactions during the administration of Pimozide have been reported frequently, often during the first few days of treatment. In most patients, these reactions involved Parkinson-like symptoms which, when first observed, were usually mild to moderately severe and usually reversible.

Other types of neuromuscular reactions (motor restlessness, dystonia, akathisia, hyperreflexia, opisthotonos, oculogyric crises) have been reported far less frequently. Severe extrapyramidal reactions have been reported to occur at relatively low doses. Generally the occurrence and severity of most extrapyramidal symptoms are dose related since they occur at relatively high doses and have been shown to disappear or become less severe when the dose is reduced. Administration of antiparkinson drugs such as benztropine mesylate or trihexyphenidyl hydrochloride may be required for control of such reactions. It should be noted that persistent extrapyramidal reactions have been reported and that the drug may have to be discontinued in such cases.

Withdrawal Emergent Neurological Signs: Generally, patients receiving short term therapy experience no problems with abrupt discontinuation of antipsychotic drugs. However, some patients on maintenance treatment experience transient dyskinetic signs after abrupt withdrawal. In certain of these cases the dyskinetic movements are indistinguishable from the syndrome described below under "Tardive Dyskinesia" except for duration. It is not known whether gradual withdrawal of antipsychotic drugs will reduce the rate of occurrence of withdrawal emergent neurological signs but until further evidence becomes available, it seems reasonable to gradually withdraw use of Pimozide.

Tardive Dyskinesia: Pimozide may be associated with persistent dyskinesias. Tardive dyskinesias. Tardive dyskinesia, a syndrome consisting of potentially irreversible, involuntary, dyskinetic movements, may appear in some patients on long-term therapy or may occur after drug therapy has been discontinued. The risk appears to be greater in elderly patients on long-term therapy or may occur after drug therapy has been discontinued. The risk appears to be greater in elderly patients on high-dose therapy, especially females. The symptoms are persistent and in some patients appear irreversible. The syndrome is characterized by rhythmical involuntary movements of tongue, face, mouth or jaw (*e.g.,* protrusion of tongue, puffing of cheeks, puckering of mouth, chewing movements). Sometimes these may be accompanied by involuntary movements of extremities and the trunk.

There is no known effective treatment for tardive dyskinesia; antiparkinson agents usually do not alleviate the symptoms of this syndrome. It is suggested that all antipsychotic agents be discontinued if these symptoms appear. Should it be necessary to reinstitute treatment, or increase the dosage of the agent, or switch to a different antipsychotic agent, this syndrome may be masked.

It has been reported that fine vermicular movement of the tongue may be an early sign of tardive dyskinesia and if the medication is stopped at that time the full syndrome may not develop.

Electrocardiographic Changes: Electrocardiographic changes have been observed in clinical trials of Pimozide in Tourette's Disorder and schizophrenia. These have included prolongation of the QT interval, flattening, notching and inversion of the T wave and the appearance of U waves. Sudden, unexpected deaths and grand mal seizure have occurred at doses above 20 mg/day.

Neuroleptic Malignant Syndrome: Neuroleptic malignant syndrome (NMS) has been reported with Pimozide. (See WARNINGSfor further information concerning NMS.)

Hyperpyrexia: Hyperpyrexia has been reported with other antipsychotic drugs.

Clinical Trials: The following adverse reaction tabulation (TABLE 1) was derived from 20 patients in a 6 week long placebo controlled clinical trial of Pimozide in Tourette's Disorder.

The following adverse event tabulation was derived from 36 children (age 2 to 12) in a 24 week open trial of Pimozide in Tourette's Disorder. (See TABLE 2)

Because clinical investigational experience with Pimozide in Tourette's Disorder is limited, uncommon adverse reactions may not have been detected. The physician should consider that other adverse reactions associated with antipsychotics may occur.

OTHER ADVERSE REACTIONS

In addition to the adverse reactions listed above, those listed below have been reported in U.S. clinical trials of Pimozide in conditions other than Tourette's Disorder.

Body as a Whole: Asthenia, chest pain, periorbital edema

Cardiovascular/Respiratory: Postural hypotension, hypotension, hypertension, tachycardia, palpitations

Gastrointestinal: Increased salivation, nausea, vomiting anorexia, GI distress

Endocrine: Loss of libido

Metabolic/Nutritional: Weight gain, weight loss

Central Nervous System: Dizziness, tremor, parkinsonism, fainting, dyskinesia

Psychiatric: Excitement

Skin: Rash, sweating, skin irritation

Special Senses: Blurred vision, cataracts

ADVERSE REACTIONS: *(cont'd)*

TABLE 1

Body System/ Adverse Reaction	Pimozide (N = 20)	Placebo (N = 20)
Body as a Whole		
Headache	1	2
Gastrointestinal		
Dry Mouth	5	1
Diarrhea	1	0
Nausea	0	2
Vomiting	0	1
Constipation	4	2
Eructations	0	1
Thirsty	1	0
Appetite increase	1	0
Endocrine		
Menstrual disorder	0	1
Breast secretions	0	1
Musculoskeletal		
Muscle cramps	0	1
Muscle tightness	3	0
Stooped posture	2	0
CNS		
Drowsiness	7	3
Sedation	14	5
Insomnia	2	2
Dizziness	0	1
Akathisia	8	0
Rigidity	2	0
Speech disorder	2	0
Handwriting change	1	0
Akinesia	8	0
Psychiatric		
Depression	2	3
Excitement	0	1
Nervous	1	0
Adverse behavior effect	5	0
Special Senses		
Visual disturbance	4	0
Taste change	1	0
Sensitivity of eyes to light	1	0
Decreased accommodation	4	1
Spots before eyes	0	1
Urogenital		
Impotence	3	0

TABLE 2 Pimozide, Adverse Reactions

Body System/Adverse Reaction	Number of Patients Experiencing Each Event (%)	
	All Events (N=36)	Drug-Related Events (N=36)
Body as a Whole		
Asthenia	9 (25.0)	5 (13.8)
Headache	8 (22.2)	1 (2.7)
Gastrointestinal		
Dysphagia	1 (2.7)	1 (2.7)
Increased Salivation	5 (13.8)	2 (5.5)
Musculoskeletal		
Myalgia	1 (2.7)	1 (2.7)
Central Nervous System		
Dreaming Abnormal	1 (2.7)	1 (2.7)
Hyperkinesia	2 (5.5)	1 (2.7)
Somnolence	10 (27.7)	9 (25.0)
Torticollis	1 (2.7)	1 (2.7)
Tremor, Limbs	1 (2.7)	1 (2.7)
Psychiatric		
Adverse Behavior Effect	10 (27.7)	8 (22.2)
Nervous	3 (8.3)	2 (5.5)
Skin		
Rash	3 (8.3)	1 (2.7)
Special Senses		
Visual Disturbances	2 (5.5)	1 (2.7)
Cardiovascular		
ECG Abnormal	1 (2.7)	1 (2.7)

Urogenital: Nocturia, urinary frequency

POSTMARKETING REPORTS

The following experiences were described in spontaneous postmarketing reports. These reports do not provide sufficient information to establish a clear causal relationship with the use of Pimozide.

Hematologic: Hemolytic anemia

Other: Seizure has been reported in one patient.

OVERDOSAGE:

In general, the signs and symptoms of overdosage with Pimozide would be an exaggeration of known pharmacologic effects and adverse reactions, the most prominent of which would be: 1) electrocardiographic abnormalities, 2) severe extrapyramidal reactions, 3) hypotension, 4) a comatose state with respiratory depression.

In the event of overdosage, gastric lavage, establishment of a patent airway and, if necessary, mechanically-assisted respiration are advised. Electrocardiographic monitoring should commence immediately and continue until the ECG parameters are within the normal range. Hypotension and circulatory collapse may be counteracted by use of intravenous fluids, plasma, or concentrated albumin, and vasopressor agents such as metaraminol, phenylephrine and norepinephrine. Epinephrine should not be used. In case of severe extrapyramidal reactions, antiparkinson medication should be administered. Because of the long half-life of Pimozide, patients who take an overdose should be observed for at least 4 days. As with all drugs, the physician should consider contacting a poison control center for additional information on the treatment of overdose.

DOSAGE AND ADMINISTRATION:

General: The suppression of tics by Pimozide requires a slow and gradual introduction of the drug. The patient's dose should be carefully adjusted to a point where the suppression of tics and the relief afforded is balanced against the untoward side effects of the drug.

An ECG should be done at baseline and periodically thereafter, especially during the period of dose adjustment (see WARNINGSand PRECAUTIONS, Laboratory Tests.)

DOSAGE AND ADMINISTRATION: *(cont'd)*

Periodic attempts should be made to reduce the dosage of Pimozide to see whether or not tics persist at the level and extent first identified. In attempts to reduce the dosage of Pimozide, consideration should be given to the possibility that increases of tic intensity and frequency may represent a transient, withdrawal related phenomenon rather than a return of disease symptoms. Specifically, one to two weeks should be allowed to elapse before one concludes that an increase in tic manifestations is a function of the underlying disease syndrome rather than a response to drug withdrawal. A gradual withdrawal recommended in any case.

Children: Reliable dose response data for the effects of Pimozide on tic manifestations in Tourette's Disorder patients below the age of twelve are not available. Treatment should be initiated at a dose of 0.05 mg/kg preferably taken once at bedtime. The dose may be increased every third day to a maximum of 0.2 mg/kg not to exceed 10 mg/day.

Adults: In general, treatment with Pimozide should be initiated with a dose of 1 to 2 mg a day in divided doses. The dose may be increased thereafter every other day. Most patients are maintained at less than 0.2 mg/kg per day, or 10 mg/day, whichever is less. Doses greater than 0.2 mg/kg/day or 10 mg/day are not recommended.

ANIMAL PHARMACOLOGY:

A chronic study in dogs indicated that Pimozide caused gingival hyperplasia when administered for several months at about 5 times the maximum recommended human dose. This condition was reversible after withdrawal. This condition has not been observed following chronic administration of Pimozide to man.

HOW SUPPLIED:

Pimozide 2 mg tablets, white, scored, debossed "LEMMON" and "ORAP 2" bottles of 100.

Dispense in a tight, light-resistant container as defined in the official compendium.

Pharmacist: Dispense in child resistant container.

(Lemmon Company, Rev D 8/94)

HOW SUPPLIED - EQUIVALENTS NOT AVAILABLE:

Tablet, Uncoated - Oral - 2 mg

100's	$70.70	ORAP, Gate Pharms	57844-0187-01

PINDOLOL *(002039)*

CATEGORIES: Antihypertensives; Beta Adrenergic Blocking Agents; Beta Blockers; Cardiovascular Drugs; Hypertension; Pregnancy Category B; FDA Approved 1982 Sep; Patent Expiration 1992 Sep

BRAND NAMES: *Apo-Pindolol*; *Barbloc*; *Bedrenal*; *Betadren*; *Betapindol*; *Blocklin*; *Carvisken* (Japan); *Cinbloc* (Japan); *Cocaserin*; *Decreten*; *ID IMPLIED*; *Dolopin*; *Dranolis*; *Durapindol* (Germany); *Hexapindol*; *Marles* (Japan); *Nonspi* (Germany); *Novo-Pindol* (Canada); *Osnon* (Japan); *Pidol*; *Pinbetol* (Germany); *Pinden*; *Pindol*; *Pindomex*; *Pinloc*; *Pynastin* (Japan); *Pinsken*; *Symphol* (Japan); *Syn-Pindolol* (Canada); *Treparasen*; *Viskeen*; *Viskeen Retard*; **Visken**; *Viskene*; *Vypen*
(International brand names outside U.S. in italics)

FORMULARIES: Aetna; BC-BS; Medi-Cal; PCS

COST OF THERAPY: $169.72 (Hypertension; Tablet; 5 mg; 2/day; 365 days) vs. Potential Cost of $24,027.04 (Coronary Bypass)

PRIMARY ICD9: 401.1 (Essential Hypertension, Benign)

DESCRIPTION:

Pindolol, a synthetic beta-adrenergic receptor blocking agent with intrinsic sympathomimetic activity is 4-(2-hydroxy-3-isopropylamino-propoxy)-indole.

Pindolol is a white to off-white odorless powder soluble in organic solvents and aqueous acids. Pindolol is intended for oral administration.

5 MG AND 10 MG TABLETS

Active Ingredient: Pindolol

Inactive Ingredients: colloidal silicon dioxide, magnesium stearate, microcrystalline cellulose, and pregelatinized starch.

CLINICAL PHARMACOLOGY:

Pindolol is a non-selective beta-adrenergic antagonist (beta-blocker) which possesses intrinsic sympathomimetic activity (ISA) in therapeutic dosage ranges but dose not possess quinidine-like membrane stabilizing activity.

PHARMACODYNAMICS

In standard pharmacologic tests in humans and animals, Pindolol attenuates increases in heart rate, systolic blood pressure, and cardiac output resulting from exercise and isoproterenol administration, thus confirming its beta-blocking properties. The ISA or partial agonist activity of Pindolol is mediated blocked by other beta-blockers. In catecholamine depleted animal experiments, ISA is manifested as an increase in the inotropic and chronotropic activity of the myocardium. In man, ISA is manifested by a smaller reduction in the resting heart rate (4-8 beats/min) than is seen with drugs lacking ISA. There is also a smaller reduction in resting cardiac output. The clinical significance of this observation has not been evaluated and there is no evidence, or reason to believe, that exercise cardiac output is less affected by Pindolol.

Pindolol has been shown in controlled, double-blind clinical studies to be an effective antihypertensive agent when used as monotherapy, or when added to therapy with thiazide-type diuretics. Divided dosages in the range of 10 mg-60 mg daily has been shown to be effective. As monotherapy Pindolol is an effective as propranolol, α-methyldopa, hydrochlorothiazide and chlorthalidone in reducing systolic and diastolic blood pressure. The effect on blood pressure is not orthostatic, i.e. Pindolol was equally effective in reducing the supine and standing blood pressure.

In open, long term studies up to four (4) years, no evidence of diminution of the blood pressure lowering response was observed.

An average 3 pound increase in body weight has been noted in patients treated with Pindolol alone, a larger increase than was observed with propranolol or placebo. The weight gain appeared unrelated to blood pressure response and was not associated with an increased risk of heart failure, although edema was more common than in control patients. Pindolol does not have a consistent effect on plasma renin activity.

The mechanism of the antihypertensive effects of beta-blocking agents has not been established, but several mechanisms have been postulated: 1) an effect on the central nervous system resulting in a reduced sympathetic outflow to the periphery, 2) competitive antagonism of catecholamines at peripheral (especially cardiac) adrenergic receptor sites, leading to

CLINICAL PHARMACOLOGY: *(cont'd)*

decreased cardiac output, 3) an inhibition of renin release. These mechanisms appear less likely for pindolol than other beta-blockers in view of the modest effect on resting cardiac output and renin.

Beta-blockade therapy is useful when it is necessary to suppress the effects of beta-adrenergic agonists in order to achieve therapeutic goals. However, in certain clinical situation, (*e.g.*, cardiac failure, heart block, bronchospasm) the preservation of an adequate sympathetic tone may be necessary to maintain vital functions. Although a beta-antagonist with ISA such as Pindolol does not eliminate sympathetic tone entirely, there is no controlled evidence that it is safer other beta-blockers in such conditions as heart failure, heart block, or bronchospasm or is less likely to cause those conditions. In single dose studies of the effects of beta-blockers on FEV_1, Pindolol was indistinguishable from other non-cardioselective agents in its reduction of FEV_1, and its reduction in the effectiveness of an exogenous beta agonist.

Exacerbation of angina and, in some cases, myocardial infarction and ventricular dysrhythmias have been reported after abrupt discontinuation of therapy with beta-adrenergic blocking agents in patients with coronary artery disease. Abrupt withdrawal of these agents in patients with out coronary artery disease has resulted in transient symptoms, including tremulousness, sweating, palpitation, headache, and malaise. Several mechanisms have been proposed to explain these phenomena, among them increased sensitivity to catecholamines because of increase numbers of beta receptors.

PHARMACOKINETICS AND METABOLISM

Pindolol is rapidly and reproducibly absorbed (greater than 95%) achieving peak plasma concentrations within one hour of drug administration. Pindolol has no significant first-pass effect. The blood concentrations are proportional in a linear manner to the administered dose in the range of 5-20 mg. Upon repeated administration to the same subject, carnation is minimal. After a single dose, intersubject variation for peak plasma concentrations was about 4 fold (*e.g.*, 45-167 ng/ml for a 20 mg dose). Upon multiple dosing, intersubject variation decreased to 2-2.5 fold. Pindolol is only 40% bound to plasma proteins and is evenly distributed between plasma and red cells. The volume of distribution in healthy subjects is about 2 L/kg.

Pindolol undergoes extensive metabolism in animals and man. In man, 35-40% is excreted unchanged in the urine and 60-65% is metabolized primarily to hydroxy-metabolites which are excreted as glucuronides and ethereal sulfates. The polar metabolites are excreted with a half-life of approximately 8 hours multiple dosing, therapy (q.8H) results in a less than 50% accumulation in plasma. About 6-9% of an administered intravenous dose is excreted by the bile into the feces.

The disposition of Pindolol after oral administration is monophasic is monophasic with a half-life in healthy subjects or hypertensive patients with normal renal function of approximately 3-4 hours. Following t.i.d. administration (q.8H), no significant accumulation of Pindolol is observed.

In elderly hypertensive patients with normal renal function the half-life of Pindolol is more variable, averaging about 7 hours, but with values as high as 15 hours.

In hypertensive patients with renal disease, the half-life is within the range expected for healthy subjects. However, a significant decrease (50%) in volume of distribution (V_D) is observed in uremic patients and V_D appears to be directly correlated to creatinine clearance. Therefore, renal drug clearance is significantly reduced in uremic patients, resulting in a significant decrease in urinary excretion of unchanged drug. Uremic patients with a creatinine clearance of less than 20 ml/min generally excreted less than 15% of the administered dose an changed in the urine.

In patients with histologically diagnosed cirrhosis of the liver, the elimination of Pindolol was more variable in rate and generally significantly slower than in healthy subjects. The total body clearance of Pindolol in cirrhotic patients ranged from about 50 ml/min to 300 ml/min and was directly correlated to antipyrine clearance. The half-life ranged from 2.5 hours to greater than 30 hours. These findings strongly suggest that caution should be exercised in dosage adjustments of Pindolol in such patients.

The bioavailability of Pindolol is not significantly affected by co-administration of food, hydralazine, hydrochlorothiazide or aspirin. Pindolol has no effect on warfarin activity or the clinical effectiveness of digoxin, although small transient decreases in plasma digoxin concentrations were noted.

INDICATIONS AND USAGE:

Pindolol is indicated in the management of hypertension. It may be used alone or concomitantly with other antihypertensive agents, with a thiazide type diuretic.

CONTRAINDICATIONS:

Pindolol is contraindicated in: 1) bronchial asthma; 2) overt cardiac failure; 3) cardiogenic shock; 4) second and third degree heart block; 5) severe bradycardia; (see WARNINGS.)

WARNINGS:

CARDIAC FAILURE

Sympathetic stimulation may be a vital component supporting circulatory function in patients with congestive heart failure, and its inhibition by beta-blockade may precipitate more severe failure. Although beta-blockers should be avoided in overt congestive heart failure, if necessary, Pindolol can be used with caution in patients with a history of failure who are well-compensated, usually with digitalis and diuretics. Beta-adrenergic blocking agents do not abolish the inotropic action of digitalis on heart muscle.

IN PATIENTS WITHOUT A HISTORY OF CARDIAC FAILURE

In patients with latent cardiac insufficiency, continued depression of the myocardium with beta-blocking agents over a period of time can in some cases lead to cardiac failure. At the first sign or symptom of impending cardiac failure, patients should be fully digitalized and/or be given a diuretic, and the response observed closely. If cardiac failure continues, despite adequate digitalization and diuretic, Pindolol therapy should be withdrawn (gradually if possible).

Exacerbation of Ischemic Heart Disease Following Abrupt Withdrawal: Hypersensitivity to catecholamines has been observed in patients withdrawn from beta-blockers therapy; exacerbation of angina and, in some cases, myocardial infarction have occurred after abrupt discontinuation of such therapy. When discontinuing chronically administered Pindolol, particularly in patients with ischemic heart disease, the dosage should be gradually reduced over a period of one to two weeks and the patient should be carefully monitored. If angina markedly worsens or acute coronary insufficiency develops. Pindolol administration should be reinstituted promptly, at least temporarily, and other measures appropriate for the management of unstable angina should be taken. Patients should be warned against interruption or discontinuation of therapy without the physician's advice. Because coronary artery disease is common and may be unrecognized, it may be present not to discontinue Pindolol therapy abruptly even in patients treated only for hypertension.

Nonallergic Bronchospasm (*e.g.*, chronic bronchitis, emphysema)-Patients with Bronchospastic Disease Should in General Not Receive Beta-Blockers: Pindolol should be administered with caution since it may block bronchodilation produced by endogenous or exogenous catecholamine stimulation of $beta_2$ receptors.

WARNINGS: *(cont'd)*

MAJOR SURGERY

Because beta Blockade impairs the ability of the heart to respond to reflex stimuli and may increase, the risks of general anesthesia and surgical procedures, resulting in protracted hypotension or low cardiac output, it has generally been suggested that such therapy should be withdrawn several days prior to surgery. Recognition of the increased sensitivity to catecholamines of patients of patients recently withdrawn from beta-blocker therapy, however, has made this recommendation controversial. If possible, beta-blockers should be withdrawn well before surgery takes place. In the event of emergency surgery, the anesthesiologist should be informed that the patients is one beta-blockers therapy. The effects of Pindolol can be reversed by administration of beta-receptor agonists such as isoproterenol, dopamine, dobutamine, or levarterenol. Difficulty in restarting and maintaining the heart beat also been reported with beta-adrenergic receptor blocking agents.

DIABETES AND HYPOGLYCEMIA

Beta-adrenergic blockade may prevent the appearance of premonitory signs and symptoms (*e.g.,* tachycardia and blood pressure changes) of acute hypoglycemia. This is especially important with labile diabetic. Beta-blockade also reduces the release of insulin in response to hyperglycemia; therefore, it may be necessary to adjust the dose of antidiabetic drugs.

THYROTOXICOSIS

Beta-adrenergic blockade may mask certain clinical signs (*e.g.,* tachycardia) of hyperthyroidism. Patients suspected of developing thyrotoxicosis should be managed carefully to avoid abrupt withdrawal of beta-blockade which might precipitate a thyroid crisis.

PRECAUTIONS:

IMPAIRED RENAL OR HEPATIC FUNCTION

Beta-blocking agents should be used with caution in patients with impaired hepatic or renal function. Poor renal function has only minor effects on Pindolol clearance, but poor hepatic function may cause blood levels of Pindolol to increase substantially.

INFORMATION FOR THE PATIENT

Patients, especially those with evidence of coronary artery insufficiency, should be warned against interruption or discontinuation of Pindolol therapy without the physician's advice. Although cardiac failure rarely occurs in properly selected patients, patients being treated with beta-adrenergic blocking agents should be advised to consult the physician at the first sign or symptom of impending failure.

CARCINOGENESIS, MUTAGENESIS, AND IMPAIRMENT OF FERTILITY

In chronic oral toxicologic studies (one to two years) in mice, rats, and dogs, Pindolol did not produce any significant toxic effect. In two-year oral carcinogenicity studies in rats and mice in dose as high as 59 mg/kg/day and 124 mg/kg/day (50 and 100 times the maximum recommended human dose), respectively, Pindolol did not produce any neoplastic, preneoplastic, or nonneoplastic pathologic lesions. In fertility and general reproductive performance studies in rats, Pindolol caused no adverse effects at a dose of 10 mg/kg.

In the male fertility and general reproductive performance test in rats, definite toxicity characterized by mortality and decreased weight gain was observed in the group given 100 mg/kg/day. At 30 mg/kg/day, decreased mating was associated with testicular atrophy and/or decreased spermatogenesis. This response is not clearly drug related, however, as there was not dose response relationship within this experiment and no similar effect on testes of rats administered Pindolol as a dietary admixture for 104 weeks. There appeared to be an increase in prenatal mortality in males given 100 mg/kg but development of offspring was not impaired.

In females administered Pindolol prior to mating through day 21 of lactation, mating behavior was decreased at 100 mg/kg and 30 mg/kg. At these dosage there also was increased mortality of offspring. Prenatal mortality was increased at 10 mg/kg but there was not a clear dose response relationship in this experiment. There was an increased resorption rate at 100 mg/kg observed in females necropsied on the 15th day of gestation.

PREGNANCY CATEGORY B

Studies in rats and rabbits exceeding 100 times the maximum recommended human doses, revealed no embryotoxicity or teratogenicity. Since there are no adequate and well-controlled studies in pregnant women, and since animal reproduction studies are not always predictive of human response, Pindolol, as with any drug, should be employed during pregnancy only if the potential benefit justifies the potential risk of the fetus.

NURSING MOTHERS

Since Pindolol is secreted in human milk, nursing should not be undertaken by mothers receiving the drug.

PEDIATRIC USE

Safety and effectiveness in children have not been established.

CLINICAL LABORATORY

Minor persistent elevations in serum transaminases (SGOT, SGPT) have been noted in 7% of patients during Pindolol administration, but progressive elevations were not observed. These elevations were not associated with other abnormalities that would suggest hepatic impairment, such as decreased serum albumin and total proteins. During more than a decade of worldwide marketing, there have been no reports in the medical literature of overt hepatic injury. Alkaline phosphatase, lactic acid dehydrogenase (LDH), and uric acid are also elevated on rare occasions. The significance of these findings is unknown.

DRUG INTERACTIONS:

Catecholamine-depleting drugs (*e.g.,* reserpine) may have an additive effect when given with beta-blocking agents. Patients receiving Pindolol plus a catecholamine depleting agent should, therefore, be closely observed for evidence of hypotension and/or marked bradycardia which may produce vertigo, syncope, or postural hypotension.

Pindolol has been used with a variety of antihypertensive agents, including hydrochlorothiazide, hydralazine, and guanethidine without unexpected adverse interactions.

Pindolol has been shown to increase serum thioridazine levels when both drugs are coadministered. Pindolol levels may also be increased with this combination.

Risk of Anaphylactic Reaction: While taking beta blockers, patients with a history of severe anaphylactic reaction to a variety of allergens may be more reactive to repeated challenge, either accidental, diagnostic, or therapeutic. Such patients may be unresponsive to the usual doses of epinephrine used to treat allergic reaction.

ADVERSE REACTIONS:

Most adverse reactions have been mild. The incidences listed in the following table are derived from 12 week comparative double-blind, parallel design trails in hypertensive patients given Pindolol as monotherapy, given various active control drugs as monotherapy, or given placebo. Data for Pindolol and the positive controls were pooled from several trials because no striking differences were seen in the individual studies, with one exception. The frequency of edema was noticeably higher in positive control trials (16% Pindolol vs 9% positive control) than in placebo controlled trials (6% Pindolol) vs 3% placebo). The table, (TABLE 1), includes adverse reactions reported in greater than 2% of Pindolol patients and other selected important reactions.

ADVERSE REACTIONS: *(cont'd)*

TABLE 1 ADVERSE REACTIONS WERE VOLUNTEERED OR ELICITED (AND AT LEAST POSSIBLY DRUG RELATED)

Body System/ Adverse Reaction	Pindolol (N = 322) %	Active Controls* (N = 188) %	Placebo (N = 78) %
Central Nervous System			
Bizarre or Many Dreams	5	O	6
Dizziness	9	11	1
Fatigue	8	4	4
Hallucinations	<1	0	0
Insomnia	10	3	10
Nervousness	7	3	5
Weakness	4	2	1
Autonomic Nervous System			
Paresthesia	3	1	6
Cardiovascular			
Dyspnea	5	4	6
Edema	6	3	1
Heart Failure	<1	<1	0
Palpitations	<1	1	0
Musculoskeletal			
Chest Pain	3	1	3
Joint Pain	7	4	4
Muscle Cramps	3	1	0
Muscle Pain	10	9	8
Gastrointestinal			
Abdominal Discomfort	4	4	5
Nausea	5	2	1
Skin			
Pruritus	1	<1	0
Rash	<1	<1	1

* Acute Controls: Patients received either propranolol, α- methyldopa or a diuretic (hydrochlorothiazide or chlorthalidone).

The following selective (potentially important) adverse reactions were seen in 2% or fever patients and their relationship to Pindolol is uncertain.

Central Nervous System: anxiety, lethargy;

Autonomic Nervous System: visual disturbances, hyperhidrosis;

Cardiovascular: bradycardia, claudication, cold extremities, heart block, hypotension, syncope, tachycardia; weight gain;

Gastrointestinal: diarrhea, vomiting;

Respiratory: wheezing;

Urogenital: impotence, pollakiuria;

Miscellaneous: eye discomfort or burning eyes.

POTENTIAL ADVERSE EFFECTS

In addition, other adverse effects not listed above have been reported with other beta-adrenergic blocking agents and should be considered potential adverse effects of Pindolol.

CENTRAL NERVOUS SYSTEM

Reversible mental depression progressing to catatonia; an acute reversible syndrome characterized by disorientation for time and place, short-term memory loss, emotional lability, slightly clouded sensorium, and decreased performance on neuropsychometrics.

Cardiovascular: Intensification of AV block. See CONTRAINDICATIONS.

Allergic: Erythematous rash; fever combined with aching and sore throat; laryngospasm; respiratory distress.

Hematologic: Agranulocytosis, thrombocytopenic and nonthrombocytopenic purpura.

Gastrointestinal: Mesenteric arterial thrombosis; ischemic colitis.

MISCELLANEOUS:

Reversible alopecia; Peyronie's disease.

The oculomucocutaneous syndrome associated with the beta-blocker practolol has not been reported with Pindolol during investigational use and extensive foreign experience amounting to over 4 million patient-years.

OVERDOSAGE:

No specific information on emergency treatment of overdosage is available. Therefore, on the basis of the pharmacologic actions of Pindolol, the following general measures should be employed as appropriate in addition to gastric lavage:

Excessive Bradycardia: administer atropine: if there is no response to vagal blockade, administer isoproterenol cautiously.

Cardiac Failure: digitalize the patient and/or administer diuretic. It has been reported that glucagon may be useful in this situation.

Hypotension: administer vasopressors, e.g. epinephrine or levarterenol, with serial monitoring of blood pressure. (There is evidence that epinephrine may be the drug of choice.)

Bronchospasm: administer a beta$_2$stimulating agent such as isoproterenol and/or a theophylline derivative.

A case of an acute overdosage has been reported with an intake of 500 mg of Pindolol by a hypertensive patient. Blood pressure increased and heart rate was ≥ 80 beat/min. Recovery was uneventful. In another case 250 mg of Pindolol was taken with 150 mg diazepam and 50 mg nitrazepam, producing coma and hypotension. The patient recovered in 24 hours.

DOSAGE AND ADMINISTRATION:

The dose of Pindolol should be individualized. The recommended initial dose of Pindolol is 5 mg b.i.d. alone or in combination with other antihypertensive agents. An antihypertensive response usually occurs within the first week of treatment. Maximal response, however, may take as long as or occasionally longer than two weeks. If a satisfactory reduction in blood pressure does not occur within 3-4 weeks, the dose may be adjusted in increments of 10 mg per day at these intervals up to a maximum of 60 mg per day.

HOW SUPPLIED - RATED THERAPEUTICALLY EQUIVALENT:

Tablet - Oral - 5 mg

100's	$64.25	Pindolol, Duramed Pharms	51285-0905-02
500's	$320.00	Pindolol, Duramed Pharms	51285-0905-04

Tablet - Oral - 10 mg

100's	$93.27	Pindolol, Duramed Pharms	51285-0906-02
500's	$465.10	Pindolol, Duramed Pharms	51285-0906-04

HOW SUPPLIED - RATED THERAPEUTICALLY EQUIVALENT: *(cont'd)*

Tablet, Uncoated - Oral - 5 mg

30's	$6.97	Pindolol, H.C.F.A. F F P	99999-2039-01
100's	$23.25	Pindolol, United Res	00677-1457-01
100's	$23.25	Pindolol, Geneva Pharms	00781-1168-01
100's	$23.25	Pindolol, H.C.F.A. F F P	99999-2039-02
100's	$40.16	Pindolol, Vangard Labs	00615-3547-13
100's	$58.00	Pindolol, Par Pharm	49884-0442-01
100's	$59.98	Pindolol, Qualitest Pharms	00603-5220-21
100's	$60.45	Pindolol, Mutual Pharm	53489-0430-01
100's	$60.65	Pindolol, Novopharm (US)	55953-0088-40
100's	$61.05	Pindolol, Aligen Independ	00405-4804-01
100's	$61.16	Pindolol, Purepac Pharm	00228-2534-10
100's	$62.25	Pindolol, Rugby	00536-4243-01
100's	$62.80	Pindolol, Martec Pharms	52555-0545-01
100's	$65.25	Pindolol, Zenith Labs	00172-4217-60
100's	$65.25	Pindolol, Goldline Labs	00182-1946-01
100's	$65.25	Pindolol, Major Pharms	00904-7893-60
100's	$66.95	Pindolol, HL Moore Drug Exch	00839-7761-06
100's	$67.20	Pindolol, Schein Pharm (US)	00364-2547-01
100's	$71.98	Pindolol, Mylan	00378-0052-01
100's	**$79.98**	**VISKEN, Novartis**	**00078-0111-05**
500's	$116.25	Pindolol, H.C.F.A. F F P	99999-2039-03
500's	$283.49	Pindolol, HL Moore Drug Exch	00839-7761-12
500's	$284.75	Pindolol, Zenith Labs	00172-4217-70
500's	$288.00	Pindolol, Novopharm (US)	55953-0088-70

Tablet, Uncoated - Oral - 10 mg

30's	$10.12	Pindolol, H.C.F.A. F F P	99999-2039-04
100's	$33.75	Pindolol, United Res	00677-1458-01
100's	$33.75	Pindolol, Geneva Pharms	00781-1169-01
100's	$33.75	Pindolol, H.C.F.A. F F P	99999-2039-05
100's	$62.02	Pindolol, Vangard Labs	00615-3506-13
100's	$79.51	Pindolol, Qualitest Pharms	00603-5221-21
100's	$79.90	Pindolol, Par Pharm	49884-0443-01
100's	$80.30	Pindolol, Mutual Pharm	53489-0431-01
100's	$80.45	Pindolol, Novopharm (US)	55953-0093-40
100's	$81.24	Pindolol, Purepac Pharm	00228-2535-10
100's	$82.28	Pindolol, Martec Pharms	52555-0546-01
100's	$82.41	Pindolol, Rugby	00536-4244-01
100's	$84.11	Pindolol, Aligen Independ	00405-4805-01
100's	$86.45	Pindolol, Zenith Labs	00172-4218-60
100's	$86.45	Pindolol, Goldline Labs	00182-1947-01
100's	$86.50	Pindolol, Major Pharms	00904-7894-60
100's	$89.63	Pindolol, HL Moore Drug Exch	00839-7762-06
100's	$91.50	Pindolol, Schein Pharm (US)	00364-2548-01
100's	$95.30	Pindolol, Mylan	00378-0127-01
100's	**$105.90**	**VISKEN, Novartis**	**00078-0073-05**
500's	$168.75	Pindolol, H.C.F.A. F F P	99999-2039-06
500's	$364.49	Pindolol, HL Moore Drug Exch	00839-7762-12
500's	$377.60	Pindolol, Zenith Labs	00172-4218-70
500's	$382.15	Pindolol, Novopharm (US)	55953-0093-70

PIPECURONIUM BROMIDE *(003025)*

CATEGORIES: Anesthesia; Autonomic Drugs; Endotracheal Intubation; Intubation; Muscle Relaxants; Neuromuscular Blocking Agents; Non-Depolarizing Muscle Relaxants; Skeletal Muscle Relaxants; Pregnancy Category C; FDA Class 1C ("Little or No Therapeutic Advantage"); FDA Approved 1990 Jun

BRAND NAMES: **Arduan**

> WARNING:
> This drug should be administered by adequately-trained individuals familiar with its actions, characteristics, and hazards.

DESCRIPTION:

Pipecuronium bromide for injection is a long-acting non-depolarizing neuromuscular blocking agent, chemically designated as piperazinium, 4, 4'-((2β, 3α, 5α, 16β, 17β)-3, 17-bis (acetyloxy) androstane-2, 16-diyl] bis [1, 1-dimethyl]-, dibromide, dihydrate.

The chemical formula is $C_{35}H_{62}N_4O_4Br_2{\cdot}2H_2O$ with a molecular weight of 798.74. At normal physiological states, the compound exists primarily in the ionized form and is poorly soluble in fat.

Arduane is supplied as a sterile nonpyrogenic freeze-dried cake, for intravenous injection only. Each 10 ml vial contains 10 mg pipecuronium bromide, and 380 mg mannitol, USP (to adjust tonicity). When necessary, pH is adjusted with sodium hydroxide and/or hydrochloric acid (pH 6).

Bacteriostatic water for injection, USP, when supplied, contains 0.9% w/v BENZYL ALCOHOL, WHICH IS NOT FOR USE IN NEWBORNS.

CLINICAL PHARMACOLOGY:

Pipecuronium bromide for injection is a long-acting non-depolarizing neuromuscular blocking agent possessing all of the characteristic pharmacological actions of this class of drugs (curariform). It acts by competing for cholinergic receptors at the motor end-plate. This action is antagonized by acetylcholinesterase inhibitors, such as neostigmine.

Pharmacodynamics: The individual cumulative ED_{95} (dose required to produce 95% suppression of T_1 of the train-of-four or 95% suppression of single twitch response) during balanced anesthesia has averaged 41 mcg/kg actual body weight (ABW) (range 20-91 mcg/kg). Maximum blockade is achieved in approximately 5 minutes following single doses of 70 to 85 mcg/kg ABW. Under balanced anesthesia, following single doses of 70 mcg/kg ABW in 4 clinical trials (n=65), the mean times to recovery to 25% of control (clinical duration) were 47-98 minutes (range 30-175 min.). The mean times to recovery following 80-85 mcg/kg ABW single doses in 4 clinical trials (n=69) were 80-124 minutes (range 40-211 min.). Pipecuronium bromide was shown to have an onset time and clinical duration (range and variability) similar to those of pancuronium bromide at comparable doses (historic data and limited comparisons).

Individualization of Dosages: Pipecuronium bromide like other long-acting neuromuscular blocking agents, displays a great deal of variability in the clinical duration of its effect. With experience, anesthesiologists will determine when and how to modify dosage on individual patients based on clinical factors like age, sex, weight/degree of obesity, renal, hepatic and/or other diseases, etc., much as they do with pancuronium. TABLE 1 is included to assist those physicians who may wish to adjust dosage based on ideal body weight and renal function, two factors which were identified in controlled clinical trials that may warrant dosage adjustment. Although the tables differ in approach, and thus appear different, i.e., one derives the total dose in mg and the other presents it in mcg/kg IBW, they ultimately suggest the same dose for patients with the same height, weight, age, and serum creatinine level.

It should be noted from the tables that for small patients with decreased renal function the suggested initial dose is less than 70 to 85 mcg/kg IBW, i.e., less than 2x the average ED_{95} dose which is generally the recommended intubating dose for neuromuscular blocking agents. A review of 80 patients who received initial doses < 70 mcg/kg IBW compared with 202 who received > 70 mcg/kg doses in controlled clinical trials showed neither longer mean time to intubation nor any problems during intubation. **HOWEVER, PHYSICIANS SHOULD USE EXTRA CARE DURING INTUBATION OF ANY PATIENT IN WHOM, IN ORDER TO DECREASE THE POSSIBILITY OF PROLONGED CLINICAL DURATION, THEY ELECT TO USE LESS THAN 70 mcg/KG IBW FOR INTUBATION.**

Dosing in accordance with the following tables may reduce the variability in clinical duration to bring approximately 20% more patients to within ± 30 minutes of the duration predicted by the dose adjusted by IBW and calculated creatinine clearance. It should be emphasized, however, that it will not entirely eliminate the variability associated with the use of long acting neuromuscular blocking agents and physicians must be prepared to monitor patients carefully during surgery and recovery to support them until they have adequate return of muscular function.

TABLE 1 Calculated Dose in mg Based on Ideal Body Weight in kg (*) and Estimated Creatinine Clearance ** (mg = ml if 10 mg vial is reconstituted with 10 ml)

Creatinine Clearance (ml/min)	IDEAL BODY WEIGHT IN KG 50 kg	60 kg	70 kg	80 kg	90 kg	100 kg
< = 40	(2.5)	(3.0)	(3.5)	(4.0)	(4.5)	(5.0)
60	(2.5)	(3.0)	3.8	4.9	6.2	7.7
80	2.6	3.7	5.0	6.5	8.3	[10.0]
> = 100	3.2	4.6	6.3	8.2	[9.0]	[10.0]

Calculated Dose in mcg/kg Ideal Body Weight (*) Adjusted for Renal Function (Estimated Creatinine Clearance)**

Creatinine Clearance in ml/min >/=

< 40	60	80	100	> 100
(50)	55	70	85	[100]

——— mcg/kg ideal body wt ———-

() Minimum calculated dose for adequate intubation - in these patients prolonged clinical blockade should be anticipated.

[ ] Maximum calculated dose for intubation - in these patients use of maintenance doses should be anticipated.

* IBW men in kg = [106 + (6 lbs./inch in ht > 5 feet)] ÷ 2.2

IBW women in kg = [100 + (5 lbs./inch in ht > 5 feet)] ÷ 2.2

NOTE: Use actual body weight in the calculation if it is less than ideal body weight.

** Est CRcl = [(140 - age in years) × IBW (kg)* × (0.85 for females only)] ÷ [72 × serum creatinine in mg/100 ml]

Hemodynamics: Administration of pipecuronium bromide doses up to and including 100 mcg/kg (=2.5 X ED_{95}) as a rapid bolus over 5 sec. to healthy patients during stable state balanced anesthesia produced no dose-related effects on heart-rate or blood pressure.

In patients undergoing surgery for coronary artery bypass grafting, hemodynamic studies were performed using higher than currently recommended pipecuronium bromide doses, i.e., 100 mcg/kg ABW and 200 mcg/kg ABW. Pipecuronium bromide was administered during induction of anesthesia with a narcotic or etomidate/narcotic combination, respectively. Observed hemodynamic effects were small and included reductions in mean systolic and mean arterial pressures (down 10-14%), ventricular stroke-work index (down 8-25%) and cardiac output (down 20%); sustained increases in pulmonary capillary wedge and central venous pressures and changes in mean heart rate were not observed. Pipecuronium bromide has not been studied in patients with hemodynamic dysfunction secondary to cardiac valvular disease.

Pipecuronium bromide has not been found to influence the cardiovascular depression or stimulations associated with other drugs administered during anesthesia or with surgical stimulation. The most common observations, comparing vital signs immediately prior to initial dosage with pipecuronium bromide and two minutes after injection, are a slight decrease in heart rate, systolic blood pressure and diastolic blood pressure.

Human plasma histamine concentrations, following effective initial doses of pipecuronium bromide, have not been studied. However, clinical experience with more than 1000 patients indicated hypersensitivity reactions such as bronchospasm, tachycardia, and other reactions commonly associated with histamine release are unlikely to occur.

Pharmacokinetics: Only limited information is available, at the present time, regarding the pharmacokinetics of pipecuronium bromide in humans.

CLINICAL STUDIES:

An analysis of 282 cases in U.S. clinical trials, utilizing a variety of premedications, varying lengths of surgery, and various anesthetic agents, indicates that two thirds of the patients had clinical durations within 30 minutes of the duration predicted by the dose adjusted by ideal body weight (IBW) and calculated creatinine clearance (there is an inverse relationship between renal function and clinical duration such that the mean clinical duration more than doubles when the calculated creatinine clearance goes from 100 to 40 ml/min).

The likelihood of prolonged clinical duration may be decreased by calculating creatinine clearance based on serum creatinine and ideal body weight based on height, or by using doses at the lower end of the recommended dosage range for intubation in patients with moderate decreases in renal function. In patients with renal failure the drug should be used with extra caution (see TABLE 1, INDICATIONS AND USAGE, and PRECAUTIONS).

In 333 of nearly 600 cases in U.S. clinical trials with evaluable clinical duration data, clinical durations greater than 120 minutes for the dose of 70 mcg/kg ABW or greater than 150 minutes for doses of 80 mcg/kg ABW or more were reported in approximately 8% (27/333) of cases. In about one-third (10/27) of such cases, dosage was administered to obese patients (defined as 30% or more above ideal body weight for height) based on actual body weight. Prolonged clinical duration was approximately 2 times more common in obese patients (10/73 cases) than among non-obese (17/260 cases) patients. Therefore, in calculating dosage on a mg/kg basis, ideal body weight can also be used to decrease the variability in clinical duration and to reduce the possibility of overdosage in the obese population (see CLINICAL PHARMACOLOGY, Individualization of Dosages.)

Limited data (3 studies, n=29) are available on the administration of single doses of 100 mcg/kg ABW of pipecuronium bromide. No significant differences were observed in mean clinical duration compared to that seen with doses of 80 - 85 mcg/kg ABW. Doses above 100 mcg/kg based of actual or ideal body weight are not recommended because of the possibility of even longer duration of action for individual patients.

CLINICAL STUDIES: *(cont'd)*

The mean time for spontaneous recovery from 25% to 50% of control T_1 based on 90 patients in 6 studies in whom the final dose produced a T_1 of less than 25% of control, is approximately 24 minutes (range 8-131 minutes). Because of the use of antagonism following surgery, there are insufficient data to report the time required for greater than 50% spontaneous recovery of T1.

Pipecuronium bromide can be administered following recovery from succinylcholine, when the latter is used to facilitate endotracheal intubation. Preliminary data (from 1 study in 25 patients) suggest that, if a single dose of 50 mcg/kg ABW pipecuronium bromide is administered under these conditions, prolongation in clinical duration may be noted (range of 23 - 95 minutes following succinylcholine versus 8 - 50 minutes without it). Prior use of succinylcholine has not been shown to alter the clinical duration of larger doses of pipecuronium bromide (80 or more mcg/kg ABW administered after recovery from succinylcholine, n=53).

Initial pipecuronium bromide doses of 70 to 85 mcg/kg ABW, used without succinylcholine (from 3 studies, in 43 patients), have produced good to excellent intubation conditions within 2.5 to 3.0 minutes of injection (which is before maximum blockade). Review of the time (range from 2 - 6 minutes) to intubation and any comments about the quality of intubation in patients receiving up to 100 mcg/kg ABW indicated no reports of problems in intubating such patients.

The mean clinical duration of first maintenance doses of 10-15 mcg/kg ABW pipecuronium bromide administered at 25% recovery of control T_1 is approximately 50 minutes (range 17-175 minutes; 6 studies, 148 patients).

Preliminary pharmacokinetic results from 4 normal subjects and 7 subjects undergoing cadaver renal transplant is reproduced in TABLE 2. These results tend to indicate that some prolongation of plasma levels can be expected in patients with severe impairment of renal function which may in turn significantly extend recovery time. A clear relationship between plasma levels and the degree or extent of muscle twitch suppression has not been determined at this time.

TABLE 2 Preliminary [1] Pharmacokinetic Parameters of Arudan

	Mean (range)[2] Normal Renal and Hepatic Function n=4	Renal Transplant n=7
Clearance (L/hr/kg)	0.12 (0.10-0.14)	0.08 (0.02-0.12)
Vol. of Distribution at Steady State (L/kg)	0.25 (0.12-0.37)	0.37 (0.28-0.51)
$t_{1/2}$ distribution (min)	6.22 (1.34-10.66)	4.33 (1.69-6.17)
$t_{1/2}$ elimination (hr)	1.7 (0.9-2.7)	4.0 (2.0-8.2)

[1]Due to the small number of subjects represented by these data, and the interpatient variation seen with Arudan this information is being provided to the clinician as a general guide only. Definitive concentration-effect and pharmacokinetic relationships have not yet been established for Arduan.

[2]Determined following rapid administration of a single bolus dose of 70 mcg/kg ABW, in patients with normal renal and hepatic function, or with renal failure undergoing cadaver renal transplant surgery under halothane anesthesia, who have been adequately dialyzed prior to surgery.

Studies of distribution, metabolism, and excretion in animals (rats, dogs, and cats), indicate that pipecuronium bromide is eliminated primarily by the kidneys (more than 75% of drug recovered in the urine, primarily as the unchanged drug). The 3-deacetyl, 17- deacetyl, and 3,17-dideacetyl derivatives of pipecuronium bromide have been identified in urine collected from dogs; these metabolites account for approximately 20% of the administered dose. The 3-deacetyl derivative is the only metabolite with substantial neuromuscular blocking activity, manifesting approximately 40-50% of the activity of the parent drug in the cat and the dog. On the basis of experience gained with other agents in this category it is most probable that similar metabolites exist in other animal species and in humans.

At the present time only the 3-deacetyl metabolite of pipecuronium bromide has been detected in the urine of humans undergoing coronary artery bypass surgery. Following administration of 200 mcg/kg ABW, 56% of the administered dose was recovered in the urine, of which 41% was unchanged drug and the remaining 15% was the 3-deacetyl metabolite of pipecuronium bromide. In the same study no metabolites of pipecuronium were found in the plasma.

INDICATIONS AND USAGE:

Pipercuronium bromide for injection is a long-acting neuromuscular blocking agent, indicated as an adjunct to general anesthesia, to provide skeletal muscle relaxation during surgery. Arudan can also be used to provide skeletal muscle relaxation for endotracheal intubation.

CONTRAINDICATIONS:

None known.

WARNINGS:

PIPECURONIUM BROMIDE FOR INJECTION SHOULD BE ADMINISTERED IN CAREFULLY ADJUSTED DOSAGES BY OR UNDER THE SUPERVISION OF EXPERIENCED CLINICIANS WHO ARE FAMILIAR WITH THE DRUG'S ACTIONS AND THE POSSIBLE COMPLICATIONS OF ITS USE. THE DRUG SHOULD NOT BE ADMINISTERED UNLESS FACILITIES FOR INTUBATION, ARTIFICIAL RESPIRATION, OXYGEN THERAPY, AND AN ANTAGONIST ARE WITHIN IMMEDIATE REACH. IT IS RECOMMENDED THAT CLINICIANS ADMINISTERING LONG-ACTING NEUROMUSCULAR BLOCKING AGENTS SUCH AS PIPECURONIUM BROMIDE EMPLOY A PERIPHERAL NERVE STIMULATOR TO MONITOR DRUG RESPONSE, NEED FOR ADDITIONAL RELAXANT, AND ADEQUACY OF SPONTANEOUS RECOVERY OR ANTAGONISM.

In patients with myasthenia gravis or myasthenic (Eaton-Lambert) syndrome, small doses of non-depolarizing neuromuscular blocking agents may have profound effects. Shorter acting muscle relaxants than pipecuronium bromide may be more suitable for these patients.

PRECAUTIONS:

General: Since pipecuronium bromide for injection has little or no effect on the heart rate, the drug will not counteract the bradycardia produced by many opioid anesthetic agents or vagal stimulation.

Renal Failure: Pipecuronium bromide in the dose of 70 mcg/kg ABW, has been studied in a limited number of patients (n = 20) undergoing renal transplant surgery, recently dialyzed in preparation for cadaver renal transplant. The mean clinical duration (injection to 25% recovery) of 103 minutes was not judged prolonged, however, there was a wide individual

PRECAUTIONS: *(cont'd)*

variation (30 to 267 minutes). Pipecuronium bromide has not otherwise been studied in patients with renal failure (for elective or emergency non-renal surgery). Because it is primarily excreted by the kidney, pipecuronium bromide should be used with caution in patients with renal failure (see TABLE 2).

Increased Volume of Distribution: Conditions associated with an increased volume of distribution, e.g., slower circulation time in cardiovascular disease, old age or edematous states, may be associated with a delay in onset time. Because higher doses of pipecuronium bromide may produce a longer duration of action, the initial dosage should not usually be increased in these patients to enhance onset time; instead, more time should be allowed for the drug to achieve maximum effect.

Hepatic Diseases: There are no data on dosage requirements, onset, duration or pharmacokinetics in patients with moderate or severe hepatic dysfunction and/or biliary obstruction. This should be considered in selection of muscle relaxants for use in these patients.

Obesity: The most common patient condition associated with prolonged clinical duration was obesity, defined as 30% or more over ideal body weight (see CLINICAL PHARMACOLOGY). Clinical study subjects were dosed on the basis of actual body weight, which may have contributed to the higher incidence of prolonged duration. It is therefore recommended that dosage be based upon ideal body weight for height in obese patients (see DOSAGE AND ADMINISTRATION).

Malignant Hyperthermia (MH): Human malignant hyperthermia has not been reported with the administration of pipecuronium bromide. Because pipecuronium bromide is never used alone, and because the occurrence of malignant hyperthermia during anesthesia is possible even in the absence of known triggering agents, clinicians should be familiar with early signs, confirmatory diagnosis and treatment of malignant hyperthermia prior to the start of any anesthetic. In an animal study in MH-susceptible swine (n=7), the administration of pipecuronium bromide was not associated with the development of malignant hyperthermia.

Long-Term Use in the Intensive Care Unit (ICU): No data are available on the long-term use of pipecuronium bromide in patients undergoing mechanical ventialtion in the I.C.U.

Central Nervous System: Pipecuronium bromide has no known effect on consciousness, the pain threshold or cerebration. Therefore, administration must be accompanied by adequate anesthesia.

Drug/Laboratory Test Interactions: None known.

Carcinogenesis, Mutagenesis, and Impairment of Fertility: Studies in animals have not been performed to evaluate carcinogenic potential or impairment of fertility. Mutagenicity studies (Ames test, Sister Chromatid Exchange) conducted with pipecuronium bromide revealed no mutagenic potential.

Pregnancy Category C: A teratogenicity study has been conducted in rats using intravenously administered doses of pipecuronium bromide approximating the clinical dose in humans (50 mcg/kg). No teratogenic effects were observed in this study. An embryotoxic effect (secondary to maternal toxicity) was observed at the highest dose administered (50 mcg/kg) as demonstrated by an increase in earlier fetal resorptions. There are no adequate and well-controlled studies in pregnant women. Arudan should be used during pregnancy only if the potential benefit justifies the potential risk to the fetus.

Use in Obstetrics (Cesarean Section): There are insufficient data on placental transfer of pipecuronium bromide and possible related effect(s) upon the neonate following Cesarean section delivery. In addition, the duration of action of pipecuronium exceeds the duration of operative obstetrics (Cesarean section). Therefore pipecuronium bromide is not recommended for use in patients undergoing C-section.

Pediatric Use: Infants (3 months to 1 year) under balanced anesthesia (2 studies in 52 infants), or halothane anesthesia (1 study in 29 infants), manifest similar dose response to pipecuronium bromide as do adults on a mcg/kg ABW basis. Children (1 to 14 years) under balanced anesthesia (4 studies in 57 children), or halothane anesthesia (2 studies in 29 children), may be less sensitive than adults. These conclusions come from studies involving titrating patient response, by the incremental method, to approximately 1.2 times ED_{95}. There are no data on either onset time or clinical duration of larger doses in infants or children. There are no data on maintenance dosing in infants and children.

Pharmacokinetic studies in infants and children have not been performed, therefore no pharmacokinetic modeling of incremental dosing can be attempted. The use of pipecuronium bromide in neonates and infants below 3 months of age has not been investigated. Antagonism has not been systematically studied in infants or children, however, usual clinical doses of neostigmine administered following significant levels of spontaneous recovery (recovery of $T_1$to more than 50% of control) produced complete antagonism residual neuromuscular block in less than 10 minutes in the majority of cases.

DRUG INTERACTIONS:

Pipecuronium bromide can be administered following recovery from succinylcholine when the latter is used to facilitate endotracheal intubation (see DOSAGE AND ADMINISTRATION and CLINICAL PHARMACOLOGY).

The use of pipecuronium bromide before succinylcholine, in order to attenuate some of the side effects of succinylcholine is not recommended because it has not been studied.

There are no clinical data on concomitant use of pipecuronium bromide and other non-depolarizing neuromuscular blocking agents.

Inhalation Anesthetics: Use of volatile inhalation anesthetics have been shown to enhance the activity of other neuromuscular blocking agents on the order of enflurane > isoflurane > halothane.

Since the neuromuscular blocking agents are routinely administered before or shortly after the administration of the inhalation anesthetic, minimal effects are generally observed on onset time and peak effect. In routine use of neuromuscular blocking agents, only clinical duration is generally affected (prolonged). No definite interaction between pipecuronium bromide and halothane, as used clinically, has been demonstrated. Use of isoflurane in one study of 25 patients resulted in an increase in mean clinical duration by 12%. In another study of 25 patients first anesthetized with enflurane for 5 minutes or more, the mean clinical duration was increased by 50%. Therefore, a prolonged clinical duration following initial or maintenance doses and prolonged recovery from neuromuscular blocking effect of Pipecuronium should generally be anticipated, with enflurane > isoflurane > halothane.

Antibiotics: Parenteral/intraperitoneal administration of high doses of certain antibiotics may intensify or produce neuromuscular block on their own.

The following antibiotics have been associated with various degrees of paralysis: aminoglycosides (such as neomycin, streptomycin, kanamycin, gentamycin, and dihydrostreptomycin); tetracyclines; bacitracin; polymyxin B; colistin; and sodium colistimethate. If these or other newly introduced antibiotics are used in conjunction with pipecuronium bromide during surgery, prolongation of neuromuscular block should be considered a possibility.

Other: Experience concerning injection of quinidine during recovery from use of other muscle relaxants suggests that recurrent paralysis may occur. This possibility must also be considered for pipecuronium bromide.

DRUG INTERACTIONS: *(cont'd)*

Pipecuronium bromide-induced neuromuscular blockade has been counteracted by alkalosis and enhanced by acidosis in experimental animals (cat). In addition, experience with other drugs has suggested that acute (*e.g.,* diarrhea) or chronic (*e.g.,* adrenocortical insufficiency) electrolyte imbalance may alter the neuromuscular blockade. Since electrolyte imbalance and acid-base imbalance are usually mixed, either enhancement or inhibition may occur. Magnesium salts, administered for the management of toxemia of pregnancy, may enhance neuromuscular blockade.

ADVERSE REACTIONS:

The most frequent side effect of non-depolarizing blocking agents, as a class, is an extension of the drug's pharmacological action beyond the time period needed for surgery and anesthesia (see CLINICAL PHARMACOLOGY). Clinical signs may vary from skeletal muscle weakness to profound and prolonged skeletal muscle paralysis resulting in respiratory insufficiency or apnea. This may be due to the drug's effect or inadequate antagonism.

The following listings are based upon U.S. clinical studies involving nearly 600 patients, utilizing a variety of premedications, varying lengths of surgical procedures and various anesthetic agents.

Adverse experiences in greater than 1% of cases and judged by the investigator to have a possible causal relationship:

Clinically significant hypotension (2.5% of cases).

Clinically significant bradycardia (1.4% of cases).

Adverse experiences in less than 1% of cases and judged by the investigator to have a possible causal relationship:

Cardiovascular: hypertension, myocardial ischemia, cerebrovascular accident, thrombosis, atrial fibrillation, ventricular extrasystole

Metabolic and Nutritional: increased creatinine, hypoglycemia, hyperkalemia

Musculoskeletal: muscle atrophy, difficult intubation

Nervous: hypesthesia, CNS depression

Respiratory: dyspnea, respiratory depression, laryngismus, atelectasis

Skin and Appendages: rash, urticaria

Urogenital System: anuria

OVERDOSAGE:

No cases of significant accidental or intentional gross overdose have been reported. In foreign clinical studies with doses up to 200 mcg/kg ABW, no non-musculoskeletal effects were seen that could be attributed to the higher dosage.

In case of relative or absolute overdosage ventilation must be supported by artificial means until no longer required. Intensified monitoring of vital organ function is required for the period of paralysis and during an extended period post recovery.

Antagonism of Neuromuscular Blockade: ANTAGONISTS (SUCH AS NEOSTIGMINE) SHOULD NOT BE ADMINISTERED PRIOR TO THE DEMONSTRATION OF SOME SPONTANEOUS RECOVERY FROM NEUROMUSCULAR BLOCKADE. THE USE OF A NERVE STIMULATOR TO DOCUMENT RECOVERY AND ANTAGONISM OF NEUROMUSCULAR BLOCKADE IS RECOMMENDED.

In an analysis (across U.S. studies) of different degrees of spontaneous recovery prior to antagonism among patients antagonized by neostigmine (usual dose 0.04 mg/kg ABW), approximately 75% of patients antagonized at a T_1 of approximately 25% and approximately 42% of patients antagonized at a T_1 of approximately 10% manifested a T_4/T_1 of 0.7 or greater within 10 minutes. When T_1 had recovered to at least 10 or 25% of the preblock value, T_4/T_1 was often zero; antagonism with neostigmine 0.04 mg/kg ABW was usually inadequate 10 minutes after intravenous dosing in these cases. If train-of-four monitoring is available, T_4/T_1 should be > zero before antagonism with neostigmine is attempted. However, if T_1 has recovered to at least 10% of the preblock value, additional time (more than 10 minutes) or additional neostigmine dosing usually resulted in adequate antagonism.

Patients should be evaluated for adequate clinical evidence of antagonism, e.g., 5 second head lift, adequate phonation, ventilation and upper airway maintenance. Ventilation must be supported until no longer required. As with other neuromuscular blocking agents, physicians should be alert to the possibility that the action of drugs used to antagonize neuromuscular blockade may wear off before plasma levels of pipecuronium bromide have declined sufficiently.

Antagonism may be delayed in the presence of debilitation, carcinomatosis, and concomitant use of certain broad spectrum antibiotics, or anesthetic agents and other drugs which enhance neuromuscular blockade or separately cause respiratory depression. Under such circumstances the management is the same as that of prolonged neuromuscular blockade.

In clinical trials, edrophonium doses of 0.5 mg/kg ABW were not as effective as neostigmine doses of 0.04 mg/kg ABW in antagonizing pipecuronium bromide-induced neuromuscular block, and were often inadequate. Therefore, the use of edrophonium 0.5 mg/kg ABW is not recommended to antagonize pipecuronium bromide-induced neuromuscular blockade. The use of greater (1.0 mg/kg ABW) doses of edrophonium or of pyridostigmine has not been investigated.

DOSAGE AND ADMINISTRATION:

PIPECURONIUM BROMIDE FOR INJECTION IS FOR INTRAVENOUS USE ONLY. THIS DRUG SHOULD BE ADMINISTERED BY OR UNDER THE SUPERVISION OF EXPERIENCED CLINICIANS FAMILIAR WITH THE USE OF NEUROMUSCULAR BLOCKING AGENTS. DOSAGE MUST BE INDIVIDUALIZED IN EACH CASE.

The dosage information which follows is derived from studies based upon units of drug per unit of body weight. It is expressed in this section in units of mg/kg (instead of mcg/kg) to assist the clinician in calculating the individual patient dosage requirements relative to the product as supplied for clinical use. It is intended to serve as an initial guide to clinicians familiar with other neuromuscular blocking agents to acquire experience with pipecuronium bromide. The monitoring of twitch response is recommended to evaluate recovery from pipecuronium bromide and decrease the hazards of overdosage if additional doses are administered (see CLINICAL PHARMACOLOGY, and Maintenance Dosing).

It is recommended that the clinicians administering long-acting neuromuscular blocking agents such as pipecuronium bromide employ a peripheral nerve stimulator to monitor drug response, need for additional relaxant and adequacy of spontaneous recovery or antagonism.

Dose for Endotracheal Intubation: The recommended initial dose of pipecuronium bromide for injection under balanced anesthesia, halothane, isoflurane, or enflurane anesthesia in patients with normal renal function who were not obese is 0.07-0.085 mg/kg (70-85 mcg/kg) (see CLINICAL PHARMACOLOGY). Good to excellent intubating conditions are generally provided within 2.5 to 3 minutes. Maximum blockade, usually > 95%, is achieved in approximately 5 minutes. Doses in this range provide approximately 1-2 hours of clinical relaxation under balanced anesthesia (47-124 minutes). Under halothane, isoflurane and enflurane anesthesia, extension of the period of clinical relaxation should be expected (see DRUG INTERACTIONS, Inhalational Anesthetics.)

DOSAGE AND ADMINISTRATION: *(cont'd)*

For obese patients (30% or more above ideal body weight for height) it is particularly important that a dosage adjustment be considered and the dosage administered according to ideal body weight (see CLINICAL PHARMACOLOGY, Individualization of Dosage).

Use Following Succinylcholine: If succinylcholine is used to facilitate endotracheal intubation, pipecuronium bromide may be administered after recovery from succinylcholine paralysis. In patients with normal renal function who are not obese starting at doses of 0.05 mg/kg (50 mcg/kg) of pipecuronium bromide are recommended and will provide approximately 45 minutes of clinical relaxation. (See CLINICAL PHARMACOLOGY.) In patients with normal renal function who are not obese higher pipecuronium bromide doses of 0.07-0.85 mg/kg (70-85 mcg/kg), if administered after recovery from succinylcholine, are associated with approximately the same clinical duration as pipecuronium bromide without prior administration of succinylcholine.

Maintenance Dosing: Maintenance doses of 0.010-0.015 mg/kg (10-15 mcg/kg) pipecuronium bromide administered at 25% recovery of control T_1, provide approximately 50 minutes (range 17 to 175 minutes) clinical duration under balanced anesthesia (see CLINICAL PHARMACOLOGY.) A lower dose should be considered in patients receiving inhalation anesthetics (see DRUG INTERACTIONS.) In all cases, dosing should be guided based on the clinical duration following initial dose or prior maintenance dose and not administered until signs of neuromuscular function are evident.

Use in Pediatrics: Infants (3 months to 1 year) under balanced anesthesia (2 studies in 52 infants), or halothane anesthesia (1 study in 20 infants), manifest similar dose response to pipecuronium bromide as do adults on a mcg/kg ABW basis, children (1 to 14 years) under balanced anesthesia (4 studies in 57 children), or halothane anesthesia (2 studies in 29 children), may be less sensitive than adults. The clinical duration of doses averaging 0.04 mg/kg ABW (40 mcg/kg) in infants, and 0.057 mg/kg ABW, (57 mcg/kg) in children, ranged from 10 to 44 minutes, and from 18 to 52 minutes, respectively. These doses were approximately 1.2 times ED_{95}. There are no data on maintenance dosing in infants or children. The use of pipecuronium bromide in neonates and infants below 3 months of age has not been investigated.

Compatibility: Pipecuronium bromide is compatible with, and can be reconstituted using the following commonly used IV solutions:

0.9% NaCl solution, lactated ringer's, 5% glucose in saline, sterile water for injection, 5% glucose in water, bacteriostatic water for injection.

Pipecuronium bromide is not recommended for dilution into and/or administration from large volume IV solutions.

Use within 24 hours of mixing with the above solutions.

Parenteral drug products should be inspected visually for particulate matter and discoloration prior to administration, whenever solution and container permit.

Storage: 2°-30°C (35°-86°F). Protect from light.

After Reconstitution: When reconstituted with bacteriostatic water for injection, USP; CONTAINS BENZYL ALCOHOL WHICH IS NOT INTENDED FOR USE IN NEWBORNS. Use within 5 days. May be stored at room temperature or refrigerated.

When reconstituted with sterile water for injection or other compatible IV solutions: Refrigerate vial. Use within 24 hours. Single use only. Discard unused portion.

HOW SUPPLIED - EQUIVALENTS NOT AVAILABLE:

Injection, Lyphl-Soln - Intravenous - 1 mg/ml

10 ml x 6 $266.93 ARDUAN, Organon 00052-0446-36

PIPERACILLIN SODIUM *(002042)*

CATEGORIES: Anti-Infectives; Antibiotics; Antimicrobials; Broad Spectrum Penicillins; Bone Infections; Cellulitis; Gynecologic Infections; Intra-Abdominal Infections; Joint Infections; Pelvic Inflammatory Disease; Penicillins; Perioperative Prophylaxis; Respiratory Tract Infections; Septicemia; Skin Infections; Urethritis; Urinary Tract Infections; Pregnancy Category B; FDA Approval Pre 1982

BRAND NAMES: *Acopex*; *Avocin*; *Cypercil*; *Ivacin*; *Ledercil*; *Picillin*; *Pipcil*; *Piperacin*; *Piperilline* (France); **Pipracil**; *Pipril* (Australia, England, Germany); *Piprilin*; *Pitamycin*
(International brand names outside U.S. in italics)

FORMULARIES: BC-BS

DESCRIPTION:

Piperacillin sodium is a semisynthetic broad-spectrum penicillin for parenteral use derived from D(-)-α-aminobenzylpenicillin. The chemical name of piperacillin sodium is (2S-(2α,5α,6β (S*)))-6-(((((4-ethyl-2,3 -dioxo-1- piperazinyl) carbonyl)amino)phenylacetyl)amino)-3, 3-dimethyl-7-oxo-4-thia-1 -azabicyclo (3.2.0)heptane-2-carboxylic acid, monosodium salt.

Piperacillin sodium is a white to off-white hygroscopic cryodesiccated crystalline powder which is readily soluble in water and gives a colorless to pale-yellow solution. The pH of the aqueous solution is 5.5 to 7.5 One g contains 1.85mEq (42.5mg) of sodium (Na+).

CLINICAL PHARMACOLOGY:

INTRAVENOUS ADMINISTRATION

In healthy adult volunteers, mean serum levels immediately after a two to three minute intravenous injection of 2, 4 or 6 g were 305, 412, and 775 mcg/ml. Serum levels lack dose proportionally (TABLE 1A and 1B and TABLE 2A and 2B).

TABLE 1A Piperacillin Serum Levels in Adults (mcg/ml) After a Two - Three Minute IV Injection

DOSE	0	10 min	20 min	30 min	1 h	1.5 h
2	305	202	156	67	40	24
	(159-615)	(164-225)	(52-165)	(41-88)	(25-57)	(18-31)
4	412	344	295	117	93	60
	(389-484)	(315-379)	(269-330)	(98-138)	(78-110)	(50-67)
6	775	609	563	325	208	138
	(695-849)	(530-670)	(492-630)	(292-363)	(180-239)	(115-175)

A 30 minute infusion of 6 g every 6 h gave, on the fourth day, a mean peak serum concentration of 420 mcg/ml.

INTRAMUSCULAR ADMINISTRATION

Piperacillin sodium is rapidly absorbed after intramuscular injection. In healthy volunteers, the mean peak serum concentration occurs approximately 30 minutes after a single dose of 2 g and is about 36 mcg/ml. The oral administration of 1 g probenecid before injection produces an increase in piperacillin peak serum level of about 30%. The area under the curve (AUC) is increased by approximately 60%.

CLINICAL PHARMACOLOGY: *(cont'd)*

TABLE 1B

DOSE	2 h	3 h	4 h	6 h	8 h
2	20 (14-24)	8 (3-11)	3 (2-4)	2 (<0.6-3)	-
4	36 (26-51)	20 (17-24)	8 (7-11)	4 (3.7-4.1)	0.9 (0.7-1)
6	90 (71-113)	38 (29-53)	33 (25-44)	8 (3-19)	3.2 (<2-6)

TABLE 2A Piperacillin Serum Levels in Adults (mcg/ml) After a 30-minute IV Infusion

DOSE	0	5 min	10 min	15 min	30 min
4	244 (155-298)	215 (169-247)	186 (140-209)	177 (142-213)	141 (122-156)
6	353 (324-371)	298 (242-339)	298 (232-331)	272 (219-314)	229 (185-249)

TABLE 2B

DOSE	45 min	1h	1.5 h	2h	4 h	6 h	7.5 h
4	146 (110-265)	105 (85-133)	72 (53-105)	53 (36-69)	15 (6-24)	4 (1-9)	2 (0.5-3)
6	180 (144-209)	149 (117-171)	104 (89-113)	73 (66-94)	22 (12-39)	1 (5-49)	- -

GENERAL

Piperacillin sodium is not absolved when given orally. Peak serum concentrations ate attained approximately 30 minutes after intramuscular injections and immediately after completion of intravenous injection or infusion. The serum half-life in healthy volunteers ranges from 36 minutes to one hours and 12 minutes. The mean elimination half-life of piperacillin sodium in healthy adult volunteers is 54 minutes following administration of 2 g and 63 minutes following 6 g. As with other penicillins, piperacillin sodium is eliminated primarily by glomerular filtration and tubular secretion; it is excreted rapidly as unchanged drug in high concentration in the urine. Approximately 60% to 80% of the administered dose is excreted in the urine in the first 24 hours. Piperacillin urine concentrations, determined by microbioassay, were as high as 14,100 mcg/ml following a 6 g intravenous dose and 8,500 mcg/ml following a 4 g intravenous dose. These urine drug concentrations remained well above 1,000 mcg/ml throughout the dosing interval. The elimination half-life is increased twofold in mild to moderate renal impairment and fivefold to sixfold in severe impairment. Piperacillin sodium binding to human serum proteins is 16%. The drug is widely distributed in human tissues and body fluids, including bone, prostate, and heart and reaches high concentrations in bile. After a 4 gram bolus, maximum biliary concentrations averaged 3,205 mcg/ml. It penetrates into the cerebrospinal fluid in the presence of inflamed meninges. Because piperacillin sodium is excreted by the biliary route as well as by the renal route, it can be used safely in appropriate dosage (see DOSAGE AND ADMINISTRATION) in patients with severely restricted kidney function, and can be used effectively in treatment of hepatobiliary infections.

MICROBIOLOGY

Piperacillin sodium is an antibiotic which exerts its bactericidal activity by inhibiting both septum and cell wall synthesis. It is active against a variety of gram-positive and gram-negative aerobic and anaerobic bacteria. *In vitro*, piperacillin is active against most strains of clinical isolates of the following microorganisms (TABLE 3).

TABLE 3

Aerobic and facultatively anaerobic organisms

Gram-negative bacteria	
Escherichia coli	*Salmonella* species*
Proteus mirabilis	*Shigella* species*
Proteus vulgaris	*Pseudomonas aeruginosa*
Morganella morganii	*Pseudomonas* species
(formerly*Proteus morganii*)	including*P cepacia*,*
Providencia rettgeri	*P maltophilia*,* *P fluorescens*
(formerly*Proteus rettgeri*)	*Acinetobacter* species
Serratia species including	(formerly*Mima-herellea*)
S marcescens and *S liquefaciens*	*Haemophilus influenzae*
	(non-β-lactamase-producing strains)
Klebsiella pneumoniae	*Neisseria gonorrhoeae*
Klebsiella species	*Neisseria meningitidis**
Enterobacter species including	*Moraxella* species*
E aerogenes and *E cloacae*	*Yersinia* species*
Citrobacter species including	(formerly*pasteurella*)
C freundii and *C diversus*	*Streptococcus pneumoniae*
Gram-positive bacteria	*Streptococcus viridans*
Group D streptococci including	*Staphylococcus aureus*
Enterococci (Streptococcus faecalis,	(non-penicillinase-producing)*
S faucium)	*Staphylococcus epidermidis*
Non-enterococci*	(non-penicillinase-producing)*
β-hemolytic streptococci including	*Clostridium* species including
Group A*Streptococcus (S pyogenes)*	*C perfringens* and *C difficile**
Group B*Streptococcus (S agalactiae)*	*Eubacterium* species
Anaerobic bacteria	*Fusobacterium* species
Actinomyces species*	*F nucleatum* and *F necrophorum*
Bacteroides species including	*Peptococcus* species
B fragilis group (*B fragilis*,	*Peptostreptococcus* species
including*B vulgatus*)	*Veillonella* species
Non-*B fragilis* group	
(*B melaninogenicus*)	
*B asaccharolyticus**	

* Piperacillin has been shown to be active *in vitro* against these organisms; however, clinical efficacy has not yet been established.

In vitro, piperacillin sodium is inactivated by staphylococcal β-lactamase and β-lactamase produced by gram-negative bacteria. However, it is active against β-lactamase-producing gonococci. Many strains of gram-negative organisms resistant to certain antibiotics have been found to be susceptible to piperacillin sodium.

Piperacillin sodium has excellent activity against gram-positive organisms, including enterococci (*S faecalis*). It is active against obligate anaerobes such as *Bacteroides* species and also against *C difficile* (which has been associated with pseudomembranous colitis).

Piperacillin is active against many gram-negative bacteria including *Enterobacteriaceae, klebsiella, Serratia, Pseudomonas, E coli, Proteus*, and *Citrobacter*, and, in addition, it is active against anaerobes and enterococci.

CLINICAL PHARMACOLOGY: *(cont'd)*

In vitro tests show piperacillin to act synergistically with aminoglycoside antibiotics against most isolates of *P aeruginosa*.

SUSCEPTIBILITY TESTING

The use of a 100 mcg piperacillin antibiotic disk with susceptibility test methods which measure zone diameter gives an accurate estimation of susceptibility of organisms to piperacillin sodium. The following standard procedure† has been recommended for use with disks for testing antimicrobials. †NCCLS Approved Standard; M2-A2 (Formerly ASM-2) Performance Standards for Antimicrobic Disk Susceptibility Tests, Second Edition, available from the National Committee of Clinical Laboratory Standards.

With this type of procedure, a report of "susceptible" from the laboratory indicates that the infecting organism is likely to respond to therapy. A report of "intermediate susceptibility" suggests that the organism would be susceptible if high dosage is used or if the infection is confined to tissues and fluids (*e.g.*, urine) in which high antibiotic levels are obtained. A report of "resistant" indicates that the infecting organism is not likely to respond to therapy. With the piperacillin disk, a zone of 18 mm or greater indicates susceptibility, zone sizes of 14 mm or less indicate resistance, and zone sizes of 15 to 17 mm indicate intermediate susceptibility.

Haemophilus and *Neisseria* species which give zones of ≥ 29mm are susceptible; resistant strains give zones of ≤ 28 mm. The above interpretive criteria are based on the use of the standardized procedure. Antibiotic susceptibility testing requires carefully prescribed procedures. Susceptibility tests are biased to a considerable degree when different methods are used.

The standardized procedure requires the use of control organisms. The 100 mcg piperacillin disk should give zone diameters between 24 and 30 mm for *E coli* ATCC No. 25922 and between 25 and 33 mm for *pseudomonas aeruginosa*ATCC No. 27853.

Dilution methods such as those described in the International Collaborative study‡ have been used to determine susceptibility of organisms to piperacillin sodium.

‡*Acta Pathol Microbial Scand* (B) 1971; suppl 217.

Enterobacteriaceae, Pseudomonas species and *Acinetobacter* sp. are considered susceptible if the minimal inhibitory concentration (MIC) of piperacillin is no greater than 64 mcg/ml and are considered resistant if the MIC is greater than 128 mcg/ml.

Haemophilus and *Neisseria* species are considered susceptible if the MIC of piperacillin is ≤ to 1 mcg/ml.

When anaerobic organisms are isolated from infection sites, it is recommended that other tests such as the modified Broth-Disk Method (Wilkins TD and Thiel T: *Antimicrob Agents Chemother* 1973; 3:350-356) be used to determine the antibiotic susceptibility of these slowly growing organisms.

INDICATIONS AND USAGE:

Therapeutic: Piperacillin sodium is indicated for the treatment of serious infections caused by susceptible strains of the designated organisms in the conditions as listed below.

Intra-Abdominal Infections including hepatobiliary and surgical infections caused by *E coli, P aeruginosa*, enterococci,*Clostridium* sp., anaerobic cocci, and *Bacteroides* sp., including *B fragilis.*

Urinary Tract infections caused by *E coli, Klebsiella* sp., *P aeruginosa, Proteus* sp., including*P mirabilis*, and enterococci.

Gynecologic Infections including endometritis, pelvic inflammatory disease, pelvic cellulitis caused by *Bacteroides* sp. including *B fragilis*, anaerobic cocci, *Neisseria gonorrhoeae*, and enterococci (*S faecalis*).

Septicemia, including bacteremia caused by *E coli, Klebsiella* sp., *Enterobacter* sp., *Serratia* sp., *P mirabilis, S pneumoniae*, enterococci, *P aeruginosa, Bacteroides* sp. and anaerobic cocci.

Lower Respiratory Tract Infections caused by *E coli, Klebsiella* sp.,*Enterobacter* sp., *Pseudomonas aeruginosa, Serratia* sp.,*H influenzae, Bacteroides* sp., and anaerobic cocci. Although improvement has been noted in patients with cystic fibrosis, lasting bacterial eradication may not necessarily be achieved.

Skin and Skin Structure Infections caused by *E coli, Klebsiella* sp., *Serratia* sp., *Acinetobacter* sp., *Enterobacter* sp., *Pseudomonas aeruginosa*, indole-positive *Proteus* sp., *proteus mirabilis, Bacteroides* sp., including *B fragilis*, anaerobic cocci, and enterococci.

Bone and Joint Infections: caused by *P aeruginosa*, enterococci, *Bacteroides* sp., and anaerobic cocci.

Gonococcal Infections: Piperacillin sodium has been effective in the treatment of uncomplicated gonococcal urethritis.

Piperacillin sodium has also been shown to be clinically effective for the treatment of infections at various sites caused by *Streptococcus* species including Group A β-hemolytic *Streptococcus* and *S. pneumoniae*; however, infections caused by these organisms are ordinarily treated with more narrow spectrum penicillins. Because of its broad spectrum of bactericidal activity against gram-positive and gram-negative aerobic and anaerobic bacteria, piperacillin sodium is particularly useful for the treatment of mixed infections and presumptive therapy prior to the identification of the causative organisms.

Also piperacillin sodium may be administered as single drug therapy in some situations where normally two antibiotics might be employed.

Piperacillin has been successfully used with aminoglycosides, especially in patients with impaired host defenses. Both drugs should be used in full therapeutic doses.

Appropriate cultures should be made for susceptibility testing before initiating therapy and therapy adjusted, if appropriate, once the results are known.

Prophylaxis: Piperacillin sodium is indicated for prophylactic use in surgery including intra-abdominal (gastrointestinal and biliary) procedures, vaginal hysterectomy, abdominal hysterectomy, and cesarean section. Effective prophylactic use depends on the time of administration and piperacillin sodium should be given one-half to one hour before the operation so that effective levels can be achieved in the site prior to the procedure.

The prophylactic use of piperacillin should be stopped within 24 hours, since continuing administration of any antibiotic increased the possibility of adverse reactions, but in the majority of surgical procedures, does not reduce the incidence of subsequent infections. If there are signs of infection, specimens for culture should be obtained for identification of the causative organism so that appropriate therapy can be instituted.

CONTRAINDICATIONS:

A history of allergic reactions to any of the penicillins and/or cephalosporins.

WARNINGS:

Serious and occasionally fatal hypersensitivity (anaphylactic) reactions have been reported in patients receiving therapy with penicillins. These reactions are more apt to occur in persons with a history of sensitivity to multiple allergens.

There have been reports of patients with a history of penicillin hypersensitivity who have experienced severe hypersensitivity reactions when treated with a cephalosporin. Before initiating therapy with piperacillin sodium, careful inquiry should be made concerning

WARNINGS: *(cont'd)*

previous hypersensitivity reactions to penicillins, cephalosporins, and other allergens. If an allergic reaction occurs during therapy with piperacillin sodium, the antibiotic should be discontinued. The usual agents (antihistamines, pressor amines, and corticosteroids) should be readily available. SERIOUS ANAPHYLACTOID REACTIONS REQUIRE IMMEDIATE EMERGENCY TREATMENT WITH EPINEPHRINE. OXYGEN AND INTERVENOUS CORTICOSTEROIDS AND AIRWAY MANAGEMENT INCLUDING INTUBATION SHOULD ALSO BE ADMINISTERED AS NECESSARY.

PRECAUTIONS:

GENERAL

While piperacillin possesses the characteristic low toxicity of the penicillin group of antibiotics, periodic assessment of organ system functions including renal, hepatic, and hematopoietic during prolonged therapy is advisable.

Bleeding manifestations have occurred in some patients receiving β-lactam antibiotics, including piperacillin. These reactions have sometimes been associated with abnormalities of coagulation tests such as clotting time, platelet aggregation and prothrombin time and are more likely to occur in patients with renal failure.

If bleeding manifestations occur, the antibiotic should be discontinued and appropriate therapy instituted.

The possibility of the emergence of resistant organisms which might cause superinfections should be kept in mind, particularly during prolonged treatment. If this occurs, appropriate measures should be taken.

As with other penicillins, patients may experience neuromuscular excitability or convulsions if higher than recommended doses are given intravenously.

Piperacillin sodium is a monosodium salt containing 1.85 mEq of Na + per g. This should be considered when treating patients requiring restricted salt intake. Periodic electrolyte determinations should be made in patients with low potassium reserves, and the possibility of hypokalemia should be kept in mind with patients who have potentially low potassium reserves and who are receiving cytotoxic therapy or diuretics.

Antimicrobials used in high doses for short periods to treat gonorrhea may mask or delay the symptoms of incubating syphilis. Therefore, prior to treatment, patients with gonorrhea should also be evaluated for syphilis. Specimens for darkfield examination should be obtained from patients with any suspected primary lesion, and serologic tests should be performed. In all cases where concomitant syphilis is suspected, monthly serological tests should be made for a minimum of 4 months.

As with other semisynthetic penicillins, piperacillin sodium therapy has been associated with an increased incidence of fever and rash in cystic fibrosis patients.

PREGNANCY CATEGORY B

Although reproduction studies in mice and rats performed at doses up to 4 times the human dose have shown no evidence of impaired fertility or harm to the fetus, safety of piperacillin sodium use in pregnant women has not been determined by adequate and well-controlled studies. Because animal reproduction studies are not always predictive of human response, this drug should be used during pregnancy only if clearly needed. It has been found to cross the placenta in rats.

NURSING MOTHERS

Caution should be exercised when piperacillin sodium is administered to nursing mothers. It is excreted in low concentrations in milk.

PEDIATRIC USE

Dosages for children under age of 12 have not been established. The safety of piperacillin sodium in neonates is not known. In dog neonates dilated renal tubules and peritubular hyalinization occurred following administer of piperacillin sodium.

DRUG INTERACTIONS:

The mixing of piperacillin with an aminoglycoside *in vitro* can result in substantial inactivation of the aminoglycosides.

ADVERSE REACTIONS:

Piperacillin sodium is generally well tolerated. The most common adverse reactions have been local in nature, following intravenous or intramuscular injection. The following adverse reactions may occur.

Local Reactions: In clinical trials thrombophlebitis was noted in 4% of patients. Pain, erythema, and/or induration at the injection site occurred in 2% of patients. Less frequent reactions including ecchymosis, deep vein thrombosis and hematomas have also occurred.

Gastrointestinal: Diarrhea and loose stools were noted in 2% of patients. Other less frequent reactions included vomiting, nausea, increases in liver enzymes, (LDH, SGOT, SGPT), hyperbilirubinemia, cholestatic hepatitis, bloody diarrhea and, rarely, pseudomembranous colitis.

Hypersensitivity Reactions. Anaphylactoid Reactions, see WARNINGS.

Rash was noted in 1% patients. Other less frequent findings included pruritus, vesicular eruptions, positive Coombs tests.

Other dermatologic manifestations, such as erythema multiforme and Stevens-Johnson syndrome have been reported rarely.

Renal: Elevations of creatinine or BUN, and rarely, interstitial nephritis.

Central Nervous System: Headache, dizziness, fatigue.

Hemic and Lymphatic: Reversible leukopenia, leukopenia, thrombocytopenia and/or eosinophilia have been reported. As with other β-lactam antibiotics, reversible leukopenia (neutropenia) is more apt to occur in patients prolonged therapy at high dosages or in association with drugs known to cause this reaction.

Serum Electrolytes: Individuals with liver disease or individuals receiving cytotoxic therapy or diuretics were reported rarely to demonstrate a decrease in serum potassium concentrations with high of piperacillin.

Skeletal: Rarely, prolonged muscle relaxation.

Other: Superinfection, including candidiasis. Hemorrhagic manifestations.

DOSAGE AND ADMINISTRATION:

Piperacillin sodium may be administered by the intramuscular route (see NOTE) or intravenously or given in a three to five minute intravenous injection. The usual dosage of piperacillin sodium for serious infections is 3-to 4-g given every four to six hours as a 20-to 30-minute infusion. For serious infections, the intravenous route should be used.

Piperacillin sodium should not be mixed with an aminoglycoside in a syringe or infusion bottle since this can result in inactivation of the aminoglycoside.

The maximum daily dose for adults is usually 24 g/day, although higher doses have been used. Intramuscular injections (see NOTE) should be limited to 2 g per injection site. This route of administration has been used primarily in the treatment of patients with uncomplicated gonorrhea and urinary tract infections.[1]

DOSAGE AND ADMINISTRATION: *(cont'd)*

NOTE: THE ADD-VANTAGE VAIL IS *NOT*FOR IM USE (TABLE 4).

TABLE 4 Dosage Recommendations

Type of Infection	Used Total Daily Dose
Serious infections such as septicemia, nosocomial pneumonia, intraabdominal infections, aerobic and anaerobic gynecologic infections, and skin and soft tissue infections	12 - 18 g/d IV (200 - 300 mg/kg/d) in divided doses every 4 to 6 h
Completed urinary tract infections	8 - 16 g/d IV (125 - 200 mg/kg/d) in divided doses every 6 to 8 h
Uncomplicated urinary tract infections and most community-acquired pneumonia	6 - 8 g/d IM or IV (100 - 125 mg/kg/d) in divided doses every 6 to 12 h
Uncomplicated gonorrhea infections	2 g IM* as a one-time dose

* One g of probenecid given orally one-half hour prior to injection.

The average duration of piperacillin sodium treatment is from seven to ten days, except in the treatment of gynecologic infections, in which it is from three to ten days; the duration should be guided by the patient's clinical and bacteriological progress. For most acute infections, treatment should be continued for at least 48 to 72 hours after the patient becomes asymptomatic. Antibiotic therapy for group A β-hemolytic streptococcal infections should be maintained for at least ten days to reduce the risk of rheumatic fever or glomerulonephritis.

When piperacillin sodium is given concurrently with aminoglycosides, both drugs should be used in full therapeutic doses.

Dosage for Impaired Renal Function: (TABLE 5)

TABLE 5 Dosage in Renal Impairment

Creatinine Clearance ml/min	Urinary Tract Infection (uncomplicated)	Urinary Tract Infection (complicated)	Serious Systemic Infection
>40	No dosage adjustment necessary		
20-40	No dosage adjustment necessary	9 g/day 3 g every 8 h	12 g/day 4 g every 8 h
<20	6 g/day 3 g every 12 h	6 g/day 3 g every 12 h	8 g/day 4 g every 12 h

For patients on hemodialysis the maximum daily dose is 6 g/day (2 g every 8 h). In addition, because hemodialysis removes 30%-50% of piperacillin in 4 hours, 1 g additional dose should be administered following each dialysis period.

For patients with renal failure and hepatic insufficiency, measurement of serum level of piperacillin sodium will provide additional guidance for adjusting dosage.

PROPHYLAXIS

When possible, piperacillin sodium should be administered as a 20-30 minute infusion just prior to anesthesia. Administration while the patient is awake will facilitate identification of possible adverse reactions during drug infusion (TABLE 6).

TABLE 6

INDICATION	1st Dose	2nd Dose	3rd Dose
Intra-abdominal Surgery	2g IV just prior to surgery	2g during surgery	2g every 6 h Post-Op for no more than 24 h
Vaginal Hysterectomy	2g IV just prior to surgery	2g 6 h after 1st dose	2g 12 h after 1st dose
Cesarean Section	2g IV after cord is clamped	2g 4 h after 1st dose	2g 8 h after 1st dose
Abdominal Hysterectomy	2g IV just prior to surgery	2g on return to recovery room	2g after 6 h

Infants and Children . Dosage in infants and children under 12 years of age have not been established.

PRODUCT RECONSTITUTION/DOSAGE PREPARATION

Conventional Vials: (TABLE 7).

TABLE 7 Diluents for Reconstitution

Sterile Water for Injection Bacteriostatic Water for Injection Chloride Either Parabens or Benzyl Alcohol	Sodium Chloride Injection Bacteriostatic Sodium Injection Dextrose 5% in Water Dextrose 5% and 0.9% Sodium Chloride *Lidocaine HCl 0.5-1% (without epinephrine)

* For Intramuscular Use Only. Lidocaine is contraindicated in patients with a known history of hypersensitivity to local anesthetics of the amide type.

Conventional Vials: (TABLE 8)

TABLE 8

Intravenous Solutions	Intravenous Admixtures
Dextrose 5% in Water	Normal Saline (+ KCl 40 mEq)
0.9% Sodium Chloride	5% Dextrose in Water (+ KCl 40mEq)
Dextrose 5% and 0.9% Sodium Chloride	5% Dextrose/Normal Saline (+ KCl 40mEq)
Lactated Ringer's Injection	Ringer's Injection (+ KCl 40mEq)
Dextran 6% in 9% Sodium Chloride	Lactated Ringer's Injection (+ KCl 40 mEq)

ADD-VANTAGEVIALS**

ADD-Vantage System Admixtures: Dextrose 5% in Water (50 or 100 ml); 0.9% Sodium Chloride (50 or 100 ml)

**(ADD-Vantage is the registered trademark of Abbott Laboratories)

DOSAGE AND ADMINISTRATION: *(cont'd)*

INTRAVENOUS ADMINISTRATION

Reconstitution Directions for Conventional Vials: Reconstitute each gram of piperacillin sodium with at least 5 ml of a suitable diluent (except Lidocaine HCl 0.5%-1% without epinephrine) listed above.

Shake well until dissolved. Reconstituted solution may be further diluted to the desired volume (*e.g.,* 50 or 100 ml) in the above listed intravenous solutions and admixtures.

Reconstitution Directions for ADD-Vantage Vials: See Instruction Sheet provided in box.

Reconstitution Directions for Pharmacy Bulk Vial: Reconstitute the 40 g vial with 172 ml of a suitable diluent (except Lidocaine HCL 0.5%-1% without epinephrine) listed above to achieve a concentration of 1 g per 5 ml.

DIRECTION OF ADMINISTRATION

Intermittent IV Infusion: Infuse diluted solution over period of about 30 minutes. During infusion it is desirable to discontinue the primary intravenous solution.

Intravenous Injection (Bolus): Reconstituted solution should be injected slowly over a 3-to 5-minute period to help avoid vein irritation.

Intramuscular Administration (Conventional Vials Only): *Reconstitution Direction:* Reconstitute each gram of piperacillin sodium with 2 ml of a suitable diluent listed above to achieve a concentration of 1 g per 2.5 ml. Shake well until dissolved.

Direction for Administration: When indicated by clinical and bacteriological findings, intramuscular administration of 6 to 8 g daily of piperacillin sodium, in divided doses, may be utilized for initiation of therapy. In addition, intramuscular administration of the drug may be considered for maintenance therapy after clinical and bacteriologic improvement has been obtained with intravenous piperacillin sodium treatment. Intramuscular administration should not exceed 2 g per injection at any one site.

The preferred site is the upper outer quadrant of the buttock (*i.e.,* gluteus maximus).

The deltoid area should be used only if well-developed, and then caution to avoid radial nerve injury. Intramuscular injections should not be made into the lower or mid-third of the upper arm.

STABILITY OF PIPERACILLIN SODIUM FOLLOWING RECONSTITUTION

Piperacillin sodium is stable in both glass and plastic when reconstituted with recommended diluents when diluted with the intravenous solutions and intravenous admixtures indicated above.

Extensive stability studies have demonstrated chemical stability (potency, pH, and clarity) through 24 hours at room temperature, up to one week refrigerated, and up to one month frozen (-10° to -20°). (Note: The 40 g Pharmacy Bulk vial should not be frozen after reconstitution.) Appropriate consideration of aseptic technique and individual hospital policy, however, may recommend discarding unused portions after storage for 48 hours under refrigeration and discarding after 24 hours storage at room temperature.

ADD-VANTAGE SYSTEM

Stability studies with the ad-mixed ADD-Vantage system have demonstrated chemical stability (potency, pH and clarity) through 24 hours at room temperature. (Note: The ad-mixed ADD-Vantage should not be refrigerated or frozen after reconstitution.)

Additional stability data available upon request.

This product should be stored at controlled room temperature 15-30°C (59-86°F).

HOW SUPPLIED - EQUIVALENTS NOT AVAILABLE:

Injection, Lyphl-Soln - Intramuscular; - 2 gm/vial

2 gm x 10	$110.15	PIPRACIL, Lederle Piperacillin	00206-3879-16
2gm x 10	$113.11	PIPRACIL, Lederle Piperacillin	00206-3879-27

Injection, Lyphl-Soln - Intramuscular; - 3 gm/vial

3 gm x 10	$165.20	PIPRACIL, Lederle Piperacillin	00206-3882-55
3 gm x 10	$169.68	PIPRACIL, Lederle Piperacillin	00206-3882-28
3 gm x 10	$176.36	PIPRACIL, Lederle Piperacillin	00206-3882-65

Injection, Lyphl-Soln - Intramuscular; - 4 gm/vial

4 gm x 10	$220.28	PIPRACIL, Lederle Piperacillin	00206-3880-25
4 gm x 10	$235.16	PIPRACIL, Lederle Piperacillin	00206-3880-66
4gm x 10	$226.24	PIPRACIL, Lederle Piperacillin	00206-3880-29

Injection, Solution - Intramuscular; - 40 gm/vial

40 gm	$190.51	PIPRACIL 40, Lederle Piperacillin	00206-3877-60

PIPERACILLIN SODIUM; TAZOBACTAM SODIUM *(003186)*

CATEGORIES: Anti-Infectives; Antibiotics; Antimicrobials; Appendicitis; Beta-Lactam Antibiotics; Endometriosis; Gynecologic Infections; Intra-Abdominal Infections; Penicillins; Pneumonia; Respiratory Tract Infections; Skin Infections; FDA Class 1S ("Standard Review"); FDA Approved 1993 Oct

BRAND NAMES: *Tazobac* (Germany); *Tazocel*; *Tazocilline* (France); *Tazocin* (England, Mexico); Tazosyn; **Zosyn**
(International brand names outside U.S. in italics)

DESCRIPTION:

Zosyn (Piperacillin sodium) is an injectable antibacterial combination product consisting of the semisynthetic antibiotic piperacillin sodium and the beta-lactamase inhibitor tazobactam sodium for intravenous administration.

Piperacillin sodium is derived from D(-)-α-aminobenzylpenicillin. The chemical name of piperacillin sodium is sodium (2*S*,5*R*,6*R*)-6-[(*R*)-2-(4-ethyl-2,3-dioxo-1-piperazine-carboxyamido)-2-phenylacetamido]-3,3-dimethyl-7-oxo-4-thia-1- azabicyclo[3.2.0]-heptane-2-carboxylate. The chemical formula is $C_{23}H_{26}N_5NaO_7S$ and the molecular weight is 539.5.

Tazobactam sodium, a derivative of the penicillin nucleus, is a penicillinic acid sulfone. Its chemical name is sodium (2*S*,3*S*,5*R*)-3-methyl-7-oxo-3-(1*H*-1,2,3- triazol-1-ylmethyl)-4-thia-1-azabicyclo-[3.2.0]heptane-2-carboxylate-4,4-dioxide. The chemical formula is $C_{10}H_{11}N_4NaO_5S$ and the molecular weight is 322.3.

Piperacillin/tazobactam parenteral combination, is a white to off- white sterile, cryodesiccated powder consisting of piperacillin and tazobactam as their sodium salts packaged in glass vials. The product does not contain excipients or preservatives.

Each Zosyn 2.25 g single dose vial contains an amount of drug sufficient for withdrawal of piperacillin sodium equivalent to 2 grams of piperacillin and tazobactam sodium equivalent to 0.25 g of tazobactam.

Each Zosyn 3.375 g single dose vial contains an amount of drug sufficient for withdrawal of piperacillin sodium equivalent to 3 grams of piperacillin and tazobactam sodium equivalent to 0.375 g of tazobactam.

DESCRIPTION: *(cont'd)*

Each Zosyn 4.5 single dose vial contains an amount of drug sufficient for withdrawal of piperacillin sodium equivalent to 4 grams of piperacillin and tazobactam sodium equivalent to 0.5 g of tazobactam.

Zosyn is a monosodium salt of piperacillin and a monosodium salt of tazobactam containing a total of 2.35 mEq (54 mg) of Na+ per gram of piperacillin in the combination product.

CLINICAL PHARMACOLOGY:

Peak plasma concentrations of piperacillin and tazobactam are attained immediately after completion of an intravenous infusion of Zosyn. Piperacillin plasma concentrations, following a 30-minute infusion of Zosyn, were similar to those attained when equivalent doses of piperacillin were administered alone, with mean peak plasma concentrations of approximately 134, 142, and 298 mcg/ml for the 2.25 g, 3.375 g, and 4.5 g Zosyn (piperacillin/tazobactam) doses, respectively. The corresponding mean peak plasma concentrations of tazobactam were 15, 24, and 34 mcg/ml, respectively.

Following a 30-minute IV infusion of 3.375 g Piperacillin STS every 6 hours, steady- state plasma concentrations of piperacillin and tazobactam were similar to those attained after the first dose. In like manner, steady-state plasma concentrations were not different from those attained after the first dose when 2.25 g or 4.5 g doses of Piperacillin STS were administered via 30- minute infusion every 6 hours.

Steady-state plasma concentrations after 30-minute infusions every 6 hours are provided in TABLE 1.

Following single or multiple Piperacillin STS doses to healthy subjects, the plasma half-life of piperacillin and of tazobactam ranged from 0.7 to 1.2 hours and were unaffected by dose or duration of infusion.

Piperacillin is metabolized to a minor microbiologically active desethyl metabolite. Tazobactam is metabolized to a single metabolite that lacks pharmacological and antibacterial activities. Both piperacillin and tazobactam are eliminated via the kidney by glomerular filtration and tubular secretion. Piperacillin is excreted rapidly as unchanged drug with 68% of the administered dose excreted in the urine. Tazobactam and its metabolite are eliminated primarily by renal excretion with 80% of the administered dose excreted as unchanged drug and the remainder as the single metabolite. Piperacillin, tazobactam, and desethyl piperacillin are also secreted into the bile.

Both piperacillin and tazobactam are approximately 30% bound to plasma proteins. The protein binding of either piperacillin or tazobactam is unaffected by the presence of the other compound. Protein binding of the tazobactam metabolite is negligible.

Piperacillin and tazobactam are widely distributed into tissues and body fluids including intestinal mucosa, gallbladder, lung, female reproductive tissues (uterus, ovary, and fallopian tube), interstitial fluid, and bile. Mean tissue concentrations are generally 50-100% of those in plasma. Distribution of piperacillin and tazobactam into cerebrospinal fluid is low in subjects with non-inflamed meninges, as with other penicillins.

After the administration of single doses of piperacillin/tazobactam to subjects with renal impairment, the half-life of piperacillin and of tazobactam increases with decreasing creatinine clearance. At creatinine clearance below 20 ml/min, the increase in half-life is twofold for piperacillin and fourfold for tazobactam compared to subjects with normal renal function. Dosage adjustments for Piperacillin STS are recommended when creatinine clearance is below 40 ml/min in patients receiving the usual recommended daily dose of Piperacillin STS. (See DOSAGE AND ADMINISTRATION section for specific recommendations for the treatment of patients with renal insufficiency.)

Hemodialysis removes 30-40% of a piperacillin/tazobactam dose with an additional 5% of the tazobactam dose removed as the tazobactam metabolite. Peritoneal dialysis removes approximately 6% and 21% of the piperacillin and tazobactam doses, respectively, with up to 16% of the tazobactam dose removed as the tazobactam metabolite. For dosage recommendation for patients undergoing hemodialysis, see DOSAGE AND ADMINISTRATION section.

The half-life of piperacillin and of tazobactam increases by approximately 25% and 18%, respectively, in patients with hepatic cirrhosis compared to healthy subjects. However, this difference does not warrant dosage adjustment of Piperacillin STS due to hepatic cirrhosis.

TABLE 1 Sterile Piperacillin Sodium & Tazobactam Sodium, Clinical Pharmacology STEADY STATE MEAN PLASMA CONCENTRATIONS IN ADULTS AFTER 30-MINUTE INTRAVENOUS INFUSION OF PIPERACILLIN/TAZOBACTAM EVERY 6 HOURS PIPERACILLIN

		Plasma Concentrations ** (mcg/ml)			AUC ** (mcg°hr/ml)
Piperacillin/ Tazobactam[c] Dose	No. of Evaluable Subjects	30 min	1 hr	2 hr	AUC_{0-6}
2.25 g	8	134(14)	57(14)	17.1(23)	131(14)
3.375 g	6	242(12)	106 (8)	34.6(20)	242(10)
4.5 g	8	298(14)	141(19)	46.6(28)	322(16)

[c]Piperacillin and tazobactam were given in combination.

TABLE 1A - PIPERACILLIN, cont.

		Plasma Concentrations ** (mcg/ml)			AUC ** (mcg°hr/ml)
Piperacillin/ Tazobactam[c] Dose	No. of Evaluable Subjects	3 hr	4 hr	6 hr	AUC_{0-6}
2.25 g	8	5.2(32)	2.5(35)	0.9(14)[a]	131(14)
3.375 g	6	11.5(19)	5.1(22)	1.0(10)	242(10)
4.5 g	8	16.4(29)	6.9(29)	1.4(30)	322(16)

[a]N=4
[c]Piperacillin and tazobactam were given in combination.

TABLE 1B- TAZOBACTAM

		Plasma Concentrations ** (mcg/ml)			AUC ** (mcg°hr/ml)
Piperacillin/ Tazobactam[c] Dose	No. of Evaluable Subjects	30 min	1 hr	2 hr	AUC_{0-6}
2.25 g	8	14.8(14)	7.2(22)	2.6(30)	16.0(21)
3.375 g	6	24.2(14)	10.7 (7)	4.0(18)	25.0 (8)
4.5 g	8	33.8(15)	17.3(16)	6.8(24)	39.8(15)

[c]Piperacillin and tazobactam were given in combination.

CLINICAL PHARMACOLOGY: *(cont'd)*

TABLE 1C -TAZOBACTAM

Piperacillin/ Tazobactam[c] Dose	No. of Evaluable Subjects	Plasma Concentrations ** (mcg/ml) 3 hr	4 hr	6 hr	AUC ** (mcg°hr/ml) AUC_{0-6}
2.25 g	8	1.1(35)	0.7 (6)[b]	<0.5	16.0(21)
3.375 g	6	1.4(21)	1.4(16)[a]	<0.5	25.0 (8)
4.5 g	8	2.8(25)	1.3(30)	<0.5	39.8(15)

[a]N=4
[b]N=3
[c]Piperacillin and tazobactam were given in combination.

Microbiology: Piperacillin sodium exerts bactericidal activity by inhibiting septum formation and cell wall synthesis. *In vitro*, piperacillin is active against a variety of gram-positive and gram- negative aerobic and anaerobic bacteria. Tazobactam sodium, which has very little intrinsic microbiologic activity due to its very low level of binding to penicillin-binding proteins, is a β-lactamase inhibitor of the Richmond-Sykes class III (Bush class 2b & 2b') penicillinases and cephalosporinases. It varies in its ability to inhibit class II and IV (2a & 4) penicillinases. Tazobactam does not induce chromosomally- mediated β-lactamases at tazobactam levels achieved with the recommended dosing regimen.

Piperacillin/tazobactam has been shown to be active against most strains of the following piperacillin resistant β-lactamase producing microorganisms both *in vitro* and in clinical infections as described in the INDICATIONS AND USAGE section.

Gram-Positive Aerobes:
Staphylococcus aureus (NOT methicillin-resistant strains)
Gram-Negative Aerobes:
Escherichia coli
Haemophilus influenzae (NOT ampicillin-resistant β-lactamase negative strains)
Gram-Negative Anaerobes:
*Bacteroides fragilis*group (*B. fragilis, B. ovatus, B. thetaiotaomicron* or *B. vulgatus)*

The following *in vitro* data are available; **but their clinical significance is unknown.**

Piperacillin/tazobactam exhibits *in vitro*minimal inhibitory concentrations (MIC's) of 16 mcg/ml or less against most (≥90%) strains of the following microorganisms (or MIC's of 1 mcg/ml or less against *Haemophilus* species or *Neisseria* species or MIC's of 8 μg/ml or less against *Staphylococcus* species); however, the safety and effectiveness of piperacillin/tazobactam in treating clinical infections due to these microorganisms have not been established in adequate and well-controlled clinical trials.

Gram-Positive Aerobes:
Enterococcus faecalis†
Staphylococcus epidermis (NOT methicillin/oxacillin-resistant strains)
Streptococcus agalactiae †
Streptococcus pneumoniae†
Streptococcus pyogenes†
*Viridans*group *streptococci*†
Gram-Negative Anaerobes:
Klebsiella oxytoca
Klebsiella pneumoniae
Klebsiella catarrhalis
Morganella morganii
Neisseria gonorrhoeae
Neisseria meningitidis
Proteus mirabilis
Proteus vulgaris
Serratia marcescens
Gram-Positive Anaerobes:
Bacteroides distasonis
Fusobacterium nucleatum
Prevotella melaninogenica (formerly *Bacteroides melaninogenicus*)

† These are not beta-lactamase producing strains and, therefore, are susceptible to piperacillin alone.

Susceptibility Tests: *Dilution Techniques:* Quantitative methods that are used to determine minimum inhibitory concentrations provide reproducible estimates of the susceptibility of bacteria to antimicrobial compounds. One such standardized procedure uses a dilution method[1] (broth, agar, or microdilution) or equivalent with piperacillin and tazobactam standard powders. MIC values should be determined using serial dilutions of piperacillin combined with a fixed concentration of 4 mcg/ml tazobactam. The MIC values obtained should be interpreted according to the criteria found in TABLE 2.

TABLE 2 Sterile Piperacillin Sodium & Tazobactam Sodium, Clinical Pharmacology

For*Enterobacteriaceae:* MIC (mcg/ml)	Interpretation
≤16	Susceptible (S)
32-64	Intermediate (I)
≤128	Resistant (R)

TABLE 2A Sterile Piperacillin Sodium & Tazobactam Sodium, Clinical Pharmacology

For*Haemophilus* species: MIC (mcg/ml)	Interpretation
≤1	Susceptible (S)
≥2	Resistant (R)

TABLE 2B Sterile Piperacillin Sodium & Tazobactam Sodium, Clinical Pharmacology

For*Staphylococcus* species: MIC (mcg/ml)	Interpretation
≤8	Susceptible (S)
≥16	Resistant (R)

CLINICAL PHARMACOLOGY: *(cont'd)*

A report of "Susceptible" indicates that the pathogen is likely to be inhibited by usually achievable concentrations of the antimicrobial compound in the blood. A report of "Intermediate" indicates that the result should be considered equivocal, and, if the microorganism is not fully susceptible to alternative, clinically feasible drugs, the test should be repeated. This category implies clinical applicability in body sites where the drug is physiologically concentrated or in situations where high dosage of drug can be used. This category also provides a buffer zone that prevents small uncontrolled technical factors from causing major discrepancies in interpretation. A report of "Resistant" indicates that usually achievable concentrations of the antimicrobial compound in the blood are unlikely to be inhibitory and other therapy should be selected.

Measurement of MIC or MBC and achieved compound concentrations may be appropriate to guide therapy in some infections. (See CLINICAL PHARMACOLOGY section for further information on drug concentrations achieved in infected body sites and other pharmacokinetic properties of this antimicrobial product.)(TABLE 3).

TABLE 3 Sterile Piperacillin Sodium & Tazobactam Sodium, Clinical Pharmacology

Microorganism	Zone Diameter (mm)
Escherichia coli ATCC 25922	1-4
Escherichia coli ATCC 35218	0.5-2
Haemophilus influenzae ATCC 49247	0.06-0.5
Staphylococcus aureus ATCC 29213	0.25-2

Anaerobic Techniques: For anaerobic bacteria, the susceptibility to piperacillin/tazobactam can be determined by the reference agar dilution method or by alternate standardized test methods.[2]

For *Bacteroides* species, the dilution and zone diameters should be interpreted as seen in TABLE 4.

TABLE 4 Sterile Piperacillin Sodium & Tazobactam Sodium, Clinical Pharmacology

MIC (mcg/ml)	Interpretation
≤ 16	Susceptible (S)
≥ 32	Resistant (R)

Serial dilutions of piperacillin combined with a fixed concentration of 4 mcg/ml tazobactam should provide the MIC values found in TABLE 5.

TABLE 5 Sterile Piperacillin Sodium & Tazobactam Sodium, Clinical Pharmacology

Microorganism	MIC (mcg/ml)
Bacteroides fragilis ATCC 25285	0.12 - 0.5
Bacteroides thetaiotaomicron ATCC 29741	4-16

Diffusion techniques: Quantitative methods that require measurement of zone diameters provide reproducible estimates of the susceptibility of bacteria to antimicrobial compounds. One such standardized procedure[3] that has been recommended for use with disks to test the susceptibility of microorganisms to piperacillin/tazobactam uses the 100 mcg/10 mcg piperacillin/tazobactam disk. Interpretation involves correlation of the diameter obtained in the disk test with the MIC for piperacillin/tazobactam.

Reports from the laboratory giving results of the standard single-disk susceptibility test 100 mcg/10 mcg piperacillin/tazobactam disk should be interpreted according to the criteria found in TABLE 6.

TABLE 6 Sterile Piperacillin Sodium & Tazobactam Sodium, Clinical Pharmacology

For Enterobacteriaceae: Zone Diameter (mm)	Interpretation
≥ 21	Susceptible (S)
18-20	Intermediate (I)
≤ 17	Resistant (R)

TABLE 6A Sterile Piperacillin Sodium & Tazobactam Sodium, Clinical Pharmacology

***For Staphylococcus* species:** Zone Diameter (mm)	Interpretation
≥ 20	Susceptible (S)
≤ 19	Resistant (R)

Interpretation is as stated above for results using dilution techniques.

As with standardized dilution techniques, diffusion susceptibility test procedures require the use of laboratory control microorganisms. The 100 mcg/10 mcg piperacillin/tazobactam disk should give the following zone diameters in these laboratory test quality control strains (TABLE 7).

TABLE 7 Sterile Piperacillin Sodium & Tazobactam Sodium, Clinical Pharmacology

Microorganism	Zone Diameter (mm)
Escherichia coli ATCC 25922	24-30
Escherichia coli ATCC 35218	24-30
Staphylococcus aureus ATCC 25923	27-36

INDICATIONS AND USAGE:

Piperacillin STS is indicated for the treatment of patients with moderate to severe infections caused by piperacillin resistant, piperacillin/tazobactam susceptible, β-lactamase producing strains of the designated microorganisms in the specified conditions listed below:

Appendicitis (complicated by rupture or abscess) and peritonitis caused by piperacillin resistant, β-lactamase producing strains of*Escherichia coli* or the following members of the *Bacteroides fragilis* group: *B. fragilis, B. ovatus, B. thetaiotaomicron,*or *B. vulgatus.* The individual members of this group were studied in less than 10 cases.

Uncomplicated and complicated skin and skin structure infections, including cellulitis, cutaneous abscesses, and ischemic/diabetic foot infections caused by piperacillin resistant, β-lactamase producing strains of *Staphylococcus aureus.*

Postpartum endometritis or pelvic inflammatory disease caused by piperacillin resistant, β-lactamase producing strains of*Escherichia coli.*

Community-acquired pneumonia (moderate severity only) caused by piperacillin resistant, β-lactamase producing strains of*Haemophilus influenzae.*

INDICATIONS AND USAGE: *(cont'd)*

Clinical trial data for the treatment of complicated urinary tract infections demonstrated inadequate efficacy at the dosage regimen of Piperacillin STS studied (*i.e.,* 3.375 g every 8 hours). There are no other adequate and well controlled trial data to support the use of this product in the treatment of complicated urinary tract infections.

A study for the treatment of nosocomial lower respiratory tract infections was initiated with Piperacillin STS as monotherapy at 3.375 g every 6 hours. This study was terminated because of an unacceptable level of efficacy at this dosage.

As a combination product, Piperacillin STS is indicated only for the specified conditions listed above. Infections caused by piperacillin susceptible organisms for which piperacillin has been shown to be effective are also amenable to Piperacillin STS treatment due to its piperacillin content. The tazobactam component of this combination product does not decrease the activity of the piperacillin component against piperacillin susceptible organisms. Therefore, the treatment of mixed infections caused by piperacillin susceptible organisms and piperacillin resistant, β- lactamase producing organisms susceptible to Piperacillin STS should not require the addition of another antibiotic.

Piperacillin STS is useful as presumptive therapy in the indicated conditions prior to the identification of causative organisms because of its broad spectrum of bactericidal activity against gram-positive and gram-negative anaerobic organisms.

Appropriate cultures should usually be performed before initiating antimicrobial treatment in order to isolate and identify the organisms causing infection and to determine their susceptibility to Piperacillin STS. Antimicrobial therapy should be adjusted, if appropriate, once the results of culture(s) and antimicrobial susceptibility testing are known.

CONTRAINDICATIONS:

Piperacillin STS is contraindicated in patients with a history of allergic reactions to any of the penicillins, cephalosporins, or β-lactamase inhibitors.

WARNINGS:

SERIOUS AND OCCASIONALLY FATAL HYPERSENSITIVITY (ANAPHYLACTIC) REACTIONS HAVE BEEN REPORTED IN PATIENTS IN PENICILLIN THERAPY. THESE REACTIONS ARE MORE LIKELY TO OCCUR IN INDIVIDUALS WITH A HISTORY OF PENICILLIN HYPERSENSITIVITY OR A HISTORY OF SENSITIVITY TO MULTIPLE ALLERGENS. THERE HAVE BEEN REPORTS OF INDIVIDUALS WITH A HISTORY OF PENICILLIN HYPERSENSITIVITY WHO HAVE EXPERIENCED SEVERE REACTIONS WHEN TREATED WITH CEPHALOSPORINS. BEFORE INITIATING THERAPY WITH PIPERACILLIN STS, CAREFUL INQUIRY SHOULD BE MADE CONCERNING PREVIOUS HYPERSENSITIVITY REACTIONS TO PENICILLINS, CEPHALOSPORINS, OR OTHER ALLERGENS. IF AN ALLERGIC REACTION OCCURS, PIPERACILLIN STS SHOULD BE DISCONTINUED AND APPROPRIATE THERAPY INSTITUTED.**SERIOUS ANAPHYLACTIC REACTIONS REQUIRE IMMEDIATE EMERGENCY TREATMENT WITH EPINEPHRINE. OXYGEN, INTRAVENOUS STEROIDS, AND AIRWAY MANAGEMENT, INCLUDING INTUBATION, SHOULD ALSO BE ADMINISTERED AS INDICATED.**

Pseudomembranous colitis has been reported with nearly all antibacterial agents, including piperacillin/tazobactam, and may range in severity from mild to life-threatening. Therefore, it is important to consider this diagnosis in patients who present with diarrhea subsequent to the administration of antibacterial agents.

Treatment with antibacterial agents alters the normal flora of the colon and may permit overgrowth of clostridia. Studies indicate that a toxin produced by *Clostridium difficile* is one primary cause of "antibiotic-associated colitis."

After the diagnosis of pseudomembranous colitis has been established, therapeutic measures should be initiated. Mild cases of pseudomembranous colitis usually respond to drug discontinuation alone. In moderate to severe cases, consideration should be given to management with fluids and electrolytes, protein supplementation, and treatment with an antibacterial drug clinically effective against *Clostridium difficile* colitis.

PRECAUTIONS:

GENERAL

Bleeding manifestations have occurred in some patients receiving β-lactam antibiotics, including piperacillin. These reactions have sometimes been associated with abnormalities of coagulation tests such as clotting time, platelet aggregation, and prothrombin time and are more likely to occur in patients with renal failure. If bleeding manifestations occur, Piperacillin STS should be discontinued and appropriate therapy instituted.

The possibility of the emergence of resistant organisms that might cause superinfections should be kept in mind. If this occurs, appropriate measures should be taken.

As with other penicillins, patients may experience neuromuscular excitability or convulsions if higher than recommended doses are given intravenously (particularly in the presence of renal failure).

Piperacillin STS is a monosodium salt of piperacillin and a monosodium salt of tazobactam and contains a total of 2.35 mEq (54 mg) of Na+ per gram of piperacillin in the combination product. This should be considered when treating patients requiring restricted salt intake. Periodic electrolyte determinations should be performed in patients with low potassium reserves, and the possibility of hypokalemia should be kept in mind with patients who have potentially low potassium reserves and who are receiving cytotoxic therapy for diuretics.

As with other semisynthetic penicillins, piperacillin therapy has been associated with an increased incidence of fever and rash in cystic fibrosis patients.

LABORATORY TESTS

Periodic assessment of hematopoietic function should be performed, especially with prolonged therapy, (*i.e.,* ≥ 21 days). (See ADVERSE REACTIONS, Adverse Laboratory Events.)

DRUG/LABORATORY TEST INTERACTIONS

As with other penicillins, the administration of Piperacillin STS may result in a false-positive reaction for glucose in the urine using a copper-reduction method (Clinitest[†]). It is recommended that glucose tests based on enzymatic glucose oxidase reactions (such as Diastix[†]or Tes-Tape[†]) be used.

CARCINOGENESIS, MUTAGENESIS, AND IMPAIRMENT OF FERTILITY

Long term carcinogenicity studies in animals have not been conducted with piperacillin/tazobactam, piperacillin, or tazobactam.

Piperacillin/Tazobactam: was negative in microbial mutagenicity assays at concentrations up to 14.84/1.86 mcg/plate. Piperacillin/tazobactam was negative in the unscheduled DNA synthesis (UDS) test at concentrations up to 5689/711 mcg/ml. Piperacillin/tazobactam was negative in a mammalian point mutation (Chinese hamster ovary cell HPRT) assay at concentrations up to 8000/1000 mcg/ml. Piperacillin/tazobactam was negative in a mammalian cell (BALB/c-3T3) transformation assay at concentrations up to 8/1 mcg/ml.*In vivo,* piperacillin/tazobactam did not induce chromosomal aberrations in rats dosed IV with 1500/187.5 mg/kg; this dose is similar to the maximum recommended human daily dose on a body-surface-area basis (mg/m^2).

PRECAUTIONS: *(cont'd)*

Piperacillin: was negative in microbial mutagenicity assays at concentrations up to 50 mcg/plate. There was no DNA damage in bacteria (Rec assay) exposed to piperacillin at concentrations up to 200 mcg/disk. Piperacillin was negative in the UDS test at concentrations up to 10,000 mcg/ml. In a mammalian point mutation (mouse lymphoma cells) assay, piperacillin was positive at concentrations ≥2500 mcg/ml. Piperacillin was negative in a cell (BALB/c-3T3) transformation assay at concentrations up to 3000 mcg/ml. *In vivo,* piperacillin did not induce chromosomal aberrations in mice at IV doses up to 1500 mg/kg/day. These doses are half (mice) or similar (rats) to the maximum recommended human daily dose based on body-surface area (mg/m^2). In another *in vivo* test, there was no dominant lethal effect when piperacillin was administered to rats at IV doses up to 2000 mg/kg/day, which is similar to the maximum recommended human daily dose based on body-surface area (mg/m^2). When mice were administered piperacillin at IV doses up to 2000 mg/kg/day, which is half the maximum recommended human daily dose based on body-surface area (mg/m^2), urine from these animals was not mutagenic when tested in a microbial mutagenicity assay. Bacteria injected into the peritoneal cavity of mice administered piperacillin at IV doses up to 2000 mg/kg/day did not show increased mutation frequencies.

Tazobactam: was negative in microbial mutagenicity assays at concentrations up to 330 mcg/plate. Tazobactam was negative in the UDS test at concentrations up to 2000 mcg/ml. Tazobactam was negative in a mammalian point mutation (Chinese hamster ovary cell HPRT) assay at concentrations up to 5000 mcg/ml. In another mammalian point mutation (mouse lymphoma cells) assay, tazobactam was positive at concentrations ≥3000 mcg/ml. Tazobactam was negative in a cell (BALB/c-3T3) transformation assay at concentrations up to 900 mcg/ml. In an *in vitro* cytogenetics (Chinese hamster lung cells) assay, tazobactam was negative at concentrations up to 3000 mcg/ml. *In vivo,* tazobactam did not induce chromosomal aberrations in rats at IV doses up to 5000 mg/kg, which is 23 times the maximum recommended human daily dose based on body-surface area (mg/m^2).

PREGNANCY, TERATOGENIC EFFECTS, PREGNANCY CATEGORY B

Piperacillin/Tazobactam; Reproduction studies have performed in rats and have revealed no evidence of impaired fertility due to piperacillin/tazobactam administered up to a dose which is similar to the maximum recommended human daily dose based on body-surface area (mg/m^2).

Teratology studies have been performed in mice and rats and have revealed no evidence of harm to the fetus due to piperacillin/tazobactam administered up to a dose which is 1 to 2 times and 2 to 3 times the human dose of piperacillin and tazobactam, respectively, based on body- surface area (mg/m^2).

Piperacillin: Reproduction and teratology studies have been performed in mice and rats and have revealed no evidence of impaired fertility or harm to the fetus due to piperacillin administered up to a dose which is half (mice) or similar (rats) to the maximum recommended human daily dose based on body-surface area (mg/m^2).

Tazobactam: Reproduction studies have been performed in rats and have revealed no evidence of harm to the fetus due to tazobactam administered at doses up to 3 times the maximum recommended human daily dose based on body-surface area (mg/m^2).

Teratology studies have been performed in mice and rats and have revealed no evidence of harm to the fetus due to tazobactam administered at doses up to 6 and 14 times, respectively, the human dose based on body-surface area (mg/m^2). In rats, tazobactam crosses the placenta. Concentrations in the fetus are less than or equal to 10% of that found in maternal plasma.

There are, however, no adequate and well-controlled studies with the piperacillin/tazobactam combination or with piperacillin or tazobactam alone in pregnant women. Because animal reproduction studies are not always predictive of the human response, this drug should be used during pregnancy only if clearly needed.

NURSING MOTHERS

Piperacillin is excreted in low concentrations in human milk; tazobactam concentrations in human milk have not been studied. Caution should be exercised when Piperacillin STS is administered to a nursing woman.

PEDIATRIC USE

Safety and efficacy in children below the age of 12 years have not been established.

GERIATRIC USE

Patients over 65 years are **not** at an increased risk of developing adverse effects solely because of age. However, dosage should be adjusted in the presence of renal insufficiency. (See DOSAGE AND ADMINISTRATION.)

DRUG INTERACTIONS:

Aminoglycosides: The mixing of Piperacillin STS with an aminoglycoside *in vitro* can result in substantial inactivation of the aminoglycoside. (See DOSAGE AND ADMINISTRATION, Compatible Intravenous Diluents.)

When Piperacillin STS is co-administered with tobramycin, the area under the curve, renal clearance, and urinary recovery of tobramycin were decreased by 11%, 32%, and 38%, respectively. The alterations in the pharmacokinetics of tobramycin when administered in combination with piperacillin/tazobactam may be due to *in vivo* and *in vitro* inactivation of tobramycin in the presence of piperacillin/tazobactam. The inactivation of aminoglycosides in the presence of penicillin class drugs has been recognized. It has been postulated that penicillin-aminoglycoside complexes form; these complexes are microbiologically inactive and of unknown toxicity. In patients with severe renal dysfunction (*i.e.,* chronic hemodialysis patients), the pharmacokinetics of tobramycin are significantly altered when tobramycin is administered in combination with piperacillin.[4] The alteration of tobramycin pharmacokinetics and the potential toxicity of the penicillin-aminoglycoside complexes in patients with mild to moderate renal dysfunction who are administered an aminoglycoside in combination with piperacillin/tazobactam is unknown.

Probenecid: Probenecid administered concomitantly with Piperacillin STS prolongs the half-life of piperacillin by 21% and of tazobactam by 71%.

Vancomycin: No pharmacokinetic interactions have been noted between Piperacillin STS and vancomycin.

Heparin: Coagulation parameters should be tested more frequently and monitored regularly during simultaneous administration of high doses of heparin, oral anticoagulants, or other drugs that may affect the blood coagulation system or the thrombocyte function.

Vecuronium: Piperacillin when used concomitantly with vecuronium has been implicated in the prolongation of the neuromuscular blockade of vecuronium. Piperacillin STS (piperacillin/tazobactam) could produce the same phenomenon if given along with vecuronium. Due to their similar mechanism of action, it is expected that the neuromuscular blockade produced by any of the non-depolarizing muscle relaxants could be prolonged in the presence of piperacillin (See monograph for vecuronium bromide).

ADVERSE REACTIONS:

During the clinical investigations, 2621 patients worldwide were treated with Piperacillin STS in phase 3 trials. In the key North American clinical trials (n=830 patients), 90% of the adverse events reported were mild to moderate in severity and transient in nature. However, in 3.2% of the patients treated worldwide, Piperacillin STS was discontinued because of adverse events primarily involving the skin (1.3%), including rash and pruritus; the gastrointestinal system (0.9%), including diarrhea, nausea, and vomiting; and allergic reactions (0.5%).

Adverse local reactions that were reported, irrespective of relationship to therapy with Piperacillin STS, were phlebitis (1.3%), injection site reaction (0.5%), pain (0.2%), inflammation (0.2%), thrombophlebitis (0.2%), and edema (0.1%).

Adverse Clinical Events: Based on patients from the North American trials (n=1063), the events with the highest incidence in patients, irrespective of relationship to Piperacillin STS therapy, were diarrhea (11.3%); headache (7.7%); constipation (7.7%); nausea (6.9%); insomnia (6.6%); rash (4.2%), including maculopapular, bullous, urticarial, and eczematoid; vomiting (3.3%); dyspepsia (3.3%); pruritus (3.1%); stool changes (2.4%); fever (2.4%); agitation (2.1%); pain (1.7%); moniliasis (1.6%); hypertension (1.6%); dizziness (1.4%); abdominal pain (1.3%); chest pain (1.3%); edema (1.2%); anxiety (1.2%); rhinitis (1.2%); and dyspnea (1.1%).

Additional adverse systemic clinical events reported in 1.0% or less of the patients are listed below within each body system:

Autonomic Nervous System: hypotension, ileus, syncope

Body as a Whole: rigors, back pain, malaise

Cardiovascular: tachycardia, including supraventricular and ventricular; bradycardia; arrhythmia, including atrial fibrillation, ventricular fibrillation, cardiac arrest, cardiac failure, circulatory failure, myocardial infarction

Central Nervous System: tremor, convulsions, vertigo

Gastrointestinal: melena, flatulence, hemorrhage, gastritis, hiccough, ulcerative stomatitis

Pseudomembranous colitis was reported in one patient during the clinical trials. The onset of pseudomembranous colitis symptoms may occur during or after antibacterial treatment. (See WARNINGS.)

Hearing: tinnitus

Hypersensitivity: anaphylaxis

Metabolic and Nutritional: symptomatic hypoglycemia, thirst

Musculoskeletal: myalgia, arthralgia

Platelet, Bleeding, Clotting: mesenteric embolism, purpura, epistaxis, pulmonary embolism (see PRECAUTIONS, General).

Psychiatric: confusion, hallucination, depression

Reproductive, Female: leukorrhea, vaginitis

Respiratory: pharyngitis, pulmonary edema, bronchospasm, coughing

Skin and Appendages: genital pruritus, diaphoresis

Special Senses: taste perversion

Urinary: retention, dysuria, oliguria, hematuria, incontinence

Vision: photophobia

Vascular (Extracardiac): flushing

ADVERSE LABORATORY EVENTS

Changes in laboratory parameters, without regard to drug relationship, include:

Hematologic: Decreases in hemoglobin and hematocrit, thrombocytopenia, increases in platelet count, eosinophilia, leukopenia, neutropenia. The leukopenia/neutropenia associated with Piperacillin STS administration appears to be reversible and most frequently associated with prolonged administration, (*i.e.,* ≥ 21 days of therapy). These patients were withdrawn from therapy; some had accompanying systemic symptoms (*e.g.,* fever, rigors, chills).

Coagulation: Positive direct Coombs' test, prolonged prothrombin time, prolonged partial thromboplastin time

Hepatic: Transient elevations of AST (SGOT), ALT (SGPT), alkaline phosphatase, bilirubin

Renal: Increases in serum creatinine, blood urea nitrogen

Urinalysis: Proteinuria, hematuria, pyuria

Additional laboratory events include abnormalities in electrolytes (*i.e.,* increases and decreases in sodium, potassium, and calcium), hyperglycemia, decreases in total protein or albumin

The following adverse reactions have also been reported for Pipracil (sterile piperacillin sodium):

Skin and appendages: Erythema multiforme and Stevens-Johnson syndrome, rarely reported

Gastrointestinal: Cholestatic hepatitis

Renal: Rarely, interstitial hepatitis

Skeletal: Prolonged muscle relaxation (See DRUG INTERACTIONS)

OVERDOSAGE:

Information on overdosage of Piperacillin STS in humans is not available.

Excessive serum levels of either piperacillin or tazobactam may be reduced by hemodialysis. (See CLINICAL PHARMACOLOGY.) No specific antidote is known. As with other penicillins, neuromuscular excitability or convulsions have occurred following large intravenous doses, primarily in patients with impaired renal function.

In the case of motor excitability or convulsions, general supportive measures, including administration of anticonvulsive agents (*e.g.,* diazepam or barbiturates) may be considered.

DOSAGE AND ADMINISTRATION:

Piperacillin STS should be administered by intravenous administration over 30 minutes.

The usual total daily dose of Piperacillin STS for adults is 12 g/1.5 g, given as 3.375 g every six hours.

Renal Insufficiency: In patients with renal insufficiency, the intravenous dose should be adjusted to the degree of actual renal function impairment. The recommended daily doses are as in TABLE 8.

TABLE 8 Sterile Piperacillin Sodium & Tazobactam Sodium, DOSAGE AND ADMINISTRATION Piperacillin STS Dosage Recommendations

Creatinine Clearance (ml/min)	Recommended Dosage Regimen
>40	12 g/1.5 g/day in divided doses of 3.375 g q6h
20-40	8 g/1.0 g/day in divided doses of 2.25 g q6h
<20	6 g/0.75 g/day in divided doses of 2.25 g q8h

DOSAGE AND ADMINISTRATION: *(cont'd)*

For patients on hemodialysis, the maximum dose is 2.25 g Piperacillin STS q eight hours. In addition, because hemodialysis removes 30%-40% of a Piperacillin STS dose in four hours, one additional dose of 0.75 g Piperacillin STS should be administered following each dialysis period. For patients with renal failure, measurement of serum levels of piperacillin and tazobactam will provide additional guidance for adjusting dosage.

Duration of Therapy: The usual duration of Piperacillin STS treatment is from seven to ten days. The duration should be guided by the severity of the infection and the patient's clinical and bacteriological progress.

Intravenous Administration: Reconstitute Piperacillin STS per gram of piperacillin with 5 ml of a compatible reconstitution diluent from the list provided below. Shake well until dissolved. Single dose vials should be used immediately after reconstitution. Discard any unused portion after 24 hours if stored at room temperature, or after 48 hours if stored at refrigerated temperature [2 to 8°C (36 to 46°F)].

Compatible Intravenous Diluents: 0.9% Sodium Chloride for Injection

Sterile Water for Injection

Dextrose 5%

Bacteriostatic Saline/Parabens

Bacteriostatic Water/Parabens

Bacteriostatic Saline/Benzyl Alcohol

Bacteriostatic Water/Benzyl Alcohol

Reconstituted Piperacillin STS solution should be further diluted (recommended volume per dose of 50 ml to 150 ml) in a compatible intravenous diluent solution listed below. Administer by infusion over a period of at least 30 minutes. During the infusion it is desirable to discontinue the primary infusion solution.

COMPATIBLE INTRAVENOUS DILUENT SOLUTIONS

0.9% Sodium Chloride for Injection

Sterile Water for Injection‡

Dextrose 5%

Dextran 6% in Saline

‡Maximum recommended volume per dose of Sterile Water for Injection is 50 ml.

LACTATED RINGERS SOLUTION IS NOT COMPATIBLE WITH PIPERACILLIN STS

When concomitant therapy with aminoglycosides is indicated, Piperacillin STS and the aminoglycoside should be reconstituted and administered separately, due to the *in vitro* inactivation of aminoglycoside by the penicillin. (See DRUG INTERACTIONS.)

Piperacillin STS can be used in ambulatory intravenous infusion pumps.

Stability of Piperacillin STS Following Reconstitution: Piperacillin STS is stable in glass and plastic containers (plastic syringes, IV bags, and tubing) when reconstituted with acceptable diluents.

Stability studies in the IV bags have demonstrated chemical stability [potency, pH of reconstituted solution, and clarity of solution] for up to 24 hours at room temperature and up to one week at refrigerated temperature. Piperacillin STS contains no preservatives. Appropriate consideration of aseptic technique should not be used.

Stability of Piperacillin STS in an ambulatory intravenous infusion pump has been demonstrated for a period of 12 hours at room temperature. Each dose was reconstituted and diluted to a volume of 37.5 ml or 25 ml. One day supplies of dosing solution were aseptically transferred into the medication reservoir (IV bags or cartridge). The reservoir was fitted to a preprogrammed ambulatory intravenous infusion pump per the manufacturer's instructions. Stability of Piperacillin STS is not affected when administered using an ambulatory intravenous infusion pump.

Parenteral drug products should be inspected visually for particulate matter and discoloration prior to administration, whenever solution and container permit.

REFERENCES:

1. National Committee for Clinical Laboratory Standards, Methods for Dilution Antimicrobial Tests for Bacteria that Grow Aerobically - Third Edition. Approved Standard NCCLS Document M7-A3, Vol. 13, No. 25, NCCLS, Villanova, PA, December, 1993. **2.** National Committee for Clinical Laboratory Standards, Methods for Antimicrobial Susceptibility Testing for Anaerobic Bacteria - Third Edition. Approved Standard NCCLS Document M11-A3, Vol. 13, No. 26, NCCLS, Villinova, PA, December, 1993. **3.** National Committee for Clinical Laboratory Standards, Performance Standard for Antimicrobial Disk Susceptibility Tests - Fifth Edition. Approved Standard NCCLS Document M2-A5, Vol. 13, No.24, NCCLS, Villanova, PA, December, 1993. **4.** Halstenson CE, Hirata CAI, Heim-Duthoy KL, Abraham PA, and Matzke GR. Effect of concomitant administration of piperacillin on the dispositions of netilmicin and tobramycin in patients with end-stage renal disease. Antimicrob Agents Chemother 34(1):128-133, 1990.† Clinitest and Diastix are registered trademarks of Ames Division, Miles Laboratories, Inc.† Tes-Tape is a registered trademark of Eli Lilly and Company.

HOW SUPPLIED:

Piperacillin STS (sterile piperacillin sodium and tazobactam sodium) is supplied in the following sizes:

Each Zosyn 2.25 g vial provides piperacillin sodium equivalent to 2 grams of piperacillin and tazobactam sodium equivalent to 0.25 gram of tazobactam. Each vial contains 4.69 mEq (108 mg) of sodium.

Each Zosyn 3.375 g vial provides piperacillin sodium equivalent to 3 grams piperacillin and tazobactam sodium equivalent to 0.375 gram of tazobactam. Each vial contains 7.04 mEq (162 mg) of sodium.

Each Zosyn 4.5 g vial provides piperacillin sodium equivalent to 4 grams of piperacillin and tazobactam sodium equivalent to 0.5 gram of tazobactam. Each vial contains 9.37 mEq (216 mg) of sodium.

Zosyn vials should be stored at controlled room temperature 15 to 30°C (59 to 86°F) prior to reconstitution.

HOW SUPPLIED - EQUIVALENTS NOT AVAILABLE:

Injection, Solution - Intravenous - 2 gm/0.25 mg

10's $98.71 ZOSYN, Lederle Piperacillin 00206-8452-16

Injection, Solution - Intravenous - 3 gm/0.375 mg

10's $148.06 ZOSYN, Lederle Piperacillin 00206-8454-55

Injection, Solution - Intravenous - 4 gm/0.5 mg

10's $197.43 ZOSYN, Lederle Piperacillin 00206-8455-25

Injection, Solution - Intravenous - 36 gm/4.5 mg

1's $177.70 ZOSYN, Lederle Piperacillin 00206-8620-11

PIRBUTEROL ACETATE *(002046)*

CATEGORIES: Airway Obstruction; Antiasthmatics/Bronchodilators; Asthma; Autonomic Drugs; Beta Adrenergic Stimulators; Bronchial Dilators; Bronchospasm; Respiratory & Allergy Medications; Sympathomimetic Agents; Sympathomimetics, Beta Agonist; Pregnancy Category C; FDA Approved 1986 Dec

BRAND NAMES: *Exirel*; **Maxair**; *Spirolair*; *Zeisin*; *Zeisin Autohaler* (Germany)
(International brand names outside U.S. in italics)

FORMULARIES: Aetna; BC-BS; FHP; Foundation; Medi-Cal; PCS

COST OF THERAPY: (Asthma; Aerosol; 0.2 mg; 1.6/day; 365 days) (DRG 96)

PRIMARY ICD9: 493.90 (Asthma, Unspecified, Without Mention of Status Asthmaticus)

DESCRIPTION:

The active component of Maxair Inhaler is α^6-(((1,1-dimethylethyl)amino)methy)-3-hydroxy-2,6-pyridine-di methanol monoacetate salt.

Pirbuterol acetate is a white, crystalline powder, freely soluble in water, with a molecular weight of 300.3 and empirical formula of $C_{12}H_{20}N_2O_3{\cdot}C_2H_4O_2$.

Maxair Inhaler is a metered dose aerosol unit for oral inhalation. It provides a fine-particle suspension of pirbuterol acetate in the propellant mixture of trichloromonofluoromethane and dichlorodifluoromethane, with sorbitan trioleate. Each actuation delivers from the mouthpiece pirbuterol acetate equivalent to 0.2 mg of pirbuterol with the majority of particles less than 5 microns in diameter. Each canister provides at least 300 inhalations.

CLINICAL PHARMACOLOGY:

In vitro studies and *in vivo* pharmacologic studies have demonstrated that pirbuterol acetate has preferential effect on beta-2 adrenergic receptors compared with isoproterenol. While it is recognized that beta-2 adrenergic receptors are the predominant receptors in bronchial smooth muscle, recent data indicate that there is a population of beta-2 receptors in the human heart, existing in a concentration between 10-50%. The precise function of these, however, is not yet established (see WARNINGS.)

The pharmacologic effects of beta adrenergic agonist drugs, including pirbuterol acetate, are at least in part attributable to stimulation through beta adrenergic receptors of intracellular adenyl cyclase, the enzyme which catalyzes the conversion of adenosine triphosphate (ATP) to cyclic-3'5'-adenosine monophosphate (c-AMP). Increased c-AMP levels are associated with relaxation of bronchial smooth muscle and inhibition of release of mediators of immediate hypersensitivity from cells, especially from mast cells.

Bronchodilator activity of pirbuterol acetate was manifested clinically by an improvement in various pulmonary function parameters (FEV_1, MMF, PEFR, airway resistance (RAW) and conductance (GA/V_{tg}).

In controlled double-blind single dose clinical trials, the most of improvement in pulmonary function occurred within 5 minutes in most patients as determined by forced expiratory volume in one second (FEV_1) FEV_1 and MMF measurements also showed that maximum improvement in pulmonary function generally occurred 30-60 minutes following one (1) or two (2) inhalations of pirbuterol (0.2-0.4 mg).

The duration of action of pirbuterol acetate is maintained for 5 hours (the time at which the last observations were made) in a substantial number of patients, based on a 15% or greater increase in FEV_1. In controlled repetitive dose studies of 12 weeks duration, 74% of 156 patients on pirbuterol and 62% of 141 patients on metaproterenol showed a clinically significant improvement based on a 15% or greater increase in FEV_1, on at least half of the days. Onset and duration were equivalent to that seen in single dose studies. Continued effectiveness was demonstrated over the 12-week period in the majority (94%) of responding patients; however, chronic dosing was associated with the development of tachyphylaxis (tolerance) to the bronchodilator effect in some patients in both treatment groups.

A placebo-controlled double-blind single dose study (24 patients per treatment group), utilizing continuous Holter monitoring for 5 hours after drug administration, showed no significant difference in ectopic activity between the placebo control group and pirbuterol acetate at the recommended dose (0.2-0.4 mg), and twice the recommended dose (0.8 mg). As with other inhaled beta adrenergic agonists, supraventricular and ventricular ectopic beats have been seen with pirbuterol acetate (see WARNINGS.)

Recent studies in laboratory animals (minipigs, rodents, and dogs) recorded the occurrence of cardiac arrhythmias and sudden death (with histologic evidence of myocardial necrosis) when beta agonists and methylxanthines were administered concurrently. The significance of these findings when applied to humans is currently unknown.

PHARMACOKINETICS

As expected by extrapolation from oral data, systemic blood levels of pirbuterol are below the limit of assay sensitivity (2-5 ng/ml) following inhalation of doses up to 0.8 mg (twice the maximum recommended dose). A mean of 51% of the dose is recovered in urine as pirbuterol plus its sulfate conjugate following administration by aerosol. Pirbuterol is not metabolized by catechol-O methyltransferase. The percent of administered dose recovered as pirbuterol plus its sulfate conjugate does not change significantly over the range of 0.4 mg to 0.8 mg and is not significantly different from that after oral administration of pirbuterol. the plasma half-life measured after oral administration is about two hours.

INDICATIONS AND USAGE:

Pirbuterol acetateis indicated for the prevention and reversal of bronchospasm in patients with reversible bronchospasm including asthma. It may be used with or without concurrent theophylline and/or steroid therapy.

CONTRAINDICATIONS:

Pirbuterol acetate is contraindicated in patients with a history of hypersensitivity to any of its ingredients.

WARNINGS:

As with other beta adrenergic aerosols, pirbuterol acetate should not be used in excess. Controlled clinical studies and other clinical experience have shown that pirbuterol acetate like other inhaled beta adrenergic agonists can produce a significant cardiovascular effect in some patients, as measured by pulse rate, blood pressure, symptoms, and/or ECG changes. As with other beta adrenergic aerosols, the potential for paradoxical bronchospasm (which can be life threatening) should be kept in mind. If it occurs, the preparation should be discontinued immediately and alternative therapy instituted.

Fatalities have been reported in association with excessive use of inhaled sympathomimetic drugs.

The contents of Pirbuterol acetate are under pressure. Do not puncture. Do not use or store near heat or open flame. Exposure to temperature above 120°F may cause bursting. Never throw container into fire or incinerator. Keep out of reach of children.

PRECAUTIONS:

GENERAL

Since pirbuterol is a sympathomimetic amine, it should be used with caution in patients with cardiovascular disorders, including ischemic heart disease, hypertension, or cardiac arrhythmias, in patients with hyperthyroidism or diabetes mellitus, and in patients who are unusually responsive to sympathomimetic amines or who have convulsive disorders. Significant changes in systolic and diastolic blood pressure could be expected to occur in some patients after use of any beta adrenergic aerosol bronchodilator.

INFORMATION FOR THE PATIENT

pirbuterol acetate effects may last up to five hours or longer. It should not be used more often than recommended and the patient should not increase the number of inhalations or frequency of use without first asking the physician. If symptoms of asthma get worse, adverse reactions occur, or the patient does not respond to the usual dose, the patient should be instructed to contact the physician immediately. The patient should be advised to see the illustrated directions for Use.

CARCINOGENESIS, MUTAGENESIS AND IMPAIRMENT OF FERTILITY

Pirbuterol hydrochloride administered in the diet to rats for 24 months and to mice for 18 months was free of carcinogenic activity at doses corresponding to 200 times the maximum human inhalation dose. In addition, the intragastric intubation of the drug at doses corresponding to 6250 times the maximum recommended human daily inhalation dose resulted in no increase in tumors in a 12-month rat study. Studies with pirbuterol revealed no evidence of mutagenesis. Reproduction studies in rats revealed no evidence of impaired fertility.

TERATOGENIC EFFECTS - PREGNANCY CATEGORY C

Reproductions studies have been performed in rats and rabbits by the inhalation route at doses up to 12 times (rat) and 16 times (rabbit) the maximum human inhalation dose and have revealed no significant findings. Animal reproduction studies in rats at oral doses up to 300 mg/kg and in rabbits at oral doses up to 100 mg/kg have shown no adverse effect on reproductive behavior, fertility, litter size, peri- and postnatal viability or fetal development. In rabbits at the highest dose level given, 300 mg/kg, abortions and fetal mortality were observed. There are no adequate and well controlled studies in pregnant women and pirbuterol acetate should be used during pregnancy only if the potential benefit justifies that potential risk to the fetus.

NURSING MOTHERS

It is not known whether pirbuterol acetate is excreted in human milk. Therefore, pirbuterol acetate should be used during nursing only if the potential benefit justifies the possible risk to the newborn.

PEDIATRIC USE

Pirbuterol acetate is not recommended for patients under the age of 12 years because of insufficient clinical data to establish safety and effectiveness.

DRUG INTERACTIONS:

Other beta adrenergic aerosol bronchodilators should not be used concomitantly with pirbuterol acetate because they may have additive effects. Beta adrenergic agonists should be administered with caution to patients being treated with monoamine oxidase inhibitors or tricyclic antidepressants, since the action of beta adrenergic agonists on the vascular system may be potentiated.

ADVERSE REACTIONS:

The following rates of adverse reactions to pirbuterol are based on single and multiple dose clinical trials involving 761 patients, 400 of whom received multiple doses (mean duration of treatment was 2.5 months and maximum was 19 months).

The following were the adverse reactions reported more frequently than 1 in 100 patients:

CNS: nervousness (6.9%), tremor (6.0%), headache (2.0%), dizziness (1.2%).

Cardiovascular: palpitations (1.7%), tachycardia (1.2%).

Respiratory: Cough (1.2%).

Gastrointestinal: nausea (1.7%).

The following adverse reactions occurred less frequently than 1 in 100 patients and there may be a causal relationship with pirbuterol.

CNS: depression, anxiety, confusion, insomnia, weakness, hyperkinesia, syncope.

Cardiovascular: hypotension, skipped beats, chest pain.

Gastrointestinal: dry mouth, glossitis, abdominal pain/cramps, anorexia, diarrhea, stomatitis nausea and vomiting.

Ear, Nose and Throat: smell/taste changes, sore throat.

Dermatological: rash, pruritus.

Other: numbness in extremities, alopecia, bruising, fatigue, edema, weight gain, flushing.

Other adverse reactions were reported with a frequency of less than 1 in 100 patients but a causal relationship between pirbuterol and the reaction could not be determined: migraine, productive cough, wheezing, and dermatitis.

The following rates of adverse reactions during three-month controlled clinical trials involving 310 patients are noted. the table does not include mild reactions (TABLE 1).

TABLE 1 Percent of Patients with Moderate to Severe Adverse Reactions

Adverse Reaction	Pirbuterol N=157	Metaproterenol N-153
Central Nervous System		
tremors	1.3%	3.3%
nervousness	4.5%	2.6%
headache	1.3%	2.0%
weakness	0%	1.3%
drowsiness	0%	0.7%
dizziness	0.6%	0%
Cardiovascular		
palpitations	1.3%	1.3%
tachycardia	1.3%	2.0%
Respiratory		
chest pain/tightness	1.3%	0%
cough	0%	0.7%
Gastrointestinal		
nausea	1.3%	2.0%
diarrhea	1.3%	0.7%
dry mouth	1.3%	1.3%
vomiting	0%	0.7%
Dermatological		
skin reaction	0%	0.7%
rash	0%	1.3%
Other		
bruising	0.6%	0%
smell/taste change	0.6%	.0%
backache	0%	0.7%
fatigue	0%	0.7%
hoarseness	0%	0.7%
nasal congestion	0%	0.7%

OVERDOSAGE:

The expected symptoms with overdosage are those of excessive beta-stimulation and/or any of the symptoms listed under adverse reactions e.g., angina, hypertension or hypotension, arrhythmias, nervousness, headache, tremor, dry mouth, palpitation, nausea, dizziness, fatigue, malaise, and insomnia.

Treatment consists of discontinuation of pirbuterol together with appropriate symptomatic therapy.

The oral acute lethal dose in male and female rats and mice was greater than 2000 mg base/kg. The aerosol acute lethal dose was not determined.

DOSAGE AND ADMINISTRATION:

The usual dose for adults and children 12 years and older is two inhalations (0.4 mg) repeated every 4-6 hours. One inhalation (0.2 mg) repeated every 4-6 hours may be sufficient for some patients.

A total daily dose of 12 inhalations should not be exceeded.

If a previously effective dosage regimen fails to provide the usual relief, medical advice should be sought immediately as this is often a sign of seriously worsening asthma which would require reassessment of therapy.

Store between 15 and 30°C (59 to 86°F).

HOW SUPPLIED - EQUIVALENTS NOT AVAILABLE:

Aerosol - Inhalation - 0.2 mg

2.8 gm	$9.60	MAXAIR AUTOHALER, 3M Pharms	00089-0817-10
14 gm	$34.14	MAXAIR AUTOHALER, 3M Pharms	00089-0815-21
25.6 gm	$24.42	MAXAIR, 3M Pharms	00089-0790-21

PIROXICAM *(002047)*

CATEGORIES: Analgesics; Anti-Inflammatory Agents; Antiarthritics; Antipyretics; Arthritis; Central Nervous System Agents; NSAIDS; Nonsteroidal Anti-Inflammatory; Osteoarthritis; Pain; Sales > $500 Million; FDA Approved 1982 Apr; Patent Expiration 1992 Apr

BRAND NAMES: *Abdicam*; *Antiflog*; *Apo-Piroxicam* (Canada); *Arpyrox*; *Atidem*; *Baxo* (Japan); *Benoxicam*; *Brexic*; *Brexin*; *Butacinon*; *Candyl-D*; *Dacam*; *Desinflam*; *Dixonal* (Mexico); *Doblexan*; *Dolonex*; *Facicam* (Mexico); *Felcam*; *Felden* (Germany); **Feldene**; *Feldine*; *Feline*; *Felxicam*; *Felrox*; *Feroden*; *Flogosan* (Mexico); *Focus*; *Hotemin*; *Indene*; *Infeld*; *Inflamene*; *Inflavan*; *Konshien*; Lampoflex; *Larapam* (England); *Medoptil*; *Mepirox*; *Movon-20*; *Novopirocam* (Canada); *Nu-Pirox* (Canada); *Osteral* (Mexico); *Paldon*; *Pericam*; *Piraldene*; *Piram*; *Piram-D*; *Pirax*; *Piricam*; *Pirkam*; *Pirocam*; *Pirocaps*; *Pirom*; *Pirox*; *Piroxan* (Mexico); *Piroxedol*; *Piroxicam*; *Piroxim*; *Posidene*; *Pyrocaps*; *Pyroxy*; *Rexicam*; *Rocam*; *Rogal* (Mexico); *Rosic*; *Rosiden*; *Roxicam*; *Ruvamed*; *Scandene*; *Sinalgico*; *Sotilen*; *Stopen*; *Toldin*; *Unicam*; *Xicam*; *Xycam*; *Yucam*; *Zitumex*; *Zunden*
(International brand names outside U.S. in italics)

FORMULARIES: Aetna; BC-BS; Medi-Cal

COST OF THERAPY: $51.20 (Arthritis; Capsule; 20 mg; 1/day; 365 days)

PRIMARY ICD9: 715.99 (Osteoarthritis, Unspecified, Without Mention of Status Asthmaticus)

DESCRIPTION:

Piroxicam is 4-Hydroxy-2-methyl-*N*-2-pyridinyl-2*H*-1,2-benzothiazine-3-c arboxamide 1,1-dioxide, an oxicam. Members of the oxicam family are not carboxylic acids, but they are acidic by virtue of the enolic 4-hydroxy substituent. Piroxicam occurs as a white crystalline solid, sparingly soluble in water, dilute acid and most organic solvents. It is slightly soluble in alcohols and in aqueous alkaline solution. It exhibits a weakly acidic 4-hydroxy proton (pKa 5.1) and a weakly basic pyridyl nitrogen (pKa 1.8).

Molecular Formula: $C_{15}H_{13}N_3O_4S$ *Molecular Weight:* 331.35

Inert Ingredients in the Formulations Are: hard gelatin capsules (which may contain Blue 1, Red 3, and other inert ingredients); lactose; magnesium stearate; sodium lauryl sulfate; starch.

CLINICAL PHARMACOLOGY:

Piroxicam has shown anti-inflammatory, analgesic and antipyretic properties in animals. Edema, erythema, tissue proliferation, fever, and pain can all be inhibited in laboratory animals by the administration of Piroxicam. It is effective regardless of the etiology of the inflammation. The mode of action of Piroxicam is not fully established at this time. However, a common mechanism for the above effects may exist in the ability of Piroxicam to inhibit the biosynthesis of prostaglandins, known mediators of inflammation.

It is established that Piroxicam does not act by stimulating the pituitary-adrenal axis.

Piroxicam is well absorbed following oral administration. Drug plasma concentrations are proportional for 10 and 20 mg doses, generally peak within three to five hours after medication, and subsequently decline with a mean half-life of 50 hours (range of 30 to 86 hours, although values outside of this range have been encountered).

This prolonged half-life results in the maintenance of relatively stable plasma concentrations throughout the day on once daily doses and to significant drug accumulation upon multiple dosing. A single 20 mg dose generally produces peak piroxicam plasma levels of 1.5 to 2 mcg/ml, while maximum drug plasma concentrations, after repeated daily ingestion of 20 mg Piroxicam, usually stabilize at 3-8 mcg/ml. Most patients approximate steady state plasma levels within 7 to 12 days. Higher levels, which approximate steady state at two to three weeks, have been observed in patients in whom longer plasma half-lives of piroxicam occurred.

Piroxicam and its biotransformation products are excreted in urine and feces, with about twice as much appearing in the urine as the feces. Metabolism occurs by hydroxylation at the 5 position of the pyridyl side chain and conjugation of this product; by cyclodehydration; and by a sequence of reactions involving hydrolysis of the amide linkage, decarboxylation, ring contraction, and N-demethylation. Less than 5% of the daily dose is excreted unchanged.

Concurrent administration of aspirin (3900 mg/day) and Piroxicam (20 mg/day), resulted in a reduction of plasma levels of piroxicam to about 80% of their normal values. The use of Piroxicam in conjunction with aspirin is not recommended because data are inadequate to demonstrate that the combination produces greater improvement than that achieved with aspirin alone and the potential for adverse reactions is increased. Concomitant administration of antacids had no effect on Piroxicam plasma levels. The effects of impaired renal function or hepatic disease on plasma levels have not been established.

Piroxicam, like salicylates and other nonsteroidal anti-inflammatory agents, is associated with symptoms of gastrointestinal tract irritation (see ADVERSE REACTIONS.) However, in a study utilizing ^{51}Cr-tagged red blood cells, 20 mg of Piroxicam administered as a single dose for four days did not result in a significant increase in fecal blood loss and did not detectably

CLINICAL PHARMACOLOGY: *(cont'd)*

affect the gastric mucosa. In the same study a total daily dose of 3900 mg of aspirin, i.e., 972 mg q.i.d., caused a significant increase in fecal blood loss and mucosal lesions as demonstrated by gastroscopy.

In controlled clinical trials, the effectiveness of Piroxicam has been established for both acute exacerbations and long-term management of rheumatoid arthritis and osteoarthritis.

The therapeutic effects of Piroxicam are evident early in the treatment of both diseases with a progressive increase in response over several (8-12) weeks. Efficacy is seen in terms of pain relief and, when present, subsidence of inflammation.

Doses of 20 mg/day Piroxicam display a therapeutic effect comparable to therapeutic doses of aspirin, with a lower incidence of minor gastrointestinal effects and tinnitus.

Piroxicam has been administered concomitantly with fixed doses of gold and corticosteroids. The existence of a "steroid-sparing" effect has not been adequately studied to date.

INDICATIONS AND USAGE:

Piroxicam is indicated for acute or long-term use in the relief of signs and symptoms of the following:

1. Osteoarthritis
2. Rheumatoid arthritis

Dosage recommendations for use in children have not been established.

CONTRAINDICATIONS:

Piroxicam should not be used in patients who have previously exhibited hypersensitivity to it, or in individuals with the syndrome comprised of bronchospasm, nasal polyps, and angioedema precipitated by aspirin or other nonsteroidal anti-inflammatory drugs.

WARNINGS:

RISK OF GI ULCERATION, BLEEDING AND PERFORATION WITH NSAID THERAPY

Serious gastrointestinal toxicity such as bleeding, ulceration, and perforation can occur at any time, with or without warning symptoms, in patients treated chronically with NSAID therapy. Although minor upper gastrointestinal problems, such as dyspepsia, are common, usually developing early in therapy, physicians should remain alert for ulceration and bleeding in patients treated chronically with NSAIDs even in the absence of previous GI tract symptoms. In patients observed in clinical trials of several months to two years duration, symptomatic upper GI ulcers, gross bleeding or perforation appear to occur in approximately 1% of patients treated for 3-6 months, and in about 2-4% of patients treated for one year. Physicians should inform patients about the signs and/or symptoms of serious GI toxicity and what steps to take if they occur.

Studies to date have not identified any subset of patients not at risk of developing peptic ulceration and bleeding. Except for a prior history of serious GI events and other risk factors known to be associated with peptic ulcer disease, such as alcoholism, smoking, etc., no risk factors (*e.g.,* age, sex) have been associated with increased risk. Elderly or debilitated patients seem to tolerate ulceration or bleeding less well than other individuals and most spontaneous reports of fatal GI events are in this population. Studies to date are inconclusive concerning the relative risk of various NSAIDs in causing such reactions. High doses of any NSAID probably carry a greater risk of these reactions, although controlled clinical trials showing this do not exist in most cases. In considering the use of relatively large doses (within the recommended dosage range), sufficient benefit should be anticipated to offset the potential increased risk of GI toxicity.

PRECAUTIONS:

RENAL EFFECTS

As with other nonsteroidal anti-inflammatory drugs, long-term administration of piroxicam to animals has resulted in renal papillary necrosis and other abnormal renal pathology. In humans, there have been reports of acute interstitial nephritis with hematuria, proteinuria, and occasionally, nephrotic syndrome.

A second form of renal toxicity has been seen in patients with prerenal conditions leading to a reduction in renal blood flow or blood volume, where the renal prostaglandins have a supportive role in the maintenance of renal perfusion. In these patients administration of an NSAID may cause a dose-dependent reduction in prostaglandin formation and may precipitate overt renal decompensation. Patients at greatest risk of this reaction are those with impaired renal function, heart failure, liver dysfunction, those taking diuretics, and the elderly. Discontinuation of NSAID therapy is typically followed by recovery to the pretreatment state.

Because of extensive renal excretion of piroxicam and its biotransformation products (less than 5% of the daily dose excreted unchanged, see CLINICAL PHARMACOLOGY, lower doses of piroxicam should be anticipated in patients with impaired renal function, and they should be carefully monitored.

Although other nonsteroidal anti-inflammatory drugs do not have the same direct effects on platelets that aspirin does, all drugs inhibiting prostaglandin biosynthesis do interfere with platelet function to some degree; therefore, patients who may be adversely affected by such an action should be carefully observed when Piroxicam is administered.

Because of reports of adverse eye findings with nonsteroidal anti-inflammatory agents, it is recommended that patients who develop visual complaints during treatment with Piroxicam have ophthalmic evaluation.

As with other nonsteroidal anti-inflammatory drugs, borderline elevations of one or more liver tests may occur in up to 15% of patients. These abnormalities may progress, may remain essentially unchanged, or may be transient with continued therapy. The SGPT (ALT) test is probably the most sensitive indicator of liver dysfunction. Meaningful (3 times the upper limit of normal) elevations of SGPT or SGOT (AST) occurred in controlled clinical trials in less than 1% of patients. A patient with symptoms and/or signs suggesting liver dysfunction, or in whom an abnormal liver test has occurred, should be evaluated for evidence of the development of more severe hepatic reaction while on therapy with Piroxicam. Severe hepatic reactions, including jaundice and cases of fatal hepatitis, have been reported with Piroxicam. Although such reactions are rare, if abnormal liver tests persist or worsen, if clinical signs and symptoms consistent with liver disease develop, or if systemic manifestations occur (*e.g.,* eosinophilia, rash, etc.), Piroxicam should be discontinued. (See also ADVERSE REACTIONS.)

Although at the recommended dose of 20 mg/day of Piroxicam increased fecal blood loss due to gastrointestinal irritation did not occur (see CLINICAL PHARMACOLOGY), in about 4% of the patients treated with Piroxicam alone or concomitantly with aspirin, reductions in hemoglobin and hematocrit values were observed. Therefore, these values should be determined if signs or symptoms of anemia occur.

Peripheral edema has been observed in approximately 2% of the patients treated with Piroxicam. Therefore, as with other nonsteroidal anti-inflammatory drugs, Piroxicam should be used with caution in patients with heart failure, hypertension or other conditions predisposing to fluid retention, since its usage may be associated with a worsening of these conditions.

PRECAUTIONS: *(cont'd)*

A combination of dermatological and/or allergic signs and symptoms suggestive of serum sickness have occasionally occurred in conjunction with the use of Piroxicam. These include arthralgias, pruritus, fever, fatigue, and rash including vesiculo bullous reactions and exfoliative dermatitis.

INFORMATION FOR THE PATIENT

Piroxicam, like other drugs of its class, is not free of side effects. The side effects of these drugs can cause discomfort and, rarely, there are more serious side effects, such as gastrointestinal bleeding, which may result in hospitalization and even fatal outcomes.

NSAIDs (Nonsteroidal Anti-Inflammatory Drugs) are often essential agents in the management of arthritis, but they also may be commonly employed for conditions which are less serious.

Physicians may wish to discuss with their patients the potential risks (see WARNINGS, PRECAUTIONS, and ADVERSE REACTIONS) and likely benefits of NSAID treatment, particularly when the drugs are used for less serious conditions where treatment without NSAIDs may represent an acceptable alternative to both the patient and physician.

LABORATORY TESTS

Because serious GI tract ulceration and bleeding can occur without warning symptoms, physicians should follow chronically treated patients for the signs and symptoms of ulceration and bleeding and should inform them of the importance of this follow-up (see Risk of GI Ulceration, Bleeding and Perforation with NSAID Therapy.)

CARCINOGENESIS, MUTAGENESIS, AND IMPAIRMENT OF FERTILITY

Subacute and chronic toxicity studies have been carried out in rats, mice, dogs, and monkeys.

The pathology most often seen was that characteristically associated with the animal toxicology of anti-inflammatory agents: renal papillary necrosis (see PRECAUTIONS) and gastrointestinal lesions.

In classical studies in laboratory animals piroxicam did not show any teratogenic potential.

Reproductive studies revealed no impairment of fertility in animals.

PREGNANCY:

Like other drugs which inhibit the synthesis and release of prostaglandins, piroxicam increased the incidence of dystocia and delayed parturition in pregnant animals when piroxicam administration was continued late into pregnancy. Gastrointestinal tract toxicity was increased in pregnant females in the last trimester of pregnancy compared to nonpregnant females or females in earlier trimesters of pregnancy.

Nursing Mothers: Piroxicam is not recommended for use in nursing mothers or in pregnant women because of the animal findings and since safety for such use has not been established in humans.

PEDIATRIC USE

Dosage recommendations and indications for use in children have not been established.

DRUG INTERACTIONS:

Piroxicam is highly protein bound, and, therefore, might be expected to displace other protein-bound drugs. Although this has not occurred in *in vitro* studies with coumarin-type anticoagulants, interactions with coumarin-type anticoagulants have been reported with Piroxicam since marketing, therefore, physicians should closely monitor patients for a change in dosage requirements when administering Piroxicam to patients on coumarin-type anticoagulants and other highly protein-bound drugs.

Plasma levels of piroxicam are depressed to approximately 80% of their normal values when Piroxicam is administered in conjunction with aspirin (3900 mg/day), but concomitant administration of antacids has no effect on piroxicam plasma levels (see CLINICAL PHARMACOLOGY).

Nonsteroidal anti-inflammatory agents, including Piroxicam, have been reported to increase steady state plasma lithium levels. It is recommended that plasma lithium levels be monitored when initiating, adjusting and discontinuing Piroxicam.

ADVERSE REACTIONS:

The incidence of adverse reactions to piroxicam is based on clinical trials involving approximately 2300 patients, about 400 of whom were treated for more than one year and 170 for more than two years. About 30% of all patients receiving daily doses of 20 mg of Piroxicam experienced side effects. Gastrointestinal symptoms were the most prominent side effects - occurring in approximately 20% of the patients, which in most instances did not interfere with the course of therapy. Of the patients experiencing gastrointestinal side effects, approximately 5% discontinued therapy with an overall incidence of peptic ulceration of about 1%.

Other than the gastrointestinal symptoms, edema, dizziness, headache, changes in hematological parameters, and rash have been reported in a small percentage of patients. Routine ophthalmoscopy and slit-lamp examinations have revealed no evidence of ocular changes in 205 patients followed from 3 to 24 months while on therapy.

INCIDENCE GREATER THAN 1%

The following adverse reactions occurred more frequently than 1 in 100.

Gastrointestinal: Stomatitis, anorexia, epigastric distress*, nausea*, constipation, abdominal discomfort, flatulence, diarrhea, abdominal pain, indigestion

Hematological: Decreases in hemoglobin* and hematocrit* (see PRECAUTIONS), anemia, leucopenia, eosinophilia

Dermatologic: Pruritus, rash

Central Nervous System: Dizziness, somnolence, vertigo

Urogenital: BUN and creatinine elevations (see PRECAUTIONS)

Body as a Whole: Headache, malaise

Special Senses: Tinnitus

Cardiovascular/Respiratory: Edema (see PRECAUTIONS)

*Reactions occurring in 3% to 9% of patients treated with Piroxicam. Reactions occurring in 1-3% of patients are unmarked.

INCIDENCE LESS THAN 1% (CAUSAL RELATIONSHIP PROBABLE)

The following adverse reactions occurred less frequently than 1 in 100. The probability exists that there is a causal relationship between Piroxicam and these reactions.

Gastrointestinal: Liver function abnormalities, jaundice, hepatitis (see PRECAUTIONS), vomiting, hematemesis, melena, gastrointestinal bleeding, perforation and ulceration (see WARNINGS), dry mouth

Hematological: Thrombocytopenia, petechial rash, ecchymosis, bone marrow depression including aplastic anemia, epistaxis

Dermatologic: Sweating, erythema, bruising, desquamation, exfoliative dermatitis, erythema multiforme, toxic epidermal necrolysis, Stevens-Johnson syndrome, vesiculobullous reaction, photoallergic skin reactions

Central Nervous System: Depression, insomnia, nervousness

Urogenital: Hematuria, proteinuria, interstitial nephritis, renal failure, hyperkalemia, glomerulitis, papillary necrosis, nephrotic syndrome (see PRECAUTIONS)

ADVERSE REACTIONS: *(cont'd)*

Body as a Whole: Pain (colic), fever, flu-like syndrome (see PRECAUTIONS)

Special Senses: Swollen eyes, blurred vision, eye irritations

Cardiovascular/Respiratory: Hypertension, worsening of congestive heart failure (see PRECAUTIONS), exacerbation of angina

Metabolic: Hypoglycemia, hyperglycemia, weight increase, weight decrease

Hypersensitivity: Anaphylaxis, bronchospasm, urticaria/angioedema, vasculitis, "serum sickness" (see PRECAUTIONS)

INCIDENCE LESS THAN 1% (CAUSAL RELATIONSHIP UNKNOWN)

Other adverse reactions were reported with a frequency of less than 1 in 100, but a causal relationship between Piroxicam and the reaction could not be determined.

Gastrointestinal: Pancreatitis

Dermatologic: Onycholysis, loss of hair

Central Nervous System: Akathisia, hallucinations, mood alterations, dream abnormalities, mental confusion, paresthesias

Urogenital System: Dysuria

Body as a Whole: Weakness

Cardiovascular/Respiratory: Palpitations, dyspnea

Hypersensitivity: Positive ANA

Special Senses: Transient hearing loss

Hematological: Hemolytic anemia

OVERDOSAGE:

In the event treatment for overdosage is required the long plasma half-life (see CLINICAL PHARMACOLOGY) of piroxicam should be considered. The absence of experience with acute overdosage precludes characterization of sequelae and recommendation of specific antidotal efficacy at this time. It is reasonable to assume, however, that the standard measures of gastric evacuation and general supportive therapy would apply. In addition to supportive measures, the use of activated charcoal may effectively reduce the absorption and reabsorption of piroxicam. Experiments in dogs have demonstrated that the use of multiple-dose treatments with activated charcoal could reduce the half-life of piroxicam elimination from 27 hours (without charcoal) to 11 hours and reduce the systemic bioavailability of piroxicam by as much as 37% when activated charcoal is given as late as 6 hours after administration of piroxicam.

DOSAGE AND ADMINISTRATION:

RHEUMATOID ARTHRITIS, OSTEOARTHRITIS

It is recommended that Piroxicam therapy be initiated and maintained at a single daily dose of 20 mg. If desired the daily dose may be divided. Because of the long half-life of Piroxicam, steady-state blood levels are not reached for 7-12 days. Therefore although the therapeutic effects of Piroxicam are evident early in treatment, there is a progressive increase in response over several weeks and the effect of therapy should not be assessed for two weeks.

Dosage recommendations and indications for use in children have not been established.

HOW SUPPLIED - RATED THERAPEUTICALLY EQUIVALENT:

Capsule, Gelatin - Oral - 10 mg

100's	$11.25	Piroxicam, H.C.F.A. F F P	99999-2047-01
100's	$11.63	Piroxicam, United Res	00677-1430-01
100's	$80.00	Piroxicam, Roxane	00054-2660-25
100's	$113.50	Piroxicam, Harber Pharm	51432-0666-03
100's	$118.77	Piroxicam, Qualitest Pharms	00603-5222-21
100's	$118.77	Piroxicam, Rosemont	00832-0109-00
100's	$119.00	Piroxicam, Mutual Pharm	53489-0441-01
100's	$119.36	Piroxicam, SCS Pharm	00905-5752-31
100's	$119.36	Piroxicam, West Point Pharma	59591-0617-68
100's	$120.15	Piroxicam, HL Moore Drug Exch	00839-7734-06
100's	$120.28	Piroxicam, Schein Pharm (US)	00364-2545-01
100's	$120.94	Piroxicam, Royce	51875-0335-01
100's	$120.94	Piroxicam, Royce	51875-0355-01
100's	$121.50	Piroxicam, Rexall Rexall	60814-0701-01
100's	$123.28	Piroxicam, Rugby	00536-5558-01
100's	$124.00	Piroxicam, Sidmak Labs	50111-0853-01
100's	$125.75	Piroxicam, Goldline Labs	00182-1933-01
100's	$125.75	Piroxicam, Aligen Independ	00405-4807-01
100's	$125.75	Piroxicam, Par Pharm	49884-0440-01
100's	$126.30	Piroxicam, Martec Pharms	52555-0972-01
100's	$127.00	Piroxicam, Major Pharms	00904-7697-60
100's	$127.00	Piroxicam, Major Pharms	00904-7845-60
100's	$127.00	Piroxicam, Novopharm (US)	55953-0617-40
100's	$128.60	Piroxicam, Teva	00093-0756-01
100's	$130.93	Piroxicam, Lederle Pharm	00005-3327-43
100's	**$131.02**	**FELDENE, Pfizer Pharm**	**00663-3220-66**
100's	$132.03	Piroxicam, HL Moore Drug Exch	00839-7773-06
100's	$140.02	Piroxicam, Mylan	00378-1010-01
100's	**$150.33**	**FELDENE, Pfizer Labs**	**00069-3220-66**
500's	$56.25	Piroxicam, H.C.F.A. F F P	99999-2047-02
500's	$569.69	Piroxicam, HL Moore Drug Exch	00839-7734-12
500's	$580.92	Piroxicam, Rosemont	00832-0109-50

Capsule, Gelatin - Oral - 20 mg

100's	$14.03	Piroxicam, United Res	00677-1431-01
100's	$14.03	Piroxicam, H.C.F.A. F F P	99999-2047-03
100's	$78.17	Piroxicam, Vangard Labs	00615-0389-13
100's	$130.00	Piroxicam, Roxane	00054-2661-25
100's	$194.50	Piroxicam, Harber Pharm	51432-0699-03
100's	$203.90	Piroxicam, Mova Pharms	55370-0170-07
100's	$203.92	Piroxicam, Qualitest Pharms	00603-5223-21
100's	$204.00	Piroxicam, Mutual Pharm	53489-0442-01
100's	$204.21	Piroxicam, West Point Pharma	59591-0640-68
100's	$204.24	Piroxicam, SCS Pharm	00905-5762-31
100's	$205.05	Piroxicam, HL Moore Drug Exch	00839-7774-06
100's	$205.82	Piroxicam, Schein Pharm (US)	00364-2546-01
100's	$207.00	Piroxicam, Dupont Pharma	00056-0260-70
100's	$207.87	Piroxicam, Royce	51875-0336-01
100's	$207.87	Piroxicam, Royce	51875-0356-01
100's	$208.75	Piroxicam, Rexall Rexall	60814-0700-01
100's	$210.00	Piroxicam, Rosemont	00832-0110-00
100's	$210.00	Piroxicam, Sidmak Labs	50111-0854-01
100's	$210.25	Piroxicam, Rugby	00536-5559-01
100's	$215.19	Piroxicam, Goldline Labs	00182-1934-01
100's	$215.19	Piroxicam, Aligen Independ	00405-4808-01
100's	$215.19	Piroxicam, Par Pharm	49884-0441-01
100's	$217.50	Piroxicam, Major Pharms	00904-5063-60
100's	$217.50	Piroxicam, Major Pharms	00904-7698-60
100's	$217.50	Piroxicam, Major Pharms	00904-7812-60

HOW SUPPLIED - RATED THERAPEUTICALLY EQUIVALENT:

(cont'd)

100's	$217.50	Piroxicam, Novopharm (US)	55953-0640-40
100's	$219.83	Piroxicam, Martec Pharms	52555-0973-01
100's	**$224.20**	**FELDENE, Pfizer Pharm**	**00663-3230-66**
100's	$224.23	Piroxicam, Lederle Pharm	00005-3328-43
100's	**$232.92**	**FELDENE, Pfizer Pharm**	**00663-3230-41**
100's	$239.60	Piroxicam, Mylan	00378-2020-01
100's	$241.30	Piroxicam, Teva	00093-0757-01
100's	$241.37	Piroxicam, HL Moore Drug Exch	00839-7735-06
100's	**$257.24**	**FELDENE, Pfizer Labs**	**00069-3230-66**
100's	**$267.25**	**FELDENE, Pfizer Labs**	**00069-3230-41**
500's	$70.15	Piroxicam, United Res	00677-1431-05
500's	$70.15	Piroxicam, H.C.F.A. F F P	99999-2047-04
500's	$670.00	Piroxicam, Roxane	00054-2661-29
500's	$800.00	Piroxicam, Rugby	00536-5559-05
500's	$969.21	Piroxicam, Aligen Independ	00405-4808-02
500's	$997.50	Piroxicam, Rosemont	00832-0110-50
500's	$999.20	Piroxicam, Mova Pharms	55370-0170-08
500's	$999.21	Piroxicam, Qualitest Pharms	00603-5223-28
500's	$999.50	Piroxicam, Mutual Pharm	53489-0442-05
500's	$999.60	Piroxicam, Dupont Pharma	00056-0260-85
500's	$999.91	Piroxicam, SCS Pharm	00905-5762-51
500's	$999.99	Piroxicam, Royce	51875-0336-02
500's	$999.99	Piroxicam, Royce	51875-0356-02
500's	$1022.65	Piroxicam, Major Pharms	00904-5063-40
500's	$1022.65	Piroxicam, Major Pharms	00904-7698-40
500's	$1022.65	Piroxicam, Major Pharms	00904-7812-40
500's	$1025.15	Piroxicam, Rexall Rexall	60814-0700-50
500's	$1026.52	Piroxicam, Schein Pharm (US)	00364-2546-05
500's	$1030.00	Piroxicam, Sidmak Labs	50111-0854-02
500's	$1033.10	Piroxicam, Novopharm (US)	55953-0640-70
500's	$1053.47	Piroxicam, Goldline Labs	00182-1934-05
500's	$1053.47	Piroxicam, Par Pharm	49884-0441-05
500's	$1054.10	Piroxicam, Teva	00093-0757-05
500's	$1054.28	Piroxicam, Lederle Pharm	00005-3328-31
500's	$1068.20	Piroxicam, Martec Pharms	52555-0973-05
500's	$1076.42	Piroxicam, HL Moore Drug Exch	00839-7735-12
500's	**$1097.59**	**FELDENE, Pfizer Pharm**	**00663-3230-73**
500's	$1172.99	Piroxicam, Mylan	00378-2020-05
500's	**$1259.32**	**FELDENE, Pfizer Labs**	**00069-3230-73**
750's	$1523.97	Piroxicam, Glasgow Pharm	60809-0302-55
750's	$1523.97	Piroxicam, Glasgow Pharm	60809-0302-72
1000's	$140.30	Piroxicam, H.C.F.A. F F P	99999-2047-05
1000's	$1962.95	Piroxicam, Novopharm (US)	55953-0640-80
1000's	$2009.49	Piroxicam, HL Moore Drug Exch	00839-7774-16
1000's	$2100.00	Piroxicam, Par Pharm	49884-0441-10

PLAGUE VACCINE *(002050)*

CATEGORIES: Immunologic; Serums, Toxoids and Vaccines; Vaccines; Pregnancy Category C; FDA Pre 1938 Drugs

BRAND NAMES: Bubonic Plague Vaccine; *Plague Vaccine*
(International brand names outside U.S. in italics)

Prescribing information not available at time of publication.

HOW SUPPLIED - EQUIVALENTS NOT AVAILABLE:

Injection, Solution - Intramuscular

20 ml	$31.20	Plague Vaccine, Miles	00161-0060-17

PLICAMYCIN *(002053)*

CATEGORIES: Antimetabolites; Antineoplastics; Calcium Metabolism; Homeostatic & Nutrient; Hypercalcemia; Hypercalciuria; Oncologic Drugs; Testicular Carcinoma; Tumors; Pregnancy Category X; FDA Approval Pre 1982

BRAND NAMES: **Mithracin**; *Mithraline* (France); Mithramycin
(International brand names outside U.S. in italics)

FORMULARIES: BC-BS; Medi-Cal

WARNING:
FOR INTRAVENOUS USE
WARNING - IT IS RECOMMENDED THAT PLICAMYCIN BE ADMINISTERED ONLY TO HOSPITALIZED PATIENTS BY OR UNDER THE SUPERVISION OF A QUALIFIED PHYSICIAN WHO IS EXPERIENCED IN THE USE OF CANCER CHEMOTHERAPEUTIC AGENTS, BECAUSE OF THE POSSIBILITY OF SEVERE REACTIONS. FACILITIES FOR THE DETERMINATION OF NECESSARY LABORATORY STUDIES MUST BE MADE AVAILABLE.
SEVERE THROMBOCYTOPENIA, A HEMORRHAGIC TENDENCY AND EVEN DEATH MAY RESULT FROM THE USE OF MITHRACIN. ALTHOUGH SEVERE TOXICITY IS MORE APT TO OCCUR IN PATIENTS WHO HAVE FAR-ADVANCED DISEASE OR ARE OTHERWISE CONSIDERED POOR RISKS FOR THERAPY, SERIOUS TOXICITY MAY ALSO OCCASIONALLY OCCUR EVEN IN PATIENTS WHO ARE IN RELATIVELY GOOD CONDITION.
IN THE TREATMENT OF EACH PATIENT, THE PHYSICIAN MUST WEIGH CAREFULLY THE POSSIBILITY OF ACHIEVING THERAPEUTIC BENEFIT VERSUS THE RISK OF TOXICITY WHICH MAY OCCUR WITH MITHRACIN THERAPY. THE FOLLOWING DATA CONCERNING THE USE OF MITHRACIN IN THE TREATMENT OF TESTICULAR TUMORS, HYPERCALCEMIC AND/OR HYPERCALCIURIC CONDITIONS ASSOCIATED WITH VARIOUS ADVANCED MALIGNANCIES SHOULD BE THOROUGHLY REVIEWED BEFORE ADMINISTERING THIS COMPOUND.

DESCRIPTION:

Plicamycin is a yellow crystalline compound which is produced by a microorganism, *Streptomyces plicatus.* Plicamycin is available as a freeze-dried, sterile preparation for IV administration. Each vial contains 2500 mcg of Plicamycin with 100 mg of mannitol and disodium phosphate to adjust pH 7. After reconstitution with sterile water for injection, the solution has a pH of 7. The drug is unstable in acid solutions with a pH below 4.

Plicamycin is an antineoplastic agent. It has an empirical formula of $C_{52}H_{76}O_{24}$.

CLINICAL PHARMACOLOGY:

Although the exact mechanism by which plicamycin is not yet known, studies have indicated that this compound forms a complex deoxyribonucleic acid (DNA) and inhibits cellular ribonucleic acid (RNA) and enzymatic RNA synthesis. The binding of Plicamycin to DNA in the presence of Mg^{++} (or other divalent cations) is responsible for the inhibition of DNA-dependent or DNA-directed RNA synthesis. This action presumably accounts for the biological properties of Plicamycin.

Plicamycin shows potent cytotoxicity against malignant cells of human origin (Hela cells) growing in tissue culture. Plicamycin is lethal to Hela cells in 48 hours at concentrations as low as 0.5 mcg per ml of tissue culture medium. Plicamycin has shown significantly anti-tumor activity against experimental leukemia in mice when administered intraperitoneally.

Plicamycin may lower serum calcium levels: the exact mechanism (or mechanisms) by which the drug exerts this effect is unknown. It appears that plicamycin may block the hypercalcemic action of pharmacologic doses of vitamin D. It has also been suggested that plicamycin may lower calcium serum levels by inhibiting the effect of parathyroid hormone upon osteoclasts. Plicamycin's inhibition of DNA-dependent RNA synthesis appears to render osteoclasts unable to fully respond to parathyroid hormone with the biosynthesis necessary for osteolysis. Decreases in serum phosphate levels and urinary calcium excretion accompany the lower serum calcium concentrations.

Radioautography studies[1] with ^{3}H-labeled plicamycin in C3H mice show that the greatest concentrations of the isotope are in the Kupffer cells of the liver and cells of the renal tubules. Plicamycin is rapidly cleared from the blood within the first 2 hours and excretion is also rapid. Sixty-seven percent of measured excretion occurs within 4 hours, 75% within 8 hours and 90% is recovered in the first 24 hours after injection. There is no evidence of protein binding, nor is there any evidence of metabolism of the carbohydrate moiety of the drug to carbon dioxide and water with loss through respiration. Plicamycin crosses the blood-brain barrier; the concentration found in brain tissue is low but it persists longer than other tissues. The experimental results in animals correlate closely with results achieved in man.[2]

CLINICAL STUDIES:

TREATMENT OF PATIENTS WITH INOPERABLE TESTICULAR TUMORS

In a combined series of 305 patients with inoperable testicular tumors treated with Mithracin (plicamycin), 33 patients (10.8%) showed a complete disappearance of tumor masses and an additional 80 patients (26.2%) responded with significant partial regression of tumor masses. The longest duration of a continuing-complete response is now over 8 1/2 years. The therapeutic responses in this series of patients have been summarized by type of testicular tumor in the following table (TABLE 1):

TABLE 1 Results In 305 Testicular Tumor Cases By Tumor Type

TYPE OF TUMOR	TOTAL	COMPLETE RESPONSE	PARTIAL RESPONSE	NO RESPONSE
EMBRYONAL CELL	173	26	42	105
TERATOMA	5	0	1	4
TERATOCARCINOMA	23	0	5	18
SEMINOMA	18	0	7	11
CHORIOCARCINOMA	13	1	6	6
MIXED TUMORS	73	6	19	48
TOTALS	305	33	80	192

Mithracin may be useful in the treatment of patients with testicular tumors which are resistant to other chemotherapeutic agents. Prior radiation therapy or prior chemotherapy did not alter the responsive rate with Mithracin. This suggests that there is no significant cross resistant between Mithracin and other chemotherapeutic agents.

TREATMENT OF PATIENTS WITH HYPERCALCEMIA AND HYPERCALCIURIA

A limited number of patients with hypercalcemia (range: 12.0 - 25.8 mg%) and patients with hypercalciuria (range 215-492 mg/day) associated with malignant disease were treated with Mithracin. Hypercalcemia and hypercalciuria were promptly reversed in all patients. In some patients, the primary malignancy was of non-testicular origin.

INDICATIONS AND USAGE:

Plicamycin is a potent antineoplastic agent which has been shown to be useful in the treatment of carefully selected hospitalized patients with malignant tumors of the testis in whom successful treatment by surgery and/or radiation is impossible. Also, on the basis of limited clinical experience to date, it may be considered in the treatment of certain symptomatic patients with hypercalcemia and hypercalciuria with a variety of advanced neoplasms.

The use of Plicamycin in other types of neoplastic disease is not recommended at the present time.

CONTRAINDICATIONS:

Plicamycin is contraindicated in patients with thrombocytopenia, thrombocytopathy, coagulation disorder or an increased susceptibility to bleeding due to other causes. Plicamycin should not be administered to any patient with impairment of blood marrow function.

Plicamycin may cause fetal harm when administered to pregnant women. Plicamycin is contraindicated in women who are or may become pregnant. If this drug is used during pregnancy, or if the patient becomes pregnant while taking the drug, the patient should be apprised of the potential hazard to the fetus.

WARNINGS:

See BOXED WARNING at beginning of monograph.

PRECAUTIONS:

General: Plicamycin should be administered only to patients who are hospitalized and who can be observed carefully and frequently during and after therapy.

Severe thrombocytopenia, a hemorrhagic tendency and even death may result from the use of this drug. Although severe toxicity is more apt to occur in patients who have far-advanced disease or are otherwise considered poor risk for therapy, serious toxicity may also occasionally occur even in patients who are in relatively good condition.

PRECAUTIONS: *(cont'd)*

Electrolyte imbalance, especially hypocalcemia, hypokalemia, and hypophosphatasemia, should be corrected with appropriate electrolyte therapy prior to treatment with Plicamycin.

Plicamycin should be used with extreme caution in patients with significant impairment of renal or hepatic function.

Plicamycin should not be administered to patients who are pregnant or to mothers who are breast feeding.

In the treatment of each patient, the physician must weigh carefully the possibility of achieving therapeutic benefit versus the risk of toxicity which may occur with Plicamycin therapy.

Laboratory Tests: The following laboratory studies should be obtained frequently during therapy and for several days following the last dose; platelet count, prothrombin time, bleeding time. The occurrence of thrombocytopenia or a significant prolongation of prothrombin time or bleeding time is an indication for the termination of therapy.

Carcinogenesis, Mutagenesis, and Impairment of Fertility: No long- term studies in animals have been performed to evaluate the carcinogenic potential of Plicamycin. Histologic evidence of inhibition of spermatogenesis was observed in a substantial number of male rats receiving doses of 0.6 mg/kg/day and above.

Pregnancy Category X: See CONTRAINDICATIONS.

Nursing Mothers: It is not known whether this drug is excreted in human milk. Because many drugs are excreted in human milk and because of the potential for serious adverse reactions in nursing infants from Plicamycin, a decision should be made whether to discontinue the drug, taking into account the importance of the drug to the mother.

ADVERSE REACTIONS:

THE MOST IMPORTANT FORM OF TOXICITY ASSOCIATED WITH THE USE OF MITHRACIN CONSISTS OF A BLEEDING SYNDROME WHICH USUALLY BEGINS WITH AN EPISODE OF EPISTAXIS. This bleeding tendency may only consist of a single or several episodes of epistaxis and progress no further. However, in some cases, this hemorrhagic syndrome can start with an episode of hematemesis which may progress to more widespread hemorrhage in the gastrointestinal tract or to a more generalized bleeding tendency. This hemorrhagic diathesis is most likely due to abnormalities in multiple clotting factors.

A detailed analysis of clinical data in 1,160 patients treated with Mithracin (plicamycin) indicates that the hemorrhagic syndrome is dose- related. With doses of 30 mcg/kg/day or less for 10 or fewer doses, the incidence of bleeding episodes has been 5.4% with an associated drug- related mortality rate of 1.6%. With doses greater than 30 mcg /kg/day and/or for more than 10 doses, a significantly large number of bleeding episodes, occurred (11.9%) and the associated drug-related mortality rate was also significantly higher (5.7%).

The most common side effects reported with the use of Mithracin (plicamycin) consists of gastrointestinal symptoms; anorexia, nausea, vomiting, diarrhea, and stomatitis. Other less frequently reported side effects include fever, drowsiness, weakness, lethargy, malaise, headache, depression, phlebitis, facial flushing, and skin rash.

The following laboratory abnormalities have been reported during therapy with Mithracin and in most instances were reversible following cessation of treatment:

Hematologic Abnormalities: Depression of platelet count, white count, hemoglobin and prothrombin content; elevation of clotting time, bleeding time; abnormal clot retraction.

Thrombocytopenia may be rapid in onset and may occur at anytime during therapy or within several days following the last dose. With the occupance of severe thrombocytopenia, the infusion of platelet concentrates of platelet-rich plasma may be helpful in elevating the platelet count.

The occupance of leukopenia with the use of Mithracin (plicamycin) is relatively uncommon, occurring in approximately 6% of patients.

It has been uncommon for abnormalities in clotting time or clot retraction to be demonstrated prior to the onset of an overt bleeding episode noted in some patients treated with Mithracin. Nevertheless, the performance of these tests in patients periodically is recommended because in a few instances, an abnormality in one of these studies may have served as a warning to terminate therapy because of impending serious toxicity.

Abnormal Liver Function Tests: Increased levels of serum glutamic oxaloacetic transaminase, serum glutamic pyruvic transaminase, lactic dehydrogenase, alkaline phosphatase, serum bilirubin, ornithine carbamyl transferase, isocitric dehydrogenase, and increased retention of bromsulphalein.

Increased Renal Function Tests: Increased blood urea nitrogen and serum creatinine; proteinuria.

Abnormalities in Electrolyte Concentrations: Depression of serum calcium, phosphorus, and potassium.

OVERDOSAGE:

Generally, adverse effects following the use of Mithracin (plicamycin), especially the hemorrhagic syndrome, are dose related. Therefore, following administration of an overdose, patients can be expected to experience an exaggeration of the usual adverse effects. Close monitoring of the hematologic function, including factors involved un the clotting mechanism, hepatic and renal functions, and serum electrolytes, is necessary. No specific antidote for Mithracin is known. Management of overdosage would include general supportive measures to sustain the patient through the period of toxicity.

DOSAGE AND ADMINISTRATION:

The daily dose of Mithracin (plicamycin) is based on the patient's body weight. If a patient has abnormal fluid retention such as edema, hydrothorax or ascites, if the patient's ideal weight rather than actual body weight than actual body weight should calculate the dose.

TREATMENT OF TESTICULAR TUMORS

In the treatment of patients with testicular tumors the recommended daily dose of Mithracin (plicamycin) is 25 to 30 mcg per kilogram of body weight. Therapy should be continued for a period of 8 to 10 days unless significant side effects or toxicity occur during therapy. A course of therapy consisting of more than 10 daily doses is not recommended. Individuals daily doses should not exceed 30 mcg per kilogram of body weight.

In those patients with responsive tumors, some degree of regression is usually evident within 3 or 4 weeks following the initial course of therapy. If tumors masses remain unchanged following an initial course of therapy, additional courses of therapy at monthly intervals are warranted.

When a significant tumor regression is obtained, it is suggested that additional courses of therapy be given at monthly intervals until a complete regression of tumor masses is achieved or until definite tumor progression of new tumor masses occur in spite of continued therapy.

TREATMENT OF HYPERCALCEMIA AND HYPERCALCIURIA

Reversal of hypercalcemia and hypercalciuria associated with advanced malignancy the recommended course of treatment with Mithracin (plicamycin) is 25 mcg per kilogram of body weight per day for 3 or 4 days.

DOSAGE AND ADMINISTRATION: *(cont'd)*

If the desired degree of reversal of hypercalcemia or hypercalciuria is not achieved with the initial course of therapy, additional courses of therapy may be administrated at intervals of one week or more to achieve the desired result or to maintain serum calcium and urinary calcium excretion at normal levels. It may be possible to maintain normal calcium balance with single, weekly doses or with a schedule of 2 or 3 doses per week.

NOTE: BECAUSE OF THE DRUG'S TOXICITY AND THE LIMITED CLINICAL EXPERIENCE TO DATE IN THESE INDICATIONS, THE FOLLOWING RECOMMENDATIONS SHOULD BE KEPT IN MIND BY THE PHYSICIAN.

1. CONSIDER CASES OF HYPERCALCEMIA AND HYPERCALCIURIA NOT RESPONSIVE TO CONVENTIONAL TREATMENT.

2. APPLY THE SAME CONTRAINDICATIONS AND PRECAUTIONARY MEASURES AS IN ANTITUMOR TREATMENT.

3. RENAL FUNCTION SHOULD BE CAREFULLY MONITORED BEFORE, DURING, AND AFTER TREATMENT.

4. BENEFITS OF USE DURING PREGNANCY OR IN WOMEN OF CHILDBEARING AGE SHOULD BE WEIGHED AGAINST THE POTENTIAL TOXICITY TO EMBRYO OR FETUS.

ADMINISTRATION

By IV administration only. The appropriate daily dose of Mithracin (plicamycin) should be diluted in one liter of 5% Dextrose Injection, USP or Sodium Chloride Injection, USP and administered by slow IV infusion over a period of 4 to 6 hours. Rapid direct IV injection of Mithracin should be avoided as it may be associated with a higher incidence and greater severity of gastrointestinal side effects. Extravasation of solutions of Mithracin may cause local irritation and cellulitis at injection sites. Should thrombophlebitis or perivascular cellulitis occur, the infusion should be terminated and reinstituted at another site. The application of moderate heat to the site of extravasation may help to disperse the compound and minimize discomfort and local tissue irritation. The use of antiemetic compounds prior to and during treatment with Mithracin may be helpful in relieving nausea and vomiting.

Procedures for proper handling and disposal of anti-cancer drugs should be considered. Several guidelines on this subject have been published.[3-8] There is no general agreement that all procedures recommended in the guidelines are necessary or appropriate.

ANIMAL PHARMACOLOGY:

In mice, the average intravenous LD_{50} of Mithracin (plicamycin) is 2,000 mcg/kg of body weight. When administered orally, it is not toxic to mice at doses 100 times greater than the intravenous LD_{50}. In rats the average intravenous $LD_{50}$of Mithracin is 1,700 mcg/kg of body weight. It is not toxic to rats when administered orally at doses 17 times greater than the intravenous LD_{50}. In dogs and monkeys Mithracin is essentially non-toxic when administered intravenously for 24 days at doses as high as 50 and 24 mcg/kg of body weight, respectively. However, at higher doses of 100 mcg/kg/day intravenously it is lethal to dogs and monkeys. Signs of toxicity in dogs and monkeys included anorexia, vomiting, listlessness, melena, anemia, lymphopenia, elevated alkaline phosphatase, serum glutamic oxaloacetic transaminase, serum glutamic pyruvic transaminase values, hypochloremia, and azotemia. Dogs also showed marked thrombocytopenia, hyponatremia, hypokalemia, hypocalcemia, and decreased prothrombin consumption. Necropsy findings consisted of necrosis of lymphoid tissue and multiple generalized hemorrhages. Mithracin (plicamycin) was only mildly irritating when injected intramuscularly in rabbits and subcutaneously in guinea pigs. Histologic evidence of inhibition of spermatogenesis was observed in a substantial number of male rats receiving doses of 0.6 mg/kg/day and above. This preclinical finding of selective drug effect constituted the scientific rationale for clinical trials in testicular tumors.

REFERENCES:

1. Kennedy, B.D. et al.: Cancer Res. *27*:1534, 1967. **2.** Randsohoff, J. et al: Cancer Chemother. Rep. *49*:51, 1965. **3.** Recommendations for the Safe Handling of Parenteral Antineoplastic Drugs, NIH Publication No. 83-2621. For sale by the superintendent of Documents, U.S. Gov't Printing Office, Washington, D.C. 20402. **4.** AMA Council Report. Guidelines for Handling Parenteral Antineoplastics. JAMA, March 15, 1985. **5.** National Study Commission on Cytotoxic Exposure- Recommendations for Handling Cytotoxic Agents. Available from Louis P. Jeffrey, Sc.D., Director of Pharmacy Services, Rhode Island Hospital, 593 Eddy Street, Providence, Rhode Island 02902. **6.** Clinical Oncological Society of Australia; Guidelines and recommendations for safe handling of antineoplastic agents. Med J Australia *1*: 426-428, 1983. **7.** Jones, R.B. et al. Safe handling of chemotherapeutic agents: a report from the Mount Sinai Medical center. Ca-A Cancer Journal for Clinicians, Sept/Oct, 258-263, 1983. **8.** American Society of Hospital Pharmacists technical assistance bulletin on handling cytotoxic drugs in hospitals. Am J Hosp Pharm *42*:131- 137, 1985.

HOW SUPPLIED - EQUIVALENTS NOT AVAILABLE:

Injection, Lyphl-Soln - Intravenous - 500 mcg

5 ml $822.71 MITHRACIN, Bayer **00026-8161-15**

PNEUMOCOCCAL VACCINE *(002055)*

CATEGORIES: Bacteremia; Biologicals; Diabetes; Diabetes Mellitus; Hodgkin's Disease; Immunologic; Influenza; Nephrotic Syndrome; Pneumococcal Disease; Pneumonia; Renal Failure; Serums, Toxoids and Vaccines; Sickle Cell Disease; Streptococcal Infection; Vaccines; Pregnancy Category C; FDA Approval Pre 1982

BRAND NAMES: *Moniarix*; *Pneumo 23*; *Pneumo 23 Imovax*; *Pneumovax* (Japan); Pneumovax 23; **Pnu-Imune 23**
(International brand names outside U.S. in italics)

FORMULARIES: Medi-Cal

DESCRIPTION:

Pneumococcal Vaccine Polyvalent, is a sterile, liquid vaccine for intramuscular or subcutaneous injection. It consists of a mixture of highly purified capsular polysaccharides from the 23 most prevalent or invasive pneumococcal types accounting for at least 90% of pneumococcal blood isolates and at least 85% of all pneumococcal isolates from sites which are generally sterile as determined by ongoing surveillance of U.S. data.[1]

Pneumococcal Vaccine Polyvalent is manufactured according to methods developed by the Merck Sharp & Dohme Research Laboratories. Each 0.5 ml dose of vaccine contains 25 mcg of each polysaccharide type dissolved in isotonic saline solution containing 0.25% phenol as preservative.

Type 6B pneumococcal polysaccharide exhibits somewhat greater stability in purified form than does Type 6A.[1] A high degree of cross-reactivity between the two types has been demonstrated in adult volunteers.[2,3] Therefore, Type 6B has replaced Type 6A, which had been used in the 14-valent vaccine. Although contained in the 14-valent vaccine, Type 25 is not included in Pneumococcal Vaccine Polyvalent because it has recently become a rare isolate in many parts of the world including the United States, Canada and Europe.[2] (see TABLE 1.)

TABLE 1 Pneumococcal Vaccine Polyvalent, Description 23 Pneumococcal Capsular Types Included in PNEUMOVAX 23	
Nomenclature	**Pneumococcal Types**
Danish	1 2 3 4 5 6B 7F 8 9N 9V 10A 11A 12F 14 15B 17F 18C 19F 19A 20 22F 23F 33F
U.S.	1 2 3 4 5 26 51 8 9 68 34 43 12 14 54 17 56 19 57 20 22 23 70

CLINICAL PHARMACOLOGY:

Pneumococcal infection is a leading cause of death throughout the world[4] and a major cause of pneumonia, meningitis, and otitis media. The emergence of strains of pneumococci with increased resistance to one or more of the common antibiotics[5] and recent isolations of pneumococci with multiple antibiotic resistance[6]emphasize the importance of vaccine prophylaxis against pneumococcal disease. Based on projection from limited observations[7]in the United States, it has been estimated that 400,000 to 500,000 cases of pneumococcal pneumonia may occur annually. The overall case fatality rate ranges from 5 - 10%.[7] Populations at high risk are the elderly; individuals with immune deficiencies; patients with asplenia or splenic deficiencies, including sickle cell anemia and other severe hemoglobinopathies; alcoholics; and patients with the following diseases: Hodgkin's disease, multiple myeloma and nephrotic syndrome.[8] About 25% of all persons with pneumococcal pneumonia develop bacteremia. Death occurs in about 28% of these bacteremic patients over 50 years of age.[9]Of all patients with pneumococcal bacteremia who died despite treatment with penicillin or tetracycline, as many as 60% died within five days of onset of the illness.[9]

The annual incidence of pneumococcal meningitis is approximately 1.5 to 2.5 per 100,000 population. One-half of the cases occur in children, in whom the fatality rate is about 40%.[7] Children with sickle cell disease have been estimated to have a risk of pneumococcal meningitis nearly 600 times greater than normal children.[10]Other illnesses caused by pneumococci include acute exacerbations of chronic bronchitis, sinusitis, arthritis and conjunctivitis.

Invasive pneumococcal disease causes high morbidity and mortality in spite of effective antimicrobial control by a antibiotics.[9] These effects of pneumococcal disease appear due to irreversible physiologic damage caused by the bacteria during the first 5 days following onset of illness,[11,12] and occur irrespective of antimicrobial therapy.[5,11] Vaccination offers an effective means of further reducing the mortality and morbidity of this disease.

At present, there are 83 known pneumococcal capsular types. However, the preponderance of pneumococcal diseases is caused by only some capsular types.[5,9,13,14] For example, a 10-year (1952-1962) surveillance at a New York medical center,[9] showed that 56% of all deaths due to pneumococcal pneumonia were caused by 6 capsular types and that approximately 78% of all pneumococcal pneumonias were caused by 12 capsular types. Such unequal distribution of pneumococcal capsular types causing disease has been shown throughout the world.[5,13,14]It is on the basis of this information that the pneumococcal vaccine is composed of 23 capsular types, designed to provide coverage of approximately 90% of the most frequently reported types.

It has been established that the purified pneumococcal capsular polysaccharides induce antibody production and that such antibody is effective in preventing pneumococcal disease.[2,12] Studies in humans have demonstrated the immunogenicity (antibody-stimulating capability) of each of the 23 capsular types when tested in polyvalent vaccines. Adults of all ages responded immunologically to the vaccines.[2] Earlier studies with 12- and 14-valent pneumococcal vaccines in children two years of age and older and in adults showed immunogenic responses.[15-18] Protective capsular type-specific antibody levels develop by the third week following vaccination.[17]

The protective efficacy of pneumococcal vaccines containing 6 and 12 capsular polysaccharides was investigated in controlled studies of gold miners in South Africa, in whom there is a high attack rate for pneumococcal pneumonia.[1] Capsular type-specific attack rates for pneumococcal pneumonia were observed for the period from 2 weeks through about 1 year after vaccination. The rates for pneumonia caused by the same capsular types represented in the vaccines are given in the table (TABLE 2). Protective efficacy was 76% and 92%, respectively, in the two studies for the capsular types represented.

TABLE 2 Pneumococcal Vaccine Polyvalent, Clinical Pharmacology

Number of Capsular Types in Pneumococcal Vaccine	Rate/1000 for Pneumonia Caused by Homologous Capsular Types: Vaccinated Group	Control Group	Protective Efficacy
6	9.2	38.3	76%
12	1.8	22.0	92%

In similar studies carried out by Dr. R. Austrian and Associates[13] using similar pneumococcal vaccines prepared for the National Institute of Allergy and Infectious Diseases, the reduction in pneumonia caused by the capsular types contained in the vaccines was 79%. Reduction in type-specific pneumococcal bacteremia was 82%. A preliminary report[19] suggests that in patients with sickle cell anemia and/or anatomical or functional asplenia, the vaccine was highly effective in persons over two years of age in preventing severe pneumococcal disease and bacteremia.

The duration of protective effect of Pneumococcal Vaccine Polyvalent is presently unknown, but it has been shown in previous studies[12,20] with other pneumococcal vaccines that antibody induced by the vaccine may persist for as long as 5 years. Type-specific antibody levels induced by Pneumococcal Vaccine Polyvalent (14-valent) have been observed to decline over a 42-month period of observation, but remain significantly above prevaccination levels in almost all recipients who manifest an initial response.[21]

INDICATIONS AND USAGE:

Pneumococcal Vaccine Polyvalent is indicated for immunization against pneumococcal disease caused by those pneumococcal types included in the vaccine. Effectiveness of the vaccine in the prevention of pneumococcal pneumonia and pneumococcal bacteremia has been demonstrated in controlled trials.

Pneumococcal Vaccine Polyvalent *will not immunize against capsular types of pneumococcus other than those contained in the vaccine.*

Use in selected individuals over 2 years of age as follows: (1) patients who have anatomical asplenia or who have splenic dysfunction due to sickle cell disease or other causes; (2) persons with chronic illnesses in which there is an increased risk of pneumococcal disease, such as functional impairment of cardiorespiratory, hepatic and renal systems; (3) persons 50 years of age or older; (4) patients with other chronic illnesses who may be at greater risk of developing pneumococcal infection or experiencing more severe pneumococcal illness as a result of alcohol abuse or coexisting diseases including diabetes mellitus, chronic cerebrospinal fluid leakage, or conditions associated with immunosuppression;[22] (5) patients with Hodgkin's disease if immunization can be given at least 10 days prior to treatment. For maximal

INDICATIONS AND USAGE: *(cont'd)*

antibody response immunization should be given at least 14 days prior to the start of treatment with radiation or chemotherapy. Immunization of patients less than 10 days prior to or during treatment is not recommended.[23] (See CONTRAINDICATIONS.)

Use in communities. Persons over 2 years of age as follows: (1) closed groups such as those in residential schools, nursing homes and other institutions. (To decrease the likelihood of acute outbreaks of pneumococcal disease in closed institutional populations where there is increased risk that the disease may be severe, vaccination of the entire closed population should be considered where there are no other contraindications.[22]); (2) groups epidemiologically at risk in the community when there is a generalized outbreak in the population due to a single pneumococcal type included in the vaccine; (3) patients at high risk of influenza complications, particularly pneumonia.[7]

Pneumococcal Vaccine Polyvalent may not be effective in preventing infection resulting from basilar skull fracture or from external communication with cerebrospinal fluid.

Simultaneous administration of pneumococcal polysaccharide vaccine and whole-virus influenza vaccine give satisfactory antibody response with out increasing the occurrence of adverse reactions.[24] Simultaneous administration of the pneumococcal vaccine and split-virus influenza vaccine may also be expected to yield satisfactory results.[25]

REVACCINATION

Routine revaccination of adults previously vaccinated with PNEUMOVAX 23 is not recommended because an increased incidence and severity of adverse reactions have been reported among healthy adults revaccinated with pneumococcal vaccines at intervals under three years.[2,15] This was probably due to sustained high antibody levels.[26]

Based on a clinical study, revaccination with PNEUMOVAX 23 is recommended for adults at highest risk of fatal pneumococcal infection who were initially vaccinated with PNEUMOVAX (Pneumococcal Vaccine Polyvalent, MSD) (14-valent) without serious or severe reaction four or more years previously.[30]**

Children at highest risk for pneumococcal infection (*e.g.,* children with asplenia, sickle cell disease or nephrotic syndrome) may have lower peak antibody levels and/or more rapid antibody decline than do healthy adults.[27,31] There is evidence that some of these high-risk children, (*e.g.,* asplenic children) benefit from revaccination with vaccine containing antigen types 7F, 8, 19F.[33,34] The Immunization Practices Advisory Committee (ACIP) recommends that revaccination after three to five years should be considered for children at highest risk for pneumococcal infection (*e.g.,* children with asplenia, sickle cell disease or nephrotic syndrome) who would be ten years old or younger at revaccination.[35]

**NOTE: The Immunization Practices Advisory Committee (ACIP) has stated that, without more information: persons who received the 14-valent pneumococcal vaccine should not be routinely revaccinated with the 23-valent vaccine, as increased coverage is modest and duration of protection is not well defined. However, revaccination with the 23-valent vaccine should be strongly considered for persons who received the 14-valent vaccine if they are at highest risk of fatal pneumococcal infection (*e.g.,* asplenic patients). Revaccination should also be considered for adults at highest risk who received the 23-valent vaccine ≥ 6 years before and for those shown to have rapid decline in pneumococcal antibody levels (*e.g.,* patients with nephrotic syndrome, renal failure, or transplant recipients).[35]

CONTRAINDICATIONS:

Hypersensitivity to any component of the vaccine. Epinephrine injection (1:1000) must be immediately available should an acute anaphylactoid reaction occur due to any component of the vaccine.

Revaccination of adults with Pneumococcal Vaccine Polyvalent is contraindicated except as described under **INDICATIONS AND USAGE.**

Patients with Hodgkin's disease immunized less than 7 to 10 days prior to immunosuppressive therapy have in some instances been found to have post-immunization antibody levels below their pre-immunization levels.[23] Because of these results, immunization less than 10 days prior to or during treatment is contraindicated.

Patients with Hodgkin's disease who have received extensive chemotherapy and/or nodal irradiation have been shown to have an impaired antibody response to a 12-valent pneumococcal vaccine.[28] Because, in some intensively treated patients, administration of that vaccine depressed pre-existing levels of antibody to some pneumococcal types, Pneumococcal Vaccine Polyvalent is not recommended at this time for patients who have received these forms of therapy for Hodgkin's disease.

WARNINGS:

If the vaccine is used in persons receiving immunosuppressive therapy, the expected serum antibody response may not be obtained.

Intradermal administration may cause severe local reactions.

PRECAUTIONS:

GENERAL

Caution and appropriate care should be exercised in administering Pneumococcal Vaccine Polyvalent to individuals with severely compromised cardiac and/or pulmonary function in whom a systemic reaction would pose a significant risk.

Any febrile respiratory illness or other active infection is reason for delaying use of Pneumococcal Vaccine Polyvalent, except when, in the opinion of the physician, withholding the agent entails even greater risk.

In patients who require penicillin (or other antibiotic) prophylaxis against pneumococcal infection, such prophylaxis should not be discontinued after vaccination with Pneumococcal Vaccine Polyvalent.

PREGNANCY CATEGORY C

Animal reproduction studies have not been conducted with Pneumococcal Vaccine Polyvalent. It is also not known whether Pneumococcal Vaccine Polyvalent can cause fetal harm when administered to a pregnant woman or can affect reproduction capacity. Pneumococcal Vaccine Polyvalent should be given to a pregnant woman only if clearly needed.

NURSING MOTHERS

It is not known whether this drug is excreted in human milk. Because many drugs are excreted in human milk, caution should be exercised when Pneumococcal Vaccine Polyvalent is administered to a nursing woman.

PEDIATRIC USE

Children less than 2 years of age do not respond satisfactorily to the capsular types of Pneumococcal Vaccine Polyvalent that are most often the cause of pneumococcal disease in this age group. Safety and effectiveness in children below the age of 2 years have not been established. Accordingly, Pneumococcal Vaccine Polyvalent is not recommended in this age group.

ADVERSE REACTIONS:

Local reactions including local injection site soreness, erythema and swelling, usually of less than 48 hours duration, occurs commonly; local induration occurs less commonly. In a study of Pneumococcal Vaccine Polyvalent (containing 22 capsular types) in 29 adults, 21 (71%) showed local reaction characterized principally by local soreness and/or induration at the injection site within 2 days after vaccination.[2]

Rash, urticaria, arthritis, arthralgia, serum sickness, and adenitis have been reported rarely.

Low grade fever (less than 100.9°F) occurs occasionally and is usually confined to the 24-hour period following vaccination. Although rare, fever over 102°F has been reported. Malaise, myalgia, headache, and asthenia also have been reported.

Patients with otherwise stabilized idiopathic thrombocytopenic purpura have, on rare occasions, experienced a relapse in their thrombocytopenia, occurring 2 to 14 days after vaccination, and lasting up to 2 weeks.[29]

Reactions of greater severity, duration, or extent are unusual. Neurological disorders such as paresthesias and acute radiculoneuropathy including Guillain-Barr̀e syndrome have been rarely reported in temporal association with administration of pneumococcal vaccine. No cause and effect relationship has been established. Rarely, anaphylactoid reactions have been reported.

DOSAGE AND ADMINISTRATION:

Do not inject intravenously. Intradermal administration should be avoided.

Parenteral drug products should be inspected visually for particulate matter and discoloration prior to administration, whenever solution and container permit. Pneumococcal Vaccine Polyvalent is a clear, colorless solution.

Administer a single 0.5 ml dose of Pneumococcal Vaccine Polyvalent subcutaneously or intramuscularly (preferably in the deltoid muscle or lateral mid-thigh), with appropriate precautions to avoid intravascular administration.

SINGLE-DOSE AND 5-DOSE VIALS

For Syringe Use Only: Withdraw 0.5 ml from the vial using a sterile needle and syringe free of preservatives, antiseptics and detergents.

It is important to use a separate sterile syringe and needle for each individual patient to prevent transmission of hepatitis B and other infectious agents from one person to another.

Store unopened and opened vials at 2 - 8°C (36 - 46°F). The vaccine is used directly as supplied. No dilution or reconstitution is necessary. Phenol 0.25% added as preservative. All vaccine must be discarded after the expiration date.

REFERENCES:

1. Robbins, J.B.; Lee, C.J.; Schiffman, G.; Austrian, R.; Henrichsen, J.; M̈akel̈a, P.H.; Broome, C.V.; Facklam, R.R.; Tiesjema, R.H.; Rastogi, S.C.: Considerations for formulating the second-generation pneumococcal capsular polysaccharide vaccine with emphasis on the cross-reactive types within groups, J. Infect. Dis. *148:* 1136-1159, 1983. **2.** Unpublished data; files of Merck Sharp & Dohme Research Laboratories. **3.** Robbins, J.B.; Lee, C.J.; Rastogi, S.C.; Schiffman, G.; Henrichsen, J.: Comparative immunogenicity of group 6 pneumococcal type 6A (6) and type 6B (26) capsular polysaccharides, Infect. Immun. *26:* 1116-1122, 1979. **4.** WHO: Vital statistics and causes of death, World Health Statistics Annual, 1, 1976. **5.** Mufson, M.A.; Kruss, D.M.; Wasil, R.E.; Metzger, W.I.: Capsular types and outcome of bacteremic pneumococcal disease in the antibiotic era, Arch. Intern. Med. *134:* 505-510, 1974. **6.** Multiple-antibiotic resistance of pneumococci—South Africa, Morbidity and Mortality Weekly Report *26* (35): 285, September 2, 1977. **7.** Recommendation of the Public Health Service Advisory Committee on Immunization Practices: Pneumococcal polysaccharide vaccine. Morbidity and Mortality Weekly Report *27* (4): 25, January 27, 1978. **8.** Mufson, M.A.: Pneumococcal infections, J. Am. Med. Assoc. *246* (17): 1942-1948, 1981. **9.** Austrian, R.; Gold, J.: Pneumococcal bacteremia with especial reference to bacteremic pneumococcal pneumonia, Ann. Intern. Med.*60:* 759-776, 1964. **10.** Barrett-Connor, E.: Bacterial infection and sickle cell anemia: an analysis of 250 infections in 166 patients and a review of the literature, Medicine *50:* 97-112, 1971. **11.** Austrian, R.: Random gleanings from a life with the pneumococcus, J. Infect. Dis. *131:* 474-484, 1975. **12.** Austrian, R.: Vaccines of pneumococcal capsular polysaccharides and the prevention of pneumococcal pneumonia in, "The role of immunological factors in infectious, allergic and autoimmune processes", R.F. Beers, Jr. and E.G. Bassett (eds.), New York, Raven Press: 79-89. 1976. **13.** Austrian, R.; Douglas, R.M.; Schiffman, G.; Coetzee, A.M.; Koornhof, H.J.; Hayden-Smith, S.; Reid, R.D.W.: Prevention of pneumococcal pneumonia by vaccination, Trans. Assoc. Am. Physicians *89:* 184-194, 1976. **14.** Lund, E.: Distribution of pneumococcus types at different times in different areas, in "Bayer symposium III. bacterial infections: changes in their causative agents, trends, and possible basis," M.Finland, W. Marget and K. Bartmann (eds.), Berlin, Springer-Verlag, 1971, 49-56. **15.** Borgono, J.M.; McLean, A.A.; Vella, P.P.; Woodhour, A.F.; Canepa, I.; Davidson, W.L.; Hilleman, M.R.: Vaccination and revaccination with polyvalent pneumococcal polysaccharide vaccines in adults and infants (40010), Proc. Soc. Exper. Biol. & Med. *157:* 148-154, 1978. **16.** Hilleman, M.R.; McLean, A.A.; Vella, P.P.; Weibel, R.E.; Woodhour, A.F.: Polyvalent pneumococcal polysaccharide vaccines, Bull. World Health Organ. *56:* 371-375, 1978. **17.** Smit, P.; Oberholzer, D.; Hayden-Smith, S.; Koornof, H.J.; Hilleman, M.R.: Protective efficacy of pneumococcal polysaccharide vaccines, J.A.M.A. *238:* 2613-2616, 1977. **18.** Weibel, R.E.; Vella, P.P.; McLean, A.A.; Woodhour, A.F.; Hilleman, M.R.: Studies in human subjects of polyvalent pneumococcal vaccines (39894), Proc. Soc. Exper. Biol. & Med. *156:* 144-150, 1977. **19.** Ammann, A.J.; Addiego, J.; Wara, D.W.; Lubin, B.; Smith, W.B.; and Mentzer, W.C.: Polyvalent pneumococcal-polysaccharide immunization of patients with sickle-cell anemia and patients with splenectomy, New Engl. J. Med. *297:* 897-900, 1977. **20.** Heidelberger, M.; DiLapi, M.M.; Siegel, M.; Walter, A.W.: Persistence of antibodies in human subjects injected with pneumococcal polysaccharides, J. Immunol. *65:* 535-541, 1950. **21.** Vella, P.P., McLean, A.A.; Woodhour, A.F.; Weibel, R.E.; Hilleman, M.R.: Persistence of pneumococcal antibodies in human subjects following vaccination, Proc. Soc. Exper. Biol. & Med. *164:* 435-538, 1980. **22.** Recommendation of the Immunization Practices Advisory Committee, Pneumococcal polysaccharide vaccine, Morbidity and Mortality Weekly Report *30* (33): 410-412, 417-419, August 28, 1981. **23.** Siber, G.R.; Weitzman, S.A.; Aisenberg, A.C.: Antibody response of patients with Hodgkin's disease to protein and polysaccharide antigens, Rev. Inf. Dis. 3 (suppl.): S144-S159, 1981. **24.** Carlson, A.J.; Davidson, W.L.; McLean, A.A.; Vella, P.P.; Weibel, R.E.; Woodhour, A.F.; Hilleman, M.R.: Pneumococcal vaccine dose, revaccination, and coadministration with influenza vaccine (40596), Proc. Soc. Exp. Biol. & Med. *161:* 558-563, 1979. **25.** Recommendation of the Immunization Practices Advisory Committee — General recommendations on immunization, Morbidity and Mortality Weekly Report *32* (1): 7, January 14, 1983. **26.** Hilleman, M.R.; Carlson, A.J., Jr.; McLean, A.A.; Vella, P.P.; Weibel, R.E.; Woodhour, A.F.: *Streptococcus pneumoniae* polysaccharide vaccine: age and dose responses, safety, persistence of antibody, revaccination, and simultaneous administration of pneumococcal and influenza vaccines, Rev. Inf. Dis. *3* (Suppl.): S31-S42, 1981. **27.** Kaplan, J.; Frost, H.; Sarnaik, S.; Schiffman, G.: Type-specific antibodies in children with sickle cell anemia given polyvalent pneumococcal vaccine, J. Pediatr. *100:*404-406, 1982. **28.** Siber, G.R.; et al: Impaired antibody response after treatment for Hodgkin's Disease, N. Engl. J. Med. *299:* 442-448, 1978. **29.** Kelton, J.G.: Vaccination-associated relapse of immune thrombocytopenia, J. Am. Med. Assoc. *245* (4): 369-371, 1981. **30.** Unpublished data; files of Merck Sharp and Dohme Research Laboratories. **31.** Giebink, G.S.; Le, C.T.; Schiffman, G.: Decline of serum antibody in splenectomized children after vaccination with pneumococcal capsular polysaccharides, J. Pediatrics *105:*576-582, Oct. 1984. **32.** Giebink, G.S.: Preventing pneumococcal disease in children: recommendations for using pneumococcal vaccine, Ped. Inf. Dis. *4:* 343-348, July 1985. **33.** Rigau-Peraz, J.G.; Overturf, G.D.; Chan, L.S.; et al.: Reactions to booster pneumococcal revaccination in patients with sickle cell disease, Ped. Inf. Dis. *2:* 199-202, 1983. **34.** Weintraub, P.S.; Schiffman, G.; Addiego, J.E.; et al.: Long-term follow-up and booster immunization with polyvalent pneumococcal polysaccharide in patients with sickle cell anemia, Journal of Ped.*105:* 261-263, 1984. **35.** Recommendation of the Immunization Practices Advisory Committee — Pneumococcal polysaccharide vaccine, Morbidity and Mortality Weekly Report *38* (5): 64-68, 73-76, February 10, 1989.*Registered trademark of MERCK & CO., INC.

HOW SUPPLIED - EQUIVALENTS NOT AVAILABLE:

Injection, Solution - Intramuscular - 700 mcg

0.5 ml x 5	**$79.83**	**PNU-IMUNE 23, SYRINGE, Lederle Pharm**	**00005-2309-33**
2.5 ml	**$71.18**	**PNU-IMUNE 23, Lederle Pharm**	**00005-2309-31**

Injection, Solution - Intramuscular; - 25 mcg/0.5ml

0.5 ml x 5	$47.60	PNEUMOVAX 23, Merck	00006-4741-00
2.5 ml	$42.43	PNEUMOVAX 23, Merck	00006-4739-00

PODOFILOX *(003018)*

CATEGORIES: Antimitotics; Genital Warts; Topical; Warts; Pregnancy Category C; FDA Approved 1990 Dec

BRAND NAMES: *Condyline* (England, France); *Condyline Liquid*; *Condyline Paint*; **Condylox**; *Podofilox*; *Warix*; *Wartec*; *Warticon* (England)
(International brand names outside U.S. in italics)

FORMULARIES: PCS

DESCRIPTION:

Podofilox is an antimitotic drug which can be chemically synthesized or purified from the plant families Coniferae and Berberidaceae (*e.g.*, species of Juniperus and Podophyllum). Podofilox 0.5% solution is formulated for topical administration. Each milliliter of solution contains 5 mg of podofilox, in a vehicle containing lactic acid and sodium lactate in alcohol 95%, USP.

Podofilox has a molecular weight of 414.4 daltons, and is soluble in alcohol and sparingly soluble in water. Its chemical name is 5,8,8a,9-Tetrahydro-9-hydroxy-5-(3,4,5-trimethoxylphenyl)furo (3',4':6,7)naphtho (2,3,d)-1, 3-dioxol-6(5aH)-one.

CLINICAL PHARMACOLOGY:

Mechanism of Action: Treatment of genital warts with podofilox results in necrosis of visible wart tissue. The exact mechanism of action is unknown.

Pharmacokinetics: In systemic absorption studies in 52 patients, topical applications of 0.05 ml of 0.5% podofilox solution to external genitalia did not result in detectable serum levels. Applications of 0.1 to 1.5 ml resulted in peak serum levels of 1 to 17 ng/ml one to two hours after application. The elimination half-life ranged from 1.0 to 4.5 hours. The drug was not found to accumulate after multiple treatments.

CLINICAL STUDIES:

In clinical studies with Podofilox solution, the test product and its vehicle were applied in a double-blind fashion to comparable patient groups.

Patients were treated for two to four weeks, and reevaluated at a two-week follow-up examination. Although the number of patients and warts evaluated at each time were varied, the results among investigators were relatively consistent.

The following table represents the responses noted in terms of frequency of response by lesions treated and the overall response by patients.

Data are presented for the 2-week follow-up only for those patients evaluated at that time point.

TABLE 1 Podofilox, Clinical Pharmacology

	INITIALLY CLEARED	RECURRED AFTER CLEARING	CLEARED AT 2-Weeks FOLLOW-UP(*)
% Warts (n= 524)	79% (412/524)	35% (146/412)	60% (269/449)
% Patients (n = 70)	50% (35/70)	60% (21/35)	25% (14/57)

* Cleared and clearing mean no visible wart tissue remaine at the treated sites.

INDICATIONS AND USAGE:

Podofilox 0.5% solution is indicated for the topical treatment of external and genital warts (Condyloma acuminatum). This product is not indicated in the treatment of perianal or mucous membrane warts (see PRECAUTIONS.)

Diagnosis: Although genital warts have a characteristic appearance, histopathologic confirmation should be obtained if there is any doubt of the diagnosis. Differentiating warts from squamous cell carcinoma (so-called "Bowenoid papulosis") is of particular concern. Squamous cell carcinoma may also be associated with human papillomavirus but should not be treated with podofilox 0.5% solution.

CONTRAINDICATIONS:

Podofilox 0.5% solution is contraindicated for patients who develop hypersensitivity or intolerance to any component of the formulation.

WARNINGS:

Correct diagnosis of the lesions to be treated is essential. See the "Diagnosis" subsection of the INDICATIONS AND USAGEstatement.

Podofilox 0.5% solution is intended for cutaneous use only.

AVOID CONTACT WITH THE EYE. IF EYE CONTACT OCCURS, PATIENTS SHOULD IMMEDIATELY FLUSH THE EYE WITH COPIOUS QUANTITIES OF WATER AND SEEK MEDICAL ADVICE.

PRECAUTIONS:

GENERAL

Data are not available of the safe and effective use of this product for the treatment of warts occurring in the perianal area or mucous membranes of the genital area (including the urethra, rectum, and vagina). The recommended method of application, frequency of application, and duration of usage should not be exceeded (see DOSAGE AND ADMINISTRATION.)

INFORMATION FOR THE PATIENT

The patient should be provided with a Patient Information leaflet when a Podofilox prescription is filled.

CARCINOGENESIS, MUTAGENESIS, AND IMPAIRMENT OF FERTILITY

Reports of lifetime carcinogenicity studies in mice are not available. Published animal studies, in general, have not shown the drug substance, podofilox, to be carcinogenic. There are published reports that, in mouse studies, crude podophyllin resin (containing podofilox) applied topically to the cervix produced changes resembling carcinoma in situ. These changes were reversible at five weeks after cessation of treatment. In one reported experiment, epidermal carcinoma of the vagina and cervix was found in 1 out of 18 mice after 120 applications of podophyllin (the drug was applied twice weekly over a 15-month period).

Podofilox was not mutagenic in the Ames plate reverse mutation assay at concentrations up to 5 mg/plate, with and without metabolic activation. No cell transformation related to potential oncogenicity was observed in BABL/3T3 cells after exposure to podofilox at concentrations up to 0.008 micrograms/ml without metabolic activation and 12 micrograms/ml podofilox with metabolic activation. Results from the mouse micronucleus *in vivo* assay using podofilox 0.5% solution in concentrations up to 25 mg/kg, indicate that podofilox should be considered a potential clastogen (a chemical that induces disruption and breakage of chromosomes).

Daily topical applications of Podofilox 0.5% solution at doses up to the equivalent of 0.2 mg/kg (5 times the recommended maximum human dose) to rats throughout gametogenesis, mating gestation, parturition and lactation for two generations demonstrated no impairment of fertility.

PRECAUTIONS: *(cont'd)*

PREGNANCY CATEGORY C

Podofilox was not teratogenic in the rabbit following topical application of up to 0.21 mg/kg (5 times the maximum human dose) once daily for 13 days. The scientific literature contains references that podofilox is embryotoxic in rats when administered systemically in a dose approximately 250 times the recommended maximum human dose. Teratogenicity and embryotoxicity have not been studied with intravaginal application. Many antimitotic drug products are known to be embryotoxic. There are no adequate and well-controlled studies in pregnant women. Podofilox should be used in pregnancy only if the potential benefit justifies the potential risk to the fetus.

NURSING MOTHERS

It is not known whether this drug is excreted in human milk. Because of the potential for serious adverse reactions in nursing infants from podofilox, a decision should be made whether to discontinue nursing or to discontinue the drug, taking into account the importance of the drug to the mother.

PEDIATRIC USE

Safety and effectiveness in children have not been established.

ADVERSE REACTIONS:

In clinical trials, local adverse reactions were reported at some point during treatment (TABLE 2).

TABLE 2 Podofilox, Adverse Reactions

ADVERSE EXPERIENCE	MALES	FEMALES
Burning	64%	78%
Pain	50%	72%
Inflammation	71%	63%
Erosion	67%	67%
Itching	50%	65%

Reports of burning and pain were more frequent and of greater severity in women than in men.

Adverse effects reported in less than 5% of the patients included pain with intercourse, insomnia, tingling, bleeding, tenderness, chafing, malodor, dizziness, scarring, vesicle formation, crusting edema, dryness/peeling, foreskin irretraction, hematuria, vomiting and ulceration.

OVERDOSAGE:

Topically applied podofilox may be absorbed systemically (see CLINICAL PHARMACOLOGY). Toxicity reported following systemic administration of podofilox in investigational use for cancer treatment included: nausea, vomiting, fever, diarrhea, bone marrow depression, and oral ulcers. Following 5 to 10 daily intravenous doses of 0.5 to 1 mg/kg/day, significant hematological toxicity occurred but was reversible. Other toxicities occurred at lower doses. Toxicity reported following systemic administration of podophyllum resin included: nausea, vomiting, fever, diarrhea, peripheral neuropathy, altered mental status, lethargy, coma, tachypnea, respiratory failure, leukocytosis, pancytosis, hematuria, renal failure, and seizures. Treatment of topical overdosage should include washing the skin free of any remaining drug and symptomatic and supportive therapy.

DOSAGE AND ADMINISTRATION:

In order to insure that the patient is fully aware of the correct method of therapy and to identify which specific warts should be treated, the technique for initial application of medication should be demonstrated by the prescriber.

Apply twice daily morning and evening (every 12 hours), for 3 consecutive days, then withhold use for 4 consecutive days. This one week cycle of treatment may be repeated up to four times until there is no visible wart tissue. **IF THERE IS INCOMPLETE RESPONSE AFTER FOUR TREATMENT WEEKS, ALTERNATIVE TREATMENT SHOULD BE CONSIDERED. SAFETY AND EFFECTIVENESS OF MORE THAN FOUR TREATMENT WEEKS HAVE NOT BEEN ESTABLISHED.**

Podofilox 0.5% solution is applied to the warts with a cotton-tipped applicator supplied with the drug. The drug dampened applicator should be touched to the wart to be treated, applying the minimum amount of solution necessary to cover the lesion. **TREATMENT SHOULD BE LIMITED TO LESS THAN 10 SQUARE CM OF WART TISSUE AND TO NO MORE THAN 0.5 ML OF THE SOLUTION PER DAY.** There is no evidence to suggest that more frequent application will increase efficacy, but additional applications would be expected to increase the rate of local adverse reactions and systemic absorption.

Care should be taken to allow the solution to dry before allowing the return of opposing skin surfaces to their normal positions. After each treatment, the used applicator should be carefully disposed of and the patient should wash his or her hands.

Store at controlled room temperature between 15° and 30° C (59° and 86° F). **AVOID EXCESSIVE HEAT. DO NOT FREEZE.**

(Oclassen)

HOW SUPPLIED - EQUIVALENTS NOT AVAILABLE:

Solution - Topical - 5 mg/ml

3.5 ml	**$52.44**	**CONDYLOX, Oclassen Pharms**	**55515-0101-01**

PODOPHYLLUM RESIN *(002057)*

CATEGORIES: Keratolytic Agents; Skin/Mucous Membrane Agents; FDA Pre 1938 Drugs

BRAND NAMES: *Condil* (Mexico); Podoben; Podocon-25; Pododerm; *Podofilia No. 2* (Mexico); Podofin
(International brand names outside U.S. in italics)

FORMULARIES: WHO

Prescribing information not available at time of publication.

HOW SUPPLIED - EQUIVALENTS NOT AVAILABLE:

Liquid - Topical - 25 %

5 ml	$6.95	PODOBEN, Americal Pharm	54945-0590-21
5 ml	$17.00	PODODERM, Liquipharm	54198-0131-05
15 ml	$26.00	PODODERM, Liquipharm	54198-0131-15
15 ml	$35.00	PODOCON-25 TOPICAL, Paddock Labs	00574-0601-15
30 ml	$55.00	PODODERM, Liquipharm	54198-0131-30

HOW SUPPLIED - EQUIVALENTS NOT AVAILABLE: *(cont'd)*

Powder

25 gm	$86.67	Podophyllum, Paddock Labs	00574-0600-25
30 gm	$36.00	Podophyllum Resin, Millgood	53118-0318-01
30 gm	$59.10	Podophyllum Resin, Mallinckrodt	00406-7700-34
100 gm	$261.67	Podophyllum, Paddock Labs	00574-0600-01
120 gm	$120.00	Podophyllum Resin, Millgood	53118-0318-04
125 gm	$236.39	Podophyllum Resin, Mallinckrodt	00406-7700-01

POISON IVY EXTRACT *(002058)*

CATEGORIES: Dermatitis; Diagnostic Agents; Immunologic; Poison Ivy; Serums, Toxoids and Vaccines; Vaccines; FDA Pre 1938 Drugs

BRAND NAMES: Rhus Tox Antigen

DESCRIPTION:

Poison Ivy Extract consists of the toluene-absolute alcohol soluble irritating principle from the leaves of Rhus toxicodendron (poison ivy, poison oak) dissolved in sterile almond oil. Chloretone (chlorobutanol), 0.6%, is included as a preservative. The activity is controlled by biological assay.

The toxic oil "urushiol" is not separated from the natural waxes in this extract, as it is desired to retain such glucosides and other compounds as may be necessary for full antigenic response.

This phenolic substance, urushiol, is also found in Rhus vernicifera, Rhus diversilobia, and other related ivies and is believed to be the vesicant substance in the poison ivies, oaks and sumacs.

INDICATIONS AND USAGE:

Poison Ivy Extract is indicated for the prevention of Rhus dermatitis.

DOSAGE AND ADMINISTRATION:

PROPHYLACTIC

It has been found that the intramuscular injection of 1 ml of the extract will protect many sensitive persons. Where the hazard of exposure is great, or in persons who have had repeated attacks, three 1-ml doses at weekly intervals may be given as additional protection. Preventive treatment may be started at any time, even in mid-season.

The use of Poison Ivy Extract for treatment of individuals already suffering from Rhus dermatitis or in persons having a history of kidney damage is not recommended.

ADMINISTRATION

Injections of Poison Ivy Extract should be made deep in the muscle tissue rather than in subcutaneous tissue. This aids in avoiding local skin reactions.

A separate heat-sterilized syringe and needle should be used for each individual patient to prevent transmission of homologous serum hepatitis and other infectious agents from one person to another.

It is important that the extract does not come in contact with the skin. The sides of the needle should be cleansed of adhering extract solution by wiping with alcohol or acetone. The use of a second clean sterile needle for injection obviates this difficulty. The point of injection may be covered with adhesive tape or sealed with collodion. The patient should avoid exercise that would produce a massage-like action of the injected area as, even if sealed, the back-seepage of the fluid may then cause irritation and vesiculation at the point of injection.

If, by any chance, the extract comes into contact with the skin, it should be sponged off by repeated swabbing with undiluted alcohol, or other solvent, using fresh cotton each time.

REFERENCES:

Hill, Mattacotti and Graham: J. Am. Chem. Soc. 56, 2736, 1934.Majima: Ber 55B, 172, 1922.McNair: J. Am. Chem. Soc. 38, 1417, 1916. Ibid. 43, 159, 1921.Toyama: J. Cut. Dis. 36, 157, 1918. Ber 55B, 208, 1922.Blank, J.M. and Coca, A.F.: J. Allergy 7:552, 1936.Molitch, M. and Poliakoff, S.: J. Allergy 9:270, 1938.Clarke, J.R. and Hanna, C.M.: J. Allergy 13:599-605, 1942.Baer, R.L. and Leider, M.: Annals of Allergy 8:128, 1950.Clemens and Prokesch: Archives of Pediatrics 67:267, 1950.Rytand, D.A.: Am. J. Med., 5:548, Oct. 1948.Shaffer, B.: Burgoon, C.F. and Gosman, J.H.: J.A.M.A. 146:1570, (Aug. 25) 1951.Stevens, F.A.: Status of Poison Ivy Extracts, report of the Council on Pharmacy and Chemistry, J.A.M.A. 127, 912 (April 7) 1945.

HOW SUPPLIED - EQUIVALENTS NOT AVAILABLE:

Injection, Solution - Intramuscular

1 ml	$8.54	Poison Ivy Extract, Parke-Davis	00071-4397-03

POLIO VACCINE, INACTIVATED *(002060)*

CATEGORIES: Immunologic; Poliomyelitis; Serums, Toxoids and Vaccines; Vaccines; Pregnancy Category C; FDA Approval Pre 1982

BRAND NAMES: *Imovax Polio*; **Ipol**; *Polio Salk "Sero"*; Poliovax
(International brand names outside U.S. in italics)

DESCRIPTION:

Poliovirus Vaccine Inactivated, produced by Pasteur Merieux Serums & Vaccins S.A., is a sterile suspension of three types of poliovirus: Type 1 (Mahoney), Type 2 (MEF-1), and Type 3 (Saukett). The viruses are grown in cultures of VERO cells, a continuous line of monkey kidney cells, by the microcarrier technique. The viruses are concentrated, purified, and made noninfectious by inactivation with formaldehyde. Each sterile immunizing dose (0.5 ml) of trivalent vaccine is formulated to contain 40 D antigen units of Type 1, 8 D antigen units of Type 2, and 32 D antigen units of Type 3 poliovirus, determined by comparison to a reference preparation. The poliovirus vaccine is dissolved in phosphate buffered saline. Also present are 0.5% of 2-phenoxyethanol and a maximum of 0.02% of formaldehyde per dose as preservatives. Neomycin, streptomycin and polymyxin B are used in vaccine production, and although purification procedures eliminate measurable amounts, less than 5 ng neomycin, 200 ng streptomycin and 25 ng polymyxin B per dose may still be present. The vaccine is clear and colorless and should be administered subcutaneously.

CLINICAL PHARMACOLOGY:

Poliovirus Vaccine Inactivated is a highly purified, inactivated poliovirus vaccine produced by microcarrier culture.[1,2] This culture technique and improvements in purification, concentration and standardization of poliovirus antigen have resulted in a more potent and more consistently immunogenic vaccine than the Poliovirus Vaccine Inactivated which was available in the U.S. prior to 1988. These new methods allow for the production of vaccine that induces antibody responses in most children after administering fewer doses[3] than with vaccine available prior to 1988.

CLINICAL PHARMACOLOGY: *(cont'd)*

Studies in developed[3] and developing[4,5] countries with a similar inactivated poliovirus vaccine produced by the same technology have shown that a direct relationship exists between the antigenic content of the vaccine, the frequency of seroconversion, and resulting antibody titer.

A study in the U.S. was carried out, which involved 219 two-month-old infants who had received three doses of a Poliovirus Vaccine Inactivated manufactured by the same process as Poliovirus Vaccine Inactivated except the cell substrate was primary monkey kidney cells. Seroconversion to all three Types of poliovirus was demonstrated in 99% of these infants after two doses of vaccine. Following a third dose of vaccine at 18 months of age, high titers of neutralizing antibody were present in 99.1% of children to Type 1 and 100% of children to Types 2 and 3 polioviruses.[6]

Additional studies were carried out in the U.S. with Poliovirus Vaccine Inactivated. Results were reported for 120 infants who received two doses of Poliovirus Vaccine Inactivated at 2 and 4 months of age. Of these 120 children, detectable serum neutralizing antibody was induced after two doses of vaccine in 98.3% (Type 1), 100% (Type 2) and 97.5% (Type 3) of the children. In 83 children receiving three doses at 2, 4, and 12 months of age detectable serum neutralizing antibodies were detected in 97.6% (Type 1) and 100% (Types 2 and 3) of the children.[7,8]

Poliovirus Vaccine Inactivated reduces pharyngeal excretion of poliovirus.[9-12] Field studies in Europe have demonstrated immunity in populations thoroughly immunized with another IPV.[13-17] A survey of Swedish children and young adults given a Swedish IPV demonstrated persistence of circulating antibodies for at least 10 years to all three types of poliovirus.[13]

PARALYTIC POLIO HAS NOT BEEN REPORTED IN ASSOCIATION WITH ADMINISTRATION OF POLIOVIRUS VACCINE INACTIVATED.

INDICATIONS AND USAGE:

Poliovirus Vaccine Inactivated is indicated for active immunization of infants, children and adults for the prevention of poliomyelitis. Recommendations on the use of live and inactivated poliovirus vaccines are described in the ACIP Recommendations[18,19] and the 1988 American Academy of Pediatrics Red Book.[20]

INFANTS, CHILDREN, AND ADOLESCENTS

General Recommendations: It is recommended that all infants, unimmunized children and adolescents not previously immunized be vaccinated routinely against paralytic poliomyelitis.[18] Poliovirus Vaccine Inactivated should be offered to individuals who have refused Poliovirus Vaccine Live Oral Trivalent (OPV) or in whom OPV is contraindicated. Parents should be adequately informed of the risks and benefits of both inactivated and oral polio vaccines so that they can make an informed choice (Report of An Evaluation of Poliomyelitis Vaccine Policy Options, Institute of Medicine, National Academy of Sciences, Washington, D.C., 1988).

OPV should not be used in households with immunodeficient individuals because OPV is excreted in the stool by healthy vaccinees and can infect an immunocompromised household member, which may result in paralytic disease. In a household with an immunocompromised member, only Poliovirus Vaccine Inactivated should be used for all those requiring poliovirus immunization.[20]

Children Incompletely Immunized: Children of all ages should have their immunization status reviewed and be considered for supplemental immunization as follows for adults. Time intervals between doses longer than those recommended for routine primary immunization do not necessitate additional doses as long as a final total of four doses is reached (See DOSAGE AND ADMINISTRATION.)

Previous clinical poliomyelitis (usually due to only a single poliovirus type) or incomplete immunization with OPV are not contraindications to completing the primary series of immunization with Poliovirus Vaccine Inactivated.

ADULTS

General Recommendations: Routine primary poliovirus vaccination of adults (generally those 18 years of age or older) residing in the U.S. is not recommended. Adults who have increased risk of exposure to either vaccine or wild poliovirus and have not been adequately immunized should receive polio vaccination in accordance with the schedule given in the DOSAGE AND ADMINISTRATION section.[16]

The following categories of adults run an increased risk of exposure to wild polioviruses:[19]

- Travelers to regions or countries where poliomyelitis is endemic or epidemic.
- Health care workers in close contact with patients who may be excreting polioviruses.
- Laboratory workers handling specimens that may contain polioviruses.
- Members of communities or specific population groups with disease caused by wild polioviruses.
- Incompletely vaccinated or unvaccinated adults in a household (or other close contacts) with children given OPV provided that the immunization of the child can be assured and not unduly delayed. The adult should be informed of the small OPV related risk to the contact.

IMMUNODEFICIENCY AND ALTERED IMMUNE STATUS

Patients with recognized immunodeficiency are at greater risk of developing paralysis when exposed to live poliovirus than persons with a normal immune system. Under no circumstances should oral live poliovirus vaccine be used in such patients or introduced into a household where such a patient resides.[18]

Poliovirus Vaccine Inactivated should be used in all patients with immunodeficiency diseases and members of such patients' households when vaccination of such persons is indicated. This includes patients with asymptomatic HIV infection, AIDS or AIDS Related Complex, severe combined immunodeficiency, hypogammaglobulinemia, or agammaglobulinemia; altered immune states due to diseases such as leukemia, lymphoma, or generalized malignancy; or an immune system compromised by treatment with corticosteroids, alkylating drugs, antimetabolites or radiation. Patients with an altered immune state may or may not develop a protective response against paralytic poliomyelitis after administration of Poliovirus Vaccine Inactivated.[21]

CONTRAINDICATIONS:

Poliovirus Vaccine Inactivated is contraindicated in persons with a history of hypersensitivity to any component of the vaccine, including neomycin, streptomycin and polymyxin B.

If anaphylaxis or anaphylactic shock occurs within 24 hours of administration of a dose of vaccine, no further doses should be given.

Vaccination of persons with any acute, febrile illness should be deferred until after recovery; however, minor illnesses such as mild upper respiratory infections are not in themselves reasons for postponing vaccine administration.

WARNINGS:

Neomycin, streptomycin, and polymyxin B are used in the production of this vaccine. Although purification procedures eliminate measurable amounts of these substances, traces may be present (see DESCRIPTION) and allergic reactions may occur in persons sensitive to these substances.

PRECAUTIONS:

General: Before injection of the vaccine, the physician should carefully review the recommendations for product use and the patient's medical history including possible hypersensitivities and side effects that may have occurred following previous doses of the vaccine.

Epinephrine hydrochloride (1:1000) and other appropriate agents should be available to control immediate allergic reactions.

Concerns have been raised that stimulation of the immune system of a patient with HIV infection by immunization with inactivated vaccines might cause deterioration in immunologic function. However, such effects have not been noted thus far among children with AIDS or among immunosuppressed individuals after immunizations with inactivated vaccines. The potential benefits of immunization of these children outweigh the undocumented risk of such adverse events.[18]

Carcinogenesis, Mutagenesis, and Impairment of Fertility: Long term studies in animals to evaluate carcinogenic potential or impairment of fertility have not been conducted.

Pregnancy: REPRODUCTIVE STUDIES—PREGNANCY CATEGORY C: Animal reproduction studies have not been conducted with Poliovirus Vaccine Inactivated. It is also not known whether Poliovirus Vaccine Inactivated can cause fetal harm when administered to a pregnant woman or can affect reproduction capacity. Poliovirus Vaccine Inactivated should be given to a pregnant woman only if clearly needed.

Pediatric Use: Safety and efficacy of Poliovirus Vaccine Inactivated have been shown in children 6 weeks of age and older.[6,8] (See DOSAGE AND ADMINISTRATION.)

DRUG INTERACTIONS:

There are no known interactions of Poliovirus Vaccine Inactivated with drugs or foods. Simultaneous administration of other parenteral vaccines is not contraindicated.

ADVERSE REACTIONS:

In earlier studies with the vaccine grown in primary monkey kidney cells, transient local reactions at the site of injection were observed during a clinical trial.[6] Erythema, induration and pain occurred in 3.2%, 1% and 13%, respectively, of vaccinees within 48 hours post-vaccination. Temperatures ≥ 39°C (≥ 102°F) were reported in up to 38% of vaccinees. Other symptoms noted included sleepiness, fussiness, crying, decreased appetite, and spitting up of feedings. Because Poliovirus Vaccine Inactivated was given in a different site but concurrently with Diphtheria and Tetanus Toxoids and Pertussis Vaccine Adsorbed (DTP), systemic reactions could not be attributed to a specific vaccine. However, these systemic reactions were comparable in frequency and severity to that reported for DTP given without IPV.

In another study using Poliovirus Vaccine Inactivated in the United States, there were no significant local or systemic reactions following injection of the vaccine. There were 7% (6/86), 12% (8/65) and 4% (2/45) of children with temperatures over 100.6°F, following the first, second and third doses respectively. Most of the children received DTP at the same time as IPV and therefore it was not possible to attribute reactions to a particular vaccine; however, such reactions were not significantly different than when DTP is given alone.

Although no causal relationship between Poliovirus Vaccine Inactivated and Guillain-Barre Syndrome (GBS) has been established,[22] GBS has been temporally related to administration of another Poliovirus Vaccine Inactivated.

NOTE: The National Childhood Vaccine Injury Act of 1986 requires the keeping of certain records and the reporting of certain events occurring after the administration of vaccine, including the occurrence of any contraindicating reaction. Poliovirus Vaccines are listed vaccines covered by this Act and health care providers should ensure that they comply with the terms thereof.[23]

DOSAGE AND ADMINISTRATION:

Parenteral drug products should be inspected visually for particulate matter and/or discoloration prior to administration. If these conditions exist, vaccine should not be administered.

After preparation of the injection site, immediately administer the vaccine subcutaneously. In infants and small children, the mid-lateral aspect of the thigh is the preferred site. In adults the vaccine should be administered in the deltoid area.

Care should be taken to avoid administering the injection into or near blood vessels and nerves. After aspiration, if blood or any suspicious discoloration appears in the syringe, do not inject but discard contents and repeat procedures using a new dose of vaccine administered at a different site. DO NOT ADMINISTER VACCINE INTRAVENOUSLY.

CHILDREN

Primary Immunization: A primary series of Poliovirus Vaccine Inactivated consists of three 0.5 ml doses administered subcutaneously. The interval between the first two doses should be at least four weeks, but preferably eight weeks. The first two doses are usually administered with DTP immunization and are given at two and four months of age. The third dose should follow at least six months but preferably 12 months after the second dose. It may be desirable to administer this dose with MMR and other vaccines, but at a different site, in children 15-18 months of age. All children who received a primary series of Poliovirus Vaccine Inactivated, or a combination of IPV and OPV, should be given a booster dose of OPV or IPV before entering school, unless the final (third dose) of the primary series was administered on or after the fourth birthday.[18]

The need to routinely administer additional doses is unknown at this time.[18]

A final total of four doses is necessary to complete a series of primary and booster doses. Children and adolescents with a previously incomplete series of IPV should receive sufficient additional doses to reach this number.

ADULTS

Unvaccinated Adults: For unvaccinated adults at increased risk of exposure to poliovirus, a primary series of Poliovirus Vaccine Inactivated is recommended. While the responses of adults to primary series have not been studied, the recommended schedule for adults is two doses given at a 1 to 2 month interval and a third dose given 6 to 12 months later. If less than 3 months but more than 2 months are available before protection is needed, 3 doses of Poliovirus Vaccine Inactivated should be given at least 1 month apart. Likewise, if only 1 or 2 months are available, two doses of Poliovirus Vaccine Inactivated should be given at least 1 month apart. If less than 1 month is available, a single dose of either OPV or IPV is recommended.

Incompletely Vaccinated Adults: Adults who are at an increased risk of exposure to poliovirus and who have had at least one dose of OPV, fewer than 3 doses of conventional IPV or a combination of conventional IPV or OPV totalling fewer than 3 doses should receive at least 1 dose of OPV or Poliovirus Vaccine Inactivated. Additional doses needed to complete a primary series should be given if time permits.

Completely Vaccinated Adults: Adults who are at an increased risk of exposure to poliovirus and who have previously completed a primary series with one or a combination of polio vaccines can be given a dose of either OPV or IPV.[19]

Storage: The vaccine is stable if stored in the refrigerator between 2°C and 8°C (35°F to 46°F). *The vaccine must not be frozen.*

REFERENCES:

1. van Wezel, A.L., et al: Inactivated poliovirus vaccine: Current production methods and new developments. Rev Infect Dis 6 (Suppl 2): S335-S340, 1984 **2.** Montagnon, B.J., et al: Industrial scale production of inactivated poliovirus vaccine prepared by culture of Vero cells on microcarrier. Rev Infect Dis 6 (Suppl 2): S341-S344, 1984 **3.** Salk, J., et al: Antigen content of inactivated poliovirus vaccine for use in a one- or two-dose regimen. Ann Clin Res 14: 204-212, 1982 **4.** Salk, J., et al: Killed poliovirus antigen titration in humans. Develop Biol Standard 41: 110-132, 1978 **5.** Salk, J., et al: Theoretical and practical considerations in the application of killed poliovirus vaccine for the control of paralytic poliomyelitis. Develop Biol Standard 47: 181-198, 1981 **6.** McBean, A.M., et al: Serologic response to oral polio vaccine and enhanced-potency inactivated polio vaccines. Am J Epidemiol 128: 615-628, 1988 **7.** Unpublished data available from Pasteur Merieux Serums & Vaccins S.A. **8.** Faden, H., et al: Comparative evaluation of immunization with live attenuated and enhanced potency inactivated trivalent poliovirus vaccines in childhood: Systemic and local immune responses. J Infect Dis 162: 1291-1297, 1990 **9.** Marine, W.M., et al: Limitation of fecal and pharyngeal poliovirus excretion in Salk-vaccinated children. A family study during a Type 1 poliomyelitis epidemic. Amer J Hyg 76: 173-175, 1962 **10.** Bottiger, M., et al: Vaccination with attenuated Type 1 poliovirus, the Chat strain. II. Transmission of virus in relation to age. Acta Paed Scand 55: 416-421, 1966 **11.** Dick, G.W.A., et al: Vaccination against poliomyelitis with live virus vaccines. Effect of previous Salk vaccination on virus excretion. Brit Med J 2: 266-269, 1961 **12.** Wehrle, P.F., et al: Transmission of poliovirus; III. Prevalence of polioviruses in pharyngeal secretions of infected household contacts of patients with clinical disease. Pediatrics 27: 762-764, 1961 **13.** Bottiger, M: Long-term immunity following vaccination with killed poliovirus vaccine in Sweden, a country with no circulating poliovirus. Rev Infect Dis 6 (Suppl 2): S545-551, 1984 **14.** Chin, T.D.Y.: Immunity induced by inactivated poliovirus vaccine and excretion of virus. Rev Infect Dis 6 (Suppl 2): S369-S370, 1984 **15.** Salk, D.: Herd effect and virus eradication with use of killed poliovirus vaccine. Develop Biol Standard 47: 247-255, 1981 **16.** Bijerk, H.: Surveillance and control or poliomyelitis in the Netherlands. Rev Infect Dis 6 (Suppl 2): S451-S456, 1984 **17.** Lapinleimu, K.: Elimination or poliomyelitis in Finland. Rev Infect Dis 6 (Suppl 2): S457-S460, 1984 **18.** Immunization Practices Advisory Committee (ACIP), Poliomyelitis Prevention: Enhanced-Potency Inactivated Poliomyelitis Vaccine Supplementary Statement. MMWR 36: 795-798, 1987 **19.** ACIP: Poliomyelitis Prevention, MMWR 31: 22-26 and 31-34, 1982 **20.** Report of the Committee on Infectious Diseases, American Academy of Pediatrics, 21st ed: 334-342, 1988 **21.** ACIP: Immunization of children infected with human T-lymphotropic virus type III/lymphadenopathy-associated virus. MMWR 35: 595-606, 1986 **22.** WHO: Weekly Epidemiology Record 54: 82-83, 1979 **23.** National Childhood Vaccine Injury Act: Requirements for permanent vaccination records and for reporting of selected events after vaccination. MMWR 37: 197-200, 1988

HOW SUPPLIED - EQUIVALENTS NOT AVAILABLE:

Injection, Solution - Intravenous

0.5 ml	**$24.35**	**IPOL, Connaught Labs**	**49281-0860-51**
0.5 ml x 5	$107.69	POLIOVAX, Connaught Merieux	11793-8603-01
0.5 ml x 10	**$231.09**	**IPOL, Connaught Labs**	**49281-0860-52**

POLIO VACCINE, ORAL LIVE *(002061)*

CATEGORIES: Biologicals; Immunologic; Poliomyelitis; Serums, Toxoids and Vaccines; Vaccines; Pregnancy Category C; FDA Approval Pre 1982

BRAND NAMES: *Buccapol Berna*; *Imovax Polio Sabin*; *OPV-Merieux*; *Oral Polio Vaccine*; *Oral Poliomyelitis Vaccine-Sabine*; *Oral Virelon* (Germany); **Orimune**; *Polio Sabin* (Mexico); *Polio Sabin Oral*; *Polio "Sabin" Oral Vaccine*; *Polio Sabin OS*; *Polio Sabin-S* (Germany); *Polio-Kovax*; *Polioral*; *Poliovax*; *Tri-Polio*
(International brand names outside U.S. in italics)

FORMULARIES: WHO

DESCRIPTION:

Poliovirus vaccine live oral trivalent is a mixture of three types of attenuated polioviruses that have been propagated in monkey kidney cell culture. The cells are grown in the presence of Eagle's basal medium consisting of Earle's balanced salt solution containing amino acids, antibiotics, and calf serum. After cell growth, the medium is removed and replaced with fresh medium containing the inoculating virus but no calf serum. The final vaccine is diluted with a modified cell- culture maintenance medium containing sorbitol. Each dose (0.5 ml) contains less than 25 micrograms of each of the antibiotics, streptomycin and neomycin.

Potency of the vaccine is expressed in terms of the amount of virus (log10) contained in the recommended dose as tissue culture infective doses (TCID50). The human dose of vaccine containing all three virus types shall be constituted to have infectivity titers in the final container material of (10 to power 5.4) to (10 to power 6.4) for Type 1, (10 to power 4.5) to (10 to power 5.5) for Type 2, and (10 to power 5.2) to (10 to power 6.2) for Type 3, when the primary monkey kidney tube titration method is used. If the more sensitive Hep-2 microtitration procedure is employed to determine the infectivity titers in each human dose, then equivalent vaccine is achieved with numerical infectivity titers of (10 to power 6.0) to (10 to power 7.0) for Type 1, (10 to power 5.1) to (10 to power 6.1) for Type 2, and (10 to power 5.8) to (10 to power 6.8) for Type 3.

CLINICAL PHARMACOLOGY:

Administration of attenuated, live oral poliovirus vaccine (OPV) simulates natural infection, inducing active mucosal and systemic immunity without producing symptoms of disease. For optimal mucosal immunity to occur, it is necessary for the viruses to multiply in the intestinal tract. A primary series of trivalent vaccine is designed to produce an antibody response to poliovirus Types 1, 2, and 3. This response is comparable to the immunity induced by the natural disease. The antibodies thus formed help protect the individual against clinical poliomyelitis infection by any of the three types of poliovirus. Multiple sequential doses of OPV are administered to ensure that immunity to all three types of poliovirus has been achieved. When used in the prescribed manner for immunization, type-specific neutralizing antibodies will be induced in 95% or more of susceptibles.

INDICATIONS AND USAGE:

THIS VACCINE IS INDICATED FOR USE IN THE PREVENTION OF POLIOMYELITIS CAUSED BY POLIOVIRUS TYPES 1, 2, and 3.

INFANTS FROM 6 TO 12 WEEKS OF AGE, ALL UNIMMUNIZED CHILDREN, AND ADOLESCENTS up to age 18 are the usual candidates for routine prophylaxis.

The Immunization Practices Advisory Committee (ACIP) of the Public Health Service states that trivalent oral poliovirus vaccine (OPV) and inactivated poliovirus vaccine (IPV) are both effective in preventing poliomyelitis.

The choice of OPV as the preferred poliovirus vaccine for primary administration to children in the United States has been made by the ACIP, the Committee on Infectious Diseases of the American Academy of Pediatrics, and a special expert committee of the Institute of Medicine, National Academy of Science. OPV is preferred because it induces intestinal immunity, is simple to administer, is well accepted by patients, results in immunization of some contacts of vaccinated persons, and has a record of having essentially eliminated disease associated with wild poliovirus in this country. OPV is also recommended for control of epidemic poliomyelitis.

IPV is specifically indicated for use in immunodeficient individuals, their household contacts, or in certain adults (See CONTRAINDICATIONS and INDICATIONS AND USAGE: USE IN ADULTS for details).

Prior to immunization, the parent, guardian, or adult patient should be informed of the two types of poliovirus vaccines available, the risks and benefits of each to the individual and to the community, and the reasons why recommendations are made for giving specific vaccines under certain circumstances.

Past history of clinical poliomyelitis or prior vaccination with IPV in otherwise healthy individuals does not preclude the administration of OPV when otherwise indicated.

INDICATIONS AND USAGE: *(cont'd)*

The simultaneous administration of OPV, diphtheria and tetanus toxoids and pertussis vaccine (DTP), and/or measles-mumps-rubella vaccine (MMR), has resulted in seroconversion rates and rates of side effects similar to those observed when the vaccines are administered separately.

Administration of Immune Globulin (IG), if necessary, within 7 days prior to immunization with OPV does not reduce the antibody response to OPV based on a study conducted in Peace Corps volunteers.

Use In Adults: Routine primary poliovirus immunization of adults (generally those 18 years of age or older), residing in the United States, is not recommended by the Immunization Practices Advisory Committee (ACIP). Immunization is recommended by the ACIP for certain adults who are at greater risk of exposure to wild polioviruses than the general population, including travelers to areas where poliomyelitis is endemic or epidemic, members of communities or specific population groups with disease caused by wild polioviruses, laboratory workers handling specimens that may contain polioviruses, and health care workers in close contact with patients who might be excreting polioviruses as follows: UNIMMUNIZED ADULTS-primary immunization with enhanced-potency IPV is recommended. However, if less than 1 month is available before protection is needed, a single dose of either OPV or enhanced- potency IPV is recommended, with the remaining doses given later if the person remains at increased risk. INCOMPLETELY IMMUNIZED ADULTS who have had 1) at least one dose OPV, 2) fewer than three doses of conventional IPV, or 3) a combination of conventional IPV and OPV totaling fewer than three doses, should receive at least one dose of OPV or enhanced-potency IPV. Additional doses needed to complete a primary series should be given prior to exposure, if time permits. ADULTS WHO HAVE COMPLETED A PRIMARY SERIES with any one or a combination of polio vaccines may be given a dose of OPV or enhanced-potency IPV. Immunization with IPV may be undertaken in unimmunized or inadequately immunized adults in households in which children are to be given OPV (See ADVERSE REACTIONS.)

Epidemic Control: Poliovirus Vaccine Live Oral trivalent has been recommended for epidermic control. Within an epidemic are, OPV should be provided for all persons over 6 weeks of age who have not been completely immunized or whose immunization status is unknown, with the exceptions noted under immunodeficiency. (See CONTRAINDICATIONS.)

In certain tropical endemic areas, where poliomyelitis has been increasing in recent years, the physician may wish to administer OPV to the infant at birth. Because successful immunization is less likely in new born infants, a complete series of OPV should follow the neonatal dose beginning when the infants are 2 months old. If the physician elects to immunize the infant at birth, it may be prudent to wait until the child is 3 days old, and to recommend abstention from breast-feeding for 2 to 3 hours before and after oral immunization to minimize exposure of the vaccine viruses to colostrum and to permit the establishment of the vaccine viruses in the gut.

CONTRAINDICATIONS:

UNDER NO CIRCUMSTANCES SHOULD THIS VACCINE BE ADMINISTERED PARENTERALLY.

Poliovirus vaccine liver oral trivalent must not be administered to patients with immune deficiency diseases such as combined immunodeficiency, hypogammaglobulinemia and agammaglobulinemia. Further, poliovirus vaccine live oral trivalent must not be administered to patients with altered immune states, such as those occurring in human immunodeficiency virus (hiv) infection, thymic abnormalities, leukemia, lymphoma, generalized malignancy or advanced debilitating conditions, or by lowered resistance from therapy with corticosteroids, alkylating drugs, antimetabolites, or radiation. Because vaccine viruses are excreted by the vaccinee, and may spread to contacts, poliovirus vaccine live oral trivalent should not be used in families with immunodeficient members.

Recipients of the vaccine should avoid close household-type contact with all persons with altered immune status for at least 6 to 8 weeks.

Because of the possibility of immunodeficiency in other children born to a family in which there has been one such case, opv should not be given to a member of a household in which there is a family history of immunodeficiency until the immune status of the intended recipient and other children in the family is determined to be normal.

Immunization of all persons in the above described circumstances should be with ipv.

WARNINGS:

UNDER NO CIRCUMSTANCES SHOULD THIS VACCINE BE ADMINISTERED PARENTERALLY.

Immunization should be deferred during the course of any febrile illness or acute infection. In addition, immunization should be deferred in the presence of persistent vomiting or diarrhea, or suspected gastroenteritis infection. Other viruses (including poliovirus and other enteroviruses) may compromise the desired response to this vaccine, since their presence in the intestinal tract may interfere with the replication of the attenuated strains of poliovirus.

PRECAUTIONS:

The vaccine is not effective in modifying or preventing cases of existing and/or incubating poliomyelitis.

RECORDS REQUIRED BY THE NATIONAL CHILDHOOD VACCINE INJURY ACT

This act requires that the manufacturer and lot number of the vaccine administered be recorded by the health care provider in the vaccine recipient's permanent record, along with the date of administration of the vaccine and the name, address, and title of the person administering the vaccine.

The act further requires that the health care provider report to a health department or to the FDA the occurrence, following immunization, of any event set forth in the Vaccine Injury Table including: paralytic poliomyelitis - in a nonimmunodeficient recipient within 30 days of vaccination, - in an immunodeficient recipient within 6 months of vaccination; any vaccine-associated community case of paralytic poliomyelitis; or any acute complication or sequela (including death) of above events.

PREGNANCY CATEGORY C

Animal reproduction studies have not been conducted with Poliovirus Vaccine Live Oral Trivalent. It is also not known whether OPV can cause fetal harm when administered to a pregnant woman or can affect reproduction capacity.

Although there is no convincing evidence documenting adverse effects of either OPV or IPV on the developing fetus or pregnant women, it is prudent on theoretical grounds to avoid vaccinating pregnant women. However, if immediate protection against poliomyelitis is needed, OPV is recommended. (See CONTRAINDICATIONS and ADVERSE REACTIONS.)

ADVERSE REACTIONS:

Paralytic disease following the ingestion of live poliovirus vaccines has been, on rare occasion, reported in individuals receiving the vaccine, and in persons who were in close contact with vaccinees. The vaccine viruses are shed in the vaccinee's stools up to 6 to 8 weeks as well as via the pharyngeal route. Most reports of paralytic disease following

ADVERSE REACTIONS: *(cont'd)*

ingestion of the vaccine or contact with a recent vaccinee are based on epidemiological analysis and temporal association between vaccination or contact and the onset of symptoms and most authorities believe that a causal relationship exists.

A retrospective study of a large population given opv suggests that this vaccine may also be temporally associated with guillain-barre syndrome. A causal relationship has not been established.

Prior to administration of the vaccine, the attending physician should warn or specifically direct personnel acting under their authority to convey the WARNINGS to the vaccinee, parent, guardian, or other responsible person of the possibility of vaccine- associated paralysis, particularly to the recipient, susceptible family members and other close personal contacts.

The centers for disease control report that during the years 1973 through 1984 approximately 274.1 million opv doses were distributed in the united states. During this same period, 105 vaccine- associated cases were reported (1 case per 2.6 million doses distributed). Of these 105 cases, 35 occurred in vaccine recipients (1 case per 7.8 million doses distributed), 50 occurred in household and nonhousehold contacts of vaccinees (1 case per 5.5 million doses distributed), 14 occurred in immunodeficient recipients or contacts, and 6 occurred in persons with no history of vaccine exposure, from whom vaccine-like viruses were isolated. Thirty-three (94%) of the recipient cases, 41 (82%) of the contact cases, and 5 (35%) of the immune deficient cases were associated with the recipient's first dose of opv. Because most cases of vaccine-associated paralysis have occurred in association with the first dose, the cdc has estimated the likelihood of paralysis in association with first v subsequent doses of opv, using the number of births during 1973-1984 to estimate the number of first doses distributed, and subtracting this from the total distribution to estimate the number of subsequent doses distributed. This method estimates a frequency of paralysis for recipients of one case per 1.2 million first doses v one case per 25.9 million subsequent doses; with an overall frequency of 1 case per 520,000 first doses v one case per 12.3 million subsequent doses.

Other methods of estimating the likelihood of paralysis in association with opv have been described. Because the number of susceptible vaccine recipients or contacts of recipients is not known, the true risk of vaccine-associated poliomyelitis is impossible to determine precisely.

When the attenuated vaccine strains are to be introduced into a household with adults who are unimmunized or whose immune status cannot be determined, the risk of vaccine-associated paralysis can be reduced by giving these adults two doses of enhanced potency ipv a month apart before the children receive poliovirus vaccine live oral trivalent. The children may receive the first dose of poliovirus vaccine live oral trivalent at the same visit that the adults receive the second dose of enhanced potency ipv. For partially immunized adult contacts, a booster dose of enhanced potency ipv can be given at the same visit that the first dose of opv is given to the child.

The responsible adult should also be informed of PRECAUTIONS to be taken such as handwashing after diaper changes. The acip states: "because of the overriding importance of ensuring prompt and complete immunization of the child and the extreme rarity of opv-associated disease in contacts, the committee recommends the administration of opv to a child regardless of the poliovirus-vaccine status of adult household contacts. This is the usual practice in the united states. The responsible adult should be informed of the small risk involved. An acceptable alternative, if there is a strong assurance that ultimate, full immunization of the child will not be jeopardized or unduly delayed, is to immunize adults (with ipv) before giving opv to the child."

The American Academy of Pediatrics and the American College of Physicians have made similar recommendations.

DOSAGE AND ADMINISTRATION:

Poliovirus Vaccine Live Oral trivalent is to be administered ORALLY, UNDER THE SUPERVISION OF A PHYSICIAN. UNDER NO CIRCUMSTANCES SHOULD THIS VACCINE BE ADMINISTERED PARENTERALLY. For convenience, the vaccine is supplied in a disposable pipette containing a single dose of 0.5 ml which should be administered directly into the mouth of the vaccinee. Breast feeding does not interfere with successful immunization when OPV is administered according to the following schedule.

PRIMARY SERIES

The primary series consists of three doses.

Infants: The ACIP and AAP recommend that the first dose of OPV be administered when the infant is approximately 2 months (6-12 weeks) of age. The second dose should be given not less than 6 and preferably 8 weeks later, commonly at 4 months of age. A third dose of OPV should be given when the child is approximately 15 to 18 months of age to complete the primary series, but may be given at any time between 12 and 24 months of age. In endemic areas an additional dose administered 2 months after the second dose is desirable.

Older Children and Adolescents (up to 18 years of age): Unimmunized children and adolescents should receive two doses given not less than 6 and preferably 8 weeks apart, followed by a third dose 6 to 12 months after the second dose. If there is substantial risk of exposure to polio, the third dose should be given 6 to 8 weeks after the second dose.

Children at any age who are unimmunized or partially immunized should receive the number of doses necessary to complete the required series of three doses. If the schedule has been interrupted, the series does not need to be reinitiated.

Adults: See INDICATIONS AND USAGE and ADVERSE REACTIONS. Where OPV is given to unimmunized adults the dosage regimen is ad indicated for older children and adolescents.

Supplemental Doses / School Entry: On entering elementary school, all children who have completed the primary series should be given a single follow-up dose of OPV (all others should complete the primary series). The fourth supplemental dose is not required in those who received the third primary dose on or after their fourth birthday. The ACIP and AAP do not recommend routine booster doses of vaccine beyond that given at the time of entering school. It has been shown that over 95% of children studied 5 years after full immunization with oral polio vaccine had protective antibodies to all three types of poliovirus.

INCREASED RISK: If an individual who has completed a primary series is subjected to a substantially increased risk because of personal contact, travel, or occupation, a single dose of OPV may be given.

SIMULTANEOUS ADMINISTRATION WITH OTHER VACCINE

The simultaneous administration of OPV, diphtheria and tetanus toxoids and pertussis vaccine (DTP) and/or measles-mumps-rubella vaccine (MMR), has resulted in seroconversion rates and rates of side effects similar to those observed when the vaccines are administered separately. The AAP states that OPV, DTP, MMR and/or Haemophilus b conjugate vaccines may be given concomitantly.

Storage: To maintain potency of poliovirus vaccine live oral trivalent, it is necessary to store this vaccine at a temperature which will maintain ice continuously in a solid state (below 0°c, or 32°f). However, since the vaccine contains sorbitol it may remain fluid at temperature above -14°c (+7°f). Ice cubes that remain frozen continuously when stored in the same freezer compartment will confirm that the temperature is appropriate for storage of poliovirus vaccine live oral trivalent. If frozen, the vaccine must be completely thawed prior to use. A container of vaccine that has been frozen and then is thawed may be carried through a maximum of 10 freeze-thaw cycles, provided the temperature does not exceed 8 °c (46 °f) during the periods of thaw, and provided the total cumulative duration of thaw does not exceed 24 hours. If the 24-hour period is exceeded, the vaccine must be used within 30 days, during which time it must be stored at a temperature between 2 deg. C to 8°c (36°f to 46°f). Ideally, a poliovirus vaccine live oral trivalent dispette should be removed from the freezer and thawed immediately prior to use.

Color Change: This vaccine contains phenol red as a pH indicator. The usual color of the vaccine is pink, although some containers of vaccine, shipped or stored in dry ice, may exhibit a yellow coloration due to the very low temperature or possible absorption of carbon dioxide. The color of the vaccine prior to use (red- pink-yellow) has no effect on the virus or efficacy of the vaccine.

Directions For Use: Pull off the protective cap and squeeze to expel contents into the vaccinee's mouth.

HOW SUPPLIED - EQUIVALENTS NOT AVAILABLE:

Liquid - Oral - 3 unit

10's	$155.30	POLIOVIRUS VACCINELIVE, Lederle Pharm	00005-2084-08
50's	$723.69	POLIOVIRUS VACCINELIVE, Lederle Pharm	00005-2084-12

POLYETHYLENE GLYCOL 3350; POTASSIUM CHLORIDE; SODIUM BICARBONATE; SODIUM CHLORIDE; SODIUM SULFATE

(002065)

CATEGORIES: Bowel Evacuants; Cathartics & Laxatives; Electrolyte Solutions; Gastrointestinal Drugs; Laxatives; Pregnancy Category C; FDA Approved 1986 Apr

BRAND NAMES: Colav; Colovage; Colyte; E-Z-Em Prep Lyte; Glycoprep; Go-Evac; **Golytely**; Nulytely; Ocl; Peg 3350 Electrolyte

FORMULARIES: BC-BS; FHP

DESCRIPTION:

Note: The brand name of this drug has been left in, in order to avoid confusion.

Golytely is a white powder in a 4 liter jug for reconstitution, containing 236 g polyethylene glycol 3350, 22.74 g sodium sulfate (anhydrous), 6.74 g sodium bicarbonate, 5.86 g sodium chloride and 2.97 g potassium chloride. When dissolved in water to a volume of 4 liters, Golytely is an isosmotic solution having a mildly salty taste. Golytely is administered orally or via nasogastric tube.

CLINICAL PHARMACOLOGY:

Golytely induces a diarrhea which rapidly cleanses the bowel, usually within four hours. The osmotic activity of polyethylene glycol 3350 and the electrolyte concentration result in virtually no net absorption or excretion of ions or water. Accordingly, large volumes may be administered without significant changes in fluid or electrolyte balance.

INDICATIONS AND USAGE:

Golytely is indicated for bowel cleansing prior to colonoscopy and barium enema x-ray examination.

CONTRAINDICATIONS:

Golytely is contraindicated in patients with gastrointestinal obstruction, gastric retention, bowel perforation, toxic colitis, toxic megacolon or ileus.

WARNINGS:

No additional ingredients, e.g., flavorings, should be added to the solution. Golytely should be used with caution in patients with severe ulcerative colitis.

PRECAUTIONS:

General: Patients with impaired gag reflex, unconscious, or semiconscious patients, and patients prone to regurgitation or aspiration should be observed during the administration of Golytely, especially if it is administered via nasogastric tube. If a patient experiences severe bloating, distention or abdominal pain, administration should be slowed or temporarily discontinued until the symptoms abate. If gastrointestinal obstruction or perforation is suspected, appropriate studies should be performed to rule out these conditions before administration of Golytely.

Information for the Patient: Golytely produces a watery stool which cleanses the bowel before examination. Prepare the solution according to the instructions on the bottle. It is more palatable if chilled. For best results, no solid food should be consumed during the 3 to 4 hour period before drinking the solution, but in no case should solid foods be eaten within 2 hours of taking Golytely.

Drink 240 ml (8 oz.) every 10 minutes. Rapid drinking of each portion is better than drinking small amounts continuously. The first bowel movement should occur approximately one hour after the start of Golytely administration. You may experience some abdominal bloating and distention before the bowels start to move. If severe discomfort or distention occur, stop drinking temporarily or drink each portion at longer intervals until these symptoms disappear. Continue drinking until the watery stool is clear and free of solid matter. This usually requires at least 3 liters and is best to drink all the solution. Any unused portion should be discarded.

Carcinogenesis, Mutagenesis, and Impairment of Fertility: Carcinogenic and reproductive studies with animals have not been performed.

Pregnancy: Category C. Animal reproduction studies have not been conducted with Golytely. It is also not known whether Golytely can cause fetal harm when administered to a pregnant woman or can affect reproductive capacity. Golytely should be given to a pregnant woman only if clearly needed.

Pediatric Use: Safety and effectiveness in children have not been established.

DRUG INTERACTIONS:

Oral medication administered within one hour of the start of administration of Golytely may be flushed from the gastrointestinal tract and not absorbed.

ADVERSE REACTIONS:

Nausea, abdominal fullness and bloating are the most common adverse reactions (occurring in up to 50% of patients) to administration of Golytely. Abdominal cramps, vomiting and anal irritation occur less frequently. These adverse reactions are transient and subside rapidly. Isolated cases of urticaria rhinorrhea, dermatitis and (rarely) anaphylactic reaction have been reported which may represent allergic reactions.

DOSAGE AND ADMINISTRATION:

The recommended dose for adults is 4 liters of Golytely solution prior to gastrointestinal examination, as ingestion of this dose produces a satisfactory preparation in over 95% of patients. Ideally the patient should fast for approximately three or four hours prior to Golytely administration, but in no case should solid food be given for at least two hours before the solution is given.

Golytely is usually administered orally, but may be given via nasogastric tube to patients who are unwilling or unable to drink the solution. **Oral administration** is at a rate of 240 ml (8 oz.) every 10 minutes, until 4 liters are consumed or the rectal effluent is clear. Rapid drinking of each portion is preferred to drinking small amounts continuously. **Nasogastric tube administration** is at the rate of 20-30 ml per minute (1.2-1.8 liters per hour). The first bowel movement should occur approximately one hour after the start of Golytely administration. Various regimens have been used. One method is to schedule patients for examination in midmorning or later, allowing the patients three hours for drinking and an additional one hour period for complete bowel evacuation. Another method is to administer Golytely on the evening before the examination, particularly if the patient is to have a barium enema.

Preparation of the solution: Golytely solution is prepared by filling the container to the 4 liter mark with water and shaking vigorously several times to ensure that the ingredients are dissolved. Dissolution is facilitated by using lukewarm water. The solution is more palatable if chilled before administration. The reconstituted solution should be refrigerated and used within 48 hours. Discard any unused portion.

Storage: Store in sealed container at 59°-86°F. When reconstituted, keep solution refrigerated. Use within 48 hours. Discard unused portion.

HOW SUPPLIED - RATED THERAPEUTICALLY EQUIVALENT:

Powder, Reconstitution - Oral

1 gallon	$8.68	COLYTE FLAVORED, Schwarz Pharma (US)	00091-4403-13
4 liter	$13.94	COLYTE FLAVORED, Schwarz Pharma (US)	00091-4403-05
3785 ml	$7.68	COLYTE, Schwarz Pharma (US)	00091-4401-49
3840 ml	**$7.80**	**GOLYTELY, Braintree**	**52268-0700-01**
4000 ml	$12.00	Co-Lav, Goldline Labs	00182-7026-86
4000 ml	$12.25	GO-EVAC, Rugby	00536-2776-90
4000 ml	$12.32	COLYTE, Schwarz Pharma (US)	00091-4401-23
4000 ml	$12.48	Peg 3350/Electrolyte, Stafford Miller	55372-4460-01
4000 ml	$13.24	COLAV, Copley Pharm	38245-0688-18
4000 ml	$13.24	Go-Evac, Copley Pharm	38245-0690-18
4000 ml	**$15.04**	**GOLYTELY, Braintree**	**52268-0100-01**

HOW SUPPLIED - NOT RATED EQUIVALENT:

Powder, Reconstitution - Oral

6's	$61.69	PREPLYTE, E Z Em	10361-0308-01
3840 ml	$13.32	COLOVAGE, Dynapharm	55516-0101-01
4000 ml	$15.64	NULYTELY, Braintree	52268-0300-01

Solution - Oral - 6 gm/75 mg/168

1350 ml	$23.77	OCL, Abbott	00074-9099-16
4000 ml	$17.12	NULYTELY, Braintree	52268-0301-01

POLYMYXIN B SULFATE *(002066)*

CATEGORIES: Anti-Infectives; Antibiotics; Antimicrobials; Bacteremia; Meningitis; Polymyxins; Infections; Ocular Infections; Skin/Mucous Membrane Agents; Urinary Tract Infections; FDA Approval Pre 1982

BRAND NAMES: **Aerosporin**; *Polymyxin B* (Germany); Poly-Rx
(International brand names outside U.S. in italics)

> WARNING:
> When this drug is given intramuscularly and/or intrathecally, it should be given only to hospitalized patients, so as to provide constant supervision by a physician.
> Renal function should be carefully determined and patients with renal damage and nitrogen retention should have reduced dosage. Patients with nephrotoxicity due to polymyxin B sulfate usually show albuminuria, cellular casts, and azotemia. Diminishing urine output and a rising BUN are indications for discontinuing therapy with this drug.
> Neurotoxic reactions may be manifested by irritability, weakness, drowsiness, ataxia, perioral paresthesia, numbness of the extremities, and blurring of vision. These are usually associated with high serum levels found in patients with impaired renal function and/or nephrotoxicity. The concurrent use of other nephrotoxic and neurotoxic drugs, particularly kanamycin, streptomycin, cephaloridine, paromomycin, tobramycin, polymyxin E (colistin), neomycin, gentamicin, and viomycin, should be avoided.
> The neurotoxicity of polymyxin B sulfate can result in respiratory paralysis from neuromuscular blockade, especially when the drug is given soon after anesthesia and/or muscle relaxants.
> Usage in pregnancy: The safety of this drug in human pregnancy has not been established.

DESCRIPTION:

Polymyxin B sulfate is one of a group of basic polypeptide antibiotics derived from *B polymyxa (B aerosporous).*

Polymyxin B sulfate is in powder form suitable for preparation of sterile solutions for intramuscular, intravenous drip, intrathecal, or ophthalmic use.

In the medical literature, dosages have frequently been given in terms of equivalent weight of pure polymyxin B base. Each milligram of pure polymyxin B base is equivalent to 10,000 units of polymyxin B and each microgram of pure polymyxin B base is equivalent to 10 units of polymyxin B.

DESCRIPTION: *(cont'd)*

Aqueous solutions of polymyxin B sulfate may be stored up to 12 months without significant loss of potency if kept under refrigeration. In the interest of safety, solutions for parenteral use should be stored under refrigeration and any unused portion should be discarded after 72 hours. Polymyxin B sulfate should not be stored in alkaline solutions since they are less stable.

CLINICAL PHARMACOLOGY:

Polymyxin B sulfate has a bactericidal action against almost all gram-negative bacilli except the Proteus group. Polymyxins increase the permeability of bacterial cell wall membranes. All gram-positive bacteria, fungi, and the gram-negative cocci, *N gonorrhoeae* and *N meningitidis*, are resistant.

Susceptibility plate testing: If the Kirby-Bauer method of disc susceptibility testing is used, a 300-unit polymyxin B disc should give a zone of over 11 mm when tested against a polymyxin B-susceptible bacterial strain.

Polymyxin B sulfate is not absorbed from the normal alimentary tract. Since the drug loses 50 percent of its activity in the presence of serum, active blood levels are low. Repeated injections may give a cumulative effect. Levels tend to be higher in infants and children. The drug is excreted slowly by the kidneys. Tissue diffusion is poor and the drug does not pass the blood brain barrier into the cerebrospinal fluid. In therapeutic dosage, polymyxin B sulfate causes some nephrotoxicity with tubule damage to a slight degree.

INDICATIONS AND USAGE:

Acute Infections Caused by Susceptible Strains of *Pseudomonas aeruginosa.* Polymyxin B sulfate is a drug of choice in the treatment of infections of the urinary tract, meninges, and bloodstream caused by susceptible strains of *Ps aeruginosa.* It may also be used topically and subconjunctivally in the treatment of infections of the eye caused by susceptible strains of *Ps aeruginosa.*

It may be indicated in serious infections caused by susceptible strains of the following organisms, when less potentially toxic drugs are ineffective or contraindicated:

H influenzae, specifically meningeal infections.

Escherichia coli, specifically urinary tract infections.

Aerobacter aerogenes, specifically bacteremia.

Klebsiella pneumoniae, specifically bacteremia.

Note: In Meningeal Infections, polymyxin B sulfate Should Be Administered Only by the Intrathecal Route.

CONTRAINDICATIONS:

This drug is contraindicated in persons with a prior history of hypersensitivity reactions to the polymyxins.

PRECAUTIONS:

See BOXED WARNING.

Baseline renal function should be done prior to therapy, with frequent monitoring of renal function and blood levels of the drug during parenteral therapy.

Avoid concurrent use of a curariform muscle relaxant and other neurotoxic drugs (ether, tubocurarine, succinylcholine, gallamine, decamethonium and sodium citrate) which may precipitate respiratory depression. If signs of respiratory paralysis appear, respiration should be assisted as required, and the drug discontinued.

As with other antibiotics, use of this drug may result in overgrowth of nonsusceptible organisms, including fungi. If superinfection occurs, appropriate therapy should be instituted.

ADVERSE REACTIONS:

See BOXED WARNING.

Nephrotoxic Reactions: Albuminuria, cylinduria, azotemia, and rising blood levels without any increase in dosage.

Neurotoxic Reactions: Facial flushing, dizziness progressing to ataxia, drowsiness, peripheral paresthesias (circumoral and stocking-glove), apnea due to concurrent use of curariform muscle relaxants and other neurotoxic drugs or inadvertent overdosage, and signs of meningeal irritation with intrathecal administration; e.g., fever, headache, stiff neck, and increased cell count and protein cerebrospinal fluid.

Other Reactions Occasionally Reported: Drug fever, urticarial rash, pain (severe) at intramuscular injection sites, and thrombophlebitis at intravenous injection sites.

DOSAGE AND ADMINISTRATION:

PARENTERAL

Intravenous: Dissolve 500,000 units polymyxin B sulfate in 300-500 cc of 5 percent dextrose in water for continuous intravenous drip.

Adults and Children: 15,000-25,000 units/kg body weight/day in individuals with normal kidney function. This amount should be reduced from 15,000 units/kg downward for individuals with kidney impairment. Infusions may be given every 12 hours; however, the total daily dose must not exceed 25,000 units/kg/day.

Infants: Infants with normal kidney function may receive up to 40,000 units/kg/day without adverse effects.

Intramuscular. Not recommended routinely because of severe pain at injection sites, particularly in infants and children. Dissolve 500,000 units polymyxin B sulfate in 2 cc sterile distilled water (Water for Injection, U.S.P.) or sterile physiologic saline (Sodium Chloride Injection, U.S.P.) or 1 percent procaine hydrochloride solution.

Adults and Children: 25,000-30,000 units/kg/day. This should be reduced in the presence of renal impairment. The dosage may be divided and given at either 4-or 6-hour intervals.

Infants: Infants with normal kidney function may receive up to 40,000 units/kg/day without adverse effects.

Note: Doses as high as 45,000 units/kg/day have been used in limited clinical studies in treating prematures and newborn infants for sepsis caused by *Ps aeruginosa.*

Intrathecal: A treatment of choice for *Ps aeruginosa* meningitis. Dissolve 500,000 units polymyxin B sulfate in 10 cc of sterile physiologic saline (Sodium Chloride Injection, U.S.P.) for 50,000 units per ml dosage unit.

Adults and Children Over 2 Years of Age: Dosage is 50,000 units once daily intrathecally for 3-4 days, then 50,000 units once every other day for at least 2 weeks after cultures of the cerebrospinal fluid are negative and sugar content has returned to normal.

Children Under 2 Years of Age: 20,000 units once daily, intrathecally for 3-4 days or 25,000 units once every other day. Continue with a dose of 25,000 units once every other day for at least 2 weeks after cultures of the cerebrospinal fluid are negative and sugar content has returned to normal.

DOSAGE AND ADMINISTRATION: *(cont'd)*

IN THE INTEREST OF SAFETY, SOLUTIONS FOR PARENTERAL USE SHOULD BE STORED UNDER REFRIGERATION, AND ANY UNUSED PORTIONS SHOULD BE DISCARDED AFTER 72 HOURS.

TOPICAL

Ophthalmic: Dissolve 500,000 units polymyxin B sulfate in 20-50 cc sterile distilled water (Water for Injection, U.S.P.) or sterile physiologic saline (Sodium Chloride Injection, U.S.P.) for a 10,000-25,000 units per cc concentration.

For the treatment of *Ps aeruginosa* infections of the eye, a concentration of 0.1 percent to 0.25 percent (10,000 units to 25,000 units per cc) is administered 1-3 drops every hour, increasing the intervals as response indicates.

Subconjunctival injection of up to 10,000 units/day may be used for the treatment of *Ps aeruginosa* infections of the cornea and conjunctiva.

Note: Avoid total systemic and ophthalmic instillation over 25,000 units/kg/day.

Store at 15 to 25°C (59 to 77°F).

HOW SUPPLIED - RATED THERAPEUTICALLY EQUIVALENT:

Each - 100 mmunit

1's	$155.00	Polymyxin B Sulfate, Paddock Labs	00574-0402-10

Injection, Dry-Soln - Intramuscular; - 500000 unit/via

1's	$4.48	Polymyxin B Sulfate, Roerig	00049-0500-28

POLYMYXIN B SULFATE; TRIMETHOPRIM SULFATE *(002067)*

CATEGORIES: Anti-Infectives; Antibiotics; Blepharoconjunctivitis; Conjunctivitis; EENT Drugs; Eye, Ear, Nose, & Throat Preparations; Infections; Ocular Infections; Ocular Blepharitis; Ophthalmics; Pregnancy Category C; FDA Approved 1988 Oct

BRAND NAMES: **Polytrim**

FORMULARIES: Aetna; BC-BS; PCS

DESCRIPTION:

Polytrim Ophthalmic Solution (trimethoprim sulfate and polymyxin B sulfate) is a sterile antimicrobial solution for topical ophthalmic use. Each ml contains trimethoprim sulfate equivalent to 1 mg trimethoprim and polymyxin B sulfate 10,000 units. The vehicle contains benzalkonium chloride 0.004% (added as a preservative) and the inactive ingredients sodium chloride, sodium hydroxide or sulfuric acid (added to adjust pH), and Water for Injection.

Trimethoprim sulfate, 2,4-diamino-5-(3,4,5-trimethoxybenzyl)pyrimidine sulfate (2:1), is a white, odorless, crystalline powder with a molecular weight of 678.72.

Polymyxin B sulfate is the sulfate salt of polymyxin B_1 and B_2, which are produced by the growth of *Bacillus polymyxa* (Prazmowski) Migula (Fam. Bacillaceae). It has a potency of not less than 6,000 Polymyxin B units per mg, calculated on an anhydrous basis.

CLINICAL PHARMACOLOGY:

Trimethoprim is a synthetic antibacterial drug active against a wide variety of aerobic gram-positive and gram-negative ophthalmic pathogens. Trimethoprim blocks the production of tetrahydrofolic acid from dihydrofolic acid by binding to and reversibly inhibiting the enzyme dihydrofolate reductase. This binding is very much stronger for the bacterial enzyme than for the corresponding mammalian enzyme. For that reason, trimethoprim selectively interferes with bacterial biosynthesis of nucleic acids and proteins.

Polymyxin B, a cyclic lipopeptide antibiotic, is rapidly bactericidal for a variety of gram-negative organisms, especially *Pseudomonas aeruginosa.* It increases the permeability of the bacterial cell membrane by interacting with the phospholipid components of the membrane.

When used topically, trimethoprim and polymyxin B absorption through intact skin and mucous membranes is insignificant.

Blood samples were obtained from 11 human volunteers at 20 minutes, 1 hour and 3 hours following instillation in the eye of 2 drops of ophthalmic solution containing 1 mg trimethoprim and 10,000 units polymyxin B per ml. Peak serum concentrations were approximately 0.03 mcg/ml trimethoprim and 1 unit/ml polymyxin B.

Microbiology: *In vitro* studies have demonstrated that the anti-infective components of Polymyxin B-S-T-S are active against the following bacterial pathogens that are capable of causing external infections of the eye:

Trimethoprim: *Staphylococcus aureus* and *Staphylococcus epidermidis, Streptococcus pyogenes, Streptococcus faecalis, Streptococcus pneumoniae, Haemophilus influenzae, Haemophilus aegyptius, Escherichia coli, Klebsiella pneumoniae, Proteus mirabilis* (indole-negative), *Proteus vulgaris* (indole-positive), *Enterobacter aerogenes,* and *Serratia marcescens.*

Polymyxin B: *Pseudomonas aeruginosa, Escherichia coli, Klebsiella pneumoniae, Enterobacter aerogenes* and *Haemophilus influenzae.*

INDICATIONS AND USAGE:

Polymyxin B/Trimethoprim Ophthalmic Solution is indicated in the treatment of surface ocular bacterial infections, including acute bacterial conjunctivitis, and blepharoconjunctivitis, caused by susceptible strains of the following microorganisms: *Staphylococcus aureus, Staphylococcus epidermidis, Streptococcus pneumoniae, Streptococcus viridans, Haemophilus influenzae* and *Pseudomonas aeruginosa.**

* Efficacy for this organism in this organ system was studied in fewer than 10 infections.

CONTRAINDICATIONS:

Polymyxin B/Trimethoprim Ophthalmic Solution is contraindicated in patients with known hypersensitivity to any of its components.

WARNINGS:

NOT FOR INJECTION INTO THE EYE. If a sensitivity reaction to Polymyxin B/ Trimethoprim occurs, discontinue use. Polymyxin B/Trimethoprim Ophthalmic Solution is not indicated for the prophylaxis or treatment of ophthalmia neonatorum.

PRECAUTIONS:

GENERAL

As with other antimicrobial preparations, prolonged use may result in overgrowth of non-susceptible organisms, including fungi. If superinfection occurs, appropriate therapy should be initiated.

INFORMATION FOR THE PATIENT

Avoid contaminating the applicator tip with material from the eye, fingers, or other source. This precaution is necessary if the sterility of the drops is to be maintained.

PRECAUTIONS: *(cont'd)*

If redness, irritation, swelling or pain persists or increases, discontinue use immediately and contact your physician.

CARCINOGENESIS, MUTAGENESIS, AND IMPAIRMENT OF FERTILITY

Carcinogenesis: Long-term studies in animals to evaluate carcinogenic potential have not been conducted with polymyxin B sulfate or trimethoprim.

Mutagenesis: Trimethoprim was demonstrated to be non-mutagenic in the Ames assay. In studies at two laboratories no chromosomal damage was detected in cultured Chinese hamster ovary cells at concentrations approximately 500 times human plasma levels after oral administration; at concentrations approximately 1000 times human plasma levels after oral administration in these same cells a low level of chromosomal damage was induced at one of the laboratories. Studies to evaluate mutagenic potential have not been conducted with polymyxin B sulfate.

Impairment of Fertility: Polymyxin B sulfate has been reported to impair the motility of equine sperm, but its effects on male or female fertility are unknown.

No adverse effects on fertility or general reproductive performance were observed in rats given trimethoprim in oral dosages as high as 70 mg/kg/day for males and 14 mg/kg/day for females.

PREGNANCY, TERATOGENIC EFFECTS, PREGNANCY CATEGORY C

Animal reproduction studies have not been conducted with polymyxin B sulfate. It is not known whether polymyxin B sulfate can cause fetal harm when administered to a pregnant woman or can affect reproduction capacity.

Trimethoprim has been shown to be teratogenic in the rat when given in oral doses 40 times the human dose. In some rabbit studies, the overall increase in fetal loss (dead and resorbed and malformed conceptuses) was associated with oral doses 6 times the human therapeutic dose.

While there are no large well-controlled studies on the use of trimethoprim in pregnant women, Brumfitt and Pursell, in a retrospective study, reported the outcome of 186 pregnancies during which the mother received either placebo or oral trimethoprim in combination with sulfamethoxazole. The incidence of congenital abnormalities was 4.5% (3 of 66) in those who received placebo and 3.3% (4 of 120) in those receiving trimethoprim and sulfamethoxazole. There were no abnormalities in the 10 children whose mothers received the drug during the first trimester. In a separate survey, Brumfitt and Pursell also found no congenital abnormalities in 35 children whose mothers had received oral trimethoprim and sulfamethoxazole at the time of conception or shortly thereafter.

Because trimethoprim may interfere with folic acid metabolism, trimethoprim should be used during pregnancy only if the potential benefit justifies the potential risk to the fetus.

Nonteratogenic Effects: The oral administration of trimethoprim to rats at a dose of 70 mg/kg/day commencing with the last third of gestation and continuing through parturition and lactation caused no deleterious effects on gestation or pup growth and survival.

NURSING MOTHERS

It is not known whether this drug is excreted in human milk. Because many drugs are excreted in human milk, caution should be exercised when Polymyxin B/Trimethoprim Opthalmic Solution is administered to a nursing woman.

PEDIATRIC USE

Safety and effectiveness in children below the age of 2 months have not been established (see WARNINGS.)

ADVERSE REACTIONS:

The most frequent adverse reaction to Polymyxin B/Trimethoprim Ophthalmic Solution is local irritation consisting of increased redness, burning, stinging, and/or itching. This may occur on instillation, within 48 hours, or at any time with extended use. There are also multiple reports of hypersensitivity reactions consisting of lid edema, itching, increased redness, tearing, and/or circumocular rash.

Photosensitivity has been reported in patients taking oral trimethoprim.

DOSAGE AND ADMINISTRATION:

Adults: In mild to moderate infections, instill one drop in the affected eye(s) every three hours (maximum of 6 doses per day) for a period of 7 to 10 days.

Pediatric Use: Clinical studies have shown Polymyxin B/Trimethoprim to be safe and effective for use in children over two months of age. The dosage regimen is the same as for adults.

HOW SUPPLIED:

A sterile ophthalmic solution, each ml contains trimethoprim sulfate equivalent to 1 mg trimethoprim and polymyxin B sulfate 10,000 units in a plastic dropper bottle of 10 ml.

Store at 15°-25° C (59°-77° F) and protect from light.

(Allergan, Inc., 10/92, 70307 30-11/S)

HOW SUPPLIED - EQUIVALENTS NOT AVAILABLE:

Solution - Ophthalmic; Top - 10000 unit

10 ml	**$16.49**	**POLYTRIM OPTHALMIC, Allergan**	**00023-7824-10**

POLYRIBONUCLEOTIDE *(003085)*

CATEGORIES: AIDS Related Complex; Antivirals; Chronic Fatigue Syndrome; Hepatitis B; Lung Cancer; Melanoma; Myalgic Encephalomyelitis; Orphan Drugs; Renal Carcinoma; Recombinant DNA Origin; FDA Unapproved

BRAND NAMES: **Ampligen**

Prescribing information not available at time of publication.

POLYTHIAZIDE *(002068)*

CATEGORIES: Antihypertensives; Cardiovascular Drugs; Cirrhosis; Congestive Heart Failure; Diuretics; Edema; Electrolytic, Caloric-Water Balance; Glomerulonephritis; Heart Failure; Hypertension; Nephrotic Syndrome; Pregnancy; Renal Drugs; Renal Failure; Thiazides; FDA Approval Pre 1982

BRAND NAMES: *Drenusil* (Germany); *Nephril* (England); **Renese**
(International brand names outside U.S. in italics)

FORMULARIES: Medi-Cal

DESCRIPTION:

Polythiazide is designated generically as polythiazide, and chemically as 2*H*-1,2,4-Benzothiadiazine-7-sulfonamide, 6-chloro-3,4-dihydro-2- methyl-3-(((2,2,2-trifluoroethyl)thio) methyl)-, 1,1-dioxide. It is a white crystalline substance, insoluble in water but readily soluble in alkaline solution.

Inert Ingredients: dibasic calcium phosphate; lactose; magnesium stearate; polyethylene glycol; sodium laurel sulfate; starch; vanillin. The 2 mg tablets also contain: Yellow 6; Yellow 10.

CLINICAL PHARMACOLOGY:

The mechanism of action results in an interference with the renal tubular mechanism of electrolyte reabsorption. At maximal therapeutic dosage all thiazides are approximately equal in their diuretic potency. The mechanism whereby thiazides function in the control of hypertension is unknown.

INDICATIONS AND USAGE:

Polythiazide is indicated as adjunctive therapy in edema associated with congestive heart failure, hepatic cirrhosis, and corticosteroid and estrogen therapy.

Polythiazide has also been found useful in edema due to various forms of renal dysfunction as: Nephrotic syndrome; Acute glomerulonephritis; and Chronic renal failure.

Polythiazide is indicated in the management of hypertension either as the sole therapeutic agent or to enhance the effectiveness of other antihypertensive drugs in the more severe forms of hypertension.

Usage in Pregnancy: The routine use of diuretics in an otherwise healthy woman is inappropriate and exposes mother and fetus to unnecessary hazard. Diuretics do not prevent development of toxemia of pregnancy, and there is no satisfactory evidence that they are useful in the treatment of developed toxemia.

Edema during pregnancy may arise from pathological causes or from the physiologic and mechanical consequences of pregnancy. Thiazides are indicated in pregnancy when edema is due to pathologic causes, just as they are in the absence of pregnancy (however, see WARNINGS, below). Dependent edema in pregnancy, resulting from restriction of venous return by the expanded uterus, is properly treated through elevation of the lower extremities and use of support hose; use of diuretics to lower intravascular volume in this case is illogical and unnecessary. There is hypervolemia during normal pregnancy which is harmful to neither the fetus nor the mother (in the absence of cardiovascular disease), but which is associated with edema, including generalized edema, in the majority of pregnant women. If this edema produces discomfort, increased recumbency will often provide relief. In rare instances, this edema may cause extreme discomfort which is not relieved by rest. In these cases, a short course of diuretics may provide relief and may be appropriate.

CONTRAINDICATIONS:

Anuria. Hypersensitivity to this or other sulfonamide derived drugs.

WARNINGS:

Thiazides should be used with caution in severe renal disease. In patients with renal disease, thiazides may precipitate azotemia. Cumulative effects of the drug may develop in patients with impaired renal function.

Thiazides should be used with caution in patients with impaired hepatic function or progressive liver disease, since minor alterations of fluid and electrolyte balance may precipitate hepatic coma.

Thiazides may add to or potentiate the action of other antihypertensive drugs. Potentiation occurs with ganglionic or peripheral adrenergic blocking drugs.

Sensitivity reactions may occur in patients with a history of allergy or bronchial asthma.

The possibility of exacerbation or activation of systemic lupus erythematosus has been reported.

Usage in Pregnancy: Thiazides cross the placental barrier and appear in cord blood. The use of thiazides in pregnant women requires that the anticipated benefit be weighed against possible hazards to the fetus. These hazards include fetal or neonatal jaundice, thrombocytopenia, and possibly other adverse reactions which have occurred in the adult.

Nursing Mothers: Thiazides appear in breast milk. If use of the drug is deemed essential, the patient should stop nursing.

PRECAUTIONS:

Periodic determination of serum electrolytes to detect possible electrolyte imbalance should be performed at appropriate intervals.

All patients receiving thiazide therapy should be observed for clinical signs of fluid or electrolyte imbalance; namely, hyponatremia, hypochloremic alkalosis, and hypokalemia. Serum and urine electrolyte determinations are particularly important when the patient is vomiting excessively or receiving parenteral fluids. Medication such as digitalis may also influence serum electrolytes. Warning signs, irrespective of cause, are: dryness of mouth, thirst, weakness, lethargy, drowsiness, restlessness, muscle pains or cramps, muscular fatigue, hypotension, oliguria, tachycardia, and gastrointestinal disturbances such as nausea and vomiting.

Hypokalemia may develop with thiazides as with any other potent diuretic, especially with brisk diuresis, when severe cirrhosis is present, or during concomitant use of corticosteroids or ACTH.

Interference with adequate oral electrolyte intake will also contribute to hypokalemia. Digitalis therapy may exaggerate metabolic effects of hypokalemia especially with reference to myocardial activity.

Any chloride deficit is generally mild and usually does not require specific treatment except under extraordinary circumstances (as in liver disease or renal disease). Dilutional hyponatremia may occur in edematous patients in hot weather; appropriate therapy is water restriction, rather than administration of salt except in rare instances when the hyponatremia is life threatening. In actual salt depletion, appropriate replacement is the therapy of choice.

Hyperuricemia may occur or frank gout may be precipitated in certain patients receiving thiazide therapy.

Insulin requirements in diabetic patients may be increased, decreased, or unchanged. Latent diabetes mellitus may become manifest during thiazide administration.

Thiazide drugs may increase the responsiveness to tubocurarine.

The antihypertensive effects of the drug may be enhanced in the postsympathectomy patient.

Thiazides may decrease arterial responsiveness to norepinephrine. This diminution is not sufficient to preclude effectiveness of the pressor agent for therapeutic use.

If progressive renal impairment becomes evident, as indicated by a rising nonprotein nitrogen or blood urea nitrogen, a careful reappraisal of therapy is necessary with consideration given to withholding or discontinuing diuretic therapy.

Thiazides may decrease serum PBI levels without signs of thyroid disturbance.

ADVERSE REACTIONS:

GASTROINTESTINAL SYSTEM REACTIONS: anorexia, gastric irritation, nausea, vomiting, cramping, diarrhea, constipation, jaundice (intrahepatic cholestatic jaundice), pancreatitis

CENTRAL NERVOUS SYSTEM REACTIONS: dizziness, vertigo, paresthesias, headache, xanthopsia

HEMATOLOGIC REACTIONS: leukopenia, agranulocytosis, thrombocytopenia, aplastic anemia

DERMATOLOGIC/HYPERSENSITIVITY REACTIONS: purpura, photosensitivity, rash, urticaria, necrotizing angiitis, (vasculitis), (cutaneous vasculitis)

Cardiovascular Reaction: Orthostatic hypotension may occur and may be aggravated by alcohol, barbiturates or narcotics.

OTHER: hyperglycemia, glycosuria, hyperuricemia, muscle spasm, weakness, restlessness

Whenever adverse reactions are moderate or severe, thiazide dosage should be reduced or therapy withdrawn.

DOSAGE AND ADMINISTRATION:

Therapy should be individualized according to patient response. This therapy should be titrated to gain maximal therapeutic response as well as the minimal dose possible to maintain that therapeutic response. The usual dosage of Polythiazide tablets for diuretic therapy is 1 to 4 mg daily, and for antihypertensive therapy is 2 to 4 mg daily.

HOW SUPPLIED:

Polythiazide (polythiazide) tablets are available as:

1 mg white, scored tablets in bottles of 100.

2 mg yellow, scored tablets in bottles of 100

4 mg white, scored tablets in bottles of 100

HOW SUPPLIED - EQUIVALENTS NOT AVAILABLE:

Tablet, Uncoated - Oral - 1 mg

100's	$35.94	RENESE, Pfizer Labs	00069-3750-66

Tablet, Uncoated - Oral - 2 mg

100's	$47.04	RENESE, Pfizer Labs	00069-3760-66

Tablet, Uncoated - Oral - 4 mg

100's	$78.63	RENESE, Pfizer Labs	00069-3770-66

POLYTHIAZIDE; PRAZOSIN HYDROCHLORIDE *(002069)*

CATEGORIES: Antihypertensives; Cardiovascular Drugs; Diuretics; Hypertension; Renal Drugs; Thiazides; Pregnancy Category C; FDA Approval Pre 1982

BRAND NAMES: **Minizide**

FORMULARIES: Aetna

> WARNING:
> This fixed combination drug is not indicated for initial therapy of hypertension. Hypertension requires therapy titrated to the individual patient. If the fixed combination represents the dose so determined, its use may be more convenient in patient management. The treatment of hypertension is not static, but must be re-evaluated as conditions in each patient warrant.

DESCRIPTION:

FOR COMPLETE PRESCRIBING INFORMATION REFER TO THE INDIVIDUAL DRUG MONOGRAPHS (POLYTHIAZIDE; PRAZOSIN HYDROCHLORIDE).

DOSAGE AND ADMINISTRATION:

PRAZOSIN HYDROCHLORIDE/POLYTHIAZIDE

Dosage: as determined by individual titration of prazosin HCl and polythiazide. (See BOXED WARNING.)

Usual Polythiazide; Prazosin HCl dosage is one capsule two or three times daily, the strength depending upon individual requirement following titration.

The following is a general guide to the administration of the individual components of Polythiazide; Prazosin HCl:

PRAZOSIN HCL

Initial Dose: 1 mg two or three times a day.

Maintenance Dose: Dosage may be slowly increased to a total daily dose of 20 mg given in divided doses. The therapeutic dosages most commonly employed have ranged from 6 mg to 15 mg daily given in divided doses. Doses higher than 20 mg usually do not increase efficacy, however a few patients may benefit from further increases up to a daily dose of 40 mg given in divided doses. After initial titration some patients can be maintained adequately on a twice daily dosage regimen.

Use With Other Drugs: When adding a diuretic or other antihypertensive agent, the dose of prazosin HCl should be reduced to 1 mg or 2 mg three times a day and retitration then carried out.

POLYTHIAZIDE

The usual dose of polythiazide for antihypertensive therapy is 2 to 4 mg daily.

HOW SUPPLIED:

HOW SUPPLIED - EQUIVALENTS NOT AVAILABLE:

Capsule, Gelatin - Oral - 0.5 mg

100's	$53.59	MINIZIDE 1, Pfizer Pharm	00663-4300-66
100's	$67.47	MINIZIDE 2, Pfizer Pharm	00663-4320-66
100's	$102.34	MINIZIDE 5, Pfizer Pharm	00663-4360-66

POLYTHIAZIDE; RESERPINE *(002070)*

CATEGORIES: Antihypertensives; Cardiovascular Drugs; Diuretics; Hypertension; Renal Drugs; Thiazides; Vascular Disorders, Cerebral/Peripheral*; FDA Approval Pre 1982

* Indication not approved by the FDA

TABLE 1				
Strength	Components	Color	Capsule Code	Pkg. Size
Minizide 1	1 mg prazosin + 0.5 mg polythiazide	Blue-Green	430	.100's
Minizide 2	2 mg prazosin + 0.5 mg polythiazide	Blue-Green/ Pink	432	100's
Minizide 5	5 mg prazosin + 0.5 mg polythiazide	Blue-Green/ Blue	436	100's

BRAND NAMES: **Renese-R**

FORMULARIES: Medi-Cal

WARNING:
This fixed combination drug is not indicated for initial therapy of hypertension. Hypertension requires therapy titrated to the individual patient. If the fixed combination represents the dosage so determined, its use may be more convenient in patient management. The treatment of hypertension is not static, but must be reevaluated as conditions in each patient warrant.

DESCRIPTION:

FOR COMPLETE PRESCRIBING INFORMATION REFER TO THE INDIVIDUAL DRUG MONOGRAPHS (POLYTHIAZIDE; RESERPINE).

INDICATIONS AND USAGE:

Hypertension.

DOSAGE AND ADMINISTRATION:

As determined by individual titration.

Initial dosages of the combination should conform to those dosages of the individual components established during titration.

Maintenance dosages range from 1/2 tablet to 2 tablets daily. Dosage of other antihypertensive agents, particularly ganglionic blockers, that are used concomitantly should be reduced.

HOW SUPPLIED:

Renese-R tablets (2 mg polythiazide-0.25 mg reserpine) are available as blue scored tablets, tablet code 446, in bottles of 100 and 1,000. Polythiazide;Resperine should be stored at room temperature. Dispense in tight, light resistant container.

HOW SUPPLIED - EQUIVALENTS NOT AVAILABLE:

Tablet, Uncoated - Oral - 2 mg/0.25 mg

100's $68.22 RENESE R, Pfizer Labs 00069-4460-66

PORFIMER SODIUM *(003228)*

CATEGORIES: Antineoplastics; Cancer; Cytotoxic Agents; Chemotherapy; Esophageal Cancer; Pregnancy Category C; FDA Approved 1995 Dec

BRAND NAMES: **Photofrin**

DESCRIPTION:

Photofrin (Porfimer Sodium) for Injection is a photosensitizing agent used in the photodynamic therapy (PDT) of tumors. Following reconstitution of the freeze-dried product with 5% Dextrose Injection (USP) or 0.9% Sodium Chloride Injection (USP), it is injected intravenously. This is followed 40-50 hours later by illumination of the tumor with laser light (630 nm wavelength). Porfimer sodium is not a single chemical entity; it is a mixture of oligomers formed by ether and ester linkages of up to eight porphyrin units. It is a dark red to reddish brown cake or powder. Each vial of Photofrin contains 75 mg of porfimer sodium as a sterile freeze-dried cake or powder. Hydrochloric Acid and/or Sodium Hydroxide may be added during manufacture to adjust pH. There are no preservatives or other additives.

CLINICAL PHARMACOLOGY:

PHARMACOLOGY

The cytotoxic and antitumor actions of porfimer sodium are light and oxygen dependent. Photodynamic therapy (PDT) with porfimer sodium is a two-stage process. The first stage is the intravenous injection of porfimer sodium. Clearance from a variety of tissues occurs over 40-72 hours, but tumors, skin, and organs of the reticuloendothelial system (including liver and spleen) retain porfimer sodium for a longer period. Illumination with 630 nm wavelength laser light constitutes the second stage of therapy. Tumor selectivity in treatment occurs through a combination of selective retention of porfimer sodium and selective delivery of light. Cellular damage caused by porfimer sodium PDT is a consequence of the propagation of radical reactions. Radical initiation may occur after porfimer sodium absorbs light to form a porphyrin excited state. Spin transfer from porfimer sodium to molecular oxygen may then generate singlet oxygen. Subsequent radical reactions can form superoxide and hydroxyl radicals. Tumor death also occurs through ischemic necrosis secondary to vascular occlusion that appears to be partly mediated by thromboxane A_2 release. The laser treatment induces a photochemical, not a thermal, effect.

PHARMACOKINETICS

Following a 2 mg/kg dose of porfimer sodium to 4 male cancer patients, the average peak plasma concentration was 15 ± 3 mcg/mL, the elimination half-life was 250 ± 285 hours, the steady-state volume of distribution was 0.49 ± 0.28 L/kg, and the total plasma clearance was 0.051 ± 0.035 mL/min/kg. The mean plasma concentration at 48 hours was 2.6 ± 0.4 mcg/mL. The influence of impaired hepatic function on porfimer sodium disposition has not been evaluated.

Porfimer sodium was approximately 90% protein bound in human serum, studied *in vitro*. The binding was independent of concentration over the concentration range of 20-100 mcg/mL.

CLINICAL STUDIES:

PDT with porfimer sodium was utilized in a multicenter, single-arm study in 17 patients with completely obstructing esophageal carcinoma. Each course of PDT with porfimer sodium consisted of one injection of the drug (2 mg/kg administered as a slow intravenous injection over 3-5 minutes) followed by up to two nonthermal laser light applications (630 nm administered at a dose of 300 J/cm of tumor), the first application of light occurring 40-50 hours after injection. Debridement of residua was performed via endoscopy 96-120 hours after injection, after which any residual tumor could be retreated with a second laser light application at the same dose used for the initial treatment. Additional courses of PDT with porfimer sodium were allowed after 1 month, up to a total of 3. Assessments were made at 1 week and 1 month after the last treatment procedure. As shown in TABLE 1, after a single course of therapy, 94% of patients obtained an objective tumor response and 76% of patients experienced some palliation of their dysphagia. On average, before treatment these patients had difficulty swallowing liquids, even saliva. After one course of therapy, there was a statistically significant improvement in mean dysphagia grade (1.5 units, $p < 0.05$) and 13 of 17 patients could swallow liquids without difficulty 1 week and/or 1 month after treatment. Based on all courses, three patients achieved a complete tumor response (CR). In two of these patients, the CR was documented only at Week 1 as they had no further assessments. The third patient achieved a CR after a second course of therapy, which was supported by negative histopathology and maintained for the entire follow-up of 6 months.

Of the 17 treated patients, 11 (65%) received clinically important benefit from PDT. Clinically important benefit was defined hierarchically as a complete tumor response (3 patients), achievement of normal swallowing (2 patients went from Grade 5 dysphagia to Grade 1), or achievement of a marked improvement of two or more grades of dysphagia with minimal adverse reactions (6 patients). The median duration of benefit in these patients was 69 + days. Duration of benefit was calculated only for the period with documented evidence of improvement. All of these patients were still in response at their last assessment and, therefore, the estimate of 69 days is conservative. The median survival for these 11 patients was 115 days.

TABLE 1 Course 1 Efficacy Results in Patients with Completely Obstructing Esophagel Cancer

	PDT n=17
IMPROVEMENT[a] IN DYSPHAGIA	
Week 1	71%
Month 1	47%
Any assessment[b]	76%
MEAN DYSPHAGIA GRADE[c] AT BASELINE	4.6
MEAN IMPROVEMENT[c] IN DYSPHAGIA GRADE (units)	
Week 1	1.4
Month 1	1.5
OBJECTIVE TUMOR RESPONSE[d]	
Week 1	82%
Month 1	35%[e]
Any assessment[b]	94%
MEAN NUMBER OF LASER APPLICATIONS PER PATIENT	1.4

a Patients with at least a one-grade improvement in dysphagia grade
b Week 1 or Month 1
c Dysphagia Scale: Grade 1 = normal swallowing, Grade 2 = difficulty swallowing some hard solids; can swallow semisolids, Grade 3 = unable to swallow any solids; can swallow liquids, Grade 4 = difficulty swallowing liquids, Grade 5 = unable to swallow saliva.
d CR + PR, CR = complete response (absence of endoscopically visible tumor), PR = partial response (appearance of a visible lumen)
e Eight of the 17 treated patients did not have assessments at Month 1.

INDICATIONS AND USAGE:

Photodynamic therapy with porfimer sodium is indicated for palliation of patients with completely obstructing esophageal cancer, or of patients with partially obstructing esophageal cancer who, in the opinion of their physician, cannot be satisfactorily treated with Nd:YAG laser therapy.

CONTRAINDICATIONS:

Porfimer sodium is contraindicated in patients with porphyria or in patients with known allergies to porphyrins.

PDT is contraindicated in patients with an existing tracheoesophageal or bronchoesophageal fistula.

PDT is contraindicated in patients with tumors eroding into a major blood vessel.

WARNINGS:

If the esophageal tumor is eroding into the trachea or bronchial tree, the likelihood of tracheoesophageal or bronchoesophageal fistula resulting from treatment is sufficiently high that PDT is not recommended.

Following injection with porfimer sodium precautions must be taken to avoid exposure of skin and eyes to direct sunlight or bright indoor light (see PRECAUTIONS, General Precautions and Information for Patients).

PRECAUTIONS:

GENERAL PRECAUTIONS AND INFORMATION FOR PATIENTS

Photosensitivity: All patients who receive porfimer sodium will be photosensitive and must observe precautions to avoid exposure of skin and eyes to direct sunlight or bright indoor light (from examination lamps, including dental lamps, operating room lamps, unshaded light bulbs at close proximity, etc.) for 30 days. The photosensitivity is due to residual drug which will be present in all parts of the skin. Exposure of the skin to ambient indoor light is, however, beneficial because the remaining drug will be inactivated gradually and safely through a photobleaching reaction. Therefore, patients should not stay in a darkened room during this period and should be encouraged to expose their skin to ambient indoor light. The level of photosensitivity will vary for different areas of the body, depending on the extent of previous exposure to light. Before exposing any area of skin to direct sunlight or bright indoor light, the patient should test it for residual photosensitivity. A small area of skin should be exposed to sunlight for 10 minutes. If no photosensitivity reaction (erythema, edema, blistering) occurs within 24 hours, the patient can gradually resume normal outdoor activities, initially continuing to exercise caution and gradually allowing increased exposure. If some photosensitivity reaction occurs with the limited skin test, the patient should continue precautions for another 2 weeks before retesting. The tissue around the eyes may be more sensitive, and therefore, it is not recommended that the face be used for testing. If patients travel to a different geographical area with greater sunshine, they should retest their level of photosensitivity. **UV (ultraviolet) sunscreens are of no value in protecting against photosensitivity reactions because photoactivation is caused by visible light.**

OCULAR SENSITIVITY

Ocular discomfort, commonly described as sensitivity to sun, bright lights, or car headlights, has been reported in patients who received porfimer sodium. For 30 days, when outdoors, patients should wear dark sunglasses which have an average white light transmittance of < 4%.

PRECAUTIONS: *(cont'd)*

CHEST PAIN

As a result of PDT treatment, patients may complain of substernal chest pain because of inflammatory responses within the area of treatment. Such pain may be of sufficient intensity to warrant the short-term prescription of opiate analgesics.

AVOIDANCE OF PREGNANCY

Women of childbearing potential should practice an effective method of contraception during therapy (see Pregnancy).

CARCINOGENESIS, MUTAGENESIS, AND IMPAIRMENT OF FERTILITY

No long-term studies have been conducted to evaluate the carcinogenic potential of porfimer sodium. *In vitro*, porfimer sodium PDT did not cause mutations in the Ames test, nor did it cause chromosome aberrations or mutations (HGPRT locus) in Chinese hamster ovary (CHO) cells. Porfimer sodium caused < 2-fold, but significant, increases in sister chromatid exchange in CHO cells irradiated with visible light and a 3-fold increase in Chinese hamster lung fibroblasts irradiated with near UV light. Porfimer sodium PDT caused an increase in thymidine kinase mutants and DNA-protein cross-links in mouse L5178Y cells, but not mouse LYR83 cells. Porfimer sodium PDT caused a light-dose dependent increase in DNA-strand breaks in malignant human cervical carcinoma cells, but not in normal cells. The mutagenicity of porfimer sodium without light has not been adequately determined.*In vivo*, porfimer sodium did not cause chromosomal aberrations in the mouse micronucleus test.

Porfimer sodium given to male and female rats intravenously, at 4 mg/kg/d (0.32 times the clinical dose on a mg/m^2 basis) before conception and through Day 7 of pregnancy caused no impairment of fertility. In this study, long-term dosing with porfimer sodium caused discoloration of testes and ovaries and hypertrophy of the testes. Porfimer sodium also caused decreased body weight in the parent rats.

PREGNANCY CATEGORY C

There are no adequate and well-controlled studies in pregnant women. Porfimer sodium should be used during pregnancy only if the potential benefit justifies the potential risk to the fetus.

Porfimer sodium given to rat dams during fetal organogenesis intravenously at 8 mg/kg/d (0.64 times the clinical dose on a mg/m^2basis) for 10 days caused no major malformations or developmental changes. This dose caused maternal and fetal toxicity resulting in increased resorptions, decreased litter size, delayed ossification, and reduced fetal weight. Porfimer sodium caused no major malformations when given to rabbits intravenously during organogenesis at 4 mg/kg/d (0.65 times the clinical dose on a mg/m^2basis) for 13 days. This dose caused maternal toxicity resulting in increased resorptions, decreased litter size, and reduced fetal body weight.

Porfimer sodium given to rats during late pregnancy through lactation intravenously at 4 mg/kg/d (0.32 times the clinical dose on a mg/m^2basis) for at least 42 days caused a reversible decrease in growth of offspring. Parturition was unaffected.

NURSING MOTHERS

It is not known whether this drug is excreted in human milk. Because many drugs are excreted in human milk and because of the potential for serious adverse reactions in nursing infants from porfimer sodium, women receiving porfimer sodium must not breast feed.

PEDIATRIC USE

Safety and effectiveness in children have not been established.

USE IN ELDERLY PATIENTS

Almost 80% of the patients treated with PDT using porfimer sodium in clinical trials were over 60 years of age. There was no apparent difference in effectiveness or safety in these patients compared to younger people. Dose modification based upon age is not required.

DRUG INTERACTIONS:

There have been no formal interaction studies of porfimer sodium and any other drugs. However, it is possible that concomitant use of other photosensitizing agents (*e.g.*, tetracyclines, sulfonamides, phenothiazines, sulfonylurea, hypoglycemic agents, thiazide diuretics, and griseofulvin) could increase the photosensitivity reaction.

Porfimer sodium PDT causes direct intracellular damage by initiating radical chain reactions that damage intracellular membranes and mitochondria. Tissue damage also results from ischemia secondary to vasoconstriction, platelet activation and aggregation and clotting. Research in animals and in cell culture has suggested that many drugs could influence the effects of PDT, possible examples of which are described below. There are no human data that support or rebut these possibilities.

Compounds that quench active oxygen species or scavenge radicals, such as dimethyl sulfoxide, b-carotene, ethanol, formate and mannitol would be expected to decrease PDT activity. Preclinical data also suggest that tissue ischemia, allopurinol, calcium channel blockers and some prostaglandin synthesis inhibitors could interfere with porfimer sodium PDT. Drugs that decrease clotting, vasoconstriction or platelet aggregation, e.g., thromboxane A2 inhibitors, could decrease the efficacy of PDT. Glucocorticoid hormones given before or concomitant with PDT may decrease the efficacy of the treatment.

ADVERSE REACTIONS:

Systemically induced effects associated with PDT with porfimer sodium consist of photosensitivity and mild constipation. All patients who receive porfimer sodium will be photosensitive and must observe precautions to avoid sunlight and bright indoor light (see PRECAUTIONS). Photosensitivity reactions (mostly mild erythema on the face and hands) occurred in approximately 20% of patients treated with porfimer sodium.

Most toxicities associated with this therapy are local effects seen in the region of illumination and occasionally in surrounding tissues. The local adverse reactions are characteristic of an inflammatory response induced by the photodynamic effect.

ESOPHAGEAL CARCINOMA

The following adverse events were reported in at least 5% of patients treated with porfimer sodium PDT, who had completely or partially obstructing esophageal cancer. Table 2 presents data from 88 patients who received the currently marketed formulation. The relationship of many of these adverse events to PDT with porfimer sodium is uncertain.

Location of the tumor was a prognostic factor for three adverse events: upper-third of the esophagus (esophageal edema), middle-third (atrial fibrillation), and lower-third, the most vascular region (anemia). Also, patients with large tumors (> 10 cm) were more likely to experience anemia. Two of 17 patients with complete esophageal obstruction from tumor experienced esophageal perforations which were considered to be possibly treatment associated; these perforations occurred during subsequent endoscopies.

Serious and other notable adverse events observed in less than 5% of PDT-treated patients in the clinical studies include the following; their relationship to therapy is uncertain. In the gastrointestinal system, esophageal perforation, gastric ulcer, ileus, jaundice, and peritonitis have occurred. Sepsis has been reported occasionally. Cardiovascular events have included angina pectoris, bradycardia, myocardial infarction, sick sinus syndrome, and supraventricular tachycardia. Respiratory events of bronchitis, bronchospasm, laryngotracheal edema, pneumonitis, pulmonary hemorrhage, pulmonary edema, respiratory failure, and stridor have occurred. The temporal relationship of some gastrointestinal, cardiovascular and respiratory

ADVERSE REACTIONS: *(cont'd)*

TABLE 2 Adverse Events Reported in 5% or More of Patients with Obstructing Esophageal Cancer

BODY SYSTEM/ Adverse Event	PDT n=88	
Patients with at Least One Adverse Event	84	(95)
AUTONOMIC NERVOUS SYSTEM		
Hypertension	5	(6)
Hypotension	6	(7)
BODY AS A WHOLE		
Asthenia	5	(6)
Back pain	10	(11)
Chest pain	19	(22)
Chest pain (substernal)	4	(5)
Edema generalized	4	(5)
Edema peripheral	6	(7)
Fever	27	(31)
Pain	19	(22)
Surgical complication	4	(5)
CARDIOVASCULAR		
Cardiac failure	6	(7)
GASTROINTESTINAL		
Abdominal pain	18	(20)
Constipation	21	(24)
Diarrhea	4	(5)
Dyspepsia	5	(6)
Dysphagia	9	(10)
Eructation	4	(5)
Esophageal edema	7	(8)
Esophageal tumor bleeding	7	(8)
Esophageal stricture	5	(6)
Esophagitis	4	(5)
Hematemesis	7	(8)
Melena	4	(5)
Nausea	21	(24)
Vomiting	15	(17)
HEART RATE / RHYTHM		
Atrial fibrillation	9	(10)
Tachycardia	5	(6)
METABOLIC & NUTRITIONAL		
Dehydration	6	(7)
Weight decrease	8	(9)
PSYCHIATRIC		
Anorexia	7	(8)
Anxiety	6	(7)
Confusion	7	(8)
Insomnia	12	(14)
RED BLOOD CELL		
Anemia	28	(32)
RESISTANCE MECHANISM		
Moniliasis	8	(9)
RESPIRATORY		
Coughing	6	(7)
Dyspnea	18	(20)
Pharyngitis	10	(11)
Pleural effusion	28	(32)
Pneumonia	16	(18)
Respiratory insufficiency	9	(10)
Tracheoesophageal fistula	5	(6)
SKIN & APPENDAGES		
Photosensitivity reaction	17	(19)
URINARY		
Urinary tract infection	6	(7)

events to the administration of light was suggestive of mediastinal inflammation in some patients. Vision-related events of abnormal vision, diplopia, eye pain and photophobia have been reported.

LABORATORY ABNORMALITIES

PDT with porfimer sodium may result in anemia due to tumor bleeding. No consistent effects were observed for other parameters.

OVERDOSAGE:

There is no information on overdosage situations involving porfimer sodium. Effects of overdosage on the duration of photosensitivity are unknown. Laser treatment should not be given if an overdose of porfimer sodium is administered. In the event of an overdose, patients should protect their eyes and skin from direct sunlight or bright indoor lights for 30 days. At this time, patients should test for residual photosensitivity (see PRECAUTIONS). Porfimer sodium is not dialyzable.

OVERDOSE OF LASER LIGHT FOLLOWING PORFIMER SODIUM INJECTION

There is no information on overdose of laser light following porfimer sodium injection in patients with esophageal carcinoma. Increased symptoms and damage to normal tissue might be expected following an overdose of light.

DOSAGE AND ADMINISTRATION:

Photodynamic therapy with porfimer sodium is a two-stage process requiring administration of both drug and light. Practitioners should be trained in the safe and efficacious treatment of esophageal cancer using photodynamic therapy with porfimer sodium and associated light delivery devices. The first stage of PDT is the intravenous injection of porfimer sodium at 2 mg/kg. Illumination with laser light 40-50 hours following injection with porfimer sodium constitutes the second stage of therapy. A second laser light application may be given 96-120 hours after injection, preceded by gentle debridement of residual tumor (see Administration of Laser Light). In clinical studies, debridement via endoscopy was required 2 days after the initial light application. More recently, experienced investigators have indicated that mandatory debridement may not be necessary due to natural sloughing action in the esophagus, and may needlessly traumatize the area.

Patients may receive a second course of PDT a minimum of 30 days after the initial therapy; up to three courses of PDT (each separated by a minimum of 30 days) can be given. Before each course of treatment, patients should be evaluated for the presence of a tracheoesophageal or bronchoesophageal fistula (see CONTRAINDICATIONS).

PORFIMER SODIUM ADMINISTRATION

Porfimer sodium should be administered as a single slow intravenous injection over 3 to 5 minutes at 2 mg/kg body weight. Reconstitute each vial of porfimer sodium with 31.8 mL of either 5% Dextrose Injection (USP) or 0.9% Sodium Chloride Injection (USP), resulting in a final concentration of 2.5 mg/mL. Shake well until dissolved. Do not mix porfimer sodium with other drugs in the same solution. Porfimer sodium, reconstituted with 5% Dextrose Injection (USP) or with 0.9% Sodium Chloride Injection (USP), has a pH in the range of 7 to

DOSAGE AND ADMINISTRATION: *(cont'd)*

8. Porfimer sodium has been formulated with an overage to deliver the 75 mg labeled quantity. The reconstituted product should be protected from bright light and used immediately. Reconstituted porfimer sodium is an opaque solution, in which detection of particulate matter by visual inspection is extremely difficult. Reconstituted porfimer sodium, however, like all parenteral drug products, should be inspected visually for particulate matter and discoloration prior to administration whenever solution and container permit.

Precautions should be taken to prevent extravasation at the injection site. If extravasation occurs, care must be taken to protect the area from light. There is no known benefit from injecting the extravasation site with another substance.

ADMINISTRATION OF LASER LIGHT

Initiate 630 nm wavelength laser light delivery to the patient 40-50 hours following injection with porfimer sodium. A second laser light treatment may be given as early as 96 hours or as late as 120 hours after the initial injection with porfimer sodium. No further injection of porfimer sodium should be given for such retreatment with laser light. Before providing a second laser light treatment, the residual tumor should be debrided. Vigorous debridement may cause tumor bleeding.

The laser system must be approved for delivery of a stable power output at a wavelength of 630 ± 3 nm. Light is delivered to the tumor by cylindrical Optiguide fiber optic diffusers passed through the operating channel of an endoscope. Instructions for use of the fiber optic and the selected laser system should be read carefully before use. Photoactivation of porfimer sodium is controlled by the total light dose delivered. In the treatment of esophageal cancer, a light dose of 300 joules/cm of tumor length should be delivered. Optiguide cylindrical diffusers are available in several lengths. The choice of diffuser tip length depends on the length of the tumor. Diffuser length should be sized to avoid exposure of nonmalignant tissue to light and to prevent overlapping of previously treated malignant tissue. The total power output at the fiber tip is set to deliver the appropriate light dose using exposure times of 12 minutes and 30 seconds. Refer to the Optiguide instructions for use for complete instructions concerning the fiber optic diffuser.

HOW SUPPLIED:

Photofrin (porfimer sodium) for Injection is supplied as a freeze-dried cake or powder as 75 mg vial Photofrin freeze-dried cake or powder should be stored at Controlled Room Temperature 20-25°C (68-77°F).

SPILLS AND DISPOSAL

Spills of porfimer sodium should be wiped up with a damp cloth. Skin and eye contact should be avoided due to the potential for photosensitivity reactions upon exposure to light; use of rubber gloves and eye protection is recommended. All contaminated materials should be disposed of in a polyethylene bag in a manner consistent with local regulations.

ACCIDENTAL EXPOSURE

Porfimer sodium is neither a primary ocular irritant nor a primary dermal irritant. However, because of its potential to induce photosensitivity, porfimer sodium might be an eye and/or skin irritant in the presence of bright light. It is important to avoid contact with the eyes and skin during preparation and/or administration. As with therapeutic overdosage, any overexposed person must be protected from bright light.

HOW SUPPLIED - EQUIVALENTS NOT AVAILABLE:

Injection - Intravenous - 75 mg

10's	$2573.43	PHOTOFRIN, Sanofi Winthrop	00024-1550-01

POTASSIUM *(002073)*

CATEGORIES: Electrolyte Solutions*; Caloric-Water Balance*; FDA Pre 1938 Drugs*; Homeostatic & Nutrient*; Hypokalemia*; Potassium Supplements*; Pregnancy Category C*; Replacement Solutions*
* Indication not approved by the FDA

BRAND NAMES: Bio-K; Double K; Duo-K; Effer-K; Gen-K; K-Effervesent; K-Electrolyte; **K-Lyte**; K-Vesent; Klor-Con/EF; Kolyum; Potassium Bicarbonate; Tri-K; Trikates

Prescribing information not available at time of publication.

HOW SUPPLIED - EQUIVALENTS NOT AVAILABLE:

Liquid - Oral - 20 meq/15 ml

480 ml	$6.44	DUO-K, Rugby	00536-0680-85

Liquid - Oral - 45 meq/15 ml

480 ml	$8.85	Tri-K, Century Pharms	00436-0501-16
480 ml	$8.85	TRI-K, Century Pharms	00436-0537-16
480 ml	$11.74	TRIKATES, Lilly	00002-2463-05

Tablet, Effervescent - Oral - 25 mEq

30's	$4.25	EFFER-K, ORANGE FLAVORED, Nomax	51801-0001-30
30's	$5.31	EFFER-K, LIME FLAVORED, Nomax	51801-0002-30
30's	$5.85	K+ CAREET, 25 MEQ ORANGE, Alra Labs	51641-0135-03
30's	$6.06	Potassium Bicarbonate, HL Moore Drug Exch	00839-6619-19
30's	$6.69	K-Electrolyte, Aligen Independ	00405-4812-30
30's	$6.95	Potassium (Orange), Bajamar Chem	44184-0016-02
30's	$6.95	Potassium (Lime), Bajamar Chem	44184-0024-02
30's	$7.43	Potassium, United Res	00677-0819-07
30's	$7.46	K Effervesent, Qualitest Pharms	00603-4170-16
30's	$7.98	Potassium, Geneva Pharms	00781-1525-31
30's	$8.50	Potassium, Harber Pharm	51432-0355-08
30's	$8.70	K-Vescent, Major Pharms	00904-2720-46
30's	$9.15	GEN-K 25 MEQ, Goldline Labs	00182-1497-17
30's	$9.81	KLOR-CON/EF, Upsher Smith	00245-0039-30
30's	$45.94	K LYTE DS LIME FLAVOR, Bristol Myers Squibb	00087-0772-41
100's	$17.50	EFFER-K, ORANGE FLAVORED, Nomax	51801-0001-40
100's	$17.71	K+ CAREET, 25 MEQ ORANGE, Alra Labs	51641-0135-01
100's	$18.00	Potassium (Orange), Bajamar Chem	44184-0016-04
100's	$18.00	Potassium (Lime), Bajamar Chem	44184-0024-04
100's	$18.95	K-Vescent, Major Pharms	00904-2720-60
100's	$30.74	KLOR-CON/EF, Upsher Smith	00245-0039-01
100's	$137.80	K LYTE DS LIME FLAVOR, Bristol Myers Squibb	00087-0772-42
250's	$32.00	EFFER-K, ORANGE FLAVORED, Nomax	51801-0001-18
250's	$42.75	K+ CAREET, 25 MEQ LIME FLAVOR, Alra Labs	51641-0125-25
250's	$44.00	Potassium (Orange), Bajamar Chem	44184-0016-06
250's	$44.00	Potassium (Lime), Bajamar Chem	44184-0024-06
250's	$46.10	Potassium Bicarbonate, HL Moore Drug Exch	00839-6619-09
250's	$67.12	Potassium, Rugby	00536-3777-02

POTASSIUM (GLUCONATE AND CITRATE)
(002074)

CATEGORIES: Electrolyte Solutions; Electrolytic, Caloric-Water Balance; Homeostatic & Nutrient; Potassium Supplements; Replacement Solutions; FDA Pre 1938 Drugs

BRAND NAMES: Kem-K; **Twin-K**

Prescribing information not available at time of publication.

HOW SUPPLIED - EQUIVALENTS NOT AVAILABLE:

Liquid - Oral - 20 meq/15 ml

480 ml	$24.25	TWIN-K, Knoll Pharms	00048-0021-16

POTASSIUM ACETATE *(002075)*

CATEGORIES: Electrolyte Solutions; Electrolytic, Caloric-Water Balance; Homeostatic & Nutrient; Hypokalemia; Potassium Supplements; Replacement Solutions; Pregnancy Category C; FDA Approved 1984 Jul

DESCRIPTION:

Potassium Acetate Injection, USP, 40 mEq (2 mEq/ml) is a sterile, nonpyrogenic, CONCENTRATED SOLUTION of potassium acetate in water for injection. The solution is administered after dilution by the intravenous route as an electrolyte replenisher. IT MUST NOT BE ADMINISTERED UNDILUTED.

Each 20 ml vial contains 3.93 g of potassium acetate which provides 40 mEq each of potassium (K+) and acetate (CH3COO-). It contains no bacteriostat, antimicrobial agent or added buffer. The pH is adjusted to 6.2 (approx.) with acetic acid. The osmolar concentration is 4.0 mOsm/ml (calc.).

The solution is intended as an alternative to potassium chloride to provide potassium ion (K+) for addition to large volume infusion fluids for intravenous use.

Potassium acetate, USP is chemically designated CH2COOK, colorless crystals or white crystalline powder very soluble in water.

The semi-rigid vial is fabricated from a specially formulated polyolefin. It is a copolymer of ethylene and propylene. The safety of the plastic has been confirmed by tests in animals according to USP biological standards for plastic containers. The container requires no vapor barrier to maintain the proper drug concentration.

CLINICAL PHARMACOLOGY:

As the principal cation of the intracellular fluid, potassium plays an important role in fluid and electrolyte balance. The normal potassium concentration in the intracellular fluid compartment is about 160 mEq/liter. The kidney normally regulates potassium balance but does not conserve potassium as well or as promptly as it conserves sodium. The daily turnover of potassium in the normal adult averages 50 to 150 mEq (milliequivalents) and represents 1.5 to 5% of the total potassium content of the body.

Acetate (CH3COO-) a source of hydrogen ion acceptors, is an alternate source of bicarbonate (HCO3-) by metabolic conversion in the liver. This has been shown to proceed readily, even in the presence of sever liver disease.

INDICATIONS AND USAGE:

Potassium Acetate Injection, USP, 40 mEq is indicated as a source of potassium, for addition to large volume intravenous fluids, to prevent or correct hypokalemia in patients with restricted or no oral intake. It is also useful as an additive for preparing specific intravenous fluid formulas when the needs of the patient cannot be met by standard electrolyte or nutrient solutions.

CONTRAINDICATIONS:

Potassium administration is contraindicated in patients with severe renal insufficiency or adrenal insufficiency and in diseases where high potassium levels maybe encountered.

WARNINGS:

Potassium Acetate Injection, USP, 40 mEq must be diluted before use.

To avoid potassium intoxication, infuse potassium-containing solutions slowly. Potassium replacement therapy should be monitored whenever possible by continuous or serial electrocardiography (ECG). Serum potassium levels are not necessarily dependable indicators of tissue potassium levels.

Solutions which contain potassium ions should be used with great care, if at all, in patients with hyperkalemia, severe renal failure and in conditions in which potassium retention is present.

In patients with diminished renal function, administration of solutions containing potassium ions may result in potassium retention.

Solutions containing acetate ion should be used with great care in patients with metabolic or respiratory alkalosis. Acetate should be administered with great care in those conditions in which there is an increased level or an impaired utilization of this ion, such as severe hepatic insufficiency.

PRECAUTIONS:

GENERAL

Do not administer unless solution is clear and seal is intact. Discard unused portion.

Potassium replacement therapy should be guided primarily by ECG monitoring and secondarily by the serum potassium level.

High plasma concentrations of potassium may cause death by cardiac depression, arrhythmias or arrest.

Use with caution in the presence of cardiac disease, particularly in digitalized patients or in the presence of renal disease.

Solutions containing acetate ion should be used with caution as excess administration may result in metabolic alkalosis.

PREGNANCY CATEGORY C

Animal reproduction studies have not been conducted with potassium acetate. It is also not known whether potassium acetate can cause fetal harm when administered to a pregnant woman or can affect reproduction capacity. Potassium acetate should be given to a pregnant woman only if clearly needed.

ADVERSE REACTIONS:

Adverse reactions involve the possibility of potassium intoxication. The signs and symptoms of potassium intoxication include paresthesias of the extremities, flaccid paralysis, listlessness, mental confusion, weakness and heaviness of the legs, hypotension, cardiac arrhythmias, heart block electrocardiographic abnormalities such as disappearance of P waves, spreading and slurring of the QRS complex with development of a biphasic curve and cardiac arrest. See WARNINGS and PRECAUTIONS.

OVERDOSAGE:

In the event of overdosage, discontinue infusion containing potassium acetate immediately and institute corrective therapy as indicated to reduce elevated serum potassium levels and restore acid-base balance if necessary. See WARNINGS, PRECAUTIONS and ADVERSE REACTIONS.

DOSAGE AND ADMINISTRATION:

Potassium Acetate Injection, USP, 40 mEq is administered intravenously ONLY AFTER DILUTION IN A LARGE VOLUME OF FLUID. The dose and rate of administration are dependent upon the individual needs of the patient. ECG and serum potassium should be monitored as a guide to dosage. Using aseptic technique, all or part of the contents of one or more vials may be added to other intravenous fluids to provide any desired number of milliequivalents (mEq) of potassium (K+) with an equal number of milliequivalents of acetate (CH3COO-).

Parenteral drug products should be inspected visually for particulate matter and discoloration prior to administration, whenever container and solution permit. See PRECAUTIONS.

Protect from freezing and extreme heat.

Do not store above 40°C (104°F).

HOW SUPPLIED - EQUIVALENTS NOT AVAILABLE:

Granules

500 gm	$18.20	Potassium Acetate, Mallinckrodt	00406-6696-03

Injection, Solution - Intravenous - 2 meq/ml

20 ml	$4.75	Potassium Acetate, Abbott	00074-8183-01
20 ml	$41.25	Potassium Acetate, Fujisawa USA	00469-7600-40
20 ml x 25	$32.73	Potassium Acetate, Fujisawa USA	00469-0158-25
20 ml x 25	$59.69	Potassium Acetate, Am Regent	00517-2053-25
20 ml x 50	$98.00	Potassium Acetate, Raway	00686-2053-25
30 ml	$2.28	Potassium Acetate, McGaw	00264-3023-57
50 ml	$7.93	POTASSIUM ACETATE 2 MEQ/ML, Abbott	00074-3294-05
50 ml	$9.36	Potassium Acetate, Abbott	00074-3294-51
50 ml	$87.50	Potassium Acetate, Fujisawa USA	00469-7600-60
100 ml	$8.00	Potassium Acetate, Intl Medication	00548-6540-00
100 ml	$15.68	POTASSIUM ACETATE 2 MEQ/ML, Abbott	00074-3294-06
100 ml x 25	$174.38	Potassium Acetate, Am Regent	00517-2400-25
100 ml x 40	$312.48	Potassium Acetate, Fujisawa USA	00469-7600-63

Injection, Solution - Intravenous - 4 meq/ml

50 ml	$136.56	Potassium Acetate, Fujisawa USA	00469-3300-60
50 ml x 25	$150.00	Potassium Acetate, Raway	00686-5024-25
50 ml x 25	$156.25	Potassium Acetate, Am Regent	00517-5024-25

POTASSIUM ACID PHOSPHATE *(002076)*

CATEGORIES: Acidifying Agents; Antagonists and Antidotes; Antibacterials; Antidotes; Electrolytic, Caloric-Water Balance; Urinary Tract Infections; Pregnancy Category C; FDA Pre 1938 Drugs

BRAND NAMES: **K-Phos Original**

FORMULARIES: BC-BS

DESCRIPTION:

PHOSPHATE URINARY ACIDIFIER

Supplies 114 mg of phosphorus per tablet. Each tablet contains potassium acid phosphate 500 mg. Each tablet yields approximately 114 mg of phosphorus and 144 mg of potassium or 3.7 mEq.

CLINICAL PHARMACOLOGY:

Potassium acid phosphate (sodium free) is a highly effective urinary acidifier.

INDICATIONS AND USAGE:

For use in patients with elevated urinary pH. Helps keep calcium soluble and reduces odor and rash caused by ammoniacal urine. Also, by acidifying the urine, it increases the antibacterial activity of methenamine mandelate and methenamine hippurate.

CONTRAINDICATIONS:

This product is contraindicated in patients with infected phosphate stones; in patients with severely impaired renal function (less than 30% of normal) and in the presence of hyperphosphatemia and hyperkalemia.

PRECAUTIONS:

GENERAL

This product contains potassium and should be used with caution if regulation of this element is desired. Occasionally, some individuals may experience a mild laxative effect during the first few days of phosphate therapy. If laxation persists to an unpleasant degree, reduce the daily dosage until this effect subsides or, if necessary, discontinue the use of this product.

Caution should be exercised when prescribing this product in the following conditions: Cardiac disease (particularly in digitalized patients); severe adrenal insufficiency (Addison's disease); acute dehydration; severe renal insufficiency or chronic renal disease; extensive tissue breakdown (such as severe burns); myotonia congenita; hypoparathyroidism; and acute pancreatitis. Rickets may benefit from phosphate therapy, but caution should be exercised. High serum phosphate levels may increase the incidence of extraskeletal calcification.

INFORMATION FOR THE PATIENT

Patients with kidney stones may pass old stones when phosphate therapy is started and should be warned of this possibility. Patients should be advised to avoid the use of antacids containing aluminum, calcium, or magnesium which may prevent the absorption of phosphate. To assure against gastrointestinal injury associated with oral ingestion of concentrated potassium salt preparations, patients should be instructed to dissolve tablets completely in an appropriate amount of water before taking.

PRECAUTIONS: *(cont'd)*

LABORATORY TESTS

Careful monitoring of renal function and serum electrolytes (calcium, phosphorus, potassium) may be required at periodic intervals during potassium phosphate therapy. Other tests may be warranted in some patients, depending on conditions.

CARCINOGENESIS, MUTAGENESIS, AND IMPAIRMENT OF FERTILITY

There have been no studies in animals or humans to evaluate the carcinogenesis, mutagenesis, or impairment of fertility for this product.

PREGNANCY

Pregnancy Category C. Animal reproduction studies have not been conducted with this product. It is also not known whether this product can cause fetal harm when administered to a pregnant woman or can affect reproductive capacity. This product should be given to a pregnant woman only if clearly needed.

NURSING MOTHERS

It is not known whether this drug is excreted in human milk. Because many drugs are excreted in human milk, caution should be exercised when this product is administered to a nursing woman.

DRUG INTERACTIONS:

The use of antacids containing magnesium, calcium, or aluminum in conjunction with phosphate preparations may bind the phosphate and prevent its absorption. Potassium-containing medications or potassium- sparing diuretics may cause hyperkalemia when used concurrently with potassium salts. Patients should have serum potassium level determinations at periodic intervals. Concurrent use of salicylates may lead to increased serum salicylate levels since excretion of salicylates is reduced in acidified urine. Serum salicylate levels should be closely monitored to avoid toxicity.

ADVERSE REACTIONS:

Gastrointestinal upset (diarrhea, nausea, stomach pain, and vomiting) may occur with the use of potassium phosphate. Also, bone and joint pain (possible phosphate-induced osteomalacia) could occur. The following adverse effects may be observed with potassium administration: irregular heartbeat; dizziness; mental confusion; weakness or heaviness of legs; unusual tiredness; muscle cramps; numbness, tingling, pain, or weakness in hands or feet; numbness or tingling around lips; shortness of breath or troubled breathing.

DOSAGE AND ADMINISTRATION:

Two tablets dissolved in 6-8 oz. of water 4 times daily with meals and at bedtime. For best results, let the tablets soak in water for 2 to 5 minutes, or more if necessary, and stir. If any tablet particles remain undissolved, they may be crushed and stirred vigorously to speed dissolution.

Dispense in tight, light resistant containers with child-resistant closures.

Storage: Keep tightly closed. Store at controlled room temperature, 15-30° (59 -86°F). Protect from light.

(Beach Pharm., 7/90, K-5 R7/90)

HOW SUPPLIED - EQUIVALENTS NOT AVAILABLE:

Tablet, Uncoated - Oral - 500 mg

100's	$8.35	K PHOS ORIGINAL, Beach Pharms	00486-1111-01
500's	$40.50	K PHOS ORIGINAL, Beach Pharms	00486-1111-05

POTASSIUM ACID PHOSPHATE; SODIUM ACID PHOSPHATE *(002077)*

CATEGORIES: Acidifying Agents; Alkalinizing Agents; Antagonists and Antidotes; Antibacterials; Antidotes; Electrolytic, Caloric-Water Balance; Phosphorus Preparations; Urinary Acidifiers; Urinary Tract Infections; Pregnancy Category C; FDA Pre 1938 Drugs

BRAND NAMES: **K-Phos M.F.**

DESCRIPTION:

K-Phos M.F.: Each tablet contains potassium acid phosphate 155 mg and sodium acid phosphate, anhydrous 350 mg. Each tablet yields approximately 125.6 mg of phosphorus, 44.5 mg of potassium or 1.1 mEq and 67 mg of sodium or 2.9 mEq. *K-Phos No.2:* Each tablet contains potassium acid phosphate 305 mg and sodium acid phosphate, anhydrous, 700 mg. Each tablet yields approximately 250 mg of phosphorus, 88 mg of potassium or 2.3 mEq and 134 mg of sodium or 5.8 mEq.

CLINICAL PHARMACOLOGY:

Phosphorus has a number of important functions in the biochemistry of the body. The bulk of the body's phosphorus is located in the bones, where it plays a key role in osteoblastic and osteoclastic activities. Enzymatically catalyzed phosphate-transfer reactions are numerous and vital in the metabolism of carbohydrate, lipid and protein, and a proper concentration of the anion is of primary importance in assuring an orderly biochemical sequence. In addition, phosphorus plays an important role in modifying steady-state tissue concentration of calcium. Phosphate ions are important buffers of the intracellular fluid, and also play a primary role in the renal excretion of hydrogen ion.

In general, in adults, about two thirds of the ingested phosphate is absorbed from the bowel, most of which is rapidly excreted into the urine.

Mechanism of Action: These products are highly effective urinary acidifiers.

INDICATIONS AND USAGE:

For use in patients with elevated urinary pH. These products help keep calcium soluble and reduce odor and rash caused by ammoniacal urine. Also, by acidifying the urine they increase the antibacterial activity of methenamine mandelate and methenamine hippurate.

CONTRAINDICATIONS:

These products are contraindicated in patients with infected phosphate stones; in patients with severely impaired renal function (less than 30% of normal) and in the presence of hyperphosphatemia.

PRECAUTIONS:

General: Contains potassium and sodium and should be used with caution if regulation of these elements is desired. Occasionally, some individuals may experience a mild laxative effect during the first few days of phosphate therapy. If laxation persists to an unpleasant degree, reduce the daily dosage until this effect subsides or, if necessary, discontinue the use of this product. Use of this medication should be carefully considered when the following medical problems exist: Cardiac disease (particularly in digitalized patients), Addison's dis-

PRECAUTIONS: *(cont'd)*
ease, acute dehydration, extensive tissue breakdown, myotonia congenita, cardiac failure, cirrhosis of the liver or severe hepatic disease, peripheral and pulmonary edema, hypernatremia, hypertension, toxemia of pregnancy, hypoparathyroidism, and acute pancreatitis. Rickets may benefit from phosphate therapy but caution should be observed. High serum phosphate levels increase the risk of extraskeletal calcification.

Information for the Patient: Patients with kidney stones may pass old stones when phosphate therapy is started and should be warned of this possibility. Patients should be advised to avoid the use of antacids containing aluminum, magnesium, or calcium which may prevent the absorption of phosphate.

Laboratory Tests: Careful monitoring of renal function and serum electrolytes (calcium, phosphorus, potassium, sodium) may be required at periodic intervals. Other tests may be warranted in some patients, depending on conditions.

Carcinogenesis, Mutagenesis, and Impairment of Fertility: Long term animal studies to evaluate the carcinogenic, mutagenic, or teratogenic potential of these products have not been performed.

Pregnancy Category C: Animal reproduction studies have not been conducted with these products. It is also not known whether these products can cause fetal harm when administered to a pregnant woman or can affect reproductive capacity. These products should be given to a pregnant woman only if clearly needed.

Nursing Mothers: It is not known whether these drugs are excreted in human milk. Because many drugs are excreted in human milk, caution should be exercised when these products are administered to a nursing woman.

DRUG INTERACTIONS:

Use of antacids containing magnesium, aluminum or calcium in conjunction with phosphate preparations may bind the phosphate and prevent its absorption. Concurrent use of antihypertensives, especially diazoxide, guanethidine, hydralazine, methyldopa or rauwolfia alkaloid; or corticosteroids, especially mineralocorticoids or corticotropin, with sodium phosphate may result in hypernatremia. Potassium-containing medications or potassium-sparing diuretics may cause hyperkalemia when used with potassium phosphate. Patients should have serum potassium level determinations at periodic intervals. Plasma levels of salicylates may be increased since salicylate excretion is decreased in acidified urine; administration of monobasic phosphates to patients stabilized on salicylates may lead to toxic salicylate levels.

ADVERSE REACTIONS:

Gastrointestinal upset (diarrhea, nausea, stomach pain and vomiting) may occur with phosphate therapy. Also, bone and joint pain (possible phosphate-induced osteomalacia) could occur. The following adverse effects may be observed (primarily from sodium or potassium): headaches; dizziness; mental confusion; seizures; weakness or heaviness of legs; unusual tiredness or weakness; muscle cramps; numbness, tingling, pain, or weakness of hands or feet; numbing or tingling around lips; fast or irregular heartbeat; shortness of breath or troubled breathing; swelling of feet or lower legs; unusual weight gain; low urine output; unusual thirst.

DOSAGE AND ADMINISTRATION:

K-Phos M.F.: Two tablets four times daily with a full glass of water.

K-Phos No.2: One tablet four times daily with a full glass of water. When the urine is difficult to acidify administer one tablet every two hours not to exceed eight tablets in a 24 hour period.

Dispense in tight, light-resistant containers with child-resistant closures.

Storage: Keep tightly closed. Store at controlled room temperature, 15-30°C (59 - 86°F).
(Beach Pharmaceuticals, R10/90)

HOW SUPPLIED - EQUIVALENTS NOT AVAILABLE:

Tablet, Coated - Oral - 155 mg/350 mg

100's	**$8.35**	**K-PHOS M.F., Beach Pharms**	**00486-1135-01**
500's	**$40.50**	**K-PHOS, Beach Pharms**	**00486-1135-05**

Tablet, Coated - Oral - 305 mg/700 mg

100's	$13.45	K-PHOS NO 2, Beach Pharms	00486-1134-01
500's	$65.20	K-PHOS NO 2, Beach Pharms	00486-1134-05

POTASSIUM BICARBONATE *(002078)*

CATEGORIES: Caloric Agents; Electrolytic, Caloric-Water Balance; FDA Pre 1938 Drugs

BRAND NAMES: K-Lyte; *Kalinor*; *Kalitrans* (Germany); *Neo-K*; *Sando-K*
(International brand names outside U.S. in italics)

FORMULARIES: Aetna

Prescribing information not available at time of publication.

HOW SUPPLIED - EQUIVALENTS NOT AVAILABLE:

Tablet, Effervescent - Oral - 25 mEq

30's	$5.85	K+CARE ET, 25 MEQ LIME FLAVOR, Alra Labs	51641-0125-03
30's	$8.35	Potassium, Orange Flavor, Schein Pharm (US)	00364-0635-30
30's	$10.07	POTASSIUM, ORANGE FLAVOR, Rugby	00536-3777-07
30's	$28.00	K-LYTE LIME FLAVORED, Bristol Myers Squibb	00087-0760-01
30's	$28.00	K-LYTE ORANGE FLAVOR, Bristol Myers Squibb	00087-0761-01
30's	$50.41	K-LYTE DS ORANGE FLAVOR, Bristol Myers Squibb	00087-0771-41
100's	$17.71	K+CARE ET, 25 MEQ LIME FLAVOR, Alra Labs	51641-0125-01
100's	$25.18	Potassium, Schein Pharm (US)	00364-0635-01
100's	$88.61	K-LYTE LIME FLAVORED, Bristol Myers Squibb	00087-0760-43
100's	$88.61	K-LYTE ORANGE FLAVOR, Bristol Myers Squibb	00087-0761-43
100's	$151.19	K-LYTE DS ORANGE FLAVOR, Bristol Myers Squibb	00087-0771-42
250's	$42.75	K + CARE ET, 25 MEQ ORANGE, Alra Labs	51641-0135-25
250's	$209.77	K-LYTE ORANGE FLAVOR, Bristol Myers Squibb	00087-0761-02

POTASSIUM CHLORIDE *(002081)*

CATEGORIES: Antihypertensives; Bleeding; Caloric Agents; Diuretics; Electrolyte Solutions; Electrolytic, Caloric-Water Balance; Homeostatic & Nutrient; Hypertension; Hypokalemia; Metabolic Acidosis; Nephropathy; Neuromuscular; Paralysis; Potassium Supplements; Renal Drugs; Replacement Solutions; Skeletal Muscle Hyperactivity; Vitamins; Pregnancy Category C; Sales > $100 Million; FDA Approval Pre 1982; Top 200 Drugs

BRAND NAMES: *Acronitol*; *Addi-K*; *Apo-K* (Canada); *Celeka*; Cena-K; *Chloropotassuril*; *Chlorvescent*; *Clor-K-Zaf* (Mexico); *Diffu-K* (France); *Durekal*; *Durules*; *Durules-K*; *Enpott*; Gen-K; K Tab; K-10; K-Care; *K-Contin*; K-Dur; *K-Grad*; K-Ide; K-Lease; K-Lor; K-Lyte Cl; K-Norm; K-Sol; *K-SR*; *K-Tab*; K-Ten; *Kadalex*; *Kaleorid* (France); *Kaliduron*; *Kaliglutol*; *Kalilente*; *Kalinor-Retard P* (Germany); *Kalinorm*; *Kalinorm Depottab*; *Kaliolite* (Mexico); *Kalipor*; *Kalipoz*; *Kalitabs*; *Kalitrans Retard* (Germany); *Kalium*; *Kalium-Durettes*; *Kalium Duriles* (Germany); *Kalium Durules* (Canada); *Kalium-R*; *Kalium Retard*; *Kalium SR*; *Kalium S.R.*; Kaochlor; *Kaon* (Canada); Kaon Cl; Kaon-Cl; Kato; *Kay-Cee-L* (England); Kay Ciel; *Kayciel*; *Kay-Ciel*; *KCL Retard* (Germany); *Keylyte*; Klor-Con; Klorvess; Klotrix; *Kolyum*; *KSR*; *Lento-K*; *Lento-Kalium*; *Leo-K* (England); Micro-K; *Micro-K Extentcaps*; *Micro-Kalium Retard*; *Miopotasio*; *Nu-K* (England); *Plus Kalium Retard*; Potasalan; *Potasion*; *Potasol*; *Rekawan* (Germany); *Rekawan Retard*; Rum-K; **Slow-K**; *Span-K* (Australia); Ten-K; *Ultra-K-Chlor*
(International brand names outside U.S. in italics)

FORMULARIES: Aetna; BC-BS; CIGNA; DoD; FHP; Humana; Kaiser; Medco; Medi-Cal; PCS; PruCare; United; WHO

DESCRIPTION:

Extended-Release Capsules and Tablets: Potassium chloride extended-release capsules, USP are a solid oral dosage form of potasium chloride containing 10 mEq (750 mg) of potassium chloride [equivalent to 10 mEq (390 mg) of potassium and 10 mEq (360 mg) of chloride] in a microencapsulated capsule. This formulation is intended to slow the release of potassium so that the likelihood of a high localized concentration of potassium chloride within the gastrointestinal tract is reduced.

Potassium chloride extended-release capsules are an electrolyte replenisher. The chemical name is potassium chloride, and the structural formula is KCl. Potassium chloride, USP occurs as a white, granular powder or as colorless crystals. It is odorless and has a saline taste. Its solutions are neutral to litmus. It is freely soluble in water and insoluble in alcohol.

Inactive ingredients: Calcium stearate, gelatin, pharmaceutical glaze, povidone, sugar spheres, talc.

Klor-Con Extended-release Tablets, USP are a solid oral dosage form of potassium chloride. Each contains 600 or 750 mg of potassium chloride equivalent to 8mEq or 10mEq of potassium in a wax matrix tablet.

Extended-Release Formulation for Liquid Suspension: Potassium chloride liquid suspension is an oral dosage form of microencapsulated potassium chloride. Each packet contains 1.5 g of potassium chloride, USP equivalent to 20 mEq of potassium. Potassium chloride liquid suspension is comprised of specially formulated granules. After reconstituting with 2-6 fl oz of water and 1 minute of stirring, the suspension is odorless and tasteless.

Each crystal of potassium chloride (KCl) is microencapsulated with an insoluble polymeric coating which functions as a semipermeable membrane; it allows for the controlled release of potassium and chloride ions over an eight-ten hour period. The controlled release of K+ ions by the microcapsular membrane is intended to reduce the likelihood of a high localized concentration of potassium chloride at any point on the mucosa of the gastrointestinal tract. Fluids pass through the membrane and gradually dissolve the potassium chloride within the microcapsules. The resulting potassium chloride solution slowly diffuses outward through the membrane.

Potassium chloride liquid suspension is an electrolyte replenisher. The chemical name of the active ingredient is potassium chloride and the structural formula is KCI. Potassium Chloride, USP occurs as a white, granular powder or as colorless crystals. It is odorless and has a saline taste. Its solutions are neutral to litmus. It is freely soluble in water and insoluble in alcohol.

Inactive Ingredients: Docusate Sodium, Ethylcellulose, Povidone, Silicon Dioxide, Sucrose, and another ingredient.

CLINICAL PHARMACOLOGY:

The potassium ion is the principal intracellular cation of most body tissues. Potassium ions participate in a number of essential physiological processes, including the maintenance of intracellular tonicity, the transmission of nerve impulses, the contraction of cardiac, skeletal and smooth muscle and the maintenance of normal renal function.

The intracellular concentration of potassium is approximately 150 to 160 mEq per liter. The normal adult plasma concentration is 3.5 to 5 mEq per liter. An active ion transport system maintains this gradient across the plasma membrane.

Potassium is a normal dietary constituent and under steady state conditions the amount of potassium absorbed from the gastrointestinal tract is equal to the amount excreted in the urine. The usual dietary intake of potassium is 50 to 100 mEq per day.

Potassium depletion will occur whenever the rate of potassium loss through renal excretion and/or loss from the gastrointestinal tract exceeds the rate of potassium intake. Such depletion usually develops as a consequence of therapy with diuretics, primary or secondary hyperaldosteronism, diabetic ketoacidosis, or inadequate replacement of potassium in patients on prolonged parenteral nutrition. Depletion can develop rapidly with severe diarrhea, especially if associated with vomiting. Potassium depletion due to these causes is usually accompanied by a concomitant loss of chloride and is manifested by hypokalemia and metabolic alkalosis. Potassium depletion may produce weakness, fatigue, disturbances of cardiac rhythm (primarily ectopic beats), prominent U- waves in the electrocardiogram, and, in advanced cases, flaccid paralysis and/or impaired ability to concentrate urine.

If potassium depletion associated with metabolic alkalosis cannot be managed by correcting the fundamental cause of the deficiency, e.g., where the patient requires long term diuretic therapy, supplemental potassium in the form of high potassium food or potassium chloride may be able to restore normal potassium levels.

In rare circumstances (*e.g.,* patients with renal tubular acidosis) potassium depletion may be associated with metabolic acidosis and hyperchloremia. In such patients potassium replacement should be accomplished with potassium salts other than the chloride, such as potassium bicarbonate, potassium citrate, potassium acetate, or potassium gluconate.

INDICATIONS AND USAGE:

EXTENDED-RELEASE CAPSULES AND TABLETS: BECAUSE OF REPORTS OF INTESTINAL AND GASTRIC ULCERATION AND BLEEDING WITH EXTENDED-RELEASE POTASSIUM CHLORIDE PREPARATIONS, THESE DRUGS SHOULD BE RESERVED FOR THOSE PATIENTS WHO CANNOT TOLERATE OR REFUSE TO TAKE LIQUID OR EFFERVESCENT POTASSIUM PREPARATIONS OR FOR PATIENTS IN WHOM THERE IS A PROBLEM OF COMPLIANCE WITH THESE PREPARATIONS.

1. For the treatment of patients with hypokalemia, with or without metabolic alkalosis; in digitalis intoxication; and in patients with hypokalemic familial periodic paralysis. If hypokalemia is the result of diuretic therapy, consideration should be given to the use of a lower dose of diuretic therapy, which may be sufficient without leading to hypokalemia.

INDICATIONS AND USAGE: *(cont'd)*

2. For the prevention of hypokalemia in patients who would be at particular risk if hypokalemia were to develop (*e.g.,* digitalized patients or patients with significant cardiac arrhythmias).

The use of potassium salts in patients receiving diuretics for uncomplicated essential hypertension is often unnecessary when such patients have a normal dietary pattern and when low doses of the diuretic are used. Serum potassium levels should be checked periodically, however, and if hypokalemia occurs, dietary supplementation with potassium-containing foods may be adequate to control milder cases. In more severe cases, and if dose adjustment of the diuretic is ineffective or unwarranted, supplementation with potassium salts may be indicated.

EXTENDED-RELEASE FORMULATION FOR LIQUID SUSPENSION: BECAUSE OF REPORTS OF INTESTINAL AND GASTRIC ULCERATION AND BLEEDING WITH CONTROLLED RELEASE POTASSIUM CHLORIDE PREPARATIONS, THESE DRUGS SHOULD BE RESERVED FOR THOSE PATIENTS WHO CANNOT TOLERATE OR REFUSE TO TAKE IMMEDIATE RELEASE LIQUIDS/EFFERVESCENT POTASSIUM PREPARATIONS OR FOR PATIENTS IN WHOM THERE IS A PROBLEM OF COMPLIANCE WITH THESE PREPARATIONS.

1. For the treatment of patients with hypokalemia, with or without metabolic alkalosis; in digitalis intoxication; and in patients with hypokalemic familial periodic paralysis. If hypokalemia is the result of diuretic therapy, consideration should be given to the use of a lower dose of diuretic, which may be sufficient without leading to hypokalemia.

2. For the prevention of hypokalemia in patients who would be at particular risk if hypokalemia were to develop (*e.g.,* digitalized patients or patients with significant cardiac arrhythmias, hepatic cirrhosis with ascites, states of aldosterone excess with normal renal function, potassium losing nephropathy, and certain diarrheal states).

The use of potassium salts in patients receiving diuretics for uncomplicated essential hypertension is often unnecessary when such patients have a normal dietary pattern and when low doses of the diuretic are used. Serum potassium should be checked periodically, however, and if hypokalemia occurs, dietary supplementation with potassium-containing foods may be adequate to control milder cases. In more severe cases, and if dose adjustment of the diuretic is ineffective or unwarranted, supplementation with potassium salts may be indicated.

CONTRAINDICATIONS:

Potassium supplements are contraindicated in patients with hyperkalemia, since a further increase in serum potassium concentration in such patients can produce cardiac arrest. Hyperkalemia may complicate any of the following conditions: chronic renal failure, systemic acidosis such as diabetic acidosis, acute dehydration, heat cramps - Extended-Release Capsules, extensive tissue breakdown as in severe burns, adrenal insufficiency, or the administration of a potassium-sparing diuretic (*e.g.,* spironolactone, triamterene, amiloride) (see OVERDOSAGE).

Extended and controlled release formulations of potassium chloride have produced esophageal ulceration in certain cardiac patients with esophageal compression due to an enlarged left atrium. Potassium supplementation, when indicated in such patients, should be given as a liquid preparation/an immediate release liquid preparation.

All solid oral dosage forms of potassium chloride are contraindicated in any patient in whom there is structural, pathological (*e.g.,* diabetic gastroparesis) or pharmacologic (use of anticholinergic agents or other agents with anticholinergic properties at sufficient doses to exert anticholinergic effects) cause for arrest or delay in tablet or capsule-passage through the gastrointestinal tract; an oral liquid preparation should be used when indicated in these patients.

WARNINGS:

Hyperkalemia: (see OVERDOSAGE) In patients with impaired mechanisms for excreting potassium, the administration of potassium salts can produce hyperkalemia and cardiac arrest. This occurs most commonly in patients given potassium by the intravenous route but may also occur in patients given potassium orally. Potentially fatal hyperkalemia can develop rapidly and be asymptomatic. The use of potassium salts in patients with chronic renal disease, or any other condition which impairs potassium excretion, requires particularly careful monitoring of the serum potassium concentration and appropriate dosage adjustment.

Interaction with Potassium Sparing Diuretics: Hypokalemia should not be treated by the concomitant administration of potassium salts and a potassium-sparing diuretic (*e.g.,* spironolactone, triamterene or amiloride) since the simultaneous administration of these agents can produce severe hyperkalemia.

Interaction with Angiotensin Converting Enzyme Inhibitors: Angiotensin converting enzyme (ACE) inhibitors (*e.g.,* captopril, enalapril) will produce some potassium retention by inhibiting aldosterone production. Potassium supplements should be given to patients receiving ACE inhibitors only with close monitoring.

Gastrointestinal Lesions: Solid oral dosage forms of potassium chloride can produce ulcerative and/or stenotic lesions of the gastrointestinal tract and deaths. Based on spontaneous adverse reaction reports, enteric coated preparations of potassium chloride are associated with an increased frequency of small bowel lesions (40-50 per 100,000 patient years) compared to extended and sustained release wax matrix formulations (less than one per 100,000 patient years). Because of the lack of extensive marketing experience with microencapsulated products, a comparison between such products and wax matrix or enteric coated products is not available.

Extended-Release Capsules and Tablets: Potassium chloride capsules and tablets are microencapsulated capsules formulated to provide a controlled rate of release of potassium chloride and thus to minimize the possibility of a high local concentration of potassium near the gastrointestinal wall.

Extended-Release Formulation for Liquid Suspension: Potassium chloride liquid suspension is administered as a liquid suspension of microencapsulated potassium chloride formulated to provide a controlled rate of release of potassium chloride and thus to minimize the possibility of a high local concentration of potassium near the gastrointestinal wall.

Diarrhea or Dehydration: Potassium chloride liquid suspension contains, as a dispersing agent, docusate sodium, which also increases stool water and is used as a stool softener. Clinical studies with Potassium chloride liquid suspension indicate that minor changes in stool consistency may be common, although usually are well- tolerated. However, rarely patients may experience diarrhea or cramping abdominal pain. Patients with severe or chronic diarrhea or who are dehydrated ordinarily should not be prescribed potassium chloride liquid suspension.

Extended-Release Capsules and Tablets and Extended-Release Formulation for Liquid Suspension: Prospective trials have been conducted in normal human volunteers in which the upper gastrointestinal tract was evaluated by endoscopic inspection before and after one week of solid oral potassium chloride therapy. The ability of this model to predict events occurring in usual clinical practice is unknown. Trials which approximated usual clinical practice did not reveal any clear differences between the wax matrix and microencapsulated dosage forms. In contrast, there was a higher incidence of gastric and duodenal lesions in subjects receiving a high dose of a wax matrix extended and controlled release formulation under conditions which did not resemble usual or recommended clinical practice (*i.e.,* 96 mEq per day in divided doses of potassium chloride administered to fasted patients, in the presence of an anticholinergic drug to delay gastric emptying). The upper gastrointestinal lesions observed by endoscopy were asymptomatic and were not accompanied by evidence of bleeding (hemoccult testing). The relevance of these findings to the usual conditions (*i.e.,* non-fasting, no anticholinergic agent, smaller doses) under which extended and controlled release potassium chloride products are used is uncertain; epidemiologic studies have not identified an elevated risk, compared to microencapsulated products, for upper gastrointestinal lesions in patients receiving wax matrix formulations. Potassium chloride extended- release capsules, USP and potassium chloride liquid suspension should be discontinued immediately and the possibility of ulceration, obstruction or perforation considered if severe vomiting, abdominal pain, distention, or gastrointestinal bleeding occurs.

Metabolic Acidosis: Hypokalemia in patients with metabolic acidosis should be treated with an alkalinizing potassium salt such as potassium bicarbonate, potassium citrate, potassium acetate, or potassium gluconate.

PRECAUTIONS:

GENERAL

The diagnosis of potassium depletion is ordinarily made by demonstrating hypokalemia in a patient with a clinical history suggesting some cause for potassium depletion. In interpreting the serum potassium level, the physician should bear in mind that acute alkalosis per se can produce hypokalemia in the absence of a deficit in total body potassium while acute acidosis per se can increase the serum potassium concentration into the normal range even in the presence of a reduced total body potassium.

The treatment of potassium depletion, particularly in the presence of cardiac disease, renal disease, or acidosis requires careful attention to acid-base balance and appropriate monitoring of serum electrolytes, the electrocardiogram, and the clinical status of the patient.

Extended-Release Capsules and Tablets: Regular serum potassium determinations are recommended.

Potassium should generally not be given in the immediate postoperative period until urine flow is established.

INFORMATION FOR THE PATIENT

Physicians should consider reminding the patient of the following:

To take this medicine following the frequency and amount prescribed by the physician. This is especially important if the patient is also taking diuretics and/or digitalis preparations.

To check with the physician at once if tarry stools or other evidence of gastrointestinal bleeding is noticed.

Extended-Release Capsules and Tablets

To take each dose with meals and with a full glass of water or other liquid.

To check with the physician if there is trouble swallowing capsules or if the capsules seem to stick in the throat.

Extended-Release Formulation for Liquid Suspension

To take each dose with meals mixed in water or other suitable liquid.

To inform patients that this product contains as a dispersing agent the stool softener, docusate sodium, which may change stool consistency, or rarely produce diarrhea or cramps.

CARCINOGENESIS, MUTAGENESIS, AND IMPAIRMENT OF FERTILITY

Carcinogenicity, mutagenicity and fertility studies in animals have not been performed. Potassium is a normal dietary constituent.

LABORATORY TESTS

Extended-Release Capsules and Tablets: When blood is drawn for analysis of plasma potassium it is important to recognize that artifactual elevations can occur after improper venipuncture technique or as a result of *in vitro* hemolysis of the sample.

PREGNANCY, TERATOGENIC EFFECTS, PREGNANCY CATEGORY C

Animal reproduction studies have not been conducted with potassium chloride capsules and tablets and potassium chloride liquid suspension. It is unlikely that potassium supplementation that does not lead to hyperkalemia would have an adverse effect on the fetus or would affect reproductive capacity.

NURSING MOTHERS

The normal potassium ion content of human milk is about 13 mEq per liter. Since oral potassium becomes part of the (body) potassium pool, so long as body potassium is not excessive, the contribution of potassium chloride supplementation should have little or no effect on the level in human milk.

PEDIATRIC USE

Safety and effectiveness in pediatric patients/children have not been established.

Extended-Release Formulation for Liquid Suspension: Regular serum potassium determinations are recommended, especially in patients with renal insufficiency or diabetic nephropathy.

When blood is drawn for analysis of plasma potassium, it is important to recognize that artifactual elevations can occur after improper venipuncture technique or as a result of *in vitro* hemolysis of the sample.

DRUG INTERACTIONS:

Potassium-sparing diuretic, angiotensin converting enzyme inhibitors: see WARNINGS.

ADVERSE REACTIONS:

One of the most severe adverse effects is hyperkalemia (see CONTRAINDICATIONS, WARNINGS, and OVERDOSAGE).

The most common adverse reactions to the oral potassium salts are nausea, vomiting, flatulence, abdominal pain/discomfort, and diarrhea.

Skin rash has been reported rarely.

Extended-Release Capsules and Tablets: There also have been reports of upper and lower gastrointestinal conditions including obstruction, bleeding, ulceration, and perforation (see CONTRAINDICATIONS and WARNINGS).

These symptoms are due to irritation of the gastrointestinal tract and are best managed by diluting the preparation further, taking the dose with meals, or reducing the amount taken at one time.

Extended-Release Formulation for Liquid Suspension: Gastrointestinal bleeding and ulceration have been reported in patients treated with microencapsulated KCI (see WARNINGS).

In addition to bleeding and ulceration, perforation and obstruction have been reported in patients treated with solid KCI dosage forms, and may occur with potassium chloride liquid suspension.

These symptoms are due to irritation of the gastrointestinal tract and are best managed by taking the dose with meals, or reducing the amount taken at one time.

ADVERSE REACTIONS: *(cont'd)*

In a controlled clinical study, potassium chloride liquid suspension was associated with an increased frequency of gastrointestinal intolerance (*e.g.*, diarrhea, loose stools, abdominal pain, etc.) compared to equal doses (100 mEq/day) of Micro-K Extencaps (see WARNINGS), Diarrhea or Dehydration). This finding was attributed to an inactive ingredient used in the Micro- K LS formulation that is not present in the Micro-K Extencaps formulation.

OVERDOSAGE:

The administration of oral potassium salts to persons with normal excretory mechanisms for potassium rarely causes serious hyperkalemia. However, if excretory mechanisms are impaired, or if potassium is administered too rapidly intravenously, potentially fatal hyperkalemia can result (see CONTRAINDICATIONS and WARNINGS). It is important to recognize that hyperkalemia is usually asymptomatic and may be manifested only by an increased serum potassium concentration (6.5-8.0 mEq/l) and characteristic electrocardiographic changes (peaking of T- waves, loss of P-wave, depression of S-T segment, prolongation of the QT interval), and widening and slurring of the QRS complex (Extended- Release Capsules). Late manifestations include muscle paralysis and cardiovascular collapse from cardiac arrest (9-12 mEq/l).

Treatment measures for hyperkalemia include the following:

1. Elimination of foods and medications containing potassium and of any agents with potassium-sparing properties;

2. Intravenous administration of 300 to 500 ml/hr of 10% dextrose solution containing 10-20 units of crystalline insulin per 1,000 ml;

3. Correction of acidosis, if present, with intravenous sodium bicarbonate;

4. Use of exchange resins, hemodialysis, or peritoneal dialysis.

In treating hyperkalemia, it should be recalled that in patients who have been stabilized on digitalis, too rapid a lowering of the serum potassium concentration can produce digitalis toxicity.

DOSAGE AND ADMINISTRATION:

The usual dietary potassium intake by the average adult is 50 to 100 mEq per day. Potassium depletion sufficient to cause hypokalemia usually requires the loss of 200 or more mEq of potassium from the total body store.

Dosage must be adjusted to the individual needs of each patient. The dose for the prevention of hypokalemia is typically in the range of 20 mEq per day. Doses of 40-100 mEq per day or more are used for the treatment of potassium depletion. Dosage should be divided if more than 20 mEq per day is given such that no more than 20 mEq is given in a single dose.

Extended-Release Capsules and Tablets K-Norm Capsules provide 10 mEq of potassium chloride. K-Norm Capsules should be taken with meals and with a glass of water or other liquid. This product should not be taken on an empty stomach because of its potential for gastric irritation (see WARNINGS). Those patients having difficulty swallowing the capsules may be advised to sprinkle the contents onto a spoonful of soft food to facilitate ingestion.

Each Klor-Con Extended-Release Tablet provides 8mEq or 10mEq of potassium chloride. Klor-Con Extended-release Tablets should be taken with meals and with a glass of water or other liquid.

EXTENDED-RELEASE FORMULATION FOR LIQUID SUSPENSION *Usual Adult Dose:* One potassium chloride liquid suspension 20 mEq packet 1 to 5 times daily, depending on the requirements of the patient. This product must be suspended in a liquid, preferably water, or sprinkled on food prior to ingestion.

Suspension in Water: Pour contents of packet slowly into approximately 2-6 fluid ounces (1/4 - 3/4 glassful) of water. Stir thoroughly for approximately 1 minute until slightly thickened, then drink. The entire contents of the packet must be used immediately and not stored for future use. Any microcapsule/water mixture should be used immediately and not stored for future use.

Suspension in Liquids other than Water: Studies conducted using orange juice, tomato juice, apple juice and milk as the suspending liquid have shown that the quantity of fluid used to suspend one potassium chloride liquid suspension packet MUST be limited to **2 fluid ounces (1/4 glassful).** The use of volumes greater than 2 fluid ounces substantially reduces the dose of potassium chloride delivered. If a liquid other than water is used to suspend potassium chloride liquid suspension then the contents of the packet should be slowly poured into **2 fluid ounces (1/4 glassful)** of liquid. Stir thoroughly for approximately 1 minute, then drink. The entire contents of the packet must be used immediately and not stored for future use. Any microcapsule/liquid mixture should be used immediately and not stored for future use.

Sprinkling Contents on Food: Potassium chloride liquid suspension may be given on soft food that may be swallowed easily without chewing, such as applesauce or pudding. After sprinkling the contents of the packet on the food, it should be swallowed immediately without chewing and followed with a glass of cool water, milk, or juice to ensure complete swallowing of all the microcapsules. Do not store microcapsule/food mixture for future use.

PATIENT INFORMATION:

Potassium chloride is used to treat hypokalemia, a condition where the potassium levels are low. This often happens in patients who are taking diuretics (*i.e.,* water pills). This medication is available in tablets, liquids, powders and capsules. Some products are extended release formulations. These should not be broken or crushed. This medication can irritate the stomach and cause some bleeding. If you notice black tarry stools, call your physician immediately. Capsules and tablets should be taken with meals and with a full glass of water or other liquid. Liquids can also be taken with meals. Some tablet forms are actually permeable capsules that allow the potassium to seep out. You may see an empty capsule or tablet in your stool. If you mix potassium with something other than water, limit the liquid quantity to 2 ounces. This will provide more potassium for your body to absorb. The level of potassium in your blood should be checked regularly to make sure it is not too high or too low.

HOW SUPPLIED:

Extended-Release Capsules and Tablets: K-Norm Capsules are clear/clear hard gelatin capsules, containing 10 mEq (750 mg) of potassium chloride [equivalent to 10 mEq (390 mg) of potassium and 10 mEq (360 mg) of chloride]. Each capsule is imprinted with "K-Norm" on one side and "10" on the other side.

Film coated Klor-Con 8 (blue), imprinted round tablets containing: 600 mg potassium chloride (equivalent to 8 mEq).

Film coated Klor-Con 10 (yellow), imprinted round tablets containing: 750 mg potassium chloride (equivalent to 10 mEq).

Mico-K 8 Extencaps are pale orange capsules monogrammed Mick-K and AHR/5720, each containing 600 mg potassium chloride (equivalent to 8 mEq).

Mico-K 10 Extencaps are pale orange and opaque white capsules monogrammed Mick-K and AHR/5730, each containing 750 mg potassium chloride (equivalent to 10 mEq).

Store at controlled room temperature 15°-30°C (59°-86°F). Dispense in container with child-resistant closure.

HOW SUPPLIED: *(cont'd)*

Extended-Release Formulation for Liquid Suspension: Micro-K LS containing 1.5 g microencapsulated potassium chloride (equivalent to 20 mEq K) per packet in cartons of 30 and 100 packets.

Store at controlled room temperature, between 15°C and 30°C (59°F and 86°F).

HOW SUPPLIED - RATED THERAPEUTICALLY EQUIVALENT:

Capsule, Gelatin, Sustained Action - Oral - 8 meq

100's	$9.23	Potassium Chloride, Geneva Pharms	00781-2092-01
100's	$16.30	MICRO-K EXTENCAPS, AH Robins	00031-5720-63
100's	$19.21	MICRO-K EXTENCAPS, AH Robins	00031-5720-64
500's	$43.75	Potassium Chloride, Geneva Pharms	00781-2092-05
500's	$73.06	MICRO-K EXTENCAPS, AH Robins	00031-5720-70

Capsule, Gelatin, Sustained Action - Oral - 10 meq

100's	$14.20	Potassium Chloride, Major Pharms	00904-2295-60
100's	$15.50	Potassium Chloride, ESI Lederle	59911-5899-01
100's	$15.61	Potassium Chloride CR, Major Pharms	00904-2295-61
100's	$15.82	Potassium Chloride, Caremark	00339-5646-12
100's	$16.18	Potassium Chloride Extended Release, Ethex	58177-0001-04
100's	$16.31	K-NORM 10, Medeva Pharms	53014-0010-71
100's	$17.91	MICRO-K 10 EXTENCAPS, AH Robins	00031-5730-63
100's	$17.96	MICRO-K 10 EXTENCAPS, AH Robins	00031-5730-68
100's	$20.21	MICRO-K 10 EXTENCAPS, AH Robins	00031-5730-64
500's	$62.95	Potassium Chloride, Major Pharms	00904-2295-40
500's	$71.50	Potassium Chloride, ESI Lederle	59911-5899-02
500's	$73.06	Potassium Chloride Extended Release, Ethex	58177-0001-08
500's	$73.75	K-NORM 10, Medeva Pharms	53014-0010-85
500's	$80.85	MICRO-K 10 EXTENCAPS, AH Robins	00031-5730-70

Injection, Conc-Soln - Intravenous - 1.5 meq/ml

5 ml	$3.40	Potassium Chloride 10 Meq, Abbott	00074-4931-01
10 ml	$5.19	Potassium Chloride, Abbott	00074-1497-01
15 ml	$5.43	Potassium Chloride 30 Meq, Abbott	00074-1498-01
20 ml	$5.93	Potassium Chloride Inj. 40 Meq, Abbott	00074-1499-01
30 ml x 25	$30.62	Potassium Chloride, Fujisawa USA	00469-0067-15
150 ml x 12	$11.94	Potassium Chloride, McGaw	00264-1940-30
200 ml	$7.81	Potassium Chloride, Intl Medication	00548-6557-00
250 ml	$43.85	Potassium Chloride, Abbott	00074-1513-02
250 ml x 12	$40.64	Potassium Chloride, McGaw	00264-1940-20
500 ml x 12	$40.64	Potassium Chloride, McGaw	00264-1940-10
1000 ml	$25.19	POTASSIUM CHLORIDE/0.9% SODIUM CHLO, Abbott	00074-7115-09

Injection, Conc-Soln - Intravenous - 2 meq/ml

5 ml	$2.65	Potassium Chloride, Abbott	00074-6635-01
5 ml	$7.39	Potassium Chloride 10 Meq, Abbott	00074-4991-01
10 ml	$2.74	Potassium Chloride, Abbott	00074-6651-06
10 ml	$3.21	Potassium Chloride 20 Meq Inj., Abbott	00074-3907-03
10 ml	$3.65	Potassium Chloride 20 Meq, Abbott	00074-4932-01
10 ml	$7.59	Potassium Chloride, Abbott	00074-4992-18
10 ml x 25	$19.69	Potassium Chloride, Am Regent	00517-2110-25
10 ml x 25	$22.19	Potassium Chloride, Am Regent	00517-2210-25
10 ml x 25	$25.31	Potassium Chloride, Fujisawa USA	00469-0965-10
10 ml x 25	$35.00	Potassium Chloride, Consolidated Midland	00223-8330-10
10 ml x 100	$95.00	POTASSIUM CHLORIDE, Raway	00686-2110-25
10 ml x 100	$120.00	Potassium Chloride, Consolidated Midland	00223-8330-01
15 ml	$2.98	Potassium Chloride, Abbott	00074-6636-01
15 ml	$3.24	Potassium Chloride, Abbott	00074-4938-01
15 ml x 25	$27.19	Potassium Chloride, Fujisawa USA	00469-0965-15
20 ml	$3.03	Potassium Chloride, Abbott	00074-6653-05
20 ml	$3.71	Potassium Chloride, Abbott	00074-4939-01
20 ml	$3.91	Potassium Chloride 40 Meq, Abbott	00074-3934-02
20 ml	$8.81	Potassium Chloride, Abbott	00074-4994-19
20 ml x 25	$24.69	Potassium Chloride, Am Regent	00517-2120-25
20 ml x 25	$28.75	Potassium Chloride, Fujisawa USA	00469-0965-20
20 ml x 25	$30.94	Potassium Chloride, Am Regent	00517-2220-25
20 ml x 25	$40.00	Potassium Chloride, Consolidated Midland	00223-8331-20
30 ml x 25	$27.19	Potassium Chloride, Am Regent	00517-2130-25
30 ml x 25	$50.00	Potassium Chloride, Consolidated Midland	00223-8322-30
30 ml x 25	$50.00	Potassium Chloride, Consolidated Midland	00223-8332-30
50 ml	$14.63	Potassium Chloride, Concentrated, Baxter Hlthcare	00338-0703-41
50 ml	$14.63	Potassium Chloride, Concentrated, Baxter Hlthcare	00338-0705-41
50 ml	$18.58	POTASSIUM CHLORIDE, Abbott	00074-7075-36
50 ml	$18.60	POTASSIUM CHLORIDE, Abbott	00074-7075-14
100 ml	$14.63	Potassium Chloride, Concentrated, Baxter Hlthcare	00338-0703-48
100 ml	$14.63	Potassium Chloride, Baxter Hlthcare	00338-0705-48
100 ml	$14.63	Potassium Chloride, Baxter Hlthcare	00338-0709-48
100 ml	$18.58	POTASSIUM CHLORIDE, Abbott	00074-7074-37
100 ml	$18.58	POTASSIUM CHLORIDE, Abbott	00074-7075-37
100 ml	$18.60	POTASSIUM CHLORIDE, Abbott	00074-7074-26
100 ml	$18.60	POTASSIUM CHLORIDE, Abbott	00074-7075-26
500 ml	$27.37	Potassium Cl In D5W & Sodium, Abbott	00074-7902-03
500 ml x 12	$24.46	5% DEXTROSE/SODIUM/KCL, McGaw	00264-1235-10
1000 ml	$24.68	NORMAL SALINE W/POTASSIUM CL, McGaw	00264-7865-00
1000 ml plastic	$17.46	KCL/5 % DEXTROSE/0.45 % SODIUM I, McGaw	00264-7634-00
1000 ml x 10	$15.42	5% DEXTROSE/SODIUM CHLORIDE/POT, McGaw	00264-1636-00
1000 ml x 12	$17.46	KCL/5% DEXTROSE/0.45% SODIUM INJEC, McGaw	00264-7636-00
1000 ml x12	$17.46	KCL/5% DEXTOE/0. 45% SODIUM INJECT, McGaw	00264-7638-00
10000 mlx 12	$17.42	KCL/5% DEXTROSE IN 0.45% SODIUM INJECT, McGaw	00264-7635-00

Injection, Conc-Soln - Intravenous - 3 meq/ml

100 ml	$14.63	Potassium Chloride, Concentrated, Baxter Hlthcare	00338-0707-48
1000 ml	$16.79	Sodium Chloride & KCl, Baxter Hlthcare	00338-0695-04
1000 ml	$25.42	POTASSIUM CHLORIDE/0.9% SODIUM CHLO, Abbott	00074-7116-09

Tablet, Coated, Sustained Action - Oral - 8 meq

100's	$7.88	Potassium Chloride, United Res	00677-1096-01
100's	$7.88	Potassium Chloride, H.C.F.A. F F P	99999-2081-01
100's	$9.02	Potassium Chloride, Harber Pharm	51432-0341-03
100's	$9.44	Potassium Chloride, HL Moore Drug Exch	00839-7736-06
100's	$10.05	Potassium Chloride, Martec Pharms	52555-0481-01
100's	$10.25	Potassium Chloride, HL Moore Drug Exch	00839-7193-06
100's	$10.36	Potassium Chloride, Qualitest Pharms	00603-5238-21
100's	$10.44	Potassium Chloride, Geneva Pharms	00781-1516-01
100's	$10.50	Potassium Chloride Extended-Release, Goldline Labs	00182-1839-01
100's	$10.60	Potassium Chloride, Schein Pharm (US)	00364-0861-01
100's	$10.85	Potassium Chloride, Major Pharms	00904-2300-60
100's	$10.85	Potassium Chloride Extended Release, Copley Pharm	38245-0225-10
100's	$11.35	KLOR-CON 8, Upsher Smith	00245-0040-11
100's	$11.40	Potassium Chloride Extended-Release, Goldline Labs	00182-1319-01
100's	$12.39	Potassium Chloride, Rugby	00536-4322-01

HOW SUPPLIED - RATED THERAPEUTICALLY EQUIVALENT: *(cont'd)*

100's	$13.98	KLOR-CON 8, Upsher Smith	00245-0040-01
100's	**$16.96**	**SLOW-K, Novartis**	**57267-0165-30**
100's	**$205.46**	**SLOW-K, Novartis**	**57267-0165-65**
500's	$37.45	Potassium Chloride 8 Meq, Major Pharms	00904-3360-40
500's	$39.07	Potassium Chloride, HL Moore Drug Exch	00839-7736-12
500's	$39.40	Potassium Chloride, H.C.F.A. F F P	99999-2081-02
500's	$43.50	Potassium Chloride Extended-Release, Goldline Labs	00182-1839-05
500's	$53.57	KLOR-CON 8, Upsher Smith	00245-0040-15
1000's	$78.80	Potassium Chloride, United Res	00677-1096-10
1000's	$78.80	Potassium Chloride, H.C.F.A. F F P	99999-2081-03
1000's	$89.40	Potassium Chloride, Qualitest Pharms	00603-5238-32
1000's	$90.20	Potassium Chloride, Harber Pharm	51432-0341-06
1000's	$95.90	Potassium Chloride, Major Pharms	00904-2300-80
1000's	$95.93	Potassium Chloride, Rugby	00536-4322-10
1000's	$99.12	Potassium Chloride, Geneva Pharms	00781-1516-10
1000's	$100.70	Potassium Chloride, Schein Pharm (US)	00364-0861-02
1000's	$102.75	Potassium Chloride Extended Release, Copley Pharm	38245-0225-20
1000's	$157.01	Potassium Chloride, HL Moore Drug Exch	00839-7193-16
1000's	**$167.77**	**SLOW-K, Novartis**	**57267-0165-40**

HOW SUPPLIED - NOT RATED EQUIVALENT:

Injection, Conc-Soln - Intravenous - 1.5 meq/ml

10 ml	$4.36	10 ML POTASSIUM CHLORIDE, Intl Medication	00548-6056-00
20 ml	$7.97	Potassium Chloride, Abbott	00074-4993-01
1000 ml	$12.39	5% DEXTROSE & 0.15% KCL 20 MEQ INJ., Abbott	00074-1580-05
1000 ml	$16.79	Sodium Chloride & KCl, Baxter Hlthcare	00338-0691-04

Injection, Conc-Soln - Intravenous - 2 meq/ml

1000 ml	$17.80	5% DEXTROSE/0.45% SODIUM/0.75% KCL 10, Abbott	00074-7993-09

Liquid - Oral - 10 %

11.25 ml x 100	$41.64	Potassium Chloride, Roxane	00054-8711-04
22.5 ml x 100	$41.63	Potassium Chloride, Roxane	00054-8712-04
30 ml x 100	$41.64	Potassium Chloride, Roxane	00054-8713-04
120 ml	$11.74	KAY CIEL, Forest Pharms	00456-0661-04
480 ml	$2.20	Potassium Chloride, HR Cenci	00556-0150-16
480 ml	$2.45	Potassium Chloride, Goldline Labs	00182-6120-40
480 ml	$2.45	Potassium Chloride, HR Cenci	00556-0424-16
480 ml	$2.48	Potassium Chloride, HR Cenci	00556-0317-16
480 ml	$2.48	PC-10, HR Cenci	00556-0422-16
480 ml	$2.52	KAOCHLOR S-F, Savage Labs	00281-3093-51
480 ml	$2.55	Potassium Chloride, Major Pharms	00904-1007-16
480 ml	$2.60	Potassium Chloride, HL Moore Drug Exch	00839-5025-69
480 ml	$2.75	Potassium Chloride, Consolidated Midland	00223-6589-01
480 ml	$2.78	Potassium Chloride, Geneva Pharms	00781-6040-16
480 ml	$2.86	Potassium Chloride, Alpharma	00472-1000-16
480 ml	$3.00	Potassium Chloride, Aligen Independ	00405-3576-16
480 ml	$3.00	Potassium Chloride Liquid, Halsey Drug	00879-0224-16
480 ml	$3.19	Potassium Chloride Yellow, Alpharma	00472-1005-16
480 ml	$3.40	Potassium Chloride, Major Pharms	00904-1005-16
480 ml	$3.40	Potassium Chloride, Morton Grove	60432-0095-16
480 ml	$3.40	Potassium Chloride, Morton Grove	60432-0492-16
480 ml	$3.45	Potassium Cl (Sugar-Free), Schein Pharm (US)	00364-7047-16
480 ml	$3.64	Potassium Chloride Sugar Free, H N Norton Co.	50732-0625-16
480 ml	$3.65	Potassium Chloride, HL Moore Drug Exch	00839-5421-69
480 ml	$3.80	Potassium Chloride, Goldline Labs	00182-6099-40
480 ml	$3.80	Potassium Chloride, H N Norton Co.	50732-0627-16
480 ml	$3.80	Potassium Chloride, Morton Grove	60432-0250-16
480 ml	$3.90	Potassium Chloride, Qualitest Pharms	00603-1534-58
480 ml	$3.90	Potassium Chloride, Qualitest Pharms	00603-1535-58
480 ml	$4.03	Potassium Chloride, Purepac Pharm	00228-2318-16
480 ml	$4.27	Potassium Chloride, United Res	00677-0540-33
480 ml	$4.34	Potassium Chloride, Aligen Independ	00405-3575-16
480 ml	$4.40	Potassium Chloride, Rugby	00536-1630-85
480 ml	$4.70	Potassium Chloride, United Res	00677-0541-33
480 ml	$22.32	KLORVESS, Novartis	00078-0207-33
480 ml	$23.29	KAOCHLOR, Savage Labs	00281-3103-51
480 ml	$46.62	KAY CIEL, Forest Pharms	00456-0661-16
500 ml	$6.83	Potassium Chloride, Roxane	00054-3716-63
1000 ml	$11.26	Potassium Chloride, Roxane	00054-3716-68
3840 ml	$9.91	Potassium Chloride, Rugby	00536-0700-90
3840 ml	$10.37	Potassium Chloride, Goldline Labs	00182-6120-41
3840 ml	$10.87	Potassium Chloride, Major Pharms	00904-1006-28
3840 ml	$11.60	Potassium Chloride, Rugby	00536-1680-90
3840 ml	$11.79	Potassium Chloride, HR Cenci	00556-0150-28
3840 ml	$11.99	Potassium Chloride, Alpharma	00472-1000-28
3840 ml	$12.02	Potassium Chloride, HR Cenci	00556-0317-28
3840 ml	$12.02	PC-10, HR Cenci	00556-0422-28
3840 ml	$12.75	Potassium Chloride, Balan	00304-0369-99
3840 ml	$13.48	Potassium Chloride, Major Pharms	00904-1005-28
3840 ml	$13.48	Potassium Chloride, Major Pharms	00904-1007-28
3840 ml	$13.56	Potassium Chloride, HL Moore Drug Exch	00839-5421-70
3840 ml	$13.67	Potassium Chloride, Lederle Pharm	00005-3269-73
3840 ml	$13.94	Potassium Chloride, Consolidated Midland	00223-6589-02
3840 ml	$17.74	Potassium Chloride-Sugar Free, H N Norton Co.	50732-0625-28
3840 ml	$18.00	Potassium Chloride Liquid, Halsey Drug	00879-0224-28
3840 ml	$19.39	Potassium Chloride, H N Norton Co.	50732-0627-28
3840 ml	$337.11	KAY CIEL, Berlex Labs	50419-0145-28
3840 ml	$354.00	KAY CIEL, Forest Pharms	00456-0661-28

Liquid - Oral - 20 %

15 ml x 100	$41.64	Potassium Chloride, Roxane	00054-8714-04
30's	$5.70	Potassium Chloride, United Res	00677-1035-07
480 ml	$2.52	Potassium Chloride, Caremark	00339-5959-53
480 ml	$2.60	Potassium Chloride 20%, HR Cenci	00556-0103-16
480 ml	$2.60	Potassium Chloride, Harber Pharm	51432-0650-20
480 ml	$2.80	Potassium Chloride, HR Cenci	00556-0425-16
480 ml	$2.80	Potassium Chloride, HR Cenci	00556-0442-16
480 ml	$3.00	Potassium Chloride, Consolidated Midland	00223-6592-01
480 ml	$3.41	Potassium Chloride, Alpharma	00472-1001-16
480 ml	$3.43	Potassium Chloride, Aligen Independ	00405-3550-16
480 ml	$3.50	Potassium Chloride, Major Pharms	00904-1001-16
480 ml	$3.51	Potassium Chloride, Purepac Pharm	00228-2320-16
480 ml	$3.75	Potassium Chloride, Geneva Pharms	00781-6790-16
480 ml	$3.95	Potassium Chloride, Goldline Labs	00182-6121-40
480 ml	$3.97	Potassium Chloride-Sugar Free, H N Norton Co.	50732-0626-16
480 ml	$4.02	Potassium Chloride, HL Moore Drug Exch	00839-5420-69
480 ml	$4.25	Potassium Chloride, Qualitest Pharms	00603-1536-58
480 ml	$4.34	Potassium Chloride, Morton Grove	60432-0005-16
480 ml	$4.40	Potassium Chloride 10%, Rugby	00536-1700-85
480 ml	$4.41	Potassium Chloride, United Res	00677-0542-33
480 ml	$5.60	Potassium Chloride, Rugby	00536-1690-85

HOW SUPPLIED - NOT RATED EQUIVALENT: *(cont'd)*

480 ml	$16.95	RUM-K, Fleming	00256-0160-01
480 ml	$26.94	KAON-CL, Savage Labs	00281-3113-51
500 ml	$9.23	Potassium Chloride, Roxane	00054-3714-63
1000 ml	$15.47	Potassium Chloride, Roxane	00054-3714-68
3840 ml	$10.29	Potassium Chloride, Harber Pharm	51432-0650-21
3840 ml	$10.87	CENA K, Century Pharms	00436-0523-28
3840 ml	$13.75	Potassium Chloride 10%, Rugby	00536-1700-90
3840 ml	$13.86	Potassium Chloride 20%, HR Cenci	00556-0103-28
3840 ml	$14.67	Potassium Chloride, HR Cenci	00556-0442-28
3840 ml	$15.48	Potassium Chloride, Consolidated Midland	00223-6592-02
3840 ml	$16.44	Potassium Chloride, Major Pharms	00904-1001-28
3840 ml	$17.47	Potassium Chloride, Alpharma	00472-1001-28
3840 ml	$17.93	Potassium Chloride, Goldline Labs	00182-0882-41
3840 ml	$21.47	Potassium Chloride-Sugar Free, H N Norton Co.	50732-0626-28
3840 ml	$91.97	RUM-K, Fleming	00256-0160-02

Powder, Reconstitution - Oral - 15 meq

30's	$6.06	Potassium Chloride 20 Meq, HL Moore Drug Exch	00839-6715-19
30's	$6.17	Potassium Chloride, Geneva Pharms	00781-8010-30
30's	$6.23	Potassium Chloride 20 Meq, Rugby	00536-3773-07
30's	$23.31	MICRO-K LS, AH Robins	00031-5760-56
100's	$73.96	MICRO-K LS, AH Robins	00031-5760-63
100's	$89.55	K-LOR, 15 MEQ, Abbott	00074-3633-11

Powder, Reconstitution - Oral - 20 meq/pkg

as ordered	$354.09	K+ CARE PO., ORANGE, Alra Labs	51641-0120-99
bulk	$354.09	K+ CARE, 20 MEQ, FRUIT, Alra Labs	51641-0140-99
2.6 gm x 30	$6.00	GEN-K 20 MEQ, Goldline Labs	00182-1451-17
30's	$3.95	Potassium Chloride, Bajamar Chem	44184-0017-02
30's	$4.38	Potassium Chloride, Aligen Independ	00405-3580-30
30's	$4.44	K+ CARE PO., ORANGE, Alra Labs	51641-0120-03
30's	$4.44	K+ CARE, 20 MEQ, FRUIT, Alra Labs	51641-0140-03
30's	$4.92	K-Sol, Major Pharms	00904-1899-46
30's	$5.96	Potassium Chloride, Roxane	00054-8716-13
30's	$6.15	Potassium Chloride, Schein Pharm (US)	00364-7378-30
30's	$6.26	KLOR-CON, Upsher Smith	00245-0035-30
30's	$21.18	KLORVESS, Novartis	00078-0205-15
30's	$31.05	K LOR, Abbott	00074-3611-01
30's	$31.05	K-LOR, Abbott	00074-7349-30
30's	$50.71	KAY CIEL, Forest Pharms	00456-0662-70
100's	$11.95	K-Sol, Major Pharms	00904-1899-60
100's	$12.00	Potassium Chloride, Bajamar Chem	44184-0017-04
100's	$14.28	K+ CARE PO., ORANGE, Alra Labs	51641-0120-01
100's	$14.28	K+ CARE, 20 MEQ, FRUIT, Alra Labs	51641-0140-01
100's	$16.00	Potassium Chloride, Aligen Independ	00405-3580-01
100's	$18.78	KLOR-CON, Upsher Smith	00245-0035-01
100's	$100.40	K LOR, Abbott	00074-3611-02
100's	$100.40	K-LOR, Abbott	00074-7349-11
100's	$124.57	KAY CIEL, Forest Pharms	00456-0662-71
1000's	$0.39	Potassium Chloride, Century Pharms	00436-0702-10
1000's	$100.00	Potassium Chloride, Bajamar Chem	44184-0017-09

Powder, Reconstitution - Oral - 25 meq/pkg

30's	$7.41	KLOR-CON/25, Upsher Smith	00245-0037-30
100's	$22.23	KLOR-CON/25, Upsher Smith	00245-0037-01
225 gm	$9.76	K-LYTE/CL, Bristol Myers Squibb	00087-0763-01
250's	$55.58	KLOR-CON/25, Upsher Smith	00245-0037-25

Tablet, Coated, Sustained Action - Oral - 6.7 meq

100's	$28.00	KAON-CL, Savage Labs	00281-3071-17
250's	$67.64	KAON-CL, Savage Labs	00281-3071-19
1000's	$265.49	KAON-CL, Savage Labs	00281-3071-23

Tablet, Coated, Sustained Action - Oral - 8 meq

100's	$7.28	Potassium Chloride, Qualitest Pharms	00603-5237-21
100's	$10.00	Potassium Chloride Extended-Relaease, Abbott	00074-7767-13
100's	$15.50	Potassium Chloride, Goldline Labs	00182-1839-89
100's	$15.87	Potassium Chloride Extended Release, Warner Chilcott	00047-0951-24
500's	$32.70	Potassium Chloride, Qualitest Pharms	00603-5237-28
1000's	$39.00	Potassium Chloride, Calvin Scott	17224-0415-10
1000's	$85.74	Potassium Chloride, Abbott	00074-7767-19
1000's	$157.00	Potassium Chloride Extended Release, Warner Chilcott	00047-0951-32

Tablet, Coated, Sustained Action - Oral - 10 meq

100's	$7.80	K PLUS 10, Alra Labs	51641-0177-01
100's	$9.92	Potassium Chloride, HL Moore Drug Exch	00839-7194-06
100's	$10.11	Potassium Chloride, HL Moore Drug Exch	00839-7737-06
100's	$11.23	Potassium Chloride, United Res	00677-1097-01
100's	$11.25	Potassium Chloride Extended Release, Goldline Labs	00182-1840-01
100's	$12.07	Potassium Chloride, Qualitest Pharms	00603-5241-21
100's	$13.04	Potassium Chloride Extended Release, Rugby	00536-4311-01
100's	$13.55	KLOR-CON 10, Upsher Smith	00245-0041-11
100's	$15.65	KLOR-CON 10, Upsher Smith	00245-0041-01
100's	$16.66	Potassium Chloride, Warner Chilcott	00047-0784-24
100's	$17.00	Potassium Chloride, Goldline Labs	00182-1840-89
100's	$21.56	K-DUR 10, Schering	00085-0263-01
100's	$22.00	ED K+10, Edwards Pharms	00485-0064-01
100's	$22.34	K-DUR 10, Schering	00085-0263-81
100's	$23.39	KLOTRIX, Bristol Myers Squibb	00087-0770-41
100's	$24.15	KAON-CL 10, Savage Labs	00281-3131-17
100's	$26.83	KAON-CL 10, Savage Labs	00281-3131-18
100's	$28.24	KLOTRIX, Bristol Myers Squibb	00087-0770-43
100's	$33.75	Potassium Chloride, Abbott	00074-7763-13
100's	$33.75	K-TAB, Abbott	00074-7804-13
100's	$35.05	K PLUS 10, Alra Labs	51641-0177-11
100's	$35.53	Potassium Chloride ER, Abbott	00074-7763-11
100's	$35.53	K-TAB, Abbott	00074-7804-11
500's	$37.49	Potassium Chloride, Balan	00304-1725-05
500's	$38.99	Potassium Chloride, Qualitest Pharms	00603-5241-28
500's	$40.49	Potassium Chloride, HL Moore Drug Exch	00839-7737-12
500's	$47.25	Potassium Chloride 10 Meq, Major Pharms	00904-3361-40
500's	$47.40	Potassium Chloride Extended Release, Goldline Labs	00182-1840-05
500's	$49.25	Potassium Chloride, Warner Chilcott	00047-0784-30
500's	$61.56	KLOR-CON 10, Upsher Smith	00245-0041-15
500's	$68.00	K PLUS 10, Alra Labs	51641-0177-05
500's	$116.96	KAON-CL 10, Savage Labs	00281-3131-21
500's	$160.25	Potassium Chloride, Abbott	00074-7763-53
1000's	$12.75	K PLUS 10, Alra Labs	51641-0177-10
1000's	$89.00	Potassium Chloride, United Res	00677-1097-10
1000's	$98.40	Potassium Chloride Extended Release, Rugby	00536-4311-10
1000's	$226.75	KLOTRIX, Bristol Myers Squibb	00087-0770-42
1000's	$229.23	KAON-CL 10, Savage Labs	00281-3131-23
1000's	$320.61	K-TAB, Abbott	00074-7804-19
5000's	$613.60	Potassium Chloride Extended-Release, Abbott	00074-7763-59
5000's	$1477.15	K-TAB, Abbott	00074-7804-59
25000's	$7164.25	K-TAB, Abbott	00074-7804-25

HOW SUPPLIED - NOT RATED EQUIVALENT: *(cont'd)*

Tablet, Coated, Sustained Action - Oral - 20 meq

100's	$39.21	K-DUR 20, Schering	00085-0787-01
100's	$42.49	K-DUR 20, Schering	00085-0787-81
500's	$190.95	K-DUR, Schering	00085-0787-06
1000's	$373.66	K-DUR 20, Schering	00085-0787-10

Tablet, Effervescent - Oral - 20 meq

30's	$5.13	K+ Potassium, Qualitest Pharms	00603-4173-16
30's	$17.75	Potassium-Cl, 25 Meq Fruit Punch, HL Moore Drug Exch	00839-7174-19
30's	$18.53	POTASSIUM-CL/25 MEQ FRUIT PUNCH, Rugby	00536-3815-07
30's	$19.00	GEN-K/CL, Goldline Labs	00182-1901-17
30's	$28.00	K-LYTE/CL CITRUS FLAVOR, Bristol Myers Squibb	00087-0766-41
30's	$28.00	K-LYTE/CL FRUIT PUNCH FLAVOR, Bristol Myers Squibb	00087-0767-41
100's	$88.61	K-LYTE/CL CITRUS FLAVOR, Bristol Myers Squibb	00087-0766-43
100's	$88.61	K-LYTE/CL FRUIT PUNCH FLAVOR, Bristol Myers Squibb	00087-0767-43
250's	$191.18	K-LYTE/CL CITRUS FLAVOR, Bristol Myers Squibb	00087-0766-42
1000's	$260.22	KLORVESS, Novartis	00078-0206-19

Tablet, Effervescent - Oral - 25 meq

30's	$7.09	Potassium Chloride, HL Moore Drug Exch	00839-7278-19
30's	$17.48	Potassium Chloride, Qualitest Pharms	00603-3508-16

Tablet, Effervescent - Oral - 50 meq

30's	$50.41	K-LYTE/CL 50 CITRUS FLAVORED, Bristol Myers Squibb	00087-0758-41
100's	$137.80	K-LYTE/CL 50 FRUIT PUNCH FLAVORED, Bristol Myers Squibb	00087-0757-42

POTASSIUM CITRATE *(002082)*

CATEGORIES: Alkalinizing Agents; Antagonists and Antidotes; Antidotes; Electrolytic, Caloric-Water Balance; Hypocitraturia; Lithiasis; Nephrolithiasis; Orphan Drugs; Renal Stones; Urinary Alkalinizers; FDA Approved 1985 Aug

BRAND NAMES: *Cystopurin* (England); *Kajos*; *Kation*; Urocrit-K
(International brand names outside U.S. in italics)

FORMULARIES: BC-BS

Prescribing information not available at time of publication.

HOW SUPPLIED - EQUIVALENTS NOT AVAILABLE:

Tablet, Uncoated, Sustained Action - Oral - 5 meq

100's	$152.40	UROCIT-K, Mission Pharma	00178-0600-01

Tablet, Uncoated, Sustained Action - Oral - 10 meq

100's	$194.04	UROCIT-K, Mission Pharma	00178-0610-01

POTASSIUM CITRATE; SODIUM CITRATE *(002083)*

CATEGORIES: Alkalinizing Agents; Antagonists and Antidotes; Antidotes; Electrolyte Solutions; Electrolytic, Caloric-Water Balance; Homeostatic & Nutrient; FDA Pre 1938 Drugs

BRAND NAMES: Citrolith

Prescribing information not available at time of publication.

HOW SUPPLIED - EQUIVALENTS NOT AVAILABLE:

Tablet, Coated - Oral - 50 mg/950 mg

100's	$12.20	CITROLITH, Beach Pharms	00486-1136-01

POTASSIUM GLUCONATE *(002084)*

CATEGORIES: Acidosis; Alkalosis; Diuretics; Electrolyte Solutions; Electrolytic, Caloric-Water Balance; Homeostatic & Nutrient; Hypertension; Hypokalemia; Metabolic Acidosis; Nephropathy; Paralysis; Potassium Supplements; Renal Function; Replacement Solutions; Pregnancy Category C; FDA Pre 1938 Drugs

BRAND NAMES: Glu-K; K-G; **Kaon**; Kaylixir; *Kolyum*; *Potasoral* (Mexico); *Potassium-Rongier* (Canada); *Potasoral*; *Ultra-K*
(International brand names outside U.S. in italics)

DESCRIPTION:

Each 15 ml (tablespoonful) supplies 20 mEq of potassium (as potassium gluconate, 4.68 g) with saccharin and aromatics and alcohol 5%. The chemical name of the drug is gluconic acid potassium salt.

CLINICAL PHARMACOLOGY:

Potassium ion is the principal intracellular cation of most body tissues. Potassium ions participate in a number of essential physiological processes including the maintenance of intracellular tonicity, the transmission of nerve impulses, the contraction of cardiac, skeletal and smooth muscle and the maintenance of normal renal function.

Potassium depletion may occur whenever the rate of potassium loss through renal excretion and/or loss from the gastrointestinal tract exceeds the rate of potassium intake. Potassium depletion sufficient to cause hypokalemia usually requires the loss of 200 or more mEq of potassium from the total body store. Such depletion usually develops slowly as a consequence of prolonged therapy with oral diuretics, primary or secondary hyperaldosteronism, diabetic ketoacidosis, or inadequate replacement of potassium in patients on prolonged parenteral nutrition. Such depletion can develop rapidly with severe diarrhea, especially if associated with vomiting. Potassium depletion may produce weakness, fatigue, disturbances of cardiac rhythm (primarily ectopic beats), prominent U-waves in the electrocardiogram, and in advanced cases, flaccid paralysis and/or impaired ability to concentrate urine.

INDICATIONS AND USAGE:

1. For therapeutic use in patients with hypokalemia with or without metabolic alkalosis, in digitalis intoxication and in patients with hypokalemic familial periodic paralysis.

INDICATIONS AND USAGE: *(cont'd)*

2. For the prevention of potassium depletion when the dietary intake is inadequate in the following conditions: Patients receiving digitalis and diuretics for congestive heart failure; hepatic cirrhosis with ascites, states of aldosterone excess with normal renal function, potassium- losing nephropathy, and with certain diarrheal states.

3. The use of potassium salts in patients receiving diuretics for uncomplicated essential hypertension is often unnecessary when such patients have a normal dietary pattern. Serum potassium should be checked periodically, however, and if hypokalemia occurs, dietary supplementation with potassium- containing foods may be adequate to control milder cases. In more severe cases supplementation with potassium salts may be indicated.

4. Hypokalemia in patients with metabolic acidosis should be treated with an alkalinizing potassium salt such as potassium gluconate.

CONTRAINDICATIONS:

Potassium supplements are contraindicated in patients with hyperkalemia since a further increase in serum potassium concentration in such patients can produce cardiac arrest. Hyperkalemia may complicate any of the following conditions: Chronic renal failure, systemic acidosis such as diabetic acidosis, acute dehydration, extensive tissue breakdown as in severe burns, adrenal insufficiency, or the administration of a potassium-sparing diuretic (*e.g.*, spironolactone, triamterene, amiloride).

WARNINGS:

DO NOT ADMINISTER FULL STRENGTH. Potassium Gluconate Elixir may cause gastrointestinal irritation if administered undiluted. For details regarding adequate dilution, see DOSAGE AND ADMINISTRATION.

Hyperkalemia: In patients with impaired mechanisms for excreting potassium, the administration of potassium salts can produce hyperkalemia and cardiac arrest. This occurs most commonly in patients given potassium by the intravenous route but may also occur in patients given potassium orally. Potentially fatal hyperkalemia can develop rapidly and be asymptomatic. The use of potassium salts in patients with chronic renal disease, or any other condition which impairs potassium excretion, requires particularly careful monitoring of the serum potassium concentration and appropriate dosage adjustment.

Interaction with Potassium Sparing Diuretics: Hypokalemia should not be treated by the concomitant administration of potassium salts and a potassium-sparing diuretic (*e.g.*, spironolactone, triamterene, amiloride) since the simultaneous administration of these agents can produce severe hyperkalemia.

PRECAUTIONS:

GENERAL

The diagnosis of potassium depletion is ordinarily made by demonstrating hypokalemia in a patient with a clinical history suggesting some cause for potassium depletion.

In hypokalemic states, especially in patients on a low-salt diet, hypochloremic alkalosis is a possibility that may require chloride as well as potassium supplementation. In these circumstances, potassium replacement with potassium chloride may be more advantageous than with other potassium salts However, Potassium Gluconate Elixir can be supplemented with chloride. Ammonium chloride is an excellent source of chloride ion (18.7 mEq per gram) but it should not be used in patients with hepatic cirrhosis where ammonium salts are contraindicated.

LABORATORY TESTS

In interpreting the serum potassium level, the physician should bear in mind that acute alkalosis Per Se can produce hypokalemia in the absence of a deficit in total body potassium while acute acidosis Per Se can increase the serum potassium concentration into the normal range even in the presence of a reduced total body potassium.

The treatment of potassium depletion, particularly in the presence of cardiac disease, renal disease, or acidosis, requires careful attention to acid- base balance and appropriate monitoring of serum electrolytes, the electrocardiogram, and the clinical status of the patient.

It is important to recognize that hyperkalemia is usually asymptomatic and may be manifested only by an increased serum potassium concentration and characteristic electrocardiographic changes (peaking of T-waves, loss of P-wave, depression of S-T segment, and prolongation of the QT interval). (See CONTRAINDICATIONS, WARNINGS, and OVERDOSAGE.)

The use of potassium salts in patients with chronic renal disease, or any other condition which impairs potassium excretion, requires particularly careful monitoring of the serum potassium concentration and appropriate dosage adjustment.

When blood is drawn for analysis of plasma potassium levels, it is important to recognize that artifactual elevations do occur after repeated fist clenching to make veins more prominent during application of a tourniquet.

CARCINOGENESIS, MUTAGENESIS, AND IMPAIRMENT OF FERTILITY

There have been no studies in animals or humans to evaluate the carcinogenesis, mutagenesis or impairment of fertility for potassium.

PREGNANCY CATEGORY C

Animal reproduction studies have not been conducted with Potassium Gluconate Elixir. It is also not known whether Potassium Gluconate Elixir can cause fetal harm when administered to a pregnant woman or can affect reproduction capacity. Potassium Gluconate Elixir should be given to a pregnant woman only if clearly needed.

NURSING MOTHERS

It is not known whether this drug is excreted in human milk. Because many drugs are excreted in human milk, caution should be exercised when Potassium Gluconate Elixir is administered to a nursing woman.

PEDIATRIC USE

Safety and effectiveness in children have not been established.

ADVERSE REACTIONS:

The most severe adverse effect is hyperkalemia (see CONTRAINDICATIONS, WARNINGS, and OVERDOSAGE).

The most common adverse reactions to oral potassium salts are nausea, vomiting, abdominal discomfort, and diarrhea. These symptoms are due to irritation of the gastrointestinal tract and are best managed by diluting the preparation further, taking the dose with meals, or reducing the dose.

OVERDOSAGE:

The administration of oral potassium salts to persons with normal excretory mechanisms for potassium rarely causes serious hyperkalemia. However, if excretory mechanisms are impaired or if potassium is administered too rapidly intravenously, potentially fatal hyperkalemia can result (see CONTRAINDICATIONS and WARNINGS.)

OVERDOSAGE: *(cont'd)*

It is important to recognize that hyperkalemia is usually asymptomatic and may be manifested only by an increased serum potassium concentration and characteristic electrocardiographic changes (peaking of T-Waves, loss of P-wave, depression of S-T segment, and prolongation of the QT interval). Late manifestations include muscle-paralysis and cardiovascular collapse from cardiac arrest.

Treatment for hyperkalemia includes the following:

1. Elimination of foods and medications containing potassium and potassium-sparing diuretics.

2. Intravenous administration of 300 to 500 ml/hr of 10% dextrose solution containing 10-20 units of crystalline insulin per 1,000 ml.

3. Correction of acidosis, if present, with intravenous sodium bicarbonate.

4. Use of exchange resins, hemodialysis, or peritoneal dialysis.

In treating hyperkalemia, it should be recalled that in patients who have been stabilized on digitalis, too rapid a lowering of the serum potassium concentration can produce digitalis toxicity.

DOSAGE AND ADMINISTRATION:

The usual dietary intake of potassium by the average adult is 40 to 80 mEq per day. Potassium depletion sufficient to cause hypokalemia usually requires the loss of 200 or more mEq of potassium from the total body store.

Dosage must be adjusted to the individual needs of each patient but is typically in the range of 20 mEq per day for the prevention of hypokalemia to 40-100 mEq per day or more for the treatment of potassium depletion.

To minimize gastrointestinal irritation, patients must follow directions regarding dilution. Each tablespoonful (15 ml) should be diluted with one fluid ounce or more of water or other liquid.

One tablespoonful twice daily (after morning and evening meals) supplies 40 mEq of potassium.

Deviations from this recommendation may be indicated, since no average total daily dose can be defined but must be governed by close observation for clinical effects. However, potassium intoxication may result from any therapeutic dosage. See OVERDOSAGE and PRECAUTIONS.

HOW SUPPLIED - RATED THERAPEUTICALLY EQUIVALENT:

Tablet, Coated - Oral - 99 mg

100's	$2.96	Potassium, HL Moore Drug Exch	00839-7310-06

HOW SUPPLIED - NOT RATED EQUIVALENT:

Elixir - Oral - 20 mEq/15ml

480 ml	$5.00	Potassium Gluconate, Consolidated Midland	00223-6295-01
480 ml	$5.49	Potassium Gluconate, Qualitest Pharms	00603-1537-58
480 ml	$6.08	K-G, Geneva Pharms	00781-6846-16
480 ml	$7.45	Potassium Gluconate, Major Pharms	00904-1459-16
480 ml	$8.69	Potassium Gluconate, H N Norton Co.	50732-0628-16
480 ml	**$27.34**	**KAON, Savage Labs**	**00281-3203-51**
3840 ml	$29.91	Potassium Gluconate, Major Pharms	00904-1459-28
3840 ml	$31.18	Potassium Gluconate, Rugby	00536-1710-90
3840 ml	$32.49	Potassium Gluconate, Consolidated Midland	00223-6295-02
3840 ml	$47.69	Potassium Gluconate, H N Norton Co.	50732-0628-28

Injection, Susp - Intramuscular; - 4.68 gm/15ml

473 ml	$6.00	Potassium Gluconate, Goldline Labs	00182-0245-40

POTASSIUM IODIDE *(002085)*

CATEGORIES: Airway Obstruction; Antifungals; Antimicrobials; Antitussives/Expectorants/Mucolytics; Asthma; Bronchitis; Cough Preparations; Expectorants; Hormones; Iodide Salts; Mucolytic Agents; Pulmonary Emphysema; Respiratory & Allergy Medications; Thyroid Preparations; FDA Pre 1938 Drugs

BRAND NAMES: *Jodid* (Germany); *Kalium Jodatum* (Germany); Pima; SSKI; Strong Iodine; Yodefan

(International brand names outside U.S. in italics)

FORMULARIES: Aetna; FHP; WHO

COST OF THERAPY: (Asthma; Solution; 15 gm/15 ml; 1.2/day; 365 days) (DRG 96)

Prescribing information not available at time of publication.

HOW SUPPLIED - EQUIVALENTS NOT AVAILABLE:

Granules

125 gm	$12.38	Potassium Iodide, Mallinckrodt	00406-1112-01
125 gm	$17.69	Potassium Iodide, Mallinckrodt	00406-1123-01
500 gm	$34.05	Potassium Iodide, Mallinckrodt	00406-1112-03
500 gm	$34.05	POTASSIUM IODIDE, Mallinckrodt	00406-1115-03
2500 gm	$144.70	Potassium Iodide, Mallinckrodt	00406-1112-05

Solution - Oral - 15 gm/15ml

30 ml	$2.25	Potassium Iodide, Lyne Labs	00374-0100-01
30 ml	$5.25	Potassium Iodide, Raway	00686-0100-01
30 ml	$5.87	POTASSIUM IODIDE, Roxane	00054-3717-44
30 ml	$12.10	SSKI, Upsher Smith	00245-0003-31
100 ml	$37.25	Potassium Iodide, Roxane	00054-8718-04
118 ml	$6.90	YODEFAN, Norega Labs	51724-0432-04
240 ml	$29.31	POTASSIUM IODIDE, Roxane	00054-3717-58
240 ml	$56.31	SSKI, Upsher Smith	00245-0003-08
480 ml	$15.00	PIMA, Fleming	00256-0139-01
480 ml	$34.69	Potassium Iodide Saturated, Rugby	00536-1730-85
480 ml	$47.50	Potassium Iodide, Consolidated Midland	00223-6298-00
480 ml	$54.90	Potassium Iodide Saturated, Harber Pharm	51432-0652-20
500 ml	$15.00	STRONG IODINE, Amend Drug Chem	17317-0334-01
3840 ml	$72.00	PIMA, Fleming	00256-0139-02

POTASSIUM IODIDE; THEOPHYLLINE ANHYDROUS *(002086)*

CATEGORIES: Airway Obstruction; Antiasthmatics/Bronchodilators; Asthma; Bronchial Dilators; Bronchitis; Bronchospasm; Iodide Salts; Pulmonary Emphysema; Respiratory & Allergy Medications; Respiratory Muscle Relaxant; Smooth Muscle Relaxants; Xanthine Derivatives; FDA Pre 1938 Drugs

BRAND NAMES: Elixophyllin KI; Theophylline KI

FORMULARIES: Aetna

Prescribing information not available at time of publication.

HOW SUPPLIED - EQUIVALENTS NOT AVAILABLE:

Elixir - Oral - 130 mg/80 mg

237 ml	$84.47	ELIXOPHYLLIN KI, Forest Pharms	00456-0645-08
240 ml	$51.85	ELIXOPHYLLIN-KI, Berlex Labs	50419-0124-08
480 ml	$3.19	Theophylline K1, Rugby	00536-2120-85
480 ml	$4.60	Theophylline Ki, Qualitest Pharms	00603-1742-58
480 ml	$4.75	Theophylline Ki, Harber Pharm	51432-0680-20
480 ml	$20.22	Theophylline/Potassium Iodide, Geneva Pharms	00781-6602-16
3840 ml	$19.16	Theophylline K1, Rugby	00536-2120-90
3840 ml	$27.49	Theophylline Ki, Harber Pharm	51432-0680-21
3840 ml	$125.53	ELIXOPHYLLIN-KI, Berlex Labs	50419-0124-28

POTASSIUM PERMANGANATE *(002090)*

CATEGORIES: Anti-Infectives; Disinfectants; Local Infections; Skin/Mucous Membrane Agents; FDA Pre 1938 Drugs

FORMULARIES: Medi-Cal; WHO

Prescribing information not available at time of publication.

HOW SUPPLIED - EQUIVALENTS NOT AVAILABLE:

Granules

120 gm	$5.60	Potassium Permanganate, Millgood	53118-0722-04
500 gm	$20.06	Potassium Permanganate, Mallinckrodt	00406-7056-03
2500 gm	$74.43	Potassium Permanganate, Mallinckrodt	00406-7056-05

POTASSIUM PHOSPHATE *(002091)*

CATEGORIES: Electrolyte Solutions; Electrolytic, Caloric-Water Balance; Homeostatic & Nutrient; Replacement Solutions; FDA Pre 1938 Drugs

Prescribing information not available at time of publication.

HOW SUPPLIED - EQUIVALENTS NOT AVAILABLE:

Injection, Conc-Soln - Intravenous - 236 mg/224 mg

5 ml	$3.27	Potassium Phosphate, Abbott	00074-4952-01
5 ml	$3.50	Potassium Phosphate 15 Mm, Abbott	00074-7296-01
5 ml in 10 ml v	$24.06	Potassium Phosphates, Fujisawa USA	00469-8600-30
5 ml x 25	$20.94	Potassium Phosphate, Am Regent	00517-2305-25
15 ml	$5.58	Potassium Phosphate 45 Mm, Abbott	00074-7295-01
15 ml in 30 ml	$37.50	Potassium Phosphates, Fujisawa USA	00469-8600-50
15 ml x 25	$32.18	Potassium Phosphate, Am Regent	00517-2315-25
15 ml x 25	$35.40	Potassium Phosphates, Gensia Labs	00703-5350-04
50 ml	$17.68	Potassium Phosphate Inj., Usp 150 Mm, Abbott	00074-4201-01
50 ml	$133.75	Potassium Phosphates, Fujisawa USA	00469-8600-60
50 ml x 10	$33.00	Potassium Phosphates, Gensia Labs	00703-5357-03
50 ml x 25	$85.94	Potassium Phosphates, Am Regent	00517-2350-25
150 ml x 12	$14.60	SUPER-VIAL POTASSIUM PHOSPHATE, McGaw	00264-1944-30

POTASSIUM PHOSPHATE; SODIUM PHOSPHATE *(002092)*

CATEGORIES: Antagonists and Antidotes; Antidotes; Electrolyte Solutions; Electrolytic, Caloric-Water Balance; Homeostatic & Nutrient; Phosphorus Preparations; Replacement Solutions; Urinary Acidifiers; Pregnancy Category C; FDA Pre 1938 Drugs

BRAND NAMES: **K-Phos Neutral**; Uro-Kp-Neutral

FORMULARIES: BC-BS

DESCRIPTION:

Each tablet contains 852 mg dibasic sodium phosphate, anhydrous, 155 mg monobasic potassium phosphate, and 130 mg monobasic sodium phosphate monohydrate. Each tablet yields approximately 250 mg of phosphorus, 298 mg of sodium (13.0 mEq) and 45 mg of potassium (1.1 mEq). The components of K-Phos Neutral have the following chemical names and molecular formulae:

Dibasic Sodium Phosphate, Anhydrous: *Molecular Formula:* Na_2HPO_4, *Molecular Weight:* 141.96.

Monobasic Potassium Phosphate: *Molecular Formula:* KH_2PO_4,*Molecular Weight:* 136.09.

Monobasic Sodium Phosphate, Monohydrate: *Molecular Formula:* $NaH_2PO_4{\cdot}H_2O$, *Molecular Weight:* 1 37.98.

CLINICAL PHARMACOLOGY:

Phosphorus has a number of important functions in the biochemistry of the body. The bulk of the body's phosphorus is located in the bones, where it plays a key role in osteoblastic and osteoclastic activities. Enzymatically catalyzed phosphate-transfer reactions are numerous and vital in the metabolism of carbohydrate, lipid and protein, and a proper concentration of the anion is of primary importance in assuring an orderly biochemical sequence. In addition, phosphorus plays an important role in modifying steady-state tissue concentrations of calcium. Phosphate ions are important buffers of the intracellular fluid, and also play a primary role in the renal excretion of hydrogen ion.

Oral administration of inorganic phosphates increase serum phosphate levels. Phosphates lower urinary calcium levels in idiopathic hypercalciuria.

In general, in adults, about two thirds of the ingested phosphate is absorbed from the bowel, most of which is rapidly excreted into the urine.

INDICATIONS AND USAGE:

Potassium phosphate and sodium phosphate increases urinary phosphate and pyrophosphate. As a phosphorus supplement, each tablet supplies 25% of the U.S. Recommended Daily Allowance (U.S. RDA) of phosphorus for adults.

CONTRAINDICATIONS:

This product is contraindicated in patients with infected phosphate stones, in patients with severely impaired renal function (less than 30% of normal) and in the presence of hyperphosphatemia.

PRECAUTIONS:

General: This product contains potassium and sodium and should be used with caution if regulation of these elements is desired. Occasionally, some individuals may experience a mild laxative effect during the first few days of phosphate therapy. If laxation persists to an unpleasant degree, reduce the daily dosage until this effect subsides or, if necessary, discontinue the use of this product.

Caution should be exercised when prescribing this product in the following conditions: Cardiac disease (particularly in digitalized patients); severe adrenal insufficiency (Addison's disease); acute dehydration; severe renal insufficiency; renal function impairment or chronic renal disease; extensive tissue breakdown (such as severe burns); myotonia congenita; cardiac failure; cirrhosis of the liver or severe hepatic disease; peripheral or pulmonary edema; hypernatremia; hypertension; toxemia of pregnancy; hypoparathyroidism; and acute pancreatitis. Rickets may benefit from phosphate therapy, but caution should be exercised. High serum phosphate levels may increase the incidence of extra-skeletal calcification.

Information for the Patient: Patients with kidney stones may pass old stones when phosphate therapy is started and should be warned of this possibility. Patients should be advised to avoid the use of antacids containing aluminum, magnesium, or calcium which may prevent the absorption of phosphate.

Laboratory Tests: Careful monitoring of renal function and serum electrolytes (calcium, phosphorus, potassium, sodium) may be required at periodic intervals during phosphate therapy. Other tests may be warranted in some patients depending on conditions.

Carcinogenesis, Mutagenesis, and Impairment of Fertility: There have been no studies in animals or humans to evaluate the carcinogenesis, mutagenesis or impairment of fertility for this product.

Pregnancy Category C: Animal reproduction studies have not been conducted with this product. It is also not known whether this product can cause fetal harm when administered to a pregnant woman or can affect reproductive capacity. This product should be given to a pregnant woman only if clearly needed.

Nursing Mothers: It is not known whether this drug is excreted in human milk. Because many drugs are excreted in human milk, caution should be exercised when this product is administered to a nursing woman.

DRUG INTERACTIONS:

The use of antacids containing magnesium, aluminum, or calcium in conjunction with phosphate preparations may bind the phosphate and prevent its absorption. Concurrent use of antihypertensives, especially diazoxide, guanethidine, hydralazine, methyldopa or rauwolfia alkaloid; or corticosteroids, especially mineralocorticoids or corticotropin, with sodium phosphate may result in hypernatremia. Calcium-containing preparations and/or Vitamin D may antagonize the effects of phosphates in the treatment of hypercalcemia. Potassium-containing medications or potassium-sparing diuretics may cause hyperkalemia. Patients should have serum potassium level determinations at periodic intervals.

ADVERSE REACTIONS:

Gastrointestinal upset (diarrhea, nausea, stomach pain and vomiting) may occur with phosphate therapy. Also, bone and joint pain (possible phosphate-induced osteomalacia) could occur. The following adverse effects may be observed (primarily from sodium or potassium): headaches; dizziness; mental confusion; seizures; weakness or heaviness of legs; unusual tiredness or weakness; muscle cramps; numbness, tingling, pain, or weakness of hands or feet; numbing or tingling around lips; fast or irregular heartbeat; shortness of breath or troubled breathing; swelling of feet or lower legs; unusual weight gain; low urine output; unusual thirst.

DOSAGE AND ADMINISTRATION:

One or two tablets four times a day with a full glass of water with meals and at bedtime.

Dispense in tight, light-resistant containers with child-resistant closures.

Storage: Keep tightly closed. Store at controlled room temperature, 15 - 30°C (59 - 86°F).

(Beach Pharm. R8/90)

HOW SUPPLIED - EQUIVALENTS NOT AVAILABLE:

Tablet, Coated - Oral - 155 mg/852 mg/1

100's	**$12.20**	**K-PHOS NEUTRAL, Beach Pharms**	**00486-1125-01**
500's	**$59.20**	**K-PHOS NEUTRAL, Beach Pharms**	**00486-1125-05**

POVIDONE-IODINE *(002094)*

CATEGORIES: Anti-Infectives; Local Infections; Skin/Mucous Membrane Agents; FDA Approved 1986 Dec

BRAND NAMES: *Alphadine*; *Alphadine Mouth Wash*; *Asepta*; *Bacterodine*; *Bactroderm*; *Bactroderm Bucofaringeo*; *Benodin*; *Bernadine*; Betadine; *Betadine Mouth Wash*; *Betaisodona* (Germany); *Betascrub*; *Betaseptic*; *Better-Iodine*; *Biocil*; *Biodyne*; *Braunol*; *Braunol 2000* (Germany); *Braunosan*; *Braunovidan*; *Braunovidon* (Germany); *Brush Off*; *Cavodine*; *Dansepta*; *Dermofax*; *E.D.P.*; *Floridin*; *Igiol*; *Iodo-Vit*; *Iovidine*; *Iso-Betadine*; *Isodine*; *Isodine Bucofaringeo* (Mexico); *Isodine Espuma* (Mexico); *Isodine Pessaries*; *Isodine Solucion Antiseptica* (Mexico); *Lombocid*; *Minidine*; *Oxisept*; *Pevidine*; *Piodin*; *Podin*; *Podine*; *Polydine*; *Potadine*; *Povidine Ointment*; *Povidine Mouth Wash*; *Povidyne*; *Qualidine*; *Septadine*; Septisol; *Singtodine*; *Torvidone*; *Viodine* (Australia); *Wokadine* ; *Wokadine Gargle*; *Yodine* (Mexico); *Yodine B F* (Mexico); *Yodine Espuma* (Mexico); *Yodine J* (Mexico); *Yodine SH Shampoo* (Mexico); *Yovidona Bucofaringeo*; *Yovidona Espuma*
(International brand names outside U.S. in italics)

Prescribing information not available at time of publication.

HOW SUPPLIED - EQUIVALENTS NOT AVAILABLE:

Solution - Ophthalmic - 5%

50 ml	$208.80	BETADINE, Purdue Frederick	00034-0410-20

Solution - Topical - 7.5 %

3840 ml	$13.82	SEPTISOL, SURGICAL SCRUB, HL Moore Drug Exch	00839-6057-70

PRAVASTATIN SODIUM *(003064)*

CATEGORIES: Antilipemic Agents; Cardiovascular Drugs; Cholesterol; HMG-COA Reductase Inhibitors; Heart Disease; Homeostatic & Nutrient; Hypercholesterolemia; Hyperlipidemia; Hyperlipoproteinemia; Hypolipidemics; Obesity; Vascular Disease; Pregnancy Category X; FDA Class 1C ("Little or No Therapeutic Advantage"); Sales > $500 Million; Top 200 Drugs; FDA Approved 1991 Oct; Top 200 Drugs

BRAND NAMES: *Elisor* (France); *Lipidal*; *Lipostat* (England); *Mevalotin*; **Pravachol**; *Pravacol*; *Pravaselect*; *Pravasin* (Germany); *Pravasine*; *Pravastatin Natrium "Mayrho Fer"*; *Selectin*; *Selektine*; *Selipran*
(International brand names outside U.S. in italics)

FORMULARIES: FHP; Medco; Medi-Cal; PCS

COST OF THERAPY: $616.08 (Hypercholesterolemia; Tablet; 10 mg; 1/day; 365 days)

DESCRIPTION:

Pravachol (pravastatin sodium) is one of a new class of lipid-lowering compounds, the HMG-CoA reductase inhibitors, which reduce cholesterol biosynthesis. These agents are competitive inhibitors of 3-hydroxy-3-methylglutaryl-co-enzyme A (HMG-CoA) reductase, the enzyme catalyzing the early rate-limiting step in cholesterol biosynthesis, conversion of HMG-CoA to mevalonate.

Pravastatin sodium is designated chemically as 1-Naphthalene-heptanoic acid, 1,2,6,7,8,8a-hexahydro-β, Δ,6-trihydroxy-2-methyl -8-(2-methyl -1- oxobutoxy)-, monosodium salt,[1*S*-[1α (β*S**, Δ *S**),2α,6α,8β(*R**),8aα]]-. Formula $C_{23}H_{35}NaO_7$, Molecular Weight is 446.52.

Pravastatin sodium is an odorless, white to off-white, fine or crystalline powder. It is a relatively polar hydrophilic compound with a partition coefficient (octanol/water) of 0.59 at a pH of 7.0. It is soluble in methanol and water (>300 mg/ml), slightly soluble in isopropanol, and practically insoluble in acetone, acetonitrile, chloroform, and ether.

Pravachol is available for oral administration as 10 mg, 20 mg and 40 mg tablets. Inactive ingredients include: croscarmellose sodium, lactose, magnesium oxide, magnesium stearate, microcrystalline cellulose, and povidone. The 10 mg tablet also contains Red Ferric Oxide, the 20 mg tablet also contains Yellow Ferric Oxide, and the 40 mg tablet also contains Green Lake Blend (mixture of D&C Yellow No. 10-Aluminum Lake and FD&C Blue No. 1-Aluminum Lake).

CLINICAL PHARMACOLOGY:

Cholesterol and triglycerides in the bloodstream circulate as part of lipoprotein complexes. These complexes can be separated by density ultracentrifugation into high (HDL), intermediate (IDL), low (LDL), and very low (VLDL) density lipoprotein fractions. Triglycerides (TG) and cholesterol synthesized in the liver are incorporated into very low density lipoproteins (VLDLs) and released into the plasma for delivery to peripheral tissues. In a series of subsequent steps, VLDLs are transformed into intermediate density lipoproteins (IDLs), and cholesterol-rich low density lipoproteins (LDLs). High density lipoproteins (HDLs), containing apolipoprotein A, are hypothesized to participate in the reverse transport of cholesterol from tissues back to the liver.

Pravastatin sodium produces its lipid-lowering effect in two ways. First, as a consequence of its reversible inhibition of HMG-CoA reductase activity, it effects modest reductions in intracellular pools of cholesterol. This results in an increase in the number of LDL-receptors on cell surfaces and enhanced receptor-mediated catabolism and clearance of circulating LDL. Second, pravastatin inhibits LDL production by inhibiting hepatic synthesis of VLDL, the LDL precursor.

Clinical and pathologic studies have shown that elevated levels of total cholesterol (Total-C), low density lipoprotein cholesterol (LDL-C), and apolipoprotein B (a membrane transport complex for LDL) promote human atherosclerosis. Similarly, decreased levels of HDL-cholesterol (HDL-C) and its transport complex, apolipoprotein A, are associated with the development of atherosclerosis. Epidemiologic investigations have established that cardiovascular morbidity and mortality vary directly with the level of Total-C and LDL-C and inversely with the level of HDL-C. In multicenter clinical trials, those pharmacologic and/or non-pharmacologic interventions that simultaneously lowered LDL-C and increased HDL-C reduced the rate of cardiovascular events (both fatal and nonfatal myocardial infarctions). In both normal volunteers and patients with hypercholesterolemia, treatment with pravastatin sodium reduced Total-C, LDL-C, and apolipoprotein B. Pravastatin also modestly reduced VLDL-C and TG while producing increases of variable magnitude in HDL-C and apolipoprotein A. The effects of pravastatin on Lp (a), fibrinogen, and certain other independent biochemical risk markers for coronary heart disease are unknown. The effect of pravastatin-induced changes in lipoprotein levels, including reduction or serum cholesterol, on cardiovascular morbidity or mortality has not been established. Although pravastatin is relatively more hydrophilic than other HMG-CoA reductase inhibitors, the effect of relative hydrophilicity, if any, on either efficacy or safety has not been established.

In the Pravastatin Primary Prevention Study (West of Scotland Coronary Prevention Study - WOS), the effect of improving lipoprotein levels with pravastatin on fatal and non-fatal coronary heart disease (CHD) was assessed in 6595 men, without a previous myocardial infarction, and with LDL-C levels between 156-254 mg/dl (4-6.7 mmol/l). The patients were followed for a median of 4.8 years. In this randomized, double-blind, placebo-controlled study, pravastatin reduced the risk of a first coronary event [either CHD death or non-fatal myocardial infarction (MI)] by 31% [7.9% placebo vs pravastatin, p = 0.0001 : 248 events in the placebo group (CHD death = 44, non-fatal MI = 204) vs 174 events in the pravastatin group (CHD death = 31, non-fatal MI = 143)]. Pravastatin also decreased the risk for undergoing myocardial revascularization procedures (coronary artery bypass graft surgery or coronary angioplasty) by 37% (2.5% vs 1.7%, p = 0.009) and coronary angiography by 31% (4.2% vs 2.8%, p = 0.007). Cardiovascular deaths were decreased by 32% (2.3% vs 1.6%, p = 0.03), and there was no increase in death from non-cardiovascular causes.

PHARMACOKINETICS AND METABOLISM

Pravastatin sodium is administered orally in the active form. In clinical pharmacology studies in man, pravastatin is rapidly absorbed, with peak plasma levels of parent compound attained 1 to 1.5 hours following ingestion. Based on urinary recovery of radiolabeled drug, the average oral absorption of pravastatin is 34% and absolute bioavailability is 17%. While the presence of food in the gastrointestinal tract reduces systemic bioavailability, the lipid-lowering effects of the drug are similar whether taken with, or 1 hour prior, to meals.

Pravastatin undergoes extensive first-pass extraction in the liver (extraction ratio 0.66), which is its primary site of action, and the primary site of cholesterol synthesis and of LDL-C clearance. *In vitro* studies demonstrated that pravastatin is transported into hepatocytes with substantially less uptake into other cells. In view of pravastatin's apparently extensive first-pass hepatic metabolism, plasma levels may not necessarily correlate perfectly with lipid-lowering efficacy. Pravastatin plasma concentrations [including: area under the concentration-time curve (AUC), peak (C_{max}), and steady-state minimum (C_{min})] are directly proportional to administered dose. Systemic bioavailability of pravastatin administered following a bedtime dose was decreased 60% compared to that following an AM dose. Despite this decrease in

CLINICAL PHARMACOLOGY: *(cont'd)*

systemic bioavailability, the efficacy of pravastatin administered once daily in the evening, although not statistically significant, was marginally more effective than that after a morning dose. This finding of lower systemic bioavailability suggests greater hepatic extraction of the drug following the evening dose. Steady-state AUCs, C_{max} and C_{min} plasma concentrations showed no evidence of pravastatin accumulation following once or twice daily administration of pravastatin sodium. Approximately 50% of the circulating drug is bound to plasma proteins. Following single dose administration of ^{14}C-pravastatin, the elimination half-life (t1/2) for total radioactivity (pravastatin plus metabolites) in humans is 77 hours.

Pravastatin, like other HMG-CoA reductase inhibitors, has variable bioavailability. The coefficient of variation, based on between-subject variability, was 50% to 60% for AUC.

Approximately 20% of a radiolabeled oral dose is excreted in urine and 70% in the feces. After intravenous administration of radiolabeled pravastatin to normal volunteers, approximately 47% of total body clearance was via renal excretion and 53% by non-renal routes (*i.e.,* biliary excretion and biotransformation). Since there are dual routes of elimination, the potential exists both for compensatory excretion by the alternate route as well as for accumulation of drug and/or metabolites in patients with renal or hepatic insufficiency.

In a study comparing the kinetics of pravastatin in patients with biopsy confirmed cirrhosis (N=7) and normal subjects (N=7), the mean AUC varied 18-fold in cirrhotic patients and 5-fold in healthy subjects. Similarly, the peak pravastatin values varied 47-fold for cirrhotic patients compared to 6-fold for healthy subjects.

Biotransformation pathways elucidated for pravastatin include: (a) isomerization to 6-epi pravastatin and the 3α-hydroxyisomer of pravastatin (SQ 31,906), (b) enzymatic ring hydroxylation to SQ 31,945, (c) ω-1 oxidation of the ester side chain, (d) β-oxidation of the carboxy side chain, (e) ring oxidation followed by aromatization, (f) oxidation of a hydroxyl group to a keto group, and (g) conjugation. The major degradation product is the 3α-hydroxy isomeric metabolite, which has one-tenth to one-fortieth the HMG-CoA reductase inhibitory activity of the parent compound.

CLINICAL STUDIES:

Pravastatin is highly effective in reducing Total-C and LDL-C in patients with heterozygous familial, presumed familial combined, and non-familial (non-FH) forms of primary hypercholesterolemia. A therapeutic response is seen within 1 week, and the maximum response usually is achieved within 4 weeks. This response is maintained during extended periods of therapy. In addition, pravastatin is effective in reducing the risk of acute coronary events in hypercholesterolemic patients with and without previous myocardial infarction.

A single daily dose administered in the evening (the recommended dosing) is as effective as the same total daily dose given twice a day. Once daily administration in the evening appears to be marginally more effective than once daily administration in the morning, perhaps because hepatic cholesterol is synthesized mainly at night. In multicenter, double-blind, placebo-controlled studies of patients with primary hypercholesterolemia, treatment with pravastatin in daily doses ranging from 10 mg to 40 mg consistently and significantly decreased Total-C, LDL-C, and Total-C/HDL-C and LDL-C/HDL-C ratios; modestly decreased VLDL-C and plasma TG levels; and produced increases in HDL-C of variable magnitude.

TABLE 1 Primary Hypercholesterolemia Study Dose Response of Pravastatin Once Daily Administration At Bedtime

Dose	Total-C	LDL-C	HDL-C	TG
10 mg	-16%	-22%	+ 7%	-15%
20 mg	-24%	-32%	+ 2%	-11%
40 mg	-25%	-34%	+12%	-24%

* Mean percent change from baseline after 8 weeks.

In another clinical trial, patients treated with pravastatin in combination with cholestyramine (70% of patients were taking cholestyramine 20 or 24 g per day) had reductions equal to or greater than 50% in LDL-C. Furthermore, pravastatin attenuated cholestyramine-induced increases in TG levels (which are themselves of uncertain clinical significance).

Prevention of Coronary Heart Disease: In the Pravastatin Primary Prevention Study (West of Scotland Coronary Prevention Study- WOS)[1], the effect of pravastatin sodium on fatal and non-fatal coronary heart disease (CHD) was assessed in 6595 men 45-64 years of age, without a previous MI, and with LDL-C levels between 156–254 mg/dL (4-6.7 mmol/l). In this randomized, double-blind, placebo-controlled study, patients were treated with standard care, including dietary advice, and either pravastatin sodium 40 mg daily (N=3302) or placebo (N=3293) and followed for a median duration of 4.8 years.

Pravastatin sodium significantly reduced the rate of first coronary events (either CHD death or non-fatal MI) by 31% [248 events in the placebo group (CHD death = 44, non-fatal MI = 204) vs. 174 events in the pravastatin group (CHD death = 31, non-fatal MI = 143), p = 0.0001]. The risk reduction with pravastatin sodium was similar and significant throughout the entire range of baseline LDL cholesterol levels. This reduction was also similar and significant across the age range studied with a 40% risk reduction for patients younger than 55 years and a 27% risk reduction for patients 55 years and older. The Pravastatin Primary Prevention Study included only men and therefore it is not clear to what extent these data can be extrapolated to a similar population of female patients.

Pravastatin sodium also significantly decreased the risk for undergoing myocardial revascularization procedures (coronary artery bypass graft surgery or coronary angioplasty) by 37% (80 vs. 51 patients, p = 0.009) and coronary angiography by 31 % (128 vs. 90, p = 0.007). Cardiovascular deaths were decreased by 32% (73 vs. 50, p = 0.03), and there was no increase in death from non-cardiovascular causes.

Atherosclerosis and Myocardial Infarction: In the Pravastatin Limitation of Atherosclerosis in the Coronary Arteries (PLAC I[2]) study, the effect of pravastatin therapy on coronary atherosclerosis was assessed by coronary angiography in patients with coronary disease and moderate hypercholesterolemia (baseline LDL-C range = 130-190 mg/dl). In this double-blind, multicenter, controlled clinical trial, angiograms were evaluated at baseline and at three years in 264 patients. Although the difference between pravastatin and placebo for the primary endpoint (per-patient change in mean coronary artery diameter), and one of two secondary endpoints (change in percent lumen diameter stenosis) did not reach statistical significance, for the secondary endpoint of change in minimum lumen diameter, statistically significant slowing of disease was seen in the pravastatin treatment group (p=0.02).

In the Regression Growth Evaluation Statin Study (REGRESS)[3], the effect of pravastatin on coronary atherosclerosis was assessed by coronary angiography in 885 patients with angina pectoris, angiographically documented coronary artery disease and hypercholesterolemia (baseline total cholesterol range = 160–310 mg/dL). In this double-blind, multicenter, controlled clinical trial, angiograms were evaluated at baseline and at two years in 653 patients (323 treated with pravastatin). progression of coronary atherosclerosis was significantly slowed in the pravastatin group as assessed by changes in mean segment diameter (p = 0.037) and minimum obstruction diameter (p = 0.001).

CLINICAL STUDIES: *(cont'd)*

Analysis of pooled events from PLAC I, the Pravastatin, Lipids, and Atherosclerosis in the Carotids Study (PLAC II)[4], REGRESS, and in the Kuopio Atherosclerosis Prevention Study (KAPS)[5] (combined N = 1,891) showed that treatment with pravastatin was associated with a significant reduction in the composite event rate of fatal and non-fatal myocardial infarction (46 events or 6.4% for placebo versus 21 events or 2.4% fro pravastatin, p = 0.001). The predominant effect of pravastatin sodium was to reduce the rate of non-fatal myocardial infarction.

INDICATIONS AND USAGE:

Therapy with lipid-altering agents should be considered a component of multiple risk factor intervention in those individuals at increased risk for atherosclerotic vascular disease due to hypercholesterolemia. Lipid-altering agents should be used in addition to a diet restricted in saturated fat and cholesterol when the response to diet and other nonpharmacological measures alone has been inadequate (see NCEP Guidelines).

Primary Prevention of Coronary Events: In hypercholesterolemic patients without clinically evident coronary heart disease, pravastatin sodium is indicated to:

Reduce the risk of myocardial infarction

Reduce the risk of undergoing myocardial revascularization procedures

Reduce the risk of cardiovascular mortality with no increase in death from non-cardiovascular causes.

ATHEROSCLEROSIS: In hypercholesterolemic patients with clinically evident coronary artery disease, including prior MI, pravastatin sodium is indicated to:

Slow the progression of coronary atherosclerosis

Reduce the risk of acute coronary events

HYPERCHOLESTEROLEMIA: Pravastatin sodium is indicated for the reduction of elevated total and LDL-cholesterol levels in patients with primary hypercholesterolemia (Type IIa and IIb)[6].

TABLE 2 Classification of Hyperlipoproteinemias

Type	Lipoproteins Elevated	Lipid Elevations major	Lipid Elevations minor
I (rare)	chylomicrons	TG	↑→C
II a	LDL	C	-
II b	LDL VLDL	C	TG
III (rare)	IDL	C/TG	-
IV	VLDL	TG	↑→ C
V (rare)	chylomicrons, VLDL	TG	↑→ C

C =cholesterol, TG=triglycerides
LDL =low density
VLDL =very low density lipoprotein
IDL =intermediate density lipoprotein

For discussion of efficacy results, see CLINICAL STUDIES.

Prior to initiating therapy with pravastatin, secondary causes for hypercholesterolemia (*e.g.,* poorly controlled diabetes mellitus, hypothyroidism, nephrotic syndrome, dysproteinemia, obstructive liver disease, other drug therapy, alcoholism) should be excluded, and a lipid profile performed to measure Total-C, HDL-C, and TG. For patients with triglycerides (TG) <400 mg/dl (<4.5 mmol/l), LDL-C can be estimated using the following equation:

LDL-C = Total-C - HDL-C - 1/5 TG

For TG levels >400 mg/dl (>4.5 mmol/l), this equation is less accurate and LDL-C concentrations should be determined by ultracentrifugation. In many hypertriglyceridemic patients, LDL-C may be low or normal despite elevated Total-C. In such cases, HMG-CoA reductase inhibitors are not indicated.

Lipid determinations should be performed at intervals of no less than four weeks and dosage adjusted according to the patient's response to therapy.

The National Cholesterol Education Program's Treatment Guidelines are summarized in TABLE 3.

TABLE 3

Definite Atherosclerotic Disease*	Two or More Other Risk Factors**	LDL Cholesterol mg/dl (mmol/l) Initiation Level	LDL Cholesterol mg/dl (mmol/l) Goal
NO	NO	≥190 (>4.9)	<160 (<4.1)
NO	YES	≥160 (≥4.1)	<130 (<3.4)
YES	YES or NO	≥130 (≥3.4)	≤100 (≤2.6)

* Coronary heart disease or peripheral vascular disease (including symptomatic carotid artery disease).
** Other risk factors for coronary heart disease (CHD) include: age (males ≥45 years; females: ≥55 years or premature menopause without estrogen replacement therapy); family history of premature CHD; current cigarette smoking; hypertension; confirmed HDL-C <35 mg/dl (<0.91 mmol/l); and diabetes mellitus. Subtract one risk factor if HDL-C is ≥60 mg/dl (≥1.6 mmol/l).

Since the goal of treatment is to lower LDL-C, the NCEP recommends that LDL-C levels be used to initiate and assess treatment response. Only if LDL-C levels are not available, should the Total-C be used to monitor therapy.

As with other lipid-lowering therapy, pravastatin sodium is not indicated when hypercholesterolemia is due to hyperalphalipoproteinemia (elevated HDL-C). The efficacy of pravastatin has not been evaluated in patients with combined elevated Total-C and hypertriglyceridemia [>500 mg/dl (>5.7 mmol/l)] or in patients with elevated intermediate density lipoproteins as their primary lipid abnormality.

CONTRAINDICATIONS:

Hypersensitivity to any component of this medication.

Acute liver disease or unexplained, persistent elevations in liver function tests (see WARNINGS).

Pregnancy and Lactation: Atherosclerosis is a chronic process and discontinuation of lipid-lowering drugs during pregnancy should have little impact on the outcome of long-term therapy of primary hypercholesterolemia. Cholesterol and other products of cholesterol biosynthesis are essential components for fetal development (including synthesis of steroids and cell membranes). Since HMG-CoA reductase inhibitors decrease cholesterol synthesis and possibly the synthesis of other biologically active substances derived from cholesterol, they

CONTRAINDICATIONS: *(cont'd)*

may cause fetal harm when administered to pregnant women. Therefore, HMG-CoA reductase inhibitors are contraindicated during pregnancy and in nursing mothers. **Pravastatin should be administered to women of childbearing age only when such patients are highly unlikely to conceive and have been informed of the potential hazards.** If the patient becomes pregnant while taking this class of drug, therapy should be discontinued and the patient apprised of the potential hazard to the fetus.

WARNINGS:

Liver Enzymes: HMG-CoA reductase inhibitors, like some other lipid-lowering therapies, have been associated with biochemical abnormalities of liver function. Increases of serum transaminase (ALT, AST) values to more than 3 times the upper limit of normal occurring on 2 or more (not necessarily sequential) occasions have been reported in 1.3% of patients treated with pravastatin in the U.S. over an average period of 18 months. These abnormalities were not associated with cholestasis and did not appear to be related to treatment duration. In those patients in whom these abnormalities were believed to be related to pravastatin and who were discontinued from therapy, the transaminase levels usually fell slowly to pretreatment levels. These biochemical findings are usually asymptomatic although worldwide experience indicates that anorexia, weakness, and/or abdominal pain may also be present in rare patients.

It is recommended that liver function tests be performed before the initiation of treatment, at 6 and 12 weeks after initiation of therapy or elevation in dose, and periodically thereafter (*e.g.,* semiannually). Patients who develop increased transaminase levels should be monitored with a second liver function evaluation to confirm the finding and be followed thereafter with frequent liver function tests until the abnormality(ies) return to normal. Should an increase in AST or ALT of three times the upper limit of normal or greater persist, withdrawal of pravastatin therapy is recommended.

Active liver disease or unexplained transaminase elevations are contraindications to the use of pravastatin (see CONTRAINDICATIONS). Caution should be exercised when pravastatin is administered to patients with a history of liver disease or heavy alcohol ingestion (see CLINICAL PHARMACOLOGY, Pharmacokinetics/Metabolism). Such patients should be closely monitored, started at the lower end of the recommended dosing range, and titrated to the desired therapeutic effect.

SKELETAL MUSCLE: Rare cases of rhabdomyolysis with acute renal failure secondary to myoglobinuria have been reported with pravastatin and other drugs in this class. Uncomplicated myalgia has also been reported in pravastatin-treated patients (see ADVERSE REACTIONS). Myopathy, defined as muscle aching or muscle weakness in conjunction with increases in creatine phosphokinase (CPK) values to greater than 10 times the upper normal limit, was rare (<0.1%) in pravastatin clinical trials. Myopathy should be considered in any patient with diffuse myalgias, muscle tenderness or weakness, and/or marked elevation of CPK. Patients should be advised to report promptly unexplained muscle pain, tenderness or weakness, particularly if accompanied by malaise or fever. **Pravastatin therapy should be discontinued if markedly elevated CPK levels occur or myopathy is diagnosed or suspected. Pravastatin therapy should also be temporarily withheld in any patient experiencing an acute or serious condition predisposing to the development of renal failure secondary to rhabdomyolysis, e.g., sepsis; hypotension; major surgery; trauma; severe metabolic, endocrine, or electrolyte disorders; or uncontrolled epilepsy.**

The risk of myopathy during treatment with another HMG-CoA reductase inhibitor is increased with concurrent therapy with either erythromycin, cyclosporine, niacin, or fibrates. However, neither myopathy nor significant increases in CPK levels have been observed in three reports involving a total of 100 post-transplant patients (24 renal and 76 cardiac) treated for up to two years concurrently with pravastatin 10-40 mg of cyclosporine. Some of these patients also received other concomitant immunosuppressive therapies. In one single-dose study, pravastatin levels were found to be increased in cardiac transplant patients receiving cyclosporine. Further, in clinical trials involving small numbers of patients who were treated concurrently with pravastatin and niacin, there were no reports of myopathy. Also, myopathy was not reported in a trial of combination pravastatin (40 mg/day) and gemfibrozil (1200 mg/day), although 4 of 75 patients on the combination showed marked CPK elevations versus one of 73 receiving placebo. There was a trend toward more frequent CPK elevations and patient withdrawals due to musculoskeletal symptoms in the group receiving combined treatment as compared with the groups receiving placebo, gemfibrozil, or pravastatin monotherapy. (See DRUG INTERACTIONS.) **The use of fibrates alone may occasionally be associated with myopathy. The combined use of pravastatin and fibrates should be avoided unless the benefit of further alterations in lipid levels is likely to outweigh the increased risk of this drug combination.**

PRECAUTIONS:

GENERAL

Pravastatin may elevate creatine phosphokinase and transaminase levels (see ADVERSE REACTIONS.) This should be considered in the differential diagnosis of chest pain in a patient on therapy with pravastatin.

Homozygous Familial Hypercholesterolemia: Pravastatin has not been evaluated in patients with rare homozygous familial hypercholesterolemia. In this group of patients, it has been reported that HMG-CoA reductase inhibitors are less effective because the patients lack functional LDL receptors.

Renal Insufficiency: A single 20 mg oral dose of pravastatin was administered to 24 patients with varying degrees of renal impairment (as determined by creatinine clearance). No effect was observed on the pharmacokinetics of pravastatin or its 3α-hydroxy isomeric metabolite (SQ 31,906). A small increase was seen in mean AUC values and half-life (t1/2) for the inactive enzymatic ring hydroxylation metabolite (SQ 31,945). Given this small sample size, the dosage administered, and the degree of individual variability, patients with renal impairment who are receiving pravastatin should be closely monitored.

INFORMATION FOR THE PATIENT

Patients should be advised to report promptly unexplained muscle pain, tenderness or weakness, particularly if accompanied by malaise or fever.

Endocrine Function HMG-CoA reductase inhibitors interfere with cholesterol synthesis and lower circulating cholesterol levels and, as such, might theoretically blunt adrenal or gonadal steroid hormone production. Results of clinical trials with pravastatin in males and post-menopausal females were inconsistent with regard to possible effects of the drug on basal steroid hormone levels. In a study of 21 males, the mean testosterone response to human chorionic gonadotropin was significantly reduced (p<0.004) after 16 weeks of treatment with 40 mg of pravastatin. However, the percentage of patients showing a ≥50% rise in plasma testosterone after human chorionic gonadotropin stimulation did not change significantly after therapy in these patients. The effects of HMG-CoA reductase inhibitors on spermatogenesis and fertility have not been studied in adequate numbers of patients. The effects, if any, of pravastatin on the pituitary-gonadal axis in pre-menopausal females are unknown. Patients treated with pravastatin who display clinical evidence of endocrine dysfunction should be evaluated appropriately. Caution should also be exercised if an HMG-CoA

PRECAUTIONS: *(cont'd)*

reductase inhibitor or other agent used to lower cholesterol levels is administered to patients also receiving other drugs (*e.g.,* ketoconazole, spironolactone, cimetidine) they may diminish the levels or activity of steroid hormones.

CNS Toxicity: CNS vascular lesions, characterized by perivascular hemorrhage and edema and mononuclear cell infiltration of perivascular spaces, were seen in dogs treated with pravastatin at a dose of 25 mg/kg/day, a dose that produced a plasma drug level about 50 times higher than the mean drug level in humans taking 40 mg/day. Similar CNS vascular lesions have been observed with several other drugs in this class.

A chemically similar drug in this class produced optic nerve degeneration (Wallerian degeneration of retinogeniculate fibers) in clinically normal dogs in a dose-dependent fashion starting at 60 mg/kg/day, a dose that produced mean plasma drug levels about 30 times higher than the mean drug level in humans taking the highest recommended dose (as measured by total enzyme inhibitory activity). This same drug also produced vestibulocochlear Wallerian-like degeneration and retinal ganglion cell chromatolysis in dogs treated for 14 weeks at 180 mg/kg/day, a dose which resulted in a mean plasma drug level similar to that seen with the 60 mg/kg/day dose.

CARCINOGENESIS, MUTAGENESIS, AND IMPAIRMENT OF FERTILITY

In a 2-year study in rats fed pravastatin at doses of 10, 30, or 100 mg/kg body weight, there was an increased incidence of hepatocellular carcinomas in males at the highest dose (p <0.01). Although rats were given up to 125 times the human dose (HD) on a mg/kg body weight basis, serum drug levels were only 6 to 10 times higher than those measured in humans given 40 mg pravastatin as measured by AUC.

The oral administration of 10, 30, or 100 mg/kg (producing plasma drug levels approximately 0.5 to 5.0 times the human drug levels at 40 mg) of pravastatin to mice for 22 months resulted in a statistically significant increase in the incidence of malignant lymphomas in treated females when all treatment groups were pooled and compared to controls (p <0.05). The incidence was not dose-related and male mice were not affected.

A chemically similar drug in this class was administered to mice for 72 weeks at 25, 100, and 400 mg/kg body weight, which resulted in mean serum drug levels approximately 3, 15, and 33 times higher than the mean human serum drug concentration (as total inhibitory activity) after a 40 mg oral dose. Liver carcinomas were significantly increased in high-dose females and mid- and high-dose males, with a maximum incidence of 90 percent in males. The incidence of adenomas of the liver was significantly increased in mid- and high-dose females. Drug treatment also significantly increased the incidence of lung adenomas in mid- and high-dose males and females. Adenomas of the eye Harderian gland (a gland of the eye of rodents) were significantly higher in high-dose mice than in controls.

No evidence of mutagenicity was observed *in vitro,* with or without rat-liver metabolic activation, in the following studies: microbial mutagen tests, using mutant strains of *Salmonella typhimurium* or *Escherichia coli;* a forward mutation assay in L5178Y TK +/- mouse lymphoma cells; a chromosomal aberration test in hamster cells; and a gene conversion assay using *Saccharomyces cerevisiae.* In addition, there was no evidence of mutagenicity in either a dominant lethal test in mice or a micronucleus test in mice.

In a study in rats, with daily doses up to 500 mg/kg, pravastatin did not produce any adverse effects on fertility or general reproductive performance. However, in a study with another HMG-CoA reductase inhibitor, there was decreased fertility in male rats treated for 34 weeks at 25 mg/kg body weight, although this effect was not observed in a subsequent fertility study when this same dose was administered for 11 weeks (the entire cycle of spermatogenesis, including epididymal maturation). In rats treated with this same reductase inhibitor at 180 mg/kg/day, seminiferous tubule degeneration (necrosis and loss of spermatogenic epithelium) was observed. Although not seen with pravastatin, two similar drugs in this class caused drug-related testicular atrophy, decreased spermatogenesis, spermatocytic degeneration, and giant cell formation in dogs. The clinical significance of these findings is unclear.

PREGNANCY CATEGORY X

See CONTRAINDICATIONS. Safety in pregnant women has not been established. Pravastatin was not teratogenic in rats at doses up to 1000 mg/kg daily or in rabbits at doses of up to 50 mg/kg daily. These doses resulted in 20x (rabbit) or 240x (rat) the human exposure based on surface area ($mg/meter^2$). However, in studies with another HMG-CoA reductase inhibitor, skeletal malformations were observed in rats and mice. There has been one report of severe congenital bony deformity, tracheo-esophageal fistula, and anal atresia (Vater association) in a baby born to a woman who took another HMG-CoA reductase inhibitor with dextroamphetamine sulfate during the first trimester of pregnancy. Pravastatin sodium should be administered to women of child-bearing potential only when such patients are highly unlikely to conceive and have been informed of the potential hazards. If the woman becomes pregnant while taking pravastatin sodium, it should be discontinued and the patient advised again as to the potential hazards to the fetus.

NURSING MOTHERS

A small amount of pravastatin is excreted in human breast milk. Because of the potential for serious adverse reactions in nursing infants, women taking pravastatin sodium should not nurse (see CONTRAINDICATIONS.)

PEDIATRIC USE

Safety and effectiveness in individuals less than 18 years old have not been established. Hence, treatment in patients less than 18 years old is not recommended at this time.

DRUG INTERACTIONS:

Immunosuppressive Drugs: *Gemfibrozil, Niacin (Nicotinic Acid), Erythromycin* (See WARNINGS, Skeletal Muscle.

Antipyrine: Since concomitant administration of pravastatin had no effect on the clearance of antipyrine, interactions with other drugs metabolized via the same hepatic cytochrome isozymes are not expected.

Cholestyramine/Colestipol: Concomitant administration resulted in an approximately 40 to 50% decrease in the mean AUC of pravastatin. However, when pravastatin was administered 1 hour before or 4 hours after cholestyramine or 1 hour before colestipol and a standard meal, there was no clinically significant decrease in bioavailability or therapeutic effect. See DOSAGE AND ADMINISTRATION, Concomitant Therapy.

Warfarin: In a study involving 10 healthy male subjects given pravastatin and warfarin concomitantly for 6 days, bioavailability parameters at steady state for pravastatin (parent compound) were not altered. Pravastatin did not alter the plasma protein-binding of warfarin. Concomitant dosing did increase the AUC and C_{max} of warfarin but did not produce any changes in its anticoagulant action (*i.e.,* no increase was seen in mean prothrombin time after 6 days of concomitant therapy). However, bleeding and extreme prolongation of prothrombin time has been reported with another drug in this class. Patients receiving warfarin-type anticoagulants should have their prothrombin times closely monitored when pravastatin is initiated or the dosage of pravastatin is changed.

Cimetidine: The $AUC_{0\text{-}12hr}$ for pravastatin when given with cimetidine was not significantly different from the AUC for pravastatin when given alone. A significant difference was observed between the AUCs for pravastatin when given with cimetidine compared to when administered with antacid.

DRUG INTERACTIONS: *(cont'd)*

Digoxin: In a crossover trial involving 18 healthy male subjects given pravastatin and digoxin concurrently for 9 days, the bioavailability parameters of digoxin were not affected. The AUC of pravastatin tended to increase, but the overall bioavailability of pravastatin plus its metabolites SQ 31,906 and SQ 31,945 was not altered.

Cyclosporine: Some investigators have measured cyclosporine levels in patients on pravastatin, and to date, these results indicate no clinically meaningful elevations in cyclosporine levels. In one single-dose study, pravastatin levels were found to be increased in cardiac transplant patients receiving cyclosporine.

Gemfibrozil: In a crossover study in 20 healthy male volunteers given concomitant single doses of pravastatin and gemfibrozil, there was a significant decrease in urinary excretion and protein binding of pravastatin. In addition, there was a significant increase in AUC, C_{max}, and T_{max} for the pravastatin metabolite SQ 31,906. Combination therapy with pravastatin and gemfibrozil is generally not recommended.

In interaction studies with *aspirin, antacids* (1 hour prior to pravastatin), *cimetidine, nicotinic acid,* or *probucol,*no statistically significant differences in bioavailability were seen when pravastatin sodium was administered.

Other Drugs: During clinical trials, no noticeable drug interactions were reported when pravastatin was added to: diuretics, antihypertensives, digitalis, ACE inhibitors, calcium channel blockers, beta-blockers, or nitroglycerin.

ADVERSE REACTIONS:

Pravastatin is generally well tolerated; adverse reactions have usually been mild and transient. In 4-month long placebo-controlled trials, 1.7% of pravastatin-treated patients and 1.2% of placebo-treated patients were discontinued from treatment because of adverse experiences attributed to study drug therapy; this difference was not statistically significant. In long-term studies, the most common reasons for discontinuation were asymptomatic serum transaminase increases and mild, non-specific gastrointestinal complaints. During clinical trials the overall incidence of adverse events in the elderly was not different from the incidence observed in younger patients.

Adverse Clinical Events: All adverse clinical events (regardless of attribution) reported in more than 2% of pravastatin-treated patients in the placebo-controlled trials are identified in TABLE 4; also shown are the percentages of patients in whom these medical events were believed to be related or possibly related to the drug.

TABLE 4

Body System/Event	All Events Pravastatin (N=900) %	All Events Placebo (N=411) %	Events Attributed to Study Drug Pravastatin (N=900) %	Events Attributed to Study Drug Placebo (N=411) %
Cardiovascular				
Cardiac Chest Pain	4.0	3.4	0.1	0.0
Dermatologic				
Rash	4.0*	1.1	1.3	0.9
Gastrointestinal				
Nausea/Vomiting	7.3	7.1	2.9	3.4
Diarrhea	6.2	5.6	2.0	1.9
Abdominal Pain	5.4	6.9	2.0	3.9
Constipation	4.0	7.1	2.4	5.1
Flatulence	3.3	3.6	2.7	3.4
Heartburn	2.9	1.9	2.0	0.7
General Fatigue	3.8	3.4	1.9	1.0
Chest Pain	3.7	1.9	0.3	0.2
Influenza	2.4*	0.7	0.0	0.0
Musculoskeletal				
Localized Pain	10.0	9.0	1.4	1.5
Myalgia	2.7	1.0	0.6	0.0
Nervous System				
Headache	6.2	3.9	1.7*	0.2
Dizziness	3.3	3.2	1.0	0.5
Renal/Genitourinary				
Urinary Abnormality	2.4	2.9	0.7	1.2
Respiratory				
Common Cold	7.0	6.3	0.0	0.0
Rhinitis	4.0	4.1	0.1	0.0
Cough	2.6	1.7	0.1	0.0

* Statistically significantly different from placebo.

In the Pravastatin Primary Prevention Study (West of Scotland Coronary Prevention Study) (see CLINICAL STUDIES) involving 6595 patients treated with pravastatin sodium (n=3302) or placebo (n=3293), the adverse event profile in the pravastatin sodium group was comparable to that of the placebo group over the median 4.8 years of the study.

The following effects have been reported with drugs in this class; not all the effects listed below have necessarily been associated with pravastatin sodium therapy:

Skeletal: myopathy, rhabdomyolysis, arthralgia.

Neurological: dysfunction of certain cranial nerves (including alteration of taste, impairment of extra-ocular movement, facial paresis), tremor, vertigo, memory loss, paresthesia, peripheral neuropathy, peripheral nerve palsy, anxiety, insomnia, depression.

Hypersensitivity Reactions: An apparent hypersensitivity syndrome has been reported rarely which has included one or more of the following features: anaphylaxis, angioedema, lupus erythematous-like syndrome, polymyalgia rheumatica, dermatomyositis, vasculitis, purpura, thrombocytopenia, leukopenia, hemolytic anemia, positive ANA, ESR increase, eosinophilia, arthritis, arthralgia, urticaria, asthenia, photosensitivity, fever, chills, flushing, malaise, dyspnea, toxic epidermal necrolysis, erythema multiforme, including Stevens-Johnson syndrome.

Gastrointestinal: pancreatitis, hepatitis, including chronic active hepatitis, cholestatic jaundice, fatty change in liver, and, rarely, cirrhosis, fulminant hepatic necrosis, and hepatoma; anorexia, vomiting.

Skin: alopecia, pruritus. A variety of skin changes (*e.g.,* nodules, discoloration, dryness of skin/mucous membranes, changes to hair/nails) have been reported.

Reproductive: gynecomastia, loss of libido, erectile dysfunction.

Eye: progression of cataracts (lens opacities), ophthalmoplegia.

Laboratory Abnormalities: elevated transaminase, alkaline phosphatase, and bilirubin; thyroid function abnormalities.

Laboratory Test Abnormalities: Increases in serum transaminase (ALT, AST) values and CPK have been observed (see WARNINGS.)

Transient, asymptomatic eosinophilia has been reported. Eosinophil counts usually returned to normal despite continued therapy. Anemia, thrombocytopenia, and leukopenia have been reported with HMG-CoA reductase inhibitors.

ADVERSE REACTIONS: *(cont'd)*

Concomitant Therapy: Pravastatin has been administered concurrently with cholestyramine, colestipol, nicotinic acid, probucol and gemfibrozil. Preliminary data suggest that the addition of either probucol or gemfibrozil to therapy with lovastatin or pravastatin is **not** associated with greater reduction in LDL-cholesterol than that achieved with lovastatin or pravastatin alone. No adverse reactions unique to the combination or in addition to those previously reported for each drug alone have been reported. Myopathy and rhabdomyolysis (with or without acute renal failure) have been reported when another HMG-CoA reductase inhibitor was used in combination with immunosuppressive drugs, gemfibrozil, erythromycin, or lipid-lowering doses of nicotinic acid. Concomitant therapy with HMG-CoA reductase inhibitors and these agents is generally not recommended. See WARNINGS, Skeletal Muscle and DRUG INTERACTIONS.

OVERDOSAGE:

To date, there are two reported cases of overdosage with pravastatin, both of which were asymptomatic and not associated with clinical laboratory abnormalities. If an overdose occurs, it should be treated symptomatically and supportive measures should be instituted as required.

DOSAGE AND ADMINISTRATION:

The patient should be placed on a standard cholesterol-lowering diet before receiving pravastatin and should continue on this diet during treatment with pravastatin (see NCEP Treatment Guidelines for details on dietary therapy).

The recommended starting dose is 10 or 20 mg once daily at bedtime. In primary hypercholesterolemic patients with a history of significant renal or hepatic dysfunction, and in the elderly, a starting dose of 10 mg daily at bedtime is recommended. Pravastatin may be taken without regard to meals.

Since the maximal effect of a given dose is seen within 4 weeks, periodic lipid determinations should be performed at this time and dosage adjusted according to the patient's response to therapy and established treatment guidelines. The recommended dosage range is generally 10 to 40 mg administered once a day at bedtime. In the elderly, maximum reductions in LDL-cholesterol may be achieved with daily doses of 20 mg or less.

In patients taking immunosuppressive drugs such as cyclosporine (see WARNINGS, Skeletal Muscle) concomitantly with pravastatin, therapy should begin with 10 mg of pravastatin once-a-day at bedtime and titration to higher doses should be done with caution. Most patients treated with this combination received a maximum pravastatin dose of 20 mg/day.

Concomitant Therapy: The lipid-lowering effects of pravastatin on total and LDL cholesterol are enhanced when combined with a bile-acid-binding resin. When administering a bile-acid-binding resin (*e.g.,* cholestyramine, colestipol) and pravastatin, pravastatin should be given either 1 hour or more before or at least 4 hours following the resin. See also ADVERSE REACTIONS: Concomitant Therapy.

Storage: Do not store above 86° F (30° C). Keep tightly closed (protect from moisture). Protect from light.

REFERENCES:

1. Shepard, J, et al. Prevention of coronary heart disease with pravastatin in men with hypercholesterolemia. *N Engl J Med*1995; 333:1301-7. **2.** Pitt, B, et al. Design and recruitment in the United States of a multicenter quantitative angiographic trial of pravastatin to limit atherosclerosis in the coronary arteries (PLAC I). *Am J Cardiol*72:31, 1993. **3.** Jukema JW, et al. Effects of Lipid Lowering by Pravastatin on Progression and Regression of Coronary Artery Disease in Symptomatic Man With Normal to Moderately Elevated Serum Cholesterol Levels. The Regression Growth Evaluation Study (REGRESS). *Circulation* 1995, 91:2528–2540. **4.** Crouse, JR, et al. Pravastatin, lipids, and atherosclerosis in the carotid arteries; design features of a clinical trial with carotid atherosclerosis outcome.*Controlled Clinical Trials* 13:495, 1992. **5.** Salonen R., et al. Kuopio Atherosclerosis Prevention Study (KAPS). A population-based primary preventive trial of the effect of LDL lowering on atherosclerotic progression in carotid and femoral arteries. Research Institute of Public Health, University of Kuopio, Finland. *Circulation* 92: 1758, 1995. **6.** Fredrickson classification: Type IIa-elevation of LDL; Type IIb-elevation of LDL and VLDL. Type III (familial dysbetalipoproteinemia)-elevation of IDL. Fredrickson, DS, Fat transport in lipoproteins - an integrated approach to mechanism and disorders. *N Engl J Med*276:34, 1967.

PATIENT INFORMATION:

This drug is used to lower cholesterol and to prevent heart attacks.

Do not take if you are pregnant or nursing, or have active liver disease.

This medication can interact with many other drugs. Inform your doctor of any other medications, including over-the-counter medications, that you are taking.

Inform your physician if you experience any unexplained muscle pain, tenderness, or weakness, especially if accompanied by fever or tiredness.

Follow a low cholesterol diet. This medication may be given with or without meals.

This medication may cause nausea vomiting, diarrhea, rash, or muscle tenderness. Inform your physician or pharmacist if these effects occur.

HOW SUPPLIED:

10 mg tablets: Pink to peach, rounded, rectangular-shaped, biconvex with a P embossed on one side and PRAVACHOL 10 engraved on the opposite side.

20 mg tablets: Yellow, rounded, rectangular-shaped, biconvex with a P embossed on one side and PRAVACHOL 20 engraved on the opposite side.

40 mg tablets: Green, rounded, rectangular-shaped, biconvex with a P embossed on one side and PRAVACHOL 40 engraved on the opposite side.

HOW SUPPLIED - EQUIVALENTS NOT AVAILABLE:

Tablet, Uncoated - Oral - 10 mg

90's	$157.99	PRAVACHOL, Bristol Myers Squibb	00003-5154-05
100's	$168.79	PRAVACHOL, Bristol Myers Squibb	00003-0154-50
100's	$178.66	PRAVACHOL, Bristol Myers Squibb	00003-5154-06

Tablet, Uncoated - Oral - 20 mg

90's	$170.11	PRAVACHOL, Bristol Myers Squibb	00003-5178-05
100's	$192.41	PRAVACHOL, Bristol Myers Squibb	00003-5178-06
1000's	$1890.20	PRAVACHOL, Bristol Myers Squibb	00003-5178-75

Tablet, Uncoated - Oral - 40 mg

90's	$287.57	PRAVACHOL, Bristol Myers Squibb	00003-5194-10

PRAZIQUANTEL *(002099)*

CATEGORIES: Anthelmintics; Anti-Infectives; Antiparasitics; Helminths; Infections; Parasiticidal; Trematodes; Pregnancy Category B; FDA Approved 1982 Dec

BRAND NAMES: **Biltricide**; *Cesol*; *Cisticid* (Mexico); *Distocide*; *Ehliten* (Mexico); *Flukacide*; *Kalcide*; *Opticide*; *Pontel*; *Prazite*; *Tecprazin* (Mexico); *Teniken* (Mexico)
(International brand names outside U.S. in italics)

FORMULARIES: WHO

DESCRIPTION:

Biltricide (praziquantel) is a trematodicide provided in tablet form for the oral treatment of schistosome infections.

Biltricide (praziquantel) is 2-(cyclohexylcarbonyl-1,2,3,6,7 11b-hexahydro4H-pyrazino (2,1-a) isoquinolin-4-one with the molecular formula:

$C_{19}H_{24}N_2O_2$

Praziquantel is a colorless crystalline powder of bitter taste. The compound is stable under normal conditions and melts at 136-140°C with decomposition. The active substance is hygroscopic. Praziquantel is easily soluble in chloroform and dimethylsulfoxide, soluble in ethanol and very slightly soluble in water.

Biltricide lacquered tablets contain 600 mg of praziquantel.

CLINICAL PHARMACOLOGY:

Biltricide induces a rapid contraction of schistosomes by a specific effect on the permeability of the cell membrane. The drug further results in vacuolization & disintegration of the schistosome tegument.

After oral administration Biltricide is rapidly absorbed (80%), subjected to a first pass effect, metabolized and eliminated by the kidneys. Maximal serum concentration is achieved 1-3 hours after dosing. The half-life of praziquantel in serum is 0.8 - 1.5 hours.

INDICATIONS AND USAGE:

Biltricide is indicated for the treatment of infections due to *Schistosoma mekongi; Schistosoma japonicum, Schistosoma mansoni and Schistosoma hematobium.*

CONTRAINDICATIONS:

Biltricide should not be given to patients who previously have shown hypersensitivity to the drug.

PRECAUTIONS:

Information for the patient. Patients should be warned not to drive a car and not to operate machinery on the day of Biltricide treatment and the following day.

Minimal increases in liver enzymes have been reported in 3.31 to 27% of treated patients.

Mutagenesis, Carcinogenesis: Mutagenic effects in Salmonella tests found by one laboratory have not been confirmed in the same tested strain by other laboratories. A long term carcinogenicity study in rats did not reveal any carcinogenic effect. Results from a similar carcinogenicity study are incomplete.

Pregnancy Category B: Reproduction studies have been performed in rats and rabbits at doses up to 40 times the human dose and have revealed no evidence of impaired fertility or harm to the fetus due to Biltricide. There are, however, no adequate and well-controlled studies, in pregnant women. An increase of the abortion rate was found in rats at three times the single human therapeutic dose. While animal reproduction studies are not always predictive of human response this drug should be used during pregnancy only if clearly needed.

Nursing Mothers: Biltricide appeared in the milk of nursing women at a concentration of about 1/4 that of maternal serum. Woman should not nurse on the day of Biltricide treatment and during the subsequent 72 hours.

Pediatric Use: Safety in children under 4 years of age has not been established.

DRUG INTERACTIONS:

No data are available regarding interaction of Biltricide with other drugs.

ADVERSE REACTIONS:

In general Biltricide is very well tolerated. Side effects are usually mild and transient and do not require treatment. The following side effects were observed malaise-headache-dizziness-abdominal discomfort with or without nausea in 90% of treated cases and more rarely rising temperature and urticaria. In patients with liver impairment caused by the infection, no adverse effects of Biltricide have occurred which would necessitate restriction in use.

OVERDOSAGE:

In rats and mice the acute LD_{50} was about 2,500 mg/kg. No data are available in humans. In the event of overdose a fact-acting laxative should be given.

DOSAGE AND ADMINISTRATION:

The dosage recommended for the treatment of schistosomiasis is: 3 x 20 mg/kg bodyweight as a one day treatment. The tablets should be washed down unchewed with some liquid during meals. Keeping the tablets or segments thereof in the mouth can reveal a bitter taste which can promote gagging or vomiting. The interval between the individual doses should not be less than 4 and not more than 6 hours. Dosage for children under four years has not been established.

STORAGE CONDITIONS

Store below 86°F (30°C) avoid freezing.

HOW SUPPLIED - EQUIVALENTS NOT AVAILABLE:

Tablet, Plain Coated - Oral - 600 mg

6's $61.88 BILTRICIDE, Bayer 00026-2521-06

PRAZOSIN HYDROCHLORIDE *(002100)*

CATEGORIES: Alpha Adrenergic Receptor Inhibitors; Alpha Blockers; Antihypertensives; Cardiovascular Drugs; Hypertension; Renal Drugs; Benign Prostatic Hyperplasia*; Prostate Enlargement*; Pregnancy Category C; Sales > $100 Million; FDA Approval Pre 1982

* Indication not approved by the FDA

BRAND NAMES: *Decliten*; *Duramipress* (Germany); *Eurex* (Germany); *Hexapress*; *Hypotens*; *Hypovase* (England); *Hyprosin*; *Lopres*; *Lopress*; *Minima*; *Minipres* (Mexico); **Minipress**; *Minison*; *Mysial*; *Patsolin*; *Peripress*; *Polypress*; *Pratisol*; *Pratsiol*; *Prazac*; *Prazopress*; *Pressin*; *Rexibet*
(International brand names outside U.S. in italics)

FORMULARIES: Aetna; BC-BS; CIGNA; FHP; Foundation; Humana; Kaiser; Medco; Medi-Cal; PCS; PruCare; United

COST OF THERAPY: $45.55 (Hypertension; Capsule; 1 mg; 2/day; 365 days)

PRIMARY ICD9: 401.1 (Essential Hypertension, Benign)

DESCRIPTION:

Prazosin hydrochloride (abbreviated here as prazosin HCl), a quinazoline derivative, is the first of a new chemical class of antihypertensives. It is the hydrochloride salt of 1-(4-amino-6,7-dimethoxy-2-quinazolinyl)-4-(2-furoyl) piperazine.

It is a white, crystalline substance, slightly soluble in water and isotonic saline, and has a molecular weight of 419.87. Each 1 mg capsule of prazosin HCl for oral use contains drug equivalent to 1 mg free base.

Inert ingredients in the formulations are: hard gelatin capsules (which may contain Blue 1, Red 3, Red 28, Red 40, and other inert ingredients); magnesium stearate; sodium lauryl sulfate; starch; sucrose.

CLINICAL PHARMACOLOGY:

The exact mechanism of the hypotensive action of prazosin is unknown. Prazosin causes a decrease in total peripheral resistance and was originally thought to have a direct relaxant action on vascular smooth muscle. Recent animal studies, however, have suggested that the vasodilator effect of prazosin is also related to blockade of postsynaptic *alpha*-adrenoceptors. The results of dog forelimb experiments demonstrate that the peripheral vasodilator effect of prazosin is confined mainly to the level of the resistance vessels (arterioles). Unlike conventional *alpha*-blockers, the antihypertensive action of prazosin is usually not accompanied by a reflex tachycardia. Tolerance has not been observed to develop in long term therapy.

Hemodynamic studies have been carried out in man following acute single dose administration and during the course of long term maintenance therapy. The results confirm that the therapeutic effect is a fall in blood pressure unaccompanied by a clinically significant change in cardiac output, heart rate, renal blood flow and glomerular filtration rate. There is no measurable negative chronotropic effect.

In clinical studies to date, prazosin HCl has not increased plasma renin activity.

In man, blood pressure is lowered in both the supine and standing positions. This effect is most pronounced on the diastolic blood pressure.

Following oral administration, human plasma concentrations reach a peak at about three hours with a plasma half-life of two to three hours. The drug is highly bound to plasma protein. Bioavailability studies have demonstrated that the total absorption relative to the drug in a 20% alcoholic solution is 90%, resulting in peak levels approximately 65% of that of the drug in solution. Animal studies indicate that prazosin HCl is extensively metabolized, primarily by demethylation and conjugation, and excreted mainly via bile and feces. Less extensive human studies suggest similar metabolism and excretion in man.

In clinical studies in which lipid profiles were followed, there were generally no adverse changes noted between pre- and post-treatment lipid levels.

INDICATIONS AND USAGE:

Prazosin HCl is indicated in the treatment of hypertension. It can be used alone or in combination with other antihypertensive drugs such as diuretics or beta-adrenergic blocking agents.

CONTRAINDICATIONS:

None known.

WARNINGS:

Prazosin HCl may cause syncope with sudden loss of consciousness. In most cases this is believed to be due to an excessive postural hypotensive effect, although occasionally the syncopal episode has been preceded by a bout of severe tachycardia with heart rates of 120-160 beats per minute. Syncopal episodes have usually occurred within 30 to 90 minutes of the initial dose of the drug; occasionally they have been reported in association with rapid dosage increases or the introduction of another antihypertensive drug into the regimen of a patient taking high doses of prazosin HCl. The incidence of syncopal episodes is approximately 1% in patients given an initial dose of 2 mg or greater. Clinical trials conducted during the investigational phase of this drug suggest that syncopal episodes can be minimized by limiting the initial dose of the drug to 1 mg, by subsequently increasing the dosage slowly, and by introducing any additional antihypertensive drugs into the patient's regimen with caution (see DOSAGE AND ADMINISTRATION). **Hypotension may develop in patients given prazosin HCl who are also receiving a beta-blocker such as propranolol.**

If syncope occurs, the patient should be placed in the recumbent position and treated supportively as necessary. This adverse effect is self-limiting and in most cases does not recur after the initial period of therapy or during subsequent dose titration.

Patients should always be started on the 1 mg capsules of prazosin HCl. The 2 and 5 mg capsules are not indicated for initial therapy.

More common than loss of consciousness are the symptoms often associated with lowering of the blood pressure, namely, dizziness and lightheadedness. The patient should be cautioned about these possible adverse effects and advised what measures to take should they develop. The patient should also be cautioned to avoid situations where injury could result should syncope occur during the initiation of prazosin HCl therapy.

PRECAUTIONS:

INFORMATION FOR THE PATIENT

Dizziness or drowsiness may occur after the first dose of this medicine. Avoid driving or performing hazardous tasks for the first 24 hours after taking this medicine or when the dose is increased. Dizziness, lightheadedness or fainting may occur, especially when rising from a lying or sitting position. Getting up slowly may help lessen the problem. These effects may also occur if you drink alcohol, stand for long periods of time, exercise, or if the weather is hot. While taking prazosin HCl, be careful in the amount of alcohol you drink. Also, use extra care during exercise or hot weather, or if standing for long periods. Check with your physician if you have any questions.

DRUG/LABORATORY TEST INTERACTIONS

In a study on five patients given from 12 to 24 mg of prazosin per day for 10 to 14 days, there was an average increase of 42% in the urinary metabolite of norepinephrine and an average increase in urinary VMA of 17%. Therefore, false positive results may occur in screening tests for pheochromocytoma in patients who are being treated with prazosin. If an elevated VMA is found, prazosin should be discontinued and the patient retested after a month.

LABORATORY TESTS

In clinical studies in which lipid profiles were followed, there were generally no adverse changes noted between pre- and post-treatment lipid levels.

CARCINOGENESIS, MUTAGENESIS, AND IMPAIRMENT OF FERTILITY

No carcinogenic potential was demonstrated in an 18 month study in rats with prazosin HCl at dose levels more than 225 times the usual maximum recommended human dose of 20 mg per day. prazosin HCl was not mutagenic in *in vivo* genetic toxicology studies. In a fertility and general reproductive performance study in rats, both males and females, treated with 75

PRECAUTIONS: *(cont'd)*

mg/kg (225 times the usual maximum recommended human dose), demonstrated decreased fertility while those treated with 25 mg/kg (75 times the usual maximum recommended human dose) did not.

In chronic studies (one year or more) of prazosin HCl in rats and dogs, testicular changes consisting of atrophy and necrosis occurred at 25 mg/kg/day (75 times the usual maximum recommended human dose). No testicular changes were seen in rats or dogs at 10 mg/kg/day (30 times the usual maximum recommended human dose). In view of the testicular changes observed in animals, 105 patients on long term prazosin HCl therapy were monitored for 17-ketosteroid excretion and no changes indicating a drug effect were observed. In addition, 27 males on prazosin HCl for up to 51 months did not have changes in sperm morphology suggestive of drug effect.

PREGNANCY CATEGORY C

Prazosin HCl has been shown to be associated with decreased litter size at birth, 1, 4, and 21 days of age in rats when given doses more than 225 times the usual maximum recommended human dose. No evidence of drug-related external, visceral, or skeletal fetal abnormalities were observed. No drug-related external, visceral, or skeletal abnormalities were observed in fetuses of pregnant rabbits and pregnant monkeys at doses more than 225 times and 12 times the usual maximum recommended human dose respectively.

The use of prazosin and a beta-blocker for the control of severe hypertension in 44 pregnant women revealed no drug-related fetal abnormalities or adverse effects. Therapy with prazosin was continued for as long as 14 weeks[1].

Prazosin has also been used alone or in combination with other hypotensive agents in severe hypertension of pregnancy by other investigators. No fetal or neonatal abnormalities have been reported with the use of prazosin[2].

There are no adequate and well controlled studies which establish the safety of prazosin HCl in pregnant women. Prazosin HCl should be used during pregnancy only if the potential benefit justifies the potential risk to the mother and fetus.

NURSING MOTHERS

Prazosin HCl has been shown to be excreted in small amounts in human milk. Caution should be exercised when prazosin HCl is administered to a nursing woman.

PEDIATRIC USE

Safety and effectiveness in children have not been established.

DRUG INTERACTIONS:

Prazosin HCl has been administered without any adverse drug interaction in limited clinical experience to date with the following: (1) cardiac glycosides—digitalis and digoxin; (2) hypoglycemics—insulin, chlorpropamide, phenformin, tolazamide, and tolbutamide; (3) tranquilizers and sedatives—chlordiazepoxide, diazepam, and phenobarbital; (4) antigout—allopurinol, colchicine, and probenecid; (5) antiarrhythmics—procainamide, propranolol (see WARNINGS however), and quinidine; and (6) analgesics, antipyretics and anti— inflammatories-propoxyphene, aspirin, indomethacin, and phenylbutazone.

Addition of a diuretic or other antihypertensive agent to prazosin HCl has been shown to cause an additive hypotensive effect. This effect can be minimized by reducing the prazosin HCl dose to 1 to 2 mg three times a day, by introducing additional antihypertensive drugs cautiously and then by retitrating prazosin Hcl based on clinical response.

ADVERSE REACTIONS:

Clinical trials were conducted on more than 900 patients. During these trials and subsequent marketing experience, the most frequent reactions associated with prazosin HCl therapy are: dizziness 10.3%, headache 7.8%, drowsiness 7.6%, lack of energy 6.9%, weakness 6.5%, palpitations 5.3%, and nausea 4.9%. In most instances side effects have disappeared with continued therapy or have been tolerated with no decrease in dose of drug.

Less Frequent Adverse Reactions Which Are Reported To Occur In 1-4% Of Patients Are:

Gastrointestinal: vomiting, diarrhea, constipation.

Cardiovascular: edema, orthostatic hypotension, dyspnea, syncope.

Central Nervous System: vertigo, depression, nervousness.

Dermatologic: rash.

Genitourinary: urinary frequency.

EENT: blurred vision, reddened sclera, epistaxis, dry mouth, nasal congestion.

In Addition, Fewer Than 1% Of Patients Have Reported The Following (In Some Instances, Exact Causal Relationships Have Not Been Established):

Gastrointestinal: abdominal discomfort and/or pain, liver function abnormalities, pancreatitis.

Cardiovascular: tachycardia.

Central Nervous System: paresthesia, hallucinations.

Dermatologic: pruritus, alopecia, lichen planus.

Genitourinary: incontinence, impotence, priapism.

EENT: tinnitus.

Other: diaphoresis, fever, positive ANA titer, arthralgia.

Single reports of pigmentary mottling and serous retinopathy, and few reports of cataract development or disappearance have been reported. In these instances, the exact causal relationship has not been established because the baseline observations were frequently inadequate.

In more specific slit-lamp and funduscopic studies, which included adequate baseline examinations, no drug-related abnormal ophthalmological findings have been reported.

Literature reports exist associating prazosin HCl therapy with a worsening of pre-existing narcolepsy. A causal relationship is uncertain in these cases.

OVERDOSAGE:

Accidental ingestion of at least 50 mg of prazosin HCl in a two year old child resulted in profound drowsiness and depressed reflexes. No decrease in blood pressure was noted. Recovery was uneventful.

Should overdosage lead to hypotension, support of the cardiovascular system is of first importance. Restoration of blood pressure and normalization of heart rate may be accomplished by keeping the patient in the supine position. If this measure is inadequate, shock should first be treated with volume expanders. If necessary, vasopressors should then be used. Renal function should be monitored and supported as needed. Laboratory data indicate prazosin HCl is not dialyzable because it is protein bound.

DOSAGE AND ADMINISTRATION:

The dose of prazosin HCl should be adjusted according to the patient's individual blood pressure response. The following is a guide to its administration:

INITIAL DOSE

1 mg two or three times a day. (See WARNINGS)

DOSAGE AND ADMINISTRATION: *(cont'd)*

MAINTENANCE DOSE

Dosage may be slowly increased to a total daily dose of 20 mg given in divided doses. The therapeutic dosages most commonly employed have ranged from 6 mg to 15 mg daily given in divided doses. Doses higher than 20 mg usually do not increase efficacy, however a few patients may benefit from further increases up to a daily dose of 40 mg given in divided doses. After initial titration some patients can be maintained adequately on a twice daily dosage regimen.

USE WITH OTHER DRUGS

When adding a diuretic or other antihypertensive agent, the dose of prazosin HCl should be reduced to 1 mg or 2 mg three times a day and retitration then carried out.

REFERENCES:

1. Lubbe, W F, and Hodge, J V: *New Zealand Med J* 94 (691) 169-172, 1981. **2.** Davey, D A, and Dommisse, J: *S.A. Med J*, Oct. 4, 1980 (551-556).

HOW SUPPLIED - RATED THERAPEUTICALLY EQUIVALENT:

Capsule, Gelatin - Oral - 1 mg

60's	$3.74	Prazosin HCl, H.C.F.A. F F P	99999-2100-01
100's	$6.24	Prazosin HCl, H.C.F.A. F F P	99999-2100-02
100's	$10.04	Prazosin Hcl, US Trading	56126-0463-11
100's	$20.45	Prazosin Hcl, Amer Preferred	53445-1920-01
100's	$23.34	Prazosin Hcl, HL Moore Drug Exch	00839-7554-06
100's	$23.51	Prazosin, Lederle Pharm	00005-3473-43
100's	$24.11	Prazosin Hcl, Geneva Pharms	00781-2211-01
100's	$24.15	Prazosin Hcl, Schein Pharm (US)	00364-2389-01
100's	$24.77	Prazosin Hcl, Purepac Pharm	00228-2500-10
100's	$24.80	Prazosin Hydrochloride, Aligen Independ	00405-4816-01
100's	$26.00	Prazosin Hcl, Qualitest Pharms	00603-5286-21
100's	$26.05	Prazosin Hcl, Zenith Labs	00172-4067-60
100's	$26.05	Prazosin Hcl, Goldline Labs	00182-1255-01
100's	$26.07	Prazosin Hcl, Schein Pharm (US)	00364-2389-90
100's	$26.85	Prazosin Hcl, Martec Pharms	52555-0279-01
100's	$26.90	Prazosin Hcl, Mylan	00378-1101-01
100's	$28.48	Prazosin Hcl, Medirex	57480-0384-01
100's	$41.55	Prazosin Hcl, Goldline Labs	00182-1255-89
100's	$41.55	Prazosin Hcl, Goldline Labs	00182-1920-89
100's	**$41.87**	**MINIPRESS, Pfizer Pharm**	**00663-4310-41**
100's	$43.63	Prazosin Hcl 1, Vangard Labs	00615-0386-13
250's	$15.60	Prazosin HCl, H.C.F.A. F F P	99999-2100-03
250's	$47.56	Prazosin Hcl, Mova Pharms	55370-0817-25
250's	$51.19	Prazosin HCl, Bristol Myers Squibb	00003-3630-04
250's	$52.92	Prazosin Hcl, HL Moore Drug Exch	00839-7554-09
250's	$52.93	Prazosin Hcl, Purepac Pharm	00228-2500-25
250's	$55.95	Prazosin Hcl, Rugby	00536-4845-02
250's	$55.99	Prazosin, Lederle Pharm	00005-3473-27
250's	$56.91	Prazosin Hcl, Schein Pharm (US)	00364-2389-04
250's	$57.40	Prazosin Hcl, Geneva Pharms	00781-2211-25
250's	$59.70	Prazosin Hcl, Major Pharms	00904-1040-70
250's	$59.70	Prazosin Hcl, Major Pharms	00904-5095-70
250's	$63.01	Prazosin Hcl, Qualitest Pharms	00603-5286-24
250's	$63.10	Prazosin Hcl, Zenith Labs	00172-4067-65
250's	$63.10	Prazosin Hcl, Goldline Labs	00182-1255-02
250's	$63.20	Prazosin Hydrochloride, Aligen Independ	00405-4816-04
250's	$63.60	Prazosin Hcl, Mylan	00378-1101-25
250's	**$90.25**	**MINIPRESS, Pfizer Pharm**	**00663-4310-71**
250's	**$103.54**	**MINIPRESS, Pfizer Labs**	**00069-4310-71**
500's	$31.20	Prazosin HCl, H.C.F.A. F F P	99999-2100-04
500's	$100.58	Prazosin Hcl, Schein Pharm (US)	00364-2389-05
600's	$162.40	Prazosin Hcl, Medirex	57480-0384-06
1000's	$62.40	Prazosin HCl, H.C.F.A. F F P	99999-2100-05
1000's	$132.54	Prazosin Hcl, Rugby	00536-4845-10
1000's	$168.95	Prazosin, Lederle Pharm	00005-3473-34
1000's	$202.50	Prazosin HCl, Bristol Myers Squibb	00003-3630-03
1000's	$203.11	Prazosin Hcl, HL Moore Drug Exch	00839-7554-16
1000's	$211.23	Prazosin Hcl, Geneva Pharms	00781-2211-10
1000's	$216.49	Prazosin Hcl, Purepac Pharm	00228-2500-96
1000's	$234.15	Prazosin Hcl, Major Pharms	00904-1040-80
1000's	$246.90	Prazosin Hcl, Zenith Labs	00172-4067-80
1000's	$247.00	Prazosin Hcl, Mylan	00378-1101-10
1000's	**$353.84**	**MINIPRESS, Pfizer Pharm**	**00663-4310-82**

Capsule, Gelatin - Oral - 2 mg

60's	$4.32	Prazosin HCl, H.C.F.A. F F P	99999-2100-06
60's	$19.43	Prazosin Hcl, Schein Pharm (US)	00364-2390-06
60's	$31.20	Prazosin Hcl, Major Pharms	00904-1041-52
100's	$7.20	Prazosin HCl, H.C.F.A. F F P	99999-2100-07
100's	$12.92	Prazosin Hcl, US Trading	56126-0464-11
100's	$29.50	Prazosin Hcl, Harber Pharm	51432-0498-03
100's	$29.80	Prazosin Hcl, Martec Pharms	52555-0280-01
100's	$29.96	Prazosin Hcl, HL Moore Drug Exch	00839-7555-06
100's	$31.18	Prazosin, Lederle Pharm	00005-3474-43
100's	$32.17	Prazosin Hcl, Purepac Pharm	00228-2501-10
100's	$32.80	Prazosin Hydrochloride, Aligen Independ	00405-4817-01
100's	$33.58	Prazosin Hcl, Geneva Pharms	00781-2212-01
100's	$33.62	Prazosin Hcl, Geneva Pharms	00781-2212-13
100's	$33.71	Prazosin Hcl, Schein Pharm (US)	00364-2390-01
100's	$34.30	Prazosin Hcl, Zenith Labs	00172-4068-60
100's	$34.30	Prazosin Hcl, Goldline Labs	00182-1256-01
100's	$34.40	Prazosin Hcl, Qualitest Pharms	00603-5287-21
100's	$35.10	Prazosin Hcl, Mylan	00378-2302-01
100's	$37.55	Prazosin Hcl, Schein Pharm (US)	00364-2390-90
100's	$39.35	Prazosin Hcl, Medirex	57480-0385-01
100's	$57.55	Prazosin Hcl, Goldline Labs	00182-1256-89
100's	$57.55	Prazosin Hcl, Goldline Labs	00182-1921-89
100's	**$57.99**	**MINIPRESS, Pfizer Pharm**	**00663-4370-41**
100's	$60.42	Prazosin Hydrochoride, Vangard Labs	00615-0387-13
100's	**$61.81**	**MINIPRESS, Pfizer Labs**	**00069-4370-41**
250's	$18.00	Prazosin HCl, H.C.F.A. F F P	99999-2100-08
250's	$49.88	Prazosin Hcl, HL Moore Drug Exch	00839-7555-09
250's	$64.57	Prazosin Hcl, Martec Pharms	52555-0280-02
250's	$65.97	Prazosin Hcl, Mova Pharms	55370-0818-25
250's	$70.63	Prazosin HCl, Bristol Myers Squibb	00003-3640-04
250's	$70.63	Prazosin Hcl, Amer Preferred	53445-1921-02
250's	$72.13	Prazosin Hcl, Purepac Pharm	00228-2501-25
250's	$73.50	Prazosin Hcl, Harber Pharm	51432-0498-05
250's	$77.96	Prazosin, Lederle Pharm	00005-3474-27
250's	$78.03	Prazosin Hydrochloride Capsules 2 Mg, Aligen Independ	00405-4817-04
250's	$79.00	Prazosin Hcl, Schein Pharm (US)	00364-2390-04
250's	$79.95	Prazosin HCl, Rugby	00536-4846-02
250's	$83.15	Prazosin Hcl, Major Pharms	00904-1041-70
250's	$83.15	Prazosin Hcl, Major Pharms	00904-5096-70

HOW SUPPLIED - RATED THERAPEUTICALLY EQUIVALENT: *(cont'd)*

250's	$83.60	Prazosin Hcl, Qualitest Pharms	00603-5287-24
250's	$83.65	Prazosin Hcl, Zenith Labs	00172-4068-65
250's	$83.65	Prazosin Hcl, Goldline Labs	00182-1256-02
250's	$83.65	Prazosin Hcl, Geneva Pharms	00781-2212-25
250's	$85.60	Prazosin Hcl, Mylan	00378-2302-25
250's	**$125.64**	**MINIPRESS, Pfizer Pharm**	**00663-4370-71**
250's	**$133.91**	**MINIPRESS, Pfizer Labs**	**00069-4370-71**
500's	$36.00	Prazosin HCl, H.C.F.A. F F P	99999-2100-09
500's	$140.10	Prazosin Hcl, Schein Pharm (US)	00364-2390-05
600's	$224.00	Prazosin Hcl, Medirex	57480-0385-06
1000's	$72.00	Prazosin HCl, H.C.F.A. F F P	99999-2100-10
1000's	$174.80	Prazosin Hcl, Rugby	00536-4846-10
1000's	$224.36	Prazosin Hcl, HL Moore Drug Exch	00839-7555-16
1000's	$225.47	Prazosin, Lederle Pharm	00005-3474-34
1000's	$280.00	Prazosin HCl, Bristol Myers Squibb	00003-3640-03
1000's	$294.35	Prazosin Hcl, Purepac Pharm	00228-2501-96
1000's	$325.90	Prazosin Hcl, Major Pharms	00904-1041-80
1000's	$326.00	Prazosin Hcl, Geneva Pharms	00781-2212-10
1000's	$329.20	Prazosin Hcl, Zenith Labs	00172-4068-80
1000's	$330.00	Prazosin Hcl, Mylan	00378-2302-10
1000's	**$492.53**	**MINIPRESS, Pfizer Pharm**	**00663-4370-82**
1000's	**$524.99**	**MINIPRESS, Pfizer Labs**	**00069-4370-82**

Capsule, Gelatin - Oral - 5 mg

60's	$7.15	Prazosin HCl, H.C.F.A. F F P	99999-2100-11
60's	$38.00	Prazosin Hcl, Schein Pharm (US)	00364-2391-06
100's	$11.93	Prazosin HCl, H.C.F.A. F F P	99999-2100-12
100's	$17.69	Prazosin Hcl, US Trading	56126-0465-11
100's	$45.35	Prazosin Hcl, HL Moore Drug Exch	00839-7556-06
100's	$49.80	Prazosin Hcl, Purepac Pharm	00228-2502-10
100's	$52.19	Prazosin Hydrochloride, Aligen Independ	00405-4818-01
100's	$53.16	Prazosin, Lederle Pharm	00005-3475-43
100's	$55.45	Prazosin Hcl, Martec Pharms	52555-0281-01
100's	$56.83	Prazosin Hcl, Geneva Pharms	00781-2213-13
100's	$57.60	Prazosin Hcl, Qualitest Pharms	00603-5288-21
100's	$57.70	Prazosin Hcl, Schein Pharm (US)	00364-2391-01
100's	$57.85	Prazosin Hcl, Geneva Pharms	00781-2213-01
100's	$60.00	Prazosin Hcl, Zenith Labs	00172-4069-60
100's	$60.00	Prazosin Hcl, Goldline Labs	00182-1257-01
100's	$60.25	Prazosin Hcl, Mylan	00378-3205-01
100's	$66.52	Prazosin Hcl, Medirex	57480-0386-01
100's	$87.00	Prazosin Hcl, Schein Pharm (US)	00364-2391-90
100's	$87.90	Prazosin Hcl, Goldline Labs	00182-1257-89
100's	$87.90	Prazosin Hcl, Goldline Labs	00182-1922-89
100's	$90.53	Prazosin Hcl, Vangard Labs	00615-0388-13
100's	**$98.03**	**MINIPRESS, Pfizer Pharm**	**00663-4380-41**
250's	$29.82	Prazosin HCl, H.C.F.A. F F P	99999-2100-13
250's	$90.44	Prazosin Hcl, HL Moore Drug Exch	00839-7556-09
250's	$123.75	Prazosin HCl, Bristol Myers Squibb	00003-3650-04
250's	$124.28	Prazosin Hcl, Mova Pharms	55370-0819-25
250's	$124.51	Prazosin Hcl, Purepac Pharm	00228-2502-25
250's	$132.88	Prazosin, Lederle Pharm	00005-3475-27
250's	$133.00	Prazosin Hcl, Schein Pharm (US)	00364-2391-04
250's	$133.73	Prazosin Hydrochloride, Aligen Independ	00405-4818-04
250's	$140.75	Prazosin HCl, Rugby	00536-4815-02
250's	$141.60	Prazosin Hcl, Geneva Pharms	00781-2213-25
250's	$141.69	Prazosin Hcl, Qualitest Pharms	00603-5288-24
250's	$141.70	Prazosin Hcl, Major Pharms	00904-1042-70
250's	$141.70	Prazosin Hcl, Major Pharms	00904-5097-70
250's	$142.00	Prazosin Hcl, Zenith Labs	00172-4069-65
250's	$142.00	Prazosin Hcl, Goldline Labs	00182-1257-02
250's	$142.50	Prazosin Hcl, Mylan	00378-3205-25
250's	**$214.16**	**MINIPRESS, Pfizer Pharm**	**00663-4380-71**
500's	$59.65	Prazosin HCl, H.C.F.A. F F P	99999-2100-14
500's	$198.21	Prazosin, Lederle Pharm	00005-3475-31
500's	$200.87	Prazosin Hcl, HL Moore Drug Exch	00839-7556-12
500's	$245.00	Prazosin HCl, Bristol Myers Squibb	00003-3650-02
500's	$264.50	Prazosin Hcl, Qualitest Pharms	00603-5288-28
500's	$264.64	Prazosin Hcl, Purepac Pharm	00228-2502-50
500's	$272.16	Prazosin Hcl, Geneva Pharms	00781-2213-05
500's	$280.55	Prazosin Hcl, Major Pharms	00904-1042-40
500's	$282.60	Prazosin Hcl, Zenith Labs	00172-4069-70
500's	$282.95	Prazosin Hcl, Mylan	00378-3205-05
500's	**$423.96**	**MINIPRESS, Pfizer Pharm**	**00663-4380-73**
600's	$379.00	Prazosin Hcl, Medirex	57480-0386-06

PREDNICARBATE *(003070)*

CATEGORIES: Adrenal Corticosteroids; Anti-Inflammatory Agents; Dermatoses; Skin/Mucous Membrane Agents; Steroids; FDA Class 2C ("Little or No Therapeutic Advantage"); FDA Approved 1991 Sep

BRAND NAMES: **Dermatop**

DESCRIPTION:

Dermatop Emollient Cream (prednicarbate emollient cream) 0.1% contains the following nonhalogenated prednisolone derivative, prednicarbate. Topical corticosteroids constitute a class of primarily synthetic steroids used topically as anti-inflammatory and antipruritic agents.

Each gram of Dermatop Emollient Cream 0.1% contains 1.0 mg of prednicarbate in a base consisting of white petrolatum USP, purified water USP, isopropyl myristate NF, lanolin alcohols NF, mineral oil USP, cetostearyl alcohol NF, aluminum stearate, edetate disodium USP, lactic acid USP, and magnesium stearate DAB 9.

The chemical name of prednicarbate is 11β, 17, 21-trihydroxypregna 1,4-diene-3,20-dione 17-(ethyl carbonate) 21-propionate. Prednicarbate has the empirical formula $C_{27}H_{36}O_8$ and a molecular weight of 488.58.

The CAS Registry Number is 73771-04-7.

CLINICAL PHARMACOLOGY:

In common with other topical corticosteroids, prednicarbate has anti-inflammatory, antipruritic, and vasoconstrictive properties. In general, the mechanism of the anti-inflammatory activity of topical steroids is unclear. However, corticosteroids are thought to act by the induction of phospholipase A_2 inhibitory proteins, collectively called lipocortins. It is postulated that these proteins control the biosynthesis of potent mediators of inflammation such as prostaglandins and leukotrienes by inhibiting the release of their common precursor arachidonic acid. Arachidonic acid is released from membrane phospholipids by phospholipase A_2.

CLINICAL PHARMACOLOGY: *(cont'd)*

PHARMACOKINETICS

The extent of percutaneous absorption of topical corticosteroids is determined by many factors, including the vehicle and the integrity of the epidermal barrier. Use of occlusive dressings with hydrocortisone for up to 24 hours has not been shown to increase penetration; however, occlusion of hydrocortisone for 96 hours does markedly enhance penetration. Topical corticosteroids can be absorbed from normal intact skin, whereas inflammation and/or other disease processes in the skin increase percutaneous absorption.

Studies performed with Dermatop Emollient Cream (prednicarbate emollient cream) 0.1% indicate that the drug is in the medium range of potency compared with other topical corticosteroids.

CLINICAL STUDIES:

Dermatop Emollient Cream was studied in vehicle controlled clinical trials in psoriasis and atopic dermatitis. In both studies, patients were to be treated twice daily for 21 days. Improvement in erythema, induration and scaling were studied in the psoriasis protocol. At Endpoint (*i.e.,* patient's last visit), the mean total sign scores for patients had decreased from baseline (*i.e.,* improved) by 37% and were significantly better than vehicle ($p<0.001$).

Improvement in erythema, induration and pruritus were studied in the atopic dermatitis protocol. At Endpoint (*i.e.,* patient's last visit), the mean total sign/symptom scores for patients had decreased from baseline (*i.e.,* improved) by 76% and were significantly better than vehicle ($p<0.001$).

The evaluations were performed in separate protocols by different panels of investigators. Different sets of signs/symptoms were evaluated in each protocol. These data are presented for comparison purposes only

TABLE 1 Overall Improvement of Disease at Endpoint—% of Patients

Indication	Scale Number 0	1	2	3	4	5
Psoriasis (n=105)	1%	16%	17%	51%	13%	1%
Atopic Dermatitis (n=98)	31%	42%	9%	12%	2%	4%

Scale:
0 = Cleared, 100% clearance of signs except for residual discoloration
1 = Excellent improvement; at least 75%, but less 100% clearance of signs monitored
2 = Moderate improvement; at least 50%, but less than 75% clearance of signs monitored
3 = Slight improvement; less than 50% clearance of signs monitored
4 = No change; no detectable improvement from baseline condition
5 = Exacerbation; flare of sites under study

INDICATIONS AND USAGE:

Dermatop Emollient Cream 0.1% is a medium-potency corticosteroid indicated for the relief of the inflammatory and pruritic manifestations of corticosteroid-responsive dermatoses.

CONTRAINDICATIONS:

Dermatop Emollient Cream 0.1% is contraindicated in those patients with a history of hypersensitivity to any of the components of the preparations.

PRECAUTIONS:

GENERAL

Systemic absorption of topical corticosteroids can produce reversible hypothalamic-pituitary-adrenal (HPA) axis suppression with the potential for glucorticosteroid insufficiency after withdrawal of treatment. Manifestations of Cushing's syndrome, hyperglycemia, and glucosuria can also be produced in some patients by systemic absorption of topical corticosteroids while on treatment.

Patients receiving a large dose of a higher-potency topical steroid applied to a large surface area or under occlusion should be evaluated periodically for evidence of HPA-axis suppression. This may be done by using the ACTH stimulation, AM plasma cortisol, and urinary free cortisol tests.

Dermatop Emollient Cream 0.1% did not produce significant HPA-axis suppression when used at a dose of 30 g/day for a week in 10 patients with extensive psoriasis or atopic dermatitis.

If HPA axis-suppression is noted, an attempt should be made to withdraw the drug, to reduce the frequency of application, or to substitute a less potent corticosteroid. Recovery of HPA-axis function is generally prompt and complete upon discontinuation of topical corticosteroids. Infrequently, signs and symptoms of glucocorticoid insufficiency may occur, requiring supplemental systemic corticosteroids. For information on systemic supplementation, see prescribing information for those products.

Children may be more susceptible to systemic toxicity from equivalent doses due to their larger skin surface to body mass ratios. (See PRECAUTIONS, Pediatric Use.)

If irritation develops, Dermatop Emollient Cream (prednicarbate emollient cream) 0.1% should be discontinued and appropriate therapy instituted. Allergic contact dermatitis with corticosteroids is usually diagnosed by observing failure to heal rather than noting a clinical exacerbation, as observed with most topical products not containing corticosteroids. Such an observation should be corroborated with appropriate diagnostic patch testing.

If concomitant skin infections are present or develop, an appropriate antifungal or antibacterial agent should be used. If a favorable response does not occur promptly, use of Dermatop Emollient Cream 0.1% should be discontinued until the infection has been adequately controlled.

INFORMATION FOR THE PATIENT

Patients using topical corticosteroids should receive the following information and instructions:

1. This medication is to be used as directed by the physician. It is for external use only. Avoid contact with the eyes.

2. This medication should not be used for any disorder other than that for which it was prescribed.

3. The treated skin area should not be bandaged or otherwise covered or wrapped so as to be occlusive, unless directed by the physician.

4. Patients should report any signs of local adverse reactions to their physician.

LABORATORY TESTS

The following tests may be helpful in evaluating patients for HPA-axis suppression:

ACTH stimulation test
AM plasma cortisol test
Urinary free cortisol test

PRECAUTIONS: *(cont'd)*

CARCINOGENESIS, MUTAGENESIS, AND IMPAIRMENT OF FERTILITY

In a study of the effect of prednicarbate on fertility, pregnancy, and postnatal development in rats, no effect was noted on the fertility or pregnancy of the parent animals or postnatal development of the offspring after administration of up to 0.80 mg/kg of prednicarbate subcutaneously.

Prednicarbate has been evaluated in the Salmonella reversion test (Ames test) over a wide range of concentrations in the presence and absence of an S-9 liver microsomal fraction, and did not demonstrate mutagenic activity. Similarly, prednicarbate did not produce any significant changes in the numbers of micronuclei seen in erythrocytes when mice were given doses ranging from 1 to 160 mg/kg of the drug.

PREGNANCY, TERATOGENIC EFFECTS, PREGNANCY CATEGORY C

Corticosteroids have been shown to be teratogenic in laboratory animals when administered systemically at relatively low dosage levels. Some corticosteroids have been shown to be teratogenic after dermal application in laboratory animals.

Prednicarbate has been shown to be teratogenic and embryotoxic in Wistar rats and Himalayan rabbits when given subcutaneously during gestation at doses 1900x and 45x the recommended topical human dose, assuming a percutaneous absorption of approximately 3%.

In the rats, slightly retarded fetal development and an incidence of thickened and wavy ribs higher than the spontaneous rate were noted.

In rabbits, increased liver weights and slight increase in the fetal intrauterine death rate were observed. The fetuses that were delivered exhibited reduced placental weight, increased frequency of cleft palate, ossification disorders in the sternum, omphalocele, and anomalous posture of the forelimbs.

There are no adequate and well-controlled studies in pregnant women on teratogenics of prednicarbate. Therefore, Dermatop Emollient Cream (prednicarbate emollient cream) 0.1% should be used during pregnancy only if the potential benefit justifies the potential risk to the fetus.

NURSING MOTHERS

Systemically administered corticosteroids appear in human milk and could suppress growth, interfere with endogenous corticosteroid production, or cause other untoward effects. It is not known whether topical administration of corticosteroids could result in sufficient systemic absorption to produce detectable quantities in human milk. Because many drugs are excreted in human milk, caution should be exercised when Dermatop Emollient Cream 0.1% is administered to a nursing woman.

PEDIATRIC USE

Safety and effectiveness of Dermatop Emollient Cream 0.1% in persons below the age of 18 years have not been established. Because of a higher ratio of skin surface area to body mass, children are at a greater risk than adults of HPA-axis suppression when they are treated with topical corticosteroids. They are therefore also at greater risk of glucocorticosteroid insufficiency after withdrawal of treatment and at greater risk of Cushing's syndrome while on treatment. Adverse effects including striae have been reported with inappropriate use of topical corticosteroids in infants and children (see PRECAUTIONS.)

HPA-axis suppression, Cushing's syndrome, and intracranial hypertension have been reported in children receiving topical corticosteroids. Manifestations of adrenal suppression in children include linear growth retardation, delayed weight gain, low plasma cortisol levels, and absence of response to ACTH stimulation. Manifestations of intracranial hypertension include bulging fontanelles, headaches, and bilateral papilledema.

ADVERSE REACTIONS:

In controlled clinical studies, the incidence of adverse reactions probably or possibly associated with the use of Dermatop Emollient Cream (prednicarbate emollient cream) 0.1%, was approximately 4%. Reported reactions included mild signs of skin atrophy in 1% of treated patients, as well as the following reactions which were reported in less than 1% of patients: pruritus, edema, paresthesia, urticaria, burning, allergic contact dermatitis and rash.

The following additional local adverse reactions are reported infrequently with topical corticosteroids, but may occur more frequently with the use of occlusive dressings and especially with higher potency corticosteroids. These reactions are listed in an approximate decreasing order of occurrence: dryness, folliculitis, acneiform eruptions, hypopigmentation, perioral dermatitis, secondary infection, striae, and miliaria.

OVERDOSAGE:

Topically applied corticosteroids can be absorbed in sufficient amounts to produce systemic effects (See PRECAUTIONS.)

DOSAGE AND ADMINISTRATION:

Apply a film of Dermatop Emollient Cream (prednicarbate emollient cream) 0.1% to the affected skin areas twice daily. Rub in gently.

HOW SUPPLIED:

Dermatop Emollient Cream 0.1% is supplied in 15 g (NDC 0039-0088-15), and 60 g (NDC 0039-0088-60) tubes.

Store between 41° and 77°F (5° and 25°C).

HOW SUPPLIED - EQUIVALENTS NOT AVAILABLE:

Cream - Topical - 0.1 %

15 gm	$10.75	DERMATOP, Hoechst Marion Roussel	00039-0088-15
60 gm	$28.30	DERMATOP, Hoechst Marion Roussel	00039-0088-60

PREDNISOLONE *(002102)*

CATEGORIES: Adrenal Corticosteroids; Adrenal Hyperplasia; Adrenocortical Insufficiency; Allergic Reactions; Allergies; Anemia; Ankylosing Spondylitis; Antiarthritics; Antineoplastics; Arthritis; Aspiration Pneumonitis; Asthma; Atopic Dermatitis; Bursitis; Cancer; Carditis; Chemotherapy; Choroiditis; Colitis; Conjunctivitis; Dermatitis; Dermatologicals; Dermatomyositis; Diuresis; Drug Hypersensitivity; Enteritis; Epicondylitis; Erythema Multiforme; Erythroblastopenia; Gouty Arthritis; Herpes; Herpes Zoster; Hormones; Hypercalcemia; Inflammation; Iridocyclitis; Keratitis; Leukemia; Lupus Erythematosus; Meningitis; Mycosis Fungoides; Nephrotic Syndrome; Neuritis; Oncologic Drugs; Ophthalmics; Osteoarthritis; Pain; Pemphigus; Pharmaceutical Adjuvants; Pneumonitis; Proteinuria; Psoriasis; Purpura; Rhinitis; Sarcoidosis; Serum Sickness; Spondylitis; Synovitis; Synovitis of Osteoarthritis; Tenosynovitis; Thyroiditis; Trichinosis; Ulcerative Colitis; Uveitis; FDA Approval Pre 1982; Top 200 Drugs; Top 200 Drugs

BRAND NAMES: *Adnisolone*; Cortalone; Cotolone; **Delta-Cortef**; *Deltacortril*; *Deltasolone*; *Deltastab*; *Di-Adreson F*; *Encortolone*; *Hydrocortancyl*; *Medisolone*; *Meticortelone*; *Opredsone*; *Panafcortelone*; *Precortisyl*; *Prednisolona*; Prelone; *Scherisolona*; *Scherisolone*
(International brand names outside U.S. in italics)

FORMULARIES: Aetna; BC-BS; FHP; Medi-Cal; PCS; WHO

COST OF THERAPY: $11.13 (Asthma; Tablet; 5 mg; 1/day; 365 days)

PRIMARY ICD9: 493.90 (Asthma, Unspecified, Without Mention of Status Asthmaticus)

DESCRIPTION:

Glucocorticoids are adrenocortical steroids, both naturally occurring and synthetic, which are readily absorbed from the gastrointestinal tract. Prednisolone is a white to practically white, odorless crystalline powder. It is very slightly soluble in water; soluble in methanol and in dioxane; sparingly soluble in acetone and in alcohol; slightly soluble in chloroform.

The chemical name for prednisolone is pregna-1,4-diene-3, 20-dione, 11, 17,21-trihydroxy-(11 beta)- and the molecular weight is 360.45 (anhydrous).

Each Prednisolone tablet contains 5 mg of the anti-inflammatory adrenocortical steroid, prednisolone.

CLINICAL PHARMACOLOGY:

Naturally occurring glucocorticoids (hydrocortisone & cortisone), which also have salt-retaining properties, are used as replacement therapy in adrenocortical deficiency states. Their synthetic analogs are primarily used for their potent anti-inflammatory effects in disorders of many organ systems.

Glucocorticoids cause profound and varied metabolic effects. In addition, they modify the body's immune responses to diverse stimuli.

INDICATIONS AND USAGE:

Prednisolone tablets are indicated in the following conditions:

1. Endocrine Disorders: Primary or secondary adrenocortical insufficiency (hydrocortisone or cortisone is the first choice; synthetic analogs may be used in conjunction with mineralocorticoids where applicable; in infancy mineralocorticoid supplementation is of particular importance.)

Congenital adrenal hyperplasia

Nonsuppurative thyroiditis

Hypercalcemia associated with cancer

2. rheumatic Disorders: As adjunctive therapy for short-term administration (to tide the patient over an acute episode or exacerbation) in: Psoriatic arthritis, Rheumatoid arthritis, including juvenile rheumatoid arthritis (selected cases may require low-dose maintenance therapy), Ankylosing spondylitis, Acute gouty arthritis, Acute and subacute bursitis, Post-traumatic osteoarthritis, Acute nonspecific tenosynovitis, Synovitis of osteoarthritis, Epicondylitis

3. Collagen Diseases: During an exacerbation or as maintenance therapy in selected cases of:

Systemic lupus erythematosus

Acute rheumatic carditis

Systemic dermatomyositis (polymyositis)

4. Dermatologic Diseases: Pemphigus, Exfoliative dermatitis, Bullous dermatitis herpetiformis, Mycosis Fungoides, Severe psoriasis, Severe erythema multiforme (Stevens-Johnson Syndrome), Severe seborrheic dermatitis

5. Allergic States: Control of severe or incapacitating allergic conditions intractable to adequate trials of conventional treatment: Seasonal or perennial allergic rhinitis, Contact Dermatitis, Atopic dermatitis, Serum sickness, Drug hypersensitivity reaction, Bronchial asthma

6. Ophthalmic Diseases: Severe acute and chronic allergic and inflammatory processes involving the eye and its adnexa such as: Allergic conjunctivitis, Chonoretinitis, Keratitis, Anterior segment inflammation, Allergic corneal marginal ulcers, Difuse posterior uveitis and choroiditis, Herpes zoster ophthalmicus, Optic neuritis, Iritis and iridocyclitis, Sympathetic ophthalmia

7. Respiratory Diseases: Symptomatic sarcoidosis, Loeffler's syndrome not manageable by other means, Berylliosis, Fulminating or disseminated pulmonary tuberculosis when used with appropriate antituberculous chemotherapy, Aspiration pneumonitis

8. Hematologic Disorders: Idiopathic thrombocytopenic purpura in adults, Secondary thrombocytopenia in adults, Acquired (autoimmune) hemolytic anemia, Erythroblastopenia (RBC anemia), Congenital (erythroid) hypoplastic anemia

9. Neoplastic Diseases: For palliative management of: Leukemias and lymphomas in adults, Acute leukemia of childhood

10. Edematous States: To induce a diuresis or remission of proteinuria in the nephrotic syndrome, without uremia, of the idiopathic type of that due to lupus erythematosus

11. Gastrointestinal Diseases: To tide the patient over a critical period of the disease in: Ulcerative colitis, Regionalent enteritis

12 Miscellaneous: Tuberculous meningitis with subarachnoid block or impending block when used concurrently with appropriate antituberculous chemotherapy, Trichinosis with neurologic or myocardial involvement

CONTRAINDICATIONS:

Systemic fungal infections.

WARNINGS:

In patients on corticosteroid therapy subjected to unusual stress, increased dosage of rapidly acting corticosteroids before, during, and after the stressful situation is indicated.

Corticosteroids may mask some signs of infection and new infections may appear during their use. There may be decreased resistance and inability to localize infection when corticosteroids are used.

Prolonged use of corticosteroids may produce posterior subcapsular cataracts, glaucoma with possible damage to the optic nerves, and may enhance the establishment of secondary ocular infections due to fungi or viruses.

Usage in pregnancy: Since adequate human reproduction studies have not been done with corticosteroids, the use of these drugs in pregnancy, nursing mothers or women of childbearing potential requires that the possible benefits of the drug be weighed against the potential hazards to the mother and embryo or fetus. Infants born of mothers who have received substantial doses of corticosteroids during pregnancy should be carefully observed for signs of hypoadrenalism.

WARNINGS: *(cont'd)*

Average and large doses of hydrocortisone or cortisone can cause elevation of blood pressure, salt and water retention, and increased excretion of potassium. These effects are less likely to occur with the synthetic derivatives except when used in large doses. Dietary salt restriction and potassium supplementation may be necessary. All corticosteroids increase calcium excretion.

WHILE ON CORTICOSTEROID THERAPY PATIENTS SHOULD NOT BE VACCINATED AGAINST SMALLPOX. OTHER IMMUNIZATION PROCEDURES SHOULD NOT BE UNDERTAKEN IN PATIENTS WHO ARE ON CORTICOSTEROIDS, ESPECIALLY ON HIGH DOSE, BECAUSE OF POSSIBLE HAZARDS OF NEUROLOGICAL COMPLICATIONS AND A LACK OF ANTIBODY RESPONSE.

The use of Prednisolone in active tuberculosis should be restricted to those cases of fulminating or disseminated tuberculosis in which the corticosteroid is used for the management of the disease in conjunction with an appropriate antituberculous regimen.

If corticosteroids are indicated in patients with latent tuberculosis or tuberculin reactivity, close observation is necessary as reactivation of the disease may occur. During prolonged corticosteroid therapy, these patients should receive chemoprophylaxis.

PRECAUTIONS:

Drug-induced secondary adrenocortical insufficiency may be minimized by gradual reduction of dosage. This type of relative insufficiency may persist for months after discontinuation of therapy; therefore, in any situation of stress occurring during that period, hormone therapy should be reinstituted. Since mineralocorticoid secretion may be impaired, salt and/or a mineralocorticoid should be administered concurrently.

There is an enhanced effect of corticosteroids on patients with hypothyroidism and in those with cirrhosis.

Corticosteroids should be used cautiously in patients with ocular herpes simplex because of possible corneal perforation.

The lowest possible dose of corticosteroid should be used to control the condition under treatment, and when reduction in dosage is possible, the reduction should be gradual.

Psychic derangements may appear when corticosteroids are used, ranging rom euphoria, insomnia, mood swings, personality changes, and severe depression, to frank psychotic manifestations. Also, existing emotional instability or psychotic tendencies may be aggravated by corticosteroids.

Aspirin should be used cautiously in conjunction with corticosteroids in hypoprothrombinemia.

Steroids should be used with caution in nonspecific ulcerative colitis, if there is a probability of impending perforation, abscess or other pyogenic infection; diverticulitis; fresh intestinal anastomoses; active or latent peptic ulcer; renal insufficiency; hypertension; osteoporosis; and myasthenia gravis.

Growth and development of infants and children on prolonged corticosteroid therapy should be carefully observed.

ADVERSE REACTIONS:

See below for Adverse Reactions

DOSAGE AND ADMINISTRATION:

Fluid and Electrolyte Disturbances: Sodium retention, Fluid retention, Congestive heart failure in susceptible patients, Potassium loss, Hypokalemic alkalosis, Hypertension

Musculoskeletal: Muscle weakness, Steroid myopathy, Loss of muscle mass, Osteoporosis, Vertebral compression fractures, Aseptic necrosis of femoral and humeral heads, Pathological fracture of long bones

Gastrointestinal: Peptic ulcer with possible perforation; hemorrhage, Pancreatitis, Abdominal distention, Ulcerative esophagitis

Dermatologic: Impaired wound healing, Thin, fragile skin, Petechiae and ecchymoses, Facial erythema, Increased sweating, May supress reactions to skin tests

Metabolic: Negative nitrogen balance due to protein catabolism

Neurological: Increased intracranial pressure with papilledema (pseudotumor cerebri) usually after treatment, Convulsions, Vertigo, Headache

Endocrine: Menstrual irregularities, Development of cushingoid state, Secondary adrenocortical and pituitary unresponsiveness, particularly in times of stress, as in trauma, surgery, or illness, Suppression of growth in children, Decreased carbohydrate tolerance, Manifestations of latent mellitus, Increased requirements for insulin or oral hypoglycemic agents in diabetics

Ophthalmic: Posterior subscapular cataracts, Increased intraocular pressure, Glaucoma, Exophthalmos

The initial dosage of prednisolone may vary from 5 mg to 60 mg per day depending on the specific disease entity being treated. In situations of less severity lower doses will generally suffice while in selected patients higher initial doses may be required. The initial dosage should be maintained or adjusted until a satisfactory clinical response, Prednisolone should be discontinued and the patient transferred to other appropriate therapy. IT SHOULD BE EMPHASIZED THAT DOSAGE REQUIREMENTS ARE VARIABLE AND MUST BE INDIVIDUALIZED ON THE BASIS OF THE DISEASE UNDER TREATMENT AND THE RESPONSE OF THE PATIENT. After a favorable response is noted, the proper maintenance dosage should be determined by decreasing the initial drug dosage in small decrements at appropriate time intervals until the lowest dosage which will maintain an adequate clinical response is reached. It should be kept in mind that constant monitoring is needed in regard to drug dosage. Included in the situations which may make dosage adjustments necessary are changes in clinical status secondary to remissions or exacerbations in the disease process, the patient's individual drug responsiveness, and the effect of patient exposure to stressful situations not directly related to the disease entity under treatment; in this latter situation it may be necessary to increase the dosage of Prednisolone for a period of time consistent with the patient's condition. If after long-term therapy the drug is stopped, it is recommended that it be withdrawn gradually rather than abruptly.

ALTERNATE-DAY THERAPY (ADT)

ADT is a corticosteroid dosing regimen in which twice the usual daily dose of corticoid is administered every other morning. The purpose of this mode of therapy is to provide the patient requiring long-term, pharmacologic-dose treatment with the beneficial effects of corticoids while minimizing certain undesirable effects, including pituitary-adrenal suppression, the cushingoid state, corticoid withdrawal symptoms, and growth suppression in children.

The rationale for this treatment schedule is based on two major premises: (a) the anti-inflammatory or therapeutic effect of corticoids persists longer than their physical presence and metabolic effects and (b) administration of the corticosteroid every other morning allows for reestablishment of more nearly normal hypothalamic-pituitary- adrenal (HPA) activity on the off- steroid day.

A brief review of the HPA physiology may be helpful in understanding this rationale. Acting primarily through the hypothalamus a fall in free cortisol stimulates the pituitary gland to produce increasing amounts of corticotropin (ACTH) while a rise in free cortisol inhibits

DOSAGE AND ADMINISTRATION: *(cont'd)*

ACTH secretion. Normally the HPA system is characterized by diurnal (circadian) rhythm. Serum levels of ACTH rise from a low point about 10 pm to a peak level about 6 am. Increasing levels of ACTH stimulate adrenocortical activity resulting in a rise in plasma cortisol with maximal levels occurring between 2am and 8am. This rise in cortisol dampens ACTH production and in turn adrenocortical activity. There is a gradual fall in plasma corticoids during the day with lowest levels occurring about midnight.

The diurnal rhythm of the HPA axis is lost in Cushing's disease, a syndrome of adrenocortical hyperfunction characterized by obesity with centripetal fat distribution, thinning of the skin with easy bruisability, muscle wasting with weakness, hypertension, latent diabetes, osteoporosis, electrolyte imbalance, etc. The same clinical findings of hyperadrenocorticism may be noted during long- term, pharmacologic dose corticoid therapy administered in conventional daily divided doses. It would appear, then, that a disturbance in the diurnal cycle with maintenance of elevated corticoid values during the night may play a significant role in the development of undesirable corticoid effects. Escape from these constantly elevated plasma levels for even short periods of time may be instrumental in protecting against undesirable pharmacologic effects.

During conventional pharmacologic-dose corticosteroid therapy, ACTH production is inhibited with subsequent suppression of cortisol production by the adrenal cortex. Recovery time for normal HPA activity is variable depending upon the dose and duration of treatment. During this time the patient is vulnerable to any stressful situation. Although it has been shown that there is considerably less adrenal suppression following a single morning dose of prednisolone (10 mg) as opposed to a quarter of that dose administered every 6 hours, there is evidence that some suppressive effect on adrenal activity may be carried over in to the following day when pharmacologic doses are used. Further, it has been shown that a single dose of certain corticosteroids will produce adrenocortical suppression for two or more days. Other corticoids, including methylprednisolone, hydrocortisone, prednisone, and prednisolone, are considered to be short acting (producing adrenocortical suppression for 1-1/4 to 1-1/2 days following a single dose) and thus are recommended for alternate-day therapy.

The following should be kept in mind when considering alternate-day therapy:

1) Basic principles and indications for corticosteroid therapy should apply. The benefits of ADT should not encourage the indiscriminate use of steroids.

2) ADT is a therapeutic technique primarily designed for patients in whom long-term pharmacologic corticoid therapy is anticipated.

3) In less severe disease processes in which corticoid therapy is indicated, it may be possible to initiate treatment with ADT. More severe disease states usually will require daily divided high dose therapy for initial control of the disease process. The initial suppressive dose level should be continued until satisfactory clinical response is obtained, usually four to ten days in the case of many allergic and collagen diseases. It is important to keep the period of initial suppressive dose as brief as possible particularly when subsequent use of alternate-day therapy is intended.

4) Because of the advantages of ADT, is may be desirable to try patients on this form of therapy who have been on daily corticoids for long periods of time (*e.g.,* patients with rheumatoid arthritis). Since these patients may already have a suppressed HPA axis, establishing them on ADT may be difficult and not always successful, however, it is recommended that regular attempts be made to change them over. It may be helpful to triple or even quadruple the daily maintenance dose and administer this every other day rather than just doubling the daily dose if difficulty is encountered. Once the patient is again controlled, an attempt should be made to reduce this dose to a minimum.

5) As indicated above, certain corticosteroids, because of their prolonged suppressive effect on adrenal activity, are not recommended for alternate-day therapy (*e.g.,* dexamethasone and betamethasone).

6) The maximal activity of the adrenal cortex is between 2 am and 8 am and it is minimal between 4 pm and midnight. Exogenous corticosteroids suppress adrenocortical activity the lease when given at the time of maximal activity (am).

7) In using ADT it is important, as in all therapeutic situations, to individualize and tailor the therapy to each patient. Complete control of symptoms will not be possible in all patients. An explanation of the benefits of ADT will help the patient to understand and tolerate the possible flare-up in symptoms which may occur in the latter part of the off-steroid day. Other symptomatic therapy may be added or increased at this time if needed.

8) In the event of an acute flare-up of the disease process, it may be necessary to return to a full suppressive daily divided corticoid dose for control. Once control is again established alternate-day therapy may be reinstituted.

9) Although many of the undesirable features of corticosteroid therapy can be minimized by ADT, as in any therapeutic situation, the physician must carefully weigh the benefit-risk ratio for each patient in whom corticoid therapy is being considered.

PATIENT INFORMATION:

Prednisolone is a glucocorticoid steroid used to treat arthritis conditions, severe allergies, Lupus, and inflammatory conditions of the eye or airways, some cancer conditions and other rare conditions. This drug supplements normal chemical hormones in your body to help fight off diseases conditions. This drug does suppress the immune system and therefore should not be used by those with severe fungal infections. This drug can also mask signs of infection and with long term use cause cataracts. This drug should be monitored closely by a physician if taken for a long period of time. The dose must also be decreased slowly over time (*i.e.,* tapered) to avoid the body going into withdrawal. The most common side effects include water retention, muscle weakness, stomach irritation, and visual disturbances. Stomach irritation can be alleviated by taking this medication with food. It is important to take this medication as prescribed and to be assessed by your physician on a regular basis.

HOW SUPPLIED - EQUIVALENTS NOT AVAILABLE:

Powder

5 gm	$6.50	Prednisolone, Millgood	53118-0210-05
10 gm	$12.50	Prednisolone, Millgood	53118-0210-10
25 gm	$29.00	Prednisolone, Millgood	53118-0210-25

Syrup - Oral - 15 mg/5ml

240 ml	$52.17	PRELONE, Muro Pharm	00451-1500-08
480 ml	$83.47	PRELONE, Muro Pharm	00451-1500-16

Tablet, Uncoated - Oral - 5 mg

100's	$3.05	Prednisolone, Qualitest Pharms	00603-5310-21
100's	$3.95	Prednisolone, Consolidated Midland	00223-1512-01
100's	$4.04	Prednisolone, HL Moore Drug Exch	00839-5076-06
100's	$4.60	Prednisolone, Aligen Independ	00405-4823-01
100's	$4.95	Prednisolone, Schein Pharm (US)	00364-0217-01
100's	$4.95	Prednisolone, Major Pharms	00904-2155-60
1000's	$19.95	Prednisolone, Harber Pharm	51432-0354-06
1000's	$20.40	COTOLONE, C O Truxton	00463-6071-10
1000's	$21.35	CORTALONE, Halsey Drug	00879-0128-10
1000's	$21.59	Prednisolone, HL Moore Drug Exch	00839-5076-16
1000's	$22.50	Prednisolone, Consolidated Midland	00223-1512-02
1000's	$25.58	Prednisolone, Rugby	00536-4346-10

HOW SUPPLIED - EQUIVALENTS NOT AVAILABLE: *(cont'd)*

1000's	$28.45	Prednisolone, Schein Pharm (US)	00364-0217-02
1000's	$28.45	Prednisolone, Major Pharms	00904-2155-80

PREDNISOLONE ACETATE *(002103)*

CATEGORIES: Adrenal Corticosteroids; Anti-Inflammatory Agents; Antiarthritics; Antineoplastics; Conjunctivitis; Corneal Inflammation; Corneal Injury; EENT Drugs; Eye, Ear, Nose, & Throat Preparations; Herpes; Herpes Zoster; Hormones; Keratoconjunctivitis; Ocular Blepharitis; Ocular Infections; Oncologic Drugs; Ophthalmics; Pain; Pharmaceutical Adjuvants; Pregnancy Category C; FDA Approval Pre 1982

BRAND NAMES: Ak-Tate; Articulose-50; Cotolone; Econopred; Ed-Pred 25; Key-Pred; Medicort 50; Ocu-Pred-A; **Pred Forte**; Pred Mild; Predair-A; Predaject-50; Predalone 50; Predate-50; Predcor-50; Predicort-50; Pri-Cortin; Sholone; Spectro-Tate; Uad Pred

FORMULARIES: Aetna; BC-BS; PCS

DESCRIPTION:

Prednisolone Acetate is an adrenocortical steroid prepared as a sterile ophthalmic suspension.

Established name: Prednisolone Acetate

Chemical name: Pregna-1,4-diene-3,20-dione, 21-(acetyloxy)-11,17-dihydroxy-, (11β)-.

Each Pred Forte ml contains: *Active:* Prednisolone Acetate 0.125% or 1.0%. Preservative: Benzalkonium Chloride 0.01%. *Vehicle:* Hydroxypropyl Methylcellulose. *Inactive:* Dried Sodium Phosphate, Polysorbate 80, Edetate Disodium, Glycerin, Citric Acid and/or Sodium Hydroxide (to adjust pH), Purified Water.

CLINICAL PHARMACOLOGY:

This drug causes inhibition of the inflammatory response to inciting agents of a mechanical, chemical, or immunological nature. No generally accepted explanation of this steroid property has been advanced.

INDICATIONS AND USAGE:

For use in the treatment of inflammatory and allergic conditions: allergic, nonpurulent catarrhal, and vernal conjunctivitis; acute iritis; catarrhal corneal ulcer; corneal injuries; nonpurulent blepharitis; herpes zoster ophthalmicus; nonspecific superficial keratitis; non-purulent phlyctenular keratoconjunctivitis. 1% may be indicated to suppress graft reaction after keratoplasty.

CONTRAINDICATIONS:

Contraindicated in acute superficial herpes simplex keratitis (dendritic keratitis), vaccinia, varicella, and most other viral diseases of the cornea and conjunctiva; tuberculosis; fungal diseases; acute purulent untreated infections which, like other diseases caused by microorganisms, may be masked or enhanced by the presence of the steroid.

WARNINGS:

Employment of steroid medication in the treatment of stromal herpes simplex requires great caution; frequent slit lamp microscopy is mandatory. Prolonged use may result in glaucoma, damage to the optic nerve, defects in visual acuity and visual field, posterior subcapsular cataract formation; or may aid in the establishment of secondary ocular infection from pathogens liberated from ocular tissue. In those diseases causing thinning of the cornea, or sclera, perforation has been known to occur with the use of topical steroids.

PRECAUTIONS:

During the course of the therapy, if the inflammatory reaction does not respond within a reasonable period, other forms of therapy should be instituted. As fungal infections of the cornea are particularly prone to develop coincidentally with long-term local steroid application, fungus invasion must be considered in any persistent corneal ulceration where a steroid has been used or is in use. Intraocular pressure should be checked frequently. Steroids should be used with caution in glaucoma. This product should not be used without continuing medical supervision.

Usage in Pregnancy: Safety of intensive or protracted use of topical steroids during pregnancy has not been substantiated.

ADVERSE REACTIONS:

Glaucoma with optic nerve damage, visual acuity and field defects, posterior subcapsular cataract formation, secondary ocular infections from pathogens including herpes simplex liberated from ocular tissues, perforation of the globe. Viral and fungal infections of the cornea may be exacerbated by the application of steroids.

DOSAGE AND ADMINISTRATION:

Two drops topically in the eye(s) four times daily. In cases of bacterial infections, concomitant use of antibiotics or chemotherapeutic agents is mandatory.

HOW SUPPLIED - RATED THERAPEUTICALLY EQUIVALENT:

Suspension - Ophthalmic - 1 %

1 ml	**$4.69**	**PRED FORTE STERILE OPHTHALMIC, Allergan-Amer**	**11980-0180-01**
5 ml	$12.00	Prednisolone Acetate, Falcon Ophthalmics	61314-0637-05
5 ml	**$13.15**	**PRED FORTE STERILE OPHTHALMIC, Allergan-Amer**	**11980-0180-05**
5 ml	$15.63	1% ECONOPRED PLUS, Alcon-PR	00998-0637-05
10 ml	$22.00	Prednisolone Acetate, Falcon Ophthalmics	61314-0637-10
10 ml	$23.13	1% ECONOPRED PLUS, Alcon-PR	00998-0637-10
10 ml	**$23.50**	**PRED FORTE STERILE OPHTHALMIC, Allergan-Amer**	**11980-0180-10**
15 ml	**$34.04**	**PRED FORTE STERILE OPHTHALMIC, Allergan-Amer**	**11980-0180-15**

HOW SUPPLIED - NOT RATED EQUIVALENT:

Injection, Susp - Intramuscular - 25 mg/ml

10 ml	$2.48	Prednisolone Acetate, Lannett	00527-0187-55
10 ml	$5.50	Prednisolone Acetate, Consolidated Midland	00223-8345-10
10 ml	$6.90	KEY-PRED, Hyrex Pharms	00314-0695-70
30 ml	$6.50	Prednisolone Acetate, Consolidated Midland	00223-8345-30
30 ml	$7.75	Cotolone, C O Truxton	00463-1019-30
30 ml	$9.97	Prednisolone Acetate, Steris Labs	00402-0073-30
30 ml	$10.91	Prednisolone Acetate, HL Moore Drug Exch	00839-5617-36
30 ml	$11.50	Prednisolone Acetate, Schein Pharm (US)	00364-6626-56

HOW SUPPLIED - NOT RATED EQUIVALENT: *(cont'd)*

30 ml	$12.96	KEY-PRED, Hyrex Pharms	00314-0695-30
30 ml	$12.98	Prednisolone Acetate, IDE-Interstate	00814-6255-46

Injection, Susp - Intramuscular - 50 mg/ml

10 ml	$3.74	Prednisolone Acetate, Balan	00304-1319-56
10 ml	$4.89	Prednisolone Acetate, McGuff	49072-0581-10
10 ml	$5.25	COTOLONE, C O Truxton	00463-1020-10
10 ml	$5.90	Prednisolone Acetate, Geneva Pharms	00781-3078-70
10 ml	$6.40	Prednisolone Acetate, Major Pharms	00904-0891-10
10 ml	$6.50	Prednisolone Acetate, Consolidated Midland	00223-8346-10
10 ml	$7.81	UAD PRED, UAD Labs	00785-8015-10
10 ml	$8.58	Prednisolone Acetate, Steris Labs	00402-0249-10
10 ml	$10.00	PREDICORT-50, Dunhall Pharms	00217-8404-08
10 ml	$10.00	PREDALONE, Forest Pharms	00456-0924-10
10 ml	$10.10	Sterile Prednisolone Acetate, Schein Pharm (US)	00364-6627-54
10 ml	$10.26	KEY-PRED, Hyrex Pharms	00314-0697-70
10 ml	$18.30	PREDAJECT-50, Mayrand Pharms	00259-0310-10
30 ml	$7.49	Prednisolone Acetate, Balan	00304-1319-59
30 ml	$9.50	Prednisolone Acetate, Consolidated Midland	00223-8341-30
30 ml	$13.73	Prednisolone Acetate, HL Moore Drug Exch	00839-5120-36
30 ml	$14.00	Prednisolone Acetate, Steris Labs	00402-0249-30
30 ml	$15.00	Sterile Prednisolone Acetate, Schein Pharm (US)	00364-6627-56
30 ml	$18.55	Sterile Prednisolone Acetate, Goldline Labs	00182-0939-66

Powder

5 gm	$6.50	Prednisolone Acetate, Millgood	53118-0211-05
10 gm	$12.50	Prednisolone Acetate, Millgood	53118-0211-10
25 gm	$29.00	Prednisolone Acetate, Millgood	53118-0211-25

Suspension - Ophthalmic - 0.125 %

5 ml	$14.06	1/8% ECONOPRED, Alcon-PR	00998-0635-05
10 ml	$21.25	1/8% ECONOPRED, Alcon-PR	00998-0635-10

Suspension - Ophthalmic; Top - 0.12 %

5 ml	$13.84	PRED MILD STERILE OPHTHALMIC, Allergan-Amer	11980-0174-05
10 ml	$19.70	PRED MILD STERILE OPHTHALMIC, Allergan-Amer	11980-0174-10

PREDNISOLONE ACETATE; SULFACETAMIDE SODIUM *(002104)*

CATEGORIES: Adrenal Corticosteroids; Anti-Infectives; Antibacterials; Antihypertensives; Antimicrobials; Burns; Conjunctivitis; Corneal Inflammation; Corneal Injury; Corneal Ulcer; EENT Drugs; Edema; Eye, Ear, Nose, & Throat Preparations; Hormones; Inflammatory Conditions; Ocular Infections; Ophthalmics; Steroids; Sulfonamides; Uveitis; FDA Approval Pre 1982

BRAND NAMES: Ak-Cide; *Blefamide*; Blephamide; Cetapred; *Deltamid*; I-Sulfalone; Isopto Cetapred; Kainair; Medasulf; **Metimyd**; Ocu-Lone C; Ophtha P/S; Optimyd; Or-Toptic-M; *Plascetamid*; Pred-Ide; Predamide; *Prednistyle*; Predsulfair; Spectro-Cide; Sulfacetamide W/Prednisolone; Sulfacort; Sulfalone; Sulfamide; *Sulfapred*; Sulphrin; Sulpred; Sulster; Supred; Vasocidin
(International brand names outside U.S. in italics)

FORMULARIES: Aetna; FHP; Medi-Cal

DESCRIPTION:

Prednisolone acetate and sulfacetamide sodium ophthalmic suspension is a steroid/anti-infective sterile preparation having a pH range of 7.0 to 7.4 Each ml contains: 5 mg prednisolone acetate, USP, 100 mg sulfacetamide sodium, USP; sodium phosphate dibasic, sodium phosphate monobasic, tyloxapol, sodium thiosulfate, edetate disodium, and purified water; 5 mg phenylethyl alcohol and 0.25 mg benzalkonium chloride as preservatives.

Prednisolone acetate and sulfacetamide sodium ophthalmic ointment is a steroid/anti-infective sterile preparation containing in each gram: 5 mg prednisolone acetate. USP and 100 mg sulfacetamide sodium, USP; 0.5 methylparaben and 0.1 mg propylparaben as preservatives, in a bland, unctuous base of mineral oil and white petrolatum.

The empirical formula for prednisone acetate, a 1-unsaturated analog of hydrocortisone acetate, is $C_{23}H_{30}O_6$. The molecular weight is 402.49. Chemically it is 11β,17,21-trihydroxy-pregna-1,4-diene-3,20-dione 21-acetate.

Prednisolone acetate is a nearly odorless, white to practically white, crystalline powder, It is slightly soluble in acetone, alcohol, and chloroform, and practically insoluble in water.

Sulfacetamide sodium, $C_8H_9N_2NaO_3S \cdot H_2O$, is a sulfonamide antibacterial agent with a molecular weight of 254.24. Chemically it is *N*-((4-aminophenyl)sulfonyl)-, acetamide, monosodium salt, monohydrate.

Sulfacetamide sodium is an odorless, white, crystalline powder. It is freely soluble in water, sparingly soluble in alcohol, and practically insoluble in benzene, chloroform, and ether.

CLINICAL PHARMACOLOGY:

Corticosteroids suppress the inflammatory response to a variety of agents, and they probably delay or slow healing. Since corticosteroids may inhibit the body's defense mechanism against infection a concomitant antimicrobial drug may be used when this inhibition is considered to be clinically significant in a particular case.

The anti-infective component in the combination is included to provide action against specific organisms susceptible to it.

When a decision is made to administer both a corticoid and an antimicrobial, the administration of such drugs in combination has the advantages of greater patient compliance and convenience and added assurance that the appropriate dosage of both drugs is administered. There is also assured compatibility of ingredients when both types of drug are in the same formulation and particularly, that the correct volume of drug is delivered and retained.

The relative potency of corticosteroids depends on the molecular structure, concentration, and release from the vehicle.

INDICATIONS AND USAGE:

Prednisolone acetate and sulfacetamide sodium ophthalmic suspension or ointment is indicated for steroid-responsive inflammatory ocular conditions for which a corticosteroid is indicated and where bacterial infection or a risk of bacterial ocular infection exists.

Ocular steroids are indicated in inflammatory conditions of the palpebral and bulbar conjunctivae, cornea, and anterior segment of the globe where the inherent risk of steroid use in certain infective conjunctivitises is accepted to obtain a diminution in edema and inflammation. They are also indicated in chronic anterior uveitis and corneal injury from chemical, radiation or thermal burns, or penetration of foreign bodies.

INDICATIONS AND USAGE: *(cont'd)*

The use of a combination drug with an anti-infective component is indicated where the risk of infection is high or where there is an expectation that potentially dangerous numbers of bacteria will be present in the eye.

The particular anti-infective drug in this product is active against the following common bacterial eye pathogens: *Pseudomonas* species, *Hemophilus influenzae, Klebsiella* species, *Staphylococcus aureus, Streptococcus pneumoniae, Streptococcus* (Viridans group), *Escherichia coli* and *Enterobacter* species.

This product does not provide adequate coverage against. *Neisseria* species and *Serratia marcescens.*

CONTRAINDICATIONS:

Prednisolone acetate and sulfacetamide sodium is contraindicated in: epithelial herpes simplex keratitis (dendritic keratitis), vaccinia, varicella and many other viral diseases of the cornea or conjunctiva; mycobacterial infection of the eye; and fungal diseases of ocular structures. Prednisolone acetate and sulfacetamide sodium is contraindicated in individuals with known or suspected hypersensitivity to any of the ingredients of the preparation, or to other sulfonamides, or other corticosteroids. (Hypersensitivity to the antibacterial component occurs at a higher rate than for other components). The use of these combinations is always contraindicated after uncomplicated removal of a corneal foreign body.

WARNINGS:

Prolonged use may result in glaucoma, with damage to the optic nerve, defects in visual acuity and fields of vision, and in posterior subcapsular cataract formation. Prolonged use may suppress the host response and thus increase the hazard of secondary ocular infections. In those diseases causing thinning of the cornea or sclera, perforations have been known to occur with the use of topical steroids. In acute purulent conditions of the eye, steroids may mask infection or enhance existing infection. If these products are used for ten days or longer, intraocular pressure should be routinely monitored even though this may be difficult in children and uncooperative patients.

Employment of steroid medication in the treatment of herpes simplex requires great caution.

A significant percentage of staphylococcal isolates are completely resistant to sulfonamides.

PRECAUTIONS:

The initial prescription and renewal of the medication order beyond 20 ml of prednisolone acetate and sulfacetamide sodium ophthalmic suspension or beyond 8 g of the ointment should be made by a physician only after examination of the patient with the aid of magnification, such as slitlamp biomicroscopy and where appropriate, fluorescein staining.

The possibility of fungal infections of the cornea should be considered after prolonged steroid dosing.

Sensitization may recur when a sulfonamide is read ministered irrespective of the route of administration, and cross-sensitivity among different sulfonamides may occur. (See ADVERSE REACTIONS.) Cross-allergenicity among corticosteroids has been demonstrated. If signs of hypersensitivity or other untoward reactions occur, discontinue use of the preparation.

ADVERSE REACTIONS:

Adverse reactions have occurred which can be attributed to the steroid component, the anti-infective component, or the combination. Exact incidence figures are not available since no denominator of treated patients is available.

Reactions occurring most often from the presence of the anti-infective ingredient are allergic sensitizations. Instances of Stevens-Johnson syndrome and systemic lupus erythematosus (in one case producing a fatal outcome) have been reported following the use of ophthalmic sulfonamide containing preparations.

The reactions due to the steroid component in decreasing order of frequency are: elevation of intraocular pressure (IOP) with possible development of glaucoma, and infrequent optic nerve damage; posterior subcapsular cataract formation; and delayed wound healing.

Corticosteroid-containing preparations can also cause acute anterior uveitis or perforation of the globe. Mydriasis, loss of accommodation, and ptosis have occasionally been reported following local use of corticosteroids.

Secondary Infection: The development of secondary infection has occurred after use of combinations containing steroids and antimicrobials. Fungal infections of the cornea are particularly prone to develop coincidentally with long-term applications of the steroid. The possibility of fungal invasion must be considered in any persistent corneal ulceration where steroid treatment has been used.

Secondary bacterial ocular infection following suppression of host responses also occurs.

DOSAGE AND ADMINISTRATION:

Prednisolone Acetate and Sulfacetamide Sodium Ophthalmic Suspension: Two or three drops should be instilled into the conjunctival sac every one to two hours during the day and at bedtime until a favorable response is obtained.

Prednisolone Acetate and Sulfacetamide Sodium Ophthalmic Ointment: A thin film should be applied three or four times daily and once at bedtime until a favorable response is obtained.

The initial prescription of Prednisolone acetate and sulfacetamide sodium ophthalmic should *not* be more than 20 ml of the Suspension or 8 g of the ointment and the prescription should not be refilled without further evaluation as outlined in the PRECAUTIONS.

Dosage should be adjusted according to the specific needs of the patient. Prednisolone acetate and Sulfacetamide sodium ophthalmic suspension or ointment dosage may be reduced, but care should be taken not to discontinue therapy prematurely. In chronic conditions, withdrawal of treatment should be carried out by gradually decreasing the frequency of application.

Store between 2 and 30°C (36 and 86°F). Clumping may occur on long standing at high temperatures. Shake well before using.

Protect from light.

HOW SUPPLIED - RATED THERAPEUTICALLY EQUIVALENT:

Ointment - Ophthalmic - 0.5 %/10 %

3.5 gm	$9.60	Ak-Cide, Akorn	17478-0276-35
3.5 gm	$11.58	VASOCIDIN STERILE OPHTHALMIC, Ciba Vision	00058-3095-01
3.5 gm	**$23.58**	**METIMYD OPHTHALMIC, Schering**	**00085-0695-05**

Suspension - Ophthalmic - 0.2 %/10 %

5 ml	$8.93	SULFACORT, Rugby	00536-3650-65
5 ml	$8.95	Sulpred, Qualitest Pharms	00603-7325-37

Suspension - Ophthalmic - 0.25 %/10 %

5 ml	$7.44	Supred, Ocusoft	54799-0516-05
5 ml	$12.46	Sulfacetamide W/Prednisolone, Aligen Independ	00405-6138-05
10 ml	$8.69	Supred, Ocusoft	54799-0516-10
10 ml	$15.79	Sulfacetamide W/Prednisolone, Aligen Independ	00405-6138-10

HOW SUPPLIED - RATED THERAPEUTICALLY EQUIVALENT: *(cont'd)*

Suspension - Ophthalmic - 0.5 %/10 %

5 ml	$5.93	PREDACET/SULF SOD, Rugby	00536-3705-65
5 ml	$7.45	SUPRED OPHTHALMIC, Ocusoft	54799-0517-10
5 ml	$9.60	AK-CIDE OPHTHALMIC, Akorn	17478-0275-10
5 ml	**$26.83**	**METIMYD OPHTHALMIC, Schering**	**00085-0074-05**
15 ml	$7.43	PREDACET/SULF SOD, Rugby	00536-3705-72

HOW SUPPLIED - NOT RATED EQUIVALENT:

Ointment - Ophthalmic - 10 %

3.5 gm	$15.94	CETAPRED, Alcon	00065-0607-35

Ointment - Ophthalmic; Top - 0.2 %/10 %

3.5 gm	$14.42	BLEPHAMIDE S.O.P., Allergan	00023-0313-04

Suspension - Ophthalmic - 0.2 %/10 %

2.5 ml	$3.95	BLEPHAMIDE STERILE OPHTHALMIC, Allergan-Amer	11980-0022-03
5 ml	$9.00	Prednisolone/Sulfacetamide Sodium, Goldline Labs	00182-7050-62
5 ml	$15.03	BLEPHAMIDE STERILE OPHTHALMIC, Allergan-Amer	11980-0022-05
10 ml	$21.46	BLEPHAMIDE STERILE OPHTHALMIC, Allergan-Amer	11980-0022-10

Suspension - Ophthalmic - 0.25 %/10 %

5 ml	$15.94	ISOPTO CETAPRED, Alcon-PR	00998-0613-05
15 ml	$27.50	ISOPTO CETAPRED, Alcon-PR	00998-0613-15

Suspension - Ophthalmic - 0.5 %/10 %

3.5 ml	$2.50	Prednisolone W/Sulfacetamide, Harber Pharm	51432-0868-35
15 ml	$7.00	Sulfacetamide W/Prednisolone, Harber Pharm	51432-0869-15

PREDNISOLONE SODIUM PHOSPHATE

(002105)

CATEGORIES: Adrenal Corticosteroids; Adrenal Hyperplasia; Adrenal Insufficiency; Adrenocortical Insufficiency; Airway Obstruction; Allergies; Alopecia; Alopecia Areata; Anemia; Ankylosing Spondylitis; Anti-Inflammatory Agents; Antihypertensives; Antimicrobials; Arthritis; Asthma; Atopic Dermatitis; Burns; Berylliosis; Bursitis; Cancer; Carditis; Chemotherapy; Chorioretinitis; Choroiditis; Colitis; Conjunctivitis; Corneal Inflammation; Corneal Injury; Corneal Ulcer; Dermatitis; Dermatitis Herpetiformis; Dermatomyositis; Diuresis; Drug Hypersensitivity; Endocrine Disorders; EENT Drugs; Enteritis; Epicondylitis; Erythema Multiforme; Eye, Ear, Nose, & Throat Preparations; Gastrointestinal Drugs; Glucocorticoids; Gouty Arthritis; Granuloma Annulare; Herpes; Herpes Zoster; Hormones; Hypercalcemia; Inflammatory Lesions; Iridocyclitis; Keloids; Keratitis; Laryngeal Edema; Lesions; Leukemia; Lichen Planus; Lichen Simplex Chronicus; Lupus Erythematosus; Lymphoma; Meningitis; Multiple Sclerosis; Mycosis Fungoides; Necrobiosis Lipoidica; Nephrotic Syndrome; Neuritis; Ocular Acne; Ocular Infections; Ophthalmic Corticosteroids; Ophthalmics; Osteoarthritis; Pemphigus; Pneumoconiosis; Proteinuria; Psoriasis; Purpura; Renal Drugs; Retinochoroiditis; Rhinitis; Sarcoidosis; Serum Sickness; Spondylitis; Steroids; Sulfonamides; Synovitis; Synovitis of Osteoarthritis; Tenosynovitis; Thrombocytopenia; Thyroiditis; Transfusion Reactions; Trichinosis; Tuberculosis; Tumors; Ulcerative Colitis; Urticaria; Uveitis; FDA Approval Pre 1982

BRAND NAMES: Ak-Pred; **Hydeltrasol**; I-Pred; Inflamase; Isolone Forte; Key-Pred Sp; Metreton; Nor-Pred S; Ocu-Pred; Pediapred; Predair; Predair-A; Predate-S; Predicort-Rp; Prednisol; Spectro-Pred

FORMULARIES: PCS

DESCRIPTION:

INJECTION

Prednisolone sodium phosphate, a synthetic adrenocortical steroid, is a white or slightly yellow powder that is slightly hygroscopic and is freely soluble in water. The molecular weight is 484.39. It is designated chemically as 11β, 17-dihydroxy-21-(phosphonooxy) pregna-1,4-diene-3,20-dione disodium salt. The empirical formula is $C_{21}H_{27}Na_2O_8P$.

Hydeltrasol* (Prednisolone Sodium Phosphate) injection is a sterile solution (pH 7.0 to 8.0), sealed under nitrogen, for intravenous, intramuscular, intra-articular, intralesional, and soft tissue administration.

Each milliliter contains prednisolone sodium phosphate equivalent to 20 mg prednisolone phosphate. Inactive ingredients per ml: niacinamide, 25 mg; sodium hydroxide to adjust pH; disodium edetate, 0.5 mg; Water for Injection, q.s. 1 ml. Sodium bisulfite, 1 mg, and phenol, 5 mg, added as preservatives.

* Registered trademark of Merck & Co., Inc.

ORAL LIQUID

Pediapred Oral Liquid is a dye free, colorless to light straw colored, raspberry flavored solution. Each 5 ml (teaspoonful) of Pediapred contains 6.7 mg prednisolone sodium phosphate (5 mg prednisolone base) in a palatable, aqueous vehicle.

Inactive Ingredients: Dibasic sodium phosphate, edetate disodium, methylparaben, purified water, sodium biphosphate, sorbitol, natural and artificial raspberry flavor.

Prednisolone sodium phosphate occurs as white or slightly yellow, friable granules or powder. It is freely soluble in water; soluble in methanol; slightly soluble in alcohol and in chloroform; and very slightly soluble in acetone and in dioxane. The chemical name of prednisolone sodium phosphate is pregna-1,4-diene-3,20-dione, 11, 17-dihydroxy-21-(phosphonooxy)-, disodium salt, (11β)-. The empirical formula is $C_{21}H_{27}Na_2O_8P$; the molecular weight is 484.39.

Pharmacological Category: Glucocorticoid

OPHTHALMIC SOLUTION

Inflamase Mild and Inflamase Forte (prednisolone sodium phosphate) ophthalmic solutions are sterile solutions for ophthalmic administration having the following compositions:

INFLAMASE MILD

Prednisolone Sodium Phosphate............ 1.25 mg/ml

(adrenocortical steroid/anti-inflammatory)

(equivalent to Prednisolone Phosphate 1.1 mg/ml)

INFLAMASE FORTE

Prednisolone Sodium Phosphate............ 10 mg/ml

(adrenocortical steroid/anti-inflammatory)

(equivalent to Prednisolone Phosphate 9.1 mg/ml)

DESCRIPTION: *(cont'd)*

in buffered, Isotonic solutions containing sodium biphosphate, sodium phosphate anhydrous, sodium chloride, edetate disodium and purified water; preserved with benzalkonium chloride 0.1 mg/ml.

The chemical name for prednisolone sodium phosphate is Pregna-1,4-diene-3,20-dione, 11,17-dihydroxy-21-(phosphonooxy)-, disodium salt, (11 β)-. The empirical formula is $C_{21}H_{27}Na_2O_8P$; the molecular weight is 484.39.

CLINICAL PHARMACOLOGY:

INJECTION

Hydeltrasol injection has a rapid onset but short duration of action when compared with less soluble preparations. Because of this, it is suitable for the treatment of acute disorders responsive to adrenocortical steroid therapy.

Naturally occurring glucocorticoids (hydrocortisone and cortisone), which also have salt-retaining properties, are used as replacement therapy in adrenocortical deficiency states. Their synthetic analogs, including prednisolone, are primarily used for their potent anti-inflammatory effects in disorders of many organ systems.

Glucocorticoids cause profound and varied metabolic effects. In addition, they modify the body's immune responses to diverse stimuli.

At equipotent anti-inflammatory doses, prednisolone has less tendency to cause salt and water retention than either hydrocortisone or cortisone.

ORAL LIQUID

Prednisolone is a synthetic adrenocortical steroid drug with predominantly glucocorticoid properties. Some of these properties reproduce the physiological actions of endogenous glucocorticosteroids, but others do not necessarily reflect any of the adrenal hormones' normal functions; they are seen only after administration of large therapeutic doses of the drug. The pharmacological effects of prednisolone which are due to its glucocorticoid properties include: promotion of gluconeogenesis; increased deposition of glycogen in the liver; inhibition of the utilization of glucose; anti-insulin activity; increased catabolism of protein; increased lipolysis; stimulation of fat synthesis and storage; increased glomerular filtration rate and resulting increase in urinary excretion of urate (creatinine excretion remains unchanged); and increased calcium excretion.

Decreased production of eosinophils and lymphocytes occurs, but erythropoieses and production of polymorphonuclear leukocytes are stimulated. Anti-inflammatory processes (edema, fibrin deposition, capillary dilatation, migration of leukocytes and phagocytosis) and the later stages of wound healing (capillary proliferation, deposition of collagen, cicatrization) are inhibited. Prednisolone can stimulate secretion of various components of gastric juice. Stimulation of the production of corticotropin may lead to suppression of endogenous corticosteroids. Prednisolone has slight mineralocorticoid activity, whereby entry of sodium into cells and loss of intracellular potassium is stimulated. This is particularly evident in the kidney, where rapid ion exchange leads to sodium retention and hypertension.

Prednisolone is rapidly and well absorbed from the gastrointestinal tract following oral administration. Pediapred Oral Liquid produces a 20% higher peak plasma level of prednisolone which occurs approximately 15 minutes earlier than the peak seen with tablet formulations. Prednisolone is 70-90% protein-bound in the plasma and it is eliminated from the plasma with a half-life of 2 to 4 hours. It is metabolized mainly in the liver and excreted in the urine as sulfate and glucuronide conjugates.

OPHTHALMIC SOLUTION

Prednisolone sodium phosphate causes inhibition of the inflammatory response to inciting agents of a mechanical, chemical or immunological nature. No generally accepted explanation of this steroid property has been advanced.

INDICATIONS AND USAGE:

INJECTION

By intravenous or intramuscular injection: when oral therapy is not feasible:

Endocrine Disorders: Primary or secondary adrenocortical insufficiency (hydrocortisone or cortisone is the drug of choice; synthetic analogs may be used in conjunction with mineralocorticoids where applicable; in infancy, mineralocorticoid supplementation is of particular importance)

Acute adrenocortical insufficiency (hydrocortisone or cortisone is the drug of choice; mineralocorticoid supplementation may be necessary, particularly when synthetic analogs are used)

Preoperatively, and in the event of serious trauma or illness, in patients with known adrenal insufficiency or when adrenocortical reserve is doubtful

Congenital adrenal hyperplasia; Nonsuppurative thyroiditis; Hypercalcemia associated with cancer

Rheumatic Disorders: As adjunctive therapy for short-term administration (to tide the patient over an acute episode or exacerbation) in: Post-traumatic osteoarthritis; Synovitis of osteoarthritis; Rheumatoid arthritis, including juvenile rheumatoid arthritis (selected cases may require low-dose maintenance therapy)

Acute and subacute bursitis; Epicondylitis; Acute nonspecific tenosynovitis; Acute gouty arthritis; Psoriatic arthritis; Ankylosing spondylitis

Collagen Diseases: During an exacerbation or as maintenance therapy in selected cases of: Systemic lupus erythematosus; Acute rheumatic carditis; Systemic dermatomyositis (polymyositis)

Dermatologic Diseases: Pemphigus; Severe erythema multiforme (Stevens-Johnson syndrome); Exfoliative dermatitis; Bullous dermatitis herpetiformis; Severe seborrheic dermatitis; Severe psoriasis; Mycosis fungoides

Allergic States: Control of severe or incapacitating allergic conditions intractable to adequate trials of conventional treatment in: Bronchial asthma; Contact dermatitis; Atopic dermatitis; Serum sickness; Seasonal or perennial allergic rhinitis; Drug hypersensitivity reactions; Urticarial transfusion reactions; Acute noninfectious laryngeal edema (epinephrine is the drug of first choice)

Ophthalmic Diseases: Severe acute and chronic allergic and inflammatory processes involving the eye, such as: Herpes zoster ophthalmicus; Iritis, iridocyclitis; Chorioretinitis; Diffuse posterior uveitis and choroiditis; Optic neuritis; Sympathetic ophthalmia; Anterior segment inflammation; Allergic conjunctivitis; Keratitis; Allergic corneal marginal ulcers

Gastrointestinal Diseases: To tide the patient over a critical period of the disease in: Ulcerative colitis (Systemic therapy); Regional enteritis (Systemic therapy)

Respiratory Diseases: Symptomatic sarcoidosis; Berylliosis; Fulminating or disseminated pulmonary tuberculosis when used concurrently with appropriate antituberculous chemotherapy; Loeffler's syndrome not manageable by other means; Aspiration pneumonitis

Hematologic Disorders: Acquired (autoimmune) hemolytic anemia

Idiopathic thrombocytopenic purpura in adults (IV only; IM administration is contraindicated); Secondary thrombocytopenia in adults; Erythroblastopenia (RBC anemia); Congenital (erythroid) hypoplastic anemia

Neoplastic Diseases: For palliative management of: Leukemias and lymphomas in adults; Acute leukemia of childhood

INDICATIONS AND USAGE: *(cont'd)*

Edematous States: To induce diuresis or remission of proteinuria in the nephrotic syndrome, without uremia, of the idiopathic type, or that due to lupus erythematosus

Miscellaneous: Tuberculous meningitis with subarachnoid block or impending block when used concurrently with appropriate antituberculous chemotherapy; Trichinosis with neurologic or myocardial involvement.

By Intra-Articular Or Soft Tissue Injection: As adjunctive therapy for short-term administration (to tide the patient over an acute episode or exacerbation) in: Synovitis of osteoarthritis; Rheumatoid arthritis; Acute and subacute bursitis; Acute gouty arthritis; Epicondylitis; Acute nonspecific tenosynovitis; Post-traumatic osteoarthritis.

By Intralesional Injection: Keloids; Localized hypertrophic, infiltrated, inflammatory lesions of: lichen planus, psoriatic plaques, granuloma annulare, and lichen simplex chronicus (neurodermatitis); Discoid lupus erythematosus; Necrobiosis lipoidica diabeticorum; Alopecia areata

May also be useful in cystic tumors of an aponeurosis or tendon (ganglia).

ORAL LIQUID

Pediapred Oral Liquid is indicated in the following conditions:

Endocrine Disorders: Primary or secondary adrenocortical insufficiency (hydrocortisone or cortisone is the first choice; synthetic analogs may be used in conjunction with mineralocorticoids where applicable; in infancy mineralocorticoid supplementation is of particular importance); congenital adrenal hyperplasia; hypercalcemia associated with cancer; non-suppurative thyroiditis.

Rheumatic Disorders: As adjunctive therapy for short term administration (to tide the patient over an acute episode or exacerbation) in: psoriatic arthritis; rheumatoid arthritis, including juvenile rheumatoid arthritis (selected cases may require low dose maintenance therapy); ankylosing spondylitis; acute and subacute bursitis; acute nonspecific tenosynovitis; acute gouty arthritis; post- traumatic osteoarthritis; synovitis of osteoarthritis; epicondylitis.

Collagen Diseases: During an exacerbation or as maintenance therapy in selected cases of: systemic lupus erythematosus; systemic dermatomyositis (polymyositis); acute rheumatic carditis.

Dermatologic Diseases: Pemphigus; bullous dermatitis herpetiformis; severe erythema multiforme (Stevens-Johnson syndrome); exfoliative dermatitis; mycosis fungoides; severe psoriasis; severe seborrheic dermatitis.

Allergic States: Control of severe or incapacitating allergic conditions intractable to adequate trials of conventional treatment in: seasonal or perennial allergic rhinitis; bronchial asthma; contact dermatitis; atopic dermatitis; serum sickness; drug hypersensitivity reactions.

Ophthalmic Diseases: Severe acute and chronic allergic and inflammatory processes involving the eye and its adnexa such as: allergic conjunctivitis; keratitis; allergic corneal marginal ulcers; herpes zoster ophthalmicus; iritis and iridocyclitis; chorioretinitis; anterior segment inflammation; diffuse posterior uveitis and choroiditis; optic neuritis; sympathetic ophthalmia.

Respiratory Diseases: Symptomatic sarcoidosis; Loeffler's syndrome not manageable by other means; berylliosis; fulminating or disseminated pulmonary tuberculosis when used concurrently with appropriate antituberculous chemotherapy; aspiration pneumonitis.

Hematologic Disorders: Idiopathic thrombocytopenic purpura in adults; secondary thrombocytopenia in adults; acquired (autoimmune) hemolytic anemia; erythroblastopenia (RBC anemia); congenital (erythroid) hypoplastic anemia.

Neoplastic Diseases: For palliative management of: leukemias and lymphomas in adults; acute leukemia of childhood.

Edematous States: To induce a diuresis or remission of proteinuria in the nephrotic syndrome, without uremia, of the idiopathic type or that due to lupus erythematosus.

Gastrointestinal Diseases: To tide the patient over a critical period of the disease in: ulcerative colitis; regional enteritis.

Nervous System: Acute exacerbations of multiple sclerosis.

Miscellaneous: Tuberculous meningitis with subarachnoid block or impending block when used concurrently with appropriate antituberculous chemotherapy; trichinosis with neurologic or myocardial involvement.

OPHTHALMIC SOLUTION

Inflamase Mild and Inflamase Forte Ophthalmic Solutions are indicated for the treatment of the following conditions: steroid responsive inflammatory conditions of the palpebral and bulbar conjunctiva, cornea, and anterior segment of the globe, such as allergic conjunctivitis, acne rosacea, superficial punctate keratitis, herpes zoster keratitis, iritis, cyclitis, selected infective conjunctivitis when the inherent hazard of steroid use is accepted to obtain an advisable diminution in edema and inflammation; corneal injury from chemical, radiation, or thermal burns, or penetration of foreign bodies.

Inflamase Forte Ophthalmic Solution is recommended for moderate to severe inflammations, particularly when unusually rapid control is desired. In stubborn cases of anterior segment eye disease, systemic adrenocortical hormone therapy may be required. When the deeper ocular structures are involved, systemic therapy is necessary.

CONTRAINDICATIONS:

Injection: Systemic fungal infections (see WARNINGS) regarding amphotericin B

Hypersensitivity to any component of this product, including sulfites(see WARNINGS.)

Oral Liquid: Systemic fungal infections.

Ophthalmic Solution: The use of these preparations is contraindicated in the presence of acute superficial herpes simplex, keratitis, fungal diseases of the ocular structures, acute infectious stages of vaccinia, varicella and most other viral diseases of the cornea and conjunctiva, tuberculosis of the eye and hypersensitivity to a component of this preparation.

The use of these preparations is always contraindicated after uncomplicated removal of a superficial corneal foreign body.

WARNINGS:

INJECTION

Because rare instances of anaphylactoid reactions have occurred in patients receiving parenteral corticosteroid therapy, appropriate precautionary measures should be taken prior to administration, especially when the patient has a history of allergy to any drug. Anaphylactoid and hypersensitivity reactions have been reported for Injection Hydeltrasol (see ADVERSE REACTIONS.)

Injection Hydeltrasol contains sodium bisulfite, a sulfite that may cause allergic-type reactions including anaphylactic symptoms and life-threatening or less severe asthmatic episodes in certain susceptible people. The overall prevalence of sulfite sensitivity in the general population is unknown and probably low. Sulfite sensitivity is seen more frequently in asthmatic than in nonasthmatic people.

WARNINGS: *(cont'd)*

Corticosteroids may exacerbate systemic fungal infections and therefore should not be used in the presence of such infections unless they are needed to control drug reactions due to amphotericin B. Moreover, there have been cases reported in which concomitant use of amphotericin B and hydrocortisone was followed by cardiac enlargement and congestive failure.

In patients on corticosteroid therapy subjected to any unusual stress, increased dosage of rapidly acting corticosteroids before, during, and after the stressful situation is indicated.

Drug-induced secondary adrenocortical insufficiency may result from too rapid withdrawal of corticosteroids and may be minimized by gradual reduction of dosage. This type of relative insufficiency may persist for months after discontinuation of therapy; therefore, in any situation of stress occurring during that period, hormone therapy should be reinstituted. If the patient is receiving steroids already, dosage may have to be increased. Since mineralocorticoid secretion may be impaired, salt and/or a mineralocorticoid should be administered concurrently.

Corticosteroids may mask some signs of infection, and new infections may appear during their use. There may be decreased resistance and inability to localize infection when corticosteroids are used. Moreover, corticosteroids may affect the nitroblue-tetrazolium test for bacterial infection and produce false negative results.

In cerebral malaria, a double-blind trial has shown that the use of corticosteroids is associated with prolongation of coma and a higher incidence of pneumonia and gastrointestinal bleeding.

Corticosteroids may activate latent amebiasis. Therefore, it is recommended that latent or active amebiasis be ruled out before initiating corticosteroid therapy in any patient who has spent time in the tropics or any patient with unexplained diarrhea.

Prolonged use of corticosteroids may produce posterior subcapsular cataracts, glaucoma with possible damage to the optic nerves, and may enhance the establishment of secondary ocular infections due to fungi or viruses.

Usage In Pregnancy: Since adequate human reproduction studies have not been done with corticosteroids, use of these drugs in pregnancy or in women of childbearing potential requires that the anticipated benefits be weighed against the possible hazards to the mother and embryo or fetus. Infants born of mothers who have received substantial doses of corticosteroids during pregnancy should be carefully observed for signs of hypoadrenalism.

Corticosteroids appear in breast milk and could suppress growth, interfere with endogenous corticosteroid production, or cause other unwanted effects. Mothers taking pharmacologic doses of corticosteroids should be advised not to nurse.

Average and large doses of cortisone or hydrocortisone can cause elevation of blood pressure, salt and water retention, and increased excretion of potassium. These effects are less likely to occur with the synthetic derivatives except when used in large doses. Dietary salt restriction and potassium supplementation may be necessary. All corticosteroids increase calcium excretion.

Administration of live virus vaccines, including smallpox, is contraindicated in individuals receiving immunosuppressive doses of corticosteroids. If inactivated viral or bacterial vaccines are administered to individuals receiving immunosuppressive doses of corticosteroids, the expected serum antibody response may not be obtained. However, immunization procedures may be undertaken in patients who are receiving corticosteroids as replacement therapy, e.g., for Addison's disease.

Patients who are on drugs which suppress the immune system are more susceptible to infections than healthy individuals. Chickenpox and measles, for example, can have a more serious or even fatal course in non-immune children or adults on corticosteroids. In such children or adults who have not had these diseases, particular care should be taken to avoid exposure. The risk of developing a disseminated infection varies among individuals and can be related to the dose, route and duration of corticosteroid administration as well as to the underlying disease. If exposed to chickenpox, prophylaxis with varicella zoster immune globulin (VZIG) may be indicated. If chickenpox develops, treatment with antiviral agents may be considered. If exposed to measles, prophylaxis with immune globulin (IG) may be indicated. (See the respective package inserts for VZIG and IG for complete prescribing information.)

The use of Hydeltrasol injection in active tuberculosis should be restricted to those cases of fulminating or disseminated tuberculosis in which the corticosteroid is used for the management of the disease in conjunction with appropriate antituberculous regimen.

If corticosteroids are indicated in patients with latent tuberculosis or tuberculin reactivity, close observation is necessary as reactivation of the disease may occur. During prolonged corticosteroid therapy, these patients should receive chemoprophylaxis.

Literature reports suggest an apparent association between use of corticosteroids and left ventricular free wall rupture after a recent myocardial infarction; therefore, therapy with corticosteroids should be used with great caution in these patients.

ORAL LIQUID

In patients on corticosteroid therapy subjected to unusual stress, increased dosage of rapidly acting corticosteroids before, during and after the stressful situation is indicated.

Corticosteroids may mask some signs of infection, and new infections may appear during their use. There may be decreased resistance and inability to localize infection when corticosteroids are used.

Prolonged use of corticosteroids may produce posterior subcapsular cataracts, glaucoma with possible damage to the optic nerves, and may enhance the establishment of secondary ocular infections due to fungi or viruses.

Average and large doses of hydrocortisone or cortisone can cause elevation of blood pressure, salt and water retention, and increased excretion of potassium. These effects are less likely to occur with the synthetic derivatives except when used in large doses. Dietary salt restriction and potassium supplementation may be necessary. All corticosteroids increase calcium excretion. **While on corticosteroid therapy patients should not be vaccinated against smallpox. Other immunization procedures should not be undertaken in patients who are on corticosteroids, especially on high doses, because of possible hazards of neurological complications and a lack of antibody response.**

The use of prednisolone in active tuberculosis should be restricted to those cases of fulminating or disseminated tuberculosis in which the corticosteroid is used for the management of the disease in conjunction with an appropriate antituberculous regimen.

If corticosteroids are indicated in patients with latent tuberculosis or tuberculin reactivity, close observation is necessary as reactivation of the disease may occur. During prolonged corticosteroid therapy these patients should receive chemoprophylaxis.

Persons who are on drugs which suppress the immune system are more susceptible to infections than healthy individuals. Chicken pox and measles, for example, can have a more serious or even fatal course in non-immune children or adults on corticosteroids. In such children or adults who have not had these diseases, particular care should be taken to avoid exposure. How the dose, route and duration of corticosteroid administration affects the risk of developing a disseminated infection is not known. The contribution of the underlying disease and/or prior corticosteroid treatment to the risk is also not known. If exposed to chicken pox, prophylaxis with varicella zoster immune globulin (VZIG) may be indicated. If exposed to measles, prophylaxis with pooled intramuscular immunoglobulin (IG) may be indicated. (See the respective package inserts for complete VZIG and IG prescribing information.) If chicken pox develops, treatment with antiviral agents may be considered.

OPHTHALMIC SOLUTION

NOT FOR INJECTION INTO THE EYE - FOR TOPICAL USE ONLY.

Employment of steroid medication in the treatment of herpes simplex, keratitis involving the stroma requires great caution; frequent slit lamp microscopy is mandatory.

Prolonged use may result in elevated intraocular pressure and/or glaucoma, damage to the optic nerve, defects in visual acuity and fields of vision, posterior subcapsular cataract formation, or may result in secondary ocular infections. Viral, bacterial and fungal infections of the cornea may be exacerbated by the application of steroids. In those diseases causing thinning of the cornea or sclera, perforation has been known to occur with the use of topical steroids. Acute purulent untreated infection of the eye may be masked or activity enhanced by the presence of steroid medication.

These drugs are not effective in mustard gas keratitis and Sjogren's keratoconjunctivitis.

If irritation persists or develops, the patient should be advised to discontinue use and consult prescribing physician.

PRECAUTIONS:

INJECTION

This product, like many other steroid formulations, is sensitive to heat. Therefore, it should not be autoclaved when it is desirable to sterilize the exterior of the vial.

Following prolonged therapy, withdrawal of corticosteroids may result in symptoms of the corticosteroid withdrawal syndrome including fever, myalgia, arthralgia, and malaise. This may occur in patients even without evidence of adrenal insufficiency.

There is an enhanced effect of corticosteroids in patients with hypothyroidism and in those with cirrhosis.

Corticosteroids should be used cautiously in patients with ocular herpes simplex for fear of corneal perforation.

The lowest possible dose of corticosteroid should be used to control the condition under treatment, and when reduction in dosage is possible, the reduction must be gradual.

Psychic derangements may appear when corticosteroids are used, ranging from euphoria, insomnia, mood swings, personality changes, and severe depression to frank psychotic manifestations. Also, existing emotional instability or psychotic tendencies may be aggravated by corticosteroids.

Aspirin should be used cautiously in conjunction with corticosteroids in hypoprothrombinemia.

Steroids should be used with caution in nonspecific ulcerative colitis, if there is a probability of impending perforation, abscess, or other pyogenic infection, also in diverticulitis, fresh intestinal anastomoses, active or latent peptic ulcer, renal insufficiency, hypertension, osteoporosis, and myasthenia gravis. Signs of peritoneal irritation following gastrointestinal perforation in patients receiving large doses of corticosteroids may be minimal or absent. Fat embolism has been reported as a possible complication of hypercortisonism.

When large doses are given, some authorities advise that antacids be administered between meals to help to prevent peptic ulcer.

Growth and development of infants and children on prolonged corticosteroid therapy should be carefully followed.

Steroids may increase or decrease motility and number of spermatozoa in some patients.

Phenytoin, phenobarbital, ephedrine, and rifampin may enhance the metabolic clearance of corticosteroids, resulting in decreased blood levels and lessened physiologic activity, thus requiring adjustment in corticosteroid dosage.

The prothrombin time should be checked frequently in patients who are receiving corticosteroids and coumarin anticoagulants at the same time because of reports that corticosteroids have altered the response to these anticoagulants. Studies have shown that the usual effect produced by adding corticosteroids is inhibition of response to coumarins, although there have been some conflicting reports of potentiation not substantiated by studies.

When corticosteroids are administered concomitantly with potassium-depleting diuretics, patients should be observed closely for development of hypokalemia.

Intra-articular injection of a corticosteroid may produce systemic as well as local effects.

Appropriate examination of any joint fluid present is necessary to exclude a septic process.

A marked increase in pain accompanied by local swelling, further restriction of joint motion, fever, and malaise is suggestive of septic arthritis. If this complication occurs and the diagnosis of sepsis is confirmed, appropriate antimicrobial therapy should be instituted.

Injection of a steroid into an infected site is to be avoided.

Corticosteroids should not be injected into unstable joints.

Patients should be impressed strongly with the importance of not overusing joints in which symptomatic benefit has been obtained as long as the inflammatory process remains active.

Frequent intra-articular injection may result in damage to joint tissues.

The slower rate of absorption by intramuscular administration should be recognized.

GENERAL

Oral Liquid: Drug-Induced secondary adrenocortical insufficiency may be minimized by general reduction of dosage. This type of relative insufficiency may persist for months after discontinuation of therapy; therefore, in any situation of stress occurring during that period, hormone therapy should be reinstituted. Since mineralocorticoid secretion may be impaired, salt and/or a mineralocorticoid should be administered concurrently.

There is an enhanced effect of corticosteroids in patients with hypothyroidism and in those with cirrhosis.

Corticosteroids should be used cautiously in patients with ocular herpes simplex because of possible corneal perforation.

The lowest possible dose of corticosteroid should be used to control the condition under treatment, and when reduction in dosage is possible, the reduction should be gradual.

Psychic derangements may appear when corticosteroids are used, ranging from euphoria, insomnia, mood swings, personality changes, and severe depression, to frank psychotic manifestations. Also, existing emotional instability or psychotic tendencies may be aggravated by corticosteroids.

Aspirin should be used cautiously in conjunction with corticosteroids in hypoprothrombinemia.

Steroids should be used with caution in nonspecific ulcerative colitis, if there is a probability of impending perforation, abscess or other pyogenic infection; diverticulitis; fresh intestinal anastomoses; active or latent peptic ulcer; renal insufficiency; hypertension; osteoporosis; and myasthenia gravis.

Growth and development of infants and children on prolonged corticosteroid therapy should be carefully observed.

PRECAUTIONS: *(cont'd)*

Although controlled clinical trials have shown corticosteroids to be effective in speeding the resolution of acute exacerbations of multiple sclerosis, they do not show that they affect the ultimate outcome or natural history of the disease. The studies do show that relatively high doses of corticosteroids are necessary to demonstrate a significant effect. (See DOSAGE AND ADMINISTRATION.)

Since complications of treatment with glucocorticoids are dependent on the size of the dose and the duration of treatment, a risk/benefit decision must be made in each individual case as to dose and duration of treatment and as to whether daily or intermittent therapy should be used.

Ophthalmic Solution: As fungal infections of the cornea are particularly prone to develop coincidentally with long-term local steroid applications, fungus invasion must be suspected in any persistent corneal ulceration where a steroid has been used or is in use.

Intraocular pressure should be checked frequently.

INFORMATION FOR THE PATIENT

Injection: Susceptible patients who are on immunosuppressant doses of corticosteroids should be warned to avoid exposure to chickenpox or measles. Patients should also be advised that if they are exposed, medical advice should be sought without delay.

Oral Liquid: Patients should be warned not to discontinue the use of Pediapred abruptly or without medical supervision, to advise any medical attendants that they are taking Pediapred and to seek medical advice at once should they develop fever or other signs of infection.

Persons who are on immunosuppressant doses of corticosteroids should be warned to avoid exposure to chicken pox or measles. Patients should also be advised that if they are exposed, medical advice should be sought without delay.

Ophthalmic Solution: Do not touch dropper tip to any surface as this may contaminate the solution.

PREGNANCY CATEGORY C

Oral Liquid: Prednisolone has been shown to be teratogenic in many species when given in doses equivalent to the human dose. There are no adequate and well controlled studies in pregnant women. Pediapred should be used during pregnancy only if the potential benefit justifies the potential risk to the fetus. Animal studies in which prednisolone has been given to pregnant mice, rats, and rabbits have yielded an increased incidence of cleft palate in the offspring.

Ophthalmic Solution: Animal reproductive studies have not been conducted with prednisolone sodium phosphate. It is also not known whether prednisolone sodium phosphate can cause fetal harm when administered to a pregnant woman or can affect reproductive capacity. Prednisolone sodium phosphate should be given to a pregnant woman only if clearly needed.

The effect of prednisolone sodium phosphate on the later growth, development and functional maturation of the child is unknown.

NURSING MOTHERS

Oral Liquid: Prednisolone is excreted in breast milk, but only to a small (less than 1% of the administered dose) and probably clinically insignificant extent. Caution should be exercised when Pediapred is administered to a nursing woman.

Ophthalmic Solution: It is not known whether this drug is excreted in human milk. Because many drugs are excreted in human milk, caution should be exercised when prednisolone sodium phosphate is administered to a nursing woman.

PEDIATRIC USE

Safety and effectiveness in children have not been established.

DRUG INTERACTIONS:

ORAL LIQUID

Drugs such as barbiturates which induce hepatic microsomal drug metabolizing enzyme activity may enhance metabolism of prednisolone and require that the dosage of Pediapred be increased.

ADVERSE REACTIONS:

INJECTION

Fluid And Electrolyte Disturbances: Sodium retention; Fluid retention; Congestive heart failure in susceptible patients; Potassium loss; Hypokalemic alkalosis; Hypertension

Musculoskeletal: Muscle weakness; Steroid myopathy; Loss of muscle mass; Osteoporosis; Vertebral compression fractures; Aseptic necrosis of femoral and humeral heads; Pathologic fracture of long bones; Tendon rupture

Gastrointestinal: Peptic ulcer with possible subsequent perforation and hemorrhage; Perforation of the small and large bowel, particularly in patients with inflammatory bowel disease; Pancreatitis; Abdominal distention; Ulcerative esophagitis

Dermatologic: Impaired wound healing; Thin fragile skin; Petechiae and ecchymoses; Erythema; Increased sweating; May suppress reactions to skin tests; Burning or tingling, especially in the perineal area (after IV injection); Other cutaneous reactions, such as allergic dermatitis, urticaria, angioneurotic edema

Neurologic: Convulsions; Increased intracranial pressure with papilledema (pseudotumor cerebri) usually after treatment; Vertigo; Headache; Psychic disturbances

Endocrine: Menstrual irregularities; Development of cushingoid state; Suppression of growth in children; Secondary adrenocortical and pituitary unresponsiveness, particularly in times of stress, as in trauma, surgery, or illness; Decreased carbohydrate tolerance; Manifestations of latent diabetes mellitus; Increased requirements for insulin or oral hypoglycemic agents in diabetics; Hirsutism

Ophthalmic: Posterior subcapsular cataracts; Increased intraocular pressure; Glaucoma; Exophthalmos

Metabolic: Negative nitrogen balance due to protein catabolism

Cardiovascular: Myocardial rupture following recent myocardial infarction (see WARNINGS.)

Other: Anaphylactoid or hypersensitivity reactions; Thromboembolism; Weight gain; Increased appetite; Nausea; Malaise

The following *additional* adverse reactions are related to parenteral corticosteroid therapy:

Rare instances of blindness associated with intralesional therapy around the face and head; Hyperpigmentation or hypopigmentation; Subcutaneous and cutaneous atrophy; Sterile abscess; Postinjection flare (following intra-articular use); Charcot-like arthropathy.

ORAL LIQUID

Fluid and Electrolyte Disturbances: Sodium retention; fluid retention; congestive heart failure in susceptible patients; potassium loss; hypokalemic alkalosis; hypertension.

Musculoskeletal: Muscle weakness; steroid myopathy; loss of muscle mass; osteoporosis; vertebral compression fractures; aseptic necrosis of femoral and humeral heads; pathologic fracture of long bones.

Gastrointestinal: Peptic ulcer with possible perforation and hemorrhage; pancreatitis; abdominal distention; ulcerative esophagitis.

ADVERSE REACTIONS: *(cont'd)*

Dermatologic: Impaired wound healing; thin fragile skin; petechiae and ecchymoses; facial erythema; increased sweating; may suppress reactions to skin tests.

Metabolic: Negative nitrogen balance due to protein catabolism.

Neurological: Convulsions; increased intracranial pressure with papilledema (pseudotumor cerebri) usually after treatment; vertigo; headache.

Endocrine: Menstrual irregularities; development of cushingoid state; secondary adrenocortical and pituitary unresponsiveness, particularly in times of stress, as in trauma, surgery or illness; suppression of growth in children; decreased carbohydrate tolerance; manifestations of latent diabetes mellitus; increased requirements for insulin or oral hypoglycemic agents in diabetes.

Ophthalmic: Posterior subcapsular cataracts; increased intraocular pressure; glaucoma; exophthalmos.

OPHTHALMIC SOLUTION

The following adverse reactions have been reported: glaucoma with optic nerve damage, visual acuity and field defects, posterior subcapsular cataract formation, secondary ocular infections from pathogens including herpes simplex and fungi, and perforation of the globe.

Rarely, filtering blebs have been reported when topical steroids have been used following cataract surgery.

Rarely, stinging or burning may occur.

OVERDOSAGE:

INJECTION AND OPHTHALMIC SOLUTION

Reports of acute toxicity and/or death following overdosage of glucocorticoids are rare. In the event of overdosage, no specific antidote is available; treatment is supportive and symptomatic.

The intraperitoneal LD_{50} of prednisolone phosphate disodium in female mice was 1190 mg/kg.

ORAL LIQUID

The effects of accidental ingestion of large quantities of prednisolone over a very short period of time have not been reported, but prolonged use of the drug can produce mental symptoms, moon face, abnormal fat deposits, fluid retention, excessive appetite, weight gain, hypertrichosis, acne, striae, ecchymosis, increased sweating, pigmentation, dry scaly skin, thinning scalp hair, increased blood pressure, tachycardia, thrombophlebitis, decreased resistance to infection, negative nitrogen balance with delayed bone and wound healing, headache, weakness, menstrual disorders, accentuated menopausal symptoms, neuropathy, fractures, osteoporosis, peptic ulcer, decreased glucose tolerance, hypokalemia, and adrenal insufficiency. Hepatomegaly and abdominal distention have been observed in children.

Treatment of acute overdosage is by immediate gastric lavage or emesis. For chronic overdosage in the face of severe disease requiring continuous steroid therapy the dosage of prednisolone may be reduced only temporarily, or alternate day treatment may be introduced.

DOSAGE AND ADMINISTRATION:

INJECTION

For intravenous, intramuscular, intra-articular, intralesional, and soft tissue injection. DOSAGE REQUIREMENTS ARE VARIABLE AND MUST BE INDIVIDUALIZED ON THE BASIS OF THE DISEASE AND THE RESPONSE OF THE PATIENT.

Intravenous and Intramuscular Injection: Hydeltrasol injection can be given directly from the vial, or it can be added to Sodium Chloride Injection or Dextrose Injection and given by intravenous drip.

Benzyl alcohol as a preservative has been associated with toxicity in premature infants. Solutions used for intravenous administration or further dilution of this product should be preservative-free when used in the neonate, especially the premature infant.

When it is mixed with an infusion solution, sterile precautions should be observed. Since infusion solutions generally do not contain preservatives, mixtures should be used within 24 hours.

The initial dosage varies from 4 to 60 mg a day depending on the disease being treated. In less severe diseases doses lower than 4 mg may suffice, while in severe diseases doses higher than 60 mg may be required. Usually the daily parenteral dose of Hydeltrasol injection is the same as the daily oral dose of prednisolone and the dosage interval is every 4 to 8 hours.

The initial dosage should be maintained or adjusted until the patient's response is satisfactory. If a satisfactory clinical response does not occur after a reasonable period of time, discontinue Hydeltrasol injection and transfer the patient to other therapy.

After a favorable initial response, the proper maintenance dosage should be determined by decreasing the initial dosage in small amounts to the lowest dosage that maintains an adequate clinical response.

Patients should be observed closely for signs that might require dosage adjustment, including changes in clinical status resulting from remissions or exacerbations of the disease, individual drug responsiveness, and the effect of stress (*e.g.,* surgery, infection, trauma). During stress it may be necessary to increase dosage temporarily.

If the drug is to be stopped after more than a few days of treatment, it usually should be withdrawn gradually.

Intra-articular, Intralesional, and Soft Tissue Injection: Intra-articular, intralesional, and soft tissue injections are generally employed when the affected joints or areas are limited to one or two sites. Dosage and frequency of injection vary depending on the condition being treated and the site of injection. The usual dose is from 2 to 30 mg. The frequency usually ranges from once every three to five days to once every two to three weeks. Frequent intra-articular injection may result in damage to joint tissues. Some of the usual single doses are (TABLE 1):

TABLE 1

Site of Injection	Doses: Amount of Injection (ml)	Doses: Amount of Prednisolone Phosphate (mg)
Large Joints (*e.g.,* Knee)	0.5 to 1	10 to 20
Small Joints (*e.g.,* Interphalangeal, Temporomandibular)	0.2 to 0.25	4 to 5
Bursae	0.5 to 0.75	10 to 15
Tendon Sheaths	0.1 to 0.25	2 to 5
Soft Tissue Infiltration	0.5 to 1.5	10 to 30
Ganglia	0.25 to 0.5	5 to 10

Hydeltrasol injection is particularly recommended for use in conjunction with one of the less soluble, longer-acting steroids, such as Hydeltra- T.B.A.* (Prednisolone Tebutate) suspension or Hydrocortone* Acetate (Hydrocortisone Acetate) sterile suspension, available for intra-articular and soft tissue injection.

* Registered trademark of Merck & Co., Inc.

DOSAGE AND ADMINISTRATION: *(cont'd)*

ORAL LIQUID

The initial dosage of Pediapred may vary from 5 ml to 60 ml (5 to 60 mg prednisolone base) per day depending on the specific disease entity being treated. In situations of less severity lower doses will generally suffice while in selected patients higher initial doses may be required. The initial dosage should be maintained or adjusted until a satisfactory response is noted. If after a reasonable period of time there is a lack of satisfactory clinical response, Pediapred should be discontinued and the patient transferred to other appropriate therapy. **IT SHOULD BE EMPHASIZED THAT DOSAGE REQUIREMENTS ARE VARIABLE AND MUST BE INDIVIDUALIZED ON THE BASIS OF THE DISEASE UNDER TREATMENT AND THE RESPONSE OF THE PATIENT.** After a favorable response is noted, the proper maintenance dosage should be determined by decreasing the initial drug dosage in small decrements at appropriate time intervals until the lowest dosage which will maintain an adequate clinical response is reached. It should be kept in mind that constant monitoring is needed in regard to drug dosage. Included in the situations which may make dosage adjustments necessary are changes in clinical status secondary to remissions or exacerbations in the disease process, the patient's individual drug responsiveness, and the effect of patient exposure to stressful situations not directly related to the disease entity under treatment; in this latter situation it may be necessary to increase the dosage of Pediapred for a period of time consistent with the patient's condition. If after long term therapy the drug is to be stopped, it is recommended that it be withdrawn gradually rather than abruptly.

In the treatment of acute exacerbations of multiple sclerosis daily doses of 200 mg of prednisolone for a week followed by 80 mg every other day or 4 to 8 mg dexamethasone every other day for one month have been shown to be effective.

For the purpose of comparison, the following is the equivalent milligram dosage of the various glucocorticoids: cortisone, 25; hydrocortisone, 20; prednisolone, 5; prednisone, 5; methylprednisolone, 4; triamcinolone, 4; paramethasone, 2; betamethasone, 0.75; dexamethasone, 0.75. These dose relationships apply only to oral or intravenous administration of these compounds. When these substances or their derivatives are injected intramuscularly or into joint spaces, their relative properties may be greatly altered.

OPHTHALMIC SOLUTION

Depending on the severity of inflammation, instill one or two drops of solution into the conjunctival sac up to every hour during the day and every two hours during the night as necessary as initial therapy.

When a favorable response is observed, reduce dosage to one drop every four hours.

Later, further reduction in dosage to one drop three to four times daily may suffice to control symptoms.

The duration of treatment will vary with the type of lesion and may extend from a few days to several weeks, according to therapeutic response. Relapses, more common in chronic active lesions than in self- limiting conditions, usually respond to retreatment.

HOW SUPPLIED:

INJECTION

No. 7577X — Injection Hydeltrasol, 20 mg prednisolone phosphate equivalent per ml, is a clear, colorless to slightly yellow solution, and is supplied as follows: 2 ml vials; 5 ml vials; 20 mg/ml 5 ml vial).

Storage: Sensitive to heat. Do not autoclave. Protect from light. Store container in carton until contents have been used.

ORAL LIQUID

Pediapred Oral Liquid is a colorless to light straw colored solution containing 6.7 mg prednisolone sodium phosphate (5 mg prednisolone base) per 5 ml (teaspoonful).

Store at 4°-25°C (39°-77°F). May be refrigerated. Keep tightly closed and out of the reach of children.

OPHTHALMIC SOLUTION

STORE AT CONTROLLED ROOM TEMPERATURE, 59°-86°F (15°-30°C). Protect from light. Keep out of the reach of children.

(Injection - Merck & Co., Inc., 2/93, 7407227) (Oral Liquid - Fisons Pharmaceuticals, 9/94, RF024F) (Ophthalmic Solution - Iolab Corporation, 9/92, 6020-L)

HOW SUPPLIED - RATED THERAPEUTICALLY EQUIVALENT:

Injection, Solution - Intravenous - 20 mg/ml

10 ml	$7.00	Prednisolone Sodium Phosphate, Consolidated Midland	00223-8347-10
10 ml	$12.00	Predicort-Rp, Dunhall Pharms	00217-8410-08

Solution - Ophthalmic - 0.11 %

5 ml	$7.22	Prednisolone Sodium Phosphate, H.C.F.A. F F P	99999-2105-01

Solution - Ophthalmic - 0.125 %

5 ml	$5.00	AK-PRED OPHTHALMIC, Akorn	17478-0218-10
5 ml	$5.65	Prednisolone Sodium Phosphate, Steris Labs	00402-0856-05
5 ml	$6.55	Prednisol, Ocusoft	54799-0551-05
5 ml	$7.25	Prednisolone Sodium Phosphate, Schein Pharm (US)	00364-3017-53
5 ml	$12.66	INFLAMASE MILD 1/8%, Ciba Vision	00058-2875-05
10 ml	$18.30	INFLAMASE MILD 1/8%, Ciba Vision	00058-2875-10

Solution - Ophthalmic - 0.9 %

5 ml	$5.63	Prednisolone Sodium Phosphate, H.C.F.A. F F P	99999-2105-03
10 ml	$11.25	Prednisolone Sodium Phosphate, H.C.F.A. F F P	99999-2105-04
15 ml	$16.88	Prednisolone Sodium Phosphate, H.C.F.A. F F P	99999-2105-05

Solution - Ophthalmic - 1 %

5 ml	$5.48	Prednisolone Sodium Phosphate, HL Moore Drug Exch	00839-6685-85
5 ml	$5.67	Prednisolone Sodium Phosphate, Aligen Independ	00405-6127-05
5 ml	$5.69	AK-PRED, Akorn	17478-0219-10
5 ml	$6.15	Prednisolone Sodium Phosphate, Rugby	00536-2635-65
5 ml	$6.80	Prednisolone Sodium Phosphate, Qualitest Pharms	00603-7266-37
5 ml	$7.35	Isolone Forte, Major Pharms	00904-3002-05
5 ml	$7.72	Prednisolone Sodium Phosphate, Steris Labs	00402-0857-05
5 ml	$7.95	Prednisolone Sodium Phosphate, Goldline Labs	00182-7048-62
5 ml	$8.45	Prednisol Ophthalmic, Ocusoft	54799-0550-10
5 ml	$8.88	Prednisolone Sodium Phosphate, Schein Pharm (US)	00364-3018-53
5 ml	$12.60	INFLAMASE FORTE 1.0 % OPHTHALMIC, Ciba Vision	00058-2877-05
10 ml	$9.20	Prednisolone Sodium Phosphate, Steris Labs	00402-0857-10
10 ml	$10.61	Prednisolone Sodium Phosphate, Schein Pharm (US)	00364-3018-54
10 ml	$18.48	INFLAMASE FORTE 1.0 % OPHTHALMIC, Ciba Vision	00058-2877-10
15 ml	$6.60	Prednisolone Sodium Phosphate, Aligen Independ	00405-6127-15
15 ml	$7.58	Prednisolone Sodium Phosphate, Rugby	00536-2635-72
15 ml	$8.11	AK-PRED, Akorn	17478-0219-12
15 ml	$8.84	Prednisolone Sodium Phosphate, Qualitest Pharms	00603-7266-41
15 ml	$9.43	Prednisolone Sodium Phosphate, Steris Labs	00402-0857-15
15 ml	$10.96	Prednisolone Sodium Phosphate, Schein Pharm (US)	00364-3018-72

HOW SUPPLIED - RATED THERAPEUTICALLY EQUIVALENT: *(cont'd)*

15 ml	$11.30	PREDNISOL OPHTHALMIC, Ocusoft	54799-0550-12
15 ml	$25.56	INFLAMASE FORTE 1.0 % OPHTHALMIC, Ciba Vision	00058-2877-15

HOW SUPPLIED - NOT RATED EQUIVALENT:

Injection, Solution - Intravenous - 20 mg/ml

2 ml	**$16.25**	**HYDELTRASOL, Merck**	**00006-7577-02**
5 ml	**$35.64**	**HYDELTRASOL, Merck**	**00006-7577-03**

Liquid - Oral - 5 mg/5ml

120 ml	$15.49	PEDIAPRED, Fisons	00585-2250-01

Solution - Ophthalmic - 0.125 %

5 ml	$2.70	Predair, Major Pharms	00904-3005-05

PREDNISOLONE SODIUM PHOSPHATE; SULFACETAMIDE SODIUM *(002106)*

CATEGORIES: Anti-Inflammatory Agents; Antibiotics; Burns; Corneal Injury; EENT Drugs; Edema; Eye, Ear, Nose, & Throat Preparations; Inflammation; Inflammatory Conditions; Ocular Infections; Ophthalmics; Steroids; Uveitis; Pregnancy Category C; FDA Approved 1988 Aug

BRAND NAMES: Optimyd; **Vasocidin**

FORMULARIES: Aetna; PCS

DESCRIPTION:

Vasocidin is a sterile topical ophthalmic combining an anti-infective and an adrenocortical steroid having the following composition:

Sulfacetamide Sodium (bacteriostatic antibacterial) - 100 mg/ml

Prednisolone Sodium Phosphate - 2.5 mg/ml (equivalent to Prednisolone Phosphate 2.3 mg/ml) (adrenocortical steroid/anti-inflammatory)

In a solution containing edetate disodium, poloxamer 407, boric acid, purified water, preserved with thimerosal 0.1 mg/ml. Hydrochloric acid and/or sodium hydroxide added to adjust pH.

The chemical name for sulfacetamide is Acetamide, N-((4-aminophenyl) sulfonyl)-, monosodium, salt, monohydrate.

The chemical name for prednisolone sodium phosphate is 11β, 17, 21- trihydroxypregna-1,4-diene-diene-3,20-ione, 21-(disodium phosphate)

CLINICAL PHARMACOLOGY:

Corticosteroids suppress the inflammatory response to a variety of agents and they delay or slow healing. Since corticosteroids may inhibit the body's defense mechanism against infection, a concomitant drug may be used when this inhibition is considered to be clinically significant in a particular case.

When a decision to administer both a corticosteroid and antimicrobial is made, the administration of such drugs in combination has the advantage of greater patient compliance and convenience and convenience, with the added assurance that the appropriate dosage of both drugs is administered, plus assured compatibility of ingredients when both types of drugs are the same in the same formulation and, particularly, that the correct volume of the drug is delivered and retained.

The relative potency of corticosteroids depends on the molecular structure, concentration, and release from the vehicle.

MICROBIOLOGY

Sulfacetamide sodium exerts a bacteriostatic effect against susceptible bacteria by restricting the synthesis of folic acid required for growth through competition with p-aminobenzoic acid.

Some strains of bacteria may be resistant to sulfacetamide or resistant strains may emerge *in vitro.*

The anti-infective component in Vasocidin ophthalmic solution is included to provide against specific organisms susceptible to it. Sulfacetamide sodium is active *in-vitro* against susceptible strains of the following organisms:*Escherichia coli, Staphylococcus aureus, Streptococcus (viridans group), Haemophilus influenza, Klebsiella/Enterobacter* species. This product does not provide adequate coverage against *Pseudomonas* species , *Serratia marcescens.* See INDICATIONS AND USAGE.

INDICATIONS AND USAGE:

Vasocidin is indicated for the corticosteroid-responsive inflammatory ocular conditions for which a corticosteroid is indicated and where superficial bacterial ocular infection or a risk of bacterial ocular infection exists.

Ocular corticosteroids are indicated in inflammatory conditions of the palpebral and bulbar conjunctiva, cornea, and anterior segment of the globe where the inherent risk of corticosteroid use in certain infective conjunctivitises is accepted to obtain diminution in edema and inflammation. They are also indicated in chronic anterior uveitis and corneal injury from chemical, radiation, or thermal burns or penetration of foreign bodies.

The use of a combination drug with an anti-infective component is indicated where the risk of superficial ocular infection is high or where there is an expectation that potentially dangerous numbers of bacteria will be present in the eye.

The particular anti-infective drug in this product is active against the following common bacterial eye pathogens:*Escherichia coli, Staphylococcus aureus, Streptococcus pneumoniae, Streptococcus (viridans group), Haemophilus influenzae, Klebsiella* species and *Enterobacter* species.

This product does not provide adequate coverage against:*Neisseria* species, *Species marcescens.*

A significant percentage of staphylococcal isolates are completely resistent to sulfa drugs.

CONTRAINDICATIONS:

Vasocidin Ophthalmic Solution is contraindicated in most viral diseases of the cornea and conjunctiva including epithermal herpes simplex keratitis (dendritic keratitis), vaccina, and varicella, and also in mycobacterial infection of the eye and fungal diseases of ocular structures. Vasocidin is also contraindicated in individuals with known or suspected hypersensitivity to any of the ingredients of this preparation, to other sulfonamides, or to other corticosteroids. (Hypersensitivity to the antimicrobial components occurs at a higher rate then for other components).

WARNINGS:

NOT FOR INJECTION INTO THE EYE. Prolonged use of corticosteroids may result in ocular hypertension/glaucoma with damage to the optic nerve, defects in visual acuity and fields of vision, and in posterior subcapsular cataract formation.

Acute anterior uveitis may occur in susceptible individuals, primarily blacks.

Prolonged use of Vasocidin may suppress the host response and thus increase the secondary ocular infections. In those diseases causing thinning of the cornea or sclera, perforations have been known to occur with the use of topical corticosteroids. In acute purulent conditions of the eye, corticosteroids may mask infection or enhance existing infection.

If this product is used for 10 days or longer, intraocular pressure should be routinely monitored even though it may be difficult in children and uncooperative patients. Corticosteroids should be used with caution in the presence of glaucoma. Intraocular pressure should be checked frequently.

The use of ocular corticosteroids may prolong the course and may exacerbate the severity of many viral infections of the eye (including herpes simplex). Employment of corticosteroid medication in the treatment of herpes simplex requires great caution.

A significant percentage of staphylococcol isolates are completely resistant to sulfonamides.

Topical corticosteroids are not effective in mustard gas keratitis and Sjogren's keratoconjunctivitis.

Fatalities have occurred, although rarely, due to severe reactions to sulfonamides including Steven-Johnson syndrome, toxic epidermal necrolysis, fulminant hepatic necrosis, agranulocytosis, apastic anemia, and other blood dyscrasias. Sensitization may recur when a sulfonamide is readministered irrespective of the route of administration. If signs of hypersensitivity or other serious reactions occur, discontinue use of this preparation. Cross-sensitivity among corticosteroids have been demonstrated (see ADVERSE REACTIONS.)

Do not administer this product to patients who are sensitive/allergic to thimerosal or any other mercury-containing ingredient.

PRECAUTIONS:

GENERAL

The initial prescription and renewal of the medication order beyond 20 ml of Vasocidin Ophthalmic Solution should be made by a physician only after examination of the patient wit the aid of magnification, such as slit-lamp biomicroscopy and, where appropriate, fluorescin staining. If signs and symptoms fail to improve after two days, the patient should return to the office for further evaluation.

The possibility of fungal infections of the cornea should be considered after prolonged corticosteroid. Fungal cultures should be taken when appropriate.

The p-aminobenzoic acid present in purulent exudates competes with sulfonamides and can reduce their effectiveness.

Sulfonamide solutions darken on prolonged standing and exposure to heat and light. Do not use if solution has darkened. Yellowing does not effect activity.

INFORMATION TO THE PATIENT

If inflammation or pain persists longer than 48 hours or becomes aggravated, the patient should be advised to discontinue use of the medication and consult a physician.

This product is sterile when packaged. To prevent contamination, care should be taken to avoid touching dropper tip to eyelids or to any other surface. The use of this dispenser by more than one person may spread infection. Keep bottle tightly closed when not in use. Protect from light. Sulfonamide solutions darken on prolonged standing and exposure to heat and light. Do not use if solution has darkened. Yellowing does not effect activity. Keep out of reach of children.

LABORATORY TESTS

Eyelid cultures and tests to determine the susceptibility of organisms to sulfacetamide may be indicated if signs and symptoms persist to recur in spite of the recommended course of treatment with Vasocidin ophthalmic solution.

CARCINOGENESIS, MUTAGENESIS AND IMPAIRMENT OF FERTILITY

Prednisolone has been reported to be non-carcinogenic. Long-term animal studies for carcinogenic potential have not been performed with prednisolone or sulfacetamide.

One author detected chromosomal nondisjunction in the yeast*Saccharomyces cerevisiae* following application of sulfacetamide sodium. The significance of this finding to the topical ophthalmic use of sulfacetamide sodium in the human is unknown.

Mutagenic studies with prednisolone have been negative. Studies on reproduction and fertility have not been performed with sulfacetamide. A long-term chronic toxicity study in dogs showed that high oral doses of prednisolone prevented estrus. A decrease in fertility was seen in male and female rats that were mated following oral dosing with another glucocorticosteroid.

PREGNANCY, TERATOGENIC EFFECTS, PREGNANCY CATEGORY C

Prednisolone has been shown to be teratogenic when given in doses 1 to 10 times the human ocular dose. Dexamethasone, hydrocortisone and prednisolone were ocularly applied to both eyes of pregnant mice five times per day on days 10 through 13 of gestation. A significant increase in the incidence of cleft palate was observed in the fetuses of the treated mice. There are no adequate, well controlled studies whether sulfacetamide sodium can cause fetal harm when administered to a pregnant woman or whether it can affect reproductive capacity.

Vasocidin ophthalmic solution should only be used in pregnancy if the potential benefit justifies the potential risk to the fetus.

NURSING MOTHERS

It is not known whether topical administration of corticosteroids could result in sufficient systemic absorption to produce detectable quantities in human milk. Systemically administered corticosteroid appear in human milk and could suppress growth, interfere with endogenous corticosteroid production, or cause other untoward effects. Systemically administered sulfonamides are capable of producing kernicterus in infants or lactating women. Because of the potential for serious adverse reactions in nursing infants from Vasocidin, a decision should be made whether to discontinue nursing or to discontinue medication.

PEDIATRIC USE

Safety and effectiveness in children below the age if six years have not yet been established.

DRUG INTERACTIONS:

Vasocidin ophthalmic solution is incompatible with silver preparations. Local anesthetics related to p-aminobenzoic may antagonize the action of the sulfonamides.

ADVERSE REACTIONS:

Adverse reactions have occurred with corticosteroid/anti-infective combination drugs which can be attributed to the corticosteroid component, the anti-infective component, or the combination. Exact incidence figures are not available since no denominator of treated patients is available.

ADVERSE REACTIONS: *(cont'd)*

Reactions occurring most often from the presence of the anti-infective ingredient are allergic sensitizations. Fatalities have occurred, although rarely, due to severe reactions to sulfonamides including Stevens-Johnson syndrome, toxic epidermal necrolysis, fulminant hepatic necrosis, agranulocytosis, aplastic amenia, and other blood dyscrasias (see WARNINGS.)

Sulfacetamide sodium may cause local irritation.

The reactions due to corticosteroid component in decreasing order of frequency are: elevation of IOP with possible of glaucoma, and infrequent optic nerve damage; posterior subcapsular cataract formulation; a delayed wound healing.

Although systemic effects are extremely uncommon, there have been rare occurrences of systemic hypercorticoidism after use of topical corticosteroids.

Corticosteroid-containing preparations can also cause acute anterior uveitis or perforation of the globe. Mydriasis, loss of accommodation and ptosis have occasionally been reported following local use of corticosteroids.

SECONDARY INFECTION

The development of secondary infection has occurred after use of combinations containing corticosteroids and antimicrobials. Fungal and viral infections of the cornea are particularly prone to develop coincidentally with long-term applications of corticosteroid. The possibility of fungal invasion must be considered in any persistent corneal ulceration where corticosteroid treatment has been used.

Secondary bacterial ocular infection following suppression of host responses also occurs.

DOSAGE AND ADMINISTRATION:

Instill two drops of Vasocidin ophthalmic solution topically in the eye(s) every four hours.

No more than 20 ml should be prescribed initially. If signs and symptoms fail to improve after two days, patients should be re-evaluated (see PRECAUTIONS.)

Care should be taken not to discontinue therapy prematurely. In chronic conditions, withdrawal of treatment should be carried out by gradually decreasing the frequency of the application.

To be dispensed only in original, unopened container. Store at controlled room temperature 15 to 30°C (59 to 86°F). Keep from freezing. PROTECT FROM LIGHT.

Sulfonamide solutions darken on prolonged standing and exposure to heat and light. Do not use if solution has darkened. Yellowing does not affect activity.

HOW SUPPLIED - RATED THERAPEUTICALLY EQUIVALENT:

Solution - Ophthalmic - 0.23 %/10 %

5 ml	$8.25	Sulfacetamide W/Prednisolone, H.C.F.A. F F P	99999-2106-01
10 ml	$16.50	Sulfacetamide W/Prednisolone, H.C.F.A. F F P	99999-2106-02

Suspension - Ophthalmic - 0.25 %/10 %

5 ml	$11.25	Sulfacetamide W/Prednisolone, Steris Labs	00402-0952-05
5 ml	$11.25	Sulster, Akorn	17478-0116-10
5 ml	$11.81	Sulfacetamide W/Prednisolone, Schein Pharm (US)	00364-3038-53
5 ml	$12.15	Sulfacetamide W/Prednisolone, HL Moore Drug Exch	00839-7930-85
10 ml	$14.13	Sulster, Akorn	17478-0116-11
10 ml	$15.00	Sulfacetamide W/Prednisolone, Schein Pharm (US)	00364-3038-54
10 ml	$15.00	Sulfacetamide W/Prednisolone, Steris Labs	00402-0952-10
10 ml	$15.73	Sulfacetamide W/Prednisolone, HL Moore Drug Exch	00839-7930-90

HOW SUPPLIED - NOT RATED EQUIVALENT:

Solution - Ophthalmic - 2.5 mg/100 mg

5 ml	**$13.50**	**VASOCIDIN OPHTHALMIC, Ciba Vision**	**00058-2887-05**
10 ml	**$18.06**	**VASOCIDIN OPHTHALMIC, Ciba Vision**	**00058-2887-10**

Solution - Ophthalmic - 5.5 mg/100 mg

5 ml	$22.57	OPTIMYD OPHTHALMIC, Schering	00085-0010-05

Suspension - Ophthalmic - 0.25 %/10 %

5 ml	$11.00	Sulfalone, Cooper Vision Pharm	59426-0335-05
10 ml	$14.70	Sulfalone, Cooper Vision Pharm	59426-0335-10

PREDNISOLONE TEBUTATE *(002108)*

CATEGORIES: Adrenal Corticosteroids; Anti-Inflammatory Agents; Arthritis; Bursitis; Epicondylitis; Glucocorticoids; Gouty Arthritis; Hormones; Osteoarthritis; Steroids; Synovitis; Synovitis of Osteoarthritis; Tenosynovitis; Tumors; FDA Approval Pre 1982

BRAND NAMES: Cotolone La; **Hydeltra-T.B.A.**; Nor-Pred T.B.A.; Predalone T.B.A.; Predate-T.B.A.; Predcor-Tba

WARNING:
For intra-articular, intralesional, and soft tissue injection only.

DESCRIPTION:

NOT FOR INTRAVENOUS USE

PREDNISOLONE TEBUTATE, A SYNTHETIC ADRENOCORTICAL STEROID, IS A WHITE TO SLIGHTLY YELLOW POWDER SPARINGLY SOLUBLE IN ALCOHOL, FREELY SOLUBLE IN CHLOROFORM, AND VERY SLIGHTLY SOLUBLE IN WATER. THE MOLECULAR WEIGHT IS 476.61 (MONOHYDRATE). IT IS DESIGNATED CHEMICALLY AS 11 , 17-DIHYDROXY-21-((3,3-DIMETHYL-1-OXO-BUTYL)OXY) PREGNA-1,4-DIENE-3,20-DIONE. THE EMPIRICAL FORMULA IS $C_{27}H_{38}O_6$.

PREDNISOLONE TEBUTATE STERILE SUSPENSION IS A WHITE TO SLIGHTLY YELLOW SUSPENSION (PH 6.0 TO 8.0) THAT SETTLES UPON STANDING. EACH ML CONTAINS PREDNISOLONE TEBUTATE, 20 MG. INACTIVE INGREDIENTS PER ML: SODIUM CITRATE, 1 MG; POLYSORBATE 80, 1 MG; SORBITOL SOLUTION, 0.5 ML (EQUAL TO 450 MG D-SORBITOL); WATER FOR INJECTION, Q.S., 1 ML. BENZYL ALCOHOL, 9 MG, ADDED AS PRESERVATIVE.

CLINICAL PHARMACOLOGY:

Prednisolone Tebutate has a slow onset but long duration of action when compared with more soluble preparations. Because of its slight solubility, it is suitable for intra-articular, intralesional, and soft tissue injection where its anti-inflammatory effects are confined mainly to the area in which it has been injected, although it is capable of producing systemic hormonal effects.

Naturally occurring glucocorticoids (hydrocortisone and cortisone), which also have salt-retaining properties, are used as replacement therapy in adrenocortical deficiency states. Their synthetic analogs, including prednisolone, are primarily used for their potent anti-inflammatory effects in disorders of many organ systems.

CLINICAL PHARMACOLOGY: *(cont'd)*

Glucocorticoids cause profound and varied metabolic effects. In addition, they modify the body's immune responses to diverse stimuli.

INDICATIONS AND USAGE:

A. By intra-articular or soft tissue injection: As adjunctive therapy for short-term administration (to tide the patient over an acute episode or exacerbation) in: Synovitis of osteoarthritis, Rheumatoid arthritis, Acute and subacute bursitis, Acute gouty arthritis, Epicondylitis, Acute nonspecific tenosynovitis, Post-traumatic osteoarthritis

B. By intralesional injection: May be useful in cystic tumors of an aponeurosis or tendon (ganglia).

CONTRAINDICATIONS:

Systemic fungal infections.

Hypersensitivity to any component of this product.

WARNINGS:

Because rare instances of anaphylactoid reactions have occurred in patients receiving parenteral corticosteroid therapy, appropriate precautionary measures should be taken prior to administration, especially when the patient has a history of allergy to any drug. Anaphylactoid and hypersensitivity reactions have been reported for Sterile Suspension Prednisolone Tebutate (see ADVERSE REACTIONS.)

In patients on corticosteroid therapy subjected to any unusual stress, increased dosage of rapidly acting corticosteroids before, during, and after the stressful situation is indicated.

Drug-induced secondary adrenocortical insufficiency may result from too rapid withdrawal of corticosteroids and may be minimized by gradual reduction of dosage. This type of relative insufficiency may persist for months after discontinuation of therapy; therefore, in any situation of stress occurring during that period, hormone therapy should be reinstituted. If the patient is receiving steroids already, dosage may have to be increased. Since mineralocorticoid secretion may be impaired, salt and/or a mineralocorticoid should be administered concurrently.

Corticosteroids may mask some signs of infection, and new infections may appear during their use. There may be decreased resistance and inability to localize infection when corticosteroids are used. Moreover, corticosteroids may affect the nitroblue-tetrazolium test for bacterial infection and produce false negative results.

In cerebral malaria, a double-blind trial has shown that the use of corticosteroids is associated with prolongation of coma and a higher incidence of pneumonia and gastrointestinal bleeding.

Corticosteroids may activate latent amebiasis. Therefore, it is recommended that latent or active amebiasis be ruled out before initiating corticosteroid therapy in any patient who has spent time in the tropics or any patient with unexplained diarrhea.

Prolonged use of corticosteroids may produce posterior subcapsular cataracts, glaucoma with possible damage to the optic nerves, and may enhance the establishment of secondary ocular infections due to fungi or viruses.

Usage in Pregnancy: Since adequate human reproduction studies have not been done with corticosteroids, use of these drugs in pregnancy or in women of childbearing potential requires that the anticipated benefits be weighed against the possible hazards to the mother and embryo or fetus. Infants born of mothers who have received substantial doses of corticosteroids during pregnancy should be carefully observed for signs of hypoadrenalism.

Corticosteroids appear in breast milk and could suppress growth, interfere with endogenous corticosteroid production, or cause other unwanted effects. Mothers taking pharmacologic doses of corticosteroids should be advised not to nurse.

Average and large doses of cortisone or hydrocortisone can cause elevation of blood pressure, salt and water retention, and increased excretion of potassium. These effects are less likely to occur with the synthetic derivatives except when used in large doses. Dietary salt restriction and potassium supplementation may be necessary. All corticosteroids increase calcium excretion.

Administration of live virus vaccines, including smallpox, is contraindicated in individuals receiving immunosuppressive doses of corticosteroids. If inactivated viral or bacterial vaccines are administered to individuals receiving immunosuppressive doses of corticosteroids, the expected serum antibody response may not be obtained.

If corticosteroids are indicated in patients with latent tuberculosis or tuberculin reactivity, close observation is necessary as reactivation of the disease may occur. During prolonged corticosteroid therapy, these patients should receive chemoprophylaxis.

Literature reports suggest an apparent association between use of corticosteroids and left ventricular free wall rupture after a recent myocardial infarction; therefore, therapy with corticosteroids should be used with great caution in these patients.

PRECAUTIONS:

This product, like many other steroid formulations, is sensitive to heat. Therefore, it should not be autoclaved when it is desirable to sterilize the exterior of the vial.

Following prolonged therapy, withdrawal of corticosteroids may result in symptoms of the corticosteroid withdrawal syndrome including fever, myalgia, arthralgia, and malaise. This may occur in patients even without evidence of adrenal insufficiency.

There is an enhanced effect of corticosteroids in patients with hypothyroidism and in those with cirrhosis.

Corticosteroids should be used cautiously in patients with ocular herpes simplex for fear of corneal perforation.

Psychic derangements may appear when corticosteroids are used, ranging from euphoria, insomnia, mood swings, personality changes, and severe depression to frank psychotic manifestations. Also, existing emotional instability or psychotic tendencies may be aggravated by corticosteroids.

Aspirin should be used cautiously in conjunction with corticosteroids in hypoprothrombinemia.

Steroids should be used with caution in nonspecific ulcerative colitis, if there is a probability of impending perforation, abscess, or other pyogenic infection, also in diverticulitis, fresh intestinal anastomoses, active or latent peptic ulcer, renal insufficiency, hypertension, osteoporosis, and myasthenia gravis. Signs of peritoneal irritation following gastrointestinal perforation in patients receiving large doses of corticosteroids may be minimal or absent. Fat embolism has been reported as a possible complication of hypercortisonism.

When large doses are given, some authorities advise that antacids be administered between meals to help to prevent peptic ulcer.

Growth and development of infants and children on prolonged corticosteroid therapy should be carefully followed.

Steroids may increase or decrease motility and number of spermatozoa in some patients.

PRECAUTIONS: *(cont'd)*

Phenytoin, phenobarbital, ephedrine, and rifampin may enhance the metabolic clearance of corticosteroids, resulting in decreased blood levels and lessened physiologic activity, thus requiring adjustment in corticosteroid dosage.

The prothrombin time should be checked frequently in patients who are receiving corticosteroids and coumarin anticoagulants at the same time because of reports that corticosteroids have altered the response to these anticoagulants. Studies have shown that the usual effect produced by adding corticosteroids is inhibition of response to coumarins, although there have been some conflicting reports of potentiation not substantiated by studies.

When corticosteroids are administered concomitantly with potassium-depleting diuretics, patients should be observed closely for development of hypokalemia.

Intra-articular injection of a corticosteroid may produce systemic as well as local effects.

Appropriate examination of any joint fluid present is necessary to exclude a septic process.

A marked increase in pain accompanied by local swelling, further restriction of joint motion, fever, and malaise is suggestive of septic arthritis. If this complication occurs and the diagnosis of sepsis is confirmed, appropriate antimicrobial therapy should be instituted.

Injection of a steroid into an infected site is to be avoided.

Corticosteroids should not be injected into unstable joints.

Patients should be impressed strongly with the importance of not overusing joints in which symptomatic benefit has been obtained as long as the inflammatory process remains active.

Frequent intra-articular injection may result in damage to joint tissues.

ADVERSE REACTIONS:

Fluid And Electrolyte Disturbances: Sodium retention, Congestive heart failure in susceptible patients, Fluid retention, Hypokalemic alkalosis, Hypertension

Musculoskeletal: Muscle weakness, Steroid myopathy, Loss of muscle mass, Osteoporosis, Vertebral compression fractures, Aseptic necrosis of femoral and humeral heads, Pathologic fracture of long bones, Tendon rupture

Gastrointestinal: Peptic ulcer with possible subsequent perforation and hemorrhage, Perforation of the small and large bowel, particularly in patients with inflammatory bowel disease, Pancreatitis, Abdominal distention, Ulcerative esophagitis

Dermatologic: Impaired wound healing, Thin fragile skin, Petechiae and ecchymoses, Erythema, Increased sweating, May suppress reactions to skin tests, Other cutaneous reactions such as allergic dermatitis, urticaria, angioneurotic edema

Neurologic: Convulsions, Increased intracranial pressure with papilledema (pseudotumor cerebri) usually after treatment, Vertigo, Headache, Psychic disturbances

Endocrine: Menstrual irregularities, Development of cushingoid state, Suppression of growth in children, Secondary adrenocortical and pituitary unresponsiveness, particularly in times of stress, as in trauma, surgery, or illness, Decreased carbohydrate tolerance, Manifestations of latent diabetes mellitus, Increased requirements for insulin or oral hypoglycemic agents in diabetics, Hirsutism

Ophthalmic: Posterior subcapsular cataracts, Increased intraocular pressure, Glaucoma, Exophthalmos

Metabolic: Negative nitrogen balance due to protein catabolism

Cardiovascular: Myocardial rupture following recent myocardial infarction (see WARNINGS.)

Other: Anaphylactoid or hypersensitivity reactions, Thromboembolism, Weight gain, Increased appetite, Nausea, Malaise

Foreign body granulomatous reactions involving the synovium have been reported with repeated injections of Prednisolone Tebutate.

Localized pain and swelling, sometimes distal to the site of injection and persisting for several days, have been reported.

The following *additional* adverse reactions are related to injection of corticosteroids:

Rare instances of blindness associated with intralesional therapy around the face and head, Hyperpigmentation or hypopigmentation, Subcutaneous and cutaneous atrophy, Sterile abscess, Postinjection flare (following intra-articular use), Charcot-like arthropathy

DOSAGE AND ADMINISTRATION:

For intra-articular, intralesional, and soft tissue injection only.

NOT FOR INTRAVENOUS USE

DOSAGE AND FREQUENCY OF INJECTION ARE VARIABLE AND MUST BE INDIVIDUALIZED ON THE BASIS OF THE DISEASE AND THE RESPONSE OF THE PATIENT.

The initial dose varies from 4 to 40 mg depending on the disease being treated and the size of the area to be injected. Frequency of injection depends on symptomatic response, and usually is once every two or three weeks. Severe conditions may require injection once a week. Frequent intra-articular injection may result in damage to joint tissues. If satisfactory clinical response does not occur after a reasonable period of time, discontinue Prednisolone Tebutate sterile suspension and transfer the patient to other therapy.

Patients should be observed closely for signs that might require dosage adjustment, including changes in clinical status resulting from remissions or exacerbations of the disease, and individual drug responsiveness.

For rapid onset of action, a soluble adrenocortical hormone preparation, such as Dexamethasone Sodium Phosphate injection or Prednisolone Sodium Phosphate injection, may be given with Prednisolone Tebutate.

If desired, a local anesthetic may be used, and may be injected before Prednisolone Tebutate, or mixed in a syringe with Prednisolone Tebutate and given simultaneously.

If used prior to intra-articular injection of the steroid, inject most of the anesthetic into the soft tissues of the surrounding area and instill a small amount into the joint.

If given together, mixing should be done in the injection syringe by drawing the steroid in *first,* then the anesthetic. In this way, the anesthetic will not be introduced inadvertently into the vial of steroid. The *mixture must be used immediately and any unused portion discarded.*

Some of the usual single doses are (TABLE 1):

TABLE 1

Large Joints (*e.g.,* Knee)	20 mg (1 ml), occasionally 30 mg (1.5 ml). Doses over 40 mg (2 ml) not recommended.
Small Joints (*e.g.,* Interphalangeal, Temporomandibular)	8 to 10 mg (0.4 to 0.5 ml).
Bursae	20 to 30 mg (1 to 1.5 ml).
Tendon Sheaths	4 to 10 mg (0.2 to 0.5 ml).
Ganglia	10 to 20 mg (0.5 to 1 ml).

DOSAGE AND ADMINISTRATION: *(cont'd)*

Storage: Sensitive to heat. Do not autoclave. Protect from freezing. Protect from light. Store container in carton until contents have been used.

HOW SUPPLIED - EQUIVALENTS NOT AVAILABLE:

Injection, Susp - Intra-Articular - 20 mg/ml

5 ml	$16.99	Prednisolone Tebutate, Insource	58441-1125-05
10 ml	$8.00	Prednisolone Tebutate, Consolidated Midland	00223-8339-10
10 ml	$9.90	Prednisolone Tebutate, Hyrex Pharms	00314-0441-10

PREDNISONE *(002109)*

CATEGORIES: Adrenal Corticosteroids; Adrenal Hyperplasia; Adrenal Insufficiency; Adrenocortical Insufficiency; Airway Obstruction; Allergies; Anemia; Ankylosing Spondylitis; Antiarthritics; Antineoplastics; Arthritis; Aspiration Pneumonitis; Asthma; Atopic Dermatitis; Bursitis; Cancer; Carditis; Chemotherapy; Chorioretinitis; Choroiditis; Colitis; Conjunctivitis; Corneal Ulcer; Dermatitis; Dermatitis Herpetiformis; Dermatomyositis; Diuresis; Drug Hypersensitivity; Enteritis; Epicondylitis; Erythema Multiforme; Erythroblastopenia; Gouty Arthritis; Herpes; Herpes Zoster; Hormones; Hypercalcemia; Inflammation; Iridocyclitis; Keratitis; Leukemia; Lupus Erythematosus; Lymphoma; Meningitis; Multiple Sclerosis; Mycosis Fungoides; Nephrotic Syndrome; Oncologic Drugs; Osteoarthritis; Pain; Pemphigus; Pharmaceutical Adjuvants; Philip; Pneumoconiosis; Pneumonitis; Proteinuria; Psoriasis; Purpura; Retinochoroiditis; Rhinitis; Sarcoidosis; Serum Sickness; Spondylitis; Synovitis; Synovitis of Osteoarthritis; Tenosynovitis; Thrombocytopenia; Thrombocytopenic Purpura; Thyroiditis; Trichinosis; Tuberculosis; Ulcerative Colitis; Uveitis; Pneumocystis Carinii Pneumonia*; FDA Approval Pre 1982; Top 200 Drugs

* Indication not approved by the FDA

BRAND NAMES: *Apo-Prednisone* (Canada); *Adasone*; *Cartancyl*; *Colisone*; Cordrol; Cortan; *Cortancyl* (France); *Dacortin*; *Dacorten*; *Decortin* (Germany); *Decortisyl* (England); *Delcortin*; *Dellacort*; *Dellacort A*; Delta-Dome; *Deltacortene*; *Deltacortone* (Japan); **Deltasone**; *Deltison*; *Deltisona*; *Di-Adreson* (Japan); *DiAdreson*; *Econosone*; *Encorton*; Fernisone; *Hostacortin*; Liquid Pred; *Me-Korti*; Meticorten; *Nisona*; *Novoprednisone* (Canada); Orasone; *Origen Prednisone*; *Panafcort*; Panasol; *Paracort*; *Parmenison*; *Pehacort*; *Predeltin*; Prednicen-M; *Prednicorm* (Germany); *Prednicort*; Prednicot; *Prednidib* (Mexico); *Predniment*; *Prednitone*; *Rectodelt*; *Sone*; Sterapred; *Ultracorten* (Germany); *Winpred* (Canada)

(International brand names outside U.S. in italics)

FORMULARIES: Aetna; BC-BS; CIGNA; DoD; FHP; Humana; Kaiser; Medco; Medi-Cal; PCS; PruCare; United

COST OF THERAPY: $9.59 (Asthma; Tablet; 5 mg; 1/day; 365 days) vs. Potential Cost of $3,576.99 (Bronchitis & Asthma)

PRIMARY ICD9: 493.90 (Asthma, Unspecified, Without Mention of Status Asthmaticus)

DESCRIPTION:

Prednisone tablets contain prednisone which is a glucocorticoid. Glucocorticoids are adrenocortical steroids, both naturally occurring and synthetic, which are readily absorbed from the gastrointestinal tract. Prednisone is a white to practically white, odorless, crystalline powder. It is very slightly soluble in water; slightly soluble in alcohol, in chloroform, in dioxane, and in methanol.

The chemical name for prednisone is pregna-1,4-diene-3,11,20-trione, 17,21-dihydroxy- and its molecular weight is 358.43.

Deltasone are available in 5 strengths: 2.5 mg, 5 mg, 10 mg, 20 mg and 50 mg. *Inactive Ingredients: 2.5 mg:* Calcium Stearate, Corn Starch, Erythrosine Sodium, Lactose, Mineral Oil, Sorbic Acid and Sucrose. *5 mg:* Calcium Stearate, Corn Starch, Lactose, Mineral Oil, Sorbic Acid and Sucrose. *10 mg:* Calcium Stearate, Corn Starch, Lactose, Sorbic Acid and Sucrose. *20 mg:* Calcium Stearate, Corn Starch, FD&C Yellow No. 6, Lactose, Sorbic Acid and Sucrose. *50 mg:* Corn Starch, Lactose, Magnesium Stearate, Sorbic Acid, Sucrose, and Talc.

CLINICAL PHARMACOLOGY:

Naturally occurring glucocorticoids (hydrocortisone and cortisone), which also have salt-retaining properties, are used as replacement therapy in adrenocortical deficiency states. Their synthetic analogs are primarily used for their potent anti-inflammatory effects in disorders of many organ systems.

Glucocorticoids cause profound and varied metabolic effects. In addition, they modify the body's immune responses to diverse stimuli.

INDICATIONS AND USAGE:

Prednisone tablets are indicated in the following conditions:

Endocrine Disorders: Primary or secondary adrenocortical insufficiency (hydrocortisone or cortisone is the first choice; synthetic analogs may be used in conjunction with mineralocorticoids where applicable; in infancy mineralocorticoid supplementation is of particular importance);

Congenital adrenal hyperplasia; Hypercalcemia associated with cancer;

Nonsuppurative thyroiditis

Rheumatic Disorders: As adjunctive therapy for short- term administration (to tide the patient over an acute episode or exacerbation) in: Psoriatic arthritis; Rheumatoid arthritis, including juvenile rheumatoid arthritis (selected cases may require low-dose maintenance therapy); Ankylosing spondylitis; Acute and subacute bursitis; Acute nonspecific tenosynovitis; Acute gouty arthritis; Post- traumatic osteoarthritis; Synovitis of osteoarthritis; Epicondylitis

Collagen Diseases: During an exacerbation or as maintenance therapy in selected cases of: Systemic lupus erythematosus; Systemic dermatomyositis (polymyositis); Acute rheumatic carditis

Dermatologic Diseases: Pemphigus; Bullous dermatitis herpetiformis; Severe erythema multiforme (Stevens-Johnson syndrome); Exfoliative dermatitis; Mycosis fungoides; Severe psoriasis; Severe seborrheic dermatitis

Allergic States: Control of severe or incapacitating allergic conditions intractable to adequate trials of conventional treatment: Seasonal or perennial allergic rhinitis; Bronchial asthma; Contact dermatitis; Atopic dermatitis; Serum sickness; Drug hypersensitivity reactions

INDICATIONS AND USAGE: *(cont'd)*

Ophthalmic Diseases: Severe acute and chronic allergic and inflammatory processes involving the eye and its adnexa such as: Allergic corneal marginal ulcers; Herpes zoster ophthalmicus; Anterior segment inflammation; Diffuse posterior uveitis and choroiditis; Sympathetic ophthalmia; Allergic conjunctivitis; Keratitis; Chorioretinitis; Optic neuritis; Iritis and iridocyclitis

Respiratory Diseases: Symptomatic sarcoidosis; Loeffler's syndrome not manageable by other means; Berylliosis; Fulminating or disseminated pulmonary tuberculosis when used concurrently with appropriate antituberculous chemotherapy; Aspiration pneumonitis

Hematologic Disorders: Idiopathic thrombocytopenic purpura in adults; Secondary thrombocytopenia in adults; Acquired (autoimmune) hemolytic anemia; Erythroblastopenia (RBC anemia); Congenital (erythroid) hypoplastic anemia

Neoplastic Diseases: For palliative management of: Leukemias and lymphomas in adults; Acute leukemia of childhood

Edematous States: To induce a diuresis or remission of proteinuria in the nephrotic syndrome, without uremia, of the idiopathic type or that due to lupus erythematosus

Gastrointestinal Diseases: To tide the patient over a critical period of the disease in: Ulcerative colitis; Regional enteritis

Nervous System: Acute exacerbations of multiple sclerosis

Miscellaneous: Tuberculous meningitis with subarachnoid block or impending block when used concurrently with appropriate antituberculous chemotherapy; Trichinosis with neurologic or myocardial involvement

CONTRAINDICATIONS:

Systemic fungal infections and known hypersensitivity to components.

WARNINGS:

In patients on corticosteroid therapy subjected to unusual stress, increased dosage of rapidly acting corticosteroids before, during, and after the stressful situation is indicated.

Corticosteroids may mask some signs of infection, and new infections may appear during their use. Infections with any pathogen including viral, bacterial, fungal, protozoan or helminthic infections, in any location of the body, may be associated with the use of corticosteroids alone or in combination with other immunosuppressive agents that affect cellular immunity, humoral immunity, or neutrophil function.[1]

These infections may be mild, but can be severe and at times fatal. With increasing doses of corticosteroids, the rate of occurrence of infectious complications increases.[2] There may be decreased resistance and inability to localize infection when corticosteroids are used.

Prolonged use of corticosteroids may produce posterior subcapsular cataracts, glaucoma with possible damage to the optic nerves, and may enhance the establishment of secondary ocular infections due to fungi or viruses.

Usage in pregnancy: Since adequate human reproduction studies have not been done with corticosteroids, the use of these drugs in pregnancy, nursing mothers or women of childbearing potential requires that the possible benefits of the drug be weighed against the potential hazards to the mother and embryo or fetus. Infants born of mothers who have received substantial doses of corticosteroids during pregnancy, should be carefully observed for signs of hypoadrenalism.

Average and large doses of hydrocortisone or cortisone can cause elevation of blood pressure, salt and water retention, and increased excretion of potassium. These effects are less likely to occur with the synthetic derivatives except when used in large doses. Dietary salt restriction and potassium supplementation may be necessary. All corticosteroids increase calcium excretion.

Administration of live or live, attenuated vaccines is contraindicated in patients receiving immunosuppressive doses of corticosteroids. Killed or inactivated vaccines may be administered to patients receiving immunosuppressive doses of corticosteroids; however, the response to such vaccines may be diminished. Indicated immunization procedures may be undertaken in patients receiving nonimmunosuppressive doses of corticosteroids.

The use of prednisone tablets in active tuberculosis should be restricted to those cases of fulminating or disseminated tuberculosis in which the corticosteroid is used for the management of the disease in conjunction with an appropriate anti-tuberculous regimen.

If corticosteroids are indicated in patients with latent tuberculosis or tuberculin reactivity, close observation is necessary as reactivation of the disease may occur. During prolonged corticosteroid therapy, these patients should receive chemoprophylaxis.

Persons who are on drugs which suppress the immune system are more susceptible to infections than healthy individuals. Chicken pox and measles, for example, can have a more serious or even fatal course in non-immune children or adults on corticosteroids. In such children or adults who have not had these diseases, particular care should be taken to avoid exposure. How the dose, route and duration of corticosteroid administration affects the risk of developing a disseminated infection is not known. The contribution of the underlying disease and/or prior corticosteroid treatment to the risk is also not known. If exposed to chicken pox, prophylaxis with varicella zoster immune globulin (VZIG) may be indicated. If exposed to measles, prophylaxis with pooled intramuscular immunoglobulin (IG) may be indicated. (See the respective package inserts for complete VZIG and IG prescribing information.) If chicken pox develops, treatment with antiviral agents may be considered.

PRECAUTIONS:

INFORMATION FOR THE PATIENT

Persons who are on immunosuppressant doses of corticosteroids should be warned to avoid exposure to chicken pox or measles. Patients should also be advised that if they are exposed, medical advice should be sought without delay.

GENERAL PRECAUTIONS

Drug-induced secondary adrenocortical insufficiency may be minimized by gradual reduction of dosage. This type of relative insufficiency may persist for months after discontinuation of therapy; therefore, in any situation of stress occurring during that period, hormone therapy should be reinstituted. Since mineralocorticoid secretion may be impaired, salt and/or a mineralocorticoid should be administered concurrently.

There is an enhanced effect of corticosteroids on patients with hypothyroidism and in those with cirrhosis.

Corticosteroids should be used cautiously in patients with ocular herpes simplex because of possible corneal perforation.

The lowest possible dose of corticosteroid should be used to control the condition under treatment, and when reduction in dosage is possible, the reduction should be gradual.

Psychic derangements may appear when corticosteroids are used, ranging from euphoria, insomnia, mood swings, personality changes, and severe depression, to frank psychotic manifestations. Also, existing emotional instability or psychotic tendencies may be aggravated by corticosteroids.

PRECAUTIONS: *(cont'd)*

Steroids should be used with caution in nonspecific ulcerative colitis, if there is a probability of impending perforation, abscess or other pyogenic infection; diverticulitis; fresh intestinal anastomoses; active or latent peptic ulcer; renal insufficiency; hypertension; osteoporosis; and myasthenia gravis.

Growth and development of infants and children on prolonged corticosteroid therapy should be carefully observed.

Kaposi's sarcoma has been reported to occur in patients receiving corticosteroid therapy. Discontinuation of corticosteroids may result in clinical remission.

Although controlled clinical trials have shown corticosteroids to be effective in speeding the resolution of acute exacerbations of multiple sclerosis, they do not show that corticosteroids affect the ultimate outcome or natural history of the disease. The studies do show that relatively high doses of corticosteroids are necessary to demonstrate a significant effect. (See DOSAGE AND ADMINISTRATION.)

Since complications of treatment with glucocorticoids are dependent on the size of the dose and the duration of treatment, a risk/benefit decision must be made in each individual case as to dose and duration of treatment and as to whether daily or intermittent therapy should be used.

Convulsions have been reported with concurrent use of methylprednisolone and cyclosporin. Since concurrent use of these agents results in a mutual inhibition of metabolism, it is possible that adverse events associated with the individual use of either drug may be more apt to occur.

DRUG INTERACTIONS:

The pharmacokinetic interactions listed below are potentially clinically important. Drugs that induce hepatic enzymes such as phenobarbital, phenytoin and rifampin may increase the clearance of corticosteroids and may require increases in corticosteroid dose to achieve the desired response. Drugs such as troleandomycin and ketoconazole may inhibit the metabolism of corticosteroids and thus decrease their clearance. Therefore, the dose of corticosteroid should be titrated to avoid steroid toxicity. Corticosteroids may increase the clearance of chronic high dose aspirin. This could lead to decreased salicylate serum levels or increase the risk of salicylate toxicity when corticosteroid is withdrawn. Aspirin should be used cautiously in conjunction with corticosteroids in patients suffering from hypoprothrombinemia. The effect of corticosteroids on oral anticoagulants is variable. There are reports of enhanced as well as diminished effects of anticoagulants when given concurrently with corticosteroids. Therefore, coagulation indices should be monitored to maintain the desired anticoagulant effect.

ADVERSE REACTIONS:

Fluid and Electrolyte Disturbances: Sodium retention; Fluid retention; Congestive heart failure in susceptible patients; Potassium loss; Hypokalemic alkalosis; Hypertension

Musculoskeletal: Muscle weakness; Steroid myopathy; Loss of muscle mass; Osteoporosis; Tendon rupture, particularly of the Achilles tendon; Vertebral compression fractures; Aseptic necrosis of femoral and humeral heads; Pathologic fracture of long bones

Gastrointestinal: Peptic ulcer with possible perforation and hemorrhage; Pancreatitis; Abdominal distention; Ulcerative esophagitis

Increases in alanine transaminase (ALT, SGPT), aspartate transaminase (AST, SGOT) and alkaline phosphatase have been observed following corticosteroid treatment. These changes are usually small, not associated with any clinical syndrome and are reversible upon discontinuation.

Dermatologic: Impaired wound healing; Thin fragile skin; Petechiae and ecchymoses; Facial erythema; Increased sweating; May suppress reactions to skin tests

Metabolic: Negative nitrogen balance due to protein catabolism

Neurological: Increased intracranial pressure with papilledema (pseudo-tumor cerebri) usually after treatment; Convulsions; Vertigo; Headache

Endocrine: Menstrual irregularities; Development of Cushingoid state; Secondary adrenocortical and pituitary unresponsiveness, particularly in times of stress, as in trauma, surgery or illness; Suppression of growth in children; Decreased carbohydrate tolerance; Manifestations of latent diabetes mellitus; Increased requirements for insulin or oral hypoglycemic agents in diabetics

Ophthalmic: Posterior subcapsular cataracts; Increased intraocular pressure; Glaucoma; Exophthalmos

Metabloic: Negative nitrogen balance due to protein catabolism.

Additional Reactions: Urticaria and other allergic, anaphylactic or hypersensitivity reactions

DOSAGE AND ADMINISTRATION:

The initial dosage of prednisone tablets may vary from 5 mg to 60 mg of prednisone per day depending on the specific disease entity being treated. In situations of less severity lower doses will generally suffice while in selected patients higher initial doses may be required. The initial dosage should be maintained or adjusted until a satisfactory response is noted. If after a reasonable period of time there is a lack of satisfactory clinical response, Prednisone should be discontinued and the patient transferred to other appropriate therapy. **IT SHOULD BE EMPHASIZED THAT DOSAGE REQUIREMENTS ARE VARIABLE AND MUST BE INDIVIDUALIZED ON THE BASIS OF THE DISEASE UNDER TREATMENT AND THE RESPONSE OF THE PATIENT.**After a favorable response is noted, the proper maintenance dosage should be determined by decreasing the initial drug dosage in small decrements at appropriate time intervals until the lowest dosage which will maintain an adequate clinical response is reached. It should be kept in mind that constant monitoring is needed in regard to drug dosage. Included in the situations which may make dosage adjustments necessary are changes in clinical status secondary to remissions or exacerbations in the disease process, the patients's individual drug responsiveness, and the effect of patient exposure to stressful situations not directly related to the disease entity under treatment; in this latter situation it may be necessary to increase the dosage of Prednisone for a period of time consistent with the patient's condition. If after long-term therapy the drug is to be stopped, it is recommended that it be withdrawn gradually rather than abruptly.

MULTIPLE SCLEROSIS

In the treatment of acute exacerbations of multiple sclerosis daily doses of 200 mg of prednisolone for a week followed by 80 mg every other day for 1 month have been shown to be effective. (Dosage range is the same for prednisone and prednisolone.)

ADT (ALTERNATE DAY THERAPY)

ADT is a corticosteroid dosing regimen in which twice the usual daily dose of corticoid is administered every other morning. The purpose of this mode of therapy is to provide the patient requiring long-term pharmacologic dose treatment with the beneficial effects of corticoids while minimizing certain undesirable effects, including pituitary-adrenal suppression, the Cushingoid state, corticoid withdrawal symptoms, and growth suppression in children.

DOSAGE AND ADMINISTRATION: *(cont'd)*

The rationale for this treatment schedule is based on two major premises: (a) the anti-inflammatory or therapeutic effect of corticoids persists longer than their physical presence and metabolic effects and (b) administration of the corticosteroid every other morning allows for re-establishment of more nearly normal hypothalamic-pituitary-adrenal (HPA) activity on the off-steroid day.

A brief review of the HPA physiology may be helpful in understanding this rationale. Acting primarily through the hypothalamus a fall in free cortisol stimulates the pituitary gland to produce increasing amounts of corticotropin (ACTH) while a rise in free cortisol inhibits ACTH secretion. Normally the HPA system is characterized by diurnal (circadian) rhythm. Serum levels of ACTH rise from a low point about 10 pm to a peak level about 6 am. Increasing levels of ACTH stimulate adrenocortical activity resulting in a rise in plasma cortisol with maximal levels occurring between 2 am and 8 am. This rise in cortisol dampens ACTH production and in turn adrenocortical activity. There is a gradual fall in plasma corticoids during the day with lowest levels occurring about midnight.

The diurnal rhythm of the HPA axis is lost in Cushing's disease, a syndrome of adrenocortical hyperfunction characterized by obesity with centripetal fat distribution, thinning of the skin with easy bruisability, muscle wasting with weakness, hypertension, latent diabetes, osteoporosis, electrolyte imbalance, etc. The same clinical findings of hyperadrenocorticism may be noted during long-term pharmacologic dose corticoid therapy administered in conventional daily divided doses. It would appear, then, that a disturbance in the diurnal cycle with maintenance of elevated corticoid values during the night may play a significant role in the development of undesirable corticoid effects. Escape from these constantly elevated plasma levels for even short periods of time may be instrumental in protecting against undesirable pharmacologic effects.

During conventional pharmacologic dose corticosteroid therapy, ACTH production is inhibited with subsequent suppression of cortisol production by the adrenal cortex. Recovery time for normal HPA activity is variable depending upon the dose and duration of treatment. During this time the patient is vulnerable to any stressful situation. Although it has been shown that there is considerably less adrenal suppression following a single morning dose of prednisolone (10 mg) as opposed to a quarter of that dose administered every 6 hours, there is evidence that some suppressive effect on adrenal activity may be carried over into the following day when pharmacologic doses are used. Further, it has been shown that a single dose of certain corticosteroids will produce adrenocortical suppression for two or more days. Other corticoids, including methylprednisolone, hydrocortisone, prednisone, and prednisolone, are considered to be short acting (producing adrenocortical suppression for 1 1/4 to 1 1/2 days following a single dose) and thus are recommended for alternate day therapy.

The following should be kept in mind when considering alternate day therapy:

1) Basic principles and indications for corticosteroid therapy should apply. The benefits of ADT should not encourage the indiscriminate use of steroids.

2) ADT is a therapeutic technique primarily designed for patients in whom long-term pharmacologic corticoid therapy is anticipated.

3) In less severe disease processes in which corticoid therapy is indicated, it may be possible to initiate treatment with ADT. More severe disease states usually will require daily divided high dose therapy for initial control of the disease process. The initial suppressive dose level should be continued until satisfactory clinical response is obtained, usually four to ten days in the case of many allergic and collagen diseases. It is important to keep the period of initial suppressive dose as brief as possible particularly when subsequent use of alternate day therapy is intended. Once control has been established, two courses are available: (a) change to ADT and then gradually reduce the amount of corticoid given every other day **or** (b) following control of the disease process reduce the daily dose of corticoid to the lowest effective level as rapidly as possible and then change over to an alternate day schedule. Theoretically, course (a) may be preferable.

4) Because of the advantages of ADT, it may be desirable to try patients on this form of therapy who have been on daily corticoids for long periods of time (*e.g.,* patients with rheumatoid arthritis). Since these patients may already have a suppressed HPA axis, establishing them on ADT may be difficult and not always successful. However, it is recommended that regular attempts be made to change them over. It may be helpful to triple or even quadruple the daily maintenance dose and administer this every other day rather than just doubling the daily dose if difficulty is encountered. Once the patient is again controlled, an attempt should be made to reduce this dose to a minimum.

5) As indicated above, certain corticosteroids, because of their prolonged suppressive effect on adrenal activity, are not recommended for alternate day therapy (*e.g.,* dexamethasone and betamethasone).

6) The maximal activity of the adrenal cortex is between 2 am and 8 am, and it is minimal between 4 pm and midnight. Exogenous corticosteroids suppress adrenocortical activity the least, when given at the time of maximal activity (am).

7) In using ADT it is important, as in all therapeutic situations to individualize and tailor the therapy to each patient. Complete control of symptoms will not be possible in all patients. An explanation of the benefits of ADT will help the patient to understand and tolerate the possible flare-up in symptoms which may occur in the latter part of the off-steroid day. Other symptomatic therapy may be added or increased at this time if needed.

8) In the event of an acute flare-up of the disease process, it may be necessary to return to a full suppressive daily divided corticoid dose for control. Once control is again established alternate day therapy may be re-instituted.

9) Although many of the undesirable features of corticosteroid therapy can be minimized by ADT, as in any therapeutic situation, the physician must carefully weigh the benefit-risk ratio for each patient in whom corticoid therapy is being considered.

Store at controlled room temperature 15° to 30° C (59° to 86° F).

REFERENCES:

1. Fekety R. Infections associated with corticosteroids and immunosuppressive therapy. In: Gorbach SL, Bartlett JG, Blacklow NR, eds. *Infectious Diseases.* Philadelphia: WB Saunders Company 1992:1050-1. **2.** Stuck AE, Minder CE, Frey FJ. Risk of infectious complications in patients taking glucocorticoids. *Rev Infect Dis*1989:11 (6):954-63.(The Upjohn Company, 12/94, 810 342 016, 691015)

PATIENT INFORMATION:

Prednisone is a glucocorticoid steroid used to treat inflammatory conditions of the body, breathing difficulties, some cancers, allergies, psoriasis and other conditions. This drug does suppress the immune system and those taking this medicine should avoid exposure to chicken pox or measles. If you are exposed, contact your physician immediately. This drug can also mask signs of infection and with long term use cause cataracts. This drug should be monitored closely by a physician if taken for a long period of time. The dose must also be decreased slowly over time (*i.e.,* tapered) to avoid the body going into withdrawal. The most common side effects include water retention, muscle weakness, stomach irritation, and visual disturbances. Stomach irritation can be alleviated by taking this medication with food. It is important to take this medication as prescribed and to be assessed by your physician on a regular basis. The dose of medication will be specific to you and your condition.

HOW SUPPLIED - RATED THERAPEUTICALLY EQUIVALENT:

Solution - Oral - 5 mg/5ml

480 ml	$11.90	Prednisone, Geneva Pharms	00781-6705-16

Tablet, Uncoated - Oral - 1 mg

100's	$3.25	Prednisone, Roxane	00054-4741-25
100's	$3.39	Prednisone, H.C.F.A. F F P	99999-2109-01
100's	$3.72	ORASONE, Solvay Pharms	00032-2808-01
100's	$6.47	Prednisone, Roxane	00054-8739-25
100's	$16.00	METICORTEN, Schering	00085-0843-03
1000's	$23.81	Prednisone, Roxane	00054-4741-31
1000's	$33.90	Prednisone, H.C.F.A. F F P	99999-2109-02
1000's	$34.01	ORASONE, Solvay Pharms	00032-2808-10

Tablet, Uncoated - Oral - 2.5 mg

100's	**$2.98**	**DELTASONE, Pharmacia & Upjohn**	**00009-0032-01**
100's	$5.02	Prednisone, Roxane	00054-4742-25
100's	$8.19	Prednisone, Roxane	00054-8740-25

Tablet, Uncoated - Oral - 5 mg

21's	$.55	Prednisone, H.C.F.A. F F P	99999-2109-03
21's	$3.25	Prednisone, Horizon Pharms	60904-0286-20
21's	**$3.33**	**DELTASONE, Pharmacia & Upjohn**	**00009-0045-04**
21's	$3.90	Prednisone 5, Major Pharms	00904-2157-19
21's	$3.95	Prednisone, Qualitest Pharms	00603-5332-15
21's	$6.25	STERAPRED, Mayrand Pharms	00259-0390-21
21's	$6.95	PREDNICEN M, Schwarz Pharma (US)	00131-2228-81
30's	$.78	Prednisone, H.C.F.A. F F P	99999-2109-04
30's	$1.95	Prednisone 5 Mg Tablets, Major Pharms	00904-2157-46
48's	$13.40	STERAPRED, Mayrand Pharms	00259-0391-48
60's	$1.57	Prednisone, H.C.F.A. F F P	99999-2109-05
60's	$2.55	Prednisone 5 Mg Tablets, Major Pharms	00904-2157-52
100's	$2.63	Prednisone, H.C.F.A. F F P	99999-2109-06
100's	$3.03	ORASONE, Solvay Pharms	00032-2810-01
100's	$3.25	CORTAN, Halsey Drug	00879-0129-01
100's	**$3.33**	**DELTASONE, Pharmacia & Upjohn**	**00009-0045-01**
100's	$3.40	Prednisone, Qualitest Pharms	00603-5332-21
100's	$3.50	Prednisone, West Ward Pharm	00143-1475-01
100's	$3.50	Prednisone, Consolidated Midland	00223-1515-01
100's	$3.50	Prednisone 5, Major Pharms	00904-2157-60
100's	$4.10	Prednisone, United Res	00677-0117-01
100's	$4.10	Prednisone, Mutual Pharm	53489-0138-01
100's	$4.20	Prednisone, Aligen Independ	00405-4828-01
100's	$4.43	Prednisone, IDE-Interstate	00814-6285-14
100's	$4.51	Prednisone, Roxane	00054-4728-25
100's	$4.59	Prednisone, HL Moore Drug Exch	00839-5143-06
100's	$4.89	Prednisone, Schein Pharm (US)	00364-0218-01
100's	$5.08	Prednisone, Geneva Pharms	00781-1495-01
100's	$5.65	Prednisone, Goldline Labs	00182-0201-89
100's	$7.10	Prednisone, Medirex	57480-0351-01
100's	$7.71	Prednisone, Roxane	00054-8724-25
100's UD	$7.50	Prednisone, Schein Pharm (US)	00364-0218-90
500's	**$8.37**	**DELTASONE, Pharmacia & Upjohn**	**00009-0045-02**
500's	$13.15	Prednisone, H.C.F.A. F F P	99999-2109-07
600's	$45.60	Prednisone, Medirex	57480-0351-06
1000's	**$15.88**	**DELTASONE, Pharmacia & Upjohn**	**00009-0045-16**
1000's	$18.00	PREDNICOT, C O Truxton	00463-6155-10
1000's	$18.50	CORTAN, Halsey Drug	00879-0129-10
1000's	$19.25	Prednisone, West Ward Pharm	00143-1475-10
1000's	$20.00	Prednisone, Goldline Labs	00182-0201-10
1000's	$20.00	Prednisone, Major Pharms	00904-2157-80
1000's	$22.46	Prednisone, Purepac Pharm	00228-2336-96
1000's	$22.50	Prednisone, Consolidated Midland	00223-1515-02
1000's	$22.58	Prednisone, Parmed Pharms	00349-8933-10
1000's	$23.08	Prednisone, Qualitest Pharms	00603-5332-32
1000's	$23.25	Prednisone, IDE-Interstate	00814-6285-30
1000's	$24.00	Prednisone, United Res	00677-0117-10
1000's	$24.00	Prednisone, Mutual Pharm	53489-0138-10
1000's	$26.30	Prednisone, H.C.F.A. F F P	99999-2109-08
1000's	$26.45	ORASONE, Solvay Pharms	00032-2810-10
1000's	$27.81	Prednisone, Roxane	00054-4728-31
1000's	$29.50	Prednisone, Schein Pharm (US)	00364-0218-02
1000's	$29.50	Prednisone, Aligen Independ	00405-4828-03
1000's	$29.97	Prednisone, HL Moore Drug Exch	00839-5143-16
1000's	$29.98	Prednisone, Rugby	00536-4324-10
1000's	$29.98	Prednisone, Geneva Pharms	00781-1495-10
1000's	$39.95	Prednisone, Harber Pharm	51432-0360-06
5000's	$131.50	Prednisone, H.C.F.A. F F P	99999-2109-09
5000's	$142.40	Prednisone, Rugby	00536-4324-50

Tablet, Uncoated - Oral - 10 mg

21's	$1.02	Prednisone, H.C.F.A. F F P	99999-2109-10
21's	$10.95	STERAPRED DS, UNIPAK, Mayrand Pharms	00259-0364-21
48's	$2.34	Prednisone, H.C.F.A. F F P	99999-2109-11
48's	$15.65	STERAPRED DS, Mayrand Pharms	00259-0389-48
100's	**$4.19**	**DELTASONE, Pharmacia & Upjohn**	**00009-0193-01**
100's	$4.88	Prednisone, United Res	00677-0698-01
100's	$4.88	Prednisone, H.C.F.A. F F P	99999-2109-12
100's	$4.95	ORASONE, Solvay Pharms	00032-2812-01
100's	$5.25	Prednisone, Major Pharms	00904-2141-60
100's	$5.30	Prednisone, Qualitest Pharms	00603-5333-21
100's	$5.30	Prednisone, Harber Pharm	51432-0356-03
100's	$5.35	Prednisone, Parmed Pharms	00349-8934-01
100's	$5.37	Prednisone, Purepac Pharm	00228-2338-10
100's	$5.75	Prednisone, West Ward Pharm	00143-1473-01
100's	$5.75	Prednisone, Mutual Pharm	53489-0139-01
100's	$6.51	Prednisone, Roxane	00054-4730-25
100's	$6.62	Prednisone, HL Moore Drug Exch	00839-1520-06
100's	$6.98	Prednisone, IDE-Interstate	00814-6288-14
100's	$7.05	Prednisone, Goldline Labs	00182-1334-01
100's	$7.05	Prednisone, Schein Pharm (US)	00364-0461-01
100's	$7.05	Prednisone, Rugby	00536-4325-01
100's	$7.05	Prednisone, Geneva Pharms	00781-1500-01
100's	$7.10	Prednisone, Goldline Labs	00182-1334-89
100's	$7.76	Prednisone, Aligen Independ	00405-4829-01
100's	$9.48	Prednisone, Roxane	00054-8725-25
100's	$10.00	Prednisone, Medirex	57480-0352-01
100's	$11.10	Prednisone, Geneva Pharms	00781-1500-13
100's UD	$11.50	Prednisone, Schein Pharm (US)	00364-0461-90
500's	**$14.60**	**DELTASONE, Pharmacia & Upjohn**	**00009-0193-02**
500's	$22.20	Prednisone, Aligen Independ	00405-4829-02
500's	$22.75	Prednisone, Mutual Pharm	53489-0139-05
500's	$24.40	Prednisone, United Res	00677-0698-05
500's	$24.40	Prednisone, H.C.F.A. F F P	99999-2109-13
500's	$26.75	Prednisone, Parmed Pharms	00349-8934-05
500's	$26.85	Prednisone, Purepac Pharm	00228-2338-50

HOW SUPPLIED - RATED THERAPEUTICALLY EQUIVALENT: (cont'd)

500's	$26.93	Prednisone, IDE-Interstate	00814-6288-28
500's	$27.65	Prednisone, Schein Pharm (US)	00364-0461-05
500's	$28.89	Prednisone, HL Moore Drug Exch	00839-1520-12
500's	$30.07	Prednisone, Roxane	00054-4730-29
600's	$75.80	Prednisone, Medirex	57480-0352-06
1000's	$37.75	Prednisone, Major Pharms	00904-2141-80
1000's	$38.00	Prednisone, West Ward Pharm	00143-1473-10
1000's	$43.02	Prednisone, Qualitest Pharms	00603-5333-32
1000's	$43.50	Prednisone, Mutual Pharm	53489-0139-10
1000's	$46.35	ORASONE, Solvay Pharms	00032-2812-10
1000's	$47.38	Prednisone, Aligen Independ	00405-4829-03
1000's	$48.80	Prednisone, United Res	00677-0698-10
1000's	$48.80	Prednisone, H.C.F.A. F F P	99999-2109-14
1000's	$48.85	Prednisone, Geneva Pharms	00781-1500-10
1000's	$49.40	Prednisone, Goldline Labs	00182-1334-10
1000's	$50.00	Prednisone, Schein Pharm (US)	00364-0461-02
1000's	$51.57	Prednisone, Rugby	00536-4325-10
1000's	$51.57	Prednisone, HL Moore Drug Exch	00839-1520-16
1000's	$53.00	Prednisone, Harber Pharm	51432-0356-06

Tablet, Uncoated - Oral - 20 mg

100's	**$7.31**	**DELTASONE, Pharmacia & Upjohn**	**00009-0165-01**
100's	$7.43	Prednisone, H.C.F.A. F F P	99999-2109-15
100's	$8.25	Prednisone, West Ward Pharm	00143-1477-01
100's	$8.25	Prednisone, Major Pharms	00904-2140-60
100's	$8.56	ORASONE, Solvay Pharms	00032-2814-01
100's	$8.95	Prednisone, Parmed Pharms	00349-8935-01
100's	$9.23	Prednisone, Purepac Pharm	00228-2337-10
100's	$9.48	Prednisone, Qualitest Pharms	00603-5334-21
100's	$9.50	Prednisone, Harber Pharm	51432-0358-03
100's	$10.50	Prednisone, United Res	00677-0427-01
100's	$10.50	Prednisone, Mutual Pharm	53489-0140-01
100's	$10.60	Prednisone, Goldline Labs	00182-1086-01
100's	$10.88	Prednisone, Aligen Independ	00405-4830-01
100's	$11.10	Prednisone, IDE-Interstate	00814-6290-14
100's	$11.75	Prednisone, Geneva Pharms	00781-1485-01
100's	$11.80	Prednisone, Goldline Labs	00182-1086-89
100's	$12.58	Prednisone, Roxane	00054-4729-25
100's	$12.59	Prednisone, Schein Pharm (US)	00364-0442-01
100's	$12.89	Prednisone, Rugby	00536-4326-01
100's	$12.89	Prednisone, HL Moore Drug Exch	00839-1517-06
100's	$14.09	Prednisone, Roxane	00054-8726-25
100's	$17.00	Prednisone, Schein Pharm (US)	00364-0442-90
500's	**$27.37**	**DELTASONE, Pharmacia & Upjohn**	**00009-0165-02**
500's	$34.00	Prednisone, West Ward Pharm	00143-1477-05
500's	$37.15	Prednisone, H.C.F.A. F F P	99999-2109-16
500's	$39.50	Prednisone, Mutual Pharm	53489-0140-05
500's	$40.86	Prednisone, Aligen Independ	00405-4830-02
500's	$44.10	Prednisone, United Res	00677-0427-05
500's	$44.93	Prednisone, IDE-Interstate	00814-6290-28
500's	$45.21	Prednisone, Schein Pharm (US)	00364-0442-05
500's	$46.15	Prednisone, Purepac Pharm	00228-2337-50
500's	$61.76	Prednisone, Roxane	00054-4729-29
500's	$63.45	Prednisone, HL Moore Drug Exch	00839-1517-12
500's	$77.12	Prednisone, Rugby	00536-4326-05
1000's	$61.75	Prednisone, West Ward Pharm	00143-1477-10
1000's	$72.12	Prednisone, Qualitest Pharms	00603-5334-32
1000's	$74.30	Prednisone, H.C.F.A. F F P	99999-2109-17
1000's	$74.55	Prednisone, Major Pharms	00904-2140-80
1000's	$74.81	Prednisone, Schein Pharm (US)	00364-0442-02
1000's	$75.00	Prednisone, United Res	00677-0427-10
1000's	$75.00	Prednisone, Mutual Pharm	53489-0140-10
1000's	$75.60	ORASONE, Solvay Pharms	00032-2814-10
1000's	$81.15	Prednisone, Goldline Labs	00182-1086-10
1000's	$95.00	Prednisone, Harber Pharm	51432-0358-06

Tablet, Uncoated - Oral - 25 mg

100's	$15.49	Prednisone, Roxane	00054-8747-25

Tablet, Uncoated - Oral - 50 mg

100's	**$16.66**	**DELTASONE, Pharmacia & Upjohn**	**00009-0388-01**
100's	$16.95	Prednisone, Harber Pharm	51432-0359-03
100's	$17.63	Prednisone, Caremark	00339-5296-12
100's	$18.45	ORASONE 50, Solvay Pharms	00032-2816-01
100's	$19.98	Prednisone, H.C.F.A. F F P	99999-2109-18
100's	$26.95	Prednisone, Rugby	00536-4328-01
100's	$26.95	Prednisone, Major Pharms	00904-0527-60
100's	$27.69	Prednisone, Roxane	00054-4733-25
100's	$31.32	Prednisone, Roxane	00054-8729-25

HOW SUPPLIED - NOT RATED EQUIVALENT:

Solution - Oral - 5 mg/ml

30 ml	$14.02	Prednisone Intensol, Roxane	00054-3721-44

Solution - Oral - 5 mg/5ml

5 ml x 40	$20.87	Prednisone, Roxane	00054-8722-16
500 ml	$17.22	Prednisone, Roxane	00054-3722-63

Syrup - Oral - 5 mg/5ml

120 ml	$13.30	LIQUID PRED, Muro Pharm	00451-1201-04
240 ml	$26.02	LIQUID PRED, Muro Pharm	00451-1201-08

Tablet, Uncoated - Oral - 1 mg

100's	$3.16	Prednisone, Caremark	00339-5775-12

Tablet, Uncoated - Oral - 5 mg

100's	$2.90	Prednisone, Squibb-Mark	57783-6870-01
100's	$3.03	Prednisone, Caremark	00339-5293-12
100's	$7.08	Prednisone, Vangard Labs	00615-0536-13
500's	$7.10	Prednisone, Squibb-Mark	57783-6870-02
1000's	$13.75	Prednisone, H & H Labs	46703-0007-10
1000's	$29.95	PREDNISONE-5, Quality Res Pharms	52765-1252-00

Tablet, Uncoated - Oral - 10 mg

100's	$4.95	Prednisone, Caremark	00339-5295-12

Tablet, Uncoated - Oral - 20 mg

100's	$7.90	Prednisone, Squibb-Mark	57783-6950-01
100's	$8.56	Prednisone, Caremark	00339-5777-12
100's	$9.50	Prednisone, Consolidated Midland	00223-1516-01
100's	$9.95	CORTAN, Halsey Drug	00879-0438-01
100's	$10.95	PREDNISONE, Raway	00686-1542-13
500's	$38.25	Prednisone, Squibb-Mark	57783-6950-02
500's	$43.25	CORTAN, Halsey Drug	00879-0438-05
1000's	$79.95	CORTAN, Halsey Drug	00879-0438-10

PRENATAL FORMULA *(002111)*

CATEGORIES: Anemia; Blood Formation/Coagulation; Calcium Preparations; Deficiency Anemias; Hematinics; Homeostatic & Nutrient; Multivitamins; Multivitamins W/Minerals; Prenatal Vitamins; Prenatal Vitamins w/ Folic Acid; Vitamins; FDA Pre 1938 Drugs

BRAND NAMES: Carnate B; Filibon F.A.; Furonatal Fa; Lactocal-F; Lanatal Rx; Marnatal; **Materna**; Matinex; Mynatal; Natabec Rx; Natafort; Natalins Rx; Natarex; Natavite; Nestabs Fa; Niferex Pn; Norlac Rx; Omninatal; Pan Ob Forte; Par-F; Par-Natal; Pramilet-Fa; Precare; Prelan F.A.; Previte 90; Secran Prenatal; Stuart-natal 1 Plus 1; Uni-Natal Plus 1; Vernate; Vitamed; Vynatal-Fa; Zenate; Zetavite

FORMULARIES: Aetna; BC-BS; FHP

DESCRIPTION:

Table 1

Each tablet contains:	For Pregnant or Lactating Women	Percentage of U.S. Recommended Daily Allowance (U.S. RDA)
Vitamin A (as Acetate)	5,000 I.U.	(62.5%)
Vitamin D	400 I.U.	(100%)
Vitamin E (as Dl-Alpha Tocopheryl Acetate)	30 I.U.	(100%)
Vitamin C (Ascorbic Acid)	100 mg	(167%)
Folic Acid	1 mg	(125%)
Vitamin B1 (as Thiamine Mononitrate)	3 mg	(224%)
Vitamin B2 (as Riboflavin)	3.4 mg	(170%)
Vitamin B6 (as Pyridoxine Hydrochloride)	10 mg	(400%)
Niacinamide	20 mg	(100%)
Vitamin B12 (Cyanocobalamin)	12 mcg	(150%)
Biotin	30 mcg	(10%)
Pantothenic Acid (as Calcium Pantothenate)	10 mg	(100%)
Calcium (as Calcium Carbonate)	250 mg	(19%)
Iodine (as Potassium Iodide)	150 mcg	(100%)
Iron (as Ferrous Fumarate)	60 mg	(333%)
Magnesium (as Magnesium Oxide)	25 mg	(6%)
Copper (as Cupric Oxide)	2 mg	(100%)
Zinc (as Zinc Oxide)	25 mg	(167%)
Chromium (as Chromium Chloride)	25 mcg*	
Molybdenum (as Sodium Molybdate)	25 mcg*	
Manganese (as Manganese Sulfate)	5 mg*	

* Recognized as essential in human nutrition, but no U.S. RDA established.

Inactive Ingredients: Gelatin, Hydrolyzed Protein Hydroxypropyl Methylcellulose, Lactose, Magnesium Stearate, Methylparaben, Modified Food Starch, Mono- and Di-glycerides, Polacrilin, Potassium Sorbate, Povidone, Propylparaben, Silica Gel, Sodium Benzoate, Sodium Lauryl Sulfate, Sodium Starch Glycolate, Sorbic Acid, Stearic Acid, Sucrose, Titanium Dioxide.

Contains no Color or Dyes from Artificial Sources.

CAUTION: Federal law prohibits dispensing without prescription.

WARNINGS:

Keep out of the reach of children.

Notice: Contact with moisture may produce surface discoloration or erosion of the tablet.

PRECAUTIONS:

Folic Acid may obscure pernicious anemia in that the peripheral blood picture may revert to normal while neurological manifestations remain progressive.

Allergic sensitization has been reported following both oral and parenteral administration of Folic Acid.

DOSAGE AND ADMINISTRATION:

Recommended Intake: 1 daily with or without food or as prescribed by physician.

HOW SUPPLIED - EQUIVALENTS NOT AVAILABLE:

Capsule, Gelatin - Oral

100's	$22.42	NATABEC RX, Parke-Davis	00071-0547-24
500's	$45.65	Mynatal, ME Pharm	58607-0103-50

Tablet, Uncoated - Oral

30's	$5.30	PRENATE 90, Bock Pharma	00563-1726-30
100's	$5.50	Prenatin-F, Consolidated Midland	00223-1412-01
100's	$5.55	Prenatal, Raway	00686-0111-10
100's	$6.00	SECRAN PRENATAL, Scherer	00274-3290-01
100's	$6.00	Prenatal 1+ Improved, Jerome Stevens	50564-0485-01
100's	$6.06	Prenatal W/Folic Acid & Iron, Rugby	00536-4335-01
100's	$6.15	Prenatal 2, IDE-Interstate	00814-6302-14
100's	$6.33	Prenatal + Iron 1, HL Moore Drug Exch	00839-7400-06
100's	$7.20	Prenatal Rx, Qualitest Pharms	00603-5359-21
100's	$7.20	PRENATAL RX, Copley Pharm	38245-0169-10
100's	$7.25	Prenatal Rx, Harber Pharm	51432-0361-03
100's	$7.28	PAR-NATAL PLUS ONE IMPROVED, Parmed Pharms	00349-8427-01
100's	$7.45	UNI-NATAL IMPROVED, United Res	00677-1299-01
100's	$7.48	Prenatal 1+Iron, Qualitest Pharms	00603-5357-21
100's	$7.50	Prenatal W/Zinc Improved, Geneva Pharms	00781-1459-01
100's	$7.80	PRENATAL-1 VITAMINS & MINERALS, Major Pharms	00904-0515-60
100's	$7.87	Prenatal 1+1 W/Iron, Aligen Independ	00405-4838-01
100's	$7.87	Prenatal Rx, Aligen Independ	00405-4839-01
100's	$7.90	Prenatal Rx, HL Moore Drug Exch	00839-6576-06
100's	$8.05	NATAREX PRENTAL, Major Pharms	00904-0512-60
100's	$8.30	PRENATAL FA, Copley Pharm	38245-0170-10
100's	$8.45	Prenatal 1+1, Goldline Labs	00182-4457-01
100's	$8.95	PRENTAL ONE TABLETS, Eon Labs Mfg	00185-0259-01
100's	$8.95	Prenatal 1, Parmed Pharms	00349-8586-01
100's	$9.21	Prenatal Plus, Aligen Independ	00405-4837-01
100's	$9.50	Prenatal 1+1, ESI Lederle	59911-5804-01
100's	$9.52	Prenatal Fa, HL Moore Drug Exch	00839-6577-06
100's	$9.60	Prenatal 1/1, Schein Pharm (US)	00364-2253-01
100's	$9.69	MISSION PRENATAL RX, Mission Pharma	00178-0007-01
100's	$9.70	Prenatal Rx, Goldline Labs	00182-4456-01
100's	$9.78	PRENATAL-RX, Balan	00304-0809-01
100's	$10.15	Prenatal 1+Beta Carotene, Major Pharms	00904-5057-60
100's	$10.46	Prenatal Plus W/Betacarotene, HL Moore Drug Exch	00839-7922-06

HOW SUPPLIED - EQUIVALENTS NOT AVAILABLE: *(cont'd)*

100's	$10.50	Gladesnatal Plus, Glades Pharms	59366-2455-01
100's	$10.74	Mynatal Fc, ME Pharm	58607-0102-59
100's	$10.74	Mynatal Rx, ME Pharm	58607-0103-10
100's	$10.74	MYNATAL, ME Pharm	58607-0103-59
100's	$10.74	Mynatal Pn, ME Pharm	58607-0104-58
100's	$10.74	Mynatal Pn Forte, ME Pharm	58607-0104-59
100's	$10.91	Prenatal 1 Vitamin, Vangard Labs	00615-3540-13
100's	$11.42	Prenatal Plus Improved, Rugby	00536-4339-01
100's	$12.20	Prenatal Rx, Rugby	00536-4371-01
100's	$13.25	Vitamed Tablets, Med Tek Pharms	52349-0290-10
100's	$13.74	Prenatal Z, HL Moore Drug Exch	00839-7663-06
100's	$14.00	Prenatal Z, Aligen Independ	00405-4832-01
100's	$14.00	Prenatal Z, Copley Pharm	38245-0192-10
100's	$14.00	Prenatal Z, Harber Pharm	51432-0750-03
100's	$14.25	Prenatal Rx, Ethex	58177-0216-04
100's	$14.55	Vernate Advanced, Rugby	00536-5736-01
100's	$15.00	Prenatal Rx, Schein Pharm (US)	00364-0845-01
100's	$15.34	PRENATAL PLUS, Qualitest Pharms	00603-5358-21
100's	$16.08	Equi-Natal Rx, Equipharm	57779-0109-04
100's	$16.20	MARNATAL F, Marnel Pharceut	00682-1560-01
100's	$16.38	Equi-Natal Plus, Equipharm	57779-0108-04
100's	$16.50	Equi-Natal M, Equipharm	57779-0142-04
100's	$16.50	Equi-Natal Care, Equipharm	57779-0143-04
100's	$16.53	Hi-Nate 90, Highland Pkging	55782-0090-01
100's	$16.60	Prenatal Z, Ethex	58177-0218-04
100's	$16.95	Prenatal 1Mg And Iron, Goldline Labs	00182-4463-01
100's	$16.95	Prenatal Plus, Pecos	59879-0103-01
100's	$17.75	Prenatal 1/1, Copley Pharm	38245-0111-10
100's	**$17.94**	**Maternal 90, HL Moore Drug Exch**	**00839-7843-06**
100's	$18.00	Prenatal, Geneva Pharms	00781-1474-01
100's	$18.00	Equi-Natal Z, Equipharm	57779-0107-04
100's	$18.06	Z+PRENATAL, Qualitest Pharms	00603-6475-21
100's	$18.50	Prenatal, Goldline Labs	00182-4462-01
100's	$18.55	Z+Prenatal, Qualitest Pharms	00603-6476-21
100's	$18.60	PAR-F, Pharmics	00813-0076-01
100's	**$18.70**	**Maternal Vitamin & Mineral, Major Pharms**	**00904-7755-60**
100's	$18.85	Maternity, Qualitest Pharms	00603-4304-21
100's	$18.95	Prenatal-Z, Pecos	59879-0104-01
100's	$19.65	Prenatal Plus, Rugby	00536-5683-01
100's	$19.73	Prenatal Plus, United Res	00677-1533-01
100's	$20.24	Prenatal Z, HL Moore Drug Exch	00839-7975-06
100's	$20.30	ZITAMIN, Econolab	55053-0950-01
100's	$20.95	PRETERNA, Econolab	55053-0890-01
100's	$21.10	Femnatal, Rugby	00536-5594-01
100's	$21.20	Prenatal-M, Rugby	00536-5593-01
100's	$21.45	NATALINS RX, Bristol Myers Squibb	00087-0702-01
100's	$21.57	PRENATAL-Z, Aligen Independ	00405-4840-01
100's	**$22.00**	**Maternal Vitamins with Minerals, HL Moore Drug Exch**	**00839-7911-06**
100's	**$22.00**	**Maternal Vit/Mineral Formula, Pecos**	**59879-0101-01**
100's	$22.34	PRENATAL Z, Ethex	58177-0224-04
100's	**$22.90**	**Maternal Vit/Mineral Formula, Goldline Labs**	**00182-4386-01**
100's	$23.24	STUARTNATAL PLUS, Wyeth Labs	00008-0811-01
100's	$24.83	ZENATE, Solvay Pharms	00032-1148-01
100's	$25.16	PRAMILET FA, Abbott	00074-0121-01
100's	**$25.50**	**MATERNA, Lederle Pharm**	**00005-5560-23**
100's	$26.08	NATAFORT, Parke-Davis	00071-0282-24
100's	$26.31	PRENATE 90, Bock Pharma	00563-1726-01
100's	$78.50	NATAL PLUS ONE, Harber Pharm	51432-0362-03
120's	$9.48	Ob-20 Rx, Bio-Tech Pharm	53191-0017-12
240's	$13.20	SECRAN PRENATAL, Scherer	00274-3290-24
240's	$17.64	Ob-20 Rx, Bio-Tech Pharm	53191-0017-24
500's	$23.44	Prenatal W/Folic Acid & Iron, Rugby	00536-4335-05
500's	$25.35	Prenatal 2, IDE-Interstate	00814-6302-28
500's	$28.50	Prenatal 1+ Improved, Jerome Stevens	50564-0485-05
500's	$29.95	Prenatal 1+1, Major Pharms	00904-0511-40
500's	$33.75	Prenatal W/Zinc Improved, Geneva Pharms	00781-1459-05
500's	$35.00	PRENATAL RX, Copley Pharm	38245-0169-50
500's	$35.85	Prenatal 1+1, Major Pharms	00904-0515-40
500's	$38.00	Prenatal 1/1, Schein Pharm (US)	00364-2253-05
500's	$40.45	NATAREX PRENTAL, Major Pharms	00904-0512-40
500's	$47.50	Prenatal 1+Beta Carotene, Major Pharms	00904-5057-40
500's	$48.93	PRENATAL PLUS IMPROVED, Rugby	00536-4339-05
500's	$68.00	Equi-Natal Rx, Equipharm	57779-0109-06
500's	$70.00	Equi-Natal Plus, Equipharm	57779-0108-06
500's	$79.85	Prenatal 1/1, Copley Pharm	38245-0111-50
500's	$82.95	Prenatal, Geneva Pharms	00781-1474-05
500's	$92.50	Prenatal, Goldline Labs	00182-4462-05
500's	$93.33	Prenatal Plus, Rugby	00536-5683-05
1000's	$47.50	Prenatin-F, Consolidated Midland	00223-1412-02
1000's	$87.50	PRENTAL ONE TABLETS, Eon Labs Mfg	00185-0259-10
1000's	$191.03	NATALINS RX, Bristol Myers Squibb	00087-0702-02
1200's	$71.24	Mission Prenatal Srx, Mission Pharma	00178-0163-01

PRILOCAINE HYDROCHLORIDE *(002112)*

CATEGORIES: Anesthesia; Dental; Local Anesthetics; Pregnancy Category B; FDA Approval Pre 1982

BRAND NAMES: **Citanest**

DESCRIPTION:

For Local Anesthesia in Dentistry

Prilocaine solutions are sterile nonpyrogenic isotonic solutions that contain a local anesthetic agent with and without epinephrine (as bitartrate) and are administered parenterally by injection. See INDICATIONS AND USAGE for specific uses. The quantitative composition of each available solution is shown in Table 1.

Prilocaine HCl is chemically designated as propanamide, N-2-(2-methyl-phenyl)-2-(propylamino)-, monohydrochloride.

Epinephrine is (-) -3,4-Dihydroxy-α-[(methylamino)methyl]benzyl alcohol. Parenteral drug products should be inspected visually for particulate matter and discoloration prior to administration. The specific quantitative composition of each available solution is shown in TABLE 1.

CLINICAL PHARMACOLOGY:

Mechanism of Action: Prilocaine stabilizes the neuronal membrane by inhibiting the ionic fluxes required for the initiation and conduction of impulses, thereby effecting local anesthetic action.

CLINICAL PHARMACOLOGY: *(cont'd)*

TABLE 1 Composition Of Available Injections

Product I.D.:	Prilocaine HCl	Epinephrine (as the bitartrate)	Citric Acid	Sodium Metabisulfite	pH
	Formula (mg/ml)				
Prilocaine HCl Injection	40.0	None	None	None	6.0-7.0
Prilocaine HCl Injection with Epinephrine	40.0	0.005	0.2	0.5	3.3-5.5

Note: Sodium hydroxide and/or hydrochloric acid may be used to adjust the pH of prilocaine Solutions. Filled under nitrogen.

Onset and Duration of Action: When used for infiltration injection in dental patients, the time of onset of anesthesia with prilocaine HCl injection and prilocaine HCl with epinephrine injection averages less than 2 minutes with an average duration of soft tissue anesthesia of approximately 2 hours with prilocaine HCl injection and approximately 2 1/4 hours with prilocaine HCl with epinephrine injection.

Based on electrical stimulation studies, prilocaine HCl injection provides a duration of pulpal anesthesia of approximately 10 minutes in maxillary infiltration injections. In clinical studies, this has been found to provide complete anesthesia for procedures lasting an average of 20 minutes.

When used for inferior alveolar nerve block, the time of onset of prilocaine HCl injection and prilocaine HCl with epinephrine injection averages less than three minutes with an average duration of soft tissue anesthesia of approximately 2 1/2 hours with prilocaine HCl injection and approximately 3 hours with prilocaine HCl with epinephrine injection.

Hemodynamics: Excessive blood levels may cause changes in cardiac output, total peripheral resistance, and mean arterial pressure. These changes may be attributable to a direct depressant effect of the local anesthetic agent on various components of the cardiovascular system and/or the beta-adrenergic receptor stimulating action of epinephrine when present.

Pharmacokinetics and Metabolism: Information derived from diverse formulations, concentrations and usages reveals that prilocaine is completely absorbed following parenteral administration, its rate of absorption depending, for example, upon such factors as the site of administration and the presence or absence of a vasoconstrictor agent. Prilocaine is metabolized in both the liver and the kidney and excreted via the kidney. It is not metabolized by plasma esterases. Hydrolysis of prilocaine by amidases yields ortho-toluidine and N-propylalanine. Both of these compounds may undergo ring hydroxylation.

O-toluidine has been found to produce methemoglobin, both *in vitro* and *in vivo* (see ADVERSE REACTIONS.)

Because prilocaine is metabolized in both the liver and kidneys, hepatic and renal dysfunction may alter prilocaine kinetics.

As with other local anesthetic agents, the plasma binding of prilocaine may be dependent on drug concentration. At 0.5-1.0 mcg/ml it is 55% protein bound.

Prilocaine crosses the blood-brain and placental barriers, presumably by passive diffusion.

Factors such as acidosis and the use of CNS stimulants and depressants affect the CNS levels of prilocaine required to produce overt systemic effects. In the rhesus monkey, arterial blood levels 20 mcg/ml have been shown to the threshold for convulsive activity.

INDICATIONS AND USAGE:

Prilocaine HCl 4% and 4% prilocaine HCl with epinephrine injections are indicated for the production of local anesthesia in dentistry by nerve block or infiltration techniques. Only accepted procedures for these techniques as described in standard text books are recommended.

CONTRAINDICATIONS:

Prilocaine is contraindicated in patients with a known history of hypersensitivity to local anesthetics of the amide type and in those rare patients with congenital or idiopathic methemoglobinemia.

WARNINGS:

DENTAL PRACTITIONERS WHO EMPLOY LOCAL ANESTHETIC AGENTS SHOULD BE WELL VERSED IN DIAGNOSIS AND MANAGEMENT OF EMERGENCIES THAT MAY ARISE FROM THEIR USE. RESUSCITATIVE EQUIPMENT, OXYGEN AND OTHER RESUSCITATIVE DRUGS SHOULD BE AVAILABLE FOR IMMEDIATE USE.

To minimize the likelihood of intravascular injection, aspiration should be performed before the local anesthetic solution is injected. If blood is aspirated, the needle must be repositioned until no return blood can be elicited by aspiration. Note, however, that the absence of blood in the syringe does not assure that intravascular injection will be avoided.

Prilocaine with epinephrine injections contain sodium metabisulfite, a sulfite that may cause allergic-type reactions including anaphylactic symptoms and life-threatening or less severe asthmatic episodes in certain susceptible people. The overall prevalence of sulfite sensitivity in the general population is unknown and probably low. Sulfite sensitivity is seen more frequently in asthmatic than in nonasthmatic people.

PRECAUTIONS:

GENERAL

The safety and effectiveness of prilocaine depend on proper dosage, correct technique, adequate precautions, and readiness for emergencies. Standard textbooks should be consulted for specific techniques and precautions for various regional anesthetic procedures. Resuscitative equipment, oxygen, and other resuscitative drugs should be available for immediate use. (See WARNINGS and ADVERSE REACTIONS). The lowest dosage that results in effective anesthesia should be used to avoid high plasma levels and serious adverse effects. Repeated doses of prilocaine may cause significant increases in blood levels with each repeated dose because of slow accumulation of the drug or its metabolites. Tolerance to elevated blood levels varies with the status of the patient. Debilitated, elderly patients, acutely ill patients, and children should be given reduced doses commensurate with their age and physical status. Prilocaine should also be used with caution in patients with severe shock or heart block.

Local anesthetic injections containing a vasoconstrictor should be used cautiously in areas of the body supplied by end arteries or having otherwise compromised blood supply. Patients with peripheral vascular disease and those with hypertensive vascular disease may exhibit exaggerated vasoconstrictor response. Ischemic injury or necrosis may result. Preparations

PRECAUTIONS: *(cont'd)*

containing a vasoconstrictor should be used with caution in patients during or following the administration of potent general anesthetic agents, since cardiac arrhythmias may occur under such conditions.

Cardiovascular and respiratory (adequacy of ventilation) vital signs and the patient's state of consciousness should be monitored after each local anesthetic injection. Restlessness, anxiety, tinnitus, dizziness, blurred vision, tremors, depression or drowsiness should alert the practitioner to the possibility of central nervous system toxicity. Signs and symptoms of depressed cardiovascular function may commonly result from a vasovagal reaction, particularly if the patient is in an upright position (See ADVERSE REACTIONS, Cardiovascular System.)

Since amide-type local anesthetics are metabolized by the liver, prilocaine should be used with caution in patients with hepatic disease.

Patients with severe hepatic disease, because of the inability to metabolize local anesthetics normally, are at greater risk of developing toxic plasma concentrations. Prilocaine should also be used with caution in patients with impaired cardiovascular function since they may be less able to compensate for functional changes associated with the prolongation of A-V conduction produced by these drugs.

Many drugs used during the conduct of anesthesia are considered potential triggering agents for familial malignant hyperthermia. Since it is not known whether amide-type local anesthetics may trigger this reaction and since the need for supplemental general anesthesia cannot be predicted in advance, it is suggested that a standard protocol for the management of malignant hyperthermia should be available. Early unexplained signs of tachycardia, tachypnea, labile blood pressure and metabolic acidosis may precede temperature elevation. Successful outcome is dependent on early diagnosis, prompt discontinuance of the suspect triggering agent(s)and institution of treatment, including oxygen therapy, indicated supportive measures and dantrolene (consult dantrolene sodium intravenous package insert before using).

Prilocaine should be used with caution in persons with known drug sensitivities. Patients allergic to para-aminobenzoic acid derivatives (procaine, tetracaine, benzocaine, etc.) have not shown cross sensitivity to prilocaine.

Use in the Head and Neck Area: Small doses of local anesthetics injected into the head and neck area, including retrobulbar, dental and stellate ganglion blocks, may produce adverse reactions similar to systemic toxicity seen with unintentional intravascular injections of larger doses. Confusion, convulsions, respiratory depression and/or respiratory arrest, and cardiovascular stimulation or depression have been reported. These reactions maybe due to intra-arterial injection of the local anesthetic with retrograde flow to the cerebral circulation. Patients receiving these blocks should have the circulation and respiration monitored and be constantly observed. Resuscitative equipment and personnel for treating adverse reactions should be immediately available. Dosage recommendation should not be exceeded. (See DOSAGE AND ADMINISTRATION.)

DRUG/LABORATORY TEST INTERACTIONS

The intramuscular injection of prilocaine may result in an increase in creatine phosphokinase levels. Thus, the use of this enzyme determination, without isoenzyme separation, as a diagnostic test for the presence of acute myocardial infarction may be compromised by the intramuscular injection of prilocaine.

INFORMATION FOR THE PATIENT

The patient should be informed of the possibility of temporary loss of sensation and muscle function following infiltration or nerve block injections.

The patient should be advised to exert caution to avoid inadvertent trauma to the lips, tongue, cheek mucosae or soft palate when these structures are anesthetized. The ingestion of food should therefore be postponed until normal function returns.

The patient should be advised to consult the dentist if anesthesia persists, or if a rash develops.

Carcinogenesis, Mutagenesis, and Impairment of Fertility

Studies of prilocaine in animals to evaluate the carcinogenic and mutagenic potential or the effect on fertility have not been conducted.

Chronic oral toxicity studies of ortho-toluidine, a metabolite of prilocaine, in mice (150-800 mg/kg) and rats (150-800 mg/kg) have shown that ortho-toluidine is a carcinogen in both species. The lowest dose corresponds to approximately 50 times the maximum amount of ortho-toluidine to which a 50 kg subject would be expected to be exposed following a single injection (8 mg/kg) of prilocaine.

Ortho-toluidine (0.5 mcg/ml) showed positive results in *Escherichia coli* DNA repair and phage-induction assays. Urine concentrates from rats treated with ortho-toluidine (300 mg/kg,orally) were mutagenic for *Salmonella typhimurium* with metabolic activation. Several other tests, including reverse mutations in five different*Salmonella typhimurium* strains with or without metabolic activation and single strand breaks in DNA of V79 Chinese hamster cells, were negative.

PREGNANCY CATEGORY B:

Teratogenic Effects: Reproduction studies have been performed in rats at doses up to 30 times the human dose and revealed no evidence of impaired fertility or harm to the fetus due to prilocaine. There are, however, no adequate and well-controlled studies in pregnant women. Animal reproduction studies are not always predictive of human response. General consideration should be given to this fact before administering prilocaine to women of childbearing potential, especially during early pregnancy when maximum organogenesis takes place.

NURSING MOTHERS

It is not known whether this drug is excreted in human milk. Because many drugs are excreted in human milk, caution should be exercised when prilocaine is administered to a nursing woman.

PEDIATRIC USE

Dosages in children should be reduced, commensurate with age, body weight, and physical condition. (See DOSAGE AND ADMINISTRATION.)

DRUG INTERACTIONS:

Clinically Significant Drug Interactions: The administration of local anesthetic solutions containing epinephrine or norepinephrine to patients receiving monoamine oxidase inhibitors, tricyclic antidepressants or phenothiazines may produce severe, prolonged hypotension or hypertension. Concurrent use of these agents should generally be avoided. In situations when concurrent therapy is necessary, careful patient monitoring is essential.

Concurrent administration of vasopressor drugs and ergot-type oxytocic drugs may cause severe, persistent hypertension or cerebrovascular accidents.

ADVERSE REACTIONS:

Swelling and persistent paresthesia of the lips and oral tissues may occur. Persistent paresthesia lasting weeks to months, and in rare instances paresthesia lasting greater than one year have been reported.

Adverse experiences following the administration of prilocaine are similar in nature to those observed with other amide local anesthetic agents. These adverse experiences are, in general, dose-related and may result from high plasma levels caused by excessive dosage, rapid

ADVERSE REACTIONS: *(cont'd)*

absorption or unintentional intravascular injection, or may result from a hypersensitivity, idiosyncrasy or diminished tolerance on the part of the patient. Serious adverse experiences are generally systemic in nature. The following types are those most commonly reported:

Central Nervous System: CNS manifestations are excitatory and/or depressant and may be characterized by lightheadedness, nervousness, apprehension, euphoria, confusion, dizziness, drowsiness, tinnitus, blurred or double vision, vomiting, sensations of heat, cold or numbness, twitching, tremors, convulsions, unconsciousness, respiratory depression and arrest. The excitatory manifestations may be very brief or may not occur at all, in which case the first manifestation of toxicity may be drowsiness merging into unconsciousness and respiratory arrest.

Drowsiness following the administration of prilocaine is usually a nearly sign of a high blood level of the drug and may occur as a consequence of rapid absorption.

Cardiovascular System: Cardiovascular manifestations are usually depressant and are characterized by bradycardia, hypotension, and cardiovascular collapse, which may lead to cardiac arrest.

Signs and symptoms of depressed cardiovascular function may commonly result from a vasovagal reaction, particularly if the patient is in an upright position. Less commonly, they may result from a direct effect of the drug. Failure to recognize the premonitory signs such as sweating, a feeling of faintness, changes in pulse or sensorium may result in progressive cerebral hypoxia and seizure or serious cardiovascular catastrophe. Management consists of placing the patient in the recumbent position and ventilation with oxygen. Supportive treatment of circulatory depression may require the administration of intravenous fluids, and, when appropriate, a vasopressor (*e.g.*, ephedrine) as directed by the clinical situation.

Allergic: Allergic reactions are characterized by cutaneous lesions, urticaria, edema or anaphylactoid reactions. Allergic reactions as a result of sensitivity to prilocaine are extremely rare and, if they occur, should be managed by conventional means. The detection of sensitivity by skin testing is of doubtful value.

Neurologic: The incidences of adverse reactions (*e.g.*, persistent neurologic deficit) associated with the use of local anesthetics may be related to the technique employed, the total dose of local anesthetic administered, the particular drug used, the route of administration, and the physical condition of the patient.

OVERDOSAGE:

Acute emergencies from local anesthetics are generally related to high plasma levels encountered during therapeutic use of local anesthetics(See ADVERSE REACTIONS, WARNINGS, and PRECAUTIONS).

Management of Local Anesthetic Emergencies: The first consideration is prevention, best accomplished by careful and constant monitoring of cardiovascular and respiratory vital signs and the patient's state of consciousness after each local anesthetic injection. At the first sign of change, oxygen should be administered.

The first step in the management of convulsions consists of immediate attention to the maintenance of a patent airway and assisted or controlled ventilation with oxygen and a delivery system capable of permitting immediate positive airway pressure by mask. Immediately after the institution of these ventilatory measures, the adequacy of the circulation should be evaluated, keeping in mind that drugs used to treat convulsions sometimes depress the circulation when administered intravenously. Should convulsions persist despite adequate respiratory support, and if the status of the circulation permits, small increments of an ultra-short acting barbiturate (such as thiopental or thiamylal) ora benzodiazepine (such as diazepam) may be administered intravenously. The clinician should be familiar, prior to use of local anesthetics, with these anticonvulsant drugs. Supportive treatment of circulatory depression may require administration of intravenous fluids and, when appropriate, a vasopressor as directed by the clinical situation (*e.g.*, ephedrine).

If not treated immediately, both convulsions and cardiovascular depression can result in hypoxia, acidosis, bradycardia, arrhythmias and cardiac arrest. If cardiac arrest should occur, standard cardiopulmonary resuscitative measures should be instituted.

Endotracheal intubation, employing drugs and techniques familiar to the clinician, may be indicated, after initial administration of oxygen by mask, if difficulty is encountered in the maintenance of a patent airway or if prolonged ventilatory support (assisted or controlled) is indicated.

Dialysis is of negligible value in the treatment of acute overdosage with prilocaine.

Administration of prilocaine in doses exceeding 400 mg has been associated with methemoglobinemia in adult patients and with proportionately lower doses in children. While methemoglobin values of less than 20% do not generally produce any clinical symptoms, the appearance of cyanosis at 2-4 hours following administration should be evaluated in terms of the general health status of the patient.

Methemoglobinemia can be reversed when indicated by intravenous administration of methylene blue at a dosage of 1-2 mg/kg given over a five minute period.

The subcutaneous LD_{50} of prilocaine HCl in female mice is 550 (359-905) mg/kg.

DOSAGE AND ADMINISTRATION:

The dosage of prilocaine HCl injection and prilocaine HCl with epinephrine injection varies and depends on the physical status of the patient, the area of the oral cavity to be anesthetized, the vascularity of the oral tissues, and the technique of anesthesia. The least volume of solution that results in effective local anesthesia should be administered. For specific techniques and procedures of local anesthesia in the oral cavity, refer to standard textbooks.

Inferior Alveolar Block: There are no practical clinical differences between prilocaine with and without epinephrine when used for inferior alveolar blocks.

Maxillary Infiltration: Prilocaine HCl is recommended for use in maxillary infiltration anesthesia for procedures in which the painful aspects can be completed within 15 minutes after the injection. Prilocaine HCl is therefore especially suited to short procedures in the maxillary anterior teeth. For long procedures, or those involving maxillary posterior teeth where soft tissue numbness is not troublesome to the patient, prilocaine HCl with epinephrine is recommended.

For most routine procedures, initial dosages of 1 to 2 ml of prilocaine HCl injection or prilocaine HCl with epinephrine injection will usually provide adequate infiltration or major nerve block anesthesia. No more than 600 mg (15 ml; 8 cartridges) should ever be administered within a two hour period in normal healthy adults.

In children under 10 years of age it is rarely necessary to administer more than one-half cartridge (40 mg) of prilocaine HCl injection or prilocaine HCl with epinephrine injection per procedure to achieve local anesthesia for a procedure involving a single tooth. In maxillary infiltration, this amount will often suffice to the treatment of two or even three teeth. In the mandibular block, however, satisfactory anesthesia achieved with this amount of drug will allow treatment of the teeth in an entire quadrant.

Aspiration Prior to Injection is Recommended, since it reduces the possibility of intravascular injection, thereby keeping the incidence of side effects and anesthetic failure to a minimum.

DOSAGE AND ADMINISTRATION: *(cont'd)*

NOTE: Parenteral drug products should be inspected visually for particulate matter and discoloration prior to administration whenever the solution and container permit. Solutions that are discolored and/or contain particulate matter should not be used. **Any unused portion of a cartridge of prilocaine HCl or prilocaine HCl with epinephrine injection should be discarded.**

Maximum Recommended Dosages Normal Healthy Adults: No more than 600 mg (8 mg/kg or 4 mg/lb) of prilocaine HCl should be administered as a single injection.

Children: It is difficult to recommend a maximum dose of any drug for children since this varies as a function of age and weight. For children of less than ten years who have a normal lean body mass and normal body development, the maximum dose may be determined by the application of one of the standard pediatric drug formulas (*e.g.*, Clark's rule). For example, in a child of five years weighing 50 lbs., the dose of prilocaine hydrochloride should not exceed 150-200 mg (6.6-8.8 mg/kg or 3-4 mg/lb of body weight) when calculated according to Clark's rule.

STERILIZATION, STORAGE AND TECHNICAL PROCEDURES

1. Cartridges of prilocaine HCl injection and prilocaine HCl with epinephrine injection should not be autoclaved, because solutions of epinephrine and the closures employed in cartridges cannot withstand autoclaving temperatures and pressures.

2. If chemical disinfection of anesthetic cartridges is desired, either 91% isopropyl alcohol or 70% ethyl alcohol is recommended. Many commercially available brands of rubbing alcohol, as well as solutions of ethyl alcohol not of U.S.P. grade, contain denaturants that are injurious to rubber and, therefore, are not to be used. It is recommended that chemical disinfection be accomplished by wiping the cartridge cap thoroughly with a pledget of cotton that has been moistened with the recommended alcohol just prior to use. IMMERSION IS NOT RECOMMENDED.

3. Certain metallic ions (mercury, zinc, copper etc.) have been related to swelling and edema after local anesthesia in dentistry. Therefore, chemical disinfectants containing or releasing these ions are not recommended. Antirust tablets usually contain metal ions. Accordingly, aluminum sealed cartridges should not be kept in such solutions.

4. Quaternary ammonium salts, such as benzalkonium chloride, are electrolytically incompatible with aluminum. Cartridges of prilocaine HCl injection and prilocaine HCl with epinephrine injection are sealed with aluminum caps and therefore should not be immersed in any solution containing salts.

5. To avoid leakage of solutions during injection, be sure to penetrate the center of the rubber diaphragm when loading the syringe. An off-center penetration produces an oval shaped puncture that allows leakage around the needle.

Other causes of leakage and breakage include badly worn syringes, aspirating syringes with bent harpoons, the use of syringes not designed to take 1.8 ml cartridges, and inadvertent freezing.

6. Cracking of glass cartridges is most often the result of any attempt to use a cartridge with an extruded plunger. An extruded plunger loses its lubrication and can be forced back into the cartridge only with difficulty. Cartridges with extruded plungers should be discarded.

7. Store at controlled room temperature 25°C (77°F).

8. Solutions containing epinephrine should be protected from light.

HOW SUPPLIED - EQUIVALENTS NOT AVAILABLE:

Injection, Solution - Dental; Infiltr - 4 %

1.8 ml cartridg	**$35.00**	**CITANEST PLAIN, Astra USA**	**00186-0520-14**

Injection, Solution - Dental; Infiltr - 5 mcg/40 mg

1.8 ml cartridg	**$35.00**	**CITANEST FORTE/EPINEPHRINE 1:200000, Astra USA**	**00186-0540-14**

PRIMAQUINE PHOSPHATE *(002113)*

CATEGORIES: Aminoquinolines; Anti-Infectives; Antimalarial Agents; Antiprotozoals; Malaria; Parasiticidal; FDA Approval Pre 1982

BRAND NAMES: *Neo-Quipenyl*; *Palum*; Primaquine
(International brand names outside U.S. in italics)

FORMULARIES: Aetna; Medi-Cal; PCS; WHO

> **WARNING:**
> PHYSICIANS SHOULD COMPLETELY FAMILIARIZE THEMSELVES WITH THE COMPLETE CONTENTS OF THIS MONOGRAPH BEFORE PRESCRIBING PRIMAQUINE PHOSPHATE.

DESCRIPTION:

Primaquine phosphate, USP, is an 8-aminoquinoline synthetic compound for oral administration. Each tablet contains 26.3 mg of primaquine phosphate (equivalent to 15 mg of primaquine base). The dosage is expressed in terms of the base.

Primaquine phosphate is an antimalarial drug.

Chemically, the drug is 8-[(4-Amino-1-methylbutyl)amino]-6- methoxy-quinoline phosphate. *Inactive Ingredients:* Acacia, Carnauba Wax, Gelatin, Kaolin, Lactose, Magnesium Stearate, Pharmaceutical Glaze, Precipitated Calcium Carbonate, Starch, Sucrose, Talc, Titanium Dioxide, Yellow Wax.

CLINICAL PHARMACOLOGY:

Primaquine is readily absorbed and rapidly metabolized after ingestion, and only a small proportion of the administered dose is excreted as the parent drug. The plasma concentration reaches a maximum in about 1 to 2 hours, after a single oral dose (15 mg base) of primaquine. However, the exact mechanism of primaquine is not known.

MICROBIOLOGY

Primaquine is an 8-aminoquinoline compound which eliminates tissue (exo-erythrocytic) infection. Thereby, it prevents the development of the blood (erythrocytic) forms of the parasite which are responsible for relapses in vivax malaria. Primaquine phosphate is also active against gametocytes of Plasmodium falciparum.

CLINICAL STUDIES:

Malariologists agree that malaria produced by Plasmodium vivax is the most difficult form to treat. This is ascribed to the ability of the parasite to develop extremely resistant tissue forms which are not eradicated by ordinary antimalarial compounds.

Thus, persons with acute attacks of vivax malaria, provoked by the release of erythrocytic forms of the parasite, respond readily to therapy, particularly to chloroquine phosphate. However, prior to the discovery of primaquine, no antimalarial drug was available that could

CLINICAL STUDIES: *(cont'd)*

be relied on to eliminate tissue (exo-erythrocytic) infection and to prevent relapses. The various investigations made with primaquine in experimentally induced vivax malaria in human volunteers and in persons with naturally occurring infections have demonstrated that the drug is a valuable adjunct to conventional therapy in this refractory form of the disease.

INDICATIONS AND USAGE:

Primaquine is indicated for the radical cure (prevention or relapse) of vivax malaria.

CONTRAINDICATIONS:

Primaquine is contraindicated in acutely ill patients suffering from systemic disease manifested by tendency to granulocytopenia, such as rheumatoid arthritis and lupus erythematosus, and in all patients with known hypersensitivity to it.

Primaquine is also contraindicated in patients receiving concurrently other potentially hemolytic drugs or depressants of myeloid elements of the bone marrow.

Because quinacrine hydrochloride appears to potentiate the toxicity of antimalarial compounds which are structurally related to primaquine, the use of quinacrine in patients receiving primaquine is contraindicated. Similarly, primaquine should not be administered to patients who have received quinacrine recently, as toxicity is increased.

WARNINGS:

Primaquine should be discontinued immediately if signs of hemolytic anemia occur (darkening of the urine, marked decrease in hemoglobin or erythrocytic count).

Hemolytic reactions (moderate to severe) may occur in glucose- 6-phosphate dehydrogenase (G-6-PD) deficient Caucasians (particularly in Sardinians, Asians and Mediterranean peoples, and in individuals with a family or personal history of favism). Dark-skinned persons (Negroes, for example) have a great tendency to develop hemolytic anemia (due to congenital deficiency of erythrocytic glucose-6-phosphate dehydrogenase) while receiving primaquine and related drugs.

PRECAUTIONS:

General: If primaquine is prescribed for (1) an individual who has shown a previous idiosyncrasy to primaquine (as manifested by hemolytic anemia, methemoglobinemia, or leukopenia), (2) an individual with a personal or family history of favism, or (3) an individual with erythrocytic glucose-6-phosphate dehydrogenase (G-6-PD) deficiency or nicotinamide adenine dinucleotide (NADH) methemoglobin reductase deficiency, the person should be observed closely for tolerance. The drug should be discontinued immediately if marked darkening of the urine or sudden decrease in hemoglobin concentration or leukocyte count occurs.

Since anemia, methemoglobinemia, and leukopenia have been observed following administration of large doses of primaquine, the adult dosage of 1 tablet (= 15 mg base) daily for fourteen days should not be exceeded.

Laboratory Tests: It is advisable to make routine blood examinations (particularly blood cell counts and hemoglobin determinations) during therapy.

Nursing Mothers: Caution should be exercised when primaquine is administered to a nursing woman.

Pediatric Use: Safety and effectiveness in children have not been established.

DRUG INTERACTIONS:

Potentially hemolytic drugs (*e.g.,* sulfonamides, nitrofurans) or depressants of myeloid elements of the bone marrow (*eg.,* methotrexate, phenylbutazone, chloramphenicol) should not be given concurrently with primaquine. (See CONTRAINDICATIONS.)

Primaquine should not be administered to patients who have recently received quinacrine, as toxicity is increased. (See CONTRAINDICATIONS.)

ADVERSE REACTIONS:

Gastrointestinal: Nausea, vomiting, epigastric distress, and abdominal cramps.

Hematologic: Leukopenia, Hemolytic anemia in glucose-6-phosphate dehydrogenase (G-6-PD) deficient individuals, and methemoglobinemia in nicotinamide adenine dinucleotide (NADH) methemoglobin reductase deficient individuals.

OVERDOSAGE:

Symptoms of overdosage of primaquine may occur if the single dose administered is more than 15 mg (base). They include abdominal cramps, vomiting, burning epigastric distress, central nervous system and cardiovascular disturbances, cyanosis, methemoglobinemia, moderate leukocytosis or leukopenia, and anemia. The most striking symptoms are granulocytopenia and acute hemolytic anemia in sensitive persons. Acute hemolysis occurs, but patients recover completely if the dosage is discontinued.

Treatment is symptomatic and supportive. Evacuate the stomach by emesis or gastric lavage promptly. If shock with hypotension or vascular collapse occurs, an appropriate potent vasopressor should be administered.

DOSAGE AND ADMINISTRATION:

Primaquine phosphate is recommended only for the radical cure of vivax malaria, the prevention of relapse in vivax malaria, or following the termination of chloroquine phosphate suppressive therapy in an area where vivax malaria is endemic.

Patients suffering from an attack of vivax malaria or having parasitized red blood cells should receive a course of chloroquine phosphate, which quickly destroys the erythrocytic parasites and terminates the paroxysm. Primaquine should be administered concurrently in order to eradicate the exo-erythrocytic paracytes in a dosage of 1 tablet (equivalent to 15 mg base) daily for 14 days in adults.

Storage: Store at room temperature.

HOW SUPPLIED - EQUIVALENTS NOT AVAILABLE:

Tablet, Uncoated - Oral - 26.3 mg

100's	$64.84	PRIMAQUINE, Sanofi Winthrop	00024-1596-01

PRIMIDONE *(002114)*

CATEGORIES: Anticonvulsants; Barbiturate Anticonvulsants; Central Nervous System Agents; Convulsions; Epilepsy; Neuromuscular; Seizures; Tonic-Clonic Seizures; FDA Approval Pre 1982

BRAND NAMES: *Midone*; Myidone; *Mylepsin*; **Mysoline**; *PMS Primidone*; *Prysoline* *(International brand names outside U.S. in italics)*

FORMULARIES: Aetna; BC-BS; DoD; FHP; Medi-Cal; PCS

DESCRIPTION:

Chemical name: 5-ethyldihydro-5-phenyl-4,6 (1H, 5H)-pyrimidinedione.

Primadone is a white, crystalline, highly stable substance, M.P. 279-284°C. It is poorly soluble in water (60 mg per 100 ml at 37° C) and in most organic solvents. It possesses no acidic properties, in contrast to its barbiturate analog.

Mysoline 50 mg and 250 mg tablets contain the following inactive ingredients: Microcrystalline Cellulose, NF; Lactose, USP; Methylcellulose, USP; Sodium Starch Glycolate, NF; Talc, USP; Sodium Lauryl Sulfate, NF; Magnesium Stearate, NF; Water, USP, Purified. Primadone 250 mg tablets also contain Yellow Iron Oxide, NF.

Mysoline suspension contains these inactive ingredients: Ammonia Solution, Diluted; Citric Acid, USP; D&C Yellow No. 10; FD&C Yellow No. 6; Magnesium Aluminum Silicate; Methylparaben, NF; Propylparaben, NF; Saccharin Sodium, NF; Sodium Alginate; Sodium Citrate; Sodium Hypochlorite Solution, USP; Sorbic Acid, NF; Sorbitan Monolaurate; Water, USP, Purified; Flavors.

CLINICAL PHARMACOLOGY:

Primadone raises electro- or chemoshock seizure thresholds or alters seizure patterns in experimental animals. The mechanism(s) of primidone's antiepileptic action is not known.

Primidone *per se* has anticonvulsant activity as do its two metabolites, phenobarbital and phenylethylmalonamide (PEMA). In addition to its anticonvulsant activity, PEMA potentiates the anticonvulsant activity of phenobarbital in experimental animals.

INDICATIONS AND USAGE:

Primadone, used alone or concomitantly with other anticonvulsants, is indicated in the control of grand mal, psychomotor, and focal epileptic seizures. It may control grand mal seizures refractory to other anticonvulsant therapy.

CONTRAINDICATIONS:

Primidone is contraindicated in: 1) patients with porphyria and 2) patients who are hypersensitive to phenobarbital (see CLINICAL PHARMACOLOGY).

WARNINGS:

The abrupt withdrawal of antiepileptic medication may precipitate status epilepticus.

The therapeutic efficacy of a dosage regimen takes several weeks before it can be assessed.

Usage In Pregnancy: The effects of primadone in human pregnancy and nursing infants are unknown. Recent reports suggest an association between the use of anticonvulsant drugs by women with epilepsy and an elevated incidence of birth defects in children born to these women. Data are more extensive with respect to diphenylhydantoin and phenobarbital, but these are also the most commonly prescribed anticonvulsants; less systematic or anecdotal reports suggest a possible similar association with the use of all known anticonvulsant drugs.

The reports suggesting an elevated incidence of birth defects in children of drug-treated epileptic women cannot be regarded as adequate to prove a definite cause-and-effect relationship. There are intrinsic methodologic problems in obtaining adequate data on drug teratogenicity in humans: the possibility also exists that other factors leading to birth defects, e.g., genetic factors or the epileptic condition itself, may be more important than drug therapy. The majority of mothers on anticonvulsant medication deliver normal infants. It is important to note that anticonvulsant drugs should not be discontinued in patients in whom the drug is administered to prevent major seizures because of the strong possibility of precipitating status epilepticus with attendant hypoxia and threat to life. In individual cases where the severity and frequency of the seizure disorders are such that the removal of medication does not pose a serious threat to the patient, discontinuation of the drug may be considered prior to and during pregnancy, although it cannot be said with any confidence that even minor seizures do not pose some hazard to the developing embryo or fetus.

The prescribing physician will wish to weigh these considerations in treating or counseling epileptic women of childbearing potential.

Neonatal hemorrhage, with a coagulation defect resembling vitamin K deficiency, has been described in newborns whose mothers were taking primidone and other anticonvulsants. Pregnant women under anticonvulsant therapy should receive prophylactic vitamin K_1 therapy for one month prior to, and during, delivery.

PRECAUTIONS:

The total daily dosage should not exceed 2 g. Since primadone therapy generally extends over prolonged periods, a complete blood count and a sequential multiple analysis-12 (SMA-12) test should be made every six months.

Nursing Mothers: There is evidence that in mothers treated with primidone, the drug appears in the milk in substantial quantities. Since tests for the presence of primidone in biological fluids are too complex to be carried out in the average clinical laboratory, it is suggested that the presence of undue somnolence and drowsiness in nursing newborns of primadone-treated mothers be taken as an indication that nursing should be discontinued.

ADVERSE REACTIONS:

The most frequently occurring early side effects are ataxia and vertigo. These tend to disappear with continued therapy, or with reduction of initial dosage. Occasionally, the following have been reported: nausea, anorexia, vomiting, fatigue, hyperirritability, emotional disturbances, sexual impotency, diplopia, nystagmus, drowsiness, and morbilliform skin eruptions. Granulocytopenia, and red-cell hypoplasia and aplasia, have been reported rarely. These and, occasionally, other persistent or severe side effects may necessitate withdrawal of the drug. Megaloblastic anemia may occur as a rare idiosyncrasy to primadone and to other anticonvulsants. The anemia responds to folic acid without necessity of discontinuing medication.

DOSAGE AND ADMINISTRATION:

Adult Dosage: Patients 8 years of age and older who have received no previous treatment may be started on primadone according to the following regimen using either 50 mg or scored 250 mg primadone tablets:

Days 1 to 3: 100 to 125 mg at bedtime.

Days 4 to 6: 100 to 125 mg b.i.d.

Days 7 to 9: 100 to 125 mg t.i.d.

Day 10 to maintenance: 250 mg t.i.d.

For most adults and children 8 years of age and over, the usual maintenance dosage is three to four 250 mg primadone tablets daily in divided doses (250 mg t.i.d. or q.i.d.). If required, an increase to five or six 250 mg tablets daily may be made but daily doses should not exceed 500 mg q.i.d. (TABLE 1):

Dosage should be individualized to provide maximum benefit. In some cases, serum blood level determinations of primidone may be necessary for optimal dosage adjustment. The clinically effective serum level for primidone is between 5 to 12 mcg/ml.

DOSAGE AND ADMINISTRATION: *(cont'd)*

TABLE 1 Initial: Adults And Children Over 8

DAY	AM	NOON	PM
1			2 × 50 mg
2			2 × 50 mg
3			2 × 50 mg
4	2 × 50 mg		2 × 50 mg
5	2 × 50 mg		2 × 50 mg
6	2 × 50 mg		2 × 50 mg
7	2 × 50 mg	2 × 50 mg	2 × 50 mg
8	2 × 50 mg	2 × 50 mg	2 × 50 mg
9	2 × 50 mg	2 × 50 mg	2 × 50 mg
10	250 mg	250 mg	250 mg
11	Adjust to Maintenance		
12	Adjust to Maintenance		

In Patients Already Receiving Other Anticonvulsants: Primadone should be started at 100 to 125 mg at bedtime and gradually increased to maintenance level as the other drug is gradually decreased. This regimen should be continued until satisfactory dosage level is achieved for the combination, or the other medication is completely withdrawn. When therapy with primadone alone is the objective, the transition from concomitant therapy should not be completed in less than two weeks.

PEDIATRIC DOSAGE

For children under 8 years of age, the following regimen may be used:

Days 1 to 3: 50 mg at bedtime.

Days 4 to 6: 50 mg b.i.d.

Days 7 to 9: 100 mg b.i.d.

Day 10 to maintenance: 125 mg t.i.d. to 250 mg t.i.d.

For children under 8 years of age, the usual maintenance dosage is 125 to 250 mg three times daily or, 10 to 25 mg/kg/day in divided doses.

Store at room temperature, approximately 25° C (77° F).

HOW SUPPLIED - RATED THERAPEUTICALLY EQUIVALENT:

Tablet, Uncoated - Oral - 250 mg

100's	$7.95	Primidone, Consolidated Midland	00223-1414-01
100's	$15.00	Primidone, US Trading	56126-0289-11
100's	$30.30	Primidone, H.C.F.A. F F P	99999-2114-01
100's	$31.50	Primidone, Harber Pharm	51432-0364-03
100's	$34.88	Primidone, Major Pharms	00904-0560-61
100's	$35.85	Primidone 250, Major Pharms	00904-0560-60
100's	$35.98	Primidone, United Res	00677-0354-01
100's	$36.03	Primidone, HL Moore Drug Exch	00839-1552-06
100's	$36.91	Primidone, Caremark	00339-5659-12
100's	$37.98	Primidone, Qualitest Pharms	00603-5370-21
100's	$38.55	Primidone, Goldline Labs	00182-0701-01
100's	$38.55	Primidone, Schein Pharm (US)	00364-0366-01
100's	$41.25	Primidone Tablets 250 Mg, Aligen Independ	00405-4836-01
100's	$41.25	Primidone, Lannett	00527-1231-01
100's	$41.25	Primidone, Rugby	00536-4373-01
1000's	$67.50	Primidone, Consolidated Midland	00223-1414-02
1000's	$225.00	Primidone, Harber Pharm	51432-0364-06
1000's	$303.00	Primidone, H.C.F.A. F F P	99999-2114-02
1000's	$307.38	Primidone, HL Moore Drug Exch	00839-1552-16
1000's	$320.70	Primidone 250, Major Pharms	00904-0560-80
1000's	$326.32	Primidone Tablets 250 Mg, Aligen Independ	00405-4836-03
1000's	$351.95	Primidone, Rugby	00536-4373-10
1000's	$375.00	Primidone, Goldline Labs	00182-0701-10
1000's	$375.00	Primidone, Schein Pharm (US)	00364-0366-02
1000's	$387.50	Primidone, Lannett	00527-1231-10

HOW SUPPLIED - NOT RATED EQUIVALENT:

Suspension - Oral - 250 mg/5ml

240 ml	**$38.96**	**MYSOLINE, Ayerst**	**00046-3850-08**

Tablet, Uncoated - Oral - 50 mg

100's	**$17.09**	**MYSOLINE, Ayerst**	**00046-0431-81**
500's	**$81.33**	**MYSOLINE, Ayerst**	**00046-0431-85**

Tablet, Uncoated - Oral - 250 mg

100's	**$49.75**	**MYSOLINE, Ayerst**	**00046-0430-81**
100's	**$53.25**	**MYSOLINE, Ayerst**	**00046-0430-99**
1000's	**$473.68**	**MYSOLINE, Ayerst**	**00046-0430-91**

PROBENECID *(002115)*

CATEGORIES: Antiarthritics; Antigout; Arthritis; Electrolytic, Caloric-Water Balance; Gout; Gouty Arthritis; Hyperuricemia; Pain; Penicillin Adjuvant; Uricosuric Agents; FDA Approval Pre 1982

BRAND NAMES: *Bencid*; *Benecid*; **Benemid**; *Benuryl*; *Panuric*; Probalan; *Probecid*; *Probenemid*; *Probenid*; *Procid*; *Solpurin*; *Urocid*
(International brand names outside U.S. in italics)

FORMULARIES: Aetna; BC-BS; DoD; FHP; Medi-Cal; PCS

DESCRIPTION:

Probenecid is a uricosuric and renal tubular transport blocking agent.

Probenecid is the generic name for 4-((di-propylamino)sulfonyl) benzoic acid (molecular weight 285.36).

Probenecid is a white or nearly white, fine, crystalline powder. Probenecid is soluble in dilute alkali, in alcohol, in chloroform, and in acetone; it is practically insoluble in water and in dilute acids.

Each tablet contains 0.5 g probenecid and the following inactive ingredients: calcium stearate, D&C Yellow 10, gelatin, hydroxypropyl methylcellulose, iron oxide, magnesium carbonate, polyethylene glycol, starch, talc, and titanium dioxide.

CLINICAL PHARMACOLOGY:

Probenecid is a uricosuric and renal tubular blocking agent. It inhibits the tubular reabsorption of urate, thus increasing the urinary excretion of uric acid and decreasing serum urate levels. Effective uricosuria reduces the miscible urate pool, retards urate deposition, and promotes resorption of urate deposits.

CLINICAL PHARMACOLOGY: *(cont'd)*

Probenecid inhibits the tubular secretion of penicillin and usually increases penicillin plasma levels by any route the antibiotic is given. A 2-fold to 4-fold elevation has been demonstrated for various penicillins.

Probenecid also has been reported to inhibit the renal transport of many other compounds including aminohippuric acid (PAH), aminosalicylic acid (PAS), indomethacin, sodium iodomethamate and related iodinated organic acids, 17-ketosteroids, pantothenic acid, phenolsulfonphthalein (PSP), sulfonamides, and sulfonylureas. See also DRUG INTERACTIONS.

Probenecid decreases both hepatic and renal excretion of sulfobromophthalein (BSP). The tubular reabsorption of phosphorus is inhibited in hypoparathyroid but not in euparathyroid individuals.

Probenecid does not influence plasma concentrations of salicylates, nor the excretion of streptomycin, chloramphenicol, chlortetracycline, oxytetracycline, or neomycin.

INDICATIONS AND USAGE:

For treatment of the hyperuricemia associated with gout and gouty arthritis.

As an adjuvant to therapy with penicillin or with ampicillin, methicillin, oxacillin, cloxacillin, or nafcillin, for elevation and prolongation of plasma levels by whatever route the antibiotic is given.

CONTRAINDICATIONS:

Hypersensitivity to this product.

Children under 2 years of age.

Not recommended in persons with known blood dyscrasias or uric acid kidney stones.

Therapy with probenecid should not be started until an acute gouty attack has subsided.

WARNINGS:

Exacerbation of gout following therapy with probenecid may occur; in such cases colchicine or other appropriate therapy is advisable.

Probenecid increases plasma concentrations of methotrexate in both animals and humans. In animal studies, increased methotrexate toxicity has been reported. If probenecid is given with methotrexate, the dosage of methotrexate should be reduced and serum levels may need to be monitored.

In patients on probenecid the use of salicylates in either small or large doses is contraindicated because it antagonizes the uricosuric action of probenecid. The biphasic action of salicylates in the renal tubules accounts for the so-called "paradoxical effect" of uricosuric agents. In patients on probenecid who require a mild analgesic agent the use of a acetaminophen rather than small doses of salicylates would be preferred.

Rarely, severe allergic reactions and anaphylaxis have been reported with the use of probenecid. Most of these have been reported to occur within several hours after readministration following prior usage of the drug.

The appearance of hypersensitivity reactions requires cessation of therapy with probenecid.

Use in Pregnancy: Probenecid crosses the placental barrier and appears in cord blood. The use of any drug in women of childbearing potential requires that the anticipated benefit be weighed against possible hazards.

PRECAUTIONS:

General: Hematuria, renal colic, costovertebral pain, and formation of uric acid stones associated with the use of probenecid in gouty patients may be prevented by alkalization of the urine and a liberal fluid intake (*see* DOSAGE AND ADMINISTRATION). In these cases when alkali is administered, the acid-base balance of the patient should be watched.

Use with caution in patients with a history of peptic ulcer.

Probenecid has been used in patients with some renal impairment but dosage requirements may be increased. Probenecid may not be effective in chronic renal insufficiency particularly when the glomerular filtration rate is 30 ml/minute or less. Because of its mechanism of action, probenecid is not recommended in conjunction with a penicillin in the presence of *known* renal impairment.

A reducing substance may appear in the urine of patients receiving probenecid. This disappears with discontinuance of therapy. Suspected glycosuria should be confirmed by using a test specific for glucose.

DRUG INTERACTIONS:

When probenecid is used to elevate plasma concentrations of penicillin or other beta-lactams, or when such drugs are given to patients taking probenecid therapeutically, high plasma concentrations of the other drug may increase the incidence of adverse reactions associated with that drug. In the case of penicillin or other beta-lactams, psychic disturbances have been reported.

The use of salicylates antagonizes the uricosuric action of probenecid (see WARNINGS). The uricosuric action of probenecid is also antagonized by pyrazinamide.

Probenecid produces an insignificant increase in free sulfonamide plasma concentrations but a significant increase in total sulfonamide plasma levels. Since probenecid decreases the renal excretion of conjugated sulfonamides, plasma concentrations of the latter should be determined from time to time when a sulfonamide and probenecid are coadministered for prolonged periods. Probenecid may prolong or enhance the action of oral sulfonylureas and thereby increase the risk of hypoglycemia.

It has been reported that patients receiving probenecid require significantly less thiopental for induction of anesthesia. In addition, ketamine and thiopental anesthesia were significantly prolonged in rats receiving probenecid.

The concomitant administration of probenecid increases the mean plasma elimination half-life of a number of drugs which can lead to increased plasma concentrations. These include agents such as indomethacin, acetaminophen, naproxen, ketoprofen, meclofenamate, lorazepam, and rifampin. Although the clinical significance of this observation has not been established, a lower dosage of the drug may be required to produce a therapeutic effect, and increases in dosage of the drug in question should be made cautiously and in small increments when probenecid is being co-administrated. Although specific instances of toxicity due to this potential interaction have not been observed to date, physicians should be alert to this possibility.

Probenecid given concomitantly with sulindac has only a slight effect on plasma sulfide levels, while plasma levels of sulindac and sulfone were increased. Sulindac was shown to produce a modest reduction in the uricosuric action of probenecid, which probably is not significant under most circumstances.

In animals and in humans, probenecid has been reported to increase plasma concentrations of methotrexate (see WARNINGS).

Falsely high readings for theophylline have been reported in an *in vitro* study, using the Schack and Waxler technic, when therapeutic concentrations of theophylline and probenecid were added to human plasma.

ADVERSE REACTIONS:

The following adverse reactions have been observed and within each category are listed in order of decreasing severity.

Central Nervous System: headache, dizziness.

Metabolic: precipitation of acute gouty arthritis.

Gastrointestinal: hepatic necrosis, vomiting, nausea, anorexia, sore gums.

Genitourinary: nephrotic syndrome, uric acid stones with or without hematuria, renal colic, costovertebral pain, urinary frequency.

Hypersensitivity: anaphylaxis, fever, urticaria, pruritus.

Hematologic: aplastic anemia, leukopenia, hemolytic anemia which in some patients could be related to genetic deficiency of glucose -6-phosphate dehydrogenase in red blood cells, anemia.

Integumentary: dermatitis, alopecia, flushing.

DOSAGE AND ADMINISTRATION:

GOUT

Therapy with probenecid should not be *started* until an acute gouty attack has subsided. However, if and acute attack is precipitated *during* therapy, probenecid may be continued without changing the dosage, and full therapeutic dosage of colchicine or other appropriate therapy should be given to control the acute attack.

The recommended adult dosage is 0.25 g (1/2 tablet of probenecid) twice a day for one week, followed by 0.5 g (1 tablet) twice a day thereafter.

Some degree of renal impairment may be present in patients with gout. A daily dosage of 1 g may be adequate. However, if necessary, the daily dosage may be increased by 0.5 g increments every 4 weeks within tolerance (and usually not above 2 g per day) if symptoms of gouty arthritis are not controlled or the 24 hour uric acid excretion is not above 700 mg. As noted, probenecid may not be effective in chronic renal insufficiency particularly when the glomerular filtration rate is 30 ml/minute or less.

PENICILLIN THERAPY (GONORRHEA)*

1) Uncomplicated gonococcal infection in men and women (urethral, cervical, rectal)

Recommended Regimens:** 4.8 million units of aqueous procaine penicillin G† IM, in at least 2 doses injected at different sites at one visit + 1 g of probenecid orally just before injections.

or 3.5 g of ampicillin† orally + 1 g probenecid orally given simultaneously

Remarks: Follow-up: Obtain urethral and other appropriate cultures from men, and cervical, anal, and other appropriate cultures from women, 7 to 14 days after completion of treatment.

Treatment of sexual partners: Persons with known recent exposure to gonorrhea should receive same treatment as those known to have gonorrhea. Examination and treatment of male sex partners of persons with gonorrhea are essential because of high prevalence of non-symptomatic urethral gonococcal infection in such men.

2) Pharyngeal gonococcal infection in men and women

Recommended Regimens:** 4.8 million units of aqueous procaine penicillin G† IM, in at least 2 doses injected at different sites at one visit + 1 g probenecid orally just before injections.

Remarks: Pharyngeal gonococcal infections may be more difficult to treat than anogenital gonorrhea. Post treatment cultures are essential.

3) Uncomplicated gonorrhea in pregnant patients

Recommended Regimens:** 4.8 million units of aqueous procaine penicillin G† IM, in at least 2 doses injected at different sites at one visit *or* 3.5 g of ampicillin† orally + 1 g of probenecid orally given simultaneously

4) Acute gonococcal salpingitis

Recommended Regimens:** *Outpatients:* Aqueous procaine penicillin G† or ampicillin† with probenecid as for gonorrhea in pregnancy, followed by 500 mg of ampicillin 4 times a day for 10 days

Hospitalized Patients: See details in CDC recommendations

Remarks: Follow-up of patients with acute salpingitis is essential. All patients should receive repeat pelvic examinations and cultures for *Neisseria gonorrhoeae* after treatment. Examination and appropriate treatment of male sex partners are essential because of high prevalence of non-symptomatic urethral gonorrhea in such men.

5) Disseminated gonococcal infection (arthritis-dermatitis syndrome)

Recommended Regimens:** 10 million units of aqueous crystalline penicillin G IV a day for 3 days or till significant clinical improvement occurs. May be followed with 500 mg of ampicillin† 4 times a day orally to complete 7 days of treatment *or* 3.5 g of ampicillin† orally with 1 g of probenecid, followed by 500 mg of ampicillin† 4 times a day for at least 7 days

6) Gonococcal infection in children

Recommended Regimens:** For postpubertal children and/or those weighing over 45 kg (100 lb) use the dosage regimens given above for adults.

Uncomplicated vulvovaginitis and urethritis: aqueous procaine penicillin G† 75,000 — 100,000 units/kg IM, with probenecid 23 mg/kg orally

Remarks: See CDC recommendations for detailed information about prevention and treatment of neonatal gonococcal infection and gonococcal ophthalmia.

Note: Before treating gonococcal infections in patients with suspected primary or secondary syphilis, perform proper diagnostic procedures including darkfield examinations. If concomitant syphilis is suspected, perform monthly serological tests for at least 4 months.

* Recommended by Venereal Disease Control Advisory Committee, Center for Disease Control, U.S. Department of Health, Education, and Welfare, Public Health Service (Morbidity and Mortality Weekly Report, Vol. *23:* 341, 342, 347, 348, Oct. 11, 1974).

** See CDC recommendations for definition of regimens of choice, alternative regimens, treatment of hypersensitive patients, and other aspects of therapy.

† See prescribing information for detailed information about contraindications, warnings, precautions, and adverse reactions.

Gastric intolerance may be indicative of overdosage, and may be corrected by decreasing the dosage.

As uric acid tends to crystallize out of an acid urine, a liberal fluid intake is recommended, as well as sufficient sodium bicarbonate (3 to 7.5 g daily) or potassium citrate (7.5 g daily) to maintain an alkaline urine (see PRECAUTIONS).

Alkalization of the urine is recommended until the serum urate level returns to normal limits and tophaceous deposits disappear, i.e., during the period when urinary excretion of uric acid is at a high level. Thereafter, alkalization of the urine and the usual restriction of purine-producing foods may be somewhat relaxed.

Probenecid should be continued at the dosage that will maintain normal serum urate levels. When acute attacks have been absent for 6 months or more and serum urate levels remain within normal limits, the daily dosage may be decreased by 0.5 g every 6 months. The maintenance dosage should not be reduced to the point where serum urate levels tend to rise.

DOSAGE AND ADMINISTRATION: *(cont'd)*

PROBENECID AND PENICILLIN THERAPY (GENERAL)

Adults: The recommended dosage is 2 g (4 tablets of probenecid) daily in divided doses. This dosage should be reduced in older patients in whom renal impairment may be present.

Children 2-14 Years of Age: *Initial dose:* 25 mg/kg body weight (*or* 0.7 g/square meter body surface).

Maintenance Dose: 40 mg/kg body weight (*or* 1.2 g/square meter body surface) per day, divided into 4 doses.

For children weighing more than 50 kg (110 lb) the adult dosage is recommended.

Probenecid is contraindicated in children under 2 years of age.

The PSP excretion test may be used to determine the effectiveness of probenecid in retarding penicillin excretion and maintaining therapeutic levels. The renal clearance of PSP is reduced to about one-fifth the normal rate when dosage of probenecid is adequate.

PENICILLIN THERAPY (GONORRHEA)

See information above.

(Merck 8/88, 7399021)

HOW SUPPLIED - RATED THERAPEUTICALLY EQUIVALENT:

Tablet, Plain Coated - Oral - 500 mg

100's	$11.54	Probenecid, H.C.F.A. F F P	99999-2115-01
100's	$12.20	Probenecid, Harber Pharm	51432-0366-03
100's	$13.97	Probenecid, HL Moore Drug Exch	00839-5081-06
100's	$15.36	Probenecid, Rugby	00536-4366-01
100's	$15.85	Probenecid, Zenith Labs	00172-2190-60
100's	$15.85	Probenecid, Goldline Labs	00182-0600-01
100's	$15.85	Probenecid Tablets 500 Mg, Aligen Independ	00405-4841-01
100's	$15.90	Probenecid, United Res	00677-0355-01
100's	$15.95	Probenecid, Major Pharms	00904-2190-60
100's	$16.30	Probenecid, Qualitest Pharms	00603-5381-21
100's	$17.50	Probenecid, Consolidated Midland	00223-1472-01
100's	$17.70	Probenecid, Schein Pharm (US)	00364-0314-01
100's	$17.70	Probenecid, Mylan	00378-0156-01
100's	$17.70	Probenecid, Geneva Pharms	00781-1021-01
100's	$22.58	Probenecid, US Trading	56126-0383-11
100's	**$30.60**	**BENEMID, Merck**	**00006-0501-68**
500's	$129.44	Probenecid Tablets 500 Mg, Aligen Independ	00405-4841-03
1000's	$115.40	Probenecid, H.C.F.A. F F P	99999-2115-02
1000's	$121.50	Probenecid, United Res	00677-0355-10
1000's	$137.21	Probenecid, Rugby	00536-4366-10
1000's	$140.30	Probenecid, Major Pharms	00904-2190-80
1000's	$144.75	Probenecid, Zenith Labs	00172-2190-80
1000's	$144.75	Probenecid, Goldline Labs	00182-0600-10
1000's	$145.06	Probenecid, Schein Pharm (US)	00364-0314-02
1000's	$167.50	Probenecid, Consolidated Midland	00223-1472-02
1000's	**$290.45**	**BENEMID, Merck**	**00006-0501-82**

PROCAINAMIDE HYDROCHLORIDE *(002117)*

CATEGORIES: Anesthesia; Antiarrhythmic Agents; Arrhythmia; Cardiovascular Drugs; Local Anesthetics; Tachycardia; Vascular Disorders, Cerebral/Peripheral; Pregnancy Category C; FDA Approval Pre 1982

BRAND NAMES: *Amisalin*; *Biocoryl*; Procamide Sr; Procan Sr; Promine; **Pronestyl**; *Ritmocamid*
(International brand names outside U.S. in italics)

FORMULARIES: Aetna; BC-BS; CIGNA; FHP; Humana; Kaiser; Medco; Medi-Cal; PruCare; United; WHO; PCS

COST OF THERAPY: $216.95 (Arrhythmia; Capsule; 375 mg; 8/day; 365 days)

The prolonged administration of procainamide often leads to the development of a positive anti-nuclear antibody (ANA) test, with or without symptoms of a lupus erythematosus-like syndrome. If a positive ANA titer develops, the benefits versus risks of continued procainamide therapy should be assessed.

DESCRIPTION:

Note: This monograph contains information on Procainamide Hydrochloride (Procainamide HCl) tablets, extended release tablets, capsules, and injection.

Procainamide HCl, a Group 1A cardiac antiarrhythmic drug, is p-amino-N-(2-(diethylamino) ethyl)-benzamide monohydrochloride, molecular weight 271.79.

It differs from procaine which is the p-aminobenzoyl *ester* of 2-(diethylamino)-ethanol. Procainamide as the free base has a pK_a of 9.23; the monohydrochloride is very soluble in water. Procainamide HCl is supplied for oral administration as capsules and tablets in potencies of 250, 375, and 500 mg.

INACTIVE INGREDIENTS

Pronestyl Tablets: calcium silicate, microcrystalline cellulose, colorants (FD&C Yellow No. 5 (tartrazine) and Yellow No. 6), flavor, povidone, starch, stearic acid, and other ingredients.

Pronestyl Capsules: colorants (D&C Yellow No. 10, except 375 mg; FD&C Yellow No. 6), gelatin, lactose (except 500 mg), magnesium stearate, talc, and titanium dioxide.

Pronestyl extended-release tablets are available for oral administration as green, film-coated tablets containing 250 mg procainamide HCl, as yellow scored, film-coated tablets containing 500 mg procainamide HCl; as orange, scored, film coated tablets containing 750 mg procainamide HCl; and as red, scored, film-coated tablets containing 1000 mg procainamide HCl.

All strengths of Pronestyl extended release tablets contain candeilla wax, FCC; colloidal silicon dioxide, NF; magnesium stearate, NF; titanium dioxide, vanillin NF; and other ingredients. The individual strengths contain additional ingredients as follows: *250 mg:* D&C yellow No. 10 Al lake; FD&C Blue No. 1 Al lake; FD&C yellow NO.6 Al lake; lactose, NF; may also contain methylparaben, NF; or simethicone emulsion and polysorbate 80. *500 mg:* D&C yellow No.10 Al lake; FD &C blue No.2 Al lake; FD&C yellow No. 6 Al lake; sucrose, NF; may also contain methylparaben, NF; and propylparaben, NF; or simethicone and emulsion and polysorbate 80. *750 mg:* FD&C yellow No. 6 Al lake; may also contain propylene glycol, USP; or simethicone emulsion and polysorbate 80. *1000 mg:* D&C red No.7 calcium lake; FD&C yellow NO.6 Al lake; propylene glycol, USP.

Procainamide HCl is available for parenteral use a sterile, aqueous solution providing 100 mg or 500 mg per ml. Th 100 mg/ml concentration in each ml procainamide HCl 100 mg, benzyl alcohol 0.009 ml and sodium metabisulfite 0.9 mg in Water for Injection. The 500 mg/ml concentration contains in each ml procainamide HCl 500 mg, benzyl alcohol 0.009 ml and sodium metabisulfite 2 mg in Water for Injection. For both concentrations, pH is 4.0 to 6.0; sodium hydroxide and/or hydrochloric acid added, if needed, for pH adjustment. Vials are sealed under nitrogen.

CLINICAL PHARMACOLOGY:

Procainamide (PA) increases the effective refractory period of the atria, and to a lesser extent the bundle of His-Purkinje system and ventricles of the heart. It reduces impulse conduction velocity in the atria, His-Purkinje fibers, and ventricular muscle, but has variable effects on the atrioventricular (A-V) node, a direct slowing action and a weaker vagolytic effect which may speed A-V conduction slightly. Myocardial excitability is reduced in the atria, Purkinje fibers, papillary muscles, and ventricles by an increase in the threshold for excitation, combined with inhibition of ectopic pacemaker activity by retardation of the slow phase of diastolic depolarization, thus decreasing automaticity especially in ectopic sites. Contractility of the undamaged heart is usually not affected by therapeutic concentrations, although slight reduction of cardiac output may occur, and may be significant in the presence of myocardial damage. Therapeutic levels of PA may exert vagolytic effects and produce slight acceleration of heart rate, while high or toxic concentrations may prolong A-V conduction time or induce A-V block, or even cause abnormal automaticity and spontaneous firing, by unknown mechanisms.

The electrocardiogram may reflect these effects by showing slight sinus tachycardia (due to the anticholinergic action) and widened QRS complexes and, less regularly, prolonged Q-T and P-R intervals (due to longer systole and slower conduction), as well as some decrease in QRS and T wave amplitude. These direct effects of PA on electrical activity, conduction, responsiveness, excitability and automaticity are characteristic of a Group 1A antiarrhythmic agent, the prototype for which is quinidine; PA effects are very similar. However, PA has weaker vagal blocking action than does quinidine, does not induce alpha-adrenergic blockade, and is less depressing to cardiac contractility.

Ingested PA is resistant to digestive hydrolysis, and the drug is well absorbed from the entire small intestinal surface, but individual patients vary in their completeness of absorption of PA. Following oral administration of, plasma PA levels reach about 50 percent of peak in 30 minutes, 90 percent at an hour, and peak at about 90 to 120 minutes. About 15 to 20 percent of PA is reversibly bound to plasma proteins, and considerable amounts are more slowly and reversibly bound to tissues of the heart, liver, lung, and kidney. The apparent volume of distribution eventually reaches about 2 liters per kilogram body weight with a half-time of approximately five minutes. While PA has been shown in the dog to cross the blood-brain barrier, it did not concentrate in the brain at levels higher than in plasma. It is not known if PA crosses the placenta. Plasma esterases are far less active in hydrolysis of PA than of procaine. The half-time for elimination of PA is three to four hours in patients with normal renal function, but reduced creatinine clearance and advancing age each prolong the half-time of elimination of PA.

A significant fraction of the circulating PA may be metabolized in hepatocytes to N-acetylprocainamide (NAPA), ranging from 16 to 21 percent of an administered dose in "slow acetylators" to 24 to 33 percent in "fast-acetylators". Since NAPA also has significant antiarrhythmic activity and somewhat slower renal clearance than PA, both hepatic acetylation rate capability and renal function, as well as age, have significant effects on the effective biologic half-time of therapeutic action of administered PA and the NAPA derivative. Trace amounts may be excreted in the urine as free and conjugated p-aminobenzoic acid, 30 to 60 percent as unchanged PA, and 6 to 52 percent as the NAPA derivative. Both PA and NAPA are eliminated by active tubular secretion as well as by glomerular filtration. Action of PA on the central nervous system is not prominent, but high plasma concentrations may cause tremors. While therapeutic plasma levels for PA have been reported to be 3 to 10 mcg/ml, certain patients such as those with sustained ventricular tachycardia, may need higher levels for adequate control. This may justify the increased risk of toxicity (see OVERDOSAGE.) Where programmed ventricular stimulation has been used to evaluate efficacy of PA in preventing recurrent ventricular tachyarrhythmias, higher plasma levels (mean, 13.6 mcg/ml) of PA were found necessary for adequate control.

Additional information for Procainamide HCl Injection: Following IM injection, this drug is rapidly absorbed into the blood stream, and, plasma levels peak in about 15 to 60 minutes, considerably faster than orally administered forms. IV administration of Procainamide HCl can produce therapeutic procainamide levels within minutes after the infusion is started.

INDICATIONS AND USAGE:

Procainamide HCl is indicated for the treatment of documented ventricular arrhythmias, such as sustained ventricular tachycardia, that, in the judgement of the physician, are life-threatening. Because of the proarrhythmic effects of procainamide HCl, its use with lesser arrythmias is generally not recommended. Treatment of patients with asymptomatic ventricular premature contractions should be avoided.

Initiation of procainamide HCl treatment, as with other antiarrhythmic agents used to treat life-threatening arrythmias, should be carried out in the hospital.

Antiarrhythmic drugs have not been shown to enhance survival in patients with ventricular arrythmias.

Because procainamide has the potential to produce serious hematological disorders (0.5 percent) particularly leukopenia or agranulocytosis (sometimes fatal), its use should be reserved for patients in whom, in the opinion of the physician, the benefits of treatment clearly outweigh the risks. (See WARNINGS and BOXED WARNING.)

CONTRAINDICATIONS:

Complete Heart Block: Procainamide should not be administered to patients with complete heart block because of its effects in suppressing nodal or ventricular pacemakers and the hazard of asystole. It may be difficult to recognize complete heart block in patients with ventricular tachycardia, but if significant slowing of ventricular rate occurs during PA treatment without evidence of A-V conduction appearing, PA should be stopped. In cases of second degree A-V block or various types of hemiblock, PA should be avoided or discontinued because of the possibility of increased severity of block, unless the ventricular rate is controlled by an electrical pacemaker.

Idiosyncratic Hypersensitivity: In patients sensitive to procaine or other ester-type local anesthetics, cross sensitivity to PA is unlikely; however, it should be borne in mind, and PA should not be used if it produces acute allergic dermatitis, asthma, or anaphylactic symptoms.

Lupus Erythematosus: An established diagnosis of systemic lupus erythematosus is a contraindication to PA therapy, since aggravation of symptoms is highly likely.

Torsades de Pointes: In the unusual ventricular arrhythmia called "les torsades de pointes" (Twistings of the points), characterized by alternation of one or more ventricular premature beats in the directions of the QRS complexes on ECG in persons with prolonged Q-T and often enhanced U waves, Group 1A antiarrhythmic drugs are contraindicated. Administration of PA in such cases may aggravate this special type of ventricular extrasystole or tachycardia instead of suppressing it.

WARNINGS:

MORTALITY

In the National Heart, Lung and Blood Institute's Cardiac Arrythmia Suppression Trial (CAST), a long-term, multicentered, randomized, double-blind study in patients with asymptomatic non-life-threatening ventricular arrythmias who had had myocardial infarctions more than six days but less than two years previously, an excessive mortality or non- fatal cardiac arrest rate was seen in patients treated with encainide or flecainide (56/730) compared with that seen in patients assigned to matched placebo-treated groups (22/725). The average duration of treatment with encainide or flecainide in this study was ten months.

The applicability of these results to other populations (*e.g.*, those without recent myocardial infarctions) or to other antiarrhythmic drugs is uncertain, but at present it is prudent to consider any antiarrhythmic agent to have a significant risk in patients with structural heart disease.

BLOOD DYSCRASIAS: Agranulocytosis, bone marrow depression, neutropenia, hypoplastic anemia and thrombocytopenia in patients receiving procainamide hydrochloride have been reported at a rate of approximately 0.5 percent. Most of these patients received procainamide within the recommended dosage range. Fatalities have occurred (with approximately 20-25 percent mortality in reported cases of agranulocytosis). Since most of these events have been noted during the first 12 weeks of therapy, it is recommended that complete blood counts including white cell, differential and platelet counts be performed at weekly intervals for the first three months of therapy, and periodically thereafter. Complete blood counts should be performed promptly if the patient develops any signs of infection (such as fever, chills, sore throat or stomatitis), bruising or bleeding. If any of these hematologic disorders are identified, procainamide therapy should be discontinued. Blood counts usually return to normal within one month of discontinuation. Caution should be used in patients with pre-existing marrow failure or cytopenia of any type (see ADVERSE REACTIONS.)

DIGITALIS INTOXICATION

Caution should be exercised in the use of procainamide in arrhythmias associated with digitalis intoxication. Procainamide can suppress digitalis-induced arrhythmias; however, if there is concomitant marked disturbance of atrioventricular conduction, additional depression of conduction and ventricular asystole or fibrillation may result. Therefore, use of procainamide should be considered only if discontinuation of digitalis, and therapy with potassium, lidocaine, or phenytoin are ineffective.

FIRST DEGREE HEART BLOCK

Caution should be exercised also if the patient exhibits or develops first degree heart block while taking PA, and dosage reduction is advised in such cases. If the block persists despite dosage reduction, continuation of PA administration must be evaluated on the basis of current benefit versus risk of increased heart block.

PREDIGITALIZATION FOR ATRIAL FLUTTER OR FIBRILLATION

Patients with atrial flutter or fibrillation should be cardioverted or digitalized prior to PA administration to avoid enhancement of A-V conduction which may result in ventricular rate acceleration beyond tolerable limits. Adequate digitalization reduces but does not eliminate the possibility of sudden increase in ventricular rate as the atrial rate is slowed by PA in these arrhythmias.

CONGESTIVE HEART FAILURE

For patients in congestive heart failure, and those with acute ischemic heart disease or cardiomyopathy, caution should be used in PA therapy, since even slight depression of myocardial contractility may further reduce cardiac output of the damaged heart.

CONCURRENT OTHER ANTIARRHYTHMIC AGENTS

Concurrent use of PA with other Group 1A antiarrhythmic agents such as quinidine or disopyramide may produce enhanced prolongation of conduction or depression of contractility and hypotension, especially in patients with cardiac decompensation. Such use should be reserved for patients with serious arrhythmias unresponsive to a single drug and employed only if close observation is possible.

RENAL INSUFFICIENCY

Renal insufficiency may lead to accumulation of high plasma levels from conventional oral doses of PA, with effects similar to those of overdosage (see OVERDOSAGE), unless dosage is adjusted for the individual patient.

MYASTHENIA GRAVIS

Patients with myasthenia gravis may show worsening of symptoms from PA due to its procaine-like effect on diminishing acetylcholine release at skeletal muscle motor nerve endings, so that PA administration may be hazardous without optimal adjustment of anticholinesterase medications and other precautions.

Additional information for the injection: This contains sodium metabisulfite, a sulfite that may cause allergic-type reactions including anaphylactic symptoms and life-threatening or less severe asthmatic episodes in certain susceptible people. The overall prevalence of sulfite sensitivity in the general population is unknown and probably low. Sulfite sensitivity is seen more frequently in asthmatic than in non-asthmatic people.

PRECAUTIONS:

GENERAL

Immediately after initiation of PA therapy, patients should be closely observed for possible hypersensitivity reactions, especially if procaine or local anesthetic sensitivity is suspected, and for muscular weakness if myasthenia gravis is a possibility.

In conversion of atrial fibrillation to normal sinus rhythm by any means, dislodgement of mural thrombi may lead to embolization, which should be kept in mind.

After a day or so, steady state plasma PA levels are produced following regular oral administration of a given dose of Procainamide HCl Tablets; Procainamide HCl Capsules at set intervals, with peak plasma concentrations at about 90 to 120 minutes after each dose. After achieving and maintaining therapeutic plasma concentrations and satisfactory electrocardiographic and clinical responses, continued frequent periodic monitoring of vital signs and electrocardiograms is advised. If evidence of QRS widening of more than 25 percent or marked prolongation of the Q-T interval occurs, concern for overdosage is appropriate, and reduction in dosage is advisable if a 50 percent increase occurs. Elevated serum creatinine or urea nitrogen, reduced creatinine clearance, or history of renal insufficiency, as well as use in older patients (over age 50), provide grounds to anticipate that less than the usual dosage and longer time intervals between doses may suffice, since the urinary elimination of PA and NAPA may be reduced, leading to gradual accumulation beyond normally-predicted amounts. If facilities are available for measurement of plasma PA and NAPA, or acetylation capability, individual dose adjustment for optimal therapeutic levels may be easier, but close observation of clinical effectiveness is the most important criterion.

In the longer term, periodic complete blood counts are useful to detect possible idiosyncratic hematologic effects of PA on neutrophil, platelet or red cell homeostasis; agranulocytosis has been reported to occur occasionally in patients on long-term PA therapy. A rising titer of serum ANA may precede clinical symptoms of the lupoid syndrome (see BOXED WARNING and ADVERSE REACTIONS). If the lupus erythematosus-like syndrome develops in a patient with recurrent life-threatening arrhythmias not controlled by other agents, cortico-

PRECAUTIONS: *(cont'd)*

steroid suppressive therapy may be used concomitantly with PA. Since the PA-induced lupoid syndrome rarely includes the dangerous pathologic renal changes, PA therapy may not necessarily have to be stopped unless the symptoms of serositis and the possibility of further lupoid effects are of greater risk than the benefit of PA in controlling arrhythmias. Patients with rapid acetylation capability are less likely to develop the lupoid syndrome after prolonged PA therapy.

Procainamide HCl Tablets contain FD&C Yellow No. 5 (tartrazine) which may cause allergic-type reactions (including bronchial asthma) in certain susceptible individuals. Although the overall incidence of FD&C Yellow No. 5 (tartrazine) sensitivity in the general population is low, it is frequently seen in patients who also have aspirin hypersensitivity.

Additional information for the injection: Blood pressure should be monitored with the patient supine during parenteral, especially intravenous, administration of Procainamide (see DOSAGE AND ADMINISTRATION.) There is a possibility that relatively high, although transient, plasma levels of procainamide may be attained and cause hypotension before the procainamide can be disturbed from the plasma volume to its full apparently volume to its full apparent volume of distribution, which is approximately 50 times greater. Therefore, caution should be exercised to avoid overly rapid administration of procainamide. If the blood pressure falls 15 mm Hg or more, procainamide administration should be temporarily discontinued. ECG monitoring is advisable as well, both for observation of the progress and response of the arrhythmia under treatment, and for early detection of any tendency to excessive widening of the QRS complex, prolongation of the P-R interval or any signs of the heat block (see OVERDOSAGE.) Parenteral therapy with procainamide should be limited to use in hospitals in which monitoring and intensive supportive care are available or to emergency situations in which equivalent observation and treatment can be provided.

INFORMATION FOR THE PATIENT

The physician is advised to explain to the patient that close cooperation in adhering to the prescribed dosage schedule is of great importance in controlling the cardiac arrhythmia safely. The patient should understand clearly that more medication is not necessarily better and may be dangerous, that skipping doses or increasing intervals between doses to suit personal convenience may lead to loss of control of the heart problem, and that "making up" missed doses by doubling up later may be hazardous.

The patient should be encouraged to disclose any past history of drug sensitivity, especially to procaine or other local anesthetic agents, or aspirin, and to report any history of kidney disease, congestive heart failure, myasthenia gravis, liver disease, or lupus erythematosus.

The patient should be counseled to report promptly any symptoms of arthralgia, myalgia, fever, chills, skin rash, easy bruising, sore throat or sore mouth, infections, dark urine or icterus, wheezing, muscular weakness, chest or abdominal pain, palpitations, nausea, vomiting, anorexia, diarrhea, hallucinations, dizziness, or depression.

LABORATORY TESTS

Laboratory tests such as complete blood count (CBC), electrocardiogram, and serum creatinine or urea nitrogen may be indicated, depending on the clinical situation, and periodic rechecking of the CBC and ANA may be helpful in early detection of untoward reactions.

DRUG/LABORATORY TEST INTERACTIONS

Suprapharmacologic concentrations of lidocaine and meprobamate may inhibit fluorescence of PA and NAPA, and propranolol shows a native fluorescence close to the PA/NAPA peak wavelengths, so that tests which depend on fluorescence measurement may be affected.

CARCINOGENESIS, MUTAGENESIS, AND IMPAIRMENT OF FERTILITY

Long term studies in animals have not been performed.

PREGNANCY, TERATOGENIC EFFECTS, PREGNANCY CATEGORY C

Animal reproduction studies have not been conducted with PA. It also is not known whether PA can cause fetal harm when administered to a pregnant woman or can affect reproduction capacity. PA should be given to a pregnant woman only if clearly needed.

NURSING MOTHERS

Both PA and NAPA are excreted in human milk, and absorbed by the nursing infant. Because of the potential for serious adverse reactions in nursing infants, a decision to discontinue nursing or the drug should be made, taking into account the importance of the drug to the mother.

PEDIATRIC USE

Safety and effectiveness in children have not been established.

DRUG INTERACTIONS:

If other antiarrhythmic drugs are being used, additive effects on the heart may occur with PA administration, and dosage reduction may be necessary (see WARNINGS.)

Anticholinergic drugs administered concurrently with PA may produce additive antivagal effects on A-V nodal conduction, although this is not as well documented for PA as for quinidine.

Patients taking PA who require neuromuscular blocking agents such as succinylcholine may require less than usual doses of the latter, due to PA effects on reducing acetylcholine release.

ADVERSE REACTIONS:

Cardiovascular: Hypotension following oral PA administration is rare. Hypotension and serious disturbances of cardiorhythm such as ventricular asystole or fibrillation are more common after intravenous administration (see OVERDOSAGE, WARNINGS.) Second degree heart block has been reported in 2 of almost 500 patients taking PA orally.

Multisystem: A lupus erythematosus-like syndrome of arthralgia, pleural or abdominal pain, and sometimes arthritis, pleural effusion, pericarditis, fever, chills, myalgia, and possibly related hematologic or skin lesions is fairly common after prolonged PA administration, perhaps more often in patients who are slow acetylators(see BOXED WARNING and PRECAUTIONS). While some series have reported less than 1 in 500, others have reported the syndrome in up to 30 percent of patients on long term oral PA therapy. If discontinuation of PA does not reverse the lupoid symptoms, corticosteroid treatment may be effective.

Hematologic: Neutropenia, thrombocytopenia, or hemolytic anemia may rarely be encountered. Agranulocytosis has occurred after repeated use of PA, and deaths have been reported. (See BOXED WARNING,WARNINGS).

Skin: Angioneurotic edema, urticaria, pruritus, flushing, and maculopapular rash have also occurred occasionally.

Gastrointestinal: Anorexia, nausea, vomiting, abdominal pain, bitter taste, or diarrhea may occur in 3 to 4 percent of patients taking oral procainamide. Hepatomegaly with increased serum aminotransferase activity have been reported after a single oral dose.

Nervous System: Dizziness or giddiness, weakness, mental depression, and psychosis with hallucinations have been reported occasionally.

OVERDOSAGE:

Progressive widening of the QRS complex, prolonged Q-T and P-R intervals, lowering of the R and T waves, as well as increasing A-V block, may be seen with doses which are excessive for a given patient. Increased ventricular extrasystoles, or even ventricular tachycardia or

OVERDOSAGE: *(cont'd)*

fibrillation may occur. After intravenous administration but seldom after oral therapy, transient high plasma levels of PA may induce hypotension, affecting systolic more than diastolic pressures, especially in hypertensive patients. Such high levels may also produce central nervous depression, tremor, and even respiratory depression.

Plasma levels above 10 mcg/ml are increasingly associated with toxic findings, which are seen occasionally in the 10 to 12 mcg/ml range, more often in the 12 to 15 mcg/ml range, and commonly in patients with plasma levels greater than 15 mcg/ml. Overdosage symptoms may result following a single 2 g dose; while 3 g may be dangerous, especially if the patient is a slow acetylator, has decreased renal function, or underlying organic heart disease.

Treatment of overdosage or toxic manifestations includes general supportive measures, close observation, monitoring of vital signs and possibly intravenous pressor agents and mechanical cardiorespiratory support. If available, PA and NAPA plasma levels may be helpful in assessing the potential degree of toxicity and response to therapy. Both PA and NAPA are removed from the circulation by hemodialysis but not peritoneal dialysis. No specific antidote for PA is known.

DOSAGE AND ADMINISTRATION:

Oral Forms: The oral dose and interval of administration should be adjusted for the individual patient, based on clinical assessment of the degree of underlying myocardial disease, the patient's age, and renal function.

As a general guide, for younger adult patients with normal renal function, an initial total daily oral dose of up to 50 mg/kg of body weight of Capsules or Tablets may be used, given in divided doses, every three hours, to maintain therapeutic blood levels. For older patients, especially those over 50 years of age, or for patients with renal, hepatic, or cardiac insufficiency, lesser amounts or longer intervals may produce adequate blood levels, and decrease the probability of occurrence of dose related adverse reactions.For the tablets and capsules, the total daily dose should be administered in divided doses at three, four, or six hour intervals and adjusted according to the patient's response (TABLES 1 and 2):

TABLE 1 Capsules and Tablets; To provide up to 50 mg per kg of body weight per day:*

Patients weighing lb	kg	
88-110	40-50	250 mg q3 hrs to 500 mg q6 hrs
132-154	60-70	375 mg q3 hrs to 750 mg q6 hrs
176-198	80-90	500 mg q3 hrs to 1 g q6 hrs
>220	>100	625 mg q3 hrs to 1.25 g q6 hrs

TABLE 2 Extended Release Tablets; To provide up to 50 mg per kg of body weight per day:*

Patients weighing lb	kg	
88-110	40-50	500 mg q6 hrs
132-154	60-70	750 mg q6 hrs
176-198	80-90	1 g q6 hrs
>220	>100	1.25 g q6 hrs

* Initial dosage schedule guide only, to be adjusted for each patient individually, based on age, cardiorenal function, blood level (if available), and clinical response.

Injection: Procainamide HCl Injection is useful for arrhythmias which require immediate suppression and for maintenance of arrhythmia control. IV therapy allows most rapid control of serious arrhythmias, including those following myocardial infarction; it should be carried out in circumstances where close observation and monitoring of the patient are possible, such as hospital or emergency facilities. IM administration is less opt to produce temporary high plasma levels but therapeutic plasma levels are not obtained as rapidly as with IV administration. Oral procainamide dosage forms are preferable for less urgent arrhythmias as well as long-term maintenance after initial parenteral procainamide therapy.

IM administration may be used as an alternative to the oral route for patients with less threatening arrhythmias but who are nauseated or vomiting, who are ordered to receive nothing by mouth preoperatively or who may have malabsorptive problems. An initial dose of 50 mg per kg body weight may be estimated. This amount should be divided into fractional doses of one eighth to one quarter to be injected by the IM route every three ti six hours until oral therapy is possible. If more than three injections are given, the physician may wish to assess the patient factors such as age and renal function, clinical response, and if available, blood levels of procainamide and NAPA in adjusting further doses for that individual. For treatment of arrhythmias associated with anesthesia or surgical operation, the suggested dose is 100 to 500 mg by IM injection.

IV administration for Procainamide HCl Injection should be done cautiously to avoid a possible hypotensive response (see PRECAUTIONSand OVERDOSAGE). Initial arrhythmia control, under ECG monitoring, may usually be accomplished safely within a half-hour by either of the two methods which follow:

A) Direct Injection into a vein or tubing an established infusion line should be done slowly at a rate not to exceed 50 mg per minute. It is advisable to dilute either the 100 mg/ml or the 500 mg/ml concentrations of Procainamide HCl Injection prior to IV injection to facilitate control of dosage rate. Doses of 100 mg may be administered every 5 minutes at this rate until the arrhythmia is suppressed or until 500 mg has been administered, after which it is advisable to wait 10 minutes or longer to allow for more distribution into tissues before resuming.

B) Alternatively, a loading infusion containing 20 mg of Procainamide HCl per ml (1 g diluted to 50 ml with 5% Dextrose Injection, USP) may be administered at a constant rate of 1 ml per minute for 25 to 30 minutes to deliver 500 to 600 mg of procainamide. Some effects may be seen after the infusion of the first 100 or 200 mg; it is unusual to require more than 600 mg to achieve satisfactory antiarrhythmic effects.

The maximum advisable dosage to be given either by repeated bolus injections or such loading infusion is 1 g.

To maintain therapeutic levels, a more dilute IV infusion ata concentration of 2 mg/ml is convenient (1 g Procainamide HCl in 500 ml of 5% Dextrose Injection, USP), and may be administered at 1 to 3 ml/minute. If daily total fluid intake must be limited, a 4 mg/ml concentration (1 g Procainamide HCl Injection, USP in 250 ml of 5% Dextrose Injection, USP) administered at 0.5 to 1.5 ml/minute will deliver an equivalent 2 to 6 mg per minute. The amount needed in a given patient to maintain therapeutic level should be assessed principally from the clinical response and will depend upon the patient's weight and age, renal elimination, hepatic acetylation rate and cardiac status, but should be adjusted for each patient based upon close observation. A maintenance infusion rate of 50 mcg/min/kg body weight to a person with a normal renal procainamide elimination half-time of three hours may be expected to produce a plasma level of approximately 6.5 mcg/ml (see TABLE 3.)

DOSAGE AND ADMINISTRATION: *(cont'd)*

Since the principle route for elimination of procainamide and NAPA is renal excretion, reduced excretion will prolong the half-life of elimination and lower the dose rate needed to maintain therapeutic levels. Advancing age reduces the renal excretion of procainamide and NAPA independently of reductions in creatine clearance; compared to normal young adults, there is approximately 25 percent reduction at age 50 and 50 percent at age 75.

IV therapy should be terminated if persistent conduction disturbances or hypotension develop. As soon as the patient's basic cardiac rhythm appears to be stabilized, oral antiarrhythmic maintenance therapy is preferable, if indicated and possible. A period of about three to fours (one half-time for renal elimination, ordinarily) should elapse after the last IV dose before administering the first dose of procainamide tablets or capsules.

TABLE 3 DILUTIONS AND RATES FOR IV INFUSIONS* PROCAINAMIDE HCl INJECTION

	Final Concentration	Infusion Volume†	Procainamide to be added	Infusion Rate
Initial Loading Infusion	20 mg/ml	50 ml	1000 mg	1 ml/min (for up to 25-30 min*)
Maintenance Infusion	2 mg/ml or 4 mg/ml	500 ml 250 ml	1000 mg 1000 mg	1 to 3 ml/min 0.5 to 1.5 ml/min

The maintenance infusion rates are calculated to deliver 2 to 6 mg per minute depending on body weight, renal elimination rate and steady-state plasma level needed to maintain control of the arrhythmia*.
The 4 mg/ml maintenance concentration may be preferred if total infusion volume is to be limited.
* Please see text under DOSAGE AND ADMINISTRATIONfor further details. The flow rate of any IV Procainamide infusion must be monitored closely to avoid transiently high plasma levels and possible hypotension (see PRECAUTIONS).
† All infusions should be made up to final volume with 5% Dextrose Injection, USP.

Parenteral drug products should be inspected visually for particulate matter and discoloration prior to administration, whenever solution and container permit.

Store at controlled room temperature 15-30°C (59-86°F).

Discard solution if darker than slightly yellow or otherwise discolored.

Storage (oral forms):

Store at room temperature; avoid excessive heat (104° F); protect from moisture.

(Tablets and Capsules: Apothecon, 8/91, P1902-00)

(Extended-Release Tablets: Princeton, 8/91, J4-104E)

(Injection: Princeton, 8/91, J4-423)

HOW SUPPLIED - RATED THERAPEUTICALLY EQUIVALENT:

Capsule, Gelatin - Oral - 250 mg

100's	$6.83	Procainamide HCl, H.C.F.A. F F P	99999-2117-01
100's	$7.20	Procainamide Hcl, United Res	00677-0450-01
100's	$7.85	Procainamide Hcl, Raway	00686-3567-13
100's	$8.30	Procainamide Hcl, Harber Pharm	51432-0370-03
100's	$8.35	Procainamide Hydrochloride, Aligen Independ	00405-4851-01
100's	$8.90	Procainamide Hcl, Qualitest Pharms	00603-5404-21
100's	$9.10	Procainamide HCl, Rugby	00536-4367-01
100's	$9.15	Procainamide Hcl, Zenith Labs	00172-2345-60
100's	$9.15	Procainamide Hcl, Goldline Labs	00182-0705-01
100's	$9.15	Procainamide Hcl, Parmed Pharms	00349-2179-01
100's	$9.17	Procainamide HCl, HL Moore Drug Exch	00839-5224-06
100's	$9.90	Procainamide Hcl, Vangard Labs	00615-0342-13
100's	$11.99	Procainamide HCl, Schein Pharm (US)	00364-0219-01
100's	$14.50	Procainamide Hcl, Consolidated Midland	00223-1456-01
100's	$15.50	Procainamide HCl, Schein Pharm (US)	00364-0219-90
100's	**$45.01**	**PRONESTYL, Bristol Myers Squibb**	**00003-0758-53**
100's	**$53.93**	**PRONESTYL, Bristol Myers Squibb**	**00003-0758-50**
250's	$17.07	Procainamide HCl, H.C.F.A. F F P	99999-2117-02
250's	$17.80	Procainamide Hcl 250, Major Pharms	00904-2345-70
500's	$49.06	Procainamide Hydrochloride, Aligen Independ	00405-4851-03
1000's	$52.50	Procainamide Hcl, Consolidated Midland	00223-1456-02
1000's	$64.15	Procainamide Hcl 250, Major Pharms	00904-2345-80
1000's	$68.30	Procainamide HCl, H.C.F.A. F F P	99999-2117-03
1000's	$72.50	Procainamide Hcl, Rugby	00536-4367-10
1000's	$75.00	Procainamide Hcl, Zenith Labs	00172-2345-80
1000's	$75.00	Procainamide Hcl, Schein Pharm (US)	00364-0219-02
1000's	$75.00	Procainamide Hcl, Harber Pharm	51432-0370-06
1000's	**$404.86**	**PRONESTYL, Bristol Myers Squibb**	**00003-0758-80**

Capsule, Gelatin - Oral - 375 mg

100's	$7.43	Procainamide HCl, H.C.F.A. F F P	99999-2117-04
100's	$9.30	Procainamide Hcl, Major Pharms	00904-2346-60
100's	$9.59	Procainamide Hcl, Qualitest Pharms	00603-5405-21
100's	$9.60	Procainamide Hydrochloride, Aligen Independ	00405-4852-01
100's	$9.74	Procainamide Hcl, United Res	00677-0667-01
100's	$9.80	Procainamide HCl, Schein Pharm (US)	00364-0343-01
100's	$9.86	Procainamide HCl, HL Moore Drug Exch	00839-1563-06
100's	$9.90	Procainamide Hcl, Zenith Labs	00172-2346-60
100's	$9.90	Procainamide Hcl, Goldline Labs	00182-0925-01
100's	$9.90	Procainamide HCl, Rugby	00536-4377-01
100's	$9.90	Procainamide Hcl, Harber Pharm	51432-0372-03
100's	$11.70	Procainamide Hcl, US Trading	56126-0291-11
100's	$18.00	Procainamide HCl, Schein Pharm (US)	00364-0343-90
100's	**$65.54**	**PRONESTYL, Bristol Myers Squibb**	**00003-0756-53**
100's	**$74.79**	**PRONESTYL, Bristol Myers Squibb**	**00003-0756-50**
1000's	$60.60	Procainamide Hcl, Rugby	00536-4377-10
1000's	$74.30	Procainamide HCl, H.C.F.A. F F P	99999-2117-05
1000's	$84.70	Procainamide Hcl, Zenith Labs	00172-2346-80
1000's	$84.70	Procainamide Hcl, Harber Pharm	51432-0372-06

Capsule, Gelatin - Oral - 500 mg

100's	$8.48	Procainamide HCl, H.C.F.A. F F P	99999-2117-06
100's	$9.70	Procainamide Hcl, United Res	00677-0470-01
100's	$9.72	Procainamide Hcl, Qualitest Pharms	00603-5406-21
100's	$11.00	Procainamide Hcl, Zenith Labs	00172-2347-60
100's	$11.00	Procainamide Hcl, Goldline Labs	00182-0521-01
100's	$11.00	Procainamide HCl, HL Moore Drug Exch	00839-5050-06
100's	$11.00	Procainamide Hcl, Harber Pharm	51432-0374-03
100's	$11.20	Procainamide Hydrochloride, Aligen Independ	00405-4853-01
100's	$12.00	Procainamide Hcl, Raway	00686-0102-20
100's	$12.70	Procainamide HCl, Rugby	00536-4368-01
100's	$12.71	Procainamide HCl, Schein Pharm (US)	00364-0344-01
100's	$12.95	Procainamide Hcl, Raway	00686-3584-13
100's	$16.17	Procainamide Hcl, Vangard Labs	00615-0343-13
100's	$16.95	Procainamide Hcl, Consolidated Midland	00223-1457-01
100's	$22.00	Procainamide HCl, Schein Pharm (US)	00364-0344-90

HOW SUPPLIED - RATED THERAPEUTICALLY EQUIVALENT: *(cont'd)*

100's	**$81.05**	**PRONESTYL, Bristol Myers Squibb**	**00003-0757-53**
100's	**$97.10**	**PRONESTYL, Bristol Myers Squibb**	**00003-0757-50**
250's	$21.20	Procainamide HCl, H.C.F.A. F F P	99999-2117-07
250's	$21.40	Procainamide Hcl 500, Major Pharms	00904-2347-70
1000's	$69.97	Procainamide Hcl, Aligen Independ	00405-4853-03
1000's	$72.50	Procainamide Hcl, Consolidated Midland	00223-1457-02
1000's	$84.80	Procainamide HCl, H.C.F.A. F F P	99999-2117-08
1000's	$92.46	Procainamide Hcl, HL Moore Drug Exch	00839-5050-16
1000's	$92.85	Procainamide Hcl, Rugby	00536-4368-10
1000's	$93.00	Procainamide Hcl 500, Major Pharms	00904-2347-80
1000's	$94.34	Procainamide HCl, Schein Pharm (US)	00364-0344-02
1000's	$95.85	Procainamide Hcl, Zenith Labs	00172-2347-80
1000's	$95.85	Procainamide Hcl, Harber Pharm	51432-0374-06

Injection, Solution - Intramuscular; - 100 mg/ml

10 ml	$4.00	Procainamide Hcl, Consolidated Midland	00223-8353-10
10 ml	$11.61	Procainamide Hcl, Elkins Sinn	00641-2587-41
10 ml	$11.94	Procainamide Hcl, Fujisawa USA	00469-2230-30
10 ml	$14.44	Procainamide Hcl, Intl Medication	00548-1199-00
10 ml	$22.09	Procainamide Hcl, Abbott	00074-1902-01
10 ml	**$36.44**	**PRONESTYL, Bristol Myers Squibb**	**00003-0759-20**

Injection, Solution - Intramuscular; - 500 mg/ml

2 ml	$4.00	Procainamide Hcl, Consolidated Midland	00223-8354-02
2 ml	$11.61	Procainamide Hcl, Elkins Sinn	00641-0489-21
2 ml	$11.94	Procainamide Hcl, Fujisawa USA	00469-2220-10
2 ml	$22.09	Procainamide Hcl, Abbott	00074-1903-01
2 ml	**$36.44**	**PRONESTYL, Bristol Myers Squibb**	**00003-1443-04**
2 ml x 10	$50.59	Procainamide HCl, Sanofi Winthrop	00024-1526-02
4 ml	$27.19	Procainamide Hcl, Intl Medication	00548-6201-00

Tablet, Coated, Sustained Action - Oral - 250 mg

100's	$8.37	Procainamide Hcl, US Trading	56126-0332-11
100's	$11.81	Procainamide HCl, Bristol Myers Squibb	00003-0726-50
100's	$12.35	Procainamide Hcl, Lederle Pharm	00005-3195-23
100's	$13.67	Procainamide Hcl, Medirex	57480-0353-01
100's	$13.75	Procainamide Hcl, Sidmak Labs	50111-0339-01
100's	$14.76	Procainamide Hcl, HL Moore Drug Exch	00839-7027-06
100's	$15.00	Procainamide Hcl, United Res	00677-0986-01
100's	$16.40	Procainamide HCl, H.C.F.A. F F P	99999-2117-09
100's	$25.99	Procainamide HCl ER, Schein Pharm (US)	00364-0715-01
120's	$34.98	PROCAN SR, Parke-Davis	00071-0202-25
500's	$57.75	Procainamide HCl, Bristol Myers Squibb	00003-0726-60
500's	$67.32	Procainamide Hcl, Sidmak Labs	50111-0339-02
500's	$82.00	Procainamide HCl, H.C.F.A. F F P	99999-2117-10
500's	$146.00	PROCAN SR, Parke-Davis	00071-0202-30
600's	$164.60	Procainamide Hcl, Medirex	57480-0353-06
1000's	$113.33	Procainamide Hcl, HL Moore Drug Exch	00839-7027-16
1000's	$164.00	Procainamide HCl, H.C.F.A. F F P	99999-2117-11

Tablet, Coated, Sustained Action - Oral - 500 mg

100's	$10.70	Procainamide Hcl, US Trading	56126-0333-11
100's	$15.53	Procainamide Hcl, United Res	00677-0987-01
100's	$15.53	Procainamide HCl, H.C.F.A. F F P	99999-2117-12
100's	$17.78	Procainamide, Rugby	00536-4357-01
100's	$22.44	Procainamide Hcl, Sidmak Labs	50111-0340-01
100's	$22.85	Procainamide Hcl S.R. 500, Major Pharms	00904-2368-60
100's	$25.00	Procainamide Hcl, Goldline Labs	00182-1708-89
100's	$26.22	Procainamide Hcl Sustained Release, Purepac Pharm	00228-2372-10
100's	$26.70	Procainamide HCl, Rugby	00536-5576-01
100's	$26.90	Procainamide Hcl, Qualitest Pharms	00603-5411-21
100's	$26.95	Procainamide Hcl S.R., Invamed	52189-0201-24
100's	$26.99	Procainamide Hcl, Goldline Labs	00182-1708-01
100's	$28.40	Procainamide Hcl, Medirex	57480-0354-01
100's	$29.75	Procainamide Hcl SR, Copley Pharm	38245-0188-10
100's	$29.77	Procainamide HCl Sr, HL Moore Drug Exch	00839-7028-06
100's	$29.89	Procainamide HCl ER, Schein Pharm (US)	00364-0716-01
100's	$29.95	Procainamide Hcl, Parmed Pharms	00349-8978-01
100's	$63.72	PROCAN SR, Parke-Davis	00071-0204-24
120's	$59.52	PROCAN SR, Parke-Davis	00071-0204-25
500's	$77.65	Procainamide HCl, H.C.F.A. F F P	99999-2117-13
500's	$92.50	Procainamide HCl, Major Pharms	00904-2368-40
500's	$107.25	Procainamide Hcl, Sidmak Labs	50111-0340-02
500's	$111.85	Procainamide Hcl, Qualitest Pharms	00603-5411-28
500's	$112.60	Procainamide HCl, Rugby	00536-5576-05
500's	$117.98	Procainamide Hcl, Goldline Labs	00182-1708-05
500's	$117.98	Procainamide Hcl, Parmed Pharms	00349-8395-05
500's	$130.75	Procainamide Hcl S.R., Invamed	52189-0201-29
500's	$131.00	Procainamide HCl ER, Schein Pharm (US)	00364-0716-05
500's	$133.00	Procainamide Hcl Er, Copley Pharm	38245-0188-50
500's	$139.95	Procainamide SR, Parmed Pharms	00349-8978-05
500's	$158.00	Procainamide Hcl SR, Aligen Independ	00405-4859-02
500's	$248.03	PROCAN SR, Parke-Davis	00071-0204-30
600's	$170.40	Procainamide Hcl, Medirex	57480-0354-06
1000's	$155.30	Procainamide HCl, H.C.F.A. F F P	99999-2117-14
1000's	$211.30	Procainamide Hcl ER, Schein Pharm (US)	00364-0716-02

Tablet, Coated, Sustained Action - Oral - 750 mg

100's	$24.38	Procainamide Hcl, United Res	00677-0988-01
100's	$24.38	Procainamide HCl, H.C.F.A. F F P	99999-2117-15
100's	$29.75	Procainamide HCl, Bristol Myers Squibb	00003-0777-50
100's	$29.90	Procainamide Hcl Sr 750, Major Pharms	00904-2369-60
100's	$34.70	Procainamide Hcl, Qualitest Pharms	00603-5412-21
100's	$34.75	Procainamide Hcl, Goldline Labs	00182-1709-01
100's	$34.75	Procainamide, Rugby	00536-4358-01
100's	$37.40	Procainamide Hcl Sr, HL Moore Drug Exch	00839-7029-06
100's	$39.39	Procainamide Hcl Sr 750, Major Pharms	00904-2369-61
100's	$40.95	Procainamide Hcl SR, Copley Pharm	38245-0114-10
100's	$40.95	Procainamide Hcl, Martec Pharms	52555-0456-01
100's	$44.95	Procainamide Hcl Sr, Parmed Pharms	00349-8396-01
100's	$94.60	PROCAN SR, Parke-Davis	00071-0205-24
120's	$88.24	PROCAN SR, Parke-Davis	00071-0205-25
250's	$50.50	Procainamide Hcl Sr 750, Major Pharms	00904-2369-70
500's	$121.90	Procainamide HCl, H.C.F.A. F F P	99999-2117-16
500's	$144.38	Procainamide HCl, Bristol Myers Squibb	00003-0777-60
500's	$170.00	Procainamide, Rugby	00536-4358-05
500's	$184.00	Procainamide Hcl SR, Copley Pharm	38245-0114-50
500's	$368.23	PROCAN SR, Parke-Davis	00071-0205-30

Tablet, Coated, Sustained Action - Oral - 1000 mg

100's	$121.04	PROCAN SR, Parke-Davis	00071-0207-24
120's	$113.00	PROCAN SR, Parke-Davis	00071-0207-25

HOW SUPPLIED - NOT RATED EQUIVALENT:

Tablet, Coated, Sustained Action - Oral - 500 mg

100's	$20.13	Procainamide HCl, Bristol Myers Squibb	00003-0742-50
100's	$20.15	Procainamide Hcl Sr, Harber Pharm	51432-0373-03
100's	$29.75	Procainamide Hcl, Martec Pharms	52555-0480-01
100's	**$56.81**	**PRONESTYL-SR, Bristol Myers Squibb**	**00003-0775-51**
100's	**$64.49**	**PRONESTYL-SR, Bristol Myers Squibb**	**00003-0775-50**
500's	$98.00	Procainamide HCl, Bristol Myers Squibb	00003-0742-60
500's	$100.25	Procainamide Hcl, Harber Pharm	51432-0373-06
500's	$130.85	Procainamide Hcl, Martec Pharms	52555-0480-05

Tablet, Sugar Coated - Oral - 250 mg

100's	$12.70	Procainamide Hcl Sr, Harber Pharm	51432-0371-03
100's	**$53.93**	**PRONESTYL, Bristol Myers Squibb**	**00003-0431-50**

Tablet, Sugar Coated - Oral - 375 mg

100's	**$74.79**	**PRONESTYL, Bristol Myers Squibb**	**00003-0434-50**

Tablet, Sugar Coated - Oral - 500 mg

100's	**$97.10**	**PRONESTYL 500, Bristol Myers Squibb**	**00003-0438-50**

PROCAINE HYDROCHLORIDE *(002118)*

CATEGORIES: Anesthesia; Local Anesthetics; Pregnancy Category C; FDA Approval Pre 1982

BRAND NAMES: **Novocain**; Ravocaine-Novocain-Levophed

DESCRIPTION:

LOCAL ANESTHETIC

Local Anesthetic for Major Infiltration and Peripheral Nerve Block:

These Solutions Are Not Intended For Spinal Or Epidural Anesthesia Or Dental Use

Procaine Hydrochloride (abbreviated here as Procaine HCl), is a benzoic acid, 4-amino-, 2-(diethylamino) ethyl ester, monohydrochloride, the ester of diethylaminoethanol and para-aminobenzoic acid.

It is a white crystalline, odorless powder that is freely soluble in water, but less soluble in alcohol an has a molecular weight of 272.77

(TABLE 1 shows the composition of solutions).

TABLE 1 Composition of Available Solutions

Each ml contains	1% Ampul	1% Vial	2% Vial
Procaine HCl	10 mg	10 mg	20 mg
Acetone sodium bisulfite	≤ 1 mg	≤ 2 mg	≤ 2 mg
Chlorobutanol	—	≤ 2.5 mg	≤ 2.5 mg

Acetone sodium bisulfite is added as an antioxidant in all products, and is added as an antimicrobial preservative in the multiple-dose vial.

The solutions are made isotonic with sodium chloride and the pH is adjusted between 3 and 5.5 with sodium hydroxide and/or hydrochloric acid.

Procaine HCl is available as sterile solutions in concentrations of 1% and 2% for injection via local infiltration and peripheral nerve block.

SPINAL INJECTION

Procaine Hydrochloride (abbreviated here as Procaine HCl), is a benzoic acid, 4-amino-, 2-(diethylamino) ethyl ester, monohydrochloride, the ester of diethylaminoethanol and para-aminobenzoic acid.

It is a white crystalline, odorless powder that is freely soluble in water but less soluble in alcohol. Each ml contains 100 mg Procaine HCl

and 4 mg acetone sodium bisulfite as antioxidant. DO NO NOT USE SOLUTIONS IF CRYSTALS, CLOUDINESS, OR DISCOLORATION IS OBSERVED EXAMINE SOLUTIONS CAREFULLY BEFORE USE. REAUTOCLAVING INCREASES LIKELIHOOD OF CRYSTAL FORMATION.

CLINICAL PHARMACOLOGY:

LOCAL ANESTHETIC

Local anesthetics block the generation and the conduction of nerve impulses, presumably by increasing the threshold for electrical excitation in the nerve, by slowing the propagation of the nerve impulse, and by reducing the rate of rise of the action potential. In general, the progression of anesthesia is related to the diameter, myelination, and conduction velocity of affected nerve fibers. Clinically, the order of loss of nerve function is as follows: pain, temperature, touch, proprioception, and skeletal muscle tone. Procaine HCl lacks topical anesthetic activity.

Systemic absorption of local anesthetics produces effects on the cardiovascular and the central nervous systems. At blood concentrations achieved with normal therapeutic doses, changes in cardiac conduction, excitability, refractoriness, contractility, and peripheral vascular resistance are minimal. However, toxic blood concentrations depress cardiac conduction and excitability, which may lead to atrioventricular block and ultimately to cardiac arrest. In addition, myocardial contractility is depressed and peripheral vasodilation occurs, leading to decreased cardiac output and arterial blood pressure.

Following systemic absorption, local anesthetics can produce central nervous system stimulation, depression, or both. Apparent central stimulation is manifested as restlessness, tremors and shivering, progressing to convulsions, followed by depression, and coma progressing ultimately to respiratory arrest. However, the local anesthetics have a primary depressant effect on the medulla and on higher centers. The depressed stage may occur without a prior exited stage.

Pharmacokinetics: The rate system absorption of local anesthetics is dependant upon the total dose and concentration of drug administered, the route of administration, the vascularity of the administration site, and the presence or absence of epinephrine in the anesthetic solution. A dilute concentration of epinephrine (1:200,000 or 5 mcg/ml) usually reduces the rate of absorption and plasma concentration of Procaine HCl. It also will promote local hemostasis and increase the duration of anesthesia.

Onset of anesthesia with Procaine HCl is rapid, the time of onset for sensory block ranging from about two to five minutes depending upon such factors as the anesthetic technique, the type of block, the concentration of the solution, and the individual patient. The degree of motor blockade produced is dependent on the concentration of the solution.

The duration of anesthesia also varies depending upon the technique and type of block, the concentration, and the individual. Procaine HCl will normally provide anesthesia which is adequate for one hour.

The duration of anesthesia also varies depending upon the technique and type of block, the concentration, and the individual. Procaine HCl will normally provide anesthesia which is adequate for one hour.

CLINICAL PHARMACOLOGY: *(cont'd)*

Local anesthetics are bound to plasma proteins in varying degrees. Generally, the lower the plasma concentration of the drug, the higher the percentage of drug bound to plasma.

Local anesthetics appear to cross the placenta by passive diffusion. The rate and degree of diffusion is governed by the degree of plasma protein binding, the degree of ionization, and the degree of lipid solubility. Fetal/maternal ratios of local anesthetics appear to be inversely related to the degree of plasma protein binding, because only the free, unbound drug is available for placental transfer. The extent of placental transfer is also determined by the degree of ionization and lipid solubility of the drug. Lipid, soluble nonionized drugs readily enter the fetal blood from the maternal circulation.

Depending upon the route of administration, local anesthetics are distributed to some extent to all body tissues, with high concentrations found in highly perfused organs such as the liver, lungs, heart, and brain.

Various pharmacokinetics parameters of the local anesthetics can be significantly altered by the presence of hepatic or renal disease, addition of epinephrine, factors affecting urinary pH, renal blood flow, the route of drug administration, and the age of patient. The *in vitro* plasma half-life of Procaine HCl in adults is 40 ± 9 seconds and in neonates 84 ± 30 seconds.

Procaine HCl is readily absorbed following parenteral administration and is rapidly hydrolyzed by plasma cholinesterase to para-aminobenzoic acid and diethylaminoethanol.

The para-aminobenzoic acid metabolite inhibits the action of the sulfonamides. (see PRECAUTIONS.)

For Procaine HCl, approximately 90% of the para-aminobenzoic acid metabolite and its conjugates and 33% of the diethylaminoethanol metabolite are recovered in the urine, while less than 2% of the administered dose is recovered unchanged in the urine.

SPINAL INJECTION

Procaine HCl stabilizes the neuronal membrane an prevents the initiation and transmission of nerve impulses, thereby effecting local anesthesia. Procaine HCl lacks surface anesthetic activity. The onset of action is rapid (2 to 5 minutes) and the duration of action is relatively short (average 1 to 1 1/2 hours), depending upon the anesthetic technique, the type of block, the concentration, and the individual patient.

Procaine HCl is readily absorbed following parenteral administration and is rapidly hydrolyzed by plasma cholinesterase to aminobenzoic acid and diethylaminoethanol.

A vasoconstrictor maybe added to the solution of Procaine HCl to promote local hemostasis, delay systemic absorption, and increase duration of anesthesia.

INDICATIONS AND USAGE:

Local Anesthetic: Procaine HCl is indicated for the production of local or regional analgesia and anesthesia by local infiltration and peripheral nerve block techniques.

The routes of administration and concentrations are: for local infiltration use 0.25% to 0.5% (via dilution) and for peripheral nerve blocks use 0.5% (via dilution), 1% and 2% (see DOSAGE AND ADMINISTRATIONfor additional information.)

Standard textbooks should be consulted to determine the accepted procedures and techniques for the administration of Procaine HCl.

Spinal Injection: Procaine HCl is indicated for spinal anesthesia.

CONTRAINDICATIONS:

Local Anesthetic: Procaine HCl is contraindicated in patients with a known hypersensitivity to procaine, drugs of a similar chemical configuration, or a para-aminobenzoic acid or its derivatives.

It is also contraindicated in patients with a known hypersensitivity to other components of solutions of Procaine HCl.

Spinal Injection: Spinal anesthesia with Procaine HCl is contraindicated in patients with generalized septicemia: sepsis at the proposed injection site; certain diseases of the cerebrospinal system, e.g., meningitis, syphilis; and a known hypersensitivity to the drug, drugs of a similar chemical configuration, or aminobenzoic acid or its derivatives.

The decision as to whether or not spinal anesthesia should be used in an individual case should be made by the physician after weighing the advantages with the risks and possible complications.

WARNINGS:

LOCAL ANESTHETIC

Contains acetone sodium bisulfite, a sulfite that may cause allergic-type reactions including anaphylactic symptoms and life-threatening or less severe asthmatic episodes in certain susceptible people. The overall prevalence of sulfite sensitivity in the general population is unknown and probably low. Sulfite sensitivity is seen more frequently in asthmatic than in non-asthmatic people.

LOCAL ANESTHETICS SHOULD ONLY BE EMPLOYED BY CLINICIANS WHO ARE WELL VERSED IN DIAGNOSIS AND MANAGEMENT OF DOSE-RELATED TOXICITY AND OTHER ACUTE EMERGENCIES WHICH MIGHT ARISE FROM THE BLOCK TO BE EMPLOYED AND THEN ONLY AFTER INSURING THE IMMEDIATE AVAILABILITY OF OXYGEN, OTHER RESUSCITATIVE DRUGS, CARDIOPULMONARY RESUSCITATIVE EQUIPMENT, AND THE PERSONNEL RESOURCES NEEDED FOR PROPER MANAGEMENT OF TOXIC REACTIONS AND RELATED EMERGENCIES (see also ADVERSE REACTIONS and PRECAUTIONS.)**DELAY IN PROPER MANAGEMENT OF DOSE-RELATED TOXICITY, UNDERVENTILATION FROM ANY CAUSE, AND/OR ALTERED SENSITIVITY MAY LEAD TO THE DEVELOPMENT OF ACIDOSIS, CARDIAC ARREST, AND, POSSIBLY DEATH.**

It is essential that aspiration for blood or cerebrospinal fluid, where applicable, be done prior to injecting any local anesthetic, both the original dose and all subsequent doses, to avoid intravascular or subarachnoid injection.

Reactions resulting in fatality have occurred on rare occasions with the use of local anesthetics, even in the absence of a history of hypersensitivity. Large doses of local anesthetics should not be used in patients with heartblock.

Procaine HCl with epinephrine or other vasopressors should not be used concomitantly with ergot-type oxytocic drugs, because a severe persistent hypertension may occur. Likewise, solutions of Procaine HCl containing a vasoconstrictor, such as epinephrine, should be used with extreme caution in patients receiving monoamine oxidase inhibitors (MAOI) or antidepressants of the triptyline or imipramine types, because severe prolonged hypertension or disturbances of cardiac rhythm may occur.

Local anesthetic procedures should be used with caution when there is inflammation and/or sepsis in the region of the proposed injection.

Mixing or the prior or intercurrent use of any local anesthetic with Procaine HCl cannot be recommended because of insufficient data on the clinical use of such mixtures.

WARNINGS: *(cont'd)*

SPINAL INJECTION

RESUSCITATIVE EQUIPMENT AND DRUGS SHOULD BE IMMEDIATELY AVAILABLE WHENEVER ANY LOCAL ANESTHETIC DRUG IS USED. Spinal anesthesia should not.only be administered by those qualified to do so.

Large doses of local anesthetics should not be used in patients with heartblock.

Reactions resulting in fatality have occurred on rare occasions with the use of local anesthetics, even in the absence of a history of hypersensitivity.

Usage in Pregnancy: Safe use of Procaine HCl has not been established with respect to adverse effects on fetal development. Careful consideration should be given to this fact before administering this drug to women of childbearing potential particularly during early pregnancy. This does not exclude the use of the drug at term for obstetrical analgesia. Vasopressor agents (administered for the treatment of hypotension or added to the anesthetic solution for vasoconstriction) should be used with extreme caution in the presence of of oxytocic drugs as they may produce severe, persistent hypertension with possible rupture of a cerebral blood vessel.

Solutions which contain a vasoconstrictor should be used with extreme caution in patients receiving drugs known to produce alterations in blood pressure (*i.e.,* monoamine oxidase inhibitors (MAOI). tricyclic antidepressants, phenothiazines, etc), as either severe sustained hypertension or hypotension may occur.

Local anesthetic procedures should be used with caution when there is inflammation and/or sepsis in the region of the proposed injection.

Contains acetone sodium bisulfite, a sulfite that may cause allergic-type reactions including anaphylactic symptoms and life-threatening or less severe asthmatic episodes in certain susceptible people. The overall prevalence of sulfite sensitivity in the general population in unknown and probably low. Sulfite sensitivity is seen more frequently in asthmatic than in non asthmatic people.

PRECAUTIONS:

GENERAL

The safety and effectiveness of local and a spinal anesthetic depend on proper dosage, correct technique, adequate precautions, and readiness for emergencies. Resuscitative equipment, oxygen, and other resuscitative drugs should be available for immediate use (see WARNINGS and ADVERSE REACTIONS). During major regional nerve blocks, the patient should have IV fluids running via an indwelling catheter to assure a functioning intravenous pathway. The lowest dosage of local anesthetic that results in effective anesthesia should be used to avoid high plasma levels and serious adverse effects. Injections should be made slowly, with frequent aspirations before and during the injection to avoid intravascular injection. Current opinion favors fractional administration with constant attention to the patient, rather than rapid bolus injection. Syringe aspirations should also be performed before and during each supplemental injection in continuous (intermittent) catheter techniques. An intramuscular injection is still possible even if aspirations for blood are negative.

Injection of repeated doses of local anesthetics may cause significant increases in plasma levels with each repeated dose due to slow accumulation of the drug or its metabolites or to slow metabolic degradation. Tolerance to alleviated blood levels varies with the status of the patient. Debilitated, elderly patients and acutely ill patients should be given reduced doses commensurate with their age and physical status. Local anesthetics should also be used with caution in patients with severe disturbances of cardiac rhythm, shock, heartblock, or hypotension.

Careful and constant monitoring of cardiovascular and respiratory (adequacy of ventilation) vital signs and the patient's state of consciousness should be performed after each local anesthetic injection. It should be kept in mind at such times that restlessness, anxiety, incoherent speech, light-headedness, numbness, and tingling of the mouth and lips, metallic taste, tinnitus, dizziness, blurred vision, tremors, twitching, depression, or drowsiness may be early warning signs of central nervous system toxicity.

Local anesthetic solutions containing a vasoconstrictor should be used cautiously and in carefully circumscribed quantities in the areas of the body supplied by end arteries, or those areas having otherwise compromised blood supply such as digits, nose, external ear, penis. Patients with peripheral vascular disease and hypertensive vascular disease may exhibit an exaggerated vasoconstrictor response. Ischemic injury or necrosis may result.

Procaine HCl should be used with caution in patients with known allergies and sensitivities. A thorough history of the patient's prior experience with Procaine HCl or other local anesthetics as well as concomitant or recent drug use should be taken (see CONTRAINDICATIONS and WARNINGS.)

Because ester-type local anesthetics such as Procaine HCl are hydrolyzed by plasma cholinesterase produced by the liver and excreted by the kidneys, these drugs, especially repeat doses, should be used cautiously in patients with hepatic disease. Because of their inability to metabolize local anesthetics normally, patients with severe hepatic disease are at a greater risk of developing toxic plasma concentrations. Local anesthetics should also be used with caution in patients with impaired cardiovascular function because they be less able to compensate for functional changes associated with the prolongation of AV conduction produced by these drugs.

Serious dose-related cardiac arrhythmias may occur if preparations containing a vasoconstrictor such as epinephrine are employed in patients during or following the administration of potent inhalation anesthetics. In deciding whether to use these products concurrently in the same patient, the combined action of both agents upon the myocardium, the concentration and volume of vasoconstrictor used, and the time since injection, when applicable, should be taken into account.

Many drugs used during the conduction of anesthesia are considered potential triggering agents for familial malignant hyperthermia. Because it is not known whether ester-type local anesthetics may trigger this reaction and because the need for supplemental general anesthesia cannot be predicted in advance, it is suggested that a standard protocol for management should be available. Early unexplained signs if tachycardia, tachypnea, labile blood pressure, and metabolic acidosis may precede temperature elevation. Successful outcome is dependant on early diagnosis, prompt discontinuance of the suspect triggering agent(s), and institution of treatment, including oxygen therapy, indicated supportive measures, and dantrolene. (Consult dantrolene sodium IV package insert before using).

Uses in Head and Neck Area: Small doses of local anesthetics injected into the head and neck area may produce adverse reactions similar to systemic toxicity seen with unintentional IV injections of larger doses. Confusion, convulsions, respiratory depression and/or respiratory arrest and cardiovascular stimulation or depression have been reported.

These reactions may be due to intra-arterial injection of the local anesthetic with retrograde flow to cerebral circulation. Patients receiving these blocks should have their circulation and respiration monitored and be constantly observed. Resuscitative equipment and personnel for treating adverse reactions should be immediately available. Dosage recommendation should not be exceeded.

PRECAUTIONS: *(cont'd)*

INFORMATION FOR THE PATIENT

When appropriate, patients should be informed, in advance, that they may experience temporary loss of sensation and motor activity following proper administration of regional anesthesia. Also, when appropriate, the physician should discuss other information including adverse reactions in the package inserts.

CARCINOGENESIS, MUTAGENESIS, AND IMPAIRMENT OF FERTILITY

Long-term studies in animals of most local anesthetics, including Procaine HCl, to evaluate the carcinogenic potentials have not been conducted. Mutagenic potential or the effect on fertility have not been determined. There is no evidence from human data that Procaine HCl may be carcinogenic, or mutagenic, or that it impairs fertility.

PREGNANCY CATEGORY C

Animal reproduction studies have not been conducted with Procaine HCl. It is not known whether procaine can cause fetal harm when administered to a pregnant woman or can affect reproduction capacity. Procaine HCl should be given to a pregnant women only if clearly needed and the potential benefits outweigh the risk. This does not exclude the use of Procaine HCl at term for obstetrical anesthesia or analgesia (see Labor and Delivery.)

LABOR AND DELIVERY

Local anesthetics rapidly cross the placenta, and when used for paracervical or pudendal block anesthesia can cause varying degrees of maternal, fetal, and neonatal toxicity (see CLINICAL PHARMACOLOGY.) The incidence and degree of toxicity depend upon the procedure performed, the type and amount of drug used, and the technique of drug administration. Adverse reactions in the parturient, fetus, and neonate involve alterations of the central nervous system, peripheral vascular tone, and cardiac function.

Maternal hypotension has resulted from regional anesthesia. Local aesthetics produce vasodilation by blocking by blocking sympathetic nerves. Elevating the patient's legs and positioning her on her left side will help prevent decreases in blood pressure. The heart rate also should be monitored continuously and electric fetal monitoring is highly advisable.

Paracervical or pudendal anesthesia may alter the forces of parturition through changes in uterine contractility or maternal expulsive efforts. In one study, paracervical block anesthesia was associated with a decrease in the mean duration of first stage labor and facilitation of cervical dilation. The use of obstetrical anesthesia may increase the need for forceps assistance.

The use of some local anesthetic drug products during labor and delivery may be followed by diminished muscle strength and tone for the first day or two of life. The long-term significance of these observations is unknown.

Fetal bradycardia which infrequently follows paracervical block may be indicative of high fetal blood concentrations and procaine with resultant fetal acidosis. Fetal heart rate should be monitored prior to and during paracervical block. Added risk appears to be present in prematurity, toxemia of pregnancy, and fetal distress. The physician should weigh the considering paracervical block in these in these conditions. Careful adherence to recommended dosage is of the utmost importance in paracervical block. Failure to achieve adequate analgesia with these doses should arouse suspicion of intravascular or fetal injection.

Cases compatible with unintended fetal intracranial injection of local anesthetic solution have been reported following intended paracervical or pudendal block or both. Babies so affected present with unexplained neonatal depression at birth, which correlates with high local anesthetic serum levels, and usually manifest seizures within six hours. Prompt use of supportive measures combined with forced urinary excretion of the local anesthetic has been used successfully to manage this complication.

Case reports of maternal convulsions and cardiovascular collapse following use of some local anesthetics for paracervical block in early pregnancy (as anesthesia for elective abortion) suggest that systemic absorption under these circumstances may be rapid. The recommended maximum dose of the local anesthetic should not be exceeded. Injection should be made slowly and with frequent aspiration. Allow a five-minute interval between sides.

It is extremely important to avoid aortocaval compression by the gravid uterus during administration of regional block to parturients. To do this, the patient must be maintained in the left lateral decubitus position or a blanket roll or sandbag may be placed beneath the right hip and the gravid uterus displaced to the left.

NURSING MOTHERS

It is not known whether local anesthetic drugs are excreted in human milk. Because many drugs are excreted in human milk, caution should be exercised when local anesthetics to a nursing woman.

PEDIATRIC USE

(see DOSAGE AND ADMINISTRATION.)

SPINAL INJECTION

Standard textbooks should be consulted for specific techniques and precautions for various spinal anesthetic procedures. The safety and effectiveness of a spinal anesthetic depend upon proper dosage, correct technique, adequate precautions, and readiness for emergencies. The lowest dosage that results in effective anesthesia should be used to avoid high plasma levels and possible adverse effects. Tolerance varies with the status of the patient. Debilitated, elderly patients, or acutely ill patients should be given reduced doses commensurate with their weight and physical status. Reduced dosages are also indicated for obstetric delivery and patients with increased intra-abdominal pressure.

The decision whether or not to use spinal anesthesia in the following disease states depends on the physician's appraisal of the advantages as opposed to the risk: cardiovascular disease (*i.e.,* shock, hypertension, anemia, etc), pulmonary disease, renal impairment, metabolic or endocrine disorders, gastrointestinal disorders (*i.e.,* intestinal obstruction, peritonitis, etc), or complicated obstetrical deliveries.

PROCAINE HCl SHOULD BE USED WITH CAUTION IN PATIENTS KNOWN WITH DRUG ALLERGIES AND SENSITIVES. A thorough history of patient's prior experience with Procaine HCl or local anesthetics as well as concomitant or recent drug use of should be taken (see CONTRAINDICATIONS.) Procaine HCl should not be used in any condition in which a sulfonamide drug is being employed since aminobenzoic acid inhibits the action of sulfonamides.

Solutions containing a vasopressor should be used with caution in the presence of diseases which may adversely affect the cardiovascular system.

Procaine HCl should be used with caution in patients with severe disturbances of cardiac rhythm, shock or heartblock.

DRUG INTERACTIONS:

The administration of local anesthetic solutions containing epinephrine or norepinephrine to patients receiving Monoamine oxidase inhibitors tricyclic antidepressants may produce severe, prolonged hypertension. Concurrent use of these agents should generally be avoided. In situations when concurrent therapy is necessary, careful patient monitoring is essential.

Concurrent administration of vasopressor drugs and of ergot-type oxytocic drugs may cause severe, persistent hypertension or cerebrovascular accidents.

Phenothiazines and butyrophenones may reduce or reverse the pressor effect of epinephrine.

DRUG INTERACTIONS: *(cont'd)*

The clinical observation has been made that despite adequate sulfonamide therapy local infections have occurred in areas infiltrated with Procaine HCl prior to diagnostic punctures and drainage procedures. Therefore, Procaine HCl should not be used in any condition in which a sulfonamide drug is being employed since para-aminobenzoic acid inhibits the action of sulfonamide.

ADVERSE REACTIONS:

Reactions to procaine are characteristic of those associated with other ester-type local anesthetics. A major cause of adverse reactions to this group of drugs is excessive plasma levels which may be due to overdosage, rapid absorption, inadvertent intravascular injection, or slow metabolic degradation.

A small number of reactions may result from hypersensitivity, idiosyncrasy, or diminished tolerance to normal dosage.

Systemic: The most commonly encountered acute adverse experiences which demand immediate countermeasures are related to the central nervous system and the cardiovascular system. These adverse experiences are generally dose related and due to high plasma levels, which may result from overdosage, rapid absorption from the injection site, diminished tolerance, or from unintentional intravascular injection of the local anesthetic solution. In addition to systemic dose-related toxicity, unintentional subarachnoid injection or drug during the intended performance of nerve blocks near the vertebral column (especially in the head and neck region), may result in underventilation or apnea ("Total or High Spinal"). Factors influencing plasma protein binding, such as acidosis, systemic diseases which alter protein production, or competition of other drugs for protein binding sites may diminish individual tolerance.

Plasma cholinesterase deficiency may also account for diminished tolerance to ester-type local anesthetics.

Central Nervous System Reactions: These are characterized by excitation and/or depression. Restlessness, anxiety, dizziness, tinnitus, blurred vision, or tremors may occur, possibly proceeding to convulsions. However, excitement may be transient or absent, with depression being the first manifestation of an adverse reaction. This may quickly be followed by drowsiness merging into unconsciousness and respiratory arrest.

The incidence of convulsions associated with the use of local anesthetics varies with the procedure used and the total dose administered.

Cardiovascular Reactions: High doses or inadvertent intravascular injection may lead to high plasma levels and related depression of the myocardium, decreased cardiac output, heartblock, hypotension (or sometimes hypotension), bradycardia, ventricular arrhythmias, and cardiac arrest. (See WARNINGS, PRECAUTIONS, and OVERDOSAGE).

Allergic: Allergic-type reactions are rare and may occur as a result of sensitivity to the local anesthetic or to other formulation ingredients, such as the antimicrobial preservative-chlorobutanol contained in multiple-dose vials. These reactions are characterized by signs such urticaria, pruritus, erythema, angioneurotic edema (including laryngeal edema), tachycardia, sneezing, nausea, vomiting, dizziness, syncope, excessive sweating, elevated temperature and, possibly, anaphylactoid-like symptomatology (including severe hypotension). Cross sensitivity among members of the ester-type local anesthetic group has been reported. The usefulness of screening for sensitivity has not been definitely established.

Neurologic: The incidences of adverse neurologic reactions associated with the use of local anesthetics may be related to the total dose of local anesthetic administered, and are also dependent upon the particular drug used, the route of administration, and the physical status of the patient. Many of these effects may be related to local anesthetic techniques, with or without a contribution from the drug.

Treatment of Reactions: Toxic effects of local anesthetics require symptomatic treatment: There is no specific cure. The physician should be prepared to maintain an airway and to support ventilation with oxygen and assisted or controlled respiration as required. Supportive treatment of the cardiovascular system includes intravenous fluids and, when appropriate, vasopressors (preferably those that stimulate the myocardium, such as ephedrine). Convulsions may be controlled with oxygen and by the intravenous administration of diazepam or ultra-short acting barbiturates or a short-acting muscle relaxant (succinylcholine). Intravenous anticonvulsant agents and muscle relaxants should only be administered by those familiar with their use and only when ventilation and oxygenation are assured. In spinal and epidural anesthesia, sympathetic blockade also occurs as a pharmacological reaction, resulting in peripheral vasodilation and often *hypotension*. The extent of the hypotension will usually depend on the number of dermatomes blocked. The blood pressure should therefore be monitored in the early phases of anesthesia. If hypotension occurs, it is readily controlled by vasoconstrictors administered wither by the intramuscular or the intravenous route, the dosage of which would depend on the severity of the hypotension and the response to treatment.

OVERDOSAGE:

Acute emergencies from local anesthetics are generally related to high plasma levels encountered during therapeutic use of local anesthetics or to unintended subarachnoid injection of local anesthetic solution (See ADVERSE REACTIONS, WARNINGS, and PRECAUTIONS).

Management of Local Anesthetics Emergencies: The first consideration is prevention, best accomplished by careful and constant monitoring of cardiovascular and respiratory vital signs, and the patient's state of consciousness after each local anesthetic injection. At the first sign of change, oxygen should be administered.

The first step in the management of systemic toxic reactions, as well as underventilations or apnea due to unintentional subarachnoid injection of drug solution, consists of immediate attention to the establishment and maintenance of a patient airway, and effective assisted or controlled ventilation with 100% oxygen with a delivery system capable of permitting immediate positive airway pressure by mask. This may prevent convulsions if they have not already occurred.

If necessary, use of drugs to control the convulsions. A 50 mg to 100 mg bolus IV injection of succinylcholine will paralyze the patient without depressing the central nervous or cardiovascular systems and facilitate ventilation. A bolus IV dose of 5 mg to 10 mg of diazepam or 50 mg to 100 mg of thiopental will permit ventilation and counteract central nervous system stimulation, but these drugs also depress central nervous system, respiratory and cardiac function, add to postictal depression, and may result in apnea. IV barbiturates, anticonvulsants agents, or muscle relaxants should only be administered by those familiar with their use. Immediately after the institution of these ventilatory measures, the adequacy of the circulation should be evaluated. Supportive treatment of circulatory depression may require administration of IV fluids and, when appropriate, a vasopressor dictated by the clinical situation (such as ephedrine or epinephrine to enhance myocardial contractile force).

Endotracheal intubation, employing drugs and techniques familiar to the clinician, may be indicated, after initial administration of oxygen by mask, if difficulty is encountered in the maintenance of a patent airway or if prolonged ventilatory support (assisted or controlled) is indicated.

Recent clinical data from patients experiencing local anesthetic-induced convulsions demonstrated rapid development hypoxia, hypercarbia, and acidosis within a minute of the onset of convulsions. These observations suggest that oxygen consumption and carbon dioxide

OVERDOSAGE: *(cont'd)*

production are greatly increased during local anesthetic convulsions, and emphasize the importance of immediate and effective ventilation with oxygen which may avoid cardiac arrest.

If not treated immediately, convulsions with simultaneous hypoxia, hypercarbia, and acidosis plus myocardial depression from the direct effects of the local anesthetic may result in cardiac arrhythmias, bradycardia, asystole, ventricular fibrillation, or cardiac arrest. Respiratory abnormalities, including apnea, may occur. Underventilation or apnea due to unintentional subarachnoid injection of local anesthetic solution may produce these same signs and also lead to cardiac arrest if ventilatory support is not instituted. If cardiac arrest should occur, standard cardiopulmonary resuscitative measures should be instituted and maintained for a prolonged period if necessary. Recovery has been reported after prolonged resuscitative efforts.

The supine position is dangerous in pregnant women at term because of aortocaval compression by the gravid uterus. Therefore, during treatment of systemic toxicity, maternal hypotension, or fetal bradycardia following regional block, the parturient should be maintained in left lateral decubitus position if possible, or manual displacement of the uterus off the great vessels be accomplished.

The IV and subcutaneous and intraperitoneal LD_{50} of Procaine HCl in mice is 46 mg/kg to 80 mg/kg and 400 mg/kg and 200 mg/kg respectively.

DOSAGE AND ADMINISTRATION:

LOCAL ANESTHETIC

The dose of any local anesthetic administered varies with the anesthetic procedure, the area to be anesthetized, the vascularity of the tissue, the number of neuronal segments to be blocked, the depth of anesthesia and degree of muscle relaxation required, the duration of anesthesia desired, individual tolerance, and the physical condition of the patient. The smallest dose and concentration required to produce the desired result should be administered. Dosages of Procaine HCl should be reduced for elderly and debilitated patients and patients with cardiac and/or liver disease. The rapid injection of a large volume of local anesthetic solution should be avoided and fractional doses should be used when feasible.

For specific techniques and procedures, refer to standard textbooks.

For infiltration anesthesia, 0.25% or 0.5% solution; 350 mg to 600 mg is generally considered to be a single safe total dose. To prepare 60 ml of 0.5% solution (5 mg/ml), dilute 30 ml of the 1% solution with 30 ml sodium chloride injection 0.9%. To prepare 60 ml of a 0.25% solution (2.5 mg/ml), dilute 15 ml of 1% solution with 45 ml sodium chloride injection 0.9%. An anesthetic solution of 0.5 ml to 1 ml of epinephrine 1:1,000 per 100 ml may be added for vasoconstrictive effect (1:200,000 to 1:000,000).(See WARNINGS and PRECAUTIONS).

For peripheral nerve block 0.5% solution (up to 200 ml), 1% solution (up to 100 ml), or 2% solution (up to 50 ml). The use of 2% solution should usually be limited to cases requiring a small volume of anesthetic solution (10 ml to 25 ml). An anesthetic solution of 0.5% ml to 1 ml of epinephrine 1:1,000 per 100 ml may be added for vasoconstrictive effect (1:200,000 to 1:000,000). (See WARNINGS and PRECAUTIONS).

THE USUAL TOTAL DOSE DURING ONE TREATMENT SHOULD NOT EXCEED 1,000 MG.

This product should be inspected visually for particulate matter and discoloration prior to administration whenever solution and container permit. Do not use solutions if crystals, cloudiness, or discoloration is observed. Examine solution carefully before use. Reautoclaving increases likelihood of crystal formation. Solutions which are discarded or which contain particulate matter should be administered.

Unused portions of solutions not containing preservatives should be discarded.

Pediatric Use: In children 15 mg/kg of a 0.5% solution for local infiltration is the maximum recommended dose.

SPINAL INJECTION

As with all local anesthetics, the dose of Procaine HCl varies and depends upon the area to be anesthetized, the vascularity of the tissues, the number of neuronal segments to be blocked, individual tolerance, and the technique of anesthesia. The lowest dose needed to provide effective anesthesia should be administered. For specific techniques and procedures, refer to standard textbooks (TABLE 2).

TABLE 2 Recommended Dosage For Spinal Anesthesia

Procaine HCl 10% Solution

Extent of Anesthesia	Volume of 10% Solution (ml)	Volume of Diluent (ml)	Total Dose (mg)	Site of Inj. (lumbar interspace)
Perineum	0.5	0.5	50	4th
Perineum and lower extremities	1	1	100	3rd or 4th
Up to costal margin	2	1	200	2nd, 3rd or 4th

The diluent may be sterile normal saline, sterile distilled water, spinal fluid; and for hyperbaric technique, sterile dextrose solution.

The first rate of injection is 1 ml per 5 seconds. Full anesthesia and fixation usually occurs in 5 minutes.

Sterilization: The drug in intact ampules is sterile. The preferred method of destroying bacteria on the exterior of ampules before opening is heat sterilization (autoclaving). Immersion in antiseptic solution is not recommended.

Autoclave at 15-pound pressure, at 121°C (250°F), for 15 minutes. The diluent dextrose may show some brown discoloration due to carmelization.

Protect solutions from Light.

The air in the ampuls has been displaced by nitrogen gas.

HOW SUPPLIED - RATED THERAPEUTICALLY EQUIVALENT:

Injection, Solution - Infiltration - 1 %

2 ml x 25	**$76.88**	**NOVOCAIN, Sanofi Winthrop**	**00024-1381-25**
6 ml x 50	**$284.46**	**NOVOCAIN, Sanofi Winthrop**	**00024-1381-05**
30 ml	$0.88	Procaine Hcl, Lannett	00527-0188-58
30 ml	$3.50	1% PROCAINE HCL, Abbott	00074-1923-04
30 ml	**$14.13**	**NOVOCAIN, Sanofi Winthrop**	**00024-1385-01**
100 ml	$1.30	Procaine Hcl, Lannett	00527-0188-59

Injection, Solution - Infiltration - 2 %

30 ml	$0.68	Procaine Hcl, Lannett	00527-0112-58
30 ml	$2.39	Procaine Hcl, McGuff	49072-0587-30
30 ml	$3.40	Procaine Hcl, Pasadena	00418-2211-61
30 ml	$3.50	2% PROCAINE HCL INJ., Abbott	00074-1953-04
30 ml	$4.00	Procaine Hcl, Consolidated Midland	00223-8362-30
30 ml	$4.13	Procaine Hcl, Schein Pharm (US)	00364-2371-56
30 ml	$4.13	Procaine Hcl, Steris Labs	00402-0527-30

HOW SUPPLIED - RATED THERAPEUTICALLY EQUIVALENT: *(cont'd)*

30 ml	$4.20	Procaine Hydrochloride Injection, IDE-Interstate	00814-6354-46
30 ml	**$14.13**	**NOVOCAIN, Sanofi Winthrop**	**00024-1386-01**
100 ml	$1.30	Procaine Hcl, Lannett	00527-0112-59
100 ml	$3.75	Procaine 2 %, C O Truxton	00463-1052-01

HOW SUPPLIED - NOT RATED EQUIVALENT:

Injection, Solution - Dental

1.8 ml x 10	$104.64	RAVOCAINE-NOVOCAIN-LEVOPHED, Cook-Waite Labs	00961-0035-04
1.8 ml x 10	$104.64	RAVOCAINE-NOVOCAIN W/NEO-COBEF, Cook-Waite Labs	00961-0045-04

Injection, Solution - Intravenous - 10 %

2 ml x 25	**$171.81**	**NOVOCAIN, Sanofi Winthrop**	**00024-1384-25**

Powder

30 gm	$8.48	Procaine Hcl, Mallinckrodt	00406-8836-01
125 gm	$21.71	Procaine Hcl, Mallinckrodt	00406-8836-03

PROCAINE HYDROCHLORIDE; TETRACYCLINE HYDROCHLORIDE *(003118)*

BRAND NAMES: **Achromycin**; Tetracyn

Prescribing information not available at time of publication.

PROCARBAZINE HYDROCHLORIDE *(002119)*

CATEGORIES: Antineoplastics; Cancer; Chemotherapy; Cytotoxic Agents; Hodgkin's Disease; Oncologic Drugs; Pregnancy Category D; FDA Approval Pre 1982

BRAND NAMES: **Matulane**; *Natulan*
(International brand names outside U.S. in italics)

FORMULARIES: Aetna; BC-BS; Medi-Cal; WHO

> WARNING:
> It is recommended that procarbazine be given only by or under the supervision of a physician experienced in the use of potent antineoplastic drugs. Adequate clinical and laboratory facilities should be available to patients for proper monitoring of treatment.

DESCRIPTION:

Procarbazine hydrochloride, a hydrazine derivative antineoplastic agent, is available as capsules containing the equivalent of 50 mg procarbazine as the hydrochloride. Each capsule also contains corn starch, mannitol and talc. Gelatin capsule shells contain parabens (methyl and propyl), potassium sorbate, titanium dioxide, FD & C Yellow No. 6 and D & C Yellow No. 10.

Chemically, procarbazine hydrochloride is*N*-isopropyl-α-(2-methylhydrazino)-*p*-toluamide monohydrochloride. It is a white to pale yellow crystalline powder which is soluble but unstable in water or aqueous solutions. The molecular weight of procarbazine hydrochloride is 257.76.

CLINICAL PHARMACOLOGY:

The precise mode of cytotoxic action of procarbazine has not been clearly defined. There is evidence that the drug may act by inhibition of protein, RNA and DNA synthesis. Studies have suggested that procarbazine may inhibit transmethylation of methyl groups of methionine into t-RNA. The absence of functional t-RNA could cause the cessation of protein synthesis and consequently DNA and RNA synthesis. In addition, procarbazine may directly damage DNA. Hydrogen peroxide, formed during the auto-oxidation of the drug, may attack protein sulfhydryl groups contained in residual protein which is tightly bound to DNA.

Procarbazine is metabolized primarily in the liver and kidneys. The drug appears to be auto-oxidized to the azo derivative with the release of hydrogen peroxide. The azo derivative isomerizes to the hydrazone, and following hydrolysis splits into a benzylaldehyde derivative and methylhydrazine. The methylhydrazine is further degraded to $CO_2$and CH_4 and possibly hydrazine, whereas the aldehyde is oxidized to *N*-isopropylterephthalamic acid, which is excreted in the urine.

Procarbazine is rapidly and completely absorbed. Following oral administration of 30 mg of ^{14}C-labeled procarbazine, maximum peak plasma radioactive concentrations were reached within 60 minutes.

After intravenous injection, the plasma half-life of procarbazine is approximately 10 minutes. Approximately 70% of the radioactivity is excreted in the urine as *N*-isopropylterephthalamic acid within 24 hours following both oral and intravenous administration of^{14}C-labeled procarbazine.

Procarbazine crosses the blood-brain barrier and rapidly equilibrates between plasma and cerebrospinal fluid after oral administration.

INDICATIONS AND USAGE:

Procarbazine is indicated for use in combination with other anticancer drugs for the treatment of Stage III and IV Hodgkin's disease. Procarbazine HCl is used as part of the MOPP (nitrogen mustard, vincristine, procarbazine, prednisone) regimen.

CONTRAINDICATIONS:

Procarbazine is contraindicated in patients with known hypersensitivity to the drug or inadequate marrow reserve as demonstrated by bone marrow aspiration. Due consideration of this possible state should be given to each patient who has leukopenia, thrombocytopenia or anemia.

WARNINGS:

To minimize CNS depression and possible potentiation, barbiturates, antihistamines, narcotics, hypotensive agents or phenothiazines should be used with caution. Ethyl alcohol should not be used since there may be a disulfiram (Antabuse)-like reaction. Because procarbazine HCl exhibits some monoamine oxidase inhibitory activity, sympathomimetic drugs, tricyclic antidepressant drugs (*e.g.,* amitriptyline HCl, imipramine HCl) and other drugs and foods with known high tyramine content, such as wine, yogurt, ripe cheese and bananas, should be avoided. A further phenomenon of toxicity common to many hydrazine derivatives is hemolysis and the appearance of Heinz-Ehrlich inclusion bodies in erythrocytes.

WARNINGS: *(cont'd)*

PREGNANCY CATEGORY D

Teratogenic Effects: Procarbazine hydrochloride can cause fetal harm when administered to a pregnant woman. While there are no adequate and well-controlled studies with procarbazine hydrochloride in pregnant women, there are case reports of malformations in the offspring of women who were exposed to procarbazine hydrochloride in combination with other antineoplastic agents during pregnancy. Procarbazine HCl should be used during pregnancy only if the potential benefit justifies the potential risk to the fetus. If this drug is used during pregnancy, or if the patient becomes pregnant while taking this drug, the patient should be apprised of the potential hazard to the fetus. Women of childbearing potential should be advised to avoid becoming pregnant. Procarbazine hydrochloride is teratogenic in the rat when given at doses approximately 4 to 13 times the maximum recommended human therapeutic dose of 6 mg/kg/day.

Nonteratogenic Effects: Procarbazine hydrochloride has not been adequately studied in animals for its effects on peri- and postnatal development. However, neurogenic tumors were noted in the offspring of rats given intravenous injections of 125 mg/kg of procarbazine hydrochloride on day 22 of gestation. Compounds which inhibit DNA, RNA and protein synthesis might be expected to have adverse effects on peri- and postnatal development.

CARCINOGENESIS, MUTAGENESIS AND IMPAIRMENT OF FERTILITY

Carcinogenesis: The carcinogenicity of procarbazine hydrochloride in mice, rats and monkeys has been reported in a considerable number of studies. Instances of a second nonlymphoid malignancy, including acute myelocytic leukemia, have been reported in patients with Hodgkin's disease treated with procarbazine in combination with other chemotherapy and/or radiation. The International Agency for Research on Cancer (IARC) considers that there is "sufficient evidence" for the human carcinogenicity of procarbazine hydrochloride when it is given in intensive regimens which include other antineoplastic agents but that there is inadequate evidence of carcinogenicity in humans given procarbazine hydrochloride alone.

Mutagenesis: Procarbazine hydrochloride has been shown to be mutagenic in a variety of bacterial and mammalian test systems.

Impairment of Fertility: Azoospermia and antifertility effects associated with procarbazine hydrochloride administration in combination with other chemotherapeutic agents for treating Hodgkin's disease have been reported in human clinical studies. Since these patients received multicombination therapy, it is difficult to determine to what extent procarbazine hydrochloride alone was involved in the male germ-cell damage. The usual Segment I fertility/reproduction studies in laboratory animals have not been carried out with procarbazine hydrochloride. However, compounds which inhibit DNA, RNA and/or protein synthesis might be expected to have adverse effects on gametogenesis. Unscheduled DNA synthesis in the testis of rabbits and decreased fertility in male mice treated with procarbazine hydrochloride have been reported.

PRECAUTIONS:

GENERAL

Undue toxicity may occur if procarbazine HCl is used in patients with impairment of renal and/or hepatic function. When appropriate, hospitalization for the initial course of treatment should be considered.

If radiation or a chemotherapeutic agent known to have marrow-depressant activity has been used, an interval of one month or longer without such therapy is recommended before starting treatment with procarbazine HCl. The length of this interval may also be determined by evidence of bone marrow recovery based on successive bone marrow studies.

Prompt cessation of therapy is recommended if any one of the following occurs:

Central Nervous System: signs or symptoms such as paresthesias, neuropathies or confusion.

Leukopenia: (white blood count under 4000).

Thrombocytopenia: (platelets under 100,000).

Hypersensitivity Reaction

Stomatitis: The first small ulceration or persistent spot soreness around the oral cavity is a signal for cessation of therapy.

Diarrhea: Frequent bowel movements or watery stools.

Hemorrhage: or bleeding tendencies.

Bone marrow depression often occurs 2 to 8 weeks after the start of treatment. If leukopenia occurs, hospitalization of the patient may be needed for appropriate treatment to prevent systemic infection.

INFORMATION FOR THE PATIENT

Patients should be warned not to drink alcoholic beverages while on procarbazine HCl therapy since there may be an disulfiram (Antabuse)-like reaction. They should also be cautioned to avoid foods with known high tyramine content such as wine, yogurt, ripe cheese and bananas. Over-the-counter drug preparations which contain antihistamines or sympathomimetic drugs should also be avoided. Patients taking procarbazine HCl should also be warned against the use of prescription drugs without the knowledge and consent of their physician.

LABORATORY TESTS

Baseline laboratory data should be obtained prior to initiation of therapy. The hematologic status as indicated by hemoglobin, hematocrit, white blood count (WBC), differential, reticulocytes and platelets should be monitored closely - at least every 3 or 4 days.

Hepatic and renal evaluation are indicated prior to beginning therapy. Urinalysis, transaminase, alkaline phosphatase and blood urea nitrogen tests should be repeated at least weekly.

CARCINOGENESIS, MUTAGENESIS AND IMPAIRMENT OF FERTILITY

See WARNINGS.

PREGNANCY CATEGORY D

See WARNINGS.

NURSING MOTHERS

It is not known whether procarbazine HCl is excreted in human milk. Because of the potential for tumorigenicity shown for procarbazine hydrochloride in animal studies, mothers should not nurse while receiving this drug.

DRUG INTERACTIONS:

See WARNINGS.

No cross-resistance with other chemotherapeutic agents, radiotherapy or steroids has been demonstrated.

ADVERSE REACTIONS:

Leukopenia, anemia and thrombopenia occur frequently. Nausea and vomiting are the most commonly reported side effects.

Other adverse reactions are:

Hematologic: Pancytopenia; eosinophilia; hemolytic anemia; bleeding tendencies such as petechiae, purpura, epistaxis and hemoptysis.

ADVERSE REACTIONS: *(cont'd)*

Gastrointestinal: Hepatic dysfunction, jaundice, stomatitis, hematemesis, melena, diarrhea, dysphagia, anorexia, abdominal pain, constipation, dry mouth.

Neurologic: Coma, convulsions, neuropathy, ataxia, paresthesia, nystagmus, diminished reflexes, falling, foot drop, headache, dizziness, unsteadiness.

Cardiovascular: Hypotension, tachycardia, syncope.

Ophthalmic: Retinal hemorrhage, papilledema, photophobia, diplopia, inability to focus.

Respiratory: Pneumonitis, pleural effusion, cough.

Dermatologic: Herpes, dermatitis, pruritus, alopecia, hyperpigmentation, rash, urticaria, flushing.

Allergic: Generalized allergic reactions.

Genitourinary: Hematuria, urinary frequency, nocturia.

Musculoskeletal: Pain, including myalgia and arthralgia; tremors.

Psychiatric: Hallucinations, depression, apprehension, nervousness, confusion, nightmares.

Endocrine: Gynecomastia in prepubertal and early pubertal boys.

Miscellaneous: Intercurrent infections, hearing loss, pyrexia, diaphoresis, lethargy, weakness, fatigue, edema, chills, insomnia, slurred speech, hoarseness, drowsiness.

Second nonlymphoid malignancies, including acute myelocytic leukemia and malignant myelosclerosis, and azoospermia have been reported in patients with Hodgkin's disease treated with procarbazine in combination with other chemotherapy and/or radiation.

OVERDOSAGE:

The major manifestations of overdosage with procarbazine HCl would be anticipated to be nausea, vomiting, enteritis, diarrhea, hypotension, tremors, convulsions and coma. Treatment should consist of either the administration of an emetic or gastric lavage. General supportive measures such as intravenous fluids are advised. Since the major toxicity of procarbazine hydrochloride is hematologic and hepatic, patients should have frequent complete blood counts and liver function tests throughout their period of recovery and for a minimum of two weeks thereafter. Should abnormalities appear in any of these determinations, appropriate measures for correction and stabilization should be immediately undertaken.

The estimated mean lethal dose of procarbazine hydrochloride in laboratory animals varied from approximately 150 mg/kg in rabbits to 1300 mg/kg in mice.

DOSAGE AND ADMINISTRATION:

The following doses are for administration of the drug as a single agent. When used in combination with other anticancer drugs, the procarbazine HCl dose should be appropriately reduced, e.g., in the MOPP regimen, the procarbazine HCl dose is 100 mg/m^2 daily for 14 days. All dosages are based on the patient's actual weight. However, the estimated lean body mass (dry weight) is used if the patient is obese or if there has been a spurious weight gain due to edema, ascites or other forms of abnormal fluid retention.

Adults: To minimize the nausea and vomiting experienced by a high percentage of patients beginning procarbazine HCl therapy, single or divided doses of 2 to 4 mg/kg/day for the first week are recommended. Daily dosage should then be maintained at 4 to 6 mg/kg/day until maximum response is obtained or until the white blood count falls below 4000/cmm or the platelets fall below 100,000/cmm. When maximum response is obtained, the dose may be maintained at 1 to 2 mg/kg/day. Upon evidence of hematologic or other toxicity (see PRECAUTIONS), the drug should be discontinued until there has been satisfactory recovery. After toxic side effects have subsided, therapy may then be resumed at the discretion of the physician, based on clinical evaluation and appropriate laboratory studies, at a dosage of 1 to 2 mg/kg/day.

Children: Very close clinical monitoring is mandatory. Undue toxicity, evidenced by tremors, coma and convulsions, has occurred in a few cases. Dosage, therefore, should be individualized. The following dosage schedule is provided as a guideline only.

Fifty (50) mg per square meter of body surface per day is recommended for the first week. Dosage should then be maintained at 100 mg per square meter of body surface per day until maximum response is obtained or until leukopenia or thrombocytopenia occurs. When maximum response is attained, the dose may be maintained at 50 mg per square meter of body surface per day. Upon evidence of hematologic or other toxicity (see PRECAUTIONS), the drug should be discontinued until there has been satisfactory recovery, based on clinical evaluation and appropriate laboratory tests. After toxic side effects have subsided, therapy may then be resumed.

Procedures for proper handling and disposal of anticancer drugs should be considered. Several guidelines on this subject have been published.[1-6] There is no general agreement that all of the procedures recommended in the guidelines are necessary or appropriate.

REFERENCES:

1. Recommendations for the safe handling of parenteral antineoplastic drugs. Washington, DC, U.S. Government Printing Office (NIH Publication No. 83-2621). **2.** AMA Council Report. Guidelines for handling parenteral antineoplastics. *JAMA 253*: 1590-1592, Mar 15, 1985. **3.** National Study Commission on Cytotoxic Exposure: Recommendations for handling cytotoxic agents. Available from Louis P.Jeffrey, ScD, Director of Pharmacy Services, Rhode Island Hospital, 593 Eddy Street, Providence, Rhode Island 02902. **4.** Clinical Oncological Society of Australia: Guidelines and recommendations for safe handling of antineoplastic agents. *Med JAust 1*: 426-428, Apr 30,1983. **5.** Jones RB, Frank R, Mass T: Safe handling of chemotherapeutic agents: a report from the Mount Sinai Medical Center. *CA 33*: 258-263, Sept-Oct 1983. **6.** ASHP technical assistance bulletin on handling cytotoxic drugs in hospitals. *Am J Hosp Pharm 42*: 131-137, Jan 1985.

HOW SUPPLIED - EQUIVALENTS NOT AVAILABLE:

Capsule, Gelatin - Oral - 50 mg

100's $68.25 MATULANE, Roche 00004-0053-01

PROCHLORPERAZINE *(002120)*

CATEGORIES: Analeptics; Anesthesia; Antiemetics; Antipsychotics/Antimanics; Anxiety; Central Nervous System Agents; Gastrointestinal Drugs; Nausea; Nausea and Vomiting; Neuroleptics; Phenothiazine Tranquilizers; Psychotherapeutic Agents; Psychotic Disorders; Tranquilizers; Vertigo/Motion Sickness/Vomiting; Vomiting; FDA Approval Pre 1982

BRAND NAMES: *Buccastem*; Compa-Z; **Compazine**; Cotranzine; *Nautisol*; *Nibromin*; *Normalmin*; *Novamin*; *Novomit*; *Pasotomin*; Prochlorperazine Edisylate; Prochlorperazine Maleate; *Stella*; *Stemetil*; *Steremal*; *Tementil*; Ultrazine-10; *Vertigon*
(International brand names outside U.S. in italics)

FORMULARIES: Aetna; BC-BS; CIGNA; FHP; Humana; Kaiser; Medco; Medi-Cal; PCS; PruCare; United

COST OF THERAPY: $52.11 (Nausea; Tablet; 5 mg; 3/day; 30 days)

DESCRIPTION:

Tablets: Each round, yellow-green, coated tablet contains prochlorperazine maleate equivalent to prochlorperazine as follows: 5 mg imprinted SKF and C66; 10 mg imprinted SKF and C67. *5 mg and 10 mg Tablets: Modified Formulation:* Inactive ingredients consist of cellulose, lactose, magnesium stearate, polyethylene glycol, sodium croscarmellose, titanium dioxide, D&C Yellow No. 10, FD&C Blue No. 2, FD&C Yellow No. 6, FD&C Red No. 40, iron oxide, starch, stearic acid and trace amounts of other inactive ingredients.

NOTE: Compazine 5 mg and 10 mg tablets have been changed from yellow-green sugar-coated tablets to yellow-green film-coated tablets. The film-coated tablets are smaller in size than the sugar-coated tablets. The inactive ingredients have changed, but the drug content remains unchanged.

Spansule Sustained Release Capsules: Each Prochlorperazine Spansule capsule is so prepared that an initial dose is released promptly and the remaining medication is released gradually over a prolonged period.

Each capsule, with black cap and natural body, contains prochlorperazine maleate equivalent to prochlorperazine as follows: 10 mg imprinted SKF and C44; 15 mg imprinted SKF and C46. Inactive ingredients consist of benzyl alcohol, cetylpyridinium chloride, D&C Green No. 5, D&C Yellow No. 10, FD&C Blue No. 1, FD&C Red No. 40, FD&C Yellow No. 6, gelatin, glyceryl monostearate, sodium lauryl sulfate, starch, sucrose, wax and trace amounts of other inactive ingredients.

Vials: 2 ml (5 mg/ml) and 10 ml (5 mg/ml)—Each ml contains, in aqueous solution, 5 mg prochlorperazine as the edisylate, 5 mg sodium biphosphate, 12 mg sodium tartrate, 0.9 mg sodium saccharin and 0.75% benzyl alcohol as preservative.

Disposable Syringes: 2 ml (5 mg/ml)—Each ml contains, in aqueous solution, 5 mg prochlorperazine as the edisylate, 5 mg sodium biphosphate, 12 mg sodium tartrate, 0.9 mg sodium saccharin, and 0.75% benzyl alcohol as preservative.

Suppositories: Each suppository contains 2 1/2 mg, 5 mg or 25 mg of prochlorperazine; with glycerin, glyceryl monopalmitate, glyceryl monostearate, hydrogenated cocoanut oil fatty acids and hydrogenated palm kernel oil fatty acids.

Syrup: Each 5 ml (1 teaspoonful) of clear, yellow-orange, fruit-flavored liquid contains 5 mg of prochlorperazine as the edisylate. Inactive ingredients consist of FD&C Yellow No. 6, flavors, polyoxyethylene polyoxypropylene glycol, sodium benzoate, sodium citrate, sucrose and water.

INDICATIONS AND USAGE:

For control of severe nausea and vomiting.

For management of the manifestations of psychotic disorders.

Prochlorperazine is effective for the short-term treatment of generalized nonpsychotic anxiety. However, Prochlorperazine is not the first drug to be used in therapy for most patients with non-psychotic anxiety, because certain risks associated with its use are not shared by common alternative treatments (*e.g.,* benzodiazepines).

When used in the treatment of non-psychotic anxiety, Prochlorperazine should not be administered at doses of more than 20 mg per day or for longer than 12 weeks, because the use of Prochlorperazine at higher doses or for longer intervals may cause persistent tardive dyskinesia that may prove irreversible (see WARNINGS.)

The effectiveness of Prochlorperazine as treatment for non-psychotic anxiety was established in 4-week clinical studies of outpatients with generalized anxiety disorder. This evidence does not predict that Prochlorperazine will be useful in patients with other non-psychotic conditions in which anxiety, or signs that mimic anxiety, are found (*e.g.,* physical illness, organic mental conditions, agitated depression, character pathologies, etc.).

Prochlorperazine has not been shown effective in the management of behavioral complications in patients with mental retardation.

CONTRAINDICATIONS:

Do not use in patients with known hypersensitivity to phenothiazines.

Do not use in comatose states or in the presence of large amounts of central nervous system depressants (alcohol, barbiturates, narcotics, etc.).

Do not use in pediatric surgery.

Do not use in children under 2 years of age or under 20 lbs. Do not use in children for conditions for which dosage has not been established.

WARNINGS:

The extrapyramidal symptoms which can occur secondary to prochlorperazine may be confused with the central nervous system signs of an undiagnosed primary disease responsible for the vomiting, e.g., Reye's syndrome or other encephalopathy. The use of Prochlorperazine and other potential hepatotoxins should be avoided in children and adolescents whose signs and symptoms suggest Reye's syndrome.

TARDIVE DYSKINESIA

Tardive dyskinesia, a syndrome consisting of potentially irreversible, involuntary, dyskinetic movements, may develop in patients treated with neuroleptic (antipsychotic) drugs. Although the prevalence of the syndrome appears to be highest among the elderly, especially elderly women, it is impossible to rely upon prevalence estimates to predict, at the inception of neuroleptic treatment, which patients are likely to develop the syndrome. Whether neuroleptic drug products differ in their potential to cause tardive dyskinesia is unknown.

Both the risk of developing the syndrome and the likelihood that it will become irreversible are believed to increase as the duration of treatment and the total cumulative dose of neuroleptic drugs administered to the patient increase. However, the syndrome can develop, although much less commonly, after relatively brief treatment periods at low doses.

There is no known treatment for established cases of tardive dyskinesia, although the syndrome may remit, partially or completely, if neuroleptic treatment is withdrawn. Neuroleptic treatment itself, however, may suppress (or partially suppress) the signs and symptoms of the syndrome and thereby may possibly mask the underlying disease process.

The effect that symptomatic suppression has upon the long-term course of the syndrome is unknown.

Given these considerations, neuroleptics should be prescribed in a manner that is most likely to minimize the occurrence of tardive dyskinesia. Chronic neuroleptic treatment should generally be reserved for patients who suffer from a chronic illness that, 1) is known to respond to neuroleptic drugs, and 2) for whom alternative, equally effective, but potentially less harmful treatments are *not* available or appropriate. In patients who do require chronic treatment, the smallest dose and the shortest duration of treatment producing a satisfactory clinical response should be sought. The need for continued treatment should be reassessed periodically.

If signs and symptoms of tardive dyskinesia appear in a patient on neuroleptics, drug discontinuation should be considered. However, some patients may require treatment despite the presence of the syndrome.

For further information about the description of tardive dyskinesia and its clinical detection, please refer to the sections on PRECAUTIONSand ADVERSE REACTIONS.

WARNINGS: *(cont'd)*

NEUROLEPTIC MALIGNANT SYNDROME (NMS)

A potentially fatal symptom complex sometimes referred to as Neuroleptic Malignant Syndrome (NMS) has been reported in association with antipsychotic drugs. Clinical manifestations of NMS are hyperpyrexia, muscle rigidity, altered mental status and evidence of autonomic instability (irregular pulse or blood pressure, tachycardia, diaphoresis and cardiac dysrhythmias).

The diagnostic evaluation of patients with this syndrome is complicated. In arriving at a diagnosis, it is important to identify cases where the clinical presentation includes both serious medical illness (*e.g.,* pneumonia, systemic infection, etc.) and untreated or inadequately treated extrapyramidal signs and symptoms (EPS). Other important considerations in the differential diagnosis include central anticholinergic toxicity, heat stroke, drug fever and primary central nervous system (CNS) pathology.

The management of NMS should include 1) immediate discontinuation of antipsychotic drugs and other drugs not essential to concurrent therapy, 2) intensive symptomatic treatment and medical monitoring, and 3) treatment of any concomitant serious medical problems for which specific treatments are available. There is no general agreement about specific pharmacological treatment regimens for uncomplicated NMS.

If a patient requires antipsychotic drug treatment after recovery from NMS, the potential reintroduction of drug therapy should be carefully considered. The patient should be carefully monitored, since recurrences of NMS have been reported.

An encephalopathic syndrome (characterized by weakness, lethargy, fever, tremulousness and confusion, extrapyramidal symptoms, leukocytosis, elevated serum enzymes, BUN and FBS) has occurred in a few patients treated with lithium plus a neuroleptic. In some instances, the syndrome was followed by irreversible brain damage. Because of a possible causal relationship between these events and the concomitant administration of lithium and neuroleptics, patients receiving such combined therapy should be monitored closely for early evidence of neurologic toxicity and treatment discontinued promptly if such signs appear. This encephalopathic syndrome may be similar to or the same as neuroleptic malignant syndrome (NMS).

Patients with bone marrow depression or who have previously demonstrated a hypersensitivity reaction (*e.g.,* blood dyscrasias, jaundice) with a phenothiazine should not receive any phenothiazine, including Prochlorperazine, unless in the judgment of the physician the potential benefits of treatment outweigh the possible hazards.

Prochlorperazine may impair mental and/or physical abilities, especially during the first few days of therapy. Therefore, caution patients about activities requiring alertness (*e.g.,* operating vehicles or machinery).

Phenothiazines may intensify or prolong the action of central nervous system depressants (*e.g.,* alcohol, anesthetics, narcotics).

USAGE IN PREGNANCY

Safety for the use of Prochlorperazine during pregnancy has not been established. Therefore, Prochlorperazine is not recommended for use in pregnant patients except in cases of severe nausea and vomiting that are so serious and intractable that, in the judgment of the physician, drug intervention is required and potential benefits outweigh possible hazards.

There have been reported instances of prolonged jaundice, extrapyramidal signs, hyperreflexia or hyporeflexia in newborn infants whose mothers received phenothiazines.

NURSING MOTHERS

There is evidence that phenothiazines are excreted in the breast milk of nursing mothers. Caution should be exercised when Prochlorperazine is administered to a nursing woman.

PRECAUTIONS:

The antiemetic action of Prochlorperazine may mask the signs and symptoms of overdosage of other drugs and may obscure the diagnosis and treatment of other conditions such as intestinal obstruction, brain tumor and Reye's syndrome (see WARNINGS.)

When Prochlorperazine is used with cancer chemotherapeutic drugs, vomiting as a sign of the toxicity of these agents may be obscured by the antiemetic effect of Prochlorperazine.

Because hypotension may occur, large doses and parenteral administration should be used cautiously in patients with impaired cardiovascular systems. To minimize the occurrence of hypotension after injection, keep patient lying down and observe for at least 1/2 hour. If hypotension occurs after parenteral or oral dosing, place patient in head-low position with legs raised. If a vasoconstrictor is required, Levophed* and Neo-Synephrine† are suitable. Other pressor agents, including epinephrine, should not be used because they may cause a paradoxical further lowering of blood pressure.

Aspiration of vomitus has occurred in a few post-surgical patients who have received Prochlorperazine as an antiemetic. Although no causal relationship has been established, this possibility should be borne in mind during surgical aftercare.

Deep sleep, from which patients can be aroused, and coma have been reported, usually with overdosage.

Neuroleptic drugs elevate prolactin levels; the elevation persists during chronic administration. Tissue culture experiments indicate that approximately one third of human breast cancers are prolactin-dependent *in vitro*, a factor of potential importance if the prescribing of these drugs is contemplated in a patient with a previously detected breast cancer. Although disturbances such as galactorrhea, amenorrhea, gynecomastia and impotence have been reported, the clinical significance of elevated serum prolactin levels is unknown for most patients. An increase in mammary neoplasms has been found in rodents after chronic administration of neuroleptic drugs. Neither clinical nor epidemiologic studies conducted to date, however, have shown an association between chronic administration of these drugs and mammary tumorigenesis; the available evidence is considered too limited to be conclusive at this time.

Chromosomal aberrations in spermatocytes and abnormal sperm have been demonstrated in rodents treated with certain neuroleptics.

As with all drugs which exert an anticholinergic effect, and/or cause mydriasis, prochlorperazine should be used with caution in patients with glaucoma.

Because phenothiazines may interfere with thermoregulatory mechanisms, use with caution in persons who will be exposed to extreme heat.

Phenothiazines can diminish the effect of oral anticoagulants.

Phenothiazines can produce alpha-adrenergic blockade.

Thiazide diuretics may accentuate the orthostatic hypotension that may occur with phenothiazines.

Antihypertensive effects of guanethidine and related compounds may be counteracted when phenothiazines are used concomitantly.

Concomitant administration of propranolol with phenothiazines results in increased plasma levels of both drugs.

Phenothiazines may lower the convulsive threshold; dosage adjustments of anticonvulsants may be necessary. Potentiation of anticonvulsant effects does not occur. However, it has been reported that phenothiazines may interfere with the metabolism of Dilantin‡ and thus precipitate Dilantin toxicity.

PRECAUTIONS: *(cont'd)*

The presence of phenothiazines may produce false-positive phenylketonuria (PKU) test results.

LONG-TERM THERAPY

Given the likelihood that some patients exposed chronically to neuroleptics will develop tardive dyskinesia, it is advised that all patients in whom chronic use is contemplated be given, if possible, full information about this risk. The decision to inform patients and/or their guardians must obviously take into account the clinical circumstances and the competency of the patient to understand the information provided.

To lessen the likelihood of adverse reactions related to cumulative drug effect, patients with a history of long-term therapy with Prochlorperazine and/or other neuroleptics should be evaluated periodically to decide whether the maintenance dosage could be lowered or drug therapy discontinued.

Children with acute illnesses (*e.g.,* chickenpox, CNS infections, measles, gastroenteritis) or dehydration seem to be much more susceptible to neuromuscular reactions, particularly dystonias, than are adults. In such patients, the drug should be used only under close supervision.

Drugs which lower the seizure threshold, including phenothiazine derivatives, should not be used with metrizamide (AmipaqueS). As with other phenothiazine derivatives, Prochlorperazine should be discontinued at least 48 hours before myelography, should not be resumed for at least 24 hours postprocedure, and should not be used for the control of nausea and vomiting occurring either prior to myelography with Amipaque, or postprocedure.

ADVERSE REACTIONS:

Drowsiness, dizziness, amenorrhea, blurred vision, skin reactions and hypotension may occur. Neuroleptic Malignant Syndrome (NMS) has been reported in association with antipsychotic drugs (see WARNINGS.)

Cholestatic jaundice has occurred. If fever with grippe-like symptoms occurs, appropriate liver studies should be conducted. If tests indicate an abnormality, stop treatment. There have been a few observations of fatty changes in the livers of patients who have died while receiving the drug. No causal relationship has been established.

Leukopenia and agranulocytosis have occurred. Warn patients to report the sudden appearance of sore throat or other signs of infection. If white blood cell and differential counts indicate leukocyte depression, stop treatment and start antibiotic and other suitable therapy.

NEUROMUSCULAR (EXTRAPYRAMIDAL) REACTIONS

These symptoms are seen in a significant number of hospitalized mental patients. They may be characterized by motor restlessness, be of the dystonic type, or they may resemble parkinsonism.

Depending on the severity of symptoms, dosage should be reduced or discontinued. If therapy is reinstituted, it should be at a lower dosage. Should these symptoms occur in children or pregnant patients, the drug should be stopped and not reinstituted. In most cases barbiturates by suitable route of administration will suffice. (Or, injectable Benadryl may be useful.) In more severe cases, the administration of an anti-parkinsonism agent, except levodopa (see prescribing information for levodopa), usually produces rapid reversal of symptoms. Suitable supportive measures such as maintaining a clear airway and adequate hydration should be employed.

MOTOR RESTLESSNESS

Symptoms may include agitation or jitteriness and sometimes insomnia. These symptoms often disappear spontaneously. At times these symptoms may be similar to the original neurotic or psychotic symptoms. Dosage should not be increased until these side effects have subsided.

If these symptoms become too troublesome, they can usually be controlled by a reduction of dosage or change of drug. Treatment with antiparkinsonian agents, benzodiazepines or propranolol may be helpful.

DYSTONIAS

Symptoms may include spasm of the neck muscles, sometimes progressing to torticollis; extensor rigidity of back muscles, sometimes progressing to opisthotonos; carpopedal spasm, trismus, swallowing difficulty, oculogyric crisis and protrusion of the tongue.

These usually subside within a few hours, and almost always within 24 to 48 hours, after the drug has been discontinued.

In mild cases: reassurance or a barbiturate is often sufficient. *In moderate cases:* barbiturates will usually bring rapid relief. *In more severe adult cases:* the administration of an anti-parkinsonism agent, except levodopa (see prescribing information for levodopa), usually produces rapid reversal of symptoms. *In children:* reassurance and barbiturates will usually control symptoms. (Or, injectable Benadryl may be useful. Note: See Benadryl prescribing information for appropriate *children's* dosage.) If appropriate treatment with anti-parkinsonism agents or Benadryl fails to reverse the signs and symptoms, the diagnosis should be reevaluated.

PSEUDO-PARKINSONISM

Symptoms may include: mask-like facies; drooling; tremors; pillrolling motion; cogwheel rigidity; and shuffling gait. Reassurance and sedation are important. In most cases these symptoms are readily controlled when an anti-parkinsonism agent is administered concomitantly. Anti-parkinsonism agents should be used only when required. Generally, therapy of a few weeks to 2 or 3 months will suffice. After this time patients should be evaluated to determine their need for continued treatment. (Note: Levodopa has not been found effective in pseudo-parkinsonism.) Occasionally it is necessary to lower the dosage of Prochlorperazine or to discontinue the drug.

TARDIVE DYSKINESIA

As with all antipsychotic agents, tardive dyskinesia may appear in some patients on long-term therapy or may appear after drug therapy has been discontinued. The syndrome can also develop, although much less frequently, after relatively brief treatment periods at low doses. This syndrome appears in all age groups. Although its prevalence appears to be highest among elderly patients, especially elderly women, it is impossible to rely upon prevalence estimates to predict at the inception of neuroleptic treatment which patients are likely to develop the syndrome. The symptoms are persistent and in some patients appear to be irreversible. The syndrome is characterized by rhythmical involuntary movements of the tongue, face, mouth or jaw (*e.g.,* protrusion of tongue, puffing of cheeks, puckering of mouth, chewing movements). Sometimes these may be accompanied by involuntary movements of extremities. In rare instances, these involuntary movements of the extremities are the only manifestations of tardive dyskinesia. A variant of tardive dyskinesia, tardive dystonia, has also been described.

There is no known effective treatment for tardive dyskinesia; anti-parkinsonism agents do not alleviate the symptoms of this syndrome. It is suggested that all antipsychotic agents be discontinued if these symptoms appear.

Should it be necessary to reinstitute treatment, or increase the dosage of the agent, or switch to a different antipsychotic agent, the syndrome may be masked.

It has been reported that fine vermicular movements of the tongue may be an early sign of the syndrome and if the medication is stopped at that time the syndrome may not develop.

ADVERSE REACTIONS: *(cont'd)*

CONTACT DERMATITIS

Avoid getting the Injection solution on hands or clothing because of the possibility of contact dermatitis.

ADVERSE REACTIONS REPORTED WITH PROCHLORPERAZINE OR OTHER PHENOTHIAZINE DERIVATIVES

Adverse reactions with different phenothiazines vary in type, frequency and mechanism of occurrence, i.e., some are dose-related, while others involve individual patient sensitivity. Some adverse reactions may be more likely to occur, or occur with greater intensity, in patients with special medical problems, e.g., patients with mitral insufficiency or pheochromocytoma have experienced severe hypotension following recommended doses of certain phenothiazines.

Not all of the following adverse reactions have been observed with every phenothiazine derivative, but they have been reported with 1 or more and should be borne in mind when drugs of this class are administered: extrapyramidal symptoms (opisthotonos, oculogyric crisis, hyperreflexia, dystonia, akathisia, dyskinesia, parkinsonism) some of which have lasted months and even years—particularly in elderly patients with previous brain damage; grand mal and petit mal convulsions, particularly in patients with EEG abnormalities or history of such disorders; altered cerebrospinal fluid proteins; cerebral edema; intensification and prolongation of the action of central nervous system depressants (opiates, analgesics, antihistamines, barbiturates, alcohol), atropine, heat, organophosphorus insecticides; autonomic reactions (dryness of mouth, nasal congestion, headache, nausea, constipation, obstipation, adynamic ileus, ejaculatory disorders/impotence, priapism, atonic colon, urinary retention, miosis and mydriasis); reactivation of psychotic processes, catatonic-like states; hypotension (sometimes fatal); cardiac arrest; blood dyscrasias (pancytopenia, thrombocytopenic purpura, leukopenia, agranulocytosis, eosinophilia, hemolytic anemia, aplastic anemia); liver damage (jaundice, biliary stasis); endocrine disturbances (hyperglycemia, hypoglycemia, glycosuria, lactation, galactorrhea, gynecomastia, menstrual irregularities, false-positive pregnancy tests); skin disorders (photosensitivity, itching, erythema, urticaria, eczema up to exfoliative dermatitis); other allergic reactions (asthma, laryngeal edema, angioneurotic edema, anaphylactoid reactions); peripheral edema; reversed epinephrine effect; hyperpyrexia; mild fever after large IM doses; increased appetite; increased weight; a systemic lupus erythematosus-like syndrome; pigmentary retinopathy; with prolonged administration of substantial doses, skin pigmentation, epithelial keratopathy, and lenticular and corneal deposits.

EKG changes-particularly nonspecific, usually reversible Q and T wave distortions-have been observed in some patients receiving phenothiazine tranquilizers.

Although phenothiazines cause neither psychic nor physical dependence, sudden discontinuance in long-term psychiatric patients may cause temporary symptoms, e.g., nausea and vomiting, dizziness, tremulousness.

Note: There have been occasional reports of sudden death in patients receiving phenothiazines. In some cases, the cause appeared to be cardiac arrest or asphyxia due to failure of the cough reflex.

OVERDOSAGE:

See also ADVERSE REACTIONS.

Symptoms: Primarily involvement of the extrapyramidal mechanism producing some of the dystonic reactions described above.

Symptoms of central nervous system depression to the point of somnolence or coma. Agitation and restlessness may also occur. Other possible manifestations include convulsions, EKG changes and cardiac arrhythmias, fever and autonomic reactions such as hypotension, dry mouth and ileus.

Treatment: It is important to determine other medications taken by the patient since multiple-dose therapy is common in overdosage situations. Treatment is essentially symptomatic and supportive. Early gastric lavage is helpful. Keep patient under observation and maintain an open airway, since involvement of the extrapyramidal mechanism may produce dysphagia and respiratory difficulty in severe overdosage. **Do not attempt to induce emesis because a dystonic reaction of the head or neck may develop that could result in aspiration of vomitus.** Extrapyramidal symptoms may be treated with anti-parkinsonism drugs, barbiturates, or Benadryl. See Physicians GenRx prescribing information for these products. Care should be taken to avoid increasing respiratory depression.

If administration of a stimulant is desirable, amphetamine, dextroamphetamine or caffeine with sodium benzoate is recommended.

Stimulants that may cause convulsions (*e.g.,* picrotoxin or pentylenetetrazol) should be avoided.

If hypotension occurs, the standard measures for managing circulatory shock should be initiated. If it is desirable to administer a vasoconstrictor, Levophed and Neo-Synephrine are most suitable. Other pressor agents, including epinephrine, are not recommended because phenothiazine derivatives may reverse the usual elevating action of these agents and cause a further lowering of blood pressure.

Limited experience indicates that phenothiazines are *not* dialyzable.

Special note on Spansule capsules: Since much of the Spansule capsule medication is coated for gradual release, therapy directed at reversing the effects of the ingested drug and at supporting the patient should be continued for as long as overdosage symptoms remain. Saline cathartics are useful for hastening evacuation of pellets that have not already released medication.

DOSAGE AND ADMINISTRATION:

NOTES ON INJECTION

Stability: This solution should be protected from light. This is a clear, colorless to pale yellow solution; a slight yellowish discoloration will not alter potency. If markedly discolored, solution should be discarded.

Compatibility: It is recommended that Prochlorperazine (prochlorperazine) Injection not be mixed with other agents in the syringe.

ADULTS

(For children's dosage and administration, see below.) Dosage should be increased more gradually in debilitated or emaciated patients.

Elderly Patients: In general, dosages in the lower range are sufficient for most elderly patients. Since they appear to be more susceptible to hypotension and neuromuscular reactions, such patients should be observed closely. Dosage should be tailored to the individual, response carefully monitored and dosage adjusted accordingly. Dosage should be increased more gradually in elderly patients.

To Control Severe Nausea and Vomiting

Adjust dosage to the response of the individual. Begin with the lowest recommended dosage.

Oral Dosage *Tablets:* Usually one 5 mg or 10 mg tablet 3 or 4 times daily. Daily dosages above 40 mg should be used only in resistant cases. *Spansule capsules:* Initially, usually one 15 mg capsule on arising or one 10 mg capsule q12h. Daily doses above 40 mg should be used only in resistant cases.

Rectal Dosage: 25 mg twice daily.

DOSAGE AND ADMINISTRATION: *(cont'd)*

IM Dosage: Initially 5 to 10 mg (1 to 2 ml) injected *deeply* into the upper outer quadrant of the buttock. If necessary, repeat every 3 or 4 hours. Total IM dosage should not exceed 40 mg per day.

IV Dosage: 2 1/2 to 10 mg (1/2 to 2 ml) by slow IV injection or infusion at a rate not to exceed 5 mg per minute. Prochlorperazine Injection may be administered either undiluted or diluted in isotonic solution. A single dose of the drug should not exceed 10 mg; total IV dosage should not exceed 40 mg per day. When administered IV, do not use bolus injection. Hypotension is a possibility if the drug is given by IV injection or infusion.

Subcutaneous administration is not advisable because of local irritation.

Adult Surgery (for severe nausea and vomiting)

Total parenteral dosage should not exceed 40 mg per day. Hypotension is a possibility if the drug is given by IV injection or infusion.

IM Dosage: 5 to 10 mg (1 to 2 ml) 1 to 2 hours before induction of anesthesia (repeat once in 30 minutes, if necessary), or to control acute symptoms during and after surgery (repeat once if necessary).

IV Dosage: 5 to 10 mg (1 to 2 ml) as a slow IV injection or infusion 15 to 30 minutes before induction of anesthesia, or to control acute symptoms during or after surgery. Repeat once if necessary. Prochlorperazine may be administered either undiluted or diluted in isotonic solution, but a single dose of the drug should not exceed 10 mg. The rate of administration should not exceed 5 mg per minute. When administered IV, do not use bolus injection.

In Adult Psychiatric Disorders

Adjust dosage to the response of the individual and according to the severity of the condition. Begin with the lowest recommended dose. Although response ordinarily is seen within a day or 2, longer treatment is usually required before maximal improvement is seen.

Oral Dosage

Non-Psychotic Anxiety: Usual dosage is 5 mg 3 or 4 times daily; by Spansule capsule, usually one 15 mg capsule on arising or one 10 mg capsule q12h. Do not administer in doses of more than 20 mg per day or for longer than 12 weeks.

Psychotic Disorders—In relatively mild conditions, as seen in private psychiatric practice or in outpatient clinics, dosage is 5 or 10 mg 3 or 4 times daily.

In moderate to severe conditions, for hospitalized or adequately supervised patients, usual starting dosage is 10 mg 3 or 4 times daily. Increase dosage gradually until symptoms are controlled or side effects become bothersome. When dosage is increased by small increments every 2 or 3 days, side effects either do not occur or are easily controlled. Some patients respond satisfactorily on 50 to 75 mg daily.

In more severe disturbances, optimum dosage is usually 100 to 150 mg daily.

IM Dosage

For immediate control of severely disturbed adults, inject an initial dose of 10 to 20 mg (2 to 4 ml) *deeply* into the upper outer quadrant of the buttock. Many patients respond shortly after the first injection. If necessary, however, repeat the initial dose every 2 to 4 hours (or, in resistant cases, every hour) to gain control of the patient. More than three or four doses are seldom necessary. After control is achieved, switch patient to an oral form of the drug at the same dosage level or higher. If, in rare cases, parenteral therapy is needed for a prolonged period, give 10 to 20 mg (2 to 4 ml) every 4 to 6 hours. Pain and irritation at the site of injection have seldom occurred.

Subcutaneous administration is not advisable because of local irritation.

CHILDREN

Do not use in pediatric surgery. Children seem more prone to develop extrapyramidal reactions, even on moderate doses. Therefore, use lowest effective dosage. Tell parents not to exceed prescribed dosage, since the possibility of adverse reactions increases as dosage rises.

Occasionally the patient may react to the drug with signs of restlessness and excitement; if this occurs, do not administer additional doses. Take particular precaution in administering the drug to children with acute illnesses or dehydration; see under Dystonias.

When writing a prescription for the 2 1/2 mg size suppository, write "2 1/2," not "2.5"; this will help avoid confusion with the 25 mg adult size.

Severe Nausea and Vomiting in Children

Prochlorperazine should not be used in children under 20 pounds in weight or 2 years of age. It should not be used in conditions for which children's dosages have not been established. Dosage and frequency of administration should be adjusted according to the severity of the symptoms and the response of the patient. The duration of activity following intramuscular administration may last up to 12 hours. Subsequent doses may be given by the same route if necessary.

Oral or Rectal Dosage: More than 1 day's therapy is seldom necessary.

IM Dosage: Calculate each dose on the basis of 0.06 mg of the drug per lb of body weight; give by deep IM injection. Control is usually obtained with one dose.

TABLE 1

Weight	Usual Dosage	Not to Exceed
under 20 lbs not recommended		
20 to 29 lbs	2 1/2 mg 1 or 2 times a day	7.5 mg per day
30 to 39 lbs	2 1/2 mg 2 or 3 times a day	10 mg per day
40 to 85 lbs	2 1/2 mg 3 times a day or 5 mg 2 times a day	15 mg per day

In Psychotic Children

Oral or Rectal Dosage: For children 2 to 12 years, starting dosage is 2 1/2 mg 2 or 3 times daily. Do not give more than 10 mg the first day. Then increase dosage according to patient's response. *For Ages 2 to 5,* total daily dosage usually does not exceed 20 mg. *For Ages 6 to 12,* total daily dosage usually does not exceed 25 mg.

IM Dosage: For ages under 12, calculate each dose on the basis of 0.06 mg of Prochlorperazine per lb of body weight; give by deep IM injection. Control is usually obtained with one dose. After control is achieved, switch the patient to an oral form of the drug at the same dosage level or higher. *For Ages 2 to 5,* total daily dosage usually does not exceed 20 mg. *For Ages 6 to 12,* total daily dosage usually does not exceed 25 mg.

HOW SUPPLIED:

Storage: Store Prochlorperazine vials and syringes below 86°F. Do not freeze.

HOW SUPPLIED - RATED THERAPEUTICALLY EQUIVALENT:

Injection, Solution - Intramuscular; - 5 mg/ml

2 ml	$65.00	Prochlorperazine Edisylate, Solopak Labs	39769-0076-02
2 ml x 1	**$13.80**	**COMPAZINE (DISPOSABLE SYRINGE), SKB Pharms**	**00007-3351-01**
2 ml x 10	$25.88	Prochlorperazine Edisylate, Sanofi Winthrop	00024-1598-01
2 ml x 10	$29.88	Prochlorperazine Edisylate, Sanofi Winthrop	00024-1598-04

HOW SUPPLIED - RATED THERAPEUTICALLY EQUIVALENT: *(cont'd)*

2 ml x 10	**$59.70**	**COMPAZINE 10, SKB Pharms**	**00007-3342-11**
2 ml x 25	$54.69	Prochlorperazine Edisylate, Elkins Sinn	00641-0491-25
2 ml x 25	$126.55	Prochlorperazine Edisylate, Schein Pharm (US)	00364-2231-42
2 ml x 25	**$178.65**	**COMPAZINE, SKB Pharms**	**00007-3352-16**
2 ml x 100	**$531.95**	**COMPAZINE 10, SKB Pharms**	**00007-3342-20**
2 ml x 100	**$531.95**	**COMPAZINE 10, SKB Pharms**	**00007-3342-76**
2 ml x 100	**$557.95**	**COMPAZINE, SKB Pharms**	**00007-3352-20**
2 ml x 100	**$1185.65**	**COMPAZINE (DISPOSABLE SYRINGE), SKB Pharms**	**00007-3351-20**
5 mg	$31.45	Prochlorperazine Edisylate, Wyeth Labs	00008-0542-01
10 ml	$9.03	Prochlorperazine Edisylate, HL Moore Drug Exch	00839-7409-30
10 ml	$12.75	Prochlorperazine Edisylate, Rugby	00536-2152-70
10 ml	$13.00	Prochlorperazine Edisylate, Schein Pharm (US)	00364-2231-54
10 ml	$13.00	Prochlorperazine Edisylate, Steris Labs	00402-0830-10
10 ml	$14.25	PROCHLOPERAZINE EDISYLATE, Goldline Labs	00182-3049-63
10 ml	**$34.65**	**COMPAZINE, SKB Pharms**	**00007-3343-01**
10 ml	$309.38	Prochlorperazine Edisylate, Solopak Labs	39769-0076-10
10 ml x 20	**$533.40**	**COMPAZINE, SKB Pharms**	**00007-3343-12**
10 ml x 100	**$2103.05**	**COMPAZINE, SKB Pharms**	**00007-3343-20**

Suppository - Rectal - 25 mg

12's	$23.12	Prochlorperazine Maleate, GW Labs	00713-0135-12
12's	$32.15	Prochlorperazine Maleate, HL Moore Drug Exch	00839-7985-92
12's	**$34.30**	**COMPAZINE, SKB Pharms**	**00007-3362-03**

Tablet, Plain Coated - Oral - 5 mg

100's	**$57.90**	**COMPAZINE, SKB Pharms**	**00007-3366-20**
100's	**$60.35**	**COMPAZINE, SKB Pharms**	**00007-3366-21**

Tablet, Plain Coated - Oral - 10 mg

100's	**$86.95**	**COMPAZINE, SKB Pharms**	**00007-3367-20**
100's	**$89.45**	**COMPAZINE, SKB Pharms**	**00007-3367-21**

HOW SUPPLIED - NOT RATED EQUIVALENT:

Capsule, Gelatin, Sustained Action - Oral - 10 mg

50's	**$53.05**	**COMPAZINE, SKB Pharms**	**00007-3344-15**

Capsule, Gelatin, Sustained Action - Oral - 15 mg

50's	**$78.85**	**COMPAZINE, SKB Pharms**	**00007-3346-15**

Suppository - Rectal - 2.5 mg

12's	**$24.90**	**COMPAZINE, SKB Pharms**	**00007-3360-03**

Suppository - Rectal - 5 mg

12's	**$27.70**	**COMPAZINE, SKB Pharms**	**00007-3361-03**

Syrup - Oral - 5mg/5ml

120 ml	**$18.95**	**COMPAZINE, SKB Pharms**	**00007-3363-44**

Tablet, Plain Coated - Oral - 5 mg

100's	$34.43	Prochlorperazine, HL Moore Drug Exch	00839-6301-06
100's	$38.00	Prochlorperazine, United Res	00677-0615-01

Tablet, Plain Coated - Oral - 10 mg

100's	$51.98	Prochlorperazine, HL Moore Drug Exch	00839-6302-06
100's	$56.00	Prochlorperazine, United Res	00677-0616-01

Tablet, Plain Coated - Oral - 25 mg

100's	**$104.85**	**COMPAZINE, SKB Pharms**	**00007-3369-20**

PROCYCLIDINE HYDROCHLORIDE *(002121)*

CATEGORIES: Akathisia; Anticholinergic Agents; Antiparkinson Agents; Autonomic Drugs; Extrapyramidal Movement Disorders; Fatigue; Mydriasis; Neuromuscular; Parkinsonism; Salivation; Sialorrhea; Tremor; FDA Approval Pre 1982

BRAND NAMES: *Apricolin*; *Kemadren*; **Kemadrin**; *Osnervan*
(International brand names outside U.S. in italics)

FORMULARIES: Medi-Cal

COST OF THERAPY: $334.63 (Parkinsonism; Tablet; 5 mg; 2/day; 365 days)

DESCRIPTION:

Kemadrin (procyclidine hydrochloride) is a synthetic antispasmodic compound of relatively low toxicity. It has been shown to be useful for the symptomatic treatment of parkinsonism (paralysis agitans) and extrapyramidal dysfunction caused by tranquilizer therapy. Procyclidine hydrochloride was developed at The Wellcome Research Laboratories as the most promising of a series of antiparkinsonism compounds produced by chemical modification of antihistamines. Procyclidine hydrochloride is a white crystalline substance which is soluble in water and almost tasteless. It is known chemically as α-cyclohexyl-α-phenyl-1-pyrrolidinepropanol hydrochloride.

Kemadrin (procyclidine hydrochloride) is available in tablet form for oral administration. Each scored tablet contains 5 mg procyclidine hydrochloride and the inactive ingredients corn and potato starch, lactose, and magnesium stearate.

CLINICAL PHARMACOLOGY:

Pharmacologic tests have shown that procyclidine hydrochloride has an atropine-like action and exerts an antispasmodic effect on smooth muscle. It is a potent mydriatic and inhibits salivation. It has no sympathetic ganglion blocking activity in doses as high as 4 mg/kg, as measured by the lack of inhibition of the response of the nictitating membrane to preganglionic electrical stimulation.

The intravenous LD_{50} in mice was about 60 mg/kg. Subcutaneously, doses of 300 mg/kg were not toxic. In dogs the intraperitoneal administration of procyclidine hydrochloride in doses of 5 mg/kg caused maximal dilation of the pupil and inhibition of salivation, but had not toxic action. When the dose was increased to 20 mg/kg the same symptoms occurred, and in addition there were tremors and ataxia lasting 4 to 5 hours. In one animal convulsions occurred which were controlled by pentobarbital. In all animals behavior returned to normal within 24 hours.

Chronic toxicity tests in rats showed that the compound caused only a very slight retardation in growth, and no change in the erythrocyte count or the histological appearance of the lungs, liver, spleen and kidney when as much as 10 mg/kg body weight was given subcutaneously daily for 9 weeks.

INDICATIONS AND USAGE:

Kemadrin (procyclidine hydrochloride) is indicated in the treatment of parkinsonism including the postencephalitic, arteriosclerotic and idiopathic types. Partial control of the parkinsonism symptoms is the usual therapeutic accomplishment. Procyclidine hydrochloride is usually more efficacious in the relief of rigidity than tremor; but tremor, fatigue, weakness and sluggishness are frequently beneficially influenced. It can be substituted for all the previous medications in mild and moderate cases. For the control of more severe cases other drugs may be added to procyclidine therapy as indications warrant.

Clinical reports indicate that procyclidine often successfully relieves the symptoms of extrapyramidal dysfunction (dystonia, dyskinesia, akathisia, and parkinsonism) which accompany the therapy of mental disorders with phenothiazine and rauwolfia compounds. In addition to minimizing the symptoms induced by tranquilizing drugs, the drug effectively controls sialorrhea resulting from neuroleptic medication. At the same time freedom from the side effects induced by tranquilizer drugs, as provided by the administration of procyclidine, permits a more sustained treatment of the patient's mental disorder.

Clinical results in the treatment of parkinsonism indicate that most patients experience subjective improvement characterized by a feeling of well-being and increased alertness, together with diminished salivation and a marked improvement in muscular coordination as demonstrated by objective tests of manual dexterity and by increased ability to carry out ordinary self-care activities. While the drug exerts a mild atropine-like action and therefore causes mydriasis, this may be kept minimal by careful adjustment of the daily dosage.

CONTRAINDICATIONS:

Procyclidine hydrochloride should not be used in angle-closure glaucoma although simple type glaucomas do not appear to be adversely affected.

WARNINGS:

Usage in Children: Safety and efficacy have not been established in the pediatric age group, therefore, the use of procyclidine hydrochloride in this age group requires that the potential benefits be weighed against the possible hazards to the child.

Pregnancy Warning: The safe use of this drug in pregnancy has not been established; therefore, the use of procyclidine hydrochloride in pregnancy, lactation or in women of childbearing age requires that the potential benefits be weighed against the possible hazards to the mother and child.

PRECAUTIONS:

Conditions in which inhibition of the parasympathetic nervous system is undesirable such as tachycardia and urinary retention (such as may occur with marked prostatic hypertrophy) require special care in the administration of the drug. Hypotensive patients who receive the drug should be observed closely. Occasionally, particularly in older patients, mental confusion and disorientation may occur with the development of agitation, hallucinations and psychotic-like symptoms.

Patients with mental disorders occasionally experience a precipitation of a psychotic episode when the dosage of antiparkinsonism drugs is increased to treat the extrapyramidal side effects of phenothiazine and rauwolfia derivatives.

ADVERSE REACTIONS:

Anticholinergic effects can be produced by therapeutic doses although these can frequently be minimized or eliminated by careful dosage. They include: dryness of the mouth, mydriasis, blurring of vision, giddiness, lightheadedness and gastrointestinal disturbances such as nausea, vomiting, epigastric distress and constipation. Occasionally an allergic reaction such as a skin rash may be encountered. Feelings of muscular weakness may occur. Acute suppurative parotitis as a complication of dry mouth has been reported.

DOSAGE AND ADMINISTRATION:

For Parkinsonism: The dosage of the drug for the treatment of parkinsonism depends upon the age of the patient, the etiology of the disease, and individual responsiveness. Therefore, the dosage must remain flexible to permit adjustment to the individual tolerance and requirements of each patient. In general, younger and postencephalitic patients require and tolerate a somewhat higher dosage than older patients and those with arteriosclerosis.

For Patients Who Have Received No Other Therapy: The usual dose of procyclidine hydrochloride for initial treatment is 2.5 mg administered three times daily after meals. If well tolerated, this dose may be gradually increased to 5 mg three times a day and occasionally 5 mg given before retiring. In some cases smaller doses may be employed with good therapeutic results.

Occasionally a patient is encountered who cannot tolerate a bedtime dose of the drug. In such cases it may be desirable to adjust dosage so that the bedtime dose is omitted and the total daily requirement is administered in three equal daytime doses. It is best administered during or after meals to minimize the development of side reactions.

To Transfer Patients to Kemadrin (procyclidine hydrochloride) from Other Therapy: Patients who have been receiving other drugs may be transferred to procyclidine hydrochloride. This is accomplished gradually by substituting 2.5 mg three times a day for all or part of the original drug. The dose of procyclidine is then increased as required while that of the other drug is correspondingly omitted or decreased until complete replacement is achieved. The total daily dosage may then be adjusted to the level which produces maximum benefit.

For Drug-Induced Extrapyramidal Symptoms: For treatment of symptoms of extrapyramidal dysfunction induced by tranquilizer drugs during the therapy of mental disorders, the dosage of procyclidine hydrochloride will depend on the severity of side effects associated with tranquilizer administration. In general the larger the dosage of the tranquilizer the more severe will be the associated symptoms, including rigidity and tremors. Accordingly, the drug dosage should be adjusted to suit the needs of the individual patient and to provide maximum relief of the induced symptoms. A convenient method to establish the daily dosage of procyclidine is to begin with the administration of 2.5 mg three times daily. This may be increased by 2.5 mg daily increments until the patient obtains relief of symptoms. In most cases excellent results will be obtained with 10 to 20 mg daily.

HOW SUPPLIED:

White, scored tablets containing 5 mg procyclidine hydrochloride, imprinted with "Kemadrin" and "S3A".

Store at 15° to 25°C (59° to 77°F) in a dry place.

HOW SUPPLIED - EQUIVALENTS NOT AVAILABLE:

Tablet, Uncoated - Oral - 5 mg

100's	**$45.84**	**KEMADRIN, Glaxo Wellcome**	**00173-0604-55**

PROGESTERONE *(002122)*

CATEGORIES: Amenorrhea; Antineoplastics; Contraceptives; Hormones; Infertility; Menorrhagia; Oncologic Drugs; Progestins; Uterine Bleeding; FDA Approval Pre 1982

BRAND NAMES: Gesterol 50; Lutolin-S; Progestaject-50; **Progestasert**; Progestrone; Rogest 50

FORMULARIES: BC-BS; Medi-Cal

COST OF THERAPY: $75.00 (Contraceptive; Insert; 38 mg; 1/day; 1 days) vs. Potential Cost of $2,351.94 (Pregnancy)

WARNING:
THE USE OF PROGESTERONE INJECTION DURING THE FIRST FOUR MONTHS OF PREGNANCY IS NOT RECOMMENDED.
Progestational agents have been used beginning with the first trimester of pregnancy in an attempt to prevent habitual abortion. There is no adequate evidence that such use is effective when such drugs are given during the first 4 months of pregnancy. Furthermore, in the vast majority of women, the cause of abortion is a defective ovum, which progestational agents could not be expected to influence. In addition, the use of progestational agents, with their uterine-relaxant properties, in patients with fertilized defective ova may cause a delay in spontaneous abortion. Therefore, the use of such drugs during the first 4 months of pregnancy is not recommended.
Several reports suggest an association between intrauterine exposure to progestational drugs in the first trimester of pregnancy and genital abnormalities in male and female fetuses. The risk of hypospadias, 5 to 8 per 1,000 male births in the general population, may be approximately doubled with exposure to these drugs. There are insufficient data to quantify the risk to exposed female fetuses, but insofar as some of these drugs induce mild virilization of the external genitalia of the female fetus, and because of the increased association of hypospadias in the male fetus, it is prudent to avoid the use of these drugs during the first trimester of pregnancy.
If the patient is exposed to Progesterone Injection during the first four months of pregnancy or if she becomes pregnant while taking this drug, she should be apprised of the potential risks to the fetus.

INTRAMUSCULAR INJECTION

Important Advice To Physicians: You are required (in conformance with federal regulations) to give a PATIENT PACKAGE INSERT to each premenopausal woman, except those in whom childbearing is impossible, receiving this drug.

DESCRIPTION:

NOTE: This monograph includes information for the Intramuscular Injection, USP and the Intrauterine System.

Progesterone injection is a sterile solution of progesterone in a suitable vegetable oil available for intramuscular use.

Progesterone occurs as a white or creamy white, crystalline powder. It is odorless and is stable in air. Practically insoluble in water, it is soluble in alcohol, acetone, and dioxane and sparingly soluble in vegetable oils.

Each ml contain: Progesterone 50 mg, Benzyl Alcohol 10% as preservative in Sesame Oil q.s.

INTRAUTERINE SYSTEM

(Note: For complete graphic illustrations, please refer to original package insert)

NOTICE

You have received Patient Information Leaflets that Federal Regulations (21 CFR 310.502) require you to furnish to each patient who is considering the use of the Progestasert system.

The Patient Information Leaflet contains information on the safety and efficacy of the system. It also contains the Informed Choice Statement. You must not insert the Progestasert system until:

You have read this physician prescription labeling and are familiar with all the information it contains.

You and the patient have read and she had initialed each section of the Patient Information Leaflet.

You have counseled the patient and answered her questions about contraception, the Progestasert system, and the material in the Leaflet.

You and the patient have reviewed and signed the Informed Choice Statement.

The completely initialed and signed Leaflet, including the signed Informed Choice Statement, should be retained in the patient's records and a second copy of the initialed and signed leaflet given to the patient for her records.

The Leaflet is also available in Spanish should your practice require it. Address requests to: Customer Service Department, ALZA Corporation (Please refer to the Supplier Profile section for the address and phone number).

SYSTEM

The Progestasert system is a white, T-shaped unit constructed of ethylene/vinyl acetate copolymer (EVA) containing titanium dioxide. The 36-mm tubular vertical stem of the T contains a reservoir of 38 mg of progesterone, together with barium sulfate for radiopacity; both are dispersed in medical grade silicone fluid. The 32-mm horizontal crossarms are solid EVA. Two monofilament blue-black nylon indicator/retrieval threads are fastened to the base of the T stem.

The tip of the shorter indicator thread is 9 cm from the top or leading end of the system and is used to ascertain correct placement at insertion. The long thread extends the length of the inserter, to which it is anchored by a plug that retains the system in the inserter.

INSERTER

The inserter is a malleable, curved tube designed to conform to the anatomical configuration of most cervical-uterine cavities. The horizontal arms of the T are positioned outside of the inserter and are folded by an arm-cocker attachment immediately prior to insertion. The inserter does not contain a plunger.

DO NOT REMOVE ANY COMPONENT FROM THE INSERTER BEFORE INSERTION OF THE SYSTEM INTO THE UTERUS.

The Progestasert system inserter permits determination of the depth of uterine placement of the Progestasert system. The curvature of the inserter conforms with the usual orientation of the uterus; however, in cases of extreme flexion, the malleable inserter may need to be gently shaped to the desired curvature prior to insertion.

The Progestasert system is packaged sterile within its inserter. Progesterone is released from the system *in situ* at an average rate of 65 mcg/day for one year by membrane-controlled diffusion from the reservoir. Inert ingredients of the reservoir or membrane - barium sulfate, silicone fluid, titanium dioxide, or EVA - are not released.

CLINICAL PHARMACOLOGY:

INTRAMUSCULAR INJECTION

Transforms proliferative endometrium into secretory endometrium.

Inhibits (at the usual dosage) the secretion of pituitary gonadotropins, which in turn prevents follicular maturation and ovulation.

May also demonstrate some estrogenic, anabolic, or androgenic activity but should not be relied upon.

INTRAUTERINE SYSTEM

Available data indicate that the contraceptive effectiveness of the Progestasert system is enhanced by its continuous release of progesterone into the uterine cavity. The mechanism by which progesterone enhances the contraceptive effectiveness of the T is local, not systemic. The concentration of luteinizing hormone, estradiol, and progesterone in systemic venous plasma follow regular cyclic patterns indicative of ovulation during use of the Progestasert system. Blood chemistry studies related to liver, kidney, and thyroid function also reveal no clinically meaningful changes.

During use of the Progestasert system, the endometrium shows progestational influence. Progesterone released from the system at an average rate of 65 mcg/day suppresses endometrial proliferation (an anti-estrogenic effect.) Following system removal, the cyclic endometrial pattern rapidly returns to normal. The local mechanism by which continuously released progesterone enhances the contraceptive effectiveness of the T has not been conclusively demonstrated. Two hypotheses have been offered: progesterone-induced inhibition of sperm capacitation or survival; and alteration of the uterine milieu so as to prevent nidation.

CLINICAL STUDIES:

Different event rates have been reported with the use of different IUDS. Inasmuch as these rates are usually derived from separate studies conducted by different investigators in several population groups, they cannot be compared with precision. Clinical trials of the Progestasert system were conducted by ALZA and the World Health Organization from 1970 to 1981; use - effectiveness was determined from combined data as tabulated by the life table method. (Rates are expressed as events per 100 women through 12 months of use.) This experience is based on 5104 women who completed 12 months of use (TABLE 2):

TABLE 2

	Parous*	12 Months Nulliparous*
Pregnancy		
Intrauterine	1.3	2.1
Extrauterine (ectopic)	0.5	0.4
Total	1.8	2.5
Expulsion	2.7	7.6
Medical Removals	9.3	12.0
Continuation Rate	81.2	73.4

* Columns do not total 100 because rates are not included for the following: scheduled removals, removals for planned pregnancy, release from studies, and lost-to-follow-up.

The lowest expected and typical rates during the first year of continuous use of all contraceptive methods are listed in TABLE 3.[9]

TABLE 3 Percentage of Women Experiencing an Accidental Pregnancy in the First Year of Continuous Use

Method	Lowest Expected*	Typical**
No Contraception	85.0	85.0
Oral Contraceptives	3.0	
combined	0.1	N/A***
progestin only	0.5	N/A>***
Diaphragm with spermicidal cream or jelly	6.0	18.0
Spermicides alone (foam, creams, jellies and vaginal suppositories)	3.0	21.0
Vaginal Sponge		
nulliparous	6.0	18.0
multiparous	>9.0	28.0
IUD (medicated)	2.0	3.0†
Condom without spermicides	2.0	12.0
Periodic abstinence (all methods)	1.0-9.0	20.0
Female sterilization	0.2	0.4
Male sterilization	0.1	0.15
Norplant	0.04	0.04

* The authors' best guess of the percentage of women expected to experience an accidental pregnancy among couples who initiate a method (not necessarily for the first time) and use it consistently and correctly during the first year if they do not stop for any other reason.
** This term represents "typical" couples who initiate use of a method (not necessarily for the first time), who experience an accidental pregnancy during the first year if they do not stop use for any other reason.
*** N/A - Data not available.
† Combined typical rate for both the Progestasert and Copper T 380A. The typical rate for the Progestasert system alone is not available.

INDICATIONS AND USAGE:

INTRAMUSCULAR INJECTION

This drug is indicated in amenorrhea and abnormal uterine bleeding due to hormonal imbalance in the absence of organic pathology, such as submucous fibroids or uterine cancer.

INTRAUTERINE SYSTEM

The Progestasert system is indicated for intrauterine contraception in women who have had at least one child, are in a stable, mutually monogamous relationship, and have no history of pelvic inflammatory disease. The Progestasert system must be replaced every 12 months for continued contraceptive effect.

CONTRAINDICATIONS:

INTRAMUSCULAR INJECTION

1. Thrombophlebitis, thromboembolic disorders, cerebral apoplexy or patients with a past history of these secretions.

2. Known or suspected carcinoma of the breast.

3. Undiagnosed vaginal bleeding.

4. Missed abortion.

5. As a diagnostic test for pregnancy (see BOXED WARNING.)

INTRAUTERINE SYSTEM

The Progestasert system is contraindicated when one or more of the following conditions exist:

1. Pregnancy or suspected pregnancy.

CONTRAINDICATIONS: *(cont'd)*

2. History of ectopic pregnancy or a condition that predisposes to ectopic pregnancy (see WARNINGS, Ectopic Pregnancy.)

3. Presence of - or a history of - pelvic inflammatory disease (PID) or factors that predispose to PID (see WARNINGS, Pelvic Infection.)

4. Patient or her partner has multiple sexual partners.

5. Presence of, or a history of, sexually transmitted disease (one or more episodes), including but not limited to gonorrhea or chlamydial infections of the genital tract.

6. Postpartum endometritis or infected abortion.

7. Incomplete involution of the uterus following abortion or childbirth.

8. A previously inserted IUD is still in place.

9. History of pelvic surgery that may be associated with an increased risk of ectopic pregnancy, such as surgery of the fallopian tubes or surgery for pelvic adhesions or endometriosis.

10. Abnormalities of the uterus resulting in distortion of the uterine cavity or uteri that measure less than 6 cm or greater than 10 cm by sounding.

11. Known or suspected uterine or cervical malignancy including an unresolved, abnormal Pap smear.

12. Genital bleeding of unknown etiology.

13. Vaginitis or cervicitis unless and until infection has been eradicated and has been shown to be non-gonococcal and non-chlamydial.

14. Genital actinomycosis.

15. Conditions or treatments associated with increased susceptibility to infections with microorganisms. Such conditions include, but are not limited to, leukemia, diabetes, history of endocarditis or certain types of heart disease that are associated with an increased risk of endocarditis, acquired immune deficiency syndrome (AIDS), and conditions requiring chronic corticosteroid therapy.

16. IV drug abuse.

WARNINGS:

INTRAMUSCULAR INJECTION

1. Discontinue medication pending examination if there is a sudden partial or complete loss of vision, or if there is sudden onset of proptosis, diplopia, or migraine. If examination reveals papilledema or retinal vascular lesions, medication should be withdrawn.

2. Detectable amounts of progestogens have been identified in the milk of mothers receiving them. The effect of this on the nursing infant has not been determined.

3. Because of the occasional occurrence of thrombophlebitis and pulmonary embolism in patients taking progestogens, the physician should be alert to the earliest manifestation of the disease.

4. Masculinization of the female fetus has occurred when progestogens have been used in pregnant women.

INTRAUTERINE SYSTEM

Ectopic Pregnancy

The Progestasert system is contraindicated in patients who, in the physician's judgment, are at special risk of having an ectopic pregnancy. Ectopic pregnancy is potentially fatal and appears to occur more frequently with Progestasert system use than with other IUDs and other contraceptives. Therefore, the possibility of ectopic pregnancy must always be considered in Progestasert system users - including those lacking the specific risk factors described below.

The material that follows is intended to aid the physician in the following:

Understanding the risks of ectopic pregnancy in Progestasert system users (Section 1a).

Proper selection of women for Progestasert system use by identifying and excluding those at special risk to ectopic pregnancy (see Women at special risk to ectopic pregnancy.)

Diagnosing and managing ectopic pregnancy in IUD users (see Diagnosis of ectopic pregnancy and Management of diagnosed or suspected ectopic pregnancy).

Informing patients of ectopic pregnancy risks (see Ectopic pregnancy warning to Progestasert system users).

Risks of ectopic pregnancy with Progestasert system use: Should a woman become pregnant while using the Progestasert system, the pregnancy is more likely to be ectopic than a pregnancy in a woman using no contraception, ovulation-suppressing oral contraception, or barrier methods.[1,2] This is because the Progestasert system acts in the uterus to prevent uterine pregnancy, but it does not prevent either ovulation or ectopic pregnancy. Thus, each month that the Progestasert system is used there is protection against uterine pregnancy but not against ectopic pregnancy. In clinical trials of the Progestasert system 1 of 3.6 pregnancies in parous women and 1 of 6.2 pregnancies in nulliparous women were ectopic.

The per-year risk of ectopic pregnancy in Progestasert system users is approximately 5 per 1,000 or 1 ectopic pregnancy in 200 users per year. This risk is approximately the same as in noncontracepting, sexually active women. In contrast, barrier contraceptives, which prevent fertilization, or oral contraceptives that prevent ovulation, reduce the risk of ectopic pregnancy to a few percent of the risk in noncontracepting, sexually active women.

Two clinical studies conducted by the World Health Organization compared the risk of ectopic pregnancies among 2,239 women wearing a progesterone-releasing IUD similar to the Progestasert system with the risk in 3,303 women wearing a copper-releasing IUD. For the first year the risk of ectopic pregnancy was approximately 6 times higher among women using progesterone system than among women using copper systems. Over the two years that the studies ran, the risk of an ectopic pregnancy with the progesterone-releasing IUD was about 10 times higher than that with copper-releasing IUDs.

Women at special risk to ectopic pregnancy: Several factors have been identified as placing a woman at special risk to ectopic pregnancy. The presence of any of these factors contraindicates use of the Progestasert system. Factors indicating high risk to ectopic pregnancy include a history of ectopic pregnancy or a history or presence of a condition predisposing to ectopic pregnancy such as PID. A prospective clinical study was conducted over 9.5 years in 415 women who had verified PID and 100 healthy control subjects. The ratio between ectopic and intrauterine pregnancies after PID was 1/24. In contrast, the ratio in the controls was 1/147. Further analysis of these data suggests that women who have had PID subsequently have an 8-to 10-fold greater risk of ectopic pregnancy than sexually active noncontracepting women who have never had PID.

Factors other than PID may also indicate a high risk to ectopic pregnancy. These factors include multiple sexual partners or a partner with multiple sexual partners, pelvic surgery of certain types, retrograde menstruation, endometritis, and endometriosis.

Diagnosis of ectopic pregnancy: The absence of risk factors for ectopic pregnancy described above does not rule out ectopic pregnancy. In every instance of pregnancy occurring in a Progestasert system user it is essential that proper measures be taken to determine if the pregnancy is ectopic.

To determine whether ectopic pregnancy has occurred, special attention should be directed to patients with any of the following symptoms or conditions: unusual, abnormal, or irregular vaginal bleeding; delayed or missed menses; pelvic pain, usually unilateral, which may be associated with fainting or the urge to defecate; unexplained pain in the shoulder; or pain associated with bleeding if not part of the usual menstrual cycle. Ectopic pregnancy should be strongly suspected in patients with positive pregnancy test or elevated B-HCG values but who lack ultrasonographic or other evidence of intrauterine pregnancy.

Management of diagnosed or suspected ectopic pregnancy: When ectopic pregnancy is suspected, diagnostic uncertainty should be resolved as quickly as possible, in view of the life-threatening risk of ruptured ectopic pregnancy. When ectopic pregnancy is diagnosed, immediate surgery is often required because a ruptured ectopic pregnancy may occur at any time.

Ectopic pregnancy warning to Progestasert system users: All women who choose the Progestasert system must be informed before insertion that a pregnancy occurring in a Progestasert system user is more likely to be ectopic than one occurring in users of ovulation-preventing oral contraceptives, barrier modes or other IUDs. They should be taught to recognize and report to their physician promptly any symptoms of ectopic pregnancy. Women should also be informed that ectopic pregnancy has been associated with complications leading to loss of fertility.

Intrauterine Pregnancy

Intrauterine pregnancy can occur during use of the Progestasert system (see CLINICAL STUDIES for pregnancy rates).

Long-term effects and congenital anomalies: When pregnancy occurs or proceeds with the Progestasert system in place, long-term effects on the offspring are unknown. Congenital anomalies have occurred under such conditions. Their relationship to the Progestasert system has not been established. Systemically administered sex steroids, including progestational agents, have been associated with an increased risk of congenital anomalies. It is not known whether an increased risk of such anomalies exists when pregnancy continues with a Progestasert system in place. The decision to continue or terminate pregnancy should take into account this unknown risk.

Septic abortion: Reports have indicated an increased incidence of septic abortion - with septicemia, septic shock, and death - in patients becoming pregnant with an IUD in place. Most of these reports have been associated with, but are not limited to, the mid-trimester of pregnancy. In some cases, the initial symptoms have been insidious and not easily recognized. If pregnancy should occur with a Progestasert system *in situ*, the system should be removed if the thread is visible and removal is easily accomplished. Removal or manipulation of the Progestasert system may precipitate abortion. If removal would be or proves to be difficult, or if threads are not visible, termination of the pregnancy should be considered and offered to the patient as an option, bearing in mind that the risks associated with an elective abortion increase with gestational age.

Continuation of pregnancy: If the patient chooses to continue the pregnancy with the system in place, she must be warned that this increases the risk of spontaneous abortion and sepsis, which may cause death. In addition, she is at increased risk of premature labor and delivery. As a consequence of premature birth, the fetus is at increased risk of damage. She should be followed more closely than the usual obstetrical patient. She must be advised to report immediately all symptoms such as flu-like syndrome, fever, chills, abdominal cramping and pain, bleeding, or vaginal discharge, because generalized symptoms of septicemia may be insidious.

Pelvic Infection (Pelvic Inflammatory Disease)

The Progestasert system is contraindicated in the presence of PID or suspected PID or in women with a history of PID.Use of all IUDs, including the Progestasert system, has been associated with an increased incidence of PID. In a hospital-based, case-control study done in the United States in 1976-1978, women using IUD's had a relative risk of PID of 1.6 compared with women using no method.[3]Therefore a decision to use the Progestasert system must include consideration of the risks of PID. The highest rate of PID occurs shortly after insertion and up to four months thereafter. Administration of prophylactic antibiotics may be useful, but the utility of this treatment is still under consideration (see Insertion Precautions.) PID can necessitate hysterectomy; can lead to tubo-ovarian abscesses, tubal occlusion and infertility, and tubal damage that predisposes to ectopic pregnancy; can result in peritonitis; and can cause death in infrequent cases. The effect of PID on fertility is especially important for women who may wish to have children at a later date.

Women at special risk to PID: PID is usually a sexually transmitted disease, and the Progestasert system does not protect against sexually transmitted disease. The risk of PID appears to be greater for women who have multiple sexual partners and also for women whose sexual partner(s) have multiple sexual partners. Women who have ever had PID are at high risk for a recurrence or re-infection.

PID warning to Progestasert system users: All women who choose the Progestasert system must be informed prior to insertion that IUD use has been associated with an increased incidence of PID and that PID can necessitate hysterectomy, can cause tubal damage leading to ectopic pregnancy or infertility, or in infrequent cases can cause death. Patients must be taught to recognize and report to their physician promptly any symptoms of pelvic inflammatory disease. These symptoms include development of menstrual disorders (prolonged or heavy bleeding), unusual vaginal discharge, abdominal or pelvic pain or tenderness, dyspareunia, chills, and fever.

Asymptomatic PID: PID may be asymptomatic but still result in tubal damage and its sequelae.[4,5]

Treatment of PID: Following diagnosis of PID, or suspected PID, bacteriological specimens should be obtained and antibiotic therapy should be initiated promptly. Removal of the Progestasert intrauterine progesterone contraceptive system after initiation of antibiotic therapy is required.

Guidelines for PID treatment are available from the Center for Disease Control (CDC), Atlanta, Georgia. A copy of the printed guidelines has been provided to you by ALZA Corporation. The guidelines were established after deliberation by a group of experts and staff of the CDC but they should not be construed as rules suitable for use in all patients. Adequate PID treatment requires the application of current standards of therapy prevailing at the time of occurrence of the infection with reference to the specific antibiotics' prescription labeling.

Genital actinomycosis has been associated primarily with long-term IUD use. If it occurs, promptly institute appropriate antibiotic therapy and remove the Progestasert system.

Embedment

Partial penetration or embedment of the Progestasert system in the endometrium or myometrium may decrease contraceptive effectiveness and can result in difficult removals. In some cases, this can result in fragmentation of the IUD, necessitating surgical removal.

Fragmentation

If fragmentation of the Progestasert system occurs, all pieces should be removed if possible. Verification or removal should take into account that the horizontal cross-arms are not radiopaque.

Perforation

Partial or total perforation of the uterine wall or cervix may occur with use of a uterine sound or the Progestasert system. It is generally believed that perforations, if they occur, happen at the time of insertion, although the perforation may not be detected until some time later. The possibility of perforation must be kept in mind during insertion and at the

WARNINGS: *(cont'd)*

time of any subsequent examination. It is recommended that the Progestasert system insertion be postponed postpartum, or post abortion until involution of the uterus is complete since the incidence of perforation and expulsion is greater if involution is not complete. Involution may be delayed in nursing mothers; there is an increased risk of perforation in women who are lactating. If perforation occurs, the Progestasert system should be removed. A surgical procedure may be required. Adhesions, foreign body reactions, peritonitis, cystic masses in the pelvis, intestinal penetrations, intestinal obstruction and local inflammatory reactions with abscess formation and erosion of adjacent viscera may result if an IUD is left in the peritoneal cavity.

Risks of Mortality

The available data from a variety of sources have been analyzed to estimate the risk of death associated with various methods of contraception. The estimates of risk of death include the combined risk of the contraceptive method plus the risk of pregnancy or abortion in the event of method failure. The findings of the analysis are shown in TABLE 1.[6]

TABLE 4 Annual Number of Birth-Related or Method-Related Deaths Associated with Control of Fertility per 100,000 Nonsterile Women, by Fertility Control Method According to Age.

Method control and outcome	15-19	20-24	25-29	30-34	35-39	40-44
No fertility control methods*	7.0	7.4	9.1	14.8	25.7	28.2
Oral contraceptives/non-smokers**	0.3	0.5	0.9	1.9	13.8	31.6
Oral contraceptives/ smokers**	2.2	3.4	6.6	13.5	51.1	117.2
IUD**	0.8	0.8	1.0	1.0	1.4	1.4
Condom*	1.1	1.6	0.7	0.2	0.3	0.4
Diaphragm/ Spermicide*	1.9	1.2	1.2	1.3	2.2	2.8
Periodic abstinence	2.5	1.6	1.6	1.7	2.9	3.6

* Deaths are birth related
** Deaths are method related

PRECAUTIONS:

GENERAL

Intramuscular Injection: The pretreatment physical examination should include special reference to the breast and pelvic organs, as well as Papanicolaou smear.

Because this drug may cause some degree of fluid retention, conditions which might be influenced by this factor, such as epilepsy, migraines, asthma, cardiac, or renal dysfunction, require careful observation.

In cases of breakthrough bleeding, as in all cases of irregular bleeding*per vaginum,* non-functional causes should be borne in mind. In cases of undiagnosed vaginal bleeding, adequate diagnostic measures are indicated.

Patients who have a history of psychic depression should be carefully observed and the drug discontinued if the depression recurs to a serious degree.

Any possible influence of prolonged progestin therapy on pituitary, ovarian, adrenal, hepatic, or uterine functions awaits further study.

A decrease in glucose tolerance has been observed in a small percentage of patients on estrogen-progestin combination drugs. The mechanism of this decrease is obscure. For this reason, diabetic patients should be carefully observed while receiving progestin therapy.

The age of the patient constitutes no absolute limiting factor although treatment with progestins may mask the onset of climacteric.

The pathologist should be advised of progestin therapy when relevant specimens are submitted.

Studies of the addition of a progestin product to an estrogen replacement regimen for seven or more days of a cycle of estrogen administration have reported a lowered incidence of endometrial hyperplasia. Morphological and biochemical studies of endometrium suggest that 10 to 13 days of a progestin are needed to provide maximal maturation of the endometrium and to eliminate any hyperplastic changes. Whether this will provide protection from endometrial carcinoma has not been clearly established. There are possible additional risks which may be associated with the inclusion of progestin in estrogen replacement regimens. The potential risks include adverse effects on carbohydrate and lipid metabolism. The dosage used may be important in minimizing these adverse effects.

INFORMATION FOR THE PATIENT

See Text of PATIENT PACKAGE INSERT.

LABORATORY TESTS

The following laboratory results may be altered by the concomitant use of an estrogen and a progestogen:

Hepatic function: increased sulfobromophthalein retention and other tests.

Coagulation tests: increase in prothrombin Factors VII, VIII, IX and X.

Thyroid function: increase in PBI and BEI and a decrease in T_3 uptake values.

CARCINOGENESIS, MUTAGENESIS, AND IMPAIRMENT OF FERTILITY

Metyrapone test: In dogs, the experimental administration of the progestational agent medroxyprogesterone acetate increased the frequency of mammary nodules. Although nodules occasionally appeared in control animal, they were intermittent in nature, whereas nodules in treated animals were larger, more numerous, persistent, and there were some breast malignancies with metastases. Their significance with respect to humans has not been established.

PREGNANCY

Pregnancy Category D: See WARNINGS and information in the box at the start of this literature.

Nursing Mothers: Detectable amounts of progesterone have been identified in the milk of mothers receiving the steroid. Its effect on the nursing infant has not been determined.

Because of the potential for tumorigenicity shown for progesterone in animal studies, a decision should be made whether to discontinue nursing or to discontinue the drug, taking into account the importance of the drug to the mother.

Pediatric Use: Safety and effectiveness in children have not been established.

INTRAUTERINE SYSTEM

Patient Counseling

a. Patients should be counseled that this product does not protect against HIV infection (AIDS) and other sexually transmitted diseases.

b. Patients must be informed of the availability, effectiveness, and risks of the Progestasert system and other forms of contraception. They should also be informed of the health risks associated with pregnancy resulting from failure to use any contraception.

PRECAUTIONS: *(cont'd)*

c. Prior to insertion of the Progestasert system, the physician, nurse, or other trained health professional must provide the patient with the Patient Information Leaflet. The patient must read the leaflet in its entirety and discuss fully any questions she has concerning the Progestasert system and other methods of contraception. She must then initial and sign the leaflet, including the informed Choice Statement, where indicated.

Patient Evaluation and Clinical Considerations

a. A complete medical and social history should be obtained to determine conditions that might influence the selection of the Progestasert system or contraindicate its use (see CONTRAINDICATIONS.) Physical examination should include a pelvic examination, Pap smear, N. gonorrhea and Chlamydia culture (or other specific tests for these organisms) and, if indicated, appropriate tests for other forms of venereal disease. **Special attention must be given to ascertaining whether the woman is at increased risk of ectopic pregnancy or PID. The Progestasert system is contraindicated in these women.**

b. The Progestasert system is not intended for immediate postabortion or postpartum insertion. It should not be inserted until involution of the uterus is complete. (Involution may be delayed in nursing mothers.) The incidence of perforation and expulsion is greater if involution is not completed. Data also suggest there may be an increased risk of perforation and expulsion if the woman is lactating.[7,8]

c. The physician should determine that the patient is not pregnant. The possibility of insertion in the presence of an existing undetermined pregnancy is reduced if insertion is performed during or shortly following a menstrual period.

d. Patients with certain types of valvular heart disease and surgically constructed systemic-pulmonary shunts have an increased risk of infective endocarditis. Use of a Progestasert system in these patients may represent a potential source of septic emboli and is contraindicated. Other conditions predisposing to infection (see CONTRAINDICATIONS) are also contraindications to Progestasert system insertion.

e. IUDs should be used with caution in those patients who have an anemia or a history of menorrhagia or hypermenorrhea. Patients experiencing menorrhagic and/or metrorrhagia following IUD insertion may be at risk for the development of hypochromic microcytic anemia. Also, IUDs should be used with caution in patients who have a coagulopathy or are receiving anticoagulants.

f. Use of the Progestasert system in patients with vaginitis or cervicitis should be postponed until proper treatment has cleared up the infection and until the cervicitis has been shown not to be due to gonorrhea or chlamydia (see CONTRAINDICATIONS.)

Insertion Precautions

a. Because the presence of organisms capable of establishing PID cannot be determined by appearance, and because IUD insertion may be associated with introduction of vaginal bacteria into the uterus, administration of prophylactic antibiotics may be considered, but the utility of this treatment is still under evaluation. Regimens include doxycycline 200 mg orally 1 hour before insertion or erythromycin 500 mg orally 1 hour before insertion and 500 mg orally 6 hours after insertion. The use of antibiotics in nursing mothers is not recommended. Before prescribing the above mentioned antibiotics, refer to their prescription drug labeling, and make certain that the patient is a suitable candidate for the drug.

b. The uterus should be carefully sounded prior to insertion to determine the degree of patency of the endocervical canal and the internal os, and the direction and depth of the uterine cavity. In occasional cases, severe cervical stenosis may be encountered. Do not use excessive force to overcome this resistance.

c. The uterus should sound to a depth of 6 to 10 centimeters (cm). Insertion of the Progestasert system into a uterine cavity measuring less than 6.5 cm by sounding may increase the incidence of expulsion, bleeding, and pain.

d. Syncope, bradycardia, or other neurovascular episodes may occur during insertion or removal of the Progestasert system, especially in patients with a previous disposition to these conditions or cervical stenosis. If decreased pulse, perspiration, or pallor are observed, the patient should remain supine until these signs have disappeared.

e. The patient should be told that some bleeding and/or cramps may occur during the first few weeks after insertion. If her symptoms continue or are severe she should report them to her physician. She should also be given instructions on what other symptoms require her to call her physician. She should be instructed on how to check after her menstrual period to make certain that the thread still protrudes from the cervix and cautioned not to pull on the thread and displace the Progestasert system. She should be informed that there is no contraceptive protection if the Progestasert system is displaced or expelled. If a partial expulsion occurs, removal is indicated.

f. The patient must be told to return within 3 months for a checkup and at 12 months after insertion for removal of the Progestasert system. Patient reminder cards should be properly completed and given to the patient.

Requirements for Continuation and Removal

a. The Progestasert system must be replaced every 12 months. There is no evidence of decreasing contraceptive efficacy with time before 12 months, but contraceptive effectiveness after 12 months decreases; therefore, the patient should be informed of the known duration of contraceptive efficacy and be advised to return in 12 months for removal and possible insertion of a new Progestasert system.

b. The Progestasert system should be removed for the following medical reasons: menorrhagic-and/or metrorrhagic-producing anemia; acquired immune deficiency syndrome (AIDS); sexually transmitted disease; pelvic infection; endometritis; genital actinomycosis; intractable pelvic pain; dyspareunia; pregnancy; endometrial or cervical malignancy; uterine or cervical perforation; increase in length of the threads extending from the cervix, or any other indication of partial expulsion.

c. If the retrieval threads are not visible, they may have retracted into the uterus or have been broken, or the Progestasert system may have been broken, perforated the uterus, or have been expelled. Location may be determined by feeling with a probe, X-ray or sonography.

Continuing Care of Patients Using the Progestasert system

a. Any inquiries regarding pain, odorous discharge, bleeding, fever, genital lesions or sores, or a missed period should be promptly responded to and prompt examination recommended.

b. If examination during visits subsequent to insertion reveals that the length of the threads had visibly or palpably changed from the length at time of insertion, the system should be considered displaced and should be removed. A new system may be inserted at that time or during the next menses if it is certain that conception hasn't occurred. When the thread cannot be seen by the physician, further investigation is necessary.

c. Since the Progestasert system may be expelled or displaced, patients should be reexamined and evaluated shortly after the first postinsertion menses, but definitely within 3 months after insertion. **The Progestasert system must be removed every 12 months because of diminished contraceptive effectiveness thereafter.**At the time of reinsertion, appropriate medical and laboratory examinations should be carried out.

d. In the event a pregnancy is confirmed during Progestasert system use, the following steps should be taken:

Determine whether pregnancy is ectopic and take appropriate measures if it is.

PRECAUTIONS: *(cont'd)*

Inform patient of the risks of leaving an IUD *in situ* or removing it during pregnancy and of the lack of data on the Progestasert system's long-term effects on the offspring of women who have had it *in utero* during conception or gestation (see WARNINGS.)

If possible the Progestasert system should be removed after the patient has been warned of the risks of removal. If removal is difficult, the patient should be counseled about and offered pregnancy termination.

If the Progestasert system is left in place, the patient's course should be followed closely.

e. Should the patient's relationship cease to be mutually monogamous, or should her partner become HIV positive, or acquire a sexually transmitted disease, she should be instructed to report this change and see her physician immediately.

ADVERSE REACTIONS:

INTRAMUSCULAR INJECTION

The following adverse reactions have been observed in women taking progestogens: Break through bleeding, spotting, change in menstrual flow, amenorrhea, edema, changes in weight (increase or decrease), changes in cervical erosion and cervical secretions, cholestatic jaundice, rash (allergic) with and without pruritus, melasma or chloasma, and mental depression.

A small percentage of patients have local reactions at the site of injection.

The administration of large doses of progesterone (50 to 100 mg daily) may result in a moderate catabolic effect and a transient increase in sodium and chloride excretion.

The result of a pregnanediol determination may be altered if a patient is being treated with a progestogen.

A STATISTICALLY SIGNIFICANT ASSOCIATION HAS BEEN DEMONSTRATED BETWEEN THE USE OF ESTROGEN-PROGESTIN COMBINATION DRUGS AND THE FOLLOWING SERIOUS ADVERSE REACTIONS:

Thrombophlebitis; pulmonary embolism and cerebral thrombosis and embolism. For this reason patients on progestin therapy should be carefully observed.

ALTHOUGH AVAILABLE EVIDENCE IS SUGGESTIVE OF AN ASSOCIATION, SUCH A RELATIONSHIP HAS BEEN NEITHER CONFIRMED NOR REFUTED FOR THE FOLLOWING SERIOUS, ADVERSE REACTIONS:

Beuro-Ocular lesions, e.g. retinal thrombosis and optic neuritis.

THE FOLLOWING ADVERSE REACTIONS HAVE BEEN OBSERVED IN PATIENTS RECEIVING ESTROGEN-PROGESTIN COMBINATION DRUGS:

Rise in blood pressure in susceptible individuals; premenstrual-like syndrome; changes in libido, changes in appetite, cystitis-like syndrome, headache, nervousness, dizziness, fatigue, backache, hirsutism, loss of scalp hair, erythema multiforme, erythema nodosum, hemorrhagic eruption, and itching.

In view of these observation, patients on progestin therapy should be carefully observed for their occurrence.

INTRAUTERINE SYSTEM

These adverse reactions are not listed in any order of frequency or severity.

Reported adverse reactions with intrauterine contraceptives include: endometritis; spontaneous abortion; septic abortion; septicemia; perforation of the uterus and cervix; embedment; fragmentation of the IUD; pelvic infection; tubo-ovarian abscess; tubal damage; vaginitis; leukorrhea; cervical erosion; pregnancy; ectopic pregnancy; fetal damage and congenital anomalies; difficult removal; complete or partial expulsion of the IUD; intermenstrual spotting; prolongation of menstrual flow; anemia; amenorrhea or delayed menses; pain and cramping; dysmenorrhea; backaches; dyspareunia; neurovascular episodes, including bradycardia and syncope secondary to insertion. Uterine perforation and IUD displacement into the abdomen have been followed by peritonitis, abdominal adhesions, intestinal penetration, intestinal obstruction, local inflammatory reaction with abscess formation and erosion of adjacent viscera, and cystitic masses in the pelvis. Certain of these adverse reactions can lead to loss of fertility, partial or total removal of reproductive organs, hormonal imbalance, or death.

DOSAGE AND ADMINISTRATION:

INTRAMUSCULAR INJECTION

Progesterone is administered by intramuscular injection. It differs from other commonly used steroids in that it is irritating at the place of injection. This is true whether the preparation is in an oil or an aqueous vehicle. The latter is particularly painful.

AMENORRHEA

Five to 10 mg are given for six to eight consecutive days. If there has been sufficient ovarian activity to produce a proliferative endometrium, one can expect withdrawal bleeding forty-eight to seventy hours after the last injection. This may be followed by spontaneous normal cycles.

FUNCTIONAL UTERINE BLEEDING

Five to 10 mg are given daily for six doses. Bleeding may be expected to cease within six days. When estrogen is given as well, the administration of progesterone is begun after two weeks of estrogen therapy. If menstrual flow begins during the course of injections of progesterone, they are discontinued.

Store at controlled room temperature 15-30°C (59-86°F)

INTRAUTERINE SYSTEM

Directions For Use A single Progestasert system is to be inserted into the uterine cavity (see PRECAUTIONS.) The system must be removed 12 months after insertion and replaced for continued contraceptive effectiveness. See INSERTION AND REMOVAL INSTRUCTIONS.

INSERTION AND REMOVAL INSTRUCTIONS

NOTE: Physicians are cautioned to become thoroughly familiar with the insertion instructions in their entirety before attempting placement of the Progestasert intrauterine progesterone contraceptive system.

There is debate as to how many IUD insertions constitute adequate training for a clinician. It is probably wise to have done 15-25 insertions under supervision prior to inserting an IUD unsupervised. A practitioner with only 4-6 insertions would probably not have had adequate experience with difficult insertions.

The insertion technique for Progestasert is different in several respects from that used with other intrauterine contraceptives and the physician should pay particular attention to the drawing and commentary accompanying these instructions.

The usual time of insertion is during the latter part of the menstrual period, or one or two days thereafter.

The Progestasert system retains its efficacy for 12 months. Therefore, it must be removed and a new one inserted no more than 12 months after insertion for continued contraceptive efficacy.

PRELIMINARY PREPARATION

1. Before insertion, the patient must read and initial each section of the Patient Information Leaflet; the medical and social history and counseling of the patient must be completed; and the Informed Choice Statement must be signed by the patient and by the doctor.

DOSAGE AND ADMINISTRATION: *(cont'd)*

2. Refer to CONTRAINDICATIONS, WARNINGS, and PRECAUTIONS.

3. Prior to insertion of the Progestasert system, a cervical Pap smear, N. gonorrhea and Chlamydia cultures (or other specific tests for these organisms), and pelvic examination are to be performed.

4. If appropriate, commence antibiotic prophylaxis one hour before insertion.

5. Use of aseptic technique during insertion is essential.

6. The cervix should be cleansed with an antiseptic solution and a tenaculum applied to the cervix with downward traction for stabilization of the cervix and correction of angulation.

7. Prior to insertion, determine by uterine sounding the depth and position of the uterus and the patency of the cervical canal. Insertion into a uterus that sounds less that 6 cm or more than 10 cm is contraindicated. Great care must be exercised during the preinsertion sounding and subsequent insertion. No attempt should be made to force the insertion.

8. THE PROGESTASERT SYSTEM MUST BE USED ONLY WITH ITS SPECIALLY DESIGNED INSERTER. This inserter will facilitate fundal placement and is designed to decrease the possibility of uterine perforation. No component should be removed from the inserter before insertion of the system into the uterus.

NOTE: Any intrauterine procedure can result in severe pain, bradycardia, and syncope.

SYSTEM INSERTION

1. Place the pouch on a hard, flat surface. Peel the clear cover back completely. Inspect the inserter to make sure the thread-retaining plug is secure at the end of the inserter with 2.5-5.0 cm. of the long "retainer" thread protruding. Do not insert the system if the plug cannot be easily secured. Remove the system and inserter by grasping the inserter at a point between the two sets of graduations. DO NOT CONTAMINATE THE END CONTAINING THE SYSTEM.

2. IMMEDIATELY PRIOR TO INSERTION, cock the arms of the Progestasert system by holding the inserter vertically with the arm cocker flat on the sterile interior of the pouch. Press down firmly to cock the arms. This will cause the arms to fold against the sides of the inserter. *NOTE:*To avoid alteration of system shape, do not leave the system cocked for more than five minutes.

3. Examine the curvature of the inserter. Make any necessary adjustments to the curvature of the inserter to fit the flexion of the uterus, maintaining aseptic technique. For an anteverted uterus, the black numbers on the inserter should face up; they should face down for a retroverted uterus. Be certain that the thread-retaining plug is still secure in the end of the inserter, then introduce the inserter into the cervical canal. The feet of the arm-cocker will rest centered on the cervical os as you push the inserter gently but steadily through the cervical canal.

4. When the fundus is reached, the number on the inserter at the base of the arm-cocker should equal the previously sounded uterine depth.

5. DO NOT PULL BACK ON THE ARMCOCKER OR INSERTER. Release the Progestasert intrauterine progesterone contraceptive system by squeezing the wings of the thread-retaining plug and removing it.

6. Slowly withdraw the inserter. The Progestasert system remains in the uterus as the inserter is withdrawn. After insertion is complete, check to make certain that no components of the inserter are in the uterus. Dispose of the inserter shaft with attached armcocker, as well as the thread-retaining plug.

CORRECT FUNDAL PLACEMENT

To be fully effective, the Progestasert system must be placed at the fundus. To confirm the correct position of the Progestasert system, measure the length of the short "indicator" thread against the graduations on the thread-retaining end of the inserter. The length of this short thread should be the difference between 9 cm and the uterine depth.

For example, if the uterus was sounded to 7 cm., the short "indicator" thread should extend out of the cervix 9 cm -7 cm = 2 cm.

Cut the long "retainer" thread to a standard length of your choice - at least 3 cm from the cervix. This can be used for future reference in determining if fundal placement is being maintained. (If pregnancy, displacement, or perforation occurs, the thread may be drawn up through the cervix.) Record the uterine depth and length of cut "retain" thread in the patient's chart.

SYSTEM REMOVAL

To remove the Progestasert system, pull gently on the exposed threads. The arms of the system will fold upward as it is withdrawn from the uterus. Even if removal proves difficult, the system should not remain in the uterus after one year.

PATIENT PACKAGE INSERT:

INTRAMUSCULAR INJECTION

PATIENT LABELING FOR PROGESTATIONAL DRUG PRODUCTS

WARNING FOR WOMEN

Progesterone or progesterone-like drugs have been used to prevent miscarriage in the first few months of pregnancy. No adequate evidence is available to show that they are effective for this purpose. Furthermore, most cases of early miscarriage are due to causes which could not be helped by these drugs.

There is an increased risk of minor birth defects in children whose mothers take this drug during the first 4 months of pregnancy. Several reports suggest an association between mothers who take these drugs in the first trimester of pregnancy and genital abnormalities in male and female babies. The risk to the male baby is the possibility of being born with a condition in which the opening of the penis is on the underside rather than the tip of the penis (hypospadias). Hypospadia occurs in about 5 to 8 per 1,000 male births and is about doubled with exposure to these drugs. There is not enough information to quantify the risk to exposed female fetuses, but enlargement of the clitoris and fusion of the labia may occur, although rarely.

Therefore, since drugs of this type may induce mild masculinization of the external genitalia of the female fetus, as well as hypospadia in the male fetus, it is wise to avoid using the drug during the first trimester of pregnancy.

These drugs have been used as a test for pregnancy but such use is no longer considered safe because of possible damage to a developing baby. Also, more rapid methods for testing for pregnancy are now available.

If you are taking progesterone or a progesterone-like drug and later find you were pregnant when you took it, be sure to discuss this with your doctor as soon as possible.

REFERENCES:

Intrauterine System 1. World Health Organization's Special Programme of Research, Development and Research Training in Human Reproduction: A multi-national case-control study of ectopic pregnancy. "Clin. Reprod. Fertil." 1985; 3: 131 - 143. **2.** Ory, H.W.: Women's Health Study: Ectopic pregnancy and intrauterine contraceptive devices: New perspectives. "Obstet. Gynecol." 1981; 57: 137-144. **3.** Lee, N.C. Rubin, G.L., and Borucki, R.: The Intrauterine Device and Pelvic Inflammatory Disease Revisited: New Results From the Women's Health Study. "Obstet. Gynecol." 1988; 72: 1-6. **4.** Cramer, D.W. et al: Tubal infertility and the intrauterine device. "N. Engl. J. Med." 1985; 312:941-947. **5.** Daling, J.R. et al: Primary tubal infertility in relation to the use of an intrauterine device. "N Engl. J. Med." 1985; 312: 937-941. **6.** Ory, H.W.: Mortality associated with fertility and fertility control. "Family Planning Perspectives" 1983; 15: 57-63. **7.** Heartwell, S.F., Schlesselman, S.: Risk of uterine perforation among users of intrauterine devices. "Obstet. Gynecol." 1983; 61: 31-36. **8.** Chi, I.C. Kelly,

REFERENCES: *(cont'd)*

E.: Is lactation a risk factor of IUD and sterilization-related uterine perforations. A hypothesis. "Int. J. Gynaecol. Obstet." 1984; 22: 315-317. 9. Trussel, J., Kost, K.: Contraceptive failure in the United States: A critical review of the literature. "Studies in Family Planning" 1987; 18: 237-283.

HOW SUPPLIED - RATED THERAPEUTICALLY EQUIVALENT:

Injection, Solution - Intramuscular - 50 mg/ml

10 ml	$8.99	Progesterone, McGuff	49072-0589-10
10 ml	$9.51	Progesterone (in Oil), Pasadena	00418-0631-41
10 ml	$13.00	Progesterone In Oil, Consolidated Midland	00223-8381-10
10 ml	$13.55	Progesterone, Paddock Labs	00574-0704-10
10 ml	$13.90	Progesterone, Hyrex Pharms	00314-0060-10
10 ml	$14.95	Progesterone, United Res	00677-0301-21
10 ml	$14.95	Rogest 50, Robar	54171-0379-10
10 ml	$16.36	Progesterone Oil, HL Moore Drug Exch	00839-5165-30
10 ml	$18.00	Progesterone, Steris Labs	00402-0379-10
10 ml	$19.50	Progesterone In Oil, Rugby	00536-7400-70
10 ml	$20.30	Progesterone, Goldline Labs	00182-0862-63
10 ml	$21.60	Progesterone, Schein Pharm (US)	00364-6683-54
10 ml	$26.80	Progesterone In Oil, Eveready Drugs	57548-0379-10
10 ml	$36.30	Progesterone, Lilly	00002-1438-01

HOW SUPPLIED - NOT RATED EQUIVALENT:

Crystals

100 gm	$44.00	Progesterone, Millgood	53118-0201-01
1000 gm	$370.00	Progesterone, Millgood	53118-0201-02

Insert, Sustained Action - Intrauterine - 38 mg

6's	**$450.00**	**PROGESTASERT, Alza**	**17314-4231-01**

Powder

10 gm	$13.80	Progesterone, Micronized, Paddock Labs	00574-0430-10
10 gm	$13.80	Progesterone Wettable Microcrystal, Paddock Labs	00574-0431-10
25 gm	$25.00	Progesterone, Micronized, Paddock Labs	00574-0430-25
25 gm	$25.00	Progesterone Wettable Microcrystal, Paddock Labs	00574-0431-25
100 gm	$44.00	Progesterone, Millgood	53118-0200-01
100 gm	$82.10	Progesterone, Micronized, Paddock Labs	00574-0430-01
100 gm	$82.10	Progesterone Wettable Microcrystal, Paddock Labs	00574-0431-01
100 gm	$453.00	Progesterone, Milled, Paddock Labs	00574-0432-00
100 gm	$566.25	Progesterone, Paddock Labs	00574-0431-11
1000 gm	$370.00	Progesterone, Millgood	53118-0200-02
1000 gm	$453.00	Progesterone, Micronized, Paddock Labs	00574-0430-00
1000 gm	$453.00	Progesterone Wettable Microcrystal, Paddock Labs	00574-0431-00

PROMAZINE HYDROCHLORIDE *(002124)*

CATEGORIES: Central Nervous System Agents; Phenothiazine Tranquilizers; Psychotherapeutic Agents; Psychotic Disorders; Tranquilizers; Vertigo/Motion Sickness/Vomiting; FDA Approval Pre 1982

BRAND NAMES: *Liranol*; *Prazine*; Primazine; *Protactyl*; Prozine-50; *Savamine*; **Sparine**; *Talofen*
(International brand names outside U.S. in italics)

DESCRIPTION:

With any compound, it is well to review carefully not only its therapeutic efficacy but also the possibilities of the occurrence of undesirable side effects. The physician, therefore, should be thoroughly familiar with the data presented in this report prior to prescribing Promazine.

Promazine is a member of the group of phenothiazines containing an acyclic aliphatic moiety at the 10 position.

Promazine tablets contain 25 mg, 50 mg, or 100 mg promazine hydrochloride. The inactive ingredients present are acacia, calcium carbonate, confectioner's sugar, gelatin magnesium stearate, pharmaceutical glaze, sucrose, and titanium dioxide. Each dosage strength also contains the following:

25 mg: FD & C Yellow 5 and FD & C Yellow 6
50 mg: FD & C Yellow 6
100 mg: FD & C Red 3 and sorbitol.

CLINICAL PHARMACOLOGY:

Promazine has actions at all levels of the central nervous system, as well as on multiple-organ systems. The mechanism whereby its therapeutic action takes place is not known.

INDICATIONS AND USAGE:

Promazine is effective in the management of manifestations of psychotic disorders.

Promazine has not been shown effective in the management of behavioral complications in patients with mental retardation.

CONTRAINDICATIONS:

Promazine should not be used in comatose states due to central nervous system depressants (alcohol, barbiturates, opiates, etc.). In patients with cerebral arteriosclerosis, coronary heart disease, severe hypotension, or other conditions where a drop in blood pressure may be undesirable, promazine should be used with caution.

Intra-arterial injection of promazine is contraindicated.

Promazine is contraindicated in patients known to be sensitive to promazine.

Bone-marrow depression is also a contraindication.

WARNINGS:

The drug is not recommended for use in children under 12 years of age.

The use of alcohol should be avoided, since there may be additive effects and hypotension.

The sedative effect of promazine is a desirable action under most circumstances; however, in certain cases the drug may cause undesirable drowsiness. Drowsiness will usually disappear on continued therapy or can be controlled by decreasing the dose.

Promazine may impair the mental and/or physical abilities required for the performance of potentially hazardous tasks, such as driving a car or operating machinery, especially during the first few days of therapy.

The preferred parenteral route of administration is by intramuscular injection. Routine use of the intravenous route of administration is not recommended. When intravenous administration is deemed preferable, it should be reserved only for those patients who are hospitalized. The intravenous route of medication is not without hazards. Among the hazards are extravasation into surrounding tissues and/or intraarterial injection due to the close proximity of artery and vein. Spasm of digital vessels with resulting gangrene, requiring amputation of the digits, is a possibility. Under no circumstances should intraarterial injection be given.

WARNINGS: *(cont'd)*

Care should be exercised during intravenous administration not to allow perivascular extravasation, since under such circumstances chemical irritation may be severe.

Promazine, when used intravenously, should be used in a concentration no greater than 25 mg per ml. The injection should be given slowly.

Tardive Dyskinesia: Tardive dyskinesia, a syndrome consisting of potentially irreversible, involuntary, dyskinetic movements, may develop in patients treated with neuroleptic (antipsychotic) drugs. Although the prevalence of the syndrome appears to be highest among the elderly, especially elderly women, it is impossible to rely upon prevalence estimates to predict, at the inception of neuroleptic treatment, which patients are likely to develop the syndrome. Whether neuroleptic drug products differ in their potential to cause tardive dyskinesia is unknown.

Both the risk of developing the syndrome and the likelihood that it will become irreversible are believed to increase as the duration of treatment and the total cumulative dose of neuroleptic drugs administered to the patient increase. However, the syndrome can develop, although much less commonly, after relatively brief treatment periods at low doses.

There is no known treatment for established cases of tardive dyskinesia, although the syndrome may remit, partially or completely, if neuroleptic treatment is withdrawn. Neuroleptic treatment itself, however, may suppress (or partially suppress) the signs and symptoms of the syndrome and thereby may possibly mask the underlying disease process. The effect that symptomatic supression has upon the long-term course of the syndrome is unknown.

Given these considerations, neuroleptics should be prescribed in a manner that is most likely to minimize the occurrence of tardive dyskinesia. Chronic neuroleptic treatment should generally be reserved for patients who suffer from a chronic illness that 1) is known to respond to neuroleptic drugs and 2) for whom alternative, equally effective, but potentially less harmful treatments are NOT available or appropriate. In patients who do require chronic treatment, the smallest dose and the shortest duration of treatment producing a satisfactory clinical response should be sought. The need for continued treatment should be reassessed periodically.

If signs and symptoms of tardive dyskinesia appear in a patient on neuroleptics, drug discontinuation should be considered. However, some patients may require treatment despite the presence of the syndrome.

(for further information about the description of tardive dyskinesia and its clinical detection, please refer to the section on ADVERSE REACTIONS.)

Usage In Pregnancy: Safe use of promazine in pregnancy has not been established; therefore, it should be given to pregnant patients, nursing mothers, or women of childbearing potential only when the expected benefits outweigh the possible hazards to mother and child. Adequate animal reproduction studies have not been done.

PRECAUTIONS:

Patients with history of epilepsy should be treated with phenothiazine compounds only when such therapy is absolutely necessary. In such cases adequate anticonvulsant therapy should be given concomitantly.

Promazine may potentiate the effects of organic phosphates found in certain insecticides.

Promazine must be used with caution in persons exposed to extreme heat and administered cautiously to persons with cardiovascular or liver disease.

It should be kept in mind that the antiemetic effect may mask toxicity of other drugs or obscure other diagnoses, such as gastrointestinal obstruction.

Promazine should be given with caution to patients who are suffering from respiratory impairment due to acute pulmonary infections or chronic respiratory disorders, such as severe asthma or emphysema.

Additive Effect: Promazine prolongs and intensifies the central nervous system depressant action of anesthetic barbiturates and narcotics; 1/4 to 1/2 the usual dose of these drugs is required when promazine is administered concomitantly. When the additive effect is not desired, such depressants should be discontinued before starting promazine therapy.

Promazine should also be used with caution in persons receiving atropine or related drugs, since phenothiazines have occasionally been shown to potentiate anticholinergic drugs.

Abrupt Withdrawal: In general, phenothiazines (including promazine) do not produce psychic dependence. However, gastritis, nausea and vomiting, dizziness, and tremulousness have been reported following abrupt cessation of high-dose therapy. Reports suggest that these symptoms can be reduced if concomitant antiparkinson agents are continued for several weeks after the phenothiazine is withdrawn.

Promazine 25 mg tablets contain FD&C Yellow 5 (tartrazine) which may cause allergic-type reactions (including bronchial asthma) in certain susceptible individuals. Although the overall incidence of FD&C Yellow 5 (tartrazine) sensitivity in the general population is low, it is frequently seen in patients who also have aspirin hypersensitivity.

ADVERSE REACTIONS:

NOTE: Not all of the following adverse reactions have occurred with this specific drug, but pharmacological similarities among the various phenothiazine derivatives require that each be considered when promazine is administered.

NOTE: Sudden death has occasionally been reported in patients who have received phenothiazines. In some cases, death was apparently due to cardiac arrest. In others, the cause appeared to be asphyxia due to the failure of the cough reflex. In others, the cause could not be determined, nor could it be established that death was due to the administration of the phenothiazine.

Drowsiness: The sedative effect of promazine is a desirable action under most circumstances; however, in certain cases the drug may cause undesirable drowsiness. Drowsiness will usually disappear on continued therapy or can be controlled by decreasing the dose.

Jaundice: Overall incidence is low. This is generally regarded as a sensitivity reaction and usually occurs during the early weeks of therapy. The clinical picture resembles infectious hepatitus, but the liver-function test results mimic those of hepatic obstruction. There is no conclusive evidence that preexisting liver disease makes patients more susceptible to jaundice. It is usually reversible on withdrawal of the phenothiazine, though chronic jaundice has been reported.

Hematologic Disorders: Include agranulocytosis, eosinophilia, leukopenia, hemolytic anemia, thrombocytopenic purpura, and pancytopenia; though rare, have been reported.

Agranulocytosis: Most cases have occurred between the 4th and the 10th week of therapy. Patients should be watched closely during that period for the sudden appearance of signs of infection, such as sore throat. If white-blood-cell count and differential smears give an indication of significant cellular depression, discontinue the drug and start appropriate therapy. However, a slightly lowered white count in itself is not necessarily an indication for immediate discontinuance of the drug.

CARDIOVASCULAR: TRANSITORY POSTURAL HYPOTENSION HAS BEEN NOTED IN A FEW PATIENTS, USUALLY FOLLOWING THE FIRST PARENTERAL DOSE, PARTICULARLY WHEN GIVEN INTRAVENOUSLY AND RELATED TO THE RATE OF ADMINISTRATION. WHEN THIS HAPPENED, RECOVERY WAS SPONTANEOUS AND THE SYMPTOMS OF WEAKNESS AND DIZZINESS DISAPPEARED. RARELY,

ADVERSE REACTIONS: *(cont'd)*

PARTICULARLY IN ALCOHOLICS, THE DOSAGE HAD TO BE DECREASED OR THE DRUG DISCONTINUED. IT IS DESIRABLE TO KEEP PATIENTS UNDER OBSERVATION (PREFERABLY IN BED) FOR A SHORT TIME AFTER THE INITIAL DOSE.

Should hypotension occur, it can usually be controlled by placing the patient in a recumbent position with head lowered and legs elevated. Administration of oxygen may also be advisable. Occasionally the effects are severe and prolonged, producing a shocklike condition.

IF IT IS DESIRABLE TO ADMINISTER A VASOPRESSOR DRUG, NOREPINEPHRINE APPEARS TO BE THE MOST SUITABLE. EPINEPHRINE SHOULD NOT BE USED, BECAUSE PROMAZINE HYDROCHLORIDE MAY REVERSE ITS ACTION, CAUSING A FURTHER LOWERING OF BLOOD PRESSURE INSTEAD OF ITS USUAL ELEVATING EFFECT.

EKG changes, nonspecific, usually reversible, have been observed in some patients recieving phenothiazines. The relationship to myocardial damage has not been confirmed. When the patient's blood pressure has returned to normal, promazine therapy may be resumed at a lower dosage level.

CNS Effect: Extrapyramidal symptoms, including pseudoparkinsonism, dysarthria, and dyskinetic disturbances, have been reported following the use of large doses of promazine, as in hospitalized mental patients. These symptoms are reversible and may be managed by reducing the dose or the addition of antiparkinsonism drugs—if severe, promazine therapy should be discontinued.

In rare instances, persistent dyskinesia, usually involving the face, tongue and jaw, has been reported to be irreversible, particularly in elderly patients with previous brain damage. Hyperreflexia has been reported in the newborn when a phenothiazine was used in pregnancy.

Adverse Behavioral Effects: Paradoxical exacerbation of psychotic symptoms.

Other CNS Effects: Cerebral edema, abnormality of CSF protein, convulsive seizures, particularly in patients with EEG abnormalities or a history of seizures.

Allergic Reactions: Allergic skin reactions, including dermatitis, dry skin, and edema, have been reported in rare instances during the use of promazine. The incidence is considerably lower than that reported for chlorpromazine.

Mild urticaria and photosensitivity are seen. To minimize, avoid undue exposure to sunlight. Nursing personnel sensitive to phenothiazines should exercise caution when handling these compounds and thus avoid contact dermatitis.

Evidence has become available to indicate a relationship between phenothiazine therapy and the occurrence of systemic lupus erythematosus-like syndrome.

Endocrine Disorders: Lactation, moderate breast engorgement, and amenorrhea in females and gynecomastia in males may necessitate a lower dosage or withdrawal of the drug. False-positive pregnancy tests have been reported, but are less likely to occur when a serum test is used. Hyperglycemia, hypoglycemia, and glycosuria have been reported.

Autonomic Reactions: Autonomic reactions, such as dryness of the mouth, may occur, particularly when large oral doses are administered over prolonged period of time.

Nasal congestion, constipation, adynamic ileus, miosis, and mydriasis have been reported with other phenothiazines.

Persistent Tardive Dyskinesia: As with all antipsychotic agents, tardive dyskinesia may appear in some patients on long-term therapy or may occur after drug therapy has been discontinued. However, the syndrome can develop, although much less commonly, after relatively brief treatment periods at low dose. The risk appears to be greater in elderly patients on high-dose therapy, especially females. The symptoms are persistant and in some patients appear irreversible. The syndrome is characterized by rhythmical involuntary movements of the tongue, face, face, mouth, or jaw (*e.g.,* protrusion of tongue, puffing of cheeks, puckering of mouth, chewing movements). Sometimes these may be accompanied by involuntary movements of extremities.

There is no known effective treatment for tardive dyskinesia; antiparkinsonism agents usually do not alleviate the symptoms of this syndrome. It is suggested that all antipsychotic agents be discontinued if these symptoms appear. Should it be necessary to reinstitute treatment, or increase the dosage of the agent, or switch to a different antipsychotic agent, this syndrome may be masked.

It has been reported that fine, vermicular movements of the tongue may be an early sign of the syndrome, and if the medication is stopped at that time the syndrome may not develop.

Other Adverse Reactions: Mild fever may occur after large intramuscular doses. Increase in appetite and weight sometimes occurs.

Reactions occurring with other phenothiazines have included ocular changes and changes related to skin pigmentation; such reactions should be kept in mind during the administration of promazine even though they have not been noted with this agent to date. The etiology of these reactions is not clear, but exposure to light, along with dosage/duration of therapy, appears to be the most significant factor. If any of these reactions is observed, the physician should weigh the benefits of continued therapy against the possible risks and, on the merits of the individual case, determine whether or not to continue present therapy, lower the dosage, or withdraw the drug.

OVERDOSAGE:

One of three clinical pictures may be seen:

1. Extreme somnolence; patient can usually be roused with prodding, but if permitted will fall asleep. General condition is usually satisfactory. The skin, though pale, is warm and dry. Slight blood pressure, respiratory, and pulse changes may occur but are not problems.

2. Mild-to moderate drop in blood pressure (whether the patient is conscious or unconscious). Skin is markedly gray but warm and dry. Nail beds are pink. Respiration is slow and regular. Pulse is Strong but rate slightly increased.

3. Severe hypotension, possibly accompanied by weakness, cyanosis, perspiration, rapid thready pulse, and respiratory depression.

Treatment is essentially symptomatic and supportive. Early gastric lavage and intestinal purges may help. Centrally acting emetics will not help because of the antiemetic effect of promazine. Give hot coffee or tea.

Severe hypotension usually responds to measures described under hypotensive effects. Additional measures include pressure bandages to lower limbs, oxygen, and IV fluids.

Avoid stimulants that may cause convulsion (*e.g.,* picrotoxin and pentylenetetrazol).

Limited experience with dialysis indicates that it is not helpful.

DOSAGE AND ADMINISTRATION:

The amount, route of administration, and frequency of dose should be governed by the severity of the condition treated and the response of the patient. For maximal therapeutic benefit, dosage must be individualized for the patient. The oral route of administration should be used whenever possible, but when it is thought that the effect obtained by oral dosage would not produce a sufficient response, it may be given parenterally, as for instance when nausea, vomiting, or lack of cooperation is evident.

DOSAGE AND ADMINISTRATION: *(cont'd)*

The preferred parenteral route of administration is by intramuscular injection. In general, parenteral administration should be reserved for bedfast patients, although acute states in ambulatory patients may also be treated by intramuscular injection, provided proper precautions are taken to eliminate the possibility of postural hypotension. It is important to make sure that intramuscular injections are given deeply into large muscle masses, i.e., gluteal region.

The intravenous route of medication is not without hazards. Routine use of the intravenous route of administration is not recommended. When intravenous administration is deemed preferable, it should be reserved only for those patients who are hospitalized. (See WARNINGS.) Under no circumstances should intraarterial injections be given.

The intravenous injection, when indicated, should be given slowly in diluted solution (25 mg/ml or less).

The whole contents of the syringe should be injected into the lumen of the vein and injections be made only into vessels previously undamaged by multiple injections or trauma.

Mental And Emotional Disturbances: The dosage of Promazine for either acute or chronic mental disease wil vary with the severity of the condition.

In the management of severely agitated patients, it is recommended that Promazine be given intramuscularly in initial doses of 50 mg to 150 mg, depending on the degree of excitation. In general, these doses are sufficient, but if the desired calming effect is not apparent within thirty minutes, additional doses up to a total of 300 mg may be given. Once the desired control is obtained, Promazine may then be given orally. The oral or intramuscular dose is 10 mg to 200 mg at 4 to 6 hour intervals, depending on the response of the patient.

In severe disturbances, dosage should be adjusted downward. Maintenance dosage may range from 10 mg to 200 mg, given at 4 to 6 hour intervals.

The degree of central nervous system depression induced by Promazine has not been great; however, in the acutely inebriated patient the initial dose should not exceed 50 mg, to be sure that the depressant effect of alcohol is not enhanced.

NOTE: THE PERCENTAGE OF EFFECTIVE RESULTS DOES NOT APPEAR TO BE MATERIALLY AFFECTED BY THE ADMINISTRATION OF DOSES IN EXCESS OF 800 MG TO 1000 MG PER DAY. IT IS THEREFORE RECOMMENDED THAT THE TOTAL DAILY DOSE OF PROMAZINE NOT EXCEED ONE (1) GRAM (1,000 MG).

Dosage In Children: In acute episodes of chronic psychotic disease in children over 12, 10 to 25 mg every 4 to 6 hours.

HOW SUPPLIED - RATED THERAPEUTICALLY EQUIVALENT:

Injection, Solution - Intramuscular - 25 mg/ml

2 ml	**$7.08**	**SPARINE, Wyeth Labs**	**00008-0040-01**
10 ml	**$27.66**	**SPARINE, Wyeth Labs**	**00008-0040-02**

Injection, Solution - Intramuscular - 50 mg/ml

1 ml x 10	**$27.63**	**SPARINE, Wyeth Labs**	**00008-0236-01**
10 ml	$4.13	Promazine, Schein Pharm (US)	00364-6668-54
10 ml	$5.25	Promazine Hcl, Consolidated Midland	00223-8398-10

HOW SUPPLIED - NOT RATED EQUIVALENT:

Injection, Solution - Intramuscular - 25 mg/ml

10 ml	$4.80	Promazine Hcl, Consolidated Midland	00223-8397-10

Tablet, Enteric Coated - Oral - 25 mg

50's	**$20.59**	**SPARINE, Wyeth Labs**	**00008-0029-01**

Tablet, Enteric Coated - Oral - 50 mg

50's	**$25.04**	**SPARINE, Wyeth Labs**	**00008-0028-01**

PROMETHAZINE HYDROCHLORIDE *(002125)*

CATEGORIES: Allergic Reactions; Allergies; Analeptics; Analgesics; Anaphylactic Reactions; Anesthesia; Angioedema; Antiasthmatics/Bronchodilators; Antiemetics; Antihistamines; Antitussives/Expectorants/Mucolytics; Anxiolytics, Sedatives, Hypnotic; Central Nervous System Agents; Conjunctivitis; Cough Preparations; Dermatographism; Expectorants; Motion Sickness; Nasal Congestion; Nausea; Nausea and Vomiting; Pain; Psychotherapeutic Agents; Respiratory & Allergy Medications; Rhinitis; Sedation; Sedatives; Tranquilizers; Urticaria; Vertigo/Motion Sickness/Vomiting; Pregnancy Category C; DEA Class CV; FDA Approval Pre 1982; Top 200 Drugs

BRAND NAMES: Adgan; *Allerfen*; Anergan; *Antiallersin*; *Atosil* (Germany); *Avomine*; *Bonnox* (Germany); *Camergan*; *Closin* (Germany); Edrex-25; *Eusedon Mono* (Germany); *Fargan*; *Farganesse*; *Fenergan*; *Goodnight*; *Hibechin* (Japan); *Hiberna* (Japan); *Histantil* (Canada); *Lergigan*; *Metaryl*; Mymethazine Fortis; Or-Phen-50; *Pelpica*; Pentazine; Phena-Plex; Phenameth; Phenazine; Phencen-50; Phenerex; **Phenergan**; Phenerzine; Phenoject-50; Pherazine; *Pilothia*; *Pipolphene*; *PMS Promethazine* (Canada); Pro-50; Promacot; *Prome*; *Promergan*; *Promesan*; Prometh; Promethacon; Promethapar; Promethazine Hcl; Promethegan; Prorex; Prothazine; *Prothiazine*; *Prozine*; *Pyrethia* (Japan); Remsed; *Sayomol*; Shogan; V-Gan; *Xepagan*

(International brand names outside U.S. in italics)

FORMULARIES: Aetna; BC-BS; CIGNA; FHP; Humana; Kaiser; Medco; Medi-Cal; PCS; PruCare; United; WHO

COST OF THERAPY: $0.76 (Rhinitis; Tablet; 25 mg; 1/day; 30 days)

PRIMARY ICD9: 477.9 (Allergic Rhinitis, Cause Unspecified)

DESCRIPTION:

Promethazine hydrochloride is a racemic compound; the empirical formula is $C_{17}H_{20}N_2S{\cdot}HCl$ and its molecular weight is 320.88.

Promethazine hydrochloride, a phenothiazine derivative, is designated chemically as N,N,α-trimethyl-10H-phenothiazine-10-ethanamine monohydrochloride.

Promethazine hydrochloride occurs as a white to faint yellow, practically odorless, crystalline powder which slowly oxidizes and turns blue on prolonged exposure to air. It is soluble in water and freely soluble in alcohol.

Injection: Each ml of the Tubex and Tubex Blunt Pointe Sterile Cartridge Units contains either 25 or 50 mg promethazine hydrochloride with 0.1 mg edetate disodium, 0.04 mg calcium chloride, not more than 5 mg monothioglycerol and 5 mg phenol with sodium acetate-acetic acid buffer. Sealed under nitrogen.

DESCRIPTION: *(cont'd)*

Syrup: Each teaspoon (5 ml) of Phenergan Syrup Plain contains 6.25 mg promethazine hydrochloride in a flavored syrup base with a pH between 4.7 and 5.2. Alcohol 7%. The inactive ingredients present are artificial and natural flavors, citric acid, D&C Red 33, D&C Yellow 10, FD&C Blue 1, FD&C Yellow 6, glycerin, saccharin sodium, sodium benzoate, sodium citrate, sodium propionate, water, and other ingredients.

Each teaspoon (5 ml) of Phenergan Syrup Fortis contains 25 mg promethazine hydrochloride in a flavored syrup base with a pH between 5.0 and 5.5. Alcohol 1.5%. The inactive ingredients present are artificial and natural flavors, citric acid, saccharin sodium, sodium benzoate, sodium propionate, water, and other ingredients.

Tablets and Suppositories: Each tablet of Phenergan contains 12.5 mg, 25 mg, or 50 mg promethazine hydrochloride. The inactive ingredients present are lactose, magnesium stearate, and methylcellulose. Each dosage strength also contains the following: 12.5 mg—FD&C Yellow 6 and saccharin sodium; 25 mg—saccharin sodium; 50 mg—FD&C Red 40.

Each rectal suppository of Phenergan contains 12.5 mg, 25 mg, or 50 mg promethazine hydrochloride with ascorbyl palmitate, silicon dioxide, white wax, and cocoa butter.

CLINICAL PHARMACOLOGY:

Injection: Promethazine hydrochloride, a phenothiazine derivative, possesses antihistaminic, sedative, antimotion-sickness, antiemetic, and anticholinergic effects. The duration of action is generally from four to six hours. The major side reaction of this drug is sedation. As an antihistamine, it acts by competitive antagonism but does not block the release of histamine. It antagonizes in varying degrees most but not all of the pharmacological effects of histamine.

Syrup, Tablets and Suppositories: Promethazine is a phenothiazine derivative which differs structurally from the antipsychotic phenothiazines by the presence of a branched side chain and no ring substitution. It is thought that this configuration is responsible for its relative lack (1/10 that of chlorpromazine) of dopaminergic (CNS) action.

Promethazine is an H_1 receptor blocking agent. In addition to its antihistaminic action, it provides clinically useful sedative and antiemetic effects. In therapeutic dosage, promethazine produces no significant effects on the cardiovascular system.

Promethazine is well absorbed from the gastrointestinal tract. Clinical effects are apparent within 20 minutes after oral administration and generally last four to six hours, although they may persist as long as 12 hours. Promethazine is metabolized by the liver to a variety of compounds; the sulfoxides of promethazine and N-demethylpromethazine are the predominant metabolites appearing in the urine.

INDICATIONS AND USAGE:

INJECTION

The injectable form of promethazine hydrochloride is indicated for the following conditions:

1. Amelioration of allergic reactions to blood or plasma.

2. In anaphylaxis as an adjunct to epinephrine and other standard measures after the acute symptoms have been controlled.

3. For other uncomplicated allergic conditions of the immediate type when oral therapy is impossible or contraindicated.

4. Active treatment of motion sickness.

5. Preoperative, postoperative, and obstetric (during labor) sedation.

6. Prevention and control of nausea and vomiting associated with certain types of anesthesia and surgery.

7. As an adjunct to analgesics for the control of postoperative pain.

8. For sedation and relief of apprehension and to produce light sleep from which the patient can be easily aroused.

9. Intravenously in special surgical situations, such as repeated bronchoscopy, ophthalmic surgery, and poor-risk patients, with reduced amounts of meperidine or other narcotic analgesic as an adjunct to anesthesia and analgesia.

SYRUP, TABLETS AND SUPPOSITORIES

Promethazine is useful for:

Perennial and seasonal allergic rhinitis.

Vasomotor rhinitis.

Allergic conjunctivitis due to inhalant allergens and foods.

Mild, uncomplicated allergic skin manifestations of urticaria and angioedema.

Amelioration of allergic reactions to blood or plasma.

Dermographism.

Anaphylactic reactions, as adjunctive therapy to epinephrine and other standard measures, after the acute manifestations have been controlled.

Preoperative, postoperative, or obstetric sedation.

Prevention and control of nausea and vomiting associated with certain types of anesthesia and surgery.

Therapy adjunctive to meperidine or other analgesics for control of postoperative pain.

Sedation in both children and adults, as well as relief of apprehension and production of light sleep from which the patient can be easily aroused.

Active and prophylactic treatment of motion sickness.

Antiemetic therapy in postoperative patients.

CONTRAINDICATIONS:

Injection: Promethazine is contraindicated in comatose states, in patients who have received large amounts of central-nervous-system depressants (alcohol, sedative hypnotics, including barbiturates, general anesthetics, narcotics, narcotic analgesics, tranquilizers, etc.), and in patients who have demonstrated an idiosyncrasy or hypersensitivity to promethazine.

Under no circumstances should promethazine be given by intra-arterial injection due to the likelihood of severe arteriospasm and the possibility of resultant gangrene (see WARNINGS.)

Promethazine HCl injection should not be given by the subcutaneous route; evidence of chemical irritation has been noted, and necrotic lesions have resulted on rare occasions following subcutaneous injection. The preferred parenteral route of administration is by deep intramuscular injection.

Syrup, Tablets and Suppositories: Promethazine is contraindicated in individuals known to be hypersensitive or to have had an idiosyncratic reaction to promethazine or to other phenothiazines.

Antihistamines are contraindicated for use in the treatment of lower respiratory tract symptoms including asthma.

WARNINGS:

INJECTION

Promethazine may impair the mental and/or physical abilities required for the performance of potentially hazardous tasks, such as driving a vehicle or operating machinery. The concomitant use of alcohol, sedative hypnotics (including barbiturates), general anesthetics, narcotics, narcotic analgesics, tranquilizers or other central-nervous-system depressants may have an additive sedative effect. Patients should be warned accordingly.

Usage In Pregnancy: The safe use of promethazine has not been established with respect to the possible adverse effects upon fetal development. Therefore, the need for the use of this drug during pregnancy should be weighted against the possible but unknown hazards to the developing fetus.

Usage in Children: Excessively large dosages of antihistamines, including promethazine, in children may cause hallucinations, convulsions, and sudden death. In children who are acutely ill associated with dehydration, there is an increased susceptibility to dystonias with the use of promethazine hydrochloride injection.

CAUTION SHOULD BE EXERCISED WHEN ADMINISTERING Promethazine HCl TO CHILDREN. ANTIEMETICS ARE NOT RECOMMENDED FOR TREATMENT OF UNCOMPLICATED VOMITING IN CHILDREN, AND THEIR USE SHOULD BE LIMITED TO PROLONGED VOMITING OF KNOWN ETIOLOGY. THE EXTRAPYRAMIDAL SYMPTOMS WHICH CAN OCCUR SECONDARY TO Promethazine HCl ADMINISTRATION MAY BE CONFUSED WITH THE CNS SIGNS OF UNDIAGNOSED PRIMARY DISEASE, e.g., ENCEPHALOPATHY OR REYE'S SYNDROME. THE USE OF Promethazine HCl SHOULD BE AVOIDED IN CHILDREN WHOSE SIGNS AND SYMPTOMS MAY SUGGEST REYE'S SYNDROME, OR OTHER HEPATIC DISEASES.

Use In The Elderly (Approximately 60 Years Or Older): Since therapeutic requirements for sedative drugs tend to be less in elderly patients, the dosage of promethazine HCl should be reduced for these patients.

Other Considerations: Drugs having anticholinergic properties should be used with caution in patients with asthmatic attack, narrow- angle glaucoma, prostatic hypertrophy, stenosing peptic ulcer, pyloroduodenal obstruction, and bladder-neck obstruction.

Promethazine HCl should be used with caution in patients with bone-marrow depression. Leukopenia and agranulocytosis have been reported, usually when promethazine HCl has been used in association with other known toxic agents.

Inadvertent Intra-Arterial Injection: Due to the close proximity of arteries and veins in the areas most commonly used for intravenous injection, extreme care should be exercised to avoid perivascular extravasation or inadvertent intra-arterial injection. Reports compatible with inadvertent intra-arterial injection of promethazine, usually in conjunction with other drugs intended for intravenous use, suggest that pain, severe chemical irritation, severe spasm of distal vessels, and resultant gangrene requiring amputation are likely under such circumstances. Intravenous injection was intended in all cases reported, but perivascular extravasation or arterial placement of the needle is now suspect. There is no proven successful management of this condition after it occurs, although sympathetic block and heparinization are commonly employed during the acute management because of the results of animal experiments with other known arteriolar irritants. Aspiration of dark blood does not preclude intra-arterial needle placement, because blood is discolored upon contact with promethazine. Use of syringes with rigid plungers or of small bore needles might obscure typical arterial backflow if this is relied upon alone.

When used intravenously, promethazine hydrochloride should be given in a concentration no greater than 25 mg per ml and at a rate not to exceed 25 mg per minute. When administering any irritant drug intravenously, it is usually preferable to inject it through the tubing of an intravenous infusion set that is known to be functioning satisfactorily. In the event that a patient complains of pain during intended intravenous injection of promethazine, the injection should immediately be stopped to provide for evaluation of possible arterial placement or perivascular extravasation.

SYRUP, TABLETS AND SUPPOSITORIES

Promethazine may cause marked drowsiness. Ambulatory patients should be cautioned against such activities as driving or operating dangerous machinery until it is known that they do not become drowsy or dizzy from promethazine therapy.

The sedative action of promethazine hydrochloride is additive to the sedative effects of central nervous system depressants; therefore, agents such as alcohol, narcotic analgesics, sedatives, hypnotics, and tranquilizers should either be eliminated or given in reduced dosage in the presence of promethazine hydrochloride. When given concomitantly with promethazine hydrochloride, the dose of barbiturates should be reduced by at least one-half, and the dose of analgesic depressants, such as morphine or meperidine, should be reduced by one-quarter to one-half.

Promethazine may lower seizure threshold. This should be taken into consideration when administering to persons with known seizure disorders or when giving in combination with narcotics or local anesthetics which may also affect seizure threshold.

Sedative drugs or CNS depressants should be avoided in patients with a history of sleep apnea.

Antihistamines should be used with caution in patients with narrow-angle glaucoma, stenosing peptic ulcer, pyloroduodenal obstruction, and urinary bladder obstruction due to symptomatic prostatic hypertrophy and narrowing of the bladder neck.

Administration of promethazine has been associated with reported cholestatic jaundice.

PRECAUTIONS:

INJECTION

Promethazine may significantly affect the actions of other drugs. It may increase, prolong, or intensify the sedative action of central-nervous-system depressants, such as alcohol, sedative hypnotics (including barbiturates), general anesthetics, narcotics, narcotic analgesics, tranquilizers, etc. When given concomitantly with promethazine hydrochloride, the dose of barbiturates should be reduced by at least one-half, and the dose of narcotics should be reduced by one-quarter to one-half. Dosage must be individualized. Excessive amounts of promethazine relative to a narcotic may lead to restlessness and motor hyperactivity in the patient with pain; these symptoms usually disappear with adequate control of the pain. Promethazine should be used cautiously in persons with cardiovascular disease or impairment of liver function.

Although reversal of the vasopressor effect of epinephrine has not been reported with promethazine, the possibility should be considered in case of promethazine overdose.

SYRUP, TABLETS AND SUPPOSITORIES

General: Promethazine should be used cautiously in persons with cardiovascular disease or with impairment of liver function.

Information for the Patient: Promethazine HCl may cause marked drowsiness or impair the mental and/or physical abilities required for the performance of potentially hazardous tasks, such as driving a vehicle or operating machinery. Ambulatory patients should be told to avoid engaging in such activities until it is known that they do not become drowsy or dizzy from promethazine HCl therapy. Children should be supervised to avoid potential harm in bike riding or in other hazardous activities.

PRECAUTIONS: *(cont'd)*

The concomitant use of alcohol or other central nervous system depressants, including narcotic analgesics, sedatives, hypnotics, and tranquilizers, may have an additive effect and should be avoided or their dosage reduced.

Patients should be advised to report any involuntary muscle movements or unusual sensitivity to sunlight.

Drug/Laboratory Test Interactions: The following laboratory tests may be affected in patients who are receiving therapy with promethazine hydrochloride:

Pregnancy Tests: Diagnostic pregnancy tests based on immunological reactions between HCG and anti-HCG may result in false-negative or false-positive interpretations.

Glucose Tolerance Test: An increase in blood glucose has been reported in patients receiving promethazine.

Carcinogenesis, Mutagenesis, and Impairment of Fertility: Long-term animal studies have not been performed to assess the carcinogenic potential of promethazine, nor are there other animal or human data concerning carcinogenicity, mutagenicity, or impairment of fertility with this drug. Promethazine was nonmutagenic in the *Salmonella* test system of Ames.

Pregnancy Category C: *Teratogenic Effects:* Teratogenic effects have not been demonstrated in rat-feeding studies at doses of 6.25 and 12.5 mg/kg of promethazine. These doses are from approximately 2.1 to 4.2 times the maximum recommended total daily dose of promethazine for a 50-kg subject, depending upon the indication for which the drug is prescribed. Specific studies to test the action of the drug on parturition, lactation, and development of the animal neonate were not done, but a general preliminary study in rats indicated no effect on these parameters. Although antihistamines, including promethazine, have been found to produce fetal mortality in rodents, the pharmacological effects of histamine in the rodent do not parallel those in man. There are no adequate and well-controlled studies of promethazine in pregnant women. Promethazine HCl should be used during pregnancy only if the potential benefit justifies the potential risk to the fetus. *Nonteratogenic Effects:* Promethazine taken within two weeks of delivery may inhibit platelet aggregation in the newborn.

Labor and Delivery: Promethazine HCl, in appropriate dosage form, may be used alone or as an adjunct to narcotic analgesics during labor and delivery. (See INDICATIONS AND USAGE and DOSAGE AND ADMINISTRATION.) See also Nonteratogenic Effects.

Nursing Mothers: It is not known whether promethazine is excreted in human milk. Caution should be exercised when promethazine is administered to a nursing woman.

Pediatric Use: This product should not be used in children under 2 years of age because safety for such use has not been established.

DRUG INTERACTIONS:

INJECTION

Narcotics And Barbiturates: The CNS-depressant effects of narcotics are additive with promethazine hydrochloride.

Monoamine Oxidase Inhibitors (Maoi): Drug interactions, including an increased incidence of extrapyramidal effects, have been reported when some MAOI and phenothiazines are used concomitantly. Although such a reaction has not been reported with promethazine, the possibility should be considered.

SYRUP, TABLETS AND SUPPOSITORIES

The sedative action of promethazine is additive to the sedative effects of other central nervous system depressants, including alcohol, narcotic analgesics, sedatives, hypnotics, tricyclic antidepressants, and tranquilizers; therefore, these agents should be avoided or administered in reduced dosage to patients receiving promethazine.

ADVERSE REACTIONS:

INJECTION

Cns Effects: Drowsiness is the most prominent CNS effect of this drug. Extrapyramidal reactions may occur with high doses; this is almost always responsive to a reduction in dosage. Other reported reactions include dizziness, lassitude, tinnitus, incoordination, fatigue, blurred vision, euphoria, diplopia, nervousness, insomnia, tremors, convulsive seizures, oculogyric crises, excitation, catatonic-like states, and hysteria.

Cardiovascular Effects: Tachycardia, bradycardia, faintness, dizziness, and increases and decreases in blood pressure have been reported following the use of promethazine hydrochloride injection. Venous thrombosis at the injection site has been reported. INTRA-ARTERIAL INJECTION MAY RESULT IN GANGRENE OF THE AFFECTED EXTREMITY (see WARNINGS.)

Gastrointestinal: Nausea and vomiting have been reported, usually in association with surgical procedures and combination drug therapy.

Allergic Reactions: These include urticaria, dermatitis, asthma, and photosensitivity. Angioneurotic edema has been reported.

Other Reported Reactions: Leukopenia and agranulocytosis, usually when promethazine HCl has been used in association with other known toxic agents, have been reported. Thrombocytopenic purpura and jaundice of the obstructive type have been associated with the use of promethazine. The jaundice is usually reversible on discontinuation of the drug. Subcutaneous injection has resulted in tissue necrosis. Nasal stuffiness may occur. Dry mouth has been reported.

Laboratory Tests: The following laboratory tests may be affected in patients who are receiving therapy with promethazine hydrochloride:

Pregnancy Tests: Diagnostic pregnancy tests based on immunological reactions between HCG and anti-HCG may result in false-negative or false-positive interpretations.

Glucose Tolerance Test: An increase in blood glucose has been reported in patients receiving promethazine.

Paradoxical Reactions (Overdosage): Hyperexcitability and abnormal movements, which have been reported in children following a single administration of promethazine, may be manifestations of relative overdosage, in which case, consideration should be given to the discontinuation of the promethazine and to the use of other drugs. Respiratory depression, nightmares, delirium, and agitated behavior have also been reported in some of these patients.

SYRUP, TABLETS AND SUPPOSITORIES

Nervous System: Sedation, sleepiness, occasional blurred vision, dryness of mouth, dizziness; rarely confusion, disorientation, and extrapyramidal symptoms such as oculogyric crisis, torticollis, and tongue protrusion (usually in association with parenteral injection or excessive dosage).

Cardiovascular: Increased or decreased blood pressure.

Dermatologic: Rash, rarely photosensitivity.

Hematologic: Rarely leukopenia, thrombocytopenia; agranulocytosis (1 case).

Gastrointestinal: Nausea and vomiting.

OVERDOSAGE:

Signs and symptoms of overdosage range from mild depression of the central nervous system and cardiovascular system to profound hypotension, respiratory depression, and unconsciousness.

Stimulation may be evident, especially in children and geriatric patients.

Atropine-like signs and symptoms—dry mouth, fixed, dilated pupils, flushing, etc., as well as gastrointestinal symptoms, may occur.

Convulsions may rarely occur. A paradoxical reaction has been reported in children receiving single doses of 75 mg to 125 mg orally, characterized by hyperexcitability and nightmares.

Treatment: The treatment of overdosage is essentially symptomatic and supportive. Early gastric lavage may be beneficial if promethazine has been taken orally. Centrally acting emetics are of little use.

Treatment of overdosage is essentially symptomatic and supportive. Only in cases of extreme overdosage or individual sensitivity do vital signs, including respiration, pulse, blood pressure, temperature, and EKG, need to be monitored. Activated charcoal orally or by lavage may be given, or sodium or magnesium sulfate orally as a cathartic. Attention should be given to the reestablishment of adequate respiratory exchange through provision of a patent airway and institution of assisted or controlled ventilation. Diazepam may be used to control convulsions. Acidosis and electrolyte losses should be corrected. Note that any depressant effects of promethazine are not reversed by naloxone.

Avoid analeptics, which may cause convulsions.

Limited experience with dialysis indicates that it is not helpful.

Syrup, Tablets and Suppositories: Severe hypotension usually responds to the administration of norepinephrine or phenylephrine. EPINEPHRINE SHOULD NOT BE USED, since its use in patients with partial adrenergic blockage may further lower the blood pressure.

Injection: Severe hypotension usually responds to the administration of levarterenol or phenylephrine. EPINEPHRINE SHOULD NOT BE USED, since its use in a patient with partial adrenergic blockage may further lower the blood pressure.

Extrapyramidal reactions may be treated with anticholinergic antiparkinson agents, diphenhydramine, or barbiturates. Additional measures include oxygen and intravenous fluids.

DOSAGE AND ADMINISTRATION:

INJECTION

The preferred parenteral route of administration for promethazine hydrochloride is by deep intramuscular injection. The proper intravenous administration of this product is well tolerated, but use of this route is not without some hazard.

INADVERTENT INTRA-ARTERIAL INJECTION CAN RESULT IN GANGRENE OF THE AFFECTED EXTREMITY (see WARNINGS.) SUBCUTANEOUS INJECTION IS CONTRAINDICATED, AS IT MAY RESULT IN TISSUE NECROSIS (see CONTRAINDICATIONS.) When used intravenously, promethazine hydrochloride should be given in concentration no greater than 25 mg/ml at a rate not to exceed 25 mg per minute; it is preferable to inject through the tubing of an intravenous infusion set that is known to be functioning satisfactorily.

The Tubex Blunt Pointe Sterile Cartridge Unit is suitable for substances to be administered intravenously only. It is intended for use with injection sets specifically manufactured as "needle-less" injection systems. Tubex Blunt Pointe is compatible with Abbott's LifeShield prepierced reseal injection site, Baxter's InterLink injection Site, and B. Braun Medical's SafSite Reflux Valve. Consult manufacturer's recommendations regarding "Directions for Use" of the "needle-less" system. It is also intended for admixture with, and convenient administration of, various medicaments when using Drug Vial Adapters for "needle-less" injection systems.

The Tubex Sterile Cartridge-Needle Unit is suitable for substances to be administered intravenously or intramuscularly.

Allergic Conditions: The average adult dose is 25 mg. This dose may be repeated within two hours if necessary, but continued therapy, if indicated, should be via the oral route as soon as existing circumstances permit. After initiation of treatment, dosage should be adjusted to the smallest amount adequate to relieve symptoms. The average adult dose for amelioration of allergic reactions to blood or plasma is 25 mg.

Sedation: In hospitalized adult patients, nighttime sedation may be achieved by a dose of 25 to 50 mg of promethazine hydrochloride.

Pre- And Postoperative Use: As an adjunct to pre- or postoperative medication, 25 to 50 mg of promethazine hydrochloride in adults may be combined with appropriately reduced doses of analgesics and atropine-like drugs as desired. Dosage of concomitant analgesic or hypnotic medication should be reduced accordingly.

Nausea And Vomiting: For control of nausea and vomiting, the usual adult dose is 12.5 to 25 mg, not to be repeated more frequently than every four hours. When used for control of postoperative nausea and vomiting, the medication may be administered either intramuscularly or intravenously and dosage of analgesics and barbiturates reduced accordingly.

Obstetrics: Promethazine HCl in doses of 50 mg will provide sedation and relieve apprehension in the early stages of labor. When labor is definitely established, 25 to 75 mg (average dose, 50 mg) promethazine hydrochloride may be given intramuscularly or intravenously with an appropriately reduced dose of any desired narcotic. Amnesic agents may be administered as necessary. If necessary, promethazine HCl with a reduced dose of analgesic may be repeated once or twice at four-hour intervals in the course of a normal labor. A maximum total dose of 100 mg of promethazine HCl may be administered during a 24-hour period to patients in labor.

Children: In children under the age of 12 years, the dosage should not exceed half that of the suggested adult dose. As an adjunct to premedication, the suggested dose is 0.5 mg per lb. of body weight in combination with an equal dose of narcotic or barbiturate and the appropriate dose of an atropine-like drug.

Antiemetics should not be used in vomiting of unknown etiology in children.

Parenteral drug products should be inspected visually for particulate matter and discoloration prior to administration, whenever solution and container permit.

Store at room temperature, between 15°-25° C (59°-77° F). Protect from light. Use carton to protect contents from light. Do not use if solution is discolored or contains a precipitate.

SYRUP, TABLETS AND SUPPOSITORIES

Allergy: The average oral dose is 25 mg taken before retiring; however, 12.5 mg may be taken before meals and on retiring, if necessary. Children tolerate this product well. Single 25-mg doses at bedtime or 6.25 to 12.5 mg taken three times daily will usually suffice. After initiation of treatment in children or adults, dosage should be adjusted to the smallest amount adequate to relieve symptoms.

Promethazine HCl Rectal Suppositories may be used if the oral route is not feasible, but oral therapy should be resumed as soon as possible if continued therapy is indicated.

The administration of promethazine hydrochloride in 25-mg doses will control minor transfusion reactions of an allergic nature.

DOSAGE AND ADMINISTRATION: *(cont'd)*

Motion Sickness: The average adult dose is 25 mg taken twice daily. The initial dose should be taken one-half to one hour before anticipated travel and be repeated 8 to 12 hours later, if necessary. On succeeding days of travel, it is recommended that 25 mg be given on arising and again before the evening meal. For children, promethazine HCl tablets, syrup, or rectal suppositories, 12.5 to 25 mg, twice daily, may be administered.

Nausea And Vomiting: The average effective dose of promethazine HCl for the active therapy of nausea and vomiting in children or adults is 25 mg. When oral medication cannot be tolerated, the dose should be given parenterally (cf. promethazine HCl injection) or by rectal suppository. 12.5- to 25-mg doses may be repeated, as necessary, at 4- to 6-hour intervals.

For nausea and vomiting in children, the usual dose is 0.5 mg per pound of body weight, and the dose should be adjusted to the age and weight of the patient and the severity of the condition being treated.

For prophylaxis of nausea and vomiting, as during surgery and the postoperative period, the average dose is 25 mg repeated at 4- to 6-hour intervals, as necessary.

Sedation: This product relieves apprehension and induces a quiet sleep from which the patient can be easily aroused. Administration of 12.5 to 25 mg promethazine HCl by the oral route or by rectal suppository at bedtime will provide sedation in children. Adults usually require 25 to 50 mg for nighttime, presurgical, or obstetrical sedation.

Pre- And Postoperative Use: Promethazine HCl in 12.5- to 25-mg doses for children and 50-mg doses for adults the night before surgery relieves apprehension and produces a quiet sleep.

For preoperative medication children require doses of 0.5 mg per pound of body weight in combination with an equal dose of meperidine and the appropriate dose of an atropinelike drug.

Usual adult dosage is 50 mg promethazine HCl with an equal amount of meperidine and the required amount of a belladonna alkaloid.

Postoperative sedation and adjunctive use with analgesics may be obtained by the administration of 12.5 to 25 mg in children and 25- to 50-mg doses in adults.

Phenergan Syrup Plain and Phenergan Syrup Fortis are not recommended for children under 2 years of age. **Keep bottles tightly closed. Store at Room Temperature, between 15° C and 25° C (59° F and 77° F). Protect from light. Dispense in light-resistant, glass, tight containers.**

Phenergan Tablets and Phenergan Rectal Suppositories are not recommended for children under 2 years of age. **Keep tightly closed. Store at room temperature, between 15° C and 25° C (59° F and 77° F). Protect from light. Dispense in light-resistant, tight container. Use carton to protect contents from light.**

Suppositories **Store refrigerated between 2°-8° C (36°-46° F). Dispense in well-closed container.**

(Injection - Wyeth Laboratories Inc., 6/94, CI 3727-5)

(Syrup - Wyeth Laboratories Inc., 7/91, CI 3913-3)

(Tablets and Suppositories - Wyeth Laboratories Inc., 2/94, CI 3759-9)

PATIENT INFORMATION:

Promethazine hydrochloride is used to treat allergic symptoms, to prevent nausea and vomiting, with other medicines to treat pain, prevent motion sickness. The major side reaction of this drug is sedation. Promethazine can cause significant sedation. It is advised that you not drink alcohol or take other medications that may make you drowsy or uncoordinated. Care should be taken while driving until it is known that the drug effects will not interfere. This medication can be taken with food to prevent stomach irritation. If this drug is taken to prevent motion sickness it should be taken 30 minutes prior to the event.

HOW SUPPLIED - RATED THERAPEUTICALLY EQUIVALENT:

Injection, Solution - Intramuscular; - 25 mg/ml

1 ml	$1.00	PROMETHAZINE HCL, Raway	00686-1495-35
1 ml x 10	**$15.53**	**PHENERGAN, Wyeth Labs**	**00008-0416-01**
1 ml x 25	$12.74	Promethazine Hcl, Elkins Sinn	00641-1495-35
1 ml x 25	**$19.24**	**PHENERGAN, Wyeth Labs**	**00008-0063-01**
1 ml x 25	$20.00	Promethazine Hcl, Consolidated Midland	00223-8393-01
10 ml	$1.80	Promethazine Hcl, Lannett	00527-0146-55
10 ml	$2.10	Promethazine Hcl, Lannett	00527-0152-55
10 ml	$4.00	Promethazine Hcl, Consolidated Midland	00223-8393-10
10 ml	$4.10	Promethazine Hcl 25, Pasadena	00418-0961-10
10 ml	$6.90	PROREX, Hyrex Pharms	00314-0684-70
10 ml	$6.90	Promethazine Hcl, Steris Labs	00402-0258-10
10 ml	$8.25	Promethazine Hcl, IDE-Interstate	00814-6421-40
10 ml	$9.75	Promethazine Hydrochlorine, Rugby	00536-8451-70
10 ml	$10.38	Promethazine HCl, Schein Pharm (US)	00364-6570-54
10 ml	$10.60	Promethazine Hcl, Goldline Labs	00182-0774-63

Injection, Solution - Intramuscular; - 50 mg/ml

1 ml	$1.10	PROMETHAZINE HCL, Raway	00686-1496-35
1 ml x 10	**$18.68**	**PHENERGAN, Wyeth Labs**	**00008-0417-01**
1 ml x 25	$16.00	Promethazine Hcl, Elkins Sinn	00641-1496-35
1 ml x 25	**$23.79**	**PHENERGAN, Wyeth Labs**	**00008-0746-01**
1 ml x 25	$25.00	Promethazine Hcl, Consolidated Midland	00223-8394-01
10 ml	$4.25	Promethazine Hcl, Consolidated Midland	00223-8394-10
10 ml	$4.50	Promethazine Hcl 50, Pasadena	00418-0971-10
10 ml	$4.70	Promethazine Hcl, Geneva Pharms	00781-3088-70
10 ml	$4.97	Promethazine Hcl, Insource	58441-0114-10
10 ml	$5.77	ADGAN, UAD Labs	00785-8090-10
10 ml	$6.00	PHENERZINE 50, Bolan Pharm	44437-0259-10
10 ml	$6.50	PROMACOT, C O Truxton	00463-1095-10
10 ml	$6.57	Promethazine Hcl, General Inj & Vac	52584-0259-10
10 ml	$7.10	PROREX, Hyrex Pharms	00314-0685-70
10 ml	$8.87	Promethazine Hcl, Steris Labs	00402-0259-10
10 ml	$8.87	Promethazine Hcl, HL Moore Drug Exch	00839-5158-30
10 ml	$9.00	Promethazine Hcl, IDE-Interstate	00814-6424-40
10 ml	$10.25	ANERGAN, Forest Pharms	00456-1009-10
10 ml	$11.65	Promethazine Hcl, Goldline Labs	00182-0501-63
10 ml	$11.79	Promethazine, Schein Pharm (US)	00364-6571-54
10 ml	$11.85	Promethazine HCl, Rugby	00536-8460-70
10 ml	$14.95	PHENOJECT-50, Mayrand Pharms	00259-0308-10
10 ml	$18.25	PHENACEN, Schwarz Pharma (US)	00131-1166-05

Syrup - Oral - 6.25 mg/5ml

5 ml x 100	$56.60	Promethazine Hcl, Xactdose	50962-0100-05
118 ml	$2.91	Promethazine Syrup Plain, Rugby	00536-1745-97
118 ml	$3.00	PHENAMETH PLAIN SYRUP 6.25, Major Pharms	00904-1508-00
120 ml	$.84	Promethazine Hcl, H.C.F.A. F F P	99999-2125-01
120 ml	$2.10	Promethazine Hcl, Consolidated Midland	00223-6345-01
120 ml	$2.10	Promethazine Plain, HR Cenci	00556-0365-04
120 ml	$2.20	Promethazine Hcl, Morton Grove	60432-0608-04
120 ml	$2.40	Prometh Syrup Plain, Alpharma	00472-1504-04
120 ml	$2.50	Promethazine Hcl, Halsey Drug	00879-0539-04
120 ml	$3.00	Phenameth, Major Pharms	00904-1508-20
120 ml	$3.04	Promethazine Hcl, HL Moore Drug Exch	00839-6314-65
480 ml	$3.36	Promethazine HCl, H.C.F.A. F F P	99999-2125-02
480 ml	$4.50	Promethazine Hcl, Consolidated Midland	00223-6343-01

HOW SUPPLIED - RATED THERAPEUTICALLY EQUIVALENT: *(cont'd)*

480 ml	$4.50	Promethazine Plain, HR Cenci	00556-0365-16
480 ml	$4.95	Promethazine Hcl, Consolidated Midland	00223-6345-02
480 ml	$5.49	Promethazine Hcl, Aligen Independ	00405-3600-16
480 ml	$5.70	Prometh Syrup Plain, Goldline Labs	00182-1737-40
480 ml	$5.80	Promethazine Syrup Plain, Schein Pharm (US)	00364-0733-16
480 ml	$6.00	Promethazine Hcl, ESI Lederle	59911-5818-03
480 ml	$6.21	Promethazine, HL Moore Drug Exch	00839-6314-69
480 ml	$6.50	Phenameth Plain Syrup 6.25, Major Pharms	00904-1508-16
480 ml	$6.85	Promethazine Hcl, Qualitest Pharms	00603-1580-58
480 ml	$7.28	Promethazine Hcl, Morton Grove	60432-0608-16
480 ml	$7.45	Promethazine Hcl, Halsey Drug	00879-0539-16
480 ml	$7.50	Prometh Syrup Plain, Alpharma	00472-1504-16
480 ml	$7.50	Promethazine Syrup Plain, Rugby	00536-1745-85
480 ml	$7.50	PROMETAZINE PLAIN, Geneva Pharms	00781-6575-16
3785 ml	$31.49	Prometh Syrup Plain, Goldline Labs	00182-1737-41
3840 ml	$26.88	Promethazine Hcl, H.C.F.A. F F P	99999-2125-03
3840 ml	$27.49	Promethazine Hcl, Consolidated Midland	00223-6345-03
3840 ml	$28.80	Promethazine Plain, HR Cenci	00556-0365-28
3840 ml	$31.15	Promethazine Syrup Plain, Rugby	00536-1745-90
3840 ml	$32.99	Promethazine Hcl, HL Moore Drug Exch	00839-6314-70
3840 ml	$35.90	Prometh Syrup Plain, Alpharma	00472-1504-28
3840 ml	$36.83	Promethazine Hcl, Halsey Drug	00879-0539-28
3840 ml	$41.89	Promethazine Hcl, Major Pharms	00904-1508-28
4000 ml	$28.00	Promethazine Hcl, H.C.F.A. F F P	99999-2125-04

Syrup - Oral - 25 mg/5ml

480 ml	$11.00	Promethazine Hcl, Consolidated Midland	00223-6344-01
3840 ml	$77.49	Promethazine Hcl, Consolidated Midland	00223-6344-02

HOW SUPPLIED - NOT RATED EQUIVALENT:

Suppository - Rectal - 12.5 mg

12's	**$27.21**	**PHENERGAN, Wyeth Labs**	**00008-0498-01**

Suppository - Rectal - 25 mg

12's	**$31.22**	**PHENERGAN, Wyeth Labs**	**00008-0212-01**

Suppository - Rectal - 50 mg

1's	$25.00	PROMETHEGAN, GW Labs	00713-0132-12
12's	$26.50	Promethazine Hcl, Harber Pharm	51432-0415-12
12's	$36.80	Promethazine Hcl, Rugby	00536-7405-12
12's	$37.45	Promethazine Hcl, Major Pharms	00904-1290-12
12's	**$39.98**	**PHENERGAN, Wyeth Labs**	**00008-0229-01**
12's	$45.00	Promethazine Hcl, HL Moore Drug Exch	00839-7492-92
25's	$46.10	PROMETHEGAN, GW Labs	00713-0132-25

Syrup - Oral - 6.25 mg/5ml

120 ml x 24	**$140.49**	**PHENERGAN PLAIN, Wyeth Labs**	**00008-0549-02**
480 ml	**$21.83**	**PHENERGAN PLAIN, Wyeth Labs**	**00008-0549-03**

Syrup - Oral - 25 mg/5ml

480 ml	**$45.47**	**PHENERGAN, Wyeth Labs**	**00008-0231-01**

Tablet, Uncoated - Oral - 12.5 mg

100's	$6.50	Promethazine Hcl, ESI Lederle	59911-5871-01
100's	**$18.11**	**PHENERGAN, Wyeth Labs**	**00008-0019-01**

Tablet, Uncoated - Oral - 25 mg

100's	$2.55	Promethazine Hcl, HL Moore Drug Exch	00839-1535-06
100's	$3.15	PHENAMETH, Major Pharms	00904-2329-60
100's	$3.69	Promethazine HCl, Schein Pharm (US)	00364-0222-01
100's	$3.70	Promethazine Hcl, United Res	00677-0481-01
100's	$3.96	Promethazine HCl, Geneva Pharms	00781-1830-01
100's	$3.96	Promethazine Hcl, ESI Lederle	59911-5872-01
100's	$4.25	Promethazine Hcl, Consolidated Midland	00223-1521-01
100's	$6.15	Promethazine Hcl, Raway	00686-1540-13
100's	$6.80	Promethazine Hcl, Martec Pharms	52555-0318-01
100's	$9.49	Promethazine Hcl 25, Vangard Labs	00615-1540-13
100's	**$31.99**	**PHENERGAN, Wyeth Labs**	**00008-0027-02**
100's	**$32.53**	**PHENERGAN, Wyeth Labs**	**00008-0027-07**
1000's	$14.43	Promethazine Hcl, HL Moore Drug Exch	00839-1535-16
1000's	$18.75	PHENAMETH, Major Pharms	00904-2329-80
1000's	$24.72	Promethazine HCl, Schein Pharm (US)	00364-0222-02
1000's	$26.15	Promethazine Hcl, United Res	00677-0481-10
1000's	$28.80	Promethazine HCl, Geneva Pharms	00781-1830-10
1000's	$39.50	Promethazine Hcl, Consolidated Midland	00223-1521-02
1000's	$47.30	Promethazine Hcl, Martec Pharms	52555-0318-10

Tablet, Uncoated - Oral - 50 mg

100's	$4.65	PHENAMETH, Major Pharms	00904-2330-60
100's	$5.96	Promethazine HCl, Schein Pharm (US)	00364-0345-01
100's	$5.96	Promethazine Hcl, ESI Lederle	59911-5873-01
100's	$5.98	Promethazine HCl, Geneva Pharms	00781-1832-01
100's	$12.75	Promethazine Hcl, Martec Pharms	52555-0319-01
100's	**$49.03**	**PHENERGAN, Wyeth Labs**	**00008-0227-01**

PROPAFENONE HYDROCHLORIDE *(002127)*

CATEGORIES: Antiarrhythmic Agents; Arrhythmia; Cardiovascular Drugs; Tachycardia; Pregnancy Category C; FDA Class 1C ("Little or No Therapeutic Advantage"); FDA Approved 1989 Nov

BRAND NAMES: *Arythmol*; *Norfenon*; *Normorytmin*; *Rythmex*; **Rythmol**; *Rytmonorm*
(International brand names outside U.S. in italics)

FORMULARIES: Aetna; BC-BS; PCS

COST OF THERAPY: $917.82 (Arrhythmia; Tablet; 150 mg; 3/day; 365 days)

DESCRIPTION:

Propafenone HCl is an antiarrhythmic drug supplied in scored film-coated tablets of 150, 225 and 300 mg for oral administration. Propafenone has some structural similarities to beta blocking agents.

The chemical formula for propafenone HCl is $C_{21}H_{27}NO_3HCl$, 2'-(2-Hydroxy -3- (propylamino)- propyl))-3-phenylpropiophenone hydroxide, with a molecular weight of 377.92.

Propafenone HCl occurs as colorless, crystals or white crystalline powder with a very bitter taste. It is slight, soluble in water (20°C) chloroform and ethanol. The following inactive ingredients are contained in the tablet: corn starch, hydroxypropyl, methyl cellulose, magnesium stearate, polyethylene glycol, polysorbate povidone, propylene glycol, sodium starch glycolate, and titanium dioxide.

CLINICAL PHARMACOLOGY:

MECHANISM OF ACTION

Propafenone HCl is a Class IC antiarrhythmic drug with local anesthetic effects, and a direct stabilizing action on myocardial membranes. The electrophysiological effect of propafenone HCl manifests itself in a reduction of upstroke velocity (Phase O) of the monophasic action potential. In Purkinje fibers, and to a lesser extent myocardial fibers, propafenone HCl reduces the fast inward current carried by sodium ions. Diastolic excitability threshold is increased and effective refractory period prolonged. Propafenone reduces spontaneous automaticity and depresses triggered activity.

Studies in anesthetized dogs and isolated organ preparations show that propafenone HCl has beta-sympatholytic activity at about 1/50 the potency of propranolol. Clinical studies employing isoproterenol challenge and exercise testing after single doses of propafenone indicate a beta adrenergic blocking potency (per mg) about 1/40 that of propranolol in man. In clinical trials, resting heart rate decreases of about 8% were noted at the higher end of the therapeutic plasma concentration range. At very high concentrations *in vitro*, propafenone can inhibit the slow inward current carried by calcium but this calcium antagonist effect probably does not contribute to antiarrhythmic efficacy. Propafenone has local anesthetic activity approximately equal to procaine.

ELECTROPHYSIOLOGY

Electrophysiology studies in patients with ventricular tachycardia have shown that propafenone HCl prolongs atrioventricular conduction while having little or no effect on sinus node function. Both AV nodal conduction time (AH interval) and His-Purkinje conduction time (HV interval) are prolonged. Propafenone has little or no effect on the atrial functional refractory period, but AV nodal functions and effective refractory periods are prolonged. In patients with WPW, propafenone HCl reduces conduction and increases the effective refractory period of the accessory pathway in both directions. Propafenone slows conduction and consequently produces dose related changes in the PR interval and QRS duration QT_C interval does not change (TABLE 1).

TABLE 1 Mean Changes in ECG Intervals* Total Daily Dose (mg)

Interval	337.5 mg msec	337.5 mg %	450 mg msec	450 mg %	675 mg msec	675 mg %	990 mg msec	990 mg %
RR	-14.5	-1.8	30.6	3.8	31.5	3.9	41.7	5.1
PR	3.6	2.1	19.1	11.6	28.9	17.8	35.6	21.9
QRS	5.6	6.4	5.5	6.1	7.7	8.4	15.6	17.3
QT_c	2.7	0.7	-7.5	-1.8	5.0	1.2	14.7	3.7

* Change and percent change based on mean baseline values for each treatment group.

In any individual patient, the above ECG changes cannot be readily used to predict either efficacy or plasma concentration.

Propafenone HCl causes a dose-related and concentration related decrease in the rate of single and multiple PVCs and can suppress recurrence of ventricular tachycardia. Based on the percent of patients attaining substantial (80-90%) suppression of ventricular ectopic activity if appears that trough plasma levels of 0.2 to 1.5 mcg/ml can provide good suppression with higher concentrations giving a greater rate of good response.

HEMODYNAMICS

Sympathetic stimulation may be a vital component supporting circulatory function in patients with congestive heart failure and its inhibition by the beta blockade produced by propafenone HCl may in itself aggravate congestive heart failure.

Additionally, like other Class IC antiarrhythmic drugs studies in humans have shown that propafenone HCl exerts a negative inotropic effect on the myocardium. Cardiac catheterization studies in patients with moderately impaired ventricular function (mean C.I.=2.61 L/min/m^2) utilizing intravenous propafenone infusions (2 mg/kg over 10 min + 2 mg/min for 30 min) that gave mean plasma concentrations of 30 mcg/ml (well above the therapeutic range of 0.2-1.5 mcg/ml) showed significant increases in pulmonary capillary wedge pressure systemic and pulmonary vascular resistances and depression of cardiac output and cardiac index.

PHARMACOKINETICS AND METABOLISM

Propafenone HCl is nearly completely absorbed after oral administration with peak plasma levels occurring approximately 3-5 hours after administration in most individuals. Propafenone exhibits extensive saturable presystemic biotransformation (first pass effect) resulting in a dose dependent and dosage form dependent absolute bioavailability (*e.g.,* a 150 mg tablet had absolute bioavailability of 3-4% while a 300 mg tablet had absolute bioavailability of 10.6%). A 300 mg solution which was rapidly absorbed had absolute bioavailability of 21.4%. At still larger doses above those recommended bioavailability increases still further. Decreased liver function also increases bioavailability is inversely related to indocyanine green clearance reaching 60-70% at clearances of 7 ml/min and below. The clearance of propafenone is reduced and the elimination half-life increased in patients with significant hepatic dysfunction (see PRECAUTIONS.)

Propafenone HCl follows a nonlinear pharmacokinetic disposition presumably due to saturation of first pass hepatic metabolism as the liver is exposed to higher concentrations of propafenone and shows a very high degree of interindividual variability. For example, for a three-fold increase in daily dose from 300 to 900 mg/day there is a ten-fold increase in steady-state plasma concentration. The top 25% of patients given 375 mg/day, however, had a mean concentration of propafenone larger than the bottom 25%, and about equal to the second 25%, of patients given a dose of 900 mg. Although food increased peak blood level and bioavailability in a single dose study, during multiple dose administration of propafenone to healthy volunteers food did not change bioavailability significantly.

There are two genetically determined patterns of propafenone metabolism. In over 90% of patients the drug is rapidly and extensively metabolized with an elimination half life from 2-10 hours. These patients metabolize propafenone into two active metabolites 5-hydroxypropafenone and N-depropylpropafenone. *In vitro* preparations have shown these two metabolites to have antiarrhythmic activity comparable to propafenone but in man they both are usually present in concentrations less than 20% of propafenone. Nine additional metabolites have been identified most in only trace amounts. It is the saturable hydroxylation pathway that is responsible for the nonlinear pharmacokinetic disposition.

In less than 10% of patients (and in any patient also receiving Quinidine (see PRECAUTIONS) metabolism of propafenone is slower because the 5-hydroxy metabolite is not formed or is minimally formed. The estimated propafenone elimination half life ranges from 10-32 hours. Decreased ability to form the 5-hydroxy metabolite of propafenone is associated with a diminished ability to metabolize debrisoquine and a variety of other drugs (encainide, metoprolol, dextromethorphan). In these patients, the N-depropyl-propafenone occurs in quantities comparable to the levels occurring in extensive metabolizers. In slow metabolizers propafenone pharmacokinetics are linear.

There are significant differences in plasma concentrations of propafenone in slow and extensive metabolizers the former achieving concentrations 15 to 20 times those of the extensive metabolizers at daily doses of 675-900 mg/day. At low doses the differences are greater with slow metabolizers attaining concentrations more than five times that of extensive metabolizers. Because the difference decreases at high doses and is mitigated by the lack of

CLINICAL PHARMACOLOGY: *(cont'd)*

the active 5-hydroxy metabolite in the slow metabolizers and because steady state conditions are achieved after 4-5 days of dosing in all patients the recommended dosing regimen is the same for all patients. The greater variability in blood levels require that the drug be titrated carefully in all patients with close attention to clinical and ECG evidence of toxicity (See DOSAGE AND ADMINISTRATION.)

INDICATIONS AND USAGE:

Propafenone HCl is indicated for the treatment of documented ventricular arrhythmias such as sustained ventricular tachycardia that in the judgement of the physician, are life threatening. Because of the proarrhythmic effects of propafenone HCl, its use should be reserved for patients in whom, in the opinion of the physician, the benefits of treatment outweighs the risks. The use of propafenone HCl is not recommended in patients with less severe ventricular arrhythmias, even if the patients are symptomatic.

Use of propafenone HCl for the treatment of sustained ventricular tachycardia, like other antiarrhythmics, should be initiated in the hospital.

The effects of propafenone HCl in patients with recent myocardial infarction and in patients with supraventricular tachycardia have not been adequately studied. As is the case for other antiarrhythmic agents, there is no evidence from controlled trials that the use of propafenone HCl favorably affects survival or the incidence of sudden death.

CONTRAINDICATIONS:

Propafenone HCl is contraindicated in the presence of uncontrolled congestive heart failure cardiogenic shock sinoatrial, atrioventricular and intraventricular disorders of impulse generation and/or conduction (*e.g.,* sick sinus node syndrome, atrioventricular block) in the absence of an artificial pacemaker, bradycardia, marked hypotension, bronchospastic disorders, manifest electrolyte imbalance, and known hypersensitivity to the drug.

WARNINGS:

Mortality: In the National Heart Lung and Blood Institute's Cardiac Arrhythmia Suppression Trial (CAST), a long-term, multi-center, randomized, double blind study in patients with asymptomatic non-life-threatening ventricular ectopy who had a myocardial infarction more than six days but less than two years previously, an excessive mortality or non-fatal cardiac arrest rate was seen in patients treated with encainide or flecainide (56/730) compared with that seen in patients assigned to carefully matched placebo-treated groups (22/725). The average duration of treatment with encainide or flecainide in this study was ten months.

The applicability of these results to other populations (*e.g.,* those without recent myocardial infarction and to other antiarrhythmic drugs) is uncertain, but at present it is prudent (1) to consider any IC agent (especially one documented to provoke new serious arrhythmias) to have a similar risk and (2) to consider the risks of Class IC agents, coupled with the lack of any evidence of improved survival generally unacceptable in patients without life-threatening ventricular arrhythmias, even if the patients are experiencing unpleasant but not life-threatening, symptoms or signs.

Proarrhythmic Effects: Propafenone HCl like other antiarrhythmic agents may cause new or worsened arrhythmias. Such proarrhythmic effects range from an increase in frequency of PVCs to the development of more severe ventricular tachycardia, ventricular fibrillation or torsade de pointes; i.e., tachycardia that is more sustained or more rapid which may lead to fatal consequences. It is therefore essential that each patient given propafenone HCl be evaluated electrocardiographically and clinically prior to, and during therapy to determine whether the response to propafenone HCl supports continued treatment.

Overall in clinical trials with propafenone 4.7% of all patients had new or worsened ventricular arrhythmia possibly representing a proarrhythmic event (0.7% was an increase in PVCs; 4.0% a worsening or new appearance of VT or VF). Of the patients who had worsening of VT (4%), 92% had a history of VT and/or VT/VF. 71% had coronary artery disease, and 68% had a prior myocardial infarction. The incidence of proarrhythmias, which include patients with less serious or benign arrhythmias, which include patients with an increase in frequency of PVCs, was 1.6%. Although most proarrhythmic events occurred during the first week of therapy, late events were also seen and the CAST study (see WARNINGS, Proarrhythmic Effects) suggests that an increased risk is present throughout treatment.

Nonallergic Bronchospasm (*e.g.,*chronic bronchitis, emphysema): PATIENTS WITH BRONCHOSPASTIC DISEASE SHOULD, IN GENERAL, NOT RECEIVE PROPAFENONE or other agents with beta adrenergic blocking activity.

Congestive Heart Failure: During treatment with oral propafenone in patients with depressed baseline function (mean EF=33.5%), no significant decreases in ejection fraction were seen. In clinical trial experience, new or worsened CHF has been reported in 3.7% of patients; of those 0.9% were considered probably or definitely related to propafenone HCl. Of the patients with congestive heart failure probably related to propafenone, 80% had preexisting heart failure and 85% had coronary artery disease. CHF attributable to propafenone HCl developed rarely (<0.2%) in patients who had no previous history of CHF.

As propafenone HCl exerts both beta blockade and a (dose-related) negative inotropic effect on cardiac muscle, patients with congestive heart failure should be fully compensated before receiving propafenone HCl. If congestive heart failure worsens, propafenone HCl should be discontinued (unless congestive hart failure is due to the cardiac arrhythmia) and, if indicated, restarted at a lower dosage only after adequate cardiac compensation has been established.

Conduction Disturbances: Propafenone HCl slows atrioventricular conduction and also causes first degree AV block. Average PR interval prolongation and increases in CRS duration are close, correlated with dosage increases and concomitant increases in propafenone plasma concentrations. The incidence of first degree, second degree, and third degree AV block observed in 2,127 patients was 2.5% 0.6% and 0.2% respectively. Development of second or third degree AV block requires a reduction dosage or discontinuation of propafenone HCl. Bundle branch block (1.2%) and intraventricular conduction delay (1.1%) have been reported in patients receiving propafenone. Bradycardia has also been reported (1.5%). Experience in patients with sick sinus node syndrome is limited and these patients should not be treated with propafenone.

Effects on Pacemaker Threshold: Propafenone HCl may alter both pacing and sensing thresholds of artificial pacemakers. Pacemakers should be monitored and programmed accordingly during therapy.

Hematologic Disturbances: One case of agranulocytosis with fever and sepsis, probably related to the use of propafenone, was seen in U.S. clinical trials. The agranulocytosis appeared after 8 weeks of therapy. Propafenone therapy was stopped and the white count had normalized by 14 days. The patient recovered. In the course of over 800,000 patient years of exposure during marketing outside the U.S. since 1978, seven additional cases have been reported. In one of these, concomitant captopril, a drug known to cause agranulocytosis, was used. Unexplained fever and/or decrease in white cell count, particularly during the first three months of therapy, warrant consideration of possible agranulocytosis/granulocytopenia. Patients should be instructed to promptly report the development of any signs of infection such as fever, sore throat, or chills.

PRECAUTIONS:

GENERAL

Hepatic Dysfunction: Propafenone is highly metabolized by the liver and should, therefore, be administered cautiously to patients with impaired hepatic function. Severe liver dysfunction increases the bioavailability of propafenone to approximately 70% compared to 3-40% for patients with normal liver function. In eight patients with moderate to severe liver disease, the mean half-life was approximately 9 hours. As a result, the dose of propafenone given to patients with impaired hepatic function should be approximately 20-30% of the dose given to patients with normal hepatic function (see DOSAGE AND ADMINISTRATION.) Careful monitoring for excessive pharmacological effects (see OVERDOSAGE) should be carried out.

Renal Dysfunction: A considerable percentage of propafenone metabolites (18.5%-38% of the dose 48/hours) are excreted in the urine.

Until further data are available propafenone HCl should be administered cautiously to patients with impaired renal function. These patients should be carefully monitored for signs of overdosage (see OVERDOSAGE.)

Elevated ANA Titers: Positive ANA titers have been reported in patients receiving propafenone. They have been reversible upon cessation of treatment and may disappear even in the face of continued propafenone therapy. These laboratory findings were usually not associated with clinical symptoms but there is one published case of drug induced lupus erythematosus (positive rechallenge); it resolved completely upon discontinuation of therapy. Patients who develop an abnormal ANA test should be carefully evaluated and if persistent or worsening elevation of ANA titers is detected, consideration should be given to discontinuing therapy.

Impaired Spermatogenesis: Reversible disorders of spermatogenesis have been demonstrated in monkeys, dogs and rabbits after high dose intravenous administration. Evaluation of the effects of short term propafenone administration on spermatogenesis in 11 normal subjects suggests that propafenone produced a reversible short-term drop (within normal range) in sperm count. Subsequent evaluation in 11 patients receiving propafenone chronically have suggested no effect of propafenone on sperm count.

CARCINOGENESIS, MUTAGENESIS, AND IMPAIRMENT OF FERTILITY

Lifetime maximally tolerated oral dose studies in mice (up to 360 mg/kg/day) and rats (up to 270 mg/kg/day) provided no evidence of a carcinogenic potential for propafenone.

Propafenone HCl was not mutagenic when assayed for genotoxicity in 1) mouse Dominant Lethal test 2) rat bone marrow Chromosome Analysis 3) Chinese hamster bone marrow and spermatogonia chromosome analysis 4) Chinese hamster micronucleus test, and 5) Ames bacterial test.

Propafenone administered intravenously to rabbits, dogs, and monkeys has been shown to decrease spermatogenesis. These effects were reversible, were not found following oral dosing of propafenone, were seen only at lethal or sublethal dose levels and, were not seen in rats treated either orally or intravenously (see PRECAUTIONS, Impaired Spermatogenesis). Propafenone did not effect either male or female fertility rates when administered intravenously to rats and rabbits at dose levels up to 18 times the maximum recommended daily human dose of 900 mg (based on 60 kg human body weight).

PREGNANCY CATEGORY C

Teratogenic Effects: Propafenone has been shown to be embryotoxic in rabbits and rats when given in doses 10 and 40 times, respectively, the maximum recommended human dose. No teratogenic potential was apparent in either species. There are no adequate and well-controlled studies in pregnant women. Propafenone should be used during pregnancy only if the potential benefit justifies the potential risk to the fetus.

Nonteratogenic Effects: In a perinatal and postnatal study in rats, propafenone, at dose levels of 6 or more times the maximum recommended human dose, produced dose dependent increases in maternal and neonatal mortality, decreased maternal and pup body weight gain and reduced neonatal physiological development.

LABOR AND DELIVERY

It is not known whether the use of propafenone during labor or delivery has immediate or delayed adverse effects on the fetus or whether it prolongs the duration of labor or increases the need for forceps delivery or other obstetrical intervention.

NURSING MOTHERS

It is not known whether this drug is excreted in human milk. Because many drugs are excreted in human milk and because of the potential for serious adverse reactions in nursing infants from propafenone HCl, a decision should be made whether to discontinue nursing or to discontinue the drug taking into account the importance of the drug to the mother.

PEDIATRIC USE

The safety and efficacy of propafenone HCl in children has not been established.

GERIATRIC USE

There do not appear to be any age-related differences in adverse reaction rates in the most commonly reported adverse reactions. Because of the possible increased risk of impaired hepatic or renal function in this age group, propafenone HCl should be used with caution. The effective dose may be lower in these patients.

DRUG INTERACTIONS:

Quinidine: Small doses of quinidine completely inhibit the hydroxylation metabolic pathway, making all patients in effect show metabolizers (see CLINICAL PHARMACOLOGY.) There is, as yet, too little information to recommend concomitant use of propafenone and quinidine.

Local Anesthetics: Concomitant use of local anesthetics (*i.e.,* during pacemaker implantations, surgery, or dental use) may increase the risks of central nervous system side effects.

Digitalis: Propafenone HCl produces dose related increases in serum digoxin levels ranging from about 35% at 450 mg/day to 85% at 900 mg/day of propafenone without affecting digoxin renal clearance. These elevations of digoxin levels were maintained for up to 16 months during concomitant administration. Plasma digoxin levels of patients on concomitant therapy should be measured, and digoxin dosage should ordinarily be reduced when propafenone is started, especially if a relatively large digoxin dose is used or if plasma concentrations are relatively high.

Beta-Antagonists: In a study involving healthy subjects concomitant administration of propafenone and propranolol has resulted in substantial increases in propranolol plasma concentration and elimination half-life with no change in propafenone plasma levels from control values. Similar observations have been reported with metoprolol. (Propafenone appears to inhibit the hydroxylation pathway for the two beta antagonists just as quinidine inhibits propafenone metabolism). Increased plasma concentrations of metoprolol could overcome its relative cardioselectivity. In propafenone clinical trials, patients who were receiving beta-blockers concurrently did not experience an increased incidence of side effects. While the therapeutic range for beta-blockers is wide, a reduction in dosage may be necessary during concomitant administration with propafenone.

Warfarin: In a study of eight healthy subjects receiving propafenone and warfarin concomitantly, mean steady-state warfarin plasma concentrations increased 39% with a corresponding increase in prothrombin times of approximately 25%. It is therefore recommended that prothrombin times be routinely monitored and the dose of warfarin be adjusted if necessary.

DRUG INTERACTIONS: *(cont'd)*

Cimetidine: Concomitant administration of propafenone and cimetidine in 12 healthy subjects resulted in a 20% increase in steady-state plasma concentrations of propafenone with no detectable changes in electrocardiographic parameters beyond that measured on propafenone alone.

Other: Limited experience with propafenone combined with calcium antagonists and diuretics has been reported without evidence of clinically significant adverse reactions.

ADVERSE REACTIONS:

Adverse reactions associated with propafenone HCl occur most frequently in the gastrointestinal cardiovascular and central nervous systems. About 20% of patients discontinued due to adverse reactions. Results of controlled trials comparing adverse reaction rates on propafenone and placebo and on propafenone and quinidine are shown in the following table. Adverse reactions appearing in TABLE 2 were reported for ≥1% of the patients receiving propafenone. The most common events were dizziness, unusual taste, first degree AV block, intraventricular conduction, nausea and/or vomiting, and constipation. Headache was relatively common also, but was not increased compared to placebo.

TABLE 2 Adverse Reactions Reported for ≥ 1% of the Patients

	Prop/Placebo Trials		Prop/Quinidine Trial	
	Prop (N=247)	Placebo (N=111)	Prop (N=53)	Quinidine (N=52)
Unusual Taste	7.3%	0.9%	22.6%	0.0%
Dizziness	6.5%	5.4%	15.1%	9.6%
First Degree AV Block	4.5%	0.9%	1.9%	0.0%
Headache(s)	4.5%	4.5%	1.9%	7.7%
Constipation	4.0%	0.0%	5.7%	1.9%
Intraventricular Conduction Delay	4.0%	0.0%	-	-
Nausea and/or Vomiting	2.8%	0.9%	5.7%	15.4%
Fatigue	-	-	3.8%	1.9%
Palpitations	2.4%	0.9%	-	-
Blurred vision	2.0%	0.9%	5.7%	1.9%
Dry Mouth	2.0%	0.9%	5.7%	5.8%
Dyspnea	2.0%	2.7%	3.8%	0.0%
Abdominal Pain/Cramps	-	-	1.9%	7.7%
Dyspepsia	-	-	1.9%	7.7%
Congestive Heart Failure	-	-	1.9%	0.0%
Fever	-	-	1.9%	9.6%
Tinnitus	-	-	1.9%	1.9%
Vision Abnormal	-	-	1.9%	1.9%
Esophagitis	-	-	1.9%	0.0%
Gastroenteritis	-	-	1.9%	0.0%
Anxiety	2.0%	1.8%	-	-
Anorexia	1.6%	0.9%	-	1.9%
Proarrhythmia	1.2%	0.0%	1.9%	0.0%
Flatulence	1.2%	0.0%	1.9%	0.0%
Angina	1.2%	0.0%	1.9%	3.8%
Second Degree AV Block	1.2%	0.0%	-	-
Bundle Branch Block	1.2%	0.0%	1.9%	1.9%
Loss of Balance	1.2%	0.0%	-	-
Diarrhea	1.2%	0.9%	5.7%	38.5%

Adverse reactions reported for ≥ 1% of 2,127 patients who received propafenone in U.S clinical trials are presented in the following table by propafenone daily dose. The most common adverse reactions in controlled clinical trials appeared dose related (but note that most patients spent more time at the larger doses), especially dizziness, nausea and/or vomiting, unusual taste, constipation, and blurred vision. Some less common reactions may also have been dose related such as first degree AV Block, congestive heart failure, dyspepsia, and weakness. The principal causes of discontinuation were the most common events and are shown in TABLE 3.

In addition the following adverse reactions were reported less frequently than 1% either in clinical trials or in marketing experience (*adverse events for marketing experience are given in italics*). Causality and relationship to propafenone therapy cannot necessarily be judged from these events.

Cardiovascular System: Atrial flutter, AV dissociation cardiac arrest, flushing, hot flashes, sick sinus syndrome, sinus pause, or arrest supraventricular tachycardia.

Nervous System: Abnormal dreams, abnormal speech, abnormal vision, *apnea*, *coma*, confusion, depression, memory loss, numbness, paresthesias, psychosis/mania seizures (0.3%), tinnitus, unusual small sensation, vertigo.

Gastrointestinal: A number of patients with lever abnormalities associated with propafenone therapy have been reported in foreign post marketing experience. Some appeared due to hepatocellular injury, some were cholestatic and some showed a mixed picture. Some of these reports were simply discovered through clinical chemistries, others because of clinical symptoms. One case was rechallenged with a positive outcome. Cholestasis (0.1%) elevated liver enzymes (alkaline phosphatase serum, transaminases) (0.2%), gastroenteritis, hepatitis (0.03%).

Hematologic: Agranulocytosis, amenia, bruising, granulocytopenia, *increased bleeding time,*leukopenia, purpura, thrombocytopenia.

Other: Alopecia, eye irritation, *hyponatremia/inappropriate ADH secretion*, impotence, increased glucose, *kidney failure*, positive ANA (0.7%), *lupus erythematosus*, muscle cramps, muscle weakness, nephrotic syndrome, pain, pruritus.

OVERDOSAGE:

The symptoms of overdosage, which are usually most severe within 3 hours of ingestion, may include hypotension, somnolence, bradycardia, intra-atrial and intraventricular conduction disturbances, and rarely convulsions and high grade ventricular arrhythmias. Defibrillation as well as infusion of dopamine and isoproterenol have been effective in controlling rhythm and blood pressure. Convulsions have been alleviated with intravenous diazepam. General supportive measures such as mechanical respiratory assistance and external cardiac massage may be necessary.

DOSAGE AND ADMINISTRATION:

The dose of propafenone HCl must be individually titrated on the basis of response and tolerance. It is recommended that therapy be initiated with 150 mg propafenone given every eight hours (450 mg/day). Dosage may be increased at a minimum of 3 to 4 day intervals to 225 mg every 8 hours (675 mg/day) and, if necessary, to 300 mg every 8 hours (900 mg/day). The usefulness and safety of dosages exceeding 900 mg per day have not been established. In those patients in whom significant widening of the QRS complex or second or third degree AV block occurs dose reduction should be considered.

As with other antiarrhythmic agents, in the elderly or in patients with marked previous myocardial damage, the dose of propafenone HCl should be increased more gradually during the initial phase of treatment.

TABLE 3 Adverse Reactions Reported for ≥ 1% of the Patients N = 2127

	Incidence by Total Daily Dose 450 mg (N=1430)	500 mg (N=1337)	≥ 900 mg (N=1333)	Total Incidence (N=2127)	% of Pts. Who Discont.
Dizziness	3.6%	6.6%	11.0%	12.5%	2.4%
Nausea and/or Vomiting	2.4%	6.1%	8.9%	10.7%	3.4%
Unusual Taste	2.5%	4.9%	6.3%	8.8%	0.7%
Constipation	2.0%	4.1%	5.3%	7.2%	0.5%
Fatigue	1.8%	2.8%	4.1%	6.0%	1.0%
Dyspnea	2.2%	2.3%	3.6%	5.3%	1.6%
Proarrhythmia	2.0%	2.1%	2.9%	4.7%	4.7%
Angina	1.7%	2.1%	3.2%	4.6%	0.5%
Headache(s)	1.5%	2.5%	2.8%	4.5%	1.0%
Blurred Vision	0.6%	2.4%	3.1%	3.8%	0.8%
CHF	0.8%	2.2%	2.6%	3.7%	1.4%
Ventricular Tachycardia	1.4%	1.6%	2.9%	3.4%	1.2%
Dyspepsia	1.3%	1.7%	2.5%	3.4%	0.9%
Palpitations	0.6%	1.6%	2.6%	3.4%	0.5%
Rash	0.6%	1.4%	1.9%	2.6%	0.8%
AV Block First Degree	0.8%	1.2%	2.1%	2.5%	0.3%
Diarrhea	0.5%	1.6%	1.7%	2.5%	0.6%
Weakness	0.6%	1.6%	1.7%	2.4%	0.7%
Dry Mouth	0.9%	1.0%	1.4%	2.4%	0.2%
Syncope Near Syncope	0.8%	1.3%	1.4%	2.2%	0.7%
ORS Duration Increased	0.5%	0.9%	1.7%	1.9%	0.5%
Chest Pain	0.5%	0.7%	1.4%	1.8%	0.2%
Anorexia	0.5%	0.7%	1.6%	1.7%	0.4%
Abdominal Pain Cramps	0.8%	0.9%	1.1%	1.7%	0.4%
Ataxia	0.3%	0.6%	1.5%	1.6%	0.2%
Insomnia	0.3%	1.3%	0.7%	1.5%	0.3%
Premature Ventricular Contraction(s)	0.6%	0.6%	1.1%	1.5%	0.1%
Anxiety	0.7%	0.5%	0.9%	1.5%	0.6%
Edema	0.6%	0.4%	1.0%	1.4%	0.2%
Tremor(s)	0.3%	0.8%	1.1%	1.4%	0.3%
Diaphoresis	0.6%	0.4%	1.1%	1.4%	0.3%
Bundle Branch Block	0.3%	0.7%	1.0%	1.2%	0.5%
Drowsiness	0.6%	0.5%	0.7%	1.2%	0.2%
Atrial Fibrillation	0.7%	0.7%	0.5%	1.2%	0.4%
Flatulence	0.3%	0.7%	0.9%	1.2%	0.1%
Hypotension	0.1%	0.5%	1.0%	1.1%	0.4%
Intraventricular Conduction delay	0.2%	0.7%	0.9%	1.1%	0.1%
Pain, joints	0.2%	0.4%	0.9%	1.0%	0.1%

ANIMAL PHARMACOLOGY:

Animal Toxicology: Renal changes have been observed in the rat following 6 months of oral administration of propafenone at doses of 180 and 360 mg/kg/day, (12-24 times the maximum recommended human dose) but not 90 mg/kg/day. Both inflammatory and non-inflammatory changes in the renal tubules with accompanying interstitial nephritis were observed. These lesions were reversible in that they were not found in rats treated at these dosage levels and allowed to recover for 6 weeks. Fatty degenerative changes of the liver were found in rats following chronic administration of propafenone at dose levels 19 times the maximum recommended human dose.

HOW SUPPLIED:

Propafenone HCl tablets are supplied as scored, round, film-coated tablets containing either 150 mg, 225 mg or 300 mg of propafenone HCl and embossed with 150, 225 or 300 and an arched triangle on the same side.

Storage: 59 to 86°F (15-30°C) Dispense in tight, light-resistant container as defined in U.S.P.

HOW SUPPLIED - EQUIVALENTS NOT AVAILABLE:

Tablet, Coated - Oral - 150 mg

100's	$83.82	RHYTHMOL, Knoll Labs	00044-5022-02
100's	$88.00	RHYTHMOL, Knoll Labs	00044-5022-10

Tablet, Coated - Oral - 225 mg

100's	**$119.48**	**RYTHMOL, Knoll Labs**	**00044-5024-02**
100's	**$125.41**	**RYTHMOL, Knoll Labs**	**00044-5024-10**

Tablet, Coated - Oral - 300 mg

10 x10's	$159.68	RHYTHMOL, Knoll Labs	00044-5023-10
100's	$152.08	RHYTHMOL, Knoll Labs	00044-5023-02

PROPANTHELINE BROMIDE *(002128)*

CATEGORIES: Anticholinergic Agents; Antihypertensives; Antimuscarinics/Antispasmodics; Autonomic Drugs; Gastrointestinal Drugs; Peptic Ulcer; Urinary Incontinence*; Pregnancy Category C; FDA Approval Pre 1982

* Indication not approved by the FDA

BRAND NAMES: *Bropantil*; *Corrigast*; *Ercoril*; *Ercotina*; *Norproban*; *Pantheline*; **Pro-Banthine**; Probamide; *Probanthine*; *Propantel*
(International brand names outside U.S. in italics)

FORMULARIES: Aetna; FHP; Medi-Cal; PCS

DESCRIPTION:

Propantheline Bromide oral tablets contain 15 mg or 7 1/2 mg of the anticholinergic propantheline bromide, (2-hydroxyethyl) diisopropylmethylammonium bromide xanthene-9-carboxylate.

Propantheline bromide is very soluble in water, alcohol, and chloroform, but it is practically insoluble in ether and in benzene. Its molecular weight is 448.40.

Inactive ingredients include calcium carbonate, corn starch, edible ink, flavor, lactose, magnesium carbonate, magnesium stearate, sucrose, talc, titanium dioxide, and waxes, The 15-mg tablet also contains red oxide and yellow oxide as coloring agents.

CLINICAL PHARMACOLOGY:

Propantheline Bromide inhibits gastrointestinal motility and diminishes gastric acid secretion. The drug also inhibits the action of acetylcholine at the postganglionic nerve endings of the parasympathetic nervous system.

Propantheline bromide is extensively metabolized in man primarily by hydrolysis to the inactive materials xanthene-9-carboxylic acid and (2-hydroxyethyl) diisopropylmethylammonium bromide. After a single 30-mg oral dose given as two 15-mg tablets the mean peak plasma concentration of propantheline was 21 ng/ml at one hour in six healthy subjects.

The plasma elimination half-life of propantheline is about 1.6 hours. Approximately 70% of the dose is excreted in the urine, mostly as metabolites. The urinary excretion of propantheline is about 3% after oral tablet administration.

INDICATIONS AND USAGE:

Propantheline Bromide is effective as adjunctive therapy in the treatment of peptic ulcer.

CONTRAINDICATIONS:

Propantheline Bromide is contraindicated in patients with:

1. Glaucoma, since mydriasis is to be avoided.

2. Obstructive disease of the gastrointestinal tract (pyloroduodenal stenosis, achalasia, paralytic ileus, etc).

3. Obstructive uropathy (*e.g.,* bladder-neck obstruction due to prostatic hypertrophy).

4. Intestinal atony of elderly or debilitated patients.

5. Severe ulcerative colitis or toxic megacolon complicating ulcerative colitis.

6. Unstable cardiovascular adjustment in acute hemorrhage.

7. Myasthenia gravis.

WARNINGS:

In the presence of a high environmental temperature, heat prostration (fever and heat stroke due to decreased sweating) can occur with the use of Propantheline Bromide.

Diarrhea may be an early symptom of incomplete intestinal obstruction, especially in patients with ileostomy or colostomy. In this instance treatment with Propantheline Bromide would be inappropriate and possibly harmful.

With overdosage, a curare-like action may occur (*i.e.,* neuromuscular blockade leading to muscular weakness and possible paralysis).

Propantheline Bromide may cause increased heart rate and, therefore should be used with caution in patients with heart disease.

PRECAUTIONS:

GENERAL

Propantheline Bromide should be used with caution in the elderly and in all patients with autonomic neuropathy, hepatic or renal disease, hyperthyroidism, coronary heart disease, congestive heart failure, cardiac tachyarrhythmias, hypertension, or hiatal hernia associated with reflux esophagitis, since anticholinergics may aggravate this condition.

In patients with ulcerative colitis, large, doses of Propantheline Bromide may suppress intestinal motility to the point of producing paralytic ileus and, for this reason, may precipitate or aggravate toxic megacolon, a serious complication of the disease.

INFORMATION FOR THE PATIENT

Propantheline Bromide may produce drowsiness or blurred vision. The patient should be cautioned regarding activities requiring mental alertness, such as operating a motor vehicle or other machinery or performing hazardous work, while taking this drug.

CARCINOGENESIS, MUTAGENESIS, AND IMPAIRMENT OF FERTILITY

No long-term fertility, carcinogenicity, or mutagenicity studies have been done with Propantheline Bromide.

PREGNANCY CATEGORY C

Animal reproduction studies have not been conducted with Propantheline Bromide. It is also not known whether Propantheline Bromide can cause fetal harm when administered to a pregnant woman or can affect reproduction capacity. Propantheline Bromide should be given to a pregnant woman only if clearly needed.

NURSING MOTHERS

It is not known whether this drug is excreted in human milk. Because many drugs are excreted in human milk, caution should be exercised when Propantheline Bromide is administered to a nursing woman. Suppression of lactation may occur with anticholinergic drugs.

PEDIATRIC USE

Safety and effectiveness in children have not been established.

DRUG INTERACTIONS:

Anticholinergics may delay absorption of other medication given concomitantly.

Excessive cholinergic blockade may occur if Propantheline Bromide is given concomitantly with belladonna alkaloids, synthetic or semisynthetic anticholinergic agents, narcotic analgesics such as meperidine, Type 1 antiarrhythmic drugs (*e.g.,* disopyramide, procainamide, or quinidine), antihistamines, phenothiazines, tricyclic antidepressants, or other psychoactive drugs. Propantheline Bromide may also potentiate the sedative effect of phenothiazines. Increased intraocular pressure may result from concurrent administration of anticholinergics and corticosteroids.

Concurrent use of Propantheline Bromide with slow-dissolving tablets of digoxin may cause increased serum digoxin levels. This interaction can be avoided by using only those digoxin tablets that rapidly dissolve by USP standards.

ADVERSE REACTIONS:

Varying degrees of drying of salivary secretions may occur as well as decreased sweating. Ophthalmic side effects include blurred vision, mydriasis, cycloplegia, and increased ocular tension. Other reported adverse reactions include urinary hesitancy and retention, tachycardia, palpitations, loss of the sense of taste, headache, nervousness, mental confusion, drowsiness, weakness, dizziness, insomnia, nausea, vomiting, constipation, bloated feeling, impotence, suppression of lactation, and allergic reactions or drug idiosyncrasies, including anaphylaxis, urticaria, and other dermal manifestations.

OVERDOSAGE:

The symptoms of overdosage with Propantheline Bromide progress from an intensification of the usual side effects to CNS disturbances (from restlessness and excitement to psychotic behavior), circulatory changes (flushing, fall in blood pressure, circulatory failure), respiratory failure, paralysis, and coma.

Measures to be taken are (1) immediate induction of emesis or lavage of the stomach, (2) injection of physostigmine 0.5 to 2 mg intravenously, repeated as necessary up to a total of 5 mg, and (3) monitoring of vital sings and managing as necessary.

OVERDOSAGE: *(cont'd)*

Fever may be treated symptomatically (cooling blanket or alcohol sponging). Excitement of a degree which demands attention may be managed with thiopental sodium 2% solution given slowly intravenously, or diazepam, 5 to 10 mg intravenously or 10 mg intramuscularly. In the event of progression of the curare-like effect to paralysis of the respiratory muscles, mechanical respiration should be instituted and maintained until effective respiratory action returns.

The oral LD_{50} of propantheline bromide is 780 mg/kg in the mouse and 370 mg/kg in the rat.

DOSAGE AND ADMINISTRATION:

The usual initial adult dosage of Propantheline Bromide tablets is 15 mg taken 30 minutes before each meal and 30 mg at bedtime (a total of 75 mg daily). Subsequent dosage adjustment should be made according to the patient's individual response and tolerance. The administration of one 7 1/2-mg tablet three times a day is convenient for patients with mild manifestations, for geriatric patients, and for those of small stature.

Store below 86°F (30°C).

HOW SUPPLIED - RATED THERAPEUTICALLY EQUIVALENT:

Tablet, Sugar Coated - Oral - 15 mg

100's	$15.56	Propantheline, US Trading	56126-0393-11
100's	$22.22	Propantheline, H.C.F.A. F F P	99999-2128-01
500's	$111.10	Propantheline, H.C.F.A. F F P	99999-2128-02
1000's	$222.20	Propantheline, H.C.F.A. F F P	99999-2128-03

HOW SUPPLIED - NOT RATED EQUIVALENT:

Tablet, Sugar Coated - Oral - 7.5 mg

100's	**$46.29**	**PRO-BANTHINE, Roberts Labs**	**54092-0073-01**

Tablet, Sugar Coated - Oral - 15 mg

100's	$17.15	Propantheline, Roxane	00054-8737-25
100's	$19.93	Propantheline, Roxane	00054-4721-25
100's	$20.25	Propantheline Bromide, Major Pharms	00904-2344-60
100's	$22.20	Propantheline, Goldline Labs	00182-1858-01
100's	$22.95	Propantheline Bromide, Par Pharm	49884-0118-01
100's	$23.75	Propantheline Bromide, Harber Pharm	51432-0384-03
100's	$24.10	Propantheline Bromide, HL Moore Drug Exch	00839-1545-06
100's	**$70.51**	**PRO-BANTHINE TABLETS, Roberts Labs**	**54092-0074-01**
100's	**$76.46**	**PRO-BANTHINE, Roberts Labs**	**54092-0074-52**
500's	$94.50	Propantheline Bromide, Major Pharms	00904-2344-40
500's	$100.76	Propantheline Bromide, Aligen Independ	00405-4879-02
500's	$108.00	Propantheline Bromide, Par Pharm	49884-0118-05
500's	**$330.95**	**PRO-BANTHINE TABLETS, Roberts Labs**	**54092-0074-05**
1000's	$149.73	Propantheline, Roxane	00054-4721-31
1000's	$202.05	Propantheline Bromide, Harber Pharm	51432-0384-05

PROPARACAINE HYDROCHLORIDE *(002129)*

CATEGORIES: Anesthesia; EENT Drugs; Eye, Ear, Nose, & Throat Preparations; Local Anesthetics; Ophthalmic Anesthetics; Ophthalmics; Topical; Vascular Disorders, Cerebral/Peripheral; Pregnancy Category C; FDA Approval Pre 1982

BRAND NAMES: Ak-Taine; Alcaine; *Chibro-Kerakain*; I-Paracaine; Infi-Cain; Kainair; Ocu-Caine; Ophthaine; **Ophthetic**; Parcaine; Spectro-Caine
(International brand names outside U.S. in italics)

FORMULARIES: Medi-Cal

DESCRIPTION:

Proparacaine hydrochloride solution is a local anesthetic for ophthalmic instillation. Each ml of sterile aqueous solution contains 5 mg proparacaine HCl with glycerin as a stabilizer, sodium hydroxide or hydrochloric acid to adjust the pH, and 2 mg chlorobutanol (chloral derivative) and benzalkonium chloride as antimicrobial preservatives. At the time of manufacture, the air in the container is replaced by nitrogen.

Proparacaine HCl is designated chemically as 2-(Diethylamino)ethyl 3-amino-4-propoxybenzoate monohydrochloride.

$C_{16}H_{26}N_2O_3$·HCl. Molecular Weight is 330.85 (CAS-5875-06-9).

CLINICAL PHARMACOLOGY:

Proparacaine HCl solution is a rapid acting local anesthetic suitable for ophthalmic use. With a single drop, the onset of anesthesia occurs in approximately 13 seconds and persists for 15 minutes or longer.

The main site of anesthetic action is the nerve cell membrane where proparacaine interferes with the large transient increase in the membrane permeability to sodium ions that is normally produced by a slight depolarization of the membrane. As the anesthetic action progressively develops in a nerve, the threshold for electrical stimulation gradually increases and the safety factor for conduction decreases; when this action is sufficiently well developed, block of conduction is produced.

The exact mechanism whereby proparacaine and other local anesthetics influence the permeability of the cell membrane is unknown; however, several studies indicate that local anesthetics may limit sodium ion permeability by closing the pores through which the ions migrate in the lipid layer of the nerve cell membrane. This limitation prevents the fundamental change necessary for the generation of the action potential.

INDICATIONS AND USAGE:

Proparacaine HCl ophthalmic solution is indicated for topical anesthesia in ophthalmic practice. Representative ophthalmic procedures in which the preparation provides good local anesthesia include measurement of intraocular pressure (tonometry), removal of foreign bodies and sutures from the cornea, conjunctival scraping in diagnosis and gonioscopic examination; it is also indicated for use as a topical anesthetic prior to surgical operations such as cataract extraction.

CONTRAINDICATIONS:

This preparation is contraindicated in patients with known hypersensitivity to any component of the solution.

WARNINGS:

For topical ophthalmic use only.

Prolonged use of a topical ocular anesthetic may produce permanent corneal opacification with accompanying loss of vision.

PRECAUTIONS:

General: Proparacaine should be used cautiously and sparingly in patients with known allergies, cardiac disease, or hyperthyroidism. The long-term toxicity of proparacaine is unknown; prolonged use may possibly delay wound healing. Although exceedingly rare with ophthalmic application of local anesthetics, it should be borne in mind that systemic toxicity (manifested by central nervous system stimulation followed by depression) may occur.

Protection of the eye from irritating chemicals, foreign bodies and rubbing during the period of anesthesia is very important. Tonometers soaked in sterilizing or detergent solutions should be thoroughly rinsed with sterile distilled water prior to use. Patients should be advised to avoid touching the eye until the anesthesia has worn off.

Carcinogenesis, Mutagenesis, and Impairment of Fertility: Long-term studies in animals have not been performed to evaluate carcinogenic potential, mutagenicity, or possible impairment of fertility in males or females.

Pregnancy, Teratogenic Effects, Pregnancy Category C: Animal reproduction studies have not been conducted with proparacaine HCl ophthalmic solution. It is also not known whether proparacaine HCl can cause fetal harm when administered to a pregnant woman or can affect reproduction capacity. Proparacaine HCl should be administered to a pregnant woman only if clearly needed.

Nursing Mothers: It is not known whether this drug is excreted in human milk. Because many drugs are excreted in human milk, caution should be exercised when proparacaine HCl is administered to a nursing woman.

Pediatric Use: Controlled clinical studies have not been performed with proparacaine HCl ophthalmic solution to establish safety and effectiveness in children; however, the literature cites the use of proparacaine HCl as a topical ophthalmic anesthetic agent in children.

ADVERSE REACTIONS:

Pupillary dilation or cycloplegic effects have rarely been observed with proparacaine HCl. The drug appears to be safe for use in patients sensitive to other local anesthetics, but local or systemic sensitivity occasionally occurs. Instillation of proparacaine in the eye at recommended concentration and dosage usually produces little or no irritation, stinging, burning, conjunctival redness, lacrimation or increased winking. However, some local irritation and stinging may occur several hours after the instillation.

Rarely, a severe, immediate-type, apparently hyperallergic corneal reaction may occur which includes acute, intense and diffuse epithelial keratitis; a gray, ground-glass appearance; sloughing of large areas of necrotic epithelium; corneal filaments and, sometimes, iritis with descemetitis.

Allergic contact dermatitis with drying and fissuring of the fingertips has been reported.

Softening and erosion of the corneal epithelium and conjunctival congestion and hemorrhage have been reported.

DOSAGE AND ADMINISTRATION:

Deep Anesthesia as in Cataract Extraction: Instill 1 drop every 5 to 10 minutes for 5 to 7 doses.

Removal of Sutures: Instill 1 or 2 drops 2 or 3 minutes before removal of stitches.

Removal of Foreign Bodies: Instill 1 or 3 drops prior to operating.

Tonometry: Instill 1 or 2 drops immediately before measurement.

Storage: Refrigerate at 2° to 8°C. Keep bottle tightly closed. Store bottle in carton until empty o protect from light. If solution shows more than a faint yellow color, it should not be used.

HOW SUPPLIED - RATED THERAPEUTICALLY EQUIVALENT:

Solution - Ophthalmic - 0.5 %

2 ml	$1.00	Proparacaine Hcl, H.C.F.A. F F P	99999-2129-01
2 ml	$3.90	Parcaine, Ocusoft	54799-0500-02
2 ml	$3.95	SPECTRO CAINE, Spectrum Scitfc	53268-0331-59
2 ml	$4.06	Ak-Taine, Akorn	17478-0263-20
15 ml	$5.75	SPECTRO CAINE, Spectrum Scitfc	53268-0331-12
15 ml	$6.55	PARCAINE OPHTHALMIC, Ocusoft	54799-0500-12
15 ml	$7.49	Proparacaine Hcl, H.C.F.A. F F P	99999-2129-02
15 ml	$7.81	Ak-Taine, Akorn	17478-0263-12
15 ml	**$11.89**	**OPHTHETIC STERILE OPHTHALMIC, Allergan-Amer**	**11980-0048-15**
15 ml	$13.13	ALCAINE, Alcon-PR	00998-0016-15
15 ml	$16.52	OPHTHAINE, Bristol Myers Squibb	00003-0646-30

HOW SUPPLIED - NOT RATED EQUIVALENT:

Solution - Ophthalmic - 0.5 %

2 ml	$2.44	Infi-Cain, Infinity Pharm	58154-0730-01
15 ml	$4.29	INFI-CAIN, Infinity Pharm	58154-0730-06
15 ml	$6.74	Proparacaine Hcl, HL Moore Drug Exch	00839-6686-31

PROPIOMAZINE HYDROCHLORIDE *(002131)*

CATEGORIES: Analgesics; Antianxiety Drugs; Anxiolytics, Sedatives, Hypnotic; Central Nervous System Agents; Labor; Psychotherapeutic Agents; Tranquilizers; FDA Approval Pre 1982

BRAND NAMES: **Largon**

DESCRIPTION:

As with any new synthetic compound, it is well to review carefully not only the therapeutic efficacy of Largon (propiomazine hydrochloride) but also the possibilities of the occurrence of undesirable side effects. The physician, therefore, should be thoroughly familiar with the following data before prescribing Largon.

In the ampul each ml contains 20 mg propiomazine hydrochloride with sodium acetate buffer and not more than 1 mg sodium formaldehyde sulfoxylate. Sealed under nitrogen.

INDICATIONS AND USAGE:

As a sedative for the relief of restlessness and apprehension, preoperatively or during surgery. As an adjunct to analgesics for the relief of restlessness and apprehension during labor.

CONTRAINDICATIONS:

The intra-arterial injection of propiomazine hydrochloride is contraindicated because of the possible occurrence of arterial or arteriolar spasm with resultant local impairment of circulation.

WARNINGS:

Largon Injection contains sodium formaldehyde sulfoxylate as an antioxidant. Upon oxidation or decomposition, sodium formaldehyde sulfoxylate can produce sulfites, the quantities of which have not been determined. Sulfites may cause allergic-type reactions, including

WARNINGS: *(cont'd)*

anaphylactic symptoms and life-threatening or less severe asthmatic episodes, in certain susceptible people. The overall prevalence of sulfite sensitivity in the general population is unknown and probably low. Sulfite sensitivity is seen more frequently in asthmatic than in nonasthmatic people.

NEUROLEPTIC MALIGNANT SYNDROME (NMS)

A potentially fatal symptom complex sometimes referred to as Neuroleptic Malignant Syndrome (NMS) has been reported in association with antipsychotic drugs. Clinical manifestations of NMS are hyperpyrexia, muscle rigidity, altered mental status, and evidence of autonomic instability (irregular pulse or blood pressure, tachycardia, diaphoresis, and cardiac dysrhythmias).

The diagnostic evaluation of patients with this syndrome is complicated. In arriving at a diagnosis, it is important to identify cases where the clinical presentation includes both serious medical illness (e.g. pneumonia, systemic infection, etc.) and untreated or inadequately treated extrapyramidal signs and symptoms (EPS). Other important considerations in the differential diagnosis include central anticholinergic toxicity, heat stroke, drug fever, and primary central nervous system (CNS) pathology.

The management of NMS should include 1) immediate discontinuation of antipsychotic drugs and other drugs not essential to concurrent therapy, 2) intensive symptomatic treatment and medical monitoring, and 3) treatment of any concomitant serious medical problems for which specific treatments are available. There is no general agreement about specific pharmacological treatment regimens for uncomplicated NMS.

If a patient requires antipsychotic drug treatment after recovery from NMS, the potential reintroduction of drug therapy should be carefully considered. The patient should be carefully monitored, since recurrences of NMS have been reported.

Do not use if solution is cloudy or contains a precipitate.

PRECAUTIONS:

PROPIOMAZINE HYDROCHLORIDE ENHANCES THE EFFECTS OF CENTRAL NERVOUS SYSTEM DEPRESSANTS; THEREFORE, THE DOSE OF BARBITURATES SHOULD BE ELIMINATED OR REDUCED BY AT LEAST 1/2 IN THE PRESENCE OF LARGON THE DOSES OF MEPERIDINE, MORPHINE, AND OTHER ANALGESIC DEPRESSANTS SHOULD BE REDUCED BY 1/4 TO 1/2.

Because of the possible occurrence of thrombophlebitis from any irritant substance, it is important that intravenous injection of Largon be made only into vessels previously undamaged by multiple injections or trauma. Care should be exercised not to allow perivascular extravasation, since under such circumstances chemical irritation may be severe.

Largon is a premedicant of marked potency, with a shorter duration of action than other agents of its type.

Because of the sedative action attendant to the use of propiomazine hydrochloride in full therapeutic doses, it should be administered with caution to ambulatory patients.

Ambulatory patients should be cautioned against driving automobiles or operating dangerous machinery until it is known that they do not become drowsy or dizzy from propiomazine hydrochloride.

Safety for use of Largon in the first trimester of pregnancy has not yet been established.

ADVERSE REACTIONS:

Autonomic reactions are rare, and the dryness of mouth which may occur is usually considered desirable in patients undergoing anesthesia.

Cardiovascular effects reported include a moderate elevation in blood pressure and rarely hypotension. The moderate increase in blood pressure seen during surgical procedures is considered desirable in many instances. Tachycardia has also been reported.

Among vasopressor drugs, norepinephrine appears to be most suitable if it is necessary to administer this type drug to patients receiving propiomazine hydrochloride. The pressor response to epinephrine is usually reduced and may even be reversed in the presence of propiomazine hydrochloride.

Neuroleptic Malignant Syndrome (NMS): (See WARNINGS.)

DOSAGE AND ADMINISTRATION:

Parenteral drug products should be inspected visually for particulate matter and discoloration prior to administration, whenever solution and container permit. Do not use if solution is cloudy or contains a precipitate.

The usual adult dosage for preoperative medication is 20 mg of Largon with 50 mg of meperidine, both intravenously or intramuscularly. Although 20 mg of Largon is sufficient for most patients, for adequate sedation some will require as much as 40 mg, IV or IM, at the discretion of the physician. The desired amount of belladonna alkaloids may be added as required.

Sedation during surgery with local, nerve block, or spinal anesthesia may be obtained by the IM or IV administration of 10 to 20 mg doses of Largon.

OBSTETRICS

The IM or IV administration of Largon in doses of 20 mg will provide sedation and relieve apprehension in the early stages of labor. Some patients may require up to 40 mg of Largon. When labor is definitely established, administer 20 to 40 mg of Largon, IM or IV, with 25 to 75 mg of meperidine (average dose: 50 mg). Amnesic agents may be administered as necessary. If the average doses of Largon and meperidine are used, it is seldom necessary to repeat the medication during normal labor. If necessary, additional doses may be repeated at 3-hour intervals. Neither prolongation of labor nor significant maternal or fetal depression has been observed.

PEDIATRICS

Propiomazine hydrochloride has been used in children as a sedative the night before surgery and for preanesthetic and postoperative medication. In children under 60 pounds of body weight, dosage of propiomazine hydrochloride should be calculated on a basis of 0.25 mg to 0.5 mg per pound of body weight. The higher dosage recommendation should be necessary only in the extremely nervous, excitable child. In a clinical evaluation of Largon (propiomazine hydrochloride), satisfactory results were obtained, utilizing the dosage schedule in TABLE 1.

TABLE 1

Ages	Single Dosage
2 to 4 years	10 mg
4 to 6 years	15 mg
6 to 12 years	25 mg

Store at controlled room temperature. Protect from light.

HOW SUPPLIED - EQUIVALENTS NOT AVAILABLE:

Injection, Solution - Intramuscular; - 20 mg/ml

1 ml x 25 $103.65 LARGON, Wyeth Labs 00008-0245-01

PROPOFOL *(002132)*

CATEGORIES: Anesthesia; Central Nervous System Agents; Endotracheal Intubation; General Anesthetics; Hypnotics; Injectable Anesthetics; Intubation; Sedation; Ischemia*; Pregnancy Category B; Sales > $100 Million; FDA Approved 1989 Oct; Patent Expiration 1996 Nov

* Indication not approved by the FDA

BRAND NAMES: **Diprivan**

DESCRIPTION:

Diprivan Injectable Emulsion is a sterile, nonpyrogenic emulsion containing 10 mg/ml of propofol suitable for intravenous administration. Propofol is chemically described as 2,6-diisopropylphenol and has a molecular weight of 178.27.

Propofol is very slightly soluble in water and, thus, is formulated in a white, oil-in-water emulsion. The pKa is 11. The octanol/water partition coefficient for propofol 6761:1 at physiologic pH. In addition to the active component, propofol, the formulation also contains soybean oil (100 mg/ml), glycerol (22.5 mg/ml) and egg lecithin (12 mg/ml); with sodium hydroxide to adjust pH. The Propofol Injectable Emulsion emulsion is isotonic and has a pH of 7-8.5.

STRICT ASEPTIC TECHNIQUE MUST ALWAYS BE MAINTAINED DURING HANDLING. PROPOFOL INJECTABLE EMULSION IS A SINGLE-USE PARENTERAL PRODUCT, CONTAINS NO ANTIMICROBIAL PRESERVATIVES, AND CAN SUPPORT RAPID GROWTH OF MICRO ORGANISMS. DISCARD UNUSED PORTIONS AS DIRECTED WITHIN THE REQUIRED TIME LIMITS (SEE DOSAGE AND ADMINISTRATION, HANDLING PROCEDURES). THERE HAVE BEEN REPORTS IN WHICH FAILURE TO USE ASEPTIC TECHNIQUE WHEN HANDLING PROPOFOL INJECTABLE EMULSION WAS ASSOCIATED WITH MICROBIAL CONTAMINATION OF THE PRODUCT AND WITH FEVER, INFECTION/SEPSIS, OTHER LIFE-THREATENING ILLNESS, AND/OR DEATH. DO NOT USE IF CONTAMINATION IS SUSPECTED.

CLINICAL PHARMACOLOGY:

General: Propofol is an intravenous sedative hypnotic agent for use in the induction and maintenance of anesthesia or sedation. Intravenous injection of a therapeutic dose of propofol produces hypnosis rapidly with minimal excitation, usually within 40 seconds from the start of an injection (the time for one arm-brain circulation). As with other rapidly acting intravenous anesthetic agents, the half-time of the blood- brain equilibration is approximately 1 to 3 minutes, and this accounts for the rapid induction of anesthesia.

Pharmacodynamics: Pharmacodynamic properties of propofol are dependent upon the therapeutic blood propofol concentrations. Steady state propofol blood concentrations are generally proportional to infusion rates, especially within an individual patient. Undesirable side effects such as cardiorespiratory depression are likely to occur at higher blood concentrations which result from bolus dosing or rapid increase in infusion rate. An adequate interval (3 to 5 minutes) must be allowed between clinical dosage adjustments in order to assess drug effects.

The hemodynamic effects of propofol during induction of anesthesia vary. If spontaneous ventilation is maintained, the major cardiovascular effects are arterial hypotension (sometimes greater than a 30% decrease) with little or no change in heart rate and no appreciable decrease in cardiac output. If ventilation is assisted or controlled (positive pressure ventilation), the degree and incidence of decrease in cardiac output are accentuated. Addition of a potent opioid (*e.g.,* fentanyl) when used as a premedicant further decreases cardiac output and respiratory drive.

If anesthesia is continued by infusion of propofol, the stimulation of endotracheal intubation and surgery may return arterial pressure towards normal. However, cardiac output may remain depressed. Comparative clinical studies have shown that the hemodynamic effects of propofol during induction of anesthesia are generally more pronounced than with other IV induction agents traditionally used for this purpose.

Clinical and preclinical studies suggest that propofol is rarely associated with elevation of plasma histamine levels.

Induction of anesthesia with propofol is frequently associated with apnea in both adults and children. In 1573 patients who received propofol (2 to 2.5 mg/kg), apnea lasted less than 30 seconds in 7% of patients, 30-60 seconds in 24% of patients, and more than 60 seconds in 12% of patients. In the 213 pediatric patients between the ages of 3 and 12 years assessable for apnea who received propofol (1 to 3.6 mg/kg), apnea lasted less than 30 seconds in 12% of patients, 30-60 seconds in 10% of patients, and more than 60 seconds in 5% of patients.

During maintenance, propofol causes a decrease in ventilation usually associated with an increase in carbon dioxide tension which may be marked depending upon the rate of administration and other concurrent medications (*e.g.,* opioids, sedatives, etc.).

During monitored anesthesia care (MAC) sedation, attention must be given to the cardiorespiratory effects of propofol. Hypotension, oxyhemoglobin desaturation, apnea, airway obstruction, and/or oxygen desaturation can occur, especially following a rapid bolus of propofol. During initiation of MAC sedation, slow infusion or slow injection techniques are preferable over rapid bolus administration, and during maintenance of MAC sedation, a variable rate infusion is preferable over intermittent bolus administration in order to minimize undesirable cardiorespiratory effects. In the elderly, debilitated, or ASA III/IV patients, rapid (single or repeated) bolus dose administration should not be used for MAC sedation. (See WARNINGS.) propofol is not recommended for MAC Sedation in children because safety and effectiveness have not been established.

Clinical studies in humans and studies in animals show that propofol does not suppress the adrenal response to ACTH.

Preliminary findings in patients with normal intraocular pressure indicate that propofol anesthesia produces a decrease in intraocular pressure which may be associated with a concomitant decrease in systemic vascular resistance.

Animal studies and limited experience in susceptible patients have not indicated any propensity of propofol to induce malignant hyperthermia.

Studies to date indicate that propofol when used in combination with hypocarbia increases cerebrovascular resistance and decreases cerebral blood flow, cerebral metabolic oxygen consumption, and intracranial pressure. Propofol does not affect cerebrovascular reactivity to changes in arterial carbon dioxide tension. See CLINICAL STUDIES, Neuroanesthesia.

Pharmacokinetics: *The proper use of propofol requires an understanding of the disposition and elimination characteristics of propofol.*

The pharmacokinetics of propofol are well described by a three compartment linear model with compartments representing the plasma, rapidly equilibrating tissues, and slowly equilibrating tissues.

CLINICAL PHARMACOLOGY: *(cont'd)*

Following an IV bolus dose, there is rapid equilibration between the plasma and the highly perfused tissue of the brain, thus accounting for the rapid onset of anesthesia. Plasma levels initially decline rapidly as a result of both rapid distribution and high metabolic clearance. Distribution accounts for about half of this decline following a bolus of propofol.

However, distribution is not constant over time, but decreases as body tissues equilibrate with plasma and become saturated. The rate at which equilibration occurs is a function of the rate and duration of the infusion. When equilibration occurs there is no longer a net transfer of propofol between tissues and plasma.

Discontinuation of the recommended doses of propofol after the maintenance of anesthesia for approximately one-hour, or for sedation in the ICU for one-day, results in a prompt decrease in blood propofol concentrations and rapid awakening. Longer infusions (10 days of ICU sedation) result in accumulation of significant tissue stores of propofol, such that the reduction in circulating propofol is slowed and the time to awakening is increased.

By daily titration of propofol dosage to achieve only the minimum effective therapeutic concentration, rapid awakening within 10 to 15 minutes will occur even after long term administration. If, however, higher than necessary infusion levels have been maintained for a long time, propofol will be redistributed from fat and muscle to the plasma, and this return of propofol from peripheral tissues will slow recovery.

The large contribution of distribution (about 50%) to the fall of propofol plasma levels following brief infusions means that after very long infusions (at steady state), about half the initial rate will maintain the same plasma levels. Failure to reduce the infusion rate in patients receiving propofol for extended periods may result in excessively high blood concentrations of the drug. Thus, titration to clinical response and daily evaluation of sedation levels are important during the use of propofol infusion for ICU sedation, especially of long duration.

Adults: Propofol clearance ranges from 23-50 ml/kg/min (1.6 to 3.4 l/min in 70 kg adults). It is chiefly eliminated by hepatic conjugation to inactive metabolites which are excreted by the kidney. A glucuronide conjugate accounts for about 50% of the administered dose. Propofol has a steady state volume of distribution (10-day infusion) approaching 60 l/kg in healthy adults. A difference in pharmacokinetics due to gender has not been observed. The terminal half-life of propofol after a 10-day infusion is 1 to 3 days.

Geriatrics: With increasing age, the dose of propofol needed to achieve a defined anesthetic endpoint (dose-requirement) decreases. This does not appear to be an age related change of pharmacodynamics or brain sensitivity, as measured by EEG burst suppression. With increasing age pharmacokinetic changes are such that for a given IV bolus dose, higher peak plasma concentrations occur, which can explain the decreased dose requirement. These higher peak plasma concentrations in the elderly can predispose patients to cardiorespiratory effects including hypotension, apnea, airway obstruction and/or oxygen desaturation. The higher plasma levels reflect an age-related decrease in volume of distribution and reduced intercompartmental clearance. Lower doses are thus recommended for initiation and maintenance of sedation/anesthesia in elderly patients. See CLINICAL STUDIES, Individualization of Dosage.

Pediatrics: The pharmacokinetics of propofol were studied in 53 children between the ages of 3 and 12 years who received propofol for periods of approximately 1-2 hours. The observed distribution and clearance of propofol in these children was similar to adults.

Organ Failure: The pharmacokinetics of propofol do not appear to be different in people with chronic hepatic cirrhosis or chronic renal impairment compared to adults with normal hepatic and renal function. The effects of acute hepatic or renal failure on the pharmacokinetics of propofol have not been studied.

CLINICAL STUDIES:

Anesthesia and Monitored Anesthesia Care (MAC) Sedation: propofol was compared to intravenous and inhalational anesthetic or sedative agents in 91 trials involving a total of 5,135 patients. Of these 3,354 received propofol and comprised the overall safety database for anesthesia and MAC sedation. Fifty-five of these trials, 20 for anesthesia induction and 35 for induction and maintenance of anesthesia or MAC sedation, were carried out in the US or Canada and provided the basis for dosage recommendations and the adverse event profile during anesthesia or MAC sedation.

Pediatric Anesthesia: propofol was compared to standard anesthetic agents in 12 clinical trials involving 534 patients receiving propofol. Of these, 349 were from US/Canadian clinicals trials and comprised the overall safety database for Pediatric Anesthesia.

TABLE 1 Patients Receiving Propofol Median and (Range)

	Induction Only	Induction and Maintenance
Number of Patients*	243	105
Induction Bolus Dosages	2.5 mg/kg (1-3.5)	3 mg/kg (2-3.6)
Injection Duration	20 sec (6-45)	
Maintenance Dosage	—	181 mcg/kg/min (107-418)
Maintenance Duration	—	78 min (29-268)

* Body weight not recorded for one patient.

Neuroanesthesia: propofol was studied in 50 patients undergoing craniotomy for supratentorial tumors in two clinical trials. The mean lesion size (anterior/posterior and lateral) was 31 and 32 mm in one trial and 55 and 42 mm in the other trial respectively.

TABLE 2 Neuroanesthesia Clinical Studies Patients Receiving Propofol Median and (Range)

Patient Type	No. of Patients	Induction Bolus Dosages	Main- tenance Dosage	Main- tenance Duration
		(mg/kg)	(mcg/kg/min)	(min)
Craniotomy patients	50	1.36 (0.9-6.9)	146 (68-425)	285 (48-622)

In ten of these patients, propofol was administered by infusion in a controlled clinical trial to evaluate the effect of propofol on cerebrospinal fluid pressure (CSFP). The mean arterial pressure was maintained relatively constant over 25 minutes with a change from baseline of -4% ± 17% (mean ± SD), whereas the percent change in cerebrospinal fluid pressure (CSFP) was -46% ± 14%. As CSFP is an indirect measure of intracranial pressure (ICP), when given by infusion or slow bolus, propofol, in combination with hypocarbia, is capable of decreasing ICP independent of changes in arterial pressure.

CLINICAL STUDIES: *(cont'd)*

Intensive Care Unit (ICU) Sedation: Propofol was compared to benzodiazepines and/or opioids in 14 clinical trials involving a total of 550 ICU patients. Of these, 302 received propofol and comprise the overall safety database for ICU sedation. Six of these studies were carried out in the US or Canada and provide the basis for dosage recommendations and the adverse event profile.

Information from 193 literature reports of propofol used for ICU sedation in over 950 patients and information from the clinical trials are summarized in TABLE 3.

TABLE 3 ICU Sedation Clinical Studies And Literature Patients Receiving Propofol Median and (Range)

Number of Patients: Trials	Literature	Sedation Dose: mcg/kg/min	mg/kg/h	Sedation Duration Hours
ICU Patient Type: Post-CABG				
41	-	11 (0.1-30)	.66 (.006-1.8)	10 (2-14)
-	334	(5-100)	(0.3-6)	(4-24)
Post-Surgical				
60	-	20 (6-53)	1.2 (0.4-3.2)	18 (0.3-187)
—	142	(23-82)	(1.4-4.9)	(6-96)
Neuro/Head Trauma				
7	—	25 (13-37)	1.5 (0.8-2.2)	168 (112-282)
—	184	(8.3-87)	(0.5-5.2)	(8 hr-5 days)
Medical				
49	—	41 (9-131)	2.5 (0.5-7.9)	72 (0.4-337)
—	76	(3.3-62)	(0.2-3.7)	(4-96)
Special Patients				
ARDS/Resp. Failure				
—	56	(10-142)	(0.6-8.5)	(1 hr -8 days)
COPD/Asthma				
—	49	(17-75)	(1-4.5)	(1-8 days)
Status Epilepticus				
—	15	(25-167)	(1.5-10)	(1-21 days)
Tetanus				
—	11	(5-100)	(0.3-6)	(1-25 days)

Trials (Individual patients from clinical studies)
Literature (Individual patients from published reports)
CABG (Coronary Artery Bypass Graft)
ARDS (Adult Respiratory Distress Syndrome)

Cardiac Anesthesia: Propofol was evaluated in 5 clinical trials conducted in the US and Canada, involving a total of 569 patients undergoing coronary artery bypass graft (CABG). Of these, 301 patients received propofol. They comprise the safety database for cardiac anesthesia and provide the basis for dosage recommendations in this patient population, in conjunction with reports in the published literature.

INDIVIDUALIZATION OF DOSAGE

GENERAL: STRICT ASEPTIC TECHNIQUE MUST ALWAYS BE MAINTAINED DURING HANDLING. PROPOFOL IS A SINGLE-USE PARENTERAL PRODUCT, CONTAINS NO ANTIMICROBIAL PRESERVATIVES, AND CAN SUPPORT RAPID GROWTH OF MICRO ORGANISMS. DISCARD UNUSED PORTIONS AS DIRECTED WITHIN THE REQUIRED TIME LIMITS (SEE DOSAGE AND ADMINISTRATION, HANDLING PROCEDURES). THERE HAVE BEEN REPORTS IN WHICH FAILURE TO USE ASEPTIC TECHNIQUE WHEN HANDLING PROPOFOL WAS ASSOCIATED WITH MICROBIAL CONTAMINATION OF THE PRODUCT AND WITH FEVER, INFECTION/SEPSIS, OTHER LIFE-THREATENING ILLNESS, AND/OR DEATH. DO NOT USE IF CONTAMINATION IS SUSPECTED.

Propofol blood concentrations at steady state are generally proportional to infusion rates, especially in individual patients. Undesirable effects such as cardiorespiratory depression are likely to occur at higher blood concentrations which result from bolus dosing or rapid increases in the infusion rate. An adequate interval (3 to 5 minutes) must be allowed between clinical dosage adjustments in order to assess drug effects.

When administering propofol by infusion, syringe pumps or volumetric pumps are recommended to provide controlled infusion rates. When infusing propofol to patients undergoing magnetic resonance imaging, metered control devices may be utilized if mechanical pumps are impractical.

Changes in vital signs (increases in pulse rate, blood pressure, sweating and/or tearing) that indicate a response to surgical stimulation or lightening of anesthesia may be controlled by the administration of propofol 25 mg (2.5 ml) to 50 mg (5 ml) incremental boluses and/or by increasing the infusion rate.

For minor surgical procedures (*e.g.,* body surface) nitrous oxide (60%-70%) can be combined with a variable rate propofol infusion to provide satisfactory anesthesia. With more stimulating surgical procedures (*e.g.,*intra-abdominal), or if supplementation with nitrous oxide is not provided, administration rate(s) of propofol and/or opioids should be increased in order to provide adequate anesthesia.

Infusion rates should always be titrated downward in the absence of clinical signs of light anesthesia until a mild response to surgical stimulation is obtained in order to avoid administration of propofol at rates higher than are clinically necessary. Generally, rates of 50 to 100 mcg/kg/min in adults, should be achieved during maintenance in order to optimize recovery times.

Other drugs that cause CNS depression (hypnotics/sedatives, inhalational anesthetics and opioids) can increase CNS depression induced by propofol. Morphine premedication (0.15 mg/kg) with nitrous oxide 67% in oxygen has been shown to decrease the necessary propofol maintenance infusion rate and therapeutic blood concentrations when compared to non-narcotic (lorazepam) premedication.

INDUCTION OF GENERAL ANESTHESIA

Adult Patients: Most adult patients under 55 years of age and classified ASA I/II require 2 to 2.5 mg/kg of propofol for induction when unpremedicated or when premedicated with oral benzodiazepines or intramuscular opioids. For induction, propofol should be titrated (approximately 40 mg every 10 seconds) against the response of the patient until the clinical signs show the onset of anesthesia. As with other sedative hypnotic agents, the amount of intravenous opioid and/or benzodiazepine premedication will influence the response of the patient to an induction dose of propofol.

Elderly, Debilitated, or ASA III/IV Patients: It is important to be familiar and experienced with the intravenous use of propofol before treating elderly, debilitated or ASA III/IV patients. Due to the reduced clearance and higher blood concentrations, most of these patients require approximately 1 to 1.5 mg/kg (approximately 20 mg every 10 seconds) of propofol for induction of anesthesia according to their condition and responses. A rapid bolus

CLINICAL STUDIES: *(cont'd)*

should not be used as this will increase the likelihood of undesirable cardiorespiratory depression including hypotension, apnea, airway obstruction and/or oxygen desaturation. (See DOSAGE AND ADMINISTRATION.)

Neurosurgical Patients: Slower induction is recommended using boluses of 20 mg every 10 seconds. Slower boluses or infusions of propofol for induction of anesthesia, titrated to clinical responses, will generally result in reduced induction dosage requirements (1 to 2 mg/kg). (See PRECAUTIONS and DOSAGE AND ADMINISTRATION.)

Cardiac Anesthesia: Propofol has been well studied in patients with coronary artery disease, but experience in patients with hemodynamically significant valvular or congenital heart disease is limited. As with other anesthetic and sedative-hypnotic agents, propofol in healthy patients causes a decrease in blood pressure that is secondary to decreases in preload (ventricular filling volume at the end of the diastole) and afterload (arterial resistance at the beginning of the systole). The magnitude of these changes is proportional to the blood and effect site concentrations achieved. These concentrations depend upon the dose and speed of the induction and maintenance infusion rates.

In addition, lower heart rates are observed during maintenance with propofol, possibly due to reduction of the sympathetic activity and/or resetting of the baroreceptor reflexes. Therefore, anticholinergic agents should be administered when increases in vagal tone are anticipated.

As with other anesthetic agents, propofol reduces myocardial oxygen consumption. Further studies are needed to confirm and delineate the extent of these effects on the myocardium and the coronary vascular system.

Morphine premedication (0.15 mg/kg) with nitrous oxide 67% in oxygen has been shown to decrease the necessary propofol maintenance infusion rates and therapeutic blood concentrations when compared to non- narcotic (lorazepam) premedication. The rate of propofol administration should be determined based on the patient's premedication and adjusted according to clinical responses.

A rapid bolus induction should be avoided. A slow rate of approximately 20 mg every 10 seconds until induction onset (0.5 to 1.5 mg/kg) should be used. In order to assure adequate anesthesia, when propofol is used as the primary agent, maintenance infusion rates should not be less than 100 mcg/kg/min and should be supplemented with analgesic levels of continuous opioid administration. When an opioid is used as the primary agent, propofol maintenance rates should not be less than 50 mcg/kg/min and care should be taken to insure amnesia with concomitant benzodiazepines. Higher doses of propofol will reduce the opioid requirements (see TABLE 4). When propofol is used as the primary anesthetic, it should not be administered with the high dose opioid technique as this may increase the likelihood of hypotension (see PRECAUTIONS, Cardiac Anesthesia.)

TABLE 4 Cardiac Anesthesia Techniques

Primary Agent	Rate	Secondary Agent/Rate
DIPRIVAN		(Following Induction with Primary Agent) Opioid[a]/0.05-0.075 mcg/kg/min (no bolus)
Preinduction anxiolysis	25 mcg/kg/min	
Induction	0.5-1.5 mg/kg over 60 sec	
Maintenance (Titrated to Clinical Response)	100-150 mcg/kg/min	
OPIOID[b]		Diprivan/50-100 mcg/kg/min (no bolus)
Induction	25-50 mcg/kg	
Maintenance	0.2-0.3 mcg/kg/min	

[a]Opioid is defined in terms of fentanyl equivalents, i.e., 1 mcg of fentanyl = 5 mcg of alfentanil (for bolus) = 10 mcg of alfentanil (for maintenance) or = 0.1 mcg of sufentanil
[b]Care should be taken to ensure amnesia with concomitant benzodiazepine therapy

Maintenance of General Anesthesia: In adults, anesthesia can be maintained by administering propofol by infusion or intermittent IV bolus injection. The patient's clinical response will determine the infusion rate or the amount and frequency of incremental injections.

Continuous Infusion: Propofol 100 to 200 mcg/kg/min administered in a variable rate infusion with 60%-70% nitrous oxide and oxygen provides anesthesia for patients undergoing general surgery. Maintenance by infusion of propofol should immediately follow the induction dose in order to provide satisfactory or continuous anesthesia during the induction phase. During this initial period following the induction dose higher rates of infusion are generally required (150 to 200 mcg/kg/min) for the first 10 to 15 minutes. Infusion rates should subsequently be decreased 30%-50% during the first half-hour of maintenance.

Other drugs that cause CNS depression (hypnotics/sedatives, inhalational anesthetics and opioids) can increase the CNS depression induced by propofol.

Intermittent Bolus: Increments of propofol 25 mg (2.5 ml) to 50 mg (5 ml) may be administered with nitrous oxide in adult patients undergoing general surgery. The incremental boluses should be administered when changes in vital signs indicate a response to surgical stimulation or light anesthesia.

Propofol has been used with a variety of agents commonly used in anesthesia such as atropine, scopolamine, glycopyrrolate, diazepam, depolarizing and nondepolarizing muscle relaxants, and opioid analgesics, as well as with inhalational and regional anesthetic agents.

In the elderly, debilitated or ASA III/IV patients, rapid bolus doses should not be used as this will increase cardiorespiratory effects including hypotension, apnea, airway obstruction and/or oxygen desaturation.

PEDIATRIC ANESTHESIA

Induction of General Anesthesia: Most pediatric patients 3 years of age or older and classified ASA I or II require 2.5 to 3.5 mg/kg of propofol for induction when unpremedicated or when lightly premedicated with oral benzodiazepines or intramuscular opioids. Within this dosage range, younger children may require larger induction doses than older children. As with other sedative hypnotic agents, the amount of intravenous opioid and/or benzodiazepine premedication will influence the response of the patient to an induction dose of propofol. In addition, a lower dosage is recommended for children ASA III or IV. Attention should be paid to minimize pain on injection when administering propofol to pediatric patients. Rapid boluses of propofol may be administered if small veins are pretreated with lidocaine or when antecubital or larger veins are utilized (see PRECAUTIONS, General.

Propofol administered in a variable rate infusion with nitrous oxide 60-70% provides satisfactory anesthesia for most pediatric patients 3 years of age or older, ASA I or II, undergoing general anesthesia.

Maintenance of General Anesthesia: Maintenance by infusion of propofol at a rate of 200-300 mcg/kg/min should immediately follow the induction dose. Following the first half hour of maintenance, if clinical signs of light anesthesia are not present, the infusion rate should be decreased; during this period, infusion rates of 125-150 mcg/kg/min are typically needed. However, younger children (5 years of age or less) may require larger maintenance infusion rates than older children.

CLINICAL STUDIES: *(cont'd)*

MONITORED ANESTHESIA CARE (MAC) SEDATION IN ADULTS

When propofol is administered for MAC sedation, rates of administration should be individualized and titrated to clinical response. In most patients the rates of propofol administration will be in the range of 25-75 mcg/kg/min.

During initiation of MAC sedation, slow infusion or slow injection techniques are preferable over rapid bolus administration. During maintenance of MAC sedation, a variable rate infusion is preferable over intermittent bolus dose administration. In the elderly, debilitated, or ASA III/IV patients, rapid (single or repeated) bolus dose administration should not be used for MAC sedation. (See WARNINGS.) **A rapid bolus injection can result in undesirable cardiorespiratory depression including hypotension, apnea, airway obstruction and/or oxygen desaturation.**

Initiation of MAC Sedation: For initiation of MAC sedation, either an infusion or a slow injection method may be utilized while closely monitoring cardiorespiratory function. With the infusion method, sedation may be initiated by infusing propofol at 100 to 150 mcg/kg/min (6 to 9 mg/kg/h) for a period of 3 to 5 minutes and titrating to the desired level of sedation while closely monitoring respiratory function. With the slow injection method for initiation, patients will require approximately 0.5 mg/kg administered over 3 to 5 minutes and titrated to clinical responses. When propofol is administered slowly over 3 to 5 minutes, most patients will be adequately sedated and the peak drug effect can be achieved while minimizing undesirable cardiorespiratory effects occurring at high plasma levels.

In the elderly, debilitated, or ASA III/IV patients, rapid (single or repeated) bolus dose administration should not be used for MAC sedation. (See WARNINGS.) The rate of administration should be over 3-5 minutes and the dosage of propofol should be reduced to approximately 80% of the usual adult dosage in these patients according to their condition, responses, and changes in vital signs. (See DOSAGE AND ADMINISTRATION.)

Maintenance of MAC Sedation: For maintenance of sedation, a variable rate infusion method is preferable over an intermittent bolus dose method. With the variable rate infusion method, patients will generally require maintenance rates of 25 to 75 mcg/kg/min (1.5 to 4.5 mg/kg/h) during the first 10 to 15 minutes of sedation maintenance. Infusion rates should subsequently be decreased over time to 25 to 50 mcg/kg/min and adjusted to clinical responses. In titrating to clinical effect, allow approximately 2 minutes for onset of peak drug effect.

Infusion rates should always be titrated downward in the absence of clinical signs of light sedation until mild responses to stimulation are obtained in order to avoid sedative administration of propofol at rates higher than are clinically necessary.

If the intermittent bolus dose method is used, increments of propofol 10 mg (1 ml) or 20 mg (2 ml) can be administered and titrated to desired level of sedation. With the intermittent bolus method of sedation maintenance there is the potential for respiratory depression, transient increases in sedation depth, and/or prolongation of recovery.

In the elderly, debilitated, or ASA III/IV patients, rapid (single or repeated) bolus dose administration should not be used for MAC sedation. (See WARNINGS.) The rate of administration and the dosage of propofol should be reduced to approximately 80% of the usual adult dosage in these patients according to their condition, responses, and changes in vital signs. (See DOSAGE AND ADMINISTRATION.)

Propofol can be administered as the sole agent for maintenance of MAC sedation during surgical/diagnostic procedures. When propofol sedation is supplemented with opioid and/or benzodiazepine medications, these agents increase the sedative and respiratory effects of propofol and may also result in a slower recovery profile.(See DRUG INTERACTIONS.)

ICU SEDATION

See WARNINGS and DOSAGE AND ADMINISTRATION, Handling Procedures. For intubated, mechanically ventilated adult patients, Intensive Care Unit (ICU) sedation should be initiated slowly with a continuous infusion in order to titrate to desired clinical effect and minimize hypotension. (See DOSAGE AND ADMINISTRATION.)

Across all 6 US/Canadian clinical studies, the mean infusion maintenance rate for all propofol patients was 27 ± 21 mcg/kg/min. The maintenance infusion rates required to maintain adequate sedation ranged from 2.8 mcg/kg/min to 130 mcg/kg/min. The infusion rate was lower in patients over 55 years of age (approximately 20 mcg/kg/min) compared to patients under 55 years of age (approximately 38 mcg/kg/min). In these studies, morphine or fentanyl was used as needed for analgesia.

Most adult ICU patients recovering from the effects of general anesthesia or deep sedation will require maintenance rates of 5 to 50 mcg/kg/min (0.3 to 3 mg/kg/h) individualized and titrated to clinical response. (See DOSAGE AND ADMINISTRATION.)With medical ICU patients or patients who have recovered from the effects of general anesthesia or deep sedation, the rate of administration of 50 mcg/kg/min or higher may be required to achieve adequate sedation. These higher rates of administration may increase the likelihood of patients developing hypotension.

Although there are reports of reduced analgesic requirements, most patients received opioids for analgesia during maintenance of ICU sedation. Some patients also received benzodiazepines and/or neuromuscular blocking agents. During long term maintenance of sedation, some ICU patients were awakened once or twice every 24 hours for assessment of neurologic or respiratory function. See TABLE 3.

In post-CABG (coronary artery bypass graft) patients, the maintenance rate of propofol administration was usually low (median 11 mcg/kg/min) due to the intraoperative administration of high opioid doses. Patients receiving propofol required 35% less nitroprusside than midazolam patients; this difference was statistically significant ($P<0.05$). During initiation of sedation in Post-CABG patients, a 15% to 20% decrease in blood pressure was seen in the first 60 minutes. It was not possible to determine cardiovascular effects in patients with severely compromised ventricular function. See TABLE 3.

In Medical or Postsurgical ICU studies comparing propofol to benzodiazepine infusion or bolus, there were no apparent differences in maintenance of adequate sedation, mean arterial pressure, or laboratory findings. Like the comparators, propofol reduced blood cortisol during sedation while maintaining responsivity to challenges with adrenocorticotropic hormone (ACTH). Case reports from the published literature generally reflect that propofol has been used safely in patients with a history of porphyria or malignant hyperthermia.

In hemodynamically stable head trauma patients ranging in age from 19-43 years, adequate sedation was maintained with propofol or morphine (N=7 in each group). There were no apparent differences in adequacy of sedation, intracranial pressure, cerebral perfusion pressure, or neurologic recovery between the treatment groups. In literature reports from Neurosurgical ICU and severely head injured patients propofol infusion with or without diuretics and hyperventilation controlled intracranial pressure while maintaining cerebral perfusion pressure. In some patients bolus doses resulted in decreased blood pressure and compromised cerebral perfusion pressure. See TABLE 3.

Propofol was found to be effective in status epilepticus which was refractory to the standard anticonvulsant therapies. For these patients as well as for ARDS/respiratory failure and tetanus patients sedation maintenance dosages were generally higher than those for other critically ill patient populations. See TABLE 3.

CLINICAL STUDIES: *(cont'd)*

Abrupt discontinuation of propofol prior to weaning or for daily evaluation of sedation levels should be avoided. This may result in rapid awakening with associated anxiety, agitation and resistance to mechanical ventilation. Infusions of propofol should be adjusted to maintain a light level of sedation through the weaning process or evaluation of sedation level. (See PRECAUTIONS.)

INDICATIONS AND USAGE:

Propofol is an IV sedative-hypnotic agent that can be used for both induction and/or maintenance of anesthesia as part of a balanced anesthetic technique for inpatient and outpatient surgery in adults and in children 3 years of age or older.

Propofol, when administered intravenously as directed, can be used to initiate and maintain monitored anesthesia care (MAC) sedation during diagnostic procedures in adults. Propofol may also be used for MAC sedation in conjunction with local/regional anesthesia in patients undergoing surgical procedures. (See PRECAUTIONS.)

Propofol should only be administered to intubated, mechanically ventilated adult patients in the Intensive Care Unit (ICU) to provide continuous sedation and control of stress responses. In this setting, propofol should be administered only by persons skilled in the medical management of critically ill patients and trained in cardiovascular resuscitation and airway management.

Propofol is not recommended for obstetrics, including cesarean section deliveries. Propofol crosses the placenta, and as with other general anesthetic agents, the administration of propofol may be associated with neonatal depression. (See PRECAUTIONS.)

Propofol is not recommended for use in nursing mothers because propofol has been reported to be excreted in human milk and the effects of oral absorption of small amounts of propofol are not known. (See PRECAUTIONS.)

Propofol is not recommended for anesthesia in children below the age of 3 years because safety and effectiveness have not been established. Propofol is not recommended for MAC sedation in children because safety and effectiveness have not been established.

Propofol is not recommended for pediatric ICU sedation because safety and effectiveness have not been established.

CONTRAINDICATIONS:

Propofol is contraindicated in patients with a known hypersensitivity to propofol or its components, or when general anesthesia or sedation are contraindicated.

WARNINGS:

For general anesthesia or monitored anesthesia care (MAC) sedation, propofol should be administered only by persons trained in the administration of general anesthesia and not involved in the conduct of the surgical/diagnostic procedure. Patients should be continuously monitored, and facilities for maintenance of a patent airway, artificial ventilation, and oxygen enrichment and circulatory resuscitation must be immediately available.

For sedation of intubated, mechanically ventilated adult patients in the Intensive Care Unit (ICU), propofol should be administered only by persons skilled in the management of critically ill patients and trained in cardiovascular resuscitation and airway management.

In the elderly, debilitated or ASA III/IV patients, rapid (single or repeated) bolus administration should not be used during general anesthesia or MAC sedation in order to minimize undesirable cardiorespiratory depression including hypotension, apnea, airway obstruction and/or oxygen desaturation.

MAC sedation patients should be continuously monitored by persons not involved in the conduct of the surgical or diagnostic procedure; oxygen supplementation should be immediately available and provided where clinically indicated; and oxygen saturation should be monitored in all patients. Patients should be continuously monitored for early signs of hypotension, apnea, airway obstruction and/or oxygen desaturation. These cardiorespiratory effects are more likely to occur following rapid initiation (loading) boluses or during supplemental maintenance boluses, especially in the elderly, debilitated, or ASA III/IV patients.

Propfol Injection should not be coadministered through the same IV catheter with blood or plasma because compatibility has not been established. *In vitro* tests have shown that aggregates of the globular component of the emulsion vehicle have occurred with blood/plasma/serum from humans and animals. The clinical significance is not known.

STRICT ASEPTIC TECHNIQUE MUST ALWAYS BE MAINTAINED DURING HANDLING. PROPOFOL IS A SINGLE-USE PARENTERAL PRODUCT, CONTAINS NO ANTIMICROBIAL PRESERVATIVES, AND CAN SUPPORT RAPID GROWTH OF MICRO ORGANISMS. DISCARD UNUSED PORTIONS AS DIRECTED WITHIN THE REQUIRED TIME LIMITS (SEE DOSAGE AND ADMINISTRATION, HANDLING PROCEDURES). THERE HAVE BEEN REPORTS IN WHICH FAILURE TO USE ASEPTIC TECHNIQUE WHEN HANDLING PROPOFOL WAS ASSOCIATED WITH MICROBIAL CONTAMINATION OF THE PRODUCT AND WITH FEVER, INFECTION/SEPSIS, OTHER LIFE-THREATENING ILLNESS, AND/OR DEATH. DO NOT USE IF CONTAMINATION IS SUSPECTED.

PRECAUTIONS:

GENERAL

A lower induction dose and a slower maintenance rate of administration should be used in elderly, debilitated, or ASA III/IV patients. See CLINICAL STUDIES, Individualization of Dosage. Patients should be continuously monitored for early signs of significant hypotension and/or bradycardia. Treatment may include increasing the rate of intravenous fluid, elevation of lower extremities, use of pressor agents, or administration of atropine. Apnea often occurs during induction and may persist for more than 60 seconds. Ventilatory support may be required. Because propofol is an emulsion, caution should be exercised in patients with disorders of lipid metabolism such as primary hyperlipoproteinemia, diabetic hyperlipemia, and pancreatitis.

The clinical criteria for discharge from the recovery/day surgery area established for each institution should be satisfied before discharge of the patient from the care of the anesthesiologist.

When propofol is administered to an epileptic patient, there may be a risk of seizure during the recovery phase.

In adults and children, attention should be paid to minimize pain on administration of Propfol Injection. Transient local pain can be minimized if the larger veins of the forearm or antecubital fossa are used. Pain during intravenous injection may also be reduced by prior injection of IV lidocaine (1 ml of a 1% solution). Pain on injection occurred frequently in pediatric patients (45%) when a small vein of the hand was utilized without lidocaine pretreatment. With lidocaine pretreatment or when antecubital veins were utilized, pain was minimal (incidence less than 10%) and well tolerated.

Venous sequelae (phlebitis or thrombosis) have been reported rarely (<1%). In two well-controlled clinical studies using dedicated intravenous catheters, no instances of venous sequelae were reported up to 14 days following induction. Accidental clinical extravasation and intentional injection into subcutaneous or perivascular tissues of animals caused minimal tissue reaction.

PRECAUTIONS: *(cont'd)*

Intra-arterial injection in animals did not induce local tissue effects. Accidental intra-arterial injection has been reported in patients, and other than pain, there were no major sequelae.

Perioperative myoclonia, rarely including convulsions and opisthotonus, has occurred in temporal relationship in cases in which propofol has been administered.

Clinical features of anaphylaxis, which may include bronchospasm, erythema and hypotension, occur rarely following propofol administration, although use of other drugs in most instances makes the relationship to propofol unclear.

There have been rare reports of pulmonary edema in temporal relationship to the administration of propofol, although a causal relationship is unknown.

Very rarely, cases of unexplained postoperative pacreatitis (requiring hospital admission) have been reported after anesthesia in which propofol was one of the induction agents used. Due to a variety of confounding factors in these cases, including concomitant medications, a causal relationship to propofol is unclear.

Propofol has no vagolytic activity. Reports of bradycardia, asystole, and rarely, cardiac arrest have been associated with propofol. The intravenous administration of anticholinergic agents (*e.g.,* atropine or glycopyrrolate) should be considered to modify potential increases in vagal tone due to concomitant agents (*e.g.,* succinylcholine) or surgical stimuli.

Intensive Care Unit Sedation: See WARNINGSand DOSAGE AND ADMINISTRATION, Handling Procedures.The administration of propofol should be initiated as a continuous infusion and changes in the rate of administration made slowly (>5 min) in order to minimize hypotension and avoid acute overdosage. See CLINICAL STUDIES, Individualization of Dosage.

Patients should be monitored for early signs of significant hypotension and/or cardiovascular depression, which may be profound. These effects are responsive to discontinuation of propofol, IV fluid administration, and/or vasopressor therapy.

As with other sedative medications, there is wide interpatient variability in propofol dosage requirements, and these requirements may change with time.

Failure to reduce the infusion rate in patients receiving propofol for extended periods may result in excessively high blood concentrations of the drug. Thus, titration to clinical response and daily evaluation of sedation levels are important during use of propofol infusion for ICU sedation, especially of long duration.

Opioids and paralytic agents should be discontinued and respiratory function optimized prior to weaning patients from mechanical ventilation. Infusions of propofol should be adjusted to maintain a light level of sedation prior to weaning patients from mechanical ventilatory support. Throughout the weaning process this level of sedation may be maintained in the absence of respiratory depression. Because of the rapid clearance of propofol, abrupt discontinuation of a patient's infusion may result in rapid awakening of the patient with associated anxiety, agitation, and resistance to mechanical ventilation, making weaning from mechanical ventilation difficult. It is therefore recommended that administration of propofol be continued in order to maintain a light level of sedation throughout the weaning process until 10-15 minutes prior to extubation at which time the infusion can be discontinued.

Since propofol is formulated in an oil-in-water emulsion, elevations in serum triglycerides may occur when propofol is administered for extended periods of time. Patients at risk of hyperlipidemia should be monitored for increases in serum triglycerides or serum turbidity. Administration of propofol should be adjusted if fat is being inadequately cleared from the body. A reduction in the quantity of concurrently administered lipids is indicated to compensate for the amount of lipid infused as part of the propofol formulation; 1 ml of propofol contains approximately 0.1 g of fat (1.1 kcal).

The long-term administration of propofol to patients with renal failure and/or hepatic insufficiency has not been evaluated.

Neurosurgical Anesthesia: When propofol is used in patients with increased intracranial pressure or impaired cerebral circulation, significant decreases in mean arterial pressure should be avoided because of the resultant decreases in cerebral perfusion pressure. To avoid significant hypotension and decreases in cerebral perfusion pressure, an infusion or slow bolus of approximately 20 mg every 10 seconds should be utilized instead of rapid, more frequent, and/or larger boluses of propofol. Slower induction titrated to clinical responses, will generally result in reduced induction dosage requirements (1 to 2 mg/kg). When increased ICP is suspected, hyperventilation and hypocarbia should accompany the administration of propofol. (See DOSAGE AND ADMINISTRATION.)

Cardiac Anesthesia: Slower rates of administration should be utilized in premedicated patients, geriatric patients, patients with recent fluid shifts, or patients who are hemodynamically unstable. Any fluid deficits should be corrected prior to administration of propofol. In those patients where additional fluid therapy may be contraindicated, other measures, e.g., elevation of lower extremities, or use of pressor agents, may be useful to offset the hypotension which is associated with the induction of anesthesia with propofol.

INFORMATION FOR PATIENTS

Patients should be advised that performance of activities requiring mental alertness, such as operating a motor vehicle, or hazardous machinery or signing legal documents may be impaired for some time after general anesthesia or sedation.

CARCINOGENESIS, MUTAGENESIS, IMPAIRMENT OF FERTILITY

Animal carcinogenicity studies have not been performed with propofol.

In vitro and *in vivo* animal tests failed to show any potential for mutagenicity by propofol. Tests for mutagenicity included the Ames (using *Salmonella* sp) mutation test, gene mutation/gene conversion using *Saccharomyces cerevisiae, in vitro*cytogenetic studies in Chinese hamsters and a mouse micronucleus test.

Studies in female rats at intravenous doses up to 15 mg/kg/day (6 times the maximum recommended human induction dose) for 2 weeks before pregnancy to day 7 of gestation did not show impaired fertility. Male fertility in rats was not affected in a dominant lethal study at intravenous doses up to 15 mg/kg/day for 5 days.

PREGNANCY CATEGORY B

Reproduction studies have been performed in rats and rabbits at intravenous doses of 15 mg/kg/day (6 times the recommended human induction dose) and have revealed no evidence of impaired fertility or harm to the fetus due to propofol. Propofol, however, has been shown to cause maternal deaths in rats and rabbits and decreased pup survival during the lactating period in dams treated with 15 mg/kg/day (or 6 times the recommended human induction dose). The pharmacological activity (anesthesia) of the drug on the mother is probably responsible for the adverse effects seen in the offspring. There are, however, no adequate and well-controlled studies in pregnant women. Because animal reproduction studies are not always predictive of human responses, this drug should be used during pregnancy only if clearly needed.

LABOR AND DELIVERY

Propofol is not recommended for obstetrics, including cesarean section deliveries. Propofol crosses the placenta, and as with other general anesthetic agents, the administration of propofol may be associated with neonatal depression.

PRECAUTIONS: *(cont'd)*

NURSING MOTHERS

Propofol is not recommended for use in nursing mothers because propofol has been reported to be excreted in human milk and the effects of oral absorption of small amounts of propofol are not known.

PEDIATRICS

Propofol is not recommended for use in pediatric patients for ICU or MAC sedation. In addition, propofol is not recommended for general anesthesia for children below the age of 3 years because safety and effectiveness have not been established.

Although no causal relationship has been established, serious adverse events (including fatalities) have been reported in children given propofol for ICU sedation. These events were seen most often in children with respiratory tract infections given doses in excess of those recommended for adults.

DRUG INTERACTIONS:

The induction dose requirements of propofol may be reduced in patients with intramuscular or intravenous premedication, particularly with narcotics (*e.g.*, morphine, meperidine, and fentanyl, etc.) and combinations of opioids and sedatives (*e.g.*, benzodiazepines, barbiturates, chloral hydrate, droperidol, etc.). These agents may increase the anesthetic or sedative effects of propofol and may also result in more pronounced decreases in systolic, diastolic, and mean arterial pressures and cardiac output.

During maintenance of anesthesia or sedation, the rate of propofol administration should be adjusted according to the desired level of anesthesia or sedation and may be reduced in the presence of supplemental analgesic agents (*e.g.*, nitrous oxide or opioids). The concurrent administration of potent inhalational agents (*e.g.*, isoflurane, enflurane, and halothane) during maintenance with propofol has not been extensively evaluated. These inhalational agents can also be expected to increase the anesthetic or sedative and cardiorespiratory effects of propofol.

Propofol does not cause a clinically significant change in onset, intensity or duration of action of the commonly used neuromuscular blocking agents (*e.g.*, succinylcholine and nondepolarizing muscle relaxants).

No significant adverse interactions with commonly used premedications or drugs used during anesthesia or sedation (including a range of muscle relaxants, inhalational agents, analgesic agents, and local anesthetic agents) have been observed.

ADVERSE REACTIONS:

General: Adverse event information is derived from controlled clinical trials and worldwide marketing experience. In the description below, rates of the more common events represent US/Canadian clinical study results. Less frequent events are also derived from publications and marketing experience in over 8 million patients; there are insufficient data to support an accurate estimate of their incidence rates. These studies were conducted using a variety of premedicants, varying lengths of surgical/diagnostic procedures and various other anesthetic/sedative agents. Most adverse events were mild and transient.

Anesthesia and MAC Sedation in Adults: The following estimates of adverse events for propofol include data from clinical trials in general anesthesia/MAC sedation (N = 2889 adult patients). The adverse events listed below as probably causally related are those events in which the actual incidence rate in patients treated with propofol was greater than the comparator incidence rate in these trials. Therefore, incidence rates for anesthesia and MAC sedation in adults generally represent estimates of the percentage of clinical trial patients which appeared to have probable causal relationship.

The adverse experience profile from reports of 150 patients in the MAC sedation clinical trials is similar to the profile established with propofol during anesthesia. During MAC sedation clinical trials, significant respiratory events included cough, upper airway obstruction, apnea, hypoventilation, and dyspnea.

Anesthesia in Children: Generally the adverse experience profile from reports of 349 propofol pediatric patients between the ages of 3 and 12 years in the US/Canadian anesthesia clinical trials is similar to the profile established with propofol during anesthesia in adults (see Pediatric percentages [Peds %]). Although not reported as an adverse event in clinical trials, apnea is frequently observed in pediatric patients.

ICU Sedation in Adults: The following estimates of adverse events include data from clinical trials in ICU sedation (N=159) patients. Probably related incidence rates for ICU sedation were determined by individual case report form review. Probable causality was based upon an apparent dose response relationship and/or positive responses to rechallenge. In many instances the presence of concomitant disease and concomitant therapy made the causal relationship unknown. Therefore, incidence rates for ICU sedation generally represent estimates of the percentage of clinical trial patients which appeared to have a probable causal relationship.

DRUG ABUSE AND DEPENDENCE:

Rare cases of self administration of propofol by health care professionals have been reported, including some fatalities. Propofol should be managed to prevent the risk of diversion, including restriction of access and accounting procedures as appropriate to the clinical setting.

OVERDOSAGE:

If overdosage occurs, propofol administration should be discontinued immediately. Overdosage is likely to cause cardiorespiratory depression. Respiratory depression should be treated by artificial ventilation with oxygen. Cardiovascular depression may require repositioning of the patient by raising the patient's legs, increasing the flow rate of intravenous fluids and administering pressor agents and/or anticholinergic agents.

DOSAGE AND ADMINISTRATION:

Dosage and rate of administration should be individualized and titrated to the desired effect, according to clinically relevant factors including preinduction and concomitant medications, age, ASA physical classification and level of debilitation of the patient.

The following is abbreviated dosage and administration information which is only intended as a general guide in the use of propofol. Prior to administering propofol, it is imperative that the physician review and be completely familiar with the specific dosage and administration information detailed in the CLINICAL STUDIES, Individualization of Dosage.

IN THE ELDERLY, DEBILITATED, OR ASA III/IV PATIENTS, RAPID BOLUS DOSES SHOULD NOT BE THE METHOD OF ADMINISTRATION. (SEE WARNINGS.)

INTENSIVE CARE UNIT SEDATION: Strict aseptic techniques must be followed when handling propofol as the vehicle is capable of supporting rapid growth of microorganisms. See DOSAGE AND ADMINISTRATION, Handling Procedures. Propofol should be individualized according to the patient's condition and response, blood lipid profile, and vital signs. See PRECAUTIONS, ICU sedation. For intubated, mechanically ventilated adult patients, Intensive Care Unit (ICU) sedation should be initiated slowly with a continuous infusion in order to titrate to desired clinical effect and minimize hypotension. When indicated, initiation of sedation should begin at 5 mcg/kg/min (0.3 mg/kg/h). The infusion rate should be increased

DOSAGE AND ADMINISTRATION: *(cont'd)*

TABLE 5

Incidence Greater Than 1%-Probably Causally Related	
Anesthesia/MAC Sedation	**ICU Sedation**
Cardiovascular	
Bradycardia, Hypotension* [Peds: 17%] [Hypertension Peds: 8%] (see alsoCLINICAL PHARMACOLOGY)	Bradycardia, Decreased Cardiac Output, Hypotension* 26%
Central Nervous System	
Movement* [Peds: 17%]	
Injection Site	
Burning/Stinging or Pain, 17.6% [Peds: 10%]	
Metabolic/Nutritional	
	Hyperlipemia*
Respiratory	
Apnea (see alsoCLINICAL PHARMACOLOGY)	Respiratory Acidosis during Weaning
Skin and Appendages	
Rash [Peds: 5%]	
Events without an * or % had an incidence of 1%-3%	
Incidence Less Than 1%-Probably Causally Related	
Body as a Whole	
Anaphylaxis/Anaphylactoid Reaction, Perinatal Disorder	
Cardiovascular	
Premature Atrial Contractions, Syncope	
Central Nervous System	
Hypertonia/Dystonia, Paresthesia	Agitation
Digestive	
Hypersalivation	
Musculoskeletal	
Myalgia	
Respiratory	
Wheezing	Decreased lung function
Skin and Appendages	
Flushing, Pruritus, Amblyopia	
Urogenital	
Cloudy Urine	Green Urine
Incidence Less Than 1%-Probably Causally Related	
Body as a Whole	
Asthenia, Awareness, Chest Pain, Extremities Pain, Fever, Increased Drug Effect, Neck Rigidity/Stiffness, Trunk Pain	Fever, Sepsis, Trunk Pain, Whole body Weakness
Cardiovascular	
Arrhythmia, Atrial Fibrillation, Atrioventricular Heart Block, Bigeminy, Bleeding, Bundle Branch Block, Cardiac Arrest, ECG Abnormal, Edema, Extrasystole, Heart Block, Hypertenion, Myocardial Infarction, Myocardial Ischemia, Premature Ventricular Contractions, ST Segment Depression, Supraventricular Tachycardia, Tachycardia, Ventricular Fibrillation	Arrhythmia, Atrial Fibrillation, Bigeminy, Cardiac Arrest, Extrasystole, Right Heart Failure, Ventricular Tachycardia
Central Nervous System	
Abnormal Dreams, Agitation, Amorous Behavior, Anxiety, Bucking/Jerking/Thrashing, Chills/Shivering, Clonic/ Myoclonic Movement, Combativeness, Confusion, Delerium, Depression, Dizziness, Emotional Lability, Euphoria, Fatigue, Hallucinations, Headache, Hypotonia, Hysteria, Insomnia, Moaning, Neuropathy, Opisthotonos, Rigidity, Seizures, Somnolence, Tremor, Twitching	Chills/Shivering, Intracranial Hypertension, Seizures, Somnolence, Thinking Abnormal
Digestive	
Cramping, Diarrhea, Dry Mouth, Enlarged Parotid, Nausea, Swallowing, Vomiting	Ileus, Liver Function Abnormal
Hematologic/Lymphatic	
Caogulation Disorder, Leukocytosis	
Injection Site	
Hives/Itching, Phlebitis, Redness, Discoloration	
Metabolic/Nutritional	
Hyperkalemia, Hyperlipemia	BUN Increased, Creatnine Increased, Dehydration, Hyperglycemia, Metabolic Acidosis, Osmolity Increased
Respiratory	
Bronchospasm, Burning in Throat, Cough Dyspnea, Hiccough, Hyperventilation, Hypoventilation, Hypoxia, Laryngospasm, Pharyngitis, Sneezing, Tachypnea, Upper Airway Obstruction	Hypoxia
Skin and Appendages	
Conjunctival Hyperemia, Diaphoresis, Urticaria	Rash
Special Senses	
Diplopia, Ear Pain, Eye Pain, Nystagmus, taste Perversion, Tinnitus	
Urogenital	
Oliguria, Urine Retention	Kidney Failure

by increments of 5 to 10 mcg/kg/min (0.3 to 0.6 mg/kg/h) until the desired level of sedation is achieved. A minimum period of 5 minutes between adjustments should be allowed for onset of peak drug effect. Most adult patients require maintenance rates of 5 to 50 mcg/kg/min (0.3 to 3 mg/kg/h) or higher. Dosages of propofol should be reduced in patients who have received large doses of narcotics. Conversely, the propofol dosage requirement may be reduced by adequate management of pain with analgesic agents. As with other sedative medications, there is interpatient variability in dosage requirements, and these requirements may change with time. See Dosage Guide. EVALUATION OF LEVEL OF SEDATION AND ASSESSMENT OF CNS FUNCTION SHOULD BE CARRIED OUT DAILY THROUGHOUT MAINTENANCE TO DETERMINE THE MINIMUM DOSE OF propofol REQUIRED FOR SEDATION (see PRECAUTIONS, ICU sedation. Bolus administration of 10 or 20 mg should only be used to rapidly increase depth of sedation in patients where hypotension is not likely to occur. Patients with compromised myocardial function, intravascular volume depletion, or abnormally low vascular tone (*e.g.*, sepsis) may be more susceptible to hypotension. (See PRECAUTIONS.)

Summary Of Dosage Guidelines: Dosages and rates of administration in the following list should be individualized and titrated to clinical response. Safety and dosage requirements in Pediatric patients have only been established for induction and maintenance of anesthesia. For complete dosage information, see CLINICAL STUDIES, Individualization of Dosage.

Induction Of General Anesthesia

Healthy Adults Less Than 55 Years of Age: 40 mg every 10 seconds until induction onset (2 to 2.5 mg/kg).

DOSAGE AND ADMINISTRATION: *(cont'd)*

Elderly, Debilitated, or ASA III/IV Patients: 20 mg every 10 seconds until induction onset (1 to 1.5 mg/kg).

Cardiac Anesthesia: 20 mg every 10 seconds until induction onset (0.5 to 1.5 mg/kg).

Neurosurgical Patients: 20 mg every 10 seconds until induction onset (1 to 2 mg/kg)

Pediatric-healthy, 3 years of age or older: 2.5 to 3.5 mg/kg administered over 20-30 seconds.

Maintenance of General Anesthesia: Infusion

Healthy Adults Less Than 55 Years of Age: 100 to 200 mcg/kg/min (6 to 12 mg/kg/h).

Elderly, Debilitated, ASA III/IV Patients: 50 to 100 mcg/kg/min (3 to 6 mg/kg/h).

Cardiac Anesthesia: Most patients require: Primary propofol with Secondary Opioid - 100 - 150 mcg/kg/min

Low dose propofol with Primary Opioid - 50 - 100 mcg/kg/min (See TABLE 4)

Neurosurgical Patients: 100 to 200 mcg/kg/min (6 to 12 mg/kg/h).

Pediatric-healthy, 3 years of age or older: 125 to 300 mcg/kg/min (7.5 to 18 mg/kg/h)

Maintenance of General Anesthesia: Intermittent Bolus

Healthy Adults Less Than 55 Years of Age: Increments of 20 to 50 mg as needed.

Initiation of MAC Sedation

Healthy Adults Less Than 55 Years of Age: Slow infusion or slow injection techniques are recommended to avoid apnea or hypotension. Most patients require an infusion of 100 to 150 mcg/kg/min (6 to 9 mg/kg/h) for 3 to 5 minutes or a slow injection of 0.5 mg/kg over 3 to 5 minutes followed immediately by a maintenance infusion.

Elderly, Debilitated, Neurosurgical, or ASA III/IV Patients: Most patients require dosages similar to healthy adults. Rapid boluses are to be avoided. (See WARNINGS.)

Maintenance of MAC Sedation

Healthy Adults Less Than 55 Years of Age: A variable rate infusion technique is preferable over an intermittent bolus technique. Most patients require an infusion of 25 to 75 mcg/kg/min (1.5 to 4.5 mg/kg/h) or incremental bolus doses of 10 mg or 20 mg.

In Elderly, Debilitated, Neurosurgical, or ASA III/IV Patients: Most patients require 80% of the usual adult dose. A rapid (single or repeated) bolus dose should not be used. (See WARNINGS.)

Initiation and Maintenance of ICU Sedation in Intubated, Mechanically Ventilated

Adult Patients: Because of the lingering effects of previous anesthetic or sedative agents, in most patients the initial infusion should be 5 mcg/kg/min (0.3 mg/kg/h) for at least 5 minutes. Subsequent increments of 5 to 10 mcg/kg/min (0.3 to 0.6 mg/kg/h) over 5 to 10 minutes may be used until desired level of sedation is achieved.

Maintenance rates of 5 to 50 mcg/kg/min (0.3 to 3 mg/kg/h) or higher may be required. Evaluation of level of sedation and assessment of CNS function should be carried out daily throughout maintenance to determine the minimum dose of propofol required for sedation. The tubing and any unused portions of propofol should be discarded after 12 hours because propofol contains no preservatives and is capable of supporting rapid growth of microorganisms (See WARNINGS, and DOSAGE AND ADMINISTRATION.)

Compatibility and Stability: Propofol should not be mixed with other therapeutic agents prior to administration.

Dilution Prior to Administration: When propofol is diluted prior to administration, it should only be diluted with 5% Dextrose Injection, USP, and it should not be diluted to a concentration less than 2 mg/ml because it is an emulsion. In diluted form it has been shown to be more stable when in contact with glass than with plastic (95% potency after 2 hours of running infusion in plastic).

Administration with Other Fluids: Compatibility of propofol with the coadministration of blood/serum/plasma has not been established. (See WARNINGS.) propofol has been shown to be compatible when administered with the following intravenous fluids.

5% Dextrose Injection, USP

Lactated Ringers Injection, USP

Lactated Ringers and 5% Dextrose Injection

5% Dextrose and 0.45% Sodium Chloride Injection, USP

5% Dextrose and 0.2% Sodium Chloride Injection, USP

HANDLING PROCEDURES

General: Parenteral drug products should be inspected visually for particulate matter and discoloration prior to administration whenever solution and container permit. Propofol must not be administered through filters with a pore size less than 5 µm because this could restrict the flow of propofol and/or cause the breakdown of the emulsion.

Do not use if there is evidence of separation of the phases of the emulsion.

Rare cases of self administration of propofol, by health care professionals have been reported, including some fatalities (See DRUG ABUSE AND DEPENDENCE.)

STRICT ASEPTIC TECHNIQUE MUST ALWAYS BE MAINTAINED DURING HANDLING. PROPOFOL IS A SINGLE-USE PARENTERAL PRODUCT, CONTAINS NO ANTIMICROBIAL PRESERVATIVES, AND CAN SUPPORT RAPID GROWTH OF MICRO ORGANISMS. DISCARD UNUSED PORTIONS AS DIRECTED WITHIN THE REQUIRED TIME LIMITS. (SEE DOSAGE AND ADMINISTRATION, HANDLING PROCEDURES). THERE HAVE BEEN REPORTS IN WHICH FAILURE TO USE ASEPTIC TECHNIQUE WHEN HANDLING PROPOFOL WAS ASSOCIATED WITH MICROBIAL CONTAMINATION OF THE PRODUCT AND WITH FEVER, INFECTION/SEPSIS, OTHER LIFE-THREATENING ILLNESS, AND/OR DEATH. DO NOT USE IF CONTAMINATION IS SUSPECTED.

Aseptic Guidelines for General Anesthesia/MAC Sedation: Propofol should be prepared for use just prior to initiation of each individual anesthetic/sedative procedure. The ampule neck surface or vial rubber stopper should be disinfected using 70% isopropyl alcohol. Propofol should be drawn into sterile syringes immediately after ampules or vials are opened. When withdrawing propofol from vials, a sterile vent spike should be used. The syringe(s) should be labeled with appropriate information including the data and time the ampule or vial was opened. Administration should commence promptly and be completed within 6 hours after the ampules or vials have been opened.

Propofol should be prepared for single patient use only. Any unused portions of propofol, reservoirs, dedicated administration tubing and/or solutions containing propofol must be discarded at the end of the anesthetic procedure or at 6 hours, whichever occurs sooner. The IV line should be flushed every 6 hours and at the end of the anesthetic procedure to remove residual propofol.

Aseptic Guidelines for ICU Sedation: When propofol is administered directly from the vial, strict aseptic techniques must be followed. The vial rubber stopper should be disinfected using 70% isopropyl alcohol. A sterile vent spike and sterile tubing must be used for administration of propofol. As with other lipid emulsions the number of IV line manipulations should be minimized. Administration should commence promptly and must be completed within 12 hours after the vial has been spiked. The tubing and any unused portions of propofol must be discarded after 12 hours.

DOSAGE AND ADMINISTRATION: *(cont'd)*

If propofol is transferred to a syringe or other container prior to administration, the handling procedures for General anesthesia/MAC sedation should be followed and the product should be discarded and administration lines changed after 6 hours.

HOW SUPPLIED:

Dipravin is available in ready to use 20 ml ampules, 50 ml infusion vials, and 100 ml infusion vials containing 10 mg/ml of propofol.

Propofol undergoes oxidative degradation, in the presence of oxygen, and is therefore packaged under nitrogen to eliminate this degradation path.

Storage: Store below 22°C (72°F). Do not store below 4°C (40°F). Refrigeration is not recommended. Shake well before use.

HOW SUPPLIED - EQUIVALENTS NOT AVAILABLE:

Injection, Emulsion - Intravenous - 10 mg/ml

20 ml x 5	$64.25	DIPRIVAN, Zeneca Pharms	00310-0290-20
20 ml x 5	$64.25	DIPRIVAN, Zeneca Pharms	00310-0290-62
50 ml	$32.12	DIPRIVAN, Zeneca Pharms	00310-0290-50
50 ml	$32.12	DIPRIVAN, Zeneca Pharms	00310-0290-65
100 ml	$64.25	DIPRIVAN, Zeneca Pharms	00310-0290-11
100 ml	$64.25	DIPRIVAN, Zeneca Pharms	00310-0290-61

PROPOXYPHENE HYDROCHLORIDE *(002133)*

CATEGORIES: Analgesics; Antipyretics; Central Nervous System Agents; Narcotic Analgesics; Narcotics, Synthetics & Combinations; Opiate Agonists (Controlled); Pain; DEA Class CIV; FDA Approval Pre 1982

BRAND NAMES: *Algafan*; *Antalvic*; Darvon; *Deprancol*; *Depronal*; *Develin*; Dolene; *Dolotard*; *Doloxene*; *Dolpoxene*; Kesso-Gesic; *Liberen*; Margesic; *Novopropoxyn*; *Parvon*; Prophene 65; Propoxycon
(International brand names outside U.S. in italics)

FORMULARIES: Aetna; BC-BS; FHP

DESCRIPTION:

Propoxyphene hydrochloride, USP is an odorless, white crystalline powder with a bitter taste. It is freely soluble in water. Chemically, it is (2*S*,3*R*)-(+)-4-(Dimethylamino)-3-methyl-1,2-diphenyl-2-butanol propionate (ester) hydrochloride.

Each capsule contains 65 mg (172.9 mcmol)(No. 65) propoxyphene hydrochloride. It also contains D&C Red No. 33, FD&C Yellow No.6, gelatin, magnesium stearate, silicone, starch, titanium dioxide, and other inactive ingredients.

CLINICAL PHARMACOLOGY:

Propoxyphene is a centrally acting narcotic analgesic agent. Equimolar doses of propoxyphene hydrochloride or napsylate provide similar plasma concentrations. Following administration of 65, 130, or 195 mg of propoxyphene hydrochloride, the bioavailability of propoxyphene is equivalent to that of 100, 200, or 300 mg respectively of propoxyphene napsylate. Peak plasma concentrations of propoxyphene are reached in 2 to 2 1/2 hours. After a 65-mg oral dose of propoxyphene hydrochloride, peak plasma levels of 0.05 to 0.1 mcg/ml are achieved.

Repeated doses of propoxyphene at 6-hour intervals lead to increasing plasma concentrations, with a plateau after the ninth dose at 48 hours.

Propoxyphene is metabolized in the liver to yield norpropoxyphene. Propoxyphene has a half-life of 6 to 12 hours, whereas that of norpropoxyphene is 30 to 36 hours.

Norpropoxyphene has substantially less central-nervous-system-depressant effect than propoxyphene but a greater local anesthetic effect, which is similar to that of amitriptyline and antiarrhythmic agents, such as lidocaine and quinidine.

In animal studies in which propoxyphene and norpropoxyphene were continuously infused in large amounts, intracardiac conduction time (P-R and QRS intervals) was prolonged. Any intracardiac conduction delay attributable to high concentrations of norpropoxyphene may be of relatively long duration.

Propoxyphene is a mild narcotic analgesic structurally related to methadone. The potency of propoxyphene hydrochloride is from two-thirds to equal that of codeine.

INDICATIONS AND USAGE:

For the relief of mild to moderate pain.

CONTRAINDICATIONS:

Hypersensitivity to propoxyphene.

WARNINGS:

Do not prescribe propoxyphene for patients who are suicidal or addiction-prone.

Prescribe propoxyphene with caution for patients taking tranquilizers or antidepressant drugs and patients who use alcohol in excess.

Tell your patients not to exceed the recommended dose and to limit their intake of alcohol.Propoxyphene products in excessive doses, either along or in combination with other CNS depressants, including alcohol, are a major cause of drug-related deaths. Fatalities within the first hour of overdosage are not uncommon. In a survey of deaths due to overdosage conducted in 1975, in approximately 20% of the fatal cases, death occurred within the first hours (5% occurred within 15 minutes). Propoxyphene should not be taken in doses higher than those recommended by the physician. The judicious prescribing of propoxyphene is essential to the safe use of this drug. With patients who are depressed or suicidal, considerations should be given to the use of non-narcotic analgesics. Patients should be cautioned about the concomitant use of propoxyphene products and alcohol because of potentially serious CNS-additive effects of these agents. Because of its added depressant effects, propoxyphene should be prescribed with caution for those patients whose medical condition requires the concomitant administration of sedatives, tranquilizers, muscle relaxants, antidepressants, or other CNS-depressant drugs. Patients should be advised of the additive depressant effects of these combinations.

Many of the propoxyphene-related deaths have occurred in patients with previous histories of emotional disturbances or suicidal ideation or attempts as well as histories of misuse of tranquilizers, alcohol, and other CNS-ac-

WARNINGS: *(cont'd)*

tive drugs. Some deaths have occurred as a consequence of the accidental ingestion of excessive quantities of propoxyphene alone or in combination with other drugs. Patients taking propoxyphene should be warned not to exceed the dosage recommended by the physician.

Usage in Ambulatory Patients: Propoxyphene may impair the mental and/or physical abilities required for the performance of potentially hazardous tasks, such as driving a car or operating machinery. The patient should be cautioned accordingly.

PRECAUTIONS:

General: Propoxyphene should be administered with caution to patients with hepatic or renal impairment since higher serum concentrations or delayed elimination may occur.

Usage in Pregnancy: Safe use in pregnancy has not been established relative to possible adverse effects on fetal development. Instances of withdrawal symptoms in the neonate have been reported following usage during pregnancy. Therefore, propoxyphene should not be used in pregnant women unless, in the judgment of the physician, the potential benefits outweigh the possible hazards.

Usage in Nursing Mothers: Low levels of propoxyphene have been detected in human milk. In postpartum studies involving nursing mothers who were given propoxyphene, no adverse effects were noted in infants receiving mother's milk.

Usage in Children: Propoxyphene is not recommended for use in children, because documented clinical experience has been insufficient to establish safety and a suitable dosage regimen in the pediatric age group.

Geriatric Use: The rate of propoxyphene metabolism may be reduced in some patients. Increased dosing interval should be considered.

DRUG INTERACTIONS:

The CNS-depressant effect of propoxyphene is additive with that of other CNS depressants, including alcohol.

As is the case with many medicinal agents, propoxyphene may slow the metabolism of a concomitantly administered drug. Should this occur, the higher serum concentrations of that drug may result in increased pharmacologic or adverse effects of that drug. Such occurrences have been reported when propoxyphene was administered to patients on antidepressants, anticonvulsants, or warfarin-like drugs. Sever neurologic signs, including coma, have occurred with concurrent use of carbamazepine.

ADVERSE REACTIONS:

In a survey conducted in hospitalized patients, less than 1% of patients taking propoxyphene hydrochloride at recommended doses experienced side effects. The most frequently reported have been dizziness, sedation, nausea, and vomiting. Some of these adverse reactions may be alleviated if the patient lies down.

Other adverse reactions include constipation, abdominal pain, skin rashes, lightheadedness, headache, weakness, euphoria, dysphoria, and minor visual disturbances.

Propoxyphene therapy has been associated with abnormal liver function tests, and, more rarely, with instances of reversible jaundice (including cholestatic jaundice).

Subacute painful myopathy has occurred following chronic propoxyphene overdosage.

DRUG ABUSE AND DEPENDENCE:

Propoxyphene, when taken in higher-than-recommended doses over long periods of time, can produce drug dependence characterized by psychic dependence and, less frequently, physical dependence and tolerance. Propoxyphene will only, partially suppress the withdrawal syndrome in individuals physically dependent on morphine or other narcotics. The abuse liability of propoxyphene is qualitatively similar to that of codeine although quantitatively less, and propoxyphene should be prescribed with the same degree of caution appropriate to the use of codeine.

OVERDOSAGE:

In all cases of suspected overdosage, call your regional Poison Control Center to obtain the most up-to-date information about the treatment of overdosage. This recommendation is made because, in general, information regarding the treatment of overdosage may change more rapidly than do package inserts.

Initial consideration should be given to the management of the CNS effects of propoxyphene overdosage. Resuscitative measures should be initiated promptly.

Symptoms of Propoxyphene Overdosage: The manifestations of acute overdosage with propoxyphene are those of narcotic overdosage. The patient is usually somnolent but may be stuporous or comatose and convulsing. Respiratory depression is characteristic. The ventilatory rate and/or tidal volume is decreased, which results in cyanosis and hypoxia. Pupils, initially pinpoint, may become dilated as hypoxia increases. Cheyne-Stokes respiration and apnea may occur. Blood pressure and heart rate are usually normal initially, but blood pressure falls and cardiac performance deteriorates, which ultimately results in pulmonary edema and circulatory collapse, unless the respiratory depression is corrected and adequate ventilation is restored promptly, Cardiac arrhythmias and conduction delay may be present. A combined respiratory-metabolic acidosis occurs owing to retained CO_2 (hypercapnia) and to lactic acid formed during anaerobic glycolysis. Acidosis may be severe if large amounts of salicylates have also been ingested. Death may occur.

Treatment of Propoxyphene Overdosage: Attention should be directed first to establish a patent airway and to restoring ventilation. Mechanically assisted ventilation, with or without oxygen, may be required, and positive pressure respiration may be desirable if pulmonary edema is present. The narcotic antagonist naloxone will markedly reduce the degree of respiratory depression, and 0.4 to 2 mg should be administered promptly, preferably intravenously. If the desired degree of counteraction with improvement in respiratory functions is not obtained, naloxone should be repeated at 2 to 3-minute intervals. The duration of action of the antagonist may be brief. If no response is observed after 10 mg of naloxone have been administered, the diagnosis of propoxyphene toxicity should be questioned. Naloxone may also be administered by continuous intravenous infusion.

Treatment of Propoxyphene Overdosage in Children: The usual initial dose of naloxone in children is 0.01 mg/kg body weight given intravenously, If this dose does not result in the desired degree of clinical improvement, a subsequent increased dose of 0.1 mg/kg body weight may be administered. If an IV route of administration is not available, naloxone may be administered IM or subcutaneously in divided doses. If necessary, naloxone can be diluted with sterile water for injection.

Blood gases, pH, and electrolytes should be monitored in order that acidosis and any electrolyte disturbance present may be corrected promptly. Acidosis, hypoxia, and generalized CNS depression predispose to the development of cardiac arrhythmias. Ventricular fibrillation or cardiac arrest may occur and necessitate the full complement of cardiopulmonary resuscitation (CPR) measures. Respiratory acidosis rapidly subsides as ventilation is restored and hypercapnia eliminated, but lactic acidosis may require intravenous bicarbonate for prompt correction.

OVERDOSAGE: *(cont'd)*

Electrocardiographic monitoring is essential. Prompt correction of hypoxia, acidosis, and electrolyte disturbance (when present) will help prevent these cardiac complications and will increase the effectiveness of agents administered to restore normal cardiac function.

In addition to the use of a narcotic antagonist, the patient may require careful titration with an anticonvulsant to control convulsions. Analeptic drug (for example, caffeine or amphetamine) should not be used because of their tendency to precipitate convulsions.

General supportive measures, in addition to oxygen, include, when necessary, intravenous fluids, vasopressor-inotropic compounds, and, when infection is likely, anti-infective agents. Gastric lavage may be useful, and activated charcoal can adsorb a significant amount of ingested propoxyphene. Dialysis is of little value in poisoning due to propoxyphene. Efforts should be made to determine whether other agents, such as alcohol, barbiturates, tranquilizers, or other CNS depressants, were also ingested, since these increase CNS depressions as well as cause specific toxic effects.

Store at controlled room temperature, 59° to 86°F (15° to 30°C).

DOSAGE AND ADMINISTRATION:

Propoxyphene hydrochloride is given orally. The usual dosage is 65 mg propoxyphene hydrochloride every 4 hours as needed for pain. The maximum recommended dose of propoxyphene hydrochloride is 390 mg/day.

Consideration should be given to a reduced total daily dosage in patients with hepatic or renal impairment.

HOW SUPPLIED - RATED THERAPEUTICALLY EQUIVALENT:

Capsule, Gelatin - Oral - 65 mg

100's	$2.25	Propoxyphene Hydrochloride, Anabolic	00722-5374-01
100's	$2.50	Propoxyphene HCl, West Ward Pharm	00143-3235-01
100's	$4.88	Propoxyphene HCl, H.C.F.A. F F P	99999-2133-01
100's	$5.48	Propoxyphene Hcl, Geneva Pharms	00781-2140-01
100's	$6.10	BLUE CROSS PROPHENE 65, Halsey Drug	00879-0155-01
100's	$6.61	Propoxyphene Hcl, Qualitest Pharms	00603-5459-21
100's	$6.65	Propoxyphene Hcl, Major Pharms	00904-7700-60
100's	$6.65	Propoxyphene Hcl, Harber Pharm	51432-0388-03
100's	$7.32	Propoxyphene Hcl, Geneva Pharms	00781-2140-13
100's	$7.35	Propoxyphene HCl, Teva	00093-0741-01
100's	$7.35	Propoxyphene Hcl, United Res	00677-0356-01
100's	$7.40	Propoxyphene Hcl, Zenith Labs	00172-2186-60
100's	$7.40	Propoxyphene Hcl, Goldline Labs	00182-0698-01
100's	$7.40	Propoxyphene Hcl, Purepac Pharm	00228-2082-10
100's	$7.48	Propoxyphene Hcl, Aligen Independ	00405-0175-01
100's	$8.35	Propoxyphene HCl, Rugby	00536-4382-01
100's	$8.37	Propoxyphene Hcl, HL Moore Drug Exch	00839-5098-06
100's	$8.60	Propoxyphene HCl, Schein Pharm (US)	00364-0312-01
100's	$8.60	Propoxyphene Hcl, Mylan	00378-0129-01
100's	$8.63	Propoxyphene Hcl, IDE-Interstate	00814-6457-14
100's	$9.30	Propoxyphene Hcl, Vangard Labs	00615-0439-13
100's	$29.96	Propoxyphene Hcl, Major Pharms	00904-7700-61
100's	**$34.38**	**DARVON, Lilly**	**00002-0803-02**
100's	**$38.76**	**DARVON, Lilly**	**00002-0803-33**
250's	$36.73	Propoxyphene Hcl, Roxane	00054-8732-11
500's	$8.95	Propoxyphene Hydrochloride, Anabolic	00722-5374-02
500's	$9.50	Propoxyphene HCl, West Ward Pharm	00143-3235-05
500's	$21.25	Propoxyphene Hcl, Harber Pharm	51432-0388-05
500's	$21.75	Propoxyphene Hcl, Major Pharms	00904-7700-40
500's	$22.80	Propoxyphene Hcl, United Res	00677-0356-05
500's	$22.94	Propoxyphene Hcl, HL Moore Drug Exch	00839-5098-12
500's	$23.11	Propoxyphene Hcl, Qualitest Pharms	00603-5459-28
500's	$24.40	Propoxyphene HCl, H.C.F.A. F F P	99999-2133-02
500's	$25.60	Propoxyphene Hcl, Zenith Labs	00172-2186-70
500's	$25.60	Propoxyphene Hcl, Goldline Labs	00182-0698-05
500's	$26.60	BLUE CROSS PROPHENE 65, Halsey Drug	00879-0155-05
500's	$26.95	Propoxyphene HCl, Rugby	00536-4382-05
500's	$27.30	Propoxyphene HCl, Teva	00093-0741-05
500's	$30.23	Propoxyphene Hcl, IDE-Interstate	00814-6457-28
500's	$33.40	Propoxyphene HCl, Schein Pharm (US)	00364-0312-05
500's	$33.50	Propoxyphene Hcl, Mylan	00378-0129-05
500's	$34.78	Propoxyphene Hcl, Aligen Independ	00405-0175-02
500's	$37.00	Propoxyphene Hcl, Purepac Pharm	00228-2082-50
500's	**$163.34**	**DARVON, Lilly**	**00002-0803-46**
500's	**$164.20**	**DARVON, Lilly**	**00002-0803-03**
1000's	$18.00	Propxyphene HCl, West Ward Pharm	00143-3235-10
1000's	$39.75	Propoxyphene Hcl, Major Pharms	00904-7700-80
1000's	$44.00	Propoxyphene Hcl, United Res	00677-0356-10
1000's	$46.56	Propoxyphene Hcl, Geneva Pharms	00781-2140-10
1000's	$47.75	Propoxyphene HCl, Rugby	00536-4382-10
1000's	$48.40	Propoxyphene HCl, Teva	00093-0741-10
1000's	$48.80	Propoxyphene HCl, H.C.F.A. F F P	99999-2133-03
1000's	$48.87	Propoxyphene Hcl, HL Moore Drug Exch	00839-5098-16
1000's	$48.90	Propoxyphene Hcl, Zenith Labs	00172-2186-80
1000's	$48.90	Propoxyphene Hcl, Goldline Labs	00182-0698-10
1000's	$49.20	BLUE CROSS PROPHENE 65, Halsey Drug	00879-0155-10

PROPOXYPHENE NAPSYLATE *(002134)*

CATEGORIES: Analgesics; Antipyretics; Central Nervous System Agents; Narcotic Analgesics; Narcotics, Synthetics & Combinations; Opiate Agonists (Controlled); Pain; DEA Class CIV; FDA Approval Pre 1982

BRAND NAMES: **Darvon-N**; *Doloxene*
(International brand names outside U.S. in italics)

FORMULARIES: Aetna; BC-BS

DESCRIPTION:

Propoxyphene napsylate, USP is an odorless, white crystalline powder with a bitter taste. It is very slightly soluble in water and soluble in methanol, ethanol, chloroform, and acetone. Chemically, it is (αS,1*R*)-α-[2- (Dimethylamino) -1-methylethyl] -α- phenylphenethyl propionate compound with 2-naphthalenesulfonic acid (1:1) monohydrate. Its molecular weight is 565.72.

Propoxyphene napsylate differs from propoxyphene hydrochloride in that it allows more stable liquid dosage forms and tablet formulations. Because of differences in molecular weight, a dose of 100 mg (176.8 μmol) of propoxyphene napsylate is required to supply an amount of propoxyphene equivalent to that present in 65 mg (172.9 μmol) of propoxyphene hydrochloride.

Each tablet of propoxyphene napsylate contains 100 mg (176.8 μmol) propoxyphene napsylate. The tablet also contains cellulose, cornstarch, iron oxides, lactose, magnesium stearate, silicon dioxide, stearic acid, and titanium dioxide.

CLINICAL PHARMACOLOGY:

Propoxyphene is a centrally acting narcotic analgesic agent. Equimolar doses of propoxyphene hydrochloride or napsylate provide similar plasma concentrations. Following administration of 65, 130, or 195 mg of propoxyphene hydrochloride, the bioavailability of propoxyphene is equivalent to that of 100, 200, or 300 mg respectively of propoxyphene napsylate. Peak plasma concentrations of propoxyphene are reached in 2 to 2 1/2 hours. After a 100-mg oral dose of propoxyphene napsylate, peak plasma levels of 0.05 to 0.1 mcg/ml are achieved. The napsylate salt tends to be absorbed more slowly than the hydrochloride. At or near therapeutic doses, this difference is small when compared with that among subjects and among doses.

Because of this several hundredfold difference in solubility, the absorption rate of very large doses of the napsylate salt is significantly lower than that of equimolar doses of the hydrochloride.

Repeated doses of propoxyphene at 6-hour intervals lead to increasing plasma concentrations, with a plateau after the ninth dose at 48 hours.

Propoxyphene is metabolized in the liver to yield norpropoxyphene. Propoxyphene has a half-life of 6 to 12 hours, whereas that of norpropoxyphene is 30 to 36 hours.

Norpropoxyphene has substantially less central-nervous-system-depressant effect than propoxyphene but a greater local anesthetic effect, which is similar to that of amitriptyline and antiarrhythmic agents, such as lidocaine and quinidine.

In animal studies in which propoxyphene and norpropoxyphene were continuously infused in large amounts, intracardiac conduction time (PR and QRS intervals) was prolonged. Any intracardiac conduction delay attributable to high concentrations of norpropoxyphene may be of relatively long duration.

Propoxyphene is a mild narcotic analgesic structurally related to methadone. The potency of propoxyphene napsylate is from two thirds to equal that of codeine.

INDICATIONS AND USAGE:

For the relief of mild to moderate pain.

CONTRAINDICATIONS:

Hypersensitivity to propoxyphene.

WARNINGS:

Do not prescribe propoxyphene for patients who are suicidal or addiction-prone.

Prescribe propoxyphene with caution for patients taking tranquilizers or antidepressant drugs and patients who use alcohol in excess.

Tell your patients not to exceed the recommended dose and to limit their intake of alcohol.

Propoxyphene products in excessive doses, either alone or in combination with other CNS depressants, including alcohol, are a major cause of drug-related deaths. Fatalities within the first hour of overdosage are not uncommon. In a survey of deaths due to overdosage conducted in 1975, in approximately 20% of the fatal cases, death occurred within the first hour (5% occurred within 15 minutes). Propoxyphene should not be taken in doses higher than those recommended by the physician. The judicious prescribing of propoxyphene is essential to the safe use of this drug. With patients who are depressed or suicidal, consideration should be given to the use of non-narcotic analgesics. Patients should be cautioned about the concomitant use of propoxyphene products and alcohol because of potentially serious CNS-additive effects of these agents. Because of its added depressant effects, propoxyphene should be prescribed with caution for those patients whose medical condition requires the concomitant administration of sedatives, tranquilizers, muscle relaxants, antidepressants, or other CNS-depressant drugs. Patients should be advised of the additive depressant effects of these combinations.

Many of the propoxyphene-related deaths have occurred in patients with previous histories of emotional disturbances or suicidal ideation or attempts as well as histories of misuse of tranquilizers, alcohol, and other CNS-active drugs. Some deaths have occurred as a consequence of the accidental ingestion of excessive quantities of propoxyphene alone or in combination with other drugs. Patients taking propoxyphene should be warned not to exceed the dosage recommended by the physician.

Drug Dependence: Propoxyphene, when taken in higher-than -recommendeddoses over long periods of time, can produce drug dependence characterized by psychic dependence and, less frequently, physical dependence and tolerance. Propoxyphene will only partially suppress the withdrawal syndrome in individuals physically dependent on morphine or other narcotics. The abuse liability of propoxyphene is qualitatively similar to that of codeine although quantitatively less, and propoxyphene should be prescribed with the same degree of caution appropriate to the use of codeine.

Usage in Ambulatory Patients: Propoxyphene may impair the mental and/or physical abilities required for the performance of potentially hazardous tasks, such as driving a car or operating machinery. The patient should be cautioned accordingly.

PRECAUTIONS:

General: Propoxyphene should be administered with caution to patients with hepatic or renal impairment since higher serum concentrations or delayed elimination may occur.

Usage in Pregnancy: Safe use in pregnancy has not been established relative to possible adverse effects on fetal development. Instances of withdrawal symptoms in the neonate have been reported following usage during pregnancy. Therefore, propoxyphene should not be used in pregnant women unless, in the judgment of the physician, the potential benefits outweigh the possible hazards.

Usage in Nursing Mothers: Low levels of propoxyphene have been detected in human milk. In postpartum studies involving nursing mothers who were given propoxyphene, no adverse effects were noted in infants receiving mother's milk.

Usage in Children: Propoxyphene is not recommended for use in children, because documented clinical experience has been insufficient to establish safety and a suitable dosage regimen in the pediatric age group.

Geriatric Use: The rate of propoxyphene metabolism may be reduced in some patients. Increased dosing interval should be considered.

A Patient Information Sheet is available for this product. See PATIENT PACKAGE INSERT below.

DRUG INTERACTIONS:

The CNS-depressant effect of propoxyphene is additive with that of other CNS depressants, including alcohol.

As is the case with many medicinal agents, propoxyphene may slow the metabolism of a concomitantly administered drug. Should this occur, the higher serum concentrations of that drug may result in increased pharmacologic or adverse effects of that drug. Such occurrences have been reported when propoxyphene was administered to patients on antidepressants, anticonvulsants, or warfarin-like drugs. Severe neurologic signs, including coma, have occurred with concurrent use of carbamazepine.

ADVERSE REACTIONS:

In a survey conducted in hospitalized patients, less than 1% of patients taking propoxyphene hydrochloride at recommended doses experienced side effects. The most frequently reported were dizziness, sedation, nausea, and vomiting. Some of these adverse reactions may be alleviated if the patient lies down.

Other adverse reactions include constipation, abdominal pain, skin rashes, lightheadedness, headache, weakness, euphoria, dysphoria, hallucinations, and minor visual disturbances.

Propoxyphene therapy has been associated with abnormal liver function tests and, more rarely, with instances of reversible jaundice (including cholestatic jaundice).

Subacute painful myopathy has occurred following chronic propoxyphene overdosage.

OVERDOSAGE:

In all cases of suspected overdosage, call your regional Poison Control Center to obtain the most up-to-date information about the treatment of overdose. Telephone numbers of certified poison control centers are listed at the beginning of Physicians GenRx. This recommendation is made because, in general, information regarding the treatment of overdosage may change more rapidly than do package inserts.

Initial consideration should be given to the management of the CNS effects of propoxyphene overdosage. Resuscitative measures should be initiated promptly.

Symptoms of Propoxyphene Overdosage: The manifestations of acute overdosage with propoxyphene are those of narcotic overdosage. The patient is usually somnolent but may be stuporous or comatose and convulsing. Respiratory depression is characteristic. The ventilatory rate and/or tidal volume is decreased, which results in cyanosis and hypoxia. Pupils, initially pinpoint, may become dilated as hypoxia increases. Cheyne-Stokes respiration and apnea may occur. Blood pressure and heart rate are usually normal initially, but blood pressure falls and cardiac performance deteriorates, which ultimately results in pulmonary edema and circulatory collapse, unless the respiratory depression is corrected and adequate ventilation is restored promptly. Cardiac arrhythmias and conduction delay may be present. A combined respiratory-metabolic acidosis occurs owing to retained CO_2(hypercapnia) and to lactic acid formed during anaerobic glycolysis. Acidosis may be severe if large amounts of salicylates have also been ingested. Death may occur.

Treatment of Propoxyphene Overdosage: Attention should be directed first to establishing a patent airway and to restoring ventilation. Mechanically assisted ventilation, with or without oxygen, may be required, and positive pressure respiration may be desirable if pulmonary edema is present. The narcotic antagonist naloxone will markedly reduce the degree of respiratory depression, and 0.4 to 2 mg should be administered promptly, preferably intravenously. If the desired degree of counteraction with improvement in respiratory functions is not obtained, naloxone should be repeated at 2- to 3- minute intervals. The duration of action of the antagonist may be brief. If no response is observed after 10 mg of naloxone have been administered, the diagnosis of propoxyphene toxicity should be questioned. Naloxone may also be administered by continuous intravenous infusion.

Treatment of Propoxyphene Overdosage in Children: The usual initial dose of naloxone in children is 0.01 mg/kg body weight given intravenously. If this dose does not result in the desired degree of clinical improvement, a subsequent increased dose of 0.1 mg/kg body weight may be administered. If an IV route of administration is not available, naloxone may be administered IM or subcutaneously in divided doses. If necessary, naloxone can be diluted with Sterile Water for Injection.

Blood gases, pH, and electrolytes should be monitored in order that acidosis and any electrolyte disturbance present may be corrected promptly. Acidosis, hypoxia, and generalized CNS depression predispose to the development of cardiac arrhythmias. Ventricular fibrillation or cardiac arrest may occur and necessitate the full complement of cardiopulmonary resuscitation (CPR) measures. Respiratory acidosis rapidly subsides as ventilation is restored and hypercapnia eliminated, but lactic acidosis may require intravenous bicarbonate for prompt correction.

Electrocardiographic monitoring is essential. Prompt correction of hypoxia, acidosis, and electrolyte disturbance (when present) will help prevent these cardiac complications and will increase the effectiveness of agents administered to restore normal cardiac function.

In addition to the use of a narcotic antagonist, the patient may require careful titration with an anticonvulsant to control convulsions. Analeptic drugs (for example, caffeine or amphetamine) should not be used because of their tendency to precipitate convulsions.

General supportive measures, in addition to oxygen, include, when necessary, intravenous fluids, vasopressor-inotropic compounds, and, when infection is likely, anti-infective agents. Gastric lavage may be useful, and activated charcoal can adsorb a significant amount of ingested propoxyphene. Dialysis is of little value in poisoning due to propoxyphene. Efforts should be made to determine whether other agents, such as alcohol, barbiturates, tranquilizers, or other CNS depressants, were also ingested, since these increase CNS depression as well as cause specific toxic effects.

DOSAGE AND ADMINISTRATION:

Propoxyphene napsylate is given orally. The usual dosage is 100 mg propoxyphene napsylate every 4 hours as needed for pain. The maximum recommended dose of propoxyphene napsylate is 600 mg per day.

Consideration should be given to a reduced total daily dosage in patients with hepatic or renal impairment.

Store at controlled room temperature, 59° to 86°F (15° to 30°C).

ANIMAL PHARMACOLOGY:

Animal Toxicology: The acute lethal doses of the hydrochloride and napsylate salts of propoxyphene were determined in 4 species. The results shown in (TABLE 1) indicate that, on a molar basis, the napsylate salt is less toxic than the hydrochloride. This may be due to the relative insolubility and retarded absorption of propoxyphene napsylate.

Some indication of the relative insolubility and retarded absorption of propoxyphene napsylate was obtained by measuring plasma propoxyphene levels in 2 groups of 4 dogs following oral administration of equimolar doses of the 2 salts. The peak plasma concentration observed with propoxyphene hydrochloride was much higher than that obtained after administration of the napsylate salt.

ANIMAL PHARMACOLOGY: *(cont'd)*

TABLE 1 Acute Oral Toxicity of Propoxyphene

Species	LD50(mg/kg) ± SE LD50(mmol/kg) Propoxyphene Hydrochloride	Propoxyphene Napsylate
Mouse	282 ± 39 0.75	915 ± 163 1.62
Rat	230 ± 44 0.61	647 ± 95 1.14
Rabbit	ca 82 0.22	>183 >0.32
Dog	*ca* 100 0.27	>183 >0.32

Although none of the animals in this experiment died, 3 of the 4 dogs given propoxyphene hydrochloride exhibited convulsive seizures during the time interval corresponding to the peak plasma levels. The 4 animals receiving the napsylate salt were mildly ataxic but not acutely ill.

PATIENT PACKAGE INSERT:

Patient Information Sheet

YOUR PRESCRIPTION FOR A PROPOXYPHENE PRODUCT

Summary: Products containing propoxyphene napsylate are used to relieve pain.

LIMIT YOUR INTAKE OF ALCOHOL WHITE TAKING THIS DRUG. Make sure your doctor knows if you are taking tranquilizers, sleep aids, antidepressants, antihistamines, or any other drugs that make you sleepy. Combining propoxyphene with alcohol or these drug in excessive doses is dangerous.

Use care while driving a car or using machines until you see how the drug affects you because propoxyphene can make you sleepy. Do not take more of the drug than your doctor prescribed. Dependence has occurred when patients have taken propoxyphene for a long period of time at doses greater than recommended.

The rest of this leaflet gives you more information about propoxyphene. Please read it and keep it for future use.

Uses of Propoxyphene Napsylate: Products containing propoxyphene napsylate are used for the relief of mild to moderate pain. Products which contain propoxyphene napsylate plus aspirin or acetaminophen are prescribed for the relief of pain or pain associated with fever.

Before Taking Propoxyphene Napsylate: Make sure your doctor knows if you have ever had an allergic reaction to propoxyphene, aspirin, or acetaminophen. Some forms of propoxyphene products contain aspirin to help relieve the pain. Your doctor should be advised if you have a history of ulcers or if you are taking an anticoagulant ("blood thinner"). The aspirin may irritate the stomach lining and may cause bleeding, particularly if an ulcer is present. Also, bleeding may occur if you are taking an anticoagulant. In a small group of people, aspirin may cause an asthma attack. If you are one of these people, be sure your drug does not contain aspirin.

The effect of propoxyphene in children under 12 has not been studied. Therefore, use of the drug in this age group is not recommended.

Also, due to the possible association between aspirin and Reye Syndrome, those propoxyphene products containing aspirin should not be given to children, including teenagers, with chicken pox or flu unless prescribed by a physician. The following propoxyphene product contains aspirin: Darvon Compound-65 (Propoxyphene Hydrochloride, Aspirin, and Caffeine, USP)

How to Take Propoxyphene Napsylate: Follow your doctor's directions exactly. Do not increase the amount you take without your doctor's approval. If you miss a dose of the drug, do not take twice as much the next time.

Pregnancy: Do not take propoxyphene during pregnancy unless your doctor knows you are pregnant and specifically recommends its use. Cases of temporary dependence in the newborn have occurred when the mother has taken propoxyphene consistently in the weeks before delivery. As a general principle, no drug should be taken during pregnancy unless it is clearly necessary.

General Cautions: Heavy use of alcohol with propoxyphene is hazardous and may lead to overdosage symptoms (see OVERDOSAGE.) THEREFORE, LIMIT YOUR INTAKE OF ALCOHOL WHILE TAKING PROPOXYPHENE.

Combinations of excessive doses of propoxyphene, alcohol, and tranquilizers are dangerous. Make sure your doctor knows you are taking tranquilizers, sleep aids, antidepressant drugs, antihistamines, or any other drugs that make you sleepy. The use of these drugs with propoxyphene increases their sedative effects and may lead to overdosage symptoms, including death (see OVERDOSAGE).

Propoxyphene may cause drowsiness or impair your mental and/or physical abilities; therefore, use caution when driving a vehicle or operating dangerous machinery. DO NOT perform any hazardous task until you have seen your response to this drug.

Propoxyphene may increase the concentration in the body of medications, such as anticoagulants ("blood thinners"), antidepressants, or drugs used for epilepsy. The result may be excessive or adverse effects of these medications. Make sure your doctor knows if your are taking any of these medications.

Dependence: You can become dependent on propoxyphene if you take it in higher than recommended doses over a long period of time. Dependence is a feeling of need for the drug and a feeling that you cannot perform normally without it.

Overdose: An overdose of propoxyphene napsylate, alone or in combination with other drugs, including alcohol, may cause weakness, difficulty in breathing, confusion, anxiety, and more severe drowsiness and dizziness. Extreme overdosage may lead to unconsciousness and death.

If the propoxyphene product contains acetaminophen, the overdosage symptoms include nausea, vomiting, lack of appetite, and abdominal pain. Liver damage may occur.

When the propoxyphene product contains aspirin, symptoms of taking too much of the drug are headache, dizziness, ringing in the ears, difficulty in hearing, dim vision, confusion, drowsiness, sweating, thirst, rapid breathing, nausea, vomiting, and, occasionally, diarrhea.

In any suspected overdosage situation, contact your doctor or nearest hospital emergency room. GET EMERGENCY HELP IMMEDIATELY. KEEP THIS DRUG AND ALL DRUGS OUT OF THE REACH OF CHILDREN.

Possible Side Effects: When propoxyphene is taken as directed, side effects are infrequent. Among those reported are drowsiness, dizziness, nausea, and vomiting. If these effects occur, it may help if you lie down and rest.

Less frequently reported side effects are constipation, abdominal pain, skin rashes, lightheadedness, headache, weakness, hallucinations, minor visual disturbances, and feelings of elation or discomfort.

If side effects occur and concern you, contact your doctor.

PATIENT PACKAGE INSERT: *(cont'd)*

Other Information: The safe and effective use of propoxyphene depends on your taking it exactly as directed. This drug has been prescribed specifically for you and your present condition. Do not give this drug to others who may have similar symptoms. Do not use it for any other reason.

If you would like more information about propoxyphene, ask your doctor or pharmacist. They have a more technical leaflet (professional labeling) you may read.

HOW SUPPLIED:

Darvon: 100 mg, buff (No. 1883)

HOW SUPPLIED - RATED THERAPEUTICALLY EQUIVALENT:

Tablet, Uncoated - Oral - 50 mg

500's	$65.00	Propoxyphene Napsylate/APAP, Halsey Drug	00879-0610-05
1000's	$123.00	Propoxyphene Napsylate And APAP Tabl, Halsey Drug	00879-0610-10

HOW SUPPLIED - NOT RATED EQUIVALENT:

Tablet, Uncoated - Oral - 100 mg

100's	**$50.03**	**DARVON-N, Lilly**	**00002-0353-02**
100's	**$54.41**	**DARVON-N, Lilly**	**00002-0353-33**
500's	**$236.50**	**DARVON-N, Lilly**	**00002-0353-03**

PROPRANOLOL HYDROCHLORIDE *(002135)*

CATEGORIES: Anesthesia; Angina; Antianginals; Antiarrhythmic Agents; Antihypertensives; Arrhythmia; Atherosclerosis; Beta Adrenergic Blocking Agents; Beta Blockers; Bradycardia; Cardiovascular Drugs; Headache; Heart Flutter; Hypertension; Migraine; Myocardial Infarction; Neuromuscular; Pheochromocytoma; Tachyarrhythmias; Tachycardia; Tremor; Alcohol Withdrawal*; Agoraphobia*; Anxiety*; Depression*; Dementia*; Extrapyramidal Movement Disorders*; Panic Disorder*; Performance Anxiety*; Psychotic Disorders*; Shock*; Stenosis*; Syncope*; Thyrotoxicosis*; Vertigo/Motion Sickness/Vomiting*; Pregnancy Category C; Sales > $500 Million; FDA Approval Pre 1982

* Indication not approved by the FDA

BRAND NAMES: *Acifol*; *Angilol*; *Apsolol*; *Arcablock*; *Artensol*; *Atensin*; *Beprane*; *Berkolol*; *Betabloc*; *Biocard*; *Blocaryl*; *Cardinol*; *Caridolol*; *Cinlol*; *Ciplar*; *Corbeta*; *Deralin*; *Detensol*; *Dibudinate*; *Dociton*; *Duranol*; *Elbrol*; *Emforal*; *Farprolol*; *Herzul*; *Impral*; **Inderal**; Inderal LA; *Inderex*; *Indobloc*; *Indon*; *Kidoral*; Lorol; *Nelderal*; *Noloten*; *Novopranol*; *Oposim*; *Procor*; *Prolol*; Pronol; *Propadex*; *Propalong*; *Propayerst*; *Prosin*; *Pylapron*; *Rexigen*; *Sagittol*; *Sawatol*; *Scandrug*; *Sinal*; *Sloprolol*; *Sudenol*; *Sumial*; *Tensiflex*; *Tesnol*

(International brand names outside U.S. in italics)

FORMULARIES: Aetna; BC-BS; CIGNA; DoD; FHP; Foundation; Humana; Kaiser; Medco; Medi-Cal; PCS; PruCare; United; WHO

COST OF THERAPY: $14.89 (Hypertension; Tablet; 40 mg; 2/day; 365 days) vs. Potential Cost of $24,027.04 (Coronary Bypass)

PRIMARY ICD9: 401.1 (Essential Hypertension, Benign)

DESCRIPTION:

Propranolol hydrochloride (abbreviated here as Propranolol HCl) is a synthetic beta-adrenergic receptor blocking agent chemically described as 1- (Isopropylamino)-3-(1-naphthyloxy)-2-propanol hydrochloride.

Propranolol hydrochloride is a stable, white, crystalline solid which is readily soluble in water and ethanol. Its molecular weight is 295.81.

Propranolol HCl is available as 10 mg, 20 mg, 40 mg, 60 mg, and 80 mg tablets for oral administration and as a 1 mg/ml sterile injectable solution for intravenous administration.

The inactive ingredients contained in Propranolol HCl Tablets are: lactose, magnesium stearate, microcrystalline cellulose, and stearic acid. In addition, Propranolol HCl 10 mg and 80 mg Tablets contain FD&C Yellow No. 6 and D&C Yellow No. 10; Propranolol HCl 20 mg Tablets contain FD&C Blue No. 1; Propranolol HCl 40 mg Tablets contain FD&C Blue No. 1, FD&C Yellow No. 6, and D&C Yellow No. 10; Propranolol HCl 60 mg Tablets contain D&C Red No. 30.

CLINICAL PHARMACOLOGY:

Propranolol HCl is a nonselective beta-adrenergic receptor blocking agent possessing no other autonomic nervous system activity. It specifically competes with beta-adrenergic receptor stimulating agents for available receptor sites. When access to beta-receptor sites is blocked by Propranolol HCl, the chronotropic, inotropic, and vasodilator responses to beta-adrenergic stimulation are decreased proportionately.

Propranolol is almost completely absorbed from the gastrointestinal tract, but a portion is immediately bound by the liver. Peak effect occurs in one to one-and-one-half hours. The biologic half-life is approximately four hours.

There is no simple correlation between dose or plasma level and therapeutic effect, and the dose-sensitivity range as observed in clinical practice is wide. The principal reason for this is that sympathetic tone varies widely between individuals. Since there is no reliable test to estimate sympathetic tone or to determine whether total beta blockade has been achieved, proper dosage requires titration.

The mechanism of the antihypertensive effect of Propranolol HCl has not been established. Among the factors that may be involved in contributing to the antihypertensive action are (1) decreased cardiac output, (2) inhibition of renin release by the kidneys, and (3) diminution of tonic sympathetic nerve outflow from vasomotor centers in the brain. Although total peripheral resistance may increase initially, it readjusts to or below the pretreatment level with chronic use. Effects on plasma volume appear to be minor and somewhat variable. Propranolol HCl has been shown to cause a small increase in serum potassium concentration when used in the treatment of hypertensive patients.

In angina pectoris, propranolol generally reduces the oxygen requirement of the heart at any given level of effort by blocking the catecholamine-induced increases in the heart rate, systolic blood pressure, and the velocity and extent of myocardial contraction. Propranolol may increase oxygen requirements by increasing left ventricular fiber length, end diastolic pressure, and systolic ejection period. The net physiologic effect of beta-adrenergic blockade is usually advantageous and is manifested during exercise by delayed onset of pain and increased work capacity.

Propranolol exerts its antiarrhythmic effects in concentrations associated with beta-adrenergic blockade, and this appears to be its principal antiarrhythmic mechanism of action. In dosages greater than required for beta blockade, Propranolol HCl also exerts a quinidine-like or anesthetic-like membrane action, which affects the cardiac action potential. The significance of the membrane action in the treatment of arrhythmias is uncertain.

CLINICAL PHARMACOLOGY: *(cont'd)*

The mechanism of the antimigraine effect of propranolol has not been established. Beta-adrenergic receptors have been demonstrated in the pial vessels of the brain.

The specific mechanism of Propranolol HCl's antitremor effects has not been established, but beta-2 (noncardiac) receptors may be involved. A central effect is also possible. Clinical studies have demonstrated that Propranolol HCl is of benefit in exaggerated physiological and essential (familial) tremor.

Beta-receptor blockade can be useful in conditions in which, because of pathologic or functional changes, sympathetic activity is detrimental to the patient. But there are also situations in which sympathetic stimulation is vital. For example, in patients with severely damaged hearts, adequate ventricular function is maintained by virtue of sympathetic drive, which should be preserved. In the presence of AV block greater than first degree, beta blockade may prevent the necessary facilitating effect of sympathetic activity on conduction. Beta blockade results in bronchial constriction by interfering with adrenergic bronchodilator activity, which should be preserved in patients subject to bronchospasm.

Propranolol is not significantly dialyzable.

The Beta-Blocker Heart Attack Trial (BHAT) was a National Heart, Lung and Blood Institute-sponsored multicenter, randomized, double-blind, placebo-controlled trial conducted in 31 U.S. centers (plus one in Canada) in 3,837 persons without history of severe congestive heart failure or presence of recent heart failure; certain conduction defects; angina since infarction, who had survived the acute phase of myocardial infarction. Propranolol was administered at either 60 or 80 mg t.i.d. based on blood levels achieved during an initial trial of 40 mg t.i.d. Therapy with Propranolol HCl, begun 5 to 21 days following infarction, was shown to reduce overall mortality up to 39 months, the longest period of follow-up. This was primarily attributable to a reduction in cardiovascular mortality. The protective effect of Propranolol HCl was consistent regardless of age, sex, or site of infarction. Compared with placebo, total mortality was reduced 39% at 12 months and 26% over an average follow-up period of 25 months. The Norwegian Multicenter Trial in which propranolol was administered at 40 mg q.i.d. gave overall results which support the findings in the BHAT.

Although the clinical trials used either t.i.d. or q.i.d. dosing, clinical, pharmacologic, and pharmacokinetic data provide a reasonable basis for concluding that b.i.d. dosing with propranolol should be adequate in the treatment of postinfarction patients.

Clinical: In the BHAT, patients on Propranolol HCl were prescribed either 180 mg/day (82% of patients) or 240 mg/day (18% of patients). Patients were instructed to take the medication 3 times a day at mealtimes. This dosing schedule would result in an overnight dosing interval of 12 to 14 hours, which is similar to the dosing interval for a b.i.d. regimen. In addition, blood samples were drawn at various times and analyzed for propranolol. When the patients were grouped into tertiles based on the blood levels observed and the mortality in the upper and lower tertiles was compared, there was no evidence that blood levels affected mortality.

Pharmacologic: Studies in normal volunteers have shown that a 90 mg b.i.d. regimen maintains beta blockade at, or above, the minimum for 60 mg t.i.d. dosing for 24 hours even though differences occurred at two time intervals. At 10 to 12 hours after the first dose of the day, t.i.d. dosing gave more beta blockade than b.i.d. dosing; at 20 to 24 hours the trend of the relationship was reversed. These relationships were similar in direction to those observed for plasma propranolol levels. (See Pharmacokinetics)

Pharmacokinetics: A bioavailability study in normal volunteers showed that the blood levels produced by 180 mg/day given b.i.d. are below those provided by the same daily dosage given t.i.d. at 10 to 12 hours after the first dose of the day, but above those of a t.i.d. regimen at 20 to 24 hours. However, the blood levels produced by b.i.d. dosing were always equivalent to or above the minimum for t.i.d. dosing throughout the 24 hours. In addition, the mean AUC on the fourth day for the b.i.d. regimen was about 17% greater than for the t.i.d. regimen (1,194 *vs.* 1,024 ng/ml/hr).

INDICATIONS AND USAGE:

HYPERTENSION

Propranolol HCl is indicated in the management of hypertension. It may be used alone or used in combination with other antihypertensive agents, particularly a thiazide diuretic. Propranolol HCl is not indicated in the management of hypertensive emergencies.

ANGINA PECTORIS DUE TO CORONARY ATHEROSCLEROSISA

Propranolol HCl is indicated for the long-term management of patients with angina pectoris.

CARDIAC ARRHYTHMIAS

Supraventricular arrhythmias:

a) Paroxysmal atrial tachycardias, particularly those arrhythmias induced by catecholamines or digitalis or associated with the Wolff-Parkinson-White syndrome. (See WARNINGS)

b) Persistent sinus tachycardia which is noncompensatory and impairs the well-being of the patient.

c) Tachycardias and arrhythmias due to thyrotoxicosis when causing distress or increased hazard and when immediate effect is necessary as adjunctive, short-term (2 to 4 weeks) therapy. May be used with, but not in place of, specific therapy. (See WARNINGS)

d) Persistent atrial extrasystoles which impair the well-being of the patient and do not respond to conventional measures.

e) Atrial flutter and fibrillation when ventricular rate cannot be controlled by digitalis alone, or when digitalis is contraindicated.

Ventricular tachycardias:

Ventricular arrhythmias do not respond to propranolol as predictably as do the supraventricular arrhythmias.

a) Ventricular tachycardias: With the exception of those induced by catecholamines or digitalis, Propranolol HCl is not the drug of first choice. In critical situations when cardioversion techniques or other drugs are not indicated or are not effective, Propranolol HCl may be considered. If, after consideration of the risks involved, Propranolol HCl is used, it should be given intravenously in low dosage and very slowly. (See DOSAGE AND ADMINISTRATION.) *Care in the administration of Propranolol HCl with constant electrocardiographic monitoring is essential as the failing heart requires some sympathetic drive for maintenance of myocardial tone.*

b) Persistent premature ventricular extrasystoles which do not respond to conventional measures and impair the well-being of the patient.

Tachyarrhythmias of digitalis intoxication: If digitalis-induced tachyarrhythmias persist following discontinuance of digitalis and correction of electrolyte abnormalities, they are usually reversible with *oral* Propranolol HCl. Severe bradycardia may occur. (See OVERDOSAGE) Intravenous propranolol hydrochloride is reserved for life-threatening arrhythmias. Temporary maintenance with oral therapy may be indicated. (See DOSAGE AND ADMINISTRATION.)

Resistant tachyarrhythmias due to excessive catecholamine action during anesthesia: Tachyarrhythmias due to excessive catecholamine action during anesthesia may sometimes arise because of release of endogenous catecholamines or administration of catecholamines. When usual measures fail in such arrhythmias, Propranolol HCl may be given intravenously to abolish them. All general inhalation anesthetics produce some degree of myocardial depression. Therefore, when Propranolol HCl is used to treat arrhythmias during anesthesia, it should be used with extreme caution and constant ECG and central venous pressure monitoring. (See WARNINGS)

MYOCARDIAL INFARCTION

Propranolol HCl is indicated to reduce cardiovascular mortality in patients who have survived the acute phase of myocardial infarction and are clinically stable.

MIGRAINE

Propranolol HCl is indicated for the prophylaxis of common migraine headache. The efficacy of propranolol in the treatment of a migraine attack that has started has not been established, and propranolol is not indicated for such use.

ESSENTIAL TREMOR

Propranolol HCl is indicated in the management of familial or hereditary essential tremor. Familial or essential tremor consists of involuntary, rhythmic, oscillatory movements, usually limited to the upper limbs. It is absent at rest but occurs when the limb is held in a fixed posture or position against gravity and during active movement. Propranolol HCl causes a reduction in the tremor amplitude but not in the tremor frequency. Propranolol HCl is not indicated for the treatment of tremor associated with Parkinsonism.

HYPERTROPHIC SUBAORTIC STENOSIS

Propranolol HCl is useful in the management of hypertrophic subaortic stenosis, especially for treatment of exertional or other stress-induced angina, palpitations, and syncope. Propranolol HCl also improves exercise performance. The effectiveness of propranolol hydrochloride in this disease appears to be due to a reduction of the elevated outflow pressure gradient, which is exacerbated by beta-receptor stimulation. Clinical improvement may be temporary.

PHEOCHROMOCYTOMA

After primary treatment with an alpha-adrenergic blocking agent has been instituted, Propranolol HCl may be useful as *adjunctive* therapy if the control of tachycardia becomes necessary before of during surgery.

It is hazardous to use Propranolol HCl unless alpha-adrenergic blocking drugs are already in use, since this would predispose to serious blood pressure elevation. Blocking only the peripheral dilator (beta) action of epinephrine leaves its constrictor (alpha) action unopposed. In the event of hemorrhage or shock, there is a disadvantage in having both beta and alpha blockade since the combination prevents the increase in heart rate and peripheral vasoconstriction needed to maintain blood pressure.

With inoperable or metastatic pheochromocytoma, Propranolol HCl may be useful as an adjunct to the management of symptoms due to excessive beta-receptor stimulation.

CONTRAINDICATIONS:

Propranolol HCl is contraindicated in 1) cardiogenic shock, 2) sinus bradycardia and greater than first degree block, 3) bronchial asthma, 4) congestive heart failure (see WARNINGS) unless the failure is secondary to a tachyarrhythmia treatable with Propranolol HCl.

WARNINGS:

Cardiac Failure: Sympathetic stimulation may be a vital component supporting circulatory function in patients with congestive heart failure, and its inhibition by beta blockade may precipitate more severe failure. Although beta blockers should be avoided in overt congestive heart failure, if necessary, they can be used with close follow-up in patients with a history of failure who are well compensated and are receiving digitalis and diuretics. Beta-adrenergic blocking agents do not abolish the inotropic action of digitalis on heart muscle.

In Patients without a History of Heart Failure: Continued use of beta blockers can, in some cases, lead to cardiac failure. Therefore, at the first sign or symptom of heart failure, the patient should be digitalized and/or treated with diuretics, and the response observed closely, or Propranolol HCl should be discontinued (gradually, if possible).

In Patients With Angina Pectoris: There have been reports of exacerbation of angina and, in some cases, myocardial infarction, following *abrupt* discontinuance of Propranolol HCl therapy. Therefore, when discontinuance of Propranolol HCl is planned, the dosage should be gradually reduced over at least a few weeks and the patient should be cautioned against interruption or cessation of therapy without the physician's advice. If Propranolol HCl therapy is interrupted and exacerbation of angina occurs, it usually is advisable to reinstitute Propranolol HCl therapy and take other measures appropriate for the management of unstable angina pectoris. Since coronary artery disease may be unrecognized, it may be prudent to follow the above advice in patients considered at risk of having occult atherosclerotic heart disease who are given propranolol for other indications.

Nonallergic Bronchospasm: (*e.g.* chronic bronchitis, emphysema) PATIENTS WITH BRONCHOSPASTIC DISEASES SHOULD IN GENERAL NOT RECEIVE BETA BLOCKERS. Propranolol HCl should be administered with caution since it may block bronchodilation produced by endogenous and exogenous catecholamine stimulation of beta receptors.

Major Surgery: The necessity or desirability of withdrawal of beta-blocking therapy prior to major surgery is controversial. It should be noted, however, that the impaired ability of the heart to respond to reflex adrenergic stimuli may augment the risks of general anesthesia and surgical procedures.

Propranolol HCl, like other beta blockers, is a competitive inhibitor of beta-receptor agonists, and its effects can be reversed by administration of such agents, (*e.g.,* dobutamine or isoproterenol). However, such patients may be subject to protracted severe hypotension. Difficulty in starting and maintaining the heartbeat has also been reported with beta blockers.

Diabetes and Hypoglycemia: Beta blockers should be used with caution in diabetic patients if a beta-blocking agent is required. Beta blockers may mask tachycardia occurring with hypoglycemia, but other manifestations such as dizziness and sweating may not be significantly affected. Following insulin-induced hypoglycemia, propranolol may cause a delay in the recovery of blood glucose to normal levels.

Thyrotoxicosis: Beta blockade may mask certain clinical signs of hyperthyroidism. Therefore, abrupt withdrawal of propranolol may be followed by an exacerbation of symptoms of hyperthyroidism, including thyroid storm. Propranolol may change thyroid-function tests, increasing T_4 and reverse T_3 and decreasing T_3.

In Patients with Wolf-Parkinson-White Syndrome: Several cases have been reported in which, after propranolol, the tachycardia was replaced by a severe bradycardia requiring a demand pacemaker. In one case this resulted after an initial dose of 5 mg propranolol.

PRECAUTIONS:

General: Propranolol should be used with caution in patients with impaired hepatic or renal function. Propranolol HCl is not indicated for the treatment of hypertensive emergencies.

PRECAUTIONS: *(cont'd)*

Beta-adrenoreceptor blockade can cause reduction of intraocular pressure. Patients should be told that Propranolol HCl may interfere with the glaucoma screening test. Withdrawal may lead to a return of increased intraocular pressure.

Clinical Laboratory Test: Elevated blood urea levels in patients with severe heart disease, elevated serum transaminase, alkaline phosphatase, lactate dehydrogenase.

Carcinogenesis, Mutagenesis, and Impairment of Fertility: Long-term studies in animals have been conducted to evaluate toxic effects and carcinogenic potential. In 18-month studies, in both rats and mice, employing doses up to 150 mg/kg/day, there was no evidence of significant drug-induced toxicity. There were no drug-related tumorigenic effects at any of the dosage levels. Reproductive studies in animals did not show any impairment of fertility that was attributable to the drug.

Pregnancy Category C: In a series of reproduction and developmental toxicology studies, propranolol was given to rats at doses up to 150 mg/kg/day by gavage or in the diet throughout pregnancy and through lactation. In rats given 150 mg/kg/day (about 10 times the maximum recommended human dose) propranolol was embryotoxic (reduced litter sizes and increased resorption sites). In addition, an unexplained increase in neonatal toxicity (death) was noted at all dosage groups in some of the studies. Maternal toxicity (decreased body weight) was evident at 150 mg/kg/day. Propranolol also was given to rabbits at dosages up to 250 mg/kg/day (approximately 20 times the maximum recommended human dose) throughout pregnancy. No evidence of embryotoxicity was noted.

Teratogenicity was not noted in either species.

There are no adequate and well-controlled studies in pregnant women. Intertwine growth retardation has been reported in neonates whose mothers received propranolol during pregnancy. Neonates whose mothers are receiving propranolol at parturition have exhibited bradycardia, hypoglycemia and respiratory depression. Adequate facilities for monitoring these infants at birth should be available. Propranolol HCl should be used during pregnancy only if the potential benefit justifies the potential risk to the fetus.

Nursing Mothers: Propranolol HCl is excreted in human milk. Caution should be exercised when Propranolol HCl is administered to a nursing woman.

Pediatric Use: High serum propranolol levels have been noted in patients with Down's syndrome (trisomy 21), suggesting that the bioavailability of propranolol may be increased in patients with this condition. Evaluation of the effects of propranolol in children, relative to the drug's efficacy and safety, has not been as systematically performed as in adults. Information is available in the medical literature to allow fair estimates, and specific dosing information has been reasonably studied.

Cardiovascular diseases that are common to adults and children are generally as responsive to propranolol intervention in children as they are in adults.

Adverse reactions are also similar: for example, bronchospasm and congestive heart failure related to propranolol therapy have been reported in children and occur through the same mechanisms as previously described in adults.

The normal echocardiogram evolves through a series of changes as the heart matures during growth and development in children. Should echocardiography be used to monitor propranolol therapy in children, the age-related changes in the echocardiogram need to be borne in mind.

DRUG INTERACTIONS:

Patients receiving catecholamine-depleting drugs such as reserpine should be closely observed if Propranolol HCl is administered. The added catecholamine-blocking action may produce an excessive reduction of resting sympathetic nervous activity, which may result in hypotension, marked bradycardia, vertigo, syncopal attacks, or orthostatic hypotension.

Caution should be exercised when patients receiving a beta blocker are administered a calcium-channel blocking drug, especially intravenous verapamil, for both agents may depress myocardial contractility or atrioventricular conduction. On rare occasions, the concomitant intravenous use of a beta blocker and verapamil has resulted in serious adverse reactions, especially in patients with severe cardiomyopathy, congestive heart failure, or recent myocardial infarction.

Blunting of the antihypertensive effect of beta-adrenoceptor blocking agents by nonsteroidal anti-inflammatory drugs has been reported.

Hypotension and cardiac arrest have been reported with the concomitant use of propranolol and haloperidol.

Aluminum hydroxide gel: Greatly reduces intestinal absorption of propranolol.

Ethanol: Slows the rate of absorption of propranolol.

Phenytoin, phenobarbitone: and **rifampin** accelerate propranolol clearance.

Chlorpromazine: When used concomitantly with propranolol, results in increased plasma levels of both drugs.

Antipyrine: and **lidocaine** have reduced clearance when used concomitantly with propranolol.

Thyroxine: May result in a lower than expected T_3 concentration when used concomitantly with propranolol.

Cimetidine Decreases the hepatic metabolism of propranolol, delaying elimination and incre: asing blood levels.

Theophylline: Clearance is reduced when used concomitantly with propranolol.

ADVERSE REACTIONS:

Most adverse effects have been mild and transient and have rarely required the withdrawal of therapy.

Cardiovascular: Bradycardia; congestive heart failure; intensification of AV block; hypotension; paresthesia of hands; thrombocytopenic purpura; arterial insufficiency, usually of the Raynaud type.

Central Nervous System: Light-headedness; mental depression manifested by insomnia, lassitude, weakness, fatigue; reversible mental depression progressing to catatonia; visual disturbances; hallucinations, vivid dreams, an acute reversible syndrome characterized by disorientation for time and place, short-term memory loss, emotional lability, slightly clouded sensorium, and decreased performance on neuropsychometrics. Total daily doses above 160 mg (when administered as divided doses of greater than 80 mg each) may be associated with an increased incidence of fatigue, lethargy, and vivid dreams.

Gastrointestinal: Nausea, vomiting, epigastric distress, abdominal cramping, diarrhea, constipation, mesenteric arterial thrombosis, ischemic colitis.

Allergic: Pharyngitis and agranulocytosis, erythematous rash, fever combined with aching and sore throat, laryngospasm, and respiratory distress.

Respiratory: Bronchospasm.

Hematologic: Agranulocytosis, nonthrombocytopenic purpura, thrombocytopenic purpura.

Autoimmune: In extremely rare instances, systemic lupus erythematosus has been reported.

ADVERSE REACTIONS: *(cont'd)*

Miscellaneous: Alopecia, LE-like reactions, psoriasiform rashes, dry eyes, male impotence, and Peyronie's disease have been reported rarely. Oculomucocutaneous reactions involving the skin, serous membranes and conjunctivae reported for a beta blocker (practolol) have not been associated with propranolol.

OVERDOSAGE:

Propranolol HCl is not significantly dialyzable. In the event of overdosage or exaggerated response, the following measures should be employed:

General: If ingestion is or may have been recent, evacuate gastric contents, taking care to prevent pulmonary aspiration.

Bradycardia: ADMINISTER ATROPINE (0.25 mg to 1.0 mg); IF THERE IS NO RESPONSE TO VAGAL BLOCKADE, ADMINISTER ISOPROTERENOL CAUTIOUSLY.

Cardiac Failure: DIGITALIZATION AND DIURETICS.

Hypotension: VASOPRESSORS, (*e.g.,*LEVARTERENOL OR EPINEPHRINE (THERE IS EVIDENCE THAT EPINEPHRINE IS THE DRUG OF CHOICE)).

Bronchospasm: ADMINISTER ISOPROTERENOL AND AMINOPHYLLINE.

DOSAGE AND ADMINISTRATION:

ORAL

The dosage range for Propranolol HCl is different for each indication.

Hypertension: *Dosage must be individualized.* The usual initial dosage is 40 mg Propranolol HCl twice daily, whether used alone or added to a diuretic. Dosage may be increased gradually until adequate blood pressure control is achieved. The usual maintenance dosage is 120 mg to 240 mg per day. In some instances a dosage of 640 mg a day may be required. The time needed for full antihypertensive response to a given dosage is variable and may range from a few days to several weeks.

While twice-daily dosing is effective and can maintain a reduction in blood pressure throughout the day, some patients, especially when lower doses are used, may experience a modest rise in blood pressure toward the end of the 12-hour dosing interval. This can be evaluated by measuring blood pressure near the end of the dosing interval to determine whether satisfactory control is being maintained throughout the day. If control is not adequate, a larger dose, or 3-times-daily therapy may achieve better control.

Angina Pectoris: *Dosage must be individualized.*

Total daily doses of 80 mg to 320 mg, when administered orally, twice a day, three times a day, or four times a day, have been shown to increase exercise tolerance and to reduce ischemic changes in the ECG. If treatment is to be discontinued, reduce dosage gradually over a period of several weeks. (See WARNINGS)

Arrhythmias: 10 mg to 30 mg three or four times daily, before meals and at bedtime.

Myocardial Infarction: The recommended daily dosage is 180 mg to 240 mg per day in divided doses. Although a t.i.d. regimen was used in the Beta-Blocker Heart Attack Trial and a q.i.d. regimen in the Norwegian Multicenter Trial, there is a reasonable basis for the use of either a t.i.d. or b.i.d. regimen (see CLINICAL PHARMACOLOGY.) The effectiveness and safety of daily dosages greater than 240 mg for prevention of cardiac mortality have not been established. However, higher dosages may be needed to effectively treat coexisting diseases such as angina or hypertension (See DOSAGE AND ADMINISTRATION).

Migraine: *Dosage must be individualized.*

The initial oral dose is 80 mg Propranolol HCl daily in divided doses. The usual effective dose range is 160 mg to 240 mg per day. The dosage may be increased gradually to achieve optimum migraine prophylaxis. If a satisfactory response is not obtained within four to six weeks after reaching the maximum dose, Propranolol HCl therapy should be discontinued. It may be advisable to withdraw the drug gradually over a period of several weeks.

Essential Tremor: *Dosage must be individualized.*

The initial dosage is 40 mg Propranolol HCl twice daily. Optimum reduction of essential tremor is usually achieved with a dose of 120 mg per day. Occasionally, it may be necessary to administer 240 mg to 320 mg per day.

Hypertrophic Subaortic Stenosis: 20 mg to 40 mg three or four times daily, before meals and at bedtime.

Pheochromocytoma: *Preoperatively*—60 mg daily in divided doses for three days prior to surgery, concomitantly with an alpha-adrenergic blocking agent.

Management of inoperable tumor: 30 mg daily in divided doses.

Use in Children: Intravenous administration of Propranolol HCl is not recommended in children. Oral dosage for treating hypertension requires individual titration, beginning with a 1.0 mg per kg (body weight) per day dosage regimen (*i.e.,* 0.5 mg per kg b.i.d.).

The usual pediatric dosage range is 2 mg to 4 mg per kg per day in two equally divided doses (*i.e.,* 1.0 mg per kg b.i.d. to 2.0 mg per kg b.i.d.). Pediatric dosage calculated by weight (recommended) generally produces propranolol plasma levels in a therapeutic range similar to that in adults. On the other hand, pediatric doses calculated on the basis of body surface area (*not*recommended) usually result in plasma levels above the mean adult therapeutic range. Doses above 16 mg per kg per day should not be used in children. If treatment with Propranolol HCl is to be discontinued, a gradually decreasing dose titration over a 7- to 14-day period is necessary.

INTRAVENOUS

Parenteral drug products should be inspected visually for particulate matter and discoloration prior to administration, whenever solution and container permit. Intravenous administration is reserved for life-threatening arrhythmias or those occurring under anesthesia. The usual dose is from 1 mg to 3 mg administered under careful monitoring, (*e.g.,* electrocardiographic, central venous pressure). The rate of administration should not exceed 1 mg (1 ml) per minute to diminish the possibility of lowering blood pressure and causing cardiac standstill. Sufficient time should be allowed for the drug to reach the site of action even when a slow circulation is present. If necessary, a second dose may be given after two minutes. Thereafter, additional drug should not be given in less than four hours. Additional Propranolol HCl should not be given when the desired alteration in rate and/or rhythm is achieved.

Transference to oral therapy should be made as soon as possible.

The intravenous administration of Propranolol HCl has not been evaluated adequately in the management of hypertensive emergencies.

Store at room temperature (approximately 25° C). Dispense in well-closed, light-resistant containers.

HOW SUPPLIED - RATED THERAPEUTICALLY EQUIVALENT:

Capsule, Gelatin, Sustained Action - Oral - 60 mg

100's	$53.40	Propranolol Hcl, United Res	00677-1363-01
100's	$53.40	Propranolol HCl, H.C.F.A. F F P	99999-2135-01
100's	$62.55	Propranolol Hcl, Major Pharms	00904-0421-60
100's	$64.91	Propranolol Hcl, Qualitest Pharms	00603-5497-21
100's	$64.92	Propranolol ER Caps, HL Moore Drug Exch	00839-7572-06
100's	$65.00	Propranolol Hcl, ESI Lederle	59911-5470-01

HOW SUPPLIED - RATED THERAPEUTICALLY EQUIVALENT:
(cont'd)

100's	$65.75	Propranolol Hcl, Caremark	00339-5753-12
100's	$66.68	Propranolol Hcl, Schein Pharm (US)	00364-2413-01
100's	$66.80	Propranolol, Goldline Labs	00182-1926-01
100's	$66.85	Propranolol HCl, Teva	00093-0691-01
100's	$67.18	Propranolol Hcl, Inwood Labs	00258-3609-01
100's	$67.19	Propranolol, Parmed Pharms	00349-8699-01
100's	$67.36	Propranolol Hcl, Aligen Independ	00405-4890-01
100's	$68.99	Propranolol HCl, Rugby	00536-4911-01
100's	$68.99	Propranolol HCl, Geneva Pharms	00781-2061-01
100's	**$80.50**	**INDERAL-LA, Ayerst**	**00046-0470-81**
1000's	$527.75	Propranolol Hcl, ESI Lederle	59911-5470-02
1000's	$534.00	Propranolol HCl, H.C.F.A. F F P	99999-2135-02
1000's	**$772.77**	**INDERAL-LA, Ayerst**	**00046-0470-91**

Capsule, Gelatin, Sustained Action - Oral - 80 mg

100's	$63.75	Propranolol, United Res	00677-1364-01
100's	$63.75	Propranolol HCl, H.C.F.A. F F P	99999-2135-03
100's	$73.55	Propranolol Hcl 80, Major Pharms	00904-0422-60
100's	$77.28	Propranolol Hcl, Qualitest Pharms	00603-5498-21
100's	$77.30	Propranolol, Goldline Labs	00182-1927-01
100's	$77.34	Propranolol Hcl, HL Moore Drug Exch	00839-7573-06
100's	$77.52	Propranolol HCl, Teva	00093-0692-01
100's	$77.54	Propranolol Hcl, Schein Pharm (US)	00364-2414-01
100's	$77.90	Propranolol Hcl, Parmed Pharms	00349-8700-01
100's	$78.96	Propranolol Hcl, Caremark	00339-5755-12
100's	$80.00	Propranolol Hcl, ESI Lederle	59911-5471-01
100's	$80.65	Propranolol HCl, Geneva Pharms	00781-2062-01
100's	$81.17	BETACHRON, Inwood Labs	00258-3610-01
100's	$81.17	Propranolol HCl, Rugby	00536-4912-01
100's	$81.36	Propranolol Hcl, Aligen Independ	00405-4891-01
100's	**$94.11**	**INDERAL LA, Ayerst**	**00046-0471-81**
100's	**$95.74**	**INDERAL LA, Ayerst**	**00046-0471-99**
250's	$159.37	Propranolol HCl, H.C.F.A. F F P	99999-2135-04
250's	$182.75	Propranolol Hcl, Rugby	00536-4912-02
1000's	$617.00	Propranolol Hcl, ESI Lederle	59911-5471-02
1000's	$637.50	Propranolol HCl, H.C.F.A. F F P	99999-2135-05
1000's	**$903.62**	**INDERAL LA, Ayerst**	**00046-0471-91**

Capsule, Gelatin, Sustained Action - Oral - 120 mg

100's	$80.25	Propranolol, United Res	00677-1365-01
100's	$80.25	Propranolol HCl, H.C.F.A. F F P	99999-2135-06
100's	$90.90	Propranolol Hcl 120, Major Pharms	00904-0423-60
100's	$95.50	Propranolol HCl, Teva	00093-0693-01
100's	$95.75	Propranolol Hcl, Caremark	00339-5757-12
100's	$95.90	Propranolol Hcl, Qualitest Pharms	00603-5499-21
100's	$96.24	Propranolol Hcl, HL Moore Drug Exch	00839-7574-06
100's	$96.38	Propranolol Hcl, Schein Pharm (US)	00364-2415-01
100's	$96.50	Propranolol, Goldline Labs	00182-1928-01
100's	$96.50	Propranolol Hcl, Parmed Pharms	00349-8701-01
100's	$98.00	Propranolol Hcl, ESI Lederle	59911-5473-01
100's	$99.98	Propranolol HCl, Geneva Pharms	00781-2063-01
100's	$101.06	BETACHRON, Inwood Labs	00258-3611-01
100's	$101.06	Propranolol HCl, Rugby	00536-4913-01
100's	**$116.66**	**INDERAL LA, Ayerst**	**00046-0473-81**
100's	**$117.84**	**INDERAL LA, Ayerst**	**00046-0473-99**
100's	$132.63	Propranolol Hcl, Aligen Independ	00405-4892-01
1000's	$764.90	Propranolol Hcl, ESI Lederle	59911-5473-02
1000's	$802.50	Propranolol HCl, H.C.F.A. F F P	99999-2135-07
1000's	**$1119.97**	**INDERAL LA, Ayerst**	**00046-0473-91**

Capsule, Gelatin, Sustained Action - Oral - 160 mg

100's	$106.73	Propranolol, United Res	00677-1366-01
100's	$106.73	Propranolol HCl, H.C.F.A. F F P	99999-2135-08
100's	$118.90	Propranolol, Major Pharms	00904-0424-60
100's	$125.80	Propranolol Hcl, Qualitest Pharms	00603-5500-21
100's	$125.83	Propranolol HCl, Teva	00093-0694-01
100's	$126.00	Propranolol, Goldline Labs	00182-1929-01
100's	$126.02	Propranolol, HL Moore Drug Exch	00839-7575-06
100's	$127.27	Propranolol Hcl, Schein Pharm (US)	00364-2416-01
100's	$129.76	Propranolol Hcl, Caremark	00339-5759-12
100's	$130.00	Propranolol Hcl, ESI Lederle	59911-5479-01
100's	$130.90	Propranolol HCl, Geneva Pharms	00781-2064-01
100's	$132.31	BETACHRON, Inwood Labs	00258-3612-01
100's	$137.34	Propranolol Hcl, Parmed Pharms	00349-8707-01
100's	$137.34	Propranolol, Rugby	00536-4914-01
100's	$137.63	Propranolol Hcl, Aligen Independ	00405-4893-01
100's	**$152.75**	**INDERAL LA, Ayerst**	**00046-0479-81**
100's	**$153.28**	**INDERAL LA, Ayerst**	**00046-0479-99**
1000's	$1067.30	Propranolol HCl, H.C.F.A. F F P	99999-2135-09
1000's	**$1466.41**	**INDERAL LA, Ayerst**	**00046-0479-91**

Injection, Solution - Intravenous - 1 mg/ml

1 ml	$156.25	Propranolol Hcl Inj 1, Solopak Labs	39769-0075-02
1 ml x 10	**$43.14**	**INDERAL, Ayerst**	**00046-3265-10**

Tablet, Uncoated - Oral - 10 mg

60's	**$17.18**	**INDERAL, Ayerst**	**00046-0421-60**
90's	**$24.67**	**INDERAL, Ayerst**	**00046-0421-61**
100's	$1.43	Propranolol Hcl, United Res	00677-1041-01
100's	$1.43	Propranolol HCl, H.C.F.A. F F P	99999-2135-10
100's	$2.25	Propranolol Hcl, Consolidated Midland	00223-2550-01
100's	$3.53	Propranolol Hcl, US Trading	56126-0321-11
100's	$3.90	Propranolol Hcl, Voluntary Hosp	53258-0153-01
100's	$4.50	Propranolol Hcl, Major Pharms	00904-0411-60
100's	$4.55	Propranolol Hcl, Qualitest Pharms	00603-5489-21
100's	$4.95	Propranolol Hcl, Am Generics	58634-0001-01
100's	$5.40	Propranolol Hcl, Caremark	00339-5315-12
100's	$5.45	Propranolol HCl, Rugby	00536-4309-01
100's	$6.00	Propranolol Hcl, Purepac Pharm	00228-2327-10
100's	$6.11	Propranolol Hcl, Talbert Phcy	44514-0756-88
100's	$6.12	Propranolol Hcl, Voluntary Hosp	53258-0153-13
100's	$6.38	Propranolol Hydrochloride, Aligen Independ	00405-4884-01
100's	$6.38	Propranolol Hcl, Sidmak Labs	50111-0467-01
100's	$6.83	Propranolol Hcl, Goldline Labs	00182-1758-01
100's	$6.95	Propranolol Hcl, Watson Labs	52544-0305-01
100's	$8.41	Propranolol HCl, Schein Pharm (US)	00364-0756-01
100's	$8.94	Propranolol HCl, Geneva Pharms	00781-1344-01
100's	$8.95	Propranolol HCl, Warner Chilcott	00047-0070-24
100's	$8.95	Propranolol Hcl, Mylan	00378-0182-01
100's	$16.46	Propranolol Hcl, Major Pharms	00904-0411-61
100's	$16.70	Propranolol HCl, Schein Pharm (US)	00364-0756-90
100's	$16.93	Propranolol Hcl, Medirex	57480-0355-01
100's	$17.55	Propranolol Hcl, Goldline Labs	00182-1812-89
100's	$18.42	Propranolol Hcl, Vangard Labs	00615-2561-13

HOW SUPPLIED - RATED THERAPEUTICALLY EQUIVALENT:
(cont'd)

100's	**$32.83**	**INDERAL, Ayerst**	**00046-0421-81**
100's	**$37.15**	**INDERAL, Ayerst**	**00046-0421-99**
120's	**$32.19**	**INDERAL, Ayerst**	**00046-0421-62**
500's	$7.15	Propranolol HCl, H.C.F.A. F F P	99999-2135-11
500's	$23.00	Propranolol Hcl, Rugby	00536-4309-05
500's	$30.00	Propranolol Hcl, Purepac Pharm	00228-2327-50
500's	$43.11	Propranol Hcl, Lederle Pharm	00005-3109-31
500's	$61.05	Propranolol Hcl, Goldline Labs	00182-1758-10
600's	$94.60	Propranolol Hcl, Medirex	57480-0355-06
750's	$130.50	Propranolol Hcl, Glasgow Pharm	60809-0141-55
750's	$130.50	Propranolol Hcl, Glasgow Pharm	60809-0141-72
1000's	$12.50	Propranolol Hcl, Consolidated Midland	00223-2550-02
1000's	$14.30	Propranolol Hcl, United Res	00677-1041-10
1000's	$14.30	Propranolol Hcl, Sidmak Labs	50111-0467-03
1000's	$14.30	Propranolol HCl, H.C.F.A. F F P	99999-2135-12
1000's	$37.12	Propranolol Hcl, Qualitest Pharms	00603-5489-32
1000's	$37.80	Propranolol Hcl, Major Pharms	00904-0411-80
1000's	$40.70	Propranolol Hcl, HL Moore Drug Exch	00839-7114-16
1000's	$41.42	Propranolol Hcl, Am Generics	58634-0001-02
1000's	$42.63	Propranolol Hcl, Roxane	00054-4758-31
1000's	$48.82	Propranolol Hcl, Purepac Pharm	00228-2327-96
1000's	$59.45	Propranolol Hcl, Parmed Pharms	00349-8936-10
1000's	$61.20	Propranolol Hydrochlorides 10, Aligen Independ	00405-4884-03
1000's	$65.99	Propranolol Hcl, Watson Labs	52544-0305-10
1000's	$65.99	Propranolol Hcl, Martec Pharms	52555-0343-10
1000's	$66.10	Propranolol HCl, Geneva Pharms	00781-1344-10
1000's	$66.81	Propranolol Hcl, Amer Preferred	53445-1758-00
1000's	$69.51	Propranolol HCl, Schein Pharm (US)	00364-0756-02
1000's	$72.75	Propranolol HCl, Bristol Myers Squibb	00003-0729-75
1000's	$73.00	Propranolol HCl, Warner Chilcott	00047-0070-32
1000's	$73.00	Propranolol Hcl, Mylan	00378-0182-10
1000's	$73.00	Propranolol HCl, Rugby	00536-4309-10
1000's	**$320.61**	**INDERAL, Ayerst**	**00046-0421-91**
1080's	$25.61	Propranolol Hcl, Rugby	00536-4309-11
5000's	$71.50	Propranolol HCl, H.C.F.A. F F P	99999-2135-13
5000's	$117.75	Propranolol Hcl, Interpharm	53746-0218-79
5000's	$296.18	Propranolol Hcl, Sidmak Labs	50111-0467-07
5000's	**$1583.15**	**INDERAL, Ayerst**	**00046-0421-95**
50000's	**$13005.39**	**INDERAL, Ayerst**	**00046-0421-98**

Tablet, Uncoated - Oral - 20 mg

90's	**$33.79**	**INDERAL, Ayerst**	**00046-0422-61**
100's	$1.65	Propranolol Hcl, United Res	00677-1042-01
100's	$1.65	Propranolol HCl, H.C.F.A. F F P	99999-2135-14
100's	$2.50	Propranolol Hcl, Consolidated Midland	00223-2551-01
100's	$2.50	Pronol 20, H & H Labs	46703-0095-01
100's	$3.70	Propranolol Hcl, Interpharm	53746-0217-01
100's	$3.74	Propranolol Hcl, US Trading	56126-0322-11
100's	$4.62	Propranolol Hcl, Voluntary Hosp	53258-0154-01
100's	$4.95	Propranolol Hcl, Talbert Phcy	44514-0757-88
100's	$5.74	Propranolol Hcl, Qualitest Pharms	00603-5490-21
100's	$6.00	Propranolol Hcl, Major Pharms	00904-0412-60
100's	$6.99	Propranolol Hcl, Am Generics	58634-0002-01
100's	$7.62	Propranolol Hcl, Voluntary Hosp	53258-0154-13
100's	$7.84	Propranolol Hcl, Caremark	00339-5317-12
100's	$7.85	Propranolol Hcl, Rugby	00536-4313-01
100's	$8.17	Propranolol Hcl, Purepac Pharm	00228-2329-10
100's	$8.97	Propranolol Hcl, Goldline Labs	00182-1759-01
100's	$8.97	Propranolol Hydrochloride, Aligen Independ	00405-4885-01
100's	$8.97	Propranolol Hcl, Sidmak Labs	50111-0468-01
100's	$9.10	Propranolol HCl, Schein Pharm (US)	00364-0757-01
100's	$9.95	Propranolol Hcl, Watson Labs	52544-0306-01
100's	$12.23	Propranolol Hcl, Lederle Pharm	00005-3110-23
100's	$12.59	Propranolol HCl, Geneva Pharms	00781-1354-01
100's	$12.85	Propranolol HCl, Warner Chilcott	00047-0071-24
100's	$12.85	Propranolol Hcl, Mylan	00378-0183-01
100's	$21.57	Propranolol Hcl, Medirex	57480-0356-01
100's	$23.98	Propranolol Hcl, Major Pharms	00904-0412-61
100's	$25.00	Propranolol HCl, Schein Pharm (US)	00364-0757-90
100's	$26.60	Propranolol Hcl, Goldline Labs	00182-1813-89
100's	$27.93	Propranolol Hcl, Vangard Labs	00615-2562-13
100's	**$35.10**	**INDERAL, Ayerst**	**00046-0422-80**
100's	**$46.06**	**INDERAL, Ayerst**	**00046-0422-81**
100's	**$50.39**	**INDERAL, Ayerst**	**00046-0422-99**
120's	**$44.27**	**INDERAL, Ayerst**	**00046-0422-62**
500's	$8.25	Propranolol HCl, H.C.F.A. F F P	99999-2135-15
500's	$14.25	Propranolol Hydrochloride, Interpharm	53746-0217-05
500's	$31.25	Propranolol Hcl, Rugby	00536-4313-05
500's	$40.85	Propranolol Hcl, Purepac Pharm	00228-2329-50
600's	$114.80	Propranolol Hcl, Medirex	57480-0356-06
1000's	$7.95	Pronol 20, H & H Labs	46703-0095-10
1000's	$15.00	Propranolol Hcl, Consolidated Midland	00223-2551-02
1000's	$16.50	Propranolol Hcl, United Res	00677-1042-10
1000's	$16.50	Propranolol HCl, H.C.F.A. F F P	99999-2135-16
1000's	$28.45	Propranolol Hcl, Interpharm	53746-0217-10
1000's	$49.53	Propranolol Hcl, HL Moore Drug Exch	00839-7115-16
1000's	$49.70	Propranolol Hcl, Qualitest Pharms	00603-5490-32
1000's	$49.90	Propranolol Hcl, Major Pharms	00904-0412-80
1000's	$59.95	Propranolol Hcl, Am Generics	58634-0002-02
1000's	$66.34	Propranolol Hcl, Purepac Pharm	00228-2329-96
1000's	$73.83	Propranolol Hcl, Parmed Pharms	00349-8937-10
1000's	$85.91	Propranolol Hcl, Goldline Labs	00182-1759-10
1000's	$85.91	Propranolol Hcl, Sidmak Labs	50111-0468-03
1000's	$85.98	Propranolol Hydrochloride, Aligen Independ	00405-4885-03
1000's	$90.14	Propranolol Hcl, Amer Preferred	53445-1759-00
1000's	$94.50	Propranolol HCl, Schein Pharm (US)	00364-0757-02
1000's	$94.50	Propranolol Hcl, Watson Labs	52544-0306-10
1000's	$94.50	Propranolol Hcl, Martec Pharms	52555-0344-10
1000's	$94.95	Propranolol HCl, Warner Chilcott	00047-0071-32
1000's	$94.95	Propranolol Hcl, Mylan	00378-0183-10
1000's	$94.95	Propranolol HCl, Rugby	00536-4313-10
1000's	$94.95	Propranolol HCl, Geneva Pharms	00781-1354-10
1000's	$102.35	Propranolol HCl, Bristol Myers Squibb	00003-0731-75
1000's	**$451.11**	**INDERAL, Ayerst**	**00046-0422-91**
1080's	$31.30	Propranolol Hcl, Rugby	00536-4313-11
5000's	$82.50	Propranolol HCl, H.C.F.A. F F P	99999-2135-17
5000's	$140.25	Propranolol Hcl, Interpharm	53746-0217-79
5000's	$196.20	Propranolol Hcl, Roxane	00054-4759-33
5000's	$416.65	Propranolol Hcl, Sidmak Labs	50111-0468-07
5000's	**$2227.55**	**INDERAL, Ayerst**	**00046-0422-95**
50000's	**$18298.93**	**INDERAL, Ayerst**	**00046-0422-98**

HOW SUPPLIED - RATED THERAPEUTICALLY EQUIVALENT:
(cont'd)

Tablet, Uncoated - Oral - 40 mg

60's	**$27.72**	**INDERAL, Ayerst**	**00046-0424-60**
100's	$2.04	Propranolol HCl, H.C.F.A. F F P	99999-2135-18
100's	$2.10	Propranolol Hcl, United Res	00677-1043-01
100's	$2.95	Pronol 40, H & H Labs	46703-0096-01
100's	$3.00	Propranolol Hcl, Consolidated Midland	00223-2552-01
100's	$3.69	Propranolol Hcl, US Trading	56126-0323-11
100's	$5.65	Propranolol Hcl, Interpharm	53746-0219-01
100's	$6.09	Propranolol Hcl, Voluntary Hosp	53258-0155-01
100's	$7.65	Propranolol Hcl, HL Moore Drug Exch	00839-7116-06
100's	$8.60	Propranolol Hcl 40, Major Pharms	00904-0414-60
100's	$9.00	Propranolol Hcl, Voluntary Hosp	53258-0155-13
100's	$11.53	Propranolol Hcl, Caremark	00339-5319-12
100's	$12.25	LOROL, Embrex Economed	38130-0051-01
100's	$12.38	Propranolol Hcl, Talbert Phcy	44514-0758-88
100's	$12.75	Propranolol HCl, Rugby	00536-4314-01
100's	$12.78	Propranolol Hcl, Purepac Pharm	00228-2331-10
100's	$12.87	Propranolol Hcl, Goldline Labs	00182-1760-01
100's	$12.87	Propanolol Hcl, Sidmak Labs	50111-0469-01
100's	$12.89	Propranolol Hydrochloride, Aligen Independ	00405-4886-01
100's	$13.95	Propranolol Hcl, Watson Labs	52544-0307-01
100's	$15.95	Propranolol HCl, Geneva Pharms	00781-1364-01
100's	$18.00	Propranolol HCl, Schein Pharm (US)	00364-0758-01
100's	$18.34	Propranolol HCl, Warner Chilcott	00047-0072-24
100's	$18.34	Propranolol Hcl, Mylan	00378-0184-01
100's	$29.28	Propranolol Hcl, Am Generics	58634-0003-01
100's	$29.75	Propranolol Hcl, Medirex	57480-0357-01
100's	$30.72	Propranolol Hcl 40, Major Pharms	00904-0414-61
100's	$34.00	Propranolol HCl, Schein Pharm (US)	00364-0758-90
100's	$40.00	Propranolol Hcl, Goldline Labs	00182-1814-89
100's	$42.00	Propranolol Hcl, Vangard Labs	00615-2563-13
100's	**$59.78**	**INDERAL, Ayerst**	**00046-0424-81**
100's	**$64.06**	**INDERAL, Ayerst**	**00046-0424-99**
120's	**$58.01**	**INDERAL, Ayerst**	**00046-0424-62**
400's	$45.90	LOROL, Embrex Economed	38130-0051-04
500's	$10.20	Propranolol HCl, H.C.F.A. F F P	99999-2135-19
500's	$17.25	Propranolol Hydrochloride, Interpharm	53746-0219-05
500's	$37.60	Propranolol Hcl, Rugby	00536-4314-05
500's	$63.90	Propranolol Hcl, Purepac Pharm	00228-2331-50
500's	$84.75	Propranolol Hcl, Lederle Pharm	00005-3111-31
500's	$123.75	Propranolol Hcl, Goldline Labs	00182-1760-10
600's	$147.80	Propranolol Hcl, Medirex	57480-0357-06
1000's	$8.75	Pronol 40, H & H Labs	46703-0096-10
1000's	$20.40	Propranolol HCl, H.C.F.A. F F P	99999-2135-20
1000's	$21.00	Propranolol Hcl, United Res	00677-1043-10
1000's	$22.50	Propranolol Hcl, Consolidated Midland	00223-2552-02
1000's	$34.45	Propranolol Hcl, Interpharm	53746-0219-10
1000's	$57.76	Propranolol Hcl, Qualitest Pharms	00603-5491-32
1000's	$58.75	Propranolol Hcl 40, Major Pharms	00904-0414-80
1000's	$64.25	Propranolol Hcl, HL Moore Drug Exch	00839-7116-16
1000's	$73.95	Propranolol Hcl, Am Generics	58634-0003-02
1000's	$86.44	Propranolol Hcl, Purepac Pharm	00228-2331-96
1000's	$90.90	Propranolol Hcl, Parmed Pharms	00349-8938-10
1000's	$120.70	Propranolol Hcl, Amer Preferred	53445-1760-00
1000's	$123.75	Propanolol Hcl, Sidmak Labs	50111-0469-03
1000's	$123.82	Propranolol Hydrochloride, Aligen Independ	00405-4886-03
1000's	$132.50	Propranolol Hcl, Watson Labs	52544-0307-10
1000's	$132.50	Propranolol Hcl, Martec Pharms	52555-0345-10
1000's	$132.95	Propranolol HCl, Geneva Pharms	00781-1364-10
1000's	$134.03	Propranolol HCl, Bristol Myers Squibb	00003-0745-75
1000's	$134.29	Propranolol HCl, Schein Pharm (US)	00364-0758-02
1000's	$134.30	Propranolol HCl, Warner Chilcott	00047-0072-32
1000's	$134.30	Propranolol Hcl, Mylan	00378-0184-10
1000's	$134.30	Propranolol HCl, Rugby	00536-4314-10
1000's	**$585.46**	**INDERAL, Ayerst**	**00046-0424-91**
1080's	$46.18	Propranolol Hcl, Rugby	00536-4314-11
5000's	$102.00	Propranolol HCl, H.C.F.A. F F P	99999-2135-21
5000's	$170.25	Propranolol Hcl, Interpharm	53746-0219-79
5000's	$247.50	Propranolol Hcl, Roxane	00054-4760-33
5000's	$600.15	Propanolol Hcl, Sidmak Labs	50111-0469-07
5000's	**$2890.80**	**INDERAL, Ayerst**	**00046-0424-95**
50000's	**$23750.46**	**INDERAL, Ayerst**	**00046-0424-98**

Tablet, Uncoated - Oral - 60 mg

100's	$2.55	Propranolol HCl, H.C.F.A. F F P	99999-2135-22
100's	$3.50	Propranolol Hcl, Consolidated Midland	00223-2553-01
100's	$5.58	Propranolol Hcl, US Trading	56126-0392-11
100's	$7.30	Propranolol Hcl, Qualitest Pharms	00603-5492-21
100's	$8.91	Propranolol Hcl, HL Moore Drug Exch	00839-7117-06
100's	$9.00	Propranolol Hcl, Major Pharms	00904-0416-60
100's	$13.58	Propranolol Hcl, Caremark	00339-5320-12
100's	$14.40	Propranolol HCl, Schein Pharm (US)	00364-0759-01
100's	$15.30	Propranolol Hcl, Purepac Pharm	00228-2321-10
100's	$15.95	Propranolol Hcl, Watson Labs	52544-0352-01
100's	$17.60	Propranolol Hcl, Goldline Labs	00182-1761-01
100's	$17.66	Propranolol HCl, Warner Chilcott	00047-0073-24
100's	$17.66	Propranolol HCl, Geneva Pharms	00781-1374-01
100's	$17.66	Propranolol Hcl, Sidmak Labs	50111-0470-01
100's	$19.10	Propranolol HCl, Bristol Myers Squibb	00003-0750-50
100's	$22.80	Propranolol Hcl, Am Generics	58634-0004-01
100's	$24.88	Propranolol Hcl, Lederle Pharm	00005-3102-23
100's	$24.88	Propranolol HCl, Rugby	00536-4315-01
100's	**$82.70**	**INDERAL, Ayerst**	**00046-0426-81**
500's	$12.75	Propranolol Hcl, Sidmak Labs	50111-0470-02
500's	$12.75	Propranolol HCl, H.C.F.A. F F P	99999-2135-23
500's	$36.12	Propranolol Hcl, Qualitest Pharms	00603-5492-28
500's	$38.25	Propranolol Hcl, Major Pharms	00904-0416-40
500's	$49.95	Propranolol Hcl, Am Generics	58634-0004-02
500's	$75.76	Propranolol Hcl, Watson Labs	52544-0352-05
500's	$111.96	Propranolol Hcl, Lederle Pharm	00005-3102-31
1000's	$25.50	Propranolol HCl, H.C.F.A. F F P	99999-2135-24
1000's	$30.00	Propranolol Hcl, Consolidated Midland	00223-2553-02
1000's	**$794.85**	**INDERAL, Ayerst**	**00046-0426-91**

Tablet, Uncoated - Oral - 80 mg

90's	**$68.04**	**INDERAL, Ayerst**	**00046-0428-61**
100's	$2.63	Propranolol Hcl, United Res	00677-1044-01
100's	$2.63	Propranolol HCl, H.C.F.A. F F P	99999-2135-25
100's	$3.25	Pronol 80, H & H Labs	46703-0097-01
100's	$3.75	Propranolol Hcl, Consolidated Midland	00223-2554-01
100's	$4.40	Propranolol Hcl, US Trading	56126-0324-11
100's	$7.45	Propranolol Hcl, Interpharm	53746-0220-01
100's	$9.75	Propranolol Hcl, Voluntary Hosp	53258-0156-01

HOW SUPPLIED - RATED THERAPEUTICALLY EQUIVALENT:
(cont'd)

100's	$11.22	Propranolol Hcl, Talbert Phcy	44514-0759-88
100's	$11.90	Propranolol Hcl, Major Pharms	00904-0418-60
100's	$11.94	Propranolol Hcl, Qualitest Pharms	00603-5493-21
100's	$14.95	Propranolol Hcl, Am Generics	58634-0005-01
100's	$16.20	Propranolol Hcl, Voluntary Hosp	53258-0156-13
100's	$17.23	Propranolol Hcl, Caremark	00339-5321-12
100's	$17.50	Propranolol HCl, Rugby	00536-4316-01
100's	$18.94	Propranolol Hcl, Purepac Pharm	00228-2333-10
100's	$21.45	Propranolol Hcl, Goldline Labs	00182-1762-01
100's	$21.45	Propranolol HCl, Schein Pharm (US)	00364-0760-01
100's	$21.45	Propranolol Hcl, Sidmak Labs	50111-0471-01
100's	$21.48	Propranolol Hydrochloride, Aligen Independ	00405-4888-01
100's	$21.50	Propranolol Hcl, Watson Labs	52544-0308-01
100's	$21.76	Propranolol HCl, Geneva Pharms	00781-1384-01
100's	$21.95	Propranolol HCl, Warner Chilcott	00047-0074-24
100's	$23.26	Propranolol HCl, Bristol Myers Squibb	00003-0765-50
100's	$30.95	Propranolol Hcl, Mylan	00378-0185-01
100's	$44.60	Propranolol Hcl, Goldline Labs	00182-1815-89
100's	**$91.79**	**INDERAL, Ayerst**	**00046-0428-81**
120's	**$89.05**	**INDERAL, Ayerst**	**00046-0428-62**
500's	$11.25	Pronol, H & H Labs	46703-0097-05
500's	$13.15	Propranolol Hcl, United Res	00677-1044-05
500's	$13.15	Propranolol Hcl, H.C.F.A. F F P	99999-2135-26
500's	$15.00	Propranolol Hcl, Interpharm	53746-0220-05
500's	$50.92	Propranolol Hcl, HL Moore Drug Exch	00839-7118-12
500's	$54.90	Propranolol Hcl, Major Pharms	00904-0418-40
500's	$58.15	Propranolol Hcl, Qualitest Pharms	00603-5493-28
500's	$63.95	Propranolol Hcl, Am Generics	58634-0005-02
500's	$67.29	Propranolol Hcl, Purepac Pharm	00228-2333-50
500's	$77.38	Propranolol Hcl, Parmed Pharms	00349-8952-05
500's	$80.25	Propranolol HCl, Rugby	00536-4316-05
500's	$93.80	Propranolol HCl, Schein Pharm (US)	00364-0760-05
500's	$101.95	Propranolol Hcl, Watson Labs	52544-0308-05
500's	$103.18	Propranolol HCl, Warner Chilcott	00047-0074-30
500's	$103.18	Propranolol Hcl, Goldline Labs	00182-1762-05
500's	$103.18	Propranolol Hcl, Sidmak Labs	50111-0471-02
500's	$103.22	Propranolol Hydrochloride, Aligen Independ	00405-4888-02
500's	$103.95	Propranolol HCl, Geneva Pharms	00781-1384-05
500's	$139.82	Propranolol Hcl, Amer Preferred	53445-1762-05
500's	$145.95	Propranolol Hcl, Mylan	00378-0185-05
1000's	$26.30	Propranolol HCl, H.C.F.A. F F P	99999-2135-27
1000's	$29.25	Propranolol Hcl, Interpharm	53746-0220-10
1000's	$37.50	Propranolol Hcl, Consolidated Midland	00223-2554-02
1000's	**$899.00**	**INDERAL, Ayerst**	**00046-0428-91**
5000's	$131.50	Propranolol HCl, H.C.F.A. F F P	99999-2135-28
5000's	$530.00	Propranolol Hcl, Interpharm	53746-0220-79
5000's	**$4440.85**	**INDERAL, Ayerst**	**00046-0428-95**
50000's	**$36497.40**	**INDERAL, Ayerst**	**00046-0428-98**

Tablet, Uncoated - Oral - 90 mg

100's	$16.25	Propranolol Hcl, H.C.F.A. F F P	99999-2135-29
100's	$23.16	Propranolol Hcl, Sidmak Labs	50111-0472-01
500's	$81.25	Propranolol Hcl, Sidmak Labs	50111-0472-02
500's	$81.25	Propranolol Hcl, H.C.F.A. F F P	99999-2135-30

HOW SUPPLIED - NOT RATED EQUIVALENT:

Solution - Oral - 20 mg/5ml

5 ml x 40	$50.74	Propranolol Hcl, Roxane	00054-8764-16
500 ml	$31.50	Propranolol Hcl, Roxane	00054-3727-63

Solution - Oral - 40 mg/5ml

5 ml x 40	$72.57	Propranolol Hcl, Roxane	00054-8765-16
500 ml	$45.01	Propranolol Hcl, Roxane	00054-3730-63

Solution - Oral - 80 mg/ml

30 ml	$30.48	Propranolol Hcl Intensol, Roxane	00054-3728-44

PROPYLENE GLYCOL *(002136)*

CATEGORIES: Emollients; Skin/Mucous Membrane Agents

BRAND NAMES: Vehicle/N

Prescribing information not available at time of publication.

HOW SUPPLIED - EQUIVALENTS NOT AVAILABLE:

Solution - Topical

50 ml	$5.00	VEHICLE/N, Neutrogena	10812-9100-01

PROPYLTHIOURACIL *(002138)*

CATEGORIES: Antithyroid Agents; Graves' Disease; Hormones; Hyperthyroidism; Thyroid Agents; Thyroid Preparations; Pregnancy Category D; FDA Approval Pre 1982

BRAND NAMES: *Propacil; Propycil; Propyl-Thyracil; Tiotil*
(International brand names outside U.S. in italics)

FORMULARIES: Aetna; BC-BS; DoD; FHP; Medi-Cal; WHO; PCS

COST OF THERAPY: $52.45 (Hyperthyroidism; Tablet; 50 mg; 3/day; 365 days) vs. Potential Cost of $3,804.44 (Thyroid Procedures)

DESCRIPTION:

Propylthiouracil (6-propyl-2-thiouracil) is one of the thiocarbamide compounds. It is a white, crystalline substance that has a bitter taste and is slightly soluble in water.

Each tablet contains propylthiouracil, 50 mg (293.7 µmol), lactose, sodium lauryl sulfate, starch, stearic acid, and talc.

Propylthiouracil is an antithyroid drug administered orally. The molecular weight is 170.23. The empirical formula is $C_7H_{10}N_2OS$.

CLINICAL PHARMACOLOGY:

Propylthiouracil inhibits the synthesis of thyroid hormones and thus is effective in the treatment of hyperthyroidism. The drug does not inactivate existing thyroxine and triiodothyronine that are stored in the thyroid or circulating in the blood nor does it interfere with the effectiveness of thyroid hormones given by mouth or by injection.

CLINICAL PHARMACOLOGY: *(cont'd)*

Propylthiouracil is readily absorbed from the gastrointestinal tract. It is metabolized rapidly and requires frequent administration. Approximately 35% of the drug is excreted in the urine, intact and in conjugated forms, within 24 hours.

In laboratory animals, various interventions, including propylthiouracil administration, that continuously suppress thyroid function and thereby increase TSH secretion result in thyroid tissue hypertrophy.

INDICATIONS AND USAGE:

Propylthiouracil is indicated in the medical treatment of hyperthyroidism. Long-term therapy may lead to remission of the disease. Propylthiouracil may also be used to ameliorate hyperthyroidism in preparation for subtotal thyroidectomy or in radioactive iodine therapy. Propylthiouracil is also used when thyroidectomy is contraindicated or not advisable.

CONTRAINDICATIONS:

Propylthiouracil is contraindicated in the presence of hypersensitivity to the drug and, in nursing mothers, because the drug is excreted in milk.

WARNINGS:

Agranulocytosis is potentially the most serious side effect of propylthiouracil therapy. Patients should be instructed to report any symptoms of agranulocytosis, such as fever or sore throat. Leukopenia, thrombocytopenia, and aplastic anemia (pancytopenia) may also occur. The drug should be discontinued in the presence of agranulocytosis, aplastic anemia (pancytopenia), hepatitis, fever, or exfoliative dermatitis. The patient's bone marrow function should be monitored.

Propylthiouracil can cause fetal harm when administered to a pregnant woman. Because the drug readily crosses placental membranes and can induce goiter and even cretinism in the developing fetus, it is important that a sufficient, but not excessive, dose be given. In many pregnant women, the thyroid dysfunction diminishes as the pregnancy proceeds; consequently, a reduction of dosage may be possible. In some instances, propylthiouracil can be withdrawn 2 or 3 weeks before delivery.

If this drug is used during pregnancy, or if the patient becomes pregnant while taking this drug, the patient should be warned of the potential hazard to the fetus.

Postpartum patients receiving propylthiouracil should not nurse their babies.

Rare reports exist of severe hepatic reactions including encephalopathy fulminant hepatic necrosis, and death in patients receiving propylthiouracil. Symptoms suggestive of hepatic dysfunction (anorexia, pruritus, right upper quadrant pain, etc) should prompt evaluation of liver function. Treatment with propylthiouracil should be discontinued promptly in the event of clinically significant evidence of liver abnormality, including hepatic transaminases in excess of 3 times the upper limit of normal.

PRECAUTIONS:

General: Patients who receive propylthiouracil should be under close surveillance and should be impressed with the necessity of reporting immediately any evidence of illness, particularly sore throat, skin eruptions, fever, headache, or general malaise. In such cases, white-blood-cell and differential counts should be made to determine whether agranulocytosis has developed. Particular care should be exercised with patients who are receiving additional drugs known to cause agranulocytosis.

Laboratory Tests: Because propylthiouracil may cause hypoprothrombinemia and bleeding, prothrombin time should be monitored during therapy with the drug, especially before surgical procedures. Thyroid function tests should be monitored periodically during therapy. Once clinical evidence of hyperthyroidism has resolved, the finding of an elevated serum TSH indicates that a lower maintenance dose of propylthiouracil should be employed.

Carcinogenesis, Mutagenesis, and Impairment of Fertility: Laboratory animals treated with propylthiouracil for > 1 year have demonstrated thyroid hyperplasia and carcinoma formation. Such animal findings are seen with continuous suppression of thyroid function by sufficient doses of a variety of antithyroid agents, as well as in dietary iodine deficiency, subtotal thyroidectomy, and implantation of autonomous thyrotropic hormone-secreting pituitary tumors. Pituitary adenomas have also been described.

Usage in Pregnancy: Pregnancy Category D—See WARNINGS.

Nursing Mothers: The drug appears in human milk and is contraindicated in nursing mothers. See WARNINGS.

Pediatric Use: See DOSAGE AND ADMINISTRATION.

DRUG INTERACTIONS:

The activity of anticoagulants may be potentiated by anti-vitamin-K activity attributed to propylthiouracil.

ADVERSE REACTIONS:

Major adverse reactions (much less common than the minor adverse reactions) include inhibition of myelopoiesis (agranulocytosis, granulopenia, and thrombocytopenia) aplastic anemia, drug fever, a lupus-like syndrome including splenomegaly, hepatitis, periarteritis, and hypoprothrombinemia and bleeding. Nephritis, interstitial pneumonitis, and erythema nodosum have been reported. Minor adverse reactions include skin rash, urticaria, nausea, vomiting, epigastric distress, arthralgia, paresthesia, loss of taste, abnormal loss of hair, myalgia, headache, pruritus, drowsiness, neuritis, edema, vertigo, skin pigmentation, jaundice, sialadenopathy, and lymphadenopathy. It should be noted that about 10% of patients with untreated hyperthyroidism have leukopenia (white-blood-cell count of less than 4,000/cubic mm), often with relative granulopenia.

OVERDOSAGE:

Signs and Symptoms: Nausea, vomiting, epigastric distress, headache, fever, arthralgia, pruritus, edema, and pancytopenia. Agranulocytosis is the most serious effect. Rarely,exfoliative dermatitis, hepatitis, neuropathies, or CNS stimulation or depression may occur. No information is available on the following: LD 50; concentration of propylthiouracil in biologic fluids associated this toxicity and/or death; the amount of drug in a single dose usually associated with symptoms of overdosage; or the amount of propylthiouracil in a single dose likely to be life-threatening.

Treatment: To obtain up-to-date information about the treatment of overdose, a good resource is your certified Regional Poison Control Center. In managing overdose, consider the possibility of multiple drug overdoses, interaction among drugs, and unusual drug kinetics in your patient. Protect the patient's airway and support ventilation and perfusion. Meticulously monitor and maintain, within acceptable limits, the patient's vital signs, blood gases, serum electrolytes, etc. The patient's marrow function should be monitored. Absorption of drugs from the gastrointestinal tract may be decreased by giving activated charcoal, which, in many cases, is more effective than emesis or lavage; consider charcoal instead of or in addition to gastric emptying. Repeated doses of charcoal over time may hasten elimination of some drugs that have been absorbed. Safeguard the patient's airway when employing gastric emptying or charcoal. Forced diuresis, peritoneal dialysis, hemodialysis, or charcoal hemoperfusion have not been established as beneficial for an overdose of propylthiouracil.

DOSAGE AND ADMINISTRATION:

Propylthiouracil is administered orally. The total daily dosage is usually given in 3 equal doses at approximately 8-hour intervals.

Adult: The initial dosage is 300 mg daily. In patients with severe hyperthyroidism, very large goiters, or both, the beginning dosage usually should be 400 mg daily; an occasional patient will require 600 to 900 mg/day initially. The usual maintenance dosage is 100 to 150 mg daily.

Pediatric: For children 6 to 10 years of age, the initial dosage is 50 to 150 mg daily. For children 10 years and over, the initial dosage is 150 to 300 mg daily. The maintenance dosage is determined by the response of the patient.

Store at controlled room temperature, 59 to 86°F (15 to 30°C).

HOW SUPPLIED - EQUIVALENTS NOT AVAILABLE:

Tablet, Uncoated - Oral - 50 mg

100's	$4.79	Propylthiouracil, Harber Pharm	51432-0394-03
100's	$5.33	Propylthiouracil, Purepac Pharm	00228-2348-10
100's	$5.53	Propylthiouracil, Lederle Pharm	00005-4609-23
100's	$8.75	Propylthiouracil, Consolidated Midland	00223-1540-01
100's	$9.51	Propylthiouracil, US Trading	56126-0441-11
1000's	$32.39	Propylthiouracil, HL Moore Drug Exch	00839-5093-16
1000's	$36.10	Propylthiouracil, Halsey Drug	00879-0130-10
1000's	$39.07	Propylthiouracil, Lederle Pharm	00005-4609-34
1000's	$44.10	Propylthiouracil, Goldline Labs	00182-0598-10
1000's	$47.50	Propylthiouracil, United Res	00677-0118-10
1000's	$77.50	Propylthiouracil, Consolidated Midland	00223-1540-02

PROTAMINE SULFATE *(002139)*

CATEGORIES: Anticoagulants; Anticoagulants/Thrombolytics; Antidotes; Antiheparin Agents; Blood Formation/Coagulation; Coagulants and Anticoagulants; Heparin Overdose; Pregnancy Category C; FDA Approval Pre 1982

FORMULARIES: Medi-Cal; WHO

DESCRIPTION:

Protamines are simple proteins of low molecular weight that are rich in arginine and strongly basic. They occur in the sperm of salmon and certain other species of fish.

Protamine sulfate occurs as fine white or off-white amorphous or crystalline powder. It is sparingly soluble in water. The pH is between 6 and 7. The cationic hydrogenated protamine at a pH of 6.8 to 7.1 reacts with anionic heparin at a pH of 5.0 to 7.5 to form an inactive complex.

Protamine sulfate Injection, USP is a sterile, isotonic solution of Protamine sulfate. It acts as a heparin antagonist. It is also a weak anticoagulant.

Each ml contains Protamine sulfate 10 mg and sodium chloride 9 mg in Water for Injection. pH 6.5-7.5; dibasic sodium phosphate, anhydrous and/or sulfuric acid used, if needed, for pH adjustment. It contains no preservative.

Protamine sulfate is administered intravenously.

CLINICAL PHARMACOLOGY:

When administered alone, protamine has an anticoagulant effect. However, when it is given in the presence of heparin (which is strongly acidic), a stable salt is formed and the anticoagulant activity of both drugs is lost.

Protamine sulfate has a rapid onset of action. Neutralization of heparin occurs within five minutes after intravenous administration of an appropriate dose of Protamine sulfate. Although the metabolic fate of the heparin-protamine complex has not been elucidated, it has been postulated that Protamine sulfate in the heparin-protamine complex may be partially metabolized or may be attacked by fibrinolysin, thus freeing heparin.

INDICATIONS AND USAGE:

Protamine sulfate is indicated in the treatment of heparin overdosage.

CONTRAINDICATIONS:

Protamine sulfate is contraindicated in patients who have shown previous intolerance to the drug.

WARNINGS:

Hyperheparinemia or bleeding has been reported in experimental animals and in some patients 30 minutes to 18 hours after cardiac surgery (under cardiopulmonary bypass) in spite of complete neutralization of heparin by adequate doses of Protamine sulfate at the end of the operation. It is important to keep the patient under close observation after cardiac surgery. Additional doses of Protamine sulfate should be administered if indicated by coagulation studies, such as the heparin titration test with protamine and the determination of plasma thrombin time.

Too-rapid administration of Protamine sulfate can cause severe hypotensive and anaphylactoid reactions (see DOSAGE AND ADMINISTRATION and WARNINGS). Facilities to treat shock should be available.

PRECAUTIONS:

General: Because of the anticoagulant effect of protamine, it is unwise to give more than 100 mg over a short period unless a larger dose is clearly needed.

Patients with a history of allergy to fish may develop hypersensitivity reactions to protamine, although to date no relationship has been established between allergic reactions to protamine and fish allergy.

Previous exposure to protamine through use of protamine-containing insulins or during heparin neutralization may predispose susceptible individuals to the development of untoward reactions from the subsequent use of this drug. Reports of the presence of antiprotamine antibodies in the serums of infertile or vasectomized men suggest that some of these individuals may react to use of Protamine sulfate.

Carcinogenesis, Mutagenesis, and Impairment of Fertility: Studies have not been performed to determine potential for carcinogenicity, mutagenicity or impairment of fertility.

Pregnancy Category C: Animal reproduction studies have not been conducted with Protamine sulfate. It is also not known whether Protamine sulfate can cause fetal harm when administered to a pregnant woman or can affect reproduction capacity. Protamine sulfate should be given to a pregnant woman only if clearly needed.

PRECAUTIONS: *(cont'd)*

Nursing Mothers: It is not known whether this drug is excreted in human milk. Because many drugs are excreted in human milk, caution should be exercised when Protamine sulfate is administered to a nursing woman.

Pediatric Use: Safety and effectiveness in children have not been established.

DRUG INTERACTIONS:

Protamine sulfate has been shown to be incompatible with certain antibiotics, including several of the cephalosporins and penicillins (see DOSAGE AND ADMINISTRATION.)

ADVERSE REACTIONS:

Intravenous injections of protamine may cause a sudden fall in blood pressure, bradycardia, pulmonary hypertension, dyspnea, or transitory flushing and a feeling of warmth. There have been reports of anaphylaxis that resulted in severe respiratory embarrassment (see WARNIN-GSand PRECAUTIONS). Other reported adverse reactions include systemic hypertension, nausea, vomiting and lassitude. Back pain has been reported rarely in conscious patients undergoing such procedures as cardiac catheterization.

Because fatal reactions often resembling anaphylaxis have been reported after administration of Protamine sulfate, the drug should be given only when resuscitation techniques and treatment of anaphylactoid shock are readily available.

High-protein, noncardiogenic pulmonary edema associated with the use of protamine has been reported in patients on cardiopulmonary bypass who are undergoing cardiovascular surgery. The etiologic role of protamine in the pathogenesis of this condition is uncertain, and multiple possible causative factors have been present in most cases. This condition has also been reported in association with administration of certain blood products, other drugs, cardiopulmonary bypass alone and other etiologic factors. Although rare, it is potentially life threatening.

OVERDOSAGE:

Signs and Symptoms: Overdose of Protamine sulfate may cause bleeding. Protamine has a weak anticoagulant effect due to an interaction with platelets and with many proteins including fibrinogen. This effect should be distinguished from the rebound anticoagulation that may occur 30 minutes to 18 hours following the reversal of heparin with protamine.

Rapid administration of protamine is more likely to result in bradycardia, dyspnea, a sensation of warmth, flushing and severe hypotension. Hypertension has also occurred.

The median lethal dose of Protamine sulfate is 100 mg/kg in mice. Serum concentrations of Protamine sulfate are not clinically useful. Information is not available on the amount of drug in a single dose that is associated with overdosage or is likely to be life threatening.

Treatment: To obtain up-to-date information about the treatment of overdose, a good resource is your certified Regional Poison Control Center. Telephone numbers of certified poison control centers are listed in the at the beginning of *GenRx*. In managing overdosage, consider the possibility of multiple drug overdoses, interaction among drugs and unusual drug kinetics in your patient.

Replace blood loss with blood transfusions or fresh frozen plasma.

If the patient is hypotensive, consider fluids, epinephrine, dobutamine or dopamine.

DOSAGE AND ADMINISTRATION:

Each mg of Protamine sulfate neutralizes approximately 90 USP units of heparin activity derived from lung tissue or about 115 USP units of heparin activity derived from intestinal mucosa.

Protamine sulfate Injection should be given by very slow intravenous injection over a 10-minute period in doses not to exceed 50 mg (see WARNINGS.)

Protamine sulfate is intended for injection without further dilution; however, if further dilution is desired, D5-W or normal saline may be used. Diluted solutions should not be stored since they contain no preservative.

Protamine sulfate should not be mixed with other drugs without knowledge of their compatibility, because Protamine sulfate has been shown to be incompatible with certain antibiotics, including several of the cephalosporins and penicillins.

Because heparin disappears rapidly from the circulation, the dose of Protamine sulfate required also decreases rapidly with the time elapsed following intravenous injection of heparin. For example, if the Protamine sulfate is administered 30 minutes after the heparin, one-half the usual dose may be sufficient.

The dosage of Protamine sulfate should be guided by blood coagulation studies (see WARNINGS.)

Parenteral drug products should be inspected visually for particulate matter and discoloration prior to administration, whenever solution and container permit.

Store at controlled room temperature 15-30°C (59-86°F). Avoid freezing.

CAUTION—The total dose of Protamine sulfate contained in the 25 ml vial (250 mg in 25 ml) is five times greater than that in the 5 ml ampul (50 mg in 5 ml).

The large-size vials, 25 ml, are designed for antiheparin treatment only when large doses of heparin have been given during surgery and are to be neutralized by large doses of Protamine sulfate after surgical procedures.

HOW SUPPLIED - RATED THERAPEUTICALLY EQUIVALENT:

Injection, Solution - Intravenous - 10 mg/ml

1's	$11.04	Protamine Sulfate, Voluntary Hosp	53258-2290-50
5 ml	$104.06	Protamine Sulfate, Fujisawa USA	00469-2290-20
5 ml x 6	$28.22	Protamine Sulfate, Lilly	00002-1691-16
5 ml x 25	$101.56	Protamine Sulfate Inj 10, Elkins Sinn	00641-1494-35
5 ml x 25	$114.78	Protamine Sulfate, Lilly	00002-1691-25
25 ml	$12.49	Protamine Sulfate, Fujisawa USA	00469-2290-50
25 ml	$19.25	Protamine Sulfate, Lilly	00002-1462-01
25 ml x 1	$17.01	Protamine Sulfate Inj 10, Elkins Sinn	00641-2554-41

PROTEINASE INHIBITOR (HUMAN), A *(002141)*

CATEGORIES: Blood Components/Substitutes; Blood Formation/Coagulation; Emphysema; Orphan Drugs; Pregnancy Category C; FDA Pre 1938 Drugs

BRAND NAMES: **Prolastin**

DESCRIPTION:

Alpha$_1$-Proteinase Inhibitor (Human), is a sterile, stable, lyophilized preparation of purified human Alpha$_1$-Proteinase Inhibitor (alpha$_1$-PI) also known as alpha$_1$- antitrypsin. Alpha$_1$-Proteinase Inhibitor (Human) is intended for use in therapy of congenital alpha$_1$-antitrypsin deficiency.

DESCRIPTION: *(cont'd)*

Alpha$_1$-Proteinase Inhibitor (Human) is prepared from pooled human plasma of normal donors by modification and refinements of the cold ethanol method of Cohn. Each unit of plasma has been tested and found nonreactive for hepatitis B surface antigen (HBsAg) and negative for antibody to human immunodeficiency virus (HIV) by FDA approved tests. In addition, in order to reduce the potential risk of transmission of infectious agents, Alpha$_1$-Proteinase Inhibitor (Human) has been heat-treated in solution at 60 +/- 0.5 °C for not less than 10 hours. However, no procedure has been found to be totally effective in removing viral infectivity from plasma fractionation products.

The specific activity of Alpha$_1$-Proteinase Inhibitor (Human) is greater than or equal to 0.35 mg functional alpha$_1$-PI/mg protein and when reconstituted, the concentration of alpha$_1$-PI is greater than or equal to 20 mg/ml. When reconstituted, Alpha$_1$-Proteinase Inhibitor (Human) has a pH of 6.6-7.4, a sodium content of 100-210 mEq/L, a chloride content of 60-180 mEq/L, a sodium phosphate content of 0.015-0.025 M, a polyethylene glycol content of NMT 5 ppm, and NMT 0.1% sucrose. Alpha$_1$-Proteinase Inhibitor (Human) contains small amounts of other plasma proteins including alpha2-plasmin inhibitor, alpha$_1$-antichymotrypsin, C1-esterase inhibitor, haptoglobin, antithrombin III,

Alpha$_1$-lipoprotein, albumin, and IgA. Each vial of Alpha$_1$-Proteinase Inhibitor (Human) contains the labeled amount of functionally active alpha$_1$-PI in milligrams per vial (mg/vial), as determined by capacity to neutralize porcine pancreatic elastase. Alpha$_1$-Proteinase Inhibitor (Human) contains no preservative and must be administered by the intravenous route.

CLINICAL PHARMACOLOGY:

Alpha$_1$-antitrypsin deficiency is a chronic hereditary, usually fatal, autosomal recessive disorder in which a low concentration of alpha$_1$-PI (alpha$_1$-antitrypsin) is associated with slowly progressive, severe, panacinar emphysema that most often manifests itself in the third to fourth decades of life. (Although the terms "Alpha$_1$-Proteinase Inhibitor" and "alpha$_1$-antitrypsin" are used interchangeably in the scientific literature, the hereditary disorder associated with a reduction in the serum level of alpha$_1$-PI is conventionally referred to as "alpha$_1$-antitrypsin deficiency" while the deficient protein is referred to as "Alpha$_1$-Proteinase Inhibitor." The emphysema is typically worse in the lower lung zones. The pathogenesis of development of emphysema in alpha$_1$-antitrypsin deficiency is not well understood at this time.

It is believed, however, to be due to a chronic biochemical imbalance between elastase (an enzyme capable of degrading elastin tissues, released by inflammatory cells, primarily neutrophils, in the lower respiratory tract) and alpha$_1$-PI (the principal inhibitor of neutrophil elastase) which is deficient in alpha$_1$-antitrypsin disease.

As a result, it is believed that alveolar structures are unprotected from chronic exposure to elastase released from a chronic, low level burden of neutrophils in the lower respiratory tract, resulting in progressive degradation of elastin tissues. The eventual outcome is the development of emphysema. Neonatal hepatitis with cholestatic jaundice appears in approximately 10% of newborns with alpha$_1$-antitrypsin deficiency. In some adults, alpha$_1$-antitrypsin deficiency is complicated by cirrhosis.

A large number of phenotypic variants of alpha$_1$-antitrypsin deficiency exists. The most severely affected individuals are those with the PiZZ variant, typically characterized by alpha$_1$- PI serum levels <35% normal. Epidemiologic studies of individuals with various phenotypes of alpha$_1$-antitrypsin deficiency have demonstrated that individuals with endogenous serum levels of alpha$_1$-PI less than or equal to 50 mg/dL (based on commercial standards) have a risk of >80% of developing emphysema over a lifetime. However, individuals with endogenous alpha$_1$-PI levels >80 mg/dL, in general, do not manifest an increased risk for development of emphysema above the general population background risk. From these observations, it is believed that the "threshold" level of alpha$_1$-PI in the serum required to provide adequate anti-elastase activity in the lung of individuals with alpha$_1$-antitrypsin deficiency is about 80 mg/dL (based on commercial standards for immunologic assay of alpha$_1$-PI). In clinical studies of Alpha$_1$-Proteinase Inhibitor (Human), 23 subjects with the PiZZ variant of congenital deficiency of alpha$_1$-antitrypsin deficiency and documented destructive lung disease participated in a study of acute and/or chronic replacement therapy with Alpha$_1$-Proteinase Inhibitor (Human). The mean *in vivo* recovery of alpha$_1$-PI was 4.2 mg (immunologic) dL per mg (functional)/kg body weight administered. The half-life of alpha$_1$-PI In Vivo was approximately 4.5 days.

Based on these observations, a program of chronic replacement therapy was developed. Nineteen of the subjects in these studies received Alpha$_1$-Proteinase Inhibitor (Human) replacement therapy, 60 mg/kg body weight, once weekly for up to 26 weeks (average 24 weeks of therapy). With this schedule of replacement therapy, blood levels of alpha$_1$-PI were maintained above 80 mg/dL (based on the commercial standards for alpha$_1$-PI immunologic assay). Within a few weeks of commencing this program, bronchoalveolar lavage studies demonstrated significantly increased levels of alpha$_1$-PI and functional antineutrophil elastase capacity in the epithelial lining fluid of the lower respiratory tract of the lung, as compared to levels prior to commencing the program of chronic replacement therapy with Alpha$_1$-Proteinase Inhibitor (Human).

All 23 individuals who participated in the investigations were immunized with Hepatitis B Vaccine and received a single dose of Hepatitis B Immune Globulin (Human) on entry into the investigation. Although no other steps were taken to prevent hepatitis, neither hepatitis B nor non-A, non-B hepatitis occurred in any of the subjects. All subjects remained seronegative for HIV antibody. None of the subjects developed any detectable antibody to alpha$_1$-PI or other serum protein.

Long-term controlled clinical trials to evaluate the effect of chronic replacement therapy with Alpha$_1$-Proteinase Inhibitor (Human), on the development of, or progression of, emphysema in patients with congenital alpha$_1$-antitrypsin deficiency, have not been performed. Estimates of the sample size required of this rare disorder and the slow progressive nature of the clinical course have been considered impediments in the ability to conduct such a trial. Studies to monitor the long term effects will continue as part of the post approval process.

INDICATIONS AND USAGE:

CONGENITAL ALPHA$_1$-Antitrypsin Deficiency

Alpha$_1$-Proteinase Inhibitor (Human) is indicated for chronic replacement therapy of individuals having congenital deficiency of alpha$_1$-PI (alpha$_1$-antitrypsin deficiency) with clinically demonstrable panacinar emphysema. Clinical and biochemical studies have demonstrated that with such therapy, it is possible to increase plasma levels of alpha$_1$-PI, and that levels of functionally active alpha$_1$-PI in the lung epithelial lining fluid are increased proportionately. As some individuals with alpha$_1$-antitrypsin deficiency will not go on to develop panacinar emphysema, only those with early evidence of such disease should be considered for chronic replacement therapy with Alpha$_1$-Proteinase Inhibitor (Human). Subjects with the PiMZ or PiMS phenotypes of alpha$_1$-antitrypsin deficiency should not be considered for such treatment as they appear to be at small risk for panacinar emphysema.

Clinical data are not available as to the long-term effects derived from chronic replacement therapy of individuals with alpha$_1$-antitrypsin deficiency with Alpha$_1$-Proteinase Inhibitor (Human). Only adult subjects have received Alpha$_1$-Proteinase Inhibitor (Human) to date.

ALPHA$_1$-PROTEINASE INHIBITOR (HUMAN) IS NOT INDICATED FOR USE IN PATIENTS OTHER THAN THOSE WITH PIZZ, PIZ(NULL), OR PI(NULL) (NULL) PHENOTYPES.

CONTRAINDICATIONS:

Individuals with selective IgA deficiencies who have known antibody against IgA (anti-IgA antibody) should not receive $Alpha_1$-Proteinase Inhibitor (Human), since these patients may experience severe reactions, including anaphylaxis, to IgA which may be present.

WARNINGS:

$Alpha_1$-Proteinase Inhibitor (Human) is purified from large pools of fresh human plasma obtained from many paid donors. Although each unit of plasma has been found nonreactive for hepatitis B surface antigen (HBsAg) using an FDA approved test, the presence of viruses in such pools must be assumed.

$Alpha_1$-Proteinase Inhibitor (Human) has been heat-treated in solution at 60 deg C for 10 hours in order to reduce the potential for transmission of infectious agents. No procedure has been found to be totally effective in removing viral infectivity from plasma products. No cases of hepatitis, either hepatitis B or non-A, non-B hepatitis have been recorded to date in individuals receiving $Alpha_1$-Proteinase Inhibitor (Human). However, as all individuals received prophylaxis against hepatitis B, no conclusion can be drawn at this time regarding potential transmission of hepatitis B virus.

PRECAUTIONS:

GENERAL

1. Administer within 3 hours after reconstitution. Do not refrigerate after reconstitution.

2. Administer only by the intravenous route.

3. As with any colloid solution there will be an increase in plasma volume following intravenous administration of $Alpha_1$-Proteinase Inhibitor (Human). Caution should therefore be used in patients at risk for circulatory overload.

4. It is recommended that in preparation for receiving $Alpha_1$-Proteinase Inhibitor (Human) recipients be immunized against hepatitis B using a licensed Hepatitis B Vaccine according to the manufacturer's recommendations. Should it become necessary to treat an individual with $Alpha_1$-Proteinase Inhibitor (Human), and time is insufficient for adequate antibody response to vaccination, individuals should receive a single dose of Hepatitis B Immune Globulin (Human), 0.06 ml/kg body weight, intramuscularly, at the time of administration of the initial dose of Hepatitis B Vaccine.

5. $Alpha_1$-Proteinase Inhibitor (Human) should be given alone, without mixing with other agents or diluting solutions.

6. Administration equipment and any reconstituted $Alpha_1$-Proteinase Inhibitor (Human) not used should be appropriately discarded.

CARCINOGENESIS, MUTAGENESIS, IMPAIRMENT OF FERTILITY

Long-term studies in animals to evaluate carcinogenesis, mutagenesis or impairment of fertility have not been conducted.

PREGNANCY CATEGORY C

Animal reproduction studies have not been conducted with $Alpha_1$-Proteinase Inhibitor (Human). It is also not known whether $Alpha_1$-Proteinase Inhibitor (Human) can cause fetal harm when administered to a pregnant woman or can affect reproduction capacity. $Alpha_1$-Proteinase Inhibitor (Human) should be given to a pregnant woman only if clearly needed.

PEDIATRIC USE

Safety and effectiveness in children have not been established.

ADVERSE REACTIONS:

Therapeutic administration of $Alpha_1$-Proteinase Inhibitor (Human), 60 mg/kg weekly, has been demonstrated to be well tolerated. In clinical studies, 6 reactions were observed with 517 infusions of $Alpha_1$-Proteinase Inhibitor (Human), or 1.16%. None of the reactions was severe.

The adverse reactions reported included delayed fever (maximum temperature rise was 38.9 deg C, resolving spontaneously over 24 hours) occurring up to 12 hours following treatment (0.77%), lightheadedness (0.19%), and dizziness (0.19%). Mild transient leukocytosis and dilutional anemia several hours after infusion have also been noted.

DOSAGE AND ADMINISTRATION:

Each bottle of $Alpha_1$-Proteinase Inhibitor (Human) has the functional activity, as determined by inhibition of porcine pancreatic elastase, stated on the label of the bottle.

The "threshold" level of $alpha_1$-PI in the serum believed to provide adequate anti-elastase activity in the lung of individuals with $alpha_1$-antitrypsin deficiency is 80 mg/dL (based on commercial standards for $alpha_1$-PI immunologic assay). However, assays of $alpha_1$-PI based on commercial standards measure antigenic activity of $alpha_1$-PI, whereas the labeled potency value of $alpha_1$-PI is expressed as actual functional activity, i.e., actual capacity to neutralize porcine pancreatic elastase. As functional activity may be less than antigenic activity serum levels of $alpha_1$-PI determined using commercial immunologic assays may not accurately reflect actual functional $alpha_1$-PI levels. Therefore, although it may be helpful to monitor serum levels of $alpha_1$-PI in individuals receiving $Alpha_1$-Proteinase Inhibitor (Human), using currently available commercial assays of antigenic activity, results of these assays should not be used to determine the required therapeutic dosage.

The recommended dosage of $Alpha_1$-Proteinase Inhibitor (Human) is 60 mg/kg body weight administered once weekly. This dose is intended to increase and maintain a level of functional $alpha_1$-PI in the epithelial lining of the lower respiratory tract providing adequate anti- elastase activity in the lung of individuals with $alpha_1$-antitrypsin deficiency.

$Alpha_1$-Proteinase Inhibitor (Human) may be given at a rate of 0.08 ml/kg/min or greater and must be administered intravenously. The recommended dosage of 60 mg/kg takes approximately 30 minutes to infuse.

Parenteral drug products should be inspected visually for particulate matter and discoloration prior to administration, whenever solution and container permit.

RECONSTITUTION

1. Warm the unopened diluent and concentrate to room temperature (NMT 37 °C, 99°F).

2. After removing the plastic flip-top caps, aseptically cleanse rubber stoppers of both bottles.

3. Remove the protective cover from the plastic transfer needle cartridge with tamper-proof seal and penetrate the stopper of the diluent bottle.

4. Remove the remaining portion of the plastic cartridge. Invert the diluent bottle and penetrate the rubber seal on the concentrate bottle with the needle at an angle.

5. The vacuum will draw the diluent into the concentrate bottle. For best results, and to avoid foaming, hold the diluent bottle at an angle to the concentrate bottle in order to direct the jet of diluent against the wall of the concentrate bottle.

6. After removing the diluent bottle and transfer needle, gently swirl the concentrate bottle until the powder is completely dissolved.

7. Swab top of reconstituted bottle of $Alpha_1$-Proteinase Inhibitor (Human), again.

8. Attach the sterile filter needle provided to syringe. With filter needle in place, insert syringe into reconstituted bottle of $Alpha_1$-Proteinase Inhibitor (Human) and withdraw $Alpha_1$-Proteinase Inhibitor (Human) solution into syringe.

DOSAGE AND ADMINISTRATION: *(cont'd)*

9. To administer $Alpha_1$-Proteinase Inhibitor (Human), replace filter needle with appropriate injection needle and follow procedure for I.V. administration.

10. The contents of more than one bottle of $Alpha_1$-Proteinase Inhibitor (Human) may be drawn into the same syringe before administration. If more than one bottle of $Alpha_1$-Proteinase Inhibitor (Human) is used, withdraw contents from bottles using aseptic technique. Place contents into an administration container (plastic minibag or glass bottle) using a syringe (for a patient of average weight (about 70 kg), the volume needed will exceed the limit of one syringe). Avoid pushing an I.V. administration set spike into the product container stopper as this has been known to force the stopper into the vial, with a resulting loss of sterility.

HOW SUPPLIED - EQUIVALENTS NOT AVAILABLE:

Injection, Solution - Intravenous - 500 mg

1's $95.00 PROLASTIN, Bayer Pharm 00192-0601-30

Injection, Solution - Intravenous - 1000 mg

1's $190.00 PROLASTIN, Bayer Pharm 00192-0601-35

PROTRIPTYLINE HYDROCHLORIDE *(002143)*

CATEGORIES: Antidepressants; Central Nervous System Agents; Depression; Psychotherapeutic Agents; Tricyclics; Tricyclic Antidepressants; FDA Approval Pre 1982

BRAND NAMES: *Concordin*; *Triptil*; **Vivactil**
(International brand names outside U.S. in italics)

FORMULARIES: Aetna; BC-BS; Medi-Cal

COST OF THERAPY: $125.52 (Depression; Tablet; 5 mg; 3/day; 90 days) vs. Potential Cost of $2,456.15 (Depression)

PRIMARY ICD9: 311 (Depressive Disorder, Not Elsewhere Classified)

DESCRIPTION:

Protriptyline HCl is *N*- methyl-5*H*-dibenzo(*a,d*)-cycloheptene -5- propanamine hydrochloride. Its empirical formula is $C_{19}H_{21}N°HCl$.

Protriptyline HCl, a dibenzocycloheptene derivative, has a molecular weight of 299.84. It is a white to yellowish powder that is freely soluble in water and soluble in dilute HCl.

Vivactil (Protriptyline HCl) is supplied as 5 mg and 10 mg film coated tablets. Inactive ingredients are calcium phosphate, cellulose, guar gum, hydroxypropyl cellulose, hydroxypropyl methylcellulose, lactose, magnesium stearate, starch, talc, and titanium dioxide. Tablets Vivactil 5 mg and 10 mg also contain FD&C Yellow 6. Tablets Vivactil 10 mg also contain D&C Yellow 10.

CLINICAL PHARMACOLOGY:

Protriptyline HCl is an antidepressant agent. The mechanism of its antidepressant action in man is not known. It is not a monoamine oxidase inhibitor, and it does not act primarily by stimulation of the central nervous system.

Protriptyline HCl has been found in some studies to have a more rapid onset of action than imipramine or amitriptyline. The initial clinical effect may occur within one week. Sedative and tranquilizing properties are lacking. The rate of excretion is slow.

METABOLISM

Metabolic studies indicate that protriptyline is well absorbed from the gastrointestinal tract and is rapidly sequestered in tissues. Relatively low plasma levels are found after administration, and only a small amount of unchanged drug is excreted in the urine of dogs and rabbits. Preliminary studies indicate that demethylation of the secondary amine moiety occurs to a significant extent, and that metabolic transformation probably takes place in the liver. It penetrates the brain rapidly in mice and rats, and moreover that which is present in the brain is almost all unchanged drug.

Studies on the disposition of radioactive protriptyline in human test subjects showed significant plasma levels within 2 hours, peaking at 8 to 12 hours, then declining gradually.

Urinary excretion studies in the same subjects showed significant amounts of radioactivity in 2 hours. The rate of excretion was slow. Cumulative urinary excretion during 16 days accounted for approximately 50% of the drug. The fecal route of excretion did not seem to be important.

INDICATIONS AND USAGE:

Protriptyline HCl is indicated for the treatment of symptoms of mental depression in patients who are under close medical supervision. Its activating properties make it particularly suitable for withdrawn and anergic patients.

CONTRAINDICATIONS:

Protriptyline HCl is contraindicated in patients who have shown prior hypersensitivity to it.

It should not be given concomitantly with a monoamine oxidase inhibiting compound. Hyperpyretic crises, severe convulsions, and deaths have occurred in patients receiving tricyclic antidepressant and monoamine oxidase inhibiting drugs simultaneously. When it is desired to substitute protriptyline HCl for a monoamine oxidase inhibitor, a minimum of 14 days should be allowed to elapse after the latter is discontinued. Protriptyline HCl should then be initiated cautiously with gradual increase in dosage until optimum response is achieved.

This drug should not be used during the acute recovery phase following myocardial infarction.

WARNINGS:

Protriptyline HCl may block the antihypertensive effect of guanethidine or similarly acting compounds.

Protriptyline HCl should be used with caution in patients with a history of seizures, and, because of its autonomic activity, in patients with a tendency to urinary retention, or increased intraocular tension.

Tachycardia and postural hypotension may occur more frequently with protriptyline HCl than with other antidepressant drugs. Protriptyline HCl should be used with caution in elderly patients and patients with cardiovascular disorders; such patients should be observed closely because of the tendency of the drug to produce tachycardia, hypotension, arrhythmias and prolongation of the conduction time. Myocardia infarction and stroke have occurred with drugs of this class.

On rare occasions, hyperthyroid patients or those receiving thyroid medication may develop arrhythmias when this drug is given.

WARNINGS: *(cont'd)*

In patients who may use alcohol excessively, it should be borne in mind that the potentiation may increase the danger inherent in any suicide attempt of overdosage.

USAGE IN CHILDREN

This drug is not recommended for use in children because safety and effectiveness in the pediatric age group have not been established.

USAGE IN PREGNANCY

Safe use in pregnancy and lactation has not been established; therefore, use in pregnant women, nursing mothers or women who may become pregnant requires that possible benefits be weighed against possible hazards to mother and child.

In mice, rats, and rabbits, doses about ten times greater than the recommended human doses had no apparent adverse effects on reproduction.

PRECAUTIONS:

When protriptyline HCl is used to treat the depressive component of schizophrenia, psychotic symptoms may be aggravated. Likewise, in manic-depressive psychosis, depressed patients may experience a shift toward the manic phase if they are treated with an antidepressant drug. Paranoid delusions, with or without associated hostility, may be exaggerated. In any of these circumstances, it may be advisable to reduce the dose of protriptyline HCl or to use a major tranquilizing drug concurrently.

Symptoms, such as anxiety or agitation, may be aggravated in overactive or agitated patients.

When protriptyline HCl is given with anticholinergic agents or sympathomimetic drugs, including epinephrine combined with local anesthetics, close supervision and careful adjustment of dosages are required.

Hyperpyrexia has been reported when tricyclic antidepressants are administered with anticholinergic agents or with neuroleptic drugs, particularly during hot weather.

Cimetidine is reported to reduce hepatic metabolism of certain tricyclic antidepressants, thereby delaying elimination and increasing steady-state concentrations of these drugs. Clinically significant effects have been reported with the tricyclic antidepressants when used concomitantly with cimetidine. Increases in plasma levels of tricyclic antidepressants, and in the frequency and severity of side effects, particularly anticholinergic, have been reported when cimetidine was added to the drug regimen. Discontinuation of cimetidine in well-controlled patients receiving tricyclic antidepressants and cimetidine may decrease the plasma levels and efficacy of the antidepressants.

It may enhance the response to alcohol and the effects of barbiturates and other CNS depressants.

The possibility of suicide in depressed patients remains during treatment and until significant remission occurs. This type of patient should not have access to large quantities of the drug.

Concurrent administration of protriptyline HCl and electroshock therapy may increase the hazards of therapy. Such treatment should be limited to patients for whom it is essential.

Discontinue the drug several days before elective surgery, if possible.

Both elevation and lowering of blood sugar levels have been reported.

INFORMATION FOR THE PATIENT

While on therapy with protriptyline HCl, patients should be advised as to the possible impairment of mental and/or physical abilities required for performance of hazardous tasks, such as operating machinery or driving a motor vehicle.

ADVERSE REACTIONS:

Within each category the following adverse reactions are listed in order of decreasing severity. Included in the listing are a few adverse reactions which have not been reported with this specific drug. However, the pharmacological similarities among the tricyclic antidepressant drugs require that each of the reactions be considered when protriptyline is administered. Protriptyline HCl is more likely to aggravate agitation and anxiety and produce cardiovascular reactions such as tachycardia and hypotension.

Cardiovascular: Myocardial infarction; stroke; heart block; arrhythmias; hypotension, particularly orthostatic hypotension; hypertension; tachycardia; palpitation.

Psychiatric: Confusional states (especially in the elderly) with hallucinations, disorientation, delusions, anxiety, restlessness, agitation; hypomania; exacerbation of psychosis; insomnia, panic, and nightmares.

Neurological: Seizures; incoordination; ataxia; tremors; peripheral neuropathy; numbness, tingling, and paresthesias of extremities; extrapyramidal symptoms; drowsiness; dizziness; weakness and fatigue; headache; syndrome of inappropriate ADH (antidiuretic hormone) secretion; tinnitus; alteration in EEG patterns.

Anticholinergic: Paralytic ileus; hyperpyrexia; urinary retention, delayed micturition, dilatation of the urinary tract; constipation; blurred vision, disturbance of accommodation, increased intraocular pressure, mydriasis; dry mouth and rarely associated sublingual adenitis.

Allergic: Drug fever; petechiae, skin rash, urticaria, itching, photosensitization (avoid excessive exposure to sunlight); edema (general, or of face and tongue).

Hematologic: Agranulocytosis; bone marrow depression; leukopenia; thrombocytopenia; purpura; eosinophilia.

Gastrointestinal: Nausea and vomiting; anorexia; epigastric distress; diarrhea; peculiar taste; stomatitis; abdominal cramps; black tongue.

Endocrine: Impotence, increased or decreased libido; gynecomastia in the male; breast enlargement and galactorrhea in the female; testicular swelling; elevation or depression of blood sugar levels.

Other: Jaundice (simulating obstructive); altered liver function; parotid swelling; alopecia; flushing; weight gain or loss; urinary frequency, nocturia; perspiration.

Withdrawal Symptoms: Though not indicative of addiction, abrupt cessation of treatment after prolonged therapy may produce nausea, headache, and malaise.

OVERDOSAGE:

MANIFESTATIONS

High doses may cause temporary confusion, disturbed concentration, or transient visual hallucinations. Overdosage may cause drowsiness; hypothermia; tachycardia and other arrhythmic abnormalities, for example, bundle branch block; ECG evidence of impaired conduction; congestive heart failure; dilated pupils; convulsions; severe hypotension; stupor; and coma. Other symptoms may be agitation, hyperactive reflexes, muscle rigidity, vomiting, hyperpyrexia, or any of those listed underADVERSE REACTIONS.

Experience in the management of overdosage with protriptyline is limited. The following recommendations are based on the management of overdosage with other tricyclic antidepressants.

All patients suspected of having taken an overdosage should be admitted to a hospital as soon as possible. Treatment is symptomatic and supportive. Empty the stomach as quickly as possible by emesis followed by gastric lavage upon arrival at the hospital. Following gastric lavage, activated charcoal may be administered. Twenty to 30 g of activated charcoal may be given every four to six hours during the first 24 to 48 hours after ingestion. An ECG should be taken and close monitoring of cardiac function instituted if there is any sign of abnormality. Maintain an open airway and adequate fluid intake; regulate body temperature.

The intravenous administration of 1-3 mg of physostigmine salicylate is reported to reverse the symptoms of other tricyclic antidepressant poisoning in humans. Because physostigmine is rapidly metabolized, the dosage of physostigmine should be repeated as required particularly if life threatening signs such as arrhythmias, convulsions, and deep coma recur or persist after the initial dosage of physostigmine. Because physostigmine itself may be toxic, it is not recommended for routine use.

Standard measures should be used to manage circulatory shock and metabolic acidosis. Cardiac arrhythmias may be treated with neostigmine, pyridostigmine, or propranolol. Should cardiac failure occur, the use of digitalis should be considered. Close monitoring of cardiac function for not less than five days is advisable.

Anticonvulsants may be given to control convulsions.

Dialysis is of no value because of low plasma concentrations of the drug.

Since overdosage is often deliberate, patients may attempt suicide by other means during the recovery phase.

Deaths by deliberate or accidental overdosage have occurred with this class of drugs.

DOSAGE AND ADMINISTRATION:

Dosage should be initiated at a low level and increased gradually, noting carefully the clinical response and any evidence of intolerance.

Usual Adult Dosage: Fifteen to 40 mg a day divided into 3 or 4 doses. If necessary, dosage may be increased to 60 mg a day. Dosages above this amount are not recommended. Increases should be made in the morning dose.

Adolescent and Elderly Patients: In general, lower dosages are recommended for these patients. Five mg 3 times a day may be given initially, and increased gradually if necessary. In elderly patients, the cardiovascular system must be monitored closely if the daily dose exceeds 20 mg.

When satisfactory improvement has been reached, dosage should be reduced to the smallest amount that will maintain relief of symptoms.

Minor adverse reactions require reduction in dosage. Major adverse reactions or evidence of hypersensitivity require prompt discontinuation of the drug.

Usage in Children: This drug is not recommended for use in children because safety and effectiveness in the pediatric age group have not been established.

Storage: Store protriptyline HCl in a tightly closed container. Avoid storage at temperatures above 40°C (104°F).

HOW SUPPLIED - RATED THERAPEUTICALLY EQUIVALENT:

Tablet, Plain Coated - Oral - 5 mg

100's	$46.49	VIVACTIL, Merck	00006-0026-68

Tablet, Plain Coated - Oral - 10 mg

100's	$67.36	VIVACTIL, Merck	00006-0047-68
100's	$72.36	VIVACTIL, Merck	00006-0047-28

PSEUDOEPHEDRINE HYDROCHLORIDE

(002144)

CATEGORIES: Antiasthmatics/Bronchodilators; Autonomic Drugs; Common Cold; Congestion; Decongestants; Nasal Congestion; Respiratory & Allergy Medications; Sympathomimetic Agents; FDA Approval Pre 1982

BRAND NAMES: *Bronalin Decongestant*; Cenafed; Chlordrine; *Maxiphed*; **Novafed**; Pseudogest; Slofed-60; Sufedrin
(International brand names outside U.S. in italics)

FORMULARIES: Aetna

DESCRIPTION:

Each Novafed capsule contains 120 mg of pseudoephedrine hydrochloride in specially formulated pellets designed to provide continuous therapeutic effect for 12 hours. About one-half of the active ingredient is released soon after administration and the rest slowly over the remaining time period. Each capsule also contains as inactive ingredients: corn starch, FD&C Blue No. 1, FD&C Red No. 3, FD&C Yellow No. 6, gelatin, sucrose, titanium dioxide, and other ingredients.

CLINICAL PHARMACOLOGY:

Pseudoephedrine (a sympathomimetic) is an orally effective nasal decongestant with peripheral effects similar to epinephrine and central effects similar to, but less intense than, amphetamines. It has the potential for excitatory side effects. At the recommended oral dosage, it has little or no pressor effect in normotensive adults. Patients have not been reported to experience the rebound congestion sometimes experienced with frequent, repeated use of topical decongestants.

INDICATIONS AND USAGE:

Relief of nasal congestion or eustachian tube congestion. May be given concomitantly with analgesics, antihistamines, expectorants and antibiotics.

CONTRAINDICATIONS:

Patients with severe hypertension, severe coronary artery disease, and patients on MAO inhibitor therapy. Also contraindicated in patients with hypersensitivity or idiosyncrasy to sympathomimetic amines which may be manifested by insomnia, dizziness, weakness, tremor or arrhythmias.

Children under 12: Should not be used by children under 12 years.

Nursing Mothers: Contraindicated because of the higher than usual risk for infants from sympathomimetic amines.

WARNINGS:

Use judiciously and sparingly in patients with hypertension, diabetes mellitus, ischemic heart disease, increased intraocular pressure, hyperthyroidism, or prostatic hypertrophy. See, however, CONTRAINDICATIONS. Sympathomimetics may produce central nervous stimulation with convulsions or cardiovascular collapse with accompanying hypotension.

Do not exceed recommended dosage.

Use in Pregnancy: Safety in pregnancy has not been established.

WARNINGS: *(cont'd)*

Use in Elderly: The elderly (60 years and older) are more likely to have adverse reactions to sympathomimetics. Overdosage of sympathomimetics in the elderly may cause hallucinations, convulsions, CNS depression, and death. Safe use of a short-acting sympathomimetic should be demonstrated in the individual elderly patient before considering the use of a sustained-action formulation.

PRECAUTIONS:

Patients with diabetes, hypertension, cardiovascular disease and hyper-reactivity to ephedrine.

DRUG INTERACTIONS:

MAO inhibitors and beta adrenergic blockers increase the effects of pseudoephedrine. Sympathomimetics may reduce the antihypertensive effects of methyldopa, mecamylamine, reserpine and veratrum alkaloids.

ADVERSE REACTIONS:

Hyper-reactive individuals may display ephedrine-like reactions such as tachycardia, palpitations, headache, dizziness or nausea. Sympathomimetics have been associated with certain untoward reactions including fear, anxiety, tenseness, restlessness, tremor, weakness, pallor, respiratory difficulty, dysuria, insomnia, hallucinations, convulsions, CNS depression, arrhythmias, and cardiovascular collapse with hypotension.

DOSAGE AND ADMINISTRATION:

One capsule every 12 hours. Do not give to children under 12 years of age.

HOW SUPPLIED - EQUIVALENTS NOT AVAILABLE:

Syrup - Oral - 30 mg/5ml

480 ml	$6.40	PSEUDOGEST, Major Pharms	00904-1517-16

Tablet, Uncoated - Oral - 60 mg

100's	$3.36	Pseudoephedrine Hcl, HL Moore Drug Exch	00839-1543-06
100's	$3.60	Pseudoephedrine Hcl, Harber Pharm	51432-0400-03
100's	$4.35	Pseudoephedrine HCl, UDL	51079-0012-20
100's	$4.90	Pseudoephedrine Hcl, Major Pharms	00904-0101-60
100's	$24.95	Pseudoephedrine Hcl, Harber Pharm	51432-0400-06
1000's	$25.00	Pseudoephedrine HCl, Geneva Pharms	00781-1535-10
1000's	$26.80	Pseudoephedrine Hcl, Major Pharms	00904-0101-80

PSEUDOEPHEDRINE HYDROCHLORIDE; TERFENADINE *(003062)*

CATEGORIES: Allergies; Antihistamines; Decongestants; Lacrimation; Nasal Congestion; Non-Sedating Antihistamines; Pruritus; Respiratory & Allergy Medications; Rhinitis; Rhinorrhea; Sneezing; Pregnancy Category C; FDA Class 4C ("Little or No Therapeutic Advantage"); FDA Approved 1991 Aug; Top 200 Drugs

BRAND NAMES: **Seldane-D**; *Seldane Decongestant*; *Teldane-D* (Mexico); *Teldane D*
(International brand names outside U.S. in italics)

FORMULARIES: BC-BS

COST OF THERAPY: $63.54 (Rhinitis; Tablet; 120 mg/60 mg; 2/day; 30 days)

PRIMARY ICD9: 477.9 (Allergic Rhinitis, Cause Unspecified)

DESCRIPTION:

FOR COMPLETE PRESCRIBING INFORMATION, REFER TO THE INDIVIDUAL DRUG MONOGRAPHS (PSEUDOEPHEDRINE HYDROCHLORIDE; TERFENADINE).

INDICATIONS AND USAGE:

Seldane-D is indicated for the relief of symptoms associated with seasonal allergic rhinitis such as sneezing, rhinorrhea, pruritus, lacrimation, and nasal congestion. It should be administered when both the antihistaminic properties of Seldane (terfenadine) and the nasal decongestant activity of pseudoephedrine hydrochloride are desired.

Seldane-D has not been studied for effectiveness in relieving symptoms of the common cold.

DOSAGE AND ADMINISTRATION:

Adults and pediatric patients 12 years and older: one tablet swallowed whole, morning and night.

USE OF DOSES IN EXCESS OF ONE TABLET B.I.D. IS NOT RECOMMENDED BECAUSE OF THE INCREASED POTENTIAL FOR QT INTERVAL PROLONGATION AND ADVERSE CARDIAC EVENTS. USE OF SELDANE-D IN PATIENTS WITH SIGNIFICANT HEPATIC DYSFUNCTION AND IN PATIENTS TAKING KETOCONAZOLE, ITRACONAZOLE, CLARITHROMYCIN, ERYTHROMYCIN, OR TROLEANDOMYCIN IS CONTRAINDICATED.

PATIENT INFORMATION:

Pseudoephedrine HCl; terfenadine is a combination product containing a decongestant (pseudoephedrine hydrochloride) and an antihistamine (terfenadine). This medication is indicated for the relief of allergies and symptoms such as sneezing, runny nose, itching, watery eyes and nasal congestion. This medication has not been studied for its effectiveness against the common cold. The antihistamine in this medication can interact with several drugs and product severe effects on the heart. This medication should therefore only be taken as prescribed. This medication should be taken with caution by patients with high blood pressure. Consult with your pharmacist or physician to determine the effects with your medications.

HOW SUPPLIED:

Seldane-D Tablets containing 60 mg of terfenadine and 10 mg of pseudoephedrine hydrochloride in an outer press-coat for immediate release and 110 mg of pseudoephedrine hydrochloride in an extended- release core.

Tablets are white to off-white, biconvex capsule-shaped; debossed "Seldane-D".

Store at controlled room temperature (59-86°F) (15-30°C). Protect from moisture.

HOW SUPPLIED - EQUIVALENTS NOT AVAILABLE:

Tablet, Coated, Sustained Action - Oral - 120 mg/60 mg

100's	**$105.90**	**SELDANE-D, Hoechst Marion Roussel**	**00068-0722-61**

PSEUDOEPHEDRINE HYDROCHLORIDE; TRIPROLIDINE HYDROCHLORIDE *(002145)*

CATEGORIES: Allergies; Antihistamines; Common Cold; Congestion; Cough Preparations; Respiratory & Allergy Medications; Rhinitis; Pregnancy Category B; FDA Approved 1983 May

BRAND NAMES: A-Rex; Actahist; Actamine; *Actifed*; Allerfed; Allerfrin; Aprodine; Atridine; Corphed; Harber-Fed; Histafed; Myfed; Pseudocot-T; Tri-Sudo; Triacin; Triaphed; Trifed; Trilitron; **Triphed**; Triprolidine W/Pseudoephedrine; Trofedrin; Vi-Sudo
(International brand names outside U.S. in italics)

FORMULARIES: DoD

DESCRIPTION:

Each tablet for oral administration contains Triprolidine Hydrochloride, USP 2.5 mg and Pseudoephedrine Hydrochloride, USP 60 mg.

Triprolidine HCl is Pyridine, 2-(1-(4-methylphenyl)-3-(1-pyrrolidinyl)-1-propenyl)-, monohydrochloride, monohydrate, (E)-, a potent antihistamine. It is virtually tasteless and lacking in topical anesthetic effect.

Pseudoephedrine HCl is Benzenemethanol α-(1-(methylamino)ethyl)-,(S-(R*,R*))-, hydrochloride, a naturally occurring dextrostereo isomer of ephedrine. The compound is classified as a sympathomimetic amine.

Triprolidine HCl: $C_{19}H_{22}N_2{\cdot}HCl{\cdot}H_2O$

M.W. 332.87

Pseudoephedrine HCl: $C_{10}H_{15}NO{\cdot}HCl$

M.W. 201.70

Inactive ingredients include hydrous lactose, magnesium stearate, povidone and sodium starch glycolate.

CLINICAL PHARMACOLOGY:

Triprolidine HCl acts as an antagonist of the H_1histamine receptor. Consequently, it prevents histamine from eliciting typical immediate hypersensitivity responses in the nose, eye, lungs and skin.

Pseudoephedrine acts as an indirect sympathomimetic agent by stimulating sympathetic (adrenergic) nerve endings to release norepinephrine. Norepinephrine in turn stimulates alpha and beta receptors throughout the body. The action of Pseudoephedrine HCl is apparently more specific on the blood vessels of the systemic circulation. The vasoconstriction elicited at these sites results in the shrinkage of tissues in the sinuses and nasal passages.

INDICATIONS AND USAGE:

For the treatment of the symptoms of seasonal and perennial allergic rhinitis, and vasomotor rhinitis, including nasal obstruction (congestion).

CONTRAINDICATIONS:

Use in New born and Premature Infants: Triprolidine HCl and Pseudoephedrine HCl should not be used in newborn or premature infants.

Use in Lower Respiratory Disease: This drug is contraindicated for the treatment of lower respirator symptoms, including asthma.

Also Contraindicated in the Following Conditions: Hypersensitivity to: 1) Triprolidine HCl and other antihistamines of similar chemical structure; and/or 2) sympathomimetic amines including pseudoephedrine.

Monoamine oxidase (MAO) inhibitor therapy (see DRUG INTERACTIONS).

WARNINGS:

Triprolidine HCl and Pseudoephedrine HCl should be used with considerable caution in patients with: Increased intraocular pressure (narrow angle glaucoma) stenosing peptic ulcer; pyloroduodenal obstruction; symptomatic prostatic hypertrophy; bladder neck obstruction; hypertension; diabetes mellitus; ischemic heart disease and hyperthyroidism.

Use in Elderly (approximately 60 years of older): Antihistamines are more likely to cause dizziness, sedation and hypotension in elderly patients. This age group is also more likely to have adverse reactions to sympathomimetics.

PRECAUTIONS:

General: Triprolidine and Pseudoephedrine should be used with caution in patients with a history of bronchial asthma.

Information to Patients: Patients should be cautious about engaging in activities requiring mental alertness such as driving a car or operating appliances, machinery, etc. Triprolidine HCl has additive effects with alcohol and other Central Nervous System (CNS) depressants (hypnotic, sedatives, tranquilizers, etc.)

Carcinogenesis, Mutagenesis, and Impairment of Fertility: Long term studies in animals have not been performed to evaluate carcinogenic potential of the active ingredients of Pseudoephedrine and Triprolidine.

Pregnancy, Teratogenic Effects, Pregnancy Category B: Reproduction studies consisting of teratology studies have been performed in rats and rabbits at doses up to 70 times the human dose and have revealed no evidence of impaired fertility or harm to the fetus due to the combination of Triprolidine and Pseudoephedrine. There are, however, no adequate and well-controlled studies in pregnant women. Because animal reproduction studies are not always predictive of human response, this drug should be used during pregnancy only if clearly needed.

Nursing Mothers: Because of the higher risk of antihistamine and sympathomimetic amines for infants generally and for newborn and premature infants in particular, therapy with Triprolidine and Pseudoephedrine is contraindicated in nursing mothers.

Pediatric Use: See CONTRAINDICATIONS.

DRUG INTERACTIONS:

MAO inhibitors prolong and intensify the anticholinergic (drying) effects of antihistamines and overall effects of sympathomimetics.

Triprolidine HCl has additive effects with alcohol and other Central Nervous System (CNS) depressants (hypnotic, sedatives, tranquilizers, etc.)

Sympathomimetics may reduce the antihypertensive effects of methyldopa, guanethidine, reserpine, decamylamine, and veratrum alkaloids.

ADVERSE REACTIONS:

The most frequent adverse reactions are underlined:

1. General: Dryness of mouth, dryness of nose, and dryness of throat, urticaria, drug rash, anaphylactic shock, photosensitivity, excessive perspiration, chills.

2. Cardiovascular System: Hypotension, headache, palpitations, tachycardia, extrasystoles.

3. Hematologic System: Hemolytic anemia, thrombocytopenia, agranulocytosis.

4. Nervous System: Sedation, sleepiness, dizziness, disturbed coordination, fatigue, confusion, restlessness, excitation, nervousness, tremor, irritability, insomnia, euphoria, paresthesia, blurred vision, diplopia, vertigo, tinnitus, acute labyrinthitis, hysteria, neuritis, convulsions, CNS depression, hallucination.

5. G.I. System: Epigastric distress, anorexia, nausea, vomiting, diarrhea, constipation.

6. G.U. System: Urinary frequency, difficult urination, urinary retention, early menses.

7. Respiratory System: Thickening of bronchial secretions, tightness of chest and wheezing, nasal stuffiness.

OVERDOSAGE:

Since triprolidine and pseudoephedrine is comprised of two pharmacologically different components, it is difficult to predict how an overdose will be manifested in a given individual. Reaction to an overdose may vary from CNS depression to stimulation. Stimulation is particularly likely in children. A detailed description of symptoms which are likely to appear after ingestion of an excess of the individual components follows:

Overdosage with Pseudoephedrine can cause CNS stimulation, resulting in such manifestations as excitement, nervousness, anxiety, tremor, restlessness and insomnia. Other effects include tachycardia, hypertension, pallor, mydriasis, hyperglycemia and urinary retention. Severe overdosage may cause tachypnea or hyperpnea, hallucinations, convulsions, or delirium, but in some individuals, there may be CNS depression, with somnolence, stupor or respiratory depression. Arrhythmias (including ventricular fibrillation) may lead to hypotension and circulatory collapse. Severe hypokalemia can occur, probably due to compartmental shift rather than depletion of potassium.

Overdosage of Triprolidine may produce reactions varying from depression to stimulation of the CNS; the latter is particularly likely in children. Atropine-like signs and symptoms, dry mouth, fixed dilated pupils, flushing, tachycardia, hallucinations, convulsions, urinary retention, cardiac arrhythmias and coma may occur.

The mean LD_{50} (single, oral dose) of pseudoephedrine is 726 mg/kg in the mouse, 2206 mg/kg in the rat, and 1177 mg/kg in the rabbit. The toxic and lethal concentrations in human biologic fluids are not known. Excretion rates increase with acidification of urine and decrease with alkalinization.

The mean LD_{50} (single, oral dose) or Triprolidine is 163 to 308 mg/kg in the mouse (depending on strain) and 840 mg/kg in the rat.

Insufficient data are available to estimate the toxic and lethal doses of either compound in man. Few reports of toxicity due to Pseudoephedrine HCl have been published and no cases of fetal overdosage is known. No reports of acute poisoning with Triprolidine have appeared.

Adrenergic-receptor blocking agents are antidotes to pseudoephedrine. In practice, the most useful is the beta-blocker propanolol, which is indicated when there are signs of cardiac toxicity. There is no specific antidote to triprolidine. Histamine should not be given. Administration of activated charcoal will help reduce the absorption of Triprolidine if given within 1 hour of ingestion. If instituted within 4 hours of overdosage, therapy is initially aimed at reducing further absorption of the drugs. If vomiting has not occurred spontaneously, the patient should be induced to vomit. This is best done by having him drink a glass of water or milk, then making him gag. Centrally acting emetics are likely to be less effective than usual in view of the antiemetic action of antihistamines. Gastric aspiration and lavage may be carried out up to 4 hours after ingestion if large amounts of milk were given beforehand. Either isotonic or half isotonic saline may be used for lavage.

Saline cathartic such as Milk of Magnesia, by drawing water into the gut, help to dilute the concentration of the drug into the bowel and hasten its elimination.

In severe cases of overdosage, it is essential to monitor both the heart (by electrocardiography) and plasma electrolytes and to give intravenous potassium as indicated by these continuous controls. Vasopressors may be used to treat hypotension, and excessive CNS stimulation may be counteracted with parenteral diazepam. Stimulants should not be used.

DOSAGE AND ADMINISTRATION:

DOSAGE SHOULD BE INDIVIDUALIZED ACCORDING TO THE NEEDS AND THE RESPONSE OF THE PATIENT.

USUAL DOSE

Adults and children 12 years and older: 1 tablet 3 or 4 times a day.

Children 6 to 12 years: 1/2 tablet 3 or 4 times a day.

For children under 6 years: Triprolidine HCl and Pseudoephedrine HCl syrup should be used for greater ease and flexibility in administering doses smaller than 1/2 tablet.

Store at controlled room temperature 15 - 30°C(59 - 86°F). Protect from moisture.

HOW SUPPLIED - RATED THERAPEUTICALLY EQUIVALENT:

Syrup - Oral - 30 mg/1.25 mg/5

10 ml x 100	$26.59	Triprolidine/Pseudoephedrine, Roxane	00054-8745-04
16 oz	$4.86	Actamine, HL Moore Drug Exch	00839-5123-69
120 ml	$0.86	Triprolidine/Pseudoephedrine, H.C.F.A. F F P	99999-2145-02
120 ml	$2.49	Harber-Fed, Harber Pharm	51432-0684-18
120 ml	$2.92	Allerfrin, Rugby	00536-0510-97
128 oz	$31.99	Actahist, HR Cenci	00556-0173-28
180 ml	$1.30	Triprolidine/Pseudoephedrine, H.C.F.A. F F P	99999-2145-04
240 ml	$1.73	Triprolidine/Pseudoephedrine, H.C.F.A. F F P	99999-2145-05
480 ml	$3.24	TRIACIN SYRUP, Harber Pharm	51432-0684-20
480 ml	$3.46	Triprolidine/Pseudoephedrine, H.C.F.A. F F P	99999-2145-01
480 ml	$5.20	ACTAHIST, HR Cenci	00556-0173-16
480 ml	$9.21	Allerfrin, Rugby	00536-0510-85
500 ml	$3.60	Triprolidine/Pseudoephedrine, H.C.F.A. F F P	99999-2145-06
500 ml	$3.83	Triprolidine/Pseudoephedrine, Roxane	00054-3733-63
3840 ml	$19.05	TRIACIN SYRUP, Harber Pharm	51432-0684-21
3840 ml	$25.50	ACTAMINE, HL Moore Drug Exch	00839-5123-70
3840 ml	$27.65	Triprolidine/Pseudoephedrine, H.C.F.A. F F P	99999-2145-03

Tablet, Uncoated - Oral - 60 mg/2.5 mg

12's	$.34	Triprolidine/Pseudoephedrine, H.C.F.A. F F P	99999-2145-07
24's	$.69	Triprolidine/Pseudoephedrine, H.C.F.A. F F P	99999-2145-08
24's	$3.45	Allerfrim, Rugby	00536-3021-35
30's	$.87	Triprolidine/Pseudoephedrine, H.C.F.A. F F P	99999-2145-09
48's	$1.39	Triprolidine/Pseudoephedrine, H.C.F.A. F F P	99999-2145-10
50's	$1.45	Triprolidine/Pseudoephedrine, H.C.F.A. F F P	99999-2145-11
100's	$2.91	Triprolidine/Pseudoephedrine, H.C.F.A. F F P	99999-2145-12
100's	$4.25	Triprolidine W/Pseudoephedrine, Consolidated Midland	00223-2115-01
100's	$4.50	APRODINE, Major Pharms	00904-0250-60

HOW SUPPLIED - RATED THERAPEUTICALLY EQUIVALENT: *(cont'd)*

100's	$5.95	Triprolidine W/Pseudoephedrine, Raway	00686-0046-20
100's	$7.40	Triprolidine/Pseudoephedrine, Roxane	00054-8746-25
100's	$8.90	Allerfrim, Rugby	00536-3021-01
100's	$8.96	TRIFED, Geneva Pharms	00781-1663-01
1000's	$18.75	Trifed, H & H Labs	46703-0025-10
1000's	$21.78	Triprolidine/Pseudoephedrine, Roxane	00054-4746-31
1000's	$25.15	APRODINE, Major Pharms	00904-0250-80
1000's	$29.10	Triprolidine/Pseudoephedrine, H.C.F.A. F F P	99999-2145-13
1000's	$29.50	Triprolidine W/Pseudoephedrine, Consolidated Midland	00223-2115-02
1000's	$40.71	Allerfrim, Rugby	00536-3021-10
1000's	$45.50	TRIFED, Geneva Pharms	00781-1663-10

HOW SUPPLIED - NOT RATED EQUIVALENT:

Syrup - Oral - 30 mg/1.25 mg/5

120 ml	$1.50	Triacin, Apotheca	12634-0204-04
120 ml	$2.25	Triacin, Consolidated Midland	00223-6199-01
480 ml	$5.50	Triacin, Consolidated Midland	00223-6199-02
3840 ml	$27.49	Triacin, Consolidated Midland	00223-6199-03

PYRAZINAMIDE *(002150)*

CATEGORIES: Anti-Infectives; Antimicrobials; Antimycobacterials; Antituberculosis Agents; Tuberculosis; FDA Approval Pre 1982

BRAND NAMES: *Braccopiral*; *Corsazinmid*; *Dipimide*; *Isopas*; *Lynamide*; *Pezetamid*; *Pharozinamide*; *Piraldina*; *Pirazinamida*; *Pirilene*; *Prazina*; *Pyramide*; *Pyrazide*; *Pyzamed*; *Rozide*; *Tebrazio*; *Zinamide*; *Zinastat*
(International brand names outside U.S. in italics)

FORMULARIES: Aetna; BC-BS; FHP; Medi-Cal; WHO

COST OF THERAPY: $606.85 (Tuberculosis; Tablet; 500 mg; 3/day; 180 days)

PRIMARY ICD9: 011.93 (Pulmonary Tuberculosis, Unspecified, Tubercle Bacilli Found)

DESCRIPTION:

Pyrazinamide, the pyrazine analogue of nicotinamide, is a white crystalline powder, stable at room temperature, and sparingly soluble in water. Pyrazinamide Tablets contain 500 mg of pyrazinamide and the following inactive ingredients: Corn Starch, Magnesium Stearate, Modified Food Starch and Stearic Acid.

CLINICAL PHARMACOLOGY:

Bacteriostatic against Mycobacterium tuberculosis.

INDICATIONS AND USAGE:

Failure after adequate treatment with primary drugs (that is, isoniazid, streptomycin, aminosalicylic acid) in any form of active tuberculosis. Pyraminazide should only be given with other effective antituberculous agents.

CONTRAINDICATIONS:

Severe hepatic damage.

WARNINGS:

Pyrazinamide should be used only when close observation of the patient is possible and when laboratory facilities are available for performing frequent reliable liver function tests and blood uric acid determinations.

Pyraminazide should be discontinued and not be resumed if signs of hepatocellular damage or hyperuricemia accompanied by an acute gouty arthritis become manifest.

USAGE IN CHILDREN: Safe use of this drug in children has not been established. Because of its potential toxicity, its use in children should be avoided unless crucial to therapy.

PRECAUTIONS:

Pretreatment examinations should include *in vitro* susceptability tests of recent cultures of M. tuberculosis from the patient as measured against pyrazinamide and the usual primary drugs; however, there is no reliable *in vitro* test for pyraminazide resistance.

Liver function tests (especially SGPT, SGOT determinations) should be carried out prior to, and every 2 to 4 weeks during therapy.

This drug should be used with caution in patients with a history of gout or diabetes mellitus, as management may be more difficult.

ADVERSE REACTIONS:

The principal untoward effect is a hepatic reaction. This varies from a symptomless abnormality of hepatic cell function, detectable only by laboratory tests, through a mild syndrome of fever, anorexia, malaise, liver tenderness, hepatomegaly and splenomegaly to more serious reactions such as clinical jaundice and rare cases of progressive fulminating acute yellow atrophy and death.

Other reactions are active gout, sideroblastica anemia, and adverse effects on the blood-clotting mechanism or vascular integrity.

DOSAGE AND ADMINISTRATION:

Pyraminazide should be administered with at least one other effective antituberculous drug.

Usual adult dose: 20 to 35 milligrams per kilogram per day in 3 to 4 divided doses; 3.0 grams per day should not be exceeded.

Store at Controlled Room Temperature 15-30 deg. C (59-86 deg. F)

HOW SUPPLIED - RATED THERAPEUTICALLY EQUIVALENT:

Tablet, Uncoated - Oral - 500 mg

100's	$112.38	Pyrazinamide, Lederle Pharm	00005-5093-23
100's	$116.88	Pyrazinamide, UDL	51079-0691-20
500's	$541.99	Pyrazinamide, Lederle Pharm	00005-5093-31

PYRIDOSTIGMINE BROMIDE *(002151)*

CATEGORIES: Autonomic Drugs; Muscle Relaxants; Myasthenia Gravis; Neuromuscular; Parasympathomimetic Agents; Respiratory Depression; FDA Approval Pre 1982

BRAND NAMES: **Mestinon**; Regonol

FORMULARIES: Aetna; BC-BS; Medi-Cal; WHO

DESCRIPTION:

Pyridostigmine bromide is an orally active cholinesterase inhibitor. Chemically, pyridostigmine bromide is 3-hydroxy-1-methylpyridinium bromide dimethylcarbamate.

Mestinon is available in the following forms: *Syrup:* containing 60 mg pyridostigmine bromide per teaspoonful in a vehicle containing 5% alcohol, glycerin, lactic acid, sodium benzoate, sorbitol, sucrose, FD&C Red No. 40, FD&C Blue No. 1, flavors and water. *Tablets:* containing 60 mg pyridostigmine bromide; each tablet also contains lactose, silicondioxide and stearic acid. *Timespan Tablets:* containing 180 mg pyridostigmine bromide; each tablet also contains carnauba wax, corn-derived proteins, magnesium stearate, silica gel and tribasic calcium phosphate. *Injectable:* : Each ml contains 5 mg pyridostigmine bromide compounded with 0.2% parabens (methyl and propyl) as preservatives, 0.02% sodium citrate and pH adjusted to approximately 5.0 with citric acid and, if necessary, sodium hydroxide.

CLINICAL PHARMACOLOGY:

Pyridostigmine bromide inhibits the destruction of acetylcholine by cholinesterase and thereby permits freer transmission of nerve impulses across the neuromuscular junction. Pyridostigmine is an analog of neostigmine (Prostigmin), but differs from it in certain clinically significant respects; for example, pyridostigmine is characterized by a longer duration of action and fewer gastrointestinal side effects.

Injection: Animal studies using the injectable form of pyridostigmine and human studies using the oral preparation have indicated that pyridostigmine has a longer duration of action than does neostigmine measured under similar circumstances.

INDICATIONS AND USAGE:

Oral Forms: Pyridostigmine bromide is useful in the treatment of myasthenia gravis.

Injection: Pyridostigmine bromide injectable is useful in the treatment of myasthenia gravis and as a reversal agent or antagonist to nondepolarizing muscle relaxants such as curariform drugs and gallamine triethiodide.

CONTRAINDICATIONS:

Oral Forms: Pyridostigmine bromide is contraindicated in mechanical intestinal or urinary obstruction, and particular caution should be used in its administration to patients with bronchial asthma. Care should be observed in the use of atropine for counteracting side effects, as discussed below.

Injection: Known hypersensitivity to anticholinesterase agents; intestinal and urinary obstructions of the mechanical type.

WARNINGS:

Although failure of patients to show clinical improvement may reflect underdosage, it can also be indicative of overdosage. As is true of all cholinergic drugs, overdosage of pyridostigmine bromide may result in cholinergic crisis, a state characterized by increasing muscle weakness which, through involvement of the muscles of respiration, may lead to death. Myasthenic crisis due to an increase in the severity of the disease is also accompanied by extreme muscle weakness, and thus may be difficult to distinguish from cholinergic crisis on a symptomatic basis. Such differentiation is extremely important, since increases in doses of pyridostigmine bromide or other drugs of this class in the presence of cholinergic crisis or of a refractory or "insensitive" state could have grave consequences. Osserman and Genkins[1] indicate that the differential diagnosis of the two types of crisis may require the use of Tensilon (edrophonium chloride) as well as clinical judgment. The treatment of the two conditions obviously differs radically. Whereas the presence of myasthenic crisis suggests the need for more intensive anticholinesterase therapy, the diagnosis of cholinergic crisis, according to Osserman and Genkins,[1] calls for the prompt *withdrawal* of all drugs of this type. The immediate use of atropine in cholinergic crisis is also recommended.

Atropine may also be used to abolish or obtund gastrointestinal side effects or other muscarinic reactions; but such use, by masking signs of overdosage, can lead to inadvertent induction of cholinergic crisis.

For detailed information on the management of patients with myasthenia gravis, the physician is referred to one of the excellent reviews such as those by Osserman and Genkins,[2] Grob[3] or Schwab.[4,5]

Usage in Pregnancy: The safety of pyridostigmine bromide during pregnancy or lactation in humans has not been established. Therefore, use of pyridostigmine bromide in women who may become pregnant requires weighing the drug's potential benefits against its possible hazards to mother and child.

Injection: Pyridostigmine bromide injectable should be used with particular caution in patients with bronchial asthma or cardiac dysrhythmias. Transient bradycardia may occur and be relieved by atropine sulfate. Atropine should also be used with caution in patients with cardiac dysrhythmias. When large doses of pyridostigmine bromide are administered, as during reversal of muscle relaxants, the prior or simultaneous injection of atropine is advisable. Because of the possibility of hypersensitivity in an occasional patient. atropine and antishock medication should always be readily available.

A syringe containing 1 mg of atropine sulfate should be immediately available to be given in aliquots intravenously to counteract severe cholinergic reactions.

When used as an antagonist to nondepolarizing muscle relaxants, adequate recovery of voluntary respiration and neuromuscular transmission must be obtained prior to discontinuation of respiratory assistance and there should be continuous patient observation. Satisfactory recovery may be defined by a combination of clinical judgment, respiratory measurements and observation of the effects of peripheral nerve stimulation. If there is any doubt concerning the adequacy of recovery from the effects of the nondepolarizing muscle the relaxant, artificial ventilation should be continued until all doubt has been removed.

ADVERSE REACTIONS:

The side effects of pyridostigmine bromide are most commonly related to overdosage and generally are of two varieties, muscarinic and nicotinic. Among those in the former group are nausea, vomiting, diarrhea, abdominal cramps, increased peristalsis, increased salivation, increased bronchial secretions, miosis and diaphoresis. Nicotinic side effects are comprised chiefly of muscle cramps, fasciculation and weakness. Muscarinic side effects can usually be counteracted by atropine, but for reasons shown in the preceding section the expedient is not without danger. As with any compound containing the bromide radical, a skin rash may be

ADVERSE REACTIONS: *(cont'd)*

seen in an occasional patient. Such reactions usually subside promptly upon discontinuance of the medication. (Thrombophlebitis has been reported subsequent to intravenous administration).

DOSAGE AND ADMINISTRATION:

Pyridostigmine bromide is available in three oral dosage forms:

Mestinon Syrup: Raspberry-flavored, containing 60 mg pyridostigmine bromide per teaspoonful (5 ml). This form permits accurate dosage adjustment for children and "brittle" myasthenic patients who require fractions of 60-mg doses. It is more easily swallowed, especially in the morning, by patients with bulbar involvement.

Conventional Tablets: Each containing 60 mg pyridostigmine bromide.

Timespan Tablets: Each containing 180 mg pyridostigmine bromide. This form provides uniformly slow release, hence prolonged duration of drug action; it facilitates control of myasthenic symptoms with fewer individual doses daily. The immediate effect of a 180-mg Timespan tablet is about equal to that of a 60-mg conventional tablet; however, its duration of effectiveness, although varying in individual patients, averages 2.5 times that of a 60-mg dose.

DOSAGE

The size and frequency of the dosage must be adjusted to the needs of the individual patient.

Oral

Syrup And Conventional Tablets: The average dose is ten 60-mg tablets or ten 5-ml teaspoonfuls daily, spaced to provide maximum relief when maximum strength is needed. In severe cases as many as 25 tablets or teaspoonfuls a day may be required, while in mild cases one to six tablets or teaspoonfuls a day may suffice.

Timespan Tablets: One to three 180-mg tablets, once or twice daily, will usually be sufficient to control symptoms; however, the needs of certain individuals may vary markedly from this average. The interval between doses should be at least six hours. For optimum control, it may be necessary to use the more rapidly acting regular tablets or syrup in conjunction with Timespan therapy.

Injection

For Myasthenia Gravis: To supplement oral dosage, pre-and postoperatively, during labor and post-partum, during myasthenic crisis, or whenever oral therapy is impractical, approximately 1/30th of the oral dose of pyridostigmine bromide may be given parenterally, either by intramuscular or *very slow* intravenous injection. *The patient must be closely observed for cholinergic reactions, particularly if the intravenous route is used.*

For details regarding the management of the myasthenic patients who are to undergo major surgical procedures, see the article by Foldes.[3]

Neonates of myasthenic mothers may have transient difficulty in swallowing, sucking and breathing. Injectable pyridostigmine may be indicated-by symptomology and use of edrophonium chloride (Tensilon)-until pyridostigmine bromide syrup can be taken. To date the world literature consists of less than 100 neonate patients.[7] Of these only 5 were treated with injectable pyridostigmine, with the vast majority of the remaining neonates receiving neostigmine. Dosage requirements of injectable pyridostigmine are minute, ranging from 0.05 mg to 0.15 mg/kg of body weight given intramuscularly. It is important to differentiate between cholinergic and myasthenic crises in neonates (see WARNINGS).

Pyridostigmine bromide given parenterally one hour before completion of the second stage of labor enables patients to have adequate strength during labor and provides protection to infants in the immediate postnatal state. For further information on the use of pyridostigmine bromide injectable in neonates of myasthenic mothers, see the article by Namba.[7]

For Reversal of Nondepolarizing Muscle Relaxants: When pyridostigmine bromide injectable is given intravenously to reverse the action of

muscle relaxant drugs, it is recommended that atropine sulfate (0.6 to 1.2 mg) also to be given intravenously immediately prior to the pyridostigmine bromide. Side effects, notably excessive secretions and bradycardia, are thereby minimized. Usually 10 or 20 mg of pyridostigmine bromide will be sufficient for antagonism of the effects of the nondepolarizing muscle relaxants. Although full recovery may occur within 15 minutes in most patients, others may require a half hour or more. Satisfactory reversal can be evident by adequate voluntary respiration, respiratory measurements and use of a peripheral nerve stimulator device. It is recommended that the patient be well ventilated and a patent airway maintained until complete recovery of normal respiration is assured. Once satisfactory reversal has been attained, recuraization has not been reported. For additional information on the use of pyridostigmine bromide for antagonism of nondepolarizing muscle relaxants see the article by Katz[8] and McNall[9].

Failure of pyridostigmine bromide injectable to provide prompt (within 30 minutes) reversal may occur, *e.g.*, in the presence of extreme debilitation, carcinomatosis, or within the concomitant use of certain broad spectrum antibiotics or anesthetic agents, notably ether. Under these circumstances ventilation must be supported by artificial means until the patient has resumed control of his respiration.

Note: For information on a diagnostic test for myasthenia gravis, and for the evaluation and stabilization of therapy, please see product literature on edrophonium chloride (Tensilon).

Note: Because of the hygroscopic nature of the Timespan tablets, mottling may occur. This does not affect their efficacy.

REFERENCES:

1. K.E. Osserman & G. Genkins, *J.A.M.A., 183*:97, 1963. **2.** K.E. Osserman & G. Genkins, *New York State J. Med., 61*:2076, 1961. **3.** D. Grob, *Arch. Intern. Med., 108*:615, 1961. **4.** R.S. Schwab, *New Eng. J. Med., 268*:596, 1963. **5.** R.S. Schwab, *New Eng. J. Med., 268*:717, 1963. **6.** F.F. Foldes and P. McNall, *Anesthesiology,* 23:837. 1962. **7.** T.Namba *et al., Pediatrics,* 45:488, 1970. **8.** R.L. Katz, *Anesthesiology,* 28:528, 1967. **9.** P.McNall *et al. Anesthesia and Analgesia,* 48:1026, 1969.

HOW SUPPLIED - RATED THERAPEUTICALLY EQUIVALENT:

Injection, Solution - Intramuscular; - 5 mg/ml

2 ml x 10	**$52.50**	**MESTINON 10, ICN Pharms**	**00187-3011-10**
2 ml x 25	$32.95	REGONOL, Organon	00052-0460-02
5 ml x 25	$82.50	REGONOL, Organon	00052-0460-05

HOW SUPPLIED - NOT RATED EQUIVALENT:

Syrup - Oral - 60 mg/5ml

480 ml	**$33.43**	**MESTINON, ICN Pharms**	**00187-3012-20**

Tablet, Coated, Sustained Action - Oral - 180 mg

100's	**$85.75**	**MESTINON TIMESPAN, ICN Pharms**	**00187-3013-50**

Tablet, Uncoated - Oral - 60 mg

100's	**$39.19**	**MESTINON 60, ICN Pharms**	**00187-3010-30**
500's	**$193.31**	**MESTINON 60, ICN Pharms**	**00187-3010-40**

PYRIDOXINE HYDROCHLORIDE *(002152)*

CATEGORIES: Anemia; Blood Formation/Coagulation; Convulsions; Deficiency Anemias; Homeostatic & Nutrient; Pyridoxine Deficiency; Vitamin B Complex; Vitamins; Pregnancy Category A; FDA Approval Pre 1982

BRAND NAMES: *B(6)-Vicotrat*; Beesix; *Godabion B6*; **Hexa-Betalin**; Rodex; Vitabee 6; Vitamin B-6
(International brand names outside U.S. in italics)

FORMULARIES: Aetna; Medi-Cal; DoD; WHO

DESCRIPTION:

Pyridoxine Hydrochloride, Injection, USP, a sterile solution of pyridoxine hydrochloride in Water for Injection with a pH between 2 and 3.8.

Each vial is preserved with chlorobutanol (chloroform derivative), 0.5%. Sodium hydroxide and/or hydrochloric acid may have been added during manufacture to adjust the pH.

Pyridoxine hydrochloride is a colorless or white crystal or a white crystalline powder. One g dissolves in 5 ml of water. It is stable in air and slowly affected by sunlight. Its chemical name is 2-methyl-3-hydroxy-4,5-bis(hydroxymethyl) pyridine hydrochloride.

CLINICAL PHARMACOLOGY:

Natural substances that have vitamin B6 activity are pyridoxine in plants and pyridoxal or pyridoxamine in animals. All 3 are converted to pyridoxal phosphate by the enzyme pyridoxal kinase. The physiologically active forms of vitamin B6 are pyridoxal phosphate (codecarboxylase) and pyridoxamine phosphate. Riboflavin is required for the conversion of pyridoxine phosphate to pyridoxal phosphate.

Vitamin B6 acts as a coenzyme in the metabolism of protein, carbohydrate, and fat. In protein metabolism, it participates in the decarboxylation of amino acids, conversion of tryptophan to niacin or to serotonin (5-hydroxytryptamine), deamination, and transamination and transulfuration of amino acids. In carbohydrate metabolism, it is responsible for the breakdown of glycogen to glucose-1-phosphate.

The total adult body pool consists of 16 to 25 mg of pyridoxine. Its half-life appears to be 15 to 20 days. Vitamin B6 is degraded to 4-pyridoxic acid in the liver. This metabolite is excreted in the urine.

The need for pyroxidine increases with the amount of protein the diet. The tryptophan load test appears to uncover early vitamin B6 deficiency by detecting xanthinuria. The average adult minimum daily requirement is about 1.25 mg. The "Recommended Dietary Allowance" of the National Academy of Sciences is estimated to be as much as 2 mg for adults and 2.5 mg for pregnant and lactating women. The requirements are more in persons having certain genetic defects or those being treated with isonicotinic acid hydrazide (INH) or oral contraceptives.

INDICATIONS AND USAGE:

Pyridoxine hydrochloride injection is effective for the treatment of pyridoxine deficiency as seen in the following:

Inadequate dietary intake

Drug-induced deficiency, as from isoniazid (INH) or oral contraceptives

Inborn errors of metabolism, e.g., vitamin-B6-dependent convulsions or vitamin-B6-responsive anemia.

The parenteral route is indicated when oral administration is not feasible, as in anorexia, nausea and vomiting, and preoperative and postoperative conditions. It is also indicated when gastrointestinal absorption is impaired.

CONTRAINDICATIONS:

A history of sensitivity to pyridoxine or to any of the ingredients in pyridoxine is a contraindication.

PRECAUTIONS:

General: Single deficiency, as of pyridoxine alone, is rare. Multiple vitamin deficiency is to be expected in any inadequate diet. Patients treated with levodopa should avoid supplemental vitamins that contain more than 5 mg pyridoxine in the daily dose.

Women taking oral contraceptives may exhibit increased pyridoxine requirements.

Pregnancy Category A: The requirement for pyridoxine appears to be increased during pregnancy. Pyridoxine is sometimes of value in the treatment of nausea and vomiting of pregnancy.

Nursing Mothers: The need for pyridoxine is increased during lactation.

It is not known whether this drug is excreted in human milk. Because many drugs are excreted in human milk, caution should be exercised when Pyridoxine is administered to a nursing woman.

Pediatric Use: Safety and effectiveness in children have not been established.

DRUG INTERACTIONS:

Pyridoxine supplements should not be given to patients receiving levodopa, because the action of the latter drug is antagonized by pyridoxine. However, this vitamin may be used concurrently in patients receiving a preparation containing both carbidopa and levodopa.

ADVERSE REACTIONS:

Paresthesia, somnolence, and low serum folic acid levels have been reported.

DRUG ABUSE AND DEPENDENCE:

Symptoms of dependence have been noted in adults given only 200 mg daily, followed by withdrawal.

OVERDOSAGE:

Pyridoxine given to animals in amounts of 3 to 4 g/kg of body weight produces convulsions and death. In man, a dose of 25 mg/kg of body weight is well tolerated. Two patients were reported to have received extremely large doses of pyridoxine for mushroom poisoning. Each received 2700 mg/kg of pyridoxine and 135 mg/kg of chlorobutanol (the preservative) within a period of 48 hours. Both patients developed profound bulbar and other muscle weakness along with respiratory insufficiency.

DOSAGE AND ADMINISTRATION:

In cases of dietary deficiency, the dosage is 10 to 20 mg daily for 3 weeks. Follow-up treatment is recommended daily for several weeks with an oral therapeutic multivitamin preparation containing 2 to 5 mg pyridoxine. Poor dietary habits should be corrected, an adequate, well-balanced diet should be prescribed.

DOSAGE AND ADMINISTRATION: *(cont'd)*

The vitamin-B6-dependency syndrome may require a therapeutic dosage of as much as 600 mg a day and a daily intake of 30 mg for life.

In deficiencies due to INH, the dosage is 100 mg daily for 3 weeks, followed by a 30-mg maintenance dose daily.

In poisoning caused by ingestion of more than 10 g of INH, an equal amount of pyroxidine should be given—4 g intravenously followed by 1 g intramuscularly every 30 minutes.

This product should be protected from exposure to light.

HOW SUPPLIED - RATED THERAPEUTICALLY EQUIVALENT:

Injection, Solution - Intramuscular; - 100 mg/ml

1 ml x 25	$46.88	Pyridoxine Hcl, Fujisawa USA	00469-0018-25
10 ml	$2.80	Pyridoxine Hcl, Lannett	00527-0144-55
10 ml	$3.40	Pyridoxine Hcl (B-6), Pasadena	00418-2661-41
10 ml	$3.40	Pyridoxine Hcl, Major Pharms	00904-0828-10
10 ml	$4.70	Pyridoxine Hcl, Steris Labs	00402-0077-10
10 ml	$4.92	Pyridoxine Hcl, Hyrex Pharms	00314-0758-70
10 ml	$5.50	Pyridoxine Hcl, Consolidated Midland	00223-8403-10
10 ml	$5.66	Pyridoxine Hcl, United Res	00677-0319-21
10 ml	$5.88	Pyridoxine HCl, Schein Pharm (US)	00364-6644-54
10 ml	$6.45	Pyridoxine Hcl, Goldline Labs	00182-0500-63
10 ml	**$6.74**	**HEXA-BETALIN, Lilly**	**00002-1694-01**
30 ml	$3.09	Pyridoxine Hcl, McGuff	49072-0597-30
30 ml	$3.10	Pyridoxine Hcl, Americal Pharm	54945-0553-53
30 ml	$3.75	Pyridoxine Hcl, Consolidated Midland	00223-8410-30
30 ml	$5.15	Pyridoxine Hcl (B-6), Pasadena	00418-2661-61
30 ml	$5.50	Pyridoxine Hcl, Steris Labs	00402-0077-30
30 ml	$6.50	Pyridoxine Hcl, Consolidated Midland	00223-8404-30
30 ml	$7.10	Pyridoxine HCl, Schein Pharm (US)	00364-6644-56
30 ml	$9.90	Vitamin B-6, Rugby	00536-3350-75

PYRIMETHAMINE *(002155)*

CATEGORIES: Anti-Infectives; Antimalarial Agents; Antiparasitics; Antiprotozoals; Malaria; Parasiticidal; Protozoal Agents; Toxoplasma; Toxoplasmosis; Pregnancy Category C; FDA Approval Pre 1982

BRAND NAMES: **Daraprim**; *Erbaprelina*; *Malocide*; *Pirimecidan*
(International brand names outside U.S. in italics)

FORMULARIES: Aetna; Medi-Cal

DESCRIPTION:

Daraprim is an antiparasitic available in tablet form for oral administration. Each scored tablet contains 25 mg pyrimethamine and the inactive ingredients are corn and potato starch, lactose, and magnesium stearate.

Pyrimethamine is known chemically as 5-(4-chlorophenyl)-6-ethyl-2,4-pyrimidinediamine. The empirical formula is $C_{12}H_{13}ClN_4$, and has a molecular weight of 248.71

CLINICAL PHARMACOLOGY:

Pyrimethamine is well absorbed, with peak levels occurring between 2 to 6 hours following administration. It is eliminated slowly & has a plasma half-life of approximately 96 hours. Pyrimethamine is 87% bound to human plasma proteins.

Microbiology: Pyrimethamine is a folic acid antagonist and the rationale for its therapeutic action is based on the differential requirement between host and parasite for nucleic acid precursors involved in growth. This activity is highly selective against plasmodia and *Toxoplasma gondii*.

Pyrimethamine possesses blood schizonticidal and some tissue schizonticidal activity against malaria parasites of man. However, its blood schizonticidal activity may be slower than that of 4-aminoquinoline compounds. It does not destroy gametocytes, but arrests sporogony in the mosquito.

The action of pyrimethamine against *Toxoplasma gondii* is greatly enhanced when used in conjunction with sulfonamides. This was demonstrated by Eyles and Coleman[1] in the treatment of experimental toxoplasmosis in the mouse. Jacobs et al[2] demonstrated that combination of the two drugs effectively prevented the development of severe uveitis in most rabbits following the inoculation of the anterior chamber of the eye with toxoplasma.

INDICATIONS AND USAGE:

Pyrimethamine is indicated for the chemoprophylaxis of malaria due to susceptible strains of plasmodia. It should not be used alone to treat an acute attack of malaria. Fast-acting schizonticides such as chloroquine or quinine are indicated and preferable for the treatment of acute attacks. However, conjoint use of pyrimethamine will initiate *transmission control* and *suppressive cure* for susceptible strains of plasmodia.

Pyrimethamine is also indicated for the treatment of toxoplasmosis. For this purpose the drug should be used conjointly with a sulfonamide since synergism exists with this combination.

CONTRAINDICATIONS:

Use of pyrimethamine is contraindicated in patients with known hypersensitivity to pyrimethamine. Use of the drug is also contraindicated in patients with documented megaloblastic anemia due to folate deficiency.

WARNINGS:

The dosage of pyrimethamine required for the treatment of toxoplasmosis is 10 to 20 times the recommended antimalaria dosage and approaches the toxic level. If signs of folate deficiency develop (see ADVERSE REACTIONS), reduce the dosage or discontinue the drug according to the response of the patient. Folinic acid (leucovorin) should be administered in a dosage of 5 to 15 mg daily (orally, IV or IM) until normal hematopoiesis restored.

Pyrimethamine should be kept out of the reach of children as children and infants are extremely susceptible to adverse effects from an overdose. Deaths in pediatric patients have been reported after accidental ingestion.

PRECAUTIONS:

GENERAL

The recommended dosage for chemoprophylaxis of malaria should not be exceeded. A small "starting" dose for toxoplasmosis is recommended in patients with convulsive disorders to avoid the potential nervous system toxicity of pyrimethamine.

Pyrimethamine should be used with caution in patients with impaired renal or hepatic function or in patients with possible folate deficiency, such as individuals with malabsorption syndrome, alcoholism, or pregnancy, and those receiving therapy, such as phenytoin, affecting folate levels (see Teratogenic Effects.)

PRECAUTIONS: *(cont'd)*

INFORMATION FOR THE PATIENT

Patients should be warned that at the first appearance of a skin rash they should stop use of pyrimethamine and seek medical attention immediately. Patients should also be warned that the appearance of sore throat, pallor, purpura, or glossitis may be early indications of serious disorders which require prophylactic treatment to be stopped, and medical treatment to be sought. Patients should be warned to keep pyrimethamine out of the reach of children.

Patients should be warned that if anorexia and vomiting occur, they may be minimized by taking the drug with meals.

LABORATORY TESTS

In patients receiving high dosage, as for the treatment of toxoplasmosis, semiweekly blood counts, including platelet counts, should be done.

CARCINOGENESIS, MUTAGENESIS, IMPAIRMENT OF FERTILITY

Carcinogenesis: Pyrimethamine has been reported to produce a significant increase in the number of lung tumors per mouse when given intraperitoneally at high doses (0.025 g/kg).[3] There have been two reports of cancer associated with pyrimethamine administration: a 51-year-old female who developed chronic granulocytic leukemia after taking pyrimethamine for two years for toxoplasmosis,[4] and a 56-year-old patient who developed reticulum cell sarcoma after 14 months of pyrimethamine for toxoplasmosis.[5]

Mutagenesis: Pyrimethamine has been shown to be non-mutagenic in the following *in vitro* assays: the Ames point mutation assay, the Rec assay and the*E. Coli* WP2 assay. It was positive in the L5178Y/TK +/- mouse lymphoma assay in the absence of exogenous metabolic activation.[6] Human blood lymphocytes cultured *in vitro* had structural chromosome aberrations induced by pyrimethamine.

In vivo, chromosomes analyzed from the bone marrow of rats dosed with pyrimethamine showed an increased number of structural and numerical aberrations.

Impairment of Fertility: The effects of pyrimethamine on rat pregnancy seem to indicate that the fertility index of rats treated with pyrimethamine is lowered only when the higher dosage is used, suggesting a possible toxic effect upon the whole organism and/or the conceptuses.[7]

PREGNANCY, TERATOGENIC EFFECTS, PREGNANCY CATEGORY C

Pyrimethamine has been shown to be teratogenic in rats, hamsters, and Goettingen miniature pigs. There are no adequate and well-controlled studies in pregnant women. Pyrimethamine should be used during pregnancy only if the potential benefit justifies the potential risk to the fetus. Concurrent administration of folinic acid is strongly recommended when used for the treatment of toxoplasmosis during pregnancy.

Thiersch[8] reported that when rats were given an oral dose of pyrimethamine of 12.5 mg/kg from day 7 to 9 of the gestation period, there was 66.2% resorption and 32.8% of the live fetuses were stunted. When lower doses of 1 mg/kg and 0.5 mg/kg were given for 10 days, days 4 to 13 of gestation, there was 15% and 8.5% resorption, respectively, and 16.6% and 6.9% of the live fetuses were stunted. A daily oral dose as low as 0.3 mg/kg given for days 7 to 16 of gestation still resulted in 2.7% of the fetuses being stunted.

Sullivan and Takacs[9] found that less than 10% of hamster fetuses died or were malformed following single doses of 20 mg to the mother, which on a mg/kg basis was eight to nine times greater than that given to rats.

Hayama and Kokue[10] reported on the administration of pyrimethamine to pregnant female Goettingen miniature pigs. Sows given 0.9 mg/kg/day, during days 11 to 35 of pregnancy, i.e., the period of organogenesis in the pig, delivered normal offspring. Sows administered a high dose 3.6 mg/kg/day during the same gestational period delivered offspring with a high incidence of malformations including cleft palate, club foot, and micrognathia.

NURSING MOTHERS

Pyrimethamine is excreted in human milk. Milk samples obtained from lactating mothers after treatment with pyrimethamine were found to have measurable concentrations of the drug, with peak concentration at 6 hours postadministration. It is estimated that after a single 75 mg dose of oral pyrimethamine, approximately 3 to 4 mg of the drug would be passed on to the feeding child over a 48-hour period.

Because of the potential for serious adverse reactions in nursing infants from pyrimethamine, a decision should be made whether to discontinue nursing or to discontinue the drug, taking into account the importance of the drug to the mother.

See Carcinogenesis, Mutagenesis, and Impairment of Fertility and Pregnancy, Teratogenic Effects.

PEDIATRIC USE

See DOSAGE AND ADMINISTRATION.

DRUG INTERACTIONS:

Pyrimethamine may be used with sulfonamides, quinine, and other antimalarials, and with other antibiotics. However, the concomitant use of other antifolic drugs, such as sulfonamides or trimethoprim-sulfamethoxazole combinations, while the patient is receiving pyrimethamine for antimalarial prophylaxis, may increase the risk of bone marrow suppression. If signs of folate deficiency develop, pyrimethamine should be discontinued. Folinic acid (leucovorin) should be administered until normal hematopoiesis restored (see WARNINGS). Mild hepatotoxicity has been reported in some patients when lorazepam and pyrimethamine were administered concomitantly.

ADVERSE REACTIONS:

Hypersensitivity reactions, occasionally severe, can occur at any dose, particularly when pyrimethamine is administered concomitantly with a sulfonamide. With large doses of pyrimethamine, anorexia and vomiting may occur. Vomiting may be minimized by giving the medication with meals; it usually disappears promptly upon reduction of dosage. Doses used in toxoplasmosis may produce megaloblastic anemia, leukopenia, thrombocytopenia, pancytopenia, atrophic glossitis, hematuria, and disorders of cardiac rhythm. Hematologic effects, however, may also occur at low doses in certain individuals (see PRECAUTIONS, General.)

Insomnia, diarrhea, headache, light-headedness, dryness of the mouth or throat, fever, malaise, dermatitis, abnormal skin pigmentation, depression, seizures, pulmonary eosinophilia, and hyperphenylalaninemia have been reported rarely.

OVERDOSAGE:

Acute intoxication may follow the ingestion of an excessive amount of pyrimethamine. Gastrointestinal and/or central nervous system signs may be present, including convulsions. The initial symptoms are usually gastrointestinal and may include abdominal pain, nausea, severe and repeated vomiting, possibly including hematemesis. Central nervous system toxicity maybe manifest by initial excitability, generalized and prolonged convulsions which may be followed by respiratory depression, circulatory collapse and death within a few hours. Neurological symptoms appear rapidly (30 minutes to 2 hours after drug ingestion), suggesting that in gross overdosage pyrimethamine has a direct toxic effect on the central nervous system.

OVERDOSAGE: *(cont'd)*

The fatal dose is variable, with the smallest reported fatal single dose being 250 mg to 300 mg. There are, however, reports of pediatric patients who have recovered after taking 375 mg to 625 mg.

There is no specific antidote to acute pyrimethamine poisoning. Gastric lavage is recommended and is effective if carried out very soon after drug ingestion. A parenteral barbiturate may be indicated to control convulsions. Folinic acid may also be given to counteract effects on the hematopoietic system (see WARNINGS).

DOSAGE AND ADMINISTRATION:

FOR CHEMOPROPHYLAXIS OF MALARIA

Adults and pediatric patients over 10 years: 25 mg (1 tablet) once weekly.

Children 4 through 10 years: 12.5 mg (1/2 tablet) once weekly.

Infants and children under 4 years: 6.25 mg (1/4 tablet) once weekly.

Regimens planned to include *suppressive cure* should be extended through any characteristic periods of early recrudescence and late relapse for at least 10 weeks in each case.

For Treatment of Acute Attacks: Pyrimethamine is recommended in areas where only susceptible plasmodia exist. This drug is not recommended alone in the treatment of acute attacks of malaria in nonimmune persons. Fast-acting schizonticides such as chloroquine or quinine are indicated for treatment of acute attacks.

However, conjoint pyrimethamine dosage of 25 mg daily for 2 days will initiate*transmission control* and *suppressive cure.* Should circumstances arise where in pyrimethamine must be used alone in semi-immune persons, the adult dosage for an acute attack is 50 mg for 2 days; children 4 through 10 years old may be given 25 mg daily for 2 days. In any event, clinical cure should be followed by the once-weekly regimen described above.

FOR TOXOPLASMOSIS

The dosage of pyrimethamine for the treatment of toxoplasmosis must be carefully adjusted so as to provide maximum therapeutic effect and a minimum of side effects. At the high dosage required, there is a marked variation in the tolerance to the drug. Young patients may tolerate higher doses than older individuals.

The adult *starting* dose is 50 to 75 mg of the drug daily, together with 1 to 4 g daily of a sulfonamide of the sulfapyrimidine type, e.g., sulfadiazine. This dosage is ordinarily continued for 1 to 3 weeks, depending on the response of the patient and his tolerance of the therapy. The dosage may then be reduced to about one-half that previously given for each drug and continued for an additional 4 to 5 weeks.

The pediatric dosage of pyrimethamine is 1 mg/kg per day divided into 2 equal daily doses; after 2 to 4 days this dose may be reduced to one-half and continued for approximately one month. The usual pediatric sulfonamide dosage is used in conjunction with pyrimethamine.

HOW SUPPLIED:

White, scored tablets containing 25 mg pyrimethamine, imprinted with "Daraprim" and "A3A".

Storage: Store at 15° to 25°C (59° to 77°F) in a dry place and protect from light.

REFERENCES:

1. Eyles DE, Coleman N. Synergistic effect of sulfadiazine and Daraprim against experimental toxoplasmosis in the mouse.*Antibiot Chemother.* 1953;3:483-490. **2.** Jacobs L, Melton ML, Kaufman HE. Treatment of experimental ocular toxoplasmosis.*Arch Ophthalmol.* 1964;71:111-118. **3.** Bahna L. Pyrimethamine. *LARC Monogr Eval Carcinog Risk Chem.* 1977;13:233-242. **4.** Jim RTS, Elizaga FV. Development of chronic granulocytic leukemia in a patient treated with pyrimethamine.*Hawaii Med J.* 1977;36:173-176. **5.** Sadoff L. Antimalarial drugs and Burkitt's lymphoma.*Lancet.*1973;2:1262-1263. **6.** Clive D, Johnson KO, Spector JKS, et al. Validation and characterization of the L5178Y/TK +/- mouse lymphoma mutagen assay system.*Mut Res.* 1979;59:61-108. **7.** Andrade ATL, Guerra MO, Silva NOG, et al. Antifertility effects of pyrimethamine.*Excerpta Med Int Cong Ser.*1976;370:317-321. **8.** Thiersch JB. Effects of certain 2, 4-diaminopyrimidine antagonists of folic acid on pregnancy and rat fetus.*Proc Soc Exp Biol Med.* 1954;87:571-577. **9.** Sullivan GE, Takacs E. Comparative teratogenicity of pyrimethamine in rats and hamsters.*Teratology.* 1971;4:205-210. **10.** Hayama T, Kokue E. Use of Goettingen miniature pigs for studying pyrimethamine teratogenesis.*CRC Crit Rev Toxicol.* 1985;14:403-421.

HOW SUPPLIED - EQUIVALENTS NOT AVAILABLE:

Tablet, Uncoated - Oral - 25 mg

100's $41.29 DARAPRIM, Glaxo Wellcome 00173-0201-55

PYRIMETHAMINE; SULFADOXINE *(002156)*

CATEGORIES: Anti-Infectives; Antimalarial Agents; Antiparasitics; Antiprotozoals; Malaria; Parasiticidal; Protozoal Agents; Pregnancy Category C; FDA Approval Pre 1982

BRAND NAMES: *Cryodoxin*; **Fansidar**; *Malocide*; *Methipox*
(International brand names outside U.S. in italics)

FORMULARIES: Aetna; WHO

> WARNING:
> FATALITIES ASSOCIATED WITH THE ADMINISTRATION OF PYRIMETHAMINE HAVE OCCURRED DUE TO SEVERE REACTIONS, INCLUDING STEVENS-JOHNSON SYNDROME AND TOXIC EPIDERMAL NECROLYSIS. PYRIMETHAMINE PROPHYLAXIS SHOULD BE DISCONTINUED AT THE FIRST APPEARANCE OF SKIN RASH, IF A SIGNIFICANT REDUCTION IN THE COUNT OF ANY FORMED BLOOD ELEMENTS IS NOTED, OR UPON THE OCCURRENCE OF ACTIVE BACTERIAL OR FUNGAL INFECTIONS.

DESCRIPTION:

Fansidar is an antimalarial agent, each tablet containing 500 mg N^1-(5,6-dimethoxy-4-pyrimidinyl) sulfanilamide (sulfadoxine) and 25 mg 2,4-diamino-5-(p-chlorophenyl)-6-ethylpyrimidine (pyrimethamine). Each tablet also contains corn starch, gelatin, lactose, magnesium stearate and talc.

CLINICAL PHARMACOLOGY:

Pyrimethamine is an antimalarial agent which acts by reciprocal potentiation of its two components, achieved by a sequential blockade of two enzymes involved in the biosynthesis of folinic acid within the parasites. Pyrimethamine is effective against certain strains of *Plasmodium falciparum* that are resistant to chloroquine.

Both the sulfadoxine and the pyrimethamine of pyrimethamine are absorbed orally and are excreted mainly by the kidney. Following a single tablet administration, sulfadoxine peak plasma concentrations of 51 to 76 mcg/ml were achieved in 2.5 to 6 hours and the pyrimethamine peak plasma concentrations of 0.13 to 0.4 mcg/ml were achieved in 1.5 to 8

CLINICAL PHARMACOLOGY: *(cont'd)*

hours. The apparent half-life of elimination of sulfadoxine ranged from 100 to 231 hours with a mean of 169 hours, whereas pyrimethamine half-lives ranged from 54 to 148 hours with a mean of 111 hours. Both drugs appear in breast milk of nursing mothers.

INDICATIONS AND USAGE:

Pyrimethamine is indicated for the treatment of *P. falciparum* malaria for those patients in whom chloroquine resistance is suspected. Malaria prophylaxis with pyrimethamine is indicated for travelers to areas where chloroquine-resistant *P. falciparum* malaria is endemic. However, strains of *P. falciparum* may be encountered which have developed resistance to pyrimethamine.

CONTRAINDICATIONS:

Prophylactic (repeated) use of pyrimethamine is contraindicated in patients with severe renal insufficiency, marked liver parenchymal damage or blood dyscrasias. Hypersensitivity to pyrimethamine or sulfonamides. Patients with documented megaloblastic anemia due to folate deficiency. Infants less than two months of age. Pregnancy at term and during the nursing period because sulfonamides pass the placenta and are excreted in the milk and may cause kernicterus.

WARNINGS:

FATALITIES ASSOCIATED WITH THE ADMINISTRATION OF PYRIMETHAMINE HAVE OCCURRED DUE TO SEVERE REACTIONS, INCLUDING STEVENS-JOHNSON SYNDROME AND TOXIC EPIDERMAL NECROLYSIS. PYRIMETHAMINE PROPHYLAXIS SHOULD BE DISCONTINUED AT THE FIRST APPEARANCE OF SKIN RASH, IF A SIGNIFICANT REDUCTION IN THE COUNT OF ANY FORMED BLOOD ELEMENTS IS NOTED, OR UPON THE OCCURRENCE OF ACTIVE BACTERIAL OR FUNGAL INFECTIONS.

Fatalities associated with the administration of sulfonamides, although rare, have occurred due to severe reactions, including fulminant hepatic necrosis, agranulocytosis, aplastic anemia and other blood dyscrasias. Pyrimethamine prophylactic regimen has been reported to cause leukopenia during a treatment of two months or longer. This leukopenia is generally mild and reversible.

PRECAUTIONS:

GENERAL

Pyrimethamine should be given with caution to patients with impaired renal or hepatic function, to those with possible folate deficiency and to those with severe allergy or bronchial asthma. As with some sulfonamide drugs, in glucose-6-phosphate dehydrogenase-deficient individuals, hemolysis may occur. Urinalysis with microscopic examination and renal function tests should be performed during therapy of those patients who have impaired renal function.

INFORMATION FOR THE PATIENT

Patients should be warned that at the first appearance of a skin rash, they should stop use of pyrimethamine and seek medical attention immediately. Adequate fluid intake must be maintained in order to prevent crystalluria and stone formation.

Patients should also be warned that the appearance of sore throat, fever, arthralgia, cough, shortness of breath, pallor, purpura, jaundice or glossitis may be early indications of serious disorders which require prophylactic treatment to be stopped and medical treatment to be sought.

Females should be cautioned against becoming pregnant and should not breast feed their infants during pyrimethamine therapy or prophylactic treatment.

Patients should be warned to keep pyrimethamine out of reach of children.

LABORATORY TESTS

Periodic blood counts and analysis of urine for crystalluria are desirable during prolonged prophylaxis.

CARCINOGENESIS, MUTAGENESIS, IMPAIRMENT OF FERTILITY

Pyrimethamine was not found carcinogenic in female mice or in male and female rats. The carcinogenic potential of pyrimethamine in male mice could not be assessed from the study because of markedly reduced life-span. Pyrimethamine was found to be mutagenic in laboratory animals and also in human bone marrow following 3 or 4 consecutive daily doses totaling 200 mg to 300 mg. Pyrimethamine was not found mutagenic in the Ames test. Testicular changes have been observed in rats treated with 105 mg/kg/day of pyrimethamine and with 15 mg/kg/day of pyrimethamine alone. Fertility of male rats and the ability of male or female rats to mate were not adversely affected at dosages of up to 210 mg/kg/day of pyrimethamine. The pregnancy rate of female rats was not affected following their treatment with 10.5 mg/kg/day, but was significantly reduced at dosages of 31.5 mg/kg/day or higher, a dosage approximately 30 times the weekly human prophylactic dose or higher.

PREGNANCY CATEGORY C

Teratogenic Effects: Pyrimethamine has been shown to be teratogenic in rats when given in weekly doses approximately 12 times the weekly human prophylactic dose. Teratology studies with pyrimethamine plus sulfadoxine (1:20) in rats showed the minimum oral teratogenic dose to be approximately 0.9 mg/kg pyrimethamine plus 18 mg/kg sulfadoxine. In rabbits, no teratogenic effects were noted at oral doses as high as 20 mg/kg pyrimethamine plus 400 mg/kg sulfadoxine.

There are no adequate and well-controlled studies in pregnant women. However, due to the teratogenic effect shown in animals and because pyrimethamine plus sulfadoxine may interfere with folic acid metabolism, pyrimethamine therapy should be used during pregnancy only if the potential benefit justifies the potential risk to the fetus. Women of childbearing potential who are traveling to areas where malaria is endemic should be warned against becoming pregnant.

Nonteratogenic Effects: See CONTRAINDICATIONS.

NURSING MOTHERS

See CONTRAINDICATIONS.

PEDIATRIC USE

Pyrimethamine should not be given to infants less than two months of age because of inadequate development of the glucuronide-forming enzyme system.

DRUG INTERACTIONS:

There have been reports which may indicate an increase in incidence and severity of adverse reactions when chloroquine is used with pyrimethamine as compared to the use of pyrimethamine alone. Pyrimethamine is compatible with quinine and with antibiotics. However, antifolic drugs such as sulfonamides or trimethoprim-sulfamethoxazole combinations should not be used while the patient is receiving pyrimethamine for antimalarial prophylaxis. Pyrimethamine has not been reported to interfere with antidiabetic agents.

If signs of folic acid deficiency develop, pyrimethamine should be discontinued. Folinic acid (leucovorin) may be administered in doses of 5 mg to 15 mg intramuscularly daily, for 3 days or longer, for depressed platelet or white blood cell counts in patients with drug-induced folic acid deficiency when recovery is too slow.

ADVERSE REACTIONS:

For completeness, all major reactions to sulfonamides and to pyrimethamine are included below, even though they may not have been reported with pyrimethamine. See WARNINGS and PRECAUTIONS, Information for the Patient.

Blood dyscrasias: Agranulocytosis, aplastic anemia, megaloblastic anemia, thrombopenia, leukopenia, hemolytic anemia, purpura, hypoprothrombinemia, methemoglobinemia and eosinophilia.

Allergic reactions: Erythema multiforme, Stevens-Johnson syndrome, generalized skin eruptions, toxic epidermal necrolysis, urticaria, serum sickness, pruritus, exfoliative dermatitis, anaphylactoid reactions, periorbital edema, conjunctival and scleral injection, photosensitization, arthralgia and allergic myocarditis.

Gastrointestinal Reactions: Glossitis, stomatitis, nausea, emesis, abdominal pains, hepatitis, hepatocellular necrosis, diarrhea and pancreatitis.

C.N.S. Reactions: Headache, peripheral neuritis, mental depression, convulsions, ataxia, hallucinations, tinnitus, vertigo, insomnia, apathy, fatigue, muscle weakness and nervousness.

Respiratory Reactions: Pulmonary infiltrates.

Miscellaneous Reactions: Drug fever, chills, and toxic nephrosis with oliguria and anuria. Periarteritis nodosa and L.E. phenomenon have occurred.

The sulfonamides bear certain chemical similarities to some goitrogens, diuretics (acetazolamide and the thiazides) and oral hypoglycemic agents. Diuresis and hypoglycemia have occurred rarely in patients receiving sulfonamides. Cross-sensitivity may exist with these agents. Rats appear to be especially susceptible to the goitrogenic effects of sulfonamides, and long-term administration has produced thyroid malignancies in the species.

OVERDOSAGE:

Acute intoxication may be manifested by anorexia, vomiting and central nervous system stimulation (including convulsions), followed by megaloblastic anemia, leukopenia, thrombocytopenia, glossitis and crystalluria. In acute intoxication, emesis and gastric lavage followed by purges may be of benefit. The patient should be adequately hydrated to prevent renal damage. The renal and hematopoietic systems should be monitored for at least one month after an overdosage. If the patient is having convulsions, the use of a parenteral barbiturate is indicated. For depressed platelet or white blood cell counts, folinic acid (leucovorin) should be administered in a dosage of 5 mg to 15 mg intramuscularly daily for 3 days or longer.

DOSAGE AND ADMINISTRATION:

(See INDICATIONS AND USAGE)

(a) Treatment of acute attack of malaria: A single dose of the following number of pyrimethamine tablets is used in sequence with quinine or alone (TABLE 1):

TABLE 1

Adults	2 to 3 tablets
9 to 14 years	2 tablets
4 to 8 years	1 tablet
Under 4 years	1/2 tablet

(b) Malaria prophylaxis: The first dose of pyrimethamine should be taken one or two days before departure to an endemic area; administration should be continued during the stay and for four to six weeks after return.(TABLE 2)

TABLE 2

	Once Weekly	Once Every Two Weeks
Adults	1 tablet	2 tablets
9 to 14 years	3/4 tablet	1 1/2 tablets
4 to 8 years	1/2 tablet	1 tablet
Under 4 years	1/4 tablet	1/2 tablet

HOW SUPPLIED:

Scored tablets, containing 500 mg sulfadoxine and 25 mg pyrimethamine—Tel-E-Dose packages of 25. Imprint on tablets: FANSIDAR ROCHE.

HOW SUPPLIED - EQUIVALENTS NOT AVAILABLE:

Tablet, Uncoated - Oral - 25 mg/500 mg

25's $84.27 FANSIDAR, Roche 00004-0161-03

QUAZEPAM *(002160)*

CATEGORIES: Anxiolytics, Sedatives, Hypnotic; Benzodiazepines; Central Nervous System Agents; Hypnotics; Insomnia; Pregnancy Category X; DEA Class CIV; FDA Class 1C ("Little or No Therapeutic Advantage"); FDA Approved 1985 Dec

BRAND NAMES: **Doral**; Dormalin; *Oniria*; *Pamerex*; *Quazium*; *Quiedorm*; *Selepam*; *Temodal*
(International brand names outside U.S. in italics)

COST OF THERAPY: $9.59 (Insomnia; Tablet; 15 mg; 1/day; 7 days)

DESCRIPTION:

Doral (quazepam) Tablets contain quazepam, a trifluoroethyl benzodiazepine hypnotic agent, having the chemical name 7-chloro-5- (o-fluorophenyl)-1,3-dihydro-1-(2,2,2-trifluoroethyl)-2*H*-1,4-benzo-diazepine-2-thione.

Quazepam has the empirical formula $C_{17}H_{11}ClF_4N_2S$, and a molecular weight of 386.8. It is a white crystalline compound, soluble in ethanol and insoluble in water. Each Doral Tablet contains either 7.5 or 15 mg of quazepam. The inactive ingredients for Doral Tablets 7.5 or 15 mg include cellulose, corn starch, FD&C Yellow No. 6 Al Lake, lactose, magnesium stearate, silicon dioxide, and sodium lauryl sulfate.

CLINICAL PHARMACOLOGY:

Central nervous system agents of the 1,4-benzodiazepine class presumably exert their effects by binding to stereo-specific receptors at several sites within the central nervous system (CNS). Their exact mechanism of action is unknown.

In a sleep laboratory study, quazepam significantly decreased sleep latency & total wake time, and significantly increased total sleep time and percent sleep time, for one or more nights. Quazepam 15 mg was effective on the first night of administration. Sleep latency, total wake time and wake time after sleep onset were still decreased and percent sleep time was still increased for several nights after the drug was discontinued. Percent slow wave sleep was decreased, and REM sleep was essentially unchanged. No transient sleep disturbance, such as "rebound insomnia," was observed after withdrawal of the drug in sleep laboratory studies in 12 patients using 15 mg doses.

In outpatient studies, quazepam improved all subjective measures of sleep including sleep induction time, duration of sleep, number of nocturnal awakenings, occurrence of early morning awakening, and sleep quality. Some effects were evident on the first night of administration of quazepam (sleep induction time, number of nocturnal awakenings, and duration of sleep). Residual medication effects ("hangover") were minimal.

Quazepam is rapidly (absorption half-life of about 30 minutes) and well absorbed from the gastrointestinal tract. The peak plasma concentration of quazepam is approximately 20 ng/ml after a 15 mg dose and is obtained at about 2 hours. Quazepam, the active parent compound, is extensively metabolized in the liver; two of the plasma metabolites are 2-oxoquazepam and N-desalkyl-2-oxoquazepam. All three compounds show pharmacological central nervous system activity in animals.

Following administration of ^{14}C-quazepam, approximately 31% of the dose appears in the urine and 23% in the feces over a five-day period; only trace amounts of unchanged drug are present in the urine.

The mean elimination half-life of quazepam and 2-oxoquazepam is 39 hours and that of N-desalkyl-2-oxoquazepam is 73 hours. Steady-state levels of quazepam and 2-oxoquazepam are attained by the seventh daily dose and that of N-desalkyl-2-oxoquazepam by the thirteenth daily dose.

The pharmacokinetics of quazepam and 2-oxoquazepam in geriatric subjects are comparable to those seen in young adults; as with desalkyl metabolites of other benzodiazepines, the elimination half-life of N-desalkyl-2-oxoquazepam in geriatric patients is about twice that of young adults.

The degree of plasma protein binding for quazepam and its two major metabolites is greater than 95%. The absorption, distribution, metabolism, and excretion of benzodiazepines may be altered in various disease states including alcoholism, impaired hepatic function, and impaired renal function.

The type and duration of hypnotic effects and the profile of unwanted effects during administration of benzodiazepine drugs may be influenced by the biologic half-life of administered drug and any active metabolites formed. When half-lives are long, drug or metabolites may accumulate during periods of nightly administration and be associated with impairments of cognitive and/or motor performance during waking hours; the possibility of interaction with other psychoactive drugs or alcohol will be enhanced. In contrast, if half-lives are short, drug and metabolites will be cleared before the next dose is ingested, and carry-over effects related to excessive sedation or CNS depression should be minimal or absent. However, during nightly use for an extended period, pharmacodynamic tolerance or adaptation to some effects of benzodiazepine hypnotics may develop. If the drug has a short half-life of elimination, it is possible that a relative deficiency of the drug or its active metabolites (*i.e.,* in relationship to the receptor site) may occur at some point in the interval between each night's use. This sequence of events may account for two clinical findings reported to occur after several weeks of nightly use of rapidly eliminated benzodiazepine hypnotics, namely, increased wakefulness during the last third of the night, and the appearance of increased signs of daytime anxiety in selected patients.

Quazepam crosses the placental barrier of mice. Quazepam, 2-oxoquazepam and N-desalkyl-2-oxoquazepam are present in breast milk of lactating women, but the total amount found in the milk represents only about 0.1% of the administered dose.

INDICATIONS AND USAGE:

Quazepam is indicated for the treatment of insomnia characterized by difficulty in falling asleep, frequent nocturnal awakenings, and/or early morning awakenings. The effectiveness of quazepam has been established in placebo-controlled clinical studies of 5 nights duration in acute and chronic insomnia. The sustained effectiveness of quazepam has been established in chronic insomnia in a sleep lab (polysomnographic) study of 28 nights duration.

Because insomnia is often transient and intermittent, the prolonged administration of quazepam is generally not necessary or recommended. Since insomnia may be a symptom of several other disorders, the possibility that the complaint may be related to a condition for which there is a more specific treatment should be considered.

CONTRAINDICATIONS:

Quazepam is contraindicated in patients with known hypersensitivity to this drug or other benzodiazepines, and in patients with established or suspected sleep apnea.

Usage in Pregnancy: Benzodiazepines may cause fetal damage when administered during pregnancy. An increased risk of congenital malformations associated with the use of diazepam and chlordiazepoxide during the first trimester of pregnancy has been suggested in several studies. Transplacental distribution has resulted in neonatal CNS depression following the ingestion of therapeutic doses of a benzodiazepine hypnotic during the last weeks of pregnancy.

Quazepam are contraindicated in pregnancy because the potential risks outweigh the possible advantages of their use during this period. If there is a likelihood of the patient becoming pregnant while receiving quazepam, she should be warned of the potential risk to the fetus. Patients should be instructed to discontinue the drug prior to becoming pregnant. The possibility that a woman of childbearing potential may be pregnant at the time of institution of therapy should be considered. See Pregnancy, Teratogenic Effects.

WARNINGS:

Patients receiving benzodiazepines should be cautioned about possible combined effects with alcohol and other CNS depressants. Also, caution patients that an additive effect may occur if alcoholic beverages are consumed during the day following the use of benzodiazepines for nighttime sedation. The potential for this interaction continues for several days following their discontinuance until serum levels of psychoactive metabolites have declined.

Patients should also be cautioned about engaging in hazardous occupations requiring complete mental alertness, such as operating machinery or driving a motor vehicle, after ingesting benzodiazepines, including potential impairment of the performance of such activities which may occur the day following ingestion.

Withdrawal symptoms of the type associated with sedatives/hypnotics (*e.g.,* barbiturates, bromides, etc.) and alcohol have been reported after the discontinuation of benzodiazepines. While these symptoms have been more frequently reported after the discontinuation of excessive benzodiazepine doses, there have also been controlled studies demonstrating the

WARNINGS: *(cont'd)*

occurrence of such symptoms after discontinuation of therapeutic doses of benzodiazepines, generally following prolonged use (but in some instances after periods as brief as six weeks). It is generally believed that the gradual reduction of dosage will diminish the occurrence of such symptoms (see DRUG ABUSE AND DEPENDENCE.)

PRECAUTIONS:

GENERAL

Impaired motor and/or cognitive performance attributable to the accumulation of benzodiazepines and their active metabolites following several days of repeated use at their recommended doses is a concern in certain vulnerable patients (*e.g.,* those especially sensitive to the effects of benzodiazepines or those with a reduced capacity to metabolize and eliminate them). Consequently, elderly or debilitated patients and those with impaired renal or hepatic function should be cautioned about the risk and advised to monitor themselves for signs of excessive sedation or impaired coordination.

The possibility of respiratory depression in patients with chronic pulmonary insufficiency should be considered.

When benzodiazepines are administered to depressed patients, there is a risk that the signs and symptoms of depression may be intensified. Consequently, appropriate precautions (*e.g.,* limiting the total prescription size and increased monitoring for suicidal ideation) should be considered.

INFORMATION FOR THE PATIENT

It is suggested that physicians discuss the following information with patients. This information is intended to aid in the safe and effective use of this medication. It is not a disclosure of all possible adverse or intended effects.

1. Inform your physician about any alcohol consumption and medicine you are taking now, including drugs you may buy without a prescription. Alcohol should generally not be used during treatment with hypnotics.

2. Inform your physician if you are planning to become pregnant, if you are pregnant, or if you become pregnant while you are taking this medicine.

3. Inform your physician if you are nursing.

4. Until you experience how this medicine affects you, do not drive a car or operate potentially dangerous machinery, etc.

5. Benzodiazepines may cause daytime sedation, which may persist for several days following drug discontinuation.

6. Patients should be told not to increase the dose on their own and should inform their physician if they believe the drug "does not work anymore".

7. If benzodiazepines are taken on a prolonged and regular basis (even for periods as brief as six weeks), patients should be advised not to stop taking them abruptly or to decrease the dose without consulting their physician, because withdrawal symptoms may occur.

LABORATORY TESTS

Laboratory tests are not ordinarily required in otherwise healthy patients when quazepam is used as recommended.

CARCINOGENESIS, MUTAGENESIS, AND IMPAIRMENT OF FERTILITY

Quazepam showed no evidence of carcinogenicity or other significant pathology in oral oncogenicity studies in mice and hamsters.

Quazepam was tested for mutagenicity using the L5178Y TK +/-Mouse Lymphoma Mutagenesis Assay and Ames Test. The L5178Y TK +/-Assay was equivocal and the Ames Test did not show mutagenic activity.

Reproduction studies in mice conducted with quazepam at doses equal to 60 and 180 times the human dose of 15 mg, and with diazepam at 67 times the human dose, produced slight reductions in the pregnancy rate. Similar reduction in pregnancy rates have been reported in mice dosed with other benzodiazepines, and is believed to be related to the sedative effects of these drugs at high doses.

PREGNANCY CATEGORY X

Teratogenic Effects: (See CONTRAINDICATIONS, Usage in Pregnancy.) Reproduction studies of quazepam in mice at doses up to 400 times the human dose revealed no major drug-related malformations. Minor developmental variations that occurred were delayed ossification of the sternum, vertebrae, distal phalanges and supraoccipital bones, at doses of 66 and 400 times the human dose. Studies with diazepam at 200 times the human dose showed a similar or greater incidence than quazepam. A reproduction study of quazepam in New Zealand rabbits at doses up to 134 times the human dose demonstrated no effect on fetal morphology or development of offspring.

Nonteratogenic Effects: The child born of a mother who is taking benzodiazepines may be at some risk of withdrawal symptoms from the drug during the postnatal period. Neonatal flaccidity has been reported in children born of mothers who had been receiving benzodiazepines.

LABOR AND DELIVERY

Quazepam has no established use in labor or delivery.

NURSING MOTHERS

Quazepam and its metabolites are excreted in the milk of lactating women. Therefore, administration of quazepam to nursing women is not recommended.

PEDIATRIC USE

Safety and effectivenes in children below the age of 18 years have not been established.

DRUG INTERACTIONS:

The benzodiazepines, including quazepam, produce additive CNS depressant effects when co-administered with psychotropic medications, anticonvulsants, antihistaminics, ethanol, and other drugs which produce CNS depression.

ADVERSE REACTIONS:

Adverse events most frequently encountered in patients treated with quazepam are drowsiness and headache.

Accurate estimates of the incidence of adverse events associated with the use of any drug are difficult to obtain. Estimates are influenced by drug dose, detection technique, setting, physician judgments, etc. Consequently, the table below is presented solely to indicate the relative frequency of adverse events reported in representative controlled clinical studies conducted to evaluate the safety and efficacy of quazepam. The figures cited cannot be used to predict precisely the incidence of such events in the course of usual medical practice. These figures, also, cannot be compared with those obtained from other clinical studies involving related drug products and placebo.

The figures cited below (TABLE 1) are estimates of untoward clinical event incidences of 1% or greater among subjects who participated in the relatively short duration placebo-controlled clinical trials of quazepam.

ADVERSE REACTIONS: *(cont'd)*

TABLE 1

Number Of Patients	Quazepam 15 mg 267	Placebo 268
	% Of Patients Reporting	
Central Nervous System		
Daytime Drowsiness	12.0	3.3
Headache	4.5	2.2
Fatigue	1.9	0
Dizziness	1.5	<1
Autonomic Nervous System		
Dry Mouth	1.5	<1
Gastrointestinal System		
Dyspepsia	1.1	<1

The following incidences of laboratory abnormalities occurred at a rate of 1% or greater in patients receiving quazepam and the corresponding placebo group. None of these changes were considered to be of physiological significance (TABLE 2).

TABLE 2

Number Of Patients % of Patients Reporting	Low	Quazepam 234 High	Low	Placebo 244 High
Hematology				
Hemoglobin	1.4	0	1.2	0
Hematocrit	1.5	0	1.7	0
Lymphocyte	1.3	1.6	1.2	1.9
Eosinophil	*	1.5	*	1.3
SEG	1.1	*	1.6	*
Monocyte	*	1.1	*	*
Blood Chemistry				
Glucose	*	*	*	1.2
SGOT	*	1.3	*	1.1
Urinalysis				
Specific Gravity	*	*	*	1.1
WBC	0	2.6	0	3.0
RBC	0	*	0	1.1
Epithelial Cells	0	2.5	0	3.2
Crystals	0	*	0	1.0

* These laboratory abnormalities occurred in less than 1% of patients. In addition, abnormalities in the following laboratory tests were observed in less than 1% of the patients evaluated: WBC count, platelet count, total protein, albumin, BUN, creatinine, total bilirubin, alkaline phosphatase, and SGPT.

The following additional events occurred among individuals receiving quazepam at doses equivalent to or greater than those recommended during its clinical testing and development. There is no way to establish whether or not the administration of quazepam caused these events.

Hypokinesia, ataxia, confusion, incoordination, hyperkinesia, speech disorder, and tremor were reported.

Also, depression, nervousness, agitation, amnesia, anorexia, anxiety, apathy, euphoria, impotence, decreased libido, paranoid reaction, nightmares, abnormal thinking, abnormal taste perception, abnormal vision, and cataract were reported.

Also reported were urinary incontinence, palpitations, nausea, constipation, diarrhea, abdominal pain, pruritus, rash, asthenia, and malaise.

The following list provides an overview of adverse experiences that have been reported and are considered to be reasonably related to the administration of benzodiazepines: incontinence, slurred speech, urinary retention, jaundice, dysarthria, dystonia, changes in libido, irritability, and menstrual irregularities.

As with all benzodiazepines, paradoxical reactions such as stimulation, agitation, increased muscle spasticity, sleep disturbances, hallucinations, and other adverse behavioral effects may occur in rare instances and in a random fashion. Should these occur, use of the drug should be discontinued.

There have been reports of withdrawal signs and symptoms of the type associated with withdrawal from CNS depressant drugs following the rapid decrease or the abrupt discontinuation of benzodiazepines (see DRUG ABUSE AND DEPENDENCE.)

DRUG ABUSE AND DEPENDENCE:

Controlled Substance: Quazepam is a controlled substance under the Controlled Substance Act and has been assigned by the Drug Enforcement Administration to Schedule IV.

Abuse and Dependence: Withdrawal symptoms, similar in character to those noted with barbiturates and alcohol (*e.g.,* convulsions, tremor, abdominal and muscle cramps, vomiting and sweating), have occurred following abrupt discontinuance of benzodiazepines. The more severe withdrawal symptoms have usually been limited to those patients who received excessive doses over an extended period of time. Generally milder withdrawal symptoms (*e.g.,* dysphoria and insomnia) have been reported following abrupt discontinuance of benzodiazepines taken continuously at therapeutic levels for several months. Consequently, after extended therapy, abrupt discontinuation should generally be avoided and a gradual dosage tapering schedule followed. Addiction-prone individuals (such as drug addicts or alcoholics) should be under careful surveillance when receiving quazepam or other psychotropic agents because of the predisposition of such patients to habituation and dependence.

OVERDOSAGE:

Manifestations of overdosage seen with other benzodiazepines include somnolence, confusion, and coma. In the event that an overdose occurs, the following is the recommended treatment. Respiration, pulse, and blood pressure should be monitored, as in all cases of drug overdosage. General supportive measures should be employed, along with immediate gastric lavage. Intravenous fluids should be administered and an adequate airway maintained. Hypotension may be treated with the use of norepinephrine bitartrate or metaraminol bitartrate. Dialysis is of limited value. Animal experiments suggest that forced diuresis or hemodialysis are probably of little value in treating overdosage. As with the management of intentional overdosing with any drug, it should be borne in mind that multiple agents may have been ingested.

The oral LD_{50} in mice was greater than 5,000 mg/kg.

DOSAGE AND ADMINISTRATION:

Adults: Initiate therapy at 15 mg until individual responses are determined. In some patients, the dose may then be reduced to 7.5 mg.

DOSAGE AND ADMINISTRATION: *(cont'd)*

Elderly and debilitated patients: Because the elderly and debilitated may be more sensitive to benzodiazepines, attempts to reduce the nightly dosage after the first one or two nights of therapy are suggested.

Store quazepam tablets between 2 and 30°C (36 and 86°F).

Protect unit doses from excessive moisture.

HOW SUPPLIED - EQUIVALENTS NOT AVAILABLE:

Tablet, Coated - Oral - 7.5 mg

100's $125.36 DORAL, Wallace Labs 00037-9000-01
100's $125.36 DORAL, Wallace Labs 00037-9000-02

Tablet, Coated - Oral - 15 mg

100's $137.00 DORAL, Wallace Labs 00037-9002-01
100's $137.00 DORAL, Wallace Labs 00037-9002-02

QUINAPRIL HYDROCHLORIDE *(003069)*

CATEGORIES: ACE Inhibitors; Angiotensin Converting Enzyme Inhibitors; Antihypertensives; Cardiovascular Drugs; Congestive Heart Failure; Heart Failure; Hypertension; Pregnancy Category D; FDA Class 1C ("Little or No Therapeutic Advantage"); Sales > $100 Million; FDA Approved 1991 Nov; Top 200 Drugs

BRAND NAMES: **Accupril**; *Accuprin*; *Accupro* (England); *Accupron*; *Acequin*; *Acuitel* (France); *Acuprel*; *Acupril* (Mexico); *Asig*; *Korec* (France); *Quinazil*
(International brand names outside U.S. in italics)

FORMULARIES: Medi-Cal; PCS

COST OF THERAPY: $331.82 (Hypertension; Tablet; 10 mg; 1/day; 365 days)

PRIMARY ICD9: 401.1 (Essential Hypertension, Benign)

WARNING:
Use In Pregnancy: When used in pregnancy during the second and third trimesters, ACE inhibitors can cause injury and even death to the developing fetus. When pregnancy is detected, quinapril HCl should be discontinued as soon as possible. (See WARNINGS, Fetal/Neonatal Morbidity and Mortality).

DESCRIPTION:

Quinapril hydrochloride is the hydrochloride salt of quinapril, the ethyl ester of a nonsulfhydryl, angiotensin-converting enzyme (ACE) inhibitor, quinaprilat.

Quinapril hydrochloride is chemically described as (3S-(2(R*(R*)), 3R*))-2-(2-((1-(ethoxycarbonyl)-3-phenylpropyl)amino)-1-oxopropyl)-1,2,3, 4-tetrahydro-3-isoquinolinecarboxylic acid, monohydrochloride. Its empirical formula is $C_{25}H_{30}N_2O_5$·HCl.

Quinapril hydrochloride is a white to off-white amorphous powder that is freely soluble in aqueous solvents.

Accupril tablets contain 5 mg, 10 mg, 20 mg, or 40 mg of quinapril for oral administration. Each tablet also contains candelilla wax, crospovidone, gelatin, lactose, magnesium carbonate, magnesium stearate, synthetic red iron oxide, and titanium dioxide.

CLINICAL PHARMACOLOGY:

MECHANISM OF ACTION

Quinapril is deesterified to the principal metabolite, quinaprilat, which is an inhibitor of ACE activity in human subjects and animals. ACE is a peptidyl dipeptidase that catalyzes the conversion of angiotensin I to the vasoconstrictor, angiotensin II. The effect of quinapril in hypertension appears to result primarily from the inhibition of circulating and tissue ACE activity, thereby reducing angiotensin II formation. Quinapril inhibits the elevation in blood pressure caused by intravenously administered angiotensin I, but has no effect on the pressor response to angiotensin II, norepinephrine or epinephrine. Angiotensin II also stimulates the secretion of aldosterone from the adrenal cortex, thereby facilitating renal sodium and fluid reabsorption. Reduced aldosterone secretion by quinapril may result in a small increase in serum potassium. In controlled hypertension trials, treatment with quinapril HCl alone resulted in mean increases in potassium of 0.07 mmol/L(see PRECAUTIONS.) Removal of angiotensin II negative feedback on renin secretion leads to increased plasma renin activity (PRA).

While the principal mechanism of antihypertensive effect is thought to be through the renin-angiotensin-aldosterone system, quinapril exerts antihypertensive actions even in patients with low renin hypertension. Quinapril HCl was an effective antihypertensive in all races studied, although it was somewhat less effective in blacks (usually a predominantly low renin group) than in nonblacks. ACE is identical to kininase II, an enzyme that degrades bradykinin, a potent peptide vasodilator; whether increased levels of bradykinin play a role in the therapeutic effect of quinapril remains to be elucidated.

Pharmacokinetics and Metabolism

Following oral administration, peak plasma quinapril concentrations are observed within one hour. Based on recovery of quinapril and its metabolites in urine, the extent of absorption is at least 60%. The rate and extent of quinapril absorption are diminished moderately (approximately 25-30%) when quinapril HCl tablets are administered during a high-fat meal. Following absorption, quinapril is deesterified to its major active metabolite, quinaprilat (about 38% of oral dose), and to other minor inactive metabolites. Following multiple oral dosing of quinapril HCl, there is an effective accumulation half-life of quinaprilat of approximately 3 hours, and peak plasma quinaprilat concentrations are observed approximately 2 hours post-dose. Quinaprilat is eliminated primarily by renal excretion, up to 96% of an IV dose, and has an elimination half-life in plasma of approximately 2 hours and a prolonged terminal phase with a half-life of 25 hours. The pharmacokinetics of quinapril and quinaprilat are linear over a single-dose range of 5-80 mg doses and 40-160 mg in multiple daily doses. Approximately 97% of either quinapril or quinaprilat circulating in plasma is bound to proteins.

In patients with renal insufficiency, the elimination half-life of quinaprilat increases as creatinine clearance decreases. There is a linear correlation between plasma quinaprilat clearance and creatinine clearance. In patients with end-stage renal disease, chronic hemodialysis or continuous ambulatory peritoneal dialysis has little effect on the elimination of quinapril and quinaprilat. Elimination of quinaprilat is reduced in elderly patients (≥65 years) and in those with heart failure; this reduction is attributable to decrease in renal function (see DOSAGE AND ADMINISTRATION), and not to age itself. Quinaprilat concentrations are reduced in patients with alcoholic cirrhosis due to impaired deesterification of quinapril. Studies in rats indicate that quinapril and its metabolites do not cross the blood-brain barrier.

CLINICAL PHARMACOLOGY: *(cont'd)*

PHARMACODYNAMICS AND CLINICAL EFFECTS

Hypertension: Single doses of 20 mg of quinapril HCl provide over 80% inhibition of plasma ACE for 24 hours. Inhibition of the pressor response to angiotensin I is shorter-lived, with a 20 mg dose giving 75% inhibition for about 4 hours, 50% inhibition for about 8 hours, and 20% inhibition at 24 hours. With chronic dosing, however, there is substantial inhibition of angiotensin II levels at 24 hours by doses of 20-80 mg.

Administration of 10 to 80 mg of quinapril HCl to patients with mild to severe hypertension results in a reduction of sitting and standing blood pressure to about the same extent with minimal effect on heart rate. Symptomatic postural hypotension is infrequent although it can occur in patients who are salt- and/or volume-depleted (see WARNINGS.) Antihypertensive activity commences within 1 hour with peak effects usually achieved by 2 to 4 hours after dosing. During chronic therapy, most of the blood pressure lowering effect of a given dose is obtained in 1-2 weeks. In multiple-dose studies, 10-80 mg per day in single or divided doses lowered systolic and diastolic blood pressure throughout the dosing interval, with a trough effect of about 5-11/3-7 mm Hg. The trough effect represents about 50% of the peak effect. While the dose-response relationship is relatively flat, doses of 40-80 mg were somewhat more effective at trough than 10-20 mg, and twice daily dosing tended to give a somewhat lower trough blood pressure than once daily dosing with the same total dose. The antihypertensive effect of quinapril HCl continues during long-term therapy, with no evidence of loss of effectiveness.

Hemodynamic assessments in patients with hypertension indicate that blood pressure reduction produced by quinapril is accompanied by a reduction in total peripheral resistance and renal vascular resistance with little or no change in heart rate, cardiac index, renal blood flow, glomerular filtration rate, or filtration fraction.

Use of quinapril HCl with a thiazide diuretic gives a blood-pressure lowering effect greater than that seen with either agent alone.

In patients with hypertension, quinapril HCl 10-40 mg was similar in effectiveness to captopril, enalapril, propranolol, and thiazide diuretics.

Therapeutic effects appear to be the same for elderly (≥65 years of age) and younger adult patients given the same daily dosages, with no increase in adverse events in elderly patients.

Heart Failure: In a placebo-controlled trial involving patients with congestive heart failure treated with digitalis and diuretics, parenteral quinaprilat, the active metabolite of quinapril, reduced pulmonary capillary wedge pressure, and systemic vascular resistance and increased cardiac output/index. Similar favorable hemodynamic effects were seen with oral quinapril, and such effects appeared to be maintained during chronic oral quinapril therapy. Quinapril reduced renal hepatic vascular resistance and increased renal and hepatic blood flow with glomerular filtration rate remaining unchanged.

A significant dose response relationship for improvement in maximal exercise tolerance has been observed with quinapril HCl therapy. Beneficial effects on the severity of heart failure as measured by New York Heart Association (NYHA) classification and Quality of Life and on symptoms of dyspnea, fatigue, and edema were evident after 6 months in a double blind, placebo controlled study. Favorable effects were maintained for up to two years of open label therapy. The effects of quinapril on long-term mortality in heart failure have not been evaluated.

INDICATIONS AND USAGE:

Hypertension: Quinapril HCl is indicated for the treatment of hypertension. It may be used alone or in combination with thiazide diuretics.

Heart Failure: Quinapril HCl is indicated in the management of heart failure as adjunctive therapy when added to conventional therapy including diuretics and/or digitalis.

In using quinapril HCl, consideration should be given to the fact that another angiotensin converting enzyme inhibitor, captopril, has caused agranulocytosis, particularly in patients with renal impairment or collagen vascular disease. Available data are insufficient to show that quinapril HCl does not have a similar risk (see WARNINGS.)

CONTRAINDICATIONS:

Quinapril HCl is contraindicated in patients who are hypersensitive to this product and in patients with a history of angioedema related to previous treatment with an ACE inhibitor.

WARNINGS:

Anaphylactoid and Possibly Related Reactions: Presumably because angiotensin-converting inhibitors affect the metabolism of eicosanoids and polypeptides, including endogenous bradykinin, patients receiving ACE inhibitors (including quinapril HCl) may be subject to a variety of adverse reactions, some of them serious.

Angioedema: Angioedema of the face, extremities, lips, tongue, glottis, and larynx has been reported in patients treated with ACE inhibitors and has been seen in 0.1% of patients receiving quinapril HCl. Angioedema associated with laryngeal edema can be fatal. If laryngeal stridor or angioedema of the face, tongue, or glottis occurs, treatment with quinapril HCl should be discontinued immediately, the patient treated in accordance with accepted medical care, and carefully observed until the swelling disappears. In instances where swelling is confined to the face and lips, the condition generally resolves without treatment; antihistamines may be useful in relieving symptoms. **Where there is involvement of the tongue, glottis, or larynx likely to cause airway obstruction, emergency therapy including, but not limited to, subcutaneous epinephrine solution 1:1000 (0.3 to 0.5 ml), should be promptly administered** (see ADVERSE REACTIONS.)

Patients with a history of angioedema unrelated to ACE inhibitor therapy may be at increased risk of angioedema while receiving an ACE inhibitor (see also CONTRAINDICATIONS).

Anaphylactoid reactions during desensitization: Two patients undergoing desensitizing treatment with hymenoptera venom while receiving ACE inhibitors sustained life-threatening anaphylactoid reactions. In the same patients, these reactions were avoided when ACE inhibitors were temporarily withheld, but they reappeared upon inadvertent rechallenge.

Anaphylactoid reactions during membrane exposure: Anaphylactoid reactions have been reported in patients dialyzed with high-flux membranes and treated concomitantly with an ACE inhibitor. Anaphylactoid reactions have also been reported in patients undergoing low-density lipoprotein apheresis with dextran sulfate absorption (a procedure dependent upon devices not approved in the United States).

Hepatic Failure: Rarely, ACE inhibitors have been associates with a syndrome that starts with cholestatic jaundice and progresses to fulminant hepatic necrosis and (sometimes) death. The mechanism of this syndrome is not understood. Patients receiving ACE inhibitors who develop jaundice or marked elevations of hepatic enzymes should discontinue the ACE inhibitor and receive appropriate medical follow-up.

Hypotension: Excessive hypotension is rare in patients with uncomplicated hypertension treated with quinapril HCl alone. Patients with heart failure given quinapril HCl commonly have some reduction in blood pressure, but discontinuation of therapy because of continuing symptomatic hypotension usually is not necessary when dosing instructions are followed. Caution should be observed when initiating therapy in patients with heart failure (see

WARNINGS: *(cont'd)*

DOSAGE AND ADMINISTRATION.) In controlled studies, syncope was observed in 0.4% of patients (N=3203); this incidence was similar to that observed for captopril (1%) and enalapril (0.8%).

Patients at a risk of excessive hypotension, sometimes associated with oliguria and/or progressive azotemia, and rarely with acute renal failure and/or death, include patients with the following conditions or characteristics: heart failure, hyponatremia, high dose diuretic therapy, recent intensive diuresis or increase in diuretic dose, renal dialysis, or severe volume and/or salt depletion of any etiology. It may be advisable to eliminate the diuretic (except in patients with heart failure), reduce the diuretic dose or cautiously increase salt intake (except in patients with heart failure) before initiating therapy with quinapril HCl in patients at risk for excessive hypotension who are able to tolerate such adjustments.

In patients at risk of excessive hypotension, therapy with quinapril HCl should be started under close medical supervision. Such patients should be followed closely for the first two weeks of treatment and whenever the dose of quinapril HCl and/or diuretic is increased. Similar considerations may apply to patients with ischemic heart or cerebrovascular disease in whom an excessive fall in blood pressure could result in a myocardial infarction or a cerebrovascular accident.

If excessive hypotension occurs, the patient should be placed in the supine position and, if necessary, receive an intravenous infusion of normal saline. A transient hypotensive response is not a contraindication to further doses of quinapril HCl, which usually can be given without difficulty once the blood pressure has stabilized. If symptomatic hypotension develops, a dose reduction or discontinuation of quinapril HCl or concomitant diuretic may be necessary.

Neutropenia/Agranulocytosis: Another ACE inhibitor, captopril, has been shown to cause agranulocytosis and bone marrow depression rarely in patients with uncomplicated hypertension, but more frequently in patients with renal impairment, especially if they also have a collagen vascular disease, such as systemic lupus erythematosus or scleroderma. Agranulocytosis did occur during quinapril HCl treatment in one patient with a history of neutropenia during previous captopril therapy. Available data from clinical trials of quinapril HCl are insufficient to show that, in patients without prior reactions to other ACE inhibitors, quinapril HCl does not cause agranulocytosis at similar rates. As with other ACE inhibitors, periodic monitoring of white blood cell counts in patients with collagen vascular disease and/or renal disease should be considered.

Fetal/Neonatal Morbidity and Mortality: ACE inhibitors can cause fetal and neonatal morbidity and death when administered to pregnant women. Several dozen cases have been reported in the world literature. When pregnancy is detected, ACE inhibitors should be discontinued as soon as possible.

The use of ACE inhibitors during the second and third trimesters of pregnancy has been associated with fetal and neonatal injury, including hypotension, neonatal skull hypoplasia, anuria, reversible or irreversible renal failure, and death. Oligohydramnios has also been reported, presumably resulting from decreased fetal renal function; oligohydramnios in this setting has been associated with fetal limb contractures, craniofacial deformation, and hypoplastic lung development. Prematurity, intrauterine growth retardation, and patent ductus arteriosus have also been reported, although it is not clear whether these occurrences were due to the ACE inhibitor exposure.

These adverse effects do not appear to have resulted from intrauterine ACE inhibitor exposure that has been limited to he first trimester. Mothers whose embryos and fetuses are exposed to ACE inhibitors only during the first trimester should be so informed. Nonetheless, when patients become pregnant, physicians should make every effort to discontinue the use of quinapril HCl as soon as possible.

Rarely (probably less often than once in every thousand pregnancies), no alternative to ACE inhibitors will be found. In these rare cases, the mothers should be apprised of the potential hazards to their fetuses, and serial ultrasound examinations should be performed to assess the intramniotic environment.

If oligohydramnios is observed, quinapril HCl should be discontinued unless it is considered life-saving for the mother. Contraction stress testing (CST), a non-stress test (NST), or biophysical profiling (BPP) may be appropriate, depending upon the week of pregnancy. Patients and physicians should be aware, however, that oligohydramnios may not appear until after the fetus has sustained irreversible injury.

Infants with histories of *in utero*exposure to ACE inhibitors should be closely observed for hypotension, oliguria, and hyperkalemia. If oliguria occurs, attention should be directed toward support of blood pressure and renal perfusion. Exchange transfusion or dialysis may be required as a means of reversing hypotension and/or substituting for disordered renal function. Removal of quinapril HCl, which crosses the placenta, from the neonatal circulation is not significantly accelerated by these means.

No teratogenic effects of quinapril HCl were seen in studies of pregnant rats and rabbits. On a mg/kg basis, the doses used were up to 180 times (in rats) and one time (in rabbits) the maximum recommended human dose.

PRECAUTIONS:

GENERAL

Impaired Renal Function: As a consequence of inhibiting the renin-angiotensin-aldosterone system, changes in renal function may be anticipated in susceptible individuals. In patients with severe heart failure whose renal function may depend on the activity of the renin-angiotensin-aldosterone system, treatment with ACE inhibitors, including quinapril HCl, may be associated with oliguria and/or progressive azotemia and rarely acute renal failure and/or death.

In clinical studies in hypertensive patients with unilateral or bilateral renal artery stenosis, increases in blood urea nitrogen and serum creatinine have been observed in some patients following ACE inhibitor therapy. These increases were almost always reversible upon discontinuation of the ACE inhibitor and/or diuretic therapy. In such patients, renal function should be monitored during the first few weeks of therapy.

Some patients with hypertension or heart failure with no apparent preexisting renal vascular disease have developed increases in blood urea and serum creatinine, usually minor and transient, especially when quinapril HCl has been given concomitantly with a diuretic. This is more likely to occur in patients with preexisting renal impairment. Dosage reduction and/or discontinuation of any diuretic and/or quinapril HCl may be required.

Evaluation of patients with hypertension or heart failure should always include assessment of renal function (see DOSAGE AND ADMINISTRATION.)

Hyperkalemia and potassium-sparing diuretics: In clinical trials, hyperkalemia (serum potassium ≥5.8 mmol/L) occurred in approximately 2% of patients receiving quinapril HCl. In most cases, elevated serum potassium levels were isolated values which resolved despite continued therapy. Less than 0.1% of patients discontinued therapy due to hyperkalemia. Risk factors for the development of hyperkalemia include renal insufficiency, diabetes mellitus, and the concomitant use of potassium-sparing diuretics, potassium supplements, and/or potassium-containing salt substitutes, which should be used cautiously, if at all, with quinapril HCl (see DRUG INTERACTIONS.)

PRECAUTIONS: *(cont'd)*

Cough: Presumably due to the inhibition of the degradation of endogenous bradykinin, persistant non-productive cough has been reported with all ACE inhibitors, always resolving after disconinuation of therapy. ACE inhibitor-induced cough should be considered in the differential diagnosis of cough.

Surgery/anesthesia: In patients undergoing major surgery or during anesthesia with agents that produce hypotension, quinapril HCl will block angiotensin II formation secondary to compensatory renin release. If hypotension occurs and is considered to be due to this mechanism, it can be corrected by volume expansion.

INFORMATION FOR THE PATIENT

Pregnancy: Female patients of childbearing age should be told about the consequences of second- and third-trimester exposure to ACE inhibitors, and they should also be told that these consequences do not appear to have resulted from intrauterine ACE-inhibitor exposure that has been limited to the first trimester. These patients should be asked to report pregnancies to their physicians as soon as possible.

Angioedema: Angioedema, including laryngeal edema can occur with treatment with ACE inhibitors, especially following the first dose. Patients should be so advised and told to report immediately any signs or symptoms suggesting angioedema (swelling of face, extremities, eyes, lips, tongue, difficulty in swallowing or breathing) and to stop taking the drug until they have consulted with their physician (see WARNINGS.)

Symptomatic hypotension: Patients should be cautioned that lightheadedness can occur, especially during the first few days of quinapril HCl therapy, and that it should be reported to a physician. If actual syncope occurs, patients should be told to not take the drug until they have consulted with their physician (see WARNINGS.)

All patients should be cautioned that inadequate fluid intake or excessive perspiration, diarrhea, or vomiting can lead to an excessive fall in blood pressure because of reduction in fluid volume, with the same consequences of lightheadedness and possible syncope.

Patients planning to undergo any surgery and/or anesthesia should be told to inform their physician that they are taking an ACE inhibitor.

Hyperkalemia: Patients should be told not to use potassium supplements or salt substitutes containing potassium without consulting their physician (see PRECAUTIONS.)

Neutropenia: Patients should be told to report promptly any indication of infection (*e.g.*, sore throat, fever) which could be a sign of neutropenia.

NOTE: As with many other drugs, certain advice to patients being treated with quinapril HCl is warranted. This information is intended to aid in the safe and effective use of this medication. It is not a disclosure of all possible adverse or intended effects.

CARCINOGENESIS, MUTAGENESIS, AND IMPAIRMENT OF FERTILITY

Quinapril hydrochloride was not carcinogenic in mice or rats when given in doses up to 75 or 100 mg/kg/day (50 to 60 times the maximum human daily dose, respectively, on an mg/kg basis and 3.8 to 10 times the maximum human daily dose when based on an mg/m^2 basis) for 104 weeks. Female rats given the highest dose level had an increased incidence of mesenteric lymph node hemangiomas and skin/subcutaneous lipomas. Neither quinapril nor quinaprilat were mutagenic in the Ames bacterial assay with or without metabolic activation. Quinapril was also negative in the following genetic toxicology studies: *in vitro* mammalian cell point mutation, sister chromatid exchange in cultured mammalian cells, micronucleus test with mice, *in vitro* chromosome aberration with V79 cultured lung cells, and in an *in vivo* cytogenetic study with rat bone marrow. There were no adverse effects on fertility or reproduction in rats at doses up to 100 mg/kg/day (60 and 10 times the maximum daily human dose when based on mg/kg and mg/m^2, respectively).

PREGNANCY

Pregnancy Category C (first trimester) and D (second and third trimesters): See WARNINGS, Fetal/Neonatal Morbidity and Mortality.

NURSING MOTHERS

It is not known if quinapril or its metabolites are secreted in human milk. Quinapril is secreted to a limited extent, however, in milk of lactating rats (5% or less of the plasma drug concentration was found in rat milk). Because many drugs are secreted in human milk, caution should be exercised when quinapril HCl is given to a nursing mother.

GERIATRIC USE

Elderly patients exhibited increased area under the plasma concentration time curve (AUC) and peak levels for quinaprilat compared to values observed in younger patients; this appeared to relate to decreased renal function rather than to age itself. In controlled and uncontrolled studies of quinapril HCl where 918 (21%) patients were 65 years and older, no overall differences in effectiveness or safety were observed between older and younger patients. However, greater sensitivity of some older individual patients cannot be ruled out.

PEDIATRIC USE

The safety and effectiveness of quinapril HCl in children have not been established.

DRUG INTERACTIONS:

Concomitant diuretic therapy: As with other ACE inhibitors, patients on diuretics, especially those on recently instituted diuretic therapy, may occasionally experience an excessive reduction of blood pressure after initiation of therapy with quinapril HCl. The possibility of hypotensive effects with quinapril HCl may be minimized by either discontinuing the diuretic or cautiously increasing salt intake prior to initiation of treatment with quinapril HCl. If it is not possible to discontinue the diuretic, the starting dose of quinapril should be reduced (see DOSAGE AND ADMINISTRATION.)

Agents increasing serum potassium: Quinapril can attenuate potassium loss caused by thiazide diuretics and increase serum potassium when used alone. If concomitant therapy of quinapril HCl with potassium-sparing diuretics (*e.g.*, spironolactone, triamterene, or amiloride), potassium supplements, or potassium-containing salt substitutes is indicated, they should be used with caution along with appropriate monitoring of serum potassium (see PRECAUTIONS.)

Tetracycline and other drugs that interact with magnesium: Simultaneous administration of tetracycline with quinapril HCl reduced the absorption of tetracycline by approximately 28% to 37%, possibly due to the high magnesium content in quinapril HCl tablets. This interaction should be considered if coprescribing quinapril HCl and tetracycline or other drugs that interact with magnesium.

Lithium: Increased serum lithium levels and symptoms of lithium toxicity have been reported in patients receiving concomitant lithium and ACE inhibitor therapy. These drugs should be coadministered with caution and frequent monitoring of serum lithium levels is recommended. If a diuretic is also used, it may increase the risk of lithium toxicity.

Other agents: Drug interaction studies of quinapril HCl with other agents showed:

Multiple dose therapy with propranolol or cimetidine has no effect on the pharmacokinetics of single doses of quinapril HCl.

The anticoagulant effect of a single dose of warfarin (measured by prothrombin time) was not significantly changed by quinapril coadministration twice-daily.

Quinapril HCl treatment did not affect the pharmacokinetics of digoxin.

No pharmacokinetic interaction was observed when single doses of quinapril HCl and hydrochlorothiazide were administered concomitantly.

ADVERSE REACTIONS:

HYPERTENSION

Quinapril HCl has been evaluated for safety in 4960 subjects and patients. Of these, 3203 patients, including 655 elderly patients, participated in controlled clinical trials. Quinapril HCl has been evaluated for long-term safety in over 1400 patients treated for 1 year or more.

Adverse experiences were usually mild and transient.

In placebo-controlled trials, discontinuation of therapy because of adverse events was required in 4.7% of patients with hypertension.

Adverse experiences probably or possibly related to therapy or of unknown relationship to therapy occurring in 1% or more of the 1563 patients in placebo-controlled hypertension trials who were treated with quinapril HCl are shown in TABLE 1.

TABLE 1 Adverse Events in Placebo-Controlled Trials

	Quinapril HCl (N=1563) Incidence (Discontinuance)	Placebo (N=579) Incidence (Discontinuance)
Headache	5.6 (0.7)	10.9 (0.7)
Dizziness	3.9 (0.8)	2.6 (0.2)
Fatigue	2.6 (0.3)	1.0
Coughing	2.0 (0.5)	0.0
Nausea and/or Vomiting	1.4 (0.3)	1.9 (0.2)
Abdominal Pain	1.0 (0.2)	0.7

HEART FAILURE

Quinapril HCl has been evaluated for safety in 1222 quinapril HCl treated patients. Of these, 632 patients participated in controlled clinical trials. In placebo-controlled trials, discontinuation of therapy because of adverse events was required in 6.8% of patients with congestive heart failure.

Adverse experiences probably or possibly related or of unknown relationship to therapy occurring in 1% or more of the 585 patients in placebo-controlled congestive heart failure trials who were treated with quinapril HCl are shown below (TABLE 2).

TABLE 2

	Quinapril HCl (N=585) Incidence (Discontinuance)	Placebo (N=295) Incidence (Discontinuance)
Dizziness	7.7 (0.7)	5.1 (1.0)
Coughing	4.3 (0.3)	1.4
Fatigue	2.6 (0.2)	1.4
Nausea and/or vomiting	2.4 (0.2)	0.7
Chest Pain	2.4	1.0
Hypotension	2.9 (0.5)	1.0
Dyspnea	1.9 (0.2)	2.0
Diarrhea	1.7	1.0
Headache	1.7	1.0 (0.3)
Myalgia	1.5	2.0
Rash	1.4 (0.2)	1.0
Back Pain	1.2	0.3

See PRECAUTIONS, Cough.

HYPERTENSION AND/OR HEART FAILURE

Clinical adverse experiences probably, possibly, or definitely related, or of uncertain relationship to therapy occurring in 0.5% to 1.0% (except as noted) of the patients treated with quinapril HCl (with or without concomitant diuretic) in controlled or uncontrolled trials (N=4847) and less frequent, clinically significant events seen in clinical trials or post-marketing experience (the rarer events are in italics) include (listed by body system):

General: back pain, malaise, viral infections

Cardiovascular: palpitation, vasodilation, tachycardia, *heart failure, hyperkalemia, myocardial infarction, cerebrovascular accident, hypertensive crisis, angina pectoris, orthostatic hypotension, cardiac rhythm disturbances, cardiogenic shock*

Hematology: *hemolytic anemia*

Gastrointestinal: dry mouth or throat, constipation, *gastrointestinal hemorrhage, pancreatitis, abnormal liver function tests*

Nervous/Psychiatric: somnolence, vertigo, syncope, nervousness, depression

Integumentary: increased sweating, pruritus, *exfoliative dermatitis, photosensitivity reaction, dermatopolymiositis*

Urogenital: acute renal failure, worsening renal failure

Other: amblyopia, pharyngitis, sinusitis, bronchitis, *agranulocytosis, thrombocytopenia*

FETAL/NEONATAL MORBIDITY AND MORTALITY

See WARNINGS, Fetal/Neonatal Morbidity and Mortality.

ANGIOEDEMA

Angioedema has been reported in patients receiving quinapril HCl (0.1%). Angioedema associated with laryngeal edema may be fatal. If angioedema of the face, extremities, lips, tongue, glottis, and/or larynx occurs, treatment with quinapril HCl should be discontinued and appropriate therapy instituted immediately. (See WARNINGS.)

CLINICAL LABORATORY TEST FINDINGS

Hematology: (See WARNINGS)

Hyperkalemia: (See PRECAUTIONS)

Creatinine and Blood Urea Nitrogen: Increases (>1.25 times the upper limit of normal) in serum creatinine and blood urea nitrogen were observed in 2% and 2%, respectively, of patients treated with quinapril HCl alone. Increases are more likely to occur in patients receiving concomitant diuretic therapy than in those on quinapril HCl alone. These increases often remit on continued therapy. In controlled studies of heart failure, increases in blood urea nitrogen and serum creatinine were observed in 11% and 8%, respectively, of patients treated with quinapril HCl; most often these patients were receiving diuretics with or without digitalis.

OVERDOSAGE:

No data are available with respect to overdosage in humans. Doses of 1440 to 4280 mg/kg of quinapril cause significant lethality in mice and rats.

The most likely clinical manifestation would be symptoms attributable to severe hypotension.

Laboratory determinations of serum levels of quinapril and its metabolites are not widely available, and such determinations have, in any event, no established role in the management of quinapril overdose.

OVERDOSAGE: *(cont'd)*

No data are available to suggest physiological maneuvers (*e.g.*, maneuvers to change pH of the urine) that might accelerate elimination of quinapril and its metabolites.

Hemodialysis and peritoneal dialysis have little effect on the elimination of quinapril and quinaprilat. Angiotensin II could presumably serve as a specific antagonist-antidote in the setting of quinapril overdose, but angiotensin II is essentially unavailable outside of scattered research facilities. Because the hypotensive effect of quinapril is achieved through vasodilation and effective hypovolemia, it is reasonable to treat quinapril overdose by infusion of normal saline solution.

DOSAGE AND ADMINISTRATION:

HYPERTENSION

Monotherapy: The recommended initial dosage of quinapril HCl in patients not on diuretics is 10 mg once daily. Dosage should be adjusted according to blood pressure response measured at peak (2-6 hours after dosing) and trough (predosing). Generally, dosage adjustments should be made at intervals of at least 2 weeks. Most patients have required dosages of 20, 40, or 80 mg/day, given as a single dose or in 2 equally divided doses. In some patients treated once daily, the antihypertensive effect may diminish toward the end of the dosing interval. In such patients an increase in dosage or twice daily administration may be warranted. In general, doses of 40-80 mg and divided doses give a somewhat greater effect at the end of the dosing interval.

Concomitant Diuretics: If blood pressure is not adequately controlled with quinapril HCl monotherapy, a diuretic may be added. In patients who are currently being treated with a diuretic, symptomatic hypotension occasionally can occur following the initial dose of quinapril HCl. To reduce the likelihood of hypotension, the diuretic should, if possible, be discontinued 2 to 3 days prior to beginning therapy with quinapril HCl (see WARNINGS.) Then, if blood pressure is not controlled with quinapril HCl alone, diuretic therapy should be resumed.

If the diuretic cannot be discontinued, an initial dose of 5 mg quinapril HCl should be used with careful medical supervision for several hours and until blood pressure has stabilized.

The dosage should subsequently be titrated (as described above) to the optimal response (see WARNINGS, PRECAUTIONS, and DRUG INTERACTIONS).

Dosage for Impaired Renal Function: Kinetic data indicate that the apparent elimination half-life of quinaprilat increases as creatinine clearance decreases. Recommended starting doses, based on clinical and pharmacokinetic data from patients with renal impairment, are as follows (TABLE 3):

TABLE 3

Creatinine Clearance	Maximum Recommended Initial Dose
>60 ml/min	10 mg
30-60 ml/min	5 mg
10-30 ml/min	2.5 mg
<10 ml/min	Insufficient data for dosage recommendation

Patients should subsequently have their dosage titrated (as described above) to the optimal response.

Elderly (≥65 years): The recommended initial dosage of quinapril HCl in elderly patients is 10 mg given once daily followed by titration (as described above) to the optimal response.

HEART FAILURE

Quinapril HCl is indicated as adjunctive therapy when added to conventional therapy including diuretics and/or digitalis. The recommended starting dose is 5 mg twice daily. This dose may improve symptoms of heart failure, but increases in exercise duration have generally required higher doses. Therefore, if the initial dosage of quinapril HCl is well tolerated, patients should then be titrated at weekly intervals until an effective dose, usually 20 to 40 mg daily given in two equally divided doses, is reached or undesirable hypotension, orthostatis, azotemia (see WARNINGS) prohibit reaching this dose.

Following the initial dose of quinapril HCl, the patient should be observed under medical supervision for at least two hours for the presence of hypotension or orthostatis and, if present, until blood pressure stabilizes. The appearance of hypotension or orthostatis, or azotemia early in dose titration should not preclude further careful dose titration. Consideration should be given to reducing the dose of concomitant diuretics.

DOSE ADJUSTMENTS IN PATIENTS WITH HEART FAILURE AND RENAL IMPAIRMENT OR HYPONATREMIA

Pharmacokinetic data indicate that quinapril elimination is dependent on level of renal function. In patients with heart failure and renal impairment, the recommended initial dose of quinapril HCl is 5 mg in patients with a creatinine clearance above 30 ml/min and 2.5 mg in patients with a creatinine clearance of 10 to 30 ml/min. There is insufficient data for dosage recommendation in patients with a creatinine clearance less than 10 ml/min. See DOSAGE AND ADMINISTRATION, Heart Failure, WARNINGS and DRUG INTERACTIONS.

If the initial dose is well tolerated, quinapril HCl may be administered the following day as a twice daily regimen. In the absence of excessive hypotension or significant deterioration of renal function, the dose may be increased at weekly intervals based on clinical and hemodynamic response.

PATIENT INFORMATION:

Quinapril HCl is used to treat high blood pressure and some forms of heart failure alone or in combination with other medications. This medication should not be used during pregnancy and should be discontinued when pregnancy is determined. A nonproductive, persistent cough has been reported with the use of ACE inhibitors. The cough normally disappears when the medication is discontinued. A rare condition called angioedema can occur with ACE inhibitors, especially following the first dose. If you experience swelling of the face, eyes, lips, or tongue, difficulty in breathing) do not take additional medication and contact your physician immediately. Dizziness and lightheadedness can result when the mediation is first started. If this persists longer than one week, contact your physician. Signs of infections (sore throat or fever) should be reported to your physician as well to assure these are not drug related. Your blood pressure should be checked regularly to assure adequate control.

HOW SUPPLIED:

Acupril tablets are supplied as follows:

5-mg tablets: brown, film-coated, elliptical scored tablets, coded "PD 527" on one side and "5" on the other.

10-mg tablets: brown, film-coated, triangular tablets, coded "PD 530" on one side and "10" on the other.

20-mg tablets: brown, film-coated, round tablets, coded "PD 532" on one side and "20" on the other.

40-mg tablets: brown, film coated, elliptical tablets, coated "PD 535" on one side and "40" on the other.

HOW SUPPLIED: *(cont'd)*

Dispense in well-closed containers as defined in the USP.

Storage: Store at controlled room temperature 15-30°C (59-86°F).

HOW SUPPLIED - EQUIVALENTS NOT AVAILABLE:

Tablet, Uncoated - Oral - 5 mg

90's	$81.82	ACCUPRIL, Parke-Davis	00071-0527-23
100's	$90.91	ACCUPRIL, Parke-Davis	00071-0527-40

Tablet, Uncoated - Oral - 10 mg

90's	$81.82	ACCUPRIL, Parke-Davis	00071-0530-23
100's	$90.91	ACCUPRIL, Parke-Davis	00071-0530-40

Tablet, Uncoated - Oral - 20 mg

90's	$81.82	ACCUPRIL, Parke-Davis	00071-0532-23
100's	$90.91	ACCUPRIL, Parke-Davis	00071-0532-40

Tablet, Uncoated - Oral - 40 mg

90's	$81.82	ACCUPRIL, Parke-Davis	00071-0535-23
100's	$78.54	ACCUPRIL, Parke-Davis	00071-0535-40

QUINIDINE GLUCONATE *(002165)*

CATEGORIES: Antiarrhythmic Agents; Arrhythmia; Cardiovascular Drugs; Fibrillation; Heart Flutter; Quinidines; Renal Drugs; Tachycardia; Pregnancy Category C; FDA Approval Pre 1982

BRAND NAMES: Duraquin; Quin-G; Quinact; Quinagen Duratab; **Quinaglute**; Quinalan; Quinatime

FORMULARIES: Aetna; BC-BS; CIGNA; DoD; FHP; Humana; Kaiser; Medco; Medi-Cal; PruCare; United

COST OF THERAPY: $125.92 (Arrhythmia; Tablet; 324 mg; 2/day; 365 days)

DESCRIPTION:

TABLETS

Each quinidine gluconate sustained-release tablet contains 324 mg quinidine gluconate (equivalent to 202 mg quinidine base) in a tablet matrix specially designed for the sustained-release (8 to 12 hours) of the drug in the gastrointestinal tract. Quinidine gluconate sustained release tablets are to be administered orally.

Quinidine gluconate is the gluconate salt of quinidine (6-methoxy-α-(5-vinyl -2-quinuclidinyl)-4-quinoline-methanol), a dextrorotatory isomer of quinine.

Quinidine gluconate contains 62.3% of the anhydrous quinidine alkaloid, whereas quinidine sulfate contains 82.86%. In prescribing, Quinidine gluconate sustained release tablets, this factor should be considered.

Therapeutic Category: Type I antiarrhythmic.

Each Quinaglute sustained release tablet also contains the following inactive ingredients: confectioner's sugar, magnesium stearate, starch (corn), and other ingredient(s).

INJECTION

Quinidine gluconate Injection, USP, a myocardial depressant, is a sterile, white dextrorotary salt containing 62.3% anhydrous quinidine and 37.7% glucuronic acid. It is suitable for parenteral use because of its high efficacy, local tolerance, and stability in solution. It may be administered intramuscularly or intravenously.

Chemically, it is cinchonan-9-ol. 6'-methoxy-, (9*S*)-, mono-D- gluconate (salt). Quinidine gluconate has the empirical formula $C_{20}H_{24}N_2O_2 \cdot C_6H_{12}O_7$, representing a molecular weight of 520.58

Each vial contains 800 mg (1.5 mmol) of the salt of the alkaloid in 10 ml of Sterile Water for Injection, with 0.005% edetate disodium and 0.25% phenol. Glucono delta lactone may have been added during manufacture to adjust the pH. This quantity of quinidine gluconate represents 500 mg (0.96 mmol) of anhydrous quinidine.)

CLINICAL PHARMACOLOGY:

TABLETS

The antiarrhythmic activity consists of the following basic actions:

1. In arrhythmias due to enhanced automaticity, quinidine decreases the rate of rise of low diastolic (Phase 4) depolarization, thereby depressing automaticity, particularly in ectopic foci.

2. In addition to the above, quinidine slows depolarization, repolarization and amplitude of the action potential, thus increasing its duration leading to an increase in the refractoriness of atrial and ventricular tissue. Prolongation of the effective refractory period and an increase in conduction time may prevent the recently phenomenon.

3. Quinidine exerts an indirect anticholinergic effect through blockade of vagal innervation. This anticholinergic effect may facilitate conduction in the atrioventricular junction.

Quinidine absorption from quinidine gluconate sustained release tablets proceeds at a slower rate then the immediate-release products. In the single-dose pharmacokinetic study conducted in normal volunteers, the time of peak quinidine serum concentration was 1.6 hours for quinidine sulfate tablets and 3.6 hours for quinidine gluconate sustained release tablets.

The apparent elimination half-life or quinidine ranges from 4 to 10 hours in healthy persons with a usual mean value of 6 to 7 hours. The half-life may be prolonged in elderly persons. From 60% to 80% of the dose is metabolized by the liver. Renal excretion of the intact drug comprises the remainder of the total clearance. Quinidine is approximately 75% bound to serum proteins.

In the past, plasma levels of 1.5 to 5 mcg/ml have been reported as therapeutic,[1] based on non-specific assay methodology that quantitates quinidine metabolites as well as intact quinidine. The therapeutic plasma level range using newer, more specific assays has not been definitively established, however, effective reduction of premature ventricular contractions has been reported with blood levels less than 1.0 mcg/ml[2]. In general, plasma quinidine levels are lower using specific assays. Clinicians requesting serum quinidine determinations should therefore also ask that the method of analysis be specified.

Due to the wide individual variation in response to quinidine therapy, the usefulness of serum quinidine levels in the planning of optimal quinidine therapy has not been clearly established. A serum quinidine concentration within the reported therapeutic range may not necessarily be the optimal concentration for some patients. In the absence of toxicity, such patients may warrant an increase in dose to achieve the desired therapeutic effect. However, for these patients in whom a high blood level has been achieved without significant therapeutic response, increasing the dose to potentially toxic levels is not warranted and consideration should be given to combination or alternate therapy. In all cases, the physician should carefully consider patient response and evidence of toxicity along with blood levels in determining optimal quinidine therapy.

CLINICAL PHARMACOLOGY: *(cont'd)*

INJECTION

Quinidine is generally regarded as a myocardial depressant drug, because it depresses excitability, conduction velocity, and contractility of the myocardium. Besides these direct effects, quinidine exerts some indirect activity on the heart through an anticholinergic action. Large oral doses may reduce the arterial pressure by means of peripheral vasodilation. Hypotension of a serious degree is more likely with the parenteral use of the drug.

The maximum effects of quinidine gluconate occur 30 to 90 minutes after intramuscular administration. the onset of action is more rapid after intravenous administration, and activity persists for 6 to 8 hours or more. Quinidine is metabolized in the liver and excreted by the kidney. Ten percent to 50% of quinidine is excreted in the urine as unchanged drug within 24 hours. The degree of protein binding is 80% to 90%.

Plasma levels of quinidine can be measured. Values vary according to the assay employed. Traditionally, plasma concentrations for effective use of quinidine have been reported to range from 2 to 5 mcg/ml; levels of greater than 5 mcg/ml are associated with toxicity. This information is based on less specific analytic methods, which quantitate metabolites as well as intact quinidine. However, with the use of more specific assays plasma quinidine concentrations will be lower. Therefore, clinicians requesting serum quinidine determinations should be aware of the method of analysis. there is a wide individual variation in response to quinidine therapy. In all cases, the physician should carefully consider patient response and evidence of toxicity along with blood levels in determining optimal quinidine therapy.

INDICATIONS AND USAGE:

TABLETS

Quinidine gluconate sustained release tablets are indicated in the prevention and/or treatment of:

Ventricular arrhythmias

Premature ventricular contractions

Ventricular tachycardia (when not associated with complete heartblock)

Junctional (nodal) arrhythmias

AV junctional premature complexes

Paroxysmal junctional tachycardia

Supraventricular (atrial) arrhythmias

Premature atrial contractions

Paroxysmal atrial tachycardia

Atrial flutter

Atrial fibrillation (chronic and paroxysmal)

INJECTION

Parenteral administration of quinidine is indicated in the treatment of the following condition when oral therapy is not feasible or when rapid therapeutic effect is required:

Premature atrial and ventricular contractions

Paroxysmal atrial tachycardia

Paroxysmal atrioventricular junctional rhythm

Atrial flutter

Paroxysmal atrial fibrillation

Established atrial-fibrillation when therapy is appropriate

Paroxysmal ventricular tachycardia when not associated with complete heart block.

Maintenance therapy after electrical conversion of atrial fibrillation and or flutter.

Life-threatening *Plasmodium falciparum*malaria - Unless impossible, therapy should be undertaken in an intensive care setting with continuous monitoring of the electrocardiogram, frequent monitoring of blood pressure, and periodic monitoring of parasitemia (see PRECAUTIONS).

CONTRAINDICATIONS:

TABLETS

1. Idiosyncrasy or hypersensitivity to quinidine.

2. Complete AV block.

3. Complete bundle branch block or other severe intraventricular conduction defects, especially those exhibiting a marked grade of QRS widening.

4. Digitalis intoxication manifested by AV conduction disorders.

5. Myasthenia gravis.

6. Aberrant impulses and abnormal rhythms due to escape mechanisms.

INJECTION

Hypersensitivity or idiosyncrasy to the drug, history of thrombocytopenic purpura associated with previous quinidine administration.

Digitalis Intoxication manifested by AV conduction disorders, complete AV block with an AV nodal or idioventricular pacemaker, left bundle branch block or other severe intraventricular conduction defects with marked widening of QRS complex. Ectopic impulses and abnormal rhythms due to escape mechanisms. Also, myasthenia gravis.

WARNINGS:

TABLETS

1. In the treatment of atrial flutter, reversion to sinus rhythm may be preceded by a progressive reduction in the degree of AV block to a 1:1 ratio resulting in an extremely rapid ventricular rate. This possible hazard may be reduced by digitalization prior to administration of quinidine.

2. Recent reports indicate that plasma concentrations of digoxin increase and may even double when quinidine is administered concurrently. Patients on concomitant therapy should be carefully monitored. Reduction of digoxin dosage may have to be considered.

3. Manifestations of quinidine cardiotoxicity, such a excessive prolongation of the Q-T interval, widening of the QRS complex and ventricular tachyarrhythmias mandate immediate discontinuation of the drug and/or close clinical and electrocardiographic monitoring.

4. In susceptible individuals, such as those with marginally compensated cardiovascular disease, quinidine may produce clinically important depression of cardiac function such as hypotension, bradycardia or heartblock. Quinidine therapy should be carefully monitored in such individuals.

5. Quinidine should be used with extreme caution in patients with incomplete AV block since complete block and asystole may be produced. Quinidine may cause abnormalities of cardiac rhythm in digitalized patients and therefore should be used with caution in the presence of digitalis intoxication.

6. Quinidine should be used with caution in patients exhibiting renal, cardiac or hepatic insufficiency because of potential accumulation of quinidine in plasma leading to toxicity.

WARNINGS: *(cont'd)*

7. Patients taking quinidine occasionally have syncopal episodes, usually resulting from ventricular tachycardia or fibrillation. This syndrome has not been shown to be related to dose of plasma levels. Syncopal episodes frequently terminate spontaneously or in response to treatment but sometimes are fatal.

8. A few cases of hepatotoxicity, including granulomatous hepatitis, due to quinidine hypersensitivity have been reported in patients taking quinidine. Unexplained lever and/or elevation of hepatic enzymes, particularly in the early stages of therapy, warrant consideration of possible hepatotoxicity. Monitoring liver function during the first 4 to 8 weeks should be considered. Cessation of quinidine in these cases usually results in the disappearance of toxicity.

INJECTION

In the treatment of atrial flutter, reversion to sinus rhythm may be preceded by a progressive reduction in the degree of AV block to a 1:1 ratio, which results in extremely rapid ventricular rate. This possible hazard may be decreased by digitalization prior to administration of quinidine.

In susceptible individuals, such as those with marginally compensated cardiovascular disease, quinidine may produce clinically important depression of cardiac function, such as hypotension, bradycardia, or heart block. Quinidine therapy should be carefully monitored in such individuals.

Evidence of quinidine cardiotoxicity (excessive prolongation of Q-T interval, 50% widening of QRS complex, frequent ventricular ectopic beats) mandates immediate discontinuation of the drug and subsequent close observation (electrocardiographic monitoring) of the patient.

Quinidine should be used with extreme caution when there is incomplete AV block, since complete block and asystole may result. The drug may cause unpredictable abnormalities of rhythm in digitalized hearts, and it should be used with special caution in the presence of digitalis intoxication.

The effect of quinidine is enhanced by potassium and reduced if hypokalemia is present.

The depressant actions of quinidine on cardiac contractility and arterial blood pressure limit its use in congestive heart failure and in hypotensive states unless these conditions are due to or aggravated by the arrhythmia. The potential disadvantages and benefits must be weighed.

Patients taking quinidine occasionally have syncopal episodes, which usually result from ventricular tachycardia or fibrillation. This syndrome has not been shown to be related to dose or plasma levels. Syncopal episodes frequently terminate spontaneously or in response to treatment but sometimes are fatal.

Recent reports have described increased, potentially toxic, digoxin plasma levels when quinidine is administered concurrently. When concurrent use is necessary, digoxin dosage should be reduced, its plasma concentration monitored, and the patient observed closely for digitalis intoxication.

Caution should be used when quinidine is administered concurrently with coumarin anticoagulants. This combination may reduce prothrombin levels and cause bleeding.

PRECAUTIONS:

GENERAL

The precautions to be observed include all those applicable to quinidine. A preliminary test dose of a single tablet of quinidine sulfate may be administered to determine if the patient has an idiosyncrasy to quinidine. Hypersensitivity to quinidine, although rare, should constantly be considered, especially during the first weeks of therapy.

Hospitalization for close clinical observation, electrocardiographic monitoring, and possible determination of plasma quinidine levels is indicated when large doses are used, or with patients who present an increased risk.

INFORMATION FOR THE PATIENT

As with all solid oral dosage medications, quinidine gluconate sustained release tablets should be taken with an adequate amount of fluid, preferably in an upright position, to facilitate swallowing.

CARCINOGENESIS, MUTAGENESIS, AND IMPAIRMENT OF FERTILITY

Long-term studies in animals have not been performed to evaluate the carcinogenic potential of quinidine. There is currently no evidence of quinidine-induced mutagenesis or impairment of fertility.

PREGNANCY CATEGORY C

Teratogenic Effects: Animal reproduction studies have not been conducted with quinidine. There are no adequate and well-controlled studies in pregnant women. Quinidine gluconate sustained release tablets should be administered to a pregnant women only if clearly indicated.

Nonteratogenic Effects: Like quinine, quinidine has been reported to have oxytocic properties. The significance of this property in the clinical setting has not been established.

NURSING MOTHERS

Because of passage of the drug into breast milk, caution should be exercised when quinidine gluconate sustained release tablets are administered to a nursing woman.

PEDIATRIC USE

There ar no adequate and well-controlled studies establishing the safety and effectiveness of quinidine gluconate sustained release tablets in children.

DRUG INTERACTIONS:

See TABLE 1

TABLE 1

Drug	Effect
Quinidine with anti-cholinergic drugs	Additive vagolytic effect
Quinidine with cholinergic drugs	Antagonism of cholinergic effects
Quinidine with carbonic anhydrase inhibitors, sodium bicarbonate, thiazide diuretics	Alkalinization of urine resulting in decreased excretion of quinidine
Quinidine with coumarin anticoagulants	Reduction of clotting factor concentrations
Quinidine with tubocurate, succinylcholine and decamethonium	Potentiation of neuro-muscular blockade
Quinidine with pheno-thiazines and reserpine	Additive cardiac depressive effects
Quinidine with hepatic enzyme-inducing drugs (phenobarbital, phenytoin, rifampin)	Potential for reduction or quinidine plasma levels.
Quinidine with cimetidine	Potential for elevation of quinidine plasma levels.
Quinidine with digoxin	Increased plasma concentrations of digoxin (SeeWARNINGS)

ADVERSE REACTIONS:

Symptoms of cinchonism, ringing in ears, headache, nausea and/or disturbed vision may appear in sensitive patients after a single dose of the drug.

The most frequently encountered side effects to quinidine are gastrointestinal in nature. These gastrointestinal effects include nausea, vomiting, abdominal pain, diarrhea, and rarely, esophagitis.

Less frequently encountered adverse reactions:

Cardiovascular: Widening of QRS complex, cardiac asystole, ventricular ectopic beats, idioventricular rhythms including ventricular tachycardia and fibrillation, paradoxical tachycardia, arterial embolism and hypotension.

Hematologic: Acute hemolytic anemia, hypoprothrombinemia, thrombocytopenia (purpura), agranulocytosis.

Central Nervous System: Headache, fever, vertigo, apprehension, excitement, confusion, delirium and syncope, disturbed hearing (tinnitus, decreased auditory acuity), disturbed vision (mydriasis, blurred vision, disturbed color perception, reduced vision field, photophobia, diplopia, night blindness, scotomata), optic neuritis.

Dermatologic: Rash, cutaneous flushing with intense pruritus, urticaria. Photosensitivity has also been reported.

Hypersensitivity Reactions: Angioedema, acute asthmatic episode, vascular collapse, respiratory arrest, hepatotoxicity, including granulomatous hepatitis (see WARNINGS).

Although rare, there have been reports of lupus erythematosus in patients taking quinidine.

OVERDOSAGE:

TABLETS

If ingestion of quinidine is recent, gastric lavage, emesis and/or administration of activated charcoal may reduce absorption. Management of overdosage includes symptomatic treatment, ECG and blood pressure monitoring, cardiac pacing if indicated and acidification of the urine. Artificial respiration and other supportive measures may be required.

IV infusion of 1/6 molar sodium lactate reportedly reduces the cardiotoxic effects of quinidine. Since marked CNS depression may occur even in the presence of convulsions, CNS depressants should not be administered. Hypotension may be treated, if necessary, with metaraminol or norepinephrine after adequate fluid volume replacement. Hemodialysis has been reported to be effective in the treatment of quinidine overdosage in adults and children but is rarely warranted.

INJECTION

Signs and Symptoms: Manifestations of quinidine overdose include nausea, vomiting, diarrhea, tinnitus, vertigo headache, paresthesia, and quinidine concentrations exceed the therapeutic range of 2 to 5 mcg/ml. More serious manifestations include syncope, hypotension, heart block, prolongation of QRS and QT_c intervals. ST depression, T inversion, torsades de pointes, ventricular tachycardia, other cardiac dysrhythmias, heart failure, respiratory depression, coma and death.

Treatment: To obtain up-to-date information about the treatment of overdose, a good resource is your certified Regional Poison Control Center. Telephone numbers of certified poison control Center. Telephone numbers of certified poison control centers are listed in the front of this publication. In managing overdosage, consider the possibility of multiple drug overdoses, interaction among drugs, and unusual drug kinetics in your patient.

Protect the patient's airway and support ventilation and perfusion. Meticulously monitor and maintain, within acceptable limits, the patient's vital signs, blood gases, serum electrolytes, etc.

Hypotension may be best managed with α-adrenergic agonists such as norepinephrine. Heart block may be treated with a pacemaker. Tachydysrhythmias should respond to phenytoin or lidocaine.

Forced diuresis or dialysis can aid in the removal of quinidine. Alkalinization of the urine should be avoided as this will result in decreased quinidine excretion.

Procainamide and disopyramide, which also can prolong the QRS and QT_c intervals, are contraindicated. Verapamil and amiodarone may decrease quinidine clearance.

DOSAGE AND ADMINISTRATION:

TABLETS

The dosage varies considerably depending upon the general condition and cardiovascular state of the patient. The quantity and frequency of administration of quinidine gluconate sustained release tablets that will achieve the desired clinical results, must be determined for each patient.

The ideal dosage is the minimum amount of total dose and frequency of daily administration that will prevent premature contractions, paroxysmal tachycardias and maintain normal sinus rhythm.

Prevention of premature atrial, nodal or ventricular contractions: 1 to 2 tablets every 8 or 12 hours.

Maintenance of normal sinus rhythm following conversion of paroxysmal tachycardias: 2 tablets every 12 hours or 1.5 to 2 tablets every 8 hours usually are required.

Although most patients may be maintained in normal rhythm on a dosage of 1 quinidine gluconate sustained release tablet every 8 or 12 hours, other patients may require larger doses or more frequent administration (*i.e.,* every 6 hours) than the usually recommended schedule. Such increased dosage should be instituted only after careful clinical and laboratory evaluation of the patient, including monitoring of plasma quinidine levels and, if possible, serial electrocardiograms.

Quinidine gluconate sustained release tablets are generally well tolerated. Gastrointestinal disturbance, if they occur, may be minimized by administering the drug with food.

It is frequently desirable to determine if a patient can tolerate maintenance quinidine therapy prior to electrical conversion. Therefore, maintenance therapy may be initiated 2 to 3 days before electrical conversion if attempted. Quinidine gluconate sustained release tablets are well suited for such a program and can be administered at a maintenance dose felt necessary for a given patient as indicated above.

Note: Dosage may be titrated by breaking the tablet in half. Do not crush or chew since sustained-release properties will be lost.

Store at controlled room temperature, between 15 and 30°C (59 and 86°F).

INJECTION

If the patient's condition is not critical, quinidine gluconate should be given intramuscularly. On the other hand, extreme palpitation, dyspepsia, vomiting, and a shock-like state in patients with ventricular tachycardia are signs that the intravenous administration of quinidine may be required as a lifesaving measure when D-C cardioversion is not available.

The patient must be under close clinical observation. Frequent or continuous electrocardiograms and frequent measurement of blood pressure are desirable, especially during intravenous injection, to detect an change in rate or rhythmn. Administration of the drug must be stopped when any of the following occurs: (1) side effects of more than trivial nature (2) restoration of

DOSAGE AND ADMINISTRATION: *(cont'd)*

sinus rhythm (3) prolongation of QRS complex in excess of 25% beyond that observed prior to the injection (4) disappearance of P waves (5) decrease in heart rate to 120 beats/min (6) significant hypotension.

In the treatment of cardiac arrhythmias with quinidine, therapy should be regulated in such a way that the drug is accumulated in the heart in sufficient quantities to abolish ectopic rhythm without disturbing the normal mechanism of the heartbeat. *The effective dose must be determined for each patient.*

If the patient has not received quinidine before and time permits, and initial dose of 200 mg of quinidine gluconate may be given intramuscularly as a test for idiosyncrasy. The test dose is given intramuscularly, regardless of whether subsequent administration is to be intramuscular or intravenous (see PRECAUTIONS).

Intramuscular: In the treatment of acute tachycardia, the recommended initial dose is 600 mg. Subsequently, the injection of 400 mg of quinidine gluconate can be repeated as often as every 2 hours. The amount of each dose must be gauged by the effect of the preceding one.

Intravenous: It has been shown that in about 50% of patients who respond successfully to quinidine, the arrhythmia can be terminated by 330 mg or less of quinidine gluconate (or its equivalent in other salts). In some cases, the intravenous administration of as much as 500 to 750 mg may be required.

The quinidine gluconate solution must be injected *slowly*. It is advisable to dilute 10 ml of the preparation to 50 ml, using 5% Dextrose Injection, USP as the diluent. The resulting solution may be stored refrigerated for time periods up to 48 hours or at room temperature up to 24 hours. It has been suggested that the diluted quinidine gluconate be given at a rate of 1 ml/min for maximum safety.

P. Falciparum Malaria: Two regimens have been empirically shown to be effective, with or without concomitant exchange transfusions. As soon as practical, standard oral antiplasmodial therapy should be instituted.

a) Loading,15 mg/kg of base (24 mg/kg of quinidine gluconate) in a volume of 250 ml normal saline infused over 4 hours followed by Maintenance, beginning 8 hours after the beginning of the loading dose, 7.5 mg/kg of base (12 mg/kg of quinidine gluconate) infused over 4 hours, every 8 hours for 7 days or until oral therapy can be instituted.

b) Loading, 6.25 mg/kg of base (10 mg/kg of quinidine gluconate) in an appropriate volume of normal saline infused over 1 to 2 hours (*e.g.,* 250 ml of normal saline for an otherwise healthy 50 kg person), followed immediately by Maintenance, 0.0125 mg/kg/min of base (0.02 mg/kg/min of quinidine gluconate) for up to 72 hours or until parasitemia decreases to less than 1% or oral therapy can be instituted.

Prior to administration, parenteral drug products should be inspected visually for particulate matter whenever solution and container permit.

CLINICAL REPORTS (Injection): Intramuscular administration of quinidine gluconate was found by various investigators to be satisfactory in treating acute arrhythmias. Characteristic quinidine effect was observed as early as 15 minutes after injection, and conversion occurred within 2 hours. The maximum concentration of quinidine in the blood occurred within 2 hours. The maximum peak level was higher with a single dose of quinidine gluconate than with an equivalent intramuscular dose of quinidine sulfate in urea- antipyrine or in propylene glycol.

It has been repeatedly reported that the intravenous use of quinidine was successful in the treatment of urgent cases of tachycardias, particularly ventricular tachycardias. Normal rhythm was restored as quickly as 4 to 6 minutes after injection.

REFERENCES:

1 Koch-Wooer, *Arch. Int. Med.*1972, 129: 763-772. **2** Carliner et al, *Am, Heart J.*1980, 100: 483-489.

HOW SUPPLIED - RATED THERAPEUTICALLY EQUIVALENT:

Tablet, Uncoated, Sustained Action - Oral - 324 mg

100's	$17.25	Quinidine Gluconate, H.C.F.A. F F P	99999-2165-01
100's	$27.50	Quinidine Gluconate, Major Pharms	00904-2202-60
100's	$28.96	Quinidine Gluconate, Qualitest Pharms	00603-5598-21
100's	$29.00	Quinidine Gluconate, Goldline Labs	00182-1382-01
100's	$29.00	Quinidine Gluconate, United Res	00677-0675-01
100's	$29.00	Quinidine Gluconate, Mutual Pharm	53489-0141-01
100's	$30.82	Quinidine Gluconate, Parmed Pharms	00349-7040-01
100's	$31.56	Quinidine Gluconate SA, Aligen Independ	00405-4910-01
100's	$34.63	Quinidine Gluconate, HL Moore Drug Exch	00839-6473-06
100's	$35.49	Quinidine Gluconate, Rugby	00536-4434-01
100's	$35.49	Quinidine Gluconate, Geneva Pharms	00781-1804-01
100's	$35.54	Quinidine Gluconate, Schein Pharm (US)	00364-0604-01
100's	$43.02	Quinidine Gluconate, Vangard Labs	00615-1583-13
100's	$43.11	Quinidine Gluconate, Medirex	57480-0388-01
100's	$45.81	QUINIDINE GLUCONATE 324, Major Pharms	00904-2202-61
100's	$45.99	Quinidine Gluconate, Geneva Pharms	00781-1804-13
100's	**$56.16**	**QUINAGLUTE DURA-TABS, Berlex Labs**	**50419-0101-10**
100's	**$58.68**	**QUINAGLUTE DURA-TABS, Berlex Labs**	**50419-0101-11**
250's	$43.12	Quinidine Gluconate, H.C.F.A. F F P	99999-2165-02
250's	$57.94	Quinidine Gluconate SA, Aligen Independ	00405-4910-04
250's	$61.85	Quinidine Gluconate, Halsey Drug	00879-0582-25
250's	$61.85	Quinidine Gluconate, Major Pharms	00904-2202-70
250's	$65.19	Quinidine Gluconate, HL Moore Drug Exch	00839-6473-09
250's	$72.10	Quinidine Gluconate, Goldline Labs	00182-1382-02
250's	$72.10	Quinidine Gluconate, United Res	00677-0675-03
250's	$72.10	Quinidine Gluconate, Geneva Pharms	00781-1804-25
250's	$72.10	Quinidine Gluconate, Mutual Pharm	53489-0141-03
250's	$74.85	Quinidine Gluconate, Parmed Pharms	00349-7040-25
250's	$76.91	Quinidine Gluconate, Schein Pharm (US)	00364-0604-04
250's	$80.30	Quinidine Gluconate, Rugby	00536-4434-02
250's	**$136.44**	**QUINAGLUTE DURA-TABS, Berlex Labs**	**50419-0101-25**
500's	$86.25	Quinidine Gluconate, Mutual Pharm	53489-0141-05
500's	$86.25	Quinidine Gluconate, H.C.F.A. F F P	99999-2165-03
500's	$113.54	Quinidine Gluconate, Halsey Drug	00879-0582-05
500's	$114.50	Quinidine Gluconate, Major Pharms	00904-2202-40
500's	$132.96	Quinidine Gluconate, HL Moore Drug Exch	00839-6473-12
500's	$136.80	Quinidine Gluconate, Qualitest Pharms	00603-5598-28
500's	$137.49	Quinidine Gluconate, Geneva Pharms	00781-1804-05
500's	$137.50	Quinidine Gluconate, Goldline Labs	00182-1382-05
500's	$137.50	Quinidine Gluconate, United Res	00677-0675-05
500's	$143.80	Quinidine Gluconate ER, Schein Pharm (US)	00364-0604-05
500's	$143.80	Quinidine Gluconate, Rugby	00536-4434-05
500's	$144.40	Quinidine Gluconate, Parmed Pharms	00349-7040-05
500's	**$255.78**	**QUINAGLUTE DURA-TABS, Berlex Labs**	**50419-0101-50**
600's	$242.20	Quinidine Gluconate, Medirex	57480-0388-06
1000's	$257.60	Quinidine Gluconate, Parmed Pharms	00349-7040-10

HOW SUPPLIED - NOT RATED EQUIVALENT:

Injection, Solution - Intramuscular; - 80 mg/ml

10 ml	$13.77	Quinidine Gluconate, Lilly	00002-1407-01

HOW SUPPLIED - NOT RATED EQUIVALENT: *(cont'd)*

Tablet, Uncoated, Sustained Action - Oral - 324 mg

100's	$29.34	Quinidine Gluconate, Caremark	00339-5327-12
100's	$30.00	Quinidine Gluconate, Voluntary Hosp	53258-0157-01
100's	$33.84	Quinidine Gluconate, Lederle Pharm	00005-3113-23
100's	$34.50	Quinidine Gluconate, Voluntary Hosp	53258-0157-13
250's	$52.43	Quinidine Gluconate, IDE-Interstate	00814-6522-22
250's	$82.11	Quinidine Gluconate, Lederle Pharm	00005-3113-27

QUINIDINE POLYGALACTURONATE *(002166)*

CATEGORIES: Antiarrhythmic Agents; Arrhythmia; Atrial Fibrillation; Cardiovascular Drugs; Fibrillation; Heart Flutter; Quinidines; Renal Drugs; Tachycardia; FDA Approval Pre 1982

BRAND NAMES: **Cardioquin**

FORMULARIES: BC-BS

COST OF THERAPY: $752.63 (Arrhythmia; Tablet; 275 mg; 2/day; 365 days)

DESCRIPTION:

Quinidine Polygalacturonate, an antiarrhythmic, is a polymer of quinidine and polygalacturonic acid which occurs as a creamy white, amorphous powder and is sparingly soluble in water, and freely soluble in hot 40% alcohol.

Chemically, quinidine polygalacturonate is $C_{20}H_{24}N_2O_2C_6H_{10}O_7H_2O$.

Cardioquin Tablets, for oral administration, contain 275 mg quinidine polygalacturonate equivalent in content to 200 mg (3 grains) of quinidine sulfate.

Cardioquin Inactive components include: Corn starch, Lactose, Magnesium stearate, Povidone and Talc.

CLINICAL PHARMACOLOGY:

The quinidine component slows conduction time, prolongs the refractory period, and depresses the excitability of heart muscle. Polygalacturonate slows ionization of the drug and protects the gastrointestinal tract by its demulcent effect.

INDICATIONS AND USAGE:

Quinidine polygalacturonate is indicated as maintenance therapy after spontaneous and electrical conversion of atrial tachycardia, flutter or fibrillation and in the treatment of:

Premature atrial and ventricular contractions.

Paroxysmal atrial tachycardia.

Paroxysmal A-V junctional rhythm.

Atrial flutter.

Paroxysmal atrial fibrillation.

Established atrial fibrillation when therapy is appropriate.

Paroxysmal ventricular tachycardia when not associated with complete heartblock.

CONTRAINDICATIONS:

1. History of hypersensitivity to quinidine manifested by thrombocytopenia, skin eruptions, febrile reactions, etc.

2. Complete A-V block.

3. Complete bundle branch block or other severe intraventricular conduction defects exhibiting marked QRS widening or bizarre complexes.

4. Myasthenia gravis.

5. Arrhythmias associated with digitalis toxicity.

WARNINGS:

In the treatment of atrial fibrillation with rapid ventricular response, ventricular rate should be controlled with digitalis glycosides *prior* to administration of quinidine.

In the treatment of atrial flutter with quinidine, reversion to sinus rhythm may be preceded by progressive reduction in the degree of A-V block to a 1:1 ratio resulting in an extremely high ventricular rate. This potential hazard may be reduced by digitalization prior to administration of quinidine.

Recent reports have described increased, potentially toxic, digoxin plasma levels when quinidine is administered concurrently. When concurrent use is necessary, digoxin in dosage should be reduced and plasma concentration should be monitored and patients observed closely for digitalis intoxication.

Quinidine cardiotoxicity may be manifested by increased P-R and Q-T intervals, 50% widening of QRS, and/or ventricular ectopic beats or tachycardia. Appearance of these toxic signs during quinidine administration mandates immediate discontinuation of the drug and/or close clinical and electrocardiographic monitoring. Note: Quinidine effect is enhanced by potassium and reduced in the presence of hypokalemia.

Quinidine syncope may occur as a complication of long-term therapy. It is manifested by sudden loss of consciousness and by ventricular arrhythmias with bizarre QRS complexes. This syndrome does not appear to be related to dose or plasma levels, but occurs more often with prolonged Q-T intervals.

Because quinidine antagonizes the effect of vagal excitation upon the atrium and the A-V node, the administration of parasympathomimetic drugs (choline esters) or the use of any other procedure to enhance vagal activity may fail to terminate paroxysmal supraventricular tachycardia in patients receiving quinidine.

Quinidine should be used with extreme caution in:

a) The presence of incomplete A-V block, since a complete block and asystole may result.

b) Quinidine may cause unpredictable abnormalities of rhythm in digitalized hearts. Therefore, it should be used with caution in the presence of digitalis intoxication (see WARNINGS, 2).

c) Partial bundle branch block.

d) Severe congestive heart failure and hypotensive states due to the depressant effects of quinidine on myocardial contractility and arterial pressure.

e) Poor renal function, especially renal tubular acidosis, because of the potential accumulation of quinidine in plasma leading to toxic concentrations.

PRECAUTIONS:

Test Dose: A preliminary test dose of a single tablet of quinidine sulfate should be administered prior to the initiation of treatment with quinidine polygalacturonate to determine whether the patient has an idiosyncrasy to the quinidine molecule.

PRECAUTIONS: *(cont'd)*

Hypersensitivity: During the first weeks of therapy, hypersensitivity to quinidine, although rare, should be considered (*e.g.,* angioedema, purpura, acute asthmatic episode, vascular collapse).

Long-Term Therapy: Periodic blood counts and liver and kidney function tests should be performed during long-term therapy, and the drug should be discontinued if blood dyscrasias or signs of hepatic or renal disorders occur.

Large Doses: ECG monitoring and determination of plasma quinidine levels are recommended when doses greater than 2.5 g/day are administered.

Usage in Pregnancy: The use of quinidine in pregnancy should be reserved only for those cases where the benefits outweigh the possible hazards to the patient and fetus.

Nursing Mothers: The drug should be used with extreme caution in nursing mothers because the drug is excreted in breast milk.

General: In patients exhibiting asthma, muscle weakness and infection with fever *prior* to quinidine administration, hypersensitivity reactions to the drug may be masked.

DRUG INTERACTIONS:

1. Caution should be used when quinidine and its analogs are administered concurrently with coumarin anticoagulants. This combination may reduce prothrombin levels and cause bleeding.

2. Quinidine, a weak base, may have its half-life prolonged in patients who are concurrently taking drugs that can alkalize the urine, such as thiazide diuretics, sodium bicarbonate, and carbonic anhydrase inhibitors. Quinidine and drugs which alkalize the urine should be used together cautiously.

3. Quinidine exhibits a distinct anticholinergic activity in the myocardial tissues. An additive vagolytic effect may be seen when quinidine and drugs having anticholinergic blocking activity are used together. Drugs having cholinergic activity may be antagonized by quinidine.

4. Quinidine and other antiarrhythmic agents may produce additive cardiac depressant effects when administered together.

5. Quinidine interaction with cardiac glycosides (digoxin). See WARNINGS.

6. Antacids may delay absorption of quinidine but appear unlikely to cause incomplete absorption.

7. Phenobarbital and phenytoin may reduce plasma half-life of quinidine by 50%.

8. Quinidine may potentiate the neuromuscular blocking effect in ventilatory depression of patients receiving decamethonium, tubocurare or succinylcholine.

ADVERSE REACTIONS:

Symptoms of cinchonism (ringing in the ears, headache, disturbed vision) may appear in sensitive patients after a single dose of the drug.

Gastrointestinal: The most common side effects encountered with quinidine are referable to this system. Diarrhea frequently occurs, but it rarely necessitates withdrawal of the drug. Nausea, vomiting and abdominal pain also occur. Some of these effects may be minimized by administering the drug with meals.

Cardiovascular: Widening of QRS complex, cardiac asystole, ventricular ectopic beats, idioventricular rhythms including ventricular tachycardia and fibrillation; paradoxical tachycardia, arterial embolism, and hypotension.

Hematologic: Acute hemolytic anemia hypoprothrombinemia, thrombocytopenic purpura, agranulocytosis.

CNS: Headache, fever, vertigo, apprehension, excitement, confusion, delirium, and syncope, disturbed hearing (tinnitus, decreased auditory acuity), disturbed vision (mydriasis, blurred vision, disturbed color perception, photophobia, diplopia, night blindness, scotomata), optic neuritis.

Dermatologic: Cutaneous flushing with intense pruritus.

Hypersensitivity Reactions: Angioedema, acute asthmatic episode, vascular collapse, respiratory arrest, hepatic dysfunction.

OVERDOSAGE:

Cardiotoxic effects of quinidine may be reversed in part by molar sodium lactate; the hypotension may be reversed by vasoconstrictors and by catecholamines (since vasodilation is partly due to alpha-adrenergic blockage).

DOSAGE AND ADMINISTRATION:

Each Cardioquin tablet contains 275 mg quinidine polygalacturonate, equivalent to 3-grain tablet of quinidine sulfate. Dosage must be adjusted to individual patients's needs, both for conversion and maintenance. An initial dose of 1 to 3 tablets may be used to terminate arrhythmia, and may be repeated in 3-4 hours. If normal sinus rhythm is not restored after 3 or 4 equal doses, the dose may be increased by 1/2 to 1 tablet (137.5 to 275 mg) and administered three to four times before any further dosage increase. For maintenance, one tablet may be used two to three times a day.

REFERENCES:

1. Schwartz, G.: Angiology 10:115 (Apr.) 1959. **2.** Tricot, R., Nogrette, P.: ***Presse med.***68:1085 (June 4) 1960. **3.** Schaftel, N., Halpern, A.: ***Am. J. Med. Sci.***236:184 (Aug.) 1958.

HOW SUPPLIED:

Cardioquin 275 mg scored, uncoated Tablets are supplied in white-opaque plastic bottles containing 100 tablets and 500 tablets. Each round tablet bears the symbol "PF" on one side and is marked "C275" on the other.

Store tablets at controlled room temperature 15° to 30°C (59°-86°F).

HOW SUPPLIED - EQUIVALENTS NOT AVAILABLE:

Tablet, Uncoated - Oral - 275 mg

100's	**$103.10**	**CARDIOQUIN, Purdue Frederick**	**00034-5470-80**
500's	**$492.45**	**CARDIOQUIN, Purdue Frederick**	**00034-5470-90**

QUINIDINE SULFATE *(002167)*

CATEGORIES: Antiarrhythmic Agents; Arrhythmia; Atrial Fibrillation; Cardiovascular Drugs; Fibrillation; Heart Flutter; Quinidines; Renal Drugs; Tachycardia; Pregnancy Category C; FDA Approval Pre 1982

BRAND NAMES: *Biquin Durules*; *Cardine*; *Cardioquin*; Cin-Quin; *Galactoquin*; *Gluquine*; *Kiditard*; *Kinidin*; *Naticardina*; *Quinaglute*; *Quinate*; *Quinicardina*; Quinidex; *Quinidina*; *Quinidoxin*; **Quinora**; *Ritmocor*; *Sulfas-Chinidin*
(International brand names outside U.S. in italics)

FORMULARIES: Aetna; BC-BS; CIGNA; DoD; FHP; Humana; Kaiser; Medco; Medi-Cal; PruCare; United; WHO

COST OF THERAPY: $82.12 (Arrhythmia; Tablet; 200 mg; 3/day; 365 days)

DESCRIPTION:

Immediate-Release Tablets: Quinidine sulfate as minute needle-like white crystals (frequently cohering in masses) or fine white powder. It is odorless, has a very bitter taste, and darkness on exposure to light. It is slightly soluble in water, soluble in alcohol and in chloroform, and insoluble ether.

Quinidine sulfate is the sulfate salt of quinidine (cinchonan-9-ol, 6'-methoxy-, (9S)-sulfate (2: 1) dihydrate), a diastereomer of quinidine sulfate.

Each quinidine sulfate 300 mg tablet contains 300 mg quinidine sulfate (equivalent to 249 mg of quinidine base).

Extended-Release Tablets: Quinidine sulfate extended-release are constructed to release one-third of their alkaloidal salt, quinidine sulfate (100 mg), on reaching the stomach, to begin absorption in the upper intestinal tract. The remaining two-thirds of the active drug (200 mg) is evenly distributed throughout a homogenous core which slowly dissolves as it moves along the intestinal tract, releasing the quinidine sulfate for continuous absorption over an 8-12 hour period.

Each quinidine sulfate extended-release tablet contains 300 mg of quinidine sulfate, the equivalent of 248.6 mg of the anhydrous quinidine alkaloid. *Quinora Inactive Ingredients:* Acacia, Acetylated Monoglycerides, Calcium Sulfate, Carnauba Wax, Edible Tax, FD&C Blue 2, Gelatin, Guar Gum, Magnesium Oxide, Magnesium Stearate, Polysorbates, Shellac, Sucrose, Titanium Dioxide, White Wax and other ingredients, one of which is a corn derivative. May contain FD&C Red 40 and Yellow 6 Aluminum Lakes.

Chemically, quinidine sulfate is cinchonan-9-ol,6'-methoxy-,(9s)- sulfate (2:1) (salt) dihydrate.

CLINICAL PHARMACOLOGY:

The action of quinidine in preventing aberrant cardiac rhythms of atrial and ventricular origin resides in its ability to (a) depress excitability of cardiac muscle, (b) now the rate of spontaneous rhythm, (c) decrease vagal tone, and (d) prolong conduction of effective refractory period.

Immediate-Release Tablets: Besides these direct effects, quinidine exerts some indirect activity on the heart through an anticholinergic action. Large oral doses may reduce the arterial pressure by means of peripheral vasodilation. Hypotension of a serious degree is more likely with the parenteral use of the drug.

Quinidine is rapidly absorbed from the gastrointestinal tract. The peak concentrations in serum are attained in 60 to 90 minutes and activity persists 6 to 8 hours or more. Quinidine is metabolized in the liver and excreted by the kidney. Ten to 50% of quinidine is excreted in the urine as unchanged drug within 24 hours.

Serum levels of quinidine can be measured. Values vary according to the assay employed. Traditionally, plasma concentrations for effective use of quinidine have been reported to range from 2-7 mcg/ml and levels of 8 mcg/ml or greater are associated with toxicity. This information is based upon less specific analytic methods which quantitate metabolites as well as intact quinidine. However, plasma quinidine concentrations will be lower using more specific assays. Therefore, clinicians requesting serum quinidine determinations should be aware of the method analysis. There is a wide individual variation in response to quinidine therapy. In all cases, the physician should carefully consider patient response and evidence of toxicity along with blood levels in determining optimal therapy.

INDICATIONS AND USAGE:

Quinidine sulfate is indicated in the treatment of:

1. Premature atrial and ventricular contractions
2. Paroxysmal atrial tachycardia
3. Paroxysmal atrioventricular (A-V) junctional rhythm
4. Atrial flutter
5. Paroxysmal atrial fibrillation
6. Established atrial fibrillation when therapy is appropriate
7. Paroxysmal ventricular tachycardia when not associated with complete heartblock
8. Maintenance therapy after electrical conversion of atrial fibrillation and/or flutter.

CONTRAINDICATIONS:

Immediate-Release Tablets: Hypersensitivity or idiosyncrasy to the drug, digitals intoxication manifested by A-V condition disorders, complete A-V block with an A-V nodal or idioventricular pacemaker, left bundle branch block or other severe intraventricular condition defects with marked QRS widening. Ectopic impulses and abnormal rhythms due to escape mechanisms. Also, myasthenia gravis.

Extended-Release Tablets: Intraventricular conduction defects. Complete A-V block, A-V conduction disorders caused by digitalis intoxication. Aberrant impulses and abnormal rhythms due to escape mechanisms. Idiosyncrasy or hypersensitivity to quinidine or related cinchona derivatives. Myasthenia gravis.

WARNINGS:

In the treatment of atrial flutter, reversion to sinus rhythm may be preceded by a progressive reduction in the degree of A-V block to a 1:1 ratio, which results in extremely rapid ventricular rate. This possible hazard may be reduced by digitalization prior to administration of quinidine.

In susceptible individuals, such as those with marginally compensated cardiovascular disease, quinidine may produce clinically important depression of cardiac function manifested by hypotension, bradycardia, or heart block. Quinidine, therapy should be carefully monitored in such individuals.

Evidence of quinidine cardiotoxicity (excessive prolongation of Q-T interval, widening of QRS complex, and ventricular tachyarrhythmias) mandates immediate discontinuation of the drug and subsequent close clinical and electrocardiographic monitoring of the patient.

Quinidine should be used with extreme caution when there is incomplete A-V block, since complete block and asystole may result. The drug may cause unpredictable abnormalities of rhythm in digitalized hearts, and it should be used with special caution in the presence of digitalis intoxication.

The cardiotoxic effect of quinidine is increased by hyperkalemia and decreased by hypokalemia.

Patients taking quinidine occasionally have syncopal episodes which usually result from ventricular tachycardia or fibrillation. This syndrome has not been shown to be related to dose or serum levels. Syncopal episodes frequently terminate spontaneously or in response to treatment, but sometimes are fetal.

WARNINGS: *(cont'd)*

Recent reports have described increased, potentially toxic, digoxin serum levels when quinidine is administered concurrently. When concurrent use is necessary, reduction of digoxin dosage may have to be considered, its serum concentration should be monitored and the patient observed closely for digitalis intoxication.

Caution should be used when quinidine is administered concurrently with coumarin anticoagulants. This combination may reduce prothrombin levels and cause bleeding.

Quinidine should be used with caution in patients exhibition renal, cardiac or hepatic insufficiency because of potential accumulation of quinidine in serum leading to toxicity.

Cases of hepatotoxicity, including granulomatous hepatitis, due to quinidine hypersensitivity have been reported. Unexplained fever and/or elevation of hepatic enzymes, particularly in the early stages of therapy, warrant consideration of possible hepatotoxicity. Monitoring liver function during the first 4-8 weeks should be considered. Cessation of quinidine in these cases usually results in the disappearance of toxicity.

PRECAUTIONS:

GENERAL

A preliminary test dose of a single tablet of quinidine sulfate may be administered to determine if the patient has an idiosyncrasy to quinidine. Hypersensitivity to quinidine, although rare, should constantly be considered, especially during the first weeks of therapy. Hospitalization for close clinical observation, electrocardiographic monitoring, and possible determination of serum quinidine levels is indicated when large doses are used, or with patients who present an increased risk.

Extended-Release Tablets: As with all solid dosage medications, quinidine sulfate extended-release tablets should be taken with an adequate amount of fluid, preferably with the patient in an upright position to facilitate swallowing. They should be swallowed whole in order to preserve the controlled-release mechanism.

LABORATORY TESTS

Periodic blood counts and liver and kidney function tests should be performed during long-term therapy; the drug should be discontinued if blood dyscrasias or evidence of hepatic or renal dysfunction occurs.

Immediate-Release Tablets: Continuous electrocardiographic monitoring and determination of serum quinidine levels are indicated when large doses (more than 2 g/day) are used.

CARCINOGENESIS, MUTAGENESIS AND IMPAIRMENT OF FERTILITY

Studies in animals have not been performed to evaluate the carcinogenic potential of quinidine.

PREGNANCY CATEGORY C

Teratogenic Effects: Animal reproduction studies have not been conducted with quinidine. There are no adequate and well-controlled studies in pregnant women. Quinidine should be given to a pregnant woman only if clearly needed.

Nonteratogenic Effects: Like quinine, quinidine has been reported to have oxytocic properties. The significance of this property in the clinical setting has not been established.

LABOR AND DELIVERY

There is no known use of quinidine sulfate in labor and delivery. However, quinidine has been reported to have oxytocic properties. The significance of this property in the clinical setting has not been established.

NURSING MOTHERS

Caution should be exercised when quinidine is administered to a nursing mother due to passage of the drug into breast milk.

PEDIATRIC USE

There are no adequate and well-controlled studies establishing the safety and effectiveness of quinidine sulfate in children.

DRUG INTERACTIONS:

TABLE 1

Drug	Effect
Quinidine with:	
Anticholinergics	Additive vagolytic effect
Cholinergics	Antagonism of cholinergic effect
Carbonic anhydrase inhibitors, sodium bicarbonate thiazide diuretics	Alkalinization of urine resulting in decrease excretion of quinidine
Coumarin anticoagulants	Reduction of clotting factor concentrations (seeWARNINGS)
Tubocurarine, succinylcholine, decamethonium and pancuronium	Potentiation of neuromuscular blockage
Phenothiazines and reserpine	Additive cardiac depressive effects
Hepatic enzyme-inducing drugs (phenobarbital, phenytoin, rifampin)	Decreased plasma half-life of quinidine
Digoxin	Increased serum concentrations of digoxin (seeWARNINGS)
Amiodarone	Increased serum concentration of quinidine
Cimetidine	Prolonged quinidine half-life and an increase in serum quinidine level
Ranitidine	Premature ventricular contractions and/or bigeminy
Verapamil	Increased quinidine half-life and an increase in serum quinidine level; potential hypotensive reactions
Nifedipine	Decreased serum concentrations of quinidine

ADVERSE REACTIONS:

Symptoms of cinchonism, such as ringing in ears, loss of hearing, dizziness, light-headedness, headache, nausea, and/or disturbed vision may appear in sensitive patients after a single dose of the drug. The most frequently encountered side effects to quinidine are gastrointestinal.

Gastrointestinal: Nausea, vomiting, abdominal pain, diarrhea, anorexia, granulomatous hepatitis (which may be preceded by fever), esophagitis.

Cardiovascular: Ventricular extrasystoles occurring at a rate of one or more every 6 normal beats; widening of the QRS complex and prolonged Q-T interval; complete A-V block; ventricular tachycardia and fibrillation; ventricular flutter; torsade de pointes; arterial embolism; hypotension, syncope.

Central Nervous System: Headache, vertigo, apprehension, excitement, confusion, delirium, dementia, ataxia, depression.

Ophthalmologic and Otologic: Disturbed hearing (tinnitus, decreased auditory acuity), disturbed vision (mydriasis, blurred vision, disturbed color perception, photophobia, diplopia, night blindness, scotomata), optic neuritis, reduced visual field.

Dermatologic: Cutaneous flushing with intense pruritus, photosensitivity, urticaria, rash, eczema, exfoliative eruptions, psoriasis, abnormalities of pigmentation.

ADVERSE REACTIONS: *(cont'd)*

Hypersensitivity: Angioedema, acute asthmatic arrest, hepatotoxicity, granulomatous hepatitis (see WARNINGS), purpura, vasculitis.

Hematologic: Thrombocytopenia, thrombocytopenic purpura, agranulocytosis, acute hemolytic anemia, shift to left in WBC differential, neutropenia.

Immunologic: Systemic lupus erythematosus, lupus nephritis.

Miscellaneous: Fever, increase in serum skeletal muscle creatine phosphokinase, arthralgia, myalgia.

OVERDOSAGE:

SYMPTOMS

Overdosage of quinidine can lead to accelerated idioventricular rhythm, morphologic appearance of QRS complexes, prolonged QT intervals, intermittent sinus capture beats, paroxysms of tachycardia, ventricular arrhythmias, hypotension, oliguria, respiratory depression, pulmonary edema, acidosis, seizures, and coma.

TREATMENT

Early treatment to empty the stomach using syrup of ipecac and/or gastric lavage is recommended. Administration of activated charcoal may reduce absorption. Other general supportive measures should be employed as indicated by patient response in severe cases, circulation should be stabilized and measurements of pulmonary capillary wedge pressure should be performed to assure adequate left ventricular filling pressure. Electrolyte and blood gas abnormalities should be corrected. In quinidine-induced vasodilation, catecholamines and other alpha-adrenergic agonists may be tried. Arrhythmias may be treated with lidocaine, pacing, and cardioversion. Administration of sodium lactate reportedly reduces the cardiotoxicity of quinidine; however sodium lactate is contraindicated in the presence of alkalosis as increased urinary pH can lead to an increase in the renal tubular absorption of quinidine. Acidification of the urine may enhance the urinary excretion of quinidine.

Extended-Release Tablets: Since quinidine sulfate extended-release tablets cannot be removed through a nasogastric tube, gastric lavage should be followed by saline cathartics.

DOSAGE AND ADMINISTRATION:

IMMEDIATE-RELEASE TABLETS

A preliminary test dose of a single tablet of quinidine sulfate should be administered to determine whether the patient has an idiosyncrasy to it. Continuous electrocardiographic monitoring is recommended in all cases in which quinidine is used in large doses.

Usual Adult Dose

Premature Atrial and Ventricular contraction: 200 to 300 mg, 3 or 4 times daily.

Paroxysmal Supraventricular Tachycardias: 400 to 600 mg, every 2 or 3 hours until the paroxysm is terminated.

Atrial Flutter: Quinidine should be administered after digitalization of this indication. Doses is to be individualized.

Conversion of Atrial Fibrillation: Various schedules of quinidine administration have been in clinical use. A widely used technique is to give 200 mg of quinidine sulfate orally every 2 or 3 hours for 5 to 8 doses, with subsequent daily increases of the individual dose until sinus rhythm is restored or toxic effect occur. The total daily dose should not exceed 3 to 4 grams in any regimen. Prior to quinidine administration, the ventricular rate and congestive heart failure (if present) should be brought under control by digitalis therapy.

Usual Maintenance Therapy: 200 to 300 mg, 3 or 4 times daily.

Although most patients may be maintained in normal rhythm on a dosage of 200 to 300 mg of quinidine sulfate every 6 to 8 hours, other patients may require larger doses or more frequent administration than the usually recommended schedule. Such increased dosage should be instituted only after careful clinical and laboratory evaluation of the patient, including monitoring of serum quinidine levels and, if possible, serial electrocardiograms.

Gastrointestinal disturbances, if they occur, may be minimized by administering the drug with food.

EXTENDED-RELEASE TABLETS

One or two quinidine sulfate extended-release tablets every 8 to 12 hours as may be required to achieve the desired therapeutic effect.

Storage Conditions: Tablets must be dispensed in tight, light-resistant containers as defined in the USP. Tablets must be stored at controlled room temperature between 15 and 30°C (59 and 86°F).

(Extended-Release Tablets: A.H. Robins, 10/87)

HOW SUPPLIED - RATED THERAPEUTICALLY EQUIVALENT:

Tablet, Coated, Sustained Action - Oral - 300 mg

100's	$64.85	Quinidine Sulfate, Qualitest Pharms	00603-5596-21
100's	$66.78	Quinidine Sulfate, Goldline Labs	00182-1997-01
100's	$66.81	Quinidine Sulfate, HL Moore Drug Exch	00839-7949-06
100's	$71.05	Quinidine Sulfate, Rugby	00536-5695-01
100's	$74.50	Quinidine Sulfate, Copley Pharm	38245-0175-10
100's	$82.81	QUINIDEX, AH Robins	00031-6649-63
100's	$84.61	QUINIDEX, AH Robins	00031-6649-64
250's	$178.15	Quinidine Sulfate, Copley Pharm	38245-0175-25
250's	$198.01	QUINIDEX, AH Robins	00031-6649-67
1000's	$159.69	Quinidine Sulfate, HL Moore Drug Exch	00839-7949-09

Tablet, Uncoated - Oral - 200 mg

100's	$7.50	Quinidine Sulfate, Eon Labs Mfg	00185-4346-01
100's	$9.25	Quinidine Sulfate, Major Pharms	00904-2201-60
100's	$9.62	Quinidine Sulfate, H.C.F.A. F F P	99999-2167-01
100's	$10.50	Quinidine Sulfate, Raway	00686-0031-20
100's	$11.00	Quinidine Sulfate, Lederle Pharm	00005-3558-23
100's	$11.03	Quinidine Sulfate, Parmed Pharms	00349-2149-01
100's	$11.27	Quinidine Sulfate, HL Moore Drug Exch	00839-5063-06
100's	$11.64	Quinidine Sulfate, Lederle Pharm	00005-3558-60
100's	$11.65	Quinidine Sulfate, Goldline Labs	00182-0144-01
100's	$11.65	Quinidine Sulfate, United Res	00677-0122-01
100's	$11.65	Quinidine Sulfate, Mutual Pharm	53489-0461-01
100's	$12.55	Quinidine Sulfate, Geneva Pharms	00781-1900-01
100's	$12.56	Quinidine Sulfate, Purepac Pharm	00228-2356-10
100's	$12.56	Quinidine Sulfate, Schein Pharm (US)	00364-0229-01
100's	$12.56	Quinidine Sulfate, Aligen Independ	00405-4916-01
100's	$12.56	Quinidine Sulfate, Rugby	00536-4432-01
100's	$12.98	Quinidine Sulfate, Schein Pharm (US)	00364-0229-90
100's	$14.04	Quinidine Sulfate, Vangard Labs	00615-0515-13
100's	$16.50	Quinidine Sulfate, Voluntary Hosp	53258-0158-13
100's	$17.76	Quinidine Sulfate, Roxane	00054-8733-25
100's	$17.91	Quinidine Sulfate, Major Pharms	00904-2201-61
100's	$22.66	Quinidine Sulfate, Lilly	00002-1020-02
120's	$9.06	Quinidine Sulfate, Talbert Phcy	44514-0784-90
1000's	$65.00	Quinidine Sulfate, Eon Labs Mfg	00185-4346-10
1000's	$75.75	Quinidine Sulfate, Major Pharms	00904-2201-80

HOW SUPPLIED - RATED THERAPEUTICALLY EQUIVALENT: *(cont'd)*

1000's	$86.00	Quinidine Sulfate, Lederle Pharm	00005-3558-34
1000's	$87.50	Quinidine Sulfate, United Res	00677-0122-10
1000's	$87.75	Quinidine Sulfate, Goldline Labs	00182-0144-10
1000's	$88.80	Quinidine Sulfate, Qualitest Pharms	00603-5594-32
1000's	$89.85	Quinidine Sulfate, Mutual Pharm	53489-0461-10
1000's	$89.95	Quinidine Sulfate, Halsey Drug	00879-0358-10
1000's	$94.10	Quinidine Sulfate, Parmed Pharms	00349-2149-10
1000's	$96.20	Quinidine Sulfate, H.C.F.A. F F P	99999-2167-02
1000's	$98.77	Quinidine Sulfate, Schein Pharm (US)	00364-0229-02
1000's	$98.81	Quinidine Sulfate, Aligen Independ	00405-4916-03
1000's	$98.96	Quinidine Sulfate, HL Moore Drug Exch	00839-5063-16
1000's	$99.95	Quinidine Sulfate, Geneva Pharms	00781-1900-10
1000's	$111.62	Quinidine Sulfate, Rugby	00536-4432-10
1000's	$165.79	Quinidine Sulfate, Roxane	00054-4736-31

Tablet, Uncoated - Oral - 300 mg

100's	$13.50	Quinidine Sulfate, Eon Labs Mfg	00185-1047-01
100's	$14.93	Quinidine Sulfate, United Res	00677-1209-01
100's	$14.93	Quinidine Sulfate, H.C.F.A. F F P	99999-2167-03
100's	$16.65	Quinidine Sulfate, Harber Pharm	51432-0407-03
100's	$18.62	Quinidine Sulfate, HL Moore Drug Exch	00839-6605-06
100's	$18.70	Quinidine Sulfate, Qualitest Pharms	00603-5595-21
100's	$20.00	Quinidine Sulfate, Goldline Labs	00182-1724-01
100's	$20.00	Quinidine Sulfate, Mutual Pharm	53489-0460-01
100's	$20.15	Quinidine Sulfate, Major Pharms	00904-2203-60
100's	$20.32	Quinidine Sulfate, Aligen Independ	00405-4917-01
100's	$22.95	Quinidine Sulfate, Geneva Pharms	00781-1902-13
100's	$23.00	Quinidine Sulfate, Schein Pharm (US)	00364-0582-90
100's	$23.20	Quinidine Sulfate, Goldline Labs	00182-1724-89
100's	$23.23	Quinidine Sulfate, Rugby	00536-4429-01
100's	$23.23	Quinidine Sulfate, Geneva Pharms	00781-1902-01
100's	$26.99	Quinidine Sulfate, Schein Pharm (US)	00364-0582-01
100's	$29.84	Quinidine Sulfate, Roxane	00054-4735-25
100's	$31.62	Quinidine Sulfate, Roxane	00054-8735-25
1000's	$125.00	Quinidine Sulfate, Eon Labs Mfg	00185-1047-10
1000's	$149.30	Quinidine Sulfate, H.C.F.A. F F P	99999-2167-04
1000's	$155.00	Quinidine Sulfate, Mutual Pharm	53489-0460-10
1000's	$167.05	Quinidine Sulfate, Major Pharms	00904-2203-80
1000's	$248.28	Quinidine Sulfate, Roxane	00054-4735-31

QUININE SULFATE *(002168)*

CATEGORIES: Analgesics; Anti-Infectives; Antimalarial Agents; Antiprotozoals; Antipyretics; Antitussives/Expectorants/Mucolytics; Central Nervous System Agents; Muscle Relaxants; Parasiticidal; Leg Cramps*; Pregnancy Category X; FDA Pre 1938 Drugs

* Indication not approved by the FDA

BRAND NAMES: *Adaquin*; *Chinine*; *Genin*; *Novoquinine*; Qm-260; Quin-Amino; Quinaminoph; **Quinamm**; Quinasul; *Quinate*; Quindan; Quinite; *Quinoctal*; *Quinsan*; *Quinsul*; Quiphile

(International brand names outside U.S. in italics)

FORMULARIES: Aetna; BC-BS; FHP; WHO

DESCRIPTION:

Quinine Sulfate (hereafter referred to as Quinine) is available as tablets for oral administration. Each tablet contains 260 mg quinine sulfate. Also contains, as inactive ingredients: corn starch, pregelatinized starch, sodium starch glycolate, sucrose, and zinc stearate.

Neuromuscular Agent.

Quinine sulfate occurs as a white, crystalline powder, which darkens on exposure to light. It is odorless and has a persistent, very bitter taste. It is slightly soluble in water, alcohol, chloroform, and ether.

CLINICAL PHARMACOLOGY:

Quinine, a cinchona alkaloid, acts on skeletal muscle by three mechanisms: it increases the refractory period by direct action on the muscle fiber, it decreases the excitability of the motor end-plate, an action similar to that of curare, and it affects the distribution of calcium within the muscle fiber.

Quinine is readily absorbed when given orally. Absorption occurs mainly from the upper part of the small intestine, and is almost complete even in patients with marked diarrhea.

The cinchona alkaloids in large measure are metabolically degraded in the body, especially in the liver; less than 5% of an administered dose is excreted unaltered in the urine. It is reported that there is no accumulation of the drugs in the body upon continued administration. The metabolic degradation products are excreted in the urine, where many of them have been identified as hydroxy derivatives, but small amounts also appear in the feces, gastric juice, bile, and saliva. Renal excretion of quinine is twice as rapid when the urine is acidic as when it is alkaline, due to the greater tubular reabsorption of the alkaloidal base that occurs in an alkaline media. Excretion is also limited by the binding of a large fraction of cinchona alkaloids to plasma proteins.

Peak plasma concentrations of cinchona alkaloids occur within 1 to 3 hours after a single oral dose. The half-life is 4 to 5 hours. After chronic administration of total daily doses of 1 g of drug, the average plasma quinine concentration is approximately 7 mcg/ml. After termination of quinine therapy, the plasma level falls rapidly and only a negligible concentration is detectable after 24 hours.

A large fraction (approximately 70%) of the plasma quinine is bound to proteins. This explains in part why the concentration of the alkaloid in cerebrospinal fluid is only 2 to 5% of that in the plasma. However, it can traverse the placental membrane and readily reach fetal tissues.

Tinnitus and impairment of hearing rarely should occur at plasma quinine concentrations of less than 10 mcg/ml. While this level would not be anticipated from use of 1 or 2 tablets of quinine daily, an occasional patient may have some evidence of cinchonism on this dosage, such as tinnitus. (See WARNINGS.)

INDICATIONS AND USAGE:

For the prevention and treatment of nocturnal recumbency leg muscle cramps.

CONTRAINDICATIONS:

Quinine may cause fetal harm when administered to a pregnant woman. Congenital malformations in the human have been reported with the use of quinine, primarily with large doses (up to 30 g) for attempted abortion. In about half of these reports, the malformation was deafness related to auditory nerve hypoplasia. Among the other abnormalities reported were limb anomalies, visceral defects, and visual changes. In animal tests, teratogenic effects

CONTRAINDICATIONS: *(cont'd)*

were found in rabbits and guinea pigs and were absent in mice, rats, dogs, and monkeys. Quinine is contraindicated in women who are or may become pregnant. If this drug is used during pregnancy, or if the patient becomes pregnant while taking this drug, the patient should be apprised of the potential hazard to the fetus.

Quinine is contraindicated in patients with known quinine hypersensitivity and in patients with glucose-6-phosphate dehydrogenase (G-6-PD) deficiency.

Since thrombocytopenic purpura may follow the administration of quinine in highly sensitive patients, a history of this occurrence associated with previous quinine ingestion contraindicates its further use. Recovery usually occurs following withdrawal of the medication and appropriate therapy.

This drug should not be used in patients with tinnitus or optic neuritis or in patients with a history of blackwater fever.

WARNINGS:

Repeated doses or overdosage of quinine in some individuals may precipitate a cluster of symptoms referred to as cinchonism. Such symptoms, in the mildest form, include ringing in the ears, headache, nausea, and slightly disturbed vision; however, when medication is continued or after large single doses, symptoms also involve the gastrointestinal tract, the nervous and cardiovascular systems, and the skin.

Hemolysis (with the potential for hemolytic anemia) has been associated with a G-6-PD deficiency in patients taking quinine. Quinine should be stopped immediately if evidence of hemolysis appears.

If symptoms occur, drug should be discontinued and supportive measures instituted. In case of overdosage, see OVERDOSAGE.

PRECAUTIONS:

GENERAL

Quinine should be discontinued if there is any evidence of hypersensitivity. (See CONTRAINDICATIONS.) Cutaneous flushing, pruritus, skin rashes, fever, gastric distress, dyspnea, ringing in the ears, and visual impairment are the usual expressions of hypersensitivity, particularly if only small doses of quinine have been taken. Extreme flushing of the skin accompanied by intense, generalized pruritus is the most common form. Hemoglobinuria and asthma from quinine are rare types of idiosyncrasy.

In patients with atrial fibrillation, the administration of quinine requires the same precautions as those for quinidine. (See DRUG INTERACTIONS.)

DRUG/LABORATORY INTERACTIONS

Quinine may produce an elevated value for urinary 17-ketogenic steroids when the Zimmerman method is used.

CARCINOGENESIS, MUTAGENESIS, AND IMPAIRMENT OF FERTILITY

A study of quinine sulfate administered in drinking water (0.1%) to rats for periods up to 20 months showed no evidence of neoplastic changes.

Mutation studies of quinine (dihydrochloride) in male and female mice gave negative results by the micronucleus test. Intraperitoneal injections (0.5 mM/kg) were given twice, 24 hours apart. Direct *Salmonella typhimurium* tests were negative; when mammalian liver homogenate was added, positive results were found.

Mutation studies of quinine hydrochloride, 100 mg/kg, p.o. in Chinese hamsters showed no genotoxic activity in the sister chromatid exchange (SCE) test, micronucleus test, or chromosome aberration test. In mice given quinine hydrochloride, 100 mg/kg, p.o., the micronucleus test and chromosome aberration test were negative; the SCE test exhibited an increase of SCEs/cell. Tests were repeated in two inbred strains of mice using 55, 75, and 110 mg/kg p.o. The effect was more pronounced in these mice and the increase in SCEs/cell demonstrated a linear dose relationship. One of the inbred strains had positive micronucleus test findings. The chromosome aberration test also revealed an increase of chromatid breaks. The Ames test system results were negative for point mutation.

No information relating to the effect of quinine upon fertility in animal or in man has been found.

PREGNANCY CATEGORY X

See CONTRAINDICATIONS.

Nonteratogenic Effects: Because quinine crosses the placenta in humans, the potential for fetal effects is present. Stillbirths in mothers taking quinine have been reported in which no obvious cause for the fetal deaths was shown. Quinine in toxic amounts has been associated with abortion. Whether this action is always due to direct effect on the uterus is questionable.

NURSING MOTHERS

Caution should be exercised when quinine is given to nursing women because quinine is excreted in breast milk (in small amounts).

DRUG INTERACTIONS:

Increased plasma levels of digoxin have been demonstrated in individuals after concomitant quinine administration. Increased plasma levels of digitoxin have been demonstrated in individuals after concomitant quinidine administration. It is therefore recommended that plasma levels of digoxin or digitoxin be determined periodically for those individuals taking either of these glycosides and quinine concomitantly.

Concurrent use of aluminum-containing antacids may delay or decrease absorption of quinine.

Cinchona alkaloids, including quinine, have the potential to depress the hepatic enzyme system that synthesizes the vitamin K-dependent factors. The resulting hypoprothrombinemic effect may enhance the action of warfarin and other oral anticoagulants.

The effects of neuromuscular blocking agents (particularly pancuronium, succinylcholine, and tubocurarine) may be potentiated with quinine, and result in respiratory difficulties.

Urinary alkalizers (such as acetazolamide and sodium bicarbonate) may increase quinine blood levels with potential for toxicity.

ADVERSE REACTIONS:

The following adverse reactions have been reported with quinine in therapeutic or excessive dosage. (Individual or multiple symptoms may represent cinchonism or hypersensitivity.)

Hematologic: acute hemolysis, disseminated intravascular coagulation thrombocytopenic purpura, agranulocytosis, hypoprothrombinemia

CNS: visual disturbances, including blurred vision with scotomata, photophobia, diplopia, diminished visual fields, and disturbed color vision; tinnitus, deafness, and vertigo; headache, nausea, vomiting, fever, apprehension, restlessness, confusion, and syncope.

Dermatologic/allergic: cutaneous rashes (urticarial, the most frequent type of allergic reaction, papular, or scarlatinal), pruritus, flushing of the skin, sweating, occasional edema of the face

Respiratory: asthmatic symptoms

Cardiovascular: anginal symptoms

Gastrointestinal: nausea and vomiting (may be CNS-related), epigastric pain, hepatitis

DRUG ABUSE AND DEPENDENCE:

Tolerance, abuse, or dependence with quinine has not been reported.

OVERDOSAGE:

The more common signs and symptoms of quinine overdosage are tinnitus, dizziness, skin rash, and gastrointestinal disturbance (intestinal cramping). With higher doses, cardiovascular and CNS effects may occur, including headache, fever, vomiting, apprehension, confusion, and convulsions. Blindness and deafness, (with partial to total recovery, although persistent visual and/or auditory nerve damage have been reported) and hypoglycemia and hypokalemia may also occur. Other potential adverse effects are listed in the ADVERSE REACTIONS.

Fatalities with quinine have been reported from single oral doses of 2 to 8 grams; a single fatality reported with 1.5 grams may reflect an idiosyncratic effect.

Treatment: Gastrointestinal decontamination should be considered for the treatment of quinine overdosage. Vital signs, electrocardiogram (ECG), blood glucose and serum electrolytes should be monitored. Supportive measures should be instituted as necessary. Caution should be used in administering antiarrhythmics since quinine has Class 1 antiarrhythmic properties that can be potentiated by such agents. It is theoretically likely that mild hypokalemia may protect the heart from the toxic effects of quinine, and so the correction of only severe hypokalemia is advisable.

Fluid and electrolyte balance should be maintained with intravenous fluids. Although acidification of the urine will promote renal excretion of quinine, forced acid diuresis has had little impact on quinine elimination by the kidney. In addition, peritoneal dialysis, hemodialysis, hemoperfusion, exchange transfusion and plasmapharesis have not been shown to effectively treat quinine overdosage.

Stellate ganglion block has not been shown to effectively treat quinine-induced blindness, and may result in complications.

DOSAGE AND ADMINISTRATION:

One tablet upon retiring. If needed, 2 tablets may be taken nightly — 1 following the evening meal and 1 upon retiring.

After several consecutive nights in which recumbency leg cramps do not occur, Quinamm may be discontinued in order to determine whether continued therapy is needed.

Store at room temperature, below 86°F (30°C).

HOW SUPPLIED - EQUIVALENTS NOT AVAILABLE:

Capsule, Gelatin - Oral - 200 mg

100's	$17.50	Quinine Sulfate, Consolidated Midland	00223-1559-01
1000's	$140.00	Quinine Sulfate, Consolidated Midland	00223-1559-02

Capsule, Gelatin - Oral - 300 mg

100's	$17.13	Quinine Sulfate, H N Norton Co.	50732-0663-01
1000's	$157.74	Quinine Sulfate, H N Norton Co.	50732-0663-10

Capsule, Gelatin - Oral - 325 mg

100's	$8.20	Quinine Sulfate, Aligen Independ	00405-4922-01
100's	$12.50	Quinine Sulfate, United Res	00677-0123-01
100's	$14.15	Quinine Sulfate, Zenith Labs	00172-2184-60
100's	$15.50	Quinine Sulfate, Major Pharms	00904-2184-60
100's	$17.85	Quinine Sulfate, Voluntary Hosp	53258-0428-01
100's	$27.84	Quinine Sulfate, Voluntary Hosp	53258-0428-13
500's	$44.95	Quinine Sulfate, Major Pharms	00904-2184-40
500's	$55.00	Quinine Sulfate, United Res	00677-0123-05
1000's	$93.87	Quinine Sulfate, Aligen Independ	00405-4922-03
1000's	$106.00	Quinine Sulfate, United Res	00677-0123-10
1000's	$130.60	Quinine Sulfate, Zenith Labs	00172-2184-80

Tablet, Uncoated - Oral - 260 mg

100's	$9.95	Quinine Sulfate, Eon Labs Mfg	00185-0988-01
100's	$10.20	QUIPHILE, Geneva Pharms	00781-1926-01
100's	$10.45	Quinine Sulfate, Major Pharms	00904-0604-60
100's	$10.48	Quinine Sulfate, Aligen Independ	00405-4923-01
100's	$10.91	Quinine Sulfate, Vintage Pharms	00254-5401-28
100's	$11.50	Quinine Sulfate, Mutual Pharm	53489-0462-01
100's	$11.54	Quinine Sulfate, HL Moore Drug Exch	00839-6504-06
100's	$11.95	QUININE SULFATE 260, Major Pharms	00904-0564-60
100's	$13.35	Quinine Sulfate, Harber Pharm	51432-0411-03
100's	$14.17	Quinine Sulfate, Zenith Labs	00172-3001-60
100's	$14.17	Quinine Sulfate, Goldline Labs	00182-1213-01
100's	$14.17	Quinine Sulfate, H N Norton Co.	50732-0670-01
100's	$14.58	Quinine Sulfate, Royce	51875-0384-01
100's	$20.99	QUININE SULFATE 260, Major Pharms	00904-0564-61
100's	$21.00	Quinine Sulfate, Goldline Labs	00182-8615-89
250's	$24.50	Quinine Sulfate, Eon Labs Mfg	00185-0988-52
250's	$24.55	Quinine Sulfate, Major Pharms	00904-0564-70
500's	$44.95	Quinine Sulfate, Major Pharms	00904-0564-40
500's	$47.50	Quinine Sulfate, Eon Labs Mfg	00185-0988-05
500's	$49.55	Quinine Sulfate, Vintage Pharms	00254-5401-35
500's	$49.62	Quinine Sulfate, Aligen Independ	00405-4923-02
500's	$53.00	Quinine Sulfate, Mutual Pharm	53489-0462-05
500's	$67.21	Quinine Sulfate, Zenith Labs	00172-3001-70
500's	$67.21	Quinine Sulfate, Goldline Labs	00182-1213-05
500's	$67.21	Quinine Sulfate, H N Norton Co.	50732-0670-05
500's	$67.80	Quinine Sulfate, Royce	51875-0384-02
1000's	$128.82	Quinine Sulfate, Royce	51875-0384-04
1000's	$130.89	Quinine Sulfate, H N Norton Co.	50732-0670-10
1000's	$144.72	Quinine Sulfate, HL Moore Drug Exch	00839-7998-16

RABIES IMMUNE GLOBULIN *(002172)*

CATEGORIES: Bites; Immune Globulin; Immunologic; Rabies; Serums, Toxoids and Vaccines; Vaccines; Wound Care; Pregnancy Category C; FDA Pre 1938 Drugs

BRAND NAMES: *Bayer Bayrab Rabies Immune Globulin*; **Hyperab**; *Imogam*; Imogam Rabies; *Imogan Rabia*; *Rabigam*; *Rabuman Berna*
(International brand names outside U.S. in italics)

FORMULARIES: WHO

DESCRIPTION:

Rabies Immune Globulin (Human), USP (RIGH), is a sterile solution of antirabies immunoglobulin for intramuscular administration. This product is prepared from human plasma. It is prepared by cold alcohol fractionation from the plasma of donors hyperimmunized with rabies vaccine. RIGH is a 15%-18% solution of human protein stabilized in 0.21-0.32 M glycine. The pH of the solution has been adjusted to 6.4-7.2 with sodium carbonate. RIGH contains the mercurial preservative sodium ethylmercurithiosalicylate (thimerosal), 80-120

DESCRIPTION: *(cont'd)*

mcg/ml as measured by mercury assay. The product is standardized against the U.S. Standard Rabies Immune Globulin to contain an average potency value of 150 IU/ml. The U.S. unit of potency is equivalent to the international unit (IU) for rabies antibody.

CLINICAL PHARMACOLOGY:

The usefulness of prophylactic rabies antibody in preventing rabies in man when administered immediately after exposure was dramatically demonstrated in a group of persons bitten by a rabid wolf in Iran.[1,2] Similarly, beneficial results were later reported from the U.S.S.R.[3] Studies coordinated by WHO helped determine the optimal conditions under which antirabies serum of equine origin and rabies vaccine can be used in man.[4,7] These studies showed that serum can interfere to a variable extent with the active immunity induced by the vaccine, but could be minimized by booster doses of vaccine after the end of the usual dosage series.

Preparation of rabies immune globulin of human origin with adequate potency was reported by Cabasso et al.[8] In carefully controlled clinical studies, this globulin was used in conjunction with rabies vaccine of duck-embryo origin (DEV).[8,9] These studies determined that a human globulin dose of 20 IU/kg of rabies antibody, given simultaneously with the first DEV dose, resulted in amply detectable levels of passive rabies antibody 24 hours after injection in all recipients. The injections produced minimal, if any, interference with the subject's endogenous antibody response to DEV.

More recently, human diploid cell rabies vaccines (HDCV) prepared from tissue culture fluids containing rabies virus have received substantial clinical evaluation in Europe and the United States.[10-16] In a study in adult volunteers, the administration of Rabies Immune Globulin (Human) did not interfere with antibody formation induced by HDCV when given in a dose of 20 IU per kilogram body weight simultaneously with the first dose of vaccine.[15]

INDICATIONS AND USAGE:

Rabies vaccine and Rabies Immune Globulin (Human), USP (RIGH), should be given to all persons suspected of exposure to rabies with one exception: persons who have been previously immunized with rabies vaccine and have a confirmed adequate rabies antibody titer should receive only vaccine. RIGH should be administered as promptly as possible after exposure, but can be administered up to the eighth day after the first dose of vaccine is given.

Recommendations for use of passive and active immunization after exposure to an animal suspected of having rabies have been detailed by the U.S. Public Health Service Immunization Practices Advisory Committee (ACIP).[17]

Every exposure to possible rabies infection must be individually evaluated. The following factors should be considered before specific antirabies treatment is initiated:

SPECIES OF BITING ANIMAL

Carnivorous wild animals (especially skunks, foxes, coyotes, raccoons, and bobcats) and bats are the animals most commonly infected with rabies and have caused most of the indigenous cases of human rabies in the United States since 1960.[18] Unless the animal is tested and shown not to be rabid, postexposure prophylaxis should be initiated upon bite or nonbite exposure to these animals (See INDICATIONS AND USAGE, Type of Exposure). If treatment has been initiated and subsequent testing in a competent laboratory shows the exposing animal is not rabid, treatment can be discontinued.

In the United States, the likelihood that a domestic dog or cat is infected with rabies varies from region to region; hence, the need for postexposure prophylaxis also varies. However, in most of Asia and all of Africa and Latin America, the dog remains the major source of human exposure; exposures to dogs in such countries represent a special threat. Travelers to those countries should be aware that > 50% of the rabies cases among humans in the United States result from exposure to dogs outside the United States.

Rodents (such as squirrels, hamsters, guinea pigs, gerbils, chipmunks, rats, and mice) and lagomorphs (including rabbits and hares) are rarely found to be infected with rabies and have not been known to cause human rabies in the United States. However, from 1971 through 1988, woodchucks accounted for 70% of the 179 cases of rabies among rodents reported to CDC.[19] In these cases, the state or local health department should be consulted before a decision is made to initiate postexposure antirabies prophylaxis.

CIRCUMSTANCES OF BITING INCIDENT

An unprovoked attack is more likely to mean that the animal is rabid. (Bites during attempts to feed or handle an apparently healthy animal may generally be regarded as provoked.)

TYPE OF EXPOSURE

Rabies is transmitted only when the virus is introduced into open cuts or wounds in skin or mucous membranes. If there has been no exposure (as described in this section), postexposure treatment is not necessary. Thus, the likelihood that rabies infection will result from exposure to a rabid animal varies with the nature and extent of the exposure. Two categories of exposure should be considered:

Bite: any penetration of the skin by teeth. Bites to the face and hands carry the highest risk, but the site of the bite should not influence the decision to begin treatment.[20]

Nonbite: scratches, abrasions, open wounds or mucous membranes contaminated with saliva or any potentially infectious material, such as brain tissue, from a rabid animal constitute nonbite exposures. If the material containing the virus is dry, the virus can be considered noninfectious. Casual contact, such as petting a rabid animal and contact with the blood, urine, or feces (*e.g.,* guano) of a rabid animal, does not constitute an exposure and is not an indication for prophylaxis. Instances of airborne rabies have been reported rarely. Adherence to respiratory precautions will minimize the risk of airborne exposure.[21]

The only documented cases of rabies from human-to-human transmission have occurred in patients who received corneas transplanted from persons who died of rabies undiagnosed at the time of death. Stringent guidelines for acceptance of donor corneas have reduced this risk.

Bite and nonbite exposures from humans with rabies theoretically could transmit rabies, although no cases of rabies acquired this way have been documented.

VACCINATION STATUS OF BITING ANIMAL

A properly immunized animal has only a minimal chance of developing rabies and transmitting the virus.

PRESENCE OF RABIES IN REGION

If adequate laboratory and field records indicate that there is no rabies infection in a domestic species within a given region, local health officials are justified in considering this in making recommendations on antirabies treatment following a bite by that particular species. Such officials should be consulted for current interpretations.

RABIES POSTEXPOSURE PROPHYLAXIS

The following recommendations are only a guide. In applying them, take into account the animal species involved, the circumstances of the bite or other exposure, the vaccination status of the animal, and presence of rabies in the region. Local or state public health officials should be consulted if questions arise about the need for rabies prophylaxis.

INDICATIONS AND USAGE: *(cont'd)*

Local Treatment of Wounds: Immediate and thorough washing of all bite wounds and scratches with soap and water is perhaps the most effective measure for preventing rabies. In experimental animals, simple local wound cleansing has been shown to reduce markedly the likelihood of rabies.

Tetanus prophylaxis and measures to control bacterial infection should be given as indicated.

Active Immunization: Active immunization should be initiated as soon as possible after exposure (within 24 hours). Many dosage schedules have been evaluated for the currently available rabies vaccines and their respective manufacturers' literature should be consulted.

Passive Immunization: A combination of active and passive immunization (vaccine and immune globulin) is considered the acceptable postexposure prophylaxis except for those persons who have been previously immunized with rabies vaccine and who have documented adequate rabies antibody titer. These individuals should receive vaccine only. For passive immunization, Rabies Immune Globulin (Human) is preferred over antirabies serum, equine.[16,17] It is recommended both for treatment of all bites by animals suspected of having rabies and for nonbite exposure inflicted by animals suspected of being rabid. Rabies Immune Globulin (Human) should be used in conjunction with rabies vaccine and can be administered through the seventh day after the first dose of vaccine is given. Beyond the seventh day, Rabies Immune Globulin (Human) is not indicated since an antibody response to cell culture vaccine is presumed to have occurred.

TABLE 1 Rabies Postexposure Prophylaxis Guide [17]

Animal Species	Condition of animal at time of Attack	Treatment of exposed person [1]
Dog and cat	Healthy and available for 10 days of observation	None, unless animal develops rabies [2]
	Rabid or suspected rabid	RIGH [3] and HDCV
	Unknown (escaped)	Consult public health officials
Skunk, bat, fox, coyote, raccoon, bobcat, and other carnivores; woodchuck	Regard as rabid unless geographic area is known to be free of rabies or proven negative by laboratory tests [4]	RIGH [3] and HDCV
Livestock, rodents, and lagomorphs (rabbits and hares)	Consider individually. Local and state public health officials should be consulted on questions about the need for rabies prophylaxis. In most geographical areas bites of squirrels, hamsters, guinea pigs, gerbils, chipmunks, rats, mice, other rodents, rabbits, and hares almost never call for antirabies prophylaxis.	

[1] ALL BITES AND WOUNDS SHOULD IMMEDIATELY BE THOROUGHLY CLEANSED WITH SOAP AND WATER. If antirabies treatment is indicated, both Rabies Immune Globulin (Human) [RIGH] and human diploid cell rabies vaccine (HDCV) should be given as soon as possible, REGARDLESS of the interval from exposure.
[2] During the usual holding period of 10 days, begin treatment with RIGH and vaccine (HDCV) at first sign of rabies in a dog or cat that has bitten someone. The symptomatic animal should be killed immediately and tested.
[3] If RIGH is not available, use antirabies serum, equine (ARS). Do not use more than the recommended dosage.
[4] The animal should be killed and tested as soon as possible. Holding for observation is not recommended. Discontinue vaccine if immunofluorescence test results of the animal are negative.

CONTRAINDICATIONS:

None known.

WARNINGS:

Rabies Immune Globulin (Human), USP (RIGH), should be given with caution to patients with a history of prior systemic allergic reactions following the administration of human immunoglobulin preparations or in patients who are known to have had an allergic response to thimerosal.

The attending physician who wishes to administer RIGH to persons with isolated immunoglobulin A (lgA) deficiency must weigh the benefits of immunization against the potential risks of hypersensitivity reactions. Such persons have increased potential for developing antibodies to IgA and could have anaphylactic reactions to subsequent administration of blood products that contain IgA.[22]

As with all preparations administered by the intramuscular route, bleeding complications may be encountered in patients with thrombocytopenia or other bleeding disorders.

PRECAUTIONS:

GENERAL

Rabies Immune Globulin (Human), USP (RIGH), should **not** be administered intravenously because of the potential for serious reactions. Although systemic reactions to immunoglobulin preparations are rare, epinephrine should be available for treatment of acute anaphylactoid symptoms.

PREGNANCY CATEGORY C

Animal reproduction studies have not been conducted with RIGH. It is also not known whether RIGH can cause fetal harm when administered to a pregnant woman or can affect reproduction capacity. RIGH should be given to a pregnant woman only if clearly needed.

DRUG INTERACTIONS:

Repeated doses of RIGH should not be administered once vaccine treatment has been initiated as this could prevent the full expression of active immunity expected from the rabies vaccine.

Other antibodies in the RIGH preparation may interfere with the response to live vaccines such as measles, mumps, polio or rubella. Therefore, immunization with live vaccines should not be given within 3 months after RIGH administration.

ADVERSE REACTIONS:

Soreness at the site of injection and mild temperature elevations may be observed at times. Sensitization to repeated injections has occurred occasionally in immunoglobulin-deficient patients. Angioneurotic edema, skin rash, nephrotic syndrome, and anaphylactic shock have rarely been reported after intramuscular injection, so that a causal relationship between immunoglobulin and these reactions is not clear.

DOSAGE AND ADMINISTRATION:

The recommended dose for RIGH is 20 IU/kg (0.133 ml/kg) of body weight given preferably at the time of the first vaccine dose.[8,9] It may also be given through the seventh day after the first dose of vaccine is given. If anatomically feasible, up to one-half the dose of RIGH should be thoroughly infiltrated in the area around the wound and the rest should be administered intramuscularly in the gluteal area. Because of risk of injury to the sciatic nerve,

DOSAGE AND ADMINISTRATION: *(cont'd)*

the central region of the gluteal area MUST be avoided; only the upper, outer quadrant should be used.[23] Rabies Immune Globulin (Human), USP (RIGH), should never be administered in the same syringe or into the same anatomical site as vaccine.

Parenteral drug products should be inspected visually for particulate matter and discoloration prior to administration, whenever solution and container permit.

REFERENCES:

1. Baltazard M, Bahmanyar M, Ghodssi M, et al: Essai pratique du serum antirabique chez les mordus par loups enrages. *Bull WHO*13:747-72, 1955. **2.** Habel K, Koprowski H: Laboratory data supporting the clinical trial of antirabies serum in persons bitten by a rabid wolf. *Bull WHO* 13:773-9, 1955. **3.** Selimov M, Boltucij L, Semenova E, et al: [The use of antirabies gamma globulin in subjects severely bitten by rabid wolves or other animals.]*J Hyg Epidemiol Microbiol Immunol (Praha)* 3:168-80, 1959. **4.** Atanasiu P, Bahmanyar M, Baltazard M, et al: Rabies neutralizing antibody response to different schedules of serum and vaccine inoculations in non-exposed persons. *Bull WHO* 14:593-611, 1956. **5.** Atanasiu P, Bahmanyar M, Baltazard M, et al: Rabies neutralizing antibody response to different schedules of serum and vaccine inoculations in non-exposed persons: Part II. *Bull WHO*17:911-32, 1957. **6.** Atanasiu P, Cannon DA, Dean DJ, et al: Rabies neutralizing antibody response to different schedules of serum and vaccine inoculations in non-exposed persons: Part 3. *Bull WHO* 25: 103-14, 1961. **7.** Atanasiu P, Dean DJ, Habel K, et al: Rabies neutralizing antibody response to different schedules of serum and vaccine inoculations in non-exposed persons: Part 4. *Bull WHO* 36:361-5, 1967. **8.** Cabasso VJ, Loofbourow JC, Roby RE, et al: Rabies immune globulin of human origin: preparation and dosage determination in non-exposed volunteer subjects. *Bull WHO*45:303-15, 1971. **9.** Loofbourow JC, Cabasso VJ, Roby RE, et al: Rabies immune globulin (human): clinical trials and dose determination.*JAMA* 217(13): 1825-31, 1971. **10.** Plotkin SA: New rabies vaccine halts disease—without severe reactions. *Mod Med*45(20):45-8, 1977. **11.** Plotkin SA, Wiktor TJ, Koprowski H, et al: Immunization schedules for the new human diploid cell vaccine against rabies. *Am J Epidemiol* 103(1):75-80, 1976. **12.** Hafkin B, Hattwick MA, Smith JS, et al: A comparison of a WI-38 vaccine and duck embryo vaccine for preexposure rabies prophylaxis. *Am J Epidemiol* 107(5):439-43, 1978. **13.** Kuwert EK, Marcus I, Hoher PG; Neutralizing and complement-fixing antibody responses in pre- and post-exposure vaccinees to a rabies vaccine produced in human diploid cells. *J Biol Stand*4(4):249-62, 1976. **14.** Grandien M: Evaluation of tests for rabies antibody and analysis of serum responses after administration of three different types of rabies vaccines. *J Clin Microbiol* 5(3):263-7, 1977. **15.** Kuwert EK, Marcus I, Werner J, et al: Postexpositionelle Schutzimpfung des Menschen gegen Tollwut mit einer nuentwickelten Gewebekulturvakzine (HDCS-Impfstoff). *Zentralbl Bakteriol* [A] 239(4):437-58, 1977. **16.** Bahmanyar M, Fayaz A, Nour-Salehi S, et al: Successful protection of humans exposed to rabies infection: postexposure treatment with the new human diploid cell rabies vaccine and antirabies serum. *JAMA* 236(24):2751-4, 1976. **17.** Recommendations of the Immunization Practices Advisory Committee (ACIP): Rabies prevention—United States, 1991. *MMWR*40(RR-3):1-19, 1991. **18.** Reid-Sanden FL, Dobbins JG, Smith JS, et al: Rabies surveillance in the United States during 1989. *J Am Vet Med Assoc* 197(12):1571-83, 1990. **19.** Fishbein DB, Belotto AJ, Pacer RE, et al: Rabies in rodents and lagomorphs in the United States, 1971-1984: increased cases in the woodchuck (*Marmota monax*) in mid-Atlantic states. *J Wildl Dis* 22(2):151-5, 1986. **20.** Hattwick MAW: Human rabies. *Public Health Rev*3(3):229-74, 1974. **21.** Garner JS, Simmons BP: Guideline for isolation precautions in hospitals. *Infect Control.* **22.** Fudenberg HH: Sensitization to immunoglobulins and hazards of gamma globulin therapy. In: Merler E (ed.): Immunoglobulins: biologic aspects and clinical uses. Washington, DC, Nat Acad Sci, 1970, pp 211-20. **23.** Recommendations of the Immunization Practices Advisory Committee (ACIP): General recommendations on immunization. *MMWR*38 (13):205-14; 219-27, 1989.

HOW SUPPLIED:

STORAGE

RIGH should be stored under refrigeration (2°- 8°C, 35°-46°F). Solution that has been frozen should not be used.

HOW SUPPLIED - EQUIVALENTS NOT AVAILABLE:

Injection, Solution - Intramuscular - 150 unit/ml

2 ml	**$87.50**	**HYPERAB, Bayer Pharm**	**00192-0608-02**
2 ml	$111.94	Imogam Rabies, Connaught Labs	49281-0180-02
2 ml	$128.50	Imogam Rabies, Connaught Labs	49281-0180-20
10 ml	**$345.00**	**HYPERAB, Bayer Pharm**	**00192-0608-10**
10 ml	$538.63	Imogam Rabies, Connaught Labs	49281-0180-10

RABIES VACCINE *(002173)*

CATEGORIES: Immunologic; Serums, Toxoids and Vaccines; Vaccines; FDA Pre 1938 Drugs

BRAND NAMES: Imogam Rabies; *Imovax Rabbia*; Imovax Rabies; *Lyssavac N Berna*; *Rabies-Imovax*; *Rabipur* (Germany); *Rabuman Berna*; *Rasilvax*; *Vacuna Antirrabica Humana*
(International brand names outside U.S. in italics)

FORMULARIES: WHO

Prescribing information not available at time of publication.

HOW SUPPLIED - EQUIVALENTS NOT AVAILABLE:

Injection, Solution - Intradermal - 0.25 unit

1's	$59.50	IMOVAX RABIES I.D., Connaught Labs	49281-0251-20

Injection, Solution - Intradermal

1's	$119.45	RABIES VACCINE ADSORBED, SKB Pharms	00007-4840-01

Injection, Solution - Intramuscular - 2.5 unit

1's	$133.88	IMOVAX RABIES VACCINE, Connaught Labs	49281-0250-10

RAMIPRIL *(003032)*

CATEGORIES: ACE Inhibitors; Angiotensin Converting Enzyme Inhibitors; Antihypertensives; Cardiovascular Drugs; Hypertension; Pregnancy Category D; FDA Class 1C ("Little or No Therapeutic Advantage"); FDA Approved 1991 Jan; Top 200 Drugs

BRAND NAMES: **Altace**; *Cardace*; *Delix* (Germany); *Hytren*; *Pramace*; *Quark*; *Ramace* (Mexico); *Triatec* (France); *Tritace* (Australia, England, Mexico, England); *Unipril*
(International brand names outside U.S. in italics)

FORMULARIES: Aetna; BC-BS; CIGNA; FHP; Humana; Kaiser; Medco; Medi-Cal; PruCare; United

COST OF THERAPY: $252.98 (Hypertension; Capsule; 2.5 mg; 1/day; 365 days)

PRIMARY ICD9: 401.1 (Essential Hypertension, Benign)

> **WARNING:**
> **USE IN PREGNANCY:** When used in pregnancy during the second and third trimesters, ACE inhibitors can cause injury and even death to the developing fetus. When pregnancy is detected, ramipril should be discontinued as soon as possible. See WARNINGS: Fetal/neonatal morbidity and mortality.

DESCRIPTION:

Ramipril is a 2-aza-bicyclo [3.3.0]-octane-3-carboxylic acid derivative. It is a white, crystalline substance soluble in polar organic solvents and buffered aqueous solutions. Ramipril melts between 105°C and 112°C. The CAS Registry Number is 87333-19-5. Ramipril's chemical name is (2*S*,3a*S*,6a*S*)-1[(*S*)-*N*-[(*S*)-1-Carboxy-3-phenylpropyl]alanyl]octahydrocyclopenta[*b*]pyrrole- 2-carboxylic acid, 1-ethyl ester.

Its empiric formula is $C_{23}H_{32}N_2O_5$, and its molecular weight is 416.5.

Ramiprilat, the diacid metabolite of ramipril, is a non-sulfhydryl angiotensin converting enzyme inhibitor. Ramipril is converted to ramiprilat by hepatic cleavage of the ester group.

Altace (ramipril) is supplied as hard shell capsules for oral administration containing 1.25 mg, 2.5 mg, 5 mg, and 10 mg of ramipril. The inactive ingredients present are pregelatinized starch NF, gelatin, and titanium dioxide. The 1.25 mg capsule shell contains yellow iron oxide, the 2.5 mg capsule shell contains D&C yellow #10 and FD&C red #40, the 5 mg capsule shell contains FD&C blue #1 and FD&C red #40, and the 10 mg capsule shell contains FD&C blue #1.

CLINICAL PHARMACOLOGY:

MECHANISM OF ACTION

Ramipril and ramiprilat inhibit angiotensin-converting enzyme (ACE) in human subjects and animals. ACE is a peptidyl dipeptidase that catalyzes the conversion of angiotensin I to the vasoconstrictor substance, angiotensin II. Angiotensin II also stimulates aldosterone secretion by the adrenal cortex. Inhibition of ACE results in decreased plasma angiotensin II, which leads to decreased vasopressor activity and to decreased aldosterone secretion. The latter decrease may result in a small increase of serum potassium. In hypertensive patients with normal renal function treated with ramipril alone for up to 56 weeks, approximately 4% of patients during the trial has an abnormally high serum potassium and an increase from baseline greater than 0.75 mEq/l, and none of the patients had an abnormally low potassium and a decrease from baseline greater than 0.75 mEq/l. In the same study, approximately 2% of patients treated with ramipril and hydrochlorothiazide for up to 56 weeks had abnormally high potassium values and an increase from baseline of 0.75 mEq/l or greater, and approximately 2% had abnormally low values and decreases from baseline of 0.75 mEq/l or greater. (See PRECAUTIONS.) Removal of angiotensin II negative feedback on renin secretion leads to increased plasma renin activity.

The effect of ramipril on hypertension appears to result at least in part from inhibition of both tissue and circulating ACE activity, thereby reducing angiotensin II formation in tissue and plasma.

ACE is identical to kininase, an enzyme that degrades bradykinin. Whether increased levels of bradykinin, a potent vasodepressor peptide, play a role in the therapeutic effects of ramipril remains to be elucidated.

While the mechanism through which ramipril lowers blood pressure is believed to be primarily suppression of the renin-angiotensin-aldosterone system, ramipril has an antihypertensive effect even in patients with low-renin hypertension. Although ramipril was antihypertensive in all races studied, black hypertensive patients (usually a low renin-hypertensive population) had a smaller average response to monotherapy than non-black patients.

PHARMACOKINETICS AND METABOLISM

Following oral administration of ramipril, peak plasma concentrations of ramipril are reached within one hour. The extent of absorption is at least 50-60% and is not significantly influenced by the presence of food in the GI tract, although the rate of absorption is reduced.

In a trial in which subjects received ramipril capsules or the contents of identical capsules dissolved in water, dissolved in apple juice, or suspended in apple sauce, serum ramiprilat levels were essentially unrelated to the use or nonuse of the concomitant liquid or food.

Cleavage of the ester group (primarily in the liver) converts ramipril to its active diacid metabolite, ramiprilat. Peak plasma concentrations of ramiprilat are reached 2-4 hours after drug intake. The serum protein binding of ramipril is about 73% and that of ramiprilat about 56%; *in vitro*, these percentages are independent of concentration over the range of 0.01 to 10 mcg/ml.

Ramipril is almost completely metabolized to ramiprilat, which has about 6 times the ACE inhibitory activity of ramipril, and to the diketopiperazine ester, the diketopiperazine acid, and the glucuronides of ramipril and ramiprilat, all of which are inactive. After oral administration of ramipril, about 60% of the parent drug and its metabolites are eliminated in the urine, and about 40% is found in the feces. Drug recovered in the feces may represent both biliary excretion of metabolites and/or unabsorbed drug, however the proportion of a dose eliminated by the bile has not been determined. Less than 2% of the administered dose is recovered in urine as unchanged ramipril.

Blood concentrations of ramipril and ramiprilat increase with increased dose, but are not strictly dose-proportional. The 24-hour AUC for ramiprilat, however, is dose-proportional over the 2.5-20 mg dose range. The absolute bioavailabilities of ramipril and ramiprilat were 28% and 44%, respectively, when 5 mg of oral ramipril was compared with the same dose of ramipril given intravenously.

Plasma concentrations of ramiprilat decline in a triphasic manner (initial rapid decline, apparent elimination phase, terminal elimination phase). The initial rapid decline, which represents distribution of the drug into a large peripheral compartment and subsequent binding to both plasma and tissue ACE, has a half-life of 2-4 hours. Because of its potent binding to ACE and slow dissociation from the enzyme, ramiprilat shows two elimination phases. The apparent elimination phase corresponds to the clearance of free ramiprilat and has a half-life of 9-18 hours. The terminal elimination phase has a prolonged half-life (>50 hours) and probably represents the binding/dissociation kinetics of the ramiprilat/ACE complex. It does not contribute to the accumulation of the drug. After multiple daily doses of ramipril 5-10 mg, the half-life of ramiprilat concentrations within the therapeutic range was 13-17 hours.

After once-daily dosing, steady-state plasma concentrations of ramiprilat are reached by the fourth dose. Steady-state concentrations of ramiprilat are somewhat higher than those seen after the first dose of ramipril, especially at low doses (2.5 mg), but the difference is clinically insignificant.

In patients with creatinine clearance less than 40 ml/min/1.73m^2, peak levels of ramiprilat are approximately doubled, and trough levels may be as much as quintupled. In multiple- dose regimens, the total exposure to ramiprilat (AUC) in these patients is 3-4 times as large as it is in patients with normal renal function who receive similar doses.

The urinary excretion of ramipril, ramiprilat, and their metabolites is reduced in patients with impaired renal function. Compared to normal subjects, patients with creatinine clearance less than 40 ml/min/1.73m^2 had higher peak and trough ramiprilat levels and slightly longer times to peak concentrations. (See DOSAGE AND ADMINISTRATION.)

In patients with impaired liver function, the metabolism of ramipril to ramiprilat appears to be slowed, possibly because of diminished activity of hepatic esterases, and plasma ramipril levels in these patients are increased about 3-fold. Peak concentrations of ramiprilat in these patients, however, are not different from those seen in subjects with normal hepatic function, and the effect of a given dose of plasma ACE activity does not vary with hepatic function.

CLINICAL PHARMACOLOGY: *(cont'd)*

PHARMACODYNAMICS

Single doses of ramipril of 2.5-20 mg produce approximately 60-80% inhibition of ACE activity 4 hours after dosing with approximately 40-60% inhibition after 24 hours. Multiple oral doses of ramipril of 2.0 mg or more cause plasma ACE activity to fall by more than 90% 4 hours after dosing, with over 80% inhibition of ACE activity remaining 24 hours after dosing. The more prolonged effect of even small multiple doses presumably reflects saturation of ACE binding sites by ramiprilat and relatively slow release from those sites.

PHARMACODYNAMICS AND CLINICAL EFFECTS

Hypertension: Administration of ramipril to patients with mild to moderate hypertension results in a reduction of both supine and standing blood pressure to about the same extent with no compensatory tachycardia. Symptomatic postural hypotension is infrequent, although it can occur in patients who are salt- and/or volume-depleted. (See WARNINGS.) Use of ramipril in combination with thiazide diuretics gives a blood pressure lowering effect greater than that seen with either agent alone.

In single-dose studies, doses of 5-20 mg of ramipril lowered blood pressure within 1-2 hours, with peak reductions achieved 3-6 hours after dosing. The antihypertensive effect of a single dose persisted for 24 hours. In longer term (4-12 weeks) controlled studies, once-daily doses of 2.5-10 mg were similar in their effect, lowering supine or standing systolic and diastolic blood pressures 24 hours after dosing by about 6/4 mm Hg more than placebo. In comparisons of peak vs. trough effect, the trough effect represented about 50-60% of the peak response. In a titration study comparing divided (bid) vs. qd treatment, the divided regimen was superior, indicating that for some patients the antihypertensive effect with once-daily dosing is not adequately maintained. (See DOSAGE AND ADMINISTRATION.)

In most trials, the antihypertensive effect of ramipril increased during the first several weeks of repeated measurements. The antihypertensive effect of ramipril has been shown to continue during long-term therapy for at least 2 years. Abrupt withdrawal of ramipril has not resulted in a rapid increase in blood pressure.

Ramipril has been compared with other ACE inhibitors, beta-blockers, and thiazide diuretics. It was approximately as effective as other ACE inhibitors and as atenolol. In both caucasians and blacks, hydrochlorothiazide (25 or 50 mg) was significantly more effective than ramipril.

Except for thiazides, no formal interaction studies of ramipril with other antihypertensive agents have been carried out. Limited experience in controlled and uncontrolled trials combining ramipril with a calcium channel blocker, a loop diuretic, or triple therapy (beta-blocker, vasodilator, and a diuretic) indicate no unusual drug-drug interactions. Other ACE inhibitors have had less than additive effects with beta adrenergic blockers, presumably because both drugs lower blood pressure by inhibiting parts of the renin-angiotensin system.

Ramipril was less effective in blacks than in caucasians. The effectiveness of ramipril was not influenced by age, sex, or weight.

In a baseline controlled study of 10 patients with mild essential hypertension, blood pressure reduction was accompanied by a 15% increase in renal blood flow. In healthy volunteers, glomerular filtration rate was unchanged.

Heart Failure post myocardial infarction: Ramipril was studied in the Acute Infarction Ramipril Efficacy (AIRE) trial. This was a multinational (mainly European) 161-center, 2006-patient, double- blind, randomized, parallel-group study comparing ramipril to placebo in stable patients, 2-9 days after an acute myocardial infarction (MI), who had shown clinical signs of congestive heart failure (CHF) at any time after the MI. Patients in severe (NYHA class IV) heart failure, patients with unstable angina, patients with heart failure of congenital or valvular etiology, and patients with contraindications to ACE inhibitors were all excluded. The majority of patients had received thrombolytic therapy at the time of the index infarction, and the average time between infarction and initiation of treatment was 5 days.

Patients randomized to ramipril treatment were given an initial dose of 2.5 mg twice daily. If the initial regimen caused undue hypotension, the dose was reduced to 1.25 mg, but in either event doses were titrated upward (as tolerated) to a target regimen (achieved in 77% of patients randomized to ramipril) of 5 mg twice daily. Patients were then followed for an average of 15 months (range 6-46).

The use of ramipril was associated with a 27% reduction (p=0.002), in the risk of death from any cause; about 90% of the deaths that occurred were cardiovascular, mainly sudden death. The risks of progression to severe heart failure and of CHF-related hospitalization were also reduced, by 23% (p=0.017) and 26% (p=0.011), respectively. The benefits of ramipril therapy were seen in both genders, and they were not affected by the exact timing of the initiation of therapy, but older patients may have had a greater benefit than those under 65. The benefits were seen in patients on, and not on, various concomitant medications; at the time of randomization these included aspirin (about 80% of patients), diuretics (about 60%), organic nitrates (about 55%), beta-blockers (about 20%), calcium channel blockers (about 15%), and digoxin (about 12%).

INDICATIONS AND USAGE:

Hypertension: Ramipril is indicated for the treatment of hypertension. It may be used alone or in combination with thiazide diuretics.

In using ramipril, consideration should be given to the fact that another angiotensin converting enzyme inhibitor, captopril, has caused agranulocytosis, particularly in patients with renal impairment or collagen-vascular disease. Available data are insufficient to show that ramipril does not have a similar risk. (See WARNINGS.)

In considering use of ramipril, it should be noted that in controlled trials ACE inhibitors have an effect on blood pressure that is less in black patients than in non-blacks. In addition, ACE inhibitors (for which adequate data are available) cause a higher rate of angioedema in black than in non-black patients (see WARNINGS, Angioedema.)

Heart Failure Post-Myocardial Infarction: Ramipril is indicated in stable patients who have demonstrated clinical signs of congestive heart failure within the first few days after sustaining acute myocardial infarction. Administration of ramipril to such patients has been shown to decrease the risk of death (principally cardiovascular death) and to decrease the risks of failure-related hospitalization and progression to severe/resistant heart failure (See CLINICAL PHARMACOLOGY, Heart Failure post myocardial infarction for details and limitations of the survival trial.)

CONTRAINDICATIONS:

Ramipril is contraindicated in patients who are hypersensitive to this product and in patients with a history of angioedema related to previous treatment with an angiotensin converting enzyme inhibitor.

WARNINGS:

Anaphylactoid and Possibly Related Reactions: Presumably because angiotensin-converting enzyme inhibitors affect the metabolism of eicosanoids and polypeptides, including endogenous bradykinin, patients receiving ACE inhibitors (including ramipril) may be subject to a variety of adverse reactions, some of the serious.

Angioedema: Patients with a history of angioedema unrelated to ACE inhibitor therapy may be at increased risk of angioedema while receiving an ACE inhibitor (See also CONTRAINDICATIONS.)

WARNINGS: *(cont'd)*

Angioedema of the face, extremities, lips, tongue, glottis, and larynx has been reported in patients treated with angiotensin converting enzyme inhibitors. Angioedema associated with laryngeal edema can be fatal. If laryngeal stridor or angioedema of the face, tongue, or glottis occurs, treatment with ramipril should be discontinued and appropriate therapy instituted immediately. **When there is involvement of the tongue, glottis, or larynx, likely to cause airway obstruction, appropriate therapy, e.g., subcutaneous epinephrine solution 1:1,000 (0.3 ml to 0.5 ml) should be promptly administered**. (See ADVERSE REACTIONS.)

In a large U.S. postmarketing study, angioedema (defined as reports of angio, face, larynx, tongue, or throat edema) was reported in 3/1523 (0.20%) of black patients and in 8/8680 (0.09%) of white patients. These rates were not different statistically.

Anaphylactoid reactions during desensitization: Two patients undergoing desensitizing treatment with hymenoptera venom while receiving ACE inhibitors sustained life-threatening anaphylactoid reactions. In the same patients, these reactions were avoided when ACE inhibitors were temporarily withheld, but they reappeared upon inadvertent rechallenge.

Anaphylactoid reactions during membrane exposure: Anaphylactoid reactions have been reported in patients dialyzed with high-flux membranes and treated concomitantly with an ACE inhibitor. Anaphylactoid reactions have also been reported in patients undergoing low-density lipoprotein apheresis with dextran sulfate absorption (a procedure dependent upon devises not approved in the United States).

Hypotension: Ramipril can cause symptomatic hypotension, after either the initial dose or a later dose when the dosage has been increased. Like other ACE inhibitors, ramipril has been only rarely associated with hypotension in uncomplicated hypertensive patients. Symptomatic hypotension is most likely to occur in patients who have been volume- and/or salt-depleted as a result of prolonged diuretic therapy, dietary salt restriction, dialysis, diarrhea, or vomiting. Volume and/or salt depletion should be corrected before initiating therapy with ramipril.

In patients with congestive heart failure, with or without associated renal insufficiency, ACE inhibitor therapy may cause excessive hypotension, which may be associated with oliguria or azotemia and, rarely, with acute renal failure and death. In such patients, ramipril therapy should be started under close medical supervision; they should be followed closely for the first 2 weeks of treatment and whenever the dose of ramipril or diuretic is increased.

If hypotension occurs, the patient should be placed in a supine position and, if necessary, treated with intravenous infusion of physiological saline. Ramipril treatment usually can be continued following restoration of blood pressure and volume.

Hepatic Failure: Rarely, ACE inhibitors have been associated with a syndrome that starts with cholestatic jaundice and progresses to fulminant hepatic necrosis and (sometimes) death. The mechanism of this syndrome is not understood. Patients receiving ACE inhibitors who develop jaundice or marked elevations of hepatic enzymes should discontinue the ACE inhibitor and receive appropriate medical follow-up.

Neutropenia/Agranulocytosis: Another angiotensin converting enzyme inhibitor, captopril, has been shown to cause agranulocytosis and bone marrow depression, rarely in uncomplicated patients, but more frequently in patients with renal impairment, especially if they also have a collagen-vascular disease such as systemic lupus erythematosus or scleroderma. Available data from clinical trials of ramipril are insufficient to show that ramipril does not cause agranulocytosis at similar rates. Monitoring of white blood cell counts should be considered in patients with collagen-vascular disease, especially if the disease is associated with impaired renal function.

Fetal/Neonatal Morbidity and Mortality: ACE inhibitors can cause fetal and neonatal morbidity and death when administered to pregnant women. Several dozen cases have been reported in the world literature. When pregnancy is detected, ACE inhibitors should be discontinued as soon as possible.

The use of ACE inhibitors during the second and the third trimesters of pregnancy has been associated with fetal and neonatal injury, including hypotension, neonatal skull hypoplasia, anuria, reversible or irreversible renal failure, and death. Oligohydramnios has also been reported, presumably resulting from decreased fetal renal function; oligohydramnios in this setting has been associated with fetal limb contractures, craniofacial deformation, and hypoplastic lung development. Prematurity, intrauterine growth retardation, and patent ductus arteriosus have also been reported, although it is not clear whether these occurrences were due to the ACE-inhibitor exposure.

These adverse effects do not appear to have resulted from intrauterine ACE-inhibitor exposure that has been limited to the first trimester. Mothers whose embryos and fetuses are exposed to ACE inhibitors only during the first trimester should be so informed. Nonetheless, when patients become pregnant, physicians should make every effort to discontinue the use of ramipril as soon as possible.

Rarely (probably less often than once in every thousand pregnancies), no alternative to ACE inhibitors will be found. In these rare cases, the mothers should be apprised of the potential hazards to their fetuses, and serial ultrasound examinations should be performed to assess the intraamniotic environment.

If oligohydramnios is observed, ramipril should be discontinued unless it is considered life-saving for the mother. Contraction stress testing (CST), a non-stress test (NST), or biophysical profiling (BPP) may be appropriate, depending upon the week of pregnancy. Patients and physicians should be aware, however, that oligohydramnios may not appear until after the fetus has sustained irreversible injury.

Infants with histories of *in utero* exposure to ACE inhibitors should be closely observed for hypotension, oliguria, and hyperkalemia. If oliguria occurs, attention should be directed toward support of blood pressure and renal perfusion. Exchange transfusion or dialysis may be required as means of reversing hypotension and/or substituting for disordered renal function. Ramipril which crosses the placenta can be removed from the neonatal circulation by these means, but limited experience has not shown that such removal is central to the treatment of these infants.

No teratogenic effects of ramipril were seen in studies of pregnant rats, rabbits, and cynomolgus monkeys. On a body surface area basis, the doses used were up to approximately 400 times (in rats and monkeys) and 2 times (in rabbits) the recommended human dose.

PRECAUTIONS:

GENERAL

Impaired Renal Function: As a consequence of inhibiting the renin-angiotensin-aldosterone system, changes in renal function may be anticipated in susceptible individuals. In patients with severe congestive heart failure whose renal function may depend on the activity of the renin-angiotensin-aldosterone system, treatment with angiotensin converting enzyme inhibitors, including ramipril, may be associated with oliguria and/or progressive azotemia and (rarely) with acute renal failure and/or death.

In hypertensive patients with unilateral or bilateral renal artery stenosis, increases in blood urea nitrogen and serum creatinine may occur. Experience with another angiotensin converting enzyme inhibitor suggests that these increases are usually reversible upon discontinuation of ramipril and/or diuretic therapy. In such patients renal function should be monitored during the first few weeks of therapy. Some hypertensive patients with no apparent pre-existing renal vascular disease have developed increases in blood urea nitrogen and serum creatinine, usually minor and transient, especially when ramipril has been given concomi-

PRECAUTIONS: *(cont'd)*

tantly with a diuretic. This is more likely to occur in patients with pre-existing renal impairment. Dosage reduction of ramipril and/or discontinuation of the diuretic may be required.

Evaluation of the hypertensive patient should always include assessment of renal function. (See DOSAGE AND ADMINISTRATION.)

Hyperkalemia: In clinical trials, hyperkalemia (serum potassium greater than 5.7 mEq/l) occurred in approximately 1% of hypertensive patients receiving ramipril. In most cases, these were isolated values, which resolved despite continued therapy. None of these patients was discontinued from the trials because of hyperkalemia. Risk factors for the development of hyperkalemia include renal insufficiency, diabetes mellitus, and the concomitant use of potassium-sparing diuretics, potassium supplements, and/or potassium-containing salt substitutes, which should be used cautiously, if at all, with ramipril. (See DRUG INTERACTIONS.)

Cough: Presumably due to the inhibition of the degradation of endogenous bradykinin, persistent nonproductive cough has been reported with all ACE inhibitors, always resolving after discontinuation of therapy. ACE inhibitor-induced cough should be considered in the differential diagnosis of cough.

Impaired Liver Function: Since ramipril is primarily metabolized by hepatic esterases to its active moiety, ramiprilat, patients with impaired liver function could develop markedly elevated plasma levels of ramipril. No formal pharmacokinetic studies have been carried out in hypertensive patients with impaired liver function.

Surgery/Anesthesia: In patients undergoing surgery or during anesthesia with agents that produce hypotension, ramipril may block angiotensin II formation that would otherwise occur secondary to compensatory renin release. Hypotension that occurs as a result of this mechanism can be corrected by volume expansion.

INFORMATION FOR THE PATIENT

Pregnancy: Female patients of childbearing age should be told about the consequences of second- and third-trimester exposure to ACE inhibitors, and they should also be told that these consequences do not appear to have resulted from intrauterine ACE-inhibitor exposure that has been limited to the first trimester. These patients should be asked to report pregnancies to their physicians as soon as possible.

Angioedema: Angioedema, including laryngeal edema, can occur with treatment with ACE inhibitors, especially following the first dose. Patients should be so advised and told to report immediately any signs or symptoms suggesting angioedema (swelling of face, eyes, lips, or tongue, or difficulty in breathing) and to take no more drug until they have consulted with the prescribing physician.

Symptomatic Hypotension: Patients should be cautioned that lightheadedness can occur, especially during the first days of therapy, and it should be reported. Patients should be told that if syncope occurs, ramipril should be discontinued until the physician has been consulted.

All patients should be cautioned that inadequate fluid intake or excessive perspiration, diarrhea, or vomiting can lead to an excessive fall in blood pressure, with the same consequences of lightheadedness and possible syncope.

Hyperkalemia: Patients should be told not to use salt substitutes containing potassium without consulting their physician.

Neutropenia: Patients should be told to promptly report any indication of infection (*e.g.,* sore throat, fever), which could be a sign of neutropenia.

CARCINOGENESIS, MUTAGENESIS, AND IMPAIRMENT OF FERTILITY

No evidence of a tumorigenic effect was found when ramipril was given by gavage to rats for up to 24 months at doses of up to 500 mg/kg/day or to mice for up to 18 months at doses of up to 1000 mg/kg/day. (For- either species, these doses are about 200 times the maximum recommended human dose when compared on the basis of body surface area.) No mutagenic activity was detected in the Ames test in bacteria, the micronucleus test in mice, unscheduled DNA synthesis in a human cell line, or a forward gene-mutation assay in a Chinese hamster ovary cell line. Several metabolites and degradation products of ramipril were also negative in the Ames test. A study in rats with dosages as great as 500 mg/kg/day did not produce adverse effects on fertility.

PREGNANCY

Pregnancy Categories C (first trimester) and D (second and third trimesters): See WARNINGS: Fetal/neonatal morbidity and mortality.

NURSING MOTHERS

Ingestion of single 10 mg oral dose of ramipril resulted in undetectable amounts of ramipril and its metabolites in breast milk. However, because multiple doses may produce low milk concentrations that are not predictable from single doses, women receiving ramipril should not breast feed.

GERIATRIC USE

Of the total number of patients who received ramipril in US clinical studies of ramipril 11.0% were 65 and over while 0.2% were 75 and over. No overall differences in effectiveness or safety were observed between these patients and younger patients, and other reported clinical experience has not identified differences in responses between the elderly and younger patients, but greater sensitivity of some older individuals cannot be ruled out.

One pharmacokinetic study conducted in hospitalized elderly patients indicated that peak ramiprilat levels and area under the plasma concentration time curve (AUC) for ramiprilat are higher in older patients.

PEDIATRIC USE

Safety and effectiveness in pediatric patients have not been established.

DRUG INTERACTIONS:

With diuretics: Patients on diuretics, especially those in whom diuretic therapy was recently instituted, may occasionally experience an excessive reduction of blood pressure after initiation of therapy with ramipril. The possibility of hypotensive effects with ramipril can be minimized by either discontinuing the diuretic or increasing the salt intake prior to initiation of therapy with ramipril. If this is not possible, the starting dose should be reduced. (See DOSAGE AND ADMINISTRATION.)

With potassium supplements and potassium-sparing diuretics: Ramipril can attenuate potassium loss caused by thiazide diuretics. Potassium-sparing diuretics (spironolactone, amiloride, triamterene, and others) or potassium supplements can increase the risk of hyperkalemia. Therefore, if concomitant use of such agents is indicated, they should be given with caution, and the patient's serum potassium should be monitored frequently.

With lithium: Increased serum lithium levels and symptoms of lithium toxicity have been reported in patients receiving ACE inhibitors during therapy with lithium. These drugs should be coadministered with caution, and frequent monitoring of serum lithium levels is recommended. If a diuretic is also used, the risk of lithium toxicity may be increased.

Other: Neither ramipril nor its metabolites have been found to interact with food, digoxin, antacid, furosemide, cimetidine, indomethacin, and simvastatin. The combination of ramipril and propranolol showed no adverse effects on dynamic parameters (blood pressure and heart rate). The co-administration of ramipril and warfarin did not adversely affect the anticoagulant effects of the latter drug. Additionally, co- administration of ramipril with phenprocoumon did not affect minimum phenprocoumon levels or interfere with the subjects' state of anti- coagulation.

ADVERSE REACTIONS:

Hypertension: Ramipril has been evaluated for safety in over 4,000 patients with hypertension; of these, 1,230 patients were studied in US controlled trials, and 1,107 were studied in foreign controlled trials. Almost 700 of these patients were treated for at least one year. The overall incidence of reported adverse events was similar in ramipril and placebo patients. The most frequent clinical side effects (possibly or probably related to study drug) reported by patients receiving ramipril in US placebo-controlled trials were: headache (5.4%), "dizziness" (2.2%) and fatigue or asthenia (2.0%), but only the last was more common in ramipril patients than in patients given placebo. Generally, the side effects were mild and transient, and there was no relation to total dosage within the range of 1.25 to 20 mg. Discontinuation of therapy because of a side effect was required in approximately 3% of US patients treated with ramipril. The most common reasons for discontinuation were: cough (1.0%), "dizziness" (0.5%), and impotence (0.4%).

The side effects considered possibly or probably related to study drug that occurred in US placebo-controlled trials in more than 1% of patients treated with ramipril are shown below (TABLE 1).

TABLE 1 Patients In U.S. Placebo Controlled Studies

	Altace (N=651)		Placebo (N=286)	
	n	%	n	%
Headache	35	5.4	17	5.9
"Dizziness"	14	2.2	9	3.1
Asthenia (Fatigue)	13	2.0	2	0.7
Nausea/Vomiting	7	1.1	3	1.0

In placebo-controlled trials, there was also an excess of upper respiratory infection and flu syndrome in the ramipril group. As these studies were carried out before the relationship of cough to ACE inhibitors was recognized, some of these events may represent ramipril-induced cough. In a later 1-year study, increased cough was seen in almost 12% of ramipril patients, with about 4% of these patients requiring discontinuation of treatment.

Heart Failure post myocardial infarction: Adverse reactions (except laboratory abnormalities) considered possibly/probably related to study drug that occurred in more than one percent of patients with heart failure treated with ramipril are shown below (TABLE 2). the incidences represent the experiences from the AIRE study. the follow-up time was between 6 and 46 months for this study.

TABLE 2 Percentage of Patients with Adverse Events Possibly/Probably Related to Study Placebo-Controlled (AIRE) Mortality StudyDrug

Adverse Event	Ramipril (N=1004)	Placebo (N=982)
Hypotension	10.7	4.7
Cough Increased	7.6	3.7
Dizziness	4.1	3.2
Angina Pectoris	2.9	2.0
Nausea	2.2	1.4
Postural Hypotension	2.2	1.4
Syncope	2.1	1.4
Heart Failure	2.0	2.2
Severe/Resistance Heart Failure	2.0	3.0
Myocardial Infarct	1.7	1.7
Vomiting	1.6	0.5
Vertigo	1.5	0.7
Headache	1.2	0.8
Kidney Function	1.2	0.5
Abnormal Chest Pain	1.1	0.9
Diarrhea	1.1	0.4
Asthenia	0.3	0.8

Other adverse experiences reported in controlled clinical trials (in less than 1% of ramipril patients), or rarer events seen in postmarketing experience, include the following (in some, a causal relationship to drug use is uncertain.):

Body As a Whole: Anaphylactoid reactions. (See WARNINGS.)

Cardiovascular: Symptomatic hypotension (reported in 0.5% of patients in US trials) (See WARNINGSand PRECAUTIONS), syncope (not reported in US trials), angina pectoris, arrhythmia, chest pain, palpitations, myocardial infarction, and cerebrovascular events.

Hematologic: Pancytopenia, hemolytic anemia and thrombocytopenia.

Renal: Some hypertensive patients with no apparent pre-existing renal disease have developed minor, usually transient, increases in blood urea nitrogen and serum creatinine when taking ramipril, particularly when ramipril was given concomitantly with a diuretic. (See WARNINGS.)

Angioneurotic Edema: Angioneurotic edema has been reported in 0.3% of patients in US clinical trials. (See WARNINGS.)

Cough: A tickling, dry, persistent, nonproductive cough has been reported with the use of ACE inhibitors. Approximately 1% of patients treated with ramipril have required discontinuation because of cough. The cough disappears shortly after discontinuation of treatment. (See PRECAUTIONS, Cough.)

Gastrointestinal: Pancreatitis, abdominal pain (sometimes with enzyme changes suggesting pancreatitis), anorexia, constipation, diarrhea, dry mouth, dyspepsia, dysphagia, gastroenteritis, hepatitis, nausea, increased salivation, taste disturbance, and vomiting.

Dermatologic: Apparent hypersensitivity reactions (manifested by urticaria, pruritus, or rash, with or without fever), erythema multiforme, photosensitivity, and purpura.

Neurologic and Psychiatric: Anxiety, amnesia, convulsions, depression, hearing loss, insomnia, nervousness, neuralgia, neuropathy, paresthesia, somnolence, tinnitus, tremor, vertigo, and vision disturbances.

Miscellaneous: As with other ACE inhibitors, a symptom complex has been reported which may include a positive ANA, an elevated erythrocyte sedimentation rate, arthralgia/arthritis, myalgia, fever, vasculitis, eosinophilia, photosensitivity, rash and other dermatologic manifestations.

Fetal/neonatal morbidity and mortality: See WARNINGS: Fetal/neonatal morbidity and mortality.

Other: Arthralgia, arthritis, dyspnea, edema, epistaxis, impotence, increased sweating, malaise, myalgia, and weight gain.

ADVERSE REACTIONS: *(cont'd)*

Clinical Laboratory Test Findings: Creatinine and Blood Urea Nitrogen: Increases in creatinine levels occurred in 1.2% of patients receiving ramipril alone, and in 1.5% of patients receiving ramipril and a diuretic. Increases in blood urea nitrogen levels occurred in 0.5% of patients receiving ramipril alone and in 3% of patients receiving ramipril with a diuretic. None of these increases required discontinuation of treatment. Increases in these laboratory values are more likely to occur in patients with renal insufficiency or those pretreated with a diuretic and, based on experience with other ACE inhibitors, would be expected to be especially likely in patients with renal artery stenosis. (See WARNINGS and PRECAUTIONS.) Since ramipril decreases aldosterone secretion, elevation of serum potassium can occur. Potassium supplements and potassium-sparing diuretics should be given with caution, and the patient's serum potassium should be monitored frequently. (See WARNINGSand PRECAUTIONS.)

Hemoglobin and Hematocrit: Decreases in hemoglobin or hematocrit (a low value and a decrease of 5 g/dl or 5% respectively) were rare, occurring in 0.4% of patients receiving ramipril alone and in 1.5% of patients receiving ramipril plus a diuretic. No US patients discontinued treatment because of decreases in hemoglobin or hematocrit.

Other (causal relationships unknown): Clinically important changes in standard laboratory tests were rarely associated with ramipril administration. Elevations of liver enzymes, serum bilirubin, uric acid, and blood glucose have been reported, as have cases of hyponatremia and scattered incidents of leukopenia, eosinophilia, and proteinuria. In US trials, less than 0.2% of patients discontinued treatment for laboratory abnormalities: all of these were cases of proteinuria or abnormal liver-function tests.

OVERDOSAGE:

Single oral doses in rats and mice of 10-11 g/kg resulted in significant lethality. In dogs, oral doses as high as 1 g/kg induced only mild gastrointestinal distress. Limited data on human overdosage are available. The most likely clinical manifestations would be symptoms attributable to hypotension.

Laboratory determinations of serum levels of ramipril and its metabolites are not widely available, and such determinations have, in any event, no established role in the management of ramipril overdose.

No data are available to suggest physiological maneuvers (*e.g.*, maneuvers to change the pH of the urine) that might accelerate elimination of ramipril and its metabolites. Similarly, it is not known which, if any, of these substances can be usefully removed from the body by hemodialysis.

Angiotensin II could presumably serve as a specific antagonist-antidote in the setting of ramipril overdose, but angiotensin II is essentially unavailable outside of scattered research facilities. Because the hypotensive effect of ramipril is achieved through vasodilation and effective hypovolemia, it is reasonable to treat ramipril overdose by infusion of normal saline solution.

DOSAGE AND ADMINISTRATION:

Hypertension: The recommended initial dose for patients not receiving a diuretic is 2.5 mg once a day. Dosage should be adjusted according to the blood pressure response. The usual maintenance dosage range is 2.5 to 20 mg per day administered as a single dose or in two equally divided doses. In some patients treated once daily, the antihypertensive effect may diminish toward the end of the dosing interval. In such patients, an increase in dosage or twice daily administration should be considered. If blood pressure is not controlled with ramipril alone, a diuretic can be added.

Heart Failure post myocardial infarction: For the treatment of post-infarction patients who have shown signs of congestive failure, the recommended starting dose of ramipril is 2.5 mg twice daily. A patient who becomes hypotensive at this dose may be switched to 1.25 mg twice daily, but all patients should then be titrated (as tolerated) toward a target dose of 5 mg twice daily.

After the initial dose of ramipril, the patient should be observed under medical supervision for at least two hours and until blood pressure has stabilized for at least an additional hour. (See WARNINGSand DRUG INTERACTIONS.) If possible, the dose of any concomitant diuretic should be reduced which may diminish the likelihood of hypotension. The appearance of hypotension after the initial dose of ramipril does not preclude subsequent careful dose titration with the drug, following effective management of the hypotension.

The ramipril capsule is usually swallowed whole. The ramipril capsule can also be opened and the contents sprinkled on a small amount (about 4 oz.) of apple sauce or mixed in 4 oz. (120 ml) of water or apple juice. To be sure that ramipril is not lost when such a mixture is used, the mixture should be consumed in its entirety. The described mixtures can be pre-prepared and stored for up to 24 hours at room temperature or up to 48 hours under refrigeration.

Concomitant administration of ramipril with potassium supplements, potassium salt substitutes, or potassium-sparing diuretics can lead to increases of serum potassium. (See PRECAUTIONS.)

In patients who are currently being treated with a diuretic, symptomatic hypotension occasionally can occur following the initial dose of ramipril. To reduce the likelihood of hypotension, the diuretic should, if possible, be discontinued two to three days prior to beginning therapy with ramipril (See WARNINGS.) Then, if blood pressure is not controlled with ramipril alone, diuretic therapy should be resumed.

If the diuretic cannot be discontinued, an initial dose of 1.25 mg ramipril should be used to avoid excess hypotension.

Dosage Adjustment in Renal Impairment: In patients with creatinine clearance <40 ml/min/1.73m^2 (serum creatinine approximately >2.5 mg/dl) doses only 25% of those normally used should be expected to induce full therapeutic levels of ramiprilat. (See CLINICAL PHARMACOLOGY.)

Hypertension: For patients with hypertension and renal impairment, the recommended initial dose is 1.25 mg ramipril once daily. Dosage may be titrated upward until blood pressure is controlled or to a maximum total daily dose of 5 mg.

Heart Failure post myocardial infarction: For patients with heart failure and renal impairment, the recommended initial dose is 1.25 mg ramipril once daily. The dose may be increased to 1.25 mg b.i.d. and up to a maximum dose of 2.5 mg b.i.d. depending upon clinical response and tolerability.

PATIENT INFORMATION:

Ramipril is considered an ACE-inhibitor and is used to treat high blood pressure alone or in combination with other medications. It can also be used to treat some forms of heart failure afer a heart attack. This medication should not be used during pregnancy and should be discontinued when pregnancy is determined. A nonproductive, persistent cough has been reported with the use of ACE inhibitors. The cough normally disappears when the medication is discontinued. A rare condition called angioedema can occur with ACE inhibitors, especially following the first dose. If you experience swelling of the face, eyes, lips, or tongue, difficulty in breathing) do not take additional medication and contact your physician immediately. Dizziness and lightheadedness can result when the mediation is first started. If this persists longer than one week, contact your physician. Signs of infections (sore throat or fever) should be reported to your physician as well to assure these are not drug related. Your blood pressure should be checked regularly to assure adequate control.

HOW SUPPLIED:

Altace is available in potencies of 1.25 mg, 2.5 mg, 5 mg, and 10 mg in hard gelatin capsules, packaged in bottles of 100 capsules. Altace is also supplied in blister packages (10 capsules/blister card).

Dispense in well-closed container with safety closure.

Store at controlled room temperature (59 to 86°F).

HOW SUPPLIED - EQUIVALENTS NOT AVAILABLE:

Capsule, Gelatin - Oral - 1.25 mg

100's	$59.08	ALTACE, Hoechst Marion Roussel	00039-0103-10
100's	$59.08	ALTACE, Hoechst Marion Roussel	00039-0103-11

Capsule, Gelatin - Oral - 2.5 mg

100's	$69.31	ALTACE, Hoechst Marion Roussel	00039-0104-10
100's	$69.31	ALTACE, Hoechst Marion Roussel	00039-0104-11

Capsule, Gelatin - Oral - 5 mg

100's	$74.18	ALTACE, Hoechst Marion Roussel	00039-0105-10
100's	$74.18	ALTACE, Hoechst Marion Roussel	00039-0105-11

Capsule, Gelatin - Oral - 10 mg

100's	$86.00	ALTACE, Hoechst Marion Roussel	00039-0106-10

RANITIDINE HYDROCHLORIDE *(002174)*

CATEGORIES: Acid/Peptic Disorders; Adenoma; Antacids; Antiulcer Drugs; Duodenal Ulcer; Endocrine Adenomas; Esophagitis; GERD; Gastric Ulcer; Gastrointestinal Drugs; Histamine H2 Receptor Antagonists; Hypersecretory Conditions; Mastocytosis; Ulcer; Zollinger-Ellison Syndrome; Pregnancy Category B; Sales > $1 Billion; FDA Approved 1983 Jun; Patent Expiration 2002 Dec; Top 200 Drugs

BRAND NAMES: *Achedos*; *Acidex*; *Aciloc*; *Acloral* (Mexico); *Anistal* (Mexico); *Apo-Ranitidine* (Canada); *Atural*; *Axoban* (Japan); *Azantac* (France, Mexico); *Consec*; *Coralen*; *Curan*; *Danitin*; *Duractin*; *Ezopta*; *Galidrin* (Mexico); *Gastrial*; *Gastridin*; *Gastrosedol*; *Histac*; *Istomar*; *Logast*; *Lydin*; *Mauran*; *Microtid* (Mexico); *Nodol*; *Ptinolin*; *Quantor*; *Quicran*; *Radinat*; *Ranacid*; *Randin*; *Ranial*; *Raniben*; *Ranidil*; *Ranidine*; *Ranimed*; *Ranimex*; *Ranin*; *Raniogas*; *Raniplex* (France); *Ranisen* (Mexico); *Ranital*; *Raniter*; *Ranitiget*; *Ranix*; *Rantac*; *Rantacid*; *Rantin*; *Ratic*; *Raticina*; *Rosimol*; *RND*; *Sampep*; *Sostril* (Germany); *Taural*; *Ul-Pep*; *Ulceran*; *Ulceranin*; *Ulcex*; *Ulsal*; *Ultac*; *Urantac*; *Verlost*; *Vesyca*; *Vizerul*; *Weichilin*; *Weidos*; *Xanidine*; *Zantab*; **Zantac**; *Zantadin*; *Zantic* (Germany); *Zinetac*
(International brand names outside U.S. in italics)

FORMULARIES: BC-BS; Kaiser; Foundation

COST OF THERAPY: $93.96 (Duodenal Ulcer; Tablet; 150 mg; 2/day; 28 days)

DESCRIPTION:

The active ingredient in Zantac 150 Tablets, Zantac 300 Tablets, Zantac 150 GELdose Capsules, Zantac 300 GELdose Capsules, Zantac 150 EFFERdose Tablets, Zantac 150 EFFERdose Granules, Zantac Syrup, Zantac Injection, Zantac Injection Premixed, and Zantac Injection Pharmacy Bulk Package—(Not for Direct Infusion), is ranitidine hydrochloride (HCl), a histamine H_2-receptor antagonist.

Chemically it is N[2-[[[5-[(dimethylamino)methyl]-2-furanyl]methyl]thio]ethyl]-N'-methyl-2 -nitro-1,1-ethenediamine, hydrochloride.

The empirical formula is $C_{13}H_{22}N_4O_3S{\cdot}HCl$, representing a molecular weight of 350.87.

Ranitidine HCl is a white to pale yellow, granular substance that is soluble in water.

It has a slightly bitter taste and sulfurlike odor.

Each Zantac 150 Tablet for oral administration contains 168 mg of ranitidine HCl equivalent to 150 mg of ranitidine. Each tablet also contains the inactive ingredients FD&C Yellow No. 6 Aluminum Lake, hydroxypropyl methylcellulose, magnesium stearate, microcrystalline cellulose, titanium dioxide, triacetin, and yellow iron oxide.

Each Zantac 300 Tablet for oral administration contains 336 mg of ranitidine HCl equivalent to 300 mg of ranitidine. Each tablet also contains the inactive ingredients croscarmellose sodium, D&C Yellow No. 10 Aluminum Lake, hydroxypropyl methylcellulose, magnesium stearate, microcrystalline cellulose, titanium dioxide, and triacetin.

Zantac 150 GELdose Capsules and Zantac 300 GELdose Capsules for oral administration are soft gelatin capsules containing 168 mg of ranitidine HCl equivalent to 150 mg of ranitidine and 336 mg of ranitidine HCl equivalent to 300 mg of ranitidine, respectively, in a nonaqueous matrix of synthetic coconut oil and synthetic triglycerides. The soft gelatin capsule shell contains gelatin, Sorbitol Special (sorbitol and sorbitol anhydrides), glycerin, purified water, titanium dioxide, FD&C Yellow No. 6, FD&C Blue No. 1, and FD&C Red No. 40. The capsule shell may also contain mineral oil and soybean lecithin. The capsules are printed with edible ink.

Zantac 150 EFFERdose Tablets and Zantac 150 EFFERdose Granules for oral administration are effervescent formulations of ranitidine that must be dissolved in water before use. Each individual tablet or the contents of a packet contain 168 mg of ranitidine HCl equivalent to 150 mg of ranitidine and the following inactive ingredients: aspartame, monosodium citrate anhydrous, povidone, and sodium bicarbonate. Each tablet also contains sodium benzoate. The total sodium content of each tablet is 183.12 mg (7.96 mEq) per 150 mg of ranitidine, and the total sodium content of each packet of granules is 173.54 mg (7.55 mEq) per 150 mg of ranitidine.

Each 1 ml of Zantac Syrup contains 16.8 mg of ranitidine HCl equivalent to 15 mg of ranitidine. Zantac Syrup also contains the inactive ingredients alcohol (7.5%), butylparaben, dibasic sodium phosphate, hydroxypropyl methylcellulose, peppermint flavor, monobasic potassium phosphate, propylparaben, purified water, saccharin sodium, sodium chloride, and sorbitol.

INJECTION, INJECTION PREMIXED, AND INJECTION PHARMACY BULK PACKAGE—NOT FOR DIRECT INFUSION

ZANTAC INJECTION IS A CLEAR, COLORLESS TO YELLOW, NONPYROGENIC LIQUID. THE YELLOW COLOR OF THE LIQUID TENDS TO INTENSIFY WITHOUT ADVERSELY AFFECTING POTENCY. THE PH OF THE INJECTION SOLUTION IS 6.7 TO 7.3.

DESCRIPTION: *(cont'd)*

STERILE INJECTION FOR INTRAMUSCULAR OR INTRAVENOUS ADMINISTRATION OR INJECTION PHARMACY BULK PACKAGE: Each 1 ml of aqueous solution contains ranitidine 25 mg (as the hydrochloride); phenol 5 mg as preservative; and 0.96 mg of monobasic potassium phosphate and 2.4 mg of dibasic sodium phosphate as buffers.**Injection Pharmacy Bulk Package—Not for Direct Infusion**

A pharmacy bulk package is a container of a sterile preparation for parenteral use that contains many single doses. The contents are intended for use in a pharmacy admixture program and are restricted to the preparation of admixtures for intravenous (IV) infusion.

Sterile, Premixed Solution for Intravenous Administration in Single- Dose, Flexible Plastic Containers: Each 50 ml contains ranitidine HCl equivalent to 50 mg of ranitidine, sodium chloride 225 mg, and citric acid 15 mg and dibasic sodium phosphate 90 mg as buffers in water for injection. It contains no preservatives. The osmolarity of this solution is 180 mOsm/l (approx.), and the pH is 6.7 to 7.3.

The flexible plastic container is fabricated from a specially formulated, nonplasticized, thermoplastic co-polyester (CR3). Water can permeate from inside the container into the overwrap but not in amounts sufficient to affect the solution significantly. Solutions inside the plastic container also can leach out certain of the chemical components in very small amounts before the expiration period is attained. However, the safety of the plastic has been confirmed by tests in animals according to USP biological standards for plastic containers.

CLINICAL PHARMACOLOGY:

Ranitidine HCl is a competitive, reversible inhibitor of the action of histamine at the histamine H_2-receptors, including receptors on the gastric cells. Ranitidine HCl does not lower serum Ca++ in hypercalcemic states. Ranitidine HCl is not an anticholinergic agent.

ANTISECRETORY ACTIVITY: EFFECTS ON ACID SECRETION

Oral

Ranitidine HCl inhibits both daytime and nocturnal basal gastric acid secretions as well as gastric acid secretion stimulated by food, betazole, and pentagastrin, as shown in the following table (TABLE 1):

TABLE 1 Effect of Oral Ranitidine HCl on Gastric Acid Secretion

	Time After Dose, h	% Inhibition of Gastric Acid Output by Intravenous Dose, mg			
		75-80	100	150	200
Basal	Up to 4		99	95	
Nocturnal	Up to 13	95	96	92	
Betazole	Up to 3		97	99	
Pentagastrin	Up to 5	58	72	72	80
Meal	Up to 3		73	79	95

It appears that basal-, nocturnal-, and betazole-stimulated secretions are most sensitive to inhibition by ranitidine HCl, responding almost completely to doses of 100 mg or less, while pentagastrin- and food-stimulated secretions are more difficult to suppress.

Injection, Injection Premixed, and Injection Pharmacy Bulk Package—Not for Direct Infusion

Ranitidine HCl injection inhibits basal gastric acid secretion as well as gastric acid secretion stimulated by betazole and pentagastrin, as shown in the following table (TABLE 2):

TABLE 2 Effect of Intravenous Ranitidine HCl on Gastric Acid Secretion

	Time After Dose, h	% Inhibition of Gastric Acid Output by Intravenous Dose, mg		
		20 mg	60 mg	100 mg
Betazole	Up to 2	93	99	99
Pentagastrin	Up to 3	47	66	77

In a group of 10 known hypersecretors, ranitidine plasma levels of 71, 180, and 376 ng/ml inhibited basal acid secretion by 76%, 90%, and 99.5%, respectively.

It appears that basal- and betazole-stimulated secretions are most sensitive to inhibition by ranitidine HCl, while pentagastrin-stimulated secretion is more difficult to suppress.

EFFECTS ON OTHER GASTROINTESTINAL SECRETIONS

Pepsin: Ranitidine HCl does not affect pepsin secretion. Total pepsin output is reduced in proportion to the decrease in volume of gastric juice.

Intrinsic Factor: Ranitidine HCl has no significant effect on pentagastrin-stimulated intrinsic factor secretion.

Serum Gastrin: Ranitidine HCl has little or no effect on fasting or postprandial serum gastrin.

Other Pharmacologic Actions

a. Gastric bacterial flora: increase in nitrate-reducing organisms, significance not known.

b. Prolactin levels: no effect in recommended oral or (IV) dosage, but small, transient, dose-related increases in serum prolactin have been reported after IV bolus injections of 100 mg or more.

c. Other pituitary hormones: no effect on serum gonadotropins, TSH, or GH. Possible impairment of vasopressin release.

d. No change in cortisol, aldosterone, androgen, or estrogen levels.

e. No antiandrogenic action.

f. No effect on count, motility, or morphology of sperm.

PHARMACOKINETICS

Oral: Ranitidine HCl is 50% absorbed after oral administration, compared to an IV injection with mean peak levels of 440 to 545 ng/ml occurring at 2 to 3 hours after a 150-mg dose. The syrup, capsule, and effervescent formulations are bioequivalent to the tablets. In a pharmacodynamic comparison of the effervescent with the ranitidine HCl Tablets, during the first hour after administration, the effervescent tablet formulation gave a significantly higher intragastric pH, by approximately 1 pH unit, compared to the ranitidine HCl Tablets. The elimination half-life is 2.5 to 3 hours.

Absorption is not significantly impaired by the administration of food or antacids. Propantheline slightly delays and increases peak blood levels of ranitidine HCl, probably by delaying gastric emptying and transit time. In one study, simultaneous administration of high-potency antacid (150 mmol) in fasting subjects has been reported to decrease the absorption of ranitidine HCl.

Serum concentrations necessary to inhibit 50% of stimulated gastric acid secretion are estimated to be 36 to 94 ng/ml. Following a single oral dose of 150 mg, serum concentrations of ranitidine HCl are in this range up to 12 hours. However, blood levels bear no consistent relationship to dose or degree of acid inhibition.

The principal route of excretion is the urine, with approximately 30% of the orally administered dose collected in the urine as unchanged drug in 24 hours. Renal clearance is about 410 ml per minute, indicating active tubular excretion. Four patients with clinically significant renal function impairment (creatinine clearance 25 to 35 ml per minute) administered 50 mg of ranitidine intravenously had an average plasma half-life of 4.8 hours, a ranitidine clearance of 29 ml per minute, and a volume of distribution of 1.76 l/kg. In general, these parameters appear to be altered in proportion to creatinine clearance (see DOSAGE AND ADMINISTRATION).

CLINICAL PHARMACOLOGY: *(cont'd)*

In man, the N-oxide is the principal metabolite in the urine; however, this amounts to < 4% of the dose. Other metabolites are the S-oxide (1%) and the desmethyl ranitidine (1%). The remainder of the administered dose is found in the stool. Studies in patients with hepatic dysfunction (compensated cirrhosis) indicate that there are minor, but clinically insignificant, alterations in ranitidine half-life, distribution, clearance, and bioavailability.

The volume of distribution is about 1.4 l/kg. Serum protein binding averages 15%.

Injection, Injection Premixed, and Injection Pharmacy Bulk Package: Not for Direct Infusion Serum concentrations necessary to inhibit 50% of stimulated gastric acid secretion are estimated to be 36 to 94 ng/ml. Following single IV or intramuscular (IM) 50-mg doses, serum concentrations of ranitidine HCl are in this range for 6 to 8 hours.

Following IV injection, approximately 70% of the dose is recovered in the urine as unchanged drug. Renal clearance averages 530 ml per minute, with a total clearance of 760 ml per minute. The volume of distribution is 1.4 l/kg, and the elimination half-life is 2 to 2.5 hours.

Four patients with clinically significant renal function impairment (creatinine clearance 25 to 35 ml per minute) administered 50 mg of ranitidine intravenously had an average plasma half-life of 4.8 hours, a ranitidine clearance of 29 ml per minute, and a volume of distribution of 1.76 l/kg. In general, these parameters appear to be altered in proportion to creatinine clearance (see DOSAGE AND ADMINISTRATION).

Ranitidine HCl is absorbed very rapidly after IM injection. Mean peak levels of 576 ng/ml occur within 15 minutes or less following a 50-mg IM dose. Absorption from IM sites is virtually complete, with a bioavailability of 90% to 100% compared with IV administration. Following oral administration, the relative bioavailability of ranitidine HCl Tablets is 50%.

In man, the N-oxide is the principal metabolite in the urine; however, this amounts to less than 4% of the dose. Other metabolites are the S-oxide (1%) and the desmethyl ranitidine (1%). The remainder of the administered dose is found in the stool.

Studies in patients with hepatic dysfunction (compensated cirrhosis) indicate that there are minor, but clinically insignificant, alterations in ranitidine half-life, distribution, clearance, and bioavailability.

Serum protein binding averages 15%.

CLINICAL STUDIES:

Active Duodenal Ulcer: In a multicenter, double-blind, controlled, US study of endoscopically diagnosed duodenal ulcers, earlier healing was seen in the patients treated with ranitidine HCl as shown in (TABLE 3).

TABLE 3

	Ranitidine HCl* Number Entered	Ranitidine HCl* Healed/ Evaluable	Placebo* Number Entered	Placebo* Healed/ Evaluable
Outpatients				
Week 2	195	69/182 (38%)†	188	31/164 (19%)
Week 4		137/187 (73%)†	76/168	(45%)

* All patients were permitted p.r.n. antacids for relief of pain.
† $p<0.0001$.

In these studies, patients treated with ranitidine HCl reported a reduction in both daytime and nocturnal pain, and they also consumed less antacid than the placebo-treated patients (TABLE 4).

TABLE 4 Mean Daily Doses of Antacid

	Ulcer Healed	Ulcer Not Healed
Zantac	0.06	0.71
Placebo	0.71	1.43

ORAL

Foreign studies have shown that patients heal equally well with 150 mg b.i.d. and 300 mg h.s. (85% versus 84%, respectively) during a usual 4-week course of therapy. If patients require extended therapy of 8 weeks, the healing rate may be higher for 150 mg b.i.d. as compared to 300 mg h.s. (92% versus 87%, respectively).

Studies have been limited to short-term treatment of acute duodenal ulcer. Patients whose ulcers healed during therapy had recurrences of ulcers at the usual rates.

Maintenance Therapy in Duodenal Ulcer: Ranitidine has been found to be effective as maintenance therapy for patients following healing of acute duodenal ulcers. In two independent, double-blind, multicenter, controlled trials, the number of duodenal ulcers observed was significantly less in patients treated with ranitidine HCl (150 mg h.s.) than in patients treated with placebo over a 12-month period (TABLE 5).

TABLE 5 Duodenal Ulcer Prevalence Double-blind, Multicenter, Placebo-Controlled Trials

Multicenter Trial	Drug	Duodenal Ulcer Prevalence 0-4 Months	0-8 Months	0-12 Months	No. of Patients
USA	RAN	20%*	24%*	35%*	138
	PLC	44%	54%	59%	139
Foreign	RAN	12%*	21%*	28%*	174
	PLC	56%	64%	68%	165

RAN=ranitidine (Zantac).
PLC=placebo.
% =Life table estimate. * $=p<0.05$ (Zantac vs comparator).

As with other H_2-antagonists, the factors responsible for the significant reduction in the prevalence of duodenal ulcers include prevention of recurrence of ulcers, more rapid healing of ulcers that may occur during maintenance therapy, or both.

Gastric Ulcer: In a multicenter, double-blind, controlled US study of endoscopically diagnosed gastric ulcers, earlier healing was seen in the patients treated with ranitidine HCl as shown in the following table (TABLE 6):

In this multicenter trial, significantly more patients treated with ranitidine HCl became pain free during therapy.

CLINICAL STUDIES: *(cont'd)*

TABLE 6

	Ranitidine HCl*		Placebo*	
	Number Entered	Healed/ Evaluable	Number Entered	Healed/ Evaluable
Outpatients				
Week 2	92	16/83 (19%)	94	10/83 (12%)
Week 6		50/73 (68%)†		35/69 (51%)

* All patients were permitted p.r.n. antacids for relief of pain.
† p=0.009.

Maintenance of Healing of Gastric Ulcers: In two multicenter, double-blind, randomized, placebo-controlled, 12-month trials conducted in patients whose gastric ulcers had been previously healed, ranitidine HCl 150 mg h.s. was significantly more effective than placebo in maintaining healing of gastric ulcers.

Tablets, Capsules, Granules, Syrup, Injection, Injection Premixed, and Injection Pharmacy Bulk Package—Not for Direct Infusion

Pathological Hypersecretory Conditions (such as Zollinger-Ellison syndrome): Ranitidine HCl inhibits gastric acid secretion and reduces occurrence of diarrhea, anorexia, and pain in patients with pathological hypersecretion associated with Zollinger-Ellison syndrome, systemic mastocytosis, and other pathological hypersecretory conditions (*e.g.,* postoperative, "short-gut" syndrome, idiopathic). Use of ranitidine HCl was followed by healing of ulcers in 8 of 19 (42%) patients who were intractable to previous therapy.

In a retrospective review of 52 Zollinger-Ellison patients given ranitidine HCl as a continuous IV infusion for up to 15 days, no patients developed complications of acid-peptic disease such as bleeding or perforation. Acid output was controlled to ≤10 mEq per hour.

Gastroesophageal Reflux Disease (GERD): In two multicenter, double-blind, placebo-controlled, 6-week trials performed in the United States and Europe, ranitidine HCl 150 mg b.i.d. was more effective than placebo for the relief of heartburn and other symptoms associated with GERD. Ranitidine-treated patients consumed significantly less antacid than did placebo-treated patients.

The US trial indicated that ranitidine HCl 150 mg b.i.d. significantly reduced the frequency of heartburn attacks and severity of heartburn pain within 1 to 2 weeks after starting therapy. The improvement was maintained throughout the 6-week trial period. Moreover, patient response rates demonstrated that the effect on heartburn extends through both the day and night time periods.

Erosive Esophagitis: In two multicenter, double-blind, randomized, placebo-controlled, 12-week trials performed in the United States, ranitidine HCl 150 mg q.i.d. was significantly more effective than placebo in healing endoscopically diagnosed erosive esophagitis and in relieving associated heartburn. The erosive esophagitis healing rates were as follows (TABLE 7):

TABLE 7 Erosive Esophagitis Patient Healing Rates

	Healed/Evaluable	
	Placebo* n=229	Ranitidine HCl 150 mg q.i.d.* n=215
Week 4	43/198 (22%)	96/206 (47%)†
Week 8	63/176 (36%)	142/200 (71%)†
Week 12	92/159 (58%)	162/192 (84%)†

* All patients were permitted p.r.n. antacids for relief of pain.
† p<0.001 versus placebo.

No additional benefit in healing of esophagitis or in relief of heartburn was seen with a ranitidine dose of 300 mg q.i.d.

Maintenance of Healing of Erosive Esophagitis: In two multicenter, double-blind, randomized, placebo-controlled, 48-week trials conducted in patients whose erosive esophagitis had been previously healed, ranitidine HCl 150 mg b.i.d. was significantly more effective than placebo in maintaining healing of erosive esophagitis.

INDICATIONS AND USAGE:

Oral ranitidine HCl is indicated in:

1. Short-term treatment of active duodenal ulcer. Most patients heal within 4 weeks. Studies available to date have not assessed the safety of ranitidine in uncomplicated duodenal ulcer for periods of more than 8 weeks.
2. Maintenance therapy for duodenal ulcer patients at reduced dosage after healing of acute ulcers. No placebo-controlled comparative studies have been carried out for periods of longer than 1 year.
3. The treatment of pathological hypersecretory conditions (*e.g.,* Zollinger-Ellison syndrome and systemic mastocytosis).
4. Short-term treatment of active, benign gastric ulcer. Most patients heal within 6 weeks and the usefulness of further treatment has not been demonstrated. Studies available to date have not assessed the safety of ranitidine in uncomplicated, benign gastric ulcer for periods of more than 6 weeks.
5. Maintenance therapy for gastric ulcer patients at reduced dosage after healing of acute ulcers. Placebo-controlled studies have been carried out for 1 year.
6. Treatment of GERD. Symptomatic relief commonly occurs within 1 or 2 weeks after starting therapy with ranitidine HCl 150 mg b.i.d.
7. Treatment of endoscopically diagnosed erosive esophagitis. Symptomatic relief of heartburn commonly occurs within 24 hours of therapy initiation with ranitidine HCl 150 mg q.i.d.
8. Maintenance of healing of erosive esophagitis. Placebo-controlled trials have been carried out for 48 weeks.

Concomitant antacids should be given as needed for pain relief to patients with active duodenal ulcer; active, benign gastric ulcer; hypersecretory states; GERD; and erosive esophagitis.**Injection, Injection Premixed, and Injection Pharmacy Bulk Package—Not for Direct Infusion**

Injection: Ranitidine HCl injection is indicated in some hospitalized patients with pathological hypersecretory conditions or intractable duodenal ulcers, or as an alternative to the oral dosage form for short-term use in patients who are unable to take oral medication.

CONTRAINDICATIONS:

Ranitidine HCl is contraindicated for patients known to have hypersensitivity to the drug or any of the ingredients (see PRECAUTIONS).

PRECAUTIONS:

GENERAL

1. Symptomatic response to ranitidine HCl therapy does not preclude the presence of gastric malignancy.
2. Since ranitidine HCl is excreted primarily by the kidney, dosage should be adjusted in patients with impaired renal function (see DOSAGE AND ADMINISTRATION). Caution should be observed in patients with hepatic dysfunction since ranitidine HCl is metabolized in the liver.
3. Rare reports suggest that ranitidine HCl may precipitate acute porphyric attacks in patients with acute porphyria. Ranitidine HCl should therefore be avoided in patients with a history of acute porphyria.
4. In controlled studies in normal volunteers, elevations in SGPT have been observed when H_2-antagonists have been administered intravenously at greater than recommended dosages for 5 days or longer. Therefore, it seems prudent in patients receiving IV ranitidine at dosages ≥100 mg q.i.d. for periods of 5 days or longer to monitor SGPT daily (from day 5) for the remainder of IV therapy.
5. Bradycardia in association with rapid administration of ranitidine HCl injection has been reported rarely, usually in patients with factors predisposing to cardiac rhythm disturbances. Recommended rates of administration should not be exceeded (see DOSAGE AND ADMINISTRATION).

INFORMATION FOR THE PATIENT

Phenylketonurics: Ranitidine HCl 150 effervescent Tablets and ranitidine HCl 150 effervescent Granules contain phenylalanine 16.84 mg per 150 mg of ranitidine.

LABORATORY TESTS

False-positive tests for urine protein with Multistix may occur during ranitidine HCl therapy, and therefore testing with sulfosalicylic acid is recommended.

CARCINOGENESIS, MUTAGENESIS, AND IMPAIRMENT OF FERTILITY

There was no indication of tumorigenic or carcinogenic effects in life-span studies in mice and rats at dosages up to 2,000 mg/kg per day.

Ranitidine was not mutagenic in standard bacterial tests *(Salmonella, Escherichia coli)* for mutagenicity at concentrations up to the maximum recommended for these assays.

In a dominant lethal assay, a single oral dose of 1,000 mg/kg to male rats was without effect on the outcome of two matings per week for the next 9 weeks.

PREGNANCY, TERATOGENIC EFFECTS, PREGNANCY CATEGORY B

Reproduction studies have been performed in rats and rabbits at doses up to 160 times the human dose and have revealed no evidence of impaired fertility or harm to the fetus due to ranitidine HCl. There are, however, no adequate and well-controlled studies in pregnant women. Because animal reproduction studies are not always predictive of human response, this drug should be used during pregnancy only if clearly needed.

NURSING MOTHERS

Ranitidine HCl is secreted in human milk. Caution should be exercised when ranitidine HCl is administered to a nursing mother.

PEDIATRIC USE

Safety and effectiveness in pediatric patients/children have not been established.

GERIATRIC USE

Ulcer healing rates in elderly patients (65 to 82 years of age) were no different from those in younger age-groups. The incidence rates for adverse events and laboratory abnormalities were also not different from those seen in other age- groups.

DRUG INTERACTIONS:

Although ranitidine HCl has been reported to bind weakly to cytochrome P-450 *in vitro,* recommended doses of the drug do not inhibit the action of the cytochrome P-450-linked oxygenase enzymes in the liver. However, there have been isolated reports of drug interactions that suggest that ranitidine HCl may affect the bioavailability of certain drugs by some mechanism as yet unidentified (*e.g.,* a pH-dependent effect on absorption or a change in volume of distribution).

Increased or decreased prothrombin times have been reported during concurrent use of ranitidine and warfarin. However, in human pharmacokinetic studies with dosages of ranitidine up to 400 mg per day, no interaction occurred; ranitidine had no effect on warfarin clearance or prothrombin time. The possibility of an interaction with warfarin at dosages of ranitidine higher than 400 mg per day has not been investigated.

ADVERSE REACTIONS:

Injection, Injection Premixed, and Injection Pharmacy Bulk Package—Not for Direct Infusion

Transient pain at the site of IM injection has been reported. Transient local burning or itching has been reported with IV administration of ranitidine HCl.

The following have been reported as events in clinical trials or in the routine management of patients treated with ranitidine HCl. The relationship to ranitidine HCl therapy has been unclear in many cases. Headache, sometimes severe, seems to be related to ranitidine HCl administration.

Central Nervous System: Rarely, malaise, dizziness, somnolence, insomnia, and vertigo. Rare cases of reversible mental confusion, agitation, depression, and hallucinations have been reported, predominantly in severely ill elderly patients. Rare cases of reversible blurred vision suggestive of a change in accommodation have been reported. Rare reports of reversible involuntary motor disturbances have been received.

Cardiovascular: As with other H_2-blockers, rare reports of arrhythmias such as tachycardia, bradycardia, asystole (injection only), atrioventricular block, and premature ventricular beats.

Gastrointestinal: Constipation, diarrhea, nausea/vomiting, abdominal discomfort/pain, and rare reports of pancreatitis.

Hepatic: In normal volunteers, SGPT values were increased to at least twice the pretreatment levels in 6 of 12 subjects receiving 100 mg q.i.d. intravenously for 7 days, and in 4 of 24 subjects receiving 50 mg q.i.d. intravenously for 5 days. There have been occasional reports of hepatitis, hepatocellular or hepatocanalicular or mixed, with or without jaundice. In such circumstances, ranitidine should be immediately discontinued. These events are usually reversible, but in exceedingly rare circumstances death has occurred.

Musculoskeletal: Rare reports of arthralgias and myalgias.

Hematologic: Blood count changes (leukopenia, granulocytopenia, and thrombocytopenia) have occurred in a few patients. These were usually reversible. Rare cases of agranulocytosis, pancytopenia, sometimes with marrow hypoplasia, and aplastic anemia and exceedingly rare cases of acquired immune hemolytic anemia have been reported.

Endocrine: Controlled studies in animals and man have shown no stimulation of any pituitary hormone by ranitidine HCl and no antiandrogenic activity, and cimetidine-induced gynecomastia and impotence in hypersecretory patients have resolved when ranitidine HCl has been substituted. However, occasional cases of gynecomastia, impotence, and loss of libido have been reported in male patients receiving ranitidine HCl, but the incidence did not differ from that in the general population.

ADVERSE REACTIONS: *(cont'd)*

Integumentary: Rash, including rare cases of erythema multiforme, and, rarely, alopecia.

Other: Rare cases of hypersensitivity reactions (*e.g.*, bronchospasm, fever, rash, eosinophilia), anaphylaxis, angioneurotic edema, and small increases in serum creatinine.

OVERDOSAGE:

There has been virtually no experience with overdosage with ranitidine HCl injection and limited experience with oral doses of ranitidine. Reported acute ingestions of up to 18 g orally have been associated with transient adverse effects similar to those encountered in normal clinical experience (see ADVERSE REACTIONS). In addition, abnormalities of gait and hypotension have been reported.

When overdosage occurs, the usual measures to remove unabsorbed material from the gastrointestinal tract, clinical monitoring, and supportive therapy should be employed.

Studies in dogs receiving dosages of ranitidine HCl in excess of 225 mg/kg per day have shown muscular tremors, vomiting, and rapid respiration. Single oral doses of 1,000 mg/kg in mice and rats were not lethal. Intravenous LD_{50} values in mice and rats were 77 and 83 mg/kg, respectively.

DOSAGE AND ADMINISTRATION:

ORAL

Active Duodenal Ulcer: The current recommended adult oral dosage of ranitidine HCl for duodenal ulcer is 150 mg or 10 ml (2 teaspoonfuls equivalent to 150 mg of ranitidine) twice daily. An alternative dosage of 300 mg or 20 ml (4 teaspoonfuls equivalent to 300 mg of ranitidine) once daily after the evening meal or at bedtime can be used for patients in whom dosing convenience is important. The advantages of one treatment regimen compared to the other in a particular patient population have yet to be demonstrated (see CLINICAL STUDIES, Active Duodenal Ulcer). Smaller doses have been shown to be equally effective in inhibiting gastric acid secretion in US studies, and several foreign trials have shown that 100 mg b.i.d. is as effective as the 150-mg dose.

Antacid should be given as needed for relief of pain (see CLINICAL PHARMACOLOGY, Pharmacokinetics.)

Maintenance of Healing of Duodenal Ulcers: The current recommended adult oral dosage is 150 mg or 10 ml (2 teaspoonfuls equivalent to 150 mg of ranitidine) at bedtime.

Pathological Hypersecretory Conditions (such as Zollinger-Ellison syndrome): The current recommended adult oral dosage is 150 mg or 10 ml (2 teaspoonfuls equivalent to 150 mg of ranitidine) twice a day. In some patients it may be necessary to administer ranitidine HCl 150-mg doses more frequently. Dosages should be adjusted to individual patient needs, and should continue as long as clinically indicated. Dosages up to 6 g per day have been employed in patients with severe disease.

Benign Gastric Ulcer: The current recommended adult oral dosage is 150 mg or 10 ml (2 teaspoonfuls equivalent to 150 mg of ranitidine) twice a day.

Maintenance of Healing of Gastric Ulcers: The current recommended adult oral dosage is 150 mg or 10 ml (2 teaspoonfuls equivalent to 150 mg of ranitidine) at bedtime.

GERD: The current recommended adult oral dosage is 150 mg or 10 ml (2 teaspoonfuls equivalent to 150 mg of ranitidine) twice a day.

Erosive Esophagitis: The current recommended adult oral dosage is 150 mg or 10 ml (2 teaspoonfuls equivalent to 150 mg of ranitidine) four times a day.

Maintenance of Healing of Erosive Esophagitis: The current recommended adult oral dosage is 150 mg or 10 ml (2 teaspoonfuls equivalent to 150 mg of ranitidine) twice a day.

Dosage Adjustment for Patients With Impaired Renal Function: On the basis of experience with a group of subjects with severely impaired renal function treated with ranitidine HCl, the recommended dosage in patients with a creatinine clearance < 50 ml per minute is 150 mg or 10 ml (2 teaspoonfuls equivalent to 150 mg of ranitidine) every 24 hours. Should the patient's condition require, the frequency of dosing may be increased to every 12 hours or even further with caution. Hemodialysis reduces the level of circulating ranitidine. Ideally, the dosing schedule should be adjusted so that the timing of a scheduled dose coincides with the end of hemodialysis.

Preparation of Ranitidine HCl 150 effervescent Tablets and Ranitidine HCl 150 effervescent Granules: Dissolve each dose in approximately 6 to 8 oz of water before drinking.

INJECTION

Injection, Injection Premixed, and Injection Pharmacy Bulk Package—Not for Direct Infusion

Parenteral Administration: In some hospitalized patients with pathological hypersecretory conditions or intractable duodenal ulcers, or in patients who are unable to take oral medication, ranitidine HCl may be administered parenterally according to the following recommendations:

Intramuscular Injection: 50 mg (2 ml) every 6 to 8 hours. (No dilution necessary.)

Intermittent Intravenous Injection

a. Intermittent Bolus: 50 mg (2 ml) every 6 to 8 hours. Dilute ranitidine HCl injection, 50 mg, in 0.9% sodium chloride injection or other compatible IV solution (see DOSAGE AND ADMINISTRATION, Stability) to a concentration no greater than 2.5 mg/ml (20 ml). Inject at a rate no greater than 4 ml per minute (5 minutes).

b. Intermittent Infusion: 50 mg (2 ml) every 6 to 8 hours. Dilute ranitidine HCl injection, 50 mg, in 5% dextrose injection or other compatible IV solution (see DOSAGE AND ADMINISTRATION, Stability) to a concentration no greater than 0.5 mg/ml (100 ml). Infuse at a rate no greater than 5 to 7 ml per minute (15 to 20 minutes).

Ranitidine HCl injection premixed solution, 50 mg, in 0.45% sodium chloride, 50 ml, requires no dilution and should be infused over 15 to 20 minutes.

In some patients it may be necessary to increase dosage. When this is necessary, the increases should be made by more frequent administration of the dose, but it generally should not exceed 400 mg per day.

Continuous Intravenous Infusion

Add ranitidine HCl injection to 5% dextrose injection or other compatible IV solution (see DOSAGE AND ADMINISTRATION, Stability). Deliver at a rate of 6.25 mg per hour (*e.g.*, 150 mg [6 ml] ranitidine HCl injection in 250 ml of 5% dextrose injection at 10.7 ml per hour).

For Zollinger-Ellison patients, dilute ranitidine HCl injection in 5% dextrose injection or other compatible IV solution (see DOSAGE AND ADMINISTRATION, Stability) to a concentration no greater than 2.5 mg/ml. Start the infusion at a rate of 1.0 mg/kg per hour. If after 4 hours either a measured gastric acid output is > 10 mEq per hour or the patient becomes symptomatic, the dose should be adjusted upward in 0.5-mg/kg per hour increments, and the acid output should be remeasured. Dosages up to 2.5 mg/kg per hour and infusion rates as high as 220 mg per hour have been used.

Zantac Injection Premixed in Flexible Plastic Containers: Instructions for use: To Open tear outer wrap at notch and remove solution container. Check for minute leaks by squeezing container firmly. If leaks are found, discard unit as sterility may be impaired.

Preparation for Administration: Use aseptic technique.

1. Close flow control clamp of administration set.

DOSAGE AND ADMINISTRATION: *(cont'd)*

2. Remove cover from outlet port at bottom of container.
3. Insert piercing pin of administration set into port with a twisting motion until the pin is firmly seated. NOTE: See full directions on administration set carton.
4. Suspend container from hanger.
5. Squeeze and release drip chamber to establish proper fluid level in chamber during infusion of Zantac Injection Premixed.
6. Open flow control clamp to expel air from set. Close clamp.
7. Attach set to venipuncture device. If device is not indwelling, prime and make venipuncture.
8. Perform venipuncture.
9. Regulate rate of administration with flow control clamp.

Caution: Zantac Injection Premixed in flexible plastic containers is to be administered by slow IV drip infusion only.**Additives should not be introduced into this solution.** If used with a primary IV fluid system, the primary solution should be discontinued during Zantac Injection Premixed infusion.

Do not administer unless solution is clear and container is undamaged.

Warning: Do not use flexible plastic container in series connections.

Dosage Adjustment for Patients With Impaired Renal Function: The administration of ranitidine as a continuous infusion has not been evaluated in patients with impaired renal function. On the basis of experience with a group of subjects with severely impaired renal function treated with ranitidine HCl, the recommended dosage in patients with a creatinine clearance < 50 ml per minute is 50 mg every 18 to 24 hours. Should the patient's condition require, the frequency of dosing may be increased to every 12 hours or even further with caution. Hemodialysis reduces the level of circulating ranitidine. Ideally, the dosing schedule should be adjusted so that the timing of a scheduled dose coincides with the end of hemodialysis.

Stability: Undiluted, ranitidine HCl injection tends to exhibit a yellow color that may intensify over time without adversely affecting potency. Ranitidine HCl injection is stable for 48 hours at room temperature when added to or diluted with most commonly used IV solutions, e.g., 0.9% sodium chloride injection, 5% dextrose injection, 10% dextrose injection, lactated ringer's injection, or 5% sodium bicarbonate injection.

Ranitidine HCl injection premixed in flexible plastic containers is sterile through the expiration date on the label when stored under recommended conditions.

Note: Parenteral drug products should be inspected visually for particulate matter and discoloration before administration whenever solution and container permit.

Directions for Dispensing: Pharmacy Bulk Package—Not for Direct Infusion. The pharmacy bulk package is for use in a pharmacy admixture service only under a laminar flow hood. The closure should be penetrated only once with a sterile transfer set or other sterile dispensing device, which allows measured distribution of the contents, and the contents dispensed in aliquots using aseptic technique. CONTENTS SHOULD BE USED AS SOON AS POSSIBLE FOLLOWING INITIAL CLOSURE PUNCTURE. DISCARD ANY UNUSED PORTION WITHIN 24 HOURS OF FIRST ENTRY. Following closure puncture, container should be maintained below 30°C (86°F) under a laminar flow hood until contents are dispensed.

PATIENT INFORMATION:

Ranitidine is known as a histamine blocker or an H2-receptor blocker. It is used to treat ulcers and heartburn. Although this drug blocks histamine in the stomach, it cannot be used in place of antihistamine used to treat runny noses and watery eyes. This drug works primarily in the stomach and intestines. In most cases therapy is needed for 4-8 weeks to produce ulcer healing. Some patients may need long term preventative therapy with lower doses taken at bedtime. Ranitidine has no clinically significant drug interactions and few side effects. The most common side effects reported include headache and abdominal pain. This medication must be taken as prescribed for ulcers to heal. You may be asked to follow a certain diet that will not aggravate your ulcer or cause a new one. If you choose to also take antacids, take them two hours before or after taking this medication. Phenylketonurics should be aware that the Zantac EFFERdose tablets and granules contain phenylalanine.

HOW SUPPLIED:

ORAL

Zantac 150 Tablets (ranitidine HCl equivalent to 150 mg of ranitidine) are peach, film-coated, five-sided tablets embossed with "Zantac 150" on one side and "Glaxo" on the other.

Zantac 300 Tablets (ranitidine HCl equivalent to 300 mg of ranitidine) are yellow, film-coated, capsule-shaped tablets embossed with "Zantac 300" on one side and "Glaxo" on the other.

Store between 15° and 30°C (59° and 86°F) in a dry place. Protect from light. Replace cap securely after each opening.

Zantac 150 GELdose Capsules (ranitidine HCl equivalent to 150 mg of ranitidine) are beige, soft gelatin capsules imprinted with "Zantac 150" on one side and "Glaxo" on the other.

Zantac 300 GELdose Capsules (ranitidine HCl equivalent to 300 mg of ranitidine) are beige, soft gelatin capsules imprinted with "Zantac 300" on one side and "Glaxo" on the other.

Store between 2° and 25°C (36° and 77°F) in a dry place. Protect from light. Replace cap securely after each opening.

Zantac 150 EFFERdose Tablets (ranitidine HCl equivalent to 150 mg of ranitidine) are white to pale yellow, round, flat-faced, bevel-edged tablets embossed with "Zantac 150" on one side and "427" on the other.

Zantac 150 EFFERdose Granules (ranitidine HCl equivalent to 150 mg of ranitidine) are white to pale yellow granules. Each 150-mg dose of granules (approximately 1.44 g) is packaged in individual foil packets.

Store between 2° and 30°C (36° and 86°F).

Zantac Syrup, a clear, peppermint-flavored liquid, contains 16.8 mg of ranitidine HCl equivalent to 15 mg of ranitidine per 1 ml in bottles of 16 fluid ounces (one pint).

Store between 4° and 25°C (39° and 77°F). Dispense in tight, light-resistant containers as defined in the USP/NF.

Zantac Injection, 25 mg/ml, contains phenol 0.5% as preservative.**Store between 4° and 30°C (39° and 86°F). Protect from light.**

Zantac Injection Premixed, 50 mg/50 ml, in 0.45% sodium chloride, contains no preservatives. **Store between 2° and 25°C (36° and 77°F). Protect from light.**

Exposure of pharmaceutical products to heat should be minimized. Avoid excessive heat; however, brief exposure up to 40°C does not adversely affect the product. Protect from freezing. **Injection Pharmacy Bulk Package—Not for Direct Infusion**

Zantac Injection, 25 mg/ml, containing phenol 0.5% as preservative, in a 40-ml pharmacy bulk package. **Store between 4° and 30°C (39° and 86°F). Protect from light. Store vial in carton until time of use.**

HOW SUPPLIED - EQUIVALENTS NOT AVAILABLE:

Capsule, Gelatin - Oral - 150 mg

60's	$95.66	ZANTAC 150, GELDOSE, Glaxo Wellcome	00173-0428-00
60's	$97.10	ZANTAC 150, GELDOSE, Glaxo Wellcome	00173-0428-02

Capsule, Gelatin - Oral - 300 mg

30's	$86.27	ZANTAC 300, GELDOSE, Glaxo Wellcome	00173-0429-00
30's	$86.99	ZANTAC 300, GELDOSE, Glaxo Wellcome	00173-0429-02

Granule, Effervescent - Oral - 150 mg

30's	$47.83	ZANTAC 150, EFFERDOSE, Glaxo Wellcome	00173-0451-00
60's	$95.66	ZANTAC 150, EFFERDOSE, Glaxo Wellcome	00173-0451-01

Injection, Solution - Intramuscular; - 25 mg/ml

2 ml x 10	$39.91	ZANTAC, Glaxo Wellcome	00173-0362-38
6 ml	$9.26	ZANTAC, Glaxo Wellcome	00173-0363-01
40 ml	$60.54	ZANTAC, Glaxo Wellcome	00173-0363-00

Injection, Solution - Intravenous - 50 mg/50 ml

50 ml x 24	$141.86	ZANTAC, Glaxo Wellcome	00173-0441-00

Syrup - Oral - 15 mg/ml

10 ml x 10	$544.60	RANITIDINE HCL SYRUP 150, Xactdose	50962-0203-10
10 ml x 50	$279.98	RANITIDINE HCL SYRUP 150, Xactdose	50962-0202-10
480 ml	$186.74	ZANTAC, Glaxo Wellcome	00173-0383-54

Tablet, Coated - Oral - 150 mg

60's	$99.20	ZANTAC, Glaxo Wellcome	00173-0344-42
100's	$167.80	ZANTAC, Glaxo Wellcome	00173-0344-47
500's	$826.69	ZANTAC, Glaxo Wellcome	00173-0344-14

Tablet, Coated - Oral - 300 mg

30's	$90.06	ZANTAC 300, Glaxo Wellcome	00173-0393-40
100's	$302.51	ZANTAC 300, Glaxo Wellcome	00173-0393-47
250's	$750.53	ZANTAC, Glaxo Wellcome	00173-0393-06

Tablet, Effervescent - Oral - 150 mg

30's	$47.83	ZANTAC 150, EFFERDOSE, Glaxo Wellcome	00173-0427-00
60's	$95.66	ZANTAC 150, EFFERDOSE, Glaxo Wellcome	00173-0427-02

RAUWOLFIA SERPENTINA *(002176)*

CATEGORIES: Antihypertensives; Cardiovascular Drugs; Hypertension; Psychotic Disorders; Rauwolfia Alkaloids; Schizophrenia; Vascular Disorders, Cerebral/Peripheral; Pregnancy Category C; FDA Approval Pre 1982

BRAND NAMES: Hiwolfia; *Hypercal*; **Raudixin**; Rauneed; Rauval; Rauverid; Rauwolfemms; Serfolia; Wolfina
(International brand names outside U.S. in italics)

FORMULARIES: Medi-Cal

COST OF THERAPY: $562.02 (Schizophrenia; Tablet; 100 mg; 2/day; 365 days)

DESCRIPTION:

Powdered Rauwolfia Serpentina USP is a hypotensive agent prepared from the whole root of *Rauwolfia serpentina* Benth. The Powder contains not less than 0.15% and not more than 0.2% of reserpine-rescinnamine group alkaloids, calculated as reserpine.

CLINICAL PHARMACOLOGY:

Rauwolfia serpentina probably produces its antihypertensive effects through depletion of tissue stores of catecholamines (epinephrine and norepinephrine) from peripheral sites. By contrast, its sedative and tranquilizing properties are thought to be related to depletion of 5-hydroxytryptamine from the brain. Rauwolfia serpentina is characterized by slow onset of action and sustained effect. Both its cardiovascular and central nervous system effects may persist following withdrawal of the drug.

INDICATIONS AND USAGE:

Mild essential hypertension; also useful as adjunctive therapy with other antihypertensive agents in the more severe forms of hypertension. Relief of symptoms in agitated psychotic states (*e.g.,* schizophrenia), primarily in those individuals unable to tolerate phenothiazine derivatives or those who also require antihypertensive medication.

CONTRAINDICATIONS:

Demonstrated hypersensitivity to rauwolfia, mental depression (especially with suicidal tendencies), active peptic ulcer, ulcerative colitis, and in patients receiving electroconvulsive therapy.

WARNINGS:

Extreme caution should be exercised in treating patients with a history of mental depression. Discontinue the drug at first sign of despondency, early morning insomnia, loss of appetite, impotence, or self-deprecation. Drug-induced depression may persist for several months after drug withdrawal and may be severe enough to result in suicide.

In co-therapy, MAO inhibitors should be avoided or used with extreme caution.

Usage in Pregnancy: The safety or rauwolfia preparations for use during pregnancy or lactation has not been established; therefore, the drug should be used in pregnant patients or in women of childbearing potential only when, in the judgement of the physician, it is essential to the welfare of the patient. Increased respiratory tract secretions, nasal congestion, cyanosis, and anorexia may occur in infants born to rauwolfia-treated mothers since the drug crosses the placental barrier and appears in cord blood.

Usage in Nursing: Rauwolfia appears in breast milk.

PRECAUTIONS:

Because rauwolfia preparations increase gastrointestinal motility and secretion, this drug should be used cautiously in patients with a history of peptic ulcer, ulcerative colitis, or gallstones (biliary colic may be precipitated). Patients on high dosage should be checked regularly for possible reactivation of peptic ulcer. Caution should be used when treating hypertensive patients with renal insufficiency since they adjust poorly to lowered blood pressure levels.

Use rauwolfia serpentina cautiously with digitalis and quinidine since cardiac arrhythmias have occurred with rauwolfia preparations.

Preoperative withdrawal of rauwolfia serpentina does not assure that circulatory instability will not occur. It is important that the anesthesiologist be aware of the patient's drug intake and consider this in the overall management since hypotension has occurred in patients receiving rauwolfia preparations. Anticholinergic and/or adrenergic drugs (*e.g.,* metaraminol, norepinephrine) have been employed to treat adverse vagocirculatory effects.

PRECAUTIONS: *(cont'd)*

Animal tumorigenicity: Rodent studies have shown that reserpine is an animal tumorigen, causing an increased incidence of mammary fibroadenomas in female mice, malignant tumors of the seminal vesicles in male mice, and malignant adrenal medullary tumors in male rats. These findings arose in 2 year studies in which the drug was administered in the feed at concentrations of 5 and 10 ppm—about 100 to 300 times the usual human dose. The breast neoplasms are though to be related to reserpine's prolactin-elevating effect. Several other prolactin-elevating drugs have also been associated with an increased incidence of mammary neoplasia in rodents.

The extent to which these findings indicate a risk to humans in uncertain. Tissue culture experiments show that about one-third of human breast tumors are prolactin-dependent in vitro, a factor of considerable importance if the use of the drug is contemplated in a patient with previously detected breast cancer.

The possibility of an increased risk of breast cancer in reserpine users has been studied extensively; however, non firm conclusion has emerged. Although a few epidemiologic studies have suggested a slightly increased risk (less than twofold in all studies except one) in women who have used reserpine, other studies of generally similar design have not confirmed this. Epidemiologic studies conducted using other drug's (neuroleptic agents) that, like reserpine, increase prolactin levels and therefore would be considered rodent mammary carcinogens, have not shown an association between chronic administration of the drug and human mammary tumorigenesis. While long-term clinical observation has not suggested such an association, the available evidence is considered too limited to be conclusive at this time. An association of reserpine intake with pheochromocytoma or tumors of the seminal vesicles has not been explored.

ADVERSE REACTIONS:

Gastrointestinal: hypersecretion, nausea, vomiting, anorexia, and diarrhea.

Central Nervous System: drowsiness, depression, nervousness, paradoxical anxiety, nightmares, rare Parkinsonian syndrome and other extrapyramidal tract symptoms, and CNS sensitization manifested by dull sensorium deafness, glaucoma, uveitis, and optic atrophy.

Cardiovascular: angina-like symptoms, arrhythmias (particularly when used concurrently with digitalis or quinidine), and bradycardia.

Other: nasal congestion (frequent), pruritus, rash, dryness of mouth, dizziness, headache, dyspnea, syncope, epistaxis, purpura and other hematologic reactions, impotence or decreased libido, dysuria, muscular aches, conjunctival injection, weight gain, breast engorgement, pseudolactation, and gynecomastia have been reported. These reactions are usually reversible and usually disappear after the drug is discontinued.

Water retention with edema in patients with hypertensive vascular disease may occur rarely, but the condition generally clears with cessation of therapy, or with the administration of a diuretic agent.

OVERDOSAGE:

Signs & Symptoms: Consciousness may be impaired, ranging from drowsiness to coma, depending on severity of overdosage. Flushing of the skin, conjunctival injection, and pupillary constriction are to be expected. Hypotension, hypothermia, central respiratory depression, and bradycardia may develop in severe cases. Diarrhea may also occur.

Treatment: Evacuate stomach contents, with precaution against aspiration and for protection of airway; instill activated charcoal slurry. Treat symptomatically. If hypotension requires treatment with a vasopressor, use one having a direct action upon vascular smooth muscle (*e.g.,* phenylephrine, levarterenol, metaraminol). Since this drug is long-acting, observe the patient for at least this drug is long-acting, observe the patient for at least 72 hours, administering treatment as required.

DOSAGE AND ADMINISTRATION:

For adults, the average oral dose is 200 to 400 mg daily, given in divided doses in the morning and evening. Higher doses should be used cautiously because serious mental depression and other side effects may be considerably increased. (Orally, 200 to 300 mg of powdered whole root is equivalent to 0.5 mg of reserpine.) Maintenance doses may vary from 50 to 300 mg per day given as a single dose or as two divided doses. Concomitant use of rauwolfia serpentina and ganglionic blocking agents, guanethidine, veratrum, hydralazine, methyldopa, chlorthalidone, or thiazides necessitates careful titration of dosage with each agent.

HOW SUPPLIED - EQUIVALENTS NOT AVAILABLE:

Tablet, Uncoated - Oral - 50 mg

100's	**$46.19**	**RAUDIXIN, Bristol Myers Squibb**	**00003-0713-50**
1000's	$17.75	Rauwolfia Serpentina, United Res	00677-0124-10
1000's	$17.80	Rauwolfia Serpentina, Major Pharms	00904-2195-80
1000's	**$416.58**	**RAUDIXIN, Bristol Myers Squibb**	**00003-0713-80**
5000's	$45.80	Rauwolfia Serpentina, Rugby	00536-4436-50

Tablet, Uncoated - Oral - 100 mg

100's	**$76.99**	**RAUDIXIN, Bristol Myers Squibb**	**00003-0776-50**
1000's	$21.50	Rauwolfia Serpentina, United Res	00677-0125-10
1000's	$22.00	Rauwolfia Serpentina, Major Pharms	00904-2196-80
5000's	$52.15	Rauwolfia Serpentina, Rugby	00536-4440-50

REMIFENTANIL HYDROCHLORIDE *(003300)*

CATEGORIES: Analgesics; Anesthesia; Central Nervous System Agents; DEA Class CII; FDA Approved 1996 Sep; Narcotic Analgesics; Narcotics, Synthetics & Combinations; Opiate Agonists (Controlled); Pain; Pregnancy Category C

BRAND NAMES: **Ultiva**

DESCRIPTION:

Remifentanil HCl for injection is a [micro]-opioid agonist chemically designated as a 3-[4-methoxycarbonyl-4-[(1-oxopropyl)phenylamino]-1-piperidine]propanoic acid methyl ester, hydrochloride salt, $C_{20}H_{28}N_2O_5$·HCl, with a molecular weight of 412.91.

Ultiva is a sterile, nonpyrogenic, preservative-free, white to off-white lyophilized powder for intravenous (IV) administration after reconstitution and dilution. Each vial contains 1, 2, or 5 mg of remifentanil base; 15 mg glycine; and hydrochloric acid to buffer the solutions to a nominal pH of 3 after reconstitution. When reconstituted as directed, solutions of Ultiva are clear and colorless and contain remifentanil HCl equivalent to 1 mg/ml of remifentanil base. The pH of reconstituted solutions of remifentanil HCl ranges from 2.5 to 3.5. Remifentanil HCl has a pKa of 7.07. Remifentanil HCl has an n-octanol:water partition coefficient of 17.9 at pH 7.3.

CLINICAL PHARMACOLOGY:

Remifentanil HCl is a [micro]-opioid agonist with rapid onset and peak effect, and short duration of action. The [micro]-opioid activity of remifentanil HCl is antagonized by opioid antagonists such as naloxone.

Unlike other opioids, remifentanil HCl is rapidly metabolized by hydrolysis of the propanoic acid-methyl ester linkage by nonspecific blood and tissue esterases. Remifentanil HCl is not a substrate for plasma cholinesterase (pseudocholinesterase) and, therefore, patients with atypical cholinesterase are expected to have a normal duration of action.

Pharmacodynamics: The analgesic effects of remifentanil HCl are rapid in onset and offset. Its effects and side effects are dose dependent and similar to other [micro]-opioids. Remifentanil HCl in humans has a rapid blood-brain equilibration half-time of 1 ± 1 minutes (mean ± SD) and a rapid onset of action. The pharmacodynamic effects of remifentanil HCl closely follow the measured blood concentrations, allowing direct correlation between dose, blood levels, and response. Blood concentration decreases 50% in 3 to 6 minutes after a 1–minute infusion or after prolonged continuous infusion due to rapid distribution and elimination processes and is independent of duration of drug administration. Recovery from the effects of remifentanil HCl occurs rapidly (within 5 to 10 minutes). New steady-state concentrations occur within 5 to 10 minutes after changes in infusion rate. When used as a component of an anesthetic technique, remifentanil HCl can be rapidly titrated to the desired depth of anesthesia/analgesia (*e.g.*, as required by varying levels of intraoperative stress) by changing the continuous infusion rate or by administering an IV bolus injection.

Hemodynamics: In premedicated patients undergoing anesthesia, 1–minute infusions of <2 μ/kg of remifentanil HCl cause dose-dependent hypotension and bradycardia. While additional doses >2 μ/kg (up to 30 μ/kg) do not produce any further decreases in heart rate or blood pressure, the duration of the hemodynamic change is increased in proportion to the blood concentrations achieved. Peak hemodynamic effects occur within 3 to 5 minutes of a single dose of remifentanil HCl or an infusion rate increase. Glycopyrrolate, atropine, and vagolytic neuromuscular blocking agents attenuate the hemodynamic effects associated with remifentanil HCl. When appropriate, bradycardia and hypotension can be reversed by reduction of the rate of infusion of remifentanil HCl, or the dose of concurrent anesthetics, or by the administration of fluids or vasopressors.

Respiration: Remifentanil HCl depresses respiration in a dose-related fashion. Unlike other fentanyl analogs, the duration of action of remifentanil HCl at a given dose does not increase with increasing duration of administration, due to lack of drug accumulation. When remifentanil HCl and alfentanil were dosed to equal levels of respiratory depression, recovery of respiratory drive after 3–hour infusions was more rapid and less variable with remifentanil HCl.

Spontaneous respiration occurs at blood concentrations of 4 to 5 ng/ml in the absence of other anesthetic agents; for example, after discontinuation of a 0.25–μ/kg/min infusion of remifentanil, these blood concentrations would be reached in 2 to 4 minutes. In patients undergoing general anesthesia, the rate of respiratory recovery depends upon the concurrent anesthetic; N_20 < propofol < isoflurane (see CLINICAL STUDIES, Recovery).

Muscle Rigidity: Skeletal muscle rigidity can be caused by remifentanil HCl and is related to the dose and speed of administration. Remifentanil HCl may cause chest wall rigidity (inability to ventilate) after single doses of >1 μ/kg administered over 30 to 60 seconds or infusion rates >0.1 μ/kg/min; peripheral muscle rigidity may occur at lower doses. Administration of doses <1 μ/kg may cause chest wall rigidity when given concurrently with a continuous infusion of remifentanil HCl. Prior or concurrent administration of a hypnotic (propofol or thiopental) or a neuromuscular blocking agent may attenuate the development of muscle rigidity. Excessive muscle rigidity can be treated by decreasing the rate of discontinuing the infusion of remifentanil HCl or by administering a neuromuscular blocking agent.

Histamine Release: Assays of histamine in patients and normal volunteers have shown no elevation in plasma histamine levels after administration of remifentanil HCl in doses up to 30 μ/kg over 60 seconds.

Analgesia: Infusions of 0.05 to 0.1 μ/kg/min, producing blood concentrations of 1 to 3 ng/ml, are typically associated with analgesia with minimal decrease in respiratory rate. Supplemental doses of 0.5 to 1 μ/kg, incremental increases in infusion rate >0.05 μ/kg/min, and blood concentrations exceeding 5 ng/ml (typically produced by infusions of 0.2 μ/kg/min) have been associated with transient and reversible respiratory depression, apnea, and muscle rigidity.

Anesthesia: Remifentanil HCl is synergistic with the activity of hypnotics (propofol and thiopental), inhaled anesthetics, and benzodiazepines (see CLINICAL STUDIES, PRECAUTIONS, and DOSAGE AND ADMINISTRATION).

Age: The pharmacodynamic activity of remifentanil HCl (as measured by the EC_{50} for development of delta waves on the EEG) increases with increasing age. The $EC_{50}$of remifentanil for this measure was 50% less in patients over 65 years of age when compared to healthy volunteers (25 years of age) (see DOSAGE AND ADMINISTRATION).

Gender: No differences have been shown in the pharmacodynamic activity (as measured by the EEG) of remifentanil HCl between men and women.

Drug Interactions: In animals the duration of muscle paralysis from succinylcholine is not prolonged by remifentanil.

Interocular Pressure: There was no change in intraocular pressure after the administration of remifentanil HCl prior to ophthalmic surgery under monitored anesthesia care.

Cerebrodynamics: Under isoflurane-nitrous oxide anesthesia ($PaCO_2$<30 mmHg), a 1–minute infusion of remifentanil HCl (0.5 or 1.0 μ/kg) produced no change in intracranial pressure. Mean arterial pressure and cerebral perfusion decreased as expected with opioids. In patients receiving remifentanil HCl and nitrous oxide anesthesia, cerebrovascular reactivity to carbon dioxide remained intact. In humans, no epileptiform activity was seen on the EEG (n = 44) at remifentinal doses up to 8 μ/kg/min.

Renal Dysfunction: The pharmacodynamics of remifentanil HCl (ventilatory response to hypercarbia) are unaltered in patients with end stage renal disease (creatinine clearance <10 ml/min).

Hepatic Dysfunction: The pharmacodynamics of remifentanil HCl (ventilatory response to hypercarbia) are unaltered in patients with severe hepatic dysfunction awaiting liver transplant.

Pharmacokinetics: After IV doses administered over 60 seconds the pharmacokinetics of remifentanil fit a three-compartment model with a rapid distribution half-life of 1 minute, a slower distribution half-life of 6 minutes, and a terminal elimination half-life of 10 to 20 minutes. Since the terminal elimination component contributes less than 10% of the overall area under the concentration versus time curve (AUC), the effective biological half-life of remifentanil HCl is 3 to 10 minutes. This is similar to the 3- to 10-minute half-life measured after termination of prolonged infusions (up to 4 hours) and correlates with recovery times observed in the clinical setting after infusions up to 12 hours. Concentrations of remifentanil are proportional to the dose administered throughout the recommended dose range. The pharmacokinetics of remifentanil are unaffected by the presence of renal or hepatic impairment.

Distribution: The initial volume of distribution (V_d) of remifentanil is approximately 100 ml/kg and represents distribution throughout the blood and rapidly perfused tissues. Remifentanil subsequently distributes into peripheral tissues with a steady-state volume of distribution of approximately 350 ml/kg. These two distribution volumes generally correlate with total body weight (except in severely obese patients when they correlate better with ideal body weight [IBW]). Remifentanil is approximately 70% bound to plasma proteins of which two-thirds is binding to alpha 1-acid-glycoprotein.

CLINICAL PHARMACOLOGY: *(cont'd)*

Metabolism: Remifentanil is an esterase-metabolized opioid. A labile ester linkage renders this compound susceptible to hydrolysis by nonspecific esterases in blood and tissues. This hydrolysis results in the production of the carboxylic acid metabolite (3-[4-methoxycarbonyl-4-[(1- oxopropyl) phenylamino]-1-piperidine]propanoic acid), and represents the principal metabolic pathway for remifentanil (>95%). The carboxylic acid metabolite is essentially inactive (1/4600 as potent as remifentanil in dogs) and is excreted by the kidneys with an elimination half-life of approximately 90 minutes. Remifentanil is not metabolized by plasma cholinesterase (pseudocholinesterase) and is not appreciably metabolized by the liver or lung.

Elimination: The clearance of remifentanil in young, healthy adults is approximately 40 ml/min/kg. Clearance generally correlates with total body weight (except in severely obese patients when it correlates better with IBW). The high clearance of remifentanil combined with a relatively small volume of distribution produces a short elimination half-life of approximately 3 to 10 minutes. This value is consistent with the time taken for blood or effect site concentrations to fall by 50% (context-sensitive half-times) which is approximately 3 to 6 minutes. Unlike other fentanyl analogs, the duration of action does not increase with prolonged administration.

Titration to Effect: The rapid elimination of remifentanil permits the titration of infusion rate without concern for prolonged duration. In general every 0.1-μ/kg/min change in the IV infusion rate will lead to a corresponding 2.5 ng/ml change in blood remifentanil concentration within 5 to 10 minutes. In intubated patients only, a more rapid increase (within 3 to 5 minutes) to a new steady state can be achieved with a 1.0-μ/kg bolus dose in conjunction with an infusion rate increase.

SPECIAL POPULATIONS

Children: In children 2 to 12 years of age (n = 13), the blood concentrations of remifentanil after a 1-minute infusion of 5.0 μ/kg were similar to those seen in adults receiving the same dose. The pharmacokinetic parameters of remifentanil in children (volume of distribution, clearance, and half-life) were similar to adults after correcting for differences in weight. The pharmacokinetics of remifentanil have not been studied in patients under 2 years of age.

Renal Impairment: The pharmacokinetic profile of remifentanil HCl is not changed in patients with end stage renal disease (creatinine clearance <10 ml/min). In anephric patients, the half-life of the carboxylic acid metabolite increases from 90 minutes to 30 hours. The metabolite is removed by hemodialysis with a dialysis extraction ratio of approximately 30%.

Hepatic Impairment: The pharmacokinetics of remifentanil and its carboxylic acid metabolite are unchanged in patients with severe hepatic impairment.

Elderly: The clearance of remifentanil is reduced (approximately 25%) in the elderly (>65 years of age) compared to young adults (average 25 years of age). However, remifentanil blood concentrations fall as rapidly after termination of administration in the elderly as in young adults.

Gender: There is no significant difference in the pharmacokinetics of remifentanil in male and female patients after correcting for differences in weight.

Obesity: There is no difference in the pharmacokinetics of remifentanil in non-obese versus obese (greater than 30% over IBW) patients when normalized to IBW.

Cardiopulmonary Bypass (CPB): Remifentanil clearance is reduced by approximately 20% during hypothermic CPB.

Drug Interactions: Remifentanil clearance is not altered by concomitant administration of thiopental, isoflurane, propofol, or temazepam during anesthesia. *In vitro* studies with atracurium, mivacurium, esmolol, echothiophate, neostigmine, physostigmine, and midazolam revealed no inhibition of remifentanil hydrolysis in whole human blood by these drugs.

CLINICAL STUDIES:

Remifentanil HCl was evaluated in 2808 patients undergoing general anesthesia (n = 2169) and monitored anesthesia care (n = 639). These patients were evaluated in the following settings: inpatient (n = 1573) which included cardiovascular (n = 225), and neurosurgical (n = 61), and outpatient (n = 1235). Three hundred seventy-seven (377) elderly patients (age range 66 to 90 years) and 68 pediatric patients received remifentanil HCl. Of the general anesthesia patients, 682 also received remifentanil HCl as an IV analgesic agent during the immediate postoperative period.

Induction and Maintenance of General Anesthesia-Inpatient/Outpatient: The efficacy of remifentanil HCl was investigated in 1562 patients in 15 randomized, controlled trials as the analgesic component for the induction and maintenance of general anesthesia. Eight of these studies compared remifentanil HCl to alfentanil and two studies compared remifentanil HCl to fentanyl. In these studies, doses of remifentanil HCl up to the ED_{90}were compared to recommended doses (approximately ED_{50}) of alfentanil or fentanyl. If alfentanil or fentanyl were administered in doses equipotent to the ED_{90} of remifentanil HCl, an intraoperative profile similar to the results below for remifentanil HCl could be expected.

Induction of Anesthesia: Remifentanil HCl was administered with isoflurane, propofol, or thiopental for the induction of anesthesia (n = 1562). The majority of patients (80%) received propofol as the concurrent agent. Remifentanil HCl reduced the propofol and thiopental requirements for loss of consciousness. Compared to alfentanil and fentanyl, a higher relative dose of remifentanil HCl resulted in fewer responses to intubation (TABLE 1). Overall, hypotension occurred in 5% of patients receiving remifentanil HCl compared to 2% of patients receiving the other opioids.

Remifentanil HCl has been used as a primary agent for the induction of anesthesia; however, it should not be used as a sole agent because loss of consciousness cannot be assured and because of a high incidence of apnea, muscle rigidity, and tachycardia. The administration of an induction dose of propofol or thiopental or a paralyzing dose of a muscle relaxant prior to or concurrently with remifentanil HCl during the induction of anesthesia markedly decreased the incidence of muscle rigidity from 20% to <1%.

Use During Maintenance of Anesthesia: Remifentanil HCl was investigated in 929 patients in seven well-controlled general surgery studies in conjunction with nitrous oxide, isoflurane, or propofol in both inpatient and outpatient settings. These studies demonstrated that remifentanil HCl could be dosed to high levels of opioid effect and rapidly titrated to optimize analgesia intraoperatively without delaying or prolonging recovery.

Compared to alfentanil and fentanyl, these higher relative doses (ED_{90}) of remifentanil HCl resulted in fewer responses to intraoperative stimuli (TABLE 2A and TABLE 2B) and a higher frequency of hypotension (16% compared to 5% for the other opioids). Remifentanil HCl was infused to the end of surgery while alfentanil was discontinued 5 to 30 minutes before the end of surgery as recommended. The mean final infusion rates of remifenanil HCl were between 0.25 and 0.48 μ/kg/min.

In three randomized controlled studies (n = 407) during general anesthesia, remifentanil HCl attenuated the signs of light anesthesia within a median time of 3 to 6 minutes after bolus doses of 1 μ/kg with or without infusion rate increases of 50% to 100% (up to a maximum rate of 2 μ/kg/min).

CLINICAL STUDIES: *(cont'd)*

TABLE 1 Response to Intubation (Propofol/Opioid Induction*)

Opioid Treatment Group/(No. of Patients)	Initial Dose (μ/kg)	Pre-Intubation Rate (μ/kg/min)	No. (%) Muscle Rigidity	No. (%) Hypotension During Induction	No. (%) Response to Intubation
Study 1:					
Remifentanil HCl (35)	1	0.1	1 (3%)	0	27 (77%)
Remifentanil HCl (35)	1	0.4	3 (9%)	0	11 (31%)†
Alfentanil (35)	20	1.0	2 (6%)	0	26 (74%)
Study 2:					
Remifentanil HCl (116)	1	0.5	9 (8%)	5 (4%)	17 (15%)†
Alfentanil (118)	25	1.0	6 (5%)	5 (4%)	33 (28%)
Study 3:					
Remifentanil HCl (134)	1	0.5	2 (1%)	4 (3%)	25 (19%)
Alfentanil (66)	20	2.0	0	0	19 (29%)
Study 4:					
Remifentanil HCl (98)	1	0.2	11 (11%)†	2 (2%)	35 (36%)
Remifentanil HCl (91)	2‡	0.4	11 (12%)†	2 (2%)	12 (13%)†
Fentanyl (97)	3	NA	1 (1%)	1 (1%)	29 (30%)

* Propofol was titrated to loss of consciousness. **Not all doses of remifentanil HCl were equipotent to the comparator opioid.**
† Differences were statistically significant ($P < 0.02$).
‡ Initial doses greater than 1 mcg/kg are not recommended.

TABLE 2A Intraoperative Responses*

Opioid Treatment Group/(No. of Patients)	Concurrent Anesthetic	Post-Intubation Infusion Rate (μ/kg/min)	No. (%) With Intraoperative Hypotension
Study 1:			
Remifentanil HCl (35)		0.1	0
Remifentanil HCl (35)	Nitrous oxide	0.4	0
Alfentanil (35)		1.0	0
Study 2:			
Remifentanil HCl (116)	Isoflurane +	0.25	35 (30%)†
Alfentanil (118)	Nitrous oxide	0.5	12 (10%)
Study 3:			
Remifentanil HCl (134)	Propofol	0.5	3 (2%)
Alfentanil (66)		2.0	2 (3%)
Study 4:			
Remifentanil HCl (98)		0.2	13 (13%)
Remifentanil HCl (91)	Isoflurane	0.4	16 (18%)†
Fentanyl (97)		1.5-3 mcg/kg prn	7 (7%)

* **Not all doses of remifentanil HCl were equipped to the comparator opioid.**† Differences were statistically significant ($P < 0.05$).

TABLE 2B Intraoperative Responses*

Opioid Treatment Group/(No. of Patients)	No. (%) With Response to Skin Incision	No. (%) With Signs of Light Anesthesia	No. (%) With Response to Skin Closure
Study 1:			
Remifentanil HCl (35)	20 (57%)	33 (94%)	6 (17%)
Remifentanil HCl (35)	3 (9%)†	12 (34%)†	2 (6%)†
Alfentanil (35)	24 (69%)	33 (94%)	12 (34%)
Study 2:			
Remifentanil HCl (116)	9 (8%)†	66 (57%)†	19 (16%)
Alfentanil (118)	20 (17%)	85 (72%)	25 (21%)
Study 3:			
Remifentanil HCl (134)	14 (11%)†	70 (52%)†	25 (19%)
Alfentanil (66)	21 (32%)	47 (71%)	13 (20%)
Study 4:			
Remifentanil HCl (98)	12 (12%)†	67 (68%)†	7 (7%)
Remifentanil HCl (91)	4 (4%)†	44 (48%)†	3 (3%)†
Fentanyl (97)	32 (33%)	84 (87%)	11 (11%)

* **Not all doses of remifentanil HCl were equipotent to the comparator opioid.**
† Differences were statistically significant ($P < 0.05$).

In an additional double-blind, randomized study (n = 103), a constant rate (0.25 μ/kg/min) of remifentanil HCl was compared to doubling the rate to 0.5 μ/kg/min approximately 5 minutes before the start of the major surgical stress event. Doubling the rate decreased the incidence of signs of light anesthesia from 67% to 8% in patients undergoing abdominal hysterectomy and from 19% to 10% in patients undergoing radical prostatectomy. In patients undergoing laminectomy the lower dose was adequate.

Recovery: In 2169 patients receiving remifentanil HCl for periods up to 16 hours, recovery from anesthesia was rapid, predictable, and independent of the duration of the infusion of remifentanil HCl. In the seven controlled, general surgery studies, extubation occurred in a median of 5 minutes (range: -3 to 17 minutes in 95% of patients) in outpatient anesthesia and 10 minutes (range: 0 to 32 minutes in 95% of patients) in inpatient anesthesia. Recovery in studies using nitrous oxide or propofol was faster than in those using isoflurane as the concurrent anesthetic. There was no case of remifentanil-induced delayed respiratory depression occurring more than 30 minutes after discontinuation of remifentanil (see PRECAUTIONS).

In a double-blind, randomized study, administration of morphine sulfate (0.15 mg/kg) intravenously 20 minutes before the anticipated end of surgery to 98 patients did not delay recovery of respiratory drive in patients undergoing major surgery with remifentanil-propofol total IV anesthesia.

Spontaneous Ventilation Anesthesia: Two randomized, dose-ranging studies (n = 127) examined the administration of remifentanil HCl to outpatients undergoing general anesthesia with a laryngeal mask. Starting infusion rates of remifentanil HCl of ≤0.05 μ/kg/min provided supplemental analgesia while allowing spontaneous ventilation with propofol or isoflurane. **Bolus doses of remifentanil HCl during spontaneous ventilation lead to transient periods of apnea, respiratory depression, and muscle rigidity.**

Pediatric Anesthesia: Remifentanil HCl has been evaluated in one clinical trial (n = 68) in children 2 to 12 years of age undergoing strabismus surgery. After induction of anesthesia which included the administration of atropine, remifentanil HCl was administered as an initial infusion of 1 μ/kg/min with 70% nitrous oxide. The infusion rate required during maintenance of anesthesia was 0.73 to 1.95 μ/kg/min. Time to extubation and to purposeful movement was a median of 10 minutes (range 1 to 24 minutes).

Coronary Artery Bypass Surgery: In preliminary investigations of cardiac anesthesia remifentanil HCl was administered to 217 patients undergoing elective coronary artery bypass graft (CABG) surgery in two dose-finding studies without active comparators. In both studies, patients were preloaded with fluid to PAOP 10 to 15 mmHg and all had preoperative stroke volume >50 ml.

In the total IV anesthesia study (n = 132), patients received diazepam or midazolam preoperatively and randomly received remifentanil HCl (1,1.5, or 2 μ/kg/min) plus propofol (0.5 mg/kg followed by 50 μ/kg/min) and muscle relaxant for the induction and maintenance of anesthesia. Overall response to sternotomy/maximal sternal spread was 12% with no relationship to dose of remifentanil HCl. Thirty-nine percent (39%) of patients had treated hypotension reported as an adverse event.

In the other study, remifentanil HCl (administered at initial doses of 1,2,3 μ/kg/min and then titrated to effect) was administered to 76 patients as a sole agent following a large preoperative dose of lorazepam (40 to 80 μ/kg). Muscle rigidity at induction occurred in 49% of the patients. Responses at sternotomy occurred in 22% of patients with no relationship to dose of remifentanil HCl. Most patients (75%) required intermittent isoflurane supplementation for signs of light anesthesia; significantly more patients in the 1-μ/kg/min group required isoflurane.

In both of these CABG studies, remifentanil HCl was continued at a rate of 1 μ/kg/min in the intensive care unit (ICU) for up to 6 hours after surgery. The transition from remifentanil HCl to other analgesics (IV morphine sulfate; 0.1 to 0.15 mg/kg) was initiated prior to extubation. This transition usually occurred over 30 to 90 minutes with additional morphine, midazolam, and/or propofol administered as needed. Seventy-one percent (71 %) of patients were eligible for early (<6 hours after entry into the ICU) extubation. Sixty-two percent (62%) of eligible patients were actually extubated early (range of times to extubation: 1.4 to 5.9 hours). The rate of major adverse cardiac events was 5.1% (myocardial infarction, 3.7%; ventricular failure, 0.5%; and death due to cardiac causes, 0.9%).

Neurosurgery: Remifentanil HCl was administered to 61 patients undergoing craniotomy for removal of a supratentorial mass lesion. In these studies, ventilation was controlled to maintain a predicted $PaCO_2$ of approximately 28 mmHg. In one study (n = 30) with remifentanil HCl and 66% nitrous oxide, the median time to extubation and to patient response to verbal commands was 5 minutes (range -1 to 19 minutes). Intracranial pressure and cerebrovascular responsiveness to carbon dioxide were normal (see CLINICAL PHARMACOLOGY).

A randomized, controlled study compared remifentanil HCl (n = 31) to fentanyl (n = 32). Remifentanil HCl (1 μ/kg/min) and fentanyl (2 μ/kg/min) were administered after induction with thiopental and pancuronium. A similar number of patients (6%) receiving remifentanil HCl and fentanyl had hypotension during induction. Anesthesia was maintained with nitrous oxide and remifentanil HCl at a mean infusion rate of 0.23 μ/kg/min (range 0.1 to 0.4) compared with a fentanyl mean infusion rate of 0.04 μ/kg/min (range 0.02 to 0.07). Supplemental isoflurane was administered as needed. The patients receiving remifentanil HCl required a lower mean isoflurane dose (0.07 MAC-hours) compared with 0.64 MAC-hours for the fentanyl patients (P= 0.04). Remifentanil HCl was discontinued at the end of anesthesia, whereas fentanyl was discontinued at the time of bone flap replacement (a median time of 44 minutes before the end of surgery). Median time to extubation was similar (5 and 3.5 minutes, respectively, with remifentanil HCl and fentanyl). None of the patients receiving remifentanil HCl required naloxone compared to seven of the fentanyl patients (P= 0.01). Eighty-one percent (81%) of patients receiving remifentanil HCl recovered (awake, alert, and oriented) within 30 minutes after surgery compared with 59% of fentanyl patients (P= 0.06). At 45 minutes, recovery rates were similar (81% and 69% respectively for remifentanil HCl and fentanyl, P= 0.27). Patients receiving remifentanil HCl required an analgesic for headache sooner than fentanyl patients (median of 35 minutes compared with 136 minutes, respectively [P= 0.04]). No adverse cerebrovascular effects were seen in this study (see CLINICAL PHARMACOLOGY).

Continuation of Analgesic Use into the Immediate Postoperative Period: Analgesia with remifentanil HCl in the immediate postoperative period (until approximately 30 minutes after extubation) was studied in 401 patients in four dose-finding studies and in 281 patients in two efficacy studies. In the dose-finding studies, the use of bolus doses of remifentanil HCl and incremental infusion rate increases ≥0.05 μ/kg/min led to respiratory depression and muscle rigidity. **Bolus doses of remifentanil HCl to treat postoperative pain are not recommended and incremental infusion rate increases should not exceed 0.025 μ/kg/min at 5-minute intervals.**

In two efficacy studies, remifentanil HCl 0.1 μ/kg/min was started immediately after discontinuing anesthesia. Incremental infusion rate increases of 0.025 μ/kg/min every 5 minutes were given to treat moderate to severe postoperative pain. In Study 1, 50% decreases in infusion rate were made if respiratory rate decreased below 12 breaths/min and in Study 2, the same decreases were made if respiratory rate was below 8 breaths/min. With this difference in criteria for infusion rate decrease, the incidence of respiratory depression was lower in Study 1 (4%) than in Study 2 (12%). In both studies, remifentanil HCl provided effective analgesia (no or mild pain with respiratory rate ≥8 breaths/min) in approximately 60% of patients at mean final infusion rates of 0.1 to 0.125 μ/kg/min.

Study 2 was a double-blind, randomized, controlled study in which patients received either morphine sulfate (0.15 mg/kg administered 20 minutes before the anticipated end of surgery plus 2-mg bolus doses for supplemental analgesia) or remifentanil HCl (as described above). Emergence from anesthesia was similar between groups; median time to extubation was 5 to 6 minutes for both. Remifentanil HCl provided effective analgesia in 58% of patients compared to 33% of patients who received morphine. Respiratory depression occurred in 12% of patients receiving remifentanil HCl compared to 4% of morphine patients. For patients who received remifentanil HCl, morphine sulfate (0.15 mg/kg) was administered in divided doses 5 and 10 minutes before discontinuing remifentanil HCl. Within 30 minutes after discontinuation of remifentanil HCl, the percentage of patients with effective analgesia decreased to 34%.

Monitored Anesthesia Care: Remifentanil HCl has been studied in the monitored anesthesia care setting in 609 patients in eight clinical trials. Nearly all patients received supplemental oxygen in these studies. Two early dose-finding studies demonstrated that use of sedation as an endpoint for titration of remifentanil HCl led to a high incidence of muscle rigidity (69%) and respiratory depression. Subsequent trials titrated remifentanil HCl to specific clinical endpoints of patient comfort, analgesia, and adequate respiration (respiratory rate >8 breaths/min) with a corresponding lower incidence of muscle rigidity (3%) and respiratory depression. With doses of midazolam >2 mg (4 to 8 mg), the dose of remifentanil HCl could be decreased by 50%, but the incidence of respiratory depression rose to 32%.

The efficacy of a single dose of remifentanil HCl (1.0 μ/kg over 30 seconds) was compared to alfentanil (7 μ/kg over 30 seconds) in patients undergoing ophthalmic surgery. More patients receiving remifentanil HCl were pain free at the time of the nerve block (77% versus 44% P= 0.02) and more experienced nausea (12% versus 4%) than those receiving alfentanil.

CLINICAL STUDIES: *(cont'd)*

In a randomized, controlled study (n =118), remifentanil HCl 0.5 µ/kg over 30 to 60 seconds followed by a continuous infusion of 0.1 µ/kg/min, was compared to a propofol bolus (500 µ/kg) followed by a continuous infusion (50 µ/kg/min) in patients who received a local or regional anesthetic nerve block 5 minutes later. The incidence of moderate or severe pain during placement of the block was similar between groups (2% with remifentanil HCl and 8% with propofol, $P= 0.2$) and more patients receiving remifentanil HCl experienced nausea (26% versus 2% $P< 0.001$). The final mean infusion rate of remifentanil HCl was 0.08 µ/kg/min.

In a randomized, double-blind study, remifentanil HCl with or without midazolam was evaluated in 159 patients undergoing superficial surgical procedures under local anesthesia. Remifentanil HCl was administered without midazolam as a 1-µ/kg dose over 30 seconds followed by a continuous infusion of 0.1 µ/kg/min. In the group of patients that received midazolam, remifentanil HCl was administered as a 0.5-µ/kg dose over 30 seconds followed by a continuous infusion of 0.05 µ/kg/min and midazolam 2 mg was administered 5 minutes later. The occurrence of moderate or severe pain during the local anesthetic injection was similar between groups (16% and 20%). Other effects for remifentanil HCl alone and remifentanil HCl/midazolam were: respiratory depression with oxygen desaturation (SPO_2<90%), 5% and 2%; nausea 8% and 2%; and pruritus, 23% and 12%. Titration of remifentanil HCl resulted in prompt resolution of respiratory depression (median 3 minutes range 0 to 6 minutes). The final mean infusion rate of remifentanil HCl was 0.12 µ/kg/min (range 0.03 to 0.3) for the group receiving remifentanil HCl alone and 0.07 µ/kg/min (range 0.02 to 0.2) for the group receiving remifentanil HCl/midazolam.

Because of the risk for hypoventilation, the infusion rate of remifentanil HCl should be decreased to 0.5 µ/kg/min following placement of the local or regional block and titrated thereafter in increments of 0.025 µ/kg/min at 5-minute intervals. Bolus doses of remifentanil HCl administered simultaneously with a continuous infusion of remifentanil HCl to spontaneously breathing patients are not recommended.

INDICATIONS AND USAGE:

Remifentanil HCl is indicated for IV administration:

1. as an analgesic agent for use during the induction and maintenance of general anesthesia for inpatient and outpatient procedures, and for continuation as an analgesic into the immediate postoperative period under the direct supervision of an anesthesia practitioner in a postoperative anesthesia care unit or intensive care setting.

2. as an analgesic component of monitored anesthesia care.

CONTRAINDICATIONS:

Due to the presence of glycine in the formulation, remifentanil HCl is contraindicated for epidural or intrathecal administration. Remifentanil HCl is also contraindicated in patients with known hypersensitivity to fentanyl analogs.

WARNINGS:

Continuous infusions of remifentanil HCl should be administered only by an infusion device. **IV bolus administration of remifentanil HCl should be used only during the maintenance of general anesthesia.**In nonintubated patients, single doses of remifentanil HCl should be administered over 30 to 60 seconds.

Interruption of an infusion of remifentanil HCl will result in rapid offset of effect. Rapid clearance and lack of drug accumulation result in rapid dissipation of respiratory depressant and analgesic effects upon discontinuation of remifentanil HCl at recommended doses. Discontinuation of an infusion of remifentanil HCl should be preceded by the establishment of adequate postoperative analgesia.

Injections of remifentanil HCl should be made into IV tubing at or close to the venous cannula. Upon discontinuation of remifentanil HCl, the IV tubing should be cleared to prevent the inadvertent administration of remifentanil HCl at a later point in time. **Failure to adequately clear the IV tubing to remove residual remifentanil HCl has been associated with the appearance of respiratory depression, apnea, and muscle rigidity upon the administration of additional fluids or medications through the same IV tubing.**

USE OF REMIFENTANIL HCl IS ASSOCIATED WITH APNEA AND RESPIRATORY DEPRESSION. REMIFENTANIL HCl SHOULD BE ADMINISTERED ONLY BY PERSONS SPECIFICALLY TRAINED IN THE USE OF ANESTHETIC DRUGS AND THE MANAGEMENT OF THE RESPIRATORY EFFECTS OF POTENT OPIOIDS, INCLUDING RESPIRATORY AND CARDIAC RESUSCITATION OF PATIENTS IN THE AGE GROUP BEING TREATED. SUCH TRAINING MUST INCLUDE THE ESTABLISHMENT AND MAINTENANCE OF A PATENT AIRWAY AND ASSISTED VENTILATION.

REMIFENTANIL HCl SHOULD NOT BE USED IN DIAGNOSTIC OR THERAPEUTIC PROCEDURES OUTSIDE THE MONITORED ANESTHESIA CARE SETTING. PATIENTS RECEIVING MONITORED ANESTHESIA CARE SHOULD BE CONTINUOUSLY MONITORED BY PERSONS NOT INVOLVED IN THE CONDUCT OF THE SURGICAL OR DIAGNOSTIC PROCEDURE. OXYGEN SATURATION SHOULD BE MONITORED ON A CONTINUOUS BASIS. RESUSCITATIVE AND INTUBATION EQUIPMENT, OXYGEN, AND AN OPIOID ANTAGONIST MUST BE READILY AVAILABLE.

Respiratory depression in spontaneously breathing patients is generally managed by decreasing the rate of the infusion of remifentanil HCl by 50% or by temporarily discontinuing the infusion.

Skeletal muscle rigidity can be caused by remifentanil HCl and is related to the dose and speed of administration. Remifentanil HCl may cause chest wall rigidity (inability to ventilate) after single doses of >1 µ/kg administered over 30 to 60 seconds, or after infusion rates >0.1 µ/kg/min. Single doses <1 µ/kg may cause chest wall rigidity when given concurrently with a continuous infusion of remifentanil HCl.

Muscle rigidity induced by remifentanil HCl should be managed in the context of the patient's clinical condition. Muscle rigidity occurring during the induction of anesthesia should be treated by the administration of a neuromuscular blocking agent and the concurrent induction medications.

Muscle rigidity seen during the use of remifentanil HCl in spontaneously breathing patients may be treated by stopping or decreasing the rate of administration of remifentanil HCl. Resolution of muscle rigidity after discontinuing the infusion of remifentanil HCl occurs within minutes. In the case of life-threatening muscle rigidity, a rapid onset neuromuscular blocker or naloxone may be administered.

Remifentanil HCl should not be administered into the same IV tubing with blood due to potential inactivation by nonspecific esterases in blood products.

PRECAUTIONS:

Vital signs and oxygenation must be continually monitored during the administration of remifentanil HCl.

General: Bradycardia has been reported with remifentanil HCl and is responsive to ephedrine or anticholinergic drugs, such as atropine and glycopyrrolate.

PRECAUTIONS: *(cont'd)*

Hypotension has been reported with remifentanil HCl and is responsive to decreases in the administration of remifentanil HCl or to IV fluids or catecholamine (ephedrine, epinephrine, norepinephrine, etc.) administration.

Intraoperative awareness has been reported in patients under 55 years of age when remifentanil HCl has been administered with propofol infusion rates of ≤75 µ/kg/min.

Rapid Offset of Action: Within 5 to 10 minutes after the discontinuation of remifentanil hcl, no residual analgesic activity will be present. However, respiratory depression may occur in some patients up to 30 minutes after termination of infusion due to residual effects of concomitant anesthetics. Standard monitoring should be maintained in the postoperative period to ensure adequate recovery without stimulation. For patients undergoing surgical procedures where postoperative pain is generally anticipated, other analgesics should be administered prior to the discontinuation of remifentanil HCl.

Pediatric Use: Remifentanil HCl has not been studied in pediatric patients under 2 years of age. For clinical experience and recommendations for use in pediatric patients 2 to 12 years of age (see CLINICAL PHARMACOLOGYand DOSAGE AND ADMINISTRATION).

Use In Elderly Patients: While the effective biological half-life of remifentanil is unchanged, elderly patients have been shown to be twice as sensitive as the younger population to the pharmacodynamic effects of remifentanil. The recommended starting dose of remifentanil HCl should be decreased by 50% in patients over 65 years of age (see CLINICAL PHARMACOLOGYand DOSAGE AND ADMINISTRATION).

Use in Morbidly Obese Patients: As for all potent opioids, caution is required with use in morbidly obese patients because of alterations in cardiovascular and respiratory physiology (see DOSAGE AND ADMINISTRATION).

Long-term Use in the ICU: No data are available on the long-term (longer than 16 hours) use of remifentanil HCl as an analgesic in ICU patients.

Carcinogenesis, Mutagenesis, Impairment of Fertility: Animal carcinogenicity studies have not been performed with remifentanil.

Remifentanil did not induce gene mutation in prokaryotic cells *in vitro* and was not genotoxic in the *in vivo* rat hepatocyle unscheduled DNA synthesis assay. No clastogenic effect was seen in cultured Chinese hamster ovary cells or in the *in vivo* mouse micronucleus test. In the *in vitro* mouse lymphoma assay, mutagenicity was seen only with metabolic activation.

Remifentanil has been shown to reduce fertility in male rats when tested after 70+ days of daily IV administration of 0.5 mg/kg, or approximately 40 times the maximum recommended human dose (MRHD) in terms of mg/m^2 of body surface area. The fertility of female rats was not affected at IV doses as high as 1 mg/kg when administered for at least 15 days before mating.

Pregnancy Category C: Teratogenic effects were not observed following administration of remifentanil at doses up to 5 mg/kg in rats and 0.8 mg/kg in rabbits. These doses are approximately 400 times and 125 times the MRHD, respectively, in terms of mg/m^2 of body surface area. Administration of radiolabeled remifentanil to pregnant rabbits and rats demonstrated significant placental transfer to fetal tissue. There are no adequate and well-controlled studies in pregnant women. Remifentanil HCl should be used during pregnancy only if the potential benefit justifies the potential risk to the fetus.

Administration of remifentanil to rats throughout late gestation and lactation at IV doses up to 5 mg/kg, or approximately 400 times the MRHD in terms of mg/m^2 of body surface area, had no significant effect on the survival, development, or reproductive performance of the F_1 generation.

Labor and Delivery: Respiratory depression and other opioid effects may occur in newborns whose mothers are given remifentanil HCl shortly before delivery. The safety of remifentanil HCl during labor or delivery has not been demonstrated. Placental transfer studies in rats and rabbits showed that pups are exposed to remifentanil and its metabolites. In a human clinical trial, the average maternal remifentanil concentrations were approximately twice those seen in the fetus. In some cases, however, fetal concentrations were similar to those in the mother. The umbilical arteriovenous ratio of remifentanil concentrations was approximately 30% suggesting metabolism of remifentanil in the neonate.

Nursing Mothers: It is not known whether remifentanil is excreted in human milk. After receiving radioactive-labeled remifentanil, the radioactivity was present in the milk of lactating rats. Because fentanyl analogs are excreted in human milk, caution should be exercised when remifentanil HCl is administered to a nursing woman.

ADVERSE REACTIONS:

Remifentanil HCl produces adverse events that are characteristic of µ-opioids, such as respiratory depression, bradycardia, hypotension, and skeletal muscle rigidity. These adverse events dissipate within minutes of discontinuing or decreasing the infusion rate of remifentanil HCl. (See CLINICAL PHARMACOLOGY, WARNINGS, and PRECAUTIONS.)

Adverse event information is derived from controlled clinical trials that were conducted in a variety of surgical procedures of varying duration, using a variety of premedications and other anesthetics, and in patient populations with diverse characteristics including underlying disease.

Approximately 2,492 patients were exposed to remifentanil HCl in controlled clinical trials. The frequencies of adverse events during general anesthesia with the recommended doses of remifentanil HCl are given in TABLE 3A AND TABLE 3B. Each patient was counted once for each type of adverse event.

In the elderly population (>65 years), the incidence of hypotension is higher, whereas the incidence of nausea and vomiting is lower.

The frequencies of adverse events from the clinical studies at the recommended doses of remifentanil HCl in monitored anesthesia care are given in TABLE 5.

Other Adverse Events: The frequencies of less commonly reported adverse clinical events from all controlled general anesthesia and monitored anesthesia care studies are presented below.

Event frequencies are calculated as the number of patients who were administered remifentanil HCl and reported an event divided by the total number of patients exposed to remifentanil HCl in all controlled studies including cardiac and neurosurgery studies (n = 1,883 general anesthesia, n = 609 monitored anesthesia care).

Incidence Less than 1%:

Digestive: constipation, abdominal discomfort, xerostomia, gastro-esophageal reflux, dysphagia, diarrhea, heartburn, ileus.

Cardiovascular: various atrial and ventricular arrhythmias, heart block, ECG change consistent with myocardial ischemia, elevated CPK-MB level, syncope.

Musculoskeletal: muscle stiffness, musculoskeletal chest pain.

Respiratory: cough, dyspnea, bronchospasm, laryngospasm, rhonchi, stridor, nasal congestion, pharyngitis, pleural effusion, hiccup(s), pulmonary edema, rales, bronchitis, rhinorrhea.

Nervous: anxiety, involuntary movement, prolonged emergence from anesthesia, confusion, awareness under anesthesia without pain, rapid awakening from anesthesia, tremors, disorientation, dysphoria, nightmare(s), hallucinations, paresthesia, nystagmus, twitch, sleep disorder, seizure, amnesia.

ADVERSE REACTIONS: *(cont'd)*

TABLE 3A Adverse Events Reported in ≥1% of Patients in General Anesthesia Studies at the Recommended Doses of Remifentanil HCl

Adverse Event	Induction/Maintenance Remifentanil HCl (n = 921)	Induction/Maintenance Alfentanil/Fentanyl (n = 466)	Postoperative Analgesia Remifentanil HCl (n = 281)	Postoperative Analgesia Morphine (n = 98)
Nausea	8 (<1%)	0	61 (22%)	15 (15%)
Hypotension	178 (19%)	30 (6%)	0	0
Vomiting	4 (<1%)	1 (<1%)	22 (8%)	5 (5%)
Muscle rigidity	98 (11%)†	37 (8%)	7 (2%)	0
Bradycardia	62 (7%)	24 (5%)	3 (1%)	3 (3%)
Shivering	3 (<1%)	0	15 (5%)	9 (9%)
Fever	1 (<1%)	0	2 (<1%)	0
Dizziness	0	0	1 (<1%)	0
Visual disturbance	0	0	0	0
Headache	0	0	1 (<1%)	1 (1%)
Respiratory depression	1 (<1%)	0	19 (7%)	4 (4%)
Apnea	0	1 (<1%)	9 (3%)	2 (2%)
Pruritus	2 (<1%)	0	7 (2%)	1 (1%)
Tachycardia	6 (<1%)	7 (2%)	0	0
Postoperative pain	0	0	7 (2%)	0
Hypertension	10 (<1%)	7 (2%)	5 (2%)	3 (3%)
Agitation	2 (<1%)	0	3 (1%)	1 (1%)
Hypoxia	0	0	1 (<1%)	0

* See TABLE 6for recommended doses. **Not all doses of remifentanil HCl were equipotent to the comparator opioid. Administration of remifentanil HCl in excess of the recommended dose (*i.e.,* doses >1 and up to 20 μ/kg) resulted in a higher incidence of some adverse events: muscle rigidity (37%), bradycardia (12%), hypertension (4%), and tachycardia (4%).**
† Included in the muscle rigidity incidence is chest wall rigidity (5%). The overall muscle rigidity incidence is <1% when remifentanil is administered concurrently or after a hypnotic induction agent.

TABLE 3B Adverse Events Reported in ≤1% of Patients in General Anesthesia Studies at the Recommended Doses of Remifentanil HCl*

Adverse Event	After Discontinuation Remifentanil HCl (n = 929)	After Discontinuation Alfentanil/Fentanyl (n = 466)
Nausea	339 (36%)	202 (43%)
Hypotension	16 (2%)	9 (2%)
Vomiting	150 (16%)	91 (20%)
Muscle rigidity	2 (<1%)	1 (<1%)
Bradycardia	11 (1%)	6 (1%)
Shivering	49 (5%)	10 (2%)
Fever	44 (5%)	9 (2%)
Dizziness	27 (3%)	9 (2%)
Visual disturbance	24 (3%)	14 (3%)
Headache	21 (2%)	8 (2%)
Respiratory depression	17 (2%)	20 (4%)
Apnea	2 (<1%)	1 (<1%)
Pruritus	22 (2%)	7 (2%)
Tachycardia	10 (1%)	8 (2%)
Postoperative pain	4 (<1%)	5 (1%)
Hypertension	12 (1%)	8 (2%)
Agitation	6 (<1%)	1 (<1%)
Hypoxia	10 (1%)	7 (2%)

* See TABLE 6 for recommended doses. **Not all doses of remifentanil HCl were equipotent to the comparator opioid. Administration of remifentanil HCl in excess of the recommended dose (*i.e.,* doses >1 and up to 20 μ/kg) resulted in a higher incidence of some adverse events: muscle rigidity (37%), bradycardia (12%), hypertension (4%), and tachycardia (4%).**
† Included in the muscle rigidity incidence is chest wall rigidity (5%). The overall muscle rigidity incidence is <1% when remifentanil is administered concurrently or after a hypnotic induction agent.

TABLE 4A Incidence (%) of Most Common Adverse Events by Gender in General Anesthesia Studies at the Recommended Dose* of Remifentanil HCl

Adverse Event	Induction/Maintenance Remifentanil HCl		Induction/Maintenance Alfentanil/Fentanyl	
n	Male 326	Female 595	Male 183	Female 283
Nausea	2%	<1%	0	0
Hypotension	29%	14%	7%	6%
Vomiting	<1%	<1%	0	<1%
Muscle rigidity	17%	7%	14%	4%

* See TABLE 6 for recommended doses. **Not all doses of remifentanil HCl were equipotent to the comparator opioid.**

TABLE 4B Incidence (%) of Most Common Adverse Events by Gender in General Anesthesia Studies at the Recommended Dose* of Remifentanil HCl

Adverse Event	Postoperative Analgesia Remifentanil HCl		Postoperative Analgesia Morphine	
n	Male 85	Female 196	Male 36	Female 62
Nausea	12%	26%	8%	19%
Hypotension	0	0	0	0
Vomiting	4%	10%	0	8%
Muscle rigidity	6%	1%	0	0

* See TABLE 6 for recommended doses. **Not all doses of remifentanil HCl were equipotent to the comparator opioid.**

Body as a Whole: decreased body temperature, anaphylactic reaction, delayed recovery from neuromuscular block.

Skin: rash, urticaria.

Urogenital: urine retention, oliguria, dysuria, urine incontinence.

Infusion Site Reaction: erythema, pruritus, rash.

Metabolic and Nutrition: abnormal liver function, hyperglycemia, electrolyte disorders, increased CPK level.

Hematologic and Lymphatic: anemia, lymphopenia, leukocytosis, thrombocytopenia.

TABLE 4C Incidence (%) of Most Common Adverse Events by Gender in General Anesthesia Studies at the Recommended Dose* of Remifentanil HCl

Adverse Event	After Discontinuation Remifentanil HCl		After Discontinuation Afentanil/Fentanyl	
n	Male 332	Female 597	Male 183	Female 283
Nausea	22%	45%	30%	52%
Hypotension	2%	2%	2%	2%
Vomiting	5%	22%	8%	27%
Muscle rigidity	<1%	<1%	0	<1%

* See TABLE 6 for recommended doses. **Not all doses of remifentanil HCl were equipotent to the comparator opioid.**

TABLE 5 Adverse Events Reported in ≥1% of Patients in Monitored Anesthesia Care Studies at the Recommended Doses of Remifentanil HCl*

Adverse Event	Remifentanil HCl (n = 159)	Remifentanil HCl + 2 mg Midazolam† (n = 103)	Propofol (0.5 mg/kg/min then 50 mg μ/kg/min) (n = 63)
Nausea	70 (44%)	19 (18%)	20 (32%)
Vomiting	35 (22%)	5 (5%)	13 (21%)
Pruritus	28 (18%)	16 (16%)	0
Headache	28 (18%)	12 (12%)	6 (10%)
Sweating	10 (6%)	0	1 (2%)
Shivering	8 (5%)	1 (<1%)	1 (2%)
Dizziness	8 (5%)	5 (5%)	1 (2%)
Hypotension	7 (4%)	0	6 (10%)
Bradycardia	6 (4%)	0	7 (11%)
Respiratory depression	4 (3%)	1 (<1%)*	0
Muscle rigidity	4 (3%)	0	1 (2%)
Chills	2 (1%)	0	2 (3%)
Flushing	2 (1%)	0	0
Warm sensation	2 (1%)	0	0
Pain at study IV site	2 (1%)	0	11 (17%)

* See TABLE 7 for recommended doses. **Administration of remifentanil HCl in excess of the recommended infusion rate (*i.e.,* starting doses >0.1 μ/kg/min) resulted in a higher incidence of some adverse events: nausea (60%), apnea (8%), and muscle rigidity (5%).**
† With higher midazolam doses, higher incidences of respiratory depression and apnea were observed.

DRUG ABUSE AND DEPENDENCE:

Remifentanil HCl is a Schedule II controlled drug substance that can produce drug dependence of the morphine type and has the potential for being abused.

OVERDOSAGE:

As with all potent opioid analgesics, overdosage would be manifested by an extension of the pharmacological actions of remifentanil HCl. Expected signs and symptoms of overdosage include: apnea, chest-wall rigidity, seizures, hypoxemia, hypotension, and bradycardia.

In case of overdosage or suspected overdosage, discontinue administration of remifentanil HCl, maintain a patent airway, initiate assisted or controlled ventilation with oxygen, and maintain adequate cardiovascular function. If depressed respiration is associated with muscle rigidity, a neuromuscular blocking agent or a μ-opioid antagonist may be required to facilitate assisted or controlled respiration. Intravenous fluids and vasopressors for the treatment of hypotension and other supportive measures may be employed. Glycopyrrolate or atropine may be useful for the treatment of bradycardia and/or hypotension.

Intravenous administration of an opioid antagonist such as naloxone may be employed as a specific antidote to manage severe respiratory depression or muscle rigidity. Respiratory depression from overdosage with remfentanil HCl is not expected to last longer than the opioid antagonist, naloxone. Reversal of the opioid effects may lead to acute pain and sympathetic hyperactivity.

DOSAGE AND ADMINISTRATION:

Remifentanil HCl is for IV use only. **Continuous infusions of remifentanil HCl should be administered only by an infusion device. The injection site should be close to the venous cannula and all IV tubing should be cleared at the time of discontinuation of infusion.**

During General Anesthesia: Remifentanil HCl is not recommended as the sole agent in general anesthesia because loss of consciousness cannot be assured and because of a high incidence of apnea, muscle rigidity, and tachycardia. Remifentanil HCl is synergistic with other anesthetics and doses of thiopental, propofol, isoflurane, and midazolam have been reduced by up to 75% with the coadministration of remifentanil HCl. The administration of remifentanil HCl must be individualized based on the patient's response.

TABLE 6 summarizes the recommended doses in adult patients, predominately ASA physical status I, II, or III. Recommendations for maintenance anesthesia with nitrous oxide also apply to pediatric patients ≥2 years.

TABLE 6 Dosing Guidlines-General Anesthesia and Continuing as an Analgesic into the Postoperative Care Unit or Intensive Care Setting*

Phase	Continuous IV Infusion of Remifentanil HCl (μ/kg/min)	Infusion Dose Range of Remifentanil HCl (μ/kg/min)	Supplemental IV Bolus Dose of Remifentanil HCl (μ/kg)
Induction of Anesthesia (through intubation)	0.5 - 1*	-	-
Maintenance of anesthesia with:			
Nitrous oxide (66%)	0.4	0.1 - 2	1
Isoflurane (0.4 to 1.5 MAC)	0.25	0.05 - 2	1
Propofol (100 to 200 μ/kg/min)	0.25	0.05 - 2	1
Continuation as an analgesic into the immediate postoperative period	0.1	0.025 - 0.2	not recommended

* An initial dose of 1 μ/kg may be administered over 30 to 60 seconds.

During Induction of Anesthesia: Remifentanil HCl should be administered at an infusion rate of 0.5 to 1 μ/kg/min with a hypnotic or volatile agent for the induction of anesthesia. If endotracheal intubation is to occur less than 8 minutes after the start of the infusion of remifentanil HCl, then an initial dose of 1 μ/kg may be administered over 30 to 60 seconds.

During Maintenance of Anesthesia: After endotracheal intubation, the infusion rate of remifentanil HCl should be decreased in accordance with the dosing guidelines in TABLE 6. Due to the fast onset and short duration of action of remifentanil HCl, the rate of

DOSAGE AND ADMINISTRATION: *(cont'd)*

administration during anesthesia can be titrated upward in 25% to 100% increments or downward in 25% to 50% decrements every 2 to 5 minutes to attain the desired level of μ-opioid effect. In response to light anesthesia or transient episodes of intense surgical stress supplemental bolus doses of 1 μ/kg may be administered every 2 to 5 minutes. At infusion rates >1 μ/kg/min, increases in the concomitant anesthetic agents should be considered to increase the depth of anesthesia. *Continuation as an Analgesic into the Immediate Postoperative Period Under the Direct Supervision of an Anesthesia Practitioner:* **Infusions of Remifentanil HCl may be continued into the immediate postoperative period for select patients for whom later transition to longer acting analgesics may be desired. The use of bolus injections of remifentanil HCl to treat pain during the postoperative period is not recommended.** When used as an IV analgesic in the immediate postoperative period, remifentanil HCl should be initially administered by continuous infusion at a rate of 0.1 μ/kg/min. The infusion rate may be adjusted every 5 minutes in 0.025-μ/kg/min increments to balance the patient's level of analgesia and respiratory rate. Infusion rates greater than 0.2 μ/kg/min are associated with respiratory depression (respiratory rate less than 8 breaths/min).

Guidelines for Discontinuation: Upon discontinuation of remifentanil HCl the IV tubing should be cleared to prevent the inadvertent administration of remifentanil HCl at a later time.

Due to the rapid offset of action of remifentanil HCl, no residual analgesic activity will be present within 5 to 10 minutes after discontinuation. For patients undergoing surgical procedures where postoperative pain is generally anticipated, alternative analgesics should be administered prior to discontinuation of remifentanil HCl. The choice of analgesic should be appropriate for the patient's surgical procedure and the level of follow-up care (see CLINICAL STUDIES).

Analgesic Component of Monitored Anesthesia Care: It is strongly recommended that supplemental oxygen be supplied to the patient whenever remifentanil HCl is administered.

TABLE 7 summarizes the recommended doses for monitored anesthesia care in adult patients, predominately ASA physical status I, II or III.

TABLE 7 Dosing Guidelines-Monitored Anesthesia Care

Timing	Remifentanil HCl Alone	Remifentanil HCl + 2 mg Midazolam
Single IV Dose		
Given 90 seconds before local anesthetic	1 μ/kg over 30 to 60 seconds	0.5 μ/kg over 30 to 60 seconds
Continuous IV Infusion		
Beginning 5 minutes before local anesthetic	0.1 μ/kg/min	0.05 μ/kg/min
After local anesthetic	0.05 μ/kg/min (Range: 0.025 - 0.2 μ/kg/min)	0.025 μ/kg/min (Range: 0.025 - 0.2 μ/kg/min)

Single Dose: A single IV dose of 0.5 to 1 μ/kg over 30 to 60 seconds of remifentanil HCl may be given 90 seconds before the placement of the local or regional anesthetic block (see PRECAUTIONS).

Continuous Infusion: When used alone as an IV analgesic component of monitored anesthesia care, remifentanil HCl should be initially administered by continuous infusion at a rate of 0.1 μ/kg/mm beginning 5 minutes before placement of the local or regional anesthetic block. **Because of the risk for hypoventilation, the infusion rate of remifentanil HCl should be decreased to 0.05 μ/kg/min following placement of the block.** Thereafter, rate adjustments of 0.025. μ/kg/min at 5-minute intervals may be used to balance the patient's level of analgesia and respiratory rate. Rates greater than 0.2 μ/kg/min are generally associated with respiratory depression (respiratory rates less than 8 breaths/min). **Bolus doses of remifentanil HCl administered simultaneously with a continuous infusion of remifentanil HCl to spontaneously breathing patients are not recommended.**

Individualization of Dosage: *Use in Elderly Patients:* The starting doses of remifentanil HCl should be decreased by 50% in elderly patients (>65 years). Remifentanil HCl should then be cautiously titrated to effect.

Use in Pediatric Patients: No data are available on the use of remifentanil HCl in pediatric patients under 2 years of age. The same doses (per kg) as adults are recommended for pediatric patients 2 years of age and older.

Use in Obese Patients: The starting doses of remifentanil HCl should be based on ideal body weight (IBW) in obese patients (greater than 30% over their IBW).

Preanesthetic Medication: The need for premedication and the choice of anesthetic agents must be individualized. In clinical studies, patients who received remifentanil HCl frequently received a benzodiazepine premedication.

Preparation for Administration: To reconstitute solution, add 1 ml of diluent per mg of remifentanil. Shake well to dissolve. When reconstituted as directed, the solution contains approximately 1 mg of remifentanil activity per 1 ml. **Remifentanil HCl should be diluted to a recommended final concentration of 25, 50, or 250 μ/ml prior to administration (TABLE 8). Remifentanil HCl should not be administered without dilution.**

TABLE 8 Reconstitution and Dilution of Remifentanil HCl

Final Concentration	Amount of Remifentanil HCl in Each Vial	Final Volume After Reconstitution and Dilution
25 μ/ml	1mg	40 ml
	2mg	80 ml
	5mg	200 ml
50 μ/ml	1 mg	40 ml
	2 mg	20 ml
	5 mg	100 ml
250 μ/ml	5 mg	20 ml

Continuous IV infusions of remifentanil HCl should be administered only by an infusion device. Infusion rates of remifentanil HCl can be individualized for each patient using TABLE 9.

When remifentanil HCl is used as an analgesic component of monitored analgesia care or for pediatric patients ≥2 years of age, a final concentration of 25 μ/ml is recommended. TABLE 10A and TABLE 10B are guidelines for milliliter-per-hour delivery for a solution of 25 μ/ml with an infusion device.

TABLE 11A and TABLE 11B are guidelines for milliliter-per-hour delivery for a solution of 50 μ/ml with an infusion device.

TABLE 12A and TABLE 12B are guidelines for milliliter-per-hour delivery for a solution of 250 μ/ml with an infusion device.

COMPATIBILITY AND STABILITY:

Reconstitution and Dilution Prior to Administration: Remifentanil HCl is stable for 24 hours at room temperature after reconstitution and further dilution to concentrations of 20 to 250 μ/ml with the IV fluids listed below.

DOSAGE AND ADMINISTRATION: *(cont'd)*

TABLE 9 IV Infusion Rates of Remifentanil HCl (ml/kg/h)

Drug Delivery Rate (μ/kg/min)	Infusion Delivery Rate (ml/kg/h) 25 μ/ml	50 μ/ml	250 μ/ml
0.0125	0.03	0.015	not recommended
0.025	0.06	0.03	not recommended
0.05	0.12	0.06	0.012
0.075	0.18	0.09	0.018
0.1	0.24	0.12	0.024
0.15	0.36	0.18	0.036
0.2	0.48	0.24	0.048
0.25	0.6	0.3	0.06
0.5	1.2	0.6	0.12
0.75	1.8	0.9	0.18
1.0	2.4	1.2	0.24
1.25	3.0	1.5	0.3
1.5	3.6	1.8	0.36
1.75	4.2	2.1	0.42
2.0	4.8	2.4	0.48

TABLE 10A IV Infusion Rates of Remifentanil HCl (ml/h) for a 25–μ/ml Solution

Infusion Rate (μ/kg/min)	Patient Weight (kg) 10	20	30	40	50
0.0125	0.3	0.6	0.9	1.2	1.5
0.025	0.6	1.2	1.8	2.4	3.0
0.05	1.2	2.4	3.6	4.8	6.0
0.075	1.8	3.6	5.4	7.2	9.0
0.1	2.4	4.8	7.2	9.6	12.0
0.15	3.6	7.2	10.8	14.4	18.0
0.2	4.8	9.6	14.4	19.2	24.0

TABLE 10B IV Infusion Rates of Remifentanil HCl (ml/h) for a 25–μ/ml Solution

Infusion Rate (μ/kg/min)	Patient Weight (kg) 60	70	80	90	100
0.0125	1.8	2.1	2.4	2.7	3.0
0.025	3.6	4.2	4.8	5.4	6.0
0.05	7.2	8.4	9.6	10.8	12.0
0.075	10.8	12.6	14.4	16.2	18.0
0.1	14.4	16.8	19.2	21.6	24.0
0.15	21.6	25.2	28.8	32.4	36.0
0.2	28.8	33.6	38.4	43.2	48.0

TABLE 11A IV Infusion Rates of Remifentanil HCl (ml/h) for a 50–μ/ml Solution

Infusion Rate (μ/kg/min)	Patient Weight (kg) 30	40	50	60	70
0.025					2.1
0.05		2.4	3.0	3.6	4.2
0.075	2.7	3.6	4.5	5.4	6.3
0.1	3.6	4.8	6.0	7.2	8.4
0.15	5.4	7.2	9.0	10.8	12.6
0.2	7.2	9.6	12.0	14.4	16.8
0.25	9.0	12.0	15.0	18.0	21.0
0.5	18.0	24.0	30.0	36.0	42.0
0.75	27.0	36.0	45.0	54.0	63.0
1.0	36.0	48.0	60.0	72.0	84.0
1.25	45.0	60.0	75.0	90.0	105.0
1.5	54.0	72.0	90.0	108.0	126.0
1.75	63.0	84.0	105.0	126.0	147.0
2.0	72.0	96.0	120.0	144.0	168.0

TABLE 11B IV Infusion Rates of Remifentanil HCl (ml/h) for a 50–μ/ml Solution

Infusion Rate (μ/kg/min)	Patient Weight (kg) 80	90	100
0.025	2.4	2.7	3.0
0.05	4.8	5.4	6.0
0.075	7.2	8.1	9.0
0.1	9.6	10.8	12.0
0.15	14.4	16.2	18.0
0.2	19.2	21.6	24.0
0.25	24.0	27.0	30.0
0.5	48.0	54.0	60.0
0.75	72.0	81.0	90.0
1.0	96.0	108.0	120.0
1.25	120.0	135.0	150.0
1.5	144.0	162.0	180.0
1.75	168.0	189.0	210.0
2.0	192.0	216.0	240.0

TABLE 12A IV Infusion Rates of Remifentanil HCl (ml/h) for a 250–μ/ml Solution

Infusion Rate (μ/kg/min)	Patient Weight (kg) 30	40	50	60
0.1	0.72	0.96	1.20	1.44
0.15	1.08	1.44	1.80	2.16
0.2	1.44	1.92	2.40	2.88
0.25	1.80	2.40	3.00	3.60
0.5	3.60	4.80	6.00	7.20
0.75	5.40	7.20	9.00	10.80
1.0	7.20	9.60	12.00	14.40
1.25	9.00	12.00	15.00	18.00
1.5	10.80	14.40	18.00	21.60
1.75	12.60	16.80	21.00	25.20
2.0	14.40	19.20	24.00	28.80

DOSAGE AND ADMINISTRATION: *(cont'd)*

TABLE 12B IV Infusion Rates of Remifentanil HCl (ml/h) for a 250–μ/ml Solution

Infusion Rate (μ/kg/min)	Patient Weight (kg) 70	80	90	100
0.1	1.68	1.92	2.16	2.40
0.15	2.52	2.88	3.24	3.60
0.2	3.36	3.84	4.32	4.80
0.25	4.20	4.80	5.40	6.00
0.5	8.40	9.60	10.80	12.00
0.75	12.60	14.40	16.20	18.00
1.0	16.80	19.20	21.60	24.00
1.25	21.00	24.00	27.00	30.00
1.5	25.20	28.80	32.40	36.00
1.75	29.40	33.60	37.80	42.00
2.0	33.60	38.40	43.20	48.00

Sterile Water for Injection, USP
5% Dextrose Injection, USP
5% Dextrose and 0.9% Sodium Chloride Injection, USP
0.9% Sodium Chloride Injection, USP
0.45% Sodium Chloride Injection, USP
Lactated Ringer's and 5% Dextrose Injection, USP

Remifentanil HCl is stable for 4 hours at room temperature after reconstitution and further dilution to concentrations of 20 to 250 μ/ml with Lactated Ringer's Injection, USP.

Remifentanil HCl has been shown to be compatible with these IV fluids when coadministered into a running IV administration set.

Compatibility With Other Therapeutic Agents: Remifentanil HCl has been shown to be compatible with Diprivan (propofol) Injection when coadministered into a running IV administration set. The compatibility of remifentanil HCl with other therapeutic agents has not been evaluated.

Incompatibilities: Nonspecific esterases in blood products may lead to the hydrolysis of remifentanil to its carboxylic acid metabolite. Therefore, administration of remifentanil HCl into the same IV tubing with blood is not recommended.

Note: Parenteral drug products should be inspected visually for particulate matter and discoloration prior to administration whenever solution and container permit. Product should be a clear, colorless liquid after reconstitution and free of visible particulate matter.

Remifentanil HCl does not contain any antimicrobial preservative and thus care must be taken to assure the sterility of prepared solutions.

ANIMAL PHARMACOLOGY:

Animal Toxicology: Intrathecal administration of the glycine formulation without remifentanil to dogs caused agitation, pain, hind limb dysfunction, and incoordination. These effects are believed to be caused by the glycine. Glycine is a commonly used excipient in IV products and this finding has no relevance for IV administration of remifentanil HCl.

HOW SUPPLIED:

Ultiva should be stored at 2° to 25°C (36° to 77°F). Ultiva for IV use is supplied as remifentanil base lyophilized powder.

HOW SUPPLIED - EQUIVALENTS NOT AVAILABLE:

Injection, Solution - Intramuscular, - 1 mg
3 ml vial $117.00 ULTIVA, Glaxo Wellcome 00173-0483-00

Injection, Solution - Intramuscular, - 2 mg
5 ml vial $228.00 ULTIVA, Glaxo Wellcome 00173-0484-00

Injection Solution - Intramuscular, - 5 mg
10 ml vials $540.00 ULTIVA, Glaxo Wellcome 00173-0485-00

RESERPINE *(002179)*

CATEGORIES: Antihypertensives; Cardiovascular Drugs; Hypertension; Renal Drugs; Vascular Disorders, Cerebral/Peripheral; Pregnancy Category C; FDA Approval Pre 1982

BRAND NAMES: *Anserpin*; *Apoplon*; *Inerpin*; *Maviserpin*; *Novoreserpine*; *Rauverid*; Resa; *Reserfia*; Reserpaneed; *Sedaraupin*; Serpalan; **Serpasil**; *Serpasol*; Serpatabs; Serpate; Serpivite; *Tionsera*
(International brand names outside U.S. in italics)

FORMULARIES: Aetna; FHP; Medi-Cal; WHO

COST OF THERAPY: $12.77 (Hypertension; Tablet; 0.25 mg; 1/day; 365 days) vs. Potential Cost of $24,027.04 (Coronary Bypass)

PRIMARY ICD9: 401.1 (Essential Hypertension, Benign)

DESCRIPTION:

Reserpine USP is an antihypertensive, available as 0.1 mg and 0.25 mg tablets for oral administration. Its chemical name is methyl 18β- hydroxy-11, 17α- dimethoxy-3β,20α-yohimban-16β-carboxylate 3,4,5- trimethoxybenzoate (ester).

Reserpine USP, a pure crystalline alkaloid of rauwolfia, is a white or pale buff to slightly yellowish, odorless crystalline powder. It darkens slowly on exposure to light, but more rapidly when in solution. It is insoluble in water, freely soluble in acetic acid and in chloroform, slightly soluble in benzene, and very slightly soluble in alcohol and in ether. It molecular weight is 608.69.

Inactive Ingredients. Lactose, magnesium stearate, polyethylene glycol, starch, sucrose, talc, and tragacanth (0.1 mg tablets).

CLINICAL PHARMACOLOGY:

Reserpine depletes stores of catecholamines and 5-hydroxytryptamine in many organs, including the brain and adrenal medulla. Most of its pharmacological effects have been attributed to this action. Depletion is slower and less complete in the adrenal medulla than in other tissues.

The depression of sympathetic nerve function results in a decreased heart rate and a lowering of arterial blood pressure. The sedative and tranquilizing properties of Reserpine are thought to be related to depletion of catecholamines and 5-hydroxytryptamine from the brain.

Reserpine, like other rauwolfia compounds, is characterized by slow onset of action and sustained effects. Both cardiovascular and central nervous system effects may persist for a period of time following withdrawal of the drug.

CLINICAL PHARMACOLOGY: *(cont'd)*

Mean maximum plasma levels of 1.54 ng/ml were attained after a median of 3.5 hours in six normal subjects receiving a single oral dose of four 0.25 mg Reserpine tablets. Bioavailability was approximately 50% of that of a corresponding intravenous dose. Plasma levels of reserpine after intravenous administration declined with a mean half-life of 33 hours. Reserpine is extensively bound (96%) to plasma proteins. No definitive studies on the human metabolism of reserpine have been made.

INDICATIONS AND USAGE:

Mild essential hypertension; also useful as adjunctive therapy with other antihypertensive agents in the more severe forms of hypertension; relief of symptoms in agitated psychotic states (*e.g.,* schizophrenia), primarily in those individuals unable to tolerate phenothiazine derivatives or in those who also require antihypertensive medication.

CONTRAINDICATIONS:

Known hypersensitivity, mental depression or history of mental depression (especially with suicidal tendencies), active peptic ulcer, ulcerative colitis, and patients receiving electroconvulsive therapy.

WARNINGS:

Reserpine may cause mental depression. Recognition of depression may be difficult because this condition may often be disguised by somatic complaints. The drug should be discontinued at first signs of depression such as despondency, early morning insomnia, loss of appetite, impotence, or self-deprecation. Drug-induced depression may persist for several months after drug withdrawal and may be severe enough to result in suicide.

PRECAUTIONS:

GENERAL

Since Reserpine increases gastrointestinal motility and secretion, it should be used cautiously in patients with a history of peptic ulcer, ulcerative colitis, or gallstones (biliary colic may be precipitated).

Caution should be exercised when treating hypertensive patients with renal insufficiency, since they adjust poorly to lowered blood pressure levels.

Preoperative withdrawal of Reserpine does not assure that circulatory instability will not occur. It is important that the anesthesiologist be aware of the patient's drug intake and consider this in the overall management, since hypotension has occurred in patients receiving rauwolfia preparations. Anticholinergic and/or adrenergic drugs (*e.g.,* metaraminol, norepinephrine) have been employed to treat adverse vagocirculatory effects.

INFORMATION FOR THE PATIENT

Patients should be informed of possible side effects and advised to take the mediation regularly and continuously as directed.

DRUG INTERACTIONS:

MAO inhibitors should be avoided or used with extreme caution.

Reserpine should be used cautiously with digitalis and quinidine, since cardiac arrhythmias have occurred with rauwolfia preparations.

Concurrent use of Reserpine with other antihypertensive agents necessitates careful titration of dosage with each agent.

Concurrent use of tricyclic antidepressants may decrease the antihypertensive effect of Reserpine (see CONTRAINDICATIONS.)

Concurrent use of Reserpine and direct or indirect-acting sympathomimetics should be closely monitored. The action of direct-acting amines (epinephrine, isoproterenol, phenylephrine, metaraminol) may be prolonged when given to patients taking Reserpine. The action of indirect acting amines (ephedrine, tyramine, amphetamines) is inhibited.

CARCINOGENESIS, MUTAGENESIS, IMPAIRMENT OF FERTILITY

Animal Tumorigenicity: Rodent studies have shown that Reserpine is an animal tumorigen, causing an increased incidence of mammary fibroadenomas in female mice, malignant tumors of the seminal vesicles in male mice, and malignant adrenal medullary tumors in male rats. These findings arose in 2-year studies in which the drug was administered in the feed at concentrations of 5 and 10 ppm - about 100 to 300 times the usual human dose. The breast neoplasms are thought to be related to Reserpine's prolactin elevating effect. Several other prolactin-elevating drugs have also been associated with an increased incidence of mammary neoplasia in rodents.

The extent to which these findings indicate a risk to humans is uncertain. Tissue culture experiments show that about one third of human breast tumors are prolactin-dependent *in vitro*, a factor of considerable importance if the use of the drug is contemplated in a patient with previously detected breast cancer. The possibility of an increased risk of breast cancer in Reserpine users has been studied extensively; however, no firm conclusion has emerged. Although a few epidemiologic studies have suggested a slightly increased risk (less than twofold in all studies except one) in women who have used reserpine, other studies of generally similar design ave not confirmed this. Epidemiologic studies conducted using other drugs (neuroleptic agents) that, like Reserpine, increase prolactin levels and therefore would be considered rodent mammary carcinogens have not shown an association between chronic administration of the drug and human mammary tumorigenesis. While long-term clinical observation has not suggested such an association, the available evidence is considered too limited to be conclusive at this time. An association of reserpine intake with pheochromocytoma or tumors of the seminal vesicles has not been explored.

PREGNANCY CATEGORY C

Reserpine administered parenterally has been shown to be teratogenic in rats at doses up to 2 mg/kg and to have an embryocidal effect in guinea pigs given dosages of 0.5 mg daily.

There are no adequate and well-controlled studies of Reserpine in pregnant women. Reserpine should be used during pregnancy only if the potential benefit justifies the potential risk to the fetus.

Nonteratogenic Effects: Reserpine crosses the placental barrier, and increased respiratory tract secretions, nasal congestion, cyanosis, and anorexia may occur in neonates of reserpine-treated mothers.

DRUG INTERACTIONS: *(cont'd)*

NURSING MOTHERS

Reserpine is excreted in maternal breast milk, and increased respiratory tract secretions, nasal congestion, cyanosis, and anorexia may occur in breast-fed infants. Because of the potential for adverse reactions in nursing infants and the potential for adverse reactions in nursing infants and the potential for tumorigenicity shown for Reserpine in animal studies, a decision should be made whether to discontinue nursing or to discontinue the drug, taking into account the importance of the drug to the mother.

PEDIATRIC USE

Safety and effectiveness in children have not been established by means of controlled clinical trials, although there is experience with the use of Reserpine in children. (See DOSAGE AND ADMINISTRATION.) Because of adverse effects such as emotional depression and lability, sedation, and stuffy nose, Reserpine is not usually recommended as a step-2 drug in the treatment of hypertension in children.

ADVERSE REACTIONS:

The following adverse reactions have been observed with rauwolfia preparations, but there has not been enough systematic collection of data to support an estimate of their frequency. Consequently the reactions are categorized by organ systems and are listed in decreasing order of severity and not frequency.

Digestive: Vomiting, diarrhea, nausea, anorexia, dryness of mouth, hypersecretion.

Cardiovascular: Arrhythmias (particularly when used concurrently with digitalis or quinidine), syncope, angina-like symptoms, bradycardia, edema.

Respiratory: Dyspnea, epistaxis, nasal congestion.

Neurologic: Rare parkinsonian syndrome and other extrapyramidal tract symptoms; dizziness; headache; paradoxical anxiety; depression; nervousness; night-mares; dull sensorium; drowsiness.

Musculoskeletal: Muscular aches.

Genitourinary: Pseudolactation, impotence, dysuria, gynecomastia, decreased libido, breast engorgement.

Metabolic: Weight gain.

Special Sense: Deafness, optic atrophy, glaucoma, uveitis, conjunctival injection.

Hypersensitive Reactions: Purpura, rash, pruritus.

OVERDOSAGE:

ACUTE TOXICITY

No deaths due to acute poisoning with reserpine have been reported. Highest known doses survived: children, 1000 mg (age and sex not specified); young children 200 mg (20 month-old boy).

The oral LD_{50}'s in animals (mg/kg):rat, 2993; mouse, 47 and 500.

SIGNS AND SYMPTOMS

The clinical picture of acute poisoning is characterized chiefly by signs and symptoms due to the reflex parasympathomimetic effect of reserpine.

Impairment of consciousness may occur and may range from drowsiness to coma, depending upon the severity of overdosage. Flushing of the skin, conjunctival injection, and pupillary constriction are to be expected. Hypotension, hypothermia, central respiratory depression, and bradycardia may develop in cases of severe overdosage. Increased salivary and gastric secretion and diarrhea may also occur.

TREATMENT

There is no specific antidote.

Stomach contents should be evacuated, taking adequate precautions against aspiration and for protection of the airway. Activated charcoal slurry should be instilled.

The effects of Reserpine overdosage should be treated symptomatically. If hypotension is severe enough to require treatment with a vasopressor, one having a direct action upon vascular smooth muscle (*e.g.*, phenylephrine, levarterenol, metaraminol) should be used. Since Reserpine is long- acting, the patient should be observed carefully for at least 72 hours, and treatment administered as required.

DOSAGE AND ADMINISTRATION:

HYPERTENSION

In the average patient not receiving other antihypertensive agents, the usual initial dosage is 0.5 mg daily for 1 or 2 weeks. For maintenance, reduce to 0.1 - 0.25 mg daily. Higher dosages should be used cautiously, because occurrence of serious mental depression and other side effects may increase considerably.

PSYCHIATRIC DISORDERS

The initial dosage is 0.5 mg daily, but may range from 0.1 mg to 1.0 mg. Adjust dosage upward or downward according to the patient's response.

CHILDREN

Reserpine is not recommended for use in children (see PRECAUTIONS, Pediatric Use). If it is to be used in treating a child, the usual recommended starting dose is 20 mcg/kg daily. The maximum recommended dose is 0.25 mg (total) daily.

Protect from light. Dispense in tight, light-resistant container (USP).

HOW SUPPLIED - EQUIVALENTS NOT AVAILABLE:

Tablet, Uncoated - Oral - 0.1 mg

100's	$2.95	Reserpine, Consolidated Midland	00223-1590-01
100's	$5.50	Reserpine, Eon Labs Mfg	00185-0032-01
1000's	$19.95	Reserpine, Consolidated Midland	00223-1590-02
1000's	$29.95	Reserpine, Harber Pharm	51432-0414-06
1000's	$31.27	Reserpine, Geneva Pharms	00781-1086-10
1000's	$40.45	Reserpine, Major Pharms	00904-2198-80
1000's	$42.00	Reserpine, C O Truxton	00463-6167-10
1000's	$42.05	Reserpine, Aligen Independ	00405-4925-03
1000's	$43.95	Reserpine, Eon Labs Mfg	00185-0032-10
1000's	$44.42	Reserpine, Rugby	00536-4454-10
1000's	$52.64	Reserpine, HL Moore Drug Exch	00839-1585-16

Tablet, Uncoated - Oral - 0.25 mg

100's	$3.50	Reserpine, Consolidated Midland	00223-1591-01
100's	$7.65	Reserpine, Eon Labs Mfg	00185-0134-01
1000's	$22.50	Reserpine, Consolidated Midland	00223-1591-02
1000's	$49.00	Reserpine, C O Truxton	00463-6168-10
1000's	$49.84	Reserpine, Geneva Pharms	00781-1096-10
1000's	$57.90	Reserpine, Aligen Independ	00405-4926-03
1000's	$57.96	Reserpine, United Res	00677-0126-10
1000's	$59.95	Reserpine, Harber Pharm	51432-0416-06
1000's	$60.50	Reserpine, Eon Labs Mfg	00185-0134-10
1000's	$64.45	Reserpine, Major Pharms	00904-2199-80
1000's	$69.80	Reserpine, Rugby	00536-4458-10
1000's	$121.22	Reserpine, HL Moore Drug Exch	00839-5128-16

RESERPINE; TRICHLORMETHIAZIDE *(002180)*

CATEGORIES: Antihypertensives; Cardiovascular Drugs; Diuretics; Hypertension; Renal Drugs; Vascular Disorders, Cerebral/Peripheral; FDA Approval Pre 1982

BRAND NAMES: **Metatensin**; Naquival; Ropres

FORMULARIES: Medi-Cal

> WARNING:
> This fixed combination drug is not indicated for initial therapy of hypertension. Hypertension requires therapy titrated to the individual patient. If the fixed combination represents the dosage so determined, its use may be more convenient in patient management. The treatment of hypertension is not static, but must be reevaluated as conditions in each patient warrant.

DESCRIPTION:

Each yellow tablet contains trichlormethiazide 2 mg and reserpine 0.1 mg. The tablet also contains inactive ingredients: corn starch, FD&C Yellow No. 5 tartrazine (see PRECAUTIONS), lactose, magnesium stearate, and pregelatinized corn starch.

Each lavender tablet contains trichlormethiazide 4 mg and reserpine 0.1 mg. The tablet also contains inactive ingredients: corn starch, D&C Red No. 33, FD&C Blue No. 1, lactose, magnesium stearate, and pregelatinized corn starch.

Trichlormethiazide is an orally effective diuretic and antihypertensive of the thiazide class. Chemically trichlormethiazide is 2*H*-1,2,4- benzothiadiazine-7-sulfonamide, 6-chloro-3-(dichloromethyl)-3,4-dihydro-,1,1-dioxide, differing from other thiazides by the inclusion of a dichloromethyl radical at the 3 position on the benzothiadiazine structure.

Reserpine is a pure crystalline alkaloid derived from the root of*Rauwolfia serpentina.* Chemically reserpine is methyl 18β- hydroxy-11, 17α-dimethoxy-3β, 20α-yohimban-16β-carboxylate 3,4,5-trimethoxybenzoate.

CLINICAL PHARMACOLOGY:

Trichlormethiazide: The mechanism of action involves interference with the renal tubular mechanism of electrolyte reabsorption. At maximal therapeutic dosage, all thiazides are approximately equal in their diuretic potency. The mechanism whereby thiazides function in the control of hypertension is unknown.

Reserpine: Reserpine probably produces its antihypertensive effects through depletion of tissue stores of epinephrine and norepinephrine from peripheral sites. By contrast, its sedative and tranquilizing properties are thought to be related to depletion of 5-hydroxytryptamine from the brain.

Reserpine is characterized by slow onset of action and sustained effect. Both its cardiovascular and central nervous system effects may persist following withdrawal of the drug.

INDICATIONS AND USAGE:

Hypertension (See BOXED WARNING.)

CONTRAINDICATIONS:

Trichlormethiazide: Trichlormethiazide is contraindicated in patients with anuria and in patients known to be hypersensitive to this or other sulfonamide derivatives.

Reserpine: Reserpine is contraindicated in patients with hypersensitivity to the drug, history of mental depression (especially with suicidal tendencies), active peptic ulcer, or ulcerative colitis.

WARNINGS:

GENERAL

Trichlormethiazide: Use with caution in severe renal disease. In patients with renal disease, thiazides may precipitate azotemia. Cumulative effects of the drug may develop in patients with impaired renal function.

Thiazides should be used with caution in patients with impaired hepatic function or progressive liver disease, since minor alterations of fluid and electrolyte balance may precipitate hepatic coma.

Thiazides may add to or potentiate the action of other antihypertensive drugs. Potentiation occurs with ganglionic or peripheral adrenergic- blocking drugs.

Sensitivity reactions may occur in patients with a history of allergy or bronchial asthma. Exacerbation or activation of systemic lupus erythematosus has been reported.

Reserpine: Reserpine may cause mental depression. Recognition of depression may be difficult because this condition may often be disguised by somatic complaints (masked depression). The drug should be discontinued at the first signs of depression, such as despondency, early morning insomnia, loss of appetite, impotence, or self-deprecation. Drug-induced depression may persist for several months after drug withdrawal and may be severe enough to result in suicide.

Reserpine may induce peptic ulceration; discontinue use if peptic ulcer develops.

Electroshock therapy should not be given to patients taking reserpine, since severe and even fatal reactions have been reported. The drug should be discontinued for two weeks before giving electroshock therapy.

Monoamine oxidase (MAO) inhibitors should be avoided or used with extreme caution.

USAGE IN PREGNANCY

Trichlormethiazide: Thiazides cross the placental barrier and appear in cord blood. The use of thiazides in pregnant women requires that the anticipated benefit be weighed against possible hazards to the fetus. These hazards include fetal or neonatal jaundice, thrombocytopenia, and possibly other adverse reactions which have occurred in the adult.

Reserpine: The safety of reserpine for use during pregnancy has not been established; therefore, the drug should be used in pregnant patients or in women of childbearing potential only when, in the judgement of the physician, it is essential to the welfare of the patient. Increased respiratory secretions, nasal congestion, cyanosis, and anorexia may occur in infants born to reserpine-treated mothers, since reserpine crosses the placental barrier and appears in maternal breast milk.

NURSING MOTHERS

Thiazides and reserpine appear in breast milk. If use of Metatensin is deemed essential, the patient should stop nursing.

PRECAUTIONS:

Metatensin #2 tablets contain FD&C Yellow No. 5 (tartrazine), which may cause allergic-type reactions (including bronchial asthma) in certain susceptible individuals. Although the overall incidence of tartrazine sensitivity in the general population is low, it is frequently seen in patients who also have aspirin hypersensitivity.

PRECAUTIONS: *(cont'd)*

Trichlormethiazide

Periodic determinations of serum electrolytes to detect possible electrolyte imbalance should be performed at appropriate intervals.

All patients receiving thiazide therapy should be observed for clinical signs of fluid or electrolyte imbalance; namely, hyponatremia, hypochloremic alkalosis, and hypokalemia. Serum and urine electrolyte determinations are particularly important when the patient is vomiting excessively or receiving parenteral fluids.

Medication, such as digitalis, may also influence serum electrolytes. Warning signs, irrespective of cause, are: dryness of the mouth, thirst, weakness, lethargy, drowsiness, restlessness, muscle pains or cramps, muscular fatigue, hypotension, oliguria, tachycardia, and gastrointestinal disturbances, such as nausea and vomiting.

Hypokalemia may develop with thiazides as with any other potent diuretic, especially with brisk diuresis, when severe cirrhosis is present, or during concomitant use of corticosteroids or ACTH.

Interference with adequate oral electrolyte intake will also contribute to hypokalemia. Digitalis therapy may exaggerate metabolic effects of hypokalemia, especially with reference to myocardial activity.

Any chloride deficit is generally mild and usually does not require specific treatment except under extraordinary circumstances (as in liver disease or renal disease). Dilutional hyponatremia may occur in edematous patients in hot weather; appropriate therapy is water restriction rather than administration of salt, except in rare instances when the hyponatremia is life threatening. In actual salt depletion, appropriate replacement is the therapy of choice. Hyperuricemia may occur or frank gout may be precipitated in certain patients receiving thiazide therapy.

Insulin requirements in diabetic patients may be increased, decreased, or unchanged. Latent diabetes mellitus may become manifest during thiazide administration.

Thiazide drugs may increase the responsiveness to tubocurarine.

The antihypertensive effects of the drug may be enhanced in the postsympathectomy patient.

Thiazides may decrease arterial responsiveness to norepinephrine. This diminution is not sufficient to preclude effectiveness of the pressor agent for therapeutic use.

If progressive renal impairment becomes evident, as indicated by a rising nonprotein nitrogen or blood urea nitrogen, a careful reappraisal of therapy is necessary with consideration given to withholding or discontinuing diuretic therapy.

Thiazides may decrease serum PBI levels without signs of thyroid disturbance.

Reserpine

Caution should be used in treating hypertensive patients with renal insufficiency.

Cardiac arrhythmias have occurred in patients receiving digitalis and quinidine with reserpine.

Reserpine potentiates many anesthetic agents; hypotension and bradycardia have been noted during anesthesia. In addition, a relative sensitivity to norepinephrine or other pressor agents may exist due to the previous action of reserpine; thus, usual amounts of the pressor agent may be excessive.

Use with caution in patients with a history of depression, peptic ulcer or other gastrointestinal disorders, and in hypertensive patients with functionally severe coronary artery disease.

ANIMAL TUMORIGENICITY

Rodent studies have shown that reserpine is an animal tumorigen, causing an increased incidence of mammary fibroadenomas in female mice, malignant tumors of the seminal vesicles in male mice, and malignant adrenal medullary tumors in male rats. These findings arose in 2 year studies in which the drug was administered in the feed at concentrations of 5 and 10 ppm (about 100 to 300 times the usual human dose). The breast neoplasms are thought to be related to reserpine's prolactin-elevating effect. Several other prolactin-elevating drugs have also been associated with an increased incidence of mammary neoplasia in rodents.

The extent to which these findings indicate a risk to humans is uncertain. Tissue culture experiments show that about one-third of human breast tumors are prolactin-dependent in vitro, a factor of considerable importance if the use of the drug is contemplated in a patient with previously detected breast cancer. The possibility of an increased risk of breast cancer in reserpine users has been studied extensively; however, no firm conclusion has emerged. Although a few epidemiologic studies have suggested a slightly increased risk (less than twofold in all studies except one) in women who have used reserpine, other studies of generally similar design have not confirmed this. Epidemiologic studies conducted using other drugs (neuroleptic agents) like reserpine that increase prolactin levels and, therefore, would be considered rodent mammary carcinogens, have not shown an association between chronic administration of the drug and human mammary tumorigenesis. While long- term clinical observation has not suggested such an association, the available evidence is considered too limited to be conclusive at this time. An association of reserpine intake with pheochromocytoma or tumors of the seminal vesicles has not been explored.

ADVERSE REACTIONS:

Trichlormethiazide

1. Gastrointestinal: anorexia, gastric irritation, nausea, diarrhea, constipation, jaundice (intrahepatic cholestatic jaundice), vomiting, cramping, pancreatitis.

2. Central Nervous System: dizziness, vertigo, paresthesia, headache, xanthopsia.

3. Hematologic: leukopenia, agranulocytosis, thrombocytopenia, aplastic anemia.

4. Dermatologic-Hypersensitivity: purpura, photosensitivity, rash, urticaria, necrotizing angiitis (vasculitis), cutaneous vasculitis.

5. Cardiovascular: orthostatic hypotension (possibly aggravated by alcohol, barbiturates, or narcotics).

6. Other: hyperglycemia, glycosuria, hyperuricemia, muscle spasm, weakness, restlessness.

Reserpine: Gastric hypersecretion; vomiting; nervousness; paradoxical anxiety; CNS sensitization manifested by deafness, glaucoma, uveitis, and optic atrophy; purpura; nasal stuffiness; loose stools; reversible parkinsonism; muscular fatigue and weakness; and nightmares. Mental depression has been reported, particularly when reserpine doses of over 1 mg daily are used. Other side effects of reserpine reported include anorexia, nausea, dizziness, headaches, impotence, flushing of the skin, dryness of the mouth, biliary colic, blurred vision, muscular aches, and pruritus. Hypotension, including the orthostatic variety, may occur in some patients. Angina pectoris, arrhythmias, and congestive heart failure have also been reported but are uncommon.

After the onset of therapy with reserpine, a turbulent phase of short duration may occur. Very rare additional adverse effects that have been observed in association with reserpine therapy include epistaxis, skin eruptions, and edema due to sodium retention. Bradycardia may occur as an exaggerated response related to the pharmacodynamic effect of reserpine.

DOSAGE AND ADMINISTRATION:

As determined by individual titration. (See BOXED WARNING.)

In the stabilized hypertensive patient, administration may be continued on a once-daily basis administered in the morning. The maximum single effective dose of Metatensin is 8 mg (in some patients 4 mg). Doses in excess of 8 mg normally will not produce any increase in sodium and water excretion and in refractory patients may increase excretion of potassium.

Store at room temperature, preferably below 86°F (30°C).

(Marion Merrell Dow, 5/87)

HOW SUPPLIED - EQUIVALENTS NOT AVAILABLE:

Tablet, Uncoated - Oral - 0.1 mg/2 mg

100's	$58.56	METATENSIN #2, Hoechst Marion Roussel	00068-0064-01

Tablet, Uncoated - Oral - 0.1 mg/4 mg

100's	$87.18	METATENSIN #4, Hoechst Marion Roussel	00068-0065-01

RESPIRATORY SYNCYTIAL VIRUS IMMUNE GLOBULIN *(003188)*

CATEGORIES: Antiserum; Biologicals; Immunologic; Serums, Toxoids and Vaccines; Vaccines; FDA Approved 1996 Jan

BRAND NAMES: **RespiGam**; Respivir

DESCRIPTION:

RespiGam, Respiratory Syncytial Virus Immune Globulin Intravenous (Human) (RSV-IGIV) is a sterile liquid immunoglobulin G containing neutralizing antibody to Respiratory Syncytial Virus (RSV). Each lot of RSV-IGIV meets the minimum potency specifications when compared to the validated Reference Standard. The globulin is stabilized with 5% sucrose and 1% Albumin (Human). RSV-IGIV contains no preservative. The immunoglobulin is purified from pooled adult human plasma selected for high titers of neutralizing antibody against RSV using a proprietary patented screening assay (1). Source material for fractionated may be obtained from another U.S.-licensed manufacturer. Pooled plasma is fractionated by ethanol precipitation of the proteins according to Cohn Method 6 and Oncley Method 9, with additional steps to yield a product suitable for intravenous administration. A widely utilized solvent-detergent viral inactivation process is used to decrease the possibility of transmission of bloodborne pathogens (2). Certain manufacturing operations may be performed by other firms. Each milliliter contains 50 ± 10 mg immunoglobulin, primarily IgG, and trace amounts of IgA and IgM; 50 mg sucrose; and 10 mg Albumin (Human). The sodium content is 20-30 mEq per liter, i.e., 1.0-1.5 mEq per 50 ml. The solution should appear colorless and translucent.

CLINICAL PHARMACOLOGY:

Respiratory Syncytial Virus Immune Globulin Intravenous (Human) (RSV-IGIV) contains IgG antibodies representative of the large number of normal healthy persons who contributed to the plasma pools from which the product was derived. The immune globulin contains a high concentration of neutralizing and protective antibodies directed against RSV (3). In vitro tests demonstrated that RSV-IGIV neutralized each of 62 different RSV clinical isolates of both subgroup A (n=39) and subgroup B (n=23). In the PREVENT study monthly doses of 750 mg/kg of RSV-IGIV attained trough geometric mean serum RSV neutralization antibody titers of 1:297 ± 38 (SE) one month after the first infusion, 1:477 ± 85 one month after the second infusion, 1:490 ± 61 one month after the third infusion and 1:429 ± 23 one month after the fourth infusion. The mean half-life of serum RSV neutralizing antibodies after RSV-IGIV infusion is 22-28 days (4).

CLINICAL STUDIES:

In randomized, controlled studies of RSV disease prophylaxis, monthly doses of 750 mg/kg of RSV-IGIV were effective in reducing the incidence of RSV hospitalization in high-risk children. Children with BPD may be at high risk for serious RSV disease up to 60 months of age (5). Children born prematurely may be at high risk for serious RSV disease during the first year of life (6). Summarized below are the results of the pivotal trial and three additional studies supportive of the safety and efficacy of RSV-IGIV.

Prevent Trial: The pivotal trial known as the PREVENT trial was a 54 center, randomized, placebo-controlled, double-blind study of the safety and effectiveness of RSV-IGIV in the prophylaxis of RSV disease in infants and children with BPD ≤ 24 months of age or premature birth (≤ 35 weeks gestation) ≤ 6 months of age at study entry. The age of premature infants at the end of the study ranged from 4.8 to 11.4 months. In this trial, 510 patients were randomized to receive monthly infusions in November through April of either 750 mg/kg (15 ml/kg) RSV-IGIV or 15 ml/kg 1% Albumin (Human) serum as a control. The efficacy analyses of this study were conducted on an 'intent-to-treat' basis that included all randomized patients. The prospectively defined endpoints for the study are shown in TABLE 1. RSV-IGIV reduced the incidence of RSV hospitalization by 41% (p=0.047) total days of RSV hospitalization by 53%, (p=0.045) total RSV hospital days with increased supplemental oxygen requirement by 60%, (p=0.007) and total RSV hospital days with a moderate or severe lower respiratory tract infection by 54% (p=0.049). A trend in reduction in total intensive care unit (ICU) days (44%) was observed although it was not statistically significant (p=0.407).

Two additional endpoints were evaluated. The incidence of any hospitalization due to respiratory illness was compared between placebo control and children receiving RSV-IGIV. The incidence in placebo controls was 69/260 (26.5%) versus 41/250 (16.4%) in the RSV-IGIV recipients. This represents a 38% reduction (p=0.005) in the incidence of respiratory hospitalization for RSV-IGIV recipients. The total days of hospitalization for respiratory illness per 100 randomized children were compared between placebo controls and RSV-IGIV recipients. There were 317 days per 100 control children and 170 days per 100 RSV-IGIV children. This represents a 46% reduction (p=0.005) in the total days of hospitalization for respiratory illness per 100 randomized children for RSV-IGIV recipients.

PREVENT was not designed nor powered to detect treatment differences among subsets of participants. Reductions in RSV hospitalization ranging from 17% to 58% were observed in RSV-IGIV treated subgroups defined by gender, categorical age (< or > 6 months at entry) and diagnosis. The largest reductions were seen in children > 6 months of age, all of whom had BPD. The smallest observed reduction was seen among children age < 6 months. This subgroup also had a low incidence of RSV hospitalization which limited the ability to quantify the magnitude of the treatment effect. Consequently, the effectiveness of RSV-IGIV in the subgroup of premature infants without BPD could not be definitively established in this study. Analyses using weight as a categorical variable revealed that children with entry weight below the median (4.3 kg) had a 49% observed reduction in the incidence of RSV hospitalization.

RSV-IGIV has not been investigated for its effect in the prevention of RSV related apnea or RSV related apnea-hypothermia-sepsis syndrome.

CLINICAL STUDIES: *(cont'd)*

TABLE 1 Summary of PREVENT Trial Results

Clinical Endpoint	Control N=260	RSV-IGIV (750 mg/kg) N=250	% Reduction
Incidence of RSV Hospitalization	35 (13.5%)	20 (8.0%)	41%
RSV Hospital Days/100 Children	129	60	53%
RSV Hospital Days with Increased Supplemental 02/100 Children	85	34	60%
RSV Hospital Days with Moderate to Severe LRI*/100 Children	106	49	54%
RSV ICU Days/100 Children	50	28	44%
Days of RSV Mechanical Ventilation/100 Children	20	18	10%

* Lower Respiratory Tract Infection/Illness

NIAID Trial: The NIAID study was a supportive, multi-center, randomized, non-placebo controlled, single-blind study of the safety and effectiveness of RSV-IGIV in the prophylaxis of RSV disease in 274 infants and children at high risk of RSV disease due to chronic pulmonary disease (principally BPD), congenital heart disease (CHD), or premature birth (≤ 35 weeks gestation) (7, 8, 9). Compared to control children (n=90), children randomized to receive 750 mg/kg RSV-IGIV, Respiratory Syncytial Virus Immune Globulin Intravenous (Human) (RSV-IGIV) (n=92) showed a 57% (p=0.029) reduction in the incidence of RSV hospitalization, a 59% (p=0.030) reduction in total days of RSV hospitalization per 100 children, a 97% (p=0.049) reduction in RSV ICU days per 100 children and 100% reduction in mechanical ventilation per 100 children.

Cardiac Trial: The CARDIAC trial was a supportive multi-center, randomized non-placebo controlled, single-blind study conducted to further assess the safety and efficacy of RSV-IGIV in 429 children with congenital heart disease (CHD) of less than 48 months of age at enrollment. The mean age of children at entry was 9 months and ranged from 0 to 47 months. Although trends toward RSV-IGIV efficacy were observed, the data were not statistically significant. The efficacy and safety of RSV-IGIV has not been established in children with CHD (See WARNING SECTION).

Open Label Trial: A third supportive clinical trial was conducted to determine the safety and pharmacokinetics of monthly 750 mg/kg doses of RSV-IGIV in 68 children with BPD or prematurity. This multi-center study was open-label in design. During the study, seven children (10.3%) were hospitalized for RSV. RSV hospital days were 54 per 100 children (mean = 5.3 days, n=7) and RSV ICU days were 15 per 100 children (mean = 10 days, n=1).

RSV-IGIV has not been demonstrated to be effective for the treatment of RSV infection.

INDICATIONS AND USAGE:

Respiratory Syncytial Virus Immune Globulin Intravenous (Human) (RSV-IGIV) is indicated for the prevention of serious lower respiratory tract infection caused by RSV in children under 24 months of age with bronchopulmonary dysplasia (BPD) or a history of premature birth (≤ 35 weeks gestation). RSV-IGIV has been demonstrated to be safe and effective in reducing the incidence and duration of RSV hospitalization and the severity of RSV illness in these high risk infants.

CONTRAINDICATIONS:

RSV-IGIV should not be used in patients with a history of a severe prior reaction associated with the administration of RSV-IGIV or other human immunoglobulin preparations. Patients with selective IgA deficiency have the potential for developing antibodies to IgA and could have anaphylactic or allergic reactions to subsequent administration of blood products that contain IgA, including RSV-IGIV.

WARNINGS:

Infants with underlying pulmonary disease may be sensitive to extra fluid volume. Infusion of RSV-IGIV, particularly in children with BPD, may precipitate symptoms of fluid overload. Overall, 8.4% of participants (1% premature and 13% BPD) received new or extra diuretics during the period 24 hours before through 48 hours after at least one of their infusions in the PREVENT trial. The reason for this use was not recorded (*e.g.,* prophylaxis, treatment, or part of routine care during a clinical visit). RSV-IGIV - related fluid overload was reported in 3 patients (1.2%) and RSV-IGIV - related respiratory distress was reported in 4 patients (1.6%); all had underlying BPD. With the exception of one child with respiratory distress (part of an acute allergic reaction) for whom RSV-IGIV was discontinued, these children were managed with diuretics and/or modification of the infusion rate and went on to receive subsequent infusions. Complications related to fluid volume were recorded as a reason for incomplete or prolonged infusion in 2.0% of children receiving RSV-IGIV (2.5% BPD and 1.1% premature) and in 1.5% of children receiving placebo in the PREVENT trial. Children with clinically apparent fluid overload should not be infused with RSV-IGIV.

RSV-IGIV should be administered cautiously (see DOSAGE AND ADMINISTRATION). During administration, a patient's vital signs should be monitored frequently, and a patient should be observed for increases in heart rate, respiratory rate, retractions, and rales. **A loop diuretic such as furosemide or bumetanide should be available for management of fluid overload.**

Severe reactions, such as anaphylaxis or angioneurotic edema, have been reported in association with intravenous immunoglobulins even in patients not known to be sensitive to human immunoglobulins or blood products. Serious allergic reaction was noted in 2 patients in the PREVENT trial. These reactions were manifest as an acute episode of cyanosis, mottling and fever in one patient and respiratory distress in the other. The rate of allergic reaction appears to be low and consistent with rates observed for other Immune Globulin Intravenous (Human)[IGIV] products. **If hypotension, anaphylaxis, or severe allergic reaction occurs, discontinue infusion and administer epinephrine (1:1000), as required.**

The safety and efficacy of RSV-IGIV in children with CHD has not been established. Although equivalent proportions of children in the RSV-IGIV and control groups in the CARDIAC trial had adverse events, a larger number of RSV-IGIV recipients had severe or life-threatening adverse events. These events were most frequently observed in infants with CHD with right to left shunts who underwent cardiac surgery.

PRECAUTIONS:

Except for hypersensitivity reactions, adverse reactions to IGIVs may be related to the rate of administration. Careful adherence to the infusion rate outlined under DOSAGE AND ADMINISTRATION is therefore important. Loop diuretics should be available for the management of patients who are at risk for fluid overload. Although systemic allergic reactions are rare (see ADVERSE REACTIONS), epinephrine and diphenhydramine should be available for treatment of acute allergic symptoms.

PRECAUTIONS: *(cont'd)*

Rare occurrences of aseptic meningitis syndrome (AMS) have been reported in association with Immune Globulin Intravenous (Human) (IGIV) treatment (10, 11, 12, 13). AMS usually begins within several hours to two days following IGIV treatment and is characterized by symptoms and signs including severe headache, drowsiness, fever, photophobia, painful eye movements, muscle rigidity, and nausea and vomiting. Cerebrospinal fluid studies generally demonstrate pleocytosis, predominantly granulocytic, and elevated protein levels. Patients exhibiting such symptoms and signs should be thoroughly evaluated to rule out other causes of meningitis. AMS may occur more frequently in association with high dose (2 g/kg) IGIV treatment. Discontinuation of IGIV treatment has resulted in remission of AMS within several days without sequelae.

RSV-IGIV is made from human plasma and, like other plasma products, carries the possibility for transmission of bloodborne pathogenic agents. The risk of transmission of recognized bloodborne viruses is considered to be low because of screening of plasma donors, an added viral inactivation step and removal properties in the Cohn-Oncley cold ethanol precipitation procedure used for purification of immune globulin products (14, 15, 16). Until 1993, cold ethanol manufactured immune globulins licensed in the United States had not been documented to transmit any viral agent. However, during a brief period in late 1993 to early 1994, intravenous immune globulin made by one U.S. manufacturer was associated with transmission of Hepatitis C virus (17). To further guard against possible transmission of bloodborne viruses, RSV-IGIV is treated with a solvent-detergent viral inactivation procedure (2) known to inactivate a wide spectrum of lipid enveloped viruses, including HIV-1, HIV-2, Hepatitis B Virus and Hepatitis C Virus (18). However, because new bloodborne agents may yet emerge, some of which may not be inactivated or eliminated by the manufacturing process or by solvent-detergent treatment. RSV-IGIV, like any other blood product, should be given only if a benefit is expected.

RSV-IGIV does not contain a preservative. The single-use vial should be entered only once for administration purposes and the infusion should begin within 6 hours. The infusion schedule should be adhered to closely (see DOSAGE AND ADMINISTRATION). Do not use if the solution is turbid.

Pregnancy Category C: Animal reproduction studies have not been conducted with RSV-IGIV, Respiratory Syncytial Virus Immune Globulin Intravenous (Human) (RSV-IGIV). It is also not known whether RSV-IGIV can cause fetal harm when administered to a pregnant woman or could affect reproduction capacity. RSV-IGIV should be given to a pregnant woman only if clearly indicated.

DRUG INTERACTIONS:

Antibodies present in immune globulin preparations may interfere with the immune response to live virus vaccines, such as mumps, rubella, and particularly measles. If such vaccines are given during or within 10 months after RSV-IGIV infusion, reimmunization is recommended, if appropriate (19). Studies have suggested that responses to non-live childhood vaccines (*e.g.,* DPT) are not substantially influenced by IGIVs administration (20). Limited information available from infants who received RSV-IGIV concurrently with one or more doses of their primary immunization series indicates that antibody responses to diphtheria, tetanus, pertussis, and H. Influenza b may be lower in RSV-IGIV recipients than in controls. It is not known whether antibody responses to trivalent oral polio vaccine might be affected by concurrent RSV-IGIV. Physicians may wish to consider giving a booster dose of these vaccines three or four months after the last dose of RSV-IGIV in order to ensure immunity to DPT (diphtheria, pertussis, tetanus), DaPT (Diphtheria, acellular pertussis, tetanus), Hib (hemophilus influenza b) and OPV (oral poliovirus). The effect of human immunoglobulin on immunization with eIPV (enhanced, inactivated poliovirus vaccine) has not been evaluated. Admixtures of RSV-IGIV with other drugs have not been studied; however, it is recommended that RSV-IGIV be administered separately from other drugs or medications that the patient may be receiving (see DOSAGE AND ADMINISTRATION).

ADVERSE REACTIONS:

RSV-IGIV is generally well tolerated. In the PREVENT trial of RSV-IGIV in children with BPD or prematurity, there was no difference in the proportion of children in the RSV-IGIV and placebo groups who reported adverse events.

Table 2 illustrates adverse events which the investigator judged potentially related to study drug (RSV-IGIV or Placebo) and which were reported at an incidence of 1% or greater in the RSV-IGIV group in the PREVENT trial. The number of children reporting one or more of these adverse events were evenly distributed between the two treatment groups (35 of 260 in placebo, and 43 of 250 in RSV-IGIV patients, p=0.269). In addition, the distribution of severity of adverse events was not significantly different between the two groups (p=0.216). Respiratory distress occurred in 2% (6 of 250) of children receiving RSV-IGIV. Patients in the RSV-IGIV group reported a slightly higher incidence of fever compared to the placebo group.

TABLE 2 Potentially Drug Related* Adverse Events Reported at an incidence of 1% in the RSV-IGIV Group in the PREVENT Clinical Study of RSV-IGIV

Number in study	Placebo N=260		RSV-IGIV N =250	
	N	%	N	%
Number of children with any drug related adverse event	**35**	**13**	**43**	**15**
Number of children with drug related [1]:				
fever/pyrexia	6	2%	15	6%
respiratory distress	1	<1%	6	2%
vomiting/emesis	3	1%	5	2%
wheezing	4	2%	4	2%
diarrhea	1	<1%	3	1%
rales	0	0%	3	1%
fluid overload	0	0%	3	1%
tachycardia/increased pulse rate	0	0%	3	1%
rash	5	2%	3	1%
hypertension	0	0%	2	1%
hypoxia/hypoxemia	2	1%	2	1%
tachypnea	1	<1%	2	1%
gastroenteritis	1	<1%	2	1%
injection site inflammation	2	1%	2	1%
overdose effect	1	<1%	2	1%

* = events possibly, probably, or definitely related to study drug.
[1] a child may be represented in more than one category

The incidence of serious adverse events potentially related to study drug was equivalent for both treatment groups with 2% of children in the placebo group and 2% of children in the RSV-IGIV group reporting such events (p=0.538). The rate of serious adverse events is similar to the rate reported for other IGIVs.

ADVERSE REACTIONS: *(cont'd)*

Infrequent adverse reactions were reported (rate of less than one percent) in the PREVENT trial as potentially related to the use of RSV-IGIV including: edema, pallor, hypotension, heart murmur, gagging, cyanosis, sleepiness, cough, rhinorrhea, eczema, skin cold and clammy, and conjunctival hemorrhage. Adverse events occurring only in the placebo group are not listed.

Reactions similar to those reported with other IGIVs may occur with RSV-IGIV. These include dizziness, flushing, blood pressure changes, anxiety, palpitations, chest tightness, dyspnea, abdominal cramps, pruritus, myalgia or arthralgia (see WARNINGS). Such reactions are often related to the rate of infusion. Immediate allergic, anaphylactic, or hypersensitivity reactions may be observed (see CONTRAINDICATIONS). Rarely, aseptic meningitis syndrome (AMS) has been reported in association with IGIV treatment, particularly at high dosage (2 g/kg)(10-13) (see PRECAUTIONS). In the PREVENT trial, 3 children developed aseptic meningitis of unknown etiology: one had a presumptive diagnosis of enteroviral infection, another child had an unconfirmed diagnosis of Herpes simplex meningitis which improved in association with acyclovir treatment and a third child developed fever, vomiting and malaise associated with 21 cells/mm3 in cerebrospinal fluid. Also, one child was initially reported to have hepatitis but was subsequently diagnosed with hemosiderosis judged unrelated to RSV-IGIV.

Other Safety Experience: In the single-blind, controlled NIAID trial in children with BPD, CHD or prematurity, adverse reactions were reported in 3% of all RSV-IGIV infusions. Five of 160 children were considered to have had mild fluid overload associated with infusion. The remaining adverse reactions consisted of mild decreases in oxygen saturation (n=8) and fever (n=5).

In the Open-label study in children with BPD or prematurity (n=68) infusion-associated adverse reactions were noted in 14 of 294 (4.8%) infusions. Six adverse events were considered related to infusion, including 4 mild and 2 moderate events.

In the CARDIAC study, children with CHD with right to left shunts appeared to have an increased frequency of cardiac surgery and had a greater frequency of severe and life-threatening adverse events associated with cardiac surgery (See WARNINGS).

OVERDOSAGE:

Although few data are available, clinical experience with other immune globulin preparations suggests that the major manifestations would be those related to fluid volume overload.

DOSAGE AND ADMINISTRATION:

The maximum recommended total dosage per monthly infusion is 750 mg/kg, administered according to the following schedule:

TABLE 3

Time After Start of Infusion	Rate of Infusion (ml/kg of Body Mass per Hour)
0 - 15 minutes	1.5 ml/kg/hr
15 - 30 minutes	3.0 ml/kg/hr
30 minutes to end of infusion	6.0 ml/kg/hr

Administer RSV-IGIV intravenously at 1.5 ml/kg/hr for 15 minutes. It the clinical condition does not contraindicate a higher rate, increase the rate to 3.0 ml/kg/hr for 15 minutes and finally increase to a maximum rate of 6.0 ml/kg/hr. DO NOT EXCEED THIS RATE OF ADMINISTRATION. Monitor the patient closely during and after each rate change. In especially ill children with BPD, slower rates of infusion may be indicated.

A physician may want to consider factors such as other clinical illness, how well the child has grown and the risk of exposure from siblings or daycare when determining whether to use RSV-IGIV. Respiratory Syncytial Virus Immune Globulin Intravenous (Human) (RSV-IGIV). The first dose should be administered prior to commencement of the RSV season and subsequent doses should be administered monthly throughout the RSV season in order to maintain protection. In the Northern Hemisphere the RSV season typically commences in November and runs through April. Children should be infused from early November through April, unless RSV activity begins earlier or persists later in a community. It is recommended that RSV-IGIV be administered separately from other drugs or medications that the patient may be receiving. It is recommended that children infected with RSV continue to receive monthly doses of RSV-IGIV for the duration of the RSV season.

PREPARATION FOR ADMINISTRATION

Remove the tab portion of the vial cap and clean the rubber stopper with 70% alcohol or equivalent. RSV-IGIV, like all parenteral drug products, should be inspected for particulate matter and discoloration prior to administration. Infuse the solution only if it is colorless and not turbid. DO NOT SHAKE VIAL; AVOID FOAMING.

INFUSION

Infusion should begin within 6 hours and should be completed within 12 hours after the single-use vial is entered. The patient's vital signs and cardiopulmonary status should be assessed prior to infusion, before each rate increase, and thereafter at 30-minute intervals until 30 minutes following completion of the infusion. RSV-IGIV should be administered through an intravenous line using a constant infusion pump (*i.e.,* IVAC pump or equivalent). Predilution of RSV-IGIV before infusion is not recommended. If possible, RSV-IGIV should be administered through a separate intravenous line, although it may be 'piggy-backed' into a pre-existing line if that line contains one of the following dextrose solutions (with or without sodium chloride): 2.5%, 5%, 10%, or 20% dextrose in water. If a pre-existing line must be used, the RSV-IGIV should not be diluted more than 1:2 with any other of the above-named solutions. Admixtures of RSV-IGIV with any other solutions have not been evaluated. While filters are not necessary, an in-line filter with a pore size larger than 15 micrometers may be used for the infusion of RSV-IGIV.

To prevent the transmission of hepatitis viruses or infectious agents from one person to another, sterile disposable syringes and needles should be used. Do not reuse syringes and needles.

HOW SUPPLIED:

RespiGam, Respiratory Syncytial Virus Immune Globulin Intravenous (Human) is supplied in a single-use vial containing:

Respiratory Syncytial Virus Immune Globulin:

Total Quantity of Immunoglobulin = 2500 mg ± 500 mg, Concentration 50 mg ± 10 mg/ml

Storage: RSV-IGIV should be stored between 2°C and 8° C (35.6° F and 46.4° F). Do not freeze.

REFERENCES:

1. Siber GR, Leszczynski J, Pena-Cruz V, et al. Protective Activity of a Human Respiratory Syncytial Virus Immune Globulin Prepared from Donors Screened by Microneutralization Assay. J. Infect. Dis.: 165:456-463, 1992. **2.** Horowitz B, Wiebe ME, Lippin A, et al. Inactivation of Viruses in Labile Blood Derivatives. Transfusion: 25:516-522, 1985. **3.** Siber GR, Leombruno D, Leszczynski J, et al. Comparison of Antibody Concentrations and Protective Activity of Respiratory Syncytial Virus (RSV) Immune Globulin and Conventional Immune Globulin. J. Infect. Dis.: 169:1368-1373, 1994. **4.** Groothuis JR, Simoes EAF, Lehr MV, et al. Safety and

REFERENCES: *(cont'd)*

Bioequivalency of Three Formulations of Respiratory Syncytial Virus-enriched Immunoglobulin. Antimicrob. Agents Chemother: 39:668-671, 1995. **5.** Groothuis JR, Gutierrez M, Lauer B. Respiratory Syncytial Virus Infection in Children with Bronchopulmonary Dysplasia. Pediatrics: 82: 199-203, 1988. **6.** Green, Brayer, Schenkman and Wald. Ped. Inf. Dis. J.: 8:601-605, 1989. **7.** Groothuis JR, Simoes EAF, Hemming VG, et al. Prophylactic Administration of Respiratory Syncytial Virus (RSV) Immune Globulin in High Risk Infants and Young Children. N. Engl. J. Med.: 329:1524-30, 1993. **8.** Ellenberg SS, Epstein JS, Fratantoni JC, et al. A Trial of RSV Immune Globulin in Infants and Young Children; The FDA's View. N. Engl. J. Med.: 331:203-204, 1994. **9.** Groothuis JR, Hemming VR, Siber GR, et al. Reply to ibid. N. Engl. J. Med.: 331:204-205, 1994. **10,** Sekul E, Culper E, Daiaks M. Aseptic Meningitis Associated with High-dose Intravenous Immunoglobulin Therapy: Frequency and Risk Factors. Ann. Int. Med.: 123:259-262, 1994. **11.** Kato E, Shindo S, Eto Y, et al. Administration of Immune Globulin Associated with Aseptic Meningitis. JAMA: 3269-3270, 1988. **12.** Casteels Van Daele M, Wijndaele L, Hunnick K, et al. Intravenous Immunoglobulin and Acute Aseptic Meningitis. N. Engl. J. Med.: 323:614-615, 1990. **13.** Scribner C, Kapit R, Phillips E, et al. Aseptic Meningitis and Intravenous Immunoglobulin Therapy. Ann. Int. Med.: 121:305-306, 1994. **14.** Bossell J. Safety of Therapeutic Immune Globulin Preparations with Respect to Transmission of Human T-lymphotropic Virus Type III/ Lymphadenopathy-Associated Virus Infection. MMWR: 35:231-233, 1986. **15.** Wells MA, Wittek AE, Epstein JS, et al. Inactivation and Partition of Human T-cell Lymphotrophic Virus. Type III. During Ethanol Fractionation of Plasma. Transfusion: 26:210-213, 1986. **16.** McIver J, Grady G. Immunoglobulin Preparations. In: Churchill WH and Kurtz S R, (ed): Transfusion Medicine. Boston: Blackwell: 1988. **17.** Schneider L, Geha R. Outbreak of Hepatitis C Associated with Intravenous Immunoglobulin Administration - United States October 1993 - June 1994. MMWR: 43:505-509, 1994. **18.** Edwards CA, Piet MPJ, Chin S, et al. Tri(n Butyl) Phosphate Detergent Treatment of Licensed Therapeutic and Experimental Blood Derivatives. Vox Sang: 52:53-59, 1987. **19.** Siber GR, Werner BG, Halsey NA, et al. Interference of Immune Globulin with Measles and Rubella Immunization. J. Pediatrics: 122:204-211, 1993. **20.** General Recommendations on Immunization. Recommendations of the Advisory Committee on Immunization Practices. MMWR: 43:1-38, 1994.

HOW SUPPLIED - EQUIVALENTS NOT AVAILABLE:

Injection - Intravenous - 50 ml

Vial $599.21 RESPIGAM, Medimmune 60574-2101-01

RESPIRATORY VACCINE, MIXED *(002181)*

CATEGORIES: Serums, Toxoids and Vaccines; Toxoids; Vaccines; FDA Pre 1938 Drugs

BRAND NAMES: Mrv

Prescribing information not available at time of publication.

HOW SUPPLIED - EQUIVALENTS NOT AVAILABLE:

Injection, Solution - Intramuscular

20 ml $43.24 MRV, Miles Spokane 00118-9978-01

RETEPLASE *(003334)*

CATEGORIES: Anticoagulants/Thrombolytics; Blood Formation/Coagulation; Embolism; Congestive Heart Failure; Enzymes; Heart Failure; Myocardial Infarction; Pulmonary Embolism; Thrombolytic Agents; Pregnancy Category C; FDA Approved 1996 Nov

BRAND NAMES: **Retavase**

DESCRIPTION:

Reteplase is a non-glycosylated deletion mutein of tissue plasminogen activator (tPA)[1] containing the kringle 2 and the protease domains of human tPA. Reteplase contains 355 of the 527 amino acids of native tPA (amino acids 1-3 and 176-527), reteplase is produced by recombinant DNA technology in *E. coli.* The protein is isolated as inactive inclusion bodies from *E. coli*, converted into its active form by an *in vitro* folding process and purified by chromatographic separation. The molecular weight of reteplase is 39,571 daltons.

Potency is expressed in units (U) using a reference standard which is specific for reteplase and is not comparable with units used for other thrombolytic agents.

Reteplase is a sterile, white lyophilized powder for intravenous bolus injection after reconstitution with Sterile Water for Injection, USP (without preservatives) provided as part of a kit. Following reconstitution, the pH is 7.2 ± 0.2. Retavase is supplied as a 10.8 U vial to ensure sufficient drug for administration of each 10 U dose. Each single vial dose contains: Reteplase 18.8 mg, L-Arginine 940.7 mg, Phosphoric Acid 290.1 mg, Polysorbate 20 1.1 mg.

CLINICAL PHARMACOLOGY:

Reteplase is a recombinant plasminogen activator which catalyzes the cleavage of endogenous plasminogen to generate plasmin. Plasmin in turn degrades the fibrin matrix of the thromus, thereby exerting its thrombolytic action.[1,2] In a controlled trial, 35 of 68 patients treated for an acute myocaridal infarction (AMI) had a decrease in fibrogen levels to below 100 mg/dl by 2 hours following the administration of reteplase as a double-bolus intravenous injection (10 + 10 U) in which 10 U (17.4 mg) was followed 30 minutes later by a second bolus of 10 U (17.4 mg).[3] The mean fibrinogen level returned to the baseline value by 48 hours.

Pharmacokinetics: Based on the measurement of thrombolytic activity, reteplase is cleared from plasma at a rate of 250-450 ml/min, with an effective half-life of 13-16 minutes. Reteplase is cleared primarily by the liver and kidney.

CLINICAL STUDIES:

The safety and efficacy of reteplase were evaluated in three controlled clinical trials in which reteplase was compared to other thrombolytic agents. The INJECT study was designed to assess the relative effects of reteplase or the Streptase brand of streptokinase upon mortality rates at 35 days following an AMI. The other studies (RAPID 1 and RAPID 2) were arteriorgraphic studies which compared the effect on coronary potency of reteplase to two regimens of alteplase (a tissue plasminogen activator; Activase in the USA and Actilyse in Europe) in patients with an AMI. In all three studies, patients were treated with aspirin (initial doses of 160 mg to 350 mg and subsequent doses of 75 mg to 350 mg) and heparin (a 5000 U IV bolus prior to the administration of reteplase, followed by a 1000 U/hr continuous IV infusion for at least 24 hours). [2,8,11] The safety and efficacy of reteplase have not been evaluated using antithrombotic or antiplatelet regimens other than those described above.

Reteplase (10+10U) was compared to streptokinase (1.5 million units over 60 minutes) in a double-blind, randomized, European study (INJECT), which studied 6010 patients treated within 12 hours of the onset of symptoms of AMI. To be eligible for enrollment, patients had to have chest pain consistent with coronary ischemia and ST segment elevation, or a bundle branch block pattern on the EKG. Patients with known cerebrovascular or other bleeding risks or those with a systolic blood pressure >200 mm Hg or a diastolic blood pressure >100 mm Hg were excluded from enrollment. The results of the primary endpoint (mortality at 35 days), six month mortality and selected other 35 day endpoints are shown in TABLE 1 for patients receiving study medications.

For mortality, stroke and the combined outcome of mortality or stroke, the95% confidence intervals in TABLE 1reflect the range within which the true difference in outcomes probably lies and includes the possibility of no difference. The incidences of congestive heart failure and of cardiogenic shock were significantly lower among patients treated with reteplase.

CLINICAL STUDIES: *(cont'd)*

TABLE 1 INJECT Trial: Incidence of Selected Outcomes

Endpoint	Reteplase (n=2985)	Streptokinase (n=2971)	Reteplase, Streptokinase Difference (95% CI)	P- Value
35 Day mortality	8.9%	9.4%	-0.5 (-2.0,0.9)	0.49*
6 Month mortality†	11.0%	12.1%	-1.1 (-2.7, 0.5)	0.22
Combined outcome of 35 day mortality or nonfatal stroke within 35 days	9.5%	10.2%	-0.6 (-2.1, 1.0)	0.47
Heart failure	24.8%	28.1%	-3.3 (-5.6, -1.1)	0.004
Cardiogenic shock	4.6%	5.8%	-1.2 (-2.4, -0.1)	0.03
Any stroke	1.4%	1.1%	0.3 (-0.3, 0.8)	0.34
Intracranial hemorrhage	0.8%	0.4%	0.4 (0.0, 0.8)	0.04

* p value for the exploratory analysis comparing reteplase versus streptokinase.
† Kaplan-Meier estimates.

The total incidence of stroke was similar between the groups. However, more patients treated with reteplase experienced hemorrhagic strokes than patients treated with streptokinase. An exploratory analysis indicated that the incidence of intracranial hemorrhage was higher among older patients or those with elevated blood pressure. The incidence of intracranial hemorrhage among the 698 patients treated with reteplase who were older than 70 years was 2.2%. Intracranial hemorrhage occurred in 8 of the 332 (2.4%) patients treated with reteplase who had an initial systolic blood pressure >160 mm Hg and in 15 of the 2629 (0.6%) reteplase patients who had an initial systolic blood pressure <160 mm Hg.

Two arteriographic studies (RAPID 1and RAPID 2) were performed utilizing open-label administration of the study agents and a blinded review of the arteriograms. In RAPID 1, patients were treated within 6 hours of the onset of symptoms, and in RAPID 2, patients were treated within 12 hours of the onset of symptoms. Both studies evaluated coronary artery perfusion through the infarct-related artery 90 minutes after the initiation of therapy as the primary endpoint. Some patients in each study also had perfusion through the infarct-related artery evaluated at 60 minutes after the initiation of therapy. In RAPID 1, reteplase (in doses of 10+10 U, 15 U, or 10+5 U) was compared to a 3 hour regimen of alteplase (100 mg administered over 3 hours). In RAPID 2, reteplase (10+10 U) was compared to an accelerated regimen of alteplase (100 mg administered over 1.5 hours). The percentages of patients with partial or complete flow (TIMI grades 2 or 3) and complete flow (TIMI grade 3), are shown along with ventricular function assessments in TABLE 2A and TABLE 2B. The follow-up arteriogram was performed at a median of 8 (RAPID 1) and 5 (RAPID 2) days following the administration of the thrombolytics. In RAPID 1 the best potency results were obtained with the 10+10 U dose. In RAPID 2, the percentage of patients with partial or complete flow and the percentage of patients with complete flow was significantly higher with reteplase than with alteplase at 90 minutes after the intiation of therapy. In both clinical trials the inclusion rates were similar for reteplase and alteplase.

TABLE 2A RAPID 2 Trial: Arteriographic Results

Outcome	Reteplase (10+10 U)	Alteplase (Accelerated regimen)	p
90 minute potency rates	n=157	n=146	
TIMI 2 or 3	83%	73%	0.03
TIMI 3	60%	45%	0.01
Follow-up potency rates	n=128	n=113	
TIMI 2 or 3	89%	90%	0.76
TIMI 3	75%	77%	0.72
Follow-up	n=89	n=77	
ejection fraction mean %	52%	54%	0.25
Follow-up regional wall motion	n=87	n=72	
standard deviation from mean normal value	-2.3	-2.3	0.96

* p values represent one of the multiple dose comparisons

TABLE 2B RAPID 1 Trial: Arteriographic Results

Outcome	Reteplase (10+10 U)	Alteplase (Accelerated regimen)	p
90 minute potency rates	n=142	n=145	
TIMI 2 or 3	85%	77%	0.08
TIMI 3	63%	49%	0.02
Follow-up potency rates	n=123	n=123	
TIMI 2 or 3	95%	88%	0.04
TIMI 3	88%	71%	0.001
Follow-up	n=91	n=84	
ejection fraction mean %	53%	49%	0.03
Follow-up regional wall motion	n=84	n=80	
standard deviation from mean normal value	-2.2	-2.6	0.02

* p values represent one of the multiple dose comparisons

Approximately 70% (RAPID 1) and 78% (RAPID 2) of the patients in the arteriographic studies underwent optional arteriography at 60 minutes following the administration of the study agents. In both trials the percentage of patients with complete flow at 60 minutes was significantly higher with reteplase than with alteplase. Neither RAPID clinical trial was designed nor powered to compare the efficacy or safety of reteplase and alteplase with respect to the outcomes of mortality and stroke.

INDICATIONS AND USAGE:

Reteplase is indicated for the use in the management of acute myocardial infarction (AMI) in adults for the improvement of ventricular function following AMI, the reduction of the incidence of congestive heart failure and the reduction of mortality associated with AMI. Treatment should be initiated as soon as possible after the inset of AMI symptoms (see CLINICAL PHARMACOLOGY).

CONTRAINDICATIONS:

Because thrombolytic therapy increases the risk of bleeding, reteplase is contraindicated in the following situations:

Active internal bleeding

CONTRAINDICATIONS: *(cont'd)*

History of cerebrovascular accident

Recent intracranial or intraspinal surgery or trauma (see WARNINGS).

Intracranial neoplasm, arteriovenous malformation or aneurysm

Known bleeding diarhesis

Severe uncontrolled hypertension

WARNINGS:

BLEEDING

The most common complication encountered during reteplase therapy is bleeding. The sites of bleeding include both internal bleeding sites (intracranial, retroperitoneal, gastrointestinal, genitourinary, or respiratory) and superficial bleeding sites (venous cutdowns, arterial punctures, sites of recent surgical intervention). The concomitant use of heparin anticoagulation may contribute to bleeding. In clinical trials some of the hemorrhage episodes occurred one or more days after the effects of reteplase had dissipated, but while heparin therapy was continuing.

As fibrin is lysed during reteplase therapy, bleeding from recent puncture sites may occur. Therefore, thrombolytic therapy requires careful attention to all potential bleeding sites (including catheter insertion sites, arterial and venous puncture sites, cutdown sites, and needle puncture sites). Noncompressible arterial puncture must be avoided and internal jugular and subclavian venous punctures should be avoided to minimize bleeding from noncompressible sites. Should an arterial puncture be necessary during the administration of reteplase, it is preferable to use an upper extremity vessel that is accessible to natural compression. Pressure should be applied for at least 30 minutes, a pressure dressing applied, and the puncture site checked frequently for evidence of bleeding.

Intramuscular injections and nonessential handling of the patient should be avoided during treatment with reteplase. Venipuncture should be performed carefully and only as required.

Should serious bleeding (not controllable by local pressure) occur, concomitant anticoagulant therapy should be terminated immediately. In addition, the second bolus of reteplase should not be given if serious bleeding occurs before it is administered.

Each patient being considered for therapy with reteplase should be carefully evaluated and anticipated benefits weighed against the potential risks associated with therapy. In the following conditions, the risks of reteplase therapy may be increased and should be weighed against the anticipated benefits:

Recent major surgery *e.g.,* coronary artery bypass graft, obstetrical delivery, organ biopsy)

Previous puncture of noncompressible vessels

Cerebrovascular disease

Recent gastrointestinal or genitourinary bleeding

Recent trauma

Hypertension: systolic BP ≥180 mm Hg and/or diastolic BP ≥110 mm Hg

High likelihood of left heart thrombus (*e.g.,* mitral stonosis with atrial fibrillation)

Acute pericarditis

Subacute bacterial endocarditis

Hemostatic defects including those secondary to severe hepatic or renal disease

Severe hepatic or renal dysfunction

Pregnancy

Diabetic hemorrhagic retinopathy or other hemorrhagic ophthalmic conditions

Septic thrombophlebitis or occluded AV cannula at a seriosly infected site

Advanced age

Patients currently receiving oral anticoagulants (*e.g.,* warfarin sodium)

Any other condition in which bleeding constitutes a significant hazard or would be particularly difficult to manage because of its location

CHOLESTEROL EMBOLIZATION

Cholesterol embolization has been reported rarely in patients treated with thrombolytic agents; the true incidence is unknown. This serious condition, which can be lethal, is also associated with invasive vascular procedures (*e.g.,* cardiac catherization, angiography, vascular surgery) and/or anticoagulant therapy. Clinical features of cholesterol embolism may include livedo reticularis, "purple toe" syndrome, acute renal failure, gangrenous digits, hypertension, pancreatitis, myocardial infarction, cerebral infarction, spinal cord infarction, retinal artery occlusion, bowel infarction, and rhabdomyolysis

ARRHYTHMIAS

Coronary thrombolysis may result in arrhythmias associated with reperfusion. These arrhythmias (such as sinus bradycardia, accelerated idioventricular rhythm, ventricular premature depolarizations, ventricular tachycardia) are not different from those often seen in the ordinary course of acute myocardial infarction and should be managed with standard antiarrhythmic measures. It is recommended that antiarrhythmic therapy for bradycardia and/or ventricular irritability be available when reteplase is administered.

PRECAUTIONS:

GENERAL

Standard management of myocardial infarction should be implemented concomitantly with reteplase treatment. Arterial and venous punctures should be minimized (see WARNINGS). In addition, the second bolus of reteplase should not be given if serious bleeding occurs before it is administered. In the event of serious bleeding, any concomitant heparin should be terminated immediately. Heparin effects can be reversed by proamitine.

READMINISTRATION

There is no experience with patients receiving repeat courses of therapy with reteplase. Reteplase did not induce the formation of reteplase specific antibodies in any of the approximately 2400 patients who were tested for antibody formation in clinical trials. If an anaphylactoid reaction occurs, the second bolus of reteplase should not be given, and the appropriate therapy should be initiated.

DRUG/LABORATORY TEST INTERACTIONS

Administration of reteplase may cause decreases in plasminogen and fibrinogen. During reteplase therapy, if coagulation test and/or measurements of fibrinolytic activity are performed, the results may be unreliable unless specific precautions are taken to prevent *in vitro* artifacts. Reteplase is an enzyme that when present in blood in pharmacologic concentrations remains active under *in vitro* conditions. This can lead to degradation of fibrinogen in blood samples removed for analysis. Collection of blood samples in the presence of PPACK (chloromethylkotons) at 2 μM concentrations was used in clinical trials to prevent *in vitro* fibrinolytic artifacts.

USE OF ANTITHROMBOLYTICS

Heparin and aspirin have been administered concomitantly with and following the administration of reteplase in the management of acute myocardial infarction. Because heparin, aspirin, or reteplase may cause bleeding complications, careful monitoring for bleeding is advised, especially at atrial puncture sites.

PRECAUTIONS: *(cont'd)*

CARCINOGENESIS, MUTAGENESIS, AND IMPAIRMENT OF FERTILITY

Long-term studies in animals have not been performed to evaluate the carcinogenic potential of reteplase. Studies to determine mutagenicity, chromosomal aberrations, gene mutations, and micronucleic induction were negative at all concentrations tested. Reproductive toxicity studies in rats revealed no effects on fertility at doses up to 15 times the human dose (4.31 U/kg).

PREGNANCY CATEGORY C

Reteplase has been shown to have an abortifacient effect in rabbits when given in doses 3 times the human dose (0.86 U/kg). Reproduction studies performed in rats at doses up to 15 times the human dose (4.31 U/kg) revealed no evidence of fetal anomalies; however, reteplase administered to pregnant rabbits resulted in hemorrhaging in the genital tract, leading to abortions in mid-gestation. There are no adequate and well-controlled studies in pregnant women. The most common complication of thrombolytic therapy is bleeding and certain conditions, including pregnancy, can increase this risk. Reteplase should be used during pregnancy only if the potential benefit justifies the potential risk to the fetus.

NURSING MOTHERS

It is not known whether reteplase is excreted in human milk. Because many drugs are excreted in human milk, caution should be exercised when reteplase is administered to a nursing woman.

PEDIATRIC USE

Safety and effectiveness in pediatric patients have not been established.

DRUG INTERACTIONS:

The interaction of reteplase with other cardioactive drugs has not been studied. In addition to bleeding associated with heparin and vitamin K antagonists, drugs that alter platelet function (such as aspirin, dipyridamole, and abciximab) may increase the risk of bleeding if administered prior to or after reteplase therapy.

ADVERSE REACTIONS:

BLEEDING

The most frequent adverse reaction associated with reteplase is bleeding (see WARNINGS). The types of bleeding events associated with thrombolytic therapy may be broadly categorized as either intracranial hemorrhage or other types of hemorrhage.

Intracranial Hemorrhage: (See CLINICAL PHARMACOLOGY) In the INJECT clinical trial the rate of in-hospital, intracranial hemorrhage among all patients treated with reteplase was 0.8% (23 of 2965 patients). As seen with reteplase and other thrombolytic agents, the risk for intracranial hemorrhage is increased in patients with advanced age or with elevated blood pressure.

Other Types of Hemorrhage: The incidence of other types of bleeding events in clinical studies of reteplase varied depending upon the use of arterial catherization or other invasive procedures and whether the study was performed in Europe or the USA. The overall incidence of any bleeding event in patients treated with reteplase in clinical studies (n=3805) was 21.1%. The rates for bleeding events, regardless of severity, for the 10+10 U reteplase regimen from controlled clinical studies are summarized in TABLE 3.

TABLE 3 Reteplase Hemorrhage Rates

Bleeding Site	INJECT Europe (n=2965)	RAPID 1 and RAPID 2 USA (n=218)	RAPID 1 and RAPID 2 Europe (n=113)
Injection Site*	4.6%	48.6%	19.5%
Gastrointestinal	2.5%	9.0%	1.8%
Genitourinary	1.6%	9.5%	0.9%
Anemia, site unknown	2.8%	1.4%	0.9%

* Includes the arterial catherization site (all patients in the RAPID studies underwent arterial catherization).

In those studies the severity and sites of bleeding events were comparable for reteplase and the comparison thrombolytic agents.

Should serious bleeding in a critical location (intracranial, gastrointestinal, retroperitoneal, pericardial) occur, any contcomitant heparin should be terminated immediately. In addition, the second bolus of reteplase should not be given if the serious bleeding occurs before it is administered. Death and permanent disability are not uncommonly reported in patients who have experienced stroke (including intracranial bleeding) and other serious bleeding episodes.

Fibrin, which is part of the hemostatic plug formed at needle puncture sites will be lysed during reteplase therapy. Therefore, reteplase therapy requires careful attention to potential bleeding sites (*e.g.,* catheter insertion sites, arterial puncture sites).

ALLERGIC REACTIONS

Among the 2965 patients receiving reteplase in the INJECT trial, serious allergic reactions were noted in 3 patients, with one patient experiencing dyspnea and hypotension. No anaphylactoid reactions were observed among the 3856 patients treated with reteplase in initial clinical trials. In an ongoing clinical trial two anaphylactoid reactions have been reported among approximately 2500 patients receiving reteplase.

OTHER ADVERSE REACTIONS

Patients adminsitered reteplase as treatment for myocardial infarction have experienced many events which are frequent sequelae of myocardial infarction and may or may not be attributable to reteplase therapy. These events include cardiogenic shock, arrhythmias (*e.g.,* sinus bradycardia, accelerated idioventricular rhythm, ventricular premature depolarization, supraventricular tachycardia, ventricular tachycardia, ventricular fibrillation), AV block, pulmonary edema, heart failure, cardiac arrest, recurrent ischemia, reinfarction, myocardial rupture, mitral regurgitation, pericardial effusion, pericarditis, cardiac tamponade, venous thrombosis and embolism, and electromechanical dissociation. These events can be life-threatening and may lead to death. Other adverse events have been reported, including nausea and/or vomiting, hypotension, and fever.

DOSAGE AND ADMINISTRATION:

Reteplase is for intravenous administration only. Reteplase is administered as a 10+10 U double-bolus injection. Each bolus is administered as an intravenous injection over 2 minutes. The second bolus is given 30 minutes after initiation of the first bolus injection. Each bolus injection should be given via an intravenous line in which no other medication is being simultaneously injected or infused. No other medication should be added to the injection solution containing reteplase. There is no experience with patients receiving repeat courses of therapy with reteplase.

Heparin and reteplase are incompatible when combined in solution. Do not administer heparin and reteplase simultaneously in the same intravenous line. If reteplase is to be injected through an intravenous line containg heparin, a normal saline or 5% dextrose (DSW) solution should be flushed through the line prior to and following the retevase injection.

DOSAGE AND ADMINISTRATION: *(cont'd)*

Although the value of anticoagulants and antiplatelt drugs during and following administration of reteplase has not been studied, heparin has been administered concomitantly in more than 99% of patients. Aspirin has been given either during and/or following heparin treatment. Studies assessing the safety and efficacy of reteplase without adjunctive therapy with heparin and aspirin have not been performed.

RECONSTITUTION

Reconstitution should be carried out using the diluent, syringe, needle and dispensing pin provided with reteplase. It is important that reteplase be reconstituted only with Sterile Water for injection, USP (without preservative). The reconstituted preparation results in a colorless solution containing reteplase 1 U/ml. Slight foaming upon reconstitution is not unusual; allowing the vial to stand undisturbed for several minutes is ususally sufficient to allow dissipation of any large bubbles.

Because retavase contains no antibacterial preservatives, it should be reconstituted immediately before use. When reconstituted as directed, the solution may be used within 4 hours when stored at 2°-30°C (35°-86°F). Prior to administration, the product should be visually inspected for particulate matter and discoloration.

RECONSTITUTION INSTRUCTIONS

Use aseptic technique throughout.

Step 1: Remove the protective flip-cap from one vial of Sterile Water for Injection, USP (SWFI). Open the package containing the 10 cc syringe with attached needle. Remove the protective cap from the needle and withdraw 10 ml of SWFI from the vial.

Step 2: Open the package containing the dispensing pin. Remove the needle from the syringe, discard the needle. Remove the protective cap from the lock port of the dispensing pin and connect the syringe to the dispensing pin. Remove the protective flip-cap from one vial of Retavase.

Step 3: Remove the protective cap from the spike end of the dispensing pin, and insert the spike into the vial of Retavase. Transfer the 10 ml of SWFI through the dispensing pin into the vial of Retavase.

Step 4: With the dispensing pin and syringe still attached to the vial, swirl the vial gently to dissolve the Retavase. **DO NOT SHAKE.**

Step 5: Withdraw 10 ml of retavase reconstituted solution back into the syringe. A small amount of solution (0.7 ml) will remain in the vial due to overfill.

Step 6: Detach the syringe from the dispensing pin, and attach the sterile 20 gauge needle provided.

Step 7: The 10 ml bolus is now ready for administration.

Safely discard all used reconstitution components and the empty Retavase vial according to institutional procedures.

REFERENCES:

1. Martin U, Spooner G, Strein K. Evaluation of thrombolutic and systemic effects of the novel recombinant plasminogen activator BM 06.022 compared with alteplase, anistreptase, streptokinase and urokinase in a canine model of coronary artery thrombosis; *JACC.* 1992;19:433-440 **2.** Kohnert U, Rudolph R, Verheijen JH. Biochemical properties of the kringle 2 and protease domains are maintained in the unfolded t-PA deletion variant BM 06.022. *Protein Engineering.* 1992:5;93-100. **3.** Smalling R, Bode C, Kalbfleisch J, et al. More rapid, complete, and stable coronary thrombolysis with bolus administration of reteplase compared with alteplase infusion in acute myocardial infarction. *Circulation.* 1995:91;2725-2732. **4.** Bode C, Smalling R, Gunther B, et al. Randomized comparsion of coronary thrombolysis achieved with double bolus reteplase (recombinant plasminogen activator) and front-loaded, accelerated alteplase (recombinant tissue plasminogen activator) in patients with acute myocardial infarction. *Circulation.* 1996:94;891-898. **5.** INJECT Study Group. Randomized, double-blind comparison of reteplase double-bolus administration with streptokinase in acute myocardial infarction (INJECT): trial to investigate equivalence. *Lancet.* 1995:546;329-336. **6.** Martin U, Gartner D, Markl HJ, et al. D-PHE-PRO-ARGCHLOROMETHYLKETONE prevents *in vitro* fibrinogen reduction by the novel recombinant plasminogen activator BM 06.022. *Ann Hematol.* 1992;64(suppl)A47.

HOW SUPPLIED:

Retavase is supplied as a sterile, preservative-free, lyophilized powder in 10.8 U (18.8 mg) vials without a vacuum, in a kit with components for reconstitution. Each kit contains a package insert, 2 single-use Retavase vials 10.8 U (18.8 mg), 2 single-use diluent vials for reconstitution (10 ml Sterile Water for Injection, USP), 2 sterile 10 cc syringes with 20 G needle attached, 2 steirle dispensing pins, 2 sterile 20 G needles for dose administration, and 2 alcohol swabs.

Storage: Store the kit containing retaplase at 2°-25°C (36°-77°F). Kit should remain sealed until use to protect the lyophilisate from exposure to light. Do not use beyond expiration date printed on the kit.

RHO (D) IMMUNE GLOBULIN *(002184)*

CATEGORIES: Abortion; Blood Components/Substitutes; Blood Formation/Coagulation; Hemolytic Disease; Hemorrhage; Immune Globulin; Immunologic; Orphan Drugs; Pregnancy; Red Blood Cells; Serums, Toxoids and Vaccines; Vaccines; Pregnancy Category C; FDA Pre 1938 Drugs

BRAND NAMES: *Anti Rho (D)* (Mexico); *Bay Rho-D*; *Cutter Hyperab*; *Cutter Hyprho-D*; Gamulin Rh; **Hyprho-D**; *IGRHO*; Mini-Gamulin Rh; *Partobulin*; *Partogloman*; *Probi RHO (D)* (Mexico); *Rhesogam* (Germany); *Rhesogamma*; Rhesonativ; *Rhesugam*; *Rhesuman*; *Rhesuman Berna*; *Rhogam*; Winrho Sd
(International brand names outside U.S. in italics)

DESCRIPTION:

Rh_o(D) Immune Globulin (Human) Gamulin Rh, is a sterile immunoglobulin solution containing Rh_o(D) antibodies for intramuscular use only. It is obtained by alcohol fractionation of plasma from human blood donors, concentrated and standardized to give a total globulin content of 11.5 ± 1.5 percent. All lots are assayed for Rh_o(D) antibody content by a serological method (anti-globulin titer). The Rh_o(D) antibody level in each vial or syringe of Gamulin Rh is equal to or greater than that of the Office of Biologics Research and Review Reference Rh_o(D) Immune Globulin (Human). This dose has been shown to effectively inhibit the immunizing potential of up to 15 ml of Rh-positive packed red blood cells.

The final product contains 0.3 molar glycine as a stabilizer and 0.01% thimerosal (mercury derivative) as a preservative.

Mini-Gamulin Rh: Mini-Gamulin Rh contains one-sixth the quantity of Rh_o(D) Immune Globulin (Human). The contents of one vial or syringe of Mini-Gamulin Rh will suppress the immunizing potential of 5 ml of whole blood or 2.5 ml of packed red blood cells.

CLINICAL PHARMACOLOGY:

Gamulin Rh effectively suppresses the immune response of non-sensitized Rh_o(D) negative individuals who receive Rh_o(D) positive blood as the result of a fetomaternal hemorrhage or a transfusion accident. The administration of Rh_o(D) antibody to an Rh_o(D) negative mother or to the Rh negative recipient of Rh positive red cells suppresses the antibody response and the formation of anti-Rh_o(D). Clinical studies indicated that the administration of Rh_o(D) immune globulin within 72 hours of a full term delivery of an Rh_o(D) positive infant to an Rh_o(D) negative mother reduces the incidence of Rh isoimmunization from 12-13% to 1-2%.

CLINICAL PHARMACOLOGY: *(cont'd)*

Data have been reported to indicate that 1.5 to 1.8% of Rh_o(D) negative mothers, carrying Rh_o(D) positive fetuses, who are given Rh immune globulin postpartum may be immunized to Rh during the latter part of their pregnancies or after delivery. Bowman reported that the incidence of immunization can be further reduced from approximately 1.6% to less than 0.1% by administering Rh_o(D) immune globulin in two doses to Rh negative primigravida or multigravida patients. One antepartum at 28 weeks gestation and another following delivery.

INDICATIONS AND USAGE:

GAMULIN RH

Full Term Delivery: Rh_o(D) Immune Globulin (Human) Gamulin Rh is used to prevent sensitization to the Rh_o(D) factor and thus to prevent hemolytic disease of the newborn (Erythroblastosis fetalis) in a pregnancy that follows the injection of Gamulin Rh. It effectively suppresses the immune response of non-sensitized Rh-negative mothers after delivery of an Rh-positive infant.

Criteria for an Rh-incompatible pregnancy requiring administration of: Rh_o(D) Immune Globulin (Human) Gamulin Rh are:

1. The mother must be Rh_o(D) negative.

2. The mother should not have been previously sensitized to the Rh_o(D) factor.

3. The infant must be Rh_o(D) positive and direct antiglobulin negative.

Other Obstetric Conditions: Gamulin Rh should be administered to all non-sensitized Rh-negative women after spontaneous or induced abortions after ruptured tubal pregnancies, amniocentesis, and other abdominal trauma, or any occurrence of transplacental hemorrhage unless the blood type of the fetus has been determined to be Rh_o(D) negative.

If Rh_o(D) Immune Globulin (Human) Gamulin Rh is administered antepartum, it is essential that the mother receive another dose of Gamulin Rh after the delivery of an Rh_o(D) positive infant.

NOTE: In a case of abortion or ectopic pregnancy when Rh typing of the fetus is not possible, the fetus must be assumed to be Rh_o(D) positive. In such an instance the patient should be considered a candidate for administration of Rh_o(D) Immune Globulin (Human) Gamulin Rh.

If the father can be determined to be Rh_o(D) negative, Gamulin Rh need not be given.

Gamulin Rh should be given within 72 hours following an Rh-incompatible delivery, miscarriage or abortion.

Transfusions: Gamulin Rh can be used to prevent Rh_o(D) sensitization in Rh_o(D) negative patients accidentally transfused with Rh_o(D) positive RBC or blood components containing RBC.

It should be administered within 72 hours following an Rh-incompatible transfusion.

MINI-GAMULIN RH

Rh sensitization may occur in nonsensitized Rh_o(D) negative women following transplacental hemorrhage resulting from spontaneous or induced abortions. sensitization occurs more frequently in women undergoing induced abortions than those aborting spontaneously.

Rh_o(D) Immune Globulin, at the dosage level contained in one vial or syringe of Mini-Gamulin Rh prevents the formation of anti-Rh_o(D) antibodies in nonsensitized Rh_o(D) negative women who receive Rh_o(D) positive blood during transplacental hemorrhage resulting from spontaneous or induced abortion up to 12 weeks' gestation.

For spontaneous or induced abortions occurring after 12 weeks' gestation, an appropriate dose of standard Rh_o(D) Immune Globulin (Gamulin Rh) sufficient to suppress the immunizing potential of ml of Rh-positive packed red blood cells, should be given.

NOTE: Mini-Gamulin Rh Prophylaxis is not indicated if the fetus or the father can be determined to be Rh negative. If Rh typing of the fetus is not possible, the fetus must be assumed to be Rh_o(D) positive and the patient should be considered a candidate for treatment.

Mini-Gamulin Rh should be administered promptly following spontaneous or induced abortion. If prompt administration is not possible, Mini-Gamulin Rh should be given within 72 hours following termination of the pregnancy. However, if Mini-Gamulin is not given within this time period, administration of this product should be considered.

CONTRAINDICATIONS:

None known.

WARNINGS:

Gamulin Rh
Gamulin Rh must not be given to the Rho(D) positive postpartum infant.
Do not give intravenously.
Mini-Gamulin Rh
Do not inject intravenously.

PRECAUTIONS:

GENERAL

Gamulin Rh: Before administering Gamulin Rh, it is desirable that all diagnostic laboratory criteria be met, as outlined in the Preadministration Laboratory Procedures section below.

Babies born of women given Rh immune globulin antepartum may have a weakly positive antiglobulin test at birth.

Passively acquired anti-Rh_o(D) may be detected in maternal serum if antibody screening tests are performed subsequent to antepartum or postpartum administration of Gamulin Rh status, Gamulin Rh should be administered.

Mini-Gamulin Rh: A Separate, sterile syringe and needle should be used for each individual patient to avoid transmission of hepatitis B and other infectious agents from one person to another.

The possibility of hypersensitivity reaction is very remote but should be borne in mind. Epinephrine should be available for immediate use should hypersensitivity reaction occur.

PREGNANCY CATEGORY C

Animal reproduction studies have not been conducted with Rh_o(D) Immune Globulin (Human) Gamulin Rh. It is also not known whether Gamulin Rh can cause fetal harm when administered to a pregnant woman or can affect reproduction capacity. Gamulin Rh should be given to a pregnant woman only if clearly needed. However, use of Rh antibody during the third trimester in full doses of antibody has been reported to produce no evidence of hemolysis in the infant.

The presence of passively administered Rh antibody in the maternal blood sample can however, affect the interpretation of laboratory tests to identify the patient as a candidate for Rh_o(D) Immune Globulin (Human) Gamulin Rh. A large fetomaternal hemorrhage late in pregnancy or following delivery may cause a weak, mixed field positive D test result. If there is any doubt about the mother's Rh type, she should be given Rh_o(D) Immune Globulin (Human) Gamulin Rh. A screening test for fetal red blood cells may help in such cases. If more than 15 ml of Rh_o(D) positive fetal red blood cells are present in the mother's circulation, more than a single dose of Rh_o(D) Immune Globulin (Human) Gamulin Rh is required. Failure to recognize this may result in the administration of inadequate dose. In case of doubt as to the patient's Rh group of Immune status, Gamulin Rh should be administered.

ADVERSE REACTIONS:

Gamulin Rh: Since Gamulin Rh is an Rh_o(D) immune globulin derived from homologous human serum proteins, allergic reactions are not expected but the possibility cannot be ruled out. Such reactions have been reported following extensive use of immune serum globulin in hypogammaglobulinemic patients. On occasion a patient has shown a systemic reaction manifested by a low-grade fever but, generally, reactions have been mild, infrequent and confined to the site of injection.

Rh_o(D) negative patients inadvertently transfused with Rh_o(D) positive blood have received from 15 to 33 vials of Gamulin Rh with no adverse reaction other than soreness at the injection site. A 1°F temperature elevation in one patient which could have been due to the underlying illness has been reported.

Mini-Gamulin Rh: Reactions following intramuscular injection of Mini-Gamulin Rh, as with any immune globulin preparation, are infrequent, usually mild in nature, and confined to the site of injection. An occasional patient may react more strongly with localized tenderness, erythema, or low-grade fever. Rh_o(D) Immune Globulin and other immune globulins rarely cause systemic reactions or induce sensitization upon repeated injections.

DOSAGE AND ADMINISTRATION:

GAMULIN RH

Preadministration Laboratory Procedure

Infant: Immediately postpartum determine the infant's blood group (ABO Rh_o(D)) and perform a direct antiglobulin test. Umbilical cord, venous or capillary blood may be used.

Mother: Confirm that the mother is Rh_o(D) negative.

Dosage

Postpartum Prophylaxis Miscarriage, Abortion, Or Ectopic Pregnancy: One vial or syringe of Rh_o(D) Immune Globulin (Human) Gamulin Rh is sufficient to prevent maternal sensitization to the Rh factor if the fetal packed red blood cell volume which entered the mother's blood due to fetomaternal hemorrhage is less than 15 ml (30 ml of whole blood). When the fetomaternal hemorrhage exceeds 15 ml of packed cells or 30 ml of whole blood, more than one vial or syringe of Gamulin Rh should be administered.

Antepartum Prophylaxis: The Contents of one vial or syringe of Gamulin Rh injected intramuscularly at 28 weeks gestation and the contents of one vial or syringe within 72 hours after an Rh incompatible delivery is highly effective in preventing Rh iso-immunization during pregnancy.

To determine the number of vials or syringes required, the volume of packed fetal red blood cells must be determined by an approved laboratory assay, such as the Kleihauer-Betke Acid Elution Technic or the Clayton Modification. The volume of fetomaternal hemorrhage divided by two gives the volume of packed fetal red blood cells in the maternal blood. The number of vials or syringes of Gamulin Rh to be administered is determined by dividing the volume (ml) of packed red blood cells by 15.

Transfusion Accidents: The number of vials or syringes of Rh_o(D) Immune Globulin (Human) Gamulin Rh to be administered is dependent on the volume of packed red cells or whole blood transfused. The method to determine the number of vials or syringes of Gamulin Rh required to prevent sensitization is outlined below. If the dose calculation results in a fraction, administer the next whole number of vials or syringes of Gamulin Rh.

Procedure

a. Multiply the volume (in ml) of Rh-positive whole blood administered by the hematocrit of the donor unit. This value equals the volume of packed red blood cells transfused.

b. Divide the volume (in ml) of packed red blood cells by 15 to obtain the number of vials or syringes of Gamulin Rh to be administered.

Administration

Single Vial Or Syringe Dose: Inject intramuscularly the entire contents of the vial or syringe of Rh_o(D) Immune Globulin (Human) Gamulin Rh.

Multiple Vial Or Syringe Dose: The contents of the total number of vials or syringes may be injected as a divided dose at different injection sites at the same time or the total dosage may be divided and injected at intervals provided the total dosage to be given is injected within 72 hours postpartum or after a transfusion accident.

This product should be administered within 72 hours after Rh-incompatible delivery or transfusion.

Do not inject intravenously.

Parenteral drug products should be inspected visually for particulate matter and discoloration prior to administration, whenever solution and container permit. The following information should be included in the patient's records:

1. Patient's complete identification.

2. Patient's ABO and Rh group, and date determined.

3. Result of test for prior Rh sensitization.

4. Infant's ABO and Rh group, when known, and result of direct antiglobulin test, or in the case of transfusion accident, the ABO and Rh groups of the donor blood and the volume transfused.

5. Notification of patient concerning nature of medication, date and reason for giving it.

6. Lot number of Rh_o(D) Immune Globulin (Human) Gamulin Rh and date and time of injection and the number of vials or syringes injected.

7. Adequate documentation, if medication is refused by the patient.

Keep refrigerated at 2 to 8°C (36 to 46°F). Do not freeze.

MINI-GAMULIN RH

Do not inject intravenously

The contents of one vial or syringe of Mini-Gamulin Rh provides protection from Rh immunization for women with transplacental hemorrhage resulting from spontaneous or induced abortion up to 12 weeks' gestation. Inject intramuscularly the entire contents of the vial or syringe.

Mini-Gamulin Rh should be administered promptly following spontaneous or induced abortion. If prompt administration is not possible, Mini-Gamulin Rh should be given 72 hours following termination of pregnancy.

Parenteral drug products should be inspected visually for particulate matter and discoloration prior to administration whenever solution and container permit.

REFERENCES:

Rh_0(D) Immune Globulin (Human). *The Medical Letter On Drugs and Therapeutics* 16:3-4, 1974.Public Health Services Advisory Committee on Immunization Practices. *MMWR* 21:15 (April 21), 1972.Prevention of Rh sensitization. WHO Technical Report Series No. 468, 1971.Eich F.G., Tripodi D. Screening and quantitating fetal maternal hemorrhages *Amer J Clin Path* 61.192-198, 1974.Bowman J.M., Chown B. Prevention of Rh immunization after massive Rh-positive transfusion *Can Med J* 99:385-388, 1968.Keith L. Anti-Rh therapy after transfusion. *J Reprod Med* 8:293-298, 1972.Pollack W., et al. Studies of Rh prophylaxis. II Rh immune prophylaxis after transfusion with Rh-positive blood. *Transfusion* 11:340-344, 1971.Henny C.S., Ellis E.F. Antibody production to aggregated human γ G-globulin in acquired hypogammaglobulinemia *New England J Med* 278:1144-46, 1968.Walker R.H. Fetomaternal hemorrhage. A summary *American Association of Blood Banks - Technical Workshop* Chicago, September 12, 1971. pp 17-29.Chalos M.K. Detection of fetomaternal hemorrhage *American Association of Blood Banks - Technical Workshop* Chicago, September 12, 1971. pp 12-16Bowman J.M., Pollock J.M. Antenatal prophylaxis of Rh isoimmunization 28 weeks-gestation service program *Can Med J* 118:627-630, 1978.Zipursky A. and Israels L.G. The paibogenesis and prevention of Rh immunization. *Can Med J* 97:1245, 1967.Pollack W. Rh hemolytic disease of the newborn: its cause and prevention *Reprod Immunol.* Alan R. Liss, New York 1981.Bowman J.M., et al. Rh isoimmunization during pregnancy antenatal prophylaxis *Canad Med Assoc J* 118(6):623-627, 1971.Queenan JT, et al. Role of induced abortion in *Rhesus*immunization. *Lancet* 1.815-817, 1971Parmley, TH et al: Transplacental hemorrhage in patients subjected to therapeutic abortion. *Am J Obstet Gynecol* 106.540-542, 1970Grimes DA et al:Rh immunoglobulin utilization after spontaneous and induced abortion. *Obstet Gynecol* 50.261-263, 1977American College of Obstetricians and Gynecologists: Current use of Rh_0 immune globulin and detection of antibodies. *Technical Bulletin* 35, 1976World Health Organization: Prevention of Rh sensitization. *Technical Series* 468, 1971Scott JR:Report on Rh immune globulin therapy. *Cont Ob Gyn* 8;27-30. 1976Keith L. Bozorgi N. Small dose anti-Rh therapy after first trimester abortion. *Intern J. Gynecol Obstet* 15;235-237,1977

HOW SUPPLIED - EQUIVALENTS NOT AVAILABLE:

Injection, Solution - Intramuscular

single vial	$16.00	RHO, Centeon	00053-7591-02
1's	**$45.00**	**HYPRHO-D, Miles**	**00161-0621-15**
1's	**$45.00**	**Hyprho-D, Bayer Pharm**	**00192-0621-01**
5's	**$210.00**	**HYPRHO-D, Miles**	**00161-0621-25**
6's	$168.00	MINI-GAMULIN RH, Centeon	00053-7591-04
6's	$400.00	RH., Centeon	00053-7590-02
10's	**$268.75**	**Hyprho-D, Bayer Pharm**	**00192-0621-05**
10's	$280.00	MINI-GAMULIN RH, Centeon	00053-7591-06
10's	**$450.00**	**Hyprho-D, Bayer Pharm**	**00192-0621-10**
10's	**$450.00**	**HYPRHO-D, Bayer Pharm**	**00192-0621-22**
10's	$600.00	GAMULIN RH, Centeon	00053-7590-06
25 vials	$700.00	RHO, Centeon	00053-7591-03
25's	$1333.75	RH., Centeon	00053-7590-03

RIBAVIRIN *(002186)*

CATEGORIES: Anti-Infectives; Antimicrobials; Antivirals; Infections; Respiratory Syncytial Virus; Respiratory Tract Infections; Respiratory Tract Secretions; Viral Agents; Hepatitis C*; Pregnancy Category X; FDA Approved 1985 Dec
* Indication not approved by the FDA

BRAND NAMES: *Viramid*; *Virazid*; **Virazole**
(International brand names outside U.S. in italics)

COST OF THERAPY: $4,124.53 (Respiratory Syncytial Virus; Aerosol; 6 gm; 1/day; 3 days)

WARNING:
WARNINGS: USE OF AEROSOLIZED Ribavirin PATIENTS REQUIRING MECHANICAL VENTILATOR ASSISTANCE SHOULD BE UNDERTAKEN ONLY BY PHYSICIANS AND SUPPORT STAFF FAMILIAR WITH THE SPECIFIC VENTILATOR BEING USED AND THIS MODE OF ADMINISTRATION OF THE DRUG. STRICT ATTENTION MUST BE PAID TO PROCEDURES THAT HAVE BEEN SHOWN TO MINIMIZE THE ACCUMULATION OF DRUG PRECIPITATE, WHICH CAN RESULT IN MECHANICAL VENTILATOR DYSFUNCTION AND ASSOCIATED INCREASED PULMONARY PRESSURES (SEE WARNINGS).
SUDDEN DETERIORATION OF RESPIRATORY FUNCTION HAS BEEN ASSOCIATED HAS BEEN ASSOCIATED WITH INITIATION OF AEROSOLIZED Ribavirin USE IN INFANTS. RESPIRATORY FUNCTION SHOULD BE CAREFULLY MONITORED DURING TREATMENT. IF INITIATION OF AEROSOLIZED Ribavirin TREATMENT APPEARS TO PRODUCE SUDDEN DETERIORATION OF RESPIRATORY FUNCTION, TREATMENT SHOULD BE STOPPED AND REINSTITUTED ONLY WITH EXTREME CAUTION, CONTINUOUS MONITORING AND CONSIDERATION OF CONCOMITANT ADMINISTRATION OF BRONCHODILATORS (SEE WARNINGS).
Ribavirin IS NOT INDICATED FOR USE IN ADULTS. PHYSICIANS AND PATIENTS SHOULD BE AWARE THAT RIBAVIRIN HAS BEEN SHOWN TO PRODUCE TESTICULAR LESIONS IN RODENTS AND TO BE TERATOGENIC IN ALL ANIMAL SPECIES IN WHICH ADEQUATE STUDIES HAVE BEEN CONDUCTED (RODENTS AND RABBITS); (SEE CONTRAINDICATIONS).

DESCRIPTION:

Ribavirin is a synthetic, nucleoside with antiviral activity. Ribavirin for inhalation solution is a sterile, lyophilized powder to be reconstituted for aerosol administration. Each 100 ml glass vial contains 6 grams of ribavirin, and when reconstituted to the recommended volume of 300 ml with sterile water for injection sterile water for inhalation (no preservatives added), will contain 20 mg of ribavirin per ml, pH approximately 5.5. Aerosolization is to be carried out in a Small Particle Aerosol Generator (SPAG-2) nebulizer only.

Ribavirin is 1-beta-D-ribofuranosyl-1H-1,2,4-triazole-3-carboxamide.

Ribavirin is a stable, white crystalline compound with a maximum solubility in water of 142 mg/ml at 25°C and with only a slight solubility in ethanol. The empirical formula is $C_8H_{12}N_4O_5$ and the molecular weight is 244.21.

CLINICAL PHARMACOLOGY:

Mechanism of Action: In cell cultures the inhibitory activity of ribavirin for respiratory syncytial virus (RSV) is selective. The mechanism of action is unknown. Reversal of the *in vitro* antiviral activity by guanosine or xanthosine suggests ribavirin may act as an analogue of these cellular metabolites.

Microbiology: Ribavirin has demonstrated antiviral activity against RSV *in vitro*[1]and experimentally infected cotton rats.[2] Several clinical isolates of RSV were evaluated for ribavirin susceptibility by plaque reduction in tissue culture. Plaques were reduced 85-98% by 16 µG/Ml; however, results may vary with the test system. The development of resistance has not been evaluated *in vitro* or in clinical trials.

CLINICAL PHARMACOLOGY: *(cont'd)*

In addition to the above, ribavirin has been shown to have an *in vitro* activity against influenza A and B viruses and herpes simplex virus, but the clinical significance of these data is unknown.

Immunologic Effects: Neutralizing antibody responses to RSV were decreased in aerosolized Ribavirin treated infants compared to placebo treated infants.[3] One study decreased in patients treated with aerosolized Ribavirin. In rats, ribavirin administration resulted in lymphoid atrophy of the thymus, spleen, and lymph nodes. Humoral immunity was reduced in guinea pigs and ferrets. Cellular immunity was also mildly depressed in animal studies. The clinical significance of these observations is unknown.

Pharmacokinetics: Assay for Ribavirin in human materials is by a radioimmunoassay which detects ribavirin and at least one metabolite.

Ribavirin brand of ribavirin, when administered by aerosol, is absorbed systematically. Four pediatric patients inhaling Ribavirin aerosol administered by face mask for 2.5 hours each day for 3 days had plasma concentrations ranging from 0.44 to 1.55 µm, with a mean concentration of 0.76 µm. The plasma half-life was reported to be 9.5 hours. Three pediatric patients inhaling aerosolized Ribavirin administered by face mask or mist tent for 20 hours each day for 5 days had plasma concentrations ranging from 1.5 to 14.3 µm, with a mean concentration of 6.8 µm.

The bioavailability of aerosolized Ribavirin is unknown and may depend on the mode of aerosol delivery. After aerosol treatment, peak plasma concentrations of ribavirin are 85% to 98% less than the concentration that reduced RSV plaque formation in tissue culture. After aerosol treatment, respiratory tract secretions are likely to contain ribavirin in concentrations many fold higher than those required to reduce plaque formation. However, RSV is an intracellular virus and it is unknown whether plasma concentrations or respiratory secretion concentrations of the drug better reflect intracellular concentrations in the respiratory tract.

In man, rats, and rhesus monkeys, accumulation of ribavirin and/or metabolites in the red blood cells has been noted, plateauing in red cells in man in about 4 days and gradually declining with an apparent half-life of 40 days (the half-life of erythrocytes). The extent of accumulation of ribavirin following inhalation therapy is not well defined.

Animal Toxicology: Ribavirin, when administered orally or as an aerosol, produced cardiac lesions in mice, rats, and monkeys when given at doses of 30, 36 and 120 mg/kg or greater for 4 weeks or more (estimated human equivalent doses of 4.8, 12.3 and 111.4 mg/kg for a 5 kg child, or 2.5, 5.1 and 40 mg/kg for 60 kg adult, based on body surface area adjustment). Aerosolized ribavirin administered to developing ferrets at 60 mg/kg for 10 to 30 days resulted in inflammatory and possibly emphysematous changes in the lungs. Proliferative changes were seen in the lungs following exposure at 131 mg/kg for 30 days. The significance of these findings to human administration is unknown.

CLINICAL STUDIES:

DESCRIPTION OF STUDIES

Non-Mechanically-Ventilated Infants: In two placebo controlled trials in infants hospitalized with RSV lower respiratory tract infection, aerosolized Ribavirin treatment had a therapeutic effect, as judged by the reduction in severity of clinical manifestations of disease by treatment day.[3,4] Treatment was most effective when instituted within the first 3 days of clinical illness. Virus titers in respiratory secretions were also significantly reduced with Ribavirin in one of these original studies.[4] Additional controlled studies conducted since these initial trials of aerosolized Ribavirin in the treatment of RSV infection have supported these data.

Mechanically-Ventilated Infants: A randomized, double-blind, placebo controlled evaluation of aerosolized Ribavirin at the recommended dose was conducted in 28 infants requiring mechanical ventilation for respiratory failure caused by documented RSV infection.[6] Mean age was 1.4 months (SD, 1.7 months). Seven patients had underlying diseases predisposing them to severe infection and 21 were previously normal. Aerosolized Ribavirin treatment significantly decreased the duration of mechanical ventilation required (4.9 vs. 9.9 days, p=0.01) and duration of required supplemental oxygen (8.7 vs. 13.5 days, p=0.01). Intensive patient management and monitoring techniques were employed in this study. These included endotracheal tube suctioning every 1 to 2 hours; recording of proximal airway pressure, ventilatory rate, and F_1O_2 every hour; and arterial blood gas monitoring every 2 to 6 hours. To reduce the risk of Ribavirin precipitation and ventilator malfunction, heated wire tubing, two bacterial filters connected in series in the expiratory limb of the ventilator (with filter changes every 4 hours), and water column pressure release valves to monitor internal ventilator pressures were used in connecting ventilator circuits to the SPAG-2.

Employing these techniques, no technical difficulties with Ribavirin administration were encountered during the study. Adverse events consisted of bacterial pneumonia in one case, staphyloccus bacteremia in one case and two cases of post-extubation stridor. None were felt to be related to Ribavirin administration.

INDICATIONS AND USAGE:

Ribavirin is indicated for the treatment of hospitalized infants and young children with severe lower respiratory tract infections due to respiratory syncytial virus. Treatment early in the course of severe lower respiratory tract infection may be necessary to achieve efficacy.

Only severe RSV lower respiratory tract infection should be treated with Ribavirin. The vast majority of infants and children with RSV infection have disease that is mild, self-limited, and does not require hospitalization or antiviral treatment. Many children with mild lower respiratory tract involvement will require shorter hospitalization than would be required for a full course of Ribavirin aerosol (3 to 7 days) and should not be treated with the drug. Thus the decision to treat with Ribavirin should be based on the severity of the RSV infection. The presence of an underlying condition such as prematurity, immunosuppression or cardiopulmonary disease may increase the severity of clinical manifestations and complications of RSV infection.

Use of aerosolized Ribavirin in patients requiring mechanical ventilator assistance should be undertaken only by physicians and support staff familiar with this mode of administration and the specific ventilator being used (see WARNINGS, and DOSAGE AND ADMINISTRATION).

Diagnosis: RSV infection should be documented by a rapid diagnostic method such as demonstration of viral antigen in respiratory tract secretions by immunofluorescence[3,4] or ELISA[5]before or during the first 24 hours of treatment. Treatment may be initiated while awaiting rapid diagnostic test results. However, treatment should not be continued without documentation of RSV infection. Non-culture antigen detection techniques may have false positives or false negative results. Assessment of the clinical situation, the time of year and other parameters may warrant reevaluation of the laboratory diagnosis.

CONTRAINDICATIONS:

Ribavirin is contraindicated in individuals who have shown hypersensitivity to the drug or its components, and in women who are or may become pregnant during exposure to the drug. Ribavirin has demonstrated significant teratogenic and/or embryocidal potential in all animal species in which adequate studies have been conducted (rodents and rabbits). Therefore, although clinical studies have not been performed, it should be assumed that Ribavirin may

CONTRAINDICATIONS: *(cont'd)*

cause fetal harm in humans. Studies in which the drug has been administered systematically demonstrate that ribavirin is concentrated in the red blood cells and persists for the life of the erythrocyte.

WARNINGS:

SUDDEN DETERIORATION OF RESPIRATORY FUNCTION HAS BEEN ASSOCIATED WITH INITIATION OF AEROSOLIZED Ribavirin USE IN INFANTS. Respiratory function should be carefully monitored during treatment. If initiation of aerosolized Ribavirin treatment appears to produce sudden deterioration of respiratory function, treatment should be stopped and reinstituted only with extreme caution, continuous monitoring, and consideration of concomitant of bronchodilators.

Use with Mechanical Ventilators: USE OF AEROSOLIZED Ribavirin IN PATIENTS REQUIRING MECHANICAL VENTILATOR ASSISTANCE SHOULD BE UNDERTAKEN ONLY BY PHYSICIANS AND SUPPORT STAFF FAMILIAR WITH THIS MODE OF ADMINISTRATION AND THE SPECIFIC VENTILATOR BEING USED. Strict attention must be paid to procedures that have been shown to minimize the accumulation of drug precipitate, which can result in mechanical ventilator dysfunction and associated increased pulmonary pressures. These procedures include the use of bacteria filters in series in the expiratory limb of the ventilator circuit with frequent changes (every 4 hours), water column pressure release valves to indicate elevated ventilator pressures, frequent monitoring of these devices and verification that ribavirin crystals have not accumulated within the ventilator circuitry, and frequent suctioning and monitoring of the patient (see CLINICAL STUDIES).

Those administering aerosolized Ribavirin in conjunction with mechanical ventilator use should be thoroughly familiar with detailed descriptions of these procedures as outlined in the SPAG-2 manual.

PRECAUTIONS:

General: Patients with severe lower respiratory tract infection due to respiratory syncytial virus require optimum monitoring and attention to respiratory and fluid status (SPAG, 2 manual.)

Carcinogenesis and Mutagenesis: Ribavirin increased the incidence of cell transformations and mutations in mouse Balb/c 3T3 (fibroblasts) and L5178Y (lymphoma) cells at concentrations of 0.015 and 0.03-5.0 mg/ml, respectively (without metabolic activation). Modest increases in mutation rates (3-4x) were observed at concentrations between 3.75-10.0 mg/ml in L5178Y cells *in vitro* with the addition of a metabolic activation fraction. In the mouse micronucleus assay, ribavirin was clastogenic at intravenous doses of 20-200 mg/kg, (estimated human equivalent of 1.67-16.7 mg/kg, based on body surface area adjustment for a 60 kg adult). Ribavirin was not mutagenic in a dominant lethal assay in rats at intraperitoneal doses between 50-200 mg/kg when administered for 5 days (estimated human equivalent of 7.14-28.6 mg/kg, based on body surface area adjustment; see Pharmacokinetics).

In vivo carcinogenicity studies with ribavirin are incomplete. However, results of a chronic feeding study with ribavirin in rats, at doses of 16-100 mg/kg/day (estimated human equivalent of 2.3-14.3 mg/kg/day, based on body surface area adjustment for the adult), suggest that ribavirin may induce benign mammary, pancreatic, pituitary and adrenal tumors. Preliminary results of 2 oral gavage oncogenicity studies in the mouse and rat (18-24 months; doses of 20-75 and 10-40 mg/kg/day, respectively [estimated human equivalent of 1.67-6.25 and 1.43-5.71 mg/kg/day, respectively, based on body surface area adjustment for the adult]) are inconclusive as to the carcinogenic potential of ribavirin(see Pharmacokinetics.) However, these studies have demonstrated a relationship between chronic ribavirin exposure and increased incidences of vascular lesions (microscopic hemorrhages in mice) and retinal degeneration (in rats).

Impairment of Fertility: The fertility of ribavirin-treated animals (male or female) has not been fully investigated. However, in the mouse, administration of ribavirin at doses between 35-150 mg/kg/day (estimated human equivalent of 2.92-12.5 mg/kg/day, based on body surface area adjustment for the adult) resulted in significant seminiferous tubule atrophy, decreased sperm concentrations, and increased numbers of sperm with abnormal morphology. Partial recovery of sperm production was apparent 3-6 months following dose cessation in several additional toxicology studies, ribavirin has been shown to cause testicular lesions (tubular atrophy) in adult rats at oral dose levels as low as 16 mg/kg/day (estimated human equivalent of 2.29 mg/kg/day, based on body surface area adjustment; see Pharmacokinetics). Lower doses were not tested. The reproductive capacity of treated male animals has not been studied.

Pregnancy Category X: Ribavirin has demonstrated significant teratogenic and/or embryocidial potential in all animal species in which adequate studies have been conducted. Teratogenic effects were evident after single oral doses of 2.5 mg/kg or greater in the hamster, and after daily oral doses of 0.3 and 1.0 mg/kg in the rabbit and rat, respectively (estimated human equivalent doses of 0.12 and 0.14 mg/kg, based on body surface area adjustment for the adult). Malformations of the skull, palate, eye, jaw, limbs, skeleton, and gastrointestinal tract were noted. The incidence and severity of teratogenic effects increased with escalation of the drug dose. Survival of fetuses and offspring was reduced. Ribavirin caused embryolethality in the rabbit at daily oral dose levels as low as 1 mg/kg. No teratogenic effects were evident in the rabbit and rat administered daily oral doses of 0.1 and 0.3 mg/kg, respectively with estimated human equivalent doses of 0.01 and 0.04 mg/kg, based on body surface area adjustment (see Pharmacokinetics). These doses are considered to define the "No Observable Teratogenic Effects Level" (NOTEL) for ribavirin in the rabbit and rat.

Following oral administration of ribavirin in the pregnant rat (1.0 mg/kg) and rabbit (0.3 mg/kg) mean plasma levels of drug ranged from 0.10-0.20 µm[0.024-0.049 mcg/ml] at 1 hour after dosing, to undetectable levels at 24 hours. At 1 hour following the administration of 0.3 or 0.1 mg/kg in the rat and rabbit (NOTEL), respectively, mean plasma levels of drug in both species were near or below the limit of detection (0.05 µm; see Pharmacokinetics).

Although clinical studies have not been performed, Ribavirin may cause fetal harm in humans. As noted previously, ribavirin is concentrated in red blood cells and persists for the life of the cell. Thus the terminal half-life for the systemic elimination of ribavirin is essentially that of the half-life of circulating erythrocytes. The minimum interval following exposure to Ribavirin before pregnancy may be safely initiated is unknown (see CONTRAINDICATIONS, WARNINGS and PRECAUTIONS, Information for Health Care Personnel).

Nursing Mothers: Ribavirin has been shown to be toxic to lactating animals and their offspring. It is not known if Ribavirin is excreted in human milk.

Information for Health Care Personnel: Health care workers directly providing care to patients receiving aerosolized Ribavirin should be aware that ribavirin has been shown to be teratogenic in all animal species in which adequate studies have been conducted (rodents and rabbits). Although no reports of teratogenesis in offspring of mothers who were exposed to aerosolized Ribavirin during pregnancy have been confirmed, no controlled studies have been conducted in pregnant women. Studies of environmental exposure in treatment settings have shown that the drug can disperse into the immediate bedside area during routine patient care activities with highest ambient levels closest to the patient and extremely low levels outside of the immediate bedside area. Adverse reactions resulting from actual occupational exposure in adults are described below (see ADVERSE REACTIONS, Adverse Events in Health Care

PRECAUTIONS: *(cont'd)*

Workers). Some studies have documented ambient drug concentrations at the bedside that could potentially lead to systemic exposures above those considered safe for exposure during pregnancy (1/1000 of the NOTEL dose in the most sensitive animal species)[7,8,9]

A 1992 study conducted by the National Institute of Occupational Safety and Health (NIOSH) demonstrated measurable urine levels of ribavirin in health care workers exposed to aerosol in the course of direct patient care.[7] Levels were lowest in workers caring for infants receiving aerosolized Ribavirin with mechanical ventilation and highest in those caring for patients being administered the drug via an oxygen tent or hood. This study employed a more sensitive assay to evaluate ribavirin levels in urine than was available for several previous studies of environmental exposure that failed to detect measurable ribavirin levels in exposed workers. Creatinine adjusted urine levels in the NIOSH study ranged from less than 0.001 to 0.140 µm of ribavirin per gram of creatine in exposed workers. However, the relationship between urinary ribavirin levels exposed workers, plasma levels in animal studies, and the specific risk of teratogenesis in exposed pregnant women is unknown.

It is good practice to avoid unnecessary occupational exposure to chemicals wherever possible. Hospitals are encouraged to conduct training programs to minimize potential occupational exposure to Ribavirin. Health care workers who are pregnant should consider avoiding direct care of patients receiving aerosolized Ribavirin. If close patient contact cannot be avoided, precautions to limit exposure should be taken. These include administration of Ribavirin in negative pressure rooms; adequate room ventilation (at least six air exchanges per hour); the use of Ribavirin aerosol scavenging devices; turning off the SPAG-2 device for 5 to 10 minutes prior to prolonged patient contact; and wearing appropriately fitted minutes prior to prolonged patient contact; and wearing appropriately fitted respirator masks. Surgical masks do not provide adequate filtration of Ribavirin particles. Further information is available from NIOSH's Hazard Evaluation and Technical Assistance Branch and additional recommendations have been published in an Aerosol Consensus Statement by the American Respiratory Care Foundation and the American Association for Respiratory Care.[10]

ADVERSE REACTIONS:

The description of adverse reactions is based on events from clinical studies (approximately 200 patients) conducted prior to 1986, and the controlled trial of aerosolized Ribavirin conducted in 1989-1990. Additional data from spontaneous post-marketing reports of adverse events in individual patients have been available since 1986.

Deaths: Deaths during or shortly after treatment with aerosolized Ribavirin have been reported in 20 cases of patients treated with Ribavirin (12 of these patients were being treated for RSV infections). Several cases have been characterized as "possibly related" to Ribavirin by the treating physician; these were in infants who experienced worsening respiratory status related to bronchospasm while being treated with the drug. Several other cases have been attributed to mechanical ventilator malfunction in which Ribavirin precipitation within the ventilator apparatus led to excessively high pulmonary pressures and diminished oxygenation. In these cases the monitoring procedures described in the current package insert were not employed (see CLINICAL STUDIES, Description of Studies and DOSAGE AND ADMINISTRATION).

Pulmonary and Cardiovascular: Pulmonary function significantly deteriorated during aerosolized Ribavirin treatment in six of adults with chronic obstructive lung disease and in four of six asthmatic adults. Dyspnea and chest soreness were also reported in the latter group. Minor abnormalities in pulmonary function were also seen in healthy adult volunteers.

In the original study population of approximately 200 infants who received aerosolized Ribavirin, several serious adverse events occurred in severely ill infants with life-threatening underlying diseases, many of whom required assisted ventilation. The role of Ribavirin in these events is indeterminate. Since the drugs approval in 1986, additional reports of similar serious, through non-fatal, events have been filed infrequently. Events associated with aerosolized Ribavirin use have included the following:

Pulmonary: Worsening of respiratory status, bronchospasm, pulmonary edema, hypoventilation, cyanosis, dyspnea, bacterial pneumonia, pneumothorax, apnea, atelectasis and ventilator dependence.

Cardiovascular: Cardiac arrest, hypotension, bradycardia and digitalis toxicity. Bigeminy, bradycardia and tachycardia have been described in patients with underlying congenital heart disease.

Some subjects requiring assisted ventilation experienced serious difficulties, due to inadequate ventilation and gas exchange. Precipitation of drug within the ventilatory apparatus, including the endotracheal tube, has resulted in increased positive end expiratory pressure and increased positive inspiratory pressure. Accumulation of fluid in tubing ("rain out") has also been noted. Measures to avoid these complications should be followed carefully (see DOSAGE AND ADMINISTRATION).

Hematologic: Although anemia was not reported with use of aerosolized Ribavirin in controlled clinical trials, most infants treated with the aerosol have not been evaluated 1 to 2 weeks post-treatment when anemia is likely to occur. Anemia has been shown to occur frequently with experimental oral and intravenous Ribavirin in humans. Also, cases of anemia (type unspecified), reticulocytosis and hemolytic anemia associated with aerosolized Ribavirin use have been reported through post- marketing reporting systems. All have been reversible with discontinuation of the drug.

Other: Rash and conjunctivitis have been associated with the use of aerosolized Ribavirin. These usually resolve within hours of discontinuing therapy. Seizures and asthenia associated with experimental intravenous Ribavirin therapy have also been reported.

Adverse Events in Health Care Workers: Studies of environmental exposure to aerosolized Ribavirin in health care workers administering care to patients receiving the drug have not detected adverse signs or symptoms related to exposure. However, 152 health care workers have reported experiencing adverse events through post-marketing surveillance. Nearly all were in individuals providing direct care to infants receiving aerosolized Ribavirin. Of 358 events from these 152 individual health care worker reports, the most common signs and symptoms were headache (51% of reports), conjunctivitis (32%), and rhinitis, nausea, rash, dizziness, pharyngitis, or lacrimation (10-20% each). Several cases of bronchospasm and/or chest pain were also reported, usually individuals with known underlying reactive airway disease. Several case reports of damage to contact lenses after prolonged close exposure to aerosolized Ribavirin have been reported. Most signs and symptoms reported as having occurred in exposed health care workers resolved within minutes to hours of discontinuing close exposure to aerosolized Ribavirin (also see Information for Health Care Personnel).

The symptoms of RSV in adults can include headache, conjunctivitis, sore throat and/or cough, fever, hoarseness, nasal congestion and wheezing, although RSV infections in adults are typically mild and transient. Such infections represent a potential hazard to a potential hazard to uninfected hospital patients. It is unknown whether certain symptoms cited in reports from health care workers were due to exposure to the drug or infection with RSV. Hospitals should implement appropriate infection control procedures.

OVERDOSAGE:

No overdosage with Ribavirin by aerosol administration has been reported in humans. The LD_{50} in mice is 2 gm orally and is associated with hypoactivity and gastrointestinal symptoms (estimated human equivalent dose of 0.17 gm/kg, based on body surface area conversion). The mean plasma half-life after administration of aerosolized Ribavirin for pediatric patients is 9.5 hours. Ribavirin is concentrated and persists on red blood cells for the life of the erythrocyte (see Pharmacokinetics).

DOSAGE AND ADMINISTRATION:

BEFORE USE, READ THOROUGHLY THE VIRATEK SMALL PARTICLE AEROSOL GENERATOR (SPAG) MODEL SPAG-2 OPERATORS MANUAL FOR SMALL PARTICLE AEROSOL GENERATOR OPERATING INSTRUCTIONS. AEROSOLIZED Ribavirin SHOULD NOT BE ADMINISTERED WITH ANY OTHER AEROSOL GENERATING DEVICE.

The recommended treatment regimens is 20/ mg/ml Ribavirin as the starting solution in the drug reservoir of the SPAG-2 unit, with continuous Aerosol administration for 12-18 hours per day for 3 to 7 days. Using the recommended drug concentration of 20 mg/ml the average aerosol concentration for a 12 hour delivery period would be 190 micrograms/liter of air. Aerosolized Ribavirin should not be administered in a mixture for combined aerosolization or simultaneously with other aerosolized medications.

Non-mechanically ventilated infants: Ribavirin should be delivered to an infant oxygen hood from the SPAG-2 aerosol generator. Administration by face mask or oxygen tent may necessary if a hood cannot be employed (SPAG, 2 manual.) However, the volume and condensation area are larger in a tent and this may alter delivery dynamics of the drug.

Mechanically ventilated infants: The recommended dose and administration schedule for infants who require mechanical ventilation is the same as for those who do not. Either a pressure or volume cycle ventilator may be used in conjunction with the SPAG-2. In either case, patients should have their endotracheal tubes suctioned every 1-2 hours, and their pulmonary pressures monitored frequently (every 2-4 hours). For both pressure and volume ventilators, heated wire connective tubing bacteria filters in series in the expiratory limb of the system (which must be changed frequently, i.e., every 4 hours) must be used to minimize the risk of Ribavirin precipitation in the system and the subsequent risk of ventilator dysfunction. Water column pressure release valves should be used in the ventilator circuit for pressure cycled ventilators, and may be utilized with volume cycled ventilators (SPAG, 2 MANUAL FOR DETAILED INSTRUCTIONS).

Method of Preparation: Ribavirin brand of ribavirin is supplied as 6 grams of lyophilized powder per 100 ml vial for aerosol administration only. By sterile technique, reconstitute drug with a minimum of 75 ml of **sterile USP water for injection or inhalation** in the original 100 ml glass vial. Shake well. Transfer to the clean, sterilized 500 ml SPAG-2 reservoir and further dilute to a final volume of 300 with Sterile Water for Injection, USP, or Inhalation. The final concentration should be 20 mg/ml. **Important:** This water should NOT have had any antimicrobial agent or other substance added. The solution should be inspected visually for particulate matter and discoloration prior to administration. Solutions that have been placed in the SPAG-2 unit should be discarded at least every 24 hours and when the liquid level is low before adding newly reconstituted solution.

REFERENCES:

1. Hruska JF Bernstein JM, Douglas Jr., RG, and Hall CB. Effects of Ribavirin on respiratory syncytial virus *in vitro*. Antimicrob Agents Chemother 17:770-775, 1 1980. **2.** Hruska JF, Morrow PE, Suffin SC, and Douglas Jr., RG. *In vivo* inhibition of respiratory syncytial virus by Ribavirin. Antimicrob Agents Chemother 21:125-130, 1982. **3.** Taber LH, Knight V, Gilbert BE, McClung HW et al. Ribavirin aerosol treatment of bronchiolitis associated with respiratory tract infection in infants. Pediatrics 72:613-618, 1983. **4.** Hall CB, McBride JT, Walsh EE, Bell DM et al. Aerosolized Ribavirin treatment of infants with respiratory syncytial viral infection. N. Engl J Med 308:1443-7, 1983. **5.** Hendry RM, McIntosh K, Fahnestock ML, and Pierik LT. Enzyme-linked immunosorbent assay for detection of respiratory syncytial virus infection J Clin Microbiol 16:329-33, 1982. **6.** Smith, David W., Frankel, Lorry R., Mather, Larry H., Tang, Allen T.S., Ariagno, Ronald L., Prober, Charles G. A Controlled Trial of Aerosolized Ribavirin in Infants Receiving Mechanical Ventilation for Severe Respiratory Syncytial Virus Infection. The New England Journal of Medicine 1991; 325:24-29. **7.** Decker, John, Schultz, Ruth A., Health Hazard Evaluation Report: Florida Hospital, Orlando, Florida. Cincinnati OH: U.S. Department of Health and Human Services, Public Health Service, Centers for NIOSH Report No. HETA 91-104-2229.* **8.** Barnes, D.J. and Doursew, M. Reference dose: Description and use in health risk assessments. Regul Tox. and Pharm. Vol. 8; p. 471-486, 1988. **9.** Federal Register Vol. 53 No. 126 Thurs. June 30, 1988 p. 24834-24847. **10.** American Association for Respiratory Care [1991]. Aerosol Consensus Statement-1991. Respiratory Care 36(9): 916- 921.*Copies of the Report may be purchased from national technical Information Service, 5285 Port Royal Road, Springfield, VA 22161; Ask for Publication PB 93119-345.

HOW SUPPLIED:

Ribavirin for inhalation solution is supplied in 100 ml glass vials with 6 grams of sterile, lyophilized drug which is to be reconstituted with 300 ml Sterile Water for Injection or Sterile Water for Inhalation (no preservatives added) and administered only by a small particle aerosol generator (SPAG-2). Vials containing the lyophilized drug powder should be stored in a dry place at 15-25°C (59- 78°F). Reconstituted solutions may be stored under sterile conditions, at room temperature (20-30°C, 68-86°F) for 24 hours. Solutions which have been placed in the SPAG-2 unit should be discarded at least every 24 hours.

HOW SUPPLIED - EQUIVALENTS NOT AVAILABLE:

Aerosol, Solution - Inhalation - 6 gm

4's $5499.38 VIRAZOLE, Viratek 53095-0007-14

RIFABUTIN *(003135)*

CATEGORIES: AIDS Related Complex; Anti-Infectives; Antibacterials; Antibiotics; Antituberculosis Agents; HIV Infection; Macrolide; Mycobacterium Avium Complex; Orphan Drugs; Tuberculosis*; FDA Class 1P ("Priority Review"); Sales > $100 Million; FDA Approved 1992 Dec

* Indication not approved by the FDA

BRAND NAMES: Ansamycin; **Mycobutin**

FORMULARIES: PCS

COST OF THERAPY: $2,704.65 (AIDS MAC; Capsule; 150 mg; 2/day; 365 days)

DESCRIPTION:

Mycobutin is the brand name for the antimycobacterial agent rifabutin. It is a semisynthetic ansamycin antibiotic derived from rifamycin S. Mycobutin capsules for oral administration contain 150 mg of rifabutin, USP per capsule, along with the inactive ingredients microcrystalline cellulose, magnesium stearate, red iron oxide, silica gel, sodium lauryl sulfate, titanium dioxide, and edible white ink.

The chemical name for rifabutin is 1',4-didehydro-1-deoxy-1,4-dihydro-5'- (2-methylpropyl)-1-oxorifamycin XIV (Chemical Abstracts Service, 9th Collective Index) or (9*S*, 12*E*, 14*S*, 15*R*, 16*S*, 17*R*, 18*R*, 19*R*, 20*S*, 21*S*, 22*E*, 24*Z*)-6,16, 18,20 -tetrahydroxy-1'- isobutyl-14-methoxy - 7, 9, 15, 17, 19, 21, 25- heptamethyl-spiro [9,4- (epoxypentadeca[1, 11, 13]trienimino)-2*H*-furo[2',3':7,8]naphth[1,2-*d*]imidazole-2,4'-piperidine]-5,10,26- (3*H*,9*H*)-trione-16-acetate. Rifabutin has a molecular formula of $C_{46}H_{62}N_4O_{11}$, a molecular weight of 847.02.

DESCRIPTION: *(cont'd)*

Rifabutin is a red-violet powder soluble in chloroform and methanol, sparingly soluble in ethanol, and very slightly soluble in water (0.19 mg/ml). Its log P value (the base 10 logarithm of the partition coefficient between n-octanol and water) is 3.2 (n-octanol/water).

CLINICAL PHARMACOLOGY:

PHARMACOKINETICS

Following a single oral dose of 300 mg to nine healthy adult volunteers, rifabutin was readily absorbed from the gastrointestinal tract with mean (± SD) peak plasma levels (C_{max}) of 375 (± 267) ng/ml (range: 141 to 1033 ng/ml) attained in 3.3 (± 0.9) hours (T_{max} range: 2 to 4 hours). Plasma concentrations post-C_{max} declined in an apparent biphasic manner. Kinetic dose-proportionality has been established over the 300 to 600 mg dose range in nine healthy adult volunteers (crossover design) and in 16 early symptomatic human immunodeficiency virus (HIV)-positive patients over a 300 to 900 mg dose range. Rifabutin was slowly eliminated from plasma in seven healthy adult volunteers, presumably because of *distribution-limited elimination*, with a mean terminal half-life of 45 (± 17) hours (range: 16 to 69 hours). Although the systemic levels of rifabutin following multiple dosing decreased by 38%, its terminal half-life remained unchanged. Rifabutin, due to its high lipophilicity, demonstrates a high propensity for distribution and intracellular tissue uptake. Estimates of apparent steady-state distribution volume (9.3 ± 1.5 l/kg) in five HIV-positive patients, following I.V. dosing, exceed total body water by approximately 15-fold. Substantially higher intracellular tissue levels than those seen in plasma have been observed in both rat and man. The lung to plasma concentration ratio, obtained at 12 hours, was found to be approximately 6.5 in four surgical patients administered an oral dose. Mean rifabutin steady-state trough levels ($C_{p,min}^{ss}$; 24-hour post-dose) ranged from 50 to 65 ng/ml in HIV-positive patients and in healthy adult volunteers. About 85% of the drug is bound in a concentration-independent manner to plasma proteins over a concentration range of 0.05 to 1 mcg/ml. Binding does not appear to be influenced by renal or hepatic dysfunction.

Mean systemic clearance (Cl_s/F) in healthy adult volunteers following a single oral dose was 0.69 (± 0.32) l/hr/kg (range: 0.46 to 1.34 l/hr/kg). Renal and biliary clearance of unchanged drug each contribute approximately 5% to Cl_s/F. About 30% of the dose is excreted in the feces. A mass-balance study in three healthy adult volunteers with ^{14}C-labeled drug has shown that 53% of the oral dose was excreted in the urine, primarily as metabolites. Of the five metabolites that have been identified, 25-O-desacetyl and 31-hydroxy are the most predominant, and show a plasma metabolite:parent area under the curve ratio of 0.10 and 0.07, respectively. The former has an activity equal to the parent drug and contributes up to 10% to the total antimicrobial activity.

Absolute bioavailability assessed in five HIV-positive patients, who received both oral and I.V. doses, averaged 20%. Total recovery of radioactivity in the urine indicates that at least 53% of the orally administered rifabutin dose is absorbed from the G.I. tract. The bioavailability of rifabutin from the capsule dosage form, relative to a solution, was 85% in 12 healthy adult volunteers. High-fat meals slow the rate without influencing the extent of absorption from the capsule dosage form. The overall pharmacokinetics of rifabutin are modified only slightly by alterations in hepatic function or age. Rifabutin steady- state kinetics in early symptomatic HIV-positive patients are similar to healthy volunteers. Compared to healthy volunteers, steady-state kinetics of rifabutin are more variable in elderly patients (>70 years) and in symptomatic HIV-positive patients. Somewhat reduced drug distribution and faster elimination of rifabutin in patients with compromised renal function may result in decreased drug concentrations. The clinical implications of this are unknown.

No rifabutin disposition information is currently available in children or adolescents under 18 years of age.

MICROBIOLOGY

Mechanism of Action: Rifabutin inhibits DNA-dependent RNA polymerase in susceptible strains of *Escherichia coli* and *Bacillus subtilis* but not in mammalian cells. In resistant strains of *E. coli*, rifabutin, like rifampin, did not inhibit this enzyme. It is not known whether rifabutin inhibits DNA-dependent RNA polymerase in *Mycobacterium avium* or in *M. intracellulare* which comprise *M. avium* complex (MAC).

SUSCEPTIBILITY TESTING

In vitro susceptibility testing methods and diagnostic products used for determining minimum inhibitory concentration (MIC) values against *M. avium* complex (MAC) organisms have not been standardized. Breakpoints to determine whether clinical isolates of MAC and other mycobacterial species are susceptible or resistant to rifabutin have not been established.

In Vitro Studies Rifabutin has demonstrated *in vitro* activity against *M. avium* complex (MAC) organisms isolated from both HIV-positive and HIV-negative people. While gene probe techniques may be used to identify these two organisms, many reported studies did not distinguish between these two species. The vast majority of isolates from MAC-infected, HIV-positive people are *M. avium*, whereas in HIV-negative people, about 40% of the MAC isolates are *M. intracellulare*.

Various *in vitro* methodologies employing broth or solid media, with and without polysorbate 80 (Tween 80), have been used to determine rifabutin MIC values for mycobacterial species. In general, MIC values determined in broth are several fold lower than that observed with methods employing solid media. Utilization of Tween 80 in these assays had been shown to further lower MIC values. However, MIC values were substantially higher for egg based compared to agar based solid media.

Rifabutin activity against 211 MAC isolates from HIV-positive people was evaluated *in vitro* utilizing a radiometric broth and an agar dilution method. Results showed that 78% and 82% of these isolates had MIC_{99} values of ≤0.25 mcg/ml and ≤1.0 mcg/ml, respectively, when evaluated by these two methods. Rifabutin was also shown to be active against phagocytized, *M. avium* complex in a mouse macrophage cell culture model.

Rifabutin has *in vitro* activity against many strains of*Mycobacterium tuberculosis*. In one study, utilizing the radiometric broth method, each of 17 and 20 rifampin-naive clinical isolates tested from the United States and Taiwan, respectively, were shown to be susceptible to rifabutin concentrations of ≤0.125 mcg/ml.

Cross-resistance between rifampin and rifabutin is commonly observed with*M. tuberculosis* and *M. avium* complex isolates. Isolates of *M. tuberculosis* resistant to rifampin are likely to be resistant to rifabutin. Rifampicin and rifabutin MIC_{99} values against 523 isolates of *M. avium* complex were determined utilizing the agar dilution method (Ref. Heifets, Leonid B. and Iseman, Michael D. 1985. Determination of *in vitro* susceptibility of Mycobacteria to Ansamycin. Am. Rev. Respir. Dis. 132 (3):710-711). (TABLE 1)

Rifabutin *in vitro* MIC_{99} values of ≤0.5 mcg/ml, determined by the agar dilution method, for *M. kansasii, M. gordonae* and *M. marinum* have been reported; however, the clinical significance of these results is unknown.

CLINICAL STUDIES:

Two randomized, double-blind clinical trials (study 023 and study 027) compared rifabutin (300 mg/day) to placebo in patients with CDC-defined AIDS and CD4 counts ≤200 cells/µl. These studies accrued patients from 2/90 through 2/92. Study 023 enrolled 590 patients, with a median CD4 cell count at study entry of 42 cells/µl (mean 61). Study 027 enrolled 556 patients, with a median CD4 cell count at study entry of 40 cells/µl (mean 58).

Endpoints included the following:

CLINICAL STUDIES: *(cont'd)*

TABLE 1 Susceptibility Of *M. avium* Complex Strains To Rifampin And Rifabutin

		% of Strains Susceptible/Resistant to Different Concentrations of Rifabutin			
Susceptibility to Rifampin (mcg/ml)	**Number of Strains**	**Susceptible to 0.5**	**Resistant to 0.5 only**	**Resistant to 1.0**	**Resistant to 2.0**
Susceptible to 1.0	30	100.0	0.0	0.0	0.0
Resistant to 1.0 only	163	88.3	11.7	0.0	0.0
Resistant to 5.0	105	38.0	57.1	2.9	2.0
Resistant to 10.0	225	20.0	50.2	19.6	10.2
TOTAL	523	49.5	36.7	9.0	4.8

(1) MAC bacteremia, defined as at least one blood culture positive for *M. avium* complex bacteria.

(2) Clinically significant disseminated MAC disease, defined as MAC bacteremia accompanied by signs or symptoms of serious MAC infection, including one or more of the following: fever, night sweats, rigors, weight loss, worsening anemia, and/or elevations in alkaline phosphatase.

(3) Survival *MAC bacteremia* Participants who received rifabutin were one-third to one-half as likely to develop MAC bacteremia as were participants who received placebo. These results were statistically significant (study 023: $p<0.001$; study 027: $p = 0.002$).

In study 023, the one-year cumulative incidence of MAC bacteremia, on an intent to treat basis, was 9% for patients randomized to rifabutin and 22% for patients randomized to placebo. In study 027, these rates were 13% and 28% for rifabutin-treated and placebo-treated patients, respectively.

Most cases of MAC bacteremia (approximately 90% in these studies) occurred among participants whose CD4 count at study entry was ≤ 100 cells/µl. The median and mean CD4 counts at onset of MAC bacteremia were 13 cells/µl and 24 cells/µl, respectively. These studies did not investigate the optimal time to begin MAC prophylaxis.

Clinically significant disseminated MAC disease: In association with the decreased incidence of bacteremia, patients on **Rifabutin showed reductions in the signs and symptoms of disseminated MAC disease, including fever, night sweats, weight loss, fatigue, abdominal pain, anemia, and hepatic dysfunction.**

Survival: The one year survival rates in study 023 were 77% for the rifabutin group and 77% for the placebo group. In study 207, the one year survival rates were 77% for the rifabutin group and 70% for the placebo group. These differences were not statistically significant.

INDICATIONS AND USAGE:

Rifabutin is indicated for the prevention of disseminated *Mycobacterium avium* complex (MAC) disease in patients with advanced HIV infection.

CONTRAINDICATIONS:

Rifabutin is contraindicated in patients who have had clinically significant hypersensitivity to this drug, or to any other rifamycins.

WARNINGS:

Rifabutin prophylaxis must not be administered to patients with active tuberculosis. Tuberculosis in HIV-positive patients is common and may present with atypical or extrapulmonary findings. Patients are likely to have a nonreactive purified protein derivative (PPD) despite active disease. In addition to chest X-ray and sputum culture, the following studies may be useful in the diagnosis of tuberculosis in the HIV-positive patient: blood culture, urine culture, or biopsy of a suspicious lymph node.

Patients who develop complaints consistent with active tuberculosis while on rifabutin prophylaxis should be evaluated immediately, so that those with active disease may be given an effective combination regimen of anti-tuberculosis medications. Administration of single-agent rifabutin to patients with active tuberculosis is likely to lead to the development of tuberculosis that is resistant both to rifabutin and to rifampin.

There is no evidence that rifabutin is effective prophylaxis against *M. tuberculosis.* Patients requiring prophylaxis against both *M. tuberculosis* and *Mycobacterium avium* complex may be given isoniazid and rifabutin concurrently.

PRECAUTIONS:

Because rifabutin may be associated with neutropenia, and more rarely thrombocytopenia, physicians should consider obtaining hematologic studies periodically in patients receiving rifabutin prophylaxis.

INFORMATION FOR THE PATIENT

Patients should be advised of the signs and symptoms of both MAC and tuberculosis, and should be instructed to consult their physicians if they develop new complaints consistent with either of these diseases. In addition, since rifabutin may rarely be associated with myositis and uveitis, patients should be advised to notify their physicians if they develop signs or symptoms suggesting either of these disorders.

Urine, feces, saliva, sputum, perspiration, tears, and skin may be colored brown-orange with rifabutin and some of its metabolites. Soft contact lenses may be permanently stained. Patients to be treated with rifabutin should be made aware of these possibilities.

CARCINOGENESIS, MUTAGENESIS, AND IMPAIRMENT OF FERTILITY

Long term carcinogenicity studies were conducted with rifabutin in mice and in rats. Rifabutin was not carcinogenic in mice at doses up to 180 mg/kg/day, or approximately 36 times the recommended human daily dose. Rifabutin was not carcinogenic in the rat at doses up to 60 mg/kg/day, about 12 times the recommended human dose.

Rifabutin was not mutagenic in the bacterial mutation assay (Ames Test) using both rifabutin-susceptible and resistant strains. Rifabutin was not mutagenic in *Schizosaccharomyces pombe P₁* and was not genotoxic in V-79 Chinese hamster cells, human lymphocytes *in vitro*, or mouse bone marrow cells *in vivo*.

Fertility was impaired in male rats given 160 mg/kg (32 times the recommended human daily dose).

PREGNANCY CATEGORY B

Reproduction studies have been carried out in rats and rabbits given rifabutin using dose levels up to 200 mg/kg (40 times the recommended human daily dose). No teratogenicity was observed in either species. In rats, given 200 mg/kg/day, there was a decrease in fetal viability. In rats, at 40 mg/kg/day (8 times the recommended human daily dose), rifabutin caused an increase in fetal skeletal variants. In rabbits, at 80 mg/kg/day (16 times the recommended human daily dose), rifabutin caused maternotoxicity and increase in fetal skeletal anomalies. There are no adequate and well-controlled studies in pregnant women. Because animal reproduction studies are not always predictive of human response, rifabutin should be used in pregnant women only the potential benefit justifies the potential risk to the fetus.

PRECAUTIONS: *(cont'd)*

NURSING MOTHERS

It is not known whether rifabutin is excreted in human milk. Because many drugs are excreted in human milk and because of the potential for serious adverse reactions in nursing infants, a decision should be made whether to discontinue nursing or discontinue the drug, taking into account the importance of the drug to the mother.

PEDIATRIC USE

Safety and effectiveness of rifabutin for prophylaxis of MAC in children have not been established. Limited safety data are available from treatment use in 22 HIV-positive children with MAC who received rifabutin in combination with at least two other antimycobacterials for periods from 1 to 183 weeks. Mean doses (mg/kg) for these children were: 18.5 (range 15.0 to 25.0) for infants one year of age; 8.6 (range 4.4 to 18.8) for children 2 to 10 years of age; and 4.0 (range 2.8 to 5.4) for adolescents 14 to 16 years of age. There is no evidence that doses greater than 5 mg/kg daily are useful. Adverse experiences were similar to those observed in the adult population, and included leukopenia, neutropenia and rash. Doses of rifabutin may be administered mixed with foods such as applesauce.

DRUG INTERACTIONS:

In 10 healthy adult volunteers and 8 HIV-positive patients, steady-state plasma levels of zidovudine (ZDV), an antiretroviral agent which is metabolized mainly through glucuronidation, were decreased after repeated rifabutin dosing; the mean decrease in C_{max} and AUC was 48% and 32%, respectively. *In vitro* studies have demonstrated that rifabutin does not affect the inhibition of HIV by ZDV.

Steady-state kinetics in 12 HIV-positive patients show that both the rate and extent of systemic availability of didanosine (ddI), was not altered after repeated dosing of rifabutin.

Rifabutin has liver enzyme-inducing properties. The related drug rifampin is known to reduce the activity of a number of other drugs, including dapsone, narcotics (including methadone), anticoagulants, corticosteroids, cyclosporine, cardiac glycoside preparations, quinidine, oral contraceptives, oral hypoglycemic agents (sulfonylureas), and analgesics. Rifampin has also been reported to decrease the effects of concurrently administered ketoconazole, barbiturates, diazepam, verapamil, beta-adrenergic blockers, clofibrate, progestins, disopyramide, mexiletine, theophylline, chloramphenicol, and anticonvulsants. Because of the structural similarity of rifabutin and rifampin, rifabutin may be expected to have some effect on these drugs as well. However, unlike rifampin, rifabutin appears not to affect the acetylation of isoniazid. When rifabutin was compared with rifampin in a study with 8 healthy normal volunteers, rifabutin appeared to be a less potent enzyme inducer than rifampin. The significance of this finding for clinical drug interactions is not known.

Dosage adjustment of drugs listed above may be necessary if they are given concurrently with rifabutin.

Patients using oral contraceptives should consider changing to nonhormonal methods of birth control.

ADVERSE REACTIONS:

Rifabutin was generally well tolerated in the controlled clinical trials. Discontinuation of therapy due to an adverse event was required in 16% of patients receiving rifabutin compared to 8% of patients receiving placebo in these trials. Primary reasons for discontinuation of rifabutin were rash (4% of treated patients), gastrointestinal intolerance (3%), and neutropenia (2%).

The following table (TABLE 2) enumerates adverse experiences that occurred at a frequency of 1% or greater, among the patients treated with rifabutin in studies 023 and 027.

TABLE 2 Clinical Adverse Experiences Reported In ≥ 1% Of Patients Treated With Rifabutin

Adverse Event	MYCOBUTIN (n = 566) %	PLACEBO (n = 580) %
Body As A Whole		
Abdominal Pain	4	3
Asthenia	1	1
Chest Pain	1	1
Fever	2	1
Headache	3	5
Pain	1	2
Digestive System		
Anorexia	2	2
Diarrhea	3	3
Dyspepsia	3	1
Eructation	3	1
Flatulence	2	1
Nausea	6	5
Nausea and Vomiting	3	2
Vomiting	1	1
Musculoskeletal System		
Myalgia	2	1
Nervous System		
Insomnia	1	1
Skin And Appendages		
Rash	11	8
Special Senses		
Taste Perversion	3	1
Urogenital System		
Discolored Urine	30	6

Clinical Adverse Events Reported In <1% Of Patients Who Received Rifabutin Considering data from the 023 and 027 pivotal trials, and from other clinical studies, rifabutin appears to be a likely cause of the following adverse events which occurred in less than 1% of treated patients: flu-like syndrome, hepatitis, hemolysis, arthralgia, myositis, chest pressure or pain with dyspnea, and skin discoloration.

The following adverse events have occurred in more than one patient receiving rifabutin, but an etiologic role has not been established: seizure, paresthesia, aphasia, confusion, and nonspecific T wave changes on electrocardiogram.

When rifabutin was administered at doses from 1050 mg/day to 2400 mg/day, generalized arthralgia and uveitis were reported. These adverse experiences abated when rifabutin was discontinued.

The following table (TABLE 3) enumerates the changes in laboratory values that were considered as laboratory abnormalities in studies 023 and 027.

The incidence of neutropenia in patients treated with rifabutin was significantly greater than in patients treated with placebo ($p = 0.03$). Although thrombocytopenia was not significantly more common among rifabutin treated patients in these trials, rifabutin has been clearly linked to thrombocytopenia in rare cases. One patient in study 023 developed thrombotic thrombocytopenic purpura, which was attributed to rifabutin.

ADVERSE REACTIONS: *(cont'd)*

TABLE 3 Percentage Of Patients With Laboratory Abnormalities

Laboratory Abnormalities	Rifabutin (n = 566) %	Placebo (n = 580) %
Chemistry:		
Increased Alkaline Phosphatase[1]	<1	3
Increased SGOT[2]	7	12
Increased SGPT[2]	9	11
Hematology:		
Anemia[3]	6	7
Eosinophilia	1	1
Leukopenia[4]	17	16
Neutropenia[5]	25	20
Thrombocytopenia[6]	5	4

1 all values >450 U/l
2 all values >150 U/l
3 all hemoglobin values < 8.0 g/dl
4 all WBC values < 1,500/mm^3
5 all ANC values < 750/mm^3
6 all platelet count values < 50,000/mm^3
Includes Grade 3 Or 4 Toxicities As Specified:

Uveitis is rare when rifabutin is used as a single agent at 300 mg/day for prophylaxis of MAC in HIV-infected persons, even with the concomitant use of fluconazole and/or macrolide antibiotics. However, if higher doses of rifabutin are administered in combination with these agents, the incidence of uveitis is higher.

Patients who developed uveitis had mild to severe symptoms that resolved after treatment with corticosteroids and/or mydriatic eye drops; in some severe cases, however, resolution of symptoms occurred after several weeks.

When uveitis occurs, temporary discontinuance of rifabutin and ophthalmologic evaluation are recommended. In most mild cases, rifabutin may be restarted; however, if signs or symptoms recur, use of rifabutin should be discontinued (Morbidity and Mortality Weekly Report, September 9, 1994).

OVERDOSAGE:

No information is available on accidental overdosage in humans.

Treatment: While there is no experience in the treatment of overdose with rifabutin, clinical experience with rifamycins suggest that gastric lavage to evacuate gastric contents (within a few hours of overdose), followed by instillation of an activated charcoal slurry into the stomach, may help absorb any remaining drug from the gastrointestinal tract.

Rifabutin is 85% protein bound and distributed extensively into tissues (Vss:8 to 9 l/kg). It is not primarily excreted via the urinary route (less than 10% as unchanged drug), therefore, neither hemodialysis nor forced diuresis is expected to enhance the systemic elimination of unchanged rifabutin from the body in a patient with rifabutin overdose.

DOSAGE AND ADMINISTRATION:

It is recommended that 300 mg of rifabutin be administered once daily. For those patients with propensity to nausea, vomiting, or other gastrointestinal upset, administration of rifabutin at doses of 150 mg twice daily taken with food may be useful.

ANIMAL PHARMACOLOGY:

Liver abnormalities, (increased bilirubin and liver weight), occurred in all species tested, in rats at doses 5 times, in monkeys at doses 8 times, and in mice at doses 6 times the recommended human daily dose. Testicular atrophy occurred in baboons at doses 4 times the recommended human dose, and in rats at doses 40 times the recommended human daily dose.

HOW SUPPLIED:

Mycobutin Capsules, USP is supplied as hard gelatin capsules having an opaque red-brown cap and body, imprinted with Mycobutin/Pharmacia in white ink, each containing 150 mg of Rifabutin, USP.

Keep tightly closed and dispense in a tight container as defined in the USP. Store at controlled room temperature, 15° to 30°C (59° to 86°F).

HOW SUPPLIED - EQUIVALENTS NOT AVAILABLE:

Capsule, Gelatin - Oral - 150 mg

100's $370.50 MYCOBUTIN, Pharmacia & Upjohn 00013-5301-17

RIFAMPIN *(002188)*

CATEGORIES: Anti-Infectives; Antibiotics; Antimicrobials; Antimycobacterials; Antituberculosis Agents; Orphan Drugs; Tuberculosis; Pregnancy Category C; FDA Approval Pre 1982

BRAND NAMES: *Abrifam*; *Aptecin*; *Corifam*; *Fenampicin*; *Finamicina*; *Kalrifam*; *Medifam*; *Ramfin*; *Ramicin*; *Rifacilin*; **Rifadin**; *Rifagen*; *Rifaldin*; Rifamate; *Rifamed*; Rifampicin; *Rifamycin*; *Rifapiam*; *Rifarad*; *Rifasynt*; *Rifocina*; *Rifodex*; *Rifoldin-E*; *Rifumycin*; Rimactane; *Rimpacin*; *Rimpin*; *Rimycin*; *Ripin*; *Ripolin*; *Rofact*; *Syntaxil*; *Syntoren*; *Tibirim*; *Visedan*
(International brand names outside U.S. in italics)

FORMULARIES: Aetna; BC-BS; DoD; FHP; Medi-Cal; PCS; WHO

COST OF THERAPY: $578.98 (Tuberculosis; Capsule; 300 mg; 2/day; 180 days)

PRIMARY ICD9: 011.93 (Pulmonary Tuberculosis, Unspecified, Tubercle Bacilli Found)

DESCRIPTION:

Rifampin capsules for oral administration contain 150 mg or 300 mg rifampin per capsule. The 150 and 300 mg capsules also contain, as inactive ingredients: corn starch, D&C Red No. 28, FD&C Blue No. 1, FD&C Red No. 40, gelatin, magnesium stearate, and titanium dioxide.

Rifampin IV (rifampin for injection) contains rifampin 600 mg, sodium formaldehyde sulfoxylate 10 mg, and sodium hydroxide to adjust pH.

Rifampin is a semisynthetic antibiotic derivative of rifamycin B. The chemical name for rifampin is 3-(4-methyl-1-piperazinyl-iminomethyl)- rifamycin SV.

Rifampin USP is a red-brown crystalline powder very slightly soluble in water, freely soluble in chloroform, and soluble in ethyl acetate and in methanol. Its molecular weight is 822.95.

CLINICAL PHARMACOLOGY:

HUMAN PHARMACOLOGY - ORAL

Rifampin is readily absorbed from the gastrointestinal tract. Peak blood levels in normal adults vary widely from individual to individual. The peak level averages 7 mcg/ml but may vary from 4 to 32 mcg/ml. Absorption of rifampin is reduced when the drug is ingested with food.

In normal subjects, the biological half-life of rifampin in serum averages about 3 hours after a 600 mg oral dose, with increases up to 5.1 hours reported after a 900 mg dose. With repeated administration, the half-life decreases and reaches average values of approximately 2-3 hours. It does not differ in patients with renal failure at doses not exceeding 600 mg daily and, consequently, no dosage adjustment is required. Refer to WARNINGSfor information regarding patients with hepatic insufficiency.

After absorption, rifampin is rapidly eliminated in the bile, and an enterohepatic circulation ensues. During this process, rifampin undergoes progressive deacetylation so that nearly all the drug in the bile is in this form in about 6 hours. This metabolite is microbiologically active. Intestinal reabsorption is reduced by deacetylation, and elimination is facilitated. Up to 30% of a dose is excreted in the urine, with about half of this being unchanged drug.

Rifampin is widely distributed throughout the body. It is present in effective concentrations in many organs and body fluids, including cerebrospinal fluid. Rifampin is about 80% protein bound. Most of the unbound fraction is not ionized and therefore diffuses freely into tissues.

Serum Levels in Children

In one recent study, children 6-58 months old were given rifampin suspended in simple syrup or as dry powder mixed with applesauce at a dose of 10 mg/kg body weight. Peak serum levels of 10.7 and 11.5 mcg/ml were obtained 1 hour after preprandial ingestion of the drug suspension and the applesauce mixture, respectively. The calculated $t_{1/2}$ for both preparations was 2.9 hrs. It should be noted that in other studies in children, at doses of 10 mg/kg body weight, mean peak serum levels of 3.5 mcg/ml to 15 mcg/ml have been reported.

HUMAN PHARMACOLOGY - IV

After intravenous administration of a 300 or 600 mg dose of rifampin infused over 30 minutes to healthy male volunteers (n=11), mean peak plasma concentrations were 9.0 and 17.5 mcg/ml, respectively. The average plasma concentrations in these volunteers remained detectable for 8 and 12 hours, respectively (see TABLE 1.)

TABLE 1

Rifampin Dosage IV	Plasma Concentrations (mcg/ml) 30 min	1 hr	2 hr	4 hr	8 hr	12 hr
300 mg	8.9	4.9	4.0	2.5	< 2	< 2
600 mg	17.4	11.7	9.4	6.4	3.5	< 2

Plasma concentrations after the 600 mg dose, which were disproportionately higher (up to 50% greater than expected) than those found after the 300 mg dose, indicated that the elimination of larger doses was not as rapid.

After repeated once-a-day infusions (3 hr duration) of 600 mg in patients (n=5) for 7 days, concentrations of IV rifampin decreased from 5.8 mcg/ml 8 hours after the infusion on day 1 to 2.6 mcg/ml 8 hours after the infusion on day 7.

The rifampin dose is widely distributed throughout the body. It is present in effective concentrations in many organs and body fluids, including cerebrospinal fluid. Rifampin is about 80% protein bound. Most of the unbound fraction is not ionized and therefore diffuses freely into tissues.

Rifampin is rapidly eliminated in the bile and undergoes progressive enterohepatic circulation and deacetylation to the primary metabolite, 25-desacetyl-rifampin. This metabolite is microbiologically active. Less than 30% of the dose is excreted as rifampin or metabolites. Serum concentrations do not differ in patients with renal failure and, consequently, no dosage adjustment is required.

Serum Concentrations of Rifampin in Children

In patients 0.25 to 12.8 years old (n=12), the mean peak serum concentration of rifampin at the end of a 30 minute infusion of approximately 300 mg/m^2 was 26 mcg/ml. In these patients, peak concentrations 1 to 4 days after initiation of therapy ranged from 11.7 to 41.5 mcg/ml; peak concentrations 5 to 14 days after initiation of therapy were 13.6 to 37.4 mcg/ml. The serum half-life of rifampin decreased significantly from 1.34 to 3.24 hours early in therapy to 1.17 to 3.19 hours 5 to 14 days after therapy was initiated.

MICROBIOLOGY

Rifampin inhibits DNA-dependent RNA polymerase activity in susceptible cells. Specifically, it interacts with bacterial RNA polymerase but does not inhibit the mammalian enzyme. Rifampin is particularly active against rapidly growing extracellular organisms but has been demonstrated to have intracellular bactericidal activity against susceptible organisms as well.

Cross-resistance to rifampin has been shown only with other rifamycins.

Rifampin has bactericidal activity against slow and intermittently growing *M. tuberculosis*. It also has significant activity against*Neisseria meningitidis* (see INDICATIONS AND USAGE.)

In the treatment of both tuberculosis and the meningococcal carrier state (see INDICATIONS AND USAGE), **the small number of resistant cells present within large populations of susceptible cells can rapidly become predominant. In addition, resistance to rifampin has been determined to occur as single-step mutations of the DNA-dependent RNA polymerase. Since resistance can emerge rapidly, appropriate susceptibility tests should be performed in the event of persistent positive cultures.**

Rifampin has been shown to have initial *in vitro* activity against the following organisms; however, clinical efficacy has not been established (see INDICATIONS AND USAGE): *Mycobacterium leprae, Haemophilus influenzae, Staphylococcus aureus,* and *Staphylococcus epidermidis.* Both penicillinase-producing and non-penicillinase- producing strains, and β-lactam resistant staphylococci (Methicillin Resistant *S. aureus*/MRSA) are initially susceptible to rifampin*in vitro.*

SUSCEPTIBILITY TESTING

Use only diagnostic products and methods approved by the Food and Drug Administration for rifampin susceptibility testing of *Mycobacterium tuberculosis* and *Neisseria meningitidis.* Consult the Food and Drug Administration-approved labeling of the diagnostic products for interpretation criteria and quality control parameters.

For the other organisms listed in the microbiology subsection of the labeling, *in vitro* susceptibility testing should be assessed by standardized methodsdeveloped by the National Committee for Clinical Laboratory Standards.

INDICATIONS AND USAGE:

Tuberculosis: Rifampin is indicated in the treatment of all forms of tuberculosis. Rifampin must always be used in conjunction with at least one other antituberculosis drug. Frequently used regimens are rifampin and isoniazid; rifampin, isoniazid, and pyrazinamide; rifampin, isoniazid, and ethambutol; and rifampin and ethambutol.

INDICATIONS AND USAGE: *(cont'd)*

Rifampin IV is indicated for the initial treatment and retreatment of tuberculosis when the drug cannot be taken by mouth.

Meningococcal Carriers: Rifampin is indicated for the treatment of asymptomatic carriers of *N. meningitidis* to eliminate meningococci from the nasopharynx. *Rifampin is not indicated for the treatment of meningococcal infection because of the possibility of the rapid emergence of resistant organisms.* (See WARNINGS.)

Rifampin should not be used indiscriminately, and therefore diagnostic laboratory procedures, including serotyping and susceptibility testing, should be performed for establishment of the carrier state and the correct treatment. So that the usefulness of rifampin in the treatment of asymptomatic meningococcal carriers is preserved, the drug should be used only when the risk of meningococcal disease is high.

In the treatment of both tuberculosis and the meningococcal carrier state, the small number of resistant cells present within large populations of susceptible cells can rapidly become predominant. Since resistance can emerge rapidly, susceptibility tests should be performed in the event of persistent positive cultures.

CONTRAINDICATIONS:

Rifampin is contraindicated in patients with a history of hypersensitivity to any of the rifamycins. (See WARNINGS.)

WARNINGS:

Rifampin has been shown to produce liver dysfunction. Fatalities associated with jaundice have occurred in patients with liver disease and in patients taking rifampin with other hepatotoxic agents. Patients with impaired liver function should only be given rifampin in cases of necessity and then with caution and under strict medical supervision.

In these patients, careful monitoring of liver function, especially serum glutamic pyruvic transaminase (SGPT) and serum glutamic oxaloacetic transaminase (SGOT) should be carried out prior to therapy and then every two to four weeks during therapy. If signs of hepatocellular damage occur, rifampin should be withdrawn.

In some cases, hyperbilirubinemia resulting from competition between rifampin and bilirubin for excretory pathways of the liver at the cell level can occur in the early days of treatment. An isolated report showing a moderate rise in bilirubin and/or transaminase level is not in itself an indication for interrupting treatment; rather, the decision should be made after repeating the tests, noting trends in the levels, and considering them in conjunction with the patient's clinical condition.

Rifampin has enzyme-inducing properties, including induction of delta amino levulinic acid synthetase. Isolated reports have associated porphyria exacerbation with rifampin administration.

The possibility of rapid emergence of resistant meningococci restricts the use of Rifampin to short-term treatment of the asymptomatic carrier state. *Rifampin is not to be used for the treatment of meningococcal disease.*

PRECAUTIONS:

GENERAL

For the treatment of tuberculosis, rifampin is usually administered on a daily basis. High doses of rifampin (greater than 600 mg) given once or twice weekly have resulted in a high incidence of adverse reactions, including the "flu syndrome" (fever, chills and malaise), hematopoietic reactions (leukopenia, thrombocytopenia, or acute hemolytic anemia), cutaneous, gastrointestinal, and hepatic reactions, shortness of breath, shock and renal failure. Recent studies indicate that regimens using twice-weekly doses of rifampin 600 mg plus isoniazid 15 mg/kg are much better tolerated.

Intermittent therapy may be used if the patient cannot or will not self-administer drugs on a daily basis. Patients on intermittent therapy should be closely monitored for compliance and cautioned against intentional or accidental interruption of prescribed therapy because of the increased risk of serious adverse reactions.

Rifampin IV: For intravenous infusion only. Must not be administered by intramuscular or subcutaneous route. Avoid extravasation during injection; local irritation and inflammation due to extravascular infiltration of the infusion have been observed. If these occur, the infusion should be discontinued and restarted at another site.

INFORMATION FOR THE PATIENT

The patient should be told that this medication may cause the urine, feces, saliva, sputum, sweat and tears to turn red-orange. Permanent discoloration of soft contact lenses may occur.

The patient should be advised that the reliability of oral contraceptives may be affected; consideration should be given to using alternative contraceptive measures.

LABORATORY TESTS

A complete blood count (CBC) should be obtained prior to instituting therapy and periodically throughout the course of therapy. Because of a possible transient rise in transaminase and bilirubin values, blood for baseline clinical chemistries should be obtained before rifampin dosing.

DRUG/LABORATORY INTERACTIONS

Therapeutic levels of rifampin have been shown to inhibit standard microbiological assays for serum folate and Vitamin B_{12}. Thus, alternate assay methods should be considered. Transient abnormalities in liver function tests (*e.g.,* elevation in serum bilirubin, abnormal bromsulphalein (BSP) excretion, alkaline phosphatase and serum transaminases), and reduced biliary excretion of contrast media used for visualization of the gallbladder have also been observed. Therefore, these tests should be performed before the morning dose of rifampin.

CARCINOGENESIS, MUTAGENESIS, AND IMPAIRMENT OF FERTILITY

There are no known human data on long-term potential for carcinogenicity, mutagenicity, or impairment of fertility. A few cases of accelerated growth of lung carcinoma have been reported in man, but a causal relationship with the drug has not been established. An increase in the incidence of hepatomas in female mice (of a strain known to be particularly susceptible to the spontaneous development of hepatomas) was observed when rifampin was administered in doses 2 to 10 times the average daily human dose for 60 weeks followed by an observation period of 46 weeks. No evidence of carcinogenicity was found in male mice of the same strain, mice of a different strain, or rats, under similar experimental conditions.

Rifampin has been reported to possess immunosuppressive potential in rabbits, mice, rats, guinea pigs, human lymphocytes *in vitro,* and humans. Antitumor activity *in vitro* has also been shown with rifampin.

There was no evidence of mutagenicity in bacteria, *Drosophila melanogaster,* or mice, nor did rifampin induce chromosome aberrations in human lymphocytes treated *in vitro.* However, an increase in chromatid breaks was noted when whole-blood cell cultures were treated with rifampin.

PREGNANCY, TERATOGENIC EFFECTS, PREGNANCY CATEGORY C

Rifampin has been shown to be teratogenic in rodents given oral doses of rifampin 15 to 25 times the human dose. Although rifampin has been reported to cross the placental barrier and appear in cord blood, the effect of rifampin, alone or in combination with other antituberculosis drugs, on the human fetus is not known. Neonates of rifampin-treated mothers should be carefully observed for any evidence of adverse effects. Isolated cases of fetal malformations have been reported; however, there are no adequate and well-controlled studies in pregnant women. Rifampin should be used during pregnancy only if the potential benefit justifies the potential risk to the fetus. Rifampin in oral doses of 150 to 250 mg/kg produced teratogenic effects in mice and rats. Malformations were primarily cleft palate in the mouse and spina bifida in the rat. The incidence of these anomalies was dose-dependent. When rifampin was given to pregnant rabbits in doses up to 20 times the usual daily human dose, imperfect osteogenesis and embryotoxicity were reported.

When administered during the last few weeks of pregnancy, rifampin can cause post-natal hemorrhages in the mother and infant for which treatment with Vitamin K may be indicated.

NURSING MOTHERS

Because of the potential for tumorigenicity shown for rifampin in animal studies, a decision should be made whether to discontinue nursing or discontinue the drug, taking into account the importance of the drug to the mother.

PEDIATRIC USE

See CLINICAL PHARMACOLOGY, Serum Levels in Children; see also DOSAGE AND ADMINISTRATION.

DRUG INTERACTIONS:

Rifampin has liver enzyme-inducing properties and may reduce the activity of a number of drugs, including anticoagulants, corticosteroids, cyclosporine, cardiac glycoside preparations, quinidine, oral contraceptives, oral hypoglycemic agents (sulfonylureas), dapsone, narcotics and analgesics. Rifampin also has been reported to diminish the effects of concurrently administered methadone, barbiturates, diazepam, verapamil, beta-adrenergic blockers, clofibrate, progestins, disopyramide, mexiletin, theophylline, chloramphenicol and anticonvulsants. It may be necessary to adjust the dosages of these drugs if they are given concurrently with rifampin.

Patients using oral contraceptives should be advised to change to nonhormonal methods of birth control during rifampin therapy. Also, diabetes may become more difficult to control.

When rifampin is taken with paraaminosalicylic acid (PAS), rifampin levels in the serum may decrease. Therefore, the drugs should be taken at least 8 hours apart.

Probenecid has been reported to increase rifampin blood levels. Halothane, when given concomitantly with rifampin, has been reported to increase the hepatotoxicity of both drugs.

Ketoconazole, when given concomitantly with rifampin, has been reported to diminish the serum concentrations of both drugs. Dosage should be adjusted if indicated by the patient's clinical condition. An interaction has also been reported with rifampin-isoniazid and Vitamin D.

ADVERSE REACTIONS:

Gastrointestinal: Heartburn, epigastric distress, anorexia, nausea, vomiting, jaundice, flatulence, cramps and diarrhea have been noted in some patients. Although *C. difficile* has been shown *in vitro* to be sensitive to rifampin, pseudomembranous colitis has been reported with the use of rifampin (and other broad spectrum antibiotics). Therefore, it is important to consider this diagnosis in patients who develop diarrhea in association with antibiotic use. Rarely, hepatitis or a shock-like syndrome with hepatic involvement and abnormal liver function tests has been reported.

Hematologic: Thrombocytopenia has occurred primarily with high dose intermittent therapy, but has also been noted after resumption of interrupted treatment. It rarely occurs during well supervised daily therapy. This effect is reversible if the drug is discontinued as soon as purpura occurs. Cerebral hemorrhage and fatalities have been reported when rifampin administration has been continued or resumed after the appearance of purpura.

Transient leukopenia, hemolytic anemia and decreased hemoglobin have been observed.

Central Nervous System: Headache, fever, drowsiness, fatigue, ataxia, dizziness, inability to concentrate, mental confusion, behavioral changes, muscular weakness, pains in extremities and generalized numbness have been observed.

Rare reports of myopathy have also been observed.

Ocular: Visual disturbances have been observed.

Endocrine: Menstrual disturbances have been observed.

Renal: Elevations in BUN and serum uric acid have been reported. Rarely, hemolysis, hemoglobinuria, hematuria, interstitial nephritis, renal insufficiency and acute renal failure have been noted. These are generally considered to be hypersensitivity reactions. They usually occur during intermittent therapy or when treatment is resumed following intentional or accidental interruption of a daily dosage regimen, and are reversible when rifampin is discontinued and appropriate therapy instituted.

Dermatologic: Cutaneous reactions are mild and self-limiting and do not appear to be hypersensitivity reactions. Typically, they consist of flushing and itching with or without a rash. More serious cutaneous reactions which may be due to hypersensitivity occur but are uncommon.

Hypersensitivity Reactions: Occasionally, pruritus, urticaria, rash, pemphigoid reaction, eosinophilia, sore mouth, sore tongue and conjunctivitis have been observed.

Miscellaneous: Edema of the face and extremities has been reported. Other reactions reported to have occurred with intermittent dosage regimens include "flu" syndrome (such as episodes of fever, chills, headache, dizziness and bone pain), shortness of breath, wheezing, decrease in blood pressure and shock. The "flu" syndrome may also appear if rifampin is taken irregularly by the patient or if daily administration is resumed after a drug free interval.

OVERDOSAGE:

SIGNS AND SYMPTOMS

Nausea, vomiting and increasing lethargy will probably occur within a short time after ingestion; unconsciousness may occur when there is severe hepatic disease. Brownish-red or orange discoloration of the skin, urine, sweat, saliva, tears and feces will occur, and its intensity is proportional to the amount ingested.

Liver enlargement, possibly with tenderness, may develop within a few hours after severe overdosage; jaundice may develop rapidly. Hepatic involvement may be more marked in patients with prior impairment of hepatic function. Other physical findings remain essentially normal.

Bilirubin levels may increase rapidly with severe overdosage; hepatic enzyme levels may be affected, especially with prior impairment of hepatic function. A direct effect upon the hematopoietic system, electrolyte levels, or acid-base balance is unlikely.

ACUTE TOXICITY

In animal studies, the LD_{50} of rifampin is approximately 885 mg/kg in the mouse, 1720 mg/kg in the rat, and 2120 mg/kg in the rabbit.

Non-fatal overdoses with as high as 12 g of rifampin have been reported. In one patient who swallowed 12 g of rifampin, vomiting occurred four times within 1 hour of ingestion. Gastric lavage with 20 liters of water was initiated 5 hours after ingestion. Twelve hours after ingestion of rifampin, a plasma concentration of 400 mcg of rifampin/ml was measured by

OVERDOSAGE: *(cont'd)*

microbiological assay. The plasma concentration fell to 64 mcg/ml on the following day, and to 0.1 mcg/ml on the third day. Urinary rifampin concentration was 313 mcg/ml approximately 30 hours after ingestion of the drug, 625 mcg/ml after 36 hours, and 78 mcg/ml after 40 hours. By the fourth day following the dose, only 0.1 mcg/ml rifampin was present in the urine. There was biochemical evidence of mild impairment of liver function. Liver function tests had returned to normal within 5 days, and the patient's recovery was described as uneventful.

One case of fatal overdose is known: A 26-year-old man died after self-administering 60 g of rifampin.

TREATMENT

Since nausea and vomiting are likely to be present, gastric lavage is probably preferable to induction of emesis. Following evacuation of the gastric contents, the instillation of activated charcoal slurry into the stomach may help absorb any remaining drug from the gastrointestinal tract. Antiemetic medication may be required to control severe nausea and vomiting.

Active diuresis (with measured intake and output) will help promote excretion of the drug. Hemodialysis may be of value in some patients. In patients with previously adequate hepatic function, reversal of liver enlargement and of impaired hepatic excretory function probably will be noted within 72 hours, with a rapid return toward normal thereafter.

DOSAGE AND ADMINISTRATION:

Rifampin can be administered by the oral route or by IV infusion (see INDICATIONS AND USAGE.)

TUBERCULOSIS

Adults: 600 mg in a single daily administration, oral or IV.

Children: 10-20 mg/kg not to exceed 600 mg/day, oral or IV.

It is recommended that oral rifampin be administered once daily, either one hour before, or two hours after a meal.

In the treatment of tuberculosis, rifampin should always be administered with at least one other antituberculosis drug.

In general, therapy for tuberculosis should be continued for 6 to 9 months or until at least 6 months have elapsed from conversion of sputum to culture negativity. In patients who cannot be relied on for compliance, intermittent therapy with 600 mg/day two or three times/week under close supervision may be prescribed and substituted for the daily regimen after 1-2 months of an initial daily phase of therapy.

The 9-Month Regimen: ordinarily consists of rifampin and isoniazid, usually supplemented during the initial phase by pyrazinamide, streptomycin or ethambutol.

The 6-Month Regimen: ordinarily consists of an initial *2- month* phase of rifampin, isoniazid and pyrazinamide, and, if clinically indicated, streptomycin or ethambutol; followed by *4 months* of rifampin and isoniazid.

Either of the above regimens is recommended as standard therapy.

The above recommendations apply to patients with drug-susceptible organisms. Patients with drug-resistant organisms may require longer treatment with other drug regimens.

MENINGOCOCCAL CARRIERS

Adults: For adults, it is recommended that 600 mg rifampin be administered twice daily for two days.

Infants and Children: *Children 1 month of age or older:* 10 mg/kg every 12 hours for two days. *Children under 1 month of age:* 5 mg/kg every 12 hours for two days.

PREPARATION OF SOLUTION FOR IV INFUSION

Reconstitute the lyophilized powder by transferring 10 ml of sterile water for injection to a vial containing 600 mg of rifampin for injection. Swirl vial gently to completely dissolve the antibiotic. The reconstituted solution contains 60 mg rifampin per ml and is stable at room temperature for 24 hours. Immediately prior to administration, withdraw from the reconstituted solution a volume equivalent to the amount of rifampin calculated to be administered and add to 500 ml of infusion medium. Mix well and infuse at a rate allowing for complete infusion in 3 hours. In some cases, the amount of rifampin calculated to be administered may be added to 100 ml of infusion medium and infused in 30 minutes. The 500 ml and 100 ml infusion solutions should be prepared and used within a total 4 hour period. Precipitation of rifampin from the infusion solution may occur beyond this time.

CAUTION: Dextrose 5% for injection is the recommended infusion medium. Sterile saline may be used when dextrose is contraindicated, but the stability of rifampin is slightly reduced. Other infusion media are not recommended.

PREPARATION OF EXTEMPORANEOUS ORAL SUSPENSION

For pediatric and adult patients in whom capsule swallowing is difficult or where lower doses are needed, a liquid suspension may be prepared as follows:

Rifampin 1% w/v suspension (10 mg/ml) can be compounded using one of five syrups — Simple Syrup (Syrup NF), Simple Syrup (Humco Laboratories), Simple Syrup (Whiteworth Inc.), Wild Cherry Syrup (Eli Lilly and Company), and Syrpalta Syrup (Emerson Laboratories).

1. Empty contents of four Rifampin 300 mg capsules or eight Rifampin 150 mg capsules onto a piece of weighing paper.

2. If necessary, gently crush the capsule contents with a spatula to produce a fine powder.

3. Transfer rifampin powder blend to a 4-ounce amber glass prescription bottle.

4. Rinse the paper and spatula with 20 ml of one of the above-mentioned syrups and add the rinse to the bottle. Shake vigorously.

5. Add 100 ml of syrup to the bottle and shake vigorously.

This compounding procedure results in a 1% w/v suspension containing 10 mg rifampin/ml. Stability studies indicate that the suspension is stable when stored at room temperature (25 ± 3°C) or in a refrigerator (2-8°C) for four weeks. This extemporaneously prepared suspension must be shaken well prior to administration.

STORAGE

Keep tightly closed. Store in a dry place. Avoid excessive heat.

I.V.: Avoid excessive heat (temperatures above 40°C or 104°F). Protect from light.

REFERENCES:

1. National Committee for Clinical Laboratory Standards, Approved Standard: Performance Standards for Antimicrobial Disk Susceptibility Tests (M7-A2), Second Edition; Approved Standard (1990). **2.** National Committee for Clinical Laboratory Standards, Approved Standard: Methods for Dilution Antimicrobial Susceptibility Tests for Bacteria that Grow Aerobically (M2-A4), Fourth Edition; Approved Standard (1990).

HOW SUPPLIED - RATED THERAPEUTICALLY EQUIVALENT:

Capsule, Gelatin - Oral - 300 mg

30's	**$63.36**	**RIFADIN, Hoechst Marion Roussel**	**00068-0508-30**
60's	$89.24	RIMACTANE, Novartis	00083-0154-29
60's	**$126.66**	**RIFADIN, Hoechst Marion Roussel**	**00068-0508-60**
100's	$160.83	RIMACTANE, Novartis	00083-0154-30
100's	**$211.20**	**RIFADIN, Hoechst Marion Roussel**	**00068-0508-61**

HOW SUPPLIED - NOT RATED EQUIVALENT:

Capsule, Gelatin - Oral - 150 mg

30's	**$44.70**	**RIFADIN, Hoechst Marion Roussel**	**00068-0510-30**

Injection, Solution - Intravenous - 600 mg/vial

600 mg	**$79.38**	**RIFADIN IV, Hoechst Marion Roussel**	**00068-0597-01**

RILUZOLE *(003281)*

CATEGORIES: Amyotrophic Lateral Sclerosis; Antiglutamate; Beuzothiazole

BRAND NAMES: **Rilutek**

DESCRIPTION:

Riluzole is a member of the benzothiazole class. Chemically, riluzole is 2-amino-6-(trifluoromethoxylbenzothiazole). Its molecular formula is $C_8H_5F_3N_2OS$ and its molecular weight is 234.2.

Riluzole is a white to slightly yellow powder that is very soluble in dimethylformamide, dimethylsulfoxide and methanol, freely soluble in dichloromethane, sparingly soluble in 0.1 N HCl and very slightly soluble in water and in 0.1 N NaOH.

Rilutek Inactive Ingredients: *Core:* anhydrous dibasic calcium phosphate, USP; microcrystalline cellulose, NF; anhydrous colloidal silica, NF; magnesium stearate, NF; croscarmellose sodium, NF. *Film coating:* hydroxypropyl methylcellulose, USP; polyethylene glycol 6000; titanium dioxide

CLINICAL PHARMACOLOGY:

MECHANISM OF ACTION

The etiology and pathogenesis of amyotrophic lateral sclerosis (ALS) are not known, although a number of hypotheses have been advanced. One hypothesis is that motor neurons, made vulnerable through either genetic predisposition or environmental factors, are injured by glutamate. In some cases of familial ALS the enzyme superoxide dismutase has been found to be defective.

The mode of action of riluzole is unknown. Its pharmacological properties include the following, some of which may be related to its effect:

1. an inhibitory effect on glutamate release,

2. inactivation of voltage-dependent sodium channels, and

3. ability to interfere with intracellular events that follow transmitter binding at excitatory amino acid receptors.

Riluzole has also been shown, in a single study, to delay median time to death in a transgenic mouse model of ALS. These mice express human superoxide dismutase bearing one of the mutations found in one of the familial forms of human ALS.

It is also neuroprotective in various *in vivo* experimental models of neuronal injury involving excitotoxic mechanisms. In *in vitro* tests, riluzole protected cultured rat motor neurons from the excitotoxic effects of glutamic acid and prevented the death of cortical neurons induced by anoxia.

Due to its blockade of glutametergic neurotransmission, riluzole also exhibits myorelaxant and sedative properties in animal models at doses of 30 mg/kg (about 20 times the recommended human daily dose) and anticonvulsant properties at a dose of 2.5 mg/kg (about 2 times the recommended human daily dose).

PHARMACOKINETICS

Riluzole is well-absorbed (approximately 90%), with average absolute oral bioavailability of about 60% (CV=30%). Pharmacokinetics are linear over a dose range of 25-100 mg given every 12 hours. A high fat meal decreases absorption, reducing AUC by about 20% and peak blood levels by about 45%. The mean elimination half-life of riluzole is 12 hours (CV=35%) after repeated doses. With multiple-dose administration, riluzole accumulates in plasma by about 2 fold and steady-state is reached in less than 5 days. Riluzole is 96% bound to plasma proteins, mainly to albumin and lipoproteins over the clinical concentration range.

The 50 mg market tablet was equivalent, with respect to AUC, to the tablet used in the dose ranging clinical trials, while the C_{max} was approximately 30% higher. Both tablets have been used in clinical trials. However, if doses greater than those recommended are given, it is likely that higher plasma levels will be achieved, the safety of which has not been established (see DOSAGE AND ADMINISTRATION.)

METABOLISM AND ELIMINATION

Riluzole is extensively metabolized to six major and a number of minor metabolites, not all of which have been identified. Some metabolites appear pharmacologically active in *in vitro* assays. The metabolism of riluzole is mostly hepatic and consists of cytochrome P450-dependent hydroxylation and glucuronidation.

There is marked inter-individual variability in the clearance of riluzole, probably attributable to variability of CYP 1A2 activity, the principal isozyme involved in N-hydroxylation.

In vitro studies using liver microsomes show that hydroxylation of the primary amino group producing N-hydroxyriluzole is the main metabolic pathway in human, monkey, dog and rabbit. In humans, cytochrome P450 1A2 is the principal isozyme involved in N-hydroxylation. *In vitro* studies predict that CYP 2D6, CYP 2C19, CYP 3A4 and CYP 2E1 are unlikely to contribute significantly to riluzole metabolism in humans. Whereas direct glucuroconjugation of riluzole (involving the glucurotransferase isoform UGT HP4) is very slow in human liver microsomes, N-hydroxyriluzole is readily conjugated at the hydroxylamine group resulting in the formation of O- (>90%) and N-glucuronides.

Following a single 150 mg dose of ^{14}C-riluzole to 6 healthy males, 90% and 5% of the radioactivity was recovered in the urine and feces respectively over a period of 7 days. Glucuronides accounted for more than 85% of the metabolites in urine. Only 2% of a riluzole dose was recovered in the urine as unchanged drug.

SPECIAL POPULATIONS

The pharmacokinetics of riluzole have not been studied in renally and hepatically impaired subjects, nor is there information about the effects of smoking, age and gender on the pharmacokinetics of riluzole but certain differences in population subsets should be anticipated (see PRECAUTIONS.)

Hepatic and Renal Disease: Since riluzole is extensively metabolized and subsequently excreted in the urine, it is likely that functional hepatic and renal impairment will reduce the clearance of riluzole and its metabolites and give higher plasma levels (see PRECAUTIONSand WARNINGS).

Age: Age-related decreased renal function would be expected to give higher plasma levels of riluzole and metabolites. However, in controlled clinical trials, in which approximately 30% of patients were over 65, there were no differences in adverse events between younger and older patients (see PRECAUTIONS.)

Gender: CYP 1A2 activity has been reported to be lower in women than in men. Therefore, a gender effect on riluzole kinetics may be expected in women, resulting in higher blood concentrations of riluzole and its metabolites (see PRECAUTIONS.) No gender effect on favorable or adverse effects of riluzole was seen in controlled trials, however.

CLINICAL PHARMACOLOGY: *(cont'd)*

Smoking: Cigarette smoking is known to induce CYP 1A2. Patients who smoke cigarettes would be expected to eliminate riluzole faster. There is no information, however, on the effect of, or need for, dosage adjustment in these patients.

Race: Clearance of riluzole in Japanese subjects native to Japan was found to be 50% lower as compared to Caucasians after normalizing for body weight. Although it is not clear if this difference is due to genetic or environmental factors (*e.g.*, smoking, alcohol, coffee, and dietary preferences), it is possible that Japanese subjects may possess a lower capacity (oxidative and/or conjugative) for metabolizing riluzole. There are no studies, however, of lower doses in Japanese subjects (see PRECAUTIONS.)

CLINICAL STUDIES:

The efficacy of riluzole as a treatment of ALS was established in two adequate and well-controlled trials in which the time to tracheostomy or death was longer for patients randomized to riluzole than for those randomized to placebo.

These studies admitted patients with either familial or sporadic ALS, a disease duration of less than 5 years, and a baseline forced vital capacity greater than or equal to 60%.

In one study, performed in France and Belgium, the 155 ALS patients were followed for at least 13 months (maximum duration 18 months) after being randomized to either 100 mg/day (given 50 mg BID) of riluzole or placebo.

Although the survival curves were not statistically significantly different when evaluated specified in the study protocol (Logrank test p=0.12), the difference was found to be significant by another appropriate analysis (Wilcoxon test p=0.05). The study showed an early increase in survival in patients given riluzole. Among the patients in whom treatment failed during the study (tracheostomy or death) there was a difference between the treatment groups in median survival of approximately 90 days. There was no statistically significant difference in mortality at the end of the study.

In the second study, performed in both Europe and North America, 959 ALS patients were followed for at least one year (North American centers) and up to 18 months (European centers) after being randomized to either 50, 100, 200 mg/day of riluzole or placebo. Although the survival curves were not statistically significantly different when evaluated specified in the study protocol (Logrank test p=0.076), the difference was found to be significant by another appropriate analysis (Wilcoxon test p=0.05). The results of the 50 mg/day of riluzole could not be statistically distinguished from placebo. The results of the 200 mg/day are essentially identical to 100 mg/day. The study showed an early increase in survival in patients given riluzole. Among the patients in whom treatment failed during the study (tracheostomy or death) there was a difference between the treatment groups in median survival of approximately 60 days. There was no statistically significant difference in mortality at the end of the study.

Although riluzole improved early survival in both studies, measures of muscle strength and neurological function did not show a benefit.

INDICATIONS AND USAGE:

Riluzole is indicated for the treatment of patients with amyotrophic lateral sclerosis (ALS). Riluzole extends survival and/or time to tracheostomy.

CONTRAINDICATIONS:

Riluzole is contraindicated in patients who have a history of severe hypersensitivity reactions to riluzole or any of the tablet components.

WARNINGS:

Liver Injury/Monitoring Liver Chemistries: Riluzole should be prescribed with care in patients with current evidence or history of abnormal liver function indicated by significant abnormalities in serum transaminase (ALT/SGPT; AST/SGOT), bilirubin, and/or gamma-glutemate transferase (GGT) levels (see PRECAUTIONS and DOSAGE AND ADMINISTRATION). Baseline elevations of several LFTs (especially elevated bilirubin) should preclude the use of riluzole.

Riluzole, even in patients without a prior history of liver disease, causes serum aminotransferase elevations. Experience in almost 800 ALS patients indicates that about 50% of riluzole-treated patients will experience at least one ALT/SGPT level above the upper limit of normal, about 8% will have elevations > 3 X ULN, and about 2% of patients will have elevations > 5 X ULN. A single non-ALS patient with epilepsy treated with concomitant carbamazepine and phenobarbital experienced marked, rapid elevations of liver enzymes with jaundice (ALT 26 X ULN, AST 17 X ULN, and bilirubin 11 X ULN) four months after starting riluzole; these returned to normal 7 weeks after treatment discontinuation.

Maximum increases in serum ALT usually occurred within 3 months after the start of riluzole therapy and were usually transient when < 5 times ULN. In trials, if ALT levels were < 5 times ULN, treatment continued and ALT levels usually returned to below 2 times ULN within 2 to 6 months. Treatment in studies was discontinued, however, if ALT levels exceeded 5 X ULN, so that there is no experience with continued treatment of ALS patients once ALT values exceed 5 times ULN (see PRECAUTIONS, Laboratory Tests.) There were rare instances of jaundice.

Liver chemistries should be monitored (see PRECAUTIONS.)

Neutropenia: Among approximately 4000 patients given riluzole for ALS, there were three cases of marked neutropenia (absolute neutrophil count less than 500/mm^3), all seen within the first 2 months of riluzole treatment. In one case, neutrophil counts rose on continued treatment. In a second case, neutrophil counts rose after therapy was stopped. A third case was more complex, with marked anemia as well as neutropenia and the etiology of both is uncertain. Patients should be warned to report any febrile illness to their physicians. The report of a febrile illness should prompt treating physicians to check white blood cell counts.

PRECAUTIONS:

Use in Patients with Concomitant Disease: Riluzole should be used with caution in patients with concomitant liver and/or renal insufficiency (see WARNINGSand CLINICAL PHARMACOLOGY). In particular, in cases of riluzole-induced hepatic injury manifested by elevated liver enzymes, the effect of the hepatic injury on riluzole metabolism is unknown.

Special Populations: Riluzole should be used with caution in elderly patients whose hepatic or renal functions may be compromised due to age. Also, females and Japanese patients may possess a lower metabolic capacity to eliminate riluzole compared to males and Caucasian subjects, respectively (see CLINICAL PHARMACOLOGY, Special Populations.)

Information for the Patient: Patients should be advised to report any febrile illness to their physicians WARNINGS, Neutropenia.

Patients and caregivers should be advised that riluzole should be taken on a regular basis and at the same time of the day (*e.g.*, in the morning and in the evening) each day. If a dose is missed, take the next tablet as originally planned (see DOSAGE AND ADMINISTRATION.)

Whether alcohol increases the risk of serious hepatotoxicity with riluzole is unknown; therefore, patients being treated with riluzole should be discouraged from drinking excessive amounts of alcohol.

PRECAUTIONS: *(cont'd)*

Patients should also be made aware that riluzole should be stored at room temperatures between 20°-25°C (68°-77°F) and protected from the bright light.

Riluzole must be kept out of the reach of children.

Laboratory Tests: It is recommended that serum aminotransferases including ALT levels be measured before and during riluzole therapy. Serum ALT levels should be evaluated every month during the first 3 months of treatment, every 3 months during the remainder of the first year, and periodically thereafter. Serum ALT levels should be evaluated more frequently in patients who develop elevations (see WARNINGS.)

As noted in WARNINGS, there is no experience with continued treatment of patients once ALT exceeds 5 X ULN. If a decision is made to continue to treat these patients, frequent monitoring (at least weekly) of complete liver function is recommended. Treatment should be discontinued if ALT exceeds 10 X ULN or if clinical jaundice develops. Because there is no experience with rechallenge of patients who have had riluzole discontinued for ALT > 5 X ULN, no recommendations about restarting riluzole can be made.

In the two controlled trials in patients with ALS, the frequency with which values for hemoglobin, hematocrit, and erythrocyte counts fell below the lower limit of normal was greater in riluzole-treated patients than in placebo-treated patients; however, these changes were mild and transient. The proportions of patients observed with abnormally low values for these parameters showed a dose-response relationship. Only one patient was discontinued from treatment because of severe anemia. The significance of this finding is unknown.

Carcinogenesis, Mutagenesis, and Impairment of Fertility: Long-term studies to determine the carcinogenic potential of riluzole have not yet been completed.

The genotoxic potential of riluzole was evaluated in the bacterial mutagenicity (Ames) test, the mouse lymphoma mutation assay in L5178Y cells, the *in vivo* rat cytogenetic assay and *in vivo* mouse micronucleus assay in bone marrow. There was no evidence of mutagenic or clastogenic potential in the Ames test, the mouse lymphoma assay, or the *in vivo* assays in the mouse and rat. There was an equivocal clastogenic response in the *in vitro* lymphocyte chromosomal aberration assay.

Riluzole impaired fertility when administered to male and female rats prior to and during mating at an oral dose of 15 mg/kg or 1.5 times the maximum daily dose on a mg/m^2 basis (see PRECAUTIONS, Pregnancy for effects on fertility).

Pregnancy Category C: Oral administration of riluzole to pregnant animals during the period of organogenesis caused embryotoxicity in rats and rabbits at doses of 27 mg/kg and 60 mg/kg, respectively, or 2.6 and 11.5 times, respectively, the recommended maximum human daily dose on a mg/m^{2}basis. Evidence of maternal toxicity was also observed at these doses.

When administered to rats prior to and during mating (males and females) and throughout gestation and lactation (females), riluzole produced adverse effects on pregnancy (decreased implantations, increased intrauterine death) and offspring viability and growth at an oral dose of 15 mg/kg or 1.5 times the maximum daily dose on a mg/m^2 basis.

There are no adequate and well-controlled studies in pregnant women. Riluzole should be used during pregnancy only if the potential benefit justifies the potential risk to the fetus.

Nursing Women: In rat studies, C-riluzole was detected in maternal milk. It is not known whether riluzole is excreted in human breast milk. Because many drugs are excreted in human milk, and because of the potential for serious adverse reactions in nursing infants from riluzole is unknown, women should be advised not to breastfeed during treatment with riluzole.

Geriatric Use: Age-related compromised renal and hepatic function may cause a decrease in clearance of riluzole (see CLINICAL PHARMACOLOGY, Special Populations.) In controlled clinical trials, about 30% of patients were over 65. There were no differences in adverse effects between younger and older patients.

Pediatric Use: The safety and the effectiveness of riluzole in pediatric patients have not been established.

DRUG INTERACTIONS:

There have been no clinical studies designed to evaluate the interaction of riluzole with other drugs.

As with all drugs, the potential for interaction by a variety of mechanisms is a possibility.

Hepatotoxic Drugs: The clinical trials in ALS excluded patients on concomitant medications which were potentially hepatotoxic, (*e.g.*, allopurinol, methyldopa, sulfasalazine). Accordingly, there is no information about the safety of administering riluzole in conjunction with such medications. If the practitioner chooses to prescribe such a combination, caution should be exercised.

Drugs Highly Bound to Plasma Proteins: Riluzole is highly bound (96%) to plasma proteins, binding mainly to serum albumin and to lipoproteins. The effect of riluzole (up to 5 mcg/mL) on warfarin (5 mcg/mL) binding did not show any displacement of warfarin. Conversely, riluzole binding was unaffected by the addition of warfarin, digoxin, imipramine and quinine at high therapeutic concentrations.

Effect of Other Drugs on Riluzole Metabolism: *In vitro* studies using human liver microsomal preparations suggest that CYP 1A2 is the principal isozyme involved in the initial oxidative metabolism of riluzole and, therefore, potential interactions may occur when riluzole is given concurrently with agents that affect CYP 1A2 activity. Potential inhibitors of CYP 1A2 (*e.g.*, caffeine, phenacetin, theophylline, amitriptyline, and quinolones) could decrease the rate of riluzole elimination, while inducers of CYP 1A2 (*e.g.* cigarette smoke, charcoal-broiled food, rifampicin, and omeprazole) could increase the rate of riluzole elimination.

Effect of Riluzole On the Metabolism of Other Drugs: CYP 1 A2 is the principle isoenzyme inolved in the initial oxidative metabolism of riluzole; potential interactions may occur when riluzole is given concurrently with other agents which are also metabolized primarily by CYP 1A2 (*e.g.*, theophylline, caffeine and tacrine). Currently, it is not known whether riluzole has any potential for enzyme induction in humans.

Drug Laboratory Test Interactions: None known.

ADVERSE REACTIONS:

The most commonly observed AEs associated with the use of riluzole more frequently than placebo treated patients, were: asthenia, nausea, dizziness, decreased lung function, diarrhea, abdominal pain, pneumonia, vomiting, vertigo, circumoral paresthesia, anorexia, and somnolence. Asthenia, nausea, dizziness, diarrhea, anorexia, vertigo, somnolence, and circumoral paresthesia were dose related.

Approximately 14% (n=141) of the 982 individuals with ALS who received riluzole in premarketing clinical trials discontinued treatment because of an adverse experience. Of those patients who discontinued due to adverse events, the most commonly reported were: nausea, abdominal pain, constipation, and ALT elevations. In a dose response study in ALS patients, the rates of discontinuation of riluzole for asthenia, nausea, abdominal pain, and ALT elevation were dose related.

ADVERSE REACTIONS: *(cont'd)*

INCIDENCE IN CONTROLLED ALS CLINICAL STUDIES

Table 1 lists treatment emergent signs and symptoms that occurred in at least 2% of patients with ALS treated with riluzole (n=794) participating in placebo-controlled trials and were numerically greater in the patients treated with riluzole 100 mg/day than with placebo or for which a dose response relationship is suggested.

The prescriber should be aware that these figures cannot be used to predict the frequency of adverse experiences in the course of usual medical practice where patient characteristics and other factors may differ from those prevailing during clinical studies. Inspection of these frequencies, however, does provide the prescriber with one basis to estimate the relative contribution of drug and non-drug factors to the AE incidences in the population studied.

TABLE 1 Adverse Events Occurring in Placebo-Controlled Clinical Trials (Percentage of patients reporting events*)

Body System/ Adverse Event*	Riluzole 50 mg/day (N=237)	Riluzole 100 mg/day (N=313)	Riluzole 200 mg/day (N=244)	Placebo (N=320)
Body as a Whole				
Asthenia	14.8	19.2	20.1	12.2
Headache	8.0	7.3	7.0	6.6
Abdominal Pain	6.8	5.1	7.8	3.8
Back pain	1.7	3.2	4.1	2.5
Aggravation reaction	0.4	1.3	2.0	0.9
Malaise	0.4	0.6	1.2	0.0
Digestive				
Nausea	12.2	16.3	20.5	10.6
Vomiting	4.2	4.2	4.5	1.6
Dyspepsia	2.5	3.8	6.1	5.0
Anorexia	3.8	3.2	8.6	3.8
Diarrhea	5.5	2.9	9.0	3.1
Flatulence	2.5	2.6	2.0	1.9
Stomatitis	0.8	1.0	1.2	0.0
Tooth disorder	0.0	1.0	1.2	0.3
Oral Moniliasis	0.4	0.6	1.2	0.3
Nervous				
Hypertonia	6.9	6.1	5.3	5.9
Depression	4.2	4.5	6.1	5.0
Dizziness	5.1	3.8	12.7	2.5
Dry mouth	3.0	3.5	2.0	3.4
Insomnia	2.1	3.5	2.9	3.4
Somnolence	0.8	1.9	4.1	1.3
Vertigo	2.5	1.9	4.5	0.9
Circumoral paresthesia	1.3	1.6	3.3	0.0
Skin and Appendages				
Pruritus	3.8	3.8	2.5	3.1
Eczema	0.8	1.6	1.6	0.6
Alopecia	0.0	1.0	1.2	0.0
Exfoliative dermatitis	0.0	0.6	1.2	0.0
Respiratory				
Decreased lung function	13.1	10.2	16.0	9.4
Rhinitis	8.9	6.4	7.8	6.3
Increased cough	2.1	2.6	3.7	1.6
Sinusitis	0.4	1.0	1.6	0.9
Cardiovascular				
Hypertension	6.8	5.1	3.3	4.1
Tachycardia	1.3	2.6	2.0	1.3
Phlebitis	0.4	1.0	0.8	0.3
Palpitation	0.4	0.6	1.2	0.9
Postural hypotension	0.8	0.0	1.6	0.6
Metabolic and Nutritional Disorders				
Weight loss	4.6	4.8	3.7	4.7
Peripheral edema	4.2	2.9	3.3	2.2
Musculoskeletal System				
Arthralgia	5.1	3.5	1.6	3.4
Urogenital System				
Urinary tract infection	2.5	2.6	4.5	2.2
Dysuria	0.0	1.0	1.2	0.3

OTHER ADVERSE EVENTS OBSERVED

Other events which occurred in more than 2% of patients treated with riluzole 100 mg/day but equally or more frequently in the placebo group included: accidental injury, apnea, bronchitis, constipation, death, dysphagia, dyspnea, flu syndrome, heart arrest, increased sputum, pneumonia, and respiratory disorder.

The overall adverse event profile for riluzole was similar between females and males, and was independent of age. Because the largest non-white racial subgroup was only 2% of patients exposed to riluzole (18/794) in placebo-controlled trials, there are insufficient data to support a statement regarding the distribution of adverse experience reports by race. In ALS studies, dizziness did occur more commonly in females (11%) than in males (4%). There was not a difference between females and males in the rates of discontinuation of riluzole for individual adverse experiences.

OTHER ADVERSE EVENTS OBSERVED DURING ALL CLINICAL TRIALS

Riluzole has been administered to 1713 individuals during all clinical trials, some of which were placebo-controlled. During these trials, all adverse events were recorded by the clinical investigators using terminology of their own choosing. To provide a meaningful estimate of the proportion of individuals having adverse events, similar types of events were grouped into a smaller number of standardized categories using modified COSTART dictionary terminology. The frequencies presented represent the proportion of the 1713 individuals exposed to riluzole who experienced an event of the type cited on at least one occasion while receiving riluzole. All reported events are included except those already listed in the previous table, those too general to be informative, and those not reasonably associated with the use of the drug.

Events are further classified within body system categories and enumerated in order of decreasing frequency using the following definitions: *frequent* adverse events are defined as those occurring in at least 1/100 patients; *infrequent* adverse events are those occurring in 1/100 to 1/1000 patients; *rare* adverse events are those occurring in fewer than 1/1000 patients.

* =AE frequency ≤ to placebo

Body as a Whole: *Frequent:*Hostility*.*Infrequent:*Abscess*, sepsis*, photosensitivity reaction*, cellulitis, face edema*, hernia, peritonitis, attempted suicide, injection site reaction, chills*, flu syndrome, intentional injury, enlarged abdomen, neoplasm.*Rare:*Acrodynia, hypothermia, moniliasis*, rheumatoid arthritis.

Digestive System: *Infrequent:*Increased appetite; intestinal obstruction*,fecal impaction, gastrointestinal hemorrhage, gastrointestinal ulceration,gastritis*, fecal incontinence, jaundice, hepatitis, glossitis, gum hemorrhage*, pancreatitis, tenesmus, esophageal stenosis. *Rare:* Cheilitis*, cholecystitis, hematemesis, melena*, biliary pain, proctitis, pseudomembranous enterocolitis, enlarged salivary gland, tongue discoloration, tooth caries.

ADVERSE REACTIONS: *(cont'd)*

Nervous System: *Frequent:*Agitation*, tremor.*Infrequent:*Hallucinations, personality disorder*, abnormal thinking*, coma, paranoid reaction*, manic reaction, ataxia, extrpyramidal syndrome, hypokinesia, urinary retention, emotional liability, delusions, apathy, hypesthesia, incoordination, confusion*, convulsion, leg cramps, amnesia, dysarthria, increased libido, stupor, subdural hematoma, abnormal gait, delirium, depersonalization, facial paralysis, hemiplegia, decreased libido, myoclonus. *Rare:*Abnormal dreams, acute brain syndrome, CNS depression, dementia, cerebral embolism, euphoria*, hypotonia, ileus*, peripheral neuritis, psychosis*, psychotic depression, schizophrenic reaction, trismus, wristdrop.

Skin and Appendages: *Infrequent:*Skin ulceration, urticaria, psoriasis, seborrhea*, skin disorder, fungal dermatitis*.*Rare:*Angioedema, contact dermatitis,erythema multiforme,furunculosis*, skin moniliasis,skin granuloma, skin nodule.

Respiratory System: *Infrequent:*Hiccup, pleural disorder*, asthma, epistaxis, hemoptysis, yawn, hyperventilation*, lung edema*, hypoventilation*, lung carcinoma, hypoxia, laryngitis, pleural effusion, pneumothorax*, respiratory moniliasis, stridor.

Cardiovascular System: *Infrequent:*Syncope*, hypotension, heart failure, migraine, peripheral vascular disease, angina pectoris*, myocardial infarction*, ventricular extrasystoles, cerebral hemorrhage, atrial fibrillation*, bundle branch block, congestive heart failure, pericarditis, lower extremity embolus, myocardial ischemia*, shock*. *Rare:*Bradycardia, cerebral ischemia, hemorrhage, mesenteric artery occlusion, subarachnoid hemorrhage, supraventricular tachycardia*, thrombosis, ventricular fibrillation, ventricular tachycardia.

Metabolic and Nutritional Disorders: *Infrequent:*Gout*, respiratory acidosis, edema, thirst*, hypokalemia, hyponatremia, weight gain*. *Rare:*Generalized edema, hypercalcemia, hypercholestermia.

Endocrine System: *Infrequent:*Diabetes mellitus,thyroid neoplasia. *Rare:*Diabetes insipidus, parathyroid disorder.

Hemic and Lymphatic System: *Infrequent:*Anemia*, leukocytosis, leukopenia,ecchymosis. *Rare:*Neutropenia, aplastic anemia, cyanosis, hypochromic anemia, iron deficiency anemia,lymphadenopathy, petechiae*, purpura.

Musculoskeletal System: *Infrequent:*Arthrosis, myasthenia*, bone neoplasm. *Rare:*Bone necrosis,osteoporosis, tetany.

Special Senses: *Infrequent:*Amblyopia, ophthalmitis. *Rare:*Blepharitis, cataract, deafness, diplopia*, ear pain, glaucoma, hyperacusis, photophobia, taste loss, vestibular disorder.

Urogenital System: *Infrequent:*Urinary urgency, urine abnormality,urinary incontinence,kidney calculus,hematuria, impotence, prostate carcinoma, kidney pain, metrorrhagia, priapism. *Rare:*Amenorrhea, breast abscess, breast pain, nephritis*, nocturia, pyelonephritis, enlarged uterine fibroids, uterine hemorrhage, vaginal moniliasis.

Laboratory Tests: *Infrequent:*Increased gamma glutamyl transferase, abnormal liver function/ tests, increased alkaline phosphatase, positive direct Coombs test, increased gamma globulins. *Rare:*increased lactic dehydrogenase.

OVERDOSAGE:

There have been no reports of overdose with riluzole. No specific antidote or information on treatment of overdosage with riluzole is available. In the event of overdose, riluzole therapy should be discontinued immediately. Treatment should be supportive and directed toward alleviating symptoms.

The estimated oral median lethal dose is 94 mg/kg and 39 mg/kg for male mice and rats, respectively.

DOSAGE AND ADMINISTRATION:

The recommended dose for riluzole is 50 mg every 12 hours. No increased benefit can be expected from higher daily doses, but adverse events are increased.

Riluzole tablets should be taken at least an hour before, or two hours after, a meal to avoid a food-related decrease in bioavailability.

SPECIAL POPULATIONS

Patients with Impaired Renal or Hepatic Function: Studies have not yet been completed in these populations (see WARNINGS, PRECAUTIONS and CLINICAL PHARMACOLOGY).

PATIENT INFORMATION:

Riluzole is used for the treatment of amyotrophic lateral sclerosis (ALS), also known as Lou Gehrig's Disease.. Do not use if you are nursing. Inform your doctor if you have a history of liver or kidney disease or are pregnant or have a fever. Take every 12 hours. Be sure to take at least one hour before, or 2 hours after, a meal. Take at the same times every day. Avoid alcohol and smoking. May cause dizziness, vertigo, nausea, diarrhea, breathing problems and pneumonia. Inform your doctor or pharmacist if these effects occur.

HOW SUPPLIED:

Rilutek is available as a capsule-shaped, white, film-coated tablet for oral administration containing 50 mg of riluzole. Each tablet is engraved with "RPR 202" on one side.

STORE AT CONTROLLED ROOM TEMPERATURE 20°-25°C (68°-77°F) AND PROTECT FROM BRIGHT LIGHT. KEEP OUT OF REACH OF CHILDREN.

HOW SUPPLIED - EQUIVALENTS NOT AVAILABLE:

Tablet - Oral - 50 mg

60's $727.75 RILUTEK, Rhone-Poulenc Rorer 00075-7700-60

RIMANTADINE HYDROCHLORIDE *(003182)*

CATEGORIES: Anti-Infectives; Antimicrobials; Antivirals; Autonomic Drugs; Influenza; Viral Agents; FDA Class 1P ("Priority Review"); FDA Approved 1993 Sep

BRAND NAMES: **Flumadine**; *Ruflual*
(International brand names outside U.S. in italics)

DESCRIPTION:

Rimantadine hydrochloride is a synthetic antiviral drug available as a 100 mg film-coated tablet and as syrup for oral administration. Each film-coated tablet contains 100 mg of rimantadine hydrochloride plus hydroxypropyl methylcellulose, magnesium stearate, microcrystalline cellulose, sodium starch glycolate, FD&C Yellow No. 6 Lake and FD&C Yellow No. 6. The film coat contains hydroxypropyl methylcellulose and polyethylene glycol. Each teaspoonful (5 ml) of the syrup contains 50 mg of rimantadine hydrochloride in an aqueous solution containing citric acid, parabens (methyl and propyl), saccharin sodium, sorbitol, D&C Red No. 33 and flavors.

Rimantadine hydrochloride is a white to off-white crystalline powder which is freely soluble in water (50 mg/ml at 20°C). Chemically, rimantadine hydrochloride is alpha-methytricyclo-(3.3.1.1/.7)decane-1-methanamine hydrochloride, with an empirical formula $C_{12}H_{21}N$°HCl, and a molecular weight of 215.7.

CLINICAL PHARMACOLOGY:

MECHANISM OF ACTION

The mechanism of action of rimantadine is not fully understood. Rimantadine appears to exert its inhibitory effect early in the viral replicative cycle, possibly inhibiting the uncoating of the virus. Genetic studies suggest that a virus protein specified by the virion M_2 gene plays an important role in the susceptibility of influenza A virus to inhibition by rimantadine.

MICROBIOLOGY

Rimantadine is inhibitory to the *in vitro*replication of influenza A virus isolates from each of the three antigenic subtypes, i.e., H1N1, H2H2 and H3N2., that have been isolated from man. Rimantadine has little or no activity against influenza B virus (Ref 1,2,). Rimantadine does not appear to interfere with the immunogenicity of inactivated influenza A vaccine.

A quantitative relationship between the *in vitro* susceptibility of influenza A virus to rimantadine and clinical response to therapy has not been established.

Susceptibility test results, expressed as the concentration of the drug required to inhibit virus replication by 50%, or more in a cell culture system, vary greatly (from 4 ng/ml to 20 mcg/ml) depending upon the assay protocol used, size of the virus inoculum, isolates of the influenza A virus strains tested, and the cell types used (Ref. 2).

Rimantadine-resistant strains of influenza A virus have emerged among freshly isolated epidemic strains in closed settings where rimantadine hs been used. Resistant viruses have been shown to be transmissible and to cause typical influenza illness (Ref. 3).

PHARMACOKINETICS

Although the pharmacokinetic profile of rimantadine HCl has been described, no pharmacodynamic data establishing a correlation between plasma concentration and its antiviral effect are available.

The tablet and syrup formulations of rimantadine HCl are equally absorbed after oral administration. The mean ± SD peal plasma concentration after a single 100 mg dose of rimantadine HCl was 74 ± 22 ng/ml (range: 45 to 138 ng/ml). The time to peak concentration was 6 ± 1 hours in healthy adults (age 20 to 44 years.) The single dose elimination half-life in this population was 25.4 ± 6.3 hours (range: 13 to 65 hours). The single dose elimination half-life in a group of healthy 71 to 79 year- old subjects was 32 ± 16 hours (range: 20 to 65 hours).

After the administration of rimantadine 1000 mg twice daily to healthy volunteers (age 18 to 70 years) for 10 days, area under the curve (AUC) values were approximately 30% greater than predicted from a single dose. Plasma trough levels at steady state ranged between 188 and 468 ng/ml. In these patients no age-related differences in pharmacokinetics were detected. However, in a comparison of three groups of healthy older subjects (age 50-60), 61-70, 71-79 years), the 71 to 79 year-old group had average AUC values, peak concentrations and elimination half-life values at steady-state that were 20 to 30% higher than the outer two groups. Steady-state concentrations in elderly nursing home patients (age 68 to 102 years) were 2- to 4-fold higher than those seen in healthy young and elderly adults.

The pharmacokinetic profile of rimantadine in children has not been established. In a group (n=10) of children 4 to 8 years old who were given a single dose (6.6 mg/kg) of rimantadine HCl syrup, plasma concentrations of rimantadine ranged from 446 to 988 ng/ml at 5 to 6 hours and from 170 to 424 ng/ml at 24 hours. In some children drug was detected in plasma 72 hours after the last dose.

Following oral administration, rimantadine is extensively metabolized in the liver with less than 25% of the dose excreted in the urine as unchanged drug. Three hydroxylated metabolites have been found in plasma. These metabolites, an additional conjugated metabolites and parent drug account for 74 ± 10% (n=4) of a single 200 mg dose of rimantadine excreted in urine over 72 hours.

In a group (n=14) of patients with chronic liver disease, the majority of whom were stabilized cirrhotics, the pharmacokinetics of rimantadine were not appreciably altered following a single 200 mg oral dose compared to 6 healthy subjects who were sex, age and weight matched to 6 of the patients with liver disease. After administration of a single 200 mg dose to patients (n=10) with severe hepatic dysfunction, AUC was approximately 3-fold larger, elimination half-life was approximately 2-fold longer and apparent clearance was about 50% lower when compared to historic data from healthy subjects.

Studies of the effects of renal insufficiency on the pharmacokinetics of rimantadine have given inconsistent results. Following administration of a single 200 mg oral dose of rimantadine to 8 patients with a creatinine clearance (CLcr) of 31-50 ml/min and 6 patients with a CLcr of 11-30 ml/min, the apparent clearance was 37% and 16% lower, respectively, and plasma metabolite concentrations were higher when compared to weight-, age-, and 16% lower, respectively, and plasma metabolite concentrations were higher when compared to weight-, age-, and sex-matched healthy subjects (n=9, CLcr > 50 ml/min). After a single 200 mg oral dose of rimantadine was given to 8 hemodialysis patients (CLcr 0-10 ml/min); there was a 1.6-fold increase in the elimination half-life and a 40% decrease in apparent clearance compared to age-matched healthy subjects. Hemodialysis did not contribute to the clearance of rimantadine.

The *in vitro* human plasma protein binding of rimantadine is about 40% over typical plasma concentrations. Albumin is the major binding protein.

INDICATIONS AND USAGE:

Rimantadine HCl is indicated for the prophylaxis and treatment of illness caused by various strains of influenza A virus in adults.

Rimantadine HCl is indicated for prophylaxis against influenza A virus in children.

PROPHYLAXIS

In controlled studies of children over the age of 1 year, healthy adults and elderly patients, Rimantadine HCl has been shown to be safe and effective in preventing signs and symptoms of infection caused by various strains of influenza A virus. Early vaccination on an annual basis as recommended by the Centers for Disease Control's Immunization Practices Advisory Committee is the method of choice in the prophylaxis of influenza unless vaccination is contraindicated, not available or not feasible. Since rimantadine HCl does not completely prevent the host immune response to influenza A infection, individuals who take this drug mat still develop immune responses to natural disease or vaccination and may be protected when later exposed to antigenically-related viruses. Following vaccination during an influenza outbreak, rimantadine HCl prophylaxis should be considered for the 2 to 4 week time period required to develop an antibody response. However, the safety and effectiveness of rimantadine HCl prophylaxis have not been demonstrated for longer than 6 weeks.

TREATMENT

Rimantadine HCl therapy should be considered for adults who develop an influenza-like illness during known or suspected influenza A infection in the community. When administered within 48 hours after onset of signs and symptoms of infection caused by influenza A virus strains, rimantadine HCl has been shown to reduce the duration of fever and systemic symptoms.

CONTRAINDICATIONS:

Rimantadine HCl is contraindicated in patients with known hypersensitivity to drugs of the adamantine class, including rimantadine and amantadine.

PRECAUTIONS:

GENERAL

An increased incidence of seizures has been reported in patients with a history of epilepsy who received the related drug amantadine. In clinical trials of rimantadine HCl, the occurrence of seizure-like activity was observed in a small number of patients with a history of seizures who were not receiving anticonvulsant medication while taking rimantadine HCl. If seizures develop, rimantadine HCl should be discontinued.

The safety and pharmacokinetics of rimantadine in renal and hepatic insufficiency have only been evaluated after single dose administration. In a single dose study of patients with anuric renal failure, the apparent clearance of rimantadine was approximately 40% lower and the elimination half-life was 1.6-fold greater than that in healthy age-matched controls. In a study of 14 persons with chronic liver disease (mostly stabilized cirrhotics), no alterations in the pharmacokinetics were observed after the administration of a single dose of rimantadine. However, the apparent clearance of rimantadine following a single dose to 10 patients with severe liver dysfunction was 50% lower than reported for healthy subjects. Because of the potential for accumulation of rimantadine and its metabolites in plasma, caution should be exercised when patients with renal or hepatic insufficiency are treated with rimantadine.

Transmission of rimantadine resistant virus should be considered when treating patients whose contacts are at high risk for influenza A illness. Influenza A virus strains resistant to rimantadine can emerge during treatment and such resistant strains have been shown to be transmissible and to cause typical influenza illness (Ref. 3). Although the frequency, rapidity, and clinical significance of the mergence of drug-resistant virus are not yet established, several small studies have demonstrated that 10% to 30% of patients with initially sensitive virus, upon treatment with rimantadine, shed rimantadine resistant virus (Ref. 3,4,5,6).

Clinical response to rimantadine, although slower in those patients who subsequently shed resistant virus, was not significantly different from those who did not shed resistant virus (Ref. 3) No Data are available in humans that address the activity or effectiveness of rimantadine therapy in subjects infected with resistant virus.

CARCINOGENESIS, MUTAGENESIS, AND IMPAIRMENT OF FERTILITY

Carcinogenesis: Carcinogenicity studies in animals have not been performed.

Mutagenesis: No mutagenic effects were seen when rimantadine was evaluated in several standard assays for mutagenicity.

Impairment of Fertility: A reproduction study in male and female rats did not show detectable impairment of fertility at dosages up to 60 mg/kg/day (3 times the maximum human dose based on body surface area comparisons).

PREGNANCY CATEGORY C

Teratogenic Effects: There are no adequate and well-controlled studies in pregnant women. Rimantadine is reported to cross the placenta in mice. Rimantadine has been shown to be embryotoxic in rats when given at a dose of 200 mg/kg/day (11 times the recommended human dose based on body surface area comparisons). At this dose the embryotoxic effect consisted of increased fetal absorption in rats; this dose also produced a variety of maternal effects including ataxia, tremors, convulsions and significantly reduced weight gain. No embryotoxicity was observed when rabbits were given doses up to 50 mg/kg/day (5 times the recommended human dose based on body surface area comparisons). However, there was evidence of a developmental abnormality in the form of a change in the ratio of fetuses with 12 or 12 ribs. This ratio is normally about 50:500 in a liter but was 80:20 after rimantadine treatment.

Nonteratogenic Effects: Rimantadine was administered to pregnant rats in a peri- and postnatal reproduction toxicity study at doses of 30, 60 and 120 mg/kg/day (1.7, 3.4 and 6.8 times the recommended human dose based on body surface area comparisons). Maternal toxicity during gestation was noted at the two higher doses of rimantadine, and at the highest dose, 120 mg/kg/day, there was an increase in pup mortality during the first 2 to 4 days postpartum. Decreased fertility of the F1 generation was also noted for the two higher doses.

For these reasons, rimantadine HCl should be used during pregnancy only if the potential benefit justifies the risk to the fetus.

NURSING MOTHERS

Rimantadine HCl should not be administered to nursing mothers because of the adverse effects noted in offspring of rats treated with rimantadine during the nursing period. Rimantadine is concentrated in rat milk in a dose-related manner: 2 to 3 hours folling administration of rimantadine, rat breast milk levels were approximately twice those observed in the serum.

PEDIATRIC USE

In children, rimantadine HCl is recommended for the prophylaxis of influenza A. The safety and effectiveness of rimantadine HCl in the treatment of symptomatic influenza infection in children have not been established. Prophylaxis studies with rimantadine HCl have not been performed in children below the age of 1 year.

DRUG INTERACTIONS:

Cimetidine: The effects of chronic cimetidine use on the metabolism of rimantadine are not known. When a single 100 mg dose of rimantadine HCl was administered one hour after the initiation of Cimetidine (300 mg four times a day), the apparent total rimantadine clearance of this single dose in normal healthy adults was reduced by 18% (compared to the apparent total rimantadine clearance in the same subjects in the absence of cimetidine).

Acetaminophen: Rimantadine HCl, 100 mg, was given twice daily for 13 days to 12 healthy volunteers. On day 11, acetaminophen (650 mg four times daily) was started and continued for 8 days. The pharmacokinetics of rimantadine were assessed on days 11 and 13. Coadministration with acetaminophen reduced the peak concentration and AUC values for rimantadine by approximately 11%.

Aspirin: Rimantadine HCl, 100 mg, was given twice daily fro 13 days to 12 healthy volunteers. On day 11, aspirin (650 mg, four times daily) was started and continued for 8 days. The pharmacokinetics of rimantadine were assessed on days 11 and 13. Peak plasma concentrations and AUC of rimantadine were reduced approximately 10% in the presence of aspirin.

ADVERSE REACTIONS:

In 1,027 patients treated with rimantadine HCl in controlled clinical trials at the recommended dose of 200 mg daily, the most frequently reported adverse events involved the gastrointestinal and nervous systems.

Incidence > 1%: Adverse events reported most frequently (1-3%) at the recommended dose in controlled clinical trials are shown in the table below (TABLE 1).

Less frequent adverse events (0.3 to 1%) at the recommended dose in controlled clinical trials were:

Gastrointestinal System: diarrhea, dyspepsia

Nervous System: impairment of concentration, ataxia, somnolence, agitation, depression

Skin and Appendages: rash

Hearing and Vestibular: tinnitus

Respiratory: dyspepsia

ADVERSE REACTIONS: *(cont'd)*

TABLE 1

	Rimantadine (n=1027)	Control (n=986)
Nervous System		
Insomnia	2.1%	0.9%
Dizziness	1.9%	1.1%
Headache	1.4%	1.3%
Nervousness	1.3%	0.6%
Fatigue	1.0%	0.9%
Gastrointestinal System		
Nausea	2.8%	1.6%
Vomiting	1.7%	0.6%
Anorexia	1.6%	0.8%
Dry Mouth	1.5%	0.6%
Abdominal Pain	1.4%	0.8%
Body as a Whole		
Asthenia	1.4%	0.5%

Additional adverse events (less than 0.3%) reported at recommended doses in controlled clinical trials were:

Nervous System: gait abnormality, euphoria, hyperkinesia, tremor, hallucination, confusion, convulsions

Respiratory: bronchospasm, cough

Cardiovascular: pallor, palpitation, hypertension, cerebrovascular disorder, cardiac failure, pedal edema, heart block, tachycardia, syncope

Reproduction: non-pleural lactation

Special Senses: taste loss/chance, parosmia

Rates of adverse events, particularly those involving the gastrointestinal and nervous systems, increased significantly in controlled studies using higher than recommended dose of rimantadine HCl. In most cases, symptoms resolved rapidly with discontinuation of treatment. In addition to the adverse events reported above, the following were also reported at higher than recommended doses: increased lacrimation, increased micturition frequency, fever, rigors, agitation, constipation, diaphoresis, dysphagia, stomatitis, hypesthesia and eye pain.

Adverse Reactions in Trials of Rimantadine and Amantadine: In a six-week prophylaxis study of 436 healthy adults comparing rimantadine with amantadine and placebo, the following adverse reactions were reported with an incidence > 1% (TABLE 2).

TABLE 2

	Rimantadine 200 mg/day (n=145)	Placebo (n=143)	Amantadine 200 mg/day (n=148)
Nervous System			
Insomnia	3.4%	0.7%	7.0%
Nervousness	2.1%	0.7%	2.8%
Impaired Concentration	2.1%	1.4%	2.1%
Dizziness	0.7%	0.0%	2.1%
Depression	0.7%	0.7%	3.5%
Total % of subjects with adverse reactions	6.9%	4.1%	14.7%
Total % of subjects withdrawn due to adverse reactions	6.9%	3.4%	14.0%

USAGE IN THE ELDERLY

In general, the incidence of adverse events in controlled clinical trials in the elderly was higher in both the rimantadine HCl and placebo-treated groups compared to younger adults and children. Most of these patients had other chronic illnesses. In a placebo-controlled study of 83 nursing home patients with influenza, 10.6% of those treated with rimantadine HCl compared with 8.3% in the placebo group experienced events related to the central nervous system. The profile of these events was similar to that for the most frequent adverse events reported in other controlled trials (see TABLE 2).

Pooled data from controlled studies of prophylaxis and treatment of influenza with rimantadine HCl in persons over 65 years of age showed an increase in adverse clinical events associated with the recommended dose of rimantadine HCl (100 mg twice a day) compared to controls as follows: central and peripheral nervous systems, 12.5% for rimantadine HCl versus 8.7% for control patients; gastrointestinal systems, 17.0% for rimantadine HCl versus 11.3% for controls.

OVERDOSAGE:

As with any overdose, supportive therapy should be administered as indicated. Overdoses of a related rug, amantadine, have been reported with adverse reactions consisting of agitation, hallucinations, cardiac arrhythmia and death. The administration of intravenous physostigmine (a cholinergic agent) at doses of 1 to 2 mg in adults (Ref. 7) and 0.5 mg in children (Ref. 8) repeated as needed as long as the dose did not exceed 2 mg/hour has been reported anecdotally to be beneficial in patients with central nervous system effects from overdoses of amantadine.

DOSAGE AND ADMINISTRATION:

FOR PROPHYLAXIS IN ADULTS AND CHILDREN

Adults: The recommended adult dose of rimantadine HCl is 100 mg twice a day. In patients with severe hepatic dysfunction, renal failure (CrCl ≤ 10 ml/min.) and elderly nursing home patients, a dose reduction to 100 mg daily is recommended. There are currently no data available regarding the safety of rimantadine during multiple dosing in subjects with renal or hepatic impairment. Because of the potential for accumulation of rimantadine metabolites during multiple dosing, patients with any degree of renal insufficiency should be monitored for adverse effects, with dosage adjustments being made as necessary.

Children: In children less than 10 years of age, rimantadine HCl should be administered once a day, at a dose of 5 mg/kg but not exceeding 150 mg. For children 10 years of age or older, use the adult dose.

FOR TREATMENT IN ADULTS

The recommended adult dose of rimantadine HCl is 100 mg twice a day. In patients with severe hepatic dysfunction, renal failure (CrCl ≤ 10 ml/min) and elderly nursing home patients, a dose reduction to 100 mg daily is recommended. There are currently no data available regarding the safety of rimantadine during multiple dosing in subjects with renal or hepatic impairment. Because of the potential for accumulation of rimantadine metabolites during multiple dosing, patients with any degree of renal insufficiency should be monitored for adverse effect, with dosage adjustments being made as necessary. rimantadine HCl therapy should be initiated as soon as possible, preferably within 48 hours after onset of signs and symptoms of influenza A infection. Therapy should be continued for approximately seven days from the initial onset of symptoms.

DOSAGE AND ADMINISTRATION: *(cont'd)*

STORAGE

Tablets and syrup should be stored at 15-30°C (59-86°F).

REFERENCES:

1. Belshe, R.B., Burk, B., Newman, F., Cerruti, R.L. and Sim, I.S. (1989) J. Infect. Dis. 159, 430-435. **2.** Sim, I.S., Cerruti, R.L. and Connell, E.V., (1989) J. Resp. Dis. (Suppl.), S46-S51. **3.** Hayden, F.G., Belshe, R.B., Clover, R.D. et al (1989) N. Engl. J. Med. 321 (25), 1696-1702. **4.** Hall, C.B., Dolin, R., Gaja, C.L., eta l (1987) Pediatrics 80, 275-282. **5.** Thompson, J., Fleet, W., Lawrence, E., et al (1987) J. Med. Vir. 21, 249-255. **6.** Belshe, R.B., Smith, M.H., Hall, C.B., et al (1988) J. Virol. 62, 1508-1512. **7.** Casey, D.F. N. Engl. J. Med. 1978:298: 516. **8.** Berkowitz, C.D. J. Pediatrics 1979:95:144.

HOW SUPPLIED - EQUIVALENTS NOT AVAILABLE:

Syrup - Oral - 50 mg/5ml

240 ml $30.28 FLUMADINE, Forest Pharms 00456-0527-08

Tablet, Plain Coated - Oral - 100 mg

100's $149.76 FLUMADINE, Forest Pharms 00456-0521-01

RIMEXOLONE *(003240)*

CATEGORIES: Anti-Inflammatory Agents; Corneal Inflammation; EENT Drugs; Eye, Ear, Nose, & Throat Preparations; Ophthalmic Corticosteroids; Ophthalmics; Uveitis; FDA Class 1P ("Priority Review"); FDA Approved 1994 Dec

BRAND NAMES: **Vexol**

FORMULARIES: PCS

DESCRIPTION:

Vexol 1% Ophthalmic Suspension is a sterile, multi-dose topical ophthalmic suspension containing the corticosteroid, rimexolone. Rimexolone is a white, water-insoluble powder with an empirical formula of $C_{24}H_{34}O_3$ and a molecular weight of 370.53. Its chemical name is 11β-Hydroxy-16a, 17a-dimethyl-17-propionylandrosta-1,4-diene-3-one.

Each ml contains: Active ingredient: rimexolone 10 mg (1%). *Preservative:* benzalkonium chloride 0.01% *Inactive ingredients:* mannitol, carbomer 934P, polysorbate 80, sodium chloride, edetate disodium, sodium hydroxide and/or hydrochloride acid (to adjust pH) and purified water.

The pH of the suspension is 6.0 to 8.0 and the tonicity is 260 to 320 mOsmol/kg.

CLINICAL PHARMACOLOGY:

Corticosteroids suppress the inflammatory response to a variety of inciting agents of a mechanical, chemical, or immunological nature. They inhibit edema, cellular infiltration capillary dilatation, fibroblastic proliferation, deposition of collagen and scar formation associated with inflammation.

Placebo-controlled clinical studies demonstrated that rimexolone is efficacious for the treatment of anterior chamber inflammation following cataract surgery.

In two controlled clinical trials rimexolone demonstrated clinical equivalence to 1% prednisolone acetate in reducing uveitic inflammation.

In a controlled 6-week study of steroid responsive subjects, the time to raise intraocular pressure was similar for rimexolone and 0.1% fluorometholone given four times daily.

As with other topically administered ophthalmic drugs, rimexolone is absorbed systemically. Studies in normal volunteers dosed bilaterally once every hour during waking hours for one week have demonstrated serum concentrations ranging from less than 80 pg/ml to 470 pg/ml. The mean serum concentrations were approximately 130 pg/ml. Serum concentrations were at one or near steady state after 5 to 7 hourly doses. After decreasing the dosing frequency to once every two hours while awake during the second week of administration, mean serum concentrations were approximately 100 pg/ml. The serum half-life of rimexolone could not be reliably estimated due to the large number of samples below the quantitation limit of the assay (80 pg/ml). However, based on the time required to reach steady-state, the half-life appears to be short (1-2 hours).

Based in *in vivo* and *in vitro* preclinical metabolism studies, and on *in vivo* results with human liver preparations, rimexolone undergoes extensive metabolism. Following IV administration of radio-labeled rimexolone to rats, greater than 80% of the dose is excreted via the feces as rimexolone and metabolites. Metabolites have been shown to be less active than parent drug, or inactive in human glucocorticoid receptor binding assays.

INDICATIONS AND USAGE:

Rimexolone is indicated for the treatment of postoperative inflammation following ocular surgery and in the treatment of anterior uveitis.

CONTRAINDICATIONS:

Rimexolone is contraindicated in epithelial herpes simplex keratitis (dendritic keratitis), vaccinia, varicella, and most other viral diseases of the cornea and conjunctiva; mycobacterial infection of the eye; fungal diseases of the eye, acute purulent untreated infections which, like other diseases caused by microorganisms, may be masked or enhanced by the presence of a steroid; and in those persons with hypersensitivity to any component of the formulation.

WARNINGS:

Not for injection. Use in the treatment of herpes simplex infection requires great caution and frequent slit-lamp examinations. Prolonged use may result in ocular hypertension/glaucoma, damage to the optic nerve, defects in visual acuity and visual fields, and posterior subcapsular cataract formation. Prolonged use may also result in secondary ocular infections due to suppression of host response. Acute purulent infections of the eye may be masked or exacerbated by the presence of corticosteroid medication. In those diseases causing thinning of the cornea or sclera, perforation has been known to occur with topical steroids. It is advisable that the intraocular pressure be checked frequently.

PRECAUTIONS:

General: Fungal infections of the cornea are particularly prone to develop coincidentally with long-term corticosteroid application. Fungal invasion must be considered in any persistent corneal ulceration where a steroid has been or is in use.

Information for the Patient: Do not touch dropper tip to any surface, as this may contaminate the suspension.

Carcinogenesis, Mutagenesis, and Impairment of Fertility: Rimexolone has been shown to be non-mutagenic in a battery of *in vitro* and *in vivo* mutagenicity assays. Fertility and reproductive capability were not impaired in a study in rats with plasma levels (42 ng/ml) approximately 200 times those obtained in clinical studies after topical administration (<0.2 ng/ml). Long-term studies have not been conducted in animals or humans to evaluate the carcinogenic potential of rimexolone.

PRECAUTIONS: *(cont'd)*

Pregnancy Category C: Rimexolone has been shown to be teratogenic and embryotoxic in rabbits following subcutaneous administration at the lowest dose tested (0.5 mg/kg/day, approximately 2 times the recommended human ophthalmic dose). Corticosteroids are recognized to cause fetal resorptions and malformations in animals. There are no adequate and well-controlled studies in pregnant women. Rimexolone should be used in pregnant women only if potential benefits to the mother justifies the potential risk to the fetus.

Nursing Mothers: It is not known whether topical ophthalmic administration of corticosteroids could result in sufficient systemic absorption to produce detectable quantities in human breast milk. Nevertheless, caution to produce detectable quantities in human breast milk. Nevertheless, caution should be exercised when topical corticosteroids are administered to a nursing woman; a decision should be made whether to discontinue nursing or discontinue therapy, taking into consideration the importance of the drug to the mother.

Pediatric Use: Safety and effectiveness in children have not been established.

ADVERSE REACTIONS:

Reactions associated with ophthalmic steroids include elevated intraocular pressure, which may be associated with optic nerve damage, visual acuity and field defects, posterior subcapsular cataract formation, secondary ocular infection from pathogens including herpes simplex, and perforation of the globe where there is thinning of the cornea or sclera.

Ocular adverse reactions occurring in 1-5% of patients in clinical studies of rimexolone included blurred vision, discharge, discomfort, ocular pain, increased intraocular pressure, foreign body sensation, hyperemia and pruritus. Other ocular adverse reactions occurring in less than 1% of patients included sticky sensation, increased fibrin, dry eye, conjunctival edema, corneal staining, keratitis, tearing, photophobia, edema, irritation, corneal ulcer, browache, lid margin crusting, corneal edema, infiltrate, and corneal erosion.

Non-ocular adverse reactions occurred in less than 2% of patients. These included headache, hypotension, rhinitis, pharyngitis, and taste perversion.

DOSAGE AND ADMINISTRATION:

Post-operative Inflammation: Apply one-two drops of rimexolone into the conjunctival sac of the affected eye four times daily beginning 24 hours after surgery and continuing throughout the first 2 weeks of the postoperative period.

Anterior Uveitis: Apply one-two drops of rimexolone into the conjunctival sac of the affected eye every hour during waking hours for the first week, one drop every two hours during waking hours of the second week and then taper until uveitis is resolved.

HOW SUPPLIED:

5 ml and 10 ml in plastic DROP-TAINER dispensers.

Storage: Store upright between 4° and 30°C (40°and 86°F).

Shake well before using.

HOW SUPPLIED - EQUIVALENTS NOT AVAILABLE:

Powder - Ophthalmic - 1 %

5 ml	**$16.13**	**VEXOL, Alcon**	**00065-0626-06**
10 ml	**$27.00**	**VEXOL, Alcon**	**00065-0626-10**

RISPERIDONE *(003165)*

CATEGORIES: Antipsychotics/Antimanics; Behavior Problems; Central Nervous System Agents; Psychotherapeutic Agents; Psychotic Disorders; Schizophrenia; Sedatives/Hypnotics; Tranquilizers; FDA Class 1P ("Priority Review"); Sales > $100 Million; FDA Approved 1993 Dec; Patent Expiration 2006 Feb; Top 200 Drugs

BRAND NAMES: **Risperdal**

FORMULARIES: Aetna; BC-BS; PCS

DESCRIPTION:

Risperidone is an antipsychotic agent belonging to a new chemical class, the benzisoxazole derivatives. The chemical designation is 3-[2-[4-(6-fluoro-1,2-benzisoxazol-3-yl)-1-piperidinyl]ethyl]-6,7,8,9-tetrahydro-2-methyl-4*H*-pyrido[1,2-a]pyrimidin-4-one. Its molecular formula is $C_{23}H_{27}FN_4O_2$ and its molecular weight is 410.49.

Risperidone is a white to slightly beige powder. It is practically insoluble in water, freely soluble in methylene chloride, and soluble in methanol and 0.1 N HCl.

Risperidone for oral use is available in tablets of 1 mg (white, scored), 2 mg (orange), 3 mg (yellow), and 4 mg (green). Inactive ingredients are colloidal silicon dioxide, hydroxypropyl methylcellulose, lactose, magnesium stearate, microcrystalline cellulose, propylene glycol, sodium lauryl sulfate, and starch (corn). Tablets of 2, 3, and 4 mg also contain talc and titanium dioxide. The 2 mg tablets contain FD&C Yellow No. 6 Aluminum Lake; the 3 mg and 4 mg tablets contain D&C Yellow No. 10; the 4 mg tablets contain FD&C Blue No. 2 Aluminum Lake.

CLINICAL PHARMACOLOGY:

PHARMACODYNAMICS

The mechanism of action of Risperidone, as with other antipsychotic drugs, is unknown. However, it has been proposed that this drug's antipsychotic activity is mediated through a combination of dopamine type 2 (D_2) and serotonin type 2 ($5HT_2$) antagonism. Antagonism at receptors other than D_2 and $5HT_2$ may explain some of the other effects of Risperidone.

Risperidone is a selective monoaminergic antagonist with high affinity (Ki of 0.12 to 7.3 nM) for the serotonin type 2 ($5HT_2$), dopamine type 2 (D_2), $\alpha_1$and α_2 adrenergic, and H_1histaminergic receptors. Risperidone antagonizes other receptors, but with lower potency. Risperidone has low to moderate affinity (Ki of 47 to 253 nM) for the serotonin $5HT_{1C}$, $5HT_{1D}$, and $5HT_{1A}$receptors, weak affinity (Ki of 620 to 800 nM) for the dopamine $D_1$and haloperidol-sensitive sigma site, and no affinity (when tested at concentrations $>10^{-5}$M) for cholinergic muscarinic or β_1 and $\beta_2$adrenergic receptors.

PHARMACOKINETICS

Risperidone is well absorbed, as illustrated by a mass balance study involving a single 1 mg oral dose of ^{14}C- risperidone as a solution in three healthy male volunteers. Total recovery of radioactivity at one week was 85%, including 70% in the urine and 15% in the feces.

Risperidone is extensively metabolized in the liver by cytochrome $P_{450}IID_6$ to a major active metabolite, 9-hydroxy-risperidone, which is the predominant circulating specie, and appears approximately equi-effective with risperidone with respect to receptor binding activity and some effects in animals. (A second minor pathway is*N*-dealkylation). Consequently, the clinical effect of the drug likely results from the combined concentrations of risperidone plus 9- hydroxyrisperidone. Plasma concentrations of risperidone, 9- hydroxyrisperidone, and risperidone plus 9-hydroxyrisperidone are dose proportional over the dosing range of 1 to 16 mg daily (0.5 to 8 mg BID). The relative oral bioavailability of risperidone from a tablet was 94% (CV=10%) when compared to a solution. Food does not affect either the rate or extent of risperidone. Thus, risperidone can be given with or without meals. The absolute oral bioavailability of risperidone was 70% (CV=25%).

The enzyme catalyzing hydroxylation of risperidone to 9- hydroxyrisperidone is cytochrome $P_{450}IID_6$, also called debrisoquin hydroxylase, the enzyme responsible for metabolism of many neuroleptics, antidepressants, antiarrhythmics, and other drugs. Cytochrome $P_{450}IID_6$ is subject to genetic polymorphism (about 6-8% of caucasians, and a very low percent of Asians have little or no activity and are "poor metabolizers") and to inhibition by a variety of substrates and some non-substrates, notably quinidine. Extensive metabolizers convert risperidone rapidly into 9- hydroxyrisperidone, while poor metabolizers convert it much more slowly. Extensive metabolizers, therefore, have lower risperidone and higher 9- hydroxyrisperidone concentrations than poor metabolizers. Following oral administration of solution or tablet, mean peak plasma concentrations occurred at about 1 hour. Peak 9-hydroxyrisperidone occurred at about 3 hours in extensive metabolizers, and 17 hours in poor metabolizers. The apparent half-life of risperidone was three hours (CV=30%) in extensive metabolizers and 20 hours (CV=40%) in poor metabolizers. The apparent half-life of 9-hydroxyrisperidone was about 21 hours (CV=20%) in extensive metabolizers and 30 hours (CV=25%) in poor metabolizers. Steady-state concentrations of risperidone are reached in 1 day in extensive metabolizers and would be expected to reach steady state in about 5 days in poor metabolizers. Steady-state concentrations of 9- hydroxyrisperidone are reached in 5-6 days (measured in extensive metabolizers).

Because risperidone and 9-hydroxyrisperidone are approximately equi-effective, the sum of their concentrations is pertinent. The pharmacokinetics of the sum of risperidone and 9-hydroxyrisperidone, after single and multiple doses, were similar in extensive and poor metabolizers, with an overall mean elimination half-life of about 20 hours. In analyses comparing adverse reaction rates in extensive and poor metabolizers in controlled and open studies, no important differences were seen.

Risperidone could be subject to two kinds of drug-drug interactions. First, inhibitors of cytochrome $P_{450}IID_6$ could interfere with conversion of risperidone to 9-hydroxyrisperidone. This in fact occurs with quinidine, giving essentially all recipients a risperidone pharmacokinetic profile typical of poor metabolizers. The favorable and adverse effects of risperidone in patients receiving quinidine have not been evaluated, but observations in a modest number (n=70) of poor metabolizers given risperidone do not suggest important differences between poor and extensive metabolizers. It would also be possible for risperidone to interfere with metabolism of other drugs metabolized by cytochrome $P_{450}IID_6$. Relatively weak binding of risperidone to the enzyme suggests this is unlikely (See PRECAUTIONS and DRUG INTERACTIONS).

The plasma protein binding of risperidone was about 90% over the *in vitro* concentration range of 0.5 to 200 ng/ml and increased with increasing concentrations of α_1-acid glycoprotein. The plasma binding of 9-hydroxyrisperidone was 77%. Neither the parent nor the metabolite displaced each other from the plasma binding sites. High therapeutic concentrations of sulfamethazine (100 mcg/ml), warfarin (10 mcg/ml) and carbamazepine (10 mcg/ml) caused only a slight increase in the free fraction of risperidone at 10 ng/ml and 9-hydroxyrisperidone at 50 ng/ml, changes of unknown clinical significance.

SPECIAL POPULATIONS

Renal Impairment: In patients with moderate to severe renal disease, clearance of the sum of risperidone and its active metabolite decreased by 60% compared to young healthy subjects. Risperidone doses should be reduced in patients with renal disease (See PRECAUTIONS and DOSAGE AND ADMINISTRATION).

Hepatic Impairment: While the pharmacokinetics of risperidone in subjects with liver disease were comparable to those in young healthy subjects, the mean free fraction of risperidone in plasma was increased by about 35% because of the diminished concentration of both albumin and α_1-acid glycoprotein. Risperidone doses should be reduced in patients with liver disease (See PRECAUTIONS and DOSAGE AND ADMINISTRATION).

Elderly: In healthy elderly subjects renal clearance of both risperidone and 9-hydroxyrisperidone was decreased, and elimination half-lives were prolonged compared to young healthy subjects. Dosing should be modified accordingly in the elderly patients (See DOSAGE AND ADMINISTRATION.)

Race and Gender Effects: No specific pharmacokinetic study was conducted to investigate race and gender effects, but a population pharmacokinetic analysis did not identify important differences in the disposition of risperidone due to gender (whether corrected for body weight or not) or race.

CLINICAL STUDIES:

The efficacy of Risperidone in the management of the manifestations of psychotic disorders was established in three short-term (6- to 8-week) controlled trials of psychotic inpatients who met DSM III-R criteria for schizophrenia.

Several instruments were used for assessing psychiatric signs and symptoms in these studies, among them the Brief Psychiatric Rating Scale (BPRS), a multi-item inventory of general psychopathology traditionally used to evaluate the effects of drug treatment in psychosis. The BPRS psychosis cluster (conceptual disorganization, hallucinatory behavior, suspiciousness, and unusual thought content) is considered a particularly useful subset for assessing actively psychotic schizophrenic patients. A second traditional assessment, the Clinical Global Impression (CGI), reflects the impression of a skilled observer, fully familiar with the manifestations of schizophrenia, about the overall clinical state of the patient. In addition, two more recently developed, but less well evaluated scales, were employed; these included the Positive and Negative Syndrome Scale (PANSS) and the Scale for Assessing Negative Symptoms (SANS).

The results of the trials follow:

(1) In a 6-week, placebo-controlled trial (n=160) involving titration of Risperidone in doses up to 10 mg/day (BID schedule), Risperidone was generally superior to placebo on the BPRS total score, on the BPRS psychosis cluster, and marginally superior to placebo on the SANS.

(2) In an 8-week, placebo-controlled trial (n=513) involving 4 fixed doses of Risperidone (2, 6, 10, and 16 mg/day, on a BID schedule), all 4 Risperidone groups were generally superior to placebo on the BPRS total score, BPRS psychosis cluster, and CGI severity score; the 3 highest Risperidone dose groups were generally superior to placebo on the PANSS negative subscale. The most consistently positive responses on all measures were seen for the 6 mg dose group, and there was no suggestion of increased benefit from larger doses.

(3) In an 8-week, dose comparison trial (n=1356) involving 5 fixed doses of Risperidone (1, 4, 8, 12, and 16 mg/day, on a BID schedule), the four highest Risperidone dose groups were generally superior to the 1 mg Risperidone dose group on BPRS total score, BPRS psychosis cluster, and CGI severity score. None of the dose groups were superior to the 1 mg group on the PANSS negative subscale. The most consistently positive responses were seen for the 4 mg dose group.

INDICATIONS AND USAGE:

Risperidone is indicated for the management of the manifestations of psychotic disorders.

The antipsychotic efficacy of Risperidone was established in short-term (6 to 8 weeks) controlled trials of schizophrenic inpatients (See CLINICAL PHARMACOLOGY.)

INDICATIONS AND USAGE: *(cont'd)*

The effectiveness of Risperidone in long-term use, that is, more than 6 to 8 weeks, has not been systematically evaluated in controlled trials. Therefore, the physician who elects to use Risperidone for extended periods should periodically re-evaluate the long-term usefulness of the drug for the individual patient (See DOSAGE AND ADMINISTRATION.)

CONTRAINDICATIONS:

Risperidone is contraindicated in patients with a known hypersensitivity to the product.

WARNINGS:

Neuroleptic Malignant Syndrome (NMS): A potentially fatal symptom complex sometimes referred to as Neuroleptic Malignant Syndrome (NMS) has been reported in association with antipsychotic drugs. Clinical manifestations of NMS are hyperpyrexia, muscle rigidity, altered mental status and evidence of autonomic instability (irregular pulse or blood pressure, tachycardia, diaphoresis and cardiac dysrhythmia). Additional signs may include elevated creatinine phosphokinase, myoglobinuria (rhabdomyolysis), and acute renal failure.

The diagnostic evaluation of patients with this syndrome is complicated. In arriving at a diagnosis, it is important to identify cases where the clinical presentation includes both serious medical illness (*e.g.,* pneumonia, systemic infection, etc.) and untreated or inadequately treated extrapyramidal signs and symptoms (EPS). Other important considerations in the differential diagnosis include central anticholinergic toxicity, heat stroke, drug fever, and primary central nervous system pathology.

The management of NMS should include: 1) immediate discontinuation of antipsychotic drugs and other drugs not essential to concurrent therapy; 2) intensive symptomatic treatment and medical monitoring; and 3) treatment of any concomitant serious medical problems for which specific treatments are available. There is no general agreement about specific pharmacological treatment regimens for uncomplicated NMS.

If a patient requires antipsychotic drug treatment after recovery from NMS, the potential reintroduction of drug therapy should be carefully considered. The patient should be carefully monitored, since recurrences of NMS have been reported.

Tardive Dyskinesia: A syndrome of potentially irreversible, involuntary, dyskinetic movements may develop in patients treated with antipsychotic drugs. Although the prevalence of the syndrome appears to be highest among the elderly, especially elderly women, it is impossible to rely upon prevalence estimates to predict, at the inception of antipsychotic treatment, which patients are likely to develop the syndrome. Whether antipsychotic drug products differ in their potential to cause tardive dyskinesia is unknown.

The risk of developing tardive dyskinesia and the likelihood that it will become irreversible are believed to increase as the duration of treatment and the total cumulative dose of antipsychotic drugs administered to the patient increase. However, the syndrome can develop, although much less commonly, after relatively brief treatment periods at low doses.

There is no known treatment for established cases of tardive dyskinesia, although the syndrome may remit, partially or completely, if antipsychotic treatment is withdrawn. Antipsychotic treatment, itself, however, may suppress (or partially suppress) the signs and symptoms of the syndrome and thereby may possibly mask the underlying process. The effect that symptomatic suppression has upon the long-term course of the syndrome is unknown.

Given these considerations, risperidone should be prescribed in a manner that is most likely to minimize the occurrence of tardive dyskinesia. Chronic antipsychotic treatment should generally be reserved for patients who suffer from a chronic illness that (1) is known to respond to antipsychotic drugs, and (2) for whom alternative, equally effective, but potentially less harmful treatments are not available or appropriate. In patients who do require chronic treatment, the smallest dose and the shortest duration of treatment producing a satisfactory clinical response should be sought. The need for continued treatment should be reassessed periodically.

If signs and symptoms of tardive dyskinesia appear in a patient on Risperidone, drug discontinuation should be considered. However, some patients may require treatment with Risperidone despite the presence of the syndrome.

Potential for Proarrhythmic Effects: Risperidone and/or 9-hydroxyrisperidone appears to lengthen the QT interval in some patients, although there is no average increase in treated patients, even at 12-16 mg/day, well above the recommended dose. Other drugs that prolong the QT interval have been associated with the occurrence of torsades de pointes, a life-threatening arrhythmia. Bradycardia, electrolyte imbalance, concomitant use with other drugs that prolong QT, or the presence of congenital prolongation in QT can increase the risk for occurrence of this arrhythmia.

PRECAUTIONS:

GENERAL

Orthostatic Hypotension: Risperidone may induce orthostatic hypotension associated with dizziness, tachycardia, and in some patients, syncope, especially during the initial dose-titration period, probably reflecting its alpha-adrenergic antagonistic properties. Syncope was reported in 0.2% (6/2607) of Risperidone treated patients in phase 2-3 studies. The risk of orthostatic hypotension and syncope may be minimized by limiting the initial dose to 1 mg BID in normal adults and 0.5 mg BID in the elderly and patients with renal or hepatic impairment (see DOSAGE AND ADMINISTRATION). A dose reduction should be considered if hypotension occurs. Risperidone should be used with particular caution in patients with known cardiovascular disease (history of myocardial infarction or ischemia, heart failure, or conduction abnormalities), cerebrovascular disease, and conditions which would predispose patients to hypotension (dehydration, hypovolemia, and treatment with antihypertensive medications).

Seizures: During premarketing testing, seizures occurred in 0.3% (9/2607) of Risperidone treated patients, two in association with hyponatremia. Risperidone should be used cautiously in patients with a history of seizures.

Hyperprolactinemia: As with other drugs that antagonize dopamine D_2 receptors, risperidone elevates prolactin levels and the elevation persists during chronic administration. Tissue culture experiments indicate that approximately one-third of human breast cancers are prolactin dependent *in vitro*, a factor of potential importance if the prescription of these drugs is contemplated in a patient with previously detected breast cancer. Although disturbances such as galactorrhea, amenorrhea, gynecomastia, and impotence have been reported with prolactin-elevating compounds, the clinical significance of elevated serum prolactin levels is unknown for most patients. As is common with compounds which increase prolactin release, an increase in pituitary gland, mammary gland, and pancreatic islet cell hyperplasia and/or neoplasia was observed in the risperidone carcinogenicity studies conducted in mice and rats (See Carcinogenesis). However, neither clinical studies nor epidemiologic studies conducted to date have shown an association between chronic administration of this class of drugs and tumorigenesis in humans; the available evidence is considered too limited to be conclusive at this time.

Potential for Cognitive and Motor Impairment: Somnolence was a commonly reported adverse event associated with Risperidone treatment, especially when ascertained by direct questioning of patients. This adverse event is dose related, and in a study utilizing a checklist to detect adverse events, 41% of the high dose patients (Risperidone 16 mg/day) reported somnolence compared to 16% of placebo patients. Direct questioning is more sensitive for

PRECAUTIONS: *(cont'd)*

detecting adverse events than spontaneous reporting, by which 8% of Risperidone 16 mg/day patients and 1% of placebo patients reported somnolence as an adverse event. Since Risperidone has the potential to impair judgment, thinking, or motor skills, patients should be cautioned about operating hazardous machinery, including automobiles, until they are reasonably certain that Risperidone therapy does not affect them adversely.

Priapism: Rare cases of priapism have been reported. While the relationship of the events to Risperidone use has not been established, other drugs with alpha-adrenergic blocking effects have been reported to induce priapism, and it is possible that Risperidone may share this capacity. Severe priapism may require surgical intervention.

Thrombotic Thrombocytopenic Purpura (TTP): A single case of TTP was reported in a 28 year-old female patient receiving Risperidone in a large, open premarketing experience (approximately 1300 patients). She experienced jaundice, fever, and bruising, but eventually recovered after receiving plasmapheresis. The relationship to Risperidone therapy is unknown.

Antiemetic effect: Risperidone has an antiemetic effect in animals; this effect may also occur in humans, and may mask signs and symptoms of overdosage with certain drugs or of conditions such as intestinal obstruction, Reye's syndrome, and brain tumor.

Body Temperature Regulation: Disruption of body temperature regulation has been attributed to antipsychotic agents. Caution is advised when prescribing for patients who will be exposed to temperature extremes.

Suicide: The possibility of a suicide attempt is inherent in schizophrenia, and close supervision of high risk patients should accompany drug therapy. Prescriptions for Risperidone should be written for the smallest quantity of tablets consistent with good patient management, in order to reduce the risk of overdose.

Use in Patients with Concomitant Illness: Clinical experience with Risperidone in patients with certain concomitant systemic illnesses is limited. Caution is advisable in using Risperidone in patients with diseases or conditions that could affect metabolism or hemodynamic responses.

Risperidone has not been evaluated or used to any appreciable extent in patients with a recent history of myocardial infarction or unstable heart disease. Patients with these diagnoses were excluded from clinical studies during the product's premarket testing. The electrocardiograms of approximately 380 patients who received Risperidone and 120 patients who received placebo in two double-blind, placebo-controlled trials were evaluated and the data revealed one finding of potential concern, i.e., 8 patients taking Risperidone whose baseline QTc interval was less than 450 msec were observed to have QTc intervals greater than 450 msec during treatment; no such prolongations were seen in the smaller placebo group. There were 3 such episodes in the approximately 125 patients who received haloperidol. Because of the risks of orthostatic hypotension and QT prolongation, caution should be observed in cardiac patients (see WARNINGS and PRECAUTIONS).

Increased plasma concentrations of risperidone and 9-hydroxyrisperidone occur in patients with severe renal impairment (creatinine clearance <30 ml/min/1.73 m^2), and an increase in the free fraction of the risperidone is seen in patients with severe hepatic impairment. A lower starting dose should be used in such patients (see DOSAGE AND ADMINISTRATION).

Information for Patients Physicians are advised to discuss the following issues with patients for whom they prescribe Risperidone.

Orthostatic Hypotension: Patients should be advised of the risk of orthostatic hypotension, especially during the period of initial dose titration.

Interference With Cognitive and Motor Performance: Since Risperidone has the potential to impair judgment, thinking, or motor skills, patients should be cautioned about operating hazardous machinery, including automobiles, until they are reasonably certain that Risperidone therapy does not affect them adversely.

Pregnancy: Patients should be advised to notify their physician if they become pregnant or intend to become pregnant during therapy.

Nursing: Patients should be advised not to breast feed an infant if they are taking Risperidone.

Concomitant Medication: Patients should be advised to inform their physicians if they are taking, or plan to take, any prescription or over-the-counter drugs, since there is a potential for interactions.

Alcohol: Patients should be advised to avoid alcohol while taking Risperidone.

Laboratory Tests No specific laboratory tests are recommended.

CARCINOGENESIS, MUTAGENESIS, IMPAIRMENT OF FERTILITY

Carcinogenesis: Carcinogenicity studies were conducted in Swiss albino mice and Wistar rats. Risperidone was administered in the diet at doses of 0.63, 2.5, and 10 mg/kg for 18 months to mice and for 25 months to rats. These doses are equivalent to 2.4, 9.4, and 37.5 times the maximum human dose (16 mg/day) on a mg/kg basis or 0.2, 0.75 and 3 times the maximum human dose (mice) or 0.4, 1.5, and 6 times the maximum human dose (rats) on a mg/m^2 basis. A maximum tolerated dose was not achieved in male mice. There were statistically significant increases in pituitary gland adenomas, endocrine pancreas adenomas and mammary gland adenocarcinomas. The following table (TABLE 1) summarizes the multiples of the human dose on a mg/m^2 (mg/kg) basis at which these tumors occurred.

TABLE 1

Tumor Type	Species	Sex	Multiple Of Maximum Human Dose In mg/m^2 (mg/kg) Lowest Effect Level	Highest No Effect Level
Pituitary adenomas	mouse	female	0.75*(9.4)*	0.2*(2.4)*
Endocrine pancreas adenomas	rat	male	1.5*(9.4)*	0.4*(2.4)*
Mammary gland adenocarcinomas	mouse	female	0.2*(2.4)*	none
	rat	female	0.4*(2.4)*	none
	rat	male	6*(37.5)*	1.5*(9.4)*
Mammary gland neoplasms, Total	rat	male	1.5*(9.4)*	0.4*(2.4)*

Antipsychotic drugs have been shown to chronically elevate prolactin levels in rodents. Serum prolactin levels were not measured during the risperidone carcinogenicity studies; however, measurements during subchronic toxicity studies showed that risperidone elevated serum prolactin levels 5 to 6 fold in mice and rats at the same doses used in the carcinogenicity studies. An increase in mammary, pituitary, and endocrine pancreas neoplasms has been found in rodents after chronic administration of other antipsychotic drugs and is considered to be prolactin mediated. The relevance for human risk of the findings of prolactin-mediated endocrine tumors in rodents is unknown (see Hyperprolactinemia under General).

PRECAUTIONS: *(cont'd)*

Mutagenesis: No evidence of mutagenic potential for risperidone was found in the Ames reverse mutation test, mouse lymphoma assay, *in vitro* rat hepatocyte DNA-repair assay, *in vivo* micronucleus test in mice, the sex-linked recessive lethal test in Drosophila, or the chromosomal aberration test in human lymphocytes or Chinese hamster cells.

Impairment of Fertility: Risperidone (0.16 to 5 mg/kg) was shown to impair mating, but not fertility, in Wistar rats in three reproductive studies (two Segment I and a multigenerational study) at doses 0.1 to 3 times the maximum recommended human dose on a mg/m^2 basis. The effect appeared to be in females since impaired mating behavior was not noted in the Segment I study in which males only were treated. In a subchronic study in Beagle dogs in which risperidone was administered at doses of 0.31 to 5 mg/kg, sperm motility and concentration were decreased at doses 0.6 to 10 times the human dose on a mg/m^2 basis. Dose-related decreases were also noted in serum testosterone at the same doses. Serum testosterone and sperm parameters partially recovered but remained decreased after treatment was discontinued. No no-effect doses were noted in either rat or dog.

PREGNANCY CATEGORY C

The teratogenic potential of risperidone was studied in three Segment II studies in Sprague-Dawley and Wistar rats and in one Segment II study in New Zealand rabbits. The incidence of malformations was not increased compared to control in offspring of rats or rabbits given 0.4 to 6 times the human dose on a mg/m^2 basis. In three reproductive studies in rats (two Segment III and a multigenerational study), there was an increase in pup deaths during the first 4 days of lactation at doses 0.1 to 3 times the human dose on a mg/m^2 basis. It is not known whether these deaths were due to a direct effect on the fetuses or pups or to effects on the dams. There was no no-effect dose for increased rat pup mortality. In one Segment III study, there was an increase in stillborn rat pups at a dose 1.5 times higher than the human dose on a mg/m^2 basis.

Placental transfer of risperidone occurs in rat pups. There are no adequate and well-controlled studies in pregnant women. However, there was one report of a case of agenesis of the corpus callosum in an infant exposed to risperidone *in utero.* The causal relationship to Risperidone therapy is unknown.

Risperidone should be used during pregnancy only if the potential benefit justifies the potential risk to the fetus.

LABOR AND DELIVERY

The effect of Risperidone on labor and delivery in humans is unknown.

NURSING MOTHERS

It is not known whether or not risperidone is excreted in human milk. In animal studies, risperidone and 9- hydroxyrisperidone were excreted in breast milk. Therefore, women receiving Risperidone should not breast feed.

PEDIATRIC USE

Safety and effectiveness in children have not been established.

GERIATRIC USE

Clinical studies of Risperidone did not include sufficient numbers of patients aged 65 and over to determine whether they respond differently from younger patients. In general, a lower starting dose is recommended for an elderly patient, reflecting a decreased pharmacokinetic clearance in the elderly, as well as a greater frequency of decreased hepatic, renal, or cardiac function, and a greater tendency to postural hypotension (See CLINICAL PHARMACOLOGY and DOSAGE AND ADMINISTRATION).

DRUG INTERACTIONS:

The interactions of Risperidone and other drugs have not been systematically evaluated. Given the primary CNS effects of risperidone, caution should be used when Risperidone is taken in combination with other centrally acting drugs and alcohol.

Because of its potential for inducing hypotension, Risperidone may enhance the hypotensive effects of other therapeutic agents with this potential. Risperidone may antagonize the effects of levodopa and dopamine agonists.

Chronic administration of carbamazepine with risperidone may increase the clearance of risperidone.

Chronic administration of clozapine with risperidone may decrease the clearance of risperidone.

Drugs that Inhibit Cytochrome $P_{450}IID_6$ and Other P_{450} Isozymes: Risperidone is metabolized to 9- hydroxyrisperidone by cytochrome $P_{450}IID_6$, an enzyme that is polymorphic in the population and that can be inhibited by a variety of psychotropic and other drugs (see CLINICAL PHARMACOLOGY). Drug interactions that reduce the metabolism of risperidone to 9- hydroxyrisperidone would increase the plasma concentrations of risperidone and lower the concentrations of 9-hydroxyrisperidone. Analysis of clinical studies involving a modest number of poor metabolizers (n=70) does not suggest that poor and extensive metabolizers have different rates of adverse effects. No comparison of effectiveness in the two groups has been made.

In vitro studies showed that drugs metabolized by other P_{450} isozymes, including 1A1, 1A2, IIC9, MP, and IIIA4, are only weak inhibitors of risperidone metabolism.

Drugs Metabolized by Cytochrome $P_{450}IID_6$: *In vitro* studies indicate that risperidone is a relatively weak inhibitor of cytochrome $P_{450}IID_6$. Therefore, Risperidone is not expected to substantially inhibit the clearance of drugs that are metabolized by this enzymatic pathway. However, clinical data to confirm this expectation are not available.

ADVERSE REACTIONS:

Associated with Discontinuation of Treatment: Approximately 9% percent (244/2607) of Risperidone (risperidone)-treated patients in phase 2-3 studies discontinued treatment due to an adverse event, compared with about 7% on placebo and 10% on active control drugs. The more common events (≥ 0.3%) associated with discontinuation and considered to be possibly or probably drug-related included (TABLE 2):

TABLE 2

Adverse Event	Risperdal	Placebo
Extrapyramidal symptoms	2.1%	0%
Dizziness	0.7%	0%
Hyperkinesia	0.6%	0%
Somnolence	0.5%	0%
Nausea	0.3%	0%

Suicide attempt was associated with discontinuation in 1.2% of Risperidone treated patients compared to 0.6% of placebo patients, but, given the almost 40-fold greater exposure time in Risperidone compared to placebo patients, it is unlikely that suicide attempt is a Risperidone related adverse event (See PRECAUTIONS.) Discontinuation for extrapyramidal symptoms was 0% in placebo patients but 3.8% in active-control patients in the phase 2-3 trials.

ADVERSE REACTIONS: *(cont'd)*

Incidence in Controlled Trials: *Commonly Observed Adverse Events in Controlled Clinical Trials:* In two 6- to 8-week placebo-controlled trials, spontaneously-reported, treatment-emergent adverse events with an incidence of 5% or greater in at least one of the Risperidone groups and at least twice that of placebo were: anxiety, somnolence, extrapyramidal symptoms, dizziness, constipation, nausea, dyspepsia, rhinitis, rash, and tachycardia.

Adverse events were also elicited in one of these two trials (*i.e.*, in the fixed-dose trial comparing Risperidone at doses of 2, 6, 10, and 16 mg/day with placebo) utilizing a checklist for detecting adverse events, a method that is more sensitive than spontaneous reporting. By this method, the following additional common and drug-related adverse events were present at least 5% and twice the rate of placebo: increased dream activity, increased duration of sleep, accommodation disturbances, reduced salivation, micturition disturbances, diarrhea, weight gain, menorrhagia, diminished sexual desire, erectile dysfunction, ejaculatory dysfunction, and orgastic dysfunction.

Adverse Events Occurring at an Incidence of 1% or More Among Risperidone Treated Patients: The table that follows (TABLE 3) enumerates adverse events that occurred at an incidence of 1% or more, and were at least as frequent among Risperidone treated patients treated at doses of ≤ 10 mg/day than among placebo-treated patients in the pooled results of two 6- to 8-week controlled trials. Patients received Risperidone doses of 2, 6, 10, or 16 mg/day in the dose comparison trial, or up to a maximum dose of 10 mg/day in the titration study. This table (TABLE 3) shows the percentage of patients in each dose group (≤ 10 mg/day or 16 mg/day) who spontaneously reported at least one episode of an event at some time during their treatment. Patients given doses of 2, 6, or 10 mg did not differ materially in these rates. Reported adverse events were classified using the World Health Organization preferred terms.

The prescriber should be aware that these figures cannot be used to predict the incidence of side effects in the course of usual medical practice where patient characteristics and other factors differ from those which prevailed in this clinical trial. Similarly, the cited frequencies cannot be compared with figures obtained from other clinical investigations involving different treatments, uses and investigators. The cited figures, however, do provide the prescribing physician with some basis for estimating the relative contribution of drug and nondrug factors to the side effect incidence rate in the population studied.

TABLE 3 Treatment-Emergent Adverse Experience Incidence in 6- to 8-Week Controlled Clinical Trials[1]

Body System/Preferred Term	Risperdal ≤10 mg/day (N=324)	Risperdal 16 mg/day (N=77)	Placebo (N=142)
Psychiatric Disorders			
Insomnia	26%	23%	19%
Agitation	22%	26%	20%
Anxiety	12%	20%	9%
Somnolence	3%	8%	1%
Aggressive reaction	1%	3%	1%
Nervous System			
Extrapyramidal symptoms[2]	17%	34%	16%
Headache	14%	12%	12%
Dizziness	4%	7%	1%
Gastrointestinal System			
Constipation	7%	13%	3%
Nausea	6%	4%	3%
Dyspepsia	5%	10%	4%
Vomiting	5%	7%	4%
Abdominal pain	4%	1%	0%
Saliva increased	2%	0%	1%
Toothache	2%	0%	0%
Respiratory System			
Rhinitis	10%	8%	4%
Coughing	3%	3%	1%
Sinusitis	2%	1%	1%
Pharyngitis	2%	3%	0%
Dyspnea	1%	0%	0%
Body as a Whole			
Back pain	2%	0%	1%
Chest pain	2%	3%	1%
Fever	2%	3%	0%
Dermatological			
Rash	2%	5%	1%
Dry skin	2%	4%	0%
Seborrhea	1%	0%	0%
Infections			
Upper respiratory	3%	3%	1%
Visual			
Abnormal vision	2%	1%	1%
Musculo-Skeletal			
Arthralgia	2%	3%	0%
Cardiovascular			
Tachycardia	3%	5%	0%

[1] Events reported by at least 1% of patients treated with Risperdal ≤ 10 mg/day are included, and are rounded to the nearest %. Comparative rates for Risperdal 16 mg/day and placebo are provided as well. Events for which the Risperdal incidence (in both dose groups) was equal to or less than placebo are not listed in the table, (TABLE 3), but included the following: nervousness, injury, and fungal infection.

[2] Includes tremor, dystonia, hypokinesia, hypertonia, hyperkinesia, oculogyric crisis, ataxia, abnormal gait, involuntary muscle contractions, hyporeflexia, akathisia, and extrapyramidal disorders. Although the incidence of extrapyramidal symptoms does not appear to differ for the ≤ 10 mg/day group and placebo, the data for individual dose groups in fixed dose trials do suggest a dose/response relationship (see ADVERSE REACTIONS, Dose Dependency).

Dose Dependency of Adverse Events: *Extrapyramidal symptoms:* Data from two fixed dose trials provided evidence of dose-relatedness for extrapyramidal symptoms associated with risperidone treatment.

Two methods were used to measure extrapyramidal symptoms (EPS) in an 8-week trial comparing four fixed doses of risperidone (2, 6, 10, and 16 mg/day), including (1) a parkinsonism score (mean change from baseline) from the Extrapyramidal Symptom Rating Scale and (2) incidence of spontaneous complaints of EPS (TABLE 4):

TABLE 4

Dose Groups	Placebo	Ris 2	Ris 6	Ris 10	Ris 16
Parkinsonism	1.2	0.9	1.8	2.4	2.6
EPS Incidence	13%	13%	16%	20%	31%

Similar methods were used to measure extrapyramidal symptoms (EPS) in an 8-week trial comparing five fixed doses of risperidone (1, 4, 8, 12, and 16 mg/day) (TABLE 5):

ADVERSE REACTIONS: *(cont'd)*

TABLE 5

Dose Groups	Ris 1	Ris 4	Ris 8	Ris 12	Ris 16
Parkinsonism	0.6	1.7	2.4	2.9	4.1
EPS Incidence	7%	12%	18%	18%	21%

Other Adverse Events: Adverse event data elicited by a checklist for side effects from a large study comparing 5 fixed doses of Risperidone (1, 4, 8, 12, and 16 mg/day) were explored for dose-relatedness of adverse events. A Cochran-Armitage Test for trend in these data revealed a positive trend ($p<0.05$) for the following adverse events: sleepiness, increased duration of sleep, accommodation disturbances, orthostatic dizziness, palpitations, weight gain, erectile dysfunction, ejaculatory dysfunction, orgastic dysfunction, asthenia/lassitude/increased fatigability, and increased pigmentation.

Vital Sign Changes: Risperidone is associated with orthostatic hypotension and tachycardia (see PRECAUTIONS).

Weight Changes: The proportions of Risperidone and placebo-treated patients meeting a weight gain criterion of ≥ 7% of body weight were compared in a pool of 6- to 8-week placebo-controlled trials, revealing a statistically significantly greater incidence of weight gain for Risperidone (18%) compared to placebo (9%).

Laboratory Changes: A between group comparison for 6- to 8-week placebo-controlled trials revealed no statistically significant Risperidone/placebo differences in the proportions of patients experiencing potentially important changes in routine serum chemistry, hematology, or urinalysis parameters. Similarly, there were no Risperidone/placebo differences in the incidence of discontinuations for changes in serum chemistry, hematology, or urinalysis. However, Risperidone administration was associated with increases in serum prolactin (see PRECAUTIONS).

ECG Changes: The electrocardiograms of approximately 380 patients who received Risperidone and 120 patients who received placebo in two double-blind, placebo-controlled trials were evaluated and revealed one finding of potential concern (*i.e.,* 8 patients taking Risperidone whose baseline QTc interval was less than 450 msec were observed to have QTc intervals greater than 450 msec during treatment) (see WARNINGS). Changes of this type were not seen among about 120 placebo patients, but were seen in patients receiving haloperidol (3/126).

Other Events Observed During the Pre-Marketing Evaluation of Risperidone: During its premarketing assessment, multiple doses of Risperidone were administered to 2607 patients in phase 2 and 3 studies. The conditions and duration of exposure to Risperidone varied greatly, and included (in overlapping categories) open and double-blind studies, uncontrolled and controlled studies, inpatient and outpatient studies, fixed-dose and titration studies, and short-term or longer-term exposure. In most studies, untoward events associated with this exposure were obtained by spontaneous report and recorded by clinical investigators using terminology of their own choosing. Consequently, it is not possible to provide a meaningful estimate of the proportion of individuals experiencing adverse events without first grouping similar types of untoward events into a smaller number of standardized event categories. In two large studies, adverse events were also elicited utilizing the UKU (direct questioning) side effect rating scale, and these events were not further categorized using standard terminology (**Note:**These events are marked with an asterisk in the listings that follow).

In the listings that follow, spontaneously reported adverse events were classified using World Health Organization (WHO) preferred terms. The frequencies presented, therefore, represent the proportion of the 2607 patients exposed to multiple doses of Risperidone who experienced an event of the type cited on at least one occasion while receiving Risperidone. All reported events are included except those already listed in TABLE 3, those events for which a drug cause was remote, and those event terms which were so general as to be uninformative. It is important to emphasize that, although the events reported occurred during treatment with Risperidone, they were not necessarily caused by it.

Events are further categorized by body system and listed in order of decreasing frequency according to the following definitions: frequent adverse events are those occurring in at least 1/100 patients (only those not already listed in the tabulated results from placebo controlled trials appear in this listing); infrequent adverse events are those occurring in 1/100 to 1/1000 patients; rare events are those occurring in fewer than 1/1000 patients.

Psychiatric Disorders: *Frequent:* increased dream activity*, diminished sexual desire*, nervousness. *Infrequent:* impaired concentration, depression, apathy, catatonic reaction, euphoria, increased libido, amnesia. *Rare:* emotional lability, nightmares, delirium, withdrawal syndrome, yawning.

Central and Peripheral Nervous System Disorders: *Frequent:* increased sleep duration*. *Infrequent:* dysarthria, vertigo, stupor, paraesthesia, confusion. *Rare:* aphasia, cholinergic syndrome, hypoesthesia, tongue paralysis, leg cramps, torticollis, hypotonia, coma, migraine, hyperreflexia, choreoathetosis.

Gastro-intestinal Disorders: *Frequent:* anorexia, reduced salivation*. *Infrequent:* flatulence, diarrhea, increased appetite, stomatitis, melena, dysphagia, hemorrhoids, gastritis.*Rare:*fecal incontinence, eructation, gastroesophageal reflux, gastroenteritis, esophagitis, tongue discoloration, cholelithiasis, tongue edema, diverticulitis, gingivitis, discolored feces, GI hemorrhage, hematemesis.

Body as a Whole/General Disorders: *Frequent:* fatigue. *Infrequent:* edema, rigors, malaise, influenza-like symptoms. *Rare:* pallor, enlarged abdomen, allergic reaction, ascites, sarcoidosis, flushing.

Respiratory System Disorders: *Infrequent:* hyperventilation, bronchospasm, pneumonia, stridor. *Rare:* asthma, increased sputum, aspiration.

Skin and Appendage Disorders: *Frequent:* increased pigmentation*, photosensitivity*. *Infrequent:* increased sweating, acne, decreased sweating, alopecia, hyperkeratosis, pruritus, skin exfoliation. *Rare:* bullous eruption, skin ulceration, aggravated psoriasis, furunculosis, verruca, dermatitis lichenoid, hypertrichosis, genital pruritus, urticaria.

Cardiovascular Disorders: *Infrequent:* palpitation, hypertension, hypotension, AV block, myocardial infarction.*Rare:* ventricular tachycardia, angina pectoris, premature atrial contractions, T wave inversions, ventricular extrasystoles, ST depression, myocarditis.

Vision Disorders: *Infrequent:* abnormal accommodation, xerophthalmia. *Rare:* diplopia, eye pain, blepharitis, photopsia, photophobia, abnormal lacrimation.

Metabolic and Nutritional Disorders: *Infrequent:* hyponatremia, weight increase, creatine phosphokinase increase, thirst, weight decrease, diabetes mellitus. *Rare:* decreased serum iron, cachexia, dehydration, hypokalemia, hypoproteinemia, hyperphosphatemia, hypertriglyceridemia, hyperuricemia, hypoglycemia.

Urinary System Disorders: *Frequent:* polyuria/polydipsia*. *Infrequent:* urinary incontinence, hematuria, dysuria. *Rare:* urinary retention, cystitis, renal insufficiency.

Musculo-skeletal System Disorders: *Infrequent:* myalgia. *Rare:* arthrosis, synostosis, bursitis, arthritis, skeletal pain.

Reproductive Disorders, Female: *Frequent:* menorrhagia*, orgastic dysfunction*, dry vagina*. *Infrequent:* nonpuerperal lactation, amenorrhea, female breast pain, leukorrhea, mastitis, dysmenorrhea, female perineal pain, intermenstrual bleeding, vaginal hemorrhage.

ADVERSE REACTIONS: *(cont'd)*

Liver and Biliary System Disorders: *Infrequent:* increased SGOT, increased SGPT. *Rare:* hepatic failure, cholestatic hepatitis, cholecystitis, cholelithiasis, hepatitis, hepatocellular damage.

Platelet, Bleeding and Clotting Disorders: *Infrequent:* epistaxis, purpura. *Rare:* hemorrhage, superficial phlebitis, thrombophlebitis, thrombocytopenia.

Hearing and Vestibular Disorders: *Rare:* tinnitus, hyperacusis, decreased hearing.

Red Blood Cell Disorders: *Infrequent:* anemia, hypochromic anemia. *Rare:*normocytic anemia.

Reproductive Disorders, Male: *Frequent:* erectile dysfunction*. *Infrequent:* ejaculation failure.

White Cell and Resistance Disorders: *Rare:* leukocytosis, lymphadenopathy, leukopenia, Pelger-Huet anomaly.

Endocrine Disorders: *Rare:* gynecomastia, male breast pain, antidiuretic hormone disorder.

Special Senses: *Rare:* bitter taste.

* Incidence based on elicited reports.

Postintroduction Reports: Adverse events reported since market introduction which were temporally (but not necessarily causally) related to Risperidone therapy, include the following: anaphylactic reaction, angioedema, atrial fibrillation, cerebrovascular disease, diabetes mellitus aggravated, hypothermia, intestinal obstruction, jaundice, mania, Parkinson's disease aggravated, pulmonary embolism, sudden death.

DRUG ABUSE AND DEPENDENCE:

Controlled Substance Class: Risperidone is not a controlled substance.

Physical and Psychologic Dependence: Risperidone has not been systematically studied in animals or humans for its potential for abuse, tolerance or physical dependence. While the clinical trials did not reveal any tendency for any drug-seeking behavior, these observations were not systematic and it is not possible to predict on the basis of this limited experience the extent to which a CNS-active drug will be misused, diverted and/or abused once marketed. Consequently, patients should be evaluated carefully for a history of drug abuse, and such patients should be observed closely for signs of Risperidone misuse or abuse (*e.g.,* development of tolerance, increases in dose, drug-seeking behavior).

OVERDOSAGE:

Human Experience: Experience with Risperidone in acute overdosage was limited in the premarketing database (8 reports), with estimated doses ranging from 20 to 300 mg and no fatalities. In general, reported signs and symptoms were those resulting from an exaggeration of the drug's known pharmacological effects, i.e., drowsiness and sedation, tachycardia and hypotension, and extrapyramidal symptoms. One case, involving an estimated overdose of 240 mg, was associated with hyponatremia, hypokalemia, prolonged QT, and widened QRS. Another case, involving an estimated overdose of 36 mg, was associated with a seizure.

Management of Overdosage: In case of acute overdosage, establish and maintain an airway and ensure adequate oxygenation and ventilation. Gastric lavage (after intubation, if patient is unconscious) and administration of activated charcoal together with a laxative should be considered. The possibility of obtundation, seizures or dystonic reaction of the head and neck following overdose may create a risk of aspiration with induced emesis. Cardiovascular monitoring should commence immediately and should include continuous electrocardiographic monitoring to detect possible arrhythmias. If antiarrhythmic therapy is administered, disopyramide, procainamide and quinidine carry a theoretical hazard of QT-prolonging effects that might be additive to those of risperidone. Similarly, it is reasonable to expect that the alpha-blocking properties of bretylium might be additive to those of risperidone, resulting in problematic hypotension.

There is no specific antidote to Risperidone. Therefore appropriate supportive measures should be instituted. The possibility of multiple drug involvement should be considered. Hypotension and circulatory collapse should be treated with appropriate measures such as intravenous fluids and/or sympathomimetic agents (epinephrine and dopamine should not be used, since beta stimulation may worsen hypotension in the setting of risperidone-induced alpha blockade). In cases of severe extrapyramidal symptoms, anticholinergic medication should be administered. Close medical supervision and monitoring should continue until the patient recovers.

DOSAGE AND ADMINISTRATION:

Usual Initial Dose: Risperidone should be administered on a BID schedule, generally beginning with 1 mg BID initially, with increases in increments of 1 mg BID on the second and third day, as tolerated, to a target dose of 3 mg BID by the third day. In some patients, slower titration may be medically appropriate. Further dosage adjustments, if indicated, should generally occur at intervals of not less than 1 week, since steady state for the active metabolite would not be achieved for approximately 1 week in the typical patient. When dosage adjustments are necessary, small dose increments/decrements of 1 mg BID are recommended.

Antipsychotic efficacy was demonstrated in a dose range of 4 to 16 mg/day in the clinical trials supporting effectiveness of Risperidone, however, maximal effect was generally seen in a range of 4 to 6 mg/day. Doses above 6 mg/day were not demonstrated to be more efficacious than lower doses, were associated with more extrapyramidal symptoms and other adverse effects, and are not generally recommended. The safety of doses above 16 mg/day has not been evaluated in clinical trials.

Dosage in Special Populations: The recommended initial dose is 0.5 mg BID in patients who are elderly or debilitated, patients with severe renal or hepatic impairment, and patients either predisposed to hypotension or for whom hypotension would pose a risk. Dosage increases in these patients should be in increments of no more than 0.5 mg BID. Increases to dosages above 1.5 mg BID should generally occur at intervals of at least 1 week. In some patients, slower titration may be medically appropriate.

Elderly or debilitated patients, and patients with renal impairment, may have less ability to eliminate Risperidone than normal adults. Patients with impaired hepatic function may have increases in the free fraction of the risperidone, possibly resulting in an enhanced effect (See CLINICAL PHARMACOLOGY.) Patients with a predisposition to hypotensive reactions or for whom such reactions would pose a particular risk likewise need to be titrated cautiously and carefully monitored (See PRECAUTIONS.)

Maintenance Therapy: While there is no body of evidence available to answer the question of how long the patient treated with Risperidone should remain on it, the effectiveness of maintenance treatment is well established for many other antipsychotic drugs. It is recommended that responding patients be continued on Risperidone, but at the lowest dose needed to maintain remission. Patients should be periodically reassessed to determine the need for maintenance treatment.

Reinitiation of Treatment in Patients Previously Discontinued: Although there are no data to specifically address reinitiation of treatment, it is recommended that when restarting patients who have had an interval off Risperidone, the initial titration schedule should be followed.

Switching from Other Antipsychotics: There are no systematically collected data to specifically address switching from other antipsychotics to Risperidone, or concerning concomitant administration with other antipsychotics. While immediate discontinuation of the previous

DOSAGE AND ADMINISTRATION: *(cont'd)*

antipsychotic treatment may be acceptable for some patients, more gradual discontinuation may be most appropriate for other patients. In all cases, the period of overlapping antipsychotic administration should be minimized. When switching patients from depot antipsychotics, if medically appropriate, initiate Risperidone therapy in place of the next scheduled injection. The need for continuing existing EPS medication should be reevaluated periodically.

PATIENT INFORMATION:

This medication is used to treat schizophrenia and other disorders of the psyche. This medication may cause dizziness when you first stand up. Stand up slowly until your body adjusts to the new medication. Risperidone affects the central nervous system and has the potential to impair judgment, thinking, or motor skills. Use caution when driving or using machinery. This medication should not be taken by pregnant or nursing women. Risperidone has several drug interactions, please consult your pharmacist or physician for special information. Avoid drinking alcohol.

HOW SUPPLIED:

Risperdal (risperidone) tablets are imprinted "Janssen", and "R" and the strength "1", "2", "3", or "4".

Storage and Handling: Risperdal should be stored at room temperature (59°-86°F/15°-30°C). Risperdal should be protected from light and moisture.

HOW SUPPLIED - EQUIVALENTS NOT AVAILABLE:

Tablet, Coated - Oral - 1 mg

60's	$113.76	RISPERDAL, Janssen Phar	50458-0300-06
100's	$189.60	RISPERDAL, Janssen Phar	50458-0300-01

Tablet, Coated - Oral - 2 mg

60's	$189.36	RISPERDAL, Janssen Phar	50458-0320-06
100's	$315.60	RISPERDAL, Janssen Phar	50458-0320-01

Tablet, Coated - Oral - 3 mg

60's	$236.88	RISPERDAL, Janssen Phar	50458-0330-06
100's	$394.80	RISPERDAL, Janssen Phar	50458-0330-01

Tablet, Coated - Oral - 4 mg

60's	$315.36	RISPERDAL, Janssen Phar	50458-0350-06
100's	$525.60	RISPERDAL, Janssen Phar	50458-0350-01

RITODRINE HYDROCHLORIDE *(002190)*

CATEGORIES: Autonomic Drugs; Hormones; Labor; Pregnancy; Relaxants/Stimulants, Uterine; Sympathomimetic Agents; Uterine Relaxants; Pregnancy Category B; FDA Approval Pre 1982

BRAND NAMES: *Pre-Par, Ritopar, Utemerin*; **Yutopar**
(International brand names outside U.S. in italics)

FORMULARIES: Aetna; BC-BS

DESCRIPTION:

Ritodrine Hydrochloride which contains the betamimetic (beta sympathomimetic amine) ritodrine hydrochloride, is available in two dosage forms. Ritodrine HCl for parenteral (intravenous) use is a clear, colorless, sterile, aqueous solution, each milliliter contains either 10 mg or 15 mg of ritodrine hydrochloride, 4.35 mg of acetic acid, 2.4 mg of sodium hydroxide, 1 mg of sodium metabisulfite, and 2.9 mg of sodium chloride in Water for Injection USP. Hydrochloric acid and/or additional sodium hydroxide is used to adjust pH. Filled under nitrogen.

FOR INTRAVENOUS USE ONLY. MUST BE DILUTED BEFORE USE. FOR DOSAGE AND ADMINISTRATION INSTRUCTIONS, SEE PRODUCT INFORMATION BELOW. DO NOT USE IF INJECTION IS DISCOLORED OR CONTAINS A PRECIPITATE.

Each Ritodrine HCl tablet contains 10 mg of ritodrine hydrochloride and the following inactive ingredients (in alphabetical order): corn starch, iron oxide yellow synthetic, lactose, magnesium stearate, povidone, and talc.

Ritodrine HCL is a white, odorless crystalline powder, freely soluble in water, with a melting point between 196° and 205°C. The chemical name of ritodrine hydrochloride is erythro-p-hydroxy-α-[1- [(p-hydroxyphenethyl)-amino]ethyl] benzyl alcohol hydrochloride.

CLINICAL PHARMACOLOGY:

Ritodrine HCl is a beta-receptor agonist, which has been shown by *in vitro* and *in vivo*pharmacologic studies in animals to exert a preferential effect of the β2 adrenergic receptors such as those in the uterine smooth muscle. Stimulation of the β2 receptors inhibits contractility of the uterine smooth muscle.

In humans, intravenous infusions of 0.05 to 0.30 mg/min or single oral doses of 10 to 20 mg decreased the intensity and frequency of uterine contractions. These effects were antagonized by beta-blocking compounds. Intravenous administration induced an immediate dose-related elevation of heart rate with maximum mean increases between 19 and 40 beats per minute. Widening of the pulse pressure was also observed; the average increase in systolic blood pressure was 4.0 mm Hg, and the average decrease in diastolic pressure was 12.3 mm Hg. With oral intake, the increase in heart rate was mild and delayed.

During intravenous infusion in humans, transient elevations of blood glucose, insulin, and free fatty acids have been observed. Decreased serum potassium has also been found, but effects on other electrolytes have not been reported.

Serum kinetics in humans (non-pregnant females) of an intravenous infusion of 60 minutes duration were determined by measuring serum ritodrine levels by a radioimmunoassay technique. The distribution half- life was found to be 6 to 9 minutes, and the effective half-life 1.7 to 2.6 hours. In a study of serum kinetics after oral ingestion (male subjects), the decline of serum drug levels could be described in terms of a two-phase decay with an initial half-life of 1.3 hours and a final half-life of 12 hours. With either route of administration, 90% of the excretion was compieted within 24 hours after the dose.

Comparison of ritodrine serum levels after intravenous administration with those after oral dosage indicates the oral bioavailability is about 30%. Intravenous infusion at a rate of 0.15 mg/min for 1 hour yielded maximum serum levels ranging between 32 and 52 ng/ml in a group of 6 nonpregnant female volunteers, maximum serum levels following single and repeated (4 x 10 mg/24 hr) 10 mg oral doses ranged between 5 and 15 ng/ml and were obtained within 30 to 60 minutes after ingestion.

Placental transfer was confirmed by measurement of drug concentrations in cord blood showing that ritodrine and its conjugates reach the fetal circulation.

INDICATIONS AND USAGE:

Ritodrine HCl is indicated for the management of preterm labor in suitable patients.

Administered intravenously, the drug will decrease uterine activity and thus prolong gestation in the majority of such patients. After intravenous Ritodrine HCl has arrested the acute episode, oral administration may help to avert relapse. Additional acute episodes may be treated by repeating the intravenous infusion. The incidence of neonatal mortality and respiratory distress syndrome increases when the normal gestation period is shortened.

Since successful inhibition of labor is more likely with early treatment, therapy with Ritodrine HCl should be instituted as soon as the diagnosis of preterm labor is established and contraindications ruled out in pregnancies of 20 or more weeks gestation. The efficacy and safety of Ritodrine HCl in advanced labor, that is, when cervical dilatation is more than 4 cm or effacement is more than 80%, have not been established.

CONTRAINDICATIONS:

Ritodrine HCl is contraindicated before the 20th week of pregnancy.

Ritodrine HCl is also contraindicated in those conditions of the mother or fetus in which continuation of pregnancy is hazardous; specific contraindications include:

1. Antepartum hemorrhage which demands immediate delivery
2. Eclampsia and severe preeclampsia
3. Intrauterine fetal death
4. Chorioamnionitis
5. Maternal cardiac disease
6. Pulmonary hypertension
7. Maternal hyperthyroidism
8. Uncontrolled maternal diabetes mellitus (See PRECAUTIONS.)
9. Pre-existing maternal medical conditions that would be seriously affected by the known pharmacologic properties of a betamimetic drug; such as: hypovolemia, cardiac arrhythmias associated with tachycardia or digitalis intoxication, uncontrolled hypertension, pheochromocytoma, bronchial asthma already treated by betamimetics and/or steroids
10. Known hypersensitivity to any component of the product

WARNINGS:

WARNING
Maternal pulmonary edema has been reported in patients treated with Ritodrine HCl, sometimes after delivery. It has occurred more often when patients were treated concomitantly with corticosteroids. Maternal death from this condition has been reported with or without corticosteroids given concomitantly with drugs of this class.
Patients so treated must be closely monitored in the hospital. The patient's state of hydration should be carefully monitored; fluid overload must be avoided. (See DOSAGE AND ADMINISTRATION.) Intravenous fluid loading may be aggravated by the use of betamimetics with or without corticosteroids and may turn into manifest circulatory overloading with subsequent pulmonary edema. If pulmonary edema develops during administration, the drug should be discontinued. Edema should be managed by conventional means.

Intravenous administration of Ritodrine HCl should be supervised by persons having knowledge of the pharmacology of the drug and who are qualified to identify and manage complications of drug administration and pregnancy. Beta-adrenergic drugs increase cardiac output, and even in a normal healthy heart this added myocardial oxygen demand can sometimes lead to myocardial ischemia. Complications may include: myocardial necrosis, which may result in death; arrhythmias, including premature atrial and ventricular contractions, ventricular tachycardia, and bundle branch block; anginal pain, with or without ECG changes. **Because cardiovascular responses are common and more pronounced during intravenous administration of Ritodrine HCl, cardiovascular effects, including maternal pulse rate and blood pressure and fetal heart rate, should be closely monitored. Care should be exercised for maternal signs and symptoms of pulmonary edema. A persistent high tachycardia (over 140 beats per minute) may be one of the signs of impending pulmonary edema with drugs of this class. Occult cardiac disease may be unmasked with the use of Ritodrine HCl. If the patient complains of chest pain or tightness of chest, the drug should be temporarily discontinued and an ECG should be done as soon as possible.**

The drug should not be administered to patients with mild to moderate preeclampsia, hypertension, or diabetes unless the attending physician considers that the benefits clearly outweigh the risks.

Ritodrine HCl Injection contains sodium metabisulfite, a sulfite that may cause allergic-type reactions including anaphylactic symptoms and life threatening or less severe asthmatic episodes in certain susceptible people. The overall prevalence of sulfite sensitivity in the general population in unknown and probably low. Sulfite sensitivity is seen more frequently in asthmatic than in nonasthmatic people.

PRECAUTIONS:

When Ritodrine HCl is used for the management of preterm labor in a patient with premature rupture of the membranes, the benefits of delaying delivery should be balanced against the potential risks of development of chorioamnionitis.

Among low birth weight infants, approximately 9% may be growth retarded for gestational age. Therefore, Intra-Uterine Growth Retardation (IUGR) should be considered in the differential diagnosis of preterm labor; this is especially important when the gestational age is in doubt. The decision to continue or reinitiate the administration of Ritodrine HCl will depend on an assessment of fetal maturity. In addition to clinical parameters, other studies, such as sonography or amniocentesis, may be helpful in establishing the state of fetal maturity if it is in doubt.

BASELINE EKG

This should be done to rule out occult maternal heart disease.

LABORATORY TESTS

Because intravenous administration of Ritodrine HCl has been shown to elevate plasma insulin and glucose and to decrease plasma potassium concentrations, monitoring of glucose and electrolyte levels is recommended during protracted infusions. Decrease of plasma potassium concentrations is usually transient, returning to normal within 24 hours. Special attention should be paid to biochemical variables when treating diabetic patients or those receiving potassium-depleting diuretics.

Serial hemograms may be helpful as an index of state of hydration.

MIGRAINE HEADACHE

Transient cerebral ischemia associated with beta sympathomimetic therapy has been reported in two patients with migraine headache.

PRECAUTIONS: *(cont'd)*

CARCINOGENESIS, MUTAGENESIS, AND IMPAIRMENT OF FERTILITY

In rats given oral doses of 1, 10, and 150 mg/kg/day of ritodrine hydrochloride for 82 weeks, benign and malignant tumors were found in the various dosage groups. Since there were no important differences between untreated controls and treated groups and no dose-related trends, it was concluded that there was no evidence of tumorigenicity. The incidence (2- 4%) of tumors of the type found in this study is not unusual in this species.

Reproduction studies in rats and rabbits have revealed no evidence of impaired fertility due to ritodrine hydrochloride.

PREGNANCY, TERATOGENIC EFFECTS, PREGNANCY CATEGORY B

Reproduction studies were performed in rats and rabbits. The doses employed intravenously were 1/9 (1 mg/kg), 1/3(3 mg/kg), and 1 (9 mg/kg) times the maximum human daily intravenous dose (but given to the animals as a bolus rather than by infusion). The oral doses, 10 and 100 mg/kg represented 5 and 50 times the maximum human daily oral maintenance dose. The results of these studies have revealed no evidence of impaired fertility of harm to the fetus due to Ritodrine HCl. No adverse fetal effects were encountered when single intravenous doses of 1,3, and 9 mg/kg/day or oral doses of 10 and 100 mg/kg/day were given to rats and rabbits on Days 6 through 15 and 6 through 18 of gestation, respectively. Intravenous doses of 1 and 8 mg/kg/day or oral doses of 10 and 100 mg/kg/day administered to the mother from Day 15 of pregnancy to Day 21 postpartum did not affect perinatal or postnatal development in rats. A slight increase in fetal weight in the rat was observed. Oral administration to both sexes did not impair fertility or reproductive performance. Lethal doses to pregnant rats did not cause immediate fetal demise. There are no adequate and well-controlled studies of Ritodrine HCl effects in pregnant women before 20 weeks gestation; therefore, this drug should not be used before the 20th week of pregnancy. Studies of Ritodrine HCl administered to pregnant women from the 20th week of gestation have not shown increased risk of fetal abnormalities. Follow-up of selected variables in a small number of children for up to 2 years has not revealed harmful effects on growth, developmental or functional maturation. Nonetheless, although clinical studies did not demonstrate a risk of permanent adverse fetal effects from Ritodrine HCl, the possibility cannot be excluded; therefore, Ritodrine HCl should be used only when clearly indicated.

Some studies indicate that infants born before 26 weeks gestation make up less than 10% of all births but account for as many as 75% of perinatal deaths and one-half of all neurologically handicapped infants. There are data available indicating that infants born at any time prior to full term may manifest a higher incidence of neurologic or other handicaps that occurs in the total population of infants born at or after full term. In delaying or preventing preterm labor, the use of Ritodrine HCl should result in an overall increase in neonatal survival. Handicapped infants who might not have otherwise survived may survive.

DRUG INTERACTIONS:

Corticosteroids used concomitantly may lead to pulmonary edema. (See WARNINGS.)

Cardiovascular effects of Ritodrine HCl Injection (especially cardiac arrhythmia or hypotension) may be potentiated by concomitant use of the following drugs:

1. magnesium sulfate
2. diazoxide
3. meperidine
4. potent general anesthetic agents

Systemic hypertension may be exaggerated in the presence of parasympatholytic agents such as atropine.

The effects of other sympathomimetic amines may be potentiated when concurrently administered and these effects may be additive. A sufficient time interval should elapse prior to administration of another sympathomimetic drug. With either oral or intravenous administration, 90% of the excretion of Ritodrine HCl is completed within 24 hours after the dose. (See CLINICAL PHARMACOLOGY.)

Beta-adrenergic blocking drugs inhibit the action of Ritodrine HCl, coadministration of these drugs should, therefore, be avoided.

With anesthetics used in surgery, the possibility that hypotensive effects may be potentiated should be considered.

ADVERSE REACTIONS:

The unwanted effects of Ritodrine HCl are related to its betamimetic activity and usually are controlled by suitable dosage adjustment.

EFFECTS ASSOCIATED WITH INTRAVENOUS ADMINISTRATION

Usual effects (80-100% of patients): Intravenous infusion of Ritodrine HCl leads almost invariably to dose related alterations in maternal and fetal heart rates and in maternal blood pressure. During clinical studies in which the maximum infusion rate was limited to 0.35 mg/min (one patient received 0.40 mg/min), the maximum maternal and fetal heart rates averaged, respectively, 130 (range 60 to 180) and 164 (range 130 to 200) beats per minute. The maximum maternal systolic blood pressures averaged 128 mm Hg (range 96 to 162 mm Hg), an average increase of 12 mm Hg from pretreatment levels. The minimum maternal diastolic blood pressures averaged 48 mm Hg (range 0 to 76 mm Hg), an average decrease of 23 mm Hg from pretreatment levels. While the more severe effects were usually managed effectively by dosage adjustments, in less than 1% of patients, persistent maternal tachycardia or decreased diastolic blood pressure required withdrawal of the drug. A persistent high tachycardia (over 140 beats per minute) may be one of the sings of impending pulmonary edema. (See WARNINGS.)

Ritodrine HCl infusion is associated with transient elevation of blood glucose and insulin, which decreases toward normal values after 48 to 72 hours despite continued infusion. Elevation of free fatty acids and cAMP has been reported. Reduction of potassium levels should be expected; other biochemical effects have not been reported.

Frequent Effects (10-50% of patients): Intravenous Ritodrine HCl, in about one-third of the patients, was associated with palpitation. Tremor, nausea, vomiting, headache, or erythema was observed in 10 to 15% of patients.

Occasional Effects (5-10% of patients): Nervousness, jitteriness, restlessness, emotional upset, or anxiety was reported in 5 to 6% of patients and malaise in similar numbers.

Infrequent Effects (1-3% of patients): Cardiac symptoms including chest pain or tightness (rarely associated with abnormalities of ECG) and arrhythmia were reported in 1 to 2% of patients. (See WARNINGS.)

Other infrequently reported maternal effects included: anaphylactic shock, rash, heart murmur, epigastric distress, ileus, bloating, constipation, diarrhea, dyspnea, hyperventilation, hemolytic icterus, glycosuria, lactic acidosis, sweating, chills, drowsiness, and weakness.Impaired liver function (*i.e.,* increased transaminase levels and hepatitis) has also be reported infrequently (less than 1%) with the use of ritodrine and other beta sympathomimetics.

Neonatal Effects: Infrequently reported neonatal symptoms include hypoglycemia and ileus. In addition, hypocalcemia and hypotension have been reported in neonates whose mothers were treated with other betamimetic agents.

ADVERSE REACTIONS: *(cont'd)*

EFFECTS ASSOCIATED WITH ORAL ADMINISTRATION

Frequent Effects (<50% of patients): Oral ritodrine in clinical studies was often associated with small increases in maternal heart rate, but little or no effect upon either maternal systolic or diastolic blood pressure or upon fetal heart rate was found.

Oral ritodrine in 10 to 15% of patients was associated with palpitation or tremor. Nausea and jitteriness were less frequent (5 to 8%), while rash was observed in some patients (3 to 4%), and arrhythmia was infrequent (about 1%). Impaired liver function (*i.e.,* increased transaminase levels and hepatitis) have also been reported infrequently (less than 1%) with the use of ritodrine and other beta sympathomimetics.

OVERDOSAGE:

The symptoms of overdosage are those of excessive beta-adrenergic stimulation including exaggeration of the known pharmacologic effects, the most prominent being tachycardia (maternal and fetal), palpitation, cardiac arrhythmia, hypotension, dyspnea, nervousness, tremor, nausea, and vomiting. If an excess of ritodrine tablets is ingested, gastric lavage or induction of emesis should be carried out followed by administration of activated charcoal. When symptoms of overdose occur as a result of intravenous administration, ritodrine should be discontinued; an appropriate beta-blocking agent may be used as an antidote. Ritodrine hydrochloride is dialyzable.

Acute intravenous toxicity was studied in rats and rabbits and acute oral toxicity in mice, rats, guinea pigs, and dogs. The LD_{50} values in the most sensitive of the species used were 64 mg/kg intravenously in the nonpregnant rabbit and 540 mg/kg orally in the nonpregnant mouse. The intravenous LD_{50} value in the pregnant rat was 85 mg/kg. The amount of drug required to produce symptoms of overdose in humans is individually variable. No reports of human mortality due to overdose have been received.

DOSAGE AND ADMINISTRATION:

In the management of preterm labor, the initial intravenous treatment should usually be followed by oral administration. The optimum dose of Ritodrine HCl is determined by a clinical balance of uterine response and unwanted effects.

INTRAVENOUS THERAPY

Do not use intravenous Ritodrine HCl if the solution is discolored or contains any precipitate or particulate matter.

Ritodrine HCl Injection should be used promptly after preparation, but in no case after 48 hours of preparation.

Method of Administration: To minimize the risks of hypotension, the patient should be maintained in the left lateral position throughout infusion and careful attention given to her state of hydration, but fluid overload must be avoided.

For appropriate control and dose titration, a controlled infusion device is recommended to adjust the rate of flow in drops/minute. An IV microdrop chamber (60 drops/ml) can provide a convenient range of infusion rates within the recommended dose range for Ritodrine HCl.

Recommended Dilution: 150 mg ritodrine hydrochloride in 500 ml fluid yielding a final concentration of 0.3 mg/ml*. Ritodrine for intravenous infusion should be diluted with 5% w/v dextrose solution. Because of the increased probability of pulmonary edema, saline diluents such as:

0.9% w/v sodium chloride solution

compound sodium chloride solution (Ringer's solution)

and Hartmann's solution, should be reserved for cases where dextrose solution is medically undesirable, e.g., diabetes mellitus.

* In those cases where fluid restriction is medically desirable, a more concentrated solution may be prepared.

Intravenous therapy should be started as soon as possible after diagnosis. The usual initial dose is 0.05 mg/minute (0.17 ml/min, 10 drops/min using a microdrip chamber at the recommended dilution), to be gradually increased by 0.05 mg/min (0.17 ml/min, 10 drops/min using a microdrip chamber at the recommended dilution) every 10 minutes until the desired result is obtained, or the maternal heart rate reaches 130 beats per minute. The effective dosage usually lies between 0.15 and 0.35 mg/minute (0.50 to 1.17 ml/min, 30-70 drops/min using a microdrip chamber at the recommended dilution).

Frequent monitoring of maternal uterine contractions, heart rate, and blood pressure, and of fetal heart rate is required, with dosage individually titrated according to response. If other drugs need to be given intravenously, the use of "piggyback" or other site of intravenous administration permits the continued independent control of the rate of infusion of the Ritodrine HCl.

The infusion should generally be continued for at least 12 hours after uterine contractions cease. With the recommended dilution, the maximum volume of fluid that might be administered after 12 hours at the highest dose (0.35 mg/min) will be approximately 840 ml.

The amount of IV fluids administered and the rate of administration should be monitored to avoid circulatory fluid overload (over-hydration). (See PRECAUTIONS, Laboratory Tests.)

ORAL MAINTENANCE

One tablet (10 mg) may be given approximately 30 minutes before the termination of intravenous therapy. The usual dosage schedule for the first 24 hours of oral administration is 1 tablet (10 mg) every two hours. Thereafter, the usual maintenance is 1 or 2 tablets (10 to 20 mg) every four to six hours, the dose depending on uterine activity and unwanted effects. The total daily dose or oral ritodrine should not exceed 120 mg. The treatment may be continued as long as the physician considers it desirable to prolong pregnancy.

Recurrence of unwanted preterm labor may be treated with repeated infusion of Ritodrine HCl.

Both the tablet and intravenous dosage forms should be stored at room temperature, preferably below 86°F (30°C). Protect from excessive heat.

HOW SUPPLIED - RATED THERAPEUTICALLY EQUIVALENT:

Injection, Solution - Intravenous - 10 mg/ml

5 ml	$35.40	Ritodrine Hcl, Abbott	00074-3193-01
5 ml	$391.88	Ritodrine Hcl, Fujisawa USA	00469-2450-20
5 ml x 10	$225.00	Ritodrine Hcl, Voluntary Hosp	53258-2450-20
5 ml x 10	**$912.08**	**YUTOPAR, Astra USA**	**00186-0569-13**
5 ml x 10	**$966.79**	**YUTOPAR, Astra USA**	**00186-0599-03**

Injection, Solution - Intravenous - 15 mg/ml

10 ml	$127.43	Ritodrine Hcl, Abbott	00074-3195-01
10 ml	$1046.88	Ritodrine Hcl, Fujisawa USA	00469-2460-30
10 ml x 10	$700.00	Ritodrine Hcl, Voluntary Hosp	53258-2460-30

Injection, Solution - Intravenous - 150 mg/syringe

10 ml x 1	**$233.34**	**YUTOPAR, Astra USA**	**00186-0644-01**

Injection, Solution - Intravenous - 150 mg/vial

10 ml x 1	**$237.84**	**YUTOPAR, Astra USA**	**00186-0597-12**

HOW SUPPLIED - NOT RATED EQUIVALENT:

Injection, Solution - Intravenous - 0.3 mg/ml

500 ml	$106.88	RITODRINE IN DEXTROSE 5%, Abbott	00074-7001-01
500 ml	$127.43	RITODRINE IN 5% DEXTROSE, Abbott	00074-7001-03

RITONAVIR *(003251)*

CATEGORIES: AIDS Related Complex; Anti-Infectives; Antimicrobials; Antivirals; HIV Infection; Infections; Protease Inhibitors; Viral Agents; FDA Approved 1996 Mar

BRAND NAMES: **Norvir**

FORMULARIES: PCS

COST OF THERAPY: $2,708.38 (HIV; Capsule; 600 mg; 2/day; 365 days)

WARNING:
Co-administration of ritonavir with certain nonsedating antihistamines, sedative hypnotics, or antiarrhythmics may result in potentially serious and/or life-threatening adverse events due to possible effects of ritonavir on the hepatic metabolism of certain drugs. See CONTRAINDICATIONS and DRUG INTERACTIONS.

DESCRIPTION:

Ritonavir is an inhibitor of HIV protease with activity against the Human Immunodeficiency Virus (HIV).

Ritonavir is chemically designated as 10-Hydroxy-2-methyl-5- (1-methylethyl)-1-[2-(1-methylethyl)-4-thiazolyl]-3, 6-dioxo-8, 11-bis(phenylmethyl)-2, 4, 7, 12-tetraazatridecan-13-oic acid, 5-thiazolylmethyl ester, [5S-(5R*,8R*,10R*,11R*)]. Its molecular formula is $C_{37}H_{48}N_6O_5S_2$, and its molecular weight is 720.95. Ritonavir is a white-to-light-tan powder. Ritonavir has a bitter metallic taste. It is freely soluble in methanol and ethanol, soluble in isopropanol and practically insoluble in water.

Norvir capsules are available for oral administration in a strength of 100 mg ritonavir with the following inactive ingredients: Caprylic/capric triglycerides, polyoxyl 35 castor oil, citric acid, gelatin, ethanol, polyglycolyzed glycerides, polysorbate 80, and propylene glycol.

Norvir oral solution is available for oral administration as 80 mg/mL of ritonavir in a peppermint and caramel flavored vehicle. Each 8-ounce bottle contains 19.2 grams of ritonavir. Norvir oral solution also contains ethanol, water, polyoxyl 35 castor oil, propylene glycol, anhydrous citric acid to adjust pH, saccharin sodium, peppermint oil, creamy caramel flavoring, and FD&C Yellow No. 6.

CLINICAL PHARMACOLOGY:

MICROBIOLOGY

Mechanism of action: Ritonavir is a peptidomimetic inhibitor of both the HIV-1 and HIV-2 proteases. Inhibition of HIV protease renders the enzyme incapable of processing the *gag-pol*polyprotein precursor which leads to production of non-infectious immature HIV particles.

Antiviral activity *in vitro*: The activity of ritonavir was assessed *in vitro* in acutely infected lymphoblastoid cell lines and in peripheral blood lymphocytes. The concentration of drug that inhibits 50% (EC_{50}) of viral replication ranged from 3.8 to 153 nM depending upon the HIV-1 isolate and the cells employed. The average $EC_{50}$for low passage clinical isolates was 22 nM (n=13). In MT_4cells, ritonavir demonstrated additive effects against HIV-1 in combination with either zidovudine (ZDV) or didanosine (ddI). Studies which measured cytotoxicity of ritonavir on several cell lines showed that >20 μM was required to inhibit cellular growth by 50% resulting in an *in vitro* therapeutic index of at least 1000.

Resistance: HIV-1 isolates with reduced susceptibility to ritonavir have been selected *in vitro*. Genotypic analysis of these isolates showed mutations in the HIV protease gene at amino acid positions 84 (Ile to Val), 82 (Val to Phe), 71 (Ala to Val), and 46 (Met to Ile). Phenotypic (n=18) and genotypic (n=44) changes in HIV isolates from selected patients treated with ritonavir were monitored in phase I/II trials over a period of 3 to 32 weeks. Mutations associated with the HIV viral protease in isolates obtained from 41 patients appeared to occur in a stepwise and ordered fashion; in sequence, these mutations were position 82 (Val to Ala/Phe), 54 (Ile to Val), 71 (Ala to Val/Thr), and 36 (Ile to Leu), followed by combinations of mutations at an additional 5 specific amino acid positions. Of 18 patients for which both phenotypic and genotypic analysis were performed on free virus isolated from plasma, 12 showed reduced susceptibility to ritonavir *in vitro*. All 18 patients possessed one or more mutations in the viral protease gene. The 82 mutation appeared to be necessary but not sufficient to confer phenotypic resistance. Phenotypic resistance was defined as a ≥ 5-fold decrease in viral sensitivity *in vitro* from baseline. The clinical relevance of phenotypic and genotypic changes associated with ritonavir therapy has not been established.

Cross-resistance to other antiretrovirals: The potential for HIV cross-resistance between protease inhibitors has not been fully explored. Therefore, it is unknown what effect ritonavir therapy will have on the activity of concordantly or subsequently administered protease inhibitors. Serial HIV isolates obtained from six patients during ritonavir therapy showed a decrease in ritonavir susceptibility *in vitro* but did not demonstrate a concordant decrease in susceptibility to saquinavir *in vitro* when compared to matched baseline isolates. However, isolates from two of these patients demonstrated decreased susceptibility to indinavir *in vitro* (8-fold). Isolates from 5 patients were also tested for cross-resistance to VX-478 and nelfinavir; isolates from 2 patients had a decrease in susceptibility to nelfinavir (12 - 14-fold), and none to VX-478. Cross-resistance between ritonavir and reverse transcriptase inhibitors is unlikely because of the different enzyme targets involved. One ZDV-resistant HIV isolate tested *in vitro* retained full susceptibility to ritonavir.

PHARMACOKINETICS

The pharmacokinetics of ritonavir have been studied in healthy volunteers and HIV-infected patients ($CD_4 \geq 50$ cells/μL). See TABLE 1 for ritonavir pharmacokinetic characteristics.

The absolute bioavailability of ritonavir has not been determined. After a 600 mg dose of oral solution, peak concentrations of ritonavir were achieved approximately 2 hours and 4 hours after dosing under fasting and non-fasting (514 KCal; 9% fat, 12% protein, and 79% carbohydrate) conditions, respectively. When the oral solution was given under non-fasting conditions, peak ritonavir concentrations decreased 23% and the extent of absorption decreased 7% relative to fasting conditions. Dilution of the oral solution, within one hour ofadministration, with 240 mL of chocolate milk, Advera or Ensure did not significantly affect the extent and rate of ritonavir absorption. After a single 600 mg dose under non-fasting conditions, in two separate studies, the capsule (n=21) and oral solution (n=18) formulations yielded mean ± SD areas under the plasma concentration-time curve (AUCs) of 129.5 ± 47.1 and 129.0 ± 39.3 mcg·h/mL, respectively. Relative to fasting conditions, the extent of absorption of ritonavir from the capsule formulation was 15% higher when administered with a meal (771 KCal; 46% fat, 18% protein, and 37% carbohydrate).

CLINICAL PHARMACOLOGY: *(cont'd)*

Nearly all of the plasma radioactivity after a single oral 600 mg dose of ^{14}C-ritonavir oral solution n=5 was attributed to unchanged ritonavir. Five ritonavir metabolites have been identified in human urine and feces. The isopropylthiazole oxidation metabolite (M-2) is the major metabolite and has antiviral activity similar to that of parent drug; however, the concentrations of this metabolite in plasma are low. Studies utilizing human liver microsomes have demonstrated that cytochrome P450 3A (CYP3A) is the major isoform involved in ritonavir metabolism, although CYP2D6 also contributes to the formation of M-2.

In a study of five subjects receiving a 600 mg dose of ^{14}C-ritonavir oral solution, 11.3 ± 2.8% of the dose was excreted into the urine, with 3.5 ± 1.8% of the dose excreted as unchanged parent drug. In that study, 86.4 ± 2.9% of the dose was excreted in the feces with 33.8 ± 10.8% of the dose excreted as unchanged parent drug. Upon multiple dosing, ritonavir accumulation is less than predicted from a single dose possibly due to a time and dose-related increase in clearance.

TABLE 1 Ritonavir Pharmacokinetic Characteristics

Parameter	n	Values (Mean ± SD)
C_{max} SS†	10	11.2 ± 3.6 mcg/ml
C_{trough} SS†	10	3.7 ± 2.6 mcg/ml
V_{β}, /F‡	91	0.41 ± 0.25 L/kg
$t_{\frac{1}{2}}$		3 - 5 h
CL/F†	10	8.8 ± 3.2 L/h
CL/F‡	91	4.6 ± 1.6 L/h
CL_R	62	<1.0 L/h
RBC/ Plasma Ratio		0.14
Percent Bound*		98 to 99%

† SS= Steady State; patients taking ritonavir 600 mg q12h
‡ Single ritonavir 600 mg dose
* Primarily bound to human serum albumin and alpha-1 acid glycoprotein over the ritonavir concentration range of 0.01 to 30 mcg/ml

SPECIAL POPULATIONS

Gender, Race and Age: No age-related pharmacokinetic differences have been observed in adult patients (18 to 63 years). Ritonavir pharmacokinetics have not been studied in older patients. A study of ritonavir pharmacokinetics in healthy males and females showed no statistically significant differences in the pharmacokinetics of ritonavir. Pharmacokinetic differences due to race have not been identified.

Renal Insufficiency: Ritonavir pharmacokinetics have not been studied in patients with renal insufficiency, however since renal clearance is negligible, a decrease in total body clearance is not expected in patients with renal insufficiency.

Hepatic Insufficiency: Ritonavir pharmacokinetics have not been studied in subjects with hepatic insufficiency (see PRECAUTIONS).

CLINICAL STUDIES:

Description of Clinical Studies: The activity of ritonavir as monotherapy or in combination with nucleoside analogues has been evaluated in 1446 patients enrolled in two double-blind, randomized trials. Ritonavir therapy in combination with zidovudine and zalcitabine was also evaluated in an open-label, non-comparative study of 32 patients. The clinical studies reported here were all conducted using ritonavir oral solution.

ADVANCED PATIENTS WITH PRIOR ANTIRETROVIRAL THERAPY

Study 247 was a randomized, double-blind trial conducted in HIV-infected patients with at least nine months of prior antiretroviral therapy and baseline CD_4 cell counts ≤ 100 cells/μL. Ritonavir 600 mg b.i.d. or placebo was added to each patient's baseline antiretroviral therapy regimen, which could have consisted of up to two approved antiretroviral agents. The study accrued 1090 patients, with mean baseline CD_4cell count at study entry of 32 cells/μL. Median duration of follow-up was 6 months.

The six month cumulative incidence of clinical disease progression or death was 17% for patients randomized to ritonavir compared to 34% for patients randomized to placebo. This difference in rates was statistically significant.

The six-month cumulative mortality was 5.8% for patients randomized to ritonavir and 10.1% for patients randomized to placebo. This difference in rates was statistically significant. In addition, analyses of mean CD_4 cell count changes from baseline over the first 16 weeks of study for the first 211 patients enrolled (mean baseline CD_4cell count = 29 cells/μL) showed that ritonavir was associated with larger increases in CD_4 cell counts than was placebo.

PATIENTS WITHOUT PRIOR ANTIRETROVIRAL THERAPY

In ongoing Study 245, 356 antiretroviral-naive HIV-infected patients (mean baseline CD_4 = 364 cells/μL) were randomized to receive either ritonavir 600 mg b.i.d., zidovudine 200 mg t.i.d., or a combination of these drugs. In analyses of average CD_4cell count changes from baseline over the first 16 weeks of study, both ritonavir monotherapy and combination therapy produced greater mean increases in CD_4 cell count than did zidovudine monotherapy. The CD_4 cell count increases for ritonavir monotherapy were larger than the increases for combination therapy.

COMBINATION THERAPY WITH RITONAVIR, ZIDOVUDINE, AND ZALCITABINE IN ANTIRETROVIRAL-NAIVE PATIENTS

In Study 208, an open-label uncontrolled trial, 32 antiretroviral-naive HIV-infected patients initially received ritonavir 600 mg b.i.d. monotherapy. Zidovudine 200 mg t.i.d. and zalcitabine 0.75 mg t.i.d. were added after 14 days of ritonavir monotherapy. Results of combination therapy for the first 20 weeks of this study show median increases in CD_4cell counts from baseline levels of 83 to 106 cells/μL over the treatment period. Mean decreases from baseline in HIV RNA particle levels ranged from 1.69 to 1.92 logs.

INDICATIONS AND USAGE:

Ritonavir is indicated in combination with nucleoside analogues or as monotherapy for the treatment of HIV-infection when therapy is warranted. For patients with advanced HIV disease, this indication is based on the results from a study that showed a reduction in both mortality and AIDS-defining clinical events for patients who received ritonavir. Median duration of follow-up in this study was 6 months. The clinical benefit from ritonavir therapy for longer periods of treatment is unknown.

For patients with less advanced disease, this indication is based on changes in surrogate markers in studies evaluating patients who received ritonavir alone or in combination with other antiretroviral agents (see Description of Clinical Studies).

CONTRAINDICATIONS:

Ritonavir is contraindicated in patients with known hypersensitivity to ritonavir or any of its ingredients.

Ritonavir is expected to produce large increases in the plasma concentrations of the following drugs: amiodarone, astemizole, bepridil, bupropion, cisapride, clozapine, encainide, flecainide, meperidine, piroxicam, propafenone, propoxyphene, quinidine, rifabutin, and terfenadine. These agents have recognized risks of arrhythmias, hematologic abnormalities, seizures, or

CONTRAINDICATIONS: *(cont'd)*

other potentially serious adverse effects. These drugs should not be co-administered with ritonavir. Ritonavir co-administration is likely to produce large increases in these highly metabolized sedatives and hypnotics: alprazolam, clorazepate, diazepam, estazolam, flurazepam, midazolam, triazolam, and zolpidem. Due to the potential for extreme sedation and respiratory depression from these agents, they should not be co-administered with ritonavir.

PRECAUTIONS:

GENERAL

Ritonavir is principally metabolized by the liver. Therefore, caution should be exercised when administering this drug to patients with impaired hepatic function.

RESISTANCE/CROSS-RESISTANCE

The potential for HIV cross-resistance between protease inhibitors has not been fully explored. Therefore, it is unknown what effect ritonavir therapy will have on the activity of subsequent protease inhibitors (see MICROBIOLOGY).

INFORMATION FOR PATIENTS

Patients should be informed that ritonavir is not a cure for HIV infection and that they may continue to acquire illnesses associated with advanced HIV infection, including opportunistic infections.

Patients should be told that the long-term effects of ritonavir are unknown at this time. They should be informed that ritonavir therapy has not been shown to reduce the risk of transmitting HIV to others through sexual contact or blood contamination.

Patients should be advised to take ritonavir with food, if possible.

Patients should be informed to take ritonavir every day as prescribed. Patients should not alter the dose or discontinue ritonavir without consulting their doctor. If a dose is missed, patients should take the next dose as soon as possible. However, if a dose is skipped, the patient should not double the next dose.

Since ritonavir interacts with some drugs when taken together, patients should be advised to report to their doctor the use of any other medications, including prescription and non-prescription drugs.

LABORATORY TESTS

Ritonavir has been associated with alterations in triglycerides, SGOT, SGPT, GGT, CPK, and uric acid. Appropriate laboratory testing should be performed prior to initiating ritonavir therapy and at periodic intervals or if any clinical signs or symptoms occur during therapy. For comprehensive information concerning laboratory test alterations associated with nucleoside analogues, physicians should refer to the complete product information for each of these drugs.

CARCINOGENESIS AND MUTAGENESIS

Long-term carcinogenicity studies of ritonavir in animal systems have not been completed. However, ritonavir was not mutagenic or clastogenic in a battery of *in vitro* and *in vivo* assays including bacterial reverse mutation (Ames) using *S. typhimurium* and *E. coli*, mouse lymphoma, mouse micronucleus, and chromosome aberrations in human lymphocytes.

PREGNANCY, FERTILITY, AND REPRODUCTION

Pregnancy Category B: Ritonavir produced no effects on fertility in rats at drug exposures approximately 40% (male) and 60% (female) of that achieved with the proposed therapeutic dose. Higher dosages were not feasible due to hepatic toxicity.

No treatment-related malformations were observed when ritonavir was administered to pregnant rats or rabbits.

Developmental toxicity observed in rats (early resorptions, decreased fetal body weight and ossification delays and developmental variations) occurred at a maternally toxic dosage at an exposure equivalent to approximately 30% of that achieved with the proposed therapeutic dose. A slight increase in the incidence of cryptorchidism was also noted in rats at an exposure approximately 22% of that achieved with the proposed therapeutic dose. Developmental toxicity observed in rabbits (resorptions, decreased litter size and decreased fetal weights) also occurred at a maternally toxic dosage equivalent to 1.8 times the proposed therapeutic dose based on a body surface area conversion factor.

There are, however, no adequate and well-controlled studies in pregnant women. Because animal reproduction studies are not always predictive of human response, this drug should be used during pregnancy only if clearly needed.

NURSING MOTHERS

It is not known whether this drug is excreted in human milk. Because many drugs are excreted in human milk, caution should be exercised when ritonavir is administered to a nursing woman. However, the U.S. Public Health Service Centers for Disease Control and Prevention advises HIV-infected women not to breast-feed to avoid postnatal transmission of HIV to a child who may not be infected.

PEDIATRIC USE

The safety and effectiveness of ritonavir in children below the age of 12 have not been established.

DRUG INTERACTIONS:

Drug-Drug Interactions: TABLES 2 and 3 summarize the effects on AUC and C_{max}, with 95% confidence intervals (95 CI), of co-administration of ritonavir with a variety of drugs.

TABLE 2 Effects on AUC and C_{max} of Co-administration of Ritonavir With Other Drugs

Drug	Ritonavir Dosage	n	AUC % (95 CI)	C_{max}% (95 CI)
Clarithromycin				
500 mg q12h 4 days	200 mg q8h 4 days	22	↑12% (2,23%)	↑15% (2,28%)
Didanosine				
200 mg q12h 4 days	600 mg q12h 4 days	12	↔	↔
Fluconazole	200 mg q6h 4 days	8	↑12% (5,20%)	↑15% (7,22%)
400 mg day 1				
200 mg daily 4 days				
Fluoxetine				
30 mg q12h 8 days	600 mg single dose	16	↑19% (7,34%)	↔
Rifampin				
600 mg or 300 mg daily 10 days[2]	500 mg q12h 20 days	7, 9*	↓ 35% (7,55%)	↓ 25% (-5,46%)
Zidovudine				
200 mg q8h 4 days	300 mg q6h 4 days	10	↔	↔

Agents which increase CYP3A activity (*e.g.,* phenobarbital, carbamazepine, dexamethasone, phenytoin, rifampin, and rifabutin) would be expected to increase the clearance of ritonavir resulting in decreased ritonavir plasma concentrations. Tobacco use is associated with an 18% decrease in the AUC of ritonavir. Ritonavir can produce large increases in plasma concentrations of certain highly metabolized drugs. Ritonavir has a high affinity for several cytochrome P450 (CYP) isoforms with the following rank order: CYP3A > CYP2D6 > CYP2C9, CYP2C19 >> CYP2A6, CYP1A2, CYP2E1. There is some evidence that ritonavir may increase the activity of glucuronosyl transferases; thus, loss of therapeutic effects from directly glucuronidated agents during ritonavir therapy may signify the need for dosage alteration of these agents. A systematic review of over 200 medications prescribed to HIV-infected patients was performed to identify potential drug interactions with ritonavir. Some commonly prescribed drugs, separated by the type of metabolism and expected magnitude of interaction when co-administered with ritonavir are listed. It is advised that concomitant use of any of these agents with ritonavir should be accompanied by therapeutic drug concentration monitoring and/or increased monitoring of therapeutic and adverse effects, especially for agents with narrow therapeutic margins (*e.g.,* oral anticoagulants, immunosuppressants). Large dosage reductions (>50% reduction) may be required for those agents extensively metabolized by CYP3A.

DRUG INTERACTIONS: *(cont'd)*

TABLE 3

Drug	Ritonavir Dosage	n	AUC % (95 CI)	C_{max}% (95 CI)
Clarithromycin				
500 mg q12h 4 days	200 mg q8h 4 days	22	↑77% (56,103%)	↑31% (15,51%)
14-OH clarithromycin metabolite			↓ 100%	↓ 99%
Desipramine				
100 mg single dose	500 mg q12h 12 days	14	↑145% (103,211%)	↑22% (12,35%)
2-OH despiramine metabolite			↓ 15% (3,26%)	↓ 67% (62,72%)
Didanosine				
200 mg q12h 4 days	600 mg q12h 4 days	12	↓ 13% (0,23%)	↓ 16% (5,26%)
Ethinyl estradiol				
50 mcg single dose	500 mg q12h 16 days	23	↓ 40$ (31,49%)	↓ 32% (24,39%)
Rifabutin				
150 mg daily 16 days	500 mg q12h 10 days	5, 11*	↑4-fold (2.8,6.1X)	↑2.5-fold (1.9,3.4X)
25-O-desacetyl rifabutin metabolite			↑35-fold (25,78X)	↑16-fold (14,20X)
Sulfamethazole				
800 mg single dose[1]	500 mg q12h 12 days	15	↓20% (16,23%)	↔
Theophylline				
3 mg/kg q8h 15 days	500 mg q12h 10 days	13, 11*	↓43% (42,45%)	↓32% (29,34%)
Trimethoprim				
160 mg single dose[1]	500 mg q12h 12 days	15	↑20% (3,43%)	↔
Zidovudine				
200 mg q8h 4 days	300 mg q6h 4 days	10	↓25% (15,34%)	↓27% (4,45%)

1 Sulfamethazole and trimethoprim taken as single combination tablet
1 Preliminary Data
↑ Indicates increase
↓ Indicates decrease
Indicates no change
* Parallel group design; entries are subjects receiving combination and control regimens, respectively.

The following list provides information based on studies of the co-administration of ritonavir on the pharmacokinetic properties of several commonly prescribed medications.

Clarithromycin: The mean increase in the AUC of clarithromycin in the presence of ritonavir was 77%. Clarithromycin may be administered without dosage adjustment to patients with normal renal function. However, for patients with renal impairment the following dosage adjustments should be considered. For patients with CL_{CR} 30 to 60 mL/min the dose of clarithromycin should be reduced by 50%. For patients with CL_{CR} < 30 mL/min the dose of clarithromycin should be decreased by 75%.

Desipramine: Co-administration of ritonavir resulted in a 145% mean increase in the AUC of desipramine. Dosage reduction of desipramine should be considered in patients taking the combination.

Disulfiram/Metronidazole: Ritonavir formulations contain alcohol, which can produce reactions when co-administered with disulfiram or other drugs that produce disulfiram-like reactions (*e.g.,* metronidazole).

Oral Contraceptives: The mean AUC of ethinyl estradiol, a component in oral contraceptives, was reduced 40% during concomitant dosing with ritonavir 500 mg q12h; dosage increase or alternate contraceptive measures should be considered.

Saquinavir: Ritonavir extensively inhibits the metabolism of saquinavir resulting in greatly increased saquinavir plasma concentrations. The safety of this combination has not been established.

Theophylline: The average AUC of theophylline was reduced by 43% when co-administered with ritonavir. Increased dosage of theophylline may be required.

Ritonavir, Drug Interactions

Analgesics, narcotic

Large [1] ↑AUC[2] (CYP3A): Alfentanil, Fentanyl
Moderate [1] ↑AUC[2] (CYP2D6): Hydrocodone, Oxycodone, Tramadol
Possible ↑**AUC** [2] (unknown CYP): Methadone
Possible ↓**AUC** [2] (glucuronidation): Codeine, Hydromorphone, Morphine

Anagesics, nonsteriodal

Moderate [1] ↑ or ↓AUC[2] (CYP2C9/19): Diclofenac, Ibuprofen, Indomethacin
Possible ↑**AUC** [2] (unknown CYP): Nabumetone, Sulindac
Possible ↓**AUC** [2] (glucuronidation): Ketoprofen, Ketorolac, Naproxen

Antiarrhythmics

Large [1] ↑AUC[2] (CYP3A): Disopyramide, Lidocaine
Moderate [1] ↑AUC[2] (CYP2D6): Mexiletine
Possible ↑**AUC** [2] (unknown CYP): Tocainide, Digoxin
Possible ↓**AUC** [2] (glucuronidation):
Large [1] ↑AUC[2] (CYP3A):
Moderate [1] ↑AUC[2] (CYP2D6):
Moderate [1] ↑ or ↓AUC[2] (CYP2C9/19):

DRUG INTERACTIONS: *(cont'd)*

Possible ↑AUC [2] (unknown CYP):
Possible ↓AUC [2] (glucuronidation):

Antibiotic, macrolide
Large [1] ↑AUC[2] (CYP3A): Erythromycin

Antocoagulant
Large [1] ↑AUC[2] (CYP3A): R-Warfarin
Moderate [1] ↑ or ↓AUC[2] (CYP2C9/19): S-Warfarin

Anticonvulsants
Large [1] ↑AUC[2] (CYP3A): Carbamazepine, Clonazepam, Ethosuximide
Moderate [1] ↑ or ↓AUC[2] (CYP2C9/19): Phentoin
Possible ↑AUC [2] (unknown CYP): Phenobarbital
Possible ↓AUC [2] (glucuronidation): Divalproex, Lamotrigine

Antihistamine
Large [1] ↑AUC[2] (CYP3A): Loratadine

Antidepressants, tricyclic
Moderate [1] ↑AUC[2](CYP2D6): Amitriptyline, Clomipramine, Desipramine, Imipramine, Maprotiline, Nortriptypine
Possible ↑AUC [2] (unknown CYP): Doxepin

Antidepressants, other
Large [1] ↑AUC[2] (CYP3A):Nefrazodone, Sertraline, Trazodone
Moderate [1] ↑AUC[2](CYP2D6): Fluoxetine, Paroxetine, Venlafaxine
Possible ↑AUC [2] (unknown CYP): Fluvoxamine

Antidiarrheal
Possible ↓AUC [2] (glucuronidation): Diphenoxylate

Antiemetics
Large [1] ↑AUC[2] (CYP3A): Dronabinol, Ondansetron
Possible ↑AUC [2] (unknown CYP): Prochlorperazine, Promethazine
Possible ↓AUC [2] (glucuronidation): Metoclopramide

Antifungal agents
Possible ↑AUC [2] (unknown CYP): Itraconazole, Ketoconazole, Miconazole

Antihypertensives
Moderate [1] ↑ or ↓AUC[2] (CYP2C9/19): Losartan
Possible ↑AUC [2] (unknown CYP): Doxazosin, Prazosin, Terazosin

Antiparasitics
Large [1] ↑AUC[2] (CYP3A): Quinine
Moderate [1] ↑ or ↓AUC[2] (CYP2C9/19): Proguanil
Possible ↑AUC [2] (unknown CYP): Albendazole, Chloroquine, Metronidazole, Primaquine, Pyrimethamine
Possible ↓AUC [2] (glucuronidation): Atovaquone

Antiulcer agents
Large [1] ↑AUC[2] (CYP3A): Lansoprazole, Omeprazole
Possible ↑AUC [2] (unknown CYP): Cimetidine

β-blockers
Moderate [1] ↑AUC[2](CYP2D6): Metoprolol, Pindolol, Propanolol, Timolol
Moderate [1] ↑ or ↓AUC[2] (CYP2C9/19):
Possible ↑AUC [2] (unknown CYP): Acebutolol, Betaxolol, Penbutolol

Calcium channel blockers
Large [1] ↑AUC[2] (CYP3A): Amlodipine, Diltiazem, Felodipine, Isradipine, Nicardipine, Nifedipine, Nimodipine, Nisoldipine, Verapamil

Cancer chemotherapeutic agents
Large [1] ↑AUC[2] (CYP3A): Etoposide Paclitaxel, Tamoxifen, Vinblastine, Vincristine
Possible ↑AUC [2] (unknown CYP): Cyclophosphamide, Daunorubicin, Doxorubicin

Corticosteroids
Large [1] ↑AUC[2] (CYP3A): Dexamethasone, Prednisone

Hemorrheologic agent
Possible ↑AUC [2] (unknown CYP): Pentoxifylline

HIV protease inhibitors
Large [1] ↑AUC[2] (CYP3A): Saquinovir

Hypoglycemics
Moderate [1] ↑ or ↓AUC[2] (CYP2C9/19): Glipizide, Glyburide, Tolbutamide

Hypolipidemics
Large [1] ↑AUC[2] (CYP3A): Lovastin, Pravastin
Possible ↑AUC [2] (unknown CYP): Fluvastin, Gemfibrozil, Simvastatin
Possible ↓AUC [2] (glucuronidation): Clofibrate

Immunosuppressants
Large [1] ↑AUC[2] (CYP3A): Cyclosporine, Tacrolimus

Neuroleptics
Moderate [1] ↑AUC[2](CYP2D6): Chlorpromazine, Haloperidol, Perphenazine, Risperidone, Thioridazine

Sedative/hypnotics
Possible ↓AUC [2] (glucuronidation): Lorazepam, Oxazepam, Propofol, Temazepam

Stimulants
Moderate [1] ↑AUC[2](CYP2D6): Methamphetamine
Possible ↑AUC [2] (unknown CYP): Methylphenidate

ADVERSE REACTIONS:

The safety of ritonavir alone and in combination with nucleoside analogues was studied in 1140 patients. TABLE 4A and B lists treatment-emergent adverse events (at least possibly related and of at least moderate intensity) that occurred in 2% or greater of patients receiving ritonavir alone or in combination with nucleosides in Study 245 or Study 247. At the time of this safety assessment, the median duration of treatment in Study 245 and Study 247 was 3.7 and 2.4 months, respectively. However, safety data was collected on patients for greater than 6 months of treatment. The most frequently reported clinical adverse events, other than asthenia, among patients receiving ritonavir were gastrointestinal and neurological disturbances including nausea, diarrhea, vomiting, anorexia, abdominal pain, taste perversion, and circumoral and peripheral paresthesias. Similar adverse event profiles were reported in patients receiving ritonavir in other trials.

Adverse events occurring in less than 2% of patients receiving ritonavir in all phase II/phase III studies and considered at least possibly related or of unknown relationship to treatment and of at least moderate intensity are listed below by body system.

Body as a Whole: Abdomen enlarged, accidental injury, allergic reaction, back pain, cachexia, chest pain, chills, facial edema, facial pain, flu syndrome, hormone level altered, hypothermia, kidney pain, neck pain, neck rigidity, pain (unspecified), substernal chest pain, and photosensitivity reaction.

Cardiovascular System: Hemorrhage, hypotension, migraine, palpitation, peripheral vascular disorder, postural hypotension, syncope, and tachycardia.

Digestive System: Abnormal stools, bloody diarrhea, cheilitis, cholangitis, colitis, dry mouth, dysphagia, eructation, esophagitis, gastritis, gastroenteritis, gastrointestinal disorder, gastrointestinal hemorrhage, gingivitis, hepatitis, hepatomegaly, ileitis, liver damage, liver function tests abnormal, mouth ulcer, oral moniliasis, pancreatitis, periodontal abscess, rectal disorder, tenesmus, and thirst.

Endocrine System: Diabetes mellitus. Hemic and Lymphatic System: Anemia, ecchymosis leukopenia, lymphadenopathy, lymphocytosis, and thrombocytopenia.

Metabolic and Nutritional Disorders: Avitaminosis, dehydration, edema, glycosuria, gout, hypercholesteremia, peripheral edema, and weight loss.

Musculoskeletal System: Arthralgia, arthrosis, joint disorder, muscle cramps, muscle weakness, myositis, and twitching.

Nervous System: Abnormal dreams, abnormal gait, agitation, amnesia, anxiety, aphasia, ataxia, confusion, convulsion, depression, diplopia, emotional lability, euphoria, grand mal convulsion, hallucinations, hyperesthesia, incoordination, libido decreased, nervousness, neuralgia, neuropathy, paralysis, peripheral neuropathy, peripheral sensory neuropathy, personality disorder, tremor, urinary retention, and vertigo.

TABLE 4 Percentage of patients with treatment Emergent [1] Adverse Events of Moderate or Severe Intensity Occurring in ≥2% of Patients Receiving Ritonavir

	Study 245 Naive Patients			Study 247 Advanced Patients	
Adverse Events	Ritonavir + ZDV n=116	Ritonavir n=117	ZDV n=119	Ritonavir n=541	Placebo n=547
Body as a Whole					
Abdominal Pain	4.3	3.4	4.2	7.0	3.1
Asthenia	27.6	9.4	10.1	14.2	5.3
Fever	1.7	0.9	1.7	4.4	2.2
Headache	7.8	5.1	7.6	6.3	4.0
Malaise	4.3	1.7	3.4	0.7	0.2
Cardiovascular					
Vasodilation	2.6	1.7	0.8	1.3	0.0
Digestive					
Anorexia	7.8	0.9	3.4	6.1	2.0
Constipation	2.6	0.0	0.8	0.0	0.4
Diarrhea	21.6	12.8	0.0	18.3	6.1
Dyspepsia	1.7	0.0	1.7	4.8	0.7
Flatulence	2.6	0.9	0.8	0.9	0.6
Local Throat Irritation	1.7	1.7	0.8	2.6	0.2
Nausea	46.6	23.1	24.4	26.2	5.7
Vomiting	22.4	12.8	12.6	15.2	2.6
Metabolic and Nutritional					
Creatine Phosphokinase Increased	1.7	3.4	3.4	0.9	0.2
Hyperlipidemia	1.7	1.7	0.0	4.1	0.0
Mysculoskeletal					
Myalgia	1.7	1.7	0.8	2.2	0.9
Nervous					
Circumoral Paresthesia	5.2	2.6	0.0	5.9	0.2
Dizziness	5.2	2.6	1.7	3.3	1.1
Insomnia	3.4	2.6	0.8	1.3	0.6
Paresthesia	5.2	2.6	0.0	2.0	0.2
Peripheral Paresthesia	0.0	6.0	0.0	5.0	0.7
Smolence	2.6	2.6	0.0	2.0	0.2
Thinking Abnormal	0.9	0.0	0.8	0.7	0.2
Respiratory					
Pharyngitis	0.9	2.6	0.0	0.4	0.4
Skin and Appendages					
Rash	0.9	0.0	0.8	2.6	0.9
Sweating	3.4	2.6	1.7	1.3	0.6
Special Senses					
Taste Perversion	15.5	10.3	7.6	5.4	1.7

1 Includes those adverse events at least possibly related to study drug or of unknown relationship and excludes concurrent HIV conditions.

Respiratory System: Asthma, dyspnea, epistaxis, hiccup, hypoventilation, increased cough, interstitial pneumonia, lung disorder, and rhinitis.

Skin and Appendages: Acne, contact dermatitis, dry skin, eczema, folliculitis, maculopapular rash, molluscum contagiosum, pruritus, psoriasis, seborrhea, urticaria, and vesiculobullous rash.

Special Senses: Abnormal electro-oculogram, abnormal electroretinogram, abnormal vision, amblyopia/blurred vision, blepharitis, ear pain, eye pain, hearing impairment, increased cerumen, iritis, parosmia, photophobia, taste loss, tinnitus, uveitis, and visual field defect.

Urogenital System: Dysuria, hematuria, impotence, kidney calculus, kidney failure, nocturia, penis disorder, polyuria, pyelonephritis, urethritis, and urinary frequency.

OVERDOSAGE:

ACUTE OVERDOSAGE

Human Overdose Experience: Human experience of acute overdose with ritonavir is limited. One patient in clinical trials took ritonavir 1500 mg/day for two days. The patient reported paresthesias which resolved after the dose was decreased.

The approximate lethal dose was found to be greater than 20 times the related human dose in rats and 10 times the related human dose in mice.

OVERDOSAGE: *(cont'd)*

TABLE 5 Percentage of Patients, by Study and Treatment Group, with Marked Chemistry and Hematology Laboratory Value Abnormalities

		Study 245 Naive Patients			Study 247 Advanced Patients	
Variable	**Limit**	**Ritonavir + ZDV**	**Ritonavir**	**ZDV**	**Ritonavir**	**Placebo**
Chemistry	**High**					
Glucose	(>250 mg/dl)	2.0	-	0.9	0.4	1.1
Uric Acid	(>12 mg/dl)	-	-	-	3.6	0.2
Creatine	(>3.6 mg/dl)	-	-		0.2	0.2
Potassium	(>6.0 mEq/l)	-	-	-	0.4	0.2
Chloride	(>122 mEq/l)	-	0.9	-	-	-
Total Bilirubin	(>3.6 mg/dl)	-	-	-	1.2	0.2
Alkaline Phosphate	(550 IU/l)	-	0.9	-	1.4	1.7
GOT (AST)S	(>180 IU/l)	2.9	6.5	1.7	3.8	4.3
SGPT (ALT)	(>215 IU/l)	3.9	5.6	2.6	6.1	2.6
GGT	(>300 IU/l)	2.0	2.8	0.9	14.7	6.7
LDH	(>1170 IU/l)				1.0	0.2
Triglycerides	(>1500 mg/dl)	1.0	2.8	-	10.1	0.2
Triglycerides Fasting	(>1500 mg/dl)	2.1	1.4	-	7.9	0.4
CPK	(>1000 mg/dl)	7.0	7.5	7.1	8.6	4.5
Amalyse	(2 X ULN[1])	-	0.9	-	0.2	-
Chemistry	**Low**					
Albumin	(<2.0 g/dl)	-	-	-	0.2	0.6
Sodium	(<123 mEq/L)	-	-	-	0.2	-
Potassium	<3.0 mEq/L)	-	0.9		2.0	1.1
Chloride	<84 mEq/L)	-	0.9	-	-	0.4
Magnesium	<1.0 mEq/L)	-	-	-	0.4	0.4
Calcium	<6.9 mEq/L)	-	-	-	1.2	0.9
Hematology	**Low**					
Hemoglobin	(<8.0 g/dl)	-	-	-	2.8	2.4
Hematocrit	(<30%)	2.0	-	-	11.7	16.0
RBC	<3.0 X 10^9/L)	1.0	-	1.7	14.9	19.7
WBC	(<2.5 X 10^9/L)	-	-	3.5	25.1	51.4
Platlet Count	(<20 X 10^9/L)	-		-	0.4	0.6
Neurophils	(≤0.5 X 10^9/L)	-	-	-	4.0	6.9
Hematology	**High**					
WBC	(>25 X 10^9/L)	-	-	-	1.6	0.7
Neutrophils	(>20 X 10^9/L)	-	-	-	1.8	0.9
Eosinophils	(1.0 X 10^9/L)	-	1.9	0.9	1.8	2.6
Prothrombin Time	(1.5 X ULN[1])	1.0	-	-	1.0	1.3

1 ULN=upper limit of normal range
- Indicates no events reported

MANAGEMENT OF OVERDOSAGE

Treatment of overdose with ritonavir consists of general supportive measures including monitoring of vital signs and observation of the clinical status of the patient. There is no specific antidote for overdose with ritonavir. If indicated, elimination of unabsorbed drug should be achieved by emesis or gastric lavage; usual precautions should be observed to maintain the airway. Administration of activated charcoal may also be used to aid in removal of unabsorbed drug. Since ritonavir is extensively metabolized by the liver and is highly protein bound, dialysis is unlikely to be beneficial in significant removal of the drug. A Certified Poison Control Center should be consulted for up-to-date information on the management of overdose with ritonavir.

DOSAGE AND ADMINISTRATION:

Ritonavir is administered orally. It is recommended that ritonavir be taken with meals if possible. Patients may improve the taste of ritonavir oral solution by mixing with chocolate milk, Ensure, or Advera within one hour of dosing. The effects of antacids on the absorption of ritonavir have not been studied.

The recommended dosage of ritonavir is 600 mg twice daily by mouth. Some patients experience nausea upon initiation of 600 mg b.i.d. dosing; dose escalation may provide some relief: 300 mg b.i.d. for 1 day, 400 mg b.i.d. for 2 days, 500 mg b.i.d. for 1 day, and then 600 mg b.i.d. thereafter. In addition, patients initiating combination regimens with ritonavir and nucleosides may improve gastrointestinal tolerance by initiating ritonavir alone and subsequently adding nucleosides before completing two weeks of ritonavir monotherapy.

PATIENT INFORMATION:

Ritonavir is used in the treatment of HIV infections.

Inform your doctor if you are pregnant or nursing.

This agent interacts with many other drugs. Inform your doctor if you are taking other medications, including over-the-counter medications.

Take with meals

May cause nausea, vomiting, diarrhea, and weakness. Notify your doctor or pharacist if these occur.

HOW SUPPLIED:

Norvir (ritonavir capsules) are white capsules imprinted with the corporate logo, 100 mg, and the Abbo-Code PI.

HOW SUPPLIED: *(cont'd)*

Recommended storage: Store capsules in the refrigerator between 36°-46°F (2°-8°C). Protect from light.

Norvir (ritonavir oral solution) is an orange-colored liquid, supplied in amber-colored, multidose bottles containing 600 mg ritonavir per 7.5 mL marked dosage cup (80 mg/mL).

Recommended storage: Store ritonavir oral solution in the refrigerator between 36°-46°F (2°-8°C) until it is dispensed.

Refrigeration of ritonavir oral solution by the patient is recommended, but not required if used within 30 days and stored below 77°F (25°C). Product should be stored in the original container. Avoid exposure to excessive heat. Keep cap tightly closed.

HOW SUPPLIED - EQUIVALENTS NOT AVAILABLE:

Capsule - Oral - 600 mg

2 x 84's $311.65 NORVIR, Abbott 00074-9492-02

Solution - Oral - 80 mg/ml

240 ml $311.65 NORVIR, Abbott 00074-1940-63

ROCURONIUM BROMIDE *(003202)*

CATEGORIES: Analeptics; Anesthesia; Autonomic Drugs; Endotracheal Intubation; Muscle Relaxants; Muscles; Neuromuscular Blocking Agents; Non-Depolarizing Muscle Relaxants; Short-Acting Neuromuscular Blockers; Skeletal Muscle Relaxants; FDA Class 1S ("Standard Review"); FDA Approved 1994 Mar

BRAND NAMES: **Zemuron**

FORMULARIES: DoD; United

DESCRIPTION:

Rocuronium bromide injection is a nondepolarizing neuromuscular blocking agent with a rapid to intermediate onset depending on dose and intermediate duration. Rocuronium bromide is chemically designated as 1-[17β-(acetyloxy)-3α—hydroxy-2β-(4-morpholinyl)-5α-androstan-16β-yl]-1-(2- propenyl)pyrrolidinium bromide.

The chemical formula is $C_{32}H_{53}BrN_2O_4$ with a molecular weight of 609.70. The partition coefficient of rocuronium bromide in n-octanol/water is 0.5 at 20°C.

Rocuronium bromide injection is supplied as a sterile, nonpyrogenic, isotonic solution for intravenous injection only. Each ml contains 10 mg rocuronium bromide and 2 mg sodium acetate. The aqueous solution is adjusted to isotonicity with sodium chloride and to a pH of 4 with acetic and/or sodium hydroxide.

CLINICAL PHARMACOLOGY:

Rocuronium bromide injection is a nondepolarizing neuromuscular blocking agent with a rapid to intermediate onset depending on dose and intermediate duration. It acts by competing for cholinergic receptors at the motor end-plate. This action is antagonized by acetylcholinesterase inhibitors, such as neostigmine and edrophonium.

Pharmacodynamics: The ED_{95} (dose required to produce 95% suppression of the first [T_1] mechanomyographic [MMG] response of the adductor pollicis muscle [thumb] to indirect supramaximal train-of- four stimulation of the ulnar nerve) during opioid/nitrous oxide/oxygen anesthesia is approximately 0.3 mg/kg. Patient variability around the ED_{95} dose suggests that 50% of patients will exhibit T_1 depression of 91-97%.

TABLE 1 presents intubating conditions in patients with intubation initiated at 60 to 70 seconds.

TABLE 1 Intubating Conditions in Patients with Intubation Initiated at 60 to 70 seconds. Percent, Median (Range)

Rocuronium Bromide Dose (mg/kg) Administered over 5 sec	Percent of patients with excellent or good intubating conditions	Time to completion of intubation (min)
Adults* 18-64 yr		
0.45 (n=43)	86%	1.6 (1.0-7.0)
0.6 (n=51)	96%	1.6 (1.0-3.2)
Pediatric 3 mo-1 yr		
0.6 (n=18)	100%	1.0 (1.0-1.5)
Pediatric 1-12 yr		
0.6 (n=12)	100%	1.0 (0.5-2.3)

* Excludes patients undergoing cesarean section Excellent intubating conditions = jaw relaxed, vocal cords apart and immobile, no diaphragmatic movement. Good intubating conditions = same as excellent but with some diaphragmatic movement.

TABLE 2 presents the time to onset and clinical duration for the initial dose of rocuronium bromide under opioid/nitrous oxide/oxygen anesthesia in adults and geriatric patients, and under halothane anesthesia in children.

Once spontaneous recovery has reached 25% of control T_1, the neuromuscular block produced by rocuronium bromide is readily reversed with anticholinesterase agents, e.g., edrophonium or neostigmine.

The median spontaneous recovery from 25 to 75% T_1 was 13 minutes in adult patients. When neuromuscular block was reversed in 36 adults at a T_1 of 22-27%, recovery to a T_1 of 89 (50-132)% and T_4/T_1 of 69 (38-92)% was achieved within 5 minutes. Only five of 320 adults reversed received an additional dose of reversal agent. The median (range) dose of neostigmine was 0.04 (0.01 to 0.09) mg/kg and the median (range) dose of edrophonium was 0.5 (0.3 to 1.0) mg/kg.

In geriatric patients (n=51) reversed with neostigmine, the median T_4/T_1 increased from 40 to 88% in 5 minutes.

Children (n=27) who received 0.5 mg/kg edrophonium had increases in the median T_4/T_1 from 37% at reversal to 93% after 2 minutes. Children (n=58) who received 1 mg/kg edrophonium had increases in the median T_4/T_1 from 72% at reversal to 100% after 2 minutes. Infants (n=10) who were reversed with 0.03 mg/kg neostigmine recovered from 25% to 75% T_1 within 4 minutes.

There were no reports of less than satisfactory clinical recovery of neuromuscular function.

The neuromuscular blocking action of rocuronium bromide may be enhanced in the presence of potent inhalation anesthetics (see PRECAUTIONS, Inhalation Anesthetics.)

Hemodynamics: There were no dose-related effects on the incidence of changes from baseline (≥ 30%) in mean arterial blood pressure (MAP) or heart rate associated with rocuronium bromide injection administration over the dose range of 0.12 to 1.2 mg/kg (4 x ED_{95}) within 5 minutes after rocuronium bromide administration and prior to intubation. Increases or

CLINICAL PHARMACOLOGY: *(cont'd)*

decreases in MAP were observed in 2-5% of geriatric and other adult patients, and in about 1% of pediatric patients. Heart rate changes (≥ 30%) occurred in 0-2% of geriatric and other adult patients. Tachycardia (≥ 30%) occurred in 12 of 127 children. Most of the children developing tachycardia were from a single study where the patients were anesthetized with halothane and who did not receive atropine for induction (see CLINICAL STUDIES, Pediatric.) In U.S. studies, laryngoscopy and tracheal intubation following rocuronium bromide administration were accompanied by transient tachycardia (≥ 30% increases) in about one-third of adult patients under opioid/nitrous oxide/oxygen anesthesia. Animal studies have indicated that the ratio of vagal:neuromuscular block following rocuronium bromide administration is less than vecuronium but greater than pancuronium. The tachycardia observed in some patients may result from this vagal blocking activity.

TABLE 2 Time to Onset and Clinical Duration following Initial (intubating) Dose during Opioid/Nitrous Oxide/Oxygen Anesthesia (Adults) and Halothane Anesthesia (Children), Median (Range)

Rocuronium Bromide Dose (mg/kg) Administered over 5 sec	Time to ≥80% Block (min)	Time to Maximum Block (min)	Clinical Duration (min)
Adults 18-64 yr			
0.45 (n=50)	1.3 (0.8-6.2)	3.0 (1.3-8.2)	22 (12-31)
0.6 (n=142)	1.0 (0.4-6.0)	1.8 (0.6-13.0)	31 (15-85)
0.9 (n=20)	1.1 (0.3-3.8)	1.4 (0.8-6.2)	58 (27-111)
1.2 (n=18)	0.7 (0.4-1.7)	1.0 (0.6-4.7)	67 (38-160)
Geriatrics ≥65 yr			
0.6 (n=31)	2.3 (1.0-8.3)	3.7 (1.3-11.3)	46 (22-73)
0.9 (n=5)	2.0 (1.0-3.0)	2.5 (1.2-5.0)	62 (49-75)
1.2 (n=7)	1.0 (0.8-3.5)	1.3 (1.2-4.7)	94 (64-138)
Pediatric 3 mo-1 yr			
0.6 (n=17)	—	0.8 (0.3-3.0)	41 (24-68)
0.8 (n=9)	—	0.7 (0.5-0.8)	40 (27-70)
Pediatric 1-12 yr			
0.6 (n=27)	0.8 (0.4-2.0)	1.0 (0.5-3.3)	26 (17-39)
0.8 (n=18)	—	0.5 (0.3-1.0)	30 (17-56)

n= the number of patients who had Time to Maximum Block recorded.
Clinical duration = time until return to 25% of control T_1. Patients receiving doses of 0.45 mg/kg who achieved less than 90% block (16% of these patients) had about 12 to 15 minutes to 25% recovery.

Histamine Release: In studies of histamine release, clinically significant concentrations of plasma histamine occurred in 1 of 88 patients. Clinical signs of histamine release (flushing, rash, or bronchospasm) associated with the administration of rocuronium bromide injection were assessed in clinical trials and reported in 9 of 1137 (0.8%) patients.

Pharmacokinetics: In an effort to maximize the information gathered in the *in vivo*pharmacokinetic studies the data from the studies was used to develop population estimates of the parameters for the subpopulations represented (*e.g.,* geriatric, pediatric, renal, and hepatic insufficiency). These population based estimates and a measure of the estimate variability are contained in the following section.

Following IV administration of rocuronium bromide injection, plasma levels of rocuronium follow a three compartment open model. The rapid distribution half-life is 1-2 minutes and the slower distribution half-life is 14-18 minutes. Rocuronium is approximately 30% bound to human plasma proteins. In geriatric and other adult surgical patients undergoing either opioid/nitrous oxide/oxygen or inhalational anesthesia the observed pharmacokinetic profile was essentially unchanged.

TABLE 3 Pharmacokinetic Parameters in Adults (n=22; ages 27-58 yr) and Geriatric (n=20; ≥ 65 yr) During Opioid/Nitrous Oxide/Oxygen Anesthesia (Mean ± SD)

PK Parameters	Adults (Ages 27-58 yr)	Geriatrics (≥ 65 yr)
Clearance (l/kg/hr)	0.25 ± 0.08	0.21 ± 0.06
Volume of Distribution at Steady State (l/kg)	0.25 ± 0.04	0.22 ± 0.03
$T_{1/2}$ β Elimination (hr)	1.4 ± 0.4	1.5 ± 0.4

In general, studies with normal adult subjects did not reveal any differences in the pharmacokinetics of rocuronium due to gender.

Studies of distribution, metabolism, and excretion in cats and dogs indicate that rocuronium is eliminated primarily by the liver.

The rocuronium analog 17-desacetyl-rocuronium, a metabolite, has been rarely observed in the plasma or urine of humans administered single doses of 0.5-1 mg/kg with or without a subsequent infusion (for up to 12 hr) of rocuronium. In the cat, 17-desacetyl-rocuronium has approximately one-twentieth the neuromuscular blocking potency of rocuronium. The effects of renal failure and hepatic disease on the pharmacokinetics and pharmacodynamics of rocuronium in humans are consistent with these findings.

In general, patients undergoing cadaver kidney transplant have a small reduction in clearance which is offset pharmacokinetically by a corresponding increase in volume, such that the net effect is an unchanged plasma half-life. Patients with demonstrated liver cirrhosis have a marked increase in their volume of distribution resulting in a plasma half-life approximately twice that of patients with normal hepatic function. TABLE 4 shows the pharmacokinetic parameters in subjects with either impaired renal or hepatic function.

TABLE 4 Pharmacokinetic Parameters in Adults with Normal Renal and Hepatic Function (n=10, ages 23-65), Renal Transplant Patients (n=10, ages 21-45) and Hepatic Dysfunction Patients (n=9, ages 31-67) During Isoflurane Anesthesia (Mean ± SD)

PK Parameters	Normal Renal and Hepatic Function	Renal Transplant Patients	Hepatic Dysfunction Patients
Clearance (l/kg/hr)	0.16 ± 0.05*	0.13 ± 0.04	0.13 ± 0.06
Volume of Distribution at Steady State (l/kg)	0.26 ± 0.03	0.34 ± 0.11	0.53 ± 0.14
$T_{1/2}$ β Elimination (hr)	2.4 ± 0.8*	2.4 ± 1.1	4.3 ± 2.6

* Differences in the calculated $T_{1/2}$ β and Cl between this study and the study in young adults *vs.* geriatrics (≥ 65 years) is related to the different sample populations and anesthetic techniques.

The net result of these findings is that subjects with renal failure have clinical durations that are similar to but somewhat more variable than the duration that one would expect in subjects with normal renal function. Hepatically impaired patients, due to the large increase in volume, may demonstrate clinical durations approaching 1.5 times that of subjects with normal hepatic function. In both populations the clinician should individualize the dose to the needs of the patient (see Individualization of Dosage).

Tissue redistribution accounts for most (about 80%) of the initial amount of rocuronium administered. As tissue compartments fill with continued dosing (4-8 hours), less drug is redistributed away from the site of action and, for an infusion-only dose, the rate to maintain neuromuscular blockade falls to about 20% of the initial infusion rate. The use of a loading dose and a smaller infusion rate reduces the need for adjustment of dose.

Special Populations: *Pediatrics:* The clinical duration of effects of rocuronium bromide injection did not vary with age in patients 4 months to 8 years of age. The terminal half-life and other pharmacokinetic parameters of rocuronium in these children are presented in TABLE 5.

TABLE 5 Pharmacokinetic Parameters of Rocuronium in Pediatric Patients (ages 3- < 12 mo, n=6; 1- < 3 yr, n=5; 3- < 8 yr, n=7) During Halothane Anesthesia (Mean ± SD)

PK Parameters	Patient Age Range: 3- < 12 mo	1- < 3 yr	3- < 8 yr
Clearance (l/kg/hr)	0.35 ± 0.08	0.32 ± 0.07	0.44 ± 0.16
Volume of Distribution at Steady State (l/kg)	0.30 ± 0.04	0.26 ± 0.06	0.21 ± 0.03
$T_{1/2}$ β Elimination (hr)	1.3 ± 0.5	1.1 ± 0.7	0.8 ± 0.3

CLINICAL STUDIES:

In U.S. clinical trials a total of 1,137 patients received rocuronium bromide injection including 176 pediatric, 140 geriatric, 55 obstetric, and 766 other adults. Most patients (90%) were ASA physical status I or II, about 9% were ASA III, and 10 patients (undergoing coronary artery bypass grafting or valvular surgery) were ASA IV. In European clinical trials, a total of 1,394 patients received rocuronium bromide including 52 pediatric, 128 geriatric (≥ 65 years) and 1,214 other adults.

Adult Patients: Intubation using doses of rocuronium bromide injection 0.6 to 0.85 mg/kg was evaluated in 203 adults in 11 clinical trials. Excellent to good intubating conditions were generally achieved within 2 minutes and maximum block occurred within 3 minutes in most patients. Doses within this range provide clinical relaxation for a median (range) time of 33 (14-85) minutes under opioid/nitrous oxide/oxygen anesthesia. Larger doses (0.9 and 1.2 mg/kg) were evaluated in two trials with 19 and 16 patients under opioid/nitrous oxide/oxygen anesthesia and provided 58 (27-111) and 67 (38-160) minutes of clinical relaxation, respectively.

Cardiovascular Disease: In one clinical trial, 10 patients with clinically significant cardiovascular disease undergoing coronary artery bypass graft received an initial dose of 0.6 mg/kg rocuronium bromide injection. Neuromuscular block was maintained during surgery with bolus maintenance doses of 0.3 mg/kg. Following induction, continuous 0.008 mg/kg/min infusion of rocuronium bromide produced relaxation sufficient to support mechanical ventilation for 6 to 12 hours in the surgical intensive care unit (SICU) while the patients were recovering from surgery. Hypertension and tachycardia were reported in some patients but these occurrences were less frequent in patients receiving beta or calcium channel blocking drugs. In 7 of these 10 patients rocuronium bromide was associated with transient increases (≥ 30%) in pulmonary vascular resistance. In another clinical trial of 17 patients undergoing abdominal aortic surgery, transient increases (≥ 30%) in pulmonary vascular resistance were observed in 4 of 17 patients receiving rocuronium bromide 0.6 or 0.9 mg/kg.

Rapid Sequence Intubation: Intubating conditions were assessed in 230 patients in six clinical trials where anesthesia was induced with either thiopental (3 to 6 mg/kg) or propofol (1.5 to 2.5 mg/kg) in combination with either fentanyl (2 to 5 mcg/kg) or alfentanil (1 mg). Most of the patients also received a premedication such as midazolam or temazepam. Most patients had intubation attempted within 60 to 90 seconds of administration of rocuronium bromide injection 0.6 mg/kg or succinylcholine 1 to 1.5 mg/kg. Excellent or good intubating conditions were achieved in 119/120 (99% [95% confidence interval 95-99.9%]) patients receiving rocuronium bromide and in 108/110 (98% [94%-99.8%]) patients receiving succinylcholine. The duration of action of rocuronium bromide 0.6 mg/kg is longer than succinylcholine and at this dose is approximately equivalent to the duration of other intermediate acting neuromuscular blocking drugs.

Geriatric Patients: Rocuronium bromide injection was evaluated in 55 geriatric patients (ages 65-80 years) in six clinical trials. Doses of 0.6 mg/kg provided excellent to good intubating conditions in a median (range) time of 2.3 (1-8) minutes. Recovery time from 25% to 75% after these doses were not prolonged in geriatric patients compared to other adult patients.

Pediatric Patients: Rocuronium bromide injection 0.6 or 0.8 mg/kg was evaluated for intubation in 75 pediatric patients (n=28; age 3-12 months, n=47; age 1-12 years) in three trials using halothane (1-5%) nitrous oxide (60-70%) in oxygen. Of the children anesthetized with halothane who did not receive atropine for induction, about 80% experienced a transient increase (≥ 30%) in heart rate after intubation. One of the 19 infants anesthetized with halothane and fentanyl who received atropine for induction experienced this magnitude of change.

Obese Patients: Rocuronium bromide injection was dosed according to actual body weight (ABW) in most clinical trials. The administration of rocuronium bromide in the 47 of 330 (14%) patients who were at least 30% or more above their ideal body weight (IBW) was not associated with clinically significant differences in the onset, duration, recovery, or reversal of rocuronium bromide induced neuromuscular block.

In one clinical trial in obese patients, rocuronium bromide 0.6 mg/kg was dosed according to ABW (n=12) or IBW (n=11). Obese patients dosed according to IBW had a longer time to maximum block, a shorter clinical duration of 25 (14-29) minutes, and did not achieve intubating conditions comparable to those dosed based on ABW. These results support the recommendation that obese patients be dosed based on actual body weight.

Obstetric Patients: Rocuronium bromide injection 0.6 mg/kg was administered with thiopental, 3-4 mg/kg (n=13) or 4-6 mg/kg (n=42), for rapid sequence induction of anesthesia for cesarean section. No neonate had APGAR scores < 7 at 5 minutes. The umbilical venous plasma concentrations were 18% of maternal concentrations at delivery. Intubating conditions were poor or inadequate in 5 of 13 women receiving 3-4 mg/kg thiopental when intubation was attempted 60 seconds after drug injection. Therefore, rocuronium bromide is not recommended for rapid sequence induction in cesarean section patients.

Individualization Of Dosage: DOSES OF ROCURONIUM BROMIDE INJECTION SHOULD BE INDIVIDUALIZED AND A PERIPHERAL NERVE STIMULATOR SHOULD BE USED TO MEASURE NEUROMUSCULAR FUNCTION DURING

CLINICAL STUDIES: *(cont'd)*

ROCURONIUM BROMIDE ADMINISTRATION IN ORDER TO MONITOR DRUG EFFECT, DETERMINE THE NEED FOR ADDITIONAL DOSES, AND CONFIRM RECOVERY FROM NEUROMUSCULAR BLOCK.

Based on the known actions of rocuronium bromide, the following factors should be considered when administering rocuronium bromide.

Renal or Hepatic Impairment: No differences from patients with normal hepatic and kidney function were observed for onset time at a dose of 0.6 mg/kg rocuronium bromide injection. When compared to patients with normal renal and hepatic function, the mean clinical duration is similar in patients with end-stage renal disease undergoing renal transplant, and is about 1.5 times longer in patients with hepatic disease. Patients with renal failure may have a greater variation in duration of effect (see CLINICAL PHARMACOLOGY, Pharmacokinetics and PRECAUTIONS, Renal Failure and Hepatic Disease).

Reduced Plasma Cholinesterase Activity: No differences from patients with normal plasma cholinesterase activity is expected since rocuronium metabolism does not depend on plasma cholinesterase.

Drugs or Conditions Causing Potentiation of or Resistance to Neuromuscular Block: The neuromuscular blocking action of rocuronium bromide injection is potentiated by isoflurane and enflurane anesthesia. Potentiation is minimal when administration of the recommended dose of rocuronium bromide occurs prior to the administration of these potent inhalation agents. The median clinical duration of a dose of 0.57- 0.85 mg/kg was 34, 38, and 42 minutes under opioid/nitrous oxide/oxygen, enflurane and isoflurane maintenance anesthesia, respectively. During 1-2 hr of infusion, the infusion rate of rocuronium bromide required to maintain about 95% block was decreased by as much as 40% under enflurane and isoflurane anesthesia (see PRECAUTIONS, Inhalation Anesthetics.)

When rocuronium bromide is administered to patients chronically receiving anticonvulsant agents such as carbamazepine or phenytoin, shorter durations of neuromuscular block may occur and infusion rates may be higher due to the development of resistance to nondepolarizing muscle relaxants (see PRECAUTIONS, Anticonvulsants.)

Pulmonary Hypertension: Rocuronium bromide injection may be associated with increased pulmonary vascular resistance so caution is appropriate in patients with pulmonary hypertension or valvular heart disease (see CLINICAL STUDIES.)

Obesity: In obese patients, the initial dose of rocuronium bromide injection 0.6 mg/kg should be based upon the patient's actual body weight (see CLINICAL STUDIES, Obese Patients.)

Based on the known actions of other nondepolarizing neuromuscular blocking agents the following additional factors should be considered when administering rocuronium bromide.

Drugs or Conditions Causing Potentiation of or Resistance to Neuromuscular Block: Resistance to nondepolarizing agents, consistent with up-regulation of skeletal muscle acetylcholine receptors, is associated with burns, disuse atrophy, denervation, and direct muscle trauma. Receptor up-regulation may also contribute to the resistance to nondepolarizing muscle relaxants which sometimes develop in patients with cerebral palsy, patients chronically receiving anticonvulsant agents such as carbamazepine or phenytoin or with chronic exposure to nondepolarizing agents (see PRECAUTIONS.)

Other nondepolarizing neuromuscular blocking agents have been found to exhibit profound neuromuscular blocking effects in cachectic or debilitated patients, patients with neuromuscular diseases, and patients with carcinomatosis. In these or other patients in whom potentiation of neuromuscular block may be anticipated, a decrease from the recommended initial dose should be considered.

Certain antibiotics, magnesium salts, lithium, local anesthetics, procainamide, and quinidine have been shown to increase the duration of neuromuscular block and decrease infusion requirements of other neuromuscular blocking agents. In patients in whom potentiation of neuromuscular block may be anticipated, a decrease from the recommended initial dose should be considered (see Antibiotics and Other subsections of PRECAUTIONS).

Severe acid-base and/or electrolyte abnormalities may potentiate or cause resistance to the neuromuscular blocking action of rocuronium bromide (see PRECAUTIONS, Other.) No data are available in such patients and no dosing recommendations can be made.

Burns: Patients with burns are known to develop resistance to nondepolarizing neuromuscular blocking agents, probably due to up- regulation of post-synaptic skeletal muscle cholinergic receptors (see Individualization of Dosage).

INDICATIONS AND USAGE:

Rocuronium bromide injection is a nondepolarizing neuromuscular blocking agent with a rapid to intermediate onset depending on dose and intermediate duration and is indicated for inpatients and outpatients as an adjunct to general anesthesia to facilitate both rapid sequence and routine tracheal intubation, and to provide skeletal muscle relaxation during surgery or mechanical ventilation.

CONTRAINDICATIONS:

Rocuronium bromide injection is contraindicated in patients known to have hypersensitivity to rocuronium bromide.

WARNINGS:

ROCURONIUM BROMIDE INJECTION SHOULD BE ADMINISTERED IN CAREFULLY ADJUSTED DOSAGES BY OR UNDER THE SUPERVISION OF EXPERIENCED CLINICIANS WHO ARE FAMILIAR WITH THE DRUG'S ACTIONS AND THE POSSIBLE COMPLICATIONS OF ITS USE. THE DRUG SHOULD NOT BE ADMINISTERED UNLESS FACILITIES FOR INTUBATION, ARTIFICIAL RESPIRATION, OXYGEN THERAPY, AND AN ANTAGONIST ARE IMMEDIATELY AVAILABLE. IT IS RECOMMENDED THAT CLINICIANS ADMINISTERING NEUROMUSCULAR BLOCKING AGENTS SUCH AS ROCURONIUM BROMIDE EMPLOY A PERIPHERAL NERVE STIMULATOR TO MONITOR DRUG RESPONSE, NEED FOR ADDITIONAL RELAXANT, AND ADEQUACY OF SPONTANEOUS RECOVERY OR ANTAGONISM.

ROCURONIUM BROMIDE HAS NO KNOWN EFFECT ON CONSCIOUSNESS, PAIN THRESHOLD, OR CEREBRATION. THEREFORE, ITS ADMINISTRATION MUST BE ACCOMPANIED BY ADEQUATE ANESTHESIA OR SEDATION.

In patients with myasthenia gravis or myasthenic (Eaton-Lambert) syndrome, small doses of nondepolarizing neuromuscular blocking agents may have profound effects. In such patients, a peripheral nerve stimulator and use of a small test dose may be of value in monitoring the response to administration of muscle relaxants.

Rocuronium bromide, which has an acid pH, should not be mixed with alkaline solutions (*e.g.,* barbiturate solutions) in the same syringe or administered simultaneously during intravenous infusion through the same needle.

PRECAUTIONS:

Long-term Use in I.C.U.: Rocuronium bromide has not been studied for long term use in the I.C.U. As with other nondepolarizing neuromuscular blocking drugs, apparent tolerance to rocuronium bromide may develop rarely during chronic administration in the ICU. While

PRECAUTIONS: *(cont'd)*

the mechanism for development of this resistance is not known, receptor up-regulation may be a contributing factor. It is STRONGLY RECOMMENDED THAT NEUROMUSCULAR TRANSMISSION BE MONITORED CONTINUOUSLY DURING ADMINISTRATION AND RECOVERY WITH THE HELP OF A NERVE STIMULATOR. ADDITIONAL DOSES OF ROCURONIUM BROMIDE OR ANY OTHER NEUROMUSCULAR BLOCKING AGENT SHOULD NOT BE GIVEN UNTIL THERE IS A DEFINITE RESPONSE (ONE TWITCH OF THE TRAIN-OF-FOUR) TO NERVE STIMULATION. Prolonged paralysis and/or skeletal muscle weakness may be noted during initial attempts to wean from the ventilator patients who have chronically received neuromuscular blocking drugs in the I.C.U. Therefore, rocuronium bromide should only be used in this setting if, in the opinion of the prescribing physician, the specific advantages of the drug outweigh the risk.

Labor and Delivery: The use of rocuronium bromide in cesarean section has been studied in a limited number of patients. Rocuronium bromide is not recommended for rapid sequence induction in cesarean section patients (see CLINICAL STUDIES.)

Hepatic Disease: Since rocuronium bromide injection is primarily excreted by the liver it should be used with caution in patients with clinically significant hepatic disease. Rocuronium bromide 0.6 mg/kg has been studied in a limited number of patients (n=9) with clinically significant hepatic disease under steady-state isoflurane anesthesia. After rocuronium bromide 0.6 mg/kg, the median (range) clinical duration of 60 (35- 166) minutes was moderately prolonged compared to 42 minutes in patients with normal hepatic function. The median recovery time of 53 minutes was also prolonged in patients with cirrhosis compared to 20 minutes in patients with normal hepatic function. Four of eight patients with cirrhosis, who received rocuronium bromide 0.6 mg/kg under opioid/nitrous oxide/oxygen anesthesia, did not achieve complete block. These findings are consistent with the increase in volume of distribution at steady state observed in patients with significant hepatic disease (see CLINICAL PHARMACOLOGY, Pharmacokinetics.) If used for rapid sequence induction in patients with ascites, an increased initial dosage may be necessary to assure complete block. Duration will be prolonged in these cases. The use of doses higher than 0.6 mg/kg has not been studied.

Renal Failure: Due to the limited role of the kidney in the excretion of rocuronium bromide injection, usual dosing guidelines should be adequate. Rocuronium bromide 0.6 mg/kg has been evaluated in three single center trials (n=30), ages 19-61 years) in patients undergoing renal transplant surgery, or shunt procedures in preparation for dialysis. After rocuronium bromide 0.6 mg/kg, the time to maximum block was about 1-2 minutes and was not different from patients without renal dysfunction. The mean ± SD clinical duration of 54 ± 22 minutes was not considered prolonged compared to 46 ± 12 minutes in normal patients; however, there was substantial variation (range, 22-90 minutes). The spontaneous recovery rate from 25 to 75% of control in renal dysfunction patients of 27 ± 11 minutes was similar to 28 ± 20 minutes in normal patients (see CLINICAL PHARMACOLOGY, Pharmacokinetics.)

Malignant Hyperthermia (MH): In an animal study in MH-susceptible swine, the administration of rocuronium bromide did not appear to trigger malignant hyperthermia. Rocuronium bromide has not been studied in MH-susceptible patients. Because rocuronium bromide is always used with other agents, and the occurrence of malignant hyperthermia during anesthesia is possible even in the absence of known triggering agents, clinicians should be familiar with early signs, confirmatory diagnosis and treatment of malignant hyperthermia prior to the start of any anesthetic.

Altered Circulation Time: Conditions associated with slower circulation time, e.g., cardiovascular disease or advanced age, may be associated with a delay in onset time. Because higher doses of rocuronium bromide produce a longer duration of action, the initial dosage should usually not be increased in these patients to reduce onset time; instead, when feasible, more time should be allowed for the drug to achieve onset of effect.

Inhalation Anesthetics: Use of inhalation anesthetics has been shown to enhance the activity of other neuromuscular blocking agents, enflurane > isoflurane > halothane.

Isoflurane and enflurane may also prolong the duration of action of initial and maintenance doses of rocuronium bromide injection and decrease the average infusion requirement of rocuronium bromide by 40% compared to opioid/nitrous oxide/oxygen anesthesia. No definite interaction between rocuronium bromide and halothane has been demonstrated. In one study, use of enflurane in 10 patients resulted in a 20% increase in mean clinical duration of the initial intubating dose, and a 37% increase in the duration of subsequent maintenance doses, when compared in the same study to 10 patients under opioid/nitrous oxide/oxygen anesthesia. The clinical duration of initial doses of rocuronium bromide of 0.57-0.85 mg/kg under enflurane or isoflurane anesthesia, as used clinically, was increased by 11% and 23% respectively. The duration of maintenance doses was affected to a greater extent, increasing by 30 to 50% under either enflurane or isoflurane anesthesia. Potentiation by these agents is also observed with respect to the infusion rates of rocuronium bromide required to maintain approximately 95% neuromuscular block. Under isoflurane and enflurane anesthesia, the infusion rates are decreased by approximately 40% compared to opioid/nitrous oxide/oxygen anesthesia. The median spontaneous recovery time (from 25 to 75% of control T_1) is not affected by halothane, but is prolonged by enflurane (15% longer) and isoflurane (62% longer). Reversal-induced recovery of rocuronium bromide neuromuscular block is minimally affected by anesthetic technique.

Intravenous Anesthetics: The use of propofol for induction and maintenance of anesthesia does not alter the clinical duration or recovery characteristics following recommended doses of rocuronium bromide injection.

Anticonvulsants: In 2 of 4 patients receiving chronic anticonvulsant therapy apparent resistance to the effects of rocuronium bromide injection was observed in the form of diminished magnitude of neuromuscular block, or shortened clinical duration. As with other nondepolarizing neuromuscular blocking drugs, if rocuronium bromide is administered to patients chronically receiving anticonvulsant agents such as carbamazepine or phenytoin, shorter durations of neuromuscular block may occur and infusion rates may be higher due to the development of resistance to nondepolarizing muscle relaxants. While the mechanism for development of this resistance is not known, receptor up-regulation may be a contributing factor (see Individualization Of Dosage).

Antibiotics: Drugs which may enhance the neuromuscular blocking action of nondepolarizing agents such as rocuronium bromide injection include certain antibiotics (*e.g.,* aminoglycosides; vancomycin; tetracyclines; bacitracin; polymyxins; colistin; and sodium colistimethate). If these antibiotics are used in conjunction with rocuronium bromide, prolongation of neuromuscular block should be considered a possibility.

Other: Experience concerning injection of quinidine during recovery from use of other muscle relaxants suggests that recurrent paralysis may occur. This possibility must also be considered for rocuronium bromide injection.

Rocuronium bromide -induced neuromuscular blockade was modified by alkalosis and acidosis in experimental pigs. Both respiratory and metabolic acidosis prolonged the recovery time. The potency of rocuronium bromide was significantly enhanced in metabolic acidosis and alkalosis, but was reduced in respiratory alkalosis. In addition, experience with other drugs has suggested that acute (*e.g.,* diarrhea) or chronic (*e.g.,* adrenocortical insufficiency)

PRECAUTIONS: *(cont'd)*

electrolyte imbalance may alter neuromuscular blockade. Since electrolyte imbalance and acid-base imbalance are usually mixed, either enhancement or inhibition may occur. Magnesium salts, administered for the management of toxemia of pregnancy, may enhance neuromuscular blockade.

A local tolerance study in rabbits demonstrated that rocuronium bromide was well tolerated following intravenous, intra-arterial and perivenous administration with only a slight irritation of surrounding tissues observed after perivenous administration. In humans, if extravasation occurs it may be associated with signs or symptoms of local irritation; the injection or infusion should be terminated immediately and restarted in another vein (see DOSAGE AND ADMINISTRATION.)

Drug/Laboratory Test Interactions: None known.

Carcinogenesis, Mutagenesis, Impairment of Fertility: Studies in animals have not been performed to evaluate carcinogenic potential or impairment of fertility. Mutagenicity studies (Ames test, analysis of chromosomal aberrations in mammalian cells, and micronucleus test) conducted with rocuronium bromide injection did not suggest mutagenic potential.

Pregnancy Category B: A teratogenicity study has been conducted in rats using intravenously administered doses of rocuronium bromide injection approximating the clinical dose in humans (0.3 mg/kg). No teratogenic effects were observed in this study. There are no adequate and well-controlled studies in pregnant women. Rocuronium bromide should be used during pregnancy only if the potential benefit justifies the potential risk to the fetus.

Pediatric Use: The use of rocuronium bromide injection in children less than 3 months of age has not been studied. See CLINICAL PHARMACOLOGY, Pharmacodynamics and DOSAGE AND ADMINISTRATION, Use in Pediatrics for clinical experience and recommendations for use in infants and children 3 months to 14 years of age.

DRUG INTERACTIONS:

The use of rocuronium bromide injection before succinylcholine, for the purpose of attenuating some of the side effects of succinylcholine, has not been studied.

If rocuronium bromide is administered following administration of succinylcholine, it should not be given until recovery from succinylcholine has been observed. The median duration of action of rocuronium bromide 0.6 mg/kg administered after a 1 mg/kg dose of succinylcholine when T_1 returned to 75% of control was 36 minutes (range 14-57, n=12) vs. 28 minutes (17-51, n=12) without succinylcholine.

There are no controlled studies documenting the use of rocuronium bromide before or after other nondepolarizing muscle relaxants. Interactions have been observed when other nondepolarizing muscle relaxants have been administered in succession.

ADVERSE REACTIONS:

Clinical studies in the U.S. (n=1,137) and Europe (n=1,394) totaled 2,531 patients. Prolonged neuromuscular block is associated with neuromuscular blockers as a class. Prolonged neuromuscular block (166 minutes) occurred after 0.6 mg/kg rocuronium bromide injection in an obese 67 year-old female with hepatic dysfunction who had received gentamicin before surgery. The patients exposed in the U.S. clinical studies provide the basis for calculation of adverse reaction rates. The following adverse experiences were reported in patients administered rocuronium bromide Injection (all events judged by investigators during the clinical trials to have a possible causal relationship.

Adverse experiences in greater than 1% of patients — NONE

Adverse experiences in less than 1% of patients Probably Related or Relationship Unknown:

Cardiovascular: arrhythmia, abnormal electrocardiogram, tachycardia

Digestive: nausea, vomiting

Respiratory: asthma (bronchospasm, wheezing, or rhonchi), hiccup

Skin and Appendages: rash, injection site edema, pruritus

In the European studies, the most commonly reported adverse experiences were transient hypotension (2%) and hypertension (2%); it is in greater frequency than the U.S. studies (0.1% and 0.1%). Changes in heart rate and blood pressure were defined differently from the U.S. studies in which changes in cardiovascular parameters were not considered as adverse events unless judged by the investigator as unexpected, clinically significant, or thought to be histamine related.

OVERDOSAGE:

No cases of significant accidental or intentional overdose with rocuronium bromide have been reported. Overdosage with neuromuscular blocking agents may result in neuromuscular block beyond the time needed for surgery and anesthesia. The primary treatment is maintenance of a patent airway and controlled ventilation until recovery of normal neuromuscular function is assured. Once evidence of recovery from neuromuscular block is observed, further recovery may be facilitated by administration of an anticholinesterase agent (*e.g.,* neostigmine, edrophonium) in conjunction with an appropriate anticholinergic agent (see Antagonism of Neuromuscular Blockade).

Antagonism of Neuromuscular Blockade ANTAGONISTS (SUCH AS NEOSTIGMINE) SHOULD NOT BE ADMINISTERED PRIOR TO THE DEMONSTRATION OF SOME SPONTANEOUS RECOVERY FROM NEUROMUSCULAR BLOCKADE. THE USE OF A NERVE STIMULATOR TO DOCUMENT RECOVERY AND ANTAGONISM OF NEUROMUSCULAR BLOCKADE IS RECOMMENDED.

Patients should be evaluated for adequate clinical evidence of antagonism, e.g., 5 sec head lift, adequate phonation, ventilation, and upper airway maintenance. Ventilation must be supported until no longer required.

Antagonism may be delayed in the presence of debilitation, carcinomatosis, and concomitant use of certain broad spectrum antibiotics, or anesthetic agents and other drugs which enhance neuromuscular blockade or separately cause respiratory depression. Under such circumstances the management is the same as that of prolonged neuromuscular blockade.

DOSAGE AND ADMINISTRATION:

Rocuronium bromide injection IS FOR INTRAVENOUS USE ONLY. THIS DRUG SHOULD BE ADMINISTERED BY OR UNDER THE SUPERVISION OF EXPERIENCED CLINICIANS FAMILIAR WITH THE USE OF NEUROMUSCULAR BLOCKING AGENTS. INDIVIDUALIZATION OF DOSAGE SHOULD BE CONSIDERED IN EACH CASE (see Individualization of Dosage).

The dosage information which follows is derived from studies based upon units of drug per unit of body weight. It is expressed in this section in units of mg/kg to assist the clinician in calculating individual patient dosage requirements relative to the product as supplied for clinical use. It is intended to serve as an initial guide to clinicians familiar with other neuromuscular blocking agents to acquire experience with rocuronium bromide. The monitoring of twitch response is recommended to evaluate recovery from rocuronium bromide and decrease the hazards of overdosage if additional doses are administered (seeCLINICAL PHARMACOLOGY, Pharmacodynamics and DOSAGE AND ADMINISTRATION, Maintenance Dosing).

It is recommended that clinicians administering neuromuscular blocking agents such as rocuronium bromide employ a peripheral nerve stimulator to monitor drug response, determine the need for additional relaxant and adequacy of spontaneous recovery or antagonism.

Rapid Sequence Intubation: In appropriately premedicated and adequately anesthetized patients, rocuronium bromide injection 0.6-1.2 mg/kg will provide excellent or good intubating conditions in most patients in less than 2 minutes (see CLINICAL STUDIES.)

Doses for Tracheal Intubation: The recommended initial dose regardless of anesthetic technique is 0.6 mg/kg. Neuromuscular block sufficient for intubation (≥ 80% block) is attained in a median (range) time of 1 (0.4-6) minute(s) and most patients have intubation completed within 2 minutes. Maximum blockade is achieved in most patients in less than 3 minutes. This dose may be expected to provide 31 (15-85) minutes of clinical relaxation under opioid/nitrous oxide/oxygen anesthesia. Under halothane, isoflurane, and enflurane anesthesia, some extension of the period of clinical relaxation should be expected (see PRECAUTIONS, Inhalation Anesthetics.)

A lower dose of rocuronium bromide injection (0.45 mg/kg) may be used. Neuromuscular block sufficient for intubation (≥ 80% block) is attained in a median (range) time of 1.3 (0.8-6.2) minute(s) and most patients have intubation completed within 2 minutes. Maximum blockade is achieved in most patients in less than 4 minutes. This dose may be expected to provide 22 (12-31) minutes of clinical relaxation under opioid/nitrous oxide/oxygen anesthesia. Patients receiving this low dose of 0.45 mg/kg who achieve less than 90% block (about 16% of these patients) may have a more rapid time to 25% recovery, 12-15 minutes.

Should there be a reason for the selection of a larger bolus dose in individual patients, initial doses of 0.9 or 1.2 mg/kg can be administered during surgery under opioid/nitrous oxide/oxygen anesthesia without adverse effects to the cardiovascular system. These doses will provide ≥ 80% block in most patients in less than 2 minutes, with maximum blockade occurring in most patients in less than 3 minutes. Doses of 0.9 and 1.2 mg/kg may be expected to provide 58 (27-111) and 67 (38- 160) minutes, respectively, of clinical relaxation under opioid/nitrous oxide/oxygen anesthesia.

Maintenance Dosing: Maintenance doses of 0.1, 0.15, and 0.2 mg/kg rocuronium bromide injection, administered at 25% recovery of control T_1 (defined as 3 twitches of train-of-four), provide a median (range) of 12 (2-31), 17 (6-50) and 24 (7-69) minutes of clinical duration under opioid/nitrous oxide/oxygen anesthesia (see CLINICAL PHARMACOLOGY, Pharmacodynamics.) In all cases, dosing should be guided based on the clinical duration following initial dose or prior maintenance dose and not administered until recovery of neuromuscular function is evident. A clinically insignificant cumulation of effect with repetitive maintenance dosing has been observed (see CLINICAL PHARMACOLOGY, Pharmacodynamics.)

Use by Continuous Infusion: Infusion at an initial rate of 0.01 to 0.012 mg/kg/min of rocuronium bromide injection should be initiated only after evidence of spontaneous recovery from an intubating dose. Due to rapid distribution (see CLINICAL PHARMACOLOGY, Pharmacodynamics) and the associated rapid spontaneous recovery, initiation of the infusion after substantial return of neuromuscular function (more than 10% of control T_1) may necessitate additional bolus doses to maintain adequate block for surgery.

Upon reaching the desired level of neuromuscular block, the infusion of rocuronium bromide must be individualized for each patient. The rate of administration should be adjusted according to the patient's twitch response as monitored with the use of a peripheral nerve stimulator. In clinical trials, infusion rates have ranged from 0.004 to 0.016 mg/kg/min.

Inhalation anesthetics, particularly enflurane and isoflurane may enhance the neuromuscular blocking action of nondepolarizing muscle relaxants. In the presence of steady-state concentrations of enflurane or isoflurane, it may be necessary to reduce the rate of infusion by 30 to 50%, at 45-60 minutes after the intubating dose.

Spontaneous recovery and reversal of neuromuscular blockade following discontinuation of rocuronium bromide infusion may be expected to proceed at rates comparable to that following comparable total dose administered by repetitive bolus injections (see CLINICAL PHARMACOLOGY, Pharmacodynamics.)

Infusion solutions of rocuronium bromide can be prepared by mixing rocuronium bromide with an appropriate infusion solution such as 5% glucose in water or Lactated Ringers (see Compatibility). Unused portions of infusion solutions should be discarded.

Infusion rates of rocuronium bromide can individualized for each patient using TABLE 8 and TABLE 9 as guidelines.

TABLE 8 Infusion Rates Using Rocuronium Bromide Injection (0.5 mg/ml)*

Patient Weight (kg)	(Lbs)	Drug Delivery Rate (mcg/kg/min) 4	5	6	7	8	9	10	12	14	16
		Infusion Delivery Rate (ml/hr)									
10	22	4.8	6.0	7.2	8.4	9.6	10.8	12.0	14.4	16.8	19.2
15	33	7.2	9.0	10.8	12.6	14.4	16.2	18.0	21.6	25.2	28.8
20	44	9.6	12.0	14.4	16.8	19.2	21.6	24.0	28.8	33.6	38.4
25	55	12.0	15.0	18.0	21.0	24.0	27.0	30.0	36.0	42.0	48.0
35	77	16.8	21.0	25.2	29.4	33.6	37.8	42.0	50.4	58.8	67.2
50	110	24.0	30.0	36.0	42.0	48.0	54.0	60.0	72.0	84.0	96.0
60	132	28.8	36.0	43.2	50.4	57.6	64.8	72.0	86.4	100.8	115.2
70	154	33.6	42.0	50.4	58.8	67.2	75.6	84.0	100.8	117.6	134.4
80	176	38.4	48.0	57.6	67.2	76.8	86.4	96.0	115.2	134.4	153.6
90	198	43.2	54.0	64.8	75.6	86.4	97.2	108.0	129.6	151.2	172.8
100	220	48.0	60.0	72.0	84.0	96.0	108.0	120.0	144.0	168.0	192.0

* 50 mg rocuronium bromide in 100 ml solution

Use in Pediatrics: Initial doses at 0.6 mg/kg in children under halothane anesthesia produce excellent to good intubating conditions within 1 minute. The median (range) time to maximum block was 1 (0.5-3.3) minute(s). This dose will provide a median (range) time of clinical relaxation of 41 (24-68) minutes in 3 months-1 year pediatric patients and 27 (17-41) minutes in 1-12 year-old children. Maintenance doses of 0.075-0.125 mg/kg, administered upon return of T_1 to 25% of control, provide clinical relaxation for 7-10 minutes.

Spontaneous recovery proceeds at approximately the same rate in pediatric patients (3 months-1 year) as in adults, but is more rapid in pediatric patients (1-12 years) than adults (see TABLE 2and TABLE 4 in CLINICAL PHARMACOLOGY, Pharmacodynamics). A continuous infusion of rocuronium bromide injection initiated at a rate of 0.012 mg/kg/min upon return of T_1 to 10% of control (one twitch present in the train-of-four), may also be used to maintain neuromuscular blockade in children. The infusion of rocuronium bromide must be individualized for each patient. The rate of administration should be adjusted

DOSAGE AND ADMINISTRATION: *(cont'd)*

according to the patient's twitch response as monitored with the use of a peripheral nerve stimulator. Spontaneous recovery and reversal of neuromuscular blockade following discontinuation of rocuronium bromide infusion may be expected to proceed at rates comparable to that following similar total exposure to single bolus doses (see CLINICAL PHARMACOLOGY, Pharmacodynamics.)

TABLE 9 Infusion Rates Using Rocuronium Bromide Injection (1 mg/ml)**

Patient Weight (kg)	(Lbs)	4	5	6	7	8	9	10	12	14	16
		Drug Delivery Rate (mcg/kg/min) / Infusion Delivery Rate (ml/hr)									
10	22	2.4	3.0	3.6	4.2	4.8	5.4	6.0	7.2	8.4	9.6
15	33	3.6	4.5	5.4	6.3	7.2	8.1	9.0	10.8	12.6	14.4
20	44	4.8	6.0	7.2	8.4	9.6	10.8	12.0	14.4	16.8	19.2
25	55	6.0	7.5	9.0	10.5	12.0	13.5	15.0	18.0	21.0	24.0
35	77	8.4	10.5	12.6	14.7	16.8	18.9	21.0	25.2	29.4	33.6
50	110	12.0	15.0	18.0	21.0	24.0	27.0	30.0	36.0	42.0	48.0
60	132	14.4	18.0	21.6	25.2	28.8	32.4	36.0	43.2	50.4	57.6
70	154	16.8	21.0	25.2	29.4	33.6	38.4	43.2	48.0	57.6	67.2
80	176	19.2	24.0	28.8	33.6	38.4	43.2	48.0	57.6	67.2	76.8
90	198	21.6	27.0	32.4	37.8	43.2	48.6	54.0	64.8	75.6	86.4
100	220	24.0	30.0	36.0	42.0	48.0	54.0	60.0	72.0	84.0	96.0

** 100 mg rocuronium bromide in 100 ml solution

Use in Obese Patients: An analysis across all U.S. controlled studies indicates that the pharmacodynamics of rocuronium bromide injection are not different between obese and non-obese patients when dosed based upon their actual body weight.

Use in Geriatrics: Geriatric patients ($\geq$ 65 years) exhibited a slightly prolonged median (range) clinical duration of 46 (22-73), 62 (49-75), and 94 (64-138) minutes under opioid/nitrous oxide/oxygen anesthesia following doses of 0.6, 0.9 and 1.2 mg/kg, respectively. Maintenance doses of 0.1 and 0.15 mg/kg rocuronium bromide injection, administered at 25% recovery of T_1, provide approximately 13 and 33 minutes of clinical duration under opioid/nitrous oxide/oxygen anesthesia. The median (range) rate of spontaneous recovery of T_1 from 25 to 75% in geriatric patients is 17 (7-56) minutes which is not different from that in other adults (see CLINICAL PHARMACOLOGY, Pharmacokineticsand Pharmacodynamics).

Compatibility: Rocuronium bromide injection is compatible in solution with: 0.9% NaCl solution; 5% glucose in water; 5% glucose in saline; Sterile water for injection; Lactated Ringers

Use within 24 hours of mixing with the above solutions.

Parenteral drug products should be inspected visually for particulate matter and clarity prior to administration whenever solution and container permit. Do not use solution if particulate matter is present.

Safety and Handling: There is no specific work exposure limit for rocuronium bromide injection. In case of eye contact, flush with water for at least 10 minutes.

HOW SUPPLIED:

Zemuron Injection is available in the following forms: Zemuron 5 ml vials containing 50 mg rocuronium bromide injection (10 mg/ml). Zemuron 10 ml multiple dose vials containing 100 mg rocuronium bromide injection (10 mg/ml)

Storage: Rocuronium bromide injection should be stored under refrigeration, 2 to 8°C (36 to 46°F). DO NOT FREEZE. Upon removal from refrigeration to room temperature storage conditions (25°C/77°F), use rocuronium bromide Injection within 30 days.

HOW SUPPLIED - EQUIVALENTS NOT AVAILABLE:

Injection, Solution - Intravenous - 10 mg/ml

5 ml x 10	$179.00	ZEMURON, Organon	00052-0450-15
10 ml x 10	$343.68	ZEMURON, Organon	00052-0450-16

ROPIVACAINE HYDROCHLORIDE *(003305)*

CATEGORIES: Anesthesia; Epidural; FDA Approved 1996 Sep; Injectable Anesthetics; Local Anesthetics; Pregnancy Category B; Spinal Anesthetics

BRAND NAMES: *Narop*; **Naropin**

(International brand names outside U.S. in italics)

DESCRIPTION:

Ropivacaine HCl is a member of the amino amide class of local anesthetics. Ropivacaine HCl injections are sterile, isotonic solutions that contain the enantiomerically pure drug substance, sodium chloride for isotonicity and Water for Injection. Sodium hydroxide and/or hydrochloric acid may be used for pH adjustment. These solutions are administered parenterally.

Ropivacaine HCl is chemically described as S-(-)-1-propyl-2',6'-pipecoloxylidide hydrochloride monohydrate. The drug substance is a white crystalline powder, with a chemical formula of $C_{17}H_{26}N_2O{\cdot}HCl{\cdot}H_2O$, molecular weight of 328.89. At 25°C ropivacaine HCl has a solubility of 53.8 mg/ml in water, a distribution ratio between n-octanol and phosphate buffer at pH 7.4 of 141 and a pKa of 8.07 in 0.1 M KCl solution. The pKa of ropivacaine is approximately the same as bupivacaine (8.1) and is similar to that of mepivacaine (7.7). However, ropivacaine has an intermediate degree of lipid solubility compared to bupivacaine and mepivacaine. Naropin is preservative free and is available in single dose containers in 2.0, 5.0, 7.5 and 10.0 mg/ml concentrations. The specific gravity of Naropin solutions range from 1.002 to 1.005 at 25°C.

CLINICAL PHARMACOLOGY:

MECHANISM OF ACTION

Ropivacaine is a member of the amino amide class of local anesthetics and is supplied as the pure S-(-)-enantiomer. Local anesthetics block the generation and the conduction of nerve impulses, presumably by increasing the threshold for electrical excitation in the nerve, by slowing the propagation of the nerve impulse, and by reducing the rate of rise of the action potential. In general, the progression of anesthesia is related to the diameter, myelination and conduction velocity of affected nerve fibers. Clinically, the order of loss of nerve function is as follows: (1) pain, (2) temperature, (3) touch, (4) proprioception, and (5) skeletal muscle tone.

PHARMACOKINETICS

Absorption: The systemic concentration of ropivacaine is dependent on the total dose and concentration of drug administered, the route of administration, the patient's hemodynamic/circulatory condition and the vascularity of the administration site.

CLINICAL PHARMACOLOGY: *(cont'd)*

From the epidural space, ropivacaine shows complete and biphasic absorption. The half-lives of the two phases, (mean $\pm$ SD) are 14 $\pm$ 7 minutes and 4.2 $\pm$ 0.9 hours respectively. The slow absorption is the rate limiting factor in the elimination of ropivacaine which explains why the terminal half-life is longer after epidural than after intravenous administration. Ropivacaine shows dose-proportionality up to the highest intravenous dose studied, 80 mg, corresponding to a mean $\pm$ SD peak plasma concentration of 1.9 $\pm$ 0.3 mcg/ml.

Distribution: After intravascular infusion, ropivacaine has a steady state volume of distribution of 41 $\pm$ 7 liters. Ropivacaine is 94% protein bound, mainly to α_1-acid glycoprotein. An increase in total plasma concentrations during continuous epidural infusion has been observed, related to a postoperative increase of α_1-acid glycoprotein. Variations in unbound (*i.e.*, pharmacologically active, concentrations have been less than in total plasma concentration). Ropivacaine readily crosses the placenta and equilibrium in regard to unbound concentration will be rapidly reached (see PRECAUTIONS, Labor and Delivery).

Metabolism: Ropivacaine is extensively metabolized in the liver, predominantly by aromatic hydroxylation mediated by cytochrome P4501A to 3-hydroxy ropivacaine. Approximately 37% of the total dose is excreted in the urine as both free and conjugated 3-hydroxy ropivacaine. Low concentrations of 3-hydroxy ropivacaine have been found in the plasma. Urinary excretion of the 4-hydroxy and both the 3-hydroxy and 4-hydroxy N-dealkylated metabolites accounts for less than 3% of dose. An additional metabolite, 2-hydroxy-methyl-ropivacaine, has been identified but not quantified in the urine. Both 3-hydroxy and 4-hydroxy ropivacaine have a local anesthetic activity in animal models less than that of ropivacaine. There is no evidence of *in vivo* racemization in urine of S-(-)-ropivacaine to R-(+)-ropivacaine.

Elimination: The kidney is the main excretory organ for most local anesthetic metabolites. In total, 86% of the ropivacaine dose is excreted in the urine after intravenous administration of which only 1% relates to unchanged drug. Ropivacaine has a mean $\pm$ SD total plasma clearance of 387 $\pm$ 107 ml/min, an unbound plasma clearance of 7.2 $\pm$ 1.6 L/min, and a renal clearance of 1 ml/min. The mean $\pm$ SD terminal half-life is 1.8 $\pm$ 0.7 hour after intravascular administration and 4.2 $\pm$ 1.0 hour after epidural administration (see CLINICAL PHARMACOLOGY, Absorption).

PHARMACODYNAMICS

Studies in humans have demonstrated that, unlike most other local anesthetics, the presence of epinephrine has no major effect on either the time of onset or the duration of action of ropivacaine. Likewise, addition of epinephrine to ropivacaine has no effect on limiting systemic absorption of ropivacaine.

Systemic absorption of local anesthetics can produce effects on the central nervous and cardiovascular systems. At blood concentrations achieved with therapeutic doses, changes in cardiac conduction, excitability, refractoriness, contractility, and peripheral vascular resistance are minimal. However, toxic blood concentrations depress cardiac conduction and excitability, which may lead to atrioventricular block, ventricular arrhythmias and to cardiac arrest, sometimes resulting in fatalities. In addition, myocardial contractility is depressed and peripheral vasodilation occurs, leading to decreased cardiac output and arterial blood pressure.

Following systemic absorption, local anesthetics can produce central nervous system stimulation, depression or both. Apparent central stimulation is usually manifested as restlessness, tremors and shivering, progressing to convulsions, followed by depression and coma, progressing ultimately to respiratory arrest. However, the local anesthetics have a primary depressant effect on the medulla and on higher centers. The depressed stage may occur without a prior excited stage.

In two clinical pharmacology studies (total n=24) ropivacaine and bupivacaine were infused (10 mg/min) in human volunteers until the appearance of CNS symptoms (*e.g.*, visual or hearing disturbances, perioral numbness, tingling and others). Similar symptoms were seen with both drugs. In one study, the mean $\pm$ SD maximum tolerated intravenous dose of ropivacaine infused (124 $\pm$ 38 mg) was significantly higher than that of bupivacaine (99 $\pm$ 30 mg) while in the other study the doses were not different (115 $\pm$ 29 mg of ropivacaine and 103 $\pm$ 30 mg of bupivacaine). In the latter study, the number of subjects reporting each symptom was similar for both drugs with the exception of muscle twitching which was reported by more subjects with bupivacaine than ropivacaine at comparable intravenous doses. At the end of the infusion, ropivacaine in both studies caused significantly less depression of cardiac conductivity (less QRS widening) than bupivacaine. Ropivacaine and bupivacaine caused evidence of depression of cardiac contractility, but there were no changes in cardiac output.

In nonclinical pharmacology studies comparing ropivacaine and bupivacaine in several animal species, the cardiac toxicity of ropivacaine was less than that of bupivacaine, although both were considerably more toxic than lidocaine. Arrhythmogenic and cardiodepressant effects were seen in animals at significantly higher doses of ropivacaine than bupivacaine. The incidence of successful resuscitation was not significantly different between the ropivacaine and bupivacaine groups.

CLINICAL STUDIES:

Ropivacaine was studied as a local anesthetic both for surgical anesthesia and for acute pain management (see DOSAGE AND ADMINISTRATION). The onset, depth and duration of sensory block are, in general, similar to bupivacaine. However, the depth and duration of motor block, in general, are less than that with bupivacaine.

Epidural Administration In Surgery: There were 25 clinical studies performed in 900 patients to evaluate ropivacaine HCl epidural injection for general surgery. Ropivacaine HCl was used in doses ranging from 75 to 250 mg. In doses of 100-200 mg, the median (lst-3rd quartile) onset time to achieve a T10 sensory block was 10 (5-13) minutes and the median (lst-3rd quartile) duration at the T10 level was 4 (3-5) hours (see DOSAGE AND ADMINISTRATION).

Higher doses produced a more profound block with a greater duration of effect.

Epidural Administration In Cesarean Section: There were 8 studies performed in 218 patients to evaluate ropivacaine HCl for cesarean section. 5 mg/ml (0.5%) ropivacaine HCl was used in doses up to 150 mg. Median onset measured at T6 ranged from 11 to 26 minutes. Median duration of sensory block at T6 ranged from 1.7 to 3.2 hour, and duration of motor block ranged from 1.4 to 2.9 hour. Ropivacaine HCl provided adequate muscle relaxation for surgery in all cases.

Epidural Administration In Labor And Delivery: There were 10 double-blind clinical studies performed to evaluate ropivacaine HCl versus bupivacaine for epidural block for management of labor pain (ropivacaine HCl, n=258; bupivacaine, n=231). When administered in doses up to 278 mg as intermittent injections or as a continuous infusion, ropivacaine HCl produced adequate pain relief.

A prospective meta-analysis on 6 of these studies provided detailed evaluation of the delivered newborns and showed no difference in clinical outcomes compared to bupivacaine. There were significantly fewer instrumental deliveries in mothers receiving ropivacaine as compared to bupivacaine.

CLINICAL STUDIES: *(cont'd)*

TABLE 1 Labor And Delivery Meta-Analysis: Mode Of Delivery

Delivery Mode	Naropin n=199		Bupivacaine n=188	
	n	%	n	%
Spontaneous Vertex	116	58	92	49
Vacuum Extractor	26	>27*	33	>40
Forceps	28		42	
Cesarean Section	29	15	21	11

* p=0.004 versus bupivacaine

Epidural Administration In Postoperative Pain Management: There were 8 clinical studies performed in 382 patients to evaluate ropivacaine HCl for postoperative pain management after upper and lower abdominal surgery and after orthopedic surgery. The studies utilized intravascular morphine via PCA as a rescue medication and as an efficacy variable. Epidural anesthesia with ropivacaine HCl was used intraoperatively for each of these procedures prior to initiation of postoperative ropivacaine HCl. The incidence and intensity of the motor block were dependent on the dose rate of ropivacaine HCl and the site of injection. Cumulative doses of up to 770 mg of ropivacaine were administered over 24 hours (intraoperative block plus postoperative continuous infusion). The overall quality of pain relief, as judged by the patients, in the ropivacaine groups was rated as good or excellent (73% to 100%). The frequency of motor block was greatest at 4 hours and decreased during the infusion period in all groups. At least 80% of patients in the upper and lower abdominal studies and 42% in the orthopedic studies had no motor block at the end of the 21-hour infusion period. Sensory block was also dose rate-dependent and a decrease in spread was observed during the infusion period. Clinical studies with 2 mg/ml (0.2%) ropivacaine HCl have demonstrated that infusion rates of 6-10 ml (12-20 mg) per hour provide adequate analgesia with only slight and non-progressive motor block in cases of moderate to severe postoperative pain. In these studies, this technique resulted in a significant reduction in patients' morphine rescue dose-requirement. Clinical experience supports the use of ropivacaine HCl epidural infusions for up to 24 hours.

Epidural infusion of ropivacaine HCl has, in some cases, been associated with transient increases in temperature to >38.5°C. This occurred more frequently at doses >16 mg/h.

Peripheral Nerve Block: Ropivacaine HCl, 5 mg/ml, (0.5%), was evaluated for its ability to provide anesthesia for surgery using the techniques of Peripheral Nerve Block. There were 13 studies performed including a series of 4 pharmacodynamic and pharmacokinetic studies performed on minor nerve blocks. From these, 235 ropivacaine HCl treated patients were evaluable for efficacy. Ropivacaine HCl was used in doses up to 275 mg. When used for brachial plexus block, onset depended on technique used. Supraclavicular blocks were consistently more successful than axillary blocks. The median onset of sensory block (anesthesia) produced by ropivacaine 0.5% via axillary block ranged from 10 minutes (medial brachial cutaneous nerve) to 45 minutes (musculocutaneous nerve). Median duration ranged from 3.7 hours (medial brachial cutaneous nerve) to 8.7 hours (ulnar nerve). The 5 mg/ml (0.5%) ropivacaine HCl solution gave success rates from 56% to 86% for axillary blocks, compared with 92% for supraclavicular blocks.

Local Infiltration: There were 7 clinical studies performed to evaluate the local infiltration of ropivacaine HCl to produce anesthesia for surgery and analgesia in postoperative pain management. In these studies, 297 patients who received ropivacaine HCl in doses up to 200 mg were evaluable for efficacy. With infiltration of 100-200 mg ropivacaine HCl, the time to first request for analgesic was 2-6 hours. When compared to placebo, ropivacaine HCl produced lower pain scores and a reduction of analgesic consumption.

INDICATIONS AND USAGE:

Ropivacaine HCl is indicated for the production of local or regional anesthesia for surgery, for postoperative pain management and for obstetrical procedures.

Surgical Anesthesia: epidural block for surgery including cesarean section; major nerve block; local infiltration.

Acute Pain Management: epidural continuous infusion or intermittent bolus (*e.g.*, postoperative or labor); local infiltration.

Standard current textbooks should be consulted to determine the accepted procedures and techniques for the administration of local anesthetic agents.

CONTRAINDICATIONS:

Ropivacaine HCl is contraindicated in patients with a known hypersensitivity to ropivacaine HCl or to any local anesthetic agent of the amide type.

WARNINGS:

FOR CESAREAN SECTION, THE 5 MG/ML (0.5%) ROPIVACAINE HCl SOLUTION IN DOSES UP TO 150 MG IS RECOMMENDED. AS WITH ALL LOCAL ANESTHETICS, ROPIVACAINE HCl SHOULD BE ADMINISTERED IN INCREMENTAL DOSES. SINCE ROPIVACAINE HCl SHOULD NOT BE INJECTED RAPIDLY IN LARGE DOSES, IT IS NOT RECOMMENDED FOR EMERGENCY SITUATIONS, WHERE A FAST ONSET OF SURGICAL ANESTHESIA IS NECESSARY. HISTORICALLY, PREGNANT PATIENTS WERE REPORTED TO HAVE A HIGH RISK FOR CARDIAC ARRHYTHMIAS, CARDIAC/CIRCULATORY ARREST AND DEATH WHEN BUPIVACAINE WAS INADVERTENTLY RAPIDLY INJECTED INTRAVENOUSLY.

LOCAL ANESTHETICS SHOULD ONLY BE EMPLOYED BY CLINICIANS WHO ARE WELL VERSED IN THE DIAGNOSIS AND MANAGEMENT OF DOSE RELATED TOXICITY AND OTHER ACUTE EMERGENCIES WHICH MIGHT ARISE FROM THE BLOCK TO BE EMPLOYED, AND THEN ONLY AFTER INSURING THE **IMMEDIATE (WITHOUT DELAY)** AVAILABILITY OF OXYGEN, OTHER RESUSCITATIVE DRUGS, CARDIOPULMONARY RESUSCITATIVE EQUIPMENT, AND THE PERSONNEL RESOURCES NEEDED FOR PROPER MANAGEMENT OF TOXIC REACTIONS AND RELATED EMERGENCIES (See ADVERSE REACTIONS AND PRECAUTIONS). DELAY IN PROPER MANAGEMENT OF DOSE RELATED TOXICITY, UNDERVENTILATION FROM ANY CAUSE AND/OR ALTERED SENSITIVITY MAY LEAD TO THE DEVELOPMENT OF ACIDOSIS, CARDIAC ARREST AND, POSSIBLY, DEATH.

SOLUTIONS OF ROPIVACAINE HCl SHOULD NOT BE USED FOR THE PRODUCTION OF OBSTETRICAL PARACERVICAL BLOCK ANESTHESIA, RETROBULBAR BLOCK OR SPINAL ANESTHESIA (SUBARACHNOID BLOCK) DUE TO INSUFFICIENT DATA TO SUPPORT SUCH USE. INTRAVENOUS REGIONAL ANESTHESIA (BIER BLOCK) SHOULD NOT BE PERFORMED DUE TO A LACK OF CLINICAL EXPERIENCE AND THE RISK OF ATTAINING TOXIC BLOOD LEVELS OF ROPIVACAINE HCl.

It is essential that aspiration for blood, or cerebrospinal fluid (where applicable), be done prior to injecting any local anesthetic, both the original dose and all subsequent doses, to avoid intravascular or subarachnoid injection. However, a negative aspiration does *not* ensure against an intravascular or subarachnoid injection.

WARNINGS: *(cont'd)*

A well-known risk of epidural anesthesia may be an unintentional subarachnoid injection of local anesthetic. Two clinical studies have been performed to verify the safety of ropivacaine HCl at a volume of 3 ml injected into the subarachnoid space since this dose represents an incremental epidural volume that could be unintentionally injected. The 15 and 22.5 mg doses injected resulted in sensory levels as high as T5 and T4, respectively. Sensory analgesia started in the sacral dermatomes in 2-3 minutes, extended to the T10 level in 10-13 minutes and lasted for approximately 2 hours. The results of these two clinical studies showed that a 3 ml dose did not produce any serious adverse events when spinal anesthesia blockade was achieved.

Ropivacaine HCl should be used with caution in patients receiving other local anesthetics or agents structurally related to amide-type local anesthetics, since the toxic effects of these drugs are additive.

PRECAUTIONS:

GENERAL

The safe and effective use of local anesthetics depends on proper dosage, correct technique, adequate precautions and readiness for emergencies. Resuscitative equipment, oxygen and other resuscitative drugs should be available for immediate use (see WARNINGS and ADVERSE REACTIONS). The lowest dosage that results in effective anesthesia should be used to avoid high plasma levels and serious adverse effects. Injections should be made slowly and incrementally, with frequent aspirations before and during the injection to avoid intravascular injection. When a continuous catheter technique is used, syringe aspirations should also be performed before and during each supplemental injection. During the administration of epidural anesthesia, it is recommended that a test dose of a local anesthetic with a fast onset be administered initially and that the patient be monitored for central nervous system and cardiovascular toxicity, as well as for signs of unintended intrathecal administration before proceeding. When clinical conditions permit, consideration should be given to employing local anesthetic solutions which contain epinephrine for the test dose because circulatory changes compatible with epinephrine may also serve as a warning sign of unintended intravascular injection. An intravascular injection is still possible even if aspirations for blood are negative. Administration of higher than recommended doses of ropivacaine HCl to achieve greater motor blockade or increased duration of sensory blockade may negate the advantages of ropivacaine HCl's favorable cardiovascular depression profile in the event that an inadvertent intravascular injection occurs.

Injection of repeated doses of local anesthetics may cause significant increases in plasma levels with each repeated dose due to slow accumulation of the drug or its metabolites or to slow metabolic degradation. Tolerance to elevated blood levels varies with the physical condition of the patient. Debilitated, elderly patients, and acutely ill patients and children should be given reduced doses commensurate with their age and physical condition. Local anesthetics should also be used with caution in patients with hypotension, hypovolemia or heart block.

Careful and constant monitoring of cardiovascular and respiratory vital signs (adequacy of ventilation) and the patient's state of consciousness should be performed after each local anesthetic injection. It should be kept in mind at such times that restlessness, anxiety, incoherent speech, light headedness, numbness and tingling of the mouth and lips, metallic taste, tinnitus, dizziness, blurred vision, tremors, twitching, depression, or drowsiness may be early warning signs of central nervous system toxicity.

Because amide-type local anesthetics such as ropivacaine HCl are metabolized by the liver, these drugs, especially repeat doses, should be used cautiously in patients with hepatic disease. Patients with severe hepatic disease, because of their inability to metabolize local anesthetics normally, are at a greater risk of developing toxic plasma concentrations. Local anesthetics should also be used with caution in patients with impaired cardiovascular function because they may be less able to compensate for functional changes associated with the prolongation of A-V conduction produced by these drugs.

Many drugs used during the conduct of anesthesia are considered potential triggering agents for malignant hyperthermia. Amide-type local anesthetics are not known to trigger this reaction. However, since the need for supplemental general anesthesia cannot be predicted in advance, it is suggested that a standard protocol for management should be available.

Epidural Anesthesia: During epidural administration, ropivacaine HCl should be administered in incremental doses of 3 to 5 ml with sufficient time between doses to detect toxic manifestations of unintentional intravascular or intrathecal injection. Syringe aspirations should also be performed before and during each supplemental injection in continuous (intermittent) catheter techniques. An intravascular injection is still possible even if aspirations for blood are negative. During the administration of epidural anesthesia, it is recommended that a test dose be administered initially and the effects monitored before the full dose is given. When clinical conditions permit, the test dose should contain epinephrine (10 to 15 mcg have been suggested) to serve as a warning of unintentional intravascular injection. If injected into a blood vessel, this amount of epinephrine is likely to produce a transient "epinephrine response" within 45 seconds, consisting of an increase in heart rate and systolic blood pressure, circumoral pallor, palpitations and nervousness in the unsedated patient. The sedated patient may exhibit only a pulse rate increase of 20 or more beats per minute for 15 or more seconds. Therefore, following the test dose, the heart should be continuously monitored for a heart rate increase. Patients on beta-blockers may not manifest changes in heart rate, but blood pressure monitoring can detect a rise in systolic blood pressure. A test dose of a short-acting amide anesthetic such as 30 to 40 mg of lidocaine is recommended to detect an unintentional intrathecal administration. This will be manifested within a few minutes by signs of spinal block (*e.g.*, decreased sensation of the buttocks, paresis of the legs, or, in the sedated patient, absent knee jerk). An intravascular or subarachnoid injection is still possible even if results of the test dose are negative. The test dose itself may produce a systemic toxic reaction, high spinal or epinephrine induced cardiovascular effects.

Use in Head and Neck Area: Small doses of local anesthetics injected into the head and neck area may produce adverse reactions similar to systemic toxicity seen with unintentional intravascular injections of larger doses. The injection procedures require the utmost care. Confusion, convulsions, respiratory depression, and/or respiratory arrest, and cardiovascular stimulation or depression have been reported. These reactions may be due to intraarterial injection of the local anesthetic with retrograde flow to the cerebral circulation. Patients receiving these blocks should have their circulation and respiration monitored and be constantly observed. Resuscitative equipment and personnel for treating adverse reactions should be immediately available. Dosage recommendations should not be exceeded (see DOSAGE AND ADMINISTRATION).

Use in Ophthalmic Surgery: The use of ropivacaine HCl in retrobulbar blocks for ophthalmic surgery has not been studied. Until appropriate experience is gained, the use of ropivacaine HCl for such surgery is not recommended.

PRECAUTIONS: *(cont'd)*

INFORMATION FOR THE PATIENT

When appropriate, patients should be informed in advance that they may experience temporary loss of sensation and motor activity in the anesthetized part of the body following proper administration of lumbar epidural anesthesia. Also, when appropriate, the physician should discuss other information including adverse reactions in the ropivacaine HCl package insert.

CARCINOGENESIS, MUTAGENESIS, AND IMPAIRMENT OF FERTILITY

Long term studies in animals of most local anesthetics, including ropivacaine HCl, to evaluate the carcinogenic potential have not been conducted.

Weak mutagenic activity was seen in the mouse lymphoma test. Mutagenicity was not noted in the other assays, demonstrating that the weak signs of *in vitro* activity in the mouse lymphoma test were not manifest under diverse *in vivo* conditions.

Studies performed with ropivacaine in rats did not demonstrate an effect on fertility or general reproductive performance over two generations.

PREGNANCY CATEGORY B

Teratogenicity studies in rats and rabbits did not show evidence of any adverse effects on organogenesis or early fetal development in rats or rabbits. The doses used were approximately equal to 5 and 2.5 times, respectively, the maximum recommended human dose (250 mg) based on body weight. There were no treatment related effects on late fetal development, parturition, lactation, neonatal viability or growth of the offspring in 2 perinatal and postnatal studies in rats, at dose levels up to approximately 5 times the maximum recommended human dose based on body weight. In another study with a higher dose, 23 mg/kg, an increased pup loss was seen during the first 3 days postpartum, which was considered secondary to impaired maternal care due to maternal toxicity.

There are no adequate and well-controlled studies in pregnant women of the effects of ropivacaine HCl on the developing fetus. Ropivacaine HCl should be used during pregnancy only if clearly needed. This does not preclude the use of ropivacaine HCl after fetal organogenesis is completed or for obstetrical anesthesia or analgesia (see Labor and Delivery).

LABOR AND DELIVERY

Local anesthetics, including ropivacaine HCl, rapidly cross the placenta, and when used for epidural block can cause varying degrees of maternal, fetal and neonatal toxicity (see CLINICAL PHARMACOLOGY, Pharmacokinetics). The incidence and degree of toxicity depend upon the procedure performed, the type and amount of drug used, and the technique of drug administration. Adverse reactions in the parturient, fetus and neonate involve alterations of the central nervous system, peripheral vascular tone and cardiac function.

Maternal hypotension has resulted from regional anesthesia with ropivacaine HCl for obstetrical pain relief. Local anesthetics produce vasodilation by blocking sympathetic nerves. Elevating the patient's legs and positioning her on her left side will help prevent decreases in blood pressure. The fetal heart rate also should be monitored continuously, and electronic fetal monitoring is highly advisable.

Epidural anesthesia has been reported to prolong the second stage of labor by removing the parturient's reflex urge to bear down or by interfering with motor function. Spontaneous vertex delivery occurred more frequently in patients receiving ropivacaine HCl than in those receiving bupivacaine.

NURSING MOTHERS

Some local anesthetic drugs are excreted in human milk and caution should be exercised when they are administered to a nursing woman. The excretion of ropivacaine or its metabolites in human milk has not been studied. Based on the milk/plasma concentration ratio in rats, the estimated daily dose to a pup will be about 4% of the dose given to the mother. Assuming that the milk/plasma concentration in humans is of the same order, the total ropivacaine HCl dose to which the baby is exposed by breast feeding is far lower than by exposure *in utero* in pregnant women at term (see PRECAUTIONS).

PEDIATRIC USE

No special studies were conducted in pediatrics. Until further experience is gained in children younger than 12 years, administration of ropivacaine HCl in this age group is not recommended.

DRUG INTERACTIONS:

Ropivacaine HCl should be used with caution in patients receiving other local anesthetics or agents structurally related to amide-type local anesthetics, since the toxic effects of these drugs are additive.

In vitro studies indicate that cytochrome P4501A is involved in the formation of 3-hydroxy ropivacaine, the major metabolite. Thus agents likely to be administered concomitantly with ropivacaine HCl, which are metabolized by this isozyme family may potentially interact with ropivacaine HCl. Such interaction might be a possibility with drugs known to be metabolized by P4501A2 via competitive inhibition such as theophylline, imipramine and with potent inhibitors such as fluvoxamine and verapamil.

ADVERSE REACTIONS:

Reactions to ropivacaine HCl are characteristic of those associated with other amide-type local anesthetics. A major cause of adverse reactions to this group of drugs may be associated with excessive plasma levels, which may be due to overdosage, unintentional intravascular injection or slow metabolic degradation.

The reported adverse events are derived from controlled clinical trials in the U.S. and other countries. The reference drug was usually bupivacaine. The studies were conducted using a variety of premedications, sedatives, and surgical procedures of varying length. Most adverse events reported were mild and transient, and may reflect the surgical procedures, patient characteristics (including disease) and/or medications administered.

Of the 3558 patients enrolled in the clinical trials, 2404 were exposed to ropivacaine HCl. Each patient was counted once for each type of adverse event.

Incidence >5%: Hypotension, fetal bradycardia, nausea, bradycardia, vomiting, paresthesia, and back pain.

Incidence 1-5%: Fever, headache, pain, postoperative complications, urinary retention, dizziness, pruritus, rigors, anemia, hypertension, tachycardia, anxiety, oliguria, hypoesthesia, chest pain, fetal disorders including tachycardia and fetal distress, and neonatal disorders including jaundice, tachypnea, fever, respiratory disorder and vomiting.

A comparison has been made between ropivacaine HCl and bupivacaine for events with a frequency of 1% or greater. TABLE 1A and TABLE 1B show adverse events (number and percentage) in patients exposed to similar doses in double-blind controlled clinical trials. In the trials, ropivacaine HCl was administered as an epidural anesthetic/analgesic for surgery, labor, or cesarean section. In addition, patients that received ropivacaine HCl for peripheral nerve block or local infiltration are included.

Incidence <1%: The following list includes all adverse and intercurrent events which were recorded in more than one patient, but occurred at an overall rate of less than one percent, and were considered clinically relevant.

ADVERSE REACTIONS: *(cont'd)*

TABLE 1A Adverse Events Reported In ≥1% Of Adult Patients Receiving Regional Or Local Anesthesia (Surgery, Labor, Cesarean Section, Peripheral Nerve Block And Local Infiltration)

Adverse Reaction	Ropivacaine HCl total N = 742 N	(%)	Bupivacaine total N = 737 N	(%)
hypotension	237	(31.9)	225	(30.5)
nausea	92	(12.4)	96	(13.0)
paresthesia	51	(6.9)	44	(6.0)
vomiting	48	(6.5)	38	(5.2)
back pain	36	(4.9)	47	(6.4)
pain	39	(5.3)	40	(5.4)
bradycardia	32	(4.3)	38	(5.2)
headache	23	(3.1)	26	(3.5)
fever	25	(3.4)	20	(2.7)
chills	16	(2.2)	14	(1.9)
dizziness	18	(2.4)	10	(1.4)
pruritus	16	(2.2)	11	(1.5)
urinary retention	10	(1.3)	12	(1.6)
hypoesthesia	8	(1.1)	10	(1.4)

TABLE 1B Adverse Events Reported In ≥1% Of Fetuses Or Neonates Of Mothers Who Received Regional Anesthesia (Cesarean Section And Labor Studies)

Adverse Reaction	Ropivacaine HCl total N = 337 N	(%)	Bupivacaine total N = 317 N	(%)
fetal bradycardia	58	(17.2)	53	(16.7)
neonatal jaundice	12	(3.6)	12	(3.8)
neonatal tachypnea	8	(2.4)	11	(3.5)
fetal tachycardia	7	(2.1)	8	(2.5)
neonatal fever	6	(1.8)	8	(2.5)
fetal distress	4	(1.2)	8	(2.5)
neonatal respiratory distress	5	(1.5)	4	(1.3)
neonatal vomiting	5	(1.5)	1	(0.3)

Application Site Reactions: injection site pain.

Cardiovascular System: vasovagal reaction, syncope, postural hypotension, non-specific ECG abnormalities.

Female Reproductive: poor progression of labor, uterine atony.

Gastrointestinal System: fecal incontinence, tenesmus.

General and Other Disorders: hypothermia, malaise, asthenia, accident and/or injury.

Hearing and Vestibular: tinnitus, hearing abnormalities.

Heart Rate and Rhythm: extrasystoles, non-specific arrhythmias, atrial fibrillation.

Liver and Biliary System: jaundice.

Metabolic Disorders: hypokalemia, hypomagnesemia

Musculoskeletal System: myalgia, cramps.

Myo/Endo/Pericardium: ST segment changes, myocardial infarction.

Nervous System: tremor, Horner's syndrome, paresis, dyskinesia, neuropathy, vertigo, coma, convulsion, hypokinesia, hypotonia, ptosis, stupor.

Psychiatric Disorders: agitation, confusion, somnolence, nervousness, amnesia, hallucination, emotional lability, insomnia, nightmares.

Respiratory System: dyspnea, bronchospasm, coughing.

Skin Disorders: rash, urticaria.

Urinary System Disorders: urinary incontinence, urinary tract infection, micturition disorder.

Vascular: deep vein thrombosis, phlebitis, pulmonary embolism.

Vision: vision abnormalities.

For the indication epidural anesthesia for surgery, the 15 most common adverse events were compared between different concentrations of ropivacaine HCl and bupivacaine. TABLE 2A and TABLE 2B are based on data from trials in the U.S. and other countries where ropivacaine HCl was administered as an epidural anesthetic for surgery.

TABLE 2A Common Events (Epidural Administration)

Adverse Reaction	Ropivacaine HCl					
	5 mg/ml total N=256		7.5 mg/ml total N=297		10 mg/ml total N=207	
	N	%	N	%	N	%
hypotension	99	(38.7)	146	(49.2)	113	(54.6)
nausea	34	(13.3)	68	(22.9)		
bradycardia	29	(11.3)	58	(19.5)	40	(19.3)
back pain	18	(7.0)	23	(7.7)	34	(16.4)
vomiting	18	(7.0)	33	(11.1)	23	(11.1)
headache	12	(4.7)	20	(6.7)	16	(7.7)
fever	8	(3.1)	5	(1.7)	18	(8.7)
chills	6	(2.3)	7	(2.4)	6	(2.9)
urinary retetntion	5	(2.0)	8	(2.7)	10	(4.8)
paresthesia	5	(2.0)	10	(3.4)	5	(2.4)
pruritus			14	(4.7)	3	(1.4)

TABLE 2B Common Events (Epidural Administration)

Adverse Reaction	Bupivacaine			
	5 mg/ml total N=236		7.5 mg/ml total N=174	
	N	(%)	N	(%)
hypotension	91	(38.6)	89	(51.1)
nausea	41	(17.4)	36	(20.7)
bradycardia	32	(13.6)	25	(14.4)
back pain	21	(8.9)	23	(13.2)
vomiting	19	(8.1)	14	(8.0)
headache	13	(5.5)	9	(5.2)
fever	11	(4.7)		
chills	4	(1.7)	3	(1.7)
urinary retention	10	(4.2)		
paresthesia	7	(3.0)		
pruritus			7	(4.0)

ADVERSE REACTIONS: *(cont'd)*

Using data from the same studies, the number (%) of patients experiencing hypotension is displayed by patient age, drug and concentration in TABLE 4A and TABLE 4B. In TABLE 3, the adverse events for ropivacaine HCl are broken down by gender.

TABLE 3 Most Common Adverse Events By Gender (Epidural Administration) Total N: Females = 405, Males = 355

Adverse Reaction	Female N	Female (%)	Male N	Male (%)
hypotension	220	(54.3)	138	(38.9)
nausea	119	(29.4)	23	(6.5)
bradycardia	65	(16.0)	56	(15.8)
vomiting	59	(14.6)	8	(2.3)
back pain	41	(10.1)	23	(6.5)
headache	33	(8.1)	17	(4.8)
chills	18	(4.4)	5	(1.4)
fever	16	(4.0)	3	(0.8)
pruritus	16	(4.0)	1	(0.3)
pain	12	(3.0)	4	(1.1)
urinary retention	11	(2.7)	7	(2.0)
dizziness	9	(2.2)	4	(1.1)
hypoesthesia	8	(2.0)	2	(0.6)
paresthesia	8	(2.0)	10	(2.8)

TABLE 4A Effects Of Age On Hypotension (Epidural Administration) Total N: Ropivacaine HCl, Bupivacaine = 410

AGE	Ropivacaine HCl 5 mg/ml N	(%)	7.5 mg/ml N	(%)	10 mg/ml N	(%)
<65	68	(32.2)	99	(43.2)	87	(51.5)
≥65	31	(68.9)	47	(69.1)	26	(68.4)

TABLE 4B Effects Of Age On Hypotension (Epidural Administration) Total N: Ropivacaine HCl, Bupivacaine = 410

AGE	Bupivacaine 5 mg/ml N	(%)	7.5 mg/ml N	(%)
<65	64	(33.5)	73	(48.3)
≥65	27	(60.0)	16	(69.6)

SYSTEMIC REACTIONS

The most commonly encountered acute adverse experiences that demand immediate countermeasures are related to the central nervous system and the cardiovascular system. These adverse experiences are generally dose-related and due to high plasma levels which may result from overdosage, rapid absorption from the injection site, diminished tolerance or from unintentional intravascular injection of the local anesthetic solution. In addition to systemic dose-related toxicity, unintentional subarachnoid injection of drug during the intended performance of lumbar epidural block or nerve blocks near the vertebral column (especially in the head and neck region) may result in underventilation or apnea ("Total or High Spinal"). Also, hypotension due to loss of sympathetic tone and respiratory paralysis or underventilation due to cephalad extension of the motor level of anesthesia may occur. This may lead to secondary cardiac arrest if untreated. Factors influencing plasma protein binding, such as acidosis, systemic diseases that alter protein production or competition with other drugs for protein binding sites, may diminish individual tolerance.

Central Nervous System Reactions: These are characterized by excitation and/or depression. Restlessness, anxiety, dizziness, tinnitus, blurred vision or tremors may occur, possibly proceeding to convulsions. However, excitement may be transient or absent, with depression being the first manifestation of an adverse reaction. This may quickly be followed by drowsiness merging into unconsciousness and respiratory arrest. Other central nervous system effects may be nausea, vomiting, chills, and constriction of the pupils.

The incidence of convulsions associated with the use of local anesthetics varies with the route of administration and the total dose administered. In a survey of studies of epidural anesthesia, overt toxicity progressing to convulsions occurred in approximately 0.1 percent of local anesthetic administrations.

Cardiovascular System Reactions: High doses or unintentional intravascular injection may lead to high plasma levels and related depression of the myocardium, decreased cardiac output, heart block, hypotension, bradycardia, ventricular arrhythmias, including ventricular tachycardia and ventricular fibrillation, and possibly cardiac arrest. (see WARNINGS, PRECAUTIONS, and OVERDOSAGE)

Allergic Reactions: Allergic type reactions are rare and may occur as a result of sensitivity to the local anesthetic (see WARNINGS). These reactions are characterized by signs such as urticaria, pruritus, erythema, angioneurotic edema (including laryngeal edema), tachycardia, sneezing, nausea, vomiting, dizziness, syncope, excessive sweating, elevated temperature, and possibly, anaphylactoid symptomatology (including severe hypotension). Cross sensitivity among members of the amide-type local anesthetic group has been reported. The usefulness of screening for sensitivity has not been definitively established.

Neurologic Reactions: The incidence of adverse neurologic reactions associated with the use of local anesthetics may be related to the total dose and concentration of local anesthetic administered and are also dependent upon the particular drug used, the route of administration and the physical status of the patient. Many of these observations may be related to local anesthetic techniques, with or without a contribution from the drug.

During lumbar epidural block, occasional unintentional penetration of the subarachnoid space by the catheter or needle may occur. Subsequent adverse effects may depend partially on the amount of drug administered intrathecally and the physiological and physical effects of a dural puncture. These observations may include spinal block of varying magnitude (including high or total spinal block), hypotension secondary to spinal block, urinary retention, loss of bladder and bowel control (fecal and urinary incontinence), and loss of perineal sensation and sexual function. Signs and symptoms of subarachnoid block typically start within 2-3 minutes of injection. Doses of 15 and 22.5 mg of ropivacaine HCl resulted in sensory levels as high as T5 and T4, respectively. Sensory analgesia started in the sacral dermatomes in 2-3 minutes and extended to the T10 level in 10-13 minutes and lasted for approximately 2 hours. Other neurological effects following unintentional subarachnoid administration during epidural anesthesia may include persistent anesthesia, paresthesia, weakness, paralysis of the lower extremities and loss of sphincter control, all of which may have slow, incomplete or no recovery. Headache, septic meningitis, meningismus, slowing of labor, increased incidence of forceps delivery, or cranial nerve palsies due to traction on nerves from loss of cerebrospinal fluid have been reported (see DOSAGE AND ADMINISTRATION, Lumbar Epidural Block). A high spinal is characterized by paralysis of the arms, loss of consciousness, respiratory paralysis and bradycardia.

OVERDOSAGE:

Acute emergencies from local anesthetics are generally related to high plasma levels encountered during therapeutic use of local anesthetics or to unintended subarachnoid or intravascular injection of local anesthetic solution. (see ADVERSE REACTIONS, WARNINGS, and PRECAUTIONS).

MANAGEMENT OF LOCAL ANESTHETIC EMERGENCIES

The practitioner should be familiar with standard contemporary textbooks that address the management of local anesthetic emergencies. No specific information is available on the treatment of overdosage with ropivacaine HCl; treatment should be symptomatic and supportive. Therapy with ropivacaine HCl should be discontinued.

The first consideration is prevention, best accomplished by incremental injection of ropivacaine HCl, careful and constant monitoring of cardiovascular and respiratory vital signs and the patient's state of consciousness after each local anesthetic injection and during continuous infusion. At the first sign of change, oxygen should be administered.

The first step in the management of systemic toxic reactions, as well as underventilation or apnea due to unintentional subarachnoid injection of drug solution, consists of immediate attention to the establishment and maintenance of a patent airway and effective assisted or controlled ventilation with 100% oxygen with a delivery system capable of permitting immediate positive airway pressure by mask. This may prevent convulsions if they have not already occurred.

If necessary, use drugs to control convulsions. Intravenous barbiturates, anticonvulsant agents, or muscle relaxants should only be administered by those familiar with their use. Immediately after the institution of these ventilatory measures, the adequacy of the circulation should be evaluated. Supportive treatment of circulatory depression may require administration of intravenous fluids, and, when appropriate, a vasopressor dictated by the clinical situation (such as ephedrine or epinephrine to enhance myocardial contractile force).

The mean dosages of ropivacaine producing seizures, after intravenous infusion in dogs, nonpregnant and pregnant sheep were 4.9, 6.1 and 5.9 mg/kg, respectively. These doses were associated with peak arterial total plasma concentrations of 11.4, 4.3 and 5.0 mcg/ml, respectively. In rats, the LD_{50} is 9.9 and 12 mg/kg by the intravenous route for males and females respectively.

In human volunteers given intravenous ropivacaine HCl, the mean maximum tolerated total and free arterial plasma concentrations were 4.3 and 0.6 mcg/ml respectively, at which time moderate CNS symptoms (muscle twitching) were noted.

Clinical data from patients experiencing local anesthetic induced convulsions demonstrated rapid development of hypoxia, hypercarbia and acidosis within a minute of the onset of convulsions. These observations suggest that oxygen consumption and carbon dioxide production are greatly increased during local anesthetic convulsions and emphasize the importance of immediate and effective ventilation with oxygen which may avoid cardiac arrest.

If difficulty is encountered in the maintenance of a patent airway or if prolonged ventilatory support (assisted or controlled) is indicated endotracheal intubation, employing drugs and techniques familiar to the clinician, may be indicated after initial administration of oxygen by mask.

The supine position is dangerous in pregnant women at term because of aorta-caval compression by the gravid uterus. Therefore, during treatment of systemic toxicity maternal hypotension or fetal bradycardia following regional block, the parturient should be maintained in the left lateral decubitus position if possible, or manual displacement of the uterus off the great vessels should be accomplished. Resuscitation of obstetrical patients may take longer than resuscitation of non-pregnant patients and closed-chest cardiac compression may be ineffective. Rapid delivery of the fetus may improve the response to resuscitative efforts.

DOSAGE AND ADMINISTRATION:

The rapid injection of a large volume of local anesthetic solution should be avoided and fractional (incremental) doses should always be used. The smallest dose and concentration required to produce the desired result should be administered.

The dose of any local anesthetic administered varies with the anesthetic procedure, the area to be anesthetized, the vascularity of the tissues, the number of neuronal segments to be blocked, the depth of anesthesia and degree of muscle relaxation required, the duration of anesthesia desired, individual tolerance, and the physical condition of the patient. Patients in poor general condition due to aging or other compromising factors such as partial or complete heart conduction block, advanced liver disease or severe renal dysfunction require special attention although regional anesthesia is frequently indicated in these patients. To reduce the risk of potentially serious adverse reactions, attempts should be made to optimize the patient's condition before major blocks are performed, and the dosage should be adjusted accordingly.

Use an adequate test dose (3-5 ml of a short acting local anesthetic solution containing epinephrine) prior to induction of complete block. This test dose should be repeated if the patient is moved in such a fashion as to have displaced the epidural catheter. Allow adequate time for onset of anesthesia following administration of each test dose.

Parenteral drug products should be inspected visually for particulate matter and discoloration prior to administration, whenever solution and container permit. Solutions which are discolored or which contain particulate matter should not be administered. For specific techniques and procedures, refer to standard contemporary textbooks.

The doses in the table are those considered to be necessary to produce a successful block and should be regarded as guidelines for use in adults. Individual variations in onset and duration occur. The figures reflect the expected average dose range needed. For other local anesthetic techniques standard current textbooks should be consulted.

When prolonged blocks are used, either through continuous infusion or through repeated bolus administration, the risks of reaching a toxic plasma concentration or inducing local neural injury must be considered. Experience to date indicates that a cumulative dose of up to 770 mg ropivacaine HCl administered over 24 hours is well tolerated in adults when used for postoperative pain management.

For treatment of postoperative pain, the following technique can be recommended: If regional anesthesia was not used intraoperatively, then an epidural block with ropivacaine HCl is induced via an epidural catheter. Analgesia is maintained with an infusion of ropivacaine HCl, 2 mg/ml (0.2%). Clinical studies have demonstrated that infusion rates of 6-10 ml (12-20 mg), per hour provide adequate analgesia with only slight and nonprogressive motor block. In cases of moderate to severe postoperative pain. If patients require additional pain relief higher infusion rates of up to 14 ml (28 mg) per hour may be used. With this technique a significant reduction in the need for opioids was demonstrated. Clinical experience supports the use of ropivacaine HCl epidural infusions for up to 24 hours.

TABLE 5 Dosage Recommendations

	Conc. mg/ml(%)	Volume ml	Dose mg	Onset min	Duration hours
Surgical Anesthesia					
Lumbar Epidural Administration	5.0 (0.5%)	15-30	75-150	15-30	2-4
	7.5 (0.75%)	15-25	113-188	10-20	3-5
Surgery	10.0 (1.0%)	15-20	150-200	10-20	4-6
Lumbar Epidural Administration	5.0 (0.5%)	20-30	100-150	15-25	2-4
Cesarean Section					
Thoracic Epidural Administration	5.0 (0.5%)	5-15	25-75	10-20	n/a*
To establish block for postoperative pain relief					
Major Nerve Block (*e.g.,* brachial plexus block)	5.0 (0.5%)	35-50	175-250	15-30	5-8
Field Block (*e.g.,* minor nerve blocks and infiltration)	5.0 (0.5%)	1-40	5-200	1-15	2-6
Labor Pain Management					
Lumbar Epidural Administration					
Initial Dose	2.0 (0.2%)	10-20	20-40	10-15	0.5-1.5
Continuous infusion‡	2.0 (0.2%)	6-14 ml/h	12-28 mg/h	n/a*	n/a*
Incremental injections (top-up)†	2.0 (0.2%)	10-15 ml/h	20-30 mg/h	n/a*	n/a*
Postoperative Pain Management					
Lumbar Epidural Administration					
Continuous infusion‡	2.0(0.2%)	6-10 ml/h	12-20 mg/h	n/a*	n/a*
Thoracic Epidural Adminstration					
Continuous infusion‡	2.0(0.2%)	4-8 ml/h	8-16 mg/h	n/a*	n/a*
Infiltration (*e.g.,* minor nerve block)	2.0 (0.2%)	1-100	2-200	1-5	2-6
	5.0 (0.5%)	1-40	5-200	1-5	2-6

*Not Applicable
†Median dose of 21 mg per hour was administered by continuous infusion or by incremental injections (top-ups) over a median delivery time of 5.5 hours.
‡Cumulative doses up to 770 mg of Naropin over 24 hours for postoperative pain management have been well tolerated in adults.

HOW SUPPLIED:

The solubility of ropivacaine is limited at pH above 6. Thus care must be taken as precipitation may occur if ropivacaine HCl is mixed with alkaline solutions. Disinfecting agents containing heavy metals, which cause release of respective ions (mercury, zinc, copper, etc.) should not be used for skin or mucous membrane disinfection since they have been related to incidents of swelling and edema.

When chemical disinfection of the container surface is desired, either isopropyl alcohol (91%) or ethyl alcohol (70%) is recommended. It is recommended that chemical disinfection be accomplished by wiping the ampule or vial stopper thoroughly with cotton or gauze that has been moistened with the recommended alcohol just prior to use. When a container is required to have a sterile outside, a Sterile-Pak should be chosen. Glass containers may, as an alternative, be autoclaved once. Stability has been demonstrated using a targeted F_0 of 7 minutes at 121°C.

Solutions should be stored at controlled room temperature 20° - 25°C (68° - 77°F).

These products are intended for single use and are free from preservatives. Any solution remaining from an opened container should be discarded promptly. In addition, continuous infusion bottles should not be left in place for more than 24 hours.

HOW SUPPLIED - EQUIVALENTS NOT AVAILABLE:

Injection - Epidural - 2 mg/ml

20 ml	$6.00	NAROPIN, Astra USA	00186-0859-51
100 ml	$18.38	NAROPIN, Astra USA	00186-0859-81
200 ml	$32.25	NAROPIN, Astra USA	00186-0859-91

Injection - Epidural - 5 mg/ml

30 ml	$11.88	NAROPIN, Astra USA	00186-0863-61

Injection - Epidural - 7.5 mg/ml

5 x 10 ml	$29.55	NAROPIN, Astra USA	00186-0867-41
20 ml	$11.88	NAROPIN, Astra USA	00186-0867-51

Injection - Epidural - 10 mg/ml

5 x 10 ml	$35.63	NAROPIN, Astra USA	00186-0868-41
20 ml	$13.13	NAROPIN, Astra USA	00186-0868-51

ROSE BENGAL *(002191)*

CATEGORIES: Diagnostic Agents; EENT Drugs; Eye, Ear, Nose, & Throat Preparations; Ophthalmics; Skin Cancer*; FDA Pre 1938 Drugs
* Indication not approved by the FDA

BRAND NAMES: Rosets

Prescribing information not available at time of publication.

HOW SUPPLIED - EQUIVALENTS NOT AVAILABLE:

Strip - Ophthalmic

100's	$19.56	Rose Bengal, Vision Pharms	00077-0929-99
100's	$19.56	Rosets, Smith & Nephew	57217-9521-01
100's	$25.00	ROSE BENGAL, Raway	00686-4003-03

RUBELLA VIRUS VACCINE LIVE *(002196)*

CATEGORIES: Immunologic; Rubella; Serums, Toxoids and Vaccines; Vaccines; Pregnancy Category C; FDA Pre 1938 Drugs

BRAND NAMES: *Cendevax*; *Ervevax* (England, Germany); *Gunevax*; **Meruvax II**; *Rubavax* (England); *Rubeaten*; *Rubeaten Berna*; *Rudivax*
(International brand names outside U.S. in italics)

FORMULARIES: WHO

DESCRIPTION:

Meruvax II (Rubella Virus Vaccine Live) is a live virus vaccine for immunization against rubella (German measles).

Meruvax II is a sterile lyophilized preparation of the Wistar Institute RA 27/3 strain of live attenuated rubella virus. The virus was adapted to and propagated in human diploid cell (WI-38) culture.[1-2]

The reconstituted vaccine is for subcutaneous administration. When reconstituted as directed, the dose for injection is 0.5 ml and contains not less than the equivalent of 1,000 $TCID_{50}$ (tissue culture infectious doses) of the U.S. Reference Rubella Virus. Each dose also contains approximately 25 mcg of neomycin. The product contains no preservative. Sorbitol and hydrolyzed gelatin are added as stabilizers.

CLINICAL PHARMACOLOGY:

Meruvax II produces a modified, non-communicable rubella infection in susceptible persons.

Extensive clinical trials of rubella virus vaccines, prepared using RA 27/3 strain rubella virus, have been carried out in more than 28,000 human subjects (approximately 11,000 with Meruvax II) in the U.S.A. and more than 20 additional countries. A single injection of the vaccine has been shown to induce rubella hemagglutination-inhibiting (HI) antibodies in 97% or more of susceptible persons. The RA 27/3 rubella strain elicits higher immediate post-vaccination HI, complement-fixing and neutralizing antibody levels than other strains of rubella vaccine[3-9] and has been shown to induce a broader profile of circulating antibodies including anti-theta and anti-iota precipitating antibodies.[10,11] The RA 27/3 rubella strain immunologically simulates natural infection more closely than other rubella vaccine viruses.[11-13] The increased levels and broader profile of antibodies produced by RA 27/3 strain rubella virus vaccine appear to correlate with greater resistance to subclinical reinfection with the wild virus,[11,13-15] and provide greater confidence for lasting immunity.

Vaccine-induced antibody levels have been shown to persist for at least 10 years without substantial decline.[16] If the present pattern continues, it will provide a basis for the expectation that immunity following vaccination will be permanent. However, continued surveillance will be required to demonstrate this point.

INDICATIONS AND USAGE:

(This section is based, in part, on the recommendation for rubella vaccine use of the Immunitazation Practices Advisory Committee (AICP), MMWR Report: 33 (22): 301-310, 315-318, June 8, 1984).

Children Between 12 Months of Age and Puberty: Meruvax II is indicated for immunization against rubella (German measles) in persons from 12 months of age to puberty. A booster is not needed. It is not recommended for infants younger than 12 months because they may retain maternal rubella neutralizing antibodies that may interfere with the immune response. Children in kindergarten and the first grades of elementary school deserve priority for vaccination because often they are epidemiologically the major source of virus dissemination in the community. A history of rubella illness is usually not reliable enough to exclude children from immunization.

Previously unimmunized children of susceptible pregnant women should receive live attenuated rubella vaccine, because an immunized child will be less likely to acquire natural rubella and introduce the virus into the household.

Adolescent and Adult Males: Vaccination of adolescent or adult males may be a useful procedure in preventing or controlling outbreaks of rubella in circumscribed population groups (*e.g.,* military bases and schools).

Non-Pregnant Adolescent and Adult Females: Immunization of susceptible non-pregnant adolescent and adult females of childbearing age with live attenuated rubella virus vaccine is indicated if certain precautions are observed (see PRECAUTIONS.) Vaccinating susceptible postpubertal females confers individual protection against subsequently acquiring rubella infection during pregnancy, which in turn prevents infection of the fetus and consequent congenital rubella injury.[17]

Women of childbearing age should be advised not to become pregnant for three months after vaccination and should be informed of the reason for this precaution.*

It is recommended that rubella susceptibility be determined by serologic testing prior to immunization.** If immune, as evidenced by a specific rubella antibody titer of 1:8 or greater (hemagglutination-inhibition test), vaccination is unnecessary. Congenital malformations do occur in up to seven percent of all live births.[18] Their chance appearance after vaccination could lead to misinterpretation of the cause, particularly if the prior rubella-immune status of vaccinees is unknown.

Postpubertal females should be informed of the frequent occurrence of generally self-limited arthralgia and/or arthritis beginning 2 to 4 weeks after vaccination (see ADVERSE REACTIONS.)

Postpartum Women: It has been found convenient in many instances to vaccinate rubella susceptible women in the immediate postpartum period (see Nursing Mothers.)

International Travelers: Individuals planning travel outside the United States, if not immune can acquire measles, mumps or rubella and import these diseases to the United States. Therefore, prior to International travel, individuals known to be susceptible to one or more of these diseases can receive either a single antigen vaccine (measles, mumps or rubella), or a combined antigen vaccine as appropriate. However, M-M-R II (Measles Mumps, and Rubella Virus Vaccine Live) is preferred for persons likely to be susceptible to mumps and rubella; and if single-antigen measles vaccine is not readily available, travelers should receive M-M-R II (Measles, Mumps, and Rubella Virus Vaccine Live) regardless of their immune status to mumps or rubella.[19,20,21]

Revaccination: Children vaccinated when younger than 12 months of age should be revaccinated. Based on available evidence, there is no reason to routinely revaccinate persons who were vaccinated originally when 12 months of age or older. However, persons should be revaccinated if there is evidence to suggest that initial immunization was ineffective.

Use with Other Vaccines: Routine administration of DTP (diphtheria, tetanus, pertussis) and/or OPV (oral poliovirus vaccine) concomitantly with measles, mumps and rubella vaccines is not recommended because there are insufficient data relating to the simultaneous administration of these antigens. However, the American Academy of Pediatrics has noted that in some circumstances, particularly when the patient may not return, some practitioners prefer to administer all these antigens on a single day. If done, separate sites and syringes should be used for DTP and Meruvax II.[22]

INDICATIONS AND USAGE: *(cont'd)*

Meruvax II should not be given less than one month before or after administration of other virus vaccines.

* NOTE: The Immunization Practices Advisory Committee (ACIP) has recommended "In view of the importance of protecting this age group against rubella, reasonable precautions in a rubella immunization program include asking females if they are pregnant, excluding those who say they are, and explaining the theoretical risks to the others."[17]

**NOTE: The Immunization Practices Advisory Committee (ACIP) has stated "When practical, and when reliable laboratory services are available, potential vaccinees of childbearing age can have serologic tests to determine susceptibility to rubella.... However, routinely performing serologic tests for all females of childbearing age to determine susceptibility so that vaccine is given only to proven susceptibles is expensive and has been ineffective in some areas. Accordingly, the ACIP believes that rubella vaccination of a woman who is not known to be pregnant and has no history of vaccination is justifiable without serologic testing."[17]

CONTRAINDICATIONS:

Do not give Meruvax II to pregnant females; the possible effects of the vaccine on fetal development are unknown at this time. If vaccination of postpubertal females is undertaken, pregnancy should be avoided for three months following vaccination. (See PRECAUTIONS, Pregnancy.)

Anaphylactic or anaphylactoid reactions to neomycin (each dose of reconstituted vaccine contains approximately 25 mcg of neomycin).

Any febrile respiratory illness or other active febrile infection.

Active untreated tuberculosis.

Patients receiving immunosuppressive therapy. This contraindication does not apply to patients who are receiving corticosteroids as replacement therapy, e.g., for Addison's disease.

Individuals with blood dyscrasias, leukemia, lymphomas of any type, or other malignant neoplasms affecting the bone marrow or lymphatic systems.

Primary and acquired immunodeficiency states, including patients who are immunosuppressed in association with AIDS or other clinical manifestations of infection with human immunodeficiency viruses;[23,24] cellular immune deficiencies; and hypogammaglobulinemic and dysgammaglobulinemic states.

Individuals with a family history of congenital or hereditary immunodeficiency, until the immune competence of the potential vaccine recipient is demonstrated.[25]

PRECAUTIONS:

GENERAL

Adequate treatment provisions including epinephrine, should be available for immediate use should an anaphylactic or anaphylactoid reaction occur.

Excretion of small amounts of the live attenuated rubella virus from the nose or throat has occurred in the majority of susceptible individuals 7-28 days after vaccination. There is no confirmed evidence to indicate that such virus is transmitted to susceptible persons who are in contact with the vaccinated individuals. Consequently, transmission through close personal contact, while accepted as a theoretical possibility, is not regarded as a significant risk.[17] However, transmission of the vaccine virus to infants via breast milk has been documented (see Nursing Mothers.)

There is no evidence that live rubella virus vaccine given after exposure to natural rubella virus will prevent illness. There is, however, no contraindication to vaccinating children already exposed to natural rubella.

Children and young adults who are known to be infected with human immunodeficiency viruses but without overt clinical manifestations of immunosuppression may be vaccinated; however, the vaccinees should be monitored closely for vaccine-preventable diseases because immunization may be less effective than for uninfected persons.[23,24]

Vaccination should be deferred for at least three months following blood or plasma transfusions, or administration of human immune serum globulin. However, susceptible postpartum patients who received blood products may receive Meruvax II prior to discharge provided that a repeat HI titer is drawn 6-8 weeks after vaccination to insure seroconversion. Similarly, although studies with other live rubella virus vaccines suggest that Meruvax II may be given in the immediate postpartum period to those non-immune women who have received anti-Rho (D) globulin (human) without interfering with vaccine effectiveness, a follow-up post-vaccination HI titer should also be determined.

It has been reported that attenuated rubella virus vaccine, live, may result in a temporary depression of tuberculin skin sensitivity. Therefore, if a tuberculin test is to be done, it should be administered either before or simultaneously with Meruvax II.

As for any vaccine, vaccination with Meruvax II may not result in seroconversion in 100% of susceptible persons given the vaccine.

PREGNANCY CATEGORY C

Animal reproduction studies have not been conducted with Meruvax II. It is also not known whether Meruvax II can cause fetal harm when administered to a pregnant woman or can affect reproduction capacity. There is evidence suggesting transmission of rubella vaccine viruses to products of conception.[26] Therefore, rubella vaccine should not be administered to pregnant females (see CONTRAINDICATIONS.)

In counseling women who are inadvertently vaccinated when pregnant or who become pregnant within 3 months of vaccination, the physician should be aware of the following: In a 10 year survey involving over 700 pregnant women who received rubella vaccine within 3 months before or after conception, (of whom 189 received the Wistar RA 27/3 strain) none of the newborns had abnormalities compatible with congenital rubella syndrome.[26]

NURSING MOTHERS

Recent studies have shown that lactating postpartum women immunized with live attenuated rubella vaccine may secrete the virus in breast milk and transmit it to breast-fed infants.[27] In the infants with serological evidence of rubella infection, none exhibited severe disease; however, one exhibited mild clinical illness typical of acquired rubella.[28,29] Caution should be exercised when Meruvax II is administered to a nursing woman.

ADVERSE REACTIONS:

Burning and/or stinging of short duration at the injection site have been reported.

Symptoms of the same kind as those seen following natural rubella may occur after vaccination. These include mild regional lymphadenopathy, urticaria, rash, malaise, sore throat, fever headache, dizziness, nausea, vomiting, diarrhea, polyneuritis, and a thralgia and/or arthritis (usually transient and rarely chronic). Local pain, wheal and flare, induration, and erythema may occur at the site injection. Reactions are usually mild and transient. Erythema multiforme has also been reported rarely.

Cough and rhinitis have also been reported.

Vasculitis has been reported rarely.

Anaphylaxis and anaphylactoid reactions have been reported.

ADVERSE REACTIONS: *(cont'd)*

Moderate fever (101 - 102.9°F (38.3 - 39.4°C)) occurs occasionally, and high fever (over 103°F (39.4°C)) occurs less commonly.

Syncope, particularly at the time of mass vaccination, has been reported.

Chronic arthritis has been associated with natural rubella infection and has been related to persistent virus and/or viral antigen isolate from body tissues. Only rarely have vaccine recipients developed chronic joint symptoms.

Following vaccination in children, reactions in joints are uncommon and generally of brief duration. In women, incidence rates for arthritis and arthralgia are generally higher than those seen in children (children: 0-3%; women: 12-20%)[30] and the reactions tend to be more marked and of longer duration. Symptoms may persist for a matter of months or on rare occasions for years. In adolescent girls, the reactions appear to be intermediate in incidence between those seen in children and in adult women. Even in older women (35 - 45 years), these reactions are generally well tolerated and rarely interfere with normal activities. Myalgia and paresthesia have been reported rarely after administration of Meruvax II.

Forms of optic neuritis, including retrobulbar neuritis and papillitis, may infrequently follow viral infections, and have been reported to occur 1 to 3 weeks following inoculation with some live virus vaccines.

Isolated reports of polyneuropathy including Guillain-Barre syndrome have been reported after immunization with rubella-containing vaccines.

Clinical experience with live rubella vaccines thus far indicates that encephalitis and other nervous system reactions have occurred very rarely in subjects who were given the vaccines, but a cause and effect relationship has not been established.

Thrombocytopenia with or without purpura has been reported.

DOSAGE AND ADMINISTRATION:

FOR SUBCUTANEOUS ADMINISTRATION

Do not inject intravenously

The dosage of vaccine is the same for all persons. Inject the total volume of the single dose vial (about 0.5 ml) or 0.5 ml of the multiple dose vial of reconstituted vaccine subcutaneously, preferably into the outer aspect of upper arm. **Do not give immune globulin (IG) concurrently with** Meruvax II.

To insure that there is no loss of potency during shipment, the vaccine must be maintained at a temperature of 10°C (50°F) or less.

Before reconstitution, store Meruvax II at 2 - 8°C (36 - 46°F). Protect from light.

CAUTION: A sterile syringe free of preservatives, antiseptics, and detergents should be used for each injection and/or reconstitution of the vaccine because these substances may inactivate the live virus vaccine. A 25 gauge, 5/8" needle is recommended.

To reconstitute, use only the diluent supplied, since it is free of preservatives or other antiviral substances which might inactivate the vaccine.

Single Dose Vial: First withdraw the entire volume of diluent into the syringe to be used for reconstitution. Inject all the diluent in the syringe into the vial of lyophilized vaccine, and agitate to mix thoroughly. Withdraw the entire contents into a syringe and inject the total volume of restored vaccine subcutaneously.

It is important to use a separate sterile syringe and needle for each individual patient to prevent transmission of hepatitis B and other infectious agents from one person to another.

10 Dose Vial (available only to government agencies/institutions): Withdraw the entire contents (7 ml) of the diluent vial into the sterile syringe to be used for reconstitution, and introduce into the 10 dose vial of lyophilized vaccine. Agitate to ensure thorough mixing. The outer labeling suggests "For Jet Injector or Syringe Use". Use with separate sterile syringes is permitted for containers of 10 doses or less. The vaccine and diluent do not contain preservatives; therefore, the user must recognize the potential contamination hazards and exercise special precautions to protect the sterility and potency of the product. The use of aseptic techniques and proper storage prior to and after restoration of the vaccine and subsequent withdrawal of the individual doses is essential. Use 0.5 ml of the reconstituted vaccine for subcutaneous injection.

It is important to use a separate sterile syringe and needle for each individual patient to prevent transmission of hepatitis B and other infectious agents from one person to another.

50 Dose Vial (available only to government agencies/institutions): Withdraw the entire contents (30 ml) of diluent vial into the sterile syringe to be used for reconstitution and introduce into the 50 dose vial of lyophilized vaccine. Agitate to ensure thorough mixing. With full aseptic precautions, attach the vial to the sterilized multidose jet injector apparatus. Use 0.5 ml of the reconstituted vaccine for subcutaneous injection.

Each dose contains not less than the equivalent of 1,000 $TCID_{50}$ of the U.S. Reference Rubella Virus.

Parenteral drug products should be inspected visually for particulate matter and discoloration prior to administration. Meruvax II, when reconstituted, is clear yellow.

STORAGE

It is recommended that the vaccine be used as soon as possible after reconstitution. Protect vaccine from light at all times, since such exposure may inactivate the virus. Store reconstituted vaccine in the vaccine vial in a dark place at 2 - 8°C (36 - 46°F) and discard if not used within 8 hours.

REFERENCES:

1. Plotkin, S. A.; Cornfeld, D.; Ingalls, T. H.: Studies of immunization with living rubella virus: Trials in children with a strain cultured from an aborted fetus, Am. J. Dis. Child. *110:*381-389, 1965. **2.** Plotkin, S. A.; Farquhar, J.; Katz, M.; Ingalls, T. H.: A new attenuated rubella virus grown in human fibroblasts: Evidence for reduced nasopharyngeal excretion, Am. J. Epidemiol. *86:*468-477, 1967. **3.** Fogel, A.; Moshkowitz, A.; Rannon, L.; Gerichter, Ch. B.: Comparative trials of RA 27/3 and Cendehill rubella vaccines in adult and adolescent females, Am. J. Epidemiol. *93:* 392-398, 1971. **4.** Andzhaparidze, O. G.; Desyatskova, R. G.; Chervonski, G. I.; Pryanichnikova, L. V.: Immunogenicity and reactogenicity of live attenuated rubella virus vaccines, Am. J. Epidemiol. *91:* 527-530, 1970. **5.** Freestone, D. S.; Reynolds, G. M.; McKinnon, J. A.; Prydie, J.: Vaccination of schoolgirls against rubella. Assessment of serological status and a comparative trial of Wistar RA 27/3 and Cendehill strain live attenuated rubella vaccines in 13-year-old schoolgirls in Dudley, Br. J. Prev. Soc. Med. *29:* 258-261, 1975. **6.** Grillner, L.; Hedstrom, C. E.; Bergstrom, H.; Forssman, L.; Rigner,A.; Lycke, E.: Vaccination against rubella of newly delivered women, Scand.J. Infect. Dis. *5:* 237-241, 1973. **7.** Grillner, L.: Neutralizing antibodies after rubella vaccination of newly delivered women: a comparison between three vaccines, Scand. J. Infect. Dis. *7:* 169-172, 1975. **8.** Wallace, R. B.; Isacson, P.: Comparative trial of HPV-77, DE-5 and RA 27/3 live-attenuated rubella vaccines, Am. J. Dis. Child. *124:*536-538, 1972. **9.** Lalla, M.; Vesikari, T.; Virolainen, M.: Lymphoblast proliferation and humoral antibody response after rubella vaccination, Clin. Exp. Immunol. *15:* 193-202, 1973. **10.** LeBouvier, G. L.; Plotkin, S. A.: Precipitin responses to rubella vaccine RA 27/3, J. Infect. Dis. *123:* 220-223, 1971. **11.** Horstmann, D. M.: Rubella: the challenge of its control, J. Infect. Dis. *123:* 640-654, 1971. **12.** Ogra, P. L.; Kerr-Grant, D.; Umana, G.; Dzierba, J.; Weintraub, D.: Antibody response in serum and nasopharynx after naturally acquired and vaccine-induced infection with rubella virus, N. Engl. J. Med. *285:* 1333-1339, 1971. **13.** Plotkin, S. A.; Farquhar, J. D.; Ogra, P. L.: Immunologic properties of RA 27/3 rubella virus vaccine, J. Am. Med. Assoc. *225:*585-590, 1973. **14.** Liebhaber, H.; Ingalls, T. H.; LeBouvier, G. L.; Horstmann, D. M.: Vaccination with RA 27/3 rubella vaccine. Persistence of immunity and resistance to challenge after two years, Am. J. Dis. Child. *123:*133-136, 1972. **15.** Farquhar, J. D.: Follow-up on rubella vaccinations and experience with subclinical reinfection, J. Pediatr. *81:*460-465, 1972. **16.** Hillary, I. B.; Griffith, A. H.: Persistence of antibody 10 years after vaccination with Wistar RA 27/3 strain live attenuated rubella vaccine. Br. Med. J. *280* (6231): 1580-1581, 1980. **17.** Recommendation of the Immunization Practices Advisory Committee (ACIP), Morbidity and Mortality Weekly Report *33* (22): 301-310, 315-318, June 8, 1984. **18.** McIntosh, R.; Merritt, K. K.; Richards, M. R.; Samuels, M. H.; Bellows, M. T.: The incidence of congenital malformations: A study of 5,964 pregnancies, Pediatrics *14:* 505-521, 1954. **19.** Recommendations of the Immunization Practices Advisory Committee (ACIP), Measles Prevention, MMWR *36* (26): 409-425, July 10, 1987. **20.** Jong, E. C., The Travel and Tropical Medicine Manual, W. B. Saunders Company, p. 12-16, 1987. **21.**

REFERENCES: *(cont'd)*

Committee on Immunization Council of Medical Societies, American College of Physicians, Phila., PA, Guide for Adult Immunization, First Edition, 1985. **22.** American Academy of Pediatrics: Report of the Committee on Infectious Disease, Evanston, Ill., 1982, p. 17. **23.** Center for Disease Control: Immunization of Children Infected with Human T-Lymphotropic Virus Type III/Lymphadenopathy-Associated Virus, Annals of Internal Medicine, *106:* 75-78, 1987. **24.** Krasinski, K.; Borkowsky, W.; Krugman, S.: Antibody following measles immunization in children infected with human T-cell lymphotropic virus-type III/lymphadenopathy associated virus (HTLV-III/LAV) (Abstract). In: Program and abstracts of the International Conference on Acquired Immunodeficiency Syndrome, Paris, France, June 23-25, 1986. **25.** Recommendation of the Immunization Practices Advisory Committee (ACIP), General Recommendations on Immunization, Morbidity and Mortality Weekly Report *32* (1): 13, January 14, 1983. **26.** Rubella vaccination during pregnancy — United States, 1971-1981, Morbidity and Mortality Weekly Report *31* (35): 477-481, September 10, 1982. **27.** Losonsky, G. A.; Fishaut, J. M.; Strussenberg, J.; Ogra, P. L.: Effect of immunization against rubella on lactation products. II. Maternal-neonatal interactions, J. Infect. Dis. *145:* 661-666, 1982. **28.** Landes, R. D.; Bass, J. W.; Millunchick, E. W.; Oetgen, W. J.: Neonatal rubella following postpartum maternal immunization, J. Pediatr.*97:* 465-467, 1980. (Letter) **29.** Lerman, S. J.: Neonatal rubella following postpartum maternal immunization, J. Pediatr. *98:* 668, 1981. (Letter) **30.** Unpublished data from the files of Merck Sharp & Dohme Research Laboratories.

HOW SUPPLIED - EQUIVALENTS NOT AVAILABLE:

Injection, Lyphl-Soln - Subcutaneous - 0.5 ml/vial

0.5 ml	$11.49	MERUVAX II, Merck	00006-4747-00

Injection, Lyphl-Soln - Subcutaneous - 1000 unit

0.5 ml x 10	$97.11	MERUVAX II, Merck	00006-4673-00

SALICYLIC ACID *(002203)*

CATEGORIES: Analgesics; Antiarthritics; Dermatologicals; Hyperkeratotic Skin Disorders; Keratolytic Agents; Keratosis Palmaris; Lesions; Pityriasis Rubra Pilaris; Psoriasis; Skin/Mucous Membrane Agents; Topical; Warts; Pregnancy Category C; FDA Pre 1938 Drugs

BRAND NAMES: *Acnisal*; *Aknederm N*; Duoplant; Formalyde-10 Spray; *Freezone*; Hydrisalic; **Keralyt**; Occlusal-Hp; Salacid; Trans-Plantar; Trans-Ver-Sal; Verrex; Viranol Gel
(International brand names outside U.S. in italics)

FORMULARIES: Aetna; WHO

DESCRIPTION:

Salicylic acid is a gel for topical administration containing 6% salicylic acid in a vehicle composed of propylene glycol, alcohol (19.4%), hydroxypropyl cellulose and water. Salicylic acid is the 2-hydroxy derivative of benzoic acid.

CLINICAL PHARMACOLOGY:

Salicylic acid has been shown to produce desquamation of the horny layer of skin while not effecting qualitative or quantitative changes in the structure of the viable epidermis.[1,2] The mechanism of action has been attributed to a dissolution of intercellular cement substance.[3] In a study of the percutaneous absorption of salicylic acid from Salicylic acid gel in four patients with extensive active psoriasis, Taylor and Halprin[4] showed that the peak serum salicylate levels never exceeded 5 mg/100 ml even though more than 60% of the applied salicylic acid was absorbed. Systemic toxic reactions are usually associated with much higher serum levels (30 to 40 mg/100 ml). Peak serum levels occurred within 5 hours of the topical application under occlusion. The sites were occluded for 10 hours over the entire body surface below the neck. Since salicylates are distributed in the extracellular space, patients with a contracted extracellular space due to dehydration or diuretics have higher salicylate levels than those with a normal extracellular space.[5] (See PRECAUTIONS.)

The major metabolites identified in the urine after topical administration are salicyluric acid (52%), salicylate glucuronides (42%) and free salicylic acid (6%)[4]. The urinary metabolites after percutaneous absorption differ from those after oral salicylate administration; those derived from percutaneous absorption contain more salicylate glucuronides and less salicyluric and salicylic acid. Almost 95% of a single dose of salicylate is excreted within 24 hours of its entrance into the extracellular space.[5]

Fifty to eighty percent of salicylate is protein bound to albumin. Salicylates compete with the binding of several drugs and can modify the action of these drugs; by similar competitive mechanisms other drugs can influence the serum levels of salicylate[5]. (See PRECAUTIONS.)

INDICATIONS AND USAGE:

For Dermatologic Use: Salicylic acid gel is a topical aid in the removal of excessive keratin in hyperkeratotic skin disorders, including verrucae, and the various ichthyoses (vulgaris, sex-linked and lamellar), keratosis palmaris and plantaris, keratosis pilaris, pityriasis rubra pilaris, psoriasis (including body, scalp, palms and soles).

For Podiatric Use: Salicylic acid gel is a topical aid in the removal of excessive keratin on dorsal and plantar hyperkeratotic lesions. Salicylic acid has been reported to be useful adjunctive therapy for verrucae plantares.

CONTRAINDICATIONS:

Salicylic acid should not be used in any patient known to be sensitive to salicylic acid or any other listed ingredients. Salicylic acid should not be used in children under 2 years of age.

WARNINGS:

Prolonged use over large areas, especially in children and those patients with significant renal or hepatic impairment, could result in salicylism. Concomitant use of other drugs which may contribute to elevated serum salicylate levels should be avoided where the potential for toxicity is present. In children under 12 years of age and those patients with renal or hepatic impairment, the area to be treated should be limited and the patient monitored closely for sings of salicylate toxicity: nausea, vomiting, dizziness, loss of hearing, tinnitus, lethargy, hyperpnea, diarrhea, psychic disturbances.

In the event of salicylic acid toxicity, the use of Salicylic acid gel should be discontinued. Fluids should be administered to promote urinary excretion. Treatment with sodium bicarbonate (oral or intravenous) should be instituted as appropriate.

PRECAUTIONS:

For external use only. Avoid contact with eyes and other mucous membranes.

PREGNANCY (CATEGORY C)

Salicylic acid has been shown to be teratogenic in rats and monkeys. It is difficult to extrapolate from oral doses of acetylsalicylic acid used in these studies to topical administration as the oral dose to monkeys may represent 6 times the maximum daily human dose of salicylic acid (as supplied in one tube, 28 g, of Salicylic acid) when applied topically over a large body surface. There are no adequate and well-controlled studies in pregnant women. Salicylic acid gel should be used during pregnancy only if the potential benefit justifies the potential risk to the fetus.

PRECAUTIONS: *(cont'd)*

NURSING MOTHERS

Because of the potential for serious adverse reactions in nursing infants from the mother's use of Salicylic acid gel, a decision should be made whether to discontinue nursing or to discontinue the drug, taking into account the importance of the drug to the mother.

CARCINOGENESIS, MUTAGENESIS, AND IMPAIRMENT OF FERTILITY

No data are available concerning potential carcinogenic or reproductive effects of Salicylic acid gel. It has been shown to lack mutagenic potential in the Ames Salmonella test.

DRUG INTERACTIONS:

(The following interactions are from a published review[5] and include reports concerning both oral and topical salicylate administration. The relationship of these interactions to the use of Salicylic acid gel is not known.)

1. Due to the competition of salicylate with other drugs for binding to serum albumin the following drug interactions may occur (TABLE 1):

TABLE 1

Drug	Description of Interaction
Tolbutamide	Hypoglycemia potentiated.
Methotrexate	Decreases tubular reabsorption; clinical toxicity from methotrexate can result.

II. Drugs changing salicylate levels by altering renal tubular reabsorption (TABLE 2):

TABLE 2

Drug	Description
Corticosteroids	Decreases plasma salicylate level; tapering doses of steroids may promote salicylism.
Ammonium Sulfate	Increases plasma salicylate level.

III. Drugs with Complicated Interactions with Salicylates (TABLE 3):

TABLE 3

Drug	Description
Heparin	Salicylate decreases platelet adhesiveness and interferes with hemostasis in heparin-treated patients.
Pyrazinamide	Inhibits pyrazinamide-induced hyperuricemia.
Uricosuric Agents	Effect of probenecid, sulfinpyrazone and phenylbutazone inhibited.

The following alterations of laboratory tests have been reported during salicylate therapy.[5] (TABLE 4):

TABLE 4

Laboratory Tests	Effect of Salicylates
Thyroid Function	Decreased PBI; increased T_3 uptake.
Urinary Sugar	False negative with glucose oxidase; false positive with clinitest with high-dose salicylate therapy (2.5g q.d.).
5-Hydroxyindole acetic acid	False negative with fluorometric test.
Acetone, ketone bodies red	False positive $FeCl_3$ in Gerhardt reaction; color persists with boiling.
17-OH corticosteroids	False reduced values with > 4.8g q.d. salicylate.
Vanilmandelic acid	False reduced values.
Uric Acid	May increase or decrease depending on dose.
Prothrombin	Decreased levels; slightly increased prothrombin time.

ADVERSE REACTIONS:

Excessive erythema and scaling conceivably could result from use on open skin lesions.

OVERDOSAGE:

See WARNINGS.

DOSAGE AND ADMINISTRATION:

The preferable method of use is to apply Salicylic acid gel thoroughly to the affected area and occlude the area at night. Preferably, the skin should be hydrated for at least five minutes prior to application. The medication is washed off in the morning and if excessive drying and/or irritation is observed a bland cream or lotion may be applied. Once clearing is apparent, the occasional use of Salicylic acid gel will usually maintain the remission. In those areas where occlusion is difficult or impossible, application may be made more frequently; hydration by wet packs or baths prior to application apparently enhances the effect. Unless hands are being treated, hands should be rinsed thoroughly after application.

REFERENCES:

1. Davies, M Marks *R: Br J Dermatol*95: 187-192, 1976. **2.** Marks R., Davies M, Cattel *A: J Invest Dermatol* 64: 283, 1975. **3.** Huber C. Christophers *E: Arch Derm Res* 257: 293-297, 1977. **4.** Taylor JR, Halprin KM: *Arch Dermatol*III: 740-743, 1975. **5.** Goldsmith LA: *Int J Dermatol*18: 32-36. **6.** Wilson JG, Ritter EJ, Scott WJ, *Fradlein R: Tox Appl Pharmacol*41: 67-78, 1977.

HOW SUPPLIED - EQUIVALENTS NOT AVAILABLE:

Gel - Topical - 6 %

1 oz	**$15.56**	**KERALYT, Westwood Squibb**	**00072-6500-01**

Gel - Topical - 27 %

15 gm	$11.19	DUOPLANT, Stiefel Labs	00145-6790-05

Plaster, Adhesive - Topical - 50 %

8 strips	$3.25	SAL-ACID PLASTER, Pedinol Pharma	00884-4387-08

Solution - Topical - 17 %

10 ml	$13.92	OCCLUSAL-HP, Genderm	52761-0185-10
13.5 ml	$5.00	Maximum Strength Wart Remover, Stiefel Labs	00145-2701-45
13.5 ml	$5.00	Maximum Strength Wart Remover, Glades Pharms	59366-2701-05

SALICYLIC ACID; SODIUM THIOSULFATE

(002208)

CATEGORIES: Anti-Infectives; Antifungals; Dermatologicals; Skin/Mucous Membrane Agents; FDA Pre 1938 Drugs

BRAND NAMES: **Tinver**; Versiclear

Prescribing information not available at time of publication.

HOW SUPPLIED - EQUIVALENTS NOT AVAILABLE:

Lotion - Topical

120 ml	$16.86	VERSICLEAR, Hope Pharms	60267-0531-04
120 ml	**$17.81**	**TINVER, Vision Pharms**	**00077-0790-04**

SALMETEROL XINAFOATE *(003156)*

CATEGORIES: Airway Obstruction; Anti-Inflammatory Agents; Antiasthmatics/Bronchodilators; Asthma; Autonomic Drugs; Beta Adrenergic Stimulators; Bronchial Dilators; Bronchospasm; Respiratory & Allergy Medications; Sympathomimetic Agents; Sympathomimetics, Beta Agonist; FDA Class 1P ("Priority Review"); Sales > $100 Million; FDA Approved 1994 Feb; Top 200 Drugs

BRAND NAMES: *Salmeter*; **Serevent**; *Serevent Inhaler and Disks*; *Serobid*; Servent
(International brand names outside U.S. in italics)

FORMULARIES: Aetna; BC-BS; United; PCS

DESCRIPTION:

Salmeterol xinafoate is the racemic form of the 1-hydroxy-2-naphthoic acid salt of salmeterol. The active component of the formulation is salmeterol base, a highly selective beta$_2$-adrenergic bronchodilator. The chemical name of salmeterol xinafoate is 4-hydroxy-α^1-[[[6-(4- phenylbutoxy) hexyl] amino] methyl]-1,3-benzenedimethanol, 1-hydroxy-2- naphthalenecarboxylate.

The molecular weight of salmeterol xinafoate is 603.8, and the empirical formula is $C_{25}H_{37}NO_4 \cdot C_{11}H_8O_3$. Salmeterol xinafoate is a white to off-white powder. It is freely soluble in methanol; slightly soluble in ethanol, chloroform, and isopropanol; and sparingly soluble in water.

Serevent Inhalation Aerosol is a pressurized, metered-dose aerosol unit for oral inhalation. It contains a microcrystalline suspension of salmeterol xinafoate in a mixture of two chlorofluorocarbon propellants (trichlorofluoromethane and dichlorodifluoromethane) with lecithin. 36.25 mcg of salmeterol xinafoate is equivalent to 25 mcg of salmeterol base. Each actuation delivers 25 mcg of salmeterol base (as salmeterol xinafoate) from the valve and 21 mcg of salmeterol base (as salmeterol xinafoate) from the actuator.

CLINICAL PHARMACOLOGY:

Mechanism of Action: Salmeterol is a long-acting beta-adrenergic agonist. *In vitro* studies and *in vivo* pharmacologic studies demonstrate that salmeterol is selective for beta$_2$- adrenoceptors compared with isoproterenol, which has approximately equal agonist activity on beta$_1$- and beta$_2$-adrenoceptors.*In vitro* studies show salmeterol to be at least 50 times more selective for beta$_2$-adrenoceptors than albuterol. Although beta$_2$-adrenoceptors are the predominant adrenergic receptors in bronchial smooth muscle and beta$_1$-adrenoceptors are the predominant receptors in the heart, there are also beta$_2$- adrenoceptors in the human heart comprising 10% to 50% of the total beta- adrenoceptors. The precise function of these is not yet established, but they raise the possibility that even highly selective beta$_2$- agonists may have cardiac effects.

The pharmacologic effects of beta$_2$-adrenoceptor agonist drugs, including salmeterol, are at least in part attributable to stimulation of intracellular adenyl cyclase, the enzyme that catalyzes the conversion of adenosine triphosphate (ATP) to cyclic -3',5'-adenosine monophosphate (cyclic AMP). Increased cyclic AMP levels cause relaxation of bronchial smooth muscle and inhibition of release of mediators of immediate hypersensitivity from cells, especially from mast cells.

In vitro tests show that salmeterol is a potent and long-lasting inhibitor of the release of mast cell mediators, such as histamine, leukotrienes, and prostaglandin $D_2$from human lung. Salmeterol inhibits histamine-induced plasma protein extravasation and inhibits platelet activating factor-induced eosinophil accumulation in the lungs of guinea pigs when administered by the inhaled route. In humans, salmeterol inhibits both the early- and late-phase responses to inhaled allergens, the latter persisting for over 30 hours after a single dose when the bronchodilator effect is no longer evident. Single doses of salmeterol also attenuate allergen-induced bronchial hyper- responsiveness.

Pharmacokinetics: Salmeterol acts locally in the lung; plasma levels therefore do not predict therapeutic effect. Because of the low therapeutic dose, systemic levels of salmeterol are low or undetectable after inhalation of recommended doses (42 mcg twice daily). Following chronic administration of an inhaled dose of 42 mcg twice daily, salmeterol was detected in plasma within 5 to 10 minutes in six asthmatic patients; plasma concentrations were very low, with peak concentrations of 150 pg/ml and no accumulation with repeated doses. Larger inhaled doses gave approximately proportionally increased blood levels. In these patients, a second peak concentration of 115 pg/ml occurred at about 45 minutes, probably due to absorption of the swallowed portion of the dose (most of the dose delivered by a metered-dose inhaler is swallowed). Oral administration of 1 mg of radiolabeled salmeterol (as salmeterol xinafoate) to two healthy subjects gave peak plasma salmeterol concentrations of about 650 pg/ml at about 45 minutes; the terminal elimination half-life was about 5.5 hours (one volunteer only).

Salmeterol xinafoate, an ionic salt, dissociates in solution so that the salmeterol and 1-hydroxy-2-naphthoic acid (xinafoate) moieties are absorbed, distributed, metabolized, and excreted independently. Salmeterol base is extensively metabolized by hydroxylation, with subsequent elimination predominantly in the feces. In the two subjects discussed above, approximately 25% and 60% of orally administered radioactivity was eliminated in urine and feces, respectively, over a period of 7 days. No significant amount of unchanged salmeterol base was detected in either urine or feces.

Salmeterol is 94% to 98% bound to human plasma proteins *in vitro* over the concentration range of 8 to 7,722 ng of base per milliliter, much higher concentrations than those achieved following therapeutic doses of salmeterol.

The xinafoate moiety has no apparent pharmacologic activity, is highly protein bound (>99%), and has a long elimination half-life of 11 days.

The pharmacokinetics of salmeterol base have not been studied in elderly patients nor in patients with hepatic or renal impairment. Since salmeterol is predominantly cleared by hepatic metabolism, liver function impairment may lead to accumulation of salmeterol in plasma. Therefore, patients with hepatic disease should be closely monitored.

CLINICAL PHARMACOLOGY: *(cont'd)*

Pharmacodynamics: Inhaled salmeterol, like other beta-adrenergic agonist drugs, can in some patients produce cardiovascular effects (see PRECAUTIONS). The cardiovascular effects (heart rate, blood pressure) associated with salmeterol administration occur with similar frequency, and are of similar type and severity, as those noted following albuterol administration.

The effects of rising inhaled doses of salmeterol and standard inhaled doses of albuterol were studied in volunteers and in patients with asthma. Salmeterol doses up to 84 mcg resulted in heart rate increases of 3 to 16 beats/minute, about the same as albuterol (4 to 10 beats/minute). In two double-blind studies, patients receiving ether salmeterol (n=81) or albuterol (n=80) underwent continuous electrocardiographic monitoring during four 24-hour periods; no clinically significant dysrhythmias were noted.

Beta-agonists and methylxanthines administered concurrently in laboratory animals (minipigs, rodents, and dogs) cause cardiac arrhythmias and sudden death (with histologic evidence of myocardial necrosis). Whether these findings are relevant to humans is not known.

CLINICAL STUDIES:

In placebo- and albuterol-controlled, single-dose clinical trials with salmeterol xinafoate, the time to onset of effective bronchodilatation (> 15% improvement in forced expiratory volume in 1 second [FEV_1]) was 10 to 20 minutes after a 42-mcg dose. Maximum improvement in FEV_1generally occurred within 180 minutes, and clinically significant improvement continued for 12 hours in most patients.

In two large, randomized, double-blind studies, salmeterol xinafoate was compared with albuterol and placebo in patients with mild-to- moderate asthma, including both patients who did and who did not receive concomitant inhaled corticosteroids. The efficacy of salmeterol xinafoate was demonstrated over the 12-week period with no change in effectiveness over this period of time. There were no gender-related differences in safety or efficacy. No development of tachyphylaxis to the bronchodilator effect has been noted in these studies. FEV_1measurements (percent of predicted) from these two 12-week studies are shown in the graph in the original package insert for both the first and last treatment days.

During daily treatment with salmeterol xinafoate for 12 weeks in patients with asthma, the following treatment effects were seen (TABLE 1):

TABLE 1 Two Large 12-Week Clinical Trials: Efficacy Parameters Multicenter Study 1

Parameter	Time	Placebo	Serevent	Albuterol
Mean AM PEFR (L/min)	baseline	410	420	404
	12 weeks	409	443*	395
Mean % days with no symptoms	baseline	12	15	15
	12 weeks	17	35*	27
Mean % nights with no awakenings	baseline	71	77	70
	12 weeks	79	89†	75
Rescue medications (mean no. of inhalations per day)	baseline	3.9	3.8	4.0
	12 weeks	2.9	1.2‡	1.9
Asthma exacerbations		53%	16%	31%

* Statistically superior to placebo (p=0.002).
† Statistically superior to placebo (p=0.008).
‡ Statistically superior to placebo (p=0.001).

TABLE 2 Two Large 12-Week Clinical Trials: Efficacy Parameters Multicenter Study 2

Parameter	Time	Placebo	Serevent	Albuterol
Mean AM PEFR (L/min)	baseline	409	406	390
	12 weeks	412	451*	388
Mean % days with no symptoms	baseline	11	8	14
	12 weeks	17	36*	21
Mean % nights with no awakenings	baseline	64	59	62
	12 weeks	70	85*	74
Rescue medications (mean no. of inhalations per day)	baseline	4.7	4.3	4.0
	12 weeks	3.6	1.4*	1.8
Asthma exacerbations		57%	17%	26%

* Statistically superior to placebo (p<0.001).

Safe usage with maintenance of efficacy for periods up to 1 year has been documented.

Protection against exercise-induced bronchospasm was examined in three controlled studies. Based on median values, patients who received salmeterol xinafoate had consistently less exercise-induced fall in FEV_1than patients who received placebo, and they were protected for a longer period of time than patients who received albuterol (see TABLE 3). There were, however, some patients who were not protected from exercise-induced bronchospasm after Serevent administration and others in whom protection against exercise-induced bronchospasm decreased with continued administration over a period of 4 weeks.

TABLE 3 Exercise-Induced Bronchospasm Mean Percentage Fall in Postexercise FEV_1

Clinical Trials/Time After Dose	Placebo	Treatment Serevent	Albuterol
Study A: 1st Dose			
6 hours	37	9*	
12 hours	27	16*	
Study A: 4th Week			
6 hours	30	19	
12 hours	24	12	
Study B:			
1 hour	37	0*	2*
6 hours	37	5*†	27
12 hours	34	6*†	33
Study C:			
0.5 hour	43	16*	8*
2.5 hours	33	12*†	30
4.5 hours	-	12†	36
6.0 hours	-	19†	41

* Statistically superior to placebo (p≤0.05).
† Statistically superior to albuterol (p≤0.05).

INDICATIONS AND USAGE:

Salmeterol xinafoate is indicated for long-term, twice-daily (morning and evening) administration in the maintenance treatment of asthma and in the prevention of bronchospasm in patients 12 years of age and older with reversible obstructive airway disease, including

INDICATIONS AND USAGE: *(cont'd)*

patients with symptoms of nocturnal asthma, who require regular treatment with inhaled, short-acting $beta_2$-agonists. It should not be used in patients whose asthma can be managed by occasional use of short-acting, inhaled $beta_2$-agonists.

Salmeterol xinafoate may be used with or without concurrent inhaled or systemic corticosteroid therapy.

Salmeterol xinafoate is also indicated for prevention of exercise- induced bronchospasm in patients 12 years of age and older.

CONTRAINDICATIONS:

Salmeterol xinafoate is contraindicated in patients with a history of hypersensitivity to any of the components.

WARNINGS:

IMPORTANT INFORMATION: SALMETEROL XINAFOATE SHOULD NOT BE INITIATED IN PATIENTS WITH SIGNIFICANTLY WORSENING OR ACUTELY DETERIORATING ASTHMA, WHICH MAY BE A LIFE-THREATENING CONDITION. Serious acute respiratory events, including fatalities, have been reported, both in the US and worldwide, when salmeterol xinafoate has been initiated in this situation.

Although it is not possible from these reports to determine whether salmeterol xinafoate contributed to these adverse events or simply failed to relieve the deteriorating asthma, the use of salmeterol xinafoate in this setting is inappropriate.

SALMETEROL XINAFOATE SHOULD NOT BE USED TO TREAT ACUTE SYMPTOMS. It is crucial to inform patients of this and prescribe a short-acting, inhaled $beta_2$-agonist for this purpose as well as warn them that increasing inhaled $beta_2$-agonist use is a signal of deteriorating asthma.

SALMETEROL XINAFOATE IS NOT A SUBSTITUTE FOR INHALED OR ORAL CORTICOSTEROIDS. Corticosteroids should not be stopped or reduced when salmeterol xinafoate is initiated.

(See Information for the Patient, and PATIENT PACKAGE INSERT)

Do Not Introduce Salmeterol Xinafoate as a Treatment for Acutely Deteriorating Asthma: salmeterol xinafoate is intended for the maintenance treatment of asthma (see INDICATIONS AND USAGE) and should not be introduced in acutely deteriorating asthma, which is a potentially life-threatening condition. There are no data demonstrating that salmeterol xinafoate provides greater efficacy than or additional efficacy to short-acting, inhaled $beta_2$-agonists in patients with worsening asthma. Serious acute respiratory events, including fatalities, have been reported, both in the US and worldwide, in patients receiving salmeterol xinafoate. In most cases, these have occurred in patients with severe asthma (*e.g.,* patients with a history of corticosteroid dependence, low pulmonary function, intubation, mechanical ventilation, frequent hospitalizations, or previous life- threatening acute asthma exacerbations) and/or in some patients in whom asthma has been acutely deteriorating (*e.g.,* unresponsive to usual medications, increasing need for inhaled short-acting $beta_2$-agonists, increasing need for systemic corticosteroids, significant increase in symptoms, recent emergency room visits, sudden or progressive deterioration in pulmonary function). However, they have occurred in a few patients with less severe asthma as well. It was not possible from these reports to determine whether salmeterol xinafoate contributed to these events or simply failed to relieve the deteriorating asthma.

Do Not Use Salmeterol Xinafoate to Treat Acute Symptoms: A short-acting inhaled $beta_2$-agonist, not salmeterol xinafoate, should be used to relieve acute asthma symptoms. When prescribing salmeterol xinafoate, the physician must also provide the patient with a short-acting, inhaled $beta_2$-agonist (*e.g.,* albuterol) for treatment of symptoms that occur acutely, despite regular twice daily (morning and evening) use of salmeterol xinafoate.

When beginning treatment with salmeterol xinafoate, patients who have been taking short-acting, inhaled $beta_2$-agonists on a regular basis (*e.g.,* q.i.d.) should be instructed to discontinue the regular use of these drugs and use them only for symptomatic relief if they develop acute asthma symptoms while taking salmeterol xinafoate (see PRECAUTIONS.)

Watch for Increasing Use of Short-Acting, Inhaled $Beta_2$- Agonists, Which Is a Marker of Deteriorating Asthma: Asthma may deteriorate acutely over a period of hours or chronically over several days or longer. If the patient's short-acting, inhaled $beta_2$-agonist becomes less effective or the patient needs more inhalations than usual, this may be a marker of destabilization of asthma. In this setting, the patient requires immediate re-evaluation with reassessment of the treatment regimen, giving special consideration to the possible need for corticosteroids. If the patient uses four or more inhalations per day of a short-acting, inhaled $beta_2$-agonist for 2 or more consecutive days, or if more than one canister (200 inhalations per canister) of short-acting, inhaled $beta_2$-agonist is used in an 8- week period in conjunction with salmeterol xinafoate, then the patient should consult the physician for re-evaluation. **Increasing the daily dosage of salmeterol xinafoate in this situation is not appropriate. Salmeterol xinafoate should not be used more frequently than twice daily (morning and evening) at the recommended dose of two inhalations.**

Do Not Use Salmeterol Xinafoate as a Substitute for Oral or Inhaled Corticosteroids: There are no data demonstrating that salmeterol xinafoate has a clinical anti-inflammatory effect and could be expected to take the place of, or reduce the dose of corticosteroids. Patients who already require oral or inhaled corticosteroids for treatment of asthma should be continued on this type of treatment even if they feel better as a result of initiating salmeterol xinafoate. Any change in corticosteroid dosage should be made ONLY after clinical evaluation (see PRECAUTIONS).

Do Not Exceed Recommended Dosage: As with other inhaled $beta_2$-adrenergic drugs, salmeterol xinafoate should not be used more often or at higher doses than recommended. Fatalities have been reported in association with excessive use of inhaled sympathomimetic drugs. Large doses of inhaled or oral salmeterol (12 to 20 times the recommended dose) have been associated with clinically significant prolongation of the QT interval, which has the potential for producing ventricular arrhythmias.

Paradoxical Bronchospasm: As with other inhaled asthma medication, paradoxical bronchospasm (which can be life threatening) has been reported following the use of salmeterol xinafoate. If it occurs, treatment with salmeterol xinafoate should be discontinued immediately and alternative therapy instituted.

Immediate Hypersensitivity Reactions: Immediate hypersensitivity reactions may occur after administration of salmeterol xinafoate, as demonstrated by rare cases of urticaria, angioedema, rash, and bronchospasm.

Upper Airway Symptoms: Symptoms of laryngeal spasm, irritation, or swelling, such as stridor and choking, have been reported rarely in patients receiving salmeterol xinafoate.

PRECAUTIONS:

GENERAL

Use with Spacer or Other Devices: The safety and effectiveness of salmeterol xinafoate when used with a spacer or other devices have not been adequately studied.

Cardiovascular and Other Effects: No effect on the cardiovascular system is usually seen after the administration of inhaled salmeterol in recommended doses, but the cardiovascular and central nervous system effects seen with all sympathomimetic drugs (*e.g.,* increased blood

PRECAUTIONS: *(cont'd)*

pressure, heart rate, excitement) can occur after use of salmeterol xinafoate and may require discontinuation of the drug. Salmeterol, like all sympathomimetic amines, should be used with caution in patients with cardiovascular disorders, especially coronary insufficiency, cardiac arrhythmias, and hypertension; in patients with convulsive disorders or thyrotoxicosis; and in patients who are unusually responsive to sympathomimetic amines.

As has been described with other beta-adrenergic agonist bronchodilators, clinically significant changes in systolic and/or diastolic blood pressure, pulse rate, and electrocardiograms have been seen infrequently in individual patients in controlled clinical studies with salmeterol.

Metabolic Effects: Doses of the related $beta_2$-adrenoceptor agonist albuterol, when administered intravenously, have been reported to aggravate pre-existing diabetes mellitus and ketoacidosis. No effects on glucose have been seen with salmeterol xinafoate at recommended doses. Administration of $beta_2$-adrenoceptor agonists may cause a decrease in serum potassium, possibly through intracellular shunting, which has the potential to increase the likelihood of arrhythmias. The decrease is usually transient, not requiring supplementation.

Clinically significant changes in blood glucose and/or serum potassium were seen rarely during clinical studies with long-term administration of salmeterol xinafoate at recommended doses.

INFORMATION FOR THE PATIENT

SHAKE WELL BEFORE USING.

It is important that patients understand how to use salmeterol xinafoate appropriately and how it should be used in relation to other asthma medications they are taking. Patients should be given the following information:

1. Shake well before using.

2. The recommended dosage (two inhalations twice daily, morning and evening) should not be exceeded.

3. Salmeterol xinafoate is not meant to relieve acute asthma symptoms and extra doses should not be used for that purpose. Acute symptoms should be treated with a short-acting, inhaled $beta_2$-agonist such as albuterol (the physician should provide the patient with such medication and instruct the patient in how it should be used).

4. The physician should be notified immediately if any of the following situations occur, which may be a sign of seriously worsening asthma.

Decreasing effectiveness of short-acting, inhaled $beta_2$-agonists

Need for more inhalations than usual of short-acting, inhaled $beta_2$-agonists

Use of four or more inhalations per day of a short-acting $beta_2$-agonist for 2 or more days consecutively

Use of more than one canister of a short-acting, inhaled $beta_2$-agonist in an 8-week period (*i.e.,* canister with 200 inhalations)

5. Salmeterol xinafoate should not be used as a substitute for oral or inhaled corticosteroids. The dosage of these medications should not be changed and they should not be stopped without consulting the physician, even if the patient feels better after initiating treatment with salmeterol xinafoate.

6. Patients should be cautioned regarding potential adverse cardiovascular effects, such as palpitations or chest pain, related to the use of additional $beta_2$agonist.

7. In patients receiving salmeterol xinafoate, other inhaled medications should be used only as directed by the physician.

8. When using salmeterol xinafoate to prevent exercise-induced bronchospasm, patients should take the dose at lest 30 to 60 minutes before exercise.

CARCINOGENESIS, MUTAGENESIS, AND IMPAIRMENT OF FERTILITY

In an 18-month oral carcinogenicity study in CD-mice, salmeterol xinafoate caused a dose-related increase in the incidence of smooth muscle hyperplasia, cystic glandular hyperplasia, and leiomyomas of the uterus and a dose-related increase in the incidence of cysts in the ovaries. A higher incidence of leiomyosarcomas was not statistically significant; tumor findings were observed at oral doses of 1.4 and 10 mg/kg, which gave 9 and 63 times, respectively, the human exposure based on rodent:human AUC comparisons.

Salmeterol caused a dose-related increase in the incidence of mesovarian leiomyomas and ovarian cysts in Sprague Dawley rats in a 24-month inhalation/oral carcinogenicity study. Tumors were observed in rats receiving doses of 0.68 and 2.58 mg/kg per day (about 55 and 215 times the recommended clinical dose [mg/m^2]). These findings in rodents are similar to those reported previously for other beta-adrenergic agonist drugs. The relevance of these findings to human use is unknown.

No significant effects occurred in mice at 0.2 mg/kg (1.3 times the recommended clinical dose based on comparisons of the AUCs) and in rats at 0.21 mg/kg (15 times the recommended clinical dose on a mg/m^2 basis).

Salmeterol xinafoate produced no detectable or reproducible increases in microbial and mammalian gene mutation *in vitro.* No blastogenic activity occurred *in vitro* in human lymphocytes or *in vivo* in a rat micronucleus test. No effects on fertility were identified in male and female rats treated orally with salmeterol xinafoate at doses up to 2 mg/kg orally (about 160 times the recommended clinical dose on a mg/m^2 basis).

PREGNANCY, TERATOGENIC EFFECTS, PREGNANCY CATEGORY C

No significant effects of maternal exposure to oral salmeterol xinafoate occurred in the rat at doses up to the equivalent of about 160 times the recommended clinical dose on a mg/m^2 basis. Dutch rabbit fetuses exposed to salmeterol xinafoate *in utero* exhibited effects characteristically resulting from beta-adrenoceptor stimulation; these included precocious eyelid openings, cleft palate, sternebral fusion, limb and paw flexures, and delayed ossification of the frontal cranial bones. No significant effects occurred at 0.6 mg/kg given orally (12 times the recommended clinical dose based on comparison of the AUCs).

New Zealand White rabbits were less sensitive since only delayed ossification of the frontal bones was seen at 10 mg/kg given orally (approximately 1,600 times the recommended clinical dose on a mg/m^2basis). Extensive use of other beta-agonists has provided no evidence that these class effects in animals are relevant to use in humans. There are no adequate and well-controlled studies with salmeterol xinafoate in pregnant women. Salmeterol xinafoate should be used during pregnancy only if the potential benefit justifies the potential risk to the fetus.

USE IN LABOR AND DELIVERY

There are no well-controlled human studies that have investigated effects of salmeterol on preterm labor or labor at term. Because of the potential for beta-agonist interference with uterine contractility, use of salmeterol xinafoate during labor should be restricted to those patients in whom the benefits clearly outweigh the risks.

NURSING MOTHERS

Plasma levels of salmeterol after inhaled therapeutic doses are very low (85 to 200 pg/ml) in humans. In lactating rats dosed with radiolabeled salmeterol, levels of radioactivity were similar in plasma and milk. In rats, concentrations of salmeterol in plasma and milk were similar. The xinafoate moiety is also transferred to milk in rats at concentrations of about half the corresponding level in plasma. However, since there is no experience with use of salmeterol xinafoate by nursing mothers, a decision should be made whether to discontinue

PRECAUTIONS: *(cont'd)*

nursing or to discontinue the drug, taking into account the importance of the drug to the mother. Caution should be exercised when salmeterol xinafoate is administered to a nursing woman.

PEDIATRIC USE

The safety and effectiveness of salmeterol xinafoate in children younger than 12 years of age have not been established.

GERIATRIC USE

Of the total number of patients who received salmeterol xinafoate in all clinical studies, 241 were 65 years and older. Geriatric patients (65 years and older) with reversible obstructive airway disease were evaluated in four well-controlled studies of 3 weeks' to 3 months' duration. Two placebo-controlled, crossover studies evaluated twice-daily dosing with salmeterol for 21 to 28 days in 45 patients. An additional 75 geriatric patients were treated with salmeterol for 3 months in two large parallel-group, multicenter studies. These 120 patients experienced increases in AM and PM peak expiratory flow rate and decreases in diurnal variation in peak expiratory flow rate similar to responses seen in the total populations of the two latter studies. The adverse event type and frequency in geriatric patients were not different from those of the total populations studied.

No apparent differences in the efficacy and safety of salmeterol xinafoate were observed when geriatric patients were compared with younger patients in clinical trials. As with other $beta_2$-agonists, however, special caution should be observed when using salmeterol xinafoate in elderly patients who have concomitant cardiovascular disease that could be adversely effected by this class of drug. Based on available data, no adjustment of salmeterol dosage in geriatric patients is warranted.

ADVERSE REACTIONS:

Adverse reactions to salmeterol are similar in nature to reactions to other selective $beta_2$-adrenoceptor agonists, i.e., tachycardia; palpitations; immediate hypersensitivity reactions, including urticaria, angioedema, rash, bronchospasm (see WARNINGS; headache; tremor; nervousness; and paradoxical bronchospasm (see WARNINGS).

Two multicenter, 12-week, controlled studies have evaluated twice-daily doses of salmeterol xinafoate in patients 12 years of age and older with asthma. The following table reports the incidence of adverse event in these two studies (TABLE 4):

TABLE 4 Adverse Experience Incidence In Two Large 12-Week Clinical Trials*

Adverse Event Type	Percent of Patients Placebo n=187	Serevent 42 mcg b.i.d. n=184	Albuterol 180 mcg q.i.d. n=185
Ear, nose, and throat			
Upper respiratory tract infection	13	14	16*
Nasopharyngitis	12	14	11
Disease of nasal cavity/sinus	4	6	1
Sinus headache	2	4	<1
Gastrointestinal			
Stomachache	0	4	0
Neurological			
Headache	23	28	27
Tremor	2	4	3
Respiratory			
Cough	6	7	3
Lower respiratory infection	2	4	2

* The only adverse experience classified as serious was one case of upper respiratory tract infection in a patient treated with albuterol.

The table above (TABLE 4) includes all events (whether considered drug related or nondrug related by the investigator) that occurred at a rate of over 3% in the salmeterol xinafoate treatment group and were more common in the salmeterol xinafoate group than in the placebo group.

Pharyngitis, allergic rhinitis, dizziness/giddiness, and influenza occurred at 3% or more but were equally common on placebo. Other events occurring in the salmeterol xinafoate treatment group at a frequency of 1% to 3% were as follows:

Cardiovascular: Tachycardia, palpitations.

Ear, Nose, and Throat: Rhinitis, laryngitis.

Gastrointestinal: Nausea, viral gastroenteritis, nausea and vomiting, diarrhea, abdominal pain.

Hypersensitivity: Urticaria.

Mouth and Teeth: Dental pain.

Musculoskeletal: Pain in joint, back pain, muscle cramp/contraction, myalgia/myositis, muscular soreness.

Neurological: Nervousness, malaise/fatigue.

Respiratory: Tracheitis/bronchitis.

Skin: Rash/skin eruption.

Urogenital: Dysmenorrhea.

In small dose-response studies, tremor, nervousness, and palpitations appeared to be dose related.

Postmarketing Experience: In extensive US and worldwide postmarketing experience, serious exacerbations of asthma, including some that have been fatal, have been reported. In most cases, these have occurred in patients with severe asthma and/or in some patients in whom asthma has been acutely deteriorating (see WARNINGS), but they have occurred in a few patients with less severe asthma as well. It was not possible from these reports to determine whether salmeterol xinafoate contributed to these events or simply failed to relieve the deteriorating asthma.

Postmarketing experience includes rare reports of upper airway symptoms of laryngeal spasm, irritation, or swelling, such as stridor and choking.

OVERDOSAGE:

Overdosage with salmeterol may be expected to result in exaggeration of the pharmacologic adverse effects associated with beta-adrenoceptor agonists, including tachycardia and/or arrhythmia, tremor, headache, and muscle cramps. Overdosage with salmeterol can lead to clinically significant prolongation of the QT_c interval, which can produce ventricular arrhythmias. Other signs of overdosage may include hypokalemia and hyperglycemia.

In these cases, therapy with salmeterol xinafoate and all beta-adrenergic-stimulant drugs should be stopped, supportive therapy provided, and judicious use of a beta-adrenergic blocking agent should be considered, bearing in mind the possibility that such agents can produce bronchospasm. Cardiac monitoring is recommended in cases of overdosage.

As with all sympathomimetic pressurized aerosol medications, cardiac arrest and even death may be associated with abuse of salmeterol xinafoate.

OVERDOSAGE: *(cont'd)*

Rats and dogs survived the maximum practicable inhalation doses of salmeterol of 2.9 and 0.7 mg/kg, respectively. The maximum nonlethal oral doses in mice and rats were approximately 150 mg/kg and >1,000 mg/kg, respectively.

Dialysis is not appropriate treatment for overdosage of salmeterol xinafoate.

DOSAGE AND ADMINISTRATION:

Salmeterol xinafoate should be administered by the orally inhaled route only. For maintenance of bronchodilatation and prevention of symptoms of asthma, including the symptoms of nocturnal asthma, the usual dosage for adults and children 12 years of age and older is two inhalations (42 mcg) twice daily (morning and evening, approximately 12 hours apart). Adverse effects are more likely to occur with higher doses of salmeterol, and more frequent administration or administration of a larger number of inhalations is not recommended.

To gain full therapeutic benefit, salmeterol xinafoate should be administered twice daily (morning and evening) in the treatment of reversible airway obstruction.

If a previously effective dosage regimen fails to provide the usual response, medical advice should be sought immediately as this is often a sign of destabilization of asthma. Under these circumstances, the therapeutic regimen should be re-evaluated and additional therapeutic options, such as inhaled or systemic corticosteroids, should be considered. If symptoms arise in the period between doses, a short- acting, inhaled $beta_2$-agonist should be taken for immediate relief.

Prevention of Exercise-Induced Bronchospasm: Two inhalations at least 30 to 60 minutes before exercise have been shown to protect against exercise-induced bronchospasm in many patients for up to 12 hours. *Additional doses of salmeterol xinafoate should not be used for 12 hours after the administration of this drug. Patients who are receiving salmeterol xinafoate twice daily (morning and evening) should not use additional salmeterol xinafoate for prevention of exercise-induced bronchospasm.* If this dose is not effective, other appropriate therapy for exercise-induced bronchospasm should be considered.

Geriatric Use: In studies where geriatric patients (65 years of age or older, see PRECAUTIONS) have been treated with salmeterol xinafoate, efficacy and safety of 42 mcg given twice daily (morning and evening) did not differ from that in younger patients. Consequently, no dosage adjustment is recommended.

PATIENT INFORMATION:

Salmeterol xinzfoate is used in the treatment of asthma and other breathing disorders such as exercise related breathing difficulties. This medication does not work quickly and should not be used to provide immediate relief of symptoms. It can be used with inhaled steroid medications and is strictly a maintenance medication. Salmeterol xinafoate should not be used more than what your physician has prescribed. More frequent use can cause serious adverse reactions. If you experience symptoms of rash, itching or difficulty breathing, discontinue use and call your physician. Common adverse reactions and side effects include: increased heart rate, itching, swelling, rash or difficulty breathing, headache, tremor, and nervousness. Salmeterol xinafoate is an aerosol product that must be inhaled. Proper technique is important to get maximum benefit. Your pharmacist or physician can provide proper instruction. This medication should be shaken well before used. If more than 4 inhalations per day are needed, contact your physician. To prevent exercise-induced breathing difficulties, inhale 30 to 60 minutes before exercising.

HOW SUPPLIED:

Serevent Inhalation Aerosol is supplied in 13-g-canisters containing 120 metered actuations in boxes of one. Each actuation delivers 25 mcg of salmeterol base (as salmeterol xinafoate) from the valve and 21 mcg of salmeterol base (as salmeterol xinafoate) from the actuator. Each canister is supplied with a green plastic actuator with a teal-colored strapcap and patient's instructions. Also available, Serevent Inhalation Aerosol Refill, a 13-g canister only with patient's instructions.

Serevent Inhalation Aerosol is also supplied in a pack that consists of a 6.5-g canister containing 60 metered actuations in boxes of one. Each actuation delivers 25 mcg of salmeterol base (as salmeterol xinafoate) from the valve and 21 mcg of salmeterol base from the actuator (as salmeterol xinafoate). Each canister is supplied with a green plastic actuator with a teal-colored strapcap and patient's instructions.

For use with Serevent Aerosol actuator only. The actuator should not be used with other aerosol medications.

Store between 2° and 30°C (36° and 86°F). Store canister with nozzle end down. Protect from freezing temperatures and direct sunlight.

Avoid spraying in eyes. Contents under pressure. Do not puncture or incinerate. Do not store at temperature above 120°F. Keep out of reach of children. As with most inhaled medications in aerosol canisters, the therapeutic effect of this medication may decrease when the canister is cold; for best results, the canister should be at room temperature before use. Shake well before using.

Note: The statement below is required by the Federal government's Clean Air Act for all products containing or manufactured with chlorofluorocarbons (CFCs).

WARNING

Contains trichlorofluoromethane and dichlorodifluoromethane, substances which harm public health and environment by destroying ozone in the upper atmosphere.

HOW SUPPLIED - EQUIVALENTS NOT AVAILABLE:

Aerosol, Metered - Inhalation - 25 mcg

6.5 gm	$34.63	SEREVENT, Glaxo Wellcome	00173-0467-00
13 gm	$53.56	SEREVENT, REFILL, Glaxo Wellcome	00173-0465-00
13 gm	$55.48	SEREVENT, Glaxo Wellcome	00173-0464-00

SALSALATE *(002206)*

CATEGORIES: Analgesics; Anti-Inflammatory Agents; Antiarthritics; Antipyretics; Arthritis; Central Nervous System Agents; Nonsteroidal Anti-Inflammatory; Osteoarthritis; Pain; Salicylates; Pregnancy Category C; FDA Pre 1938 Drugs

BRAND NAMES: Amigesic; Anaflex 750; Artha-G; *Atisuril*; Carsalate; Diagen; **Disalcid**; *Disalgesic*; Marthritic; Mono-Gesic; *Nobegyl*; Ro-Salcid; Salflex; Salgesic; Salicylsalicylic Acid; *Salina*; Salsitab; *Umbradol*
(International brand names outside U.S. in italics)

FORMULARIES: Aetna; BC-BS; FHP; Medi-Cal; PCS

DESCRIPTION:

Salsalate is a nonsteroidal anti-inflammatory agent for oral administration. Chemically, salsalate (salicylsalicylic acid or 2-hydroxybenzoic acid, 2-carboxyphenyl ester) is a dimer of salicylic acid; its structural formula is shown below.

Each round, aqua, scored, film coated Salsalate tablet contains 500 mg salsalate.

DESCRIPTION: *(cont'd)*

Each aqua and white Salsalate capsule contains 500 mg salsalate. Salsalate capsules also contain: colloidal silicon dioxide, gelatin, magnesium stearate, pregelatinized starch, corn starch, titanium dioxide, FD&C blue #1, and D&C yellow #10.

Each capsule-shaped aqua, scored, film coated Salsalate tablet contains 750 mg salsalate. Salsalate tablets also contain: hydroxypropyl methylcellulose, magnesium stearate, microcrystalline cellulose, polyethylene glycol, polysorbate 80, propylene glycol. corn starch, talc, titanium dioxide, FD&C blue #1, and D&C yellow #10.

CLINICAL PHARMACOLOGY:

Salsalate is insoluble in acid gastric fluids (<0.1 mg/ml at pH 1.0), but readily soluble in the small intestine where it is partially hydrolyzed to two molecules of salicylic acid. A significant portion of the parent compound is absorbed unchanged and undergoes rapid esterase hydrolysis in the body: its half-life is about one hour. About 13% is excreted through the kidneys as a glucuronide conjugate of the parent compound, the remainder as salicylic acid and it metabolites. Thus, the amount of salicylic acid available from Salsalate is about 15% less than from aspirin, when the two drugs are administered on a salicylic acid molar equivalent basis (3.6 g salsalate/5 g aspirin). Salicylic acid biotransformation is saturated at anti-inflammatory doses of Salsalate. Such capacity-limited biotransformation results in an increase in the half-life of salicylic acid from 3.5 to 16 or more hours. Thus, dosing with Salsalate twice a day will satisfactorily maintain blood levels within the desired therapeutic range (10 to 30 mg/100 ml) throughout the 12-hour intervals. Therapeutic blood levels continue for up to 16 hours after the last dose. The parent compound does not show capacity-limited biotransformation, nor does it accumulate in the plasma on multiple dosing. Food slows the absorption of all salicylates including Salsalate.

The mode of anti-inflammatory action of Salsalate and other nonsteroidal anti-inflammatory drugs is not fully defined. Although salicylic acid (the primary metabolite of Salsalate) is a weak inhibitor of prostaglandin synthesis **in vitro**, Salsalate appears to selectively inhibit prostaglandin synthesis **in vivo**,[1]providing anti-inflammatory activity equivalent to aspirin[2] and indomethacin.[3] Unlike aspirin. Salsalate does not inhibit platelet aggregation.[4]

The usefulness of salicylic acid, the active **in vivo** product of Salsalate, in the treatment of arthritic disorders has been established.[5,6] In contrast to aspirin, Salsalate causes no greater fecal gastrointestinal blood loss than placebo.[7]

INDICATIONS AND USAGE:

Salsalate is indicated for relief of the signs and symptoms of rheumatoid arthritis, osteoarthritis and related rheumatic disorders.

CONTRAINDICATIONS:

Salsalate is contraindicated in patients hypersensitive to salsalate.

WARNINGS:

Reye's Syndrome may develop in individuals who have chicken pox, influenza, or flu symptoms. Some studies suggest a possible association between the development of Reye's Syndrome and the use of medicines containing salicylate or aspirin. Salsalate contains a salicylate and therefore is not recommended for use in patients with chicken pox, influenza, or flu symptoms.

PRECAUTIONS:

General Precautions: Patients on treatment with Salsalate should be warned not to take other salicylates so as to avoid potentially toxic concentrations. Great care should be exercised when Salsalate is prescribed in the presence of chronic renal insufficiency or peptic ulcer disease. Protein binding of salicylic acid can be influenced by nutritional status, competitive binding of other drugs, and fluctuations in serum proteins caused by disease (rheumatoid arthritis, etc.).

Although cross reactivity, including bronchospasm, has been reported occasionally with non-acetylated salicylates, including salsalate, in aspirin-sensitive patients,[8,9] salsalate is less likely than aspirin to induce asthma in such patients.[10]

Laboratory Tests: Plasma salicylic acid concentrations should be periodically monitored during long-term treatment with Salsalate to aid maintenance of therapeutically effective levels: 10 to 30 mg/100 ml. Toxic manifestations are not usually seen until plasma concentrations exceed 30 mg/100 ml (see OVERDOSAGE.) Urinary pH should also be regularly monitored: sudden acidification, as from pH 6.5 to 5.5, can double the plasma level, resulting in toxicity.

Drug/Laboratory Test Interactions: Salicylate competes with thyroid hormone for binding to plasma proteins, which may be reflected in a depressed plasma T_4 value in some patients; thyroid function and basal metabolism are unaffected.

Carcinogenesis: No long-term animal studies have been performed with Salsalate to evaluate its carcinogenic potential.

Use in Pregnancy: Pregnancy Category C: Salsalate and salicylic acid have been shown to be teratogenic and embryocidal in rats when given in doses 4 to 5 times the usual human dose. These effects were not observed at doses twice as great as the usual human dose. There are no adequate and well-controlled studies in pregnant women. Salsalate should be used during pregnancy only if the potential benefit justifies the potential risk to the fetus.

Labor and Delivery: There exist no adequate and well-controlled studies in pregnant women. Although adverse effects on mother or infant have not been reported with Salsalate use during labor, caution is advised when anti-inflammatory dosage is involved. However, other salicylates have been associated with prolonged gestation and labor, maternal and neonatal bleeding sequelae, potentiation of narcotic and barbiturate effects (respiratory or cardiac arrest in the mother), delivery problems and stillbirth.

Nursing Mothers: It is not known whether salsalate per se is excreted in human milk; salicylic acid, the primary metabolite of Salsalate, has been shown to appear in human milk in concentrations approximating the maternal blood level. Thus, the infant of a mother of Salsalate therapy might ingest in mother's milk 30 to 80% as much salicylate per kg body weight as the mother is taking. Accordingly, caution should be exercised when Salsalate is administered to a nursing woman.

Pediatric Use: Safety and effectiveness of Salsalate use in children have not been established. (See WARNINGS.)

DRUG INTERACTIONS:

Salicylates antagonize the uricosuric action of drugs used to treat gout. ASPIRIN AND OTHER SALICYLATE DRUGS WILL BE ADDITIVE TO SALSALATE AND MAY INCREASE PLASMA CONCENTRATIONS OF SALICYLIC ACID TO TOXIC LEVELS. Drugs and foods that raise urine pH will increase renal clearance and urinary excretion of salicylic acid, thus lowering plasma levels; acidifying drugs or foods will decrease urinary excretion and increase plasma levels. Salicylates given concomitantly with anticoagulant drugs may predispose to systemic bleeding. Salicylates may enhance the hypoglycemic effect of oral

DRUG INTERACTIONS: *(cont'd)*

antidiabetic drugs of the sulfonylurea class. Salicylate competes with a number of drugs for protein binding sites, notably penicillin, thiopental, thyroxine, triiodothyronine, phenytoin, sulfinpyrazone, naproxen, warfarin, methotrexate, and possibly corticosteroids.

ADVERSE REACTIONS:

In two well-controlled clinical trials, the following reversible adverse experience characteristic of salicylates were most commonly reported with Salsalate (n - 280 pts; listed in descending order of frequency): tinnitus, nausea, hearing impairment, rash, and vertigo. These common symptoms of salicylates, i.e. tinnitus or reversible hearing impairment, are often used as a guide to therapy.

Although cause-and-effect relationships have not been established, spontaneous reports over a ten-year period have include the following additional medically significant adverse experiences: abdominal pain, abnormal hepatic function, anaphylactic shock, angioedema, bronchospasm, decreased creatinine clearance, diarrhea, G.I. bleeding, hepatitis, hypotension, nephritis and urticaria.

DRUG ABUSE AND DEPENDENCE:

Drug abuse and dependence have not been reported with Salsalate.

OVERDOSAGE:

Death has followed ingestion of 10 to 30 g of salicylates in adults, but much larger amounts have been ingested without fatal outcome.

Symptoms: The usual symptoms of salicylism — tinnitus, vertigo, headache, confusion, drowsiness, sweating, hyperventilation, vomiting and diarrhea - will occur. More severe intoxication will lead to disruption of electrolyte balance and blood pH, and hyperthermia and dehydration.

Treatment: Further absorption of Salsalate from the G.I. tract should be prevented by emesis (syrup of ipecac), and, if necessary, by gastric lavage.

Fluid and electrolyte imbalance should be corrected by the administration of appropriate IV therapy. Adequate renal function should be maintained. Hemodialysis or peritoneal dialysis may be required in extreme cases.

DOSAGE AND ADMINISTRATION:

Adults: The usual dosage is 3000 mg daily, given in divided doses as follows: 1) two doses of two 750 mg tablets: 2) two doses of three 500 mg tablets/capsules; or 3) three doses of two 500 mg tablets/capsules. Some patients, e.g. the elderly, may require a lower dosage to achieve therapeutic blood concentrations and to avoid the more common side effects such as auditory.

Alleviation of symptoms is gradual, and full benefit may not be evidence for 3 to 4 days, when plasma salicylate levels have achieved steady state. There is no evidence for development of tissue tolerance (tachyphylaxis), but salicylate therapy may induce increased activity of metabolizing liver enzymes, causing a greater rate of salicyluric acid production and excretion, with a resultant increase in dosage requirement for maintenance of therapeutic serum salicylate levels.

Children: Dosage recommendations and indications for Salsalate use in children have not been established.

Store at controlled room temperature 15-30°C (59-86°F).

REFERENCES:

1. Morris HG, Sherman NA, McQuain C, et al: Effects of Salsalate (Non-Acetylated Salicylate) and Aspirin (ASA) on Serum Prostaglandins in Humans. Ther. Drug Monit. 7:435-438, 1985. **2.** April PA, Curran NJ, Exholm BP, et al: Multicenter Comparative Study of Salsalate (SSA) vs Aspirin (ASA) in Rheumatoid Arthritis (RA). Arthritis Rheumatism **30** (4 supplement): S93, 1987. **3.** Deodhar SD, McLeod MM, Dick WC, et al: A Short-Term Comparative Trial of Salsalate and Indomethacin in Rheumatoid Arthritis. Curr. Med. Res. Opin., **5**: 185-188, 1977. **4.** Estes D, Kaplan K: Lack of Platelet Effect With the Aspirin Analog, Salsalate. Arthritis and Rheumatism, **23**:1303-1307, 1980. **5.** Dick C, Dick PH, Nuki G, et al: Effect of Anti-inflammatory Drug Therapy on Clearance of ^{133}xe from Knee Joints of Patients with Rheumatoid Arthritis. British Med. J. **3**:278-280, 1969. **6.** Dick WC, Grayson MF, Woodburn A, et al: Indices of Inflammatory Activity. Ann. of the Rheum. Dis. **29**: 634-648, 1970. **7.** Cohen A: Fecal Blood Loss and Plasma Salicylate Study of Salicylsalicylic Acid and Aspirin. J. Clin. Pharmacol,**19**:242-247, 1979. **8.** Chudwin DS, Strub M. Golden HE, et al: Sensitivity to Non-Acetylated Salicylates in a Patient with Asthma, Nasal Polyps, and Rheumatoid Arthritis. Annals of Allergy **57**:133-134, 1986. **9.** Spector SL, Wangaard CH, Farr RS: Aspirin and Concomitant Idiosyncrasies in Adult Asthmatic Patients. J. Allergy Clin. Immunol.**64**:500-506, 1979.10.Stevenson DD, Schrank PJ, Hougham AJ, et al: Salsalate Cross Sensitivity in Aspirin-Sensitive Asthmatics. J. Allergy Clin. Immunol,**81**:181, 1988.

HOW SUPPLIED - RATED THERAPEUTICALLY EQUIVALENT:

Tablet - Oral - 500 mg

100's	$20.77	Salsalate, Duramed Pharms	51285-0858-02
500's	$98.66	Salsalate, Duramed Pharms	51285-0858-04

Tablet - Oral - 750 mg

100's	$26.56	Salsalate, Duramed Pharms	51285-0859-02
500's	$126.14	Salsalate, Duramed Pharms	51285-0859-04

HOW SUPPLIED - NOT RATED EQUIVALENT:

Capsule, Gelatin - Oral - 500 mg

100's	$12.59	Salsalate, Caraco Pharm	57664-0183-08
100's	**$46.86**	**DISALCID, 3M Pharms**	**00089-0148-10**
1000's	$84.12	Salsalate, Caraco Pharm	57664-0183-18

Capsule, Gelatin - Oral - 750 mg

100's	$15.10	Salsalate, Medirex	57480-0412-01
600's	$200.00	Salsalate, Medirex	57480-0412-06

Tablet, Coated - Oral - 500 mg

100's	$11.10	Salsalated, Medirex	57480-0411-01
100's	$11.75	Salsalate, Mutual Pharm	53489-0465-01
100's	$11.90	Salsalate, Qualitest Pharms	00603-5754-21
100's	$11.99	Salsalate, United Res	00677-1024-01
100's	$12.10	Salsalate 500, Major Pharms	00904-1250-60
100's	$12.10	Salsalate, Major Pharms	00904-1253-60
100's	$13.59	Salsalate, Caraco Pharm	57664-0103-08
100's	$13.59	Salsalate, Caraco Pharm	57664-0203-08
100's	$14.16	Salsalate, HL Moore Drug Exch	00839-7167-06
100's	$14.65	SALICYLSALICYLIC ACID, Goldline Labs	00182-1802-01
100's	$16.95	Salsalate, Eon Labs Mfg	00185-0761-01
100's	$16.95	Salsalate (Blue) Tablets 500 Mg, Eon Labs Mfg	00185-0856-01
100's	$17.65	Salsalate (Yellow), Rosemont	00832-1037-00
100's	$17.75	Salsalate, Schein Pharm (US)	00364-0832-01
100's	$17.75	Salsalate, Martec Pharms	52555-0560-01
100's	$18.53	SALSITAB, Upsher Smith	00245-0153-11
100's	$20.00	SALICYLSALICYLIC ACID, Goldline Labs	00182-1802-89
100's	$20.11	SALSITAB, Upsher Smith	00245-0153-01
100's	$20.77	Salsalate, Duramed Pharms	51285-0296-02
100's	$21.25	Salsalate, Aligen Independ	00405-4934-01
100's	$21.25	Salsalate, Geneva Pharms	00781-1108-01
100's	$21.25	Salsalate, Sidmak Labs	50111-0390-01
100's	$21.95	SALFLEX, Carnrick	00086-0071-10

HOW SUPPLIED - NOT RATED EQUIVALENT: *(cont'd)*

100's	$21.95	Salsalate, Eon Labs Mfg	00185-0693-01
100's	$24.46	Salsalate 500, Major Pharms	00904-1250-61
100's	$25.02	Salsalate, Alpharma	00472-0132-10
100's	$25.02	Salsalate, Rugby	00536-4522-01
100's	$30.18	Salsalate, RID	54807-0140-01
100's	**$44.94**	**DISALCID, 3M Pharms**	**00089-0149-10**
500's	$37.45	Salsalate 500, Major Pharms	00904-1250-40
500's	$37.45	Salsalate, Major Pharms	00904-1253-40
500's	$42.00	Salsalate, United Res	00677-1024-05
500's	$42.00	Salsalate, Mutual Pharm	53489-0465-05
500's	$49.80	Salsalate, Caraco Pharm	57664-0103-13
500's	$49.80	Salsalate, Caraco Pharm	57664-0203-13
500's	$53.04	Salsalate, HL Moore Drug Exch	00839-7167-12
500's	$55.00	Salsalate (Yellow), Rosemont	00832-1037-50
500's	$75.10	Salsalate, Martec Pharms	52555-0560-05
500's	$79.95	Salsalate, Eon Labs Mfg	00185-0761-05
500's	$79.95	Salsalate (Blue) Tablets 500 Mg, Eon Labs Mfg	00185-0856-05
500's	$87.82	SALSITAB, Upsher Smith	00245-0153-15
500's	$98.66	Salsalate, Duramed Pharms	51285-0296-04
500's	$99.50	Salsalate, Eon Labs Mfg	00185-0693-05
500's	$99.50	Salsalate, Aligen Independ	00405-4934-02
500's	$99.50	Salsalate, Geneva Pharms	00781-1108-05
500's	$99.50	Salsalate, Sidmak Labs	50111-0390-02
500's	$118.83	Salsalate, Alpharma	00472-0132-50
500's	**$213.06**	**DISALCID, 3M Pharms**	**00089-0149-50**
600's	$174.40	Salsalate, Medirex	57480-0411-06
1000's	$94.12	Salsalate, Caraco Pharm	57664-0103-18
1000's	$94.12	Salsalate, Caraco Pharm	57664-0203-18

Tablet, Coated - Oral - 750 mg

100's	$13.50	Salsalate 750, Major Pharms	00904-1251-60
100's	$13.50	Salsalate 750, Major Pharms	00904-1254-60
100's	$14.40	Salsalate, Qualitest Pharms	00603-5755-21
100's	$14.95	Salsalate, United Res	00677-1025-01
100's	$14.95	Salsalate, Mutual Pharm	53489-0466-01
100's	$15.12	Salsalate, Caraco Pharm	57664-0105-08
100's	$15.12	Salsalate, Caraco Pharm	57664-0184-08
100's	$15.75	SALICYLSALICYLIC ACID, Goldline Labs	00182-1803-01
100's	$15.75	Salsalate (Yellow), Rosemont	00832-1038-00
100's	$17.75	Salsalate, HL Moore Drug Exch	00839-7168-06
100's	$22.16	Salsalate, Martec Pharms	52555-0561-01
100's	$22.40	MARTHRITIC, Marnel Pharceut	00682-0810-01
100's	$22.50	Salsalate, Eon Labs Mfg	00185-0762-01
100's	$22.50	Salsalate (Blue) Tablets 750 Mg, Eon Labs Mfg	00185-0857-01
100's	$26.00	SALICYLSALICYLIC ACID, Goldline Labs	00182-1803-89
100's	$26.33	SALSITAB, Upsher Smith	00245-0154-11
100's	$26.56	Salsalate, Duramed Pharms	51285-0297-02
100's	$27.98	Salsalate, Eon Labs Mfg	00185-0694-01
100's	$28.00	Salsalate, Aligen Independ	00405-4935-01
100's	$28.00	Salsalate, Geneva Pharms	00781-1109-01
100's	$28.00	Salsalate, Sidmak Labs	50111-0391-01
100's	$28.16	MONO-GESIC, Schwarz Pharma (US)	00131-2164-37
100's	$28.33	SALSITAB, Upsher Smith	00245-0154-01
100's	$28.50	Salsalate, Schein Pharm (US)	00364-0833-01
100's	$29.84	Salsalate 750, Major Pharms	00904-1251-61
100's	$30.00	Salsalate, Vangard Labs	00615-2553-13
100's	$30.15	SALFLEX, Carnrick	00086-0072-10
100's	$32.03	Salsalate, Alpharma	00472-0133-10
100's	$32.03	Salsalate, Rugby	00536-4523-01
100's	$42.43	Salsalate, RID	54807-0141-01
100's	**$57.54**	**DISALCID, 3M Pharms**	**00089-0151-10**
500'S	$126.14	Salsalate, Duramed Pharms	51285-0297-04
500's	$58.45	Salsalate 750, Major Pharms	00904-1251-40
500's	$58.45	Salsalate 750, Major Pharms	00904-1254-40
500's	$60.00	Salsalate, United Res	00677-1025-05
500's	$60.00	Salsalate, Mutual Pharm	53489-0466-05
500's	$61.08	Salsalate, Qualitest Pharms	00603-5755-28
500's	$62.45	Salsalate, Goldline Labs	00182-1803-05
500's	$62.45	Salsalate (Yellow), Rosemont	00832-1038-50
500's	$66.54	Salsalate, HL Moore Drug Exch	00839-7168-12
500's	$70.18	Salsalate, Caraco Pharm	57664-0184-13
500's	$70.80	Salsalate, Caraco Pharm	57664-0105-13
500's	$97.50	Salsalate, Eon Labs Mfg	00185-0762-05
500's	$97.50	Salsalate (Blue) Tablets 750 Mg, Eon Labs Mfg	00185-0857-05
500's	$98.60	Salsalate, Martec Pharms	52555-0561-05
500's	$121.00	SALFLEX, Carnrick	00086-0072-50
500's	$124.11	SALSITAB, Upsher Smith	00245-0154-15
500's	$126.50	Salsalate, Eon Labs Mfg	00185-0694-05
500's	$127.25	Salsalate, Aligen Independ	00405-4935-02
500's	$127.25	Salsalate, Geneva Pharms	00781-1109-05
500's	$127.25	Salsalate, Sidmak Labs	50111-0391-02
500's	$133.83	MONO-GESIC, Schwarz Pharma (US)	00131-2164-41
500's	$151.95	Salsalate, Alpharma	00472-0133-50
500's	**$272.52**	**DISALCID, 3M Pharms**	**00089-0151-50**
1000's	$131.40	Salsalate, Caraco Pharm	57664-0105-18
1000's	$131.40	Salsalate, Caraco Pharm	57664-0184-18

Tablet, Coated, Sustained Action - Oral - 500 mg

100's	$16.80	ARGESIC-SA, Embrex Economed	38130-0711-01

SAQUINAVIR MESYLATE *(003250)*

CATEGORIES: AIDS Related Complex; Anti-Infectives; Antimicrobials; Antivirals; HIV Infection; Infections; Protease Inhibitors; Viral Agents; FDA Approval 1995 Feb

BRAND NAMES: **Invirase**

FORMULARIES: PCS

> **WARNING:**
> The indication for saquinavir mesylate for the treatment of HIV infection is based on changes in surrogate markers. At present there are no results from controlled clinical trials evaluating the effect of regimens containing saquinavir mesylate on survival or the clinical progression of HIV infection, such as the occurrence of opportunistic infections or malignancies.

DESCRIPTION:

Saquinavir mesylate is an inhibitor of the human immunodeficiency virus (HIV) protease. Saquinavir mesylate is available as light brown and green, opaque hard gelatin capsules for oral administration in a 200-mg strength (as saquinavir free base). Each capsule also contains the inactive ingredients lactose, microcrystalline cellulose, povidone K30, sodium starch glycolate, talc and magnesium stearate. Each capsule shell contains gelatin and water with the following dye systems: red iron oxide, yellow iron oxide, black iron oxide, FD&C Blue #2 and titanium dioxide. The chemical name for saquinavir mesylate is N-tert-butyl-decahydro-2-[2(R)-hydroxy -4-phenyl - 3(S)-[[N-(2-quinolylcarbonyl)-L-asparaginyl]amino]butyl]-(4aS,8aS)-isoquinoline-3(S)-carboxamide methanesulfonate with a molecular formula $C_{38}H_{50}N_6O_5\ CH_4O_3S$ and a molecular weight of 766.96. The molecular weight of the free base is 670.86.

Saquinavir mesylate is a white to off-white, very fine powder with an aqueous solubility of 2.22 mg/mL at 25°C.

CLINICAL PHARMACOLOGY:

MECHANISM OF ACTION

HIV protease cleaves viral polyprotein precursors to generate functional proteins in HIV-infected cells. The cleavage of viral polyprotein precursors is essential for maturation of infectious virus. Saquinavir mesylate, henceforth referred to as saquinavir, is a synthetic peptide-like substrate analogue that inhibits the activity of HIV protease and prevents the cleavage of viral polyproteins.

MICROBIOLOGY

Antiviral Activity *In Vitro*: The *in vitro* antiviral activity of saquinavir was assessed in lymphoblastoid and monocytic cell lines and in peripheral blood lymphocytes. Saquinavir inhibited HIV activity in both acutely and chronically infected cells. IC50 values (50% inhibitory concentration) were in the range of 1 to 30 nM. In cell culture saquinavir demonstrated additive to synergistic effects against HIV in double and triple combination regimens with reverse transcriptase inhibitors zidovudine (ZDV), zalcitabine (ddC) and didanosine (ddI), without enhanced cytotoxicity.

Resistance: HIV isolates with reduced susceptibility to saquinavir have been selected *in vitro*. Genotypic analyses of these isolates showed substitution mutations in the HIV protease at amino acid positions 48 (Glycine to Valine) and 90 (Leucine to Methionine).

Phenotypic and genotypic changes in HIV isolates from patients treated with saquinavir were also monitored in Phase 1/2 clinical trials. Phenotypic changes were defined as a tenfold decrease in sensitivity from baseline. Two viral protease mutations (L90M and/or G48V, the former predominating) were found in virus from treated, but not untreated, patients. The incidence across studies of phenotypic and genotypic changes in the subsets of patients studied for a period of 16 to 74 weeks (median observation time approximately 1 year) is shown in TABLE 1. However, the clinical relevance of phenotypic and genotypic changes associated with saquinavir therapy has not been established.

TABLE 1 Frequency of Genotypic and Phenotypic Changes in Selected Patients Treated with Saquinavir

	Genotypic *	Phenotypic †
Monotherapy	15/33 (45%)	5/11 (45%)
Combination Therapy	16/52 (31%)	11/29 (38%)

* Double mutation (G48V and L90M) has occurred in 2 of 33 patients receiving monotherapy.
† For some patients genotypic and phenotypic changes were unrelated.

Cross-resistance to Other Antiretrovirals: The potential for HIV cross- resistance between protease inhibitors has not been fully explored. Therefore, it is unknown what effect saquinavir therapy will have on the activity of subsequent protease inhibitors. Cross-resistance between saquinavir and reverse transcriptase inhibitors is unlikely because of the different enzyme targets involved. ZDV-resistant HIV isolates have been shown to be sensitive to saquinavir *in vitro*.

PHARMACOKINETICS

The pharmacokinetic properties of saquinavir have been evaluated in healthy volunteers (n=351) and HIV-infected patients (n=270) after single and multiple oral doses of 25, 75, 200 and 600 mg tid and in healthy volunteers after intravenous doses of 6, 12, 36 or 72 mg (n=21).

Absorption and Bioavailability in Adults: Following multiple dosing (600 mg tid) in HIV-infected patients (n=29), the steady-state area under the plasma concentration versus time curve (AUC) was 2.5 times (95% Cl 1.6 to 3.8) higher than that observed after a single dose. HIV-infected patients administered saquinavir 600 mg tid, with the instructions to take saquinavir after a meal or substantial snack, had AUC and maximum plasma concentration (C_{max}) values which were about twice those observed in healthy volunteers receiving the same treatment regimen. (TABLE 2).

TABLE 2 Mean (%CV) AUC and C $_{max}$ in Patients and Healthy Volunteers

	AUC_8(dose interval) (ng•h/mL)	C_{max}(ng/mL)
Healthy Volunteers (n=6)	359.0 (46)	90.39 (49)
Patients (n=113)	757.2 (84)	253.3 (99)

Absolute bioavailability averaged 4% (CV 73%, range: 1% to 9%) in 8 healthy volunteers who received a single 600 mg dose (3 x 200 mg) of saquinavir following a high fat breakfast (48 g protein, 60 g carbohydrate, 57 g fat; 1006 kcal). The low bioavailability is thought to be due to a combination of incomplete absorption and extensive first-pass metabolism.

Food Effect: The mean 24-hour AUC after a single 600 mg oral dose (6 x 100 mg) in healthy volunteers (n=6) was increased from 24 ng·h/mL (CV 33%), under fasting conditions, to 161 ng·h/mL (CV 35%) when saquinavir was given following a high fat breakfast (48 g protein, 60 g carbohydrate, 57 g fat; 1006 kcal). Saquinavir 24-hour AUC and C_{max} (n=6) following the administration of a higher calorie meal (943 kcal, 54 g fat) were on average two times higher than after a lower calorie, lower fat meal (355 kcal, 8 g fat). The effect of food has been shown to persist for up to 2 hours.

Distribution in Adults: The mean steady-state volume of distribution following intravenous administration of a 12-mg dose of saquinavir (n=8) was 700 L (CV 39%), suggesting saquinavir partitions into tissues. Saquinavir was approximately 98% bound to plasma proteins over a concentration range of 15 to 700 ng/mL. In 2 patients receiving saquinavir 600 mg tid, cerebrospinal fluid concentrations were negligible when compared to concentrations from matching plasma samples.

Metabolism and Elimination in Adults: *In vitro* studies using human liver microsomes have shown that the metabolism of saquinavir is cytochrome P450 mediated with the specific isoenzyme, CYP3A4, responsible for more than 90% of the hepatic metabolism. Based on *in vitro* studies, saquinavir is rapidly metabolized to a range of mono- and di-hydroxylated inactive compounds. In a mass balance study using 600 mg ^{14}C-saquinavir (n=8), 88% and 1% of the orally administered radioactivity, was recovered in feces and urine, respectively,

CLINICAL PHARMACOLOGY: *(cont'd)*

within 48 hours of dosing. In an additional 4 subjects administered 10.5 mg ^{14}C-saquinavir intravenously, 81% and 3% of the intravenously administered radioactivity was recovered in feces and urine, respectively, within 48 hours of dosing. In mass balance studies, 13% of circulating radioactivity in plasma was attributed to unchanged drug after oral administration and the remainder attributed to saquinavir metabolites. Following intravenous administration, 66% of circulating radioactivity was attributed to unchanged drug and the remainder attributed to saquinavir metabolites, suggesting that saquinavir undergoes extensive first-pass metabolism.

Systemic clearance of saquinavir was rapid, 1.14 L/h/kg (CV 12%) after intravenous doses of 6, 36 and 72 mg. The mean residence time of saquinavir was 7 hours (n=8).

SPECIAL POPULATIONS

Hepatic or Renal Impairment: Saquinavir pharmacokinetics in patients with hepatic or renal insufficiency has not been investigated (see PRECAUTIONS.)

Gender, Race and Age: Pharmacokinetic data were available for 17 women in the Phase 1/2 studies. Pooled data did not reveal an apparent effect of gender on the pharmacokinetics of saquinavir.

The effect of race on the pharmacokinetics of saquinavir has not been evaluated, due to the small numbers of minorities for whom pharmacokinetic data were available.

Saquinavir pharmacokinetics has not been investigated in patients >65 years of age or in pediatric patients (<16 years).

CLINICAL STUDIES:

The activity of saquinavir mesylate in combination with HIVID and/or ZDV in HIV infection has been evaluated in three double-blind, randomized trials in a total of 810 patients with advanced HIV infection.

Advanced Patients without Prior ZDV Therapy: A dose-ranging study (Italy, V13330) conducted in 92 ZDV-naive patients (mean baseline CD_4=179) studied saquinavir mesylate at doses of 75 mg, 200 mg and 600 mg tid in combination with ZDV 200 mg tid compared to saquinavir mesylate 600 mg tid alone and ZDV alone. In analyses of average CD_4 changes over 16 weeks, treatment with the combination of saquinavir mesylate 600 mg tid + ZDV produced greater CD_4 cell increases than ZDV monotherapy. The CD_4 changes of ZDV in combination with doses of saquinavir mesylate lower than 600 mg tid were no greater than that of ZDV alone.

Advanced Patients with Prior ZDV Therapy: In ACTG229/NV14255, 295 patients (mean baseline CD_4=165) with prolonged ZDV treatment (median 713 days) were randomized to receive either saquinavir mesylate 600 mg tid + HIVID + ZDV (triple combination), saquinavir mesylate 600 mg tid + ZDV or HIVID + ZDV. In analyses of average CD_4 changes over 24 weeks, the triple combination produced greater increases in CD_4 cell counts compared to that of HIVID + ZDV. There were no significant differences in CD_4 changes among patients receiving saquinavir mesylate + ZDV and HIVID + ZDV.

Study NV14256 (North America) is an ongoing, randomized, double-blind study comparing saquinavir mesylate 600 mg tid + HIVID to HIVID monotherapy and saquinavir mesylate monotherapy in patients with advanced HIV infection and at least 16 weeks of prior ZDV treatment. The study remains blinded with respect to clinical endpoints of disease progression; however, analyses of CD_4 changes over 16 weeks were conducted for a cohort of 423 patients. These analyses showed that the combination of saquinavir mesylate + HIVID was associated with greater CD_4 increases than either HIVID or saquinavir mesylate as monotherapy.

Comparisons of data across studies (NV14256 compared to ACTG229/NV14255) suggest that when saquinavir mesylate was added to a regimen of prolonged prior zidovudine, there was little activity contributed by continuing ZDV.

HIV RNA: The clinical significance of changes in HIV-RNA measurements have not been established. At present, this laboratory measure is available on an experimental basis to monitor antiviral activity in clinical trials. Table 3 compares log RNA reductions at 16 weeks among saquinavir mesylate combination treatment arms in three clinical trials. Monotherapy arms are included for reference. Overall, RNA reductions were greater in saquinavir mesylate/nucleoside combination regimens compared to nucleoside monotherapy controls.

TABLE 3A Summary of Mean Log $_{10}$Plasma RNA Results from Major Clinical Studies*

V13330 (Italy) Naive Patients	ZDV	SAQ†	ZDV+SAQ†
n enrolled	17	19	20
Prior ZDV			
n	-	-	-
Median Duration (days)	-	-	-
Log $_{10}$ Plasma RNA by PCR (copies/ml)			
n	17	19	20
Mean Baseline (n)	5.2 (13)	5.2 (15)	5.2 (15)
Mean Change from Baseline Week 16	-0.6	-0.2	-1.0
Mean Change from Baseline Week 24	-	-	-

* NOTE: THE CLINICAL SIGNIFICANCE OF CHANGES IN HIV VIRAL RNA DURING THERAPY IS UNKNOWN.
† Saquinavir (SAQ) at 600 mg tid
- Indicates not applicable

TABLE 3B Summary of Mean Log $_{10}$Plasma RNA Results from Major Clinical Studies*

NV14255/ACTG229 (USA) ZDV-experienced	ZDV + ddC	ZDV + SAQ†	ZDV + ddC + SAQ†
n enrolled	100	99	98
Prior ZDV			
n	99	98	97
Median Duration (days)	659	713	647
Log $_{10}$ Plasma RNA by PCR (copies/ml)			
n	100	97	96
Mean Baseline (n)	4.7 (100)	4.8 (97)	4.8 (96)
Mean Change from Baseline Week 16	-0.3	0.0	-0.5
Mean Change from Baseline Week 24	-0.2	0.0	-0.5

* NOTE: THE CLINICAL SIGNIFICANCE OF CHANGES IN HIV VIRAL RNA DURING THERAPY IS UNKNOWN.
† Saquinavir (SAQ) at 600 mg tid
- Indicates not applicable

INDICATIONS AND USAGE:

Saquinavir mesylate in combination with nucleoside analogues is indicated for the treatment of advanced HIV infection in selected patients (see CLINICAL STUDIES.) This indication is based on changes in surrogate markers in patients who initiated saquinavir mesylate concomitantly with either ZDV (in previously untreated patients) or HIVID (in patients previously treated with prolonged zidovudine therapy). At present, there are no results available

INDICATIONS AND USAGE: *(cont'd)*

TABLE 3C Summary of Mean Log $_{10}$ Plasma RNA Results from Major Clinical Studies*

Surrogate Marker Analysis NV14256 (North America)	ddC	SAQ†	SAQ †+ ddc
n enrolled	145	159	147
Prior ZDV			
n	134	151	136
Median Duration (days)	614	459	442
Log $_{10}$ Plasma RNA by PCR (copies/ml)			
n	114	124	119
Mean Baseline (n)	5.2 (114)	5.1 (124)	5.1 (119)
Mean Change from Baseline Week 16	-0.4	-0.1	-0.6
Mean Change from Baseline Week 24	-	-	-

* NOTE: THE CLINICAL SIGNIFICANCE OF CHANGES IN HIV VIRAL RNA DURING THERAPY IS UNKNOWN.
† Saquinavir (SAQ) at 600 mg tid
- Indicates not applicable

from trials evaluating the activity of saquinavir mesylate in combination with nucleoside analogues other than ZDV or HIVID. There are also no results available from clinical trials confirming the clinical benefit of combination therapy with saquinavir mesylate on HIV disease progression or survival.

CONTRAINDICATIONS:

Saquinavir mesylate is contraindicated in patients with clinically significant hypersensitivity to saquinavir or to any of the components contained in the capsule.

PRECAUTIONS:

GENERAL

The safety profile of saquinavir mesylate in children younger than 16 years has not been established.

If a serious or severe toxicity occurs during treatment with saquinavir mesylate, saquinavir mesylate should be interrupted until the etiology of the event is identified or the toxicity resolves. At that time, resumption of treatment with full dose saquinavir mesylate may be considered. For nucleoside analogues used in combination with saquinavir mesylate, physicians should refer to the complete product information for these drugs for dose adjustment recommendations and for information regarding drug-associated adverse reactions.

Caution should be exercised when administering saquinavir mesylate to patients with hepatic insufficiency since patients with baseline liver function tests >5 times the upper limit of normal were not included in clinical studies.

Resistance/Cross-resistance: The potential for HIV cross-resistance between protease inhibitors has not been fully explored. Therefore, it is unknown what effect saquinavir therapy will have on the activity of subsequent protease inhibitors (see CLINICAL PHARMACOLOGY, Microbiology.)

INFORMATION FOR THE PATIENT

Patients should be informed that saquinavir mesylate is not a cure for HIV infection and that they may continue to acquire illnesses associated with advanced HIV infection, including opportunistic infections. Saquinavir mesylate has not been shown to reduce the incidence or frequency of such illnesses, and patients should be advised to remain under the care of a physician while using saquinavir mesylate.

Patients should be told that the long-term effects of saquinavir mesylate are unknown at this time. They should be informed that saquinavir mesylate therapy has not been shown to reduce the risk of transmitting HIV to others through sexual contact or blood contamination.

Patients should be advised that saquinavir mesylate should be taken within 2 hours after a full meal (see Pharmacokinetics). When saquinavir mesylate is taken without food, concentrations of saquinavir in the blood are substantially reduced and may result in no antiviral activity.

LABORATORY TESTS

No consistent alterations in standard laboratory tests have been associated with the use of saquinavir mesylate. Clinical chemistry tests should be performed prior to initiating saquinavir mesylate therapy and at appropriate intervals thereafter. For comprehensive information concerning laboratory test alterations associated with use of individual nucleoside analogues, physicians should refer to the complete product information for these drugs.

CARCINOGENESIS, MUTAGENESIS AND IMPAIRMENT OF FERTILITY

Carcinogenesis: Carcinogenicity studies in rats and mice have not yet been completed.

Mutagenesis: Mutagenicity and genotoxicity studies, with and without metabolic activation where appropriate, have shown that saquinavir has no mutagenic activity *in vitro* in either bacterial (Ames test) or mammalian cells (Chinese hamster lung V79/HPRT test). Saquinavir does not induce chromosomal damage *in vivo* in the mouse micronucleus assay or *in vitro* in human peripheral blood lymphocytes, and does not induce primary DNA damage *in vitro* in the unscheduled DNA synthesis test.

Impairment of Fertility: Fertility and reproductive performance were not affected in rats at plasma exposures (AUC values) up to five times those achieved in humans at the recommended dose.

PREGNANCY, TERATOGENIC EFFECTS, PREGNANCY CATEGORY B

Reproduction studies conducted with saquinavir in rats have shown no embryotoxicity or teratogenicity at plasma exposures (AUC values) up to five times those achieved in humans at the recommended dose or in rabbits at plasma exposures four times those achieved at the recommended clinical dose. Studies in rats indicated that exposure to saquinavir from late pregnancy through lactation at plasma concentrations (AUC values) up to five times those achieved in humans at the recommended dose had no effect on the survival, growth and development of offspring to weaning. Because animal reproduction studies are not always predictive of human response, saquinavir mesylate should be used during pregnancy after taking into account the importance of the drug to the mother. Presently, there are no reports of infants being born after women receiving saquinavir mesylate in clinical trials became pregnant.

NURSING MOTHERS

It is not known whether saquinavir mesylate is excreted in human milk. Because many drugs are excreted in human milk and because of the potential for serious adverse reactions in nursing infants from saquinavir, a decision should be made whether to discontinue nursing or discontinue the drug, taking into account the importance of saquinavir mesylate to the mother.

PEDIATRIC USE

Safety and effectiveness of saquinavir mesylate in HIV-infected children or adolescents younger than 16 years of age have not been established.

DRUG INTERACTIONS:

Hivid and ZDV: Concomitant use of saquinavir mesylate with Hivid (zalcitabine, ddC) and ZDV has been studied (as triple combination) in adults. Pharmacokinetic data suggest that the absorption, metabolism and elimination of each of these drugs are unchanged when they are used together.

Ketoconazole: Concomitant administration of ketoconazole (200 mg qd) and saquinavir (600 mg tid) to 12 healthy volunteers resulted in steady-state saquinavir AUC and C_{max} values which were three times those seen with saquinavir alone. No dose adjustment is required when the two drugs are coadministered at the doses studied. Ketoconazole pharmacokinetics was unaffected by coadministration with saquinavir.

Rifampin: Coadministration of rifampin (600 mg qd) and saquinavir (600 mg tid) to 12 healthy volunteers decreased the steady-state AUC and C_{max} of saquinavir by approximately 80%.

Rifabutin: Preliminary data from 12 HIV-infected patients indicate that the steady-state AUC of saquinavir (600 mg tid) was decreased by 40% when saquinavir was coadministered with rifabutin (300 mg qd).

Metabolic Enzyme Inducers: Saquinavir mesylate should not be administered concomitantly with rifampin, since rifampin decreases saquinavir concentrations by 80%. Rifabutin also substantially reduces saquinavir plasma concentrations by 40%. Other drugs that induce CYP3A4 (*e.g.,* phenobarbital, phenytoin, dexamethasone, carbamazepine) may also reduce saquinavir plasma concentrations. If therapy with such drugs is warranted, physicians should consider using alternatives when a patient is taking saquinavir mesylate.

Other Potential Interactions: Coadministration of terfenadine or astemizole with drugs that are known to be potent inhibitors of the cytochrome P4503A pathway (*i.e.,* ketoconazole, itraconazole, etc.) may lead to elevated plasma concentrations of terfenadine or astemizole, which may in turn prolong QT intervals leading to rare cases of serious cardiovascular adverse events. Although saquinavir mesylate is not a strong inhibitor of cytochrome P4503A, pharmacokinetic interaction studies with saquinavir mesylate and terfenadine or astemizole have not been conducted. Physicians should use alternatives to terfenadine or astemizole when a patient taking saquinavir mesylate requires antihistamines. Other compounds that are substrates of CYP3A4 (*e.g.,* calcium channel blockers, clindamycin, dapsone, quinidine, triazolam) may have elevated plasma concentrations when coadministered with saquinavir mesylate; therefore, patients should be monitored for toxicities associated with such drugs.

ADVERSE REACTIONS:

(See PRECAUTIONS): The safety of saquinavir mesylate was studied in 688 patients who received the drug either alone or in combination with ZDV and/or HIVID (zalcitabine, ddC). The majority of adverse events were of mild intensity. The most frequently reported adverse events among patients receiving saquinavir mesylate (excluding those toxicities known to be associated with ZDV and HIVID when used in combinations) were diarrhea, abdominal discomfort and nausea.

Saquinavir mesylate did not alter the pattern, frequency or severity of known major toxicities associated with the use of HIVID and/or ZVD. Physicians should refer to the complete product information for these drugs (or other antiretroviral agents as appropriate) for drug-associated adverse reactions to other nucleoside analogues.

TABLE 4 lists clinical adverse events that occurred in ≥2% of patients receiving saquinavir mesylate 600 mg tid alone or in combination with ZDV and/or HIVID in two trials. Median duration of treatment in NV14255/ACTG229 (triple combination study) was 48 weeks; median duration of treatment among the surrogate analysis cohort analyzed for safety (n=451) in NV14256 was 42 weeks.

TABLE 4A Percentage of Patients, by Study Arm, with Clinical Adverse Experiences Considered at Least Possibly Related to Study Drug or of Unknown Relationship and of Moderate, Severe or Life-Threatening Intensity. Occurring in ≥2% of the Patients in NV14255/ACTG229 and N14256

	NV14255/ACTG229		
Adverse Event	**SAQ+ZDV n=99**	**SAQ+ddC+ZDV n=98**	**ddC+ZDV n=100**
Gastrointestinal			
Dirrhea	3.0	1.0	-
Abdominal Discomfort	2.0	3.1	4.0
Nausea	-	3.1	3.0
Dyspepsia	1.0	1.0	2.0
Abdominal pain	2.0	1.0	2.0
Mucosa Damage	-	-	4.0
Buccal Mucosa Ulceration	-	2.0	2.0
Central And Peripheral Nervous System			
Headeache	2.0	2.0	2.0
Paresthesia	2.0	3.1	4.0
Extremity Numbness	2.0	1.0	4.0
Dizziness	-	2.0	1.0
Peripheral Neuropathy	-	1.0	2.0
Body As A Whole			
Asthenia	6.1	9.2	10.0
Appetite Disturbances	-	1.0	2.0
Skin And Appendages			
Rash	-	-	3.0
Pruritus	-	-	2.0
Musculoskeletal Disorders			
Musculoskeletal Pain	2.0	2.0	4.0
Myalgia	1.0	-	3.0

- Indicates no events reported

Rare occurrences of the following serious adverse experiences have been reported during clinical trials of saquinavir mesylate and were considered at least possibly related to use of study drugs: confusion, ataxia and weakness; acute myeloblastic leukemia; hemolytic anemia; attempted suicide; Stevens-Johnson syndrome; seizures; severe cutaneous reaction associated with increased liver function tests; isolated elevation of transaminases, thrombophlebitis, headache and thrombocytopenia; exacerbation of chronic liver disease with Grade 4 elevated liver function tests, jaundice, ascites, and right and left upper quadrant abdominal pain.

TABLE 5 shows the percentage of patients with marked laboratory abnormalities in studies NV14255/ACTG229 and NV14256. Marked laboratory abnormalities are defined as a Grade 3 or 4 abnormality in a patient with a normal baseline value or a Grade 4 abnormality in a patient with a Grade 1 abnormality at baseline (ACTG Grading System).

Monotherapy and Combination Studies: Other clinical adverse experiences of any intensity, at least remotely related to saquinavir mesylate, including those in <2% of patients on arms containing saquinavir mesylate in studies NV14255/ACTG229 and NV14256, and those in smaller clinical trials, are listed below by body system.

Body as a Whole: Allergic reaction, chest pain, edema, fever, intoxication, parasites external, retrosternal pain, shivering, wasting syndrome, weight decrease

ADVERSE REACTIONS: *(cont'd)*

TABLE 4B Percentage of Patients, by Study Arm, with Clinical Adverse Experiences Considered at Least Possibly Related to Study Drug or of Unknown Relationship and of Moderate, Severe or Life-Threatening Intensity. Occurring in ≥2% of the Patients in NV14255/ACTG229 and N14256

	NV14256		
Adverse Event	**ddC n=145**	**SAQ n=159**	**SAQ+ddC n=147**
Gastrointestinal			
Dirrhea	1.4	3.8	3.4
Abdominal Discomfort	1.4	1.3	0.7
Nausea	0.7	1.9	0.7
Dyspepsia	2.1	-	0.7
Abdominal pain	0.7	1.9	0.7
Mucosa Damage	1.4	-	0.7
Buccal Mucosa Ulceration	9.0	2.5	4.1
Central And Peripheral Nervous System			
Headeache	4.1	0.6	0.7
Paresthesia	0.7	1.0	1.0
Extremity Numbness	-	-	0.7
Dizziness	-	-	-
Peripheral Neuropathy	5.5	-	4.8
Body As A Whole			
Asthenia	0.7	1.3	0.7
Appetite Disturbances	-	-	-
Skin And Appendages			
Rash	0.7	1.3	0.7
Pruritus	-	-	-
Musculoskeletal Disorders			
Musculoskeletal Pain	-	0.6	0.7
Myalgia	1.4	-	-

- Indicates no events reported

TABLE 5A Percentage of Patients, by Treatment Group, with Marked Laboratory Abnormalities* in NV14255/ACTG229

	NV14255/ACTG229		
Adverse Event	**SAQ+ZDV n=99**	**SAQ+ddC+ZDV n=98**	**ddC+ZDV n=100**
Biochemistry			
Calcium (high)	1	0	0
Creatine Phosphokinase	10	12	7
Glucose (low)	0	0	0
Glucose (high)	0	0	0
Phosphorus	2	1	0
Potassium (high)	0	0	0
Potassium (low)	0	0	0
Serum Amylase	2	1	1
SGOT (AST)	2	2	0
SGPT (ALT)	0	3	1
Total Bilirubin	1	0	0
Uric Acid	0	0	1
Hematology			
Neutrophols (low)	2	2	8
Hemoglobin (low)	0	0	1
Platelets (low)	0	0	2

* Marked Laboratory Abnormality defined as a shift from Grade 0 to at least Grade 3 from Grade 1 to Grade 4 (ACTG Grading System)

TABLE 5B Percentage of Patients, by Treatment Group, with Marked Laboratory Abnormalities* in N14256

	NV14256		
Adverse Event	**ddC n=145**	**SAQ n=159**	**SAQ+ddC n=147**
Biochemistry			
Calcium (high)	<1	0	0
Creatine Phosphokinase	6	4	7
Glucose (low)	4	5	4
Glucose (high)	0	<1	<1
Phosphorus	0	0	0
Potassium (high)	1	<1	<1
Potassium (low)	0	<1	0
Serum Amylase	<1	<1	2
SGOT (AST)	3	<1	<1
SGPT (ALT)	3	<1	<1
Total Bilirubin	0	<1	0
Uric Acid	not assessed	not assessed	not assessed
Hematology			
Neutrophols (low)	0	0	0
Hemoglobin (low)	0	<1	0
Platelets (low)	0	0	<1

* Marked Laboratory Abnormality defined as a shift from Grade 0 to at least Grade 3 from Grade 1 to Grade 4 (ACTG Grading System)

Cardiovascular: Cyanosis, heart murmur, heart valve disorder, hypertension, hypotension, syncope, vein distended

Endocrine/Metabolic: Dehydration, dry eye syndrome, hyperglycemia, weight increase, xerophthalmia

Gastrointestinal: Cheilitis, constipation, dysphagia, eructation, feces bloodstained, feces discolored, gastralgia, gastritis, gastrointestinal inflammation, gingivitis, glossitis, hemorrhage rectum, hemorrhoids, hepatomegaly, hepatosplenomegaly, melena, pain pelvic, painful defecation, pancreatitis, parotid disorder, salivary glands disorder, stomatitis, tooth disorder, vomiting

Hematologic: Anemia, microhemorrhages, pancytopenia, splenomegaly, thrombocytopenia

Musculoskeletal: Arthralgia, arthritis, back pain, cramps muscle, musculoskeletal disorders, stiffness, tissue changes, trauma

Neurological: Ataxia, bowel movements frequent, confusion, convulsions, dysarthria, dysesthesia, heart rate disorder, hyperesthesia, hyperreflexia, hyporeflexia, mouth dry, numbness face, pain facial, paresis, poliomyelitis, progressive multifocal leukoencephalopathy, spasms, tremor

Psychological: Agitation, amnesia, anxiety, depression, dreaming excessive, euphoria, hallucination, insomnia, intellectual ability reduced, irritability, lethargy, libido disorder, overdose effect, psychic disorder, somnolence, speech disorder

Reproductive System: Prostate enlarged, vaginal discharge

ADVERSE REACTIONS: *(cont'd)*

Resistance Mechanism: Abscess, angina tonsillaris, candidiasis, hepatitis, herpes simplex, herpes zoster, infection bacterial, infection mycotic, infection staphylococcal, influenza, lymphadenopathy, tumor

Respiratory: Bronchitis, cough, dyspnea, epistaxis, hemoptysis, laryngitis, pharyngitis, pneumonia, respiratory disorder, rhinitis, sinusitis, upper respiratory tract infection

Skin and Appendages: Acne, dermatitis, dermatitis seborrheic, eczema, erythema, folliculitis, furunculosis, hair changes, hot flushes, photosensitivity reaction, pigment changes skin, rash maculopapular, skin disorder, skin nodule, skin ulceration, sweating increased, urticaria, verruca, xeroderma

Special Senses: Blepharitis, earache, ear pressure, eye irritation, hearing decreased, otitis, taste alteration, tinnitus, visual disturbance

Urinary System: Micturition disorder, urinary tract infection

OVERDOSAGE:

No acute toxicities or sequelae were noted in 1 patient who ingested 8 grams of saquinavir mesylate as a single dose. The patient was treated with induction of emesis within 2 to 4 hours after ingestion. In an exploratory Phase 2 study of oral dosing with saquinavir mesylate at 7200 mg/day (1200 mg q4h), there were no serious toxicities reported through the first 25 weeks of treatment.

DOSAGE AND ADMINISTRATION:

The recommended dose for saquinavir mesylate in combination with a nucleoside analogue is three 200-mg capsules three times daily taken within 2 hours after a full meal. The recommended doses of HIVID (zalcitabine, ddC) or ZDV as part of combination therapy are: HIVID 0.75 mg three times daily or ZDV, 200 mg three times daily as appropriate.

Monitoring of Patients: Clinical chemistry tests should be performed prior to initiating saquinavir mesylate therapy and at appropriate intervals thereafter. For comprehensive patient monitoring recommendations for other nucleoside analogues, physicians should refer to the complete product information for these drugs.

Dose Adjustment for Combination Therapy with Saquinavir Mesylate: For toxicities that may be associated with saquinavir mesylate, the drug should be interrupted. Saquinavir mesylate at doses less than 600 mg tid are not recommended since lower doses have not shown antiviral activity. For recipients of combination therapy with saquinavir mesylate and nucleoside analogues, dose adjustment of the nucleoside analogue should be based on the known toxicity profile of the individual drug. Physicians should refer to the complete product information for these drugs for comprehensive dose adjustment recommendations and drug-associated adverse reactions of nucleoside analogues.

PATIENT INFORMATION:

Saquinavir is used in combination with other drugs for the treatment of advanced HIV infection. Saquinavir is not a cure for HIV infection. Other illnesses associated with HIV may continue to occur. Do not use if you are younger than 16 years old. Inform your doctor if you are pregnant, nursing, or taking any other medications. Take 3 times daily within 2 hours of a full meal. May cause diarrhea, stomach discomfort and nausea. Inform your doctor if these effects occur.

HOW SUPPLIED:

Invirase 200-mg capsules are light brown and green opaque capsules with Roche and 0245 imprinted on the capsule shell - bottles of 270.

The capsules should be stored at 59° to 86°F (15° to 30°C) in tightly closed bottles.

HOW SUPPLIED - EQUIVALENTS NOT AVAILABLE:

Capsule - Oral - 200 mg

270's $572.06 INVIRASE, Roche 00004-0245-15

SARGRAMOSTIM *(003050)*

CATEGORIES: Bone Marrow Transplantation; Hodgkin's Disease; Leukemia; Lymphoma; Malignancy, Lymphoid; Monoclonal Antibodies; Transplantation; Anemia*; HIV Infection*; Neutropenia, Chemotherapy*; Pregnancy Category C; Recombinant DNA Origin; FDA Approved 1991 Mar

* Indication not approved by the FDA

BRAND NAMES: GM-CSF; Granulocyte Macrophage-Colony Stimulating Factor; *Leucogen*; **Leukine**; Prokine

(International brand names outside U.S. in italics)

DESCRIPTION:

Leukine is a recombinant human granulocyte-macrophage colony stimulating factor (rhu GM-CSF) produced by recombinant DNA technology in a yeast (*S. cerevisiae*) expression system. GM-CSF is a hematopoietic growth factor which stimulates proliferation and differentiation of hematopoietic progenitor cells. Leukine is a glycoprotein of 127 amino acids characterized by 3 primary molecular species having molecular masses of 19,500, 16,800, and 15,500 daltons. The amino acid sequence of Leukine differs from the natural human GM-CSF by a substitution of leucine at position 23, and the carbohydrate moiety may be different from the native protein. Sargramostim has been selected as the proper name for yeast-derived rhu GM-CSF.

Leukine is formulated as a sterile, white, preservative-free, lyophilized powder and is intended for IV infusion following reconstitution with 1 ml of Sterile Water for Injection, USP. Each single-use vial of Leukine contains either 250 mcg or 500 mcg Sargramostim; 40 mg Mannitol, USP; 10 mg Sucrose, NF; and 1.2 mg Tromethamine, USP. The pH of the reconstituted, isotonic solution is 7.4 ± 0.3. The specific activity Leukine is approximately 5 × 10^7 colony forming units per mg in a normal human bone marrow colony formation assay.

CLINICAL PHARMACOLOGY:

General: Granulocyte-macrophage colony stimulating factor belongs to a group of growth factors termed colony stimulating factors which support survival, clonal expansion, and differentiation of hematopoietic progenitor cells. GM-CSF induces partially committed progenitor cells to divide and differentiate in the granulocyte-macrophage pathways.

GM-CSF is also capable of activating mature granulocytes and macrophages. GM-CSF is a multilineage factor and, in addition to dose- dependent effects on the myelomonocytic lineage, can promote the proliferation of megakaryocytic and erythroid progenitors.[1] However, other factors are required to induce complete maturation in these two lineages. The various cellular responses (*i.e.*, division, maturation, activation) are induced through GM-CSF binding to specific receptors expressed on the cell surface of target cells.[2]

In Vitro Studies of Sargramostim in Human Cells: The biological activity of GM-CSF is species-specific. Consequently, *in vitro* studies have been performed on human cells to characterize the pharmacological activity of sargramostim. *In vitro* exposure of human bone marrow cells to sargramostim at concentrations ranging from 1-100 ng/ml results in the proliferation of hematopoietic progenitors and in the formation of pure granulocyte, pure macrophage, and mixed granulocyte-macrophage colonies.[3] Chemotactic, anti-fungal and anti-parasitic[4] activities of granulocytes and monocytes are increased by exposure to Leukine *in vitro*. Sargramostim increases the cytotoxicity of monocytes toward certain neoplastic cell lines[3] and activates polymorphonuclear neutrophils to inhibit the growth of tumor cells.

In Vivo Primate Studies of Sargramostim: Pharmacology/toxicology studies of sargramostim were performed in cynomolgus monkeys. An acute toxicity study revealed an absence of treatment-related toxicity following a single IV bolus injection at a dose of 300 mcg/kg. Two subacute studies were performed using IV injection (maximum dose 200 mcg/kg/day x 14 days) and subcutaneous injection (maximum dose 200 mcg/kg/day x 28 days). No major visceral organ toxicity was documented. Notable histopathology findings included increased cellularity in hematologic organs, heart and lung tissues. A dose-dependent increase in leukocyte count occurred during the dosing period which consisted primarily of segmented neutrophils; increases in monocytes, basophils, eosinophils, and lymphocytes were also noted. Leukocyte counts decreased to pretreatment values over a 1-2 week recovery period.

Pharmacokinetics: Pharmacokinetic profiles have been analyzed in patients with various neoplastic diseases following intravenous administration of sargramostim. In 2 patients receiving 250 mcg/m^2 of sargramostim by 2 hour IV infusion, serum concentration ranged from 22,000 pg/ml to 23,000 pg/ml at the termination of the infusion. The pharmacokinetic profile, calculated on samples from 5 patients receiving 500-750 mcg/m^2 of sargramostim by 2 hour IV infusion, revealed a rapid initial decline in GM-CSF serum concentration ($t_{1/2\alpha}$ — 12 to 17 minutes) followed by a slower decrease ($t_{1/2\beta}$ — 2 hours). In four patients treated with sargramostim by subcutaneous injection (125 mcg/m^2 every 12 hours), sargramostim was detected in the serum within 5 minutes after administration (range 55-450 pg/ml). Peak levels were observed 2 hours after injection (range 350-3,900 pg/ml), and sargramostim remained at detectable levels 6 hours following injection (range 150-2,700 pg/ml).[5]

Antibody Formation: Serum samples collected before and after sargramostim treatment from 165 patients with a variety of underlying diseases have been examined for the presence of antibodies. Neutralizing antibodies were detected in 5 of 165 patients (3.0%) after receiving sargramostim by continuous IV infusion (3 patients) or subcutaneous injection (2 patients) for 28 to 84 days in multiple courses. All 5 patients had impaired hematopoiesis before the administration of sargramostim and consequently the effect of the development of anti-GM-CSF antibodies on normal hematopoiesis could not be assessed. Drug-induced neutropenia, neutralization of endogenous GM-CSF activity, and diminution of the therapeutic effect of sargramostim secondary to formation of neutralizing antibody remain a theoretical possibility. A systematic screening program to evaluate antibody formation is ongoing for patients enrolled in clinical trials.

CLINICAL STUDIES:

ACUTE MYELOGENOUS LEUKEMIA

The safety and efficacy of sargramostim in patients with AML who are younger than 55 years of age has not been determined. Based on phase 2 data suggesting the best therapeutic effects could be achieved in patients at highest risk for severe infections and mortality while neutropenic, the phase 3 clinical trial was conducted in older patients. The safety and efficacy of sargramostin in the treatment of AML were evaluated in a multi-center, randomized, double-blind placebo-controlled trial of 99 newly diagnosed adult patients, 55–70 years of age, receiving induction with or without consolidation. A combination of standard doses of daunorubicin (days 1–3) and ara-C (days 1–7) was administered during induction and high dose ara-C was administered days 1–6 as a single course of consolidation, if given. Bone-marrow evaluation was performed on day 10 following induction chemotherapy. If hypoplasia with <5% blasts was not achieved, patients immediately received a second cycle of induction chemotherapy. If the bone marrow was hypoplastic with <5% blasts on day 10 or 4 days following the second cycle of induction chemotherapy, sargramostim (250 mcg/m^2/day) or placebo was given IV over 4 hours each day, starting 4 days after the completion of chemotherapy. Study drug was continued until an ANC ≥ 1500/mm^3 for three consecutive days was attained or a maximum of 42 days. Sargramostin or placebo was also administered after the single course of consolidation chemotherapy if delivered (ara-C 3–6 weeks after induction following neutrophil recovery). Study drug was discontinued immediately if leukemic regrowth occurred.

Sargramostim significantly shortened the median duration of ANC <500/mm^3 by 4 days and <1000/mm^3 by 7 days following induction (see TABLE 1.) 75% of patients receiving sargramostin achieved ANC >500/mm^3 by day 16 compared to day 25 for patients receiving placebo. The proportion of patients receiving 1 cycle (70%) or 2 cycles (30%) of induction was similar in both treatment groups; sargramostim significantly shortened the median times to neutrophil recovery whether one cycle (12 versus 15 days) or two cycles (14 versus 23 days) of induction chemotherapy was administered. Median times to platelet (>20,000/mm^3) and RBC transfusion independence were not significantly different between treatment groups.

During the consolidation phase of treatment, sargramostin did not shorten the median time to recovery of ANC to 500/mm^3 (13 days) or 1000/mm^3 (14.5 days) compared to placebo. There were no significant differences in time to platelet and RBC transfusion independence.

TABLE 1 Hematologic Recovery: Induction

Dataset	Sargramostim N=52* Median (25%, 75%)	Placebo N=47 Median (25%, 75%)	p-value**
ANC>500/mm^3[a]	13 (11, 16)	17 (13, 25)	0.009
ANC>1000/mm^3[b]	14 (12, 18)	21 (13, 34)	0.003
PLT>20,000/mm^3[c]	11 (7, 14)	12 (9, >42)	0.010
RBC[d]	12 (9, 24)	14 (9, 42)	0.53

* Patients with missing data censored.
[a] 2 patients on sargramostim and 4 patients on placebo had missing values.
[b] 2 patients on sargramostim and 3 patients on placebo had missing values.
[c] 4 patients on placebo had missing values.
[d] 3 patients on sargramostim and 4 patients on placebo had missing values.
** p=Generalized Wilcoxon.

The incidence of severe infections and deaths associated with infections was significantly reduced in patients who received sargramostim. During induction or consolidation, 27 of 52 patients receiving sargramostim and 35 of 47 patients receiving placebo had at least one grade 3, 4 or 5 infection (p=0.02). Twenty-five patients receiving sargramostim and 30 patients receiving placebo experienced severe and fatal infections during induction only. There were significantly fewer deaths from infectious causes in the sargramostim arm (3 versus 11, p=0.02). The majority of deaths in the placebo group were associated with fungal infections with pneumonia as the primary infection.

Disease outcomes were not adversely affected by the use of sargramostim. The proportion of patients achieving complete remission (CR) was higher in the sargramostim group (69% as compared to 55% for the placebo group), but the difference was not significant (p=0.21). There was no significant difference in relapse rates; 12 of 36 patients who received sarg-

CLINICAL STUDIES: *(cont'd)*

ramostim and 5 of 26 patients who received placebo relapsed within 180 days of documented CR (p=0.26). The overall median survival was 378 days for patients receiving sargramostim and 268 days for those on placebo (p=0.17). The study was not sized to assess the impact of sargramostim treatment on response or survival.

MOBILIZATION OF PBPC AND ENGRAFTMENT

A retrospective review was conducted of data from patients with cancer undergoing collection of peripheral blood progenitor cells (PBPC) at a single transplant center. Mobilization of PBPC and myeloid reconstitution post-transplant were compared between four groups of patients (n=196) receiving sargramostim for mobilization and a historical control group who did not receive any mobilization treatment [progenitor cells collected by leukapheresis without mobilization (n=100)]. Sequential cohorts received sargramostim. The cohorts differed by dose (125 or 250 mcg/m²/day), route (IV over 24 hours of SC) and use of post transplant sargramostim. Leukaphereses were initiated for all mobilization groups after the WBC reached 10,000/mm³. Leukaphereses continued until both a minimum number of mononucleated cells (MNC) were collected (6.5 or 8.0 x 10^8/kg body weight) and a minimum number of phereses (5–8) were performed. Both minimum requirements varied by treatment cohort and planned conditioning regimen. If subjects failed to reach a WBC of 10,000 cells/mm³ by day 5 another cytokine was substituted for sargramostim; these subjects were all successfully leukapheresed and transplanted. The most marked mobilization and post transplant effects were seen in patients administered the higher dose of sargramostim (250 mcg/m²) either IV (n=63) or SC (n=41).

PBPCs from patients treated at the 250 mcg/m²/day dose had significantly higher number of granulocyte-macrophage colony-forming units (CFU-GM) than those collected without mobilization. The mean value after thawing was 11.41 x 10^4 CFU-GM/kg for all sargramostim mobilized patients, compared to 0.96 x 10^4/kg for the non-mobilized group. A similar difference was observed in the mean number of erythrocyte burst-forming units (BFU-E) collected (23.96 x 10^4/kg for patients mobilized with 250 mcg/m²doses of sargramostim administered SC vs. 1.63 x 10^4/kg for non-mobilized patients).

After transplantation, mobilized subjects had shorter times to myeloid engraftment, and fewer days between transplantation and the last platelet transfusion compared to non-mobilized subjects. Neutrophil recovery (ANC >500/mm³) was more rapid in patients administered sargramostim following PBPC transplantation with sargramostim-mobilized cells (See TABLE 2) Mobilized patients also had fewer days to the last platelet transfusion and last RBC transfusion, and a shorter duration of hospitalization than did non-mobilized subjects.

TABLE 2

	Route for Mobilization	Post-transplant sargramostim	ENGRAFTMENT (median value in days) ANC> 500/mm³	Last platelet transfusion
No mobilization	-	no	29	28
	IV	no	21	24
Sargramostim 250 mcg/m²	IV	yes	12	24
	SC	yes	12	17

A second retrospective review of data from patients undergoing PBPC at another single transplant center was also conducted. Sargramostin was given SC at 250 mcg/m²/day once a day (n=10) or twice a day (n=21) until completion of the aphereses. Aphereses were begun on day 5 of sargramostim administration and continued until the targeted MNC count of 9 x 10^8/kg or CD34+ cell count of 1 x 10^6/kg was reached. There was no difference in CD34+cell count in patients receiving sargramostim once or twice a day. The median time to ANC>500/mm³ was 12 days and to platelet recovery (>25,000/mm³) was 23 days.

Survival studies comparing mobilized study patients to the non-mobilized patients and to an autologous historical bone marrow transplant group showed no differences in median survival time.

AUTOLOGOUS BONE MARROW TRANSPLANTATION[7]

Following a dose- ranging Phase I/II trial in patients undergoing autologous BMT for lymphoid malignancies,[8,9] three single-center, randomized, placebo-controlled and double-blinded studies were conducted to evaluate the safety and efficacy of sargramostim for promoting hematopoietic reconstitution following autologous BMT. A total of 128 patients (65 sargramostim, 63 placebo) were enrolled in these 3 studies. The majority of the patients had lymphoid malignancy (87 NHL, 17 ALL), 23 patients had Hodgkin's disease, and 1 patient had acute myeloblastic leukemia (AML). In 72 patients with NHL or ALL, the bone marrow harvest was purged prior to storage with one several monoclonal antibodies. No chemical agent was used for *in vitro* treatment of the bone marrow. Preoperative regimens in the 3 studies included cyclophosphamide (total dose 120-150 mg/kg) and total body irradiation (total dose 1,200-1,575 rads). Other regimens used in patients with Hodgkin's disease and NHL without radiotherapy consisted of 3 or more of the following combination (expressed as total dose): cytosine arabinoside (400 mg/m²) and carmustine (300 mg/m²), cyclophosphamide (140-150 mg/kg), hydroxyurea (4.5 mg/m²) and etoposide (375-450 mg/m²).

Compared to placebo, administration of sargramostim in 2 studies (n = 44 and 47) significantly improved the following hematologic and clinical endpoints: time to neutrophil engraftment, duration of hospitalization, and infection experience or antibacterial usage. In the third study (n=37) there was a positive trend toward earlier myeloid engraftment in favor of sargramostim. This latter study differed from the other two in having enrolled a large number of patients with Hodgkin's disease who had also received extensive radiation and chemotherapy prior to harvest of autologous bone marrow. A subgroup analysis of the data from all three studies revealed that the median time to engraftment for patients with Hodgkin's disease, regardless of treatment, was 6 days longer when compared to patients with NHL and ALL, but that the overall beneficial sargramostim treatment effect was the same. In the following combined analysis of the three studies, these two subgroups (NHL and ALL vs. Hodgkin's disease) are presented separately.

Patients with Lymphoid Malignancy (Non-Hodgkin's Lymphoma and Acute Lymphoblastic Leukemia): Myeloid engraftment (absolute neutrophil count [ANC] ≥ 500 cells/cubic mm³) in 54 patients receiving sargramostim was observed 6 days earlier than in 50 patients treated with placebo (see TABLE 3) Accelerated myeloid engraftment was associated with significant clinical benefits. The median duration of hospitalization was 6 days shorter for the sargramostim group than for the placebo group. Median duration of infectious episodes (defined as fever and neutropenia; or 2 positive cultures of the same organism; or fever >38°C and 1 positive blood culture; or clinical evidence of infection) was 3 days less in the group treated with Sagramostim. The median duration of antibacterial administration in the post-transplantation period was 4 days shorter for the patients treated with sargramostim than for placebo-treated patients. The study was unable to detect a significant difference between the treatment groups in rate of disease relapse 24 months post- transplantation. As a group, leukemic subjects receiving sargramostim derived less benefit than NHL subjects. However, both the leukemic and NHL groups receiving sargramostim engrafted earlier than controls.

CLINICAL STUDIES: *(cont'd)*

TABLE 3 Autologous BMT: Combined Analysis from Placebo-Controlled Clinical Trials of Responses in Patients with NHL and ALL

	Median Values (days) ANC≥ 500/mm³	ANC 1000/mm³	Duration of Hospitaliza-tion	Duration of Infection	Duration of Antibacterial Therapy
Sargramostim (n=54)	18*#	24*#	21*	1*	21*
Placebo (n=50)	24	32	31	4	25

* p<0.05 Wilcoxon or CMH ridit chi-squared.
Note: The single AML patient was not included.

Patients with Hodgkin's Disease: If patient's with Hodgkin's disease are analyzed separately, a trend toward earlier myeloid engraftment was noted. Sargramostim-treated patients engrafted earlier (by 5 days) than the placebo-treated subjects (p=0.189, Wilcoxon) but the number of subjects was small (n=22); 1 patient (#23) from 1 site was non-controlled and was excluded from the analysis. Studies are in progress to confirm statistically the trend toward earlier engraftment of sargramostim in patients with Hodgkin's disease.

ALLOGENEIC BONE MARROW TRANSPLANTATION

A multi-center, randomized, placebo-controlled, and double-blinded study was conducted to evaluate the safety and efficacy of sargramostim for promoting hematopoietic reconstitution following allogeneic BMT. A total of 109 patients (53 sargramostim, 56 placebo) were enrolled in the study. Twenty-three patients (11 sargramostim, 12 placebo) were 18 years old or younger. Sixty-seven patients had myeloid malignancies (33 AML, 34 CML), 17 had lymphoid malignancies (12 ALL, 5 NHL), 3 patients had Hodgkin's disease, 6 had multiple myeloma, 9 had myelodysplastic disease, and 7 patients had aplastic anemia. In 22 patients at one of the seven study sites, bone marrow harvests were depleted of T cells. Preparative regimens included cyclophosphamide, busulfan, cytosine arabinoside, etoposide, methotrexate, corticosteroids, and asparaginase. Some patients also received total body, splenic, or testicular irradiation. Primary graft-versus-host disease (GVHD) prophylaxis was cyclosporine A and a corticosteroid.

Accelerated myeloid engraftment was associated with significant laboratory and clinical benefits. Compared to placebo, administration of sargramostim significantly improved the following: time to neutrophil engraftment, duration of hospitalization, number of patients with bacteremia and overall incidence of infection (see TABLE 4)

Median time to myeloid engraftment (ANC ≥ 500 cells/mm³) in 53 patients receiving sargramostim was 4 days less than in 56 patients treated with placebo (see TABLE 4) The number of patients with bacteremia and infection was significantly lower in the sargramostim group compared to the placebo group (9/53 versus 19/56 and 30/53 versus 42/56, respectively). There were a number of secondary laboratory and clinical endpoints. Of these, only the incidence of severe (grade 3/4) mucositis was significantly improved in the sargramostim group (4/53) compared to the placebo group (16/56) at p<0.05. Sargramostim treated patients also had a shorter median duration of post-transplant IV antibiotic infusions, and shorter median number of days to last platelet and RBC transfusions compared to placebo patients, but none of these differences reached statistical significance.

TABLE 4 Allogeneic BMT: Analysis of Data from Placebo-Controlled Clinical Trial

	Median Values (days or number of patients) ANC ≥ 500/mm³	ANC ≥ 1000/mm³	Number of Patients with Infections	Number of Patients with Bacteremia	Days of Hospitaliza-tion
Sargramostim (n=53)	13*	14*	30*	9**	25*
Placebo (n=56)	17	19	42	19	26

* p < 0.05 generalized Wilcoxon test
** p < 0.05 simple Chi-square test

BONE MARROW TRANSPLANTATION FAILURE OR ENGRAFTMENT DELAY

A historically-controlled study was conducted in patients experiencing graft failure following allogeneic or autologous BMT to determine whether Leukine improved survival after BMT failure.

Three categories of patients were eligible for this study:

1) patients displaying a delay in engraftment (ANC ≤ 100 cells/mm³ by day 28 post-transplantation.

2) patients displaying a delay in engraftment (ANC ≤ 100 cells/mm³by day 21 post-transplantation) and who had evidence of an active infection; and

3) patients who lost their marrow graft after a transient engraftment (manifested by an average of ANC ≥ 500 cells/mm³for at least one week followed by loss of engraftment with ANC <500 cells/mm³ for at least one week beyond day 21 post-transplantation).

A total of 140 eligible patients from 35 institutions treated with sargramostim were evaluated in comparison to 103 historical control patients from a single institution. One hundred sixty-three patients had lymphoid or myeloid leukemia, 24 patients had non-Hodgkin's lymphoma, 19 patients had Hodgkin's disease and 37 patients had other diseases, such as aplastic anemia, myelodysplasia or non-hematologic malignancy. The majority of patients (223 out of 243) had received prior chemotherapy with or without radiotherapy and/or immunotherapy prior to preparation for transplantation.

One hundred day survival was improved in favor of the patients treated with sargramostim after graft failure following either autologous or allogenic BMT. In addition, the median survival was improved by greater than 2-fold. The median survival of patients treated with Leukine after autologous failure was 474 days versus 161 days for the historical patients. Similarly, after allogeneic failure, the median survival was 97 days with sargramostim treatment and 35 days for the historical controls.

TABLE 5 Median Survival by Multiple Organ Failure (MOF) Category

	Median Survival (days) MOF < 2 Organs	MOF > 2 Organs	MOF (Composite of Both Groups)
AUTOLOGOUS BMT			
Sargramostim	474 (n=58)	78.5 (n=10)	474 (n=68)
Historical	165 (n=14)	39 (n=3)	161 (n=17)
ALLOGENEIC BMT			
Sargramostim	174 (n=50)	27 (n=22)	97 (n=72)
Historical	52.5(n=60)	15.5(n=26)	35 (n=86)

CLINICAL STUDIES: *(cont'd)*

The MOF score is a simple clinical and laboratory assessment of seven major organ systems: cardiovascular, respiratory, gastrointestinal, hematologic, renal, hepatic and neurologic.[10] Assessment of the MOF score is recommended as an additional method of determining the need to initiate treatment with sargramostim in patients with graft failure or delay in engraftment following autologous or allogeneic BMT.

Factors that Contribute to Survival: The probability of survival was relatively greater for patients with any one of the following characteristics: autologous BMT failure or delay in engraftment, exclusion of total body irradiation from the preoperative regimen, a non-leukemic malignancy or MOF score $\leq$ 2 (0, 1 or 2 dysfunctional organ systems). Sargramostim subjects derived less benefit than other subjects.

INDICATIONS AND USAGE:

Use Following Induction Chemotherapy in Acute Myelogenous Leukemia: Sargramostin is indicated for use following induction chemotherapy in older adult patients with acute myelogenous leukemia (AML) to shorten time to neutrophil recovery and to reduce the incidence of severe and life-threatening infections and infections resulting in death. The safety and efficacy of sargramostin have not been assessed in patients with AML under 55 years of age.

The term acute myelogenous leukemia, also referred to as acute non-lymphocytic leukemia (ANLL), encompasses a heterogenous group of leukemias arising from various non-lymphoid cell lines which have been defined morphologically by the French-American-British (FAB) system of classification.

Use in Mobilization and Following Transplantation of Autologous Peripheral Blood Progenitor Cells: Sargramostin is indicated for the mobilization of hematopoietic progenitor cells into peripheral blood for collection by leukapheresis. Mobilization allows for the collection of increased numbers of progenitor cells capable of engraftment as compared with collection without mobilization. After myeloablative chemotherapy, the transplantation of an increased number of progenitor cells can lead to more rapid engraftment, which may result in a decreased need for supportive care. Myeloid reconstitution is further accelerated by administration of sargramostim following peripheral blood progenitor cell transplantation.

Use in Myeloid Reconstitution After Autologous Bone Marrow Transplantation: Leukine is indicated for acceleration of myeloid recovery in patients with non-Hodgkin's lymphoma (NHL), acute lymphoblastic leukemia (ALL), and Hodgkin's disease undergoing autologous bone marrow transplantation (BMT). After autologous BMT in patients with NHL, ALL or Hodgkin's disease, sargramostim has been found to be safe and effective in accelerating myeloid engraftment, decreasing median duration of antibiotic administration, reducing the median duration of infectious episodes and shortening the median duration of hospitalization. Hematologic response to Leukine can be detected by complete blood count (CBC) with differential performed twice per week.

Insufficient data are presently available to support the efficacy of Leukine in accelerating myeloid recovery following peripheral blood stem cell transplantation.

Use in Myeloid Reconstitution after Allogeneic Bone Marrow Transplantation: Sargramostim is indicated for acceleration of myeloid recovery in patients undergoing allogeneic BMT from HLA-matched related donors. Sargramostim has been found to be safe and effective in accelerating myeloid engraftment, reducing the incidence of bacteremia and other culture positive infections, and shortening the median duration of hospitalization.

Use in Bone Marrow Transplantation Failure or Engraftment Delay: Sargramostim is indicated in patients who have undergone allogenic or autologous bone marrow transplantation (BMT) in whom engraftment is delayed or has failed. Sargramostim has been found to be safe and effective in prolonging survival of patients who are experiencing graft failure or engraftment delay, in the presence or absence of infection, following autologous or allogeneic BMT. Survival benefit may be relatively greater in those patients who demonstrate one or more of the following characteristics: autologous BMT failure or engraftment delay, no previous total body irradiation, malignancy other than leukemia or a multiple organ failure (MOF) score $\leq$2 (see CLINICAL STUDIES.) Hematologic response to sargramostim can be detected by complete blood count (CBC) with differential performed twice per week.

CONTRAINDICATIONS:

Sargramostim is contraindicated in patients with:

1 excessive leukemic myeloid blasts in the bone marrow or peripheral blood ($\geq$ 10%).

2 known hypersensitivity to GM-CSF, yeast-derived products, or any component of the product.

3 for concomitant use with chemotherapy and radiotherapy.

Due to the potential sensitivity of rapidly dividing hematopoietic progenitor cells, sargramostin should not be administered simultaneously with cytotoxic chemotherapy or radiotherapy or within 24 hours preceding or following chemotherapy or radiotherapy. In one controlled study, patients with small cell lung cancer received sargramostin and concurrent thoracic radiotherapy and chemotherapy or the identical radiotherapy and chemotherapy without sargramostin. The patients randomized to sargramostin had significantly higher adverse events, inlcuding higher mortality and a higher incidence of grade 3 and 4 infections and grade 3 and 4 thrombocytopenia.[11]

WARNINGS:

Fluid Retention: Peripheral edema, capillary leak syndrome, pleural and/or pericardial effusion have been reported in patients after sargramostim administration. In 156 patients enrolled in placebo-controlled studies using sargramostim at a dose of 250 mcg/m^2/day by 2 hour IV effusion, 1% vs. 0%; and pericardial effusion, 4% vs. 1%. Capillary leak syndrome was not observed in this limited number of studies; based on other uncontrolled studies and post-marketing reports, incidence is estimated to be less than 1%. In patients with preexisting pleural and pericardial effusions, administration of sargramostim may aggravate fluid retention; however, fluid retention associated with or worsened by sargramostim has been reversible after interruption or dose reduction of sargramostim with or without diuretic therapy. Sargramostim should be used with caution in patients with preexisting fluid retention, pulmonary infiltrates or congestive heart failure.

Respiratory Symptoms: Sequestration of granulocytes in the pulmonary circulation has been documented following sargramostim infusion[10], and dyspnea has been reported occasionally in patients treated with sargramostim. Special attention should be given to respiratory symptoms during or immediately following sargramostim infusion, especially in patients with preexisting lung disease. In patients displaying dyspnea during sargramostim administration, the rate of infusion should be reduced by half. If respiratory symptoms worsen despite infusion rate reduction, the infusion should be discontinued. Subsequent IV infusions may administered following the standard dose schedule with careful monitoring. Sargramostim should be administered with caution in patients with hypoxia. Benzyl alcohol is a constituent of Bacteriostatic Water for Injection diluent. Benzyl alcohol has been reported to be associated with a fatal "Gasping Syndrome" in premature infants (see DOSAGE AND ADMINISTRATION.)

WARNINGS: *(cont'd)*

Cardiovascular Symptoms: Occasional transient supraventricular arrhythmia has been reported in uncontrolled studies during sargramostim administration, particularly in patients with a previous history of cardiac arrhythmia. However, these arrhythmias have been reversible after discontinuation of sargramostim. Sargramostim should be used with caution in patients with preexisting cardiac disease.

Renal and Hepatic Dysfunction: In some patients with preexisting renal or hepatic dysfunction enrolled in uncontrolled clinical trials, administration sargramostim has induced elevation of serum creatinine or bilirubin and hepatic enzymes. Dose reduction or interruption of sargramostim administration has resulted in a decrease to pretreatment values. However, in controlled clinical trials the incidences of renal and hepatic dysfunction were comparable between sargramostim (250 mcg/m^2/day by 2 hour IV infusion) and placebo-treated patients. Monitoring of renal and hepatic function in patients displaying renal or hepatic dysfunction prior to initiation of treatment is recommended at least biweekly during sargramostim administration.

PRECAUTIONS:

General: Parenteral administration of recombinant proteins should be attended by appropriate precautions in case an allergic or untoward reaction occurs. Transient rashes and local injection site reactions have occasionally been observed concomitantly with sargramostim treatment. Serious allergic or anaphylactic reactions have been reported rarely. If any serious allergic or anaphylactoid reaction occurs, sargramostim therapy should immediately be discontinued and appropriate therapy initiated(see WARNINGS.)

Rarely, hypotension with flushing and syncope has been reported following the first administration of sargramostim. These signs have resolved with symptomatic treatment and have not recurred with subsequent doses in the same cycle of treatment.

Stimulation of marrow precursors with sargramostim may result in a rapid rise in white blood cell (WBC) count. If the ANC exceeds 20,000 cells/mm^3 or if the platelet count exceeds 500,000/mm^3, sargramostim administration should be interrupted or the dose reduced by half. The decision to reduce the dose or interrupt treatment should be based on the clinical condition of the patient. Excessive blood counts have returned to normal or baseline levels within 3 to 7 days following cessation of sargramostim therapy.

Twice weekly monitoring of CBC with differential (including examination for the presence of blast cells) should be performed to preclude development of excessive counts.

Growth Factor Potential: Sargramostim is a growth factor that primarily stimulates normal myeloid precursors. However, the possibility that sargramostim can act as a growth factor for any tumor type, particularly myeloid malignancies, cannot be excluded. Because of the possibility of tumor growth potentiation, precaution should be exercised when using this drug in any malignancy with myeloid characteristics.

Should disease progression be detected during sargramostim treatment, sargramostim therapy should be discontinued.

Sargramostim has been administered to patients with myelodysplastic syndromes (MDS) in uncontrolled studies without evidence of increased relapse rates.[12,13,14] Controlled studies have not been performed in patients with MDS.

Use in Patients Receiving Purged Bone Marrow: Sargramostim is effective in accelerating myeloid recovery in patients receiving bone marrow purged by anti-B lymphocyte monoclonal antibodies. Data obtained from uncontrolled studies suggest that if *in vitro* marrow purging with chemical agents causes a significant decrease in the number of responsive hematopoietic progenitors the patient may not respond to sargramostim. When the bone marrow purging process preserves a sufficient number of progenitors ($>1.2 \times 10^4$/kg), a beneficial effect of sargramostim on myeloid engraftment has been reported[15].

Use in Patients Previously Exposed to Intensive Chemotherapy/Radiotherapy: In patients who before autologous BMT, have received extensive radiotherapy to hematopoietic sites for the treatment of primary disease in the abdomen or chest, or have been exposed to multiple myelotoxic agents (alkylating agents, anthracycline antibiotics and antimetabolites), the effect of sargramostim on myeloid reconstitution may be limited.

Use in Patients with Malignancy Underoing Sargramostim-Mobilized PBPC Collection: When using sargramostim to mobilize PBPC, the limited *in vitro* data suggest that tumor cells may be released and reinfused into the patient in the leukapheresis product. The effect of reinfusion of tumor cells has not been well studied and the data are inconclusive.

Patient Monitoring: Sargramostim can induce variable increases in WBC and/or platelet counts. In order to avoid potential complications of excessive leukocytosis (WBC >50,000 cells/mm^3; ANC >20,000 cells/mm^3), a CBC is recommended twice per week during sargramostim therapy. Monitoring of renal and hepatic function in patients displaying renal or hepatic dysfunction prior to initiation of treatment is recommended at least biweekly during sargramostim administration. Body weight and hydration status should be carefully monitored during sargramostim administration.

Carcinogenesis, Mutagenesis, and Impairment of Fertility: Animal studies have not been conducted with sargramostim to evaluate the carcinogenic potential or the effect on fertility.

Pregnancy Category C: Animal reproduction studies have not been conducted with sargramostim. It is not known whether sargramostim can cause fetal harm when administered to a pregnant woman or can affect reproductive capability. Sargramostim should be given to a pregnant woman only if clearly needed.

Nursing Mothers: It is not known whether sargramostin is excreted in human milk. Because many drugs are excreted in human milk, sargramostin should be administered to a nursing woman only if clearly needed.

Pediatric Use: Safety and effectiveness in children have not been established; however, available safety data indicate that sargramostin does not exhibit any greater toxicity in children than adults. A total of 113 pediatric subjects between the ages of 4 months and 18 years have been treated with sargramostin in clinical trials at doses ranging from 60-1,000 mcg/m^2/day intravenously and 4-1,500 mcg/m^2/day subcutaneously. In 53 pediatric patients enrolled in controlled studies at a dose of 250 mcg/m^2/day by 2 hour IV infusion, the type and frequency of adverse events were comparable to those reported for the adult population. **Sargramostim reconstituted with Bacteriostatic Water for Injection, USP (0.9% benzyl alcohol) should not be administered to neonates** (see WARNINGS.)

DRUG INTERACTIONS:

Interactions between sargramostim and other drugs have not been fully evaluated. Drugs which may potentiate the myeloproliferative effects of sargramostin, such as lithium and corticosteroids, should be used with caution.

ADVERSE REACTIONS:

Sargramostin is generally well tolerated. In 3 placebo-controlled studies enrolling a total of 156 patients after autologous BMT or peripheral stem cell transplantation, events reported in at least 10% of patients in sargramostin or placebo groups were: (see TABLE 6)

No significant differences were observed between sargramostin and placebo-treated patients in the type or frequency of laboratory abnormalities, including renal and hepatic parameters. In some patients with preexisting renal or hepatic dysfunction enrolled in uncontrolled clinical trials, administration of sargramostin has induced elevation of serum creatinine or

ADVERSE REACTIONS: *(cont'd)*

TABLE 6 Percent of Patients Reporting Event

Events by Body System	Sargramostim (n=79)	Placebo (n=77)
Body, General		
Fever	95	96
Mucous membrane disorder	75	78
Asthenia	66	51
Malaise	57	51
Sepsis	11	14
Digestive System		
Nausea	90	96
Diarrhea	89	82
Vomiting	85	90
Anorexia	54	58
GI disorder	37	47
GI hemorrhage	27	33
Stomatitis	24	29
Liver damage	13	14
Skin And Appendages		
Alopecia	73	74
Rash	44	38
Metabolic/ Nutritional Disorders		
Edema	34	35
Peripheral edema	11	7
Respiratory System		
Dyspnea	28	31
Lung disorder	20	23
Hemic And Lymphatic System		
Blood dyscrasia	25	27
Cardiovascular System		
Hemorrhage	23	30
Urogenital System		
Urinary tract disorder	14	13
Kidney function abnormal	8	10
Nervous System		
CNS disorder	11	16

bilirubin and hepatic enzymes (See WARNINGS.) In addition, there was no significant difference in relapse rate and 24 month survival between the sargramostin and placebo-treated patients.

In the placebo-controlled trial of 109 patients after allogeneic BMT, events reported in at least 10% of patients who received IV sargramostim or placebo were:

There were no significant differences in the incidence or severity of GVHD, relapse rates and survival between sargramostin and placebo-treated patients.

Adverse events observed for the patients treated with sargramostim in the historically controlled BMT failure study were similar to those reported in the placebo-controlled studies. In addition, headache (26%), pericardial effusion (25%), arthralgia (21%) and myalgia (18%) were also reported in patients treated with sargramostim in the graft failure study.

In uncontrolled Phase I/II studies with sargramostim in 215 patients, the most frequent adverse events were fever, asthenia, headache, bone pain, chills, and myalgia. These systemic events were generally mild or moderate and were usually prevented or reversed by the administration of analgesics and antipyretics such as acetaminophen. In these uncontrolled trials, other infrequent events reported were dyspnea, peripheral edema, and rash.

Reports of events occurring with marketed sargramostim include arrhythmia, eosinophilia, hypotension, injection site reactions, pain (including abdominal, back, chest, and joint pain), tachycardia, thrombosis, and transient liver function abnormalities.

In patients with preexisting peripheral edema, pleural and/or pericardial effusion, administration of sargramostim may aggravate fluid retention (see WARNINGS.) Body weight and hydration status should be carefully monitored during sargramostim administration.

Adverse events observed in pediatric patients in controlled studies were comparable to those observed in adult patients.

Acute Myelogenous Leukemia: Adverse events reported in at least 10% of patients who received sargramostim or placebo were:

Nearly all patients reported leukopenia, thrombocytopenia and anemia. The frequency and type of adverse events observed following induction were similar between sargramostim and placebo groups. The only significant difference in the rates of these adverse events was an increase in skin associated events in the sargramostim group (p=0.002). No significant differences were observed in laboratory results, renal or hepatic toxicity. No significant differences were observed between the sargramostim and placebo-treated patients for adverse events following consolidation. There was no significant difference in response rate or relapse rate.

In a historically controlled study of 86 patients with acute myelogenous leukemia (AML), the sargramostim treated group exhibited an increased incidence of weight gain (p=0.007), low serum proteins and prolonged prothrombin time (p=0.02) when compared to the control group. Two sargramostim treated patients had progressive increase in circulating monocytes and promonocytes and blasts in the marrow which reversed when sargramostim was discontinued. The historical control group exhibited an increased incidence of cardiac events (p=0.018), liver function abnormalities (p=0.008), and neurocortical hemorrhagic events (p=0.025).[14]

OVERDOSAGE:

The maximum amount of sargramostim that can be safely administered in single or multiple doses has not been determined. Doses up to 100 mcg/kg/day (4,000 mcg/m^2/day or 16 times the recommended dose) were administered to 4 patients in a Phase I uncontrolled clinical study by continuous IV infusion for 7 to 18 days. Increases in WBC up to 200,000 cells/mm^3 were observed. Adverse events reported were dyspnea, malaise, nausea, fever, rash, sinus tachycardia, headache, and chills. All of these events were reversible after discontinuation of sargramostim.

In case of overdosage, sargramostim therapy should be discontinued and the patient carefully monitored for WBC increase and respiratory symptoms.

DOSAGE AND ADMINISTRATION:

Neutrophil Recovery Following Chemotherapy in Acute Myelogenous Leukemia: The recommended dose is 250 mcg/m^2/day administered intravenously over a 4 hour period starting approximately on day 11 or 4 days following the completion of induction chemotherapy, if the day 10 bone marrow is hypoplastic with <5% blasts. If a second cycle of induction chemotherapy is necessary, sargramostim should be administered approximately 4 days after the completion of chemotherapy if the bone marrow is hypoplastic with <5% blasts. Sargramostim should be discontinued immediately if leukemic regrowth occurs. If a severe adverse reaction occurs, the dose can be reduced by half if the ANC exceeds 20,000 cells/mm^3.

DOSAGE AND ADMINISTRATION: *(cont'd)*

TABLE 7 Percent of Allogeneic BMT Patients Reporting Events

Events by Body System	Sargramostim (n=53)	Placebo (n=56)
Body, General		
Fever	77	80
Abdominal pain	38	23
Headache	36	36
Chills	25	20
Pain	17	36
Asthenia	17	20
Chest pain	15	9
Back pain	9	18
Digestive System		
Diarrhea	81	66
Nausea	70	66
Vomiting	70	57
Stomatitis	62	63
Anorexia	51	57
Dyspepsia	17	20
Hematemesis	13	7
Dysphagia	11	7
GI hemorrhage	11	5
Constipation	8	11
Skin And Appendages		
Rash	70	73
Alopecia	45	45
Pruritis	23	13
Musculo-Skeletal System		
Bone pain	21	5
Arthralgia	11	4
Special Senses		
Eye hemorrhage	11	0
Cardiovascular System		
Hypertension	34	32
Tachycardia	11	9
Metabolic/Nutritional Disorders		
Bilirubinemia	30	27
Hyperglycemia	25	23
Peripheral edema	15	21
Increased creatinine	15	14
Hypomagnesemia	15	9
Increased SGPT	13	16
Edema	13	11
Increased alk. phosphatase	8	14
Respiratory System		
Pharyngitis	23	13
Epistaxis	17	16
Dyspnea	15	14
Rhinitis	11	14
Hemic And Lymphatic System		
Thrombocytopenia	19	34
Leukopenia	17	29
Petechia	6	11
Agranulocytosis	6	11
Urogenital System		
Hematuria	9	21
Nervous System		
Paresthesia	11	13
Insomnia	11	9
Anxiety	11	2
Laboratory Abnormalities*		
High Glucose	41	49
Low albumin	27	36
High BUN	23	17
Low calcium	2	7
High cholesterol	17	8

* Grade 3 and 4 laboratory abnormalities only. Denominators may vary due to missing laboratory measurements.

Mobilization of Peripheral Blood Progenitor Cells: The recommended dose is 250 mcg/m^2/day administered IV over 24 hours or SC once daily. Dosing should continue at the same dose through the period of PBPC collection. The optimal schedule for PBPC collection has not been established. In clinical studies, collection of PBPC was usually begun by day 5 and performed daily until protocol specified targets were achieved (see CLINICAL STUDIES), Mobilization of PBPC and Engraftment). If WBC > 50,000 cells/mm^3, the sargramostim dose should be reduced by 50%. If adequate numbers of progenitor cells are not collected, other mobilization therapy should be considered.

Post Peripheral Blood Progenitor Cell Transplantation: The recommended dose is 250 mcg/m2/day administered IV over 24 hours or SC once daily beginning immediately following infusion of progenitor cells and continuing until an ANC>1500 for 3 consecutive days is attained.

Myeloid Reconstitution After Autologous Bone Marrow Transplantation: The recommended dose is 250 mcg/m^2/day for 21 days as a 2 hour IV infusion, beginning 2 to 4 hours after the autologous bone marrow infusion, and not less than 24 hours after the last dose of chemotherapy and 12 hours after the last dose of radiotherapy. If a severe adverse reaction occurs, the dose can be reduced or temporarily discontinued until the reaction abates. If blast cells appear or disease progression occurs, the treatment should be discontinued.

In order to avoid potential complications of excessive leukocytosis (WBC>50,000 cells/mm^3, ANC>20,000 cells/mm^3), a CBC with differential is recommended twice per week during sargramostim therapy. Sargramostim treatment should be interrupted or the dose reduced by half if the ANC exceeds 20,000/mm^3.

Bone Marrow Transplantation Failure or Engraftment Delay: The recommended dose is 250 mcg/m^2/day for 14 days as a 2 hour IV infusion. The dose can be repeated after 7 days off therapy if engraftment still has not occurred. If engraftment has not occurred a third course of 500 mcg/m2/day for 14 days may be tried after another 7 days off therapy. If there is still no improvement, it is unlikely that further dose escalation will be beneficial. if a severe adverse reaction occurs, the dose can be reduced or temporarily discontinued until the reaction abates. If blast cells appear or disease progression occurs, the treatment should be discontinued.

In order to avoid potential complications of excessive leukocytosis (WBC>50,000 cells/mm^3, ANC>20,000 cells/mm^3) a CBC with differential is recommended twice per week during Sargramostim therapy. Sargramostim treatment should be interrupted or the dose reduced by half if the ANC exceeds 20,000 cells/mm^3.

DOSAGE AND ADMINISTRATION: *(cont'd)*

TABLE 8 Percent of AML Patients Reporting Event

Events by Body System	Sargramostim (n=52)	Placebo (n=47)
Body, General		
Fever (no infection)	81	74
Infection	65	68
Weight loss	37	28
Weight gain	8	21
Chills	19	26
Allergy	12	15
Sweats	6	13
Digestive System		
Nausea	58	55
Liver	77	83
Diarrhea	52	53
Vomiting	46	34
Stomatitis	42	43
Anorexia	13	11
Abdominal distention	4	13
Skin And Appendages		
Skin	77	45
Alopecia	37	51
Metabolic/Nutritional Disorder		
Metabolic	58	49
Edema	25	23
Respiratory System		
Pulmonary	48	64
Hemic And Lymphatic System		
Coagulation	19	21
Cardiovascular System		
Hemorrhage	29	43
Hypertension	25	32
Cardiac	23	32
Hypotension	13	26
Urogenital System		
GU	50	57
Nervous System		
Neuro-clinical	42	53
Neuro-motor	25	26
Neuro-psych	15	26
Neuro-sensory	6	11

PREPARATION OF SARGRAMOSTIM

1. Sargramostim is a sterile, white, preservative-free, lyophilized powder suitable for IV infusion upon reconstitution. Sargramostin (250 mcg or 500 mcg vials) should be reconstituted aseptically with 1.0 ml of Sterile Water for Injection, USP (without preservative). The reconstituted sargramostin solutions are clear, colorless, isotonic with a pH of 7.4 ± 0.3, and contain 250 or 500 mcg/ml of sargramostin. **The contents of vials reconstituted with different diluents should not be mixed together.** *Sterile Water for Injection, USP (without preservative):* Sargramostim vials contain no antibacterial preservative, and therefore solutions prepared with Sterile Water for Injection, USP should be administered as soon as possible, and within 6 hours following reconstitution and/or dilution for IV infusion. The vial should not be re-entered or reused. Do not save any unused portion for administration more than 6 hours following reconstitution. *Bacteriostatic Water for Injection, USP (0.9% benzyl alcohol):*Reconstituted solutions prepared with Bacteriostatic Water for Injection, USP (0.9% benzyl alcohol) may be stored for up to 20 days at 2–8°C prior to use. Discard reconstituted solution after 20 days. Previously reconstituted solutions mixed with freshly reconstituted solutions must be administered within 6 hours following mixing. **Preparations containing benzyl alcohol should not be used in neonates (see WARNINGS.)**

2. During reconstitution the Sterile Water for Injection, USP should be directed at the side of the vial and the contents gently swirled to avoid foaming during dissolution. Avoid excessive or vigorous agitation; do not shake.

3. Dilution for IV Infusion should be performed in 0.9% Sodium Chloride Injection, USP. If the final concentration of sargramostin is below 10 mcg/ml, Albumin (Human) at a final concentration of 0.1% should be added to the saline prior to addition of Leukine to prevent adsorption to the components of the drug delivery system. To obtain a final concentration of 0.1% Albumin (Human), add 1 mg Albumin (Human) per 1 ml 0.9% Sodium Chloride Injection, USP (*e.g.,* use 1 ml 5% Albumin [Human] in 50 ml 0.9% Sodium Chloride Injection, USP).

4. An in-line membrane filter should not be used for intravenous infusion of Leukine.

5. Sargramostin contains no antibacterial preservative and therefore should be administered as soon as possible, and within 6 hours following reconstitution and/or dilution for IV infusion. Store sargramostin solutions under refrigeration at 2-8°C (36-46°F); do not freeze. Sargramostin vials are intended for single use only; discard any unused solution after 6 hours.

6. In the absence of compatibility and stability information, no other medication should be added to infusion solutions containing sargramostin. Use only 0.9% Sodium Chloride Injection, USP to prepare IV infusion solutions.

7. Aseptic technique should be employed in the preparation of all sargramostin solutions. To assure correct concentration following reconstitution, care should be exercised to eliminate any air bubbles from the needle hub of the syringe used to prepare the diluent. Parental drug products should be inspected visually for particulate matter and discoloration prior to administration whenever solution and container permit.

REFERENCES:

1. Metcalf D. The molecular biology and functions of the granulocyte-macrophage colony-stimulating factors. Blood 1986; 67(2):257-267. **2.** Park LS, Friend D. Gillis S. Urdal DL. Characterization of the cell surface receptor for human granulocyte/macrophage colony stimulating factor, J Exp Med 1986; 164:251-262. **3.** Grabstein KH, Urdal DL, Tushinski RJ, *et al.* Induction of macrophage tumoricidal activity by granulocyte-macrophage colony-stimulating factors. Science 1986; 232:506-508. **4.** Reed SG, Nathan CF, Pihl DL, *et al.* Recombinant granulocyte/macrophage colony-stimulating factor activates macrophages to inhibit *Trypanosoma cruzi* and release hydrogen peroxide. J Exp Med 1987; 166:1734-1746. **5.** Data on File Immunex Corporation; Seattle, WA **6.** Shadduck RK, Waheed A, Evans C,*et al.* Serum and urinary levels of recombinant human granulocyte-macrophage colony stimulating factor: Assessment after intravenous infusion and subcutaneous injection, Exp Hem 1990; 18:601. **7.** Nemunaitis J, Rabinowe SN, Singer JW, *et al.* Recombinant human granulocyte-macrophage colony-stimulating factor after autologous bone marrow transplantation for lymphoid malignancy: Pooled results of a randomized, double-blind, placebo controlled trial, NEJM 1991; 3234(25):1773-1778. **8.** Nemunaitis J. Singer JW, Buckner CD, *et al.* Use of Recombinant human granulocyte-macrophage colony stimulating factor in autologous bone marrow transplantation for lymphoid malignancies. Blood 1988; 72(2):834-836. **9.** Nemunaitis J, Singer JW, Buckner CD, *et al.* Long-term follow-up patients who received recombinant human granulocyte-macrophage colony stimulating factor after autologous bone marrow transplantation for lymphoid malignancy. BMT 1991; 7:49-52. **10.** Goris RJA, Boekhorst TPA, Nuytinck JKS, *et al.* Multiple organ failure: Generalized auto- destructive inflammation? Arch Surg 1985; 120:1109-1115. **11.** Hermann F, Schulz G, Lindemann A, *et al.* Yeast-expressed granulocyte-macrophage colony-stimulating factor in cancer patients: A phase Ib clinical study. In Behring Institute Research Communications, Colony Stimulating Factors-CSF. International Symposium, Garmisch-partenkirchen, West Germany. 1988; 83:107-118. **12.** Bunn P, Crowley J, Kelly K, *et al.*Chemoradiotherapy with or without granulocyte-macrophage colony-stimulating factor in the treatment of limited-stage small-cell lung cancer: a prospective phase III randomized study of the southwest oncology group. JCO 1995; 13(7):1632–1641. **13.** Estey EH, Dixon D, Kantarjian H, *et al.* Treatment of poor-prognosis, newly diagnosed acute myeloid leukemia with Ara-C and recombinant human granulocyte-macrophage colony-stimulat-

REFERENCES: *(cont'd)*

ing factor. Blood 1990; (75(9):1766-1769. **14.** Vadhan-RajS, Keating M, LeMaistre A,*et al.* Effects of recombinant human granulocyte-macrophage colony-stimulating factor in patients with myelodysplastic syndromes. NEJM 1987: 317:1545-1552. **15.** Buchner T, Hiddemann W, Koenigsmann M, *et al.* Recombinant human granulocyte-macrophage colony stimulating factor after chemotherapy in patients with acute myeloid leukemia at higher age or after relapse. Blood 1991; (78(5):1190-1197. **16.** Blazar BR, Kersey JH, McGlave PB, *et al. In vivo* administration of recombinant human granulocyte/macrophage colony-stimulating factor in acute lymphoblastic leukemia receiving purged autografts. Blood 1989; 73(3):849-857. **17.** Rowe JM, Anderson JW, Mazza JJ, *et al.* A randomized placebo-controlled phase III study of granulocyte-macrophage colony-stimulating factor in adult patients (>55 to 70 years of age) with acute myelogenous leukemia: a study of the Eastern Cooperative Oncology Group (E1490). Blood 1995; 86(2):457–462.

HOW SUPPLIED:

Leukine is available as a sterile, white, preservative-free, lyophilized powder. Each dosage form is supplied packaged individually or in cartons of 10 single-use vials.

Storage: The sterile powder, the reconstituted solution and the diluted solution for injection should be refrigerated at 2-8°C (36-46°F). Do not freeze or shake. Do not use beyond the expiration date printed on the vial.

HOW SUPPLIED - EQUIVALENTS NOT AVAILABLE:

Injectable - Intravenous - 250 mcg

5 vials x 250 m $471.15 LEUKINE, Immunex 58406-0002-33

Injectable - Intravenous - 500 mcg

5 vials x 500 m $886.85 LEUKINE, Immunex 58406-0001-35

Injection, Lyphl-Soln - Intravenous; Su - 500 mcg

1 ml $177.37 LEUKINE, Immunex 58406-0001-01

Injection, Solution - Intravenous - 250 mcg

1's $94.23 LEUKINE, Immunex 58406-0002-01

SCOPOLAMINE *(002213)*

CATEGORIES: Anticholinergic Agents; Antimuscarinics/Antispasmodics; Autonomic Drugs; Motion Sickness; Nausea; Nausea and Vomiting; Otic Preparations; Otologic; Vertigo/Motion Sickness/Vomiting; Vomiting; Topical; Pregnancy Category C; Sales > $100 Million; FDA Approval Pre 1982

BRAND NAMES: *Scopoderm-TTS*; **Transderm Scop**
(International brand names outside U.S. in italics)

FORMULARIES: Aetna

COST OF THERAPY: $7.49 (Motion Sickness; Film; 0.5 mg; 1/day; 2 days)

DESCRIPTION:

The Transderm Scop system is a circular flat disc designed for continuous release of scopolamine following application to an area of intact skin on the head, behind the ear. Clinical evaluation has demonstrated that the system provides effective antiemetic and antinauseant actions when tested against motion-sickness stimuli in adults. The Transderm Scop system is a film 0.2 mm thick and 2.5 cm^2, with four layers. Proceeding from the visible surface towards the surface attached to the skin, these layers are: (1) a backing layer of tan-color, aluminized, polyester film; (2) a drug reservoir of scopolamine, mineral oil, and polyisobutylene; (3) a microporous polypropylene membrane that controls the rate of delivery of scopolamine from the system to the skin surface; and (4) an adhesive formulation of mineral oil, polyisobutylene, and scopolamine. A protective peel strip of siliconized polyester, which covers the adhesive layer, is removed before the system is used. The inactive components, mineral oil (12.4 mg) and polyisobutylene (11.4 mg) are not released from the system.

(For graphic representation of the cross section of this system, please refer to the manufacturer's original package insert).

Release-Rate Concept: The Transderm Scop system contains 1.5 mg of scopolamine. The system is programmed to deliver 0.5 mg of scopolamine at an approximately constant rate to the systemic circulation over the 3-day lifetime of the system. An initial priming dose of scopolamine, released from the adhesive layer of the system, saturates the skin binding sites and rapidly brings the plasma concentration of scopolamine to the required steady-state level. A continuous controlled release of scopolamine, which flows from the drug reservoir through the rate-controlling membrane, maintains the plasma level constant.

CLINICAL PHARMACOLOGY:

The sole active agent of Transderm Scop is scopolamine, a belladonna alkaloid with well-known pharmacological properties. The drug has a long history of oral and parenteral use for central anticholinergic activity, including prophylaxis of motion sickness. The mechanism of action of scopolamine in the central nervous system (CNS) is not definitely known but may include anticholinergic effects. The ability of scopolamine to prevent motion-induced nausea is believed to be associated with inhibition of vestibular input to the CNS, which results in inhibition of the vomiting reflex. In addition, scopolamine may have a direct action on the vomiting center within the reticular formation of the brain stem. Applied to the postauricular skin, Transderm Scop provides for a gradual release of scopolamine from an adhesive matrix of mineral oil and polyisobutylene.

INDICATIONS AND USAGE:

Transderm Scop is indicated for prevention of nausea and vomiting associated with motion sickness in adults. The disc should be applied only to skin in the postauricular area.

Clinical Results: Transderm Scop provides antiemetic protection within several hours following application of the disc behind the ear. In 195 adult subjects of different racial origins who participated in clinical efficacy studies at sea or in a controlled motion environment, there was a 75% reduction in the incidence of motion-induced nausea and vomiting. Transderm Scop provided significantly greater protection than that obtained with oral dimenhydrinate.

CONTRAINDICATIONS:

Transderm Scop should not be used in patients with known hypersensitivity to scopolamine or any of the components of the adhesive matrix making up the therapeutic system, or in patients with glaucoma.

WARNINGS:

Transderm Scop should not be used in children and should be used with special caution in the elderly. See PRECAUTIONS.

Since drowsiness, disorientation, and confusion may occur with the use of scopolamine, patients should be warned of the possibility and cautioned against engaging in activities that require mental alertness, such as driving a motor vehicle or operating dangerous machinery.

Potentially alarming idiosyncratic reactions may occur with ordinary therapeutic doses of scopolamine.

PRECAUTIONS:

General: Scopolamine should be used with caution in patients with pyloric obstruction, or urinary bladder neck obstruction. Caution should be exercised when administering an antiemetic or antimuscarinic drug to patients suspected of having intestinal obstruction.

Transderm Scop should be used with special caution in the elderly or in individuals with impaired metabolic, liver, or kidney functions, because of the increased likelihood of CNS effects.

Information for the Patient: Since scopolamine can cause temporary dilation of the pupils and blurred vision if it comes in contact with the eyes, patients should be strongly advised to wash their hands thoroughly with soap and water immediately after handling the disc.

Patients should be advised to remove the disc immediately and contact a physician in the unlikely event that they experience symptoms of acute narrow-angle glaucoma (pain in and reddening of the eyes accompanied by dilated pupils).

Patients should be warned against driving a motor vehicle or operating dangerous machinery. A patient brochure is available.

Carcinogenesis, Mutagenesis, and Impairment of Fertility: No long-term studies in animals have been performed to evaluate carcinogenic potential. Fertility studies were performed in female rats and revealed no evidence of impaired fertility or harm to the fetus due to scopolamine hydrobromide administered by daily subcutaneous injection. In the highest-dose group (plasma level approximately 500 times the level achieved in humans using a transdermal system), reduced maternal body weights were observed.

Pregnancy Category C: Teratogenic studies were performed in pregnant rats and rabbits with scopolamine hydrobromide administered by daily intravenous injection. No adverse effects were recorded in the rats. In the rabbits, the highest dose (plasma level approximately 100 times the level achieved in humans using a transdermal system) of drug administered had a marginal embryotoxic effect. Transderm Scop should be used during pregnancy only if the anticipated benefit justifies the potential risk to the fetus.

Nursing Mothers: It is not known whether scopolamine is excreted in human milk. Because many drugs are excreted in human milk, caution should be exercised when Transderm Scop is administered to a nursing woman.

Pediatric Use: Children are particularly susceptible to the side effects of belladonna alkaloids. Transderm Scop should not be used in children because it is not known whether this system will release an amount of scopolamine that could produce serious adverse effects in children.

DRUG INTERACTIONS:

Scopolamine should be used with care in patients taking drugs, including alcohol, capable of causing CNS effects. Special attention should be given to drugs having anticholinergic properties, e.g., belladonna alkaloids, antihistamines (including meclizine), and antidepressants.

ADVERSE REACTIONS:

The most frequent adverse reaction to Transderm Scop is dryness of the mouth. This occurs in about two thirds of the people. A less frequent adverse reaction is drowsiness, which occurs in less than one sixth of the people. Transient impairment of eye accommodation, including blurred vision and dilation of the pupils, is also observed.

The following adverse reactions have also been reported on infrequent occasions during the use of Transderm Scop: disorientation; memory disturbances; dizziness; restlessness; hallucinations; confusion; difficulty urinating; rashes and erythema; acute narrow-angle glaucoma; and dry itchy, or red eyes.

Drug Withdrawal: Symptoms including dizziness, nausea, vomiting, headache and disturbances of equilibrium have been reported in a few patients following discontinuation of the use of the Transderm Scop system. These symptoms have occurred most often in patients who have used the systems for more than three days.

OVERDOSAGE:

Overdosage with scopolamine may cause disorientation, memory disturbances, dizziness, restlessness, hallucinations, or confusion. Should these symptoms occur, the Transderm Scop disc should be immediately removed. Appropriate parasympathomimetic therapy should be initiated if these symptoms are severe.

DOSAGE AND ADMINISTRATION:

Initiation of Therapy: One Transderm Scop disc (programmed to deliver 0.5 mg of scopolamine over 3 days) should be applied to the hairless area behind one ear at least 4 hours before the antiemetic effect is required. Only one disc should be worn at any time.

Handling: After the disc is applied on dry skin behind the ear, the hands should be washed thoroughly with soap and water and dried. Upon removal of the disc, it should be discarded, and the hands and application site washed thoroughly with soap and water and dried, to prevent any traces of scopolamine from coming into direct contact with the eyes. (A patient brochure is available.)

Continuation of Therapy: Should be discarded, and a fresh one placed on the hairless area behind the other ear. If therapy is required for longer than 3 days, the first disc should be discarded, and a fresh one placed on the hairless area behind the other ear.

PATIENT PACKAGE INSERT:

The Transderm Scop system helps to prevent the nausea and vomiting of motion sickness for up to 3 days. It is an adhesive disc that you place behind your ear several hours before you travel. Wear only one disc at any time.

Be sure to wash your hands thoroughly with soap and water immediately after handling the disc, so that any drug that might get on your hands will not come into contact with your eyes.

Avoid drinking alcohol while using Transderm Scop. Also, be careful about driving or operating any machinery while using the system because the drug might make you drowsy.

DO NOT USE TRANSDERM SCOP IF YOU ARE ALLERGIC TO SCOPOLAMINE OR HAVE GLAUCOMA.

TRANSDERM SCOP SHOULD NOT BE USED IN CHILDREN AND SHOULD BE USED WITH SPECIAL CAUTION IN THE ELDERLY.

HOW THE TRANSDERM SCOP SYSTEM WORKS

A group of nerve fibers deep inside the ear helps people keep their balance. For some people, the motion of ships, airplanes, trains, automobiles, and buses increases the activity of these nerve fibers. This increased activity causes the *dizziness, nausea, and vomiting* of motion sickness. People may have one, some, or all these symptoms.

Transderm Scop contains the drug scopolamine, which helps reduce the activity of the nerve fibers in the inner ear. When a Transderm Scop disc is placed on the skin behind one of the ears, scopolamine passes through the skin and into the bloodstream. One disc may be kept in place for 3 days if needed.

PRECAUTIONS

PATIENT PACKAGE INSERT: *(cont'd)*

Before using Transderm Scop be sure to tell your doctor if you

Are pregnant or nursing (or planning to become pregnant)

Have (or have had) glaucoma (increased pressure in the eyeball)

Have (or have had) any metabolic, liver, or kidney disease

Have any obstructions of the stomach or intestine

Have trouble urinating or any bladder obstruction

Have any skin allergy or have had a skin reaction such as a rash or redness to any drug, especially scopolamine, or chemical or food substance.

Any of these conditions could make Transderm Scop unsuitable for you; Also tell your doctor if you are taking any other medicines.

In the unlikely event that you experience pain in the eye and reddened whites of the eye, which may be accompanied by widening of the pupil and blurred vision, remove the disc immediately and consult your physician. As indicated below under Side Effects, widening of the pupils and blurred vision without pain or reddened whites of the eye is usually temporary and not serious.

Transderm Scop should not be used in children. The safety of its use in children has not been determined. Children and the elderly may be particularly sensitive to the effects of scopolamine.

Side Effects

The most common side effect experienced by people using Transderm Scop is dryness of the mouth. This occurs in about two thirds of the people. A less frequent side effect is drowsiness, which occurs in less than one sixth of the people. Temporary blurring of vision and dilation (widening) of the pupils may occur, especially if the drug is on your hands and comes in contact with the eyes. On infrequent occasions, disorientation, memory disturbances, dizziness, restlessness, hallucinations, confusion, difficulty urinating, skin rashes or redness, dry, itchy, or red eyes and eye pain have been reported. If these effects do occur, remove the disc and call your doctor. Since drowsiness disorientation, and confusion may occur with the use of scopolamine, be careful driving or operating any dangerous machinery, especially when you first start using the drug system.

Drug Withdrawal: Symptoms including dizziness, nausea, vomiting, headache and disturbances of equilibrium have been reported in a few people following discontinuation of the Transderm Scop system. These symptoms have occurred most often in people who have used the systems for more than three days. We recommend that you consult your doctor if these symptoms occur.

HOW TO USE TRANSDERM SCOP

Transderm Scop should be stored between 59°-86°F (15°-30°C) until you are ready to use it.

1. Plan to apply one Transderm Scop disc at least 4 hours before you are ready to use it. **Wear only one disc at a time.**

2. Select a hairless area of skin behind one ear, taking care to avoid any cuts or irritations. Wipe the area with a clean, dry tissue.

3. Peel the package open and remove the disc.

4. Remove the clear plastic six-sided backing from the round system. Try not to touch the adhesive surface on the disc with your hands.

5. Firmly apply the adhesive surface (metallic side) to the dry area of the skin behind the ear so that the tan-colored side is showing. Make good contact, especially around the edge. Once you have placed the disc behind your ear, do not move it for as long you want to use it (up to 3 days).

6. ***Important:*** *After the disc is in place, be sure to wash your hands thoroughly with soap and water to remove any scopolamine. If this drug were to contact your eyes, it could cause temporary blurring of vision and dilation (widening) of the pupils (the dark circles in the center of your eyes). This is not serious unless accompanied by eye pain and redness* (see PRECAUTIONS) *, and your pupils should return to normal.*

7. Remove the disc after 3 days and throw it away. (You may remove it sooner if you are no longer concerned about motion sickness.) After removing the disc, be sure to wash your hands and the area behind your ear thoroughly with soap and water.

8. If you wish to control nausea for longer than 3 days, *remove* the first disc after 3 days and place a new one *behind the other ear*, repeating instructions 2 to 7.

9. Keep the disc dry, if possible, to prevent it from falling off. Limited contact with water, however, as in bathing or swimming, will not effect the system. In the unlikely event that the disc falls off, throw it away and put a new one behind your ear.

This leaflet presents a summary of information about Transderm Scop. If you would like more information or if you have any questions, ask your doctor or pharmacist. A more technical leaflet is available, written for you doctor. If you would like to read the leaflet, ask your pharmacist to show you a copy. You may need the help of your doctor or pharmacist to understand some of the information.

HOW SUPPLIED:

The Transderm Scop system is a tan-colored disc, 2.5 cm^2, on a clear, oversized, hexagonal peel strip, which is removed prior to use.

Each Transderm Scop system contains 1 mg of scopolamine and is programmed to deliver *in vivo* 0.5 mg of scopolamine over 3 days. Transderm Scop is available in packages of four discs. Each disc is foil wrapped. Patient instructions are included.

1 Package (4 discs): NDC 0083-4345-04

The system should be stored between 59-86°F (15-30°C).

HOW SUPPLIED - EQUIVALENTS NOT AVAILABLE:

Film, Extended Release - Transdermal - 0.5 mg

12's $44.95 TRANSDERM SCOP, Novartis 00083-4345-04

SCOPOLAMINE HYDROBROMIDE *(002215)*

CATEGORIES: Analeptics; Anesthesia; Anticholinergic Agents; Antiemetics; Antimuscarinics/Antispasmodics; Autonomic Drugs; Conjunctivitis; Corneal Ulcer; Cycloplegics/Mydriatics; EENT Drugs; Eye, Ear, Nose, & Throat Preparations; Gastrointestinal Drugs; Iridocyclitis; Mydriasis; Mydriatics; Mydriatics & Cycloplegics; Ophthalmics; Otic Preparations; Otologic; Vertigo/Motion Sickness/Vomiting; FDA Pre 1938 Drugs

BRAND NAMES: **Isopto Hyoscine**; *Minims Hyoscine Hydrobromide (International brand names outside U.S. in italics)*

FORMULARIES: Aetna; FHP; Medi-Cal

DESCRIPTION:

Scopolamine Hydrobromide is an anticholinergic prepared as a sterile topical ophthalmic solution.

DESCRIPTION: *(cont'd)*

Established Name: Scopolamine Hydrobromide

Chemical Name: Benzeneacetic acid, α-(hydroxy-methyl)-, 9-methyl-3-oxa-9-azatricyclo (3.3.1.$0^{2,4}$)non-7-yl ester, hydrobromide, trihydrate, (7(*S*)-(1α,2β,4β,5α,7β))-.

Each ml contains: Active: Scopolamine Hydrobromide 0.25%. Preservative: Benzalkonium Chloride 0.01%. Vehicle: Hydroxypropyl Methylcellulose 0.5%. Inactive: Sodium Chloride, Glacial Acetic Acid, Sodium Acetate (to adjust pH), Purified Water.

CLINICAL PHARMACOLOGY:

This anticholinergic preparation blocks the responses of the sphincter muscle of the ciliary body to cholinergic stimulation, producing pupillary dilation (mydriasis) and paralysis of accommodation (cycloplegia).

INDICATIONS AND USAGE:

For mydriasis and cycloplegia in diagnostic procedures. For some pre- and post-operative states when a mydriatic and cycloplegic is needed in the treatment of iridocyclitis.

CONTRAINDICATIONS:

Contraindicated in persons with primary glaucoma or a tendency toward glaucoma, e.g., narrow anterior chamber angle; and in those showing hypersensitivity to any component of this preparation.

WARNINGS:

For topical use only — not for injection. In infants and small children, use with extreme caution.

PRECAUTIONS:

To avoid excessive absorption, the lacrimal sac should be compressed by digital pressure for one minute after instillation. To avoid inducing angle closure glaucoma, an estimation of the depth of the angle of the anterior chamber should be made.

Patient Warning: Patient should be advised not to drive or engage in other hazardous activities when drowsy or while pupils are dilated. Patient may experience sensitivity to light and should protect eyes in bright illumination during dilation. Parents should be warned not to get this preparation in their child's mouth and to wash their own hands and the child's hands following administration.

ADVERSE REACTIONS:

Prolonged use may produce local irritation, characterized by follicular conjunctivitis, vascular congestion, edema, exudate, and an eczematoid dermatitis. Somnolence may occur.

DOSAGE AND ADMINISTRATION:

For refraction, administer one or two drops topically in the eye(s) one hour before refracting. For uveitis, administer one or two drops topically in the eye(s) up to three times daily.

HOW SUPPLIED - EQUIVALENTS NOT AVAILABLE:

Injection, Solution - Intramuscular; - 0.4 mg/ml

1 ml x 25	$30.00	Scopolamine Hydrobromide, Fujisawa USA	00469-0268-25
1 ml x 25	$35.00	Scopolamine Hydrobromide, Consolidated Midland	00223-8413-01

Injection, Solution - Intramuscular; - 1 mg/ml

1 ml x 25	$30.00	Scopolamine Hydromide, Fujisawa USA	00469-0270-25
1 ml x 25	$31.50	Scopolamine Hydrobromide, Consolidated Midland	00223-8414-25

Solution - Ophthalmic - 0.25 %

5 ml	**$11.25**	**ISOPTO HYOSCINE, Alcon-PR**	**00998-0331-05**
15 ml	**$15.62**	**ISOPTO HYOSCINE, Alcon-PR**	**00998-0331-15**

SECOBARBITAL SODIUM *(002216)*

CATEGORIES: Anesthesia; Anxiolytics, Sedatives, Hypnotic; Barbiturates; Central Nervous System Agents; Hypnotics; Insomnia; Sedatives/Hypnotics; Pregnancy Category D; DEA Class CII; FDA Approval Pre 1982

BRAND NAMES: *Immenoctal*; *Novosecobarb*; *Secanal*; **Seconal Sodium**; Sodium Secobarbital
(International brand names outside U.S. in italics)

FORMULARIES: Medi-Cal

COST OF THERAPY: $0.14 (Insomnia; Capsule; 100 mg; 1/day; 7 days) vs. Potential Cost of $3,628.44 (Psychoses)

DESCRIPTION:

WARNING: MAY BE HABIT-FORMING

The barbiturates are nonselective central-nervous-system (CNS) depressants that are primarily used as sedative-hypnotics. In subhypnotic doses, they are also used as anticonvulsants. The barbiturates and their sodium salts are subject to control under the Federal Controlled Substances Act.

Secobarbital sodium, USP, is a barbituric acid derivative and occurs as a white, odorless, bitter powder that is very soluble in water, soluble in alcohol, and practically insoluble in ether. Chemically, the drug is sodium 5-allyl-5-(1-methylbutyl)barbiturate, with the empirical formula $C_{12}H_{17}N_2NaO_3$. Its molecular weight is 260.27.

Each Seconal Sodium capsule contains 100 mg (0.38 mmol) of secobarbital sodium. These products also contain corn starch, D&C Yellow No. 10, FD&C Red No. 3, gelatin, magnesium stearate, silicone, and other inactive ingredients.

CLINICAL PHARMACOLOGY:

Barbiturates are capable of producing all levels of CNS mood alteration, from excitation to mild sedation, hypnosis, and deep coma. Overdosage can produce death. Barbiturates depress the sensory cortex, decrease motor activity, alter cerebellar function, and produce drowsiness, sedation, and hypnosis.

Barbiturate-induced sleep differs from physiologic sleep. Sleep laboratory studies have demonstrated that barbiturates reduce the amount of time spent in the rapid eye movement (REM) phase, or dreaming stage of sleep. Also, Stages III and IV sleep are decreased. Following abrupt cessation of regularly used barbiturates, patients may experience markedly increased dreaming, nightmares, and/or insomnia. Therefore, withdrawal of a single therapeutic dose over 5 or 6 days has been recommended to lessen the REM rebound and disturbed sleep that contribute to drug withdrawal syndrome (for example, decreasing the dose from 3 to 2 doses a day for 1 week).

CLINICAL PHARMACOLOGY: *(cont'd)*

In studies, secobarbital sodium and pentobarbital sodium have been found to lose most of its effectiveness for both inducing and maintaining sleep by the end of 2 weeks of continued drug administration, even with the use of multiple doses. As with secobarbital sodium and pentobarbital sodium, other barbiturates (including amobarbital) might be expected to lose their effectiveness for inducing and maintaining sleep after about 2 weeks. The short-, intermediate-, and to a lesser degree, long-acting barbiturates have been widely prescribed for treating insomnia. Although the clinical literature abounds with claims that the short-acting barbiturates are superior for producing sleep whereas the intermediate-acting compounds are more effective in maintaining sleep, controlled studies have failed to demonstrate these differential effects. Therefore, as sleep medications, the barbiturates are of limited value beyond short-term use.

Barbiturates have little analgesic action at subanesthetic doses. Rather, in subanesthetic doses, these drugs may increase the reaction to painful stimuli. All barbiturates exhibit anticonvulsant activity in anesthetic doses. However, of the drugs in this class, only phenobarbital, mephobarbital, and metharbital are effective as oral anticonvulsants in subhypnotic doses.

Barbiturates are respiratory depressants, and the degree of depression is dependent on the dose. With hypnotic doses, respiratory depression is similar to that which occurs during physiologic sleep accompanied by a slight decrease in blood pressure and heart rate.

Studies in laboratory animals have shown that barbiturates cause reduction in the tone and contractility of the uterus, ureters, and urinary bladder. However, concentrations of the drugs required to produce this effect in humans are not reached with sedative-hypnotic doses.

Barbiturates do not impair normal hepatic function, but have been shown to induce liver microsomal enzymes, thus increasing and/or altering the metabolism of barbiturates and other drugs (see DRUG INTERACTIONS).

Pharmacokinetics: Barbiturates are absorbed in varying degrees following oral or parenteral administration. The salts are more rapidly absorbed than are the acids. The rate of absorption is increased if the sodium salt is ingested as a dilute solution or taken on an empty stomach. Duration of action, which is related to the rate at which barbiturates are redistributed throughout the body, varies among persons and in the same person from time to time.

Seconal sodium is classified as a short-acting barbiturate when taken orally. Its onset of action is 10 to 15 minutes and is duration of action ranges from 3 to 4 hours.

Barbiturates are weak acids that are absorbed and rapidly distributed to all tissues and fluids, with high concentrations in the brain, liver, and kidneys. Lipid solubility of the barbiturates is the dominant factor in their distribution within the body. Barbiturates are bound to plasma and tissue proteins; the degree of binding increases as a function of lipid solubility.

Phenobarbital has the lowest lipid solubility, lowest plasma binding, lowest brain protein binding, the longest delay in onset of activity, and the longest duration of activity, and the longest duration of action. At the opposite extreme is secobarbital, which has the highest lipid solubility, highest plasma protein binding, highest brain protein binding, the shortest delay in onset of activity, and the shortest duration of action. The plasma half-life for secobarbital sodium in adults ranges between 15 to 40 hours, with a mean of 28 hours. No data are available for children and newborns.

Barbiturates are metabolized primarily by the hepatic microsomal enzyme system, and the metabolic products are excreted in the urine and, less commonly, in the feces. The excretion of unmetabolized barbiturate is 1 feature that distinguishes the long-acting category from those belonging to other categories, which are almost entirely metabolized. The inactive metabolites of the barbiturates are excreted as conjugates of glucuronic acid.

INDICATIONS AND USAGE:

A. Hypnotic, for the short-term treatment of insomnia, since barbiturates appear to lose their effectiveness for sleep induction and sleep maintenance after 2 weeks (see CLINICAL PHARMACOLOGY).

B. Preanesthetic.

CONTRAINDICATIONS:

Secobarbital sodium is contraindicated in patients who are hypersensitive to barbiturates. It is also contraindicated in patients with a history of manifest or latent porphyria, marked impairment of liver function, or respiratory disease in which dyspnea or obstruction is evident.

WARNINGS:

Habit-Forming: Secobarbital sodium may be habit-forming. Tolerance and psychologic and physical dependence may occur with continued use (see DRUG ABUSE AND DEPENDENCE and CLINICAL PHARMACOLOGY, Pharmacokinetics). Patients who have psychologic dependence on barbiturates may increase the dosage or decrease the dosage interval without consulting a physician and subsequently may develop a physical dependence on barbiturates. To minimize the possibility of overdosage or development of dependence, the prescribing and dispensing of secobarbital sodium should be limited to the amount required for the interval until the next appointment. After prolonged use, the abrupt cessation of secobarbital sodium in a person who is dependent on the drug may result in withdrawal symptoms, including delirium, convulsions, and possibly death. Secobarbital sodium should be withdrawn gradually from any patient known to be taking excessive doses over long periods (see DRUG ABUSE AND DEPENDENCE).

Acute or Chronic Pain: Caution should be exercised when barbiturates are administered to patients with acute or chronic pain, because paradoxical excitement could be induced or important symptoms could be masked.

Usage in Pregnancy: Barbiturates can cause fetal harm when administered to a pregnant woman. Retrospective, case-controlled studies have suggested that there may be a relationship between the maternal consumption of barbiturates and a higher than expected incidence of fetal abnormalities. Secobarbital sodium readily crosses the placental barrier and is distributed throughout fetal tissues; the highest concentrations are found in the placenta, liver, and brain.

Withdrawal symptoms occur in infants born to women who receive secobarbital sodium throughout the last trimester of pregnancy (*see* DRUG ABUSE AND DEPENDENCE). If secobarbital sodium is used during pregnancy or if the patient becomes pregnant while taking this drug, the patient should be apprised of the potential hazard to the fetus.

Synergistic Effects: The concomitant use of alcohol or other CNS depressants may produce additive CNS-depressant effects.

PRECAUTIONS:

GENERAL

Barbiturates may be habit-forming. Tolerance and psychologic and physical dependence may occur with continuing use (see DRUG ABUSE AND DEPENDENCE). Barbiturates should be administered with caution, if at all, to patients who are mentally depressed, have suicidal tendencies, or have a history of drug abuse.

Elderly or debilitated patients may react to barbiturates with marked excitement, depression, or confusion. In some persons, especially children, barbiturates repeatedly produce excitement rather then depression.

PRECAUTIONS: *(cont'd)*

In patients with hepatic damage, barbiturates should be administered with caution and initially in reduced doses. Barbiturates should not be administered to patients showing the premonitory signs of hepatic coma.

INFORMATION FOR PATIENTS

The following information should be given to patients receiving secobarbital sodium:

1. The use of secobarbital sodium carries with it an associated risk of psychologic and/or physical dependence. The patient should be warned against increasing the dose of the drug without consulting a physician.

2. Secobarbital sodium may impair the mental and/or physical abilities required for the performance of potentially hazardous tasks, such as driving a car or operating machinery. The patient should be cautioned accordingly.

3. Alcohol should be consumed while taking secobarbital sodium. The concurrent use of secobarbital sodium with other CNS depressants (*e.g.,* alcohol, narcotics, tranquilizers, and antihistamines) may result in additional CNS-depressant effects.

LABORATORY TESTS

Prolonged therapy with barbiturates should be accompanied by periodic evaluation of organic systems, including hematopoietic, renal, and hepatic systems (*see* General under Precautions and Adverse Reactions).

CARCINOGENESIS

Animal Data: Phenobarbital sodium is carcinogenic in mice and rats after lifetime administration. In mice, it produced benign and malignant liver cell tumors. In rats, benign liver cell tumors were observed very late in life.

Human Data: In a 29-year epidemiologic study of 9,136 patients who were treated on an anticonvulsant protocol that included phenobarbital, results indicated a higher then normal incidence of carcinoma. Previously, some of these patients had been treated with thorotrast,a drug that is known to produce hepatic carcinomas. Thus, this study did not provide sufficient evidence that phenobarbital sodium is carcinogenic in humans.

A retrospective study of 84 children with brain tumors matched to 73 normal controls and 78 cancer controls (malignant disease other than brain tumors) suggested an association between exposure to barbiturates prenatally and an increased incidence of brain tumors.

PREGNANCY CATEGORY D

Teratogenic Effects: See WARNINGS, Use in Pregnancy.

Nonteratogenic Effects: Reports of infants suffering from long-term barbiturate exposure *in utero* included the acute withdrawal syndrome of seizures and hyperirritability from birth to a delayed onset of up to 14 days (see DRUG ABUSE AND DEPENDENCE).

LABOR AND DELIVERY

Hypnotic doses of barbiturates do not appear to impair uterine activity significantly during labor. Full anesthetic doses of barbiturates decrease the force and frequency of uterine contractions. Administration of sedative-hypnotic barbiturates to the mother during labor may result in respiratory depression in the newborn. Premature infants are particularly susceptible to the depressant effects of barbiturates. If barbiturates are used during labor and delivery, resuscitation equipment should be available.

Data are not available to evaluate the effect of barbiturates when forceps delivery or other intervention is, necessary or to determine the effect of barbiturates on the later growth, development, and functional maturity of the child.

NURSING MOTHERS

Caution should be exercised when secobarbital sodium is administered to a nursing woman, because small amounts of barbiturates are excreted in the milk.

DRUG INTERACTIONS:

Most reports of clinically significant drug interactions occurring with the barbiturates have involved phenobarbital. However, the application of these data to other barbiturates appears valid and warrants serial blood level determinations of the relevant drugs when there are multiple therapies.

Anticoagulants: Phenobarbital lowers the plasma levels of dicumarol and causes a decrease in anticoagulant activity as measured by the prothrombin time. Barbiturates can induce hepatic microsomal enzymes, resulting in increased metabolism and decreased by the resulting in increased metabolism and decreased anticoagulant response of oral anticoagulants (*e.g.,* warfarin, acenocoumarol, dicumarol, and phenprocoumon). Patients stabilized on anticoagulant therapy may require dosage adjustments if barbiturates are added to or withdrawn from their dosage regimen.

Corticosteroids: Barbiturates appear to enhance the metabolism of exogenous corticosteroids, probably through the induction of hepatic microsomal enzymes. Patients stabilized on corticosteroid therapy may require dosage adjustments if barbiturates are added to or withdrawn from their dosage regimen.

Griseofulvin: Phenobarbital appears to interfere with the absorption of orally administered griseofulvin, thus decreasing its blood level. The effect of the resultant decreased blood levels of griseofulvin on therapeutic response has not been established. However, it would be preferable to avoid concomitant administration of these drugs.

Doxycycline: Phenobarbital has been shown to shorten the half-life of doxycycline for as long as 2 weeks after barbiturate therapy is discontinued.

This mechanism is probably through the induction of hepatic microsomal enzymes that metabolize the antibiotic. If barbiturates and doxycycline are administered concurrently, the clinical response to doxycycline should be monitored closely.

Phenytoin, Sodium Valproate, Valproic Acid: The effect of barbiturates on the metabolism of phenytoin appears to be variable. Some investigators report an accelerating effect, whereas others report no effect. Because the effect of barbiturates on the metabolism of phenytoin is not predictable, phenytoin and barbiturate blood levels should be monitored more frequently if these drugs are given concurrently. Sodium valproate and valproic acid increase the secobarbital sodium blood levels; therefore, secobarbital sodium blood levels should be monitored closely and appropriate dosage adjustments made as clinically indicated.

CNS Depressants: The concomitant use of other CNS depressants, including other sedatives or hypnotics, antihistamines, tranquilizers, or alcohol, may produce additive depressant effects.

Monoamine Oxidase Inhibitors (MAOIs): MAOIs prolong the effects of barbiturates, probably because metabolism of the barbiturate is inhibited.

Estradiol, Estrone, Progesterone, and Other Steroidal Hormones: Pretreatment with or concurrent administration of phenobarbital may decrease the effect of estradiol by increasing its metabolism. There have been reports of women who become pregnant while taking oral contraceptives. An alternate contraceptive method might be suggested to women taking barbiturates.

ADVERSE REACTIONS:

The following adverse reactions and their incidence were compiled from surveillance of thousands of hospitalized patients who received barbiturates. Because such patients may be less aware of some of the milder adverse effects of barbiturates, the incidence of these reactions may be somewhat higher in fully ambulatory patients.

MORE THAN 1 IN 100 PATIENTS

The most common adverse reaction estimated to occur at a rate of 1 to 3 patients per 100 is the following:

Nervous System: Somnolence

LESS THAN 1 IN 100 PATIENTS

Adverse reactions estimated to occur at a rate of less than 1 in 100 patients are listed below, grouped by organ system and by decreasing order of occurrence:

Nervous System: Agitation, confusion, hyperkinesia, ataxia, CNS depression, nightmares, nervousness, psychiatric disturbance, hallucinations, insomnia, anxiety, dizziness, abnormality in thinking

Respiratory System: Hypoventilation, apnea

Cardiovascular System: Bradycardia, hypotension, syncope

Digestive System: Nausea, vomiting, constipation

Other Reported Reactions: Headache, injection site reactions, hypersensitivity reactions (angioedema, skin rashes, exfoliative dermatitis), fever, liver damage.

DRUG ABUSE AND DEPENDENCE:

Controlled Substance: Secobarbital sodium is a Schedule II drug.

Dependence: Barbiturates may be habit-forming; tolerance, psychologic dependence, and physical dependence may occur, especially following prolonged use of high doses of barbiturates. Daily administration in excess of 400 mg of secobarbital for approximately 90 days is likely to produce some degree of physical dependence. A dosage of 600 to 800 mg for at least 35 days is sufficient to produce withdrawal seizures. The average daily dose of the barbiturate addict is usually about 1.5 g. As tolerance to barbiturates develops, the amount needed to maintain the same level of intoxication increases; tolerance to a fatal dosage, however, does not increase more than two-fold. As this occurs, the margin between intoxicating dosage and fatal dosage becomes smaller.

Symptoms of acute intoxication with barbiturates include unsteady gait, slurred speech, and sustained nystagmus. Mental signs of chronic intoxication include confusion, poor judgement, irritability, insomnia, and somatic complaints.

Symptoms of barbiturate dependence are similar to those of chronic alcoholism. If an individual appears to be intoxicated with alcohol to a degree that is radically disproportionate to the amount of alcohol in his or her blood, the use of barbiturates should be suspected. The lethal dose of a barbiturate is far less if alcohol is also ingested.

The symptoms of barbiturate withdrawal can be severe and may cause death. Minor withdrawal symptoms may appear 8 to 12 hours after the last dose of a barbiturate. These symptoms usually appear in the following order: anxiety, muscle twitching, tremor of hands and fingers progressive weakness, dizziness distortion in visual perception, nausea, vomiting, insomnia, and orthostatic hypotension. Major withdrawal symptoms (convulsions and delirium) may occur within 16 hours and last up to 5 days after abrupt cessation of barbiturates. Intensity of withdrawal symptoms gradually declines over a period of approximately 15 days. Individuals susceptible to barbiturate abuse and dependence include alcoholics and opiate abusers, as well as other sedative-hypnotic and amphetamine abusers.

Drug dependence on barbiturates arises from repeated administration on a continuous basis, generally in amounts, exceeding therapeutic dose levels. The characteristics of drug dependence on barbiturates include the following: (a) a strong desire or need to continue taking the drug; (b) a tendency to increase the dose; (c) a psychic dependence on the effects of the drug related to subjective and individual appreciation of those effects; and (d) a physical dependence on the effect of the drug, requiring its presence for maintenance of homeostasis and resulting in a definite, characteristic, and self-limited abstinence syndrome when the drug is withdrawn.

Treatment of barbiturate dependence consists of cautions and gradual withdrawal of the drug. Barbiturate-dependent patients can be withdrawn by using a number of withdrawal regimens. In all cases, withdrawal takes an extended period. One method involves substituting a 30-mg dose of phenobarbital for each 100- to 200-mg dose of barbiturate that the patient has been taking. The total daily amount of phenobarbital is then administered in 3 or 4 divided doses, not to exceed 600 mg daily. Should signs of withdrawal occur on the first day of treatment, a loading dose of 200 to 300 mg of phenobarbital may be administered IM in addition to the oral dose. After stabilization on phenobarbital, the total daily dose is decreased by 30 mg a day as long as withdrawal is proceeding smoothly. A modification of this regimen involves initiating treatment at the patient's regular dosage level and decreasing the daily dosage by 10% as tolerated by the patient. Infants that are physically dependent on barbiturates may be given phenobarbital, 3 to 10 mg/kg/day. After withdrawal symptoms (hyperactivity, disturbed sleep, tremors, and hyperreflexia) are relieved, the dosage of phenobarbital should be gradually decreased and completely withdrawn over a 2-week period.

OVERDOSAGE:

The toxic dose of barbiturates varies considerably. In general, an oral dose of 1 g of most barbiturates produces serious poisoning in an adult. Death commonly occurs after 2 to 10 g of ingested barbiturate. The sedated, therapeutic blood levels of secobarbital range between 0.5 to 5 mg/L; the usual lethal blood level ranges from 15 to 40 mg/L. Barbiturate intoxication may be confused with alcoholism, bromide intoxication, and various neurologic disorders. Potential tolerance must be considered when evaluating significance of dose and plasma concentration.

Signs and Symptoms: Symptoms of oral overdose may occur within 15 minutes and begin with central nervous system depression, under-ventilation, hypotension, and hypothermia, which may progress to pulmonary edema and death. Hemorrhagic blisters may develop, especially at pressure points.

In extreme overdose, all electrical activity in the brain may cease, in which case a "flat" EEG normally equated with clinical death cannot be accepted, as indicative of brain death. This effect is fully reversible unless hypoxic damage occurs. Consideration should be given to the possibility of barbiturate intoxication even in situations that appear to involve trauma.

Complications such as pneumonia, pulmonary edema, cardiac arrhythmias, congestive heart failure, and renal failure may occur. Uremia may increase CNS sensitivity to barbiturates if renal function is impaired. Differential diagnosis should include hypoglycemia, head trauma, cerebrovascular accidents, convulsive states, and diabetic coma.

Treatment: To obtain up-to-date information about the treatment of overdose, a good resource is your certified Regional Poison Control Center. Telephone numbers of certified poison control centers are listed in *Physicians GenRx*. In managing overdosage, consider the possibility of multiple drug overdoses, interaction among drugs, and unusual drug kinetics in your patient.

OVERDOSAGE: *(cont'd)*

Protect the patient's airway and support ventilation and perfusion. Meticulously monitor and maintain, within acceptable limits, the patient's vital signs, blood gases, serum electrolytes, etc. Absorption of drugs from the gastrointestinal tract may be decreased by giving activated charcoal, which, in many cases, is more effective than emesis or lavage; consider charcoal instead or in addition to gastric emptying. Repeated doses of charcoal over time may hasten elimination of some drugs that have been absorbed. Safeguard the patient's airway when employing gastric emptying or charcoal.

Diuresis and peritoneal dialysis are of little value; hemodialysis and hemoperfusion enhance drug clearance and should be considered in serious poisoning. If the patient has chronically abused sedatives, withdrawal reactions may be manifest following acute overdose.

DOSAGE AND ADMINISTRATION:

Dosage of barbiturates must be individualized with full knowledge of their particular characteristics. Factors of consideration are the patient's age, weight, and condition.

Adults: As a hypnotic, 100 mg at bedtime. Preoperatively, 200 to 300 mg 1 to 2 hours before surgery.

Children: Preoperatively, 2 to 6 mg/kg, with a maximum dosage of 100 mg.

Special Patient Population: Dosage should be reduced in elderly or debilitated because these patients may be more sensitive to barbiturates. Dosage should be reduced for patients with impaired renal function or hepatic disease.

Store at controlled room temperature, 15° to 30°C (59° to 86°F). Dispense in a tight container.

HOW SUPPLIED - RATED THERAPEUTICALLY EQUIVALENT:

Capsule, Gelatin - Oral - 50 mg

100's	**$10.68**	**SECONAL SODIUM, Lilly**	**00002-0642-02**

Capsule, Gelatin - Oral - 100 mg

100's	$2.00	Secobarbital Sodium, Anabolic	00722-5120-02
100's	$6.20	Secobarbital Sodium, Halsey Drug	00879-0029-01
100's	**$20.08**	**SECONAL SODIUM, Lilly**	**00002-0640-02**
100's	**$24.46**	**SECONAL SODIUM, Lilly**	**00002-0640-33**
500's	**$69.74**	**SECONAL SODIUM, Lilly**	**00002-0640-03**
1000's	$15.75	Secobarbital Sodium, Anabolic	00722-5120-03
1000's	$58.00	Secobarbital Sodium, Halsey Drug	00879-0029-10

HOW SUPPLIED - NOT RATED EQUIVALENT:

Injection, Solution - Intramuscular; - 50 mg/ml

2 ml x 10	$27.36	Sodium Secorbarbital, Wyeth Labs	00008-0305-02
2 ml x 10	$31.11	SECOBARBITAL SODIUM, Wyeth Labs	00008-0305-50

SELEGILINE HYDROCHLORIDE *(002218)*

CATEGORIES: Anticholinergic Agents; Antiparkinson Agents; Autonomic Drugs; Extrapyramidal Movement Disorders; Neuromuscular; Orphan Drugs; Parkinsonism; Alzheimer's Disease*; Sialorrhea*; Tremor*; Pregnancy Category C; Sales > $100 Million; FDA Approved 1989 Jun
* Indication not approved by the FDA

BRAND NAMES: Alzene; Carbex; Deprenyl; *Eldeprine*; **Eldepryl**; *Jumex*; *Movergan*; *Plurimen*
(International brand names outside U.S. in italics)

FORMULARIES: Aetna; BC-BS; Medi-Cal; PCS

COST OF THERAPY: $1,576.07 (Parkinsonism; Tablet; 5 mg; 2/day; 365 days)

DESCRIPTION:

Selegiline hydrochloride is a levorotatory acetylenic derivative of phenethylamine. It is commonly referred to in the clinical and pharmacological literature as L-deprenyl.

The chemical name is: (R)-(-)-N,2-dimethyl-N-2- propynylphenethylamine hydrochloride. It is a white to near white crystalline powder, freely soluble in water, chloroform, and methanol. The molecular formula is $C_{13}H_{17}N \cdot HCl$and has a molecular weight of 223.75.

Each Eldepryl white, shield shaped, unscored tablet, debossed on one side with "S" and "5" on the other side, contains 5 mg selegiline hydrochloride. Inactive ingredients are citric acid, lactose, magnesium stearate, and microcrystalline cellulose.

Each Carbex tablet for oral administration contains 5 mg selegiline hydrochloride and the following inactive ingredients: corn starch, lactose monohydrate, magnesium stearate, povidone, and talc.

CLINICAL PHARMACOLOGY:

The mechanisms accounting for selegiline's beneficial adjunctive action in the treatment of Parkinson's disease are not fully understood. Inhibition of monoamine oxidase, type B, activity is generally considered to be of primary importance; in addition, there is evidence that selegiline may act through other mechanisms to increase dopaminergic activity.

Selegiline is best known as an irreversible inhibitor of monoamine oxidase (MAO), an intracellular enzyme associated with the outer membrane of mitochondria. Selegiline inhibits MAO by acting as a 'suicide' substrate for the enzyme; that is, it is converted by MAO to an active moiety which combines irreversibly with the active site and/or the enzyme's essential FAD cofactor. Because selegiline has greater affinity for type B than for type A active sites, it can serve as a selective inhibitor of MAO type B if it is administered at the recommended dose.

MAOs are widely distributed throughout the body; their concentration is especially high in liver, kidney, stomach, intestinal wall, and brain. MAOs are currently subclassified into two types, A and B, which differ in their substrate specificity and tissue distribution. In humans, intestinal MAO is predominantly type A, while most of that in brain is type B.

In CNS neurons, MAO plays an important role in the catabolism of catecholamines (dopamine, norepinephrine and epinephrine) and serotonin. MAOs are also important in the catabolism of various exogenous amines found in a variety of foods and drugs. MAO in the GI tract and liver (primarily type A), for example, is thought to provide vital protection from exogenous amines (*e.g.,* tyramine) that have the capacity, if absorbed intact, to cause a 'hypertensive crisis,' the so-called 'cheese reaction.' (If large amounts of certain exogenous amines gain access to the systemic circulation [e.g., from fermented cheese, red wine, herring, over-the-counter cough/cold medications, etc.] they are taken up by adrenergic neurons and displace norepinephrine from storage sites within membrane bound vesicles. Subsequent release of the displaced norepinephrine causes the rise in systemic blood pressure, etc.)

In theory, therefore, because MAO A of the gut is not inhibited, patients treated with selegiline at a dose of 10 mg a day can take medications containing pharmacologically active amines and consume tyramine-containing foods without risk of uncontrolled hypertension. However, one case of hypertensive crisis has been reported in a patient taking the recom-

CLINICAL PHARMACOLOGY: *(cont'd)*

mended dose of selegiline and a sympathomimetic medication (ephedrine). The pathophysiology of the 'cheese reaction' is complicated and, in addition to its ability to inhibit MAO B selectively, selegiline's relative freedom from this reaction has been attributed to an ability to prevent tyramine and other indirect acting sympathomimetics from displacing norepinephrine from adrenergic neurons.

However, until the pathophysiology of the cheese reaction is more completely understood, it seems prudent to assume that selegiline can only be used safely without dietary restrictions at doses where it presumably selectively inhibits MAO B (*e.g.,* 10 mg/day). **In short, attention to the dose dependent nature of selegiline's selectivity is critical if it is to be used without elaborate restrictions being placed on diet and concomitant drug use although, as noted above, a case of hypertensive crisis has been reported at the recommended dose.** (See WARNINGS and PRECAUTIONS.)

It is important to be aware that selegiline may have pharmacological effects unrelated to MAO B inhibition. As noted above, there is some evidence that it may increase dopaminergic activity by other mechanisms, including interfering with dopamine re-uptake at the synapse. Effects resulting from selegiline administration may also be mediated through its metabolites. Two of its three principal metabolites, amphetamine and methamphetamine, have pharmacological actions of their own; they interfere with neuronal uptake and enhance release of several neurotransmitters (*e.g.,* norepinephrine, dopamine, serotonin). However, the extent to which these metabolites contribute to the effects of selegiline are unknown.

Rationale for the Use of a Selective Monoamine Oxidase Type B Inhibitor in Parkinson's Disease: Many of the prominent symptoms of Parkinson's disease are due to a deficiency of striatal dopamine that is the consequence of a progressive degeneration and loss of a population of dopaminergic neurons which originate in the substantia nigra of the midbrain and project to the basal ganglia or striatum. Early in the course of Parkinson's, the deficit in the capacity of these neurons to synthesize dopamine can be overcome by administration of exogenous levodopa, usually given in combination with a peripheral decarboxylase inhibitor (carbidopa).

With the passage of time, due to the progression of the disease and/or the effect of sustained treatment, the efficacy and quality of the therapeutic response to levodopa diminishes. Thus, after several years of levodopa treatment, the response, for a given dose of levodopa, is shorter, has less predictable onset and offset (*i.e.,* there is "wearing off"), and is often accompanied by side effects (*e.g.,* dyskinesia, akinesias, on-off phenomena, freezing, etc.).

This deteriorating response is currently interpreted as a manifestation of the inability of the ever decreasing population of intact nigrostriatal neurons to synthesize and release adequate amounts of dopamine.

MAO B inhibition may be useful in this setting because, by blocking the catabolism of dopamine, it would increase the net amount of dopamine available (*i.e.,* it would increase the pool of dopamine). Whether or not this mechanism or an alternative one actually accounts for the observed beneficial effects of adjunctive selegiline is unknown.

Selegiline's benefit in Parkinson's disease has only been documented as an adjunct to levodopa/carbidopa. Whether or not it might be effective as a sole treatment is unknown, but past attempts to treat Parkinson's disease with non-selective MAOI monotherapy are reported to have been unsuccessful. It is important to note that attempts to treat Parkinsonian patients with combinations of levodopa and currently marketed non-selective MAO inhibitors were abandoned because of multiple side effects including hypertension, increase in involuntary movement, and toxic delirium.

Pharmacokinetic Information (Absorption, Distribution, Metabolism and Elimination—ADME): Only preliminary information about the details of the pharmacokinetics of selegiline and its metabolites is available.

Data obtained in a study of 12 healthy subjects that was intended to examine the effects of selegiline on the ADME of an oral hypoglycemic agent, however, provides some information. Following the oral administration of a single dose of 10 mg of selegiline hydrochloride to these subjects, serum levels of intact selegiline were below the limit of detection (less than 10 ng/ml). Three metabolites, N-desmethyldeprenyl, the major metabolite (mean half-life 2.0 hours), amphetamine (mean half- life 17.7 hours), and methamphetamine (mean half-life 20.5 hours), were found in serum and urine. Over a period of 48 hours, 45% of the dose administered appeared in the urine as these 3 metabolites.

In an extension of this study intended to examine the effects of steady state conditions, the same subjects were given a 10 mg dose of selegiline hydrochloride for seven consecutive days. Under these conditions, the mean trough serum levels for amphetamine were 3.5 ng/ml and 8.0 ng/ml for methamphetamine; trough levels of N-desmethyldeprenyl were below the levels of detection.

The rate of MAO B regeneration following discontinuation of treatment has not been quantitated. It is this rate, dependent upon *de novo* protein synthesis, which seems likely to determine how fast normal MAO B activity can be restored.

INDICATIONS AND USAGE:

Selegiline hydrochloride is indicated as an adjunct in the management of Parkinsonian patients being treated with levodopa/carbidopa who exhibit deterioration in the quality of their response to this therapy. There is no evidence from controlled clinical studies that selegiline has any beneficial effect in the absence of concurrent levodopa therapy.

Evidence supporting this claim was obtained in randomized controlled clinical investigations that compared the effects of added selegiline or placebo in patients receiving levodopa/carbidopa. Selegiline was significantly superior to placebo on all three principal outcome measures employed; change from baseline in daily levodopa/carbidopa dose, the amount of 'off' time, and patient self-rating of treatment success. Beneficial effects were also observed on other measures of treatment success (*e.g.,* measures of reduced end of dose akinesia, decreased tremor and sialorrhea, improved speech and dressing ability and improved overall disability as assessed by walking and comparison to previous state).

CONTRAINDICATIONS:

Selegiline hydrochloride is contraindicated in patients with a known hypersensitivity to this drug.

Selegiline hydrochloride is contraindicated for use with meperidine. This contraindication is often extended to other opioids. (See DRUG INTERACTIONS.)

WARNINGS:

Selegiline should not be used at daily doses exceeding those recommended (10 mg/day) because of the risks associated with non-selective inhibition of MAO. (See CLINICAL PHARMACOLOGY.)

The selectivity of selegiline for MAO B may not be absolute even at the recommended daily dose of 10 mg a day and selectivity is further diminished with increasing daily doses. The precise dose at which selegiline becomes a non-selective inhibitor of all MAO is unknown, but may be in the range of 30 to 40 mg a day.

Severe CNS toxicity associated with hyperpyrexia and death have been reported with the combination of tricyclic antidepressants and non-selective MAOIs (Phenelzine, Tranylcypromine). A similar reaction has been reported for a patient on amitriptyline and selegiline.

WARNINGS: *(cont'd)*

Another patient receiving protriptyline and selegiline developed tremors, agitation, and restlessness followed by unresponsiveness and death two weeks after selegiline was added. Related adverse events including hypertension, syncope, asystole, diaphoresis, seizures, changes in behavioral and mental status, and muscular rigidity have also been reported in some patients receiving selegiline and various tricyclic antidepressants.

Serious, sometimes fatal, reactions with signs and symptoms that may include hyperthermia, rigidity, myoclonus, autonomic instability with rapid fluctuations of the vital signs, and mental status changes that include extreme agitation progressing to delirium and coma have been reported with patients receiving a combination of fluoxetine hydrochloride and non-selective MAOIs. Similar signs have been reported in some patients on the combination of selegiline (10 mg a day) and selective serotonin reuptake inhibitors including fluoxetine, sertraline, and paroxetine.

Since the mechanisms of these reactions are not fully understood, it seems prudent, in general, to avoid the combination of selegiline and tricyclic antidepressants as well as selegiline and selective serotonin reuptake inhibitors. At least 14 days should elapse between discontinuation of selegiline and initiation of treatment with a tricyclic antidepressant or selective serotonin reuptake inhibitors. Because of the long half lives of fluoxetine and its active metabolite, at least five weeks (perhaps longer, especially if fluoxetine has been prescribed chronically and/or at higher doses) should elapse between discontinuation of fluoxetine and initiation of treatment with selegiline.

PRECAUTIONS:

General: Some patients given selegiline may experience an exacerbation of levodopa associated side effects, presumably due to the increased amounts of dopamine reacting with super-sensitive post-synaptic receptors. These effects may often be mitigated by reducing the dose of levodopa/carbidopa by approximately 10 to 30%.

The decision to prescribe selegiline should take into consideration that the MAO system of enzymes is complex and incompletely understood and there is only a limited amount of carefully documented clinical experience with selegiline. Consequently, the full spectrum of possible responses to selegiline may not have been observed in pre-marketing evaluation of the drug. It is advisable, therefore, to observe patients closely for atypical responses.

Information for the Patient: Patients should be advised of the possible need to reduce levodopa dosage after the initiation of selegiline hydrochloride therapy.

Patients (or their families if the patient is incompetent) should be advised not to exceed the daily recommended dose of 10 mg. The risk of using higher daily doses of selegiline should be explained, and a brief description of the 'cheese reaction' provided. While hypertensive reactions with selegiline associated with dietary influences have not been reported, documented experience is limited.

Consequently, it may be useful to inform patients (or their families) about the signs and symptoms associated with MAOI induced hypertensive reactions. In particular, patients should be urged to report, immediately, any severe headache or other atypical or unusual symptoms not previously experienced.

Laboratory Tests: No specific laboratory tests are deemed essential for the management of patients on selegiline hydrochloride. Periodic routine evaluation of all patients, however, is appropriate.

Carcinogenesis, Mutagenesis, and Impairment of Fertility: Assesement of the carcinogenic potential of selegiline in mice and rats is ongoing.

Selegiline did not induce mutations or chromosomal damage when tested in the bacterial mutation assay in *Salmonella typhimurium*and an *in vivo* chromosomal aberration assay. While these studies provide some resurrance that selegiline is not mutagenic or clastogenic, they are not definitive because of methodological limitations. No definitive *in vitro* chromosomal aberration or *in vitro* mammalian gene mutation assays have been performed.

The effect of selegiline on fertility has not been adequately assessed.

Pregnancy, Teratogenic Effects, Pregnancy Category C: No teratogenic effects were observed in a study of embryo-fetal development in Sprague-Dawley rats at oral doses of 4, 12, and 36 mg/kg or 4, 12, and 35 times the human therapeutic dose on a mg/m^2 basis. No teratogenic effects were observed in a study of embryo-fetal development in New Zealand White rabbits at oral doses of 5, 25, and 50 mg/kg or 10, 48, and 95 times the human therapeutic dose on a mg/m^2basis; however, in this study, the number of litters produced at the two higher doses was less than recommended for assessing teratogenic potential. In the rat study, increases in total resorptions and percent post-implantation loss, and a decrease in the number of live fetuses per dam occurred at the highest dose tested. In a peri- postnatal development study in Sprague-Dawley rats oral doses of 4, 16, and 64 mg/kg or 4, 15, and 62 times the human therapeutic dose on a mg/m^2 basis, an increase in the numbers if stillbirths and decrease in the number of pups per dam, pup survival, and pup body weight (at birth and throughout the lactation period) were observed at the two highest doses. At the highest dose tested, no pups born alive survived to Day 4 postpartum. Postnatal development at the highest dose tested in dams could not be evaluated because of the lack of surviving pups. The reproductive performance of the untreated offspring was not assessed.

There are no adequate and well-controlled studies in pregnant women. Selegiline should be used during pregnancy only if the potential benefit justifies the potential risk to the fetus.

Nursing Mothers: It is not known whether selegiline hydrochloride is excreted in human milk. Because many drugs are excreted in human milk, consideration should be given to discontinuing the use of all but absolutely essential drug treatments in nursing women.

Pediatric Use: The effects of selegiline hydrochloride in pediatric patients have not been evaluated.

DRUG INTERACTIONS:

The occurrence of stupor, muscular rigidity, severe agitation, and elevated temperature has been reported in some patients receiving the combination of selegiline and meperidine. Symptoms usually resolve over days when the combination is discontinued. This is typical of the interaction of meperidine and MAOIs. Other serious reactions (including severe agitation, hallucinations, and death) have been reported in patients receiving this combination (see CONTRAINDICATIONS). Severe toxicity has also been reported in patients receiving the combination of tricyclic antidepressants and selegiline hydrochloride and selective serotonin reuptake inhibitors and selegiline hydrochloride. (See WARNINGS for details.)

ADVERSE REACTIONS:

Introduction: The number of patients who received selegiline in prospectively monitored pre-marketing studies is limited. While other sources of information about the use of selegiline are available (*e.g.,* literature reports, foreign post-marketing reports, etc.) they do not provide the kind of information necessary to estimate the incidence of adverse events. Thus, overall incidence figures for adverse reactions associated with the use of selegiline cannot be provided. Many of the adverse reactions seen have also been reported as symptoms of dopamine excess.

Moreover, the importance and severity of various reactions reported often cannot be ascertained. One index of relative importance, however, is whether or not a reaction caused treatment discontinuation. In prospective pre-marketing studies, the following events led, in

ADVERSE REACTIONS: *(cont'd)*

decreasing order of frequency, to discontinuation of treatment with selegiline: nausea, hallucinations, confusion, depression, loss of balance, insomnia, orthostatic hypotension, increased akinetic involuntary movements, agitation, arrhythmia, bradykinesia, chorea, delusions, hypertension, new or increased angina pectoris, and syncope. Events reported only once as a cause of discontinuation are ankle edema, anxiety, burning lips/mouth, constipation, drowsiness/lethargy, dystonia, excess perspiration, increased freezing, gastrointestinal bleeding, hair loss, increased tremor, nervousness, weakness, and weight loss.

Experience with selegiline hydrochloride obtained in parallel, placebo controlled, randomized studies provides only a limited basis for estimates of adverse reaction rates. The following reactions that occurred with greater frequency among the 49 patients assigned to selegiline as compared to the 50 patients assigned to placebo in the only parallel, placebo controlled trial performed in patients with Parkinson's disease are shown in TABLE 1. None of these adverse reactions led to a discontinuation of treatment.

TABLE 1 Incidence Of Treatment-Emergent Adverse Experiences In The Placebo-Controlled Clinical Trial

Adverse Event	Number of Patients Reporting Events selegiline HCl N=49	placebo N=50
Nausea	10	3
Dizziness/ Lightheaded/ Fainting	7	1
Abdominal Pain	4	2
Confusion	3	0
Hallucinations	3	1
Dry mouth	3	1
Vivid Dreams	2	0
Dyskinesias	2	5
Headache	2	1
The following events were reported once in either or both groups:		
Ache, generalized	1	0
Anxiety/Tension	1	1
Anemia	0	1
Diarrhea	1	0
Hair Loss	0	1
Insomnia	1	1
Lethargy	1	0
Leg pain	1	0
Low back pain	1	0
Malaise	0	1
Palpitations	1	0
Urinary Retention	1	0
Weight Loss	1	0

In all prospectively monitored investigations, enrolling approximately 920 patients, the following adverse events, classified by body system, were reported.

Central Nervous System: *Motor/Coordination/Extrapyramidal:* increased tremor, chorea, loss of balance, restlessness, blepharospasm, increased bradykinesia, facial grimace, falling down, heavy leg, muscle twitch*, myoclonic jerks*, stiff neck, tardive dyskinesia, dystonic symptoms, dyskinesia, involuntary movements, freezing, festination, increased apraxia, muscle cramps. *Mental Status/Behavioral/Psychiatric:* hallucinations, dizziness, confusion, anxiety, depression, drowsiness, behavior/mood change, dreams/nightmares, tiredness, delusions, disorientation, lightheadedness, impaired memory*, increased energy*, transient high*, hollow feeling, lethargy/malaise, apathy, overstimulation, vertigo, personality change, sleep disturbance, restlessness, weakness, transient irritability. *Pain/Altered Sensation:* headache, back pain, leg pain, tinnitus, migraine, supraorbital pain, throat burning, generalized ache, chills, numbness of toes/fingers, taste disturbance.

Autonomic Nervous System: dry mouth, blurred vision, sexual dysfunction.

Cardiovascular: orthostatic hypotension, hypertension, arrhythmia, palpitations, new or increased angina pectoris, hypotension, tachycardia, peripheral edema, sinus bradycardia, syncope.

Gastrointestinal: nausea/vomiting, constipation, weight loss, anorexia, poor appetite, dysphagia, diarrhea, heartburn, rectal bleeding, bruxism*, gastrointestinal bleeding (exacerbation of preexisting ulcer disease).

Genitourinary/Gynecologic/Endocrine: slow urination, transient anorgasmia*, nocturia, prostatic hypertrophy, urinary hesitancy, urinary retention, decreased penile sensation*, urinary frequency.

Skin and Appendages: increased sweating, diaphoresis, facial hair, hair loss, hematoma, rash, photosensitivity.

Miscellaneous: asthma, diplopia, shortness of breath, speech affected.

Postmarketing Reports: The following experiences were described in spontaneous post-marketing reports. These reports do not provide sufficient information to establish a clear causal relationship with the use of selegiline hydrochloride.

CNS: Seizure in dialyzed chronic renal failure patient on concomitant medications.

* indicates events reported only at doses greater than 10 mg/day.

OVERDOSAGE:

Selegiline: No specific information is available about clinically significant overdoses with selegiline hydrochloride. However, experience gained during selegiline's development reveals that some individuals exposed to doses of 600 mg d,l-selegiline suffered severe hypotension and psychomotor agitation.

Since the selective inhibition of MAO B by selegiline hydrochloride is achieved only at doses in the range recommended for the treatment of Parkinson's disease (*e.g.,* 10 mg/day), overdoses are likely to cause significant inhibition of both MAO A and MAO B. Consequently, the signs and symptoms of overdose may resemble those observed with marketed non-selective MAO inhibitors [e.g., tranylcypromine, isocarboxazide, and phenelzine].

Overdose with Non-Selective MAO Inhibition: NOTE: This section is provided for reference; it does not describe events that have actually been observed with selegiline in overdose.

Characteristically, signs and symptoms of non-selective MAOI overdose may not appear immediately. Delays of up to 12 hours between ingestion of drug and the appearance of signs may occur. Importantly, the peak intensity of the syndrome may not be reached for upwards of a day following the overdose. Death has been reported following overdosage. Therefore, immediate hospitalization, with continuous patient observation and monitoring for a period of at least two days following the ingestion of such drugs in overdose, is strongly recommended.

The clinical picture of MAOI overdose varies considerably; its severity may be a function of the amount of drug consumed. The central nervous and cardiovascular systems are prominently involved.

OVERDOSAGE: *(cont'd)*

Signs and symptoms of overdosage may include, alone or in combination, any of the following: drowsiness, dizziness, faintness, irritability, hyperactivity, agitation, severe headache, hallucinations, trismus, opisthotonus, convulsions, and coma; rapid and irregular pulse, hypertension, hypotension and vascular collapse; precordial pain, respiratory depression and failure, hyperpyrexia, diaphoresis, and cool, clammy skin.

Treatment Suggestions for Overdose: NOTE: Because there is no recorded experience with selegiline overdose, the following suggestions are offered based upon the assumption that selegiline overdose may be modeled by non-selective MAOI poisoning. In any case, up-to-date information about the treatment of overdose can often be obtained from a certified Regional Poison Control Center. Telephone numbers of certified Poison Control Centers are listed in the Physicians GenRx.

Treatment of overdose with non-selective MAOIs is symptomatic and supportive. Induction of emesis or gastric lavage with instillation of charcoal slurry may be helpful in early poisoning, provided the airway has been protected against aspiration. Signs and symptoms of central nervous system stimulation, including convulsions, should be treated with diazepam, given slowly intravenously. Phenothiazine derivatives and central nervous system stimulants should be avoided. Hypotension and vascular collapse should be treated with intravenous fluids and, if necessary, blood pressure titration with an intravenous infusion of a dilute pressor agent. It should be noted that adrenergic agents may produce a markedly increased pressor response.

Respiration should be supported by appropriate measures, including management of the airway, use of supplemental oxygen, and mechanical ventilatory assistance, as required.

Body temperature should be monitored closely. Intensive management of hyperpyrexia may be required. Maintenance of fluid and electrolyte balance is essential.

DOSAGE AND ADMINISTRATION:

Selegiline hydrochloride is intended for administration to Parkinsonian patients receiving levodopa/carbidopa therapy who demonstrate a deteriorating response to this treatment. The recommended regimen for the administration of selegiline hydrochloride is 10 mg per day administered as divided doses of 5 mg each taken at breakfast and lunch. There is no evidence that additional benefit will be obtained from the administration of higher doses. Moreover, higher doses should ordinarily be avoided because of the increased risk of side effects.

After two to three days of selegiline treatment, an attempt may be made to reduce the dose of levodopa/carbidopa. A reduction of 10 to 30% was achieved with the typical participant in the domestic placebo controlled trials who was assigned to selegiline treatment. Further reductions of levodopa/carbidopa may be possible during continued selegiline therapy.

HOW SUPPLIED:

Eldepryl tablets are available containing 5 mg of selegiline hydrochloride. Each white, shield shaped, unscored tablet is debossed with "S" on one side and "5" on the other side.

Carbex 5 mg tablets are white, oval tablets; debossed with E620 on one side and plain on the other.

Store at controlled room temperature, 59° to 86°F (15° to 30°C).

HOW SUPPLIED - EQUIVALENTS NOT AVAILABLE:

Tablet, Uncoated - Oral - 5 mg

60's	$129.54	ELDEPRYL, Somerset	39506-0011-25

SELENIUM *(002219)*

CATEGORIES: Electrolytic, Caloric-Water Balance; Homeostatic & Nutrient; Mineral Supplements; Replacement Solutions; Vitamins; FDA Pre 1938 Drugs

BRAND NAMES: Sele-Pak; Selenitrace; Selepen

Prescribing information not available at time of publication.

HOW SUPPLIED - EQUIVALENTS NOT AVAILABLE:

Injection, Solution - Intravenous - 40 mcg/ml

10 ml	$199.06	SELE-PAK, Solopak Labs	39769-0053-10
10 ml x 25	$69.69	Selenium, Am Regent	00517-6510-25
10 ml x 25	$195.31	SELEPEN, Fujisawa USA	00469-8820-30
30 ml x 10	$228.00	SELEPEN, Fujisawa USA	00469-5400-50

SELENIUM SULFIDE *(002220)*

CATEGORIES: Anti-Infectives; Antifungals; Antimicrobials; Dandruff; Dermatitis; Dermatologicals; Local Infections; Seborrhea; Shampoos; Skin/Mucous Membrane Agents; Tinea Versicolor; Pregnancy Category C; FDA Approval Pre 1982

BRAND NAMES: *Abbottselsun*; Exsel; Glo-Sel; *Lenium*; *Micalon*; *Sebo-Lenium*; Sel-Pen; *Selsum*; **Selsun**; *Selukos*; *Versel*
(International brand names outside U.S. in italics)

FORMULARIES: Aetna; BC-BS; DoD; FHP; PCS; WHO

DESCRIPTION:

Selenium Sulfide (selenium sulfide lotion) is a liquid antiseborrheic, antifungal preparation for topical application, containing selenium sulfide 2 1/2% w/v in aqueous suspension. The product also contains: bentonite, lauric diethanolamide, ethylene glycol monostearate, titanium dioxide, amphoteric-2, sodium lauryl sulfate, sodium phosphate (monobasic), glyceryl monoricinoleate, citric acid, captan, and perfume.

CLINICAL PHARMACOLOGY:

Selenium sulfide appears to have a cytostatic effect on cells of the epidermis and follicular epithelium, thus reducing corneocyte production.

INDICATIONS AND USAGE:

For the treatment of dandruff and seborrheic dermatitis of the scalp.

For treatment of tinea versicolor.

CONTRAINDICATIONS:

Selenium Sulfide should not be used by patients allergic to any of its components.

PRECAUTIONS:

General: Should not be used when acute inflammation or exudation is present as increased absorption may occur.

PRECAUTIONS: *(cont'd)*

Information For Patients: Application to skin or scalp may produce skin irritation or sensitization. If sensitivity reactions occur, use should be discontinued. May be irritating to mucous membranes of the eyes and contact with this area should be avoided. When applied to the body for treatment of tinea versicolor, Selenium Sulfide may produce skin irritation especially in the genital area and where skin folds occur.

These areas should be thoroughly rinsed after application.

Carcinogenesis: Studies in mice using dermal application of 25% and 50% solutions of 2.5% selenium sulfide lotion over an 88 week period, indicated no carcinogenic effects.

Pregnancy: WHEN USED ON BODY SURFACES FOR THE TREATMENT OF TINEA VERSICOLOR, Selenium Sulfide IS CLASSIFIED AS PREGNANCY CATEGORY C. Animal reproduction studies have not been conducted with Selenium Sulfide. It is also not known whether Selenium Sulfide can cause fetal harm when applied to body surfaces of a pregnant woman or can affect reproduction capacity. Under ordinary circumstances Selenium Sulfide should not be used for the treatment of tinea versicolor in pregnant women.

Pediatric Use: Safety and effectiveness in infants have not been established.

ADVERSE REACTIONS:

In decreasing order of severity: skin irritation; occasional reports of increase in amount of normal hair loss; discoloration of the hair (can be avoided or minimized by thorough rinsing of hair after treatment).

As with other shampoos, oiliness or dryness of hair and scalp may occur.

OVERDOSAGE:

Accidental Oral Ingestion:

Selenium Sulfide is intended for external use only.

There have been no documented reports of serious toxicity in humans resulting from acute ingestion of Selenium Sulfide; however, acute toxicity studies in animals suggest that ingestion of large amounts could result in potential human toxicity. For this reason, evacuation of the stomach contents should be considered in cases of acute oral ingestion.

DOSAGE AND ADMINISTRATION:

For Treatment Of Dandruff Or Seborrheic Dermatitis:

1. Massage about 1 or 2 teaspoonfuls of the medicated shampoo into wet scalp.

2. Allow product to remain on the scalp for 2 to 3 minutes.

3. Rinse scalp thoroughly.

4. Repeat application and rinse thoroughly.

5. After treatment wash hands well.

For the usual case, two applications each week for two weeks will afford control.

After this, the lotion may be used at less frequent intervals—weekly, every two weeks, or even every 3 or 4 weeks in some cases. The preparation should not be applied more frequently than required to maintain control.

For Treatment Of Tinea Versicolor:

Apply to affected areas and lather with a small amount of water. Allow product to remain on skin for 10 minutes, rinse the body thoroughly.

Repeat this procedure once a day for 7 days. The product may damage jewelry; jewelry should be removed before use.

HOW SUPPLIED - RATED THERAPEUTICALLY EQUIVALENT:

Lotion/Shampoo - Topical - 2.5 %

4 oz	$2.81	Selenium Sulfide 2.5%, Clay Park Labs	45802-0040-64
4 oz	$5.39	Selenium, HL Moore Drug Exch	00839-5435-65
4 oz	$5.58	Selenium, Geneva Pharms	00781-7100-04
4 oz	$6.95	Selenium, Rugby	00536-1980-97
4 oz	**$11.99**	**SELSUN, Abbott**	**00074-2660-04**
118 ml	$3.30	SEL-PEN, Major Pharms	00904-1533-00
118 ml	$4.48	Selenium, United Res	00677-0552-41
118 ml	$5.00	Selenium, Alpharma	00472-1533-04
118 ml	$6.95	Selenium, Goldline Labs	00182-6088-37
120 ml	$2.75	Selenium Sulfide, Consolidated Midland	00223-6608-00
120 ml	$3.75	Selenium Sulfide, Harber Pharm	51432-0668-18
120 ml	$3.90	Selenium, H.C.F.A. F F P	99999-2220-01
120 ml	$4.00	Selenium, Schein Pharm (US)	00364-7169-77
120 ml	$4.30	Sel-Pen, Major Pharms	00904-1533-20
120 ml	$4.50	Selenium Sulfide, Syosset Labs	47854-0605-22
120 ml	$5.51	Selenium, Qualitest Pharms	00603-1674-54
120 ml	$11.00	Selenium Sulfide, Syosset Labs	47854-0502-22
120 ml	$12.86	EXSEL, Allergan	00023-0817-99
240 ml	$3.59	Selenium Sulfide, Harber Pharm	51432-0668-19

SEPTOMONAB *(003086)*

CATEGORIES: Anti-Endotoxin; Antibacterials; Bacteremia; Igm Antibody; Monoclonal Antibodies; Sepsis, gram-Negative; Septic Shock; Recombinant DNA Origin; FDA Unapproved

BRAND NAMES: **Centoxin**; Ha-1A; Nebacumab

Prescribing information not available at time of publication.

SERTRALINE HYDROCHLORIDE *(003087)*

CATEGORIES: Antidepressants; Central Nervous System Agents; Depression; Depressive Disorder; Psychotherapeutic Agents; Selective Serotonin Reuptake Inhibitors; Obsessive-Compulsive Disorder; Panic Disorder*; Pregnancy Category B; FDA Class 1C ("Little or No Therapeutic Advantage"); Sales > $1 Billion; FDA Approved 1991 Dec; Patent Expiration 2005 Dec; Top 200 Drugs
* Indication not approved by the FDA

BRAND NAMES: *Atruline*; Lustral; **Zoloft**
(International brand names outside U.S. in italics)

FORMULARIES: Aetna; BC-BS; CIGNA; FHP; Humana; Kaiser; Medco; Medi-Cal; PCS; PruCare; WellPoint

COST OF THERAPY: $158.60 (Depression; Tablet; 50 mg; 1/day; 90 days) vs. Potential Cost of $2,456.15 (Depression)

PRIMARY ICD9: 311 (Depressive Disorder, Not Elsewhere Classified)

DESCRIPTION:

Sertraline HCl is a selective serotonin reuptake inhibitor (SSRI) for oral administration. It is chemically unrelated to other SSRIs, tricyclic, tetracyclic, or other available antidepressant agents. It has a molecular weight of 342.7. Sertraline hydrochloride has the following chemical name: (1S-cis)-4-(3,4-dichlorophenyl)-1,2,3,4-tetrahydro-N-methyl-1-nanphthalenamine hydrochloride. The empirical formula is $C_{17}H_{17}NCl_2$·HCl.

Sertraline hydrochloride is a white crystalline powder that is slightly soluble in water and isopropyl alcohol, and sparingly soluble in ethanol.

Zoloft is supplied for oral administration as scored tablets containing sertraline hydrochloride equivalent to 50 and 100 mg of sertraline and the following inactive ingredients: dibasic calcium phosphate dihydrate, FD&C Blue #2 aluminum lake (in 50 mg tablet), hydroxypropyl cellulose, hydroxypropyl methylcellulose, magnesium stearate, microcrystalline cellulose, polyethylene glycol, polysorbate 80, sodium starch glycolate, synthetic yellow iron oxide (in 100 mg tablet), and titanium dioxide.

CLINICAL PHARMACOLOGY:

PHARMACODYNAMICS

The mechanism of action of sertraline is presumed to be linked to its inhibition of CNS neuronal uptake of serotonin (5HT). Studies at clinically relevant doses in man have demonstrated that sertraline blocks the uptake of serotonin into human platelets. *In vitro* studies in animals also suggest that sertraline is a potent and selective inhibitor of neuronal serotonin reuptake and has only very weak effects on norepinephrine and dopamine neuronal reuptake. *In vitro* studies have shown that sertraline has no significant affinity for adrenergic ($alpha_1$, $alpha_2$, beta), cholinergic, GABA, dopaminergic, histaminergic, serotonergic ($5HT_{1A}$, $5HT_{1B}$, $5HT_2$), or benzodiazepine receptors; antagonism of such receptors has been hypothesized to be associated with various anticholinergic, sedative, and cardiovascular effects for other psychotropic drugs. The chronic administration of sertraline was found in animals to downregulate brain norepinephrine receptors, as has been observed with other clinically effective antidepressants. Sertraline does not inhibit monoamine oxidase.

PHARMACOKINETICS

Systemic Bioavailability: In man, following oral once-daily dosing over the range of 50 to 200 mg for 14 days, mean peak plasma concentrations (*Cmax*) of sertraline occurred between 4.5 to 8.4 hours post-dosing. The average terminal elimination half-life of plasma sertraline is about 26 hours. Based on this pharmacokinetic parameter, steady-state sertraline plasma levels should be achieved after approximately one week of once-daily dosing. Linear dose-proportional pharmacokinetics were demonstrated in a single dose study in which the *Cmax* and area under the plasma concentration time curve (AUC) of sertraline were proportional to dose over a range of 50 to 200 mg. Consistent with the terminal elimination half-life, there is an approximately two-fold accumulation, compared to a single dose, of sertraline with repeated dosing over a 50 to 200 mg dose range. The single-dose bioavailability of sertraline tablets is approximately equal to an equivalent dose of solution.

The effects of food on the bioavailability of sertraline were studied in subjects administered a single-dose with and without food. AUC was slightly increased when drug was administered with food but the *Cmax* was 25% greater, while the time to reach peak plasma concentration decreased from 8 hours post-dosing to 5.5 hours.

Metabolism: Sertraline undergoes extensive first pass metabolism. The principal initial pathway of metabolism for sertraline is N-demethylation. N-desmethylsertraline has a plasma terminal elimination half-life of 62 to 104 hours. Both *in vitro* biochemical and *in vivo* pharmacological testing have shown N-desmethylsertraline to be substantially less active than sertraline. Both sertraline and N-desmethylsertraline undergo oxidative deamination and subsequent reduction, hydroxylation, and glucuronide conjugation. In a study of radiolabeled sertraline involving two healthy male subjects, sertraline accounted for less than 5% of the plasma radioactivity. About 40-45% of the administered radioactivity was recovered in urine in 9 days. Unchanged sertraline was not detectable in the urine. For the same period, about 40-45% of the administered radioactivity was accounted for in feces, including 12-14% unchanged sertraline.

Desmethylsertraline exhibits time-related, dose dependent increases in AUC (0-24 hour), *Cmax* and *Cmin*, with about a five to nine-fold increase in these pharmacokinetic parameters between day 1 and day 14.

Protein Binding: *In vitro* protein binding studies performed with radiolabeled ^{3}H-sertraline showed that sertraline is highly bound to serum proteins (98%) in the range of 20 to 500 ng/ml. However, at up to 300 and 200 ng/ml concentrations, respectively, sertraline and N-desmethylsertraline did not alter the plasma protein binding of two other highly protein bound drugs, viz., warfarin and propranolol (see PRECAUTIONS.)

Age: Sertraline plasma clearance in a group of 16 (8 male, 8 female) elderly patients treated for 14 days at a dose of 100 mg/day was approximately 40% lower than in a similarly studied group of younger (25 to 32 years old) individuals. Steady state, therefore, should be achieved after 2 to 3 weeks in older patients. The same study showed a decreased clearance of desmethylsertraline in older males, but not in older females.

Liver Disease: As might be predicted from its primary site of metabolism, liver impairment can effect the elimination of sertraline. The elimination of half-life of sertraline was prolonged in a single dose study of patients with mild, stable cirrhosis, with a mean of 52 hours compared to 22 hours seen in subjects without liver disease. In hepatically impaired patients, it was observed that the C_{max} and AUC were increased by 1.7 and 4.4 fold, respectively, compated to healthy subjects. This suggests that the use of sertraline in patients with liver disease must be approached with caution. If sertraline HCl is administered to patients with liver disease, a lower or less frequent dose should be used (see PRECAUTIONS) and DOSAGE AND ADMINISTRATION.

Renal Disease: The pharmacokinetics of sertraline HCl in patients with significant renal dysfunction have not been determined.

CLINICAL STUDIES:

DEPRESSION

The efficacy of sertraline HCl as a treatment for depression was established in two placebo-controlled studies in adult outpatients meeting DSM-III criteria for major depression. Study 1 was an 8-week study with flexible dosing of sertraline HCl in a range of 50 to 200 mg/day: the mean dose for completers was 145 mg/day. Study 2 was a 6-week fixed-dose study, including sertraline HCl doses of 50, 100, and 200 mg/day. Overall, these studies demonstrated sertraline HCl to be superior to placebo on the Hamilton Depression Rating Scale and the Clinical Global Impression Severity and Improvement scales. Study 2 was not readily interpretable regarding a dose response relationship for effectiveness.

OBSESSIVE-COMPULSIVE DISORDER (OCD)

The effectiveness of sertraline HCl in the treatment of OCD was demonstrated in three multicenter placebo-controlled studies of adult outpatients (Studies 1-3). Patients in all studies had moderate to severe OCD (DSM-III or DSM-III-R) with mean baseline ratings on the Yale Brown Obsessive-Compulsive Scale (YBOCS) total score ranging from 23 to 25.

CLINICAL STUDIES: *(cont'd)*

Study 1 was an 8-week study with flexible dosing of sertraline HCl in a range of 50 to 200 mg/day, the mean dose for completers was 186 mg/day. Patients receiving sertraline HCl experienced a mean reduction of approximately 4 points on the YBOCS total score which was significantly greater than the mean reduction of 2 points in placebo-treated patients.

Study 2 was a 12-week fixed-dose study including sertraline HCl doses of 50, 100, and 200 mg/day. Patients receiving sertraline HCl doses of 50 and 200 mg/day experienced mean reductions of approximately 6 points on the YBOCS total score which were significantly greater than the approximately 3 point reduction in placebo-treated patients.

Study 3 was a 12-week study with flexible dosing of sertraline HCl in a range of 50 to 200 mg/day, the mean dose for completers was 185 mg/day. Patients receiving sertraline HCl experienced a mean reduction of approximately 7 points on the YBOCS total score which was significantly greater than the mean reduction of approximately 4 points in placebo-treated patients.

Analyses for age and gender effects on outcome did not suggest any differential responsiveness on the basis of age or sex.

INDICATIONS AND USAGE:

DEPRESSION

Sertraline HCl is indicated for the treatment of depression.

The efficacy of sertraline HCl in the treatment of a major depressive episode was established in six to eight week controlled trials of outpatients whose diagnoses corresponded most closely to the DSM-III category of major depressive disorder (See CLINICAL STUDIES.)

A major depressive episode implies a prominent and relatively persistent depressed or dysphoric mood that usually interferes with daily functioning (nearly every day for at least 2 weeks); it should include at least 4 of the following 8 symptoms: change in appetite, change in sleep, psychomotor agitation or retardation, loss of interest in usual activities or decrease in sexual drive, increased fatigue, feelings of guilt or worthlessness, slowed thinking or impaired concentration, and a suicide attempt or suicidal ideation.

The antidepressant action of sertraline HCl in hospitalized depressed patients has not been adequately studied.

A study of depressed outpatients who had responded to sertraline HCl during an initial eight-week open treatment phase and were then randomized to continuation on sertraline HCl or placebo demonstrated a significantly lower relapse rate over the next eight weeks for patients taking sertraline HCl compared to those on placebo. However, the effectiveness of sertraline HCl in long-term use, that is, for more than 16 weeks, has not been systematically evaluated in controlled trials of depressed patients. Therefore, the physician who elects to use sertraline HCl for extended periods should periodically reevaluate the long-term usefulness of the drug for the individual patient.

OBSESSIVE-COMPULSIVE DISORDER

Sertraline HCl is indicated for the treatment of obsessions and compulsions in patients with obsessive-compulsive disorder (OCD), as defined in the DSM-III-R (*i.e.*, the obsessions and compulsions cause marked distress, are time-consuming, or significantly interfere with social or occupational functioning.

The efficacy of sertraline HCl was established in 12-week trials with obsessive-compulsive outpatients having diagnosis of obsessive-compulsive disorder as defined according to DSM-III or DSM-III-R criteria (see CLINICAL STUDIES.)

Obsessive-compulsive disorder is characterized by recurrent and persistent ideas, thoughts, impulses, or images (obsessions) that are ego-dystonic and/or repetitive, purposeful, and intentional behaviors (compulsions) that are recognized by the person as excessive or unreasonable.

The effectiveness of sertraline HCl in long-term use for OCD (*i.e.*, for more than 12 weeks) has not been systematically evaluated in placebo-controlled trials. Therefore the physician who elects to use sertraline HCl for extended periods should periodically reevaluate the long-term usefulness of the drug for the individual patient (see DOSAGE AND ADMINISTRATION.)

CONTRAINDICATIONS:

Concomitant use in patients taking monoamine oxidase inhibitors (MAOIs) is contraindicated (see WARNINGS.)

WARNINGS:

Cases of serious, sometimes fatal, reactions have been reported in patients receiving sertraline HCl, a selective serotonin reuptake inhibitor (SSRI), in combination with a monoamine oxidase inhibitor (MAOI). Symptoms of a drug interaction between an SSRI and an MAOI include: hyperthermia, rigidity, myoclonus, autonomic instability with possible rapid fluctuations of vital signs, mental status changes that include confusion, irritability, and extreme agitation progressing to delirium and coma. These reactions have also been reported in patients who have recently discontinued an SSRI and have been started on an MAOI. Some cases presented with features resembling neuroleptic malignant syndrome. Therefore, it is recommended that sertraline HCl not be used in combination with an MAOI, or within 14 days of discontinuing treatment with an MAOI. Similarly, at least 14 days should be allowed after stopping sertraline HCl before starting an MAOI.

PRECAUTIONS:

GENERAL

Activation of Mania/Hypomania: During premarketing testing, hypomania or mania occurred in approximately 0.4% of sertraline HCl treated patients. Activation of mania/hypomania has also been reported in a small proportion of patients with Major Affective Disorder treated with other marketed antidepressants and antiobsessional drugs.

Weight Loss: Significant weight loss may be an undesirable result of treatment with sertraline for some patients, but on average, patients in controlled trials had minimal, 1 to 2 pound weight loss, versus smaller changes on placebo. Only rarely have sertraline patients been discontinued for weight loss.

Seizure: Sertraline HCl has not been evaluated in patients with a seizure disorder. These patients were excluded from clinical studies during the product's premarket testing. No seizures were observed among approximately 3000 patients treated with sertraline HCl in the development program for depression. However, 4 patients out of approximately 1800 exposed during the development program for obsessive-compulsive disorder experienced seizures, representing a crude incidence of 0.2%. Three of these patients were adolescents, two with a seizure disorder and one with a family history of seizure disorder, none of whom were receiving anticonvulsant medication. Accordingly, like other antidepressants and antiobsessional drugs, sertraline HCl should be introduced with care in patients with a seizure disorder.

Suicide: The possibility of a suicide attempt is inherent in depression and may persist until significant remission occurs. Close supervision of high risk patients should accompany initial drug therapy. Prescriptions for sertraline HCl should be written for the smallest quantity of tablets consistent with good patient management, in order to reduce the risk of overdose.

PRECAUTIONS: *(cont'd)*

Weak Uricosuric Effect: Sertraline HCl is associated with a mean decrease in serum uric acid of approximately 7%. The clinical significance of this weak uricosuric effect is unknown, and there have been no reports of acute renal failure with sertraline HCl.

Use in Patients with Concomitant Illness: Clinical experience with sertraline HCl in patients with certain concomitant systemic illness is limited. Caution is advisable in using sertraline HCl in patients with diseases or conditions that could affect metabolism or hemodynamic responses.

Sertraline HCl has not been evaluated or used to any appreciable extent in patients with a recent history of myocardial infarction or unstable heart disease. Patients with these diagnoses were excluded from clinical studies during the product's premarket testing. However, the electrocardiograms of 774 patients who received sertraline HCl in double-blind trials were evaluated and the data indicate that sertraline HCl is not associated with the development of significant ECG abnormalities.

Sertraline HCl is extensively metabolized by the liver. In subjects with mild, stable cirrhosis of the liver, the clearance of sertraline was decreased, thus increasing the elimination half-life. A lower or less frequent dose should be used in patients with cirrhosis.

Since sertraline HCl is extensively metabolized, excretion of unchanged drug in urine is a minor route of elimination. However, until the pharmacokinetics of sertraline HCl have been studied in patients with renal impairment and until adequate numbers of patients with severe renal impairment have been evaluated during chronic treatment with sertraline HCl, it should be used with caution in such patients.

Interference with Cognitive and Motor Performance: In controlled studies, sertraline HCl did not cause sedation and did not interfere with psychomotor performance.

Hyponatremia: Several cases of hyponatremia have been reported and appeared to be reversible when sertraline HCl was discontinued. Some cases were possibly due to the syndrome of inappropriate antidiuretic hormone secretion. The majority of these occurrences have been in elderly individuals, some in patients taking diuretics, or who were otherwise volume depleted.

Platelet Function: There have been rare reports of altered platelet function and/or abnormal results from laboratory studies in patients taking sertraline HCl. While there have been reports of abnormal bleeding or purpura in several patients taking sertraline HCl, it is unclear whether sertraline HCl had a causative role.

INFORMATION FOR PATIENTS

Physicians are advised to discuss the following issues with patients for whom they prescribe sertraline HCl:

Patients should be told that although sertraline HCl has not been shown to impair the ability of normal subjects to perform tasks requiring complex motor and mental skills in laboratory experiments, drugs that act upon the central nervous system may affect some individuals adversely.

Patients should be told that although sertraline HCl has not been shown in experiments with normal subjects to increase the mental and motor skill impairments caused by alcohol, the concomitant use of sertraline HCl and alcohol in depressed patients is not advised.

Patients should be told that while no adverse interaction of sertraline HCl with over-the-counter (OTC) drug products is known to occur, the potential for interaction exists. Thus, the use of any OTC product should be initiated cautiously according to the directions of use given for the OTC product.

Patients should be advised to notify their physician if they become pregnant or intend to become pregnant during therapy.

Patients should be advised to notify their physician if they are breast feeding an infant.

LABORATORY TESTS

None.

CARCINOGENESIS, MUTAGENESIS, IMPAIRMENT OF FERTILITY

Carcinogenesis: Lifetime carcinogenicity studies were carried out in CD-1 mice and Long-Evans rats at doses up to 40 mg/kg/day. These doses correspond to 1 times (mice) and 2 times (rats) the maximum recommended human dose (MRHD) on a mg/m^2 basis. There was a dose-related increase in the incidence of liver adenomas in male mice receiving sertraline at 10-40 mg/kg (0.25-1.0 times the MRHD on a mg/m^2 basis). No increase was seen in female mice or in rats of either sex receiving the same treatments, nor was there an increase in hepatocellular carcinomas. Liver adenomas have a variable rate of spontaneous occurrence in the CD-1 mouse and are of unknown significance to humans. There was an increase in follicular adenomas of the thyroid in female rats receiving sertraline at 40 mg/kg (2 times the MHRD on a mg/m^2 basis); this was not accompanied by thyroid hyperplasia. While there was an increase in uterine adenocarcinomas in rats receiving sertraline at 10-40 mg/kg (0.5-2.0 times the MHRD on a mg/m^2 basis) compared to placebo controls, this effect was not clearly drug related.

Mutagenesis: Sertraline had no genotoxic effects, with or without metabolic activation, based on the following assays: bacterial mutation assay; mouse lymphoma mutation assay; and tests for cytogenetic aberrations *in vivo* in mouse bone marrow and *in vitro* in human lymphocytes.

Impairment of Fertility: A decrease in fertility was seen in one of two rat studies at a dose of 80 mg/kg (4 times the maximum human dose on a mg/kg basis and 4 times on a mg/m^2 basis).

PREGNANCY, TERATOGENIC EFFECTS, PREGNANCY CATEGORY C

Reproduction studies have been performed in rats and rabbits at doses up to 80 mg/kg/day and 40 mg/kg/day, respectively. These doses correspond to approximately 4 times the maximum recommended human dose (MRHD) on a mg/m^2 basis. There was no evidence of teratogenicity at any dose level. When pregnant rats and rabbits were given sertraline during the period of organogenesis, delayed ossification was observed in fetuses at doses of 10 mg/kg (0.5 times the MRHD on a mg/m^{2}basis) in rats and 40 mg/kg (4 times the MRHD on a mg/m^{2}basis) in rabbits. When female rats received sertraline HCl during the last third of gestation and throughout lactation, there was an increase in the number of stillborn pups and in the number of pups dying during the first four days after birth. Pup body weights were also decreased during the first four days after birth. These effects occurred at a dose of 20 mg/kg (1 times the MRHD on a mg/m^2 basis). The no effect dose for rat pup mortality was 10 mg/kg (0.5 times the MRHD on a mg/m^{2}basis). The decrease in pup survival was shown to be due to *in utero* exposure to sertraline HCl. The clinical significance of these effects is unknown. There are no adequate and well controlled studies in pregnant women. Sertraline HCl should be used during pregnancy only if the potential benefit justifies the potential risk to the fetus.

LABOR AND DELIVERY

The effect of sertraline HCl on labor and delivery in humans is unknown.

NURSING MOTHERS

It is not known whether, and if so in what amount, sertraline or its metabolites are excreted in human milk. Because many drugs are excreted in human milk, caution should be exercised when sertraline HCl is administered to a nursing woman.

PEDIATRIC USE

Safety and effectiveness in children have not been established.

PRECAUTIONS: *(cont'd)*

GERIATRIC USE

Several hundred elderly patients have participated in clinical studies with sertraline HCl. The pattern of adverse reactions in the elderly was similar to that in younger patients.

DRUG INTERACTIONS:

Potential Effects of Coadministration of Drugs Highly Bound to Plasma Proteins: Because sertraline is tightly bound to plasma protein, the administration of sertraline HCl to a patient taking another drug which is tightly bound to protein, (*e.g.*, warfarin, digitoxin) may cause a shift in plasma concentrations potentially resulting in an adverse effect. Conversely, adverse effects may result from displacement of protein bound sertraline HCl by other tightly bound drugs.

In a study comparing prothrombin time AUC (0-120 hr) following dosing with warfarin (0.75 mg/kg) before and after 21 days of dosing with either sertraline HCl (50-200 mg/day) or placebo, there was a mean increase in prothrombin time of 8% relative to baseline for sertraline HCl compared to a 1% decrease for placebo ($p<0.02$). The normalization of prothrombin time for the sertraline HCl group was delayed compared to the placebo group. The clinical significance of this change is unknown. Accordingly, prothrombin time should be carefully monitored when sertraline HCl therapy is initiated or stopped.

Cimetidine: In a study assessing disposition of sertraline HCl (100 mg) on the second of 8 days of cimetidine administration (800 mg daily), there were significant increases in sertraline HCl mean AUC (50%), C_{max} (24%) and half-life (26%) compared to the placebo group. The clinical significance of these changes is unknown.

CNS Active Drugs: In a study comparing the disposition of intravenously administered diazepam before and after 21 days of dosing with either sertraline HCl (50 to 200 mg/day escalating dose) or placebo, there was a 32% decrease relative to baseline in diazepam clearance for the sertraline HCl group compared to a 19% decrease relative to baseline for the placebo group ($p<0.03$). There was a 23% increase in $T_{max}$for desmethyldiazepam in the sertraline HCl group compared to a 20% decrease in the placebo group ($p<0.03$). The clinical significance of these changes is unknown.

In a placebo-controlled trial in normal volunteers, the administration of two doses of sertraline HCl did not significantly alter steady-state lithium levels or the renal clearance of lithium.

Nonetheless, at this time, it is recommended that plasma lithium levels be monitored following initiation of sertraline HCl therapy with appropriate adjustments to the lithium dose.

The risk of using sertraline HCl in combination with other CNS active drugs has not been systematically evaluated. Consequently, caution is advised if the concomitant administration of sertraline HCl and such drugs is required.

There is limited controlled experience regarding the optimal timing of switching from other antidepressants to sertraline HCl. Care and prudent medical judgement should be exercised when switching, particularly from long-acting agents. The duration of an appropriate washout period which should intervene before switching from one selective serotonin reuptake inhibitor (SSRI) to another has not been established.

Monoamine Oxidase Inhibitors: (See CONTRAINDICATIONS) and WARNINGS.

Drugs Metabolized by Cytochrome P450 3A3: In two separate *in vivo* interaction studies, sertraline was co-administered with cytochrome P450 3A4 substrates, terfenadine or carbamazepine, under steady-state conditions. The results of these studies demonstrated that sertraline co-administration did not increase plasma concentrations of terfenadine or carbamazepine. These data suggest that sertraline HCl's extent of inhibition of P450 3A4 is not likely to be of clinical significance.

Drugs Metabolized by P450 2D6: Many antidepressants (*e.g.*, the SSRIs) including sertraline, and most tricyclic antidepressants inhibit the biochemical activity of the drug metabolizing isozyme cytochrome P450 2D6 (debrisoquin hydroxylase), and thus, may increase the plasma concentrations of co-administered drugs that are metabolized by P450 2D6. The drugs for which this potential interaction is of greatest concern are those metabolized primarily by 2D6 and which have a narrow therapeutic index (*e.g.*, the tricyclic antidepressants and the type 1C antiarrhythmics propafenone and flecainide). The extent to which this interaction is an important clinical problem depends on the extent of the inhibition of P450 2D6 by the antidepressant and the therapeutic index of the co-administered drug. There is variability among the antidepressants in the extent of clinically important 2D6 inhibition, and in fact sertraline at lower doses has a less prominent inhibitory effect on 2D6 than some others in the class. Nevertheless, even sertraline has the potential for clinically important 2D6 inhibition. Consequently, concomitant use of a drug metabolized by P450 2D6 with sertraline HCl may require lower doses than usually prescribed for the other drug. Furthermore, whenever sertraline is withdrawn from co-therapy, an increased dose of the co-administered drug may be required (see Tricyclic Antidepressants).

Tricyclic Antidepressants (TCAs): The extent to which SSRI TCA interactions may pose clinical problems will depend on the degree of inhibition and the pharmacokinetics of the SSRI involved. Nevertheless, caution is indicated in the co-administration of TCAs with sertraline HCl, because sertraline HCl may inhibit TCA metabolism. Plasma TCA concentrations may need to be monitored, and the dose of TCA may need to be reduced, if a TCA is co-administered with sertraline HCl (see PRECAUTIONS; Drugs Metabolized by P450 2D6.

Hypoglycemic Drugs: In a placebo-controlled trial in normal volunteers, administration of sertraline HCl for 22 days (including 200 mg/day for the final 13 days) caused a statistically significant 16% decrease from baseline in the clearance of tolbutamide following an intravenous 1000 mg dose. Sertraline HCl administration did not noticeably change either the plasma protein binding or the apparent volume of distribution of tolbutamide, suggesting that the decreased clearance was due to a change in the metabolism of the drug. The clinical significance of this decrease in tolbutamide clearance is unknown.

Atenolol: Sertraline HCl (100 mg) when administered to 10 healthy male subjects had no effect on the beta-adrenergic blocking ability of atenolol.

Digoxin: In a placebo-controlled trial in normal volunteers, administration of sertraline HCl for 17 days (including 200 mg/day for the last 10 days) did not change serum digoxin levels on digoxin renal clearance.

Microsomal Enzyme Induction: Preclinical studies have shown sertraline HCl to induce hepatic microsomal enzymes. In clinical studies, sertraline HCl was shown to induce hepatic enzymes minimally as determined by a small (5%) but statistically significant decrease in antipyrine half-life following administration of 200 mg/day for 21 days. This small change in antipyrine half-life reflects a clinically insignificant change in hepatic metabolism.

Electroconvulsive Therapy: There are no clinical studies establishing the risks or benefits of the combined use of electroconvulsive therapy (ECT) and sertraline HCl.

Alcohol: Although sertraline HCl did not potentiate the cognitive and psychomotor effects of alcohol in experiments with normal subjects, the concomitant use of sertraline HCl and alcohol in depressed patients or OCD patients is not recommended.

ADVERSE REACTIONS:

Commonly Observed: Among patients treated with sertraline HCl in placebo-controlled studies, the most commonly observed adverse events associated with the use of sertraline HCl and not seen at an equivalent incidence among placebo-treated patients were: gastrointestinal complaints, including nausea, diarrhea/loose stools and dyspepsia; tremor; dizziness; insomnia; somnolence; increased sweating; dry mouth; and male sexual dysfunction (primarily ejaculatory delay).

In placebo-controlled clinical trials for OCD, adverse events observed at an incidence of at least 5% for sertraline HCl and at an incidence that was twice or more the incidence among placebo-treated patients included: nausea, insomnia, diarrhea, decreased libido, anorexia, dyspepsia, ejaculation failure (primarily ejaculatory delay), tremor, and increased sweating.

Associated with Discontinuation of Treatment: Fifteen percent of 2710 subjects who received sertraline HCl in premarketing multiple dose clinical trials discontinued treatment due to an adverse event. The more common events (reported by at least 1% of subjects) associated with discontinuation included agitation, insomnia, male sexual dysfunction (primarily ejaculatory delay), somnolence, dizziness, headache, tremor, anorexia, diarrhea loose stools, nausea, and fatigue.

In placebo-controlled clinical trials for OCD, 10% of patients treated with sertraline HCl discontinued treatment due to an adverse event. The more common events were nausea, insomnia, and diarrhea.

Incidence in Controlled Clinical Trials: TABLE 1 enumerates adverse events that occurred at a frequency of 1% or more among sertraline HCl patients who participated in depression and other premarketing controlled trials comparing titrated sertraline HCl with placebo. Most patients received doses of 50 to 200 mg per day. The prescriber should be aware that these figures cannot be used to predict the incidence of side effects in the course of usual medical practice where patient characteristics and other factors differ from those which prevailed in the clinical trials. Similarly, the cited frequencies cannot be compared with figures obtained from other clinical investigations involving different treatments, uses, and investigators. The cited figures (TABLE 1) however, do provide the prescribing physician with some basis for estimating the relative contribution of drug and non-drug factors to the side effect incidence rate in the population studied.

TABLE 1 Treatment-Emergent Adverse Experience Incidence in Placebo-Controlled Clinical Trials*

Adverse Experience	(Percent of Patients Reporting) Sertraline HCl (N=861) %	Placebo (N=853)%
Autonomic Nervous System Disorders		
Mouth Dry	16	9
Sweating Increased	8	3
Cardiovascular		
Palpitations	4	2
Central & Peripheral Nervous System Disorders		
Headache	20	19
Dizziness	12	7
Tremor	11	3
Hypoesthesia	2	1
Twitching	1	0
Hypertonia	1	0
Gastrointestinal Disorders		
Nausea	26	12
Diarrhea/Loose Stools	18	9
Constipation	8	6
Dyspepsia	6	3
Vomiting	4	2
Anorexia	3	2
General		
Fatigue	11	8
Hot Flushes	2	1
Fever	2	1
Back Pain	2	1
Psychiatric Disorders		
Insomnia	16	9
Sexual Dysfunction - Male (†)	16	2
Somnolence	13	6
Agitation	6	4
Nervousness	3	2
Anxiety	3	1
Yawning	2	0
Sexual Dysfunction - Female (‡)	2	0
Special Senses		
Vision Abnormal	4	2
Urinary System Disorders		
Micturition Frequency	2	1

* Events reported by at least 1% of patients treated with sertraline HCl are included except for the following events which had an incidence on placebo greater than or equal to sertraline HCl: flatulence, abdominal pain, rash, rhinitis, parathesia, myalgia, thirst, tinnitus, micturation disorder, appetite increased, concentration impaired, pharyngitis, taste perversion, mentrual disorder(‡), and chest pain.
(†) Primarily ejaculatory delay: % based on male patients only; 271 sertraline HCl and 271 placebo patients
(‡) % based on female patients only: 590 sertraline HCland 582 placebo patients.

Obsessive-Compulsive Disorder: TABLE 2 enumerates adverse events that occurred at a frequency of 2% or more among patients on sertraline HCl who participated in controlled trials comparing sertraline HCl with placebo in the treatment of OCD.

Other Events Observed During the Premarketing Evaluation of Sertraline HCl: During its premarketing assessment, multiple doses of sertraline HCl were administered to approximately 2700 subjects. The conditions and duration of exposure to sertraline HCl varied greatly, and included (in overlapping categories) clinical pharmacology studies, open and double-blind studies, uncontrolled and controlled studies, inpatient and outpatient studies, fixed-dose and titration studies, and studies for indications other than depression. Untoward events associated with this exposure were recorded by clinical investigators using terminology of their own choosing. Consequently, it is not possible to provide a meaningful estimate of the proportion of individuals experiencing adverse events without first grouping similar types of untoward events into a smaller number of standardized event categories.

In the tabulations that follow, a World Health Organization dictionary of terminology has been used to classify reported adverse events. The frequencies presented, therefore, represent the proportion of the approximately 2700 individuals exposed to multiple doses of sertraline HCl who experienced an event of the type cited on at least one occasion while receiving sertraline HCl. All events are included except those already listed in the previous table and those reported in terms so general as to be uninformative. It is important to emphasize that although the events reported occurred during treatment with sertraline HCl, they were not necessarily caused by it.

ADVERSE REACTIONS: *(cont'd)*

TABLE 2 Treatment-Emergent Adverse Experiences In Placebo-Controlled Clinical Trials for Obsessive-Compulsive Disorder*

Adverse Experience	Percent of Patients Reporting Sertraline HCl (N=533)	Placebo (N=373)
Autonomic Nervous System Disoders		
Mouth Dry	14%	9%
Sweating Increased	6%	1%
Cardiovascular		
Palpitations	3%	2%
Chest Pain	3%	2%
Central & Periipheral Nervous System Disorders		
Headache	30%	24%
Dizziness	17%	9%
Tremor	8%	1%
Paresthesia	3%	1%
Hypertonia	2%	1%
Disorders of Skin and Appendages		
Rash	2%	1%
Gastrointestinal Disorders		
Nausea	30%	11%
Diarrhea	24%	10%
Anorexia	11%	2%
Dyspepsia	10%	4%
Constipation	6%	4%
Flatulence	4%	1%
Vomiting	3%	1%
Appetite Increased	3%	1%
General		
Fatigue	14%	10%
Pain	3%	1%
Hot Flushes	2%	1%
Back Pain	2%	1%
Metabolic and Nutrional Disorders		
Weight Increase	3%	0%
Psychiatric Disorders		
Insomnia	28%	12%
Somnolence	15%	8%
Libido Decreased	11%	2%
Anxiety	8%	6%
Nervousness	7%	6%
Agitation	6%	3%
Depersonalization	3%	1%
Paroniria	3%	1%
Respiratory System Disorders		
Pharyngitis	4%	2%
Special Senses		
Vision Abnormal	4%	2%
Taste Perversion	3%	1%
Urogenital		
Ejaculation Failure (*)	17%	2%
Impotence (†)	5%	1%

* Events reported by at least 2% or patients treated with sertraline HCl are included, except for the following events which had an incidence on placebo greater than or equal to sertraline HCl: abdominal pain, respiratory disorder, depression, and amnesia.

† Primarily ejaculatory delay; % based on male patients only: 296 sertraline HCl and 219 placebo patients.
‡ % based on male patients only: 296 sertraline HCl and 219 placebo patients.

Events are further categorized by body system and listed in order of decreasing frequency according to the following definitions: frequent adverse events are those occurring on one or more occasions in at least 1/100 patients (only those not already listed in the tabulated results from placebo controlled trials appear in this listing); infrequent adverse events are those occurring in 1/100 to 1/1000 patients; rare events are those occurring in fewer than 1/1000 patients. Events of major clinical importance are also described in the PRECAUTIONS section.

Autonomic Nervous System Disorders: *Infrequent:*flushing, mydriasis, increased saliva, cold clammy skin; *Rare:*pallor.

Cardiovascular: *Infrequent:*postural dizziness, hypertension, hypotension, postural hypotension, edema, dependent edema, periorbital edema, peripheral edema, peripheral ischemia, syncope, tachycardia; *Rare:*precordial chest pain, substernal chest pain, aggravated hypertension, myocardial infarction, varicose veins.

Central and Peripheral Nervous System Disorders: *Frequent:*confusion;*Infrequent:*ataxia, abnormal coordination, abnormal gait, hyperesthesia, hyperkinesia, hypokinesia, migraine, nystagmus, vertigo;*Rare:*local anesthesia, coma, convulsions, dyskinesia, dysphonia, hyporeflexia, hypotonia, ptosis.

Disorders of Skin and Appendages: *Infrequent:*acne, alopecia, pruritus, erythematous rash, maculopapular rash, dry skin;*Rare:*bullous eruption, dermatitis, erythema multiforme, abnormal hair texture, hypertrichosis, photosensitivity reaction, follicular rash, skin discoloration, abnormal skin odor, urticaria.

Endocrine Disorders: *Rare:*exophthalmos, gynecomastia.

Gastrointestinal Disorders: *Infrequent:*dysphagia, eructation; *Rare:*diverticulitis, fecal incontinence, gastritis, gastroenteritis, glossitis, gum hyperplasia, hemorrhoids, hiccup, melena, hemorrhagic peptic ulcer, proctitis, stomatitis, ulcerative stomatitis, tenesmus, tongue edema, tongue ulceration.

General: *Frequent:*asthenia; *Infrequent:*malaise, generalized edema, rigors, weight decrease, weight increase;*Rare:*enlarged abdomen, halitosis, otitis media, aphthous stomatitis.

Hematopoietic and Lymphatic: *Infrequent:*lymphadenopathy, purpura; *Rare:*anemia, anterior chamber eye hemorrhage.

Metabolic and Nutritional Disorders: *Rare:*dehydration, hypercholesterolemia, hypoglycemia.

Musculoskeletal System Disorders: *Infrequent:*arthralgia, arthrosis, dystonia, muscle cramps, muscle weakness; *Rare:*hernia.

Psychiatric Disorders: *Infrequent:*abnormal dreams, aggressive reaction, amnesia, apathy, delusion, depersonalization, depression, aggravated depression, emotional lability, euphoria, hallucination, neurosis, paranoid reaction, suicide ideation and attempt, teeth-grinding, abnormal thinking; *Rare:*hysteria, somnambulism, withdrawal syndrome.

Reproductive: *Infrequent:*dysmenorrhea (2), intermenstrual bleeding (2); *Rare:*amenorrhea (2), balanoposthitis (1), breast enlargement (2), female breast pain (2), leukorrhea (2), menorrhagia (2), atrophic vaginitis (2).

1 - % based on male subjects only: 1005.
2 - % based on female subjects only: 1705.

ADVERSE REACTIONS: *(cont'd)*

Respiratory System Disorders: *Infrequent:*bronchospasm, coughing, dyspnea, epistaxis; *Rare:* bradypnea, hyperventilation, sinusitis, stridor.

Special Senses: *Infrequent:*abnormal accommodation, conjunctivitis, diplopia, earache, eye pain, xerophthalmia; *Rare:*abnormal lacrimation, photophobia, visual field defect.

Urinary System Disorders: *Infrequent:*dysuria, face edema, nocturia, polyuria, urinary incontinence; *Rare:*oliguria, renal pain, urinary retention.

Laboratory Tests: In man, asymptomatic elevations in serum transaminases (SGOT [or AST] and SGPT [or ALT] have been reported infrequently (approximately 0.8%) in association with sertraline HCl administration. These hepatic enzyme elevations usually occurred within the first 1 to 9 weeks of drug treatment and promptly diminished upon drug discontinuation.

Sertraline HCl therapy was associated with small mean increases in total cholesterol (approximately 3%) and triglycerides (approximately 5%), and a small mean decrease in serum uric acid (approximately 7%) of no apparent clinical importance.

The safety profile observed in OCD patients treated with sertraline HCl is imilar to the safety profile in depressed patients.

Other Events Observed During the Postmarketing Evaluation of Sertraline HCl: Reports of adverse events temporarily associated with sertraline HCl that have been received since market introduction, that are not listed above and that may have no causal relationship with the drug include the following: galactorrhea, hyperprolactinemia, neuroleptic malignant syndrome-like events, pyschosis, rare reports of pancreatitis, and liver events-clinical features (which in the majority of cases appeared to be reversible with discontinuation of sertraline HCl) occurring in one or more patients include: elevated enzymes, increased bilirubin, hepatomegaly, hepatitis, jaundice, abdominal pain, vomiting, liver failure, and death.

DRUG ABUSE AND DEPENDENCE:

Controlled Substance Class: Sertraline HCl is not a controlled substance.

Physical and Psychological Dependence: Sertraline HCl has not been systematically studied, in animals or humans, for its potential for abuse, tolerance, or physical dependence. However, the premarketing clinical experience with sertraline HCl did not reveal any tendency for a withdrawal syndrome or any drug-seeking behavior. As with any new CNS active drug, physicians should carefully evaluate patients for history of drug abuse and follow such patients closely, observing them for signs of sertraline HCl misuse or abuse (*e.g.*, development of tolerance, incrementation of dose, drug-seeking behavior).

OVERDOSAGE:

Human Experience: As of November 1992, there were 79 reports of non-fatal acute overdoses involving sertraline HCl, of which 28 were overdoses of sertraline HCl alone and the remainder involved a combination of other drugs and/or alcohol in addition to sertraline HCl. In those cases of overdose involving only sertraline HCl, the reported doses ranged from 500 mg to 6000 mg. In a subset of 18 of these patients in whom sertraline HCl blood levels were determined, plasma concentrations ranged from <5 ng/ml to 554 ng/ml. Symptoms of overdose with sertraline HCl alone included somnolence, nausea, vomiting, tachycardia, ECG changes, anxiety and dilated pupils. Treatment was primarily supportive and included monitoring of and use of activated charcoal, gastric lavage or cathartics and hydration. Although there were no reports of death when sertraline HCl was taken alone, there were 4 deaths involving overdoses of sertraline HCl in combination with other drugs and/or alcohol. Therefore, any overdose should be treated aggressively.

Management of Overdoses: Establish and maintain an airway, insure adequate oxygenation and ventilation. Activated charcoal, which may be used with sorbitol, may be as or more effective than emesis or lavage, and should be considered in treating overdose.

Cardiac and vital signs monitoring is recommended along with general symptomatic and supportive measures.

There are no specific antidotes for sertraline HCl.

Due to the large volume of distribution of sertraline HCl, forced diuresis, dialysis, hemoperfusion, and exchange transfusion are unlikely to be of benefit.

In managing overdosage, consider the possibility of multiple drug involvement. The physician should consider contacting a poison control center on the treatment of any overdose.

DOSAGE AND ADMINISTRATION:

Initial Treatment: Sertraline HCl treatment should be initiated with a dose of 50 mg once daily. A relationship between dose and either antidepressant or antiobsessive effect has not been established. Patients were dosed in a range of 50-200 mg/day in the clinical trials demonstrating the antidepressant and antiobsessive effectiveness of sertraline HCl. Consequently, a dose of 50 mg, administered once daily, is recommended as the intial dose. Patients not responding to a 50 mg dose may benefit from dose increases up to a maximum of 200 mg/day. Given the 24 elimination half-life of sertraline, dose changes should not occur at intervals of less than 1 week.

Sertraline HCl should be administered once daily, either in the morning or evening.

As indicated under PRECAUTIONS, a lower or less frequent dosage should be used in patients with hepatic impairment. In addition, particular care should be used in patients with hepatic and/or renal impairment.

Maintenance/Continuation/Extended Treatment: There is evidence to suggest that depressed patients responding during an initial 8 week treatment phase will continue to benefit during an additional 8 weeks of treatment. While there are insufficient data regarding any benefits from treatment beyond 16 weeks, it is generally agreed among expert psychopharmacologists that acute episodes of depression require several months or longer of sustained pharmacological therapy. Whether the dose of antidepressant needed to induce remission is identical to the dose needed to maintain and/or sustain euthymia is unknown.

Although the efficacy of sertraline HCl beyond 12 weeks of dosing for OCD has not been documented in controlled trials, OCD is a chronic condition, and it is reasonable to consider continuation for a responding patient. Dosage adjustments may be needed to maintain the patient on the lowest effective dosage, and patients should be periodically reassessed to determine the need for continued treatment.

Switching Patients to or from a Monoamine Oxidase Inhibitor: At least 14 days should elapse between discontinuation of a MAOI and initiation of therapy with sertraline HCl. In addition, at least 14 days should be allowed after stopping sertraline HCl before starting a MAOI (see CONTRAINDICATIONS) and WARNINGS.

PATIENT INFORMATION:

Sertraline HCl is used for the treatment of Depression and Obsessive Compulsive Disorder.

Do not take this medication if you are taking MAO Inhibitors (*e.g.*, Parnate). Do not drink alcohol while taking this medication.

Inform your doctor if you are pregnant or breast feeding. Sertraline HCl may cause dizziness, use caution while driving or operating hazordous machinery.

This medication may cause stomach upset, nausea, diarrhea, dizziness, tremor, insomnia, sleepiness, sweating, dry mouth, and male sexual dysfunction. Inform your physician or pharmacist if these occur.

HOW SUPPLIED:

Zoloft capsular-shaped scored tablets containing sertraline hydrochloride equivalent to 50 and 100 mg of sertraline.

50 mg Tablets: Light blue film coated tablets engraved on the front with Zoloft and on the back scored and engraved with 50 mg.

100 mg Tablets: Light yellow film coated tablets engraved on the front with Zoloft and on the back scored and engraved with 100 mg.

Storage: Store at controlled room temperature of 59° to 86°F (15° to 30°C).

HOW SUPPLIED - EQUIVALENTS NOT AVAILABLE:

Tablet, Uncoated - Oral - 50 mg

100's	$176.23	ZOLOFT, Roerig	00049-4900-41
100's	$176.23	ZOLOFT, Roerig	00049-4900-66
500's	$881.12	ZOLOFT, Roerig	00049-4900-73

Tablet, Uncoated - Oral - 100 mg

100's	$181.33	ZOLOFT, Roerig	00049-4910-41
100's	$181.33	ZOLOFT, Roerig	00049-4910-66
500's	$906.63	ZOLOFT, Roerig	00049-4910-73

SILVER NITRATE *(002226)*

CATEGORIES: Anti-Infectives; Antiseptics/Disinfectants; Dermatologicals; Disinfectants; EENT Drugs; Eye, Ear, Nose, & Throat Preparations; Local Infections; Ocular Infections; Ophthalmics; Skin/Mucous Membrane Agents; FDA Pre 1938 Drugs

FORMULARIES: WHO

Prescribing information not available at time of publication.

HOW SUPPLIED - EQUIVALENTS NOT AVAILABLE:

Crystals

25 gm	$20.60	Silver Nitrate, Paddock Labs	00574-0653-25
30 gm	$34.69	Silver Nitrate, Mallinckrodt	00406-7992-34
30 gm	$35.10	Silver Nitrate, Mallinckrodt	00406-2169-34
100 gm	$78.64	Silver Nitrate, Paddock Labs	00574-0653-01
120 gm	$70.65	Silver Nitrate, Mallinckrodt	00406-2169-01
125 gm	$82.63	Silver Nitrate, Mallinckrodt	00406-7992-01
500 gm	$256.80	Silver Nitrate, Mallinckrodt	00406-7992-03
500 gm	$260.76	Silver Nitrate, Mallinckrodt	00406-2169-03

Each - Topical

12 x 100	$120.00	Silver Nitrate Applicators, Raway	00686-1535-10
100's	$4.98	Silver Nitrate, HL Moore Drug Exch	00839-0083-88
100's	$5.70	Silver Nitrate Applicator, Arzol Chem	12870-0001-02
100's	$6.10	Silver Nitrate Applicator, Arzol Chem	12870-0001-01
100's	$9.19	Silver Nitrate Applicator, Rugby	00536-0930-01
100's	$10.00	Silver Nitrate, Raway	00686-1590-10

Solution - Ophthalmic - 1 %

100's	$136.16	Silver Nitrate, Lilly	00002-1608-02

Solution - Topical

960 ml x 12	$63.36	Silver Nitrate, Copley Pharm	38245-0614-13

SILVER SULFADIAZINE *(002228)*

CATEGORIES: Anti-Infectives; Antibacterials; Antimicrobials; Burns; Dermatologicals; Local Infections; Sepsis; Skin/Mucous Membrane Agents; Topical; Wound Care; Pregnancy Category B; FDA Approval Pre 1982

BRAND NAMES: *Canflame*; *Dermazin*; *Flamazine*; *Flammazine*; *Geben*; Sildimac; **Silvadene**; SSD; *Silvazine*; *Silverderma*; *Silverol*; *Silvirin*; *Sofargen*; Thermazene
(International brand names outside U.S. in italics)

FORMULARIES: Aetna; BC-BS; CIGNA; FHP; Humana; Kaiser; Medco; Medi-Cal; PCS; PruCare; United; WHO

DESCRIPTION:

Silver sulfadiazine cream 1% is a soft, white, water-miscible cream containing the antimicrobial agent silver sulfadiazine in micronized form.

Each gram of silver sulfadiazine cream 1% contains 10 mg of micronized silver sulfadiazine. The cream vehicle consists of white petrolatum, stearyl alcohol, isopropyl myristate, sorbitan monooleate, polyoxyl 40 stearate, propylene glycol, and water, with methylparaben 0.3% as a preservative. Silver sulfadiazine cream 1% spreads easily and can be washed off readily with water.

CLINICAL PHARMACOLOGY:

Silver sulfadiazine has broad antimicrobial activity. It is bactericidal for many gram-negative and gram-positive bacteria as well as being effective against yeast. Results from *in vitro* testing are listed in TABLE 1.

Sufficient data have been obtained to demonstrate that silver sulfadiazine will inhibit bacteria that are resistant to other antimicrobial agents and that the compound is superior to sulfadiazine.

Studies utilizing radioactive micronized silver sulfadiazine, electron microscopy, and biochemical techniques have revealed that the mechanism of action of silver sulfadiazine on bacteria differs from silver nitrate and sodium sulfadiazine. Silver sulfadiazine acts only on the cell membrane and cell wall to produce its bactericidal effect.

Silver sulfadiazine is not a chronic anhydrase inhibitor and may be useful in situations where such agents are contraindicated.

INDICATIONS AND USAGE:

Silver sulfadiazine cream 1% is a topical antimicrobial drug indicated as an adjunct for the prevention and treatment of wound sepsis in patients with second- and third-degree burns.

CONTRAINDICATIONS:

Silver sulfadiazine cream 1% is contraindicated in patients who are hypersensitive to silver sulfadiazine or any of the other ingredients in the preparation.

Because sulfonamide therapy is known to increase the possibility of kernicterus, silver sulfadiazine cream 1% should not be used on pregnant women approaching or at term, on premature infants, or on newborn infants during the first 2 months of life.

TABLE 1 Results of *In Vitro* Testing with Silver Sulfadiazine 1% Cream Concentration of Silver Sulfadiazine Number of Sensitive Strains/Total Strains Tested

Genus & Species	50 mcg/ml	100 mcg/ml
Pseudomonas aeruginosa	130/130	130/130
Xanthomonas (Pseudomonas) maltophilia	7/7	7/7
Enterobacter species	48/50	50/50
Enterobacter cloacae	24/24	24/24
Klebsiella species	53/54	54/54
Escherichia coli	63/63	63/63
Serratia species	27/28	28/28
Proteus mirabilis	53/53	53/53
Morganella morganii	10/10	10/10
Providencia rettgeri	2/2	2/2
Providencia species	1/1	1/1
Proteus vulgaris	2/2	2/2
Citrobacter species	10/10	10/10
Acinetobacter calcoaceticus	10/11	11/11
Staphylococcus aureus	100/101	100/101
Staphylococcus epidermidis	51/51	51/51
β-Hemolytic Streptococcus	4/4	4/4
Enterococcus species	52/53	53/53
Corynebacterium diphtheriae	2/2	2/2
Clostridium perfringens	0/2	2/2
Candida albicans	43/50	50/50

WARNINGS:

There is potential cross-sensitivity between silver sulfadiazine and other sulfonamides. If allergic reactions attributable to treatment with silver sulfadiazine occur, continuation of therapy must be weighed against the potential hazards of the particular allergic reaction.

Fungal proliferation in and below the eschar may occur. However, the incidence of clinically reported fungal superinfection is low.

The use of silver sulfadiazine cream 1% in some cases of glucose-6-phosphate dehydrogenase-deficient individuals may be hazardous, as hemolysis may occur.

PRECAUTIONS:

General: If hepatic and renal functions become impaired and elimination of drug decreases, accumulation may occur and discontinuation of silver sulfadiazine cream 1% should be weighed against the therapeutic benefit being achieved.

In considering the use of topical proteolytic enzymes in conjunction with silver sulfadiazine cream 1%, the possibility should be noted that silver may inactivate such enzymes.

Laboratory Tests: In the treatment of burn wounds involving extensive areas of the body, the serum sulfa concentrations may approach adult therapeutic levels (8 mg% to 12 mg%). Therefore, in these patients it would be advisable to monitor serum sulfa concentrations. Renal function should be carefully monitored and the urine should be checked for sulfa crystals. Absorption of the propylene glycol vehicle has been reported to affect serum osmolality, which may affect the interpretation of laboratory tests.

Carcinogenesis, Mutagenesis, and Impairment of Fertility: Long-term dermal toxicity studies of 24 months' duration in rats and 18 months' in mice with concentrations of silver sulfadiazine three to ten times the concentration in silver sulfadiazine cream 1% revealed no evidence of carcinogenicity.

Pregnancy, Teratogenic Effects, Pregnancy Category B: A reproductive study has been performed in rabbits at doses up to three to ten times the concentration of silver sulfadiazine in silver sulfazdiazine cream 1% and has revealed no evidence of harm to the fetus due to silver sulfadiazine. There are, however, no adequate and well- controlled studies in pregnant women. Because animal reproduction studies are not always predictive of human response, this drug should be used during pregnancy only if clearly justified, especially in pregnant women approaching or at term. (See CONTRAINDICATIONS.)

Nursing Mothers: It is not known whether silver sulfadiazine is excreted in human milk. However, sulfonamides are known to be excreted in human milk, and all sulfonamide derivatives are known to increase the possibility of kernicterus. Because of the possibility for serious adverse reactions in nursing infants from sulfonamides, a decision should be made whether to discontinue nursing or to discontinue the drug, taking into account the importance of the drug to the mother.

Pediatric Use: Safety and effectiveness in pediatric patients have not been established. (See CONTRAINDICATIONS.)

ADVERSE REACTIONS:

Several cases of transient leukopenia have been reported in patients receiving silver sulfadiazine therapy.[1,2,3] Leukopenia associated with silver sulfadiazine administration is primarily characterized by decreased neutrophil count. Maximal white blood cell depression occurs within 2 to 4 days of initiation of therapy. Rebound to normal leukocyte levels follows onset within 2 to 3 days. Recovery is not influenced by continuation of silver sulfadiazine therapy. An increased incidence of leukopenia has been reported in patients treated concurrently with cimetidine.

Other infrequently occurring events include skin necrosis, erythema multiforme, skin discoloration, burning sensation, rashes, and interstitial nephritis.

Reduction in bacterial growth after application of topical antibacterial agents has been reported to permit spontaneous healing of deep partial-thickness burns by preventing conversion of the partial thickness to full thickness by sepsis. However, reduction in bacterial colonization has caused delayed separation, in some cases necessitating escharotomy in order to prevent contracture.

Absorption of silver sulfadiazine varies depending upon the percent of body surface area and the extent of the tissue damage. Although few have been reported, it is possible that any adverse reaction associated with sulfonamides may occur. Some of the reactions, which have been associated with sulfonamides are as follows: blood dyscrasias including agranulocytosis, aplastic anemia, thrombocytopenia, leukopenia, and hemolytic anemia; dermatologic and allergic reactions including Stevens-Johnson syndrome and exfoliative dermatitis; gastrointestinal reactions; hepatitis and hepatocellular necrosis; CNS reactions; and toxic nephrosis.

DOSAGE AND ADMINISTRATION:

Prompt institution of appropriate regimens for care of the burned patient is of prime importance and includes the control of shock and pain. The burn wounds are then cleansed and debrided, and silver sulfadiazine cream 1% is applied under sterile conditions. The burn areas should be covered with silver sulfadiazine cream 1% at all times. The cream should be applied once to twice daily to a thickness of approximately 1/16 inch. Whenever necessary, the cream should be reapplied to any areas from which it has been removed by patient activity. Administration may be accomplished in minimal time because dressings are not required. However, if individual patient requirements make dressings necessary, they may be used.

DOSAGE AND ADMINISTRATION: *(cont'd)*

Reapply immediately after hydrotherapy.

Treatment with silver sulfadiazine cream 1% should be continued until satisfactory healing has occurred, or until the burn site is ready for grafting. The drug should not be withdrawn from the therapeutic regimen while there remains the possibility of infection except if a significant adverse reaction occurs.

REFERENCES:

1. Caffee F, Bingham H. Leukopenia and silver sulfadiazine.*J. Trauma,* 1982;22:586-587. 2. Jarret F, Ellerbe S, Demling R. Acute leukopenia during topical burn therapy with silver sulfadiazine. *Amer J Surg* 1978;135:818-819. 3. Kiker RG, Carvajal HF, Micak RP, Larson DL. A controlled study of the effects of silver sulfadiazine on white blood cell counts in burned children. *J Trauma.* 1977;17:835-836.

HOW SUPPLIED - RATED THERAPEUTICALLY EQUIVALENT:

Cream - Topical - 1 %

20 gm	$3.39	Silver Sulfadiazine, H.C.F.A. F F P	99999-2228-01
20 gm	$3.70	Thermazene, Par Pharm	49884-0459-20
20 gm	$3.80	Thermazene, Sherwood-Davis & Gec	08880-9505-02
20 gm	**$4.06**	**SILVADENE, Hoechst Marion Roussel**	**00088-1050-20**
25 gm	$2.78	Silver Sulfadiazine, H.C.F.A. F F P	99999-2228-02
25 gm	$3.65	SSD 1% SILVER SULFADIAZINE, Knoll Pharms	00048-2100-77
30 gm	$3.50	Silver Sulfadiazine, Raway	00686-0521-46
30 gm	$4.75	Thermazene, Par Pharm	49884-0459-46
30 gm	$4.75	Silver Sulfadiazine, Par Pharm	49884-0521-46
30 gm	$5.08	Silver Sulfadiazine, H.C.F.A. F F P	99999-2228-03
50 gm	$4.20	Silver Sulfadiazine, Raway	00686-0521-36
50 gm	$4.90	Silver Sulfadiazine, Rugby	00536-6415-80
50 gm	$4.94	Silver Sulfadiazine, Qualitest Pharms	00603-7840-84
50 gm	$4.95	SSD RP, Geneva Pharms	00781-7680-50
50 gm	$5.35	Ssd, Knoll Labs	00044-2100-71
50 gm	$5.55	Silver Sulfadiazine, H.C.F.A. F F P	99999-2228-04
50 gm	$5.70	SSD 1% SILVER SULFADIAZINE, Knoll Pharms	00048-2100-78
50 gm	$5.74	Silver Sulfadiazine, HL Moore Drug Exch	00839-7644-81
50 gm	$5.85	Silver Sulfadiazine, Goldline Labs	00182-5055-67
50 gm	$6.00	Silver Sulfadiazine, Rugby	00536-6485-80
50 gm	$6.15	Silver Sulfadiazine, Major Pharms	00904-5108-50
50 gm	$6.15	Thermazene, Sherwood-Davis & Gec	08880-9505-05
50 gm	$6.15	Thermazene, Par Pharm	49884-0459-36
50 gm	$6.15	Silver Sulfadiazine, Par Pharm	49884-0521-36
50 gm	$6.30	Ssd Af, Knoll Labs	00044-2110-71
50 gm	**$6.63**	**SILVADENE, Hoechst Marion Roussel**	**00088-1050-50**
85 gm	$9.92	Silver Sulfadiazine, H.C.F.A. F F P	99999-2228-05
85 gm	$10.00	SSD 1% SILVER SULFADIAZINE, Knoll Pharms	00048-2100-79
85 gm	$11.00	Thermazene, Sherwood-Davis & Gec	08880-9505-85
85 gm	$11.00	Thermazene, Par Pharm	49884-0459-85
85 gm	**$11.81**	**SILVADENE, Hoechst Marion Roussel**	**00088-1050-85**
400 gm	$22.70	SSD 1% SILVER SULFADIAZINE, Knoll Pharms	00048-2100-70
400 gm	$23.09	Silver Sulfadiazine, Rugby	00536-6415-37
400 gm	$25.00	Silver Sulfadiazine, Raway	00686-0521-40
400 gm	$25.40	Silver Sulfadiazine, H.C.F.A. F F P	99999-2228-06
400 gm	$25.61	Silver Sulfadiazine, Rugby	00536-6485-37
400 gm	$25.62	Thermazene, Sherwood-Davis & Gec	08880-9505-40
400 gm	$26.00	Thermazene, Par Pharm	49884-0459-40
400 gm	$26.00	Silver Sulfadiazine, Par Pharm	49884-0521-40
400 gm	$26.70	Ssd Af, Knoll Labs	00044-2110-70
400 gm	**$28.19**	**SILVADENE, Hoechst Marion Roussel**	**00088-1050-72**
1000 gm	$45.00	Silver Sulfadiazine, Raway	00686-0521-39
1000 gm	$51.00	Thermazene, Par Pharm	49884-0459-39
1000 gm	$51.00	Silver Sulfadiazine, Par Pharm	49884-0521-39
1000 gm	$51.55	SSD 1% SILVER SULFADIAZINE, Knoll Pharms	00048-2100-73
1000 gm	$51.90	Ssd Af* Cream 1% (Boots), Knoll Pharms	00048-2110-73
1000 gm	$53.48	Thermazene, Sherwood-Davis & Gec	08880-9505-10
1000 gm	**$55.06**	**SILVADENE, Hoechst Marion Roussel**	**00088-1050-58**
1000 gm	$59.60	Silver Sulfadiazine, H.C.F.A. F F P	99999-2228-07

SIMVASTATIN *(003088)*

CATEGORIES: Antilipemic Agents; Atherosclerosis; Cardiovascular Drugs; Cholesterol; HMG-COA Reductase Inhibitors; Heart Disease; Hypercholesterolemia; Hyperlipidemia; Hyperlipoproteinemia; Hypertriglyceridemia; Hypolipidemics; Vascular Disease; Obesity*; Pregnancy Category X; FDA Class 1C ("Little or No Therapeutic Advantage"); Sales > $1 Billion; FDA Approved 1991 Dec; Patent Expiration 2001 Dec; Top 200 Drugs
* Indication not approved by the FDA

BRAND NAMES: **Denan** (Germany); *Lipex*; *Liponorm*; *Lodales* (France); *Simovil*; *Sinvacor*; *Sivastin*; **Zocor**; *Zocord*
(International brand names outside U.S. in italics)

FORMULARIES: CIGNA; FHP; Kaiser

COST OF THERAPY: $649.99 (Hypercholesterolemia; Tablet; 5 mg; 1/day; 365 days)

DESCRIPTION:

Simvastatin is a cholesterol lowering agent that is derived synthetically from a fermentation product of *Aspergillus terreus.* After oral ingestion, simvastatin, which is an inactive lactone, is hydrolyzed to the corresponding β-hydroxyacid form. This is an inhibitor of 3-hydroxy-3-methylglutaryl-coenzyme A (HMG-CoA) reductase. This enzyme catalyzes the conversion of HMG-CoA to mevalonate, which is an early and rate-limiting step in the biosynthesis of cholesterol.

Simvastatin is butanoic acid, 2,2-dimethyl-,- 1,2,3,7,8,8a-hexahydro-3,7-dimethyl-8-[2-(tetrahydro-4-hydroxy-6-oxo-2*H*-pyran-2-yl)-ethyl]- 1-naphthalenyl ester, (1*S*- [1α,3α,7β,8β (2*S**,4*S**),-8aβ]]. The empirical formula of simvastatin is $C_{25}H_{38}O_5$ and its molecular weight is 418.57.

Simvastatin is a white to off-white, nonhygroscopic, crystalline powder that is practically insoluble in water, and freely soluble in chloroform, methanol and ethanol.

Simivastatin tablets for oral administration contain either 5 mg, 10 mg, 20 mg or 40 mg of simvastatin and the following inactive ingredients: cellulose, hydroxypropyl cellulose, hydroxypropyl methylcellulose, iron oxides, lactose, magnesium stearate, starch, talc, titanium dioxide and other ingredients. Butylated hydroxyanisole is added as a preservative.

CLINICAL PHARMACOLOGY:

The involvement of low-density lipoprotein (LDL) cholesterol in atherogenesis has been well-documented in clinical and pathological studies, as well as in many animal experiments. Epidemiological studies have established that high LDL (low-density lipoprotein) cholesterol and low HDL (high-density lipoprotein) cholesterol are both risk factors for coronary heart

CLINICAL PHARMACOLOGY: *(cont'd)*

disease. The Lipid Research Clinics Coronary Primary Prevention Trial (LRC-CPPT), coordinated by the National Institutes of Health (NIH), studied men aged 35-59 with total cholesterol levels of 265 mg/dl (6.8 mmol/L) or greater, LDL cholesterol values 175 mg/dl (4.5 mmol/L) or greater, and triglyceride levels not more than 300 mg/dl (3.4 mmol/L). This seven-year, double-blind, placebo-controlled study demonstrated that lowering LDL cholesterol with diet and cholestyramine decreased the combined rate of coronary heart disease death plus non-fatal myocardial infarction.

Simivastatin has been shown to reduce both normal and elevated LDL cholesterol concentrations. The effect of simivastatin-induced changes in lipoprotein levels, including reduction of serum cholesterol, on cardiovascular morbidity or mortality has not been established.

LDL is formed from very-low-density lipoprotein (VLDL) and is catabolized predominantly by the high affinity LDL receptor. The mechanism of the LDL-lowering effect of simivastatin may involve both reduction of VLDL cholesterol concentration, and induction of the LDL receptor, leading to reduced production and/or increased catabolism of LDL cholesterol. Apolipoprotein B also falls substantially during treatment with simivastatin. Since each LDL particle contains one molecule of apolipoprotein B, and since little apolipoprotein B is found in other lipoproteins, this strongly suggests that simivastatin does not merely cause cholesterol to be lost from LDL, but also reduces the concentration of circulating LDL particles. In addition, simivastatin modestly reduces VLDL cholesterol and plasma triglycerides and can produce increases of variable magnitude in HDL cholesterol. The effects of simivastatin on Lp(a), fibrinogen, and certain other independent biochemical risk markers for coronary heart disease are unknown.

Simivastatin is a specific inhibitor of HMG-CoA reductase, the enzyme that catalyzes the conversion of HMG-CoA to mevalonate. The conversion of HMG-CoA to mevalonate is an early step in the biosynthetic pathway for cholesterol.

Pharmacokinetics: Simivastatin is a lactone that is readily hydrolyzed *in vivo* to the corresponding β-hydroxyacid, a potent inhibitor of HMG-CoA reductase. Inhibition of HMG-CoA reductase is the basis for an assay in pharmacokinetic studies of the β-hydroxyacid metabolites (active inhibitors) and, following base hydrolysis, active plus latent inhibitors (total inhibitors) in plasma following administration of simivastatin.

Following an oral dose of ^{14}C-labeled simvastatin in man, 13% of the dose was excreted in urine and 60% in feces. The latter represents absorbed drug equivalents excreted in bile, as well as any unabsorbed drug. Plasma concentrations of total radioactivity (simvastatin plus^{14}C-metabolites) peaked at 4 hours and declined rapidly to about 10% of peak by 12 hours postdose. Absorption of simvastatin, estimated relative to an intravenous reference dose, in each of two animal species tested, averaged about 85% of an oral dose. In animal studies, after oral dosing, simvastatin achieved substantially higher concentrations in the liver than in non-target tissues. Simvastatin undergoes extensive first-pass extraction in the liver, its primary site of action, with subsequent excretion of drug equivalents in the bile. As a consequence of extensive hepatic extraction of simvastatin (estimated to be > 60% in man), the availability of drug to the general circulation is low. In a single-dose study in nine healthy subjects, it was estimated that less than 5% of an oral dose of simvastatin reaches the general circulation as active inhibitors. Following administration of simvastatin tablets, the coefficient of variation, based on between-subject variability was approximately 48% for the area under the concentration-time curve (AUC) for total inhibitory activity in the general circulation.

Both simvastatin and its β-hydroxyacid metabolite are highly bound (approximately 95%) to human plasma proteins. Animal studies have not been performed to determine whether simvastatin crosses the blood-brain and placental barriers. However, when radiolabeled simvastatin was administered to rats, simvastatin-derived radioactivity crossed the blood-brain barrier.

The major active metabolites of simvastatin present in human plasma are the β-hydroxyacid of simvastatin and its 6'-hydroxy, 6'-hydroxymethyl, and 6'-exo-methylene derivatives. Peak plasma concentrations of both active and total inhibitors were attained within 1.3 to 2.4 hours postdose. While the recommended therapeutic dose range is 5 to 40 mg/day, there was no substantial deviation from linearity of AUC of inhibitors in the general circulation with an increase in dose to as high as 120 mg. Relative to the fasting state, the plasma profile of inhibitors was not affected when simvastatin was administered immediately before an A.H.A. recommended low-fat meal.

Kinetic studies with another reductase inhibitor, having a similar principal route of elimination, have suggested that for a given dose level higher systemic exposure may be achieved in patients with severe renal insufficiency (as measured by creatinine clearance).

CLINICAL STUDIES:

Simivastatin has been shown to be highly effective in reducing total and LDL cholesterol in heterozygous familial and non-familial forms of hypercholesterolemia and in mixed hyperlipidemia. A marked response was seen within 2 weeks, and the maximum therapeutic response occurred within 4-6 weeks. The response was maintained during chronic therapy.

In a multicenter, double-blind, placebo-controlled, dose-response study in patients with familial or non-familial hypercholesterolemia, simivastatin given as a single-dose in the evening (the recommended dosing) was similarly effective as when given on a twice-daily basis. Simivastatin consistently and significantly decreased total plasma cholesterol (TOTAL-C), LDL cholesterol (LDL-C), total cholesterol/HDL cholesterol (TOTAL- C/HDL-C) ratio, and LDL cholesterol/HDL cholesterol (LDL-C/HDL-C) ratio. Simivastatin also modestly decreased triglycerides (TRIG) and produced increases of variable magnitude in HDL cholesterol (HDL-C).

The results of a dose response study in patients with primary hypercholesterolemia are presented in TABLE 1:

TABLE 1 Dose Response in Patients with Primary Hypercholesterolemia (Mean Percent Change from Baseline After 8 Weeks)

Treatment	N	Total-C	LDL-C	HDL-C	LDL-C/ HDL-C	Total-C/ HDL-C	Trig.
Placebo	28	-3	-4	+2	-4	-3	+7
Zocor							
5 mg q.p.m.	28	-17	-24	+7	-27	-22	-10
10 mg q.p.m.	27	-24	-33	+9	-37	-29	-10
20 mg q.p.m.	26	-25	-33	+11	-36	-30	-19
40 mg q.p.m.	29	-28	-40	+12	-46	-36	-19

Simivastatin was compared to cholestyramine, probucol, or gemfibrozil, respectively, in double-blind parallel studies involving 1102 patients. All studies were performed in patients who were at moderate to high risk of coronary events based on serum cholesterol levels. At all dosage levels tested, simivastatin produced a significantly greater reduction of total plasma cholesterol, LDL cholesterol, VLDL cholesterol, triglycerides, and total cholesterol/HDL cholesterol ratio when compared to cholestyramine or probucol. The increase in HDL seen with simivastatin was not significantly greater than the increase seen with cholestyramine but was significantly different from the decrease seen with probucol (see TABLE 2 and TABLE 3).

CLINICAL STUDIES: *(cont'd)*

TABLE 2 Simivastatin vs. Cholestyramine (Percent Change from Baseline After 12 Weeks)

Treatment	N	Total-C (mean)	LDL-C (mean)	HDL-C (mean)	LDLC/ HDL-C (mean)	Total-C/ HDL-C (mean)	VLDL-C (median)	Trig (mean)
Zocor								
20 mg q.p.m.	84	-27	-32	+10	-36	-31	-8	-13
40 mg q.p.m.	82	-33	-41	+10	-45	-38	-28	-21
Cholestyramine								
4-24 g/day*	85	-15	-21	+8	-25	-19	+7	+15

* maximum tolerated dose (mean dose taken, 18 g/day)

TABLE 3 Simivastatin vs. Probucol (Percent Change from Baseline After 12 Weeks)

Treatment	N	Total-C (mean)	LDL-C (mean)	LDL-C/ HDL-C (mean)	Total-C/ HDL-C (mean)	HDL-C (mean)	HLDL--C (median)	TRIG (mean)
Zocor								
20 mg q.p.m.	82	-27	-34	+10	-39	-34	-18	-17
40 mg q.p.m.	86	-30	-40	+13	-45	-37	-14	-19
Probucol								
500 mg b.i.d	81	-13	-8	-27	+31	+25	+11	-0.4

In the Multicenter Anti-Atheroma Study, the effect of therapy with simvastatin on atherosclerosis was assessed by quantitative coronary angiography in hypercholesterolemic men and women with coronary heart disease. In this randomized, double-blind, controlled trial, patients with mean baseline total cholesterol value of 245 mg/dl (6.4 mmol/l) and a mean baseline LDL value of 170 mg/dl (4.4 mmol/l) were treated with conventional measures and with simvastatin 20 mg/d or placebo. Angiograms were evaluated at baseline, two and four years. A total of 347 patients had a baseline angiogram and at least one follow-up angiogram. The co- primary endpoints of the trial were mean change per patient in minimum and mean lumen diameters, indicating focal and diffuse disease, respectively. Simvastatin significantly slowed the progression of lesions as measured un the final angiogram by both these parameters (mean changes in minimum lumen diameter:-0.04 mm with simvastatin vs -0.12 mm with placebo; mean changes in mean lumen diameter:-0.03 mm with simvastatin vs -0.08 mm with placebo), as well as by change from baseline in percent diameter stenosis (0.9% simvastatin vs 3.6% placebo). After four years, the groups also differed significantly in the proportions of patients categorized with disease progression (23% simvastatin vs 33% placebo) and disease regression (18% simvastatin vs 12% placebo). In addition, simvastatin significantly decreased the proportion of patients with new lesions (13% simvastatin vs 24% placebo) and with new total occlusions (5% vs 11%). The mean change per-patient in mean and minimum lumen diameters calculated by comparing angiograms in the subset of 274 patients who had matched angiographic projections at baseline, two and four years is present in the graphs shown in the original package insert.

In a study designed to evaluate the possible effects of simvastatin on reproductive hormones and sperm characteristics in men with familial hypercholesterolemia, there was a small decrease in the mean percentage of vital sperm and a small increase in the mean percentage of abnormal forms, with these changes achieving statistical significance at week 14. However, there was no effect on numbers of concentration of motile sperm. Simvastatin had no effect on basal reproductive hormone levels (prolactin, luteinizing hormone, follicle-stimulating hormone, and plasma testosterone). Provocative testing (HCG stimulation) was not done. Treatment with another HMG-CoA reductase inhibitor resulted in a statistically significant decrease in plasma testosterone response to HCG.

In a study to evaluate the effect of simvastatin on adrenocortical function in patients with Type II hypercholesterolemia, simvastatin had no effect on basal adrenocortical function as assessed by determination of morning plasma cortisol levels, urine free cortisol, and urinary excretion of 17-hydroxy steroids. Simvastatin also had no effect on adrenocortical reserve as evaluated by the plasma cortisol response to ACTH stimulation and insulin-induced hypoglycemia.

INDICATIONS AND USAGE:

Therapy with lipid-altering agents should be a component of multiple risk factor intervention in those individuals at significantly increased risk for atherosclerotic vascular disease due to hypercholesterolemia. Simivastatin is indicated as an adjunct to diet for the reduction of elevated total and LDL cholesterol levels in patients with primary hypercholesterolemia (Types IIa and IIb***), when the response to a diet restricted in saturated fat and cholesterol and other nonpharmacological measures alone has been inadequate.

Prior to initiating therapy with simvastatin, secondary causes for hypercholesterolemia (*e.g.,* poorly controlled diabetes mellitus, hypothyroidism, nephrotic syndrome, dysproteinemias, obstructive liver disease, other drug therapy, alcoholism) should be excluded, and a lipid profile performed to measure TOTAL-C, HDL-C, and triglycerides (TG). For patients with TG less than 400 mg/dl (<4.5 mmol/L), LDL-C can be estimated using the following equation:

LDL-C = Total cholesterol - [0.20 x (triglycerides) + HDL-C]

For TG levels >400 mg/dl (>4.5 mmol/L), this equation is less accurate and LDL-C concentrations should be determined by ultracentrifugation. In many hypertriglyceridemic patients, LDL-C may be low or normal despite elevated TOTAL-C. In such cases, simivastatin is not indicated.

Lipid determinations should be performed at intervals of no less than four weeks and dosage adjusted according to the patient's response to therapy.

The National Cholesterol Education Program (NCEP) Treatment Guidelines are summarized below (TABLE 4):

Since the goal of treatment is to lower LDL-C, the NCEP recommends that LDL-C levels be used to initiate and assess treatment response. Only if LDL-C levels are not available, should the TOTAL-C be used to monitor therapy.

Although simivastatin may be useful to reduce elevated LDL cholesterol levels in patients with combined hypercholesterolemia and hypertriglyceridemia where hypercholesterolemia is the major abnormality (Type IIb hyperlipoproteinemia), it has not been studied in conditions where the major abnormality is elevation of chylomicrons VLDL or IDL (*i.e.,* hyperlipoproteinemia types I, III, IV, or V).***

The effect of simivastatin-induced changes in lipoprotein levels, including reduction of serum cholesterol, on cardiovascular morbidity or mortality has not been established.

TABLE 4

Definite Atherosclerotic Disease*	Two or More Other Risk Factors**	LDL-Cholesterol mg/dl(mmol/L) Initiation Level	Goal
NO	NO	≥190 (≥4.9)	<160 (<4.1)
NO	YES	≥160 (≥4.1)	<130 (<3.4)
YES	YES OR NO	≥130 (≥3.4)	≤100 (≤2.6)

*Coronary heart disease or peripheral vascular disease (including symptomatic carotid artery disease).

**Other risk factors for coronary heart disease (CHD) include: age (males:≥45 years; females: ≥55 years or premature menopause without estrogen replacement therapy); family history of premature CHD; cigarette smoking; hypertension; confirmed HDL-C <35 mg/dl (<0.91 mmol/l); and diabetes mellitus. Subtract one risk factor if HDL-C is ≥60 mg/dl (≥1.6 mmol/L).

TABLE 5 *** Classification of Hyperlipoproteinemias

Type I (rare)	Lipoproteins elevated chylomicrons	Lipid Elevations major TG	minor ↑→C
IIa	LDL	C	—
IIb	LDL, VLDL	C	TG
III (rare)	IDL	C/TG	—
IV	VLDL	TG	↑→C
V (rare)	chylomicrons, VLDL	TG	↑→C

C = cholesterol, TG = triglycerides, LDL = low-density lipoprotein, VLDL = very-low-density lipoprotein, IDL = intermediate-density lipoprotein.

CONTRAINDICATIONS:

Hypersensitivity to any component of this medication.

Active liver disease or unexplained persistent elevations of serum transaminase (see WARNINGS.)

Pregnancy And Lactation: Atherosclerosis is a chronic process and the discontinuation of lipid-lowering drugs during pregnancy should have little impact on the outcome of long-term therapy of primary hypercholesterolemia. Moreover, cholesterol and other products of the cholesterol biosynthesis pathway are essential components for fetal development, including synthesis of steroids and cell membranes. Because the ability of inhibitors of HMG-CoA reductase such as simivastatin to decrease by synthesis of cholesterol and possibly other products of the cholesterol biosynthesis pathway. Simivastatin may cause fetal harm when administered to a pregnant women. Therefore, simvastatin is contraindicated during pregnancy and in nursing mothers. **Simvastatin should be administered to women of childbearing age only when such patients are highly unlikely to conceive.** If the patient becomes pregnant while taking this drug, simvastatin should be discontinued and the patient should be apprised of the potential hazard to the fetus.

WARNINGS:

Liver Dysfunction: *Persistent increases (to more than 3 times the upper limit of normal) in serum transaminases have occurred in 1% of patients who received simvastatin in clinical trials.* When drug treatment was interrupted or discontinued in these patients the transaminase levels usually fell slowly to pretreatment levels. The increases were not associated with jaundice or other clinical signs or symptoms. There was no evidence of hypersensitivity.

It is recommended that liver function tests be performed before the initiation of treatment, at 6 and 12 weeks after initiation therapy or evaluation in dose, and periodically thereafter (*e.g.,* semiannually). Patients who develop increased transaminase levels should be monitored with a second liver function evaluation to confirm the finding and be followed thereafter with frequent liver function tests until the abnormality (ies) return to normal. Should an increase in AST or ALT of three times the upper limit of normal or greater persist, withdrawal of therapy with simivastatin is recommended.

The drug should be used with caution in patients who consume substantial quantities of alcohol and/or have a past history of liver disease. Active liver disease or unexplained transaminase elevations are contraindications to the use of simvastatin.

As with other lipid-lowering agents, moderate (less than three times the upper limit of normal) elevations of serum transaminases have been reported following therapy with simvastatin. These changes appeared soon after initiation of therapy with simvastatin, were often transient, were not accompanied by any symptoms and did not require interruption of treatment.

Skeletal Muscle: Rare cases of rhabdomyolysis with acute renal failure secondary to myoglobinuria have been associated with simvastatin therapy. Rhabdomyolysis has also been associated with other HMG-CoA reductase inhibitors when they were administered alone or concomitantly with 1) immunosuppressive therapy, including cyclosporine in cardiac transplant patients; 2) gemfibrozil or lipid-lowering doses (≥1 g/day) of nicotinic acid in non-transplant patients, or 3) erythromycin in seriously ill patients. Some of the patients who had rhabdomyolysis in association with the reductase inhibitors had pre-existing renal insufficiency, usually as a consequence of long-standing diabetes most subjects who have had an unsatisfactory lipid response to either simvastatin or gemfibrozil alone, the possible benefits of combined therapy with these drugs are not considered to outweigh the risk of severe myopathy, rhabdomyolysis, and acute renal failure. While it is not known whether this interaction occurs with fibrates other than gemfibrozil, myopathy and rhabdomyolysis have occasionally been associated with the use of other fibrates alone, including clofibrate. Therefore, the combined use of simvastatin with other fibrates should generally be avoided.

Muscle weakness accompanied by marked elevation of creatine phosphokinase was observed in a renal transplant patient on cyclosporine and simvastatin following the initiation of systemic itraconazole therapy. Rhabdomyolysis with renal failure has been reported in a renal transplant patient receiving cyclosporine and another HMG CoA reductase inhibitor shortly after a dose increase in the systemic antifungal agent itraconazole. The HMG CoA reductase inhibitors and the azole derivative antifungal agents inhibit cholesterol biosynthesis at different points in the biosynthetic pathway.

In patients receiving cyclosporine, simvastatin should be temporarily discontinued if systemic azole derivative antifungal therapy is required; patients not taking cyclosporine should be carefully monitored if systemic azole derivative antifungal therapy is required.

Physicians contemplating combined therapy with simvastatin and lipid-lowering doses of nicotinic acid, or with immunosuppressive drugs should carefully weigh the potential benefits and risks and should carefully monitor patients for any signs and symptoms of muscle pain, tenderness, or weakness, particularly during the initial months of therapy and during any periods of upward dosage titration of either drug. Periodic creatine phosphokinase (CPK) determinations may be considered in some situations, but there is no assurance that such monitoring will prevent the occurrence of severe myopathy.

WARNINGS: *(cont'd)*

Because of an apparent relationship between increased plasma levels of active metabolites derived from other HMG-CoA reductase inhibitors and myopathy, in patients taking cyclosporine, the daily dosage should not exceed 10 mg/day (see DOSAGE AND ADMINISTRATION.)

Simvastatin therapy should be temporarily withheld or discontinued in any patient with an acute, serious condition suggestive of a myopathy or having a risk factor predisposing to the development of renal failure secondary to rhabdomyolysis, (*e.g.,* severe acute infection, hypotension, major surgery, trauma, severe metabolic, endocrine and electrolyte disorders, and uncontrolled seizures).

Myopathy should be considered in any patient with diffuse myalgias, muscle tenderness or weakness, and/or marked elevation of CPK. Patients should be advised to report promptly unexplained muscle pain, tenderness or weakness, particularly if accompanied by malaise or fever. Simvastatin therapy should be discontinued if markedly elevated CPK levels occur or myopathy is diagnosed or suspected.

PRECAUTIONS:

General: Before instituting therapy with simivastatin, an attempt should be made to control hypercholesterolemia with appropriate diet, exercise, and weight reduction in obese patients, and to treat other underlying medical problems (see INDICATIONS AND USAGE.)

Simvastatin may cause elevation of creatine phosphokinase and transaminase levels (see WARNINGS and ADVERSE REACTIONS). This should be considered in the differential diagnosis of chest pain in a patient on therapy with simvastatin.

Homozygous Familial Hypercholesterolemia: Simivastatin is less effective in patients with the rare homozygous familial hypercholesterolemia, possibly because these patients have few functional LDL receptors.

Information for the Patient: Patients should be advised to report promptly unexplained muscle pain, tenderness, or weakness, particularly if accompanied by malaise or fever.

Endocrine Function: HMG-CoA reductase inhibitors interfere with cholesterol synthesis and as such might theoretically blunt adrenal and/or gonadal steroid production. However, clinical studies have shown that simvastatin does not reduce basal plasma cortisol concentration or impair adrenal reserve, and does not reduce basal plasma testosterone concentration (see CLINICAL STUDIES.) Another HMG-CoA reductase inhibitor has been shown to reduce the plasma testosterone response to HCG; the effect of simvastatin on HCG-stimulated testosterone secretion has not been studied.

Results of clinical trials with drugs in this class have been inconsistent with regard to drug effects on basal and reserve steroid levels. The effects of HMG-CoA reductase inhibitors on male fertility have not been studied in adequate numbers of male patients. The effects, if any, on the pituitary-gonadal axis in pre-menopausal women are unknown. Patients treated with simvastatin who develop clinical evidence of endocrine dysfunction should be evaluated appropriately. Caution should also be exercised if an HMG-CoA reductase inhibitor or other agent used to lower cholesterol levels is administered to patients also receiving other drugs (*e.g.,* ketoconazole, spironolactone, cimetidine) that may decrease the levels or activity of endogenous steroid hormones.

CNS Toxicity: Optic nerve degeneration was seen in clinically normal dogs treated with simvastatin for 14 weeks at 180 mg/kg/day, a dose that produced mean plasma drug levels about 44 times higher than the mean drug level in humans taking 40 mg/day.

A chemically similar drug in this class also produced optic nerve degeneration (Wallerian degeneration of retinogeniculate fibers) in clinically normal dogs in a dose-dependent fashion starting at 60 mg/kg/day, a dose that produced mean plasma drug levels about 30 times higher than the mean drug levels in humans taking the highest recommended dose (as measured by total enzyme inhibitory activity). The same drug also produced vestibulocochlear Wallerian-like degeneration and retinal ganglion cell chromatolysis in dogs treated for 14 weeks at 180 mg/kg/day, a dose that resulted in a mean plasma drug level similar to that seen with the 60 mg/kg/day dose.

CNS vascular lesions, characterized by perivascular hemorrhage and edema, mononuclear cell infiltration of perivascular spaces, perivascular fibrin deposits and necrosis of small vessels were seen in dogs treated with simvastatin at a dose of 360 mg/kg/day, a dose that produced plasma drug levels that were about 50 times higher than the mean drug levels in humans taking 40 mg/day. Similar CNS vascular lesions have been observed with several other drugs of this class.

There were cataracts in female rats after two years of treatment with 50 and 100 mg/kg/day (100 and 120 times the human AUC at 40 mg/day) and in dogs in three month studies at 90 and 360 mg/kg/day and at two years at 50 mg/kg/day. These treatment levels represented plasma drug levels (AUC) of approximately 42, 40, and 26 times the mean human plasma drug exposure after a 40 milligram daily dose.

Carcinogenesis, Mutagenesis, and Impairment of Fertility: In a 72-week carcinogenicity study, mice were administered daily doses of simvastatin of 25, 100, and 400 mg/kg body weight, which resulted in mean plasma drug levels approximately 3, 15, and 33 times higher than the mean human plasma drug concentration (as total inhibitory activity) after a 40 mg oral dose. Liver carcinomas were significantly increased in high-dose females and mid-and high-dose males with a maximum incidence of 90 percent in males. The incidence of adenomas of the liver was significantly increased in mid- and high-dose females. Drug treatment also significantly increased the incidence of lung adenomas in mid- and high-dose males and females. Adenomas of the Harderian gland (a gland of the eye of rodents) were significantly higher in high-dose mice than in controls. No evidence of a tumorigenic effect was observed at 25 mg/kg/day. Although mice were given up to 500 times the human dose (HD) on a mg/kg/body weight basis, blood levels of HMG-CoA reductase inhibitory activity were only 3-33 times higher in mice than in humans given 40 mg of simivastatin.

In a separate 92-week carcinogenicity study in mice at doses up to 25 mg/kg/day, no evidence of a tumorigenic effect was observed. Although mice were given up to 31 times the human dose on a mg/kg basis, plasma drug levels were only 2-4 times higher than humans given 40 mg simvastatin as measured by AUC.

In a two-year study in rats, there was a statistically significant increase in the incidence of thyroid follicular adenomas in female rats exposed to approximately 45 times higher levels of simvastatin than humans given 40 mg simvastatin (as measured by AUC).

A second two-year rat carcinogenicity study with doses of 50 and 100 mg/kg/day produced hepatocellular adenomas and carcinomas (in female rats at both doses and in males at 100 mg/kg/day). Thyroid follicular cell adenomas were increased in males and females at both doses; thyroid follicular cell carcinomas were increased in females at 100 mg/kg/day. The increased incidence of thyroid neoplasms appears to be consistent with findings from other HMG-CoA reductase inhibitors. These treatment levels represented plasma drug levels (AUC) of approximately 35 and 75 times (males) and 110 and 120 times (females) the mean human plasma drug exposure after a 40 milligram daily dose.

PRECAUTIONS: *(cont'd)*

No evidence of mutagenicity was observed in a microbial mutagen test using mutant strains of *Salmonella typhimurium* with or without rat or mouse liver metabolic activation. In addition, no evidence of damage to genetic material was noted in an *in vitro* alkaline elution assay using rat hepatocytes, a V-79 mammalian cell forward mutation study, an *in vitro* chromosome aberration study in CHO cells, or an *in vivo* chromosomal aberration assay in mouse bone marrow.

There was decreased fertility in male rats treated with simvastatin for 34 weeks at 25 mg/kg body weight (15 times the maximum human exposure level, based on AUC, in patients receiving 40 mg/day); however, this effect was not observed during a subsequent fertility study in which simvastatin was administered at this same dose level to male rats for 11 weeks (the entire cycle of spermatogenesis including epididymal maturation). No microscopic changes were observed in the testes of rats from either study. At 180 mg/kg/day, (which produces exposure levels 44 times higher than those in humans taking 40 mg/day), seminiferous tubule degeneration (necrosis and loss of spermatogenic epithelium) was observed. In dogs, there was drug-related testicular atrophy, decreased spermatogenesis, spermatocytic degeneration and giant cell formation at 10 mg/kg/day, (approximately 7 times the human exposure level, based on AUC, at 40 mg/day). The clinical significance of these findings is unclear.

Pregnancy Category X: See CONTRAINDICATIONS. Safety in pregnant women has not been established. Simvastatin was not teratogenic in rats at doses of 25 mg/kg/day or in rabbits at doses up to 10 mg/kg daily. These doses resulted in 6 times (rat) or 4 times (rabbit) the human exposure based on mg/m^2 surface area. However, in studies with another structurally-related HMG-CoA reductase inhibitor, skeletal malformations were observed in rats and mice. Rare reports of congenital anomalies have been received following intrauterine exposure to HMG-CoA reductase inhibitors. There has been one report of severe congenital bony deformity, tracheo-esophageal fistula, and anal atresia (VATER association) in a baby born to a woman who took another HMG-CoA reductase inhibitor with dextroamphetamine sulfate during the first trimester of pregnancy. Simvastatin should be administered to women of child-bearing potential only when such patients are highly unlikely to conceive and have been informed of the potential hazards. If the woman becomes pregnant while taking simvastatin, it should be discontinued and the patient advised again as to the potential hazards to the fetus.

Nursing Mothers: It is not known whether simvastatin is excreted in human milk. Because a small amount of another drug in this class is excreted in human milk and because of the potential for serious adverse reactions in nursing infants, women taking simvastatin should not nurse their infants (see CONTRAINDICATIONS.)

Pediatric Use: Safety and effectiveness in children and adolescents have not been established. Because children and adolescents are not likely to benefit from cholesterol lowering for at least a decade and because experience with this drug is limited (no studies in subjects below the age of 20 years), treatment of children or adolescents with simvastatin is not recommended at this time.

DRUG INTERACTIONS:

Immunosuppressive Drugs, Itraconazole, Gemfibrozil, Niacin (Nicotinic Acid), Erythromycin: See WARNINGS, Skeletal Muscle.

Antipyrine: Because simvastatin had no effect on the pharmacokinetics of antipyrine, interactions with other drugs metabolized via the same cytochrome isozymes are not expected.

Propranolol: In healthy male volunteers there was a significant decrease in mean C_{max}, but no change in AUC, for simvastatin total and active inhibitors with concomitant administration of single doses of simivastatin and propranolol. The clinical relevance of this finding is unclear. The pharmacokinetics of the enantiomers of propranolol were not affected.

Digoxin: Concomitant administration of a single dose of digoxin in healthy male volunteers receiving simvastatin resulted in a slight elevation (less than 0.3 ng/ml) in digoxin concentrations in plasma (as measured by a radioimmunoassay) compared to concomitant administration of placebo and digoxin. Patients taking digoxin should be monitored appropriately when simvastatin is initiated.

Warfarin: In two clinical studies, one in normal volunteers and the other in hypercholesterolemic patients, simvastatin 20-40 mg/day modestly potentiated the effect of coumarin anticoagulants: the prothrombin time, reported as International Normalized Ratio (INR), increased from a baseline of 1.7 to 1.8 and from 2.6 to 3.4 in the volunteer and patient studies, respectively. With other reductase inhibitors, clinically evident bleeding and/or increased prothrombin time has been reported in a few patients taking coumarin anticoagulants concomitantly. In such patients, prothrombin time should be determined before starting simvastatin and frequently enough during early therapy to insure that no significant alteration of prothrombin time occurs. Once a stable prothrombin time has been documented, prothrombin times can be monitored at the intervals usually recommended for patients on coumarin anticoagulants. If the dose of simvastatin is changed, the same procedure should be repeated. Simvastatin therapy has not been associated with bleeding or with changes in prothrombin time in patients not taking anticoagulants.

Other Concomitant Therapy: Although specific interaction studies were not performed, in clinical studies, simvastatin was used concomitantly with angiotensin-converting enzyme (ACE) inhibitors, beta blockers, calcium-channel blockers, diuretics and nonsteroidal anti-inflammatory drugs (NSAIDs) without evidence of clinically significant adverse interactions. The effect of cholestyramine on the absorption and kinetics of simvastatin has not been determined.

ADVERSE REACTIONS:

In the pre-marketing controlled clinical studies and their open extensions (2423 patients with mean duration of follow-up of approximately 18 months), 1.4% of patients were discontinued due to adverse experiences attributable to simivastatin. Adverse reactions have usually been mild and transient. Simivastatin has been evaluated for serious adverse reactions in more than 21,000 patients and is generally well-tolerated.

Clinical Adverse Experiences: Adverse experiences occurring at an incidence of 1 percent or greater in patients treated with simivastatin, regardless of causality, in controlled clinical studies are shown in TABLE 6.

In the Multicenter Anti-Atheroma Study, the incidence of adverse experiences was comparable in the simvastatin and placebo treatment groups over the four years of this study.

The following effects have been reported with drugs in this class. Not all the effects listed below have necessarily been associated with simvastatin therapy.

ADVERSE REACTIONS: *(cont'd)*

TABLE 6

	Zocor (N = 1583) %	Placebo (N = 157) %	Cholestyramine (N = 179) %	Probucol (N = 81) %
Body as a Whole				
Abdominal pain	3.2	3.2	8.9	2.5
Asthenia	1.6	2.5	1.1	1.2
Gastrointestinal				
Constipation	2.3	1.3	29.1	1.2
Diarrhea	1.9	2.5	7.8	3.7
Dyspepsia	1.1	—	4.5	3.7
Flatulence	1.9	1.3	14.5	6.2
Nausea	1.3	1.9	10.1	2.5
Nervous System/Psychiatric				
Headache	3.5	5.1	4.5	3.7
Respiratory				
Upper respiratory infection	2.1	1.9	3.4	6.2

Skeletal: muscle cramps, myalgia, myopathy, rhabdomyolysis, arthralgias.

Neurological: dysfunction of certain cranial nerves (including alteration of taste, impairment of extra-ocular movement, facial paresis), tremor, dizziness, vertigo, memory loss, paresthesia, peripheral neuropathy, peripheral nerve palsy, anxiety, insomnia, depression.

Hypersensitivity Reactions: An apparent hypersensitivity syndrome has been reported rarely which has included one or more of the following features: anaphylaxis, angioedema, lupus erythematous-like syndrome, polymyalgia rheumatica, vasculitis, purpura, thrombocytopenia, leukopenia, hemolytic anemia, positive ANA, ESR increase, eosinophilia, arthritis, arthralgia, urticaria, asthenia, photosensitivity, fever, chills, flushing, malaise, dyspnea, toxic epidermal necrolysis, erythema multiforme, including Stevens-Johnson syndrome.

Gastrointestinal: pancreatitis, hepatitis, including chronic active hepatitis, cholestatic jaundice, fatty change in liver, and, rarely, cirrhosis, fulminant hepatic necrosis, and hepatoma; anorexia, vomiting.

Skin: alopecia, pruritus. A variety of skin changes (e.g. nodules, discoloration, dryness of skin/mucous membranes, changes to hair/nails) has been reported.

Reproductive: gynecomastia, loss of libido, erectile dysfunction.

Eye: progression of cataracts (lens opacities), ophthalmoplegia.

Laboratory Abnormalities: elevated transaminases, alkaline phosphatase, γ-glutamyl transpeptidase, and bilirubin; thyroid function abnormalities.

Laboratory Tests: Marked persistent increases of serum transaminases have been noted (see WARNINGS, Liver Dysfunction.) About 5% of patients had elevations of creatine phosphokinase (CPK) levels of 3 or more times the normal value on one or more occasions. This was attributable to the noncardiac fraction of CPK. Muscle pain or dysfunction usually was not reported (see WARNINGS, Skeletal Muscle).

Concomitant Therapy: In controlled clinical studies in which simvastatin was administered concomitantly with cholestyramine, no adverse reactions peculiar to this concomitant treatment were observed. The adverse reactions that occurred were limited to those reported previously with simvastatin or cholestyramine. The combined use of simvastatin with fibrates should generally be avoided (see WARNINGS, Skeletal Muscle).

OVERDOSAGE:

Significant lethality was observed in mice after a single oral dose of 9 g/m^2. No evidence of lethality was observed in rats or dogs treated with doses of 30 and 100 g/m^2, respectively. No specific diagnostic signs were observed in rodents. At these doses the only signs seen in dogs were emesis and mucoid stools.

A few cases of overdosage with simivastatin have been reported; no patients had any specific symptoms, and all patients recovered without sequelae. The maximum dose taken was 450 mg. Until further experience is obtained, no specific treatment of overdosage with simivastatin can be recommended.

The dialyzability of simvastatin and its metabolites in man is not known at present.

DOSAGE AND ADMINISTRATION:

The patient should be placed on a standard cholesterol-lowering diet before receiving simivastatin and should continue on this diet during treatment with simivastatin (see NCEP Treatment Guidelines for details on dietary therapy).

The recommended starting dose is 5-10 mg once a day in the evening. The recommended dosing range is 5-40 mg/day as a single dose in the evening; the maximum recommended dose is 40 mg/day. Doses should be individualized according to base-line LDL-C levels, the recommended goal of therapy (see NCEP Guidelines) and the patient's response. A starting dose of 5 mg/day should be considered for patients with LDL-C (on diet) of ≤190 mg/dl (4.9 mmol/L) and for the elderly. Patients with LDL-C levels >190 mg/dl (4.9 mmol/L) should be started on 10 mg/day. Adjustments of dosage should be made at intervals of 4 weeks or more.

In the elderly, maximum reductions in LDL cholesterol may be achieved with daily doses of 20 mg or less.

Cholesterol levels should be monitored periodically and consideration should be given to reducing the dosage of simivastatin if cholesterol falls below the targeted range.

Concomitant Therapy: Simivastatin is effective alone or when used concomitantly with bile-acid sequestrants. Use of simivastatin with fibrate-type drugs such as gemfibrozil or clofibrate should generally be avoided (see WARNINGS, Skeletal Muscle.)

In patients taking immunosuppressive drugs concomitantly with simvastatin (see WARNINGS, Skeletal Muscle), therapy should begin with 5 mg of simivastatin and should not exceed 10 mg/day.

Dosage in Patients with Renal Insufficiency: Because simivastatin does not undergo significant renal excretion, modification of dosage should not be necessary in patients with mild to moderate renal insufficiency. However, caution should be exercised when simivastatin is administered to patients with severe renal insufficiency; such patients should be started at 5 mg/day and be closely monitored (see CLINICAL PHARMACOLOGY, Pharmacokineticsand WARNINGS, Skeletal Muscle).

PATIENT INFORMATION:

Simvastatin is called an HMG-CoA reductase inhibitor and it is used to treat high cholesterol. It is called an HMG Co-A reductase inhibitor because it inhibits an enzyme in your body that makes cholesterol. It is important to continue with dietary modification and exercise programs. This drug should not be taken by those with liver disease. You may be asked to have some tests to determine if your liver is working properly. It should not be taken by pregnant or nursing women. If pregnancy results while taking this medication, it may be necessary to discontinue the medication temporarily. Please consult your physician. If you experience any muscle pain, tenderness, weakness, or fever please inform your physician. This drug also has several drug interactions, please inform your physician or pharmacist of all medications, prescription and over-the-counter, you are taking. This medication is most effective when taken in the evening before bedtime. You should have your cholesterol checked periodically to determine if dosage adjustments are necessary.

HOW SUPPLIED:

No. 3588 - Tablets Zocor 5 mg are buff, shield-shaped, film-coated tablets, coded MSD 726.

No. 3589 - Tablets Zocor 10 mg are peach, shield-shaped, film-coated tablets, coded MSD 735 on one side and Zocor on the other.

No. 3590 - Tablets Zocor 20 mg are tan, shield-shaped, film coated tablets, coded MSD 740 on one side and Zocor on the other.

No. 3591 - Tablets Zocor 40 mg are brick-red, shield-shaped, film-coated tablets, coded MSD 749 on one side and Zocor on the other.

Storage: Store between 5-30°C (41-86°F).

HOW SUPPLIED - EQUIVALENTS NOT AVAILABLE:

Tablet, Plain Coated - Oral - 5 mg

60's	$106.84	ZOCOR, Merck	00006-0726-61
90's	$160.26	ZOCOR, Merck	00006-0726-54
100's	$178.08	ZOCOR, Merck	00006-0726-28

Tablet, Plain Coated - Oral - 10 mg

60's	$112.77	ZOCOR, Merck	00006-0735-61
90's	$169.17	ZOCOR, Merck	00006-0735-54
100's	$187.98	ZOCOR, Merck	00006-0735-28
1000's	$1879.71	ZOCOR, Merck	00006-0735-82
10000's	$17312.50	ZOCOR, Merck	00006-0735-87

Tablet, Plain Coated - Oral - 20 mg

60's	$204.38	ZOCOR, Merck	00006-0740-61
1000's	$3406.32	ZOCOR, Merck	00006-0740-82
10000's	$31372.91	ZOCOR, Merck	00006-0740-87

Tablet, Plain Coated - Oral - 40 mg

60's	$206.25	ZOCOR, Merck	00006-0749-61

SODIUM ASCORBATE *(002237)*

CATEGORIES: Homeostatic & Nutrient; Vitamin C; Vitamins; FDA Pre 1938 Drugs

BRAND NAMES: Cenolate

Prescribing information not available at time of publication.

HOW SUPPLIED - EQUIVALENTS NOT AVAILABLE:

Injection, Solution - Intramuscular; - 1 gm/1ml

2 ml	$2.90	CENOLATE 1, Abbott	00074-3397-02

Injection, Solution - Intramuscular; - 250 mg/ml

30 ml	$2.99	Sodium Ascorbate, McGuff	49072-0035-30

Injection, Solution - Intramuscular; - 500 mg/ml

1 ml	$2.24	CENOLATE, Abbott	00074-3118-02
50 ml	$4.25	Sodium Ascorbate, Pegasus Med Svs	10974-0201-50

SODIUM BICARBONATE *(002241)*

CATEGORIES: Acidosis; Alkalinizing Agents; Antacids and Adsorbents; Antagonists and Antidotes; Antidotes; Barbiturates; Cardiac Arrest; Dehydration; Diabetes; Electrolyte Solutions; Electrolytic, Caloric-Water Balance; Gastrointestinal Drugs; Homeostatic & Nutrient; Lactic Acidosis; Metabolic Acidosis; Nephrotoxicity; Pharmaceutical Aids; Poisoning; Shock; Diarrhea*; Urinary Alkalinizers; Pregnancy Category C; FDA Approved 1986 Jun

* Indication not approved by the FDA

BRAND NAMES: Baros Granules; Neut

DESCRIPTION:

Sodium bicarbonate injection, USP is a sterile, nonpyrogenic, hypertonic solution of sodium bicarbonate ($NaHCO_3$) in water for injection for administration by the intravenous route as an electrolyte replenisher and systemic alkalizer.

Solutions are offered in concentrations of 4.2%, 5.0%, 7.5% and 8.4%. Solutions in LVP container syringe has 0.9 mg/ml of edetate disodium, anhydrous added as a stabilizer.

The solutions contain no bacteriostat, antimicrobial agent or added buffer and are intended only for use as a single-dose injection. When smaller doses are required, the unused portion should be discarded with the entire unit.

Sodium bicarbonate, 84 mg is equal to one milliequivalent each of NA+ and HCO_3-. Sodium Bicarbonate, USP is chemically designated $NaHCO_3$, a white crystalline powder soluble in water.

Water for injection, USP is chemically designated H_2O.

CLINICAL PHARMACOLOGY:

Intravenous sodium bicarbonate therapy increases plasma bicarbonate, buffers excess hydrogen ion concentration, raises blood pH and reverses the clinical manifestations of acidosis.

Sodium bicarbonate in water dissociates to provide sodium (Na+) and bicarbonate (HCO_3-) ions. Sodium (Na+) is the principal cation of the extracellular fluid and plays a large part in the therapy of fluid and electrolyte disturbances. Bicarbonate (HCO_3-) is a normal constituent of body fluids and the normal plasma level ranges from 24 to 31 mEq/liter. Plasma concentration is regulated by the kidney through acidification of the urine when there is an excess. Bicarbonate anion is considered "labile" since at a proper concentration of hydrogen ion (H+) it may be converted to carbonic acid (H_2CO_3) and thence to its volatile form, carbon dioxide (CO_2) excreted by the lung. Normally a ratio of 1:20 (carbonic acid; bicarbonate) is present in the extracellular fluid. In a healthy adult with normal kidney function, practically all the glomerular filtered bicarbonate ion is reabsorbed; less than 1% is excreted in the urine.

INDICATIONS AND USAGE:

Sodium bicarbonate injection, USP is indicated in the treatment of metabolic acidosis which may occur in severe renal disease, uncontrolled diabetes, circulatory insufficiency due to shock or severe dehydration, extracorporeal circulation of blood, cardiac arrest and severe primary lactic acidosis. Sodium bicarbonate is further indicated in the treatment of certain drug intoxications, including barbiturates (where dissociation of the barbiturate-protein complex is desired), in poisoning by salicylates or methyl alcohol and in hemolytic reactions requiring alkalinization of the urine to diminish nephrotoxicity of hemoglobin and its breakdown products. Sodium bicarbonate also is indicated in severe diarrhea which is often accompanied by a significant loss of bicarbonate.

Treatment of metabolic acidosis should, if possible, be superimposed on measures designed to control the basic cause of the acidosis - e.g., insulin in uncomplicated diabetes, blood volume restoration in shock. But since an appreciable time interval may elapse before all of the ancillary effects are brought about, bicarbonate therapy is indicated to minimize risks inherent to the acidosis itself.

Vigorous bicarbonate therapy is required in any form of metabolic acidosis where a rapid increase in plasma total CO_2 content is crucial - e.g., cardiac arrest, circulatory insufficiency due to shock or severe dehydration, and in severe primary lactic acidosis or severe diabetic acidosis.

CONTRAINDICATIONS:

Sodium bicarbonate injection, USP is contraindicated in patients who are losing chloride by vomiting or from continuous gastrointestinal suction, and in patients receiving diuretics known to produce a hypochloremic alkalosis.

WARNINGS:

Solutions containing sodium ions should be used with great care, if at all, in patients with congestive heart failure, severe renal insufficiency and in clinical states in which there exists edema with sodium retention.

In patients with diminished renal function, administration of solutions containing sodium ions may result in sodium retention.

The intravenous administration of these solutions can cause fluid and/or solute overloading resulting in dilution of serum electrolyte concentrations, overhydration, congested states or pulmonary edema.

Extravascular infiltration should be avoided, (see ADVERSE REACTIONS.)

PRECAUTIONS:

The potentially large loads of sodium given with bicarbonate require that caution be exercised in the use of sodium bicarbonate in patients with congestive heart failure or other edematous or sodium-retaining states, as well as in patients with oliguria or anuria.

Caution must be exercised in the administration of parenteral fluids, especially those containing sodium ions, to patients receiving corticosteroids or corticotropin.

Potassium depletion may predispose to metabolic alkalosis and coexistent hypocalcemia may be associated with carpopedal spasm as the plasma pH rises. These dangers can be minimized if such electrolyte imbalances are appropriately treated prior to or concomitantly with bicarbonate infusion.

Rapid injection (10 ml/min) of hypertonic sodium bicarbonate injection, USP solutions into neonates and children under two years of age may produce hypernatremia, a decrease in cerebrospinal fluid pressure and possible intracranial hemorrhage. The rate of administration in such patients should therefore be limited to no more than 8 mEq/kg/day. A 4.2% solution may be preferred for such slow administration. In emergencies such as cardiac arrest, the risk of rapid infusion must be weighed against the potential for fatality due to acidosis.

Laboratory Tests: The aim of all bicarbonate therapy is to produce a substantial correction of the low total CO_2 content and blood pH, but the risks of overdosage and alkalosis should be avoided. Hence, repeated fractional doses and periodic monitoring by appropriate laboratory tests are recommended to minimize the possibility of overdosage.

Pregnancy Category C: Animal reproduction studies have not been conducted with sodium bicarbonate. It is also not known whether sodium bicarbonate can cause fetal harm when administered to a pregnant woman or can affect reproduction capacity. Sodium bicarbonate should be given to a pregnant woman only if clearly needed.

DRUG INTERACTIONS:

Additives may be incompatible; norepinephrine and dobutamine are incompatible with sodium bicarbonate solution.

The addition of sodium bicarbonate to parenteral solutions containing calcium should be avoided, except where compatibility has been previously established. Precipitation or haze may result from sodium bicarbonate/calcium admixtures. *NOTE:* Do not use the injection if it contains precipitate. Additives may be incompatible. Consult with pharmacist, if available. When introducing additives, use aseptic technique, mix thoroughly and do not store.

ADVERSE REACTIONS:

Overly aggressive therapy with sodium bicarbonate injection, USP can result in metabolic alkalosis (associated with muscular twitchings, irritability, and tetany) and hypernatremia.

Inadvertent extravasation of intravenously administered hypertonic solutions of sodium bicarbonate have been reported to cause chemical cellulitis because of their alkalinity, with tissue necrosis, ulceration or sloughing at the site of infiltration. Prompt elevation of the part, warmth and local injection of lidocaine or hyaluronidase are recommended to reduce the likelihood of tissue slough from extravasated IV infusions.

OVERDOSAGE:

Should alkalosis result, the bicarbonate should be stopped and the patient managed according to the degree of alkalosis present. 0.9% sodium chloride injection intravenous may be given; potassium chloride also may be indicated if there is hypokalemia. Severe alkalosis may be accompanied by hyperirritability or tetany and these symptoms may be controlled by calcium gluconate. An acidifying agent such as ammonium chloride may also be indicated in severe alkalosis. (See WARNINGS and PRECAUTIONS.)

DOSAGE AND ADMINISTRATION:

Sodium bicarbonate injection, USP is administered by the intravenous route.

In cardiac arrest: A rapid intravenous dose of one to two 50 ml vials (44.6 to 100 mEq) may be given initially and continued at a rate of 50 ml (44.6 to 50 mEq) every 5 to 10 minutes if necessary (as indicated by arterial pH and blood gas monitoring) to reverse the acidosis. Caution should be observed in emergencies where very rapid infusion of large quantities; of

DOSAGE AND ADMINISTRATION: *(cont'd)*

bicarbonate is indicated. Bicarbonate solutions are hypertonic and may produce an undesirable rise in plasma sodium concentration in the process of correcting the metabolic acidosis. In cardiac arrest, however, the risks from acidosis exceed those of hypernatremia.

In infants: (up to two years of age) The 4.2% solution is recommended for intravenous administration at a dose not to exceed 8 mEq/kg/day. Slow administration rates and the 4.2% solution are recommended in neonates, to guard against the possibility of producing hypernatremia, decreasing cerebrospinal fluid pressure and inducing intracranial hemorrhage.

In less urgent forms of metabolic acidosis: Sodium bicarbonate injection, USP may be added to other intravenous fluids. The amount of bicarbonate to be given to older children and adults over a four-to-eight-hour period is approximately 2 to 5 mEq/kg of body weight - depending upon the severity of the acidosis as judged by the lowering of total CO_2 content, blood pH and clinical condition of the patient. In metabolic acidosis associated with shock, therapy should be monitored by measuring blood gases, plasma osmolarity, arterial blood lactate, hemodynamics and cardiac rhythm. Bicarbonate therapy should always be planned in a stepwise fashion since the degree of response from a given dose is not precisely predictable. Initially an infusion of 2 to 5 mEq/kg body weight over a period of 4 to 8 hours will produce a measurable improvement in the abnormal acid-base status of the blood. The next step of therapy is dependent upon the clinical response of the patient. If severe symptoms have abated, then the frequency of administration and the size of the dose may be reduced.

In general, it is unwise to attempt full correction of a low total CO_2 content during the first 24 hours of therapy, since this may be accompanied by an unrecognized alkalosis because of a delay in the readjustment of ventilation to normal. Owing to this lag, the achievement of total CO_2 content of about 20 mEq/liter at the end of the first day of therapy will usually be associated with a normal blood pH. Further modification of the acidosis to completely normal values usually occurs in the presence of normal kidney function when and if the cause of the acidosis can be controlled. Values for total CO_2 which are brought to normal or above normal within the first day of therapy are very likely to be associated with grossly alkaline values for blood pH, with ensuing undesired side effects.

Parenteral drug products should be inspected visually for particulate matter and discoloration prior to administration, whenever solution and container permit. (See PRECAUTIONS.)

Do not use unless solution is clear and the container or seal is intact. Discard unused portion.

Store at controlled room temperature 15° to 30°C (59° to 86°F).

HOW SUPPLIED - EQUIVALENTS NOT AVAILABLE:

Granules, Effervescent - Oral

3 gm x 100	$180.56	BAROS GRANULES, Lafayette Pharms	59081-0651-03

Injection, Solution - Intravenous - 4.2 %

5 ml	$5.58	NEUT, Abbott	00074-6609-02
5 ml x 10	$39.40	SODIUM BICARBONATE, Astra USA	00186-0645-01
5 ml x 25	$19.93	Sodium Bicarbonate, Fujisawa USA	00469-1605-25
5 ml x 25	$61.25	Sodium Bicarbonate 4.2%, Fujisawa USA	00469-0026-25
5 ml/10ml	$5.32	NEUT, Abbott	00074-4935-01
10 ml	$7.44	Sodium Bicarbonate Injection 4.2%, Intl Medication	00548-1031-00
10 ml	$12.97	SODIUM BICARBONATE, Abbott	00074-5534-18
10 ml	$13.75	Sodium Bicarbonate, Abbott	00074-5534-23
10 ml	$14.30	SODIUM BICARBONATE, Abbott	00074-5534-34
10 ml x 10	$38.70	Sodium Bicarbonate, Voluntary Hosp	53258-9115-08
10 ml x 10	$74.36	SODIUM BICARBONATE, Astra USA	00186-0646-01
10 ml x 10	$76.88	Sodium Bicarbonate, Fujisawa USA	00469-9115-87
50 ml	$7.74	Sodium Bicarbonate, Intl Medication	00548-1002-00
50 ml	$7.74	Sodium Bicarbonate, Intl Medication	00548-1052-00
50 ml x 25	$54.69	Sodium Bicarbonate, Am Regent	00517-0639-25

Injection, Solution - Intravenous - 5 %

500 ml	$39.23	Sodium Bicarbonate, Baxter Hlthcare	00338-0374-03
500 ml	$41.18	5% SODIUM BICARBONATE, Abbott	00074-1594-03
500 ml x 6	$40.75	5% SODIUM BICARBONATE, McGaw	00264-1498-10

Injection, Solution - Intravenous - 7.5 %

50 ml	$7.46	7.5% SODIUM BICARBONATE, Abbott	00074-4103-03
50 ml	$8.11	Sodium Bicarbonate, Intl Medication	00548-2002-00
50 ml	$18.38	SODIUM BICARBONATE, Abbott	00074-4916-22
50 ml	$18.96	Sodium Bicarbonate, Abbott	00074-4916-23
50 ml	$19.38	Sodium Bicarbonate, Intl Medication	00548-3002-00
50 ml	$19.72	SODIUM BICARBONATE, Abbott	00074-4916-34
50 ml	$62.19	Sodium Bicarbonate, Fujisawa USA	00469-8400-60
50 ml x 10	$110.88	Sodium Bicarbonate, Fujisawa USA	00469-9121-87
50 ml x 10	$111.63	SODIUM BICARBONATE, Astra USA	00186-0647-01

Injection, Solution - Intravenous - 8.4 %

10 ml	$7.44	Sodium Bicarbonate, Intl Medication	00548-1032-00
10 ml	$12.79	SODIUM BICARBONATE, Abbott	00074-4900-18
10 ml	$13.59	Sodium Bicarbonate, Abbott	00074-4900-23
10 ml	$14.13	Sodium Bicarbonate, Abbott	00074-4900-34
10 ml x 10	$76.88	Sodium Bicarbonate, Fujisawa USA	00469-9125-87
10 ml x 10	$78.75	SODIUM BICARBONATE, Astra USA	00186-0656-01
50 ml	$6.70	8.4% SODIUM BICARBONATE, Abbott	00074-6625-02
50 ml	$8.11	Sodium Bicarbonate, Intl Medication	00548-2052-00
50 ml	$18.64	SODIUM BICARBONATE, Abbott	00074-6637-22
50 ml	$19.21	SODIUM BICARBONATE, Abbott	00074-6637-23
50 ml	$19.64	Sodium Bicarbonate, Intl Medication	00548-3052-00
50 ml	$19.99	SODIUM BICARBONATE, Abbott	00074-6637-34
50 ml	$64.38	Sodium Bicarbonate Injection 84/Ml, Fujisawa USA	00469-0600-60
50 ml x 10	$106.05	SODIUM BICARBONATE, Astra USA	00186-0650-01
50 ml x 10	$112.38	Sodium Bicarbonate, Fujisawa USA	00469-9124-87
50 ml x 25	$35.10	Sodium Bicarbonate, Fujisawa USA	00469-0019-25
50 ml x 25	$57.19	Sodium Bicarbonate, Am Regent	00517-1550-25

SODIUM CHLORIDE *(002243)*

CATEGORIES: Cough Preparations; EENT Drugs; Electrolyte Solutions; Electrolytic, Caloric-Water Balance; Eye, Ear, Nose, & Throat Preparations; Homeostatic & Nutrient; Irrigating Solutions; Mucolytic Agents; Pharmaceutical Adjuvants; Pharmaceutical Aids; Relaxants/Stimulants, Uterine; Replacement Solutions; Pregnancy Category C; FDA Approval Pre 1982

BRAND NAMES: Bacteriostatic Sodium Chloride; Dispos-A-Vial Respiratory Prods.; Iocare; Normal Saline; Sodium Cl For Inhalation

FORMULARIES: BC-BS; Medi-Cal; WHO

DESCRIPTION:

Sodium Chloride Injection, USP is a sterile, non-pyrogenic, isotonic solution of sodium chloride 0.9% (9 mg/ml) in Water for Injection containing no antimicrobial agent or other added substance. The pH is between 4.5 and 7.0. Its chloride and sodium ion concentrations are approximately 0.154 mEq of each per milliliter and its calculated osmolality is 0.308 milliosmols per ml.

Sodium chloride occurs as colorless cubic crystals or white crystalline powder and has a saline taste. Sodium chloride is freely soluble in water. It is soluble in glycerin and slightly soluble in alcohol.

The empirical formula for sodium chloride is NaCl, and the molecular weight is 58.44.

CLINICAL PHARMACOLOGY:

Sodium chloride comprises over 90% of the inorganic constituents of the blood serum. Sodium chloride in water dissociates to provide sodium (Na^+) and chloride (Cl^-) ions. These ions are normal constituents of the body fluids (principally extracellular) and are essential for maintaining electrolyte balance. The small volume of fluid and amount of sodium chloride provided by Sodium Chloride Injection, USP, 0.9%, when used only as a vehicle for parenteral injection of drugs, is unlikely to exert a significant effect on fluid and electrolyte balance except possibly in very small infants.

INDICATIONS AND USAGE:

Sodium Chloride Injection is used to flush intravascular catheters or as a sterile, isotonic single dose vehicle, solvent, or diluent for substances to be administered intravenously, intramuscularly or subcutaneously and for other extemporaneously prepared single dose sterile solutions according to instructions of the manufacturer of the drug to be administered.

WARNINGS:

Sodium chloride must be used with caution in the presence of congestive heart failure, circulatory insufficiency, kidney dysfunction or hypoproteinemia.

Excessive amounts of sodium chloride by any route may cause hypokalemia and acidosis. Excessive amounts by parenteral routes may precipitate congestive heart failure and acute pulmonary edema, especially seen in patients with preexisting cardiovascular disease and those receiving corticosteroids, corticotropin or other drugs that may give rise to sodium retention.

For use in newborns, when a Sodium Chloride solution is required for preparation or diluting medications, or in flushing intravenous catheters, only preservative-free Sodium Chloride Injection, USP, 0.9% should be used.

PRECAUTIONS:

General: Since Sodium Chloride Injection does not contain antimicrobial agents and is intended for single use, any unused amount must be discarded immediately following withdrawal of any portion of the contents of the vial or ampul. Do not open ampul until it is to be used.

Consult the manufacturer's instructions for choice of vehicle, appropriate dilution or volume for dissolving the drugs to be injected, including the route and rate of injection.

Pregnancy Category C: Animal reproduction studies have not been conducted with Sodium Chloride Injection. It is also not known whether Sodium Chloride Injection can cause fetal harm when administered to a pregnant woman or can affect reproduction capacity. Sodium Chloride Injection should be given to a pregnant woman only if clearly needed.

ADVERSE REACTIONS:

Reactions which may occur because of this solution, added drugs or the technique of reconstitution or administration include febrile response, local tenderness, abscess, tissue necrosis or infection at the site of injection, venous thrombosis or phlebitis extending from the site of injection and extravasation.

If an adverse reaction does occur, discontinue the infusion, evaluate the patient, institute appropriate countermeasures, and if possible, retrieve and save the remainder of the unused vehicle for examination.

OVERDOSAGE:

When used as a diluent, solvent or intravascular flushing solution, this parenteral preparation is unlikely to pose a threat of sodium chloride or fluid overload except possibly in very small infants. In the event these should occur, reevaluate the patient and institute appropriate corrective measures.

DOSAGE AND ADMINISTRATION:

Before Sodium Chloride Injection, USP, 0.9% is used as a vehicle for the administration of a drug, specific references should be checked for any possible incompatibility with sodium chloride.

The volume of the preparation to be used for diluting or dissolving any drug for injection is dependent on the vehicle concentration, dose and route of administration as recommended by the manufacturer.

Sodium Chloride Injection, USP, 0.9% is also indicated for use in flushing intravenous catheters. Prior to and after administration of the medication, the intravenous catheter should be flushed in its entirety with Sodium Chloride Injection, USP, 0.9%. Use in accord with any warnings or precautions appropriate to the medication being administered.

Parenteral drug products should be inspected visually for particulate matter and discoloration prior to administration, whenever solution and container permit.

Avoid freezing.

HOW SUPPLIED - RATED THERAPEUTICALLY EQUIVALENT:

Injection, Solution - Intravenous - 0.45 %

25 ml	$15.72	0.45% Sodium Chloride, Abbott	00074-7730-20
50 ml	$11.51	0.45% Sodium Chloride, Abbott	00074-7132-13
50 ml	$13.98	0.45% Sodium Chloride, Abbott	00074-7730-13
50 ml	$15.72	Sodium Chloride, Abbott	00074-7730-36
100 ml	$11.51	Sodium Chloride, Abbott	00074-7132-23
100 ml	$15.72	Sodium Chloride, Abbott	00074-7730-37
250 ml	$10.15	Sodium Chloride, Abbott	00074-7985-02
250 ml	$13.93	Sodium Chloride, Abbott	00074-7132-02
250 ml x 24	$10.26	5% Dextrose/0.45% Sodium Chloride, McGaw	00264-7612-20
500 ml	$7.32	Sodium Chloride, Abbott	00074-1585-03
500 ml	$9.67	Sodium Chloride, Baxter Hlthcare	00338-0043-03
500 ml	$10.38	Sodium Chloride, McGaw	00264-7802-10
500 ml x 10	$8.94	0.45% Sodium Chloride, McGaw	00264-1802-10
500 ml x 12	$10.12	0.45% Sodium Chloride, McGaw	00264-1402-10
500 ml x 24	$10.26	5% Dextrose/0.45% Sodium Chloride, McGaw	00264-7612-10
1000 ml	$8.41	Sodium Chloride, Abbott	00074-1585-05
1000 ml	$11.23	Sodium Chloride, McGaw	00264-7802-00
1000 ml	$12.24	5% Dextrose/0.45% Sodium Chloride, McGaw	00264-7612-00

HOW SUPPLIED - RATED THERAPEUTICALLY EQUIVALENT:
(cont'd)

1000 ml x 6	$11.34	0.45% Sodium Chloride, McGaw	00264-1402-00
1000 ml x 10	$10.03	0.45% Sodium Chloride, McGaw	00264-1802-00

Injection, Solution - Intravenous - 0.9 %

2 ml x 25	$21.25	Sodium Chloride, Fujisawa USA	00469-9186-02
5 ml x 25	$10.94	Sodium Chloride, Solopak Labs	39769-0112-05
10 ml	$1.45	Bacteriostatic 0.9% Sodium, Abbott	00074-1966-04
10 ml	$1.57	Sodium Chloride, Abbott	00074-4888-25
10 ml x 25	$21.25	Bacteriostatic Sodium Chloride, Fujisawa USA	00469-0248-15
10 ml x 25	$22.50	Sodium Chloride, Solopak Labs	39769-0112-10
10 ml x 25	$23.13	Sodium Chloride, Fujisawa USA	00469-9186-10
20 ml	$1.66	Bacteriostatic 0.9% Sodium, Abbott	00074-1966-05
20 ml x 25	$34.38	Sodium Chloride, Fujisawa USA	00469-9186-20
25 ml	$15.38	Sodium Chloride, McGaw	00264-1800-36
25 ml	$15.72	Sodium Chloride, Abbott	00074-7984-20
25 ml/150 ml	$11.31	Sodium Chloride, Baxter Hlthcare	00338-0049-10
30 ml	$1.84	Bacteriostatic 0.9% Sodium, Abbott	00074-1966-07
30 ml	$2.10	Sodium Chloride, C O Truxton	00463-1047-30
30 ml	$2.25	Bacteriostatic Sodium Chloride, Major Pharms	00904-0896-30
30 ml	$4.35	Bacteriostatic Sodium Chloride, Rugby	00536-2501-75
30 ml x 25	$24.89	Bacteriostatic Sodium Chloride, Gensia Labs	00703-7586-04
30 ml x 25	$29.68	Bacteriostatic Sodium Chloride, Fujisawa USA	00469-2248-15
50 ml	$3.91	0.9% Sodium Chloride Inj., Abbott	00074-1493-01
50 ml	$7.35	0.9% Sodium Chloride, Abbott	00074-7984-10
50 ml	$9.12	0.9% Sodium Chloride, Abbott	00074-7984-13
50 ml	$9.67	Sodium Chloride, Baxter Hlthcare	00338-0049-11
50 ml	$9.67	Sodium Chloride, Baxter Hlthcare	00338-0049-31
50 ml	$9.67	Sodium Chloride, Baxter Hlthcare	00338-0049-41
50 ml	$9.90	Sodium Chloride, McGaw	00264-1800-31
50 ml	$10.25	Sodium Chloride, Abbott	00074-7984-36
50 ml	$11.51	0.9% Sodium Chloride, Abbott	00074-7101-13
50 ml	$14.50	Sodium Chloride, Baxter Hlthcare	00338-0553-11
50 ml	$16.46	0.9% Sodium Chloride Inj., Abbott	00074-1584-01
50 ml in 150 ml	$7.79	Sodium Chloride, McGaw	00264-1400-31
100 ml	$4.06	0.9% Sodium Chloride Inj., Abbott	00074-1492-01
100 ml	$9.12	0.9% Sodium Chloride, Abbott	00074-7984-23
100 ml	$9.57	Sodium Chloride, Abbott	00074-7984-27
100 ml	$9.67	Sodium Chloride, Baxter Hlthcare	00338-0049-18
100 ml	$9.67	Sodium Chloride, Baxter Hlthcare	00338-0049-38
100 ml	$9.67	Sodium Chloride, Baxter Hlthcare	00338-0049-48
100 ml	$9.90	Sodium Chloride, McGaw	00264-1800-32
100 ml	$10.25	Sodium Chloride, Abbott	00074-7984-37
100 ml	$11.51	0.9% Sodium Chloride, Abbott	00074-7101-23
100 ml	$14.50	Sodium Chloride, Baxter Hlthcare	00338-0553-18
100 ml	$16.46	0.9% Sodium Chloride Inj., Abbott	00074-1584-11
100 ml in 150 m	$7.79	Sodium Chloride, McGaw	00264-1400-32
100 ml x 25	$68.75	Sodium Chloride 0.9%, Fujisawa USA	00469-0186-25
150 ml	$8.58	0.9% Sodium Chloride, Abbott	00074-7983-01
150 ml	$9.11	Sodium Chloride, Baxter Hlthcare	00338-0049-01
150 ml	$9.56	Sodium Chloride, Abbott	00074-7983-61
150 ml	$10.15	0.9% Sodium Chloride, Abbott	00074-1583-01
150 ml x 12	$5.66	Sodium Chloride, McGaw	00264-1400-30
250 ml	$9.01	Sodium Chloride, Abbott	00074-7983-53
250 ml	$9.11	Sodium Chloride, Baxter Hlthcare	00338-0049-02
250 ml	$9.56	0.9% Sodium Chloride, Abbott	00074-7983-02
250 ml	$9.58	Sodium Chloride, McGaw	00264-7800-20
250 ml	$10.15	0.9% Sodium Chloride, Abbott	00074-1583-02
250 ml	$13.93	0.9% Sodium Chloride, Abbott	00074-7101-02
250 ml x 12	$5.66	Sodium Chloride, McGaw	00264-1400-20
500 ml	$6.65	0.9% Sodium Chloride, Abbott	00074-1583-03
500 ml	$9.11	Sodium Chloride, Baxter Hlthcare	00338-0049-03
500 ml	$9.56	0.9% Sodium Chloride, Abbott	00074-7983-03
500 ml	$10.39	Sodium Chloride, McGaw	00264-7800-10
500 ml x 10	$9.06	Sodium Chloride, McGaw	00264-1800-10
500 ml x 12	$10.81	Sodium Chloride, McGaw	00264-1400-10
1000 ml	$7.61	0.9% Sodium Chloride, Abbott	00074-1583-05
1000 ml	$9.86	Sodium Chloride, Baxter Hlthcare	00338-0049-04
1000 ml	$10.35	0.9% Sodium Chloride, Abbott	00074-7983-09
1000 ml plastic	$11.23	0.9% Sodium Chloride, McGaw	00264-7800-00
1000 ml x 6	$10.26	Sodium Chloride, McGaw	00264-1400-00
1000 ml x 10	$9.06	Sodium Chloride, McGaw	00264-1800-00

Injection, Solution - Intravenous - 3 %

500 ml	$12.06	Sodium Chloride, McGaw	00264-7805-10

Injection, Solution - Intravenous - 4.5 mg/10ml

1000 ml	$10.88	Sodium Chloride In Water, Baxter Hlthcare	00338-0043-04

Injection, Solution - Intravenous - 5 %

500 ml	$12.25	Sodium Chloride, McGaw	00264-7806-10

Injection, Solution - Intravenous - 9 mg/ml

10 ml	$1.57	0.9% Sodium Chloride, Abbott	00074-4888-10
20 ml	$1.83	0.9% Sodium Chloride, Abbott	00074-4888-20
50 ml	$2.73	0.9% Sodium Chloride, Abbott	00074-4888-50
100 ml	$3.59	0.9% Sodium Chloride, Abbott	00074-4888-99

Injection, Solution - Intravenous - 20 meq

1000 ml	$25.19	Potassium Chloride/Dextrose 5%, Abbott	00074-7111-09

Injection, Solution - Intravenous - 45 mg/10ml

500 ml	$10.15	0.45% Sodium Chloride, Abbott	00074-7985-03
1000 ml	$11.42	0.45% Sodium Chloride, Abbott	00074-7985-09

Solution - Irrigation - 0.45 %

1500 ml	$20.27	0.4% Sodium Chloride, Abbott	00074-6147-06
2000 ml	$8.50	Sodium Chloride, Baxter Hlthcare	00338-0041-46

Solution - Irrigation - 0.9 %

250 ml	$11.56	Sodium Chloride, Baxter Hlthcare	00338-0048-02
250 ml	$12.14	0.9% Sodium Chloride, Abbott	00074-6138-02
500 ml	$11.56	Sodium Chloride, Baxter Hlthcare	00338-0048-03
500 ml	$12.14	0.9% Sodium Chloride, Abbott	00074-6138-03
500 ml x 12	$12.29	Sodium Chloride, McGaw	00264-2201-10
1000 ml	$4.67	Sodium Chloride, Baxter Hlthcare	00338-0047-24
1000 ml	$7.14	Sodium Chloride, Baxter Hlthcare	00338-0047-44
1000 ml	$7.49	0.9% Sodium Chloride, Abbott	00074-7972-05
1000 ml	$11.22	0.9% Sodium Chloride, Abbott	00074-6138-09
1000 ml	$14.16	Sodium Chloride, Baxter Hlthcare	00338-0048-04
1000 ml	$14.85	0.9% Sodium Chloride, Abbott	00074-7138-09
1000 ml x 12	$12.06	Sodium Chloride, McGaw	00264-2201-00
1500 ml	$8.51	Sodium Chloride, Baxter Hlthcare	00338-0046-05
1500 ml	$13.80	0.9% Sodium Chloride, Abbott	00074-7138-16
1500 ml	$15.23	0.9% Sodium Chloride, Abbott	00074-6138-06
1500 ml	$16.17	Sodium Chloride, Baxter Hlthcare	00338-0048-05
1500 ml	$20.12	Sodium Chloride, Abbott	00074-7138-06

HOW SUPPLIED - RATED THERAPEUTICALLY EQUIVALENT:
(cont'd)

2000 ml	$11.00	Sodium Chloride, Baxter Hlthcare	00338-0047-46
2000 ml	$11.54	0.9% Sodium Chloride, Abbott	00074-7972-07
2000 ml x 6	$21.04	Sodium Chloride, McGaw	00264-2201-50
3000 ml	$12.54	Sodium Chloride, Baxter Hlthcare	00338-0047-27
3000 ml	$13.29	Sodium Chloride Processing, Baxter Hlthcare	00338-0050-47
3000 ml	$16.47	Sodium Chloride, Baxter Hlthcare	00338-0047-47
3000 ml	$17.25	0.9% Sodium Chloride, Abbott	00074-7972-08
4000 ml x 4	$22.92	Sodium Chloride, McGaw	00264-2201-70
5000 ml	$20.70	Sodium Chloride, Baxter Hlthcare	00338-0047-29

HOW SUPPLIED - NOT RATED EQUIVALENT:

Injection, Conc-Soln - Intravenous - 50 meq

20 ml	$3.37	Sodium Chloride, Abbott	00074-6657-02

Injection, Conc-Soln - Intravenous - 100 meq

40 ml	$3.81	Sodium Chloride, Abbott	00074-6660-02

Injection, Solution - Intravenous - 0.9 %

1 ml x 50	$45.94	Bacteriostatic Sodium Chloride, Wyeth Labs	00008-0333-08
1 ml x 50	$65.00	SODIUM CHLORIDE, Wyeth Labs	00008-0333-51
2 ml x 25	$12.05	Sodium Chloride, Elkins Sinn	00641-0495-25
2 ml x 25	$13.50	Sodium Chloride, Gensia Labs	00703-7562-04
2 ml x 25	$24.69	Sodium Chloride, Am Regent	00517-2802-25
2 ml x 50	$38.83	Sodium Chloride, Sanofi Winthrop	00024-1815-02
2 ml x 50	$40.31	Bacteriostatic Sodium Chloride, Elkins Sinn	00641-3430-09
2 ml x 50	$49.14	Sodium Chloride, Sanofi Winthrop	00024-1816-02
2 ml x 50	$62.35	Sodium Chloride, Sanofi Winthrop	00024-1812-02
2 ml x 50	$77.65	Sodium Chloride, Sanofi Winthrop	00024-1811-20
2 ml x 50	$77.65	Sodium Chloride, Sanofi Winthrop	00024-1815-20
2 ml x 120	$193.50	Sodium Chloride, Solopak Mdcl	59747-0112-72
2 ml x 120	$193.50	Sodium Chloride, Solopak Mdcl	59747-0112-82
2 ml x 500	$850.00	Sodium Chloride, Solopak Mdcl	59747-0032-03
2.5 ml x 50	$45.94	Bacteriostatic Sodium Chloride, Wyeth Labs	00008-0333-02
2.5 ml x 50	$45.94	Bacteriostatic Sodium Chloride, Wyeth Labs	00008-0333-05
2.5 ml x 50	$65.00	Sodium Chloride, Wyeth Labs	00008-0333-50
3 ml	$1.99	Sodium Chloride, Fujisawa USA	00469-2005-86
3 ml	$2.16	Sodium Chloride, Fujisawa USA	00469-2005-88
3 ml x 25	$21.12	Sodium Chloride, Sanofi Winthrop	00024-1815-03
3 ml x 25	$33.53	Sodium Chloride, Sanofi Winthrop	00024-1816-03
3 ml x 25	$35.54	Sodium Chloride, Sanofi Winthrop	00024-1812-03
3 ml x 30	$73.80	Sodium Chloride, Marsam	00209-8864-36
3 ml x 120	$246.00	Sodium Chloride, Solopak Mdcl	59747-0112-73
3 ml x 120	$246.00	Sodium Chloride, Solopak Mdcl	59747-0112-83
3 ml x 500	$1087.50	Sodium Chloride, Solopak Mdcl	59747-0032-04
5 ml	$1.03	Sodium Chloride, Abbott	00074-2102-05
5 ml x 25	$10.80	Sodium Chloride, Elkins Sinn	00641-1500-35
5 ml x 25	$18.75	Sodium Chloride, Consolidated Midland	00223-8496-05
5 ml x 25	$22.92	Sodium Chloride, Sanofi Winthrop	00024-1811-05
5 ml x 25	$22.92	Sodium Chloride, Sanofi Winthrop	00024-1815-05
5 ml x 25	$33.53	Sodium Chloride, Sanofi Winthrop	00024-1816-05
5 ml x 25	$35.54	Sodium Chloride, Sanofi Winthrop	00024-1812-05
5 ml x 30	$80.10	Sodium Chloride, Marsam	00209-8880-36
5 ml x 30	$105.90	Sodium Chloride, Marsam	00209-8882-36
5 ml x 100	$41.51	Sodium Chloride, Elkins Sinn	00641-1500-36
5 ml x 120	$267.00	Sodium Chloride, Solopak Mdcl	59747-0112-75
5 ml x 120	$267.00	Sodium Chloride, Solopak Mdcl	59747-0112-85
5 ml x 120	$267.00	Sodium Chloride, Solopak Mdcl	59747-0112-95
5 ml x 500	$1175.00	Sodium Chloride, Solopak Mdcl	59747-0032-05
10 ml	$1.59	Sodium Chloride, Abbott	00074-7067-10
10 ml	$1.64	Sodium Chloride, Abbott	00074-2102-01
10 ml x 25	$15.00	Sodium Chloride, Harber Pharm	51432-0871-10
10 ml x 25	$15.60	Sodium Chloride, Gensia Labs	00703-7564-04
10 ml x 25	$18.75	Sodium Chloride, Consolidated Midland	00223-8497-10
10 ml x 25	$18.75	Sodium Chloride, Fujisawa USA	00469-2059-10
10 ml x 25	$24.69	Sodium Chloride, Am Regent	00517-2810-25
10 ml x 25	$25.00	Sodium Chloride, Solopak Labs	39769-0138-10
10 ml x 30	$114.00	Sodium Chloride, Marsam	00209-8881-36
10 ml x 100	$41.51	Sodium Chloride, Elkins Sinn	00641-1510-36
10 ml x 120	$379.80	Sodium Chloride, Solopak Mdcl	59747-0112-97
20 ml	$1.01	Sodium Chloride, Abbott	00074-2102-02
20 ml	$15.85	0.9% Sodium Chloride, Abbott	00074-8993-01
20 ml x 6	$14.51	Sodium Chloride, Lilly	00002-1689-16
20 ml x 25	$24.75	Sodium Chloride, P.F, S.D.V., Pasadena	00418-2191-56
20 ml x 25	$25.80	Sodium Chloride, Gensia Labs	00703-7565-04
20 ml x 25	$31.25	Sodium Chloride, Solopak Labs	39769-0138-20
25 ml fill/130	$2.40	Sodium Chloride Injection 0.9%, McGaw	00264-1400-35
30 ml	$0.78	Sodium Chloride, Insource	58441-0101-30
30 ml	$1.65	Sodium Chloride, Steris Labs	00402-0191-30
30 ml	$1.83	Bacteriostatic Sodium Chloride, Geneva Pharms	00781-3251-90
30 ml	$1.90	Bacteriostatic Sodium Chloride, Schein Pharm (US)	00364-6559-56
30 ml	$1.90	Sodium Chloride, HL Moore Drug Exch	00839-5628-36
30 ml	$1.90	Sodium Chloride, Goldline Labs	00182-0273-66
30 ml	$2.98	Bacteriostatic Sodium Chloride, United Res	00677-0291-23
30 ml	$28.32	Normal Saline With Phenol, Miles Spokane	00118-9990-10
30 ml x 25	$12.19	Bacteriostatic Sodium Chloride, Elkins Sinn	00641-2670-45
30 ml x 25	$29.68	Sodium Chloride, Fujisawa USA	00469-2059-30
30 ml x 25	$31.00	Sodium Chloride, B.A., Pasadena	00418-2221-66
30 ml x 25	$35.93	Bacteriostatic Sodium Chloride, Am Regent	00517-0648-25
30 ml x 25	$37.50	Sodium Chloride, Consolidated Midland	00223-8490-30
30 ml x 25	$37.50	Sodium Chloride, Consolidated Midland	00223-8500-30
30 ml x 25	$39.38	Sodium Chloride, Solopak Labs	39769-0138-30
30 ml x 25	$48.75	Sodium Chloride, Parabens, Pasadena	00418-2231-66
30 ml x 100	$109.98	Bacteriostatic Sodium Chloride, Raway	00686-0648-25
50 ml in 130 ml	$1.44	Sodium Chloride, McGaw	00264-1400-34
100 ml in 130 m	$1.44	Sodium Chloride, McGaw	00264-1400-33
100 ml x 10	$17.88	Sodium Chloride, Gensia Labs	00703-7568-03
150 ml fill/250	$9.83	Sodium Chloride, McGaw	00264-1400-23
250 ml	$9.67	Sodium Chloride, Baxter Hlthcare	00338-0044-02

Injection, Solution - Intravenous - 2.5 meq/ml

20 ml	$3.98	Sodium Chloride, Abbott	00074-6657-73
20 ml	$7.51	Sodium Chloride 50 Meq, Abbott	00074-4893-01
40 ml	$4.24	Sodium Chloride, Abbott	00074-6660-75
250 ml	$25.59	Sodium Chloride, Abbott	00074-4219-02

Injection, Solution - Intravenous - 3 %

500 ml	$10.77	Sodium Chloride, Baxter Hlthcare	00338-0054-03
500 ml x 12	$11.02	3% Sodium Chloride, McGaw	00264-1405-10

Injection, Solution - Intravenous - 4 mEq/ml

30 ml x 25	$36.29	Sodium Chloride, Gensia Labs	00703-5336-04
30 ml x 25	$43.13	Sodium Chloride, Fujisawa USA	00469-1187-25
50 ml	$4.96	Sodium Chloride, Abbott	00074-1141-01
100 ml	$6.28	Sodium Chloride, Abbott	00074-1141-02

HOW SUPPLIED - NOT RATED EQUIVALENT: *(cont'd)*

100 ml x 10	$41.04	Sodium Chloride, Gensia Labs	00703-5338-03
200 ml x 20	$249.48	Sodium Chloride Rapid Add, Fujisawa USA	00469-8802-00
250 ml	$8.05	Sodium Chloride, Abbott	00074-1130-02

Injection, Solution - Intravenous - 5 %

500 ml	$11.88	Sodium Chloride, Baxter Hlthcare	00338-0056-03
500 ml	$12.48	5% Sodium Chloride, Abbott	00074-1586-03
500 ml x 12	$11.20	5% Sodium Chloride, McGaw	00264-1406-10

Injection, Solution - Intravenous - 14.6 %

20 ml	$50.63	Sodium Chloride, Fujisawa USA	00469-1390-40
40 ml	$59.68	Sodium Chloride, Fujisawa USA	00469-1390-60

Injection, Solution - Intravenous - 23.4 %

25x100 ml (pharm	$93.75	Concentrated Sodium Chloride, Am Regent	00517-2900-25
30 ml x 25	$35.93	Concentrated Sodium Chloride, Am Regent	00517-2930-25
100 ml	$332.00	Sodium Chloride, Fujisawa USA	00469-8801-00
200 ml	$8.65	Sodium Chloride Additive, Intl Medication	00548-6520-00

Ointment - Ophthalmic - 5 %

3.5 gm	$9.44	Sodium Chloride, HL Moore Drug Exch	00839-7733-43

Solution - Inhalation - 0.45 %

3 ml x 100	$24.20	Sodium Chloride, Dey Labs	49502-0820-03
5 ml x 100	$24.20	Sodium Chloride, Dey Labs	49502-0820-05

Solution - Inhalation - 0.9 %

3 ml x 100	$24.20	Sodium Chloride, Dey Labs	49502-0830-03
3 ml x 250	$61.00	DEY-VIAL, SODIUM CHLORIDE, Dey Labs	49502-0030-03
5 ml x 100	$24.20	Sodium Chloride, Dey Labs	49502-0830-05
5 ml x 250	$61.00	DEY-VIAL, SODIUM CHLORIDE, Dey Labs	49502-0030-05
10 ml x 125	$61.00	DEY-VIAL, SODIUM CHLORIDE, Dey Labs	49502-0030-10
15 ml x 24	$14.10	Sodium Chloride, Dey Labs	49502-0830-15
20 ml x 100	$71.00	DEY-VIAL, SODIUM CHLORIDE, Dey Labs	49502-0030-20

Solution - Inhalation - 3 %

15 ml x 50	$51.00	Sodium Chloride, Dey Labs	49502-0640-15

Solution - Inhalation - 10 %

15 ml x 50	$51.00	Sodium Chloride, Dey Labs	49502-0641-15

Solution - Irrigation - 0.45 %

2000 ml	$11.54	Sodium Chloride, Abbott	00074-7975-07

Solution - Irrigation - 0.9 %

500 ml	$3.33	Sodium Chloride, HL Moore Drug Exch	00839-6674-83
1000 ml	$51.20	Sodium Chloride, Baxter Hlthcare	00338-0051-44

Solution - Ophthalmic - 5 %

15 ml	$9.44	Sodium Chloride, HL Moore Drug Exch	00839-7732-31

SODIUM FLUORIDE *(002244)*

CATEGORIES: Dental; Dental Caries; Fluoride Salts; Homeostatic & Nutrient; Topical; Tumors; Vasodilating Agents; Vitamins; Osteoporosis*; FDA Pre 1938 Drugs
* Indication not approved by the FDA

BRAND NAMES: Acidulated Phosphate Fluoride; Altaflor; *Audifluor*, *En-De-Kay*; *Flour-A-Day*; *Fluoen*; Fluorabon; *Fluorigard*; Fluorineed; Fluorinse; Fluoritab; Fluorodex; Flura; Karidium; Karigel; Liqui-Flur; **Luride**; Nafrinse; Neutracare; *Pedi-Dent*; Pediaflor; Perio Med; Pharmaflur; Phos-Flur; Phosphate Fluoride; Prevident; Prevident 5000 Plus; *Solu-Flur*; Thera-Flur; *Vinafluor*, *Zymafluor*
(International brand names outside U.S. in italics)

FORMULARIES: BC-BS; FHP; Medi-Cal; WHO

DESCRIPTION:

Oral Rinse: Sodium fluoride oral rinse is acidulated phosphate sodium fluoride and is an oral rinse/supplement. Each teaspoonful (5 ml) contains 1.0 mg fluoride ion (F-) from 2.2 mg sodium fluoride (NaF), in a 0.1 Molar phosphate solution at pH 4, for use as a dental caries preventive in children. Cherry, cool mint, bubble gum, grape - sugar and saccharin free. Cinnamon - contains saccharin, but is sugar free.

Dental Rinse: Sodium fluoride dental rinse provides 0.2% sodium fluoride in a mint-flavored, neutral aqueous solution containing 6% alcohol. For weekly use as caries preventive.

Brush-On Gel: Self-topical neutral fluoride containing 1.1% sodium fluoride for use as a dental caries preventive in children and adults. This prescription product is not a dentifrice.

Gel-Drops: Sodium fluoride (acidulated) gel-drops contain 0.5% fluoride ion (F-) from 1.1% sodium fluoride (NaF) in a lime-flavored aqueous solution containing 0.1 Molar Phosphate at pH 4.5. For daily self-topical use as a dental caries preventive. This form of this drug (neutral) also contains 0.5% fluoride ion (F-) from 1.1% NaF, but with no acid phosphate, nor artificial flavor or color, at neutral pH.

Drops/Tablets: Each ml contains 0.5 mg fluoride ion (F-) from 1.1 mg sodium fluoride (NaF). For use as a dental caries preventive in children. Sugar free. Saccharin-free.

Sodium fluoride lozenge-type chewable tablets for use as a dental caries preventive in children. Sugar free. Saccharin-free. Erythrosine (FD&C Red #3) Free. Each 0.25 mg F tablet (quarter-strength) contains 0.25 mg F from 0.55 mg NaF. Each 0.5 mg F tablet (half-strength) contains 0.5 mg F from 1.1 mg NaF. Each 1.0 mg F tablet (full-strength) contains 1.0 mg F from 2.2 mg NaF. Each *SF* 0.25 mg F tablet (SF for Special Formula: no artificial color or flavor) contains 0.25 mg F from 0.55 mg NaF.

CLINICAL PHARMACOLOGY:

Oral Rinse and Drops/Tablets: Sodium fluoride acts systemically, before tooth eruption and topically, post-eruption, by increasing tooth resistance to acid dissolution, by promoting remineralization, and by inhibiting the cariogenic microbial process. Acidulation provides greater topical fluoride uptake by dental enamel than neutral solutions. Phosphate protects enamel from demineralization by the acidulated formulation (common ion effect).

Dental Rinse: Topical application of sodium fluoride increases tooth resistance to acid dissolution, promotes remineralization, and inhibits the cariogenic microbial process.

Brush-On Gel/Gel Drops: Frequent topical applications to the teeth with preparations having a relatively high fluoride content increase tooth resistance to acid dissolution and enhance penetration of the fluoride ion into tooth enamel.

INDICATIONS AND USAGE:

Oral Rinse: It has been well established that ingestion of fluoridated drinking water (1 ppm F) during the period of tooth development results in a significant decrease in the incidence of dental caries. This oral rinse was developed to provide topical and systemic fluoride use as a supplement (rinse-and-swallow) in children age 3 and older living in areas where the water fluoride level does not exceed 0.6 ppm. Sodium fluoride oral rinse provides benefits as a topical fluoride dental rinse only (rinse-and-expectorate) for children age 6 and older. Pioneering clinical studies on sodium fluoride oral rinse were published by Frankel et al. and Aasenden et al. in 1972.

Dental Rinse: It has been established that weekly rinsing with a neutral 0.2% sodium fluoride solution protects against dental caries in children. Prevident Rinse was developed to provide a ready-to-use, flavored preparation for convenient administration and favorable compliance.

Brush-on Gel: It is well established that 1.1% sodium fluoride is safe and extraordinarily effective as a caries preventive when applied frequently with mouthpiece applicators. Sodium fluoride Brush-on Gel in a squeeze-tube is a particularly convenient dosage form which permits the application of a thin ribbon of gel onto a tooth brush as well as a mouth-piece tray.

Gel-Drops: It is well established that 1.1% sodium fluoride is a safe and effective caries preventive when applied frequently with mouthpiece applicators. Pioneering clinical studies with this form of sodium fluoride in school children were conducted by Englander et al.

Both neutral and acidulated phosphate fluoride gels have been effective in controlling rampant dental decay which frequently follows xerostomia-producing radiotherapy of tumors in the head and neck region.

Drops/Tablets: It has been well established that ingestion of fluoridated drinking water (1 ppm F) during the period of tooth development results in a significant decrease in the incidence of dental caries. These forms were developed to provide systemic fluoride use as a supplement in children age 6 months to 3 years living in areas where the water fluoride level does not exceed 0.3 ppm and in children age 3 to 16 years living in areas where the water fluoride level does not exceed 0.6 ppm.

CONTRAINDICATIONS:

Oral Rinse: DO NOT SWALLOW in areas where the F-content of drinking water exceeds 0.6 ppm, nor in children under the age of 3.

Dental Rinse/Brush on Gel/Gel Drops: None. (May be used whether drinking water is fluoridated or not, since **topical** fluoride cannot produce fluorosis).

Drops/Tablets: These forms are contraindicated in areas where the drinking water exceeds 0.6 ppm F and in pediatric patients under 6 months of age. The 1 mg F strength tablet is contraindicated where the drinking water exceeds 0.3 ppm F. The 0.5 mg tablets should not be administered to pediatric patients under the age of 3, and the 1 mg tablets should not be administered to pediatric patients under the age of 6.

WARNINGS:

Oral Rinse: Do not use as rinse in children under age 6. Do not use as a supplement in children under age 3, nor in areas where the drinking water exceeds 0.6 ppm F. As in the case of all medications, keep out of reach of infants and children.

Dental Rinse: DO NOT SWALLOW. Do not use in children under age 6, since younger children frequently cannot perform the rinse process without significant swallowing. As in the case of all medications, keep out of reach of children.

Brush on Gel/Gel Drops: As with all medications, keep out of reach of children. Not to be used in children under 6. The fruit sherbet flavor of the Brush-on gel contains FD&C Yellow No.6.

Drops/Tablets: (See CONTRAINDICATIONS) As in the case of all medications, keep out of reach of infants and children. The 0.5 mg/ml F drops and Orange 1.0 mg F tablets contain FD&C Yellow No. 6.

PRECAUTIONS:

Oral Rinse: (See OVERDOSAGE.) Incompatibility of systemic fluoride with dairy foods has been reported due to formation of calcium fluoride which is poorly absorbed.

Dental Rinse: Not for systemic use. (Each 5 ml contains 4.5 mg fluoride ion).

Gel-Drops: Laboratory tests indicate that the use of acidulated fluoride may cause dulling of porcelain and ceramic restorations. Therefore, the neutral formulation this form of sodium fluoride is recommended for this type of patient.

Drops/Tablets: (See OVERDOSAGE.) Incompatibility of fluoride with dairy foods has been reported due to formation of calcium fluoride which is poorly absorbed.

ADVERSE REACTIONS:

Oral Rinse and Drops/Tablets: Allergic reactions and other idiosyncrasies have been rarely reported.

Dental Rinse/Gel Drops: In patients with mucositis, gingival tissues may be hypersensitive to flavor or alcohol present in formulation or to the acidity.

OVERDOSAGE:

Oral Rinse: In the event a dose is accidentally swallowed (pediatric patients 12 years and under: one teaspoonful [5 ml]; over age 12: 2 teaspoonfuls [10 ml]), administer milk or antacid. In case more than a dose is accidentally swallowed, administer milk or antacid and seek medical attention.

Dental Rinse: In the event a dose is accidentally swallowed (pediatric patients: one teaspoonful [5 ml]; over age 12: 2 teaspoonful [10 ml]), administer milk or antacid. In case more than a dose is accidentally swallowed, administer milk or antacid and seek medical attention.

Gel-Drops: Accidental ingestion of a usual treatment dose (2-4 mg F) is not harmful.

Brush-On Gel: Accidental ingestion of a usual treatment dose (2 mg F) is not harmful.

Drops/Tablets: Prolonged daily ingestion of excessive fluoride will result in varying degrees of dental fluorosis. The total amount of sodium fluoride in a bottle of 50 ml sodium fluoride drops (25 mg F) and in a bottle of 120 tablets (all strengths) conforms with the recommendations of the American Dental Association for the maximum to be dispensed at one time for safety purposes.

DOSAGE AND ADMINISTRATION:

ORAL RINSE

As a Daily Dental Rinse: Pediatric patients age 6 to 12, use 5 ml (one teaspoonful); pediatric patients age 12 and over, use 10 ml (two teaspoonful). After thoroughly brushing teeth, preferably at bedtime, rinse vigorously around and between teeth for one minute, then expectorate.

As a Daily Supplement: In areas where the drinking water contains less than 0.3 ppm F: pediatric patients age 3-6, rinse with half a teaspoonful (2.5 ml) and swallow; age 6-16, rinse with one teaspoonful (5 ml) and swallow. When drinking water contains 0.3 to 0.6 ppm F, inclusive, reduce dosage to half a teaspoonful (2.5 ml) for age 6-16; do not use in age 3-6 when water is partially fluoridated (0.3-0.6 ppm F). Dental Rinse

DOSAGE AND ADMINISTRATION: *(cont'd)*

Children ages 6 to 12, one teaspoonful (5 ml); over age 12, 2 teaspoonfuls (10 ml). Once a week, preferably at bedtime after thoroughly brushing the teeth, rinse vigorously around and between teeth for one minute then expectorate. DO NOT SWALLOW. For maximum benefit, do not eat, drink, or rinse mouth for at least 30 minutes afterwards.

GEL-DROPS

Age 6 and older. For daily use with applicators supplied by the dentist. Apply 4 to 8 drops as required to cover inner surface of each applicator. Spread gel-drops with tip of bottle. Place applicators over upper and lower teeth at the same time. Bite down lightly for 6 minutes. Remove applicators and rinse mouth. Clean applicators with cold water.

BRUSH-ON GEL

After brushing with toothpaste, rinse as usual. Adults and children 6 years of age and older. Apply a thin ribbon of gel to the teeth with a toothbrush or mouthtrays, for at least one minute, preferably at bedtime. After use, adults expectorate gel. For best results, do not eat, drink or rinse for 30 minutes. Children age 6-16, expectorate gel and rinse mouth thoroughly.

DROPS/TABLETS

Adjustable dose gives you the flexibility to prescribe optimal DAILY dosage (based on age and F content of water), TABLE 1:

TABLE 1

F- Content of Drinking Water	Daily Dosage (Fluoride Ion)* Birth to Age 2	Age 2-3	Age 3 and Over
Less than 0.3 ppm	0.25 mg tab or 2 drops	0.5 mg tab or 4 drops	1.0 mg tab or 8 drops
0.3 to 0.7 ppm	one-half above dosage		
over 0.7 ppm	Fluoride dietary supplements contraindicated		

REFERENCES:

1. American Academy of Pediatrics, Committee on Nutrition. Vitamin and mineral supplement needs in normal children in the United States. Pediatrics 1980; 66(6): 1015-1021. **2.** Data on life, Colgate-Hoyt Labs. **3.** Aasendon R, Peebles TC. Effects of fluoride supplementation on human deciduous and permanent teeth. Arch oral Biol 1974; 19:321-326. **4.** Keyes PH, Englander HR. Fluoride therapy in the treatment of dentomicrobiol plaque diseases. J Am Soc Prev Dent 1975; 5: 36-48. **5.** Trautner K et al. Influences of milk and food on fluoride bioavailability from NaF and Na_2FPO_3 in man. J. Dent Res 1989; 68 (1): 72-77. **6.** American Dental Association, Council on Dental Therapeutics. Ed. 40, Chicago: ADA, 1984; various pages. **7.** American Academy of Pediatrics, Committee on Nutrition. Fluoride Supplementation: Pediatrics 1986; 77(5): 758-761. **8.** National Institute of Dental Research, National Caries Program. Fluoride to protect the teeth of adults. NIH Publication No. 83-2329, January, 1983. **9.** Englander HR et al, Incremental rates of dental caries after repeated topical sodium fluoride applications by mouthpieces. JADA 1967; 75(3):639-644. **10.** Englander HR et al. Incremental rates of dental caries after repeated topical fluoride applications in children with lifelong consumption of fluoride water. JADA 1971; 82(2): 354-358. **11.** Mellberg JP et al. Effects of two fluoride gels on fluoride uptake and phosphorus loss during loss during artificial caries formation. J. Dent Res 1986; 65(8): 1084-1086. **12.** DePaola P and Soparkar P. Monograph on the Proceedings of Conference Cariology for the Nineties, U. of Rochester Press 1991 (in Press). **13.** Brudevold F et al. A study of acidulated fluoride solutions- I. In vitro effects on enamel. Archs oral Biol 1963; 8; 1967-177. **14.** Frankl SN2 et al. The topical anticariogenic effect of daily rinsing with an acidulated phosphate fluoride solution. JADA 1972; 85: 882-886. **15.** Aasendon et al. Effects of fluoride solution upon dental caries and enamel fluoride. Archs oral Biol 1972; 17: 1705-1714. **16.** Hirschfield RE. Controls of decalcification by use of fluoride mouthrinse. J. Dent Child 1978; 45: 458-460. **17.** Corpron RE et al. In vivo remineralization of artificial enamel lesions by a fluoride dentifrice or mouthrinse. Caries Res 1986; 20: 48-55. **18.** Ripa LW et al. Supervised weekly rinsing with a 0.2% neutral NaF solution: final results of a demonstration program after six school years. J. Public Health Dent 1983; 43(1): 53-62. **19.** Weisz WS. The reduction of dental caries through the use of a sodium fluoride mouthwash. JADA 1960; 60: 438-456. **20.** American Dental Association, Oral Health Care Guidelines. Head and neck cancer patients receiving radiation therapy. ADA Publication No. J073, September 1989. **21.** Johansen E, Olsen TO. Topical fluorides in the prevention and arrest of dental caries. In: Johansen E, Taves DR, Olson TO eds. Continuing evaluation of the use of fluorides. Boulder, CO: Westview Press, 1979: 66.6 **22.** Drelzen S. et al. Prevention of xerostomia-related dental caries in irradiated cancer patients, J Dent Res 1977; 56: 99-104. **23.** Hirschfield RE et al. Decalcification under orthodontic bands. Angle Orthodont 1974; 44: 218-221. **24.** Renner RP et al. Overdenture sequelae: a nine-month report. J. Prost Dent 1982; 48 (4): 377-384.

HOW SUPPLIED - RATED THERAPEUTICALLY EQUIVALENT:

Solution - Dental; Oral; T - 0.2 %

500 ml	$6.75	ACIDULATED PHOSPHATE FLUORIDE, Harber Pharm	51432-0515-19

Tablet, Chewable - Oral - 2.2 mg

1000's	$14.98	Sodium Fluoride, HL Moore Drug Exch	00839-5035-16

HOW SUPPLIED - NOT RATED EQUIVALENT:

Gel - Dental - 1.1 %

0.8 oz	$2.20	PREVIDENT, BRUSH-ON GEL MINT, Colgate Oral	00126-0088-82
0.8 oz	$2.20	PREVIDENT, BERRY-FLAVORED, Colgate Oral	00126-0288-82
0.8 oz	$2.20	PREVIDENT, FRUIT SHERBERT, Colgate Oral	00126-0289-82
0.8 oz	$2.20	PREVIDENT, BING CHERRY FLAVOR, Colgate Oral	00126-0290-82
2 oz	$92.81	PREVIDENT, BRUSH-ON GEL MINT, Colgate Oral	00126-0088-02
2 oz	$92.81	PREVIDENT, BRUSH-ON GEL LIME, Colgate Oral	00126-0089-02
2 oz	$92.81	PREVIDENT, BERRY-FLAVORED, Colgate Oral	00126-0288-02
2 oz	$92.81	PREVIDENT, FRUIT SHERBERT, Colgate Oral	00126-0289-02
2 oz	$92.81	PREVIDENT, BING CHERRY FLAVOR, Colgate Oral	00126-0290-02
24 ml	$1.67	KARIGEL-N, Lorvic	00273-0131-01
24 ml	$67.50	THERA-FLUR-N, Colgate Oral	00126-0196-54
30 ml	$1.67	KARIGEL, Lorvic	00273-0103-01
56 gm	$8.50	PREVIDENT 5000 PLUS, Colgate Oral	00126-0287-02
60 ml	$51.54	NEUTRACARE HOME TOPICAL GRAPE GEL, Oral B Labs	00041-0240-22
60 ml	$51.54	NEUTRACARE HOME TOPICAL MINT GEL, Oral B Labs	00041-0241-22
125 ml	$3.97	KARIGEL-N, Lorvic	00273-0131-04
130 ml	$3.97	KARIGEL, Lorvic	00273-0103-02
250 ml	$6.63	KARIGEL, Lorvic	00273-0103-03

Liquid - Dental - 0.275 mg/ml

22.8 ml	$1.65	FLUORITAB, Fluoritab	00288-0002-01
30 ml	$2.80	Sodium Fluoride Drops, Copley Pharm	38245-0600-11
30 ml	$3.48	Sodium Fluoride Drops, HL Moore Drug Exch	00839-7315-63
30 ml	$5.76	Sodium Fluoride Drops, Rugby	00536-1981-75
50 ml	$12.86	PEDIAFLOR, Abbott	00074-0101-50

Lozenge - Oral - 1 mg

100	$1.20	FLORA-LOZ, Kirkman Sales	58223-0672-01
1000	$10.00	FLORA-LOZ, Kirkman Sales	58223-0672-04
1000's	$12.50	Flura, Kirkman Sales	58223-0672-10

Mouthwash - Dental; Topical - 0.2 %

16 oz	$89.86	FLUORINSE MINT, Oral B Labs	00041-0350-07
16 oz	$89.86	FLUORINSE CINNAMON, Oral B Labs	00041-0351-07
500 ml	$6.00	Acidulated Phosphate Fluoride Rinse, Copley Pharm	38245-0616-07

Powder

454 gm	$21.70	Sodium Fluoride, Paddock Labs	00574-0654-16
500 gm	$30.31	Sodium Fluoride, Mallinckrodt	00406-7636-03

HOW SUPPLIED - NOT RATED EQUIVALENT: *(cont'd)*

Powder - Dental - 0.125 mg/gm

16 oz	$1.50	NAFRINSE, NEUTRAL, Medcl Prods Labs	10733-0571-16

Solution - Dental; Oral; T - 0.2 %

30 ml	$4.25	Sodium Floride Drops, Major Pharms	00904-1127-30
250 ml	$66.18	PHOS-FLUR CHERRY-FLAVORED, Colgate Oral	00126-0129-99
250 ml x 12	$72.84	PREVIDENT, Colgate Oral	00126-0179-99
300 ml	$9.50	PERIO MED, Dunhall Pharms	00217-3315-35
300 ml	$9.50	PERIO MED, Dunhall Pharms	00217-3316-35
480 ml	$7.55	Liqui-Flur, Liquipharm	54198-0172-16
500 ml	$6.82	Liqui-Flur, HL Moore Drug Exch	00839-7484-79
500 ml	$111.18	PHOS-FLUR CINNAMON, Colgate Oral	00126-0126-46
500 ml	$111.18	PHOS-FLUR CHERRY-FLAVORED, Colgate Oral	00126-0129-46
500 ml	$111.18	PHOS-FLUR, Colgate Oral	00126-0451-46
500 ml	$111.18	PHOS-FLUR GRAPE, Colgate Oral	00126-0453-46
500 ml x 12	$111.18	PHOS-FLUR COOL MINT, Colgate Oral	00126-0452-46
500 ml x 12	$111.18	PHOS-FLUR BUBBLEGUM, Colgate Oral	00126-0454-46

Solution - Dental; Oral; T - 0.5 %

50 ml	$5.10	Sodium Fluoride, Qualitest Pharms	00603-1244-47
50 ml	$6.00	Altaflor, Altaire Pharm	59390-0041-23
50 ml	$6.80	Sodium Fluoride, Liquipharm	54198-0171-50
50 ml	$7.49	Sodium Fluoride, HL Moore Drug Exch	00839-7982-99
50 ml x 12	**$108.68**	**LURIDE DROPS, Colgate Oral**	**00126-0002-62**

Solution - Dental; Oral; T - 1 %

24 ml	$67.50	THERA-FLUR GEL, Colgate Oral	00126-0048-54
30 ml	$2.00	Flura-Drops, Kirkman Sales	58223-0684-30
30 ml	$4.40	Sodium Fluoride, Qualitest Pharms	00603-1244-45
30 ml	$5.25	Sodium Fluoride, Aligen Independ	00405-3720-53
30 ml	$5.25	Sodium Fluoride, Hi Tech Pharma	50383-0629-30
30 ml	$6.30	Sodium Fluoride, Goldline Labs	00182-6133-66

Solution - Dental; Oral; T - 1 mg

24 ml	$1.60	FLURA-DROPS, Kirkman Sales	58223-0684-24

Tablet - Oral - 1 mg

100	$1.00	FLORA-TAB, Kirkman Sales	58223-0671-01
1000	$8.00	FLORA-TAB, Kirkman Sales	58223-0671-04

Tablet, Chewable - Dental; Oral - 0.5 mg

120's	$1.50	NAFRINSE, Medcl Prods Labs	10733-0765-04

Tablet, Chewable - Oral - 0.25 mg

100's	$1.50	Fluoritab, Fluoritab	00288-5509-01
100's	$1.50	Fluoritab, Fluoritab	00288-5510-01
100's	$1.50	Fluoritab, Fluoritab	00288-5511-01
120's	**$7.81**	**LURIDE-SF, Colgate Oral**	**00126-0009-21**
120's	**$72.81**	**LURIDE VANILLA, Colgate Oral**	**00126-0186-21**
1000's	$9.35	Fluoritab, Fluoritab	00288-5509-10
1000's	$9.35	Fluoritab, Fluoritab	00288-5510-10
1000's	$9.35	Fluoritab, Fluoritab	00288-5511-10
5000's	$28.00	Fluoritab, Fluoritab	00288-5509-02
5000's	$28.00	Fluoritab, Fluoritab	00288-5510-02
5000's	$28.00	Fluoritab, Fluoritab	00288-5511-02

Tablet, Chewable - Oral - 0.5 mg

100's	$1.50	Fluoritab, Fluoritab	00288-1106-01
100's	$1.50	Fluoritab, Fluoritab	00288-1107-01
100's	$1.50	Fluoritab, Fluoritab	00288-1108-01
1000's	$7.32	Sodium Fluoride, Aligen Independ	00405-4938-03
1000's	$7.55	Sodium Fluoride, Qualitest Pharms	00603-3622-32
1000's	$9.35	Fluoritab, Fluoritab	00288-1106-10
1000's	$9.35	Fluoritab, Fluoritab	00288-1107-10
1000's	$9.35	Fluoritab, Fluoritab	00288-1108-10
1000's	$14.98	Sodium Fluoride, HL Moore Drug Exch	00839-6578-16
1200's	**$32.42**	**LURIDE GRAPE, Colgate Oral**	**00126-0014-81**
5000's	$28.00	Fluoritab, Fluoritab	00288-1106-02
5000's	$28.00	Fluoritab, Fluoritab	00288-1107-02
5000's	$28.00	Fluoritab, Fluoritab	00288-1108-02

Tablet, Chewable - Oral - 1 mg

100's	$1.50	Fluoritab, Fluoritab	00288-0005-01
100's	$1.50	Fluoritab, Fluoritab	00288-0007-01
100's	$1.50	Fluoritab, Fluoritab	00288-2204-01
120's	$1.50	NAFRINSE, Medcl Prods Labs	10733-0567-05
120's	**$72.81**	**LURIDE HALF-STRENGTH GRAPE, Colgate Oral**	**00126-0014-21**
120's	**$88.73**	**LURIDE-SF, Colgate Oral**	**00126-0007-21**
1000's	$7.10	Sodium Fluoride, Pharmacist Choice	54979-0455-10
1000's	$7.15	Sodium Fluoride Flavored, Copley Pharm	38245-0123-20
1000's	$7.19	Sodium Fluoride Flavored, Rugby	00536-4548-10
1000's	$7.37	Sodium Fluoride, Aligen Independ	00405-4939-03
1000's	$7.55	Sodium Fluoride, Qualitest Pharms	00603-3623-32
1000's	$8.65	Fluoride Sodium 1.1, Major Pharms	00904-1125-80
1000's	$9.35	Fluoritab, Fluoritab	00288-2201-10
1000's	$9.35	Fluoritab, Fluoritab	00288-2203-10
1000's	$9.35	Fluoritab, Fluoritab	00288-2204-10
1000's	$9.75	Pharmaflur 1.1 Chewable Tablets, Pharmics	00813-0065-10
5000's	$28.00	Fluoritab, Fluoritab	00288-2201-02
5000's	$28.00	Fluoritab, Fluoritab	00288-2203-02
5000's	$28.00	Fluoritab, Fluoritab	00288-2204-02

Tablet, Chewable - Oral - 2.2 mg

100's	$1.50	FLUORITAB, Fluoritab	00288-0003-01
100's	$2.50	Sodium Fluoride, Consolidated Midland	00223-1773-01
120's	**$88.73**	**LURIDE CHERRY FLAVORED, Colgate Oral**	**00126-0006-21**
120's	**$88.73**	**LURIDE ASSORTED FLAVORS, Colgate Oral**	**00126-0143-21**
180's	$5.50	KARIDIUM, Lorvic	00273-0101-01
1000's	$6.73	Sodium Fluoride, Geneva Pharms	00781-1816-10
1000's	$7.15	Sodium Fluoride, Copley Pharm	38245-0131-20
1000's	$7.19	Sodium Fluoride Flavored, Rugby	00536-4547-10
1000's	$7.85	Sodium Fluoride, United Res	00677-0132-10
1000's	$8.91	Sodium Fluoride Chew Tabs, Schein Pharm (US)	00364-0254-02
1000's	$9.75	PHARMAFLUR, Pharmics	00813-0066-10
1000's	$10.15	Fluoride Sodium Chewable 2.2, Major Pharms	00904-1126-80
1000's	$15.75	Sodium Fluoride, Consolidated Midland	00223-1773-02
1000's	**$32.43**	**LURIDE CHERRY FLAVORED, Colgate Oral**	**00126-0006-10**
1000's	**$32.43**	**LURIDE ASSORTED FLAVORS, Colgate Oral**	**00126-0143-10**

SODIUM HYALURONATE *(002246)*

CATEGORIES: EENT Drugs; Eye, Ear, Nose, & Throat Preparations

BRAND NAMES: *Amo Vitrax*; *Biolon* (Mexico); Duovisc; Healon; Healon Gv; *Healon Yellow*, *Healonid* (England, France); *Hyalgan* (France); *IAL*; Provisc; Viscoat; Vitrax

(International brand names outside U.S. in italics)

Prescribing information not available at time of publication.

HOW SUPPLIED - EQUIVALENTS NOT AVAILABLE:

Injection, Solution - Ophthalmic - 10 mg/ml

0.4 ml	$81.25	HEALON, Pharmacia & Upjohn	00016-0314-40
0.4 ml	$93.75	PROVISC, Alcon Surgical	08065-1830-04
0.5 ml	$123.75	VISCOAT, Alcon Surgical	08065-1839-05
0.55 ml	$118.75	HEALON, Pharmacia & Upjohn	00016-0310-55
0.55 ml	$118.75	PROVISC, Alcon Surgical	08065-1830-55
0.65 ml	$120.00	Vitrax, Allergan	00023-6663-65
0.85 ml	$156.25	HEALON, Pharmacia & Upjohn	00016-0310-85
0.85 ml	$156.25	PROVISC, Alcon Surgical	08065-1830-85
1's	$162.50	DUOVISC, Alcon Surgical	08065-1831-35

Injection, Solution - Ophthalmic - 14 mg/ml

0.55 ml	$143.75	HEALON GV, Pharmacia & Upjohn	00016-0319-55
0.85 ml	$175.00	HEALON GV, Pharmacia & Upjohn	00016-0319-85

SODIUM IODIDE, I-123 *(002248)*

CATEGORIES: Antithyroid Agents; Diagnostic Agents; Homeostatic & Nutrient; Hormones; Thyroid Function; Thyroid Preparations; Vitamins; FDA Approval Pre 1982

BRAND NAMES: Iodine; Iodo-Pak; Iodopen; Iodotope

Prescribing information not available at time of publication.

HOW SUPPLIED - EQUIVALENTS NOT AVAILABLE:

Granules

500 gm	$56.99	Sodium Iodide, Mallinckrodt	00406-1136-03

SODIUM LACTATE *(002249)*

CATEGORIES: Alkalinizing Agents; Electrolyte Solutions; Electrolytic, Caloric-Water Balance; Homeostatic & Nutrient; Metabolic Acidosis; Replacement Solutions; Urinary Alkalinizers; Pregnancy Category C; FDA Approval Pre 1982

FORMULARIES: WHO

DESCRIPTION:

For additive use only after dilution inIV fluids to correct serum-bicarbonate deficit in acidosis.

Sodium lactate injection, USP 50 mEq (5 mEq/ml), is a sterile, nonpyrogenic, concentrated solution of sodium lactate in water for injection. The solution is administered after dilution by the intravenous route as an electrolyte replenisher and systemic alkalizer. IT SHOULD NOT BE ADMINISTERED UNDILUTED. Each 10 ml vial contains sodium lactate, anhydrous 5.6 g (50 mEq each of Na+ and lactate anion). The solution contains no bacteriostat, antimicrobial agent or added buffer. The pH is adjusted with hydrochloric acid. The osmolar concentration is 10 mOsm/ml (calc.). When diluted with sterile water for injection to make a 1/6 molar solution, the pH os sodium lactate injection lies between 6.0 and 7.3.

Sodium Lactate, USP is chemically designated $CH_3CH(OH)COONa$, a 60% aqueous solution miscible in water.

The semi-rigid vial is fabricated from a specially formulated polyolefin. It is a copolymer of ethylene and propylene. The safety of the plastic has been confirmed by tests in animals according to USP biological standards for plastic containers. The container requires no vapor barrier to maintain the proper drug concentration.

CLINICAL PHARMACOLOGY:

Lactate anion ($CH_3CH(OH)COO$-) serves the important purpose of providing "raw material" for subsequent regeneration of bicarbonate (HCO_3-) and thus acts as a source (alternate) of bicarbonate when normal production and utilization of lactic acid is not impaired as a result of disordered lactate metabolism. Lactate anion is usually present in extracellular fluid at a level of less than 1 mEq/liter during exercise. It is seldom measured as such and thus is one of the "unmeasured anions" ("anion gap") in determinations of the ionic composition of plasma.

Since metabolic conversion of lactate to bicarbonate is dependent on the integrity of cellular oxidative processes, lactate may be inadequate or ineffective as a source of bicarbonate in patients suffering from acidosis associated with shock or other disorders involving reduced perfusion of body tissues. When oxidative activity is intact, one to two hours time is required for conversion of lactate to bicarbonate.

The lactate anion is in equilibrium with pyruvate and has an alkalizing effect resulting from simultaneous removal by the liver of lactate and hydrogen ions. In the liver, lactate is metabolized to glycogen which is ultimately converted to carbon dioxide and water by oxidative metabolism.

The sodium (Na+) ion combines with bicarbonate ion produced from carbon dioxide of the body and thus retains bicarbonate to combat metabolic acidosis (bicarbonate deficiency). The normal plasma level of lactate ranges from 0.9 to 1.9 mEq/liter.

Sodium is the principal cation of extracellular fluid. It comprises more than 90% of total cations at its normal plasma concentration of approximately 140 mEq/liter. The sodium ion exerts a primary role in controlling total body water and its distribution.

INDICATIONS AND USAGE:

Sodium lactate injection, USP 50 mEq (5mEq/ml), is primarily indicated, after dilution, as a source of bicarbonate for prevention or control of mild to moderate metabolic acidosis in patients with restricted oral intake whose oxidative processes are not seriously impaired. It is not intended nor effective for correcting severe acidotic states which require immediate restoration of plasma bicarbonate levels. Sodium lactate has no advantage over sodium bicarbonate and may be detrimental in the management of lactic acidosis.

CONTRAINDICATIONS:

Sodium lactate injection, USP 50 mEq is contraindicated in patients suffering from hypernatremia or fluid retention.

CONTRAINDICATIONS: *(cont'd)*

It should not be used in conditions in which lactate levels are increased (*e.g.*, shock, congestive heart failure, respiratory alkalosis) or in which utilization of lactate is diminished (*e.g.*, anoxia, beriberi).

NOT FOR USE IN THE TREATMENT OF LACTIC ACIDOSIS.

WARNINGS:

Solutions containing sodium ions should be used with great care, if at all, in patients with congestive heart failure, severe renal insufficiency and in clinical states in which there exists edema with sodium retention.

In patients with diminished renal function, administration of solutions containing sodium ions may result in sodium retention.

The intravenous administration of this solution (after appropriate dilution) can cause fluid and/or solute overloading resulting in dilution of other serum electrolyte concentrations, overhydration, congested states or pulmonary edema.

Excessive administration of potassium-free solutions may result in significant hypokalemia.

PRECAUTIONS:

Sodium lactate injection, USP 50 mEq must be suitably diluted before infusion to avoid a sudden increase in the level of sodium or lactate. Too rapid administration and overdosage should be avoided.

The potentially large loads of sodium given with lactate require that caution be exercised in patients with congestive heart failure or other edematous or sodium-retaining states, as well as in patients with oliguria or anuria.

Caution must be exercised in the administration of parenteral fluids, especially those containing sodium ions, to patients receiving corticosteroids or corticotropin.

Solutions containing lactate ions should be used with caution as excess administration may result in metabolic alkalosis.

Do not administer unless solution is clear and seal is intact. Discard unused portion.

Pregnancy Category C: Animal reproduction studies have not been conducted with sodium lactate. It is not known whether sodium lactate can cause fetal harm when administered to a pregnant woman or can affect reproduction capacity. Sodium lactate should be given to a pregnant woman only if clearly needed.

ADVERSE REACTIONS:

Adverse effects of sodium lactate are essentially limited to overdosage of either sodium or lactate ions. (See WARNINGS and PRECAUTIONS.)

OVERDOSAGE:

In the event of overdosage, discontinue infusion containing sodium lactate immediately and institute corrective therapy as indicated to reduce elevated serum sodium levels and restore acid-base balance if necessary. (See WARNINGS and PRECAUTIONS.)

DOSAGE AND ADMINISTRATION:

Sodium lactate injection, USP, 50 mEq (5 mEq/ml) is administered intravenously only after addition to a larger volume of fluid. The amount of sodium ion and lactate ion to be added to larger volume intravenous fluids should be determined in accordance with the electrolyte requirements of each individual patient.

All or part of the content(s) of one (50 mEq in 10 ml) or more vial containers may be added to other intravenous solutions to provide any desired number of milliequivalents of lactate anion (with the same number of milliequivalents of (Na+). The contents of one container (50 mEq in 10 ml) added to 290 ml of a nonelectrolyte solution or of sterile water for injection will provide 300 ml of an approximately isotonic (1/6 molar) concentration of sodium lactate (1.9%), containing 167 mEq/liter each of Na+ and lactate anion.

Parenteral drug products should be inspected visually for particulate matter and discoloration prior to administration. See CONTRAINDICATIONS.

Exposure of pharmaceutical products to heat should be minimized. Avoid excessive heat. Protect from freezing. It is recommended that the product be stored at room temperature (25 deg. C); however, brief exposure up to 40 deg. C does not adversely affect the product.

HOW SUPPLIED - RATED THERAPEUTICALLY EQUIVALENT:

Injection, Solution - Intravenous - 18.7 mg/ml

500 ml	$10.55	Sodium Lactate, Abbott	00074-1587-03
500 ml	$14.22	M/6 Sodium Lactate, Baxter Hlthcare	00338-0129-03
500 ml	$14.94	Sodium Lactate 1/6 M, Abbott	00074-7987-03
500 ml x 10	$9.38	1/6 MOLAR SODIUM LACTATE, McGaw	00264-1810-10
1000 ml	$17.98	M/6 Sodium Lactate, Baxter Hlthcare	00338-0129-04
1000 ml	$18.86	Sodium Lactate 1/6 M, Abbott	00074-7987-09
1000 ml x 10	$16.52	1/6 MOLAR SODIUM LACTATE, McGaw	00264-1810-00

HOW SUPPLIED - NOT RATED EQUIVALENT:

Injection, Solution - Intravenous - 5 meq/ml

10 ml	$4.93	Sodium Lactate 50 Meq, Abbott	00074-6664-02
10 ml	$63.13	Sodium Lactate, Fujisawa USA	00469-3750-30

Injection, Solution - Intravenous - 18.7 mg/ml

150 ml x 12	$8.00	1/6 MOLAR SODIUM LACTATE, McGaw	00264-1410-30
500 ml x 12	$9.00	1/6 MOLAR SODIUM LACTATE, McGaw	00264-1410-10
1000 ml	$18.67	Sodium Lactate, McGaw	00264-7810-00
1000 ml x 6	$12.12	1/6 MOLAR SODIUM LACTATE, McGaw	00264-1410-00

SODIUM NITROPRUSSIDE *(002254)*

CATEGORIES: Antihypertensives; Bleeding; Cardiovascular Drugs; Hypertension; Hypotension; Renal Drugs; Pregnancy Category C; FDA Approval Pre 1982

BRAND NAMES: **Nipride**; Nitropress; Nitroprusside Sodium

FORMULARIES: WHO

After reconstitution, sodium nitroprusside is not suitable for direct injection. THE RECONSTITUTED SOLUTION MUST BE FURTHER DILUTED IN STERILE 5% DEXTROSE INJECTION BEFORE INFUSION (SEE DOSAGE AND ADMINISTRATION).

Sodium nitroprusside can cause PRECIPITOUS DECREASES IN BLOOD PRESSURE (SEE DOSAGE AND ADMINISTRATION). In patients not properly Monitored, these decreases can lead to IRREVERSIBLE ISCHEMIC INJURIES OR DEATH. Sodium nitroprusside should be used only when available equipment and personnel allow blood pressure to be continuously monitored.

Except when used briefly or at low (<2 mcg/kg/min) infusion rates, sodium nitroprusside injection gives rise to important quantities of cyanide ion, which can reach TOXIC, POTENTIALLY LETHAL LEVELS (SEE WARNINGS). The usual dose rate is 0.5 to 10 mcg/kg/

min, but INFUSION AT THE MAXIMUM DOSE RATE SHOULD NEVER LAST MORE THAN 10 MINUTES. If blood pressure has not been adequately controlled after 10 minutes of infusion at the maximum rate, administration of sodium nitroprusside should be terminated immediately.

Although acid-base balance and venous oxygen concentration should be monitored and may indicate cyanide toxicity, these laboratory tests provide imperfect guidance.

This package insert should be thoroughly reviewed before administration of sodium nitroprusside infusion.

DESCRIPTION:

Sodium nitroprusside is disodium pentacyanonitrosylferrate(2-)dihydrate, an inorganic hypotensive agent whose molecular formula is $Na_2(Fe(CN)_5NO)°2H_2O$, and whose molecular weight is 297.95. Dry sodium nitroprusside is a reddish-brown powder, soluble in water. In an aqueous solution infused intravenously, sodium nitroprusside is rapid-acting vasodilator, active on both arteries and veins.

Sodium nitroprusside solution is rapidly degraded by trace contaminants, often with resulting color changes (see DOSAGE AND ADMINISTRATION). The solution is also sensitive to certain wavelengths of light, and it must be protected from light in clinical use.

Each 5-ml vial contains the equivalent of 50 mg sodium nitroprusside dihydrate.

CLINICAL PHARMACOLOGY:

The principal pharmacological action of sodium nitroprusside is relaxation of vascular smooth muscle and consequent dilatation of peripheral arteries and veins. Other smooth muscle (*e.g.*, uterus, duodenum) is not affected. Sodium nitroprusside is more active on veins than on arteries, but this selectivity is much less marked than that of nitroglycerin. Dilatation of the veins promotes peripheral pooling of blood and decreases venous return to the heart, thereby reducing left ventricular end-diastolic pressure and pulmonary capillary wedge pressure (preload). Arteriolar relaxation reduces systemic vascular resistance, systolic arterial pressure and mean arterial pressure (afterload). Dilatation of the coronary arteries also occurs.

In association with the decrease in blood pressure, sodium nitroprusside administered intravenously to hypertensive and normotensive patients produces slight increases in heart rate and a variable effect on cardiac output. In hypertensive patients, moderate doses induce renal vasodilatation roughly proportional to the decrease in systemic blood pressure, so there is no appreciable change in renal blood flow or glomerular filtration rate.

In normotensive subjects, acute reduction of mean arterial pressure to 60 to 75 mm Hg by infusion of sodium nitroprusside caused a significant increase in renin activity. In the same study, ten renovascular-hypertensive patients given sodium nitroprusside had significant increases in renin release from the involved kidney at mean arterial pressures of 90 to 137 mm Hg.

The hypotensive effect of sodium nitroprusside is seen within a minute or two after the start of an adequate infusion, and it dissipates almost as rapidly after an infusion is discontinued. The effect is augmented by ganglionic blocking agents and inhaled anesthetics.

Pharmacokinetics and Metabolism: Infused sodium nitroprusside is rapidly distributed to a volume that is approximately coextensive with the extracellular space. The drug is cleared from this volume by intraerythrocytic reaction with hemoglobin (Hgb), and sodium nitroprusside's resulting circulatory half-life is about 2 minutes.

The products of the nitroprusside/hemoglobin reaction are cyanmethemoglobin (cyanmetHgb) and cyanide ion (CN^-). Safe use of sodium nitroprusside injection must be guided by knowledge of the further metabolism of these products.

The essential features of nitroprusside metabolism are:

one molecule of sodium nitroprusside is metabolized by combination with hemoglobin to produce one molecule of cyanmethemoglobin and four CN^- ions;

methemoglobin, obtained from hemoglobin, can sequester cyanide as cyanmethemoglobin;

thiosulfate reacts with cyanide to produce thiocyanate;

thiocyanate is eliminated in the urine;

cyanide not otherwise removed binds to cytochromes; and

cyanide is much more toxic than methemoglobin or thiocyanate.

Cyanide ion is normally found in serum; it is derived from dietary substrates and from tobacco smoke. Cyanide binds avidly (but reversibly) to ferric ion (Fe^{+++}), most body stores of which are found in erythrocyte methemoglobin (metHgb) and in mitochondrial cytochromes. When CN^- is infused or generated within the bloodstream, essentially all of it is bound to methemoglobin until intraerythrocytic methemoglobin has been saturated.

When the Fe^{+++} of cytochromes is bound to cyanide, the cytochromes are unable to participate in oxidative metabolism. In this situation, cells may be able to provide for their energy needs by utilizing anaerobic pathways, but they thereby generate an increasing body burden of lactic acid. Other cells may be unable to utilize these alternate pathways, and they may die hypoxic deaths.

CN^-levels in packed erythrocytes are typically less than 1 μmol/L (less than 25 mcg/L); levels are roughly doubled in heavy smokers.

At healthy steady-state, most people have less than 1% of their hemoglobin in the form of methemoglobin. Nitroprusside metabolism can lead to methemoglobin formation (a) through dissociation of cyanmethemoglobin formed in the original reaction of sodium nitroprusside with Hgb and (b) by direct oxidation of Hgb by the released nitroso group. Relatively large quantities of sodium nitroprusside, however, are required to produce significant methemoglobinemia.

At physiologic methemoglobin levels, the CN^-binding capacity of packed red cells is a little less than 200 μmol/L (5 mg/L). Cytochrome toxicity is seen at levels only slightly higher, and death has been reported at levels from 300 to 3000 μmol/L (8 to 80 mg/L). Put another way, a patient with a normal red-cell mass (35 ml/kg) and normal methemoglobin levels can buffer about 175 mcg/kg of CN^-, corresponding to a little less than 500 mcg/kg of infused sodium nitroprusside.

Some cyanide is eliminated from the body as expired hydrogen cyanide, but most is enzymatically converted to thiocyanate (SCN^-) by thiosulfate-cyanide sulfur transferase (rhodanese, EC 2.8.1.1), a mitochondrial enzyme. The enzyme is normally present in great excess, so the reaction is rate-limited by the availability of sulfur donors, especially thiosulfate, cystine and cysteine.

Thiosulfate is a normal constituent of serum, produced from cysteine by way of β-mercaptopyruvate. Physiological levels of thiosulfate are typically about 0.1 mmol/L (11 mg/L), but they are approximately twice this level in children and in adults who are not eating. Infused thiosulfate is cleared from the body (primarily by the kidneys) with a $t_{1/2}$of about 20 minutes.

When thiosulfate is being supplied only by normal physiologic mechanisms, conversion of CN^- to SCN^-generally proceeds at about 1 mcg/kg/min. This rate of CN^-clearance corresponds to steady-state processing of a sodium nitroprusside infusion of slightly more than 2 mcg/kg/min. CN^-begins to accumulate when sodium nitroprusside infusions exceed this rate.

Thiocyanate (SCN^-) is also a normal physiological constituent of serum, with normal levels typically in the range of 50 to 250 μmol/L (3 to 15 mg/L). Clearance of SCN^- is primarily renal, with a $t_{1/2}$ of about 3 days. In renal failure, the $t_{1/2}$ can be doubled or tripled.

CLINICAL STUDIES:

Baseline-controlled clinical trials have uniformly shown that sodium nitroprusside has a prompt hypotensive effect, at least initially, in all populations. With increasing rates of infusion, sodium nitroprusside has been able to lower blood pressure without an observed limit of effect.

Clinical trials have also shown that the hypotensive effect of sodium nitroprusside is associated with reduced blood loss in a variety of major surgical procedures.

Many trials have verified the clinical significance of the metabolic pathways described above. In patients receiving unopposed infusions of sodium nitroprusside, cyanide and thiocyanate levels have increased with increasing rates of sodium nitroprusside infusion. Mild to moderate metabolic acidosis has usually accompanied higher cyanide levels, but peak base deficits have lagged behind the peak cyanide levels by an hour or more.

Progressive tachyphylaxis to the hypotensive effects of sodium nitroprusside has been reported in several trials and numerous case reports. This tachyphylaxis has frequently been attributed to concomitant cyanide toxicity, but the only evidence adduced for this assertion has been the observation that in patients treated with sodium nitroprusside and found to be resistant to its hypotensive effects, cyanide levels are often found to be elevated. In the only reported comparisons of cyanide levels in resistant and nonresistant patients, cyanide levels did not correlate with tachyphylaxis. The mechanism of tachyphylaxis to sodium nitroprusside remains unknown.

INDICATIONS AND USAGE:

Sodium nitroprusside is indicated for the immediate reduction of blood pressure of patients in hypertensive crises. Concomitant longer-acting antihypertensive medication should be administered so that the duration of treatment with sodium nitroprusside can be minimized.

sodium nitroprusside is also indicated for producing controlled hypotension in order to reduce bleeding during surgery.

CONTRAINDICATIONS:

Sodium nitroprusside should not be used in the treatment of compensatory hypertension, where the primary hemodynamic lesion is aortic coarctation or arteriovenous shunting.

sodium nitroprusside should not be used to produce hypotension during surgery in patients with known inadequate cerebral circulation or in moribund patients (A.S.A. Class 5E) coming to emergency surgery.

Patients with congenital (Leber's) optic atrophy or with tobacco amblyopia have unusually high cyanide/thiocyanate ratios. These rare conditions are probably associated with defective or absent rhodanese, and sodium nitroprusside use should be avoided in these patients.

WARNINGS:

(See BOXED WARNING at the beginning of this insert)

The principal hazards of sodium nitroprusside administration are excessive hypotension and excessive accumulation of cyanide (see OVERDOSAGEand DOSAGE AND ADMINISTRATION).

Excessive Hypotension: Small transient excesses in the infusion rate of sodium nitroprusside can result in excessive hypotension, sometimes to levels so low as to compromise the perfusion of vital organs. These hemodynamic changes may lead to a variety of associated symptoms: (see ADVERSE REACTIONS). Nitroprusside-induced hypotension will be self-limited within 1 to 10 minutes after discontinuation of the nitroprusside infusion; during these few minutes, it may be helpful to put the patient into a head-down (Trendelenburg) position to maximize venous return. **If hypotension persists more than a few minutes after discontinuation of the infusion of sodium nitroprusside, sodium nitroprusside is not the cause, and the true cause must be sought.**

Cyanide Toxicity: As described in CLINICAL PHARMACOLOGY, sodium nitroprusside infusions at rates above 2 mcg/kg/min generate cyanide ion (CN^-) faster than the body can normally dispose of it. (When sodium thiosulfate is given, as described under DOSAGE AND ADMINISTRATION, the body's capacity for CN^-elimination is greatly increased.) Methemoglobin normally present in the body can buffer a certain amount of CN^-, but the capacity of this system is exhausted by the CN^- produced from about 500 mcg/kg of sodium nitroprusside. This amount of sodium nitroprusside is administered in less than an hour when the drug is administered at 10 mcg/kg/min (the maximum recommended rate). Thereafter, the toxic effects of CN^-may be rapid, serious and even lethal.

The true rates of clinically important cyanide toxicity cannot be assessed from spontaneous reports or published data. Most patients reported to have experienced such toxicity have received relatively prolonged infusions, and the only patients whose deaths have been unequivocally attributed to nitroprusside-induced cyanide toxicity have been patients who had received nitroprusside infusions at rates (30 to 120 mcg/kg/min) much greater than those now recommended. Elevated cyanide levels, metabolic acidosis, and marked clinical deterioration, however, have occasionally been reported in patients who received infusions at recommended rates for only a few hours and even, in one case, for only 35 minutes. In some of these cases, infusion of sodium thiosulfate caused dramatic clinical improvement, supporting the diagnosis of cyanide toxicity.

Cyanide toxicity may manifest itself as venous hyperoxemia with bright red venous blood, as cells become unable to extract the oxygen delivered to them; metabolic (lactic) acidosis; air hunger; confusion; and death. Cyanide toxicity due to causes other than nitroprusside has been associated with angina pectoris and myocardial infarction; ataxia, seizures and stroke; and other diffuse ischemic damage.

Hypertensive patients, and patients concomitantly receiving other antihypertensive medications, may be more sensitive to the effects of sodium nitroprusside than normal subjects.

PRECAUTIONS:

General: Like other vasodilators, sodium nitroprusside can cause increases in intracranial pressure. In patients whose intracranial pressure is already elevated, sodium nitroprusside should be used only with extreme caution.

Hepatic: Use caution when administering sodium nitroprusside to patients with hepatic insufficiency.

Use In Anesthesia: When sodium nitroprusside (or any other vasodilator) is used for controlled hypotension during anesthesia, the patient's capacity to compensate for anemia and hypovolemia may be diminished. If possible, pre-existing anemia and hypovolemia should be corrected prior to administration of sodium nitroprusside.

Hypotensive anesthetic techniques may also cause abnormalities of the pulmonary ventilation/perfusion ratio. Patients intolerant of these abnormalities may require a higher fraction of inspired oxygen.

Extreme caution should be exercised in patients who are especially poor surgical risks (A.S.A. Classes 4 and 4E).

Laboratory Tests: The cyanide-level assay is technically difficult, and cyanide levels in body fluids other than packed red blood cells are difficult to interpret. Cyanide toxicity will lead to lactic acidosis and venous hyperoxemia, but these findings may not be present until an hour or more after the cyanide capacity of the body's red-cell mass has been exhausted.

PRECAUTIONS: *(cont'd)*

Carcinogenesis, Mutagenesis, and Impairment of Fertility: sodium nitroprusside has not undergone adequate carcinogenicity testing in animals. The mutagenic potential of sodium nitroprusside has not been assessed. Sodium nitroprusside has not been tested for effects on fertility.

Pregnancy, Teratogenic Effects, Pregnancy Category C There are no adequate or well-controlled studies of sodium nitroprusside in either laboratory animals or pregnant women. It is not known whether sodium nitroprusside can cause fetal harm when administered to a pregnant woman or can affect reproductive capacity. Sodium nitroprusside should be given to a pregnant woman only if clearly needed.

Nonteratogenic Effects: In three studies in pregnant ewes, nitroprusside was shown to cross the placental barrier. Fetal cyanide levels were shown to be dose-related to maternal levels of nitroprusside. The metabolic transformation of sodium nitroprusside given to pregnant ewes led to fatal levels of cyanide in the fetuses. The infusion of 25 mcg/kg/min of sodium nitroprusside for one hour in pregnant ewes resulted in the death of all fetuses. Pregnant ewes infused with 1 mcg/kg/min of sodium nitroprusside for one hour delivered normal lambs.

The effects of administering sodium thiosulfate in pregnancy, either by itself or as a co-infusion with sodium nitroprusside, are completely unknown.

Nursing Mothers: It is not known whether sodium nitroprusside and its metabolites are excreted in human milk. Because many drugs are excreted in human milk and because of the potential for serious adverse reactions in nursing infants from sodium nitroprusside, a decision should be made whether to discontinue nursing or to discontinue the drug, taking into account the importance of the drug to the mother.

Pediatric Use: See DOSAGE AND ADMINISTRATION.

DRUG INTERACTIONS:

The hypotensive effect of sodium nitroprusside is augmented by that of most other hypotensive drugs, including ganglionic blocking agents, negative inotropic agents and inhaled anesthetics.

ADVERSE REACTIONS:

The most important adverse reactions to sodium nitroprusside are the avoidable ones of excessive hypotension and cyanide toxicity, described above under WARNINGS. The adverse reactions described in this section develop less rapidly and, as it happens, less commonly.

Methemoglobinemia: As described in Clinical Pharmacology above, sodium nitroprusside infusions can cause sequestration of hemoglobin as methemoglobin. The back-conversion process is normally rapid, and clinically significant methemoglobinemia (>10%) is seen only rarely in patients receiving sodium nitroprusside. Even patients congenitally incapable of back-converting methemoglobin should demonstrate 10% methemoglobinemia only after they have received about 10 mg/kg of sodium nitroprusside, and a patient receiving sodium nitroprusside at the maximum recommended rate (10 mcg/kg/min) would take over 16 hours to reach this total accumulated dose.

Methemoglobin levels can be measured by most clinical laboratories. The diagnosis should be suspected in patients who have received >10 mg/kg of sodium nitroprusside and who exhibit signs of impaired oxygen delivery despite adequate cardiac output and adequate arterial pO_2. Classically, methemoglobinemic blood is described as chocolate brown, without color change on exposure to air.

When methemoglobinemia is diagnosed, the treatment of choice is 1 to 2 mg/kg of methylene blue, administered intravenously over several minutes. In patients likely to have substantial amounts of cyanide bound to methemoglobin as cyanmethemoglobin, treatment of methemoglobinemia with methylene blue must be undertaken with extreme caution.

Thiocyanate Toxicity: As described in CLINICAL PHARMACOLOGY, most of the cyanide produced during metabolism of sodium nitroprusside is eliminated in the form of thiocyanate. When cyanide elimination is accelerated by the co-infusion of thiosulfate, thiocyanate production is increased.

Thiocyanate is mildly neurotoxic (tinnitus, miosis, hyperreflexia) at serum levels of 1 mmol/L (60 mg/L). Thiocyanate toxicity is life-threatening when levels are 3 or 4 times higher (200 mg/L).

The steady-state thiocyanate level after prolonged infusions of sodium nitroprusside is increased with increased infusion rate, and the half-time of accumulation is 3 to 4 days. To keep the steady-state thiocyanate level below 1 mmol/L, a prolonged infusion of sodium nitroprusside should not be more rapid than 3 mcg/kg/min; in anuric patients, the corresponding limit is just 1 mcg/kg/min. When prolonged infusions are more rapid than these, thiocyanate levels should be measured daily.

Physiologic maneuvers (*e.g.*, those that alter the pH of the urine) are not known to increase the elimination of thiocyanate. Thiocyanate clearance rates during dialysis, on the other hand, can approach the blood flow rate of the dialyzer.

Thiocyanate interferes with iodine uptake by the thyroid.

Abdominal pain, apprehension, diaphoresis, "dizziness", headache, muscle twitching, nausea, palpitations, restlessness, retching, and retrosternal discomfort have been noted when the blood pressure was too rapidly reduced. These symptoms quickly disappeared when the infusion was slowed or discontinued, and they did not reappear with a continued (or resumed) slower infusion.

Other adverse reactions reported are:

Cardiovascular: Bradycardia, electrocardiographic changes, tachycardia.

Dermatologic: Rash.

Endocrine: Hypothyroidism.

Gastrointestinal: Ileus

Hematologic: Decreased platelet aggregation, methemoglobinemia.

Neurologic: Increased intracranial pressure.

Miscellaneous: Flushing, venous streaking, irritation at the infusion site.

OVERDOSAGE:

Overdosage of nitroprusside can be manifested as excessive hypotension or cyanide toxicity (WARNINGS) or as thiocyanate toxicity (ADVERSE REACTIONS).

The acute intravenous mean lethal doses (LD_{50}) of nitroprusside in rabbits, dogs, mice and rats are 2.8, 5.0, 8.4 and 11.2 mg/kg, respectively.

Treatment of cyanide toxicity: Cyanide levels can be measured by many laboratories, and blood-gas studies that can detect venous hyperoxemia or acidosis are widely available. **Acidosis may not appear until more than an hour after the appearance of dangerous cyanide levels, and laboratory tests should not be awaited. Reasonable suspicion of cyanide toxicity is adequate grounds for initiation of treatment.**

Treatment of cyanide toxicity consists of:

discontinuing the administration of sodium nitroprusside.

providing a buffer for cyanide by using sodium nitrite to convert as much hemoglobin into methemoglobin as the patient can safely tolerate; and then

OVERDOSAGE: *(cont'd)*

infusing sodium thiosulfate in sufficient quantity to convert the cyanide into thiocyanate.

The necessary medications for this treatment are contained in commercially available Cyanide Antidote Kits. Alternatively, discrete stocks of medications can be used.

Hemodialysis is ineffective in removal of cyanide, but it will eliminate most thiocyanate.

Cyanide Antidote Kits contain both amyl nitrite and sodium nitrite for induction of methemoglobinemia. The amyl nitrite is supplied in the form of inhalant ampuls, for administration in environments where intravenous administration of sodium nitrite may be delayed. In a patient who already has a patent intravenous line, use of amyl nitrite confers no benefit that is not provided by infusion of sodium nitrite.

Sodium nitrite is available in a 3% solution, and 4 to 6 mg/kg (about 0.2 ml/kg) should be injected over 2 to 4 minutes. This dose can be expected to convert about 10% of the patient's hemoglobin into methemoglobin; this level of methemoglobinemia is not associated with any important hazard of its own. The nitrite infusion may cause transient vasodilatation and hypotension, and this hypotension must, if it occurs, be routinely managed.

Immediately after infusion of the sodium nitrite, sodium thiosulfate should be infused. This agent is available in 10% and 25% solutions, and the recommended dose is 150 to 200 mg/kg; a typical adult dose is 50 ml of the 25% solution. Thiosulfate treatment of an acutely cyanide-toxic patient will raise thiocyanate levels, but not to a dangerous degree.

The nitrite/thiosulfate regimen may be repeated, at half the original doses, after two hours.

DOSAGE AND ADMINISTRATION:

Solution of the powder: The contents of a 50-mg sodium nitroprusside vial should be dissolved in 2 to 3 ml of dextrose in water. No other diluent should be used.

Dilution to proper strength for infusion: Depending on the desired concentration, the initially reconstituted solution containing 50 mg of sodium nitroprusside must be further diluted in 250 to 1000 ml of sterile 5% dextrose injection. The diluted solution should be protected from light by promptly wrapping with aluminum foil or other opaque material. It is not necessary to cover the infusion drip chamber or the tubing.

Verification of the chemical integrity of the product: Sodium nitroprusside solution can be inactivated by reactions with trace contaminants. The products of these reactions are often blue, green or red, much brighter than the faint brownish color of unreacted sodium nitroprusside. Discolored solutions, or solutions in which particulate matter is visible, should not be used. If properly protected from light, the freshly reconstituted and diluted solution is stable for 24 hours.

No other drugs should be administered in the same solution with sodium nitroprusside.

Avoidance of excessive hypotension: While the average effective rate in adults and children is about 3 mcg/kg/min, some patients will become dangerously hypotensive when they receive sodium nitroprusside at this rate. Infusion of sodium nitroprusside should therefore be started at a very low rate (0.3 mcg/kg/min), with gradual upward titration every few minutes until the desired effect is achieved or the maximum recommended infusion rate (10 mcg/kg/min) has been reached.

Because sodium nitroprusside's hypotensive effect is very rapid in onset and in dissipation, small variations in infusion rate can lead to wide, undesirable variations in blood pressure. **Sodium nitroprusside should not be infused through ordinary IV apparatus regulated only by gravity and mechanical clamps. Only an infusion pump, preferably a volumetric pump, should be used.**

Because sodium nitroprusside can induce essentially unlimited blood-pressure reduction, **the blood pressure of a patient receiving this drug must be continuously monitored,** using either a continually reinflated sphygmomanometer or (preferably) an intra-arterial pressure sensor. Special caution should be used in elderly patients, since they may be more sensitive to the hypotensive effects of the drug.

The table below shows the infusion rates for adults and children of various weights corresponding to the recommended initial and maximal doses (0.3 mcg/kg/min and 10 mcg/kg/min, respectively). Some of the listed infusion rates are so slow or so rapid as to be impractical, and these practicalities must be considered when the concentration to be used is selected. Note that when the concentration used in a given patient is changed, the tubing is still filled with a solution at the previous concentration.

Avoidance of cyanide toxicity: As described in CLINICAL PHARMACOLOGY, when more than 500 mcg/kg of sodium nitroprusside is administered faster than 2 mcg/kg/min, cyanide is generated faster than the unaided patient can eliminate it. Administration of sodium thiosulfate has been shown to increase the rate of cyanide processing, reducing the hazard of cyanide toxicity. Although toxic reactions to sodium thiosulfate have not been reported, the co-infusion regimen has not been extensively studied and it cannot be recommended without reservation. In one study, sodium thiosulfate appeared to potentiate the hypotensive effects of sodium nitroprusside.

TABLE 1 Infusion Rates (ml/hour) to Achieve Initial (0.3 mcg/kg/min) and Maximal (10 mcg/kg/min) Dosing of sodium nitroprusside

Volume sodium nitroprusside concentration pt weight		250 ml 50 mg 200 mcg/ml		500 ml 50 mg 100 mcg/ml		1000 ml 50 mg 50 mcg/ml	
kg	lbs	init	max	init	max	init	max
10	22	1	30	2	60	4	120
20	44	2	60	4	120	7	240
30	66	3	90	5	180	11	360
40	88	4	120	7	240	14	480
50	110	5	150	9	300	18	600
60	132	5	180	11	360	22	720
70	154	6	210	13	420	25	840
80	176	7	240	14	480	29	960
90	198	8	270	16	540	32	1080
100	220	9	300	18	600	36	1200

Co-infusions of sodium thiosulfate have been administered at rates of 5 to 10 times that of sodium nitroprusside. Care must be taken to avoid the indiscriminate use of prolonged or high doses of sodium nitroprusside with sodium thiosulfate as this may result in thiocyanate toxicity and hypovolemia. In cautious administration of sodium nitroprusside must still be avoided, and all of the precautions concerning sodium nitroprusside administration must still be observed.

Consideration of methemoglobinemia and thiocyanate toxicity: Rare patients receiving more than 10 mg/kg of sodium nitroprusside will develop methemoglobinemia; other patients, especially those with impaired renal function, will predictably develop thiocyanate toxicity after prolonged, rapid infusions. In accordance with the descriptions in ADVERSE REACTIONS, patients with suggestive findings should be tested for these toxicities.

Store the 5-ml amber-colored vials at 59 to 86°F.

HOW SUPPLIED - RATED THERAPEUTICALLY EQUIVALENT:

Injection, Lyphl-Soln - Intravenous - 50 mg/vial

1's	$8.06	NITROPRESS, Abbott	00074-3024-01
5 ml	$6.25	Sterile Sodium Nitroprusside, Elkins Sinn	00641-0125-21
5 ml	**$16.13**	**NIPRIDE 50, Roche**	**00004-1938-08**
50 mg	$4.24	NITROPRESS, Abbott	00074-3219-01
50 mg	$7.54	NITROPRESS, Abbott	00074-3019-02
50 mg	$8.53	NITROPRESS, Abbott	00074-3034-44

Injection, Solution - Intravenous - 25 mg/ml

2 ml	$5.04	NITROPRUSSIDE SODIUM, Gensia Labs	00703-1802-01

Kit - Intravenous - 50 mg

1's	$11.76	NITROPRESS, Abbott	00074-3250-01

SODIUM POLYSTYRENE SULFONATE *(002258)*

CATEGORIES: Electrolyte Solutions; Electrolytic, Caloric-Water Balance; Homeostatic & Nutrient; Hyperkalemia; Potassium-Removing Resins; Resins, Ion Exchange; Pregnancy Category C; FDA Approval Pre 1982

BRAND NAMES: **Kayexalate**; *Resinsodio*; *Resonium-A*; Sps
(International brand names outside U.S. in italics)

FORMULARIES: BC-BS; Medi-Cal

DESCRIPTION:

Sodium polystyrene sulfonate is a benzene, diethenyl-, polymer with ethenylbenzene, sulfonated, sodium salt.

The drug is a light brown to brown finely ground, powdered form of sodium polystyrene sulfonate, a cation-exchange resin prepared in the sodium phase with an *in vitro* exchange capacity of approximately 3.1 mEq (*in vivo* approximately 1 mEq) of potassium per gram. The sodium content is approximately 100 mg (4.1 mEq) per gram of the drug. It can be administered orally or in an enema.

CLINICAL PHARMACOLOGY:

As the resin passes along the intestine or is retained in the colon after administration by enema, the sodium ions are partially released and are replaced by potassium ions. For the most part, this action occurs in the large intestine, which excretes potassium ions to a greater degree than does the small intestine. The efficiency of this process is limited and unpredictably variable. It commonly approximates the order of 33 percent but the range is so large that definitive indices of electrolyte balance must be clearly monitored. Metabolic data are unavailable.

INDICATIONS AND USAGE:

Sodium polystyrene sulfonate is indicated for the treatment of hyperkalemia.

CONTRAINDICATIONS:

Sodium polystyrene sulfonate is contraindicated in patients with hypokalemia or those patients who are hypersensitive to it.

WARNINGS:

Alternative Therapy in Severe Hyperkalemia: Since effective lowering of serum potassium with sodium polystyrene sulfonate may take hours to days, treatment with this drug alone may be insufficient to rapidly correct severe hyperkalemia associated with states of rapid tissue breakdown (e.g. burns and renal failure) or hyperkalemia so marked as to constitute a medical emergency. Therefore, other definitive measures, including dialysis, should always be considered and may be imperative.

Hypokalemia: Serious potassium deficiency can occur from therapy with sodium polystyrene sulfonate. The effect must be carefully controlled by frequent serum potassium determinations within each 24 hour period. Since intracellular potassium deficiency is not always reflected by serum potassium levels, the level at which treatment with sodium polystyrene sulfonate should be discontinued must be determined individually for each patient. Important aids in making this determination are the patient's clinical condition and electrocardiogram. Early clinical signs of severe hypokalemia include a pattern of irritable confusion and delayed thought processes. Electrocardiographically, severe hypokalemia is often associated with a lengthened Q-T interval, widening, flattening, or inversion of the T wave, and prominent U waves. Also, cardiac arrhythmias may occur, such as premature atrial, nodal, and ventricular contractions, and supraventricular and ventricular tachycardias. The toxic effects of digitalis are likely to be exaggerated. Marked hypokalemia can also be manifested by severe muscle weakness, at times extending into frank paralysis.

Electrolyte Disturbances: Like all cation-exchange resins, sodium polystyrene sulfonate is not totally selective (for potassium) in its actions, and small amounts of other cations such as magnesium and calcium can also be lost during treatment. Accordingly, patients receiving sodium polystyrene sulfonate should be monitored for all applicable electrolyte disturbances.

Systemic Alkalosis: Systemic alkalosis has been reported after cation-exchange resins were administered orally in combination with nonabsorbable cation-donating antacids and laxatives such as magnesium hydroxide and aluminum carbonate. Magnesium hydroxide should not be administered with sodium polystyrene sulfonate. One case of grand mal seizure has been reported in a patient with chronic hypocalcemia of renal failure who was given sodium polystyrene sulfonate with magnesium hydroxide as laxative. (See DRUG INTERACTIONS.)

PRECAUTIONS:

Caution is advised when sodium polystyrene sulfonate is administered to patients who cannot tolerate even a small increase in sodium loads (*i.e.,* severe congestive heart failure, severe hypertension, or marked edema). In such instances compensatory restriction of sodium intake from other sources may be indicated.

If constipation occurs, patients should be treated with sorbitol (from 10 ml to 20 ml of 70 percent syrup every two hours or as needed to produce one or two watery stools daily), a measure which also reduces any tendency to fecal impaction.

Carcinogenesis, Mutagenesis, and Impairment of Fertility: Studies have not been performed.

Pregnancy Category C: Animal reproduction studies have not been conducted with sodium polystyrene sulfonate. It is also not known whether sodium polystyrene sulfonate can cause fetal harm when administered to a pregnant woman or can affect reproduction capacity. Sodium polystyrene sulfonate should be given to a pregnant woman only if clearly needed.

Nursing Mothers: It is not known whether this drug is excreted in human milk. Because many drugs are excreted in human milk, caution should be exercised when sodium polystyrene sulfonate is administered to a nursing woman.

DRUG INTERACTIONS:

Antacids: The simultaneous oral administration of sodium polystyrene sulfonate with nonabsorbable cation-donating antacids and laxatives may reduce the resin's potassium exchange capability.

Systemic alkalosis has been reported after cation-exchange resins were administered orally in combination with nonabsorbable cation-donating antacids and laxatives such as magnesium hydroxide and aluminum carbonate. Magnesium hydroxide should not be administered with sodium polystyrene sulfonate. One case of grand mal seizure has been reported in a patient with chronic hypocalcemia of renal failure who was given sodium polystyrene sulfonate with magnesium hydroxide as a laxative.

Intestinal obstruction due to concretions of aluminum hydroxide when used in combination with sodium polystyrene sulfonate has been reported.

Digitalis: The toxic effects of digitalis on the heart, especially various ventricular arrhythmias and A-V nodal dissociation, are likely to be exaggerated by hypokalemia, even in the face of serum digoxin concentrations in the "normal range". (See WARNINGS.)

ADVERSE REACTIONS:

Sodium polystyrene sulfonate may cause some degree of gastric irritation. Anorexia, nausea, vomiting, and constipation may occur especially if high doses are given. Also, hypokalemia, hypocalcemia, and significant sodium retention may occur. Occasionally diarrhea develops. Large doses in elderly individuals may cause fecal impaction (see PRECAUTIONS.) This effect may be obviated through usage of the resin in enemas as described under DOSAGE AND ADMINISTRATION. Rare instances of colonic necrosis have been reported. Intestinal obstruction due to concretions of aluminum hydroxide, when used in combination with sodium polystyrene sulfonate, has been reported.

DOSAGE AND ADMINISTRATION:

Suspension of this drug should be freshly prepared and not stored beyond 24 hours.

The average daily adult dose of the resin is 15 g to 60 g. This is best provided by administering 15 g (approximately 4 *level* teaspoons) of sodium polystyrene sulfonate one to four times daily. One gram of sodium polystyrene sulfonate contains 4.1 mEq of sodium; one level teaspoon contains approximately 3.5 g of sodium polystyrene sulfonate and 15 mEq of sodium. (A heaping teaspoon may contain as much as 10 g to 12 g of sodium polystyrene sulfonate.) Since the *in vivo* efficiency of sodium-potassium exchange resins is approximately 33 percent, about one third of the resin's actual sodium content is being delivered to the body.

In smaller children and infants, lower doses should be employed by using as a guide a rate of 1 mEq of potassium per gram of resin as the basis for calculation.

Each dose should be given as a suspension in a small quantity of water or, for greater palatability, in syrup. The amount of fluid usually ranges from 20 ml to 100 ml, depending on the dose, or may be simply determined by allowing 3 ml to 4 ml per gram of resin. Sorbitol may be administered in order to combat constipation.

The resin may be introduced into the stomach through a plastic tube and, if desired, mixed with a diet appropriate for a patient in renal failure.

The resin may also be given, although with less effective results, in an enema consisting (for adults) of 30 g to 50 g every six hours. Each dose is administered as a warm emulsion (at body temperature) in 100 ml of aqueous vehicle, such as sorbitol. The emulsion should be agitated gently during administration. The enema should be retained as long as possible and followed by a cleansing enema.

After an initial cleansing enema, a soft, large size (French 28) rubber tube is inserted into the rectum for a distance of about 20 cm, with the tip well into the sigmoid colon, and taped in place. The resin is then suspended in the appropriate amount of aqueous vehicle at body temperature and introduced by gravity, while the particles are kept in suspension by stirring. The suspension is flushed with 50 ml or 100 ml of fluid, following which the tube is clamped and left in place. If back leakage occurs, the hips are elevated on pillows or a knee-chest position is taken temporarily. A somewhat thicker suspension may be used, but care should be taken that no paste is formed, because the latter has a greatly reduced exchange surface and will be particularly ineffective if deposited in the rectal ampulla. The suspension is kept in the sigmoid colon for several hours, if possible. Then, the colon is irrigated with nonsodium containing solution at body temperature in order to remove the resin. Two quarts of flushing solution may be necessary. The returns are drained constantly through a Y tube connection. Particular attention should be paid to this cleansing enema when sorbitol has been used.

The intensity and duration of therapy depend upon the severity and resistance of hyperkalemia.

Store at room temperature.

Sodium polystyrene sulfonate should not be heated for to do so may alter the exchange properties of the resin.

HOW SUPPLIED - RATED THERAPEUTICALLY EQUIVALENT:

Powder - Oral

454 gm	**$164.58**	**KAYEXALATE, Sanofi Winthrop**	**00024-1075-01**

Powder - Oral; Rectal - 60 mg

454 gm	$52.50	Sodium Polystyrene Sulfonate, Carolina Med	46287-0012-16

Suspension - Rectal - 15 gm/60ml

60 ml	$58.50	SPS, Carolina Med	46287-0006-60
60 ml x 10	$86.49	SODIUM POLYSTRENE SULFONATE, Roxane	00054-8816-11
120 ml	$66.60	SPS, Carolina Med	46287-0006-04
120 ml enema bo	$19.67	Sodium Polystyrene Sulfonate, Roxane	00054-8815-01
200 ml enema bo	$29.50	Sodium Polystyrene Sulfonate, Roxane	00054-8817-55
480 ml	$29.70	SPS, Carolina Med	46287-0006-01
500 ml	$47.86	Sodium Polystyrene Sulfonate, Roxane	00054-3805-63

HOW SUPPLIED - NOT RATED EQUIVALENT:

Powder - Oral

454 gm	$65.00	Sodium Polystyrene Sulfonate, Raway	00686-0012-16

SODIUM SULFACETAMIDE *(003322)*

CATEGORIES: Acne Vulgaris; Acne; Anti-Infectives; Antibacterials; Antibiotics; Antimicrobials; Dermatologicals; Sulfonamides; Topical; Pregnancy Category C; FDA Approved 1996 Dec

BRAND NAMES: **Klaron**

PRIMARY ICD9: 706.1 (Acne Vulgaris)

DESCRIPTION:

Each ml of sodium sulfacetamide lotion, 10% contains 100 mg of sodium sulfacetamide in a vehicle consisting of purified water; propylene glycol; lauramide DEA (and) diethanolamine; polyethylene glycol 400, monolaurate; hydroxyethyl cellulose; sodium chloride; sodium metabisulfite; methylparaben; xanthan gum; EDTA and simethicone.

Sodium sulfacetamide is a sulfonamide with antibacterial activity. Chemically sodium sulfacetamide is N'-[(4-aminophenyl)sulfonyl]-acetamide, monosodium salt, monohydrate.

CLINICAL PHARMACOLOGY:

The most widely accepted mechanism of action of sulfonamides is the Woods-Fildes theory, based on sulfonamides acting as a competitive inhibitor of para-aminobenzoic acid (PABA) utilization, an essential component for bacterial growth. While absorption through intact skin in humans has not been determined, *in vitro* studies with human cadaver skin indicated a percutaneous absorption of about 4%. Sodium sulfacetamide is readily absorbed from the gastrointestinal tract when taken orally and excreted in the urine, largely unchanged. The biological half-life has been reported to be between 7 to 13 hours.

INDICATIONS AND USAGE:

Sodium sulfacetamide lotion indicated in the topical treatment of acne vulgaris.

CONTRAINDICATIONS:

Sodium sulfacetamide lotion contraindicated for use by patients having known hypersensitivity to sulfonamides or any other component of this preparation. (See WARNINGS.)

WARNINGS:

Fatalities have occurred, although rarely, due to severe reactions to sulfonamides including Stevens-Johnson syndrome, toxic epidermal necrolysis, fulminant hepatic necrosis, agranulocytosis, aplastic anemia, and other blood dyscrasias. Hypersensitivity reactions may occur when a sulfonamide is readministered, irrespective of the route of administration. Sensitivity reactions have been reported in individuals with no prior history of sulfonamide hypersensitivity. At the first sign of hypersensitivity, skin rash or other reactions, discontinue use of this prepartion (see ADVERSE REACTIONS).

Sodium sulfacetamide lotion contains sodium bisulfite, a sulfite that may cause allergic-type reactions including anaphylactic symptoms and life-threatening or less severe asthmatic episodes in certain susceptible people. The overall prevalence of sulfite sensitivity in the general population is unknown and probably low. Sulfite sensitivity is seen more frequently in asthmatic than in non-asthmatic people. (See CONTRAINDICATIONS.)

PRECAUTIONS:

General: For external use only. Keep away from eyes. If irritation develops, use of the product should be discontinued and appropriate therapy instituted. Patients should be carefully observed for possible local irritation or sensitization during long-term therapy. Hypersensitivity reactions may occur when a sulfonamide is readministered irrespective of the route of administration, and cross-sensitivity between different sulfonamides may occur. Sodium sulfacetamide can cause reddening and scaling of the skin. Particular caution should be employed if areas of involved skin to be treated are denuded or abraded.

Keep out of reach of children.

Carcinogenesis, Mutagenesis, and Impairment of Fertility: Long-term studies in animals have not been performed to evaluate carcinogenic potential.

Pregnancy: Pregnancy Category C: Animal reproduction studies have not been conducted with sodium sulfacetamide lotion. It is also not known whether sodium sulfacetamide lotion can cause fetal harm when administered to a pregnant woman or can affect reproduction capacity. Sodium sulfacetamide lotion should be given to a pregnant woman only if clearly needed.

Kemicterus may occur in the newborn as a result of treatment of a pregnant woman at term with orally administered sulfonamide. There are no adequate and well controlled studies of sodium sulfacetamide lotion in pregnant women, and it is not known whether topically applied sulfonamides can cause fetal harm when administered to a pregnant woman.

Nursing Mothers: It is not known whether sodium sulfacetamide is excreted in the human milk following topical use of sodium sulfacetamide lotion. Systemic administered sulfonamides are capable of producing kemicterus n the infants of lactating wome. Small amounts of orally administered sulfonamides have been reported to be eliminated in human milk. Because many drugs are excreted in human milk, caution should be exercised in prescribing for nursing women.

Pediatric Use: Safety and effectiveness in pediatric patients under the age of 12 have not been established.

ADVERSE REACTIONS:

In controlled clinical trials for the management of *acne vulgaris*, the occurrence of adverse reactions associated with the use of sodium sulfacetamide lotion was infrequent and restricted to local events. The total incidence of adverse reaction reported in these studies was less than 2%. Only one of 105 patients treated with sodium sulfacetamide lotion had adverse reactions of erythema, itching, and edema. It has been reported that sodium sulfacetamide may cause local irritation, stinging and burning. While the irritation may be transient, occasionally, the use of medication has to be discontinued.

DOSAGE AND ADMINISTRATION:

Apply a thin film to affected areas twice daily.

PATIENT INFORMATION:

Sodium sulfacetamide lotion is for the treatment of acne vulgaris.

Do not use if you are allergic to "sulfa" drugs.

Inform your physician if you are pregnant or nursing.

May cause redness, itching, edema, local irritation, stinging or burning.

Severe reactions to sulfacetamides have occured.

If signs of hypersensitivity occur (skin rash or other reactions), discontinue use and consult physician.

For external use only. Keep out of eyes.

HOW SUPPLIED:

Store at room temperature.

HOW SUPPLIED - EQUIVALENTS NOT AVAILABLE:

Lotion - Topical - 100 mg/ml

59 ml bottles	**$27.18**	**KLARON, Dermik Labs**	**00066-7500-02**

SODIUM SULFACETAMIDE; SULFUR *(002260)*

CATEGORIES: Acne; Acne Rosacea; Acne Vulgaris; Anti-Infectives; Antibacterials; Dermatitis; Dermatologicals; Keratolytic Agents; Local Infections; Rosacea; Seborrhea; Skin/Mucous Membrane Agents; Sulfonamides; Topical; Pregnancy Category C; FDA Pre 1938 Drugs

BRAND NAMES: Novacet; **Sulfacet-R**

FORMULARIES: Aetna; BC-BS

DESCRIPTION:

Each ml of sodium sulfacetamide 10% and sulfur 5% as dispensed contains 100 mg of sodium sulfacetamide and 50 mg of sulfur in a tinted lotion of purified water, alkylaryl sulfonic acid salts, hydroxyethylcellulose, propylene glycol, xanthan gum, lauric myristic diethanolamide, polyxyethylene laurate, butylparaben, methylparaben, silicone emulsion, talc, zinc oxide, titanium dioxide, attapulgite, iron oxides, sodium bisulfite, sodium chloride and 2-bromo- 2-nitropropane-1, 3 diol.

Sodium sulfacetamide is a sulfonamide with antibacterial activity while sulfur acts as a keratolytic agent. Chemically sodium sulfacetamide is N' -((4-aminophenyl) sulfonyl)-acetamide, monosodium salt, monohydrate.

CLINICAL PHARMACOLOGY:

The most widely accepted mechanism of action of sulfonamides is the Woods-Fildes theory which is based on the fact that sulfonamides act as competitive antagonists to para-aminobenzoic acid (PABA), an essential component for bacterial growth. While absorption through intact skin has not been determined sodium sulfacetamide is readily absorbed from the gastrointestinal tract when taken orally and excreted in the urine, largely unchanged. The biological half-life has variously been reported as 7 to 12.8 hours.

The exact mode of action of sulfur in the treatment of acne is unknown, but it has been reported that it inhibits the growth of *p. acnes* and the formation of free fatty acids.

INDICATIONS AND USAGE:

Sodium Sulfacetamide with Sulfur is indicated in the topical control of acne vulgaris, acne rosacea and seborrheic dermatitis.

CONTRAINDICATIONS:

Sodium Sulfacetamide with Sulfur is contraindicated for use by patients having known hypersensitivity to sulfonamides, sulfur, or any other component of this preparation. Sodium Sulfacetamide with Sulfur is not to be used by patients with kidney disease.

WARNINGS:

Although rare, sensitivity to sodium sulfacetamide may occur. Therefore, caution and careful supervision should be observed when prescribing this drug for patients who may be prone to hypersensitivity to topical sulfonamides. Systemic toxic reactions such as agranulocytosis, acute hemolytic anemia, purpura hemorrhagica, drug fever, jaundice, and contact dermatitis indicate hypersensitivity to sulfonamides. Particular caution should be employed if areas of denuded or abraded skin are involved.

Contains sodium bisulfite, a sulfite that may cause allergic-type reactions including anaphylactic symptoms and life-threatening or less severe asthmatic episodes in certain susceptible people. The overall prevalence of sulfite sensitivity in the general population is unknown and probably low. Sulfite sensitivity is seen more frequently in asthmatic than in non-asthmatic people.

PRECAUTIONS:

General: If irritation develops, use of the product should be discontinued and appropriate therapy instituted. For external use only. Keep away from eyes. Patients should be carefully observed for possible local irritation or sensitization during long-term therapy. The object of this therapy is to achieve desquamation without irritation, but sodium sulfacetamide and sulfur can cause reddening and scaling of epidermis. These side effects are not unusual in the treatment of acne vulgaris, but patients should be cautioned about the possibility. Keep out of the reach of children.

Carcinogenesis, Mutagenesis and Impairment of Fertility: Long- term studies in animals have not been performed to evaluate carcinogenic potential.

Pregnancy Category C: Animal reproduction studies have not been conducted with sodium sulfacetamide with sulfur. It is also not known whether sodium sulfacetamide with sulfur can cause fetal harm when administered to a pregnant woman or can affect reproduction capacity. Sodium sulfacetamide with sulfur should be given to a pregnant woman only if clearly needed.

Nursing Mothers: It is not known whether sodium sulfacetamide is excreted in the human milk following topical use of **sodium sulfacetamide with sulfur lotion**. However, small amounts of orally administered sulfonamides have been reported to be eliminated in human milk. In view of this and because many drugs are excreted in human milk, caution should be exercised when **sodium sulfacetamide with sulfur lotion** is administered to a nursing woman.

Pediatric Use: Safety and effectiveness in children under the age of 12 have not been established.

ADVERSE REACTIONS:

Although rare, sodium sulfacetamide may cause local irritation.

DOSAGE AND ADMINISTRATION:

Shake well before using. Apply a thin film to affected areas with light massaging to blend in each application 1 to 3 times daily. Each package contains a **Dermik Color Blender** which enables the patient to alter the basic shade of the lotion so that it matches the skin color exactly.

(Important to the Pharmacist—At the time of dispensing, add contents of vial* to the bottle. Shake well and/or stir with a glass rod to ensure uniform dispersion. Place expiration date of four (4) months on bottle label.)

*Sulfa-Pak vial contains 2.1 g of sodium sulfacetamide.

HOW SUPPLIED - EQUIVALENTS NOT AVAILABLE:

Lotion - Topical - 10% mg/5 %

25 ml	$17.34	SODIUM SULFACETAMIDE/SULFUR, Glades Pharms	59366-2762-03
25 ml	**$23.03**	**SULFACET-R, Dermik Labs**	**00066-0028-25**
30 gm	$22.51	NOVACET, Genderm Corp	29936-0530-30
30 ml	$17.34	SODIUM SULFACETAMIDE/SULFUR, Glades Pharms	59366-2762-05
30 ml	$22.51	Novacet, Genderm	52761-0530-30
60 gm	$40.50	NOVACET, Genderm Corp	29936-0530-60
60 gm	$40.50	NOVACET, Genderm	52761-0530-60

SODIUM TETRADECYL SULFATE *(002262)*

CATEGORIES: Cardiovascular Drugs; Detergents; Sclerosing Agents; Skin/Mucous Membrane Agents; Varicose Veins; Pregnancy Category C; FDA Approval Pre 1982

BRAND NAMES: **Sotradecol**

DESCRIPTION:

Sodium tetradecyl sulfate is an anionic surfactant which occurs as a white, waxy solid.

Sodium tetradecyl sulfate injection is a sterile nonpyrogenic solution for intravenous use as a sclerosing agent. Each ml contains sodium tetradecyl sulfate 10 mg or 30 mg, benzyl alcohol 0.02 ml and dibasic sodium phosphate, anhydrous 0.72 mg in Water for injection. pH 7.9; monobasic sodium phosphate and/or sodium hydroxide added, if needed, for pH adjustment.

CLINICAL PHARMACOLOGY:

Sodium tetradecyl sulfate injection is a mild sclerosing agent. Intravenous injection causes intima inflammation and thrombus formation. This usually occludes the injected vein. Subsequent formation of fibrous tissue results in partial or complete vein obliteration.

INDICATIONS AND USAGE:

Indicated in the treatment of small uncomplicated varicose veins of the lower extremities that show simple dilation with competent valves. The benefit-to-risk ratio should be considered in selected patients who are great surgical risks due to conditions such as old age.

CONTRAINDICATIONS:

Contraindicated in previous hypersensitivity reactions to the drug; in acute superficial thrombophlebitis; significant valvular or deep vein incompetence; huge superficial veins with wide open communications to deeper veins; phlebitis migrans; acute cellulitis; allergic conditions; acute infections; varicosities caused by abdominal and pelvic tumors unless the tumor has been removed; bedridden patients; such uncontrolled systemic diseases as diabetes, toxic hyperthyroidism, tuberculosis, asthma, neoplasm, sepsis, blood dyscrasias and acute respiratory or skin diseases.

WARNINGS:

Since severe adverse local effects, including tissue necrosis, may occur following extravasation, sodium tetradecyl sulfate injection, should be administered only by a physician familiar with proper injection technique. Extreme care in needle placement and using the minimal effective volume at each injection site are, therefore, important. Allergic reactions have been reported. Therefore, as a precaution against anaphylactoid shock, it is recommended that 0.5 ml of sodium tetradecyl sulfate be injected into a varicosity, followed by observation of the patient for several hours before administration of a second or larger dose. The possibility of an anaphylactoid reaction should be kept in mind, and the physician should be prepared to treat it appropriately. In extreme emergencies, 0.25 ml of 1:1000 Epinephrine Injection (0.25 mg) intravenously should be used and side reactions controlled with antihistamines.

PRECAUTIONS:

GENERAL

Venous sclerotherapy should not be undertaken if tests, such as the Trendelenburg and Perthes, and angiography show significant valvular or deep venous incompetence. The physician should bear in mind the fact that injection necrosis is likely to result from extravascular injection of sclerosing agents.

Extreme caution must be exercised in the presence of underlying arterial disease such as marked peripheral arteriosclerosis or thromboangiitis obliterans (Buerger's Disease).

The drug should only be administered by physicians who are familiar with an acceptable injection technique. Because of the danger of thrombosis extension into the deep venous system, thorough preinjection evaluation for valvular competency should be carried out and slow injections with a small amount (not over 2 ml) of the preparation should be injected into the varicosity. In particular, deep venous patency must be determined by angiography and/or the Perthes test before sclerotherapy is undertaken.

Embolism may occur as much as four weeks after injection of sodium tetradecyl sulfate.

The incidence of recurrence is low if the patient wears elastic stockings.

CARCINOGENESIS, MUTAGENESIS, IMPAIRMENT OF FERTILITY

When tested in the L5178YTK$^{+/-}$ mouse lymphoma assay, sodium tetradecyl sulfate did not induce a dose-related increase in the frequency of thymidine kinase-deficient mutants and, therefore, was judged to be nonmutagenic in this system. However, no long-term animal carcinogenicity studies with sodium tetradecyl sulfate have been performed.

PREGNANCY, TERATOGENIC EFFECTS, PREGNANCY CATEGORY C

Adequate reproduction studies have not been performed in animals to determine whether this drug affects fertility in males or females, has teratogenic potential, or has other adverse effects on the fetus. There are no well-controlled studies in pregnant women, but investigational and marketing experience does not include any positive evidence of adverse effects on the fetus. Although there is no clearly defined risk, such experience cannot exclude the possibility of infrequent or subtle damage to the human fetus.

NURSING MOTHERS

It is not known whether this drug is excreted in human milk. Because many drugs are excreted in human milk, caution should be exercised when Sodium Tetradecyl Sulfate Injection is administered to a nursing woman.

DRUG INTERACTIONS:

No well-controlled studies have been performed on patients taking antiovulatory agents. The physician must use judgment and evaluate any patient taking antiovulatory drugs prior to initiating treatment with sodium tetradecyl sulfate. (See ADVERSE REACTIONS.)

Heparin should not be included in the same syringe as sodium tetradecyl sulfate since the two are incompatible.

ADVERSE REACTIONS:

Local reactions consisting of pain, urticaria or ulceration may occur at the site of injection. A permanent discoloration, usually small and hardly noticeable but which may be objectionable from a cosmetic viewpoint, may remain along the path of the sclerosed vein segment. Sloughing and necrosis of tissue may occur following extravasation of the drug. Systemic reactions, except for allergic ones, have been slight. These include headache, nausea and vomiting. Allergic reactions such as hives, asthma, hay fever and anaphylactoid shock have been reported. (See WARNINGS.)

One death has been reported in a patient who received sodium tetradecyl sulfate and who had been receiving an antiovulatory agent.

Another death (fetal pulmonary embolism) has been reported in a 36-years-old female treated with sodium tetradecyl *acetate* and who was **not** taking oral contraceptives.

DOSAGE AND ADMINISTRATION:

For intravenous use only. Do not use if precipitated or discolored. The strength of solution required depends on the size and degree of varicosity. In general, the 1% solution will be found most useful with the 3% solution preferred for larger varicosities. The dosage should be kept small, using 0.5 to 2 ml (preferably 1 ml maximum) for each injection, and the maximum single treatment should not exceed 10 ml.

Parenteral drug products should be inspected visually for particulate matter and discoloration prior to administration, whenever solution and container permit.

Storage: Store at controlled room temperature 15-30°C (59-86°F).

ANIMAL PHARMACOLOGY:

The intravenous LD_{50} of sodium tetradecyl sulfate in mice was reported to be 90 ± 5 mg/kg. In the rat, the acute intravenous LD_{50} of sodium tetradecyl sulfate was estimated to be between 72 mg/kg and 108 mg/kg.

Purified sodium tetradecyl sulfate was found to have an LD_{50} of 2 g/kg when administered orally by stomach tube as a 25% aqueous solution to rats. In rats given 0.15 g/kg in drinking water for 30 days, no appreciable toxicity was seen although some growth inhibition was discernible.

HOW SUPPLIED - EQUIVALENTS NOT AVAILABLE:

Injection, Solution - Intravenous - 1 %

2 ml x 5	$62.50	Sotradecol, Consolidated Midland	00223-8586-02
2 ml x 5	$64.28	SOTRADECOL, Elkins Sinn	00641-1514-34

Injection, Solution - Intravenous - 3 %

2 ml x 5	$76.19	SOTRADECOL, Elkins Sinn	00641-1516-34
2 ml x 5	$80.00	Sotradecol, Consolidated Midland	00223-8587-02

SODIUM THIOSALICYLATE *(002263)*

CATEGORIES: Analgesics; Analgesics/Antipyretics; Antiarthritics; Antipyretics; Central Nervous System Agents; Pain; FDA Pre 1938 Drugs

BRAND NAMES: Asproject; Barocyl; Myosal; Pirosal; Rexolate; Thiocyl; Tusal

Prescribing information not available at time of publication.

HOW SUPPLIED - EQUIVALENTS NOT AVAILABLE:

Injection, Solution - Intramuscular; - 50 mg/ml

2 ml x 10	$110.00	PIROSAL, Teral Labs	51234-0104-10
2 ml x 15	$165.00	PIROSAL, Teral Labs	51234-0104-02
2 ml x 25	$165.00	THIOCYL, Alba Pharma	10023-0213-02
10 x 2 ml	$115.00	Thiocyl Injection 50 Mg/Ml, Alba Pharma	10023-0226-02
30 ml	$29.50	REXOLATE, Hyrex Pharms	00314-0762-30
30 ml	$150.00	PIROSAL, Teral Labs	51234-0105-30

SODIUM THIOSULFATE *(002264)*

CATEGORIES: Antagonists and Antidotes; Anti-Infectives; Antidotes; Antifungals; Heavy Metal Antagonists; Skin/Mucous Membrane Agents; FDA Pre 1938 Drugs

FORMULARIES: Medi-Cal; WHO

Prescribing information not available at time of publication.

HOW SUPPLIED - EQUIVALENTS NOT AVAILABLE:

Injection, Solution - Intravenous - 100 mg/ml

10 ml x 5	$37.50	Sodium Thiosulfate, Am Regent	00517-1019-05
10 ml x 5	$75.00	Sodium Thiosulfate, Consolidated Midland	00223-8573-05
10 ml x 25	$300.00	Sodium Thiosulfate, Consolidated Midland	00223-8573-10

Injection, Solution - Intravenous - 250 mg/ml

5 X 10 ml	$30.25	Sodium Thiosulfate, Pasadena	00418-1854-10
30 ml	$8.00	Sodium Thiosulfate, Consolidated Midland	00223-8570-30
50 ml	$12.49	Sodium Thiosulfate, Hope Pharms	60267-0823-50
50 ml	$22.50	Sodium Thiosulfate, Am Regent	00517-5019-01
50 ml	$22.50	Sodium Thiosulfate, Am Regent	00517-5019-02
50 ml	$28.60	Sodium Thiosulfate, Pasadena	00418-1861-50

SOMATREM *(002265)*

CATEGORIES: Anterior Pituitary/Hypothalmic Function; Chronic Renal Insufficiency; Growth Failure; Hormones; Human Growth Hormone; Orphan Drugs; Pituitary; AIDS Related Complex*; Turner's Syndrome*; Pregnancy Category C; Recombinant DNA Origin; Sales > $100 Million; FDA Approved 1985 Oct; Patent Expiration 1992 Oct

* Indication not approved by the FDA

BRAND NAMES: Genotropin; *Somatonorm* (France); **Somatrem**
(International brand names outside U.S. in italics)

FORMULARIES: BC-BS

COST OF THERAPY: $13,107.15 (Growth Failure; Kit; 5 mg/vial; 0.171/day; 365 days)

DESCRIPTION:

Somatrem for injection, is a polypeptide hormone produced by recombinant DNA technology. Somatrem has 192 amino acid residues and a molecular weight of about 22,000 daltons. The product contains the identical sequence of 191 amino acids constituting pituitary-derived human growth hormone plus an additional amino acid, methionine, on the N-terminus of the molecule. Somatrem is synthesized in a special laboratory strain of *E. coli* bacteria which has been modified by the addition of the gene for human growth hormone production.

Somatrem is a highly purified preparation. Biological potency is determined by measuring the increase in body weight induced in hypophysectomized rats.

Somatrem is a sterile, white, lyophilized powder intended for intramuscular or subcutaneous administration after reconstitution with Bacteriostatic Water for Injection, USP (benzyl alcohol preserved).

Each 5 mg Somatrem vial contains 5 mg (approximately 15 IU) somatrem, lyophilized with 40 mg mannitol, and 1.7 mg sodium phosphates (0.1 mg sodium phosphate monobasic and 1.6 mg sodium phosphate dibasic).

DESCRIPTION: *(cont'd)*

Each 10 mg Somatrem vial contains 10 mg (approximately 30 IU) somatrem, lyophilized with 80 mg mannitol, and 3.4 mg sodium phosphates (0.2 mg sodium phosphate monobasic and 3.2 mg sodium phosphate dibasic).

Phosphoric acid may be used for pH adjustment.

Bacteriostatic Water for Injection, USP is a sterile water containing 0.9 percent benzyl alcohol per ml as an antimicrobial preservative packaged in a multi-dose vial. The diluent pH is 4.5-7.0.

CLINICAL PHARMACOLOGY:

In vitro and in vivo preclinical, and clinical testing have demonstrated that somatrem is therapeutically equivalent to pituitary-derived human growth hormone. Treatment of children who lack adequate endogenous growth hormone secretion with somatrem resulted in an increase in growth rate and an increase in insulin-like growth factor-I levels similar to that seen with pituitary-derived human growth hormone.

Actions that have been demonstrated for Somatrem, somatropin and/or pituitary-derived human growth hormone include:

A. Tissue Growth: 1) Skeletal Growth: somatrem stimulates skeletal growth in children with growth failure due to a lack of adequate secretion of endogenous growth hormone. Skeletal growth is accomplished at the epiphyseal plates at the ends of a growing bone. Growth and metabolism of epiphyseal plate cells are directly stimulated by growth hormone and one of its mediators, insulin-like growth factor- I. Serum levels of insulin-like growth factor-I are low in children and adolescents who are growth hormone deficient, but increase during treatment with somatrem. New bone is formed at the epiphyses in response to growth hormone. This results in linear growth until these growth plates fuse at the end of puberty. 2) Cell Growth: Treatment with pituitary-derived human growth hormone results in an increase in both the number and the size of skeletal muscle cells. 3) Organ Growth: Growth hormone of human pituitary origin influences the size of internal organs, including kidneys, and increases red cell mass. Treatment of hypophysectomized or genetic dwarf rats with somatropin results in organ growth that is proportional to the overall body growth.

B. Protein Metabolism: Linear growth is facilitated in part by growth hormone-stimulated protein synthesis. This is reflected by nitrogen retention as demonstrated by a decline in urinary nitrogen excretion and blood urea nitrogen during growth hormone therapy.

C. Carbohydrate Metabolism: Growth hormone is a modulator of carbohydrate metabolism. For example, children with inadequate secretion of growth hormone sometimes experience fasting hypoglycemia that is improved by treatment with growth hormone. Somatrem therapy may decrease glucose tolerance. Administration of somatrem to normal adults and patients who lacked adequate secretion of endogenous growth hormone resulted in increases in mean serum fasting and postprandial insulin levels. However, mean glucose and hemoglobin A_{1C} levels remained in the normal range.

D. Lipid Metabolism: Acute administration of pituitary-derived human growth hormone to humans resulted in lipid mobilization. Nonesterified fatty acids increased in plasma within two hours of pituitary-derived human growth hormone administration. In growth hormone deficient patients, long-term growth hormone administration often decreases body fat. Mean cholesterol levels decreased in patients treated with growth hormone.

E. Mineral Metabolism: The retention of total body potassium in response to growth hormone administration apparently results from cellular growth. Serum levels of inorganic phosphorus may increase slightly in patients with inadequate secretion of endogenous growth hormone after growth hormone therapy due to metabolic activity associated with bone growth as well as increased tubular reabsorption of phosphate by the kidney. Serum calcium is not significantly altered in these patients. Sodium retention also occurs. (See PRECAUTIONS, Laboratory Tests.)

F. Connective Tissue Metabolism: Growth hormone stimulates the synthesis of chondroitin sulfate and collagen as well as the urinary excretion of hydroxyproline.

INDICATIONS AND USAGE:

Somatrem for injection is indicated only for the long-term treatment of children who have growth failure due to a lack of adequate endogenous growth hormone secretion. Other etiologies of short stature should be excluded.

CONTRAINDICATIONS:

Somatrem should not be used in subjects with closed epiphyses.

Somatrem should not be used in patients with active neoplasia. Growth hormone therapy should be discontinued if evidence of neoplasia develops.

Somatrem, when reconstituted with Bacteriostatic Water for Injection, USP (benzyl alcohol preserved) should not be used in patients with a known sensitivity to benzyl alcohol.

WARNINGS:

Benzyl alcohol as a preservative in Bacteriostatic Water for Injection, USP has been associated with toxicity in newborns. When administering somatrem to newborns, reconstitute with Sterile Water for Injection, USP. USE ONLY ONE DOSE PER SOMTREM VIAL AND DISCARD THE UNUSED PORTION.

PRECAUTIONS:

General: Somatrem should be prescribed by physicians experienced in the diagnosis and management of patients with growth failure.

Because somatrem may induce a state of insulin resistance, patients should be observed for evidence of glucose intolerance.

Patients with a history of an intracranial lesion should be examined frequently for progression or recurrence of the lesion.

Slipped capital femoral epiphysis may occur more frequently in patients with endocrine disorders or in patients undergoing rapid growth. Physicians and parents should be alert to the development of a limp or complaints of hip or knee pain in somatrem-treated patients.

Progression of scoliosis can occur in children who experience rapid growth. Because growth hormone increases growth rate, patients with a history of scoliosis who are treated with growth hormone should be monitored for progression of scoliosis. Growth hormone has been shown to increase the incidence of scoliosis.

Intracranial hypertension (IH) with papilledema, visual changes, headache, nausea and/or vomiting has been reported in a small number of patients treated with growth hormone products. Symptoms usually occurred within the first (8) weeks of the initiation of growth hormone therapy. In all reported cases, IH-associated signs and symptoms resolved after termination of therapy or a reduction of the growth hormone dose. Funduscopic examination of patients is recommended at the initiation and periodically during the course of growth hormone therapy.

See WARNINGS for use of Bacteriostatic Water for Injection, USP (benzyl alcohol preserved) in newborns.

PRECAUTIONS: *(cont'd)*

As with any protein, local or systemic allergic reactions may occur. Parents/Patient should be informed that such reactions are possible and that prompt medical attention should be sought if allergic reactions occur.

Laboratory Tests: Serum levels of inorganic phosphorus, alkaline phosphatase, and parathyroid hormone (PTH) may increase with somatrem therapy. Changes in thyroid hormone laboratory measurements may develop during somatrem treatment of children who lack adequate endogenous growth hormone secretion. Untreated hypothyroidism prevents optimal response to somatrem. Therefore, patients should have periodic thyroid function tests and should be treated with thyroid hormone when indicated.

Carcinogenesis, Mutagenesis, and Impairment of Fertility: Carcinogenicity, mutagenicity and reproduction studies have not been conducted with somatrem.

Pregnancy: Pregnancy (Category C). Animal reproduction studies have not been conducted with somatrem. It is also not known whether somatrem can cause fetal harm when administered to a pregnant woman or can affect reproduction capacity. Somatrem should be given to a pregnant woman only if clearly needed.

Nursing Mothers: It is not known whether this drug is excreted in human milk. Because many drugs are excreted in human milk, caution should be exercised when somatrem is administered to a nursing mother.

Information for the Patient: Patients being treated with growth hormone and/or their parents should be informed of the potential benefits and risks associated with treatment. If home use is determined to be desirable by the physician, instructions on appropriate use should be given, including a review of the contents of the Patient Information Insert. This information is intended to aid in the safe and effective administration of the medication. It is not a disclosure of all possible adverse or intended effects.

If home use is prescribed, a puncture resistant container for the disposal of used syringes and needles should be recommended to the patient. Patients and/or parents should be thoroughly instructed in the importance of proper disposal and cautioned against any reuse of needles and syringes (see Patient Information Insert.)

DRUG INTERACTIONS:

Concomitant glucocorticoid therapy may inhibit the growth promoting effect of somatrem. If glucocorticoid replacement is required, the dose should be carefully adjusted.

ADVERSE REACTIONS:

As with all protein pharmaceuticals, a small percentage of patients may develop antibodies to the protein. Growth hormone antibody binding capacities below 2 mg/l have not been associated with growth attenuation. In some cases when binding capacity exceeds 2 mg/ml, growth attenuation has been observed. In clinical studies and postmarketing experience of patients treated with somatrem, approximately 0.4 percent of patients screened for antibody production developed antibodies with binding capacities > 2 mg/l at six months. Out of approximately 26,000 patients who have been treated with somatrem, 5 patients have had growth deceleration associated with binding capacities > 2 mg/l. If growth deceleration is observed that is not attributable to another cause, the patient should be tested for antibodies to growth hormone. Although no evidence exists to indicate that the methionine on the N-terminus of somatrem causes antibodies to growth hormone, the physician should consider transferring the patient to somatropin (rDNA origin) for injection, if a patient has antibody binding capacity > 2 mg/l, and has exhibited growth attenuation.

In addition to an evaluation of compliance with the prescribed treatment program and thyroid status, testing for antibodies to human growth hormone should be carried out in any patient who fails to respond to therapy.

Additional short-term immunologic and renal function studies were carried out in a group of patients after approximately two years of treatment to detect other potential adverse effects of antibodies to growth hormone. The antibody was determined to be of the IgG class; no antibodies to growth hormone of the IgE class were detected. Testing included immune complex determination, measurement of total hemolytic complement and specific complement components, and immunochemical analyses. No adverse effects of growth hormone antibody formation were observed.

These findings are supported by a toxicity study conducted in a primate model in which a similar antibody response to growth hormone was observed. Somatrem, administered to monkeys by intramuscular injection at doses of 125 and 625 mcg/kg TIW, was compared to pituitary-human growth hormone at the same doses and with placebo over a period of 90 days. Most monkeys treated with high-dose somatrem developed persistent antibodies at week four. There were no biologically significant drug related changes in standard laboratory variables. Histopathologic examination of the kidney and other selected organs (pituitary, lungs, liver and pancreas) showed no treatment related toxicity. There was no evidence of immune complexes or immune complex toxicity when the kidney was also examined for the presence of immune complexes and possible toxic effects of immune complexes by immunohistochemistry and electron microscopy.

In studies in children treated with somatrem, injection site pain was reported infrequently.

Leukemia has been reported in a small number of growth hormone deficient patients treated with growth hormone. It is uncertain whether this increased risk is related to the pathology of growth hormone deficiency itself, growth hormone therapy, or other associated treatments such as radiation therapy for intracranial tumors. On the basis of current evidence, experts cannot conclude that growth hormone therapy is responsible for these occurrences. The risk to an individual patient, if any, remains to be established.

Other adverse drug reactions that have been reported in growth hormone-treated patients include the following: 1) Metabolic: Infrequent, mild and transient peripheral edema. 2) Musculoskeletal: Rare carpal tunnel syndrome. 3) Skin: Rare increased growth of pre-existing nevi. Malignant nevi transformation has not been reported. 4) Endocrine: Rare gynecomastia. Rare pancreatitis.

OVERDOSAGE:

The recommended dosage of up to 0.30 mg/kg (approximately 0.90 IU/kg) of body weight weekly should not be exceeded due to the potential risk of known effects of excess human growth hormone.

DOSAGE AND ADMINISTRATION:

A weekly dosage of 0.30 mg/kg (approximately 0.90 IU/kg) of body weight administered by daily intramuscular or subcutaneous injection is recommended.

The somatrem dosage and administration schedule should be individualized for each patient. Therapy should not be continued if final height is achieved or epiphyseal fusion occurs. Patients who fail to respond adequately while on somatrem therapy should be evaluated to determine the cause of unresponsiveness.

After the dose has been determined, reconstitute as follows: each 5 mg vial should be reconstituted with 1-5 ml of Bacteriostatic Water for Injection, USP (benzyl alcohol preserved); or each 10 mg vial should be reconstituted with 1-10 ml of Bacteriostatic Water for

DOSAGE AND ADMINISTRATION: *(cont'd)*

Injection, USP (benzyl alcohol preserved) only. For use in newborns see WARNINGS. The pH of somatrem after reconstitution with Bacteriostatic Water for Injection, USP (benzyl alcohol preserved) is approximately 7.8.

To prepare the somatrem solution, inject the Bacteriostatic Water for Injection, USP (benzyl alcohol preserved) into the somatrem vial, aiming the stream of liquid against the glass wall. Then swirl the product vial with a **GENTLE** rotary motion until the contents are completely dissolved. **DO NOT SHAKE**. Because somatrem is a protein, shaking can result in a cloudy solution. The somatrem solution should be clear immediately after reconstitution. Occasionally, after refrigeration, you may notice that small colorless particles of protein are present in the somatrem solution. This is not unusual for solutions containing proteins. If the solution is cloudy immediately after reconstitution or refrigeration, the contents **MUST NOT** be injected.

Before needle insertion, wipe the septum of both the somatrem and diluent vials with rubbing alcohol or an antiseptic solution to prevent contamination of the contents by microorganisms that may be introduced by repeated needle insertions. It is recommended that somatrem be administered using sterile, disposable syringes and needles. The syringes should be of small enough volume that the prescribed dose can be drawn from the vial with reasonable accuracy.

STABILITY AND STORAGE

Before Reconstitution: Somatrem (somatropin for injection), and Bacteriostatic Water for Injection, USP (benzyl alcohol preserved), must be stored at 2-8°C/36- 46°F (under refrigeration). **Avoid freezing the vials of somatrem and Bacteriostatic Water for Injection, USP (benzyl alcohol preserved).** Expiration dates are stated on the labels.

After Reconstitution: Vial contents are stable for 14 days when reconstituted with Bacteriostatic Water for Injection, USP (benzyl alcohol preserved) at 2-8°C/36-46°F (under refrigeration). Store the unused portion of Bacteriostatic Water for Injection, USP (benzyl alcohol preserved) at 2-8°C/36- 46°F (under refrigeration). **Avoid freezing the vials of somatrem and Bacteriostatic Water for Injection, USP (benzyl alcohol preserved).**

HOW SUPPLIED:

Somatrem for injection is supplied as 5 mg (approximately 15 IU) or 10 mg (approximately 30 IU) of lyophilized, sterile, somatrem per vial.

Each 5 mg carton contains two vials of Somatrem (somatrem for injection) (5 mg per vial) and one 10 ml multiple dose vial of Bacteriostatic Water for Injection, USP (benzyl alcohol preserved).

Each 10 mg carton contains two vials of somatrem for injection (10 mg per vial) and two 10 ml multiple dose vials of Bacteriostatic Water for Injection, USP (benzyl alcohol preserved). NDC 50242-016-20

HOW SUPPLIED - EQUIVALENTS NOT AVAILABLE:

Injection, Lyphl-Soln - Intramuscular; - 10 mg/vial

2's	$840.00	PROTROPIN, Genentech	50242-0016-20

Kit - Intramuscular - 5 mg/vial

2's	$420.00	PROTROPIN, 10ML WATER, Genentech	50242-0015-02

SOMATROPIN, BIOSYNTHETIC *(002266)*

CATEGORIES: Anterior Pituitary/Hypothalmic Function; Growth Failure; Hormones; Human Growth Hormone; Orphan Drugs; Pituitary; Turner's Syndrome*; Recombinant DNA Origin; Sales > $500 Million; FDA Approved 1987 Mar; Pregnancy Category B

* Indication not approved by the FDA

BRAND NAMES: Bio-Tropin; Genotropin; **Humatrope**; Norditropin; Nutropin; Saizen; Serostim

FORMULARIES: Aetna

DESCRIPTION:

Somatropin, (rDNA Origin) for Injection, is a human growth hormone (hGH) produced by recombinant DNA technology. Somatropin has 191 amino acid residues and a molecular weight of 22,125 daltons. The amino acid sequence of the product is identical to that of pituitary-derived human growth hormone. The protein is synthesized by a specific laboratory strain of *E. coli* as a precursor consisting of the rhGH molecule preceded by the secretion signal from an *E. coli* protein. This precursor is directed to the plasma membrane of the cell. The signal sequence is removed and the native protein is secreted into the periplasm so that the protein is folded appropriately as it is synthesized.

Somatropin is a highly purified preparation. Biological potency is determined by measuring the increase in body weight induced in hypophysectomized rats.

Somatropin is a sterile, white, lyophilized powder intended for subcutaneous administration after reconstitution with Bacteriostatic Water for Injection, USP (benzyl alcohol preserved). Some brand smay be administered intramuscularly.

CLINICAL PHARMACOLOGY:

GENERAL

In vitro preclinical, and clinical testing have demonstrated that somatropin is therapeutically equivalent to pituitary-derived human growth hormone. Clinical studies in normal adults also demonstrated equivalent pharmacokinetic.

Treatment of children who lack adequate endogenous growth hormone secretion with Nutropin resulted in an increase in growth rate and an increase in insulin-like growth factor-I levels similar to that seen with pituitary-derived human growth hormone.

Actions that have been demonstrated for somatropin, somatrem and/or pituitary-derived human growth hormone include:

Tissue Growth:

1) Skeletal Growth: Somatropin stimulates skeletal growth in prepubertal children with pituitary growth hormone deficiency. Skeletal growth is accomplished at the epiphyseal plates at the ends of long bone. Growth and metabolism of epiphyseal plate cells are directly stimulated by growth hormone and one of its mediators, insulin-like growth factor-I. Serum levels of insulin-like growth factor-I are low in children and adolescents who are growth hormone deficient, but increase during treatment with somatropin. Linear growth continues until these growth plates fuse at the end of puberty.

2) Cell Growth: Treatment with pituitary-derived human growth hormone results in an increase in both the number and the size of skeletal muscle cells.

3) Organ Growth: Growth hormone of human pituitary origin influences the size and function of internal organs and increases red cell mass. Somatropin has been shown to promote similar organ weight increase to pituitary human growth hormone in an adequate animal model.

CLINICAL PHARMACOLOGY: *(cont'd)*

Protein Metabolism: Linear growth is facilitated in part by growth hormone-stimulated protein synthesis. This is reflected by increased cellular uptake of amino acids and notrogen retention as demonstrated by a decline in urinary nitrogen excretion and blood urea nitrogen during growth hormone therapy.

Carbohydrate Metabolism: Growth hormone is a modulator of carbohydrate metabolism. Children with inadequate secretion of growth hormone sometimes experience fasting hypoglycemia that is improved by treatment with growth hormone. Saizen therapy may decrease glucose tolerance. Administration of Somatropin to normal adults, patients with hrowth hormone deficiency resulted in transient increases in mean serum fasting and postprandial insulin levels. However, mean glucose levels remained in the normal range.

Lipid Metabolism: Acute administration of human growth hormone to humans results in lipid mobilization. Nonesterified fatty acids increased in plasma within one hour of Somatropin administration. In growth hormone deficient patients, long-term growth hormone administration often decreases body fat. Mean cholesterol levels decreased in patients treated with Somatropin. The clinical significance of this is unknown.

Mineral Metabolism: Human growth hormone administration results in the retention of total body potassium, phosphorus, and sodium. Serum calcium levels appear to be unaffected.

Connective Tissue Metabolism: Growth hormone stimulates the synthesis of chondroitin sulfate and collagen as well as the urinary excretion of hydroxyproline.

PHARMACOKINETICS

Absorption: The absolute bioavailability of recombinant growth hormone (r-hGH) after subcutaneous administration ranges between 70-90%.

Distribution: The mean volume of distribution of r-hGH given to healthy volunteers was estimated to be 12.0 ± 1.08 L.

Metabolism: The metabolic rate of somatropin involves classical catabolism in both the liver and kidneys. In renal cells, at least a portion of the breakdown products is returned to the systemic circulation. The mean half-life of intravenous somatropin in normal males is 0.6 hours, whereas subcutaneously and intramuscularly administered somatropin has a half-life of 1.75 and 3.4 hours, respectively. The longer half-life observed after subcutaneous or intramuscular administration is due to slow absorption from the injection site.

Excretion: The mean clearance of intravenously administered r-hGH in six normal male volunteers was 14.6 ± 2.8 L/hr.

Nutropin

When compared to intravenous administration, approximately 80% of 1.5 mg somatropin for injection was systemically available following subcutaneous injection in the thigh in a study using healthy male sublects. In another study involving healthy male subjects following a subcutaneous injection dose of 0.033 mg/kg in the thigh, the extent of absorption (AUC) for 5mg/ml somatropin for injection was 35% greater than that for 1.3 mg/ml somatropin for injection. The mean (+ standard deviation) peak (C_{max}) serum levels were 35.5 (+14.5) ng/ml and 26.8 (+14.2) ng/ml, respectlvely. In a study involving children with growth hormone deficiency, 5 mg/ml somatropin for injection following a subcutaneous injection dose of 0.033 mg/kg in the thigh, had a mean AUC that was 17% greater than 1.3 mg/ml somatropin for injection. The mean (C_{max}) levels were 32.4 ng/ml and 25.2 ng/ml, respectively.

Mean (C_{max}) levels were all achieved at approximately 3 to 4 hours and the apparent terminal half-life ($T_{1/2}$) is approximately 2 hours following subcutaneous injection.

The pharmacokinetics of Nutropin have been investigated in healthy men after the subcutaneous administration of 0.1 mg/kg of body weight. A mean peak concentration (C_{max}) of 56.1 ng/ml occurred at a mean time of 7.5 hrs. The extent of absorption of Nutropin, assessed by area under the concentration versus time curve (AUC), was 626 ng·hr/ml and closely compares with that of somatrem (590 ng · hr/ml). The AUC of Nutropin is similar regardless of injection site.

Growth hormone localizes to highly perfused organs, most notably liver and kidney. In the kidney, growth hormone is filtered by the glomerulus, reabsorbed in the proximal tubule, and is broken down within renal cells into amino acids which return to the circulation.

In both normal and growth hormone deficient adults and children, the intramuscular and subcutaneous pharmacokinetic profiles of somatropin are similar regardless of type of growth hormone or dosing regimen used. The subcutaneous pharmacokinetic profile of Nutropin is comparable to estimates in the published literature. A small number of dose-ranging studies suggest that clearance and AUC of somatropin is proportional to dose in the therapeutic dose range. Consistent with the role of the liver and kidney as major elimination organs for exogenously administered human growth hormone, there is a reduction in growth hormone clearance in patients with severe liver or kidney dysfunction.

Effects of Nutropin on Growth Failure Due to Chronic Renal Insufficiency (CRI) Two multicenter, randomized, controlled clinical trials were conducted to determine whether treatment with Nutropin prior to renal transplantation in children with chronic renal insufficiency could improve their growth rates and height deficits. One study was a double-blinded, placebo-controlled trial and the other was an open-label, randomized trial. The dose of Nutropin in both controlled studies was 0.05 mg/kg/day (0.35 mg/kg/wk) administered daily by subcutaneous injection. Combining the data from those patients completing two years in the two controlled studies results in 62 children treated with Nutropin and 28 children in the control groups (either placebo-treated or untreated). The mean first growth rate was 10.8 cm/yr for Nutropin-treated patients, compared with a mean growth rate of 6.5 cm/yr for placebo/untreated controls (p<0.00005). The mean second year growth rate was 7.8 cm/yr for the Nutropin-treated group, compared with 5.5 cm/yr for controls (p<0.00005). There was a significant increase in mean height standard deviation score in the Nutropin group (-2.9 at baseline to -1.5 at Month 24, n=62) but no significant change in the controls (-2.8 at baseline to -2.9 at Month 24, n=28). The mean third year growth rate of 7.6 cm/yr in the Nutropin-treated patients (n=27) suggests that Nutropin stimulates growth beyond two years. However, there are no control data for the third year because control patients crossed over to growth hormone treatment after two years of participation. The gains in height were accompanied by appropriate advancement of skeletal age. These data demonstrate that Nutropin therapy improves growth rate and corrects the acquired height deficit associated with chronic renal insufficiency. Currently there are insufficient data regarding the benefit of treatment beyond three years. Although predicted final height was improved during Nutropin therapy, the effect of Nutropin on final adult height remains to be determined.

Post-Transplant Growth: The North American Pediatric Renal Transplant Cooperative Study (NAPRTCS) has reported data for growth post-transplant in children who did not receive growth hormone. The average change in height SD score during the initial two years post-transplant was 0.18 (n=300, J Ped 1993; 122:397-402).

Controlled studies of growth hormone treatment for the short stature associated with CRI were not designed to compare the growth of treated or untreated patients after they received renal transplants. However, growth data are available from a small number of patients who have been followed for at least 11 months. Of the 7 control patients, 4 increased their height SD score and 3 had either no significant change or a decrease in height SD score. The 13 patients treated with Nutropin prior to transplant had either no significant change or an increase in height SD score after transplantation, indicating that the individual gains achieved

CLINICAL PHARMACOLOGY: *(cont'd)*

with growth hormone therapy prior to transplant were maintained after transplantation. The differences in the height deficit narrowed between the treated and untreated groups in the post-transplant period.

SPECIAL POPULATIONS

Pediatric: The pharmacokinetics of r-hGH is similar in children and adults.

Gender: No gender studies have been performedin children. In adults, the clearance of r-hGH in both men and women tends to be similar.

Race: No data available.

Renal Insuffiency: Children and adults with chronic renal failure tend to have decreased clearance of r-hGH as compared to normals.

Hepatic Insuffiency: A reduction in r-hGH clearance has been noted in patients with hepatic dysfunction as compared with normal controls.

INDICATIONS AND USAGE:

Somatropin (rDNA origin) for injection is indicated for the long-term treatment of children who have growth failure due to a lack of adequate endogenous growth hormone secretion.

Somatropin is also indicated for the treatment of children who have growth failure associated with chronic renal insufficiency up to the time of renal transplantation. Somatropin therapy should be used in conjunction with optimal management of chronic renal insufficiency.

CONTRAINDICATIONS:

Somatropin should not be used in subjects with closed epiphyses.

Somatropin should not be used in patients with active neoplasia. Growth hormone therapy should be discontinued if evidence of neoplasia develops.

Humatrope should not be used when there is any evidence of activity of a tumor. Intracranial lesions must be inactive and antitumor therapy complete prior to the institution of therapy. Humatrope should be discontinued if there is evidence of tumor growth.

Somatropin, when reconstituted with Bacteriostatic Water for Injection, USP (benzyl alcohol preserved) should not be used in patients with a known sensitivity to benzyl alcohol.

Caution should be used if growth hormone is administered to children with diabetes mellitus.

WARNINGS:

Benzyl alcohol as a preservative in Bacteriostatic Water for Injection, USP has been associated with toxicity in newborns. If sensitivity to the dilutent occurs, somatropin may be reconstituted with Sterile Water for Injection, USP. When somatropin is reconsitiuted in this manner, the reconstituted solution should be discarded immediately and any unused solution should be discarded.

PRECAUTIONS:

General: Therapy with Humatrope should be directed by physicians who are experienced in the diagnosis and management of patients with growth hormone deficiency.

Because somatropin may induce a state of insulin resistance, patients should be monitored for evidence of glucose intolerance.

Patients with a history of an intracranial lesion taking somatropin should be examined frequently for progression or recurrence of the lesion.

Patients with growth failure secondary to chronic renal insufficiency should be examined periodically for evidence of progression of renal osteodystrophy. Slipped capital femoral epiphysis or avascular necrosis of the femoral head may be seen in children with advanced renal osteodystrophy, and it is uncertain whether these problems are affected by growth hormone therapy. X-rays of the hip should be obtained prior to initiating therapy. Physicians and parents should be alert to the development of a limp or complaints of hip or knee pain in patients treated with somatropin.

Progression of scoliosis can occur in children who experience rapid growth. Because growth hormone increases growth rate, patients with a history of scoliosis who are treated with growth hormone should be monitored for progression of scoliosis. Growth hormone has not been shown to increase the incidence of scoliosis.

Bone age should be monitored periodically during somatropin administration especially in patients who are pubertal and/or receiving concomitant thyroid replacement therapy. Under these circumstances, epiphyseal maturation may progress rapidly.

Patients with growth hormone deficiency secondary to an intracranial lesion should be examined frequently for progression or recurrence of the underlying disease process.

Because human growth hormone may induce a state of insulin resistance, patients should be observed for evidence of glucose intolerance.

Excessive glucocorticoid therapy will inhibit the growth promoting effect of human growth hormone. Patients with coexisting ACTH deficiency should have their glucocorticoid replacement dose carefully adjusted to avoid an inhibitory effect on growth.

Hypothyroidism may develop during treatment with human growth hormone, and inadequate treatment of hypothyroidism may prevent optimal response to human growth hormone. Therefore, patients should have periodic thyroid function tests and be treated with thyroid hormone when indicated.

Patients with endocrine disorders, including growth hormone deficiency, may develop slipped capital epiphyses more frequently. Any child with the onset of a limp during growth hormone therapy should be evaluated.

Intracranial hypertension (IH) with papilledema, visual changes, headache, nausea and/or vomiting has been reported in a small number of patients treated with growth hormone products. Symptoms usually occurred within the first eight weeks of the initiation of growth hormone therapy. In all reported cases, IH-associated signs and symptoms resolved after termination of therapy or a reduction of the growth hormone dose. Funduscopic examination of patients is recommended at the initiation and periodically during the course of growth hormone therapy.

When growth hormone is administered subcutaneously at the same site over a long period of time, lipodystrophy may result. This can be avoided by rotating the injection site.

As for any protein, local or systemic allergic reactions may occur. Parents/Patient should be informed that such reactions are possible and that prompt medical attention should be sought if allergic reactions occur.

See WARNINGS for use of Bacteriostatic Water for Injection, USP (benzyl alcohol preserved) in newborns.

Laboratory Tests: Serum levels of inorganic phosphorus, alkaline phosphatase, and parathyroid hormone (PTH) may increase with somatropin therapy. Changes in thyroid hormone laboratory measurements may develop during somatropin treatment in children who lack adequate endogenous growth hormone secretion. Untreated hypothyroidism prevents optimal response to somatropin. Therefore, patients should have periodic thyroid function tests and should be treated with thyroid hormone when indicated.

Serum levels of inorganic phosphorus, alkaline phosphatase, and IGF-1 may increase with Somatropin therapy.

PRECAUTIONS: *(cont'd)*

Information for the Patient: Patients being treated with growth hormone and/or their parents should be informed of the potential benefits and risks associated with treatment. If home use is determined to be desirable by the physician, instructions on appropriate use should be given, including a review of the contents of the Patient Information Insert. This information is intended to aid in the safe and effective administration of the medication. It is not a disclosure of all possible adverse or intended effects.

If home use is prescribed, a puncture resistant container for the disposal of used syringes and needles should be recommended to the patient. Patients and/or parents should be thoroughly instructed in the importance of proper disposal and cautioned against any reuse of needles and syringes.

Carcinogenesis, Mutagenesis, and Impairment of Fertility: Carcinogenicity, mutagenicity and reproduction studies have not been conducted with somatropin. No potential mutagenicity of rhGH was revealed in a battery of tests including the Ames test, induction of gene mutations in mammalian cells (LS1 78Y) in vitro and in intact bone marrow cells (rats). See Pregancy for effect on fertility.

Pregnancy Category B: Reproduction studies carried out with somatropin for injection at doses of 1, 3 and 10 IU/kg/day subcutaneously in the rat and 0.25, 1 and 4 IU/kg/day intramuscularly in the rabbit (doses approximately 80 times and 32 times the recommended human therapeutic levels, respectively) showed decreased maternal body weight gains but were not teratogenic. In rats dosed subcutaneously during gametogenesis and up to seven days of pregnancy, 10 IU/kg/day (approximately 80 times human dose) produced anestrus or extended estrus cycles in females and fewer and less motile sperm in males. When given to pregnant female rats (days 1-7 of gestation) at 10 IU/kg/day a very slight increase in fetal deaths was observed. At 3 IU/kg/day (approximately 24 times human dose) rats showed slightly extended estrus cycles whereas at 1 IU/kg/day no effects were noted. Peri- and post-natal studies in rats dosed with somatropin for injection at doses of 1, 3 and 10 IU/kg/day produced growth promoting effects in the dams but not in the fetuses of young rats at the highest dose showed increased weight gain during suckling but the effect was not apparent by 10 weeks of age. No adverse effects were observed on gestation, morphogenesis, parturition, lactation, post-natal development or reproductive capacity of the offsprings due to somatropin for injection. There are, however, no adequate and well-controlled studies in pregnant woman. Because animal reproduction studies are not always predictive of human response, this drug should be used during pregnancy only if clearly needed.

Reproduction studies have been performed in rats and rabbits at doses up to 31 and 62 times, respectively, the human (child) weekly dose based on body surface area. The results have revealed no evidence of impaired fertility or harm to the fetus due to somatropin. There are, however, no adequate and well controlled studies in pregnant women. Because animal reproduction studies are not always predictive of human response, this drug should be used during pregnancy only if clearly needed.

Nursing Mothers: It is not known whether this drug is excreted in human milk. Because many drugs are excreted in human milk, caution should be exercised when somatropin is administered to a nursing woman.

DRUG INTERACTIONS:

The use of somatropin in patients with chronic renal insufficiency receiving glucocorticoid therapy has not been evaluated. Concomitant glucocorticoid therapy may inhibit the growth promoting effect of somatropin. If glucocorticoid replacement is required, the dose should be carefully adjusted.

There was no evidence in the controlled studies of somatropin's interaction with drugs commonly used in chronic renal insufficiency patients. However, formal drug interaction studies have not been conducted.

ADVERSE REACTIONS:

Nutropin: As with all protein drugs, a small number of patients may develop antibodies to the protein. Growth hormone antibody with binding lower than 2 mg/L has not been associated with growth attenuation. In some cases, when binding capaclty is >2mg/L, interference with growth response has been observed.

In 419 patients evaluated in clinical studies with somatropin for injection, 244 had been treated previously with somatropin for injection or other growth hormone preparations and 175 patients had received no previous growth hormone therapy. Antibodies to growth hormone (anti-hGH antibodies), were present in 6 previously treated patients at baseline. Three of the six became negative for anti-hGH antibodies during 6 to 12 months of treatment with somatropin for injection. Of the remaining 413, eight (1.9%) developed detectable anti-hGH antibodies during somatropin for injection treatment, none had an antibody binding capacity > 2 mg/L. There was no evidence that the growth response to somatropin for injection was affected in these antibody positive patients. Somatropin for injection preparations contain a small amount of periplasmic *Escherichia coli* peptides (PECP). Anti-PECP antibodies are found in a small number of patients treated with somatropin for injection, but these appear to be of no clinical significance. In clinical studies with somatropin for injection, the following events were reported infrequently: injection site reactions, e.g., pain or burning associated with the injection, fibrosis, nodules, rash, inflammation, pigmentation, bleeding; lipoatrophy; headache; hematuria; hypothyroidism; mild hyperglycemia.

Leukemia has been reported in a small number of growth hormone deficient patients treated with growth hormone. It is uncertain whether this increased risk is related to the pathology of growth hormone deficiency itself, growth hormone therapy, or other associated treatments such as radiation therapy for intracranial tumors. On the basis of current evidence, experts cannot conclude that growth hormone therapy is responsible for these occurrences. There have been no reports of leukemia in growth hormone-treated CRI patients. The risk to GHI and CRI patients, if any, remains to be established.

Other adverse drug reactions that have been reported in growth hormone-treated patients include the following: *1) Metabolic:* Infrequent, mild and transient peripheral edema. *2) Musculoskeletal:* Rare, carpal tunnel syndrome. *3) Skin:* Rare, increased growth of pre-existing nevi. Malignant nevi transformation has not been reported. *4) Endocrine:* Rare, gynecomastia. Rare, pancreatitis.

Humatrope: Approximately 2% of 481 naive and previously treated clinical trial patients treated with Humatrope have developed antibodies to growth hormone, as demonstrated by a binding capacity determination threshold ≥0.02 mcg/ml. Nevertheless, even these patients experienced increases in linear growth and other salutary effects of Humatrope and did not experience any unusual adverse events. Although growth-limiting antibodies have been observed with other growth hormone preparations (including products of pituitary origin), antibodies in patients treated with Humatrope have not limited growth. The long-term implications of antibody development are uncertain at this time.

Of the 232 naive and previously treated clinical trial patients receiving Humatrope for 6 months or more, 4.7% had serum binding of radiolabeled growth hormone in excess of twice the binding observed in control sera when the serum samples were assayed at a tenfold dilution. Among these patients were 160 naive patients, of whom 6.9% had positive serum

ADVERSE REACTIONS: *(cont'd)*

binding. In comparison, 74.5% of 106 naive patients treated for 6 months or more with somatrem (produced by Lilly) in a similar clinical trial had serum binding of radiolabeled growth hormone of at least twice the binding observed in control sera.

In addition to an evaluation of compliance with the treatment program and of thyroid status, testing for antibodies to human growth hormone should be carried out in any patient who fails to respond to therapy.

In clinical studies in which high doses of Humatrope were administered to healthy adult volunteers, the following events occurred infrequently: headache, localized muscle pain, weakness, mild hyperglycemia, and glucosuria. In studies with growth-hormone-deficient children, injection site pain was reported infrequently. A mild and transient edema, which appeared in 2.5% of patients, was observed early during the course of treatment.

Leukemia has been reported in a small number of children who have been treated with growth hormone, including growth hormone of pituitary origin as well as of recombinant DNA origin (somatrem and somatropin). The relationship, if any, between leukemia and growth hormone therapy is uncertain.

Saizen: As with all protein pharmaceuticals, a small pecentage of patients may develop antibodies to the protein. Anti-growth hormone (GH) antibody capacities below 2 mg/L have not been associated with growth attentuation. In some cases when binding capacity exceeds 2 mg/L, growth attentuation has been described. In clinical studies with Saizen involving 280 patients (204 naive and 76 transfer patinets), one patient 6 months of therapy developed anti-GH antibodies with binding capacities exceeding 2 mg/L. Despite the high binding capacity, these antibodies were not growing attenuating. The patient was subsequently shown to have a hGH-N gene defect. Thus, genetic analysis should be undertaken in any patinet in whom anti-GH antibodies with high binding capacities occur. No antibodies against proteins of the host cells were detected in the sera of patinets treated up to five years.

Any patinets with well-documented growth hormone deficiency who fails to respond to therapy should be tested for antibodies to human growth hormone and for thyroid status.

In clinical studies in which Saizen was administered to growth hormone deficient patients children, the following events were infrequently seen: local reactions at the injection site (such as pain, numbness, redness and swelling), hypothyroidism, hypoglycemia, seizures, exacerbation of pre-exisitng psoriasis and disturbances in fluid bablance.

Leukemia has been reported in a small number of growth hormone deficient patients treated with growth hormone. It is uncertain whether this increased risk is related to the pathology of growth hormone deficiency itself, groeth hormone therapy, or other associated treatments such as radiation therapy for intracranial tumors. So far, epidemiological data fail to confirm the hypothesis of a relationship between growth hormone therapy and leukemia.

OVERDOSAGE:

Acute overdosage could lead initially to hypoglycemia and subsequently to hyperglycemia. Long-term overdosage could result in signs and symptoms of gigantism/acromegaly consistent with the known effects of excess human growth hormone.

DOSAGE AND ADMINISTRATION:

NUTROPIN

Somatropin for injection may be given in the thigh, buttocks or abdomen, the site of subcutaneous injections should be rotated daily in an attempt to prevent lipoatrophy.

Growth Hormone Inadequacy (GHI): A weekly dosage of 0.30 mg/kg (approximately 0.90 IU/kg) of body weight administered by daily subcutaneous injection is recommended.

The Nutropin dosage and administration schedule for GHI should be individualized for each patient. Therapy should not be continued if final height is achieved or epiphyseal fusion occurs. Patients who fail to respond adequately while on Nutropin therapy should be evaluated to determine the cause of unresponsiveness.

Chronic Renal Insufficiency (CRI): A weekly dosage of 0.35 mg/kg (approximately 1.05 IU/kg) of body weight administered by daily subcutaneous injection is recommended.

The duration of Nutropin therapy for CRI should be individualized for each patient.

Nutropin therapy may be continued up to the time of renal transplantation. Therapy should not be continued if final height is achieved or epiphyseal fusion occurs. Patients who fail to respond adequately while on Nutropin therapy should be evaluated to determine the cause of unresponsiveness.

In order to optimize therapy for patients who require dialysis, the following guidelines for injection schedule are recommended:

1. Hemodialysis patients should receive their injection at night just prior to going to sleep or at least 3-4 hours after their hemodialysis to prevent hematoma formation due to the heparin.

2. Chronic Cycling Peritoneal Dialysis (CCPD) patients should receive their injection in the morning after they have completed dialysis.

3. Chronic Ambulatory Peritoneal Dialysis (CAPD) patients should receive their injection in the evening at the time of the overnight exchange.

After the dose has been determined, reconstitute as follows: each 5 mg vial should be reconstituted with 1-5 ml of Bacteriostatic Water for Injection, USP (benzyl alcohol preserved); or each 10 mg vial should be reconstituted with 1-10 ml of Bacteriostatic Water for Injection, USP (benzyl alcohol preserved) only. For use in newborns see WARNINGS. The pH of Nutropin after reconstitution with Bacteriostatic Water for Injection, USP (benzyl alcohol preserved) is approximately 7.4.

To prepare the Nutropin solution, inject the Bacteriostatic Water for Injection, USP (benzyl alcohol preserved) into the Nutropin vial, aiming the stream of liquid against the glass wall. Then swirl the product vial with a GENTLE rotary motion until the contents are completely dissolved. DON NOT SHAKE. Because Nutropin is a protein, shaking can result in a cloudy solution. The Nutropin solution should be clear immediately after reconstitution. Occasionally, after refrigeration, you may notice that small colorless particles of protein are present in the Nutropin solution. This is not unusual for solutions containing proteins. If the solution is cloudy immediately after reconstitution or refrigeration, the contents MUST NOT be injected.

Before needle insertion, wipe the septum of both the Nutropin and diluent vials with rubbing alcohol or an antiseptic solution to prevent contamination of the contents by microorganisms that may be introduced by repeated needle insertions. It is recommended that Nutropin be administered using sterile, disposable syringes and needles. The syringes should be of small enough volume that the prescribed dose can be drawn from the vial with reasonable accuracy.

Stability And Storage

Before Reconstitution: Nutropin [somatropin (rDNA origin) for injection], and Bacteriostatic Water for Injection, USP (benzyl alcohol preserved), must be stored at 2- 8°C/36-46°F (under refrigeration). **Avoid freezing the vials of Nutropin and Bacteriostatic Water for Injection, USP (benzyl alcohol preserved).**Expiration dates are stated on the labels.

After Reconstitution: Vial contents are stable for 14 days when reconstituted with Bacteriostatic Water for Injection, USP (benzyl alcohol preserved) and stored at 2-8°C/36-46°F (under refrigeration). Store the unused portion of Bacteriostatic Water for Injection, USP (benzyl alcohol preserved) at 2-8°C/36- 46°F (under refrigeration). **Avoid freezing the reconstituted vial of Nutropin and the Bacteriostatic Water for Injection, USP (benzyl alcohol preserved).**

DOSAGE AND ADMINISTRATION: *(cont'd)*

HUMATROPE

The recommended weekly dosage is 0.18 mg/kg (0.48 IU/kg) of body weight. It should be divided into equal doses given either on 3 alternate days or 6 times per week. The maximal replacement dosage is 0.1 mg/kg (0.267 IU/kg) administered 3 times a week. The route of administration should be by subcutaneous or intramuscular injection. The dosage and administration schedule for Humatrope should be individualized for each patient.

Each 5-mg vial of Humatrope should be reconstituted with 1.5 to 5 ml of Diluent for Humatrope. The diluent should be injected into the vial of Humatrope by aiming the stream of liquid against the glass wall. Following reconstitution, the vial should be swirled with a GENTLE rotary motion until the contents are completely dissolved. DO NOT SHAKE. The resulting solution should be clear, without particulate matter. If the solution is cloudy or contains particulate matter, the contents MUST NOT be injected.

Before and after injection, the septum of the vial should be wiped with rubbing alcohol or an alcoholic antiseptic solution to prevent contamination of the contents by repeated needle insertion. Sterile disposable syringes and/or needles should be used for administration of Humatrope. The volume of the syringe should be small enough so that the prescribed dose can be withdrawn from the vial with reasonable accuracy.

Stability And Storage

Before Reconstitution: Vials of Humatrope as well as the Diluent for Humatrope are stable when refrigerated (36° to 46°F [2° to 8°C]). Avoid freezing Diluent for Humatrope. Expiration dates are stated on the labels.

After Reconstitution: Vials of Humatrope are stable for up to 14 days when reconstituted with Diluent for Humatrope and stored in a refrigerator at 36° to 46°F (2° to 8°C). Avoid freezing the reconstituted vial of Humatrope.

SAIZEN

Saizen dosage and schedule of administration should be individualized for each patient. For the treatment of growth hormone inadequacy, a dosage of 0.06 mg/kg (approximately 0.18 IU/kg) administered 3 times per week by subcutaneous or intramuscular injection is recommended.

Treatment with Saizen of growth failure due to growth hormone deficiency should be discontinued when epiphyses are fused. Patients who fail to respond adequately while on Saizen therapy should be evaluated to determine the cause of unresponsiveness.

To prevent possible contamination, wipe the rubber vial stopper with an antiseptic solution before puncturing it with the needle. It is recommended that Saizen be administered using sterile, disposable syringes and needles. The syringes should be small enough volume that the prescribed dose cn be drawn from the vial with reasonable accuracy.

After determining the appropriate patient dose, reconstitute each 5 mg vial of Saizen with 1-3 ml of Bacteriostatic Water for Injection, USP (benzlu alcohol preserved). For use in patinets sensitive to the diluent (see WARNINGS).

To reconstitute Saizen, inject the diluent into the vial of Saizen aiming the liquid against the glass wall. Swirl the vial with a GENTLE rotary motion until contents are disolved completely. DO NOT SHAKE. Because Siazen groeth hormone is a protein, shaking can result in a cloudy solution. The Saizen solution should be clear immediately after reconstitution. DO NOT INJECT Saizen if the reconstituted product is cloudy immediately after reconstitution or refrigeration. Occasionally, after refrigeration, small colorless particles may be present in the Saizen solution. This is not unusual for proteins like Saizen.

Stability And Storage

Before Reconstitution: Saizen should be store at room temperature (15°-30°C/59°-86°F). Expiration dates are stated on the labels.

After Reconstitution: When reconstiuted with the diluent provided, the reconstituted solution should be stored under refrigeration (2° to 8°C/36° to 46°F) for up to 14 days. Avoid freezing the reconstituted vials of Saizen.

HOW SUPPLIED - RATED THERAPEUTICALLY EQUIVALENT:

Injection, Dry-Soln - Intramuscular - 5 mg/vial

1's	$420.00	NUTROPIN, Genentech	50242-0072-02

Injection, Dry-Soln - Intramuscular - 10 mg/vial

1's	$840.00	NUTROPIN, Genentech	50242-0018-20

HOW SUPPLIED - NOT RATED EQUIVALENT:

Injection - Subcutaneous - 1.5 mg

1.3 mg/ml	$315.00	GENOTROPIN, Pharmacia & Upjohn	00013-2606-94

Injection - Subcutaneous - 5.8 mg

5 mg/ml x 1	$210.00	GENOTROPIN, Pharmacia & Upjohn	00013-2616-81
5 mg/ml x 5	$1050.00	GENOTROPIN, Pharmacia & Upjohn	00013-2616-94

Injection, Dry-Soln - Intramuscular - 5 mg

5 mg x 6	**$1260.05**	**HUMATROPE 5, Lilly**	**00002-7335-16**

Injection, Dry-Soln - Intramuscular - 5 mg/vial

5 mg x 7	$1050.00	SEROSTIM, Serono Labs	44087-1006-05

Powder for Injection - Subcutaneous or - 5 mg

5 mg	$210.00	SAIZEN, Serono Labs	44087-1005-02

SORBITOL *(002267)*

CATEGORIES: Electrolytic, Caloric-Water Balance; Gastrointestinal Drugs; Irrigating Solutions; FDA Approval Pre 1982

DESCRIPTION:

FOR UROLOGIC IRRIGATION ONLY

Each 100 ml contains: Sorbitol (from Sorbitol Solution USP) 3.3 g; Water for Injection USP qs; PH: 5.3

Calculated Osmolarity: Approx. 183 MOSM/liter

Sorbitol ($C_6H_{14}O_6$), an isomer of mannitol, is a hexitol naturally occurring in many fruits, and is produced synthetically for commercial purposes by catalytic reduction of glucose.

3.3% Sorbitol Irrigation is a prediluted, sterile, nonpyrogenic aqueous solution suitable for urologic irrigation. The solution is slightly hypotonic.

The plastic container is a copolymer of ethylene and propylene formulated and developed for parenteral drugs. The copolymer contains no plasticizers and exhibits virtually no leachability. The plastic container is also virtually impermeable to vapor transmission and therefore, requires no overwrap to maintain the proper drug concentration. The safety of the plastic

DESCRIPTION: *(cont'd)*

container has been confirmed by biological evaluation procedures. The material passes Class VI testing as specified in the U.S. Pharmacopeia for Biological Tests - Plastic Containers. These tests have shown that the container is nontoxic and biologically inert.

CLINICAL PHARMACOLOGY:

In humans, sorbitol is nontoxic and rapidly metabolized. It will be either metabolized 70% to carbon dioxide and 30% to dextrose and/or excreted by the kidneys.

As a 3.3% solution, sorbitol is recommended for irrigation of the urinary bladder and prostatic bed during transurethral prostatectomy. Unlike dextrose solutions, sorbitol solutions are not sticky, and if administered in the above dilution, are not hemolytic.

INDICATIONS AND USAGE:

3.3% Sorbitol Irrigation is indicated for use as a urologic irrigation fluid.

CONTRAINDICATIONS:

3.3% Sorbitol Irrigations is not for injection. It is contraindicated in patients with anuria.

WARNINGS:

Solutions for urologic irrigation must be used with caution in patients with severe cardiopulmonary or renal dysfunction.

Since irrigating fluids used during transurethral prostatectomy have been demonstrated to enter the systemic circulation in relatively large volumes, any irrigation solution must be regarded as a systemic drug. Absorption of large amounts of fluids containing sorbitol and the resultant osmotic diuresis may significantly affect cardiopulmonary and renal dynamics.

After opening container, it's contents should be used promptly to minimize the possibility of bacterial growth or pyrogen formation.

Discard unused portion of irrigating solution since it contains no preservative.

Do not warm above 150 deg. F (66 deg. C).

Hyperglycemia from metabolism of sorbitol may occur in patients with diabetes mellitus.

3.3% Sorbitol Irrigation must be used with caution in patients unable to metabolize sorbitol rapidly enough to avoid the development of hyperosmolar states.

PRECAUTIONS:

Cardiovascular status, especially in patients with cardiac disease, should be carefully determined before and during transurethral resection of the prostate when using sorbitol irrigation as an irrigant. The fluid absorbed into the systemic circulation via severed prostatic veins may produce significant extracellular fluid expansion and lead to fulminating congestive heart failure.

Shift of sodium-free intracellular fluid into the extracellular compartment following systemic absorption of 3.3% Sorbitol Irrigation may lower serum sodium concentration and aggravate pre-existing hyponatremia.

Excessive loss of water and electrolytes may lead to serious imbalances. Continuous administration of 3.3% Sorbitol Irrigation may cause loss of water in excess of electrolytes and produce hypernatremia.

Excessive loss of water and electrolytes may lead to serious imbalances. Continuous administration of 3.3% Sorbitol Irrigation may cause loss of water in excess of electrolytes and produce hypernatremia.

Sustained diuresis from transurethral irrigation with 3.3% Sorbitol Irrigation may obscure and intensify inadequate hydration or hypovolemia.

Use only if solution is clear and container and seal are intact.

ADVERSE REACTIONS:

Occasional adverse reactions may occur which include slight increases in postoperative serum glucose, inhibition of intestinal absorption of vitamin B12, fluid and electrolyte disturbances, such as acidosis, electrolyte loss, edema, dryness of the mouth, thirst and dehydration, cardiovascular/pulmonary disorders such as pulmonary congestion, hypotension, tachycardia and angina-like pains. In addition, patients unable to metabolize sorbitol rapidly enough may develop hyperosmolar states.

Should any adverse reactions occur, discontinue administration of the irrigant and reevaluate the clinical status of the patient.

DOSAGE AND ADMINISTRATION:

As required for irrigation.

This drug product should be inspected visually for particulate matter and discoloration prior to administration, whenever solution and container permit.

Exposure of pharmaceutical products to heat should be minimized. Avoid excessive heat. Protect from freezing. It is recommended that the product be stored at room temperature (25 deg. C); however, brief exposure up to 40 deg. C does not adversely affect the product.

HOW SUPPLIED - EQUIVALENTS NOT AVAILABLE:

Solution - Irrigation - 3.3 %

4000 ml x 4	$25.60	3.3% SORBITOL SOL., McGaw	00264-2301-70

Solution - Irrigation - 30 mg/ml

3000 ml	$20.34	Sorbitol Urologic, Baxter Hlthcare	00338-0295-47
5000 ml	$32.85	Sorbitol Urologic, Baxter Hlthcare	00338-0295-49

SOTALOL HYDROCHLORIDE *(003089)*

CATEGORIES: Antiarrhythmic Agents; Arrhythmia; Beta Adrenergic Blocking Agents; Beta Blockers; Cardiovascular Drugs; Orphan Drugs; Tachycardia; Hypertension*; Hypotension*; FDA Class 1P ("Priority Review"); FDA Approved 1992 Oct

* Indication not approved by the FDA

BRAND NAMES: *Beta-Cardone* (England); *Betacardone*; *Betades*; **Betapace**; *Cardol*; Sotacor; *Sotagard*; *Sotahexal* (Germany); *Sotalex* (France, Germany); *Sotapor* *(International brand names outside U.S. in italics)*

FORMULARIES: PCS

COST OF THERAPY: $1,177.85 (Arrhythmia; Tablet; 80 mg; 2/day; 365 days)

DESCRIPTION:

Sotalol hydrochloride, is an antiarrhythmic drug with Class II (beta-adrenergic blocking) and Class II (cardiac action potential duration prolongation) properties. It is supplied as a light-blue, capsule-shaped tablet for oral administration. Sotalol HCl is a white, crystalline solid with a molecular weight of 308.8. It is hydrophilic, soluble in water, propylene glycol and ethanol, but is only slightly soluble in chloroform. Chemically, sotalol hydrochloride is d,l- N-(4-(l-hydroxy-2-((l-methylethyl)amino)ethyl)phenyl)methane-sulfonamide monohydrochloride. The molecular formula is:

$C_{12}H_{20}N_2O_3S \cdot HCl$

Sotalol HCl tablets contain the following inactive ingredients: microcrystalline cellulose, lactose, starch, stearic acid, magnesium stearate, colloidal silicon dioxide, and FD&C blue color #2 (aluminum lake, conc.).

CLINICAL PHARMACOLOGY:

MECHANISM OF ACTION

Sotalol HCl has both beta-adrenoreceptor blocking (Vaughan Williams Class II) and cardiac action potential duration prolongation (Vaughan Williams Class III) antiarrhythmic properties. Sotalol HCl is a racemic mixture of d- and l-sotalol. Both isomers have similar Class III antiarrhythmic effects, while the l-isomer is responsible for virtually all of the beta-blocking activity. The beta-blocking effect of sotalol is non-cardioselective, half maximal at about 80 mg/day and maximal at doses between 320 and 640 mg/day. Sotalol does not have partial agonist or membrane stabilizing activity. Although significant beta-blockade occurs at oral doses as low as 25 mg, Class III effects are seen only at daily doses of 160 mg and above.

ELECTROPHYSIOLOGY

Sotalol HCl prolongs the plateau phase of the cardiac action potential in the isolated myocyte, as well as in isolated tissue preparations of ventricular or atrial muscle (Class III activity). In intact animals it slows heart rate, decreases AV nodal conduction and increases the refractory periods of atrial and ventricular muscle and conduction tissue.

In man, the Class II (beta-blockade) electrophysiological effects of sotalol HCl tablets are manifested by increased sinus cycle length (slowed heart rate), decreased AV nodal conduction and increased AV nodal refractoriness. The Class III electrophysiological effects in man include prolongation of the atrial and ventricular monophasic action potentials, and effective refractory period prolongation of atrial muscle, ventricular muscle, and atrioventricular accessory pathways (where present) in both the anterograde and retrograde directions. With oral doses of 160 to 640 mg/day, the surface ECG shows dose-related mean increases of 40-100 msec in QT and 10-40 msec in QT_c. (See WARNINGS for description of relationship between QT_c and torsade de pointes type arrhythmias.) No significant alteration in QRS interval is observed.

In a small study (n=25) of patients with implanted defibrillators treated concurrently with sotalol HCl tablets, the average defibrillatory threshold was 6 joules (range 2-15 joules) compared to a mean of 16 joules for a non-randomized comparative group primarily receiving amiodarone.

HEMODYNAMICS

In a study of systemic hemodynamic function measured invasively in 12 patients with a mean LV ejection fraction of 37% and ventricular tachycardia (9 sustained and 3 non-sustained), a median dose of 160 mg twice daily of sotalol HCl tablets produced a 28% reduction in heart rate and a 24% decrease in cardiac index at 2 hours post dosing at steady state. Concurrently, systemic vascular resistance and stroke volume showed non-significant increases of 25% and 8%, respectively. Pulmonary capillary wedge pressure increased significantly from 6.4 mmHg to 11.8 mmHg in the 11 patients who completed the study. One patient was discontinued because of worsening congestive heart failure. Mean arterial pressure, mean pulmonary artery pressure and stroke work index did not significantly changes. Exercise and isoproterenol induced tachycardia are antagonized by sotalol HCl tablets, and total peripheral resistance increases by a small amount.

In hypersensitive patients, sotalol HCl produces significant reductions in both systolic and diastolic blood pressures. Although sotalol HCl is usually well-tolerated hemodynamically, caution should be exercised in patients with marginal cardiac compensation as deterioration in cardiac performance may occur. See WARNINGS, Congestive Heart Failure.

CLINICAL ACTIONS

Sotalol HCl has been studied in life-threatening and less severe arrhythmias. In patients with frequent premature ventricular complexes (VPC), sotalol HCl was significantly superior to placebo in reducing AVPCs, paired VPCs and non-sustained ventricular tachycardias (NSVT); the response was dose-related through 640 mg/day with 80-85% of patients having at least 75% reduction of VPCs. Sotalol HCl was also superior, at the doses evaluated, to propranolol (40-80 mg TID) and similar to quinidine (200-400 mg QID) in reducing VPCs. In patients with life-threatening arrhythmias (sustained ventricular tachycardia/fibrillation (VT/VF), sotalol HCl was studied acutely (by suppression of programmed electrical stimulation (PES) induced VT and by suppression of Holter monitor evidence of sustained VT) and, in acute responders chronically.

In a double-blind, randomized comparison of sotalol HCl tablets and procainamide given intravenously (total of 2 mg/kg sotalol HCl tablets vs. 19 mg/kg of procainamide over 90 minutes), sotalol HCl tablets suppressed PES induction in 30% of patients vs, 20% for procainamide (p=0.2).

In a randomized clinical trial (Electrophysiological Study Versus Electrocardiographic Monitoring (ESVEM) Trial) comparing choice of antiarrhythmic therapy by PES suppression vs. Holter monitor selection (in each case followed by treadmill exercise testing) in patients with a history of sustained VT/VF who were also inducible by PES, the effectiveness acutely and chronically of sotalol HCl tablets was compared with 6 other drugs (procainamide, quinidine, mexiletin, propafenone, imipramine and pirmenol). Overall response, limited to first drug, was 39% for sotalol HCl and 30% for the pooled other drugs. Acute response rate for first drug randomized using suppression of PES induction was 36% for sotalol HCl tablets vs. a mean of 13% for the other drugs. Using the Holter monitoring endpoint (complete suppression of sustained VT, 90% suppression of NSVT, 80% suppression of sustained VPC pairs, and at least 70% suppression of VPCs), sotalol HCl tablets yielded 41% response vs. 45% for the other drugs combined. Among responders placed on long-term therapy identified acutely as effective (by either PES or Holter), sotalol HCl tablets, when compared to the pool of other drugs, had the lowest two-year mortality (13% vs. 22%), the lowest two-year VT recurrence rate (30% vs. 60%), and the lowest withdrawal rate (38% vs. about 75-80%). The most commonly used doses of sotalol HCl in this trial were 320-480 mg/day (66% of patients), with 16% receiving 240 mg/day or less and 18% receiving 640 or more.

It cannot be determined, however, in the absence of a controlled comparison of sotalol HCl tablets vs. no pharmacologic treatment (*e.g.,* in patients with implanted defibrillators whether sotalol HCl tablets response causes improved survival or identifies a population with a good prognosis.

In a large double-blind, placebo controlled secondary prevention (post-infarction) trial (n=1,456), sotalol HCl was given as a non-titrated initial dose of 320 mg once daily. Sotalol HCl tablets did not produce a significant increase in survival (7.3% mortality on sotalol HCl Tablets vs. 8.9% in placebo, p=0.3), but overall did not suggest an adverse effect on survival. There was, however, a suggestion of an early (*i.e.,* first 10 days) excess mortality (3% on sotalol HCl vs. 2% on placebo). In a second small trial (n=17 randomized to Sotalol) where sotalol was administered at high doses (*e.g.,* 320 mg twice daily) to high-risk post-infarction patients (ejection fraction <40% and either >10 VPC/hr or VT on Holter), there were 4 fatalities and 3 serious hemodynamic/electrical adverse events within two weeks of initiating sotalol HCl.

CLINICAL PHARMACOLOGY: *(cont'd)*

PHARMACOKINETICS

In healthy subjects, the oral bioavailability of sotalol HCl is 90-100%. After oral administration, peak plasma concentrations are reached in 2.5 to 4 hours and steady state plasma concentrations are attained within 2-3 days (*i.e.*, after 5-6 doses when administered twice daily). Over the dosage range 160-640 mg/day sotalol HCl displays dose proportionality with respect to plasma concentrations. Distribution occurs to a central (plasma) and to a peripheral compartment, with a mean elimination half-life of 12 hours. Dosing every 12 hours results in trough plasma concentrations which are approximately one-half of those at peak.

Sotalol HCl does not bind to plasma proteins and is not metabolized. Sotalol HCl shows very little intersubject variability in plasma levels. The pharmacokinetics of the d and the l enantiomers of sotalol are essentially identical. Sotalol HCl crosses the blood brain barrier poorly. Excretion is predominantly via the kidney in the unchanged form, and therefore lower doses are necessary in conditions of renal impairment (see DOSAGE AND ADMINISTRATION).

Age per se does not significantly alter the pharmacokinetics of sotalol HCl tablets, but impaired renal function in geriatric patients can increase the terminal elimination half-life, resulting in increased drug accumulation. The absorption of sotalol HCl was reduced by approximately 20% compared to fasting when it was administered with a standard meal. Since sotalol HCl is not subject to first pass metabolism, patients with hepatic impairment show no alteration in clearance of sotalol HCl tablets.

INDICATIONS AND USAGE:

Oral sotalol HCl is indicated for the treatment of documented ventricular arrhythmias, such as sustained ventricular tachycardia, that in the judgement of the physician are life-threatening. Because of the proarrhythmic effects of sotalol HCl Tablets (see WARNINGS), including a 1.5 to 2% rate of torsade de pointes or new VT/VF in patients with either NSVT or supraventricular arrhythmias, its use in patients with less severe arrhythmias, even if the patients are symptomatic, is generally not recommended. Treatment of patients with asymptomatic ventricular premature contractions should be avoided.

Initiation of sotalol HCl tablets treatment or increasing doses, as with other antiarrhythmic agents used to treat life-threatening arrhythmias should be carried out in the hospital. The response to treatment should then be evaluated by a suitable method (*e.g.*, PES or Holter monitoring) prior to continuing the patient on chronic therapy. Various approaches have been used to determine the response to antiarrhythmic therapy, including sotalol HCl tablets.

In the ESVEM Trial, response by Holter monitoring was tentatively defined as 100% suppression of ventricular tachycardia, 90% suppression of non-sustained VT, 80% of suppression of paired VPCs, and 75% suppression of total VPCs in patients who had at least 10 VPCs/hour at baseline; this tentative response was confirmed if VT lasting 5 or more beats was not observed during treadmill exercise testing using a standard Bruce protocol. The PES protocol utilized a maximum of three extra-stimuli at three pacing cycle lengths and two right ventricular pacing sites. Response by PES was defined as prevention of induction of the following: 1) monomorphic VT lasting over 15 beats; 2) non-sustained polymorphic VT containing more than 15 beats of monomorphic VT in patients with a history of monomorphic VT; 3) polymorphic VT or VF greater than 15 beats in patients with a history of aborted sudden death without monomorphic VT; and 4) two episodes of polymorphic VT or VF of greater than 15 beats in a patient presenting with monomorphic VT. Sustained VT or NSVT producing hypotension during the final treadmill test was considered a drug failure.

In a multicenter open-label long-term study of sotalol HCl tablets in patients with life-threatening ventricular arrhythmias which had proven refractory to other antiarrhythmic medications, response by Holter monitoring was defined as in ESVEM. Response by PES was defined as non- inducibility of sustained VT by at least double extrastimuli delivered at a pacing cycle length of 400 msec. Overall survival and arrhythmia recurrence rates in this study were similar to those seen in ESVEM, although there was no comparative group to allow a definitive assessment of outcome.

Antiarrhythmic drugs have not been shown to be enhance survival in patients with ventricular arrhythmias.

CONTRAINDICATIONS:

Sotalol HCl is contraindicated in patients with bronchial asthma, sinus bradycardia, second and third degree AV block, unless a functioning pacemaker is present, congenital or acquired long QT syndromes, cardiogenic shock, uncontrolled congestive heart failure, and previous evidence of hypersensitivity to sotalol HCl tablets.

WARNINGS:

MORTALITY

The national Heart Lung and Blood Institute conducted the Cardiac Arrhythmia Suppression Trial (CAST), a long-term multicenter, randomized, double-blind study in patients with asymptomatic nonlife-threatening ventricular ectopy who had a myocardial infarction more than six days but less than two years previously. An excessive mortality or nonfatal cardiac arrest was seen in patients treated with encainide or flecainide (56/730) compared with that seen in patients assigned to matched placebo-treated groups (22/725) and a similar excess has been seen with moricizine. The average duration of treatment with encainide or flecainide in this study was ten months.

The applicability of these results to other populations (*e.g.*, those without recent myocardial infarction) and to other than Class I antiarrhythmic agents is uncertain. Sotalol HCl is devoid of Class I effect, and in a large (n=1,456) controlled trial in patients with a recent myocardial infarction, who did not necessarily have ventricular arrhythmias, sotalol HCl tablets did not produce increased mortality at doses up to 320 mg/day (see Clinical Actions). On the other hand, in the large post-infarction study using a non-titrated initial dose of 320 mg once daily and in a second small randomized trial in high-risk post-infarction patients treated with high doses (320 mg BID), there have been suggestions of an excess of early sudden deaths.

PROARRHYTHMIA

Like other antiarrhythmic agents, sotalol HCl tablets can provoke new or worsened ventricular arrhythmias in some patients, including sustained ventricular tachycardia or ventricular fibrillation, with potentially fatal consequences. Because of its effect on cardiac repolarization (QT_c interval prolongation), torsade de pointes, a polymorphic ventricular tachycardia with prolongation of the QT interval and a shifting electrical axis is the most common form of proarrhythmias associated with sotalol HCl tablets, occurring in about 4% of high risk (history of sustained VT/VF) patients. The risk of torsade de pointes progressively increases with prolongation of the QT interval, and is worsened also by reduction in heart rate and reduction in serum potassium. See Electrolyte Disturbances.

Because of the variable temporal recurrence of arrhythmias, it is not always possible to distinguish between a new or aggravated arrhythmic event and the patient's underlying rhythm disorder. (Note, however, that torsade de pointes is usually a drug induced arrhythmias in people with an initially normal QT_c.) Thus, the incidence of drug-related events cannot be precisely determined, so that the occurrence rates provided must be considered approximations. Note also that drug-induced arrhythmias may often not be identified, particularly if they occur long after starting the drug, due to less frequent monitoring. It is clear from the NIH-sponsored CAST (see WARNINGS, Mortality) that some antiarrhythmic drugs cause increased sudden death mortality, presumably due to new arrhythmias or asystole, that do not appear early in treatment but that represent a sustained increased risk.

Overall in clinical trials with sotalol, 4.3% of 3257 patients experienced a new or worsened ventricular arrhythmias. Of this 4.3%, there was new or worsened sustained ventricular tachycardia in approximately 1% of patients and torsade de pointes in 2.4%. Additionally, in approximately 1% of patients, deaths were considered possibly drug-related; such cases, although difficult to evaluate, may have been associated with proarrhythmic events. **In patients with a history of sustained ventricular tachycardia, the incidence of torsade de pointes was 4% and worsened VT in about 1%; in patients with other, less serious, ventricular arrhythmias and supraventricular arrhythmias, the incidence of torsade de pointes was 1% and 1.4%, respectively.**

Torsade de pointes arrhythmias were dose related, as is the prolongation of QT (QT_c) interval, as shown in the table below (TABLE 1).

TABLE 1 Sotalol HCl, Warnings
Percent Incidence of Torsade de Pointes and Mean QT_c Interval by Dose For Patients with Sustained VT/VF

Daily Dose (mg)	Incidence of Torsade de pointes	Mean QT_c+ (msec)
80	0.0 (69)	463 (17)
160	0.5 (832)	467 (181)
320	1.8 (835)	473 (344)
480	4.4 (459)	483 (234)
640	3.7 (324)	490 (185)
>640	5.8 (103)	512 (62)

() Number of patients assessed
+ highest on-therapy value

In addition to dose and presence of sustained VT, other risk factors for torsade de pointes were gender (females had a higher incidence), excessive prolongation of the QT_c interval (see TABLE 2) and history of cardiomegaly or congestive heart failure. Patients with sustained ventricular tachycardia and a history of congestive heart failure appear to have the highest risk for serious proarrhythmia (7%). Of the patients experiencing torsade de pointes, approximately two-thirds spontaneously reverted to their baseline rhythm. The other were either converted electrically (D/C cardioversion or overdrive pacing) or treated with other drugs (see OVERDOSAGE). It is not possible to determine whether sudden deaths represented episodes of torsade de pointes, but in some instances sudden death did follow a documented episode of torsade de pointes. Although sotalol HCl tablets therapy was discontinued in most patients experiencing torsade de pointes, 17% were continued on lower dose. Nonetheless, sotalol HCl tablets should be used with particular caution if the QT_c is greater than 500 msec on-therapy and serious consideration should be given to reducing the dose or discontinuing therapy when the QT_c exceeds 550 msec. Due to the multiple risk-factors associated with torsade de pointes, however, caution should be exercised regardless of the QT_c interval. The table below (TABLE 2) relates the incidence of torsade de pointes to on- therapy QT_c and change in QT_c from baseline. It should be noted, however, that the on therapy QT_c was in many cases the one obtained at the time of the torsades de pointes event, so that the table (TABLE 2) overstates the predictive value of a high QT_c.

TABLE 2 Sotalol, Warnings Relationship Between QT_c Interval Prolongation and Torsade de Pointes

On-Therapy QT_c Interval(msec)	Incidence of Torsade de Pointes	Changes in QT_c Intervals from Baseline (msec)	Incidence of Torsade de pointes
less than 500	1.3% (1787)	less than 65	1.6% (1516)
500 - 525	3.4% (236)	65-80	3.2% (158)
525 - 550	5.6% (125)	80-100	4.1% (146)
> 550	10.8% (157)	100-130	5.2% (115)
		>130	7.1% (99)

() Number of patients assessed.

Proarrhythmic events must be anticipated not only initiating therapy, but with every upward dose adjustment. Proarrhythmic events most often occur during within 7 days of initiating therapy or of an increase in dose; 75% of serious proarrhythmias (torsade de points and worsened VT) occurred within 7 days of initiating sotalol HCl tablets therapy, while 60% of such events occurred within 3 days of initiation or a dosage change. Initiating therapy at 80 mg BID with gradual upward dose titration and appropriate evaluations for efficacy (*e.g.*, PES or Holter) and safety (*e.g.*, QT interval, heart rate and electrolytes) prior to dose escalation, should reduce the risk of proarrhythmia. Avoiding excessive accumulation of Sotalol in patients with diminished renal function, by appropriate dose reduction, should also reduce the risk proarrhythmias (see DOSAGE AND ADMINISTRATION).

CONGESTIVE HEART FAILURE

Sympathetic stimulation is necessary in supporting circulatory function in congestive heart failure, and beta-blockade carries the potential hazard of further depressing myocardial contractility and precipitating more severe failure. In patients who have congestive heart failure controlled by digitalis and/or diuretics, sotalol HCl tablets should be administered cautiously. Both digitalis and Sotalol slow AV conduction. As with all beta-blockers, caution is advised when initiating therapy in patients with any evidence of left ventricular dysfunction. In premarketing studies, new or worsened congestive heart failure (CHF) occurred in 3.3% (n=3257) of patients and led to discontinuation in approximately 1% of patients receiving sotalol HCl tablets. The incidence was higher in patients presenting with sustained ventricular tachycardia/fibrillation (4.6%, n=1363), or a prior history of heart failure (7.3%, n=696). Based on a life-table analysis, the one-year incidence of new or worsened CHF was 3% in patients without a prior history and 10% in patients with a prior history of CHF, NYHA Classification was also closely associated to the incidence of new or worsened heart failure while receiving sotalol HCl tablets (1.8% in 1935 Class I patients 4.95 in 1254 Class II patients and 6.1% in 278 Class III or IV patients).

Electrolyte Disturbances: Sotalol HCl tablets should not be used in patients with hypokalemia or hypomagnesemia prior to correction of imbalance, as these conditions can exaggerate the degree of QT prolongation, and increase the potential for torsade de pointes. Special attention should be given to electrolyte and acid-base balance in patients experiencing severe or prolonged diarrhea or patients receiving concomitant diuretic drugs.

Conduction Disturbances: Excessive prolonged of the QT interval (>550 msec) can promote serious arrhythmias and should be avoided (see Proarrhythmias above). Sinus bradycardia (heart rate less than 50 bpm) occurred in 13% of patients receiving sotalol HCl tablets in clinical trials, and led to discontinuation in about 3% of patients. Bradycardia itself increases the risk of torsade de pointes. Sinus pause, sinus arrest and sinus node dysfunction occur in less than 1% of patients. The incidence of 2nd- or 3rd- degree AV block is approximately 1%.

WARNINGS: *(cont'd)*

Recent Acute MI: Sotalol HCl Tablets can be used safely and effectively in the long-term treatment and life-threatening ventricular arrhythmias following a myocardial infarction. However, experience in the use of sotalol HCl tablets to treat cardiac arrhythmias in the early phase of recovery from active MI is limited and at least at high initial doses is not reassuring (see WARNINGS, Mortality). In the first 2 weeks of post-MI caution is advised and careful dose titration is especially important, particularly in patients with marked impaired ventricular function.

The following warnings are related to the beta-blocking activity of sotalol HCl tablets.

Abrupt Withdrawal: Hypersensitivity to catecholamines has been observed in patients withdrawn from beta-blocker therapy. Occasional cases of exacerbation of angina pectoris, arrhythmias and, in some cases, myocardial infarction have been reported after abrupt discontinuation of beta-blocker therapy. Therefore, it is prudent when discounting chronically administered sotalol HCl tablets, particularly in patients with ischemic heart disease, to carefully monitor the patient and consider the temporary use of an alternate beta-blocker if appropriate. If possible, the dosage of sotalol HCl tablets should be gradually reduced over a period of one to two weeks. If angina or acute coronary insufficiency develops, appropriate therapy should be instituted promptly. Patients should be warned against interruption or discontinuation of therapy without the physician's advice. Because coronary artery disease is common and may be unrecognized in patients receiving sotalol HCl tablets, abrupt discontinuation in patients with arrhythmias may unmask latent coronary insufficiency.

Non-Allergic Bronchospasm (*e.g.,* chronic bronchitis and emphysema): **PATIENTS WITH BRONCHOSPASTIC DISEASES SHOULD IN GENERAL NOT RECEIVE BETA-BLOCKERS.** It is prudent, if sotalol HCl is to be administered, to use the smallest dose, so that inhibition of bronchodilation produced by endogenous or exogenous catecholamine simulation of $beta_2$ receptors may be minimized.

Anaphylaxis: While taking beta-blockers, patients with a history of anaphylactic reaction to a variety of allergens may have a more severe reaction or repeated challenge, either accidental, diagnostic or therapeutic. Such patients may be unresponsive to the usual doses of epinephrine used to treat the allergic reaction.

Anesthesia: The management of patients undergoing major surgery who are being treated with beta-blockers is controversial. Protracted severe hypotension and difficulty in restoring and maintaining normal cardiac rhythm after anesthesia have been reported in patients receiving beta-blockers.

Diabetes: In patients with diabetes (especially labile diabetes) or with a history of episodes of spontaneous hypoglycemia, sotalol HCl tablets should be given with caution since beta-blockade may mask some important premonitory signs of acute hypoglycemia; e.g., tachycardia.

Sick Sinus Syndrome: Sotalol HCl tablets should only be used with extreme caution in patients with sick sinus syndrome associated symptomatic arrhythmias, because it may cause sinus bradycardia, sinus pauses or sinus arrest.

Thyrotoxicosis: Beta-blockade may mask certain clinical signs (*e.g.,* tachycardia) of hyperthyroidism. Patients suspended of developing thyrotoxicosis should be managed carefully to avoid abrupt withdrawal of beta-blockades which might be followed by an exacerbation of symptoms of hyperthyroidism, including thyroid storm.

PRECAUTIONS:

Renal Impairment: Sotalol HCl is mainly eliminated via the kidneys through glomerular filtration and to a small degree by tubular secretion. There is a relationship between renal function, as measured by serum creatinine or creatinine clearance, and the elimination rate of sotalol HCl tablets. Guidance for dosing in conditions of renal impairment can be found underDOSAGE AND ADMINISTRATION.

Carcinogenesis, Mutagenicity, Impairment of Fertility: No evidence of carcinogenesic potential was observed in rats during a 24-month study at 137-275 mg/kg/day (approximately 30 times the maximum recommended human oral dose (MRHD) as mg/kg or 5 times the maximum recommended as mg/m^2) or in mice, during a 24-month period at 4141-7122 mg/kg/day (approximately 450-750 times the MRHD as mg/kg or 36-63 times the MRHD as mg/m^2).

Sotalol has not been evaluated in any specific assay of mutagenicity or clastogenicity.

No significant reduction in fertility occurred in rats at oral doses of 1,000 mg/kg/day (approximately 100 times the MRHD as mg/kg or 9 times the MRHD as mg/m^2) prior to mating, except for a small reduction in the number of offspring per liter.

Pregnancy Category B: Reproduction studies in rats and rabbits during organogenesis at 100 and 22 times the MRHD as mg/kg (9 and 7 times the MRHD as mg/m^2), respectively, did not reveal any teratogenetic potential associated with sotalol HCl. In rabbits, a high dose of sotalol HCl (160 mg/kg/day) at 16 times the MRHD as mg/kg (6 times the MRHD as mg/m^2) produced a slight increase in fetal death likely due to maternal toxicity. Eight times the maximum does (80 mg/kg/day or 3 times the MHRD (18 times the MHRD as mg/m^2) increased the number of early resorptions, while at 14 times the maximum dose (2.5 times the MHRD) as mg/m^2), no increase in early resorptions was noted. However, animal reproduction studies are not always predictive of human response.

Although there are no adequate and well-controlled studies in pregnant women, sotalol HCl has been shown to cross the placenta, and is found in amniotic fluid. There has been a report of subnormal birth weight with sotalol HCl tablets. Therefore, sotalol HCl tablets should be used during pregnancy only if the potential benefit outweighs the potential risk.

Nursing Mothers: Sotalol is excreted in the milk of laboratory animals and has not been reported to be present in human milk. Because of the potential for adverse reactions in nursing infants from sotalol HCl tablets, a decision should be made whether to discontinue the drug, taking into account the importance of the drug to the mother.

Pediatric Use: The safety and effectiveness of sotalol HCl tablets in children have not been established.

DRUG INTERACTIONS:

Antiarrhythmics: Class Ia antiarrhythmic drugs, such as disopyramide, quinidine and procainamide and other Class III drugs (*e.g.,* amiodarone) are not recommended as concomitant therapy with sotalol HCl tablets because of their potential to prolong refractoriness (see WARNINGS). There is only limited experience with concomitant use of Ib or Ic antiarrhythmics. Additive Class II effects would also be anticipated with the use other beta-blocking agents concomitantly with sotalol HCl tablets.

Digoxin: Single and multiple doses of sotalol HCl tablets do not substantially affect serum digoxin levels. Proarrhythmic events were more common in sotalol HCl tablets treated patients also receiving digoxin. It is not clear whether this represents an interaction or is related to the presence of CHF, a known risk factor for proarrhythmia, in the patients receiving digoxin.

Calcium Block Drugs: Sotalol HCl tablets should be administered with caution in conjunction with calcium blocking drugs because of possible additive effects on atrioventricular conduction or ventricular function. Additionally, concomitant use of these drugs may have additive effects on blood pressure, possibly leading to hypotension.

DRUG INTERACTIONS: *(cont'd)*

Catecholamine-depleting agents: Concomitant use of catecholamine-depleting drugs, such as reserpine and guanethidine, with a beta-blocker may produce an excessive reduction of resting sympathetic nervous tone. Patients treated with sotalol HCl tablets plus a catecholamine depletor should therefore be closely monitored for evidence of hypotension and or marked bradycardia which may produce syncope.

Insulin and oral antidiabetics: Hyperglycemia may occur, and the dosage of insulin or antidiabetic drugs may require adjustments. Symptoms of hypoglycemia may be masked.

Beta-2-receptor stimulants: Beta-agonists such as salbutamol, terbutaline and isoprenaline may have to be administered in increased dosages when used concomitantly with sotalol HCl tablets.

Clonidine: Beta-blocking drugs may potentiate the rebound hypertension sometimes observed with discontinuation of clonidine; therefore, caution is advised when discontinuing clonidine in patients receiving sotalol HCl tablets.

Other: No pharmacokinetic interactions were observed with hydrochlorothiazide or warfarin.

Drugs prolonging the QT Interval: Sotalol HCl tablets should be administered with caution in conjunction with other drugs known to prolong the QT interval such as Class I antiarrhythmic agents, phenothiazides, tricyclic antidepressants, terfenadine and astemizole (see WARNINGS).

ADVERSE REACTIONS:

During premarketing trials, 3186 patients with cardiac arrhythmias (1363 with sustained ventricular tachycardia) received oral sotalol HCl tablets, of whom 2451 received the drug for at least two weeks. The most important adverse effects are torsade de points and other serious new ventricular arrhythmias (see WARNINGS), occurring at rates of almost 4% and 1%, respectively, in the VT/VF population. Overall, discontinuation because of unacceptable side effects was necessary in 17% of all patients in clinical trials, and in 13% of patients treated for at least two-weeks. The most common adverse reactions leading to discontinuation of sotalol HCl tablets are as follows: fatigue 4%, bradycardia (less than 50 bpm) 3%, dyspnea 3%, proarrhythmias 3%, asthenia 2%, and dizziness 2%.

Occasional reports of elevated serum liver enzymes have occurred with sotalol HCl tablets therapy but no cause and effect relationship has been established. One case of peripheral neuropathy which resolved on discontinuation of sotalol HCl tablets and recurred when the patient was rechallenged with the drug was reported in an early dose tolerance study. Elevated blood glucose levels and increased insulin requirements can occur in diabetic patients.

TABLE 3 lists as a function of dosage the most common (incidence of 2% or greater) adverse events, regardless of relationship to therapy and the percent of patients discontinued due to the event, as collected from clinical trials involving 1292 patients with sustained VT/VF.

POTENTIAL ADVERSE EFFECTS

Foreign marketing experience with sotalol HCl shows an adverse experience profile similar to that described above from clinical trials. Voluntary reports since introduction include rare reports (less than one report per 10,000 patients) of: emotional lability, slightly clouded sensorium, incoordination, vertigo, paralysis, thrombocytopenia, eosinophilia, leukopenia, photosensitivity reaction, fever, pulmonary edema, hyperlipidemia, myalgia, pruritus, alopecia.

The oculomucocutaneous syndrome associated with the beta-blocker practolol has not been associated with sotalol HCl tablets during investigational use and foreign marketing experience.

OVERDOSAGE:

Intentional or accidental overdosage with sotalol HCl has rarely resulted in death.

SYMPTOMS AND TREATMENT OF OVERDOSAGE

The most common signs to be expected are bradycardia, congestive heart failure, hypotension, bronchospasm and hypoglycemia. In cases of massive intentional overdosage (2-16 grams) of sotalol HCl tablets the following clinical findings were seen: hypotension, bradycardia, prolongation of QT interval, torsade de pointes, ventricular tachycardia, and premature ventricular complexes. If overdosage occurs, therapy with sotalol HCl tablets should be discontinued and the patient observed closely. Because of the lack of protein binding, hemodialysis is useful for reducing sotalol HCl tablets plasma concentrations. Patients should be carefully observed until QT intervals are normalized. In addition, if required, the following therapeutic measures are suggested:

Bradycardia: Atropine, another anticholinergic drug, a beta-adrenergic agonist or transvenous cardiac pacing.

Heart Block: (second and third degrees) transvenous cardiac pacemaker.

Hypotension: (depending on associated factors) epinephrine rather than isoproterenol or norepinephrine may be useful.

Bronchospasm: Aminophylline or aerosol beta-2-receptor stimulant.

Torsade de Pointes: DC cardioversion, transvenous cardiac pacing, epinephrine, magnesium sulfate.

DOSAGE AND ADMINISTRATION:

As with other antiarrhythmic agents, sotalol HCl tablets should be initiated and doses increased in a hospital with facilities for cardiac rhythm monitoring and assessment (see INDICATIONS AND USAGE). Sotalol HCl tablets should be administered only after appropriate clinical assessment (see INDICATIONS AND USAGE), and the dosage of sotalol HCl tablets should be administered only after appropriate clinical assessment (see INDICATIONS AND USAGE), and the dosage of sotalol HCl tablets must be individualized for each patient on the basis of therapeutic response and tolerance. Proarrhythmic events can occur not only at initiation of therapy, but also with each upward dosage adjustment.

Dosage of sotalol HCl tablets should be adjusted gradually, allowing 2-3 days between dosing increments in order to attain steady-state plasma concentrations, and to allow monitoring of QT interval. Graded dose adjustment will help prevent the usage of doses which are higher than necessary to control the arrhythmia. The recommended initial dose is 80 mg twice daily. This dose may be increased, if necessary, after appropriate evaluation to 240 or 320 mg/day. In most patients, a therapeutic response is obtained at a total daily dose of 160 to 320 mg/day, given in two or three divided doses. Some patients with life- threatening refractory ventricular arrhythmias may require doses as high as 480-640 mg/day; however, these doses should only be prescribed when the potential benefit outweighs the increased risk of adverse events, in particular proarrhythmia.

Because of the long terminal elimination half-life of sotalol HCl tablets, dosing in more than a BID regimen is usually not necessary.

Because sotalol HCl is excreted predominantly in urine and its terminal elimination half-life is prolonged in conditions of renal impairment, the dosing interval of sotalol HCl should be modified (when creatinine clearance is lower than 60 ml/min) according to TABLE 4.

DOSAGE AND ADMINISTRATION: *(cont'd)*

TABLE 3 Incidence (%) of Adverse Events and Discontinuations

Body System	Daily Dose 180mg n=832	240mg n=263	320mg n=835	480mg n=459	640mg n=324	Any Dose n=1292	% Patients Discontinued n=1292
Body as a Whole							
infection	1	2	2	2	3	4	<1
fever	1	2	3	2	2	4	<1
localized pain	1	1	2	2	2	3	<1
Cardiovascular							
dyspnea	5	8	11	15	15	21	2
bradycardia	8	8	9	7	5	16	2
chest pain	4	3	10	10	14	16	<1
palpitation	3	3	8	9	12	14	<1
edema	2	2	5	3	5	8	1
ECG abnormal	4	2	4	2	2	7	1
hypotension	3	4	3	2	3	6	2
proarrhythmia	<1	<1	2	4	5	5	3
syncope	1	1	3	2	5	5	1
heart failure	2	3	2	2	2	5	1
presyncope	1	2	2	4	3	4	<1
peripheral vascular disorder	1	2	1	1	2	3	<1
cardiovascular disorder	1	<1	2	2	2	3	<1
vasodilation	1	<1	1	2	1	3	<1
AICD discharge	<1	2	2	2	2	3	<1
hypertension	<1	1	1	1	2	2	<1
Nervous							
fatigue	5	8	12	12	13	20	2
dizziness	7	6	11	11	14	20	1
asthenia	4	5	7	8	10	13	1
light-headed	4	3	6	6	9	12	1
headache	3	2	4	4	4	8	<1
sleep-problem	1	1	5	5	6	8	<1
perspiration	1	2	3	4	5	6	<1
altered consciousness	2	3	1	2	3	4	<1
depression	1	2	2	2	3	4	<1
paresthesia	1	1	2	3	2	4	<1
anxiety	2	2	2	3	2	4	<1
mood change	<1	<1	1	3	2	3	<1
appetite disorder	1	2	2	1	3	3	<1
stroke	<1	<1	1	1	<1	1	<1
Digestive							
nausea/vomiting	5	4	4	6	6	10	1
diarrhea	2	3	3	3	5	7	<1
dyspepsia	2	3	3	3	3	6	<1
abdominal pain	<1	<1	2	2	2	3	<1
colon problem	2	1	1	<1	2	3	<1
flatulence	1	<1	1	1	2	2	<1
Respiratory							
pulmonary prob.	3	3	5	3	4	8	<1
upper respiratory tract problem	1	1	3	4	3	5	<1
asthma	1	<1	1	1	1	2	<1
Urogenital							
genitourinary disorder	1	0	1	1	2	3	<1
Sexl. Dysfunction	<1	1	1	1	3	2	<1
Metabolic							
abnorm. lab value	1	2	3	2	1	4	<1
weight change	1	1	1	<1	2	2	<1
Musculoskeletal							
extremity pain	2	2	4	5	3	7	<1
back pain	1	<1	2	2	2	3	<1
Skin + Appendages							
rash	2	3	2	3	4	5	<1
Hematologic							
bleeding	1	<1	1	<1	2	2	<1
Special Senses							
visual problem	1	1	2	4	5	5	<1

* Because patients are counted at each dose level tested, the Any Dose column cannot be determined by adding across the doses.

TABLE 4

Creatinine Clearance ml/min	Dosing Interval (hours)
> 60	12
30 - 60	24
10 - 30	36 - 48
< 10	Dose should be individualized

Since the terminal half-life of sotalol HCl is increased in patients with renal impairment, a longer duration of dosing is required to reach steady-state. Dose escalations in renal impairment should be done after administration of at least 5-6 doses at appropriate intervals (see TABLE 4).

TRANSFER TO SOTALOL HCL TABLETS

Before starting sotalol HCl tablets, previous antiarrhythmic therapy should generally be withdrawn under careful monitoring for a minimum of 2-3 plasma half-lives if the patient's clinical condition permits (see DRUG INTERACTIONS). Treatment has been initiated in some patients receiving I.V. lidocaine without ill effect. After discontinuation of amiodarone, sotalol HCl tablets should not be initiated until the QT is normalized (see WARNINGS).

Store at controlled room temperature, between 15 to 30°C (59 to 86°F).

(Berlex 60589-0. Rev. 7/92)

HOW SUPPLIED - EQUIVALENTS NOT AVAILABLE:

Tablet, Coated - Oral - 80 mg

100's	$161.35	BETAPACE, Berlex Labs	50419-0105-10
100's	$164.20	BETAPACE, Berlex Labs	50419-0105-11

HOW SUPPLIED - EQUIVALENTS NOT AVAILABLE: *(cont'd)*

Tablet, Coated - Oral - 120 mg

100's	$215.15	BETAPACE, Berlex Labs	50419-0109-10
100's	$218.00	BETAPACE, Berlex Labs	50419-0109-11

Tablet, Coated - Oral - 160 mg

100's	$269.00	BETAPACE, Berlex Labs	50419-0106-10
100's	$271.80	BETAPACE, Berlex Labs	50419-0106-11

Tablet, Coated - Oral - 240 mg

100's	$349.70	BETAPACE, Berlex Labs	50419-0107-10
100's	$352.50	BETAPACE, Berlex Labs	50419-0107-11

SPARFLOXACIN *(003324)*

CATEGORIES: Anti-Infectives; Antibacterials; Antibiotics; FDA Approved 1997 Jan; Fluoroquinolones; Pregnancy Category C; Quinolones; Respiratory Tract Infections

BRAND NAMES: *Spara* (Japan); *Sparlox*; *Torospar*; **Zagam**
(International brand names outside U.S. in italics)

PRIMARY ICD9: 482.9 (Pneumonia, bacterial)

DESCRIPTION:

Sparfloxacin is a synthetic broad-spectrum antimicrobial agent for oral administration. Sparfloxacin, an aminodifluoroquinolone, is 5-Amino-1-cyclopropyl-7-(*cis*-3,5-dimethyl-1-piperazinyl)-6,8-difluoro-1,4-dihydro-4-oxo-3-quinolinecarboxylic acid. Its empirical formula is $C_{19}H_{22}F_2N_4O_3$.

Sparfloxacin has a molecular weight of 392.41. It occurs as a yellow crystalline powder. It is sparingly soluble in glacial acetic acid or chloroform, very slightly soluble in ethanol (95%), and practically insoluble in water and ether. It dissolves in dilute acetic acid or 0.1 N sodium hydroxide.

Zagam is available as a 200 mg round, white film-coated tablet. Each 200-mg tablet contains the following inactive ingredients: microcrystalline cellulose NF, corn starch NF, L-hydroxypropylcellulose NF, magnesium stearate NF, and colloidal silicone dioxide NF. The film coating contains: methylhydroxypropylcellulose USP, polyethylene glycol 6000, and titanium dioxide USP.

CLINICAL PHARMACOLOGY:

Absorption: Sparfloxacin is well absorbed following oral administration with an absolute oral bioavailability of 92%. The mean maximum plasma sparfloxacin concentration following a single 400 mg oral dose was approximately 1.3 (±0.2) mcg/ml. The area under the curve (mean $AUC_{0\rightarrow\infty}$)following a single 400 mg oral dose was approximately 34 (±6.8) mcg·hr/ml.

Steady-state plasma concentration was achieved on the first day by giving a loading dose that was double the daily dose. Mean (±SD) pharmacokinetic parameters observed for the 24-hour dosing interval with the recommended dosing regimen are shown in TABLE 1.

TABLE 1

Dosing Regimen (mg/day)	Peak C_{max}(mcg/ml)	Trough C_{24}(mcg/ml)	AUC_{0-24} hr·mcg/ml
400 mg loading dose (day 1)	1.3 (±0.2)	0.5 (±0.1)	20.6 (±3.1)
200 mg q24 hours (steady-state)	1.1 (±0.1)	0.5 (±0.1)	18.7 (±2.6)

Maximum plasma concentrations for the initial oral 400 mg loading dose were typically achieved between 3 to 6 hours following administration with a mean value of approximately 4 hours. Maximum plasma concentrations for a 200 mg dose were also achieved between 3 to 6 hours after administration with a mean of about 4 hours.

Oral absorption of sparfloxacin is unaffected by administration with milk or food, including high fat meals. Concurrent administration of antacids containing magnesium hydroxide and aluminum hydroxide reduces the oral bioavailability of sparfloxacin by as much as 50%. (See PRECAUTIONS, Information for the Patient, and DRUG INTERACTIONS.)

Distribution: Upon reaching general circulation, sparfloxacin distributes well into the body, as reflected by the large mean steady-state volume of distribution (Vd_{ss}) of 3.9 (±0.8) L/kg. Sparfloxacin exhibits low plasma protein binding in serum at about 45%.

Sparfloxacin penetrates well into body fluids and tissues. Results of tissue and body fluid distribution studies demonstrated that oral administration of sparfloxacin produces sustained concentrations and that sparfloxacin concentrations in lower respiratory tract tissues and fluids generally exceed the corresponding plasma concentrations. The concentration of sparfloxacin in respiratory tissues (pulmonary parenchyma, bronchial wall, and bronchial mucosa) at 2 to 6 hours following standard oral dosing was approximately 3 to 6 times greater than the corresponding concentration in plasma. Concentrations in these respiratory tissues increase at up to 24 hours following dosing. Sparfloxacin is also highly concentrated into alveolar macrophages compared to plasma. Tissue or fluid to plasma sparfloxacin concentration ratios for respiratory tissues and fluids are found in TABLE 2.

TABLE 2 Tissue to Plasma Sparfloxacin Concentration Mean Ratio (%CV)*

Respiratory Tissues and Fluids	n† value	Time of Collection Postdose 2 to 6 hour	12 to 24 hour
alveolar macrophage	6/5	51.8 (88.7%)	68.1 (47.9%)
epithelial lining fluid	10/10	12.3 (26.7%)	17.6 (35.3%)
pulmonary parenchyma	8/7	5.9 (15.0%)	15.8 (32.0%)
bronchial wall	8/7	2.8 (16.0%)	5.7 (25.0%)
bronchial mucosa	6/5	2.7 (11.5%)	3.1 (11.6%)

* % CV (percent coefficient of variation)
† For tissues with two values, the first n is for 2 to 6 hours and the second n is for 12 to 24 hours.

Mean pleural effusion to plasma concentration ratios were 0.34 and 0.69 at 4 and 20 hours postdose, respectively.

Metabolism: Sparfloxacin is metabolized by the liver, primarily by phase II glucuronidation, to form a glucuronide conjugate. Its metabolism does not utilize or interfere with cytochrome-mediated oxidation, in particular cytochrome P450.

Excretion: The total body clearance and renal clearance of sparfloxacin were 11.4 (±3.5) and 1.5 (±0.5) L/hr, respectively. Sparfloxacin is excreted in both the feces (50%) and urine (50%). Approximately 10% of an orally administered dose is excreted in the urine as unchanged drug in patients with normal renal function. Following a 400 mg loading dose of

CLINICAL PHARMACOLOGY: *(cont'd)*

sparfloxacin, the mean urine concentration 4 hours postdose was in excess of 12.0 mcg/ml, and measurable concentrations of active drug persisted through six days for subjects with normal renal function.

The terminal elimination phase half-life ($t_{\frac{1}{2}}$) of sparfloxacin in plasma generally varies between 16 and 30 hours, with a mean $t_{\frac{1}{2}}$ of approximately 20 hours. The $t_{\frac{1}{2}}$ is independent of the administered dose, suggesting that sparfloxacin elimination kinetics are linear.

SPECIAL POPULATIONS

Geriatric: The pharmacokinetics of sparfloxacin are not altered in the elderly with normal renal function.

Pediatric: The pharmacokinetics of sparfloxacin in pediatric subjects have not been studied.

Gender: There are no gender differences in the pharmacokinetics of sparfloxacin.

Renal Insufficiency: In patients with renal impairment (creatinine clearance <50 ml/min), the terminal elimination half-life of sparfloxacin is lengthened. Single or multiple doses of sparfloxacin in patients with varying degrees of renal impairment typically produce plasma concentrations that are twice those observed in subjects with normal renal function. (See PRECAUTIONS, General and DOSAGE AND ADMINISTRATION.)

Hepatic Insufficiency: The pharmacokinetics of sparfloxacin are not altered in patients with mild or moderate hepatic impairment without cholestasis.

MICROBIOLOGY

Sparfloxacin has *in vitro* activity against a wide range of gram-negative and gram-positive microorganisms. Sparfloxacin exerts its antibacterial activity by inhibiting DNA gyrase, a bacterial topoisomerase. DNA gyrase is an essential enzyme which controls DNA topology and assists in DNA replication, repair, deactivation, and transcription.

Quinolones differ in chemical structure and mode of action from β-lactam antibiotics. Quinolones may, therefore, be active against bacteria resistant to β-lactam antibiotics.

Although cross-resistance has been observed between sparfloxacin and other fluoroquinolones, some microorganisms resistant to other fluoroquinolones may be susceptible to sparfloxacin.

In vitro tests show that the combination of sparfloxacin and rifampin is antagonistic against *Staphylococcus aureus.*

Sparfloxacin has been shown to be active against most strains of the following microorganisms, both *in vitro* and in clinical infections as described in INDICATIONS AND USAGE.

Aerobic gram-positive microorganisms

Staphylococcus aureus

Streptococcus pneumoniae, (penicillin-susceptible strains)

Aerobic gram-negative microorganisms

Enterobacter cloacae

Haemophilus influenzae

Haemophilus parainfluenzae

Klebsiella pneumoniae

Moraxella catarrhalis

Other microorganisms

Chlamydia pneumoniae

Mycoplasma pneumoniae

The following *in vitro* data are available, **but their clinical significance is unknown:**

Sparfloxacin exhibits *in vitro* minimal inhibitory concentrations (MIC's) of 1 mcg/ml or less against most (≥90%) strains of the following microorganisms; however, the safety and effectiveness of sparfloxacin in treating clinical infections due to these microorganisms have not been established in adequate and well controlled clinical trials.

Aerobic gram-positive microorganisms

Streptococcus agalactiae

Streptococcus pneumoniae, (penicillin-resistant strains)

Streptococcus pyogenes

Viridans group streptococci

Aerobic gram-negative microorganisms

Acinetobacter anitratus

Acinetobacter lwoffi

Citrobacter diversus

Enterobacter aerogenes

Klebsiella oxytoca

Legionella pneumophila

Morganella morganii

Proteus mirabilis

Proteus vulgaris

SUSCEPTIBILITY TESTING

Dilution Techniques: Quantitative methods are used to determine antimicrobial minimal inhibitory concentrations (MIC's). These MIC's provide estimates of the susceptibility of bacteria to antimicrobial compounds. The MIC's should be determined using a standardized procedure. Standardized procedures are based on a dilution method[1] (broth or agar) or equivalent with standardized inoculum concentrations and standardized concentrations of sparfloxacin powder. The MIC values should be interpreted according to the criteria in TABLE 3.

TABLE 3 For Testing Aerobic Microorganisms Other Than *Haemophilus influenzae*, Haemophilus parainfluenzae and *Streptococcus pneumoniae*

MIC (mcg/ml)	Interpretation
≤1	Susceptible (S)
2	Intermediate (I)
≥4	Resistant (R)

TABLE 4 For Testing *Haemophilus influenzae* and *Haemophilus parainfluenzae**

MIC (mcg/ml)	Interpretation
≤0.25	Susceptible (S)

* These interpretive standards are applicable only to broth microdilution susceptibility testing with *Haemophilus influenzae* and *Haemophilus parainfluenzae* using Haemophilus Test Medium[1].

The current absence of data on resistant strains precludes defining any categories other than "Susceptible." Strains yielding MIC results suggestive of a "nonsusceptible" category should be submitted to a reference laboratory for further testing.

CLINICAL PHARMACOLOGY: *(cont'd)*

TABLE 5 For Testing *Streptococcus Pneumoniae**

MIC (mcg/ml)	Interpretation
≤0.5	Susceptible

* These interpretive standards are applicable only to broth microdilution susceptibility tests using cation-adjusted Mueller-Hinton broth with 2-5% lysed horse blood.

The current absence of data on resistant strains precludes defining any categories other than "Susceptible." Strains yielding MIC results suggestive of a "nonsusceptible" category should be submitted to a reference laboratory for further testing.

A report of "Susceptible" indicates that the pathogen is likely to be inhibited if the antimicrobial compound in the blood reaches the concentration usually achievable. A report of "Intermediate" indicates that the result should be considered equivocal, and, if the microorganism is not fully susceptible to alternative, clinically feasible drugs, the test should be repeated. This category implies possible clinical applicability in body sites where the drug is physiologically concentrated or in situations where a high dosage of drug can be used. This category also provides a buffer zone which prevents small uncontrolled technical factors from causing major discrepancies in interpretation. A report of "Resistant" indicates that the pathogen is not likely to be inhibited if the antimicrobial compound in the blood reaches the concentration usually achievable; other therapy should be selected.

Standardized susceptibility test procedures require the use of laboratory control microorganisms to control the technical aspects of the laboratory procedures. Standard sparfloxacin powder should provide the MIC values found in TABLE 6.

TABLE 6

Microorganism	MIC Range (mcg/ml)
Enterococcus faecalis ATCC 29212	0.12-0.5
Escherichia coli ATCC 25922	0.004-0.016
Haemophilus influenzae ATCC 49247*	0.004-0.016
Staphylococcus aureaus ATCC 29213	0.03-0.12
Streptococcus pneumoniae ATCC 49619†	0.12-0.5

* This quality control range is applicable to only *H. influenzae* ATCC 49247 tested by a broth microdilution procedure using Haemophilus Test Medium (HTM).[1]
† This quality control range is applicable to only *S. pneumoniae* ATCC 49619 tested by a broth microdilution procedure using cation-adjusted Mueller-Hinton broth with 2-5% lysed horse blood.

Diffusion Techniques: Quantitative methods that require measurement of zone diameters also provide reproducible estimates of the susceptibility of bacteria to antimicrobial compounds. One such standardized procedure[2] requires the use of standardized inoculum concentrations. This procedure uses paper disks impregnated with 5 mcg sparfloxacin to test the susceptibility of microorganisms to sparfloxacin.

Reports from the laboratory providing results of the standard single-disk susceptibility test with a 5 mcg sparfloxacin disk should be interpreted according to the following criteria:

TABLE 7 For Aerobic Microorganisms Other Than *Haemophilus influenzae, Haemophilus* parainfluenzae, and *Streptococcus pneumoniae*

Zone Diameter (mm)	Interpretation
≥19	Susceptible (S)
16-18	Intermediate (I)
≤15	Resistant (R)

Haemophilus influenzae and *Haemophilus parainfluenzae* should not be tested by diffusion techniques. An MIC should be determined for these isolates.

TABLE 8 For *Streptococcus pneumoniae**

Zone Diameter	Interpretation
≥19	Susceptible (S)

* These zone diameter standards for *Streptococcus pneumoniae* apply only to tests performed using Mueller-Hinton agar supplemented with 5% sheep blood and incubated in 5% CO_2.

The current absence of data on resistant strains precludes any category other than "Susceptible." Strains yielding zone diameter results suggestive of a "nonsusceptible" category should be submitted to a reference laboratory for further testing.

Interpretation should be as stated above for results using dilution techniques. Interpretation involves correlation of the diameter obtained in the disk test with the MIC for sparfloxacin.

As with standard dilution techniques, diffusion methods require the use of laboratory control microorganisms that are used to control the technical aspects of the laboratory procedures. For the diffusion technique, the 5 mcg sparfloxacin disk should provide the zone diameters in these laboratory quality control strains found in TABLE 9.

TABLE 9

Microorganism	Zone Diameter (mm)
Escherichia coli ATCC 25922	30-38
Staphylococcus areus ATCC 25923	27-33
Streptococcus pneumoniae ATCC 49619*	21-27

* These quality control limits apply to tests conducted with *S. pneumoniae* ATCC 49619 using Mueller-Hinton agar supplemented with 5% sheep blood incubated in 5% CO_2.

CLINICAL STUDIES:

COMMUNITY-ACQUIRED PNEUMONIA STUDIES

In two controlled clinical studies of community-acquired pneumonia conducted in the United States, sparfloxacin was compared to erythromycin and cefaclor. The patient clinical success and pathogen eradication rates for sparfloxacin were equivalent to those of the comparators. In these studies, the pathogen eradication rates/presumed pathogen eradication rates were obtained and are found in TABLE 10.

Safety

TABLE 11 lists possibly and probably drug-related adverse events that occurred in these studies at an incidence of ≥2%.

ACUTE BACTERIAL EXACERBATIONS OF CHRONIC BRONCHITIS STUDY

In a controlled clinical study of acute bacterial exacerbations of chronic bronchitis conducted in the United States, sparfloxacin was compared to ofloxacin. In this study, the pathogen eradication rates were obtained and are found in TABLE 12.

CLINICAL STUDIES: *(cont'd)*

TABLE 10

Organism	Sparfloxacin	Erythromycin*	Cefaclor
C. pneumoniae	19/22 (86.4%)	3/4 (75%)	5/5 (100%)
H. influenzae	20/24 (83.3%)	0	25/31 (80.6%)
H. parainfluenzae	61/63 (96.8%)	4/4 (100%)	31/41 (75.6%)
M. catarrhalis	7/8 (87.5%)	4/4 (100%)	5/6 (83.3%)
M. pneumoniae	36/39 (92.3%)	15/15 (100%)	20/24 (83.3%)
S. pneumoniae	39/41 (95.1%)	10/11 (90%)	16/17 (94.1%)

* Pathogen numbers were smaller since many of the strains were intrinsically resistant to erythromycin.

TABLE 11

Event	Sparfloxacin n=387	Erythromycin n=209	Cefaclor n=162
Abdominal Pain	6 (1.6%)	18 (8.6%)	2 (1.2%)
Photosensitivity Reaction	16 (4.1%)	0	1 (0.6%)
QT Interval Prolonged	8 (2.1%)	2 (1.0%)	1 (0.6%)
Sinus Bradycardia	2 (0.5%)	6 (2.9%)	0
Diarrhea	15 (3.9%)	33 (15.8%)	7 (4.3%)
Flatulence	0	5 (2.4%)	0
Nausea	11 (2.8%)	32 (15.3%)	4 (2.5%)
Vomiting	10 (2.6%)	15 (7.2%)	1 (0.6%)
Insomnia	6 (1.6%)	5 (2.4%)	0

TABLE 12

Organism	Sparfloxacin	Ofloxacin
H. parinfluenzae	104/109 (95.4%)	90/95 (94.7%)
H. influenzae	51/57 (89.5%)	61/65 (93.8%)
C. pneumoniae	37/45 (82.2%)	36/40 (90%)
M. catarrhalis	36/38 (94.7%)	33/34 (97.1%)
S. pneumoniae	30/34 (88.2%)	20/22 (90.9%)
S. aureus	16/19 (84.2%)	13/14 (92.9%)
K. pneumoniae	17/17 (100%)	15/17 (88.2%)
E. cloacae	12/13 (92.3%)	12/15 (80%)

Safety

TABLE 13 lists possibly and probably drug-related adverse events that occurred in the study at an incidence of ≥2% for either compound.

TABLE 13

Event	Sparfloxacin (n=395)	Ofloxacin (n=403)
Headache	11 (2.8%)	6 (1.5%)
Photosensitivity Reaction	29 (7.3%)	3 (0.7%)
Diarrhea	6 (1.5%)	9 (2.2%)
Dyspepsia	8 (2.0%)	14 (3.5%)
Nausea	16 (4.1%)	29 (7.2%)
Dizziness	12 (3.0%)	10 (2.5%)
Insomnia	4 (1.0%)	46 (11.4%)
Taste Perversion	10 (2.5%)	10 (2.5%)

CONTRAINDICATIONS:

Sparfloxacin is contraindicated for individuals with a history of hypersensitivity or photosensitivity reactions.

Torsade de pointes has been reported in patients receiving sparfloxacin concomitantly with disopyramide and amiodarone. Consequently, sparfloxacin is contraindicated for individuals receiving these drugs as well as other QT_c-prolonging antiarrhythmic drugs reported to cause torsade de pointes, such as class Ia antiarrhythmic agents (*e.g.,* quinidine, procainamide), class III antiarrhythmic agents (*e.g.,* sotalol), and bepridil. Sparfloxacin is contraindicated in patients with known QT_c prolongation or in patients being treated concomitantly with medications known to produce an increase in the QTc interval and/or torsade de pointes (*e.g.,* terfenadine). (See WARNINGS and PRECAUTIONS.)

It is essential to avoid exposure to the sun, bright natural light, and UV rays throughout the entire duration of treatment and for 5 days after treatment is stopped. Sparfloxacin is contraindicated in patients whose life-style or employment will not permit compliance with required safety precautions concerning phototoxicity. (See WARNINGS and PRECAUTIONS.)

INDICATIONS AND USAGE:

Sparfloxacin is indicated for the treatment of adults (≥18 years of age) with the following infections caused by susceptible strains of the designated microorganisms:

Community-acquired pneumonia caused by *Chlamydia pneumoniae, Haemophilus influenzae, Haemophilus parainfluenzae, Moraxella catarrhalis, Mycoplasma pneumoniae,* or *Streptococcus pneumoniae.*

Acute bacterial exacerbations of chronic bronchitis caused by *Chlamydia pneumoniae, Enterobacter cloacae, Haemophilus influenzae, Haemophilus parainfluenzae, Klebsiella pneumoniae, Moraxella catarrhalis, Staphylococcus aureus,* or *Streptococcus pneumoniae.*

Appropriate culture and susceptibility tests should be performed before treatment in order to isolate and identify organisms causing the infection and to determine their susceptibility to sparfloxacin. Therapy with sparfloxacin may be initiated before results of these tests are known; once results become available, appropriate therapy should be selected. Culture and susceptibility testing performed periodically during therapy will provide information on the continued susceptibility of the pathogen to the antimicrobial agent and also on the possible emergence of bacterial resistance.

WARNINGS:

MODERATE TO SEVERE PHOTOTOXIC REACTIONS HAVE OCCURRED IN PATIENTS EXPOSED TO DIRECT OR INDIRECT SUNLIGHT OR TO ARTIFICIAL ULTRAVIOLET LIGHT (*e.g.,* SUNLAMPS) DURING OR FOLLOWING TREATMENT. THESE REACTIONS HAVE ALSO OCCURRED IN PATIENTS EXPOSED TO SHADED OR DIFFUSE LIGHT, INCLUDING EXPOSURE THROUGH GLASS OR DURING CLOUDY WEATHER. PATIENTS SHOULD BE ADVISED TO DISCONTINUE SPARFLOXACIN THERAPY AT THE FIRST SIGNS OR SYMPTOMS OF A PHOTOTOXICITY REACTION SUCH AS A SENSATION OF SKIN BURNING, REDNESS, SWELLING, BLISTERS, RASH, ITCHING, OR DERMATITIS.

WARNINGS: *(cont'd)*

The overall incidence of drug related phototoxicity in the 1585 patients who received sparfloxacin during clinical trials with recommended dosage was 7.9% (n=126). Phototoxicity ranged from mild 4.1% (n=65) to moderate 3.3% (n=52) to severe 0.6% (n=9), with severe defined as involving at least significant curtailment of normal daily activity. The frequency of phototoxicity reactions characterized by blister formation was 0.8% (n=13) of which 3 were severe. The discontinuation rate due to phototoxicity independent of drug relationship was 1.1% (n=17).

As with some other types of phototoxicity, there is the potential for exacerbation of the reaction on reexposure to sunlight or artificial ultraviolet light prior to complete recovery from the reaction. In a few cases, recovery from phototoxicity reactions was prolonged for several weeks. In rare cases, reactions have recurred up to several weeks after stopping sparfloxacin therapy.

EXPOSURE TO DIRECT AND INDIRECT SUNLIGHT (EVEN WHEN USING SUNSCREENS OR SUNBLOCKS) SHOULD BE AVOIDED WHILE TAKING SPARFLOXACIN AND FOR FIVE DAYS FOLLOWLNG THERAPY. SPARFLOXACIN THERAPY SHOULD BE DISCONTINUED IMMEDIATELY AT THE FIRST SIGNS OR SYMPTOMS OF PHOTOTOXICITY.

These phototoxic reactions have occurred with and without the use of sunscreens or sunblocks and have been associated with a single dose of sparfloxacin. However, a study in healthy volunteers has demonstrated that some sunscreen products, specifically those active in blocking UVA spectrum wavelengths (those containing the active ingredients octocrylene or Parsol 1789), can moderate the photosensitizing effect of sparfloxacin. However, many over-the-counter sunscreens do not provide adequate UVA protection.

Increases in the QT_c interval have been observed in healthy volunteers treated with sparfloxacin. After a single loading dose of 400 mg, a mean increase in QT_c interval of 11 msec (2.9%) is seen; at steady-state the mean increase is 7 msec (1.9%). The magnitude of the QT_c effect does not increase with repeated administration, and the QT_c returns to baseline within 48 hours of the last dose. In clinical trials involving 1489 patients with a baseline QT_c measurement, the mean prolongation at steady-state was 10 msec (2.5%); 0.7% of patients had a QT_c interval greater than 500 msec; however, no arrhythmic effects were seen.

THE SAFETY AND EFFECTIVENESS OF SPARFLOXACIN IN CHILDREN, ADOLESCENTS (UNDER THE AGE OF 18 YEARS), PREGNANT WOMEN, AND LACTATING WOMEN HAVE NOT BEEN ESTABLISHED. (See PRECAUTIONS, Pregnancy, Nursing Mothers; and Pediatric Use.)

Sparfloxacin has been shown to cause arthropathy in immature dogs when given in oral doses of 25 mg/kg/day (approximately 1.9 times the highest human dose on a mg/m^2 basis) for seven consecutive days. Examination of the weight-bearing joints of the dogs revealed small erosive lesions of the cartilage. Other quinolones also produce erosions of cartilage of weight-bearing joints and other signs of arthropathy in immature animals of various species.

Convulsions and toxic psychoses have been reported in patients receiving quinolones, including sparfloxacin. Quinolones may also cause increased intracranial pressure and central nervous system stimulation which may lead to tremors, restlessness/agitation, anxiety/nervousness, lightheadedness, confusion, hallucinations, paranoia, depression, nightmares, insomnia, and, rarely, suicidal thoughts or acts. These reactions may occur following the first dose. If these reactions occur in patients receiving sparfloxacin, the drug should be discontinued and appropriate measures instituted. As with other quinolones, sparfloxacin should be used with caution in patients with a known or suspected CNS disorder that may predispose to seizures or lower the seizure threshold (*e.g.,* severe cerebral arteriosclerosis, epilepsy) or in the presence of other risk factors that may predispose to seizures or lower the seizure threshold (*e.g.,* certain drug therapy, renal dysfunction). Cases of seizure associated with hypoglycemia have been reported. (See PRECAUTIONS, General, Information for the Patient, DRUG INTERACTIONS and ADVERSE REACTIONS.)

Serious and occasionally fatal hypersensitivity (including anaphylactoid or anaphylactic) reactions, some following the first dose, have been reported in patients receiving quinolones. Some reactions were accompanied by cardiovascular collapse, hypotension/shock, seizure, loss of consciousness, tingling, angioedema (including tongue, laryngeal, throat, or facial edema), airway obstruction (including bronchosyasm, shortness of breath, and acute respiratory distress), dyspnea, urticaria, and/or itching. Only a few patients had a history of previous hypersensitivity reactions. If an allergic reaction to sparfloxacin occurs, the drug should be discontinued immediately. Serious acute hypersensitivity reactions may require immediate treatment with epinephrine, and other resuscitative measures including oxygen, intravenous fluids, antihistamines, corticosteroids, pressor amines, and airway management, including intubation, as clinically indicated.

Serious and sometimes fatal events, some due to hypersensitivity, and some due to uncertain etiology, have been reported rarely in patients receiving therapy with quinolones. These events may be severe and generally occur following the administration of multiple doses. Clinical manifestations may include one or more of the following: fever, rash or severe dermatologic reactions (*e.g.,* toxic epidermal necrolysis, Stevens-Johnson Syndrome); vasculitis; arthralgia; myalgia; serum sickness; allergic pneumonitis; interstitial nephritis; acute renal insufficiency or failure; hepatitis; jaundice; acute hepatic necrosis or failure; anemia, including hemolytic and aplastic; thrombocytopenia, including thrombotic thrombocytopenic purpura; leukopenia; agranulocytosis; pancytopenia; and/or other hematologic abnormalities. The drug should be discontinued immediately at the first appearance of a skin rash or any other sign of hypersensitivity and supportive measures instituted. (See PRECAUTIONS, Information for the Patient and ADVERSE REACTIONS.)

Pseudomembranous colitis has been reported with nearly all antibacterial agents, including sparfloxacin, and may range in severity from mild to life-threatening. Therefore, it is important to consider this diagnosis in patients who present with diarrhea subsequent to the administration of antibacterial agents.

Treatment with antibacterial agents alters the normal flora of the colon and may permit overgrowth of clostridia. Studies indicate that a toxin produced by *Clostridium difficile* is one primary cause of "antibiotic-associated colitis."

After the diagnosis of pseudomembranous colitis has been established, therapeutic measures should be initiated. Mild cases of pseudomembranous colitis usually respond to drug discontinuation alone. In moderate to severe cases, consideration should be given to management with fluids and electrolytes, protein supplementation, and treatment with an antibacterial drug clinically effective against *C. difficile* colitis.

Ruptures of the shoulder, hand, and Achilles tendons that required surgical repair or resulted in prolonged disability have been reported with sparfloxacin and other quinolones. Sparfloxacin should be discontinued if the patient experiences pain, inflammation, or rupture of a tendon. Patients should rest and refrain from exercise until the diagnosis of tendonitis or tendon rupture has been confidently excluded. Tendon rupture can occur at any time during or after therapy with sparfloxacin.

PRECAUTIONS:

GENERAL

Adequate hydration of patients receiving sparfloxacin should be maintained to prevent the formation of a highly concentrated urine.

PRECAUTIONS: *(cont'd)*

Administer sparfloxacin with caution in the presence of renal insufficiency. Careful clinical observation and appropriate laboratory studies should be performed prior to and during therapy since elimination of sparfloxacin may be reduced. Adjustment of the dosage regimen is necessary for patients with impaired renal function-creatinine clearance <50 ml/min. (See CLINICAL PHARMACOLOGY and DOSAGE AND ADMINISTRATION.)

Avoid the concomitant prescription of medications known to prolong the QT_c interval, (*e.g.*, erythromycin, terfenadine, astemizole, cisapride, pentamidine, tricyclic antidepressants, some antipsychotics including phenothiazines). (See CONTRAINDICATIONS.) Sparfloxacin is not recommended for use in patients with pro-arrhythmic conditions (*e.g.*, hypokalemia, significant bradycardia, congestive heart failure, myocardial ischemia, and atrial fibrillation).

Moderate to severe phototoxicity reactions have been observed in patients exposed to direct sunlight while receiving drugs in this class. Excessive exposure to sunlight should be avoided. In clinical trials with sparfloxacin, phototoxicity was observed in approximately 7% of patients. Therapy should be discontinued if phototoxicity (*e.g.*, a skin eruption) occurs.

As with other quinolones, sparfloxacin should be used with caution in any patient with a known or suspected CNS disorder that may predispose to seizures or lower the seizure threshold (*e.g.*, severe cerebral arteriosclerosis, epilepsy) or in the presence of other risk factors that may predispose to seizures or lower the seizure threshold (*e.g.*, certain drug therapy, renal dysfunction). (See WARNINGS and DRUG INTERACTIONS.)

INFORMATION FOR THE PATIENT

Patients should be advised:

to avoid exposure to direct or indirect sunlight (including through glass, while using sunscreens and sunblocks, reflected sunlight, and cloudy weather) and exposure to artificial ultraviolet light (*e.g.*, sunlamps) during treatment with sparfloxacin and for five days after therapy. If brief exposure to the sun cannot be avoided, patients should cover as much of their skin as possible with clothing;

to discontinue sparfloxacin therapy at the first sign or symptom of phototoxicity reaction such as a sensation of skin burning, redness, swelling, blisters, rash, itching or dermatitis;

that a patient who has experienced a phototoxic reaction with sparfloxacin should also be advised to avoid further exposure to sunlight and artificial ultraviolet light until the phototoxicity reaction has resolved and he or she has completely recovered from the reaction or for five days whichever is longer. In rare cases, reactions have recurred up to several weeks after stopping sparfloxacin therapy;

that sparfloxacin may cause neurologic adverse effects (*e.g.*, dizziness, lightheadedness) and that patients should know how they react to sparfloxacin before they operate an automobile or machinery or engage in other activities requiring mental alertness and coordination (see WARNINGS and ADVERSE REACTIONS);

to discontinue treatment and inform their physician if they experience pain, inflammation, or rupture of a tendon, and to rest and refrain from exercise until the diagnosis of tendonitis or tendon rupture has been confidently excluded;

that sparfloxacin can be taken with food or milk or caffeine-containing products;

that mineral supplements or vitamins with iron, or zinc, or calcium may be taken 4 hours after sparfloxacin administration;

that sucralfate or magnesium- and aluminum-containing antacids may be taken 4 hours after sparfloxacin administration (see DRUG INTERACTIONS);

that sparfloxacin may be associated with hypersensitivity reactions, even following the first dose, and to discontinue the drug at the first sign of a skin rash or other allergic reaction;

to drink fluids liberally

DRUG/LABORATORY TEST INTERACTIONS

Sparfloxacin therapy may produce false-negative culture results for *Mycobacterium tuberculosis* by suppression of mycobacterial growth.

CARCINOGENESIS, MUTAGENESIS, AND IMPAIRMENT OF FERTILITY

Carcinogenesis: Sparfloxacin was not carcinogenic in mice or rats when administered for 104 weeks at daily oral doses 3.5 - 6.2 times greater than the maximum human dose (400 mg), respectively, based upon mg/m^2. These doses corresponded to plasma concentrations approximately equal to (mice) and 2.2 times greater than (rats) maximum human plasma concentrations.

Mutagenesis: Sparfloxacin was not mutagenic in *Salmonella typhimurium* TA98, TA100, TA1535, or TA1537, in *Escherichia coli* strain WP2 uvrA, nor in Chinese hamster lung cells. Sparfloxacin and other quinolones have been shown to be mutagenic in *Salmonella typhimurium* strain TA102 and to induce DNA repair in *Escherichia coli*, perhaps due to their inhibitory effect on bacterial DNA gyrase. Sparfloxacin induced chromosomal aberrations in Chinese hamster lung cells *in vitro* at cytotoxic concentrations; however, no increase in chromosomal aberrations or micronuclei in bone marrow cells was observed after sparfloxacin was administered orally to mice.

Impairment of Fertility: Sparfloxacin had no effect on the fertility or reproductive performance of male or female rats at oral doses up to 15.4 times the maximum human dose (400 mg) based upon mg/m^2 (equivalent to approximately 12 times the maximum human plasma concentration).

PREGNANCY, TERATOGENIC EFFECTS, PREGNANCY CATEGORY C

Reproduction studies performed in rats, rabbits, and monkeys at oral doses 6.2, 4.4, and 2.6 times higher than the maximum human dose, respectively, based upon mg/m^2 (corresponding to plasma concentrations 4.5- and 6.5-fold higher than in humans in the monkey and rat, respectively) did not reveal any evidence of teratogenic effects. At these doses, sparfloxacin was clearly maternally toxic to the rabbit and monkey with evidence of slight maternal toxicity observed in the rat. When administered to pregnant rats at clearly maternally toxic doses (≥9.3 times the maximum human dose based upon mg/m^2), sparfloxacin induced a dose-dependent increase in the incidence of fetuses with ventricular septal defects. Among the three species tested, this effect was specific to the rat. There are, however, no adequate and well controlled studies in pregnant women. Sparfloxacin should be used during pregnancy only if the potential benefit justifies the potential risk to the fetus. (See WARNINGS.)

NURSING MOTHERS

Sparfloxacin is excreted in human milk. Because of the potential for serious adverse reactions in infants nursing from mothers taking sparfloxacin, a decision should be made whether to discontinue nursing or to discontinue the drug, taking into account the importance of the drug to the mother. (See WARNINGS.)

PEDIATRIC USE

Safety and effectiveness have not been established in patients below the age of 18 years. Quinolones, including sparfloxacin, cause arthropathy and osteochondrosis in juvenile animals of several species. (See WARNINGS.)

DRUG INTERACTIONS:

Digoxin: Sparfloxacin has no effect on the pharmacokinetics of digoxin.

Methylxanthines: Sparfloxacin does not increase plasma theophylline concentrations. Since there is no interaction with theophylline, interaction with other methylxanthines such as caffeine is unlikely.

DRUG INTERACTIONS: *(cont'd)*

Warfarin: Sparfloxacin does not increase the anti-coagulant effect of warfarin.

Cimetidine: Cimetidine does not affect the pharmacokinetics of sparfloxacin.

Antacids and Sucralfate: Aluminum and magnesium cations in antacids and sucralfate form chelation complexes with sparfloxacin. The oral bioavailability of sparfloxacin is reduced when an aluminum magnesium suspension is administered between 2 hours before and 2 hours after sparfloxacin administration. The oral bioavailability of sparfloxacin is not reduced when the aluminum-magnesium suspension is administered 4 hours following sparfloxacin administration.

Zinc/iron salts: Absorption of quinolones is reduced significantly by these preparations. These products may be taken 4 hours after sparfloxacin administration.

Probenecid: Probenecid does not alter the pharmacokinetics of sparfloxacin.

ADVERSE REACTIONS:

In clinical trials, most of the adverse events were mild to moderate in severity and transient in nature. During clinical investigations with the recommended dosage, 1585 patients received sparfloxacin and 1331 patients received a comparator. The discontinuation rate due to adverse events was 6.6% for sparfloxacin versus 5.6% for cefaclor, 14.8% for erythromycin, 8.9% for ciprofloxacin, 7.4% for ofloxacin, and 8.3% for clarithromycin.

The most frequently reported events (remotely, possibly, or probably drug related with an incidence of ≥1%) among sparfloxacin treated patients in the U.S. phase 3 clinical trials with the recommended dosage were: photosensitivity reaction (7.9%), diarrhea (4.6%), nausea (4.3%), headache (4.2%), dyspepsia (2.3%), dizziness (2.0%), insomnia (1.9%), abdominal pain (1.8%), pruritus (1.8%), taste perversion (1.4%), and QT_c interval prolongation (1.3%), vomiting (1.3%), flatulence (1.1%) and vasodilatation (1.0%).

In US phase 3 clinical trials of shorter treatment duration than the recommended dosage, the most frequently reported events (incidence ≥1%, remotely, possibly, or probably drug related) were: headache (8.1%), nausea (7.6%), dizziness (3.8%), photosensitivity reaction (3.6%), pruritus (3.3%), diarrhea (3.2%), vaginal moniliasis (2.8%), abdominal pain (2.4%), asthenia (1.7%), dyspepsia (1.6%), somnolence (1.5%), dry mouth (1.4%), and rash (1.1%).

Additional possibly or probably related events that occurred in less than 1% of all patients enrolled in U.S. phase 3 clinical trials are listed below:

Body As A Whole: Fever, chest pain, generalized pain, allergic reaction, cellulitis, back pain, chills, face edema, malaise, accidental injury, anaphylactoid reaction, infection, mucous membrane disorder, neck pain, rheumatoid arthritis;

Cardiovascular: Palpitation, electrocardiogram abnormal, hypertension, tachycardia, sinus bradycardia, PR interval shortened, angina pectoris, arrhythmia, atrial fibrillation, atrial flutter, complete AV block, first degree AV block, second degree AV block, cardiovascular disorder, hemorrhage, migraine, peripheral vascular disorder, supraventricular extrasystoles, ventricular extrasystoles, postural hypotension;

Gastrointestinal: Constipation, anorexia, gingivitis, oral moniliasis, stomatitis, tongue disorder, tooth disorder, gastroenteritis, increased appetite, mouth ulceration, flatulence, vomiting;

Hematologic: Cyanosis, ecchymosis, lymphadenopathy;

Metabolism: Gout, peripheral edema, thirst;

Musculoskeletal: Arthralgia, arthritis, joint disorder, myalgia;

Central Nervous System: Paresthesia, hypesthesia, nervousness, somnolence, abnormal dreams, dry mouth, depression, tremor, anxiety, confusion, hallucinations, hyperesthesia, hyperkinesia, sleep disorder, hypokinesia, vertigo, abnormal gait, agitation, lightheadedness, emotional lability, euphoria, abnormal thinking, amnesia, twitching;

Respiratory: Asthma, epistaxis, pneumonia, rhinitis, pharyngitis, bronchitis, hemoptysis, sinusitis, cough increased, dyspnea, laryngismus, lung disorder, pleural disorder;

Skin/Hypersensitivity: Rash, maculopapular rash, dry skin, herpes simplex, sweating, urticaria, vesiculobullous rash, exfoliative dermatitis, acne, alopecia, angioedema, contact dermatitis, fungal dermatitis, furunculosis, pustular rash, skin discoloration, herpes zoster, petechial rash;

Special Senses: Ear pain, amblyopia, photophobia, tinnitus, conjunctivitis, diplopia, abnormality of accommodation, blepharitis, ear disorder, eye pain, lacrimation disorder, otitis media;

Urogenital: Vaginitis, dysuria, breast pain, dysmenorrhea, hematuria, menorrhagia, nocturia, polyuria, urinary tract infection, kidney pain, leukorrhea, metrorrhagia, vulvovaginal disorder.

Laboratory Changes: In the U.S. phase 3 clinical trials, with the recommended dosage, the most frequently (incidence ≥1%) reported changes in laboratory parameters listed as adverse events, regardless of relationship to drug, were: elevated ALT (SGPT) (2.0%), AST (SGOT) (2.3%) and white blood cells (1.1%).

Increases for the following laboratory tests were reported in less than 1% of all patients enrolled in clinical trials: alkaline phosphatase, serum amylase, aPTT, blood urea nitrogen, calcium, creatinine, eosinophils, serum lipase, monocytes, neutrophils, total bilirubin, urine glucose, urine protein, urine red blood cells, and urine white blood cells.

Decreases for the following laboratory tests were reported in less than 1% of all patients enrolled in clinical trials: albumin, creatinine clearance, hematocrit, hemoglobin, lymphocytes, phosphorus, red blood cells, and sodium.

Increases and decreases for the following laboratory tests were reported in less than 1% of all patients in clinical trials: blood glucose, platelets, potassium, and white blood cells.

POSTMARKETING ADVERSE EVENTS

The following are additional adverse events (regardless of relationship to drug) reported from worldwide postmarketing experience with sparfloxacin or other quinolones: acidosis, acute renal failure, agranulocytosis, albuminuria, anaphylactic shock, angioedema, anosmia, ataxia, bullous eruption, candiduria, cardiopulmonary arrest, cerebral thrombosis, convulsions, crystalluria, dysgeusia, dysphasia, ebrious feeling, embolism, erythema nodosum, exacerbation of myasthenia gravis, gastralgia, hemolytic anemia, hepatic necrosis, hepatitis, hiccough, hyperpigmentation, interstitial nephritis, interstitial pneumonia, intestinal perforation, jaundice, laryngeal or pulmonary edema, manic reaction, numbness, nystagmus, painful oral mucosa, pancreatitis, phobia, prolongation of prothrombin time, pseudomembranous colitis, Quincke's edema, renal calculi, rhabdomyolysis, sensory disturbance, Stevens-Johnson syndrome, squamous cell carcinoma, tendonitis, tendon rupture, tremor, thrombocytopenia, thrombocytopenia purpura, toxic epidermal necrolysis, toxic psychosis, urinary retention, uveitis, vaginal candidiasis, vasculitis.

Laboratory Changes: Elevation of serum triglycerides, serum cholesterol, blood glucose, serum potassium, decrease in WBC counts, RBC counts, hemoglobin level, hematocrit level, thrombocyte counts, elevation in GOT, GPT, ALP, LDH, γ-GTP, total bilirubin.

OVERDOSAGE:

In case of overdosage, the patient should be monitored in a suitably equipped medical facility and advised to avoid sun exposure for five days. ECG monitoring is recommended due to the possible prolongation of the QT_c interval. There is no known antidote for sparfloxacin overdosage.

OVERDOSAGE: *(cont'd)*

It is not known whether sparfloxacin is dialyzable.

Single doses of sparfloxacin were relatively non-toxic via the oral route of administration in mice, rats, and dogs. No deaths occurred within a 14-day post-treatment observation period at the highest oral doses tested, up to 5000 mg/kg in either rodent species, or up to 600 mg/kg in the dog. Clinical signs observed included inactivity in mice and dogs, diarrhea in both rodent species, and vomiting, salivation, and tremors in dogs.

DOSAGE AND ADMINISTRATION:

Sparfloxacin can be taken with or without food.

The recommended daily dose of sparfloxacin in patients with normal renal function is two 200 mg tablets taken on the first day as a loading dose. Thereafter, one 200 mg tablet should be taken every 24 hours for a total of 10 days of therapy (11 tablets).

The recommended daily dose of sparfloxacin in patients with renal impairment (creatinine clearance <50 ml/min) is two 200 mg tablets taken on the first day as a loading dose. Thereafter, one 200 mg tablet should be taken every 48 hours for a total of 9 days of therapy (6 tablets).

Store at controlled room temperature 20 to 25°C (68 to 77°F).

ANIMAL PHARMACOLOGY:

Sparfloxacin and other quinolones have been shown to cause arthropathy in juvenile animals of most species tested. (See WARNINGS.)

Sparfloxacin had no convulsive activity in mice when administered alone or in combination with the nonsteroidal anti-inflammatory agents ketoprofen, or naproxen.

PATIENT INFORMATION:

Sparfloxacin is an antibiotic used to treat pneumonia and chronic bronchitis.

Do not take if you are pregnant or nursing.

Do not take if you are taking certain antiarrhythmic drugs (*e.g.,* quinidine, procainamide, sotalol, bepridil) or terfenadine.

Inform physician if you have kidney disease or any CNS condition that may predispose to seizures (*e.g.,* epilepsy).

Avoid exposure to the sun, bright natural light (direct or indirect) and UV light. Discontinue sparfloxacin at the first sign of phototoxicity (sensation of skin burning, redness, swelling, blisters, rash, itching or dermatitis).

Pseudomembranous colitis (severe, possibly life-threatening diarrhea) has accurred. Inform physician if diarrhea occurs.

May cause dizziness or lightheadedness. Use caution while driving or operating hazardous machinery.

Allergic reaction may occur. Discontinue use at the first sign of skin rash or other allergic reaction.

Discontinue use if pain, inflammation or tendon rupture occurs. Rest, refrain from exercise and contact physician.

May cause photosensitivity, diarrhea, nausea, headache, dyspepsia, dizziness, insomnia, abdominal pain, pruritus, taste perversion, QT_c interval prolongation, vomiting, flatulence, and vasodilation. Inform physician if these occur.

Drink plenty of fluids.

May be taken with food, milk or caffeine-containing products.

Take vitamins or minerals containing iron, zinc or calcium at least 4 hours after taking sparfloxacin.

Take sucralfate or aluminum or magnesium-containing antacids at least 4 hours after taking sparfloxacin.

REFERENCES:

1. National Committee for Clinical Laboratory Standards. Methods for Dilution Antimicrobial Susceptibility Tests for Bacteria that Grow Aerobically-Third Edition. Approved Standard NCCLS Document M7-A3, Vol. 13, No. 25, NCCLS, Villanova, PA, December, 1993. **2.** National Committee for Clinical Laboratory Standards. Performance Standards for Antimicrobial Disk Susceptibility Tests-Fifth Edition. Approved Standard NCCLS Document M2-A5, Vol. 13, No. 24, NCCLS, Villanova, PA, December 1993.

SPECTINOMYCIN HYDROCHLORIDE *(002268)*

CATEGORIES: Anti-Infectives; Antibiotics; Antimicrobials; Gonorrhea; Infections; Proctitis; Urethritis; FDA Approval Pre 1982

BRAND NAMES: **Trobicin**

FORMULARIES: WHO

DESCRIPTION:

Trobicin Sterile Powder contains spectinomycin hydrochloride which is an aminocyclitol antibiotic produced by a species of soil microorganism designated as *Streptomyces spectabilis.* Sterile spectinomycin hydrochloride is the pentahydrated dihydrochloride salt of spectinomycin.

Spectinomycin hydrochloride is isolated as a white to pale buff crystalline dihydrochloride pentahydrate powder, molecular weight 495, and is stable in the dry state for 36 months.

CLINICAL PHARMACOLOGY:

Spectinomycin hydrochloride is an inhibitor of protein synthesis in the bacterial cell; the site of action is the 30S ribosomal subunit.

In vitro studies have shown spectinomycin hydrochloride to be active against most strains of *Neisseria gonorrhoeae* (minimum inhibitory concentration < 7.5 to 20 mcg/ml).

Definitive *in vitro* studies have shown no cross-resistance of *N. gonorrhoeae* between spectinomycin hydrochloride and penicillin. The antibiotic is not significantly bound to plasma protein.

INDICATIONS AND USAGE:

Trobicin (Spectinomycin HCl) Sterile Powder is indicated in the treatment of acute gonorrheal urethritis and proctitis in the male and acute gonorrheal cervicitis and proctitis in the female when due to susceptible strains of *Neisseria gonorrhoeae.* Men and women with known recent exposure to gonorrhea should be treated as those known to have gonorrhea.

The *in vitro* susceptibility of *Neisseria gonorrhoeae* to spectinomycin hydrochloride can be tested by agar diluted methods. Trobicin Susceptibility Powder is available for this purpose and its package insert should be consulted for details.

CONTRAINDICATIONS:

The use of Trobicin (Spectinomycin HCl) Sterile Powder is contraindicated in patients previously found hypersensitive to it.

WARNINGS:

Spectinomycin hydrochloride is not effective in the treatment of syphilis. Antibiotics used in high doses for short periods of time to treat gonorrhea may mask or delay the symptoms of incubating syphilis. Since the treatment of syphilis demands prolonged therapy with any effective antibiotic, patients being treated for gonorrhea should be closely observed clinically. All patients with gonorrhea should have a serologic test for syphilis at the time of diagnosis. Patients treated with spectinomycin hydrochloride should have a follow-up serologic test for syphilis after three months.

Usage in pregnancy: Safety for use in pregnancy has not been established.

Usage in infants and children: Safety for use in infants and children has not been established.

The diluent provided with this product contains benzylalcohol which has been associated with a fatal gasping syndrome in infants.

PRECAUTIONS:

The usual precautions should be observed with atopic individuals.

The clinical effectiveness of Trobicin (Spectinomycin HCl) Sterile Powder should be monitored to detect evidence of development of resistance by *Neisseria gonorrhoeae.*

ADVERSE REACTIONS:

The following reactions were observed during the single dose clinical trials: soreness at the injection site, urticaria, dizziness, nausea, chills, fever and insomnia.

During multiple dose subchronic tolerance studies in normal human volunteers, the following were noted: a decrease in hemoglobin, hematocrit and creatinine clearance; elevation of alkaline phosphatase, BUN and SGPT. In single and multiple dose studies in normal volunteers, a reduction in urine output was noted. Extensive renal function studies demonstrated no consistent changes indicative of renal toxicity.

A few cases of anaphylaxis or anaphylactoid reactions have been reported. If serious allergic reactions occur, the usual agents (epinephrine, corticosteroids, and/or antihistamines) should be available for emergency use. In cases of severe anaphylaxis, airway support and oxygen may also be required.

DOSAGE AND ADMINISTRATION:

PREPARATION OF DRUG FOR INTRAMUSCULAR INJECTION

Trobicin (Spectinomycin HCl) Sterile Powder, 2 grams: reconstitute with 3.2 ml of the accompanying diluent.*

Trobicin (Spectinomycin HCl) Sterile Powder, 4 grams: reconstitute with 6.2 ml of the accompanying diluent.*

Shake vials vigorously immediately after adding diluent and before withdrawing dose. It is recommended that disposable syringes and needles be used to avoid contamination with penicillin residue, especially when treating patients known to be highly sensitive to penicillin. **Use of a 20 gauge needle is recommended.**

DOSAGE

Intramuscular injections should be made deep into the upper outer quadrant of the gluteal muscle.

Adults (Men and Women)-Inject 5 ml Intramuscularly for a 2 gram dose. This is also the recommended dose for patients being treated after failure of previous antibiotic therapy.

In geographic areas where antibiotic resistance is known to be prevalent, initial treatment with 4 grams (10 ml) intramuscularly is preferred. The 10 ml injection may be divided between two gluteal injection sites.

STORAGE CONDITIONS

Store unreconstituted product at controlled room temperature 15-30° C (50-86° F). Store prepared suspension at controlled room temperature 15-30° C (59-30° F) and use within 24 hours.

HUMAN PHARMACOLOGY

Spectinomycin HCl Sterile Powder is rapidly absorbed after intramuscular injection. A single, two gram injection produces peak serum concentrations averaging about 100 mcg/ml at one hour; a single, four gram injection produces peak serum concentrations averaging 160 mcg/ml at two hours. Average serum concentrations of 15 mcg/ml for the two gram dose and 31 mcg/ml for the four gram dose were present eight hours after dosing.

*Bacteriostatic Water for Injection with Benzyl Alcohol 0.945% w/v added as preservative.

HOW SUPPLIED - EQUIVALENTS NOT AVAILABLE:

Injection, Dry-Susp - Intramuscular - 400 mg/ml

2 gm	**$16.86**	**TROBICIN, Pharmacia & Upjohn**	**00009-0566-01**

SPIRAPRIL *(003238)*

CATEGORIES: ACE Inhibitors; Angiotensin Converting Enzyme Inhibitors; Antihypertensives; Cardiovascular Drugs; Hypertension; FDA Class 1S ("Standard Review"); FDA Approved 1994 Dec

BRAND NAMES: **Renormax**

Prescribing information not available at time of publication.

SPIRONOLACTONE *(002269)*

CATEGORIES: Adrenal Hyperplasia; Antagonists and Antidotes; Antihypertensives; Cardiovascular Drugs; Cirrhosis; Congestive Heart Failure; Diuretics; Edema; Electrolytic, Caloric-Water Balance; Heart Failure; Hyperaldosteronism; Hypertension; Hypokalemia; Nephrotic Syndrome; Potassium Sparing Diuretics; Pregnancy; Renal Drugs; FDA Approval Pre 1982

BRAND NAMES: *Adultmin;* **Aldactone**; *Aldopur; Aldospirone; Almatol; Berlactone; Diatensec; Diram; Esekon; Hypazon; Idrolattone; Merabis; Novospiroton; Osiren; Osyrol; Pirolacton; Resacton; Sincomen; Spiractin; Spiroctan; Spirolacton; Spirolang; Spironex; Spirotone; Tensin; Tevaspirone; Verospiron; Xenalon Lactabs; Youlactone (International brand names outside U.S. in italics)*

FORMULARIES: Aetna; BC-BS; CIGNA; DoD; FHP; Humana; Kaiser; Medco; Medi-Cal; PCS; PruCare; United; WHO

COST OF THERAPY: $33.06 (Hypertension; Tablet; 25 mg; 2/day; 365 days)

PRIMARY ICD9: 401.1 (Essential Hypertension, Benign)

> **WARNING:**
> Spironolactone has been shown to be a tumorigen in chronic toxicity studies in rats (see WARNINGS.) Spironolactone should be used only in those conditions described under INDICATIONS AND USAGE. Unnecessary use of this drug should be avoided.

DESCRIPTION:

Spironolactone oral tablets contain 25 mg, 50 mg, or 100 mg of the aldosterone antagonist spironolactone, 17-hydroxy-7α-mercapto-3-oxo-17α-pregn-4-ene -21-carboxylic acid γ-lactone acetate.

Spironolactone is practically insoluble in water, soluble in alcohol, and freely soluble in benzene and in chloroform.

Inactive ingredients include calcium sulfate, corn starch, flavor, hydroxypropyl methylcellulose, iron oxide, magnesium stearate, polyethylene glycol, povidone, and titanium dioxide.

CLINICAL PHARMACOLOGY:

Mechanism of Action: Spironolactone is a specific pharmacologic antagonist of aldosterone, acting primarily through competitive binding of receptors at the aldosterone-dependent sodium-potassium exchange site in the distal convoluted renal tubule. Spironolactone causes increased amounts of sodium and water to be excreted, while potassium is retained. Spironolactone acts both as a diuretic and as an antihypertensive drug by this mechanism. It may be given alone or with other diuretic agents which act more proximally in the renal tubule.

Aldosterone Antagonist Activity: Increased levels of the mineralocorticoid, aldosterone, are present in primary and secondary hyperaldosteronism. Edematous states in which secondary aldosteronism is usually involved include congestive heart failure, hepatic cirrhosis, and the nephrotic syndrome. By competing with aldosterone for receptor sites, spironolactone provides effective therapy for the edema and ascites in those conditions. Spironolactone counteracts secondary aldosteronism inducted by the volume depletion and associated sodium loss caused by active diuretic therapy.

Spironolactone is effective in lowering the systolic and diastolic blood pressure in patients with primary hyperaldosteronism. It is also effective in most cases of essential hypertension, despite the fact that aldosterone secretion may be within normal limits in benign essential hypertension.

Through its action in antagonizing the effect of aldosterone, spironolactone inhibits the exchange of sodium for potassium in the distal rental tubule and helps to prevent potassium loss.

Spironolactone has not been demonstrated to elevate serum uric acid, to precipitate gout or to alter carbohydrate metabolism.

Pharmacokinetics: Spironolactone is rapidly and extensively metabolized. Sulfur-containing products are the predominant metabolites and are thought to be primarily responsible, together with spironolactone, for the therapeutic effects of the drug. The following pharmacokinetic data (TABLE 1) were obtained from 12 healthy volunteers following administration of 100 mg of spironolactone (film-coated tablets) daily for 15 days. On the 15th day, spironolactone was given immediately after a low-fat breakfast and blood was drawn thereafter (TABLE 1).

TABLE 1

	Accumulation Factor AUC (0-24 hr, day 15)/AUC (0-24 hr, day 1)	Mean Peak Serum Concentration	Mean (SD) Post-Steady State Half-Life
7-α-(thiomethyl) spirolactone (TMS)	1.25	391 ng/ml at 3.2 hr	13.8 hr (6.4) (terminal)
6-β-hydroxy-7-α-(thiomethyl) spirolactone (HTMS)	1.50	125 ng/ml at 5.1 hr	15.0 hr (4.0) (terminal)
Canrenone (C)	1.41	181 ng/ml at 4.3 hr	16.5 hr (6.3) (terminal)
Spironolactone	1.30	80 ng/ml at 2.6 hr	Approximately 1.4 hr (0.5) (β half-life)

The pharmacological activity of spironolactone metabolites in man is not known. however, in the adrenalectomized rat the antimineralocorticoid activities of the metabolites C, TMS, and HTMS, relative to spironolactone, were 1.10, 1.28, and 0.32, respectively. Relative to spironolactone, their binding affinities to the aldosterone receptors in rat kidney slices were 0.19, 0.86, and 0.06, respectively.

In humans the potencies of TMS and 7-α-thiospirolactone in reversing the effects of the synthetic mineralocorticoid, fludrocortisone, on urinary electrolyte composition were 0.33 and 0.26, respectively, relative to spironolactone. However, since the serum concentrations of these steroids were not determined, their incomplete absorption and/or first-pass metabolism could not be rules out as a reason for their reduced *in vivo* activities.

Both spironolactone and canrenone are more than 90% bound to plasma proteins. The metabolites are excreted primarily in the urine and secondarily in bile. The effect food on spironolactone absorption (two 100 mg spironolactone tablets) was assessed in a single dose study of 9 healthy, drug-free volunteers. Food increased the bioavailability of unmetabolized spironolactone by almost 100%. The clinical importance of this finding is not known.

INDICATIONS AND USAGE:

Spironolactone is indicated in the management of:

Primary hyperaldosteronism for: Establishing the diagnosis of primary hyperaldosteronism by therapeutic trial.

Short-term preoperative treatment of patients with primary hyperaldosteronism.

Long-term maintenance therapy for patients with discrete aldosterone-producing adrenal adenomas who are judged to be poor operative risk, or who decline surgery.

Long-term maintenance therapy for patients with bilateral micro- or macronodular adrenal hyperplasia (idiopathic hyperaldosteronism).

Edematous conditions for patients with:

Congestive heart failure: For the management of edema and sodium retention when the patient is only partially responsive to, or is intolerant of, other therapeutic measures. Spironolactone is also indicated for patients with congestive heart failure taking digitalis when other therapies are considered inappropriate.

Cirrhosis of the liver accompanied by edema and/or ascites: Spironolactone levels may be exceptionally high in this condition. Spironolactone is indicated for maintenance therapy together with bed rest and the restriction of fluid and sodium.

INDICATIONS AND USAGE: *(cont'd)*

The nephrotic syndrome: For nephrotic patients when treatment of the underlying disease, restriction of fluid and sodium intake, and the use of other diuretics do not provide on adequate response.

ESSENTIAL HYPERTENSION

Usually in combination with other drugs, spironolactone is indicated for patients who cannot be treated adequately with other agents or for whom other agents are considered inappropriate.

HYPOKALEMIA

For the treatment of patients with hypokalemia when other measures are considered inappropriate or inadequate. Spironolactone is also indicated for the prophylaxis of hypokalemia in patients taking digitalis when other measures are considered inadequate or inappropriate.

Usage in Pregnancy: The routine uses of diuretics in an otherwise healthy woman is inappropriate and exposes mother and fetus to unnecessary hazard. Diuretics do not prevent development of toxemia of pregnancy, and there is no satisfactory evidence that they are useful in the treatment of developing toxemia.

Edema during pregnancy may arise from pathologic causes or from the physiologic and mechanical consequences of pregnancy.

Spironolactone is indicated in pregnancy when edema is due to pathologic causes just as it is in the absence of pregnancy (however, see WARNINGS). Dependent edema in pregnancy, resulting from restriction of venous return by the expanded uterus, is properly treated through elevation of the lower extremities and use of support house; use of diuretics to lower intravascular volume in this case is unsupported and unnecessary. There is hypervolemia during normal pregnancy which is harmful to neither the fetus nor the mother (in the absence of cardiovascular disease), but which is associated with edema, including generalized edema, in the majority of pregnancy women. If this edema produces discomfort, increased recumbency will often provide relief. In rare instances, this edema may cause extreme discomfort which is not relieved by rest. In these cases, a short course of diuretics may provide relief and may be appropriate.

CONTRAINDICATIONS:

Spironolactone is contraindicated for patients with anuria, acute renal insufficiency, significant impairment of renal excretory function, or hyperkalemia.

WARNINGS:

Potassium supplementation, either in the form of medication or as a diet rich in potassium, should not ordinarily be given in association with spironolactone therapy. Excessive potassium intake may cause hyperkalemia in patients receiving spironolactone (see PRECAUTIONS.) Spironolactone should not be administered concurrently with other potassium-sparing diuretics. Spironolactone, when used with ACE inhibitors, even in the presence of a diuretic, has been associated with severe hyperkalemia. Extreme caution should be exercised when spironolactone is given concomitantly with ACE inhibitors (see DRUG INTERACTIONS.)

Spironolactone has been shown to be a tumorigen in chronic toxicity studies performed in rats, with its proliferative effects manifested on endocrine organs and the liver. In one study using 25, 75 and 250 times the usual daily human dose (2 mg/kg) there was a statistically significant dose-related increase in benign adenomas of the thyroid and testes. In female rats there was a statistically significant increase in malignant mammary tumors at the mid-dose only. In male rats there was a dose-related increase in proliferative changes in the liver. At the highest dosage level (500 mg/kg) the range of effects included hepatocytomegaly, hyperplastic nodules and hepatocellular carcinoma; the last was not statistically significant at a value of $p = 0.05$. A dose-related (above 20 mg/kg/day) incidence of myelocytic leukemia was observed in rats fed daily doses of potassium canrenoate for a period of one year. In long-term (two-year) oral carcinogenicity studies of potassium canrenoate in the rat, myelocytic leukemia and hepatic, thyroid, testicular, and mammary tumors were observed. Potassium canrenoate did not produce a mutagenic effect in tests using bacteria or yeast. It did produce a positive mutagenic effect in several *in vitro* tests in mammalian cells following metabolic activation. In an*in vivo* mammalian system potassium canrenoate was not mutagenic. Canrenone and canrenoic acid are the major metabolites of potassium canrenoate. Spironolactone is also metabolized to canrenone. An increased incidence of leukemia was not observed in chronic rat toxicity studies conducted with spironolactone at doses up to 500 mg/kg/day.

PRECAUTIONS:

General: Because of the diuretic action of spironolactone, patients should be carefully evaluated for possible disturbances of fluid and electrolyte balance. Hyperkalemia may occur in patients with impaired renal function or excessive potassium intake and can cause cardiac irregularities which may be fatal. Consequently, no potassium supplement should ordinarily be given with spironolactone. Hyperkalemia can be treated promptly by the rapid intravenous administration of glucose (20% to 50%) and regular insulin, using 0.25 to 0.5 units of insulin per gram of glucose. This is a temporary measure to be repeated as required. Spironolactone use should be discontinued and potassium intake (including dietary potassium) restricted.

Reversible hyperchloremic metabolic acidosis, usually in association with hyperkalemia, has been reported to occur in some patients with decompensated hepatic cirrhosis, even in the presence of normal renal function.

Hyperkalemia, manifested by dryness of mouth, thirst, lethargy and drowsiness, and confirmed by a low serum sodium level, may be caused or aggravated, especially when spironolactone is administered in combination with other diuretics.

Gynecomastia may develop in association with the use of spironolactone; physicians should be alert to its possible onset. The development of gynecomastia appears to be related to both dosage level and duration of therapy and is normally reversible when spironolactone is discontinued. In rare instances some breast enlargement may persist when spironolactone is discontinued.

Spironolactone therapy may cause a transient elevation of BUN, especially in patients with preexisting renal impairment. Spironolactone may cause mild acidosis.

A determination of serum electrolytes to detect possible electrolyte imbalance should be performed at periodic intervals.

Drug/Laboratory Test Interactions: Several reports of possible interference with digoxin radioimmunoassays by spironolactone, or its metabolites, have appeared in the literature. neither the extent nor the potential clinical significance of its interference (which may be assay-specific) has been fully established.

Pregnancy: Spironolactone or its metabolites may cross the placental barrier. Therefore, the use of spironolactone in pregnant women requires that the anticipated benefit be weighed against possible hazard to the fetus.

Nursing Mothers: Canrenone, a metabolite of spironolactone, appears in breast milk. If use of the drug is deemed essential, an alternative method of infant feeding should be instituted.

DRUG INTERACTIONS:

When used in combination with other diuretics or antihypertensive agents spironolactone potentiates their effects. Therefore, the dosage of such drugs, particularly the ganglionic blocking agents, should be reduced by at least 50% when spironolactone is added to the regimen.

Concomitant administration of potassium-sparring diuretics with ACE inhibitors or indomethacin has been associated with severe hyperkalemia.

Spironolactone reduces the vascular responsiveness to norepinephrine. Therefore, caution should be exercised in the management of patients subjected to regional or general anesthesia while they are being treated with spironolactone.

Spironolactone has been shown to increase the half-life of digoxin. This may result in increased serum digoxin levels and subsequent digitalis toxicity. It may be necessary to reduce the maintenance and digitalization doses when spironolactone is administered, and the patient should be carefully monitored to avoid over- or underdigitalization.

ADVERSE REACTIONS:

Gynecomastia is observed not infrequently. Other adverse reactions that have been reported in association with spironolactone are: gastrointestinal symptoms including cramping and diarrhea, drowsiness, lethargy, headache, maculopapular or erythematous cutaneous eruption, urticaria, mental confusion, drug fever, ataxia, inability to achieve or maintain erection, irregular menses or amenorrhea, postmenopausal bleeding, hirsutism and deepening of the voice. Carcinoma of the breast has been reported in patients taking spironolactone, but a cause and effect relationship has not been established.

Adverse reactions are usually reversible upon discontinuation of the drug.

DOSAGE AND ADMINISTRATION:

Primary hyperaldosteronism. Spironolactone may be employed as an initial diagnostic measure to provide presumptive evidence of primary hyperaldosteronism while patients are on normal diets.

Long test: Spironolactone is administered at a daily dosage of 400 mg for three to four weeks. Correction of hyperkalemia and of hypertension provides presumptive evidence for the diagnosis of primary hyperaldosteronism.

Short test: Spironolactone is administered at a daily dosage of 400 mg for four days. If serum potassium increased during spironolactone administration but drops when spironolactone is discontinued, a presumptive diagnosis of primary hyperaldosteronism should be considered.

After the diagnosis of hyperaldosteronism has been established by more definitive testing procedures, spironolactone may be administered in doses of 100 to 400 mg daily in preparation for surgery. For patients who are considered unsuitable for surgery, spironolactone may be employed for long-term maintenance therapy at the lowest effective dosage determined for the individual patient.

Edema in adults: *(congestive heart failure, hepatic cirrhosis or nephrotic syndrome).* An initial daily dosage of 100 mg of spironolactone administered in divided doses is recommended, but may range from one to eight tablets (25 to 200 mg) daily. When given as the sole agent for diuresis, spironolactone should be continued for at least five days at the initial dosage level, after which it may be adjusted to the optimal therapeutic or maintenance level. If, after five days, an adequate diuretic response to spironolactone has not occurred, a second diuretic which acts more proximally in the renal tubule may be asked to the regimen. Because of the additive effect of spironolactone when administered concurrently with such diuretics, an enhanced diuresis usually begins on the first day of combined treatment; combined therapy is indicated when more rapid diuresis is desired. The dosage of spironolactone should remain unchanged when other diuretic therapy is added.

Edema in children: The initial daily dosage should provide approximately 1.5 mg of spironolactone per pound of body weight (3.3 mg/kg) administered in divided doses.

Essential hypertension: For adults, an initial daily dosage of 50 to 100 mg of spironolactone administered in divided doses is recommended. Spironolactone may also be given with diuretics which act more proximally in the renal tubule or with other antihypertensive agents. Treatment with spironolactone should be continued for at least two weeks, since the maximum response may not occur before this time. Subsequently, dosage should be adjusted according to the response of the patient.

Hypokalemia: Spironolactone in a dosage ranging from 25 to 100 mg daily is useful in treating a diuretic-induced hypokalemia, when oral potassium supplements or other potassium-sparing regimens are considered inappropriate.

Storage: Store below 86°F (30°C).

HOW SUPPLIED - RATED THERAPEUTICALLY EQUIVALENT:

Tablet, Plain Coated - Oral - 25 mg

100's	$4.53	Spironolactone, H.C.F.A. F F P	99999-2269-01
100's	$5.13	Spironolactone, US Trading	56126-0304-11
100's	$5.70	Spironolactone, Voluntary Hosp	53258-0159-01
100's	$6.25	Spironolactone, Consolidated Midland	00223-1724-01
100's	$6.90	Spironolactone, Qualitest Pharms	00603-5766-21
100's	$7.15	Spironolactone, Rugby	00536-4575-01
100's	$7.25	Spironolactone, Goldline Labs	00182-1157-01
100's	$7.25	Spironolactone, Mutual Pharm	53489-0143-01
100's	$7.57	Spironolactone, Aligen Independ	00405-4940-01
100's	$7.71	Spironolactone, United Res	00677-0625-01
100's	$7.81	Spironolactone, Caremark	00339-5355-12
100's	$7.85	Spironolactone, Purepac Pharm	00228-2388-10
100's	$7.95	Spironolactone, Parmed Pharms	00349-2305-01
100's	$8.17	Spironolactone, HL Moore Drug Exch	00839-6330-06
100's	$9.35	Spironolactone, Mylan	00378-2146-01
100's	$9.85	Spironolactone, Raway	00686-3885-13
100's	$10.72	Spironolactone 25, Major Pharms	00904-0343-61
100's	$12.18	Spironolactone, Voluntary Hosp	53258-0159-13
100's	$16.12	Spironolactone, Vangard Labs	00615-1535-13
100's	$16.75	Spironolactone, Medirex	57480-0382-01
100's	**$38.64**	**ALDACTONE, Searle**	**00025-1001-31**
250's	$11.32	Spironolactone, H.C.F.A. F F P	99999-2269-02
250's	$11.60	Spironolactone 25, Major Pharms	00904-0343-70
500's	$5.80	Spironolactone 25, Major Pharms	00904-0343-60
500's	$14.95	Spirono 25, H & H Labs	46703-0057-05
500's	$21.40	Spironolactone, Major Pharms	00904-0343-40
500's	$22.65	Spironolactone, H.C.F.A. F F P	99999-2269-03
500's	$30.76	Spironolactone, Qualitest Pharms	00603-5766-28
500's	$33.20	Spironolactone, Rugby	00536-4575-05
500's	$34.85	Spironolactone, United Res	00677-0625-05
500's	$34.85	Spironolactone, Mutual Pharm	53489-0143-05
500's	$39.40	Spironolactone, Purepac Pharm	00228-2388-50
500's	$40.35	Spironolactone, Mylan	00378-2146-05
500's	$42.49	Spironolactone, Amer Preferred	53445-1157-05
500's	**$183.45**	**ALDACTONE, Searle**	**00025-1001-51**
600's	$104.40	Spironolactone, Medirex	57480-0382-06
1000's	$42.75	Spironolactone 25, Major Pharms	00904-0343-80

HOW SUPPLIED - RATED THERAPEUTICALLY EQUIVALENT:

(cont'd)

1000's	$45.30	Spironolactone, H.C.F.A. F F P	99999-2269-04
1000's	$55.00	Spironolactone, Consolidated Midland	00223-1724-02
1000's	$58.80	Spironolactone, Goldline Labs	00182-1157-10
1000's	$58.80	Spironolactone, United Res	00677-0625-10
1000's	$58.80	Spironolactone, Mutual Pharm	53489-0143-10
1000's	$61.89	Spironolactone, Aligen Independ	00405-4940-03
1000's	$64.95	Spironolactone, Parmed Pharms	00349-2305-10
1000's	$66.35	Spironolactone, HL Moore Drug Exch	00839-6330-16
1000's	$78.80	Spironolactone, Purepac Pharm	00228-2388-96
1000's	$80.00	Spironolactone, Harber Pharm	51432-0428-06
1000's	$91.80	Spironolactone, Rugby	00536-4575-10
2500's	$113.25	Spironolactone, H.C.F.A. F F P	99999-2269-05
2500's	**$862.70**	**ALDACTONE, Searle**	**00025-1001-55**

HOW SUPPLIED - NOT RATED EQUIVALENT:

Tablet, Plain Coated - Oral - 50 mg

100's	**$67.86**	**ALDACTONE, Searle**	**00025-1041-31**
100's	**$71.08**	**ALDACTONE, Searle**	**00025-1041-34**

Tablet, Plain Coated - Oral - 100 mg

100's	**$113.78**	**ALDACTONE, Searle**	**00025-1031-31**
100's	**$119.29**	**ALDACTONE, Searle**	**00025-1031-34**

STANNOUS FLUORIDE *(002270)*

CATEGORIES: Dental; FDA Pre 1938 Drugs

BRAND NAMES: Cav-X; Gel-Kam; Gel-Pro; Omni Med; Omni Perio-Med; *Omnigel*; Omnii Pm; Omnii-Gel; Perfect Choice; Perio-Rinse; Perioselect Take Home Care; Stanimax; Stop

(International brand names outside U.S. in italics)

Prescribing information not available at time of publication.

HOW SUPPLIED - EQUIVALENTS NOT AVAILABLE:

Gel - Dental - 0.4 %

4.3 oz	$49.94	HOME FLUORIDE GEL, REDBERRY, Challenge Prod	50467-0110-04
4.3 oz	$49.94	HOME FLUORIDE GEL, GRAPE, Challenge Prod	50467-0811-04
4.3 oz	$49.94	HOME FLUORIDE GEL, CINNAMON, Challenge Prod	50467-0812-04
4.3 oz	$49.94	HOME FLUORIDE GEL, CREMEDE MENTHE, Challenge Prod	50467-0813-04
4.3 oz	$49.94	HOME FLUORIDE GEL, TUTTI FRUITTI, Challenge Prod	50467-0814-04
4.3 oz	$49.94	HOME FLUORIDE STANNOUS GEL, Challenge Prod	50467-0815-04
4.3 oz	$49.94	HOME FLUORIDE GEL, BUBBLE GUM, Challenge Prod	50467-0816-04
65 gm	$4.06	GEL-KAM, Colgate Oral	00126-2328-02
65 gm	$4.06	GEL-KAM, Colgate Oral	00126-2342-02
65 gm	$4.06	GEL-KAM, Colgate Oral	00126-2350-02
65 gm	$4.06	GEL-KAM, Colgate Oral	00126-2351-02
65 gm	$4.06	GEL-KAM, Colgate Oral	00126-2352-02
65 gm	$4.06	GEL-KAM, Colgate Oral	00126-2361-02
69 gm	$2.00	OMNI MED, Dunhall Pharms	00217-4050-20
69 gm	$2.25	OMNI MED, Dunhall Pharms	00217-4010-20
69 gm	$2.25	OMNI MED, Dunhall Pharms	00217-4020-20
69 gm	$2.25	OMNI MED, Dunhall Pharms	00217-4030-20
69 gm	$2.25	OMNI MED, Dunhall Pharms	00217-4040-20
69 gm	$2.25	OMNI MED, Dunhall Pharms	00217-4060-20
69 gm	$2.25	OMNI MED, Dunhall Pharms	00217-4070-20
120 gm	$99.29	GEL-KAM, Colgate Oral	00126-2328-93
120 gm	$99.29	GEL-KAM, Colgate Oral	00126-2342-93
120 gm	$99.29	GEL-KAM, Colgate Oral	00126-2350-93
120 gm	$99.29	GEL-KAM, Colgate Oral	00126-2351-93
120 gm	$99.29	GEL-KAM, Colgate Oral	00126-2352-93
120 gm	$99.29	GEL-KAM, Colgate Oral	00126-2361-93
120 gm x 12	$72.27	STOP, Oral B Labs	00041-0700-24
120 gm x 12	$72.27	STOP, Oral B Labs	00041-0701-24
120 gm x 12	$72.27	STOP, Oral B Labs	00041-0702-24
129 gm x 12	$49.94	Perfect Choice, Challenge Prod	50467-0817-04
200 gm	$153.65	GEL-KAM, Colgate Oral	00126-2328-98
200 gm	$153.65	GEL-KAM, Colgate Oral	00126-2342-98
200 gm	$153.65	GEL-KAM, Colgate Oral	00126-2350-98
200 gm	$153.65	GEL-KAM, Colgate Oral	00126-2351-98
200 gm	$153.65	GEL-KAM, Colgate Oral	00126-2352-98
200 gm	$153.65	GEL-KAM, Colgate Oral	00126-2361-98
210 gm	$5.50	OMNI MED, Dunhall Pharms	00217-4010-30
210 gm	$5.50	OMNI MED, Dunhall Pharms	00217-4020-30
210 gm	$5.50	OMNI MED, Dunhall Pharms	00217-4040-30
210 gm	$5.50	OMNI MED, Dunhall Pharms	00217-4050-30
210 gm	$5.50	OMNI MED, Dunhall Pharms	00217-4060-30
210 gm	$5.50	OMNI MED, Dunhall Pharms	00217-4070-30

Solution - Dental - 0.63 %

283.5 ml	$8.00	OMNII PM, Dunhall Pharms	00217-3310-35
300 ml	$181.37	GEL-KAM, Colgate Oral	00126-2310-02
300 ml	$181.37	GEL-KAM, Colgate Oral	00126-2312-02

STANOZOLOL *(002271)*

CATEGORIES: Anabolic Steroids; Androgens; Angioedema; Steroids; Pregnancy Category X; DEA Class CIII; FDA Approved 1984 May

BRAND NAMES: *Menabol*; *Stromba*; **Winstrol**

(International brand names outside U.S. in italics)

DESCRIPTION:

Stanozolol, is an anabolic steroid, a synthetic derivative of testosterone. Each Winstrol tablet contains 2 mg of stanozolol. It is designated chemically as 17-methyl-2'*H*-5α-androst-2-eno (3,2-c)pyrazol-17β-ol.

Winstrol Inactive Ingredients: Dibasic Calcium Phosphate, D&C Red #28, FD&C Red #40, Lactose, Magnesium Stearate, Starch.

CLINICAL PHARMACOLOGY:

Anabolic steroids are synthetic derivatives of testosterone.

Certain clinical effects and adverse reactions demonstrate the androgenic properties of this class of drugs. Complete dissociation of anabolic and androgenic effects has not been achieved. The actions of anabolic steroids are therefore similar to those of male sex hormones with the possibility of causing serious disturbances of growth and sexual development if given to young children. They suppress the gonadotropic functions of the pituitary and may exert a direct effect upon the testes.

Stanozolol has been found to increase low-density lipoproteins and decrease high-density lipoproteins. These changes are not associated with any increase in total cholesterol or triglyceride levels and revert to normal on discontinuation of treatment.

Hereditary angioedema (HAE) is an autosomal dominant disorder caused by a deficient or nonfunctional C1 esterase inhibitor (C1 INH) and clinically characterized by episodes of swelling of the face, extremities, genitalia, bowel wall, and upper respiratory tract.

In small scale clinical studies, stanozolol was effective in controlling the frequency and severity of attacks of angioedema and in increasing serum levels of C1 INH and C4. Stanozolol is not effective in stopping HAE attacks while they are under way. The effect of stanozolol on increasing serum levels of C1 INH and C4 may be related to an increase in protein anabolism.

INDICATIONS AND USAGE:

Hereditary Angioedema: Stanozolol is indicated prophylactically to decrease the frequency and severity of attacks of angioedema.

CONTRAINDICATIONS:

The use of stanozolol is contraindicated in the following:

1. Male patients with carcinoma of the breast, or with known or suspected carcinoma of the prostate.

2. Carcinoma of the breast in females with hypercalcemia; androgenic anabolic steroids, may stimulate osteolytic resorption of bone.

3. Nephrosis or the nephrotic phase of nephritis.

4. Stanozolol can cause fetal harm when administered to a pregnant woman.

Stanozolol is contraindicated in women who are or may become pregnant. If this drug is used during pregnancy, or if the patient becomes pregnant while taking this drug, the patient should be apprised of the potential hazard to the fetus.

WARNINGS:

PELIOSIS HEPATIS, A CONDITION IN WHICH LIVER AND SOMETIMES SPLENIC TISSUE IS REPLACED WITH BLOOD-FILLED CYSTS, HAS BEEN REPORTED IN PATIENTS RECEIVING ANDROGENIC ANABOLIC STEROID THERAPY. THESE CYSTS ARE SOMETIMES PRESENT WITH MINIMAL HEPATIC DYSFUNCTION, BUT AT OTHER TIMES THEY HAVE BEEN ASSOCIATED WITH LIVER FAILURE. THEY ARE OFTEN NOT RECOGNIZED UNTIL LIFE-THREATENING LIVER FAILURE OR INTRA-ABDOMINAL HEMORRHAGE DEVELOPS. WITHDRAWAL OF DRUG USUALLY RESULTS IN COMPLETE DISAPPEARANCE OF LESIONS.

LIVER CELL TUMORS ARE ALSO REPORTED. MOST OFTEN THESE TUMORS ARE BENIGN AND ANDROGEN-DEPENDENT, BUT FATAL MALIGNANT TUMORS HAVE BEEN REPORTED. WITHDRAWAL OF DRUG OFTEN RESULTS IN REGRESSION OR CESSATION OF PROGRESSION OF THE TUMOR. HOWEVER, HEPATIC TUMORS ASSOCIATED WITH ANDROGENS OR ANABOLIC STEROIDS ARE MUCH MORE VASCULAR THAN OTHER HEPATIC TUMORS AND MAY BE SILENT UNTIL LIFE-THREATENING INTRA-ABDOMINAL HEMORRHAGE DEVELOPS.

BLOOD LIPID CHANGES THAT ARE KNOWN TO BE ASSOCIATED WITH INCREASED RISK OF ATHEROSCLEROSIS ARE SEEN IN PATIENT TREATED WITH ANDROGENS AND ANABOLIC STEROIDS. THESE CHANGES INCLUDE DECREASED HIGH-DENSITY LIPOPROTEIN AND SOMETIMES INCREASED LOW-DENSITY LIPOPROTEIN. THE CHANGES MAY BE VERY MARKED AND COULD HAVE A SERIOUS IMPACT ON THE RISK OF ATHEROSCLEROSIS AND CORONARY ARTERY DISEASE.

Cholestatic hepatitis and jaundice occur with 17-alpha-alkylated androgens at relatively low doses. If cholestatic hepatitis with jaundice appears, the anabolic steroid should be discontinued. If liver function tests become abnormal, the patients should be monitored closely and the etiology determined. Generally, the anabolic steroid should be discontinued although in cases of mild abnormalities, the physician may elect to follow the patient carefully at a reduced drug dosage.

In patients with breast cancer, anabolic steroid therapy may cause hypercalcemia by stimulating osteolysis. In this case, the drug should be discontinued.

Edema with or without congestive heart failure may be a serious complication in patients with preexisting cardiac, renal, or hepatic disease. Concomitant administration of adrenal cortical steroids or ACTH may add to the edema.

Geriatric male patients treated with androgenic anabolic steroids may be at an increased risk for the development of prostatic hypertrophy and prostatic carcinoma.

In children, anabolic steroid treatment may accelerate bone maturation without producing compensatory gain in linear growth. This adverse effect may result in compromised adult stature. The younger the child, the greater the risk of compromising final mature height. The effect on bone maturation should be monitored by assessing bone age of the wrist and hand every six months.

Anabolic steroids have not been shown to enhance athletic ability.

PRECAUTIONS:

GENERAL

Anabolic steroids may cause suppression of clotting factors II, V, VII, and X, and an increase in prothrombin time.

Women should be observed for signs of virilization (deepening of the voice, hirsutism, acne, and clitoromegaly). To prevent irreversible change, drug therapy must be discontinued, or the dosage significantly reduced when mild virilism is first detected. Such virilization is usual following androgenic anabolic steroid use of high doses. Some virilizing changes in women are irreversible even after prompt discontinuance of therapy and are not prevented by concomitant use of estrogens. Menstrual irregularities may also occur.

PRECAUTIONS: *(cont'd)*

The insulin or oral hypoglycemic dosage may need adjustment in diabetic patients who receive anabolic steroids.

INFORMATION FOR THE PATIENT

The physician should instruct patients to report any of the following side effects of androgens:

Adult or Adolescent Males: Too frequent or persistent erections of the penis, appearance or aggravation of acne.

Women: Hoarseness, acne, changes in menstrual period, or more hair on the face.

All Patients: Any nausea, vomiting, changes in skin color, or ankle swelling.

LABORATORY TESTS

Women with disseminated breast carcinoma should have frequent determination of urine and serum calcium levels during the course of androgenic anabolic steroid therapy (see WARNINGS.)

Because of the hepatotoxicity associated with the use of 17-alpha-alkylated androgens, liver function tests should be obtained periodically.

Periodic (every 6 months) x-ray examinations of bone age should be made during treatment of prepubertal patients to determine the rate of bone maturation and the effects of androgenic anabolic steroid therapy on the epiphyseal centers.

In common with other anabolic steroids, stanozolol has been reported to lower the level of high-density lipoproteins and raise the level of low-density lipoproteins. These changes usually revert to normal on discontinuation of treatment. Increased low-density lipoproteins and decreased high-density lipoproteins are considered cardiovascular risk factors. Serum lipids and high-density lipoprotein cholesterol should be determined periodically.

Hemoglobin and hematocrit should be checked periodically for polycythemia in patients who are receiving high doses of anabolic steroids.

DRUG/LABORATORY TEST INTERFERENCES

Therapy with androgenic anabolic steroids may decrease levels of thyroxine-binding globulin resulting in decreased total T_4 serum levels and increase resin uptake of T_3 and T_4. Free thyroid hormone levels remain unchanged and there is no clinical evidence of thyroid dysfunction.

CARCINOGENESIS, MUTAGENESIS, AND IMPAIRMENT OF FERTILITY

Animal Data: Testosterone has been tested by subcutaneous injection and implantation in mice and rats. The implant induced cervical-uterine tumors in mice, which metastasized in some cases. There is suggestive evidence that injection of testosterone into some strains of female mice increases their susceptibility to hepatoma. Testosterone is also known to increase the number of tumors and decrease the degree the differentiation of chemically-induced carcinomas of the liver in rats.

Human Data: There are rare reports of hepatocellular carcinoma in patients receiving long-term therapy with androgens in high doses. Withdrawal of the drugs did not lead to regression of the tumors in all cases.

Geriatric patients treated with androgens may be at an increased risk of developing prostatic hypertrophy and prostatic carcinoma although conclusive evidence to support this concept is lacking.

This compound has not been tested for mutagenic potential. However, as noted above, carcinogenic effects have been attributed to treatment with androgenic hormones. The potential carcinogenic effects likely occur through a hormonal mechanism rather than by a direct chemical interaction mechanism.

Impairment of fertility was not tested directly in animal species. However, as noted below under ADVERSE REACTIONS, oligospermia in males and amenorrhea in females are potential adverse effects of treatment with stanozolol tablets. Therefore, impairment of fertility is a possible outcome of treatment with stanozolol.

PREGNANCY CATEGORY X

See CONTRAINDICATIONS.

NURSING MOTHERS

It is not known whether anabolic steroids are excreted in human milk. Many drugs are excreted in milk and because of the potential for adverse reactions in nursing infants from stanozolol, a decision should be made whether to discontinue nursing or discontinue the drug, taking into account the importance of the drug to the mother.

PEDIATRIC USE

Anabolic agents may accelerate epiphyseal maturation more rapidly than linear growth in children, and the effect may continue for 6 months after the drug has been stopped. Therefore, therapy should be monitored by x-ray studies at 6 month intervals in order to avoid the risk of compromising the adult height. The safety and efficacy of stanozolol in children with hereditary angioedema have not been established.

DRUG INTERACTIONS:

Anabolic steroids may increase sensitivity to anticoagulants; therefore, dosage of an anticoagulant may have to be decreased in order to maintain the prothrombin time at the desired therapeutic level.

ADVERSE REACTIONS:

Hepatic: Cholestatic jaundice with, rarely, hepatic necrosis and death. Hepatocellular neoplasms and peliosis hepatis have been reported in association with long-term androgenic-anabolic steroid therapy (see WARNINGS.) Reversible changes in liver function tests also occur including increased bromsulphalein (BSP) retention and increases in serum bilirubin, glutamic oxaloacetic transaminase (SGOT), and alkaline phosphatase.

Genitourinary System: *In men. Prepubertal:* Phallic enlargement and increased frequency of erections. *Postpubertal:* Inhibition of testicular function, testicular atrophy and oligospermia, impotence, chronic priapism, epididymitis and bladder irritability. *In women:* Clitoral enlargement, menstrual irregularities. *In both sexes:* Increased or decreased libido.

CNS: Habituation, excitation, insomnia, depression.

Gastrointestinal: Nausea, vomiting, diarrhea.

Hematologic: Bleeding in patients on concomitant anticoagulant therapy.

Breast: Gynecomastia.

Larynx: Deepening of the voice in women.

Hair: Hirsutism and male pattern baldness in women.

Skin: Acne (especially in women and prepubertal boys).

Skeletal: Premature closure of epiphyses in children (see PRECAUTIONS, Pediatric Use.)

Fluid and Electrolytes: Edema, retention of serum electrolytes (sodium, chloride, potassium, phosphate, calcium).

Metabolic/Endocrine: Decreased glucose tolerance (see PRECAUTIONS), increased serum levels of low-density lipoproteins and decreased levels of high-density lipoproteins (see PRECAUTIONS, Laboratory Tests), increased creatine and creatinine excretion, increased serum levels of creatinine phosphokinase (CPK).

ADVERSE REACTIONS: *(cont'd)*

Some virilizing changes in women are irreversible even after prompt discontinuance of therapy and are not prevented by concomitant use of estrogens (see PRECAUTIONS.)

DRUG ABUSE AND DEPENDENCE:

Controlled Substance Class: Stanozolol is classified as a controlled substance under the Anabolic Steroids Control Act of 1990 and has been assigned to Schedule III.

DOSAGE AND ADMINISTRATION:

The use of anabolic steroids may be associated with serious adverse reactions, many of which are dose related; therefore, patients should be placed on the lowest possible effective dose.

Hereditary Angioedema: The dosage requirements for continuous treatment of hereditary angioedema with stanozolol should be individualized on the basis of the clinical response of the patient. It is recommended the patient be started on 2 mg, three times a day. After a favorable initial response is obtained in terms of prevention of episodes of edematous attacks, the proper continuing dosage should be determined by decreasing the dosage at intervals of one to three months to a maintenance dosage of 2 mg a day. Some patients may be successfully managed on a 2 mg alternate day schedule. During the dose adjusting phase, close monitoring of the patient's response is indicated, particularly if the patient has a history of airway involvement.

The prophylactic dose of stanozolol to be used prior to dental extraction, or other traumatic or stressful situations has not been established and may be substantially larger.

Attacks of hereditary angioedema are generally infrequent in childhood and the risks from stanozolol administration are substantially increased. Therefore, long-term prophylactic therapy with this drug is generally not recommended in children, and should only be undertaken with due consideration of the benefits and risks involved (see PRECAUTIONS, Pediatric Use.)

HOW SUPPLIED - EQUIVALENTS NOT AVAILABLE:

Tablet, Uncoated - Oral - 2 mg

100's $65.87 WINSTROL, Sanofi Winthrop 00024-2253-04

STAVUDINE *(003209)*

CATEGORIES: AIDS Related Complex; Anti-Infectives; Antivirals; HIV Infection; Nucleoside Analogue Drugs; Viral Agents; FDA Class 1P ("Priority Review"); FDA Approved 1994 Jun

BRAND NAMES: d4T; **Zerit**

FORMULARIES: Medi-Cal; PCS

> WARNING:
> Patients receiving stavudine capsules or any other antiretroviral therapy may continue to develop opportunistic infections and other complications of HIV infection, and therefore should remain under close clinical observation by physicians experienced in the treatment of patients with HIV-associated diseases.

DESCRIPTION:

Stavudine (formerly called d4T), a synthetic thymidine nucleoside analogue, active against the Human Immunodeficiency Virus (HIV). Zerit (stavudine capsules) are supplied for oral administration in strengths of 15, 20, 30, and 40 mg of stavudine. Each capsule also contains inactive ingredients microcrystalline cellulose, sodium starch glycolate, lactose, and magnesium stearate. The hard gelatin shell consists of gelatin, methylparaben, propylparaben, titanium dioxide, and iron oxides.

The chemical name for stavudine is 2',3'-didehydro-3'-deoxythymidine.

Stavudine is a white to off-white crystalline solid with the molecular formula $C_{10}H_{12}N_2O_4$ and a molecular weight of 224.2. The solubility of stavudine at 23°C is approximately 83 mg/ml in water and 30 mg/ml in propylene glycol. The n-octanol/water partition coefficient of stavudine at 23°C is 0.144.

CLINICAL PHARMACOLOGY:

MECHANISM OF ACTION

Stavudine, a nucleoside analogue of thymidine, inhibits the replication of HIV in human cells *in vitro.* Stavudine is phosphorylated by cellular kinases to stavudine triphosphate which exerts antiviral activity. Stavudine triphosphate has an intracellular half-life of 3.5 hours in CEM and peripheral blood mononuclear cells. Stavudine triphosphate inhibits HIV replication by two known mechanisms: 1) it inhibits HIV reverse transcriptase by competing with the natural substrate deoxythymidine triphosphate (K_i=0.0083 to 0.032 μM); and 2) it inhibits viral DNA synthesis by causing DNA chain termination because stavudine lacks the 3'-hydroxyl group necessary for DNA elongation. In addition to the inhibitory effect on HIV reverse transcriptase, stavudine triphosphate inhibits cellular DNA polymerase beta and gamma, and markedly reduces the synthesis of mitochondrial DNA.

MICROBIOLOGY

Antiviral Activity *In Vitro*: The antiviral activity of stavudine has been demonstrated *in vitro* in a variety of primary and continuous cell types infected with laboratory derived and clinical isolates of HIV. However, the relationship between *in vitro* susceptibility of HIV to stavudine and the inhibition of HIV replication in humans or clinical response to therapy has not been established.

PHARMACOKINETICS

The pharmacokinetics of stavudine have been evaluated in 142 HIV-infected patients following administration of oral doses ranging from 0.03 to 4 mg/kg administered as single doses and as multiple doses every 6, 8, or 12 hours. Stavudine pharmacokinetics have also been evaluated in 44 HIV-infected patients after single intravenous doses ranging from 0.0625 to 1 mg/kg administered as 1-hour infusions.

ABSORPTION AND BIOAVAILABILITY

Following oral administration to HIV-infected patients, stavudine was rapidly absorbed with the mean ± SD absolute bioavailability of 86.4 ± 18.2% (n=25). Peak plasma concentrations (C_{max}) increased in a dose-related manner for doses (n=4 to 10 per dose level) ranging from 0.03 to 4 mg/kg and occurred ≤ 1 hour after dosing. Area under the plasma concentration-time curve (AUC) increased in proportion to dose after both single and multiple doses. There was no significant accumulation of stavudine with repeated administration every 6, 8, or 12 hours.

CLINICAL PHARMACOLOGY: *(cont'd)*

When stavudine (70 mg) was administered to 16 asymptomatic HIV- infected patients under fasting conditions, 1 hour before a standardized high-fat meal (773 Kcal, 53% fat), or immediately after the meal, systemic exposure (AUC) was similar. Mean ± SD C_{max} of stavudine was reduced from 1.44 ± 0.49 mcg/ml in the fasting state to 0.75 ± 0.16 mcg/ml after the meal, and the median time to reach C_{max} was prolonged from 0.6 to 1.5 hours.

DISTRIBUTION

Following 1-hour intravenous infusions (n=44) of stavudine doses ranging from 0.0625 to 1 mg/kg, mean ± SD volume of distribution was 58 ± 21 L, suggesting that stavudine distributes into extravascular spaces. Mean ± SD apparent volume of distribution following administration of single oral doses (n=71) ranging from 0.03 to 4 mg/kg was 66 ± 22 L. Volume of distribution was independent of dose and did not correlate with body weight.

Binding of stavudine to serum proteins was negligible over the concentration range of 0.01-11.4 mcg/ml. Stavudine distributes equally between red blood cells and plasma.

METABOLISM

The metabolic fate of stavudine has not been elucidated in humans.

ELIMINATION

Plasma clearance and terminal elimination half-life were independent of dose over an intravenous dosing range of 0.0625 to 1 mg/kg and an oral dosing range of 0.03 to 4 mg/kg. Following 1-hour infusions (n=44), plasma concentrations of stavudine declined in a biphasic manner with a mean ± SD terminal elimination half-life of 1.15 ± 0.35 hours. After single oral doses (n= 115), the mean ± SD terminal elimination half-life was 1.44 ± 0.30 hours. Mean ± SD total body clearance, after intravenous infusion was 594 ± 164 ml/min (8.3 ± 2.3 ml/min/kg), and was independent of dose and body weight. Following single-dose oral administration (n=113), mean ± SD apparent oral clearance was independent of dose having a value of 559 ± 168 ml/min (8.03 ± 2.54 ml/min/kg). Renal elimination accounted for about 40% of the overall clearance regardless of the route of administration. The mean renal clearance was about twice the average endogenous creatinine clearance, indicating active tubular secretion in addition to glomerular filtration. Mean ± SD (n=88) cumulative urinary excretion of unchanged drug over 6 to 24 hours after administration of an oral dose was 39 ± 23% of the dose.

SPECIAL POPULATIONS

Pediatric: (See PRECAUTIONS, Pediatric Use.)

Renal Insufficiency: Preliminary data from 14 non-HIV-infected subjects with reduced renal function and 5 subjects with normal renal function indicated that the apparent oral clearance (CL/F) of stavudine decreased as creatinine clearance (CL_{cr}) decreased (see TABLE 1.) The terminal elimination half-life ($t_{1/2}$) was prolonged up to 8 hours. C_{max} and T_{max} were not significantly affected by reduced renal function. Based on these preliminary observations, it is recommended that stavudine dosage be modified in patients with reduced creatinine clearance (see DOSAGE AND ADMINISTRATION.)

TABLE 1 Mean ± SD Pharmacokinetic Parameter Values; Single 40-mg Oral Dose of Stavudine

	Creatinine Clearance		
	>50 ml/min (n = 10)	26-50 ml/min (n = 5)	9-25 ml/min (n = 4)
CL_{cr} (ml/min)	104 ± 28	41 ± 5	15 ± 6
CL/F (ml/min)	335 ± 57	191 ± 39	106 ± 12
CL_R (ml/min)*	167 ± 65	73 ± 18	16 ± 3
$t_{1/2}$ (h)	1.7 ± 0.4	3.5 ± 2.5	4.8 ± 0.8

* CL_R = renal clearance

Hepatic Insufficiency: Stavudine pharmacokinetics were not altered in 6 non-HIV infected patients with hepatic impairment secondary to cirrhosis (Child-Pugh classification B or C) following administration of a single 40 mg dose.

Geriatric: Stavudine pharmacokinetics have not been specifically investigated in patients >65 years of age.

Gender: Stavudine pharmacokinetics have not been studied as a function of gender.

Race: Pharmacokinetic differences due to race have not been evaluated.

CLINICAL STUDIES:

Study Al455-019 was a multi-center, randomized, double-blind trial of stavudine capsules vs. zidovudine for the treatment of HIV-infected adults with CD4 counts of 50 to 500 cells/mm^3 who had received at least six months prior zidovudine treatment. Stavudine was administered in dosages of 40 mg BID for patients weighing ≥60 kg, and 30 mg BID for those weighing <60 kg. The zidovudine dosage was 200 mg TID.

The study enrolled 822 patients with a median baseline CD4 count of 235 cells/mm^3 (range: 10 to 735 cells/mm^3), and a median duration of prior zidovudine treatment of 88 weeks (range 11 to 356 weeks). Fourteen percent of subjects had AIDS at baseline, 50% had HIV-related symptoms and 36% were asymptomatic.

TABLE 2 gives the Kaplan-Meier estimates for the time to disease progression.

TABLE 2 Incidence of Disease Progression

	First AIDS-Defining Event or Death*	
	Stavudine	Zidovudine
6 Months	4.4%	5.7%
12 Months	10.4%	14.1%
18 Months	18.5%	23.3%
24 Months	26.6%	31.8%

* Kaplan-Meier estimates; the overall difference between stavudine and zidovudine was not significant.

DRUG RESISTANCE

Preclinical Studies: The potential for development of resistance to stavudine has been investigated *in vitro.* Selection studies performed with HIV-1 strains HXB2 and IIIb have produced isolates with reduced (7- to 30-fold) sensitivity to stavudine.

Clinical Studies: Limited phenotypic and genotypic resistance studies (20 paired HIV isolates) have shown that 4- to 12-fold decreases (3/20 isolates) in stavudine susceptibility are possible; however, the genetic basis for the observed susceptibility changes has not been identified. The clinical relevance of stavudine susceptibility changes has not been established.

Five of the 11 stavudine post-treatment isolates (9 of which were from patients who had previously received zidovudine) developed moderate resistance to zidovudine (9 to 176-fold) and 3 of those 11 isolates developed moderate resistance to didanosine (7- to 29-fold). The clincal relevance of these findings has not been established.

INDICATIONS AND USAGE:

Stavudine is indicated for the treatment of HIV-infected adults who have received prolonged prior zidovudine therapy.

CONTRAINDICATIONS:

Stavudine is a contraindicated in patients with clinically significant hypersensitivity to stavudine or to any of the components contained in the formulation.

WARNINGS:

The major clinical toxicity of stavudine is peripheral neuropathy. This complication occurred in 19 to 24 percent of the 11,784 patients with advanced HIV disease who received the two dose levels of stavudine in the Parallel Track Program[1]. In patients with less advanced HIV infection in the zidovudine comparative trial, peripheral neuropathy occurred in 14 percent of zidovudine-treated patients as compared to 4 percent of zidovudine-treated patients.

Patients should be monitored for the development of neuropathy that is usually characterized by numbness, tingling, or pain in the feet or hands. Stavudine-related peripheral neuropathy may resolve if therapy is withdrawn promptly. In some cases, symptoms may worsen temporarily following discontinuation of therapy. If symptoms resolve completely, resumption of treatment may be considered at a reduced dose (see DOSAGE AND ADMINISTRATION.)

Patients with a history of peripheral neuropathy are at increased risk for the development of neuropathy. If stavudine must be administered in this clinical setting, careful monitoring is essential.

PRECAUTIONS:

INFORMATION FOR THE PATIENT

Patients should be informed that stavudine is not a cure for HIV infection, and that they may continue to acquire illnesses associated with HIV infection, including opportunistic infections. Patients should be advised to remain under the care of a physician when using stavudine.

Patients should be informed that the most common toxicity of stavudine is peripheral neuropathy. Symptoms of peripheral neuropathy usually include tingling, burning, pain, or numbness in the hands or feet. Patients should be counseled that this toxicity occurs with greater frequency in patients with a history of peripheral neuropathy. They should be advised that these symptoms should be reported to their physicians and that dose changes may be necessary. They should also be cautioned about the use of other medications that may exacerbate peripheral neuropathy.

Patients should be told that the long-term effects of stavudine capsules are unknown at this time. They should be advised that stavudine therapy has not been shown to reduce the risk of transmission of HIV to others through sexual contact or blood contamination.

Patients should be informed that the Center for Disease Control (CDC) recommends that HIV-infected mothers not nurse newborn infants to reduce the risk of postnatal transmission of HIV infection.

LABORATORY TESTS

Mild to moderate increases in AST (SGOT) and ALT (SGPT) occurred commonly in clinical trials; these did not interfere with continued therapy (see DOSAGE AND ADMINISTRATION.)

CARCINOGENESIS, MUTAGENESIS, AND IMPAIRMENT OF FERTILITY

Long-term carcinogenicity studies of stavudine in animals have not been completed. Stavudine was not mutagenic in the Ames, *E.coli* reverse mutation, or the CHO/HGPRT mammalian cell forward gene mutation assays, with and without metabolic activation. Stavudine produced positive results in the *in vitro* human lymphocyte clastogenesis and mouse fibroblast assays, and in the *in vivo* mouse micronucleus test. In the *in vitro* assays, stavudine elevated the frequency of chromosome aberrations in human lymphocytes (concentrations of 25 to 250 mcg/ml, without metabolic activation) and increased the frequency of transformed foci in mouse fibroblast cells (concentrations of 25 to 2500 mcg/ml, with and without metabolic activation). In the *in vivo*micronucleus assay, stavudine was clastogenic in bone marrow cells following oral stavudine administration to mice at dosages of 600 to 2000 mg/kg/day for 3 days.

No evidence of impaired fertility was seen in rats with exposures (based on C_{max}) up to 216 times that observed following a clinical dosage of 1 mg/kg/day.

PREGNANCY CATEGORY C

Reproduction studies have been performed in rats and rabbits with exposures (based on C_{max}) up to 399 and 183 times, respectively, of that seen at a clinical dosage of 1 mg/kg/day and have revealed no evidence or teratogenicity. The incidence in fetuses of a common skeletal variation, unossified or incomplete ossification of sternebra, was increased in rats at 399 times human exposure, while no effect was observed at 216 times human exposure. A slight post-implantation loss was noted at 216 times the human exposure with no effect noted at approximately 135 times the human exposure. An increase in early rat neonatal mortality (birth to 4 days of age) occurred at 399 times the human exposure, while survival of neonates was unaffected at approximately 135 times the human exposure. A study in rats showed that stavudine is transferred to the fetus through the placenta. The concentration in fetal tissue was approximately one-half the concentration in maternal plasma. There are no adequate and well controlled studies in pregnant women. Because animal reproduction studies are not always predictive of human response, stavudine should be used during pregnancy only if clearly needed.

NURSING MOTHERS

The Center for Disease Control (CDC) recommends that HIV-infected mothers not breast feed their infants to avoid risking postnatal transmission of HIV infection. In addition, studies in which lactating rats were administered a single dose (5 or 100 mg/kg) of stavudine demonstrated that stavudine is readily excreted into breast milk. It is not known whether stavudine is excreted in human milk. Because many drugs are excreted in human milk, and because of the potential for adverse reactions from stavudine in nursing infants, mothers should be instructed not to nurse if they are receiving stavudine.

PEDIATRIC USE

Safety and effectiveness of stavudine for the treatment of HIV infection in pediatric patients have not been established. Limited data are available from 37 pediatric patients aged 5 months to 15 years who received stavudine in doses ranging from 0.125 to 4.0 mg/kg/day for a median duration of 37 weeks (range 8 to 75 weeks). Serious adverse events that have been observed include AST(SGOT) and ALT (SGPT) elevations and one case of neuropathy.

Pharmacokinetics: Stavudine pharmacokinetics have been evaluated in 19 HIV-infected pediatric patients after single intravenous doses ranging from 0.125 to 2 mg/kg administered as 1-hour infusions. The pharmacokinetics of stavudine have been evaluated in 10 children (age 8 months to 4.5 years) who received stavudine oral solution and 8 children (age 6 to 15 years) who received stavudine capsules at oral doses ranging from 0.125 to 2 mg/kg administered every 12 hours.

Absorption: Stavudine was rapidly absorbed following oral administration to HIV-infected children with a mean ± SD absolute bioavailability of 78.5 ± 35% and 69.2 ± 23% for capsule and solution formulations, respectively. First-dose and multiple-dose (after 12 weeks of treatment) pharmacokinetic profiles were similar, indicating no accumulation of stavudine.

Distribution: Following intravenous infusions (n=19) of stavudine at doses ranging from 0.125 to 2 mg/kg, the mean ± SD volume of distribution was 13.2 ± 8.95 (0.68 ± 0.29 L/kg), suggesting that stavudine distributes into extravascular spaces. After 12 weeks of treatment, the concentration of stavudine in cerebrospinal fluid samples collected from seven patients ranged from 0.01 to 0.12 mcg/ml at times ranging from 2 to 3 hours post-dose (doses ranging from 0.125 to 1 mg/kg). The cerebrospinal fluid concentrations corresponded to 16% to 97% (mean, 55%; n=6) of the concentration in simultaneous plasma samples.

PRECAUTIONS: *(cont'd)*

Elimination: Plasma concentrations of stavudine declined with a mean ± SD terminal elimination half-life of 1.09 ± 0.28 hours following the end of a 1-hour infusion (n=19). After a single oral dose (n=18), the mean ± SD terminal half-life was 0.91 ± 0.24 hours. The mean ± SD total body clearance after intravenous infusion was 181.13 ± 98.36 ml/min (9.64 ± 3.10 ml/min/kg). The mean ± SD apparent oral clearance after administration of solution (n=10, age <6 years) and capsule (n=8, age >6 years) formulations was 16.45 ± 4.28 and 11.01 ± 2.94 ml/min/kg, respectively.

ADVERSE REACTIONS:

The major clinical toxicity of stavudine is peripheral neuropathy (see WARNINGS.) This toxicity is dose related (see TABLE 3.) Modest elevation of hepatic transaminases was observed commonly in controlled trials.

TABLE 3 Incidence of Peripheral Neuropathy Requiring Dose Modification in Controlled Clinical Trials

	%			
	Study Al455-019		Parallel Track Program	
	Stavudine (40 mg BID) N=412	Zidovudine (200 mg TID) N=402	Stavudine (40 mg BID) N=5905	Stavudine (20 mg BID) N=5879
Peripheral Neuropathy[1]				
Grade 1 - 2	11	3	20	17
Grade 3 - 4	2	1	4	2
Total	13	4	24	19
Peripheral Neurologic Symptoms[2]				
Grade 1 - 2	38	35	5	5
Grade 3 - 4	<1	-	<1	1
Total	38	35	5	6

1 Peripheral neuropathy regardless of grade leading to dose modification.
2 Peripheral neurologic symptoms not requiring dose modification.

Selected adverse events that occurred in adult patients receiving stavudine in Phase 3 controlled comparative trial (Study Al455-019) and in the Parallel Track Program Study Al455-900 are provided in TABLE 4.

TABLE 4 Selected Clinical Adverse Events in the Phase 3 Controlled Clinical Trials [1]

	%			
	Study Al455-019[2]		Parallel Track Program	
Adverse Events	Stavudine (40 mg BID) (n = 412)	Zidovudine (200 mg TID) (n = 402)	Stavudine (40 mg BID) (n =5905)	Stavudine (20 mg BID) (n = 5879)
Headache	54	49	3	4
Chills/Fever	50	51	6	6
Diarrhea	50	43	5	5
Rash	40	35	4	4
Nausea and Vomiting	38	44	6	7
Peripheral Neurologic Symptoms[3]	38	35	5	6
Abdominal Pain	34	27	4	6
Myalgia	32	35	2	2
Insomnia	29	31	2	2
Anorexia	19	22	*	1
Peripheral Neuropathy[4]	14	4	24	19
Allergic Reaction	9	8	*	*
Pacreatitis	*	*	2	2

* This event was reported in fewer than 1% of patients.
1 Includes all clinical complaints.
2 Median duration of stavudine therapy = 79 weeks; median duration of zidovudine therapy = 53 weeks.
3 Peripheral neurologic symptoms not requiring dose modification.
4 Peripheral neuropathy leading to dose modification.

Laboratory abnormalities reported in the Phase 3 controlled comparative trial (Study Al455-019) and the Parallel Track Program (Study Al455-900) are shown in TABLE 5.

TABLE 5 Controlled Clinical Trials: Incidence of Adult Laboratory Abnormalities [a]

	Study Al455-019		Parallel Track Program	
Lab Tests (units)	Stavudine (40 mg BID) (n = 412)	Zidovudine (200 mg TID) (n = 402)	Stavudine (40 mg BID) (n = 5905)	Stavudine (20 mg BID) (n = 5879)
AST (SGOT) (1.25 • ≤5.0 × ULN[c]	63	49	60	59
AST (SGOT) (>5.0 x ULN)	11	10	6	6
ALT (SGPT) (1.25 • ≤5.0 × ULN[c]	65	46	62	62
ALT (SGPT) (>5.0 x ULN)	13	11	11	10
Bilirubin (>2.5 x ULN)	2	3	N/A[d]	N/A[d]
Anemia (<8.0 g/dl)	*	3	3	4
Neutropenia (neutrophils <750/mm^3)	5	9	12	13
Thrombocytopenia (platelets <50,000/mm^3)	3	3	4	5
Amylase (>1.4 x ULN)	14	13	N/A[d]	N/A[d]

* This abnormality was reported in fewer than 1% of patients
[a]Data presented for patients for whom laboratory evaluations were performed.
[b]Median duration of stavudine therapy = 79 weeks; median duration of zidovudine therapy = 53 weeks.
[c]ULN = upper limit of normal.
d Collection of this data was not required per protocol.

OVERDOSAGE:

Experience with adults treated with 12 to 24 times the recommended daily dosage revealed no acute toxicity. Complications of chronic overdosage include peripheral neuropathy and hepatic toxicity. It is not known whether stavudine is eliminated by peritoneal dialysis or hemodialysis.

DOSAGE AND ADMINISTRATION:

Adults: The interval between oral doses should be 12 hours. C_{max} was decreased by approximately 45% when stavudine was administered with food; however, the systemic availability (AUC) was unchanged (see CLINICAL PHARMACOLOGY.) Thus, it appears that stavudine capsules may be taken without regard to meals. The recommended starting dose based on body weight is as follows:

40 mg twice daily for patients ≥ 60 kg.
30 mg twice daily for patients < 60 kg.

DOSAGE ADJUSTMENT

Patients should be monitored for the development of peripheral neuropathy, which is usually characterized by numbness, tingling, or pain in the feet or hands. If these symptoms develop on treatment, stavudine therapy should be interrupted. Symptoms may resolve if therapy is withdrawn promptly. In some cases, symptoms may worsen temporarily following discontinuation of therapy. If symptoms resolve completely, resumption of treatment may be considered using the following dosage schedule:

20 mg twice daily for patients ≥ 60 kg.
15 mg twice daily for patients < 60 kg.

Clinically significant elevations of hepatic transaminases should be managed in the same fashion.

Dosage for Impaired Renal Function: Stavudine may be administered to adult patients with impaired renal function. The schedule represented in TABLE 6 is recommended.

TABLE 6

Creatinine Clearance (ml/min)	Recommended Stavudine Dose by Patient Weight ≥ 60 kg	< 60kg
> 50	40 mg every 12 hours	30 mg every 12 hours
26-50	20 mg every 12 hours	15 mg every 12 hours
10-25	20 mg every 24 hours	15 mg every 24 hours

There are insufficient data to recommend a dose for patients with creatinine clearance < 10 ml/min or for patients undergoing dialysis.

PATIENT INFORMATION:

Stavudine is used for the treatment of HIV-infected adults. It is not a cure for HIV infection.

Inform your doctor if you are pregnant. Do not nurse while taking this drug.

Stavudine may cause peripheral neuropathy. Symptoms of peripheral neuropathy include tingling, burning, pain or numbness of the hands or feet. Inform your doctor if any of these occur.

Stavudine may be taken with or without food.

HOW SUPPLIED:

Zerit (Stavudine) capsules are available in plastic bottles with child-resistant closures. The 15 mg tablet is light yellow and dark red imprinted with "BMS 1964 15"; the 20 mg tablets is light brown and imprinted with "BMS 1965 20"; the 30 mg tablet is light orange and dark orange and imprinted with "BMS 1966 30"; the 40 mg tablet is dark orange and imprinted with "BMS 1967 40".

Storage: Stavudine capsules should be stored in tightly closed containers at controlled room temperature, 59° to 86°F (15° to 30°C).

HOW SUPPLIED - EQUIVALENTS NOT AVAILABLE:

Capsule, Gelatin - Oral - 15 mg
60's $207.47 ZERIT, Bristol Myers Squibb 00003-1964-01

Capsule, Gelatin - Oral - 20 mg
60's $215.76 ZERIT, Bristol Myers Squibb 00003-1965-01

Capsule, Gelatin - Oral - 30 mg
60's $225.10 ZERIT, Bristol Myers Squibb 00003-1966-01

Capsule, Gelatin - Oral - 40 mg
60's $233.40 ZERIT, Bristol Myers Squibb 00003-1967-01

STREPTOKINASE *(002276)*

CATEGORIES: Anticoagulants/Thrombolytics; Blood Formation/Coagulation; Congestive Heart Failure; Embolism; Heart Failure; Myocardial Infarction; Pulmonary Embolism; Thrombolytic Agents; Thrombolytic Enzymes; Thrombosis; Pregnancy Category C; FDA Pre 1938 Drugs

BRAND NAMES: Kabikinase; **Streptase**

FORMULARIES: WHO

DESCRIPTION:

Streptase is a sterile, purified preparation of a bacterial protein elaborated by group C β-hemolytic streptococci. It is supplied as a lyophilized white powder containing 25 mg cross-linked gelatin polypeptides, 25 mg sodium L-glutamate, sodium hydroxide to adjust pH, and 100 mg albumin (human) per vial as stabilizers. The preparation contains no preservatives and is intended for intravenous and intracoronary administration.

CLINICAL PHARMACOLOGY:

Streptokinase acts with plasminogen to produce an "activator complex" that converts plasminogen to the proteolytic enzyme plasmin. The $t_{1/2}$ of the activator complex is about 23 minutes; the complex is inactivated, in part, by antistreptococcal antibodies. The mechanism by which streptokinase is eliminated is by sites in the liver; however, no metabolites of streptokinase have been identified. Plasmin degrades fibrin clots as well as fibrinogen and other plasma proteins. Plasmin is inactivated by circulating inhibitors, such as α-2-plasmin inhibitor of α-2-macroglobulin. These inhibitors are rapidly consumed at high doses of streptokinase.

CLINICAL PHARMACOLOGY: *(cont'd)*

Intravenous infusion of streptokinase is followed by increased fibrinolytic activity, which decrease plasma fibrinogen levels for 24 to 36 hours. The decrease in plasma fibrinogen in associated with decreases in plasma and blood viscosity and red blood cell aggregation. The hyperfibrinolytic effect disappears within a few hours after discontinuation, but a prolonged thrombin time may persist for up to 24 hours due to the decrease in plasma levels of fibrinogen and an increase in the amount of circulating fibrin(ogen) degradation products (FDP). Depending upon the dosage and duration of infusion of streptokinase, the thrombin time will decrease less than two times the normal control value within 4 hours, and return to normal by 24 hours.

Intravenous administration has been shown to reduce blood pressure and total peripheral resistance with a corresponding reduction in cardiac afterload. These expected responses were not studied with the intracoronary administration of Streptase, Streptokinase. The quantitative benefit has not been evaluated.

Variable amounts of circulating antistreptokinase antibody are present in individuals as a result of recent streptococcal infections. The recommended dosage schedule usually obviates the need for antibody titration.

Two large randomized, placebo-controlled studies[1,2] involving almost 30,000 patients have demonstrated that a 60-minute intravenous infusion of 1,500,000 IU of Streptokinase significantly reduces mortality following a myocardial infarction. One of these studies also evaluated concomitant oral administration of low dose aspirin (160 mg/d over one month).

In the GISSI study, the reduction in mortality was time dependent. There was a 47% reduction in mortality among patients treated within one hour of the onset of chest pain, a 23% reduction among patients treated within three hours, and a 17% reduction among patients treated between three and six hours. There was also a reduction in mortality in patients treated between six and twelve hours from the onset of symptoms, but the reduction was not statistically significant.

In the ISIS-2 study the reduction in mortality was also time dependent. If Streptokinase and aspirin were administered within the first hour after symptom onset, the reduction in mortality was 44%. The reduction in the odds of death in patients treated within four hours was 53% for the combination of Streptokinase and aspirin, and 35% for Streptokinase alone. However, the reduction was still significant when treatment was started 5-24 hours after symptom onset: 33% for the combined therapy and 17% for Streptokinase alone. Overall, in the 0-24 hour time period there was a 42% reduction in the odds of death with combined treatment (Streptokinase and aspirin) versus placebo (2p<0.00001) and 25% reduction in the odds of death with Streptokinase alone versus placebo (2p<0.00001).

One of eight smaller studies using a similar dosing schedule showed a statistically significant reduction in mortality. When all of these studies were pooled, the overall decrease in mortality was approximately 23%. Results from pooling several studies using different dosages with long term infusion corroborate these observations.

In addition, studies measuring left ventricular ejection fraction (LVEF) at discharge showed the mean LVEFs were approximately 3-6 percentage points higher in the Streptokinase group than in the control group. This difference was statistically significant in some of the studies.[3,4]Furthermore, some studies reported greater improvement in LVEF among patients treated within three hours than in patients treated later.

Results from a randomized controlled trial in over 11,000 patients show that, following treatment with IV Streptokinase, there is a reduction in the number of patients with clinical congestive heart failure during the 14-21 day in-hospital period. Clinical congestive heart failure occurred in 12.8% of Streptokinase-treated patients compared with 15% of the control patients (p=0.001)[1].

The rate of reclusion of the infarct-related vessel has been reported to be approximately 15-20%. The rate of reclusion depends on dosage, additional anticoagulant therapy and residual stenosis. When the reinfarctions were evaluated in studies involving 8800 Streptokinase-treated patients, the overall rate was 3.8% (range 2-15%). In over 8500 control patients, the rate of reinfarction was 2.4%. However, the ISIS-2 study showed that a increase in reinfarction was avoided when Streptokinase was combined with lose dose aspirin. The rate of reinfarction in the combination group was 1.8% vs 1.9% in the group given aspirin alone.

Streptase, Streptokinase, administered by the intracoronary route has resulted in thrombolysis usually within one hour, and ensuing reperfusion results in limitation of infarct size, improvement of cardiac function, and reduction of mortality[5,6]. LVEF was increased in patients treated with Streptokinase when compared to patients treated with conventional therapy. When the initial LVEF was low, the Streptokinase- treated patients showed greater improvement than did the controls. Spontaneous reperfusion is known to occur and has been observed with angiography at various time points after infarction. Data from one study show that 73% of the Streptokinase-treated patients and 47% of the placebo-allocated patients reperfused during hospitalization.

Studies with thrombolytic therapy for pulmonary embolism show no significant difference in lung perfusion scan between the thrombolysis group and the heparin group at one year follow-up. However, measurements of pulmonary capillary blood volumes and diffusing capacities at two weeks and one year after therapy indicate that a more complete resolution of thrombotic obstruction and normalization of pulmonary physiology was achieved with thrombolytic therapy, thus preventing the long term sequelae of pulmonary hypertension and pulmonary failure.[7]

The long term benefit of Streptase, Streptokinase therapy for deep vein thrombosis (DVT) has been evaluated venographically.[8]The combined results of five randomized studies show no residual thrombotic material in 60-75% of patients treated with Streptokinase versus only 10% of those treated with heparin. Thrombolytic therapy also preserves venous valve function in a majority of cases, thus avoiding the pathologic venous changes that produce the clinical post-phlebitic syndrome which occurs in 90% of the DVT patients treated with heparin.

There is a time-related decrease in effectiveness when Streptase, Streptokinase is used in the management of peripheral arterial thromboembolism. When administered three to ten days after onset of obstruction, rates of clearance of 50-75% were reported.

INDICATIONS AND USAGE:

Acute Evolving Transmural Myocardial Infarction: Streptase, Streptokinase, is indicated for use in the management of acute myocardial infarction (AMI) in adults, for the lysis of intracoronary thrombi, for the improvement of ventricular function, for the reduction of mortality associated with AMI, when administered by either the intravenous or the intracoronary route, as well as for the reduction of infarct size and congestive heart failure associated with AMI when administered by the intravenous route. Earlier administration of Streptokinase is correlated with greater clinical benefit. (See CLINICAL PHARMACOLOGY.)

Pulmonary Embolism: Streptase, Streptokinase is indicated for the lysis of objectively diagnosed (angiography or lung scan) pulmonary emboli, involving obstruction of blood flow to a lobe or multiple segments, with or without unstable hemodynamics.

Deep Vein Thrombosis: Streptase, Streptokinase, is indicated for the lysis of objectively diagnosed (preferably ascending venography), acute, extensive thrombi of the deep veins such as those involving the popliteal and more proximal vessels.

INDICATIONS AND USAGE: *(cont'd)*

Arterial Thrombosis or Embolism: Streptase, Streptokinase, is indicated for the lysis of acute arterial thrombi and emboli. Streptokinase is not indicated for arterial emboli originating from the left side of the heart due to the risk of new embolic phenomena such as cerebral embolism.

Occlusion of Arteriovenous Cannulae: Streptase, Streptokinase is indicated as an alternative to surgical revision for clearing totally or partially occluded arteriovenous cannulae when acceptable flow cannot be achieved.

CONTRAINDICATIONS:

Because thrombolytic therapy increases the risk of bleeding, Streptase, Streptokinase, is contraindicated in the following situations:

active internal bleeding

recent (within 2 months) cerebrovascular accident, intracranial or intraspinal surgery (see WARNINGS)

intracranial neoplasm

severe uncontrolled hypertension

Streptokinase should not be administered to patients having experienced severe allergic reaction to the product.

WARNINGS:

Bleeding: Following intravenous high-dose brief-duration Streptokinase therapy in acute myocardial infarction, severe bleeding complications requiring transfusion are extremely rare (0.3-0.5%), and combined therapy with low dose aspirin does not appear to increase the risk of major bleeding. The addition of aspirin to Streptokinase,au cause a slight increase in the risk of minor bleeding (3.1% without aspirin vs. 3.9% with)[2].

Streptokinase will cause lysis of hemostatic fibrin deposits such as those occurring at sites of needle punctures, particularly when infused over several hours, and bleeding may occur from such sites. In order to minimize the risk of bleeding during treatment with Streptokinase, venipunctures and physical handling of the patient should be performed carefully and as infrequently as possible, and intramuscular injections must be avoided.

Should arterial puncture be necessary during intravenous therapy, upper extremity vessels are preferable. Pressure should be applied for at least 30 minutes, a pressure dressing applied, and the puncture site checked frequently for evidence of bleeding.

In the following conditions, the risks of therapy may be increased and should be weighed against the anticipated benefits.

Recent (within 10 days) major surgery, obstetrical delivery, organ biopsy, previous puncture of noncompressible vessels

Recent (within 10 days) serious gastrointestinal bleeding

Recent (within 10 days) trauma including cardiopulmonary resuscitation

Hypertension: systolic BP > 180 mm Hg and/or diastolic BP > 110 mm Hg

High likelihood of left heart thrombus, e.g., mitral stenosis with atrial fibrillation

Subacute bacterial endocarditis

Hemostatic defects including those secondary to severe hepatic or renal disease

Pregnancy

Age > 75 years

Cerebrovascular disease

Diabetic hemorrhagic retinopathy

Septic thrombophlebitis or occluded AV cannula at seriously infected site

Any other condition in which bleeding constitutes a significant hazard or would be particularly difficult to manage because of its location.

Should serious spontaneous bleeding (not controllable by local pressure) occur, the infusion of Streptase, Streptokinase should be terminated immediately and treatment instituted as described under ADVERSE REACTIONS.

Arrhythmias: Rapid lysis of coronary thrombi has been shown to cause reperfusion atrial or ventricular dysrhythmias requiring immediate treatment. Careful monitoring for arrhythmia is recommended during and immediately following administration of Streptase, Streptokinase, for acute myocardial infarction.

Hypotension: Hypotension, sometimes severe, not secondary to bleeding or anaphylaxis has been observed during intravenous Streptase, Streptokinase, infusion in 1 to 10% of patients. Patients should be monitored closely and, should symptomatic or alarming hypotension occur, appropriate treatment should be administered. This treatment may include a decrease in the intravenous Streptokinase infusion rate. Smaller hypotensive effects are common and have not required treatment.

Other: Non-cardiogenic pulmonary edema has been reported rarely in patients treated with Streptase, Streptokinase. The risk of this appears greatest in patients who have large myocardial infarctions and are undergoing thrombolytic therapy by the intracoronary route.

Rarely, polyneuropathy has been temporally related to the use of Streptase, Streptokinase.

Should pulmonary embolism or recurrent pulmonary embolism occur during Streptase, Streptokinase, therapy, the originally planned course of treatment should be completed in an attempt to lyse the embolus. While pulmonary embolism may occasionally occur during streptokinase treatment, the incidence is no greater than when patients are treated with heparin alone.

PRECAUTIONS:

GENERAL

Repeated Administration: Because of the increased likelihood of resistance, due to antistreptokinase antibody, Streptase, Streptokinase, may not be effective if administered between five days and twelve months of prior Streptokinase or Anistreplase administration or streptococcal infections, such as streptococcal pharyngitis, acute rheumatic fever, or acute glomerulonephritis secondary to a streptococcal infection.

LABORATORY TESTS

Intravenous or Intracoronary Infusion for Myocardial Infarction: Intravenous administration of Streptase, Streptokinase, will cause marked decreases in plasminogen and fibrinogen and increases in thrombin time (TT), activated partial thromboplastin time (APTT), and prothrombin time (PT), which usually normalize within 12-24 hours. These changes may also occur in some patients with intracoronary administration of Streptokinase.

Intravenous Infusion for Other Indications Before commencing thrombolytic therapy, it is desirable to obtain an activated partial thromboplastin time (APTT), a prothrombin time (PT), a thrombin time (TT), or fibrinogen levels, and a hematocrit and platelet count. If heparin has been given, it should be discontinued and the TT or APTT should be less than twice the normal control value before thrombolytic therapy is started.

PRECAUTIONS: *(cont'd)*

During the infusion, decreases in plasminogen and fibrinogen levels and an increase in the level of FDP (the latter two causing a prolongation in the clotting times of coagulation tests) will generally confirm the existence of a lytic state. Therefore, lytic therapy can be confirmed by performing the TT, APTT, PT, or fibrinogen levels approximately 4 hours after initiation of therapy.

If heparin is to be (re)instituted following the Streptase, Streptokinase, infusion, the TT or APTT should be less than twice the normal control value (see manufacturer's prescribing information for proper use of heparin).

PREGNANCY CATEGORY C

Animal reproduction studies have not been conducted with Streptase, Streptokinase. It is also not known whether streptokinase can cause fetal harm when administered to a pregnant woman or can affect reproduction capacity. Streptokinase should be given to a pregnant woman only if clearly needed.

Pediatric Use

Safety and effectiveness in children have not been established.

DRUG INTERACTIONS:

The interaction of Streptase, Streptokinase with other drugs has not been well studied.

Use of Anticoagulants and Antiplatelet Agents; Streptase, Streptokinase, alone or in combination with antiplatelet agents and anticoagulants, may cause bleeding complications. Therefore, careful monitoring is advised. In the treatment of acute MI, aspirin, when not otherwise contraindicated, should be administered with Streptokinase (See DRUG INTERACTIONS).

Anticoagulation After Treatment for Myocardial Infarction: In the treatment of acute myocardial infarction, the use of aspirin has been shown to reduce the incidence of reinfarction and stroke. The addition of aspirin to Streptokinase causes a minimal increase in the risk of minor (3.9% vs. 3.1%), but does not appear to increase the incidence of major bleeding (see ADVERSE REACTIONS)[2]. The use of anticoagulants following administration of Streptokinase increases the risk of bleeding, but has not yet been shown to be of unequivocal clinical benefit. Therefore, whereas the use of aspirin is recommended unless otherwise contraindicated, the use of anticoagulants should be decided by the treating physician.

Anticoagulation After IV Treatment for Other Indications: Continuous intravenous infusion of heparin, without a loading dose, has been recommended following termination of Streptase, Streptokinase, infusion for treatment of pulmonary embolism or deep vein thrombosis to prevent rethrombosis. The effect of Streptokinase on thrombin time (TT) and activated partial thromboplastin time (APTT) will usually diminish within 3 to 4 hours after Streptokinase therapy, and heparin therapy without a loading dose can be initiated when the TT or the APTT is less than twice the normal control value.

ADVERSE REACTIONS:

The following adverse reactions have been associated with intravenous therapy and may also occur with intracoronary artery infusion:

Bleeding: The reported incidence of bleeding (major or minor) varied widely depending on dosage, patient population and concomitant therapy.

Minor bleeding can be anticipated mainly at invaded or disturbed sites. If such bleeding occurs, local measures should be taken to control the bleeding.

Severe internal bleeding involving gastrointestinal, genitourinary, retroperitoneal, or intracerebral sites has occurred and has resulted in fatalities. In the treatment of acute myocardial infarction with intravenous Streptokinase, the GISSI and ISIS-2 studies reported a rate of major bleeding (requiring transfusion) of 0.5-0.5%. However, rates as high as 16% have been reported in studies which required administration of anticoagulants and invasive procedures.

Major bleed rates are difficult to determine for other dosages and patient populations because of the different dosing and intervals of infusions. The rates reported appear to be within the ranges reported for intravenous administration in acute myocardial infarction.

Should uncontrollable bleeding occur, Streptokinase infusion should be terminated immediately, rather than slowing the rate of administration of or reducing the dose of Streptokinase. If necessary, bleeding can be reversed and blood loss effectively managed with appropriate replacement therapy. Although the use of aminocaproic acid in humans as an antidote for Streptokinase has not been documented, it may be considered in an emergency situation.

Allergic Reactions: Fever and shivering, occurring in 1-4% of patients[1,2], are the most commonly reported allergic reactions with intravenous use of Streptase, Streptokinase, in acute myocardial infarction. Anaphylactic and anaphylactoid reactions ranging in severity from minor breathing difficulty to bronchospasm, periorbital swelling or angioneurotic edema have been observed rarely. Other milder allergic effects such as urticaria, itching, flushing, nausea, headache and musculoskeletal pain have also been observed, as have delayed hypersensitivity reactions such as vasculitis and interstitial nephritis. Anaphylactic shock is very rare, having been reported in 0-0.1% of patients[1,2,4].

Mild or moderate allergic reactions may be managed with concomitant antihistamine and/or corticosteroid therapy. Severe allergic reactions require immediate discontinuation of Streptase, Streptokinase, with adrenergic, antihistamine, and/or corticosteroid agents administered intravenously as required.

Other Adverse Reactions: Transient elevations of serum transaminases have been observed. The source of these enzyme rises and their clinical significance is not fully understood.

DOSAGE AND ADMINISTRATION:

Acute Evolving Transmural Myocardial Infarction: Administer Streptokinase as soon as possible after onset of symptoms. The greatest benefit in mortality reduction was observed when Streptokinase was observed when Streptokinase was administered within four hours, but statistically significant benefits has been reported up to 24 hours (see CLINICAL PHARMACOLOGY.) (TABLE 1):

TABLE 1

Route	Total Dose	Dosage/Duration
Intravenous infusion	1,500,000 IU	1,500,000 IU within 60 min.
Intracoronary infusion	140,000 IU	20,000 IU by bolus followed by 2,000 IU/min. for 60 min.

Pulmonary Embolism, Deep Vein Thrombosis, Arterial Thrombosis or Embolism: Streptase, Streptokinase, treatment should be instituted as soon as possible after onset of the thrombotic event, preferably within 7 days. Any delay in instituting lytic therapy to evaluate the effect of heparin therapy decreases the potential for optimal efficacy. Since human exposure to streptococci is common, antibodies to Streptokinase are prevalent. Thus, a loading dose of Streptokinase sufficient to neutralize these antibodies is required. A dose of 250,000 IU of Streptokinase infused into a peripheral vein over 30 minutes has been found appropriate in over 90% of patients. Furthermore, if the thrombin time or any other parameter of lysis after 4 hours of therapy is not significantly different from the normal control level, discontinue Streptokinase because excessive resistance is present (TABLE 2):

DOSAGE AND ADMINISTRATION: *(cont'd)*

TABLE 2		
Indication	**Loading Dose**	**IV Infusion Dosage/Duration**
Pulmonary Embolism	250,000 IU/30 min.	100,000 IU/hr for 24 hr (72 hrs if concurrent DVT is suspected).
Deep Vein Thrombosis	250,000 IU/30 min.	100,000 IU/hr for 72 hr
Arterial Thrombosis or Embolism	250,000 IU/30 min.	100,000 IU/hr for 24-72 hr

Arteriovenous Cannulae Occlusion: Before using Streptase, Streptokinase, an attempt should be made to clear the cannula by careful syringe technique, using heparinized saline solution. If adequate flow is not re-established, Streptokinase may be employed. Allow the effect of any pretreatment anticoagulants to diminish. Instill 250,000 IU streptokinase in 2 ml of solution into each occluded limb of the cannula slowly. Clamp off cannula limb(s) for 2 hours. Observe the patient closely for possible adverse effects. After treatment, aspirate contents of infused cannula limb(s), flush with saline, reconnect cannula.

Reconstitution and Dilution: The protein nature and lyophilized form of Streptase, Streptokinase require careful reconstitution and dilution. Slight flocculation (described as thin translucent fibers) of reconstituted streptokinase occurred occasionally during clinical trials but did not interfere with the safe use of the solution. The following reconstitution and dilution procedures are recommended:

Vials and Infusion Bottles

1. Slowly add 5 ml Sodium Chloride Injection, USP or 5% Dextrose Injection, USP to the Streptase, Streptokinase vial, directing the diluent at the side of the vacuum-packed vial rather than into the drug powder.

2. Roll and tilt the vial gently to reconstitute. Avoid shaking. (Shaking may cause foaming). If necessary, total volume may be increased to a maximum of 500 ml in glass or 50 ml in plastic containers, and the infusion pump rate in TABLE 3 should be adjusted accordingly.) To facilitate setting the infusion pump rate. a total volume of 45 ml, or a multiple thereof, is recommended.

3. Withdraw the entire reconstituted contents of the vial; slowly and carefully dilute further to a total volume as recommended in TABLE 3. Avoid shaking and agitation on dilution.

4. When diluting the 1,500,000 IU infusion bottle (50 ml), slowly add 5 ml Sodium Chloride Injection, USP, or 5% Dextrose Injection, USP, directing it at the side of the bottle rather than into the drug powder. Roll and tilt and bottle gently to reconstitute. Avoid shaking as it may cause foaming. Add an additional 40 ml of diluent to the bottle, avoiding shaking and agitation (Total volume = 45 ml). Administer by infusion pump at the rate indicated in TABLE 3.

5. Parenteral drug products should be inspected visually for particulate matter and discoloration prior to administration. (The Albumin (Human) may impart a slightly yellow color to the solution.)

6. The reconstituted solution can be filtered through a 0.8 µm or larger pore size filter.

7. Because Streptase, Streptokinase contains no preservatives, it should be reconstituted immediately before use. The solution may be used for direct intravenous administration within eight hours following reconstitution if stored at 2-8°C (36-46°F).

8. Do not add other medication to the container of Streptase, Streptokinase.

9. Unused reconstituted drug should be discarded.

TABLE 3 Suggested Dilutions And Infusion Rates

Dosage	**Vial Size (IU)**	**Total Solution Volume**	**Infusion Rate**
I. Acute Myocardial Infarction			
A. Intravenous Infusion	1,500,000	45 ml	Infuse 45 ml within 60 min.
B. Intracoronary Infusion	250,000	125 ml	
1. 20,000 IU bolus			1. Loading Dose of 10 ml
2. 2,000 IU/minute for 60 minutes			2. Then 60 ml/hours
II. Pulmonary Embolism, Deep Vein Thrombosis, Arterial Thrombosis or Embolism			
Intravenous Infusion			
A. 1. 250,000 IU loading dose over 30 minutes 2. 100,000 IU/hour maintenance dose	1,500,000	90 ml	1. Infuse 30 ml/hour for 30 minutes 2. Infuse 6 ml/hour
B. SAME	1,500,000 infusion bottle	45 ml	1.15 ml/hour for 30 minutes 2. Infuse 3 ml/hour

For Use In Arteriovenous Cannulae: Slowly reconstitute the contents of 250,000 IU Streptase, Streptokinase vacuum-packed vial with 2 ml Sodium Chloride Injection, USP or 5% Dextrose Injection, USP.

Store unopened vials at controlled room temperature (15-30°C or 59-86°F).

REFERENCES:

1. GISSI: Effectiveness of intravenous thrombolytic treatment in acute myocardial infarction. Lancet I: 395-402, 1986. **2.** ISIS-2 Collaborative Group: Randomized trial of streptokinase, oral aspirin, both, or neither among 17,187 cases of suspected acute myocardial infarction: ISIS-2, Lancet II:349-360, 1988. **3.** White, H., Norris, R., Brown, M., et al: Effect of intravenous streptokinase on left ventricular function and early survival after acute myocardial infarction. N Engl J Med 317: 850-5, 1987. **4.** The I.S.A.M. Study Group: A prospective trial of intravenous streptokinase in acute myocardial infarction (I.S.A.M.). N Engl J Med 314: 1465-1471, 1986. **5.** Anderson, J., Marshall, H., Bray, B., et al: A randomized trial of intracoronary streptokinase in the treatment of acute myocardial infarction. N Engl J Med 308: 1312-8, 1983. **6.** Kennedy, J., Ritchie, J., Davis, K., Fritz, J.: Western Washington randomized trial of intracoronary streptokinase in acute myocardial infarction. N Engl J Med 309: 1477-82, 1983. **7.** Sharma, G., Burleson, V., Sasahara, A.: Effect of thrombolytic therapy on pulmonary-capillary blood volume in patients with pulmonary embolism. N Engl J Med 303: 842-5, 1980. **8.** Arneson, H., Heilo, A., Jakobsen, E., et al: A prospective study of streptokinase and heparin in the treatment of venous thrombosis. Acta Med Scand 203: 457-463, 1978.

HOW SUPPLIED - EQUIVALENTS NOT AVAILABLE:

Injection, Lyphl-Soln - Intracardiac; I - 1,500,000 unit/

6.5 ml	**$511.75**	**STREPTASE, Astra USA**	**00186-1773-01**
50 ml	**$516.85**	**STREPTASE, Astra USA**	**00186-1774-01**
1500 ml	$412.00	KABIKINASE, Pharmacia & Upjohn	00016-0111-75

Injection, Lyphl-Soln - Intracardiac; I - 250,000 unit/vi

6.5 ml	**$115.93**	**STREPTASE, Astra USA**	**00186-1770-01**
250 ml	$77.25	KABIKINASE, Pharmacia & Upjohn	00016-0110-59

Injection, Lyphl-Soln - Intracardiac; I - 600,000 unit/vi

10's	$160.00	KABIKINASE, Pharmacia & Upjohn	00016-0110-67

HOW SUPPLIED - EQUIVALENTS NOT AVAILABLE: *(cont'd)*

Injection, Lyphl-Soln - Intracardiac; I - 750,000 unit/vi

6.5 ml	**$255.86**	**STREPTASE, Astra USA**	**00186-1771-01**
750 ml	$218.88	KABIKINASE, Pharmacia & Upjohn	00016-0119-35

STREPTOMYCIN SULFATE *(002277)*

CATEGORIES: Aminoglycosides; Anti-Infectives; Antibacterials; Antibiotics; Antimicrobials; Antimycobacterials; Antituberculosis Agents; Bacteremia; Chancroid; Endocarditis; Granuloma; Infections; Influenza; Plague; Pneumonia; Respiratory Tract Infections; Septicemia; Tuberculosis; Tularemia; Urinary Tract Infections; FDA Approval Pre 1982

FORMULARIES: BC-BS; Medi-Cal; WHO

COST OF THERAPY: $1,441.75 (Tuberculosis; Injection; 1 gm; 1/day; 365 days)

PRIMARY ICD9: 011.93 (Pulmonary Tuberculosis, Unspecified, Tubercle Bacilli Found)

WARNING:
THE RISK OF SEVERE NEUROTOXIC REACTIONS IS SHARPLY INCREASED IN PATIENTS WITH IMPAIRED KIDNEY FUNCTION OR PRERENAL AZOTEMIA. THESE INCLUDE DISTURBANCES OF THE AUDITORY NERVE, OPTIC NERVE, PERIPHERAL NEURITIS, ARACHNOIDITIS, AND ENCEPHALOPATHY. RENAL FUNCTION SHOULD BE CAREFULLY DETERMINED AND PATIENTS WITH RENAL DAMAGE AND NITROGEN RETENTION SHOULD HAVE REDUCED DOSAGE. THE PEAK SERUM CONCENTRATION IN INDIVIDUALS WITH KIDNEY DAMAGE SHOULD NOT EXCEED 20 TO 25 MCG PER MILLILITER.
THE CONCURRENT OR SEQUENTIAL USE OF OTHER NEUROTOXIC AND/OR NEPHROTOXIC DRUGS WITH STREPTOMYCIN SULFATE, PARTICULARLY NEOMYCIN, KANAMYCIN, GENTAMICIN, CEPHALORIDINE, PAROMOMYCIN, VIOMYCIN, POLYMYXIN B, COLISTIN, AND TOBRAMYCIN SHOULD BE AVOIDED.
THE NEUROTOXICITY OF STREPTOMYCIN CAN RESULT IN RESPIRATORY PARALYSIS FROM NEUROMUSCULAR BLOCKADE, ESPECIALLY WHEN THE DRUG IS GIVEN SOON AFTER ANESTHESIA AND THE USE OF MUSCLE RELAXANTS. THE ADMINISTRATION OF STREPTOMYCIN IN PARENTERAL FORM SHOULD BE RESERVED FOR PATIENTS WHERE ADEQUATE LABORATORY FACILITIES ARE AVAILABLE AND CONSTANT SUPERVISION OF THE PATIENT IS POSSIBLE.

DESCRIPTION:

Streptomycin is a water-soluble aminoglycoside derived from *Streptomyces griseus*. It is marketed as the sulfate salt of streptomycin.

CLINICAL PHARMACOLOGY:

Streptomycin sulfate is a bactericidal antibiotic in therapeutic dosage. The mode of action is the interference with normal protein synthesis and production of "faulty proteins."

Following intramuscular injection of 1 g of the drug, a peak serum level of 25 to 50 mcg per milliliter is reached within 1 hour, diminishing slowly to about 50 percent after 5 to 6 hours. Appreciable concentrations are found in all organ tissues except the brain. Significant amounts have been found in pleural fluid and tuberculous cavities. Streptomycin passes through the placenta with serum levels in the cord blood similar to maternal levels. Small amounts are excreted in milk, saliva, and sweat.

Streptomycin is excreted rapidly in the urine by glomerular filtration. In patients with normal kidney function, between 29 and 89 percent of a single 0.6 g dose is excreted within 24 hours. Any reduction of glomerular activity results in decreased excretion of the drug and concurrent rise in serum and tissue levels.

Sensitivity Plate Testing: If the Kirby-Bauer method of disc sensitivity is used, a 10 mcg streptomycin disc should give a zone of over 15 millimeters when tested against a streptomycin-sensitive bacterial strain.

INDICATIONS AND USAGE:

Mycobacterium tuberculosis: Streptomycin may be indicated for all forms of this infection when the infecting organisms are susceptible. It should be used only in combination with other antituberculosis drugs. The common combined drug therapy is streptomycin PAS, and, isoniazid; this combination is effective only where the organisms are susceptible to the drugs being used in combination.

Nontuberculosis infections: Streptomycin should be used only in those serious nontuberculosis infections caused by organisms shown by*in vitro* sensitivity studies to be susceptible to it and when less potentially hazardous therapeutic agents are ineffective or contraindicated.

a. *Pasteurella pestis* (plague)

b. *Pasteurella tularensis* (tularemia).

c. *Brucella*.

d. *Donovanosis* (granuloma inguinale).

e. *H. ducreyi* (chancroid).

f. *H. influenzae* (in respiratory, endocardial, and meningeal infections-concomitantly with another antibacterial agent).

g. *K. pneumoniae* pneumonia (concomitantly with another antibacterial agent).

h. *E coli, Proteus, A. aerogenes, K. pneumoniae*, and *Streptococcus faecalis* in urinary tract infections.

i. *Strep. viridans, Strep. faecalis* (in endocardial infections - concomitantly with penicillin).

j. Gram-negative bacillary bacteremia (concomitantly with another antibacterial agent).

Note: The use of streptomycin should be limited to the treatment of infections caused by bacteria which have been shown to be susceptible to the antibacterial effects of streptomycin and which are not amenable to therapy with less potentially toxic agents.

CONTRAINDICATIONS:

Streptomycin is contraindicated in those individuals who have shown previous toxic or hypersensitivity reactions to it.

WARNINGS:

Ototoxicity: Streptomycin may frequently affect the vestibular branch of the auditory nerve causing severe nausea, vomiting, and vertigo. The incidence is directly proportional to duration and amount of the drug administered. Advanced age and renal impairment predispose to ototoxicity. Symptoms subside and recovery is usually complete following discontinuance of the drug.

Loss of hearing has been reported following long term therapy; however, ototoxic effect on the auditory branch of the eighth nerve is infrequent and usually is preceded by vestibular symptoms. Hearing loss, when extensive, is usually permanent.

Usage In Pregnancy: Since streptomycin readily crosses the placental barrier, caution in use of the drug is important to prevent ototoxicity in the fetus.

PRECAUTIONS:

Baseline and periodic caloric stimulation tests and audiometric tests are advisable with extended streptomycin therapy. Tinnitus, roaring noises, or a sense of fullness in the ears indicates need for audiometric examination or termination of streptomycin therapy or both.

Care should be taken by individuals handling or preparing streptomycin for injection to avoid skin sensitivity reactions.

As with all intramuscular preparations, streptomycin sulfate injection should be injected well within the body of a relatively large muscle, ADULTS: The preferred site is the upper outer quadrant of the buttock, (*i.e.*, gluteus maximus), or the mid-lateral thigh.

Children: It is recommended that intramuscular injections be given preferably in the mid-lateral muscles of the thigh. In infants and small children the periphery of the upper outer quadrant of the gluteal region should be used only when necessary, such as in burn patients, in order to minimize the possibility of damage to the sciatic nerve.

The deltoid area should be used only if well developed such as in certain adults and older children, and then only with caution to avoid radial nerve injury. Intramuscular injections should not be made into the lower and mid-third of the upper arm. As with all intramuscular injections, aspiration is necessary to help avoid inadvertent injection into a blood vessel,

Injection sites should be alternated, and solutions of concentration greater than 500 mg/ml are not recommended.

As higher doses or more prolonged therapy with streptomycin may be indicated for more severe or fulminating infections (endocarditis, meningitis, etc.), the physician should always take adequate measures to be immediately aware of any toxic signs or symptoms occurring in the patient as a result of streptomycin therapy.

While disturbances in renal function due to streptomycin have been reported in the past, purification of the drug has minimized this side effect. In the presence of pre-existing renal insufficiency, however, extreme caution must be exercised in the administration of streptomycin. Since in severely uremic patients a single dose may produce reasonably high blood levels for several days, the cumulative effect may produce ototoxic sequelae. When streptomycin must be given for prolonged periods of time, alkalinization of the urine may minimize or prevent renal irritation.

A syndrome of apparent central nervous system depression, characterized by stupor and flaccidity, at times to the extent of coma and deep respiratory depression, has been reported in very young infants in whom streptomycin dosage had materially exceeded the recommended limits, Thus, infants should not receive streptomycin in excess of the recommended dosage.

In the treatment of venereal infections such as granuloma inguinale, and chancroid, if concomitant syphilis is suspected, suitable laboratory procedures such as a dark field examination should be performed before the start of treatment, and monthly serologic tests should be done for at least four months.

As with other antibiotics, use of this drug may result in overgrowth of nonsusceptible organisms, including fungi. If superinfection occurs, appropriate therapy should be instituted.

ADVERSE REACTIONS:

The following reactions are common: ototoxicity - nausea, vomiting and vertigo; paresthesia of face; rash; fever; urticaria; angioneurotic edema; and eosinophilia.

The following reactions are less frequent: deafness, exfoliative dermatitis, anaphylaxis, azotemia, leucopenia, thrombocytopenia, pancytopenia, hemolytic anemia, muscular weakness, and amblyopia.

Vestibular dysfunction resulting from the parenteral administration of streptomycin is cumulatively related to the total daily dose. When 1.8 to 2.0 g/day are given, symptoms are likely to develop in the large percentage of patients - especially in the elderly or patients with impaired renal function-within four weeks. Therefore, it is recommended that caloric and audiometric tests be done prior to, during, and following intensive therapy with streptomycin in order to facilitate detection of any vestibular dysfunction and/or impairment of hearing which may occur.

Vestibular symptoms generally appear early and usually are reversible with early detection and cessation of administration of the drug. After two to three months, gross vestibular symptoms usually disappear, except for the relative inability to walk in total darkness or on very rough terrain.

Clinical judgment as to termination of therapy must be exercised when side effects occur.

DOSAGE AND ADMINISTRATION:

Intramuscular Route Only

TUBERCULOSIS

All forms when organisms are known or believed to be drug susceptible.

Adult, combined therapy: Streptomycin - 1 g daily with PAS 5 g t.i.d. and isoniazid 200 to 300 mg daily. Elderly patients should have a smaller daily dose of streptomycin, based on age, renal function, and eighth nerve function. Ultimately the streptomycin should be discontinued or reduced in dosage to 1 g 2 to 3 times weekly. Therapy with streptomycin may be terminated when toxic symptoms have appeared, when impending toxicity is feared, when organisms become resistant, or when full treatment effect has been obtained. The total period of drug treatment of tuberculosis is a minimum of 1 year; however, indications for terminating therapy with streptomycin may occur at any time as noted above.

TULAREMIA

One to 2 g daily in divided doses for 7 to 10 days until the patient is afebrile for 5 to 7 days.

PLAGUE

Two to 4 g daily in divided doses until the patient is afebrile for at least 3 days.

Bacterial endocarditis: In penicillin-sensitive alpha and nonhemolytic streptococcal endocarditis (penicillin sensitive to 0.1 mcg per milliliter or less), streptomycin may be used for 2-week treatment concomitantly with penicillin. Streptomycin dosage is 1 g b.i.d. for 1 week, and 0.5 g b.i.d. for the 2d week. If the patient is over 60 years of age, the dosage should be 0.5 g b.i.d. for the entire 2-week period.

Enterococcal endocarditis: Streptomycin in doses of 1 g b.i.d. for 2 weeks and 0.5 g b.i.d. for 4 weeks is given in combination with penicillin. Ototoxicity may require termination of the streptomycin prior to completion of the 6 week course of treatment.

DOSAGE AND ADMINISTRATION: *(cont'd)*

CONCOMITANT USE

For use concomitantly with other agents to which the infecting organism is also sensitive. Streptomycin in these conditions is considered as a drug of secondary choice: gram-negative bacillary bacteremia, meningitis, and pneumonia; brucellosis; granuloma inguinale; chancroid, and urinary tract infection.

For Adults: *Severe fulminating infection:* 2 to 4 g daily, administered intramuscularly in divided doses every 6 to 12 hours. *With less severe infections and with highly susceptible organisms:* 1 to 2 daily,

For Children: 20 to 40 mg per kg of body weight daily (8 to 20 mg per pound) in divided doses every 6 to 12 hours. (Particular care should be taken to avoid excessive dosage in children.)

The dry powder is dissolved by adding Water for Injection, U.S.P. or Isotonic Sodium Chloride Solution, U.S.P. in an amount to yield the desired concentration as indicated in the following table (TABLE 1):

TABLE 1

Approx. Conc. (mg/ml)	Volume (ml) of Solvent 1 g Vial	5 g Vial
200	4.2	-
250	3.2	-
400	1.8	9.0

Sterile reconstituted solutions may be stored at room temperature for four weeks without significant loss of potency.

HOW SUPPLIED - RATED THERAPEUTICALLY EQUIVALENT:

Injection, Solution - Intramuscular - 1 gm

1's $3.95 Streptomycin Sulfate, Lilly 00002-1681-01

STREPTOZOCIN *(002278)*

CATEGORIES: Antineoplastics; Cancer; Chemotherapy; Oncologic Drugs; Pancreatic Cancer; Pregnancy Category C; FDA Approved 1982 May

BRAND NAMES: **Zanosar**

FORMULARIES: BC-BS; Medi-Cal

> WARNING:
> Zanosar Sterile Powder should be administered under the supervision of a physician experienced in the use of cancer chemotherapeutic agents.
> A patient need to be hospitalized but should have access to a facility with laboratory and supportive resources sufficient to monitor drug tolerance and to protect and maintain a patient compromised by drug toxicity. Renal toxicity is dose-related and cumulative and may be severe or fatal. Other major toxicities are nausea and vomiting which may be severe and at times treatment-limiting. In addition, liver dysfunction, diarrhea, and hematological changes have been observed in some patients. Streptozocin is mutagenic. When administered parenterally, it has been found to be tumorigenic or carcinogenic in some rodents.
> The physician must judge the possible benefit to his patient against the known toxic effects of this drug in considering the advisability of therapy with streptozocin. He should be familiar with the following text before making his judgement and beginning treatment.

DESCRIPTION:

Each vial of streptozocin sterile powder contains 1 g of the active ingredient streptozocin 2-deoxy-2[[(methylnitrosoamino)carbonyl]amino]-α(and β)-D-glucopyranose and 220 mg citric acid anhydrous. Streptozocin is available as a sterile, pale yellow, freeze-dried preparation for intravenous administration. The pH was adjusted with sodium hydroxide. When reconstituted as directed, the pH of the solution will be between 3.5 and 4.5. Streptozocin is a synthetic antineoplastic agent that is chemically related to other nitrosoureas used in cancer chemotherapy. Streptozocin is an ivory-colored crystalline powder with a molecular weight of 265.2. It is very soluble in water or physiological saline and is soluble in alcohol.

CLINICAL PHARMACOLOGY:

Streptozocin inhibits DNA synthesis in bacterial and mammalian cells. In bacterial cells, a specific interaction with cytosine moieties leads to degradation of DNA. The biochemical mechanism leading to mammalian cell death has not been definitely established; streptozocin inhibits cell proliferation at a considerably lower level than that needed to inhibit precursor incorporation into DNA or to inhibit several of the enzymes involved in DNA synthesis. Although streptozocin inhibits the progression of cells into mitosis, no specific phase of the cell cycle is particularly sensitive to its lethal effects.

Streptozocin is active in the L1210 leukemic mouse over a fairly wide range of parenteral dosage schedules. In experiments in many animal species, streptozocin induced a diabetes that resembles human hyperglycemic nonketotic diabetes mellitus. This phenomenon, which has been extensively studied, appears to be mediated through a lowering of beta cell nicotinamide adenine dinucleotide (NAD) and consequent histopathologic alteration of pancreatic islet beta cells.

The metabolism and the chemical dissociation of streptozocin that occurs under physiologic conditions has not been extensively studied. When administered intravenously to a variety of experimental animals, streptozocin disappears from the blood very rapidly. In all species tested, it was found to concentrate in the liver and kidney. As much as 20% of the drug (or metabolites containing an N-nitrosourea group) is metabolized and/or excreted by the kidney. Metabolic products have not yet been identified.

INDICATIONS AND USAGE:

Streptozocin sterile powder is indicated in the treatment of metastatic islet cell carcinoma of the pancreas. Responses have been obtained with both functional and nonfunctional carcinomas. Because of its inherent renal toxicity, therapy with this drug should be limited to patients with symptomatic or progressive metastatic disease.

WARNINGS:

Renal Toxicity: Many patients treated with streptozocin sterile powder have experienced renal toxicity, as evidenced by azotemia, anuria hypophosphatemia, glycosuria and renal tubular acidosis. **Such toxicity is dose-related and cumulative and may be severe or fatal.** Renal function must be monitored before and after each course of therapy. Serial urinalysis, blood urea

WARNINGS: *(cont'd)*

nitrogen, plasma creatinine, serum electrolytes and creatinine clearance should be obtained prior to, at least weekly during, and for four weeks after drug administration. Serial urinalysis is particularly important for the early detection of proteinuria and should be quantitated with a 24 hour collection when proteinuria is detected. Mild proteinuria is one of the first signs of renal toxicity and may herald further deterioration of renal function. Reduction of the dose of streptozocin or discontinuation of treatment is suggested in the presence of significant renal toxicity.

Use of streptozocin in patients with preexisting renal disease requires a judgment by the physician of potential benefit as opposed to the known risk of serious renal damage.

This drug should not be used in combination with or concomitantly with other potential nephrotoxins.

When exposed dermally, some rats developed benign tumors at the site of application of streptozocin. Consequently, streptozocin may pose a carcinogenic hazard following topical exposure if not properly handled(see DOSAGE AND ADMINISTRATION.)

See additional warnings at the beginning of this insert.

PRECAUTIONS:

Laboratory Tests: Patients who are treated with streptozocin sterile powder must be monitored closely, particularly for evidence of renal, hepatic, and hematopoietic toxicity. Renal function tests are described in WARNINGS. Patients should also be monitored closely for evidence of hematopoietic and hepatic toxicities. Complete blood counts and liver function tests should be done at least weekly. Dosage adjustments or discontinuance of the drug may be indicated, depending upon the degree of toxicity noted.

Mutagenesis, Carcinogenesis, Impairment of Fertility: Streptozocin is mutagenic in bacteria, plants and mammalian cells. When administered parenterally, it has been shown to induce renal tumors in rats and to induce liver tumors and other tumors in hamsters. Stomach and pancreatic tumors were observed in rats treated orally with streptozocin. Streptozocin has also been shown to be carcinogenic in mice.

Streptozocin adversely affected fertility when administered to male and female rats.

Pregnancy Category C: Reproduction studies revealed that streptozocin is teratogenic in the rat and has abortifacient effects in rabbits. When administered intravenously to pregnant monkeys, it appears rapidly in the fetal circulation. There are no studies in pregnant women. Streptozocin should be used during pregnancy only if the potential benefit justifies the potential risk to the fetus.

Nursing Mothers: It is not known whether streptozocin is excreted in human milk. Because many drugs are excreted in human milk and because of the potential for serious adverse reactions nursing infants, nursing should be discontinued in patients receiving streptozocin.

ADVERSE REACTIONS:

Renal: See WARNINGS.

Gastrointestinal: Most patients treated with streptozocin sterile powder have experienced severe nausea and vomiting, occasionally requiring discontinuation of drug therapy. Some patients experienced diarrhea. A number of patients have experienced hepatic toxicity, as characterized by elevated liver enzyme (SGOT and LDH) levels and hypoalbuminemia.

Hematological: Hematological toxicity has been rare, most often involving mild decreases in hematocrit values. However, **fatal hematological toxicity with substantial reductions in leukocyte and platelet count** has been observed.

Metabolic: Mild to moderate abnormalities of glucose tolerance have been noted in some patients treated with streptozocin. These have generally been reversible, but insulin shock with hypoglycemia has been observed.

Genitourinary: Two cases of nephrogenic diabetes insipidus following therapy with streptozocin have been reported. One had spontaneous recovery and the second responded to indomethacin.

OVERDOSAGE:

No specific antidote for streptozocin is known.

DOSAGE AND ADMINISTRATION:

Streptozocin sterile powder should be administered intravenously. It is not active orally. Although it has been administered intra-arterially, this is not recommended pending further evaluation of the possibility that adverse renal effects may be evoked more rapidly by this route of administration.

Two different dosage schedules have been employed successfully with streptozocin.

Daily Schedule: The recommended dose for daily intravenous administration is 500 mg/m^2 of body surface area for five consecutive days every six weeks until maximum benefit or until treatment-limiting toxicity is observed. Dose escalation on this schedule is not recommended.

Weekly Schedule: The recommended initial dose for weekly intravenous administration is 1000 mg/m^2 of body surface area at weekly intervals for the first two courses (weeks). In subsequent courses, drug doses may be escalated in patients who have not achieved a therapeutic response and who have not experienced significant toxicity with the previous course of treatment. However, A SINGLE DOSE OF 1500 mg/m^2BODY SURFACE AREA SHOULD NOT BE EXCEEDED as a greater dose may cause azotemia. When administrated on this schedule, the median time to onset of response is about 17 days and the median time to maximum response is about 35 days. The median **total** dose to onset of response is about 2000 mg/m^2 body surface area and the median**total** dose to maximum response is about 4000 mg/m^2 body surface area.

The ideal duration of maintenance therapy with streptozocin has not yet been clearly established for either of the above schedules.

For patients with functional tumors, serial monitoring of fasting insulin levels allows a determination of biochemical response to therapy. For patients with either functional or nonfunctional tumors, response to therapy can be determined by measurable reductions of tumor size (reduction of organomegaly, masses, or lymph nodes).

Reconstitute streptozocin with 9.5 ml of Dextrose Injection USP, or 0.9% Sodium Chloride Injection USP. The resulting pale-gold solution will contain 100 mg of streptozocin and 22 mg of citric acid per ml. Where more dilute infusion solutions are desirable, further dilution in the above vehicles is recommended. The total storage time for streptozocin after it has been placed in solution should not exceed 12 hours. This product contains no preservatives and is not intended as a multiple-dose vial.

Caution in the handling and preparation of the powder and solution should be exercised, and the use of gloves is recommended. If streptozocin sterile powder or a solution prepared from streptozocin contacts the skin or mucosae, immediately wash the affected area with soap and water.

Procedures for proper handling and disposal of anticancer drugs should be considered. Several guidelines on this subject have been published.[4-9] There is no general agreement that all of the procedures recommended in the guidelines are necessary or appropriate.

REFERENCES:

1. Broder LE and Carter SK: *Ann Int Med, 79:*101-118, 1972. **2.** Schein PS, O'Connell MJ, Blom J, Hubbard S, Magrath IT, Bergevin P, Wiernik PH, Ziegler TL, and DeVita VT: *Cancer, 34:*993-1000, 1974. **3.** Moertel CG, et al: *Cancer Chemother Rep, 55:*303-307, 1972. **4.** Recommendations for the Safe Handling of Parenteral Antineoplastic Drugs. NIH Publication No. 83-2621. For sale by the Superintendent of Documents, US Government Printing Office, Washington, DC 20402. **5.** AMA Council Report. Guidelines for Handling Parenteral Antineoplastics. JAMA, March 15, 1985. **6.** National Study Commission on Cytotoxic Exposure-Recommendations for Handling Cytotoxic Agents. Available from Louis P. Jeffrey, ScD, Director of Pharmacy Services, Rhode Island Hospital, 593 Eddy Street, Providence, Rhode Island 02902. **7.** Clinical Oncological Society of Australia: Guidelines and recommendations for safe handling of antineoplastic agents. *Med J Australia 1:*426-428, 1983. **8.** Jones RB, et al, Safe handling of chemotherapeutic agents: A report from the Mount Sinai Medical Center CA-A Cancer Journal for Clinicians Sept/Oct., 1983, pp. 258-263. **9.** American Society of Hospital Pharmacists Technical assistance bulletin on handling cytotoxic drugs in hospitals.*Amj Hosp Pharm 42:*131-137, 1985.

HOW SUPPLIED:

Zanosar Sterile Powder is supplied in 1 gram vials (NDC 0009-0844-01). Unopened vials of Zanosar should be stored at refrigeration temperatures (2° to 8° C) and protected from light (preferably stored in carton).

HOW SUPPLIED - EQUIVALENTS NOT AVAILABLE:

Injection, Lyphl-Soln - Intravenous - 1 gm/vial

1 gm $63.79 ZANOSAR, Pharmacia & Upjohn 00009-0844-01

STRONTIUM CHLORIDE, SR-89 *(003173)*

CATEGORIES: Bone Disease; Pain; Prostatic Carcinoma; Radiopharmaceuticals; FDA Class 1P ("Priority Review"); FDA Approved 1993 Jun

BRAND NAMES: **Metastron**

DESCRIPTION:

Metastron is a sterile, non-pyrogenic, aqueous solution of Strontium-89 Chloride for intravenous administration. The solution contains no preservative. Each milliliter contains:

Strontium Chloride: 10.9 - 22.6 mg

Water for Injection: q.s. to 1 ml

The radioactive concentration is 37 MBq/ml, 1mCi/ml, and the specific activity is 2.96-6.17 MGq/mg, 80-167 μCi/mg at calibration. The pH of the solution is 4 - 7.5.

Physical Characteristics: Strontium-89 decays by beta emission with a physical half-life of 50.5 days. The maximum beta energy is 1.463 MeV (100%). The maximum range of β-from Strontium-89 in tissue is approximately 8 mm.

Radioactive decay factors to be applied to the stated value for radioactive concentration at calibration, when calculating injection volumes at the time of administration, are given in TABLE 1.

TABLE 1 Strontium-89, Description Decay of Strontium-89

Day*	Factor	Day*	Factor
-24	1.39	+6	0.92
-22	1.35	+8	0.90
-20	1.32	+10	0.87
-18	1.28	+12	0.85
-16	1.25	+14	0.83
-14	1.21	+16	0.80
-12	1.18	+18	0.78
-10	1.15	+20	0.76
-8	1.12	+22	0.74
-6	1.09	+24	0.72
-4	1.06	+26	0.70
-2	1.03	+28	0.68
0	1.00		

* Days before (-) or after (+) the calibration date stated on the vial.
0 = calibration

CLINICAL PHARMACOLOGY:

Following intravenous injection, soluble strontium compounds behave like their calcium analogs, clearing rapidly from the blood and selectively localizing in bone mineral. Uptake of strontium by bone occurs preferentially in sites of active osteogenesis; thus primary bone tumors and areas of metastatic involvement (blastic lesions) can accumulate significantly greater concentrations of strontium than surrounding normal bone.

Strontium-89 Chloride is retained in metastatic bone lesions much longer than in normal bone, where turnover is about 14 days. In patients with extensive skeletal metastases, well over half of the injected dose is retained in the bones.

Excretion pathways are two-thirds urinary and one-third fecal in patients with bone metastases. Urinary excretion is higher in people without bone lesions. Urinary excretion is greatest in the first two days following injection.

Strontium-89 is a pure beta emitter and Strontium-89 Chloride selectively irradiates sites of primary and metastatic bone involvement with minimal irradiation of soft tissues distant from the bone lesions. (The maximum range in tissue is 8 mm; maximum energy is 1.463 MeV.) Mean absorbed radiation doses are listed under the Radiation Dosimetry.

Clinical trials have examined relief of pain in cancer patients who have received therapy for bone metastases (external radiation to indexed sites) but in whom persistent pain recurred. In a multi-center Canadian placebo-controlled trial of 126 patients, pain relief occurred in more patients treated with a single injection of strontium chloride, SR-89 than in patients treated with an injection of placebo. Results are given in TABLE 2 and TABLE 3.

Table 2 compares the percentage and number of patients treated with strontium chloride, SR-89 or placebo who had reduced pain and no increase in analgesic or radiotherapy re-treatment.

Table 2 comparison Of The Effects Of Strontium-89 And Placebo, As Adjunct To Radiotherapy, On Treatment Outcome Over Time

Months Post-Treatment	1	2	3	4	5	6
Metastron	71.4% (n=42)	78.9% (n=38)	60.6% (n=33)	59.3% (n=27)	36.4% (n=22)	63.6% (n=22)
Placebo	61.4% (n=44)	57.1% (n=35)	55.9% (n=34)	25.0% (n=24)	31.8% (n=22)	35.0% (n=20)

At each visit, treatment success, defined as a reduction in a patient's pain score without any increase in analgesic intake and without any supplementary radiotherapy at the index site, was more frequent among patients assigned to strontium chloride, SR-89 than to placebo.

CLINICAL PHARMACOLOGY: *(cont'd)*

Table 3 compares the number and percentage of patients treated with strontium chloride, SR-89 or placebo as an adjunct to radiotherapy who were pain free without analgesic at the intervals shown.

Table 3 comparison Of The Effects Of Strontium-89 And Placebo As Adjunct To Radiotherapy, On Reduction Of Pain Score And Analgesic Score To Zero

Months Post-Treatment	1	2	3	4	5	6	9
Metastron	6 14.3% (n=42)	5 13.2% (n=38)	5 15.2% (n=33)	3 11.1% (n=27)	4 18.2% (n=22)	4 18.2% (n=22)	2 18.2% (N=11)
Placebo	3 6.8% (n=44)	3 8.6% (N=35)	2 5.9% (n=34)	0 (n=24)	1 4.5% (n=22)	1 5% (n=20)	0 (n=17)

The number of patients classified at each visit as treatment successes who were pain free at the index site and required no analgesics was consistently higher in the strontium chloride, SR-89 group.

New pain sites were less frequent in patients treated with strontium chloride, SR-89.

In another clinical trial, pain relief was greater in a group of patients treated with strontium chloride, SR-89 compared with a group treated with non-radioactive strontium-88.

INDICATIONS AND USAGE:

Strontium chloride, SR-89 injection is indicated for the relief of bone pain in patients with painful skeletal metastases.

The presence of bone metastases should be confirmed prior to therapy.

CONTRAINDICATIONS:

None known.

WARNINGS:

Use of strontium chloride, SR-89 in patients with evidence of seriously compromised bone marrow from previous therapy or disease infiltration is not recommended unless the potential benefit of the treatment outweighs its risks. Bone marrow toxicity is to be expected following the administration of strontium chloride, SR-89, particularly white blood cells and platelets. The extent of toxicity is variable. It is recommended that the patient's peripheral blood cell counts be monitored at least once every other week. Typically, platelets will be depressed by about 30% compared to pre-administration levels. The nadir of platelet depression in most patients is found between 12 and 16 weeks following administration of strontium chloride, SR-89. White blood cells are usually depressed to a varying extent compared to pre-administration levels. Thereafter, recovery occurs slowly, typically reaching pre-administration levels six months after treatment unless the patient's disease or additional therapy intervenes.

In considering repeat administration of strontium chloride, SR-89, the patient's hematologic response to the initial dose, current platelet level and other evidence of marrow depletion should be carefully evaluated.

Verification of dose and patient identification is necessary prior to administration because strontium chloride, SR-89 delivers a relatively high dose of radioactivity.

Strontium chloride, SR-89 may cause fetal harm when administered to a pregnant woman. There are no adequate and well-controlled studies in pregnant women. If this drug is used during pregnancy, or if the patient becomes pregnant while receiving this drug, the patient should be apprised of the potential hazard to the fetus. Women of childbearing potential should be advised to avoid becoming pregnant.

PRECAUTIONS:

General: Strontium chloride, SR-89 is not indicated for use in patients with cancer not involving bone. Strontium chloride, SR-89 should be used with caution in patients with platelet counts below 60,000 and white cell counts below 2,400.

Radiopharmaceuticals should only be used by physicians who are qualified by training and experience in the safe use and handling of radionuclides and whose experience and training have been approved by the appropriate government agency authorized to license the use of radionuclides.

Strontium chloride, SR-89, like other radioactive drugs, must be handled with care and appropriate safety measures taken to minimize radiation to clinical personnel.

In view of the delayed onset of pain relief, typically 7 to 20 days post injection, administration of strontium chloride, SR-89 to patients with very short life expectancy is not recommended.

A calcium-like flushing sensation has been observed in patients following a rapid (less than 30 second injection) administration.

Special precautions, such as urinary catheterization, should be taken following administration to patients who are incontinent to minimize the risk of radioactive contamination of clothing, bed linen and the patient's environment.

Carcinogenesis, Mutagenesis, and Impairment of Fertility: Data from a repetitive dose animal study suggests that Strontium-89 Chloride is a potential carcinogen. Thirty-three of 40 rats injected with Strontium-89 Chloride in ten consecutive monthly doses of either 250 or 350 µCi/kg developed malignant bone tumors after a latency period of approximately 9 months. No neoplasia was observed in the control animals. Treatment with Strontium-89 Chloride should be restricted to patients with well documented metastatic bone disease.

Adequate studies with Strontium-89 Chloride have not been performed to evaluate mutagenic potential or effects on fertility.

Pregnancy, Teratogenic Effects, Pregnancy Category D: See WARNINGS.

Nursing Mothers: Because Strontium acts as a calcium analog, secretion of Strontium-89 Chloride into human milk is likely. It is recommended that nursing be discontinued by mothers about to receive intravenous Strontium-89. It is not known whether this drug is excreted in human milk.

Pediatric Use: Safety and effectiveness in children below the age of 18 years have not been established.

ADVERSE REACTIONS:

A single case of fatal septicemia following leukopenia was reported during clinical trials. Most severe reactions of marrow toxicity can be managed by conventional means.

A small number of patients have reported a transient increase in bone pain at 36 to 72 hours after injection. This is usually mild and self- limiting, and controllable with analgesics. A single patient reported chills and fever 12 hours after injection without long-term sequelae.

DOSAGE AND ADMINISTRATION:

The recommended dose of strontium chloride, SR-89 is 148 MBq, 4 mCi, administered by slow intravenous injection (1-2 minutes). Alternatively, a dose of 1.5 - 2.2 MBq/kg, 40-60 µCi/kg body weight may be used.

Repeated administrations of strontium chloride, SR-89 should be based on an individual patient's response to therapy, current symptoms, and hematologic status, and are generally not recommended at intervals of less than 90 days.

The patient dose should be measured by a suitable radioactivity calibration system immediately prior to administration.

Radiation Dosimetry: The estimated radiation dose that would be delivered over time by the intravenous injection of 37 MBq, 1 mCi of Strontium-89 to a normal healthy adult is given in Table 4. Data are taken from the ICRP publication "Radiation Dose to Patients from Radiopharmaceuticals" -ICRP #53, Vol. 18, No. 1-4, Page 171, Pergamon Press, 1988.

TABLE 4

Strontium-89 Dosimetry Organ	mGy/MBq	rad/mCi
Bone Surface	17.0	63.0
Red Bone Marrow	11.0	40.7
Lower Bowel Wall	4.7	17.4
Bladder Wall	1.3	4.8
Testes	0.8	2.9
Ovaries	0.8	2.9
Uterine Wall	0.8	2.9
Kidneys	0.8	2.9

When blastic osseous metastases are present, significantly enhanced localization of the radiopharmaceutical will occur with correspondingly higher doses to the metastases compared with normal bones and other organs.

The radiation dose hazard in handling Strontium-89 Chloride injection during dose dispensing and administration is similar to that from phosphorus-32. The beta emission has a range in water of about 8 mm (max.) and in glass of about 3 mm, but the bremsstrahlung radiation may augment the contact dose.

Measured values of the dose on the surface of the unshielded vial are about 65 mR/minute/mCi.

It is recommended that the vial be kept inside its transportation shield whenever possible.

Storage: The calibration date (for radioactivity content) and expiration date are quoted on the vial label. The expiration date will be 28 days after calibration. Stability studies have shown no change in any of the product characteristics monitored during routine product quality control over the period from manufacture to expiration.

HOW SUPPLIED - EQUIVALENTS NOT AVAILABLE:

Injection, Solution - Intravenous

4 ml $2020.00 METASTRON, Medi Physics 17156-0524-01

SUCCINYLCHOLINE CHLORIDE *(002279)*

CATEGORIES: Anesthesia; Autonomic Drugs; Endotracheal Intubation; Muscle Relaxants; Muscles; Neuromuscular Blocking Agents; Non-Depolarizing Muscle Relaxants; Short-Acting Neuromuscular Blockers; Skeletal Muscle Relaxants; Pregnancy Category C; FDA Approval Pre 1982

BRAND NAMES: **Anectine**; Quelicin; Sucostrin; Sux-Cert; Suxamethonium

FORMULARIES: WHO

WARNING:
RISK OF CARDIAC ARREST FROM HYPERKALEMIC RHABDOMYOLYSIS

There have been rare reports of acute rhabdomyolysis with hyperkalemia followed by ventricular dysrhythmias, cardiac arrest and death after the administration of succinylcholine to apparently healthy children who were subsequently found to have undiagnosed skeletal muscle myopathy, most frequently Duchenne's muscular dystrophy.

This syndrome often presents as peaked T-waves and sudden cardiac arrest within minutes after the administration of the drug in healthy appearing children (usually, but not exclusively, males, and most frequently 8 years of age or younger).

There have also been reports in adolescents.

Therefore, when a healthy appearing infant or child develops cardiac arrest soon after administration of succinylcholine, not felt to be due to inadequate ventilation, oxygenation or anesthetic overdose, immediate treatment for hyperkalemia should be instituted. This should include administration of intravenous calcium, bicarbonate, and glucose with insulin, with hyperventilation. Due to the abrupt onset of this syndrome, routine resuscitative measures are likely to be unsuccessful. However, extraordinary and prolonged resuscitative efforts have resulted in successful resuscitation in some reported cases. In addition, in presence of signs of malignant hyperthermia, appropriate treatment should be instituted concurrently.

Since there may be no signs or symptoms to alert the practitioner to which patients are at risk, it is recommended that the use of succinylcholine in children should be reserved for emergency intubation or instances where immediate securing of the airway is necessary (*e.g.*, laryngospasm, difficult airway, full stomach) or for intramuscular use when a suitable vein is inaccessible (see PRECAUTIONS, Pediatric Use and DOSAGE AND ADMINISTRATION).

DESCRIPTION:

The drug should be used only by individuals familiar with its actions, characteristics and hazards.

Anectine (succinylcholine chloride) is an ultra short-acting depolarizing-type, skeletal muscle relaxant for intravenous administration.

Succinylcholine chloride is a white, odorless, slightly bitter powder and very soluble in water. The drug is unstable in alkaline solutions but relatively stable in acid solutions, depending upon the concentration of the solution and the storage temperature. Solutions of succinylcholine chloride should be stored under refrigeration to preserve potency. Anectine

DESCRIPTION: *(cont'd)*

Injection is a sterile non-pyrogenic solution for intravenous injection, containing 20 mg succinylcholine chloride in each ml and made isotonic with sodium chloride. The pH is adjusted to 3.5 with hydrochloric acid. Methylparaben (0.1%) is added as a preservative. Anectine Flo-Pack is a sterile powder, containing either 500 mg or 1000 mg of succinylcholine chloride in each vial.

The chemical name for succinylcholine chloride is 2,2'-[(1,4-dioxo-1,4-butanediyl)bis(oxy)]bis[*N,N,N*-trimethylethanaminium] dichloride.

CLINICAL PHARMACOLOGY:

Succinylcholine is a depolarizing skeletal muscle relaxant. As does acetylcholine, it combines with the cholinergic receptors of the motor end plate to produce depolarization. This depolarization may be observed as fasciculations. Subsequent neuromuscular transmission is inhibited so long as adequate concentration of succinylcholine remains at the receptor site. Onset of flaccid paralysis is rapid (less than one minute after intravenous administration), and with single administration lasts approximately 4 to 6 minutes.

Succinylcholine is rapidly hydrolyzed by plasma cholinesterase to succinylmonocholine (which possesses clinically insignificant depolarizing muscle relaxant properties) and then more slowly to succinic acid and choline (see PRECAUTIONS). About 10% of the drug is excreted unchanged in the urine. The paralysis following administration of succinylcholine is progressive, with differing sensitivities of different muscles. This initially involves consecutively the levator muscles of the face, muscles of the glottis and finally the intercostals and the diaphragm and all other skeletal muscles.

Succinylcholine has no direct action on the uterus or other smooth muscle structures. Because it is highly ionized and has low fat solubility, it does not readily cross the placenta.

Tachyphylaxis occurs with repeated administration (see PRECAUTIONS).

Depending on the dose and duration of succinylcholine administration, the characteristic depolarizing neuromuscular block (Phase I block) may change to a block with characteristics superficially resembling a non- depolarizing block (Phase II block). This may be associated with prolonged respiratory muscle paralysis or weakness in patients who manifest the transition to Phase II block. When this diagnosis is confirmed by peripheral nerve stimulation, it may sometimes be reversed with anticholinesterase drugs such as neostigmine (see PRECAUTIONS). Anticholinesterase drugs may not always be effective. If given before succinylcholine is metabolized by cholinesterase, anticholinesterase drugs may prolong rather than shorten paralysis.

Succinylcholine has no direct effect on the myocardium. Succinylcholine stimulates both autonomic ganglia and muscannic receptors which may cause changes in cardiac rhythm, including cardiac arrest. Changes in rhythm, including cardiac arrest, may also result from vagal stimulation, which may occur during surgical procedures, or from hypokalemia, particularly in children (see PRECAUTIONS, Pediatric Use). These effects are enhanced by halogenated anesthetics.

Succinylcholine causes an increase in intraocular pressure immediately after its injection and during the fasciculation phase, and slight increases which may persist after onset of complete paralysis (see WARNINGS).

Succinylcholine may cause slight increases in intracranial pressure immediately after its injection and during the fasciculation phase (see PRECAUTIONS).

As with other neuromuscular blocking agents, the potential for releasing histamine mediated release such as flushing, hypotension and bronchoconstriction are, however, uncommon in normal clinical usage.

Succinylcholine has no effect on consciousness, pain threshold or cerebration. It should be used only with adequate anesthesia (see WARNINGS).

INDICATIONS AND USAGE:

Succinylcholine chloride is indicated as an adjunct to general anesthesia, to facilitate endotracheal intubation, and to provide skeletal muscle relaxation during surgery or mechanical ventilation.

CONTRAINDICATIONS:

Succinylcholine is contraindicated in persons with personal or familial history of malignant hyperthermia, skeletal muscle myopathies, and known hypersensitivity to the drug. It is also contraindicated in patients after the acute phase of injury following major burns, multiple trauma, extensive denervation of skeletal muscle, or upper motor neuron injury, because succinylcholine administered to such individuals may result in severe hyperkalemia which may result in cardiac arrest (see WARNINGS). The risk of hyperkalemia in these patients increases over time and usually peaks at 7 to 10 days after the injury. The risk is dependent on the extent and location of the injury. The precise time of onset and the duration of the risk period are not known.

Except when used for emergency tracheal intubation or in instances where immediate securing of the airway is necessary, succinylcholine is contraindicated in children and adolescent patients. Acute rhabdomyolysis with hyperkalemia can occur when used in these individuals with a skeletal muscle myopathy (diagnosed or undiagnosed) such as Duchenne's muscular dystrophy (see PRECAUTIONS, Pediatric Use).

WARNINGS:

SUCCINYLCHOLINE SHOULD BE USED ONLY BY THOSE SKILLED IN THE MANAGEMENT OF ARTIFICIAL RESPIRATION AND ONLY WHEN FACILITIES ARE INSTANTLY AVAILABLE FOR TRACHEAL INTUBATION AND FOR PROVIDING ADEQUATE VENTILATION OF THE PATIENT, INCLUDING THE ADMINISTRATION OF OXYGEN UNDER POSITIVE PRESSURE AND THE ELIMINATION OF CARBON DIOXIDE. THE CLINICIAN MUST BE PREPARED TO ASSIST OR CONTROL RESPIRATION.

TO AVOID DISTRESS TO THE PATIENT, SUCCINYLCHOLINE SHOULD NOT BE ADMINISTERED BEFORE UNCONSCIOUSNESS HAS BEEN INDUCED. IN EMERGENCY SITUATIONS. HOWEVER, IT MAY BE NECESSARY TO ADMINISTER SUCCINYLCHOLINE BEFORE UNCONSCIOUSNESS IS INDUCED.

SUCCINYLCHOLINE IS METABOLIZED BY PLASMA CHOLINESTERASE AND SHOULD BE USED WITH CAUTION, IF AT ALL. IN PATIENTS KNOWN TO BE OR SUSPECTED OF BEING HOMOZYGOUS FOR THE ATYPICAL PLASMA CHOLINESTERASE GENE.

Hyperkalemia: (see BOXED WARNING).

GREAT CAUTION should be observed if succinylcholine is administered to patients during the acute phase of injury following major burns, multiple trauma, extensive denervation of skeletal muscle, or upper motor neuron injury (see CONTRAINDICATIONS). The risk of hyperkalemia in these patients increases over time and usually peaks at 7 to 10 days after the injury. The risk is dependent on the extent and location of the injury. The precise time of onset and the duration of the risk period are undetermined. Patients with chronic abdominal infection, subarachnoid hemorrhage, or conditions causing degeneration of central and peripheral nervous systems should receive succinylcholine with **GREAT CAUTION** because of the potential for developing severe hyperkalemia.

WARNINGS: *(cont'd)*

Malignant Hyperthermia: Succinylcholine administration has been associated with acute onset of malignant hyperthermia, a potentially fatal hypermetabolic state of skeletal muscle. The risk of developing malignant hyperthermia following succinylcholine administration increases with the concomitant administration of volatile anesthetics. Malignant hyperthermia frequently presents as intractable spasm of the jaw muscles (masseter spasm) which may progress to generalized rigidity, increased oxygen demand, tachycardia, tachypnea and profound hyperpyrexia. Successful outcome depends on recognition of early signs, such as jaw muscle spasm, acidosis, or generalized rigidity to initial administration of succinylcholine for tracheal intubation, or failure of tachycardia to respond to deepening anesthesia. Skin mottling, rising temperature and coagulopathies may occur later in the course of the hypermetabolic process. Recognition of the syndrome is a signal for discontinuance of anesthesia, attention to increased oxygen consumption, correction of acidosis, support of circulation, assurance od adequate urinary output and institution of measures to control rising temperature. Intravenous dantrolene sodium is recommended as an adjunct to supportive measures in the management of the problem. Consult literature references and the dantrolene prescribing information for additional information about the management of malignant hyperthermic crisis. Continuous monitoring of temperature and expired CO_2 is recommended as an aid to early recognition of malignant hyperthermia.

Other: In both adults and children the incidence of bradycardia, which may progress to asystole, is higher following a second dose of succinylcholine. The incidence and severity of bradycardia is higher in children than adults. Pretreatment with anticholinergic agents (*e.g.*, atropine) may reduce the occurrence of bradyarrhythmias. Succinylcholine causes an increase in intraocular pressure. It should not be used in instances in which an increase in intraocular pressure is undesirable (*e.g.*, narrow angle glaucoma, penetrating eye injury) unless the potential benefit of its use outweighs the potential risk.

Succinylcholine is acidic (pH = 3.5) and should not be mixed with alkaline solutions having a pH greater than 8.5 (*e.g.*, barbiturate solutions).

PRECAUTIONS:

(See BOXED WARNING.)

GENERAL

When succinylcholine is given over a prolonged period of time, the characteristic depolarization block of the myoneural junction (Phase I block) may change to a block with characteristics superficially resembling a non-depolarizing block (Phase II block). Prolonged respiratory depression or apnea may be observed in patients manifesting this transition to Phase II block. The transition from Phase I to Phase II block has been reported in 7 of 7 patients studied under halothane anesthesia after an accumulated dose of 2 to 4 mg/kg succinylcholine (administered in repeated, divided doses). The onset of Phase II block coincided with the onset of tachyphylaxis and prolongation of spontaneous recovery. In another study, using balanced anesthesia (N_2O/O_2/narcotic-thiopental) and succinylcholine infusion, the transition was less abrupt, with great individual variability in the dose of succinylcholine required to produce Phase II block. Of 32 patients studied, 24 developed Phase II block. Tachyphylaxis was not associated with the transition to Phase II block, and 50% of the patients who developed Phase II block experienced prolonged recovery.

When Phase II block is suspected in cases of prolonged neuromuscular blockade, positive diagnosis should be made by peripheral nerve stimulation, prior to administration of any anticholinesterase drug. Reversal of Phase II block is a medical decision which must be made upon the basis of the individual clinical pharmacology and the experience and judgment of the physician. The presence of Phase II block is indicated by fade of responses to successive stimuli (preferably "train of four"). The use of anticholinesterase drugs to reverse Phase II block should be accompanied by appropriate doses of atropine to prevent disturbances of cardiac rhythm. After adequate reversal of Phase II block with an anticholinesterase agent, the patient should be continually observed for at least 1 hour for signs of return of muscle relaxation. Reversal should not be attempted unless: (1) a peripheral nerve stimulator is used to determine the presence of Phase II block (since anticholinesterase agents will potentiate succinylcholine-induced Phase I block), and (2) spontaneous recovery of muscle twitch has been observed for at least 20 minutes and has reached a plateau with further recovery proceeding slowly; this delay is to ensure complete hydrolysis of succinylcholine by pseudocholinesterase prior to administration of the anticholinesterase agent. Should the type of block be misdiagnosed, depolarization of the type initially induced by succinylcholine, that is depolarizing block, will be prolonged by an anticholinesterase agent.

Succinylcholine should be employed with caution in patients with fractures or muscle spasm because the initial muscle fasciculations may cause additional trauma.

Succinylcholine may cause a transient increase in intracranial pressure; however, adequate anesthetic induction prior to administration of succinylcholine will minimize this effect.

Succinylcholine may increase intragastric pressure, which could result in regurgitation and possible aspiration of stomach contents.

Neuromuscular blockade may be prolonged in patients with hypokalemia or hypocalcemia.

Reduced Plasma Cholinesterase Activity: Succinylcholine should be used carefully in patients with reduced plasma cholinesterase (pseudocholinesterase) activity. The likelihood of prolonged neuromuscular block following administration of succinylcholine must be considered in such patients (see DOSAGE AND ADMINISTRATION).

Plasma cholinesterase activity may be diminished in the presence of genetics abnormalities of plasma cholinesterase (*e.g.*, patients heterozygous or homozygous for atypical plasma cholinesterase gene), pregnancy, severe liver or kidney disease, malignant tumors, infections, burns, anemia, decompensated heart disease, peptic ulcer, or myxedema. Plasma cholinesterase activity may also be diminished by chronic administration of oral contraceptives, glucocorticoids, or certain monoamine oxidase inhibitors and by irreversible inhibitors of plasma cholinesterase (*e.g.*, organophosphate insecticides, echothiophate, and certain antineoplastic drugs).

Patients homozygous for atypical plasma cholinesterase gene (1 in 2500 patients) are extremely sensitive to the neuromuscular blocking effect of succinylcholine. In these patients, a 5 to 10 mg test dose of succinylcholine may be administered to evaluate sensitivity to succinylcholine, or neuromuscular blockade may be produced by the cautious administration of a 1 mg/ml solution of succinylcholine by slow intravenous infusion. Apnea or prolonged muscle paralysis should be treated with controlled respiration.

CARCINOGENESIS, MUTAGENESIS, AND IMPAIRMENT OF FERTILITY

There have been no long-term studies performed in animals to evaluate carcinogenic potential.

PREGNANCY CATEGORY C

Teratogenic Effects: Animal reproduction studies have not been conducted with succinylcholine chloride. It is also not known whether succinylcholine can cause fetal harm when administered to a pregnant woman or can affect reproduction capacity. Succinylcholine should be given to a pregnant woman only if clearly needed.

Nonteratogenic Effects: Pseudocholinesterase levels are decreased by approximately 24% during pregnancy and for several days postpartum. Therefore, a higher proportion of patients may be expected to show sensitivity (prolonged apnea) to succinylcholine when pregnant than when nonpregnant.

PRECAUTIONS: *(cont'd)*

LABOR AND DELIVERY

Succinylcholine is commonly used to provide muscle relaxation during delivery by caesarean section. While small amounts of succinylcholine are known to cross the placental barrier, under normal conditions the quantity of drug that enters fetal circulation after a single dose of 1 mg/kg to the mother will not endanger the fetus. However, since the amount of drug that crosses the placental barrier is dependent on the concentration gradient between the maternal and fetal circulations, residual neuromuscular blockade (apnea and flaccidity) may occur in the neonate after repeated high doses to, or in the presence of atypical pseudocholinesterase in, the mother.

NURSING MOTHERS

It is not known whether succinylcholine is excreted in human milk. Because many drugs are excreted in human milk, caution should be exercised following succinylcholine administration to a nursing woman.

PEDIATRIC USE

There are rare reports of ventricular dysrhythmias and cardiac arrest secondary to acute rhabdomyolysis with hyperkalemia in apparently healthy children who receive succinylcholine (see BOXED WARNING). Many of these children were subsequently found have skeletal muscle myopathy such as Duchenne's muscular dystrophy whose clinical signs were not obvious. The syndrome often presents as sudden cardiac arrest within minutes after the administration of succinylcholine. These children are usually, but not exclusive, males, and most frequently 8 years of age or younger. there have also been reports in adolescents. There may be no signs or symptoms to alert the practitioner to which patients are at risk. A careful history and physical may identify developmental delays suggestive of a myopathy. A preoperative creatine kinase could identify some but not all patients at risk. Due to the abrupt onset of this syndrome, routine resuscitative measures are likely to be unsuccessful. Careful monitoring of the electrocardiogram may alert the practitioner to peaked T-waves (an early sign). Administration of intravenous calcium, bicarbonate, and glucose with insulin, with hyperventilation have resulted in successful resuscitation in some of the reported cases. Extraordinary and prolonged resuscitative efforts have been effective in some cases. In addition, in the presence of signs of malignant hyperthermia, appropriate treatment should be initiated concurrently (see WARNINGS). Since it is difficult to identify which patients are at risk, it is recommended that the use of succinylcholine in children should be reserved for emergency intubation or instances where immediate securing of the airway is necessary, *e.g.*, laryngospasm, difficult airway, full stomach, or for intramuscular use when a suitable vein is inaccessible.

As in adults, the incidence of bradycardia in children is higher following the second dose of succinylcholine. The incidence and severity of bradycardia is higher in children than adults. Pre-treatment with anticholinergic agents (*e.g.*, atropine) may reduce the occurrence of bradyarrhythmias.

DRUG INTERACTIONS:

Drugs which may enhance the neuromuscular blocking action of succinylcholine include: promazine, oxytocin, aprotinin, certain non- penicillin antibiotics, quinidine, β-adrenergic blockers, procainamide, lidocaine, trimethaphan, lithium carbonate, magnesium salts, quinine, chloroquine, diethylether, isoflurane, desflurane, metoclopramide and terbutaline. The neuromuscular blocking effect of succinylcholine may be enhanced by drugs that reduce plasma cholinesterase activity (*e.g.*, chronically administered oral contraceptives, glucocorticoids, or certain monoamine oxidase inhibitors) or by drugs that irreversibly inhibit plasma cholinesterase (see PRECAUTIONS).

If other neuromuscular blocking agents are to be used during the same procedure, the possibility of a synergistic or antagonistic effect should be considered.

ADVERSE REACTIONS:

Adverse reactions consist primarily of an extension of its pharmacological actions. Succinylcholine causes profound muscle relaxation resulting in respiratory depression to the point of apnea; this effect may be prolonged. Hypersensitivity reactions, including anaphylaxis, may occur in rare instances. The following additional adverse reactions have been reported: cardiac arrest, malignant hyperthermia, arrhythmias, bradycardia, tachycardia, hypertension, hypotension, hyperkalemia, prolonged respiratory depression or apnea, increased intraocular pressure, muscle fasciculation, postoperative muscle pain, rhabdomyolysis with possible myoglobinuric acute renal failure, excessive salivation, and rash.

OVERDOSAGE:

Overdosage with succinylcholine may result in neuromuscular block beyond the time needed for surgery and anesthesia. This may be manifested by skeletal muscle weakness, decreased respiratory reserve, low tidal volume, or apnea. The primary treatment is maintenance a patent airway and respiratory support until recovery of respiration is assured. Depending on the dose and duration of succinylcholine administration, the characteristic depolarizing neuromuscular block (Phase I) may change to a block with characteristics superficially resembling a non-depolarizing block (Phase II) (see PRECAUTIONS).

DOSAGE AND ADMINISTRATION:

The dosage of succinylcholine should be individualized and its administration should always be determined by the clinician after careful assessment of the patient (see WARNINGS).

Parenteral drug products should be inspected visually for particulate matter and discoloration prior to administration whenever solution and container permit. Solutions which are clear and colorless should not be used.

ADULTS

Short Surgical Procedures: The average dose required to produce neuromuscular blockade and to facilitate tracheal intubation is 0.6 mg/kg Anectine (succinylcholine chloride) Injection given intravenously. The optimum dose will vary among individuals and may be from 0.3 to 1.1 mg/kg for adults. Following administration of doses in this range, neuromuscular blockade develops in about 1 minute; maximum blockade may persist for about 2 minutes, after which recovery takes place within 4 to 6 minutes. However, very large doses may result in more prolonged blockade. A5 to 10 mg test dose may be used to determine the sensitivity of the patient and the individual recovery time (see PRECAUTIONS).

For Long Surgical Procedures: The dose of succinylcholine administered by infusion depends upon the duration of the surgical procedure and the need for muscle relaxation. The average rate for an adult ranges between 2.5 and 4.3 mg per minute.

Solutions containing from 1 to 2 mg per ml succinylcholine have commonly been used for continuous infusion. The more dilute solution (1 mg per ml) is probably preferable from the standpoint of ease of control of the rate of administration of the drug and, hence, of relaxation. This intravenous solution containing 1 mg per ml may be administered at a rate of 0.5 mg (0.5 ml) to 10 mg (10 ml) per minute to obtain the required amount of relaxation. The amount required per minute will depend upon the individual response as well as the degree of relaxation required. Avoid overburdening the circulation with a large volume of fluid. It is recommended that neuromuscular function be carefully monitored with a peripheral nerve stimulator when using succinylcholine by infusion in order to avoid overdose, detect development of Phase II block, follow its rate of recovery, and assess the effects of reversing agents (see PRECAUTIONS).

DOSAGE AND ADMINISTRATION: *(cont'd)*

Intermittent intravenous injections of succinylcholine may also be used to provide muscle relaxation for long procedures. An intravenous injection of 0.3 to 1.1 mg/kg may be given initially, followed, at appropriate intervals, by further injections of 0.04 to 0.07 mg/kg to maintain the degree of relaxation required.

PEDIATRICS

For emergency tracheal intubation or in instances where immediate securing of the airway is necessary, the intravenous dose of succinylcholine is 2 mg/kg for infants and small children; for older children and adolescents the dose is 1 mg/kg (see CONTRAINDICATIONS) and PRECAUTIONS, Pediatric Use).

Rarely, IV bolus administration of succinylcholine in infants and children may result in malignant ventricular arrhythmias and cardiac arrest secondary to acute rhabdomyolysis with hyperkalemia. In such situations, an underlying myopathy should be suspected.

Intravenous bolus administration of succinylcholine in infants or children may result in profound bradycardia or, rarely, asystole. As in adults, the incidence of bradycardia in children is higher following a second dose of succinylcholine. The occurrence of bradyarrhythmias may be reduced by pretreatment with atropine (see PRECAUTIONS, Pediatric Use.

INTRAMUSCULAR USE

If necessary, succinylcholine may be given intramuscularly to infants, older children or adults when a suitable vein is inaccessible. A dose of up to 3 to 4 mg/kg may be given, but not more than 150 mg total dose should be administered by this route. The onset of effect of succinylcholine given intramuscularly is usually observed in about 2 to 3 minutes.

COMPATIBILITY AND ADMIXTURES

Succinylcholine is acidic (pH 3.5) and should not be mixed with alkaline solutions having a pH greater than 8.5 (*e.g.*, barbiturate solutions). Admixtures containing 1 to 2 mg/ml may be prepared by adding 1 g succinylcholine (the contents of one Anectine Sterile Powder Flo-Pack unit containing 1 g succinylcholine chloride) to 1000 or 500 ml sterile solution, such as 5% Dextrose Injection USP or 0.9% Sodium Chloride Injection USP. Admixtures of Anectine must be used within 24 hours after preparation. Aseptic techniques should be used to prepare the diluted product. Admixtures of Anectine should be prepared for single patient use only. The unused portion of diluted Anectine should be discarded.

HOW SUPPLIED:

Store in refrigerator at 2 to 8°C (36 to 46°F). The multi-dose vials are stable for up to 14 days at room temperature without significant loss of potency.

Anectine Flo-Pack does not require refrigeration. Store at 15 to 30°C (59 to 86°F). Solutions of succinylcholine must be used within 24 hours after preparation. Discard unused solutions.

HOW SUPPLIED - RATED THERAPEUTICALLY EQUIVALENT:

Injection, Solution - Intramuscular; - 20 mg/ml

5 ml	$10.72	QUELICIN 100, Abbott	00074-8065-01
10 ml	$3.73	QUELICIN, Abbott	00074-6629-02

Injection, Solution - Intramuscular; - 100 mg/ml

5 ml	$5.94	QUELICIN 500, Abbott	00074-4936-01
10 ml	$8.25	QUELICIN, Abbott	00074-6970-10
10 ml	$9.92	QUELICIN 1000, Abbott	00074-4937-01

HOW SUPPLIED - NOT RATED EQUIVALENT:

Injection, Conc, W/Buf - Intravenous - 50 mg/ml

10 ml	$5.34	QUELICIN, Abbott	00074-6642-02

Injection, Solution - Intramuscular; - 20 mg/ml

10 ml x 12	**$44.96**	**ANECTINE, Glaxo Wellcome**	**00173-0071-95**

Injection, Solution - Intramuscular; - 100 mg/ml

12's	**$110.40**	**ANECTINE, Glaxo Wellcome**	**00173-0085-15**
12's	**$180.25**	**ANECTINE, Glaxo Wellcome**	**00173-0086-15**

SUCRALFATE *(002280)*

CATEGORIES: Acid/Peptic Disorders; Antiulcer Drugs; Duodenal Ulcer; Duodenal Ulcer Adherent Complex; Gastrointestinal Drugs; Ulcer; Diarrhea*; Pregnancy Category B; Sales > $100 Million; FDA Approval Pre 1982; Patent Expiration 1986 Dec

* Indication not approved by the FDA

BRAND NAMES: *Adopilon* (Japan); *Alsucral*; *Andapsin*; *Antepsin* (England, Mexico); *Bisma* (Japan); *Calmidan*; **Carafate**; *Dolisec*; *Duracralfat* (Germany); *Hexagastron*; *Iselpin*; *Keal* (France); *Melicide*; *Neciblok*; *Peptonorm*; *SCF*; *Scrat*; *Sucafate*; *Succosa*; *Sucrabest* (Germany); *Sucrace*; *Sucralate*; *Sucralbene*; *Sucralfin*; *Sucramal*; *Sulcrate* (Canada); *Ufarene*; *Ulcar* (France); *Ulcekon*; *Ulcerfate*; *Ulcerlmin* (Japan); *Ulcogant* (Germany); *Ulcona*; *Ulcumaag*; *Ulcyte*; *Ulsaheal*; *Ulsanic*; *Ulsidex*; *Ulsidex Forte*; *Urbal*; *Yuwan-S*; *Yuwan S* (Japan)

(International brand names outside U.S. in italics)

FORMULARIES: Aetna; BC-BS; CIGNA; FHP; Humana; Kaiser; Medco; Medi-Cal; PCS; PruCare; United

COST OF THERAPY: $82.53 (Duodenal Ulcer; Tablet; 1 gm; 4/day; 28 days)

DESCRIPTION:

Carafate (sucralfate) is an α-D-glucopyranoside, β-D-fructofuranosyl-, octakis-(hydrogen sulfate), aluminum complex.

Tablets for oral administration contain 1 g of sucralfate.

Also contain: D&C Red #30 Lake, FD&C Blue #1 Lake, magnesium stearate, microcrystalline cellulose, and starch.

Carafate Suspension for oral administration contains 1 g of sucralfate per 10 ml. Carafate Suspension also contains: colloidal silicon dioxide NF, FD&C Red #40, flavor, glycerin USP, methylcellulose USP, methylparaben NF, microcrystalline cellulose NF, purified water USP, simethicone USP, and sorbitol solution USP.

Therapeutic category: antiulcer.

CLINICAL PHARMACOLOGY:

Sucralfate is only minimally absorbed from the gastrointestinal tract. The small amounts of the sulfated disaccharide that are absorbed are excreted primarily in the urine.

CLINICAL PHARMACOLOGY: *(cont'd)*

Although the mechanism of sucralfate's ability to accelerate healing of duodenal ulcers remains to be fully defined, it is known that it exerts its effect through a local, rather than systemic, action. The following observations also appear pertinent:

1. Studies in human subjects and with animal models of ulcer disease have shown that sucralfate forms an ulcer-adherent complex with proteinaceous exudate at the ulcer site.
2. *In vitro*, a sucralfate-albumin film provides a barrier to diffusion of hydrogen ions.
3. In human subjects, sucralfate given in doses recommended for ulcer therapy inhibits pepsin activity in gastric juice by 32%.
4. *In vitro*, sucralfate adsorbs bile salts.

These observations suggest that sucralfate's antiulcer activity is the result of formation of an ulcer-adherent complex that covers the ulcer site and protects it against further attack by acid, pepsin, and bile salts. There are approximately 14 to 16 mEq of acid-neutralizing capacity per 1-g dose of sucralfate.

CLINICAL STUDIES:

TABLETS

Acute Duodenal Ulcer: Over 600 patients have participated in well-controlled clinical trials worldwide. Multicenter trials conducted in the United States, both of them placebo-controlled studies with endoscopic evaluation at 2 and 4 weeks, showed (TABLE 1):

TABLE 1

Study 1 Treatment Groups	Ulcer Healing/No. Patients 2 wk	4 week (overall)
Sucralfate	37/105 (35.2%)	82/109 (75.2%)
Placebo	26/106 (24.5%)	68/107 (63.6%)
Study 2		
Sucralfate	8/24 (33%)	22/24 (92%)
Placebo	4/31 (13%)	18/31 (58%)

The sucralfate-placebo differences were statistically significant in both studies at 4 weeks but not at 2 weeks. The poorer result in the first study may have occurred because sucralfate was given 2 hours after meals and at bedtime rather than 1 hour before meals and at bedtime, the regimen used in international studies and in the second United States study. In addition, in the first study liquid antacid was utilized as needed, whereas in the second study antacid tablets were used.

Maintenance Therapy After Healing of Duodenal Ulcer: Two double-blind randomized placebo-controlled U.S. multicenter trials have demonstrated that sucralfate (1 g bid) is effective as maintenance therapy following healing of duodenal ulcers.

In one study, endoscopies were performed monthly for 4 months. Of the 254 patients who enrolled, 239 were analyzed in the intention-to-treat life table analysis presented in TABLE 2.

TABLE 2 Duodenal Ulcer Recurrence Rate (%); Months of Therapy

Drug	n	1	2	3	4
Carafate	122	20*	30*	38†	42†
Placebo	117	33	46	55	63

* P<0.05
† P<0.01
In this study, prn antacids were not permitted.

In the other study, scheduled endoscopies were performed at 6 and 12 months, but for-cause endoscopies were permitted as symptoms dictated. Median symptom scores between the sucralfate and placebo groups were not significantly different. A life table intention-to-treat analysis for the 94 patients enrolled in the trial had the following results (TABLE 3):

TABLE 3 Duodenal Ulcer Recurrence Rate (%)

Drug	n	6 months	12 months
Carafate	48	19*	27*
Placebo	46	54	65

* P<0.002
In this study, prn antacids were permitted.

Data from placebo-controlled studies longer than 1 year are not available.

SUSPENSION

In a multicenter, double-blind, placebo-controlled study of Carafate Suspension, a dosage regimen of 1 g (10 ml) four times daily was demonstrated to be superior to placebo in ulcer healing TABLE 4

TABLE 4 Results From Clinical Trials Healing Rates for Acute Duodenal Ulcer

Treatment	n	Week 2 Healing Rates	Week 4 Healing Rates	Week 8 Healing Rates
Carafate Suspension	145	23 (16%)*	66 (46%)†	95 (66%)‡
Placebo	147	10 (7%)	39 (27%)	58 (39%)

* P=0.016
† P=0.001
‡ P=0.0001

Equivalence of sucralfate suspension to sucralfate tablets has not been demonstrated.

INDICATIONS AND USAGE:

Tablets: Sucralfate is indicated in:

Short-term treatment (up to 8 weeks) of active duodenal ulcer. While healing with sucralfate may occur during the first week or two, treatment should be continued for 4 to 8 weeks unless healing has been demonstrated by x-ray or endoscopic examination.

Maintenance therapy for duodenal ulcer patients at reduced dosage after healing of acute ulcers.

Suspension: Sucralfate Suspension is indicated in the short-term (up to 8 weeks) treatment of active duodenal ulcer.

CONTRAINDICATIONS:

There are no known contraindications to the use of sucralfate.

PRECAUTIONS:

GENERAL

Duodenal ulcer is a chronic, recurrent disease. While short-term treatment with sucralfate can result in complete healing of the ulcer, a successful course of treatment with sucralfate should not be expected to alter the posthealing frequency or severity of duodenal ulceration.

Special Populations: *Chronic Renal Failure and Dialysis Patients:* When sucralfate is administered orally, small amounts of aluminum are absorbed from the gastrointestinal tract. Concomitant use of sucralfate with other products that contain aluminum, such as aluminum-containing antacids, may increase the total body burden of aluminum. Patients with normal renal function receiving the recommended doses of sucralfate and aluminum-containing products adequately excrete aluminum in the urine. Patients with chronic renal failure or those receiving dialysis have impaired excretion of absorbed aluminum. In addition, aluminum does not cross dialysis membranes because it is bound to albumin and transferrin plasma proteins. Aluminum accumulation and toxicity (aluminum osteodystrophy, osteomalacia, encephalopathy) have been described in patients with renal impairment. Sucralfate should be used with caution in patients with chronic renal failure.

CARCINOGENESIS, MUTAGENESIS, AND IMPAIRMENT OF FERTILITY

Chronic oral toxicity studies of 24 months' duration were conducted in mice and rats at doses up to 1 g/kg (12 times the human dose). There was no evidence of drug-related tumorigenicity. A reproduction study in rats at doses up to 38 times the human dose did not reveal any indication of impairment of fertility. Mutagenicity studies were not conducted.

PREGNANCY, TERATOGENIC EFFECTS, PREGNANCY CATEGORY B

Teratogenicity studies have been performed in mice, rats, and rabbits at doses up to 50 times the human dose and have revealed no evidence of harm to the fetus due to sucralfate. There are, however, no adequate and well-controlled studies in pregnant women. Because animal reproduction studies are not always predictive of human response, this drug should be used during pregnancy only if clearly needed.

NURSING MOTHERS

It is not known whether this drug is excreted in human milk. Because many drugs are excreted in human milk, caution should be exercised when sucralfate is administered to a nursing woman.

PEDIATRIC USE

Safety and effectiveness in pediatric patients/children have not been established.

DRUG INTERACTIONS:

Some studies have shown that simultaneous sucralfate administration in healthy volunteers reduced the extent of absorption (bioavailability) of single doses of the following: cimetidine, digoxin, fluoroquinolone antibiotics, ketoconazole, l-thyroxine, phenytoin, quinidine, ranitidine, tetracycline, and theophylline. Subtherapeutic prothrombin times with concomitant warfarin and sucralfate therapy have been reported in spontaneous and published case reports. However, two clinical studies have demonstrated no change in either serum warfarin concentration or prothrombin time with the addition of sucralfate to chronic warfarin therapy.

The mechanism of these interactions appears to be nonsystemic in nature, presumably resulting from sucralfate binding to the concomitant agent in the gastrointestinal tract. In all cases studied to date (cimetidine, ciprofloxacin, digoxin, norfloxacin, ofloxacin, and ranitidine), dosing the concomitant medication 2 hours before sucralfate eliminated the interaction. Because of the potential of sucralfate to alter the absorption of some drugs, sucralfate should be administered separately from other drugs when alterations in bioavailability are felt to be critical. In these cases, patients should be monitored appropriately.

ADVERSE REACTIONS:

Adverse reactions to sucralfate in clinical trials were minor and only rarely led to discontinuation of the drug. In studies involving over 2700 patients treated with sucralfate tablets, adverse effects were reported in 129 (4.7%).

Constipation was the most frequent complaint (2%). Other adverse effects reported in less than 0.5% of the patients are listed below by body system:

Gastrointestinal: diarrhea, dry mouth, flatulence, gastric discomfort, indigestion, nausea, vomiting

Dermatological: pruritus, rash

Nervous System: dizziness, insomnia, sleepiness, vertigo

Other: back pain, headache

Postmarketing reports of hypersensitivity reactions, including urticaria (hives), angioedema, respiratory difficulty, rhinitis, laryngospasm, and facial swelling have been reported in patients receiving sucralfate tablets. Similar events were reported with sucralfate suspension. However, a causal relationship has not been established.

Bezoars have been reported in patients treated with sucralfate. The majority of patients had underlying medical conditions that may predispose to bezoar formation (such as delayed gastric emptying) or were receiving concomitant enteral tube feedings.

Inadvertent injection of insoluble sucralfate and its insoluble excipients has led to fatal complications, including pulmonary and cerebral emboli. Sucralfate is **not** intended for intravenous administration.

OVERDOSAGE:

Due to limited experience in humans with overdosage of sucralfate, no specific treatment recommendations can be given. Acute oral toxicity studies in animals, however, using doses up to 12 g/kg body weight, could not find a lethal dose. Sucralfate is only minimally absorbed from the gastrointestinal tract. Risks associated with acute overdosage should, therefore, be minimal. In rare reports describing sucralfate overdose, most patients remained asymptomatic. Those few reports where adverse events were described included symptoms of dyspepsia, abdominal pain, nausea, and vomiting.

DOSAGE AND ADMINISTRATION:

Active Duodenal Ulcer: The recommended adult oral dosage for duodenal ulcer is 1 g (10 ml/2 teaspoonfuls) four times a day on an empty stomach.

Antacids may be prescribed as needed for relief of pain but should not be taken within one-half hour before or after sucralfate.

While healing with sucralfate may occur during the first week or two, treatment should be continued for 4 to 8 weeks unless healing has been demonstrated by x-ray or endoscopic examination.

Tablets: *Maintenance Therapy:* The recommended adult oral dosage is 1 g twice a day.

HOW SUPPLIED:

Tablets: Carafate (sucralfate) 1-g tablets are supplied in bottles of 100, 120, and 500 and in Unit Dose Identification Paks of 100. Light pink, scored, oblong tablets are embossed with Carafate on one side and 1712 on the other.

HOW SUPPLIED: *(cont'd)*

Suspension: Carafate (sucralfate) Suspension 1 g/10 ml is a pink suspension supplied in bottles of 14 fl oz. *Shake Well Before Using.* Store at controlled room temperature 59- 86°F (15-30°C). Avoid freezing.

HOW SUPPLIED - RATED THERAPEUTICALLY EQUIVALENT:

Tablet, Uncoated - Oral - 1 gm

100's	$73.69	CARAFATE, Hoechst Marion Roussel	00088-1712-47
100's	$85.63	CARAFATE, Hoechst Marion Roussel	00088-1712-49
120's	$90.13	CARAFATE, Hoechst Marion Roussel	00088-1712-53
500's	$357.63	CARAFATE, Hoechst Marion Roussel	00088-1712-55
3000's	$2146.50	CARAFATE, Hoechst Marion Roussel	00088-1712-25

HOW SUPPLIED - NOT RATED EQUIVALENT:

Suspension - Oral - 1 gm/10 ml

414 ml	$30.81	CARAFATE, Hoechst Marion Roussel	00088-1700-15

Tablet - Oral - 1 g

100's	$77.06	CARAFATE, UDL	51079-0871-20

SUFENTANIL CITRATE *(002281)*

CATEGORIES: Analgesics; Anesthesia; Antipyretics; Central Nervous System Agents; Narcotic Analgesics; Narcotics, Synthetics & Combinations; Opiate Agonists (Controlled); Pain; Pregnancy Category C; DEA Class CII; FDA Approved 1984 May; Patent Expiration 1994 May

BRAND NAMES: **Sufenta**

DESCRIPTION:

Sufenta (sufentanil citrate) is a potent opioid analgesic chemically designated as N-[4-(methoxymethyl)-1-[2-(2-thienyl)ethyl]-4- piperidinyl]-N-phenylpropanamide 2-hydroxy-1,2,3-propanetricarboxylate (1:1) with a molecular weight of 578.68.

Sufenta is a sterile, preservative free, aqueous solution containing sufentanil citrate equivalent to 50 mcg per ml of sufentanil base for intravenous injection. The solution has a pH range of 3.5-6.0.

CLINICAL PHARMACOLOGY:

Sufentanil citrate is an opioid analgesic. When used in balanced general anesthesia, sufentanil citrate has been reported to be as much as 10 times as potent as fentanyl. When administered as a primary anesthetic agent with 100% oxygen, sufentanil citrate is approximately 5 to 7 times as potent as fentanyl.

Assays of histamine in patients administered sufentanil citrate have shown no elevation in plasma histamine levels and no indication of histamine release.

(See dosage chart for more complete information on the intravenous use of sufentanil citrate).

PHARMACODYNAMICS

Intravenous use: At intravenous doses of up to 8 mcg/kg, sufentanil citrate is an analgesic is an analgesic component of general anesthesia; at intravenous doses ≥8 mcg/kg, sufentanil citrate produces a deep level of anesthesia. Sufentanil citrate produces a dose related attenuation of catecholamine release, particularly norepinephrine.

At intravenous dosages ≥8 mcg/kg, sufentanil citrate produces hypnosis and anesthesia without the use of additional anesthetic agents. A deep level of anesthesia is maintained at these dosages, as demonstrated by EEG patterns. Dosages of up to 25 mcg/kg attenuate the sympathetic response to surgical stress. The catecholamine response, particularly norepinephrine, is further attenuated at doses of sufentanil citrate of 25-30 mcg/kg, with hemodynamic stability and preservation of favorable myocardial oxygen balance.

Sufentanil citrate has an immediate onset of action, with relatively limited accumulation. Rapid elimination from tissue storage sites allows for relatively more rapid recovery as compared with equipotent dosages of fentanyl. At dosages of 1-2 mcg/kg, recovery times are comparable to those observed with fentanyl; at dosage of >2-6 mcg/kg, recovery times are comparable to enflurane, isoflurane and fentanyl. Within the anesthetic dosage range of 8-30 mcg/kg of sufentanil citrate, recovery times are more rapid compared to equipotent fentanyl dosages.

The vagolytic effects of pancuronium may produce a dose dependent elevation in heart rate during sufentanil citrate-oxygen anesthesia. The use of moderate doses of pancuronium or of a less vagolytic neuromuscular blocking agent may be used to maintain a stable lower heart rate and blood pressure during sufentanil citrate-oxygen anesthesia. The vagolytic effects of pancuronium may be reduced in patients administered nitrous oxide with sufentanil citrate.

Preliminary data suggest that in patients administered high doses of sufentanil citrate, initial dosage requirements for neuromuscular blocking agents are generally lower as compared to patients given fentanyl or halothane, and comparable to patients given enflurane.

Bradycardia is infrequently seen in patients administered sufentanil citrate-oxygen anesthesia. The use of nitrous oxide with high doses of sufentanil citrate may decrease mean arterial pressure, heart rate and cardiac output.

Sufentanil citrate at 20 mcg/kg has been shown to provide more adequate reduction in intracranial volume than equivalent doses of fentanyl, based upon requirements for furosemide and anesthesia supplementation in one study of patients undergoing craniotomy. During carotid endarterectomy, sufentanil citrate-nitrous oxide/oxygen produced reductions in cerebral blood flow comparable to those of enflurane-nitrous oxide/oxygen. During cardiovascular surgery, sufentanil citrate-oxygen produced EEG patterns similar to fentanyl-oxygen; these EEG changed were judged to be compatible with adequate general anesthesia.

The intraoperative use of sufentanil citrate at anesthetic dosages maintains cardiac output, with a slight reduction in systemic vascular resistance during the initial postoperative period. The incidence of postoperative hypertension, need for vasoactive agents and requirements for postoperative analgesics are generally reduced in patients administered moderate or high doses of sufentanil citrate as compared to patients given inhalation agents.

Skeletal muscle rigidity is related to the dose and speed of administration of sufentanil citrate. This muscular rigidity may occur unless preventative measures are taken (see WARNINGS).

Decreased respiratory drive and increased airway resistance occur with sufentanil citrate. The duration and degree of respiratory depression are dose related when sufentanil citrate is used at sub-anesthetic dosages. At high doses, a pronounced decrease in pulmonary exchange and apnea may be produced.

Epidural Use In Labor And Delivery: Onset of analgesic effect occurs within approximately 10 minutes of administration of epidural doses of sufentanil citrate and bupivacaine. Duration of analgesia following a single epidural injection of 10-15 mcg sufentanil citrate and bupivacaine 0.125% averaged 1.7 hours.

During labor and vaginal delivery, the addition of 10-15 mcg sufentanil citrate to 10 ml 0.125% bupivacaine provided an increase in the duration of analgesia compared to bupivacaine without an opioid. Analgesia from 10 mcg sufentanil citrate plus 10 ml 0.125% bupivacaine is comparable to analgesia from 10 ml of 0.25% bupivacaine alone. Apgar scores of neonates following epidural administration of both drugs to women in labor were comparable to neonates whose mothers received bupivacaine with out and opioid epidurally.

PHARMACOKINETICS

Intravenous Use: The pharmacokinetics of intravenous sufentanil citrate can be described as a three- compartment model, with a distribution time of 1.4 minutes, redistribution of 17.1 minutes and an elimination half-life of 164 minutes. The liver and small intestine are the major sites of biotransformation. Approximately 80% of the administered dose is excreted dose is excreted within 24 hours and only 2% of the dose is eliminated as unchanged drug. Plasma protein binding of sufentanil, related to the alpha, acid glycoprotein concentration, was approximately 93% in healthy males, 91% in mothers and 79% neonates.

Epidural use in Labor and Delivery: After epidural administration of incremental doses totaling 5-40 mcg sufentanil citrate during labor and delivery, maternal and neonatal sufentanil plasma concentrations were at or near the 0.05-0.1 ng/ml limit of detection, and were slightly higher in mothers than in their infants.

CLINICAL STUDIES:

EPIDURAL USE IN LABOR AND DELIVERY

Epidural sufentanil was tested in 340 patients in two (one single-center and one multicenter) double-blind, parallel studies. Doses ranged from 10-15 mcg, sufentanil and were delivered in a 10 ml volume of 0.125% bupivacaine with and without epinephrine 1:200,000. In all cases sufentanil was administered following a dose of local anesthetic to test proper catheter placement. Since epidural opioids and local anesthetics potentiate each other, these results may not reflect the dose or efficacy of epidural sufentanil by itself.

Individual doses of 10-15 mcg/kg sufentanil citrate plus bupivacaine 0.125% with epinephrine provided analgesia during the first stage of labor with a duration of 1-2 hours. Onset was rapid (within 10 minutes). Subsequent doses (equal dose) tended to have shorter duration. analgesia was profound (complete pain relief) in 80% to 100% of patients and 25% incidence of pruritus was observed. The duration of initial doses of sufentanil citrate plus bupivacaine with epinephrine is approximately 95 minutes, and of subsequent doses, 70 minutes.

There are insufficient data to critically evaluate neonatal neuromuscular and adaptive capacity following recommended doses of maternally administered epidural sufentanil with bupivacaine. However, if larger than recommended doses are used for combined local and systemic analgesia, *e.g.*, after administration of a single dose of 50 mcg epidural sufentanil during delivery, then impaired neonatal adaptation to sound and light can be detected for 1 to 4 hours and if a dose of 80 mcg is used impaired neuromuscular coordination can be detected for more than 4 hours.

INDICATIONS AND USAGE:

Sufentanil citrate is indicated for intravenous administration:

as an analgesic adjunct in the maintenance of balanced general anesthesia in patients who are intubated and ventilated.

as a primary anesthetic agent for the induction and maintenance of anesthesia with 100% oxygen in patients undergoing major surgical procedures, in patients who are intubated and ventilated, such as cardiovascular surgery or neurosurgical procedures in the sitting position, to provide favorable and cerebral oxygen balance or when extended postoperative ventilation is anticipated.

Sufentanil citrate is indicated for epidural administration asa an analgesic combined with low dose bupivacaine, usually 12.5 mg per administration, during labor and vaginal delivery.

SEE DOSAGE AND ADMINISTRATION FOR MORE COMPLETE INFORMATION ON THE USE OF SUFENTANIL CITRATE.

CONTRAINDICATIONS:

Sufentanil citrate is contraindicated in patients with known hypersensitivity to the drug.

WARNINGS:

SUFENTANIL CITRATE SHOULD BE ADMINISTERED ONLY BY PERSONS SPECIFICALLY TRAINED IN THE USE OF INTRAVENOUS ANESTHETICS AND MANAGEMENT OF THE RESPIRATORY EFFECTS OF POTENT OPIOIDS.

AN OPIOID ANTAGONIST, RESUSCITATIVE AND INTUBATION EQUIPMENT AND OXYGEN SHOULD BE READILY AVAILABLE.

PRIOR TO CATHETER INSERTION, THE PHYSICIAN SHOULD BE FAMILIAR WITH PATIENT CONDITIONS (SUCH AS INFECTION AT THE SITE, BLEEDING DIATHESIS, ANTICOAGULANT THERAPY, ETC.) WHICH CALL FOR SPECIAL EVALUATION OF THE BENEFIT VERSUS RISK POTENTIAL.

Intravenous Use: Intravenous administration or unintentional intravascular injection during epidural administration of sufentanil citrate may cause skeletal muscle rigidity, particularly of the truncal muscles. The incidence and severity of muscle rigidity is dose related. Administration of sufentanil citrate may produce muscular rigidity with a more rapid onset of action than that seen with fentanyl. Sufentanil citrate may produce muscular rigidity that involves the skeletal muscles of the neck and extremities. As with fentanyl, muscular rigidity has been reported to occur or recur infrequently in the extended postoperative period. The incidence of muscular rigidity associated with intravenous sufentanil citrate can be reduced by: 1) administration of up to 1/4 of the full paralyzing dose of a non- depolarizing neuromuscular blocking agent just prior to administration of sufentanil citrate at dosages of ip to 8 mcg/kg., 2) administration of a full paralyzing dose of a neuromuscular blocking agent following loss of consciousness when sufentanil citrate is used in anesthetic dosages (above 8 mcg/kg) titrated by slow intravenous infusion, or, 3) simultaneous administration of sufentanil citrate and a full paralyzing dose of a neuromuscular blocking agent when sufentanil citrate is used in rapidly administered anesthetic dosages (above 8 mcg/kg).

The neuromuscular blocking agents used should be compatible with the patient's cardiovascular status. Adequate facilities should be available for post-operative monitoring and ventilation of patients administered sufentanil citrate. It is essential that these facilities be fully equipped to handle all degrees of respiratory depression.

PRECAUTIONS:

GENERAL

The initial dose of sufentanil citrate should be appropriately reduced in elderly and debilitated patients. The effect of the initial dose should be considered in determining supplemental doses.

Vital signs should be monitored routinely.

Nitrous oxide may produce cardiovascular depression when given with high doses of sufentanil citrate (see CLINICAL PHARMACOLOGY).

Bradycardia has been reported infrequently with sufentanil citrate-oxygen anesthesia and has been responsive to atropine.

PRECAUTIONS: *(cont'd)*

Respiratory depression caused by opioid analgesics can be reversed by opioid antagonists such as naloxone. Because the duration of respiratory depression produced by sufentanil citrate may last longer than the duration of the opioid antagonist action, appropriate surveillance should maintained. As with all potent opioids, profound analgesia is accompanied by respiratory depression and diminished sensitivity to CO_2 stimulation which may persist into or recur in the postoperative period. Respiratory depression may be enhanced when sufentanil citrate is administered in combination with volatile inhalational agents and/or other central nervous system depressants such as barbiturates, tranquilizers, and other opioids. Appropriate postoperative monitoring should be employed to ensure that adequate spontaneous breathing is established and maintained prior to discharging the patient from the recovery area. Respiration should be closely monitored following each administration of an epidural injection of sufentanil citrate.

Proper placement of the needle or catheter in the epidural space should be verified before sufentanil citrate is injected to assure that unintentional intravascular or intrathecal administration does not occur. Unintentional intravascular injection of sufentanil citrate could result in a potentially serious overdose, including acute or intrathecal administration does not occur. Unintentional intravascular injection of sufentanil citrate could result in a potentially serious overdose, including acute truncal muscular rigidity and apnea. Unintentional intrathecal injection of the full sufentanil/bupivacaine epidural doses and volume could produce effects of high spinal anesthesia including prolonged paralysis and delayed recovery. If analgesia is inadequate, the placement and integrity of the catheter should be verified prior to the administration of any additional epidural medications. Sufentanil citrate should be administered epidurally by slow injection.

Neuromuscular Blocking Agents: The hemodynamic effects and degree of skeletal muscle relaxation required should be considered in the selection of a neuromuscular blocking agent. High doses of pancuronium may produce increases in heart rate during sufentanil citrate-oxygen anesthesia. Bradycardia and hypotension have been reported with other muscle relaxants during sufentanil citrate-oxygen anesthesia; this effect may be more pronounced in the presence of calcium channel and/or beta-blockers. Muscle relaxants with no clinically significant effect on heart rate (at recommended doses) would not counteract the vagotonic effect of sufentanil citrate, therefore a lower heart rate would be expected. Rare reports of bradycardia associated with the concomitant use of succinylcholine and sufentanil citrate have been reported.

Head Injuries: Sufentanil citrate may obscure the clinical course of patients with head injuries.

Impaired Respiration: Sufentanil citrate should be used with caution in patients with pulmonary disease, decrease respiratory reserve or potentially compromised respiration. In such patients, opioids may additionally decrease respiratory drive and increase airway resistance. During anesthesia, this can be managed by assisted or controlled respiration.

Impaired Hepatic or Renal Function: In patients with liver or kidney dysfunction, sufentanil citrate should be administered with caution due to the importance of these organs in the metabolism and excretion of sufentanil citrate.

CARCINOGENESIS, MUTAGENESIS AND IMPAIRMENT OF FERTILITY

No long-term animal studies of sufentanil citrate have been performed to evaluate carcinogenic potential. The micronucleus test in female rats revealed that single intravenous doses of sufentanil citrate as high as 80 mcg/kg (approximately 2.5 times the upper human dose) produced no structural chromosome mutations. The Ames *Salmonella typhimurium* metabolic activating test also revealed no mutagenic activity. See ANIMAL TOXICOLOGY for reproduction studies in rats and rabbits.

PREGNANCY CATEGORY C

Sufentanil citrate has been shown to have an embryocidal effect in rats and rabbits when given in doses 2.5 times the upper human dose for a period of 10 days to over 30 days. These effects were most probably due to maternal toxicity (decreased food consumption with increased mortality) following prolonged administration of the drug.

No evidence of teratogenic effects have been observed after administration of sufentanil citrate in rats or rabbits.

LABOR AND DELIVERY

The use of epidurally administered sufentanil citrate in combination with bupivacaine 0.125% with or without epinephrine is indicated for labor and delivery. (See INDICATIONS AND USAGE and DOSAGE AND ADMINISTRATION). Sufentanil citrate is not recommended for intravenous use or for use of larger epidural doses during labor and delivery because of potential risks to the newborn infant after delivery. In clinical trials,one case of severe fetal bradycardia associated with maternal hypotension was reported within 8 minutes of maternal administration of sufentanil 15 mcg plus bupivacaine 0.125% (10 ml total volume).

NURSING MOTHERS

It is not known whether this drug is excreted in human milk. Because many drugs are excreted in human milk, caution should be exercised when sufentanil citrate is administered to a nursing woman.

PEDIATRIC USE

The safety and efficacy of sufentanil citrate in children under two years of age undergoing cardiovascular surgery has been documented in a limited number of cases.

DRUG INTERACTIONS:

Interaction with Calcium Channel and Beta Blockers: The incidence and degree of bradycardia and hypotension during induction with sufentanil citrate may be greater in patients on chronic calcium channel and beta blocker therapy. (See DOSAGE AND ADMINISTRATION, Neuromuscular Blocking Agents).

Interaction with Other Central Nervous System Depressants: Both the magnitude and duration of central nervous system and cardiovascular effects may be enhanced when sufentanil citrate is administered to patients receiving barbiturates, tranquilizers, other opioids, general anesthetics or other CNS depressants. In such cases of combined treatment, the dose of sufentanil citrate and/or these agents should be reduced.

The use of benzodiazepines with sufentanil citrate during induction may result in a decrease in mean arterial pressure and systemic vascular resistance.

ADVERSE REACTIONS:

The most common adverse reactions of opioids are respiratory depression and skeletal muscle rigidity, particularly of the truncal muscles. Sufentanil citrate may produce muscular rigidity that involves the skeletal muscles of the neck and extremities. See CLINICAL PHARMACOLOGY, WARNINGS and PRECAUTIONS on the management of respiratory depression and skeletal muscle rigidity. Urinary retention has been associated with the use of epidural opioids but was not reported in the clinical trials of epidurally administered sufentanil due to the use of indwelling catheters. The incidence of urinary retention in patients without urinary catheters receiving epidural sufentanil is unknown; return of normal bladder activity may be delayed.

ADVERSE REACTIONS: *(cont'd)*

The following adverse reaction information is derived from controlled clinical trials in 320 patients who received intravenous sufentanil during surgical anesthesia and in 340 patients who received epidural sufentanil plus bupivacaine 0.125% for analgesia during labor and is presented below. Based on the observed frequency, none of the reactions occurring with an incidence less than 1% were observed during clinical trials of epidural sufentanil used during labor and delivery (n=340).

In general cardiovascular and musculoskeletal adverse experiences were not observed in clinical trials of epidural sufentanil. Hypotension was observed 7 times more frequently in intravenous trials than in epidural trials. The incidence of central nervous system, dermatological and gastrointestinal adverse experiences was approximately 4 to 25 times higher in studies of epidural use in labor delivery.

Probably Causally Related: Incidence Greater than 1% - Derived from clinical trials

Cardiovascular: bradycardia*, hypertension*, hypotension*.

Musculoskeletal: chest wall rigidity*.

Central Nervous System: somnolence*.

Dermatological: pruritus (25%).

Gastrointestinal: nausea*, vomiting*.

* Incidence 3% to 9%.

Probably Causally Related: Incidence less than 1% - Derived from clinical trials

(Adverse events reported in post-marketing surveillance, not seen in clinical trials, are *italicized.*)

Cardiovascular: arrhythmia*, tachycardia*.

Central Nervous System: chills*.

Dermatological: erythema*.

Musculoskeletal: skeletal muscle rigidity of neck and extremities.

Respiratory: apnea*, bronchospasm*, postoperative respiratory depression*.

Miscellaneous: intraoperative muscle movement*.

*0.3% to 1%.

DRUG ABUSE AND DEPENDENCE:

Sufentanil citrate is a Schedule II controlled drug substance that can produce drug dependence of the morphine type and therefore has the potential for being abused.

OVERDOSAGE:

Overdosage would be manifested by an extension of the pharmacological actions of sufentanil citrate (see CLINICAL PHARMACOLOGY) as with other potent opioid analgesics. The most serious and significant effect of overdose for both intravenous and epidural administration of sufentanil citrate is respiratory depression. Intravenous administration of an opioid antagonist such as naloxone should be employed as a specific antidote to manage respiratory depression. The duration of respiratory depression following overdosage with sufentanil citrate may be longer than the duration of action of the opioid antagonist. Administration of an opioid antagonist should not preclude more immediate counter measures. In the event of overdosage, oxygen should be administered and ventilation assisted or controlled as indicated for hypoventilation or apnea. A patent airway must be maintained, and a nasopharyngeal airway or endotracheal tube may be indicated. If depressed respiration is associated with muscular rigidity,a neuromuscular blocking agent may be required to facilitate assisted or controlled respiration. Intravenous fluids and vasopressors for the treatment of hypotension and other supportive measures may be employed.

DOSAGE AND ADMINISTRATION:

The dosage of sufentanil citrate should be individualized in each case according to body weight, physical status, underlying pathological condition, use of other drugs, and type of surgical procedure and anesthesia. In obese patients (more than 20% above ideal total body weight), the dosage of sufentanil citrate should be determined on the basis of lean body weight. Dosage should be reduced in elderly and debilitated patients (see PRECAUTIONS).

Vital signs should be monitored routinely.

Parenteral drug products should be inspected visually for particulate matter and discoloration prior to administration, whenever solution and container permit.

INTRAVENOUS USE

Sufentanil citrate may be administered intravenously by slow injection or infusion 1) in doses of up to 8 mcg/kg as an analgesic adjunct to general anesthesia, and 2) in doses $\geq$ 8 mcg/kg as a primary anesthetic agent for induction and maintenance of anesthesia. If benzodiazepines, barbiturates, inhalation agents, other opioids or other central nervous system depressants are used concomitantly, the dose of sufentanil citrate and/or these agents should be reduced (see PRECAUTIONS). In all cases dosage should be titrated to individual patient response.

Usage in Children: For induction and maintenance of anesthesia in children less than 12 years of age undergoing cardiovascular surgery, an anesthetic dose of 10-25 mcg/kg administered with 100% oxygen is generally recommended. Supplemental dosages of up to 25-50 mcg are recommended for maintenance, based on response to initial dose and as determined by changes in vital signs indicating surgical stress or lightening of anesthesia.

Premedication: The selection of preanesthetic medications should be based upon the needs of the individual patient.

Neuromuscular Blocking Agents: The neuromuscular blocking agent selected should be compatible with the patient's condition, taking into account the hemodynamic effects of a particular muscle relaxant and the degree of skeletal muscle relaxation required (see CLINICAL PHARMACOLOGY, WARNINGS, and PRECAUTIONS).

ANALGESIC DOSAGES

Total Dosage: Total dosage requirements of 1 mcg/kg/hr or less are recommended

Incremental or Infusion: 1-2 mcg/kg (expected duration of anesthesia 1-2 hours). Approximately 75% or more of the total calculated sufentanil citrate dosage may be administered prior to intubation by either slow injection or infusion titrated to individual patient response. Dosage in this range generally administered with nitrous oxide/oxygen in patients undergoing general surgery in which endotracheal intubation and mechanical ventilation are required.

MAINTENANCE DOSAGE

Maintenance Dosage: Total dosage requirements of 1 mcg/kg/hr or less are recommended

Incremental: 10-25 mcg (0.2-0.5 ml) may be administered in increments as needed when movement and/or changes in vital signs indicate surgical stress or lightening of analgesia. Supplemental dosages should be individualized and adjusted to remaining operative time anticipated.

Infusion: Sufentanil citrate may be administered as an intermittent or continuous infusion as needed in response to signs of lightening of analgesia. In absence of signs of lightening of analgesia infusion rates should always be adjusted downward until there is some response to surgical stimulation. Maintenance infusion rates should be adjusted based upon the induction

DOSAGE AND ADMINISTRATION: *(cont'd)*

dose of sufentanil citrate so that the total dose does not exceed 1 mcg/kg/hr of expected surgical time. Dosage should be individualized and adjusted to remaining operative time anticipated.

ANALGESIC DOSAGES

Total Dosage: Total dosage requirements of 1 mcg/kg/hr or less are recommended

Incremental or Infusion: 2-8 mcg/kg (expected duration of anesthesia 2-8 hours). Approximately 75% or less of the total calculated sufentanil citrate dosage may be administered by slow injection or infusion prior to intubation, titrated to individual patient response. Dosages in this range are generally administered with nitrous oxide/oxygen in patients undergoing more complicated major surgical procedures in which endotracheal intubation and mechanical ventilation are required. At dosages in this range, sufentanil citrate has been shown to provide some attenuation of sympathetic reflex activity in response to surgical stimuli, provide hemodynamic stability, and provide relatively rapid recovery.

MAINTENANCE DOSAGE

Maintenance Dosage: Total dosage requirements of 1 mcg/kg/hr or less are recommended

Incremental: 10-50 mcg(0.2 ml) may be administered in increments as needed when movement and/or changes in vital signs indicate surgical stress or lightening of analgesia. Supplemental dosages should be individualized and adjusted to remaining operative time anticipated.

Infusion: Sufentanil citrate may be administered as an intermittent or continuous infusion as needed in response to signs of lightening of analgesia. In the absence of signs of lightening of analgesia, infusion rates should always be adjusted downward until there is some response to surgical stimulation. Maintenance infusion rates should be adjusted based upon the induction dose of sufentanil citrate so that the total dose does not exceed 1 mcg/kg/hr of expected surgical time. Dosage should be individualized and adjusted to remaining operative time anticipated.

ANESTHETIC DOSAGES - TOTAL DOSAGE

Incremental or infusion: 8-30 mcg/kg (anesthetic doses). At this anesthetic dosage range sufentanil citrate is generally administered as a slow injection, as an infusion, or as an injection followed by an infusion. Sufentanil citrate with 100% oxygen and a muscle relaxant has been found to produce sleep at dosages ≥ 8 mcg/kg and to maintain a deep level of anesthesia without the use of additional anesthetic agents. The addition of N_2O to these dosages will reduce systolic blood pressure. At dosages in this range of up to 25 mcg/kg, catecholamine release is attenuated. Dosages of 25-30 mcg/kg have been shown to block sympathetic responses including catecholamine release. High doses are indicated in patients undergoing major surgical procedures, in which endotracheal intubation and mechanical ventilation are required, such as cardiovascular surgery and neurosurgery in the sitting position with maintenance of favorable myocardial and cerebral oxygen balance. Postoperative observation is essential and postoperative mechanical ventilation may be required at the higher dosage range due to extended postoperative respiratory depression. Dosage should be titrated to individual patient response.

ANESTHETIC DOSAGES - MAINTENANCE DOSAGE

Incremental: Depending on the initial dose, maintenance doses of 0.5-10 mcg/kg may be administered by slow injection in anticipation of surgical stress such as incision, sternotomy or cardiopulmonary bypass.

Infusion: Sufentanil citrate may be administered by continuous or intermittent infusion as needed in response to signs of lightening of anesthesia. In the absence of lightening of anesthesia, infusion rates should be adjusted downward until there is some response to surgical stimulation. The maintenance infusion rate for sufentanil citrate should be based upon the induction dose so that the total dose for the procedure does not exceed 30 mcg/kg.

In patients administered high doses of sufentanil citrate, it is essential that qualified personnel and adequate facilities are available for the management of postoperative respiratory depression.

Also see WARNINGS and PRECAUTIONS sections.

For purposes of administering small volumes of sufentanil citrate accurately, the use of a tuberculin syringe or equivalent is recommended.

EPIDURAL USE IN LABOR AND DELIVERY

Proper placement of the needle or catheter in the epidural space should be verified before sufentanil citrate is injected to assure that unintentional intravascular or intrathecal administration does not occur. unintentional intravascular injection of sufentanil citrate could result in a potentially serious overdose, including acute truncal muscular rigidity and apnea. Unintentional intrathecal injection of the full sufentanil, bupivacaine epidural doses and volume could produce effects of high spinal anesthesia including prolonged paralysis and delayed recovery. If analgesia is inadequate, the placement and integrity of the catheter should be verified prior to the administration of any additional epidural medication. Sufentanil citrate should be administered by slow injection. Respiration should be closely monitored following each administration of an epidural injection of sufentanil citrate.

Dosage for Labor and Delivery: The recommended dosage is sufentanil citrate 10-15 mcg administered with 10 ml bupivacaine 0.125% with or without epinephrine. Sufentanil citrate and bupivacaine should be mixed together before administration. Doses can be repeated twice (for a total of three doses) at not less than one-hour intervals until delivery.

ANIMAL PHARMACOLOGY:

Animal Toxicology: The intravenous LD_{50} of sufentanil citrate is 16.8 to 18.0 mg/kg in mice, 11.8 to 13.0 mg/kg in guinea pigs and 10.1 to 19.5 mg/kg in dogs. Reproduction studies performed in rats and rabbits given doses of up to 2.5 times the upper human dose for a period of 10 to over 30 days revealed high maternal mortality rates due to decreased food consumption and anoxia, which preclude any meaningful interpretation of the results. Epidural and intrathecal injections of sufentanil in dogs and epidural injections in rats were not associated with neurotoxicity.

HOW SUPPLIED:

Sufenta Injection is supplied as a sterile aqueous preservative-free solution for intravenous and epidural use.

Protect from light. Store at room temperature 15°-30°C (59°-86°F).

(Janssen, 3/93, 7618510M)

HOW SUPPLIED - RATED THERAPEUTICALLY EQUIVALENT:

Injection, Solution - Intramuscular; - 50 mcg/ml

1 ml x 10	$135.67	SUFENTA, Janssen Phar	50458-0050-01
2 ml x 10	$240.64	SUFENTA, Janssen Phar	50458-0050-02
5 ml x 10	$500.04	SUFENTA, Janssen Phar	50458-0050-05

SULCONAZOLE NITRATE *(002282)*

CATEGORIES: Anti-Infectives; Antifungals; Antimicrobials; Dermatologicals; Fungal Agents; Skin/Mucous Membrane Agents; Tinea Corporis; Tinea Cruris; Tinea Pedis; Tinea Versicolor; Topical; Pregnancy Category C; FDA Approved 1989 Feb

BRAND NAMES: **Exelderm**; Sulcosyn

DESCRIPTION:

Sulconazole nitrate is a white to off-white crystalline powder with a molecular weight of 460.77. It is freely soluble in pyridine: slightly soluble in ethanol, acetone, and chloroform: and very slightly soluble in water. It has a melting point of about 130°C.

Exelderm (sulconazole nitrate) Cream 1.0% and Exelderm (sulconazole nitrate) Solution 1.0% is a broad-spectrum antifungal agent intended for topical application. Sulconazole nitrate, the active ingredient in Exelderm Cream, is an imidazole derivative with in vitro antifungal and antiyeast activity. Its chemical name is (±)-1-(2.4-dichloro-β-((p- chlorobenzyl)-thio)-phenethyl) imidazole mononitrate.

Exelderm Cream contains sulconazole nitrate 10 mg/g in an emollient cream base consisting of propylene glycol, stearyl alcohol, isopropyl myristate, cetyl alcohol, polysorbate 60, sorbitan monostearate, glyceryl stearate (and) PEG-100 stearate, ascorbyl palmitate, and purified water, with sodium hydroxide and/or nitric acid added to adjust the pH.

Exelderm Solution contains sulconazole nitrate 10 mg/ml in a solution consisting of propylene glycol, poloxamer 407, polysorbate 20, butylated hydroxyanisole, and purified water, with sodium hydroxide and, if necessary, nitric acid added to adjust the pH.

CLINICAL PHARMACOLOGY:

Sulconazole nitrate is an imidazole derivative with broad-spectrum antifungal activity that inhibits the growth in vitro of the common pathogenic dermatophytes including *Trichophyton rubrum, Trichophyton mentagrophytes, Epidermophyton floccosum* and *Microsporum canis.* It also inhibits *(in vitro)* the organism responsible for tinea versicolor, *Malassezia furfur.* Sulconazole nitrate has been shown to be active *in vitro* against the following microorganisms, although clinical efficacy has not been established:*Candida albicans* and certain gram positive bacteria.

A modified Draize test showed no allergic contact dermatitis and a phototoxicity study showed no phototoxic or photoallergic reaction to sulconazole nitrate cream. Maximization tests with sulconazole nitrate cream showed no evidence of contact sensitization or irritation.

CLINICAL STUDIES:

In a vehicle-controlled study for the treatment of tinea pedis (moccasin type) due to *T. rubrum,* after 4-6 weeks of treatment 69% of patients on the active drug and 19% of patients on the drug vehicle had become KOH and culture negative. In addition, 68% of patients on the active drug and 20% of patients on the drug vehicle showed a good or excellent clinical response.

INDICATIONS AND USAGE:

Sulconazole nitrate cream, 1.0% is an antifungal agent indicated for the treatment of tinea pedis (athlete's foot), tinea cruris, and tinea corporis caused by *Trichophyton rubrum, Trichophyton mentagrophytes, Epidermophyton floccosum,* and *Microsporum canis,** and for the treatment of tinea versicolor.

CONTRAINDICATIONS:

Sulconazole nitrate cream, 1.0% is contraindicated in patients who have a history of hypersensitivity to any of its ingredients.

PRECAUTIONS:

General: Sulconazole nitrate cream, 1.0% is for external use only. Avoid contact with the eyes. If irritation develops, the cream should be discontinued and appropriate therapy instituted.

Information for the Patient: Patients should be told to use sulconazole nitrate cream as directed by the physician, to use it externally only, and to avoid contact with he eyes.

Carcinogenesis, Mutagenesis, and Impairment of Fertility: Long-term animal studies to determine carcinogenic potential have not been performed. In vitro studies have shown no mutagenic activity.

Pregnancy Category C: There are no adequate and well controlled studies in pregnant women. Sulconazole nitrate should be used during pregnancy only if clearly needed. Sulconazole nitrate has been shown to be embryotoxic in rats when given in doses of 125 times the adult human dose (in mg/kg). The drug was not teratogenic in rats or rabbits at oral doses of 50 mg/kg/day.

Sulconazole nitrate given orally to rats at a dose 125 times the human dose resulted in prolonged gestation and dystocia. Several females died during the prenatal period, most likely due to labor complications.

Nursing Mothers: It is not known whether sulconazole nitrate is excreted in human milk. Caution should be exercised when sulconazole nitrate is administered to an nursing woman.

Pediatric Use: Safety and effectiveness in children have not been established.

ADVERSE REACTIONS:

There were no systemic effects and only infrequent cutaneous adverse reactions in 1185 patient treated with sulconazole nitrate cream in controlled clinical trials. Approximately 3% of these patients reported itching, 3% burning or stinging, and 1% redness. These complaints did not usually interfere with treatment.

DOSAGE AND ADMINISTRATION:

Cream: A small amount of cream should be gently massaged into the affected and surrounding skin areas once or twice daily, except in tinea pedis, where administration should be twice daily.

Early relief of symptoms is experienced by the majority of patients and clinical improvement may be seen fairly soon after treatment is begun; however, tinea corporis/cruris and tinea versicolor should be treated for 3 weeks and tinea pedis for 4 weeks to reduce the possibility of recurrence.

If significant clinical improvement is not seen after 4 to 6 weeks of treatment, an alternate diagnosis should be considered.

Solution: A small amount of the solution should be gently massaged into the affected and surrounding skin areas once or twice daily.

Symptomatic relief usually occurs within a few days after starting sulconazole nitrate solution, 1.0% and clinical improvement usually occurs within one week. To reduce the possibility of recurrence, tinea cruris, tinea corporis, and tinea versicolor should be treated for 3 weeks.

If significant clinical improvement is not seen after 4 weeks of treatment, an alternate diagnosis should be considered.

DOSAGE AND ADMINISTRATION: *(cont'd)*

Avoid excessive heat, above 40°C (104°F).

*Efficacy for this organism in the organ system was studied in fewer than ten infections.

HOW SUPPLIED - EQUIVALENTS NOT AVAILABLE:

Cream - Topical - 10 mg/gm

15 gm	$9.76	EXELDERM, Westwood Squibb	00072-8200-15
30 gm	$17.16	EXELDERM, Westwood Squibb	00072-8200-30
60 gm	$28.43	EXELDERM, Westwood Squibb	00072-8200-60

Solution - Topical - 10 mg/ml

30 ml	$21.00	EXELDERM, Westwood Squibb	00072-8400-30

SULFABENZAMIDE; SULFACETAMIDE; SULFATHIAZOLE *(002283)*

CATEGORIES: Anti-Infectives; Antimicrobials; Dermatologicals; Local Infections; Skin/Mucous Membrane Agents; Sulfonamides; Vaginal Preparations; Vaginitis; Pregnancy Category C; FDA Approval Pre 1982

BRAND NAMES: Alba Gyn; Chero-Trisulfa-V; Dayto-Sulf; Diti-3; Gyne-Sulf; Lantrisul; Neotrizine; Romisulf; Sulfa; Sulfa-Gyn; Sulfa-Triple #2; Sulfadimidine; Sulfaloid; Sulfamethazine; Sulfose; Sulnac; **Sultrin**; Terfonyl; Triple Sulfa; Trisulfapyrimidines; Trysul; Vagilia

FORMULARIES: Aetna; BC-BS; Medi-Cal

DESCRIPTION:

Cream contains sulfathiazole (Benzenesulfonamide,4-amino-N-2-thiazolyl-N1-2-thiazolylsulfanilamide) 3.42%, sulfacetamide (Acetamide,N-((4-aminophenyl) sulfonyl)-N- Sulfanilylacetamide) 2.86%, sulfabenzamide (Benzamide,N-((4-aminophenyl) sulfonyl)-N- Sulfanilylbenzamide) 3.7% and urea (carbamide) 0.64%, compounded with glyceryl monostearate, cetyl alcohol 2%, stearic acid, cholesterol, lanolin, lecithin, peanut oil, propylparaben, propylene glycol, diethylaminoethyl stearamide, phosphoric acid, methylparaben and purified water.

Each Tablet contains sulfathiazole (Benzenesulfonamide,4-amino-N-2-thiazolyl-N1-2-thiazolylsulfanilamide) 172.5 mg, sulfacetamide (Acetamide,N-((4-aminophenyl)sulfonyl)-N-Sulfanilylacetamide) 143.75 mg and sulfabenzamide (Benzamide,N-((4-aminophenyl)sulfonyl)-N-
Sulfanilylbenzamide) 184.0 mg, compounded with urea, lactose, guar gum, starch and magnesium stearate.

Cream and Tablets are topical antibacterial preparations available for intravaginal administration.

Oral tablets also available to provide therapeutic effect of total sulfonamide content; reduces chance of precipitation in kidneys and crystalluria, as solubility of each sulfonamide is independent of others.

CLINICAL PHARMACOLOGY:

The mode of action of this drug is not completely known. Cream and Tablets are topical antibacterial preparations used intravaginally against Haemophilus (Gardnerella)

Vaginalis bacteria. Indirect effects, such as lowering the vaginal pH, may be equally important mechanisms.

INDICATIONS AND USAGE:

Cream and Tablets are indicated for the treatment of vaginitis caused by Haemophilus (Gardnerella) Vaginalis bacteria.

The diagnosis of a Haemophilus (Gardnerella) Vaginalis vaginitis should be firmly established before initiation of treatment with this drug.

CONTRAINDICATIONS:

This drug is contraindicated in the following circumstances: kidney disease; hypersensitivity to sulfonamides; in pregnancy at term and during the nursing period because sulfonamides cross the placenta, are excreted in breast milk and may cause Kernicterus.

WARNINGS:

Deaths associated with the administration of sulfonamides have been reported from hypersensitivity reactions, agranulocytosis, aplastic anemia and other blood dyscrasias.

The presence of clinical signs such as sore throat, fever, pallor, purpura or jaundice may be early indications of serious blood disorders.

PRECAUTIONS:

Because sulfonamides may be absorbed from the vaginal mucosa, the usual precautions for oral sulfonamides apply. Patients should be observed for skin rash or evidence of systemic toxicity, and if these develop, the medications should be discontinued.

Laboratory Tests: Standard office diagnostic procedures for vaginitis are usually sufficient to establish the diagnosis of Haemophilus (Gardnerella) Vaginalis and to rule out a trichomonal or monilial infection. These include noting a fish-like odor upon addition of 10% KOH to vaginal discharge and microscopic identification of "clue cells" in a wet mount preparation. If cultures are obtained, care must be taken to use appropriate media and methods for Haemophilus (Gardnerella) Vaginalis.

Carcinogenesis, Mutagenesis, and Impairment of Fertility: The sulfonamides bear certain chemical similarities to some goitrogens. Rats appear to be especially susceptible to the goitrogenic effects of sulfonamides, and long-term administration has produced thyroid malignancies in this species.

Pregnancy, Teratogenic Effects, Pregnancy Category C: The safe use of sulfonamides in pregnancy has not been established. The teratogenicity potential of most sulfonamides has not been thoroughly investigated in either animals or humans.

However, a significant increase in the incidence of cleft palate and other bony abnormalities of offspring has been observed when certain sulfonamides of the short, intermediate and long-acting types were given to pregnant rats and mice at high oral doses (7 to 25 times the human therapeutic dose).

Nursing Mothers: Because of the potential for serious adverse reactions in nursing infants from this drug, a decision should be made whether to discontinue nursing or to discontinue the drug, taking into account the importance of the drug to the mother. See CONTRAINDICATIONS.

Pediatric Use: Safety and effectiveness in children have not been established.

ADVERSE REACTIONS:

There has been one reported case of Agranulocytosis in a patient receiving this drug Cream. The most frequent adverse reactions to this drug are localized irritation and/or allergy including rare reports of Stevens Johnson syndrome which may be fatal.

DOSAGE AND ADMINISTRATION:

CREAM

One full applicator intravaginally twice daily for four to six days. This course of therapy may be repeated if necessary; the dosage may be reduced one-half to one-quarter.

VAGINAL TABLETS

One tablet intravaginally before retiring and again in the morning for ten days. This course may be repeated, if necessary.

ORAL TABLETS

Adults: 2 to 4 g initially, then 2 to 4 g daily in 3 to 6 divided doses. (1 tablet is 500 mg)

Children And Infants > 2 Months: 75 mg/kg initially, then 120 TO 150 mg/kg/day (4g/sq.m/day) in 4 to 6 divided doses. Do not exceed 6 g daily.

Recommended doses for toxoplasmosis (with pyrimethamine) for 3 to 4 weeks:

Infants: 100 mg/kg/day divided 4 times;

Children: 25 to 50 mg/kg 4 times/day.

HOW SUPPLIED - RATED THERAPEUTICALLY EQUIVALENT:

Cream - Vaginal - 3.7 %/2.86 %/3.

78 gm	$3.97	Sulfabenzamide; Sulfacetamide; Sulfathia, H.C.F.A. F F P	99999-2283-01
78 gm	$4.21	TRIPLE SULFA VAGINAL, Clay Park Labs	45802-0156-45
78 gm	$4.75	Triple Sulfa, Qualitest Pharms	00603-7880-86
78 gm	$5.33	Triple Sulfa, United Res	00677-0754-48
78 gm	$5.40	Triple Sulfa Vaginal, Major Pharms	00904-2746-67
78 gm	$5.45	TRIPLE SULFA, Goldline Labs	00182-1215-75
78 gm	$6.46	TRIPLE SULFA, HL Moore Drug Exch	00839-6329-46
78 gm	$6.54	TRIPLE SULFA VAGINAL, NMC Labs	23317-0700-78
78 gm	$13.00	Diti-3, Dunhall Pharms	00217-0810-78
78 gm	$22.00	ALBA GYN, Alba Pharma	10023-0219-27
78 gm	$23.17	TRYSUL, Savage Labs	00281-3790-47
78 gm	**$28.68**	**SULTRIN, Ortho Pharm**	**00062-5440-77**
80 gm	$3.09	GYNE-SULF, GW Labs	00713-0214-33
80 gm	$6.25	TRIPLE SULFA, Rugby	00536-5280-69
80 gm	$7.39	TRIPLE SULFA, Fougera	00168-0018-33
80 gm	$8.98	VVS VAGINAL, Embrex Economed	38130-0049-03
80 gm	$12.20	Triple Sulfa Vaginal, Schein Pharm (US)	00364-7284-37
90 gm	$4.50	Triple Sulfa Vaginal, Consolidated Midland	00223-4456-85
90 gm	$18.00	DAYTO SULF, Dayton Labs	52041-0017-31
120 gm	$4.50	VAGINAL SULFA, Consolidated Midland	00223-4455-11

Suspension - Oral - 167 mg/167 mg/1

480 ml	$23.72	TERFONYL, Bristol Myers Squibb	00003-0888-50

HOW SUPPLIED - NOT RATED EQUIVALENT:

Tablet, Uncoated - Vaginal - 184 mg/143.75 m

20's	**$31.20**	**SULTRIN, Ortho Pharm**	**00062-5441-64**

SULFACETAMIDE SODIUM *(002284)*

CATEGORIES: Anti-Infectives; Antibacterials; Antibiotics; Antimicrobials; Conjunctivitis; Corneal Ulcer; Dermatologicals; EENT Drugs; Eye, Ear, Nose, & Throat Preparations; Ocular Infections; Ophthalmics; Skin/Mucous Membrane Agents; Sulfonamides; Topical; Trachoma; Glaucoma*; FDA Approval Pre 1982

* Indication not approved by the FDA

BRAND NAMES: Ak-Sulf; *Albucid*; *Antebor*; Bleph-10; Cetamide; *Cetasil*; *Colirio Sulfacetamido Kriya*; *Covosulf*; *Dansemid*; Dayto-Sulf; I-Sulfacet; Infa-Sulf; Isopto Cetamide; *Lersa*; Ocu-Sul; Ocusulf; Ophthacet; *Optamide*; *Optin*; *Optisol*; *Prontamid*; Sebizon; **Sodium Sulamyd**; Sodium Sulfacetamide; Spectro-Sulf; *Spersacet*; Storz-Sulf; Sulf-10; Sulfac; Sulfacel-15; Sulfacet Sodium; Sulfair; Sulfamide; *Sulfex*; *Sulphacalyre*; Sulten-10

(International brand names outside U.S. in italics)

FORMULARIES: Aetna; BC-BS; DoD; FHP; Medi-Cal; PCS

DESCRIPTION:

Sulfacetamide sodium ophthalmic solution, USP, is a sterile, topical anti-bacterial agent for ophthalmic use.

Chemical name: *N*-Sulfanilylacetamide monosodium salt monohydrate.

THE PLASTIC SQUEEZE BOTTLE CONTAINS:

Active: Sulfacetamide Sodium 10% (100 mg/ml).

Preservative: Thimerosal 0.1 mg/ml

Inactives: Boric acid, hydroxypropyl methylcellulose 2208 (4000 cps) 1.0 mg/ml, sodium thiosulfate and purified water. Sodium carbonate anhydrous and/or hydrochloric acid to adjust pH (7.0-7.4) when necessary.

THE DROPPERETTES APPLICATOR CONTAINS:

Active: Sulfacetamide Sodium 10% (100 mg/ml).

Preservative: Thimerosal 0.05 mg/ml

Inactives: Boric acid, sodium thiosulfate and purified water. Sodium carbonate anhydrous and/or hydrochloric acid to adjust pH (7.0-7.4) when necessary.

CLINICAL PHARMACOLOGY:

Microbiology: The sulfonamides are bacteriostatic agents and the spectrum of activity is similar for all. Sulfonamides inhibit bacterial synthesis of dihydrofolic acid by preventing the condensation of the pteridine with aminobenzoic acid through competitive inhibition of the enzyme dihydropteroate synthetase. Resistant strains have altered dihydropteroate synthetase with reduced affinity for sulfonamides or produce increased quantities of aminobenzoic acid.

Topically applied sulfonamides do not provide adequate coverage against susceptible strains of the following common bacterial eye pathogens: *escherichia coli, Staphylococcus aureus, Streptococcus pneumoniae, Streptococcus* (viridans group), *Haemophilus influenzae, Klebsiella species*, and *Enterobacter* species.

Topically applied sulfonamides do not provide adequate coverage against *Neisseria* species, *Serratia marcescens* and *Pseudomonas aeruginosa*. A significant percentage of staphylococcal isolates are completely resistant to sulfa drugs.

INDICATIONS AND USAGE:

For the treatment of conjunctivitis and other superficial ocular infections due to susceptible microorganisms and as an adjunctive in systemic sulfonamide therapy of trachoma:

Escherichia coli, Staphylococcus aureus, Streptococcus pneumoniae, Streptococcus (viridans group), *Haemophilus influenzae, Klebsiella* species, and *Enterobacter* species.

Topically applied sulfonamides do not provide adequate coverage against *Neisseria* species, *Serratia marcescens* and *Pseudomonas aeruginosa*. A significant percentage of staphylococcal isolates are completely resistant sulfa drugs.

CONTRAINDICATIONS:

Hypersensitivity to sulfonamides or to any ingredient of the preparation.

WARNINGS:

FOR TOPICAL EYE USE ONLY - NOT FOR INJECTION. FATALITIES HAVE OCCURRED, ALTHOUGH RARELY, DUE TO SEVERE REACTIONS TO SULFONAMIDES INCLUDING STEVENS-JOHNSON SYNDROME, TOXIC EPIDERMAL NECROLYSIS, FULMINANT HEPATIC NECROSIS, AGRANULOCYTOSIS, APLASTIC ANEMIA AND OTHER BLOOD DYSCRASIAS. Sensitizations may recur when a sulfonamide is readministered, irrespective of the route of administration. Sensitivity reactions have been reported in individuals with no prior history of sulfonamide hypersensitivity. At the first sign of hypersensitivity, skin rash or other serious reaction, discontinue use of this preparation.

PRECAUTIONS:

General: Prolonged use of topical anti-bacterial agents may give rise to overgrowth of nonsusceptible organisms including fungi. Bacterial resistance to sulfonamides may also develop.

The effectiveness of sulfonamides may be reduced by the paraminobenzoic acid present in purulent exudates.

Sensitization may recur when a sulfonamide is readministered irrespective of the route of administration, and cross-sensitivity between different sulfonamides may occur.

At the first sign of hypersensitivity, increase in purulent discharge, or aggravation of inflammation or pain, the patient should discontinue use of the medication and consult a physician (see WARNINGS.)

Information for the Patient: To avoid contamination, do not touch tip of container to eye, eyelid or any surface.

Carcinogenesis, Mutagenesis, and Impairment of Fertility: No studies have been conducted in animals or in humans to evaluate the possibility of these effects with ocularly administered sulfacetamide. Rats appear to be especially susceptible to the goitrogenic effects of sulfonamides, and long-term oral administration of sulfonamides has resulted in thyroid malignancies in these animals.

Pregnancy Category C Animal reproduction studies have not been conducted with sulfonamide ophthalmic preparations. Kernicterus may occur in the newborn as a result of treatment of a pregnant woman at term with orally administered sulfonamides. There are no adequate and well controlled studies of sulfonamide ophthalmic preparation in pregnant women and it is not known whether topically applied sulfonamides can cause fetal harm when administered to a pregnant woman. This product should be used in pregnancy only if the potential benefit justifies the potential risk to the fetus.

Nursing Mothers: Systemically administered sulfonamides are capable of producing kernicterus in infants of lactating women. Because of the potential for the development of kernicterus in neonates, a decision should be made whether to discontinue nursing or discontinue the drug taking into account the importance of the drug to the mother.

Pediatric Use: Safety and effectiveness in children below the age of two months have not been established.

ADVERSE REACTIONS:

Bacterial and fungal corneal ulcers have developed during treatment with sulfonamide ophthalmic preparations.

The most frequently reported reactions are local irritation, stinging and burning. Less commonly reported reactions include non-specific conjunctivitis, conjunctival hyperemia, secondary infections and allergic reactions.

Fatalities have occurred, although rarely, due to severe reactions to sulfonamides including Stevens-Johnson syndrome, toxic epidermal necrolysis, fulminant hepatic necrosis, agranulocytosis, aplastic anemia, and other blood dyscrasias (see WARNINGS.)

DOSAGE AND ADMINISTRATION:

FOR CONJUNCTIVITIS AND OTHER SUPERFICIAL OCULAR INFECTIONS:

Instill one or two drops into the conjunctival sac(s) every two or three hours initially. Dosages may be tapered by increasing the time interval between doses as the condition responds. The usual duration if treatment is seven to ten days.

FOR TRACHOMA:

Instill two drops into the conjunctival sac(s) of the affected eye(s) every two hours. Topical administration must be accompanied by systemic administration.

KEEP BOTTLE TIGHTLY CLOSED.

STORE AT CONTROLLED ROOM TEMPERATURE

15°-30°C (59°-86°F).

Sulfonamide solutions darken on prolonged standing and exposure to heat and light. Do not use if solution has darkened. Yellowishness does not affect activity.

HOW SUPPLIED - RATED THERAPEUTICALLY EQUIVALENT:

Ointment - Ophthalmic - 10 %

3.5 gm	$1.30	Sulfair, Raway	00686-5770-02
3.5 gm	$1.85	INFA-SULF, Infinity Pharm	58154-0770-02
3.5 gm	$2.20	Sulfacetamide Sodium, Harber Pharm	51432-0770-30
3.5 gm	$2.25	Sulfacetamide Sodium, United Res	00677-0916-18
3.5 gm	$2.55	Sulfacetamide Sodium, HL Moore Drug Exch	00839-5501-43
3.5 gm	$2.75	Sulfacetamide Sodium, Consolidated Midland	00223-4430-03
3.5 gm	$2.83	Sulfacetamide Sodium, H.C.F.A. F F P	99999-2284-01
3.5 gm	$3.23	AK-SULF, Akorn	17478-0227-35
3.5 gm	$4.90	SPECTRO SULF, Spectrum Scitfc	53268-0770-55
3.5 gm	$6.37	Sulfacetamide Sodium, Fougera	00168-0079-38
3.5 gm	$12.17	BLEPH-10, Allergan	00023-0311-04
3.5 gm	$14.06	CETAMIDE, Alcon	00065-0526-35
3.5 gm	**$15.75**	**SODIUM SULAMYD OPHTHALMIC, Schering**	**00085-0066-03**
3.5 gm x 12	$24.30	Sodium Sulfacetamide, Rugby	00536-6701-91

Solution - Ophthalmic - 10 %

1 ml	$0.33	Sulfacetamide Sodium, H.C.F.A. F F P	99999-2284-02
1 ml x 12	$25.80	SULF-10 OPHTHALMIC, Ciba Vision	00058-0786-12
2 ml	$1.59	Sulfacetamide Sodium, H.C.F.A. F F P	99999-2284-03

HOW SUPPLIED - RATED THERAPEUTICALLY EQUIVALENT: *(cont'd)*

2 ml	$2.25	OCUSULF-10, Optopics	52238-0650-02
2 ml	$2.80	Sulfac, Ocusoft	54799-0782-02
2 ml	$2.93	AK-SULF, Akorn	17478-0221-20
2.5 ml	$1.99	Sulfacetamide Sodium, H.C.F.A. F F P	99999-2284-04
2.5 ml	$4.08	BLEPH-10, Allergan-Amer	11980-0011-03
5 ml	$1.65	Sulfacetamide Sodium, H.C.F.A. F F P	99999-2284-05
5 ml	$3.15	AK-SULF 10%, Akorn	17478-0221-10
5 ml	$12.24	BLEPH-10, Allergan-Amer	11980-0011-05
5 ml x 25	**$375.14**	**SODIUM SULAMYD OPHTHALMIC, Schering**	**00085-0946-03**
15 ml	$1.57	Sulfacetamide Sodium, H.C.F.A. F F P	99999-2284-06
15 ml	$2.48	Sulfacetamide Sodium Ophthalmic, IDE-Interstate	00814-7063-42
15 ml	$2.50	Sulfacetamide Sodium, Qualitest Pharms	00603-7280-41
15 ml	$2.82	Sulfacetamide Sodium, HL Moore Drug Exch	00839-5523-31
15 ml	$2.95	OCUSULF-10, Optopics	52238-0650-15
15 ml	$3.30	SULFAMIDE, Major Pharms	00904-2728-35
15 ml	$3.35	Sulfacetamide Sodium, Goldline Labs	00182-0671-64
15 ml	$3.38	Sulfacetamide Sodium, Balan	00304-0385-58
15 ml	$3.49	Sulfacetamide Sodium, Parmed Pharms	00349-8472-85
15 ml	$3.50	Sulfacetamide Sodium, Steris Labs	00402-0782-15
15 ml	$3.50	Sulfacetamide Sodium, Aligen Independ	00405-6135-15
15 ml	$3.53	AK-SULF, Akorn	17478-0221-12
15 ml	$3.55	Sulfacetamide Sodium, Geneva Pharms	00781-7120-85
15 ml	$3.82	Sulfacetamide Sodium, Fougera	00168-0220-15
15 ml	$3.85	Sulfacetamide Sodium, Martec Pharms	52555-0993-01
15 ml	$3.90	Sulfacetamide, Schein Pharm (US)	00364-7136-72
15 ml	$3.95	Sodium Sulfacetamide, Rugby	00536-3502-72
15 ml	$5.95	SPECTRO-SULF, Spectrum Scitfc	53268-0334-12
15 ml	$7.05	SULFAC 10 % OPHTHALMIC, Ocusoft	54799-0782-15
15 ml	$9.66	SULF-10 OPHTHALMIC, Ciba Vision	00058-0732-15
15 ml	$11.95	Sulfacetamide Sodium, United Res	00677-0917-30
15 ml	$17.12	BLEPH-10, Allergan-Amer	11980-0011-15
15 ml	**$19.24**	**SODIUM SULAMYD OPHTHALMIC, Schering**	**00085-0946-06**

Solution - Ophthalmic - 15 %

5 ml	$12.81	ISOPTO CETAMIDE, Alcon-PR	00998-0522-05
15 ml	$1.63	I-SULFACET, Americal Pharm	54945-0513-12
15 ml	$3.53	Sodium Sulfacetamide, Rugby	00536-3525-72
15 ml	$16.88	ISOPTO CETAMIDE, Alcon-PR	00998-0522-15

Solution - Ophthalmic - 30 %

5 ml	$1.63	I-SULFACET, Americal Pharm	54945-0514-10
15 ml	$5.06	Sodium Sulfacetamide, Geneva Pharms	00781-7130-85
15 ml	$6.00	Sulfacetamide, Schein Pharm (US)	00364-7137-72
15 ml	$6.00	Sulfacetamide Sodium, Steris Labs	00402-0783-15
15 ml	$7.10	Sulfacetamide Sodium, Rugby	00536-3520-72
15 ml	$9.00	Sulfacetamide Sodium, H.C.F.A. F F P	99999-2284-07
15 ml	**$20.42**	**SODIUM SULAMYD OPHTHALMIC, Schering**	**00085-0717-06**

HOW SUPPLIED - NOT RATED EQUIVALENT:

Lotion - Topical - 10 %

85 gm	$19.35	SEBIZON, Schering	00085-0600-05

Powder

120 gm	$19.85	Sulfacetamide Sodium, Millgood	53118-0308-04
454 gm	$49.85	Sodium Sulfacetamide, Millgood	53118-0308-10

Solution - Ophthalmic - 10 %

2 ml	$2.25	Sulfacetamide Sodium, Apotex	60505-7551-01
5 ml	$2.30	Sulfacetamide Sodium, Apotex	60505-7551-02
12 ml	$2.75	Sulfacetamide Sodium, Consolidated Midland	00223-6710-15
15 ml	$1.30	Sulfair, Raway	00686-0670-04
15 ml	$1.77	INFA-SULF, Infinity Pharm	58154-0670-04
15 ml	$1.85	Sulfacetamide Sodium, Logen Pharm	00820-0104-25
15 ml	$2.95	Sulfacetamide Sodium, Apotex	60505-7551-05
15 ml	$4.50	Dayto-Sulf, Dayton Labs	52041-0026-24

Solution - Ophthalmic - 30 %

15 ml	$6.50	Sulfacetamide Sodium, Consolidated Midland	00223-6711-15
15 ml	$7.95	Spectro-Sulf-30, Spectrum Scitfc	53268-0695-12

SULFACYTINE *(002285)*

CATEGORIES: Anti-Infectives; Antibacterials; Antimicrobials; Infections; Pyelitis; Pyelonephritis; Sulfonamides; Urinary Tract Infections; FDA Approval Pre 1982

BRAND NAMES: **Renoquid**

DESCRIPTION:

Sulfacytine, a short-acting sulfonamide, is a white crystalline solid with a melting point in the range of 168.5° to 170°C. It is slightly soluble in pH 5 buffer (109 mg/100 ml). It can be dissolved in human urine to 500 mg/100 ml at pH 6.0. One gram in 5 ml hot 70% aqueous methanol makes a clear solution.

Chemically it is 1-ethyl-N-sulfanilylcytosine.

CLINICAL PHARMACOLOGY:

The systemic sulfonamides are bacteriostatic agents having a similar spectrum of activity. Sulfonamides competitively inhibit bacterial synthesis of folic acid (pteroylglutamic acid) from aminobenzoic acid. Resistant strains are capable of utilizing folic acid precursors or preformed folic acid.

Sulfacytine is rapidly adsorbed following single oral doses of 0.5, 1.0, 2.0, and 4.0 grams. Peak blood levels occur within two to three hours. The area under the blood level curve indicates essentially complete oral absorption. The plasma half-life is 4 hours.

A sulfacytine dose of 250 mg four times daily for seven days will produce a mean total sulfonamide plasma level of 16.8 mcg/ml, mean free plasma level of 16.5 mcg/ml for days 2 to 7.

Protein binding studies indicate that the unbound fraction of sulfacytine is 14%. The binding is readily reversible. Dialysis equilibrium studies with human plasma yielded a dissociation constant of 5 x 10-5 M for sulfacytine.

Sulfacytine is rapidly excreted by the kidneys. Following a single oral dose of 500 mg, 88% was recovered in the urine at the end of 24 hours, 95% at the end of five days. Following a dose of 250 mg four times daily for seven days chromatographic analysis of the urine on the final day showed the following distribution: 79% free drug, 11% N-glucuronides, and 10% acetylated metabolite (inactive). The "free" form is considered to be therapeutically active form.

CLINICAL PHARMACOLOGY: *(cont'd)*

Following administration of 500 mg initially, then 250 mg four times daily for seven days, the mean urinary concentration of free sulfacytine for all sampling periods was 419 mcg/ml. This is over ten times the highest minimal inhibitory concentration (MIC) for sensitive strains Escherichia coli, Enterobacter, and Proteus (31 mcg/ml).

INDICATIONS AND USAGE:

Sulfacytine is indicated for the treatment of acute urinary tract infections only (primarily pyelonephritis, pyelitis, and cystitis), in the absence of obstructive uropathy or foreign bodies when due to susceptible strains of the following microorganisms: *Escherichia coli, Klebsiella-Enterobacter, Staphylococcus aureus, Proteus mirabilis,* and *Proteus vulgaris.*

IMPORTANT NOTE: *In vitro* sulfonamide sensitivity tests are not always reliable. The test must be carefully coordinated with bacteriologic and clinical response. When the patient is already taking sulfonamides, follow-up cultures should have aminobenzoic acid added to the culture media.

Currently, the increasing frequency of resistant microorganisms is a limitation of the usefulness of antibacterial agents including the sulfonamides.

CONTRAINDICATIONS:

Hypersensitivity to sulfonamides. Infants less than two months of age. Pregnancy at term and during the nursing period because sulfonamides cross the placenta and are excreted in the breast milk and may cause kernicterus.

WARNINGS:

Deaths associated with the administration of sulfonamides have been reported from hypersensitivity reactions, agranulocytosis, aplastic anemia, and other blood dyscrasias. The presence of clinical signs, such as sore throat, fever, pallor, purpura, or jaundice, may be early indications of serious blood disorders.

Complete blood counts should be done frequently in patients receiving sulfonamides.

The frequency of renal complication is considerably lower in patients receiving the more soluble sulfonamides. Urinalysis with careful microscopic examination should be performed frequently for patients receiving sulfonamides.

Due to lack of clinical experience with sulfacytine in the pediatric age group, it is not recommended for use in children under age 14.

PRECAUTIONS:

Sulfonamides should be given with caution to patients with impaired renal or hepatic function and to those with sever allergies or bronchial asthma.

Adequate fluid intake must be maintained in order to prevent crystalluria and formulation of calculi.

In glucose-6-phosphate dehydrogenase-deficient individuals, hemolysis may occur. This reaction is frequently dose-related.

Usage in Pregnancy: Reproduction studies have been performed in rats and rabbits and have revealed no evidence of impaired fertility or harm to the fetus due to sulfacytine. There are no well controlled studies in pregnant women. Therefore, sulfacytine should be used in pregnant women only when clearly needed.

ADVERSE REACTIONS:

The most common adverse reactions associated with sulfacytine are headache, gastrointestinal disturbances, and allergic reactions (rash).

The following reactions have been associated with sulfonamide therapy:

Blood Dyscrasias: agranulocytosis, aplastic anemia, thrombocytopenia, leukopenia, hemolytic anemia, purpura, hypoprothrombinemia, methemoglobinemia.

Allergic reactions: erythema multiforme (including Steven's-Johnson syndrome), generalized skin eruptions, epidermal necrolysis, urticaria, serum sickness, pruritus, exfoliative dermatitis, anaphylactoid reactions, periorbital edema, conjunctival and scleral injection, photosensitization, arthralgia, and allergic myocarditis.

Gastrointestinal reactions: Nausea, emesis, abdominal pains, hepatitis, diarrhea, anorexia, pancreatitis, and stomatitis.

CNS Reactions: headache, peripheral neuritis, mental depression, convulsions, ataxia, hallucinations, tinnitus, vertigo, and insomnia.

Miscellaneous reactions: drug fever, chills, and toxic nephrosis with oliguria and anuria. Periarteritis nodosum and lupus erythematosus phenomena have occurred.

The sulfonamide bear certain chemical similarities to some goitrogens, diuretics (acetazolamide and the thiazides), and oral hypoglycemia agents. Goiter production, diuresis, and hypoglycemia have occurred rarely in patients receiving sulfonamides.

Cross-sensitivity may exist with these agents.

Rats appear to be especially susceptible to the goitrogenic effects of sulfonamides, and long-term administration has produced thyroid malignancies in the species.

DOSAGE AND ADMINISTRATION:

The usual adult dose is 500 mg initially as a loading dose, then 250 mg four times daily for 10 days.

Due to lack of clinical experience with sulfacytine in the pediatric age group, it is not recommended for use in children under age 14.

HOW SUPPLIED - EQUIVALENTS NOT AVAILABLE:

Tablet, Uncoated - Oral - 250 mg

100's	$26.20	RENOQUID, Glenwood	00516-0081-01

SULFADIAZINE *(002286)*

CATEGORIES: Anti-Infectives; Antibacterials; Antimicrobials; Chancroid; Conjunctivitis; Fever; Hemophilus; Inclusion Conjunctivitis; Infections; Malaria; Meningitis; Nocardiosis; Orphan Drugs; Otitis Media; Pyelitis; Pyelonephritis; Rheumatic Fever; Sulfonamides; Toxoplasmosis; Trachoma; Urinary Tract Infections; FDA Approval Pre 1982

BRAND NAMES: Microsulfon; Sulfadiazine Sodium

DESCRIPTION:

Sulfadiazine is an oral sulfonamide anti-bacterial agent.

Each tablet, for oral administration, contains 500 mg sulfadiazine. In addition, each tablet contains the following inactive ingredients: croscarmellose sodium, docusate sodium, microcrystalline cellulose, povidone, sodium benzoate, sodium starch glycolate and stearic acid.

DESCRIPTION: *(cont'd)*

Sulfadiazine occurs as a white or slightly yellow powder. It is odorless, or nearly so, and slowly darkens on exposure to light. It is practically insoluble in water and slightly soluble in alcohol. The chemical name of sulfadiazine is N^1-2-pyrimidinyl sulfanilamide. The molecular formula is $C_{10}H_{10}N_4O_2S$. It has a molecular weight of 250.27.

Most sulfonamides slowly darken on exposure to light.

CLINICAL PHARMACOLOGY:

The systemic sulfonamides are bacteriostatic agents having a similar spectrum of activity. Sulfonamides competitively inhibit bacterial synthesis of folic acid (pteroylglutamic acid) from aminobenzoic acid. Resistant strains are capable of utilizing folic acid precursors or preformed folic acid.

Sulfonamides exist in the blood in 3 forms - free, conjugated (acetylated and possibly others), and protein bound. The free form is considered to be the therapeutically active one.

Sulfadiazine given orally is readily absorbed from the gastrointestinal tract. After a single 2 g oral dose, a peak of 6.04 mg/100 ml is reached in 4 hours; of this, 4.65 mg/100 ml is free drug.

When a dose of 100 mg/kg of body weight is given initially and followed by 50 mg/kg every 6 hours, blood levels of free sulfadiazine are about 7 mg/100 ml. Protein binding is 38 to 48%.

Sulfadiazine diffuses into the cerebrospinal fluid; free drug reaches 32 to 65% of blood levels and total drug 40 to 60%.

Sulfadiazine is excreted largely in the urine, where concentrations are 10 to 25 times greater than serum levels. Approximately 10% of a single oral dose is excreted in the first 6 hours, 50% within 24 hours, and 60 to 85% in 48 to 72 hours. Of the amount excreted in the urine, 15% to 40% is in the acetyl form.

INDICATIONS AND USAGE:

Sulfadiazine tablets are indicated in the following conditions:

Chancroid

Trachoma

Inclusion conjunctivitis

Nocardiosis

Urinary tract infections (primarily pyelonephritis, pyelitis, and cystitis) in the absence of obstructive uropathy or foreign bodies, when these infections are caused by susceptible strains of the following organisms: *Escherichia coli, Klebsiella species, Enterobacter species, Staphylococcus aureus, Proteus mirabilis,* and *P. vulgaris.* Sulfadiazine should be used for urinary tract infections only after use of more soluble sulfonamides has been unsuccessful.

Toxoplasmosis, as adjunctive therapy with pyrimethamine. Malaria due to chloroquine-resistant strains of *Plasmodium falciparum,* when used as an adjunctive therapy.

Prophylaxis of meningococcal meningitis when sulfonamide-sensitive group A strains are known to prevail in family groups or larger closed populations (the prophylactic usefulness of sulfonamides when group B or C infections are prevalent is not proved and may be harmful in closed population groups.)

Meningococcal meningitis, when the organism has been demonstrated to be susceptible.

Acute otitis media due to *Haemophilus influenzae,* when used concomitantly with adequate doses of penicillin.

Prophylaxis against recurrences of rheumatic fever, as an alternative to penicillin.

H. influenzae meningitis, as an adjunctive therapy with parenteral streptomycin.

Important Notes: *In vitro* sulfonamide susceptibility tests are not always reliable. The test must be carefully coordinated with bacteriologic and clinical response. When the patient is already taking sulfonamides, follow-up cultures should have aminobenzoic acid added to the culture media.

Currently, the increasing frequency of resistant organisms limits the usefulness of antibacterial agents, including the sulfonamides, especially in the treatment of recurrent and complicated urinary tract infections.

Wide variation in blood levels may result with identical doses. Blood levels should be measured in patients receiving sulfonamides for serious infections. Free sulfonamide blood levels of 5 to 15 mg per 100 ml may be considered therapeutically effective for most infections, and blood levels of 12 to 15 mg per 100 ml may be considered optimal for serious infections. Twenty mg per 100 ml should be the maximum total sulfonamide level, since adverse reactions occur more frequently above this level.

CONTRAINDICATIONS:

Sulfadiazine is contraindicated in the following circumstances: Hypersensitivity to sulfonamides.

In infants less than 2 months of age (except as adjunctive therapy with pyrimethamine in the treatment of congenital toxoplasmosis).

In pregnancy at term and during the nursing period, because sulfonamides cross the placenta and are excreted in breast milk and may cause kernicterus.

WARNINGS:

The sulfonamides should not be used for the treatment of group A beta-hemolytic streptococcal infections. In an established infection, they will not eradicate the streptococcus and, therefore, will not prevent sequelae such as rheumatic fever and glomerulonephritis.

Deaths associated with the administration of sulfonamides have been reported from hypersensitivity reactions, agranulocytosis, aplastic anemia, and other blood dyscrasias.

The presence of such clinical signs as sore throat, fever, pallor, purpura, or jaundice may be early indications of serious blood disorders.

The frequency of renal complications is considerably lower in patients receiving the more soluble sulfonamides.

PRECAUTIONS:

General: Sulfonamides should be given with caution to patients with impaired renal of hepatic function and to those with severe allergy or bronchial asthma.

Hemolysis may occur in individuals deficient in glucose-6-phosphate dehydrogenase. This reaction is dose related.

Adequate fluid intake must be maintained in order to prevent crystalluria and stone formation.

Information for the Patient: Patients should be instructed to drink an eight ounce glass of water with each dose of medication and at frequent intervals throughout the day. Caution patients to report promptly the onset of sore throat, fever, pallor, purpura, or jaundice when taking this drug, since these may be early indications of serious blood disorders.

Laboratory Tests: Complete blood counts and urinalyses with careful microscopic examinations should be done frequently in patients receiving sulfonamides.

PRECAUTIONS: *(cont'd)*

Carcinogenesis, Mutagenesis, and Impairment of Fertility: The sulfonamides bear certain chemical similarities to some goitrogens. Rats appear to be especially susceptible to the goitrogenic effects of sulfonamides, and long-term administration has produced thyroid malignancies in rats.

Pregnancy, Teratogenic Effects, Pregnancy Category C: The safe use of sulfonamides in pregnancy has not been established. The teratogenic potential of most sulfonamides has not been thoroughly investigated in either animals or humans. However, a significant increase in the incidence of cleft palate and other bony abnormalities in offspring has been observed when certain sulfonamides of the short, intermediate, and long acting types were given to pregnant rats and mice in high oral doses (7 to 25 times the human therapeutic dose).

Nursing Mothers: Sulfadiazine is contraindicated for use in nursing mothers because the sulfonamides cross the placenta, are excreted in breast milk and may cause kernicterus.

Because of the potential for serious adverse reactions in nursing infants from sulfadiazine, a decision should be made whether to discontinue nursing or to discontinue the drug, taking into account the importance of the drug to the mother. See CONTRAINDICATIONS.

Pediatric Use: Sulfadiazine is contraindicated in infants less than 2 months of age (except as adjunctive therapy with pyrimethamine in the treatment of congenital toxoplasmosis). See CONTRAINDICATIONS and DOSAGE AND ADMINISTRATION.

ADVERSE REACTIONS:

Blood Dyscrasias: Agranulocytosis, aplastic anemia, thrombocytopenia, leukopenia, hemolytic anemia, purpura, hypothrombinemia, and methemoglobinemia.

Allergic Reactions: Erythema multiforme (Stevens-Johnson syndrome), generalized skin eruptions, epidermal necrolysis, urticaria, serum sickness, pruritus, exfoliative dermatitis, anaphylactoid reactions, periorbital edema, conjunctival and scleral injection, photosensitization, arthralgia, allergic myocarditis, drug fever, and chills.

Gastrointestinal Reactions: Nausea, emesis, abdominal pains, hepatitis, diarrhea, anorexia, pancreatitis, and stomatitis.

C.N.S. Reactions: Headache, peripheral neuritis, mental depression, convulsions, ataxia, hallucinations, tinnitus, vertigo, and insomnia.

Renal: Crystalluria, stone formation, toxic nephrosis with oliguria and anuria; periarteritis nodosa and lupus erythematosus phenomenon have been noted.

Miscellaneous Reactions: The sulfonamides bear certain chemical similarities to some goitrogens, diuretics (acetazolamide and the thiazides), and oral hypoglycemic agents. Goiter production, diuresis, and hypoglycemia have occurred rarely in patients receiving sulfonamides. Cross-sensitivity may exist with these agents.

DOSAGE AND ADMINISTRATION:

SYSTEMIC SULFONAMIDES ARE CONTRAINDICATED IN INFANTS UNDER 2 MONTHS OF AGE except as adjunctive therapy with pyrimethamine in the treatment of congenital toxoplasmosis.

Usage Dosage for Infants over 2 Months of Age and Children: Initially, one-half the 24-hour dose. Maintenance, 150 mg/kg or 4 g/m^2, divided into 4 to 6 doses, every 24 hours, with a maximum of 6 g every 24 hours. Rheumatic fever prophylaxis, under 30 kg (66 pounds), 500 mg every 24 hours; over 30 kg (66 pounds), 1 g every 24 hours.

Usual Adult Dosage: Initially, 2 to 4 g. Maintenance, 2 to 4 g, divided into 3 to 6 doses, every 24 hours.

HOW SUPPLIED:

Sulfadiazine 500 mg Tablets are white, unscored, capsule-shaped tablets, imprinted 757 and are available in bottles of 100 and 1000.

Storage: Store at controlled room temperature 15°-30°C (59°-86°F).

Dispense in a tight, light-resistant container as defined in the USP.

HOW SUPPLIED - RATED THERAPEUTICALLY EQUIVALENT:

Tablet - Oral - 500 mg

100's	$55.13	Sulfadiazine, H.C.F.A. F F P	99999-2286-01

Tablet, Uncoated - Oral - 500 mg

100's	$16.50	MICROSULFON, Consolidated Midland	00223-1891-01
100's	$33.00	Sulfadiazine, Raway	00686-0757-01
100's	$37.50	Sulfadiazine, Eon Labs Mfg	00185-0757-01
100's	$39.47	Sulfadiazine, Aligen Independ	00405-4955-01
100's	$48.75	Sulfadiazine, Goldline Labs	00182-1996-01
100's	$49.75	SULFADIAZINE, Major Pharms	00904-7870-60
100's	$50.25	Sulfadiazine, Major Pharms	00904-2543-60
100's	$70.52	SULFADIAZINE, UDL	51079-0840-20
1000's	$75.00	Sulfadiazine, C O Truxton	00463-6190-10
1000's	$125.00	MICROSULFON, Consolidated Midland	00223-1891-02
1000's	$131.20	Sulfadiazine, Harber Pharm	51432-0443-06
1000's	$358.50	Sulfadiazine, Eon Labs Mfg	00185-0757-10
1000's	$365.95	Sulfadiazine, Major Pharms	00904-7870-80
1000's	$425.30	Sulfadiazine, Goldline Labs	00182-1996-10

SULFAMETHIZOLE *(002287)*

CATEGORIES: Anti-Infectives; Antibacterials; Antimicrobials; Infections; Pyelitis; Pyelonephritis; Sulfonamides; Urinary Antibacterial; Urinary Tract Infections; Pregnancy Category C; FDA Approval Pre 1982

BRAND NAMES: Microsul; Proklar; **Thiosulfil**; Thiosulfil Forte

DESCRIPTION:

Sulfamethizole is an antibacterial sulfonamide available in tablet form for oral administration.

Chemical name: N'-(5-methyl-1,3,4-thiadiazol-2-yl) sulfanilamide.

Sulfamethizole is a 5-membered heterocyclic sulfanilamide, occurring as a white or light buff-colored crystalline powder. Solubility in water is dependent upon the pH (1 g/5 ml at pH 7.5; 1 g/4000 ml at pH 6.5). It is soluble in alcohol, and practically insoluble in benzene.

Sulfamethizole Tablets contain the following inactive ingredients: gelatin, magnesium stearate, microcrystalline cellulose, starch.

CLINICAL PHARMACOLOGY:

Mechanism Of Sulfonamide Bacteriostatic Action: The primary mechanism of bacteriostatic action by Sulfamethizole is the same as that of most sulfonamides. By competing with the precursor para- aminobenzoic acid, sulfonamides inhibit bacterial synthesis of folic (pteroylglutamic) acid which is required for bacterial growth. Resistant strains are capable of utilizing folic acid precursors or preformed folic acid.

CLINICAL PHARMACOLOGY: *(cont'd)*

Antibacterial Spectrum: The antibacterial spectrum of all sulfonamides is similar. *In vitro* sensitivity of bacteria to sulfonamides does not always reflect*in vivo* sensitivity. Therefore, efficacy must be carefully evaluated with bacteriologic and clinical responses in the individual patient. See WARNINGS.

Factors Determining Efficacy: Efficacy of antimicrobial therapy is dependent upon a number of factors including the *in vivo* sensitivity of the involved organisms, the concentration of the drug required for bacteriostasis, and the achievable concentration of the sulfonamide at the desired site of action.

Because of the very rapid renal clearance of sulfamethizole, the blood levels attained are low, and accumulation of the drug in tissues outside the urinary tract is very limited. Therefore, sulfamethizole is not appropriate for treatment of systemic infections such as nocardiosis or for local lesions outside the urinary tract such as chancroid and trachoma. However, its low degree of acetylation and its rapid renal clearance permit high concentrations of active sulfamethizole to occur in the urinary tract, making it especially applicable for the treatment of infections of this tract. In addition, the possibility of crystalluria is minimized because of the high solubility of the drug in urine.

Approximately 95% of a given dose of sulfamethizole is not metabolized; less than 5% is acetylated. As a consequence, almost all of a given dose of Sulfamethizole is present in its active form in the body.

Approximately 80% of an administered dose is recoverable within eight hours; approximately 98% is cleared within 15 to 24 hours. Sulfamethizole is cleared by the kidney at a rate only 10 to 20% lower than that for creatinine.

Blood Concentrations: Following a single 2 g dose of sulfamethizole, peak total drug levels in whole blood are in the range of 6 mg %, the levels fall to about 50% in four hours, and are negligible at eight hours. Approximately the same concentrations are found in children following a single dose of 100 mg/kg.

Urine Concentrations: The following average values of free drug in mg/ml were found after a single 4 g dose of sulfamethizole (TABLE 1).

TABLE 1

0 to 2 hours	—	7.01
2 to 4 "	—	10.97
4 to 6 "	—	5.93
6 to 10 "	—	1.09
10 to 24 "	—	0.31

Following a single 2 g dose, the following average concentrations of total drug in mg/ml of urine were found (TABLE 2).

TABLE 2

0 to 4 hours	—	5.15
4 to 8 "	—	1.8
8 to 12 "	—	0.4
16 to 24 "	—	0.1

Following a single 1 g dose of sulfamethizole, the average concentration of total drug during the first 3.5 hours was 2.9 mg/ml.

Solubility In Urine: Sulfamethizole is highly soluble in urine. The solubilities of free and acetylated drug in buffered urine at 37° C at various pH's, in mg/ml, are given in TABLE 3.

TABLE 3

pH	free	acetylated
4.5	108	33
5.3	220	.....
5.6	480	278
6.0	729	310
6.5	5,650	380
7.0	8,250	1,500
7.5	54,000	.....

INDICATIONS AND USAGE:

Sulfamethizole is indicated in the treatment of urinary tract infections (primarily pyelonephritis, pyelitis, and cystitis) in the absence of obstructive uropathy or foreign bodies, when these infections are caused by susceptible strains of the following organisms: *Escherichia coli, Klebsiella-Enterobacter, Staphylococcus aureus, Proteus mirabilis,* and *Proteus vulgaris.*

Important Note: *In vitro* sulfonamide sensitivity tests are not always reliable. The test must be carefully coordinated with bacteriologic and clinical response. When the patient is already taking sulfonamides, follow-up cultures should have aminobenzoic acid added to the culture media.

Currently, the increasing frequency of resistant organisms is a limitation of the usefulness of antibacterial agents, including the sulfonamides, especially in the treatment of recurrent and complicated urinary tract infections.

Wide variation in blood levels may result with identical doses. Blood levels should be measured in patients receiving sulfonamides for serious infections. Free sulfonamide blood levels of 5-15 mg per 100 ml may be considered therapeutically effective for most infections, with blood levels of 12-15 mg per 100 ml optimal for serious infections; 20 mg per 100 ml should be the maximum total sulfonamide level, as adverse reactions occur more frequently above this level.

CONTRAINDICATIONS:

Sulfonamides should not be used in patients hypersensitive to sulfa drugs. They should not be used in infants less than two months of age, in pregnancy at term, and during the nursing period, because sulfonamides cross the placenta and are excreted in breast milk and may cause kernicterus.

WARNINGS:

Deaths associated with the administration of sulfonamides have been reported from hypersensitivity reactions, agranulocytosis, aplastic anemia, and other blood dyscrasias. The occurrence of sore throat, fever, pallor, purpura, or jaundice during sulfonamide administration may be an early indication of serious blood dyscrasias.

PRECAUTIONS:

General: The usual precautions used in sulfonamide therapy should be observed, including the maintenance of an adequate fluid intake. Sulfonamides should be used with caution in patients with impairment of hepatic or renal function, severe allergy or bronchial asthma, and in patients with glucose-6-phosphate dehydrogenase deficiency since sulfas may cause hemolysis in this latter group.

PRECAUTIONS: *(cont'd)*

Information for the Patient: Adequate fluid intake should be maintained while taking Sulfamethizole. Patients should drink a full 8 oz. glass of water with each dose of Sulfamethizole and drink additional fluids at frequent intervals throughout the day. Patients should immediately report any adverse side effects to their physician.

Laboratory Tests: Frequent blood counts and renal function tests should be carried out during sulfonamide treatment, especially during prolonged administration. Microscopic urinalyses should be done once a week when a patient is treated for longer than two weeks. Urine cultures should be made to confirm eradication of bacteriuria.

Carcinogenesis, Mutagenesis, Impairment Of Fertility: Rats appear to be especially susceptible to the goitrogenic effects of sulfonamides, and long-term administration has produced thyroid malignancies in the species.

No long-term fertility or mutagenicity studies have been conducted in animals or humans.

Pregnancy, Teratogenic Effects, Pregnancy Category C: The safe use of sulfonamides in pregnancy has not been established. The teratogenicity potential of most sulfonamides has not been thoroughly investigated in either animals or humans. However, a significant increase in the incidence of cleft palate and other bony abnormalities of offspring has been observed when certain sulfonamides of the short-, intermediate-, and long-acting types were given to pregnant rats and mice at high oral doses (7 to 25 times the human dose).

Sulfamethizole should be used during pregnancy only if the potential benefit justifies the potential risk to the fetus.

Nursing Mothers: Sulfamethizole is contraindicated in pregnant women and nursing mothers. Sulfonamides cross the placenta and are excreted in breast milk to a significant degree. Because of the potential for serious adverse reactions in nursing infants from sulfonamides, a decision should be made whether to discontinue nursing or to discontinue the drug, taking into account the importance of the drug to the mother. See CONTRAINDICATIONS.

Pediatric Use: Sulfamethizole is not indicated for use in infants less than two months old. See CONTRAINDICATIONSand DOSAGE AND ADMINISTRATION.

DRUG INTERACTIONS:

The most important interactions between the sulfonamides and other drugs involve those with oral anticoagulants, the sulfonylurea hypoglycemic agents, and the hydantoin anticonvulsants. In each case, sulfonamides can potentiate the effects of the other drug. Dosage adjustments may have to be made when these drugs are given concomitantly. Cross sensitivity may exist with these agents. PABA and certain local anesthetics such as procaine that are esters of PABA, antagonize the effects of sulfonamides and therefore decrease their effectiveness.

An insoluble precipitate may form in acidic urine when sulfamethizole is used concomitantly with methenamine mandelate.

Tolbutamide, diphenylhydantoin, phenytoin, and warfarin may have prolonged half-lives when administered with sulfamethizole.

ADVERSE REACTIONS:

Blood Dyscrasias: Agranulocytosis, aplastic anemia, thrombocytopenia, leukopenia, hemolytic anemia, purpura, hypoprothrombinemia, and methemoglobinemia.

Allergic Reactions: Drug fever, erythema multiforme (Stevens-Johnson syndrome), generalized skin eruptions, epidermal necrolysis, urticaria, serum sickness, pruritus, exfoliative dermatitis, anaphylactoid reactions, periorbital edema, conjunctival and scleral injection, photosensitization, arthralgia, and allergic myocarditis.

Nausea, emesis, abdominal pains, hepatitis, diarrhea, anorexia, pancreatitis, and stomatitis.

CNS Reactions: Headache, peripheral neuritis, mental depression, convulsions, ataxia, hallucinations, tinnitus, vertigo, and insomnia.

Renal: Crystalluria, toxic nephrosis with oliguria and anuria.

Miscellaneous Reactions: Chills, periarteritis nodosum, and LE phenomenon.

The sulfonamides bear certain chemical similarities to some goitrogens, diuretics (acetazolamide and the thiazides), and oral hypoglycemic agents. Goiter production, diuresis, and hypoglycemia have occurred rarely in patients receiving sulfonamides. Cross-sensitivity may exist with these agents. See PRECAUTIONS, Carcinogenesis, Mutagenesis, Impairment of Fertility.

OVERDOSAGE:

The maximum tolerated single dose of sulfa drug has not been established. Sulfamethoxazole has been given in single doses up to 2000 mg. The acute signs and symptoms associated with sulfonamide overdose include anorexia, nausea, colicky abdominal pain, vertigo, headache, drowsiness and unconsciousness. Pyrexia, hematuria and crystalluria have been reported. Blood dyscrasias and jaundice are late manifestations of overdosing.

General treatment of overdose for sulfonamides includes induction of emesis and gastric lavage. Urine output should be maintained by either oral or IV fluid administration in patients with normal renal function. Renal function with appropriate blood chemistries including electrolytes should be monitored closely in the acute period. Hematologic parameters should be followed over the next 10 days to two weeks after the overdose ingestion. Methemoglobinuria can be acutely reversed with intravenous 1% methylene blue. Sulfamethizole is only minimally dialyzable by hemodialysis and is not dialyzable by peritoneal dialysis. Other supportive measures should be instituted appropriate to signs and symptoms.

DOSAGE AND ADMINISTRATION:

USUAL DOSAGE

Adults: 500 mg to 1 g three or four times daily.

Children and infants (over 2 months of age): 30 to 45 mg/kg/24 hours, divided into 4 doses.

Storage: Store at room temperature (approximately 25° C.)

HOW SUPPLIED - RATED THERAPEUTICALLY EQUIVALENT:

Tablet, Uncoated - Oral - 0.5 gm

100's	$57.33	THIOSULFIL FORTE, Ayerst	00046-0786-81

SULFAMETHOXAZOLE *(002288)*

CATEGORIES: Anti-Infectives; Antibacterials; Antimicrobials; Chancroid; Conjunctivitis; Inclusion Conjunctivitis; Infections; Malaria; Meningitis; Nocardiosis; Otitis Media; Pyelitis; Pyelonephritis; Sulfonamides; Toxoplasmosis; Trachoma; Urinary Antibacterial; Urinary Tract Infections; Pregnancy Category C; FDA Approval Pre 1982

BRAND NAMES: Gamazole; **Gantanol**; *Sinomin*; Urobak
(International brand names outside U.S. in italics)

FORMULARIES: Aetna

DESCRIPTION:

Sulfamethoxazole is an intermediate-dosage antibacterial sulfonamide available in tablets and suspension. Each tablet contains 0.5 g sulfamethoxazole plus corn starch, polyvinyl acetate, polyvinyl alcohol, magnesium stearate, FD&C Blue No. 1 Lake, FD&C Yellow No. 6 Lake and D&C Yellow No. 10 Lake. Each teaspoonful (5 ml) of the suspension contains 0.5 g sulfamethoxazole in a vehicle containing carboxyvinyl polymer, citric acid, edetate disodium, methylcellulose, saccharin, saccharin sodium, simethicone, sodium benzoate, sodium citrate, sodium hydroxide, sodium lauryl sulfate, sorbitol, sucrose, FD&C Red No. 40, flavors and water.

Sulfamethoxazole isN^1-(5-methyl-3-isoxazolyl)sulfanilamide. It is an almost white, odorless, tasteless compound with a molecular weight of 253.28.

CLINICAL PHARMACOLOGY:

Sulfamethoxazole is rapidly absorbed following oral administration. It exists in the blood as unbound, protein-bound, metabolized and conjugated forms. The metabolism of sulfamethoxazole occurs predominately by N_4-acetylation, although the glucuronide conjugate has been identified. The free form is considered to be the therapeutically active form. Approximately 70% of sulfamethoxazole is bound to plasma proteins; of the unbound portion, 80% to 90% is in the nonacetylated form.

Following a single 1-g oral dose in 12 volunteer male subjects, the mean peak plasma concentration of 38 mcg/ml of intact sulfamethoxazole was achieved by 2 hours. The mean half-life of sulfamethoxazole is approximately 10 hours. However, patients with severely impaired renal function, as shown by a creatinine clearance of less than 30 ml-minute, exhibit an increase in the half-life of sulfamethoxazole, requiring dosage regimen adjustment.

Sulfamethoxazole is excreted primarily by the kidneys chiefly through glomerular filtration but also through tubular secretion. Urine concentrations of sulfamethoxazole are considerably higher than are the concentrations in blood. Eighty percent to 100 percent of the dose is excreted in the urine as total sulfamethoxazole, of which 30% is intact drug with the remaining as the N_4-acetylated metabolite.

Sulfamethoxazole diffuses into cerebrospinal fluid, with peak concentrations occurring at 8 hours and reaching approximately 14% of simultaneous plasma concentrations. The drug has also been shown to distribute to aqueous humor, vaginal fluid and middle ear fluid; it also passes the placental barrier and is excreted in breast milk.

Microbiology: The systemic sulfonamides are bacteriostatic agents and the spectrum of activity is similar for all. Sulfonamides inhibit bacterial synthesis of dihydrofolic acid by competing with*para*-aminobenzoic acid (PABA). Resistant strains are capable of utilizing folic acid precursors or preformed folic acid.

INDICATIONS AND USAGE:

Acute, recurrent or chronic urinary tract infections (primarily pyelonephritis, pyelitis and cystitis) due to susceptible organisms (usually *E. coli, Klebsiella-Enterobacter*, staphylococcus,*Proteus mirabilis* and, less frequently, *Proteus vulgaris*) in the absence of obstructive uropathy or foreign bodies.

Meningococcal meningitis prophylaxis when sulfonamide-sensitive group A strains are known to prevail in family groups or larger closed populations. (The prophylactic usefulness of sulfonamides when group B or C infections are prevalent has not been proven and in closed population groups may be harmful.)

Acute otitis media due to *Haemophilus influenzae* when used concomitantly with adequate doses of penicillin.

Trachoma. Inclusion conjunctivitis. Nocardiosis. Chancroid. Toxoplasmosis as adjunctive therapy with pyrimethamine. Malaria due to chloroquine-resistant strains of *Plasmodium falciparum*, when used as adjunctive therapy.

Important note: *In vitro* sulfonamide susceptibility tests are not always reliable. The test must be carefully coordinated with bacteriologic and clinical response. When the patient is already taking sulfonamides, follow-up cultures should have aminobenzoic acid added to the culture media.

Currently, the increasing frequency of resistant organisms is a limitation of the usefulness of antibacterial agents including the sulfonamides, especially in the treatment of chronic and recurrent urinary tract infections.

Wide variation in blood concentrations may result with identical doses. Blood concentrations should be measured in patients receiving sulfonamides for serious infections. Free sulfonamide blood concentrations of 5 to 15 mg/100 ml may be considered therapeutically effective for most infections, with blood concentrations of 12 to 15 mg/100 ml optimal for serious infections; 20 mg/100 ml should be the maximum total sulfonamide concentration, since adverse reactions occur more frequently above this concentration.

CONTRAINDICATIONS:

Hypersensitivity to sulfonamides. Infants less than 2 months of age (except in the treatment of congenital toxoplasmosis as adjunctive therapy with pyrimethamine). Pregnancy at term and during the nursing period because sulfonamides pass the placenta and are excreted in the milk and may cause kernicterus.

WARNINGS:

The sulfonamides should not be used for the treatment of group A beta-hemolytic streptococcal infections. In an established infection, they will not eradicate the streptococcus, and therefore will not prevent sequelae such as rheumatic fever and glomerulonephritis.

Deaths associated with the administration of sulfonamides have been reported from hypersensitivity reactions, hepatocellular necrosis, agranulocytosis, aplastic anemia and other blood dyscrasias.

The presence of clinical signs such as sore throat, fever, arthralgia, cough, shortness of breath, pallor, purpura or jaundice may be early indications of serious reactions, including serious blood disorders.

PRECAUTIONS:

GENERAL

Sulfonamides should be given with caution to patients with impaired renal or hepatic function and to those with severe allergy or bronchial asthma. In glucose-6-phosphate dehydrogenase-deficient individuals, hemolysis may occur. This reaction is frequently dose-related.

Information for the Patient

Patients should be instructed to maintain an adequate fluid intake in order to prevent crystalluria and stone formation.

LABORATORY TESTS

Complete blood counts should be done frequently in patients receiving sulfonamides. If a significant reduction in the count of any formed blood element is noted, sulfamethoxazole should be discontinued. Urinalyses with careful microscopic examination and renal function tests should be performed during therapy, particularly for those patients with impaired renal function.

Carcinogenesis, Mutagenesis, and Impairment of Fertility

PRECAUTIONS: *(cont'd)*

Carcinogenesis: Sulfamethoxazole has not been adequately tested in animals to permit an evaluation of its carcinogenic potential.

Mutagenesis: Bacterial mutagenic studies have not been performed with sulfamethoxazole. No chromosomal damage was observed in human leukocytes cultured *in vitro* with sulfamethoxazole; the concentrations used exceeded blood levels of sulfamethoxazole following therapy with sulfamethoxazole.

Impairment of Fertility: No adverse effects on fertility or general reproductive performance were observed in rats given sulfamethoxazole in oral dosages as high as 350 mg/kg/day.

PREGNANCY CATEGORY C

Teratogenic Effects: In rats, oral doses of 533 mg/kg of sulfamethoxazole produced teratologic effects manifested mainly as cleft palates. The highest dose which did not cause cleft palates in rats was 512 mg/kg of sulfamethoxazole. In rabbits, 150 to 350 mg/kg/day increased maternal mortality but had no deleterious effects on fetal development.

There are no adequate and well-controlled studies of sulfamethoxazole in pregnant women. Sulfamethoxazole should be used during pregnancy only if the potential benefit justifies the potential risk to the fetus.

Nonteratogenic Effects: See CONTRAINDICATIONS.

NURSING MOTHERS

See CONTRAINDICATIONS.

PEDIATRIC USE

Sulfamethoxazole is not recommended in infants under 2 months of age, except in the treatment of congenital toxoplasmosis as adjunctive therapy with pyrimethamine. (See CONTRAINDICATIONS.) At the present time there are insufficient clinical data on prolonged or recurrent therapy in chronic renal diseases of children under 6 years of age.

DRUG INTERACTIONS:

In elderly patients concurrently receiving certain diuretics, primarily thiazides, an increased incidence of thrombopenia with purpura has been reported.

It has been reported that sulfamethoxazole may prolong the prothrombin time in patients who are receiving the anticoagulant warfarin. This interaction should be kept in mind when sulfamethoxazole is given to patients already on anticoagulant therapy, and the coagulation time should be reassessed.

Sulfamethoxazole may inhibit the hepatic metabolism of phenytoin. At a 1.6-gm dose, sulfamethoxazole produced a slight but significant increase in the half-life of phenytoin but did not produce a corresponding decrease in the metabolic clearance rate. When administering these drugs concurrently, one should be alert for possible excessive phenytoin effect.

Sulfonamides can also displace methotrexate from plasma protein-binding sites, thus increasing free methotrexate concentrations.

The presence of sulfamethoxazole may interfere with the Jaffe alkaline picrate reaction assay for creatinine, resulting in overestimations of about 10% in the range of normal values.

ADVERSE REACTIONS:

Included in the listing that follows are adverse reactions that have not been reported with this specific drug; however, the pharmacologic similarities among the sulfonamides require that each of the reactions be considered with sulfamethoxazole administration.

Hematologic: Agranulocytosis, aplastic anemia, thrombocytopenia, leukopenia, hemolytic anemia, purpura, hypoprothrombinemia, methemoglobinemia, neutropenia, eosinophilia.

Allergic Reactions: Anaphylaxis, allergic myocarditis, serum sickness, conjunctival and scleral injection, generalized allergic reactions. In addition, periarteritis nodosa and systemic lupus erythematosus have been reported.

Dermatologic: Stevens-Johnson syndrome, epidermal necrolysis, erythema multiforme, exfoliative dermatitis, photosensitivity, pruritus, urticaria, rash, generalized skin eruptions.

Gastrointestinal: Hepatitis, hepatocellular necrosis, pseudomembranous enterocolitis, pancreatitis, stomatitis, glossitis, nausea, emesis, abdominal pain, diarrhea, anorexia.

Genitourinary: Creatinine elevation, toxic nephrosis with oliguria and anuria. The frequency of renal complications is considerably lower in patients receiving the more soluble sulfonamides.

Neurologic: Convulsions, peripheral neuritis, ataxia, vertigo, tinnitus, headache.

Psychiatric: Hallucinations, depression, apathy.

Endocrine: The sulfonamides bear certain chemical similarities to some goitrogens, diuretics (acetazolamide and the thiazides) and oral hypoglycemic agents. Cross-sensitivity may exist with these agents. Diuresis and hypoglycemia have occurred rarely in patients receiving sulfonamides.

Musculoskeletal: Arthralgia, myalgia.

Respiratory: Pulmonary infiltrates.

Miscellaneous: Edema (including periorbital), pyrexia, chills, weakness, fatigue, insomnia.

OVERDOSAGE:

Acute: The amount of a single dose of sulfamethoxazole that is either associated with symptoms of overdosage or is likely to be life-threatening has not been reported. Signs and symptoms of overdosage reported with sulfonamides include anorexia, colic, nausea, vomiting, dizziness, headache, drowsiness and unconsciousness. Pyrexia, hematuria and crystalluria may be noted. Blood dyscrasias and jaundice are potential late manifestations of overdosage.

General principles of treatment include the institution of gastric lavage or emesis; forcing oral fluids; and the administration of intravenous fluids if urine output is low and renal function is normal. The patient should be monitored with blood counts and appropriate blood chemistries, including electrolytes. If a significant blood dyscrasia or jaundice occurs, specific therapy should be instituted for these complications. Peritoneal dialysis is not effective and hemodialysis is only moderately effective in eliminating sulfamethoxazole.

Chronic: Use of sulfamethoxazole at high doses and/or for extended periods of time may cause bone marrow depression manifested as thrombocytopenia, leukopenia and/or megaloblastic anemia. If signs of bone marrow depression occur, the patient should be given leucovorin 3 to 6 mg intramuscularly daily for three days, or as required to restore normal hematopoiesis.

Animal Toxicity: The oral $LD_{50}$of sulfamethoxazole is 2300 mg/kg in mice, 3000 mg/kg in rats and >2000 mg/kg in rabbits.

DOSAGE AND ADMINISTRATION:

Systemic sulfonamides are contraindicated in infants under 2 months of age, except in the treatment of congenital toxoplasmosis as adjunctive therapy with pyrimethamine.

The usual dosage schedules are as follows: (TABLE 1)

Severe Infections: 4 tablets or 4 teaspoonfuls (2 gm) initially, followed by 2 tablets or 2 teaspoonfuls (1 gm) three times daily thereafter.

Patients with impaired renal function (creatinine clearance below 20 to 30 ml/min) require decreased dosage adjustment.

TABLE 1

Infants (2 Months or Older) and Children	Initial Dose (50-60 mg/kg)	Dose Morning and Evening Daily Thereafter (25-30 mg/kg)
20 lbs	1 tablet or 1 teasp (0.5 g)	1/2 tablet or 1/2 teasp (0.25 gm)
40 lbs	2 tablets or 2 teasp (1 g)	1 tablet or 1 teasp (0.5 gm)
60 lbs	3 tablets or 3 teasp (1.5 g)	1.5 tablets or 1.5 teasp (0.75 gm)
80 lbs	4 tablets or 4 teasp (2 g)	2 tablets or 2 teasp (1 gm)
(The maximum dose for children should not exceed 75 mg/kg/24 hours.)		
Adults		
Mild to Moderate Infections	4 tablets or 4 teasp (2 g)	2 tablets or 2 teasp (1 g)
Note: One teaspoonful equals 5 ml.		

HOW SUPPLIED - RATED THERAPEUTICALLY EQUIVALENT:

Tablet, Uncoated - Oral - 500 mg

100's $50.81 GANTANOL, Roche 00004-0010-01

SULFAMETHOXAZOLE; TRIMETHOPRIM

(002289)

CATEGORIES: AIDS Related Complex; Anti-Infectives; Antiarrhythmic Agents; Antibacterials; Antimicrobials; Bronchitis; Chronic Bronchitis; Diarrhea; Enteritis; HIV Infection; Infections; Otitis Media; Pneumocystis Carinii Pneumonia; Sulfonamides; Urinary Antibacterial; Urinary Tract Infections; Pregnancy Category C; FDA Approval Pre 1982; Top 200 Drugs

BRAND NAMES: *Abacin*; *Abactrim*; *Acuco*; *Alcorim-F*; *Anitrim* (Mexico); *Antrimox*; *Apo-Sulfatrim* (Canada); *Bacdan*; *Bacidal*; *Bacide*; *Bacin*; *Bacticel*; *Bactifor*; *Bactoprim*; *Bactramin* (Japan); **Bactrim**; *Bactrim DS* (Canada); *Bactrim Forte* (France, Germany); *Bactrimel*; *Baktar* (Japan); *Bencole*; Bethaprim; *Biosulten*; *Briscotrim*; *BS*; *Centrim*; *Chemitrim*; *Cidal*; Co-Trimoxizole; *Colizole*; *Colizole DS*; *Comox* (England); *Conprim*; Cotrim; *Cotrim-Diolan*; *Cotrimel*; *Deprim*; *Diseptyl*; *Dosulfin*; *Drylin*; *Duocide*; *Duratrimet* (Germany); *Ectaprim* (Mexico); *Esbesul*; *Espectrin*; *Euctrim*; *Eusaprim* (France, Germany); *Exbesul*; *Fectrim* (England); *Fermagex*; *Fortrim*; *Futin*; *Gantaprim*; *Gantrim*; *Hulin*; *Ikaprim*; *Isobac* (Mexico); *Isotrim*; *Kelfiprim*; *Kepinol* (Germany); *Lagatrim*; *Lagatrim Forte*; *Lastrim*; *Lescot*; *Lidaprim*; *Medixin*; *Metoprim*; *Microtrim* (Germany); *Missile*; *Nopil*; *Novotrimel* (Canada); *Omsat* (Germany); *Omstat*; *Oxaprim* (Japan); *Pancidim*; *Parkin*; *Protrin* (Canada); *Purbal*; *Resprim*; *Resprim Forte*; *Roubac* (Canada); *Roubal*; *Salvatrim*; Septra; *Septran*; *Septrin* (Australia, England, Mexico); *Septrin DS*; *Septrin Forte*; *Septrin S*; *Setprin*; *Sigaprim* (Germany); *Sinotrim*; Smz-Tmp; *Stopan* (Japan); *Sugaprim*; *Sulfacet* (Germany); Sulfamar; Sulfamethoprim; Sulfamethoxazole Trimethoprim; Sulfaprim; Sulfatrim; *Sulfotrimin* (Germany); Sulfoxaprim; Sulmeprim; *Sulthrim*; Sultrex; *Sumetrolim*; *Suprim*; *Suprin*; Tmp Smx; *TMS* (Germany); *Toprim*; Triazole; *Trim*; *Trimel*; *Trimetox* (Mexico); *Trimexol*; *Trimez-IFSA*; *Trimezol*; *Trimox*; *Triprim*; *Trisul*; *Trisulcom*; Trisulfam; *Trisural*; Trizole; *U-Prin*; Uro-D S; *Urobactrim*; Uroplus; *Xeroprim*; *Zamboprim*

(International brand names outside U.S. in italics)

FORMULARIES: Aetna; BC-BS; CIGNA; DoD; FHP; Foundation; Humana; Kaiser; Medco; Medi-Cal; PCS; PruCare; United; WHO

COST OF THERAPY: $2.50 (Respiratory Infections; Tablet; 800 mg/160 mg; 2/day; 14 days)

DESCRIPTION:

Tablets and Pediatric Suspension: Trimethoprim and sulfamethoxazole is a synthetic antibacterial combination product available in DS (double strength) tablets, tablets and pediatric suspension for oral administration. Each DS tablet contains 160 mg trimethoprim and 800 mg sulfamethoxazole plus magnesium stearate, pregelatinized starch and sodium starch glycolate. Each tablet contains 80 mg trimethoprim and 400 mg sulfamethoxazole plus magnesium stearate, pregelatinized starch, sodium starch glycolate, FD&C Blue No. 1 lake, FD&C Yellow No. 6 lake and D&C Yellow No. 10 lake. Each teaspoonful (5 ml) of the pediatric suspension or suspension contains 40 mg trimethoprim and 200 mg sulfamethoxazole in a vehicle containing 0.3 percent alcohol, edetate disodium, glycerin, microcrystalline cellulose, parabens (methyl and propyl), polysorbate 80, saccharin sodium, simethicone, sorbitol, sucrose, FD&C Yellow No. 6, FD&C Red No. 40, flavors and water.

Trimethoprim is 2,4-diamino-5-(3,4,5-trimethoxybenzyl)pyrimidine. It is a white to light yellow, odorless, bitter compound with a molecular weight of 290.3 and a molecular formula of $C_{14}H_{18}N_4O_3$.

Sulfamethoxazole is N^1-(5-methyl-3-isoxazolyl) sulfanilamide. It is almost white, odorless, tasteless compound with a molecular weight of 253.28 and a molecular formula of $C_{10}H_{11}N_3O_3S$.

IV Infusion: Trimethoprim and sulfamethoxazole IV Infusion, a sterile solution for intravenous infusion only, is a synthetic antibacterial combination product. Each ml contains 80 mg trimethoprim (16 mg/ml) and 400 mg sulfamethoxazole (80 mg/ml) compounded with 40% propylene glycol, 10% ethyl alcohol and 0.3% diethanolamine; 1% benzyl alcohol and 0.1% sodium metabisulfite added as preservatives, water for injection, and pH adjusted to approximately 10 with sodium hydroxide.

CLINICAL PHARMACOLOGY:

Trimethoprim and sulfamethoxazole is rapidly absorbed following oral administration. Both sulfamethoxazole and trimethoprim exist in the blood as unbound, protein-bound and metabolized forms; sulfamethoxazole also exists as the conjugated form. The metabolism of sulfamethoxazole occurs predominately by N_4-acetylation, although the glucuronide conjugate has been identified. The principal metabolites of trimethoprim are the 1-and 3-oxides and the 3'- and 4'-hydroxy derivatives. The free forms of sulfamethoxazole and trimethoprim are considered to be the therapeutically active forms. Approximately 44% of trimethoprim and 70% of sulfamethoxazole are bound to plasma proteins. The presence of 10 mg percent sulfamethoxazole in plasma decreases the protein binding of trimethoprim by an insignificant degree; trimethoprim does not influence the protein binding of sulfamethoxazole.

Peak blood levels for the individual components occur 1 to 4 hours after oral administration. The mean serum half-lives of sulfamethoxazole and trimethoprim are 10 and 8 to 10 hours, respectively. However, patients with severely impaired renal function exhibit an increase in the half-lives of both components, requiring dosage regimen adjustment (see DOSAGE AND ADMINISTRATION.) Detectable amounts of trimethoprim and sulfamethoxazole are

CLINICAL PHARMACOLOGY: *(cont'd)*

present in the blood 24 hours after drug administration. During administration of 160 mg trimethoprim and 800 mg sulfamethoxazole bid, the mean steady-state plasma concentration of trimethoprim was 1.72 mcg/ml. The steady-state mean plasma levels of free and total sulfamethoxazole were 57.4 mcg/ml and 68.0 mcg/ml, respectively. These steady-state levels were achieved after three days of drug administration.[1]

Excretion of sulfamethoxazole and trimethoprim is primarily by the kidneys through both glomerular filtration and tubular secretion. Urine concentrations of both sulfamethoxazole and trimethoprim are considerably higher than are the concentrations in the blood. The average percentage of the dose recovered in urine from 0 to 72 hours after a single oral dose of trimethoprim and sulfamethoxazole is 84.5% for total sulfonamide and 66.8% for free trimethoprim. Thirty percent of the total sulfonamide is excreted as free sulfamethoxazole, with the remaining as N_4-acetylated metabolite.[2] When administered together as trimethoprim and sulfamethoxazole, neither sulfamethoxazole nor trimethoprim affects the urinary excretion pattern of the other.

Both trimethoprim and sulfamethoxazole distribute to sputum, vaginal fluid and middle ear fluid; trimethoprim also distributes to bronchial secretion, and both pass the placental barrier and are excreted in breast milk.

Microbiology: Sulfamethoxazole inhibits bacterial synthesis of dihydrofolic acid by competing with *para*-aminobenzoic acid (PABA). Trimethoprim blocks the production of tetrahydrofolic acid from dihydrofolic acid by binding to and reversibly inhibiting the required enzyme, dihydrofolate reductase. Thus, trimethoprim and sulfamethoxazole block two consecutive steps in the biosynthesis of nucleic acids and proteins essential to many bacteria.

In vitro studies have shown that bacterial resistance develops more slowly with trimethoprim and sulfamethoxazole than with either trimethoprim or sulfamethoxazole alone.

In vitro serial dilution tests have shown that the spectrum of antibacterial activity of trimethoprim and sulfamethoxazole includes the common urinary tract pathogens with the exception of *Pseudomonas aeruginosa.* The following organisms are usually susceptible: *Escherichia coli, Klebsiella species, Enterobacter species, Morganella morganii, Proteus mirabilis,* and indole-positive *Proteus* species including *Proteus vulgaris.* The usual spectrum of antimicrobial activity of trimethoprim and sulfamethoxazole includes the following bacterial pathogens isolated from middle ear exudate and from bronchial secretions: *Haemophilus influenzae,* including ampicillin-resistant strains, and *Streptococcus pneumoniae. Shigella flexneri* and *Shigella sonnei* are usually susceptible. The usual spectrum also includes enterotoxigenic strains of *Escherichia coli* (ETEC) causing bacterial gastroenteritis.

TABLE 1 Representative Minimum Inhibitory Concentration Values for Trimethoprim and Sulfamethoxazole-Susceptible Organisms (MIC—mcg/ml)

Bacteria	TMP alone	SMX alone	TMP/SMX(1:20) TMP	SMX
Escherichia coli	0.05-1.5	1.0-245	0.05-0.5	0.95-9.5
Escherichia coli (enterotoxigenic strains)	0.015-0.15	0.285->950	0.005-0.15	0.095-2.85
Proteus species (indole positive)	0.5-5.0	7.35-300	0.05-1.5	0.95-28.5
Morganella morganii	0.5-5.0	7.35-300	0.05-1.5	0.95-28.5
Proteus mirabilis	0.5-1.5	7.35-30	0.05-0.15	0.95-2.85
Klebsiella species	0.15-5.0	2.45-245	0.05-1.5	0.95-28.5
Enterobacter species	0.15-5.0	2.45-245	0.05-1.5	0.95-28.5
Haemophilus influenzae	0.15-1.5	2.85-95	0.015-0.15	0.285-2.85
Streptococcus pneumoniae	0.15-1.5	7.35-24.5	0.05-0.15	0.95-2.85
*Shigella flexneri**	<0.01-0.04	<0.16->320	<0.002-0.03	0.04-0.625
*Shigella sonnei**	0.02-0.08	0.625->320	0.004-0.06	0.08-1.25

* Rudoy RC, Nelson JD, Haltalin KC: *Antimicrob Agents Chemother* 5:439-443, May 1974.
TMP = trimethoprim
SMX=sulfamethoxazole

The recommended quantitative disc susceptibility method may be used for estimating the susceptibility of bacteria to trimethoprim and sulfamethoxazole.[3,4,6] With this procedure, a report from the laboratory of "Susceptible to trimethoprim and sulfamethoxazole" indicates that the infection is likely to respond to therapy with trimethoprim and sulfamethoxazole. If the infection is confined to the urine, a report of "Intermediate susceptibility to trimethoprim and sulfamethoxazole" also indicates that the infection is likely to respond. A report of "Resistant to trimethoprim and sulfamethoxazole" indicates that the infection is unlikely to respond to therapy with trimethoprim and sulfamethoxazole.

ADDITIONAL INFORMATION FOR THE IV INFUSION

Following a 1-hour intravenous infusion of a single dose of 160 mg trimethoprim and 800 mg sulfamethoxazole to 11 patients whose weight ranged from 105 lbs to 165 lbs (mean 143 lbs), the peak plasma concentration of trimethoprim and sulfamethoxazole were 3.4 ± 0.3 mcg/ml and 46.3 ± 2.7 mcg/ml respectively. Following repeated intravenous admission of the same dose at eight-hour intervals, the mean plasma concentrations just prior to and immediately after each infusion at steady state were 5.6 ± 0.6 mcg/ml and 8.8 ± 0.9 mcg/ml for trimethoprim and 70.6 ± 7.3 mcg/ml and 105.6 ± 10.9 mcg/ml for sulfamethoxazole. The mean plasma half-life was 11.3 ± 0.7 hours for trimethoprim and 12.8 ± 1.8 hours for sulfamethoxazole. All of these 11 patients had normal renal function, and their ages ranged from 17 to 78 years (median 60 years)[7].

Pharmacokinetic studies in children and adults suggest an age-dependent half-life of trimethoprim, as indicated in TABLE 2.[8]

TABLE 2

Age (years)	No. of Patients	Mean TMP 1/2-life (hrs)
<1	2	7.67
1-10	9	5.59
10-20	5	8.19
20-63	6	12.82

The percent of dose excreted in urine over a 12-hour period following the intravenous administration of the first dose of 240 mg of trimethoprim and 1200 mg of sulfamethoxazole on day 1 ranged from 17% to 42.4 as free trimethoprim; 7% to 12.7% as free sulfamethoxazole and 36.7% to 56% as total (free plus the N_4-acetylated metabolite) sulfamethoxazole. When administered together, neither trimethoprim nor sulfamethoxazole affects the urinary excretion pattern of the other.

It should be noted, however, that there are little clinical data on the use of trimethoprim and sulfamethoxazole IV infusion in serious systemic infections due to *Haemophilus influenzae* and Streptococcus *pneumoniae.*

INDICATIONS AND USAGE:

TABLETS AND PEDIATRIC SUSPENSION

Urinary Tract Infections: For the treatment of urinary tract infections due to susceptible strains of the following organisms: *Escherichia coli, Klebsiella* species, *Enterobacter* species, *Morganella morganii, Proteus mirabilis* and *Proteus vulgaris.* It is recommended that initial episodes of uncomplicated urinary tract infections be treated with a single effective antibacterial agent rather than the combination.

Acute Otitis Media: For the treatment of acute otitis media in children due to susceptible strains of *Streptococcus pneumoniae* or *Haemophilus influenzae* when in the judgment of the physician trimethoprim and sulfamethoxazole offers some advantage over the use of other antimicrobial agents. To date, there are limited data on the safety of repeated use of trimethoprim and sulfamethoxazole in children under two years of age. Trimethoprim and sulfamethoxazole is not indicated for prophylactic or prolonged administration in otitis media at any age.

Acute Exacerbations of Chronic Bronchitis in Adults: For the treatment of acute exacerbations of chronic bronchitis due to susceptible strains of *Streptococcus pneumoniae* or *Haemophilus influenzae* when in the judgment of the physician trimethoprim and sulfamethoxazole offers some advantage over the use of a single antimicrobial agent.

Shigellosis: For the treatment of enteritis caused by susceptible strains of *Shigella flexneri* and *Shigella sonnei* when antibacterial therapy is indicated.

Pneumocystis Carinni Pneumonia: For the treatment of documented *Pneumocystis carinii pneumonia.*

Travelers' Diarrhea In Adults: For the treatment of travelers' diarrhea due to susceptible strains of enterotoxigenic *E. coli.*

IV INFUSION

Pneumocystis Carinni Pneumonia: Trimethoprim and sulfamethoxazole IV is indicated in the treatment of Pneumocystis carinii pneumonia in children and in adults.

Shigellosis: Trimethoprim and sulfamethoxazole IV is indicated in the treatment of enteritis caused by susceptible strains of *Shigella flexneri* and *Shigella sonnei* in children and adults.

Urinary Tract Infections: Trimethoprim and sulfamethoxazole IV is indicated in the treatment of severe or complicated urinary tract infections due to susceptible strains of *Escherichia coli, Klebsiella* species, *Enterobacter* species, *Morganella morganii* and *Proteus* species when oral administration is not feasible and when the organism is not susceptible to single-agent antibacterials effective in the urinary tract.

Although appropriate culture and susceptibility studies should be performed, therapy may be started while awaiting the results of these studies.

CONTRAINDICATIONS:

Hypersensitivity to trimethoprim or sulfonamides. Patients with documented megaloblastic anemia due to folate deficiency. Pregnancy at term and during the nursing period, because sulfonamides pass the placenta and are excreted in the milk and may cause kernicterus. Infants less than two months of age.

WARNINGS:

FATALITIES ASSOCIATED WITH THE ADMINISTRATION OF SULFONAMIDES, ALTHOUGH RARE, HAVE OCCURRED DUE TO SEVERE REACTIONS, INCLUDING STEVENS-JOHNSON SYNDROME, TOXIC EPIDERMAL NECROLYSIS, FULMINANT HEPATIC NECROSIS, AGRANULOCYTOSIS, APLASTIC ANEMIA AND OTHER BLOOD DYSCRASIAS.

TRIMETHOPRIM AND SULFAMETHOXAZOLE SHOULD BE DISCONTINUED AT THE FIRST APPEARANCE OF SKIN RASH OR ANY SIGN OF ADVERSE REACTION. Clinical signs, such as rash, sore throat, fever, arthralgia, cough, shortness of breath, pallor, purpura or jaundice may be early indications of serious reactions. In rare instances a skin rash may be followed by more severe reactions, such as Stevens-Johnson syndrome, toxic epidermal necrolysis, hepatic necrosis or serious blood disorder. Complete blood counts should be done frequently in patients receiving sulfonamides.

TRIMETHOPRIM AND SULFAMETHOXAZOLE SHOULD NOT BE USED IN THE TREATMENT OF STREPTOCOCCAL PHARYNGITIS. Clinical studies have documented that patients with group A β-hemolytic streptococcal tonsillopharyngitis have a greater incidence of bacteriologic failure when treated with trimethoprim and sulfamethoxazole than do those patients treated with penicillin, as evidenced by failure to eradicate this organism from the tonsillopharyngeal area.

IV Infusion: Trimethoprim and sulfamethoxazole IV contains sodium metabisulfite, a sulfite that may cause allergic-type reactions, including anaphylactic symptoms and life-threatening or less severe asthmatic episodes in certain susceptible people. The overall prevalence of sulfite sensitivity in the general population is unknown and probably low. Sulfite sensitivity is seen more frequently in asthmatic than in nonasthmatic people.

PRECAUTIONS:

GENERAL

Trimethoprim and sulfamethoxazole should be given with caution of patients with impaired renal or hepatic function, to those with possible folate deficiency (*e.g.,* the elderly, chronic alcoholics, patients receiving anticonvulsant therapy, patients with malabsorption syndrome, and patients in malnutrition states) and to those with severe allergies or bronchial asthma. In glucose-6-phosphate dehydrogenase deficient individuals, hemolysis may occur. This reaction is frequently dose-related.

Use in the Elderly: There may be an increased risk of severe adverse reactions in elderly patients, particularly when complicating conditions exist, *e.g.,* impaired kidney and/or liver function, or concomitant use of other drugs. Severe skin reactions, generalized bone marrow suppression (see WARNINGS and ADVERSE REACTIONS) or a specific decrease in platelets (with or without purpura) are the most frequently reported severe adverse reactions in elderly patients. In those concurrently receiving certain diuretics, primarily thiazides, an increased incidence of thrombocytopenia with purpura has been reported. Appropriate dosage adjustments should be made for patients with impaired kidney function (see DOSAGE AND ADMINISTRATION.)

Use in the Treatment of and Prophylaxis for *Pneumocystis Carinii* Pneumonia in Patients with Acquired Immunodeficiency Syndrome (AIDS): AIDS patients may not tolerate or respond to trimethoprim and sulfamethoxazole in the same manner as non-AIDS patients. The incidence of side effects, particularly rash, fever, leukopenia and elevated aminotransferase (transaminase) values, with trimethoprim and sulfamethoxazole therapy in AIDS patients who are being treated for *Pneumocystis carinii* pneumonia has been reported to be greatly increased compared with the incidence normally associated with the use of trimethoprim and sulfamethoxazole in non-AIDS patients. Adverse effects are generally less severe in patients receiving trimethoprim and sulfamethoxazole for prophylaxis. A history of mild intolerance to trimethoprim and sulfamethoxazole in AIDS patients does not appear to predict intolerance of subsequent secondary prophylaxis.[5] However, if a patient develops skin rash or any sign of adverse reaction, therapy with trimethoprim and sulfamethoxazole should be reevaluated (see WARNINGS.)

PRECAUTIONS: *(cont'd)*

IV Infusion: Local irritation and inflammation due to extravascular infiltration of the infusion have been observed with trimethoprim and sulfamethoxazole IV infusion. If these occur the infusion should be discontinued and restarted at another site.

INFORMATION FOR THE PATIENT

Patients should be instructed to maintain an adequate fluid intake in order to prevent crystalluria and stone formation.

LABORATORY TESTS

Complete blood counts should be done frequently in patients receiving trimethoprim and sulfamethoxazole; if a significant reduction in the count of any formed blood element is noted, trimethoprim and sulfamethoxazole should be discontinued. Urinalyses with careful microscopic examination and renal function tests should be performed during therapy, particularly for those patients with impaired renal function.

DRUG/LABORATORY TEST INTERACTIONS

Trimethoprim and sulfamethoxazole, specifically the trimethoprim component, can interfere with a serum methotrexate assay as determined by the competitive binding protein technique (CBPA) when a bacterial dihydrofolate reductase is used as the binding protein. No interference occurs, however, if methotrexate is measured by a radioimmunoassay (RIA).

The presence of trimethoprim and sulfamethoxazole may also interfere with the Jaffe alkaline picrate reaction assay for creatinine, resulting in overestimations of about 10% in the range of normal values.

CARCINOGENESIS, MUTAGENESIS, AND IMPAIRMENT OF FERTILITY

Carcinogenesis: Long-term studies in animals to evaluate carcinogenic potential have not been conducted with any of the forms of the drug.

Mutagenesis: Bacterial mutagenic studies have not been performed with sulfamethoxazole and trimethoprim in combination. Trimethoprim was demonstrated to be nonmutagenic in the Ames assay. No chromosomal damage was observed in human leukocytes *in vitro* with sulfamethoxazole and trimethoprim alone or in combination; the concentrations used exceeded blood levels of these compounds following therapy with trimethoprim and sulfamethoxazole. Observations of leukocytes obtained from patients treated with trimethoprim and sulfamethoxazole revealed no chromosomal abnormalities.

Impairment of Fertility: No adverse effects on fertility or general reproductive performance were observed in rats given oral dosages as high as 70 mg/kg/day trimethoprim plus 350 mg/kg/day sulfamethoxazole. *IV Infusion:* Trimethoprim and sulfamethoxazole I.V. infusion has not been studied in animals for evidence of impairment of fertility. However, studies in rats at oral dosages as high as 70 mg/kg trimethoprim plus 350 mg/kg sulfamethoxazole daily showed no adverse effects on fertility or general reproductive performance.

PREGNANCY CATEGORY C

Teratogenic Effects: In rats, oral doses of 533 mg/kg sulfamethoxazole or 200 mg/kg trimethoprim produced teratologic effects manifested mainly as cleft palates.

The highest dose which did not cause cleft palates in rats was 512 mg/kg sulfamethoxazole or 192 mg/kg trimethoprim when administered separately. In two studies in rats, no teratology was observed when 512 mg/kg of sulfamethoxazole was used in combination with 128 mg/kg of trimethoprim. In one study, however, cleft palates were observed in one litter out of 9 when 355 mg/kg of sulfamethoxazole was used in combination with 88 mg/kg of trimethoprim.

In some rabbit studies, an overall increase in fetal loss (dead and resorbed and malformed conceptuses) was associated with doses of trimethoprim 6 times the human therapeutic dose.

While there are no large, well-controlled studies on the use of trimethoprim and sulfamethoxazole in pregnant women, Brumfitt and Pursell,[5] in a retrospective study, reported the outcome of 186 pregnancies during which the mother received either placebo or trimethoprim and sulfamethoxazole. The incidence of congenital abnormalities was 4.5% (3 of 66) in those who received placebo and 3.3% (4 of 120) in those receiving trimethoprim and sulfamethoxazole. There were no abnormalities in the 10 children whose mothers received the drug during the first trimester. In a separate survey, Brumfitt and Pursell also found no congenital abnormalities in 35 children whose mothers had received oral trimethoprim and sulfamethoxazole at the time of conception or shortly thereafter.

Because trimethoprim and sulfamethoxazole may interfere with folic acid metabolism, trimethoprim and sulfamethoxazole should be used during pregnancy only if the potential benefit justifies the potential risk to the fetus.

Nonteratogenic Effects: See CONTRAINDICATIONS.

NURSING MOTHERS

See CONTRAINDICATIONS.

PEDIATRIC USE

Trimethoprim and sulfamethoxazole is not recommended for infants younger than two months of age (see INDICATIONS AND USAGEand CONTRAINDICATIONS). *IV Infusion:* Trimethoprim and sulfamethoxazole IV infusion is not recommended for infants younger than two months (see CONTRAINDICATIONS.)

DRUG INTERACTIONS:

In elderly patients concurrently receiving certain diuretics, primarily thiazides, an increased incidence of thrombocytopenia with purpura has been reported.

It has been reported that trimethoprim and sulfamethoxazole may prolong the prothrombin time in patients who are receiving the anticoagulant warfarin. This interaction should be kept in mind when trimethoprim and sulfamethoxazole is given to patients already on anticoagulant therapy, and the coagulation time should be reassessed.

Trimethoprim and sulfamethoxazole may inhibit the hepatic metabolism of phenytoin. trimethoprim and sulfamethoxazole, given at a common clinical dosage, increased the phenytoin half-life by 39% and decreased the phenytoin metabolic clearance rate by 27%. When administering these drugs concurrently, one should be alert for possible excessive phenytoin effect.

Sulfonamides can also displace methotrexate from plasma protein binding sites, thus increasing free methotrexate concentrations.

ADVERSE REACTIONS:

The most common adverse effects are gastrointestinal disturbances (nausea, vomiting, anorexia) and allergic skin reactions (such as rash and urticaria). **FATALITIES ASSOCIATED WITH THE ADMINISTRATION OF SULFONAMIDES, ALTHOUGH RARE, HAVE OCCURRED DUE TO SEVERE REACTIONS, INCLUDING STEVENS-JOHNSON SYNDROME, TOXIC EPIDERMAL NECROLYSIS, FULMINANT HEPATIC NECROSIS, AGRANULOCYTOSIS, APLASTIC ANEMIA AND OTHER BLOOD DYSCRASIAS (SEE WARNINGS).**

Hematologic: Agranulocytosis, aplastic anemia, thrombocytopenia, leukopenia, neutropenia, hemolytic anemia, megaloblastic anemia, hypoprothrombinemia, methemoglobinemia, eosinophilia.

ADVERSE REACTIONS: *(cont'd)*

Allergic Reactions: Stevens-Johnson syndrome, toxic epidermal necrolysis, anaphylaxis, allergic myocarditis, erythema multiforme, exfoliative dermatitis, angioedema, drug fever, chills, Henoch-Schoenlein purpura, serum sickness-like syndrome, generalized allergic reactions, generalized skin eruptions, photosensitivity, conjunctival and scleral injection, pruritus, urticaria and rash. In addition, periarteritis nodosa and systemic lupus erythematosus have been reported.

Gastrointestinal: Hepatitis (including cholestatic jaundice and hepatic necrosis), elevation of serum transaminase and bilirubin, pseudomembranous enterocolitis, pancreatitis, stomatitis, glossitis, nausea, emesis, abdominal pain, diarrhea, anorexia.

Genitourinary: Renal failure, interstitial nephritis, BUN and serum creatinine elevation, toxic nephrosis with oliguria and anuria, and crystalluria.

Neurologic: Aseptic meningitis, convulsions, peripheral neuritis, ataxia, vertigo, tinnitus, headache.

Psychiatric: Hallucinations, depression, apathy, nervousness.

Endocrine: The sulfonamides bear certain chemical similarities to some goitrogens, diuretics (acetazolamide and the thiazides) and oral hypoglycemic agents. Cross-sensitivity may exist with these agents. Diuresis and hypoglycemia have occurred rarely in patients receiving sulfonamides.

Musculoskeletal: Arthralgia and myalgia.

Respiratory: Pulmonary infiltrates, cough, shortness of breath.

Miscellaneous: Weakness, fatigue, insomnia.

OVERDOSAGE:

Acute: The amount of a single dose of trimethoprim and sulfamethoxazole that is either associated with symptoms of overdosage or is likely to be life-threatening has not been reported. Signs and symptoms of overdosage reported with sulfonamides include anorexia, colic, nausea, vomiting, dizziness, headache, drowsiness and unconsciousness. Pyrexia, hematuria and crystalluria may be noted. Blood dyscrasias and jaundice are potential late manifestations of overdosage.

Signs of acute overdosage with trimethoprim include nausea, vomiting, dizziness, headache, mental depression, confusion and bone marrow depression.

General principles of treatment include the institution of gastric lavage or emesis, forcing oral fluids, and the administration of intravenous fluids if urine output is low and renal function is normal. Acidification of the urine will increase renal elimination of trimethoprim. The patient should be monitored with blood counts and appropriate blood chemistries, including electrolytes. If a significant blood dyscrasia or jaundice occurs, specific therapy should be instituted for these complications. Peritoneal dialysis is not effective and hemodialysis is only moderately effective in eliminating trimethoprim and sulfamethoxazole.

Chronic: Use of trimethoprim and sulfamethoxazole at high doses and/or for extended periods of time may cause bone marrow depression manifested as thrombocytopenia, leukopenia and/or megaloblastic anemia. If signs of bone marrow depression occur, the patient should be given leucovorin 5 to 15 mg daily until normal hematopoiesis is restored.

IV INFUSION

Acute: Since there has been no extensive experience in humans with single doses of trimethoprim and sulfamethoxazole IV infusion in excess of 25 ml (400 mg trimethoprim and 2000 mg sulfamethoxazole), the maximum tolerated dos in humans is unknown.

Chronic: Use of trimethoprim and sulfamethoxazole IV infusion at high doses and/or for extended periods of any time may cause bone marrow depression manifested as thrombocytopenia,leukopenia and/or megaloblastic amenia. If signs of bone marrow depression occur, the patient should be given leucovorin 5 to 15 mg daily until normal hematopoieses is restored.

Animal Toxicity: The LD_{50} of trimethoprim and sulfamethoxazole IV infusion in mice is 700 mg/kg or 7.3 ml/kg; in rats and rabbits the LD_{50} is>500 mg/kg or>5.2 ml/kg. The vehicle produced the same LD_{50} in each of these species as the active drug.

The signs and symptoms noted in mice, rats and rabbits with the infusion or its vehicle at the high IV doses used in acute toxicity studies included ataxia, decreased motor activity, loss of righting reflex, tremors or convulsions, and/or respiratory depression.

DOSAGE AND ADMINISTRATION:

TABLETS AND PEDIATRIC SUSPENSION

Not recommended for use in infants less than two months of age.

Urinary Tract Infections and Shigellosis in Adults and Children, and Acute Otitis Media in Children

Adults: The usual adult dosage in the treatment of urinary tract infections is one trimethoprim and sulfamethoxazole DS (double strength) tablet, two trimethoprim and sulfamethoxazole tablets or four teaspoonfuls (20 ml) of trimethoprim and sulfamethoxazole Pediatric Suspension every 12 hours for 10 to 14 days. An identical daily dosage is used for 5 days in the treatment of shigellosis.

Children: The recommended dose for children with urinary tract infections or acute otitis media is 8 mg/kg trimethoprim and 40 mg/kg sulfamethoxazole per 24 hours, given in two divided doses every 12 hours for 10 days. An identical daily dosage is used for 5 days in the treatment of shigellosis. TABLE 3 is a guideline for the attainment of this dosage:

TABLE 3 Children two months of age or older:

Weight lb	Weight kg	Dose—every 12 hours Teaspoonfuls	Tablets
22	10	1 teaspoon (5 ml)	———
44	20	2 teaspoon (10 ml)	1 tablet
66	30	3 teaspoon (15 ml)	1.5 tablets
88	40	4 teaspoon (20 ml)	2 tablets or 1 DS tablet

For Patients with Impaired Renal Function: When renal function is impaired, a reduced dosage should be employed using TABLE 4.

TABLE 4 Dosage for Patients with Impaired Renal Function

Creatinine Clearance (ml/min)	Recommended Dosage Regimen
Above 30	Usual standard regimen
15-30	1/2 the usual regimen
Below 15	Use not recommended

Acute Exacerbations of Chronic Bronchitis in Adults:

The usual adult dosage in the treatment of acute exacerbations of chronic bronchitis is one trimethoprim and sulfamethoxazole DS (double strength) tablet, 2 trimethoprim and sulfamethoxazole tablets or 4 teaspoonfuls (20 ml) of trimethoprim and sulfamethoxazole Pediatric Suspension 12 hours for 14 days.

DOSAGE AND ADMINISTRATION: *(cont'd)*

***Pneumocystis Carinii* Pneumonia**

Treatment: *Adults and Children:* The recommended dosage for patients with documented *Pneumocystis carinii* pneumonia is 20 mg/kg trimethoprim and 100 mg/kg sulfamethoxazole per 24 hours given in equally divided doses every 6 hours for 14 to 21 days. TABLE 5 is a guideline for the upper limit of this dosage:

TABLE 5 Dosage for Patients with *Pneumocystis carinii*

Weight lb	Weight kg	Dose-every 6 hours Teaspoonfuls	Dose-every 6 hours Tablets
18	8	1 teasp. (5 ml)	—
35	16	2 teasp. (10 ml)	1 tablet
53	24	3 teasp. (15 ml)	1.5 tablets
70	32	4 teasp. (20 ml)	2 tablets or 1 DS tblt
88	40	5 teasp. (25 ml)	2.5 tablets
106	48	6 teasp. (30 ml)	3 tblts or 1.5 DS tblts
141	64	8 teasp. (40 ml)	4 tblts or 2 DS tblts
176	80	10 teasp. (50 ml)	5 tblts or 2.5 DS tblts

For the lower limit dose (15 mg/kg trimethoprim and 75 mg/kg sulfamethoxazole per 24 hours) administer 75% of the dose in the above table.

Prophylaxis

Adults: The recommended dosage for prophylaxis in adults is 1 trimethoprim and sulfamethoxazole DS (double strength) tablet daily.[8]

Children: For children, the recommended dose is 150 mg/m^2/day trimethoprim with 750 mg/m^2/day sulfamethoxazole given orally in equally divided doses twice a day, on 3 consecutive days per week. The total daily dose should not exceed 320 mg trimethoprim and 1600 mg sulfamethoxazole.[9] TABLE 6) is a guideline for the attainment of this dosage in children:

TABLE 6 Dosage for Patients with Prophylaxis

Body Surface Area (m^2)	Dose-every 12 hours Teaspoonfuls	Tablets
0.26	0.5(2.5 ml)	-
0.53	1 (5 ml)	.05
1.06	2 (10 ml)	1.0

Travelers' Diarrhea in Adults

For the treatment of travelers' diarrhea, the usual adult dosage is one trimethoprim and sulfamethoxazole DS (double strength) tablet; two trimethoprim and sulfamethoxazole tablets or four teaspoonfuls (20 ml) of Pediatric Suspension every 12 hours for 5 days.

TABLETS SHOULD BE STORED AT 15-30°C (59-86°F) IN A DRY PLACE AND PROTECTED FROM LIGHT.

SUSPENSION SHOULD BE STORED AT 15-30°C (59-86°F) AND PROTECTED FROM LIGHT.

IV INFUSION

Contraindicated In Infants Less Than Two Months of Age. CAUTION- TRIMETHOPRIM AND SULFAMETHOXAZOLE IV INFUSION MUST BE DILUTED IN 5% DEXTROSE IN WATER SOLUTION PRIOR TO ADMINISTRATION. DO NOT MIX THE I.V. INFUSION WITH OTHER DRUG OR SOLUTIONS. RAPID INFUSION OR BOLUS INJECTION MUST BE AVOIDED.

Dosage

Children and Adults:

Pneumocystis Carinii Pneumonia: Total daily dose is 15 to 20 mg/kg (based on the trimethoprim component) given in three of four equally divided doses every 6 to 8 hours for up to 14 days. One investigator noted that a total dose of 10 to 15 mg/kg was sufficient in 10 adult patients with normal renal function[6].

Severe Urinary Tract Infections and Shigellosis: Total daily dose is 8 to 10 mg/kg (based on the trimethoprim component) given in two to four equally divided doses every 6,8, or 12 hours for up to 14 days for severe urinary tract infections and 5 days for shigellosis. The maximum recommended daily dose is 60 ml per day.

For Patients with Impaired Renal Function: When renal function is impaired, a reduced dosage should be employed while using **TABLE 7**.

TABLE 7 Dosage for Patients with Impaired Renal Function

Creatine Clearance (ml/min)	Recommended Dosage Regimen
Above 30	Usual standard regimen
15-30	1/2 the usual regimen
Below 15	Use not recommended

Method of Preparation: Trimethoprim and sulfamethoxazole IV infusion must be diluted. EACH 5 ML SHOULD BE ADDED TO 125 ML OF 5% DEXTROSE IN WATER. After diluting with 5% dextrose in water the solution should not be refrigerated and should be used within 6 hrs. If a dilution of 5 ml per 100 ml of 5% dextrose in water is desired, it should be used within 4 hours. If upon visual inspection there is cloudiness or evidence of crystallization after mixing, the solution should be discarded and a fresh solution prepared.

Multidose Vials: After initial entry into the vial, the remaining contents must be used within 48 hours.

The following infusion systems have been tested and found satisfactory: unit-dose glass containers; unit-dose polyvinyl chloride and polyolefin. No other systems have been tested and therefore no others can be recommended.

Dilution: EACH 5 ML OF THE IV INFUSION SHOULD BE ADDED TO 125 ML OF 5% DEXTROSE IN WATER.

Note: *In those instances where fluid restriction is desirable,* each 5 ml may be added to 75 ml of 5% dextrose in water. Under these circumstances the solution should be mixed just prior to use and should be administered within two (2) hours. If upon visual inspection there is a cloudiness or evidence of crystallization after mixing, the solution should be discarded and a fresh solution prepared. DO NOT MIX SULFAMETHOXAZOLE AND TRIMETHOPRIM IV INFUSION-5% DEXTROSE IN WATER WITH DRUGS OR SOLUTIONS IN THE SAME CONTAINER.

Administration: The solution should be given by intravenous infusion over a period of 60 to 90 minutes. Rapid infusion or bolus injection must be avoided. Sulfamethoxazole and trimethoprim IV infusion should not be given intramuscularly.

STORE AT ROOM TEMPERATURE (15-30°C or 59-86°F) DO NOT REFRIGERATE.

REFERENCES:

1. Kremers P, Duvivier J, Heusghem C: Pharmacokinetic Studies of Co-Trimoxazole in Man after Single and Repeated Doses. *J Clin Pharmacol 14*:112-117, Feb-Mar 1974. **2.** Kaplan SA, *et al:* Pharmacokinetic Profile of Trimethoprim-Sulfamethoxazole in Man.*J Infect Dis 128* (Suppl): S547-S555, Nov 1973. **3.** *Federal Register 37*:

REFERENCES: *(cont'd)*

20527-20529, 1972. **4.** Bauer AW, Kirby WMM, Sherris JC, Turck M: Antibiotic Susceptibility Testing by a Standardized Single Disk Method. *Am J Clin Path 45*:493-496, Apr 1966. **5.** Brumfitt W, Pursell R: Trimethoprim/Sulfamethoxazole in the Treatment of Bacteriuria in Women. *J Infect Dis 128* (Suppl): S657-S663, Nov 1973. **6.** Approved Standard ASM-2 Performance Standards for Antimicrobial Disc Susceptibility Test: National Committee for Clinical Laboratory Standards, 771 East Lancaster Avenue, Villanova, Pennsylvania 19085. **7.** Grose WE, Bodey GP, Loo TL: Clinical Pharmacology of Intravenously Administered Trimethoprim-sulfamethoxazole. *Antimicrob Agents Chemother 15;*447-451, Mar 1979. **8.** Siber GR, Gorham C, Durbin W. Lesko L. Levin MJ: Pharmacology of Intravenously Administered Trimethoprim-Sulfamethoxazole in Children and Adults.*Current Chemotherapy and Infectious Diseases,* American Society for Microbiology. Washington D.C.,Washington D.C., 1980, Vol 1, pp.691-692 **9.** Winston DJ, Lau WK, Gale RP, Young LS: Trimethoprim-Sulfamethoxazole for the Treatment of*Pneumocystis carinii*pneumonia. *Ann Intern Med 92*:762-769,June 1980.

PATIENT INFORMATION:

Sulfamethoxazole, trimethoprim is a combination product used to treat infections of the airway such as bronchitis, sinusitis, ear infections, and urinary tract infections. This drug should not be used by those with sulfa allergies. Allergies to this medication may occur on the second or third exposure to the drug. Signs to watch for include sore throat, fever, joint pain, cough, shortness of breath, or pallor. If this occurs, stop the medication and call your physician immediately. It is very important to drink a lot of fluids while taking this medication. Each dose should be taken with a full glass of water with water being drunk throughout the day. This medication is an antibiotic. It is important to finish the full course of therapy even if your symptoms improve.

HOW SUPPLIED - RATED THERAPEUTICALLY EQUIVALENT:

Injection, Conc-Soln - Intravenous - 80 mg/16 mg/ml

5 ml x 10	$26.76	Sulfamethoxazole/Trimethoprim, Gensia Labs	00703-9503-03
5 ml x 10	$39.83	SEPTRA IV INFUSION, Glaxo Wellcome	00173-0856-44
5 ml x 10	$58.89	Sulfamethoxazole/Trimethoprim, Elkins Sinn	00641-1532-33
5 ml x 10	$64.75	Sulfamethoxazole/Trimethoprim, Elkins Sinn	00641-2764-43
5 ml x 10	**$74.05**	**BACTRIM I.V. INFUSION, Roche**	**00004-1956-01**
10 ml vials x 1	$78.05	SEPTRA IV INFUSION, Glaxo Wellcome	00173-0856-95
10 ml x 10	$59.52	Sulfamethoxazole/Trimethoprim, Gensia Labs	00703-9514-03
10 ml x 10	$79.67	SEPTRA, ADD-VANTAGE, Glaxo Wellcome	00173-0856-47
10 ml x 10	$126.91	Sulfamethoxazole/Trimethoprim, Elkins Sinn	00641-2765-43
10 ml x 10	**$155.54**	**BACTRIM IV INFUSION, Roche**	**00004-1955-01**
20 ml x 10	$144.92	SEPTRA IV INFUSION, Glaxo Wellcome	00173-0856-01
30 ml	$14.54	Sulfamethoxazole/Trimethoprim, Gensia Labs	00703-9526-01
30 ml	**$43.36**	**BACTRIM, Roche**	**00004-1958-01**
30 ml x 1	$35.35	Sulfamethoxazole/Trimethoprim, Elkins Sinn	00641-2766-41
50 ml	**$66.02**	**BACTRIM, Roche**	**00004-1958-02**

Suspension - Oral - 200 mg/40 mg/5m

10 ml x 100	$55.13	Sulfamethoxazole/Trimethoprim, Xactdose	50962-0300-10
20 ml x 50	$55.90	Sulfamethoxazole/Trimethoprim, Xactdose	50962-0302-20
20 ml x 100	$96.00	Sulfamethoxazole/Trimethoprim, Xactdose	50962-0300-20
100 ml	$3.76	Sulfamethoxazole/Trimethoprim, Teva	00332-6100-32
100 ml	$3.95	SULFATRIM PEDIATRIC, Alpharma	00472-1285-33
100 ml	$5.64	Sulfamethoxazole/Trimethoprim, H.C.F.A. F F P	99999-2289-01
100 ml x 6	$56.94	SEPTRA, Glaxo Wellcome	00173-0855-03
150 ml	$8.46	Sulfamethoxazole/Trimethoprim, H.C.F.A. F F P	99999-2289-02
200 ml	$11.28	Sulfamethoxazole/Trimethoprim, H.C.F.A. F F P	99999-2289-03
473 ml	$22.80	Sultrex, Bergmar Pharm	58173-0029-16
473 ml	$26.68	Sulfamethoxazole/Trimethoprim, H.C.F.A. F F P	99999-2289-05
480 ml	$10.29	SULFATRIM PEDIATRIC, Harber Pharm	51432-0671-20
480 ml	$10.77	TRIMETH/SULFA, Rugby	00536-1715-85
480 ml	$10.80	Sulfa/Trimethoprim Pediatric, Major Pharms	00904-0406-16
480 ml	$10.98	Sulfamethoxazole & Trimethoprim, Schein Pharm (US)	00364-2076-16
480 ml	$11.58	SULFATRIM PEDIATRIC, Qualitest Pharms	00603-1687-58
480 ml	$11.62	TRIMETH/SULFA PEDIATRIC, Rugby	00536-1725-85
480 ml	$11.65	SULFATRIM PEDIATRIC, Goldline Labs	00182-1558-40
480 ml	$11.65	SULFATRIM PEDIATRIC, Alpharma	00472-1285-16
480 ml	$11.73	Sulfamethoxazole/Trimethoprim, HL Moore Drug Exch	00839-7709-69
480 ml	$11.74	Sulfamethoxazole/Trimethoprim, Bristol Myers Squibb	00003-1201-10
480 ml	$11.78	Sulfamethoxazole & Trimethoprim, Schein Pharm (US)	00364-2077-16
480 ml	$11.95	Bethaprim, Major Pharms	00904-0405-16
480 ml	$12.04	Sulfamethoxazole/Trimethoprim, Teva	00332-6100-38
480 ml	$12.16	Sulfamethoxazole/Trimethoprim, Qualitest Pharms	00603-1688-58
480 ml	$12.18	Sulfamethoxazole/Trimethoprim, Lederle Pharm	00005-3124-65
480 ml	$12.25	COTRIM PEDIATRIC, Teva	00093-0190-16
480 ml	$12.25	Sulfamethoxazole/Trimethoprim, Teva	00093-0562-16
480 ml	$12.27	Sulfamethoxazole/Trimethoprim, Geneva Pharms	00781-6062-16
480 ml	$12.27	Sulfamethoxazole/Trimethoprim, Geneva Pharms	00781-6063-16
480 ml	$12.30	SULFATRIM, Goldline Labs	00182-1559-40
480 ml	$12.30	SULFATRIM, Alpharma	00472-1284-16
480 ml	$13.34	SMZ-TMP, Aligen Independ	00405-3675-16
480 ml	$17.28	Sulfamethoxazole/Trimethoprim, HL Moore Drug Exch	00839-6699-69
480 ml	$17.28	SULFATRIM, HL Moore Drug Exch	00839-6718-69
480 ml	$27.07	SULFATRIM, United Res	00677-0840-33
480 ml	$27.07	SULFATRIM, United Res	00677-0841-33
480 ml	$27.07	Sulfamethoxazole/Trimethoprim, H.C.F.A. F F P	99999-2289-04
480 ml	**$43.18**	**BACTRIM, Roche**	**00004-1033-28**
480 ml	$44.92	SEPTRA GRAPE, Glaxo Wellcome	00173-0854-96
480 ml	$44.92	SEPTRA, Glaxo Wellcome	00173-0855-96

Tablet, Uncoated - Oral - 400 mg/80 mg

100's	$7.11	Sulfamethoxazole/Trimethoprim, United Res	00677-0783-01
100's	$7.11	Sulfamethoxazole/Trimethoprim, H.C.F.A. F F P	99999-2289-06
100's	$7.92	Sulfamethoxazole/Trimethoprim, US Trading	56126-0139-11
100's	$11.03	SULFA-TRIMETHOPRIM, IDE-Interstate	00814-7239-14
100's	$12.00	Sulfamethoxazole/Trimethoprim, Eon Labs Mfg	00185-0111-01
100's	$12.14	Sulfamethoxazole/Trimethoprim, Roxane	00054-4800-25
100's	$12.46	Sulfamethoxazole/Trimethoprim, Geneva Pharms	00781-1062-01
100's	$12.69	UROPLUS SS, Shionogi USA	45809-0910-11
100's	$12.70	Sulfamethoxazole/Trimethoprim, Qualitest Pharms	00603-5778-21
100's	$13.40	Sulfamethoxazole/Trimethoprim, Major Pharms	00904-2726-61
100's	$13.85	Sulfamethoxazole & Trimethoprim 80, Major Pharms	00904-2726-60
100's	$14.70	Sulfamethoxazole/Trimethoprim, Voluntary Hosp	53258-0229-01
100's	$15.30	Sulfamethoxazole/Trimethoprim, Voluntary Hosp	53258-0229-13
100's	$15.30	Sulfamethoxazole/Trimethoprim, Medirex	57480-0436-01
100's	$16.57	Sulfamethoxazole & Trimethoprim, Schein Pharm (US)	00364-2068-01
100's	$16.70	Sulfamethoxazole/Trimethoprim, Roxane	00054-8800-25
100's	$18.50	Sulfamethoxazole/Trimethoprim, Mutual Pharm	53489-0145-01
100's	$18.95	Sulfamethoxazole/Trimethoprim, Martec Pharms	52555-0341-01
100's	$21.50	TRIMETH/SULFA S/S, Rugby	00536-4692-01
100's	$23.24	SULFATRIM-SS, Goldline Labs	00182-1478-01
100's	$23.24	Sulfamethoxazole/Trimethoprim, Teva	00332-2130-09
100's	$23.29	Sulfamethoxazole/Trimethoprim, HL Moore Drug Exch	00839-6487-06
100's	$24.00	Sulfamethoxazole/Trimethoprim, Teva	00093-0088-01
100's	$24.00	COTRIM, Teva	00093-0188-01
100's	$24.00	SMZ-TMP, Aligen Independ	00405-4928-01
100's	$24.00	Sulfamethoxazole/Trimethoprim, Sidmak Labs	50111-0341-01
100's	$24.40	Sulfamethoxazole/Trimethoprim, Bristol Myers Squibb	00003-0138-50
100's	$25.00	Sulfamethoxazole, Parmed Pharms	00349-2364-01
100's	$28.00	Sulfamethoxazole/Trimethoprim, Geneva Pharms	00781-1062-13

HOW SUPPLIED - RATED THERAPEUTICALLY EQUIVALENT:
(cont'd)

100's	$37.95	Sulfamethoxazole/Trimethoprim, Schein Pharm (US)	00364-2068-90
100's	$38.65	Sulfamethoxazole/Trimethoprim, Goldline Labs	00182-8843-89
100's	$40.94	SMX-TMP SINGLE STRENGTH, Vangard Labs	00615-0171-13
100's	**$74.04**	**BACTRIM, Roche**	**00004-0050-01**
100's	$77.03	SEPTRA, Glaxo Wellcome	00173-0852-55
500's	$35.55	Sulfamethoxazole/Trimethoprim, Teva	00332-2130-13
500's	$35.55	Sulfamethoxazole/Trimethoprim, United Res	00677-0783-05
500's	$35.55	Sulfamethoxazole/Trimethoprim, H.C.F.A. F F P	99999-2289-07
500's	$44.25	SULFA-TRIMETHOPRIM, IDE-Interstate	00814-7239-28
500's	$55.00	Sulfamethoxazole/Trimethoprim, Eon Labs Mfg	00185-0111-05
500's	$55.94	UROPLUS SS, Shionogi USA	45809-0910-12
500's	$58.40	Sulfamethoxazole & Trimethoprim 80, Major Pharms	00904-2726-40
500's	$67.50	Sulfamethoxazole/Trimethoprim, Mutual Pharm	53489-0145-05
500's	$67.57	Sulfamethoxazole & Trimethoprim, Schein Pharm (US)	00364-2068-05
500's	$68.95	TRIMETH/SULFA S/S, Rugby	00536-4692-05
500's	$71.60	Sulfamethoxazole, Parmed Pharms	00349-2364-05
500's	$106.00	Sulfamethoxazole/Trimethoprim, Teva	00093-0088-05
500's	$106.00	COTRIM, Teva	00093-0188-05
500's	$106.00	Sulfamethoxazole/Trimethoprim, Sidmak Labs	50111-0341-02
500's	$112.58	Sulfamethoxazole/Trimethoprim, Lederle Pharm	00005-3117-31
500's	$117.41	Sulfamethoxazole/Trimethoprim, Bristol Myers Squibb	00003-0138-60
600's	$91.80	Sulfamethoxazole/Trimethoprim, Medirex	57480-0436-06

Tablet, Uncoated - Oral - 800 mg/160 mg

20's	$1.78	Sulfamethoxazole/Trimethoprim, H.C.F.A. F F P	99999-2289-08
20's	$3.03	Sulfamethoxazole/Trimethoprim, Talbert Phcy	44514-0826-15
20's	$3.60	Sulfamethoxazole/Trimethoprim, Major Pharms	00904-2725-95
20's	$4.83	UROPLUS DS, Shionogi USA	45809-0511-24
20's	$4.83	UROPLUS DS, Shionogi USA	45809-0911-24
28's	$2.50	Sulfamethoxazole/Trimethoprim, H.C.F.A. F F P	99999-2289-09
28's	$7.52	UROPLUS DS, Shionogi USA	45809-0911-26
30's	$2.67	Sulfamethoxazole/Trimethoprim, H.C.F.A. F F P	99999-2289-10
30's	$7.52	UROPLUS DS, Shionogi USA	45809-0511-25
100's	$8.93	Sulfamethoxazole/Trimethoprim, United Res	00677-0784-01
100's	$8.93	Sulfamethoxazole/Trimethoprim, H.C.F.A. F F P	99999-2289-11
100's	$9.80	Sulfamethoxazole/Trimethoprim, US Trading	56126-0140-11
100's	$13.28	SULFA TRIMETHOPRIM 800/160, IDE-Interstate	00814-7240-14
100's	$14.77	Sulfamethoxazole/Trimethoprim, Roxane	00054-4801-25
100's	$15.00	Sulfamethoxazole/Trimethoprim, Eon Labs Mfg	00185-0112-01
100's	$16.86	Sulfamethoxazole/Trimethoprim, Roxane	00054-8801-25
100's	$17.20	Sulfamethoxazole/Trimethoprim, Qualitest Pharms	00603-5779-21
100's	$17.39	UROPLUS DS, Shionogi USA	45809-0511-21
100's	$17.39	UROPLUS DS, Shionogi USA	45809-0911-21
100's	$18.13	Sulfamethoxazole/Trimethoprim, Geneva Pharms	00781-1063-01
100's	$18.75	SULFAMETHOXAZOLE/TRIMETHOPRIM DS, Interpharm	53746-0272-01
100's	$20.45	Sulfamethoxazole & Trimethoprim 800, Major Pharms	00904-2725-60
100's	$21.74	UROPLUS DS, Shionogi USA	45809-0511-23
100's	$22.50	TRIMETHSULFA D/S, Rugby	00536-4693-01
100's	$23.70	Sulfamethoxazole/Trimethoprim, Voluntary Hosp	53258-0161-01
100's	$24.00	Sulfamethoxazole/Trimethoprim, Raway	00686-2132-10
100's	$26.10	Sulfamethoxazole/Trimethoprim, Voluntary Hosp	53258-0161-13
100's	$26.33	SMZ-TMP, HL Moore Drug Exch	00839-6406-06
100's	$26.50	Sulfamethoxazole/Trimethoprim, Martec Pharms	52555-0342-01
100's	$27.45	Sulfamethoxazole/Trimethoprim, Medirex	57480-0387-01
100's	$28.50	Sulfamethoxazole/Trimethoprim, Mutual Pharm	53489-0146-01
100's	$33.90	SMZ-TMP, Harber Pharm	51432-0422-03
100's	$34.00	Sulfamethoxazole/Trimethoprim, Parmed Pharms	00349-2336-01
100's	$36.00	Sulfamethoxazole/Trimethoprim, Geneva Pharms	00781-1063-13
100's	$38.05	Sulfamethoxazole & Trimethoprim, Schein Pharm (US)	00364-2069-01
100's	$38.14	SULFATRIM-DS, Goldline Labs	00182-1408-01
100's	$38.14	Sulfamethoxazole/Trimethoprim, Teva	00332-2132-09
100's	$38.25	Sulfamethoxazole/Trimethoprim, Teva	00093-0089-01
100's	$38.25	COTRIM DS, Teva	00093-0189-01
100's	$39.00	SMZ-TMP, Aligen Independ	00405-4929-01
100's	$39.00	Sulfamethoxazole/Trimethoprim, Sidmak Labs	50111-0342-01
100's	$40.11	Sulfamethoxazole/Trimethoprim, Bristol Myers Squibb	00003-0171-50
100's	$40.42	Sulfamethoxazole/Trimethoprim, Major Pharms	00904-2725-61
100's	$62.75	Sulfamethoxazole/Trimethoprim, Schein Pharm (US)	00364-2069-90
100's	$63.95	Sulfamethoxazole/Trimethoprim, Goldline Labs	00182-8844-89
100's	$64.13	SMX-TMP DOUBLE STRENGTH, Vangard Labs	00615-0170-13
100's	**$121.48**	**BACTRIM DS, Roche**	**00004-0117-01**
100's	$126.42	SEPTRA DS, Glaxo Wellcome	00173-0853-55
250's	$22.32	Sulfamethoxazole/Trimethoprim, H.C.F.A. F F P	99999-2289-12
250's	**$244.88**	**BACTRIM DS, Roche**	**00004-0117-04**
250's	$255.10	SEPTRA DS, Glaxo Wellcome	00173-0853-65
500's	$44.65	Sulfamethoxazole/Trimethoprim, United Res	00677-0784-05
500's	$44.65	Sulfamethoxazole/Trimethoprim, H.C.F.A. F F P	99999-2289-13
500's	$53.55	SULFA TRIMETHOPRIM 800/160, IDE-Interstate	00814-7240-28
500's	$69.95	Sulfamethoxazole/Trimethoprim, Eon Labs Mfg	00185-0112-05
500's	$73.89	UROPLUS DS, Shionogi USA	45809-0511-22
500's	$73.89	UROPLUS DS, Shionogi USA	45809-0911-22
500's	$79.95	Sulfamethoxazole/Trimethoprim, Qualitest Pharms	00603-5779-28
500's	$81.25	Sulfamethoxazole & Trimethoprim 800, Major Pharms	00904-2725-40
500's	$82.00	SULFAMETHOXAZOLE/TRIMETHOPRIM DS, Interpharm	53746-0272-05
500's	$82.43	Sulfamethoxazole/Trimethoprim, Geneva Pharms	00781-1063-05
500's	$110.00	Sulfamethoxazole/Trimethoprim, Raway	00686-2132-12
500's	$128.00	Sulfamethoxazole/Trimethoprim, Mutual Pharm	53489-0146-05
500's	$130.20	Sulfamethoxazole/Trimethoprim, Martec Pharms	52555-0342-05
500's	$133.98	Sulfamethoxazole/Trimethoprim, Parmed Pharms	00349-2336-05
500's	$145.00	TRIMETHSULFA D/S, Rugby	00536-4693-05
500's	$148.00	Sulfamethoxazole & Trimethoprim, Schein Pharm (US)	00364-2069-05
500's	$153.88	SULFATRIM-DS, Goldline Labs	00182-1408-05
500's	$153.88	Sulfamethoxazole/Trimethoprim, Teva	00332-2132-13
500's	$155.00	Sulfamethoxazole/Trimethoprim, Sidmak Labs	50111-0342-02
500's	$162.74	SMZ-TMP, HL Moore Drug Exch	00839-6406-12
500's	$162.74	Sulfamethoxazole/Trimethoprim, HL Moore Drug Exch	00839-7694-12
500's	$163.51	Sulfamethoxazole/Trimethoprim, Lederle Pharm	00005-3118-31
500's	$167.50	SMZ-TMP, Aligen Independ	00405-4929-02
500's	$168.20	Sulfamethoxazole/Trimethoprim, Teva	00093-0089-05
500's	$168.20	COTRIM DS, Teva	00093-0189-05
500's	$169.50	SMZ-TMP, Harber Pharm	51432-0422-05
500's	$190.49	Sulfamethoxazole/Trimethoprim, Bristol Myers Squibb	00003-0171-60
500's	$199.95	Sulfaprim D.S., Quality Res Pharms	52765-1305-05
500's	**$475.30**	**BACTRIM DS, Roche**	**00004-0117-14**
600's	$273.60	Sulfamethoxazole/Trimethoprim, Medirex	57480-0387-06
1000's	$89.30	Sulfamethoxazole/Trimethoprim, H.C.F.A. F F P	99999-2289-14
1000's	$120.00	Sulfamethoxazole/Trimethoprim, Interpharm	53746-0272-10

HOW SUPPLIED - NOT RATED EQUIVALENT:

Injection, Conc-Soln - Intravenous - 80 mg/16 mg/ml

5 ml x 10	$17.64	SULFAMETHOXAZOLE/TRIMETHOPRIM, Sanofi Winthrop	00024-1833-05

Suspension - Oral - 200 mg/40 mg/5m

480 ml	$12.95	Sulfatrim, Consolidated Midland	00223-6612-01
480 ml	$12.95	Sulfatrim Pediatric, Consolidated Midland	00223-6613-01

SULFANILAMIDE *(002290)*

CATEGORIES: Anti-Infectives; Antimicrobials; Dermatologicals; Local Infections; Skin/Mucous Membrane Agents; Sulfonamides; Vaginal Preparations; Vaginitis; Pregnancy Category C; FDA Approved 1985 Sep

BRAND NAMES: AVC; Avitrol Vaginal Sulfa; *Defonamid*; Vaginal Sulfa; Vagitrol *(International brand names outside U.S. in italics)*

FORMULARIES: Aetna

DESCRIPTION:

Sulfanilamide is a preparation for vaginal administration for the treatment of *Candida albicans* infections and available in the following forms:

SULFANILAMIDE CREAM

Each tube contains: Sulfanilamide 15.0% in a water-miscible, non-staining base made from lactose, propylene glycol, stearic acid, diglycol stearate, methylparaben, propylparaben, trolamine, and water; buffered with lactic acid to an acid pH of approximately 4.3.

SULFANILAMIDE SUPPOSITORIES

Each suppository contains: Sulfanilamide 1.05 g with lactose, in a base made from polyethylene glycol 400, polysorbate 80, polyethylene glycol 3350, and glycerin; buffered with lactic acid to an acid pH of approximately 4.5. Sulfanilamide suppositories have an inert, white, non-staining covering, which dissolves promptly in the vagina. The covering is composed of gelatin, glycerin, water, methylparaben, propylparaben, and coloring.

Sulfanilamide is an anti-infective agent. It is*p*-aminobenzenesulfonamide.

Sulfanilamide occurs as a white odorless crystalline powder with a slightly bitter taste and sweet aftertaste. It is slightly soluble in water, alcohol, acetone, glycerin, propylene glycol, hydrochloric acid, and solutions of potassium and sodium hydroxide. It is practically insoluble in chloroform, ether, benzene, and petroleum ether.

CLINICAL PHARMACOLOGY:

Sulfanilamide has been a useful ingredient of vaginal formulations for about four decades. It blocks certain metabolic processes essential for the growth of susceptible bacteria. The sulfanilamide is in a specially compounded base buffered to the pH (about 4.3) of the normal vagina to encourage the presence of the normally occurring Doederlein's bacilli of the vagina.

The use of sulfanilamide for the treatment of vulvovaginitis caused by *Candida albicans* is supported by three clinical investigations. The three studies show sulfanilamide to be significantly more effective ($p \leq 0.01$) than placebo as follows:

In Study I, the ratio of effectiveness was 71% for the sulfanilamide versus 49% for placebo with 30 days of treatment:

In Study II, the percentages were 48% and 24%, respectively, with 15 days of treatment;

In Study III, the percentages were 66% versus 33%, respectively, with 30 days of treatment.

INDICATIONS AND USAGE:

For the treatment of vulvovaginitis caused by *Candida albicans.* (See CLINICAL PHARMACOLOGY).

CONTRAINDICATIONS:

Sulfanilamide should not be used in patients known to be sensitive to this product or to the sulfonamides.

PRECAUTIONS:

General: Because sulfonamides are absorbed from the vaginal mucosa, the usual precautions for oral sulfonamides apply. Patients should be observed for skin rash or evidence of systemic toxicity, and if these develop, the medications should be discontinued.

Deaths associated with administration of oral sulfonamides have reportedly occurred from hypersensitivity reactions, agranulocytosis, aplastic anemia, and other blood dyscrasias.

Goiter production, diuresis, and hypoglycemia have reportedly occurred rarely in patients receiving oral sulfonamides. Cross-sensitivity may exist with these agents. Rats appear to be especially susceptible to the goitrogenic effects of sulfonamides, and long-term administration has reportedly produced thyroid malignancies in this species.

Vaginal applicators or inserters should be used with caution after the seventh month of pregnancy.

Information for the Patient: The doctor should advise the patient that in the event unusual local itching and burning occur, or other unusual symptoms develop, medication should be discontinued and not re-started without further consultation.

Carcinogenesis, Mutagenesis, and Impairment of Fertility: No data are available on long-term potential of sulfanilamide for carcinogenicity, mutagenicity, or impairment of fertility in animals or humans.

Pregnancy, Teratogenic Effects, Pregnancy Category C: Animal reproductive studies have been conducted with sulfonamides, including sulfanilamide. It is not known whether sulfanilamide can cause fetal harm when administered to a pregnant woman or can affect reproductive capacity. Sulfanilamide should be given to a pregnant woman only if clearly needed.

Sulfonamides, including sulfanilamide, readily pass through the placenta and reach fetal circulation. The concentration in the fetus is from 50-90% of that in the maternal blood and if high enough, can cause toxic effects. The safe use of sulfonamides, including sulfanilamide, in pregnancy has not been established. The teratogenic potential of most sulfonamides has not been thoroughly investigated in either animals or humans. However, a significant increase in the incidence of cleft palate and other bony abnormalities of offspring has been observed when certain sulfonamides of the short-, intermediate-, and long-acting types (including sulfanilamide) were given to pregnant rats and mice at high oral doses (seven to 25 times the human therapeutic oral dose).

Nursing Mothers: Sulfanilamide should be avoided in nursing mothers because absorbed sulfonamides will appear in maternal milk, and have caused kernicterus in the newborn. Because of the potential for serious adverse reactions in nursing infants from sulfonamides, a decision should be made whether to discontinue nursing or to discontinue the drug.

Pediatric Use: Safety and effectiveness of sulfanilamide in children have not been established.

DRUG INTERACTIONS:

Drug interactions have not been documented with sulfanilamide.

ADVERSE REACTIONS:

Local sensitivity reactions such as increased discomfort or a burning sensation have occasionally been reported following the use of topical sulfonamides. With the use of sulfanilamide Cream, sensitivity reactions (only local) were reported for 0.2% of the investigational patients.

Treatment should be discontinued if either local or systemic manifestations of sulfonamide toxicity or sensitivity occur.

DRUG ABUSE AND DEPENDENCE:

Tolerance, abuse, or dependence with sulfanilamide have not been reported.

OVERDOSAGE:

There have been no reports of accidental overdosage with sulfanilamide. The acute oral LD_{50} of sulfanilamide is 3700-4200 mg/kg in mice. The minimum human lethal dose of sulfanilamide has not been established.

It is not known if sulfanilamide is dialyzable.

DOSAGE AND ADMINISTRATION:

One applicatorful (about 6 g) or one suppository intravaginally once or twice daily. Improvements in symptoms should occur within a few days, but treatment should be continued for a period of 30 days.

Douching with a suitable solution before insertion may be recommended for hygienic purposes.

Sulfanilamide Cream: Store at room temperature, below 86°F. Protect from cold. Product darkens with age. Potency is maintained throughout labeled shelf life when stored as directed.

Sulfanilamide Suppositories: Store at room temperature, below 86°F. Protect from excessive cold and moisture.

HOW SUPPLIED - RATED THERAPEUTICALLY EQUIVALENT:

Cream - Vaginal - 15 %

120 gm	$10.52	Sulfanilamide, HL Moore Drug Exch	00839-7557-53
120 gm	$13.12	Sulfanilamide, Rugby	00536-5400-97
120 gm	$13.30	AVITROL VAGINAL, Major Pharms	00904-2264-22
120 gm	$29.46	AVC, Hoechst Marion Roussel	00068-0099-04

HOW SUPPLIED - NOT RATED EQUIVALENT:

Powder

120 gm	$21.00	Sulfanilamide, Millgood	53118-0611-04

Suppository - Vaginal - 1.05 gm

16's	$32.10	AVC, Hoechst Marion Roussel	00068-0098-16

SULFASALAZINE *(002292)*

CATEGORIES: Anti-Infectives; Anti-Inflammatory Agents; Antibacterials; Antimicrobials; Colitis; Gastrointestinal Drugs; Sulfonamides; Ulcerative Colitis; Arthritis*; Pregnancy Category B; FDA Approval Pre 1982
* Indication not approved by the FDA

BRAND NAMES: Azaline; **Azulfidine**; *Colo-Pleon*; *Salazopyrin*; *Salisulf*; *Saridine*; *Sulfazine*; *Ulcol*
(International brand names outside U.S. in italics)

FORMULARIES: Aetna; BC-BS; DoD; FHP; Medi-Cal; PCS; WHO

COST OF THERAPY: $156.80 (Ulcerative Colitis; Tablet; 500 mg; 4/day; 365 days)

DESCRIPTION:

Tablets: Azulfidine Tablets, (sulfasalazine tablets, USP), 500 mg, for Oral Administration.

Delayed Release Tablets : Azulfidine EN-tabs, (sulfasalazine delayed release tablets, USP), Enteric coated, 500 mg. for Oral Administration.

Azulfidine EN-tabs are film coated with cellulose acetate phthalate to prevent disintegration of the tablet in the stomach and thus reduce possible irritation of the gastric mucosa.

Therapeutic classification: Anti-inflammatory agent.

Chemical designation: 5-([p-(2-Pyridylsulfamoyl)phenyl]azo) salicylic acid.

CLINICAL PHARMACOLOGY:

After oral administration, sulfasalazine is partially absorbed and extensively metabolized as described below.

About one-third of a given dose of sulfasalazine (SS) is absorbed from the small intestine. The remaining two-thirds pass to the colon where the compound is split (presumably by intestinal bacteria) into its components, 5-aminosalicylic acid (5-ASA) and sulfapyridine (SP). Most of the SP thus liberated is absorbed, whereas only about one-third of the 5-ASA is absorbed, the remainder being excreted in the feces. The distribution, metabolism and excretion of SS and its two components are as follows:

SULFASALAZINE (SS)

Detectable serum concentrations of SS have been found in healthy subjects within 90 minutes after the ingestion of a single 2 g dose of sulfasalazine tablets and sulfasalazine EN-tabs. Small amounts of SS are excreted unchanged in the urine.

Tablets: Maximum concentrations of SS occur between 1.5 and 6 hours, with the mean peak concentration (14 mcg/ml) occurring at 3 hours.

Delayed Release Tablets: Maximum concentrations of SS occur between 3 and 12 hours, with the mean peak concentration (6 mcg/ml) occurring at 6 hours.

SULFAPYRIDINE (SP)

Following absorption and distribution, SP is acetylated and hydroxylated in the liver, and then conjugated with glucuronic acid.

Tablets: After ingestion of a single 2 g dose of sulfasalazine tablets by healthy subjects, SP and its various metabolites appear in the serum within 3 to 6 hours. Maximum concentrations of total SP occur between 6 and 24 hours, with the mean peak concentration (21 mcg/ml) occurring at 12 hours. The total recovery of SS and its SP metabolites from the urine of healthy subjects 3 days after administration of a single 2 g dose of sulfasalazine tablets averaged 91%.

Delayed Release Tablets : After ingestion of a single 2 g dose of sulfasalazine EN-tabs by healthy subjects peak concentrations of SP and its various metabolites appear in the serum between 12 and 24 hours, with peak concentrations (13 mcg/ml) occurring at 12 and lasting until 24 hours. The total recovery of SS and its SP metabolites from the urine of healthy subjects 3 days after the administration of a single 2 g dose of sulfasalazine EN-tabs averaged 81%.

5-aminosalicylic acid (5-ASA): The serum concentration of 5-ASA in patients with ulcerative colitis was found to range from 0 to 4μ/ml, and to exist mainly in the form of free 5-ASA. The urinary recovery of this compound was mostly in the acetylated form.

Mean serum concentrations of total SP, *i.e.*, SP and its metabolites, tend to be significantly greater in patients with a slow acetylator phenotype than in those with a fast acetylator phenotype. Total serum sulfapyridine concentrations greater than 50 μ/ml appear to be associated with an increased incidence of adverse reactions.

The mode of action of sulfasalazine is still under investigation. It may be related to the immunosuppressant properties that have been observed in animal and *in vitro* models, to its affinity for connective tissue, and/or to the relatively high concentration it reaches in serous fluids, the liver and intestinal walls, as demonstrated in autoradiographic studies in animals. Sulfasalazine has also been described as a highly efficient vehicle for carrying its principal metabolites, SP and 5-ASA, to the colon, where a local action for both of them has been postulated. Recent clinical studies utilizing rectal administration of SS, SP and 5-ASA have indicated that the major therapeutic action may reside in the 5-ASA moiety.

INDICATIONS AND USAGE:

Sulfasalazine is indicated:

a. in the treatment of mild to moderate ulcerative colitis, and as adjunctive therapy in severe ulcerative colitis.

b. for the prolongation of the remission period between acute attacks of ulcerative colitis.

Delayed Release Tablets: Sulfasalazine EN-tabs are particularly indicated in patients who cannot take the regular sulfasalazine tablet because of gastrointestinal intolerance, and in whom there is evidence that this intolerance is not primarily due to high blood levels of sulfapyridine and its metabolites, e.g. patients experiencing nausea, vomiting, etc., when taking the first few doses of the drug or patients in whom a reduction in dosage does not alleviate the gastrointestinal side effects.

CONTRAINDICATIONS:

Hypersensitivity to sulfasalazine, its metabolites, sulfonamides or salicylates. In infants under two years of age. Intestinal and urinary obstruction. Patients with porphyria should not receive sulfonamides as these drugs have been reported to precipitate an acute attack.

WARNINGS:

Only after critical appraisal should sulfasalazine be used in patients with hepatic or renal damage or blood dyscrasias. Deaths associated with the administration of sulfasalazine have been reported from hypersensitivity reactions, agranulocytosis, aplastic anemia, other blood dyscrasias, renal and liver damage, irreversible neuromuscular and CNS changes, and fibrosing alveolitis. The presence of clinical signs such as sore throat, fever, pallor, purpura or jaundice may be indications of serious blood disorders. Complete blood counts as well as a urinalysis with careful microscopic examination should be done frequently in patients receiving sulfasalazine. Oligospermia and infertility have been observed in man treated with sulfasalazine. Withdrawal of the drug appears to reverse these effects.

PRECAUTIONS:

GENERAL

Sulfasalazine should be given with caution to patients with severe allergy or bronchial asthma. Adequate fluid intake must be maintained in order to prevent crystalluria and stone formation. Patients with glucose-6 phosphate dehydrogenase deficiency should be observed closely for signs of hemolytic anemia. This reaction is frequently dose related. If toxic or hypersensitivity reactions occur, the drug should be discontinued immediately.

Delayed Release Tablets: Isolated instances have been reported when sulfasalazine EN-tabs have passed, undisintegrated. This may be due to a lack of intestinal esterases in these patients. If this is observed, the administration of sulfasalazine EN-tabs should be discontinued immediately.

INFORMATION FOR THE PATIENT

Patients should be informed of the possibility of adverse reactions and of the need for careful medical supervision. They should also be made aware that ulcerative colitis rarely remits completely, and that the risk of relapse can be substantially reduced by continued administration of sulfasalazine (at a maintenance dosage).

Patients should be instructed to take sulfasalazine in evenly divided doses preferably after meals. Additionally, patients should be advised that sulfasalazine may produce an orange-yellow discoloration of the urine or skin.

LABORATORY TESTS

The progress of the disease during treatment can be evaluated by clinical criteria, including the presence of fever, weight changes, degree and frequency of diarrhea and bleeding as well as by sigmoidoscopy and the evaluation of biopsy samples. The determination of serum sulfapyridine levels may be useful since concentrations greater than 50 mcg/ml appear to be associated with an increased incidence of adverse reactions. Complete blood counts, as well as a urinalysis with careful microscopic examination should be done frequently in patients receiving sulfasalazine.

DRUG/LABORATORY TEST INTERACTIONS

The presence of sulfasalazine or its metabolites in body fluids has not been reported to interfere with laboratory test procedures.

CARCINOGENESIS, MUTAGENESIS, AND IMPAIRMENT OF FERTILITY

There have been no long-term studies of the carcinogenic or mutagenic potential of sulfasalazine. Impairment of male fertility was observed in reproductive studies performed in rats and rabbits at doses up to six times the human dose. Oligospermia and infertility have been described in men treated with sulfasalazine. Withdrawal of the drug appears to reverse these effects(see WARNINGS.)

PREGNANCY CATEGORY B

Teratogenic Effects: Reproduction studies have been performed in rats and rabbits at doses up to 6 times the human dose and have revealed no evidence of impaired female fertility or harm to the fetus due to sulfasalazine.

There are, however, no adequate and well-controlled studies in pregnant women. Because animal reproduction studies are not always predictive of human response, this drug should be used during pregnancy only if clearly needed. A national survey evaluated the outcome of pregnancies associated with inflammatory bowel disease (IBD). In a group of 186 women treated with sulfasalazine alone or sulfasalazine and concomitant steroid therapy, the incidence of fetal morbidity and mortality was comparable to that for 245 untreated IBD pregnancies as well as with population data from the National Center for Health Statistics[1]. Another study of 1,445 pregnancies associated with exposure to sulfonamides in which sulfasalazine was included indicated that this group of drugs appeared to be devoid of any

PRECAUTIONS: *(cont'd)*

association with fetal malformation[2]. A review of the medical literature covering 1,155 pregnancies which occurred in women having ulcerative colitis suggested that the outcome was similar to what was expected in the general population[3].

No clinical studies have been performed which indicate the effect of sulfasalazine on the later growth development and functional maturation of children whose mothers received the drug during pregnancy.

Nonteratogenic Effects: Sulfasalazine and sulfapyridine pass the placental barrier. Although sulfapyridine has been shown to have a poor bilirubin displacing capacity, the potential for kernicterus in newborns should be kept in mind.

A case of agranulocytosis has been reported in an infant whose mother was taking both sulfasalazine and prednisone throughout pregnancy.

NURSING MOTHERS

Caution should be exercised when sulfasalazine is administered to a nursing woman. Sulfonamides are excreted in the milk. In the newborn, they compete with bilirubin for binding sites on the plasma proteins and may thus cause kernicterus. Insignificant amounts of uncleaved sulfasalazine have been found in milk, whereas the sulfapyridine levels in milk are about 30-60 percent of those in the serum. Sulfapyridine has been shown to have a poor bilirubin displacing capacity.

PEDIATRIC USE

Safety and effectiveness in children below the age of two years have not been established.

DRUG INTERACTIONS:

Reduced absorption of folic acid and digoxin have been reported when administered concomitantly with sulfasalazine.

ADVERSE REACTIONS:

The most common adverse reactions associated with sulfasalazine are anorexia, headache, nausea, vomiting, gastric distress and apparently reversible oligospermia. These occur in about one-third of the patients. Less frequent adverse reactions are skin rash, pruritus, urticaria, fever, Heinz body anemia, hemolytic anemia and cyanosis which may occur at a frequency of one in every thirty patients or less. Experience suggests that with a daily dosage of 4 g or more, or total serum sulfapyridine levels above 50 mcg/ml, the incidence of adverse reactions tends to increase.

Although the listing which follows includes a few adverse reactions which have not been reported with this specific drug, the pharmacological similarities among the sulfonamides require that each of these reactions be considered when sulfasalazine is administered.

Other adverse reactions which occur rarely, in approximately 1 in 1000 patients or less are:

Blood dyscrasias: aplastic anemia, agranulocytosis, leukopenia, megaloblastic (macrocytic) anemia, purpura, thrombocytopenia, hypoprothrombinemia, methemoglobinemia, congenital neutropenia, and myelodysplastic syndrome.

Hypersensitivity reactions: erythema multiforme (Stevens-Johnson syndrome), exfoliative dermatitis, epidermal necrolysis (Lyell's syndrome) with corneal damage, anaphylaxis, serum sickness syndrome, pneumonitis with or without eosinophilia, vasculitis, fibrosing alveolitis, pleuritis, pericarditis with or without tamponade, allergic myocarditis, polyarteritis nodosa, L.E. syndrome, hepatitis and hepatic necrosis with or without immune complexes, parapsoriasis varioliformis acuta (Mucha-Habermann syndrome), rhabdomyolysis, photosensitization, arthralgia, periorbital edema, conjunctival and scleral injection and alopecia.

Gastrointestinal reactions: hepatitis, pancreatitis, bloody diarrhea, impaired folic acid absorption, impaired digoxin absorption, stomatitis, diarrhea, abdominal pains, and neutropenic enterocolitis.

CNS reactions: transverse myelitis, convulsions, meningitis, transient lesions of the posterior spinal column, cauda equina syndrome, Guillain-Barre syndrome, peripheral neuropathy, mental depression, vertigo, hearing loss, insomnia, ataxia, hallucinations, tinnitus and drowsiness.

Renal reactions: toxic nephrosis with oliguria and anuria, nephritis, nephrotic syndrome, hematuria, crystalluria, proteinuria, and hemolytic-uremic syndrome.

Other reactions: urine discoloration and skin discoloration.

The sulfonamides bear certain chemical similarities to some goitrogens, diuretics (acetazolamide and the thiazides), and oral hypoglycemic agents. Goiter production, diuresis and hypoglycemia have occurred rarely in patients receiving sulfonamides. Cross-sensitivity may exist with these agents. Rats appear to be especially susceptible to the goitrogenic effects of sulfonamides and long-term administration has produced thyroid malignancies in the species.

DRUG ABUSE AND DEPENDENCE:

None reported.

OVERDOSAGE:

There is evidence that the incidence and severity of toxicity are directly related to the total serum sulfapyridine concentration. Symptoms of overdosage may include nausea, vomiting, gastric distress and abdominal pains. In more advanced cases, CNS symptoms such as drowsiness, convulsions, etc. may be observed. Serum sulfapyridine concentrations may be used to monitor the progress of recovery from overdosage.

Experience suggests that with a daily dosage of 4 g or more or total serum sulfapyridine levels above 50 mcg/ml the incidence of adverse reactions tends to increase. There are no documented reports of deaths due to ingestion of large single doses of sulfasalazine.

It has not been possible to determine the oral LD_{50}in laboratory animals such as mice, since the highest daily oral dose which can be given (12 g/kg) is not lethal. Doses of sulfasalazine of 16 g per day have been given to patients without mortality.

Instructions for overdosage: Gastric lavage or emesis plus catharsis as indicated. Alkalinize urine. If kidney function is normal, force fluids. If anuria is present, restrict fluids and salt, and treat appropriately. Catheterization of the ureters may be indicated for complete renal blockage by crystals. The low molecular weight of sulfasalazine and its metabolites may facilitate their removal by dialysis. For agranulocytosis, discontinue the drug immediately, hospitalize the patient and institute appropriate therapy.

For hypersensitivity reactions, discontinue treatment immediately. Such reactions may be controlled with antihistamines and, if necessary, systemic corticosteroids. When in the physician's opinion, reinstitution of sulfasalazine is warranted, regimens modeled upon desensitization procedures may be attempted approximately two weeks after sulfasalazine has been discontinued and symptoms have disappeared (see DOSAGE AND ADMINISTRATION.)

DOSAGE AND ADMINISTRATION:

Dosage should be adjusted to each individual's response and tolerance. The drug should be given in evenly divided doses over each 24-hour period; intervals between nighttime doses should not exceed 8 hours, with administration after meals recommended when feasible.

DOSAGE AND ADMINISTRATION: *(cont'd)*

Experience suggests that with daily dosages of 4 g or more, the incidence of adverse reactions tends to increase; hence, patients receiving these dosages should be instructed about and carefully observed for the appearance of adverse effects.

Various desensitization-like regimens have been reported to be effective in 34 of 53 patients[4], 7 of 8 patients[5] and 19 of 20 patients[6]. Upon reinstituting sulfasalazine, such regimens comprise a total daily dose of 50 to 250 mg which, every 4 to 7 days thereafter, is doubled until the desired therapeutic level is achieved. If the symptoms of sensitivity recur, sulfasalazine should be discontinued. Desensitization should not be attempted in patients who have a history of agranulocytosis or who have experienced an anaphylactoid reaction while on previous course of sulfasalazine therapy.

USUAL DOSAGE

Initial Therapy

Adults: 3-4 g daily in evenly divided doses. In some cases it is advisable to initiate therapy with a smaller dosage, *e.g.*, 1-2 g daily, to lessen adverse gastrointestinal effects. If daily doses exceeding 4 g are required to achieve desired effects, the increased risk of toxicity should be kept in mind.

Children, two years of age and older: 40-60 mg per kg body weight in each 24-hour period, divided into 3-6 doses.

Maintenance Therapy

Adults: 2 g daily.

Children, two years of age and older: 30 mg per kg body weight in each 24-hour period, divided into 4 doses.

Response to therapy and adjustment of dosage should be determined by periodic examination. It is often necessary to continue medication, even when clinical symptoms, including diarrhea, have been controlled.

When endoscopic examination confirms satisfactory improvement, dosage is reduced to a maintenance level.

If symptoms of gastric intolerance (anorexia, nausea, vomiting, etc.) occur after the first few doses of sulfasalazine, they are probably due to mucosal irritation and may be alleviated by distributing the total daily dose more evenly over the day or by giving enteric-coated EN-tabs. If diarrhea recurs, dosage should be increased to previously effective levels.

If such symptoms occur after the first few days of treatment with sulfasalazine, they are probably due to increased serum levels of total sulfapyridine, and may be alleviated by halving the dose and subsequently increasing it gradually over several days. If symptoms continue, the drug should be stopped for five to seven days, then reinstituted at a lower daily dose.

Storage: Room Temperature (15-30°C/59-86°F).

REFERENCES:

1. Pregnancy in Inflammatory Bowel Disease: Effect of Sulfasalazine and Corticosteroids on Fetal Outcome. Mogadam, M. et al, Gastroenterology, **80**: 72-76, 1981. **2.** Birth Defects and Drugs During Pregnancy, David W. Kaufman, Editor, Publishing Sciences Group Inc. **3.** Fertility, Sterility and Pregnancy in Chronic Inflammatory Bowel Disease. Jarnerot, G., Scand. J. Gastroenterology,**17**: 1-4, 1982. **4.** Korelitz B. et al: Gastroenterology**82**: 1104, 1982. **5.** Holdsworth, C.G.: Brit. Med. J.**282**:110, 1981. **6.** Taffet, S.L. and Das, K.M.: Amer. J. Med. **73**: 520-524, 1982.(Tablets: Pharmacia Inc., 7/94, 11-B-039-20)(Delayed Release Tablets: Pharmacia Inc., 7/94, 11-B-038-22)

HOW SUPPLIED - RATED THERAPEUTICALLY EQUIVALENT:

Tablet - Oral - 500 mg

100's	$12.51	Sulfasalazine, H.C.F.A. F F P	99999-2292-01

Tablet, Uncoated - Oral - 500 mg

100's	$10.74	Sulfasalazine, US Trading	56126-0306-11
100's	$11.95	Sulfasalazine 500, Harber Pharm	51432-0442-03
100's	$12.75	Sulfasalazine, Consolidated Midland	00223-1727-01
100's	$13.50	AZALINE, Major Pharms	00904-1152-60
100's	$13.50	Sulfasalazine, Mutual Pharm	53489-0147-01
100's	$14.39	Sulfasalazine, Rugby	00536-4617-01
100's	$14.40	Sulfasalazine, Goldline Labs	00182-1016-01
100's	$14.78	Sulfasalazine, HL Moore Drug Exch	00839-6098-06
100's	$14.79	Sulfasalazine, United Res	00677-0483-01
100's	$14.90	Sulfasalazine, Qualitest Pharms	00603-5802-21
100's	$15.55	Sulfasalazine, Aligen Independ	00405-4956-01
100's	**$20.50**	**AZULFIDINE, Pharmacia & Upjohn**	**00013-0101-01**
100's	**$22.94**	**AZULFIDINE, Pharmacia & Upjohn**	**00013-0101-11**
500's	$54.00	Sulfasalazine, IDE-Interstate	00814-7230-28
500's	$57.50	Sulfasalazine, Consolidated Midland	00223-1727-05
500's	$59.75	Sulfasalazine 500, Harber Pharm	51432-0442-05
500's	$60.79	Sulfasalazine, Lederle Pharm	00005-3960-31
500's	$62.00	Sulfasalazine, Mutual Pharm	53489-0147-05
500's	$62.95	AZALINE, Major Pharms	00904-1152-40
500's	$68.00	Sulfasalazine, Schein Pharm (US)	00364-0444-05
500's	$68.00	Sulfasalazine, United Res	00677-0483-05
500's	$68.30	Sulfasalazine, Qualitest Pharms	00603-5802-28
500's	$68.33	Sulfasalazine, Rugby	00536-4617-05
500's	$70.42	Sulfasalazine, Aligen Independ	00405-4956-02
500's	$73.42	Sulfasalazine, HL Moore Drug Exch	00839-6098-12
500's	$76.60	Sulfasalazine, Goldline Labs	00182-1016-05
500's	**$90.25**	**AZULFIDINE, Pharmacia & Upjohn**	**00013-0101-05**
1000's	$97.50	Sulfasalazine, Consolidated Midland	00223-1727-02
1000's	$135.00	Sulfasalazine, Rugby	00536-4617-10

HOW SUPPLIED - NOT RATED EQUIVALENT:

Tablet, Enteric Coated - Oral - 500 mg

100's	**$24.56**	**AZULFIDINE, Pharmacia & Upjohn**	**00013-0102-01**
500's	**$116.06**	**AZULFIDINE, Pharmacia & Upjohn**	**00013-0102-05**

SULFINPYRAZONE *(002293)*

CATEGORIES: Antigout; Antimicrobials; Arthritis; Electrolytic, Caloric-Water Balance; Gout; Gouty Arthritis; Pain; Sulfonamides; Uricosuric Agents; FDA Approval Pre 1982

BRAND NAMES: *Antazone*; *Antiran*; **Anturane**; *Anturano*; *Enturen*; *Falizal*; *Novopyrazone*
(International brand names outside U.S. in italics)

FORMULARIES: Aetna; Medi-Cal

DESCRIPTION:

Sulfinpyrazone USP, is a uricosuric agent available as 100-mg tablets and 200-mg capsules for oral administration. Its chemical name is 1,2-diphenyl-4-(2-(phenylsulfinyl)ethyl)-3,5-pyrazolidinedione.

DESCRIPTION: *(cont'd)*

Sulfinpyrazone USP is a white to off-white powder practically insoluble in water and in solvent hexane, soluble in alcohol and in acetone, and sparingly soluble in dilute alkali. Its molecular weight is 404.48.

Anturane Tablets Inactive Ingredients: Colloidal silicon dioxide, gelatin, lactose, magnesium stearate, starch, stearic acid, and talc.

Anturane Capsules Inactive Ingredients: D&C Red No. 33, D&C Yellow No.10, FD&C Blue No.1, gelatin, lactose, magnesium stearate, methylparaben, propylparaben, silicon dioxide, sodium lauryl sulfate, starch, stearic acid, talc, and titanium dioxide.

CLINICAL PHARMACOLOGY:

Its pharmacologic activity is the potentiation of the urinary excretion of uric acid. It is useful for reducing the blood urate levels in patients with chronic tophaceous gout and acute intermittent gout, and for promoting the resorption of tophi.

INDICATIONS AND USAGE:

Sulfinpyrazone is indicated for the treatment of:

1. Chronic gouty arthritis

2. Intermittent gouty arthritis

CONTRAINDICATIONS:

Patients with an active peptic ulcer or symptoms of gastrointestinal inflammation or ulceration should not receive the drug.

The drug is contraindicated in patients with a history or the presence of:

1. Hypersensitivity to phenylbutazone or other pyrazoles

2. Blood dyscrasias

WARNINGS:

Studies on the teratogenicity of pyrazole compounds in animals have yielded inconclusive results. Up to the present time, however, there have been no reported cases of human congenital malformation proved to be due to the use of the drug.

It is suggested that sulfinpyrazone be used with caution in pregnant women, weighing the potential risks against the possible benefits.

PRECAUTIONS:

As with all pyrazole compounds, patients receiving sulfinpyrazone should be kept under close medical supervision and periodic blood counts are recommended. It may be administered with care to patients with a history of healed peptic ulcer.

Recent reports have indicated that sulfinpyrazone potentiates the action of certain sulfonamides, such as sulfadiazine and sulfisoxazole. In addition, other pyrazole compounds (phenylbutazone) have been observed to potentiate the hypoglycemic sulfonylurea agents, as well as insulin. In view of these observations, it is suggested that sulfinpyrazone be used with caution in conjunction with sulfa drugs, the sulfonylurea hypoglycemic agents and insulin.

Because sulfinpyrazone is a potent uricosuric agent, it may precipitate urolithiasis and renal colic, especially in the initial stages of therapy. For this reason, an adequate fluid intake and alkalinization of the urine are recommended. In cases with significant renal impairment, periodic assessment of renal function is indicated. Occasional cases of renal failure have been reported; but a cause-and-effect relationship has not always been clearly established.

Salicylates antagonize the uricosuric action of sulfinpyrazone and for this reason their concomitant use is contraindicated in gouty arthritis.

Sulfinpyrazone may accentuate the action of coumarin-type anticoagulants and further depress prothrombin activity when these medications are employed simultaneously.

NOTE: Sulfinpyrazone has minimal anti-inflammatory effect and is not intended for the relief of an acute attack of gout.

In the initial stages of therapy, because of the marked ability of sulfinpyrazone to mobilize urates, acute attacks of gouty arthritis may be precipitated.

ADVERSE REACTIONS:

The most frequently reported adverse reactions with sulfinpyrazone have been upper gastrointestinal disturbances. In these patients it is advisable to administer the drug with food, milk, or antacids. Despite this precaution, sulfinpyrazone may aggravate or reactivate peptic ulcer.

Rash has been reported. In most instances, this reaction did not necessitate discontinuance of therapy. In general, sulfinpyrazone has not been observed to affect electrolyte balance.

Blood dyscrasias (anemia, leukopenia, agranulocytosis, thrombocytopenia, and aplastic anemia) have rarely been reported. There has also been a published report associating sulfinpyrazone administered concomitantly with other drugs including colchicine, with leukemia following long-term treatment of patients with gout. However, the circumstances involved in the two cases reported are such that a cause-and-effect relationship to sulfinpyrazone has not been clearly established.

OVERDOSAGE:

Symptoms: Nausea, vomiting, diarrhea, epigastric pain, ataxia, labored respiration convulsions, coma. Possible symptoms, seen after overdosage with other pyrazolone derivatives: anemia, jaundice, ulceration.

Treatment: No specific antidote. Induce emesis; gastric lavage; supportive treatment (intravenous glucose infusions, analeptics).

DOSAGE AND ADMINISTRATION:

Initial: 200-400 mg daily in two divided doses, with meals or milk, gradually increasing when necessary to full maintenance dosage in one week.

Maintenance: 400 mg daily, given in two divided doses, as above. This dosage may be increased to 800 mg daily. If necessary, and may sometimes be reduced to as low as 200 mg daily after the blood urate level has been controlled. Treatment should be continued without interruption even in the presence of acute exacerbations, which can be concomitantly treated with phenylbutazone or colchicine. Patients previously controlled with other uricosuric therapy may be transferred to sulfinpyrazone at full maintenance dosage.

HOW SUPPLIED - RATED THERAPEUTICALLY EQUIVALENT:

Capsule, Gelatin - Oral - 200 mg

100's	$16.43	Sulfinpyrazone, H.C.F.A. F F P	99999-2293-01
100's	$19.50	Sulfinpyrazone, Geneva Pharms	00781-2300-01
100's	$22.50	Sulfinpyrazone, Voluntary Hosp	53258-0419-01
100's	$23.95	Sulfinpyrazone, Harber Pharm	51432-0434-03
100's	$25.77	Sulfinpyrazone, HL Moore Drug Exch	00839-6638-06
100's	$26.06	Sulfinpyrazone, Rugby	00536-4616-01
100's	$27.80	APRAZONE, Major Pharms	00904-1187-60
100's	$28.48	Sulfinpyrazone, Barr	00555-0272-02

HOW SUPPLIED - RATED THERAPEUTICALLY EQUIVALENT: *(cont'd)*

100's	$28.62	Sulfinpyrazone, Qualitest Pharms	00603-5826-21
100's	$36.00	Sulfinpyrazone, Voluntary Hosp	53258-0419-13
100's	$38.71	Sulfinpyrazone, Schein Pharm (US)	00364-0652-01
100's	$38.75	Sulfinpyrazone, Zenith Labs	00172-2969-60
100's	$38.75	Sulfinpyrazone, Goldline Labs	00182-1544-01
100's	$38.75	Sulfinpyrazone, Aligen Independ	00405-4962-01
100's	$38.75	Sulfinpyrazone, HL Moore Drug Exch	00839-7891-06
100's	**$54.80**	**ANTURANE, Novartis**	**00083-0168-30**
500's	$82.15	Sulfinpyrazone, H.C.F.A. F F P	99999-2293-02
500's	$86.93	Sulfinpyrazone, HL Moore Drug Exch	00839-6638-12
500's	$106.80	APRAZONE, Major Pharms	00904-1187-40
500's	$109.55	Sulfinpyrazone, HL Moore Drug Exch	00839-7891-12
500's	$121.99	Sulfinpyrazone, Barr	00555-0272-04
500's	$187.50	Sulfinpyrazone, Zenith Labs	00172-2969-70
1000's	$164.30	Sulfinpyrazone, H.C.F.A. F F P	99999-2293-03
1000's	$187.50	Sulfinpyrazone, Zenith Labs	00172-2969-80

Tablet, Uncoated - Oral - 100 mg

100's	$12.10	Sulfinpyrazone, Harber Pharm	51432-0433-03
100's	$12.53	Sulfinpyrazone, HL Moore Drug Exch	00839-6604-06
100's	$13.22	Sulfinpyrazone, Barr	00555-0271-02
100's	$13.80	Sulfinpyrazone, Geneva Pharms	00781-1160-01
100's	$13.92	Sulfinpyrazone, H.C.F.A. F F P	99999-2293-04
100's	$14.65	Sulfinpyrazone, Goldline Labs	00182-1426-01
100's	$14.65	Sulfinpyrazone Tablets 100 Mg, Aligen Independ	00405-4961-01
100's	$14.75	Sulfinpyrazone, United Res	00677-0781-01
100's	$14.80	APRAZONE, Major Pharms	00904-1186-60
100's	**$34.04**	**ANTURANE, Novartis**	**00083-0041-30**
500's	$69.60	Sulfinpyrazone, H.C.F.A. F F P	99999-2293-05

SULFISOXAZOLE *(002294)*

CATEGORIES: Anti-Infectives; Antibacterials; Antimicrobials; Chancroid; Conjunctivitis; Corneal Ulcer; EENT Drugs; Eye, Ear, Nose, & Throat Preparations; Inclusion Conjunctivitis; Malaria; Meningitis; Nocardiosis; Ocular Infections; Ophthalmics; Otitis Media; Pyelitis; Pyelonephritis; Sulfonamides; Topical; Toxoplasmosis; Trachoma; Urinary Antibacterial; Urinary Tract Infections; Pregnancy Category C; FDA Approval Pre 1982

BRAND NAMES: **Gantrisin**; Gulfasin; *Isoxazine*; Lipo Gantrisin; *Novosoxazole*; *Oxazole*; Sosol; Soxa; Sulfalar; *Sulfazin*; *Sulfazole*; *Sulphafurazole*; Sulsoxin; *Thiasin*; Truxazole; *Urazole*
(International brand names outside U.S. in italics)

FORMULARIES: Aetna; BC-BS; FHP; Medi-Cal; PCS

DESCRIPTION:

Sulfisoxazole is an antibacterial sulfonamide available in tablets, pediatric suspension and syrup for oral administration. Each tablet contains 0.5 g sulfisoxazole with corn starch, gelatin, lactose and magnesium stearate. Each teaspoonful (5 ml) of the pediatric suspension contains the equivalent of approximately 0.5 g sulfisoxazole in the form of acetyl sulfisoxazole in a vehicle containing 0.3 percent alcohol, carboxymethylcellulose (sodium), citric acid, methylcellulose, parabens (methyl and propyl), partial invert sugar, sodium citrate, sorbitan monolaurate, sucrose, flavors and water. Each teaspoonful (5 ml) of the syrup contains the equivalent of approximately 0.5 g sulfisoxazole in the form of acetyl sulfisoxazole in a vehicle containing 0.9 percent alcohol, benzoic acid, carrageenan, citric acid, cocoa, sodium citrate, sorbitan monolaurate, sucrose, flavors and water.

Sulfisoxazole is N^1-(3,4-dimethyl-5-isoxazolyl) sulfanilamide. It is a white to slightly yellowish, odorless, slightly bitter, crystalline powder that is soluble in alcohol and very slightly soluble in water. Sulfisoxazole has a molecular weight of 267.30.

Acetyl sulfisoxazole, the tasteless form of sulfisoxazole, is N^1-acetyl sulfisoxazole and must be distinguished from N^4-acetyl sulfisoxazole, which is a metabolite of sulfisoxazole. Acetyl sulfisoxazole is a white or slightly yellow, crystalline powder that is slightly soluble in alcohol and practically insoluble in water. Acetyl sulfisoxazole has a molecular weight of 309.34.

CLINICAL PHARMACOLOGY:

Following oral administration, sulfisoxazole is rapidly and completely absorbed; the small intestine is the major site of absorption, but some of the drug is absorbed from the stomach. Sulfisoxazole exists in the blood as unbound, protein-bound and conjugated forms. Sulfisoxazole is metabolized primarily by acetylation and oxidation in the liver. The free form is considered to be the therapeutically active form. Approximately 85% of sulfisoxazole is bound to plasma proteins, primarily to albumin; of the unbound portion, 65% to 72% is in the nonacetylated form.

Maximum plasma concentrations of intact sulfisoxazole following a single 2-g oral dose of sulfisoxazole to healthy adult volunteers ranged from 127 to 211 mcg/ml (mean, 169 mcg/ml) and the time of peak plasma concentration ranged from 1 to 4 hours (mean, 2.5 hours). The half-life of elimination of sulfisoxazole ranged from 4.6 to 7.8 hours after oral administration. The elimination of sulfisoxazole has been shown to be slower in elderly subjects (63 to 75 years) with diminished renal function (creatinine clearance, 37 to 68 ml/min).[1] After multiple dose oral administration of 500 mg Q.I.D. to healthy volunteers, the average steady-state plasma concentrations of intact sulfisoxazole ranged from 49.9 to 88.8 mcg/ml (mean, 63.4 mcg/ml).[2]

Wide variation in blood levels may result following identical doses of a sulfonamide. Blood levels should be measured in patients receiving sulfonamides at the higher recommended doses or being treated for serious infections. Free sulfonamide blood levels of 50 to 150 mcg/ml may be considered therapeutically effective for most infections, with blood levels of 120 to 150 mcg/ml being optimal for serious infections. The maximum sulfonamide level should not exceed 200 mcg/ml, since adverse reactions occur more frequently above this concentration.

N^1-acetyl sulfisoxazole is metabolized to sulfisoxazole by digestive enzymes in the gastrointestinal tract and is absorbed as sulfisoxazole. This enzymatic splitting is presumed to be responsible for slower absorption and lower peak blood concentrations than are attained following administration of an equal oral dose of sulfisoxazole. With continued administration of acetyl sulfisoxazole, blood concentrations approximate those of sulfisoxazole. Following a single 4-g dose of acetyl sulfisoxazole to healthy volunteers, maximum plasma concentrations of sulfisoxazole ranged from 122 to 282 mcg/ml (mean, 181 mcg/ml) for the pediatric suspension and from 101 to 202 mcg/ml (mean, 144 mcg/ml) for the syrup, and occurred between 2 and 6 hours postadministration. The half-lives of elimination from plasma ranged from 5.4 to 7.4 and from 5.9 to 8.5 hours, respectively.

Sulfisoxazole and acetylated metabolites are excreted primarily by the kidneys through glomerular filtration. Concentrations of sulfisoxazole are considerably higher in the urine than in the blood. The mean urinary excretion recovery following oral administration of sulfisox-

CLINICAL PHARMACOLOGY: *(cont'd)*

azole is 97% within 48 hours, of which 52% is intact drug, with the remaining as the N^4-acetylated metabolite. Following administration of acetyl sulfisoxazole syrup or suspension, approximately 58% is excreted in the urine as total drug within 72 hours.

Sulfisoxazole is distributed only in extracellular body water. It is excreted in human milk. It readily crosses the placental barrier and enters into fetal circulation and also crosses the blood-brain barrier. In healthy subjects, cerebrospinal fluid concentrations of sulfisoxazole vary; in patients with meningitis, however, concentrations of free drug as high as 94 mcg/ml have been reported.

MICROBIOLOGY

The sulfonamides are bacteriostatic agents and the spectrum of activity is similar for all. Sulfonamides inhibit bacterial synthesis of dihydrofolic acid by preventing the condensation of the pteridine with aminobenzoic acid through competitive inhibition of the enzyme dihydropteroate synthetase. Resistant strains have altered dihydropteroate synthetase with reduced affinity for sulfonamides or produce increased quantities of aminobenzoic acid.

SUSCEPTIBILITY TESTING

Diffusion Techniques: Quantitative methods that require measurement of zone diameters give the most precise estimate of the susceptibility of bacteria to antimicrobial agents. One such standard procedure[3] which has been recommended for use with disks to test susceptibility of organisms to sulfisoxazole uses the 250- or 300-mcg sulfisoxazole disk. Interpretation involves the correlation of the diameter obtained in the disk test with the minimum inhibitory concentration (MIC) for sulfisoxazole.

Reports from the laboratory giving results of the standard single-disk susceptibility test with a 250- or 300-mcg sulfisoxazole disk should be interpreted according to the following criteria:

TABLE 1

Zone Diameter (mm)	Interpretation
≥17	Susceptible
13-16	Moderately Susceptible
≤12	Resistant

A report of "susceptible" indicates that the pathogen is likely to be inhibited by generally achievable blood levels. A report of "moderately susceptible" suggests that the organism would be susceptible if high dosage is used or if the infection is confined to tissues and fluids in which high antimicrobial levels are attained. A report of "resistant" indicates that achievable concentrations are unlikely to be inhibitory, and other therapy should be selected.

Standardized procedures require the use of laboratory control organisms. The 250- or 300-mcg sulfisoxazole disk should give the following zone diameters:

TABLE 2

Organism	Zone Diameter (mm)
E. coli ATCC 25922	16-26 mm
S. aureus ATCC 25923	24-34 mm

Dilution Techniques: Use a standard dilution method[4] (broth, agar, microdilution) or equivalent with sulfisoxazole powder. The MIC values obtained should be interpreted according to the following criteria:

TABLE 3

MIC (mcg/ml)	Interpretation
≤256	Susceptible
≥512	Resistant

As with standard diffusion techniques, dilution methods require the use of laboratory control organisms. Dilutions of standard sulfisoxazole powder should provide the following MIC values:

TABLE 4

Organism	MIC/)mcg/ml)
S. aureus ATCC 29213	32-128
E. faecalis ATCC 29212	32-128
E. coli ATCC 25922	8-32

INDICATIONS AND USAGE:

Acute, recurrent or chronic urinary tract infections (primarily pyelonephritis, pyelitis and cystitis) due to susceptible organisms (usually *Escherichia coli, Klebsiella-Enterobacter*, staphylococcus, *Proteus mirabilis* and, less frequently,*Proteus vulgaris*) in the absence of obstructive uropathy or foreign bodies.

Meningococcal meningitis where the organism has been demonstrated to be susceptible. *Haemophilus influenzae* meningitis as adjunctive therapy with parenteral streptomycin.

Meningococcal meningitis prophylaxis when sulfonamide-sensitive group A strains are known to prevail in family groups or larger closed populations. (The prophylactic usefulness of sulfonamides when group B or C infections are prevalent has not been proven and in closed population groups may be harmful.)

Acute otitis media due to *Haemophilus influenzae* when used concomitantly with adequate doses of penicillin or erythromycin (see appropriate labeling for prescribing information).

Trachoma. Inclusion conjunctivitis. Nocardiosis. Chancroid. Toxoplasmosis as adjunctive therapy with pyrimethamine. Malaria due to chloroquine-resistant strains of *Plasmodium falciparum,* when used as adjunctive therapy.

Currently, the increasing frequency of resistant organisms is a limitation of the usefulness of antibacterial agents including the sulfonamides, especially in the treatment of chronic and recurrent urinary tract infections.

Important Note: *In vitro* sulfonamide susceptibility tests are not always reliable. The test must be carefully coordinated with bacteriologic and clinical response. When the patient is already taking sulfonamides, follow-up cultures should have aminobenzoic acid added to the culture media.

CONTRAINDICATIONS:

Sulfisoxazole is contraindicated in the following patient populations: patients with a known hypersensitivity to sulfonamides; children younger than 2 months (except in the treatment of congenital toxoplasmosis as adjunctive therapy with pyrimethamine); pregnant women *at term*; and mothers nursing infants less than 2 months of age.

Use in pregnant women at term, in children less than 2 months of age and in mothers nursing infants less than 2 months of age is contraindicated because sulfonamides may promote kernicterus in the newborn by displacing bilirubin from plasma proteins.

WARNINGS:

FATALITIES ASSOCIATED WITH THE ADMINISTRATION OF SULFONAMIDES, ALTHOUGH RARE, HAVE OCCURRED DUE TO SEVERE REACTIONS, INCLUDING STEVENS-JOHNSON SYNDROME, TOXIC EPIDERMAL NECROLYSIS, FULMINANT HEPATIC NECROSIS, AGRANULOCYTOSIS, APLASTIC ANEMIA AND OTHER BLOOD DYSCRASIAS.

SULFONAMIDES, INCLUDING SULFISOXAZOLE, SHOULD BE DISCONTINUED AT THE FIRST APPEARANCE OF SKIN RASH OR ANY SIGN OF AN ADVERSE REACTION. In rare instances, a skin rash may be followed by more severe reactions such as Stevens-Johnson syndrome, toxic epidermal necrolysis, hepatic necrosis and serious blood disorders. (See PRECAUTIONS.)

Clinical signs such as rash, sore throat, fever, arthralgia, pallor, purpura or jaundice may be early indications of serious reactions.

Cough, shortness of breath and pulmonary infiltrates are hypersensitivity reactions of the respiratory tract that have been reported in association with sulfonamide treatment.

The sulfonamides should not be used for the treatment of group A beta-hemolytic streptococcal infections. In an established infection, they will not eradicate the streptococcus, and therefore, will not prevent sequelae such as rheumatic fever.

Pseudomembranous colitis has been reported with nearly all antibacterial agents, including sulfisoxazole, and may range in severity from mild to life-threatening. Therefore, it is important to consider this diagnosis in patients who present with diarrhea subsequent to the administration of antibacterial agents.

Treatment with antibacterial agents alters the normal flora of the colon and may permit overgrowth of clostridia. Studies indicate that toxin produced by *Clostridium difficile* is one primary cause of "antibiotic-associated colitis."

After the diagnosis of pseudomembranous colitis has been established, therapeutic measures should be initiated. Mild cases of pseudomembranous colitis usually respond to drug discontinuation alone. In moderate to severe cases, consideration should be given to management with fluids and electrolytes, protein supplementation, and treatment with an antibacterial drug clinically effective against*C. difficile* colitis.

PRECAUTIONS:

GENERAL

Sulfonamides should be given with caution to patients with impaired renal or hepatic function and to those with severe allergy or bronchial asthma. In glucose-6-phosphate dehydrogenase-deficient individuals, hemolysis may occur; this reaction is frequently dose-related.

The frequency of resistant organisms limits the usefulness of antibacterial agents, including the sulfonamides, as sole therapy in the treatment of urinary tract infections. Since sulfonamides are bacteriostatic and not bactericidal, a complete course of therapy is needed to prevent immediate regrowth and the development of resistant uropathogens.

INFORMATION FOR THE PATIENT

Patients should maintain an adequate fluid intake to prevent crystalluria and stone formation.

LABORATORY TESTS

Complete blood counts should be done frequently in patients receiving sulfonamides. If a significant reduction in the count of any formed blood element is noted, sulfisoxazole should be discontinued. Urinalyses with careful microscopic examination and renal function tests should be performed during therapy, particularly for those patients with impaired renal function. Blood levels should be measured in patients receiving a sulfonamide for serious infections. (See INDICATIONS AND USAGE.)

CARCINOGENESIS, MUTAGENESIS, AND IMPAIRMENT OF FERTILITY

Carcinogenesis: Sulfisoxazole was not carcinogenic in either sex when administered by gavage for 103 weeks at dosages up to approximately 18 times the highest recommended human daily dose or to rats at 4 times the highest recommended human daily dose. Rats appear to be especially susceptible to the goitrogenic effects of sulfonamides and long-term administration of sulfonamides has resulted in thyroid malignancies in this species.

Mutagenesis: There are no studies available that adequately evaluate the mutagenic potential of sulfisoxazole. Ames mutagenic assays have not been performed with sulfisoxazole. However, sulfisoxazole was not observed to be mutagenic in *E. coli* Sd-4-73 when tested in the absence of a metabolic activating system.

Impairment of Fertility: Sulfisoxazole has not undergone adequate trials relating to impairment of fertility. In a reproduction study in rats given 7 times the highest recommended human dose per day of sulfisoxazole, no effects were observed regarding mating behavior, conception rate or fertility index (percent pregnant).

PREGNANCY CATEGORY C

Teratogenic Effects: At dosages 7 times the highest recommended human daily dose, sulfisoxazole was not teratogenic in either rats or rabbits. However, in two other teratogenicity studies, cleft palates developed in both rats and mice, and skeletal defects were also observed in rats after administration of 9 times the highest recommended human daily dose of sulfisoxazole.

There are no adequate and well-controlled studies of sulfisoxazole in pregnant women. Sulfisoxazole should be used during pregnancy only if the potential benefit justifies the potential risk to the fetus.

Nonteratogenic Effects: Kernicterus may occur in the newborn as a result of treatment of a pregnant woman *at term* with sulfonamides. (See CONTRAINDICATIONS.)

NURSING MOTHERS

Sulfisoxazole is excreted in human milk. Because of the potential for the development of kernicterus in neonates due to the displacement of bilirubin from plasma proteins by sulfisoxazole, a decision should be made whether to discontinue nursing or discontinue the drug taking into account the importance of the drug to the mother. (See CONTRAINDICATIONS.)

PEDIATRIC USE

Sulfisoxazole is not recommended for use in infants younger than 2 months of age except in the treatment of congenital toxoplasmosis as adjunctive therapy with pyrimethamine. (See CONTRAINDICATIONS.)

DRUG INTERACTIONS:

It has been reported that sulfisoxazole may prolong the prothrombin time in patients who are receiving the anticoagulant warfarin. This interaction should be kept in mind when sulfisoxazole is given to patients already on anticoagulant therapy, and prothrombin time or other suitable coagulation test should be monitored.

It has been proposed that sulfisoxazole competes with thiopental for plasma protein binding. In one study involving 48 patients, intravenous sulfisoxazole reduced the amount of thiopental required for anesthesia and shortened the awakening time. It is not known whether chronic oral doses of sulfisoxazole would have a similar effect. Until more is known about this interaction, physicians should be aware that patients receiving sulfisoxazole might require less thiopental for anesthesia.

DRUG INTERACTIONS: *(cont'd)*

Sulfonamides can displace methotrexate from plasma protein-binding sites, thus increasing free methotrexate concentrations. Studies in man have shown sulfisoxazole infusions to decrease plasma protein-bound methotrexate by one-fourth.

Sulfisoxazole can also potentiate the blood sugar lowering activity of sulfonylureas, as well as cause hypoglycemia by itself.

ADVERSE REACTIONS:

The listing that follows includes adverse reactions both that have been reported with sulfisoxazole and some which have not been reported with this specific drug; however, the pharmacologic similarities among the sulfonamides require that each of the reactions be considered with the administration of any of the sulfisoxazole dosage forms.

Allergic/Dermatologic: Anaphylaxis, erythema multiforme (Stevens- Johnson syndrome), toxic epidermal necrolysis, exfoliative dermatitis, angioedema, arteritis and vasculitis, allergic myocarditis, serum sickness, rash, urticaria, pruritus, photosensitivity, and conjunctival and scleral injection, generalized allergic reactions and generalized skin eruptions. In addition, periarteritis nodosa and systemic lupus erythematosus have been reported. (See WARNINGS.)

Cardiovascular: Tachycardia, palpitations, syncope, cyanosis.

Endocrine: The sulfonamides bear certain chemical similarities to some goitrogens, diuretics (acetazolamide and thiazides) and oral hypoglycemia agents. Cross-sensitivity may exist with these agents. Development of goiter, diuresis and hypoglycemia have occurred rarely in patients receiving sulfonamides.

Gastrointestinal: Hepatitis, hepatocellular necrosis, jaundice, pseudomembranous colitis, nausea, emesis, anorexia, abdominal pain, diarrhea, gastrointestinal hemorrhage, melena, flatulence, glossitis, stomatitis, salivary gland enlargement, pancreatitis.

Onset of pseudomembranous colitis symptoms may occur during or after treatment with sulfisoxazole. (See WARNINGS.)

Sulfisoxazole has been reported to cause increased elevations of liver-associated enzymes in patients with hepatitis.

Genitourinary: Crystalluria, hematuria, BUN and creatine elevations, nephritis and toxic nephrosis with oliguria and anuria. Acute renal failure and urinary retention have also been reported. The frequency of renal complications, commonly associated with some sulfonamides, is lower in patients receiving the more soluble sulfonamides such as sulfisoxazole.

Hematologic: Leukopenia, agranulocytosis, aplastic anemia, thrombocytopenia, purpura, hemolyticanemia, anemia, eosinophilia, clotting disorders including hypoprothrombinemia, and hypofibrinogenemia, sulfhemoglobinemia, methemoglobinemia.

Musculoskeletal: Arthralgia, myalgia.

Neurologic: Headache, dizziness, peripheral neuritis, paresthesia, convulsions, tinnitus, vertigo, ataxia, intracranial hypertension.

Psychiatric: Psychosis, hallucination, disorientation, depression, anxiety, apathy.

Respiratory: Cough, shortness of breath, pulmonary infiltrates. (See WARNINGS.)

Vascular: Angioedema, arteritis, vasculitis.

Miscellaneous: Edema (including periorbital), pyrexia, drowsiness, weakness, fatigue, lassitude, rigors, flushing, hearing loss, insomnia, pneumonitis, chills.

OVERDOSAGE:

The amount of a single dose of sulfisoxazole that is either associated with symptoms of overdosage or is likely to be life-threatening has not been reported. Signs and symptoms of overdosage reported with sulfonamides include anorexia, colic, nausea, vomiting, dizziness, headache, drowsiness and unconsciousness. Pyrexia, hematuria and crystalluria may be noted. Blood dyscrasias and jaundice are potential late manifestations of overdosage.

General principles of treatment include the immediate discontinuation of the drug; institution of gastric lavage or emesis; forcing oral fluids; and the administration of intravenous fluids if urine output is low and renal function is normal. The patient should be monitored with blood counts and appropriate blood chemistries, including electrolytes. If a significant blood dyscrasia or jaundice occurs, specific therapy should be instituted for these complications. Peritoneal dialysis is not effective and hemodialysis is only moderately effective in eliminating sulfonamides.

DOSAGE AND ADMINISTRATION:

Systemic sulfonamides are contraindicated in infants under 2 months of age, except in the treatment of congenital toxoplasmosis as adjunctive therapy with pyrimethamine.

Usual Dose for Infants over 2 Months of Age and Children: *Initial Dose:* One-half of the 24-hour dose. *Maintenance Dose:* 150 mg/kg/24 hours or 4 g/M²/24 hours—dose to be divided into 4 to 6 doses/24 hours. The maximum dose should not exceed 6 g/24 hours.

Usual Adult Dose: *Initial Dose:* 2 to 4 g. *Maintenance Dose:* 4 to 8 g/24 hours, divided in 4 to 6 doses/24 hours.

REFERENCES:

1. Boisvert A, Barbeau G, Belanger PM: Pharmacokinetics of sulfisoxazole in young and elderly subjects.*Gerontology.* 1984;30 125-131. **2.** Oie S, Gambertoglio JG, Fleckenstein L: Comparison of the disposition of total and unbound sulfisoxazole after single and multiple dosing. *J Pharmacokinet Biopharm.* 1982;10:157-172. **3.** National Committee for Clinical Laboratory Standards.*Performance Standards for Antimicrobial Disk Susceptibility Tests.* 4th ed. Villanova, PA: April 1990. Approved Standard NCCLS Document M2-A4, Vol. 10, No. 7 NCCLS. **4.** National Committee for Clinical Laboratory Standards.*Methods for Dilution Antimicrobial Susceptibility Tests for Bacteria that Grow Aerobically.* 2nd ed. Villanova, PA: April 1990. Approved Standard NCCLS Document M7-A2, Vol. 10, No. 8 NCCLS.(Roche, 4/93, 13-06-73304-0493)

HOW SUPPLIED - RATED THERAPEUTICALLY EQUIVALENT:

Tablet, Uncoated - Oral - 500 mg

100's	$6.05	Sulfisoxazole, Raway	00686-1683-25
100's	$7.88	Sulfisoxazole, H.C.F.A. F F P	99999-2294-01
100's	$8.45	Sulfisoxazole, Qualitest Pharms	00603-5849-21
100's	$8.50	SULFISOCON, Consolidated Midland	00223-1980-01
100's	$10.15	Sulfisoxazole, Harber Pharm	51432-0444-03
100's	$11.55	Sulfisoxazole, Geneva Pharms	00781-1015-01
100's	$12.15	Sulfisoxazole, HL Moore Drug Exch	00839-1649-06
100's	$12.25	Sulfisoxazole, United Res	00677-0143-01
100's	$12.25	Sulfisoxazole, Martec Pharms	52555-0323-01
100's	$12.90	Sulfisoxazole, Zenith Labs	00172-2218-60
100's	$12.90	Sulfisoxazole, Goldline Labs	00182-0497-01
100's	$13.08	Sulfisoxazole, Aligen Independ	00405-4971-01
100's	$13.45	GULFASIN, Major Pharms	00904-2218-60
100's	$13.95	Sulfisoxazole, Schein Pharm (US)	00364-0265-01
100's	$13.97	Sulfisoxazole, Rugby	00536-4618-01
500's	$39.40	Sulfisoxazole, H.C.F.A. F F P	99999-2294-02
1000's	$65.00	TRUXAZOLE, C O Truxton	00463-6214-10
1000's	$72.50	SULFISOCON, Consolidated Midland	00223-1980-02
1000's	$78.80	Sulfisoxazole, H.C.F.A. F F P	99999-2294-03
1000's	$81.40	GULFASIN, Major Pharms	00904-2218-80
1000's	$109.60	Sulfisoxazole, Zenith Labs	00172-2218-80

HOW SUPPLIED - NOT RATED EQUIVALENT:

Suspension - Oral - 500 mg/5ml

120 ml	**$11.64**	**GANTRISIN PEDIATRIC, Roche**	**00004-1003-30**
480 ml	**$40.37**	**GANTRISIN PEDIATRIC, Roche**	**00004-1003-28**

SULINDAC *(002298)*

CATEGORIES: Analgesics; Ankylosing Spondylitis; Anti-Inflammatory Agents; Antiarthritics; Antigout; Antipyretics; Arthritis; Bursitis; Central Nervous System Agents; Gouty Arthritis; NSAIDS; Nonsteroidal Anti-Inflammatory; Osteoarthritis; Pain; Spondylitis; Sales > $100 Million; FDA Approval Pre 1982; Patent Expiration 1990 Apr

BRAND NAMES: *Aflodac*; *Algocetil*; *Antribid*; *Arthridex*; *Arthrocine*; *Biflace*; *Citireuma*; **Clinoril**; *Clisundac*; *Imbaral*; *Lindak*; *Lyndak*; *Mobilin*; *Reumofil*; *Sudac*; *Sulene*; *Sulic*; *Sulindal*; *Suloril*; *Sulreuma*
(International brand names outside U.S. in italics)

FORMULARIES: Aetna; BC-BS; Medi-Cal; PCS

COST OF THERAPY: $32.85 (Arthritis; Tablet; 150 mg; 2/day; 365 days)

PRIMARY ICD9: 715.99 (Osteoarthritis, Unspecified, Multiple Sites)

DESCRIPTION:

Sulindac is a non-steroidal, anti-inflammatory indene derivative designated chemically as (Z)-5-fluoro-2-methyl-1- ((*p*-(methylsulfinyl)phenyl)methylene)-1*H*-indene-3-acetic acid. It is not a salicylate, pyrazolone or propionic acid derivative. Its empirical formula is $C_{20}H_{17}FO_3S$, with a molecular weight of 356.42. Sulindac, a yellow crystalline compound, is a weak organic acid practically insoluble in water below pH 4.5, but very soluble as the sodium salt or in buffers of pH 6 or higher.

Sulindac is available in 150 and 200 mg tablets for oral administration. Each tablet contains the following inactive ingredients: cellulose, magnesium stearate, starch.

Following absorption, sulindac undergoes two major biotransformations - reversible reduction to the sulfide metabolite, and irreversible oxidation to the sulfone metabolite. Available evidence indicates that the biological activity resides with the sulfide metabolite.

CLINICAL PHARMACOLOGY:

Sulindac is a non-steroidal anti-inflammatory drug, also possessing analgesic and antipyretic activities. Its mode of action, like that of other non-steroidal, anti-inflammatory agents, is not known; however, its therapeutic action is not due to pituitary-adrenal stimulation. Inhibition of prostaglandin synthesis by the sulfide metabolite may be involved in the anti-inflammatory action of sulindac.

Sulindac is approximately 90% absorbed in man after oral administration. The peak plasma concentrations of the biologically active sulfide metabolite are achieved in about two hours when sulindac is administered in the fasting state, and in about three to four hours when sulindac is administered with food. The mean half-life of sulindac is 7.8 hours while the mean half-life of the sulfide metabolite is 16.4 hours. Sustained plasma levels of the sulfide metabolite are consistent with a prolonged anti-inflammatory action which is the rationale for a twice per day dosage schedule.

Sulindac and its sulfone metabolite undergo extensive enterohepatic circulation relative to the sulfide metabolite in animals. Studies in man have also demonstrated that recirculation of the parent drug, sulindac, and its sulfone metabolite, is more extensive than that of the active sulfide metabolite. The active sulfide metabolite accounts for less than six percent of the total intestinal exposure to sulindac and its metabolites.

The primary route of excretion in man is via the urine as both sulindac and its sulfone metabolite (free and glucuronide conjugates). Approximately 50% of the administered dose is excreted in the urine, with the conjugated sulfone metabolite accounting for the major portion. Less than 1% of the administered dose of sulindac appears in the urine as the sulfide metabolite. Approximately 25% is found in the feces, primarily as the sulfone and sulfide metabolites.

The bioavailability of sulindac, as assessed by urinary excretion, was not changed by concomitant administration of an antacid containing magnesium hydroxide 200 mg and aluminum hydroxide 225 mg per 5 ml.

Because sulindac is excreted in the urine primarily as biologically inactive forms, it may possibly affect renal function to a lesser extent than other non-steroidal anti-inflammatory drugs, however, renal adverse experiences have been reported with sulindac (see ADVERSE REACTIONS.) In a study of patients with chronic glomerular disease treated with therapeutic doses of sulindac, no effect was demonstrated on renal blood flow, glomerular filtration rate, or urinary excretion of prostaglandin $E_2$and the primary metabolite of prostacyclin, 6-keto-$PGF_{1\alpha}$. However, in other studies in healthy volunteers and patients with liver disease, sulindac was found to blunt the renal responses to intravenous furosemide, i.e., the diuresis, natriuresis, increments in plasma renin activity and urinary excretion of prostaglandins. These observations may represent a differentiation of the effects of sulindac on renal functions based on differences in pathogenesis of the renal prostaglandin dependence associated with differing dose-response relationships of different NSAIDs to the various renal functions influenced by prostaglandins. These observations need further clarification and in the interim, sulindac should be used with caution in patients whose renal function may be impaired (see PRECAUTIONS.)

In healthy men, the average fecal blood loss, measured over a two-week period during administration of 400 mg per day of sulindac, was similar to that for placebo, and was statistically significantly less than that resulting from 4800 mg per day of aspirin.

In controlled clinical studies sulindac was evaluated in the following five conditions:

Osteoarthritis: In patients with osteoarthritis of the hip and knee, the anti-inflammatory and analgesic activity of sulindac was demonstrated by clinical measurements that included: assessments by both patient and investigator of overall response; decrease in disease activity as assessed by both patient and investigator; improvement in ARA Functional Class; relief of night pain; improvement in overall evaluation of pain, including pain on weight bearing and pain on active and passive motion; improvement in joint mobility, range of motion, and functional activities; decreased swelling and tenderness; and decreased duration of stiffness following prolonged inactivity.

In clinical studies in which dosages were adjusted according to patient needs, sulindac 200 to 400 mg daily was shown to be comparable in effectiveness to aspirin 2400 to 4800 mg daily. Sulindac was generally well tolerated, and patients on it had a lower overall incidence of total adverse effects, of milder gastrointestinal reactions, and of tinnitus than did patients on aspirin. (See ADVERSE REACTIONS.)

Rheumatoid Arthritis: In patients with rheumatoid arthritis, the anti-inflammatory and analgesic activity of sulindac was demonstrated by clinical measurements that included: assessments by both patients and investigator of overall response decrease in disease activity as assessed by both patient and investigator; reduction in overall joint pain; reduction in duration and severity of morning stiffness; reduction in day and night pain; decrease in time

CLINICAL PHARMACOLOGY: *(cont'd)*

required to walk 50 feet; decrease in general pain as measured on a visual analog scale; improvement in the Ritchie articular index; decrease in proximal interphalangeal joint size; improvement in ARA Functional Class; increase in grip strength; reduction in painful joint count and score; reduction in swollen joint count and score; and increased flexion and extension of the wrist.

In clinical studies in which dosages were adjusted according to patient needs, sulindac 300 to 400 mg daily was shown to be comparable in effectiveness to aspirin 3600 to 4800 mg daily. Sulindac was generally well tolerated, and patients on it had a lower overall incidence of total adverse effects, of milder gastrointestinal reactions, and of tinnitus than did patients on aspirin. (See ADVERSE REACTIONS.)

In patients with rheumatoid arthritis, sulindac may be used in combination with gold salts at usual dosage levels. In clinical studies, sulindac added to the regimen of gold salts usually resulted in additional symptomatic relief but did not alter the course of the underlying disease.

Ankylosing Spondylitis: In patients with ankylosing spondylitis, the anti-inflammatory and analgesic activity of sulindac was demonstrated by clinical measurements that included: assessments by both patient and investigator of overall response; decrease in disease activity as assessed by both patient and investigator; improvement in ARA Functional Class; improvement in patient and investigator evaluation of spinal pain, tenderness and/or spasm; reduction in the duration of morning stiffness; increase in the time to onset of fatigue; relief of night pain; increase in chest expansion; and increase in spinal mobility evaluated by fingers-to-floor distance, occiput to wall distance, the Schober Test, and the Wright Modification of the Schober Test. In a clinical study in which dosages were adjusted according to patient need, sulindac 200 to 400 mg daily was as effective as indomethacin 75 to 150 mg daily. In a second study, sulindac 300 to 400 mg daily was comparable in effectiveness to phenylbutazone 400 to 600 mg daily. Sulindac was better tolerated than phenylbutazone. (See ADVERSE REACTIONS.)

Acute painful shoulder (Acute subacromial bursitis/supraspinatus tendinitis): In patients with acute painful shoulder (acute subacromial bursitis/supraspinatus tendinitis), the anti-inflammatory and analgesic activity of sulindac was demonstrated by clinical measurements that included: assessments by both patient and investigator of overall response; relief of night pain, spontaneous pain, and pain on active motion; decrease in local tenderness; and improvement in range of motion measured by abduction, and internal and external rotation. In clinical studies in acute painful shoulder, sulindac 300 to 400 mg daily and oxyphenbutazone 400 to 600 mg daily were shown to be equally effective and well tolerated.

Acute Gouty Arthritis: In patients with acute gouty arthritis, the anti-inflammatory and analgesic activity of sulindac was demonstrated by clinical measurements that included: assessments by both the patient and investigator of overall response; relief of weight-bearing pain; relief of pain at rest and on active and passive motion; decrease in tenderness; reduction in warmth and swelling; increase in range of motion; and improvement in ability to function. In clinical studies, sulindac at 400 mg daily and phenylbutazone at 600 mg daily were shown to be equally effective. In these short-term studies in which reduction of dosage was permitted according to response, both drugs were equally well tolerated.

INDICATIONS AND USAGE:

Sulindac is indicated for acute or long-term use in the relief of signs and symptoms of the following:

1. Osteoarthritis
2. Rheumatoid arthritis*
3. Ankylosing spondylitis
4. Acute painful shoulder (Acute subacromial bursitis/supraspinatus tendinitis)
5. Acute gouty arthritis

CONTRAINDICATIONS:

Sulindac should not be used in:

Patients who are hypersensitive to this product.

Patients in whom acute asthmatic attacks, urticaria, or rhinitis are precipitated by aspirin or other non-steroidal anti-inflammatory agents.

WARNINGS:

Gastrointestinal Effects: Peptic ulceration and gastrointestinal bleeding have been reported in patients receiving sulindac. Fatalities have occurred. Gastrointestinal bleeding is associated with higher morbidity and mortality in patients acutely ill with other conditions, the elderly and patients with hemorrhagic disorders, patients with active gastrointestinal bleeding or an active peptic ulcer, a appropriate ulcer regimen should be instituted, and the physician must weigh the benefits of therapy with sulindac against possible hazards, and careful monitor the patient's progress. When sulindac is given to patients with history of either upper or lower gastrointestinal tract disease, it should be given under close supervision and only after consulting the ADVERSE REACTIONS section.

Risk of GI Ulcerations, Bleeding and Perforation with NSAID Therapy: Serious gastrointestinal toxicity such as bleeding, ulceration, and perforation, can occur at any time, with or without warning symptoms, in patient treated chronically with NSAID therapy. Although minor upper gastrointestinal problems, such as dyspepsia, are common, usually developing early therapy, physicians should remain alert for ulceration and bleeding in patient treated chronically with NSAIDs even in the absence of previous GI tract symptoms. In patients observed in clinical trials of several months to two years duration, symptomatic upper GI ulcers, gross bleeding or perforation appear to occur in approximately 1% of patients treated for 3-6 months, and about 2-4% of patients treated for one year. Physicians should inform patient about the signs and/or symptoms of serious GI toxicity and what steps to take if they occur.

Studies to date have not identified any subset of patients not at risk on developing peptic ulceration and bleeding. Except for a prior history of serious GI events and other risk factors known to be associated with peptic ulcer disease, such as alcoholism, smoking, etc., no risk factors (*e.g.,* age, sex) have been associated with increased risk. Elderly or debilitated patients seem to tolerate ulceration or bleeding less well than other individuals and most spontaneous reports of fatal GI events are in this population. Studies to date are inconclusive concerning the relative risk of various NSAIDs in causing such reactions. High doses of any NSAID probably carry a greater risk of these reactions, although controlled clinical trials showing this do not exist in most cases. In considering the use of relatively large doses (within the recommended dosage range), sufficient benefit should be anticipated to offset the potential increased risk of GI toxicity.

Hypersensitivity: Rarely, fever and other evidence of hypersensitivity (see ADVERSE REACTIONS) including abnormalities in one or more liver function tests and severe skin reactions have occurred during therapy with sulindac. Fatalities have occurred in these patients. Hepatitis, jaundice, or both, with or without fever may occur usually within the first one to three months of therapy. Determinations of liver function should be considered whenever a patient on therapy with sulindac develops unexplained fever, rash or other dermatologic reactions or constitutional symptoms. If unexplained fever or other evidence of hypersensitivity occurs, therapy with sulindac should be discontinued. The elevated temperature and abnormalities in liver function caused by sulindac characteristically have reverted to normal after discontinuation of therapy. Administration of sulindac should not be reinstituted in such patients.

Hepatic Effects: In addition to hypersensitivity reactions involving the liver, in some patients the findings are consistent with those of cholestatic hepatitis. As with other non-steroidal anti-inflammatory drugs, borderline elevations of one or more liver tests without any other signs and symptoms may occur in up to 15% of patients. These abnormalities may progress, may remain essentially unchanged, or may be transient with continued therapy. The SGPT (ALT) test is probably the most sensitive indicator of liver dysfunction. Meaningful (3 times the upper limit of normal) elevations of SGPT or SGOT (AST) occurred in controlled clinical trials in less than 1% of patients. A patient with symptoms and/or signs suggesting liver dysfunction, or in whom an abnormal liver test has occurred, should be evaluated for evidence of the development of more severe hepatic reaction while on therapy with sulindac. Although such reactions as described above are rare, if abnormal liver tests persist or worsen, if clinical signs and symptoms consistent with liver disease develop, or if systemic manifestations occur (*e.g.,* eosinophilia, rash, etc.), sulindac should be discontinued.

In clinical trials with sulindac, the use of doses of 600 mg/day has been associated with an increased incidence of mild liver test abnormalities (see DOSAGE AND ADMINISTRATION for maximum dosage recommendation).

*The safety and effectiveness of sulindac have not been established in rheumatoid arthritis patients who are designated in the American Rheumatism Association classification as Functional Class IV (incapacitated, largely or wholly bedridden, or confined to wheelchair; little or no self-care).

PRECAUTIONS:

GENERAL

Non-steroidal anti-inflammatory drugs, including sulindac, may mask the usual signs and symptoms of infection. Therefore, the physician must be continually on alert and should use the drug with extra care in the presence of existing infection.

Although sulindac has less effect on platelet function and bleeding time than aspirin, it is an inhibitor of platelet function; therefore, patients who may be adversely affected should be carefully observed when sulindac is administered.

Pancreatitis has been reported in patients receiving sulindac (see ADVERSE REACTIONS.) Should pancreatitis be suspected, the drug should be discontinued and not restarted, supportive medical therapy instituted, and the patient monitored closely with appropriate laboratory studies (*e.g.,* serum and urine amylase, amylase/creatinine clearance ratio, electrolytes, serum calcium, glucose, lipase, etc.). A search for other causes of pancreatitis as well as those conditions which mimic pancreatitis should be conducted.

Because of reports of adverse eye findings with non-steroidal anti-inflammatory agents, it is recommended that patients who develop eye complaints during treatment with sulindac have ophthalmologic studies.

In patients with poor liver function, delayed, elevated and prolonged circulating levels of the sulfide and sulfone metabolites may occur. Such patients should be monitored closely; a reduction of daily dosage may be required.

Edema has been observed in some patients taking sulindac. Therefore, as with other non-steroidal anti-inflammatory drugs, sulindac should be used with caution in patients with compromised cardiac function, hypertension, or other conditions predisposing to fluid retention.

Sulindac may allow a reduction in dosage or the elimination of chronic corticosteroid therapy in some patients with rheumatoid arthritis. However, it is generally necessary to reduce corticosteroids gradually over several months in order to avoid an exacerbation of disease or signs and symptoms of adrenal insufficiency. Abrupt withdrawal of chronic corticosteroid treatment is generally not recommended even when patients have had a serious complication of chronic corticosteroid therapy.

RENAL EFFECTS

As with other non-steroidal anti-inflammatory drugs, long term administration of sulindac to animals has resulted in renal papillary necrosis and other abnormal renal pathology. In humans, there have been reports of acute interstitial nephritis with hematuria, proteinuria, and occasionally nephrotic syndrome.

A second form of renal toxicity has been seen in patients with prerenal and renal conditions leading to a reduction in renal blood flow or blood volume, where the renal prostaglandins have a supportive role in the maintenance of renal perfusion. In these patients administration of an NSAID may cause a dose dependent reduction in prostaglandin formation and may precipitate overt renal decompensation. Sulindac may affect renal function less than other NSAIDs in patients with chronic glomerular renal disease (see CLINICAL PHARMACOLOGY.) Until these observations are better understood and clarified, however, and because renal adverse experiences have been reported with sulindac (see ADVERSE REACTIONS), caution should be exercised when administering the drug to patients with conditions associated with increased risk of the effects of non-steroidal anti-inflammatory drugs on renal function, such as those with renal or hepatic dysfunction, diabetes mellitus, advanced age, extracellular volume depletion from any cause, congestive heart failure, septicemia, pyelonephritis, or concomitant use of any nephrotoxic drug. Discontinuation of NSAID therapy is typically followed by recovery to the pretreatment state.

Since sulindac is eliminated primarily by the kidneys, patients with significantly impaired renal function should be closely monitored; a lower daily dosage should be anticipated to avoid excessive drug accumulation.

Sulindac metabolites have been reported rarely as the major or a minor component in renal stones in association with other calculus components. Sulindac should be used with caution in patients with a history of renal lithiasis, and they should be kept well hydrated while receiving sulindac.

INFORMATION FOR THE PATIENT

Sulindac, like other drugs of its class, is not free of side effects. The side effects of these drugs can cause discomfort and, rarely, there are more serious side effects such as gastrointestinal bleeding, which may result in hospitalization and even fatal outcomes.

NSAIDs (Non-steroidal Anti-inflammatory Drugs) are often essential agents in the management of arthritis, but they also may be commonly employed for conditions which are less serious.

Physicians may wish to discuss with their patients the potential risks(see WARNINGS, PRECAUTIONS, and ADVERSE REACTIONS) and likely benefits of NSAID treatment, particularly when the drugs are used for less serious conditions where treatment without NSAIDs may represent an acceptable alternative to both the patient and physician.

LABORATORY TESTS

Because serious GI tract ulceration and bleeding can occur without warning symptoms, physicians should follow chronically treated patients for the signs and symptoms of ulceration and bleeding and should inform them of the importance of this follow-up (see WARNINGS, **Risk of GI Ulcerations, Bleeding and Perforation with NSAID Therapy**).

PRECAUTIONS: *(cont'd)*

PREGNANCY

Sulindac is not recommended for use in pregnant women, since safety for use has not been established, and because of the known effect of drugs of this class on the human fetus (closure of the ductus arteriosus, platelet dysfunction with resultant bleeding, renal dysfunction or failure with oligohydramnios, gastrointestinal bleeding or perforation, and myocardial degenerative changes) during the third trimester of pregnancy. In reproduction studies in the rat, a decrease in average fetal weight and an increase in numbers of dead pups were observed on the first day of the postpartum period at dosage levels of 20 and 40 mg/kg/day (2 1/2 and 5 times the usual maximum daily dose in humans), although there was no adverse effect on the survival and growth during the remainder of the postpartum period. Sulindac prolongs the duration of gestation in rats, as do other compounds of this class which also may cause dystocia and delayed parturition in pregnant animals. Visceral and skeletal malformations observed in low incidence among rabbits in some teratology studies did not occur at the same dosage levels in repeat studies, nor at a higher dosage level in the same species.

NURSING MOTHERS

Nursing should not be undertaken while a patient is on sulindac. It is not known whether sulindac is secreted in human milk; however, it is secreted in the milk of lactating rats.

PEDIATRIC USE

Safety and effectiveness in children have not been established.

DRUG INTERACTIONS:

DMSO should not be used with sulindac. Concomitant administration has been reported to reduce the plasma levels of the active sulfide metabolite and potentially reduce efficacy. In addition, this combination has been reported to cause peripheral neuropathy.

Although sulindac and its sulfide metabolite are highly bound to protein, studies, in which sulindac was given at a dose of 400 mg daily, have shown no clinically significant interaction with oral anticoagulants or oral hypoglycemic agents. However, patients should be monitored carefully until it is certain that no change in their anticoagulant or hypoglycemic dosage is required. Special attention should be paid to patients taking higher doses than those recommended and to patients with renal impairment or other metabolic defects that might increase sulindac blood levels.

The concomitant administration of aspirin with sulindac significantly depressed the plasma levels of the active sulfide metabolite. A double-blind study compared the safety and efficacy of sulindac 300 or 400 mg daily given alone or with aspirin 2.4 g/day for the treatment of osteoarthritis. The addition of aspirin did not alter the types of clinical or laboratory adverse experiences for sulindac; however, the combination showed an increase in the incidence of gastrointestinal adverse experiences. Since the addition of aspirin did not have a favorable effect on the therapeutic response to sulindac, the combination is not recommended.

Caution should be used if sulindac is administered concomitantly with methotrexate. Non-steroidal anti-inflammatory drugs have been reported to decrease the tubular secretion of methotrexate and to potentiate its toxicity.

Administration of non-steroidal anti-inflammatory drugs concomitantly with cyclosporine has been associated with an increase in cyclosporine-induced toxicity, possibly due to decreased synthesis of renal prostacyclin. NSAIDs should be used with caution in patients taking cyclosporine, and renal function should be carefully monitored.

The concomitant administration of sulindac and diflunisal in normal volunteers resulted in lowering of the plasma levels of the active sulindac sulfide metabolite by approximately one-third.

Probenecid given concomitantly with sulindac had only a slight effect on plasma sulfide levels, while plasma levels of sulindac and sulfone were increased. Sulindac was shown to produce a modest reduction in the uricosuric action of probenecid, which probably is not significant under most circumstances.

Neither propoxyphene hydrochloride nor acetaminophen had any effect on the plasma levels of sulindac or its sulfide metabolite.

ADVERSE REACTIONS:

The following adverse reactions were reported in clinical trials or have been reported since the drug was marketed. The probability exists of a causal relationship between sulindac and these adverse reactions. The adverse reactions which have been observed in clinical trials encompass observations in 1,865 patients, including 232 observed for at least 48 weeks.

Incidence Greater Than 1%

Gastrointestinal: The most frequent types of adverse reactions occurring with sulindac are gastrointestinal; these include gastrointestinal pain (10%), dyspepsia*, nausea* with or without vomiting, diarrhea*, constipation*, flatulence, anorexia and gastrointestinal cramps.

Dermatologic: Rash*, pruritus.

Central Nervous System: Dizziness*, headache*, nervousness.

Special Senses: Tinnitus.

Miscellaneous: Edema (see PRECAUTIONS.)

INCIDENCE LESS THAN 1 IN 100

Gastrointestinal: Gastritis, gastroenteritis or colitis. Peptic ulcer and gastrointestinal bleeding have been reported. GI perforation has been reported rarely.

Liver function abnormalities; jaundice, sometimes with fever; cholestasis; hepatitis; hepatic failure.

Pancreatitis (see PRECAUTIONS.)

Ageusia; glossitis.

There have been rare reports of sulindac metabolites in common bile duct "sludge" in patients with symptoms of cholecystitis who underwent a cholecystectomy.

Dermatologic: Stomatitis, sore or dry mucous membranes, alopecia, photosensitivity.

Erythema multiforme, toxic epidermal necrolysis, Stevens-Johnson syndrome, and exfoliative dermatitis have been reported.

Cardiovascular: Congestive heart failure, especially in patients with marginal cardiac function; palpitation; hypertension.

Hematologic: Thrombocytopenia; ecchymosis; purpura; leukopenia; agranulocytosis; neutropenia; bone marrow depression, including aplastic anemia; hemolytic anemia; increased prothrombin time in patients on oral anticoagulants (see PRECAUTIONS.)

Genitourinary: Urine discoloration; dysuria; vaginal bleeding; hematuria; proteinuria; crystalluria; renal impairment, including renal failure; interstitial nephritis; nephrotic syndrome.

Renal calculi containing sulindac metabolites have been observed rarely.

Metabolic: Hyperkalemia.

Musculoskeletal: Muscle weakness.

Psychiatric: Depression; psychic disturbances including acute psychosis.

Nervous System: Vertigo; insomnia; somnolence; paresthesia; convulsions; syncope; aseptic meningitis.

Special Senses: Blurred vision; visual disturbances; decreased hearing; metallic or bitter taste.

ADVERSE REACTIONS: *(cont'd)*

Respiratory: Epistaxis.

Hypersensitivity Reactions: Anaphylaxis; angioneurotic edema; bronchial spasm; dyspnea. Hypersensitivity vasculitis.

A potentially fatal apparent hypersensitivity syndrome has been reported. This syndrome may include constitutional symptoms (fever, chills, diaphoresis, flushing), cutaneous findings (rash or other dermatologic reactions—see above), conjunctivitis, involvement of major organs (changes in liver function including hepatic failure, jaundice, pancreatitis, pneumonitis with or without pleural effusion, leukopenia, leukocytosis, eosinophilia, disseminated intravascular coagulation, anemia, renal impairment, including renal failure), and other less specific findings (adenitis, arthralgia, arthritis, myalgia, fatigue, malaise, hypotension, chest pain, tachycardia).

CAUSAL RELATIONSHIP UNKNOWN

A rare occurrence of fulminant necrotizing fasciitis, particularly in association with Group A β- hemolytic streptococcus has been described in persons treated with non-steroidal anti-inflammatory agents, sometimes with fatal outcome (see also PRECAUTIONS, General).

Other reactions have been reported in clinical trials or since the drug was marketed, but occurred under circumstances where a causal relationship could not be established. However, in these rarely reported events, that possibility cannot be excluded. Therefore, these observations are listed to serve as alerting information to physicians.

Cardiovascular: Arrhythmia.

Metabolic: Hyperglycemia.

Nervous System: Neuritis.

Special Senses: Disturbances of the retina and its vasculature.

Miscellaneous: Gynecomastia.

OVERDOSAGE:

MANAGEMENT OF OVERDOSE

Cases of overdosage have been reported and rarely, deaths have occurred. The following signs and symptoms may be observed following overdosage stupor, coma, diminished urine output and hypotension.

In the event of overdosage, the stomach should be emptied by inducing vomiting or by gastric lavage, and the patient carefully observed and given symptomatic and supportive treatment.

Animal studies show that absorption is decreased by the prompt administration of activated charcoal and excretion is enhanced by alkalinization of the urine.

DOSAGE AND ADMINISTRATION:

Sulindac should be administered orally twice a day with food. The maximum dosage is 400 mg per day. Dosages above 400 mg per day are not recommended.

In osteoarthritis, rheumatoid arthritis, and ankylosing spondylitis, the recommended starting dosage is 150 mg twice a day. The dosage may be lowered or raised depending on the response.

A prompt response (within one week) can be expected in about one-half of patients with osteoarthritis, ankylosing spondylitis, and rheumatoid arthritis. Others may require longer to respond.

In acute painful shoulder (acute subacromial bursitis/supraspinatus tendinitis) and acute gouty arthritis, the recommended dosage is 200 mg twice a day. After a satisfactory response has been achieved, the dosage may be reduced according to the response. In acute painful shoulder, therapy for 7-14 days is usually adequate. In acute gouty arthritis, therapy for 7 days is usually adequate.

HOW SUPPLIED - RATED THERAPEUTICALLY EQUIVALENT:

Tablet, Uncoated - Oral - 150 mg

60's	$13.18	Sulindac, H.C.F.A. F F P	99999-2298-01
100's	$21.98	Sulindac, H.C.F.A. F F P	99999-2298-02
100's	$25.73	Sulindac Tablets, United Res	00677-1173-01
100's	$25.73	Sulindac, Mutual Pharm	53489-0478-01
100's	$34.00	Sulindac, Raway	00686-0666-20
100's	$68.48	Sulindac, Major Pharms	00904-3378-61
100's	$71.50	Sulindac, Qualitest Pharms	00603-5872-21
100's	$74.71	Sulindac, Lederle Pharm	00005-3550-43
100's	$75.53	Sulindac, HL Moore Drug Exch	00839-7621-06
100's	$77.50	Sulindac 150, Goldline Labs	00182-1705-01
100's	$77.50	Sulindac Tablets 150 Mg, Major Pharms	00904-3378-60
100's	$78.35	Sulindac, West Point Pharma	59591-0170-68
100's	$78.35	Sulindac, Endo Labs	60951-0780-70
100's	$78.88	Sulindac, Vangard Labs	00615-3528-13
100's	$79.00	Sulindac, Schein Pharm (US)	00364-2441-90
100's	$79.90	Sulindac Tablets 150 Mg, Aligen Independ	00405-4973-01
100's	$81.75	Sulindac, Rugby	00536-5645-01
100's	$81.82	Sulindac, Dupont Pharma	00056-0220-70
100's	$82.50	Sulindac, Harber Pharm	51432-0429-03
100's	$82.99	Sulindac, Schein Pharm (US)	00364-2441-01
100's	$83.97	Sulindac, Warner Chilcott	00047-0773-24
100's	$83.98	Sulindac, Geneva Pharms	00781-1811-01
100's	$84.95	Sulindac, Mylan	00378-0427-01
100's	$87.60	Sulindac, Geneva Pharms	00781-1811-13
100's	**$97.35**	**CLINORIL, Merck**	**00006-0941-68**
500's	$109.90	Sulindac, H.C.F.A. F F P	99999-2298-03
500's	$128.65	Sulindac, United Res	00677-1173-05
500's	$128.65	Sulindac, Mutual Pharm	53489-0478-05
500's	$302.39	Sulindac, HL Moore Drug Exch	00839-7621-12
500's	$344.65	Sulindac Tablets 150 Mg, Major Pharms	00904-3378-40
500's	$359.90	Sulindac, West Point Pharma	59591-0170-74
500's	$359.90	Sulindac, Endo Labs	60951-0780-85
500's	$372.93	Sulindac, Geneva Pharms	00781-1811-05
500's	$383.49	Sulindac, Schein Pharm (US)	00364-2441-05
500's	$383.89	Sulindac, Aligen Independ	00405-4973-02
500's	$388.60	Sulindac, Dupont Pharma	00056-0220-85
500's	$412.50	Sulindac, Harber Pharm	51432-0429-05
1000's	$219.80	Sulindac, H.C.F.A. F F P	99999-2298-04
1000's	$679.79	Sulindac, HL Moore Drug Exch	00839-7621-16
1000's	$691.08	Sulindac, Lederle Pharm	00005-3550-34
1000's	$745.98	Sulindac, Warner Chilcott	00047-0773-32

Tablet, Uncoated - Oral - 200 mg

100's	$29.63	Sulindac Tablets, United Res	00677-1174-01
100's	$29.63	Sulindac, Mutual Pharm	53489-0479-01
100's	$29.63	Sulindac, H.C.F.A. F F P	99999-2298-05
100's	$37.00	Sulindac, Raway	00686-0667-20
100's	$49.75	Sulindac, Rugby	00536-5656-01
100's	$83.47	Sulindac, Major Pharms	00904-3379-61
100's	$87.90	Sulindac, Qualitest Pharms	00603-5873-21

HOW SUPPLIED - RATED THERAPEUTICALLY EQUIVALENT: *(cont'd)*

100's	$89.91	Sulindac, Lederle Pharm	00005-3551-43
100's	$93.49	Sulindac, HL Moore Drug Exch	00839-7622-06
100's	$95.00	Sulindac, Goldline Labs	00182-1721-01
100's	$95.00	Sulindac, Aligen Independ	00405-4974-01
100's	$95.50	Sulindac, Harber Pharm	51432-0431-03
100's	$95.75	Sulindac, West Point Pharma	59591-0154-68
100's	$95.75	Sulindac, Endo Labs	60951-0781-70
100's	$96.00	Sulindac, Schein Pharm (US)	00364-2442-90
100's	$96.50	Sulindac Tablets 200 Mg, Major Pharms	00904-3379-60
100's	$99.05	Sulindac, Vangard Labs	00615-3529-13
100's	$100.35	Sulindac, Rugby	00536-5646-01
100's	$105.89	Sulindac, Schein Pharm (US)	00364-2442-01
100's	$106.50	Sulindac, Dupont Pharma	00056-0221-70
100's	$106.70	Sulindac, Geneva Pharms	00781-1812-01
100's	$106.75	Sulindac, Warner Chilcott	00047-0774-24
100's	$106.75	Sulindac, Mylan	00378-0531-01
100's	$106.75	Sulindac, Rugby	00536-4622-01
100's	$106.95	Sulindac, Geneva Pharms	00781-1812-13
100's	**$119.64**	**CLINORIL, Merck**	**00006-0942-68**
500's	$148.15	Sulindac, United Res	00677-1174-05
500's	$148.15	Sulindac, Mutual Pharm	53489-0479-05
500's	$148.15	Sulindac, H.C.F.A. F F P	99999-2298-06
500's	$276.00	Sulindac, Rugby	00536-4622-05
500's	$371.24	Sulindac, HL Moore Drug Exch	00839-7622-12
500's	$418.00	Sulindac, Major Pharms	00904-3379-40
500's	$423.00	Sulindac, Goldline Labs	00182-1706-05
500's	$430.87	Sulindac, West Point Pharma	59591-0154-74
500's	$430.87	Sulindac, Endo Labs	60951-0781-85
500's	$443.70	Sulindac, Rugby	00536-5646-05
500's	$443.70	Sulindac, Rugby	00536-5656-05
500's	$462.82	Sulindac, Schein Pharm (US)	00364-2442-05
500's	$463.26	Sulindac, Aligen Independ	00405-4974-02
500's	$463.61	Sulindac, Geneva Pharms	00781-1812-05
500's	$477.50	Sulindac, Harber Pharm	51432-0431-05
500's	$504.22	Sulindac, Dupont Pharma	00056-0221-85
1000's	$296.30	Sulindac, H.C.F.A. F F P	99999-2298-07
1000's	$790.00	Sulindac, Goldline Labs	00182-1721-10
1000's	$831.70	Sulindac, Lederle Pharm	00005-3551-34
1000's	$841.39	Sulindac, HL Moore Drug Exch	00839-7622-16
1000's	$929.06	Sulindac, Warner Chilcott	00047-0774-32

SUMATRIPTAN SUCCINATE *(003090)*

CATEGORIES: Antimigraine/Other Headaches; Autonomic Drugs; Central Nervous System Agents; Headache; Migraine; Pain; Serotonin Antagonists; Sympatholytic Agents; Cluster Headache*; Phonophobia*; Pregnancy Category C; FDA Class 1P ("Priority Review"); Sales > $500 Million; Top 200 Drugs; FDA Approved 1992 Dec

* Indication not approved by the FDA

BRAND NAMES: Imigran; *Imigrane* (France); **Imitrex**

(International brand names outside U.S. in italics)

FORMULARIES: Kaiser; PCS

COST OF THERAPY: $11.96 (Migraine; Tablet; 25 mg; 1/day; 1 days)

DESCRIPTION:

Sumatriptan (as the succinate) is a selective 5-hydroxytryptamine$_1$, receptor subtype agonist. Sumatriptan is chemically designated as 3-[2-(dimethylamino)ethyl]-N-methyl-1H-indole-5-methanesulfonamide butane-1,4-dioate (1:1).

The empirical formula is $C_{14}H_{21}N_3O_2S{\cdot}C_4H_6O_4$, representing a molecular weight of 413.5.

Sumatriptan succinate is a white to off-white powder that is readily soluble in water and in saline.

Injection: Imitrex injection is a clear, colorless to pale yellow, sterile, nonpyrogenic solution for subcutaneous injection. Each 0.5 ml of solution contains 6 mg of sumatriptan (base) as the succinate salt and 3.5 mg of sodium chloride, USP in water for injection. The pH range of the solution is approximately 4.2 to 5.3. The osmolality of the injection is 291 mOsmol.

Tablets: Each Imitrex tablet for oral administration contains 35 or 70 mg of sumatriptan succinate equivalent to 25 or 50 mg of sumatriptan, respectively. Each tablet also contains the inactive ingredients croscarmellose sodium, lactose, magnesium stearate, microcrystalline cellulose and titanium dioxide dye.

CLINICAL PHARMACOLOGY:

MECHANISM OF ACTION

Sumatriptan has been demonstrated to be a selective agonist for a vascular 5-hydroxytryptamine$_1$, receptor subtype (probably a member of the 5-HT$_{1D}$ family) with no significant affinity (as measured using standard radioligand binding assays) or pharmacological activity at 5-HT$_2$, 5-HT$_3$ receptor subtypes or at alpha$_1$ -alpha$_2$, -or beta-adrenergic; dopamine$_1$; dopamine$_2$; muscarinic; or benzodiazepine receptors.

The vascular 5-HT$_1$ receptor subtype to which sumatriptan binds selectively, and through which it presumably exerts its antimigrainous effect has been shown to be present on cranial arteries in both dog and primate, on the human basilar artery, and in the vasculature of the isolated dura mater of humans. In these tissues, sumatriptan activates this receptor to cause vasoconstriction, an action in humans correlating with the relief of migraine. In the anesthetized dog, sumatriptan selectively reduces the carotid arterial blood flow with little or no effect on arterial blood pressure or total peripheral resistance. In the cat, sumatriptan selectively constricts the carotid arteriovenous anastomoses, while having little or no effect on blood flow or resistance in cerebral or extracerebral tissues.

CORNEAL OPACITIES

Dogs receiving oral sumatriptan developed corneal opacities and defects in the corneal epithelium. Corneal opacities were seen at the lowest dosage tested, 2 mg/kg per day, and were present after 1 month of treatment. Defects in the corneal epithelium were noted in a 60-week study. Earlier examinations for these toxicities were not conducted and no-effect doses were not established; however, the relative exposure at the lowest dose tested was approximately five times the human exposure after a 100 mg oral dose or three times the human exposure after a 6 mg subcutaneous dose.

MELANIN BINDING

In rats with a single subcutaneous dose (0.5 mg/kg) [oral dose of 2 mg/kg] of radiolabeled sumatriptan, the elimination half-life of radioactivity from the eye was 15 days [oral dose was 23 days], suggesting that sumatriptan and its metabolites bind to the melanin of the eye. The clinical significance of this binding is unknown.

CLINICAL PHARMACOLOGY: *(cont'd)*

PHARMACOKINETICS

Injection: Pharmacokinetic parameters following a 6 mg subcutaneous injection into the deltoid area of the arm in nine males (mean age, 33 years; mean weight 77 kg) were systemic clearance: 1194 ± 149 ml/min (mean ± S.D.), distribution half-life: 15 ± 2 minutes, terminal half-life: 115 ± 19 minutes, and volume of distribution central compartment: 50 ± 8 liters. Of this dose, 22 ± 4% was excreted in the urine as unchanged sumatriptan and 38 ± 7% as the indole acetic acid metabolite.

After a single 6 mg subcutaneous manual injection into the deltoid area of the arm in 18 healthy males, (age, 24 ± 6 years; weight, 70 kg), the maximum serum concentration (C_{max}) was (mean ± standard deviation) 74 ± 15 ng/ml and the time to peak concentration (t_{max}) was 12 minutes after injection (range, 5 to 20 minutes). In this study, the same dose injected subcutaneously in the thigh gave a C_{max} of 61 ± 15 ng/ml by manual injection versus 52 ± 15 ng/ml by autoinjector techniques. The t_{max} or amount absorbed were not significantly altered by either the site or technique of injection.

The bioavailability of sumatriptan via subcutaneous site injection to 18 healthy male subjects was 97 ± 16% of that obtained following intravenous injection. Protein binding, determined by equilibrium dialysis over the concentration of 10 to 1000 ng/ml, is low, approximately 14% to 21%. The effect of sumatriptan on protein binding of other drugs has not yet been evaluated.

Oral: *Absorption and Elimination:* Sumatriptan succinate is rapidly absorbed after oral administration, with low absolute bioavailability, approximately 15%, primarily due to presystemic metabolism and partly due to incomplete absorption. The mean maximum concentration (C_{max}) following a 100 mg oral dose is 51 ng/ml. This compares with a C_{max} of about 75 ng/ml after a 6 mg subcutaneous dose. C_{max} is similar during a migraine attack and during a migraine-free period, but the t_{max} is slightly later during the attack, approximately 2.5 hours compared to 2.0 hours. When given as a single dose, sumatriptan displays dose proportionality in its extent of absorption (area under the curve [AUC]) over the dose range of 25 to 200 mg, but the C_{max} after 100 mg is approximately 25% less than expected (based on the 25 mg dose).

Food has no significant effect on the bioavailability of sumatriptan succinate, but delays the t_{max} slightly (by about 0.5 hours). Plasma protein binding is low (14% to 21%).

The apparent volume of distribution is 2.4 L/kg.

The elimination half-life of sumatriptan succinate is approximately 2.5 hours. Radiolabeled ^{14}C-sumatriptan succinate administered orally is largely renally excreted (about 60%) with about 40% found in the feces. Most of the radiolabeled compound excreted in the urine is the major metabolite, indole acetic acid (IAA), which is inactive, or the IAA glucuronide. Only 3% of the dose can be recovered as unchanged sumatriptan.

In vitro studies with human microsomes suggest that sumatriptan is metabolized by monoamine oxidase (MAO), predominantly the A isoenzyme, and inhibitors of that enzyme may alter sumatriptan pharmacokinetics to increase systemic exposure. No significant effect was seen with a MAO-B inhibitor (see CONTRAINDICATIONS, WARNINGS, and DRUG INTERACTIONS).

SPECIAL POPULATIONS

Renal Impairment: The effect of renal impairment on the pharmacokinetics of sumatriptan has not been examined, but little clinical effect would be expected as sumatriptan is largely metabolized to an inactive substance.

Hepatic Impairment: The effect of hepatic disease on the pharmacokinetics of subcutaneously and orally administered sumatriptan has been evaluated. There were no statistically significant differences in the pharmacokinetics of subcutaneously administered sumatriptan in hepatically impaired patients compared to healthy controls. However, the liver plays an important role in the presystemic clearance of orally administered sumatriptan. Accordingly, the bioavailability of sumatriptan following oral administration may be markedly increased in patients with liver disease. In one small study of hepatically impaired patients (n=8) matched for sex, age, and weight with healthy subjects, the hepatically impaired patients had an approximately 70% increase in AUC and C_{max} and a t_{max} 40 minutes earlier compared to the healthy subjects.

Age: *Elderly:* Sumatriptan pharmacokinetics in healthy elderly subjects were similar to those in healthy young volunteers. The pharmacokinetics of sumatriptan in the elderly (mean age, 72 years; two males and four females) and in patients with migraine (mean age, 38 years; 25 males and 155 females) were similar to that in healthy male subjects (mean age, 30 years).

Gender: In a study comparing females to males, no pharmacokinetic differences were observed between genders for AUC, C_{max}, t_{max} and half-life.

Race: The systemic clearance and C_{max} of sumatriptan were similar in black (n=34) and Caucasian (n=38) healthy male subjects. The effect of race on the pharmacokinetics of oral sumatriptan has not been examined.

PHARMACODYNAMICS

Typical Physiologic Responses from Injection:

Blood Pressure: (See WARNINGS.)

Peripheral (small) Arteries: In healthy volunteers (n=18), a study evaluating the effects of sumatriptan on peripheral (small vessel) arterial reactivity failed to detect a clinically significant increase in peripheral resistance.

Heart Rate: Transient increases in blood pressure observed in some patients in clinical studies carried out during sumatriptan's development as a treatment for migraine were not accompanied by any clinically significant changes in heart rate.

Respiratory Rate: Experience gained during the clinical development of sumatriptan as a treatment for migraine failed to detect an effect of the drug on respiratory rate.

Typical Physiologic Responses from Tablets:

Cardiovascular: *Blood Pressure:* Transient increases in systolic and diastolic blood pressure may be observed after treatment with oral sumatriptan succinate. Elderly (67 to 79 years of age) subjects given 100 or 200 mg of sumatriptan as a single oral dose had statistically significant increases in mean peak systolic blood pressure of up to 14 mmHg over the first 3 hours after dosing, with some evidence of increasing effect with dose. In the same study, however, a younger group of patients (19 to 37 years) had no chance in systolic blood pressure after doses of up to 200 mg. In this study, there were small, but statistically significant, increases in diastolic blood pressure of between 2 and 6 mmHg compared to placebo in young and elderly subjects after administration of sumatriptan (50, 100, and 200 mg), but other studies did not confirm this finding. In controlled U.S. studies in migraine patients, no consistent effects on blood pressure or heart rate were observed.

Heart and Respiratory: There have been no clinically significant effects of oral sumatriptan succinate on heart or respiratory rates.

CLINICAL STUDIES:

INJECTION

Migraine: In U.S. controlled clinical trials enrolling more than 1000 patients during migraine attacks who were experiencing moderate or severe pain and one or more of the symptoms enumerated in TABLE 2, onset of relief began as early as 10 minutes following a 6 mg

CLINICAL STUDIES: *(cont'd)*

sumatriptan succinate injection. Smaller doses of sumatriptan may also prove effective, although the proportion of patients obtaining adequate relief is decreased and the latency to that relief is greater.

In one well-controlled study where placebo (n=62) was compared to six different doses of sumatriptan succinate injection (n=30 each group) in a single attack, parallel-group design, the dose response relationship was found to be as shown in TABLE 1.

TABLE 1 Dose Response Relationship for Efficacy

Sumatriptan Dose (mg)	% Patients W/ Relief* at 10 min	30 min	1 hr	2 hrs	Adverse Events (% Incidence)
placebo	5	15	24	21	55
1	10	40	43	40	63
2	7	23	57	43	63
3	17	47	57	60	77
4	13	37	50	57	80
6	10	63	73	70	83
8	23	57	80	83	93

* Relief is defined as the reduction of moderate or severe pain to no or mild pain after dosing without use of rescue medication.

In two U.S. well-controlled trials in 1104 migraine patients with moderate and severe migraine pain, the onset of relief was rapid (less than 10 minutes). Headache relief, as evidenced by a reduction in pain from severe or moderately severe to mild or no headache, was achieved in 70% of the patients within 1 hour of a single 6 mg subcutaneous dose of sumatriptan succinate injection. Headache relief was achieved in approximately 82% of patients within 2 hours, and 65% of all patients were free of pain within 2 hours.

TABLE 2 shows the 1- and 2-hour efficacy results.

TABLE 2 Efficacy Data From U.S. Phase III Trials

One-Hour Data	Study 1 Placebo (n=190)	Study 1 Sumatriptan 6 mg (n=384)	Study 2 Placebo (n=180)	Study 2 Sumatriptan 6 mg (n=350)
Patients w/ pain relief (grade 0/1)	18%	70%*	26%	70%*
Patients with no pain	5%	48%*	13%	49%*
Patients without nausea	48%	73%*	50%	73%*
Patients without photophobia	23%	56%*	25%	58%*
Patients w/ little or no clinical disability§	34%	76%*	34%	76%*

Two-Hour Data	Study 1 Placebo†	Study 1 Sumatriptan 6 mg‡	Study 2 Placebo†	Study 2 Sumatriptan 6 mg‡
Patients w/ pain relief (grade 0/1)	31%	81%*	39%	82%*
Patients with no pain	11%	63%*	19%	65%*
Patients without nausea	56%	82%*	63%	81%*
Patients without photophobia	31%	72%*	35%	71%*
Patients w/ little or no clinical disability§	42%	85%*	49%	84%*

* $p < 0.05$ versus placebo.
† Includes patients that may have received additional placebo injection 1 hour after initial injection.
‡ Includes patients that may have received an additional 6 mg of Imitrex injection 1 hour after the initial injection.
§ A successful outcome in terms of clinical disability was defined prospectively as ability to work mildly impaired or able to work and function normally.

Sumatriptan succinate injection also relieved photophobia, phonophobia (sound sensitivity), nausea, and vomiting associated with migraine attacks. Similar efficacy was seen when patients self-administered sumatriptan succinate injection using an autoinjector.

The efficacy of sumatriptan succinate injection is unaffected by whether or not migraine is associated with aura, duration of attack, gender or age of the patient, or concomitant use of common migraine prophylactic drugs (*e.g.,* beta-blockers).

Cluster Headache: The efficacy of sumatriptan succinate injection in the acute treatment of cluster headache was demonstrated in two randomized, double-blind, placebo-controlled, two-period crossover trials. Patients age 21 to 65 were enrolled and were instructed to treat a moderate to very severe headache within 10 minutes of onset. Headache relief was defined as a reduction in headache severity to mild or no pain. In both trials, the proportion of individuals gaining relief at 10 or 15 minutes was significantly greater among patients receiving 6 mg of sumatriptan succinate injection compared to those who received placebo (see TABLE 3). One study evaluated a 12 mg dose; there was no statistically significant difference in outcome between patients randomized to the 6 and 12 mg doses.

TABLE 3 Efficacy Data From the Pivotal Cluster Headache Studies

	Study 1 Placebo (n=39)	Study 1 Sumatriptan 6 mg (n=39)	Study 2 Placebo (n=88)	Study 2 Sumatriptan 6 mg (n=92)
Patients with pain relief (no/mild)				
5 minutes postinjection	8%	21%	7%	23%*
10 minutes postinjection	10%	49%*	25%	49%*
15 minutes postinjection	26%	74%*	35%	75%*

* p<0.05
(n= Number of headaches treated.)

The Kaplan Meier (product limit) Survivorship Plot provides an estimate of the cumulative probability of a patient with a cluster headache obtaining relief after being treated with either sumatriptan or placebo.

The plot was constructed with data from patients who either experienced relief or did not require (request) rescue medication within a period of 2 hours following treatment. As a consequence, the data in the plot are derived from only a subset of the 258 headaches treated (resuce medication was required in 52 of the 127 placebo-treated headaches and 18 of the 131 sumatriptan-treated headaches).

Other data suggest that sumatriptan treatment is not associated with an increase in early recurrence of headache, and that treatment with sumatriptan has little effect on the incidence of latter occurring headaches (*i.e.,* those occurring after 2, but before 18 or 24 hours).

CLINICAL STUDIES: *(cont'd)*

TABLETS

Two U.S. controlled trials evaluated 25, 50, and 100 mg single doses of oral sumatriptan succinate in a total of 446 patients with migraine attacks who were experiencing moderate or severe pain and one or more of the symptoms enumerated in TABLE 4A. Onset relief (defined as no or mild pain) was seen as early as 1 to 1.5 hours after all three doses. Statistically significant differences from placebo were seen in the proportion of patients achieving relief at all time points starting at 1 to 2 hours and persisting out to 4 hours postdosing. There was no evidence of a dose response for pain and other measures of effectiveness. At 2 hours, approximately 54% (range, 50% to 57%) of patients on any dose of oral sumatriptan succinate had achieved relief, compared to 17% and 26% placebo response rates. By 4 hours postdosing, response rates in drug-treated patients were approximately 71% (range, 65% to 78%), compared to placebo rates of 19% and 38%. Sumatriptan succinate tablets also relieved nausea and photophobia associated with migraine attacks. TABLE 4A and TABLE 4B show the 2-4 hour efficacy results.

TABLE 4A Sumatriptan Succinate Tablets Dose Response Relationship for Efficacy

Study 1	Placebo (n=65)	Sumatriptan 25 mg (n=66)	Sumatriptan 50 mg (n=62)	Sumatriptan 100 mg (n=66)
Results at 2 Hours				
Patients with pain relief (grade 0/1)	26%	52%*	50%*	56%*
Patients with no pain	8%	21%*	16%	23%*
Patients with meaningful relief†	34%	59%*	55%*	56%*
Patients without nausea	57%	67%	68%	65%
Patients without photophobia	22%	41%*	37%*	44%*
Patients with little or no clinical disability‡	35%	58%*	60%*	59%*
Results at 4 Hours				
Patients with pain relief (grade 0/1)	38%	70%*	68%*	71%*
Patients with no pain	15%	45%*	32%*	52%*
Patients with meaningful relief†	45%	71%	71%*	79%*
Patients without nausea	60%	76%	79%*	83%*
Patients without photophobia	40%	62%*	66%*	71%*
Patients with little or no clinical disability‡	40%	68%*	71%*	71%*

* $p < 0.05$ vs. placebo. Once patients received rescue medication, they were considered treatment failures from that point onward.
† Meaningful relief is a patient assessment of when he/she felt onset of relief of headache pain.
‡ A successful outcome in terms of clinical disability was defined prospectively as ability to work mildly impaired or ability to work and function normally.

TABLE 4B Sumatriptan Succinate Tablets Dose Response Relationship for Efficacy

Study 2	Placebo (n=47)	Sumatriptan 25 mg (n=48)	Sumatriptan 50 mg (n=46)	Sumatriptan 100 mg (n=46)
Results at 2 Hours				
Patients with pain relief (grade 0/1)	17%	52%*	54%*	57%*
Patients with no pain	6%	21%*	17%	24%*
Patients with meaningful relief†	21%	54%*	54%*	57%*
Patients without nausea	40%	56%	61%	72%*
Patients without photophobia	13%	29%	26%	39%*
Patients with little or no clinical disability‡	28%	58%*	52%*	67%*
Results at 4 Hours				
Patients with pain relief (grade 0/1)	19%	65%*	72%*	78%*
Patients with no pain	11%	35%*	41%*	41%*
Patients with meaningful relief†	26%	69%*	72%*	83%*
Patients without nausea	45%	73%*	70%*	91%*
Patients without photophobia	28%	69%*	65%*	65%*
Patients with little or no clinical disability‡	23%	73%*	70%*	83%*

* $p < 0.05$ vs. placebo. Once patients received rescue medication, they were considered treatment failures from that point onward.
† Meaningful relief is a patient assessment of when he/she felt onset of relief of headache pain.
‡ A successful outcome in terms of clinical disability was defined prospectively as ability to work mildly impaired or ability to work and function normally.

The efficacy of sumatriptan succinate tablets is unaffected by whether or not migraine is associated with aura, duration of attack, gender or age of the patient, relationship to menses, or concomitant use of common migraine prophylactic drugs (*e.g.,* beta-blockers, calcium channel blockers, or tricyclic antidepressants). There was insufficient data to assess the impact of race on the efficacy of sumatriptan succinate tablets.

INDICATIONS AND USAGE:

Injection: Sumatriptan succinate injection is indicated for 1) the acute treatment of migraine attacks with or without aura and 2) the acute treatment of cluster headache episodes.

Sumatriptan succinate injection is not for use in the management of hemiplegic or basilar migraine (see CONTRAINDICATIONS).

Tablets: Sumatriptan succinate tablets are indicated for the acute treatment of migraine attacks with or without aura.

Sumatriptan succinate tablets are not for use in the management of hemiplegic or basilar migraine (see WARNINGS). Safety and effectiveness also have not been established for cluster headache, which is present in an older, predominantly male population.

CONTRAINDICATIONS:

INJECTION

Sumatriptan succinate injection should not be given intravenously because of its potential to cause coronary vasospasm.

Sumatriptan succinate injection should not be given subcutaneously to patients with ischemic heart disease (angina pectoris, history of myocardial infarction, or documented silent ischemia) or to patients with Prinzmetal's variant angina.

CONTRAINDICATIONS: *(cont'd)*

Sumatriptan succinate injection should not be given subcutaneously to patients who are determined to have symptoms or findings consistent with coronary artery vasospasm, ischemic myocardial disease, or other significant underlying cardiovascular disease (see WARNINGS).

Because sumatriptan succinate injection may increase blood pressure, it should not be given to patients with uncontrolled hypertension.

Sumatriptan succinate injection should not be used within 24 hours of treatment with an ergotamine-containing or ergot-type medication like dihydroergotamine or methysergide.

Sumatriptan succinate injection should not be administered to patients with hemiplegic or basilar migraine.

Sumatriptan succinate is contraindicated in patients with hypersensitivity to sumatriptan or any of its components.

TABLETS

Because of rare reports of coronary vasospasm, sumatriptan succinate tablets should not be given to patients with ischemic heart disease (angina pectoris, history of myocardial infarction, or documented silent ischemia) or to patients with Prinzmetal's angina. Also, patients with symptoms or signs consistent with ischemic heart disease should not receive sumatriptan succinate tablets. Because sumatriptan succinate tablets can give rise to increases in blood pressure (usually small), they should not be given to patients with uncontrolled hypertension.

Concurrent administration of MAO inhibitors or use within 2 weeks of discontinuation of MAO inhibitor therapy is contraindicated (See DRUG INTERACTIONS).

Sumatriptan succinate tablets should not be used within 24 hours of an ergotamine-containing or ergot-type medication like dihydroergotamine or methysergide.

Sumatriptan succinate tablets are contraindicated in patients with hypersensitivity to sumatriptan or any of the ingredients.

WARNINGS:

INJECTION

Sumatriptan succinate injection should only be used where a clear diagnosis migraine or cluster headache has been established.

Risk of Myocardial Ischemia and/or Infarction and Other Adverse Cardiac Events: It is strongly recommended that sumatriptan not be given to patients in whom unrecognized coronary artery disease (CAD) is predicted by the presence of risk factors (*e.g.,* hypertension, hypercholesterolemia, smoker, obesity, diabetes, strong family history of CAD, female who is surgically or physiologically postmenopausal, or male who is over 40 years of age) unless a cardiovascular evaluation provides satisfactory clinical evidence that the patient is reasonably free of coronary artery and ischemic myocardial disease or other significant underlying cardiovascular disease. The sensitivity of cardiac diagnostic procedures to detect cardiovascular disease or predisposition to coronary artery vasospasm is unknown. In considering this recommendation, it is noted that patients with cluster headache often possess one or more predictive risk factors for CAD. If, during the cardiovascular evaluation, the patient's medical history or electrocardiographic investigations reveal findings indicative of or consistent with coronary artery vasospasm or myocardial ischemia, sumatriptan should not be administered (see CONTRAINDICATIONS).

For patients with risk factors predictive of CAD who are determined to have a satisfactory cardiovascular evaluation, it is strongly recommended that administration of the first dose of sumatriptan injection take place in the setting of a physician's office or similar medically staffed and equipped facility. Because cardiac ischemia can occur in the absence of clinical symptoms, consideration should be given to obtaining on the first occasion of use an electrocardiogram (ECG) during the interval immediately following sumatriptan succinate injection, in these patients with risk factors.

It is recommended that patients who are intermittent long-term users of sumatriptan succinate injection and who have or acquire risk factors predictive of CAD, as described above, undergo periodic interval cardiovascular evaluation as they continue to use sumatriptan succinate injection. In considering this recommendation for periodic cardiovascular evaluation, it is noted that patients with cluster headache are predominantly male and over 40 years of age, which are risk factors for CAD.

The systematic approach described above is intended to reduce the likelihood that patients with unrecognized cardiovascular disease will be inadvertently exposed to sumatriptan.

Drug-Associated Cardiac Events and Fatalities: Serious adverse events, including actue myocardial infarction, life-threatening disturbances of cardiac rhythm, and death have been reported to have occurred within 1 hour following the administration of sumatriptan succinate injection. Considering the extent of use of sumatriptan in patients with migraine, the incidence of these events is extremely low. The fact that sumatriptan can cause coronary vasospasm gives credence to the possibility that at least some of the cases reported in close temporal association with the use of sumatriptan succinate may have been caused by the drug.

Premarketing Experience: Among the more than 1900 patients with migraine who participated in premarketing controlled clinical trials of sumatriptan, there were eight patients who sustained clinical events during or shortly after receiving subcutaneous sumatriptan that may have reflected coronary artery vasospasm. Six of these eight patients had ECG changes consistent with transient ischemia, but without accompanying clinical symptoms or signs. Of these eight patients, four had either findings suggestive of CAD or risk factors predictive of CAD prior to study enrollment.

Postmarketing Experience: Serious cardiovascular events, some resulting in death, have been reported in association with the use of sumatriptan succinate injection. The uncontrolled nature of postmarketing surveillance, however, makes it impossible to determine definitively the proportion of the reported cases that were actually caused by sumatriptan or to reliably assess causation in individual cases. On clinical grounds, the longer the latency between the administration of sumatriptan succinate and the onset of the clinical event, the less likely the association is to be causative. Accordingly, interest has focused on events occurring within 1 hour of the administration of sumatriptan succinate.

Cardiac events that have been observed to have onset within 1 hour of sumatriptan administration include: coronary artery vasospasm, transient ischemia, myocardial infarction, ventricular tachycardia and ventricular fibrillation, cardiac arrest, and death.

Some of these events occurred in patients who had no findings of CAD and may represent sequellae of coronary artery vasospasm. However, among domestic cases reported prior to January 1996 involving patients with serious cardiac events within 1 hour of sumatriptan administration, the majority had risk factors predictive of CAD, and use of sumatriptan may have been contraindicated. The presence of significant underlying CAD was established in most of these cases.

Drug-Associated Cerbrovascular Events and Fatalities: Cerebral hemorrhage, subarachnoid hemorrhage, stroke, and other cerebrovascular events have been reported in patients treated with oral and subcutaneous sumatriptan, and some have resulted in fatalities. In a number of cases, it appears possible that the cerebrovascular events were primary, sumatriptan having been administered in the incorrect belief the symptoms experienced were a consequence of migraine when they were not. Accordingly, sumatriptan should not be administered if the headache being experienced is atypical. In this regard, it should be noted that patients with migraine may be at increased risk of certain cerebrovascular events (*e.g.,* cerebrovascular accident, transient ischemic attack).

WARNINGS: *(cont'd)*

Increase is Blood Pressure: Significant elevation in blood pressure, including hypertensive crisis, has been reported on rare occasions in patients with and without a history of hypertension. Sumatriptan is contraindicated in patients with uncontrolled hypertension (see CONTRAINDICATIONS).

Concomitant Drug Use: In patients taking MAO-A inhibitors, sumatriptan plasma levels attained after treatment with recommended doses are nearly double those obtained under other conditions. Accordingly, the co-administration of sumatriptan and an MAO-A inhibitor is not generally recommended. If such therapy is clinically warranted, however, suitable dose adjustment and appropriate observation of the patient is advised (see CLINICAL PHARMACOLOGY).

Use in Women of Childbearing Potential: (See PRECAUTIONS.)

Hypersensitivity: Hypersensitivity (anaphylaxis/anaphylactoid) reactions have occurred on rare occasions in patients receiving sumatriptan. Such reactions can be life threatening or fatal. In general, hypersensitivity reactions to drugs are more likely to occur in individuals with a history of sensitivity to multiple allergens (see CONTRAINDICATIONS).

TABLETS

Sumatriptan succinate tablets should only be used where a clear diagnosis of migraine has been established.

Sumatriptan succinate tablets should not be administered to patients with basilar or hemiplegic migraine.

Hypersensitivity (anaphylaxis/anaphylactoid) reactions have occurred on rare occasions in patients receiving sumatriptan. Such reactions can be life threatening or fatal. In general, hypersensitivity reactions to drugs are more likely to occur in individuals with a history of sensitivity to multiple allergens.

Cardiac Events/Coronary Constriction: Serious coronary events, including some that have been fatal, following sumatriptan succinate tablets have occurred but are extremely rare. Although it is not clear how many of these can be attributed to sumatriptan succinate, because of their potential to cause coronary vasospasm, sumatriptan succinate tablets should not be given to patients in whom unrecognized coronary artery disease (CAD) is likely without a prior evaluation for underlying cardiovascular disease. Such patients include postmenopausal women, males over 40, and patients with other risk factors for CAD such as hypertension, hypercholesterolemia, obesity, diabetes, smokers, and strong family history. Following a satisfactory cardiovascular assessment, it is recommended that the first dose of sumatriptan succinate tablets be administered in the physician's office for patients with underlying risk factors for CAD unless these patients have previously received sumatriptan. If symptoms consistent with angina occur, electrocardiographic (ECG) evaluation should be carried out to look for ischemic changes.

Sumatriptan may cause coronary vasospasm in patients with a history of CAD, who are known to be more susceptible than others to coronary artery vasospasm, and, rarely, in patients without prior history suggestive of CAD. Of 6348 patients in clinical trials of oral sumatriptan, two experienced clinical adverse events shortly after receiving oral sumatriptan that may have reflected coronary vasospasm. Neither of these adverse events was associated with a serious clinical outcome.

There have been rare reports from countries where sumatriptan succinate tablets are already on the market of serious adverse events, including myocardial infarction, ECG changes suggestive of myocardial ischemia, and symptoms consistent with angina pectoris.

Drug-Associated Fatalities: In extensive worldwide postmarketing experience, deaths have been reported following the use of sumatriptan. In most cases, the deaths occurring after treatment with sumatriptan tablets occurred well after sumatriptan use (*i.e.,* 3 or more hours postdose) and probably reflect underlying disease and spontaneous events.

There have, however, been several fatalities that occurred within a few hours after the use of sumatriptan. The specific contribution of sumatriptan to most of these deaths cannot be determined, but in one case, with sumatriptan succinate injection, a 41-year-old woman with a 6-day history of unilateral headache, uncertain history of cardiovascular disease with known risk factors (positive family history, postmenopausal woman, and smoking) and a history of asthma and codeine allergy, experienced nausea, vomiting, a sense of warmth, chest pressure, and sweating within 7 minutes of dosing. This was followed by hypotension at about one-half hour, and ventricular tachycardia/ventricular fibrillation leading to death. In most other cases, death was attributed to myocardial infarctions occurring hours after drug administration.

Deaths attributed to strokes, cerebral hemorrhage, and other cerebrovascular events have been reported in patients treated with oral and subcutaneous sumatriptan. In many cases, it appears possible that the cerebrovascular events were primary, sumatriptan having been administered in the incorrect belief that the symptoms experienced were migrainous in origin when they were not. Accordingly, it is important to advise patients not to administer sumatriptan if a headache being experienced is atypical.

Use in Women of Childbearing Potential: (See PRECAUTIONS.)

PRECAUTIONS:

GENERAL

Sumatriptan succinate injection should also be administered with caution to patients with diseases that may alter the absorption, metabolism, or excretion of drugs, such as impaired hepatic or renal function. (see CLINICAL PHARMACOLOGY and DOSAGE AND ADMINISTRATION).

There have been rare reports of seizure following administration of sumatriptan.

Injection: Chest, jaw, or neck tightness is relatively common after administration of sumatriptan succinate injection, but has only rarely been associated with ischemic ECG changes. However, because sumatriptan may cause coronary artery vasospasm, patients who experience signs or symptoms suggestive of angina following sumatriptan should be evaluated for the presence of CAD or a predisposition to Prinzmetal's variant angina before receiving additional doses of sumatriptan (see WARNINGS). Similarly, patinets who experience other symptoms or sign suggestive of decreasing arterial flow (such as ischemic abdomina; syndromes or Raynaud's syndrome) following sumatriptan should be evaluated for atherosclerosis or predisposition to vasospasm.

Sumatriptan injection should also be administered with caution to patinets with diseases that may alter absorption, metabolism, or excretion of drugs, such as impaired hepatic or renal function.

There have been reports of seizure following administration of sumatriptan.

Care should be taken to exclude other potentially serious neurologic conditions before treating headache in patients not previously diagnosed with migraine or cluster headache or who experience a headache that is atypical for them. There have been rare reports where patients received sumatriptan for severe headaches that were subsequently shown to have been secondary to an evolving neurologic lesion (see WARNINGS). For a given attack, if a patient dose not respond to the first dose of sumatriptan, the diagnosis of migraine or cluster headache should be reconsidered before administration of a second dose.

PRECAUTIONS: *(cont'd)*

Oral: Atypical sensations over the precordium (tightness, pressure, heaviness) have been reported after sumatriptan succinate tablets, but have only rarely been associated with ischemic ECG changes. However, because SUM may cause coronary vasospasm, patients who experience signs or symptoms suggestive of angina following sumatriptan should be evaluated for the presence of CAD or a predisposition to Prinametal's variant angina before receiving additional doses of SUM (see WARNINGS). Similarly patinets who experience other symptoms or signs suggestive of decreased arterial flow (such as ischemic abdominal syndromes or Raynaud's syndrome) following SUM should be evaluated for atherosclerosis or predisposition to vasospasm.

Sumatriptan may cause mild, transient elevation of blood pressure (see CLINICAL PHARMACOLOGY).

As with other acute migraine therapies, before treating headaches in patients not previously diagnosed as migraineurs and in migraineurs who present with atypical symptoms, care should be taken to exclude other potentially serious neurological conditions. There have been rare reports where patients received sumatriptan for severe headaches that were subsequently shown to have been secondary to an evolving neurological lesion (cerebrovascular accident, subarachnoid hemorrhage). For a given attack, if a patient has no response to the first dose, the diagnosis of migraine should be reconsidered before administration of a second dose. In this regard, it should be noted that migraineurs may be at increased risk of certain cerebrovascular events (*e.g.,* cerebrovascular accident, transient ischemic attack).

BINDING TO MELANIN-CONTAINING TISSUES

Because sumatriptan binds to melanin, it could accumulate in melanin-rich tissues (such as the eye) over time. This raises the possibility that sumatriptan could cause toxicity in these tissues after extended use. However, no effects on the retina related to treatment with sumatriptan were noted in any of the toxicity studies. Although no systematic monitoring of ophthalmologic function was undertaken in clinical trials, and no specific recommendations for ophthalmologic monitoring are offered, prescribers should be aware of the possibility of long-term ophthalmologic effects (see CLINICAL PHARMACOLOGY).

CORNEAL OPACITIES

Sumatriptan causes corneal opacities and defects in the corneal epithelium in dogs; this raises the possibility that these changes may occur in humans. While patients were not systematically evaluated for these changes in clinical trials, and no specific recommendations for monitoring are being offered, prescribers should be aware of the possibility of these changes (see CLINICAL PHARMACOLOGY).

Injection: Although written instructions are supplied with the autoinjector, patients who are advised to self-administer sumatriptan succinate injection in medically unsupervised situations should receive instruction on the proper use of the product from the physician or other suitably qualified health care professional prior to doing so for the first time.

INFORMATION FOR THE PATIENT

(See PATIENT PACKAGE INSERT) at the end of this labeling for the text of the separate leaflet provided for patients.

LABORATORY TESTS

No specific laboratory tests are recommended for monitoring patients prior to and/or after treatment with sumatriptan succinate injection.

DRUG/LABORATORY TEST INTERACTIONS

Sumatriptan succinate is not known to interfere with commonly employed clinical laboratory tests.

CARCINOGENESIS, MUTAGENESIS, AND IMPAIRMENT OF FERTILITY

In carcinogenicity studies, rats and mice were given sumatriptan by oral gavage (rats, 104 weeks), or drinking water (mice, 78 weeks). Average exposures achieved in mice receiving the highest dose were approximately 110 times [oral 40 times] the exposure attained by humans after the maximum recommended single subcutaneous dose of 6 mg [oral 100 mg]. The highest subcutaneous dose to rats was approximately 260 times [oral 15 times]the maximum single dose on a mg/m^2 basis. There was no evidence of an increase in tumors in either species related to sumatriptan administration.

Sumatriptan was not mutagenic in the presence or absence of metabolic activation when tested in two gene mutation assays (the Ames test and the *in vitro* mammalian Chinese hamster V79/HGPRT assay). In two cytogenetics assays (the *in vitro* human lymphocyte assay and the *in vivo* rat micronucleus assay) sumatriptan was not associated with clastogenic activity.

Injection: A fertility study (Segment I) by the subcutaneous route, during which male and female rats were dosed daily with sumatriptan prior to and throughout the mating period, has shown no evidence of impaired fertility at doses equivalent to approximately 100 times the maximum recommended single human dose of 6 mg on a mg/m^2 basis. However, following oral administration, a treatment-related decrease in fertility, secondary to a decrease in mating, was seen for rats treated with 50 and 500 mg/kg per day. The no-effect dose for this finding was approximately eight times the maximum recommended single human dose of 6 mg on a mg/m^2 basis. It is not clear whether the problem is associated with the treatment of males or females or both.

Oral: In a study in which male and female rats were dosed daily with oral sumatriptan prior to and throughout the mating period, there was a treatment-related decrease in fertility secondary to a decrease in mating in animals treated with 50 and 500 mg/kg per day. The no-effect dose for tis finding was approximately one-half of the maximum recommended single human dose of 100 mg on a mg/m^2 basis. It is not clear whether the problem is associated with treatment of the males or females or both combined.

PREGNANCY CATEGORY C

To monitor fetal outcomes of pregnant women exposed to sumatriptan, Glaxo Wellcome Inc. maintains a Sumatriptan Pregnancy Registry. Physicians are encouraged to register patients by calling (800) 722-9292, ext. 58465.

Injection

Sumatriptan has been shown to be embryolethal in rabbits when given daily at a dose approximately equivalent to the maximum recommended single human subcutaneous dose of 6 mg on a mg/m^2 basis. There is no evidence that establishes that sumatriptan is a human teratogen; however, there are no adequate and well-controlled studies in pregnant women. Sumatriptan succinate injection should be used during pregnancy only if the potential benefit justifies the potential risk to the fetus.

In assessing this information, the following additional findings should be considered.

Embryolethality: When given intravenously to pregnant rabbits daily throughout the period of organogenesis, sumatriptan caused embryolethality at doses at or close to those producing maternal toxicity. The mechanism of the embryolethality is not known. These doses were approximately equivalent to the maximum single human dose of 6 mg on a mg/m^2 basis.

The intravenous administration of sumatriptan to pregnant rats throughout organogenesis at doses that are approximately 20 times a human dose of 6 mg on a mg/m^2 basis, did not cause embryolethality. Additionally, in a study of pregnant rats given subcutaneous sumatriptan daily prior to and throughout pregnancy, there was no evidence of increase embryo/fetal lethality.

PRECAUTIONS: *(cont'd)*

Teratogenicity: Term fetuses from Dutch Stride rabbits treated during organogenesis with oral sumatriptan exhibited an increased incidence of cervicothoracic vascular and skeletal abnormalities. The functional significance of these abnormalities is not known. The highest no-effect dose for these effects was 15 mg/kg per day, approximately 50 times the maximum single dose of 6 mg on a mg/m^2 basis.

In a study in rats dosed daily with subcutaneous sumatriptan prior to and throughout pregnancy, there was no evidence of teratogenicity.

Oral

In reproductive toxicity studies in rats and rabbits, oral treatment with sumatriptan was associated with embryolethality, fetal abnormalities, and pup mortality. There is no evidence that establishes that sumatriptan is a human teratogen; however, there are no adequate and well-controlled studies in pregnant women. Sumatriptan succinate tablets should be used during pregnancy only if the potential benefit justifies the potential risk to the fetus. In assessing this information, the following findings should be considered.

Embryolethality: When given orally to pregnant rabbits daily throughout the period of organogenesis, sumatriptan caused embryolethality only at a dose that clearly resulted in maternal toxicity, 100 mg/kg per day. The no-effect dose for embryolethality was 50 mg/kg per day, which is approximately nine times the maximum single human dose of 100 mg on a mg/m^2 basis.

Teratogenicity: A study in which rats were dosed daily with oral sumatriptan prior to and through gestation demonstrated fetal toxicity and a small increased incidence of a syndrome of malformations (short tail/short body and vertebral disorganization) after long-term treatment with 500 mg/kg per day. The no-effect dose for this effect was 50 mg/kg per day, approximately five times the maximum single human dose of 100 mg on a mg/m^2 basis.

Oral treatment of pregnant rats with sumatriptan during the period of organogenesis resulted in an increased incidence of blood vessel abnormalities (cervicothoracic and umbilical) at doses of approximately 250 mg/kg per day or higher. The no-effect dose for this was approximately 60 mg/kg per day, approximately six times the maximum single human dose of 100 mg on a mg/m^2 basis.

Oral treatment of pregnant rabbits with sumatriptan during the period of organogenesis resulted in an increased incidence of cervicothoracic vascular and skeletal abnormalities. The highest no-effect dose established for these effects was 15 mg/kg per day, approximately three times the human dose of 100 mg on a mg/m^2 basis.

Pup Deaths: Oral treatment of pregnant rats with sumatriptan during the period of organogenesis resulted in a decrease in pup survival between birth and postnatal day 4 at doses of approximately 250 mg/kg per day or higher. The no-effect dose for this effect was approximately 60 mg/kg per day, or six times the human dose of 100 mg on a mg/m^2 basis.

Oral treatment of pregnant rats with sumatriptan from gestational day 17 through postnatal day 21 demonstrated a decrease in pup survival measured at postnatal days 2, 4, and 20 at the dose of 1000 mg/kg per day. The no-effect dose for this finding was 100 mg/kg per day, approximately 10 times the human dose of 100 mg on a mg/m^2 basis.

NURSING MOTHERS

Sumatriptan is excreted in human breast milk. Therefore, caution should be exercised when considering the administration of sumatriptan succinate injection to a nursing woman.

PEDIATRIC USE

Safety and effectiveness of sumatriptan succinate injection in pediatric patients have not been established.

GERIATRIC USE

Although the pharmacokinetic disposition of the drug in elderly is similar to that seen in younger adults, there is no information about the safety and effectiveness of sumatriptan in this population because patients over age 65 were excluded from the controlled clinical trials.

DRUG INTERACTIONS:

INJECTION

There is no evidence that concomitant use of migraine prophylactic medications has any effect on the efficacy or unwanted effects of sumatriptan. In two Phase III trials in the US, a retrospective analysis of 282 patients who had been using prophylactic drugs (verapamil n=63, amitriptyline n=57, propranolol n=94, for 45 other drugs n=123) were compared to those who had not used prophylaxis (n=452). There were no differences in relief rates at 60 minutes postdose for sumatriptan succinate injection, whether or not prophylactic medications were used. There were also no differences in overall adverse event rates between the two groups.

Ergot-containing drugs have been reported to cause prolonged vasospastic reactions. Because there is a theoretical basis that these effects may be additive, use of ergotamine or ergot-type medications (like dihydroergotamine or methysergide) and sumatriptan within 24 hours of each other should be avoided (see CONTRAINDICATIONS).

MAO-A inhibitors reduce sumatriptan clearance, significantly increasing systemic exposure. Therefore, the use of sumatriptan in patients receiving MAO-A inhibitors is not ordinarily recommended. If the clinical situation warrants the combined use of sumatriptan and an MAOI, the dose of sumatriptan employed should be reduced (see CLINICAL PHARMACOLOGY and WARNINGS).

There have been rare postmarketing reports describing patients with weakness, hyperreflexia, and incoordination following the use of a selective serotonin reuptake inhibitor (SSRI) and sumatriptan. If concomitant treatment with sumatriptan and an SSRI (*e.g.,* fluoxetine, fluvoxamine, paroxetine, sertraline) is clinically warranted, appropriate observation of the patient is advised.

TABLETS

Note: The combined use of oral sumatriptan and MAO inhibitors in contraindicated (see CONTRAINDICATIONS).

There is no evidence that concomitant use of migraine prophylactic medications has any effect on the efficacy or unwanted effects of sumatriptan. In controlled trials, a retrospective analysis compared 199 patients who had been using sumatriptan succinate tablets and prophylactic drugs (calcium channel blockers, n=76; tricyclic antidepressants, n=43; beta blockers, n=70) to those who had not used prophylaxis (n=1220). There were no differences in overall adverse event rates between the two groups.

Ergot-containing drugs have been reported to cause prolonged vasospastic reactions. Because there is theoretical basis that these effects may be additive, use of ergot-containing or ergot-type medications (like dihydroergotamine or methysergide) and sumatriptan within 24 hours of each other should be avoided (see CONTRAINDICATIONS).

Propranolol: Pretreatment with propanolol 80 mg twice daily for 7 days had no effect on the pharmacokinetics, blood pressure, or pulse rate of oral sumatriptan administered as a single 300 mg dose.

Alcohol: Alcohol consumed 30 minutes prior to sumatriptan ingestion had no effect on the pharmacokinetics of sumatriptan.

ADVERSE REACTIONS:

INJECTION

Serious cardiac events, including some that have been fatal, have occurred following use of sumatriptan succinate injection, but are extremely rare. Events reported have included coronary artery vasospasm, transient myocardial ischemia, myocardial infarction, ventricular tachycardia, and ventricular fibrillation (see CONTRAINDICATIONS, WARNINGS, and PRECAUTIONS).

Significant hypertensive episodes, including hypertensive crises, have been reported on rare occasions in patients with or without a history of hypertension (see WARNINGS).

Among patients in clinical trials of subcutaneous sumatriptan succinate injection (n=6128), up to 3.5% of patients withdrew for reasons related to adverse events.

Incidence in Controlled Clinical Trials: TABLE 5 lists adverse events that occurred in two large U.S., Phase III, placebo-controlled clinical trials in migraine patients following either a single dose of sumatriptan succinate injection or placebo. Only events that occurred at a frequency of 1% or more in sumatriptan succinate injection treatment groups and were at least as frequent as in the placebo group are included in TABLE 5.

TABLE 5 Treatment-Emergent Adverse Experience Incidence in Two Large Placebo-Controlled Migrane Clinical Trials: Events Reported by at Least 1% of Sumatriptan Succinate Injection Patients

Adverse Event Type	Percent of Patients Reporting Sumatriptan Subcutaneous Injection 6 mg n=547	Placebo n=370
Atypical sensations	42.0	9.2
Tingling	13.5	3.0
Warm/hot sensation	10.8	3.5
Burning sensation	7.5	0.3
Feeling of heaviness	7.3	1.1
Pressure sensation	7.1	1.6
Feeling of tightness	5.1	0.3
Numbness	4.6	2.2
Feeling strange	2.2	0.3
Tight feeling in head	2.2	0.3
Cold sensation	1.1	0.5
Cardiovascular		
Flushing	6.6	2.4
Chest discomfort	4.5	1.4
Tightness in chest	2.7	0.5
Pressure in chest	1.8	0.3
Ear, nose, and throat		
Throat discomfort	3.3	0.5
Discomfort: nasal cavity/sinuses	2.2	0.3
Eye		
Vision alterations	1.1	0.0
Gastrointestinal		
Abdominal discomfort	1.3	0.8
Dysphagia	1.1	0.0
Injection site reaction	58.7	23.8
Miscellaneous		
Jaw discomfort	1.8	0.0
Mouth and teeth		
Discomfort of mouth/tongue	4.9	4.6
Musculoskeletal		
Weakness	4.9	0.3
Neck pain/stiffness	4.8	0.5
Myalgia	1.8	0.5
Muscle cramp(s)	1.1	0.0
Neurological		
Dizziness/Vertigo	11.9	4.3
Drowsiness/Sedation	2.7	2.2
Headache	2.2	0.3
Anxiety	1.1	0.5
Malaise/fatigue	1.1	0.8
Skin		
Sweating	1.6	1.1

The sum of percentages cited are greater than 100% because patients may experience more than one type of adverse event. Only events that occurred at a frequency of 1% or more in sumatriptan succinate injection treatment groups and were at least as frequent as in the placebo groups are included.

The incidence of adverse events in controlled clinical trials was not affected by gender or age of the patients. There was insufficient data to assess the impact of race on the incidence of adverse events.

Incidence in Controlled Trials of Cluster Headache: In the controlled clinical trials assessing sumatriptan's efficacy as a treatment for cluster headache, no new significant adverse events associated with the use of sumatriptan were detected that had not already been identified in association of the drug's use in migraine.

Overall, the frequency of adverse events reported in the studies of cluster headache were generally lower. Exceptions include reports of paresthesia (5% sumatriptan succinate, 0% placebo), nausea and vomiting (4% sumatriptan succinate, 0% placebo) and bronchospasm (1% sumatriptan, 0% placebo).

Other Events Observed in Association With the Administration of Sumatriptan Succinate Injection: In the paragraphs that follow, the frequencies of less commonly reported adverse clinical events are presented. Because the reports cite events observed in open and uncontrolled studies, the role of sumatriptan succinate injection in their causation cannot be reliably determined. Furthermore, variability associated with reporting requirements, the terminology used to describe the adverse events, etc., limit the value of the quantitative frequency estimates provided.

Event frequencies are calculated as the number of patients reporting an event divided by the total number of patients (n=6128) exposed to subcutaneous sumatriptan succinate injection. Given their imprecision, frequencies for specific adverse event occurrences are defined as follows: "infrequent" indicates a frequency estimated as falling between 1/1000 and 1/100; "rare", a frequency less than 1/1000.

Cardiovascular: *Infrequent:*hypertension, hypotension, bradycardia, tachycardia, palpitations, pulsating sensations, various transient ECG changes (nonspecific ST or T wave changes, prolongation of PR or QTc intervals, sinus arrhythmia, nonsustained ventricular premature beats, isolated junctional ectopic beats, atrial ectopic beats, delayed activation of the right ventricle), and syncope. *Rare:*pallor, arrhythmia, abnormal pulse, vasodilation, and Raynaud's syndrome.

Endocrine and Metabolic: *Infrequent:*thirst. *Rare:*polydipsia and dehydration.

Eye: *Infrequent:*irritation of the eye.

Gastrointestinal: *Infrequent:*gastroesophageal reflux, diarrhea, and disturbances of liver function tests. *Rare:* peptic ulcer, retching, flatulence/eructation, and gallstones.

ADVERSE REACTIONS: *(cont'd)*

Musculoskeletal: *Infrequent:*various joint disturbances (pain, stiffness, swelling, ache). *Rare:* muscle stiffness, need to flex calf muscles, backache, muscle tiredness, and swelling of the extremities.

Neurological: *Infrequent:*mental confusion, euphoria, agitation, relaxation, chills, sensation of lightness, tremor, shivering, disturbances of taste, prickling sensations, paresthesia, stinging sensations, headaches, facial pain, photophobia, and lacrimation. *Rare:*transient hemiplegia, hysteria, globus hystericus, intoxication, depression, myoclonia, monoplegia/diplegia, sleep disturbance, difficulties in concentration, disturbances of smell, hyperesthesia, dysesthesia, simultaneous hot and cold sensations, tickling sensations, dysarthria, yawning, reduced appetite, hunger, and dystonia.

Respiratory: *Infrequent:*dyspnea. *Rare:*influenza, diseases of the lower respiratory tract, and hiccoughs.

Dermatologic: *Infrequent:*erythema, pruritus, and skin rashes and eruptions. *Rare:*skin tenderness.

Urogenital: *Rare:*dysuria, frequency, dysmenorrhea, and renal calculus.

Miscellaneous: *Infrequent:*miscellaneous laboratory abnormalities, including minor disturbances in liver function tests, "seritonin agonist effect", and hypersensitivity to various agents. *Rare:*fever.

Postmarketing Experience: The following are spontaneously reported adverse events from postmarketing experience except those events already listed previously in ADVERSE REACTIONS or those too general to be informative. Because the reports cite events reported spontaneously from worldwide postmarketing experience, frequency of events and the role of sumatriptan succinate injection in their causation cannot be reliably determined.

Cardiovascular: Cerebovascular accident, ischemic colitis, Prinzmetal's variant angina, subarachnoid hemorrhage.

Dermatological: Exacerbation of sunburn, photosensitivity. Following subcutaneous administration of SUM, pain, redness, stinging, induration, swelling, confusion, subcutaneous bleeding, and, on rare occasions, lipoatrophy (depression in the skin) or lipohypertrophy (enlargement or thickening of tissue) have been reported.

Hypersensitivity reactions: Shortness of breath and urticaria. In addition, severe anaphylaxis/anaphylactoid reactions have been reported (see WARNINGS).

Neurological: Dysphasia, seizure.

Non-Site Specific: Death (see WARNINGS). Rarely, lipoathrophy (depression in the skin) or lipohypertrophy (enlargement or thickening of tissue) has been reported following subcutaneous administration of SUM.

Respiratory: Bronchospasm has been reported in patients with and without a history of asthma.

Urogenital: Acute renal failure.

TABLETS

(See also PRECAUTIONS) Sumatriptan may cause coronary vasospasm in patients with a history of CAD, known to be susceptible to coronary artery vasospasm, and, very rarely, without prior history suggestive of CAD.

There have been rare reports from countries in which sumatriptan succinate tablets have been marketed of serious and/or life-threatening arrhythmias, including atrial fibrillation, ventricular fibrillation, ventricular tachycardia; myocardial infarction; ECG changes suggestive of myocardial ischemia; and symptoms consistent with angina pectoris after oral sumatriptan. Chest discomfort, when it occurs, is usually noncardiac in origin.

Other untoward clinical events associated with the use of sumatriptan succinate tablets are: warm/hot sensations, tingling/paresthesia, pressure sensations, flushing, sensations of heaviness, chest symptoms (tightness and sensations of heaviness), dizziness/vertigo, bad taste in mouth, weakness, myalgias neck stiffness; all these untoward effects are transient, although they may be severe in occasional patients.

Incidence in Controlled Clinical Trials: TABLE 6 lists adverse events that occurred in two large U.S. placebo-controlled clinical trials. Only events that occurred at a frequency of 1% or more in the sumatriptan succinate tablets 100 mg group and that occurred more frequently in that group than the placebo group are included in TABLE 6.

TABLE 6 Treatment-Emergent Adverse Events in Controlled U.S. Clinical TRials Reported by at Least 1% of Patients With Migraine*

Placebo Adverse Event Type	Percent of Patients Reporting 25 mg (n=112)	50 mg (n=114)	Sumatriptan 100 mg (n=108)	(n=112)
Atypical Sensations				
Feeling of heaviness	<1	<1	<1	2
Feeling of tightness	0	<1	2	2
Pressure sensation	0	<1	2	2
Tingling	4	8	4	5
Warm/hot sensation	<1	2	3	3
Cardiovascular				
Flushing	<1	0	4	2
Palpitations	<1	0	<1	2
Ear, Nose, and Throat				
Discomfort: nasal	4	5	5	7
Eye				
Irritation of eye(s)	0	0	0	2
Visual disturbance	<1	0	<1	3
Musculoskeletal				
Weakness	0	2	<1	2
Neurological				
Agitation	0	0	0	2
Urogenital				
Dysuria	<1	0	0	2

* Events that occurred at a frequency of 1% or more in the sumatriptan tablets 100 mg group and that occurred more frequently in that group than the placebo group.

Other events that occurred at least as often as placebo as in the 100 mg dose group included abdominal discomfort, mouth or tongue discomfort, neck stiffness, anxiety, taste disturbance, nausea and/or vomiting, migraine, headache, drowsiness/sedation, dizziness/vertigo, and malaise/fatigue.

Sumatriptan succinate tablets are generally well tolerated. Across all doses, most adverse reactions are mild and transient and do not lead to long-lasting effects. The incidence of adverse events in controlled clinical trials was not affected by gender or age of the patients. There was insufficient data to assess the impact of race on the incidence of adverse events.

Other Events Observed in Association With the Administration of Oral Sumatriptan Succinate: In the paragraphs that follow, the frequencies of less commonly reported adverse clinical events are presented. Because the reports cite events observed in open and uncontrolled studies, the role of sumatriptan succinate tablets in their causation cannot be reliably

ADVERSE REACTIONS: *(cont'd)*

determined. Furthermore, variability associated with reporting requirements, the terminology used to describe the adverse events etc., limit the value of the quantitative frequency estimates provided.

Event frequencies are calculated as the number of patients reporting an event divided by the total number of patients (n=6348) exposed to oral sumatriptan succinate. All reported events are included except those already listed in the previous table, those too general to be informative, and those not reasonably associated with the use of the drug. Events are further classified within body system categories and enumerated in order of decreasing frequency using the following definitions: frequent adverse events are defined as those occurring in at least 1/100 patients; infrequent adverse events are those occurring in 1/100 to 1/1000 patients; rare adverse events are those occurring in fewer than 1/1000 patients.

Atypical Sensations: Frequent were burning sensation, numbness, paresthesia. *Infrequent:*tight feeling in head. Rare were dysesthesia, hot and cold sensation.

Cardiovascular: *Frequent:*chest discomfort, chest pressure/heaviness, chest tightness. *Infrequent:*arrhythmia, changes in ECG, hypertension, hypotension, pallor, pulsating sensations, tachycardia. *Rare:*angina, atherosclerosis, bradycardia, cerebral ischemia, cerebrovascular lesion, heart block, peripheral cyanosis, thrombosis, transient myocardial ischemia, vasodilation.

Ear, Nose, and Throat: *Frequent:*throat symptoms. *Infrequent:*hearing disturbances, otalgia. *Rare:*feeling of fullness in the ear(s).

Endocrine and Metabolic: *Infrequent:*thirst. *Rare:*elevated thyrotropin stimulating hormone (TSH) levels, galactorrhea, hyperglycemia, hypoglycemia, hypothyroidism, polydipsia, weight gain, weight loss.

Eye: *Rare:*disorders of sclera, mydriasis.

Gastrointestinal: *Frequent:*diarrhea, gastric symptoms. *Infrequent:*constipation, dysphagia, gastroesophageal reflux. *Rare:*gastrointestinal bleeding, hematemesis, melena, peptic ulcer.

Hematological Disorders: *Rare:*anemia.

Musculoskeletal: *Frequent:*myalgia. *Infrequent:*muscle cramps. *Rare:*tetany.

Neurological: *Frequent:*phonophobia, photophobia. *Infrequent:*confusion, depression, difficulty concentrating, disturbance of smell, dysarthria, euphoria, facial pain, heat sensitivity, incoordination, lacrimation, monoplegia, sleep disturbance, shivering, syncope, tremor. *Rare:*aggressiveness, apathy, bradylogia, cluster headache, convulsions, decreased appetite, drug abuse, dystonic reaction, facial paralysis, hallucinations, hunger, hyperesthesia, hysteria, increased alertness, memory disturbance, neuralgia, paralysis, personality change, phobia, radiculopathy, rigidity, suicide, twitching.

Respiratory: *Frequent:*dyspnea. *Infrequent:*asthma. *Rare:*hiccoughs.

Skin: *Frequent:*sweating. *Infrequent:*erythema, pruritus, rash, skin tenderness. *Rare:*dry/scaly skin, tightness of skin, wrinkling of skin.

Breasts: *Infrequent:*tenderness. *Rare:*nipple discharge.

Urogenital: *Infrequent:*dysmenorrhea, increased urination, intermenstrual bleeding. *Rare:*abortion, hematuria.

Miscellaneous: *Frequent:*hypersensitivity. *Infrequent:*cough, fever, fluid retention, overdose. *Rare:*edema, hematoma, lymphadenopathy, speech disturbance, voice disturbances.

Postmarketing Experience: The following are spontaneously reported adverse events from postmarketing experience except those events already listed previously in ADVERSE REACTIONS or those too general to be informative. Because the reports cite events reported spontaneously from worldwide postmarketing experience, frequency of events and the role of sumatriptan succinate tablets in their causation cannot be reliably determined.

Blood: Pancytopenia, thrombocytopenia.

Cardiovascular: Cardiomyopathy, cerebrovascular accident, ischemic colitis, pulmonary embolism, shock, subarachnoid hemorrhage.

Dermatological: Exacerbation of sunburn, photosensitivity.

Ear, Nose and Throat: Deafness.

Eye: Intraocular disorders, ischemic optic meuropathy, periorbital edema, retinal artery occlusion.

Gastrointestinal: Xerostomia.

Hepatic: Disturbances of liver function tests, hepatic impairment.

Hypersensitivy Reactions: Erythema, pruritis, rash, shortness of breath, and urticaria. In addition, severe anaphylaxis/anaphylactoid reactions have been reported.

Non-Site Specific: Angioneurotic edema, cyanosis, death (see WARNINGS), temporal arteritis.

Psychiatry: Panic disorder.

Urogenital: Acute renal failure.

DRUG ABUSE AND DEPENDENCE:

The abuse potential of sumatriptan succinate injection and tablets cannot be fully delineated in advance of extensive marketing experience. One clinical study with sumatriptan succinate injection enrolling 12 patients with a history of substance abuse failed to induce subjective behavior and/or physiological response ordinarily associated with drugs that have an established potential for abuse.

OVERDOSAGE:

Injection: Patients (n=269) have received single injections of 8 to 12 mg without significant adverse effects. Volunteers (n=47) have received subcutaneous doses up to 16 mg without serious adverse events.

No gross overdoses in clinical practice have been reported. Coronary vasospasm was observed after intravenous administration of sumatriptan succinate injection (see CONTRAINDICATIONS). Overdoses would be expected from animal data (dogs at 0.1 g/kg, rats at 2 g/kg) to possibly cause convulsions, tremor, inactivity, erythema of the extremities, reduced respiratory rate, cyanosis, ataxia, mydriasis, injection site reactions (desquamation, hair loss, and scab formation), and paralysis. The half-life of elimination of sumatriptan is about 2 hours (see CLINICAL PHARMACOLOGY), and therefore monitoring of patients after overdose with sumatriptan succinate injection should continue while symptoms or signs persist, and for at least 10 hours.

It is unknown what effect hemodialysis or peritoneal dialysis has on serum concentrations of sumatriptan.

Tablets: Patients (n=670) have received single oral doses of 140 to 300 mg without significant adverse effects. Volunteers (n=174) have received single oral doses of 140 to 400 mg without serious adverse events.

No gross overdoses in clinical practice have been reported. Coronary vasospasm was observed after intravenous administration of sumatriptan (see CONTRAINDICATIONS). Overdoses would be expected from animal data to possibly cause tremor, lethargy, erythema of the extremities, abnormal respiration, cyanosis, ataxia, mydriasis, and paralysis. The elimination

OVERDOSAGE: *(cont'd)*

half-life of sumatriptan succinate is about 2.5 hours (see CLINICAL PHARMACOLOGY), and therefore monitoring of patients after overdose with sumatriptan succinate tablets should continue for at least 10 hours or while symptoms or signs persist.

It is unknown what effect hemodialysis or peritoneal dialysis has on the serum concentrations of sumatriptan.

DOSAGE AND ADMINISTRATION:

Injection: The maximum single recommended adult dose of sumatriptan succinate injection is 6 mg injected subcutaneously. Controlled clinical trials have failed to show that clear benefit is associated with the administration of a second 6 mg dose in patients who have failed to respond to a first injection.

The maximum recommended dose that may be given in 24 hours is two 6 mg injections separated by at least 1 hour. Although the recommended dose is 6 mg, if side effects are dose limiting, then lower doses may be used (see CLINICAL PHARMACOLOGY). In patients receiving MAO inhibitors, decreased doses of sumatriptan should be considered (see WARNINGS and CLINICAL PHARMACOLOGY). In patients receiving doses lower than 6 mg, only the single-dose vial dosage form should be used. An autoinjection device is available for use with 6 mg prefilled syringes to facilitate self-administration in patients in whom this dose is deemed necessary. With this device, the needle penetrates approximately $\frac{1}{4}$ inch (5 to 6 mm). since the injection is intended to be given subcutaneously, intramuscular or intraveneous delivery should be avoided. Patients should be directed to use injection sites with an adequate skin and subcutaneous thickness to accomodate the length of the needle.

Parenteral drug products should be inspected visually for particulate matter and discoloration before administration whenever solution and container permit.

Tablets: The recommended adult dose of sumatriptan succinate tablets is a single 25 mg tablet taken with fluids; the maximum single dose recommended is 100 mg. There is no evidence that an initial dose of 100 mg provides substantially greater relief than 25 mg.

If a satisfactory response has not been obtained at 2 hours, a second dose of up to 100 mg may be given. Controlled trials have not examined the effectiveness of a second dose if an initial dose of 25 mg is ineffective. If headache returns, additional doses may be taken at intervals of at least 2 hours up to a daily maximum dose of 300 mg. If headache returns following an initial treatment with sumatriptan succinate injection, additional doses of single sumatriptan succinate tablets (up to 200 mg per day) may be given with an interval of at least 2 hours between tablet doses.

The maximum dose given in a 24-hour period to patients with migraine headaches has been 300 mg. This dose has been delivered either as a single 300 mg-dose, or as three 100 mg single doses given at intervals no less than every 2 hours. While these doses have been generally well tolerated, there is no evidence that these higher doses afford greater relief than the recommended dose.

Sumatriptan succinate tablets are equally effective at whatever stage of the attack they are administered, though it is advisable that sumatriptan succinate tablets be given as early as possible after the onset of an attack of migraine.

Because of the potential of MAO inhibitors to cause unpredictable elevations in the bioavailability of oral sumatriptan, their combined use is contraindicated (see CONTRAINDICATIONS).

Hepatic disease/functional impairment may also cause unpredictable elevations in the bioavailability of orally administered sumatriptan. Consequently, if treatment is deemed advisable in the presence of liver disease, the maximum single dose should in general not exceed 50 mg (see CLINICAL PHARMACOLOGY) for the basis of this recommendation.

PATIENT PACKAGE INSERT:

Please read this leaflet carefully before you take sumatriptan succinate injection or tablets. This provides a summary of the information available on your medicine. Please do not throw away this leaflet until you have finished your medicine. You may need to read this leaflet again. This leaflet does not contain all of the information on sumatriptan succinate injection or tablets. For further information or advice, ask your doctor or pharmacist.

Information About Your Medicine: The generic name of your medication is sumatriptan succinate injection or tablets. It can be obtained only with a prescription from your doctor. The decision to use sumatriptan injection or tablets is one that you and your doctor should make jointly, taking into account your individual preferences and medical circumstances. If you have risk factors for heart disease (such as high blood pressure, high cholesterol, obesity, diabetes, smoking, strong family history of heart disease, or you are postmenopausal or a male over 40), you should tell your doctor, who should evaluate you for heart disease in order to determine if sumatriptan succinate is appropriate for you. Although the vast majority of those who have taken sumatriptan succinate have not experienced any significant side effects, some individuals have experienced problems and, rarely, deaths have been reported. In all but a few instances, however, sumatriptan succinate does not appear to have been a contributory factor in these deaths.

The Purpose of Your Medicine: *Injection:* Sumatriptan succinate injection is intended to relieve your migraine or cluster headache, but not to prevent or reduce the number of attacks you experience. Use sumatriptan succinate injection only to treat an actual migraine or cluster headache attack. *Tablets:* Sumatriptan succinate tablets are intended to relieve your migraine, but not to prevent or reduce the number of attacks you experience. Use sumatriptan succinate tablets only to treat an actual migraine attack.

Important Questions to Consider Before Taking Sumatriptan Succinate Injection or Tablets: If the answer to any of the following questions is **YES** or if you do not know the answer, then please discuss with your doctor before you use sumatriptan succinate injection or tablets.

Are you pregnant? Do you think you might be pregnant? Are you trying to become pregnant? Are you using inadequate contraception? Are you breastfeeding?

Do you have any chest pain, heart disease, shortness of breath, or irregular heartbeats? Have you had a heart attack?

Do you have risk factors for heart disease (such as high blood pressure, high cholesterol, obesity, diabetes, smoking, strong family history of heart disease, or you are postmenopausal or a male over 40)?

Do you have high blood pressure?

Have you ever had to stop taking this or any other medication because of an allergy or any other problems?

Are you taking any other migraine medications, including migraine medications containing ergotamine, dihydroergotamine, or methysergide.

Are you taking any medication for depression (monoamine oxidase inhibitors or selective serotonin reuptake inhibitors [SSRIs])?

Have you had, or do you have, any disease of the liver or kidney?

Have you had, or do you have, epilepsy or seizures?

Is this headache different from your usual migraine attacks?

Remember, if you answered **YES** to any of the above questions, then discuss it with your doctor.

PATIENT PACKAGE INSERT: *(cont'd)*

The Use of Sumatriptan Succinate Injection or Tablets During Pregnancy: Do not use sumatriptan succinate injection or tablets if you are pregnant, think you might be pregnant, are trying to become pregnant, or are not using adequate contraception, unless you have discussed this with your doctor.

How to Use Sumatriptan Succinate? *Injection:* Before using the autoinjector, check with your doctor on acceptable injection sites and see the enclosed instruction pamphlet on loading your autoinjector and discarding any empty syringe cartridges.

For adults, the usual dose is a single injection given just below the skin. It should be given as soon as the symptoms of your migraine appear, but may be given at any time during an attack. A second injection may be given if your symptoms of migraine come back. If your symptoms do not improve following the first injection, do not give a second injection for the same attack without first consulting with your doctor. Do not have more than two injections in any 24 hours and allow at least 1 hour between each dose. *Tablets:* For adults, the usual dose is a single tablet taken whole with fluids. It should be given as soon as the symptoms of your migraine appear, but it may be given at any time during an attack. A second tablet may be taken if your symptoms of migraine come back, but not sooner than 2 hours following the first tablet. For a given attack, if you have no response to the first tablet, do not take a second tablet without first consulting with your doctor. Do not take more than a total of 300 mg of sumatriptan succinate tablets in any 24-hour period.

Side Effects to Watch for: Some patients experience pain or tightness in the chest or throat when using sumatriptan succinate injection or tablets. If this happens to you, then discuss it with your doctor before using any more sumatriptan succinate injection or tablets. If the chest pain is severe or does not go away, call your doctor immediately.

Shortness of breath; wheeziness; heart throbbing; swelling of eyelids, face, or lips; or a skin rash, skin lumps, or hives happen rarely. If it happens to you, then tell your doctor immediately. Do not take any more sumatriptan succinate injection or tablets unless your doctor tells you to do so.

Some people may have feelings of tingling, heat, flushing (redness of face lasting a short time), heaviness or pressure after treatment with sumatriptan succinate injection or tablets. A few people may feel drowsy, dizzy, tired or sick. Tell your doctor of these symptoms at your next visit.

If you should feel unwell in any other way or have symptoms that you do not understand, you should contact your doctor immediately.

NOTE for Injection: You may experience pain or redness at site of injection, but this usually lasts less than an hour.

What to do if an Overdose is Taken: If you have taken more medication than you have been told, contact either your doctor, hospital emergency department, or nearest poison control center immediately.

Storing Your Medicine: Keep your medicine in a safe place where children cannot reach it. It may be harmful to children. Store your medication from heat and light. Do not store at temperatures above 86°F (30°C).

If your medication has expired (the expiration date is printed on the treatment pack), throw it away as instructed. *For Injection:* Do not throw away your autoinjector.

If your doctor decides to stop treatment, do not keep any leftover medicine unless your doctor tells you to. Throw away your medicine as instructed.

HOW SUPPLIED:

Injection: Imitrex Injection 6 mg (12 mg/ml) containing sumatriptan (base) as the succinate salt is supplied as a clear, colorless to pale yellow, sterile, nonpyrogenic solution.

Protect from light.

Tablets: Imitrex Tablets, 25 and 50 mg of sumatriptan (base) as the succinate Imitrex Tablets, 25 mg are white, round, film-coated tablets embossed with "I" on one side and "25" on the other in blister packs of 9 tablets. Imitrex Tablets, 50 mg are white, capsule-shaped, film-coated tablets embossed with "Imitrex" on one side and "50" on the other.

Injection and Tablets: Store between 2° and 30°C (36° and 86°F).

(Glaxo Wellcome, Injection: 02/97, RL-393; Tablets: 02/97, RL-392)

HOW SUPPLIED - EQUIVALENTS NOT AVAILABLE:

Injection, Solution - Subcutaneous - 6 mg/0.5ml

2 x 0.5 ml	$67.19	IMITREX, Glaxo Wellcome	00173-0478-00
2 x 0.5 ml	$70.93	IMITREX, Glaxo Wellcome	00173-0479-00
5 x 0.5 ml	$198.55	IMITREX, Glaxo Wellcome	00173-0449-02

Tablet, Uncoated - Oral - 25 mg

9's	$107.72	IMITREX, Glaxo Wellcome	00173-0460-02

Tablet, Uncoated - Oral - 50 mg

9's	$122.17	IMITREX, Glaxo Wellcome	00173-0459-00

SUPROFEN *(002301)*

CATEGORIES: Anti-Inflammatory Agents; EENT Drugs; Eye, Ear, Nose, & Throat Preparations; Miosis; Miotics; Ophthalmics; FDA Approved 1988 Dec

BRAND NAMES: **Profenal**

DESCRIPTION:

Suprofen 1% ophthalmic solution is a topical nonsteroidal anti-inflammatory product for ophthalmic use. Suprofen chemically is α-methyl-4-(2-thienylcarbonyl) benzenaectic acid, with an empirical formula of $C_{14}H_{12}O_3S$, and a molecular weight of 260.3.

Profenal (Suprofen) sterile ophthalmic solution contains suprofen 1.0% (10 mg/ml), thiomersal 0.005% (0.05 mg/ml), caffeine 2% (20 mg/ml), edetate disodium, dibasic sodium phosphate, monobasic sodium phosphate. sodium chloride, sodium hydroxide and/or hydrochloric acid (to adjust pH to 7.4) and purified water.

CLINICAL PHARMACOLOGY:

Suprofen is one of a series of phenylalkanoic acids that have shown analgesic, antipyretic and anti-inflammatory activity in animal inflammatory diseases. Its mechanism of action is believed to be through inhibition of the cyclo-oxygenase enzyme that is essential in the biosynthesis of prostaglandins.

Prostaglandins have been shown in many animal models to be mediators of certain kinds of intraocular inflammation. In studies performed on animal eyes, prostaglandins have been shown to produce disruption of the blood- aqueous humor barrier, vasodilation, increased vascular permeability, leukocytosis, and increased intraocular pressure. Prostaglandins appear to play a role in the miotic response produced during ocular surgery by constricting the iris sphincter independently of cholinergic mechanisms. In clinical studies, suprofen has been shown to inhibit the miosis induced during the course of cataract surgery. Suprofen could possibly interfere with the miotic effect of intraoperatively administered acetylcholine chloride.

CLINICAL PHARMACOLOGY: *(cont'd)*

Results from clinical studies indicate that suprofen ophthalmic solution has no significant effect on intraocular pressure.

There are no data available on the systemic absorption of ocularly applied suprofen. The oral dose of suprofen is 200 mg every four to six hours. If suprofen 1% ophthalmic solution is applied as two drops (1 mg suprofen) to one eye five times on the day prior to surgery and three times on the day of surgery, the total applied dose over the two days would be about 25 times less than a single 200 mg oral dose.

INDICATIONS AND USAGE:

Suprofen ophthalmic solution is indicated for inhibition of intraoperative miosis.

CONTRAINDICATIONS:

Suprofen is contraindicated in epithelial herpes simplex keratitis (dendritic keratitis) and in individuals hypersensitive to any component of the medication.

WARNINGS:

The potential exists for cross sensitivity to acetylsalicylic acid and other nonsteroidal and anti-inflammatory drugs. Therefore, caution should be used when treating individuals who have previously exhibited sensitivities to these drugs.

With nonsteroidal anti-inflammatory drugs, the potential exists for increased bleeding time due to interference with thrombocyte aggregation. There have been reports that ocularly applied nonsteroidal anti- inflammatory drugs may cause increased bleeding tendency of ocular tissues in conjunction with ocular surgery.

PRECAUTIONS:

GENERAL

The use of oral Suprofen has been associated with a syndrome of acute flank pain and generally reversible renal insufficiency, which may present as acute uric acid nephropathy. This syndrome occurs in approximately 1 in 3500 patients and has been reported with as few as one to two doses of a 200 mg capsule. If suprofen 1% ophthalmic solution is applied as two drops (1 mg suprofen) to one eye every five times on the day prior to surgery and three times on the day prior of surgery, the total applied dose over two days would be about 25 times less than a single 200 mg oral dose. Do not touch dropper tip to any surface, as this may contaminate the solution.

Ocular: Patients with histories of herpes simplex keratitis should be monitored closely. suprofen is contraindicated in patients with active herpes simplex keratitis.

The possibility of increased ocular bleeding during surgery associated with nonsteroidal anti-inflammatory drugs should be considered.

CARCINOGENESIS, MUTAGENESIS, AND IMPAIRMENT OF FERTILITY

In an 18-month study in mice, an increased incidence of benign hepatomas occurred in females at a dose of 40 mg/kg/day. Male mice, treated at doses of 2, 5, 10 and 40 mg/kg/day, also had an increased incidence of hepatomas when compared to control animals. No evidence of carcinogenicity was found in long term studies in doses as high as 40 mg/kg/day in the rat and mouse. Based on a battery of mutagenicity tests (Ames, micronucleus, and dominant lethal) suprofen does not appear to have mutagenic potential. Reproductive studies in rats at a dose of up to 40 mg/kg/day revealed no impairment of fertility and only slight reductions of fertility at doses of 80 mg/kg/day. However, testicular atrophy/hypoplasia was observed in a six-month dog study (at 80 mg/kg/day) and a 12-month rat study (at 40 mg/kg/day).

PREGNANCY CATEGORY C

Reproductive studies have been performed in rabbits at doses up to 200 mg/kg/day and in rats at doses up to 80 mg/kg/day. In rats, doses of 40 mg/kg/day and above, and in rabbits, doses of 80 mg/kg/day and above, resulted in stillbirths and a decrease in postnatal survival in pregnant rats treated with suprofen at 2.5 mg/kg/day and above. An increased incidence of delayed parturition occurred in rats. As there are no adequate an well-controlled studies in pregnant women, this drug should be used during pregnancy only of the potential benefit justifies the potential risk to the fetus. Because of the known effect of non-steroidal anti-inflammatory drugs on the fetal cardiovascular system (closure of ductus arteriosus), use during late pregnancy should be avoided.

NURSING MOTHERS

Suprofen is excreted in human milk after a single oral dose. Based on measurements of plasma and milk levels in women taking oral Suprofen, the milk concentration is about 1% of the plasma level. Because systemic absorption may occur from topical ocular administration, a decision should be considered to discontinue nursing while receiving suprofen, since the safety of suprofen in human neonates has not been established.

PEDIATRIC USE

Safety and effectiveness in children have not been established.

DRUG INTERACTIONS:

Clinical studies with acetylcholine chloride revealed no interference, and there is no known pharmacological basis for such interaction. However, with other topical nonsteroidal anti-inflammatory products, there have been reports that acetylcholine chloride and carbachol have been ineffective when used in patients treated with these agents.

Interaction of suprofen with other topical ophthalmic medications has not been fully investigated.

ADVERSE REACTIONS:

Ocular: The most frequent adverse reactions reported are burning and stinging of short duration. Instances of discomfort, itching and redness have been reported. Other reactions in occurring less than 0.5% of patients include allergy, iritis, pain, chemosis, photophobia, irritation, and punctuate epithelial staining.

Systemic: Systemic reactions related to therapy were not reported in the clinical studies. It is known that some systemic absorption does occur with ocularly applied drugs, and that nonsteroidal anti-inflammatory drugs have been shown to increase bleeding time by interference with thrombocyte aggregation. It is recommended that suprofen be used with caution in patients with bleeding tendencies and those taking anticoagulants.

OVERDOSAGE:

Overdosage will not ordinarily cause acute problems. If accidentally ingested, ingested, drink fluids to dilute.

DOSAGE AND ADMINISTRATION:

On the day of surgery, instill two drops into the conjunctival sac at three, two and one hour prior to surgery. Two drops may be instilled into the conjunctival sac every four hours, while awake, the day proceeding surgery.

Storage: Store at room temperature.

(ALCON, 3/91, 342980)

HOW SUPPLIED - EQUIVALENTS NOT AVAILABLE:

Solution - Ophthalmic; Top - 10 mg/ml

2.5 ml $113.25 PROFENAL, Alcon 00065-0348-25

SUTILAINS *(002303)*

CATEGORIES: Burns; Decubitus Ulcer; Dermatologicals; Enzymes & Digestants; Fibrinolytic & Proteolytic; Lesions; Mucous Membrane Agents; Skin/Mucous Membrane Agents; Vascular Disease; Wound Care; Pregnancy Category B; FDA Approval Pre 1982

BRAND NAMES: **Travase**

DESCRIPTION:

Travase Ointment is a sterile topical preparation containing proteolytic enzymes, elaborated by *Bacillus subtilis,* in a hydrophobic ointment base consisting of 95% mineral oil and 5% polyethylene. One gram of ointment contains approximately 82,000 Casein Units* (see INDICATIONS AND USAGE) of proteolytic activity.

CLINICAL PHARMACOLOGY:

Sutilains ointment selectively digests necrotic soft tissues by proteolytic action, thus facilitating the removal of necrotic tissues and purulent exudates that otherwise impair formation of granulation tissue and delay wound healing.

At body temperatures these proteolytic enzymes have optimal activity in the pH range from 6.0 to 6.8.

INDICATIONS AND USAGE:

For wound debridement: sutilains ointment is indicated as an adjunct to established methods of wound care for biochemical debridement of:

Second and third degree burns,

Decubitus ulcers,

Incisional, traumatic, and pyogenic wounds,

Ulcers secondary to peripheral vascular disease.

*One UPS Casein Unit of proteolytic activity is contained in the amount of sutilains which, when incubated with 35 mg of denatured casein at 37°C, produces in one minute a hydrolysate whose absorbance at 275 nm is equal to that of a tyrosine solution containing 1.5 micrograms of USP Tyrosine Reference Standard per ml.

CONTRAINDICATIONS:

Application of sutilains ointment is contraindicated in:

Wounds communicating with major body cavities,

Wounds containing exposed major nerves or nervous tissue, and

Fungating neoplastic ulcers.

WARNINGS:

Do not permit sutilains ointment to come into contact with the eyes. In the case of inadvertent contact, the eyes should be immediately rinsed with copious amounts of preferably sterile water.

PRECAUTIONS:

A moist environment is essential for optimal activity of the enzyme.*In vitro,* several detergents and antiseptics (benzalkonium chloride, hexachlorophene, iodine, and nitrofurazone) may render the substrate indifferent to the action of the enzyme. Compounds such as thimerosal, containing metallic ions, interfere directly with enzyme activity to a slight degree, whereas neomycin, sulfamylon, streptomycin, and penicillin do not affect enzyme activity. If used concurrently with adjunctive topical therapy for 24-48 hours and no dissolution of slough occurs, then further therapy is not likely to be effective.

In cases where there is existent of threatening invasive infection, appropriate systemic antibiotic therapy should be instituted concurrently.

Although studies in humans have shown that there have may be antibody response to absorbed enzyme material, there have been no reports of systemic allergic reaction to Traverse Ointment.

Pregnancy: Pregnancy category B. Studies in rabbits at doses up to two times the maximum human dose revealed no evidence of impaired infertility or fetal harm. There are, however, no adequate and well controlled studies in women. Because animal reproductive studies are not always predicative of human response, this drug should be used during pregnancy only if no adequate alternatives are available.

Pediatric Use: Safety and effectiveness in children have not been established.

ADVERSE REACTIONS:

Adverse reactions consist of mild, transient pain, paresthesias, bleeding and transient dermatitis. Pain usually can be controlled by administration of mild analgesics. Side effects severe enough to warrant discontinuation of therapy occasionally have occurred occasionally.

If bleeding or dermatitis occurs as a result of the application of sutilains ointment (Sutilains Ointment, USP) therapy should be discontinued. No systemic toxicity has been observed as a result of the topical application of sutilains ointment.

DOSAGE AND ADMINISTRATION:

FOR TOPICAL USE ONLY - NOT FOR OPHTHALMIC USE. ADHERENCE TO THE FOLLOWING IS SUGGESTED FOR OPTIMIZING THERAPEUTIC AFFECT:

1. Thoroughly cleanse and irrigate wound area with sodium chloride or water solutions. Wound **MUST** be cleansed of antiseptics or heavy-metal antibacterials (*e.g.,* silver nitrate, thimerosal) which may alter substrate characteristics or denature the enzyme.

2. Thoroughly moisten wound area either through tubbing, showering, or wet soaks (*e.g.,* sodium chloride or tap water).

3. Apply approximately 1/8 inch (3mm) thick layer extending to 1/4 to 1/2 inch beyond the area to be debrided, assuring intimate contact with necrotic tissue.

4. Apply a dressing that provides and maintains a moist environment.

5. Repeat entire procedure 3 to 4 times per day for best results.

Refrigerate at 2 to 8° C (36° to 46° F).

HOW SUPPLIED:

Traverse Ointment (Sutilains Ointment, USP).

1/2 oz (14.2 g) tube 3P3002 NDC 0048-1500-52

Refrigerate at 2 to 8° C (36° to 46° F).

HOW SUPPLIED: *(cont'd)*

For How Supplied Information, Contact Knoll Pharms (NDA# 12828)

TACRINE HYDROCHLORIDE *(003091)*

CATEGORIES: Acetylcholine Protector; Alzheimer's Disease; Anticholinergic Agents; Autonomic Drugs; Central Nervous System Agents; Dementia; Neuromuscular; Parasympathomimetic Agents; FDA Class 1P ("Priority Review"); FDA Approved 1993 Sep

BRAND NAMES: **Cognex**; THA

FORMULARIES: Aetna; BC-BS; CIGNA; Harvard; Medi-Cal; United; PCS

DESCRIPTION:

Tacrine hydrochloride is a reversible cholinesterase inhibitor, known chemically as 1,2,3,4-tetrahydro-9-acridinamine monohydrochloride monohydrate. Tacrine hydrochloride is commonly referred to in the clinical and pharmacological literature as THA. It has an empirical formula of $C_{13}H_{14}N_2{\cdot}H_2O$ and a molecular weight of 252.74.

Tacrine hydrochloride is a white solid and is freely soluble in distilled water, 0.1N hydrochloric acid, acetate buffer (pH 4.0), phosphate buffer (pH 7.0 to 7.4), methanol, dimethylsulfoxide (DMSO), ethanol, and propylene glycol. The compound is sparingly soluble in linoleic acid and PEG 400.

Each capsule of Cognex contains tacrine as the hydrochloride. Inactive ingredients are hydrous lactose, magnesium stearate, and microcrystalline cellulose. The hard gelatin capsules contain gelatin, NF; silicon dioxide, NF; sodium lauryl sulfate,NF; and the following dyes: 10 mg: D&C Yellow #10, FD&C Green #3, titanium dioxide; 20 mg: D&C Yellow #10, FD&C Blue #1, titanium dioxide; 30 mg: D&C Yellow #10, FD&C Blue #1, FD&C Red # 40, titanium dioxide; 40 mg: D&C Yellow #10, FD&C Blue #1, FD&C Red #40, D&C Red#28; titanium dioxide.

Each 10-, 20-, 30-, and 40-mg Cognex capsule for oral administration contains 12.75, 25.50, 38.25, and 51.00 mg of tacrine HCl respectively.

CLINICAL PHARMACOLOGY:

Although widespread degeneration of multiple CNS neuronal systems eventually occurs, early pathological changes in Alzheimer's Disease involve, in a relatively selective manner, cholinergic neuronal pathways that project from the basal forebrain to the cerebral cortex and hippocampus. The resulting deficiency of cortical acetylcholine is believed to account for some the clinical manifestations of mild to moderate dementia. Tacrine, an orally bioavailable, centrally active, reversible cholinesterase inhibitor, presumably acts by elevating acetylcholine concentrations in the cerebral cortex by slowing the degradation of acetylcholine released by still intact cholinergic neurons. If this theoretical mechanism of action is correct, tacrine's effects may lessen as the disease process advances and fewer cholinergic neurons remain functionally intact. There is no evidence that tacrine alters the course of the underlying dementing process.

CLINICAL PHARMACOKINETICS (ABSORPTION, DISTRIBUTION, METABOLISM, AND ELIMINATION)

Absorption: Tacrine HCl is rapidly absorbed after oral administration; maximal plasma concentrations occur with 1 to 2 hours. The rate and extent of tacrine absorption following administration of tacrine capsules and solution are virtually indistinguishable. Absolute bioavailability of tacrine is approximately 17 (SD ± 13)%. Food reduces tacrine bioavailability by approximately 30-40%; however, there is no food effect if tacrine is administered at least an hour before meals. The effect of achlorhydria on the absorption of tacrine is unknown.

Distribution: Mean volume of distribution of tacrine is approximately 349 (SD ± 193) L. Tacrine is about 55% bound to plasma proteins. The extent and degree of tacrine's distribution within various body compartments has not been systematically studied. However, 336 hours after the administration of a single radiolabeled dose, approximately 25% of the radiolabeled dose, approximately 25% of the radiolabel was not recovered in a mass balance study, suggesting the possibility that tacrine and/or one or more of its metabolites may be retained.

Metabolism: Tacrine is extensively metabolized by the cytochrome P450 system to multiple metabolites, not all of which have been identified. The vast majority of radiolabeled species present in the plasma following a single dose of ^{14}C radiolabeled tacrine are unidentified (*i.e.,* only 5% of radioactivity in plasma has been identified (tacrine and 3-hydroxylated metabolites 1-,2-, and 4- hydroxytacrine)).

Studies utilizing human liver preparations demonstrated that cytochrome P450 1A2 is the principal isozyme involved in tacrine metabolism. These findings are consistent with the observation that tacrine and/or one of its metabolite inhibits the metabolism of theophylline in humans (see DRUG INTERACTIONS, theophylline.) Results from a study utilizing quinidine to inhibit cytochrome P450 IID6 indicate that tacrine is not metabolized extensively by this enzyme system.

Following aromatic ring hydroxylation, tacrine metabolites undergo glucuronidation. Whether tacrine and/or its metabolites undergo biliary excretion or entero-hepatic circulation is unknown.

Special Populations:

Age: Based on poled pharmacokinetic studies (n=192), there is no clinically relevant influence of age (50 to 84 years) on tacrine clearance.

Gender: Average tacrine plasma concentrations are approximately 50% higher in females than in males. This is not explained by differences in body surface area or elimination half-life. The difference is probably due to higher systemic availability after oral dosing and may reflect the known lower activity of cytochrome P450 IA2 in women.

Race: The effect of race on tacrine clearance has not been studied.

Smoking: Mean plasma tacrine concentrations in current smokers are approximately one-third the concentrations in nonsmoker. Cigarette smoking is known to induce cytochrome P450 IA2.

Renal disease: Renal disease does not appear to affect the clearance of tacrine.

Liver disease: Although studies in patients with liver disease have not been done, it is likely that functional hepatic impairment will reduce the clearance of tacrine and its metabolites.

Presystemic Clearance/Elimination/Excretion: Tacrine undergoes presystemic clearance (*i.e.,* first pass metabolism). The extent of this first pass metabolism depends upon the dose of tacrine administered. Because the enzyme system involved can be saturated at relatively low doses, a larger fraction of a high dose of tacrine will escape first pass elimination than of a smaller dose. Thus, when a 40 mg daily dose is increased by 40 mg, the average plasma concentration will be increased by 6 ng/ml. However, when a daily dose of 80 or 120 mg is increased by 40 mg, the increment in average plasma concentration is approximately 10 ng/ml.

CLINICAL PHARMACOLOGY: *(cont'd)*

Elimination of tacrine from the plasma, however, is not dose dependent (*i.e.,* the half-life is independent of dose or plasma concentration). The elimination half-life is approximately 2 to 4 hours. Following initiation of therapy or a change in daily dose, steady state tacrine plasma concentration should be attained with 24 to 36 hours.

CLINICAL STUDIES:

CLINICAL TRIAL DATA

The conclusion that tacrine HCl is an effective treatment for Alzheimer's Disease derives from two adequate and well controlled clinical investigations that evaluated tacrine's effects in patients with probable Alzheimer's disease of mild to moderate severity (NINCDS criteria, mini- Mental State Examination (MMSE) of Folstein, Folstein and McHugh scores of 10 to 26).

In each study, outcomes during treatment with tacrine and placebo were assessed on two primary measures: (1) the cognitive subscale of the Alzheimer's Disease Assessment Scale (ADAS cog) of Rosen, Mohs, and Davis and (2) a clinician's rated clinical global impression of change.

STUDY ENDPOINTS

The ADAS cog is a multi-item test battery administered by psychometrician that examines aspects of memory, attention, praxis, reason, and language. The worst possible score is 70. Elderly, normal adults may score as low as 0 or 1 unit, but individuals judged not to be demented can score higher. The mean score of patients entering each study was approximately 28 units (range 7 to 62). The ADAS cog score is reported to deteriorate at a rate of about 6 to 10 units per year for untreated patients at this stage of dementia.

The clinicians global assessments used in the two studies relied on a clinician's judgement about the overall clinical change observed in patients over the course of the study. Although the conditions for obtaining the clinical assessment differed in each study, the global assessment was rated on a 7-point scale in both studies. A rating of four (4) represents no change; lower ratings indicate improvement from baseline and higher ratings deterioration.

TWELVE-WEEK STUDY

In one study of 12 weeks duration, patients were randomized to sequences that provided a comparison between placebo, 20, 40, and 80 mg/day by study's end. Statistically significant drug-placebo differences were detected on both primary outcome measures for the group titrated to 80 mg/day. Estimates of the size of the treatment effect varied between 2 and 4 ADAS cog units. The imprecision in these estimates reflects the fact that different analyses, conducted in attempts to account for the effects of the failure of a substantial fraction of the patients randomized to complete the full 12 weeks of the study yielded different results.

The placebo-80 mg/day comparison also achieved statistical significance on the clinician's global impression of change (CGIC) with a 0.3 to 0.4 unit mean difference. The following diagram illustrates the percentages of patients falling into each global category at trial's end for the patients given placebo or 80 mg/day.)

THIRTY-WEEK STUDY

The second study was 30 weeks long. Six hundred sixty-three patients were randomized to 4 treatment sequences (placebo and 3 drug groups) that called for the daily dose of tacrine to be increased at 6-week intervals, starting with a 40-mg/day dose. By study's end, a comparison between placebo, 80, 120, and 160 mg/day was possible. Patients in the 160 mg group received this dose for the final 12 weeks; the 120 mg group received that dose for 18 weeks.

The study showed statistically significant drug-placebo differences for the 80 and 120 mg/day groups at 18 weeks and for the 120 and 160 mg/day groups at 30 weeks on both a performance-based test of cognitive function (the ADAS cog) and a clinician's assessment of global change (Clinician Interview Based Impression: CIBI). Because many patients failed to complete 30 weeks on treatment, analyses that used each patient's last on-study value or retrieved patients' 30-week value, even if they were no longer in the study ("intent-to-treat" analysis) were carried out. All analyses confirmed the effectiveness of tacrine, although the estimated mean treatment effect was different in each analysis.

Effects on ADAS cog: The results of the ADAS cog are for the subset of patients actually completing the full 30 weeks of the study. They show that individual patients, whether assigned to tacrine or to a placebo, had a wide range of responses.

Effect on CIBI: The frequency of distribution of CIBI scores was attained by patients assigned to placebo or to the 160 mg/day tacrine dose group who actually completed the full 30 weeks of the stud. The mean tacrine- placebo difference for this group of patients on the CIBI was 0.5 units and was statistically significant.

Expected Responses in Newly Treated Patients: Although the results described clearly document tacrine's effectiveness, they are based on only a fraction of the patients initially randomized to tacrine, those who could tolerate tacrine and remain on treatment uninterrupted for the full 30 weeks. In considering the expected outcome in a group of patients newly started on tacrine, account must be taken both of the likelihood of staying on therapy and the responses in patients who do so.

TABLE 1 provides 3 different estimates of the proportion of patients assigned to treatment with tacrine at 160 mg a day or with placebo who attained a particular measure of improvement (*i.e.,* a 7 point improvement from baseline in ADAS cog score). The criterion has been chosen entirely for illustrative purposes.

TABLE 1 Proportion of Patients Attaining $\geq$ 7 Unit Improvement on the ADAS Cog at the Week 30 Assessment

Treatment Group N Randomized	I N(%) of Those Randomized	II N(%) of Those Completing Week 30	III N(%) of Those With Week 30 Assessments
Placebo (N=184)	10/184 (5.4)	10/117 (8.5)	11/143[1] (7.7)
160 mg/day (N=239)	13/239 (5.4)	13/64 (20.3)	25/172[2] (14.5)

[1]13 of the 143 were receiving tacrine when evaluated.
[2]41 of the 172 were not receiving tacrine when evaluated.

The first column of the table is based on all patients participating in the study. The proportion provides an estimate of the likelihood that a patient entering the study will (1) still be on his or her assigned treatment at week 30 **and** (2) will improve 7 or more ADAS cognitive points over his or her baseline score. The estimate of response derived in this manner is conservative because the rules under which the 30-week study conducted required the withdrawal of patients with relatively low (> 3 X ULN) asymptomatic, transaminase elevations. In actual clinical practice under the conditions of treatment recommended in the DOSAGE AND ADMINISTRATIONSection, a larger fraction of these patients would be able to remain on tacrine and the proportion of those improving 7 or more points on tacrine would be expected, therefore, to be increased (the third column illustrates this.)

The second column of the table presents the proportion of 7 unit responders based on the number of patients who (1) were able to complete the full 30 weeks of the study and (2) attained and ADAS cognitive score at week 30 that was 7 or more points better than their baseline score. This analysis provides an optimistic estimate of tacrine's effects because it reflects experience gained only with the minority of patients who were able to remain on

CLINICAL STUDIES: *(cont'd)*

treatment to the study's end. The comparison between the proportions of placebo and 160 mg patients attaining a 7 or more point improvement is complicated further by the fact that a larger proportion of tacrine assigned patients withdrew prematurely.

The third column of the table presents the proportion of patients who had evaluations made at 30 weeks and had a 7-point or greater response. The analysis includes data from patients still on their assigned treatment at week 30 as well as patients who withdrew from the study prior to that time, but were retrieved for a week 30 evaluation. Because patients who withdrew prior to week 30 were permitted to receive tacrine under "open label" conditions, retrieved patients included in this analysis could be receiving either no treatment or treatment with tacrine. In this analysis, patients are considered under the treatment to which they were randomized, regardless of the treatment they were actually receiving at week 30. Thus, some placebo patients could have received tacrine and some tacrine patients could have been receiving no tacrine. Like the analysis based on percent randomized (column I), this analysis, therefore, tends to provide a conservative view of the expected effect of tacrine treatment.

Effects of Tacrine Hydrochloride Over Time: For each dose group the time course of change from baseline in ADAS cog scores for patients completing 30 weeks of treatment appears to be persistently different between groups, but all groups, after initial treatment, deteriorate with time.

Patient age, gender, and other baseline patient characteristics were not found to predict clinical outcome.

INDICATIONS AND USAGE:

Tacrine hydrochloride is indicated for the treatment of mild to moderate dementia of the Alzheimer's type.

Evidence of tacrine HCl's effectiveness in the treatment of dementia of the Alzheimer's type derives from results of two adequate and well-controlled clinical investigations that compared tacrine and placebo on both a performance based measure of cognition and clinician's global assessment of change. (See CLINICAL PHARMACOLOGY, Clinical Trial Data.)

CONTRAINDICATIONS:

Tacrine HCl is contraindicated in patients with known hypersensitivity to tacrine or acridine derivatives.

Tacrine HCl is contraindicated in patients previously treated with tacrine HCl who developed treatment-associated jaundice confirmed by elevated total bilirubin greater than 3.0 mg/dl.

WARNINGS:

ANESTHESIA

Tacrine HCl, as a cholinesterase inhibitor, is likely to exaggerate succinylcholine-type muscle relaxation during anesthesia.

CARDIOVASCULAR CONDITIONS

Because of its cholinomimetic action, tacrine HCl may have vagotonic effects on the heart rate (*e.g.,* bradycardia). This action may be particularly important to patients with conduction abnormalities, bradyarrhythmia, or a sick sinus syndrome.

GASTROINTESTINAL DISEASE AND DYSFUNCTION

Tacrine HCl is an inhibitor of cholinesterase and may be expected to increase gastric acid secretion due to increased cholinergic activity. Therefore, patients at increased risk for developing ulcers - e.g., those with a history of ulcer disease or those receiving concurrent nonsteroidal anti- inflammatory drugs (NSAIDs) - should be monitored closely for symptoms of active or occult gastrointestinal bleeding.

Tacrine HCl, also as a predictable consequence of its pharmacological properties, can cause nausea, vomiting, and loose stools at recommended doses.

LIVER DYSFUNCTION

Tacrine HCl should be prescribed with care in patients with concurrent evidence or history of abnormal liver function indicated by significant abnormalities in serum transanimase (ALT/SGPT, AST/SGOT), bilirubin, and gamma-glutamyl transpeptidase (GGT) levels (see PRECAUTIONS and DOSAGE AND ADMINISTRATION).

The use of tacrine in patients without a prior history of liver disease is commonly associated with serum transanimase elevations, some to levels ordinarily considered to indicate clinically important hepatic injury (see TABLE 2.)

Experience gained in more than 8000 patients who received tacrine in clinical studies and the treatment IND program indicated that if tacrine is promptly withdrawn following detection of these elevations, clinically evident signs and symptoms of liver injury are rare.

Long-term follow up of patients who experience transanimase elevations, however, is limited and it is impossible, therefore, to exclude, with certainty, the possibility of chronic sequelae.

CONTROLLED CLINICAL TRIALS, TREATMENT IND AND POST-MARKETING EXPERIENCE

Experience with tacrine in controlled trials and in a large, less closely monitored experience (a treatment IND) is summarized below:

Clinically evident liver toxicity: One of more than 8000 patients exposed to tacrine in clinical studies and the treatment IND program had documented elevated bilirubin (5.3 X Upper Limit of Normal, ULN) and jaundice with transanimase levels (AST/SGOT) nearly 20 X ULN.

Rare cases of liver toxicity associated with jaundice, raised serum bilirubin, pyrexia, hepatitis and liver failure have been reported in post-marketing experience. Most of these cases have been reversible but some deaths have occured. Since there was multiple pathology including infection, gallstones and carcinoma it was not possible to clearly establish the relationship to tacrine HCl treatment.

Blood chemistry signs of liver injury: Experience from the 30- week clinical study (described earlier) provides a representative estimate of the frequency of ALT/SGPT elevations expected for patients whose transaminase levels were monitored weekly and who receive tacrine HCl according to the recommended regimen for dose introduction and titration (TABLE 2). A dosing regimen employing a more rapid escalation of the daily dose of tacrine, or less frequent monitoring of liver chemistries, may be associated with more serious clinical events (see Monitoring of Liver Function and the Management of the Patient Who Develops Transanimase Elevations.)

TABLE 2 Cumulative Incidence of ALT/SGPT Elevations (Number and (%) of Patients)

Maximum ALT	Males N = 229	Females N = 250	Total N = 479
Within Normal Limits	121 (53)	100 (40)	221 (46)
> ULN	108 (47)	150 (60)	258 (54)
> 2 times ULN	77 (34)	104 (42)	181 (38)
> 3 times ULN	58 (25)	81 (32)	139 (29)
> 10 times ULN	12 (5)	19 (8)	31 (6)
> 20 times ULN	3 (1)	6 (2)	9 (2)

WARNINGS: *(cont'd)*

Experience in 2446 patients who participated in all clinical trials, including the 30-week study, indicated approximately 50% of patients treated with tacrine HCl can be expected to have at least 1 ALT/SGPT level above ULN; approximately 25% of patients are likely to develop elevations > 3 X ULN, and about 7% of patients may develop elevations > 10 X ULN. Data collected from the treatment IND program were consistent with those obtained during clinical studies, and showed 3% of 5665 patients experiencing an ALT/SGPT elevation > 10 X ULN.

In clinical trials where transanimases were monitored weekly, the median time to onset of the first ALT/SGPT elevation above ULN was approximately 6 weeks, with maximum ALT/SGPT occurring 1 week later, even in instances when tacrine HCl treatment was stopped. Under the conditions of forced slow upwards dose titration (increases of 40 mg a day every 6 weeks) employed in clinical studies, 95% of transanimase elevations > 3 X ULN occurred within the first 18 weeks of tacrine HCl therapy, and 99% of the 10-fold elevations occurred by the 12th week and on not more than 80 mg; note, however, that for most patients ALT was monitored weekly and tacrine HCl was stopped when liver enzymes exceeded 3 X ULN. A total of 276 patients were monitored for ALT/SGPT levels every other week in two double-blind clinical studies, an open-label study, and amended treatment IND. The incidence, severity, time to onset, peak and recovery of ALT/SGPT levels were similar to weekly monitoring. With less frequent monitoring or the less stringent discontinuation criteria recommended below (see DOSAGE AND ADMINISTRATION), it is possible that marked elevations might be more common. It must also be appreciated that experience with prolonged exposure to the high dose (160 mg/day) is limited. In all cases, transanimase levels returned to within normal limits upon discontinuation of tacrine HCl treatment or following dosage reduction, usually within 4 to 6 weeks.

This relatively benign experience may be the consequence of careful laboratory monitoring that facilitated the discontinuation of patients early on after the onset of their transanimase elevations. Consequently, frequent monitoring of serum transanimase levels is recommended (see DOSAGE AND ADMINISTRATION, WARNINGS, Liver Injury, Monitoring of Liver Function and the Management of the Patient Who Develops Transanimase Elevations and PRECAUTIONS, Laboratory Tests).

Liver biopsy experience: Liver biopsy results in 7 patients who received tacrine (1 in a Parke-Davis sponsored study and 6 in studies reported in the literature) revealed hepatocellular necrosis in 6 patients, and granulomatous changes in the seventh. In all cases, liver function tests returned to normal with no evidence of persisting hepatic dysfunction.

Experience with the Rechallenge of Patients with Transanimase Elevations following recovery: Two hundred and twelve patients among the 866 patients assigned to tacrine in the 12 and 30 week studies were withdrawn because they developed transanimase elevations > 3 X ULN. One hundred and forty-five of these patients were subsequently rechallenged. During their initial exposure to tacrine, 20 of these 145 had experienced initial elevations > 10 times ULN, while the remainder had experienced elevations between 3 and 10 X ULN.

Upon rechallenge with an initial dose of 40 mg/day, only 48 (33%) of the 145 patients developed transanimase elevations greater than 3 X ULN. Of these patients, 44 had elevations that were between 3 and 10 X ULN and 4 had elevations that were > 10 X ULN.

The mean time to onset of elevations occurred earlier on rechallenge than on initial exposure (22 versus 48 days). Of the 145 patients rechallenged, 127 (88%) were able to continue tacrine HCl treatment, and 91 of these 127 patients titrated to doses higher than those associated with the initial transanimase elevation.

Predictors of the risk of transanimase elevations: The incidence of transanimase elevations is higher among females. There are no other known predictors of the risk of hepatocellular injury.

MONITORING OF LIVER FUNCTION AND THE MANAGEMENT OF THE PATIENT WHO DEVELOPS TRANSANIMASE ELEVATIONS. (SEE ALSO DOSAGE AND ADMINISTRATIONand PRECAUTIONS, Laboratory Tests.

Blood chemistries: Serum transanimase levels (specifically ALT/SGPT) should be monitored every other week for at least the first 16 weeks following initiation of tacrine HCl treatment, after which monitoring may be decreased to monthly for 2 months and every 3 months thereafter. For patients who develope ALT/SGPT elevations greater than two times the upper limit of normal, the dose and monitoring regimen should be monitored as described in Table 4 (See DOSAGE AND ADMINISTRATION.)

A full monitoring sequence should be repeated in the event that a patient suspends treatment with tacrine for more than 4 weeks.

If transanimase elevations occur, the dose of tacrine HCl should be modified according to the table shown in DOSAGE AND ADMINISTRATION.

Rechallenge: Patients with clinical jaundice confirmed by a significant elevations in total bilirubin (>3 mg/dl) and/or those exhibiting clinical signs and/or symptoms of hypersensitivity (*e.g.,* rash or fever) in association with ALT/SGPT elevations should immediately and permanently discontinue tacrine HCl and not be rechallenged.Other patients who are required to discontinue tacrine HCl treatment because of transanimase elevations may be rechallenged once transanimase levels return to within normal limits. (See DOSAGE AND ADMINISTRATION.)

Rechallenge of patients with transanimase elevations less than 10 X ULN has not resulted in serious liver injury. However, because experience in the rechallenge of patients who had elevation greater than 10 X ULN is limited, the risks associated with the rechallenge of these patients are not well characterized. Careful, frequent (weekly) monitoring of serum ALT should be undertaken when rechallenging such patients.

If rechallenged, patients should be given an initial dose of 40 mg/day (10 mg QID) and transanimase levels monitored weekly. If, after 6 weeks on 40 mg/day,the patient is tolerating the dosage with no unacceptable elevations in transanimases, recommended dose-titration and transanimase monitoring may be resumed. Weekly monitoring of the ALT/SGPT levels should continue for a total of 16 weeks after which monitoring may be decreased to monthly for 2 months and every 3 months thereafter.

Liver biopsy: Liver biopsy is not indicated in cases of uncomplicated transanimase elevation.

GENITOURINARY

Cholinomimetics may cause bladder outflow obstruction.

NEUROLOGICAL CONDITIONS

Seizures: Cholinomimetics are believed to have some potential to cause generalized convulsions; seizure activity may, however, also be a manifestation of Alzheimer's Disease.

Sudden worsening of the degree of cognitive impairment: Worsening of cognitive function has been reported following abrupt discontinuation of tacrine HCl or after a large reduction in total daily dose (80 mg/day or more).

PULMONARY CONDITIONS

Because of its cholinomimetic action, tacrine HCl should be prescribed with care to patients with a history of asthma.

PRECAUTIONS:

GENERAL

Liver Injury: See WARNINGS.

PRECAUTIONS: *(cont'd)*

HEMATOLOGY

An absolute neutrophil count (ANC) less than 500/µl occurred in 4 patients who received tacrine HCl (tacrine HCl) during the course of clinical trials. Three of the 4 patients had concurrent medical conditions commonly associated with a low ANC; 2 of these patients remained on tacrine HCl. The fourth patient, who had a history of hypersensitivity (penicillin allergy), withdrew from the study as a result of a rash and also developed an ANC < 500/µl, which returned to normal; this patient was not rechallenged and, therefore, the role played by tacrine HCl in this reaction is unknown.

Six patients had an absolute neutrophil count ≤ 1500/µl, associated with an elevation of ALT/SGPT.

The total clinical experience in more than 8000 patients does not indicate a clear association between tacrine HCl treatment and serious white blood cell abnormalities.

INFORMATION FOR PATIENTS AND CAREGIVERS

Patients and caregivers should be advised that the effect of tacrine HCl therapy is thought to depend upon its administration at regular intervals, as directed.

The caregiver should be divided about the possibility of adverse effects. Two types should be distinguished: (1) those occurring in close temporal association with the initiation of treatment or an increase in dose (*e.g.,* nausea, vomiting, loose stools, diarrhea, etc) and (2) those with a delayed onset (*e.g.,* rash, jaundice, changes in the color of stool - black, very dark or light (*i.e.,* acholic)).

Patients and caregivers should be encouraged to inform the physician about the emergence of new events or any increase in the severity of existing adverse clinical events.

Caregivers should be advised that abrupt discontinuation of tacrine HCl or a large reduction in total daily dose (80 mg/day or more) may cause a decline in cognitive function and behavioral disturbances. Unsupervised increases in the dose of tacrine may also have serious consequences. Consequently, changes in dose should not be undertaken in the absence of direct instruction of a physician.

LABORATORY TESTS

(See WARNINGS, Liver Dysfunction and DOSAGE AND ADMINISTRATION.) Serum transanimase levels (specifically ALT/SGPT) should be monitored in patients given tacrine HCl (see WARNINGS, Liver Dysfunction.)

CARCINOGENESIS, MUTAGENESIS, AND IMPAIRMENT OF FERTILITY

Tacrine was mutagenic to bacteria in the Ames test. Unscheduled DNA synthesis was induced in rat and mouse hepatocytes *in vitro.* Results of cytogenic (chromosomal aberration) studies were equivocal. Tacrine was not mutagenic in an *in vitro* mammalian mutation test. Overall, the results of these tests, along with the fact that tacrine belongs to a chemical class (acridines) containing some members which are animal carcinogens, suggest that tacrine may be carcinogenic.

Studies of the effects of tacrine on fertility have not been performed.

PREGNANCY CATEGORY C

Animal reproduction studies have not been conducted with tacrine. It is also not known whether tacrine HCl can cause fetal harm when administered to a pregnant woman or can affect reproductive capacity.

NURSING MOTHERS

It is not known whether this drug is excreted in human milk.

PEDIATRIC USE

There are no adequate and well-controlled trials to document the safety and efficacy of tacrine in any dementing illness occurring in children.

DRUG INTERACTIONS:

DRUG-DRUG INTERACTIONS

Possible metabolic basis for interactions: Tacrine is primarily eliminated by hepatic metabolism via cytochrome P450 drug metabolizing enzymes. Drug-drug interactions may occur when tacrine HCl is given concurrently with agents such as theophylline that undergo extensive metabolism via cytochrome P450 IA2.

Theophylline: Coadministration of tacrine with theophylline increased theophylline elimination half-life and average plasma theophylline concentrations by approximately 2-fold. Therefore, monitoring of plasma theophylline concentrations and appropriate reduction of theophylline dose are recommended in patients receiving tacrine and theophylline concurrently. The effect of theophylline on tacrine pharmacokinetics has not been assessed.

Cimetidine: Cimetidine increased the Cmax and AUC of tacrine by approximately 54% and 64% respectively.

Anticholinergics: Because of its mechanism of action, tacrine HCl has the potential to interfere with the activity of anticholinergic medications.

Cholinomimetics and Cholinesterase Inhibitors: A synergistic effect is expected when tacrine HCl is given concurrently with succinylcholine (see WARNINGS), cholinesterase inhibitors, or cholinergic agonists such as bethanechol.

Other Interactions: Rate and extent of tacrine absorption were not influenced by the coadministration of an antacid containing magnesium and aluminum. Tacrine had no major effect on digoxin or diazepam pharmacokinetics or the anticoagulant activity of warfarin.

ADVERSE REACTIONS:

COMMON ADVERSE EVENTS LEADING TO DISCONTINUATION

In clinical trials, approximately 17% of the 2706 patients who received tacrine HCl and 5% of the 1886 patients who received placebo withdrew permanently because of adverse events. It should be noted that some the placebo-treated patients were exposed to tacrine HCl prior to receiving placebo due to the variety of study designs used, including crossover studies. Transanimase elevations were the most common reason for withdrawals during tacrine HCl treatment (8% of all tacrine HCl-treated patients, or 212 of 456 patients withdrawn). The controlled clinical trial protocols required that any patient with an ALT/SGPT elevation > 3 X ULN be withdrawn, because of concern about potential hepatotoxicity. Apart from withdrawals due to transanimase elevations, 244 patients (9%) withdrew for adverse events while receiving tacrine HCl.

Other adverse events that most frequently led to the withdrawal of tacrine-treated patients in clinical trials were nausea and/or vomiting (1.5%), agitation (0.9%), rash (0.7%), anorexia (0.7%), and confusion (0.5%). These adverse events also most frequently led to the withdrawal of placebo-treated patients, although lower frequencies (0.1% to 0.2%).

MOST FREQUENT ADVERSE CLINICAL EVENTS SEEN IN ASSOCIATION WITH THE USE OF TACRINE

The events identified here are those that occurred at an absolute incidence of at least 5% of patients treated with tacrine HCl, and at a rate at least 2-fold higher in patients treated with tacrine HCl than placebo.

The most common adverse events associated with the use of tacrine HCl were elevated transanimases, nausea and/or vomiting, diarrhea, dyspepsia, myalgia, anorexia, and ataxia. Of these events, nausea and/or vomiting, diarrhea, dyspepsia and anorexia appeared to be dose-dependent.

ADVERSE REACTIONS: *(cont'd)*

ADVERSE EVENTS REPORTED IN CONTROLLED TRIALS

The events cited in the table below (TABLE 3) reflect experience gained under closely monitored conditions of clinical trials with a highly selected patient population. In actual clinical practice or in other clinical trials, these frequency estimates may not apply, as the conditions of use, reporting behavior, and the kinds of patients treated may differ.

TABLE 3 lists treatment-emergent signs and symptoms that occurred in at least 2% of patients with Alzheimer's Disease in placebo-controlled trials and who received the recommended regimen for dose introduction and titration of tacrine HCl (see DOSAGE AND ADMINISTRATION.)

TABLE 3 Adverse Events Occurring in at Least 2% of Patients Receiving Tacrine HCl Using the Recommended Regimen for Dose Introduction and Titration in Controlled Clinical Trials
(Number (%) of Patients)

Body System/ Adverse Events	Tacrine HCl N = 634	Placebo N = 342
Laboratory Deviations		
Elevated Transanimase[a]	184 (29)	5 (20)
Body As A Whole		
Headache	67 (11)	52 (15)
Fatigue	26 (4)	9 (3)
Chest Pain	24 (4)	18 (5)
Weight Decrease	21 (3)	4 (1)
Back Pain	15 (2)	14 (4)
Asthenia	15 (2)	7 (2)
Digestive System		
Nausea and/or Vomiting	178 (28)	29 (9)
Diarrhea	99 (16)	18 (5)
Dyspepsia	57 (9)	22 (6)
Anorexia	54 (9)	11 (3)
Abdominal Pain	48 (8)	24 (7)
Flatulence	22 (4)	5 (2)
Constipation	24 (4)	8 (2)
Hemic And Lymphatic System		
Purpura	15 (2)	8 (2)
Musculoskeletal System		
Myalgia	54 (9)	18 (5)
Nervous System		
Dizziness	73 (12)	39 (11)
Confusion	42 (7)	24 (7)
Ataxia	36 (6)	12 (4)
Insomnia	37 (6)	18 (5)
Somnolence	22 (4)	11 (3)
Tremor	14 (2)	2 (<1)
Psychological Function		
Agitation	43 (7)	20 (9)
Depression	22 (4)	14 (4)
Thinking Abnormal	17 (3)	14 (4)
Anxiety	16 (3)	7 (2)
Hallucination	15 (2)	12 (4)
Hostility	15 (2)	5 (2)
Respiratory System		
Rhinitis	51 (8)	22 (6)
Upper Respiratory Infection	18 (3)	11 (3)
Coughing	17 (3)	18 (5)
Skin And Appendages		
Rash[b]	46 (7)	18 (5)
Facial Flushing, Skin Flushing	16 (3)	3 (<1)
Urogenital System		
Urination Frequency	21 (3)	12 (4)
Urinary Tract Infection	21 (3)	20 (6)
Urinary Incontinence	16 (3)	9 (3)

[a]ALT or AST value of approximately 3 X ULN or greater or that resulted in a change in patient management.
[b]Included COSTART terms: rash, rash-erythematous, rash-maculopapular, urticaria, petechial rash, rash-vesiculobullous, and pruritus.

OTHER ADVERSE EVENTS OBSERVED DURING ALL CLINICAL TRIALS

Tacrine HCl has been administered to 2706 individuals during clinical trials. A total of 1471 patients were treated for at least 3 months, 1137 for at least 6 months, and 773 for at least 1 year. Any untoward reactions that occurred during these trials were recorded as adverse events by the clinical investigators using terminology of their own choosing. To provide a meaningful estimate of the proportion of individuals having similar types of events, the events were grouped into a smaller number of standardized categories using a modified COSTART dictionary. These categories are used in the listing below. The frequencies represent the proportion of the 2706 individuals exposed to tacrine HCl who experienced that event while receiving tacrine HCl. All adverse events are included except those already listed on the previous table and those COSTART terms too general to be informative. Events are further classified by body system categories and listed using the following definitions: frequent adverse events are defined as those occurring in at least 1/100 patients; infrequent adverse events are those occurring in 1/100 to 1/1000 patients; and rare adverse events are those occurring in less than 1/1000 patients. These adverse events are not necessarily related to tacrine HCl treatment. Only rare adverse events deemed to be potentially important are included.

Body as a Whole: *Frequent:*Chill, fever, malaise, peripheral edema. *Infrequent:*Face edema, dehydration, weight increase, cachexia, edema (generalized), lipoma. *Rare:*Heat exhaustion, sepsis, cholinergic crisis, death.

Cardiovascular System: *Frequent:*Hypotension, hypertension.*Infrequent:*Heart failure, myocardial infarction, angina pectoris, cerebrovascular accident, transient ischemic attack, phlebitis, venous insufficiency, abdominal aortic aneurysm, atrial fibrillation or flutter, palpitation, tachycardia, bradycardia, pulmonary embolus, migraine, hypercholesterolemia. *Rare:*Heart arrest, premature atrial contractions, A-V block, bundle branch block.

Digestive System: *Infrequent:*Glossitis, gingivitis, mouth or throat dry, stomatitis, increased salivation, dysphagia, esophagitis, gastritis, gastroenteritis, GI hemorrhage, stomach ulcer, hiatal hernia, hemorrhoids, stools bloody, diverticulitis, fecal impaction, fecal incontinence, hemorrhage (rectum), cholelithiasis, cholecystitis, increased appetite. *Rare:*Duodenal ulcer, bowel obstruction.

Endocrine System: *Infrequent:*Diabetes. *Rare:*Hyperthyroid, hypothyroid.

Hemic and Lymphatic: *Infrequent:*Anemia, lymphadenopathy. *Rare:*Leukopenia, thrombocytopenia, hemolysis, pancytopenia.

Musculoskeletal: *Frequent:*Fracture, arthralgia, arthritis, hypertonia. *Infrequent:*Osteoporosis, tendinitis, bursitis, gout. *Rare:*Myopathy.

Nervous System: *Frequent:*Convulsions, vertigo, syncope, hyperkinesia, paresthesia. *Infrequent:* Dreaming abnormal, dysarthria, aphasia, amnesia, wandering, twitching, hypesthesia, delirium, paralysis, bradykinesia, movement disorder, cogwheel rigidity, paresis, neuritis, hemiplegia, Parkinson's disease, neuropathy, extrapyramidal syndrome, reflexes decreased/absent. *Rare:*Tardive dyskinesia, dysesthesia, dystonia, encephalitis, coma, apraxia, oculogyric crisis, akathisia, oral facial dyskinesia, Bell's palsy, exacerbation of Parkinson's disease.

Psychobiologic Function: *Frequent:*Nervousness.*Infrequent:*Apathy, increased libido, paranoia, neurosis.*Rare:*Suicidal, psychosis, hysteria.

Respiratory System: *Frequent:*Pharyngitis, sinusitis, bronchitis, pneumonia, dyspnea. *Infrequent:*Epistaxis, chest congestion, asthma, hyperventilation, lower respiratory infection. *Rare:* Hemoptysis, lung edema, lung cancer, acute epiglottis.

Skin and Appendages: *Frequent:*Sweating increased. *Infrequent:*Acne, alopecia, dermatitis eczema, skin dry, herpes zoster, psoriasis, cellulitis, cyst, furunculosis, herpes simplex, hyperkeratosis, basal cell carcinoma, skin cancer. *Rare:*Desquamation, seborrhea, squamous cell carcinoma, ulcer (skin), skin necrosis, melanoma.

Urogenital System: *Infrequent:*Hematuria, renal stone, kidney function, glycosuria, dysuria, polyuria, nocturia, pyuria, cystitis, urinary retention, urination urgency, vaginal hemorrhage, pruritus (genital), breast pain, impotence, prostate cancer. *Rare:*Bladder tumor, renal tumor, renal failure, urinary obstruction, breast cancer, epididymitis, carcinoma (ovary).

Special Senses: *Frequent:*Conjunctivitis. *Infrequent:*Cataract, eyes dry, eye pain, visual field defect, diplopia, amblyopia, glaucoma, hordeolum, deafness, earache, tinnitus, inner ear infection, otitis media, unusual taste. *Rare:*Vision loss, ptosis, blepharitis, labyrinthitis, inner ear disturbance.

POSTINTRODUCTION REPORTS

Voluntary reports of adverse events temporally with tacrine HCl that have been received since market introduction, that are not listed above, and that may have no causal relationship with the drug include the following: pancreatitis, perforated duodenal ulcer.

OVERDOSAGE:

As in any case of overdose, general supportive measures should be utilized. Overdosage with cholinesterase inhibitors can cause a cholinergic crisis characterized by severe nausea/vomiting, salivation, sweating, bradycardia, hypotension, collapse, and convulsions. Increasing muscle weakness is a possibility and may result in death if respiratory muscles are involved.

Tertiary anticholinergics such as atropine may be used as an antidote for tacrine HCl overdosage. Intravenous atropine sulfate titrated to effect is recommended: in adults, initial dose of 1.0 to 2.0 mg IV with subsequent doses base upon clinical response. In children, the usual IM or IV dose is 0.05 mg/kg, repeated every 10-30 minutes until muscarinic signs and symptoms subside and repeated if they reappear. Atypical increases in blood pressure and heart rate have been reported with other cholinomimetics when coadministered with quaternary anticholinergics such as glycopyrrolate.

It is not known whether tacrine HCl or its metabolites can be eliminated by dialysis (hemodialysis, peritoneal dialysis, or hemofiltration).

The estimated median lethal dose of tacrine following a single oral dose in rats is 40 mg/kg, or approximately 12 times the maximum recommended human dose of 160 mg/day. Dose-related signs of cholinergic stimulation were observed in animals and included vomiting, diarrhea, salivation, lacrimation; ataxia, convulsion, tremor, and stereotypic head and body movements.

DOSAGE AND ADMINISTRATION:

The recommendations for dose titration are base on experience from clinical trials. The rate of dose of escalation may be slowed if a patient is intolerant to the titration schedule recommended below. It is not advisable, however, to accelerate the dose incrementation plan.

Following initiation of therapy, or any dosage increase, patients should be observed carefully for adverse effects. Tacrine HCl should be taken between meals whenever possible; however, if minor GI upset occurs, tacrine HCl may be taken with meals to improve tolerability. Taking tacrine HCl with meals can be expected to reduce plasma levels by approximately 30% to 40%.

INITIATION OF TREATMENT

The initial dose of tacrine HCl is 40 mg/day (10 mg QID). This dose should be maintained for a minimum of 6 weeks with weekly monitoring of transaminase levels. It is important that the dose not be increased during this period because of the potential for delayed onset of transaminase elevations.

DOSE TITRATION

Following 6 weeks of treatment at 40 mg/day, the dose of tacrine HCl should then be increased to 80 mg/day (20 mg QID), providing there are no significant transanimase elevations and the patient is tolerating treatment. Patients should be titrated to higher doses (120 and 160 mg/day, in divided doses on a QID schedule) at 6-week intervals on the basis of tolerance.

DOSE ADJUSTMENT

Serum ALT/SGOT should be monitored every other week for at least the first 16 weeks following initiation of tacrine HCl treatment, after which monitoring may be decreased to monthly for 2 months and every 3 months thereafter. For patients who develope ALT/SGPT elevations greater then 2 times the upper limit of normal, the dose and monitoring regimen should be modified as described in TABLE 4.

A full monitoring and dose titration sequence must be repeated in the event that a patient suspends treatment with tacrine for more than 4 weeks.

TABLE 4 Recommended Dose Regimen Modification in Response to Transanimase Elevations

ALT/SGPT Level	Treatment and Monitoring Regimen
≤ 2 X ULN	Continue treatment according to recommended titration and monitoring schedule.
> 2 to ≤ 3 X ULN	Continue treatment according to recommended titration. Monitor ALT/SGPT levels weekly until levels return to normal limits.
> 3 to ≤ 5 X ULN	Reduce the daily dose of tacrine HCl by 40 mg/day. Monitor ALT/SGPT levels weekly. Resume dose titration and every other week monitoring when the levels of the ALT/SGPT return to normal limits.
> 5 X ULN	Stop tacrine HCl treatment. Monitor the patient closely for signs and symptoms associated with hepatitis and follow ALT/SGPT levels until within normal limits. See Rechallenge section below. Experience is limited with patients with ALT > 10 X ULN. The risk of rechallenge must be considered against demonstrated clinical benefit. **Patients with clinical jaundice confirmed by a significant elevation in total bilirubin (> 3 mg/dl) and/or symptoms of hypersensitivity (*e.g.*, rash or fever) in association with ALT/SGPT elevations should immediately and permanently discontinue tacrine HCl and not be rechallenged.**

DOSAGE AND ADMINISTRATION: *(cont'd)*

RECHALLENGE

Patients who are required to discontinue tacrine HCl treatment because of transanimase elevations may be rechallenged once transanimase levels return to within normal limits.

Rechallenge of patients exposed to transanimase elevations less than 10 X ULN has not resulted in serious liver injury. However, because experience in the rechallenge of patients who had elevations greater than 10 X ULN is limited, the risks associated with the rechallenge of these patients are not well characterized. Careful, frequent (weekly) monitoring of serum ALT should be undertaken when rechallenging such patients.

If rechallenged, patients should be given an initial dose of 40 mg/day (10 mg QID) and transanimase levels monitored weekly. If, after 6 weeks on 40 mg/day, the patient is tolerating the dosage with no unacceptable elevations in transanimases, recommended dose-titration and transaminase monitoring may be resumed. Weekly monitoring of the ALT/SGPT levels should continue for a total of 16 weeks after which monitoring may be decreased to monthly for 2 months and every 3 months thereafter.

PATIENT INFORMATION:

Tacrine is used to treat Alzheimer's disease.

Use with caution in patients with a history of ulcers or liver disease.

Inform your physician if patient is taking any other medications including over-the-counter drugs.

Do not abruptly discontinue the drug.

May cause nausea, vomiting or diarrhea.

Notify physician if rash, jaundice or changes in stool color occur.

HOW SUPPLIED:

Cognex is supplied as capsules of tacrine hydrochloride containing 10, 20, 30, 40 mg of tacrine. The capsule logo is Cognex, with the strength printed underneath and the colors as follows:

10 mg: yellow/dark green

20 mg: yellow/light blue

30 mg: yellow/swedish orange

40 mg: yellow/lavender

STORAGE

Store at controlled room temperature 15 - 30°C (59-86°F) away from moisture.

HOW SUPPLIED - EQUIVALENTS NOT AVAILABLE:

Capsule, Gelatin - Oral - 10 mg

100's $119.69 COGNEX, Parke-Davis 00071-0096-40
120's $120.48 COGNEX, Parke-Davis 00071-0096-25

Capsule, Gelatin - Oral - 20 mg

100's $119.69 COGNEX, Parke-Davis 00071-0097-40
120's $120.48 COGNEX, Parke-Davis 00071-0097-25

Capsule, Gelatin - Oral - 30 mg

100's $119.69 COGNEX, Parke-Davis 00071-0095-40
120's $120.48 COGNEX, Parke-Davis 00071-0095-25

Capsule, Gelatin - Oral - 40 mg

100's $119.69 COGNEX, Parke-Davis 00071-0098-40
120's $120.48 COGNEX, Parke-Davis 00071-0098-25

TACROLIMUS *(003138)*

CATEGORIES: Immunologic; Immunomodulators; Immunosuppressives; Renal Transplantation; FDA Class 1P ("Priority Review"); FDA Approved 1994 Apr

BRAND NAMES: **Prograf**; FK-506

FORMULARIES: Medi-Cal

COST OF THERAPY: $7,971.60 (Transplantation; Capsule; 5 mg; 2/day; 365 days)

WARNING:
Increased susceptibility to infection and the possible development of lymphoma may result from immunosuppression. Only physicians experienced in immunosuppressive therapy and management of organ transplant patients should prescribe Prograf. Patients receiving the drug should be managed in facilities equipped and staffed with adequate laboratory and supportive medical resources. The physician responsible for maintenance therapy should have complete information requisite for the follow-up of the patient.

DESCRIPTION:

Prograf is available for oral administration as capsules (tacrolimus capsules) containing the equivalent of 1 mg or 5 mg of anhydrous tacrolimus. Inactive ingredients include lactose, hydroxypropyl methylcellulose, croscarmellose sodium, and magnesium stearate. The 1-mg capsule shell contains gelatin and titanium dioxide, and the 5-mg capsule shell contains gelatin, titanium dioxide and ferric oxide.

Prograf is also available as a sterile solution (tacrolimus injection) containing the equivalent of 5 mg anhydrous tacrolimus in 1 ml for administration by intravenous infusion only. Each ml contains polyoxyl 60 hydrogenated castor oil (HCO-60), 200 mg, and dehydrated alcohol, USP, 80.0% v/v. Prograf injection must be diluted with 0.9% Sodium Chloride Injection or 5% Dextrose Injection before use.

Tacrolimus, previously known as FK506, is the active ingredient in Prograf. Tacrolimus is a macrolide immunosuppressant produced by *Streptomyces tsukubaensis.* Chemically, tacrolimus is designated as [3*S*- [3*R**[*E* (1*S**,3*S**,4*S**)], 4*S**,5*R**,8*S**,9*E*,12*R**, 14*R**,15*S**,16*R**,18*S**, 19*S**, 26a*R**]]-5, 6, 8, 11, 12, 13, 14, 15, 16, 17, 18, 19, 24, 25, 26, 26a-hexadecahydro-5,19-dihydroxy-3-[2-(4-hydroxy-3-methoxycyclohexyl)-1-methylethenyl]-14,16-dimethoxy-4,10,12,18-tetramethyl-8-(2-propenyl)- 15,19-epoxy-3H-pyrido [2,1-*c*][1,4] oxaazacyclotricosine-1, 7, 20,21(4H,23H)-tetrone, monohydrate.

Tacrolimus has an empirical formula of $C_{44}H_{69}NO_{12}{\cdot}H_2O$ and a formula weight of 822.05. Tacrolimus appears as white crystals or crystalline powder. It is practically insoluble in water, freely soluble in ethanol, and very soluble in methanol and chloroform.

CLINICAL PHARMACOLOGY:

Mechanism of Action: Tacrolimus prolongs the survival of the host and transplanted graft in animal transplant models of liver, kidney, heart, bone marrow, small bowel and pancreas, lung and trachea, skin, cornea, and limb.

In animals, tacrolimus has been demonstrated to suppress some humoral immunity and, to a greater extent, cell-mediated reactions such as allograft rejection, delayed type hypersensitivity, collagen-induced arthritis, experimental allergic encephalomyelitis, and graft versus host disease.

Tacrolimus inhibits T-lymphocyte activation, although the exact mechanism of action is not known. Experimental evidence suggests that tacrolimus binds to an intracellular protein, FKBP-12. A complex of tacrolimus-FKBP- 12, calcium, calmodulin, and calcineurin is then formed and the phosphatase activity of calcineurin inhibited. This effect may prevent the generation of nuclear factor of activated T-cells (NF-AT), a nuclear component thought to initiate gene transcription for the formation of lymphokines (interleukin-2, gamma interferon). The net result is the inhibition of T-lymphocyte activation (*i.e.,* immunosuppression).

Pharmacokinetics: Absorption of tacrolimus from the gastrointestinal tract after oral administration is variable. The absorption half-life of tacrolimus in 16 liver transplant patients averaged 5.7 hours (standard deviation 4.6 hours). Peak concentrations (C_{max}) in blood and plasma were achieved at approximately 1.5-3.5 hours. Mean (standard deviation) pharmacokinetic parameters of tacrolimus in whole blood after oral administration were:

TABLE 1

Population	No. of Subjs/ Study	Dose mg/kg/12h	C_{max} ng/ml	T_{max} hours	AUC ng/ml.h	F%
Healthy Volunteers	27	0.07 (1x5mg)	28.6 (8.6)	1.4 (0.62)	271 (122)	14.4 (6.0)
		0.07 (5x1mg)	36.2 (13.8)	1.3 (0.43)	329 (174)	17.4 (7.0)
Liver Transplant Patients	17	0.15	68.5 (30.0)	2.3 (1.5)	519 (179)	21.8 (6.3)
	11 Effect of Food	0.15 (Food)	27.1 (14.7)	3.2 (1.3)	223 (125)	-
		0.15 (Fasting)	52.4 (17.0)	1.5 (1.2)	290 (117)	-

Mean (SD)
C_{max} maximum concentration
T_{max} time to maximum concentration
AUC area under the conc-time curve
F Absolute bioavailability

The disposition of tacrolimus from whole blood was biphasic with a terminal elimination half-life of 11.7 (± 3.9) hours in liver transplant patients and 21.2 (± 8.5) hours in healthy volunteers. The volume of distribution and total body clearance for tacrolimus following intravenous administration were:

TABLE 2

Population	Number of Subjects	Dose (mg/kg/12h)	Vd (l/kg)	Cl (l/h/kg)
Healthy Volunteers	27	0.01	0.88 (0.31)	0.042 (0.016)
Liver Transplant Patients	17	0.05	0.85 (0.3)	0.053 (0.017)

Mean (SD)
Vd Volume of distribution
Cl Total body clearance

Pharmacokinetic data indicate that whole blood rather than plasma may serve as the more appropriate medium to describe the pharmacokinetic characteristics of tacrolimus.

The result of a single-dose bioequivalence study conducted in 27 healthy volunteers indicated that the absolute bioavailability of the 5-mg capsule was 14.4% and that of five 1-mg capsules was 17.4%. This study failed to establish the bioequivalence of these two formulations.

The effect of food was studied in 11 liver transplant patients. Tacrolimus was administered in the fasting state or 15 minutes after a breakfast of measured fat content (34% of 400 total calories). The results indicate that the presence of food reduces the absorption of tacrolimus (decrease in AUC and C_{max}, and increase in T_{max}). The relative oral bioavailability (whole blood) was reduced by 27.0 (± 18.2%) when compared to administration in the fasting state.

The protein-binding of tacrolimus reported in two studies was 75% and 99% over a range of concentrations of 0.1 - 100 ng/ml. Tacrolimus is bound to proteins, mainly albumin and alpha-1-acid glycoprotein, and is highly bound to erythrocytes. The distribution of tacrolimus between whole blood and plasma depends on several factors such as hematocrit, temperature of separation of plasma, drug concentration, and plasma protein concentration. In a U.S. study, the ratio of whole blood concentration to plasma concentration ranged from 12 to 67 (mean 35).

Tacrolimus trough concentrations from 10 to 60 ng/ml measured at 10-12 hours post-dose (Cmin) correlated well with the area under the plasma or whole blood concentration-time curve (AUC). In 28 liver transplant patients, the correlation coefficient was 0.94.

Pharmacokinetic studies in pediatric patients have not been conducted. However, trough concentrations obtained from 30 children (less than 12 years old) showed that children need higher doses than adults to achieve similar tacrolimus trough concentrations, suggesting that the pharmacokinetic characteristics of tacrolimus are different in children as compared to adults. (see DOSAGE AND ADMINISTRATION.)

Tacrolimus is extensively metabolized by the mixed-function oxidase system, primarily the cytochrome P-450 enzyme system (P-450 IIIA). In man, less than 1% of the dose administered is excreted unchanged in the urine. The major metabolic pathway has not been determined. Demethylation and hydroxylation were identified as the primary mechanisms of biotransformation *in vitro.* The major metabolite identified in incubations with human liver microsomes in 13-demethyl tacrolimus. Ten possible metabolites have been identified in human plasma. Two metabolites, a demethylated and a double-demethylated tacrolimus, were shown to retain 10% and 7%, respectively, of the inhibitory effect of tacrolimus on T-lymphocyte activation.

CLINICAL STUDIES:

The safety and efficacy of tacrolimus-based immunosuppression following orthotopic liver transplantation were assessed in two prospective, randomized, non-blinded multicenter studies. The active control groups were treated with a cyclosporine-based immunosuppressive regimen. Both studies used concomitant adrenal corticosteroids as part of the immunosuppressive regimens. These studies were designed to evaluate whether the two regimens were

CLINICAL STUDIES: *(cont'd)*

therapeutically equivalent, with patient and graft survival at 12 months following transplantation as the primary endpoints. The tacrolimus-based immunosuppressive regimen was found to be equivalent to the cyclosporine- based immunosuppressive regimens.

In one trial, 529 patients were enrolled at 12 clinical sites in the United States; prior to surgery, 263 were randomized to the tacrolimus- based immunosuppressive regimen and 266 to a cyclosporine-based immunosuppressive regimen (CBIR). In 10 of the 12 sites, the same CBIR protocol was used, while 2 sites used different control protocols. This trial excluded patients with renal dysfunction, fulminant hepatic failure with Stage IV encephalopathy, and cancers; pediatric patients (≤ 12 years old) were allowed.

In the second trial, 545 patients were enrolled at 8 clinical sites in Europe; prior to surgery, 270 were randomized to the tacrolimus-based immunosuppressive regimen and 275 to a CBIR. In this study, each center used its local standard CBIR protocol in the active-control arm. This trial excluded pediatric patients, but did allow enrollment of subjects with renal dysfunction, fulminant hepatic failure in Stage IV encephalopathy, and cancers other than primary hepatic with metastases.

One-year patient survival and graft survival in the tacrolimus-based treatment groups were equivalent to those in the CBIR treatment groups in both studies. The overall one-year patient survival (CBIR and tacrolimus-based treatment groups combined) was 88% in the U.S. study and 78% in the European study. The overall one-year graft survival (CBIR and tacrolimus-based treatment groups combined) was 81% in the U.S. study and 73% in the European study. In both studies, the median time to convert from IV to oral tacrolimus dosing was 2 days.

Information on secondary outcomes (incidence of acute rejection, use of OKT3 for steroid-resistant rejection, and incidence of refractory rejection) was also collected. Because of the nature of the study designs, comparisons of differences between the study arms for these secondary endpoints could not be reliably assessed.

INDICATIONS AND USAGE:

Tacrolimus is indicated for the prophylaxis of organ rejection in patients receiving allogeneic liver transplants. It is recommended that tacrolimus be used concomitantly with adrenal corticosteroids. Because of the risk of anaphylaxis, tacrolimus injection should be reserved for patients unable to take tacrolimus capsules orally.

CONTRAINDICATIONS:

Tacrolimus is contraindicated in patients with a hypersensitivity to tacrolimus. Tacrolimus injection is contraindicated in patients with a hypersensitivity to HCO-60 (polyoxyl 60 hydrogenated castor oil).

WARNINGS:

(See BOXED WARNING.)Tacrolimus can cause neurotoxicity and nephrotoxicity, particularly when used in high doses. Nephrotoxicity has been noted in 40% and 33% of liver transplantation patients receiving tacrolimus in the U.S. and European randomized trials, respectively (see ADVERSE REACTIONS.) More overt nephrotoxicity is seen early after transplantation, characterized by increasing serum creatinine and a decrease in urine output. Patients with impaired renal function should be monitored closely, and the dosage of tacrolimus may need to be reduced. In patients with persistent elevations of serum creatinine who are unresponsive to dosage adjustments, consideration should be given to changing to another immunosuppressive therapy. Care should be taken in using tacrolimus with other nephrotoxic drugs. **In particular, to avoid excess nephrotoxicity, tacrolimus should not be used simultaneously with cyclosporine. tacrolimus or cyclosporine should be discontinued at least 24 hours prior to initiating the other. In the presence of elevated tacrolimus or cyclosporine concentrations, dosing with the other drug usually should be further delayed.**

Mild to severe hyperkalemia has been noted in 44% and 10% of liver transplant recipients treated with tacrolimus in the U.S. and European randomized trials and may require treatment (see ADVERSE REACTIONS.) Serum potassium levels should be monitored and potassium-sparing diuretics should not be used during tacrolimus therapy (see PRECAUTIONS.)

Neurotoxicity, including tremor, headache, and other changes in motor function, mental status, and sensory function were reported in approximately 55% of liver transplant recipients in the two randomized studies (see ADVERSE REACTIONS.) Tremor and headache have been associated with high whole-blood concentrations of tacrolimus and may respond to dosage adjustment. Seizures have occurred in adult and pediatric patients receiving tacrolimus (see ADVERSE REACTIONS.) Coma and delirium also have been associated with high plasma concentrations of tacrolimus.

As in patients receiving other immunosuppressants, patients receiving tacrolimus are at increased risk of developing lymphomas and other malignancies, particularly of the skin. The risk appears to be related to the intensity and duration of immunosuppression rather than to the use of any specific agent. A lymphoproliferative disorder (LPD) related to Epstein-Barr Virus (EBV) infection has been reported in immunosuppressed organ transplant recipients. The risk of LPD appears greatest in young children who are at risk for primary EBV infection while immunosuppressed or who are switched to tacrolimus following long-term immunosuppression therapy. Because of the danger of oversuppression of the immune system, which can increase susceptibility to infection, tacrolimus should not be administered with other immunosuppressive agents except adrenal corticosteroids. The efficacy and safety of the use of tacrolimus in combination with other immunosuppressive agents has not been determined.

A few patients receiving tacrolimus injection have experienced anaphylactic reactions. Although the exact cause of these reactions is not known, other drugs with castor oil derivatives in the formulation have been associated with anaphylaxis in a small percentage of patients. Because of this potential risk of anaphylaxis, tacrolimus injection should be reserved for patients who are unable to take tacrolimus capsules.

Patients receiving tacrolimus injection should be under continuous observation for at least the first 30 minutes following the start of the infusion and at frequent intervals thereafter. If signs or symptoms of anaphylaxis occur, the infusion should be stopped. An aqueous solution of epinephrine 1:1000 should be available at the bedside as well as a source of oxygen.

PRECAUTIONS:

General: Hypertension is a common adverse effect of tacrolimus therapy (see ADVERSE REACTIONS.) Mild or moderate hypertension is more frequently reported than severe hypertension. Antihypertensive therapy may be required; the control of blood pressure can be accomplished with any of the common antihypertensive agents. Since tacrolimus may cause hyperkalemia, potassium-sparing diuretics should be avoided. While calcium-channel blocking agents can be effective in treating tacrolimus-associated hypertension, care should be taken since interference with tacrolimus metabolism may require a dosage reduction(see DRUG INTERACTIONS.)

Hyperglycemia was associated with the use of tacrolimus in 47% and 29% of liver transplant recipients in the U.S. and European randomized studies, respectively, and may require treatment (see ADVERSE REACTIONS.)

PRECAUTIONS: *(cont'd)*

Renally and Hepatically Impaired Patients: For patients with renal insufficiency some evidence suggests that lower doses should be used (see DOSAGE AND ADMINISTRATION.)

The use of tacrolimus in liver transplant recipients experiencing post-transplant hepatic impairment may be associated with increased risk of developing renal insufficiency related to high whole-blood levels of tacrolimus. These patients should be monitored closely and dosage adjustments should be considered. Some evidence suggests that lower doses should be used in these patients (see DOSAGE AND ADMINISTRATION.)

Information for the Patient: Patients should be informed of the need for repeated appropriate laboratory tests while they are receiving tacrolimus. They should be given complete dosage instructions, advised of the potential risks during pregnancy, and informed of the increased risk of neoplasia.

Laboratory Tests: Serum creatinine and potassium should be assessed regularly. Routine monitoring of metabolic and hematologic systems should be performed as clinically warranted.

Carcinogenesis, Mutagenesis and Impairment of Fertility: An increased incidence of malignancy is a recognized complication of immunosuppression in recipients of organ transplants. The most common forms of neoplasms are non-Hodgkin's lymphomas and carcinomas of the skin. As with other immunosuppressive therapies, the risk of malignancies in tacrolimus recipients may be higher than in the normal, healthy population. Lymphoproliferative disorders associated with Epstein-Barr Virus infection have been seen. It has been reported that reduction or discontinuation of immunosuppression may cause the lesions to regress.

No evidence of genotoxicity was seen in bacterial (Salmonella and E. coli) or mammalian (Chinese hamster lung-derived cells) *in vitro* assays of mutagenicity, the *in vitro* CHO/HGPRT assay of mutagenicity, or *in vivo* clastogenicity assays performed in mice; tacrolimus did not cause unscheduled DNA synthesis in rodent hepatocytes.

Although studies are ongoing, no adequate studies to evaluate the carcinogenic potential of tacrolimus have been completed.

No impairment of fertility was demonstrated in studies of male and female rats. Tacrolimus, given orally at 1.0 mg/kg (0.5X the recommended clinical dose based on body surface are corrections) to male and female rats, prior to and during mating, as well as to dams during gestation and lactation, was associated with embryolethality and with adverse effects on female reproduction. Effects on female reproductive function (parturition) and embryolethal effects were indicated by a higher rate of pre-implantation loss and increased numbers of undelivered and nonviable pups. When given at 3.2 mg/kg (1.5X the recommended clinical dose based on body surface are correction), tacrolimus was associated with maternal and paternal toxicity as well as reproductive toxicity including marked adverse effects on estrus cycles, parturition, pup viability, and pup malformations.

Pregnancy Category C: In reproduction studies in rats and rabbits, adverse effects on the fetus were observed mainly at dose levels that were toxic to dams. Tacrolimus at oral doses of 0.32 and 1.0 mg/kg during organogenesis in rabbits was associated with maternal toxicity as well as an increase in incidence of abortions; these doses are equivalent to 0.33X and 1.0X (based on body surface area corrections) the recommended clinical dose (0.3 mg/kg). At the higher dose only, an increased incidence of malformations and developmental variations was also seen. Tacrolimus, at oral doses of 3.2 mg/kg during organogenesis in rats, was associated with maternal toxicity and caused an increase in late resorptions, decreased numbers of live births, and decreased pup weight and viability. Tacrolimus, given orally at 1.0 and 3.2 mg/kg (equivalent to 0.5X and 1.5X the recommended clinical dose based on body surface area corrections) to pregnant rats after organogenesis and during lactation, was associated with reduced pup weights.

No reduction in male or female fertility was evident.

There are no adequate and well-controlled studies in pregnant women. Tacrolimus is transferred across the placenta. The use of tacrolimus during pregnancy has been associated with neonatal hyperkalemia and renal dysfunction. Tacrolimus should be used during pregnancy only if the potential benefit to the mother justifies potential risk to the fetus.

Nursing Mothers: Since tacrolimus is excreted in human milk, nursing should be avoided.

Pediatric Use: Successful liver transplants have been performed in pediatric patients (age less than 12 years) using tacrolimus. One of the two randomized active-controlled trials of tacrolimus in primary liver transplantation included 51 pediatric patients. Thirty patients were randomized to tacrolimus-based and 21 to cyclosporine-based therapies. Additionally, 22 pediatric patients were studied in an uncontrolled trial of tacrolimus in living related donor liver transplantation. Pediatric patients generally required higher doses of tacrolimus to maintain blood trough levels of tacrolimus similar to adult patients (see DOSAGE AND ADMINISTRATION.)

DRUG INTERACTIONS:

Drug interaction studies with tacrolimus have not been conducted. Due to the potential for additive or synergistic impairment of renal function, care should be taken when administering tacrolimus with drugs that may be associated with renal dysfunction. These include, but are not limited to, aminoglycosides, amphotericin B, and cisplatin. Initial clinical experience with the co-administration of tacrolimus and cyclosporine resulted in additive/synergistic nephrotoxicity. Patients switched from cyclosporine to tacrolimus should receive the first tacrolimus dose no sooner than 24 hours after the last cyclosporine dose. Dosing may be further delayed in the presence of elevated cyclosporine levels.

Drugs that May Alter Tacrolimus Concentrations: Since tacrolimus is metabolized mainly by the cytochrome P-450 IIIA enzyme systems, substances known to inhibit these enzymes may decrease the metabolism of tacrolimus with resultant increases in whole blood or plasm levels. Drugs known to induce these enzyme systems may result in an increased metabolism of tacrolimus and decreased whole blood or plasma levels. Monitoring of blood levels and appropriate dosage adjustments are essential when such drugs are used concomitantly.

Drugs That May Increase Tacrolimus Blood Levels

Calcium Channel Blockers: diltiazem, nicardipine, verapamil.

Antifungal Agents: clotrimazole, fluconazole, itraconazole, ketoconazole.

Other Drugs: bromocriptine, cimetidine, clarithromycin, cyclosporine, danazol, erythromycin, methylprednisolone, metoclopramide.

Drugs That May Decrease Tacrolimus Blood Levels

Anticonvulsants: carbamazepine, phenobarbital, phenytoin.

Antibiotics: rifabutin, rifampin.

Other Drug Interactions: Immunosuppressants may affect vaccination. Therefore, during treatment with tacrolimus, vaccination may be less effective. The use of live vaccines should be avoided; live vaccines may include, but are not limited to measles, mumps, rubella, oral polio, BCG, yellow fever, and TY 21a typhoid.[1]

ADVERSE REACTIONS:

The principle adverse reactions of tacrolimus are tremor, headache, diarrhea, hypertension, nausea, and renal dysfunction. These occur with oral and intravenous administration of tacrolimus and may respond to a reduction in dosing. Diarrhea was sometimes associated with other gastrointestinal complaints such as nausea and vomiting.

ADVERSE REACTIONS: *(cont'd)*

Hyperkalemia, hypomagnesemia and hyperuricemia have occurred in patients receiving tacrolimus therapy. Hyperglycemia has been noted in many patients; some may require insulin therapy.

The incidence of adverse events was determined in two randomized comparative liver transplant trials among 512 patients receiving tacrolimus and steroids and 511 patients receiving a cyclosporine-based regimen (CBIR). The proportion of patients reporting more than one adverse event was 99.8% in the tacrolimus group and 99.6% in the CBIR group. Precautions must be taken when comparing the incidence of adverse events in the U.S. study to that in the European study. Only adverse events occurring up to 12-months post-transplant in the U.S. study and up to 6-months in the European study are presented. The two studies also included different patient populations and patients were treated with immunosuppressive regimens of differing intensities. Adverse events reported in >15% in tacrolimus patients (combined study results) are presented below for the two controlled trials in liver transplantation:

TABLE 3

	U.S. Study (%) Tacrolimus (N=250)	U.S. Study (%) CBIR (N=250)	European Study (%) Tacrolimus (N=262)	European Study (%) CBIR (N=261)
Nervous System				
Headache†	64	60	31	20
Tremor †	56	46	44	30
Insomnia	64	68	29	21
Paraesthesia	40	30	15	13
Gastrointestinal				
Diarrhea	72	47	32	23
Nausea	46	37	30	22
Constipation	24	27	19	20
LFT Abnormal	36	30	5	2
Anorexia	34	24	6	4
Vomiting	27	15	12	9
Cardiovascular				
Hypertension*	47	56	31	35
Urogenital				
Kidney Function Abnormal†	40	27	33	18
Creatinine Increased†	39	25	19	16
BUN Increased†	30	22	8	7
Urinary Tract Infection	16	18	19	18
Oliguria	18	15	16	8
Metabolic And Nutritional				
Hyperkalemia†	45	26	10	7
Hypokalemia	29	34	11	14
Hyperglycemia*	47	38	29	16
Hypomagnesemia	48	45	15	8
Hemic And Lymphatic				
Anemia	47	38	4	1
Leukocytosis	32	26	8	7
Thrombocytopenia	24	20	10	14
Miscellaneous				
Abdominal Pain	59	54	26	20
Pain	63	57	19	14
Fever	48	56	15	18
Asthenia	52	48	7	4
Back Pain	30	29	13	14
Ascites	27	22	5	6
Peripheral Edema	26	26	10	11
Respiratory System				
Pleural Effusion	30	32	32	29
Atelectasis	28	30	5	4
Dyspnea	29	23	3	2
Skin And Appendages				
Pruritus	36	20	11	1
Rash	24	19	8	3

* (See PRECAUTIONS)
† (See WARNINGS)

The following adverse events, not mentioned above, were reported with greater than 3% incidence in tacrolimus-treated patients. *Nervous System:* (see WARNINGS) abnormal dreams, agitation, anxiety, confusion, convulsion, depression, dizziness, emotional lability, hallucinations, hypertonia, incoordination, myoclonus nervousness, neuropathy, psychosis, somnolence, thinking abnormal; *Special Senses:* abnormal vision, amblyopia, tinnitus; *Gastrointestinal:* cholangitis, cholestatic jaundice, dyspepsia, dysphasia, flatulence, gastrointestinal hemorrhage, GGT increase, GI perforation, hepatitis, ileus, increased appetite, jaundice, liver damage, oral moniliasis; *Cardiovascular:* chest pain, abnormal ECG, hemorrhage, hypotension, tachycardia; *Urogenital:* (see WARNINGS) hematuria, kidney failure; *Metabolic Nutritional:* acidosis, alkaline phosphatase increased, alkalosis, bilirubinemia, healing abnormal, hyperlipemia, hyperphosphatemia, hyperuricemia, hypocalcemia, hypophosphatemia, hyponatremia, hypoproteinemia, AST (SGOT) increased, ALT (SGPT) increased; *Endocrine:* (see PRECAUTIONS) diabetes mellitus; *Hemic/Lymphatic:* coagulation disorder, ecchymosis, hypochromic anemia, leukopenia, prothrombin decreased; *Miscellaneous:* abdomen enlarged, abscess, chills, hernia, peritonitis, photosensitivity reaction; *Musculoskeletal:* arthralgia, generalized spasm, leg cramps, myalgia, myasthenia, osteoporosis; *Respiratory:* asthma, bronchitis, cough increased, lung disorder, pulmonary edema, pharyngitis, pneumonia, respiratory disorder, rhinitis, sinusitis, voice alteration; *Skin:* alopecia, herpes simplex, hirsutism, skin disorder, sweating.

OVERDOSAGE:

There is minimal experience with overdosage. In patients who have received inadvertent overdosage of tacrolimus, no adverse reactions different from those reported in patients receiving therapeutic doses have been described. General supportive measures and systemic treatment should be followed in all cases of overdosage. Based on the poor aqueous solubility and extensive erythrocyte and plasma protein binding, it is anticipated that tacrolimus is not dialyzable to any significant extent.

In acute oral and intravenous toxicity studies, mortalities were seen at and above the following doses: in adult rats, 52X the recommended human oral dose; in immature rats, 16X the recommended oral dose; and in adult rats, 16X the recommended human intravenous dose (all based on body surface area corrections).

DOSAGE AND ADMINISTRATION:

TACROLIMUS INJECTION

For Intravenous Infusion Only**NOTE: Anaphylactic reactions have occurred with injectables containing castor oil derivatives. (See WARNINGS.)**

DOSAGE AND ADMINISTRATION: *(cont'd)*

In patients unable to take oral tacrolimus capsules, therapy may be initiated with tacrolimus injection. The initial dose of tacrolimus should be administered no sooner than 6 hours after transplantation. The recommended starting dose of tacrolimus injection is 0.05-0.10 mg/kg/day as a continuous intravenous infusion. Adult patients should receive doses at the lower end of the dosing range. Concomitant adrenal corticosteroid therapy is recommended early post-transplantation. Continuous intravenous infusion of tacrolimus injection should be continued only until the patient can tolerate oral administration of tacrolimus capsules.

Preparation for Administration/Stability: Tacrolimus injection must be diluted with 0.9% Sodium Chloride Injection or 5% Dextrose Injection to a concentration between 0.004 mg/ml and 0.02 mg/ml prior to use. Diluted infusion solution should be stored in glass or polyethylene containers and should be discarded after 24 hours. The diluted infusion solution should not be stored in a PVC container due to decreased stability and the potential for extraction of phthalates. Parenteral drug products should be inspected visually for particulate matter and discoloration prior to administration, whenever solution and container permit.

TACROLIMUS CAPSULES

It is recommended that patients be converted from intravenous to oral tacrolimus capsules as soon as oral therapy can be tolerated. This usually occurs within 2-3 days. The first dose of oral therapy should be given 8-12 hours after discontinuing the IV infusion. The recommended starting oral dose of tacrolimus capsules is 0.15-0.30 mg/kg/day administered in two divided daily doses every 12 hours. The initial dose of tacrolimus should be administered no sooner than 6 hours after transplantation. Adult patients should receive doses at the lower end of the dosing range.

Dosing should be titrated based on clinical assessments of rejection and tolerability. Lower tacrolimus dosages may be sufficient as maintenance therapy. Adjunct therapy with adrenal corticosteroids is recommended early post transplant.

Pediatric Patients: Pediatric patients without pre- existing renal or hepatic dysfunction have required and tolerated higher doses than adults to achieve similar blood concentrations. Therefore, it is recommended that therapy be initiated in pediatric patients at the high end of the recommended adult intravenous and oral dosing ranges (0.1 mg/kg/day intravenous and 0.3 mg/kg/day oral). Dose adjustments may be required.

Patients with Hepatic or Renal Dysfunction: Due to the potential for nephrotoxicity, patients with renal or hepatic impairment should receive doses at the lowest value of the recommended intravenous and oral dosing ranges. Further reductions in dose below these ranges may be required. Tacrolimus therapy usually should be delayed up to 48 hours or longer in patients with post-operative oliguria.

Conversion from one Immunosuppressive Regimen to Another: Tacrolimus should not be used simultaneously with cyclosporine. Tacrolimus or cyclosporine should be discontinued at least 24 hours before initiating the other. In the presence of elevated tacrolimus or cyclosporine concentrations, dosing with the other drug usually should be further delayed.

Blood Concentration Monitoring: Most study centers have found tacrolimus blood-concentration monitoring helpful in patient management. While no fixed relationship has been established, such blood monitoring may assist in the clinical evaluation of rejection and toxicity, dose adjustments, and the assessment of compliance.

Various assays have been used to measure blood concentrations of tacrolimus. Comparison of the concentrations in published literature to patient concentrations using current assays must be made with detailed knowledge of the assay methods employed.

Data from the U.S. clinical trial show that tacrolimus whole blood concentrations, as measured by ELISA, were most variable during the first week post-transplantation. After this early period, the median trough blood concentrations, measured at intervals from the second week to one year post-transplantation, ranged from 9.8 ng/ml to 19.4 ng/ml.

HOW SUPPLIED:

Prograf Capsules 1 mg: Oblong, white, branded with red "1 mg" on the capsule cap and "f 617" on the capsule body, supplied in 100-count bottles, containing the equivalent of 1 mg of anhydrous tacrolimus.

Prograf Capsules 5 mg: Oblong, grayish/red, branded with white "5 mg" on the capsule cap and "f 657" on the capsule body, supplied in 100-count bottles, containing the equivalent of 5 mg of anhydrous tacrolimus.

Store and Dispense: Store at controlled room temperature, 15°C-30°C (59°F-86°F).

Prograf injection 5 mg (for intravenous infusion only): Supplied as a sterile solution in 1-ml ampules containing the equivalent of 5 mg of anhydrous tacrolimus per ml, in boxes of 10 ampuleS.

Store and Dispense: Store between 5°C and 25°C (41°F and 77°F).

HOW SUPPLIED - EQUIVALENTS NOT AVAILABLE:

Capsule, Gelatin - Oral - 1 mg

100's $218.40 PROGRAF, Fujisawa USA 00469-0617-71

Capsule, Gelatin - Oral - 5 mg

100's $1092.00 PROGRAF, Fujisawa USA 00469-0657-71

Injection, Solution - Intravenous - 5 mg/ml

1 ml x 10 $2220.00 PROGRAF, Fujisawa USA 00469-3016-01

TAMOXIFEN CITRATE *(002306)*

CATEGORIES: Antiestrogen; Antineoplastics; Breast Carcinoma; Cancer; Oncologic Drugs; Tumors; Pregnancy Category D; Sales > $500 Million; FDA Approval Pre 1982; Patent Expiration 1993 Dec

BRAND NAMES: *Dignotamoxi; Istubol; Kessar; Mamofen; Noltam;* **Nolvadex**; *Novofen; Tamaxin; Tamifen; Tamofen; Tamoplex; Tamoxen; Valodex; Zitazonium (International brand names outside U.S. in italics)*

FORMULARIES: Aetna; BC-BS; CIGNA; FHP; Humana; Kaiser; Medco; Medi-Cal; PruCare; United; WHO

COST OF THERAPY: $1,036.35 (Ovarian Carcinoma; Tablet; 10 mg; 2/day; 365 days)

DESCRIPTION:

Tamoxifen citrate tablets, a nonsteroidal antiestrogen, are for oral administration. Each 10 mg tablet contains 15.2 mg of tamoxifen citrate which is equivalent to 10 mg of tamoxifen. Each 20 mg tablet contains 30.4 mg of tamoxifen citrate which is equivalent to 20 mg of tamoxifen. In addition, each tablet contains as inactive ingredients: carboxymethylcellulose calcium, magnesium stearate, mannitol and starch.

Chemically, tamoxifen is the trans-isomer of a triphenylethylene derivative. The chemical name is (Z)2-[4-(1,2-diphenyl-1-butenyl) phenoxy]-N, N-dimethylethanamine 2-hydroxy-1,2,3-propanetricarboxylate (1:1).

DESCRIPTION: *(cont'd)*

Tamoxifen citrate has a molecular weight of 563.62, the pKa' is 8.85, the equilibrium solubility in water at 37°C is 0.5 mg/ml and in 0.02 N HCl at 37°C, it is 0.2 mg/ml.

CLINICAL PHARMACOLOGY:

Tamoxifen citrate is a nonsteroidal agent which has demonstrated potent antiestrogenic properties in animal test systems. The antiestrogenic effects may be related to its ability to compete with estrogen for binding sites in target tissues such as breast. Tamoxifen inhibits the induction of rat mammary carcinoma induced by dimethylbenzanthracene (DMBA) and causes the regression of already established DMBA-induced tumors. In this rat model, tamoxifen appears to exert its antitumor effects by binding the estrogen receptors.

In cytosols derived from human breast adenocarcinomas, tamoxifen competes with estradiol for estrogen receptor protein.

Tamoxifen is extensively metabolized after oral administration. Studies in women receiving 20 mg of ^{14}C tamoxifen have shown that approximately 65% of the administered dose was excreted from the body over a period of 2 weeks with fecal excretion as the primary route of elimination. The drug was excreted mainly as polar conjugates, with unchanged drug and unconjugated metabolites accounting for less than 30% of the total fecal radioactivity.

N-desmethyl tamoxifen was the major metabolite found in patients' plasma. The biological activity of N-desmethyl tamoxifen appears to be similar to tamoxifen. 4-Hydroxytamoxifen and a side chain primary alcohol derivative of tamoxifen have been identified as minor metabolites in plasma.

Following a single oral dose of 20 mg tamoxifen, an average peak plasma concentration of 40 ng/ml (range 35 to 45 ng/ml) occurred approximately 5 hours after dosing. The decline in plasma concentrations of tamoxifen is biphasic with a terminal elimination half-life about 5 to 7 days. The average peak plasma concentration for N-desmethyl tamoxifen is 15 ng/ml (range 10 to 20 ng/ml). Chronic administration of 10 mg tamoxifen given twice daily for three months to patients results in average steady-state plasma concentrations of 120 ng/ml (range 67-183 ng/ml) for tamoxifen and 336 ng/ml (range 148-654 ng/ml) for N-desmethyl tamoxifen. The average steady-state plasma concentrations of tamoxifen and N-desmethyl tamoxifen after administration of 20 mg tamoxifen once daily for three months are 122 ng/ml (range 71-183 ng/ml) and 353 ng/ml (range 152-706 ng/ml), respectively. After initiation of therapy, steady state concentrations for tamoxifen are achieved in about 4 weeks and steady state concentrations for N-desmethyl tamoxifen are achieved in about 8 weeks, suggesting a half-life of approximately 14 days for this metabolite.

In a 3-month crossover steady-state bioavailability study with tamoxifen citrate 10 mg twice a day versus tamoxifen citrate 20 mg given once daily, the results demonstrated that tamoxifen citrate 20 mg taken once daily has comparable bioavailability to tamoxifen citrate 10 mg taken twice a day.

CLINICAL STUDIES:

The Early Breast Cancer Trialists' Collaborative Group (EBCTCG) conducted worldwide overviews of systemic adjuvant therapy for early breast cancer in 1985 and again in 1990. In 1992, 10-year outcome data were reported for 29,892 women in 40 randomized trials of adjuvant tamoxifen using doses of 20-40 mg/day for 1-5+ years (median 2 years). Fifty-one percent were entered into trials comparing tamoxifen to no adjuvant therapy and 49% were entered into trials of tamoxifen in combination with chemotherapy vs. the same chemotherapy alone. Twenty-nine percent were <50 years of age and 71% were ≥50 years. Fifty-seven percent were node-positive and 43% were node-negative. Fifty percent of the tumors were estrogen receptor (ER) positive (≥10 fmol/mg), 18% were ER poor (<10 fmol/mg), and 32% were ER unknown.

The overall recurrence-free survival at 10 years of follow-up was 51.2% for tamoxifen versus 44.7% for control (logrank 2p <0.00001). Overall survival at 10 years was 58.8% for tamoxifen versus 52.6% for control (logrank 2p <0.00001). Both the absolute risk of relapse and the absolute benefit of treatment with tamoxifen were greater in women with positive nodes than in women with negative nodes. In women with positive nodes, 10-year recurrence-free survival was 41.9% for tamoxifen versus 33.1% for control (logrank 1p <0.00001). Ten-year survival was 50.4% for tamoxifen versus 42.2% for control (logrank 1p <0.00001). In women with negative nodes, recurrence-free survival was 68.1% for tamoxifen versus 63.1% for control (logrank 1p <0.00001). Survival at 10 years was 74.5% for tamoxifen versus 71.0% for control (logrank 1p = 0.0002).

The reduction in the annual odds of recurrence with tamoxifen was 12% in women <50 years of age versus 29% in women ≥50 years. Similarly, the reduction in the annual odds of death was 6% versus 20%. The reduction in the annual odds of recurrence with tamoxifen was significantly greater in ER positive (32%) than in ER poor (13%) tumors (1p <0.00001). The reduction in recurrence and mortality was greater in those studies that used tamoxifen for longer (≥2 years) rather than shorter (< 2 years) periods. There was no indication that doses greater than 20 mg per day were more effective.

Two studies (Hubay and NSABP B-09) demonstrated an improved disease-free survival following radical or modified radical mastectomy in postmenopausal women or women 50 years of age or older with surgically curable breast cancer with positive axillary nodes when tamoxifen citrate was added to adjuvant cytotoxic chemotherapy. In the Hubay study, tamoxifen citrate was added to "low-dose" CMF (cyclophosphamide, methotrexate and fluorouracil). In the NSABP B-09 study, tamoxifen citrate was added to melphalan [L-phenylalanine mustard (P)] and fluorouracil (F).

In the Hubay study, patients with a positive (more than 3 fmol) estrogen receptor were more likely to benefit. In the NSABP B-09 study in women age 50-59 years, only women with both estrogen and progesterone receptor levels 10 fmol or greater clearly benefited, while there was a nonstatistically significant trend toward adverse effect in women with both estrogen and progesterone receptor levels less than 10 fmol. In women age 60-70 years, there was a trend toward a beneficial effect of tamoxifen citrate without any clear relationship to estrogen or progesterone receptor status.

Three prospective studies (ECOG-1178, Toronto, NATO) using tamoxifen citrate adjuvantly as a single agent demonstrated an improved disease-free survival following total mastectomy and axillary dissection for postmenopausal women with positive axillary nodes compared to placebo/no treatment controls. The NATO study also demonstrated an overall survival benefit.

NSABP B-14, a prospective, double-blind, randomized study evaluated tamoxifen citrate versus placebo in the treatment of women with axillary node-negative, estrogen-receptor positive (≥10 fmol/mg cytosol protein) breast cancer (as adjuvant therapy, following total mastectomy and axillary dissection, or segmental resection, axillary dissection, and breast radiation). After five years of treatment, a significant improvement in disease-free survival was demonstrated in women receiving tamoxifen citrate. This benefit was apparent both in women under age 50 and in women at or beyond age 50. In this trial women who received tamoxifen for five years and were disease-free at the end of this 5 year period were offered an additional five years of tamoxifen citrate, or placebo in a double-blind randomized scheme. With fours years of follow-up after this rerandomization, 92% of the women that received five years of tamoxifen citrate followed by the placebo are alive and disease-free, compared to 86% of the women scheduled to receive 10 years of tamoxifen citrate. This difference was not statistically significant. One additional randomized study (NATO) demonstrated improved disease-free survival for tamoxifen citrate compared to no adjuvant therapy following total mastectomy and axillary dissection in postmenopausal women with axillary node-negative breast cancer. In this study, the benefits of tamoxifen citrate appeared to be independent of estrogen receptor status.

Three prospective, randomized studies (Ingle, Pritchard, Buchanan) compared tamoxifen citrate to ovarian ablation (oophorectomy or ovarian irradiation) in premenopausal women with advanced breast cancer. Although the objective response rate, time to treatment failure, and survival were similar with both treatments, the limited patient accrual prevented a demonstration of equivalence. In an overview analysis of survival data from the three studies, the hazard ratio for death (tamoxifen citrate/ovarian ablation) was 1.00 with two-sided 95% confidence intervals of 0.73 to 1.37. Elevated serum and plasma estrogens have been observed in premenopausal women receiving tamoxifen citrate. However, the data from the randomized studies do not suggest an adverse effect. A limited number of premenopausal patients with disease progression during tamoxifen citrate therapy responded to subsequent ovarian ablation.

In a large randomized trial in Sweden of adjuvant tamoxifen citrate 40 mg/day for 2-5 years, the incidence of second primary breast tumors was reduced in the tamoxifen arm (p<0.05). In the NSABP B-14 trial in which patients were randomized to tamoxifen citrate 20 mg/day for 5 years versus placebo, the incidence of second primary breast cancers is also reduced.

Published results from 122 patients (119 evaluable) and case reports in 16 patients (13 evaluable) treated with tamoxifen citrate have shown that tamoxifen citrate is effective for the palliative treatment of male breast cancer. Sixty-six of these 132 evaluable patients responded to tamoxifen citrate which constitutes a 50% objective response rate.

INDICATIONS AND USAGE:

Adjuvant Therapy: Tamoxifen citrate is indicated for the treatment of axillary node-negative breast cancer in women following total mastectomy or segmental mastectomy, axillary dissection, and breast irradiation. Data are insufficient to predict which women are most likely to benefit and to determine if tamoxifen citrate provides any benefit in women with tumors less than 1 cm.

Tamoxifen citrate is indicated for the treatment of node-positive breast cancer in postmenopausal women following total mastectomy or segmental mastectomy, axillary dissection, and breast irradiation. In some tamoxifen citrate adjuvant studies, most of the benefit to date has been in the subgroup with 4 or more positive axillary nodes.

The estrogen and progesterone receptor values may help to predict whether adjuvant tamoxifen citrate therapy is likely to be beneficial.

Therapy for Advanced Disease: Tamoxifen citrate is effective in the treatment of metastatic breast cancer in women and men. In premenopausal women with metastatic breast cancer, tamoxifen citrate is an alternative to oophorectomy or ovarian irradiation. Available evidence indicates that patients whose tumors are estrogen receptor positive are more likely to benefit from tamoxifen citrate therapy.

CONTRAINDICATIONS:

Tamoxifen citrate is contraindicated in patients with known hypersensitivity to the drug.

WARNINGS:

Visual disturbance including corneal changes, cataracts and retinopathy have been reported in patients receiving tamoxifen citrate.

As with other additive hormonal therapy (estrogens and androgens), hypercalcemia has been reported in some breast cancer patients with bone metastases within a few weeks of starting treatment with tamoxifen citrate. If hypercalcemia does occur, appropriate measures should be taken and, if severe, tamoxifen citrate should be discontinued.

An increased incidence of endometrial changes including hyperplasia, polyps, and endometrial cancer has been reported in association with tamoxifen citrate treatment. The incidence and pattern of this increase suggest that the underlying mechanism is related to the estrogenic properties of tamoxifen citrate. Any patients receiving or having previously received tamoxifen citrate who report abnormal vaginal bleeding should be promptly evaluated.

In a large randomized trial in Sweden of adjuvant tamoxifen citrate 40 mg/day for 2-5 years, an increased incidence of uterine cancer was noted. Twenty three of 1,372 patients randomized to receive tamoxifen citrate versus 4 of 1,357 patients randomized to the observation group developed cancer of the uterus [RR = 5.6 (1.9-16.2), p<.001]. One of the patients with cancer of the uterus who was randomized to receive tamoxifen citrate never took the drug. After approximately 6.8 years of follow-up in the ongoing NSABP B-14 trial, 15 of 1,419 women randomized to receive tamoxifen citrate 20 mg/day for 5 years developed uterine cancer and 2 of the 1,424 women randomized to receive placebo, who subsequently were treated with tamoxifen citrate, also developed uterine cancer. Most of the uterine cancers were diagnosed at an early stage, but deaths from uterine cancer have been reported. Patients receiving tamoxifen citrate should have routine gynecological care and they should promptly inform their physician if they experience any menstrual irregularities, abnormal vaginal bleeding, change in vaginal discharge, or pelvic pain or pressure.

Tamoxifen citrate has been associated with changes in liver enzyme levels, and on rare occasions, a spectrum of more severe liver abnormalities including fatty liver, cholestasis, hepatitis and hepatic necrosis. A few of these serious cases included fatalities. In most reported cases the relationship to tamoxifen citrate is uncertain. However, some positive rechallenges and dechallenges have been reported.

In the Swedish trial using adjuvant tamoxifen citrate 40 mg/day for 2-5 years, 3 cases of liver cancer have been reported in the tamoxifen citrate-treated group versus 1 case in the observation group. In other clinical trials evaluating tamoxifen citrate, no other cases of liver cancer have been reported to date.

Data from the NSABP B-14 study show no increase in other (non-uterine) cancers among patients receiving tamoxifen citrate. However, a number of second primary tumors, occurring at sites other than the endometrium, have been reported following the treatment of breast cancer with tamoxifen citrate in clinical trials. Whether an increased risk for other (non-uterine) cancers is associated with tamoxifen citrate is still uncertain and continues to be evaluated.

Pregnancy Category D: Tamoxifen citrate may cause fetal harm when administered to a pregnant woman. Women should be advised not to become pregnant while taking tamoxifen citrate and should use barrier or nonhormonal contraceptive measures if sexually active. Effects on reproductive functions are expected from the antiestrogenic properties of the drug. In reproductive studies in rats at dose levels equal to or below the human dose, nonteratogenic developmental skeletal changes were seen and were found reversible. In addition, in fertility studies in rats and in teratology studies in rabbits using doses at or below those used in humans, a lower incidence of embryo implantation and a higher incidence of fetal death or retarded *in utero* growth were observed, with slower learning behavior in some rat pups when compared to historical controls. Several pregnant marmosets were dosed during organogenesis or in the last half of pregnancy. No deformations were seen and, although the dose was high enough to terminate pregnancy in some animals, those that did maintain pregnancy showed no evidence of teratogenic malformations.

WARNINGS: *(cont'd)*

In rodent models of fetal reproductive tract development, tamoxifen (at doses 0.3 to 2.4-fold the human maximum recommended dose on a mg/m² basis) caused changes in both sexes that are similar to those caused by estradiol, ethynylestradiol and diethylstilbestrol. Although the clinical relevance of these changes is unknown, some of these changes, especially vaginal adenosis, are similar to those seen in young women who were exposed to diethylstilbestrol *in utero* and who have a 1 in 1000 risk of developing clear-cell adenocarcinoma of the vagina or cervix. To date, *in utero* exposure to tamoxifen has not been shown to cause vaginal adenosis, or clear-cell adenocarcinoma of the vagina or cervix, in young women. However, only a small number of young women have been exposed to tamoxifen *in utero*, and a smaller number have been followed long enough (to age 15-20) to determine whether vaginal or cervical neoplasia could occur as a result of this exposure.

There are no adequate and well controlled trials of tamoxifen in pregnant women. There have been a small number of reports of vaginal bleeding, spontaneous abortions, birth defects, and fetal deaths in pregnant women. If this drug is used during pregnancy, or the patient becomes pregnant while taking this drug, or within approximately two months after discontinuing therapy, the patient should be apprised of the potential risks to the fetus including the potential long-term risk of a DES-like syndrome.

PRECAUTIONS:

GENERAL

Decreases in platelet counts, usually to 50,000-100,000/mm³, infrequently lower, have been occasionally reported in patients taking tamoxifen citrate for breast cancer. In patients with significant thrombocytopenia, rare hemorrhagic episodes have occurred, but it is uncertain if these episodes are due to tamoxifen citrate therapy. Leukopenia has been observed, sometimes in association with anemia and/or thrombocytopenia. There have been rare reports of neutropenia and pancytopenia in patients receiving tamoxifen citrate olvadex; this can sometimes be severe.

INFORMATION FOR THE PATIENT

Women taking or having previously taken tamoxifen citrate should be instructed to report abnormal vaginal bleeding which should be promptly investigated.

LABORATORY TESTS

Periodic complete blood counts, including platelet counts and periodic liver function tests should be obtained.

DRUG/LABORATORY TESTING INTERACTIONS

During postmarketing surveillance, T_4 elevations were reported for a few postmenopausal patients which may be explained by increases in thyroid-binding globulin. These elevations were not accompanied by clinical hyperthyroidism.

Variations in the karyopyknotic index on vaginal smears and various degrees of estrogen effect on Pap smears have been infrequently seen in postmenopausal patients given tamoxifen citrate.

In the postmarketing experience with tamoxifen citrate, infrequent cases of hyperlipidemias have been reported. Periodic monitoring of plasma triglycerides and cholesterol may be indicated in patients with pre-existing hyperlipidemias.

CARCINOGENESIS, MUTAGENESIS, AND IMPAIRMENT OF FERTILITY

Carcinogenesis: A conventional carcinogenesis study in rats (doses of 5, 20, and 35 mg/kg/day for up to 2 years) revealed hepatocellular carcinoma at all doses, and the incidence of these tumors was significantly greater among rats given 20 or 35 mg/kg/day (69%) than those given 5 mg/kg/day (14%). The incidence of these tumors in rats given 5 mg/kg/day (29.5 mg/m²) was significantly greater than in controls.

In addition, preliminary data from 2 independent reports of 6-month studies in rats reveal liver tumors which in one study are classified as malignant. (See WARNINGS.)

Endocrine changes in immature and mature mice were investigated in a 13-month study. Granulosa cell ovarian tumors and interstitial cell testicular tumors were found in mice receiving tamoxifen citrate, but not in the controls.

Mutagenesis: Although no genotoxic potential was found in a conventional battery of *in vivo* and *in vitro* tests with pro- and eukaryotic test systems with drug metabolizing systems present, increased levels of DNA adducts have been found in the livers of rats exposed to tamoxifen. Tamoxifen also has been found to increase levels of micronucleus formation *in vitro* in human lymphoblastoid cell line (MCL-5). Based on these findings, tamoxifen is genotoxic in rodent and human MCL-5 cells.

Impairment of Fertility: Fertility in female rats was decreased following administration of 0.04 mg/kg for two weeks prior to mating through day 7 of pregnancy. There was a decreased number of implantations, and all fetuses were found dead.

Following administration to rats of 0.16 mg/kg from days 7-17 of pregnancy, there were increased numbers of fetal deaths. Administration of 0.125 mg/kg to rabbits during days 6-18 of pregnancy resulted in abortion or premature delivery. Fetal deaths occurred at higher doses. There were no teratogenic changes in either rat or rabbit segment II studies. Several pregnant marmosets were dosed with 10 mg/kg/day either during organogenesis or in the last half of pregnancy. No deformations were seen, and although the dose was high enough to terminate pregnancy in some animals, those that did maintain pregnancy showed no evidence of teratogenic malformations. Rats given 0.16 mg/kg from day 17 of pregnancy to 1 day before weaning demonstrated increased numbers of dead pups at parturition. It was reported that some rat pups showed slower learning behavior, but this did not achieve statistical significance in one study, and in another study where significance was reported, this was obtained by comparing dosed animals with controls of another study.

The recommended daily human dose of 20-40 mg corresponds to 0.4-0.8 mg/kg for an average 50 kg woman.

PREGNANCY CATEGORY D

(See WARNINGS.)

NURSING MOTHERS

It is not known whether this drug is excreted in human milk. Because many drugs are excreted in human milk and because of the potential for serious adverse reactions in nursing infants from tamoxifen citrate, a decision should be made whether to discontinue nursing or to discontinue the drug, taking into account the importance of the drug to the mother.

PEDIATRIC USE

The safety and efficacy of tamoxifen citrate in pediatric patients have not been established.

DRUG INTERACTIONS:

When tamoxifen citrate is used in combination with coumarin-type anticoagulants, a significant increase in anticoagulant effect may occur. Where such coadministration exists, careful monitoring of the patient's prothrombin time is recommended.

There is an increased risk of thromboembolic events occurring when cytotoxic agents are used in combination with tamoxifen citrate.

DRUG INTERACTIONS: *(cont'd)*

Tamoxifen, N-desmethyl tamoxifen and 4-Hydroxytamoxifen have been found to be potent inhibitors of hepatic cytochrome p-450 mixed function oxidases. The effect of tamoxifen on metabolism and excretion of other antineoplastic drugs, such as cyclophosphamide and other drugs that require mixed function oxidases for activation, is not known.

One patient receiving tamoxifen citrate with concomitant phenobarbital exhibited a steady state serum level of tamoxifen lower than that observed for other patients (*i.e.*, 26 ng/ml vs. mean value of 122 ng/ml). However, the clinical significance of this finding is not known.

Concomitant bromocriptine therapy has been shown to elevate serum tamoxifen and N-desmethyltamoxifen.

ADVERSE REACTIONS:

Adverse reactions to tamoxifen citrate are relatively mild and rarely severe enough to require discontinuation of treatment.

In patients treated with tamoxifen citrate for metastatic breast cancer, the most frequent adverse reactions to tamoxifen citrate are hot flashes and nausea and/or vomiting. These may occur in up to one-fourth of patients.

Less frequently reported adverse reactions are vaginal bleeding, vaginal discharge, menstrual irregularities and skin rash. Usually these have not been of sufficient severity to require dosage reduction or discontinuation of treatment.

Increased bone and tumor pain and, also, local disease flare have occurred, which are sometimes associated with a good tumor response. Patients with increased bone pain may require additional analgesics. Patients with soft tissue disease may have sudden increases in the size of preexisting lesions, sometimes associated with marked erythema within and surrounding the lesions and/or the development of new lesions. When they occur, the bone pain or disease flare are seen shortly after starting tamoxifen citrate and generally subside rapidly.

Other adverse reactions which are seen infrequently are hypercalcemia, peripheral edema, distaste for food, pruritus vulvae, depression, dizziness, light-headedness, headache, hair thinning and/or partial hair loss, and vaginal dryness.

Tamoxifen citrate has been associated with changes in liver enzyme levels, and on rare occasions, a spectrum of more severe liver abnormalities including fatty liver, cholestasis, hepatitis and hepatic necrosis. A few of these serious cases included fatalities. In most reported cases the relationship to tamoxifen citrate is uncertain. However, some positive rechallenges and dechallenges have been reported.

There have been a few reports of endometriosis and uterine fibroids in women receiving tamoxifen citrate. The underlying mechanism may be due to the partial estrogenic effect of tamoxifen citrate. Ovarian cysts have also been observed in a small number of premenopausal patients with advanced breast cancer who have been treated with tamoxifen citrate.

Continued clinical studies have resulted in further information which better indicates the incidence of adverse reactions with tamoxifen citrate as compared to placebo.

In the ongoing NSABP study B-14, women with axillary node-negative breast cancer were randomized to 5 years of tamoxifen citrate 20 mg/day or placebo following primary surgery. The reported adverse effects are in TABLE 1 (mean follow-up of approximately 6.8 years). The incidence of hot flashes (64% v 48%), vaginal discharge (30% v 15%), and irregular menses (25% v 19%) were higher with tamoxifen citrate compared with placebo. All other adverse effects occurred with similar frequency in the two treatment groups, with the exception of thrombotic events, which although rare, were more common with tamoxifen citrate than with placebo. Two of the patients treated with tamoxifen citrate who had thrombotic events died.

TABLE 1 NSABP B-14 Study

Adverse Effect	% of Women Tamoxifen (n=1424)	Placebo (n=1440)
Hot Flashes	63.9	47.6
Weight Gain (>5%)	38.1	40.1
Fluid Retention	32.4	29.7
Vaginal Discharge	29.6	15.2
Nausea	25.7	23.9
Irregular Menses	24.6	18.8
Weight Loss (>5%)	22.6	18.0
Skin Changes	18.7	15.3
Increased BUN	18.1	20.2
Diarrhea	11.2	14.0
Increased SGOT	4.8	2.8
Increased Alkaline Phosphatase	3.0	4.6
Vomiting	2.1	1.7
Increased Bilirubin	1.8	1.2
Increased Creatinine	1.7	1.0
Thrombocytopenia*	1.5	1.2
Leukopenia**	0.4	1.1
Thrombotic Events		
Deep Vein Thrombosis	0.8	0.3
Pulmonary Embolism	0.4	0.1
Superficial Phlebitis	0.3	0.0

* Defined as a platelet count of <100,000/mm³
** Defined as a white blood cell count of <3000/mm³

In the Eastern Cooperative Oncology Group (ECOG) adjuvant breast cancer trial, tamoxifen citrate or placebo was administered for 2 years to women following mastectomy. When compared to placebo, tamoxifen citrate showed a significantly higher incidence of hot flashes (19% versus 8% for placebo). The incidence of all other adverse reactions was similar in the 2 treatment groups with the exception of thrombocytopenia where the incidence for tamoxifen citrate was 10% versus 3% for placebo, an observation of borderline statistical significance.

The other adverse reactions reported equally in the ECOG study for tamoxifen citrate and placebo include abnormal renal function tests, fatigue, dyspnea, anorexia, cough, and abdominal cramps. A relationship of these reactions to the administration of tamoxifen citrate has not been demonstrated since the frequency was not significantly different from that reported in placebo treated women.

In other adjuvant studies, Toronto and Nolvadex Adjuvant Trial Organization, women received either tamoxifen citrate or no therapy. In the Toronto study, hot flashes and nausea and/or vomiting were observed in 29% and 19% of patients, respectively, for tamoxifen citrate versus 1% and 0% in the untreated group. In the NATO trial, hot flashes, nausea and/or vomiting and vaginal bleeding were reported in 2.8%, 2.1% and 2.0% of women, respectively, for tamoxifen citrate versus 0.2% for each in the untreated group.

TABLE 2 summarizes the incidence of adverse reactions reported at a frequency of 2% or greater from clinical trials (Ingle, Pritchard, Buchanan) which compared tamoxifen citrate therapy to ovarian ablation in premenopausal patients with metastatic breast cancer.

ADVERSE REACTIONS: *(cont'd)*

TABLE 2

Adverse Reactions*	Nolvadex All Effects Number of Women (%) n = 104	OVARIAN ABLATION All Effects Number of Women (%) n = 100
Flush	34 (32.7)	46 (46)
Amenorrhea	17 (16.3)	69 (69)
Altered Menses	13 (12.5)	5 (5)
Oligomenorrhea	9 (8.7)	1 (1)
Bone Pain	6 (5.7)	6 (6)
Menstrual Disorder	6 (5.7)	4 (4)
Nausea	5 (4.8)	4 (4)
Cough/Coughing	4 (3.8)	1 (1)
Edema	4 (3.8)	1 (1)
Fatigue	4 (3.8)	1 (1)
Musculoskeletal Pain	3 (2.8)	0 (0)
Pain	3 (2.8)	4 (4)
Ovarian Cyst(s)	3 (2.8)	2 (2)
Depression	2 (1.9)	2 (2)
Abdominal Cramps	1 (1)	2 (2)
Anorexia	1 (1)	2 (2)

* Some women had more than one adverse reaction.

Tamoxifen citrate is well tolerated in males with breast cancer. Reports from the literature and case reports suggest that the safety profile of tamoxifen citrate in males is similar to that seen in women. Loss of libido and impotence have resulted in discontinuation of tamoxifen therapy in male patients. Also, in oligospermic males treated with tamoxifen, LH, FSH, testosterone and estrogen levels were elevated. No significant clinical changes were reported.

OVERDOSAGE:

Signs observed at the highest doses following studies to determine LD_{50} in animals were respiratory difficulties and convulsions.

Acute overdosage in humans has not been reported. In a study of advanced metastatic cancer patients which specifically determined the maximum tolerated dose of tamoxifen citrate in evaluating the use of very high doses to reverse multidrug resistance, acute neurotoxicity manifested by tremor, hyperreflexia, unsteady gait and dizziness were noted. These symptoms occurred within 3-5 days of beginning tamoxifen citrate and cleared within 2-5 days after stopping therapy. No permanent neurologic toxicity was noted. One patient experienced a seizure several days after tamoxifen citrate was discontinued and neurotoxic symptoms had resolved. The causal relationship of the seizure to tamoxifen citrate therapy is unknown. Doses given in these patients were all greater than 400 mg/m^2 loading dose, followed by maintenance doses of 150 mg/m^2 of tamoxifen citrate given twice a day.

In the same study, prolongation of the QT interval on the electrocardiogram was noted when patients were given doses higher than 250 mg/m^2 loading dose, followed by maintenance doses of 80 mg/m^2 of tamoxifen citrate given twice a day. For a woman with a body surface area of 1.5 m^2 the minimal loading dose and maintenance doses given at which neurological symptoms and QT changes occurred were at least 6 fold higher in respect to the maximum recommended dose.

No specific treatment for overdosage is known; treatment must be symptomatic.

DOSAGE AND ADMINISTRATION:

For patients with breast cancer, the recommended daily dose is 20–40 mg. Dosages greater than 20 mg per day should be given in divided doses (morning and evening).

In three single agent adjuvant studies in women, one 10 mg tamoxifen citrate tablet was administered two (ECOG and NATO) or three (Toronto) times a day for two years. (See CLINICAL PHARMACOLOGY.) In the EBCTCG 1990 overview, the reduction in recurrence and mortality was greater in those studies that used tamoxifen for two years or longer than in those that used tamoxifen for less than two years. There was no indication that doses greater than 20 mg per day were more effective. In B-14, the ongoing NSABP adjuvant study in women with node-negative breast cancer, one 10 mg tamoxifen citrate tablet was given twice a day for at least five years. Results of the B-14 study suggest that continuation of therapy beyond five years does not provide additional benefit. (See CLINICAL PHARMACOLOGY.)The optimal duration of adjuvant therapy remains to be determined.

PATIENT INFORMATION:

Tamoxifen is used for the treatment of breast cancer.

Do not use this drug if you are pregnant or nursing. Use a non-hormonal form of birth control (*e.g.*, condoms, diaphragm but NOT "the pill")

Patients taking this drug should have routine gynecological exams. Promptly inform your physicians if you experience menstrual irregularities, abnormal vaginal bleeding, change in vaginal discharge, or pelvic pain or pressure.

Tamoxifen may cause hot flashes, weight gain, fluid retention, vaginal discharge, nausea and vomiting. Inform your physician if these occur.

HOW SUPPLIED:

Nolvadex 10 mg Tablets containing tamoxifen as the citrate in an amount equivalent to 10 mg of tamoxifen are round, biconvex, uncoated, white tablet identified with Nolvadex 600 debossed on one side and a cameo debossed on the other side.

Nolvadex 20 mg Tablets containing tamoxifen as the citrate in an amount equivalent to 20 mg of tamoxifen are round, biconvex, uncoated, white tablet identified with Nolvadex 604 debossed on one side and a cameo debossed on the other side.

Storage: Store at controlled room temperature, 20°-25° C (68° - 77° F). Protect from heat and light.

HOW SUPPLIED - EQUIVALENTS NOT AVAILABLE:

Tablet, Uncoated - Oral - 10 mg

60's	$85.18	Tamoxifen Citrate, Barr	00555-0446-09
60's	**$89.58**	**NOLVADEX, Zeneca Pharms**	**00310-0600-60**
250's	$354.93	Tamoxifen Citrate, Barr	00555-0446-03
250's	**$373.21**	**NOLVADEX, Zeneca Pharms**	**00310-0600-25**

TAMSULOSIN HYDROCHLORIDE *(003338)*

CATEGORIES: Alpha Adrenergic Receptor Inhibitors; Benign Prostatic Hyperplasia; Pregnancy Category B; FDA Approved 1997 May

BRAND NAMES: **Flomax**

DESCRIPTION:

Flomax (tamsulosin hydrochloride) is an antagonist of $alpha_{1A}$ adrenoceptors in the prostate. Tamsulosin HCl is (-)-(*R*)-5-[2-[[2-(0-ethoxyphenoxy) ethyl]aminolpropyl]-2-methoxybenzenesulfonamide, monohydrochloride. Tamsulosin HCl occurs as white crystals that melt with decomposition at approximately 230°C. It is sparingly soluble in water and in methanol, slightly soluble in glacial acetic acid and in ethanol, and practically insoluble in ether.

The empirical formula of tamsulosin HCl is $C_{20}H_{28}N2O_5S{\cdot}HCl$. The molecular weight of tamsulosin HCl is 444.98.

Each capsule of Flomax for oral administration contains tamsulosin HCl 0.4 mg, and the following inactive ingredients: methacrylic acid copolymer, microcrystaline cellulose, triacetin, polysorbate 80, sodium lauryl sulfate, calcium stearate, talc, FD&C blue No. 2, titanium dioxide, ferric oxide, gelatin, and trace amounts of shellac, industrial methylated spirit 740P, soya lecithin, 2-ethoxyethanol, dimethylpolysiloxane, and black iron oxide E172.

CLINICAL PHARMACOLOGY:

The symptoms associated with benign prostatic hyperplasia (BPH) are related to bladder outlet obstruction, which is comprised of two underlying components: static and dynamic. The static component is related to an increase in prostate size caused, in part, by a proliferation of smooth muscle cells in the prostatic stroma. However, the severity of BPH symptoms and the degree of urethral obstruction do not correlate well with the size of the prostate. The dynamic component is a function of an increase in smooth muscle tone in the prostate and bladder neck leading to constriction of the bladder outlet. Smooth muscle tone is mediated by the sympathetic nervous stimulation of $alpha_1$ adrenoceptors, which are abundant in the prostate, prostatic capsule, prostatic urethra, and bladder neck. Blockade of these adrenoceptors can cause smooth muscles in the bladder neck and prostate to relax, resulting in an improvement in urine flow rate and a reduction in symptoms of BPH.

Tamsulosin, an $alpha_1$ adrenoceptor blocking agent, exhibits selectivity for $alpha_1$ receptors in the human prostate. At least three discrete $alpha_1$-adrenoceptor subtypes have been identified: $alpha_{1A}$, $alpha_{1B}$ and $alpha_{1D}$; their distribution differs between human organs and tissue. Approximately 70% of the $alpha_1$-receptors in human prostate are of the $alpha_{1A}$ subtype.

Tamsulosin is not intended for use as an antihypertensive drug.

PHARMACOKINETICS

The pharmacokinetics of tamsulosin have been evaluated in adult healthy volunteers and patients with BPH after single and or multiple administration with doses ranging from 0.1 mg to 1 mg.

Absorption

Absorption of tamsulosin from tamsulosin 0.4 mg is essentially complete (>90%) following oral administration under fasting conditions. Tamsulosin exhibits linear kinetics following single and multiple dosing, with achievement of steady-state concentrations by the fifth day of once-a-day dosing.

Effect of Food

The time to maximum concentration (T_{max}) is reached by four to five hours under fasting conditions and by six to seven hours when tamsulosin is administered with food. Taking tamsulosin under fasted conditions results in a 30% increase in bioavailability (AUC) and 40% to 70% increase in peak concentrations (C_{max}) compared to fed conditions.

The effects of food on the pharmacokinetics of tamsulosin are consistent regardless of whether tamsulosin is taken with a light breakfast or a high-fat breakfast (TABLE 1).

TABLE 1 Mean (± S.D.) Pharmacokinetic Parameters Following Tamsulosin 0.4 mg Once Daily or 0.8 mg Once Daily with a Light Breakfast, High-Fat Breakfast, or Fasted

Pharmacokinetic Parameter	0.4 mg, daily, to healthy volunteers; n=23 (age range 18-32 years)		0.8 mg, every day, to healthy volunteers; n=22 (age range 55-75 years)		
	Light Breakfast	Fasted	Light Breakfast	High-Fat Breakfast	Fasted
C_{min} (ng/ml)	4.0 ± 2.6	3.8 ± 2.5	12.3 ± 6.7	13.5 ± 7.6	13.3 ± 13.3
C_{max} (ng/ml)	10.1 ± 4.8	17.1 ± 17.1	29.8 ± 10.3	29.1 ± 11.0	41.6 ± 5.6
C_{max}/C_{min} Ratio	3.1 ± 1.0	5.3 ± 2.2	2.7 ± 0.7	2.5 ± 0.8	3.6 ± .1
$T\frac{1}{2}$ (hours)	-	-	-	-	14.9 ± 3.9
T_{max} (hours)	6.0	4.0	7.0	6.6	5.0
AUC (ng·hr/ml)	151 ± 81.5	199 ± 94.1	440 ± 195	449 ± 217	557 ± 257

C_{max}= observed minimum concentration
C_{min}= observed maximum tamsulosin plasma concentration
T_{max}=median time-to-maximum concentration
$T\frac{1}{2}$ = observed half-life
AUC = Area under the tamsulosin plasma time curve over the dosing interval

Distribution

The mean steady-state apparent volume of distribution of tamsulosin after intravenous administration to ten healthy male adults was 16L, which is suggestive of distribution into extracellular fluids in the body. Additionally, whole body autoradiographic studies in mice and rats and tissue distribution in rats and dogs indicate that tamsulosin is widely distributed to most tissues including kidney, prostate, liver, gall bladder, heart, aorta, and brown fat, and minimally distributed to the brain, spinal cord, and testes. Tamsulosin is extensively bound to human plasma proteins (94% to 99%), primarily $alpha_1$ acid glycoprotein (AAG), with linear binding over a wide concentration range (20 to 600 ng/ml). The results of two-way *in vitro* studies indicate that the binding of tamsulosin to human plasma proteins is not affected by amitriptyline, diclofenac, glyburide, simvastatin plus simvastatin-hydroxy acid metabolite, warfarin, diazepam, propranolol, trichlormethiazide, or chlormadinone. Likewise, tamsulosin had no effect on the extent of binding of these drugs.

Metabolism

There is no enantiometric bioconversion from tamsulosin [R(-) isomer] to the S(+) isomer in humans. Tamsulosin is extensively metabolized by cytochrome P450 enzymes in the liver and less than 10% of the dose is excreted in urine unchanged. However, the pharmacokinetic profile of the metabolites in humans has not been established. Additionally, the cytochrome P450 enzymes that primarily catalyze the Phase I metabolism of tamsulosin have not been conclusively identified. Therefore, possible interactions with other cytochrome P450 metabolized compounds cannot be discerned with current information. The metabolites of tamsulosin undergo extensive conjugation to glucuronide or sulfate prior to renal excretion.

CLINICAL PHARMACOLOGY: *(cont'd)*

Incubations with human liver microsomes showed no evidence of clinically significant metabolic interactions between tamsulosin and amitriptyline, albuterol (beta agonist), glyburide (glibenclamide) and finasteride (5alpha-reductase inhibitor for treatment of BPH). However, results of the *in vitro* testing of the tamsulosin interaction with diclofenac and warfarin were equivocal.

Exretion

On administration of the radiolabeled dose of tamsulosin to four healthy volunteers, 97% of the administered radioactivity was recovered, with urine (76%) representing the primary route of excretion compared to feces (21%) over 168 hours.

Following intravenous or oral administration of an immediate release formulation, the elimination half- life of tamsulosin in plasma range from five to seven hours. Because of absorption rate-controlled pharmacokinetics with tamsulosin the apparent half-life of tamsulosin is approximately 9 to 13 hours in healthy volunteers and 14 to 15 hours in the target population. Tamsulosin undergoes restrictive clearance in humans, with a relatively low sytemic clearance (2.88 L/h).

Special Populations

Geriatrics (Age): Cross-study comparison of tamsulosin overall exposure (AUC) and half-life indicate that the pharmacokinetic disposition of tamsulosin may be slightly prolonged in geriatric male compared to young, healthy male volunteers. Intrinsic clearance is independent of tamsulosin binding to AAG, but diminshes with age, resulting in a 40% overall higher exposure (AUC) in subjects of age 55 to 75 years compared to subjects of age 20 to 32 years.

Renal Dysfunction The pharmacokinetics of tamsulosin have been comapred in 6 subjects with mild-moderate ($30 \leq CL_{cr} < 70$ ml/min/1.73m^2) or moderate-severe ($10 \leq CL_{cr} < 30$ ml/min/1.73m^2) renal impairment and 6 normal subjects ($CL_{cr} < 90$ ml/min/1.73m^2). While a change in the overall plasma concentration of tamsulosin was observed as the result of altered binding to AAG, the unbound (active) concentration of tamsulosin, as well as the intrinsic clearance, remained relatively constant. Therefore, patients with renal impairment do not require an adjustment in tamsulosin dosing. However, patients with endstage renal disease ($CL_{cr} < 10$ ml/min/1.73m^2) have not been studied.

Hepatic Dysfunction: The pharmacokinetics of tamsulosin have been compared in 8 subjects with moderate hepatic dysfunction (Child-Pugh's classification: Grades A and B) and 8 normal subjects. While a change in the overall plasma concentration of tamsulosin was observed as the result of altered binding to AAG, the unbound (active) concentration of tamsulosin does not change significantly with only a modest (32%) change in intrinsic clearance of unbound tamsulosin. Therefore, patients with moderate hepatic dysfunction do not require an adjustment in tamsulosin dosage.

CLINICAL STUDIES:

Four placebo-controlled clinical studies and one active-controlled clinical study enrolled a total of 2296 patients (1003 received tamsulosin 0.4 mg once daily, 491 received tamsulosin 0.8 mg once daily, and 802 were control patients) in the U.S. and Europe.

In the two U.S. placebo controlled, double-blind, 13-week, multicenter studies [Study 1 (US92-03A) and Study 2 (US93-01)], 1486 men with the signs and symptoms of BPH were enrolled. In both studies, patients were randomized to either placebo, tamsulosin 0.4 mg once daily, or tamsulosin 0.8 mg once daily. Patients in tamsulosin 0.8 mg once daily treatment groups received a dose of 0.4 mg once daily for one week before increasing to the 0.8 mg once daily dose. The primary efficacy assessments included: 1) total American Urological Association (AUA) Symptom Score questionnaire, which evaluated irritative (frequency, urgency, and nocturia), and obstructive (hesitancy, incomplete emptying, intermittency, and weak stream) symptoms, where a decrease in score is consistent with improvement in symptoms and 2) peak urine flow rate where an increased peak urine flow rate value over baseline is consistent with decreased urinary obstruction.

Mean changes from baseline to week 13 in total AUA Symptom Score were significantly greater for groups treated with tamsulosin 0.4 mg and 0.8 mg once daily compared to placebo in both U.S. studies (TABLE 2). The changes from baseline to week 13 in peak urine flow rate were also significantly greater for the tamsulosin 0.4 mg and 0.8 mg once daily groups compared to placebo in Study 1, and for the tamsulosin 0.8 mg once daily group in Study 2 (TABLE 2). Overall there were no significant differences in improvement observed in total AUA Symptom Scores or peak urine flow rates between the 0.4 mg and the 0.8 mg dose groups with the exception that the 0.8 mg dose in Study 1 had a significantly greater improvement in total AUA Symptom Score compared to the 0.4 mg dose.

TABLE 2 Mean (± SD) Changes From Baseline to Week 13 in Total AUA Symptom Score ** and Peak Urine Flow Rate (ml/sec)

	Total AUA Symptom Score		Peak Urine Flow Rate	
	Mean Baseline Value	Mean Change	Mean Baseline Value	Mean Change
Study 1 †				
Tamsulosin 0.8 mg once daily	19.9 ± 4.9 n=247	-9.6* ± 6.7 n=237	9.57 ± 2.51 n=247	1.78* ± 3.35 n=247
Tamsulosin 0.4 mg once daily	19.8 ± 5.0 n=254	-8.3* ± 6.5 n=246	9.46 ± 2.49 n=254	1.75* ± 3.57 n=254
Placebo	19.6 ± 4.9 n=254	-5.5 ± 6.6 n=246	9.75 ± 2.54 n=254	0.52 ± 3.39 n=253
Study 2 ‡				
Tamsulosin 0.8 mg once daily	18.2 ± 5.6 n=244	-5.8* ± 6.4 n=238	9.96 ± 3.16 n=244	1.79* ± 3.36 n=237
Tamsulosin 0.4 mg once daily	17.9 ± 5.8 n=248	-5.1* ± 6.4 n=244	9.94 ± 3.14 n=248	1.52 ± 3.64 n=244
Placebo	19.2 ± 6.0 n=239	-3.6 ± 5.7 n=235	9.95 ± 3.12 n=239	0.93 ± 3.28 n=235

* Statistically significant difference from placebo (p-value ≤0.50; Bonferroni-Holm test procedure)
** Total AUA Symptom Scores ranged from 0 to 35
† Peak urine flow rate measured 4 to 8 hours post dose at week 13
‡ Peak urine flow rate measured 24 to 27 hours post dose at week 13
Week 13: For patients not completing the 13 week study the last observation was carried forward.

Mean total AUA Symptom Scores for both tamsulosin 0.4 mg and 0.8 mg once daily groups showed a rapid decrease starting at one week after dosing and remained decreased through 13 weeks in both studies.

In Study 1, 400 patients (53% of the originally randomized group) elected to continue in their originally assigned treatment groups in a double-blind, placebo controlled, 40 week extension trial (138 patients on 0.4 mg, 135 patients on 0.8 mg and 127 patients on placebo). Three hundred and twenty-three patients (43% of the originally randomized group) completed one year. Of these, 81% (97 patients) on 0.4 mg, 74% (75 patients) on 0.8 mg and 56% (57 patients) on placebo had a response ≥25% above baseline in total AUA Symptom Score at one year.

CLINICAL STUDIES: *(cont'd)*

Multiple testing for orthostatic hypotension was conducted in a number of studies. Such a test was considered positive if it met one or more of the following criteria: (1) a decrease in systolic blood pressure of ≥20 mmHg upon standing from the supine position during the orthostatic tests; (2) a decrease in diastolic blood pressure ≥10 mmHg upon standing, with the standing diastolic blood pressure <65 mmHg during the orthostatic test; (3) an increase in pulse rate of ≥20 bpm upon standing with a standing pulse rate ≥100 bpm during the orthostatic test and (4) the presence of clinical symptoms (faintness, lightheadedness/lightheaded, dizziness, spinning sensation, vertigo, or postural hypotension) upon standing during the orthostatic test.

Following the first dose of double-blind medication in Study 1, a positive orthostatic test result at 4 hours post-dose was observed in 7% of patients (37 of 498) who received tamsulosin 0.4 mg once daily and in 3% of the patients (8 of 253) who received placebo. At 8 hours post-dose, a positive orthostatic test result was observed for 6% of the patients (31 of 498) who received tamsulosin 0.4 mg once daily and 4% (9 of 250) who received placebo (Note: patients in the 0.8 mg group received 0.4 mg once daily for the first week of Study 1).

In Studies 1 and 2, at least one positive orthostatic test result was observed during the course of these studies for 81 of the 502 patients (16%) in the tamsulosin 0.4 mg once daily group, 92 of the 491 patients (19%) in the tamsulosin 0.8 mg once daily group and 54 of the 493 patients (11%) in the placebo group.

Because orthostasis was detected more frequently in tamsulosin-treated patients than in placebo recipients, there is a potential risk of syncope (see WARNINGS).

INDICATIONS AND USAGE:

Tamsulosin is indicated for the treatment of the signs and symptoms of benign prostatic hyperplasia (BPH). Tamsulosin is not indicated for the treatment of hypertension.

CONTRAINDICATIONS:

Tamsulosin is contraindicated in patients known to be hypersensitive to tamsulosin or any component of Flomax.

WARNINGS:

The signs and symptoms of orthostasis (postural hypotension, dizziness and vertigo) were detected more frequently in tamsulosin-treated patients than in placebo recipients. As with other alpha-adrenergic blocking agents there is a potential risk of syncope (see ADVERSE REACTIONS).

Patients beginning treatment with tamsulosin should be cautioned to avoid situations where injury could result should syncope occur.

PRECAUTIONS:

GENERAL

1) Carcinoma of the Prostate: Carcinoma of the prostate and BPH cause many of the same symptoms. These two diseases frequently co-exist. Patients should be evaluated prior to the start of tamsulosin therapy to rule out the presence of carcinoma of the prostate.

INFORMATION FOR THE PATIENT

(See PATIENT PACKAGE INSERT.) Patients should be told about the possible occurrence of symptoms related to postural hypotension such as dizziness when taking tamsulosin, and they should be cautioned about driving, operating machinery or performing hazardous tasks. Patients should be advised not to crush, chew or open the capsules of tamsulosin.

LABORATORY TESTS

No laboratory test interactions with tamsulosin are known. Treatment with tamsulosin for up to 12 months had no significant effect on prostate-specific antigen (PSA).

PREGNANCY PREGNANCY, TERATOGENIC EFFECTS, PREGNANCY CATEGORY B

Administration of tamsulosin to pregnant female rats at dose levels up to 300 mg/kg/day (approximately 50 times the human therapeutic AUC exposure) revealed no evidence of harm to the fetus. Administration of tamsulosin to pregnant rabbits at dose levels up to 50 mg/kg/day produced no evidence of fetal harm. Tamsulosin is not indicated for use in women.

CARCINOGENESIS, MUTAGENESIS, AND IMPAIRMENT OF FERTILITY

Rats administered doses up to 43 mg/kg/day in males and 52 mg/kg/day in females had no increases in tumor incidence with the exception of a modest increase in the frequency of mammary gland fibroadenomas in female rats receiving doses ≥5.4 mg/kg/day ($P < 0.015$). The highest doses of tamsulosin evaluated in the rat carcinogenicity study produced systemic exposures (AUC) in rats 3 times the exposures in men receiving the maximum therapeutic dose of 0.8 mg day.

Mice were administered doses up to 127 mg/kg/day in males and 158 mg/kg/day in females. There were no significant tumor findings in male mice. Female mice treated for 2 years with the two highest doses of 45 and 158 mg kg day had statistically significant increases in the incidence of mammary gland fibroadenomas ($P < 0.0001$) and adenocarcinomas ($P < 0.0075$). The highest dose levels of tamsulosin evaluated in the mice carcinogenicity study produced systemic exposures (AUC) in mice 8 times the exposures in men receiving the maximum therapeutic dose of 0.8 mg day.

The increased incidence of mammary gland neoplasm in female rats and mice were considered secondary to tamsulosin induced hyperprolactinemia. It is not known if tamsulosin elevates prolactin in humans. The relevance for human risk of the findings of prolactin-mediated endocrine tumors in rodents is not known.

Tamsulosin produced no evidence of mutagenic potential *in vitro* in the Ames reverse mutation test, mouse lymphoma thymidine kinase assay, unscheduled DNA repair synthesis assay, and chromosomal aberration assays in Chinese hamster ovary cells or human lymphocytes. There were no mutagenic effects in the *in vivo* sister chromatic exchange and mouse micronucleus assay.

Studies in rats revealed significantly reduced fertility in males dosed with single or multiple daily doses of 300 mg/kg/day of tamsulosin (AUC exposure in rats about 50 times the human exposure with the maximum therapeutic dose). The mechanism of decreased fertility in male rats is considered to be an effect of the compound on the vaginal plug formation possibly due to changes of semen content or impairment of ejaculation. The effects on fertility were reversible showing improvement by 3 days after a single dose and 4 weeks after multiple dosing. Effects on fertility in males were completely reversed within nine weeks of discontinuation of multiple dosing. Multiple doses of 10 and 100 mg kg day tamsulosin (15 and 16 times the anticipated human AUC exposure) did not significantly alter fertility in male rats. Effects of tamsulosin on sperm counts or sperm function have not been evaluated.

Studies in female rats revealed significant reductions in fertility after single or multiple dosing with 300 mg/kg/day of the *R*-isomer or racemic mixture of tamsulosin, respectively. In female rats, the reductions in fertility after single doses were considered to be associated with impairments in fertilization. Multiple dosing with 10 or 100 mg/kg/day of the racemic mixture did not significantly alter fertility in female rats.

NURSING MOTHERS

Tamsulosin is not indicated for use in women.

PRECAUTIONS: *(cont'd)*

PEDIATRIC USE

Tamsulosin is not indicated for use in pediatric populations.

DRUG INTERACTIONS:

Nifedipine, Atenolol, Enalapril: In three studies in hypertensive subjects (age range 47-79 years) whose blood pressure was controlled with stable doses of Procardia XL, atenolol, or enalapril for at least three months, tamsulosin 0.4 mg for seven days followed by tamsulosin 0.8 mg for another seven days (n=8 per study) resulted in no clinically significant effects on blood pressure and pulse rate compared to placebo (n=4 per study). Therefore, dosage adjustments are not necessary when tamsulosin is administered concomitantly with Procardia XL, atenolol, or enalapril.

Warfarin: A definitive drug-drug interaction study between tamsulosin and wanfarin was not conducted. Results from limited *in vitro* and *in vivo* studies are inconclusive. Therefore, caution should be exercised with concomitant administration of warfarin and tamsulosin.

Digoxin and Theopylline: In two studies in healthy volunteers (n=10 per study; age range 19-39 years) receiving Tamsulosin 0.4 mg day for two days, followed by tamsulosin 0.8 mg/day for five to eight days, single intravenous doses of digoxin 0.5 mg or theophylline 5 mg/kg resulted in no change in the pharmacokinetics of digoxin or theophylline. Therefore, dosage adjustments are not necessary when tamsulosin is administered concomitantly with digoxin or theophylline.

Furosemide: The pharmacokinetic and pharmacodynamic interaction between tamsulosin 0.8 mg day (steady-state) and furosemide 20 mg intravenously (single dose) was evaluated in ten healthy volunteers (age range 21-40 years). Tamsulosin had no effect on the pharmacodynamic (excretion of electrolytes) of furosemide. While furosemide produced an 11% to 12% reduction in tamsulosin C_{max} and AUC, these changes are expected to be clinically insignificant and do not require adjustment of the tamsulosin dosage.

Cimetidine: The effects of cimetidine at the highest recommended dose (400 mg every six hours for six days) on the pharmacokinetics of a single tamsulosin 0.4 mg dose was investigated in ten healthy volunteers (age range 21-38 years). Treatment with cimetidine resulted in a significant decrease (26%) in the clearance of tamsulosin which resulted in a moderate increase in tamsulosin AUC (44%). Therefore, tamsulosin should be used with caution in combination with cimetidine, particularly at doses higher than 0.4 mg.

Drug-Drug Interactions: The pharmacokinetics and pharmacodynamic interactions between tamsulosin and other alpha-adrenergic blocking agents have not been determined. However, interactions may be expected and tamsulosin should NOT be used in combination with other alpha-adrenergic blocking agents.

The pharmacokinetic interaction between cimetidine and tamsulosin was investigated. The results indicate significant changes in tamsulosin clearance (26% decrease) and AUC (44% increase). Therefore, tamsulosin should be used with caution in combination with cimetidine, particularly at doses higher than 0.4 mg.

Results from limited *in vitro* and *in vivo* drug-drug interaction studies between tamsulosin and warfarin are inconclusive. Therefore, caution should be exercised with concomitant administration of warfarin and tamsulosin.

ADVERSE REACTIONS:

The incidence of treatment-emergent adverse events has been ascertained from six short-term U.S. and European placebo-controlled clinical trials in which daily doses of 0.1 to 0.8 mg tamsulosin were used. These studies evaluated safety in 1783 patients treated with tamsulosin and 798 patients administered placebo. TABLE 3 summarizes the treatment-emergent adverse events that occurred in ≥2% of patients receiving either tamsulosin 0.4 mg, or 0.8 mg and at an incidence numerically higher than that in the placebo group during two 13-week U.S. trials (US92-03A and US93-01) conducted in 1487 men.

TABLE 3 Treatment Emergent [1]Adverse Events Occurring in ≥2% of Tamsulosin or Placebo Patients in Two U.S. Short-Term Placebo-Controlled Clinical Studies

Body Sytem / Adverse Event	Tamsulosin Groups 0.4 mg n=502	Tamsulosin Groups 0.8 mg n=492	Placebo n=493
Body As A Whole			
Headache	97 (19.3%)	104 (21.1%)	99 (20.1%)
Infection	45 (9.0%)	53 (10.8%)	37 (7.5%)
Asthenia	39 (7.8%)	42 (8.5%)	27 (5.5%)
Back Pain	35 (7.0%)	41 (8.3%)	27 (5.5%)
Chest Pain	20 (4.0%)	20 (4.1%)	18 (3.7%)
Nervous System			
Dizziness	75 (14.9%)	84 (17.1%)	50 (10.1%)
Somnolence	15 (3.0%)	21 (4.3%)	8 (1.6%)
Insomnia	12 (2.4%)	7 (1.4%)	3 (0.6%)
Libido Decreased	5 (1.0%)	10 (2.0%)	6 (1.6%)
Respiratory System			
Rhinitis	66 (13.1%)	88 (17.9%)	41 (8.3%)
Pharyngitis	29 (5.8%)	25 (5.1%)	23 (4.7%)
Cough Increased	17 (3.4%)	22 (4.5%)	12 (2.4%)
Sinusitis	11 (2.2%)	18 (3.7%)	8 (1.6%)
Digestive System			
Diarrhea	31 (6.2%)	21 (4.3%)	22 (4.5%)
Nausea	13 (2.6%)	19 (3.9%)	16 (3.2%)
Tooth Disorder	6 (1.2%)	10 (2.0%)	7 (1.4%)
Urogenital System			
Abnormal Ejaculation	42 (8.4%)	89 (18.1%)	1 (0.2%)
Special Senses			
Amblyopia	1 (0.2%)	10 (2.0%)	2 (0.4%)

[1]A treatment emergent adverse event was defined as any event satisfying one of the following criteria:

- **The adverse event occurred for the first time after initial dosing with double-blind study medication.**
- **The adverse event was present prior to or at the time of initial dosing with double-blind study medication and subsequently increased in severity during double-blind treatment; OR**
- **The adverse event was present prior to or at the time of initial dosing with double-blind study medication, disappeared completely, and then reappeared during double-blind treatment.**

Signs and Symptoms of Orthostasis: In the two U.S. studies, symptomatic postural hypotension was reported by 0.2% of patients (1 of 502) in the 0.4 mg group, 0.4% of patients (2 of 492) in the 0.8-mg group, and by no patients in the placebo group. Syncope was reported by 0.2% of patients (1 of 502) in the 0.4 mg group, 0.4% of patients (2 of 492) in the 0.8 mg group and 0.6% of patients (3 of 493) in the placebo group. Dizziness was reported by 15% of patients (75 of 502) in the 0.4 mg group, 17% of patients (84 of 492) in the 0.8 mg group, and 10% of patients (50 of 493) in the placebo group. Vertigo was reported by 0.6% of patients (3 of 502) in the 0.4 mg group, 1% of patients (5 of 492) in the 0.8 mg group and by 0.6% of patients (3 of 493) in the placebo group.

ADVERSE REACTIONS: *(cont'd)*

Abnormal Ejaculation: Abnormal ejaculation includes ejaculation failure, ejaculation disorder, retrograde ejaculation and ejaculation decrease. As shown in TABLE 3, abnormal ejaculation was associated with tamsulosin administration and was dose-related in the U.S. studies. Withdrawal from these clinical studies of tamsulosin because of abnormal ejaculation was also dose-dependent with 8 of 492 patients (1.6%) in the 0.8 mg group, and no patients in the 0.4 mg or placebo groups discontinuing treatment due to abnormal ejaculation.

OVERDOSAGE:

Should overdosage of tamsulosin lead to hypotension (See WARNINGS and ADVERSE REACTIONS), support of the cardiovascular system is of first importance. Restoration of blood pressure and normalization of heart rate may be accomplished by keeping the patient in the supine position. If this measure is inadequate, then administration of intravenous fluids should be considered. If necessary, vasopressors should then be used and renal function should be monitored and supported as needed. Laboratory data indicate that tamsulosin is 94% to 99% protein bound: therefore, dialysis is unlikely to be of benefit.

One patient reported an overdose of thirty 0.4 mg capsules of tamsulosin. Following the ingestion of the capsules, the patient reported a severe headache.

DOSAGE AND ADMINISTRATION:

Tamsulosin 0.4 mg once daily is recommended as the dose for the treatment of the signs and symptoms of BPH. It should be administered approximately one-half hour following the same meal each day.

For those patients who fail to respond to the 0.4 mg dose after two to four weeks of dosing, the dose of tamsulosin can be increased to 0.8 mg once daily. If tamsulosin administration is discontinued or interrupted for several days at either the 0.4 mg or 0.8 mg dose, therapy should be started again with the 0.4 mg once daily dose.

PATIENT PACKAGE INSERT:

Tamsulosin HCl is for use by men only. **It is not indicated for use in women.**

Please read the following before you start taking tamsulosin. Also, read it each time you renew your prescription, just in case new information has been added. Remember, the following information does not take the place of careful discussions with your doctor. You and your doctor should discuss tamsulosin when you start taking your medication and at regular checkups.

Why Has Your Doctor Prescribed Tamsulosin? Your doctor has prescribed tamsulosin because you have a medical condition called benign prostatic hyperplasia or BPH. This occurs only in men.

What is BPH? Benign prostatic hyperplasia is an enlargement of the prostate gland. After age 50, most men develop enlarged prostates. The prostate is located below the bladder. As the prostate enlarges, it may slowly restrict the flow of urine. This can lead to symptoms such as:

a weak or interrupted urinary stream

a feeling that you cannot empty your bladder completely

a feeling of delay or hesitation when you start to urinate

a need to urinate often, especially at night

a feeling that you must urinate right away

Since cancer of the prostate may cause similar symptoms, you should be evaluated by your doctor to rule out prostate cancer. Your doctor will likely examine your prostate gland manually to detect abnormalities and may measure prostate specific antigen (PSA) in your blood to help in evaluating for the presence of prostate cancer. Tamsulosin does not affect PSA levels.

Treatment Options for BPH: There are three main treatment options for BPH:

Program of monitoring or "Watchful Waiting". Some men have an enlarged prostate gland, but no symptoms, or symptoms that are not bothersome. If this applies, you and your doctor may decide on a program of monitoring, including regular checkups, instead of medication or surgery.

There are different kinds of medication used to treat BPH. Your doctor has prescribed tamsulosin for you. See **What Tamsulosin Does to Treat BPH.**

Surgery. Some patients may need surgery. Your doctor can describe everal different surgical procedures to treat BPH. Which procedure is best depends on your symptoms and medical condition.

What Tamsulosin Does to Treat BPH: Tamsulosin acts by relaxing muscles in the prostate and bladder neck at the site of the obstruction, resulting in improved urine flow and reduced BPH symptoms.

What You Need to Know While Taking Tamsulosin:

You must see your doctor regularly. While taking tamsulosin, you must have regular checkups. Follow your doctor's advice about when to have these checkups.

It is important for you to recognize that tamsulosin can cause a sudedn drop in blood pressure especially following the first dose or when changing doses of tamsulosin. Such a drop in blood pressure, although rare in occurrance, may be associated with fainting, dizziness, or light-headedness. Therefore, get up slowly from a chair or bed at any time until you learn how you react to tamsulosin. You should not drive or do any hazardous tasks until you are used to the side effects of tamsulosin. If you begin to feel dizzy, sit down until you feel better. Although these symptoms are unlikely, you should avoid driving or hazardous tasks for 12 hours after the initial dose or after your doctor recommends an increase in dose. If you interrupt your treatment for several days or more, resume treatment at one capsule a day, after consulting with your physician. Other side effects may include sleeplessness, runny nose, or ejaculatory problems. In some cases, side effects may decrease or disappear when you continue to take tamsulosin.

You should discuss side effects with your doctor before taking tamsulosin and anytime you think you are having a side effect.

How To Take Tamsulosin: Follow your doctor's advice about how to take tamsulosin. You should take it approximately 30 minutes following the same meal every day.

Do not share tamsulosin with anyone else; it was prescribed for only for you.

Do not crush, chew or open capsules of tamsulosin.

Keep tamsulosin and all medicines out of reach of children.

For more information about tamsulosin, and BPH, talk with your doctor. In addition, talk to your pharmacist or other healthcare provider.

HOW SUPPLIED:

Flomax capsules, 0.4 mg are hard gelatin capsules with an olive green opaque cap and orange opaque body. The capsules are imprinted on one side with "Flomax 0.4 mg" and on the other side with "BI 58."

TEMAZEPAM *(002310)*

CATEGORIES: Anxiolytics, Sedatives, Hypnotic; Benzodiazepines; Central Nervous System Agents; Hypnotics; Insomnia; Sedatives/Hypnotics; Pregnancy Category X; DEA Class CIV; FDA Approval Pre 1982; Top 200 Drugs

BRAND NAMES: *Cerepax*; *Euhypnos*; *Lenal*; *Levanxene*; *Levanxol*; *Normison*; *Planum*; **Restoril**
(International brand names outside U.S. in italics)

FORMULARIES: Aetna; BC-BS; FHP; Foundation; PCS

COST OF THERAPY: $0.27 (Insomnia; Capsule; 30 mg; 1/day; 7 days)

DESCRIPTION:

Temazepam is a benzodiazepine hypnotic agent. The chemical name is 7-chloro-1,3-dihydro-3-hydroxy-1-methyl-5-phenyl-2*H*-1,4-benzodiaz epin-2-one.

Temazepam is a white, crystalline substance, very slightly soluble in water and sparingly soluble in alcohol USP.

Temazepam capsules, 7.5 mg, 15 mg and 30 mg, are for oral administration.

Restoril 15 mg and 30 mg Capsules: *Active Ingredient:* Temazepam

Restoril 7.5 mg Capsules: *Inactive Ingredients:* FD&C Blue #1, FD&C Red #3, gelatin, lactose, magnesium stearate, sodium lauryl sulfate, synthetic red ferric oxide, and titanium dioxide. *May also include:* benzyl alcohol, butylparaben, edetate calcium disodium, methylparaben, propylparaben, silicon dioxide, sodium propionate, and another ingredient.

Restoril 15 mg Capsules: *Inactive Ingredients:* FD&C Blue #1, FD&C Red #3, gelatin, lactose, magnesium stearate, sodium lauryl sulfate, synthetic red ferric oxide, and titanium dioxide. *May also include:* benzyl alcohol, butylparaben, edetate calcium disodium, methylparaben, propylparaben, silicon dioxide, sodium propionate, and another ingredient.

Restoril 30 mg Capsules: *Inactive Ingredients:* FD&C Blue #1, FD&C Red #3, gelatin, lactose, magnesium stearate, sodium lauryl sulfate, and titanium dioxide. *May also include:* benzyl alcohol, butylparaben, edetate calcium disodium, methylparaben, propylparaben, silicon dioxide, sodium propionate, and another ingredient.

CLINICAL PHARMACOLOGY:

PHARMACOKINETICS

In a single and multiple dose absorption, distribution, metabolism, and excretion (ADME) study, using ^3H labeled drug. Temazepam was well absorbed and found to have minimal (8%) first pass metabolism. There were no active metabolites formed and the only significant metabolite present in blood was the O-conjugate. The unchanged drug was 96% bound to plasma proteins. The blood level decline of the parent drug was biphasic and the short half-life ranging from 0.4-0.6 hours and the terminal half life ranging from 3.5-18.4 hours (mean 8.8 hours), depending on the study population and the method of determination. Metabolites were formed with a half-life of 10 hours and excreted with a half-life of approximately 2 hours. Thus, formation of the major metabolite is the rate limiting step in the biodisposition of temazepam. There is no accumulation of metabolites. A dose-proportional relationship has been established for the area under the plasma concentration/time curve over the 15-30 mg dose range.

Temazepam was completely metabolized through conjugation prior to excretion: 80%-90% of the dose appeared in the urine. The major metabolite was th O-conjugate of temazepam (90%): the O-conjugate of N- desmethyl temazepam was a minor metabolite (7%).

BIOAVAILABILITY, INDUCTION, AND PLASMA LEVELS

Following ingestion of a 30 mg temazepam capsule, measurable plasma concentrations were achieved 10-20 minutes after dosing with peak plasma levels ranging from 666-982 ng/ml (mean 865 ng/ml) occurring approximately 1.2-1.6 hours (mean 1.5 hours) after dosing.

In a 7 day study, in which subjects were given a 30 mg temazepam capsule 1 hour before retiring, steady-state (as measured by the attainment of maximal trough concentrations) was achieved by the third dose. Mean plasma levels of temazepam (for days 2-7) were 260 ± 210 ng/ml at 9 hours and 75 ± 80 ng/ml at 24 hours after dosing. A slight trend toward declining 24 hour plasma levels was seen after day 4 in the study, however, the 24 hour plasma levels were quite variable.

At a dose of 30 mg once-a-day for 8 weeks, no evidence of enzyme induction was found in man.

ELIMINATION RATE OF BENZODIAZEPINE HYPNOTICS AND PROFILE OF COMMON UNTOWARD EFFECTS

The type and duration of unwanted effects during administration of benzodiazepine hypnotics may be influenced by the biologic half-life of the administered drug and for some hypnotics, the half-life of any active metabolites formed. Benzodiazepine hypnotics have a spectrum of half- lives from short (<4 hours) or long (>20 hours). When half-lives are long, drug (and for some drugs their inactive metabolites) may accumulate during periods of nightly administration and may be associated with impairments of cognitive and/or motor performance during waking hours; the possibility of interaction with other psychoactive drugs or alcohol will be enhanced. In contrast, if half-lives are shorter, drug (and for some drug their active metabolites may be accumulate during periods of nightly administration and be associated with impairments of cognitive and/or motor performance during waking hours; the possibility of interaction with other psychotropic drugs or alcohol will be enhanced. In contrast, if half-lives are shorter, drug (and, where appropriate, its active metabolites) will be cleared before the next dose is ingested, and carry-over effects related to excessive sedation or CNS depression should be minimized or absent. However, during nightly use for an extended period, pharmacodynamic tolerance or adaptation to some effects of benzodiazepine hypnotics may develop. If the drug has a short elimination half-life, it is possible that a relative deficiency of the drug, or, if appropriate, its active metabolites (*i.e.,* in relationship to the receptor site) may occur at some point in the interval between each night's use. This sequence of events may account for 2 clinical findings reported to occur after several weeks of nightly use of rapidly eliminated benzodiazepines hypnotics, namely increased wakefulness during the last third of the night, and the appearance of daytime anxiety.

CLINICAL STUDIES:

Temazepam improved sleep parameters in clinical studies. Residual medication effects ("hangover") were essentially absent. Early morning awakening, a particular problem in the geriatric patient, was significantly reduced.

CLINICAL STUDIES: *(cont'd)*

Patients with chronic insomnia were evaluated in 2 week, placebo controlled sleep laboratory studies with temazepam at doses of 7.5 mg, 15 mg, and 30 mg, given 30 minutes prior to bedtime. There was a linear dose-response improvement in total sleep time and sleep latency, with significant drug-placebo differences at 2 weeks occurring only for total sleep differences at the 2 higher doses, and for sleep latency only at the highest dose.

In these sleep laboratory studies, REM sleep was essentially unchanged and slow wave sleep was decreased. No measurable effects on daytime alertness or performance occurred following temazepam treatment or during the withdrawal period, even through a transient sleep disturbance in some sleep laboratory parameters was observed following withdrawal of the highest dose. There was no evidence of tolerance development in sleep laboratory parameters when patients were given temazepam nightly for at least 2 weeks.

In addition, normal subjects with transient insomnia associated with first night adaptation to the sleep laboratory were evaluated in 24 hour, placebo controlled sleep laboratory studies with temazepam at doses of 7.5 mg, 15 mg, and 30 mg, given 30 minutes prior to bedtime. There was a linear dose-response improvement in total sleep time, sleep latency and number of awakenings, with significant drug-placebo differences occurring for sleep latency at all doses, for total sleep time at the 2 higher doses and for number of awakenings only at the 30 mg dose.

INDICATIONS AND USAGE:

Temazepam is indicated for the short-term treatment of insomnia (generally 7-10 days). For patients in whom the drug is used for more than 2-3 weeks, periodic reevaluation is recommended to determine whether there is a continuing need. (See WARNINGS.)

For patients with short-term insomnia, instructions in the prescription should indicate that temazepam should be used for short periods of time (7-10 days).

Temazepam should not be prescribed in quantities exceeding a 1-month supply.

Insomnia is characterized by complaints of difficulty in falling asleep, frequent nocturnal awakenings, and/or early morning awakenings. Both sleep laboratory and outpatient studies provide support for the effectiveness of temazepam administered 30 minutes before bedtime in decreasing sleep latency and improving sleep maintenance in patients with chronic insomnia. In addition, sleep laboratory studies have confirmed similar effects in normal subjects with transient insomnia. (See CLINICAL PHARMACOLOGY.)

CONTRAINDICATIONS:

Benzodiazepines may cause fetal damage when administered during pregnancy. An increased risk of congenital malformations associated with the use of diazepam and chlordiazepoxide during the first trimester of pregnancy has been suggested in several studies. Transplacental distribution has resulted in neonatal CNS depression following the ingestion of therapeutic doses of a benzodiazepine hypnotic during the last weeks of pregnancy.

Reproduction studies in animals with temazepam were performed in rats and rabbits. In a perinatal-postnatal study in rats, oral doses of 60 mg/kg/day resulted in increasing nursling mortality. Teratology studies in rats demonstrated increased fetal resorptions at doses of 30 and 120 mg/kg in one study and increased occurrence of rudimentary ribs, which are considered skeletal variants, in a second study at doses of 240 mg/kg or higher. In rabbits, occasional abnormalities such as exencephaly and fusion or asymmetry of ribs were reported without dose relationship. Although these abnormalities were not found in the concurrent control group, they have been reported to occur randomly in historical controls. At doses of 40 mg/kg or higher, there was an increased incidence of the 13th rib variant when compared to the incidence in concurrent and historical controls.

Temazepam is contraindicated in pregnant women. If there is a likelihood of the patient becoming pregnant while receiving temazepam, she should be warned of the potential risk to the fetus. Patients should be instructed to discontinue the drug prior to becoming pregnant. The possibility that a woman of childbearing potential may be pregnant at the time of institution of therapy should be considered.

WARNINGS:

Sleep disturbance may be the presenting manifestation of an underlying physical and/or psychiatric disorder. Consequently, a decision to initiate symptomatic treatment of insomnia should only be made after the patient has been carefully evaluated.

The failure of insomnia to remit after 7-10 days of treatment may indicate the presence of a primary psychiatric and/or medical illness.

Worsening of insomnia may be the consequence of an unrecognized psychiatric or physical disorder as may be the emergence of new abnormalities of thinking or behavior. Such abnormalities have also been reported to occur in association with the central nervous system depressant activity, including those of the benzodiazepine class. Some of these changes may be characterized by decreased inhibition, e.g., aggressiveness and extroversion that seem out of character, similar to that seen with alcohol. Other kinds of behavioral changes can also occur, for example, bizarre behavior, agitation, hallucinations, depersonalization, and, in primarily depressed patients, the worsening of depression, including suicidal thinking. In controlled clinical trials involving 1076 patients on temazepam and 783 patients on placebo, reports of hallucinations, agitation, and overstimulation occurred at rates less than 1 in 100 patients. Hallucinations were reported in 2 temazepam patients and 1 temazepam patient; 2 temazepam patients reported overstimulation. There were no reports of worsening of depression or suicidal ideation, aggressiveness, extroversion, bizarre behavior or depersonalization in these controlled clinical trials.

It can rarely determined with certainty whether a particular instance of the abnormal behavior listed above is induced, spontaneous in origin, or a result of an underlying psychiatric or physical disorder. Nonetheless, the emergence of any new behavioral sign or symptom of concern requires careful and immediate evaluation.

Because some of the worrisome adverse effects of benzodiazepines, including temazepam, appear to be dose related (see PRECAUTIONSand DOSAGE AND ADMINISTRATION), it is important to use the lowest possible effective dose. Elderly patients are especially at risk.

Patients receiving temazepam should be cautioned about possible combined effects with alcohol and other CNS depressants. Withdrawal symptoms of the barbiturate type) have occurred after the abrupt discontinuation of benzodiazepines (see DRUG ABUSE AND DEPENDENCE).

PRECAUTIONS:

GENERAL

Since the risk of the development of over-sedation, dizziness, confusion, and/or ataxia increases substantially with larger doses of benzodiazepines in elderly and debilitated patients, 7.5 mg of temazepam is recommended as the initial dosage for such patients.

Temazepam should be administered with caution in severely depressed patients or those in whom there is any evidence of latent depression; it should be recognized that suicidal tendencies may be present and protective measures may be necessary.

The usual precautions should be observed in patients with impaired renal or hepatic function and in patients with chronic pulmonary insufficiency.

PRECAUTIONS: *(cont'd)*

If temazepam is to be combined with other drugs having known hypnotic properties or CNS-depressant effects, consideration should be given to potential additive effects.

The possibility of a synergistic effect exists with the co-administration of temazepam and diphenhydramine. One case of stillbirth at term has been reported 8 hours after a pregnant patient received temazepam and diphenhydramine. A cause and effect relationship has not yet been determined. (See CONTRAINDICATIONS)

INFORMATION FOR THE PATIENT

The text of a patient package insert is printed at the end of this insert. To assure safe and effective use of temazepam, the information and instructions provided in this patient package insert should be discussed with patients.

LABORATORY TESTS

The usual precautions should be observed in patients with impaired renal or hepatic function and in patients with chronic pulmonary insufficiency. Abnormal liver function tests as well as blood dyscrasias have been reported with benzodiazepines.

CARCINOGENESIS, MUTAGENESIS, AND IMPAIRMENT OF FERTILITY

Carcinogenicity studies were conducted in rats at dietary diazepam doses up to 160 mg/kg/day for 24 months and in mice at dietary dose of 160 mg/kg/day for 18 months. No evidence of carcinogenicity was observed although hyperplastic liver nodules were observed in female mice exposed in female mice exposed to the highest dose. The clinical significance of this finding is not known.

Fertility in male and female rats was not adversely affected by temazepam.

No mutagenicity tests have been done with temazepam.

PREGNANCY CATEGORY X

(See CONTRAINDICATIONS.)

NURSING MOTHERS

It is not known whether this drug is excreted in human milk. Because many drugs are excreted in human milk, caution should be exercised when temazepam is administered to a nursing woman.

PEDIATRIC USE

Safety and effectiveness in children below the age of 18 years have not been established.

ADVERSE REACTIONS:

During clinical studies in which 1076 patients received temazepam at bedtime, the drug was well tolerated. Side effects were usually mild and transient. Adverse reactions occurring in 1% or more of patients are presented in TABLE 1.

TABLE 1

	Temazepam % incidence (n=1076)	Placebo % incidence (n=783)
Drowsiness	9.1	5.6
Headache	8.5	9.1
Fatigue	4.8	4.7
Nervousness	4.6	8.2
Lethargy	4.5	3.4
Dizziness	4.5	3.8
Nausea	3.1	3.3
Hangover	2.5	1.1
Anxiety	2.0	1.5
Depression	1.7	1.8
Dry Mouth	1.7	2.2
Diarrhea	1.7	1.1
Abdominal Discomfort	1.5	1.9
Euphoria	1.5	0.4
Weakness	1.4	0.9
Confusion	1.3	0.5
Blurred Vision	1.3	1.3
Nightmares	1.2	1.7
Vertigo	1.2	0.8

The following adverse events have been reported less frequently (0.5-0.9%):

Central Nervous System: anorexia, ataxia, equilibrium loss, tremor, increased dreaming

Cardiovascular: dyspnea, palpitations

Gastrointestinal: vomiting

Musculoskeletal: backache

Special Senses: hyperhidrosis, burning eyes

Amnesia, hallucinations, horizontal nystagmus, and paradoxical reactions including restlessness, overstimulation and agitation were rare (less than 0.5%).

DRUG ABUSE AND DEPENDENCE:

CONTROLLED SUBSTANCE

Temazepam is a controlled substance in Schedule IV.

ABUSE AND DEPENDENCE

Withdrawal symptoms, similar in character to those noted with barbiturates and alcohol (convulsions, tremor, abdominal, and muscle cramps, vomiting, and sweating), have occurred following abrupt discontinuance of benzodiazepines. The more severe withdrawal symptoms have usually been limited to those patients who received excessive doses over an extended period of time. Generally milder withdrawal symptoms (*e.g.,* dysphoria and insomnia) have been reported following abrupt discontinuance of benzodiazepines taken continuously at therapeutic levels for several months. Consequently, after extended therapy at doses higher than 15 mg, abrupt discontinuation should generally be avoided and a gradual dosage tapering schedule followed. As with any hypnotic, caution must be exercised in administering temazepam to individuals known to be addiction-prone or to those whose history suggests they may increase the dosage on their own initiative. It is desirable to limit repeated prescriptions without adequate medical supervision.

OVERDOSAGE:

Manifestations of acute overdosage of temazepam can be expected to reflect the CNS effects of the drug and include somnolence, confusion, and coma, with reduced or absent reflexes, respiratory depression, and hypotension. If the patient is conscious, vomiting should be induced mechanically or with emetics. Gastric lavage should be employed utilizing concurrently a cuffed endotracheal tube if the patient is unconscious to prevent aspiration and pulmonary complications. Maintenance of adequate pulmonary ventilation is essential. The use of pressor agents intravenously may be necessary to combat hypotension. Fluids should be administered intravenously to encourage diuresis. The value of dialysis has not been determined. If excitation occurs, barbiturates should not be used. It should be borne in mind that multiple agents may have been ingested.

OVERDOSAGE: *(cont'd)*

Flumazenil, a specific benzodiazepine receptor antagonist, is indicated for the complete or partial reversal of the sedative effects of benzodiazepines and may be used in situations when an overdose with a benzodiazepine is known or suspected. Prior to administration of flumazenil, necessary measures should be instituted to secure airway, ventilation, and intravenous access. Flumazenil is intended as an adjunct to, not as a substitue for, proper management of benzodiazepine overdose. Patients treated with flumazenil should be monitored for re-sedation, respiratory depression, and other residual benzodiazepine effects for an appropriate period after treatment. **The prescriber should be aware of a risk of seizure in association with flumazenil treatment, particularly in long-term benzodiazepine users and in cyclic antidepressant overdose.** The complete flumazenil package insert including CONTRAINDICATIONS, WARNINGS, and PRECAUTIONS should be consulted prior to use.

The oral LD_{50} was 1963 mg/kg in mice, 1833 mg/kg in rats, and > 2400 mg/kg in rabbits.

DOSAGE AND ADMINISTRATION:

While the recommended usual adult dose is 15 mg before retiring, 7.5 mg may be sufficient for some patients, and others may need 30 mg. In transient insomnia, a 7.5 mg dose may be sufficient to improve sleep latency. In elderly and/or debilitated patients it is recommended that therapy be initiated with 7.5 mg until individual responses are determined.

PATIENT PACKAGE INSERT:

INTRODUCTION

Your doctor has prescribed temazepam to help you sleep. The following information is intended to guide you in the safe use of this medicine. It is not meant to take the place of your doctor's instructions. If you have any questions about temazepam capsules be sure to ask your doctor or pharmacist.

Temazepam is used to treat different types of sleep problems such as

trouble falling asleep

waking up too early in the morning

waking up to often during the night

Some people may have more than one of these problems.

Temazepam belongs to a group of medicines known as "benzodiazepines". There are many different benzodiazepine medicines used to help people sleep better. Sleep problems are usually temporary, requiring treatment for only a short time, usually 7-10 days. However, if your sleep problems continue, consult your doctor. He/She will determine whether other measures are needed to overcome your sleep problems. Some people have chronic sleep problems that may require prolonged use of sleep medicine. However, you should not use these medicines for long periods without taking with your doctor about the risks and benefits of prolonged use.

SIDE EFFECTS

Common Side Effects: All medicines have side effects. The most common side effects of benzodiazepine sleeping medicines include:

drowsiness

dizziness

lightheadedness

difficulty with coordination

You may find that these medicines make you sleepy during the day. How drowsy you feel depends upon how your body reacts to the medicine, which benzodiazepine sleeping medicine you are taking, and how large a dose your doctor has prescribed. Day-time drowsiness is best avoided by taking the lowest dose possible that will still help you sleep at night. Your doctor will work with you to find the dose of temazepam that is best for you.

To manage these side effects while you are taking the medicine:

Use extreme care while doing anything that requires complex alertness, such as driving a car, operating machinery, or piloting an aircraft. As with any medications used to help people sleep better, you should be very careful when you first start taking temazepam until you know how the medicine will affect you.

NEVER drink alcohol while you are being treated with temazepam or any benzodiazepine medicine. Alcohol can increase the side effects of temazepam or any other benzodiazepine medicine.

Do not take any other medicines without asking your doctor first. This includes medicines you can buy without a prescription. Some medicines can cause drowsiness and are best avoided while taking temazepam.

Always take the exact dose of temazepam prescribed by your doctor. Never change your dose without consulting your doctor first.

SPECIAL CONCERNS

There are many problems that may occur while taking benzodiazepine sleeping medicines.

MEMORY PROBLEMS

Benzodiazepine sleeping medicines may cause a special type of memory loss or "amnesia". When this occurs, a person may not remember what has happened for several hours after taking the medicine. This is usually not a problem since most people fall asleep after taking the medicine

Memory loss can be a problem, however, when sleeping medicines are taken while traveling, such as during an airplane flight and the person wakes up before the effect of the medicine is gone. This has been called "traveler's amnesia".

Memory problems were noticed in fewer than 1 in 100 patients taking temazepam in clinical trials. Memory problems can be avoided if you take temazepam only when you are able to get a full night's sleep (7-8 hours) before you need to be active again. Be sure to talk to your doctor if you think you are having memory problems.

TOLERANCE

When benzodiazepine sleeping medicines are used every night for more than a few weeks, they may lose their effectiveness to help you sleep. This is known as "tolerance".

If tolerance to the medicine develops, other effects may occur depending upon which benzodiazepine you are taking. Tolerance to benzodiazepine sleeping medicines that are shorter acting may cause you to:

wake up during the last third of the night.

become anxious or nervous when you are awake

These effects are less common with temazepam because it is intermediate acting.

DEPENDENCE

All the benzodiazepine sleeping medicines can cause dependence, especially when these medicines are used regularly for longer than a few weeks or at high doses. Some people develop a need to continue taking their medicines. This is known as dependence or "addiction".

PATIENT PACKAGE INSERT: *(cont'd)*

When people develop dependence, they may have difficulty stopping the benzodiazepine sleeping medicine. If the medicine is suddenly stopped, the body is not able to function normally and unpleasant symptoms may occur (see Withdrawal).They may find they have to keep taking the medicine either at the prescribed dose or at increasing doses just to avoid withdrawal symptoms.

All people taking benzodiazepine sleeping medicines have some risk of becoming dependent on the medicine. However, people who have been dependent on alcohol or other drugs in the past may have a higher chance of becoming addicted to benzodiazepine medicines. This possibility must be considered before using these medicines for more than a few weeks.

If you have been addicted to alcohol or drugs in the past, it is important to tell your doctor before starting temazepam or any benzodiazepine sleeping medicine.

WITHDRAWAL

Withdrawal symptoms may occur when a benzodiazepine sleeping medicine is stopped suddenly after being used for a long time. But these symptoms can occur even if the medicine has been used for a week or two.

In mild cases, withdrawal symptoms may include unpleasant feelings. In more severe cases, abdominal and muscle cramps, vomiting, sweating, shakiness, and, rarely, seizures may occur. These more severe withdrawal symptoms are very uncommon.

Another problem that may occur when taking benzodiazepine sleeping medicines are stopped is known as "rebound insomnia". This means that a person may have more trouble sleeping the first few nights after the medicine is stopped than before starting the medicine. If you should experience rebound insomnia, do not get discouraged. This problem usually goes away on its own after 1 or 2 nights.

If you have been taking temazepam or any other benzodiazepine sleeping medicine for more than 1 or 2 weeks, do not stop taking it on your own. Your doctor may give you special directions on how to gradually decrease your dose before stopping the medicine. Always follow your doctor's directions.

CHANGES IN BEHAVIOR AND THINKING

Some people using benzodiazepine sleeping medicines have experienced unusual changes in their thinking and/or behavior, including: more outgoing or aggressive behavior than normal; loss of personal identity; confusion; strange behavior; agitation; hallucinations; worsening of depression; and suicidal thoughts.

How often these effects occur depends on several factors, such as a person's general health or the use of other medicines. Clinical studies with temazepam revealed that unusual behavior changes occurred in less than 1 in 100 patients.

It is also important to realize that it is rarely clear whether these behavioral changes are caused by the medicine, an illness, or occur on their own. In fact, sleep problems that do not improve may be due to illnesses that were present before the medicine was used. If you or your family notice any changes in your behavior, or if you have any unusual or disturbing thoughts, call your doctor immediately.

PREGNANCY

Certain benzodiazepines have been linked to birth defects when taken by a pregnant woman in the early months of pregnancy. These medicines can also cause sedation of the unborn baby when used during the last weeks of pregnancy.

Temazepam should not be taken at any time during pregnancy. Be sure to tell your doctor if you are pregnant, if you ar planning to become pregnant, or if you become pregnant while taking temazepam.

SAFE USE OF BENZODIAZEPINE SLEEPING MEDICINES

To ensure the safe and effective use of temazepam or any other benzodiazepine sleeping medicine, you should observe the following cautions:

1. Temazepam is a prescription medicine and should be used ONLY as directed by your doctor. Follow your doctor's instructions about how to take, when to take, and how long to use temazepam.

2. Never use temazepam or any other benzodiazepine sleeping medicine for longer than 1 or 2 weeks without first asking your doctor.

3. If you notice any unusual or disturbing thoughts or behavior during treatment with temazepam or any other benzodiazepine sleeping medicine, contact your doctor.

4. Tell your doctor about any medicines you may be taking, including medicines you may buy without a prescription. You should also tell your doctor if you drink alcohol. DO NOT use alcohol while taking temazepam or any other benzodiazepine sleeping medicine.

5. Do not take temazepam or any other benzodiazepine sleeping medicine unless you are able to get a full night's sleep before you become active again. For example, temazepam or any other benzodiazepine sleeping medicine should not be taken on an overnight airplane flight of less than 7-8 hours since "traveler's amnesia" may occur.

6. Do not increase the prescribed dose of temazepam or any other benzodiazepine sleeping medicine unless instructed by your doctor.

7. Use extreme care while doing anything that requires complete alertness, such as driving a car, operating machinery, or piloting an aircraft, when you first start taking temazepam or any other benzodiazepine sleeping medicine until you know whether the medicine will have some carryover effect in you the next day.

8. Be aware that you may have more sleeping problems (rebound insomnia) the first night or two after stopping temazepam or any other benzodiazepine sleeping medicine.

9. Be sure to tell your doctor if you are pregnant, if you ar planning to become pregnant, or if you become pregnant while taking temazepam. Temazepam or any other benzodiazepine sleeping medicine should not be taken at any time during pregnancy.

10. As with all prescription medicines, never share temazepam or any other benzodiazepine sleeping medicine with anyone else. Always store temazepam or any other benzodiazepine sleeping medicine in the original container out of reach of children.

PATIENT INFORMATION:

Temazepam is used to treat insomnia and other sleep disorders. It should be used for a short-term period of time, for example 7-10 days. If normal sleep patterns do not return and medication is required after 3 weeks, contact your physician for additional evaluation. This medication should not be taken during pregnancy or by those intending to become pregnant. This drug is a central nervous system depressant. Alcohol should not be taken while taking temazepam. Alcohol and other depressants will have additive effects which could be dangerous. Drowsiness, headache, fatigue and nervousness were the most commonly reported side effects. These medicines are often associated with a type of amnesia where you may not remember things for several hours after taking the medication. This medication can cause dependence if taken for a long period of time. It can also cause a withdrawal type of reaction when trying to stop after taking this medicine for a long period of time. Because of the potential for side effects, talk to your pharmacist or physician about all medicine you take, prescription and non-prescription drugs.

HOW SUPPLIED - RATED THERAPEUTICALLY EQUIVALENT:

Capsule, Gelatin - Oral - 7.5 mg

100's	$46.67	Temazepam, Geneva Pharms	50752-0271-05
100's	$47.99	Temazepam, Geneva Pharms	50752-0271-06

Capsule, Gelatin - Oral - 15 mg

30's	$.94	Temazepam, H.C.F.A. F F P	99999-2310-01
100's	$3.00	Temazepam, United Res	00677-1069-01
100's	$3.15	Temazepam, H.C.F.A. F F P	99999-2310-02
100's	$17.35	Temazepam, Qualitest Pharms	00603-5895-21
100's	$17.40	Temazepam, Major Pharms	00904-2810-60
100's	$18.31	Temazepam, Bristol Myers Squibb	00003-0738-50
100's	$20.72	Temazepam, Goldline Labs	00182-1822-01
100's	$20.72	Temazepam, Purepac Pharm	00228-2076-10
100's	$21.35	Temazepam, Parmed Pharms	00349-8927-01
100's	$22.75	Temazepam, Rugby	00536-4628-01
100's	$23.75	Temazepam, HL Moore Drug Exch	00839-7164-06
100's	$23.75	Temazepam, Par Pharm	49884-0240-01
100's	$23.85	Temazepam, Voluntary Hosp	53258-0615-01
100's	$24.20	Temazepam, Martec Pharms	52555-0242-01
100's	$24.91	Temazepam, HL Moore Drug Exch	00839-7899-06
100's	$25.04	Temazepam 15 Mg Capsules, Aligen Independ	00405-0185-01
100's	$26.90	Temazepam, Goldline Labs	00182-1822-89
100's	$27.31	Temazepam, Vangard Labs	00615-0470-13
100's	$27.31	Temazepam, Vangard Labs	00615-0470-47
100's	$27.96	Temazepam, Schein Pharm (US)	00364-0815-01
100's	$29.40	RAZAPAM, Major Pharms	00904-2810-61
100's	$31.08	Temazepam, Voluntary Hosp	53258-0615-13
100's	$31.95	Temazepam, Mylan	00378-4010-01
100's	**$67.68**	**RESTORIL, Novartis**	**00078-0098-05**
100's	**$69.36**	**RESTORIL, Novartis**	**00078-0098-06**
100's	$105.24	Temazepam 15 Mg Capsules, Aligen Independ	00405-0185-02
500's	$15.75	Temazepam, H.C.F.A. F F P	99999-2310-03
500's	$60.55	Temazepam, Elkins Sinn	00641-4511-88
500's	$73.40	Temazepam, Qualitest Pharms	00603-5895-28
500's	$73.70	Temazepam, Major Pharms	00904-2810-40
500's	$99.98	Temazepam, Purepac Pharm	00228-2076-50
500's	$106.47	Temazepam, Parmed Pharms	00349-8927-05
500's	$109.95	Temazepam, Rugby	00536-4628-05
500's	$110.00	Temazepam, Amer Preferred	53445-1822-05
500's	$114.20	Temazepam, HL Moore Drug Exch	00839-7164-12
500's	$115.00	Temazepam, Goldline Labs	00182-1822-05
500's	$115.00	Temazepam, Par Pharm	49884-0240-05
500's	$120.76	Temazepam, HL Moore Drug Exch	00839-7899-12
500's	$120.99	Temazepam, Schein Pharm (US)	00364-0815-05
500's	$123.95	Temazepam, Mylan	00378-4010-05
500's	**$316.98**	**RESTORIL, Novartis**	**00078-0098-08**

Capsule, Gelatin - Oral - 30 mg

30's	$1.21	Temazepam, H.C.F.A. F F P	99999-2310-04
100's	$3.86	Temazepam, United Res	00677-1070-01
100's	$4.05	Temazepam, H.C.F.A. F F P	99999-2310-05
100's	$20.86	Temazepam, Bristol Myers Squibb	00003-0747-50
100's	$21.10	Temazepam, Qualitest Pharms	00603-5896-21
100's	$21.25	Temazepam, Major Pharms	00904-2811-60
100's	$23.74	Temazepam, Goldline Labs	00182-1823-01
100's	$23.74	Temazepam, Purepac Pharm	00228-2077-10
100's	$25.60	Temazepam, Parmed Pharms	00349-8488-01
100's	$25.80	Temazepam, Aligen Independ	00405-0186-01
100's	$25.86	Temazepam, Voluntary Hosp	53258-0616-01
100's	$26.75	Temazepam, Rugby	00536-4629-01
100's	$27.50	Temazepam, Par Pharm	49884-0241-01
100's	$28.05	Temazepam, Martec Pharms	52555-0243-01
100's	$28.88	Temazepam, HL Moore Drug Exch	00839-7900-06
100's	$30.37	Temazepam, Schein Pharm (US)	00364-0816-01
100's	$30.50	Temazepam, Goldline Labs	00182-1823-89
100's	$30.89	Temazepam, Vangard Labs	00615-0471-13
100's	$30.89	Temazepam, Vangard Labs	00615-0471-47
100's	$32.76	RAZAPAM, Major Pharms	00904-2811-61
100's	$34.29	Temazepam, Voluntary Hosp	53258-0616-13
100's	$38.95	Temazepam, Mylan	00378-5050-01
100's	**$75.66**	**RESTORIL, Novartis**	**00078-0099-05**
100's	**$77.28**	**RESTORIL, Novartis**	**00078-0099-06**
500's	$20.25	Temazepam, H.C.F.A. F F P	99999-2310-06
500's	$84.25	Temazepam, Qualitest Pharms	00603-5896-28
500's	$84.35	Temazepam, Major Pharms	00904-2811-40
500's	$85.40	Temazepam, Elkins Sinn	00641-4512-88
500's	$115.27	Temazepam, Purepac Pharm	00228-2077-50
500's	$121.33	Temazepam, Aligen Independ	00405-0186-02
500's	$124.50	Temazepam, Parmed Pharms	00349-8488-05
500's	$125.50	Temazepam, Amer Preferred	53445-1823-05
500's	$128.25	Temazepam, Rugby	00536-4629-05
500's	$128.50	Temazepam, Goldline Labs	00182-1823-05
500's	$128.50	Temazepam, Par Pharm	49884-0241-05
500's	$129.05	Temazepam, HL Moore Drug Exch	00839-7165-12
500's	$136.54	Temazepam, Schein Pharm (US)	00364-0816-05
500's	$149.11	Temazepam, HL Moore Drug Exch	00839-7900-12
500's	$151.95	Temazepam, Mylan	00378-5050-05
500's	**$367.02**	**RESTORIL, Novartis**	**00078-0099-08**

HOW SUPPLIED - NOT RATED EQUIVALENT:

Capsule, Gelatin - Oral - 7.5 mg

100's	**$60.48**	**RESTORIL, Novartis**	**00078-0140-05**
100's	**$62.22**	**RESTORIL, Novartis**	**00078-0140-06**
750's	$359.92	Temazepam, Glasgow Pharm	60809-0514-55
750's	$359.92	Temazepam, Glasgow Pharm	60809-0514-72

Capsule, Gelatin - Oral - 15 mg

100's	$24.95	Temazepam, Geneva Pharms	50752-0272-05
100's	$29.75	Temazepam, Geneva Pharms	50752-0272-06
500's	$114.95	Temazepam, Geneva Pharms	50752-0272-08
750's	$401.25	Temazepam, Glasgow Pharm	60809-0508-55
750's	$401.25	Temazepam, Glasgow Pharm	60809-0508-72
775's	$414.63	Temazepam, Glasgow Pharm	60809-0508-66
775's	$414.63	Temazepam, Glasgow Pharm	60809-0508-88

Capsule, Gelatin - Oral - 30 mg

100's	$27.50	Temazepam, Geneva Pharms	50752-0273-05
100's	$35.95	Temazepam, Geneva Pharms	50752-0273-06
500's	$128.25	Temazepam, Geneva Pharms	50752-0273-08
750's	$447.15	Temazepam, Glasgow Pharm	60809-0509-55
750's	$447.15	Temazepam, Glasgow Pharm	60809-0509-72

TENIPOSIDE *(003127)*

CATEGORIES: Acute Lymphoblastic Leukemia; Antineoplastics; Bone Marrow Transplantation; Cancer; Leukemia; Oncologic Drugs; Orphan Drugs; FDA Class 1P ("Priority Review"); FDA Approved 1992 Jul

BRAND NAMES: **Vumon**

WARNING:
Teniposide is a cytotoxic drug, which should be administered under the supervision of a qualified physician experienced in the use of cancer chemotherapeutic agents. Appropriate management of therapy and complications is possible only when adequate treatment facilities are readily available.
Severe myelosupression with resulting infection or bleeding may occur. Hypersensitivity reactions, including anaphylaxis-like symptoms, may occur with initial dosing or at repeated exposure to teniposide. Epinephrine, with or without corticosteroids and antihistamines has been employed to alleviate hypersensitivity reaction symptoms.

DESCRIPTION:

Vumon (also commonly known as VM-26), is supplied as a sterile nonpyrogenic solution in a nonaqueous medium intended for dilution with a suitable parenteral vehicle prior to intravenous infusion. Vumon is available in 50 mg (5 ml) ampules. Each ml contains 10 mg teniposide, 30 mg benzyl alcohol, 60 mg N,N-dimethylacetamide, 500 mg Cremophor EL (polyoxyethylated castor oil) and 42.7 percent (V/V) dehydrated alcohol. The pH of the clear solution is adjusted to approximately 5 with maleic acid.

Teniposide is a semisynthetic derivative of podophyllotoxin. The chemical name for teniposide is 4-demethylepipodophyllotoxin 9-(4,6-0-(R)-2- thenylidene-β-D-glucopyranoside). Teniposide differs from etoposide, another podophyllotoxin derivative, by the substitution of a thenylidene group on the glucopyranoside ring.

Teniposide is a white to off-white crystalline powder with the empirical formula $C_{32}H_{32}O_{13}S$ and a molecular weight of 656.66. It is a lipophilic compound with a partition coefficient value (octanol/water) of approximately 100. Teniposide is insoluble in water and ether. It is slightly soluble in methanol and very soluble in acetone and dimethylformamide.

CLINICAL PHARMACOLOGY:

Teniposide is a phase-specific cytotoxic drug acting in the late S or early G_2 phase of the cell cycle, thus preventing cells from entering mitosis. Teniposide causes dose-dependent single- and double-stranded breaks in DNA and DNA:protein cross-links. The mechanism of action appears to be related to the inhibition of type II topoisomerase activity since teniposide does not intercalate into DNA or bind strongly to DNA. The cytotoxic effects of teniposide are related to the relative number of double-stranded DNA breaks produced in cells, which are a reflection of the stabilization of a topoisomerase II-DNA intermediate.

Teniposide has a broad spectrum of *in vivo* antitumor activity against murine tumors, including hematologic malignancies and various solid tumors. Notably, teniposide is active against sublines of certain murine leukemias with acquired resistance to cisplatin, doxorubicin, amsacrine, daunorubicin, mitoxantrone or vincristine.

Plasma drug levels declined biexponentially following intravenous infusion (155 mg/m² over 1 to 2.5 hours) of teniposide given to eight children (4 - 11 years old) with newly diagnosed acute lymphoblastic leukemia (ALL). The observed average pharmacokinetic parameters and associated coefficients of variation (CV%) based on a two-compartmental model analysis of the data are as follows (TABLE 1):

TABLE 1

Parameter	Mean	CV%
Total body clearance (ml/min/m²)	10.3	25
Volume at steady-state (l/m²)	3.1	30
Terminal half-life (hours)	5.0	44
Volume of central compartment (l/m²)	1.5	36
Rate constant, central to peripheral (1/hours)	0.47	62
Rate constant, peripheral to central (1/hours)	0.42	37

There appears to be some association between an increase in serum alkaline phosphatase or gamma glutamyl-transpeptidase and a decrease in plasma clearance of teniposide. Therefore, caution should be exercised if teniposide is to be administered to patients with hepatic dysfunction.

In adults, at doses of 100 to 333 mg/m²/day, plasma levels increased linearly with dose. Drug accumulation in adult patients did not occur after daily administration of teniposide for 3 days. In pediatric patients, maximum plasma concentrations (Cmax) after infusions of 137 to 203 mg/m² over a period of one to two hours exceeded 40 mcg/ml; by 20 to 24 hours after infusion plasma levels were generally < 2 mcg/ml.

Renal clearance of parent teniposide accounts for about 10 percent of total body clearance. In adults, after intravenous administration of 10 mg/kg or 67 mg/m² of tritium-labeled teniposide, 44 percent of the radiolabel was recovered in urine (parent drug and metabolites) within 120 hours after dosing. From 4 to 12 percent of a dose is excreted in urine as parent drug. Fecal excretion of radioactivity within 72 hours after dosing accounted for 0 to 10 percent of the dose.

Mean steady-state volumes of distribution range from 8 to 44 l/m² for adults and 3 to 11 l/m² for children. The blood-brain barrier appears to limit diffusion of teniposide into the brain, although in a study in patients with brain tumors, CSF levels of teniposide were higher than CSF levels reported in other studies of patients who did not have brain tumors.

Teniposide is highly protein bound. *In vitro* plasma protein binding of teniposide is > 99 percent. The high affinity of teniposide for plasma proteins may be an important factor in limiting distribution of drug within the body. Steady state volume of distribution of the drug increases with a decrease in plasma albumin levels. Therefore, careful monitoring of children with hypoalbuminemia is indicated during therapy. Levels of teniposide in saliva, CSF and malignant ascites fluid are low relative to simultaneously measured plasma levels.

The pharmacokinetic characteristics of teniposide differ from those of etoposide, another podophyllotoxin. Teniposide is more extensively bound to plasma proteins, and its cellular uptake is greater. Teniposide also has a lower systemic clearance, a longer elimination half-life, and is excreted in the urine as parent drug to a lesser extent than etoposide.

In a study at St. Jude Children's Research Hospital (SJCRH), 9 children with acute lymphocytic leukemia (ALL) failing induction therapy with a cytarabine-containing regimen, were treated with teniposide for injection concentrate plus cytarabine. Three of these patients were induced into complete remission with durations of remissions of 30 weeks, 59 weeks, and 13 years. In another study at SJCRH, 16 children with ALL refractory to vincristine/prednisone-containing regimens were treated with teniposide plus vincristine and prednisone.

CLINICAL PHARMACOLOGY: *(cont'd)*

Three of these patients were induced into complete remission with durations of remission of 5.5, 37, and 73 weeks. In these two studies patients served as their own control based on the premise that long term complete remissions could not be achieved by retreatment with drugs to which they had previously failed to respond.

INDICATIONS AND USAGE:

Teniposide, in combination with other approved anticancer agents, is indicated for induction therapy in patients with refractory childhood acute lymphoblastic leukemia.

CONTRAINDICATIONS:

Teniposide is generally contraindicated in patients who have demonstrated a previous hypersensitivity to teniposide and/or Cremophor EL (polyoxyethylated castor oil).

WARNINGS:

Teniposide is a potent drug and should be used only by physicians experienced in the administration of cancer chemotherapeutic drugs. Blood counts as well as renal and hepatic function tests should be carefully monitored prior to and during therapy.

Patients being treated with teniposide should be observed frequently for myelosupression both during and after therapy. Dose-limiting bone marrow suppression is the most significant toxicity associated with teniposide therapy. Therefore, the following studies should be obtained at the start of therapy and prior to each subsequent dose of teniposide: hemoglobin, white blood cell count and differential and platelet count. If necessary, repeat bone marrow examination should be performed prior to the decision to continue therapy in the setting of severe myelosupression.

Physicians should be aware of the possible occurrence of a hypersensitivity reaction variably manifested by chills, fever, urticaria, tachycardia, bronchospasm, dyspnea, hypertension or hypotension and facial flushing. This reaction may occur with the first dose of teniposide and may be life threatening if not treated promptly with antihistamines, corticosteroids, epinephrine, intravenous fluids and other supportive measures as clinically indicated. The exact cause of these reactions is unknown. They may be due to the Cremophor EL (polyoxyethylated castor oil) component of the vehicle or to teniposide itself.[1] Patients who have experienced prior hypersensitivity reactions to teniposide are at risk for recurrence of symptoms and should only be retreated with teniposide if the antileukemic benefit already demonstrated clearly outweighs the risk of a probable hypersensitivity reaction for that patient. When a decision is made to retreat a patient with teniposide in spite of an earlier hypersensitivity reaction, the patient should be pretreated with corticosteroids and antihistamines and receive careful clinical observation during and after teniposide infusion. In the clinical experience with teniposide at SJCRH and the National Cancer Institute (NCI), retreatment of patients with prior hypersensitivity reactions has been accomplished using measures described above. To date, there is no evidence to suggest cross-sensitization between teniposide and VePesid.

One episode of sudden death, attributable to probable arrhythmia and intractable hypotension has been reported in an elderly patient receiving teniposide combination therapy for a non leukemic malignancy. (See ADVERSE REACTIONS.)**Patients receiving teniposide treatment should be under continuous observation for at least the first 60 minutes following the start of the infusion and at frequent intervals thereafter. If symptoms or signs of anaphylaxis occur, the infusion should be stopped immediately, followed by the administration of epinephrine, corticosteroids, antihistamines, pressor agents, or volume expanders at the discretion of the physician. An aqueous solution of epinephrine 1:1000 and a source of oxygen should be available at the bedside.**

For parenteral administration, teniposide should be given only by slow intravenous infusion (lasting at least 30- to 60-minutes) since hypotension has been reported as a possible side-effect of rapid intravenous injection, perhaps due to a direct effect of Cremophor EL.[2,3]If clinically significant hypotension develops, the teniposide infusion should be discontinued. The blood pressure usually normalizes within hours in response to cessation of the infusion and administration of fluids or other supportive therapy as appropriate. If the infusion is restarted, a slower administration rate should be used and the patient should be carefully monitored.

Acute central nervous system depression and hypotension have been observed in patients receiving investigational infusions of high-dose teniposide who were pretreated with anti-emetic drugs. The depressant effects of the antiemetic agents and the alcohol content of the teniposide formulation may place patients receiving higher than recommended doses of teniposide at risk for central nervous system depression.

Pregnancy Category D: Teniposide may cause fetal harm when administered to a pregnant woman. Teniposide has been shown to be teratogenic and embryotoxic in laboratory animals. In pregnant rats intravenous administration of teniposide, 0.1 -3 mg/kg (0.6 - 18 mg/m²), every second day from day 6 to day 16 post coitum caused dose-related embryotoxicity and teratogenicity. Major anomalies included spinal and rib defects, deformed extremities, anophthalmia and celosomia.

There are no adequate and well-controlled studies in pregnant women. If teniposide for injection concentrate is used during pregnancy, or if the patient become pregnant while receiving this drug, the patient should be apprised of the potential hazard to the fetus. Women of childbearing potential should be advised to avoid becoming pregnant therapy with teniposide.

PRECAUTIONS:

General: In all instances where the use of teniposide is considered for chemotherapy the physician must evaluate the need and usefulness of the drug against the risk of adverse reactions. Most such adverse reactions are reversible if detected early. If severe reactions occur, the drug should be reduced in dosage or discontinued and appropriate corrective measures should be taken according to the clinical judgement of the physician. Reinstitution of teniposide therapy should be carried out with caution, and with adequate consideration of the further need for the drug and alertness as to possible recurrence of toxicity.

Teniposide must be administered as an intravenous infusion, Care should be taken to ensure that the intravenous catheter or needle is in the proper position and functional prior to infusion. Improper administration of teniposide may result in extravasation causing local tissue necrosis and/or thrombophlebitis. In some instances, occlusion of central venous access devices has occurred during 24-hour infusion of teniposide and a concentration of 0.1 to 0.2 mg/ml. Frequent observation during these infusions is necessary to minimize this risk.[4,5]

Laboratory Tests: Periodic complete blood counts and assessments of renal and hepatic function should be done during the course of teniposide treatment. They should be performed prior to therapy and at clinically appropriate intervals during and after therapy. There should be at least one determination of hematologic status prior to therapy with teniposide.

Carcinogenesis, Mutagenesis, and Impairment of Fertility: Children at SJCRH with ALL in remission who received maintenance therapy with teniposide at weekly or twice weekly doses (plus other chemotherapeutic agents), had a relative risk of developing secondary acute non-lymphocytic leukemia (ANLL) approximately 12 times that of patients treated according to other less intensive schedules.[6] A short course of teniposide or remission-induction and/or consolidation therapy was not associated with an increased risk of secondary ANLL, but the

PRECAUTIONS: *(cont'd)*

number of patients assessed was small. The potential benefit from teniposide must be weighed on a case by case basis against the potential risk of the induction of a secondary leukemia. The carcinogenicity of teniposide has not been studies in laboratory animals. Compounds with similar mechanisms of action and mutagenicity profiles have been reported to be carcinogenic and teniposide should be considered a potential carcinogen in humans. Teniposide has been shown to be mutagenic in various bacterial and mammalian genetic toxicity tests. These include positive mutagenic effects in the Ames/Salmonella and *B. subtilis* bacterial mutagenicity assays. Teniposide caused gene mutations in both Chinese hamster ovary cells and mouse lymphoma cells and DNA damage as measured by alkaline elution in human lung carcinoma derived cell lines. In addition, teniposide induced aberrations in chromosome structure in primary cultures of human lymphocytes *in vitro* and in L5178y/TK +/- mouse lymphoma cells *in vitro*. Chromosome aberrations were observed *in vivo*in the embryonic tissue of pregnant Swiss albino mice treated with teniposide. Teniposide also caused a dose-related increase in sister-chromatid exchanges in Chinese hamster ovary cells and it has been shown to be embryotoxic and teratogenic in rats receiving teniposide during organogenesis. Treatment of pregnant rats I.V. with doses between 1.0 and 3.0 mg/kg/day on alternate days from day 6 to 16 post coitum caused retardation of embryonic development, prenatal mortality and fetal abnormalities.

Pregnancy Category D: (See WARNINGS.).

Nursing Mothers: It is not known whether this drug is excreted in human milk. Because many drugs are excreted in human milk and because of the potential for serious adverse reactions in nursing infants, a decision should be made whether to discontinue nursing or to discontinue the drug, taking into account the importance of teniposide therapy to the mother.

Patients with Down's Syndrome: Patients with both Down's Syndrome and leukemia may be especially sensitive to myelosuppressive chemotherapy, therefore, initial dosing with teniposide should be reduced in these patients. It is suggested that the first course of teniposide should be given at half the usual dose. Subsequent courses may be administered at higher dosages depending on the degree of myelosupression and mucositis encountered in earlier courses in an individual patient.

DRUG INTERACTIONS:

In a study in which 34 different drugs were tested, therapeutically relevant concentrations of tolbutamide, sodium salicylate and sulfamethizole displaced protein-bound teniposide in fresh human serum to a small but significant extent. Because of the extremely high binding of teniposide to plasma proteins, these small decreases in binding could cause substantial increases in free drug levels in plasma which could result in potentiation of drug toxicity. Therefore, caution should be used in administering teniposide to patients receiving these other agents. There was no change in the plasma kinetic of teniposide when coadministered with methotrexate. However, the plasma clearance of methotrexate was slightly increased. An increase in intracellular levels of methotrexate was observed *in vitro* in the presence of teniposide.

ADVERSE REACTIONS:

TABLE 2 presents the incidences of adverse reactions derived from an analysis of data contained within literature reports of 7 studies involving 303 pediatric patients in which teniposide was administered by injection as a single agent in a variety of doses and schedules for a variety of hematologic malignancies and solid tumors. The total number patients evaluable for a given event was not 303 since the individual studies did not address the occurrence of each event listed. Five of these seven studies assessed teniposide activity in hematologic malignancies, such as leukemia. Thus, many of these patients had abnormal hematologic status at start of therapy with teniposide and were expected to develop significant myelosupression as an endpoint of treatment.

Hematologic Toxicity: Teniposide, when used with other chemotherapeutic agents for the treatment of ALL, results in severe myelosuppression. Early onset of profound myelosuppression with delayed recovery can be expected when using the doses and schedules of teniposide necessary for treatment of refractory ALL, since bone marrow hypoplasia is a desired endpoint of therapy. The occurrence of acute non-lymphocytic leukemia (ANLL), with or without a preleukemic phase has been reported in patients treated with teniposide in combination with other antineoplastic agents. See PRECAUTIONS, Carcinogenesis, Mutagenesis, and Impairment of Fertility.

TABLE 2 Single-Agent Teniposide: Summary of Toxicity For All Evaluable Pediatric Patients

Toxicity	Incidence in Evaluable Patients (%)
Hematologic Toxicity	
Myelosupression, non-specified	75
Leukopenia (<3000 WCB/μl)	89
Neutropenia (<2000 ANC/μl)	95
Thombocytopenia (<100,000 plt/μl)	85
Anemia	88
Non-Hematologic Toxicity	
Mucositis	76
Diarrhea	33
Nausea/Vomiting	29
Infection	12
Alopecia	9
Bleeding	5
Hypersensitivity reactions	5
Rash	3
Fever	3
Hypotension/Cardiovascular	3
Neurotoxicity	<1
Hepatic dysfunction	<1
Renal Dysfunction	<1
Metabolic abnormalities	<1

Gastrointestinal Toxicity: Nausea and vomiting are the most common gastrointestinal toxicities, having occurred in 29 percent of evaluable pediatric patients. The severity of this nausea and vomiting is generally mild to moderate.

Hypotension: Transient hypotension following rapid intravenous administration has been reported in 2 percent of evaluable pediatric patients. One episode of sudden death, attributed too probable arrhythmia and intractable hypotension, has been reported in an elderly patient receiving teniposide for injection concentrate combination therapy for a non-leukemic malignancy.

No other cardiac toxicity or electrocardiographic changes have been documented. No delayed hypotension has been noted.

ADVERSE REACTIONS: *(cont'd)*

Allergic Reactions: Hypersensitivity reactions characterized by chills, fever, tachycardia, flushing, bronchospasm, dyspnea, and blood pressure changes (hypertension or hypotension) have been reported to occur in approximately 5 percent of evaluable pediatric patients receiving intravenous teniposide. The incidence of hypersensitivity reactions to teniposide appears to be increased in patients with brain tumors, and in patients with neuroblastoma.[1]

Central Nervous System: Acute central nervous system depression and hypotension have been observed in patients receiving investigational infusions of high-dose teniposide who were pretreated with antiemetic drugs. The depressant effects of the antiemetic agents and the alcohol content of the teniposide formulation may place patients receiving higher than recommended doses of teniposide at risk for central nervous system depression.

Alopecia: Alopecia, sometimes progressing to total baldness, was observed in 9 percent of evaluable pediatric patients who received teniposide as single agent therapy. It was usually reversible.

OVERDOSAGE:

There is no known antidote for teniposide overdosage. The anticipated complications of overdosage are secondary to bone marrow suppression. treatment should consist of supportive care including blood products and antibiotic as indicated.

DOSAGE AND ADMINISTRATION:

NOTE: Contact of undiluted teniposide for injection concentrate with plastic equipment or devices used to prepare solutions for infusion may result in softening or cracking and possible drug product leakage. this effect has *not* been reported with *diluted solutions* of teniposide.

In order to prevent extraction of the plasticizer DEHP (di(2- ethylhexyl)phtalate), solutions of teniposide for injection concentrate should be prepared in non-DEHP containing LVP container such as glass or Pololefin plastic bags or containers.

Teniposide solutions should be administered with non-DEHP containing IV administration sets.

In one study, childhood ALL patients failing induction therapy with a cytarabine-containing regimen were treated with the combination of teniposide 165 mg/m^2 and cytarabine 300 mg/m^2 intravenously, twice weekly for 8-9 doses. In another study, patients with childhood ALL refractory to vincristine/prednisone-containing regimens were treated with the combination of teniposide 250 mg/m^2 and vincristine 1.5 mg/m^2 intravenously, weekly for 4-8 weeks and prednisone 40 mg/m^2 orally x 28 days.

Adequate data in patients with hepatic insufficiency and/or renal insufficiency are lacking, but dose adjustments may be necessary for patients with significant renal or hepatic impairment.

PREPARATION AND ADMINISTRATION PRECAUTIONS

Teniposide is a cytotoxic anticancer drug and as with other potentially toxic compound, caution should be exercised in handling and preparing the solutions of teniposide. Skin reactions associated with accidental exposure to teniposide may occur. The use of gloves is recommended. If teniposide solution contacts the skin, immediately wash the skin thoroughly with soap and water. If teniposide contacts mucous membranes the membranes should be flushed thoroughly with water.

PREPARATION FOR INTRAVENOUS ADMINISTRATION

Teniposide must be diluted with either 5 percent Dextrose Injection, USP or 0.9 percent Sodium Chloride Injection, USP, to give final teniposide concentrations of 0.1 mg/ml, 0.2 mg/ml, 0.4 mg/ml or 1.0 mg/ml. Solutions prepared in 5 percent Dextrose Injection, USP or 0.9 percent Sodium Chloride Injection, USP at teniposide concentrations of 0.1 mg/ml, 0.2 mg/ml or 0.4 mg/ml are stable at room temperature for up to 24 hours after preparation. Teniposide solutions prepared at a final teniposide concentration of 1.0 mg/ml should be administered within 4 hours of preparation to reduce the potential for precipitation.

Refrigeration of teniposide solutions is not recommended.

Stability and use times are identical in glass and plastic parenteral solution containers.

Although solutions are chemically stable under the conditions indicated, precipitation of teniposide may occur at the recommended concentrations, especially if the diluted solution is subjected to more agitation than is recommended to prepare the drug solution for parenteral administration.[7] In addition, storage time prior to administration should be minimized and care should be taken to avoid contact of the diluted solution with other drugs or fluids. Parenteral drug products should be inspected visually for particulate matter and discoloration prior to administration whenever solution and container permit. **Precipitation has been reported during 24-hour infusions of teniposide for injection concentrate diluted to teniposide concentrations of 0.1 to 0.2 mg/ml, resulting in occlusion of central venous access catheters in several patients.[4,5]Heparin solutions can cause precipitation of teniposide, therefore, the administration apparatus should be flushed thoroughly with 5 percent Dextrose Injection or 0.9 percent Sodium Chloride Injection, USP before and after administration of teniposide.[5]**

Hypotension has been reported following rapid bolus intravenous administration; it is recommended that the teniposide solution be administered over at least as 30 to 60-minute period. **Teniposide should not be given by rapid intravenous injection.**

In a 24-hour study under simulated conditions of actual use of the product relative to dilution strength, diluent and administration rates, dilution at 0.1 to 1.0 mg/ml were chemically stable for at least 24 hours. Data collected for the presence of the extractable DEHP (di(23- ethylhexyl)phtalate) from PVC containers show that levels increased with time and concentration of the solutions. The data appeared similar for 0.9 percent Sodium Chloride Injectio, USP, and 5 percent Dextrose Injection, USP. Consequently, the use of PVC containers is not recommended.

Similarly, the use of non-DEHP IV administration sets is recommended. Lipid administration sets or low DEHP containing nitroglycerin sets will keep patients' exposure to DEHP at low levels and are suitable for use. the diluted solutions are chemically and physically compatible with the recommended IV administration sets and LVP containers of up to 24 hours at ambient room temperature and lighting conditions. **Because of the potential for precipitation, compatibility with other drugs, infusion materials or I.V. pumps cannot be assured.**

Stability: Unopened ampules of teniposide are stable until the date indicated in the package when stored under refrigeration (2-8°C) in the original package. Freezing does not adversely affect the product.

HANDLING AND DISPOSAL

Procedures for proper handling and disposal of anticancer drugs should be considered. Several guidelines on this subject have been published.[8-14] There is no general agreement that all of the procedures recommended in the guidelines are necessary or appropriate.

REFERENCES:

1. O'Dwyer PJ, King SA., Fortner CL and Leyland-Jones B: Hypersensitivity reactions to teniposide (VM-26): an analysis. *J Clin Oncol* 1986; 4(8): 1262-1269. **2.** Lorenz W., Reimannn H-J, Schmall A et al: Histamine release in dogs by Cremophor EL and its derivatives. *Agents and Actions* 19977; 7 (1):63-67. **3.** Lassus M, Scott D, and Leyland-Jones B: Allergic reactions associated with cremophor containing antineoplastic. Proc. *Am Soc Clin Oncol* 1985; 4:268 (abstract C-1042). **4.** Strong D, Morris L: Precipitation of teniposide during infusion. *Am J Hosp Pharm*; Mar 1990; Letter, 47:512, 518. **5.** Bogardus J, Kaplan M, Carpenter J: Precipitation of teniposide during infusion. *Am J Hosp Pharm*; Mar 1990: Letter, 47:518-519. **6.** Pui C-H, et al: Acute Myeloid Leukemia in Children Treated with Epipodophyllotoxins for Acute Lymphoblastic Leukemia. *N engl J med* 1991; 325: 1682-1687. **7.** Deardorff D, Schmidt C: Mixing additive in plastic LVPs. *Am J Hosp Pharm*; Dec 1980: Letter, 37:

REFERENCES: *(cont'd)*

1610, 1613. **8.** Recommendations for the safe handling of parenteral antineoplastic drugs. NIH Publication No. 83-26-21. For sale by the Superintendent of Documents, US Government Printing Office, Washington, DC 20402. **9.** AMA Council Report. Guidelines for handling parenteral antineoplastics. *JAMA* 1985; 253 (11):1590-1592. **10.** National Study Commission on Cytotoxic Exposure - Recommendations for handling cytotoxic agents. Available from Louis P. Jeffery, Chairman, National Study Commission on Cytotoxic Exposure. Massachusetts College of Pharmacy and Allied Health Sciences, 179 Longwood Avenue, Boston, MA 02115. **11.** Clinical Oncology Society of Australia: Guidelines and Recommendations for Safe Handling f Antineoplastic Agents, *Med. J. Australia* 1:425 (1983). **12.** Jones RB, et al. Safe Handling of Chemotherapeutic Agents: A report from the Mount Sinai Medical Center. *Ca- A Cancer Journal for Clinicians*, Sept/Oct. 258-263 (1983). **13.** American Society of Hospital Pharmacists Technical Assistance Bulletin on handling Cytotoxic Drugs in hospitals, *Am J. Hosp. Pharm*, **42**: 131 (1985). **14.** OSHA Work-Practice Guidelines for Personnel Dealing with Cytotoxic (antineoplastic) Drugs *Am J Hosp Pharm*, **43**: 1193 (1986).

HOW SUPPLIED - EQUIVALENTS NOT AVAILABLE:

Injection, Solution - Intravenous - 10 mg/ml

5 ml	**$150.17**	**VUMON, Mead Johnson**	**00015-3075-19**
5 ml x 10	**$1501.69**	**VUMON, Mead Johnson**	**00015-3075-97**

TERAZOSIN HYDROCHLORIDE *(002311)*

CATEGORIES: Alpha Adrenergic Receptor Inhibitors; Alpha Blockers; Antihypertensives; Benign Prostatic Hyperplasia; Cardiovascular Drugs; Hypertension; Prostate Enlargement; Pregnancy Category C; Sales > $100 Million; FDA Approved 1987 Aug; Patent Expiration 1995 Oct; Top 200 Drugs

BRAND NAMES: *Heitrin* (Germany); *Hitrin*; **Hytrin**; *Hytrine*; *Hytrinex*; *Itrin*; *Vicard*
(International brand names outside U.S. in italics)

FORMULARIES: Aetna; BC-BS; Medi-Cal; PCS

COST OF THERAPY: $463.51 (Hypertension; Capsule; 1 mg; 1/day; 365 days)

PRIMARY ICD9: 401.1 (Essential Hypertension, Benign)

DESCRIPTION:

Terazosin hydrochloride, an alpha-1-selective adrenoceptor blocking agent, is a quinazoline derivative represented by the following chemical name and structural formula: (RS)-Piperazine, 1-(4-amino-6,7-dimethoxy-2-quinazolinyl) -4-[(tetra-hydro - 2-furanyl) carbonyl]-, monohydrochloride, dihydrate.

Terazosin hydrochloride is a white, crystalline substance, freely soluble in water and isotonic saline and has a molecular weight of 459.93. Hytrin capsules (terazosin hydrochloride capsules) for oral ingestion are supplied in four dosage strengths containing terazosin hydrochloride equivalent to 1 mg, 2 mg, 5 mg, or 10 mg of terazosin.

Hytrin Inactive Ingredients: *1 mg capsules:* gelatin, glycerin, iron oxide, methylparaben, mineral oil, polyethylene glycol, povidone, propylparaben, titanium dioxide, and vanillin. *2 mg capsules:* D&C yellow No. 10, gelatin, glycerin, methylparaben, mineral oil, polyethylene glycol, povidone, propylparaben, titanium dioxide, and vanillin. *5 mg capsules:* D&C red No. 28, FD&C red No. 40, gelatin, glycerin, methylparaben, mineral oil, polyethylene glycol, povidone, propylparaben, titanium dioxide, and vanillin. *10 mg capsules:* FD&C blue No. 1, gelatin, glycerin, methylparaben, mineral oil, polyethylene glycol, povidone, propylparaben, titanium dioxide, and vanillin.

CLINICAL PHARMACOLOGY:

PHARMACODYNAMICS

Benign Prostatic Hyperplasia (BPH): The symptoms associated with BPH are related to bladder outlet obstruction, which is comprised of two underlying components: a static component and a dynamic component. The static component is a consequence of an increase in prostate size. Over time, the prostate will continue to enlarge. However, clinical studies have demonstrated that the size of the prostate does not correlate with the severity of BPH symptoms or the degree of urinary obstruction. The dynamic component is a function of an increase in smooth muscle tone in the prostate and bladder neck, leading to constriction of the bladder outlet. Smooth muscle tone is mediated by sympathetic nervous stimulation of alpha-1 adrenoceptors, which are abundant in the prostate, prostatic capsule and bladder neck. The reduction in symptoms and improvement in urine flow rates following administration of terazosin is related to relaxation of smooth muscle produced by blockade of alpha-1 adrenoceptors in the bladder neck and prostate. Because there are relatively few alpha-1 adrenoceptors in the bladder body, terazosin is able to reduce the bladder outlet obstruction without affecting bladder contractility.

Terazosin has been studied in 1222 men with symptomatic BPH. In three placebo-controlled studies, symptom evaluation and uroflowmetric measurements were performed approximately 24 hours following dosing. Symptoms were quantified using the Boyarsky Index. The questionnaire evaluated both obstructive (hesitancy, intermittency, terminal dribbling, impairment of size and force of stream, sensation of incomplete bladder emptying) and irritative (nocturia, daytime frequency, urgency, dysuria) symptoms by rating each of the 9 symptoms from 0-3, for a total score of 27 points. Results from these studies indicated that terazosin statistically significantly improved symptoms and peak urine flow rates over placebo as illustrated in TABLE 1.

TABLE 1

	Symptom Score (Range 0-27) N	Mean Baseline	Mean Change (%)	Peak Flow Rate (ml/sec) N	Mean Baseline	Mean Change (%)
Study 1 (10 mg)[a]						
Titration to fixed dose (12 wks)						
Placebo	55	9.7	-2.3 (24)	54	10.1	+1.0 (10)
Terazosin	54	10.1	-4.5 (45)*	52	8.8	+3.0 (34)*
Study 2 (2, 5, 10, 20 mg)[b]						
Titration to response (24 wks)						
Placebo	89	12.5	-3.8 (30)	88	8.8	+1.4 (16)
Terazosin	85	12.2	-5.3 (43)*	84	8.4	+2.9 (35)*
Study 3 (1, 2, 5, 10 mg)[c]						
Titration to response (24 wks)						
Placebo	74	10.4	-1.1 (11)	74	8.8	+1.2 (14)
Terazosin	73	10.9	-4.6 (42)*	73	8.6	+2.6 (30)*

[a] Highest dose 10 mg shown.
[b] 23% of patients on 10 mg, 41% of patients on 20 mg.
[c] 67% of patients on 10 mg.
* Significantly ($p \leq 0.05$) more improvement than placebo.

In all three studies, both symptom scores and peak urine flow rates showed statistically significant improvement from baseline in patients treated with terazosin from week 2 (or the first clinic visit) and throughout the study duration.

CLINICAL PHARMACOLOGY: *(cont'd)*

Analysis of the effect of terazosin on individual urinary symptoms demonstrated that compared to placebo, terazosin significantly improved the symptoms of hesitancy, intermittency, impairment in size and force of urinary stream, sensation of incomplete emptying, terminal dribbling, daytime frequency and nocturia.

Global assessments of overall urinary function and symptoms were also performed by investigators who were blinded to patient treatment assignment. In studies 1 and 3, patients treated with terazosin had a significantly ($p \leq 0.001$) greater overall improvement compared to placebo treated patients.

In a short term study (Study 1), patients were randomized to either 2, 5 or 10 mg of terazosin or placebo. Patients randomized to the 10 mg group achieved a statistically significant response in both symptoms and peak flow rate compared to placebo.

In a long-term, open-label, non-placebo controlled clinical trial, 181 men were followed for 2 years and 58 of these men were followed for 30 months. The effect of terazosin on urinary symptom scores and peak flow rates was maintained throughout the study duration.

In this long-term trial, both symptom scores and peak urinary flow rates showed statistically significant improvement suggesting a relaxation of smooth muscle cells.

Although blockade of alpha-1 adrenoceptors also lowers blood pressure in hypertensive patients with increased peripheral vascular resistance, terazosin treatment of normotensive men with BPH did not result in a clinically significant blood pressure lowering effect (TABLE 2):

TABLE 2 Mean Changes in Blood Pressure from Baseline to Final Visit in all Double-Blind, Placebo-Controlled Studies

	Group	Normotensive Patients DBP ≤ 90 mm Hg N	Mean Change	Hypertensive Patients DBP > 90 mm Hg N	Mean Change
SBP (mm Hg)	Placebo	293	-0.1	45	-5.8
	Terazosin	519	-3.3*	65	-14.4*
DBP (mm Hg)	Placebo	293	+0.4	45	-7.1
	Terazosin	519	-2.2*	65	-15.1*

* $p \leq 0.05$ vs. placebo

Hypertension: In animals, terazosin causes a decrease in blood pressure by decreasing total peripheral vascular resistance. The vasodilatory hypotensive action of terazosin appears to be produced mainly by blockade of alpha-1-adrenoceptors. Terazosin decreases blood pressure gradually within 15 minutes following oral administration.

Patients in clinical trials of terazosin were administered once daily (the great majority) and twice daily regimens with total doses usually in the range of 5-20 mg/day, and had mild (about 77%, diastolic pressure 95-105 mmHg) or moderate (23%, diastolic pressure 105-115 mmHg) hypertension. Because terazosin, like all alpha antagonists, can cause unusually large falls in blood pressure after the first dose or first few doses, the initial dose was 1 mg in virtually all trials, with subsequent titration to a specified fixed dose or titration to some specified blood pressure end point (usually a supine diastolic pressure of 90 mmHg).

Blood pressure responses were measured at the end of the dosing interval (usually 24 hours) and effects were shown to persist throughout the interval, with the usual supine responses 5-10 mmHg systolic and 3.5-8 mmHg diastolic greater than placebo. The responses in the standing position tended to be somewhat larger, by 1-3 mmHg, although this was not true in all studies. The magnitude of the blood pressure responses was similar to prazosin and less than hydrochlorothiazide (in a single study of hypertensive patients). In measurements 24 hours after dosing, heart rate was unchanged.

Limited measurements of peak response (2-3 hours after dosing) during chronic terazosin administration indicate that it is greater than about twice the trough (24 hour) response, suggesting some attenuation of response at 24 hours, presumably due to a fall in blood terazosin concentrations at the end of the dose interval. The explanation is not established with certainty, however, and is not consistent with the similarity of blood pressure response to once daily and twice daily dosing and with the absence of an observed dose-response relationship over a range of 5-20 mg, *i.e.*, if blood concentrations had fallen to the point of providing less than full effect at 24 hours, a shorter dosing interval or larger dose should have led to increased response.

Further dose response and dose duration studies are being carried out. Blood pressure should be measured at the end of the dose interval; if response is not satisfactory, patients may be tried on a larger dose or twice daily dosing regimen. The latter should also be considered if possibly blood pressure-related side effects, such as dizziness, palpitations, or orthostatic complaints, are seen within a few hours after dosing.

The greater blood pressure effect associated with peak plasma concentrations (first few hours after dosing) appears somewhat more position-dependent (greater in the erect position) than the effect of terazosin at 24 hours and in the erect position there is also a 6-10 beat per minute increase in heart rate in the first few hours after dosing. During the first 3 hours after dosing 12.5% of patients had a systolic pressure fall of 30 mmHg or more from supine to standing, or standing systolic pressure below 90 mmHg with a fall of at least 20 mmHg, compared to 4% of a placebo group.

There was a tendency for patients to gain weight during terazosin therapy. In placebo-controlled monotherapy trials, male and female patients receiving terazosin gained a mean of 1.7 and 2.2 pounds respectively, compared to losses of 0.2 and 1.2 pounds respectively in the placebo group. Both differences were statistically significant.

During controlled clinical trials, patients receiving terazosin monotherapy had a small but statistically significant decrease (a 3% fall) compared to placebo in total cholesterol and the combined low-density and very-low-density lipoprotein fractions. No significant changes were observed in high-density lipoprotein fraction and triglycerides compared to placebo.

Analysis of clinical laboratory data following administration of terazosin suggested the possibility of hemodilution based on decreases in hematocrit, hemoglobin, white blood cells, total protein and albumin. Decreases in hematocrit and total protein have been observed with alpha-blockade and are attributed to hemodilution.

PHARMACOKINETICS

Terazosin hydrochloride capsules are essentially completely absorbed in man. Administration of capsules immediately after meals had a minimal effect on the extent of absorption. The time to reach peak plasma concentration however, was delayed by about 40 minutes. Terazosin has been shown to undergo minimal hepatic first-pass metabolism and nearly all of the circulating dose is in the form of parent drug. The plasma levels peak about one hour after dosing, and then decline with a half-life of approximately 12 hours. In a study that evaluated the effect of age on terazosin pharmacokinetics, the mean plasma half-lives were 14.0 and 11.4 hours for the age group ≥ 70 years and the age group of 20-39 years, respectively. After oral administration the plasma clearance was decreased by 31.7% in patients 70 years of age or older compared to that in patients 20-39 years of age.

The drug is 90-94% bound to plasma proteins and binding is constant over the clinically observed concentration range. Approximately 10% of an orally administered dose is excreted as parent drug in the urine and approximately 20% is excreted in the feces. The remainder is

CLINICAL PHARMACOLOGY: *(cont'd)*

eliminated as metabolites. Impaired renal function had no significant effect on the elimination of terazosin, and dosage adjustment of terazosin to compensate for the drug removal during hemodialysis (approximately 10%) does not appear to be necessary. Overall, approximately 40% of the administered dose is excreted in the urine and approximately 60% in the feces. The disposition of the compound in animals is qualitatively similar to that in man.

INDICATIONS AND USAGE:

Terazosin hydrochloride is indicated for the treatment of symptomatic benign prostatic hyperplasia (BPH). There is rapid response, with approximately 70% of patients experiencing an increase in urinary flow and improvement in symptoms of BPH when treated with terazosin hydrochloride. The long-term effects of terazosin hydrochloride on the incidence of surgery, acute urinary obstruction or other complications of BPH are yet to be determined.

Terazosin hydrochloride is also indicated for the treatment of hypertension. It can be used alone or in combination with other antihypertensive agents such as diuretics or beta-adrenergic blocking agents.

CONTRAINDICATIONS:

Terazosin hydrochloride capsules are contraindicated in patients known to be hypersensitive to terazosin hydrochloride.

WARNINGS:

SYNCOPE AND "FIRST-DOSE" EFFECT

Terazosin hydrochloride capsules, like other alpha-adrenergic blocking agents, can cause marked lowering of blood pressure, especially postural hypotension, and syncope in association with the first dose or first few days of therapy. A similar effect can be anticipated if therapy is interrupted for several days and then restarted. Syncope has also been reported with other alpha-adrenergic blocking agents in association with rapid dosage increases or the introduction of another antihypertensive drug. Syncope is believed to be due to an excessive postural hypotensive effect, although occasionally the syncopal episode has been preceded by a bout of severe supraventricular tachycardia with heart rates of 120-160 beats per minute. Additionally, the possibility of the contribution of hemodilution to the symptoms of postural hypotension should be considered.

To decrease the likelihood of syncope or excessive hypotension, treatment should always be initiated with a 1 mg dose of terazosin, given at bedtime. The 2 mg, 5 mg and 10 mg capsules are not indicated as initial therapy. Dosage should then be increased slowly, according to recommendations in the DOSAGE AND ADMINISTRATION and additional antihypertensive agents should be added with caution. The patient should be cautioned to avoid situations, such as driving or hazardous tasks, where injury could result should syncope occur during initiation of therapy.

In early investigational studies, where increasing single doses up to 7.5 mg were given at 3 day intervals, tolerance to the first dose phenomenon did not necessarily develop and the "first dose" effect could be observed at all doses. Syncopal episodes occurred in 3 of the 14 subjects given terazosin at doses of 2.5, 5 and 7.5 mg, which are higher than the recommended initial dose; in addition, severe orthostatic hypotension (blood pressure falling to 50/0 mmHg) was seen in two others and dizziness, tachycardia, and lightheadedness occurred in most subjects. These adverse effects all occurred within 90 minutes of dosing.

In three placebo-controlled BPH studies 1, 2, and 3 (see CLINICAL PHARMACOLOGY), the incidence of postural hypotension in the terazosin treated patients was 5.1%, 5.2%, and 3.7% respectively.

In multiple dose clinical trials involving nearly 2000 hypertensive patients treated with terazosin, syncope was reported in about 1% of patients. Syncope was not necessarily associated only with the first dose.

If syncope occurs, the patient should be placed in a recumbent position and treated supportively as necessary. There is evidence that the orthostatic effect of terazosin is greater, even in chronic use, shortly after dosing. The risk of the events is greatest during the initial seven days of treatment, but continues at all time intervals.

PRECAUTIONS:

GENERAL

Prostatic Cancer: Carcinoma of the prostate and BPH cause many of the same symptoms. These two diseases frequently co- exist. Therefore, patients thought to have BPH should be examined prior to starting terazosin hydrochloride therapy to rule out the presence of carcinoma of the prostate.

Orthostatic Hypotension: While syncope is the most severe orthostatic effect of terazosin (see WARNINGS), other symptoms of lowered blood pressure, such as dizziness, lightheadedness and palpitations, were more common and occurred in some 28% of patients in clinical trials of hypertension. In BPH clinical trials, 21% of the patients experienced one or more of the following: dizziness, hypotension, postural hypotension, syncope, and vertigo. Patients with occupations in which such events represent potential problems should be treated with particular caution.

INFORMATION FOR THE PATIENT

Patients should be made aware of the possibility of syncopal and orthostatic symptoms, especially at the initiation of therapy, and to avoid driving or hazardous tasks for 12 hours after the first dose, after a dosage increase and after interruption of therapy when treatment is resumed. They should be cautioned to avoid situations where injury could result should syncope occur during initiation of terazosin therapy. They should also be advised of the need to sit or lie down when symptoms of lowered blood pressure occur, although these symptoms are not always orthostatic, and to be careful when rising from a sitting or lying position. If dizziness, lightheadedness, or palpitations are bothersome they should be reported to the physician, so that dose adjustment can be considered.

Patients should also be told that drowsiness or somnolence can occur with terazosin, requiring caution in people who must drive or operate heavy machinery.

LABORATORY TESTS:

Small but statistically significant decreases in hematocrit, hemoglobin, white blood cells, total protein and albumin were observed in controlled clinical trials. These laboratory findings suggested the possibility of hemodilution. Treatment with terazosin for up to 24 months had no significant effect on prostate specific antigen (PSA) levels.

CARCINOGENESIS, MUTAGENESIS, AND IMPAIRMENT OF FERTILITY

Terazosin was devoid of mutagenic potential when evaluated *in vivo* and *in vitro* (the Ames test, *in vivo* cytogenetics, the dominant lethal test in mice, *in vivo* Chinese hamster chromosome aberration test and V79 forward mutation assay).

Terazosin, administered in the feed to rats at doses of 8, 40, and 250 mg/kg/day (70, 350, and 2100 mg/m^2/day), for two years, was associated with a statistically significant increase in benign adrenal medullary tumors of male rats exposed to the 250 mg/kg dose. This dose is 175 times the maximum recommended human dose of 20 mg (12 mg/m^2). Female rats were unaffected. Terazosin was not oncogenic in mice when administered in feed for 2 years at a maximum tolerated dose of 32 mg/kg/day (110 mg/m^2; 9 times the maximum recommended human dose). The absence of mutagenicity in a battery of tests, of tumorigenicity of any cell type in the mouse carcinogenicity assay, of increased total tumor incidence in either species, and of proliferative adrenal lesions in female rats, suggests a male rat species-specific event. Numerous other diverse pharmaceutical and chemical compounds have also been associated with benign adrenal medullary tumors in male rats without supporting evidence for carcinogenicity in man.

The effect of terazosin on fertility was assessed in a standard fertility/reproductive performance study in which male and female rats were administered oral doses of 8, 30 and 120 mg/kg/day. Four of 20 male rats given 30 mg/kg (240 mg/m^2; 20 times the maximum recommended human dose) and five of 19 male rats given 120 mg/kg (960 mg/m^2; 80 times the maximum recommended human dose) failed to sire a litter. Testicular weights and morphology were unaffected by treatment. Vaginal smears at 30 and 120 mg/kg/day, however, appeared to contain less sperm than smears from control matings and good correlation was reported between sperm count and subsequent pregnancy.

Oral administration of terazosin for one or two years elicited a statistically significant increase in the incidence of testicular atrophy in rats exposed to 40 and 250 mg/kg/day (29 and 175 times the maximum recommended human dose), but not in rats exposed to 8 mg/kg/day (> 6 times the maximum recommended human dose). Testicular atrophy was also observed in dogs dosed with 300 mg/kg/day (> 500 times the maximum recommended human dose) for three months but not after one year when dosed with 20 mg/kg/day (38 times the maximum recommended human dose). This lesion has also been seen with Minipress, another (marketed) selective-alpha-1 blocking agent.

PREGNANCY CATEGORY C

Teratogenic Effects: Terazosin was not teratogenic in either rats or rabbits when administered at oral doses up to 280 and 60 times, respectively, the maximum recommended human dose. Fetal resorptions occurred in rats dosed with 480 mg/kg/day, approximately 280 times the maximum recommended human dose. Increased fetal resorptions, decreased fetal weight and an increased number of supernumerary ribs were observed in offspring of rabbits dosed with 60 times the maximum recommended human dose. These findings (in both species) were most likely secondary to maternal toxicity. There are no adequate and well-controlled studies in pregnant women and the safety of terazosin in pregnancy has not been established. Terazosin hydrochloride is not recommended during pregnancy unless the potential benefit justifies the potential risk to the mother and fetus.

Nonteratogenic Effects: In a peri- and post-natal development study in rats, significantly more pups died in the group dosed with 120 mg/kg/day (> 75 times the maximum recommended human dose) than in the control group during the three-week postpartum period.

NURSING MOTHERS

It is not known whether terazosin is excreted in breast milk. Because many drugs are excreted in breast milk, caution should be exercised when terazosin is administered to a nursing woman.

PEDIATRIC USE

Safety and effectiveness in children have not been determined.

DRUG INTERACTIONS:

In controlled trials, terazosin has been added to diuretics, and several beta-adrenergic blockers; no unexpected interactions were observed. Terazosin has also been used in patients on a variety of concomitant therapies; while these were not formal interaction studies, no interactions were observed. Terazosin has been used concomitantly in at least 50 patients on the following drugs or drug classes: 1) analgesic/anti-inflammatory (*e.g.*, acetaminophen, aspirin, codeine, ibuprofen, indomethacin); 2) antibiotics (*e.g.*, erythromycin, trimethoprim and sulfamethoxazole); 3) anticholinergic/sympathomimetics (*e.g.*, phenylephrine hydrochloride, phenylpropanolamine hydrochloride, pseudoephedrine hydrochloride); 4) antigout (*e.g.*, allopurinol); 5) antihistamines (*e.g.*, chlorpheniramine); 6) cardiovascular agents (*e.g.*, atenolol, hydrochlorothiazide, methyclothiazide, propranolol); 7) corticosteroids; 8) gastrointestinal agents (*e.g.*, antacids); 9) hypoglycemics; 10) sedatives and tranquilizers (*e.g.*, diazepam).

Use with Other Drugs: In a study (n=24) where terazosin and verapamil were administered concomitantly, terazosin's mean AUC_{0-24} increased 11% after the first verapamil dose and after 3 weeks of verapamil treatment it increased by 24% with associated increases in C_{max} (25%) and C_{min}(32%) means. Terazosin mean T_{max} decreased from 1.3 hours to 0.8 hours after 3 weeks of verapamil treatment. Statistically significant differences were not found in the verapamil level with and without terazosin. In a study (n=6) where terazosin and captopril were administered concomitantly, plasma disposition of captopril was not influenced by concomitant administration of terazosin and terazosin maximum plasma concentrations increased linearly with dose at steady-state after administration of terazosin plus captopril (see DOSAGE AND ADMINISTRATION.)

ADVERSE REACTIONS:

Benign Prostatic Hyperplasia: The incidence of treatment-emergent adverse events has been ascertained from clinical trials conducted worldwide. All adverse events reported during these trials were recorded as adverse reactions. The incidence rates presented below are based on combined data from six placebo-controlled trials involving once-a-day administration of terazosin at doses ranging from 1 to 20 mg. TABLE 3 summarizes those adverse events reported for patients in these trials when the incidence rate in the terazosin group was at least 1% and was greater than that for the placebo group, or where the reaction is of clinical interest. Asthenia, postural hypertension, dizziness, somnolence, nasal congestion/rhinitis, and impotence were the only events that were significantly ($p \leq 0.05$) more common in patients receiving terazosin than in patients receiving placebo. The incidence of urinary tract infection was significantly lower in the patients receiving terazosin than in patients receiving placebo. An analysis of the incidence rate of hypotensive adverse events (see PRECAUTIONS) adjusted for the length of drug treatment has shown that the risk of the events is greatest during the initial seven days of treatment, but continues at all time intervals (TABLE 3).

Additional adverse events have been reported, but these are, in general, not distinguishable from symptoms that might have occurred in the absence of exposure to terazosin. The safety profile of patients treated in the long-term open-label study was similar to that observed in the controlled studies.

The adverse events were usually transient and mild or moderate in intensity, but sometimes were serious enough to interrupt treatment. In the placebo-controlled clinical trials, the rates of premature termination due to adverse events were not statistically different between the placebo and terazosin groups. The adverse events that were bothersome, as judged by their being reported as reasons for discontinuation of therapy by at least 0.5% of the terazosin group and being reported more often than in the placebo group, are shown in (TABLE 4).

Hypertension: The prevalence of adverse reactions has been ascertained from clinical trials conducted primarily in the United States. All adverse experiences (events) reported during these trials were recorded as adverse reactions. The prevalence rates presented below are based on combined data from fourteen placebo-controlled trials involving once-a-day administration of terazosin, as monotherapy or in combination with other antihypertensive agents, at doses ranging from 1 to 40 mg. TABLE 5 summarizes those adverse experiences reported for patients in these trials where the prevalence rate in the terazosin group was at least 5%, where the prevalence rate for the terazosin group was at least 2% and was greater than the prevalence rate for the placebo group, or where the reaction is of particular interest. Asthenia,

ADVERSE REACTIONS: *(cont'd)*

TABLE 3 Adverse Reactions During Placebo-Controlled Trials Benign Prostatic Hyperplasia

Body System	Terazosin (N=636)	Placebo (N=360)
Body As A Whole		
†Asthenia	7.4%*	3.3%
Flu Syndrome	2.4%	1.7%
Headache	4.9%	5.8%
Cardiovascular System		
Hypotension	0.6%	0.6%
Palpitations	0.9%	1.1%
Postural Hypotension	3.9%*	0.8%
Syncope	0.6%	0.0%
Digestive System		
Nausea	1.7%	1.1%
Metabolic And Nutritional Disorders		
Peripheral Edema	0.9%	0.3%
Weight Gain	0.5%	0.0%
Nervous System		
Dizziness	9.1%*	4.2%
Somnolence	3.6%*	1.9%
Vertigo	1.4%	0.3%
Respiratory System		
Dyspnea	1.7%	0.8%
Nasal Congestion/Rhinitis	1.9%*	0.0%
Special Senses		
Blurred Vision/Amblyopia	1.3%	0.6%
Urogenital System		
Impotence	1.6%*	0.6%
Urinary Tract Infection	1.3%	3.9%*

† Includes weakness, tiredness, lassitude and fatigue.
* $p \leq 0.05$ comparison between groups.

TABLE 4 Discontinuation During Placebo-Controlled Trials Benign Prostatic Hyperplasia

Body System	Terazosin (N=636)	Placebo (N=360)
Body As A Whole		
Fever	0.5%	0.0%
Headache	1.1%	0.8%
Cardiovascular System		
Postural Hypotension	0.5%	0.0%
Syncope	0.5%	0.0%
Digestive System		
Nausea	0.5%	0.3%
Nervous System		
Dizziness	2.0%	1.1%
Vertigo	0.5%	0.0%
Respiratory System		
Dyspnea	0.5%	0.3%
Special Senses		
Blurred Vision/Amblyopia	0.6%	0.0%
Urogenital System		
Urinary Tract Infection	0.5%	0.3%

blurred vision, dizziness, nasal congestion, nausea, peripheral edema, palpitations and somnolence were the only symptoms that were significantly ($p < 0.05$) more common in patients receiving terazosin than in patients receiving placebo. Similar adverse reaction rates were observed in placebo-controlled monotherapy trials (TABLE 5).

TABLE 5 Adverse Reactions During Placebo-Controlled Trials Hypertension

Body System	Terazosin (N=859)	Placebo (N=506)
Body As A Whole		
†Asthenia	11.3%*	4.3%
Back Pain	2.4%	1.2%
Headache	16.2%	15.8%
Cardiovascular System		
Palpitations	4.3%*	1.2%
Postural Hypotension	1.3%	0.4%
Tachycardia	1.9%	1.2%
Digestive System		
Nausea	4.4%*	1.4%
Metabolic And Nutritional Disorders		
Edema	0.9%	0.6%
Peripheral Edema	5.5%*	2.4%
Weight Gain	0.5%	0.2%
Musculoskeletal System		
Pain-Extremities	3.5%	3.0%
Nervous System		
Depression	0.3%	0.2%
Dizziness	19.3%*	7.5%
Libido Decreased	0.6%	0.2%
Nervousness	2.3%	1.8%
Paresthesia	2.9%	1.4%
Somnolence	5.4%*	2.6%
Respiratory System		
Dyspnea	3.1%	2.4%
Nasal Congestion	5.9%*	3.4%
Sinusitis	2.6%	1.4%
Special Senses		
Blurred Vision	1.6%*	0.0%
Urogenital System		
Impotence	1.2%	1.4%

† Includes weakness, tiredness, lassitude and fatigue.
* Statistically significant at p=0.05 level.

Additional adverse reactions have been reported, but these are, in general, not distinguishable from symptoms that might have occurred in the absence of exposure to terazosin. The following additional adverse reactions were reported by at least 1% of 1987 patients who received terazosin in controlled or open, short- or long-term clinical trials or have been reported during marketing experience:

Body as a Whole: chest pain, facial edema, fever, abdominal pain, neck pain, shoulder pain;
Cardiovascular System: arrhythmia, vasodilation
Digestive System: constipation, diarrhea, dry mouth, dyspepsia, flatulence, vomiting;
Metabolic/Nutritional Disorders: gout

ADVERSE REACTIONS: *(cont'd)*

Musculoskeletal System: arthralgia, arthritis, joint disorder, myalgia;
Nervous System: anxiety, insomnia;
Respiratory System: bronchitis, cold symptoms, epistaxis, flu symptoms, increased cough, pharyngitis, rhinitis;
Skin and Appendages: pruritus, rash, sweating;
Special Senses: abnormal vision, conjunctivitis, tinnitus;
Urogenital System: urinary frequency, urinary incontinence primarily reported in postmenopausal women, urinary tract infection.

Post-marketing experience indicates that in rare instances patients may develop allergic reactions, including anaphylaxis, following administration of terazosin hydrochloride.

The adverse reactions were usually mild or moderate in intensity but sometimes were serious enough to interrupt treatment. The adverse reactions that were most bothersome, as judged by their being reported as reasons for discontinuation of therapy by at least 0.5% of the terazosin group and being reported more often than in the placebo group, are shown in (TABLE 6).

TABLE 6 Discontinuations During Placebo-Controlled Trials Hypertension

Body System	Terazosin (N=859)	Placebo (N=506)
Body As A Whole		
Asthenia	1.6%	0.0%
Headache	1.3%	1.0%
Cardiovascular System		
Palpitations	1.4%	0.2%
Postural Hypotension	0.5%	0.0%
Syncope	0.5%	0.2%
Tachycardia	0.6%	0.0%
Digestive System		
Nausea	0.8%	0.0%
Metabolic And Nutritional Disorders		
Peripheral Edema	0.6%	0.0%
Nervous System		
Dizziness	3.1%	0.4%
Paresthesia	0.8%	0.2%
Somnolence	0.6%	0.2%
Respiratory System		
Dyspnea	0.9%	0.6%
Nasal Congestion	0.6%	0.0%
Special Senses		
Blurred Vision	0.6%	0.0%

OVERDOSAGE:

Should overdosage of terazosin hydrochloride lead to hypotension, support of the cardiovascular system is of first importance. Restoration of blood pressure and normalization of heart rate may be accomplished by keeping the patient in the supine position. If this measure is inadequate, shock should first be treated with volume expanders. If necessary, vasopressors should then be used and renal function should be monitored and supported as needed. Laboratory data indicate that terazosin is 90-94% protein bound; therefore, dialysis may not be of benefit.

DOSAGE AND ADMINISTRATION:

If terazosin hydrochloride administration is discontinued for several days, therapy should be reinstituted using the initial dosing regimen.

BENIGN PROSTATIC HYPERPLASIA

Initial Dose: 1 mg at bedtime is the starting dose for all patients, and this dose should not be exceeded as an initial dose. Patients should be closely followed during initial administration in order to minimize the risk of severe hypotensive response.

Subsequent Doses: The dose should be increased in a stepwise fashion to 2 mg, 5 mg, or 10 mg once daily to achieve the desired improvement of symptoms and/or flow rates. Doses of 10 mg once daily are generally required for the clinical response. Therefore, treatment with 10 mg for a minimum of 4-6 weeks may be required to assess whether a beneficial response has been achieved. Some patients may not achieve a clinical response despite appropriate titration. Although some additional patients responded at a 20 mg daily dose, there was an insufficient number of patients studied to draw definitive conclusions about this dose. There are insufficient data to support the use of higher doses for those patients who show inadequate or no response to 20 mg daily. **If terazosin administration is discontinued for several days or longer, therapy should be reinstituted using the initial dosing regimen.**

Use With Other Drugs: Caution should be observed when terazosin hydrochloride is administered concomitantly with other antihypertensive agents, especially the calcium channel blocker verapamil, to avoid the possibility of developing significant hypotension. When using terazosin hydrochloride and other antihypertensive agents concomitantly, dosage reduction and retitration of either agent may be necessary (see PRECAUTIONS.)

HYPERTENSION

The dose of terazosin hydrochloride and the dose interval (12 to 24 hours) should be adjusted according to the patient's individual blood pressure response. The following is a guide to its administration:

Initial Dose: 1 mg at bedtime is the starting dose for all patients, and this dose should not be exceeded. This initial dosing regimen should be strictly observed to minimize the potential for severe hypotensive effects.

Subsequent Doses: The dose may be slowly increased to achieve the desired blood pressure response. The usual recommended dose range is 1 mg to 5 mg administered once a day; however, some patients may benefit from doses as high as 20 mg per day. Doses over 20 mg do not appear to provide further blood pressure effect and doses over 40 mg have not been studied. Blood pressure should be monitored at the end of the dosing interval to be sure control is maintained throughout the interval. It may also be helpful to measure blood pressure 2-3 hours after dosing to see if the maximum and minimum responses are similar, and to evaluate symptoms such as dizziness or palpitations which can result from excessive hypotensive response. If response is substantially diminished at 24 hours an increased dose or use of a twice daily regimen can be considered. **If terazosin administration is discontinued for several days or longer, therapy should be reinstituted using the initial dosing regimen.** In clinical trials, except for the initial dose, the dose was given in the morning.

Use With Other Drugs: See DOSAGE AND ADMINISTRATION.

PATIENT INFORMATION:

Terazosin HCl is known as an alpha-blocker. It is used to treat high blood pressure and is also used to treat enlarged prostate glands in men who experience difficulty urinating. This medication causes lightheadedness and dizziness with the first dose. It is important not to drive or partake in tasks where getting dizzy would be dangerous. For this reason, it is

PATIENT INFORMATION: *(cont'd)*

advised that the first dose be taken in the evening at home. You should be careful getting up after lying down or sitting. Fatigue and headache are the most common side effects. If you get dizzy or feel faint, sit or lie down. This effect disappears after the first 24 hours of therapy. If you are taking this medication for high blood pressure, it is important to have your blood pressure checked regularly.

HOW SUPPLIED:

Hytrin capsules (terazosin hydrochloride capsules) are available in four dosage strengths:

1 mg grey capsules (imprinted with and the Abbo-Code HH), 2 mg yellow capsules (imprinted with and the Abbo-Code HY), 5 mg red capsules (imprinted with and the Abbo-Code HK), 10 mg blue capsules (imprinted with and the Abbo-Code HN).

Abbo-Pac unit dose strip packages

Recommended Storage: Store at controlled room temperature between 20-25°C (68-77°F). See USP. Protect from light and moisture.

HOW SUPPLIED - EQUIVALENTS NOT AVAILABLE:

Capsule, Gelatin - Oral - 1 mg

100's	$126.99	HYTRIN, Abbott	00074-3805-13
100's	$135.55	HYTRIN, Abbott	00074-3805-11

Capsule, Gelatin - Oral - 2 mg

100's	$126.99	HYTRIN, Abbott	00074-3806-13
100's	$135.55	HYTRIN, Abbott	00074-3806-11

Capsule, Gelatin - Oral - 5 mg

100's	$126.99	HYTRIN, Abbott	00074-3807-13
100's	$135.55	HYTRIN, Abbott	00074-3807-11

Capsule, Gelatin - Oral - 10 mg

100's	$126.99	HYTRIN, Abbott	00074-3808-13
100's	$135.55	HYTRIN, Abbott	00074-3808-11

TERBINAFINE HYDROCHLORIDE *(003149)*

CATEGORIES: Anti-Infectives; Antibacterials; Antifungals; Antimicrobials; Dermatologicals; Fungal Agents; Infections; Skin/Mucous Membrane Agents; Tinea Corporis; Tinea Cruris; Tinea Pedis; Topical; FDA Class 1S ("Standard Review"); Sales > $100 Million; FDA Approved 1992 Dec

BRAND NAMES: **Lamisil**

FORMULARIES: PCS

DESCRIPTION:

Terbinafine hydrochloride contains the synthetic allylamine antifungal compound terbinafine hydrochloride.

Terbinafine hydrochloride is a white to off-white fine crystalline powder. It is freely soluble in methanol and methylene chloride, soluble in ethanol, and slightly soluble in water.

Each Lamsil tablet contains: *Active Ingredients:* terbenafine hydrochloride (equivalent to 250 mg base).*Inactive Ingredients:* colloidal silicon dioxide, NF; hydroxypropyl methylcellulose, USP; magnesium stearate, NF; microcrystalline cellulose, NF; sodium starch glycolate, NF.

CLINICAL PHARMACOLOGY:

PHARMACOKINETICS

Following oral administration terbinafine is well absorbed (>70%) and the bioavailability of terbinafine hydrochloride as a result of first-pass metabolism is approximately 40%. Peak plasma concentrations of 1 μ/mL appear within 2 h after a single 250 mg dose; the AUC (area under the curve) is approximately 4.56 mcg·h/mL. An increase in the AUC of terbinafine of less than 20% is observed when terbinafine hydrochloride is administered with food. No clinically relevant age-dependent changes in steady-state plasma concentrations of terbinafine have been reported. In patients with renal impairment (creatinine clearance ≤ 50 mL/min) or hepatic cirrhosis, the clearance of terbinafine is decreased by approximately 50% compared to normal volunteers. No effect of gender on the blood levels of terbinafine was detected in clinical trials. In plasma, terbinafine is >99% bound to plasma proteins and there are no specific binding sites. At steady-state, in comparison to a single dose, the peak concentration of terbinafine is 25% higher and plasma AUC increases by a factor of 2.5; the increase in plasma AUC is consistent with an effective half-life of ≈ 36 hours. Terbinafine is distributed to the sebum and skin. A terminal half-life of 200–400 h may represent the slow elimination of terbinafine from tissues such as skin and adipose. Prior to excretion, terbinafine is extensively metabolized. No metabolites have been identified that have anti-fungal activity similar to terbinafine. Approximately 70% of the administered dose is eliminated in the urine.

MICROBIOLOGY

Terbinafine hydrochloride is a synthetic allylamine derivative. Terbinafine hydrochloride exerts its antifungal effect by inhibiting squalene epoxidase, a key enzyme in sterol biosynthesis in fungi. This action results in a deficiency in ergosterol and a corresponding accumulation of sterol within the fungal cell. Depending on the concentration of the drug and the fungal species tested *in vitro*, terbinafine hydrochloride may be fungicidal; however, the clinical significance of these data is unknown. *In vitro*, mammalian squalene epoxidase is only inhibited at higher (4,000–fold) concentrations.

Terbinafine has been shown to be active against most strains of the following organisms both *in vitro* and in clinical infections of the nail.

Trichophyton rubrum
Trichophyton mentagrophytes

Blood and tissue levels of terbinafine following oral dosing with terbinafine hydrochloride 250 mg QD exceed *in vitro*MICs against most strains of the following organisms which can infect the nail; however, the efficacy of terbinafine in treating nail infections due to these organisms has not been studied in controlled clinical trials.

Epidermophyton floccosum
Microsporum gypseum
Microsporum nanum
Trichophyton verrucosum
Candida albicans
Scopulariopsis brevicaulis

CLINICAL STUDIES:

The efficacy of terbinafine hydrochloride in the treatment of onychomycosis is illustrated by the response of patients with toenail and/or fingernail infections who participated in two US/Canadian placebo-controlled clinical trials.

CLINICAL STUDIES: *(cont'd)*

Results of the toenail study, as assessed at week 48 (12 weeks of treatment with 36 weeks follow-up after completion of therapy; demonstrated mycological cure defined as simultaneous occurrence of negative KOH plus negative culture, in 70% of patients. Fifty-nine percent (59%) of patients experienced effective treatment (mycological cure plus 0% nail involvement or >5mm of new unaffected nail growth); 38% of patients demonstrated mycological cure plus clinical cure (0% nail involvement).

Results of the fingernail study, as assessed at week 24 (6 weeks of treatment with 18 weeks follow-up after completion of therapy), demonstrated mycological cure in 79% of patients, effective treatment in 75% of the patients, and mycological cure plus clinical cure in 59% of the patients.

The mean time to overall success was approximately 10 months for the toenail study and 4 months for the fingernail study. In the toenail study, for patients evaluated at least six months after achieving clinical cure and at least one year after completing terbinafine hydrochloride therapy, the clinical relapse rate was approximately 15%.

INDICATIONS AND USAGE:

Terbinafine hydrochloride is indicated for the treatment of onychomycosis of the toenail or fingernail due to dermatophytes (tinea unguium) (see DOSAGE AND ADMINISTRATION.)

CONTRAINDICATIONS:

Terbinafine hydrochloride is contraindicated in individuals with hypersensitivity to terbinafine.

WARNINGS:

Rare cases of symptomatic hepatobiliary dysfunction including cholestatic hepatitis have been reported. Treatment with terbinafine hydrochloride should be discontinued if hepatobiliary dysfunction develops (see PRECAUTIONS.) There have been isolated reports of serious skin reactions (*e.g.*, Stevens-Johnson Syndrome and toxic epidermal necrolysis). If progressive skin rash occurs, treatment with terbinafine hydrochloride should be discontinued.

PRECAUTIONS:

General: Changes in the ocular lens and retina have been reported following the use of terbinafine hydrochloride in controlled trials. The clinical significance of these changes is unknown. Hepatic function (hepatic enzyme) tests are recommended in patients administered terbinafine hydrochloride for more than six weeks (see WARNINGS.)

In patients with either pre-existing liver disease or renal impairment (creatinine clearance ≤50 mL/min), the use of terbinafine hydrochloride has not been adequately studied, and therefore, is not recommended (see CLINICAL PHARMACOLOGY, Pharmacokinetics.)

Transient decreases in absolute lymphocyte counts (ALC) have been observed in controlled clinical trials. In placebo-controlled trials, 8/465 terbinafine hydrochloride-treated patients (1.7%) and 3/137 placebo-treated patients (2.2%) had decreases in ALC to below 1000/mm^3 on two or more occasions. The clinical significance of this observation is unknown. However, in patients with known or suspected immunodeficiency, physicians should consider monitoring complete blood counts in individuals using terbinafine hydrochloride therapy for greater than six weeks.

Isolated cases of severe neutropenia have been reported. These were reversible upon discontinuation of terbinafine hydrochloride with or without supportive therapy. If clinical signs and symptoms suggestive of secondary infection occur, a complete blood count should be obtained. If the neutrophil count is ≤1,000 cells/mm^3, terbinafine hydrochloride should be discontinued and supportive management started.

Carcinogenesis, Mutagenesis, and Impairment of Fertility: In a 28–month oral carcinogenicity study in rats, a marginal increase in the incidence of liver tumors was observed in males at the highest dose level, 69 mg/kg/day [13.8 times the maximum recommended human dose (MRHD) based on body weight (BW) and 3.6 times the MRHD based on body surface area (BSA)]. There was no dose-related trend and the mid-dose male rats (20 mg/kg/day; 4.0 times the MRHD based on BW and 1.0 times the MRHD based on BSA) did not have any tumors. No increased incidence in liver tumors was noted in female rats at dose levels up to 97 mg/kg/day (19.4 times the MRHD based on BW and 4.5 times the MRHD based on BSA) or in male or female mice treated orally for 23 months at doses up to 156 mg/kg/day (31.2 times the MRHD based on BW and 3.9 times the MRHD based on BSA).

A wide range of *in vivo* studies in mice, rats, dogs, and monkeys, and *in vitro* studies using rat, monkey, and human hepatocytes suggest that the development of liver tumors in the high-dose male rats may be associated with peroxisome proliferation, and support the conclusion that this is a rat-specific finding. *In vivo* investigations included evaluations of the effects of terbinafine hydrochloride on liver weight, morphology, and ultrastructure; hepatic cytochrome P450; and peroxisome proliferation assessed morphologically and biochemically (peroxisomal enzymes) in mice, rats, dogs, and monkeys. The effects of terbinafine hydrochloride and two known metabolites on hepatic morphology and peroxisomal and P450 enzyme activities were also evaluated *in vivo* in male rats and *in vitro* in primary hepatocyte cultures from male rats and humans and from monkeys. The results of the *in vivo*investigations indicated that oral administration of terbinafine hydrochloride (500 mg/kg/day) resulted in peroxisome proliferation in rats, and that these effects did not occur in mice, dogs, or monkeys. Further, in vitro studies indicated that peroxisome proliferation occurred in rat hepatocytes, but not in monkey or human hepatocytes.

Systemic exposure to terbinafine hydrochloride, assessed by the steady-state plasma unbound fraction area under the curve (AUC) for terbinafine and metabolites, was 7.7 and 9.7 mcg·h/mL for male and female rats, respectively, and 11.2 and 13.1 mcg·h/mL for male and female mice, respectively, at doses comparable to the high doses in the carcinogenicity studies. In human subjects at the MRHD (a daily dose of 250 mg of terbinafine hydrochloride), the unbound AUC was 0.466 mcg·h/mL. The resulting safety margins for humans, based on relative systemic exposure (AUC inbound), in rats and mice were 17 to 21 and 24 to 28, respectively.

The results of a variety of *in vitro* and *in vivo* genotoxicity tests gave no evidence of a mutagenic or clastogenic potential, and demonstrated the absence of tumor-initiating or cell-proliferating activity.

Oral reproduction studies in rats at doses up to 300 mg/kg/day (60 times the MRHD based on BW and approximately 12 times the MRHD based on BSA) did not reveal any specific effects on fertility or other reproductive parameters. Intravaginal application of terbinafine hydrochloride at 150 mg/day in pregnant rabbits did not increase the incidence of abortions or premature deliveries nor affect fetal parameters.

Pregnancy Category B: Oral reproduction studies have been performed in rabbits and rats at doses up to 300 mg/kg/day (60 times the MRHD based on BW and 9 times to 12 times the MRHD, in rabbits and rats, respectively, based on BSA) and have revealed no evidence of impaired fertility or harm to the fetus due to terbinafine. There are, however, no adequate and well-controlled studies in pregnant women. Because animal reproduction studies are not always predictive of human response, and because treatment of anychomycosis can be postponed until after pregnancy is completed, it is recommended that terbinafine hydrochloride not be initiated during pregnancy.

PRECAUTIONS: *(cont'd)*

Nursing Mothers: After oral administration, terbinafine is present in breast milk of nursing mothers. The ratio of terbinafine in milk to plasma is 7:1. Treatment with terbinafine hydrochloride is not recommended in nursing mothers.

Pediatric Use: The safety and efficacy of terbinafine hydrochloride have not been established in pediatric patients.

DRUG INTERACTIONS:

In vitro studies with human liver microsomes showed that terbinafine does not inhibit the metabolism of tolbutamide, ethinylestradiol, ethoxycoumarin, and cyclosporine. *In vivo* drug-drug interaction studies conducted in normal volunteer subjects showed that terbinafine does not affect the clearance of antipyrine, digoxin, and the antihistamine terfenadine. Terbinafine does not affect the clearance of warfarin or warfarin's effect on prothrombin time. Terbinafine decreases the clearance of intravenously administered caffeine by 19%. Terbinafine increases the clearance of cyclosporine by 15%.

Terbinafine clearance is increased 100% by rifampin, a CyP450 enzyme inducer, and decreased 33% by cimetidine, a CyP450 enzyme inhibitor. Terbinafine clearance is decreased 16% by terfenadine. Terbinafine clearance is unaffected by cyclosporine.

There is no information available from prospectively conducted drug interaction studies with the following classes of drugs: oral contraceptives, hormone replacement therapies, hypoglycemics, theophyllines, phenytoins, thiazide diuretics, beta blockers, and calcium channel blockers.

ADVERSE REACTIONS:

The most frequently reported adverse events observed in the 3 US/Canadian placebo-controlled trials are listed in the table below. The adverse events reported encompass gastrointestinal symptoms (including diarrhea, dyspepsia, and abdominal pain), liver test abnormalities, rashes, urticaria, pruritus, and taste disturbances. In general, the adverse events were mild, transient, and did not lead to discontinuation from study participation.

TABLE 1

Adverse Event	Terbinafine HCl (%) n=465	Placebo (%) n=137	Discontinuation Terbinafine HCl (%) n=465	Discontinuation Placebo (%) n=137
Headache	12.9	9.5	0.2	0.0
Gastrointestinal Symptoms:				
Diarrhea	5.6	2.9	0.6	0.0
Dyspepsia	4.3	2.9	0.4	0.0
Abdominal Pain	2.4	1.5	0.4	0.0
Nausea	2.6	2.9	0.2	0.0
Flatulence	2.2	2.2	0.0	0.0
Dermatologic Symptoms:				
Rash	5.6	2.2	0.9	0.7
Pruritus	2.8	1.5	0.2	0.0
Urticaria	1.1	0.0	0.0	0.0
Liver Enzyme Abnormalities*	3.3	1.4	0.2	0.0
Taste Disturbance	2.8	0.7	0.2	0.0
Visual Disturbance	1.1	1.5	0.9	0.0

* Liver enzyme abnormalities ≥ 2x the upper limit of the normal range.

Rare adverse events, based on worldwide experience with terbinafine hydrochloride use include: symptomatic idiosyncratic hepatobiliary dysfunction (including cholestatic hepatitis) (see WARNINGS and PRECAUTIONS), serious skin reactions (see WARNINGS), severe neutropenia (see PRECAUTIONS), and allergic reactions (including anaphylaxis). Rarely, terbinafine hydrochloride may cause taste disturbance (including taste loss) which usually recovers within several weeks after discontinuation of the drug.

OVERDOSAGE:

There is no information on human overdosage with terbinafine hydrochloride. Single oral doses in rats and mice up to 400 times the therapeutic dose produce sedation, drowsiness, ataxia, dyspnea, exophthalmus, and piloerection; animal mortality was less than 50% at this level.

DOSAGE AND ADMINISTRATION:

One 250 mg tablet of terbinafine hydrochloride should be taken once daily for 6 weeks by patients with fingernail onychomycosis. One 250 mg tablet of terbinafine hydrochloride should be taken once daily for 12 weeks by patients with toenail onychomycosis. The optimal clinical effect is seen some months after mycological cure and cessation of treatment. This is related to the period required for outgrowth of healthy nail.

HOW SUPPLIED:

Lamisil supplied as white to yellow-tinged white circular, bi-convex, bevelled tablets containing 250 mg of terbinafine with "LAMISIL" in circular form on one side and code "250" on the other.

Storage: Store tablets below 25° C (77° F); in a tight container. Protect from light.

HOW SUPPLIED - EQUIVALENTS NOT AVAILABLE:

Cream - Topical - 1 %

15 gm	$25.08	LAMISIL, Novartis	00078-0170-40
30 gm	$45.00	LAMISIL, Novartis	00078-0170-46

TERBUTALINE SULFATE *(002312)*

CATEGORIES: Airway Obstruction; Antiasthmatics/Bronchodilators; Asthma; Autonomic Drugs; Beta Adrenergic Stimulators; Bronchial Dilators; Bronchitis; Bronchospasm; Emphysema; Respiratory & Allergy Medications; Sympathomimetic Agents; Sympathomimetics, Beta Agonist; Uterine Relaxants; Labor*; Pregnancy Category B; FDA Approval Pre 1982; Patent Expiration 1994 Mar

* Indication not approved by the FDA

BRAND NAMES: *Asthmasian*; *Asthmo-Kranit*; *Ataline*; Brethaire; Brethancer; Brethine; **Bricanyl**; *Brothine*; *Bucaril*; *Butaline*; *Contimit*; *Convon*; *Feevone*; *Monovent*; *Respirol*; *Syntovent*; *Terasma*; *Terbasmin*; *Vacanyl*; *Vasezorin*
(International brand names outside U.S. in italics)

FORMULARIES: Aetna; BC-BS; CIGNA; DoD; FHP; Humana; Kaiser; Medco; Medi-Cal; PCS; PruCare; United

COST OF THERAPY: $400.33 (Asthma; Tablet; 5 mg; 3/day; 365 days)

PRIMARY ICD9: 493.90 (Asthma, Unspecified, Without Mention of Status Asthmaticus)

DESCRIPTION:

Tablets: Terbutaline sulfate tablets for oral administration contain 2.5 or 5 mg of terbutaline sulfate (equivalent to 2.05 and 4.1 mg free base, respectively). Both the 2.5 and 5 mg tablets contain the following inactive ingredients: corn starch (or pregelatinized corn starch), lactose, magnesium stearate, microcrystalline cellulose, and povidone.

Terbutaline sulfate (5-(2-((1,1-dimethylethyl)amino)-1-hydroxyethyl)-1,3-benzenediol sulfate) is a β-adrenergic agonist bronchodilator.

Injection: Terbutaline sulfate subcutaneous injection is a sterile, isotonic solution. Each ml of solution contains 1 mg terbutaline sulfate (equivalent to 0.82 mg free base) and 8.9 mg sodium chloride in water for injection. Hydrochloric acid is used to adjust pH to 3.5. Filled under nitrogen.

Terbutaline sulfate (5-[2-[(1,1-dimethylethyl)amino]-1- hydroxyethyl]-1,3-benzenediol sulfate) is a β- adrenergic agonist bronchodilator.

Inhalation: A metered-dose dispenser containing micronized Terbutaline sulfate in a suspension of the following composition (TABLE 1):

TABLE 1

	7.5-ml (10.5-g) Canister
terbutaline sulfate USP	0.075 g
sorbitan trioleate	0.105 g
trichloromonofluoromethane NF	2.58 g
dichlorotetrafluoroethane NF	2.58 g
dichlorodifluoromethane NF	5.16 g

Each actuation delivers 0.20 mg of terbutaline sulfate form the mouthpiece (0.25 mg valve delivery). Each canister provides at least 300 inhalations.

Terbutaline sulfate USP is a white to gray-white crystalline powder. It is odor less or has a faint odor of acetic acid. It is soluble in water and in 0.1N hydrochloride acid, slightly soluble in methanol, and insoluble in chloroform. Its molecular weight is 548.65.

CLINICAL PHARMACOLOGY:

Terbutaline sulfate is a β-adrenergic receptor agonist which has been shown by *in vitro* and *in vivo* pharmacologic studies in animals to exert a preferential effect on β_2-adrenergic receptors, such as those located in bronchial smooth muscle. However, controlled clinical studies of patients who were administered the drug have not revealed a preferential β_2-adrenergic effect.

It has been postulated that β-adrenergic agonists produce many of their pharmacologic effects by activation of adenyl cyclase, the enzyme which catalyzes the conversion of adenosine triphosphate to cyclic adenosine monophosphate.

Terbutaline sulfate tablets have been shown in controlled clinical studies to relieve bronchospasm in chronic obstructive pulmonary disease, such as asthma, chronic bronchitis, and emphysema. This action was manifested by a clinically significant increase in pulmonary function as demonstrated by an increase of 15% or greater in FEV_1 in some patients. A measurable change in pulmonary function usually occurs within 30 minutes following oral administration. The maximum effect usually occurs within 120-180 minutes. There is a clinically significant decrease in airway and pulmonary resistance which persists for at least 4 hours or longer in most patients. Significant bronchodilator action, as measured by various pulmonary function determinations (airway resistance, MMEFR, PEFR) has been demonstrated in studies for periods up to 8 hours in many patients.

Clinical studies have evaluated the effectiveness of oral Terbutaline sulfate for periods up to 12 months and the drug continued to produce significant improvement of pulmonary function throughout the period of treatment.

Orally administered terbutaline sulfate is 30-70% absorbed in the GI tract (food reduces bioavailability by one-third). Sixty percent of the absorbed oral dose is metabolized via first pass conjugation in the gut wall and liver. There are no known active metabolites. After single oral doses, peak concentrations are found 30 minutes to 5 hours after administration. Each mg of orally administered terbutaline sulfate (in fasting adults) produces an average peak serum concentration of approximately 1 mcg/L. Terbutaline has a half-life of 3-4 hours and is excreted in the urine.

Terbutaline crosses the placenta. After single dose IV administration of terbutaline to 22 women in late pregnancy who were delivered by elective Caesarean section due to clinical reasons, umbilical blood levels of terbutaline were found to range from 11 to 48% of the maternal blood levels.

Recent studies in laboratory animals (minipigs, rodents, and dogs) recorded the occurrence of cardiac arrhythmias and sudden death (with histologic evidence of myocardial necrosis) when β agonists and methylxanthines were administered concurrently. The significance of these findings when applied to humans is currently unknown.

INDICATIONS AND USAGE:

Terbutaline sulfate is indicated as a bronchodilator for the relief of reversible bronchospasm in patients with obstructive airway diseases, such as asthma, bronchitis, and emphysema.

Inhalation: In controlled clinical trials the inset of improvement in pulmonary function was within 15 to 30 minutes. These studies also showed that maximum improvement in pulmonary function occurred at 120 minutes following two inhalations of Terbutaline sulfate and that clinically significant improvement (*i.e.,* 15% increase in FEV_1/predicted FEV_1) generally continued for 3 to 4 hours in most patients. In some studies there was a significant decrease in improvement of pulmonary function noted with continued administration of terbutaline sulfate aerosol. Continued effectiveness of terbutaline sulfate was demonstrated over a 14-week period in some patients in these clinical trials.

Some patients with asthma, in single-dose studies only, have shown a therapeutic response that was still apparent at 6 hours.

CONTRAINDICATIONS:

Terbutaline sulfate is contraindicated in patients with a history of hypersensitivity to any of its components or to sympathomimetic amines.

WARNINGS:

There have been rare reports of seizures occurring in patients receiving terbutaline, which do not recur when the drug is discontinued and have not been explained on any other basis.

Usage in Labor and Delivery: Terbutaline sulfate is not indicated and should not be used for the management of preterm labor. Serious adverse reactions have been reported following administration of terbutaline sulfate to women in labor. These reports have included transient hypokalemia, pulmonary edema (sometimes after delivery), and hypoglycemia in the mother and/or the neonatal child. Maternal death has been reported with terbutaline sulfate and other drugs of this class.

WARNINGS: *(cont'd)*

Inhalation: As with other adrenergic aerosols, the potential for paradoxical bronchospasm (which can be life-threatening) should be kept in mind. If it occurs, the preparation should be discontinued immediately and alternative therapy instituted.

Fatalities have been reported in association with excessive use of inhaled sympathomimetic drugs. The exact cause of death in unknown. As with other beta-adrenergic aerosols, terbutaline sulfate should not be use din excess. Controlled clinical studies and other clinical experience have shown that terbutaline, like other inhaled beta-adrenergic agonists, can produce a significant cardiovascular effect in some patients, as measured by pulse rate, blood pressure, symptoms, and/or ECG changes.

The contents of terbutaline sulfate inhalation are under pressure. Do not puncture the container. Do not use or store it near heat or open flame. Exposure to temperatures above 120°F may cause bursting. Never throw the container into a fire or incinerator. Keep out of children's reach.

PRECAUTIONS:

General: Terbutaline sulfate is a sympathomimetic amine and as such should be used with caution in patients with cardiovascular disorders (including arrhythmias, coronary insufficiency, and hypertension), in patients with hyperthyroidism or diabetes mellitus, history of seizures, or in patients who are unusually responsive to sympathomimetic amines. Age-related differences in the hemodynamic response to β-adrenergic receptor stimulation have been reported.

Patients susceptible to hypokalemia should be monitored because transient early falls in serum potassium levels have been reported with β agonists.

Large doses of intravenous terbutaline sulfate have been reported to aggravate preexisting diabetes and ketoacidosis. The relevance of this observation to the use of terbutaline sulfate tablets is unknown.

Immediate hypersensitivity reactions and exacerbation of bronchospasm have been reported after terbutaline administration.

Information for the Patient: The patient should be advised regarding the potential adverse reactions associated with terbutaline sulfate and that: (1) the action of terbutaline sulfate tablets may last up to 8 hours (terbutaline sulfate inhalation: up to 6 hours) and, therefore, should not be used more frequently than recommended, (2) the number or frequency of doses should not be increased without medical consultation, (3) medical consultation should be sought promptly if symptoms get worse, and (4) other medicines should not be used while taking terbutaline sulfate without consulting the physician.

Carcinogenesis, Mutagenesis, and Impairment of Fertility: A two-year, oral carcinogenesis bioassay of terbutaline sulfate (50, 500, 1000, and 2000 mg/kg, corresponding to 167, 1667, 3333, and 6667 times the recommended daily adult oral dose, respectively) in the Sprague-Dawley rat revealed drug-related changes in the female genital system. Females showed dose-related increases in leiomyomas of the mesovarium: 3 (5%) at 50 mg/kg, 17 (28%) at 500 mg/kg, 21 (35%) at 1000 mg/kg, and 23 (38%) at 2000 mg/kg, which were significant at the three highest levels. None occurred in female controls. The incidence of ovarian cysts was significantly elevated at all dose levels except at 2000 mg/kg and hyperplasia of the mesovarium was increased significantly at 500 and 2000 mg/kg. A 21-month oral study of terbutaline sulfate (5, 50, and 200 mg/kg, corresponding to 17, 167, and 667 times the recommended daily adult oral dose, respectively) in the mouse revealed no evidence of carcinogenicity.

Studies of terbutaline sulfate have not been conducted to determine mutagenic potential.

An oral reproduction study of terbutaline sulfate up to 50 mg/kg (corresponding to 167 times the human oral dose) in the rat revealed no adverse effects on fertility.

Pregnancy, Teratogenic Effects, Pregnancy Category B: Reproduction studies in mice (up to 1.1 mg/kg subcutaneously, corresponding to 4 times the human oral dose) and in rats and rabbits (up to 50 mg/kg orally, corresponding to 167 times the human oral dose) have revealed no evidence of impaired fertility or harm to the fetus due to terbutaline. There are, however, no adequate and well-controlled studies in pregnant women. Because animal reproduction studies are not always predictive of human response, this drug should be used during pregnancy only if clearly needed.

Labor and Delivery: The safe use of terbutaline sulfate for the management of preterm labor or for other uses during labor and delivery has not been established and the drug should not be used. (See WARNINGS.)

Nursing Mothers: Terbutaline is excreted in breast milk. Caution should be exercised when terbutaline sulfate is administered to a nursing woman.

Pediatric Use: Safety and effectiveness in children below the age of 12 have not been established.

DRUG INTERACTIONS:

Other sympathomimetic bronchodilators or epinephrine should not be used concomitantly with terbutaline sulfate, since their combined effect on the cardiovascular system may be deleterious to the patient. This recommendation does not preclude the judicious use of an aerosol bronchodilator of the adrenergic stimulant type in patients receiving terbutaline sulfate tablets. Such concomitant use, however, should be individualized and not given on a routine basis. If regular coadministration is required, alternative therapy should be considered. Terbutaline sulfate should be administered with caution in patients being treated with monoamine oxidase (MAO) inhibitors or tricyclic antidepressants, since the action of terbutaline sulfate on the vascular system may be potentiated.

β-Adrenergic receptor blocking agents not only block the pulmonary effect of terbutaline but may produce severe asthmatic attacks in asthmatic patients. Therefore, patients requiring treatment for both bronchospastic disease and hypertension should be treated with medication other than β-adrenergic blocking agents for hypertension.

ADVERSE REACTIONS:

The adverse reactions of terbutaline sulfate are similar to those of other sympathomimetic agents.

The most commonly observed side effects are tremor and nervousness. The frequency of these side effects appear to diminish with continued therapy. Other commonly reported reactions include increased heart rate, palpitations, and dizziness. Other reported reactions include headache, drowsiness, vomiting, nausea, sweating, and muscle cramps. These reactions are generally transient and usually do not require treatment.

OVERDOSAGE:

Overdosage information is limited. Excessive adrenergic-receptor stimulation may augment the signs and symptoms listed under ADVERSE REACTIONS and may be accompanied by other adrenergic effects.

Signs and symptoms of overdosage may include the following:

Cardiovascular: tachycardia of varying degrees, transient arrhythmias, and extrasystoles. A significant drop in blood pressure may occur due to peripheral vasodilation.

Neuromuscular: tremors of varying degrees, nervousness, drowsiness, muscle cramps, headache, and sweating.

OVERDOSAGE: *(cont'd)*

Gastrointestinal: nausea and vomiting.

Endocrine: varying degrees of hyperglycemia and rise in insulin levels which could be followed by rebound hypoglycemia. Hypokalemia in the early stages may occur. The duration of these signs and symptoms will be dependent on the degree of overdosage.

Treat the alert patient who has taken excessive oral medication by emptying the stomach by means of induced emesis, followed by gastric lavage. In the unconscious patient, secure the airway with a cuffed endotracheal tube before beginning lavage (do not induce emesis). Instillation of activated charcoal slurry may help reduce absorption of terbutaline sulfate. Maintain adequate respiratory exchange. Provide cardiac and respiratory support as needed. Continue observation until symptom-free. Careful consideration should be given to the appropriateness of any chosen therapy and possible effect on the patient's underlying disease state. (See also WARNINGS.)

Studies in mice, rats, rabbits, and dogs have established the LD_{50} of terbutaline to be 1-9 g/kg orally and 0.3-1.6 g/kg subcutaneously.

It is not known whether terbutaline is dialyzable.

DOSAGE AND ADMINISTRATION:

Tablets: *Adults:* Usual dose is 5 mg three times daily. Dosing may be initiated at 2.5 mg three or four times daily and titrated upward depending on clinical response. A total dose of 15 mg in a 24-hour period should not be exceeded. *Children (12-15 yrs):* 2.5 mg three times daily.

If a previously effective dosage regimen fails to provide the usual relief, medical advice should be sought immediately as this is often a sign of seriously worsening asthma which would require reassessment of therapy.

Store at controlled room temperature 15°-30°C (59°-86°F).

Injection: Parenteral drug products should be inspected visually for particulate matter and discoloration prior to administration, whenever solution and container permit.

The usual subcutaneous dose of terbutaline sulfate is 0.25 mg (0.25 ml, 1/4 ampul contents) injected into the lateral deltoid area. If significant clinical improvement does not occur by 15-30 minutes, a second dose of 0.25 mg may be administered. A total dose of 0.5 mg should not be exceeded within a four-hour period. If a patient fails to respond to a second 0.25 mg (0.25 ml) dose within 15-30 minutes, other therapeutic measures should be considered.

Solutions of terbutaline sulfate are sensitive to excessive heat and light. Ampuls should, therefore, be stored at controlled room temperature (15 - 30°C (59-86°F) in their original carton to provide protection from light until dispensed. Solutions should not be used if discolored.

Inhalation: The usual dosage for adults and children 12 years and older is two inhalations separated by a 60-second interval, every 4 to 6 hours. Dosing should not be repeated more often than every 4 to 6 hours. The use of terbutaline sulfate inhalator can be continued as medically indicated to control recurring bouts of bronchospasm. During this time most patients gain optimal benefit from regular use of the inhaler. Safe usage for periods extending over several years has been documented.

If a previously effective dosage regimen fails to provide the usual relief, medical advice should be sought immediately, as this is often a sign of seriously worsening asthma, which would require reassessment of therapy.

Store between 59 - 86°F (15 - 30°C). Dispense with enclosed instructions for use.

(Tablet: Marion Merrell Dow, 5/91) (Injection: Marion Merrell Dow, 8/92)

HOW SUPPLIED - RATED THERAPEUTICALLY EQUIVALENT:

Injection, Solution - Subcutaneous - 1 mg/ml

1 ml x 10	$18.58	BRETHINE AMPUL, Novartis	00028-7507-23
1 ml x 10	**$26.64**	**BRICANYL SUBCUTANEOUS, Hoechst Marion Roussel**	**00068-0702-20**
1 ml x 100	$148.02	BRETHINE AMPUL, Novartis	00028-7507-01

HOW SUPPLIED - NOT RATED EQUIVALENT:

Inhalant - Inhalation - 0.2 mg/spr

7.5 ml	$18.35	BRETHAIRE, Novartis	00028-5557-87
7.5 ml	$20.75	BRETHAIRE, Novartis	00028-5557-88

Tablet, Uncoated - Oral - 2.5 mg

100's	$25.39	BRETHINE, Novartis	00028-0072-01
100's	$27.92	BRETHINE, Novartis	00028-0072-61
100's	**$29.22**	**BRICANYL, Hoechst Marion Roussel**	**00068-0725-61**
100's	$306.18	BRETHINE, Novartis	00028-0072-65
1000's	$239.88	BRETHINE, Novartis	00028-0072-10

Tablet, Uncoated - Oral - 5 mg

100's	$36.56	BRETHINE, Novartis	00028-0105-01
100's	$39.12	BRETHINE, Novartis	00028-0105-61
100's	**$41.94**	**BRICANYL, Hoechst Marion Roussel**	**00068-0750-61**
100's	$440.60	BRETHINE, Novartis	00028-0105-65
1000's	$345.83	BRETHINE, Novartis	00028-0105-10

TERCONAZOLE *(002313)*

CATEGORIES: Anti-Infectives; Antifungals; Antimicrobials; Candidiasis; Dermatologicals; Fungal Agents; Skin/Mucous Membrane Agents; Vaginal Preparations; Vaginitis; Pregnancy Category C; FDA Approved 1987 Dec; Top 200 Drugs

BRAND NAMES: *Fungistat* (Mexico); *Fungistat 3*; *Fungistat 5*; *Gyno-Terazol*; *Gyno-Terazol 3*; **Terazol**; *Terazol 3* (Canada); *Terazol 7* (Canada); *Tercospor* (Germany) *(International brand names outside U.S. in italics)*

FORMULARIES: Aetna; BC-BS; Foundation; Medi-Cal

DESCRIPTION:

Vaginal Cream 0.4%, 0.8%: Terazol Vaginal Cream is a white to off-white, water washable cream for intravaginal administration containing 0.4% / 0.8% of the antifungal agent terconazole,*cis*-1-[4-[[2-(2,4-dichlorophenyl)-2-(1H-1,2,4-triazol-1-ylmethyl)-1,3-dioxolan-4-yl) methoxy) phenyl]-4-(1-methylethyl) piperazine, compounded in a cream base consisting of butylated hydroxyanisole, cetyl alcohol, isopropyl myristate, polysorbate 60, polysorbate 80, propylene glycol, stearyl alcohol, and purified water.

Terconazole, a triazole derivative, is a white to almost white powder with a molecular weight of 532.47. It is insoluble in water; sparingly soluble in ethanol; and soluble in butanol.

Vaginal Suppositories: Terazol 3 vaginal suppositories are white to off-white suppositories for intervaginal administration containing 80 mg of the antifungal agent terconazole,*cis*-1-[4-[[2-(2,4-dichlorophenyl)-2-(1H-1,2,4-triazol-1-ylmethyl)-1,3-ioxolan-4-yl] methoxy) phenyl)-4-(1-methylethyl) piperazine in triglycerides derived from coconut and/or palm kernel oil (a base of hydrogenated vegetable oils) and butylated hydroxyanisole.

DESCRIPTION: *(cont'd)*

Terconazole, a triazole derivative, is a white to almost white powder with a molecular weight of 532.47. It is insoluble in water; sparingly soluble in ethanol; and soluble in butanol.

CLINICAL PHARMACOLOGY:

Microbiology: Terconazole exhibits fungicidal activity *in vitro* against *Candida albicans.* Antifungal activity also has been demonstrated against other fungi. The MIC values for terconazole against most species of lactic acid bacteria typically found in the human vagina were ≥128 mcg/ml, therefore these beneficial bacteria are not affected by drug treatment.

The exact pharmacologic mode of action of terconazole is uncertain; however, it may exert its antifungal activity by the disruption of normal fungal cell membrane permeability. No resistance to terconazole has developed during successive passages of *C. albicans.*

Human Pharmacology: Following intravaginal administration of terconazole in humans, absorption ranged from 5-8% in three hysterectomized subjects with tubal ligations.

Following oral (30 mg) administration of ^{14}C-labelled terconazole, the half-life of elimination from the blood for the parent terconazole was 6.9 hours (range 4.0-11.3). Terconazole is extensively metabolized; the plasma AUC for terconazole compared to the AUC for total radioactivity was 0.6%. Total radioactivity was eliminated from the blood with a half-life of 52.2 hours (range 44-60). Excretion of radioactivity was both by renal (32-56%) and fecal (47-52%) routes.

Photosensitivity reactions were observed in some normal volunteers following repeated dermal application of terconazole, 2.0% and 0.8% creams under conditions of filtered artificial ultraviolet light. Photosensitivity reactions have not been observed in U.S. and foreign clinical trials in patients who were treated with terconazole suppositories or cream.

INDICATIONS AND USAGE:

Terconazole vaginal creams and suppositories are indicated for the local treatment of vulvovaginal candidiasis (moniliasis). As terconazole is effective only for vulvovaginitis caused by the genus *Candida*, the diagnosis should be confirmed by KOH smears and/or cultures.

CONTRAINDICATIONS:

Patients known to be hypersensitive to Terconazole or to any of its components.

WARNINGS:

None.

PRECAUTIONS:

GENERAL

Discontinue use and do not retreat with terconazole if sensitization, irritation, fever, chills or flu-like symptoms are reported during use. If there is lack of response to terconazole vaginal cream (0.4% or 0.8%), appropriate microbiological studies (standard KOH smear and/or cultures) should be repeated to confirm the diagnosis and rule out other pathogens.

CARCINOGENESIS, MUTAGENESIS, AND IMPAIRMENT OF FERTILITY

Carcinogenesis: Studies to determine the carcinogenic potential of terconazole have not been performed.

Mutagenicity: Terconazole was not mutagenic when tested *in vitro* for induction of microbial point mutations (Ames test) or for inducing cellular transformation, or *in vivo* for chromosome breaks (micronucleus test) or dominant lethal mutations in mouse germ cells.

Impairment of Fertility: No impairment of fertility occurred when female rats were administered terconazole orally up to 40 mg/kg/day.

PREGNANCY CATEGORY C

There was no evidence of teratogenicity when terconazole was administered orally up to 40 mg/kg/day (100 X the recommended intravaginal human dose) in rats, or 20 mg/kg/day in rabbits, or subcutaneously in rats up to 20 mg/kg/day.

Dosages at or below 10 mg/kg/day produced no embryotoxicity; however, there was a delay in fetal ossification at 10 mg/kg/day in rats. There was some evidence of embryotoxicity in rabbits and rats at 20-40 mg/kg. In rats this was reflected as a decrease in litter size and number of viable young and reduced fetal weight. There was also delay in ossification and an increased incidence of skeletal variants.

The no-effect oral dose of 10 mg/kg/day resulted in a mean peak plasma level of terconazole in pregnant rats of 0.176 mcg/ml which exceeds by 44 times the mean peak plasma levels (0.004 mcg/ml) seen in normal subjects after intravaginal administration of terconazole. This safety assessment does not account for possible exposure of the fetus through direct transfer of terconazole from the irritated vagina to the fetus by diffusion across amniotic membranes.

Since terconazole is absorbed from the human vagina, it should not be used in the first trimester of pregnancy unless the physician considers it essential to the welfare of the patient.

NURSING MOTHERS

It is not known whether this drug is excreted in human milk. Animal studies have shown that rat off-spring exposed via the milk of treated (40 mg/kg/orally) dams showed decreased survival during the first few post-partum days, but overall pup weight and weight gain were comparable to or greater than controls throughout lactation. Because many drugs are excreted in human milk, and because of the potential of adverse reaction in nursing infants from terconazole, a decision should be made whether to discontinue nursing or to discontinue the drug, taking into account the importance of the drug to the mother.

PEDIATRIC USE

Safety and efficacy in children have not been established.

DRUG INTERACTIONS:

The therapeutic effect of terconazole vaginal creams and suppositories are not affected by oral contraceptive usage.

ADVERSE REACTIONS:

Vaginal Cream, 0.4%: During controlled clinical studies conducted in the United States, 521 patients with vulvovaginal candidiasis were treated with terconazole 0.4% vaginal cream. Based on comparative analyses with placebo, the adverse experiences considered most likely related to terconazole 0.4% vaginal cream were headache (26% vs 17% with placebo) and body pain (2.1% vs 0% with placebo). Vulvovaginal burning (5.2%), itching (2.3%) or irritation (3.1%) occurred less frequently with terconazole 0.4% vaginal cream than with the vehicle placebo. Fever (1.7% vs 0.5% with placebo) and chills (0.4% vs 0.0% with placebo) have also been reported. The therapy-related dropout rate was 1.9%. The adverse drug experience on terconazole most frequently causing discontinuation was vulvovaginal itching (0.6%), which was lower than the incidence for placebo (0.9%).

Vaginal Cream, 0.8%: During controlled clinical studies conducted in the United States, patients with vulvovaginal candidiasis were treated with terconazole 0.8% vaginal cream for three days. Based on comparative analyses with placebo and a standard agent, the adverse experiences considered most likely related to terconazole 0.8% vaginal cream were headache (21% vs. 16% with placebo) and dysmenorrhea (6% vs. 2% with placebo). Genital complaints

ADVERSE REACTIONS: *(cont'd)*

in general, and burning and itching in particular, occurred less frequently in the terconazole 0.8% vaginal cream 3 day regimen (5% vs. 6%-9% with placebo). Other adverse experiences reported with terconazole 0.8% vaginal cream were abdominal pain (3.4% vs. 1% with placebo) and fever (1% vs. 0.3% with placebo). The therapy related dropout rate was 2.0% for the terconazole 0.8% vaginal cream. The adverse drug experience most frequently causing discontinuation of therapy was vulvovaginal itching, 0.7% with the terconazole 0.8% vaginal cream group and 0.3% with the placebo group.

Vaginal Suppositories: During controlled clinical studies conducted in the United States, 284 patients with vulvovaginal candidiasis were treated with terconazole 80 mg vaginal suppositories. Based on comparative analyses with placebo (295 patients) the adverse experiences considered adverse reactions most likely related to terconazole 80 mg vaginal suppositories were headache (30.3% vs. 20.7% with placebo) and pain of the female genitalia (4.2% vs. 0.7% with placebo). Adverse reactions that were reported but were not statistically significantly different from placebo were burning (15.2% vs. 11.2% with placebo) and body pain (3.9% vs. 1.7% with placebo). Fever (2.8% vs 1.4% with placebo) and chills (1.8% vs. 0.7% with placebo) have also been reported. The therapy-related dropout rate was 3.5% and the placebo therapy-related dropout rate was 2.7%. The adverse drug experience on terconazole most frequently causing discontinuation was burning (2.5% vs. 1.4% with placebo) and pruritus (1.8% vs 1.4% with placebo).

OVERDOSAGE:

Vaginal Cream, 0.4% and 0.8%: Overdose of terconazole in humans has not been reported to date. In the rat, the oral LD 50 values were found to be 1741 and 849 mg/kg for the male and female, respectively. The oral LD 50 values for the male and female dog were ≈/= 1280 and ≥ 640 mg/kg, respectively.

DOSAGE AND ADMINISTRATION:

Vaginal Cream, 0.4%: One full applicator (5 g) of Terazol 7 Vaginal Cream (20 mg terconazole) is administered intravaginally once daily at bedtime for seven consecutive days. Before prescribing another course of therapy, the diagnosis should be reconfirmed by smears and/or cultures and other pathogens commonly associated with vulvovaginitis ruled out. The therapeutic effect of Terazol 7 Vaginal Cream is not affected by menstruation.

Vaginal Cream, 0.8%: One full applicator (5 g) of Terazol 3 Vaginal Cream (40 mg terconazole) is administered intravaginally once daily at bedtime for three consecutive days. Before prescribing another course of therapy, the diagnosis should be reconfirmed by smears and/or cultures and other pathogens commonly associated with vulvovaginitis ruled out. The therapeutic effect of Terazol 3 Vaginal Cream is not affected by menstruation.

Vaginal Suppositories: One Terazol 3 Vaginal Suppository (80 mg terconazole) is administered intravaginally once daily at bedtime for three consecutive days. Before prescribing another course of therapy, the diagnosis should be reconfirmed by smears and/or cultures and other pathogens commonly associated with vulvovaginitis ruled out. The therapeutic effect of Terazol 3 Vaginal Suppositories is not affected by menstruation.

Store (all forms) at Controlled Room Temperature (59°F-86°F or 15°C-30°C).

PATIENT INFORMATION:

Terconazole is used to treat vaginal yeast infections caused by Candida species. It may not be effective for other vaginal infections. Terconazole is available in a cream or suppository. Terconazole has not been associated with any birth defects. However, since there is some absorption through the vagina, it should not be used during the first trimester without advice from your physiciain. Menstruation or taking oral contraceptives, the pill, does not decrease the efficacy of this drug. Terconazole is available in a 3 day regimen and a 7 day regimen. It is best administered before bedtime. Applicators should be washed after each use. It is important to complete the entire course of therapy, even if you feel relief of symptoms in the first one or two days. If the infection returns, please consult your physician.

HOW SUPPLIED - EQUIVALENTS NOT AVAILABLE:

Cream - Vaginal - 0.4 %

45 gm $23.34 TERAZOL 7, Ortho Pharm 00062-5350-01

Cream - Vaginal - 0.8 %

20 gm tube $23.34 TERAZOL 3, Ortho Pharm 00062-5356-01

Suppository - Vaginal - 80 mg

3's $23.34 TERAZOL 3, Ortho Pharm 00062-5351-01

TERFENADINE *(002314)*

CATEGORIES: Allergies; Antihistamines; Lacrimation; Non-Sedating Antihistamines; Piperidines; Pruritus; Respiratory & Allergy Medications; Rhinitis; Rhinorrhea; Sneezing; Pregnancy Category C; Sales > $500 Million; FDA Approved 1985 May; Patent Expiration 1994 Apr

BRAND NAMES: *Alergist; Allerplus; Antimin; Centerfen; Cyater; Ferdin; Hiblorex; Hisdane; Histafen; Histastop; Histerf; Hiterf; Keneter* (Mexico); *Nadane; Nodrowsy; Nunmine; Oltan; Pantadin; Pumiro; Pylitep; Rumidin;* **Seldane**; *Serden; Tafedin; Tamagon; Teldane* (Australia, France, Germany); *Teldanex; Teficor; Teranic; Terdina; Terfed; Terfen; Ternalin 40; Tofrin; Trexyl; Triludan* (England); *Vacanyl; Zenad; Zumahis*

(International brand names outside U.S. in italics)

FORMULARIES: Aetna; BC-BS

COST OF THERAPY: $56.37 (Rhinitis; Tablet; 60 mg; 2/day; 30 days)

PRIMARY ICD9: 477.9 (Allergic Rhinitis, Cause Unspecified)

WARNING:

QT INTERVAL PROLONGATION/VENTRICULAR ARRHYTHMIA

RARE CASES OF SERIOUS CARDIOVASCULAR ADVERSE EVENTS, INCLUDING DEATH, CARDIAC ARREST, TORSADES DE POINTES, AND OTHER VENTRICULAR ARRHYTHMIAS, HAVE BEEN OBSERVED IN THE FOLLOWING CLINICAL SETTINGS, FREQUENTLY IN ASSOCIATION WITH INCREASED TERFENADINE LEVELS WHICH LEAD TO ELECTROCARDIOGRAPHIC QT PROLONGATION:

1. CONCOMITANT ADMINISTRATION OF KETOCONAZOLE (NIZORAL) OR ITRACONAZOLE (SPORANOX)
2. OVERDOSE, INCLUDING SINGLE DOSES AS LOW AS 360 MG
3. CONCOMITANT ADMINISTRATION OF CLARITHROMYCIN, ERYTHROMYCIN, OR TROLEANDOMYCIN
4. SIGNIFICANT HEPATIC DYSFUNCTION

TERFENADINE IS CONTRAINDICATED IN PATIENTS TAKING KETOCONAZOLE, ITRACONAZOLE, OR ERYTHROMYCIN, CLARITHROMYCIN, OR TROLEANDOMYCIN, AND IN PATIENTS WITH SIGNIFICANT HEPATIC DYSFUNCTION.
DO NOT EXCEED RECOMMENDED DOSE.
IN SOME CASES, SEVERE ARRHYTHMIAS HAVE BEEN PRECEDED BY EPISODES OF SYNCOPE, SYNCOPE IN PATIENTS RECEIVING TERFENADINE SHOULD LEAD TO DISCONTINUATION OF TREATMENT AND FULL EVALUATION OF POTENTIAL ARRHYTHMIAS.
(See CONTRAINDICATIONS, WARNINGS, CLINICAL PHARMACOLOGY, and DRUG INTERACTIONS).

DESCRIPTION:

Seldane (terfenadine) is available as tablets for oral administration. Each tablet contains 60 mg terfenadine. Tablets also contain, as inactive ingredients: corn starch, gelatin, lactose, magnesium stearate, and sodium bicarbonate.

Terfenadine is a histamine H_1-receptor antagonist with the chemical name α-[4-(1,1-Dimethylethyl) phenyl]-4- (hydroxydiphenylmethyl) -1-piperidine-butanol (±). The molecular weight is 471.68. The molecular formula is $C_{32}H_{41}NO_2$.

Terfenadine occurs as a white to off-white crystalline powder. It is freely soluble in chloroform, soluble in ethanol, and very slightly soluble in water.

CLINICAL PHARMACOLOGY:

Terfenadine is chemically distinct from other antihistamines. Histamine skin wheal studies have shown that terfenadine in single and repeated doses of 60 mg in 64 subjects has an antihistaminic effect beginning at 1-2 hours, reaching its maximum at 3-4 hours, and lasting in excess of 12 hours. The correlation between response on skin wheal testing and clinical efficacy is unclear. The four best controlled and largest clinical trials each lasted 7 days and involved about 1,000 total patients in comparisons of terfenadine (60 mg b.i.d.) with an active drug (chlorpheniramine, 4 mg t.i.d; dexchlorpheniramine, 2 mg t.i.d, or clemastine 1 mg b.i.d.). About 50-70% of terfenadine or other antihistamine recipients had moderate to complete relief of symptoms, compared with 30- 50% of placebo recipients. The frequency of drowsiness with terfenadine was similar to the frequency with placebo and less than with other antihistamines. None of these studies showed a difference between terfenadine and other antihistamines in the frequency of anticholinergic effects. In studies which included 52 subjects in whom EEG assessments were made, no depressant effects have been observed.

Animal studies have demonstrated that terfenadine is a histamine H_1-receptor antagonist. In these animal studies, no sedative or anticholinergic effects were observed at effective antihistaminic doses. Radioactive disposition and autoradiographic studies in rats and radioligand binding studies with guinea pig brain H_1-receptors indicate that, at effective antihistamine doses, neither terfenadine nor its metabolites penetrate the blood brain barrier well.

On the basis of a mass balance study using ^{14}C labeled terfenadine the oral absorption of terfenadine was estimated to be at least 70%. Terfenadine itself undergoes extensive (99%) first pass metabolism to two primary metabolites, an active acid metabolite and an inactive dealkylated metabolite. Therefore, systematic availability of terfenadine is low under normal conditions, and parent terfenadine is not normally detectable in plasma at levels > 10 ng/ml. Although in rare cases there was measurable plasma terfenadine in apparently normal individuals without identifiable risk factors, the implications of this finding with respect to the variability of terfenadine metabolism in the normal population cannot be assessed without further study. Further studies of terfenadine metabolism in the general population are pending. From information gained in the ^{14}C study it appears that approximately forty percent of the total dose is eliminated renally (40% as acid metabolite, 30% dealkyl metabolite, and 30% minor unidentified metabolites). Sixty percent of the dose is eliminated in the feces (50% as the acid metabolite, 2% unchanged terfenadine, and the remainder as minor unidentified metabolites). Studies investigating the effect of hepatic and renal insufficiency on the metabolism and excretion of terfenadine are incomplete. Preliminary information indicates that in cases of hepatic impairment, significant concentrations of unchanged terfenadine can be detected with the rate of acid metabolite formation being decreased. A single-dose study in patients with hepatic impairment revealed increased parent terfenadine and impaired metabolism, suggesting that additional drug accumulation may occur after repetitive dosing in such patients. Terfenadine is contraindicated for use in patients with significant hepatic dysfunction. (See CONTRAINDICATIONS and WARNINGS). In subjects with normal hepatic function unchanged terfenadine plasma concentrations have not been detected. **Elevated levels of parent terfenadine, whether due to significant hepatic dysfunction, concomitant medications, or overdose, have been associated with QT interval prolongation and serious cardiac adverse events.** (See CONTRAINDICATIONS and WARNINGS).In controlled clinical trials in otherwise normal patients with rhinitis, small increases in QTc interval were observed at doses of 60 mg b.i.d. In studies at 300 mg b.i.d. a mean increase in QTc of 10% (range -4% to +30%) (mean increase of 46 msec) was observed.

Data have been reported demonstrating that compared to young subjects, elderly subjects experience a 25% reduction in clearance of the acid metabolite after single-dose oral administration of 120 mg. Further studies are necessary to fully characterize pharmacokinetics in the elderly.

In vitro studies demonstrate that terfenadine is extensively (97%) bound to human serum protein while the acid metabolite is approximately 70% bound to human serum protein. Based on data gathered from *in vitro* models of antihistaminic activity, the acid metabolite of terfenadine has approximately 30% of the H_1blocking activity of terfenadine. The relative contribution of terfenadine and the acid metabolite to the pharmacodynamic effects have not been clearly defined. Since unchanged terfenadine is usually not detected in plasma and active acid metabolite concentrations are relatively high, the acid metabolite may be the entity responsible for the majority of efficacy after oral administration of terfenadine.

In a study involving the administration of a single 60 mg terfenadine tablet to 24 subjects, mean peak plasma levels of the acid metabolite were 263 ng/ml (range 133-423 ng/ml) and occurred approximately 2.5 hours after dosing. Plasma concentrations of unchanged terfenadine were not detected. The elimination profile of the acid metabolite was biphasic in nature with an initial mean plasma half-life of 3.5 hours followed by a mean plasma half-life of 6 hours. Ninety percent of the plasma level time curve was associated with these half-lives. Although the elimination profile is somewhat complex, the effective pharmacokinetic half-life can be estimated at approximately 8.5 hours. However, receptor binding and pharmacologic effects, both therapeutic and adverse, may persist well beyond that time.

INDICATIONS AND USAGE:

Terfenadine is indicated for the relief of symptoms associated with seasonal allergic rhinitis such as sneezing, rhinorrhea, pruritus, and lacrimation.

Clinical studies conducted to date have not demonstrated effectiveness of terfenadine in the common cold.

CONTRAINDICATIONS:

CONCOMITANT ADMINISTRATION OF TERFENADINE WITH KETOCONAZOLE (NIZORAL) OR ITRACONAZOLE (SPORONOX) IS CONTRAINDICATED. TERFENADINE IS ALSO CONTRAINDICATED IN PATIENTS WITH DISEASE STATES OR OTHER CONCOMITANT MEDICATIONS KNOWN TO IMPAIR ITS METABOLISM, INCLUDING SIGNIFICANT HEPATIC DYSFUNCTION, AND CONCURRENT USE OF CLARITHROMYCIN, ERYTHROMYCIN, OR TROLEANDOMYCIN. QT PROLONGATION HAS BEEN DEMONSTRATED IN SOME PATIENTS TAKING TERFENADINE IN THESE SETTINGS, AND RARE CASES OF SERIOUS CARDIOVASCULAR EVENTS, INCLUDING DEATH, CARDIAC ARREST, AND TORSADES DE POINTES, HAVE BEEN REPORTED IN THESE PATIENT POPULATIONS. (See WARNINGS and DRUG INTERACTIONS).

Terfenadine is contraindicated in patients with a known hypersensitivity to terfenadine or any of its ingredients.

WARNINGS:

Terfenadine undergoes extensive metabolism in the liver by a specific cytochrome P-450 isoenzyme. This metabolic pathway may be impaired in patients with hepatic dysfunction (alcoholic cirrhosis, hepatitis) or who are taking drugs such as ketoconazole, itraconazole, or clarithromycin, erythromycin, or troleandomycin (macrolide antibiotics), or other potent inhibitors of this isoenzyme. Interference with this metabolism can lead to elevated terfenadine plasma levels associated with QT prolongation and increased risk of ventricular tachyarrhythmias (such as torsades de pointes, ventricular tachycardia, and ventricular fibrillation) at the recommended dose. Terfenadine is contraindicated for use by patients with these conditions (see BOXED WARNING, CONTRAINDICATIONS, and DRUG INTERACTIONS).

Other patients who may be at risk for these adverse cardiovascular events include patients who may experience new or increased QT prolongation while receiving certain drugs or having conditions which lead to QT prolongation. These include patients taking certain antiarrhythmics, bepridil, certain psychotropics, probucol, or astemizole; patients with electrolyte abnormalities such as hypokalemia or hypomagnesemia, or taking diuretics with potential for inducing electrolyte abnormalities; and patients with congenital QT syndrome. Terfenadine is not recommended for use by patients with these conditions. The relationship of underlying cardiac disease to the development of ventricular tachyarrhythmias while on terfenadine therapy is unclear; nonetheless, terfenadine should also be used with caution in these patients.

PRECAUTIONS:

INFORMATION FOR THE PATIENT

Patients taking terfenadine should receive the following information and instructions. Antihistamines are prescribed to reduce allergic symptoms. Patients should be advised to take terfenadine only as needed and NOT TO EXCEED THE PRESCRIBED DOSE. Patients should be questioned about any use of any other prescription or over-the-counter medication, and should be cautioned regarding the potential for life-threatening arrhythmias with concurrent use of ketoconazole, itraconazole, clarithromycin, erythromycin, or troleandomycin. Patients should be advised to consult the physician before concurrent use of other medications with terfenadine. Patients should be questioned about pregnancy or lactation before starting terfenadine therapy, since the drug should be used in pregnancy or lactation only if the potential benefit justifies the potential risk to the fetus or baby. Patients should also be instructed to store this medication in a tightly closed container in a cool, dry place, away from heat or direct sunlight, and away from children.

CARCINOGENESIS, MUTAGENESIS, AND IMPAIRMENT OF FERTILITY

Oral doses of terfenadine, corresponding to 63 times the recommended human daily dose, in mice for 18 months or in rats for 24 months, revealed no evidence of tumorigenicity. Microbial and micronucleus test assays with terfenadine have revealed no evidence of mutagenesis. Reproduction and fertility studies in rats showed no effects on male or female fertility at oral doses of up to 21 times the human daily dose. At 63 times the human daily dose there was a small but significant reduction in implants and at 125 times the human daily dose reduced implants and increased post-implantation losses were observed, which were judged to be secondary to maternal toxicity.

PREGNANCY CATEGORY C

There was no evidence of animal teratogenicity. Reproduction studies have been performed in rats at doses 63 times and 125 times the human daily dose and have revealed decreased pup weight gain and survival when terfenadine was administered throughout pregnancy and lactation. There are no adequate and well-controlled studies in pregnant women. Terfenadine should be used during pregnancy only if the potential benefit justifies the potential risk to the fetus.

Nonteratogenic Effects: Terfenadine is not recommended for nursing women. The drug has caused decreased pup weight gain and survival in rats given doses 63 times and 125 times the human daily dose throughout pregnancy and lactation. Effects on pups exposed to terfenadine only during lactation are not known, and there are no adequate and well-controlled studies in women during lactation.

PEDIATRIC USE

Pediatric Use Safety and effectiveness of terfenadine in children below the age of 12 years have not been established.

DRUG INTERACTIONS:

Ketoconazole: Spontaneous adverse reaction reports of patients taking concomitant ketoconazole with recommended doses of terfenadine demonstrate QT interval prolongation and rare serious cardiac events, e.g. death, cardiac arrest, and ventricular arrhythmia including torsades de pointes. Pharmacokinetic data indicate that ketoconazole markedly inhibits the metabolism of terfenadine, resulting in elevated plasma terfenadine levels. Presence of unchanged terfenadine is associated with statistically significant prolongation of the QT and QTc intervals.**Concomitant administration of ketoconazole and terfenadine is contraindicated** (see CONTRAINDICATIONS, WARNINGS, and ADVERSE REACTIONS).

Itraconazole: Torsades de pointes and elevated parent terfenadine levels have been reported during concomitant use of terfenadine and itraconazole in clinical trials of itraconazole and from foreign post-marketing sources. One death has also been reported from foreign post-marketing sources. **Concomitant administration of itraconazole and terfenadine is contraindicated** (see CONTRAINDICATIONS, WARNINGS, and ADVERSE REACTIONS).

Due to the chemical similarity of other azole-type antifungal agents (including fluconazole, metronidazole, and miconazole) to ketoconazole, and itraconazole, concomitant use of these products with terfenadine is not recommended pending full examination of potential interactions.

Macrolides: Clinical drug interaction studies indicate that erythromycin and clarithromycin can exert an effect on terfenadine metabolism by a mechanism which may be similar to that of ketoconazole, but to a lesser extent. Although erythromycin measurably decreases the clearance of the terfenadine acid metabolite, its influence on terfenadine plasma levels is still

DRUG INTERACTIONS: *(cont'd)*

under investigation. A few spontaneous accounts of QT interval prolongation with ventricular arrhythmia including torsades de pointes, have been reported in patients receiving erythromycin or troleandomycin.

Concomitant administration of terfenadine with clarithromycin, erythromycin, or troleandomycin is contraindicated: (See CONTRAINDICATIONS, WARNINGS, and ADVERSE REACTIONS.) Pending full characterization of potential interactions, concomitant administration of terfenadine with other macrolide antibiotics, including azithromycin, is not recommended. Studies to evaluate potential interactions of terfenadine with azithromycin are in progress.

ADVERSE REACTIONS:

Cardiovascular Adverse Events: Rare reports of severe cardiovascular adverse effects have been received which include ventricular tachyarrhythmias (torsades de pointes, ventricular tachycardia, ventricular fibrillation, and cardiac arrest), hypotension, palpitations, syncope, and dizziness. Rare reports of deaths resulting from ventricular tachyarrhythmias have been received (see CONTRAINDICATIONS, WARNINGS, and DRUG INTERACTIONS). Hypotension, palpitations, syncope, and dizziness could reflect undetected ventricular arrhythmia. IN SOME PATIENTS, DEATH, CARDIAC ARREST, OR TORSADES DE POINTES HAVE BEEN PRECEDED BY EPISODES OF SYNCOPE. (See BOXED WARNING). Rare reports of serious cardiovascular adverse events have been received, some involving QT prolongation and torsades de pointes, in apparently normal individuals without identifiable risk factors. There is not conclusive evidence of causal relationship of these events with terfenadine. Although in rare cases there was measurable plasma terfenadine, the implications of this finding with respect to the variability of terfenadine metabolism in the normal population cannot be assessed without further study. In controlled clinical trials in otherwise normal patients with rhinitis, small increases in QTc interval were observed at doses of 60 mg b.i.d. In studies of 300 mg b.i.d. a mean increase in QTc of 10% (range -4% to +30%) (mean increase of 46 msec) was observed.

General Adverse Events: Experience from clinical studies, including both controlled and uncontrolled studies involving more than 2,400 patients who received terfenadine, provides information on adverse experience incidence for periods of a few days up to six months. The usual dose in these studies was 60 mg twice daily, but in a small number of patients, the dose was as low as 20 mg twice a day, or as high as 600 mg daily.

In controlled clinical studies using the recommended dose of 60 mg b.i.d., the incidence of reported adverse effects in patients receiving terfenadine was similar to that reported in patients receiving placebo. (See TABLE 1).

TABLE 1 Adverse Events Reported In Clinical studies

Adverse Event	Percent of Patients Reporting — Controlled Studies*			All Clinical Studies**	
	Terfenadine n=781	Placebo n=665	Control n=626***	Terfenadine n=2462	Placebo n=1478
Central Nervous System					
Drowsiness	9.0	8.1	18.1	8.5	8.2
Headache	6.3	7.4	3.8	15.8	11.2
Fatigue	2.9	0.9	5.8	4.5	3.0
Dizziness	1.4	1.1	1.0	1.5	1.2
Nervousness	0.9	0.2	0.6	1.7	1.0
Weakness	0.9	0.6	0.2	0.6	0.5
Appetite Increase	0.6	0.0	0.0	0.5	0.0
Gastrointestinal System					
Gastrointestinal Distress (Abdominal distress, Nausea, Vomiting, Change in bowel habits)	4.6	3.0	2.7	7.6	5.4
Eye, Ear, Nose, And Throat					
Dry Mouth/Nose/Throat	2.3	1.8	3.5	4.8	3.1
Cough	0.9	0.2	0.5	2.5	1.7
Sore Throat	0.5	0.3	0.5	3.2	1.6
Epistaxis	0.0	0.8	0.2	0.7	0.4
Skin					
Eruption (including rash and urticaria) or itching	1.0	1.7	1.4	1.6	2.0

* Duration of treatment in "CONTROLLED STUDIES" was usually 7-14 days.
** Duration of treatment in "ALL CLINICAL STUDIES" was up to 6 months.
*** CONTROL DRUGS: Chlorpheniramine (291 patients), d-Chlorpheniramine (189 patients), Clemastine (146 patients)

In addition to the more frequent side effects reported in clinical trials, adverse effects have been reported at a lower incidence in clinical trials and/or spontaneously during marketing of terfenadine that warrant listing as possibly associated with drug administration. These include: alopecia (hair loss or thinning), anaphylaxis, angioedema, bronchospasm, confusion, depression, galactorrhea, insomnia, menstrual disorder (including dysmenorrhea), musculoskeletal symptoms, nightmares, paresthesia, photosensitivity, rapid flare of psoriasis, seizures, sinus tachycardia, sweating, thrombocytopenia, tremor, urinary frequency and visual disturbances.

In clinical trials, severe instances of mild, or in one case, moderate transaminase elevations were seen in patients receiving terfenadine. Mild elevations were also seen in placebo treated patients. Marketing experiences include isolated reports of jaundice, cholestatic hepatitis, and hepatitis. In most cases available information is incomplete.

OVERDOSAGE:

Signs and symptoms of overdosage may be absent or mild (*e.g.,* headache, nausea, confusion); but adverse cardiac events including cardiac arrest, ventricular arrhythmias including torsades de pointes and QT prolongation have been reported at overdoses of 360 mg or more and occur more frequently at doses in excess of 600 mg, and QTc prolongations of up to 30% have been observed at a dose of 300 mg b.i.d. Seizures and syncope have also been reported. USE OF DOSES IN EXCESS OF 60 MG B.I.D. IS NOT RECOMMENDED. (See BOXED WARNING, CLINICAL PHARMACOLOGY, and ADVERSE REACTIONS).

In overdose cases where ventricular arrhythmias are associated with significant QTc prolongation, treatment with antiarrhythmics known to prolong QTc intervals is not recommended.

Therefore, in cases of overdosage, cardiac monitoring for at least 24 hours is recommended and for as long as QTc is prolonged, along with standard measures to remove any unabsorbed drug. Limited experience with the use of hemoperfusion (n=1) or hemodialysis (n=3) was not successful in completely removing the acid metabolite of terfenadine from the blood.

Treatment of the signs and symptoms of overdosage should be symptomatic and supportive after the acute stage.

Oral LD_{50} values for terfenadine were greater than 5000 mg/kg in mature mice and rats. The oral LD_{50} was 438 mg/kg in newborn rats.

DOSAGE AND ADMINISTRATION:

One tablet (60 mg) twice daily for adults and pediatric patients 12 years and older.

USE OF DOSES IN EXCESS OF 60 MG B.I.D. IS NOT RECOMMENDED BECAUSE OF THE INCREASED POTENTIAL FOR QT INTERVAL PROLONGATIONS AND ADVERSE CARDIAC EVENTS. (See BOXED WARNING).USE OF TERFENADINE IN PATIENTS WITH SIGNIFICANT HEPATIC DYSFUNCTION AND IN PATIENTS TAKING KETOCONAZOLE, ITRACONAZOLE, CLARITHROMYCIN, ERYTHROMYCIN OR TROLEANDOMYCIN IS CONTRAINDICATED. (See CONTRAINDICATIONS, WARNINGS, and DRUG INTERACTIONS).

PATIENT PACKAGE INSERT:

This leaflet is a summary of important information about terfenadine. Be sure to ask your doctor if you have any questions or want to know more.

What is Terfenadine and What is it Used For? Terfenadine is an antihistamine. It is used to relieve symptoms of seasonal allergies or hay fever. These symptoms include runny nose, sneezing, itching of the nose or throat, and itchy watery eyes.

Clinical studies conducted to date with terfenadine have not demonstrated effectiveness in relieving the symptoms of the common cold.

How Do I Take Terfenadine? Take terfenadine only as needed when you have symptoms of seasonal allergy or hay fever.

The recommended dose of terfenadine is one tablet taken twice a day. **DO NOT TAKE MORE OFTEN THAN ONE TABLET EVERY TWELVE HOURS**

Follow any other instructions your doctor gives you.

What Are the Important Warnings About Using terfenadine? WARNING: DO NOT USE TERFENADINE IF YOU ARE USING KETOCONAZOLE (NIZORAL), ITRACONAZOLE (SPORANOX), ERYTHROMYCIN, CLARITHROMYCIN (BIAXIN), OR TROLEANDOMYCIN (TAO). IF YOU HAVE ANY LIVER OR HEART PROBLEMS, TALK TO YOUR DOCTOR BEFORE YOU USE TERFENADINE.

Do not use terfenadine with any other prescription or nonprescription medicines without first talking to your doctor and pharmacist.

If you faint, become dizzy, have any unusual heartbeats, or any other unusual symptoms while using terfenadine, contact your doctor.

If you become pregnant or are nursing a baby, talk your doctor about whether you should take terfenadine. Your doctor will decide whether you should take terfenadine based on the benefits and the risks.

What Are the Risks of Using Terfenadine? The side effects which occur most often are headaches and mild stomach or intestinal problems.

In rare cases, terfenadine has caused **IRREGULAR HEARTBEATS** which may cause serious problems like fainting, dizziness, cardiac arrest, or death. In these rare cases, this occurred when terfenadine was taken:

in more than the recommended dose (remember, do not take more often than one tablet every twelve hours);

with the antifungal drugs ketoconazole (Nizoral), or itraconazole (Sporanox);

with the antibiotic drugs erythromycin, clarithromycin (Biaxin), or troleandomycin (TAO);

by patients with serious liver disease.

How do I Store Terfenadine? Terfenadine should be stored in a tightly closed container, in a cool place, out of direct sunlight. It should be kept away from children.

HOW SUPPLIED:

Seldane Tablets are round, white, and debossed "SELDANE". Store tablets at controlled room temperature (59-86°F) (15-30°C). Protect from exposure to temperatures above 104°F (40°C) and moisture.

HOW SUPPLIED - EQUIVALENTS NOT AVAILABLE:

Tablet, Plain Coated - Oral - 60 mg

30's	$37.50	SELDANE, Hoechst Marion Roussel	00068-0723-30
100's	$93.96	SELDANE, Hoechst Marion Roussel	00068-0723-61
500's	$469.92	SELDANE, Hoechst Marion Roussel	00068-0723-65

TERODILINE HYDROCHLORIDE *(003092)*

CATEGORIES: Anticholinergic Agents; Gastrointestinal Drugs; Urinary Incontinence; FDA Unapproved

BRAND NAMES: *Mictrol*; **Micturin**
(International brand names outside U.S. in italics)

Prescribing information not available at time of publication.

TESTOLACTONE *(002317)*

CATEGORIES: Anabolic Steroids; Antineoplastics; Breast Carcinoma; Hormones; Oncologic Drugs; Pregnancy Category C; FDA Approval Pre 1982

BRAND NAMES: *Fludestrin*; **Teslac**
(International brand names outside U.S. in italics)

FORMULARIES: Aetna; Medi-Cal

Prescribing information not available at time of publication.

HOW SUPPLIED - EQUIVALENTS NOT AVAILABLE:

Tablet, Uncoated - Oral - 50 mg

100's	$129.08	TESLAC, Bristol Myers Squibb	00003-0690-50

TESTOSTERONE *(002318)*

CATEGORIES: Anabolic Steroids; Androgens; Antineoplastics; Hormones; Oncologic Drugs; Pharmaceutical Adjuvants; DEA Class CIII; FDA Approval Pre 1982

BRAND NAMES: Andro 100; Androderm; Androlan; Andronaq-50; Histerone-; Homogene-S; *Malogen*; Shotest; Testamone-100; Testoderm Transdermal; Testoject-50; Testolin; Testopel; Testro Aq; Theraderm
(International brand names outside U.S. in italics)

FORMULARIES: BC-BS; Medi-Cal; WHO

DESCRIPTION:

Androderm (testosterone transdermal system) provides continuous delivery of testosterone (the primary endogenous androgen) for 24 hours following application to intact, non-scrotal skin (*e.g.*, back, abdomen, thighs, upper arms).

Each Androderm system delivers *in vivo* 2.5 mg of testosterone per day across skin of average permeability.

Androderm has a 7.5 cm^2 central drug delivery reservoir surrounded by a peripheral adhesive area. The total contact surface area is 37 cm^2. Each system contains 12.2 mg testosterone USP, dissolved in an alcohol-based gel. Testosterone USP is a white, or creamy white crystalline powder or crystals chemically described as 17β- hydroxyandrost-4-en-3-one.

The Androderm system has six components. Proceeding from the top toward the surface attached to the skin, the system is composed of (1) a transparent ethylene vinyl acetate copolymer/polyester laminate backing film, (2) a drug reservoir of testosterone USP, alcohol USP, glycerin USP, glycerol monooleate, and methyl laurate gelled with an acrylic acid copolymer, (3) a permeable polyethylene microporous membrane, and (4) a peripheral layer of acrylic adhesive surrounding the central, active drug delivery area of the system. Prior to opening of the system and application to the skin, the central delivery surface of the system is sealed with a peelable laminate disc (5) composed of a five-layer laminate containing polyester/polyesterurethane adhesive/aluminum foil/polyesterurethane adhesive/polyethylene. Then disc is attached to and removed with the release liner (6), a silicone-coated polyester film, which is removed before the system can be used.

The active ingredient in the system is testosterone. The remaining components of the system are pharmacologically inactive.

CLINICAL PHARMACOLOGY:

Testosterone transdermal system delivers physiologic amounts of testosterone producing circulating testosterone concentrations that approximate the normal circadian rhythm of healthy young men.

Testosterone: Testosterone transdermal system delivers testosterone, the primary androgenic hormone. Testosterone is responsible for the normal growth and development of the male sex organs and for maintenance of secondary sex characteristics. These effects include the growth and maturation of the prostate, seminal vesicles, penis, and scrotum; development of male hair distribution, such as facial, pubic, chest, and axillary hair; laryngeal enlargement; vocal cord thickening; and alterations in body musculature and fat distribution.

Male hypogonadism results from insufficient secretion of testosterone and is characterized by low serum testosterone concentrations. Symptoms associated with male hypogonadism include the following: impotence and decreased sexual desire; fatigue and loss of energy; mood depression; and regression of secondary sexual characteristics.

General Androgen Effects: Androgens promote retention of nitrogen, sodium, potassium, and phosphorus, and decreased urinary excretion of calcium. Androgens have been reported to increase protein anabolism and decrease protein catabolism. Nitrogen balance is improved only when there is sufficient intake of calories and protein.

Androgens are also responsible for the growth spurt of adolescence and for the eventual termination of linear growth which is brought about by the fusion of the epiphyseal growth centers. In children, exogenous androgens accelerate linear growth rates but may cause disproportionate advancement in bone maturation. Use over long periods may result in fusion of the epiphyseal growth centers and termination of the growth process.

Androgens have been reported to stimulate the production of red blood cells by enhancing erythropoietin production.

During exogenous administration of androgens, endogenous testosterone release is inhibited through feed-back inhibition of pituitary LH secretion. With large doses of exogenous androgens, spermatogenesis may also be suppressed through feedback inhibition of pituitary follicle stimulating hormone (FSH) secretion.

There is a lack of substantial evidence that androgens are effective in accelerating fracture healing or in shortening post-surgical convalescence.

PHARMACOKINETICS

Absorption: Following testosterone transdermal system application to non-scrotal skin, testosterone is continuously absorbed during the 24-hour dosing period. Daily application of 2 systems at approximately 10 PM results in a serum testosterone concentration profile that mimics the normal circadian variation observed in healthy young men. Maximum concentrations occur in the early morning hours with minimum concentrations in the evening (TABLE 1).

TABLE 1 Steady-state serum testosterone pharmacokinetic parameters in hypogonadal men measured during continuous testosterone transdermal system treatment.

Parameter	Units	n	Mean	SD
C_{max}	ng/dl	56	753	276
C_{avg}	ng/dl	56	498	169
C_{min}	ng/dl	56	246	120
T_{max}	hr	56	7.9	2.2
$T_{1/2}$	min	29	71	32
Cl	l/day	49	1304	464

C_{max}=maximum serum concentration
Cavg=average serum concentration (AUC/24 hr)
C_{min}=minimum serum concentration
T_{max}=time of maximum serum concentration
$T_{1/2}$=elimination half-life
Cl=clearance

In a group of 34 hypogonadal men, application of two testosterone transdermal systems to the abdomen, back, thighs, or upper arms resulted in average testosterone absorption of 4 to 5 mg over 24 hours. The serum testosterone concentration profiles during application were similar for these sites (TABLE 2). Applications to the chest and shins resulted in greater inter- individual variability and average 24 hour absorption of 3 to 4 mg.

TABLE 2 Mean serum testosterone concentrations (ng/dl) measured during single-dose applications of 2 testosterone transdermal system applied at night to different sites in 34-hypogonadal men.

Sample	Abdomen		Back		Thigh		Upper Arm	
Time (hr)	Mean	SD	Mean	SD	Mean	SD	Mean	SD
0	90	82	80	74	85	76	81	69
3	286	201	429	252	271	201	308	226
6	476	236	608	250	489	254	468	245
9	570	234	613	214	592	251	534	204
12	575	244	588	233	594	247	527	199
24	352	164	403	174	367	161	332	124

CLINICAL PHARMACOLOGY: *(cont'd)*

In a steady-state study of 12 hypogonadal men, nightly application of 1, 2, or 3 testosterone transdermal systems resulted in increases in the mean morning serum testosterone concentrations. Thee concentrations averaged 424, 584, and 766 ng/dl with the application of 1, 2, and 3 systems, respectively. The mean baseline serum testosterone concentration was 76 ng/dl.

Normal range morning serum testosterone concentrations are reached during the first day of dosing. There is no accumulation of testosterone during continuous treatment.

Distribution: In serum, testosterone is bound with high affinity to sex hormone binding globulin (SHBG) and with low affinity to albumin. The albumin bound portion easily dissociates and is presumed to be bioactive. The SHBG-bound portion is not considered to be bioactive. The amount of SHBG in serum and the total testosterone concentration determine the distribution of bioactive and non-bioactive androgen.

Bioactive serum testosterone concentrations (BT) measured during testosterone transdermal system treatment paralleled the serum testosterone profile and remained within the normal reference range.

Metabolism: Inactivation of testosterone occurs primarily in the liver. Testosterone (T) is metabolized to various 17-keto steroids through two different pathways, and the major active metabolites are estradiol (E2) and dihydrotestosterone (DHT). DHT binds with greater affinity to SHBG than does testosterone. In reproductive tissues, DHT is further metabolized to 3-alpha and 3-beta androstanediol.

In many tissues, the activity of testosterone appears to depend on reduction to DHT, which binds to cytosol receptor proteins. The steroid- receptor complex is transported to the nucleus, where it initiates transcription events and cellular changes related to androgen action.

During steady-state pharmacokinetic studies in hypogonadal men treated with testosterone transdermal system, the average DHT:T and E2:T ratios were comparable to those in normal men, approximately 1:10 and 1:200, respectively.

Upon removal of the testosterone transdermal systems, serum testosterone concentrations decrease with an apparent half-life of approximately 70 minutes. Hypogonadal concentrations are reached within 24 hours following system removal.

Testosterone transdermal system therapy suppresses endogenous testosterone secretion via the pituitary/gonadal axis, resulting in a reduction in baseline serum testosterone concentrations compared to the untreated state.

Excretion: Approximately 90% of a testosterone dose given intramuscularly is excreted in the urine as glucuronide and sulfate conjugates of testosterone and its metabolites; about 6% is excreted in the feces, mostly in unconjugated form.

SPECIAL POPULATIONS

Geriatric: No age related effects on testosterone pharmacokinetics were observed in clinical trials of testosterone transdermal system in men up to 65 years of age. In a group of 9 elderly testosterone deficient men (65-79 years of age, average baseline testosterone level 184 ± 50 ng/dl), a single application of 2 testosterone transdermal systems to the back resulted in an average testosterone level of 591 ± 121 ng/dl with a T_{max} of 14.2 ± 4.2 hours. The total testosterone concentration delivered over the 24-hour application time was 3.8 ± 0.6 mg, approximately 20% less than the average amount delivered in younger patients.

Race: There is insufficient information available from testosterone transdermal system trials to compare testosterone pharmacokinetics in different racial groups.

Renal Insufficiency: There is no experience with use of testosterone transdermal system in patients with renal insufficiency.

Hepatic Insufficiency: There is no experience with use of testosterone transdermal system in patients with hepatic insufficiency.

Drug-Drug Interactions: See PRECAUTIONS.

CLINICAL STUDIES:

In clinical studies, 93% of patients were treated with two testosterone transdermal systems daily, 6% used three systems daily, and 1% used one system daily.

The hormonal effects of testosterone transdermal system as a treatment for male hypogonadism were demonstrated in four open-label trials that included 94 hypogonadal men, ages 15 to 65 years. In these trials, testosterone transdermal system produced average morning serum testosterone concentrations within the normal reference range in 92% of patients. The mean (SD) serum hormone concentrations and percentage of patients who achieved average concentrations within the normal ranges are shown in TABLE 3.

TABLE 3 Individual morning serum hormone concentrations (ng/dl) and percent of patients with mean concentrations within the normal range during continuous testosterone transdermal system treatment (n=94).

Normal Range	T (306-1031)	BT (93-420)	DHT (28-85)	E2 (0.9-3.6)
Mean	589	312	47	2.7
SD	209	127	18	1.2
% Normal	92	88	85	77
% High	1	12	2	22
% Low	7	0	13	1

A physiological suppression of the pituitary/gonadal axis occurs during continuous testosterone transdermal system treatment leading to reduced serum LH concentrations. In clinical trials, 10 of 21 (48%) of men with primary (hypergonadotropic) hypogonadism achieved normal range LH concentrations within 6 to 12 months of treatment. LH concentrations may remain elevated in some patients despite serum testosterone concentrations within the normal range.

Twenty-nine patients, previously treated with testosterone, completed 12 months of testosterone transdermal system treatment. Following an 8-week androgen withdrawal period. Testosterone transdermal system treatment produced positive effects on fatigue, mood and sexual function. The percent of patients complaining of fatigue decreased from 79% to 10% during treatment ($p<0.001$). The average patient depression score (Beck Depression Inventory) decreased from 6.9 to 3.9 ($p<0.001$). Nocturnal penile tumescence and rigidity monitoring showed an increase in mean duration of erections 0.23 to 0.39 hours per night ($p=0.01$) and an increase in penile tip rigidity from 18% to 50% ($p<0.001$). The total number of self-reported erections reported increased from 2.3 to 7.8 per week ($p<0.001$).

Comparison with Intramuscular Testosterone: Sixty-six patients, previously treated with testosterone injections, received testosterone transdermal system or intramuscular testosterone enanthate (200 mg every 2 weeks) treatment for 6 months. The percent of time that serum concentrations measured throughout the dosing interval remained within the normal range are found in TABLE 4.

Effects on Plasma Lipids: In 67 men treated for 6 to 12 months, the average (SE) serum total cholesterol and HDL concentrations were 199 (7.6) ng/dl and 46 (2.3) ng/dl.

Compared to baseline values during hypogonadal state achieved by 8 weeks of androgen withdrawal in 29 patients, the following changes in lipids were observed during 1 year of testosterone transdermal system treatment: Cholesterol decreased 1.2%; HDL decreased 8%;

CLINICAL STUDIES: *(cont'd)*

TABLE 4

	Androderm	IM	p value
T	82%	72%	0.05
BT	87%	39%	<0.001
DHT	76%	70%	0.06
E2	81%	35%	<0.001

Sexual function was comparable between groups.

Cholesterol/HDL ratio increased 9%. In these patients, lipids measured during testosterone transdermal system treatment were not significantly different from those measured during prior IM injection treatment.

Effects on the Prostate: Prostate size and serum prostate specific antigen (PSA) concentrations during treatment were comparable to values reported for eugonadal men. One case of prostate carcinoma occurred during testosterone transdermal system treatment; two cases were detected during IM treatment.

INDICATIONS AND USAGE:

Testosterone transdermal system is indicated for testosterone replacement therapy in men for conditions associated with a deficiency or absence of endogenous testosterone.

Primary hypogonadism (congenital or acquired)—Testicular failure due to cryptorchidism, bilateral torsion, orchitis, vanishing testis syndrome, or orchidectomy, Klinefelter's syndrome, chemotherapy, or toxic damage from alcohol or heavy metals. These men usually have low serum testosterone concentrations accompanied by gonadotropins (FSH, LH) above the normal range.

Secondary,(*i.e.,* hypogonadotropic hypogonadism (congenital or acquired)), idiopathic gonadotropin or luteinizing hormone-releasing hormone (LHRH) deficiency, or pituitary-hypothalamic injury from tumors, trauma, or radiation. These men have low serum testosterone concentrations without associated elevation in gonadotropins. Appropriate adrenal cortical and thyroid hormone replacement therapy may be necessary in patients with multiple pituitary or hypothalamic abnormalities.

CONTRAINDICATIONS:

Androgens are contraindicated in men with carcinoma of the breast or known or suspected carcinoma of the prostate.

Testosterone transdermal system therapy has not been evaluated in women and must not be used in women. Testosterone may cause fetal harm.

Testosterone transdermal system is contraindicated in patients with known hypersensitivity to any of its components.

WARNINGS:

Prolonged use of high doses of orally active 17-alpha-alkyl androgens (*e.g.,* methyltestosterone) has been associated with the development of peliosis hepatis, cholestatic jaundice and hepatic neoplasms, including hepatocellular carcinoma (see PRECAUTIONS, Carcinogenesis.) Peliosis hepatis can be a life-threatening or fatal complication. Testosterone is not known to produce these adverse effects.

Geriatric patients treated with androgens may be at an increased risk for the development of prostatic hyperplasia and prostatic carcinoma (see PRECAUTIONS, Carcinogenesis.)

Edema, with or without congestive heart failure, may be a serious complication of androgen treatment in patients with preexisting cardiac, renal, or hepatic disease. In addition to discontinuation of the drug, diuretic therapy may be required.

Gynecomastia frequently develops and occasionally persists in patients being treated for hypogonadism.

PRECAUTIONS:

GENERAL

The physician should instruct patients to report any of the following side effects of androgens:

Too frequent or persistent erections of the penis

Any nausea, vomiting, jaundice, or ankle swelling

Virilization of female sexual partners has been reported with male use of a topical testosterone solution. Topically applied creams leave as much as 90 mg residual testosterone on the skin. The occlusive backing film on testosterone transdermal system prevents the partner from coming in contact with the active material in the system. Transfer of the system to the partner is unlikely.

Changes in body hair distribution, significant increase in acne, or other signs of virilization of the female partner should be brought to the attention of a physician.

INFORMATION FOR THE PATIENT

An information brochure is available for patients concerning the use od testosterone transdermal system.

Advise patients of the following:

Testosterone transdermal system should not be applied to the scrotum.

Testosterone transdermal system does not have to be removed during sexual intercourse, nor while taking a shower or bath.

Testosterone transdermal systems should be applied nightly.

LABORATORY TESTS

Hemoglobin and hematocrit should be checked periodically to detect polycythemia in patients who are receiving androgen therapy.

Liver function, prostate specific antigen, total cholesterol and HDL cholesterol should be checked periodically.

DRUG/LABORATORY TEST INTERFERENCES

Androgens may decrease levels of thyroxine-binding globulin, resulting in decreased total T_4serum levels and increased resin uptake of T_3 and T_4. Free thyroid hormone levels remain unchanged, however, and there is no clinical evidence of thyroid dysfunction.

CARCINOGENESIS, MUTAGENESIS, IMPAIRMENT OF FERTILITY

Animal Data: Testosterone has been tested by subcutaneous injection and implantation in mice and rats. The implant induced cervical-uterine tumors in mice, which metastasized in some cases. There is suggestive evidence that injection of testosterone into some strains of female mice increases their susceptibility to hepatoma. Testosterone is also known to increase the number of tumors and decrease the degree of differentiation of chemically induced carcinomas of the liver in rats.

Human Data: There are rare reports of hepatocellular carcinoma in patients receiving long-term therapy with androgens in high-doses. Withdrawal of drugs did not lead to regression of the tumors in all cases.

PRECAUTIONS: *(cont'd)*

Geriatric patients treated with androgens may be at an increased risk for the development of prostatic hyperplasia and prostatic carcinoma.

PREGNANCY CATEGORY X

(See CONTRAINDICATIONS.)

Teratogenic Effects: Testosterone transdermal system must not be used in women.

NURSING MOTHERS

Testosterone transdermal system must not be used in women.

PEDIATRIC USE

Testosterone transdermal system has not been evaluated clinically in males under 15 years of age.

DRUG INTERACTIONS:

Anticoagulants: C-17 substituted derivatives of testosterone, such as methandrostenolone, have been reported to decrease the anticoagulant requirements of patients receiving oral anticoagulants. Patients receiving oral anticoagulants require close monitoring especially when androgens are started or stopped.

Oxyphenbutazone: Concurrent administration of oxyphenbutazone and androgens may result in elevated serum levels of oxyphenbutazone.

Insulin: In diabetic patients, the metabolic effects of androgens may decrease blood glucose and, therefore, insulin requirements.

ADVERSE REACTIONS:

Adverse Events Associated With Testosterone Transdermal System: In clinical studies of 122 patients treated with testosterone transdermal system, the most common adverse events reported were local effects. Transient mild to moderate erythema was observed at the site of application in the majority of patients at some time during treatment.

The adverse reactions reported by more than 1% of patients are listed in TABLE 5, shown in order of decreasing frequency.

TABLE 5

Event	Percent of Patients
pruritus at application site	37%
blister reaction under system	12%
erythema at application site	7%
vesicles at application site	6%
prostate abnormalities	5%
headache	4%
allergic contact dermatitis to the system	4%
burning at application site	3%
induration at application site	3%
depression	3%
rash	2%
gastrointestinal bleeding	2%

The following reactions occurred in less than 1% of patients: fatigue; body pain; pelvic pain; hypertension; peripheral vascular disease; increased appetite; accelerated growth; anxiety; confusion; decreased libido; paresthesia; thinking abnormalities; vertigo; acne; bullae at application site; mechanical irritation at application site; rash at application site; contamination of application site; prostate carcinoma; dysuria; hematuria; impotence; urinary incontinence; urinary tract infection; testicular abnormalities.

Chronic skin irritation caused 5% of patients to discontinue treatment. Chronic, mild irritation may be ameliorated by local treatment of application sites with over-the counter topical hydrocortisone cream or topical antihistamine products.

The five cases of localized allergic reactions to the testosterone transdermal system system occurred within 3 to 8 weeks following initiation of treatment. Rechallenge with components of the system showed ethanol sensitization in 4 patients. One reaction was attributed to testosterone. These patients experienced no adverse sequelae related to oral alcohol ingestion or injectable testosterone use. Older patients may be more prone to develop allergic contact dermatitis.

Local blister reactions, characterized by erythema and vesicles or bullae at the site of testosterone transdermal system application occurred at a rate of approximately 1 in 6,500 system applications. The majority of these reactions were associated with system application over bony prominences on the body. These reactions were self-limited and patients continued testosterone transdermal system treatment.

TESTOSTERONE TRANSDERMAL SYSTEM EVENTS ASSOCIATED WITH INJECTION OR ORAL TREATMENTS

Skin and Appendages: Hirsutism, male pattern baldness, seborrhea, and acne.

Endocrine and Urogenital: Gynecomastia and excessive frequency and duration of penile erections. Oligospermia may occur at high dosages(see CLINICAL PHARMACOLOGY.)

Fluid and Electrolyte Disturbances: Retention of sodium, chloride, water, potassium, calcium, and inorganic phosphates.

Gastrointestinal: Nausea, cholestatic jaundice, alterations in liver function tests. Rare instances of hepatocellular neoplasms and peliosis hepatis have occurred (see WARNINGS.)

Hematologic: Suppression of clotting factors II, V, VII, and X; bleeding in patients on concomitant anticoagulant therapy and polycythemia.

Nervous System: Increased or decreased libido, headache, anxiety, depression and generalized paresthesia.

Metabolic: Increased serum cholesterol.

Miscellaneous: Rarely, anaphylactoid reactions.

DRUG ABUSE AND DEPENDENCE:

Testosterone transdermal system is a Schedule III controlled substance under the Anabolic Steroids Control Act.

Oral consumption of the testosterone transdermal system or the gel contents of the system will not result in clinically significant serum testosterone concentrations in the target organs due to extensive first-pass metabolism.

OVERDOSAGE:

There is one report of acute overdosage with testosterone enanthate injection: testosterone levels of up to 11,400 ng/dl were implicated in a cerebrovascular accident.

DOSAGE AND ADMINISTRATION:

THE USUAL STARTING DOSE IS TWO TESTOSTERONE TRANSDERMAL SYSTEMS APPLIED NIGHTLY FOR 24 HOURS, PROVIDING A TOTAL DOSE OF 5 MG/DAY.

DOSAGE AND ADMINISTRATION: *(cont'd)*

THE ADHESIVE SIDE OF THE TESTOSTERONE TRANSDERMAL SYSTEM SHOULD BE APPLIED TO A CLEAN, DRY AREA OF THE SKIN ON THE BACK, ABDOMEN, UPPER ARMS, OR THIGHS. BONY PROMINENCES, SUCH AS THE SHOULDER AND HIP AREAS, SHOULD BE AVOIDED. DO NOT APPLY TO THE SCROTUM. THE SITES OF APPLICATION SHOULD BE ROTATED, WITH AN INTERVAL OF 7 DAYS BETWEEN APPLICATIONS TO THE SAME SITE. THE AREA SELECTED SHOULD NOT BE OILY, DAMAGED, OR IRRITATED. (SEE TABLE 2.)

THE SYSTEM SHOULD BE APPLIED IMMEDIATELY AFTER OPENING THE POUCH AND REMOVING THE PROTECTIVE RELEASE LINER. THE SYSTEM SHOULD BE PRESSED FIRMLY IN PLACE, MAKING SURE THERE IS GOOD CONTACT WITH THE SKIN, ESPECIALLY AROUND THE EDGES.

TO ENSURE PROPER DOSING, THE MORNING SERUM TESTOSTERONE CONCENTRATION MAY BE MEASURED FOLLOWING SYSTEM APPLICATION THE PREVIOUS EVENING. IF THE SERUM CONCENTRATION IS OUTSIDE THE NORMAL RANGE, SAMPLING SHOULD BE REPEATED WITH ASSURANCE OF PROPER SYSTEM ADHESION AS WELL AS APPROPRIATE APPLICATION TIME. CONFIRMED SERUM CONCENTRATIONS OUTSIDE THE NORMAL RANGE MAY REQUIRE INCREASING THE DOSING REGIMEN TO 3 SYSTEMS, OR DECREASING THE REGIMEN TO 1 SYSTEM, MAINTAINING NIGHTLY APPLICATION. BECAUSE OF VARIABILITY IN ANALYTICAL VALUES AMONG DIAGNOSTIC LABORATORIES, THIS LABORATORY WORK AND ANY LATER ANALYSES FOR ASSESSING THE EFFECT OF TESTOSTERONE TRANSDERMAL SYSTEM THERAPY, SHOULD BE PERFORMED AT THE SAME LABORATORY SO RESULTS CAN BE MORE EASILY COMPARED.

TESTOSTERONE TRANSDERMAL SYSTEM THERAPY FOR NON-VIRILIZED PATIENTS MAY BE INITIATED WITH ONE SYSTEM APPLIED NIGHTLY.

REFERENCES:

1. Mazer NA, et al. Mimicking the circadian pattern of testosterone and metabolite levels with an enhanced transdermal delivery system. In Gurney, Junjinger, Peppas, eds. *Pulsatile Drug Delivery: Current Applications and Future Trends.* Stuttgart: Wiss. Veri.-Ges.; 1993, 73-97.

HOW SUPPLIED:

Each system contains 12.2 mg testosterone USP for delivery of 2.5 mg of testosterone per day (see DESCRIPTION.)

Storage and Disposal: Store at room temperature, 15° to 30°C (59° to 86°F). Apply to skin immediately upon removal from the protective pouch. Do not store outside the pouch provided. Damaged systems should not be used. The drug reservoir may be burst by excessive pressure or heat. Discard systems in household trash in a manner that prevents accidental application or ingestion by children, pets or others.

HOW SUPPLIED - EQUIVALENTS NOT AVAILABLE:

Film, Continuous Release - Percutaneous - 4 mg/24 hr

30's	$59.80	TESTODERM TRANSDERMAL, Alza	17314-4608-03

Film, Continuous Release - Percutaneous - 6 mg/24 hr

30's	$59.80	TESTODERM TRANSDERMAL, Alza	17314-4609-03

Injection, Susp - Intramuscular - 25 mg/ml

10 ml	$1.60	ANDROLAN, Lannett	00527-0121-55
10 ml	$4.90	Testosterone, Major Pharms	00904-0874-10
30 ml	$4.35	Testosterone Aqueous, Rugby	00536-9100-75

Injection, Susp - Intramuscular - 50 mg/ml

10 ml	$2.40	ANDROLAN, Lannett	00527-0106-55
10 ml	$7.20	Testosterone, Major Pharms	00904-0875-10
10 ml	$8.50	Testosterone, Hyrex Pharms	00314-0083-10

Injection, Susp - Intramuscular - 100 mg/ml

10 ml	$3.80	ANDROLAN, Lannett	00527-0199-55
10 ml	$8.45	TESTOLIN, Pasadena	00418-0791-41
10 ml	$10.50	TESTRO AQ, C O Truxton	00463-1069-10
10 ml	$10.75	Testosterone, United Res	00677-0310-21
10 ml	$10.79	Testosterone, Schein Pharm (US)	00364-6607-54
10 ml	$10.79	Sterile Testosterone, Steris Labs	00402-0084-10
10 ml	$10.88	Testosterone, Hyrex Pharms	00314-0771-70
10 ml	$13.75	Testosterone, Goldline Labs	00182-0714-63
10 ml	$13.80	Testosterone, Geneva Pharms	00781-3093-70
10 ml	$15.75	Testosterone Aqueous, Rugby	00536-9500-70
10 ml	$18.38	Testosterone In Oil, Rugby	00536-8900-70
30 ml	$16.46	Testosterone, Schein Pharm (US)	00364-6607-56
30 ml	$16.46	Sterile Testosterone, Steris Labs	00402-0084-30
30 ml	$16.58	Testosterone In Oil, Rugby	00536-8900-75

Patch - Percutaneous - 2.5 mg/24 hr

60's	$97.50	ANDRODERM, SKB Pharms	00007-3155-18

Pellet - Intravenous - 75 mg

3's	$45.00	TESTOPEL, Bartor Pharcal	10116-1001-01
10's	$150.00	TESTOPEL, Bartor Pharcal	10116-1001-02
100's	$1500.00	TESTOPEL, Bartor Pharcal	10116-1001-03

Powder

5 gm	$14.20	Testosterone, Paddock Labs	00574-0460-05
25 gm	$59.60	Testosterone, Paddock Labs	00574-0460-25

TESTOSTERONE CYPIONATE *(002319)*

CATEGORIES: Anabolic Steroids; Androgens; Cryptorchidism; Hormones; Hypogonadism; Orchitis; Orchidectomy; Vanishing Testis Syndrome; Pregnancy Category X; DEA Class CIII; FDA Approval Pre 1982

BRAND NAMES: Andro-Cyp; Andronaq-La; D-Tes; Dep-Andro; **Depo-Testosterone**; Depotest; Dura-Testosterone; Duratest; Meditest; Shotest; T-Cypionate; Testa-C; Testaspan; Testoject; Testred Cypionate 200; Vigorex; Virilon Im

DESCRIPTION:

Testosterone Cypionate Sterile Solution, for intramuscular injection, contains testosterone cypionate which is the oil-soluble 17 (beta)-cyclopentylpropionate ester of the androgenic hormone testosterone.

Testosterone cypionate is a white or creamy white crystalline powder, odorless or nearly so and stable in air. It is insoluble in water, freely soluble in alcohol, chloroform, dioxane, ether, and soluble in vegetable oils.

The chemical name for testosterone cypionate is androst-4-en-3-one,

DESCRIPTION: *(cont'd)*

17-(3-cyclopentyl-1-oxopropoxy)-, (17β)-. Its molecular formula is $C_{27}H_{40}O_3$, and the molecular weight 412.61.

Testosterone Cypionate is available in two strengths, 100 mg/ml and 200 mg/ml testosterone cypionate.

Each ml of the **100 mg/ml** solution contains:
Testosterone cypionate: 100 mg
Benzyl benzoate: 0.1 ml
Cottonseed oil: 736 mg
Benzyl alcohol (as preservative): 9.45 mg

Each ml of the **200 mg/ml** solution contains:
Testosterone cypionate: 200 mg
Benzyl benzoate: 0.2 ml
Cottonseed oil: 560 mg
Benzyl alcohol (as preservative): 9.45 mg

CLINICAL PHARMACOLOGY:

Endogenous androgens are responsible for normal growth and development of the male sex organs and for maintenance of secondary sex characteristics. These effects include growth and maturation of the prostate, seminal vesicles, penis, and scrotum; development of male hair distribution, such as beard, pubic, chest, and axillary hair; laryngeal enlargement, vocal cord thickening, and alterations in body musculature and fat distribution. Drugs in this class also cause retention of nitrogen, sodium, potassium, and phosphorous, and decreased urinary excretion of calcium. Androgens have been reported to increase protein anabolism and decrease protein catabolism. Nitrogen balance is improved only when there is sufficient intake of calories and protein.

Androgens are responsible for the growth spurt of adolescence and for eventual termination of linear growth, brought about by fusion of the epiphyseal growth centers. In children, exogenous androgens accelerate linear growth rates, but may cause disproportionate advancement in bone maturation. Use over long periods may result in fusion of the epiphyseal growth centers and termination of the growth process. Androgens have been reported to stimulate production of red blood cells by enhancing production of erythropoietic stimulation factor.

During exogenous administration of androgens, endogenous testosterone release is inhibited through feedback inhibition of pituitary luteinizing hormone (LH). At large doses of exogenous androgens, spermatogenesis may also be suppressed through feedback inhibition of pituitary follicle stimulating hormone (FSH).

There is a lack of substantial evidence that androgens are effective in fractures, surgery, convalescence, and functional uterine bleeding.

Pharmacokinetics: Testosterone esters are less polar than free testosterone. Testosterone esters in oil injected intramuscularly are absorbed slowly from the lipid phase; thus, testosterone cypionate can be given at intervals of two to four weeks.

Testosterone in plasma is 98 percent bound to a specific testosterone-estradiol binding globulin, and about 2 percent is free. Generally, the amount of this sex-hormone binding globulin in the plasma will determine the distribution of testosterone between free and bound forms, and the free testosterone concentration will determine its half-life.

About 90 percent of a dose of testosterone is excreted in the urine as glucuronic and sulfuric acid conjugates of testosterone and its metabolites; about 6 percent of a dose is excreted in the feces, mostly in the unconjugated form. Inactivation of testosterone occurs primarily in the liver. Testosterone is metabolized to various 17-keto steroids through two different pathways.

The half-life of testosterone cypionate when injected intramuscularly is approximately eight days.

In many tissues the activity of testosterone appears to depend on reduction to dihydrotestosterone, which binds to cytosol receptor proteins. The steroid-receptor complex is transported to the nucleus where it initiates transcription events and cellular changes related to androgen action.

INDICATIONS AND USAGE:

Testosterone Cypionate Sterile Solution is indicated for replacement therapy in the male in conditions associated with symptoms of deficiency or absence of endogenous testosterone.

1. Primary hypogonadism (congenital or acquired)-testicular failure due to cryptorchidism, bilateral torsion, orchitis, vanishing testis syndrome; or orchidectomy.

2. Hypogonadotropic hypogonadism (congenital or acquired)-idiopathic gonadotropin or LHRH deficiency, or pituitary-hypothalamic injury from tumors, trauma, or radiation.

CONTRAINDICATIONS:

1. Known hypersensitivity to the drug
2. Males with carcinoma of the breast
3. Males with known or suspected carcinoma of the prostate gland
4. Women who are or who may become pregnant
5. Patients with serious cardiac, hepatic or renal disease

WARNINGS:

Hypercalcemia may occur in immobilized patients. If this occurs, the drug should be discontinued.

Prolonged use of high doses of androgens (principally the 17-delta alkyl-androgens) has been associated with development of hepatic adenomas, hepatocellular carcinoma, and peliosis hepatis —all potentially life-threatening complications.

Geriatric patients treated with androgens may be at an increased risk of developing prostatic hypertrophy and prostatic carcinoma although conclusive evidence to support this concept is lacking.

Edema, with or without congestive heart failure, may be a serious complication in patients with pre-existing cardiac, renal or hepatic disease.

Gynecomastia may develop and occasionally persists in patients being treated for hypogonadism.

This product contains benzyl alcohol. Benzyl alcohol has been reported to be associated with a fatal "Gasping Syndrome" in premature infants.

Androgen therapy should be used cautiously in healthy males with delayed puberty. The effect on bone maturation should be monitored by assessing bone age of the wrist and hand every 6 months. In children, androgen treatment may accelerate bone maturation without producing compensatory gain in linear growth. This adverse effect may result in compromised adult stature. The younger the child the greater the risk of compromising final mature height.

WARNINGS: *(cont'd)*

This drug has not been shown to be safe and effective for the enhancement of athletic performance. Because of the potential risk of serious adverse health effects, this drug should not be used for such purpose.

PRECAUTIONS:

GENERAL

Patients with benign prostatic hypertrophy may develop acute urethral obstruction. Priapism or excessive sexual stimulation may develop. Oligospermia may occur after prolonged administration or excessive dosage. If any of these effects appear, the androgen should be stopped and if restarted, a lower dosage should be utilized.

Testosterone cypionate should not be used interchangeably with testosterone propionate because of differences in duration of action.

Testosterone cypionate *is not* for intravenous use.

INFORMATION FOR THE PATIENT

Patients should be instructed to report any of the following: nausea, vomiting, changes in skin color, ankle swelling, too frequent or persistent erections of the penis.

LABORATORY TESTS

Hemoglobin and hematocrit levels (to detect polycythemia) should be checked periodically in patients receiving long-term androgen administration.

Serum cholesterol may increase during androgen therapy.

DRUG/LABORATORY TEST INTERFERENCES

Androgens may decrease levels of thyroxine-binding globulin, resulting in decreased total T_4 serum levels and increased resin uptake of T_3 and T_4. Free thyroid hormone levels remain unchanged, however, and there is no clinical evidence of thyroid dysfunction.

CARCINOGENESIS

Animal data. Testosterone has been tested by subcutaneous injection and implantation in mice and rats. The implant induced cervical-uterine tumors in mice, which metastasized in some cases. There is suggestive evidence that injection of testosterone into some strains of female mice increases their susceptibility to hepatoma. Testosterone is also known to increase the number of tumors and decrease the degree of differentiation of chemically- induced carcinomas of the liver in rats.

Human data. There are rare reports of hepatocellular carcinoma in patients receiving long-term therapy with androgens in high doses. Withdrawal of the drugs did not lead to regression of the tumors in all cases.

Geriatric patients treated with androgens may be at an increased risk of developing prostatic hypertrophy and prostatic carcinoma although conclusive evidence to support this concept is lacking.

PREGNANCY, TERATOGENIC EFFECTS, PREGNANCY CATEGORY X

(See CONTRAINDICATIONS.)

NURSING MOTHERS

Testosterone Cypionate is not recommended for use in nursing mothers.

PEDIATRIC USE

Testosterone Cypionate is not recommended for use in children.

DRUG INTERACTIONS:

Androgens may increase sensitivity to oral anticoagulants. Dosage of the anticoagulant may require reduction in order to maintain satisfactory therapeutic hypoprothrombinemia.

Concurrent administration of oxyphenbutazone and androgens may result in elevated serum levels of oxyphenbutazone.

In diabetic patients, the metabolic effects of androgens may decrease blood glucose and, therefore, insulin requirements.

ADVERSE REACTIONS:

The following adverse reactions in the male have occurred with some androgens:

Endocrine And Urogenital: Gynecomastia and excessive frequency and duration of penile erections. Oligospermia may occur at high dosages.

Skin And Appendages: Hirsutism, male pattern of baldness, seborrhea, and acne.

Fluid And Electrolyte Disturbances: Retention of sodium, chloride, water, potassium, calcium, and inorganic phosphates.

Gastrointestinal: Nausea, cholestatic jaundice, alterations in liver function tests, rarely hepatocellular neoplasms and peliosis hepatis (see WARNINGS.)

Hematologic: Suppression of clotting factors II, V, VII, and X, bleeding in patients on concomitant anticoagulant therapy, and polycythemia.

Nervous System: Increased or decreased libido, headache, anxiety, depression, and generalized paresthesia.

Allergic: Hypersensitivity, including skin manifestations and anaphylactoid reactions.

Miscellaneous: Inflammation and pain at the site of intramuscular injection.

DRUG ABUSE AND DEPENDENCE:

Controlled Substance Class: Testosterone is a controlled substance under the Anabolic Steroids Control Act, and Testosterone Cypionate Sterile Solution has been assigned to Schedule III.

OVERDOSAGE:

There have been no reports of acute overdosage with the androgens.

DOSAGE AND ADMINISTRATION:

Testosterone Cypionate Sterile Solution is for intramuscular use only. It should not be given intravenously. Intramuscular injections should be given deep in the gluteal muscle.

The suggested dosage for Testosterone Cypionate Sterile Solution varies depending on the age, sex, and diagnosis of the individual patient. Dosage is adjusted according to the patient's response and the appearance of adverse reactions.

Various dosage regimens have been used to induce pubertal changes in hypogonadal males; some experts have advocated lower dosages initially, gradually increasing the dose as puberty progresses, with or without a decrease to maintenance levels. Other experts emphasize that higher dosages are needed to induce pubertal changes and lower dosages can be used for maintenance after puberty. The chronological and skeletal ages must be taken into consideration, both in determining the initial dose and in adjusting the dose.

For replacement in the hypogonadal male, 50-400 mg should be administered every two to four weeks.

Parenteral drug products should be inspected visually for particulate matter and discoloration prior to administration, whenever solution and container permit. Warming and shaking the vial should redissolve any crystals that may have formed during storage at temperatures lower than recommended.

DOSAGE AND ADMINISTRATION: *(cont'd)*

Vials should be stored at controlled room temperature 15-30°C (59-86°F) and protected from light.

HOW SUPPLIED - RATED THERAPEUTICALLY EQUIVALENT:

Injection, Solution - Intramuscular - 100 mg/ml

10 ml	$6.65	ANDRONATE, Pasadena	00418-6551-41
10 ml	$6.79	Testosterone Cypionate, McGuff	49072-0711-10
10 ml	$8.20	Testosterone Cypionate, Major Pharms	00904-0872-10
10 ml	$11.80	DEPOTEST, Hyrex Pharms	00314-0815-70
10 ml	$13.00	Testosterone Cypionate, Steris Labs	00402-0255-10
10 ml	$14.80	Testosterone Cypionate, Goldline Labs	00182-0712-63
10 ml	$15.05	Testosterone Cypionate, Geneva Pharms	00781-3096-70
10 ml	$15.51	Testosterone Cypionate, Schein Pharm (US)	00364-6609-54
10 ml	$15.75	Testosterone Cypionate, Rugby	00536-9480-70
10 ml	$32.04	DEPO TESTOSTERONE CYPIONATE, Pharmacia & Upjohn	00009-0347-02

Injection, Solution - Intramuscular - 200 mg/ml

1 ml	**$10.50**	**DEPO-TESTOSTERONE CYPIONATE, Pharmacia & Upjohn**	**00009-0417-01**
10 ml	$12.65	ANDRONATE, Pasadena	00418-6561-41
10 ml	$13.50	Testosterone Cypionate, United Res	00677-0980-21
10 ml	$17.80	DEPOTEST, Hyrex Pharms	00314-0835-70
10 ml	$17.93	Testosterone Cypionate, IDE-Interstate	00814-7733-40
10 ml	$20.25	Testosterone Cypionate, Steris Labs	00402-0256-10
10 ml	$20.65	Testosterone Cypionate, Goldline Labs	00182-0713-63
10 ml	$20.75	Testosterone Cypionate, Geneva Pharms	00781-3097-70
10 ml	$26.15	Testosterone Cypionate, Schein Pharm (US)	00364-6610-54
10 ml	$26.25	Testosterone Cypionate, Rugby	00536-9490-70
10 ml	$34.88	TESTRED CYPIONATE 200, ICN Pharms	00187-0200-10
10 ml	**$57.48**	**DEPO-TESTOSTERONE CYPIONATE, Pharmacia & Upjohn**	**00009-0417-02**

TESTOSTERONE ENANTHATE *(002320)*

CATEGORIES: Anabolic Steroids; Androgens; Antiestrogen; Antineoplastics; Bilateral Torsion; Breast Carcinoma; Cancer; Delayed Puberty; Hormones; Hypogonadism; Orchidectomy; Orchitis; Oncologic Drugs; Puberty; Steroids; Tumors; Vanishing Testis Syndrome; Pregnancy Category X; DEA Class CIII; FDA Approval Pre 1982

BRAND NAMES: Andro L.A. 200; Andropository; Andryl 200; Delatest; Delatestadiol; **Delatestryl**; Durathate-200; Everone; Primotest Depot 200; Testone L.A.; Testrin-P.A.; Testro-L.A.; Tone-Tes

DESCRIPTION:

Testosterone enanthate injection provides testosterone enanthate, a derivative of the primary endogenous androgen testosterone, for intramuscular administration. In their active form, androgens have a 17-beta-hydroxy group. Esterification of the 17-beta-hydroxy group increases the duration of action of testosterone; hydrolysis to free testosterone occurs *in vivo.* Each ml of sterile, colorless to pale yellow solution provides 200 mg testosterone enanthate in sesame oil with 5 mg chlorobutanol (chloral derivative) as a preservative.

Testosterone enanthate is designated chemically as androst-4-en-3-one, 17-[(1-oxoheptyl)oxy]-, (17β)-.

$C_{26}H_{40}O_3$MW: 400.60 CAS-315-37-7

CLINICAL PHARMACOLOGY:

Endogenous androgens are responsible for the normal growth and development of the male sex organs and for maintenance of secondary sex characteristics. These effects include growth and maturation of prostate, seminal vesicles, penis, and scrotum; development of male hair distribution, such as beard, pubic, chest, and axillary hair; laryngeal enlargement; vocal chord thickening; alterations in body musculature; and fat distribution.

Androgens also cause retention of nitrogen, sodium, potassium, and phosphorus, and decreased urinary excretion of calcium. Androgens have been reported to increase protein anabolism and decrease protein catabolism. Nitrogen balance is improved only when there is sufficient intake of calories and protein.

Androgens are responsible for the growth spurt of adolescence and for the eventual termination of linear growth which is brought about by fusion of the epiphyseal growth centers. In children, exogenous androgens accelerate linear growth rates but may cause a disproportionate advancement in bone maturation. Use over long periods may result in fusion of the epiphyseal growth centers and termination of growth process. Androgens have been reported to stimulate the production of red blood cells by enhancing the production of erythropoietic stimulating factor.

During exogenous administration of androgens, endogenous testosterone release is inhibited through feedback inhibition of pituitary luteinizing hormone (LH). At large doses of exogenous androgens, spermatogenesis may also be suppressed through feedback inhibition of pituitary follicle stimulating hormone (FSH).

There is a lack of substantial evidence that androgens are effective in fractures, surgery, convalescence, and functional uterine bleeding.

Pharmacokinetics: Testosterone esters are less polar than free testosterone. Testosterone esters in oil injected intramuscularly are absorbed slowly from the lipid phase; thus testosterone enanthate can be given at intervals of two to four weeks.

Testosterone in plasma is 98 percent bound to a specific testosterone-estradiol binding globulin, and about two percent is free. Generally, the amount of this sex-hormone binding globulin in the plasma will determine the distribution of testosterone between free and bound forms, and the free testosterone concentration will determine its half-life.

About 90 percent of a dose of testosterone is excreted in the urine as glucuronic and sulfuric acid conjugates of testosterone and its metabolites; about six percent of a dose is excreted in the feces, mostly in the unconjugated form. Inactivation of testosterone occurs primarily in the liver. Testosterone is metabolized to various 17-keto steroids through two different pathways. There are considerable variations of the half-life of testosterone as reported in the literature, ranging from 10 to 100 minutes.

In responsive tissues, the activity of testosterone appears to depend on reduction to dihydrotestosterone, which binds to cytosol receptor proteins. The steroid-receptor complex is transported to the nucleus where it initiates transcription events and cellular changes related to androgen action.

INDICATIONS AND USAGE:

MALES

Testosterone enanthate injection is indicated for replacement therapy in conditions associated with a deficiency or absence of endogenous testosterone.

INDICATIONS AND USAGE: *(cont'd)*

Primary Hypogonadism (Congenital or Acquired): Testicular failure due to cryptorchidism, bilateral torsion, orchitis, vanishing testis syndrome, or orchidectomy.

Hypogonadotrophic Hypogonadism (Congenital or Acquired): Idiopathic gonadotropin or luteinizing hormone-releasing hormone (LHRH) deficiency, or pituitary-hypothalamic injury from tumors, trauma, or radiation. (Appropriate adrenal cortical and thyroid hormone replacement therapy are still necessary, however, and are actually of primary importance.) If the above conditions occur prior to puberty, androgen replacement therapy will be needed during the adolescent years for development of secondary sexual characteristics. Prolonged androgen treatment will be required to maintain sexual characteristics in these and other males who develop testosterone deficiency after puberty.

Delayed Puberty: Testosterone enanthate injection may be used to stimulate puberty in carefully selected males with clearly delayed puberty. These patients usually have a familial pattern of delayed puberty that is not secondary to a pathological disorder; puberty is expected to occur spontaneously at a relatively late date. Brief treatment with conservative doses may occasionally be justified in these patients if they do not respond to psychological support. The potential adverse effect on bone maturation should be discussed with the patient and parents prior to androgen administration. An X-ray of the hand and wrist to determine bone age should be obtained every six months to assess the effect of treatment on the epiphyseal centers (see WARNINGS).

FEMALES

Metastatic Mammary Cancer: Testosterone enanthate injection may be used secondarily in women with advancing inoperable metastatic (skeletal) mammary cancer who are one to five years postmenopausal. Primary goals of therapy in these women include ablation of the ovaries. Other methods of counteracting estrogen activity are adrenalectomy, hypophysectomy, and/or antiestrogen therapy. This treatment has also been used in premenopausal women with breast cancer who have benefited from oophorectomy and are considered to have a hormone-responsive tumor. Judgment concerning androgen therapy should be made by an oncologist with expertise in this field.

CONTRAINDICATIONS:

Androgens are contraindicated in men with carcinomas of the breast or with known or suspected carcinomas of the prostate and in women who are or may become pregnant. When administered to pregnant women, androgens cause virilization of the external genitalia of the female fetus. This virilization includes clitoromegaly, abnormal vaginal development, and fusion of genital folds to form a scrotal-like structure. The degree of masculinization is related to the amount of drug given and the age of the fetus and is most likely to occur in the female fetus when the drugs are given in the first trimester. If the patient becomes pregnant while taking androgens, she should be apprised of the potential hazard to the fetus.

This preparation is also contraindicated in patients with a history of hypersensitivity to any of its components.

WARNINGS:

In patients with breast cancer and in immobilized patients, androgen therapy may cause hypercalcemia by stimulating osteolysis. In patients with cancer, hypercalcemia may indicate progression of bony metastasis. If hypercalcemia occurs, the drug should be discontinued and appropriate measures instituted.

Prolonged use of high doses of androgens has been associated with the development of peliosis hepatis and hepatic neoplasms including hepatocellular carcinoma (see PRECAUTIONS, Carcinogenesis). Peliosis hepatis can be a life-threatening or fatal complication.

If cholestatic hepatitis with jaundice appears or if liver function tests become abnormal, the androgen should be discontinued and the etiology should be determined. Drug-induced jaundice is reversible when the medication is discontinued.

Geriatric patients treated with androgens may be at an increased risk for the development of prostatic hypertrophy and prostatic carcinoma.

Due to sodium and water retention, edema with or without congestive heart failure may be a serious complication in patients with preexisting cardiac, renal, or hepatic disease. In addition to discontinuation of the drug, diuretic therapy may be required. If the administration of testosterone enanthate is restarted, a lower dose should be used.

Gynecomastia frequently develops and occasionally persists in patients being treated for hypergonadism.

Androgen therapy should be used cautiously in healthy males with delayed puberty. The effect on bone maturation should be monitored by assessing bone age of the wrist and hand every six months. In children, androgen treatment may accelerate bone maturation without producing compensatory gain in linear growth. This adverse effect may result in compromised adult stature. The younger the child the greater the risk of compromising final mature height.

PRECAUTIONS:

GENERAL

Women should be observed for signs or virilization (deepening of the voice, hirsutism, acne, clitoromegaly, and menstrual irregularities). Discontinuation of drug therapy at the time of evidence of mild virilism is necessary to prevent irreversible virilization. Such virilization is usual following androgen use at high doses and is not prevented by concomitant use of estrogens. A decision may be made by the patient and the physician that some virilization will be tolerated during treatment for breast carcinoma.

Because androgens may alter serum cholesterol concentration, caution should be used when administering these drugs to patients with a history of myocardial infarction or coronary artery disease. Serial determinations of serum cholesterol should be made and therapy adjusted accordingly. A causal relationship between myocardial infarction and hypercholesterolemia has not been established.

INFORMATION FOR THE PATIENT

Male adolescent patients receiving androgens for delayed puberty should have bone development checked every six months.

The physician should instruct patients to report any of the following side effects of androgens:

Adult or Adolescent Males: Too frequent or persistent erections of the penis.

Women: Hoarseness, acne, changes in menstrual periods, or more facial hair.

All patients: Any nausea, vomiting, changes in skin color, or ankle swelling.

LABORATORY TESTS

Women with disseminated breast carcinoma should have frequent determination of urine and serum calcium levels during the course of androgen therapy (see WARNINGS).

Periodic (every six months) X-ray examinations of bone age should be made during treatment of prepubertal males to determine the rate of bone maturation and the effects of androgen therapy on the epiphyseal centers.

Hemoglobin and hematocrit should be checked periodically for polycythemia in patients who are receiving high doses of androgens.

PRECAUTIONS: *(cont'd)*

DRUG/LABORATORY TEST INTERFERENCES

Androgens may decrease levels of thyroxine-binding globulin, resulting in decreased total T_4 serum levels and increased resin uptake of T_3 and T_4. Free thyroid hormone levels remain unchanged, however, and there is no clinical evidence of thyroid dysfunction.

CARCINOGENESIS

Testosterone has been tested by subcutaneous injection and implantation in mice and rats. The implant induced cervical-uterine tumors in mice, which metastasized in some cases. There is suggestive evidence that injection of testosterone into some strains of female mice increases their susceptibility to hepatoma. Testosterone is also known to increase the number of tumors and decrease the degree of differentiation of chemically induced carcinomas of the liver in rats.

There are rare reports of hepatocellular carcinoma in patients receiving long-term therapy with androgens in high doses. Withdrawal of the drugs did not lead to regression of the tumors in all cases.

Geriatric patients treated with androgens may be at an increased risk for the development of prostatic hypertrophy and prostatic carcinoma.

PREGNANCY, TERATOGENIC EFFECTS, PREGNANCY CATEGORY X

(See CONTRAINDICATIONS).

NURSING MOTHERS

It is not known whether androgens are excreted in human milk. Because many drugs are excreted in human milk and because of the potential for serious adverse reactions in nursing infants from androgens, a decision should be made whether to discontinue nursing or to discontinue the drug, taking into account the importance of the drug to the mother.

PEDIATRIC USE

Androgen therapy should be used very cautiously in children and only by specialists who are aware of the adverse effects on bone maturation. Skeletal maturation must be monitored every six months by an x-ray of the hand and wrist (see INDICATIONS AND USAGE, and WARNINGS).

DRUG INTERACTIONS:

When administered concurrently, the following drugs may interact with androgens:

Anticoagulants, Oral: C-17 substituted derivatives of testosterone, such as methandrostenolone, have been reported to decrease the anticoagulant requirement. Patients receiving oral anticoagulant therapy require close monitoring especially when androgens are started or stopped.

Antidiabetic Drugs and Insulin: In diabetic patients, the metabolic effects of androgens may decrease blood glucose and insulin requirements.

ACTH and Corticosteroids: Enhanced tendency toward edema. Use caution when giving these drugs together, especially in patients with hepatic or cardiac disease.

Oxyphenbutazone: Elevated serum levels of oxyphenbutazone may result.

ADVERSE REACTIONS:

Endocrine and Urogenital, Female: The most common side effects of androgen therapy are amenorrhea and other menstrual irregularities, inhibition of gonadotropin secretion, and virilization, including deepening of the voice and clitoral enlargement. The latter usually is not reversible after androgens are discontinued. When administered to a pregnant woman, androgens cause virilization of the external genitalia of the female fetus. *Male*—Gynecomastia, and excessive frequency and duration of penile erections. Oligospermia may occur at high dosages (See CLINICAL PHARMACOLOGY).

Skin and Appendages: Hirsutism, male pattern baldness, and acne.

Fluid and Electrolyte Disturbances: Retention of sodium, chloride, water, potassium, calcium (see WARNINGS), and inorganic phosphates. Gastrointestinal—Nausea, cholestatic jaundice, alterations in liver function tests; rarely, hepatocellular neoplasms, peliosis hepatis (see WARNINGS).

Hematologic: Suppression of clotting factors II, V, VII, and X; bleeding in patients on concomitant anticoagulant therapy; polycythemia.

Nervous System: Increased or decreased libido, headache, anxiety, depression, and generalized paresthesia.

Metabolic: Increased serum cholesterol.

Miscellaneous: Rarely, anaphylactoid reactions; inflammation and pain at injection site.

DRUG ABUSE AND DEPENDENCE:

Testosterone enanthate is classified as a controlled substance under the Anabolic Steroids Control Act of 1990 and has been assigned to Schedule III.

OVERDOSAGE:

There have been no reports of acute overdosage with androgens.

DOSAGE AND ADMINISTRATION:

Dosage and duration of therapy with testosterone enanthate injection will depend on age, sex, diagnosis, patient's response to treatment, and appearance of adverse effects. When properly given, injections of testosterone enanthate are well tolerated. Care should be taken to inject the preparation deeply into the gluteal muscle following the usual precautions for intramuscular administration. In general, total doses above 400 mg per month are not required because of the prolonged action of the preparation. Injections more frequently than every two weeks are rarely indicated. NOTE: Use of a wet needle or wet syringe may cause the solution to become cloudy; however, this does not effect the potency of the material. Parenteral drug products should be inspected visually for particulate matter and discoloration prior to administration, whenever solution and container permit. Testosterone enanthate is a clear, colorless to pale yellow solution.

Male Hypogonadism: As replacement therapy, i.e., for eunuchism, the suggested dosage is 50 to 400 mg every 2 to 4 weeks.

In Males with Delayed Puberty: Various dosage regimens have been used; some call for lower dosages initially with gradual increases as puberty progresses, with or without a decrease to maintenance levels. Other regimens call for higher dosage to induce pubertal changes and lower dosage for maintenance after puberty. The chronological and skeletal ages must be taken into consideration, both in determining the initial dose and in adjusting the dose. Dosage is within the range of 50 to 200 mg every 2 to 4 weeks for a limited duration, for example, 4 to 6 months. X-rays should be taken at appropriate intervals to determine the amount of bone maturation and skeletal development (see INDICATIONS AND USAGE and WARNINGS).

Palliation of Inoperable Mammary Cancer in Women: A dosage of 200 to 400 mg every 2 to 4 weeks is recommended. Women with metastatic breast carcinoma must be followed closely because androgen therapy occasionally appears to accelerate the disease.

Storage: Testosterone enanthate should be stored at room temperature. Warming and shaking the vial will redissolve any crystals that may have formed during storage at low temperatures.

HOW SUPPLIED - RATED THERAPEUTICALLY EQUIVALENT:

Injection, Solution - Intramuscular - 200 mg/ml

10 ml	$11.10	Testosterone Enanthate, Major Pharms	00904-2455-10
10 ml	$12.50	TESTRO L A, C O Truxton	00463-1070-10
10 ml	$12.70	Testrin - P.A., Pasadena	00418-0431-41
10 ml	$13.05	Testosterone Enanthate, United Res	00677-0313-21
10 ml	$13.50	Testosterone Enanthate, Harber Pharm	51432-0775-10
10 ml	$13.54	Testosterone Enanthate, Steris Labs	00402-0356-10
10 ml	$16.55	Testosterone Enanthate, Geneva Pharms	00781-3105-70
10 ml	$16.58	ANDROPOSITORY, Rugby	00536-1670-70
10 ml	$16.59	Testosterone Enanthate, Schein Pharm (US)	00364-6617-54
10 ml	$17.25	Testosterone Enanthate, IDE-Interstate	00814-7705-40
10 ml	$17.52	EVERONE, Hyrex Pharms	00314-0652-70
10 ml	$18.50	ANDRO LA, Forest Pharms	00456-0604-10

HOW SUPPLIED - NOT RATED EQUIVALENT:

Injection, Solution - Intramuscular - 100 mg/ml

10 ml	$10.90	EVERONE, Hyrex Pharms	00314-0650-70

TESTOSTERONE PROPIONATE *(002321)*

CATEGORIES: Anabolic Steroids; Androgens; Antiestrogen; Antineoplastics; Bilateral Torsion; Breast Carcinoma; Cancer; Cryptorchidism; Delayed Puberty; Hormones; Hypogonadism; Orchidectomy; Orchitis; Oncologic Drugs; Pharmaceutical Adjuvants; Puberty; Tumors; Vanishing Testis Syndrome; Breast Engorgement*; Pregnancy Category X; DEA Class CIII; FDA Approval Pre 1982
* Indication not approved by the FDA

BRAND NAMES: Androlan; Testex

DESCRIPTION:

Testosterone is a steroid compound that is described chemically as Delta 4-androstene-17β-ol-3-one. It is the principal hormone of the testis. The ester, testosterone propionate, is a stable, white or slightly yellow crystalline substance that is insoluble in water but freely soluble in alcohol, ether, vegetable oils, and other organic solvents. Esterification of the 17 beta-hydroxy group produces compounds which have a longer duration of action and are hydrolyzed *in vivo* to free testosterone.

Testosterone Propionate injection, USP, is a sterile solution of testosterone propionate in sesame oil. It contains 0.5% phenol as a preservative.

CLINICAL PHARMACOLOGY:

Endogenous androgens are responsible for the normal growth and development of the male sex organs and for maintenance of secondary sex characteristics. These effects include the growth and maturation of the prostate, seminal vesicles, penis, and scrotum; the development of male hair distribution, such as the beard, and pubic, chest, and axillary hair; laryngeal enlargement, vocal-cord thickening; alterations in body musculature; and fat distribution. Drugs in this class also cause retention of nitrogen, sodium, potassium, and phosphorus and decreased urinary excretion of calcium. Androgens have been reported to increase protein anabolism and decrease protein catabolism. Nitrogen balance is improved only when there is sufficient intake of calories and protein.

Androgens are responsible for the growth spurt of adolescence and for the eventual termination of linear growth which is brought about by fusion of the epiphyseal growth centers. In children, exogenous androgens accelerate linear growth rates but may cause a disproportionate advancement in bone maturation. Use over long periods may result in fusion of the epiphyseal growth centers and termination of the growth process. Androgens have been reported to stimulate the production of red blood cells by enhancing the production of erythropoietic stimulating factor.

During exogenous administration of androgens, endogenous testosterone release is inhibited through feedback inhibition of pituitary luteinizing hormone (LH). At large doses of exogenous androgens, spermatogenesis may also be suppressed through feedback inhibition of pituitary follicle stimulating hormone (FSH).

There is lack of substantial evidence that androgens are effective in fractures, surgery, convalescence, and functional uterine bleeding.

Pharmacokinetics: Testosterone given orally is metabolized by the gut, and 44% is cleared by the liver in the first pass.

Testosterone propionate is less polar than free testosterone. Testosterone propionate in oil injected intramuscularly is absorbed slowly from the lipid phase; thus, it can be given at intervals of 2 to 3 times/week.

Testosterone in plasma is 98% bound to a specific testosterone-estradiol binding globulin, and about 2% is free. Generally, the amount of this sex-hormone binding globulin in the plasma will determine the distribution of testosterone between free and bound forms, and the free testosterone concentration will determine half-life.

About 90% of a dose of testosterone is excreted in the urine as glucuronic and sulfuric acid conjugates of testosterone and its metabolites; about 6% of a dose is excreted in the feces, mostly in the unconjugated form. Inactivation of testosterone occurs primarily in the liver. Testosterone is metabolized to various 17-ketosteroids through two different pathways. The half-life of testosterone as reported in the literature varies considerably; it ranges from 10 to 100 minutes.

In many tissues the activity of testosterone appears to depend on reduction to dihydrotestosterone, which binds to cytosol receptor proteins. The steroid-receptor complex is transported to the nucleus where it initiates transcription events and cellular changes related to androgen action.

INDICATIONS AND USAGE:

Males: Testosterone propionate is indicated for replacement therapy in conditions associated with a deficiency or absence of endogenous testosterone:

A. Primary hypogonadism (congenital or acquired)—testicular failure due to cryptorchidism, bilateral torsion, orchitis, vanishing testis syndrome, or orchidectomy.

B. Hypogonadotropic hypogonadism (congenital or acquired)— idiopathic gonadotropin or LHRH deficiency, or pituitary— hypothalamic injury from tumors, trauma, or radiation.

If the above conditions occur prior to puberty, androgen replacement therapy will be needed during the adolescent years for development of secondary sexual characteristics. Prolonged androgen treatment will required to maintain sexual characteristics in these and other males who develop testosterone deficiency after puberty.

C. Testosterone propionate may be used to stimulate puberty in carefully selected males with clearly delayed puberty that is not secondary to a pathologic disorder; puberty is expected to occur spontaneously at a relatively late date. Brief treatment with conservative doses may occasionally be justified in these patients if they do not respond to psychologic support. The potential adverse effect on bone maturation should be discussed with the patient and parents

INDICATIONS AND USAGE: *(cont'd)*

prior to androgen administration. An x-ray of the hand and wrist to determine bone age should be obtained every 6 months to assess the effect of treatment on the epiphyseal centers (See WARNINGS).

Females: Testosterone propionate may be used secondarily in women with advancing inoperable metastatic (skeletal) mammary cancer who are 1 to 5 years postmenopausal. Primary goals of therapy in these women include ablation of the ovaries. Other methods of counteracting estrogen activity are adrenalectomy, hypophysectomy, and/or antiestrogen therapy. This treatment has also been used in premenopausal women with breast cancer who have benefited from oophorectomy and are considered to have a hormone-responsive tumor. Judgement concerning androgen therapy should be made by an oncologist with expertise in this field.

Testosterone propionate has been used for the management of postpartum breast pain and engorgement. (There is no satisfactory evidence that this drug prevents or suppresses lactation.)

CONTRAINDICATIONS:

Testosterone propionate is contraindicated in men with carcinomas of the breast or with known or suspected carcinomas of the prostate and in women who are or may become pregnant. When administered to pregnant women, androgens cause virilization of the external genitalia of the female fetus. This virilization includes clitoromegaly, abnormal vaginal development, and fusion of genital folds to form a scrotal-like structure. The degree of masculinization is related to the amount of drug given and the age of the fetus and is most likely to occur in the female fetus when the drugs are given in the first trimester. If the patient becomes pregnant while taking these drugs, she should be apprised of the potential hazard of the fetus.

WARNINGS:

In patients with breast cancer, androgen therapy may cause hypercalcemia by stimulating osteolysis. In this case, the drug should be discontinued.

Prolonged use of high doses of androgens has been associated with the development of peliosis hepatis and hepatic neoplasms, including hepatocellular carcinoma (see PRECAUTIONS, Carcinogenesis). Peliosis hepatis can be a life-threatening or fatal complication.

Geriatric patients treated with androgens may be at an increased risk for the development of prostatic hypertrophy and prostatic carcinoma.

Edema with or without congestive heart failure may be a serious complication in patients with preexisting cardiac, renal, or hepatic disease. In addition to discontinuation of the drug, diuretic therapy may be required.

Gynecomastia frequently develops and occasionally persists in patients being treated for hypogonadism.

Androgen therapy should be used cautiously in healthy males with delayed puberty. The effect on bone maturation should be monitored by addressing bone age of the wrist and hand every 6 months. In children, androgen treatment may accelerate bone maturation without producing compensatory gain in linear growth. This adverse effect may result in compromised adult stature. The younger the child, the greater the risk of compromising final mature height.

Do not give testosterone to elderly asthenic males who may react adversely to overstimulation by androgens.

PRECAUTIONS:

GENERAL

Testosterone, through its metabolic effects, stimulates the nervous, mental, and physical activities of a patient. Therefore, it should be used with caution in the presence of cardiovascular and renal diseases, especially in the elderly male.

Prolonged administration or excessive dosage may cause inhibition of testicular function. As a result, oligospermia may develop, and there may be a decrease in ejaculatory volume.

Women should be observed for signs of virilization (deepening of the voice, hirsutism, acne, clitoromegaly, and menstrual irregularities). Discontinuation of drug therapy at the time mild virilism becomes evident is necessary to prevent irreversible virilization. Such virilization usually follows administration of androgens at high doses. A decision may be made by the patient and the physician concerning the degree of virilization that will be tolerated during treatment for breast carcinoma.

Anaphylactoid reactions, although rare, may occur, and treatment should be readily available. Hypersensitivity reactions, including rash and dermatitis, have been reported.

INFORMATION FOR THE PATIENT

The physician should instruct patients to report any of the following side effects of androgens:

Adult or Adolescent Males: Too-frequent or persistent erections of the penis.

Women: Hoarseness, acne, changes in menstrual periods, or more hair on the face.

All Patients: Any nausea, vomiting, changes in skin color, or ankle swelling.

Any male adolescent patient receiving androgens for delayed puberty should have bone development checked every 6 months.

LABORATORY TESTS

1. Women with disseminated breast carcinoma should have frequent determinations of urine and serum calcium levels during the course of androgen therapy (See WARNINGS).

2. Periodic (every 6 months) x-ray examinations of bone age should be made during treatment of prepubertal males to determine the rate of bone maturation and the effects of androgen therapy on the epiphyseal centers.

3. Hemoglobin and hematocrit should be checked periodically for polycythemia in patients who are receiving high doses of androgens.

DRUG/LABORATORY TEST INTERFERENCES

Androgens may decrease levels of thyroxine-binding globulin, resulting in decreased total T4 serum levels and increased resin uptake of T3 and T4. Free thyroid hormone levels remain unchanged, however, and there is no clinical evidence of thyroid dysfunction.

CARCINOGENESIS

Animal Data: Testosterone has been tested by subcutaneous injection and implantation in mice and rats. The implant induced cervical-uterine tumors in mice, which metastasized in some cases. There is suggestive evidence that injection of testosterone into some strains of female mice increases their susceptibility to hepatoma. Testosterone is also known to increase the number of tumors and decrease the degree of differentiation of chemically induced carcinomas of the liver in rats.

Human Data: There are rare reports of hepatocellular carcinoma in patients receiving long-term therapy with androgens in high doses. Withdrawal of the drugs did not lead to regression of the tumors in all cases.

Geriatric patients treated with androgens may be at an increased risk for the development of prostatic hypertrophy and prostatic carcinoma.

PRECAUTIONS: *(cont'd)*

PREGNANCY CATEGORY X

Teratogenic Effects: (See CONTRAINDICATIONS).

NURSING MOTHERS

It is not known whether androgens are excreted in human milk. Because many drugs are excreted in human milk and because of the potential for serious adverse reactions in nursing infants from androgens, a decision should be made whether to discontinue nursing or to discontinue the drug, taking into account the importance of the drug to the mother.

PEDIATRIC USE

Androgen therapy should be used very cautiously in children and only by specialists who are aware of the adverse effects on bone maturation. Skeletal maturation must be monitored every 6 months by an x-ray of hand and wrist (See INDICATIONS AND USAGE and WARNINGS).

DRUG INTERACTIONS:

1. Oxyphenbutazone: Concurrent administration of oxyphenbutazone and androgens may result in elevated serum levels of oxyphenbutazone.

2. Insulin: In diabetic patients, the metabolic effects of androgens may decrease blood glucose and insulin requirements.

ADVERSE REACTIONS:

Endocrine and Urogenital: *Female:* The most common side effects of androgen therapy are amenorrhea and other menstrual irregularities, inhibition of gonadotropin secretion, and virilization, including deepening of the voice and clitoral enlargement. The latter usually is not reversible after androgens are discontinued. When administered to a pregnant woman, androgens cause virilization of external genitalia of the female fetus. *Male:* Gynecomastia, and excessive frequency and duration of penile erections. Oligospermia may occur at high dosages (See CLINICAL PHARMACOLOGY).

Skin and Appendages: Hirsutism, male pattern of baldness, and acne.

Fluid and Electrolyte Disturbances: Retention of sodium, chloride, water, potassium, calcium, and inorganic phosphates.

Patients with osteolytic neoplastic lesions who are bedfast or only semiambulatory may develop nephrocalcinosis when given either estrogens or androgens.

Gastrointestinal: Nausea and, rarely, hepatocellular neoplasms and peliosis hepatis (See WARNINGS).

Hematologic: Suppression of clotting factors II, V, VII, and X, bleeding in patients on concomitant anticoagulant therapy, and polycythemia.

Nervous System: Increased or decreased libido, headache, anxiety, depression, and generalized paresthesia.

Metabolic: Increased serum cholesterol.

Miscellaneous: Inflammation and pain at the site of intramuscular injection, and, rarely, anaphylactoid reactions.

OVERDOSAGE:

There have been no reports of acute overdosage with the androgens.

DOSAGE AND ADMINISTRATION:

Testosterone propionate is administered by intramuscular injection. It must not be given intravenously. Intramuscular injections should be given deep in the gluteal muscle.

The suggested dosage varies, depending on the age, sex, and diagnosis of the individual patient. Dosage is adjusted according to the patient's response and the appearance of adverse reactions, and maintenance doses should be the minimum that produce adequate effect. This preparation is absorbed relatively slowly, and frequent injection may cause overdosage. Replacement therapy in androgen-deficient males should be in the range of 25-50 mg 2 or 3 times a week.

Various dosage regimens have been used to induce pubertal changes in hypogonadal males; some experts have advocated lower dosages initially, gradually increasing the dose as puberty progresses. With or without a decrease to maintenance levels. Other experts emphasize that higher dosages are needed to induce pubertal changes, and lower dosages can be used for maintenance after puberty. The chronologic and skeletal ages must be taken into consideration, both in determining the initial dose and in adjusting the dosage.

Dosages used in delayed puberty generally are in the lower ranges and are for a limited duration, for example, 4 to 6 months.

Carcinoma of the Breast: In inoperable carcinoma of the breast, temporary palliation may be obtained in some cases by therapy with androgens. A dosage of 50-100 mg of testosterone propionate administered intramuscularly 3 times weekly is recommended. If a response to androgen therapy is going to occur, it will be apparent within 3 months after initiation of therapy. When the disease again becomes progressive, therapy should be stopped and the patient observed for another period of improvement, known as "rebound regression." The above high dosage is likely to have masculinizing effects, particularly in young women. There may be a disturbing increase in libido, for which sedation may be helpful. It should be remembered that acceleration of tumor growth may be encountered occasionally during androgen therapy, in which case immediate cessation of the hormone is indicated. In some of these cases, the use of estrogen at this point causes regression.

Postpartum Engorgement of the Breasts: A dosage of 25 to 50 mg of testosterone propionate daily for 3 to 4 days, starting at the time of delivery, should be adequate in most cases.

HOW SUPPLIED - RATED THERAPEUTICALLY EQUIVALENT:

Injection, Solution - Intramuscular - 50 mg/ml

10 ml	$2.40	ANDROLAN, Lannett	00527-0205-55
10 ml	$15.29	Testosterone Propionate, Lilly	00002-1693-01

HOW SUPPLIED - NOT RATED EQUIVALENT:

Injection, Solution - Intramuscular - 25 mg/ml

10 ml	$1.60	ANDROLAN, Lannett	00527-0120-55

Injection, Solution - Intramuscular - 100 mg/ml

10 c	$10.50	Testosterone Propionate, C O Truxton	00463-1073-10
10 ml	$3.80	ANDROLAN, Lannett	00527-0208-55
10 ml	$8.49	Testosterone Propionate, McGuff	49072-0717-10
10 ml	$8.50	TESTEX, Pasadena	00418-0851-10
10 ml	$10.80	Testosterone Propionate, United Res	00677-0309-21
10 ml	$10.88	Testosterone, Hyrex Pharms	00314-0772-70
10 ml	$13.35	Testosterone Propionate, Major Pharms	00904-0868-10
10 ml	$13.40	Testosterone Propionate, Steris Labs	00402-0383-10
10 ml	$13.50	Testosterone Propionate, IDE-Interstate	00814-7688-40
10 ml	$15.97	Testosterone Propionate, Geneva Pharms	00781-3102-70
10 ml	$17.40	Testosterone Propionate, Goldline Labs	00182-1197-63
10 ml	$18.01	Testosterone Propionate, Schein Pharm (US)	00364-6686-54

HOW SUPPLIED - NOT RATED EQUIVALENT: *(cont'd)*

Powder

5 gm	$14.20	Testosterone Propionate, Paddock Labs	00574-0461-05
25 gm	$59.60	Testosterone Propionate, Paddock Labs	00574-0461-25

TETANUS IMMUNE GLOBULIN *(002323)*

CATEGORIES: Immunologic; Serums, Toxoids and Vaccines; Vaccines; Pregnancy Category C; FDA Pre 1938 Drugs

BRAND NAMES: Hyper-Tet; **Hypertet**

FORMULARIES: WHO

Prescribing information not available at time of publication.

HOW SUPPLIED - EQUIVALENTS NOT AVAILABLE:

Injection, Solution - Intramuscular - 250 unit/vial

1's	$12.00	HYPER-TET, Miles	00161-0614-86
1's	$24.13	HYPER-TET, Bayer Pharm	00192-0614-01
10's	$117.84	HYPER-TET, Miles	00161-0614-10
10's	$241.25	HYPER-TET, Bayer Pharm	00192-0614-70

TETANUS TOXOID *(002324)*

CATEGORIES: Biologicals; Immunologic; Serums, Toxoids and Vaccines; Tetanus; Toxoids; Vaccines; Pregnancy Category C; FDA Pre 1938 Drugs

BRAND NAMES: *Anatetall*; *Anatoxal Tetanica Berna*; *TE Anatoxal*; *TE Anatoxal Berna*; *Tetatox*; *Tetanol* (Germany, Mexico); Tetanus Toxoid Adsorbed; *Tetavax* (England, Germany)
(International brand names outside U.S. in italics)

FORMULARIES: WHO

DESCRIPTION:

Tetanus Toxoid Adsorbed, Aluminum Phosphate Adsorbed, Wyeth, is prepared by growing a suitable strain of Cl. tetani on a protein-free, semisynthetic medium (Appl. Microbiol. *10:*146, 1962). Formaldehyde is used as the toxoiding (detoxifying) agent for tetanus toxin. The final product contains no more than 0.02% free formaldehyde and contains 0.01% thimerosal (mercury derivative) as preservative.

Tetanus Toxoid Adsorbed, Wyeth, is refined by methods which eliminate at least 97% of the nontoxoid nitrogen. Adsorption of purified antigens on an optimal quantity of aluminum phosphate, a mineral adjuvant, prolongs and enhances the antigenic properties by retarding the rate of absorption. The aluminum content of the final product does not exceed 0.85 mg per 0.5 ml dose. During processing, hydrochloric acid and sodium hydroxide are used to adjust the pH. Sodium chloride is added to the finished product to control isotonicity.

INDICATIONS AND USAGE:

Tetanus Toxoid Adsorbed, Aluminum Phosphate Adsorbed, Wyeth, is indicated for active immunization against tetanus.

CONTRAINDICATIONS:

An acute respiratory infection or other active infection is reason for deferring administration of routine primary immunizing or recall (booster) doses but *not* emergency recall (booster) doses. Prolonging the interval between primary immunizing doses, for six months or longer, does not interfere with the final immunity. Any dose of tetanus toxoid an individual has received, even a decade earlier, should be counted as one of his immunizing injections.[2]

PRECAUTIONS:

Only well individuals should be injected.

If the vial is used, rather than the Tubex Sterile Cartridge-Needle Unit, a separate syringe and needle which have been adequately cleaned and sterilized should be used for each patient to prevent transmission of hepatitis B virus and other infectious agents from one person to another.

Individuals receiving therapy with corticosteroids or other immunosuppressive agents (antimetabolites, irradiation, alkylating agents) may not respond optimally to active immunization procedures. Administration of immunizing agents should be deferred in such individuals or repeated thereafter.

Before the injection of any biological, the physician should take all precautions known for prevention of allergic or any other side reactions. This should include: A review of the patient's history regarding possible sensitivity; the ready availability of epinephrine 1:1000 and other appropriate agents used for control of immediate allergic reactions; and a knowledge of the recent literature pertaining to use of the biological concerned.

ADVERSE REACTIONS:

A small area of erythema and induration surrounding the injection site, persisting for a few days, is not unusual. A nodule may be palpable at the site of injection for a few weeks.

The occurrence of significant local and systemic reactions, following administration of tetanus toxoid, either fluid or adsorbed, is not nearly as rare as once believed.[1,6-12] Severe systemic reactions, on the other hand, are extremely rare. Over the past several years, published reports from this and foreign countries have appeared describing extensive local reactions which, in some instances, were accompanied by mild-to-moderate systemic responses. A typical reaction of this type, as described in the literature, is manifested by a delayed onset (usually 12 hours or more) of erythema, boggy edema, and induration surrounding the point of injection. Pain and tenderness, if present, are usually not the primary complaints. Frequently there is itching of the edematous area, and it may resemble a giant "hive". The edema is occasionally extensive: shoulder to elbow or shoulder to wrist. Axillary lymphadenopathy has also been reported. Systemic manifestations have included low-grade fever, malaise, generalized aches and pains, flushing, generalized urticaria or pruritus, tachycardia, and hypotension. The majority of the extensive delayed-type local responses reported in the literature or to the manufacturers have occurred following BOOSTER doses in adults and especially in veterans of the armed forces, members of national guard units, employees of industries, members of hospital staffs, or others who have received routine booster doses of tetanus toxoid on a regular basis. The incidence of severe, extensive local reactions in hospital immunization programs, for instance, has been as high as five percent. Reports have also appeared concerning the occurrence of such reactions in children who have received several doses of tetanus toxoid in the past.[11,12] The increasing incidence of extensive local reactions is one of the reasons why a ten-year interval between ROUTINE booster doses is recommended by the U.S. Public Health Service, American Academy of Pediatrics, American College of Surgeons, and others. Local reactions typical of the type described above have

ADVERSE REACTIONS: *(cont'd)*

been reported from this and other countries following use of both fluid and adsorbed tetanus toxoids prepared by many different manufacturers. Although their cause is unknown, hypersensitivity to the toxin or bacillary protein of the tetanus organism itself is assumed to be a possibility in some; in others, interreaction between the injected antigen and high levels of preexisting tetanus antibody (antitoxin) from prior booster doses seems to be the most likely cause of the Arthus-type response. Edsall[1] suggests: "If doubt exists as to a patient's tolerance for toxoid and if an emergency booster dose is indicated, a small dose (*e.g.,* 0.05 to 0.1 ml) may be given subcutaneously and the rest of the dose given 12 hours later if no reaction has occurred. If a marked reaction should ensue, further toxoid injections at that time may be safely omitted since it has been shown years ago that reducing the dose of tetanus toxoid does not proportionately reduce the magnitude of the response obtained."

DOSAGE AND ADMINISTRATION:

The basic immunizing course for all age groups consists of two (primary) doses of 0.5 ml each, given at an interval of 4 to 8 weeks, followed by a third (reinforcing) dose of 0.5 ml 6 to 12 months later. The third (reinforcing) dose is an integral part of the basic immunizing course; basic immunization cannot be considered completed until the third dose has been given.[1] Prolonging the interval between primary immunizing doses, for six months or longer, does not interfere with the final immunity. Any dose of tetanus toxoid an individual has received, even a decade earlier, should be counted as one of his immunizing injections.[2] Injections should be given intramuscularly, preferably into the deltoid or midlateral muscles of the thigh. The same muscle site should not be injected more than once during the course of basic immunization.

A routine recall (booster) dose of 0.5 ml should be given at 10-year intervals throughout life to maintain immunity.[2-5]

In event of injury for which tetanus prophylaxis is indicated, an emergency recall (booster) dose of 0.5 ml should be given:

a. For clean, minor wounds: if more than TEN (10) years have elapsed since the time of administration of the last recall (booster) dose or the last (reinforcing) dose of the basic immunizing series.

b. For all other wounds: if more than FIVE (5) years have elapsed since the time of administration of the last recall (booster) dose or the last (reinforcing) dose of the basic immunizing series.

If emergency tetanus prophylaxis is indicated during the period between the second primary dose and the reinforcing dose, a 0.5 ml dose of toxoid should be given. If given before six months have elapsed, it should be counted as a primary dose; if given after six months, it should be regarded as the reinforcing dose.

A 0.5 ml dose of tetanus toxoid adsorbed *and* an appropriate dose of tetanus immune globulin (human), given with *separate* syringes and at *different* sites, are indicated at time of injury if:

a. The past immunization history with tetanus toxoid or the date of the last recall (booster) dose is unknown or of questionable validity.

b. The interval since the third (reinforcing) dose of the basic immunizing series or the last recall (booster) dose is more than 10 years; *and* a delay of more than 24 hours has occurred between the time of injury and initiation of specific tetanus prophylaxis; *and* the injury is of the type that could readily lead to fulminating tetanus[2] (for example—compound fracture; extensive burn; crushing, penetrating, or massively contaminated wound; injury causing interruption or impairment of the local blood supply).

Individuals who have received no prior injections of tetanus toxoid, or who have received only one injection of tetanus toxoid should be given an adequate dose of tetanus immune globulin (human) at time of injury.

Technic For Injection: Before injection, the skin over the site to be injected should be cleansed and prepared with a suitable germicide. After insertion of the needle, aspirate to help avoid inadvertent injection into a blood vessel. Expel the antigen slowly and terminate the dose with a small bubble of air (0.1 to 0.2 ml). Do not inject intracutaneously or into superficial subcutaneous tissues.

Keep between 2 and 8° C (35 and 46° F)

REFERENCES:

1. EDSALL, G.: Specific prophylaxis of tetanus. JAMA *171:*417, 1959. **2.** EDSALL, G.: Current status of tetanus immunization. Arch. Environ. Hlth. *8:*731, 1964. **3.** Report of the Committee on Infectious Diseases, American Academy of Pediatrics (Red Book), 1977. **4.** Control of Communicable Diseases in Man, 12th Edition, 1975, Am. Pub. Hlth. Assn. **5.** Recommendation of the Public Health Service Advisory Committee on Immunization Practices, Morbidity and Mortality Weekly Report 26 (No. 49):401, 1977, CDC, USPHS, DHEW, Atlanta, Georgia. **6.** KITTLER, F., et al.: Reactions to tetanus toxoid. Southern Med. J.*59:*149, 1966. **7.** LEVINE, L., et al.: Adult immunization: Preparation and evaluation of combined fluid tetanus and diphtheria toxoids for adult use. Am. J. Hyg.*73:*20, 1961. **8.** MCCOMB, J. and LEVINE, L.: Adult immunization: II. Dosage reduction as a solution to increasing reactions to tetanus toxoid. New Eng. J. Med.*265:*1152, 1961. **9.** EDSALL, G., et al.: Excessive use of tetanus toxoid boosters. JAMA*202:*17, 1967. **10.** FARDON, D.: Unusual reactions to tetanus toxoid. JAMA*199:*125, 1967. **11.** PEEBLES, T., et al.: Tetanus toxoid emergency boosters. A reappraisal. New Eng. J. Med. *280:*575, 1969. **12.** STEIGMAN, A.: Abuse of tetanus toxoid. J. Pediatrics *72:*753, 1968. **13.** GREEN, S. T.: Avoiding needle sticks. Lancet *1(8489):* 1096, 1986.

HOW SUPPLIED - EQUIVALENTS NOT AVAILABLE:

Injection, Solution - Intramuscular - 2 unit/ml

0.5 ml x 10	$20.33	Tetanus Toxoid Fl 0.5Ml Tubex, Wyeth Labs	00008-0340-01
0.5 ml x 10	$22.20	Tetanus Toxoid Adsorbed, Berna Prod	58337-1301-02
0.5 ml x 10	$25.03	Tetanus Toxoid Purogenated, Lederle Pharm	00005-1942-47
5 ml	$9.50	Tetanus Toxoid Adsorbed, Berna Prod	58337-1301-01
7.5 ml	$11.18	Tetanus Toxoid Fluid, Wyeth Labs	00008-0340-02
7.5 ml	$11.98	Tetanus Toxoid Purogenated, Lederle Pharm	00005-1942-33

Injection, Susp - Intramuscular - 0.5 ml

10's	$12.79	Tetanus Toxoid Adsorbed, Connaught Labs	49281-0800-83
15's	$13.09	Tetanus Toxoid Plain, Connaught Labs	49281-0812-84

Injection, Susp - Intramuscular - 0.5 ml/.5ml

0.5 ml x 10	$20.33	Tetanus Toxoid Adsorbed, Wyeth Labs	00008-0339-01
5 ml	$11.18	Tetanus Toxoid Adsorbed, Wyeth Labs	00008-0339-03

Injection, Susp - Intramuscular - 8 unit/ml

0.5 ml x 10	$31.26	Tetanus Toxoid Purogenated, Lederle Pharm	00005-1938-47
5 ml	$14.51	Tetanus Toxoid Purogenated, Lederle Pharm	00005-1938-31

TETRACAINE HYDROCHLORIDE *(002325)*

CATEGORIES: Anesthesia; Antipruritics/Local Anesthetics; EENT Drugs; Eye, Ear, Nose, & Throat Preparations; Local Anesthetics; Ophthalmics; Pharmaceutical Adjuvants; Skin/Mucous Membrane Agents; Pregnancy Category C; FDA Pre 1938 Drugs

BRAND NAMES: Ak-T-Caine; Dermacaine; *Pantocain*; **Pontocaine**; *Tedocain*; *Tetocain*; *Tetocaine*

(International brand names outside U.S. in italics)

FORMULARIES: BC-BS; WHO

DESCRIPTION:

PROLONGED SPINAL ANESTHESIA

Tetracaine hydrochloride is 2-(Dimethylamino)ethyl p-(butylamino) benzoate monohydrochloride.

It is a white crystalline, odorless powder that is readily soluble in water, physiologic saline solution, and dextrose solution.

Tetracaine hydrochloride is a local anesthetic of the ester-linkage type, related to procaine.

Pontocaine hydrochloride is supplied in two forms for prolonged spinal anesthesia: Niphanoid and 1% Solution.

Niphanoid: A sterile, instantly soluble form consisting of a network of extremely fine, highly purified particles, resembling snow.

1% Solution: A sterile, isotonic, isobaric solution, each 1 ml containing 10 mg tetracaine hydrochloride, 6.7 mg sodium chloride, and not more than 2 mg acetone sodium bisulfite. The air in the ampuls has been displaced by nitrogen gas.

The pH is 3.2 to 6.

These formulations do not contain preservatives.

CLINICAL PHARMACOLOGY:

Parenteral administration of tetracaine hydrochloride stabilizes the neuronal membrane and prevents initiation and transmission of nerve impulses thereby effecting local anesthesia.

The onset of action is rapid, and the duration prolonged (up to two or three hours or longer of surgical anesthesia).

Tetracaine hydrochloride is detoxified by plasma esterases to aminobenzoic acid and diethylaminoethanol.

INDICATIONS AND USAGE:

Tetracaine hydrochloride is indicated for the production of spinal anesthesia for procedures requiring two to three hours.

CONTRAINDICATIONS:

Spinal anesthesia with tetracaine hydrochloride is contraindicated in patients with known hypersensitivity to tetracaine hydrochloride or to drugs of a similar chemical configuration (ester-type local anesthetics), or aminobenzoic acid or its derivatives; and in patients for whom spinal anesthesia as a technique is contraindicated.

The decision as to whether or not spinal anesthesia should be used for an individual patient should be made by the physician after weighing the advantages with the risks and possible complications.

Contraindications to spinal anesthesia as a technique can be found in standard reference texts, and usually include generalized septicemia, infection at the site of injection, certain diseases of the cerebrospinal system, uncontrolled hypotension, etc.

WARNINGS:

RESUSCITATIVE EQUIPMENT AND DRUGS SHOULD BE IMMEDIATELY AVAILABLE WHENEVER ANY LOCAL ANESTHETIC DRUG IS USED.

Large doses of local anesthetics should not be used in patients with heartblock.

Reactions resulting in fatality have occurred on rare occasions with the use of local anesthetics, even in the absence of a history of hypersensitivity.

Contains acetone sodium bisulfite, a sulfite that may cause allergic-type reactions including anaphylactic symptoms and life-threatening or less severe asthmatic episodes in certain susceptible people. The overall prevalence of sulfite sensitivity in the general population is unknown and probably low. Sulfite sensitivity is seen more frequently in asthmatic than in nonasthmatic people.

PRECAUTIONS:

The safety and effectiveness of any spinal anesthetic depend upon proper dosage, correct technique, adequate precautions, and readiness for emergencies. The lowest dosage that results in effective anesthesia should be used to avoid high plasma levels and serious systemic side effects. Tolerance varies with the status of the patient; debilitated, elderly patients or acutely ill patients should be given reduced doses commensurate with their weight, age, and physical status. Reduced doses are also indicated for obstetric patients and those with increased intra-abdominal pressure.

Caution should be used in administering tetracaine hydrochloride to patients with abnormal or reduced levels of plasma esterases.

Blood pressure should be frequently monitored during spinal anesthesia and hypotension immediately corrected.

Spinal anesthetics should be used with caution in patients with severe disturbances of cardiac rhythm, shock, or heartblock.

Carcinogenesis, Mutagenesis, and Impairment of Fertility: Long-term animal studies to evaluate carcinogenic potential and reproduction studies in animals have not been performed. There is no evidence from human data that tetracaine hydrochloride may be carcinogenic or that it impairs fertility.

Pregnancy Category C: Animal reproduction studies have not been conducted with tetracaine hydrochloride. It is not known whether tetracaine hydrochloride can cause fetal harm when administered to a pregnant woman or can affect reproduction capacity. Tetracaine hydrochloride should be given to a pregnant woman only if clearly needed and the potential benefits outweigh the risk.

Labor and Delivery: Vasopressor agents administered for the treatment of hypotension resulting from spinal anesthesia may result in severe persistent hypertension and/or rupture of cerebral blood vessels if oxytocic drugs have also been administered; therefore, vasopressors should be used with extreme caution in the presence of oxytocic drugs.

Tetracaine hydrochloride has a recognized use during labor and delivery; the effect of the drug on duration of labor, incidence of forceps delivery, status of the newborn, and later growth and development of the child have not been studied.

Nursing Mothers: It is not known whether tetracaine hydrochloride is excreted in human milk; however, it is rapidly metabolized following absorption into the plasma. Because many drugs are excreted in human milk, caution should be exercised when tetracaine hydrochloride, brand of tetracaine hydrochloride, is administered to a nursing woman.

Pediatric Use: Safety and effectiveness of tetracaine hydrochloride in children have not been established.

DRUG INTERACTIONS:

Tetracaine hydrochloride should not be used if the patient is being treated with a sulfonamide because aminobenzoic acid inhibits the action of sulfonamides.

ADVERSE REACTIONS:

Systemic adverse reactions to tetracaine hydrochloride are characteristic of those associated with other local anesthetics and can involve the central nervous system and the cardiovascular system.

Systemic reactions usually result from high plasma levels due to excessive dosage, rapid absorption, or inadvertent intravascular injection.

A small number of reactions to tetracaine hydrochloride may result from hypersensitivity, idiosyncrasy or diminished tolerance to normal dosage.

Central Nervous System effects are characterized by excitation or depression. The first manifestation may be nervousness, dizziness, blurred vision, or tremors, followed by drowsiness, convulsions, unconsciousness and possibly respiratory and cardiac arrest. Since excitement may be transient or absent, the first manifestation may be drowsiness, sometimes merging into unconsciousness and respiratory and cardiac arrest. Other central nervous system effects may be nausea, vomiting, chills, constriction of the pupils, or tinnitus.

Cardiovascular system reactions include depression of the myocardium, blood pressure changes (usually hypotension), and cardiac arrest.

Allergic reactions, which may be due to hypersensitivity, idiosyncrasy, or diminished tolerance, are characterized by cutaneous lesions (eg, urticaria), edema, and other manifestations of allergy. Detection of sensitivity by skin testing is of limited value.

Severe allergic reactions including anaphylaxis have occurred rarely and are not usually dose-related.

Reactions Associated With Spinal Anesthesia Techniques: Central nervous system: post-spinal headache, meningismus, arachnoiditis, palsies, or spinal nerve paralysis. Cardiovascular: hypotension due to vasomotor paralysis and pooling of the blood in the venous bed. Respiratory: respiratory impairment or paralysis due to the level of anesthesia extending to the upper thoracic and cervical segments. Gastrointestinal: nausea and vomiting.

Treatment Of Reactions: Toxic effects of local anesthetics require symptomatic treatment; there is no specific cure. THE MOST IMPORTANT MEASURE IS OXYGENATION OF THE PATIENT BY MAINTAINING AN AIRWAY AND SUPPORTING VENTILATION. Supportive treatment of the cardiovascular system includes intravenous fluids and, when appropriate, vasopressors (preferably those that stimulate the myocardium). Convulsions are usually controlled with adequate oxygenation alone but intravenous administration in small increments of a barbiturate (preferably an ultrashort-acting barbiturate such as thiopental and thiamylal) or diazepam can be utilized. Intravenous barbiturates or anticonvulsant agents should only be administered by those familiar with their use and only if ventilation and oxygenation have first been assured. In spinal anesthesia, sympathetic blockade also occurs as a pharmacological action, resulting in peripheral vasodilation and often hypotension. The extent of the hypotension will usually depend on the number of dermatomes blocked. The blood pressure should therefore be monitored in the early phases of anesthesia. If hypotension occurs, it is readily controlled by vasoconstrictors administered either by the intramuscular or the intravenous route, the dosage of which would depend on the severity of the hypotension and the response to treatment.

DOSAGE AND ADMINISTRATION:

As with all anesthetics, the dosage varies and depends upon the area to be anesthetized, the number of neuronal segments to be blocked, individual tolerance, and the technique of anesthesia. The lowest dosage needed to provide effective anesthesia should be administered. For specific techniques and procedures, refer to standard textbooks.

TABLE 1 Suggested Dosage For Spinal Anesthesia

	Using Niphanoid		Using 1% solution		
Extent of anesthesia	**Dose of Niphanoid (mg)**	**Volume of spinal fluid (ml)**	**Dose of solution (ml)**	**Volume of spinal fluid (ml)**	**Site of injection (lumbar interspace)**
Perineum	5*	1	0.5 (=5 mg)*	0.5	4th
Perineum and lower extremities	10	2	1.0 (=10 mg)	1.0	3rd or 4th
Up to costal margin	15 to 20**	3	1.5 to 2.0 (=15 mg to 20 mg)**	1.5 to 2.0	2nd, 3rd, or 4th

* For vaginal delivery (saddle block) from 2 mg to 5 mg in dextrose.
** Doses exceeding 15 mg are rarely required and should be used only in exceptional cases.
Inject solution at rate of about 1 ml per 5 seconds.

The extent and degree of spinal anesthesia depend upon dosage, specific gravity of the anesthetic solution, volume of solution used, force of the injection, level of puncture, position of the patient during and immediately after injection, etc.

When spinal fluid is added to either the Niphanoid or solution, some turbidity results, the degree depending on the pH of the spinal fluid, the temperature of the solution during mixing, as well as the amount of drug and diluent employed. This cloudiness is due to the release of the Base from the hydrochloride. Liberation of base (which is completed within the spinal canal) is held to be essential for satisfactory results with any spinal anesthetic.

The specific gravity of spinal fluid at 25°C/ 25°C varies under normal conditions from 1.0063 to 1.0075. A solution of the instantly soluble form (Niphanoid) in spinal fluid has only a slightly greater specific gravity. The 1% concentration in saline solution has a specific gravity of 1.0060 to 1.0074 at 25°C/25°C.

A hyperbaric solution may be prepared by mixing equal volumes of the 1% Solution and Dextrose Solution 10% (which is available in ampuls of 3 ml).

If the Niphanoid form is preferred, it is first dissolved in Dextrose Solution 10% in a ratio of 1 ml dextrose to 10 mg of the anesthetic. Further dilution is made with an equal volume of spinal fluid. The resulting solution now contains 5% dextrose with 5 mg of anesthetic agent per milliliter.

A hypobaric solution may be prepared by dissolving the Niphanoid in Sterile Water for Injection, USP (1 mg per milliliter). The specific gravity of this solution is essentially the same as that of water, 1.000 at 25°C/25°C.

Examine ampuls carefully before use. Do not use solution if crystals, cloudiness, or discoloration is observed.

THESE FORMULATIONS OF TETRACAINE HYDROCHLORIDE DO NOT CONTAIN PRESERVATIVES; THEREFORE, UNUSED PORTIONS SHOULD BE DISCARDED AND THE RECONSTITUTED Niphanoid SHOULD BE USED IMMEDIATELY.

STERILIZATION OF AMPULS

The drug in intact ampuls is sterile. The preferred method of destroying bacteria on the exterior of ampuls before opening is heat sterilization (autoclaving). Immersion in antiseptic solution is not recommended.

AUTOCLAVE AT 15-POUND PRESSURE, AT 121°C (250°F), FOR 15 MINUTES. The Niphanoid form may also be autoclaved in the same way but may lose its snowlike appearance and tend to adhere to the sides of the ampul. This may slightly decrease the rate at which the drug dissolves but does not interfere with its anesthetic potency.

DOSAGE AND ADMINISTRATION: *(cont'd)*

AUTOCLAVING INCREASES LIKELIHOOD OF CRYSTAL FORMATION. UNUSED AUTOCLAVED AMPULS SHOULD BE DISCARDED. UNDER NO CIRCUMSTANCE SHOULD UNUSED AMPULS WHICH HAVE BEEN AUTOCLAVED BE RETURNED TO STOCK.

HOW SUPPLIED - EQUIVALENTS NOT AVAILABLE:

Injection, Solution - Intravenous - 1 %

2 ml x 25	**$132.45**	**PONTOCAINE, Sanofi Winthrop**	**00024-1574-25**

Injection, Solution - Intravenous - 20 mg

100's	**$1070.65**	**PONTOCAINE, Sanofi Winthrop**	**00024-1577-06**

Solution - Ophthalmic - 0.5 %

1 ml x 12	$25.80	Tetracaine HCl Ophthalmic, Ciba Vision	00058-0787-12
2 ml	$51.00	Tetracaine Hcl, Alcon	00065-0741-12
15 ml	$2.31	Tetracaine HCl 0.5%, Rugby	00536-5002-72
15 ml	$2.31	Tetracaine Hcl, Apotex	60505-7527-05
15 ml	$3.76	Tetracaine Hcl, Martec Pharms	52555-0994-01
15 ml	$4.50	Ak-T-Caine, Akorn	17478-0245-12
15 ml	$4.56	Tetracaine Hcl, Aligen Independ	00405-6139-15
15 ml	$5.30	Tetracaine, Schein Pharm (US)	00364-7138-72
15 ml	$13.13	Tetracaine Hcl, Alcon-PR	00998-0014-15
15 ml	**$16.78**	**PONTOCAINE, Sanofi Winthrop**	**00024-1583-01**
59 ml	**$32.15**	**PONTOCAINE MONODROPS, Sanofi Winthrop**	**00024-1584-01**

Solution - Topical - 2 %

30 ml	**$22.04**	**PONTOCAINE, Sanofi Winthrop**	**00024-1585-01**
118 ml	**$63.51**	**PONTOCAINE, Sanofi Winthrop**	**00024-1585-02**

TETRACYCLINE HYDROCHLORIDE *(002326)*

CATEGORIES: Acne; Amebiasis; Anti-Infectives; Antibacterials; Antibiotics; Antimicrobials; Antiprotozoals; Chlamydia; Conjunctivitis; Dental; Dermatologicals; EENT Drugs; Eye, Ear, Nose, & Throat Preparations; Gonorrhea; Granuloma; Inclusion Conjunctivitis; Lincosamides/Macrolides; Lyme Disease; Lymphogranuloma; Ocular Infections; Ophthalmics; Parasiticidal; Periodontitis; Pneumonia; Q Fever; Relapsing Fever; Respiratory Tract Infections; Rickettsial Disease; Rocky Mountain Fever; Skin/Mucous Membrane Agents; Streptococcal Infection; Syphilis; Tetracyclines; Tick Fevers; Trachoma; Urinary Tract Infections; Vincent's Infection; Yaws; H. Pylori*; Peptic Ulcer*; Ulcer*; FDA Approval Pre 1982; Top 200 Drugs
* Indication not approved by the FDA

BRAND NAMES: **Achromycin**; *Achromycin V* (Canada, Japan); *Acrimicina*; *Acromicina* (Mexico); Actisite; Ala-Tet; *Alphacycline*; *Altetra*; *Ambracyn*; *Ambramicina*; *Ambramycin*; *Apo-Tetra* (Canada); *Apocyclin*; *Austramycin*; *Bekatetracyn*; Biocycline; *Bristaciclina*; Bristacycline; Brodspec; *Calociclina*; *Carlamycin*; *Ciclotetryl*; *Cofarcilina*; *Conmycin*; *Cyclabid*; Cyclopar; *Dhatracin*; *Dicyclin*; *Dicyclin Forte*; *Dumocyclin*; *Dumocycline*; *Economycin* (England); *Egosin*; Emtet-500; *Florocycline* (France); *Grambiotico*; *Hexacycline* (France); *Hostaciclina*; *Hostaciclina P*; *Hostacyclin*; *Hostacycline*; *Hostacycline-P*; *Hydracycline*; *Hydromycin*; *Ibicyn*; *Idilin*; *Ikacyclin*; *Latycin*; *Lenocin*; *Maviciclina*; *Medocycline*; *Mysteclin*; *Nelmicyn*; Nor-Tet; *Novotetra* (Canada); *Omnaze*; *Oricyclin*; Panmycin; *Pantocycline*; *Parenciclina* (Mexico); *Pervasol*; *Polarcyclin*; *Polfamycine*; *Quimocyclar* (Mexico); *Resteclin*; *Rimatet*; Robitet; Sarocycline; *Servitet*; *Steclin* (Germany); *Steclin V*; *Subamycin*; Sumycin; *Supramycin*; *Tefilin* (Germany); Tega-Cycline; Teline; *Telmycin*; *Tetocyn*; *Tetra-Atlantis* (Mexico); *Tetrabioptal*; *Tetrablet* (Germany); Tetracap; Tetrachel; *Tetraciclina*; *Tetracitro-S*; *Tetracitro S* (Germany); Tetracon; *Tetracyclin*; Tetracyn; *Tetracyna*; Tetralan; *Tetralen*; *Tetralim*; *Tetralution* (Germany); Tetram; Tetramed; *Tetramig* (France); *Tetrana*; *Tetranovin*; *Tetrarco*; *Tetrarco L.A.*; *Tetraseptin*; *Tetrasuiss*; *Tetrex* (Mexico, Japan); *Tevacycline*; *Theracine*; Topicycline; *Triphacyclin*; *Unimycin*; *Upcyclin*; *Vemyclin*; Wesmycin; *Wintellin*; *Wintrex*; *Xepacycline*
(International brand names outside U.S. in italics)

FORMULARIES: Aetna; BC-BS; CIGNA; DoD; FHP; Humana; Kaiser; Medco; Medi-Cal; PCS; PruCare; United; WHO

COST OF THERAPY: $1.15 (Infections; Capsule; 500 mg; 2/day; 10 days)

PRIMARY ICD9: 136.9 (Unspecified Infections And Parasitic Diseases)

DESCRIPTION:

Tetracycline is a broad-spectrum antibiotic prepared from the cultures of certain streptomyces species. Chemically, Tetracycline HCl is: (4*S*-(4ß,1α,4aα,5aα,6β,12aα))-4-(dimethylamino)-1, 4,4a,5, 5a,6, 11, 12a-octahydro -3,6,10,12,12a-pentahydroxy-6-methyl-1,11-dioxo-2- naphthacenecarboxamide monohydrochloride.

CLINICAL PHARMACOLOGY:

CAPSULES

The tetracyclines are primarily bacteriostatic and are thought to exert their antimicrobial effect by the inhibition of protein synthesis. Tetracyclines are active against a wide range of gram-negative and gram-positive organisms.

The drugs in the tetracycline class have closely similar antimicrobial spectra, and cross-resistance among them is common. Micro-organisms may be considered susceptible if the MIC (minimum inhibitory concentration) is not more than 4.0 mcg/ml and intermediate if the MIC is 4.0 to 12.5 mcg/ml.

Susceptibility Testing: A tetracycline disc may be used to determine microbial susceptibility to drugs in the tetracycline class. If the Kirby-Bauer method of disc susceptibility testing is used, a 30 mcg tetracycline disc should give a zone of at least 19 mm when tested against a tetracycline-susceptible bacterial strain.

Tetracyclines are readily absorbed and are bound to plasma proteins in varying degree. They are concentrated by the liver in the bile and excreted in the urine and feces at high concentrations and in a biologically active form.

TOPICAL SOLUTION

This form delivers tetracycline to the pilosebaceous apparatus and the adjacent tissues. Tetracycline topical solution reduces inflammatory acne lesions, but its mode of actions is not fully understood.

In clinical studies, use of tetracycline topical solution on the face and neck twice daily delivered to the skin an average dose of 2.9 mg of tetracycline HCl per day. Patients who used the medication twice daily on other acne-involved areas in addition to the face and neck applied an average dose of 4.8 mg of tetracycline HCl per day.

CLINICAL PHARMACOLOGY: *(cont'd)*

Tetracycline topical solution has been formulated such that the recrystallization properties of the tetracycline on the skin greatly reduce or eliminate the yellow color after associated with topical tetracycline.

INDICATIONS AND USAGE:

CAPSULES

Tetracycline is indicated in infections caused by the following micro-organisms: Rickettsiae (Rocky Mountain spotted fever, typhus fever and the typhus group, Q fever, rickettsialpox and tick fevers),*Mycoplasma pneumoniae* (PPLO, Eaton Agent), Agents of psittacosis and ornithosis, Agents of lymphogranuloma venereum and granuloma inguinale. The spirochetal agent of relapsing fever (*Borrelia recurrentis*).

The following gram-negative micro-organisms:

Haemophilus ducreyi (chancroid)

Pasteurella pestis, Pasteurella tularensis, Bartonella bacilliformis, Bacteroides species

Vibrio comma and *Vibrio fetus, Brucella* species (in conjunction with streptomycin).

Because many strains of the following groups of micro-organisms have been shown to be resistant to tetracyclines, culture and susceptibility testing are recommended.

Tetracycline is indicated for treatment of infections caused by the following gram-negative micro-organisms, when bacteriologic testing indicates appropriate susceptibility to the drug:

Escherichia coli, Enterobacter aerogenes (formerly *Aerobacter aerogenes*)

Shigella species

Mima species and *Herellea* species

Haemophilus influenzae (respiratory infections)

Klebsiella species (respiratory and urinary infections).

Tetracycline is indicated for treatment of infections caused by the following gram-positive micro-organisms when bacteriologic testing indicates appropriate susceptibility to the drug. Streptococcus species: Up to 44 percent of strains of *Streptococcus pyogenes* and 74 percent of *Streptococcus faecalis* have been found to be resistant to tetracycline drugs. Therefore, tetracyclines should not be used for streptococcal disease unless the organism has been demonstrated to be sensitive. For upper respiratory infections due to group A beta-hemolytic streptococci, penicillin is the usual drug of choice, including prophylaxis of rheumatic fever. *Diplococcus pneumoniae, Staphylococcus aureus,* skin and soft tissue infections. Tetracyclines are not the drugs of choice in the treatment of any type of staphylococcal infections.

When penicillin is contraindicated, tetracyclines are alternative drugs in the treatment of infections due to:

Neisseria gonorrhoeae, Treponema pallidum and *Treponema pertenue* (syphilis and yaws)

Listeria monocytogenes, Clostridium species

Bacillus anthracis, Fusobacterium fusiforme (Vincent's infection)

Actinomyces species.

In acute intestinal amebiasis, the tetracyclines may be a useful adjunct to amebicides.

In severe acne, the tetracyclines may be useful adjunctive therapy.

Tetracycline HCl is indicated for the treatment of uncomplicated urethral, endocervical or rectal infections in adults caused by *Chlamydia trachomatis.*[1]

Tetracyclines are indicated in the treatment of trachoma, although the infectious agent is not always eliminated, as judged by immunofluorescence.

Inclusion conjunctivitis may be treated with oral tetracyclines or with a combination of oral and topical agents.

TOPICAL SOLUTION

Tetracycline topical solution is indicated in the treatment of acne vulgaris.

OPHTHALMIC SUSPENSION

For the treatment of superficial ocular infections susceptible to tetracycline hydrochloride.

For prophylaxis of ophthalmia neonatorum due to *Neisseria gonorrhoeae* or *Chlamydia trachomatis.* The Center for Disease Control (U.S.P.H.S.) and the Committee on Drugs, the Committee on Fetus and Newborn, and the Committee on Infectious Diseases of the American Academy of Pediatrics recommend 1 percent silver nitrate solution in single-dose ampoules or single-use tubes of an ophthalmic ointment containing 0.5 percent erythromycin or 1 percent tetracycline as "effective and acceptable regimens of prophylaxis of gonococcal ophthalmia neonatorum."[1] (For infants born to mothers with clinically apparent gonorrhea, intravenous or intramuscular injections of aqueous crystalline penicillin G should be given; a single dose of 50,000 units for term infants or 20,00 for infants of low birth weight. Topical prophylaxis alone is inadequate for these infants.[1])

The following organisms have demonstrated susceptibility to tetracycline hydrochloride:

Staphylococcus aureus,

Streptococci including *Streptococcus pneumoniae,*

E. coli

Neisseria species,

Chlamydia trachomatis.

When treating trachoma a concomitant oral tetracycline is helpful.

Other organisms, not known to cause superficial eye infections, but with demonstrated susceptibility to tetracycline hydrochloride, have been omitted from the above list.

Tetracycline hydrochloride does not provide adequate coverage against:

Haemophilus influenzae

Klebsiella/Enterobacter species

Pseudomonas aeruginosa

Serratia marcescens

CONTRAINDICATIONS:

This drug is contraindicated in persons who have shown hypersensitivity to any of the tetracyclines or to any of the other ingredients.

WARNINGS:

CAPSULES

THE USE OF DRUGS OF THE TETRACYCLINE CLASS DURING TOOTH DEVELOPMENT (LAST HALF OF PREGNANCY, INFANCY AND CHILDHOOD TO THE AGE OF 8 YEARS) MAY CAUSE PERMANENT DISCOLORATION OF THE TEETH (YELLOW-GRAY-BROWN). This adverse reaction is more common during long-term use of the drugs but has been observed following repeated short-term courses. Enamel hypoplasia has also been reported. TETRACYCLINE DRUGS, THEREFORE, SHOULD NOT BE USED IN THIS AGE GROUP UNLESS OTHER DRUGS ARE NOT LIKELY TO BE EFFECTIVE OR ARE CONTRAINDICATED.

WARNINGS: *(cont'd)*

If renal impairment exists, even usual oral or parenteral doses may lead to excessive systemic accumulation of the drug and possible liver toxicity. Under such conditions, lower than usual total doses are indicated and, if therapy is prolonged, serum level determinations of the drug may be advisable.

Photosensitivity manifested by an exaggerated sunburn reaction has been observed in some individuals taking tetracyclines. Patients apt to be exposed to direct sunlight or ultraviolet light should be advised that this reaction can occur with tetracycline drugs, and treatment should be discontinued at the first evidence of skin erythema. NOTE: Photsensitization reactions have occurred most frequently with democycline, less with chlortetracycline, and very rarely with oxytetracycline and tetracycline.

The anti-anabolic action of the tetracyclines may cause an increase in BUN. While this is not a problem in those with normal renal function, in patients with significantly impaired function, higher serum levels of tetracycline may lead to azotemia, hyperphosphatemia, and acidosis.

Usage in Pregnancy: See WARNINGSabout use during tooth development.

Results of animal studies indicate that tetracyclines cross the placenta, are found in fetal tissues and can have toxic effects on the developing fetus (often related to retardation of skeletal development). Evidence of embryotoxicity has also been noted in animals treated early in pregnancy.

Usage in Newborns, Infants, and Children: See WARNINGSabout use during tooth development.

All tetracyclines form a stable calcium complex in any bone forming tissue. A decrease in the fibula growth rate has been observed in prematures given oral tetracycline in doses of 25 mg/kg every 6 hours. This reaction was shown to be reversible when the drug was discontinued.

Tetracyclines are present in the milk of lactating women who are taking a drug in this class.

TOPICAL SOLUTION

Contains sodium bisulfite, a sulfite that may cause allergic-type reactions including anaphylactic symptoms and life threatening or less severe asthmatic episodes in certain susceptible people. The overall prevalence of sulfite sensitivity in the general population is unknown and probably low. Sulfite sensitivity is seen more frequently in asthmatic than in non-asthmatic people.

PRECAUTIONS:

GENERAL

Capsules: As with other antibiotic preparations, use of this drug may result in overgrowth of nonsusceptible organisms, including fungi. If superinfection occurs, the antibiotic should be discontinued and appropriate therapy instituted. NOTE: Superinfection of the bowel by staphylococci may be life-threatening.

In venereal diseases when coexistent syphilis is suspected, darkfield examination should be done before treatment is started and the blood serology repeated monthly for at least 4 months.

Because tetracyclines have been shown to depress plasma prothrombin activity, patients who are on anticoagulant therapy may require downward adjustment of their anticoagulant dosage.

In long-term therapy, periodic laboratory evaluation of organ systems, including hematopoietic, renal and hepatic studies should be performed.

All infections due to Group A beta-hemolytic streptococci should be treated for at least 10 days.

Since bacteriostatic drugs may interfere with the bactericidal action of penicillin, it is advisable to avoid giving tetracycline in conjunction with penicillin.

Since sensitivity reactions are more likely to occur in oersons with a history of allergy, asthma, hay fever, or urticaria, the preparation should be used with caution in such individuals.

Topical Solution: This is for external use only and care should be taken to keep it out of the eyes, nose, and mouth.

Ophthalmic Suspension: The use of antibiotics occasionally may result in overgrowth of nonsusceptible organisms. Constant observation of the patient is essential. If new infections appear during therapy, appropriate measures should be taken.

CARCINOGENESIS, MUTAGENESIS, AND IMPAIRMENT OF FERTILITY

Capsules: Long-term animal studies are currently being conducted to determine whether tetracycline HCl has carcinogenic potential. Some related antibiotics (oxytetracycline, minocycline) have shown evidence of oncogenic activity in rats.

In two *in vitro* mammalian cell assay systems (L 51784y mouse lymphoma and Chinese hamster lung cells), there was evidence of mutagenicity at tetracycline HCl concentrations of 60 and 10 mcg/ml, respectively.

Tetracycline HCl had no effect on fertility when administered in the diet to the male and female rats at a daily intake of 25 times the human dose.

Topical Solution: A two-year dermal study in mice has been performed in rats and rabbits at doses of up to 246 times the human dose (assuming the human to be 1.3 ml/40kg/day) and have revealed no evidence of impaired fertility or harm ti the fetus. There are, however, no adequate and well-controlled studies in pregnant women. Because animal reproduction studies are not always predictive of human response, this drug should be used during pregnancy only if clearly needed.

NURSING MOTHERS

It is not known whether tetracycline or any other component of tetracycline topical solution is excreted in human milk. Because many drugs are excreted in human milk, caution should be exercised when tetracycline topical solution is administered to a nursing woman.

PEDIATRIC USE

Safety and effectiveness in children below the age of eleven has not yet been established.

ADVERSE REACTIONS:

CAPSULES

Gastrointestinal: Anorexia, epigastric distress, nausea, vomiting, diarrhea, bulky loose stools, stomatitis, sore throat, glossitis, black hairy tongue, dysphagia, hoarseness, enterocolitis, and inflammatory lesions (with monilial overgrowth) in the anogenital region, including proctitus and pruritus ani. These reactions have been caused by both the oral and parenteral administration of tetracyclines.

Skin: Maculopapular and erythematous rashes. Exfoliative dermatitis has been reported but is uncommon. Photosensitivity is discussed above. (See WARNINGS.)

Renal toxicity: Rise in BUN has been reported and is apparently dose related. (See WARNINGS.)

Hepatic cholestasis has been reported rarely, and is usually associated with high dosage levels of tetracycline.

ADVERSE REACTIONS: *(cont'd)*

Hypersensitivity reactions: urticaria, angioneurotic edema, anaphylaxis, anaphylactoid purpura, pericarditis and exacerbation of systemic lupus erythematosus, and serum sickness-like reactions, as fever, rash, and arthralgia.

Bulging fontanels have been reported in young infants following full therapeutic dosage. This sign disappeared rapidly when the drug was discontinued.

Blood: anemia, hemolytic anemia, thrombocytopenia, thrombocytopenic purpura, neutropenia and eosinophilia have been reported.

Dizziness and heachache have been reported.

When given over prolonged periods, tetracyclines have been reported to produce brown-black microscopic discoloration of thyroid glands. No abnormalities of thyroid function studies are known to occur.

TOPICAL SOLUTION

Among the 838 patients treated with tetracycline topical solution under normal usage conditions during clinical evaluation, there was one instance of severe dermatitis requiring systemic steroid therapy.

About one-third of patients are likely to experience a stinging or burning sensation. The sensation ordinarily lasts no more than a few minutes, and does not occur at every application. There has been no indication that patients experience sufficient discomfort to reduce the frequency of use or to discontinue use of the product.

The kinds of side effects often associated with oral or parenteral administration of tetracyclines (*e.g.,* various gastrointestinal complaints, vaginitis, hematologic abnormalities, manifestations of systemic hypersensitivity reactions, and dental and skeletal disorders) have not been observed with tetracycline topical solution. Because this drug's topical from of administration, it is highly unlikely that such side effects will occur from its use.

OPHTHALMIC SUSPENSION

Dermatitis and allied symptomatology have been reported. If adverse reaction or idiosyncrasy occurs, discontinue medication and institute appropriate therapy.

DOSAGE AND ADMINISTRATION:

CAPSULES

Therapy should be continued for at least 24-48 hours after symptoms and fever have subsided.

Concomitant Therapy: Antacids containing aluminum, calcium, or magnesium impair absorption and should not be given to patients taking oral tetracycline.

Food and some dairy products also interfere with absorption. Oral forms of tetracycline should be given 1 hour before or 2 hours after meals. Pediatric oral dosage forms should not be given with milk formulas and should be given at least 1 hour prior to feeding.

In Patients with Renal Impairment: (See WARNINGS.) Total dosage should be decreased by reduction of recommended individual doses and/or by extending time intervals between doses.

In the treatment of streptococcal infections, a therapeutic dose of tetracycline should be administered for at least 10 days.

Adults: Usual daily dose, 1-2 g divided in two or four equal doses, depending on the severity of the infection.

For Children Above Eight Years Of Age: Usual daily dose, 10-20 mg (25-50 mg/kg) per pound of body weight divided in four equal doses.

For treatment of brucellosis, 500 mg tetracycline four times daily for 3 weeks should be accompanied by streptomycin. 1 gram intramuscularly twice daily the first week, and once daily the second week.

For treatment of syphilis, a total of 30-40 grams in equally divided doses over a period of 10-15 days should be given. Close follow up, including laboratory tests, is recommended.

Treatment of Uncomplicated Gonorrhea: When penicillin is contraindicated, tetracycline may be used for the treatment of both males and females in the following divided dosage schedule: 1.5 grams initially followed by 0.5 grams q.i.d. for a total of 9.0 grams.

For treatment of uncomplicated urethral, endocervical, or rectal infections in adults caused by *Chlamydia trachomatis*:500 mg, by mouth, 4 times a day for at least 7 days.[1]

In cases of severe acne which, in the judgment of the clinician, require long-term treatment, the recommended initial dosage is 2 g daily in the divided doses. When improvement is noted, usually within one week, dosage shoulf be gradually reduced to maintenance levels ranging from 125 mg to 500 mg daily. In some patients it may be possible to maintain adequate remission of lesions with alternate-day or intermittent therapy. Tetracycline therapy of acne should agument the other standard measures known to be of value.

Store at Controlled Room Temperature, Between 15 and 30°C (59 and 86°F).

Dispense in tight, light-resistant container.

TOPICAL SOLUTION

It is recommended that tetracycline topical solution be applied generously twice-daily to the entire affected area (not just to the individual lesions) until the skin is thoroughly wet. Instructions to the patient for proper application are provided on the bottle label. Patients may continue their normal use of cosmetics.

Concomitant use with benzoyl peroxide or oral tetracycline has been reported without observed problems.

Tetracycline topical solution should be kept at controlled room temperature 59-86°F (15-30C°) or below.

OPHTHALMIC SUSPENSION

For most susceptible bacterial infections shake well, then gently squeeze the plastic dropper bottle to instill 2 drops in the affected eye, or if necessary, in both eyes, 2 or 4 times daily, or more frequently, depending upon the severity of the infection. Very severe infections may require days of treatment, whereas other cases may be cured by instillation with much less frequency for 48 hours.

In acute and chronic trachoma instill 2 drops in each eye 2 to 4 times daily. This treatment should be continued for 1 to 3 months except that certain individual or complicated cases may require a longer duration. A concomitant oral tetracycline is helpful.

For unit dose administration and convenience, the dispenser may be used. Immediately prior to use, simultaneously roll, invert and squeeze dispenser between thumb and fingers. Repeat several times to mix contents well. Use aseptic technique to cut the tip of the dispenser, thereby maintaining sterility. Discard first two drops before instilling drops in eye(s). Instill two drops in eye(s), then discard dispenser.

Store at Controlled Room Temperature 15-30°C (59-86°F).

REFERENCES:

Capsules 1. CDC Sexually Transmitted Diseases Treatment Guidelines 1982. **Ophthalmic Suspension 1.** American Academy of Pediatrics: Prophylaxis and Treatment of Neonatal Gonococcal Infections, *Pediatrics*, 65:1047, 1980.

PATIENT INFORMATION:

Tetracycline HCl is considered a broad-spectrum antibiotic because it can be used to treat many infections. Tetracycline can be a capsule, an eye drop or a solution to put on the face. Tetracycline can discolor teeth during their formation and therefore should not be taken during the last half of pregnancy or by children under the age of 8 years. Tetracycline can also make your skin more sensitive to the sun. Adequate sunscreen and clothing protection are suggested. The solution applied to the face contains sulfites which some people are allergic to. The most common side effects involve stomach and intestines such as nausea, vomiting, diarrhea or sore throat. Wait two hours before taking any antacids. Avoid taking dairy products with tetracycline because the medication will be less effective. Because this is an antibiotic, the entire prescription should be taken as prescribed, even if your symptoms are gone and you feel better. It is important not to keep any left-overs' of this medication. It can be harmful if expired. Any unused medication should be flushed down the toilet or returned to the pharmacy for proper disposal.

HOW SUPPLIED - RATED THERAPEUTICALLY EQUIVALENT:

Capsule, Gelatin - Oral - 250 mg

40's	$1.50	Tetracycline HCl, H.C.F.A. F F P	99999-2326-01
40's	$1.72	Tetracycline Hcl, Talbert Phcy	44514-0884-25
40's	$2.16	Tetracycline Hcl, Talbert Phcy	44514-0655-28
40's	$32.20	ACHROMYCIN V, Lederle Pharm	00005-4880-61
100's	$3.75	Tetracycline HCl, H.C.F.A. F F P	99999-2326-02
100's	$3.83	ACHROMYCIN V, Lederle Pharm	00005-4880-23
100's	$4.25	Tetracycline Hcl, Eon Labs Mfg	00185-0670-01
100's	$4.50	Tetracycline Hcl, Consolidated Midland	00223-1655-01
100's	$4.79	Tetracyclilne, US Trading	56126-0362-11
100's	$5.14	Tetracycline Hcl, Purepac Pharm	00228-2404-10
100's	$5.23	PANMYCIN HCL, Pharmacia & Upjohn	00009-0782-01
100's	$5.40	SUMYCIN '250', Bristol Myers Squibb	00003-0655-40
100's	$5.60	Tetracycline Hcl, Halsey Drug	00879-0158-01
100's	$5.62	Tetracycline HCl, Rugby	00536-1820-01
100's	$5.75	Tetracycline HCl, Warner Chilcott	00047-0407-24
100's	$5.75	Tetracycline Hcl, United Res	00677-0376-01
100's	$5.75	Tetracycline Hcl, Major Pharms	00904-2416-60
100's	$5.80	Tetracycline Hcl, Zenith Labs	00172-2416-60
100's	$5.80	Tetracycline Hcl, Goldline Labs	00182-0112-01
100's	$5.85	Tetracycline Hcl, United Res	00677-0144-01
100's	$6.15	Tetracycline Hcl, Qualitest Pharms	00603-5919-21
100's	$6.21	Tetracycline HCl, HL Moore Drug Exch	00839-1656-06
100's	$6.25	Tetracycline Hcl, Schein Pharm (US)	00364-2026-01
100's	$6.30	Tetracycline Hcl, Voluntary Hosp	53258-0420-01
100's	$6.31	Tetracycline Hcl 250, Aligen Independ	00405-4981-01
100's	$7.75	Tetracycline Hcl, Schein Pharm (US)	00364-2026-90
100's	$8.00	Tetracycline Hcl, Goldline Labs	00182-0112-89
100's	$8.00	Tetram, Dunhall Pharms	00217-0803-01
100's	$8.24	Tetracycline Hcl, Vangard Labs	00615-0151-13
100's	$9.00	TETRACYCLINE HCL, Voluntary Hosp	53258-0420-13
100's	$10.47	ALA-TET, Del Ray Lab	00316-0142-01
1000's	$26.95	Tetra 250, H & H Labs	46703-0013-10
1000's	$27.50	Tetracycline Hcl, Harber Pharm	51432-0446-06
1000's	$28.00	BRODSPEC, C O Truxton	00463-5001-10
1000's	$28.03	Tetracycline Capsules 250 Mg, Labs Atral	53862-0103-03
1000's	$31.48	ACHROMYCIN V, Lederle Pharm	00005-4880-34
1000's	$32.25	Tetracycline Hcl, IDE-Interstate	00814-7756-30
1000's	$33.95	Tetracycline Hcl, Eon Labs Mfg	00185-0670-10
1000's	$37.50	Tetracycline HCl, H.C.F.A. F F P	99999-2326-03
1000's	$37.88	Tetracycline Hcl, Geneva Pharms	00781-2529-10
1000's	$38.76	Tetracycline Hcl, Purepac Pharm	00228-2404-96
1000's	$40.15	Tetracycline Hcl, Barr	00555-0011-05
1000's	$41.00	Tetracycline Hcl, Parmed Pharms	00349-8930-10
1000's	$41.00	Tetracycline Hcl, Halsey Drug	00879-0158-10
1000's	$41.95	Tetracycline Hcl, Major Pharms	00904-2416-80
1000's	$42.00	Tetracycline Hcl, Consolidated Midland	00223-1655-02
1000's	$42.90	Tetracycline Hcl, United Res	00677-0144-10
1000's	$42.95	Tetracycline Hcl, Schein Pharm (US)	00364-2026-02
1000's	$43.25	Tetracycline HCl, Rugby	00536-1820-10
1000's	$43.75	Tetracycline HCl, Warner Chilcott	00047-0407-32
1000's	$45.80	Tetracycline Hcl, Zenith Labs	00172-2416-80
1000's	$45.80	Tetracycline Hcl, Goldline Labs	00182-0112-10
1000's	$45.80	Tetracycline Hcl 250, Aligen Independ	00405-4981-03
1000's	$46.60	Tetracycline Hcl, Qualitest Pharms	00603-5919-32
1000's	$46.70	Tetracycline Hcl, Mylan	00378-0101-10
1000's	$48.96	SUMYCIN '250', Bristol Myers Squibb	00003-0655-60
1000's	$49.01	Tetracycline HCl, HL Moore Drug Exch	00839-1656-16
1200's	$44.52	ACHROMYCIN V, Lederle Pharm	00005-4880-65

Capsule, Gelatin - Oral - 500 mg

100's	$5.78	Tetracycline HCl, H.C.F.A. F F P	99999-2326-04
100's	$6.40	ACHROMYCIN V, Lederle Pharm	00005-4875-23
100's	$6.95	Tetracycline Hcl, Harber Pharm	51432-0448-03
100's	$7.40	Tetracycline Hydrochloride, US Trading	56126-0363-11
100's	$7.50	Tetracycline Hcl, Wyeth Labs	00008-0471-01
100's	$7.93	ROBITET '500', AH Robins	00031-8427-63
100's	$8.42	Tetracycline Hcl, Purepac Pharm	00228-2406-10
100's	$8.89	Tetracycline Hcl, United Res	00677-0377-01
100's	$8.90	Tetracycline Hcl, Geneva Pharms	00781-2466-01
100's	$8.95	Tetracycline Hcl, Major Pharms	00904-2407-60
100's	$8.96	EMTET, Embrex Economed	38130-0203-01
100's	$9.00	Tetracycline, IDE-Interstate	00814-7758-14
100's	$9.15	Tetracycline HCl, Warner Chilcott	00047-0697-24
100's	$9.27	Tetracycline Hcl, Schein Pharm (US)	00364-2029-01
100's	$9.45	Tetracycline Hcl, Halsey Drug	00879-0159-01
100's	$10.10	Tetracycline HCl, Rugby	00536-1870-01
100's	$10.15	Tetracycline Hcl, Barr	00555-0010-02
100's	$10.20	Tetracycline Hcl 500, Aligen Independ	00405-4976-01
100's	$10.20	Tetracycline Hcl, Qualitest Pharms	00603-5920-21
100's	$10.30	Tetracycline Hcl, Zenith Labs	00172-2407-60
100's	$10.30	Tetracycline Hcl, Goldline Labs	00182-0679-01
100's	$10.49	SUMYCIN 500, Bristol Myers Squibb	00003-0763-40
100's	$10.94	Tetracycline HCl, HL Moore Drug Exch	00839-5075-06
100's	$11.85	Tetracycline Hcl, Voluntary Hosp	53258-0421-01
100's	$11.95	Tetracycline Hcl, Mylan	00378-0102-01
100's	$14.10	Tetracycline Hcl, Voluntary Hosp	53258-0421-13
100's	$16.75	Tetracycline Hcl, Schein Pharm (US)	00364-2029-90
100's	$18.55	Tetracycline Hcl, Goldline Labs	00182-0679-89
100's	$19.02	Tetracycline Hcl, Vangard Labs	00615-0162-13
500's	$28.90	Tetracycline HCl, H.C.F.A. F F P	99999-2326-05
500's	$42.24	Tetracycline Hcl, Purepac Pharm	00228-2406-50
500's	$48.34	SUMYCIN 500, Bristol Myers Squibb	00003-0763-50
500's	$52.95	Tetracycline Hcl, Mylan	00378-0102-05
1000's	$50.34	Tetracycline Capsules 500 Mg, Labs Atral	53862-0203-04
1000's	$51.50	Tetracycline Hcl, Harber Pharm	51432-0448-06
1000's	$57.13	ACHROMYCIN V, Lederle Pharm	00005-4875-34

HOW SUPPLIED - RATED THERAPEUTICALLY EQUIVALENT: *(cont'd)*

1000's	$57.80	Tetracycline HCl, H.C.F.A. F F P	99999-2326-06
1000's	$66.75	Tetracycline Hcl, IDE-Interstate	00814-7758-30
1000's	$70.76	Tetracycline Hcl, Barr	00555-0010-05
1000's	$70.77	Tetracycline Hcl, Purepac Pharm	00228-2406-96
1000's	$74.99	Tetracycline Hcl, United Res	00677-0377-10
1000's	$75.00	Tetracycline Hcl, Schein Pharm (US)	00364-2029-02
1000's	$75.14	Tetracycline HCl, Warner Chilcott	00047-0697-32
1000's	$75.20	Tetracycline Hcl, Geneva Pharms	00781-2466-10
1000's	$77.62	Tetracycline HCl, Rugby	00536-1870-10
1000's	$77.75	Tetracycline Hcl, Major Pharms	00904-2407-80
1000's	$78.21	Tetracycline Hcl 500, Aligen Independ	00405-4976-03
1000's	$78.80	Tetracycline Hcl, Halsey Drug	00879-0159-10
1000's	$88.30	Tetracycline Hcl, Qualitest Pharms	00603-5920-32
1000's	$89.30	Tetracycline Hcl, Zenith Labs	00172-2407-80
1000's	$89.30	Tetracycline Hcl, Goldline Labs	00182-0679-10
1000's	$89.30	Tetracycline HCl, HL Moore Drug Exch	00839-5075-16

Injection, Dry-Soln - Intramuscular - 250 mg/vial

250 mg	$12.17	ACHROMYCIN IM 250, Lederle Pharm	00005-5357-95

Injection, Solution - Intravenous - 500 mg

1's	$19.77	ACHROMYCIN IV, Lederle Pharm	00005-4771-96

Syrup - Oral - 125 mg/5ml

480 ml	$8.85	Tetracycline, United Res	00677-0147-33
480 ml	$9.60	Tetracycline, Goldline Labs	00182-0678-40
480 ml	$10.00	BRODSPEC, C O Truxton	00463-5002-16
480 ml	$10.85	SUMYCIN, Bristol Myers Squibb	00003-0815-50

HOW SUPPLIED - NOT RATED EQUIVALENT:

Solution - Topical - 2.2 mg/ml

70 ml	$56.98	TOPICYCLINE, Roberts Labs	54092-0315-70

Tablet, Coated - Oral - 250 mg

100's	$5.61	SUMYCIN '250', Bristol Myers Squibb	00003-0663-45
1000's	$50.92	SUMYCIN '250', Bristol Myers Squibb	00003-0663-75

Tablet, Coated - Oral - 500 mg

100's	$10.91	SUMYCIN '500', Bristol Myers Squibb	00003-0603-43
500's	$50.28	SUMYCIN '500', Bristol Myers Squibb	00003-0603-50

TETRAHYDROZOLINE HYDROCHLORIDE

(002328)

CATEGORIES: EENT Drugs; Eye, Ear, Nose, & Throat Preparations; Nasal Congestion; Respiratory & Allergy Medications; Vasoconstrictors; Pregnancy Category C; FDA Approval Pre 1982

BRAND NAMES: **Tyzine**

DESCRIPTION:

Nasal Solution: Tetrahydrozoline nasal solution contains tetrahydrozoline hydrochloride, 2-(1,2,3,4-Tetrahydro-1-naphthyl)-2-imidazoline monohydrochloride, as a nasal decongestant. The molecular weight is 236.74.

Tetrahydrozoline nasal solution is available for topical nasal application as 0.1% nasal solution and as 0.05% pediatric nasal drops. The nasal solution is a solution of tetrahydrozoline hydrochloride in water, with sodium chloride, sodium citrate, edetate disodium, and benzalkonium chloride, with hydrochloric acid to adjust the pH.

Ophthalmic Solution: Tetrahydrozoline Hydrochloride 0.05%, Sodium Borate, Boric Acid, Sodium Chloride, Edetate Disodium 0.1%, with Benzalkonium Chloride 0.01% as preservative, in Water for Injection. Sodium Hydroxide and/or Hydrochloric Acid may have been used to adjust pH.

CLINICAL PHARMACOLOGY:

Nasal Solution: Tetrahydrozoline nasal solution, a sympathomimetic amine, possesses vasoconstrictor and decongestant actions when applied to the nasal mucosa, resulting in vasoconstriction of the smaller arterioles of the nasal passages. Information on the absorption, distribution and elimination of the drug is not available.

INDICATIONS AND USAGE:

Nasal Solution: Tetrahydrozoline nasal solution is indicated for decongestion of nasal and nasopharyngeal mucosa.

Ophthalmic Solution: Relieves redness of the eye due to minor eye irritations.

CONTRAINDICATIONS:

Nasal Solution: Tetrahydrozoline nasal solution is contraindicated for patients who have shown previous hypersensitivity to its components. The 0.1% solution is contraindicated in children under six years of age. Tetrahydrozoline Pediatric nasal solution should be used for children between the ages of 2 and 6 years (See DOSAGE AND ADMINISTRATION.) Tetrahydrozoline nasal solution should not be used by patients under treatment with Monoamine Oxidase (MAO) inhibitors.

WARNINGS:

NASAL SOLUTION

Overdosage in children may produce profound sedation. This may be accompanied by profuse sweating, hypotension or even shock (see OVERDOSAGE).

OPHTHALMIC SOLUTION

To avoid contamination, do not touch tip of container to any surface. Replace cap after using. If you experience eye pain, changes in vision, continued redness or irritation of the eye, or if the condition worsens or persists for more than 72 hours, discontinue use and consult a doctor. If you have glaucoma, do not use this product except under the advice and supervision of a doctor. Overuse of this product may produce increased redness of the eye. If solution changes color or becomes cloudy, do not use.

PRECAUTIONS:

NASAL SOLUTION

General: Avoid doses greater or more frequent than those recommended below. Excessive dosage in children may, on rare occasions, cause severe drowsiness. Profuse sweating may accompany this effect. Overdosage may also cause marked hypotension or even shock. Use cautiously in patients with cardiovascular disease (*e.g.,* coronary artery disease, hypertension), and metabolic—endocrine diseases (*e.g.,* hyperthyroidism, diabetes).

PRECAUTIONS: *(cont'd)*

Information for Patients: Patients should be advised to follow the prescribed dosage regimen. The spray should be administered with the head held upright. To spray, squeeze the bottle quickly and firmly and sniff briskly. Instillation of the nose drops can be most conveniently accomplished with the patient in the lateral head-low position.

Pregnancy Category C: Animal reproduction studies have not been conducted with tetrahydrozoline. It is also not known whether tetrahydrozoline nasal solution can cause fetal harm when administered to a pregnant woman or can affect reproduction capacity. Tetrahydrozoline nasal solution should be given to a pregnant woman only if clearly needed.

Nursing Mothers: It is not known whether this drug is secreted in human milk. Because many drugs are secreted in human milk, caution should be exercised when tetrahydrozoline nasal solution is administered to a nursing woman.

OPHTHALMIC SOLUTION

Remove contact lenses before using. Keep this and all other medication out of the reach of children. In case of accidental ingestion, seek professional assistance or contact Poison Control Center immediately.

DRUG INTERACTIONS:

NASAL SOLUTION

Drug: Monoamine Oxidase (MAO) inhibitors

Effect: Hypertension

ADVERSE REACTIONS:

Nasal Solution: Local application of tetrahydrozoline nasal solution can be associated with burning, stinging, sneezing, or dryness of the mucosa. Occasionally, systemic sympathomimetic effects can occur, including headaches, drowsiness, weakness, tremors, light-headedness, insomnia, and palpitations. Rebound congestion can also occur, and is characterized by chronic swelling of the nasal mucosa resulting in chronic redness, swelling and rhinitis. If adverse reactions occur, discontinue use.

OVERDOSAGE:

Nasal Solution: The administration or ingestion of overdoses of tetrahydrozoline HCl nasal solution may result in oversedation in young children. Overdoses have caused hypertension, bradycardia, drowsiness and rebound hypotension in adults; a shock-like syndrome with hypotension and bradycardia may also occur. In either case, the treatment of overdosage is usually that of watchful expectancy and general measures. The patient should be kept warm, fluid balance should be maintained orally, if possible, and parenterally, if necessary.

If the respiratory rate drops to 10 or below, the patient should be given oxygen, and respiration assisted. Blood pressure should be watched carefully to prevent a hypotensive crisis.

There is no known antidote for tetrahydrozoline nasal solution. the use of stimulants is contraindicated. To date, we have had no report of fatalities resulting from overdoses of tetrahydrozoline nasal solution and while the symptoms resulting from tetrahydrozoline nasal solution overdosage may be alarming, they are self-limiting and the patient recovers with no sequelae.

DOSAGE AND ADMINISTRATION:

NASAL SOLUTION

Adults and Children 6 Years and Over: It is recommended that 2 to 4 drops of tetrahydrozoline 0.1% nasal solution be instilled in each nostril as needed, never more often than every three hours. Less frequent administration is usually sufficient since relief is maintained for four hours or longer in most cases, and often for as long as eight hours. Bedtime instillation usually assures sleep undisturbed by the need for remedication before morning, or by insomnia from central stimulation.

Children 2 to 6 Years of Age: It is recommended that 2 to 3 drops of tetrahydrozoline 0.05% Pediatric Nasal Drops be instilled in each nostril as needed and never more often than every three hours. Relief usually last for several hours so that instillations are usually needed every four to six hours.

Instillation of nose drops can be most conveniently accomplished with the patient in the lateral head-low position.

Recommended Storage: Store below 86 deg. F (30 deg. C.)

OPHTHALMIC SOLUTION

Instill 1 to 2 drops in the affected eye(s) up to four times daily.

HOW SUPPLIED - EQUIVALENTS NOT AVAILABLE:

Aerosol, Spray - Nasal - 0.1 %

15 ml	**$9.01**	**TYZINE, Bradley Pharms**	**00482-4760-15**

Solution - Nasal - 0.05 %

15 ml	**$8.82**	**TYZINE - PEDIATRIC, Bradley Pharms**	**00482-4770-15**

Solution - Nasal - 0.1 %

30 ml	**$11.04**	**TYZINE, Bradley Pharms**	**00482-4760-30**

Solution - Ophthalmic - 0.05 %

30 ml	$2.50	Tetrahydrozoline Hcl, Steris Labs	00402-0900-30

THEOPHYLLINE *(002329)*

CATEGORIES: Airway Obstruction; Antiasthmatics/Bronchodilators; Antitussives/Expectorants/Mucolytics; Asthma; Bronchial Dilators; Bronchitis; Bronchospasm; Chronic Bronchitis; Emphysema; Respiratory & Allergy Medications; Respiratory Muscle Relaxant; Smooth Muscle Relaxants; Xanthine Derivatives; Pregnancy Category C; Sales > $100 Million; FDA Approval Pre 1982

BRAND NAMES: Accurbron; *Aerobin* (Germany); *Aerodyne Retard*; Aerolate; *Aldefilina*; *Almarion*; *Aloefilina*; *Amilex*; *Aminomal*; Aquaphyllin; *Armophylline* (France); Asmalix; *Asmasalon*; *Asperal*; *Asperal-T*; *Austyn*; *Bilordyl*; *Bronchoretard* (Germany); Bronkodyl; *Bronsolvan*; *Bykofilin*; *Bykofilin Retard*; Constant-T; *Cronasma* (Germany); *Diffumal*; Duraphyl; Elixicon; *Elixofilina* (Mexico); Elixomin; **Elixophyllin**; *Euphyllin Retard*; *Euphylong*; *Euphylong SR*; *Godafilin*; Hydro-Spec; Labid; Lanophyllin; *Lasma* (England); Lixolin; *Nefoben*; *Neulin-SA*; *Neulin-SR*; *Neulin SA*; *Nuelin* (Australia); *Nuelin SA*; *Nuelin SR*; *Pharphylline*; *Phyllocontin*; *Phylobid*; *PMS Theophylline* (Canada); *Provent*; *Pulmidur* (Germany); *Pulmo*; *Pulmo-Timelets* (Germany); Pulmo; *Quibran T SR*; *Quibron T SR* (Canada); Respbid; Slo-Bid; Slo-Phyllin; *Solosin* (Germany); Solu-Phyllin; *Somofillina*; Somophyllin; Sustaire; T-Phyl; *Talofren*; *Talotren* (Mexico); *Teoclear*; *Teoclear LA*; *Teofilina*; *Teofilina Retard*; *Teolixir*; *Teolong* (Mexico); *Teophyllin*; *Teosona*; *Theo-2*; Theo-24; *Theo-Bros*; Theo-Dur; Theo-Time; *Theo PA*; Theobid; Theochron; Theoclear; Theocontin; Theocot; Theolair; *Theolair S*; *Theolair S.R.* (Mexico); *Theolan*;

Theomar; *Theomax*; *Theon*; Theophyl; Theophylline Anhydrous; *Theoplus*; *Theoplus Retard*; Theosol-80; Theospan Sr; *Theospirex Retard*; *Theostat*; *Theostat LP* (France); Theostat 80; *Theotard*; *Theotrim*; Theovent; *Theovent LA*; *Theo von CT* (Germany); Theox; *Tiodilax*; Truxophyllin; *Unicontin-400 Continus*; Uni-Dur; *Unifyl*; *Unifyl Retard*; Uniphyl; *Uniphyllin*; *Uniphyllin Continus*; *Xantivent* *(International brand names outside U.S. in italics)*

FORMULARIES: Aetna; BC-BS; CIGNA; FHP; Foundation; Humana; Kaiser; Medco; Medi-Cal; PCS; PruCare; United; WHO

COST OF THERAPY: $97.78 (Asthma; Tablet; 200 mg; 3/day; 365 days)

PRIMARY ICD9: 493.40 (Asthma, Unspecified, Without Mention of Status Asthmaticus)

DESCRIPTION:

Theophylline is structurally classified as a methylxanthine. It occurs as a white, odorless, crystalline powder with a bitter taste. Anhydrous theophylline has the chemical name 1H-Purine-2,6-dione,3,7-dihydro-1,3-dimethyl-.

The molecular formula of anhydrous theophylline is $C_7H_8N_4O_2$ with a molecular weight of 180.17. (For products containing theophylline monohydrate, substitute the following: The molecular formula of theophylline monohydrate is $C_7H_8N_4O_2H_2O$ with a molecular weight of 198.18.)

The molecular formula of oxtriphylline is $C_{12}H_{21}N_5O_3$ with a molecular weight of 283.33.

Immediate-Release Oral Forms: Slo-Phyllin tablets (theophylline tablets, USP) are scored, dye-free tablets providing 100 mg or 200 mg of theophylline, anhydrous, USP.

Slo-Phyllin 80 mg Syrup (theophylline, anhydrous) is a nonalcoholic, sugar-free solution containing per 15 ml theophylline, anhydrous, USP 80 mg with sodium benzoate, NF, 18 mg and methylparaben, NF 3 mg added as preservatives.

Both tablets and syrup are intended for oral administration. Theophylline is a bronchodilator structurally classified as a xanthine derivative.

Syrup inactive ingredients are citric acid, flavors, glycerine, methylparaben, propylene glycol, saccharin sodium, sodium benzoate, sorbitol, purified water.

Tablets: 100 mg inactive ingredients are lactose, magnesium stearate, microcrystalline cellulose, sodium starch glycolate; 200 mg inactive ingredients are magnesium stearate, microcrystalline cellulose, sodium starch glycolate.

Sustained Action Capsules: Theo-Dur Sprinkle sustained action capsules contain 50 mg, 75 mg, 125 mg, or 200 mg anhydrous theophylline, a bronchodilator structurally classified as a xanthine derivative. The inactive ingredients for Theo-Dur Sprinkle are: ethylcellulose, hydroxypropylcellulose, povidone, and sucrose. Theo-Dur Sprinkle takes the form of long-acting microencapsulated beads within a hard gelatin capsule for oral administration.

The theophylline has been microencapsulated in a proprietary coating of polymers to mask the bitter taste associated with the drug while providing a prolonged effect. The entire contents of a Theo-Dur Sprinkle capsule are intended to be sprinkled on a small amount of soft food immediately prior to ingestion, or it may be swallowed whole. SUBDIVIDING THE CONTENTS OF A CAPSULE IS NOT RECOMMENDED. Each capsule is oversized to allow ease of opening.

Anhydrous theophylline is a white, odorless, crystalline powder having a bitter taste.

CLINICAL PHARMACOLOGY:

MECHANISM OF ACTION

Theophylline has two distinct actions in the airways of patients with reversible obstruction; smooth muscle relaxation (*i.e.,* bronchodilation) and suppression of the response of the airways to stimuli (*i.e.,* non-bronchodilator prophylactic effects). While the mechanisms of action of theophylline are not known with certainty, studies in animals suggest that bronchodilatation is mediated by the inhibition of two isozymes of phosphodiesterase (PDE III and, to a lesser extent, PDE IV) while non-bronchodilator prophylactic actions are probably mediated through one or more different molecular mechanisms, that do not involve inhibition of PDE III or antagonism of adenosine receptors. Some of the adverse effects associated with theophylline appear to be mediated by inhibition of PDE III (*e.g.,* hypotension, tachycardia, headache, and emesis) and adenosine receptor antagonism (*e.g.,* alterations in cerebral blood flow).

Theophylline increases the force of contraction of diaphragmatic muscles. This action appears to be due to enhancement of calcium uptake through an adenosine-mediated channel.

Serum Concentration-Effect Relationship: Bronchodilation occurs over the serum theophylline concentration range of 5-20 mcg/ml. Clinically important improvement in symptom control has been found in most studies to require peak serum theophylline concentrations > 10 mcg/ml, but patients with mild disease may benefit from lower concentrations. At serum theophylline concentrations > 20 mcg/ml, both the frequency and severity of adverse reactions increase. In general, maintaining peak serum theophylline concentrations between 10 and 15 mcg/ml will achieve most of the drug's potential therapeutic benefit while minimizing the risk of serious adverse events.

PHARMACOKINETICS

Overview: Theophylline is rapidly and completely absorbed after oral administration in solution or immediate-release solid oral dosage form. Theophylline does not undergo any appreciable pre-systemic elimination, distributes freely into fat-free tissues and is extensively metabolized in the liver.

The pharmacokinetics of theophylline vary widely among similar patients and cannot be predicted by age, sex, body weight or other demographic characteristics. In addition, certain concurrent illnesses and alterations in normal physiology (see TABLE 1) and co-administration of other drugs (see TABLE 2A and TABLE 2B) can significantly alter the pharmacokinetic characteristics of theophylline. Within-subject variability in metabolism has also been reported in some studies, especially in acutely ill patients. It is, therefore, recommended that serum theophylline concentrations be measured frequently in acutely ill patients (*e.g.,* at 24-hr intervals) and periodically in patients receiving long-term therapy, e.g., at 6-12 month intervals. More frequent measurements should be made in the presence of any condition that may significantly alter theophylline clearance (see PRECAUTIONS, Laboratory Tests).

Note: In addition to the factors listed above, theophylline clearance is increased and half-life decreased by low carbohydrate/high protein diets, parenteral nutrition, and daily consumption of charcoal-broiled beef. A high carbohydrate/low protein diet can decrease the clearance and prolong the half-life of theophylline.

Absorption: Theophylline is rapidly and completely absorbed after oral administration in solution or immediate-release solid oral dosage form. After a single dose of 5 mg/kg in adults, a mean peak serum concentration of about 10 mcg/ml (range 5-15 mcg/ml) can be expected 1-2 hr after the dose. Co-administration of theophylline with food or antacids does not cause clinically significant changes in the absorption of theophylline from immediate-release dosage forms.

CLINICAL PHARMACOLOGY: *(cont'd)*

TABLE 1 Mean and range of total body clearance and half-life of theophylline related to age and altered physiological states.*

Population Characteristics	Total Body Clearance** mean (range) †† (ml/kg/min)	Half-life mean (range) †† (hr)
PREMATURE NEONATES		
postnatal age 3-15 days	0.29 (0.09-0.49)	30 (17-43)
postnatal age 25-57 days	0.64 (0.04-1.2)	20 (9.4-30.6)
Term infants		
postnatal age 1-2 days	NR†	25.7 (25-26.5)
postnatal age 3-30 weeks	NR†	11 (6-29)
CHILDREN		
1-4 years	1.7 (0.5-2.9)	3.4 (1.2-5.6)
4-12 years	1.6 (0.8-2.4)	NR†
13-15 years	0.9 (0.48-1.3)	NR†
6-17 years	1.4 (0.2-2.6)	3.7 (1.5-5.9)
ADULTS (16-60 years) otherwise healthy non-smoking asthmatics	0.65 (0.27-1.03)	8.7 (6.1-12.8)
ELDERLY (>60 years)		
non-smokers with normal cardiac, liver, and renal function	0.41 (0.21-0.61)	9.8 (1.6-18)
Concurrent illness or altered physiological state		
Acute pulmonary edema	0.33***(0.07-2.45)	19***(3.1-82)
COPD->60 years, stable non-smoker >1 year	0.54 (0.44-0.64)	11 (9.4-12.6)
COPD with cor pulmonale	0.48 (0.08-0.88)	NR†
Cystic fibrosis (14-28 years)	1.25 (0.31-2.2)	6.0 (1.8-10.2)
Fever associated with acute viral respiratory illness (children 9-15 years)	NR†	7.0 (1.0-13)
Liver disease - cirrhosis	0.31***(0.1-0.7)	32***(10-56)
acute hepatitis	0.35 (0.25-0.45	19.2 (16.6-21.8)
cholestasis	0.65 (0.25-1.45)	14.4 (5.7-31,8)
Pregnancy - 1st trimester	NR†	8.5 (3.1-13.9)
2nd trimester	NR†	8.8 (3.8-13.8)
3rd trimester	NR†	13.0 (8.4-17.6)
Sepsis with multi-organ failure	0.47 (0.19-1.9)	18.8 (6.3-24.1)
Thyroid disease - hypothyroid	0.38 (0.13-0.57)	11.6 (8.2-25)
hyperthyroid	0.8 (0.68-0.97)	4.5 (3.7-5.6)

* For various North American patient populations from literature reports. Different rates of elimination and consequent dosage requirements have been observed among other peoples.

** Clearance represents the volume of blood completely cleared of theophylline by the liver in one minute. Values listed were generally determined at serum theophylline concentrations <20 mcg/ml; clearance may decrease and half-life may increase at higher serum concentrations due to non-linear pharmacokinetics.

†† Reported range or estimated range (mean ± 2 SD) where actual range not reported.

† NR = not reported or not reported in a comparable format.

*** Median

Distribution: Once theophylline enters the systemic circulation, about 40% is bound to plasma protein, primarily albumin. Unbound theophylline distributes throughout body water, but distributes poorly into body fat. The apparent volume of distribution of theophylline is approximately 0.45 L/kg (range 0.3-0.7 L/kg) based on ideal body weight. Theophylline passes freely across the placenta, into breast milk and into the cerebrospinal fluid (CSF). Saliva theophylline concentrations approximate unbound serum concentrations, but are not reliable for routine or therapeutic monitoring unless special techniques are used. An increase in the volume of distribution of theophylline, primarily due to reduction in plasma protein binding, occurs in premature neonates, patients with hepatic cirrhosis, uncorrected acidemia, the elderly and in women during the third trimester of pregnancy. In such cases, the patient may show signs of toxicity at total (bound + unbound) serum concentrations of theophylline in the therapeutic range (10-20 mcg/ml) due to elevated concentrations of the pharmacologically active unbound drug. Similarly, a patient with decreased theophylline binding may have a sub-therapeutic total drug concentration while the pharmacologically active unbound concentration is in the therapeutic range. If only total serum theophylline concentration is measured, this may lead to an unnecessary and potentially dangerous dose increase. In patients with reduced protein binding, measurement of unbound serum theophylline concentration provides a more reliable means of dosage adjustment than measurement of total serum theophylline concentration. Generally, concentrations of unbound theophylline should be maintained in the range of 6-12 mcg/ml.

Metabolism: Following oral dosing, theophylline does not undergo any measurable first-pass elimination. In adults and children beyond one year of age, approximately 90% of the dose is metabolized in the liver. Biotransformation takes place through demethylation to 1-methylxanthine and 3-methylxanthine and hydroxylation to 1,3-dimethyluric acid. 1-methylxanthine is further hydroxylated, by xanthine oxidase, to 1-methyluric acid. About 6% of a theophylline dose is N-methylated to caffeine. Theophylline demethylation to 3-methylxanthine is catalyzed by cytochrome P-450 1A2, while cytochromes P-450 2E1 and P-450 3A3 catalyze the hydroxylation to 1,3-dimethyluric acid. Demethylation to 1-methylxanthine appears to be catalyzed either by cytochrome P-450 1A2 or a closely related cytochrome. In neonates, the N-demethylation pathway is absent while the function of the hydroxylation pathway is markedly deficient. The activity of these pathways slowly increases to maximal levels by one year of age.

Caffeine and 3-methylxanthine are the only theophylline metabolites with pharmacologic activity. 3-methylxanthine has approximately one tenth the pharmacologic activity of theophylline and serum concentrations in adults with normal renal function are <1 mcg/ml. In patients with end-stage renal disease, 3-methylxanthine may accumulate to concentrations that approximate the unmetabolized theophylline concentration. Caffeine concentrations are usually undetectable in adults regardless of renal function. In neonates, caffeine may accumulate to concentrations that approximate the unmetabolized theophylline concentration and thus, exert a pharmacologic effect.Both the N-demethylation and hydroxylation pathways of theophylline biotransformation are capacity-limited. Due to the wide intersubject variability of the rate of theophylline metabolism, non-linearity of elimination may begin in some patients at serum theophylline concentrations <10 mcg/ml. Since this non-linearity results in more than proportional changes in serum theophylline concentrations with changes in dose, it is advisable to make increases or decreases in dose in small increments in order to achieve desired changes in serum theophylline concentrations (see TABLE 4). Accurate prediction of dose-dependency of theophylline metabolism in patients *a priori* is not possible, but patients with very high initial clearance rates (*i.e.,* low steady state serum theophylline concentrations at above average doses) have the greatest likelihood of experiencing large changes in serum theophylline concentration in response to dosage changes.

CLINICAL PHARMACOLOGY: *(cont'd)*

Excretion: In neonates, approximately 50% of the theophylline dose is excreted unchanged in the urine. Beyond the first three months of life, approximately 10% of the theophylline dose is excreted unchanged in the urine. The remainder is excreted in the urine mainly as 1,3-dimethyluric acid (35-40%), 1-methyluric acid (20-25%) and 3-methylxanthine (15-20%). Since little theophylline is excreted unchanged in the urine and since active metabolites of theophylline (*i.e.,* caffeine, 3-methylxanthine) do not accumulate to clinically significant levels even in the face of end-stage renal disease, no dosage adjustment for renal insufficiency is necessary in adults and children >3 months of age. In contrast, the large fraction of the theophylline dose excreted in the urine as unchanged theophylline and caffeine in neonates requires careful attention to dose reduction and frequent monitoring of serum theophylline concentrations in neonates with reduced renal function (See WARNINGS).

Serum Concentrations at Steady State: After multiple doses of theophylline, steady state is reached in 30-65 hours (average 40 hours) in adults. At steady state, on a dosage regimen with 6-hour intervals, the expected mean trough concentration is approximately 60% of the mean peak concentration, assuming a mean theophylline half-life of 8 hours. The difference between peak and trough concentrations is larger in patients with more rapid theophylline clearance. In patients with high theophylline clearance and half-lives of about 4-5 hours, such as children age 1 to 9 years, the trough serum theophylline concentration may be only 30% of peak with a 6-hour dosing interval. In these patients a slow release formulation would allow a longer dosing interval (8-12 hours) with a smaller peak/trough difference.

SPECIAL POPULATIONS

See TABLE 1 for mean clearance and half, life values.

Geriatric: The clearance of theophylline is decreased by an average of 30% in healthy elderly adults (>60 yrs) compared to healthy young adults. Careful attention to dose reduction and frequent monitoring of serum theophylline concentrations are required in elderly patients(see WARNINGS).

Pediatrics: The clearance of theophylline is very low in neonates(see WARNINGS). Theophylline clearance reaches maximal values by one year of age, remains relatively constant until about 9 years of age and then slowly decreases by approximately 50% to adult values at about age 16. Renal excretion of unchanged theophylline in neonates amounts to about 50% of the dose, compared to about 10% in children older than three months and in adults. Careful attention to dosage selection and monitoring of serum theophylline concentrations are required in pediatric patients (see WARNINGS and DOSAGE AND ADMINISTRATION).

Gender: Gender differences in theophylline clearance are relatively small and unlikely to be of clinical significance. Significant reduction in theophylline clearance, however, has been reported in women on the 20th day of the menstrual cycle and during the third trimester of pregnancy.

Race: Pharmacokinetic differences in theophylline clearance due to race have not been studied.

Renal Insufficiency: Only a small fraction, e.g., about 10%, of the administered theophylline dose is excreted unchanged in the urine of children greater than three months of age and adults. Since little theophylline is excreted unchanged in the urine and since active metabolites of theophylline (*i.e.,* caffeine, 3-methylxanthine) do not accumulate to clinically significant levels even in the face of end-stage renal disease, no dosage adjustment for renal insufficiency is necessary in adults and children >3 months of age. In contrast, approximately 50% of the administered theophylline dose is excreted unchanged in the urine in neonates. Careful attention to dose reduction and frequent monitoring of serum theophylline concentrations are required in neonates with decreased renal function (see WARNINGS).

Hepatic Insufficiency: Theophylline clearance is decreased by 50% or more in patients with hepatic insufficiency (*e.g.,* cirrhosis, acute hepatitis, cholestasis). Careful attention to dose reduction and frequent monitoring of serum theophylline concentrations are required in patients with reduced hepatic function (see WARNINGS).

Congestive Heart Failure (CHF): Theophylline clearance is decreased by 50% or more in patients with CHF. The extent of reduction in theophylline clearance in patients with CHF appears to be directly correlated to the severity of the cardiac disease. Since theophylline clearance is independent of liver blood flow, the reduction in clearance appears to be due to impaired hepatocyte function rather than reduced perfusion. Careful attention to dose reduction and frequent monitoring of serum theophylline concentrations are required in patients with CHF (see WARNINGS).

Smokers: Tobacco and marijuana smoking appears to increase the clearance of theophylline by induction of metabolic pathways. Theophylline clearance has been shown to increase by approximately 50% in young adult tobacco smokers and by approximately 80% in elderly tobacco smokers compared to non-smoking subjects. Passive smoke exposure has also been shown to increase theophylline clearance by up to 50%. Abstinence from tobacco smoking for one week causes a reduction of approximately 40% in theophylline clearance. Careful attention to dose reduction and frequent monitoring of serum theophylline concentrations are required in patients who stop smoking (see WARNINGS). Use of nicotine gum has been shown to have no effect on theophylline clearance.

Fever: Fever, regardless of its underlying cause, can decrease the clearance of theophylline. The magnitude and duration of the fever appear to be directly correlated to the degree of decrease of theophylline clearance. Precise data are lacking, but a temperature of 39°C (102°F) for at least 24 hours is probably required to produce a clinically significant increase in serum theophylline concentrations. Children with rapid rates of theophylline clearance (*i.e.,* those who require a dose that is substantially larger than average [e.g., >22 mg/kg/day] to achieve a therapeutic peak serum theophylline concentration when afebrile) may be at greater risk of toxic effects from decreased clearance during sustained fever. Careful attention to dose reduction and frequent monitoring of serum theophylline concentrations are required in patients with sustained fever (see WARNINGS).

MISCELLANEOUS

Other factors associated with decreased theophylline clearance include the third trimester of pregnancy, sepsis with multiple organ failure, and hypothyroidism. Careful attention to dose reduction and frequent monitoring of serum theophylline concentrations are required in patients with any of these conditions (see WARNINGS). Other factors associated with increased theophylline clearance include hyperthyroidism and cystic fibrosis.

CLINICAL STUDIES:

In patients with chronic asthma, including patients with severe asthma requiring inhaled corticosteroids or alternate-day oral corticosteroids, many clinical studies have shown that theophylline decreases the frequency and severity of symptoms, including nocturnal exacerbations, and decreases the "as needed" use of inhaled beta-2 agonists. Theophylline has also been shown to reduce the need for short courses of daily oral prednisone to relieve exacerbations of airway obstruction that are unresponsive to bronchodilators in asthmatics.

In patients with chronic obstructive pulmonary disease (COPD), clinical studies have shown that theophylline decreases dyspnea, air trapping, the work of breathing, and improves contractility of diaphragmatic muscles with little or no improvement in pulmonary function measurements.

CLINICAL STUDIES: *(cont'd)*

THEOPHYLLINE SUSTAINED ACTION CAPSULES

In two-separate single-dose studies utilizing different subjects, the following bioavailability variables were observed. Theo-Dur Sprinkle administered in a 500-mg dose as pellets on applesauce to 6 healthy adults produced mean peak theophylline serum levels of 9.03 ± 2.59 mcg/ml at 8.67 ± 1.03 hours following administration. Administration of two lots of Theo-Dur Sprinkle as intact capsules in a 600-mg dose to 6 healthy adults produced mean peak theophylline serum levels of 9.08 ±1.30 mcg/ml and 7.60 ± 0.95 mcg/ml at 8.33 ± 1.50 and 8.67 ± 3.01 hours after administration, respectively. In these studies, Theo-Dur Sprinkle exhibited complete bioavailability when compared with an immediate release product. In both of these studies, the subjects fasted for 10 hours prior to dosing and for 4 hours after dosing.

In a multiple-dose, two-way, crossover study with 18 healthy, normal adults, the bioavailability from Theo-Dur Sprinkle administered as intact capsules was evaluated using Theo-Dur Sustained Action Tablets as the reference products. Fifteen subjects received 400 mg at 7:00 AM and 7:00 PM while 3 subjects received 200 mg because of low theophylline clearance. All meals and snacks were provided to the subjects during the course of this study, with breakfast at 9:00 AM, lunch at 12:30 PM, a snack at 3:00 PM, and dinner at 9:00 PM. Theo-Dur Sprinkle produced mean Cmax and Cmin theophylline serum levels of 10.4 ± 2.6 and 6.9 ± 1.8 mcg/ml as compared with a Cmax and Cmin of 10.5 ± 2.8 and 7.5 ± 2.7 mcg/ml for Theo-Dur tablets. The mean percent fluctuation normalized to Css was 38.8± 8.5% for Theo-Dur Sprinkle and 33.4 ± 9.7% for Theo-Dur Tablets (% fluctuation = 100 (Cmax-Cmin)/Css, where Css = $AUC_{0\text{-}12}$/dosing interval). The mean percent fluctuation when normalized to Cmin was 51.9 ± 15.4% for Theo-Dur Sprinkle and 43.9 ± 17.4% for Theo-Dur Tablets (% fluctuation = 100 (Cmax-Cmin)/Cmin). The average peak-trough differences over 12 hours for Theo-Dur Sprinkle and Theo-Dur tablets were 3.5 ± 1.2 and 3.0 ± 0.7 mcg/ml, respectively. The AUC for Theo-Dur Sprinkle was 108.4 ± 26.0 while that for Theo-Dur tablets was 112.1 ± 32.5 mcg/hr/ml. In a separate study, Theo-Dur showed complete bioavailability when compared with an immediate-release product. This would suggest that bioavailability from Theo-Dur Sprinkle was complete and not statistically different from that of Theo-Dur Tablets.

INDICATIONS AND USAGE:

Theophylline is indicated for the treatment of the symptoms and reversible airflow obstruction associated with chronic asthma and other chronic lung diseases, e.g., emphysema and chronic bronchitis.

CONTRAINDICATIONS:

This product is contraindicated in individuals who have shown hypersensitivity to its components. It is also contraindicated in patients with active peptic ulcer disease, and in individuals with underlying seizure disorders (unless receiving appropriate anti-convulsant medication).

WARNINGS:

Concurrent Illness: Theophylline should be used with extreme caution in patients with the following clinical conditions due to the increased risk of exacerbation of the concurrent condition:

Active peptic ulcer disease

Seizure disorders

Cardiac arrhythmias (not including bradyarrhythmias)

Conditions That Reduce Theophylline Clearance: There are several readily identifiable causes of reduced theophylline clearance. **If the total daily dose is not appropriately reduced in the presence of these risk factors, severe and potentially fatal theophylline toxicity can occur.** Careful consideration must be given to the benefits and risks of theophylline use and the need for more intensive monitoring of serum theophylline concentrations in patients with the following risk factors:

Age: Neonates (term and premature), Children <1 year, Elderly (>60 years)

Concurrent Diseases: Acute pulmonary edema, Congestive heart failure, Cor-pulmonale, Fever; ≥102° for 24 hours or more; or lesser temperature elevations for longer periods, Hypothyroidism, Liver disease; cirrhosis, acute hepatitis, Reduced renal function in infants <3 months of age, Sepsis with multi-organ failure, Shock

WHEN SIGNS OR SYMPTOMS OF THEOPHYLLINE TOXICITY ARE PRESENT

Whenever a patient receiving theophylline develops nausea or vomiting, particularly repetitive vomiting, or other signs or symptoms consistent with theophylline toxicity (even if another cause may be suspected), additional doses of theophylline should be withheld and a serum theophylline concentration measured immediately. Patients should be instructed not to continue any dosage that causes adverse effects and to withhold subsequent doses until the symptoms have resolved, at which time the clinician may instruct the patient to resume the drug at a lower dosage (see TABLE 4).

Dosage Increases: Increases in the dose of theophylline should not be made in response to an acute exacerbation of symptoms of chronic lung disease since theophylline provides little added benefit to inhaled $beta_2$-selective agonists and systemically administered corticosteroids in this circumstance and increases the risk of adverse effects. A peak steady-state serum theophylline concentration should be measured before increasing the dose in response to persistent chronic symptoms to ascertain whether an increase in dose is safe. Before increasing the theophylline dose on the basis of a low serum concentration, the clinician should consider whether the blood sample was obtained at an appropriate time in relationship to the dose and whether the patient has adhered to the prescribed regimen (see PRECAUTIONS, Laboratory Tests).

As the rate of theophylline clearance may be dose-dependent (*i.e.,* steady-state serum concentrations may increase disproportionately to the increase in dose), an increase in dose based upon a sub-therapeutic serum concentration measurement should be conservative. In general, limiting dose increases to about 25% of the previous total daily dose will reduce the risk of unintended excessive increases in serum theophylline concentration (see TABLE 4).

Serum levels above 20 mcg/ml are rarely found after appropriate administration of the recommended doses. However, in individuals in whom theophylline plasma clearance is reduced *for any reason,* even conventional doses may result in increased serum levels and potential toxicity.

Reduced theophylline clearance has been documented in the following readily identifiable groups: 1) patients with impaired liver function; 2) patients over 55 years of age, particularly males and those with chronic lung disease; 3) those with cardiac failure from any cause; 4) patients with sustained high fever; 5) neonates and infants under 1 year of age; and 6) patients taking certain drugs (see DRUG INTERACTIONS). Frequently, such patients have markedly prolonged theophylline serum levels following discontinuation of the drug.

Reduction of dosage and laboratory monitoring is especially appropriate in the above individuals.

WARNINGS: *(cont'd)*

Serious side effects such as ventricular arrhythmias, convulsions or even death may appear as the first sign of toxicity without any previous warning. Less serious signs of theophylline toxicity (*i.e.,* nausea and restlessness) may occur frequently when initiating therapy, but are usually transient. When such signs are persistent during maintenance therapy, they are often associated with serum concentrations above 20 mcg/ml.

Stated differently, serious toxicity is not reliably preceded by less severe side effects. A serum concentration measurement is the only reliable method of predicting potentially life-threatening toxicity.

Many patients who require theophylline exhibit tachycardia due to their underlying disease process so that the cause/effect relationship to elevated serum theophylline concentrations may not be appreciated.

Theophylline products may cause dysrhythmia and/or worsen pre-existing arrhythmias and any significant change in rate and/or rhythm warrants monitoring and further investigation.

Studies in laboratory animals (minipigs, rodents, and dogs) recorded the occurrence of cardiac arrhythmias and sudden death (with histologic evidence of myocardial necrosis) when beta-agonists and methylxanthines were administered concurrently. The significance of these findings when applied to humans is currently unknown.

PRECAUTIONS:

GENERAL

Immediate Release Products

Careful consideration of the various interacting drugs and physiologic conditions that can alter theophylline clearance and require dosage adjustment should occur prior to initiation of theophylline therapy, prior to increases in theophylline dose, and during follow up (see WARNINGS). The dose of theophylline selected for initiation of therapy should be low and, **if tolerated**, increased slowly over a period of a week or longer with the final dose guided by monitoring serum theophylline concentrations and the patient's clinical response (see DOSAGE AND ADMINISTRATION).

Monitoring Serum Theophylline Concentrations: Serum theophylline concentration measurements are readily available and should be used to determine whether the dosage is appropriate. Specifically, the serum theophylline concentration should be measured as follows:

1. When initiating therapy to guide final dosage adjustment after titration.

2. Before making a dose increase to determine whether the serum concentration is sub-therapeutic in a patient who continues to be symptomatic.

3. Whenever signs or symptoms of theophylline toxicity are present.

4. Whenever there is a new illness, worsening of a chronic illness or a change in the patient's treatment regimen that may alter theophylline clearance (*e.g.,* fever >102°F sustained for ≥24 hours, hepatitis, or drugs listed in TABLE 2 are added or discontinued).

To guide a dose increase, the blood sample should be obtained at the time of the expected peak serum theophylline concentration; 1-2 hours after a dose at steady-state. For most patients, steady-state will be reached after 3 days of dosing when no doses have been missed, no extra doses have been added, and none of the doses have been taken at unequal intervals. A trough concentration (*i.e.,* at the end of the dosing interval) provides no additional useful information and may lead to an inappropriate dose increase since the peak serum theophylline concentration can be two or more times greater than the trough concentration with an immediate-release formulation. If the serum sample is drawn more than two hours after the dose, the results must be interpreted with caution since the concentration may not be reflective of the peak concentration. In contrast, when signs or symptoms of theophylline toxicity are present, the serum sample should be obtained as soon as possible, analyzed immediately, and the result reported to the clinician without delay. In patients in whom decreased serum protein binding is suspected (*e.g.,* cirrhosis, women during the third trimester of pregnancy), the concentration of unbound theophylline should be measured and the dosage adjusted to achieve an unbound concentration of 6-12 mcg/ml.

Saliva concentrations of theophylline cannot be used reliably to adjust dosage without special techniques.

Extended-Release Capsules

THE CONTENTS OF A THEO-DUR SPRINKLE CAPSULE SHOULD NOT BE CHEWED OR CRUSHED.

General: On the average, theophylline half-life is shorter in cigarette and marijuana smokers than in non-smokers, but smokers can have half-lives as long as non-smokers. Theophylline should not be administered concurrently with other xanthine medications. Use with caution in patients with hypoxemia, hypertension or those with history of peptic ulcer. Theophylline preparations should be used cautiously in patients with history of peptic ulcer. Theophylline may occasionally act as a local irritant to the GI tract; although gastrointestinal symptoms are more commonly centrally mediated and associated with serum drug concentrations over 20 mcg/ml.

LABORATORY TESTS

Immediate Release Products: As a result of its pharmacological effects, theophylline at serum concentrations within the 10-20 mcg/ml range modestly increases plasma glucose (from a mean of 88 mg% to 98 mg%), uric acid (from a mean of 4 mg/dl to 6 mg/dl), free fatty acids (from a mean of 451 q/l to 800 q/l, total cholesterol (from a mean of 140 vs 160 mg/dl), HDL (from a mean of 36 to 50 mg/dl), HDL/LDL ratio (from a mean of 0.5 to 0.7), and urinary free cortisol excretion (from a mean of 44 to 63 mcg/24 hr). Theophylline at serum concentrations within the 10-20 mcg/ml range may also transiently decrease serum concentrations of triiodothyronine (144 before, 131 after one week and 142 ng/dl after 4 weeks of theophylline). The clinical importance of these changes should be weighed against the potential therapeutic benefit of theophylline in individual patients.

Extended-Release Capsules: Serum levels should be monitored periodically to determine the theophylline level associated with observed clinical response and as the method of predicting toxicity. For such measurements, the serum sample should be obtained at the time of peak concentration, (**Immediate Release products:** 1 to 2 hours after administration) 4-8 hours when medication is taken every 12 hours, or 3-6 hours when medication is taken every 8 hours. It is important that the patient has not missed or taken additional doses during the previous 48 hours and that dosing intervals were reasonably equally spaced. DOSAGE ADJUSTMENT BASED ON SERUM THEOPHYLLINE MEASUREMENTS WHEN THESE INSTRUCTIONS HAVE NOT BEEN FOLLOWED MAY RESULT IN RECOMMENDATIONS THAT PRESENT RISK OF TOXICITY TO THE PATIENT.

INFORMATION FOR THE PATIENT

Immediate Release Products: The patient (or parent/care giver) should be instructed to seek medical advice whenever nausea, vomiting, persistent headache, insomnia or rapid heart beat occurs during treatment with theophylline, even if another cause is suspected. The patient should be instructed to contact their clinician if they develop a new illness, especially if accompanied by a persistent fever, if they experience worsening of a chronic illness, if they start or stop smoking cigarettes or marijuana, or if another clinician adds a new medication or discontinues a previously prescribed medication. Patients should be instructed to inform

PRECAUTIONS: *(cont'd)*

all clinicians involved in their care that they are taking theophylline, especially when a medication is being added or deleted from their treatment. Patients should be instructed to not alter the dose, timing of the dose, or frequency of administration without first consulting their clinician. If a dose is missed, the patient should be instructed to take the next dose at the usually scheduled time and to not attempt to make up for the missed dose.

Extended-Release Capsules: This information is intended to aid in the safe and effective use of this medication. It is not a disclosure of all possible adverse or intended effects.

The physician should reinforce the importance of taking only the prescribed dose and the time interval between doses. As with any controlled-release theophylline product, the patient should alert the physician of symptoms occur repeatedly, especially near the end of the dosing interval.

When prescribing administration by the sprinkle method, details of the proper technique should be explained to patient (see DOSAGE AND ADMINISTRATION, Sprinkling Contents on Food.)

Patients should be informed of the need to take this drug in the fasting state, and that drug administration should be 1 hour before or 2 hours after meals (see DOSAGE AND ADMINISTRATION).

CARCINOGENESIS, MUTAGENESIS, AND IMPAIRMENT OF FERTILITY

Immediate Release Products: Long term carcinogenicity studies have been carried out in mice (oral doses 30-150 mg/kg)and rats (oral doses 5-75 mg/kg). Results are pending.

Theophylline has been studied in Ames salmonella, *in vivo* and *in vitro* cytogenetics, micronucleus and Chinese hamster ovary test systems and has not been shown to be genotoxic.

In a 14 week continuous breeding study, theophylline, administered to mating pairs of $B6C3F_1$ mice at oral doses of 120, 270 and 500 mg/kg (approximately 1.0-3.0 times the human dose on a mg/m^2 basis) impaired fertility, as evidenced by decreases in the number of live pups per litter, decreases in the mean number of litters per fertile pair, and increases in the gestation period at the high dose as well as decreases in the proportion of pups born alive at the mid and high dose. In 13 week toxicity studies, theophylline was administered to F344 rats and $B6C3F_1$ mice at oral doses of 40-300 mg/kg (approximately 2.0 times the human dose on a mg/m^2 basis). At the high dose, systemic toxicity was observed in both species including decreases in testicular weight.

Extended-Release Capsules: Long-term carcinogenicity studies have not been performed with theophylline. Chromosome-breaking activity was detected in human cell cultures at concentrations of theophylline up to 50 times the therapeutic serum concentration in humans. Theophylline was not mutagenic in the dominant lethal assay in male mice given theophylline intraperitoneally in doses up to 30 times the maximum daily human oral dose.

Studies to determine the effect on fertility have not been performed with theophylline.

PREGNANCY CATEGORY C

Immediate Release Products: There are no adequate and well controlled studies in pregnant women. Additionally, there are no teratogenicity studies in non-rodents (*e.g.,* rabbits). Theophylline was not shown to be teratogenic in CD-1 mice at oral doses up to 400 mg/kg, approximately 2.0 times the human dose on a mg/m^2 basis or in CD-1 rats at oral doses up to 260 mg/kg, approximately 3.0 times the recommended human dose on a mg/m^2 basis. At a dose of 220 mg/kg, embryotoxicity was observed in rats in the absence of maternal toxicity.

Extended-Release Capsules: Animal reproduction studies have not been conducted with theophylline. It is not known whether theophylline can cause fetal harm when administered to a pregnant woman or can affect reproduction capacity. Xanthines should be given to a pregnant woman only if clearly needed.

NURSING MOTHERS

Immediate Release Products: Theophylline is excreted into breast milk and may cause irritability or other signs of mild toxicity in nursing human infants. The concentration of theophylline in breast milk is about equivalent to the maternal serum concentration. An infant ingesting a liter of breast milk containing 10-20 mcg/ml of theophylline day is likely to receive 10-20 mg of theophylline per day. Serious adverse effects in the infant are unlikely unless the mother has toxic serum theophylline concentrations.

Extended-Release Capsules: Theophylline is distributed into breast milk and may cause irritability or other signs of toxicity in nursing infants. Because of the potential of serious adverse reactions in nursing infants from theophylline, a decision should be made whether to discontinue nursing or to discontinue the drug, taking into account the importance of the drug to the mother.

PEDIATRIC USE

Immediate Release Products: Theophylline is safe and effective for the approved indications in pediatric patients (See INDICATIONS AND USAGE). The maintenance dose of theophylline must be selected with caution in pediatric patients since the rate of theophylline clearance is highly variable across the age range of neonates to adolescents (see CLINICAL PHARMACOLOGY, TABLE 1, WARNINGS, and DOSAGE AND ADMINISTRATION). Due to the immaturity of theophylline metabolic pathways in infants under the age of one year, particular attention to dosage selection and frequent monitoring of serum theophylline concentrations are required when theophylline is prescribed to pediatric patients in this age group.

Extended-Release Capsules: Safety and efficacy of Theo-Dur Sprinkle in children under 6 years of age have not been established with this product.

Safety and effectiveness of Theo-Dur Extended-Release Tablets administered:

1. Every 24 hours in children under 12 years of age, have not been established.

2. Every 12 hours in children under 6 years of age, have not been established.

GERIATRIC USE

Elderly patients are at significantly greater risk of experiencing serious toxicity from theophylline than younger patients due to pharmacokinetic and pharmacodynamic changes associated with aging. Theophylline clearance is reduced in patients greater than 60 years of age, resulting in increased serum theophylline concentrations in response to a given theophylline dose. Protein binding may be decreased in the elderly resulting in a larger proportion of the total serum theophylline concentration in the pharmacologically active unbound form. Elderly patients also appear to be more sensitive to the toxic effects of theophylline after chronic overdosage than younger patients. For these reasons, the maximum daily dose of theophylline in patients greater than 60 years of age ordinarily should not exceed 400 mg/day unless the patient continues to be symptomatic and the peak steady state serum theophylline concentration is <10 mcg/ml (see DOSAGE AND ADMINISTRATION). Theophylline doses greater than 400 mg/d should be prescribed with caution in elderly patients.

DRUG INTERACTIONS:

Theophylline interacts with a wide variety of drugs. The interaction may be pharmacodynamic, i.e., alterations in the therapeutic response to theophylline or another drug or occurrence of adverse effects without a change in serum theophylline concentration. More

DRUG INTERACTIONS: *(cont'd)*

frequently, however, the interaction is pharmacokinetic, i.e., the rate of theophylline clearance is altered by another drug resulting in increased or decreased serum theophylline concentrations. Theophylline only rarely alters the pharmacokinetics of other drugs.

The drugs listed in TABLES 2A and 2B have the potential to produce clinically significant pharmacodynamic or pharmacokinetic interactions with theophylline. The information in the "Effect" column of TABLES 2A and 2B assumes that the interacting drug is being added to a steady-state theophylline regimen. If theophylline is being initiated in a patient who is already taking a drug that inhibits theophylline clearance (*e.g.,* cimetidine, erythromycin), the dose of theophylline required to achieve a therapeutic serum theophylline concentration will be smaller. Conversely, if theophylline is being initiated in a patient who is already taking a drug that enhances theophylline clearance (*e.g.,* rifampin), the dose of theophylline required to achieve a therapeutic serum theophylline concentration will be larger. Discontinuation of a concomitant drug that increases theophylline clearance will result in accumulation of theophylline to potentially toxic levels, unless the theophylline dose is appropriately reduced. Discontinuation of a concomitant drug that inhibits theophylline clearance will result in decreased serum theophylline concentrations, unless the theophylline dose is appropriately increased.

The listing of drugs in TABLES 2A and 2B is current as of April 3, 1995. New interactions are continuously being reported for theophylline, especially with new chemical entities. **The clinician should not assume that a drug does not interact with theophylline if it is not listed in TABLES 2A and 2B.** Before addition of a newly available drug in a patient receiving theophylline, the package insert of the new drug and/or the medical literature should be consulted to determine if an interaction between the new drug and theophylline has been reported.

TABLE 2A Clinically significant drug interactions with theophylline*

Drug	Type of Interaction	Effect**
Adenosine	Theophylline blocks adenosine receptors.	Higher doses of adenosine may be required to achieve desired effect.
Alcohol	A single large dose of alcohol (3 ml/kg of whiskey) decreases theophylline clearance for up to 24 hours.	30% increase
Allopurinol	Decreases theophylline clearance at allopurinol doses ≥600 mg/day.	25% increase
Aminoglutethimide	Increases theophylline clearance by induction of microsomal enzyme activity.	25% decrease
Carbamazepine	Similar to aminoglutethimide.	30% decrease
Cimetidine	Decreases theophylline clearance by inhibiting cytochrome P450 1A2.	70% increase
Ciprofloxacin	Similar to cimetidine.	40% increase
Clarithromycin	Similar to erythromycin.	25% increase
Diazepam	Benzodiazepines increase CNS concentrations of adenosine, a potent CNS depressant, while theophylline blocks adenosine receptors.	Larger diazepam doses may be required to produce desired level of sedation. Discontinuation of theophylline without reduction of diazepam dose may result in respiratory depression.
Disulfiram	Decreases theophylline clearance by inhibiting hydroxylation and demethylation.	50% increase
Enoxacin	Similar to cimetidine.	300% increase
Ephedrine	Synergistic CNS effects	Increased frequency of nausea, nervousness, and insomnia.
Erythromycin	Erythromycin metabolite decreases theophylline clearance by inhibiting cytochrome P450 3A3.	35% increase. Erythromycin steady-state serum concentrations decreased by a similar amount.
Estrogen	Estrogen containing oral contraceptives decrease theophylline clearance in a dose-dependent fashion. The effect of progesterone on theophylline clearance is unknown.	30% increase
Flurazepam	Similar to diazepam.	Similar to diazepam.
Fluvoxamine	Similar to cimetidine myocardium to catecholamines, theophylline increases release of endogenous catecholamines.	Similar to cimetidine ventricular arrhythmias.
Interferon, human recombinant alpha-A	Decreases theophylline clearance.	100% increase
Isoproterenol (IV)	Increases theophylline clearance.	20% decrease
Ketamine	Pharmacologic	May lower theophylline seizure threshold.
Lithium	Theophylline increases renal lithium clearance.	Lithium dose required to achieve a therapeutic serum concentration increased an average of 60%.
Lorazepam	Similar to diazepam.	Similar to diazepam.

The Effect of Other Drugs on Theophylline Serum Concentration Measurements: Most serum theophylline assays in clinical use are immunoassays which are specific for theophylline. Other xanthines such as caffeine, dyphylline, and pentoxifylline are not detected by these assays. Some drugs (*e.g.,* cefazolin, cephalothin), however, may interfere with certain HPLC techniques. Caffeine and xanthine metabolites in neonates or patients with renal dysfunction may cause the reading from some dry reagent office methods to be higher than the actual serum theophylline concentration.

CESSATION OF SMOKING

Drug Interactions: Adding a drug that inhibits theophylline metabolism (*e.g.,* cimetidine, erythromycin, tacrine) or stopping a concurrently administered drug that enhances theophylline metabolism (*e.g.,* carbamazepine, rifampin). (see TABLE 2A and TABLE 2B).

TABLE 2B Clinically significant drug interactions with theophylline*

Drug	Type of Interaction	Effect**
Methotrexate (MTX)	Decreases theophylline clearance.	20% increase after low dose MTX, higher dose MTX may have a greater effect.
Mexiletine	Similar to disulfiram.	80% increase
Midazolam	Similar to diazepam.	Similar to diazepam.
Moricizine	Increases theophylline clearance.	25% decrease
Pancuronium	Theophylline may antagonize non-depolarizing neuromuscular blocking effects; possibly due to phosphodiesterase inhibition.	Larger dose of pancuronium may be required to achieve neuromuscular blockade.
Pentoxifylline	Decreases theophylline clearance.	30% increase
Phenobarbital (PB)	Similar to aminoglutethimide.	25% decrease after two weeks of concurrent PB.
Phenytoin	Phenytoin increases theophylline clearance by increasing microsomal enzyme activity. Theophylline decreases phenytoin absorption.	Serum theophyllineand phenytoin concentrations decrease about 40%.
Propafenone	Decreases theophylline clearance and pharmacologic interaction.	40% increase. Beta-2 blocking effect may decrease efficacy of theophylline.
Propranolol	Similar to cimetidine and pharmacologic interaction.	100% increase. Beta-2 blocking effect may decrease efficacy of theophylline.
Rifampin	Increases theophylline clearance by increasing cytochrome P450 1A2 and 3A3 activity.	20-40% decrease
Sulfinpyrazone	Increases theophylline clearance by increasing demethylation and hydroxylation. Decreases renal clearance of theophylline.	20% decrease
Tacrine	Similar to cimetidine, also increases renal clearance of theophylline.	90% increase
Thiabendazole	Decreases theophylline clearance.	190% increase
Ticlopidine	Decreases theophylline clearance.	60% increase
Troleandomycin	Similar to erythromycin.	33-100% increase depending on troleandomycin dose.
Verapamil	Similar to disulfiram.	20% increase

* Refer to DRUG INTERACTIONS for further information regarding table.
** Average effect on steady state theophylline concentration or other clinical effect for pharmacologic interactions. Individual patients may experience larger changes in serum theophylline concentration than the value listed.

ADVERSE REACTIONS:

Adverse reactions associated with theophylline are generally mild when peak serum theophylline concentrations are <20 mcg/ml and mainly consist of transient caffeine-like adverse effects such as nausea, vomiting, headache, and insomnia. When peak serum theophylline concentrations exceed 20 mcg/ml, however, theophylline produces a wide range of adverse reactions including persistent vomiting, cardiac arrhythmias, and intractable seizures which can be lethal (see OVERDOSAGE). The transient caffeine-like adverse reactions occur in about 50% of patients when theophylline therapy is initiated at doses higher than recommended initial doses (*e.g.,*>300 mg/day in adults and >12 mg/kg/day in children beyond >1 year of age). During the initiation of theophylline therapy, caffeine-like adverse effects may transiently alter patient behavior, especially in school age children, but this response rarely persists. Initiation of theophylline therapy at a low dose with subsequent slow titration to a predetermined age-related maximum dose will significantly reduce the frequency of these transient adverse effects (see DOSAGE AND ADMINISTRATION). In a small percentage of patients (<3% of children and <10% of adults) the caffeine-like adverse effects persist during maintenance therapy, even at peak serum theophylline concentrations within the therapeutic range (*i.e.,* 10-20 mcg/ml). Dosage reduction may alleviate the caffeine-like adverse effects in these patients, however, persistent adverse effects should result in a reevaluation of the need for continued theophylline therapy and the potential therapeutic benefit of alternative treatment.

Other adverse reactions that have been reported at serum theophylline concentrations <20 mcg/ml include diarrhea, irritability, restlessness, fine skeletal muscle tremors, and transient diuresis. In patients with hypoxia secondary to COPD, multifocal atrial tachycardia and flutter have been reported at serum theophylline concentrations ≥15 mcg/ml. There have been a few isolated reports of seizures at serum theophylline concentrations <20 mcg/ml in patients with an underlying neurological disease or in elderly patients. The occurrence of seizures in elderly patients with serum theophylline concentrations <20 mcg/ml may be secondary to decreased protein binding resulting in a larger proportion of the total serum theophylline concentration in the pharmacologically active unbound form. The clinical characteristics of the seizures reported in patients with serum theophylline concentrations <20 mcg/ml have generally been milder than seizures associated with excessive serum theophylline concentrations resulting from an overdose (*i.e.,* they have generally been transient, often stopped without anticonvulsant therapy, and did not result in neurological residua).

OVERDOSAGE:

General: The chronicity and pattern of theophylline overdosage significantly influences clinical manifestations of toxicity, management and outcome. There are two common presentations: (1) *acute overdose,* (*i.e.,* ingestion of a single large excessive dose (>10 mg/kg) as occurs in the context of an attempted suicide or isolated medication error) and (2) *chronic overdosage,* (*i.e.,* ingestion of repeated doses that are excessive for the patient's rate of theophylline clearance). The most common causes of chronic theophylline overdosage include patient or care giver error in dosing, clinician prescribing of an excessive dose or a normal dose in the presence of factors known to decrease the rate of theophylline clearance, and increasing the dose in response to an exacerbation of symptoms without first measuring the serum theophylline concentration to determine whether a dose increase is safe.

Severe toxicity from theophylline overdose is a relatively rare event. In one health maintenance organization, the frequency of hospital admissions for chronic overdosage of theophylline was about 1 per 1000 person-years exposure. In another study, among 6000 blood samples obtained for measurement of serum theophylline concentration, for any reason, from patients treated in an emergency department, 7% were in the 20-30 mcg/ml range and 3% were >30 mcg/ml. Approximately two-thirds of the patients with serum theophylline concentrations in the 20-30 mcg/ml range had one or more manifestations of toxicity while >90% of patients with serum theophylline concentrations >30 mcg/ml were clinically intoxicated. Similarly, in other reports, serious toxicity from theophylline is seen principally at serum concentrations >30 mcg/ml.

OVERDOSAGE: *(cont'd)*

TABLE 3 Manifestations Of Theophylline Toxicity.*

	Percentage of patients reported with sign or symptom			
	Acute Overdosage (Large Single Ingestion)		Chronic Overdosage (Multiple Excessive Doses)	
Sign/Symptom	**>Study 1 (n=157)**	**Study 2 (n=14)**	**Study 1 (n=92)**	**Study 2 (n=102)**
Asymptomatic	NR**	0	NR**	6
Gastrointestinal				
Vomiting	73	93	30	61
Abdominal Pain	NR**	21	NR**	12
Diarrhea	NR**	0	NR**	14
Hematemesis	NR**	0	NR**	2
Metabolic/Other				
Hypokalemia	85	79	44	43
Hyperglycemia	98	NR**	18	NR**
Acid/base disturbance	34	21	9	5
Rhabdomyolysis	NR**	7	NR**	0
Cardiovascular				
Sinus tachycardia	100	86	100	62
Other supraventricular tachycardias	2	21	12	14
Ventricular premature beats	3	21	10	19
Atrial fibrillation or flutter	1	NR**	12	NR**
Multifocal atrial tachycardia	0	NR**	2	NR**
Ventricular arrhythmias with hemodynamic instability	7	14	40	0
Hypotension/shock	NR**	21	NR**	8
Neurologic				
Nervousness	NR**	64	NR**	21
Tremors	38	29	16	14
Disorientation	NR**	7	NR**	11
Seizures	5	14	14	5
Death	3	21	10	4

* These data are derived from two studies in patients with serum theophylline concentrations >30 mcg/ml. In the first study (Study #1 - Shanon, Ann Intern Med 1993;119:1161-67), data were prospectively collected from 249 consecutive cases of theophylline toxicity referred to a regional poison center for consultation. In the second study (Study #2 - Sessler, Am J Med 1990;88:567-76), data were retrospectively collected from 116 cases with serum theophylline concentrations >30 mcg/ml among 6000 blood samples obtained for measurement of serum theophylline concentrations in three emergency departments. Differences in the incidence of manifestations of theophylline toxicity between the two studies may reflect sample selection as a result of study design #2) and different methods of reporting results.
** NR = Not reported in a comparable manner.

Several studies have described the clinical manifestations of theophylline overdose and attempted to determine the factors that predict life-threatening toxicity. In general, patients who experience an acute overdose are less likely to experience seizures than patients who have experienced a chronic overdosage, unless the peak serum theophylline concentration is >100 mcg/ml. After a chronic overdosage, generalized seizures, life-threatening cardiac arrhythmias, and death may occur at serum theophylline concentrations >30 mcg/ml. The severity of toxicity after chronic overdosage is more strongly correlated with the patient's age than the peak serum theophylline concentration; patients >60 years are at the greatest risk for severe toxicity and mortality after a chronic overdosage. Pre-existing or concurrent disease may also significantly increase the susceptibility of a patient to a particular toxic manifestation, e.g., patients with neurologic disorders have an increased risk of seizures and patients with cardiac disease have an increased risk of cardiac arrhythmias for a given serum theophylline concentration compared to patients without the underlying disease.

The frequency of various reported manifestations of theophylline overdose according to the mode of overdose are listed in TABLE 4.

Other manifestations of theophylline toxicity include increases in serum calcium, creatine kinase, myoglobin and leukocyte count, decreases in serum phosphate and magnesium, acute myocardial infarction, and urinary retention in men with obstructive uropathy.

Seizures associated with serum theophylline concentrations >30 mcg/ml are often resistant to anticonvulsant therapy and may result in irreversible brain injury if not rapidly controlled. Death from theophylline toxicity is most often secondary to cardiorespiratory arrest and/or hypoxic encephalopathy following prolonged generalized seizures or intractable cardiac arrhythmias causing hemodynamic compromise.

OVERDOSE MANAGEMENT

General Recommendations for Patients with Symptoms of Theophylline Overdose or Serum Theophylline Concentrations >30 mcg/ml (Note: Serum theophylline concentrations may continue to increase after presentation of the patient for medical care.

1. While simultaneously instituting treatment, contact a regional poison center to obtain updated information and advice on individualizing the recommendations that follow.

2. Institute supportive care, including establishment of intravenous access, maintenance of the airway, and electrocardiographic monitoring.

3. Treatment Of Seizures: Because of the high morbidity and mortality associated with theophylline-induced seizures, treatment should be rapid and aggressive. Anticonvulsant therapy should be initiated with an intravenous benzodiazepine, e.g., diazepam, in increments of 0.1-0.2 mg/kg every 1-3 minutes until seizures are terminated. Repetitive seizures should be treated with a loading dose of phenobarbital (20 mg/kg infused over 30-60 minutes). Case reports of theophylline overdose in humans and animal studies suggest that phenytoin is ineffective in terminating theophylline-induced seizures. The doses of benzodiazepines and phenobarbital required to terminate theophylline-induced seizures are close to the doses that may cause severe respiratory depression or respiratory arrest; the clinician should therefore be prepared to provide assisted ventilation. Elderly patients and patients with COPD may be more susceptible to the respiratory depressant effects of anticonvulsants. Barbiturate-induced coma or administration of general anesthesia may be required to terminate repetitive seizures or status epilepticus. General anesthesia should be used with caution in patients with theophylline overdose because fluorinated volatile anesthetics may sensitize the myocardium to endogenous catecholamines released by theophylline. Enflurane appears to less likely to be associated with this effect than halothane and may, therefore, be safer. Neuromuscular blocking agents alone should not be used to terminate seizures since they abolish the musculoskeletal manifestations without terminating seizure activity in the brain.

4. Anticipate Need for Anticonvulsants: In patients with theophylline overdose who are at high risk for theophylline-induced seizures, e.g., patients with acute overdoses and serum theophylline concentrations >100 mcg/ml or chronic overdosage in patients >60 years of age with

OVERDOSAGE: *(cont'd)*

serum theophylline concentrations >30 mcg/ml, the need for anticonvulsant therapy should be anticipated. A benzodiazepine such as diazepam should be drawn into a syringe and kept at the patient's bedside and medical personnel qualified to treat seizures should be immediately available. In selected patients at high risk for theophylline-induced seizures, consideration should be given to the administration of prophylactic anticonvulsant therapy. Situations where prophylactic anticonvulsant therapy should be considered in high risk patients include anticipated delays in instituting methods for extracorporeal removal of theophylline (*e.g.,* transfer of a high risk patient from one health care facility to another for extracorporeal removal) and clinical circumstances that significantly interfere with efforts to enhance theophylline clearance (*e.g.,* a neonate where dialysis may not be technically feasible or a patient with vomiting unresponsive to antiemetics who is unable to tolerate multiple-dose oral activated charcoal). In animal studies, prophylactic administration of phenobarbital, but not phenytoin, has been shown to delay the onset of theophylline-induced generalized seizures and to increase the dose of theophylline required to induce seizures (*i.e.,* markedly increases the LD_{50}). Although there are no controlled studies in humans, a loading dose of intravenous phenobarbital (20 mg/kg infused over 60 minutes) may delay or prevent life-threatening seizures in high risk patients while efforts to enhance theophylline clearance are continued. Phenobarbital may cause respiratory depression, particularly in elderly patients and patients with COPD.

5. Treatment Of Cardiac Arrhythmias: Sinus tachycardia and simple ventricular premature beats are not harbingers of life-threatening arrhythmias, they do not require treatment in the absence of hemodynamic compromise, and they resolve with declining serum theophylline concentrations. Other arrhythmias, especially those associated with hemodynamic compromise, should be treated with antiarrhythmic therapy appropriate for the type of arrhythmia.

6. Gastrointestinal Decontamination: Oral activated charcoal (0.5 g/kg up to 20 g and repeat at least once 1-2 hours after the first dose) is extremely effective in blocking the absorption of theophylline throughout the gastrointestinal tract, even when administered several hours after ingestion. If the patient is vomiting, the charcoal should be administered through a nasogastric tube or after administration of an antiemetic. Phenothiazine antiemetics such as prochlorperazine or perphenazine should be avoided since they can lower the seizure threshold and frequently cause dystonic reactions. A single dose of sorbitol may be used to promote stooling to facilitate removal of theophylline bound to charcoal from the gastrointestinal tract. Sorbitol, however, should be dosed with caution since it is a potent purgative which can cause profound fluid and electrolyte abnormalities, particularly after multiple doses. Commercially available fixed combinations of liquid charcoal and sorbitol should be avoided in young children and after the first dose in adolescents and adults since they do not allow for individualization of charcoal and sorbitol dosing. Ipecac syrup should be avoided in theophylline overdoses. Although ipecac induces emesis, it does not reduce the absorption of theophylline unless administered within 5 minutes of ingestion and even then is less effective than oral activated charcoal. Moreover, ipecac induced emesis may persist for several hours after a single dose and significantly decrease the retention and the effectiveness of oral activated charcoal.

7. Serum Theophylline Concentration Monitoring: The serum theophylline concentration should be measured immediately upon presentation, 2-4 hours later, and then at sufficient intervals, e.g., every 4 hours, to guide treatment decisions and to assess the effectiveness of therapy. Serum theophylline concentrations may continue to increase after presentation of the patient for medical care as a result of continued absorption of theophylline from the gastrointestinal tract. Serial monitoring of serum theophylline serum concentrations should be continued until it is clear that the concentration is no longer rising and has returned to non-toxic levels.

8. General Monitoring Procedures: Electrocardiographic monitoring should be initiated on presentation and continued until the serum theophylline level has returned to a non-toxic level. Serum electrolytes and glucose should be measured on presentation and at appropriate intervals indicated by clinical circumstances. Fluid and electrolyte abnormalities should be promptly corrected. **Monitoring and treatment should be continued until the serum concentration decreases below 20 mcg/ml.**

9. Enhance Clearance Of Theophylline: Multiple-dose oral activated charcoal (*e.g.,* 0.5 mg/kg up to 20 g, every two hours) increases the clearance of theophylline at least twofold by adsorption of theophylline secreted into gastrointestinal fluids. Charcoal must be retained in, and pass through, the gastrointestinal tract to be effective; emesis should therefore be controlled by administration of appropriate antiemetics. Alternatively, the charcoal can be administered continuously through a nasogastric tube in conjunction with appropriate antiemetics. A single dose of sorbitol may be administered with the activated charcoal to promote stooling to facilitate clearance of the adsorbed theophylline from the gastrointestinal tract. Sorbitol alone does not enhance clearance of theophylline and should be dosed with caution to prevent excessive stooling which can result in severe fluid and electrolyte imbalances. Commercially available fixed combinations of liquid charcoal and sorbitol should be avoided in young children and after the first dose in adolescents and adults since they do not allow for individualization of charcoal and sorbitol dosing. In patients with intractable vomiting, extracorporeal methods of theophylline removal should be instituted (see OVERDOSAGE, Extracorporeal Removal).

SPECIFIC RECOMMENDATIONS

Acute Overdose

A. Serum Concentration >20<30 mcg/ml

1. Administer a single dose of oral activated charcoal.

2. Monitor the patient and obtain a serum theophylline concentration in 2-4 hours to insure that the concentration is not increasing.

B. Serum Concentration >30<100 mcg/ml

1. Administer multiple dose oral activated charcoal and measures to control emesis.

2. Monitor the patient and obtain serial theophylline concentrations every 2-4 hours to gauge the effectiveness of therapy and to guide further treatment decisions.

3. Institute extracorporeal removal if emesis, seizures, or cardiac arrhythmias cannot be adequately controlled (see OVERDOSAGE, Extracorporeal Removal.)

C. Serum Concentration >100 mcg/ml

1. Consider prophylactic anticonvulsant therapy.

2. Administer multiple-dose oral activated charcoal and measures to control emesis.

3. Consider extracorporeal removal, even if the patient has not experienced a seizure (see OVERDOSAGE, Extracorporeal Removal.)

4. Monitor the patient and obtain serial theophylline concentrations every 2-4 hours to gauge the effectiveness of therapy and to guide further treatment decisions.

Chronic Overdosage

A. Serum Concentration >20<30 mcg/ml (with manifestations of theophylline toxicity)

1. Administer a single dose of oral activated charcoal.

OVERDOSAGE: *(cont'd)*

2. Monitor the patient and obtain a serum theophylline concentration in 2-4 hours to insure that the concentration is not increasing.

B. Serum Concentration >30 mcg/ml in patients <60 years of age

1. Administer multiple-dose oral activated charcoal and measures to control emesis.

2. Monitor the patient and obtain serial theophylline concentrations every 2-4 hours to gauge the effectiveness of therapy and to guide further treatment decisions.

3. Institute extracorporeal removal if emesis, seizures, or cardiac arrhythmias cannot be adequately controlled (see OVERDOSAGE, Extracorporeal Removal.)

C. Serum Concentration >30 mcg/ml in patients ≥60 years of age.

1. Consider prophylactic anticonvulsant therapy.

2. Administer multiple-dose oral activated charcoal and measures to control emesis.

3. Consider extracorporeal removal even if the patient has not experienced a seizure (see OVERDOSAGE, Extracorporeal Removal).

4. Monitor the patient and obtain serial theophylline concentrations every 2-4 hours to gauge the effectiveness of therapy and to guide further treatment decisions.

EXTRACORPOREAL REMOVAL

Increasing the rate of theophylline clearance by extracorporeal methods may rapidly decrease serum concentrations, but the risks of the procedure must be weighed against the potential benefit. Charcoal hemoperfusion is the most effective method of extracorporeal removal, increasing theophylline clearance up to six fold, but serious complications, including hypotension, hypocalcemia, platelet consumption and bleeding diatheses may occur. Hemodialysis is about as efficient as multiple-dose oral activated charcoal and has a lower risk of serious complications than charcoal hemoperfusion. Hemodialysis should be considered as an alternative when charcoal hemoperfusion is not feasible and multiple-dose oral charcoal is ineffective because of intractable emesis. Serum theophylline concentrations may rebound 5-10 mcg/ml after discontinuation of charcoal hemoperfusion or hemodialysis due to redistribution of theophylline from the tissue compartment. Peritoneal dialysis is ineffective for theophylline removal; exchange transfusions in neonates have been minimally effective.

DOSAGE AND ADMINISTRATION:

IMMEDIATE RELEASE ORAL PRODUCTS

General Considerations: The steady-state peak serum theophylline concentration is a function of the dose, the dosing interval, and the rate of theophylline absorption and clearance in the individual patient. Because of marked individual differences in the rate of theophylline clearance, the dose required to achieve a peak serum theophylline concentration in the 10-20 mcg/ml range varies fourfold among otherwise similar patients in the absence of factors known to alter theophylline clearance (*e.g.,* 400-1600 mg/day in adults <60 years old and 10-36 mg/kg/day in children 1-9 years old). For a given population there is no single theophylline dose that will provide both safe and effective serum concentrations for all patients. Administration of the median theophylline dose required to achieve a therapeutic serum theophylline concentration in a given population may result in either sub-therapeutic or potentially toxic serum theophylline concentrations in individual patients. For example, at a dose of 900 mg/d in adults <60 years or 22 mg/kg/d in children 1-9 years, the steady-state peak serum theophylline concentration will be <10 mcg/ml in about 30% of patients, 10-20 mcg/ml in about 50% and 20-30 mcg/ml in about 20% of patients. **The dose of theophylline must be individualized on the basis of peak serum theophylline concentration measurements in order to achieve a dose that will provide maximum potential benefit with minimal risk of adverse effects.**

Transient caffeine-like adverse effects and excessive serum concentrations in slow metabolizers can be avoided in most patients by starting with a sufficiently low dose and slowly increasing the dose, if judged to be clinically indicated, in small increments. Dose increases should only be made if the previous dosage is well tolerated and at intervals of no less than 3 days to allow serum theophylline concentrations to reach the new steady state. Final dosage adjustment should be guided by serum theophylline concentration measurement (see PRECAUTIONS, Laboratory Tests and TABLE 5.) Health care providers should instruct patients and care givers to discontinue any dosage that causes adverse effects, to withhold the medication until these symptoms are gone and to then resume therapy at a lower, previously tolerated dosage (see WARNINGS).

If the patient's symptoms are well controlled, there are no apparent adverse effects, and no intervening factors that might alter dosage requirements (see WARNINGS and PRECAUTIONS), serum theophylline concentrations should be monitored at 6 month intervals for rapidly growing children and at yearly intervals for all others. In acutely ill patients, serum theophylline concentrations should be monitored at frequent intervals, e.g., every 24 hours.

Theophylline distributes poorly into body fat, therefore, mg/kg dose should be calculated on the basis of ideal body weight.

The following list contains theophylline dosing titration schema recommended for patients in various age groups and clinical circumstances. TABLE 5 contains recommendations for final theophylline dosage adjustment based on serum theophylline concentrations. **Application of these general dosing recommendations to individual patients must take into account the unique clinical characteristics of each patient. In general, these recommendations should serve as the upper limit for dosage adjustments in order to decrease the risk of potentially serious adverse events associated with unexpected large increases in serum theophylline concentration.**

A. Infants <1 year old.

1. Initial Dosage.

a. Premature Neonates:

i. <24 days postnatal age; 1.0 mg/kg every 12 hr

ii. ≥24 days postnatal age; 1.5 mg/kg every 12 hr

b. Full term infants and infants up to 52 weeks of age:

Total daily dose (mg) = [(0.2 × age in weeks)+5.0] × (Kg body Wt).

i. up to age 26 weeks; divide dose into 3 equal amounts administered at 8 hour intervals.

ii. >26 Weeks of age; divide dose into 4 equal amounts administered at 6 hour intervals.

2. Final Dosage: Adjusted to maintain a peak steady-state serum theophylline concentration of 5-10 mcg/ml in neonates and 10-15 mcg/ml in older infants (see TABLE 5) Since the time required to reach steady-state is a function of theophylline half-life, up to 5 days may be required to achieve steady-state in a premature neonate while only 2-3 days may be required in a 6 month old infant without other risk factors for impaired clearance in the absence of a loading dose. **If a serum theophylline concentration is obtained before steady-state is achieved, the maintenance dose should not be increased, even if the serum theophylline concentration is < 10 mcg/ml.**

B. Children (1-15 years) and adults (16-60 years) without risk factors for impaired clearance.

C. Patients With Risk Factors For Impaired Clearance, The Elderly (>60 Years), And Those In Whom It Is Not Feasible To Monitor Serum Theophylline Concentrations: In children 1-15 years of age, the initial theophylline dose should not exceed 16 mg/kg/day up to a maximum

DOSAGE AND ADMINISTRATION: *(cont'd)*

TABLE 4 Dosing titration (as anhydrous theophylline).*,†

Titration Step	Children < 45 kg	Children > 45 kg and adults
1. Starting Dosage	12-14 mg/kg/day up to a maximum of 300 mg/day divided Q4-6 hrs*	300 mg/day divided Q6-8 hrs*
2. After 3 days, *if tolerated,* increase dose to:	16 mg/kg/day up to a maximum of 400 mg/day divided Q4-6 hrs*	400 mg/day divided Q6-8 hrs*
3. After 3 more days, *if tolerated,* increase dose to:	20 mg/kg/day up to a maximum of 600 mg/day divided Q4-6 hrs*	600 mg/day divided Q6-8 hrs*

* Patients with more rapid metabolism, clinically identified by higher than average dose requirements, should receive a smaller dose more frequently to prevent breakthrough symptoms resulting from low trough concentrations before the next dose. A reliably absorbed slow-release formulation will decrease fluctuations and permit longer dosing intervals.

† For products containing theophylline salts, the appropriate dose of the theophylline salt should be substituted for the anhydrous theophylline dose. To calculate the equivalent dose for theophylline salts, divide the anhydrous theophylline dose listed below by 0.8 for aminophylline, by 0.65 for oxtriphylline, and by 0.5 for the calcium salicylate and sodium glycinate salts.

of 400 mg/day in the presence of risk factors for reduced theophylline clearance (see WARNINGS) or if it is not feasible to monitor serum theophylline concentrations. In adolescents ≥16 years and adults, including the elderly, the initial theophylline dose should not exceed 400 mg/day in the presence of risk factors for reduced theophylline clearance (see WARNINGS) or if it is not feasible to monitor serum theophylline concentrations.

D. Loading Dose for Acute Bronchodilatation: An inhaled beta-2 selective agonist, alone or in combination with a systemically administered corticosteroid, is the most effective treatment for acute exacerbations of reversible airways obstruction. Theophylline is a relatively weak bronchodilator, is less effective than an inhaled beta-2 selective agonist and provides no added benefit in the treatment of acute bronchospasm. If an inhaled or parenteral beta agonist is not available, a loading dose of an oral immediate release theophylline can be used as a temporary measure. A single 5 mg/kg dose of theophylline, in a patient who has not received any theophylline in the previous 24 hours, will produce an average peak serum theophylline concentration of 10 mcg/ml (range 5-15 mcg/ml). If dosing with theophylline is to be continued beyond the loading dose, the guidelines in Sections A.1.b., B.3, or C., above, should be utilized and serum theophylline concentration monitored at 24 hour intervals to adjust final dosage.

TABLE 5 Final dosage adjustment guided by serum theophylline concentration.

Peak Serum Concentration	Dosage Adjustment
<9.9 mcg/ml	If symptoms are not controlled and current dosage is tolerated, increase dose about 25%. Recheck serum concentration after three days for further dosage adjustment
10 to 14.9 mcg/ml	If symptoms are controlled and current dosage is tolerated, maintain dose and recheck serum concentration at 6-12 month intervals.* If symptoms are not controlled and current dosage is tolerated consider adding additional medication(s) to treatment regimen.
15-19.9 mcg/ml	Consider 10% decrease in dose to provide greater margin of safety even if current dosage is tolerated.*
20-24.9 mcg/ml	Decrease dose by 25% even if no adverse effects are present. Recheck serum concentration after 3 days to guide further dosage adjustment.
25-30 mcg/ml	Skip next dose and decrease subsequent doses at least 25% even if no adverse effects are present. Recheck serum concentration after 3 days to guide further dosage adjustment. If symptomatic, consider whether overdose treatment is indicated (see recommendations for chronic overdosage). If theophylline is subsequently resumed, decrease dose by at least 50% and recheck serum concentration after 3 days to guide further dosage adjustment.

* Dose reduction and/or serum theophylline concentration measurement is indicated whenever adverse effects are present, physiologic abnormalities that can reduce theophylline clearance occur (*e.g.,* sustained fever), or a drug that interacts with theophylline is added or discontinued (see WARNINGS).

SUSTAINED ACTION CAPSULES: SPRINKLING CONTENTS ON FOOD

Theo-Dur Sprinkle may be administered by carefully opening the capsule and sprinkling the beaded contents on a spoonful of soft food such as applesauce or pudding. The soft food should be swallowed immediately without chewing and followed with a glass of cool water or juice to ensure complete swallowing of the beads. It is recommended that the food used should not be hot and should be soft enough to be swallowed without chewing. Any bead/food mixture should be used immediately and not stored for future use. The small amount of food (one spoonful) used to administer the dose will not alter the bioavailability of Theo-Dur Sprinkle; however, the dosing should be at least 1 hour before or 2 hours after a meal. SUBDIVIDING THE CONTENTS OF A CAPSULE IS NOT RECOMMENDED.

DOSAGE GUIDELINES

Because administration of Theo-Dur Sprinkle at the time of food ingestion has been shown to result in significantly lower peak-serum concentrations and reduced extent of absorption (bioavailability). patients should be instructed to take this medication at least 1 hour before or 2 hours after a meal (see DRUG INTERACTIONS).

Taking Theo-Dur Sprinkle at 12-hour intervals under the above restrictive recommendations in regard to food ingestion may be difficult for the patient to follow. Under such circumstances, consideration should be given to prescribing this drug every 8 hours (giving one-third of the 24-hour dosage requirement with each dose), if this regimen would more easily permit dosing under fasting conditions.

I. Acute Symptoms: NOTE: Status asthmaticus should be considered a medical emergency and is defined as that degree of bronchospasm which is not rapidly responsive to usual doses of conventional bronchodilators. Optimal therapy for such patients frequently requires both *additional medication,* Parenterally administered, and *close monitoring,* preferably in an intensive care setting. Theo-Dur Sprinkle is not intended for patients experiencing an acute episode of bronchospasm (associated with asthma, chronic bronchitis, or emphysema). Such patients require rapid relief of symptoms and should be treated with an immediate release or intravenous theophylline preparation (or other bronchodilators) and not with controlled-release products.

II. Chronic Therapy:

DOSAGE AND ADMINISTRATION: *(cont'd)*

A. Initiating Therapy with an Immediate-Release Product: It is recommended that the appropriate dosage be established sing an immediate-release preparation. Children weighing less than 25 kg should have their daily dosage requirements established with a liquid preparation to permit small dosage increments. Slow clinical titration is generally preferred to help assure acceptance and safety of the medication, and to allow the patient to develop tolerance to transient caffeine-like side effects. Then, if the total 24-hour dose can be given by use of the sustained-release product, the patient can usually be switched to Theo-Dur Sprinkle, giving one-half of the daily dose at 12-hour intervals. Patients who metabolize theophylline rapidly such as the young, smokers, and some nonsmoking adults, are the most likely candidates for dosing at 8-hour intervals. Such patients can generally be identified as having trough-serum concentrations lower than desired for repeatedly exhibiting symptoms near the end of a dosing interval.

B. Initiating Therapy with Theo-Dur Sprinkle: Alternatively, therapy can be initiated with Theo-Dur Sprinkle since it is available in dosage strengths which permit titration and adjustments of dosage in adults and older children: *Initial Dose:*16 mg/kg/24 hours or 400 mg/24 hours (whichever is less) of anhydrous theophylline in 2 divided doses, 12-hour intervals. *Increasing Dose:*The above dosage may be increased in approximately 25% increments at 3-day intervals so long as the drug is tolerated; until clinical response is satisfactory or the maximum dose as indicated in Section III (below) is reached. The serum concentration may be checked at these intervals, but at a minimum, should be checked at the end of this adjustment period.

III. III. Maintenance Dose of Theophylline where the Serum Concentration is not Measured: See TABLE 5

WARNING: DO NOT ATTEMPT TO MAINTAIN ANY DOSE THAT IS NOT TOLERATED

TABLE 6 Sustained-Release Capsules Not to exceed the following:

		Dose per 12 hours
Age 6-9 years	24 mg/kg/day	12.0 mg/kg
Age 9-12 years	20 mg/kg/day	10.0 mg/kg
Age 12-16 years	18 mg/kg/day	9.0 mg/kg
Age Over 16 years	13 mg/kg/day or 900 mg (WHICHEVER IS LESS)	6.5 mg/kg

IV. Measurement of Serum Theophylline Concentrations During Chronic Therapy: If the above maximum doses are to maintained or exceeded, serum theophylline measurement is recommended. The serum sample should be obtained at the time of peak absorption: 1 to 2 hours after administration for immediate-release products and 5 to 10 hours after dosing for Theo-Dur Sprinkle. It is important that the patient will have missed no doses during the previous 48 hours and the dosing intervals will have been reasonably typical with no added doses during that time. DOSAGE ADJUSTMENT BASED ON SERUM THEOPHYLLINE CONCENTRATION MEASUREMENTS WHEN THESE INSTRUCTIONS HAVE NOT BEEN FOLLOWED MAY RESULT IN RECOMMENDATIONS THAT PRESENT RISK OF TOXICITY TO THE PATIENT.

V. Final Adjustment of Dosage: Caution should be exercised for younger children who cannot complain of minor side effects. Those with cor pulmonale, congestive heart failure, and/or other liver disease may have unusually low dosage requirements and thus may experience toxicity at the maximum dose recommended above. It is important that no patient be maintained on any dosage that is not tolerated. In instructing patients to increase dosage according to the schedule above, they should be instructed not to take a subsequent dose if apparent side effects occur and to resume therapy at a lower dose once adverse effects have disappeared.

TABLE 7 Sustained-Release Capsules
Dosage Adjustment after serum theophylline measurement.

If serum theophylline is:		Directions
Within normal limits	10 to 20 mcg/ml	Maintain dosage of tolerated. Recheck serum theophylline concentration at 6- to 12-month intervals.*
Too High	20 to 25 mcg/ml	Decrease doses by about 10%. Serum theophylline concentrations should be checked until within normal limits. Recheck at 6 to 12 months.
	25 to 30 mcg/ml	Skip next dose and decrease subsequent doses by about 25%. Serum theophylline concentrations should be checked until within normal limits. Recheck at 6 to 12 months.
	over 30 mcg/ml	Skip next 2 doses and decrease subsequent doses by 50%. Serum theophylline should be checked until within normal limits. Recheck at 6 to 12 months.
Too Low	7.5 to 10 mcg/ml	Increase dose by about 25%.** Serum theophylline concentrations should be checked for guidance in further dosage adjustment. Recheck serum theophylline concentration at 6- to 12-month intervals.*
	5 to 7.5	Increase dose by about 25% to the nearest dose increment and recheck serum theophylline for guidance in further dosage adjustment (another increase will probably be needed, but provides a safety check).

* Finer adjustments in dosage may be needed for some patients.
** The total daily dose may need to be administered at more frequent intervals if asthma symptoms occur repeatedly at the end of a dosing interval.

STORAGE

Keep tightly closed. Store at controlled room temperature 15-30°C (59-86°F).

HOW SUPPLIED - RATED THERAPEUTICALLY EQUIVALENT:

Capsule, Elastic - Oral - 100 mg

100's	$19.61	Theophylline Anhydrous, Inwood Labs	00258-3637-01
100's	$19.76	Theophylline Anhydrous, Arcola	00070-2340-00
100's	$20.57	Theophylline Anhydrous, Qualitest Pharms	00603-5949-21
100's	$20.59	Theophylline Anhydrous, Teva	00093-0934-01

Capsule, Elastic - Oral - 125 mg

100's	$24.55	Theophylline Anhydrous, Inwood Labs	00258-3638-01
100's	$24.77	Theophylline Anhydrous, Arcola	00070-2341-00
100's	$25.75	Theophylline Anhydrous, Teva	00093-0936-01
100's	$25.75	Theophylline Anhydrous, Major Pharms	00904-7847-60
100's	$25.78	Theophylline Anhydrous, Qualitest Pharms	00603-5950-21
100's	$25.79	Theophylline Anhydrous, Schein Pharm (US)	00364-2586-01
100's	$25.84	Theophylline Anhydrous, Aligen Independ	00405-4983-01

HOW SUPPLIED - RATED THERAPEUTICALLY EQUIVALENT: *(cont'd)*

Capsule, Elastic - Oral - 200 mg

100's	$29.23	Theophylline Anhydrous, Inwood Labs	00258-3634-01
100's	$29.48	Theophylline Anhydrous, Arcola	00070-2342-00
100's	$30.60	Theophylline Anhydrous, Qualitest Pharms	00603-5951-21
100's	$30.65	Theophylline Anhydrous, Teva	00093-0938-01
100's	$30.70	Theophylline Anhydrous, Schein Pharm (US)	00364-2587-01
100's	$30.70	Theophylline Anhydrous, Major Pharms	00904-7848-60
100's	$30.77	Theophylline Anhydrous, Aligen Independ	00405-4984-01

Capsule, Elastic - Oral - 300 mg

100's	$34.82	Theophylline Anhydrous, Inwood Labs	00258-3625-01
100's	$35.10	Theophylline Anhydrous, Arcola	00070-2343-00
100's	$36.55	Theophylline Anhydrous, Teva	00093-0940-01
100's	$36.55	Theophylline Anhydrous, Major Pharms	00904-7849-60
100's	$36.56	Theophylline Anhydrous, Qualitest Pharms	00603-5952-21
100's	$36.58	Theophylline Anhydrous, Schein Pharm (US)	00364-2588-01
100's	$36.65	Theophylline Anhydrous, Aligen Independ	00405-4985-01
100's	$40.63	Theophylline Anhydrous, Rugby	00536-5634-01

Capsule, Gelatin, Sustained Action - Oral - 100 mg

100's	$20.73	Theophylline, HL Moore Drug Exch	00839-7885-06
100's	$24.25	SLO-BID, Rhone-Poulenc Rorer	00075-0100-00
100's	$25.83	SLO-BID, Rhone-Poulenc Rorer	00075-0100-62
1000's	$238.93	SLO-BID, Rhone-Poulenc Rorer	00075-0100-99

Capsule, Gelatin, Sustained Action - Oral - 125 mg

10 strip x 10	$31.16	SLO-BID 125, Rhone-Poulenc Rorer	00075-1125-62
100's	$29.74	Theophylline, HL Moore Drug Exch	00839-7886-06
100's	$30.39	SLO-BID 125, Rhone-Poulenc Rorer	00075-1125-00

Capsule, Gelatin, Sustained Action - Oral - 200 mg

60's	$18.56	THEOPHYLLINE, Talbert Phcy	44514-0903-36
100's	$35.41	Theophylline, HL Moore Drug Exch	00839-7887-06
100's	$36.16	SLO-BID, Rhone-Poulenc Rorer	00075-0200-00
100's	$36.30	SLO-BID, Rhone-Poulenc Rorer	00075-0200-62
1000's	$355.28	SLO-BID, Rhone-Poulenc Rorer	00075-0200-99

Capsule, Gelatin, Sustained Action - Oral - 300 mg

60's	$22.05	THEOPHYLLINE, Talbert Phcy	44514-0904-36
100's	$42.17	Theophylline, HL Moore Drug Exch	00839-7888-06
100's	$43.08	SLO-BID, Rhone-Poulenc Rorer	00075-0300-00
100's	$43.15	SLO-BID, Rhone-Poulenc Rorer	00075-0300-62
1000's	$421.92	SLO-BID, Rhone-Poulenc Rorer	00075-0300-99

Elixir - Oral - 80 mg/15ml

1 gal	$14.98	Theophylline, Thames Pharma	49158-0261-39
4 oz	$1.45	Theophylline, Thames Pharma	49158-0261-34
15 ml x 100	$36.65	Theophylline, Roxane	00054-8845-04
16 oz	$2.90	Theophylline, Thames Pharma	49158-0261-38
120 ml	$.66	Theophylline, H.C.F.A. F F P	99999-2329-02
480 ml	$2.50	TRUXOPHYLLIN, C O Truxton	00463-9031-16
480 ml	$2.64	Theophylline, United Res	00677-1523-33
480 ml	$2.64	Theophylline, H.C.F.A. F F P	99999-2329-03
480 ml	$3.50	ELIXOMIN, HR Cenci	00556-0149-16
480 ml	$3.50	Theophylline, HL Moore Drug Exch	00839-5029-69
480 ml	$3.60	Theophylline, Rosemont	00832-8019-16
480 ml	$3.60	Theophylline, Major Pharms	00904-1444-16
480 ml	$3.70	Theophyllin, Harber Pharm	51432-0678-20
480 ml	$3.84	Theophylline Anhydrous, Qualitest Pharms	00603-1729-58
480 ml	$3.95	Theophylline, Consolidated Midland	00223-6308-01
480 ml	$4.23	Theophylline, Morton Grove	60432-0019-16
480 ml	$4.62	Theophylline, Alpharma	00472-1444-16
480 ml	$4.70	Theophylline, Halsey Drug	00879-0226-16
480 ml	$5.45	Theophylline, Goldline Labs	00182-0226-40
480 ml	$5.50	Theophylline, Rugby	00536-2100-85
480 ml	$5.80	Theophylline, Schein Pharm (US)	00364-7060-16
480 ml	$5.82	Theophylline, Aligen Independ	00405-3825-16
480 ml	$5.94	Theophylline, Geneva Pharms	00781-6600-16
480 ml	**$75.79**	**ELIXOPHYLLIN, Forest Pharms**	**00456-0644-16**
960 ml	$5.28	Theophylline, H.C.F.A. F F P	99999-2329-04
960 ml	**$110.92**	**ELIXOPHYLLIN, Berlex Labs**	**50419-0121-32**
960 ml	**$148.65**	**ELIXOPHYLLIN, Forest Pharms**	**00456-0644-32**
1000 ml	$5.50	Theophylline, H.C.F.A. F F P	99999-2329-05
1000 ml	$7.08	Theophylline, Roxane	00054-3840-68
3785 ml	$20.62	Theophylline, Major Pharms	00904-1444-28
3785 ml	$25.34	Theophylline, Goldline Labs	00182-0226-41
3840 ml	$10.94	ASMALIX, Century Pharms	00436-0506-28
3840 ml	$15.09	Theophylline, HL Moore Drug Exch	00839-5029-70
3840 ml	$17.47	ELIXOMIN, HR Cenci	00556-0149-28
3840 ml	$18.59	Theophyllin, Harber Pharm	51432-0678-21
3840 ml	$19.47	Theophylline, Consolidated Midland	00223-6308-02
3840 ml	$19.97	Theophylline, Rosemont	00832-8019-28
3840 ml	$19.97	Theophylline, Morton Grove	60432-0019-28
3840 ml	$20.35	Theophylline, Alpharma	00472-1444-28
3840 ml	$20.74	Theophylline, Halsey Drug	00879-0226-28
3840 ml	$21.12	Theophylline, H.C.F.A. F F P	99999-2329-01
3840 ml	$26.15	Theophylline, Geneva Pharms	00781-6600-28
3840 ml	**$576.79**	**ELIXOPHYLLIN, Forest Pharms**	**00456-0644-28**

Injection, Solution - Intravenous - 0.4 mg/ml

1000 ml	$15.92	Theophylline, Abbott	00074-7662-09

Injection, Solution - Intravenous - 0.8 mg/ml

500 ml	$14.06	Theophylline, Abbott	00074-7665-03
1000 ml	$17.14	Theophylline, Abbott	00074-7665-09

Injection, Solution - Intravenous - 1.6 mg/ml

250 ml	$12.49	Theophylline, Abbott	00074-7666-02
500 ml	$15.24	Theophylline, Abbott	00074-7666-03

Injection, Solution - Intravenous - 2 mg/ml

100 ml	$13.18	Theophylline, Abbott	00074-7668-23

Injection, Solution - Intravenous - 4 mg/ml

50 ml	$13.18	Theophylline, Abbott	00074-7677-13
100 ml	$13.59	Theophylline, Abbott	00074-7677-23

Solution - Oral - 80 mg/15ml

18.75 ml x 100	$22.78	Theophylline, Roxane	00054-8848-16
30 ml x 100	$47.94	Theophylline, Roxane	00054-8846-04
480 ml	$27.48	THEOLAIR, 3M Pharms	00089-0960-16

HOW SUPPLIED - RATED THERAPEUTICALLY EQUIVALENT:
(cont'd)

500 ml	$7.31	Theophylline, Roxane	00054-3841-63
1000 ml	$12.44	Theophylline, Roxane	00054-3841-68

Syrup - Oral - 80 mg/15ml

480 ml	$13.20	THEOCLEAR-80, Schwarz Pharma (US)	00131-5098-70
480 ml	$22.48	SLO-PHYLLIN, Rhone-Poulenc Rorer	00075-3650-16
3840 ml	$78.80	THEOCLEAR-80, Schwarz Pharma (US)	00131-5098-72

Tablet, Coated, Sustained Action - Oral - 100 mg

100's	$6.30	Theophylline, H.C.F.A. F F P	99999-2329-06
100's	$6.75	Theophylline Anhydrous, United Res	00677-0845-01
100's	$7.40	THEOX 100, Carnrick	00086-0031-10
100's	$9.90	Theophylline, IDE-Interstate	00814-7801-14
100's	$10.60	Theophylline, Goldline Labs	00182-1589-01
100's	$11.19	Theophylline Anhydrous, HL Moore Drug Exch	00839-6730-06
100's	$11.19	Theophylline Anhydrous, HL Moore Drug Exch	00839-7705-06
100's	$11.25	Theophyllin Anhydrous, Schein Pharm (US)	00364-0680-01
100's	$11.50	Theophylline Anhydrous, Qualitest Pharms	00603-5944-21
100's	$11.70	Theophylline 100, Major Pharms	00904-1610-60
100's	$11.70	Theophylline, Sidmak Labs	50111-0483-01
100's	$11.70	Theophylline Anhydrous, Martec Pharms	52555-0702-01
100's	$11.85	Theophylline, Warner Chilcott	00047-0657-24
100's	$11.85	Theophylline, Inwood Labs	00258-3584-01
100's	$12.16	THEOCHRON, Teva	00093-0599-01
100's	$12.31	Theophylline CR, Aligen Independ	00405-4986-01
100's	$12.50	Theophylline Anhydrous, Parmed Pharms	00349-8280-01
100's	$12.50	Theophylline Anhydrous, Rugby	00536-4650-01
100's	$12.50	Theophylline, Geneva Pharms	00781-1003-01
100's	$12.98	Theophylline, Parmed Pharms	00349-8683-01
100's	$15.10	Theophylline, Medirex	57480-0365-01
100's	$18.32	THEO-DUR, Schering	00085-0487-01
100's	$18.50	THEOPHYLLINE ANHYDROUS, Goldline Labs	00182-1589-89
100's	$18.67	Theophylline 100, Major Pharms	00904-1610-61
100's	$27.45	THEO-DUR, Schering	00085-0487-81
500's	$31.50	Theophylline, H.C.F.A. F F P	99999-2329-07
500's	$32.75	THEOX 100, Carnrick	00086-0031-50
500's	$33.75	Theophylline, Sidmak Labs	50111-0483-02
500's	$37.95	Theophylline, Inwood Labs	00258-3584-05
500's	$38.95	Theophylline Anhydrous, Qualitest Pharms	00603-5944-28
500's	$42.70	Theophylline 100, Major Pharms	00904-1610-40
500's	$43.73	Theophylline, IDE-Interstate	00814-7801-28
500's	$45.99	Theophylline Anhydrous, HL Moore Drug Exch	00839-6730-12
600's	$87.00	Theophylline, Medirex	57480-0365-06
1000's	$63.00	Theophylline, H.C.F.A. F F P	99999-2329-08
1000's	$75.00	Theophylline, Sidmak Labs	50111-0483-03
1000's	$86.32	THEO-DUR, Schering	00085-0487-05
5000's	$167.15	THEO-DUR, Schering	00085-0487-10
5000's	$315.00	Theophylline, H.C.F.A. F F P	99999-2329-09
5000's	$789.90	THEO-DUR, Schering	00085-0487-50

Tablet, Coated, Sustained Action - Oral - 200 mg

100's	$8.93	Theophylline, H.C.F.A. F F P	99999-2329-10
100's	$9.23	Theophylline Anhydrous, United Res	00677-0846-01
100's	$10.70	THEOX 200, Carnrick	00086-0032-10
100's	$14.02	Theophylline, IDE-Interstate	00814-7802-14
100's	$17.67	Theophylline Anhydrous, HL Moore Drug Exch	00839-7706-06
100's	$17.94	Theophylline Anhydrous, Qualitest Pharms	00603-5945-29
100's	$18.65	Theophylline, Inwood Labs	00258-3583-01
100's	$18.75	Theophylline 200, Major Pharms	00904-1611-60
100's	$18.91	Theophylline Anhydrous, Qualitest Pharms	00603-5945-21
100's	$19.00	Theophylline, Goldline Labs	00182-1590-01
100's	$19.00	Theophylline, Sidmak Labs	50111-0482-01
100's	$19.00	Theophylline, Martec Pharms	52555-0703-01
100's	$19.25	Theophylline Anhydrous, Schein Pharm (US)	00364-0681-01
100's	$19.42	THEOCHRON, Teva	00093-0588-01
100's	$19.44	Theophylline Anhydrous, HL Moore Drug Exch	00839-6729-06
100's	$19.95	Theophylline Anhydrous, Parmed Pharms	00349-8281-01
100's	$19.95	Theophylline, Geneva Pharms	00781-1004-01
100's	$20.00	Theophylline CR, Aligen Independ	00405-4987-01
100's	$20.25	Theophylline, Medirex	57480-0366-01
100's	$20.78	Theophylline 200, Major Pharms	00904-1611-61
100's	$24.30	Theophylline, Rugby	00536-4651-01
100's	$25.00	Theophylline 200, Warner Chilcott	00047-0659-24
100's	$25.00	THEOPHYLLINE ANHYDROUS, Goldline Labs	00182-1590-89
100's	$27.28	THEO-DUR SUSTAINED ACTION, Schering	00085-0933-01
100's	$34.02	THEO-DUR SUSTAINED ACTION, Schering	00085-0933-81
500's	$44.65	Theophylline, H.C.F.A. F F P	99999-2329-11
500's	$46.15	Theophylline Anhydrous, United Res	00677-0846-05
500's	$49.80	THEOX 200, Carnrick	00086-0032-50
500's	$62.25	Theophylline 200, Major Pharms	00904-1611-40
500's	$62.44	Theophylline Anhydrous, HL Moore Drug Exch	00839-6729-12
500's	$62.44	Theophylline Anhydrous, HL Moore Drug Exch	00839-7706-12
500's	$66.60	Theophylline, IDE-Interstate	00814-7802-28
500's	$66.70	Theophylline Anhydrous, Qualitest Pharms	00603-5945-28
500's	$79.90	Theophylline Anhydrous, Parmed Pharms	00349-8281-05
500's	$81.95	Theophylline, Inwood Labs	00258-3583-05
500's	$82.00	Theophylline, Sidmak Labs	50111-0482-02
500's	$83.75	Theophylline, Geneva Pharms	00781-1004-05
500's	$83.79	THEOCHRON, Teva	00093-0588-05
500's	$85.75	Theophylline 200, Warner Chilcott	00047-0659-30
500's	$85.75	Theophylline Anhydrous, Schein Pharm (US)	00364-0681-05
500's	$86.32	Theophylline 200 Mg Tablets, Aligen Independ	00405-4987-02
500's	$88.30	Theophylline, Rugby	00536-4651-05
500's	$128.59	THEO-DUR SUSTAINED ACTION, Schering	00085-0933-05
600's	$107.80	Theophylline, Medirex	57480-0366-06
1000's	$89.30	Theophylline, H.C.F.A. F F P	99999-2329-12
1000's	$91.35	THEOX 200, Carnrick	00086-0032-90
1000's	$127.85	Theophylline Anhydrous, Qualitest Pharms	00603-5945-32
1000's	$149.95	Theophylline, Parmed Pharms	00349-8684-10
1000's	$150.38	Theophylline Anhydrous, HL Moore Drug Exch	00839-6729-16
1000's	$155.00	Theophylline, Goldline Labs	00182-1590-10
1000's	$155.00	Theophylline, Sidmak Labs	50111-0482-03
1000's	$155.00	Theophylline, Martec Pharms	52555-0703-10
1000's	$155.10	Theophylline Anhydrous, Major Pharms	00904-1611-80
1000's	$156.00	Theophylline, Inwood Labs	00258-3583-10
1000's	$158.95	Theophylline Anhydrous, Parmed Pharms	00349-8281-10
1000's	$158.95	Theophylline Anhydrous, Rugby	00536-4651-10
1000's	$242.81	THEO-DUR SUSTAINED ACTION, Schering	00085-0933-10

HOW SUPPLIED - RATED THERAPEUTICALLY EQUIVALENT:
(cont'd)

5000's	$446.50	Theophylline, H.C.F.A. F F P	99999-2329-13
5000's	$1178.40	THEO-DUR SUSTAINED ACTION, Schering	00085-0933-50

Tablet, Coated, Sustained Action - Oral - 300 mg

100's	$11.25	Theophylline, H.C.F.A. F F P	99999-2329-14
100's	$12.38	Theophylline, United Res	00677-0817-01
100's	$13.95	THEOX 300, Carnrick	00086-0033-10
100's	$17.30	Theophylline, Harber Pharm	51432-0453-03
100's	$18.23	Theophylline, IDE-Interstate	00814-7805-14
100's	$19.59	Theophylline Anhydrous, Qualitest Pharms	00603-5946-21
100's	$21.00	Theophylline, Goldline Labs	00182-1400-01
100's	$21.18	Theophylline Anhydrous, HL Moore Drug Exch	00839-6693-06
100's	$21.50	Theophylline Anhydrous, Schein Pharm (US)	00364-0660-01
100's	$21.90	Theophylline Anhydrous, Qualitest Pharms	00603-5946-29
100's	$21.95	Theophylline Anhydrous, Major Pharms	00904-1612-60
100's	$22.00	Theophylline, Sidmak Labs	50111-0459-01
100's	$22.00	Theophylline, Martec Pharms	52555-0704-01
100's	$22.10	Theophylline 300, Warner Chilcott	00047-0592-24
100's	$22.10	THEOCHRON, Teva	00093-0589-01
100's	$22.15	Theophylline, Geneva Pharms	00781-1005-01
100's	$22.75	Theophylline, Inwood Labs	00258-3581-01
100's	$23.16	Theophylline, Aligen Independ	00405-4988-01
100's	$23.95	Theophylline, Parmed Pharms	00349-8266-01
100's	$23.95	Theophylline, Rugby	00536-4652-01
100's	$25.90	Theophylline Anhydrous, Major Pharms	00904-1612-61
100's	$26.10	Theophylline, Medirex	57480-0367-01
100's	$30.50	THEOPHYLLINE ANHYDROUS, Goldline Labs	00182-1400-89
100's	$32.40	THEO-DUR, Schering	00085-0584-01
100's	$40.50	THEO-DUR, Schering	00085-0584-81
500's	$56.25	Theophylline, H.C.F.A. F F P	99999-2329-15
500's	$60.25	THEOX 300, Carnrick	00086-0033-50
500's	$61.90	Theophylline, United Res	00677-0817-05
500's	$75.81	Theophylline Anhydrous, Qualitest Pharms	00603-5946-28
500's	$76.90	Theophylline Anhydrous, Major Pharms	00904-1612-40
500's	$80.18	Theophylline, IDE-Interstate	00814-7805-28
500's	$86.50	Theophylline, Harber Pharm	51432-0453-05
500's	$88.03	Theophylline 300, Warner Chilcott	00047-0592-30
500's	$95.00	Theophylline, Goldline Labs	00182-1400-05
500's	$96.95	Theophylline, Parmed Pharms	00349-8266-05
500's	$98.28	Theophylline, Inwood Labs	00258-3581-05
500's	$98.50	Theophylline, Sidmak Labs	50111-0459-02
500's	$99.50	Theophylline Anhydrous, Schein Pharm (US)	00364-0660-05
500's	$99.95	Theophylline, Geneva Pharms	00781-1005-05
500's	$101.94	THEOCHRON, Teva	00093-0589-05
500's	$103.68	Theophylline Anhydrous, Aligen Independ	00405-4988-02
500's	$110.44	Theophylline, Rugby	00536-4652-05
500's	$152.73	THEO-DUR, Schering	00085-0584-05
600's	$127.80	Theophylline, Medirex	57480-0367-06
1000's	$110.55	THEOX 300, Carnrick	00086-0033-90
1000's	$112.50	Theophylline, H.C.F.A. F F P	99999-2329-16
1000's	$147.51	Theophylline Anhydrous, Qualitest Pharms	00603-5946-32
1000's	$152.81	Theophylline Cr, HL Moore Drug Exch	00839-6695-16
1000's	$152.81	Theophylline Anhydrous, HL Moore Drug Exch	00839-7707-16
1000's	$183.40	Theophylline Cr, HL Moore Drug Exch	00839-6693-16
1000's	$188.92	Theophylline, Inwood Labs	00258-3581-10
1000's	$188.95	Theophylline Anhydrous, Schein Pharm (US)	00364-0660-02
1000's	$189.00	Theophylline, Goldline Labs	00182-1400-10
1000's	$189.90	Theophylline Anhydrous, Major Pharms	00904-1612-80
1000's	$189.95	Theophylline, Parmed Pharms	00349-8266-10
1000's	$190.00	Theophylline, Sidmak Labs	50111-0459-03
1000's	$190.00	Theophylline, Martec Pharms	52555-0704-10
1000's	$198.80	Theophylline, Parmed Pharms	00349-8685-10
1000's	$198.80	Theophylline Anhydrous, Rugby	00536-4652-10
1000's	$295.52	THEO-DUR, Schering	00085-0584-10
5000's	$562.50	Theophylline, H.C.F.A. F F P	99999-2329-17
5000's	$1398.95	THEO-DUR, Schering	00085-0584-50

Tablet, Coated, Sustained Action - Oral - 450 mg

100's	$27.75	Theophylline, Sidmak Labs	50111-0518-01
100's	$27.75	Theophylline Anhydrous, Warrick Pharms	59930-1680-01
100's	$28.58	Theophylline Anhydrous, Qualitest Pharms	00603-5747-21
100's	$29.65	Theophylline Anhydrous, Martec Pharms	52555-0705-01
100's	$29.77	Theophylline CR, Aligen Independ	00405-4990-01
100's	$32.85	Theophylline, Schein Pharm (US)	00364-2490-01
100's	$32.90	Theophylline, United Res	00677-1410-01
100's	$32.95	Theophylline CR, Major Pharms	00904-1613-60
100's	$33.41	Theophylline, HL Moore Drug Exch	00839-7651-06
100's	$33.50	Theophylline Anhydrous, Goldline Labs	00182-1941-01
100's	$33.55	Theophylline Anhydrous, Geneva Pharms	00781-1928-01
100's	$35.39	Theophylline Anhydrous, Warner Chilcott	00047-0593-24
100's	$35.39	Theophylline TD, Rugby	00536-4653-01
100's	$43.01	THEO-DUR, Schering	00085-0806-01
100's	$53.77	THEO-DUR, Schering	00085-0806-81

HOW SUPPLIED - NOT RATED EQUIVALENT:

Capsule, Elastic - Oral - 100 mg

100's	$20.55	Theophylline Anhydrous, Major Pharms	00904-7846-60
100's	$20.59	Theophylline Anhydrous, Goldline Labs	00182-1311-01
100's	$20.59	Theophylline Anhydrous, Schein Pharm (US)	00364-2585-01
100's	$26.90	THEO-24, UCB Pharma	50474-0100-01

Capsule, Elastic - Oral - 125 mg

100's	$22.87	Theophylline Anhydrous, Rugby	00536-5632-01
100's	$25.79	Theophylline Anhydrous, Goldline Labs	00182-1312-01

Capsule, Elastic - Oral - 200 mg

100's	$30.69	Theophylline Anhydrous, Goldline Labs	00182-1313-01
100's	$34.12	Theophylline Anhydrous, Rugby	00536-5633-01
100's	$40.10	THEO-24, UCB Pharma	50474-0200-01
100's	**$46.70**	**ELIXOPHYLLIN, Berlex Labs**	**50419-0120-10**
100's	**$58.27**	**ELIXOPHYLLIN, Berlex Labs**	**50419-0120-11**
100's UD	$41.02	THEO-24, UCB Pharma	50474-0200-60
500's	$192.16	THEO-24, UCB Pharma	50474-0200-50
500's	**$276.05**	**ELIXOPHYLLIN, Berlex Labs**	**50419-0120-50**

Capsule, Elastic - Oral - 300 mg

100's	$36.58	Theophylline Anhydrous, Goldline Labs	00182-1314-01
100's	$47.61	THEO-24, UCB Pharma	50474-0300-01

HOW SUPPLIED - NOT RATED EQUIVALENT: *(cont'd)*

100's UD	$48.75	THEO-24, UCB Pharma	50474-0300-60
500's	$228.50	THEO-24, UCB Pharma	50474-0300-50

Capsule, Elastic - Oral - 400 mg

100's	$69.24	THEO-24, UCB Pharma	50474-0400-01

Capsule, Gelatin, Sustained Action - Oral - 50 mg

100's	$17.33	THEO-DUR SPRINKLE, Schering	00085-0928-01
100's	$20.11	SLO-BID, Rhone-Poulenc Rorer	00075-0057-00
100's	$20.91	SLO-BID, Rhone-Poulenc Rorer	00075-0057-62
1000's	$179.78	SLO-BID, Rhone-Poulenc Rorer	00075-0057-99

Capsule, Gelatin, Sustained Action - Oral - 60 mg

100's	$27.59	SLO-PHYLLIN, Rhone-Poulenc Rorer	00075-1354-00

Capsule, Gelatin, Sustained Action - Oral - 65 mg

100's	$17.00	AEROLATE III, Fleming	00256-0150-01

Capsule, Gelatin, Sustained Action - Oral - 75 mg

10 strip x 10	$23.54	SLO-BID 75, Rhone-Poulenc Rorer	00075-1075-62
100's	$19.75	THEO-DUR SPRINKLE, Schering	00085-0875-01
100's	$22.20	SLO-BID 75, Rhone-Poulenc Rorer	00075-1075-00

Capsule, Gelatin, Sustained Action - Oral - 125 mg

100's	$22.51	THEO-DUR, Schering	00085-0381-01
100's	$36.17	THEOVENT LONG ACTING, Schering	00085-0402-01
100's	$36.31	SLO-PHYLLIN 125, Rhone-Poulenc Rorer	00075-1355-00
100's	**$56.45**	**ELIXOPHYLLIN SR, Berlex Labs**	**50419-0129-10**
100's	**$58.91**	**ELIXOPHYLLIN SR, Berlex Labs**	**50419-0129-11**
1000's	**$451.34**	**ELIXOPHYLLIN SR, Berlex Labs**	**50419-0129-51**

Capsule, Gelatin, Sustained Action - Oral - 130 mg

100's	$12.89	THEOSPAN-SR, Laser	00277-0161-01
100's	$16.00	THEOCLEAR LA-130, Schwarz Pharma (US)	00131-4247-37
100's	$18.25	AEROLATE JR, Fleming	00256-0114-01

Capsule, Gelatin, Sustained Action - Oral - 200 mg

100's	$23.45	THEO-DUR SPRINKLE, Schering	00085-0620-01

Capsule, Gelatin, Sustained Action - Oral - 250 mg

100's	$45.07	THEOVENT, Schering	00085-0753-01
100's	**$62.69**	**ELIXOPHYLLIN SR, Berlex Labs**	**50419-0123-10**
100's	**$72.80**	**ELIXOPHYLLIN SR, Berlex Labs**	**50419-0123-11**

Capsule, Gelatin, Sustained Action - Oral - 260 mg

60's	$24.50	THEOBID DURACAP 260, UCB Pharma	50474-0268-12
100's	$20.00	AEROLATE SR, Fleming	00256-0115-01
100's	$23.40	THEOCLEAR LA-260, Schwarz Pharma (US)	00131-4248-37

Suspension - Oral - 300 mg/15ml

240 ml	$10.75	ELIXICON, Berlex Labs	50419-0112-08

Tablet, Coated, Sustained Action - Oral - 100 mg

100's	$10.50	Theophylline Anhydrous, US Trading	56126-0436-11
100's	$11.25	Theophylline Anhydrous, Lederle Pharm	00005-3076-43
100's	$11.70	Theophylline Anhydrous, Warrick Pharms	59930-1650-01
500's	$38.00	Theophylline Anhydrous, Warrick Pharms	59930-1650-02
1000's	$74.00	Theophylline Anhydrous, Warrick Pharms	59930-1650-03

Tablet, Coated, Sustained Action - Oral - 200 mg

100's	$15.85	Theophylline Anhydrous, Lederle Pharm	00005-3077-43
100's	$16.37	Theophylline Anhydrous, US Trading	56126-0437-11
100's	$19.00	Theophylline Anhydrous, Warrick Pharms	59930-1660-01
100's	$25.98	SLO-PHYLLIN, Rhone-Poulenc Rorer	00075-0352-68
100's	$30.06	THEOLAIR-SR, 3M Pharms	00089-0341-10
100's	$37.38	T-PHYL 200, Purdue Frederick	00034-7102-80
500's	$72.49	Theophylline Anhydrous, Lederle Pharm	00005-3077-31
500's	$82.00	Theophylline Anhydrous, Warrick Pharms	59930-1660-02
1000's	$73.44	THEOLAIR-SR, 3M Pharms	00089-0341-80
1000's	$155.00	Theophylline Anhydrous, Warrick Pharms	59930-1660-03

Tablet, Coated, Sustained Action - Oral - 250 mg

100's	$32.27	RESPBID, Boehringer Pharms	00597-0048-01
100's	$35.46	THEOLAIR-SR, 3M Pharms	00089-0345-10

Tablet, Coated, Sustained Action - Oral - 300 mg

100's	$19.58	Theophylline Anhydrous, Lederle Pharm	00005-3078-43
100's	$20.82	Theophylline Anhydrous, US Trading	56126-0438-11
100's	$22.00	Theophylline Anhydrous, Warrick Pharms	59930-1670-01
100's	$35.46	THEOLAIR-SR, 3M Pharms	00089-0343-10
100's	$37.63	QUIBRON-T/SR, Bristol Myers Squibb	00087-0519-41
100's	$39.14	QUIBRON -T, Roberts Labs	54092-0069-01
100's	$40.83	QUIBRON -T/SR, Roberts Labs	54092-0070-01
500's	$81.99	Theophylline Anhydrous, Lederle Pharm	00005-3078-31
500's	$98.00	Theophylline Anhydrous, Warrick Pharms	59930-1670-02
500's	$180.73	QUIBRON-T/SR, Bristol Myers Squibb	00087-0519-44
500's	$196.09	QUIBRON -T/SR, Roberts Labs	54092-0070-05
1000's	$88.14	THEOLAIR-SR, 3M Pharms	00089-0343-80
1000's	$190.00	Theophylline Anhydrous, Warrick Pharms	59930-1670-03

Tablet, Coated, Sustained Action - Oral - 400 mg

100's	$66.64	UNIPHYL 400, Purdue Frederick	00034-7004-80
100's	$67.26	UNIPHYL 400, Purdue Frederick	00034-7004-10
100's	$90.00	UNI-DUR, Schering	00085-0694-01
500's	$328.85	UNIPHYL 400, Purdue Frederick	00034-7004-70

Tablet, Coated, Sustained Action - Oral - 500 mg

100's	$46.68	RESPBID, Boehringer Pharms	00597-0049-01
100's	$53.04	THEOLAIR-SR, 3M Pharms	00089-0347-10
100's	$98.40	UNI-DUR, Schering	00085-0814-01

Tablet, Uncoated - Oral - 100 mg

100's	$19.56	SLO-PHYLLIN, Rhone-Poulenc Rorer	00075-0351-68
100's	$19.65	SLO-PHYLLIN, Rhone-Poulenc Rorer	00075-0351-01

Tablet, Uncoated - Oral - 125 mg

100's	$34.74	THEOLAIR, 3M Pharms	00089-0342-10

Tablet, Uncoated - Oral - 250 mg

100's	$53.88	THEOLAIR, 3M Pharms	00089-0344-10

THIABENDAZOLE *(002332)*

CATEGORIES: Anthelmintics; Anti-Infectives; Antiparasitics; Ascariasis; Ascaris; Enterobius; Fever; Helminths; Hookworm; Larva Migrans; Ocular Infections; Ophthalmics; Parasiticidal; Strongyloidiasis; Strongyloides; Trichinosis; Trichuriasis; Trichuris; Uncinariasis; Pregnancy Category C; FDA Approval Pre 1982

BRAND NAMES: **Mintezol**; Tiabendazole; *Triasox*
(International brand names outside U.S. in italics)

FORMULARIES: Aetna; Medi-Cal

DESCRIPTION:

Mintezol (Thiabendazole) is an anthelmintic provided as 500 mg chewable tablets, and as a suspension, containing 500 mg thiabendazole per 5 ml. The suspension also contains sorbic acid 0.1% added as a preservative. Inactive ingredients in the tablets are acacia, calcium phosphate, flavors, lactose, magnesium stearate, mannitol, methylcellulose, and sodium saccharin. Inactive ingredients in the suspension are an antifoam agent, flavors, polysorbate, purified water, sorbitol solution, and tragacanth.

Thiabendazole is a white to off-white odorless powder with a molecular weight of 201.26, which is practically insoluble in water but readily soluble in dilute acid and alkali. Its chemical name is 2-(4-thiazolyl)-1*H*-benzimidazole. The empirical formula is $C_{10}H_7N_3S$.

CLINICAL PHARMACOLOGY:

In man, thiabendazole is rapidly absorbed and peak plasma concentration is reached within 1 to 2 hours after the oral administration of a suspension. It is metabolized almost completely to the 5-hydroxy form which appears in the urine as glucuronide or sulfate conjugates. In 48 hours, about 5% of the administered dose is recovered from the feces and about 90% from the urine. Most is excreted in the first 24 hours.

Mechanism of Action: The precise mode of action of thiabendazole on the parasite is unknown, but it may inhibit the helminth-specific enzyme fumarate reductase.

Thiabendazole is vermicidal and/or vermifugal against *Ascaris lumbricoides* ("common roundworm"), *Strongyloides stercoralis* (threadworm), *Necator americanus,* and *Ancylostoma duodenale* (hookworm), *Trichuris trichiura* (whipworm),*Ancylostoma braziliense* (dog and cat hookworm), *Toxoicara canis* and *Toxocara cati* (ascarids), and *Enterobius vermicularis* (pinworm).

Its effect on larvae of *Trichinella spiralis* that have migrated to muscle is questionable.

Thiabendazole also suppresses egg and/or larval production and may inhibit the subsequent development of those eggs or larvae which are passed in the feces.

INDICATIONS AND USAGE:

Thiabendazole is indicated for the treatment of:

Strongyloidiasis (threadworm)

Cutaneous larva migrans (creeping eruption)

Visceral larva migrans

Trichinosis: Relief of symptoms and fever and a reduction of eosinophilia have followed the use of thiabendazole during the invasion stage of the disease.

Although not indicated as primary therapy, when enterobiasis (pinworm) occurs with any of the conditions listed above, additional therapy is not required for most patients. Thiabendazole should be used only in the following infestations when more specific therapy is not available or cannot be used or when further therapy with a second agent is desirable: Uncinariasis (hookworm: *Necator americanus* and *Ancylostoma duodenale*); Trichuriasis (whipworm); Ascariasis (large roundworm).

CONTRAINDICATIONS:

Hypersensitivity to this product.

WARNINGS:

If hypersensitivity reactions occur, the drug should be discontinued immediately and not be resumed. Erythema multiforme has been associated with thiabendazole therapy; in severe cases (Stevens-Johnson syndrome), fatalities have occurred.

Because CNS side effects may occur quite frequently, activities requiring mental alertness should be avoided.

PRECAUTIONS:

General: Thiabendazole is not suitable for the treatment of mixed infections with ascaris because it may cause these worms to migrate.

Ideally, supportive therapy is indicated for anemic, dehydrated or malnourished patients prior to initiation of the anthelmintic therapy.

In the presence of hepatic or renal dysfunction, patients should be carefully monitored.

Thiabendazole should be used only in patients in whom susceptible worm infestation has been diagnosed and should not be used prophylactically.

Information for the Patient: Because CNS side effects may occur quite frequently, activities requiring mental alertness should be avoided.

Laboratory Tests: Rarely, a transient rise in cephalin flocculation and SGOT has occurred in patients receiving thiabendazole.

Carcinogenesis, Mutagenesis, and Impairment of Fertility: Thiabendazole has been used in numerous short- and long-term studies in animals at doses up to 15 times the usual human dose and was without carcinogenic effects. It did not adversely affect fertility in the mouse at 2 1/2 times the usual human dose or in the rat at a dose equivalent to the usual human dose. Thiabendazole had no mutagenic activity in *in vitro* microbial mutagen test, the micronucleus test and the host mediated assay *in vivo.*

Pregnancy Category C: Reproduction and teratogenic studies done in the rabbit at a dose up to 15 times the usual human dose, in the rat at a dose equivalent to the human dose, and in the mouse at a dose up to 2 1/2 times the usual human dose, revealed no evidence of harm to the fetus. In an additional study in the mouse, no defects were observed when thiabendazole was given in aqueous suspension, at a dose 10 times the usual human dose; however, cleft palate and axial skeletal defects were observed when thiabendazole was suspended in olive oil and given at the same dose. There are no adequate and well controlled studies in pregnant women. Thiabendazole should be used during pregnancy only if the potential benefit justifies the potential risk to the fetus.

Nursing Mothers: It is not known whether this drug is excreted in human milk. Because of the potential for serious adverse reactions in nursing infants from thiabendazole, a decision should be made whether to discontinue nursing or to discontinue the drug, taking into account the importance of the drug to the mother.

Pediatric Use: The safety and effectiveness of thiabendazole for the treatment of Strongyloidiasis, Ascariasis, Uncinariasis, Trichuriasis and Trichinosis in children weighing less than 30 lbs has been limited.

DRUG INTERACTIONS:

Thiabendazole may compete with other drugs, such as theophylline, for sites of metabolism in the liver, thus elevating the serum levels of such compounds to potentially toxic levels. Therefore, when concomitant use of thiabendazole and xanthine derivatives is anticipated, it may be necessary to monitor blood levels and/or reduce the dosage of such compounds. Such concomitant use should be administered under careful medical supervision.

ADVERSE REACTIONS:

Gastrointestinal: anorexia, nausea, vomiting, diarrhea, epigastric distress, jaundice, cholestasis and parenchymal liver damage.

Central Nervous System: dizziness, weariness, drowsiness, giddiness, headache, numbness, hyperirritability, convulsions, collapse, psychic disturbances.

Special Senses: tinnitus, abnormal sensation in eyes, xanthopsia, blurring of vision, drying of mucous membranes (mouth, eyes, etc.).

Cardiovascular: hypotension.

Metabolic: hyperglycemia.

Hematologic: transient leukopenia.

Genitourinary: hematuria, enuresis, malodor of the urine, crystalluria.

Hypersensitivity: pruritus, fever, facial flush, chills, conjunctival injection, angioedema, anaphylaxis, skin rashes (including perianal), erythema multiforme (including Stevens-Johnson syndrome), and lymphadenopathy.

Miscellaneous: appearance of live Ascaris in the mouth and nose.

OVERDOSAGE:

Overdosage may be associated with transient disturbances of vision and psychic alterations.

There is no specific antidote in the event of overdosage. Therefore, symptomatic and supportive measures should be employed. Emesis should be induced or gastric lavage performed carefully.

The oral LD_{50} of thiabendazole is 3.6 g/kg, 3.1 g/kg and 3.8 g/kg in the mouse, rat, and rabbit respectively.

DOSAGE AND ADMINISTRATION:

The recommended maximum daily dose of Thiabendazole is 3 grams.

Thiabendazole should be given after meals if possible. Thiabendazole tablets should be chewed before swallowing. Dietary restriction, complementary medications and cleansing enemas are not needed.

The usual dosage schedule for all conditions is two doses per day. The dosage is determined by the patient's weight.

A weight-dose chart (TABLE 1):

TABLE 1

Weight	Each Dose g	Each Dose ml
30 lb	0.25 (1/2 tablet)	2.5 (1/2 teaspoon)
50 lb	0.5 (1 tablet)	5.0 (1 teaspoon)
75 lb	0.75 (1 1/2 tablets)	7.5 (1 1/2 teaspoons)
100 lb	1.0 (2 tablets)	10.0 (2 teaspoons)
125 lb	1.25 (2 1/2 tablets)	12.5 (2 1/2 teaspoons)
150 lb & over	1.5 (3 tablets)	15.0 (3 teaspoons)

The regimen for each indication is listed in TABLE 2.

TABLE 2 Therapeutic Regimens

Indication	Regimen	Comments
*Strongyloidiasis	2 doses per day for 2 successive days.	A single dose of 20 mg/lb or 50 mg/kg may be employed as an alternative schedule, but a higher incidence of side effects should be expected.
Cutaneous Larva Migrans (Creeping Eruption)	2 doses per day for 2 successive days.	If active lesions are still present 2 days after completion of therapy, a second course is recommended.
Visceral Larva Migrans	2 doses per day for 7 successive days.	Safety and efficacy data on the seven-day treatment course are limited.
*Trichinosis	2 doses per day for 2-4 successive days according to the response of the patient.	The optimal dosage for the treatment of trichinosis has not been established.
Other Indications *Intestinal roundworms (including Ascariasis, Uncinariasis and Trichuriasis)	2 doses per day for 2 successive days.	A single dose of 20 mg/lb or 50 mg/kg may be employed as an alternative schedule, but a higher incidence of side effects should be expected.

* Clinical experience with thiabendazole for treatment of each of these conditions in children weighing less than 30 lbs has been limited.

HOW SUPPLIED - EQUIVALENTS NOT AVAILABLE:

Suspension - Oral - 500 mg/5ml

120 ml	$21.06	MINTEZOL, Merck	00006-3331-60

Tablet, Chewable - Oral - 500 mg

36's	$36.25	MINTEZOL, Merck	00006-0907-36

THIAMINE HYDROCHLORIDE *(002333)*

CATEGORIES: Beriberi; Homeostatic & Nutrient; Thiamine Deficiency; Vitamin B Complex; Vitamins; Pregnancy Category A; FDA Approval Pre 1982

BRAND NAMES: *Actamin*; *Alivio*; *Anacrodyne*; *Benerva*; *Beneuril*; *Beneuron*; *Betabion*; **Betalin S**; *Betamin*; *Betatabs*; *Betaxin*; *Bevitine*; *Bewon*; Biamine; *Dumovit*; *Invite*; *Metabolin*; *Oryzanin*; *Ottovit*; *Tiamina*; Vitamin B-1; *Vitanon*; *Vitantial* *(International brand names outside U.S. in italics)*

FORMULARIES: Medi-Cal; WHO

DESCRIPTION:

Injection Thiamine HCl (Thiamine Hydrochloride Injection, USP) is a sterile solution of thiamine hydrochloride for injection. It has a pH between 2.5 and 4.5. Sodium hydroxide and/or hydrochloric acid may have been added during manufacture to adjust the pH.

Thiamine hydrochloride, or vitamin B1, occurs as small white hygroscopic crystals or crystalline powder that usually has a slight characteristic odor. One g dissolves in about 1 ml of water. Thiamine is rapidly destroyed in neutral or or alkaline solutions but is stable in the dry state. It is reasonably stable to heat in acid solution.

The chemical name of thiamine hydrochloride is 3-(4-amino-2-methylpyrimidal-5-methyl)-4-methyl-5(beta-hydroxyethyl) thiazolium chloride hydrochloride.

$C_{12}H_{17}ClN_4OS.\ HCl$

CLINICAL PHARMACOLOGY:

The water-soluble vitamins are widely distributed in both plants and animals. They are absorbed in man by both diffusion and active transport mechanisms. These vitamins are structurally diverse (derivatives of sugar, pyridine, purines, pyrimidine, organic acid complexes, and nucleotide complex) and act as coenzymes, as oxidation-reduction agents, or possibly as mitochondrial agents. Metabolism is rapid, and the excess is excreted in the urine.

Thiamine is distributed in all tissues. The highest concentrations occur in liver, brain, kidney, and heart. When thiamine intake is greatly in excess of need, tissue stores increase 2 to 3 times. If intake is insufficient, tissues become depleted of their vitamin content. Absorption of thiamine following intramuscular administration is rapid and complete.

Thiamine combines with adenosine triphosphate (ATP) to form thiamine pyrophosphate, also known as carboxylase, a coenzyme. Its role in carbohydrate metabolism is the decarboxylation of pyruvic acid and alpha-ketoacids to acetaldehyde and carbon dioxide. Increased levels of pyruvic acid in the blood indicate vitamin B1 deficiency.

The requirement for thiamine is greater when the carbohydrate content of the diet is raised. Body depletion of vitamin B1 can occur after approximately 3 weeks of total absence of thiamine in the diet.

INDICATIONS AND USAGE:

Thiamine hydrochloride injection is effective for the treatment of thiamine deficiency or beriberi. Beriberi may be manifested as the "dry" or the "wet" type.

Parenteral administration is indicated when the oral route is not feasible, as in anorexia, nausea, vomiting, or preoperative and postoperative conditions. It is also indicated when gastrointestinal absorption is impaired, as in the "malabsorption syndrome" (steatorrhea).

CONTRAINDICATIONS:

A history of sensitivity to thiamine or to any of the ingredients in Thiamine HCl is a contraindication.

WARNINGS:

Serious sensitivity reactions can occur. Deaths have resulted from intravenous use. An intradermal test dose is recommended prior to administration in patients suspected of being sensitive to the drug.

PRECAUTIONS:

General: Simple vitamin B1 deficiency is rare. Multiple vitamin deficiencies should be suspected in any case of dietary inadequacy.

Information for the Patient: The patient should be advised as to proper dietary habits during treatment so that relapses will be less likely to occur with reduction in dosage or cessation of injection therapy.

Pregnancy Category A: Studies in pregnant women have not shown that Thiamine HCl increases the risk of fetal abnormalities if administered during pregnancy. If the drug is used during pregnancy, the possibility of fetal harm appears remote. Because studies cannot rule out the possibility of harm, however, Thiamine HCl should be used during pregnancy only if clearly needed.

Nursing Mothers: It is not known whether this drug is excreted in human milk. Because many drugs are excreted in human milk, caution should be exercised when Thiamine HCl is administered to a nursing woman.

ADVERSE REACTIONS:

An occasional individual may develop a sensitivity or intolerance to thiamine, especially after repeated intravenous administration.

Some tenderness and induration may follow intramuscular use. A feeling of warmth, pruritus, urticaria, weakness, sweating, nausea, restlessness, tightness of the throat, angioneurotic edema, cyanosis, pulmonary edema, hemorrhage into the gastrointestinal tract, collapse, and deaths have been recorded.

OVERDOSAGE:

Parenteral doses of 100 to 500 mg, singly or repeated, have been administered without toxic effects. However, dosages exceeding 30 mg 3 times a day are not utilized effectively.

When the body tissues are saturated with thiamine, it is excreted in the urine as pyrimidine; as the intake of thiamine is further increased, it appears unchanged in the urine in amounts exceeding 100 mcg per 24 hours.

DOSAGE AND ADMINISTRATION:

"Wet" beriberi with myocardial failure must be treated as an emergency cardiac condition by the intravenous route.

In the treatment of beriberi, 10 to 20 mg of thiamine are given intramuscularly 3 times daily for as long as 2 weeks. An oral therapeutic multivitamin preparation containing 5 to 10 mg thiamine, administered daily for 1 month, is recommended to achieve body tissue saturation.

Poor dietary habits should be corrected, and an abundant and well-balanced dietary intake should be prescribed.

Protect from light. Store in carton until contents have been used. Store at controlled room temperature, 59 to 86°F (15 to 30°C).

HOW SUPPLIED - RATED THERAPEUTICALLY EQUIVALENT:

Injection, Solution - Intramuscular; - 100 mg/ml

1 ml x 10	$19.73	Thiamine Hcl, Wyeth Labs	00008-0302-01
1 ml x 25	$18.04	Thiamine Hcl, Elkins Sinn	00641-0610-25
1 ml x 100	$94.37	THIAMINE HCL, Lilly	00002-1663-02
2 ml x 25	$28.13	Thiamine Hcl, Fujisawa USA	00469-1013-25
10 ml	$0.88	Thiamine Hcl, Lannett	00527-0116-55
30 ml	$1.48	Thiamine Hcl, Lannett	00527-0116-58
30 ml	$2.30	Thiamine Hcl, Americal Pharm	54945-0557-53
30 ml	$3.40	Thiamine HCl, Steris Labs	00402-0085-30
30 ml	$4.00	Thiamine, C O Truxton	00463-1074-30

HOW SUPPLIED - RATED THERAPEUTICALLY EQUIVALENT: *(cont'd)*

30 ml	$4.00	VITAMIN B-1, Major Pharms	00904-0944-30
30 ml	$5.35	Thiamine Hcl, Hyrex Pharms	00314-0774-30
30 ml	$7.20	Thiamine Hcl, Rugby	00536-2900-75
30 ml	$7.50	Thiamine Hcl, Consolidated Midland	00223-8681-30
30 ml	$7.75	Vitamin B-1, Goldline Labs	00182-0567-66
30 ml	**$8.87**	**BETALIN S THIAMINE HCL, Lilly**	**00002-1662-01**

HOW SUPPLIED - NOT RATED EQUIVALENT:

Injection, Solution - Intramuscular; - 100 mg/ml

30 ml	$3.09	Thiamine HCl, McGuff	49072-0739-30

THIETHYLPERAZINE MALEATE *(002337)*

CATEGORIES: Antiemetics; Gastrointestinal Drugs; Nausea; Nausea and Vomiting; Phenothiazines; Vertigo/Motion Sickness/Vomiting; Vomiting; FDA Approval Pre 1982

BRAND NAMES: Norzine; **Torecan**; *Toresten*
(International brand names outside U.S. in italics)

FORMULARIES: Aetna; BC-BS

DESCRIPTION:

Torecan, (thiethylperazine) is a phenothiazine. Thiethylperazine is characterized by a substituted thioethyl group at position 2 in the phenothiazine nucleus, and a piperazine moiety in the side chain. The chemical designation is: 2-ethyl-mercapto-10-[3'-(1"-methyl-piperazinyl-4")-propyl-1'] phenothiazine.

TABLET, 10 MG, FOR ORAL ADMINISTRATION

ACTIVE INGREDIENT: thiethylperazine maleate USP, 10 mg.*INACTIVE INGREDIENTS:* acacia, carnauba wax, FD&C Yellow No. 5 aluminum lake (tartrazine), FD&C Yellow No. 6 aluminum lake, gelatin, lactose, magnesium stearate, povidone, sodium benzoate, sorbitol, starch, stearic acid, sucrose, talc, titanium dioxide.

AMPUL, 2 ML, FOR INTRAMUSCULAR ADMINISTRATION

ACTIVE INGREDIENT: thiethylperazine malate USP, 10 mg per 2 ml.*INACTIVE INGREDIENTS:* sodium metabisulfite NF, 0.5 mg; ascorbic acid USP, 2.0 mg; sorbitol NF, 40 mg; carbon dioxide gas q.s.; water for injection USP, q.s. to 2 ml.

SUPPOSITORY, 10 MG, FOR RECTAL ADMINISTRATION

ACTIVE INGREDIENT: thiethylperazine maleate USP, 10 mg.*INACTIVE INGREDIENT:* cocoa butter NF.

CLINICAL PHARMACOLOGY:

The pharmacodynamic action of thiethylperazine in humans in unknown. However, a direct action of thiethypersazine on both the CTZ and the vomiting center may be concluded from induced vomiting experiments in animals.

INDICATIONS AND USAGE:

Thiethyperazine is indicated for the relief of nausea and vomiting.

CONTRAINDICATIONS:

Severe central nervous system (CNS) depression and comatose states.

Use of thiethyperazine is contraindicated in patients who have demonstrated a hypersensitivity reaction (*e.g.,* blood dyscrasias, jaundice) to phenothiazines.

Because severe hypotension has been reported after the intravenous administration of phenothiazines, this route of administration is contraindicated.

Usage in Pregnancy: Thiethyperazine is contraindicated in pregnancy.

WARNINGS:

Thiethylperazine Injection contains sodium metabisulfite, a sulfite may cause allergic-type reactions including anaphylactic symptoms and life-threatening or less severe asthmatic episodes in certain susceptible people. The overall prevalence of sulfite sensitivity in the general population is unknown and probably low. Sulfite sensitivity is seen more frequently in asthmatic than in nonasthmatic people.

Phenothiazines are capable of potentiating CNS depressants (*e.g.,* barbiturates, anesthetics, opiates, alcohol, etc.) as well as atropine and phosphorous insecticides.

Since thiethylperazine may impair mental and/or physical ability required in the performance of potentially hazardous tasks such as driving a car or operating machinery, it is recommended that patients be warned accordingly.

Postoperative Nausea and Vomiting: With the use of this drug to control postoperative nausea and vomiting occurring in patients undergoing elective surgical procedures, restlessness and postoperative CNS depression during anesthesia recovery may occur. Possible postoperative complications of a severe degree of any of the known reactions of this class of drug must be considered. Postural hypotension may occur after an initial injection, rarely with the tablet or suppository.

The administration of epinephrine should be avoided in the treatment of drug induced hypotension in view of the fact that phenothiazines may induce a reversed epinephrine effect on occasion.

Should a vasoconstrictive agent be required, the most suitable are levarterenol and phenylephrine.

The use of this drug has not been studied following intracardiac and intracranial surgery.

PRECAUTIONS:

Abnormal movements such as extrapyramidal symptoms (E.P.S.) (*e.g.,* dystonia, torticollis, dysphasia, oculogyric crises, akathisia) have occurred. Convulsions have also been reported. The varied symptoms complex is more likely to occur in young adults and children. Extrapyramidal effects must be treated by reduction of dosage or cessation of medication.

Torecan tablets contain FD&C Yellow No. 5 (tartrazine) which may cause allergic-type reactions (including bronchial asthma) in certain susceptible individuals. Although the overall incidence of FD&C Yellow No. 5 (tartrazine) sensitivity in the general population is low, it is frequently seen in patients who also have aspirin hypersensitivity.

Use in patients with bone marrow depression only when potential benefits outweigh risks.

Neuroleptic Malignant Syndrome (NMS), a potentially fatal symptom complex, has been reported in association with phenothiazine drugs. Clinical manifestations include: hyperpyrexia, muscle rigidity, altered mental status and evidence of autonomic instability.

PRECAUTIONS: *(cont'd)*

The extrapyramidal symptoms which can occur secondary to thiethylperazine may be confused with the central nervous system signs of an undiagnosed primary disease responsible for the vomiting, e.g., Reye's Syndrome or other encephalopathy. The use of thiethylperazine and other potential hepatotoxins should be avoided in children and adolescents whose signs and symptoms suggest Reye's Syndrome.

Phenothiazine drugs may cause elevated prolactin levels that persist during chronic administration. Since approximately one-third of human breast cancers are prolactin-dependent *in vitro,* this elevation is of potential importance if phenothiazine drug administration is contemplated in a patient with a previously-detected breast cancer. Neither clinical nor epidemiologic studies to date, however, have shown an association between the chronic administration of phenothiazine drugs and mammary tumorigenesis.

Postoperative Nausea and Vomiting: When used in the treatment of nausea and/or vomiting associated with anesthesia and surgery, it is recommended that thiethylperazine should be administered by deep intramuscular injection at or shortly before the termination of anesthesia.

Information for the Patient: Patients receiving thiethylperazine should be cautioned about possible combined effects with alcohol and other CNS depressants. patients should be cautioned not to operate machinery or drive a motor vehicle after ingesting the drug.

Laboratory Test Interactions: The usual precautions should be observed in patients with impaired renal or hepatic function.

Nursing Mothers: Information is not available concerning the excretion of thiethylperazine in the milk of nursing should not be undertaken while the patient is on a drug, since many drugs are excreted in human milk.

Pediatric Use: The safety and efficacy of thiethylperazine in children under 12 years of age has not been established.

DRUG INTERACTIONS:

Phenothiazines are capable of potentiating CNS depressants (*e.g.,* barbiturates, anesthetics, opiates, alcohol, etc.) as well as atropine and phosphorous insecticides.

ADVERSE REACTIONS:

Central Nervous System: Serious: Convulsions have been reported. Extrapyramidal symptoms (E.P.S.) may occur, such as dystonia, torticollis, oculogyric crises, akathisia, and gait disturbances. Others: Occasional cases of dizziness, headache, fever and restlessness have been reported.

Drowsiness may occur on occasion, following an initial injection. Generally this effect tends to subside with continued therapy or is usually alleviated by a reduction in dosage.

Autonomic Nervous System: Dryness of the mouth and nose, blurred vision, tinnitus. An occasional case of sialorrhea together with altered gustatory sensation has been observed.

Endocrine System: Peripheral edema of the arms, hands and face.

Hepatotoxicity: An occasional case of cholestatic jaundice has been observed.

Other: An occasional case of cerebral vascular spasm and trigeminal neuralgia has been reported.

Phenothiazine Derivatives: The physician should be aware that the following have occurred with one or more phenothiazines and should be considered whenever one of these drugs is used:

Blood Dyscrasias: Serious - Agranulocytosis, leukopenia, thrombocytopenia, aplastic anemia, pancytopenia. Other-Eosinophilia, leukocytosis.

Autonomic Reactions: Miosis, obstipation, anorexia, paralytic ileus.

Cutaneous Reactions: Serious - Erythema, exfoliative dermatitis, contact dermatitis.

Hepatotoxicity: Serious - Jaundice, biliary stasis.

Cardiovascular Effects: Serious - Hypotension, rarely leading, to cardiac arrest; electrocardiographic (ECG) changes.

Extrapyramidal Symptoms: Serious - Akathisia, agitation, motor restlessness, dystonic reactions, trismus, torticollis, opisthotonos, oculogyric crises, tremor, muscular rigidity, akinesia - some of which have persisted for several months or years especially in patients of advanced age with brain damage.

Endocrine Disturbances: Menstrual irregularities, altered libido, gynecomastia, weight gain. False positive pregnancy tests have been reported.

Urinary Disturbances: Retention, incontinence.

Allergic Reactions: Serious - Fever laryngeal edema, angioneurotic edema, asthma.

Others: Hyperpyrexia. Behavioral effects suggestive of a paradoxical reaction have been reported. These include excitement, bizarre dreams, aggravation of psychoses and toxic confusional states. While there is no evidence at present that ECG changes observed in patients receiving phenothiazines are in any way precursors of any significant disturbances of cardiac rhythm, it should be noted that sudden and unexpected deaths apparently due to cardiac arrest have been reported in a few instances in hospitalized psychotic patients previously showing characteristic ECG changes. A peculiar skin-eye syndrome has also been recognized as a side effect following long-term treatment with certain phenothiazines. This reaction is marked by progressive pigmentation of areas of the skin or conjunctival and/or accompanied by discoloration of the exposed sclera and cornea. Opacities of the anterior lens and cornea described as irregular or stellate in shape have also been reported.

DRUG ABUSE AND DEPENDENCE:

Thiethylperazine is not a controlled substance.

OVERDOSAGE:

Manifestations of acute overdosage of thiethylperazine can be expected to reflect the CNS effects of the drug and include extrapyramidal symptoms (E.P.S.), confusion and convulsions with reduced or absent reflexes, respiratory depression and hypotension. if the patient is conscious, vomiting should be induced mechanically or with emetics. Gastric lavage should be employed utilizing concurrently a cuffed endotracheal tube if the patient is unconscious to prevent aspiration and pulmonary complications. Maintenance of adequate pulmonary ventilation is essential. The use of presser agents intravenously may be necessary to combat hypotension. the administration of epinephrine should be avoided since phenothiazines may induce a reversed epinephrine effect. The most suitable vasoconstrictive agents are norepinephrine and phenylephrine. Fluids should be administered intravenously to encourage diuresis. The value of dialysis has not been determined. If excitation occurs, barbiturates should not be used. It should be borne in mind that multiple agents may have been ingested.

DOSAGE AND ADMINISTRATION:

Adult: Usual daily dose range is 10 mg to 30 mg.*ORAL:* One tablet, one to three times daily.*INTRAMUSCULAR:* 2 ml IM, one to three times daily. (see PRECAUTIONS.) *SUPPOSITORY:* Insert suppository, one to three times daily.

Children: Appropriate dosage of thiethylperazine has not been determined in children.

HOW SUPPLIED:

Tablets: Each tablet contains 10 mg thiethylperazine maleate, USP. Bottles of 100.

Ampuls: Each 2 ml ampul contains aqueous solution 10 mg thiethylperazine malate, USP. Boxes of 10 and 100.

Storage: Below 86°F; protect from light. Administer only if clear and colorless.

Suppositories: Each containing 10 mg thiethylperazine maleate, USP. Packages of 12.

Storage: Below 77°F; tight container (sealed foil).

(Roxane Laboratories, Inc., 9/92)

HOW SUPPLIED - EQUIVALENTS NOT AVAILABLE:

Injection, Solution - Intravenous - 5 mg/ml

2 ml x 20	$105.63	TORECAN, Roxane	00054-1701-07
2 ml x 100	$447.84	TORECAN, Roxane	00054-1701-25

Tablet, Uncoated - Oral - 10 mg

100's	$54.30	TORECAN, Roxane	00054-4748-25
100's	$72.99	TORECAN, Roxane	00054-8748-25

THIOGUANINE *(002339)*

CATEGORIES: Antimetabolites; Antineoplastics; Chemotherapy; Leukemia; Oncologic Drugs; Pregnancy Category D; FDA Approval Pre 1982

BRAND NAMES: *Lanvis*; Tabloid
(International brand names outside U.S. in italics)

FORMULARIES: Aetna; BC-BS; Medi-Cal

DESCRIPTION:

CAUTION: Thioguanine is a potent drug. It should not be used unless a diagnosis of acute nonlymphocytic leukemia has been adequately established and the responsible physician is knowledgeable in assessing response to chemotherapy.

Thioguanine was synthesized and developed by Hitchings, Elion and associates at the Wellcome Research Laboratories. It is one of a large series of purine analogues which interfere with nucleic acid biosynthesis, and has been found active against selected human neoplastic diseases.[1]

Thioguanine, known chemically as 2-amino-1,7-dihydro-6*H*-purine-6-thione, is an analogue of the nucleic acid constituent guanine, and is closely related structurally and functionally to Purinethol (mercaptopurine).

Tabloid brand thioguanine is available in tablets for oral administration. Each scored tablet contains 40 mg thioguanine and the inactive ingredients gum acacia, lactose, magnesium stearate, potato starch, and stearic acid.

CLINICAL PHARMACOLOGY:

Clinical studies have shown that the absorption of an oral dose of thioguanine in man is incomplete and variable, averaging approximately 30% of the administered dose (range: 14% to 46%).[2,3] Following oral administration of ^{35}S-6-thioguanine, total plasma radioactivity reached a maximum at eight hours and declined slowly thereafter. Parent drug represented only a very small fraction of the total plasma radioactivity at any time, being virtually undetectable throughout the period of measurements.

The oral administration of radiolabeled thioguanine revealed only trace quantities of parent drug in the urine. However, a methylated metabolite, 2-amino-6-methylthiopurine (MTG), appeared very early, rose to a maximum six to eight hours after drug administration, and was still being excreted after 12 to 22 hours. Radiolabeled sulfate appeared somewhat later than MTG but was the principal metabolite after eight hours. Thiouric acid and some unidentified products were found in the urine in small amounts.[3] Intravenous administration of ^{35}S-6-thioguanine disclosed a median plasma half-disappearance time of 80 minutes (range: 25-240 minutes) when the compound was given in single doses of 65 to 300 mg/m^2. Although initial plasma levels of thioguanine did correlate with the dose level, there was no correlation between the plasma half-disappearance time and the dose.[2]

Thioguanine is incorporated into the DNA and the RNA of human bone marrow cells. Studies with intravenous ^{35}S-6-thioguanine have shown that the amount of thioguanine incorporated into nucleic acids is more than 100 times higher after five daily doses than after a single dose schedule, from one-half to virtually all of the guanine in the residual DNA was replaced by thioguanine.[2] Tissue distribution studies of ^{35}S-6-thioguanine in mice showed only traces of radioactivity in brain after oral administration. No measurements have been made of thioguanine concentrations in human cerebrospinal fluid, but observations on tissue distribution in animals, together with the lack of CNS penetration by the closely related compound, mercaptopurine, suggest that thioguanine does not reach therapeutic concentrations in the CSF.

Monitoring of plasma levels of thioguanine during therapy is of questionable value.[3] There is technical difficulty in determining plasma concentrations, which are seldom greater than 1 to 2 mcg/ml after a therapeutic oral dose. More significantly, thioguanine enters rapidly into the anabolic and catabolic pathways for purines, and the active intracellular metabolites have appreciably longer half-lives than the parent drug. The biochemical effects of a single dose of thioguanine are evident long after the parent drug has disappeared from plasma. Because of this rapid metabolism of thioguanine to active intracellular derivatives, hemodialysis would not be expected to appreciably reduce toxicity of the drug.

Thioguanine competes with hypoxanthine and guanine for the enzyme hypoxanthine-guanine phosphoribosyltransferase (HGPRTase) and is itself converted to 6-thioguanylic acid (TGMP). This nucleotide reaches high intracellular concentrations at therapeutic doses. TGMP interferes at several points with the synthesis of guanine nucleotides. It inhibits *de novo* purine biosynthesis by pseudo-feedback inhibition of glutamine-5-phosphoribosylpyrophosphate amidotransferase—the first enzyme unique to the *de novo* pathway for purine ribonucleotide synthesis. TGMP also inhibits the conversion of inosinic acid (IMP) to xanthylic acid (XMP) by competition for the enzyme IMP dehydrogenase. At one time TGMP was felt to be a significant inhibitor of ATP:GMP phosphotransferase (guanylate kinase)[4], but recent results have shown this not to be so.[5]

Thioguanylic acid is further converted to the di- and tri-phosphates, thioguanosine diphosphate (TGDP) and thioguanosine triphosphate (TGTP) (as well as their 2'-deoxyribosyl analogues) by the same enzymes which metabolize guanine nucleotides.[6] Thioguanine nucleotides are incorporated into both the RNA and the DNA by phosphodiester linkages[2] and it has been argued that incorporation of such fraudulent bases contributes to the cytotoxicity of thioguanine.

Thus, thioguanine has multiple metabolic effects and at present it is not possible to designate one major site of action. Its tumor inhibitory properties may be due to one or more of its effects on (a) feedback inhibition of *de novo* purine synthesis; (b) inhibition of purine nucleotide interconversions; or (c) incorporation into the DNA and the RNA. The net consequence of its actions is a sequential blockade of the synthesis and utilization of the purine nucleotides.[4,6,7]

CLINICAL PHARMACOLOGY: *(cont'd)*

The catabolism of thioguanine and its metabolites is complex and shows significant differences between man and the mouse.[2,3] In both humans and mice, after oral administration of ^{35}S-6-thioguanine, urine contains virtually no detectable intact thioguanine. While deamination and subsequent oxidation to thiouric acid occurs only to a small extent in man, it is the main pathway in mice. The product of deamination by guanase, 6-thioxanthene is inactive, having negligible antitumor activity. This pathway of thioguanine inactivation is not dependent on the action of xanthine oxidase, and an inhibitor of that enzyme (such as allopurinol), will not block the detoxification of thioguanine even though the inactive 6-thioxanthene is normally further oxidized by xanthine oxidase to thiouric acid before it is eliminated. In man, methylation of thioguanine is much more extensive than in the mouse. The product of methylation, 2-amino-6-methylthiopurine, is also substantially less active and less toxic than thioguanine and its formation is likewise unaffected by the presence of allopurinol. Appreciable amounts of inorganic sulfate are also found in both murine and human urine, presumably arising from further metabolism of the methylated derivatives.

In some animal tumors, resistance to the effect of thioguanine correlates with the loss of HGPRTase activity and the resulting inability to convert thioguanine to thioguanylic acid. However, other resistance mechanisms, such as increased catabolism of TGMP by a nonspecific phosphatase, may be operative. Although not invariable, it is usual to find cross-resistance between thioguanine and its close analogue, Purinethol (mercaptopurine).

INDICATIONS AND USAGE:

a) Acute Nonlymphocytic Leukemias: Thioguanine is indicated for remission induction, remission consolidation, and maintenance therapy of acute nonlymphocytic leukemias.[8,9] The response to this agent depends upon the age of the patient (younger patients faring better than older), and whether thioguanine is used in previously treated or previously untreated patients. Reliance upon thioguanine alone is seldom justified for initial remission induction of acute nonlymphocytic leukemias because combination chemotherapy including thioguanine results in more frequent remission induction and longer duration of remission than thioguanine alone.

b) Other Neoplasms: Thioguanine is not effective in chronic lymphocytic leukemia, Hodgkin's lymphoma, multiple myeloma or solid tumors. Although thioguanine is one of several agents with activity in the treatment of the chronic phase of chronic myelogenous leukemia, more objective responses are observed with Myleran (busulfan), and therefore busulfan is usually regarded as the preferred drug.

CONTRAINDICATIONS:

Thioguanine should not be used in patients whose disease has demonstrated prior resistance to this drug. In animals and man, there is usually complete cross-resistance between Purinethol (mercaptopurine) and thioguanine.

WARNINGS:

SINCE DRUGS USED IN CANCER CHEMOTHERAPY ARE POTENTIALLY HAZARDOUS, IT IS RECOMMENDED THAT ONLY PHYSICIANS EXPERIENCED WITH THE RISKS OF THIOGUANINE AND KNOWLEDGEABLE IN THE NATURAL HISTORY OF ACUTE NONLYMPHOCYTIC LEUKEMIAS ADMINISTER THIS DRUG.

The most consistent, dose-related toxicity is bone marrow suppression. This may be manifested by anemia, leukopenia, thrombocytopenia, or any combination of these. Any one of these findings may also reflect progression of the underlying disease. Since thioguanine may have a delayed effect, it is important to withdraw the medication temporarily at the first sign of an abnormally large fall in any of the formed elements of the blood.

It is recommended that evaluation of the hemoglobin concentration or hematocrit; total white blood cell count and differential count; and quantitative platelet count be obtained frequently while the patient is on thioguanine therapy. In cases where the cause of fluctuations in the formed elements in the peripheral blood is obscure, bone marrow examination may be useful for the evaluation of marrow status. The decision to increase, decrease, continue, or discontinue a given dosage of thioguanine must be based not only on the absolute hematologic values, but also upon the rapidity with which changes are occurring. In many instances, particularly during the induction phase of acute leukemia, complete blood counts will need to be done more frequently in order to evaluate the effect of the therapy. The dosage of thioguanine may need to be reduced when this agent is combined with other drugs whose primary toxicity is myelosuppression.

Myelosuppression is often unavoidable during the induction phase of adult acute nonlymphocytic leukemias if remission induction is to be successful. Whether or not this demands modification or cessation of dosage depends both upon the response of the underlying disease and a careful consideration of supportive facilities (granulocyte and platelet transfusions) which may be available. Life-threatening infections and bleeding have been observed as consequences of thioguanine-induced granulocytopenia and thrombocytopenia.

The effect of thioguanine on the immunocompetence of patients is unknown.

Pregnancy Category D: Drugs such as thioguanine are potential mutagens and teratogens. Thioguanine may cause fetal harm when administered to a pregnant woman. Thioguanine has been shown to be teratogenic in rats when given in doses five (5) times the human dose. When given to the rat on the 4th and 5th days of gestation, 13% of surviving placentas did not contain fetuses, and 19% of offspring were malformed or stunted. The malformations noted included generalized edema, cranial defects and general skeletal hypoplasia, hydrocephalus, ventral hernia, situs inversus, and incomplete development of the limbs.[10] There are no adequate and well-controlled studies in pregnant women. If this drug is used during pregnancy, or if the patient becomes pregnant while taking the drug, the patient should be apprised of the potential hazard to the fetus. Women of childbearing potential should be advised to avoid becoming pregnant.

PRECAUTIONS:

General: Although the primary toxicity of thioguanine is myelosuppression, other toxicities have occasionally been observed, particularly when thioguanine is used in combination with other cancer chemotherapeutic agents.

A few cases of jaundice have been reported in patients with leukemia receiving thioguanine. Among these were two adult male patients and four children with acute myelogenous leukemia and an adult male with acute lymphocytic leukemia who developed veno-occlusive hepatic disease while receiving chemotherapy for their leukemia.[11,12] Six patients had received cytarabine prior to treatment with thioguanine, and some were receiving other chemotherapy in addition to thioguanine when they became symptomatic. While veno-occlusive hepatic disease has not been reported in patients treated with thioguanine alone, it is recommended that thioguanine be withheld if there is evidence of toxic hepatitis or biliary stasis, and that appropriate clinical and laboratory investigations be initiated to establish the etiology of the hepatic dysfunction. Deterioration in liver function studies during thioguanine therapy should prompt discontinuation of treatment and a search for an explanation of the hepatotoxicity.

Information for the Patient: Patients should be informed that the major toxicities of thioguanine are related to myelosuppression, hepatotoxicity and gastrointestinal toxicity. Patients should never be allowed to take the drug without medical supervision and should be

PRECAUTIONS: *(cont'd)*

advised to consult their physician if they experience fever, sore throat, jaundice, nausea, vomiting, signs of local infection, bleeding from any site, or symptoms suggestive of anemia. Women of child-bearing potential should be advised to avoid becoming pregnant.

Laboratory Tests: It is advisable to monitor liver function tests (serum transaminases, alkaline phosphatase, bilirubin) at weekly intervals when first beginning therapy and at monthly intervals thereafter. It may be advisable to perform liver function tests more frequently in patients with known pre-existing liver disease or in patients who are receiving thioguanine and other hepatotoxic drugs. Patients should be instructed to discontinue thioguanine immediately if clinical jaundice is detected. (See WARNINGS.)

Carcinogenesis, Mutagenesis, and Impairment of Fertility: In view of its action on cellular DNA, thioguanine is potentially mutagenic and carcinogenic, and consideration should be given to the theoretical risk of carcinogenesis when thioguanine is administered. (See WARNINGS)

Pregnancy, Teratogenic Effects, Pregnancy Category D: See WARNINGS.

Nursing Mothers: It is not known whether this drug is excreted in human milk. Because of the potential for tumorigenicity shown for thioguanine, a decision should be made whether to discontinue nursing or to discontinue the drug, taking into account the importance of the drug to the mother.

DRUG INTERACTIONS:

There is usually complete cross-resistance between Purinethol (mercaptopurine) and thioguanine.

In one study, 12 of approximately 330 patients receiving continuous busulfan and thioguanine therapy for treatment of chronic myelogenous leukemia were found to have esophageal varices associated with abnormal liver function tests.[13] Subsequent liver biopsies were performed in four of these patients, all of which showed evidence of nodular regenerative hyperplasia. Duration of combination therapy prior to the appearance of esophageal varices ranged from 6 to 45 months. With the present analysis of the data, no cases of hepatotoxicity have appeared in the busulfan alone arm of the study. Long-term continuous therapy with thioguanine and busulfan should be used with caution.

ADVERSE REACTIONS:

The most frequent adverse reaction to thioguanine is myelosuppression. The induction of complete remission of acute myelogenous leukemia usually requires combination chemotherapy in dosages which produce marrow hypoplasia.[14] Since consolidation and maintenance of remission are also effected by multiple drug regimens whose component agents cause myelosuppression, pancytopenia is observed in nearly all patients. Dosages and schedules must be adjusted to prevent life-threatening cytopenias whenever these adverse reactions are observed.

Hyperuricemia frequently occurs in patients receiving thioguanine as a consequence of rapid cell lysis accompanying the antineoplastic effect. Adverse effects can be minimized by increased hydration, urine alkalinization, and the prophylactic administration of a xanthine oxidase inhibitor such as Zyloprim (allopurinol). Unlike Purinethol (mercaptopurine) and Imuran (azathioprine), thioguanine may be continued in the usual dosage when allopurinol is used conjointly to inhibit uric acid formation.

Less frequent adverse reactions include nausea, vomiting, anorexia and stomatitis. Intestinal necrosis and perforation have been reported in patients who received multiple drug chemotherapy including thioguanine.

Hepatic Effects: Liver enzyme and other liver function studies are occasionally abnormal. If jaundice, hepatomegaly or anorexia with tenderness in the right hypochondrium occurs, thioguanine should be withheld until the exact etiology can be determined. There have been reports of veno-occlusive liver disease occurring in patients who received combination chemotherapy including thioguanine.[11,12] Esophageal varices have been reported in patients receiving continuous busulfan and thioguanine therapy for treatment of chronic myelogenous leukemia. (See DRUG INTERACTIONS.)

OVERDOSAGE:

Signs and symptoms of overdosage may be immediate, such as nausea, vomiting, malaise, hypertension and diaphoresis; or delayed, such as myelosuppression and azotemia.[15] It is not known whether thioguanine is dialyzable. Hemodialysis is thought to be of marginal use due to the rapid intracellular incorporation of thioguanine into active metabolites with long persistence. The oral LD_{50} of thioguanine was determined to be 823 mg/kg $\pm$ 50.73 mg/kg and 740 mg/kg $\pm$ 45.24 mg/kg for male and female rats respectively.[16] Symptoms of overdosage may occur after a single dose of as little as 2.0 to 3.0 mg/kg thioguanine. As much as 35 mg/kg has been given in a single oral dose with reversible myelosuppression observed. There is no known pharmacologic antagonist of thioguanine. The drug should be discontinued immediately if unintended toxicity occurs during treatment. Severe hematologic toxicity may require supportive therapy with platelet transfusions for bleeding, and granulocyte transfusions and antibiotics if sepsis is documented. If a patient is seen immediately following an accidental overdosage of the drug, it may be useful to induce emesis.

DOSAGE AND ADMINISTRATION:

Thioguanine is administered orally. The dosage which will be tolerated and effective varies according to the stage and type of neoplastic process being treated. Because the usual therapies for adult and childhood acute nonlymphocytic leukemias involve the use of thioguanine with other agents in combination, physicians responsible for administering these therapies should be experienced in the use of cancer chemotherapy and in the chosen protocol.

Ninety-six (59%) of one hundred sixty-three children with previously untreated acute nonlymphocytic leukemia obtained complete remission with a multiple drug protocol including thioguanine, prednisone, cytarabine, cyclophosphamide, and vincristine. Remission was maintained with daily thioguanine, four-day pulses of cytarabine and cyclophosphamide, and a single dose of vincristine every 28 days. The median duration of remission was 11.5 months.[8]

Fifty-three percent of previously untreated adults with acute nonlymphocytic leukemias attained remission following use of the combination of thioguanine and cytarabine according to a protocol developed at The Memorial Sloan-Kettering Cancer Center. A median duration of remission of 8.8 months was achieved with the multiple drug maintenance regimen which included thioguanine.[9]

On those occasions when single agent chemotherapy with thioguanine may be appropriate, the usual initial dosage for children and adults is approximately 2 mg/kg of body weight per day. If, after four weeks on this dosage, there is no clinical improvement and no leukocyte or platelet depression, the dosage may be cautiously increased to 3 mg/kg per day. The total daily dose may be given at one time.

The dosage of thioguanine used does not depend on whether or not the patient is receiving Zyloprim (allopurinol); **this is in contradistinction to the dosage reduction which is mandatory when Purinethol (mercaptopurine) or Imuran (azathioprine) is given simultaneously with allopurinol.**

DOSAGE AND ADMINISTRATION: *(cont'd)*

Procedures for proper handling and disposal of anti-cancer drugs should be considered. Several guidelines on this subject have been published.[17-23]

There is no general agreement that all of the procedures recommended in the guidelines are necessary or appropriate.

Store at 15 to 25°C (59 to 77°F) in a dry place.

REFERENCES:

1. Hitchings GH, Elion GB. The chemistry and biochemistry of purine analogs. *Ann NY Acad Sci.* 1954;60:195-199. **2.** LePage GA, Whitecar JP Jr. Pharmacology of 6-thioguanine in man.*Cancer Res.* 1971;31:1627-1631. **3.** Elion GB. Biochemistry and pharmacology of purine analogues. *Fed Proc.*1967;26:898-904. **4.** Miech RP, Parks RE Jr, Anderson JH Jr, Sartorelli AC. An hypothesis on the mechanism of action of 6-thioguanine. *Biochem Pharmacol.* 1967;16: 2222-2227. **5.** Miller RL, Adamczyk DL, Spector T, Agarwal KC, Miech RP, Panks RE Jr. Reassessment of the interactions of guanylate kinase and 6-thioguanine 5'-phosphate. *Biochem Pharmacol.* 1977;26:1573-1576. **6.** Paterson ARP, Tidd DN. 6-Thiopurines. In: Sartorelli AC, Johns DG, eds.*Antineoplastic and Immunosuppressive Agents,* Part II. Berlin: Springer Verlag; 1975:384-403. **7.** Nelson JA, Carpenter JW, Rose LM, Adamson DJ. Mechanisms of action of 6-thioguanine, 6-mercaptopurine, and 8-azaguanine. *Cancer Res.* 1975;35:2872-2878. **8.** Chard RL Jr, Finklestein JZ, Sonley MJ, et al. Increased survival in childhood acute nonlymphocytic leukemia after treatment with prednisone, cytosine arabinoside, 6-thioguanine, cyclophosphamide, and oncovin (PATCO) combination therapy. *Med Ped Oncol.* 1978;4:263-273. **9.** Mertelsmann R, Drapkin RL, Gee TS, et al. Treatment of acute nonlymphocytic leukemia in adults: response to 2,2-anhydro-1-B-D-arabinofuranosyl-5-fluorocytosine and thioguanine on the L-12 protocol. *Cancer.* 1981;48:2136-2142. **10.** Thiersch JB. Effect of 2-6 diaminopurine (2-6DP): 6 chloropurine (CIP) and thioguanine (ThG) on rat litter *in utero. Proc Soc ExpBiol Med.* 1957;94:40-43. **11.** Griner PF, Elbadawi A, Packman CH. Veno-occlusive disease of the liver after chemotherapy of acute leukemia: report of two cases. *Ann Intern Med.*1976;85:578-582. **12.** Gill RA, Onstad GR, Cardamone JM, Maneval DC, Sumner HW. Hepatic veno-occlusive disease caused by 6-thioguanine.*Ann Intern Med.* 1982;96:58-60. **13.** Key NS, Kelly PMA, Emerson PM, Chapman RWG, Allan NC, McGee JO'D. Oesophageal varices associated with busulfan-thioguanine combination therapy for chronic myeloid leukaemia. *Lancet.* 1987;2:1050-1052. **14.** Clarkson BD, Dowling MD, Gee TS, Cunningham IB, Burchenal JH. Treatment of acute leukemia in adults. *Cancer.* 1975;36:775-795. **15.** Presant CA, Denes AE, Klein L, Garrett S, Metter GE. Phase I and preliminary phase II observations of high-dose intermittent 6-thioguanine. *Cancer Treat Rep.* 1980;64:1109-1113. **16.** Unpublished data on file with Burroughs Wellcome Co. **17.** Recommendations for the safe handling of parenteral antineoplastic drugs. Washington, DC: Division of Safety, National Institutes of Health; 1983. US Dept of Health and Human Services, Public Health Service publication NIH 83-2621. **18.** AMA Council on Scientific Affairs. Guidelines for handling parenteral antineoplastics.*JAMA.*1985;253:1590-1591. **19.** National Study Commission on Cytotoxic Exposure. Recommendations for handling cytotoxic agents. 1984. Available from Louis P. Jeffrey, ScD, Director of Pharmacy Services, Rhode Island Hospital, 593 Eddy Street, Providence, Rhode Island 02902. **20.** Clinical Oncological Society of Australia. Guidelines and recommendations for safe handling of antineoplastic agents. *Med J Australia.* 1983;1:426-428. **21.** Jones RB, Frank R, Mass T. Safe handling of chemotherapeutic agents: a report from the Mount Sinai Medical Center. *CA-A Cancer J forClin.*1983;33(Sept/Oct):258-263. **22.** American Society of Hospital Pharmacists. Technical assistance bulletin on handling cytotoxic drugs in hospitals. *Am J Hosp Pharm.* 1990;47:1033-1049. **23.** Yodaiken RE, Bennett D. OSHA work-practice guidelines for personnel dealing with cytotoxic (antineoplastic) drugs. *Am J Hosp Pharm.*1986;43:1193-1204.

HOW SUPPLIED - EQUIVALENTS NOT AVAILABLE:

Tablet, Uncoated - Oral - 40 mg

25's	$79.79	Thioguanine, Glaxo Wellcome	00173-0880-25

THIOPENTAL SODIUM *(002340)*

CATEGORIES: Anesthesia; Anxiolytics, Sedatives, Hypnotic; Barbiturate Anesthetics; Barbiturates; Central Nervous System Agents; General Anesthetics; Hypnotics; Injectable Anesthetics; Intracranial Pressure; Local Anesthetics; Muscle Relaxants; Narcoanalysis; Sedatives; Pregnancy Category C; DEA Class CIII; FDA Approval Pre 1982

BRAND NAMES: *Anesthal*; *Hypnostan*; *Intraval*; *Intraval Sodium*; *Nesdonal* (France); **Pentothal**; *Pentothal Sodico* (Mexico); *Pentothal Sodium*; *Sodipental* (Mexico); *Thionyl*; *Thiopental*; *Tiopental Sodico*; *Trapanal* (Germany)
(International brand names outside U.S. in italics)

FORMULARIES: WHO

DESCRIPTION:

WARNING: MAY BE HABIT FORMING.

Thiopental is a thiobarbiturate, the sulfur analogue of sodium pentobarbital.

The drug is prepared as a sterile powder and after reconstitution with an appropriate diluent is administered by the intravenous route.

Thiopental is chemically designated sodium 5-ethyl-5- (1-methylbutyl)-2-thiobarbiturate.

The drug is a yellowish, hygroscopic powder, stabilized with anhydrous sodium carbonate as a buffer (60 mg/g of thiopental sodium).

Ready-To-Mix Syringes And Vials: (For preparing solutions of Thiopental Sodium for Injection, USP). The following diluents in various container, syringe and vial sizes are provided in Pentothal Kits, Pentothal Ready-to-Mix Syringes and Vials for preparing solutions of thiopental for clinical use:

Sterile Water for Injection, USP is a sterile, nonpyrogenic preparation of water for injection which contains no bacteriostat, antimicrobial agents or added buffers. The pH is 5.7 (5.0 to 7.0). Sterile Water for Injection, USP is a pharmaceutic aid (solvent) for intravenous administration only after addition of a solute.

Water is chemically designated H_2O. 0.9% Sodium Chloride Injection, USP is a sterile, nonpyrogenic, isotonic solution of sodium chloride and water for injection. Each ml contains sodium chloride 9 mg (308 mOsmol/liter calc). It contains no bacteriostat, antimicrobial agents or added buffers except for pH adjustment. May contain hydrochloric acid and/or sodium hydroxide for pH adjustment. pH is 5.7 (4.5 to 7.0). 0.9% Sodium Chloride Injection, USP is an isotonic vehicle for intravenous administration of another solute. Sodium chloride is chemically designated NaCl, a white crystalline compound freely soluble in water. The semi-rigid vial contained in List Nos. 3329, 6418, 6419, 6420 and 6435 is fabricated from a specially formulated polyolefin. It is a copolymer of ethylene and propylene. The safety of the plastic has been confirmed by tests in animals according to USP biological standards for plastic containers. The container requires no vapor barrier to maintain the proper labeled volume.

CLINICAL PHARMACOLOGY:

Thiopental is an ultrashort-acting depressant of the central nervous system which induces hypnosis and anesthesia, but not analgesia. It produces hypnosis within 30 to 40 seconds of intravenous injection. Recovery after a small dose is rapid, with some somnolence and retrograde amnesia. Repeated intravenous doses lead to prolonged anesthesia because fatty tissues act as a reservoir; they accumulate thiopental in concentrations 6 to 12 times greater than the plasma concentration, and then release the drug slowly to cause prolonged anesthesia.

The half-life of the elimination phase after a single intravenous dose is three to eight hours. The distribution and fate of thiopental (as with other barbiturates) is influenced chiefly by its lipid solubility (partition coefficient), protein binding and extent of ionization. Thiopental has a partition coefficient of 580.

Approximately 80% of the drug in the blood is bound to plasma protein. Thiopental is largely degraded in the liver and to a smaller extent in other tissues, especially the kidney and brain. It has a pKa of 7.4. Concentration in spinal fluid is slightly less than in the plasma.

CLINICAL PHARMACOLOGY: *(cont'd)*

Biotransformation products of thiopental are pharmacologically inactive and mostly excreted in the urine.

Sterile Water for Injection, USP serves only as a pharmaceutic aid for diluting or dissolving drugs prior to administration.

Water is an essential constituent of all body tissues and accounts for approximately 70% of total body weight. Average normal adult daily requirement ranges from two to three liters (1.0 to 1.5 liters each for insensible water loss by perspiration and urine excretion). Water balance is maintained by various regulatory mechanisms. Water distribution depends primarily on the concentration of dissociated electrolytes in the body compartments and sodium (Na+) plays a major role in maintaining a physiologic equilibrium between fluid intake and output.

0.9% Sodium Chloride Injection, USP serves only as an isotonic vehicle for drugs prior to administration.

Sodium chloride in water is an electrolyte solution of sodium (Na+) and chloride (Cl-) ions. These ions are normal constituents of the body fluids (principally extracellular) and are essential for maintaining electrolyte balance.

The distribution and excretion of sodium (Na+) and chloride (Cl-) are largely under the control of the kidney which maintains a balance between intake and output of these ions.

The small volumes of fluid and amounts of sodium chloride provided by 0.9% Sodium Chloride Injection in Ready-to-Mix Syringes are unlikely to produce a significant effect on fluid or electrolyte balance.

INDICATIONS AND USAGE:

Thiopental is indicated (1) as the sole anesthetic agent for brief (15 minute) procedures, (2) for induction of anesthesia prior to administration of other anesthetic agents, (3) to supplement regional anesthesia, (4) to provide hypnosis during balanced anesthesia with other agents for analgesia or muscle relaxation, (5) for the control of convulsive states during or following inhalation anesthesia, local anesthesia, or other causes, (6) in neurosurgical patients with increased intracranial pressure, if adequate ventilation is provided, and (7) for narcoanalysis and narcosynthesis in psychiatric disorders.

CONTRAINDICATIONS:

Absolute Contraindications

(1) Absence of suitable veins for intravenous administration

(2) hypersensitivity (allergy) to barbiturates

(3) variegate porphyria (South African) or acute intermittent porphyria

Relative Contraindications

(1) Severe cardiovascular disease

(2) hypotension or shock

(3) conditions in which the hypnotic effect may be prolonged or potentiated—excessive premedication, Addison's disease, hepatic or renal dysfunction, myxedema, increased blood urea, severe anemia, asthma, myasthenia gravis

(4) status asthmaticus.

Diluents in Pentothal Kits, Ready-to-Mix Syringes or Vials should not be used for fluid or sodium chloride replacement.

WARNINGS:

KEEP RESUSCITATIVE AND ENDOTRACHEAL INTUBATION EQUIPMENT AND OXYGEN READILY AVAILABLE. MAINTAIN PATENCY of THE AIRWAY AT ALL TIMES.

THIS DRUG SHOULD BE ADMINISTERED ONLY BY PERSONS QUALIFIED IN THE USE of INTRAVENOUS ANESTHETICS.

Avoid extravasation or intra-arterial injection. WARNING: MAY BE HABIT FORMING.

Intravenous administration of Sterile Water for Injection, USP without a solute may result in hemolysis.

Use aseptic technique for preparing thiopental solutions when using Pentothal Kits, Syringes or Vials and during withdrawal from reconstituted single or multiple-use containers.

Administer only clear reconstituted solutions. Use within 24 hours after reconstitution. Discard unused portions.

PRECAUTIONS:

General: Observe aseptic precautions at all times in preparation and handling of thiopental solutions. If used in conditions involving relative contraindications, reduce dosage and administer slowly.

Care should be taken in administering the drug to patients with advanced cardiac disease, increased intracranial pressure, ophthalmoplegia plus, asthma, myasthenia gravis and endocrine insufficiency (pituitary, thyroid, adrenal, pancreas).

Nursing Mothers: Thiopental sodium readily crosses the placental barrier and small amounts may appear in the milk of nursing mothers following administration of large doses.

Pregnancy Category C: Animal reproduction studies have not been conducted with thiopental. It is also not known whether thiopental can cause fetal harm when administered to a pregnant woman or can affect reproduction capacity. Thiopental should be given to a pregnant woman only if clearly needed.

Do not use unless solution is clear and container is undamaged.

Inspect reconstituted (mixed) solutions of thiopental for clarity and freedom from precipitation or discoloration prior to administration. Use Transfer Label in each Pentothal Kit and affix to container of reconstituted solution to show concentration and time of preparation.

DRUG INTERACTIONS:

The following drug interactions have been reported with thiopental:

TABLE 1 Drug Effect

Drug	Effect
Probenecid:	Prolonged action of thiopental
Diazoxide:	Hypotension
Zimelidine:	Thiopental antagonism
Opioid analgesics:	Decreased antinociceptive action
Aminophylline:	Thiopental antagonism
Midazolam:	Synergism

ADVERSE REACTIONS:

Adverse reactions include respiratory depression, myocardial depression, cardiac arrhythmias, prolonged somnolence and recovery, sneezing, coughing, bronchospasm, laryngospasm and shivering.

ADVERSE REACTIONS: *(cont'd)*

Anaphylactic and anaphylactoid reactions to thiopental have been reported. Symptoms, (*e.g.*, urticaria, bronchospasm, vasodilation and edema) should be managed by conventional means.

Rarely, immune hemolytic anemia with renal failure and radial nerve palsy have been reported.

Reactions which may occur because of the diluents, technique of preparation or mixing, or administration of reconstituted solutions of thiopental include febrile response or infection at the site of injection, venous thrombosis or phlebitis extending from the site of injection and extravasation.

If an adverse reaction does occur, discontinue the injection, evaluate the patient, institute appropriate therapeutic countermeasures and save the remainder of unused solution (or the used container or syringe) for examination if deemed necessary.

DRUG ABUSE AND DEPENDENCE:

WARNING: MAY BE HABIT FORMING.

Thiopental sodium is classified as a Schedule III controlled substance.

OVERDOSAGE:

Overdosage may occur from too rapid or repeated injections. Too rapid injection may be followed by an alarming fall in blood pressure even to shock levels. Apnea, occasional laryngospasm, coughing and other respiratory difficulties with excessive or too rapid injections may occur. in the event of suspected or apparent overdosage, the drug should be discontinued, a patent airway established (intubate if necessary) or maintained, and oxygen should be administered, with assisted ventilation if necessary. The lethal dose of barbiturates varies and cannot be stated with certainty. Lethal blood levels may be as low as 1 mg/100 mL for short-acting barbiturates; less if other depressant drugs or alcohol are also present.

Management of Overdosage: It is generally agreed that respiratory depression or arrest due to unusual sensitivity to thiopental sodium or overdosage is easily managed if there is no concomitant respiratory obstruction. If the airway is patent, any method of ventilating the lungs (that prevents hypoxia) should be successful in maintaining other vital functions. Since depression of respiratory activity is one of the characteristic actions of the drug, it is important to observe respiration closely. Should laryngeal spasm occur, it may be relieved by one of the usual methods, such as the use of a relaxant drug or positive pressure oxygen. Endotracheal intubation may be indicated in difficult cases.

Used as diluents for preparing solutions of thiopental the small volumes of administered fluid (from Sterile Water for Injection in bottles and vials) and amounts of sodium chloride (from 0.9% Sodium Chloride Injection in Ready-to-Mix Syringes) are unlikely to pose a threat of fluid or sodium chloride overload.

DOSAGE AND ADMINISTRATION:

Thiopental is administered by the intravenous route only. Individual response to the drug is so varied that there can be no fixed dosage. The drug should be titrated against patient requirements as governed by age, sex and body weight. Younger patients require relatively larger doses than middle-aged and elderly persons; the latter metabolize the drug more slowly. Pre-puberty requirements are the same for both sexes, but adult females require less than adult males. Dose is usually proportional to body weight and obese patients require a larger dose than relatively lean persons of the same weight.

Premedication: Premedication usually consists of atropine or scopolamine to suppress vagal reflexes and inhibit secretions. in addition, a barbiturate or an opiate is often given. Sodium pentobarbital injection (Nembutal) is suggested because it provides a preliminary indication of how the patient will react to barbiturate anesthesia.

Ideally, the peak effect of these medications should be reached shortly before the time of induction.

Test Dose: It is advisable to inject a small "test" dose of 25 to 75 mg (1 to 3 mL of a 2.5% solution) of thiopental to assess tolerance or unusual sensitivity to thiopental, and pausing to observe patient reaction for at least 60 seconds. If unexpectedly deep anesthesia develops or if respiratory depression occurs, consider these possibilities: (1) the patient may be unusually sensitive to thiopental, (2) the solution may be more concentrated than had been assumed, or (3) the patient may have received too much premedication.

Use in Anesthesia: Moderately slow induction can usually be accomplished in the "average" adult by injection of 50 to 75 mg (2 to 3 mL of a 2.5% solution) at intervals of 20 to 40 seconds, depending on the reaction of the patient. Once anesthesia is established, additional injections of 25 to 50 mg can be given whenever the patient moves. Slow injection is recommended to minimize respiratory depression and the possibility of overdosage. The smallest dose consistent with attaining the surgical objective is the desired goal. Momentary apnea following each injection is typical, and progressive decrease in the amplitude of respiration appears with increasing dosage. Pulse remains normal or increases slightly and returns to normal. Blood pressure usually falls slightly but returns toward normal.

Muscles usually relax about 30 seconds after unconsciousness is attained, but this may be masked if a skeletal muscle relaxant is used. The tone of jaw muscles is a fairly reliable index. The pupils may dilate but later contract; sensitivity to light is not usually lost until a level of anesthesia deep enough to permit surgery is attained. Nystagmus and divergent strabismus are characteristic during early stages, but at the level of surgical anesthesia, the eyes are central and fixed. Corneal and conjunctival reflexes disappear during surgical anesthesia.

When thiopental is used for induction in balanced anesthesia with a skeletal muscle relaxant and an inhalation agent, the total dose of thiopental can be estimated and then injected in two to four fractional doses. With this technique, brief periods of apnea may occur which may require assisted or controlled pulmonary ventilation. As an initial dose, 210 to 280 mg (3 to 4 mg/kg) of thiopental is usually required for rapid induction in the average adult (70 kg). When thiopental is used as the sole anesthetic agent, the desired level of anesthesia can be maintained by injection of small repeated doses as needed or by using a continuous intravenous drip in a 0.2% or 0.4% concentration. (Sterile water should not be used as the diluent in these concentrations, since hemolysis will occur.) With continuous drip, the depth of anesthesia is controlled by adjusting the rate of infusion.

Use in Convulsive States: For the control of convulsive states following anesthesia (inhalation or local) or other causes, 75 to 125 mg (3 to 5 ml of a 2.5% solution) should be given as soon as possible after the convulsion begins. Convulsions following the use of a local anesthetic may require 125 to 250 mg of thiopental given over a ten minute period. If the convulsion is caused by a local anesthetic, the required dose of thiopental will depend upon the amount of local anesthetic given and its convulsant properties.

Use in Neurosurgical Patients With Increased Intracranial Pressure: In neurosurgical patients, intermittent bolus injections of 1.5 to 3.5 mg/kg of body weight may be given to reduce intraoperative elevations of intracranial pressure, if adequate ventilation is provided.

Use in Psychiatric Disorders: For narcoanalysis and narcosynthesis in psychiatric disorders, premedication with an anticholinergic agent may precede administration of thiopental. After a test dose, thiopental is injected at a slow rate of 100 mg/min (4 ml/min of a 2.5% solution) with the patient counting backwards from 100. Shortly after counting becomes confused but before actual sleep is produced, the injection is discontinued. Allow the patient to return to a

DOSAGE AND ADMINISTRATION: *(cont'd)*

semidrowsy state where conversation is coherent. Alternatively, thiopental may be administered by rapid IV drip using a 0.2% concentration in 5% dextrose and water. At this concentration, the rate of administration should not exceed 50 ml/min.

Management of Some Complications: Respiratory Depression (hypoventilation, apnea), which may result from either unusual responsiveness to thiopental or overdosage, is managed as stated above. Thiopental should be considered to have the same potential for producing respiratory depression as an inhalation agent, and patency of the airway must be protected at all times.

Laryngospasm may occur with light thiopental narcosis at intubation, or in the absence of intubation if foreign matter or secretions in the respiratory tract create irritation. Laryngeal and bronchial vagal reflexes can be suppressed, and secretions minimized by giving atropine or scopolamine premedication and a barbiturate or opiate. Use of a skeletal muscle relaxant or positive pressure oxygen will usually relieve laryngospasm. Tracheostomy may be indicated in difficult cases.

Myocardial Depression, proportional to the amount of drug in direct contact with the heart, can occur and may cause hypotension, particularly in patients with an unhealthy myocardium.

Arrhythmias may appear if PCO2 is elevated, but they are uncommon with adequate ventilation.

Management of myocardial depression is the same as for overdosage. Thiopental does not sensitize the heart to epinephrine or other sympathomimetic amines.

Extravascular Infiltration should be avoided. Care should be taken to insure that the needle is within the lumen of the vein before injection of thiopental. Extravascular injection may cause chemical irritation of the tissues varying from slight tenderness to venospasm, extensive necrosis and sloughing. This is due primarily to the high alkaline pH (10 to 11) of clinical concentrations of the drug. If extravasation occurs, the local irritant effects can be reduced by injection of 1% procaine locally to relieve pain and enhance vasodilatation. Local application of heat also may help to increase local circulation and removal of the infiltrate.

Intra-arterial Injection can occur inadvertently, especially if an aberrant superficial artery is present at the medial aspect of the antecubital fossa. The area selected for intravenous injection of the drug should be palpated for detection of an underlying pulsating vessel. Accidental intra-arterial injection can cause arteriospasm and severe pain along the course of the artery with blanching of the arm and fingers.

Appropriate corrective measures should be instituted promptly to avoid possible development of gangrene. Any patient complaint of pain warrants stopping the injection. Methods suggested for dealing with this complication vary with the severity of symptoms. The following have been suggested:

1. Dilute the injected thiopental by removing the tourniquet and any restrictive garments.

2. Leave the needle in place, if possible.

3. Inject the artery with a dilute solution of papaverine, 40 to 80 mg, or 10 mL of 1% procaine, to inhibit smooth muscle spasm.

4. If necessary, perform sympathetic block of the brachial plexus and/or stellate ganglion to relieve pain and assist in opening collateral circulation. Papaverine can be injected into the subclavian artery, if desired.

5. Unless otherwise contraindicated, institute immediate heparinization to prevent thrombus formation.

6. Consider local infiltration of an alpha-adrenergic blocking agent such as phentolamine into the vasospastic area.

7. Provide additional symptomatic treatment as required. Shivering after thiopental anesthesia, manifested by twitching face muscles and occasional progression to tremors of the arms, head, shoulder and body, is a thermal reaction due to increased sensitivity to cold. Shivering appears if the room environment is cold and if a large ventilatory heat loss has been sustained with balanced inhalation anesthesia employing nitrous oxide. Treatment consists of warming the patient with blankets, maintaining room temperature near 22°C (72°F), and administration of chlorpromazine or methylphenidate.

Preparation of Solutions: Thiopental is supplied as a yellowish, hygroscopic powder in a variety of different containers. Solutions should be prepared aseptically with one of the three following diluents: Sterile Water for Injection, USP, 0.9% Sodium Chloride Injection, USP or 5% Dextrose Injection, USP. Clinical concentrations used for intermittent intravenous administration vary between 2.0% and 5.0%. A 2.0% or 2.5% solution is most commonly used. A 3.4% concentration in sterile water for injection is isotonic; concentrations less than 2.0% in this diluent are not used because they cause hemolysis. For continuous intravenous drip administration, concentrations of 0.2% or 0.4% are used. Solutions may be prepared by adding thiopental to 5% Dextrose Injection, USP, 0.9% Sodium Chloride Injection, USP or Normosol-R pH 7.4. Since thiopental contains no added bacteriostatic agent, extreme care in preparation and handling should be exercised at all times to prevent the introduction of microbial contaminants. Solutions should be freshly prepared and used promptly; when reconstituted for administration to several patients, unused portions should be discarded after 24 hours. Sterilization by heating should not be attempted.

Warning: The 2.5 g and larger sizes contain adequate medication for several patients.

Compatibility: Any solution of thiopental with a visible precipitate should not be administered. The stability of thiopental solutions depends upon several factors, including the diluent, temperature of storage and the amount of carbon dioxide from room air that gains access to the solution. Any factor or condition which tends to lower pH (increase acidity) of thiopental solutions will increase the likelihood of precipitation of thiopental acid. Such factors include the use of diluents which are too acidic and the absorption of carbon dioxide which can combine with water to form carbonic acid.

Solutions of succinylcholine, tubocurarine or other drugs which have an acid pH should not be mixed with thiopental solutions. The most stable solutions are those reconstituted in water or isotonic saline, kept under refrigeration and tightly stoppered. The presence or absence of a visible precipitate offers a practical guide to the physical compatibility of prepared solutions of thiopental.

TABLE 2 Calculations For Various Concentrations

Concentration Desired		Amounts to Use	
%	mg/ml	Thiopental g	Diluent ml
0.2	2	1	500
0.4	4	1	250
		2	500
2.0	20	5	250
		10	500
2.5	25	1	40
		5	200
5	50	1	20
		5	100

DOSAGE AND ADMINISTRATION: *(cont'd)*

Reconstituted solutions of thiopental should be inspected visually for particulate matter and discoloration, whenever solution and container permit. Thiopental solutions should be administered only by intravenous injection and by individuals experienced in the conduct of intravenous anesthesia.

The volume and choice of diluent for preparing thiopental solutions for clinical use depends on the concentration and vehicle desired. Thiopental Kits provide only Sterile Water for Injection as the diluent for individual or multi-patient use; Thiopental Ready-to-Mix Syringes provide only 0.9% Sodium Chloride Injection, USP as the diluent for individual patient use; vials provide only Sterile Water for Injection, USP as the diluent for individual patient use.

Parenteral drug products should be inspected visually for particulate matter and discoloration prior to administration, whenever solution and container permit. (See PRECAUTIONS.)

HOW SUPPLIED - EQUIVALENTS NOT AVAILABLE:

Injection, Dry-Soln - Intravenous - 2.5 gm

1 kit	$35.55	PENTOTHAL 2.5, Abbott	00074-6260-01

Injection, Dry-Soln - Intravenous - 2.5 gm/bottle

1 kit	$16.48	PENTOTHAL 1, Abbott	00074-6244-01

Injection, Dry-Soln - Intravenous - 5 gm

5 gm	$55.88	PENTOTHAL 5, Abbott	00074-6504-01

Injection, Dry-Soln - Intravenous - 20 mg/ml

400 mg	$11.17	PENTOTHAL 400, Abbott	00074-6246-03

Injection, Solution - Intravenous - 1 gm

1 gm	$4.11	Pentothal 1 Gm Injection, Abbott	00074-6431-02
1 kit	$16.53	PENTOTHAL SODIUM, Abbott	00074-6435-01
5 gm	$19.02	Pentothal 1 Gm Injection, Abbott	00074-6431-03

Injection, Solution - Intravenous - 2 %

1 kit	$36.53	PENTOTHAL 2.5, Abbott	00074-6259-01
1 kit	$56.42	PENTOTHAL 5, Abbott	00074-6108-01

Injection, Solution - Intravenous - 250 mg

1's	$8.68	PENTOTHAL, Abbott	00074-7425-01
1's	$9.77	PENTOTHAL, Abbott	00074-3351-01
250 mg	$8.87	PENTOTHAL 250, Abbott	00074-6418-01
250 mg	$9.05	PENTOTHAL 250, Abbott	00074-6241-03

Injection, Solution - Intravenous - 400 mg

1's	$10.57	PENTOTHAL, Abbott	00074-7426-01
1's	$11.00	PENTOTHAL, Abbott	00074-6419-01
1's	$11.90	PENTOTHAL, Abbott	00074-3352-01

Injection, Solution - Intravenous - 500 mg

1 kit	$9.57	PENTOTHAL 500, Abbott	00074-3329-01
1's	$8.10	Thiopental 500, Gensia Labs	00703-2580-01
1's	$11.83	PENTOTHAL, Abbott	00074-7427-01
1's	$12.29	PENTOTHAL, Abbott	00074-6420-01
1's	$13.30	PENTOTHAL, Abbott	00074-3353-01
500 mg	$12.60	PENTOTHAL 500, Abbott	00074-6243-01

Kit - Intravenous - 1 gm

1's	$17.04	Thiopental Sodium, Gensia Labs	00703-2530-01

Kit - Intravenous - 2.5 gm

1's	$22.20	Thiopental Sodium, Gensia Labs	00703-2540-01
1's	$39.83	PENTOTHAL, Abbott	00074-6590-01

Kit - Intravenous - 5 gm

1's	$33.36	Thiopental Sodium, Gensia Labs	00703-2550-01

Kit - Intravenous - 6.25 gm

1's	$78.27	PENTOTHAL, Abbott	00074-6591-01

Suspension - Rectal - 400 mg/gm

1kit	$35.63	PENTOTHAL RECTAL, Abbott	00074-7236-04

THIORIDAZINE HYDROCHLORIDE *(002341)*

CATEGORIES: Antidepressants; Antimicrobials; Antipsychotics/Antimanics; Anxiety; Behavior Problems; Central Nervous System Agents; Depression; Neuroleptics; Phenothiazine Tranquilizers; Phenothiazines; Psychotherapeutic Agents; Psychotic Disorders; Tension; Tranquilizers; Vertigo/Motion Sickness/Vomiting; FDA Approval Pre 1982

BRAND NAMES: *Aldazine*; *Calmaril*; *Dazine*; *Mallorol*; *Meleretten*; *Meleril*; **Mellaril**; Mellaril-S; *Melleretten*; *Melleril*; *Mepiozin*; *Novoridazine*; *Ridazin*; *Sonapex*; *Thinin*; *Thiomed*; *Thioril*; *Winleril*
(International brand names outside U.S. in italics)

FORMULARIES: Aetna; BC-BS; CIGNA; FHP; Humana; Kaiser; Medco; Medi-Cal; PCS; PruCare; United

COST OF THERAPY: $8.80 (Depression; Tablet; 25 mg; 3/day; 90 days)

PRIMARY ICD9: 311 (Depressive Disorder, Not Elsewhere Classified)

DESCRIPTION:

Thioridazine is 2-methylmercapto-10-[2-(N-methyl-2-piperidyl) ethyl] phenothiazine.

The presence of a thiomethyl radical ($S\text{-}CH_3$) in position 2, conventionally occupied by a halogen, is unique and could account for the greater toleration obtained with recommended doses of thioridazine as well as a greater specificity of psychotherapeutic action.

CLINICAL PHARMACOLOGY:

Thioridazine hydrochloride is effective in reducing excitement, hypermotility, abnormal initiative, affective tension and agitation through its inhibitory effect on psychomotor functions. Successful modification of such symptoms is the prerequisite for, and often the beginning of, the process of recovery in patients exhibiting mental and emotional disturbances.

Thioridazine hydrochloride's basic pharmacological activity is similar to that of other phenothiazines, but certain specific qualities have come to light which support the observation that the clinical spectrum of this drug shows significant differences from those of the other agents of this class. Minimal antiemetic activity and minimal extrapyramidal stimulation, notably pseudoparkinsonism, are distinctive features of this drug.

INDICATIONS AND USAGE:

For the management of manifestations of psychotic disorders.

For the short-term treatment of moderate to marked depression with variable degrees of anxiety in adults patients and for the treatment of multiple symptoms such as agitation, anxiety, depressed mood, tension, sleep disturbances, and fears in geriatric patients.

For the treatment of severe behavioral problems in children marked by combativeness and/or explosive hyperexcitable behavior (out of proportion to immediate provocations), and in the short-term treatment of hyperactive children who show excessive motor activity with accompanying conduct disorders consisting of some or all of the following symptoms: impulsivity, difficulty sustaining attention, aggressivity, mood lability, and poor frustration tolerance.

CONTRAINDICATIONS:

In common with other phenothiazines, thioridazine hydrochloride is contraindicated in severe central nervous system depression or comatose states from any cause including drug induced central nervous system depression (see WARNINGS). If should also be noted that hypertensive or hypotensive heart disease of extreme degree is a contraindication of phenothiazine administration.

WARNINGS:

Tardive Dyskinesia: Tardive dyskinesia, a syndrome consisting of potentially irreversible, involuntary, dyskinetic movements may develop in patients treated with neuroleptic (antipsychotic) drugs. Although the prevalence of the syndrome appears to be highest among the elderly, especially elderly women, it is impossible to rely upon prevalence estimates to predict, at the inception of neuroleptic treatment, which patients are likely to develop the syndrome. Whether neuroleptic drug products differ in their potential to cause tardive dyskinesia is unknown.

Both the risk of developing the syndrome and the likelihood that it will become irreversible are believed to increase as the duration of treatment and the total cumulative dose of neuroleptic drugs administered to the patient increase. However, the syndrome can develop, although much less commonly, after relatively brief treatment periods at low doses.

There is no known treatment for established cases of tardive dyskinesia, although the syndrome may remit, partially or completely, if neuroleptic treatment is withdrawn. Neuroleptic treatment itself, however, may suppress (or partially suppress) the signs and symptoms of the syndrome and thereby may possibly mask the underlying disease process. The effect that symptomatic suppression has upon the long-term course of the syndrome is unknown.

Given these considerations, neuroleptics should be prescribed in a manner that is most likely to minimize the occurrence of tardive dyskinesia. Chronic neuroleptic treatment should generally be reserved for patients who suffer from a chronic illness that, 1) is known to respond to neuroleptic drugs, and, 2) for whom alternative, equally effective, but potentially less harmful treatments are *not* available or appropriate. In patients who do require chronic treatment, the smallest dose and the shortest duration of treatment producing a satisfactory clinical response should be sought. The need for continued treatment should be reassessed periodically.

If signs and symptoms of tardive dyskinesia appear in a patient on neuroleptics, drug discontinuation should be considered. However, some patients may require treatment despite the presence of the syndrome.

(For further information about the description of tardive dyskinesia and its clinical detection, please refer to the sections on Information for Patients and ADVERSE REACTIONS.)

It has been suggested in regard to phenothiazines in general, that people who have demonstrated a hypersensitivity reaction (*e.g.,* blood dyscrasias, jaundice) to one may be more prone to demonstrate a reaction to others. Attention should be paid to the fact that phenothiazines are capable of potentiating central nervous system depressants (*e.g.,* anesthetics, opiates, alcohol, etc.) as well as atropine and phosphorus insecticides. Physicians should carefully consider benefit versus risk when treating less severe disorders.

Reproductive studies in animals and clinical experience to date have failed to show a teratogenic effect with thioridazine hydrochloride. However, in view of the desirability of keeping the administration of all drugs to a minimum during pregnancy, thioridazine hydrochloride should be given only when the benefits derived from treatment exceed the possible risks to mother and fetus.

Neuroleptic Malignant Syndrome (NMS): A potentially fatal symptom complex sometimes referred to as Neuroleptic Malignant Syndrome (NMS) has been reported in association with antipsychotic drugs. Clinical manifestations of NMS are hyperpyrexia, muscle rigidity, altered mental status, and evidence of autonomic instability (irregular pulse or blood pressure, tachycardia, diaphoresis, and cardiac dysrhythmias).

The diagnostic evaluation of patients with the syndrome is complicated. In arriving at a diagnosis, it is important to identify cases where the clinical presentation includes both serious medical illness (*e.g.,* pneumonia, systemic infection, etc.) and untreated or inadequately treated extrapyramidal signs and symptoms (EPS). Other important considerations in the differential diagnosis include central anticholinergic toxicity, heat stroke, drug fever, and primary central nervous system (CNS) pathology.

The management of NMS should include, 1) immediate discontinuation of antipsychotic drugs and other drugs not essential to concurrent therapy, 2) intensive symptomatic treatment and medical monitoring, and 3) treatment of any concomitant serious medical problems for which specific treatments are available. There is no general agreement about specific pharmacological treatment regimens for uncomplicated NMS.

If a patient requires antipsychotic drug treatment after recovery from NMS, the potential reintroduction of drug therapy should be carefully considered. The patient should be carefully monitored, since recurrences of NMS have been reported.

Central Nervous System Depressants: As in the case of other phenothiazines, thioridazine hydrochloride is capable of potentiating central nervous system depressants (*e.g.,* alcohol, anesthetics, barbiturates, narcotics, opiates, other psychoactive drugs, etc.) as well as atropine and phosphorus insecticides. Severe respiratory depression and respiratory arrest have been reported when a patient was given a phenothiazine and a concomitant high dose of a barbiturate.

PRECAUTIONS:

Leukopenia and/or agranulocytosis and convulsive seizures have been reported but are infrequent. Thioridazine hydrochloride has been shown to be helpful in the treatment of behavioral disorders in epileptic patients, but anticonvulsant medication should also be maintained. Pigmentary retinopathy, which has been observed primarily in patients taking larger than recommended doses, is characterized by diminution of visual acuity, brownish coloring of vision, and impairment of night vision; examination of the fundus discloses deposits of pigment. The possibility of this complication may be reduced by remaining within the recommended limits of dosage.

Where patients are participating in activities requiring complete mental alertness (*e.g.,* driving) it is advisable to administer the phenothiazines cautiously and to increase the dosage gradually. Female patients appear to have a greater tendency to orthostatic hypotension than male patients. The administration of epinephrine should be avoided in the treatment of drug-induced hypotension in view of the fact that phenothiazines may induce a reversed epinephrine effect on occasion. Should a vasoconstrictor be required, the most suitable are levarterenol and phenylephrine.

Neuroleptic drugs elevate prolactin levels; the elevation persists during chronic administration. Tissue culture experiments indicate that approximately one third of human breast cancers are prolactin dependent *in vitro*, a factor of potential importance if the prescription of these drugs is contemplated in a patient with a previously detected breast cancer. Although disturbances such as galactorrhea, amenorrhea, gynecomastia, and impotence have been reported, the clinical significance of elevated serum prolactin levels is unknown for most patients. An increase in mammary neoplasms has been found in rodents after chronic administration of neuroleptic drugs. Neither clinical studies nor epidemiologic studies conducted to date, however, have shown an association between chronic administration of these drugs and mammary tumorigenesis; the available evidence is considered too limited to be conclusive at this time.

Concurrent administration of propanolol (100-800 mg daily) has been reported to produce increases in plasma levels of thioridazine (approximately 50%-400%) and its metabolites (approximately 80%-300%).

Pindolol: Concurrent administration of pindolol and thioridazine have resulted in moderate, dose-related increases in the serum levels of thioridazine and two of its metabolites, as well as higher than expected serum pindolol levels.

It is recommended that a daily dose in excess of 300 mg be reserved for use only in severe neuropsychiatric conditions.

Information for the Patient: Given the likelihood that some patients exposed chronically to neuroleptics will develop tardive dyskinesia, it is advised that all patients in whom chronic use is contemplated be given, if possible, full information about this risk. The decision to inform patients and/or their guardians must obviously take into account the clinical circumstances and the competency of the patient to understand the information provided.

ADVERSE REACTIONS:

In the recommended dosage ranges with thioridazine hydrochloride most side effects are mild and transient.

Central Nervous System: Drowsiness may be encountered on occasion, especially where large doses are given early in treatment. Generally, this effect tends to subside with continued therapy or a reduction in dosage. Pseudoparkinsonism and other extrapyramidal symptoms may occur but are infrequent. Nocturnal confusion, hyperactivity, lethargy, psychotic reactions, restlessness and headache have been reported but are extremely rare.

Autonomic Nervous System: Dryness or mouth, blurred vision, constipation, nausea, vomiting, diarrhea, nasal stuffiness and pallor have been seen.

Endocrine System: Galactorrhea, breast engorgement, amenorrhea, inhibition of ejaculation and peripheral edema have been described.

Skin: Dermatitis and skin eruptions of the urticarial type have been observed infrequently. Photosensitivity is extremely rare.

Cardiovascular System: ECG changes have been reported (see ADVERSE REACTIONS, Phenothiazine Derivatives, Cardiovascular Effects).

Other: Rare cases described as parotid swelling have been reported following administration of thioridazine hydrochloride.

POST INTRODUCTION REPORTS

These are voluntary reports of adverse events temporally associated with thioridazine hydrochloride that were received since marketing, and there may be no causal relationship between thioridazine hydrochloride use and these events: priapism.

PHENOTHIAZINE DERIVATIVES

It should be noted that efficacy, indications and untoward effects have varied with the different phenothiazines. It has been reported that old age lowers the tolerance for phenothiazines. The most common neurological side effects in these patients are parkinsonism and akathisia. There appears to be an increased risk of agranulocytosis and leukopenia in the geriatric population. The physician should be aware that the following have occurred with one or more phenothiazines and should be considered whenever one of these drugs is used.

Autonomic Reactions: Miosis, obstipation, anorexia, paralytic ileus.

Cutaneous Reactions: Erythema, exfoliative dermatitis, contact dermatitis.

Blood Dyscrasias: Agranulocytosis, leukopenia, eosinophilia, thrombocytopenia, anemia, aplastic anemia, pancytopenia.

Allergic Reactions: Fever, laryngeal edema, angioneurotic edema, asthma.

Hepatotoxicity: Jaundice, biliary stasis.

Cardiovascular Effects: Changes in the terminal portion of the electrocardiogram, including prolongation of the Q-T interval, lowering and inversion of the T-wave and appearance of a wave tentatively identified as a bifid T or a U wave have been observed in some patients receiving the phenothiazine tranquilizers, including thioridazine hydrochloride. To date, these appear to be due to altered repolarization and not related to myocardial damage. They appear to be reversible. While there is no evidence at present that these changes are in any way precursors of any significant disturbance of cardiac rhythm, if should be noted that several sudden and unexpected deaths apparently due to cardiac arrest have occurred in patients previously showing characteristic electrocardiographic changes while taking the drug. The use of periodic electrocardiograms has been proposed but would appear to be of questionable value as a predictive device. Hypotension, rarely resulting in cardiac arrest.

Extrapyramidal Symptoms: Akathisia, agitation, motor restlessness, dystonic reactions, trismus, torticollis, opisthotonus, oculogyric crises, tremor, muscular rigidity, akinesia.

Tardive Dyskinesia: Chronic use of neuroleptics may be associated with the development of tardive dyskinesia. The salient features of this syndrome are described in the WARNINGS section and subsequently.

The syndrome is characterized by involuntary choreoathetoid movements which variously involve the tongue, face, mouth, lips, or jaw (*e.g.,* protrusion of tongue, puffing of cheeks, puckering of the mouth, chewing movements), trunk and extremities. The severity of the syndrome and the degree of impairment produced vary widely.

The syndrome may become clinically recognizable either during treatment, upon dosage reduction, or upon withdrawal of treatment. Movements may decrease in intensity and may disappear altogether if further treatment with neuroleptics is withheld. It is generally believed that reversibility is more likely after short rather than long-term neuroleptic exposure. Consequently, early detection of tardive dyskinesia is important. To increase the likelihood of detecting the syndrome at the earliest possible time, the dosage of neuroleptic drug should be reduced periodically (if clinically possible) and the patient observed for signs of the disorder. This maneuver is critical, for neuroleptic drugs may mask the signs of the syndrome.

Neuroleptic Malignant Syndrome (NMS): Chronic use of neuroleptics may be associated with the development of Neuroleptic Malignant Syndrome. The salient features of this syndrome are described in the WARNINGS section and subsequently. Clinical manifestations of NMS are hyperpyrexia, muscle rigidity, altered mental status, and evidence of autonomic instability (irregular pulse or blood pressure, tachycardia, diaphoresis, and cardiac dysrhythmias).

ADVERSE REACTIONS: *(cont'd)*

Endocrine Disturbances: Menstrual irregularities, altered libido, gynecomastia, lactation, weight gain, edema. False positive pregnancy tests have been reported.

Urinary Disturbances: Retention, Incontinence.

Others: Hyperpyrexia. Behavioral effects suggestive of a paradoxical reaction have been reported. These include excitement, bizarre dreams, aggravation of psychoses and toxic confusional states. More recently, a peculiar skin-eye syndrome has been recognized as a side effect following long-term treatment with phenothiazines. This reaction is marked by progressive pigmentation of areas of the skin or conjunctiva and/or accompanied by discoloration of the exposed sclera and cornea. Opacities of the anterior lens and cornea described as irregular or stellate in shape have also been reported. Systemic lupus erythematosus-like syndrome.

DOSAGE AND ADMINISTRATION:

Dosage must be individualized according to the degree of mental and emotional disturbance. In all cases, the smallest effective dosage should be determined for each patient.

ADULTS

Psychotic Manifestations: The usual starting dose is 50-100 mg three times a day, with a gradual increment to a maximum of 800 mg daily if necessary. Once effective control of symptoms has been achieved, the dosage may be reduced gradually to determine the minimum maintenance dose. The total daily dosage ranges from 200-800 mg divided into two to four doses.

For the short-term treatment of moderate to marked depression with variable degrees of anxiety in adult patients and for the treatment of multiple symptoms such as agitation, anxiety, depressed mood, tension, sleep disturbances, and fears in geriatric patients: The usual starting dose is 25 mg three times a day. Dosage ranges from 10 mg two to four times a day in milder cases to 50 mg three or four times a day for more severely disturbed patients. The total daily dosage range is from 20 mg to a maximum of 200 mg.

CHILDREN

Thioridazine hydrochloride is not intended for children under 2 years of age. For children under 2-12 the dosage of thioridazine hydrochloride ranges from 0.5 mg to a maximum of 3.0 mg/kg per day. For children with moderate disorders, 10 mg two or three times a day is the usual starting dose. For hospitalized, severely disturbed, or psychotic children, 25 mg two or three times daily is the usual starting dose. Dosage may be increased gradually until optimum therapeutic effect is obtained or the maximum has been reached.

HOW SUPPLIED:

STORE AND DISPENSE

Tablets: Below 86° (30°C); tight container.

Oral Suspension and Concentrate: Below 77°F(25°C); tight, amber glass bottle. Additional information available to physicians.

(Sandoz, 06/93, 2289-42, 30160901)

HOW SUPPLIED - RATED THERAPEUTICALLY EQUIVALENT:

Concentrate - Oral - 30 mg/ml

120 ml	$11.23	Thioridazine Hcl, Copley Pharm	38245-0608-14
120 ml	$12.90	Thioridazine HCl, H.C.F.A. F F P	99999-2341-01
120 ml	$13.76	Thioridazine Hcl, HL Moore Drug Exch	00839-7056-65
120 ml	$15.24	Thioridazine, Qualitest Pharms	00603-1756-54
120 ml	$15.28	Thioridazine Hcl Intensol, Roxane	00054-3860-50
120 ml	$16.75	Thioridazine Hcl, Schein Pharm (US)	00364-2119-77
120 ml	$17.33	Thioridazine HCl, Rugby	00536-2200-97
120 ml	**$32.04**	**MELLARIL, Novartis**	**00078-0001-31**

Concentrate - Oral - 100 mg/ml

3.4 ml x 10	$96.10	Thioridazine Hcl, Xactdose	50962-0376-04
118 ml	$36.32	Thioridazine HCl, Geneva Pharms	00781-6155-04
120 ml	$36.89	Thioridazine Hcl Intensol, Roxane	00054-3861-50
120 ml	$43.05	Thioridazine HCl, Alpharma	00472-1451-94
120 ml	$55.33	Thioridazine HCl, H.C.F.A. F F P	99999-2341-02
120 ml	**$83.64**	**MELLARIL, Novartis**	**00078-0009-31**

Tablet, Coated - Oral - 10 mg

100's	$2.84	Thioridazine Hcl, United Res	00677-0823-01
100's	$3.00	Thioridazine HCl, H.C.F.A. F F P	99999-2341-03
100's	$5.56	Thioridazine Hcl, Aligen Independ	00405-4993-01
100's	$5.90	Thioridazine Hcl, Qualitest Pharms	00603-5992-21
100's	$6.25	Thioridazine Hcl, Consolidated Midland	00223-2128-01
100's	$8.00	Thioridazine HCl, Rugby	00536-4641-01
100's	$8.20	Thioridazine Hcl, Major Pharms	00904-1614-60
100's	$8.45	Thioridazine Hcl, Raway	00686-0565-20
100's	$8.49	Thioridazine Hcl, HL Moore Drug Exch	00839-6703-06
100's	$8.70	Thioridazine Hcl, Mutual Pharm	53489-0148-01
100's	$11.25	Thioridazine HCl, Geneva Pharms	00781-1604-01
100's	$11.25	Thioridazine HCl, Geneva Pharms	50752-0264-05
100's	$11.95	Thioridazine HCl, Mylan	00378-0612-01
100's	$14.97	Thioridazine Hcl, Roxane	00054-8849-25
100's	$15.41	Thioridazine Hcl, Major Pharms	00904-1793-61
100's	$17.00	Thioridazine Hcl, Vangard Labs	00615-2504-13
100's	$17.02	Thioridazine Hcl, Medirex	57480-0362-01
100's	$17.36	Thioridazine Hcl, US Trading	56126-0096-11
100's	$18.50	Thioridazine HCl, Geneva Pharms	00781-1604-13
100's	$24.53	Thioridazine HCl, Geneva Pharms	50752-0264-06
100's	**$29.64**	**MELLARIL, Novartis**	**00078-0002-05**
100's	**$31.86**	**MELLARIL, Novartis**	**00078-0002-06**
600's	$116.20	Thioridazine Hcl, Medirex	57480-0362-06
750's	$183.97	Thioridazine Hcl, Glasgow Pharm	60809-0151-55
750's	$183.97	Thioridazine Hcl, Glasgow Pharm	60809-0151-72
1000's	$28.40	Thioridazine Hcl, United Res	00677-0823-10
1000's	$30.00	Thioridazine HCl, H.C.F.A. F F P	99999-2341-04
1000's	$54.50	Thioridazine Hcl, Major Pharms	00904-1614-80
1000's	$55.00	Thioridazine Hcl, Consolidated Midland	00223-2128-02
1000's	$72.23	Thioridazine Hcl, HL Moore Drug Exch	00839-6703-16
1000's	$72.90	Thioridazine Hcl, Aligen Independ	00405-4993-03
1000's	$72.90	Thioridazine Hcl, Mutual Pharm	53489-0148-10
1000's	$76.66	Thioridazine Hcl, Schein Pharm (US)	00364-2317-02
1000's	$76.95	Thioridazine HCl, Rugby	00536-4641-10
1000's	$77.75	Thioridazine HCl, Geneva Pharms	50752-0264-09
1000's	$77.87	Thioridazine HCl, Geneva Pharms	00781-1604-10
1000's	$77.95	Thioridazine HCl, Mylan	00378-0612-10
1000's	**$285.18**	**MELLARIL, Novartis**	**00078-0002-09**

Tablet, Coated - Oral - 15 mg

100's	$3.00	Thioridazine HCl, H.C.F.A. F F P	99999-2341-05
100's	$4.97	Thioridazine Hcl, US Trading	56126-0097-11
100's	$7.75	Thioridazine Hcl, Consolidated Midland	00223-2129-01
100's	$10.50	Thioridazine Hcl, Major Pharms	00904-1794-60
100's	$10.90	Thioridazine Hcl, Raway	00686-0179-20
100's	$15.75	Thioridazine HCl, Geneva Pharms	00781-1614-01

HOW SUPPLIED - RATED THERAPEUTICALLY EQUIVALENT: *(cont'd)*

100's	$15.75	Thioridazine HCl, Geneva Pharms	50752-0265-05
100's	$15.80	Thioridazine Hcl, Aligen Independ	00405-4994-01
100's	$21.50	Thioridazine HCl, Geneva Pharms	00781-1614-13
100's	**$34.98**	**MELLARIL, Novartis**	**00078-0008-05**
750's	$201.97	Thioridazine Hcl, Glasgow Pharm	60809-0152-55
750's	$201.97	Thioridazine Hcl, Glasgow Pharm	60809-0152-72
1000's	$66.00	Thioridazine Hcl, Consolidated Midland	00223-2129-02

Tablet, Coated - Oral - 25 mg

100's	$3.26	Thioridazine Hcl, United Res	00677-0824-01
100's	$3.38	Thioridazine HCl, H.C.F.A. F F P	99999-2341-06
100's	$5.54	Thioridazine Hydrochloride, US Trading	56126-0098-11
100's	$7.31	Thioridazine Hcl, Martec Pharms	52555-0098-01
100's	$8.91	Thioridazine Hcl, Qualitest Pharms	00603-5993-21
100's	$11.35	Thioridazine Hcl, Raway	00686-0566-20
100's	$11.60	Thioridazine Hcl, Major Pharms	00904-1616-60
100's	$13.50	Thioridazine Hcl, Aligen Independ	00405-4995-01
100's	$13.50	Thioridazine HCl, Rugby	00536-4642-01
100's	$13.50	Thioridazine HCl, Geneva Pharms	50752-0266-05
100's	$13.50	Thioridazine Hcl, Mutual Pharm	53489-0149-01
100's	$13.57	Thioridazine Hcl, HL Moore Drug Exch	00839-6704-06
100's	$13.60	Thioridazine HCl, Geneva Pharms	00781-1624-01
100's	$13.65	Thioridazine Hcl, Schein Pharm (US)	00364-0662-01
100's	$13.65	Thioridazine HCl, Mylan	00378-0614-01
100's	$16.91	Thioridazine Hcl, Major Pharms	00904-1795-61
100's	$23.33	Thioridazine Hcl, Vangard Labs	00615-2506-13
100's	$23.40	Thioridazine Hcl, Medirex	57480-0363-01
100's	$25.25	Thioridazine HCl, Geneva Pharms	50752-0266-06
100's	$29.75	Thioridazine HCl, Geneva Pharms	00781-1624-13
100's	**$41.70**	**MELLARIL, Novartis**	**00078-0003-05**
100's	**$44.28**	**MELLARIL, Novartis**	**00078-0003-06**
600's	$155.20	Thioridazine Hcl, Medirex	57480-0363-06
750's	$255.90	Thioridazine Hcl, Glasgow Pharm	60809-0153-55
750's	$255.90	Thioridazine Hcl, Glasgow Pharm	60809-0153-72
1000's	$32.60	Thioridazine Hcl, United Res	00677-0824-10
1000's	$33.80	Thioridazine HCl, H.C.F.A. F F P	99999-2341-07
1000's	$73.13	Thioridazine Hcl, Martec Pharms	52555-0098-10
1000's	$82.50	Thioridazine Hcl, Major Pharms	00904-1616-80
1000's	$86.51	Thioridazine Hcl, Qualitest Pharms	00603-5993-32
1000's	$88.00	Thioridazine Hcl, Major Pharms	00904-1795-80
1000's	$105.25	Thioridazine Hcl, Aligen Independ	00405-4995-03
1000's	$105.25	Thioridazine HCl, Rugby	00536-4642-10
1000's	$105.25	Thioridazine Hcl, Mutual Pharm	53489-0149-10
1000's	$105.71	Thioridazine Hcl, HL Moore Drug Exch	00839-6704-16
1000's	$106.75	Thioridazine HCl, Geneva Pharms	50752-0266-09
1000's	$106.95	Thioridazine Hcl, Schein Pharm (US)	00364-0662-02
1000's	$106.95	Thioridazine HCl, Mylan	00378-0614-10
1000's	$163.45	Thioridazine HCl, Geneva Pharms	00781-1624-10
1000's	**$400.92**	**MELLARIL, Novartis**	**00078-0003-09**

Tablet, Coated - Oral - 50 mg

100's	$5.28	Thioridazine Hcl, United Res	00677-0825-01
100's	$5.55	Thioridazine HCl, H.C.F.A. F F P	99999-2341-08
100's	$6.77	Thioridazine Hydrochloride, US Trading	56126-0099-11
100's	$12.50	Thioridazine Hcl, Consolidated Midland	00223-2131-01
100's	$12.55	Thioridazine Hcl, Raway	00686-0567-20
100's	$15.87	Thioridazine Hcl, Qualitest Pharms	00603-5994-21
100's	$16.10	Thioridazine Hcl, Major Pharms	00904-1617-60
100's	$16.10	Thioridazine Hydrochlorides 50, Major Pharms	00904-1796-60
100's	$17.00	Thioridazine Hcl, Mutual Pharm	53489-0150-01
100's	$17.20	Thioridazine Hcl, Aligen Independ	00405-4996-01
100's	$17.75	Thioridazine HCl, Rugby	00536-4643-01
100's	$19.00	Thioridazine HCl, Geneva Pharms	50752-0267-05
100's	$19.24	Thioridazine Hcl, HL Moore Drug Exch	00839-6705-06
100's	$19.40	Thioridazine HCl, Geneva Pharms	00781-1634-01
100's	$19.45	Thioridazine Hcl, Schein Pharm (US)	00364-2318-01
100's	$19.45	Thioridazine HCl, Mylan	00378-0616-01
100's	$20.57	Thioridazine Hcl, Major Pharms	00904-1796-61
100's	$22.40	Thioridazine HCl, Amer Preferred	53445-1639-01
100's	$24.14	Thioridazine Hcl, Roxane	00054-8851-25
100's	$27.76	Thioridazine Hcl, Vangard Labs	00615-2507-13
100's	$27.80	Thioridazine Hcl, Medirex	57480-0364-01
100's	$29.75	Thioridazine HCl, Geneva Pharms	00781-1634-13
100's	$40.70	Thioridazine HCl, Geneva Pharms	50752-0267-06
100's	**$50.64**	**MELLARIL, Novartis**	**00078-0004-05**
100's	**$52.74**	**MELLARIL, Novartis**	**00078-0004-06**
500's	$27.75	Thioridazine HCl, H.C.F.A. F F P	99999-2341-09
600's	$182.40	Thioridazine Hcl, Medirex	57480-0364-06
750's	$305.25	Thioridazine Hcl, Glasgow Pharm	60809-0126-55
750's	$305.25	Thioridazine Hcl, Glasgow Pharm	60809-0126-72
1000's	$52.80	Thioridazine Hcl, United Res	00677-0825-10
1000's	$55.50	Thioridazine HCl, H.C.F.A. F F P	99999-2341-10
1000's	$97.95	Thioridazine Hcl, Martec Pharms	52555-0099-10
1000's	$120.00	Thioridazine Hcl, Consolidated Midland	00223-2131-02
1000's	$124.75	Thioridazine Hcl, Major Pharms	00904-1617-80
1000's	$135.80	Thioridazine Hcl, Qualitest Pharms	00603-5994-32
1000's	$136.00	Thioridazine Hcl, Major Pharms	00904-1796-80
1000's	$143.55	Thioridazine HCl, Geneva Pharms	00781-1634-10
1000's	$144.45	Thioridazine Hcl, HL Moore Drug Exch	00839-6705-16
1000's	$145.00	Thioridazine HCl, Rugby	00536-4643-10
1000's	$163.25	Thioridazine HCl, Geneva Pharms	50752-0267-09
1000's	$163.50	Thioridazine HCl, Mylan	00378-0616-10
1000's	$163.50	Thioridazine Hcl, Aligen Independ	00405-4996-03
1000's	$163.50	Thioridazine Hcl, Mutual Pharm	53489-0150-10
1000's	$163.51	Thioridazine Hcl, Schein Pharm (US)	00364-2318-02
1000's	**$490.14**	**MELLARIL, Novartis**	**00078-0004-09**

Tablet, Coated - Oral - 100 mg

100's	$8.55	Thioridazine Hcl, United Res	00677-0832-01
100's	$9.00	Thioridazine HCl, H.C.F.A. F F P	99999-2341-11
100's	$10.74	Thioridazine Hydrochloride, US Trading	56126-0101-11
100's	$14.64	Thioridazine Hcl, Martec Pharms	52555-0092-01
100's	$17.25	Thioridazine Hcl, Raway	00686-0580-20
100's	$19.50	Thioridazine Hcl, Consolidated Midland	00223-2132-01
100's	$20.30	Thioridazine Hcl, Qualitest Pharms	00603-5995-21
100's	$21.90	Thioridazine Hcl, Major Pharms	00904-1618-60
100's	$23.36	Thioridazine Hcl, HL Moore Drug Exch	00839-6720-06
100's	$24.00	Thioridazine Hcl, Aligen Independ	00405-4997-01
100's	$24.00	Thioridazine Hcl, Mutual Pharm	53489-0500-01
100's	$25.50	Thioridazine HCl, Geneva Pharms	50752-0268-05
100's	$25.70	Thioridazine HCl, Geneva Pharms	00781-1644-01
100's	$25.75	Thioridazine HCl, Mylan	00378-0618-01
100's	$25.81	Thioridazine, Schein Pharm (US)	00364-0670-01
100's	$25.81	Thioridazine HCl, Rugby	00536-4644-01

HOW SUPPLIED - RATED THERAPEUTICALLY EQUIVALENT: *(cont'd)*

100's	$34.06	Thioridazine Hcl, Vangard Labs	00615-2508-13
100's	$34.50	Thioridazine HCl, Geneva Pharms	00781-1644-13
100's	$35.60	Thioridazine HCl, Geneva Pharms	50752-0268-06
100's	$35.88	Thioridazine Hcl, Major Pharms	00904-1797-61
100's	$35.88	Thioridazine Hcl 100, Major Pharms	00904-1804-61
100's	**$59.46**	**MELLARIL, Novartis**	**00078-0005-05**
100's	**$61.62**	**MELLARIL, Novartis**	**00078-0005-06**
500's	$45.00	Thioridazine HCl, H.C.F.A. F F P	99999-2341-12
500's	$65.75	Thioridazine Hcl, Major Pharms	00904-1618-40
500's	$110.00	Thioridazine HCl, Rugby	00536-4644-05
750's	$356.47	Thioridazine Hcl, Glasgow Pharm	60809-0154-55
750's	$356.47	Thioridazine Hcl, Glasgow Pharm	60809-0154-72
1000's	$90.00	Thioridazine HCl, H.C.F.A. F F P	99999-2341-13
1000's	$180.70	Thioridazine Hcl, Major Pharms	00904-1618-80
1000's	$183.25	Thioridazine HCl, Geneva Pharms	50752-0268-09
1000's	$183.65	Thioridazine HCl, Geneva Pharms	00781-1644-10
1000's	$183.70	Thioridazine Hcl, Mylan	00378-0618-10
1000's	**$579.06**	**MELLARIL, Novartis**	**00078-0005-09**

Tablet, Coated - Oral - 150 mg

100's	$13.73	Thioridazine HCl, H.C.F.A. F F P	99999-2341-14
100's	$19.17	Thioridazine Hcl, US Trading	56126-0310-11
100's	$30.00	Thioridazine Hcl, Consolidated Midland	00223-2133-01
100's	$31.00	Thioridazine Hcl, Raway	00686-0177-20
100's	$31.65	Thioridazine Hcl, Rugby	00536-4654-01
100's	$31.65	Thioridazine Hcl, Major Pharms	00904-7649-60
100's	$34.42	Thioridazine Hcl, Aligen Independ	00405-4998-01
100's	$38.75	Thioridazine HCl, Geneva Pharms	00781-1664-01
100's	$38.75	Thioridazine HCl, Geneva Pharms	50752-0269-05
100's	$38.85	Thioridazine HCl, Schein Pharm (US)	00364-0723-01
100's	**$78.24**	**MELLARIL, Novartis**	**00078-0006-05**
640's	**$336.00**	**MELLARIL, Novartis**	**00078-0006-65**
1000's	$270.00	Thioridazine Hcl, Consolidated Midland	00223-2133-02
1000's	**$664.98**	**MELLARIL, Novartis**	**00078-0006-09**

Tablet, Coated - Oral - 200 mg

100's	$15.38	Thioridazine HCl, H.C.F.A. F F P	99999-2341-15
100's	$20.25	Thioridazine Hcl, US Trading	56126-0311-11
100's	$34.50	Thioridazine Hcl, Consolidated Midland	00223-2134-01
100's	$35.48	Thioridazine Hcl, Rugby	00536-4649-01
100's	$36.10	Thioridazine Hcl, Major Pharms	00904-1799-60
100's	$37.00	Thioridazine Hcl, Raway	00686-0178-20
100's	$41.95	Thioridazine Hcl, Aligen Independ	00405-4999-01
100's	$45.25	Thioridazine HCl, Geneva Pharms	50752-0270-06
100's	$49.25	Thioridazine HCl, Geneva Pharms	50752-0270-05
100's	$49.51	Thioridazine, Schein Pharm (US)	00364-0724-01
100's	$69.51	Thioridazine HCl, Geneva Pharms	00781-1674-01
100's	**$89.16**	**MELLARIL, Novartis**	**00078-0007-05**
100's	**$91.44**	**MELLARIL, Novartis**	**00078-0007-06**
500's	$76.90	Thioridazine HCl, H.C.F.A. F F P	99999-2341-16
500's	$131.63	Thioridazine Hcl, HL Moore Drug Exch	00839-7057-12
750's	$528.97	Thioridazine Hcl, Glasgow Pharm	60809-0173-55
750's	$528.97	Thioridazine Hcl, Glasgow Pharm	60809-0173-72
1000's	$153.80	Thioridazine HCl, H.C.F.A. F F P	99999-2341-17
1000's	$335.00	Thioridazine Hcl, Consolidated Midland	00223-2134-02

HOW SUPPLIED - NOT RATED EQUIVALENT:

Concentrate - Oral - 30 mg/ml

480 ml	**$50.40**	**MELLARIL-S, Novartis**	**00078-0068-33**

Concentrate - Oral - 100 mg/ml

480 ml	**$103.62**	**MELLARIL S, Novartis**	**00078-0069-33**

THIOTEPA *(002342)*

CATEGORIES: Antineoplastics; Bladder Carcinoma; Breast Carcinoma; Cancer; Chemotherapy; Hodgkin's Disease; Lymphosarcoma; Nitrogen Mustard Derivatives; Oncologic Drugs; Ovarian Carcinoma; Tumors; FDA Approval Pre 1982

BRAND NAMES: Thioplex; Triethylenethiophosphoramide

FORMULARIES: BC-BS; Medi-Cal

DESCRIPTION:

THIOTEPA IS A POLYFUNCTIONAL ALKYLATING AGENT USED IN THE CHEMOTHERAPY OF CERTAIN NEOPLASTIC DISEASES.

Thiotepa is an ethylenimine-type compound, 1,1',1"-phosphinothioylidynetris-aziridine available in powder form in vials which contain a sterile mixture of 15 mg thiotepa, 80 mg NaCl, and 50 mg $NaHCO_3$. Thiotepa has also been known as TESPA and TSPA and is not the same as TEPA. Thiotepa is stable in alkaline medium and unstable in acid medium. When reconstituted with Sterile Water for Injection, the resulting solution has a pH of approximately 7.6.

CLINICAL PHARMACOLOGY:

Thiotepa is a cytotoxic agent of the polyfunctional alkylating type (more than one reactive ethylenimine group) related chemically and pharmacologically to nitrogen mustard. Its radiomimetic action is believed to occur through the release of ethylenimine radicals which, like irradiation, disrupt the bonds of DNA. One of the principal bond disruptions is initiated by alkylation of guanine at the N-7 position, which severs the linkage between the purine base and the sugar and liberates alkylated guanines.

On the basis of tissue concentration studies, it is reported that thiotepa has no differential affinity for neoplasms. Most of the drug appears to be excreted unchanged in the urine.

INDICATIONS AND USAGE:

Thiotepa has been tried with varying results in the palliation of a wide variety of neoplastic diseases. However, the most consistent results have been seen in the following tumors:

1. Adenocarcinoma of the breast.

2. Adenocarcinoma of the ovary.

3. For controlling intracavitary effusions secondary to diffuse or localized neoplastic diseases of various serosal cavities.

4. For the treatment of superficial papillary carcinoma of the urinary bladder.

While now largely superseded by other treatments, thiotepa has been effective against other lymphomas, such as lymphosarcoma and Hodgkin's disease.

CONTRAINDICATIONS:

Therapy is probably contraindicated in cases of existing hepatic, renal, or bone marrow damage. However, if the need outweighs the risk in such patients, thiotepa may be used in low dosage, and accompanied by hepatic, renal and hemopoietic function tests.

Thiotepa is contraindicated in patients with a known hypersensitivity (allergy) to this preparation.

WARNINGS:

The administration of thiotepa to pregnant women is not recommended except in cases where the benefit to be gained outweighs the risk of teratogenicity involved.

Thiotepa is highly toxic to the hematopoietic system. A rapidly falling white blood cell or platelet count indicates the necessity for discontinuing or reducing the dosage of thiotepa. Weekly blood and platelet counts are recommended during therapy and for at least three weeks after therapy has been discontinued.

Thiotepa is a polyfunctional alkylating agent, capable of cross-linking the DNA within a cell and changing its nature. The replication of the cell is, therefore, altered, and thiotepa may be described as mutagenic. An *in vitro* study has shown that it causes chromosomal aberrations of the chromatid type and that the frequency of induced aberrations increases with the age of the subject.

Like all alkylating agents, thiotepa is carcinogenic. Carcinogenicity is shown most clearly in mouse studies, but there is strong circumstantial evidence of carcinogenicity in man.

PRECAUTIONS:

The serious complication of excessive thiotepa therapy, or sensitivity to the effects of thiotepa, is bone marrow depression. If proper precautions are not observed thiotepa may cause leukopenia, thrombocytopenia, and anemia. Death from septicemia and hemorrhage has occurred as a direct result of hematopoietic depression by thiotepa.

It is not advisable to combine simultaneously or sequentially cancer chemotherapeutic agents or a cancer chemotherapeutic agent and a therapeutic modality having the same mechanism of action. Therefore, thiotepa combined with other alkylating agents such as nitrogen mustard or cyclophosphamide or thiotepa combined with irradiation would serve to intensify toxicity rather than to enhance therapeutic response. If these agents must follow each other, it is important that recovery from the first agent, as indicated by white blood cell count, be complete before therapy with the second agent is instituted.

The most reliable guide to thiotepa toxicity is the white blood cell count. If this falls to 3000 or less, the dose should be discontinued. Another good index of thiotepa toxicity is the platelet count; if this falls to 150,000, therapy should be discontinued. Red blood cell count is a less accurate indicator of thiotepa toxicity.

Other drugs which are known to produce bone marrow depression should be avoided.

There is no known antidote for overdosage with thiotepa. Transfusions of whole blood or platelets or leukocytes have proved beneficial to the patient in combating hematopoietic toxicity.

ADVERSE REACTIONS:

Apart from its effect on the blood-forming elements, thiotepa may cause other adverse reactions. These include pain at the site of injection, nausea, vomiting, anorexia, dizziness, headache, amenorrhea, and interference with spermatogenesis.

Febrile reaction and weeping from a subcutaneous lesion may occur as the result of breakdown of tumor tissue.

Allergic reactions are rare, but hives and skin rash have been noted occasionally. One case of alopecia has been reported. In addition, a patient who has received thiotepa and other anticancer agents experienced prolonged apnea after succinylcholine was administered prior to surgery. It was theorized that this was caused by decrease of pseudocholinesterase activity caused by the anticancer drugs.

There have been rare reports of chemical cystitis or hemorrhagic cystitis following intravesical, but not parenteral administration of thiotepa.

DOSAGE AND ADMINISTRATION:

Parenteral routes of administration are most reliable since absorption of thiotepa from the gastrointestinal tract is variable.

Since thiotepa is nonvesicant, intravenous doses may be given directly and rapidly without need for slow drip or large volumes of diluent. Some physicians prefer to give thiotepa directly into the tumor mass. This may be effected transrectally, transvaginally, or intracerebrally. The technique is discussed in the appropriate section which follows. For the control of malignant effusions, thiotepa is instilled directly into the cavity involved.

Dosage must be carefully individualized. A slow response to thiotepa may be deceptive and may occasion unwarranted frequency of administration with subsequent signs of toxicity. After maximum benefit is obtained by initial therapy, it is necessary to continue patient on maintenance therapy (1 to 4 week intervals). In order to continue optimal effect, maintenance doses should be no more frequent than weekly in order to preserve correlation between dose and blood counts.

Initial and Maintenance Doses: Initially the higher dose in the given range is commonly administered. The maintenance dose should be adjusted weekly on the basis of pretreatment control blood counts and subsequent blood counts.

Intravenous Administration: Thiotepa may be given by rapid intravenous administration in doses of 0.3 - 0.4 mg/kg. Doses should be given at 1 to 4 week intervals.

For conversion of mg/kg of body weight to mg/M^2 of body surface or the reverse, a ratio of 1.30 is given as a guideline. The conversion factor varies between 1:20 and 1:40 depending on age and body build.

Intratumor Administration: Thiotepa in initial doses of 0.6 - 0.8 mg/kg may be injected directly into a tumor by means of a 22-gauge needle. A small amount of local anesthetic is injected first; then the syringe is removed and the thiotepa solution is injected through the same needle. The drug is diluted in Sterile Water for Injection, 10 mg per 1 ml. Maintenance doses at one to four week intervals range from 0.07 mg/kg to 0.8 mg/kg depending on the condition of the patient.

Intracavitary Administration: The dosage recommended is 0.6 - 0.8 mg/kg. Administration is usually effected through the same tubing which is used to remove the fluid from the cavity involved.

Intravesical Administration: Patients with papillary carcinoma of the bladder are dehydrated for 8 to 12 hours prior to treatment. Then 60 mg of thiotepa in 30 - 60 ml of Sterile Water for Injection is instilled into the bladder by catheter. For maximum effect, the solution should be retained for 2 hours. If the patient finds it impossible to retain 60 ml for 2 hours, the dose may be given in a volume of 30 ml. If desired, the patient may be positioned every 15 minutes for maximum area contact. The usual course of treatment is once a week for 4 weeks. The course may be repeated if necessary, but second and third courses must be given with caution since bone marrow depression may be increased. Deaths have occurred after intravesical administration, caused by bone marrow depression from systemically absorbed drug.

DOSAGE AND ADMINISTRATION: *(cont'd)*

Preparation of Solution: The powder should be reconstituted preferably in Sterile Water for Injection. The amount of diluent most often used is 1.5 ml resulting in a drug concentration of 5 mg in each 0.5 ml of solution. Larger volumes are usually employed for intracavitary use, intravenous drip, or perfusion therapy. The 1.5 ml reconstituted preparation may be added to larger volumes of other diluents: Sodium Chloride Injection USP, Dextrose Injection USP, Dextrose and Sodium Chloride Injection USP, Ringer's Injection USP, or Lactated Ringer's Injection USP. Reconstituted solutions should be clear to slightly opaque but solutions that are grossly opaque or precipitated should not be used.

Since the original powder form contains 15 mg thiotepa, 80 mg NaCl, and 50 mg $NaHCO_3$, reconstitution and further dilution of the powder with Sterile Water for Injection to a concentration of approximately 1 mg/ml produces an isotonic solution. Reconstitution and further dilution with other diluents may result in hypertonic solutions, which may cause mild to moderate discomfort on injection.

For local use into single or multiple sites, thiotepa may be mixed with procaine HCl 2%, epinephrine HCl 1:1000 or both.

Procedures for proper handling and disposal of anti-cancer drugs should be considered. Several guidelines on this subject have been published.[1-6] There is no general agreement that all of the procedures recommended in the guidelines are necessary or appropriate.

Whether in its original powder form or in reconstituted solution, thiotepa must be stored in the refrigerator at 2-8°C (36-46°F). Reconstituted solutions may be kept for 5 days in a refrigerator without substantial loss of potency.

REFERENCES:

1. Recommendations for the Safe Handling of Parenteral Antineoplastic Drugs. NIH Publication No. 83-2621. For sale by the Superintendent of Documents, U.S. Government Printing Office, Washington, D.C. 20402. **2.** AMA Council Report, Guidelines for Handling Parenteral Antineoplastics, *JAMA*, March 15, 1985. **3.** National Study Commission on Cytotoxic Exposure - Recommendations for Handling Cytotoxic Agents. Available from Louis P. Jeffrey, Sc. D., Director of Pharmacy Services, Rhode Island Hospital, 593 Eddy Street, Providence, Rhode Island 02902. **4.** Clinical Oncological Society of Australia: Guidelines and recommendations for safe handling of antineoplastic agents. *Med J Australia* 1983; 1:426-428. **5.** Jones R.B., et al. Safe handling of chemotherapeutic agents: A report from the Mount Sinai Medical Center. Ca - *A Cancer Journal for Clinicians* Sept/Oct 1983; 258-263. **6.** American Society of Hospital Pharmacists technical assistance bulletin on handling cytotoxic drugs in hospitals. *Am J Hosp Pharm* 1985; 42:131-137.

HOW SUPPLIED:

Whether in its original powder form or in reconstituted solution, thiotepa must stored in the refrigerator at 2-8°C (36- 46°F). Reconstituted solutions may be kept for 5 days in a refrigerator without substantial loss of potency.

HOW SUPPLIED - EQUIVALENTS NOT AVAILABLE:

Injection, Dry-Soln - Intravenous - 15 mg/vial

1's	$73.31	THIOPLEX, Immunex	58406-0661-02
6's	$402.90	THIOPLEX, Immunex	58406-0661-31

THIOTHIXENE *(002343)*

CATEGORIES: Antipsychotics/Antimanics; Central Nervous System Agents; Neuroleptics; Psychotherapeutic Agents; Psychotic Disorders; Sedatives/Hypnotics; Tranquilizers; FDA Approval Pre 1982

BRAND NAMES: **Navane**; *Orbinamon*
(International brand names outside U.S. in italics)

FORMULARIES: Aetna; BC-BS; Medi-Cal; PCS

DESCRIPTION:

Thiothixene is a thioxanthene derivative. Specifically, it is the *cis* isomer of N,N-dimethyl-9-(3-(4-methyl-1-piperazinyl)-propylidene) thioxanthene-2-sulfonamide.

The thioxanthenes differ from the phenothiazines by the replacement of nitrogen in the central ring with a carbon-linked side chain fixed in space in a rigid structural configuration. An N,N-dimethyl sulfonamide functional group is bonded to the thioxanthene nucleus.

Inert ingredients for the capsule formulations are: hard gelatin capsules (which contain gelatin and titanium dioxide; may contain Yellow 10, Yellow 6, Blue 1, Green 3, Red 3, and other inert ingredients); lactose; magnesium stearate; sodium lauryl sulfate; starch.

Inert ingredients for the oral concentrate formulation are: alcohol; cherry flavor; dextrose; passion fruit flavor; sorbitol solution; water.

Inert ingredients for the IM solution formulation are dextrose; benzyl alcohol; and propyl gallate.

CLINICAL PHARMACOLOGY:

Thiothixene is a psychotropic agent of the thioxanthene series. Thiothixene possesses certain chemical and pharmacological similarities to the piperazine phenothiazines and differences from the aliphatic group of phenothiazines.

INDICATIONS AND USAGE:

Thiothixene is effective in the management of manifestations of psychotic disorders. Thiothixene has not been evaluated in the management of behavioral complications in patients with mental retardation.

CONTRAINDICATIONS:

Thiothixene is contraindicated in patients with circulatory collapse, comatose states, central nervous system depression due to any cause, and blood dyscrasias. Thiothixene is contraindicated in individuals who have shown hypersensitivity to the drug. It is not known whether there is a cross sensitivity between the thioxanthenes and the phenothiazine derivatives, but this possibility should be considered.

WARNINGS:

Tardive Dyskinesia: Tardive dyskinesia, a syndrome consisting of potentially irreversible, involuntary, dyskinetic movements may develop in patients treated with neuroleptic (antipsychotic) drugs. Although the prevalence of the syndrome appears to be highest among the elderly, especially elderly women, it is impossible to rely upon prevalence estimates to predict, at the inception of neuroleptic treatment, which patients are likely to develop the syndrome. Whether neuroleptic drug products differ in their potential to cause tardive dyskinesia is unknown.

Both the risk of developing the syndrome and the likelihood that it will become irreversible are believed to increase as the duration of treatment and the total cumulative dose of neuroleptic drugs administered to the patient increase. However, the syndrome can develop, although much less commonly, after relatively brief treatment periods at low doses.

WARNINGS: *(cont'd)*

There is no known treatment for established cases of tardive dyskinesia, although the syndrome may remit, partially or completely, if neuroleptic treatment is withdrawn. Neuroleptic treatment, itself, however, may suppress (or partially suppress) the signs and symptoms of the syndrome and thereby may possibly mask the underlying disease process. The effect that symptomatic suppression has upon the long-term course of the syndrome is unknown.

Given these considerations, neuroleptics should be prescribed in a manner that is most likely to minimize the occurrence of tardive dyskinesia. Chronic neuroleptic treatment should generally be reserved for patients who suffer from a chronic illness that, 1) is known to respond to neuroleptic drugs, and, 2) for whom alternative, equally effective, but potentially less harmful treatments are *not* available or appropriate. In patients who do require chronic treatment, the smallest dose and the shortest duration of treatment producing a satisfactory clinical response should be sought. The need for continued treatment should be reassessed periodically.

If signs and symptoms of tardive dyskinesia appear in a patient on neuroleptics, drug discontinuation should be considered. However, some patients may require treatment despite the presence of the syndrome.

(For further information about the description of tardive dyskinesia and its clinical detection, please refer to PRECAUTIONS, Information for the Patient, and ADVERSE REACTIONS.)

Neuroleptic Malignant Syndrome (NMS): A potentially fatal symptom complex sometimes referred to as Neuroleptic Malignant Syndrome (NMS) has been reported in association with antipsychotic drugs. Clinical manifestations of NMS are hyperpyrexia, muscle rigidity, altered mental status and evidence of autonomic instability (irregular pulse or blood pressure, tachycardia, diaphoresis, and cardiac dysrhythmias).

The diagnostic evaluation of patients with this syndrome is complicated. In arriving at a diagnosis, it is important to identify cases where the clinical presentation includes both serious medical illness (*e.g.,* pneumonia, systemic infection, etc.) and untreated or inadequately treated extrapyramidal signs and symptoms (EPS). Other important considerations in the differential diagnosis include central anticholinergic toxicity, heat stroke, drug fever and primary central nervous system (CNS) pathology.

The management of NMS should include 1) immediate discontinuation of antipsychotic drugs and other drugs not essential to concurrent therapy, 2) intensive symptomatic treatment and medical monitoring, and 3) treatment of any concomitant serious medical problems for which specific treatments are available. There is no general agreement about specific pharmacological treatment regimens for uncomplicated NMS.

If a patient requires antipsychotic drug treatment after recovery from NMS, the potential reintroduction of drug therapy should be carefully considered. The patient should be carefully monitored, since recurrences of NMS have been reported.

Usage in Pregnancy: Safe use of thiothixene during pregnancy has not been established. Therefore, this drug should be given to pregnant patients only when, in the judgment of the physician, the expected benefit from the treatment exceed the possible risks to mother and fetus. Animal reproduction studies and clinical experience to date have not demonstrated any teratogenic effects.

In the animal reproduction studies with thiothixene, there was some decrease in conception rate and litter size, and an increase in resorption rate in rats and rabbits. Similar findings have been reported with other psychotropic agents. After repeated oral administration of thiothixene to rats (5 to 15 mg/kg/day), rabbits (3 to 50 mg/kg/day), and monkeys (1 to 3 mg/kg/day) before and during gestation, no teratogenic effects were seen.

Usage in Children: The use of thiothixene in children under 12 years of age is not recommended because safe conditions for its use have not been established.

As is true with many CNS drugs, thiothixene may impair the mental and/or physical abilities required for the performance of potentially hazardous tasks such as driving a car or operating machinery, especially during the first few days of therapy. Therefore, the patient should be cautioned accordingly.

As in the case of other CNS-acting drugs, patients receiving thiothixene should be cautioned about the possible additive effects (which may include hypotension) with CNS depressants and with alcohol.

PRECAUTIONS:

GENERAL

An antiemetic effect was observed in animal studies with thiothixene; since this effect may also occur in man, it is possible that thiothixene may mask signs of overdosage of toxic drugs and may obscure conditions such as intestinal obstruction and brain tumor.

In consideration of the known capability of thiothixene and certain other psychotropic drugs to precipitate convulsions, extreme caution should be used in patients with a history of convulsive disorders or those in a state of alcohol withdrawal, since it may lower the convulsive threshold. Although thiothixene potentiates the actions of the barbiturates, the dosage of the anticonvulsant therapy should not be reduced when thiothixene is administered concurrently.

Though exhibiting rather weak anticholinergic properties, thiothixene should be used with caution in patients who might be exposed to extreme heat or who are receiving atropine or related drugs.

Use with caution in patients with cardiovascular disease.

Caution as well as careful adjustment of the dosages is indicated when thiothixene is used in conjunction with other CNS depressants.

Also, careful observation should be made for pigmentary retinopathy, and lenticular pigmentation (fine lenticular pigmentation has been noted in a small number of patients treated with thiothixene for prolonged periods). Blood dyscrasias (agranulocytosis, pancytopenia, thrombocytopenic purpura), and liver damage (jaundice, biliary stasis), have been reported with related drugs.

Neuroleptic drugs elevate prolactin levels; the elevation persists during chronic administration. Tissue culture experiments indicate that approximately one-third of human breast cancers are prolactin dependent *in vitro*, a factor of potential importance if the prescription of these drugs is contemplated in a patient with a previously detected breast cancer. Although disturbances such as galactorrhea, amenorrhea, gynecomastia, and impotence have been reported, the clinical significance of elevated serum prolactin levels is unknown for most patients. An increase in mammary neoplasms has been found in rodents after chronic administration of neuroleptic drugs. Neither clinical studies nor epidemiologic studies conducted to date, however, have shown an association between chronic administration of these drugs and mammary tumorigenesis; the available evidence is considered too limited to be conclusive at this time.

INFORMATION FOR THE PATIENT

Given the likelihood that some patients exposed chronically to neuroleptics will develop tardive dyskinesia, it is advised that all patients in whom chronic use is contemplated be given, if possible, full information about this risk. The decision to inform patients and/or their guardians must obviously take into account the clinical circumstances and the competency of the patient to understand the information provided.

PRECAUTIONS: *(cont'd)*

Additional information for IM solution: As with all IM preparations, thiothixene should be injected well within the body of a relatively large muscle. The preferred sites are the upper outer quadrant of the buttock (*i.e.,* gluteus maximus) and the mid-lateral thigh.

The deltoid are should be used only if well developed such as in certain adults and older children, and then only with caution to avoid radial nerve injury. IM injections should not be made into the lower and mid- thirds of the upper arm. Aspiration is necessary to help avoid inadvertent injection into a blood vessel.

ADVERSE REACTIONS:

NOTE: Not all of the following adverse reactions have been reported with thiothixene. However, since thiothixene has certain chemical and pharmacologic similarities to the phenothiazines, all of the known side effects and toxicity associated with phenothiazine therapy should be borne in mind when thiothixene is used.

Cardiovascular Effects: Tachycardia, hypotension, lightheadedness, and syncope. In the event hypotension occurs, epinephrine should not be used as a pressor agent since a paradoxical further lowering of blood pressure may result. Nonspecific EKG changes have been observed in some patients receiving thiothixene. These changes are usually reversible and frequently disappear on continued thiothixene therapy. The incidence of these changes is lower than that observed with some phenothiazines. The clinical significance of these changes is not known.

CNS Effects: Drowsiness, usually mild, may occur although it usually subsides with continuation of thiothixene therapy. The incidence of sedation appears similar to that of the piperazine group of phenothiazines but less than that of certain aliphatic phenothiazines. Restlessness, agitation and insomnia have been noted with thiothixene. Seizures and paradoxical exacerbation of psychotic symptoms have occurred with thiothixene infrequently.

Hyperreflexia has been reported in infants delivered from mothers having received structurally related drugs.

In addition, phenothiazine derivatives have been associated with cerebral edema and cerebrospinal fluid abnormalities.

Extrapyramidal symptoms, such as pseudo-parkinsonism, akathisia and dystonia have been reported. Management of these extra-pyramidal symptoms depends upon the type and severity. Rapid relief of acute symptoms may require the use of an injectable antiparkinson agent. More slowly emerging symptoms may be managed by reducing the dosage of thiothixene and/or administering an oral antiparkinson agent.

Persistent Tardive Dyskinesia: As with all antipsychotic agents tardive dyskinesia may appear in some patients on long term therapy or may occur after drug therapy has been discontinued. The syndrome is characterized by rhythmical involuntary movements of the tongue, face, mouth or jaw (e.g. protrusion of tongue, puffing of cheeks, puckering of mouth, chewing movements). Sometimes these may be accompanied by involuntary movements of extremities.

Since early detection of tardive dyskinesia is important, patients should be monitored on an ongoing basis. It has been reported that fine vermicular movement of the tongue may be an early sign of the syndrome. If this or any other presentation of the syndrome is observed, the clinician should consider possible discontinuation of neuroleptic medication. (See WARNINGS.)

Hepatic Effects: Elevations of serum transaminase and alkaline phosphatase, usually transient, have been infrequently observed in some patients. No clinically confirmed cases of jaundice attributable to thiothixene have been reported.

Hematologic Effects: As is true with certain other psychotropic drugs, leukopenia and leucocytosis, which are usually transient, can occur occasionally with thiothixene. Other antipsychotic drugs have been associated with agranulocytosis, eosinophilia, hemolytic anemia, thrombocytopenia and pancytopenia.

Allergic Reactions: Rash, pruritus, urticaria, photosensitivity and rare cases of anaphylaxis have been reported with thiothixene. Undue exposure to sunlight should be avoided. Although not experienced with thiothixene, exfoliative dermatitis and contact dermatitis (in nursing personnel), have been reported with certain phenothiazines.

Endocrine Disorders: Lactation, moderate breast enlargement and amenorrhea have occurred in a small percentage of females receiving thiothixene. If persistent, this may necessitate a reduction in dosage or the discontinuation of therapy. Phenothiazines have been associated with false positive pregnancy tests, gynecomastia, hypoglycemia, hyperglycemia and glycosuria.

Autonomic Effects: Dry mouth, blurred vision, nasal congestion, constipation, increased sweating, increased salivation and impotence have occurred infrequently with thiothixene therapy. Phenothiazines have been associated with miosis, mydriasis, and adynamic ileus.

Other Adverse Reactions: Hyperpyrexia, anorexia, nausea, vomiting, diarrhea, increase in appetite and weight, weakness or fatigue, polydipsia, and peripheral edema.

Although not reported with thiothixene, evidence indicates there is a relationship between phenothiazine therapy and the occurrence of a systemic lupus erythematosus-like syndrome.

Neuroleptic Malignant Syndrome (NMS): Please refer to the text regarding NMS in the WARNINGS.

NOTE: Sudden deaths have occasionally been reported in patients who have received certain phenothiazine derivatives. In some cases the cause of death was apparently cardiac arrest or asphyxia due to failure of the cough reflex. In others, the cause could not be determined nor could it be established that death was due to phenothiazine administration.

OVERDOSAGE:

Manifestations include muscular twitching, drowsiness and dizziness. Symptoms of gross overdosage may include CNS depression, rigidity, weakness, torticollis, tremor, salivation, dysphagia, hypotension, disturbances of gait, or coma.

Treatment:

Essentially symptomatic and supportive. Early gastric lavage is helpful. Keep patient under careful observation and maintain an open airway, since involvement of the extrapyramidal system may produce dysphagia and respiratory difficulty in severe overdosage. If hypotension occurs, the standard measures for managing circulatory shock should be used (IV fluids and/or vasoconstrictors).

If a vasoconstrictor is needed, levarterenol and phenylephrine are the most suitable drugs. Other pressor agents, including epinephrine, are not recommended, since phenothiazine derivatives may reverse the usual pressor action of these agents and cause further lowering of blood pressure.

If CNS depression is marked, symptomatic treatment is indicated. Extrapyramidal symptoms may be treated with antiparkinson drugs.

There are no data on the use of peritoneal or hemodialysis, but they are known to be of little value in phenothiazine intoxication.

DOSAGE AND ADMINISTRATION:

Capsules: Dosage of thiothixene should be individually adjusted depending on the chronicity and severity of the condition. In general, small doses should be used initially and gradually increased to the optimal effective level, based on patient response.

Some patients have been successfully maintained on once-a-day thiothixene therapy.

The use of thiothixene in children under 12 years of age is not recommended because safe conditions for its use have not been established.

In milder conditions, an initial dose of 2 mg three times daily. If indicated, a subsequent increase to 15 mg/day total daily dose is often effective.

In more severe conditions, an initial dose of 5 mg twice daily.

The usual optimal dose is 20 to 30 mg daily. If indicated, an increase to 60 mg/day total daily dose is often effective. Exceeding a total daily dose of 60 mg rarely increases the beneficial response.

IM Injection: Dosage of thiothixene should be individually adjusted depending on the chronicity and severity of the condition. In general, small doses should be used initially and gradually increased to the optimal effective level, based on patient response. The use of thiothixene in children under 12 years of age is not recommended.

When more rapid control and treatment of acute behavior is desirable, the IM form of thiothixene may be indicated. It is also of benefit where the very nature of the patients's symptomatology, whether acute or chronic, renders oral administration impractical or even impossible.

For the treatment of acute symptomatology or in patients unable or unwilling to take oral medication, the usual dose is 4 mg of thiothixene IM administered 2 to 4 times daily. Dosage may be increased or decreased depending on response. Most patients are controlled on a total daily dosage of 16 to 20 mg. The maximum recommended dosage is 30 mg/day. An oral form should supplant the injectable as soon as possible. It may be necessary to adjust the dosage when changing from the IM to the oral dosage forms.

HOW SUPPLIED - RATED THERAPEUTICALLY EQUIVALENT:

Capsule, Gelatin - Oral - 1 mg

100's	$9.75	Thiothixene, H.C.F.A. F F P	99999-2343-01
100's	$12.23	Thiothixene, US Trading	56126-0378-11
100's	$15.75	Thiothixene, Rugby	00536-4951-01
100's	$15.77	Thiothixene, Qualitest Pharms	00603-6018-21
100's	$16.20	Thiothixene, Aligen Independ	00405-5004-01
100's	$17.50	Thiothixene, United Res	00677-1149-01
100's	$17.50	Thiothixene, Major Pharms	00904-2890-60
100's	$17.50	Thiothixene, Major Pharms	00904-2955-60
100's	$21.06	Thiothixene, HL Moore Drug Exch	00839-7288-06
100's	$21.10	Thiothixene, Schein Pharm (US)	00364-2166-01
100's	$21.50	Thiothixene, Geneva Pharms	00781-2226-01
100's	$21.95	Thiothixene, Mylan	00378-1001-01
100's	$24.92	Thiothixene, Major Pharms	00904-2955-61
100's	$28.80	Thiothixene, Vangard Labs	00615-1302-13
100's	$28.95	Thiothixene, Geneva Pharms	00781-2226-13
100's	**$33.14**	**NAVANE, Roerig**	**00049-5710-66**

Capsule, Gelatin - Oral - 2 mg

100's	$12.75	Thiothixene, H.C.F.A. F F P	99999-2343-02
100's	$15.02	Thiothixene, US Trading	56126-0379-11
100's	$20.89	Thiothixene, Qualitest Pharms	00603-6019-21
100's	$21.00	Thiothixene, Rugby	00536-4952-01
100's	$24.75	Thiothixene, United Res	00677-1150-01
100's	$24.85	Thiothixene, Major Pharms	00904-2891-60
100's	$24.85	Thiothixene, Major Pharms	00904-2956-60
100's	$25.38	Thiothixene, Aligen Independ	00405-5005-01
100's	$27.50	Thiothixene, Schein Pharm (US)	00364-2167-01
100's	$27.54	Thiothixene, HL Moore Drug Exch	00839-7289-06
100's	$28.50	Thiothixene, Geneva Pharms	00781-2227-01
100's	$28.95	Thiothixene, Mylan	00378-2002-01
100's	$31.59	Thiothixene, Major Pharms	00904-2956-61
100's	$38.05	Thiothixene, Vangard Labs	00615-1303-13
100's	$38.85	Thiothixene, Geneva Pharms	00781-2227-13
100's	**$44.68**	**NAVANE, Roerig**	**00049-5720-66**
100's	**$54.71**	**NAVANE, Roerig**	**00049-5720-41**
500's	$63.75	Thiothixene, H.C.F.A. F F P	99999-2343-03
500's	$79.75	Thiothixene, Major Pharms	00904-2891-40
500's	$79.75	Thiothixene, Major Pharms	00904-2956-40
1000's	$127.50	Thiothixene, H.C.F.A. F F P	99999-2343-04
1000's	$235.90	Thiothixene, Schein Pharm (US)	00364-2167-02
1000's	$239.71	Thiothixene, Mylan	00378-2002-10
1000's	**$397.56**	**NAVANE, Roerig**	**00049-5720-82**

Capsule, Gelatin - Oral - 5 mg

100's	$18.23	Thiothixene, H.C.F.A. F F P	99999-2343-05
100's	$18.77	Thiothixene, US Trading	56126-0380-11
100's	$36.80	Thiothixene, Major Pharms	00904-2892-60
100's	$36.80	Thiothixene, Major Pharms	00904-2957-60
100's	$37.11	Thiothixene, Qualitest Pharms	00603-6020-21
100's	$38.25	Thiothixene, Aligen Independ	00405-5006-01
100's	$38.25	Thiothixene, United Res	00677-1151-01
100's	$39.25	Thiothixene, Rugby	00536-4516-01
100's	$42.46	Tiothixene, HL Moore Drug Exch	00839-7290-06
100's	$42.50	Thiothixene, Schein Pharm (US)	00364-2168-01
100's	$43.50	Thiothixene, Geneva Pharms	00781-2228-01
100's	$43.95	Thiothixene, Mylan	00378-3005-01
100's	$46.59	Thiothixene, Major Pharms	00904-2957-61
100's	$59.50	Thiothixene, Vangard Labs	00615-1304-13
100's	$60.80	Thiothixene, Geneva Pharms	00781-2228-13
100's	**$69.87**	**NAVANE, Roerig**	**00049-5730-66**
100's	**$85.64**	**NAVANE, Roerig**	**00049-5730-41**
500's	$91.15	Thiothixene, H.C.F.A. F F P	99999-2343-06
500's	$124.68	Thiothixene, Rugby	00536-4516-05
500's	$124.95	Thiothixene, Major Pharms	00904-2892-40
500's	$124.95	Thiothixene, Major Pharms	00904-2957-40
1000's	$182.30	Thiothixene, H.C.F.A. F F P	99999-2343-07
1000's	$264.20	Thiothixene, Martec Pharms	52555-0238-10
1000's	$360.00	Thiothixene, Schein Pharm (US)	00364-2168-02
1000's	$363.20	Thiothixene, Mylan	00378-3005-10
1000's	**$621.18**	**NAVANE, Roerig**	**00049-5730-82**

Capsule, Gelatin - Oral - 10 mg

100's	$26.93	Thiothixene, H.C.F.A. F F P	99999-2343-08
100's	$27.17	Thiothixene, US Trading	56126-0381-11
100's	$41.95	Thiothixene, Martec Pharms	52555-0239-01
100's	$47.15	Thiothixene, Major Pharms	00904-2893-60
100's	$52.46	Thiothixene 10, Vangard Labs	00615-0347-13
100's	$52.70	Thiothixene, Qualitest Pharms	00603-6021-21
100's	$52.95	Thiothixene, Rugby	00536-4954-01
100's	$55.80	Thiothixene Capsules 10 Mg, Aligen Independ	00405-5007-01

HOW SUPPLIED - RATED THERAPEUTICALLY EQUIVALENT: *(cont'd)*

100's	$58.25	Thiothixene, Major Pharms	00904-2958-61
100's	$59.93	Thiothixene, HL Moore Drug Exch	00839-7291-06
100's	$60.10	Thiothixene, Schein Pharm (US)	00364-2169-01
100's	$61.50	Thiothixene, Geneva Pharms	00781-2229-01
100's	$61.95	Thiothixene, Mylan	00378-5010-01
100's	$80.10	Thiothixene, Geneva Pharms	00781-2229-13
100's	**$96.31**	**NAVANE, Roerig**	**00049-5740-66**
500's	$134.65	Thiothixene, H.C.F.A. F F P	99999-2343-09
500's	$178.15	Thiothixene, Major Pharms	00904-2893-40
500's	$217.31	Thiothixene Hcl, Rugby	00536-4954-05
1000's	$269.30	Thiothixene, H.C.F.A. F F P	99999-2343-10
1000's	$412.50	Thiothixene, Martec Pharms	52555-0239-10
1000's	$530.00	Thiothixene, Schein Pharm (US)	00364-2169-02
1000's	$530.83	Thiothixene, Mylan	00378-5010-10
1000's	**$857.18**	**NAVANE, Roerig**	**00049-5740-82**

Concentrate - Oral - 5 mg/ml

2 ml x 100	$123.11	Thiothixene Hcl, Xactdose	50962-0377-02
4 ml x 100	$162.80	Thiothixene Hcl, Xactdose	50962-0377-04
30 ml	$6.28	Thiothixene, H.C.F.A. F F P	99999-2343-11
30 ml	$11.48	Thiothixene HCl, Alpharma	00472-1457-91
120 ml	$25.12	Thiothixene Hcl, Copley Pharm	38245-0613-14
120 ml	$25.12	Thiothixene, H.C.F.A. F F P	99999-2343-12
120 ml	$31.25	Thiothixene Hcl, Qualitest Pharms	00603-1762-54
120 ml	$36.44	Intensol, Roxane	00054-3872-50
120 ml	$38.44	Thiothixene HCl, Alpharma	00472-1457-94
120 ml	$40.10	Thiothixene Hcl, Major Pharms	00904-2899-20
120 ml	$42.35	Thiothixene Hcl, Goldline Labs	00182-6112-71
120 ml	**$71.29**	**NAVANE, Roerig**	**00049-5750-47**

HOW SUPPLIED - NOT RATED EQUIVALENT:

Capsule, Gelatin - Oral - 20 mg

100's	$5.07	Thiothixene, US Trading	56126-0416-11
100's	**$135.13**	**NAVANE, Roerig**	**00049-5770-66**
100's	**$148.58**	**NAVANE, Roerig**	**00049-5770-41**
500's	**$603.84**	**NAVANE, Roerig**	**00049-5770-73**

Injection, Solution - Intramuscular - 5 mg/ml

10 mg x 10	**$29.77**	**NAVANE, Roerig**	**00049-5765-83**

THYROID *(002349)*

CATEGORIES: Cancer; Diagnostic Agents; Goiter; Hormones; Hypolipidemics; Hypothyroidism; Thyroid Agents; Thyroid Carcinoma; Thyroid Function; Thyroid Preparations; Thyroiditis; Pregnancy Category A; Sales > $100 Million; FDA Pre 1938 Drugs

BRAND NAMES: **Armour Thyroid**; *Cinetic*; Parloid Thyroid; S-P-T; *Throidine*; *Thryoboline*; *Thyradin*; *Thyreoid*; Thyro-Teric; *Tiroides*; Westhroid
(International brand names outside U.S. in italics)

FORMULARIES: Aetna; BC-BS; CIGNA; FHP; Humana; Kaiser; Medco; Medi-Cal; PruCare; United

DESCRIPTION:

Thyroid tablets, USP for oral use are natural preparations derived from porcine thyroid glands (T_3 liothyronine is approximately four times as potent as T_4 levothyroxine on a microgram for microgram basis.) They provide 38 mcg levothyroxine (T_4) and 9 mcg liothyronine (T_3) per grain of thyroid. The inactive ingredients are calcium stearate, dextrose and mineral oil.

CLINICAL PHARMACOLOGY:

The steps in the synthesis of the thyroid hormones are controlled by thyrotropin (Thyroid Stimulating Hormone, TSH) secreted by the anterior pituitary. This hormone's secretion is in turn controlled by a feedback mechanism effect by the thyroid hormones themselves and by thyrotropin releasing hormone (TRH), a tripeptide of hypothalamic origin. Endogenous thyroid hormone secretion is suppressed when exogenous hormones are administered to euthyroid individuals in excess of the normal gland's secretion.

The mechanisms by which thyroid hormone exert their physiologic action are not well understood. These hormones enhance oxygen consumption by most tissues of the body, increase the basal metabolic rate, and the metabolism of carbohydrates, lipids, and proteins. Thus, they exert a profound influence on every organ system in the body and are of particular importance in the development of the central nervous system.

The normal thyroid gland contains approximately 200 mcg of levothyroxine (T_4) per gram of gland, and 15 mcg of liothyronine (T_3) per gram. The ratio of these two hormones in the circulation does not represent the ratio in the thyroid gland, since about 80 percent of peripheral liothyronine (T_3) comes from monodeiodination of levothyroxine (T_4) at the 5 position (inner ring) also results in the formation of reverse liothyronine (T_3), which is calorigenically inactive.

Liothyronine (T_3) levels are low in the fetus and newborn, in old age, in chronic caloric deprivation, hepatic cirrhosis, renal failure, surgical stress, and chronic illnesses representing what has been called the "T_3 thyronine syndrome."

PHARMACOKINETICS

Animal studies have shown that levothyroxine (T_4) is only partially absorbed from the gastrointestinal tract. The degree of absorption is dependent on the vehicle used for its administration and by the character of the intestinal contents, the intestinal flora, including plasma protein, and soluble dietary factors, all of which bind thyroid and thereby make it unavailable for diffusion. Only 41 percent is absorbed when given in a gelatin capsules as opposed to a 74 percent absorption when given with an albumin carrier.

Depending on other factors, absorption has varied from 48 to 79 percent of the administered dose. Fasting increases absorption. Malabsorption syndromes, as well as dietary factors, (children's soybean formula, concomitant use of anionic exchange resins such as cholestyramine) cause excessive fecal loss. Liothyronine (T_3) is almost totally absorbed. 95 percent in 4 hours. The hormones contained in the natural preparations are absorbed in a manner similar to the synthetic hormones.

More than 99 percent of circulating hormones are bound to serum proteins, including thyroid-binding globulin (TBg), thyroid-binding prealbumin (TBPA), and albumin (TBa), whose capacities and affinities vary for the hormones. The higher affinity of levothyroxine (T_4) for both TBg and TBPA as compared to liothyronine (T_3) partially explains the higher serum levels and longer half-life of the former hormone. Both protein-bound hormones exist in reverse equilibrium with minute amounts of free hormone, the latter accounting for the metabolic activity.

CLINICAL PHARMACOLOGY: *(cont'd)*

Deiodination of levothyroxine (T_4) occurs at a number of sites, including liver, kidney, and other tissues. The conjugated hormone, in the form of glucuronide or sulfate, is found in the bile and gut where it may complete an enterohepatic circulation. Eighty-five percent of levothyroxine (T_4) metabolized daily is deiodinated.

INDICATIONS AND USAGE:

Thyroid tablets are indicated:

1. As replacement or supplemental therapy in patients with hypothyroidism of any etiology except transient hypothyroidism during the recovery phase of subacute thyroiditis. This category includes cretinism, myxedema and ordinary hypothyroidism in patients of any age (children, adults, the elderly) or state (including pregnancy), primary hypothyroidism resulting from functional deficiency, primary atrophy, partial or total absence of thyroid gland, or effects of surgery radiation, or drugs with or without the presence of goiter, and secondary (pituitary), or tertiary (hypothalamic) hypothyroidism (See WARNINGS.)

2. As pituitary TSH suppressants in the treatment or prevention of various types of euthyroid goiters, including thyroid nodules, subacute or chronic lymphocytic thyroiditis (Hashimoto's), multinodal goiter and in the management of thyroid cancer.

3. As a diagnostic agents in suppression tests to differentiate suspected mild hyperthyroidism or thyroid gland autonomy.

CONTRAINDICATIONS:

Thyroid hormone preparations are generally contraindicated in patients with diagnosed but as yet uncorrected adrenal cortical insufficiency, untreated thyrotoxicosis, and apparent hypersensitivity to any of their active or extraneous constituents. There is no well-documented evidence from the literature, however, of true allergic or idiosyncratic reactions to thyroid hormone.

WARNINGS:

Drugs with thyroid hormone activity, alone or together with other therapeutic agents, have been used for the treatment of obesity. In euthyroid patients, doses within the range of daily hormonal requirements are ineffective for weight reduction. Larger doses may produce serious or even life-threatening manifestations of toxicity, particularly when given in association with sympathomimetic amines such as those used for their anorectic effects.

The use of thyroid hormones in the therapy of obesity, alone or combined with other drugs, is unjustified and has been shown to be ineffective. Neither is their use justified for the treatment of male or female infertility unless this condition is accompanied by hypothyroidism.

PRECAUTIONS:

GENERAL

Thyroid hormones should be used with great caution in a number of circumstances where the integrity of the cardiovascular system, particularly the coronary arteries, is suspected. These include patients with angina pectoris or the elderly, in whom there is a greater likelihood of occult cardiac disease. In these patients therapy should be initiated with low doses, (*i.e.,* 15-30 mg thyroid). When, in such patients, a euthyroid state can only be reached at the expense of an aggravation of the cardiovascular disease, thyroid hormone dosage should be reduced.

Thyroid hormone therapy in patients with concomitant diabetes mellitus or diabetes insipidus or adrenal cortical insufficiency aggravates the intensity of their symptoms. Appropriate adjustments of the various therapeutic measures directed at these concomitant endocrine disease are required. The therapy of myxedema coma requires simultaneous administration of glucocorticoids (see DOSAGE AND ADMINISTRATION.)

Hypothyroidism decreases and hyperthyroidism increases the sensitivity to oral anticoagulants. Prothrombin time should be closely monitored in thyroid-treated patients on oral anticoagulants and dosage of the latter agents adjusted on the basis of frequent prothrombin time determinations. In infants, excessive doses of thyroid hormone preparations may produce craniosynostosis.

INFORMATION FOR THE PATIENT

Patients on thyroid hormone preparations and parents of children on thyroid therapy should be informed that:

1. Replacement therapy is to be taken essentially for life, with the exception of cases of transient hypothyroidism, usually associated with thyroiditis, and in those patients receiving a therapeutic trial of the drug.

2. They should immediately report during the course of therapy any signs or symptoms of thyroid hormone toxicity, e.g., chest pain, increased pulse rate, palpitations, excessive sweating, heat intolerance, nervousness, or any other unusual event.

3. In case of concomitant diabetes mellitus, the daily dosage of antidiabetic medication may need readjustment as thyroid hormone replacement is achieved. If thyroid medication is stopped, a downward readjustment of the dosage if insulin or oral hypoglycemic agent be necessary to avoid hypoglycemia. At all times, close monitoring of urinary glucose levels is mandatory in such patients.

4. In case of concomitant oral anticoagulant therapy, the prothrombin time should be measured frequently to determine if the dosage of oral anticoagulants is to be readjusted.

5. Partial loss of hair may be experienced by children in the first few months of thyroid therapy, but this is usually a transient phenomenon and later recovery is usually the rule.

LABORATORY TESTS

Treatment of patients with thyroid hormones requires the periodic assessment of thyroid status by means of appropriate laboratory tests besides the full clinical evaluation. The TSH suppression test can be used to test the effectiveness of any thyroid preparation bearing in mind the relative insensitivity of the infant pituitary to the negative feedback effect of thyroid hormones. Serum T_4 levels can be used to test the effectiveness of all thyroid medications except T_3. When the total serum T_4 is low but TSH is normal, a test specific to assess unbound (free) T_4 levels is warranted. Specific measurements of T_4 and T_3 by competitive protein binding or radioimmunoassay are not influenced by blood levels of organic or inorganic iodine.

DRUG/LABORATORY TEST INTERACTIONS

The following drugs or moieties are known to interfere with laboratory tests performed in patients on thyroid hormone therapy: androgens, corticosteroids, estrogens, oral contraceptives containing estrogens, iodine-containing preparations, and the numerous preparations containing salicylates.

1. Changes in TBg concentration should be taken into consideration in the interpretation of levothyroxine (T_4) and liothyronine (T_3) values. In such cases, the unbound (free) hormone should be measured. Pregnancy, estrogens, and estrogen-containing oral contraceptives increase TBg concentrations. TBg may also be increased during infectious hepatitis. Decreases

PRECAUTIONS: *(cont'd)*

in TBg concentrations are observed in nephrosis, acromegaly, and after androgen or corticosteroid therapy. Familial hyper- or hypothyroxine-binding globulinemias have been described. The incidence of TBg deficiency approximates 1 in 9,000. The binding of levothyroxine by TBPA is inhibited by salicylates.

2. Medicinal or dietary iodine interferes with all *in vivo* tests of radio-iodine uptake, producing low uptakes which may not be relative of a true decrease in hormone synthesis.

3. The persistence of clinical and laboratory evidence of hypothyroidism in spite of adequate dosage replacement indicates either poor patient compliance, poor absorption, excessive fecal loss, or inactivity of the preparation. Intracellular resistance to thyroid hormone is quite rare.

CARCINOGENESIS, MUTAGENESIS, AND IMPAIRMENT OF FERTILITY

A reportedly apparent association between prolonged thyroid therapy and breast cancer has not been confirmed and patients on thyroid for established indication should not discontinue therapy. No confirmatory long-term studies in animals have been performed to evaluate carcinogenic potential, mutagenicity, or impairment of fertility in either males or females.

PREGNANCY CATEGORY A

Thyroid hormones do not readily cross the placental barrier. The clinical experience to date does not indicate any adverse effect on fetuses when thyroid hormones are administered to pregnant women. On the basis of current knowledge, thyroid replacement therapy to hypothyroid women should not be discontinued during pregnancy.

NURSING MOTHERS

Minimal amounts of thyroid hormones are excreted in human milk. Thyroid is not associated with serious adverse reactions and does not have a known tumorigenic potential. However, caution should be exercised when thyroid is administered to a nursing woman.

PEDIATRIC USE

Pregnant mothers provide little or no thyroid hormone to the fetus. The incidence of congenital hypothyroidism is relatively high (1:4,000) and the hypothyroid fetus would not derive any benefit from the small amounts of hormone crossing the placental barrier. Routine determinations of serum T_4 and/or TSH is strongly advised in neonates in view of the deleterious effects of thyroid deficiency on growth and development.

Treatment should be initiated immediately upon diagnosis, and maintained for life, unless transient hypothyroidism is suspected, in which case, therapy may be interrupted for 2 to 8 weeks after the age of 3 years to reassess the condition. Cessation of therapy is justified in patients who have maintained a normal TSH during those 2 to 8 weeks.

DRUG INTERACTIONS:

ORAL ANTICOAGULANTS

Thyroid hormones appear to increase catabolism of vitamin K-dependent clotting factors. If oral anticoagulants are also being given, compensatory increases in clotting factor synthesis are impaired. Patients stabilized on oral anticoagulants who are found to require thyroid replacement therapy should be watched very closely when thyroid is started. If a patient is truly hypothyroid, it is likely that a reduction in anticoagulant dosage will be required. No special precautions appear to be necessary when oral anticoagulant therapy is begun in a patient already stabilized on maintenance thyroid replacement therapy.

INSULIN OR ORAL HYPOGLYCEMICS

Initiating thyroid replacement therapy may cause increases in insulin or oral hypoglycemic requirements. The effects seen are poorly understood and depend upon a variety of factors such as dose and type of thyroid preparations and endocrine status of the patient. Patients receiving insulin or oral hypoglycemics should be closely watched during initiation of thyroid replacement therapy.

CHOLESTYRAMINE OR COLESTIPOL

Cholestyramine or colestipol binds both levothyroxine (T_4) and liothyronine (T_3) in the intestine, thus impairing absorption of these thyroid hormones. *In vitro* studies indicate that the binding is not easily removed. Therefore, four to five hours should elapse between administration of cholestyramine of colestipol and thyroid hormones.

ESTROGEN ORAL CONTRACEPTIVES

Estrogens tend to increase serum thyroxine-binding globulin (TBg). In a patient with a nonfunctioning thyroid gland who is receiving thyroid replacement therapy, free levothyroxine (T_4) may be decreased when estrogens are started thus increasing thyroid requirements. However, if the patient's thyroid gland has sufficient function, the decreased free levothyroxine (T_4) will result in a compensatory increase in levothyroxine (T_4) output by the thyroid. Therefore, patients without a functioning thyroid gland who are on thyroid replacement therapy may need to increase their thyroid dose if estrogens or estrogen-containing oral contraceptives are given.

ADVERSE REACTIONS:

Adverse reactions other than those indicative of hyperthyroidism because of therapeutic overdosage, either initially or during the maintenance period, are rare (see OVERDOSAGE.)

OVERDOSAGE:

SIGNS AND SYMPTOMS

Excessive doses of thyroid result in a hypermetabolic state resembling in every respect the condition of endogenous origin. The condition may be self-induced.

TREATMENT

Dosage should be reduced or therapy temporarily discontinued if signs and symptoms of overdosage appear.

Treatment may be reinstituted at a lower dosage. In normal individuals, normal hypothalamic-pituitary-thyroid axis function is restored in 6 to 8 weeks after thyroid suppression.

Treatment of acute massive thyroid hormone overdosage is aimed at reducing gastrointestinal absorption of the drugs and counteracting central, and peripheral effect, mainly those of increased sympathetic activity. Vomiting may be induced initially if further gastrointestinal absorption can reasonably be prevented and barring contraindications such as coma, convulsions, or loss of the gagging reflex. Treatment is symptomatic and supportive. Oxygen may be administered and ventilation maintained. Cardiac glycosides may be indicated if congestive heart failure develops. Measures to control fever, hypoglycemia, or fluid loss should be instituted if needed. Antiadrenergic agents, particularly propranolol, have been used advantageously in the treatment of increased sympathetic activity. Propranolol may be administered intravenously at a dosage of 1 to 3 mg, over a 10-minute period or orally 80 to 160 mg/day, initially, especially when no contraindications exist for its use.

Other adjunctive measures may include administration of cholestyramine to interfere with thyroxine absorption, and glucocorticoids to inhibit conversion T_4 to T_3.

DOSAGE AND ADMINISTRATION:

The dosage of thyroid hormones is determined by the indication and must in every case be individualized according to patient response and laboratory findings.

DOSAGE AND ADMINISTRATION: *(cont'd)*

Thyroid hormones are given orally in acute emergency conditions. Injectable levothyroxine sodium (T_4) may be given intravenously when oral administration is not feasible or desirable as in the treatment of myxedema coma, or during total parenteral nutrition. Intramuscular administration is not advisable because of reported poor absorption.

HYPOTHYROIDISM

Therapy is usually instituted using low doses, with increments which depend on the cardiovascular status of the patient. The usual starting dose is 30 mg thyroid with increments of 15 mg every 2 to 3 weeks. A lower starting dosage, 15 mg/day, is recommended in patients with long- standing myxedema, particularly if cardiovascular impairment is suspected, in which case extreme caution is recommended. The appearance of angina is an indication for a reduction in dosage. Most patients require 60 to 120 mg/day. Failure to respond to doses of 180 mg suggests lack of compliance or malabsorption. Maintenance dosages 60 to 120 mg/day usually result in normal serum $T_4$and T_3 levels. Adequate therapy usually results in normal TSH and T_4 levels after 2 to 3 weeks of therapy.

Readjustment of thyroid hormone dosage should be made within the first four weeks of therapy, after proper clinical and laboratory evaluations, including serum levels of T_4, bound and free, and TSH.

Liothyronine (T_3) may be used in preference to levothyroxine (T_4) during radio-isotope scanning procedures, since induction of hypothyroidism in those cases is more abrupt and can be of shorter duration. It may also be preferred when impairment of peripheral conversion of levothyroxine (T_4) and liothyronine (T_3) is suspected.

MYXEDEMA COMA

Myxedema coma is usually precipitated in the hypothyroid patient of long- standing by intercurrent illness or drugs such as sedatives and anesthetics and should be considered a medical emergency. Therapy should be directed at the correction of electrolytes disturbances and possible infection besides the administration of thyroid hormones. Corticosteroids should be administered routinely. Levothyroxine (T_4) and liothyronine (T_3) may be administered via a nasogastric tube but the preferred route of administration of both hormones is intravenous. Levothyroxine sodium (T_4) is given at a starting dose of 400 mcg (100 mcg/ml) given rapidly, and is usually well tolerated, even in the elderly. This initial dose is followed by daily supplements of 100 to 200 mcg given IV. Normal T_4 levels are achieved in 24 hours followed in 3 days by threefold elevation of T_3. Oral therapy with thyroid hormone would be resumed as soon as the clinical situation has been stabilized and the patient is able to take oral medication.

THYROID CANCER

Exogenous thyroid hormone may produce regression of metastases from follicular and papillary carcinoma of the thyroid and is used as ancillary therapy of these conditions with radioactive iodine. TSH should be suppressed to low or undetectable levels. Therefore, larger amounts of thyroid hormone than those used for replacement therapy are required. Medullary carcinoma of the thyroid is usually unresponsive to this therapy.

THYROID SUPPRESSION THERAPY

Administration of thyroid hormone in doses higher than those produced physiologically by the gland results in suppression of the production of endogenous hormone. This is the basis for the thyroid suppression test and is used as an aid in the diagnosis of patients with signs of mild hyperthyroidism in whom base line laboratory tests appear normal, or to demonstrate thyroid gland autonomy in patients with Grave's ophthalmology. ^{131}I uptake is determined before and after the administration of the exogenous hormone. A 50 percent or greater suppression of uptake indicates a normal thyroid-pituitary axis and thus rules out thyroid gland autonomy.

For adults, the usual suppressive dose of levothyroxine (T_4) is 1.56 mg/kg of body weight per day given for 7 to 10 days. These doses usually yield normal serum T_4 and T_3 levels and lack of response to TSH.

Thyroid hormones should be administered cautiously to patients in whom there is strong suspicion of thyroid gland autonomy, in view of the fact that the exogenous hormone effects will be additive to the endogenous source.

PEDIATRIC DOSAGE

Pediatric dosage should follow the recommendation summarized in TABLE 1. In infants with congenital hypothyroidism, therapy with full doses should be instituted as soon as the diagnosis has been made.

TABLE 1 Recommended Pediatric Dosage for Congenital Hypothyroidism

	Thyroid Tablets	
Age	Dose Per Day	Daily dose per kg of body weight
0 - 6 months	15 - 30 mg	4.8 - 6 mg
6 - 12 months	30 - 45 mg	3.6 - 4.8 mg
1 - 5 years	45 - 60 mg	3 - 3.6 mg
6 - 12 years	60 - 90 mg	2.4 - 3 mg
Over 12 years	Over 90 mg	1.2 - 1.8

Note:(T_3 liothyronine is approximately four times as potent as T_4 levothyroxine on a microgram for microgram basis.)

Storage: Tablets should be stored at controlled room temperature, 59-86°F (15-30°).

HOW SUPPLIED - RATED THERAPEUTICALLY EQUIVALENT:

Tablet, Uncoated - Oral - 60 mg

100's	$5.89	Thyroid, Harber Pharm	51432-0458-03
1000's	$20.95	Thyroid, Harber Pharm	51432-0458-06

Tablet, Uncoated - Oral - 120 mg

100's	$3.15	Thyroid, Harber Pharm	51432-0460-03
1000's	$31.15	Thyroid, Harber Pharm	51432-0460-06

HOW SUPPLIED - NOT RATED EQUIVALENT:

Tablet, Uncoated - Oral - 15 mg

100's	**$8.28**	**ARMOUR THYROID, Forest Pharms**	**00456-0457-01**

Tablet, Uncoated - Oral - 30 mg

100's	$4.50	Thyroid, Major Pharms	00904-7865-60
100's	$4.62	Thyroid, Time-Caps Labs	49483-0021-01
100's	$5.00	Thyroid, Consolidated Midland	00223-2072-01
100's	$8.36	Thyroid, HL Moore Drug Exch	00839-7931-06
100's	**$9.71**	**ARMOUR THYROID, Forest Pharms**	**00456-0458-01**
100's	**$17.04**	**ARMOUR THYROID, Forest Pharms**	**00456-0458-63**
1000's	$8.00	Thyroid, Calvin Scott	17224-0109-10
1000's	$9.13	Thyroid, Rugby	00536-4694-10
1000's	$11.22	Thyroid, Time-Caps Labs	49483-0021-10
1000's	$11.65	Thyroid, United Res	00677-0150-10
1000's	$12.00	Thyroid, C O Truxton	00463-6199-10
1000's	$12.35	Thyroid, Qualitest Pharms	00603-6045-32
1000's	$13.45	Thyroid, Major Pharms	00904-7865-80

HOW SUPPLIED - NOT RATED EQUIVALENT: *(cont'd)*

1000's	$17.50	Thyroid, Consolidated Midland	00223-2072-02
1000's	$38.14	Thyroid, HL Moore Drug Exch	00839-7931-16
1000's	**$77.52**	**ARMOUR THYROID, Forest Pharms**	**00456-0458-00**
50000's	**$2720.28**	**ARMOUR THYROID, Forest Pharms**	**00456-0458-69**

Tablet, Uncoated - Oral - 60 mg

100's	$3.03	Thyroid, Time-Caps Labs	49483-0022-01
100's	$8.61	Thyroid, RID	54807-0891-01
100's	**$10.79**	**ARMOUR THYROID, Forest Pharms**	**00456-0459-01**
100's	**$18.12**	**ARMOUR THYROID, Forest Pharms**	**00456-0459-63**
1000's	$14.61	Thyroid, Time-Caps Labs	49483-0022-10
1000's	$18.11	Thyroid, Qualitest Pharms	00603-6046-32
1000's	$21.19	Thyroid, Rugby	00536-4706-10
1000's	**$104.23**	**ARMOUR THYROID, Forest Pharms**	**00456-0459-00**
5000's	$37.35	Thyroid, Rugby	00536-4706-50
5000's	**$404.96**	**ARMOUR THYROID, Forest Pharms**	**00456-0459-51**
50000's	**$3022.54**	**ARMOUR THYROID, Forest Pharms**	**00456-0459-69**

Tablet, Uncoated - Oral - 65 mg

10's	$14.00	Thyroid Igr Natural, Calvin Scott	17224-0113-10
100's	$4.80	Thyroid, Major Pharms	00904-0761-60
100's	$5.50	Thyroid, Consolidated Midland	00223-2074-01
1000's	$11.94	Thyroid, Rugby	00536-4702-10
1000's	$12.14	Thyroid, HL Moore Drug Exch	00839-5041-16
1000's	$14.50	Thyroid, C O Truxton	00463-6201-10
1000's	$17.00	Thyroid, Calvin Scott	17224-0110-10
1000's	$17.75	Thyroid, United Res	00677-0151-10
1000's	$18.00	Thyroid, Goldline Labs	00182-0493-10
1000's	$20.50	Thyroid, Major Pharms	00904-0761-80
1000's	$22.50	Thyroid, Consolidated Midland	00223-2074-02
5000's	$43.80	Thyroid, Rugby	00536-4702-50

Tablet, Uncoated - Oral - 90 mg

100's	**$17.04**	**ARMOUR THYROID, Forest Pharms**	**00456-0460-01**

Tablet, Uncoated - Oral - 120 mg

100's	$3.96	Thyroid, Time-Caps Labs	49483-0023-01
100's	$12.44	Thyroid, RID	54807-0892-01
100's	**$19.96**	**ARMOUR THYROID, Forest Pharms**	**00456-0461-01**
100's	**$22.60**	**ARMOUR THYROID, Forest Pharms**	**00456-0461-63**
1000's	$24.27	Thyroid, Time-Caps Labs	49483-0023-10
1000's	$26.71	Thyroid, Qualitest Pharms	00603-6047-32
1000's	**$199.57**	**ARMOUR THYROID, Forest Pharms**	**00456-0461-00**
50000's	**$5599.93**	**ARMOUR THYROID, Forest Pharms**	**00456-0461-69**

Tablet, Uncoated - Oral - 130 mg

10's	$17.00	Thyroid 2Gr Natural, Calvin Scott	17224-0123-10
100's	$5.95	Thyroid 2 Gr, Major Pharms	00904-0762-60
100's	$6.00	Thyroid, Consolidated Midland	00223-2076-01
1000's	$15.50	Thyroid, Rugby	00536-4710-10
1000's	$18.50	Thyroid, C O Truxton	00463-6203-10
1000's	$22.00	Thyroid, Calvin Scott	17224-0121-10
1000's	$24.29	Thyroid, HL Moore Drug Exch	00839-1672-16
1000's	$25.00	Thyroid, Consolidated Midland	00223-2076-02
1000's	$28.70	Thyroid 2 Gr, Major Pharms	00904-0762-80
1000's	$29.95	Thyroid, United Res	00677-0153-10
1000's	$30.00	Thyroid, Goldline Labs	00182-0494-10
1000's	$32.17	Thyroid 2 Grain, Rugby	00536-4714-10
5000's	$65.20	Thyroid, Rugby	00536-4710-50

Tablet, Uncoated - Oral - 180 mg

100's	$5.25	Thyroid, Time-Caps Labs	49483-0038-01
100's	$7.95	Thyroid, Major Pharms	00904-0763-60
100's	**$31.68**	**ARMOUR THYROID, Forest Pharms**	**00456-0462-01**
1000's	$26.93	Thyroid, Rugby	00536-4711-10
1000's	$33.30	Thyroid, Qualitest Pharms	00603-6048-32
1000's	$36.39	Thyroid, Time-Caps Labs	49483-0038-10
1000's	$36.70	Thyroid, Major Pharms	00904-0763-80
1000's	**$316.97**	**ARMOUR THYROID, Forest Pharms**	**00456-0462-00**

Tablet, Uncoated - Oral - 240 mg

100's	**$47.47**	**ARMOUR THYROID, Forest Pharms**	**00456-0463-01**

Tablet, Uncoated - Oral - 300 mg

100's	**$58.84**	**ARMOUR THYROID, Forest Pharms**	**00456-0464-01**

TICARCILLIN DISODIUM *(002352)*

CATEGORIES: Anti-Infectives; Antibiotics; Broad Spectrum Penicillins; Cystic Fibrosis; Endometritis; Genitourinary Tract Infections; Infections; Intra-Abdominal Infections; Lung Abscess; Pelvic Inflammatory Disease; Penicillins; Peritonitis; Pneumonitis; Pulmonary Abscess; Respiratory Tract Infections; Septicemia; Skin Infections; FDA Approval Pre 1982

BRAND NAMES: **Ticar**

FORMULARIES: BC-BS

DESCRIPTION:

Ticar (ticarcillin disodium) is a semisynthetic injectable penicillin derived from the penicillin nucleus, 6-aminopenicillanic acid. Chemically, it is *N*- (2-Carboxy-3,3-dimethyl-7-oxo-4-thia-1-azabicyclo (3.2.0) hept -6-yl)-3-thiophenemalonamic acid disodium salt.

It is supplied as a white to pale yellow powder for reconstitution. The reconstituted solution is clear, colorless or pale yellow, having a pH of 6.0 to 8.0. Ticarcillin is very soluble in water, its solubility is greater than 600 mg/ml.

CLINICAL PHARMACOLOGY:

Ticarcillin is not absorbed orally, therefore, it must be given intravenously or intramuscularly. Following intramuscular administration, peak serum concentrations occur within 1/2 to 1 hour. Somewhat higher and more prolonged serum levels can be achieved with the concurrent administration of probenecid.

The minimum inhibitory concentrations (MIC) for many strains of*Pseudomonas* are relatively high by usual standards; serum levels of 60 mcg/ml or greater are required. However, the low degree of toxicity of ticarcillin permits the use of doses large enough to achieve inhibitory levels for these strains in serum or tissues. Other susceptible organisms usually require serum levels in the 10-25 mcg/ml range (TABLE 1).

As with other penicillins, ticarcillin is eliminated by glomerular filtration and tubular secretion. It is not highly bound to serum protein (approximately 45%) and is excreted unchanged in high concentrations in the urine. After the administration of a 1 to 2 gram IM dose, a urine concentration of 2000 to 4000 mcg/ml may be obtained in patients with normal renal function. The serum half-life of ticarcillin in normal individuals is approximately 70 minutes.

CLINICAL PHARMACOLOGY: *(cont'd)*

TABLE 1 Ticarcillin Serum Levels mcg/ml

Dosage	Route	1/4 hr.	1/2 hr.	1 hr.	2 hr.	3 hr.	4 hr.	6 hr.
Adults:								
500 mg	IM	-	7.7	8.6	6.0	4.0	-	2.9
1 g	IM	-	31.0	18.7	15.7	9.7	-	3.4
2 g	IM	-	63.6	39.7	32.3	18.9	-	3.4
3 g	IV	190.0	140.0	107.0	52.2	31.3	13.8	4.2
5 g	IV	327.0	280.0	175.0	106.0	63.0	28.5	9.6
3 g + 1 g Probenecid	IV Oral	223.0	166.0	123.0	78.0	54.0	35.4	17.1
Neonates:		1/2 hr.	1 hr.	1 1/2 hr.	2 hr.	4 hr.	8 hr.	
50 mg/kg	IM	64.0	70.7	63.7	60.1	33.2	11.6	

An inverse relationship exists between serum half-life and creatinine clearance, but the dosage of tirarcillin disodium need only be adjusted in cases of severe renal impairment (see DOSAGE AND ADMINISTRATION). The administered ticarcillin may be removed from patients undergoing dialysis; the actual amount removed depends on the duration and type of dialysis.

Ticarcillin can be detected in tissues and interstitial fluid following parenteral administration. Penetration into the cerebrospinal fluid, bile and pleural fluid has been demonstrated.

MICROBIOLOGY

Ticarcillin is bactericidal and demonstrates substantial *in vitro* activity against both Gram-positive and Gram-negative organisms. Many strains of the following organisms were found to be susceptible to ticarcillin *in vitro*:

Pseudomonas aeruginosa (and other species); *Escherichia coli; Proteus mirabilis; Morganella morganii (formerly Proteus morganii); Providencia rettgeri (formerly Proteus rettgeri); Proteus vulgaris; Enterobacter species; Haemophilus influenzae; Neisseria* species.

Salmonella species; *Staphylococcus aureus* (non- penicillinase producing); *Staphylococcus epidermidis;* Beta- hemolytic streptococci (Group A); *Streptococcus faecalis (Enterococcus); Streptococcus pneumoniae.*

Anaerobic bacteria, including: *Bacteroides* species including*B. fragilis; Fusobacterium* species; *Veillonella* species; *Clostridium; Eubacterium* species; *Peptococcus* species;*Peptostreptococcus* species.

In vitro synergism between ticarcillin and gentamicin sulfate, tobramycin sulfate or amikacin sulfate against certain strains of *Pseudomonas aeruginosa* has been demonstrated.

Some strains of such microorganisms as *Mima-Herellea (Acinetobacter), Citrobacter* and *Serratia* have shown susceptibility.

Ticarcillin is not stable in the presence of penicillinase.

Some strains of *Pseudomonas* have developed resistance fairly rapidly.

DISK SUSCEPTIBILITY TESTS

Ticarcillin disks or powders should be used for testing susceptibility to ticarcillin. However, organisms reportedly susceptible to carbenicillin are susceptible to ticarcillin.

Diffusion Techniques: For the disk diffusion method of susceptibility testing a 75 mcg tirarcillin disodium disk should be used. The method for this test is the one outlined in NCCLS publication M2-A3* with the interpretative criteria found in TABLE 2.

TABLE 2

Culture	Susceptible	Intermediate Resistant
P. aeruginosa and *Enterobacteriaceae*	≥15 mm	12-14 mm ≤11 mm
The MIC correlates are:	Resistant > 128 mcg/ml Susceptible ≤64 mcg/ml	

Dilution Techniques: Dilution techniques for determining the MIC (minimum inhibitory concentration) are published by NCCLS for the broth and agar dilution procedures. The MIC data should be interpreted in light of the concentrations present in serum, tissue, and body fluids. Organisms with MIC ≤64 are considered susceptible when they are in tissue but organisms with MIC ≤128 would be susceptible in urine where the tirarcillin disodium concentrations are much greater. At present, only dilution methods can be recommended for testing antibiotic susceptibility of obligate anaerobes.

Susceptibility testing methods require the use of control organisms. The 75 mcg ticarcillin disk should give zone diameters between 22 and 28 mm for *P. aeruginosa* ATCC 27853 and 24 and 30 mm for *E. Coli* ATCC 25922. Reference strains are available for dilution testing of ticarcillin. 95% of the MIC's should fall within the following MIC ranges and the majority of MIC's should be at values close to the center of the pertinent range. (Reference NCCLS publication M7-A**)

S. aureus ATCC 29213, 2.0 to 8.0 mcg/ml; *S. faecalis* ATCC 29212, 16 to 64 mcg/ml; *E. coli* ATCC 25922, 2.0 to 8.0 mcg/ml; *P. aeruginosa* ATCC 27853, 8.0 to 32 mcg/ml.

*Performance standards for Antimicrobial Disk Susceptibility Tests, National Committee for Clinical Laboratory Standards, Vol. 4, No. 16, pp. 369-402, 1984.

**Methods for Dilution Antimicrobial Susceptibility Tests for Bacteria That Grow Aerobically, Vol. 5, No. 22, pp. 579-618, 1985.

INDICATIONS AND USAGE:

Tirarcillin disodium is indicated for the treatment of the following infections:

Bacterial septicemia (†)

Skin and soft-tissue infections (†)

Acute and chronic respiratory tract infections (†)(‡)

† caused by susceptible strains of *Pseudomonas aeruginosa, Proteus* species (both indole-positive and indole-negative) and *Escherichia coli.*

‡ (Though clinical improvement has been shown, bacteriological cures cannot be expected in patients with chronic respiratory disease or cystic fibrosis.)

Genitourinary tract infections (complicated and uncomplicated) due to susceptible strains of *Pseudomonas aeruginosa, Proteus* species (both indole-positive and indole-negative), *Escherichia coli, Enterobacter* and *Streptococcus faecalis* (enterococcus).

Ticarcillin is also indicated in the treatment of the following infections due to susceptible anaerobic bacteria:

1. Bacterial septicemia.

2. Lower respiratory tract infections such as empyema, anaerobic pneumonitis and lung abscess.

INDICATIONS AND USAGE: *(cont'd)*

3. Intra-abdominal infections such as peritonitis and intra-abdominal abscess (typically resulting from anaerobic organisms resident in the normal gastrointestinal tract).

4. Infections of the female pelvis and genital tract, such as endometritis, pelvic inflammatory disease, pelvic abscess and salpingitis.

5. Skin and soft-tissue infections.

Although ticarcillin is primarily indicated in gram-negative infections, its *in vitro* activity against gram-positive organisms should be considered in treating infections caused by both gram-negative and gram-positive organisms (see CLINICAL PHARMACOLOGY, Microbiology).

Based on the *in vitro* synergism between ticarcillin and gentamicin sulfate, tobramycin sulfate or amikacin sulfate against certain strains of *Pseudomonas aeruginosa*, combined therapy has been successful, using full therapeutic dosages. (For additional prescribing information, see the gentamicin sulfate, tobramycin sulfate and amikacin sulfate package inserts.)

NOTE: Culturing and susceptibility testing should be performed initially and during treatment to monitor the effectiveness of therapy and the susceptibility of the bacteria.

CONTRAINDICATIONS:

A history of allergic reaction to any of the penicillins is a contraindication.

WARNINGS:

Serious and occasionally fatal hypersensitivity (anaphylactoid) reactions have been reported in patients receiving penicillin. These reactions are more likely to occur in persons with a history of sensitivity to multiple allergens.

There are reports of patients with a history of penicillin hypersensitivity reactions who experience severe hypersensitivity reactions when treated with a cephalosporin. Before therapy with a penicillin, careful inquiry should be made about previous hypersensitivity reactions to penicillins, cephalosporins, and other allergens. If a reaction occurs, the drug should be discontinued unless, in the opinion of the physician, the condition being treated is life-threatening and amenable only to ticarcillin therapy. **Serious anaphylactoid reactions require immediate emergency treatment with epinephrine. Oxygen, intravenous steroids, airway management, including intubation, should also be administered as indicated.**

Some patients receiving high doses of ticarcillin may develop hemorrhagic manifestations associated with abnormalities of coagulation tests, such as bleeding time and platelet aggregation. On withdrawal of the drug, the bleeding should cease and coagulation abnormalities revert to normal. Other causes of abnormal bleeding should also be considered. Patients with renal impairment, in whom excretion of ticarcillin is delayed, should be observed for bleeding manifestations. Such patients should be dosed strictly according to recommendations (see DOSAGE AND ADMINISTRATION). If bleeding manifestations appear, ticarcillin treatment should be discontinued and appropriate therapy instituted.

Pseudomembranous colitis has been reported with nearly all antibacterial agents, including Ticar, and has ranged in severity from mild to life-threatening. Therefore, it is important to consider this diagnosis in patients who present with diarrhea subsequent to the administration of antibacterial agents.

Treatment with antibacterial agents alters the normal flora of the colon and may permit overgrowth of clostridia. Studies indicate that a toxin produced by *Clostridium difficile* is 1 primary cause of "antibiotic colitis."

Mild cases of pseudomembranous colitis usually respond to drug discontinuation alone. In moderate to severe cases, consideration should be given to management with fluids and electrolytes, protein supplementation and treatment with an antibacterial drug effective against *C. difficile.*

PRECAUTIONS:

Although ticarcillin disodium exhibits the characteristic low toxicity of the penicillins, as with any other potent agent, it is advisable to check periodically for organ system dysfunction (including renal, hepatic and hematopoietic) during prolonged treatment. If overgrowth of resistant organisms occurs, the appropriate therapy should be initiated.

Since the theoretical sodium content is 5.2 milliequivalents (120 mg) per gram of ticarcillin, and the actual vial content can be as high as 6.5 mEq/g, electrolyte and cardiac status should be monitored carefully.

In a few patients receiving intravenous ticarcillin, hypokalemia has been reported. Serum potassium should be measured periodically, and, if necessary, corrective therapy should be implemented.

As with any penicillin, the possibility of an allergic response, including anaphylaxis, exists, particularly in hypersensitive patients.

USAGE IN PREGNANCY

Reproduction studies have been performed in mice and rats and have revealed no evidence of impaired fertility or harm to the fetus due to ticarcillin. There are no well-controlled studies in pregnant women, but investigational experience does not include any positive evidence of adverse effects on the fetus. Although there is no clearly defined risk, such experience cannot exclude the possibility of infrequent or subtle damage to the fetus. Ticarcillin should be used in pregnant women only when clearly needed.

ADVERSE REACTIONS:

The following adverse reactions may occur:

Hypersensitivity Reactions: Skin rashes, pruritus, urticaria, drug fever.

Gastrointestinal Disturbances: Nausea and vomiting, pseudomembranous colitis symptoms may occur during or after antibiotic treatment. (See WARNINGS).

Hemic and Lymphatic Systems: As with other penicillins, anemia, thrombocytopenia, leukopenia, neutropenia and eosinophilia.

Abnormalities of Blood, Hepatic and Renal Laboratory Studies: As with other semisynthetic penicillins, SGOT and SGPT elevations have been reported. To date, clinical manifestations of hepatic or renal disorders have not been observed which could be ascribed solely to ticarcillin.

CNS: Patients, especially those with impaired renal function, may experience convulsions or neuromuscular excitability when very high doses of the drug are administered.

Other: Local reactions such as pain (rarely accompanied by induration) at the site of the injection have been reported.

Vein irritation and phlebitis can occur, particularly when undiluted solution is directly injected into the vein.

DOSAGE AND ADMINISTRATION:

Clinical experience indicates that in serious urinary tract and systemic infections, intravenous therapy in the higher doses should be used. Intramuscular injections should not exceed 2 grams per injection (TABLE 3 and TABLE 4).

NOTE: Gentamicin, tobramycin or amikacin may be used concurrently with ticarcillin for initial therapy until results of culture and susceptibility studies are known.

DOSAGE AND ADMINISTRATION: *(cont'd)*

TABLE 3

Bacterial Septicemia	200-300 mg/kg/day by IV infusion in divided doses every 4 or 6 hours.
Respiratory Tract infections	(The usual dose is 3 gm given every 4 hours (18 gm/day) or 4 gm given every 6 hours.
Skin and Soft-Tissue infections	16 gm/day) depending on weight and the severity of the infection.)
Intra-abdominal infections	
Infections of the Female Pelvis and Genital Tract	
Urinary Tract Infections	
Complicated:	150-200 mg/kg/day by IV infusion in divided doses every 4 or 6 hours. (Usual recommended dosage for average (70 kg) adults: 3 grams q.i.d.)
Uncomplicated:	1 gram IM or direct IV every 6 hours.
Infections complicated by renal insufficiency: (1)	Initial loading dose of 3 grams IV followed by IV doses, based on creatinine clearance and type of dialysis, as indicated below:
Creatinine clearance ml/min.:	
over 60	3 grams every 4 hours
30-60	2 grams every 4 hours
10-30	2 grams every 8 hours
less than 10	2 grams every 12 hours (or 1 grams IM every 6 hours)
less than 10 with hepatic dysfunction	2 grams every 24 hours (or 1 gram IM every 12 hours)
patients on peritoneal dialysis	3 grams every 12 hours
patients on hemodialysis	2 grams every 12 hours supplemented with 3 grams after each dialysis

(1) The-half-life of ticarcillin in patients with renal failure is approximately 13 hours.
To calculate creatine clearance* from a serum creatinine value use the following formula: Males: C_{cr} = [(140-Age)(wt in kg)] ÷ [72 × S_{cr} (mg/100 ml)]; Females: Value for males – 15%

* Cockcroft, D.W. et al. "Prediction of Creatinine Clearance from Serum Creatinine" Nephron16:31-41 (1976).

TABLE 4 Children: Under 40 kg (88 lbs)

The daily dose for children should not exceed the adult dosage.

Bacterial Septicemia	200-300 mg/kg/day by IV infusion in divided doses every 4 or 6 hours.
Respiratory Tract Infections	
Skin and Soft-Tissue Infections	
Intra-Abdominal Infections	
Infections of the Female Pelvis and Genital Tract	
Urinary Tract Infections	
Complicated:	150-200 mg/kg/day by IV infusion in divided doses every 4 or 6 hours.
Uncomplicated:	50-100 mg/kg/day IM or direct IV in divided doses every 6 or 8 hours.
Infections complicated by renal insufficiency:	Clinical data is insufficient to recommend optimum dose.

Children weighing more than 40 kg (88 lbs) should receive adult dosages.

Neonates: In the neonate, for severe infections (sepsis) due to susceptible strains of*Pseudomonas, Proteus,* and *E. coli*, the following ticarcillin dosages may be given IM or by 10-20 minutes IV infusion:

Infants under 2000 grams body weight:	Infants over 2000 grams body weight:
Aged 0-7 days 75 mg/kg/12 hours (150 mg/kg/day)	Aged 0-7 days 75 mg/kg/8 hours (225 mg/kg/day)
Aged over 7 days 75 mg/kg/8 hours (225 mg/kg/day)	Aged over 7 days 100 mg/kg/8 hrs. (300 mg/kg/day)

This dosage schedule is intended to produce peak serum concentrations of 125-150 mcg/ml one hour after a dose of ticarcillin and trough concentrations of 25-50 mcg/ml immediately before the next dose.

Seriously ill patients should receive the higher doses. Tirarcillin disodium has proved to be useful in infections in which protective mechanisms are impaired, such as in acute leukemia and during therapy with immunosuppressive or oncolytic drugs.

DIRECTIONS FOR USE

1 gm, 3 gm and 6 gm Standard Vials

Intramuscular Use : (Concentration of approximately 385 mg/ml).

For initial reconstitution use Sterile Water for Injection, U.S.P., Sodium Chloride Injection, U.S.P. or 1% Lidocaine Hydrochloride solution* (without epinephrine).

Each gram of ticarcillin should be reconstituted with 2 ml of Sterile Water for Injection, U.S.P., Sodium Chloride Injection, U.S.P. or 1% Lidocaine Hydrochloride solution* (without epinephrine) and used promptly. Each 2.6 ml of the resulting solution will then contain 1 gm of ticarcillin.

As with all intramuscular preparations, ticarcillin disodium should be injected well within the body of a relatively large muscle using usual techniques and precautions.

Intravenous Administration: (Concentration of approximately 200 mg/ml).

For initial reconstitution use Sodium Chloride Injection, U.S.P., Dextrose Injection 5% or Lactated Ringer's Injection.

Reconstitute each gram of ticarcillin with 4 ml of the appropriate diluent. After the addition of 4 ml of diluent per gram of ticarcillin each 1.0 ml of the resulting solution will have an approximate concentration of 200 mg. Once dissolved, further dilute if desired.

Direct Intravenous Injection: In order to avoid vein irritation, administer solution as slowly as possible.

Intravenous Infusion: Administer by continuous or intermittent intravenous drip. Intermittent infusion should be administered over a 30 minute to 2 hour period in equally divided doses.

3 g Piggyback Bottles

Direct Intravenous Injection: (Concentrations of approximately 29 mg/ml to 100 mg/ml).

The 3 gram bottle should be reconstituted with a minimum of 30 ml of the desired intravenous solution listed in TABLE 5.

In order to avoid vein irritation, the solution should be administered as slowly as possible. A dilution of approximately 50 mg/ml or more will further reduce the incidence of vein irritation.

Intravenous Infusion: Stability studies in the intravenous solutions (TABLE 6) indicate that ticarcillin disodium will provide sufficient activity at room temperature (70-75°F) within the stated time periods at concentrations between 10 mg/ml and 50 mg/ml - see TABLE 6

DOSAGE AND ADMINISTRATION: *(cont'd)*

TABLE 5

Amount of Diluent	Concentration of Solution
100 ml	1 gm/34 ml (≈29 mg/ml)
60 ml	1 gm/20 ml (50 mg/ml)
30 ml	1 gm/10 ml (100 mg/ml)

After reconstitution and prior to administration tirarcillin disodium as with other parenteral drugs should be inspected visually for particulate matter and discoloration.

TABLE 6 Stability Period

Intravenous Solution (concentration of 10 mg/ml to 100 mg/ml)21°-24°C(70°-75°F)	Room Temperature 4°C(40°F)	Refrigeration
Sodium Chloride Injection, U.S.P.	72 hours	14 days
Dextrose Injection 5%	72 hours	14 days
Lactated Ringer's Injection	48 hours	14 days

Refrigerated solutions stored longer than 72 hours should not be used for multidose purposes.

After reconstitution and dilution to a concentration of 10 mg/ml to 100 mg/ml, this solution can be frozen (0°F) and stored for up to 30 days. The thawed solution must be used within 24 hours.

Unused solutions should be discarded after the time periods mentioned above.

It is recommended that tirarcillin disodium and gentamicin sulfate, tobramycin sulfate or amikacin sulfate not be mixed together in the same IV solution due to the gradual inactivation of gentamicin sulfate, tobramycin sulfate or amikacin sulfate under these circumstances. The therapeutic effect of tirarcillin disodium and these aminoglycoside drugs remains unimpaired when administered separately.

*(For full product information, refer to lidocaine hydrochloride).

HOW SUPPLIED:

Ticar (sterile ticarcillin disodium). Each vial contains ticarcillin disodium equivalent to 1 gram, 3 grams, 6 grams of ticarcillin.

Ticar (sterile ticarcillin disodium). Each vial contains ticarcillin disodium equivalent to 20 grams, 30 grams, 3 grams of ticarcillin.

Store dry powder at room temperature or below.

HOW SUPPLIED - EQUIVALENTS NOT AVAILABLE:

Injection, Dry-Soln - Intramuscular; - 1 gm/vial

20 ml x 10	$3.68	TICAR, Beecham	00029-6550-22

Injection, Dry-Soln - Intramuscular; - 3 gm/vial

21 ml x 10	$9.60	TICAR ADD-VANTAGE, Beecham	00029-6552-40
50 ml x 10	$11.04	TICAR, Beecham	00029-6552-26
100 ml x 10	$11.82	TICAR, Beecham	00029-6552-21

Injection, Dry-Soln - Intramuscular; - 6 gm/vial

50 ml x 10	$17.50	TICAR, Beecham	00029-6555-26

Injection, Dry-Soln - Intravenous - 20 gm/vial

20 gm x 10	$67.87	TICAR, Beecham	00029-6558-21

Injection, Dry-Soln - Intravenous - 30 gm/vial

30 gm x 10	$99.69	TICAR, Beecham	00029-6559-21

TICLOPIDINE HYDROCHLORIDE *(003063)*

CATEGORIES: Antithrombotics; Cardiovascular Drugs; Platelet Aggregation Inhibitors; Stroke Prevention; Angina*; Pregnancy Category B; FDA Class 1B ("Modest Therapeutic Advantage"); FDA Approved 1991 Oct
* Indication not approved by the FDA

BRAND NAMES: *Anagregal*; *Antigreg*; *Clid*; *Declot*; *Licodin*; *Panaldine* (Japan); **Ticlid**; *Ticlidil*; *Ticlodix*; *Ticlodone*; *Ticlosan*; *Tiklid*; *Tiklyd* (Germany); *Tyklid*
(International brand names outside U.S. in italics)

FORMULARIES: PCS

DESCRIPTION:

Ticlid (ticlopidine hydrochloride) is a platelet aggregation inhibitor. Chemically it is 5-[(2-chlorophenyl)methyl]-4,5,6,7-tetrahydrothieno [3,2-c] pyridine hydrochloride.

Ticlopidine hydrochloride is a white crystalline solid. It is freely soluble in water and self buffers to a pH of 3.6. It also dissolves freely in methanol, is sparingly soluble in methylene chloride and ethanol, slightly soluble in acetone, and insoluble in a buffer solution of pH 6.3. It has a molecular weight of 300.25.

Ticlid tablets for oral administration are provided as white, oval, film coated, blue imprinted tablets containing 250 mg of ticlopidine hydrochloride. Each tablet also contains citric acid, magnesium stearate, microcrystalline cellulose, povidone, starch and stearic acid as inactive ingredients. The white film coating contains hydroxypropylmethyl cellulose, polyethylene glycol and titanium dioxide. Each tablet is printed with blue ink which includes FD&C Blue #1 aluminum lake as the colorant. The tablets are identified with "Ticlid" on one side and "250" on the reverse side.

CLINICAL PHARMACOLOGY:

Mechanism of Action: When taken orally, ticlopidine hydrochloride causes a time and dose-dependent inhibition of both platelet aggregation and release of platelet granule constituents, as well as a prolongation of bleeding time. The intact drug has no significant *in vitro* activity at the concentrations attained *in vivo*, and, although analysis of urine and plasma indicates at least twenty metabolites, no metabolite which accounts for the activity of ticlopidine has been isolated.

Ticlopidine hydrochloride, after oral ingestion, interferes with platelet membrane function by inhibiting ADP-induced platelet-fibrinogen binding and subsequent platelet-platelet interactions. The effect on platelet function is irreversible for the life of the platelet, as shown both by persistent inhibition of fibrinogen binding after washing platelets *ex vivo* and by inhibition of platelet aggregation after resuspension of platelets in buffered medium.

Pharmacokinetics and Metabolism: After oral administration of a single 250 mg dose, ticlopidine hydrochloride is rapidly absorbed, with peak plasma levels occurring at approximately 2 hours after dosing, and is extensively metabolized. Absorption is greater than 80%. Administration after meals results in a 20% increase in the AUC of ticlopidine.

CLINICAL PHARMACOLOGY: *(cont'd)*

Ticlopidine hydrochloride displays non-linear pharmacokinetics and clearance decreases markedly on repeated dosing. In older volunteers the apparent half-life of ticlopidine after a single 250 mg dose is about 12.6 hours, with repeat dosing at 250 mg BID, the terminal elimination half-life rises to 4-5 days and steady state levels of ticlopidine hydrochloride in plasma are obtained after approximately 14-21 days.

Ticlopidine hydrochloride binds reversibly (98%) to plasma proteins, mainly to serum albumin and lipoproteins. The binding to albumin and lipoproteins is nonsaturable over a wide concentration range. Ticlopidine also binds to alpha-1 acid glycoprotein. At concentrations attained with the recommended dose, only 15% or less ticlopidine in plasma is bound to this protein.

Ticlopidine hydrochloride is metabolized extensively by the liver; only trace amounts of intact drug are detected in the urine. Following an oral dose of radioactive ticlopidine hydrochloride administered in solution, 60% of the radioactivity is recovered in the urine and 23% in the feces. Approximately, 1/3 of the dose excreted in the feces is intact ticlopidine hydrochloride, possibly excreted in the bile. Ticlopidine hydrochloride is a minor component in plasma (5%) after a single dose, but at steady state is the major component (15%). Approximately 40-50% of the radioactive metabolites circulating in plasma are covalently bound to plasma proteins, probably by acylation.

Clearance of ticlopidine decreases with age. Steady state trough values in elderly patients (mean age 70 years) are about twice those in young volunteer populations.

Hepatically Impaired Patients: The effect of decreased hepatic function on the pharmacokinetics of Ticlid was studied in 17 patients with advanced cirrhosis. The average plasma concentration of ticlopidine in these subjects was slightly higher than that seen in older subjects in a separate trial. (See CONTRAINDICATIONS)

Renally Impaired Patients: Patients with mildly (Ccr 50-80 ml/min) or moderately (Ccr 20-50 ml/min) impaired renal function were compared to normal subjects (Ccr 80-150 ml/min) in a study of the pharmacokinetic and platelet pharmacodynamic effects of Ticlid (250 mg BID) for 11 days. Concentrations of unchanged Ticlid were measured after a single 250 mg dose and after the final 250 mg dose on Day 11.

AUC values of ticlopidine increased by 28 and 60% in mild and moderately impaired patients respectively and plasma clearance decreased by 37 and 52% respectively, but there were no statistically significant differences in ADP-induced platelet aggregation. In this small study (26 patients) bleeding times showed significant prolongation only in the moderately impaired patients.

Pharmacodynamics: In healthy volunteers over the age of 50 substantial inhibition (over 50%) of ADP-induced platelet aggregation is detected within 4 days after administration of ticlopidine hydrochloride 250 mg BID and maximum platelet aggregation inhibition (60-70%) is achieved after 8 to 11 days. Lower doses cause less, and more delayed, platelet aggregation inhibition, while doses above 250 mg BID give little additional effect on platelet aggregation, but an increased rate of adverse effects. The dose of 250 mg BID is the only dose that has been evaluated in controlled clinical trials.

After discontinuation of ticlopidine hydrochloride, bleeding time and other platelet function tests return to normal within two weeks in the majority of patients.

At the recommended therapeutic dose (250 mg BID), ticlopidine hydrochloride has no known significant pharmacological actions in man other than inhibition of platelet function and prolongation of the bleeding time.

CLINICAL STUDIES:

The effect of ticlopidine on the risk of stroke and cardiovascular events was studied in two multi-center randomized double-blind trials.

1. Study in patients experiencing stroke precursors: In a trial comparing ticlopidine and aspirin (The Ticlopidine Aspirin Stroke Study or TASS), 3069 patients (1987 men, 1082 women) who had experienced such stroke precursors as transient ischemic attack (TIA), transient monocular blindness (amaurosis fugax), reversible ischemic neurological deficit, or minor stroke were randomized to ticlopidine 250 mg BID or aspirin 650 mg BID. The study was designed to follow patients for at least 2 and up to 5 years.

Over the duration of the study, Ticlid significantly reduced the risk of fatal and nonfatal stroke by 24% (p =.011) from 18.1 to 13.8 per 100 patients followed for five years, compared to aspirin. During the first year, when the risk of stroke is greatest, the reduction in risk of stroke (fatal and nonfatal) compared to aspirin was 48%, the reduction was similar in men and women.

2. Study in patients who had a completed atherothrombotic stroke: In a trial comparing ticlopidine with placebo (The Canadian American Ticlopidine Study, or CATS) 1073 patients who had experienced a previous atherothrombotic stroke were treated with Ticlid 250 mg BID or placebo for up to 3 years.

Ticlid significantly reduced the overall risk of stroke by 24% (p =.017) from 24.6 to 18.6 per 100 patients followed for three years, compared to placebo. During the first year the reduction in risk of fatal and nonfatal stroke over placebo was 33%.

INDICATIONS AND USAGE:

Ticlid is indicated to reduce the risk of thrombotic stroke (fatal or nonfatal) in patients who have experienced stroke precursors, and in patients who have had a completed thrombotic stroke.

Because Ticlid is associated with a risk of neutropenia/agranulocytosis, which may be life-threatening (See WARNINGS), Ticlid should be reserved for patients who are intolerant to aspirin therapy where indicated to prevent stroke.

CONTRAINDICATIONS:

The use of Ticlid is contraindicated in the following conditions:

Hypersensitivity to the drug.

Presence of hematopoietic disorders such as neutropenia and thrombocytopenia.

Presence of a hemostatic disorder or active pathological bleeding (such as bleeding peptic ulcer or intracranial bleeding).

Patients with severe liver impairment.

WARNINGS:

Neutropenia

Neutropenia defined in these studies as an ANC <1200 neutrophils/mm3 occurred in 50 of 2,048 (2.4%) stroke patients who received ticlopidine HCl in clinical trials.

Severe Neutropenia (<450 neutrophils/mm3): Severe neutropenia and/or agranulocytosis occurred in 17 of the 2,048 (0.8%) patients who received ticlopidine HCl. When the drug was discontinued in these patients, the neutrophil counts returned to normal (>1200 neutrophils/mm3) within 1-3 weeks.

WARNINGS: *(cont'd)*

Mild to Moderate Neutropenia (451-1200 neutrophils/mm3): Mild to moderate neutropenia occurred in 33 of the 2,048 (1.6%) patients who received ticlopidine HCl. Eleven of the patients discontinued treatment and recovered within a few days. In the remaining 22 patients, the neutropenia was transient and did not require discontinuation of therapy.

The onset of severe neutropenia usually occurs 3 weeks to 3 months after the start of therapy. Nevertheless, in post-marketing experience there have been some reports of severe neutropenia beyond that time. The bone marrow typically showed a reduction in myeloid precursors. The onset of neutropenia may occur suddenly.

It is therefore essential that CBCs (including platelet count) and white cell differentials be performed every two weeks, starting at baseline before treatment is initiated to the end of the third month of therapy with ticlopidine HCl, but more frequent monitoring is necessary for patients whose absolute neutrophil counts have been consistently declining or are 30% less than the baseline count. Because of the long plasma half-life of ticlopidine HCl, it is recommended that any patient who discontinues ticlopidine HCl for any reason within the first 90 days continue to have CBC (including platelet count) monitoring and white cell differential for at least another two weeks after discontinuation of therapy.

Neutropenia (an absolute neutrophil count (ANC) of less than 1200 neutrophils/mm3) is calculated as follows: ANC = WBC x % neutrophils. If clinical evaluation and repeat laboratory testing confirm the presence of neutropenia (<1200/mm3), the drug should be discontinued.

In clinical trials, when therapy was discontinued immediately upon detection of neutropenia, the neutrophil counts typically returned to normal within 1-3 weeks. In post-marketing experience, there have been rare reports of fatalities.

After the first three months of therapy, CBCs need be obtained only for patients with signs or symptoms suggestive of infection.

Thrombocytopenia: Rarely, thrombocytopenia may occur in isolation or together with neutropenia.

If clinical evaluation and repeat laboratory testing confirm the presence of thrombocytopenia (<80,000 cells/mm^3), the drug should be discontinued. Rarely, immune thrombocytopenia (ITP) and thrombotic thrombocytopenic purpura (TTP) have been reported and some of these rare cases have been fatal. Therefore, careful attention to diagnosis should be made to guide treatment.

Other Hematological Effects: Rare cases of agranulocytosis, pancytopenia or aplastic anemia have been reported in post-marketing experience, some of which have been fatal. All forms of hematological adverse reactions are potentially fatal.

Cholesterol Evaluation: Ticlopidine HCl therapy causes increased serum cholesterol and triglycerides. Serum total cholesterol levels are increased 8-10% within one month of therapy and persist at that level. The ratios of the lipoprotein subfractions are unchanged.

Anticoagulant Drugs: The tolerance and safety of coadministration of ticlopidine HCl with heparin, oral anticoagulants, or fibrinolytic agents has not been established. If a patient is switched from an anticoagulant or fibrinolytic drug to ticlopidine HCl, the former drug should be discontinued prior to ticlopidine HCl administration.

PRECAUTIONS:

GENERAL

Ticlopidine HCl should be used with caution in patients who may be at risk of increased bleeding from trauma, surgery, or pathological conditions. If it is desired to eliminate the antiplatelet effects of ticlopidine HCl prior to elective surgery, the drug should be discontinued 10-14 days prior to surgery. Several controlled clinical studies have found increased surgical blood loss in patients undergoing surgery during treatment with ticlopidine. In TASS and CATS it was recommended that patients have ticlopidine discontinued prior to elective surgery. Several hundred patients underwent surgery during the trials, and no excessive surgical bleeding was reported.

Prolonged bleeding time is normalized within two hours after administration of 20 mg methylprednisolone IV. Platelet transfusions may also be used to reverse the effect of ticlopidine HCl on bleeding. Platelet transfusions are usually not indicated in patients with TTP on ticlopidine.

GI Bleeding: Ticlopidine HCl prolongs template bleeding time. The drug should be used with caution in patients who have lesions with a propensity to bleed (such as ulcers). Drugs that might induce such lesions should be used with caution in patients on ticlopidine HCl. (See CONTRAINDICATIONS.)

Use in Hepatically Impaired Patients: Since ticlopidine is metabolized by the liver, dosing of ticlopidine HCl or other drugs metabolized in the liver may require adjustment upon starting or stopping concomitant therapy. Because of limited experience in patients with severe hepatic disease, who may have bleeding diatheses, the use of ticlopidine HCl is not recommended in this population. (See CLINICAL PHARMACOLOGY and CONTRAINDICATIONS.)

Use in Renally Impaired Patients: There is limited experience in patients with renal impairment. Decreased plasma clearance, increased AUC values, and prolonged bleeding times can occur in renally impaired patients. In controlled clinical trials, no unexpected problems have been encountered in patients having mild renal impairment and there is no experience with dosage adjustment in patients with greater degrees of renal impairment. Nevertheless, for renally impaired patients it may be necessary to reduce the dosage of ticlopidine or discontinue it altogether, if hemorrhagic or hematopoietic problems are encountered.(See CLINICAL PHARMACOLOGY.)

INFORMATION FOR THE PATIENT

(See PATIENT PACKAGE INSERT) Patients should be told that a decrease in the number of white blood cells (neutropenia) can occur with ticlopidine HCl, especially during the first three months of treatment, and that if neutropenia is severe, it could result in an increased risk of infection. They should be told it is critically important to obtain the scheduled blood tests to detect neutropenia. Patients should also be reminded to contact their physicians if they experience any indication of infection such as fever, chill, and sore throat, all of which may be consequences of neutropenia.

All patients should be told that it may take them longer than usual to stop bleeding when they take ticlopidine HCl and that they should report any unusual bleeding to their physician. Patients should tell physicians and dentists that they are taking ticlopidine HCl before any surgery is scheduled and before any new drug is prescribed.

Patients should be told to report promptly side effects of ticlopidine HCl such as severe or persistent diarrhea, skin rashes, or subcutaneous bleeding, or any signs of cholestasis, such as yellow skin or sclera, dark urine, or light colored stools.

PRECAUTIONS: *(cont'd)*

Patients should be told to take ticlopidine HCl with food or just after eating in order to minimize gastrointestinal discomfort.

LABORATORY TESTS

Liver Function: Ticlopidine HCl therapy has been associated with elevations of alkaline phosphatase and transaminases which generally occurred within 1-4 months of therapy initiation. In controlled clinical trials, the incidence of elevated alkaline phosphatase (greater than 2 times upper limit of normal) was 7.6% in ticlopidine patients, 6.0% in placebo patients and 2.5% in aspirin patients. The incidence of elevated AST (SGOT) (greater than 2 times upper limit of normal) was 3.1% in ticlopidine patients, 4.0% in placebo patients and 2.1% in aspirin patients. No progressive increases were observed in closely monitored clinical trials (*e.g.,* no transaminase greater than 10 times the upper limit of normal was seen), but most patients with these abnormalities had therapy discontinued. Occasionally patients had developed minor elevations in bilirubin.

Based on post-marketing and clinical trials experiences, liver function testing, including SGPT and GGTP, should be considered whenever liver dysfunction is suspected, particularly during the first four months of treatment.

CARCINOGENESIS, MUTAGENESIS, AND IMPAIRMENT OF FERTILITY

In a two-year oral carcinogenicity study in rats, ticlopidine at daily doses of up to 100 mg/kg (610 mg/m^2) was not tumorigenic. For a 70 kg person (1.73 m^2 body surface area), the dose represents 14 times the recommended clinical dose on a mg/kg basis and 2 times the clinical dose on body surface area basis. In a 78 week oral carcinogenicity study in mice ticlopidine at daily doses up to 275 mg/kg (1180 mg/m^2) was not tumorigenic. The dose represents 40 times the recommended clinical dose on a mg/kg basis and 4 times the clinical dose on body surface area basis.

Ticlopidine was not mutagenic in *in vitro*Ames test, rat hepatocyte DNA- repair assay, and Chinese hamster fibroblast chromosomal aberration test and *in vivo*mouse spermatozoid morphology test, Chinese hamster micronucleus test and Chinese hamster bone marrow cell sister chromatid exchange test. Ticlopidine was found to have no effect on fertility of male and female rats at oral doses up to 400 mg/kg/day.

PREGNANCY, TERATOGENIC EFFECTS, PREGNANCY CATEGORY B

Teratology studies have been conducted in mice (doses up to 200 mg/kg/day), rats (doses up to 400 mg/kg/day) and rabbits (doses up to 200 mg/kg/day). Doses of 400 mg/kg in rats, 200 mg/kg/day in mice, and 100 mg/kg in rabbits produced maternal toxicity as well as fetal toxicity, but there was no evidence of a teratogenic potential of ticlopidine. There are, however, no adequate and well-controlled studies in pregnant women. Because animal reproduction studies are not always predictive of a human response, this drug should be used during pregnancy only if clearly needed.

NURSING MOTHERS

Studies in rats have shown ticlopidine is excreted in the milk. It is not known whether this drug is excreted in human milk. Because many drugs are excreted in human milk, and because of the potential for serious adverse reactions in nursing infants from ticlopidine, a decision should be made whether to discontinue nursing or to discontinue the drug, taking into account the importance of the drug to the mother.

PEDIATRIC USE

Safety and efficacy in patients under the age of 18 have not been established.

GERIATRIC USE

Clearance of ticlopidine is somewhat lower in elderly patients and trough levels are increased. The major clinical trials with ticlopidine HCl were conducted in an elderly population with an average age of 64 years. Of the total number of patients in the therapeutic trials, 45% of patients were over 65 years old and 12% were over 75 years old. No overall differences in effectiveness or safety were observed between these patients and younger patients, and other reported clinical experience has not identified differences in responses between the elderly and younger patients, but greater sensitivity of some older individuals cannot be ruled out.

DRUG INTERACTIONS:

Therapeutic doses of ticlopidine HCl caused a 30% increase in the plasma half-life of antipyrine and may cause analogous effects on similarly metabolized drugs. Therefore the dose of drugs metabolized by hepatic microsomal enzymes with low therapeutic ratios, or being given to patients with hepatic impairment, may require adjustment to maintain optimal therapeutic blood levels when starting or stopping concomitant therapy with ticlopidine. Studies of specific drug interactions yielded the following results:

Aspirin and other NSAIDS: Ticlopidine potentiates the effect of aspirin or other NSAIDS on platelet aggregation. The safety of concomitant use of ticlopidine with aspirin or other NSAIDS has not been established. Aspirin did not modify the ticlopidine-mediated inhibition of ADP induced platelet aggregation, but ticlopidine potentiated the effect of aspirin on collagen-induced platelet aggregation. Concomitant use of aspirin and ticlopidine is not recommended. See PRECAUTIONS, GI Bleeding.

Antacids: Administration of ticlopidine HCl after antacids resulted in an 18% decrease in plasma levels of ticlopidine.

Cimetidine: Chronic administration of cimetidine reduced the clearance of a single dose of ticlopidine HCl by 50%.

Digoxin: Co-administration of ticlopidine HCl with digoxin resulted in a slight decrease (approximately 15%) in digoxin plasma levels. Little or no change in therapeutic efficacy of digoxin would be expected.

Theophylline: In normal volunteers, concomitant administration of ticlopidine HCl resulted in a significant increase in the theophylline elimination half-life from 8.6 to 12.2 hr and a comparable reduction in total plasma clearance of theophylline.

Phenobarbital: In six normal volunteers, the inhibitory effects of ticlopidine HCl on platelet aggregation were not altered by chronic administration of phenobarbital.

Phenytoin: *In vitro* studies demonstrated that ticlopidine does not alter the plasma protein binding of phenytoin. However, the protein binding interactions of ticlopidine and its metabolites have not been studied *in vivo*. Several cases of elevated phenytoin plasma levels with associated somnolence and lethargy have been reported following co-administration with ticlopidine HCl. Caution should be exercised in coadministering this drug with ticlopidine HCl and it may be useful to remeasure phenytoin blood concentrations.

Propranolol: *In vitro* studies demonstrated that ticlopidine does not alter the plasma protein binding of propanolol. However, the protein binding interactions of ticlopidine and its metabolites have not been studied *in vivo.* Caution should be exercised in coadministering this drug with ticlopidine HCl.

Other Concomitant Therapy: Although specific interaction studies were not performed, in clinical studies, ticlopidine HCl was used concomitantly with beta blockers, calcium channel blockers, and diuretics without evidence of clinically significant adverse interactions. (See PRECAUTIONS.)

Food Interaction: The oral bioavailability of ticlopidine is increased by 20% when taken after a meal. Administration of ticlopidine HCl with food is recommended to maximize gastrointestinal tolerance. In controlled trials, ticlopidine HCl was taken with meals.

ADVERSE REACTIONS:

Adverse reactions were relatively frequent, with over 50% of patients reporting at least one. Most (30 to 40%) involved the gastrointestinal tract. Most adverse effects are mild, but 21% of patients discontinued therapy because of an adverse event, principally diarrhea, rash, nausea, vomiting, G.I. pain, and neutropenia. Most adverse effects occur early in the course of treatment, but a new onset of adverse effects can occur after several months.

The incidence rates of adverse events listed in TABLE 1 were derived from multicenter, controlled clinical trials described above comparing ticlopidine HCl, placebo, and aspirin over study periods of up to 5.8 years. Adverse events considered by the investigator to be probably drug-related that occurred in at least one percent of patients treated with ticlopidine HCl are shown in TABLE 1.

TABLE 1 Percent of Patients with Adverse Events in Controlled Studies

Event	Ticlid (n = 2048) Incidence	Aspirin (n = 1527) Incidence	Placebo (n = 536) Incidence
Any Events	60.0 (20.9)	53.2 (14.5)	34.3 (6.1)
Diarrhea	212.5 (6.3)	5.2 (1.8)	4.5 (1.7)
Nausea	7.0 (2.6)	6.2 (1.9)	1.7 (0.9)
Dyspepsia	7.0 (1.1)	9.0 (2.0)	0.9 (0.2)
Rash	5.1 (3.4)	1.5 (0.8)	0.6 (0.9)
GI Pain	3.7 (1.9)	5.6 (2.7)	1.3 (0.4)
Neutropenia	2.4 (1.3)	0.8 (0.1)	1.1 (0.4)
Purpura	2.2 (0.2)	1.6 (0.1)	0.0 (0.0)
Vomiting	1.9 (1.4)	1.4 (0.9)	0.9 (0.4)
Flatulence	1.5 (0.1)	1.4 (0.3)	0.0 (0.0)
Pruritus	1.3 (0.8)	0.3 (0.1)	0.0 (0.0)
Dizziness	1.1 (0.4)	0.5 (0.4)	0.0 (0.0)
Anorexia	1.0 (0.4)	0.5 (0.3)	0.0 (0.0)
Abnormal Liver Function test	1.0 (0.7)	0.3 (0.3)	0.0 (0.0)

Incidence of discontinuation, regardless of relationship therapy, is shown in parentheses.

Hematological: Neutropenia/thrombocytopenia (See WARNINGS), agranulocytosis, eosinophilia, pancytopenia, thrombocytosis, and bone marrow depression have been reported.

Gastrointestinal: Ticlopidine HCl therapy has been associated with a variety of gastrointestinal complaints including diarrhea and nausea. The majority of cases are mild, but about 13% of patients discontinued therapy because of these. They usually occur within 3 months of initiation of therapy and typically are resolved within 1-2 weeks without discontinuation of therapy. If the effect is severe or persistent, therapy should be discontinued. In some cases of severe or bloody diarrhea, colitis was later diagnosed.

Hemorrhagic: Ticlopidine HCl has been associated with increased bleeding, spontaneous post-traumatic bleeding, and perioperative bleeding including, but not limited to, gastrointestinal bleeding. It has also been associated with a number of bleeding complications such as ecchymosis, epistaxis, hematuria, and conjunctival hemorrhage.

Intracerebral bleeding was rare in clinical trials with ticlopidine HCl, with an incidence no greater than that seen with comparator agents (ticlopidine 0.5%, aspirin 0.6%, placebo 0.75%). It has also been reported post- marketing.

Rash: Ticlopidine has been associated with a maculopapular or urticarial rash (often with pruritus). Rash usually occurs within 3 months of initiation of therapy, with a mean onset time of 11 days. If drug is discontinued, recovery occurs within several days. Many rashes do not recur on drug rechallenge. There have been rare reports of severe rashes, including Stevens Johnson syndrome, erythema multiforme, and exfoliative dermatitis.

Less Frequent Adverse Reactions (Probably Related): Clinical adverse experiences occurring in 0.5 to 1.0 percent of patients in the controlled trials include: Digestive System: GI fullness; Skin and Appendages: urticaria; Nervous System: headache; Body as a Whole: asthenia, pain; Hemostatic System: epistaxis; Special Senses: tinnitus.

In addition, rarer, relatively serious events have also been reported from post-marketing experience: Hemolytic anemia with reticulocytosis, aplastic anemia, immune thrombocytopenia, thrombotic thrombocytopenic purpura (TTP), hepatitis, hepatocellular jaundice, cholestatic jaundice, hepatic necrosis, peptic ulcer, renal failure, nephrotic syndrome, hyponatremia, vasculitis, sepsis, angioedema, allergic pneumonitis, systemic lupus (positive ANA), peripheral neuropathy, serum sickness, arthropathy, and myositis.

OVERDOSAGE:

One case of deliberate overdosage with ticlopidine HCl has been reported by foreign postmarketing surveillance program. A 38 year old male took a single 6000 mg dose of ticlopidine HCl (equivalent to 24 standard 250 mg tablets). The only abnormalities reported were increased bleeding time and increased SGPT. No special therapy was instituted and the patient recovered without sequelae.

Single oral doses of ticlopidine at 1600 mg/kg and 500 mg/kg were lethal to rats and mice, respectively. Symptoms of acute toxicity were GI hemorrhage, convulsions, hypothermia, dyspnea, loss of equilibrium and abnormal gait.

DOSAGE AND ADMINISTRATION:

The recommended dose of ticlopidine HCl is 250 mg BID taken with food. Other doses have not been studied in controlled trials for these indications.

Store at 15-30°C (59-86°F).

PATIENT PACKAGE INSERT:

IMPORTANT INFORMATION ABOUT TICLOPIDINE HCL

The information in this leaflet is intended to help you use ticlopidine HCl safely. Please read the leaflet carefully. Although it does not contain all the detailed medical information that is provided to your doctor, it provides facts about ticlopidine HCl that are important for you to know. If you still have questions after reading this sheet or if you have questions at any time during your treatment with ticlopidine HCl, check with your doctor.

SPECIAL WARNING FOR USERS OF TICLOPIDINE HCL/NECESSARY BLOOD TESTS

Your doctor has prescribed ticlopidine HCl tablets (250 mg) to help reduce your risk of having a stroke, either because you have had a stroke already (to decrease the chance of another one) or because a stroke is threatening.

Ticlopidine HCl is recommended only for patients who cannot take aspirin, which also can decrease the risk of stroke. This is because ticlopidine HCl can on occasion, cause a serious white blood cell abnormality. A small percentage of people who take ticlopidine HCl (about 1.0%) develop a large fall in the number of their white cells (a condition called neutropenia) that can be life-threatening because it leaves them unable to fight infection. If neutropenia occurs, it typically does so during the first three months of treatment.

To make sure you don't develop this problem, your doctor will arrange for you to have your blood tested before you start taking ticlopidine HCl and then every two weeks for the first three months you are on ticlopidine HCl. If detected, neutropenia can almost always be reversed, but if left untreated, neutropenia can lead to fatal infection. It is therefore essential that you keep your appointments for the blood tests and that you call your doctor immediately if you have any sign of an infection, such as fever, chills, or sore throat, because these can mean that you have neutropenia. If you stop taking ticlopidine HCl for any reason within the first three months, you will still need to have your blood tested for an additional two weeks after you have stopped taking ticlopidine HCl.

OTHER WARNINGS AND PRECAUTIONS

A few people may develop jaundice while being treated with ticlopidine HCl. The signs of jaundice are yellowing of the skin or the whites of the eyes, or consistent darkening in the color of urine or lightening in the color of stools. **If these symptoms occur, contact your doctor immediately.**

ticlopidine HCl should be used only as directed by your doctor. Do not give ticlopidine HCl to anyone else. **Keep ticlopidine HCl out of reach of children.**

Some people may have such side effects as diarrhea, skin rash, stomach or intestinal discomfort. If any of these problems are persistent, or if you are concerned about them, bring them to your doctor's attention.

It may take longer than usual to stop bleeding when taking ticlopidine HCl. Tell your doctor if you have any more bleeding or bruising than usual, and be sure to let your doctor or dentist know that you are taking ticlopidine HCl if you have emergency surgery. Also, tell your doctor well in advance of any planned surgery (including tooth extraction), because he or she may recommend that you stop taking ticlopidine HCl temporarily.

HOW TICLOPIDINE HCL WORKS

A stroke occurs when a clot (or thrombus) forms in a blood vessel in the brain or forms in another part of the body and breaks off, then travels to the brain (an embolus). In both cases the blood supply to part of the brain is blocked and that part of the brain is damaged. Ticlopidine HCl works by making the blood less likely to clot, although not so much less that it causes you to become likely to bleed, unless you have a bleeding disorder or some injury (such as a bleeding ulcer of the stomach or intestine) that is especially likely to bleed.

WHO SHOULD NOT TAKE TICLOPIDINE HCL?

Contact your doctor immediately and do not take ticlopidine HCl if

you have an allergic reaction to ticlopidine HCl

you have a blood disorder or a serious bleeding problem, such as a bleeding stomach ulcer

you have severe liver disease or other liver problems

you are pregnant or you are planning to become pregnant

you are breast-feeding

HOW SUPPLIED:

Ticlid is available in white oval film coated 250 mg tablets, printed in blue with "TICLID" on one side and "250" on the other. They are provided in unit of use bottles of 30 tablets and 60 tablets and 500 tablets or in cartons of 100 blister packed tablets.

HOW SUPPLIED - EQUIVALENTS NOT AVAILABLE:

Tablet, Uncoated - Oral - 250 mg

30's	$43.87	TICLID, Syntex Labs	00033-0431-38
100's	$146.21	TICLID, Syntex Labs	00033-0431-53

TIMOLOL *(003263)*

CATEGORIES: Antiglaucomatous Agents; Beta Adrenergic Blocking Agents; EENT Drugs; Eye, Ear, Nose, & Throat Preparations; Glaucoma; Intraocular Pressure; Ocular Hypertension; Ophthalmics; FDA Class 2S ("Standard Review"); FDA Approved 1995 Mar

BRAND NAMES: *Apo-Timop* (Canada); *Aquanil*; **Betimol**; *Blocadren*; *Blocanol*; *Chibro-Timoptol* (Germany); *Cusimolol*; *Dispatim* (Germany); *Gen-Timolol* (Canada); *Glafemak*; *Glauco* ; *Glauco Oph*; *Glucomol*; *Hyoptol*; *Imot Ofteno Al* (Mexico); *Molotic Eye Ocupres*; *Noval*; *Ocupres*; *Ofal*; *Ofan*; *Oftan Timolol*; *Optimol*; *Temserin*; *Tenopt*; *Tiloptic*; *Timacar*; *Timoftol*; *Timohexal* (Germany); *Timoptic* (Canada, Japan); *Timoptol* (Australia, England, France, Mexico, Japan, Germany); *Timoptol-XE*; *Titol*; *Yesan*

(International brand names outside U.S. in italics)

FORMULARIES: WHO; PCS

DESCRIPTION:

Betimol (timolol ophthalmic solution), 0.25% and 0.5%, is a non-selective beta-adrenergic antagonist for ophthalmic use. The chemical name of the active ingredient is (S)-1-[(1,1-dimethylethyl)amino] -3-[[4-(4-morpholinyl) -1,2,5- thiadiazol-3-yl]oxy]-2-propanol. Timolol hemihydrate is the levo isomer. Specific rotation is $[\alpha]^{25}_{405nm}$ = -16° (C = 10% as the hemihydrate form in 1N HCl).

The molecular formula of timolol is $C_{13}H_{24}N_4O_3S$. Timolol (as the hemihydrate) is a white, odorless, crystalline powder which is slightly soluble in water and freely soluble in ethanol. Timolol hemihydrate is stable at room temperature.

Timolol is a clear, colorless, isotonic, sterile, microbiologically preserved phosphate buffered aqueous solution. It is supplied in two dosage strengths, 0.25% and 0.5%.

Each mL of timolol 0.25% contains 2.56 mg of timolol hemihydrate equivalent to 2.5 mg timolol.

Each mL of timolol 0.5% contains 5.12 mg of timolol hemihydrate equivalent to 5.0 mg timolol.

Inactive ingredients: monosodium and disodium phosphate dihydrate to adjust pH (6.5-7.5) and water for injection, benzalkonium chloride 0.01% added as preservative.

CLINICAL PHARMACOLOGY:

Timolol is a non-selective beta-adrenergic antagonist. It blocks both $beta_1$- and $beta_2$-adrenergic receptors. Timolol does not have significant intrinsic sympathomimetic activity, local anesthetic (membrane-stabilizing) or direct myocardial depressant activity.

Timolol, when applied topically in the eye, reduces normal and elevated intraocular pressure (IOP) whether or not accompanied by glaucoma. Elevated intraocular pressure is a major risk factor in the pathogenesis of glaucomatous visual field loss. The higher the level of IOP, the greater the likelihood of glaucomatous visual field loss and optic nerve damage. The predominant mechanism of ocular hypotensive action of topical beta-adrenergic blocking agents is likely due to a reduction in aqueous humor production.

In general, beta-adrenergic blocking agents reduce cardiac output both in healthy subjects and patients with heart diseases. In patients with severe impairment of myocardial function, beta-adrenergic receptor blocking agents may inhibit sympathetic stimulatory effect necessary to maintain adequate cardiac function. In the bronchi and bronchioles, beta-adrenergic receptor blockade may also increase airway resistance because of unopposed parasympathetic activity.

CLINICAL PHARMACOLOGY: *(cont'd)*

Pharmacokinetics: When given orally, timolol is well absorbed and undergoes considerable first pass metabolism. Timolol and its metabolites are primarily excreted in the urine. The half-life of timolol in plasma is approximately 4 hours.

CLINICAL STUDIES:

In two controlled multicenter studies in the U.S., timolol 0.25% and 0.5% were compared with respective timolol maleate eye drops. In these studies, the efficacy and safety profile of timolol was similar to that of timolol maleate.

INDICATIONS AND USAGE:

Timolol is indicated in the treatment of elevated intraocular pressure in patients with ocular hypertension or open-angle glaucoma.

CONTRAINDICATIONS:

Timolol is contraindicated in patients with overt heart failure, cardiogenic shock, sinus bradycardia, second- or third-degree atrioventricular block, bronchial asthma or history of bronchial asthma, or severe chronic obstructive pulmonary disease, or hypersensitivity to any component of this product.

WARNINGS:

As with other topically applied ophthalmic drugs, timolol is absorbed systemically. The same adverse reactions found with systemic administration of beta-adrenergic blocking agents may occur with topical administration. For example, severe respiratory and cardiac reactions, including death due to bronchospasm in patients with asthma, and rarely, death in association with cardiac failure have been reported following systemic or topical administration of beta-adrenergic blocking agents.

Cardiac Failure: Sympathetic stimulation may be essential for support of the circulation in individuals with diminished myocardial contractility, and its inhibition by beta-adrenergic receptor blockade may precipitate more severe cardiac failure.

In patients without a history of cardiac failure, continued depression of the myocardium with beta-blocking agents over a period of time can, in some cases, lead to cardiac failure. Timolol should be discontinued at the first sign or symptom of cardiac failure.

Obstructive Pulmonary Disease: Patients with chronic obstructive pulmonary disease (*e.g.,* chronic bronchitis, emphysema) of mild or moderate severity, bronchospastic disease, or a history of bronchospastic disease (other than bronchial asthma or a history of bronchial asthma which are contraindications) should in general not receive beta-blocking agents.

Major Surgery: The necessity or desirability of withdrawal of beta-adrenergic blocking agents prior to a major surgery is controversial. Beta-adrenergic receptor blockade impairs the ability of the heart to respond to beta-adrenergically mediated reflex stimuli. This may augment the risk of general anesthesia in surgical procedures. Some patients receiving beta-adrenergic receptor blocking agents have been subject to protracted severe hypotension during anesthesia. Difficulty in restarting and maintaining the heartbeat has also been reported. For these reasons, in patients undergoing elective surgery, gradual withdrawal of beta-adrenergic receptor blocking agents is recommended. If necessary during surgery, the effects of beta-adrenergic blocking agents may be reversed by sufficient doses of beta-adrenergic agonists.

Diabetes Mellitus: Beta-adrenergic blocking agents should be administered with caution in patients subject to spontaneous hypoglycemia or to diabetic patients (especially those with labile diabetes) who are receiving insulin or oral hypoglycemic agents. Beta-adrenergic receptor blocking agents may mask the signs and symptoms of acute hypoglycemia.

Thyrotoxicosis: Beta-adrenergic blocking agents may mask certain clinical signs (*e.g.,* tachycardia) of hyperthyroidism. Patients suspected of developing thyrotoxicosis should be managed carefully to avoid abrupt withdrawal of beta-adrenergic blocking agents which might precipitate a thyroid storm.

PRECAUTIONS:

GENERAL

Because of the potential effects of beta-adrenergic blocking agents relative to blood pressure and pulse, these agents should be used with caution in patients with cerebrovascular insufficiency. If signs or symptoms suggesting reduced cerebral blood flow develop following initiation of therapy with timolol, alternative therapy should be considered.

There have been reports of bacterial keratitis associated with the use of multiple dose containers of topical ophthalmic products. These containers had been inadvertently contaminated by patients who, in most cases, had a concurrent corneal disease or a disruption of the ocular epithelial surface. (See PRECAUTIONS, Information for Patients.)

Muscle Weakness: Beta-adrenergic blockade has been reported to potentiate muscle weakness consistent with certain myasthenic symptoms (*e.g.,* diplopia, ptosis, and generalized weakness). Beta-adrenergic blocking agents have been reported rarely to increase muscle weakness in some patients with myasthenia gravis or myasthenic symptoms.

In angle-closure glaucoma, the goal of the treatment is to reopen the angle. This requires constricting the pupil. Timolol has no effect on the pupil. Therefore, if timolol is used in angle-closure glaucoma, it should always be combined with a miotic and not used alone.

Anaphylaxis: While taking beta-blockers, patients with a history of atopy or a history of severe anaphylactic reactions to a variety of allergens may be more reactive to repeated accidental, diagnostic, or therapeutic challenge with such allergens. Such patients may be unresponsive to the usual doses of epinephrine used to treat anaphylactic reactions.

INFORMATION FOR THE PATIENT

Patients should be instructed to avoid allowing the tip of the dispensing container to contact the eye or surrounding structures.

Patients should also be instructed that ocular solutions can become contaminated by common bacteria known to cause ocular infections. Serious damage to the eye and subsequent loss of vision may result from using contaminated solutions. (See PRECAUTIONS, General.)

Patients requiring concomitant topical ophthalmic medications should be instructed to administer these at least 5 minutes apart.

Patients with bronchial asthma, a history of bronchial asthma, severe chronic obstructive pulmonary disease, sinus bradycardia, second- or third-degree atrioventricular block, or cardiac failure should be advised not to take this product. (See CONTRAINDICATIONS.)

CARCINOGENESIS, MUTAGENESIS, AND IMPAIRMENT OF FERTILITY

Carcinogenicity of timolol (as the maleate) has been studied in mice and rats. In a two-year study orally administrated timolol maleate (300 mg/kg/day) (approximately 42,000 times the systemic exposure following the maximum recommended human ophthalmic dose) in male rats caused a significant increase in the incidence of adrenal pheochromocytomas; the lower doses, 25 mg or 100 mg/kg daily did not cause any changes.

In a life span study in mice the overall incidence of neoplasms was significantly increased in female mice at 500 mg/kg/day (approximately 71,000 times the systemic exposure following the maximum recommended human ophthalmic dose). Furthermore, significant increases were observed in the incidences of benign and malignant pulmonary tumors, benign uterine polyps, as well as mammary adenocarcinomas. These changes were not seen at the daily dose

PRECAUTIONS: *(cont'd)*

level of 5 or 50 mg/kg (approximately 700 or 7,000, respectively, times the systemic exposure following the maximum recommended human ophthalmic dose). For comparison, the maximum recommended human oral dose of timolol maleate is 1 mg/kg/day.

Mutagenic potential of timolol was evaluated in vivo in the micronucleus test and cytogenetic assay and in vitro in the neoplastic cell transformation assay and Ames test. In bacterial mutagenicity test (Ames test) high concentrations of timolol maleate (5000 and 10,000 g/plate) statistically significantly increased the number of revertants in Salmonella typhimurium TA100, but not in the other three strains tested. However, no consistent dose-response was observed nor did the number of revertants reach the double of the control value, which is regarded as one of the criteria for a positive result in the Ames test. In vivo genotoxicity tests (the mouse micronucleus test and cytogenetic assay) and in vitro the neoplastic cell transformation assay were negative up to dose levels of 800 mg/kg and 100 g/mL, respectively.

No adverse effects on male and female fertility were reported in rats at timolol oral doses of up to 150 mg/kg/day (21,000 times the systemic exposure following the maximum recommended human ophthalmic dose).

PREGNANCY, TERATOGENIC EFFECTS, PREGNANCY CATEGORY C

Teratogenicity of timolol (as the maleate) after oral administration was studied in mice and rabbits. No fetal malformations were reported in mice or rabbits at a daily oral dose of 50 mg/kg (7,000 times the systemic exposure following the maximum recommended human ophthalmic dose). Although delayed fetal ossification was observed at this dose in rats, there were no adverse effects on postnatal development of offspring. Doses of 1000 mg/kg/day (142,000 times the systemic exposure following the maximum recommended human ophthalmic dose) were maternotoxic in mice and resulted in an increased number of fetal resorptions. Increased fetal resorptions were also seen in rabbits at doses of 14,000 times the systemic exposure following the maximum recommended human ophthalmic dose in this case without apparent maternotoxicity.

There are no adequate and well-controlled studies in pregnant women. Timolol should be used during pregnancy only if the potential benefit justifies the potential risk to the fetus.

NURSING MOTHERS

Because of the potential for serious adverse reactions in nursing infants from timolol, a decision should be made whether to discontinue nursing or to discontinue the drug, taking into account the importance of the drug to the mother.

PEDIATRIC USE

Safety and efficacy in pediatric patients have not been established.

DRUG INTERACTIONS:

Beta-adrenergic blocking agents: Patients who are receiving a beta-adrenergic blocking agent orally and Timolol should be observed for a potential additive effect either on the intraocular pressure or on the known systemic effects of beta-blockade.

Patients should not usually receive two topical ophthalmic beta-adrenergic blocking agents concurrently.

Catecholamine-depleting drugs: Close observation of the patient is recommended when a beta-blocker is administered to patients receiving catecholamine-depleting drugs such as reserpine, because of possible additive effects and the production of hypotension and/or marked bradycardia, which may produce vertigo, syncope, or postural hypotension.

Calcium antagonists: Caution should be used in the co-administration of beta-adrenergic blocking agents and oral or intravenous calcium antagonists, because of possible atrioventricular conduction disturbances, left ventricular failure, and hypotension. In patients with impaired cardiac function, co-administration should be avoided.

Digitalis and calcium antagonists: The concomitant use of beta-adrenergic blocking agents with digitalis and calcium antagonists may have additive effects in prolonging atrioventricular conduction time. Injectable Epinephrine: (See PRECAUTIONS, General, Anaphylaxis.).

ADVERSE REACTIONS:

The most frequently reported ocular event in clinical trials was burning/stinging on instillation and was comparable between timolol and timolol maleate (approximately one in eight patients). The following adverse events were associated with the use of timolol in frequencies of more than 5% in two controlled, double-masked clinical studies in which 184 patients received 0.25% or 0.5% timolol:

Ocular: dry eyes, itching, foreign body sensation, discomfort in the eye, eyelid erythema, conjunctival injection, headache

Body As A Whole: headache

The following side effects were reported in frequencies of 1 to 5%:

Ocular: eye pain, epiphora, photophobia, blurred or abnormal vision, corneal fluorescein staining, keratitis, blepharitis, cataract

Body As A Whole: allergic reaction, asthenia, common cold, pain in extremities

Cardiovascular: hypertension

Digestive: nausea

Metabolic/Nutritional: peripheral edema

Nervous System/Psychiatry: dizziness, dry mouth

Respiratory: respiratory infection, sinusitis

In addition, the following adverse reactions have been reported with ophthalmic use of beta blockers:

Ocular: conjunctivitis, blepharoptosis, decreased corneal sensitivity, visual disturbances including refractive changes, diplopia, retinal vascular disorder,

Body As A Whole: chest pain

Cardiovascular: arrhythmia, palpitation, bradycardia, hypotension, syncope, heart block, cerebral vascular accident, cerebral ischemia, cardiac failure, cardiac arrest

Digestive: diarrhea

Endocrine: masked symptoms of hypoglycemia in insulin dependent diabetics (see WARNINGS).

Nervous System/Psychiatry: depression, impotence, increase in signs and symptoms of myasthenia gravis, paresthesia

Respiratory: dyspnea, bronchospasm, respiratory failure, nasal congestion

Skin: alopecia, hypersensitivity including localized and generalized rash, urticaria

OVERDOSAGE:

No information is available on overdosage with timolol. Symptoms that might be expected with an overdose of a beta-adrenergic receptor blocking agent are bronchospasm, hypotension, bradycardia, and acute cardiac failure.

DOSAGE AND ADMINISTRATION:

Timolol is available in concentrations of 0.25% and 0.5%. The starting dose is one drop of timolol, 0.25% or 0.5%, twice daily in the affected eye(s).

DOSAGE AND ADMINISTRATION: *(cont'd)*

Because in some patients the pressure-lowering response to timolol may require a few weeks to stabilize, evaluation should include a determination of intraocular pressure after approximately 4 weeks of treatment with timolol.

Dosages higher than one drop of timolol 0.5% twice a day have not been studied. If the patient's intraocular pressure is still not at a satisfactory level on this regimen, concomitant therapy can be considered.

HOW SUPPLIED:

Betimol (timolol ophthalmic solution) is a clear, colorless solution.

Storage: Store between 15-30°C (59-86°F). Do not freeze. Protect from light.

HOW SUPPLIED - EQUIVALENTS NOT AVAILABLE:

Solution - Ophthalmic - 0.25 %

15 ml	$359.42	BETIMOL, Ciba Vision	58768-0898-15

Solution - Ophthalmic - 0.25%

5.0 ml	$124.27	BETIMOL, Ciba Vision	58768-0898-05
10 ml	$144.00	BETIMOL, Ciba Vision	58768-0898-10

Solution - Ophthalmic - 0.5 %

15 ml	$426.96	BETIMOL, Ciba Vision	58768-0899-15

Solution - Ophthalmic - 0.5%

5.0 ml	$147.02	BETIMOL, Ciba Vision	58768-0899-05
10 ml	$285.12	BETIMOL, Ciba Vision	58768-0899-10

TIMOLOL MALEATE *(002353)*

CATEGORIES: Antiglaucomatous Agents; Antihypertensives; Beta Adrenergic Blocking Agents; Beta Blockers; Cardiovascular Drugs; EENT Drugs; Eye, Ear, Nose, & Throat Preparations; Glaucoma; Headache; Hypertension; Intraocular Pressure; Migraine; Myocardial Infarction; Myocardial Infarction Prophylaxis; Ocular Hypertension; Ophthalmics; Renal Drugs; Pregnancy Category C; Sales > $100 Million; FDA Approval Pre 1982; Patent Expiration 1997 Mar; Top 200 Drugs

BRAND NAMES: *Apo-Timol* (Canada); *Apo-Timolol*; *Aquanil*; *Betim* (England); Blocadren; *Blocanol*; *Cardina*; *Cusimolol*; *Dispatim*; *Equiton*; *Glauco-Opu*; *Glucolol*; *Glucomol*; *Hypermol*; *Lolomit*; *Novo-Timol* (Canada); *Nyolol*; *Ocupres*; *Optimol*; *Proflax*; *Temserin* (Germany); *Tilmat*; *Tiloptic*; *Timacar*; *Timacor* (France); **Timoptic**; Timoptic-Xe; *Timoptol*; *Timpotic*
(International brand names outside U.S. in italics)

FORMULARIES: Aetna; BC-BS; CIGNA; FHP; Humana; Kaiser; Medco; Medi-Cal; PruCare; United

COST OF THERAPY: $203.45 (Hypertension; Tablet; 10 mg; 2/day; 365 days)

PRIMARY ICD9: 401.1 (Essential Hypertension, Benign)

DESCRIPTION:

Timolol maleate is a non-selective beta-adrenergic receptor blocking agent. The chemical name for timolol maleate is (*S*)-1-[(1,1-dimethylethyl)amino]-3-[[4-(4-morpholinyl)- 1,2,5-thiadiazol -3 -yl]oxy]-2-propanol, (*Z*)-butenedioate (1:1) salt. It possesses an asymmetric carbon atom in its structure and is provided as the levo isomer. Its empirical formula is $C_{13}H_{24}N_4O_3S{\cdot}C_4H_4O_4$.

Tablets: Timolol maleate has a molecular weight of 432.49. It is a white, odorless, crystalline powder which is soluble in water, methanol, and alcohol.

Ophthalmic Solution: Timoptic Ophthalmic Solution is supplied as a sterile, isotonic, buffered, aqueous solution of timolol maleate in two dosage strengths: Each ml of Timoptic 0.25% contains 2.5 mg of timolol (3.4 mg of timolol maleate). Each ml of Timoptic 0.5% contains 5.0 mg of timolol (6.8 mg of timolol maleate).

Preservative-Free Ophthalmic Solution: Timolol maleate ophthalmic solution is supplied in two formulations: Ophthalmic Solution Timoptic, which contains the preservative, benzalkonium chloride; and Ophthalmic Solution Timoptic (timolol maleate), the preservative-free formulation.

Preservative-free Ophthalmic Solution Timoptic is supplied in Ocudose, a unit dose container as a sterile, isotonic, buffered, aqueous solution of timolol maleate in two dosage strengths: Each ml of Preservative-free Timoptic in Ocudose 0.25% contains 2.5 mg of timolol (3.4 of timolol maleate). Each ml of Preservative-free Timoptic in Ocudose 0.5% contains 5.0 mg of timolol (6.8 mg of timolol maleate). Inactive ingredients: monobasic and dibasic sodium phosphate, sodium hydroxide to adjust pH, and water for injection.

CLINICAL PHARMACOLOGY:

TABLETS

Timolol maleate is a $beta_1$ and $beta_2$ (non-selective) adrenergic receptor blocking agent that does not have significant intrinsic sympathomimetic, direct myocardial depressant, or local anesthetic activity.

Pharmacodynamics: Clinical pharmacology studies have confirmed the beta-adrenergic blocking activity as shown by (1) changes in resting heart rate and response of heart rate to changes in posture; (2) inhibition of isoproterenol-induced tachycardia; (3) alteration of the response to the Valsalva maneuver and amyl nitrite administration; and (4) reduction of heart rate and blood pressure changes on exercise.

Timolol maleate decreases the positive chronotropic, positive inotropic, bronchodilator, and vasodilator responses caused by beta-adrenergic receptor agonists. The magnitude of this decreased response is proportional to the existing sympathetic tone and the concentration of timolol maleate at receptor sites.

In normal volunteers, the reduction in heart rate response to a standard exercise was dose dependent over the test range of 0.5 to 20 mg, with a peak reduction at 2 hours of approximately 30% at higher doses.

Beta-adrenergic receptor blockade reduces cardiac output in both healthy subjects and patients with heart disease. In patients with severe impairment of myocardial function beta-adrenergic receptor blockade may inhibit the stimulatory effect of the sympathetic nervous system necessary to maintain adequate cardiac function.

Beta-adrenergic receptor blockade in the bronchi and bronchioles results in increased airway resistance from unopposed parasympathetic activity. Such an effect in patients with asthma or other bronchospastic conditions is potentially dangerous.

Clinical studies indicate that timolol maleate at a dosage of 20-60 mg/day reduces blood pressure without causing postural hypotension in most patients with essential hypertension. Administration of timolol maleate to patients with hypertension results initially in a decrease in cardiac output, little immediate change in blood pressure, and an increase in calculated peripheral resistance. With continued administration of timolol maleate blood pressure

CLINICAL PHARMACOLOGY: *(cont'd)*

decreases within a few days, cardiac output usually remains reduced, and peripheral resistance falls toward pretreatment levels. Plasma volume may decrease or remain unchanged during therapy with timolol maleate. In the majority of patients with hypertension timolol maleate also decreases plasma renin activity. Dosage adjustment to achieve optimal antihypertensive effect may require a few weeks. When therapy with timolol maleate is discontinued, the blood pressure tends to return to pretreatment levels gradually. In most patients the antihypertensive activity of timolol maleate is maintained with long-term therapy and is well tolerated.

The mechanism of the antihypertensive effects of beta-adrenergic receptor blocking agents is not established at this time. Possible mechanisms of action include reduction in cardiac output, reduction in plasma renin activity, and a central nervous system sympatholytic action.

A Norwegian multi-center, double-blind study compared the effect of timolol maleate with placebo in 1,884 patients who had survived the acute phase of a myocardial infarction. Patients with systolic blood pressure below 100 mm Hg, sick sinus syndrome and contraindication to beta blockers, including uncontrolled heart failure, second or third degree AV block and bradycardia (<50 beats per minute), were excluded from the multi-center trial. Therapy with timolol maleate, begun to 28 days following infarction, was shown to reduce overall mortality; this was primarily attributable to a reduction in cardiovascular mortality. Timolol maleate significantly reduced the incidence of sudden death (deaths occurring without symptoms or within 24 hours of the onset of symptoms), including those occurring within one hour, and particularly instantaneous deaths (those occurring without preceding symptoms). The protective effect of timolol maleate was consistent regardless of age, sex or site of infarction. The effect was clearest in patients with a first infarction who were considered at a high risk of dying, defined as those with one or more of the following characteristics during the acute phase: transient left ventricular failure, cardiomegaly, newly appearing atrial fibrillation or flutter, systolic hypotension, or SGOT (ASAT) level greater than four times the upper limit of normal. Therapy with timolol maleate also reduced the incidence of non-fatal reinfarction. The mechanism of the protective effect of timolol maleate is unknown.

Timolol maleate was studied for the prophylactic treatment of migraine headache in placebo-controlled clinical trials involving 400 patients, mostly women between the ages of 18 and 66 years. Common migraine was the most frequent diagnosis. All patients had at least two headaches per month at baseline. Approximately 50 percent of patients who received timolol maleate had a reduction in the frequency of migraine headache of at least 50 percent, compared to a similar decrease in frequency in 30 percent of patients receiving placebo. The most common cardiovascular adverse effect was bradycardia (5%).

Pharmacokinetics and Metabolism: Timolol maleate is rapidly and nearly completely absorbed (about 90%) following oral ingestion. Detectable plasma levels of timolol occur within one-half hour and peak plasma levels occur in about one to two hours. The drug half-life in plasma is approximately 4 hours and this is essentially unchanged in patients with moderate renal insufficiency. Timolol is partially metabolized by the liver and timolol and its metabolites are excreted by the kidney. Timolol is not extensively bound to plasma proteins; i.e., <10% by equilibrium dialysis and approximately 60% by ultrafiltration. An *in vitro* hemodialysis study, using $_{14}C$ timolol added to human plasma or whole blood, showed that timolol was readily dialyzed from these fluids; however, a study of patients with renal failure showed that timolol did not dialyze readily. Plasma levels following oral administration are about half those following intravenous administration indicating approximately 50% first pass metabolism. The level of beta sympathetic activity varies widely among individuals, and no simple correlation exists between the dose of plasma level of timolol maleate and its therapeutic activity. Therefore, objective clinical measurements such as reduction of heart rate and/or blood pressure should be used as guides in determining the optimal dosage for each patient.

OPHTHALMIC SOLUTIONS

Timolol maleate is a $beta_1$ and $beta_2$ (non-selective) adrenergic receptor blocking agent that does not have significant intrinsic sympathomimetic, direct myocardial depressant, or local anesthetic (membrane-stabilizing) activity.

Beta-adrenergic receptor blockade reduces cardiac output in both healthy subjects and patients with heart disease. In patients with severe impairment of myocardial function beta-adrenergic receptor blockade may inhibit the stimulatory effect of the sympathetic nervous system necessary to maintain adequate cardiac function.

Beta-adrenergic receptor blockade in the bronchi and bronchioles results in increased airway resistance from unopposed parasympathetic activity. Such an effect inpatients with asthma or other bronchospastic conditions is potentially dangerous.

Timolol maleate ophthalmic solution, when applied topically in the eye, has the action of reducing elevated as well as normal intraocular pressure, whether or not accompanied by glaucoma. Elevated intraocular pressure is a major risk factor in the pathogenesis of glaucomatous visual field loss. The higher the level of intraocular pressure, the greater the likelihood of glaucomatous visual field loss and optic nerve damage.

The onset of reduction in intraocular pressure following administration of timolol maleate can usually be detected within one-half hour after a single dose. The maximum effect usually occurs in one to two hours and significant lowering of intraocular pressure can be maintained for periods as long as 24 hours with a single dose. Repeated observations over a period of one year indicate that the intraocular pressure-lowering effect of timolol maleate is well maintained.

The precise mechanism of the ocular hypotensive action of timolol maleate is not clearly established at this time. Tonography and fluorophotometry studies in man suggest that its predominant action may be related to reduced aqueous formation. However, in some studies a slight increase in outflow facility was also observed. Unlike miotics, timolol maleate reduces intraocular pressure with little or no effect on accommodation or pupil size. Thus, changes in visual acuity due to increased accommodation are uncommon, and dim or blurred vision and night blindness produced by miotics are not evident. In addition, in patients with cataracts the inability to see around lenticular opacities when the pupil is constricted is avoided.

In the clinical studies which are reported below, ocular pressure reductions to less than 22 mmHg were used as a reasonable reference point to allow comparisons between treatments. Reduction of ocular pressure to just below 22 mmHg may not be optimal for all patients; therapy should be individualized.

In controlled multiclinic studies in patients with untreated intraocular pressures of 22 mmHg or greater, timolol maleate 0.25 percent or 0.5 percent administered twice a day produced a greater reduction in intraocular pressure than 1,2,3, or 4 percent pilocarpine solution administered four times a day or 0.5, 1, or 2 percent epinephrine hydrochloride solution administered twice a day.

In the multiclinic studies comparing timolol maleate with pilocarpine, 61 percent of patients treated with timolol maleate had intraocular pressure reduced to less than 22 mmHg compared to 32 percent of patients treated with pilocarpine. For patients completing these studies, the mean reduction in pressure at the end of the study from pretreatment was 30.7 percent for patients treated with timolol maleate and 21.7 percent for patients treated with pilocarpine.

CLINICAL PHARMACOLOGY: *(cont'd)*

In the multiclinic studies comparing timolol maleate with epinephrine, 69 percent of patients treated with timolol maleate had intraocular pressure reduced to less than 22 mmHg compared to 42 percent of patients treated with epinephrine. For patients completing these studies, the mean reduction in pressure at the end of the study from pretreatment was 33.2 percent for patients treated with timolol maleate and 28.1 percent for patients treated with epinephrine.

In these studies, timolol maleate was generally well tolerated and produced fewer and less severe side effects than either pilocarpine or epinephrine. A slight reduction of resting heart rate in some patients receiving timolol maleate (mean reduction 2.9 beats/minute standard deviation 10.2) was observed.

Timolol maleate has also been used in patients with glaucoma wearing conventional (PMMA) hard contact lenses, and has generally been well tolerated. Timolol maleate has not been studied in patients wearing lenses made with materials other than PMMA. (See PRECAUTIONS, Information for the Patient.)

INDICATIONS AND USAGE:

Hypertension: *Tablets:* Timolol maleate is indicated for the treatment of hypertension. It may be used alone or in combination with other antihypertensive agents, especially thiazide-type diuretics.

Myocardial Infarction: Timolol maleate is indicated in patients who have survived the acute phase of a myocardial infarction, and are clinically stable, to reduce cardiovascular mortality and the risk of reinfarction.

Migraine: Timolol maleate is indicated for the prophylaxis of migraine headache.

OPHTHALMIC SOLUTION

Timolol maleate ophthalmic solution is indicated in the treatment of elevated intraocular pressure in patients with ocular hypertension or open-angle glaucoma.

PRESERVATIVE FREE-OPHTHALMIC SOLUTION

Timolol maleate has been shown to be effective in lowering intraocular pressure. Clinical studies have shown that the mean percent reductions in intraocular pressure with preservative-free timolol maleate and timolol maleate are similar. When a patient is sensitive to the preservative, benzalkonium chloride, or when use of a preservative- free topical medication is advisable, preservative-free timolol maleate may be used in:

Patients with chronic open-angle glaucoma; Patients with aphakic glaucoma; Some patients with secondary glaucoma; Other patients with elevated intraocular pressure who are at sufficient risk to require lowering of the ocular pressure.

OPHTHALMIC AND PRESERVATIVE-FREE OPHTHALMIC SOLUTIONS

Clinical trials have shown that in patients who respond inadequately to multiple antiglaucoma drug therapy the addition of timolol maleate may produce a further reduction of intraocular pressure.

CONTRAINDICATIONS:

Timolol maleate is contraindicated in patients with bronchial asthma or with a history of bronchial asthma, or severe chronic obstructive pulmonary disease (see WARNINGS); sinus bradycardia; second and third degree atrioventricular block; overt cardiac failure (see WARNINGS); cardiogenic shock; hypersensitivity to this product.

WARNINGS:

CARDIAC FAILURE

Tablets and Ophthalmic Solutions: Sympathetic stimulation may be essential for support of the circulation in individuals with diminished myocardial contractility, and its inhibition by beta-adrenergic receptor blockade may precipitate more severe failure.

In Patients Without a History of Cardiac Failure: continued depression of the myocardium with beta-blocking agents over a period of time can, in some cases, lead to cardiac failure.

OBSTRUCTIVE PULMONARY DISEASE

PATIENTS WITH CHRONIC OBSTRUCTIVE PULMONARY DISEASE (*e.g.,* CHRONIC BRONCHITIS, EMPHYSEMA) OF MILD OR MODERATE SEVERITY, BRONCHOSPASTIC DISEASE OR A HISTORY OF BRONCHOSPASTIC DISEASE (OTHER THAN BRONCHIAL ASTHMA OR A HISTORY OF BRONCHIAL ASTHMA, IN WHICH TIMOLOL MALEATE IS CONTRAINDICATED, see CONTRAINDICATIONS), SHOULD IN GENERAL NOT RECEIVE BETA BLOCKERS, INCLUDING TIMOLOL MALEATE. However, if timolol maleate is necessary in such patients, then the drug should be administered with caution since it may block bronchodilation produced by endogenous and exogenous catecholamine stimulation of $beta_2$ receptors.

MAJOR SURGERY

The necessity or desirability of withdrawal of beta-blocking therapy prior to major surgery is controversial. Beta-adrenergic receptor blockade impairs the ability of the heart to respond to beta-adrenergically mediated reflex stimuli. This may augment the risk of general anesthesia in surgical procedures. Some patients receiving beta-adrenergic receptor blocking agents have been subject to protracted severe hypotension during anesthesia. Difficulty in restarting and maintaining the heartbeat has also been reported. For these reasons, in patients undergoing elective surgery, some authorities recommend gradual withdrawal of beta-adrenergic receptor blocking agents.

If necessary during surgery, the effects of beta-adrenergic blocking agents may be reversed by sufficient doses of such agonists as isoproterenol, dopamine, dobutamine or levarterenol (see OVERDOSAGE.)

DIABETES MELLITUS

Timolol maleate should be administered with caution in patients subject to spontaneous hypoglycemia or to diabetic patients (especially those with labile diabetes) who are receiving insulin or oral hypoglycemia agents. Beta-adrenergic receptor blocking agents may mask the signs and symptoms of acute hypoglycemia.

THYROTOXICOSIS

Beta-adrenergic blockade may mask certain clinical signs (*e.g.,* tachycardia) of hyperthyroidism. Patients suspected of developing thyrotoxicosis should be managed carefully to avoid abrupt withdrawal of beta blockade which might precipitate a thyroid storm.

Exacerbation of Ischemic Heart Disease Following Abrupt Withdrawal: Hypersensitivity to catecholamines has been observed in patients withdrawn from beta blocker therapy; exacerbation of angina and, in some cases, myocardial infarction have occurred after abrupt discontinuation of such therapy. When discontinuing chronically administered timolol maleate, particularly in patients with ischemic heart disease, the dosage should be gradually reduced over a period of one to two weeks and the patient should be carefully monitored. If angina markedly worsens or acute coronary insufficiency develops, timolol maleate administration should be reinstituted promptly, at least temporarily, and other measures appropriate for the management of unstable angina should be taken. Patients

WARNINGS: *(cont'd)*

should be warned against interruption or discontinuation of therapy without the physician's advice. Because coronary artery disease is common and may be unrecognized, it may be prudent not to discontinue timolol maleate therapy abruptly even in patients treated only for hypertension.

Although beta blockers should be avoided in overt congestive heart failure, they can be used, if necessary, with caution in patients with a history of failure who are well-compensated, usually with digitalis and diuretics. Both digitalis and timolol maleate slow AV conduction. If cardiac failure persists, therapy with timolol maleate should be withdrawn.

At the first sign or symptom of cardiac failure, patients receiving timolol maleate should be digitalized and/or be given a diuretic, and the response observed closely. If cardiac failure continues, despite adequate digitalization and diuretic therapy, timolol maleate should be withdrawn.

IN PATIENTS WITHOUT A HISTORY OF CARDIAC FAILURE

Ophthalmic Solutions Only: At the first sign or symptom of cardiac failure timolol maleate should be discontinued,

As with other topically applied ophthalmic drugs, this drug may be absorbed systemically.

The same adverse reactions found with systemic administration of beta-adrenergic blocking agents may occur with topical administration. For example, severe respiratory reactions and cardiac reactions, including death due to bronchospasm in patients with asthma, and rarely death in association with cardiac failure, have been reported following administration of timolol maleate (see CONTRAINDICATIONS.)

PRECAUTIONS:

GENERAL

Muscle Weakness: Beta-adrenergic blockade has been reported to potentiate muscle weakness consistent with certain myasthenic symptoms (*e.g.,* diplopia, ptosis, and generalized weakness). Timolol has been reported rarely to increase muscle weakness in some patients with myasthenia gravis or myasthenic symptoms.

Ophthalmic Solutions

Patients who are receiving a beta-adrenergic blocking agent orally and timolol maleate should be observed for a potential additive effect either on the intraocular pressure or on the known systemic effects of beta blockade.

Patients should not receive two topical ophthalmic beta-adrenergic blocking agents concurrently (see DOSAGE AND ADMINISTRATION.)

Because of potential effects of beta-adrenergic blocking agents relative to blood pressure and pulse, these agents should be used with caution in patients with cerebrovascular insufficiency. If signs or symptoms suggesting reduced cerebral blood flow develop following initiation of therapy with timolol maleate, alternative therapy should be considered.

There have been reports of bacterial keratitis associated with the use of multiple dose containers of topical ophthalmic products. These containers had been inadvertently contaminated by patients who, in most cases, had a concurrent corneal disease or a disruption of the ocular epithelial surface. (See PRECAUTIONS, Information for the Patient.)

In patients with angle-closure glaucoma, the immediate objective of treatment is to reopen the angle. This requires constricting the pupil with a miotic. Timolol maleate has little or no effect on the pupil. When timolol maleate is used to reduce elevated intraocular pressure in angle-closure glaucoma, it should be used with a miotic and not alone.

As with the use of other antiglaucoma drugs, diminished responsiveness to timolol maleate after prolonged therapy has been reported in some patients. However, in one long-term study in which 96 patients have been followed for at least 3 years, no significant difference in mean intraocular pressure has been observed after initial stabilization.

Tablets

Impaired Hepatic or Renal Function: Since timolol maleate is partially metabolized in the liver and excreted mainly by the kidneys, dosage reductions may be necessary when hepatic and/or renal insufficiency is present.

Dosing in the Presence of Marked Renal Failure: Although the pharmacokinetics of timolol maleate are not greatly altered by renal impairment, marked hypotensive responses have been seen in patients with marked renal impairment undergoing dialysis after 20 mg doses. Dosing in such patients should therefore be especially cautious.

Cerebrovascular Insufficiency: Because of potential effects of beta-adrenergic blocking agents relative to blood pressure and pulse, these agents should be used with caution in patients with cerebrovascular insufficiency. If signs or symptoms suggesting reduced cerebral blood flow are observed, consideration should be given to discontinuing these agents.

INFORMATION FOR THE PATIENT

Ophthalmic Solution: Patients should be instructed to avoid allowing the tip of the dispensing container to contact the eye or surrounding structures.

Patients should also be instructed that ocular solutions, if handled improperly, cam become contaminated by common bacteria known to cause ocular infections. Serious damage to the eye and subsequent loss of vision may result from using contaminated solutions. (See PRECAUTIONS, General.)

Patients should also be advised that if they develop an intercurrent ocular condition (*e.g.,* trauma, ocular surgery or infection), they should immediately seek their physician's advice concerning the continued use of the present multidose container.

The preservative in timolol maleate, benzalkonium chloride, may be absorbed by soft contact lenses. Patients wearing soft contact lenses should be instructed to wait at least 15 minutes after instilling timolol maleate before they insert their lenses.

Preservative-Free Ophthalmic Solution: Patients should be instructed about the use of preservative-free timolol maleate in Ocudose.

Since sterility cannot be maintained after the individual unit is opened, patients should be instructed to use the product immediately after opening, and to discard the individual unit and any remaining contents immediately after use.

CARCINOGENESIS, MUTAGENESIS, AND IMPAIRMENT OF FERTILITY

In a two-year oral study of timolol maleate in rats, there was a statistically significant increase in the incidence of adrenal pheochromocytomas in male rats administered 300 mg/kg/day (250 times* the maximum recommended human dose). Similar differences were not observed in rats administered doses equivalent to approximately 20 or 80 times* the maximum recommended human dose.

In a lifetime oral study in mice, there were statistically significant increases in the incidence of benign and malignant pulmonary tumors, benign uterine polyps and mammary adenocarcinoma in female mice at 500 mg/kg/day (approximately 400 times* the maximum recommended human dose), but not at 5 or 50 mg/kg/day. In a subsequent study in female mice, in which postmortem examinations were limited to uterus and lungs, a statistically significant increase in the incidence of pulmonary tumors was again observed at 500 mg/kg/day.

PRECAUTIONS: *(cont'd)*

The increased occurrence of mammary adenocarcinomas was associated with elevations in serum prolactin that occurred in female mice administered timolol at 500 mg/kg, but not at doses of 5 or 50 mg/kg/day. An increased incidence of mammary adenocarcinomas in rodents has been associated with administration of several other therapeutic agents which elevate serum prolactin, but no correlation between serum prolactin levels and mammary tumors has been established in man. Furthermore, in adult human female subjects who received oral dosages of up to 60 mg of timolol maleate, the maximum recommended human oral dosage, there were no clinically meaningful changes in serum prolactin.

Timolol maleate was devoid of mutagenic potential when evaluated *in vivo* (mouse) in the micronucleus test and cytogenetic assay (doses up to 800 mg/kg) and *in vitro*in a neoplastic cell transformation assay (up to 100 mcg/ml). In Ames tests the highest concentrations of timolol employed, 5000 or 10,000 mcg/plate, were associated with statistically significant elevations of revertants observed with tester strain TA100 (in seven replicate assays), but not in the remaining three strains. In the assays with tester strain TA100, no consistent dose response relationship was observed, nor did the ratio of test to control revertants reach 2. A ratio of 2 is usually considered the criterion for a positive Ames test.

Reproduction and fertility studies in rats showed no adverse effect on male or female fertility at doses up to 125 times* the maximum recommended human dose.

*Based on a patient weight of 50 kg

PREGNANCY CATEGORY C

Teratogenicity studies with timolol in mice and rabbits at doses up to 50 mg/kg/day (50 times the maximum recommended human dose) showed no evidence of fetal malformations. Although delayed fetal ossification was observed at this dose in rats, there were no adverse effects on postnatal development of offspring. Doses of 1000 mg/kg/day (1,000 times the maximum recommended human dose) were maternotoxic in mice and resulted in an increased number of fetal resorptions. Increased fetal resorptions were also seen in rabbits at doses of 100 times the maximum recommended human dose, in this case without apparent maternotoxicity. There are no adequate and well-controlled studies in pregnant women. Timolol maleate should be used during pregnancy only if the potential benefit justifies the potential risk to the fetus.

NURSING MOTHERS

Because of the potential for serious adverse reactions from timolol in nursing infants, a decision should be made whether to discontinue nursing or to discontinue the drug, taking into account the importance of the drug to the mother.

PEDIATRIC USE

Safety and effectiveness in children have not been established.

ANIMAL STUDIES

No adverse ocular effects were observed in rabbits and dogs administered timolol maleate topically in studies lasting one and two years respectively.

DRUG INTERACTIONS:

Close observation of the patient is recommended when timolol maleate is administered to patients receiving catecholamine-depleting drugs such as reserpine, because of possible additive effects and the production of hypotension and/or marked bradycardia, which may produce vertigo, syncope, or postural hypotension.

Literature reports suggest that oral calcium antagonists may be used in combination with beta-adrenergic blocking agents when heart function is normal, but should be avoided in patients with impaired cardiac function. Hypotension, AV conduction disturbances, and left ventricular failure have been reported in some patients receiving beta-adrenergic blocking agents when an oral calcium antagonist was added to the treatment regimen. Hypotension was more likely to occur if the calcium antagonist were a dihydropyridine derivative, (*e.g.,* nifedipine) while left ventricular failure and AV conduction disturbances were more likely to occur with either verapamil or diltiazem.

Intravenous calcium antagonists should be used with caution in patients receiving beta-adrenergic blocking agents.

The concomitant use of beta-adrenergic blocking agents with digitalis and either diltiazem or verapamil may have additive effects in prolonging AV conduction time.

Risk from Anaphylactic Reaction: While taking beta-blockers, patients with a history of atopy or a history of severe anaphylactic reaction to a variety of allergens may be more reactive to repeated accidental, diagnostic, or therapeutic challenge with such allergens. Such patients may be unresponsive to the usual doses of epinephrine used to treat anaphylactoid reactions.

Tablets: Blunting of the antihypertensive effect of beta-adrenoceptor blocking agents by non-steroidal anti-inflammatory drugs has been reported. When using these agents concomitantly, patients should be observed carefully to confirm that the desired therapeutic effect has been obtained.

Ophthalmic Solutions: Although timolol maleate used alone has little or no effect on pupil size, mydriasis resulting from concomitant therapy with timolol maleate and epinephrine has been reported occasionally.

ADVERSE REACTIONS:

TABLETS

Timolol maleate is usually well tolerated in properly selected patients. Most adverse effects have been mild and transient.

In a multicenter (12-week) clinical trial comparing timolol maleate and placebo in hypertensive patients, the following adverse reactions were reported spontaneously and considered to be causally related to timolol maleate (TABLE 1).

These data are representative of the incidence of adverse effects that may be observed in properly selected patients treated with timolol maleate, i.e., excluding patients with bronchospastic disease, congestive heart failure or other contraindications to beta blocker therapy.

In patients with migraine the incidence of bradycardia was 5 percent.

In a coronary artery disease population studied in the Norwegian multi-center trial (see CLINICAL PHARMACOLOGY), the frequency of the principal adverse reactions and the frequency with which these resulted in discontinuation of therapy in the timolol and placebo groups (TABLE 2).

The following additional adverse effects have been reported in clinical experience with the drug:

Body as a Whole: extremity pain, decreased exercise tolerance, weight loss, fever;

Cardiovascular: cardiac arrest, cardiac failure, cerebral vascular accident, worsening of angina pectoris, worsening of arterial insufficiency, Raynaud's phenomenon, palpitations, vasodilatation;

Digestive: gastrointestinal pain, hepatomegaly, vomiting, diarrhea, dyspepsia;

Hematologic: non-thrombocytopenic purpura;

Endocrine: hyperglycemia, hypoglycemia;

Skin: rash, skin irritation, increased pigmentation, sweating, alopecia;

Musculoskeletal: arthralgia;

ADVERSE REACTIONS: *(cont'd)*

TABLE 1

		Timolol Maleate (n = 176) %	Placebo (n = 168) %
Body As A Whole			
	fatigue/tiredness	3.4	0.6
	headache	1.7	1.8
	chest pain	0.6	0
	asthenia	0.6	0
Cardiovascular			
	bradycardia	9.1	0
	arrhythmia	1.1	0.6
	syncope	0.6	0
	edema	0.6	1.2
Digestive			
	dyspepsia	0.6	0.6
	nausea	0.6	0
Skin			
	pruritus	1.1	0
Nervous System			
	dizziness	2.3	1.2
	vertigo	0.6	0
	paresthesia	0.6	0
Psychiatric			
	decreased libido	0.6	0
Respiratory			
	dyspnea	1.7	0.6
	bronchial spasm	0.6	0
	rales	0.6	0
Special Senses			
	eye irritation	1.1	0.6
	tinnitus	0.6	0

TABLE 2

	Adverse Reaction†		Withdrawal‡	
	Timolol (n = 945) %	Placebo (n = 939) %	Timolol (n = 945) %	Placebo (n = 939) %
Asthenia of Fatigue	5	1	<1	<1
Heart Rate <40 beats/minute	5	<1	4	<1
Cardiac Failure-Nonfatal	8	7	3	2
Hypotension	3	2	3	1
Pulmonary Edema-Nonfatal	2	<1	<1	<1
Claudication	3	3	1	<1
AV Block 2nd or 3rd degree	<1	<1	<1	<1
Sinoatrial Block	<1	<1	<1	<1
Cold Hands and Feet	8	<1	<1	0
Nausea or Digestive Disorders	8	6	1	<1
Dizziness	6	4	1	0
Bronchial Obstruction	2	<1	1	<1

† When an adverse reaction recurred in a patient, it is listed only once.
‡ Only principal reason for withdrawal in each patient is listed.
These adverse reactions can also occur in patients treated for hypertension.

Nervous System: local weakness, increase in signs and symptoms of myasthenia gravis;

Psychiatric: depression, nightmares, somnolence, insomnia, nervousness, diminished concentration, hallucinations;

Respiratory: cough;

Special Senses: visual disturbances, diplopia, ptosis, dry eyes;

Urogenital: impotence, urination difficulties.

There have been reports of retroperitoneal fibrosis in patients receiving timolol maleate and in patients receiving other beta-adrenergic blocking agents. A causal relationship between this condition and therapy with beta-adrenergic blocking agents has not been established.

Potential Adverse Effects: In addition, a variety of adverse effects not observed in clinical trials with timolol maleate, but reported with other beta-adrenergic blocking agents, should be considered potential adverse effects of timolol maleate:

Nervous System: Reversible mental depression progressing to catatonia; an acute reversible syndrome characterized by disorientation for time and place, short-term memory loss, emotional lability, slightly clouded sensorium, and decreased performance on neuropsychometrics;

Cardiovascular: Intensification of AV block (see CONTRAINDICATIONS);

Digestive: Mesenteric arterial thrombosis, ischemic colitis;

Hematologic: Agranulocytosis, thrombocytopenic purpura;

Allergic: Erythematous rash, fever combined with aching and sore throat, laryngospasm with respiratory distress;

Miscellaneous: Peyronie's disease.

There have been reports of a syndrome comprising psoriasiform skin rash, conjunctivitis sicca, otitis, and sclerosing serositis attributed to the beta-adrenergic receptor blocking agent, practolol. This syndrome has not been reported with timolol maleate.

Clinical Laboratory Test Findings: Clinically important changes in standard laboratory parameters were rarely associated with the administration of timolol maleate. Slight increases in blood urea nitrogen, serum potassium, uric acid, and triglycerides, and slight decreases in hemoglobin, hematocrit and HDL cholesterol occurred, but were not progressive or associated with clinical manifestations. Increases in liver function tests have been reported.

OPHTHALMIC SOLUTIONS

The following adverse reactions have been reported with timolol maleate, either in clinical trials of up to 3 years duration prior to release in 1978 or since the drug has been marketed, and may be expected to occur with preservative-free timolol maleate.

Body As A Whole: Headache, asthenia/fatigue, chest pain.

Cardiovascular: Bradycardia, arrhythmia, hypotension, syncope, heart block cerebral vascular accident, cerebral ischemia, cardiac failure, palpitation, cardiac arrest.

Digestive: Nausea, diarrhea.

Nervous System/Psychiatric: Dizziness, depression increase in signs and symptoms of myasthenia gravis, paresthesia.

Skin: Hypersensitivity, including localized and generalized rash; urticaria, alopecia.

Respiratory: Bronchospasm (predominantly in patients with pre-existing bronchospastic disease), respiratory failure, dyspnea, nasal congestion, cough.

ADVERSE REACTIONS: *(cont'd)*

Endocrine: Masked symptoms of hypoglycemia in insulin-dependent diabetics (see WARNINGS.)

Special Senses: Signs and symptoms of ocular irritation, including conjunctivitis, blepharitis, keratitis, blepharoptosis, decreased corneal sensitivity, visual disturbances including reactive changes (due to withdrawal of miotic therapy in some cases), diplopia, ptosis.

Causal Relationship Unknown: The following adverse effects have been reported, and a causal relationship to therapy with timolol maleate has not been established:

Cardiovascular: Hypertension, pulmonary edema, worsening of angina pectoris;

Digestive: Dyspepsia, anorexia, dry mouth;

Nervous System/Psychiatric: Behavioral changes including confusion, hallucinating, anxiety, disorientation, nervousness, somnolence, and other psychic disturbances;

Special Senses: Aphakic cystoid macular edema;

Urogenital: Retroperitoneal fibrosis, impotence.

The following additional adverse effects have been reported in clinical experience with oral timolol maleate, and may be considered potential effects of ophthalmic timolol maleate:

Body as a Whole: Extremity pain, decreased exercise tolerance, weight loss;

Cardiovascular: Edema, worsening of arterial insufficiency, Raynaud's phenomenon, vasodilatation;

Digestive: Gastrointestinal pain, hepatomegaly, vomiting;

Hematologic: Non-thrombocytopenic purpura;

Endocrine: Hyperglycemia, hypoglycemia;

Skin: Pruritus, skin irritation increased pigmentation, sweating, cold hands and feet;

Musculoskeletal: Arthralgia, claudication;

Nervous System/Psychiatric: Vertigo, local weakness, decreased libido, nightmares, insomnia, diminished concentration;

Respiratory: Rales, bronchial obstruction;

Special Senses: Tinnitus, dry eyes;

Urogenital: Urination difficulties.

Potential Adverse Effects: In addition, a variety of adverse effects have been reported with other beta-adrenergic blocking agents and may be considered potential effects of ophthalmic timolol maleate:

Digestive: Mesenteric arterial thrombosis, ischemic colitis;

Hematologic: Agranulocytosis, thrombocytopenic purpura;

Nervous System: Reversible mental depression progressing to catatonia; an acute reversible syndrome characterized by disorientation of time and place, short-term memory loss, emotional lability, slightly clouded sensorium and decreased performance on neuropsychometrics;

Allergic: Erythematous rash, fever combined with aching and sore throat, laryngospasm with respiratory distress;

Urogenital: Peyronie's disease.

There have been reports of a syndrome comprising psoriasiform skin rash, conjunctivitis sicca, otitis and sclerosing serositis attributed to the beta-adrenergic receptor blocking agent, practolol. This syndrome has not been reported with timolol maleate.

OVERDOSAGE:

There have been reports of inadvertent overdosage with timolol maleate ophthalmic solution resulting in systemic effects such as dizziness, headache, shortness of breath, bradycardia, bronchospasm, and cardiac arrest. Overdosage has been reported with tablets (timolol maleate). A 30 year old female ingested 650 mg of timolol maleate (maximum recommended oral daily dose is 60 mg) and experienced second and third degree heart block. She recovered without treatment but approximately two months later developed irregular heartbeat, hypertension, dizziness, tinnitus, faintness, increased pulse rate, and borderline first degree heart block.

The oral LD_{50} of the drug is 1190 and 900 mg/kg in female mice and female rats, respectively.

An *in vitro* hemodialysis study, using ^{14}C timolol added to human plasma or whole blood, showed that timolol was readily dialyzed from these fluids; however, a study of patients with renal failure showed that timolol did not dialyze readily.

The most common signs and symptoms to be expected with overdosage with a beta-adrenergic receptor blocking agent are symptomatic bradycardia, hypotension, bronchospasm, and acute cardiac failure. Therapy with timolol maleate should be discontinued and the patient observed closely. The following additional therapeutic measures should be considered:

(1) Gastric lavage.

(2) Symptomatic bradycardia: Use atropine sulfate intravenously in a dosage of 0.25 mg to 2 mg to induce vagal blockade. If bradycardia persists, intravenous isoproterenol hydrochloride should be administered cautiously. In refractory cases the use of a transvenous cardiac pacemaker may be considered.

(3) Hypotension: Use sympathomimetic pressor drug therapy, such as dopamine, dobutamine or levarterenol. In refractory cases the use of glucagon hydrochloride has been reported to be useful.

(4) Bronchospasm: Use isoproterenol hydrochloride. Additional therapy with aminophylline may be considered.

(5) Acute cardiac failure: Conventional therapy with digitalis, diuretics, and oxygen should be instituted immediately. In refractory cases the use of intravenous aminophylline is suggested. This may be followed if necessary by glucagon hydrochloride which has been reported to be useful.

(6) Heart block (second or third degree): Use isoproterenol hydrochloride or a transvenous cardiac pacemaker.

DOSAGE AND ADMINISTRATION:

TABLETS

Hypertension: The usual initial dosage of timolol maleate is 10 mg twice a day, whether used alone or added to diuretic therapy. Dosage may be increased or decreased depending on heart rate and blood pressure response. The usual total maintenance dosage is 20-40 mg per day. Increases in dosage to a maximum of 60 mg per day divided into two doses may be necessary. There should be an interval of at least seven days between increases in dosages.

Timolol maleate may be used with a thiazide diuretic or with other antihypertensive agents. Patients should be observed carefully during initiation of such concomitant therapy.

Myocardial Infarction: The recommended dosage for long-term prophylactic use in patients who have survived the acute phase of a myocardial infarction is 10 mg given twice daily (see CLINICAL PHARMACOLOGY.)

Migraine: The usual initial dosage of timolol maleate is 10 mg twice a day. During maintenance therapy the 20 mg daily dosage may be administered as a single dose. Total daily dosage may be increased to a maximum of 30 mg, given in divided doses, or decreased

DOSAGE AND ADMINISTRATION: *(cont'd)*

to 10 mg once per day depending on clinical response and tolerability. If a satisfactory response is not obtained after 6-8 weeks use of the maximum daily dosage, therapy with timolol maleate should be discontinued.

Storage: Store in a well-closed container, protected from light.

OPHTHALMIC SOLUTIONS

Timolol maleate ophthalmic solution is available in concentrations of 0.25 and 0.5 percent. The usual starting dose is one drop of 0.25 percent timolol maleate in the affected eye(s) twice a day. If the clinical response is not adequate, the dosage may be changed to one drop of 0.5 percent solution in the affected eye(s) twice a day.

Since in some patients the pressure-lowering response to timolol maleate may require a few weeks to stabilize, evaluation should include a determination of intraocular pressure after approximately 4 weeks of treatment with timolol maleate.

If the intraocular pressure is maintained at satisfactory levels, the dosage schedule may be changed to one drop once a day in the affected eye(s). Because of diurnal variations in intraocular pressure, satisfactory response to the once-a-day dose is best determined by measuring the intraocular pressure at different times during the day.

Dosages above one drop of 0.5 percent timolol maleate twice a day generally have not been shown to produce further reduction in intraocular pressure. If the patient's intraocular pressure is still not at a satisfactory level on this regimen, concomitant therapy with pilocarpine and other miotics, and/or epinephrine, and/or systemically administered carbonic anhydrase inhibitors, such as acetazolamide, can be instituted taking into consideration that the preparation(s) used concomitantly may contain one or more preservatives.

When a patient is transferred from another topical ophthalmic beta-adrenergic blocking agent, that agent should be discontinued after proper dosing on one day and treatment with timolol maleate started on the following day with 1 drop of 0.25 percent timolol maleate in the affected eye(s) twice a day. The dose may be increased to one drop of 0.5 percent timolol maleate twice a day if the clinical response is not adequate.

When a patient is transferred from a single antiglaucoma agent, other than a topical ophthalmic beta-adrenergic blocking agent, continue the agent already being used and add one drop of 0.25 percent timolol maleate in the affected eye(s) twice a day. On the following day, discontinue the previously used antiglaucoma agent completely and continue with timolol maleate. If a higher dosage of timolol maleate is required, substitute one drop of 0.5 percent solution in the affected eye(s) twice a day.

When a patient is transferred from several concomitantly administered antiglaucoma agents, individualization is required. If any of the agents is an ophthalmic beta-adrenergic blocker, it should be discontinued before starting timolol maleate. Additional adjustments should involve one agent at a time and usually should be made at intervals of not less than one week. A recommended approach is to continue the agents being used and to add one drop of 0.25 percent timolol maleate in the affected eye(s) twice a day. On the following day, discontinue one of the other antiglaucoma agents. The remaining antiglaucoma agents may be decreased or discontinued according to the patient's response to treatment. If a higher dosage of timolol maleate is required, substitute one drop of 0.5 percent solution in the affected eye(s) twice a day. The physician may be able to discontinue some or all of the other antiglaucoma agents.

PRESERVATIVE-FREE OPHTHALMIC SOLUTION

Preservative-free Timoptic in Ocudose is a sterile solution that does not contain a preservative. The solution from one individual unit is to used immediately after opening for administration to one or both eyes. Since sterility cannot be guaranteed after the individual unit is opened, the remaining contents should be discarded immediately after administration.

Preservative-free Timoptic in Ocudose is available in concentrations of 0.25 and 0.5 percent. The usual starting dose is one drop of 0.25 percent preservative-free Timoptic in Ocudose in the affected eye(s) administered twice a day. Apply enough gentle pressure on the individual container to obtain a single drop of solution. If the clinical response is not adequate, the dosage may be changed to one drop of 0.5 percent solution in the affected eye(s) administered twice a day.

PATIENT INFORMATION:

Timolol maleate is known as a beta-blocker. It is used to treat high blood pressure, treat glaucoma, prevent headaches and is given to some patients who have had a heart attack. This medication should not be used by those with breathing difficulties without the advice of a physician. It can also block signs of low blood sugar in those with diabetes. This medication should not be stopped abruptly. It should be slowly stopped over a period of days. If you are using this medication for glaucoma, you should learn to properly instill eye drops. It is important not to touch the tip of the bottle to anything, especially the skin or eye. Keeping the tip clean will prevent infections of the bottle and your eye. Wait 15 minutes after instilling the eye drops to put contact lenses in. The most common side effect of this drug is muscle weakness and feeling tired. This may subside with continued therapy. Consult your physician if this becomes a problem.

HOW SUPPLIED:

Sterile Ophthalmic Solution Timoptic is a clear, colorless to light yellow solution.

Timoptic Ophthalmic Solution, 0.25% timolol equivalent, is supplied in a white, opaque, plastic Ocumeter* ophthalmic dispenser with a controlled drop tip.

Timoptic Ophthalmic Solution, 0.5% timolol equivalent, is supplied in a white, opaque, plastic Ocumeter ophthalmic dispenser with a controlled drop tip.

Storage: Protect from light. Store at room temperature. Preservative-free Sterile Ophthalmic Solution Timoptic in Ocudose is a clear, colorless to light yellow solution.

Preservative-free Timoptic, 0.25% timolol equivalent, is supplied in Ocudose, a clearly polyethylene unit dose container. Each individual unit contains 0.45 ml of solution, and is available in a foil laminate overwrapped pouch.

Preservative-free Timoptic, 0.5% timolol equivalent, is supplied in Ocudose, a clear polyethylene unit dose container. Each individual unit contains 0.45 ml of solution, and is available in a foil laminate overwrapped pouch. Store Preservative-free Timoptic in Ocudose at room temperature.

Because evaporation can occur through the unprotected polyethylene unit dose container and prolonged exposure to direct light can modify the product, the unit dose container should be kept in the protective foil overwrap and used within one month after the foil package has been opened.

HOW SUPPLIED - RATED THERAPEUTICALLY EQUIVALENT:

Ophthalmic Solution - Topical - 0.0025%

5 ml	$14.00	Timolol Maleate, Schein Pharm (US)	00364-3077-53
10 ml	$27.00	Timolol Maleate, Schein Pharm (US)	00364-3077-54
15 ml	$40.50	Timolol Maleate, Schein Pharm (US)	00364-3077-72

Ophthalmic Solution - Topical - 0.005%

5 ml	$16.50	Timolol Maleate, Schein Pharm (US)	00364-3078-53
10 ml	$32.00	Timolol Maleate, Schein Pharm (US)	00364-3078-54
15 ml	$48.00	Timolol Maleate, Schein Pharm (US)	00364-3078-72

HOW SUPPLIED - RATED THERAPEUTICALLY EQUIVALENT:
(cont'd)

Solution - Ophthalmic - 0.25 %

2.5 ml	**$6.35**	**TIMOPTIC, Merck**	**00006-3366-32**
5 ml	**$12.45**	**TIMOPTIC, Merck**	**00006-3366-03**
10 ml	**$24.06**	**TIMOPTIC, Merck**	**00006-3366-10**
15 ml	**$36.01**	**TIMOPTIC, Merck**	**00006-3366-12**

Solution - Ophthalmic - 0.5 %

2.5 ml	**$7.57**	**TIMOPTIC, Merck**	**00006-3367-32**
5 ml	**$14.73**	**TIMOPTIC, Merck**	**00006-3367-03**
10 ml	**$28.58**	**TIMOPTIC, Merck**	**00006-3367-10**
15 ml	**$42.77**	**TIMOPTIC, Merck**	**00006-3367-12**

Tablet, Uncoated - Oral - 5 mg

100's	$20.22	Timolol Maleate, H.C.F.A. F F P	99999-2353-01
100's	$23.80	Timolol Maleate, HL Moore Drug Exch	00839-7584-06
100's	$26.45	Timolol Maleate, Novopharm (US)	55953-0961-40
100's	$26.50	Timolol Maleate, Schein Pharm (US)	00364-2357-01
100's	$26.50	Timolol Maleate, West Point Pharma	59591-0192-68
100's	$26.50	Timolol Maleate, Endo Labs	60951-0782-70
100's	$28.56	Timolol Maleate, Geneva Pharms	00781-1126-01
100's	$28.75	Timolol Maleate, Mylan	00378-0055-01
100's	$42.74	BLOCADREN, Merck	00006-0059-68

Tablet, Uncoated - Oral - 10 mg

100's	$27.87	Timolol Maleate, H.C.F.A. F F P	99999-2353-02
100's	$29.25	Timolol Maleate, Harber Pharm	51432-0569-03
100's	$30.48	Timolol Maleate, Rugby	00536-4696-01
100's	$31.80	Timolol Maleate, Qualitest Pharms	00603-6072-21
100's	$33.00	Timolol Maleate, Schein Pharm (US)	00364-2358-01
100's	$33.70	Timolol Maleate, Aligen Independ	00405-5020-01
100's	$33.70	Timolol Maleate, Novopharm (US)	55953-0972-40
100's	$33.95	Timolol Maleate, West Point Pharma	59591-0194-68
100's	$33.95	Timolol Maleate, Endo Labs	60951-0783-70
100's	$34.01	Timolol Maleate, HL Moore Drug Exch	00839-7585-06
100's	$35.30	Timolol Maleate, Geneva Pharms	00781-1127-01
100's	$35.60	Timolol Maleate, Mylan	00378-0221-01
100's	$35.71	Timolol Maleate, HL Moore Drug Exch	00839-7936-06
100's	$36.90	Timolol Maleate, Elkins Sinn	00641-4031-86
100's	$38.31	Timolol Maleate, Novopharm (US)	55953-0972-01
100's	$52.85	BLOCADREN, Merck	00006-0136-68
100's	$57.26	BLOCADREN, Merck	00006-0136-28
500's	$139.35	Timolol Maleate, H.C.F.A. F F P	99999-2353-03
500's	$167.71	Timolol Maleate, Novopharm (US)	55953-0972-70

Tablet, Uncoated - Oral - 20 mg

100's	$54.00	Timolol Maleate, Harber Pharm	51432-0571-03
100's	$56.39	Timolol Maleate, H.C.F.A. F F P	99999-2353-04
100's	$61.70	Timolol Maleate, Novopharm (US)	55953-0984-40
100's	$64.79	Timolol Maleate, HL Moore Drug Exch	00839-7586-06
100's	$64.85	Timolol Maleate, Schein Pharm (US)	00364-2359-01
100's	$66.10	Timolol Maleate, Geneva Pharms	00781-1128-01
100's	$67.50	Timolol Maleate, Mylan	00378-0715-01
100's	$68.00	Timolol Maleate, Elkins Sinn	00641-4032-86
100's	$68.03	Timolol Maleate, HL Moore Drug Exch	00839-7937-06
100's	$97.48	BLOCADREN, Merck	00006-0437-68

HOW SUPPLIED - NOT RATED EQUIVALENT:

Gel - Ophthalmic - 0.25 %

2.5 ml	**$10.25**	**TIMOPTIC-XE, Merck**	**00006-3557-32**
5 ml	**$18.09**	**TIMOPTIC-XE, Merck**	**00006-3557-03**
7.5 ml	**$36.64**	**TIMOPTIC-XE, Merck**	**00006-3557-91**

Gel - Ophthalmic - 0.5 %

2.5 ml	**$12.12**	**TIMOPTIC-XE, Merck**	**00006-3558-32**
5 ml	**$21.49**	**TIMOPTIC-XE, Merck**	**00006-3558-03**
7.5 ml	**$43.52**	**TIMOPTIC-XE, Merck**	**00006-3558-91**

Solution - Ophthalmic - 0.25 %

0.45 ml x 60	**$72.50**	**TIMOPTIC OCUDOSE, Merck**	**00006-3542-60**

Solution - Ophthalmic - 0.5 %

0.45 ml x 60	**$87.28**	**TIMOPTIC OCUDOSE, Merck**	**00006-3543-60**

TIOCONAZOLE *(003111)*

CATEGORIES: Antimycotics; Anti-infectives; Antifungals; Candidiasis; Dermatologicals; Fungal Agents; Skin/Mucous Membrane Agents; FDA Approved 1986 Dec

BRAND NAMES: *Fungibacid*; *Gino-Trosyd*; *Gyno-Trosyd* (Canada); *Trosid*; *Trosil*; *Trosy* (Japan); *Trosyd*; **Vagistat-1**; *Zoniden*
(International brand names outside U.S. in italics)

DESCRIPTION:

Tioconazole, 1-[2-l (2-chloro-3-thienyl)methoxy 1 -2(2,4-dichlorophenyl)ethyl]-1H-imidazole, is a topical antifungal agent. Its chemical formula is $C^{16}H^{13}C1^{3}N^{2}OS$ with a molecular weight of 387.7.

Vagistat-1 is formulated in a base of white, soft paraffin and aluminum magnesium silicate with butylated hydroxyanisole (BHA) added as a preservative. Each applicator-full of Vagistat-1 provides approximately 4.6 grams of ointment containing 300 mg of tioconazole.

CLINICAL PHARMACOLOGY:

Tioconazole is a broad-spectrum antifungal agent that inhibits the growth of human pathogenic yeasts. Tioconazole exhibits fungicidal activity *in vitro* against *Candida albicans*, other species of the genus *Candida* and against *Torulopsis glabrata*.

Pharmacokinetics: Systemic absorption of tioconazole after a single intravaginal application of tioconazole in non-pregnant patients is negligible.

INDICATIONS AND USAGE:

Tioconazole is indicated for the local treatment of vulvovaginal candidiasis (moniliasis). As tioconazole has been shown to be effective only for candidal vulvovaginitis, the diagnosis should be confirmed by KOH smears and/or cultures. Other pathogens commonly associated with vulvovaginitis should be ruled out by appropriate methods.

Studies have shown that women taking oral contraceptives have a cure rate similar to those not taking such agents when treated with tioconazole.

Safety and effectiveness in pregnant and diabetic patients have not been established (see PRECAUTIONS.)

CONTRAINDICATIONS:

Tioconazole is contraindicated in individuals who have been shown to be sensitive to imidazole antifungal agents or to other components of the ointment.

PRECAUTIONS:

General: Tioconazole is intended for intravaginal administration only. Applicators should be opened just prior to administration to prevent contamination. Administration of tioconazole just prior to bedtime may be preferred. The tioconazole ointment base may interact with rubber or latex products such as condoms or vaginal contraceptive diaphragms, therefore, use of such products with 72 hours following treatment is not recommended.

If clinical problems persist, appropriate microbiological tests should be repeated to rule out other pathogens and to confirm the diagnosis.

Information for the Patient: The tioconazole ointment base may interact with rubber or latex products such as condoms or vaginal contraceptive diaphragms, therefore, use of such products within 72 hours following treatment is not recommended.

Carcinogenesis, Mutagenesis, and Impairment of Fertility: No long-term studies in animals have been performed to evaluate the carcinogenic potential of tioconazole.

Tioconazole did not demonstrate mutagenic activity at the levels examined in tests at either chromosomal or subchromosomal level.

No impairment of fertility was seen in male rats administered tioconazole hydrochloride in oral doses up to 150 mg/kg/day. However, there was evidence of preimplantation loss in female rats at oral dose levels above 35 mg/kg/day.

Pregnancy Category C: Tioconazole hydrochloride had no adverse effects on fetal viability or growth when administered orally to pregnant rats at doses of 55, 110 and 165 mg/kg/day during the period of organogenesis. A drug-related increase in the incidence of dilated ureters, hydroureters, and hydronephrosis observed in the fetuses of this study was transient and no longer evident in pups raised to 21 days of age. These effects did not occur following intravaginal administration of approximately 10 mg/kg/day in a 2% cream. There was no evidence of major structural anomalies. No embryotoxic or teratogenic effects were observed in rabbits receiving oral dose levels as high as 165 mg/kg/day or daily intravaginal application of approximately 2-3 mg/kg in a 2% tioconazole cream during organogenesis. Tioconazole hydrochloride, like other azole antimycotic agents, causes dystocia in rats when treatment is extended through parturition. Associated effects in rats include prolongation of pregnancy, *in utero* deaths, and impaired pup survival. The "no-effect" level for this phenomenon is 20 mg/kg/day orally and approximately 9 mg/kg/day intravaginally. No effect on parturition in rabbits at 50 mg/kg/day orally.

There are no adequate and well-controlled studies in pregnant women. Tioconazole 6.5% should be used during pregnancy only if the potential benefit justifies the potential risk to the fetus.

Nursing Mothers: It is not known whether this drug is excreted in human milk. Because many drugs are excreted in human milk, nursing should be temporarily discontinued while tioconazole is administered.

Pediatric Use: Safety and effectiveness in children have not been established.

ADVERSE REACTIONS:

The incidence of adverse reactions to tioconazole is based on clinical trials involving 1000 patients. Burning and itching were the most frequent side effects occurring in approximately 6% and 5% of the patients, respectively. In most instances, these did not interfere with the course of therapy.

There were occasional reports (less than 1%) of other side effects including irritation, discharge, vulvar edema and swelling, vaginal pain, dysuria, nocturia, dyspareunia, dryness of vaginal secretions, desquamation, and burning sensation.

DOSAGE AND ADMINISTRATION:

Tioconazole has been found to be effective as a single-dose treatment for vulvovaginal candidiasis. Using the prefilled applicator, insert one applicator-full intravaginally. Administration of tioconazole just prior to bedtime may be preferred.

HOW SUPPLIED:

Vagistat-1 is supplied in a ready-to-use, prefilled, single dose, vaginal applicator. Each applicator-full will deliver approximately 4.6 grams of Vagistat-1 containing 65 mg of tioconazole per gram of ointment.

Storage: Store at controlled room temperature (59° to 86°F).

HOW SUPPLIED - EQUIVALENTS NOT AVAILABLE:

Ointment - Vaginal - 65 mg

4.6 gm	**$24.19**	**VAGISTAT-1, Bristol Myers Squibb**	**00087-0657-40**

TIOPRONIN *(002354)*

CATEGORIES: Cystinuria; Heavy Metal Antagonists; Nephrolithiasis; Orphan Drugs; Reducing and Complexing Agents; FDA Approved 1988 Aug

BRAND NAMES: *Acadione*; *Captimer*; Thiola
(International brand names outside U.S. in italics)

Prescribing information not available at time of publication.

HOW SUPPLIED - EQUIVALENTS NOT AVAILABLE:

Tablet, Uncoated - Oral - 100 mg

100's	$57.00	THIOLA, Mission Pharma	00178-0900-01

TIRILAZAD MESYLATE *(003093)*

CATEGORIES: Brain Damage; Central Nervous System Agents; Head Injury; Lazaroids; Spinal Cord Injury; Stroke; Subarachnoid Hemorrhage; FDA Unapproved

BRAND NAMES: **Freedox**

Prescribing information not available at time of publication.

TIZANIDINE HYDROCHLORIDE *(003321)*

CATEGORIES: Alpha Adrenoreceptor Agonists; Autonomic Drugs; Imidazolines; Multiple Sclerosis; Muscle Relaxants; Neuromuscular; Skeletal Muscle Hyperactivity; Skeletal Muscle Relaxants; Spasticity; Spinal Cord Injury

BRAND NAMES: *Sirdalud* (Europe, Mexico); *Sirdalud MR*; *Sirdalud Retard*; *Ternelax*; *Ternelin* (Japan); **Zanaflex**
(International brand names outside U.S. in italics)

DESCRIPTION:

Zanaflex is a centrally acting α_2-adrenergic agonist. Tizanidine HCl is a white to off-white fine crystalline powder, odorless or with a faint characteristic odor. Tizanidine is slightly soluble in water and methanol; solubility in water decreases as the pH increases. Its chemical name is 5-chloro-4-(2-imidazolin-2-ylamino)-2, 1,3-benzothiodiazole hydrochloride. Tizanidine's molecular formula is $C_9H_8ClN_5S{\cdot}HCl$, its molecular weight is 290.2.

Zanaflex is supplied as 4 mg tablets for oral administration. Zanaflex tablets are composed of the active ingredient tizanidine hydrochloride (4.576 mg equivalent to 4 mg tizanidine base), and the inactive ingredients, silicon dioxide colloidal, stearic acid, microcrystalline cellulose and anhydrous lactose.

CLINICAL PHARMACOLOGY:

MECHANISM OF ACTION

Tizanidine is an agonist at α_2-agonist receptor sites and presumably reduces spasticity by increasing presynaptic inhibition of motor neurons. In animal models, tizanidine has no direct effect on skeletal muscle fibers or the neuromuscular junction, and no major effect on monosynaptic spinal reflexes. The effects of tizanidine are greatest on polysynaptic pathways. The overall effect of these actions is thought to reduce facilitation of spinal motor neurons.

The imidazoline chemical structure of tizanidine is related to that of the anti-hypertensive drug clonidine and other α_2-adrenergic agonists. Pharmacological studies in animals show similarities between the two compounds, but tizanidine was found to have one-tenth to one-fiftieth (1/50) of the potency of clonidine in lowering blood pressure.

PHARMACOKINETICS

Following oral administration, tizanidine is essentially completely absorbed and has a half-life of approximately 2.5 hours (coefficient of variation [CV] = 33%). Following administration of tizanidine, peak plasma concentrations occurred at 1.5 hours (CV = 40%) after dosing. Food increases C_{max} by approximately one-third and shortens time to peak concentration by approximately 40 minutes, but the extent of tizanidine absorption is not affected. Tizanidine has linear pharmacokinetics over a dose of 1 to 20 mg. The absolute oral bioavailability of tizanidine is approximately 40% (CV = 24%), due to extensive first-pass metabolism in the liver, approximately 95% of an administered dose is metabolized. Tizanidine metabolites are not known to be active; their half-lives range from 20 to 40 hours. Tizanidine is widely distributed throughout the body; mean steady-state volume of distribution is 2.4 L/kg (CV = 21%) following intravenous administration in healthy adult volunteers.

Following single and multiple oral dosing of ^{14}C-tizanidine, an average of 60% and 20% of total radioactivity was recovered in the urine and feces, respectively.

Tizanidine is approximately 30% bound to plasma proteins, independent of concentration over the therapeutic range.

SPECIAL POPULATIONS

Age Effects: No specific pharmacokinetic study was conducted to investigate age effects. Cross study comparison of pharmacokinetic data following single dose administration of 6 mg tizanidine showed that younger subjects cleared the drug four times faster than the elderly subjects. Tizanidine has not been evaluated in children (see PRECAUTIONS).

Hepatic Impairment: Pharmacokinetic differences due to hepatic impairment have not been studied (see WARNINGS).

Renal Impairment: Tizanidine clearance is reduced by more than 50% in elderly patients with renal insufficiency (creatinine clearance < 25 ml/min) compared to healthy elderly subjects; this would be expected to lead to a longer duration of clinical effect. Tizanidine should be used with caution in renally impaired patients (see PRECAUTIONS).

Gender Effects: No specific pharmacokinetic study was conducted to investigate gender effects. Retrospective analysis of pharmacokinetic data, however, following single and multiple dose administration of 4 mg tizanidine showed that gender had no effect on the pharmacokinetics of tizanidine.

Race Effects: Pharmacokinetic differences due to race have not been studied.

CLINICAL STUDIES:

Tizanidine's capacity to reduce increased muscle tone associated with spasticity was demonstrated in two adequate and well controlled studies in patients with multiple sclerosis or spinal cord injury.

In one study, patients with multiple sclerosis were randomized to receive single oral doses of drug or placebo. Patients and assessors were blind to treatment assignment and efforts were made to reduce the likelihood that assessors would become aware indirectly of treatment assignment (*e.g.,* they did not provide direct care to patients and were prohibited from asking questions about side effects). In all, 140 patients received either placebo, 8 mg or 16 mg of tizanidine.

Response was assessed by physical examination; muscle tone was rated on a 5 point scale (Ashworth score), with a score of 0 used to describe normal muscle tone. A score of 1 indicated a slight spastic catch while a score of 2 indicated more marked muscle resistance. A score of 3 was used to describe considerable increase in tone, making passive movement difficult. A muscle immobilized by spasticity was given a score of 4.

Assignments were made at 1, 2, 3, and 6 hours after treatment. A statistically significant reduction of the Ashworth score for tizanidine compared to placebo was detected at 1, 2, and 3 hours after treatment. The greatest reduction in muscle tone was 1 to 2 hours after treatment. By 6 hours after treatment, muscle tone in the 8 and 16 mg tizanidine groups was indistinguishable from muscle tone in placebo treated patients. Within a given patient, improvement in muscle tone was correlated with plasma concentration. Plasma concentrations were variable from patient to patient at a given dose. Although 16 mg produced a larger effect, adverse events including hypotension were more common and more severe than in the 8 mg group.

In a multiple dose study, 118 patients with spasticity secondary to spinal cord injury were randomized to either placebo or tizanidine. Steps similar to those taken in the first study were employed to ensure the integrity of blinding.

Patients were titrated over 3 weeks up to a maximum tolerated dose or 36 mg daily given in three unequal doses (*e.g.,* 10 mg given in the morning and afternoon and 16 mg given at night). Patients were then maintained on their maximally tolerated dose for 4 additional weeks (*i.e.,* maintenance phase). Throughout the maintenance phase, muscle tone was assessed on the Ashworth scale within a period of 2.5 hours following either the morning or afternoon dose.

CLINICAL STUDIES: *(cont'd)*

At endpoint (the protocol-specified time of outcome assessment), there was a statistically significant reduction in muscle tone in the tizanidine treated group compared to placebo. The reduction in muscle tone was not associated with a reduction in muscle strength (a desirable outcome) but also did not lead to any consistent advantage of tizanidine treated patients on measures of activities of daily living.

INDICATIONS AND USAGE:

Tizanidine is a short-acting drug for the acute and intermittent management of increased muscle tone associated with spasticity. The reduction of muscle tone that follows the oral administration of a single dose of tizanidine has its peak effect 1 to 2 hours after dosing, and the effect dissipates between 3 to 6 hours. Use must therefore be individualized, directed to those activities and times when relief of spasticity is most important and titrated to avoid intolerance. Evidence demonstrating the effectiveness of tizanidine is derived from a single dose study and from a seven week multiple dose study conducted in patients with multiple sclerosis and spinal cord injury, respectively.

CONTRAINDICATIONS:

Tizanidine is contraindicated in patients with know hypersensitivity to tizanidine or its ingredients.

WARNINGS:

Limited Data Base For Chronic Use Of Single Doses Above 8 Mg And Multiple Doses Above 24 Mg Per Day: Clinical experience with long-term use of tizanidine at doses of 8 to 16 mg single doses or total daily doses of 24 to 36 mg (see DOSAGE AND ADMINISTRATION) is limited. Approximately 75 patients have been exposed to individual doses of 12 mg or more for at least one year or more and approximately 80 patients have been exposed to total daily doses of 30 to 36 mg/day for at least one year or more. There is essentially no long-term experience with single, daytime doses of 16 mg. Because long-term clinical study experience at high doses is limited, only those adverse events with a relatively high incidence are likely to have been identified (see WARNINGS, PRECAUTIONS, and ADVERSE REACTIONS).

Hypotension: Tizanidine is an α_2-adrenergic agonist (like clonidine) and can produce hypotension. In a single dose study where blood pressure was monitored closely after dosing, two-thirds of patients treated with 8 mg of tizanidine had a 20% reduction in either the diastolic of systolic BP. The reduction was seen within 1 hour after dosing, peaked 2 to 3 hours after dosing and was associated, at times, with bradycardia, orthostatic hypotension, light-headedness/dizziness and rarely, syncope. The hypotensive effect is dose related and has been measured following single doses of ≥2 mg.

The chance of significant hypotension may possibly be minimized by titration of the dose and by focusing attention on signs and symptoms of hypotension prior to dose advancement. In addition, patients moving from a supine to a fixed upright position may be at increased risk for hypotension and orthostatic effects.

Caution is advised when tizanidine is to be used in patients receiving concurrent antihypertensive therapy and should not be used with other α_2-adrenergic agonists.

Risk of Liver Injury: Tizanidine occasionally causes liver injury, most often hepatocellular in type. In controlled clinical studies, approximately 5% of patients treated with tizanidine had elevations of liver function tests (ALT/SGPT, AST/SGOT) to greater than 3 times the upper limit of normal (or 2 times if baseline levels were elevated) compared to 0.4% in the control patients. Most cases resolved rapidly upon drug withdrawal with no reported residual problems. In occasional symptomatic cases, nausea, vomiting anorexia and jaundice have been reported. In postmarketing experience, three deaths associated with liver failure have been reported in patients treated with tizanidine. In one case, a 49 year-old male developed jaundice and liver enlargement following 2 months of tizanidine treatment, primarily at 6 mg 3 times daily. A liver biopsy showed multiobular necrosis without eosinophilic infiltration. Treatment was discontinued and the patient died in hepatic coma 10 days later. There was no evidence of hepatitis B and C in this patient and other therapy included only oxazepam and ranitidine. There was thus no explanation, other than a reaction to tizanidine, to explain the liver injury. In the two other cases, patients were taking other drugs with known potential for liver toxicity. One patient, treated with tizanidine at a dose of 4 mg/day, was also on carbamazepine when he developed cholestatic jaundice after 2 months of treatment; this patient died with pneumonia about 20 days later. Another patient, treated with tizanidine for 11 days, was also treated with dantrolene for about 2 weeks prior to developing fatal fulminant hepatic failure.

Monitoring of aminotranferase levels is recommended during the first 6 months of treatment (*e.g.,* baseline, 1, 3, and 6 months) and periodically thereafter, based on clinical status. Because of the potential toxic hepatic effect of tizanidine, the drug should be used only with extreme caution in patients with impaired hepatic function.

Sedation: In the multiple dose, controlled clinical studies, 48% of patients receiving any dose of tizanidine reported sedation as an adverse event. In 10% of these cases, the sedation was rated as severe compared to <1% in the placebo treated patients. Sedation may interfere with every day activity.

The effect appears to be dose related. In a single dose study, 92% of the patients receiving 16 mg, when asked, reported that they were drowsy during the 6 hour study. This compares to 76% of the patients on a 8 mg and 35% of the patients on placebo. Patients began noting this effect 30 minutes following dosing. The effect peaked 1.5 hours following dosing. Of the patients who received a single dose of 16 mg, 51% continued to report drowsiness 6 hours following dosing compared to 13% in the patients receiving placebo or 8 mg of tizanidine.

In the multiple dose studies, the prevalence of patients with sedation peaked following the first week of titration and then remained stable for the duration of the maintenance phase of the study.

Hallucinations/Psychotic-Like Symptoms: Tizanidine use has been associated with hallucinations. Formed, visual hallucinations or delusions have been reported in 5 of 170 patients (3%) in two North American controlled clinical studies. These 5 cases occurred within the first 6 weeks. Most of the patients were aware that the events were unreal. One patient developed psychoses in association with the hallucinations. One patient among these 5 continued to have problems for at least 2 weeks following discontinuation of tizanidine.

PRECAUTIONS:

GENERAL

Cardiovascular: Prolongation of the QT interval and bradycardia were noted in chronic toxicity studies in dogs at doses equal to the maximum human dose on a mg/m^2 basis. ECG evaluation was not performed in the controlled clinical studies. Reduction in pulse rate has been noted in association with decreases in blood pressure in the single dose controlled study (see WARNINGS).

Ophthalmic: Dose-related retinal degeneration and corneal opacities have been found in animal studies at doses equivalent to approximately the maximum recommended dose on a mg/m^2 basis. There have been no reports of corneal opacities or retinal degeneration in the clinical studies.

PRECAUTIONS: *(cont'd)*

Use in Renally Impaired Patients: Tizanidine should be used with caution in patients with renal insufficiency (creatinine clearance <25 ml/min), as clearance is reduced by more than 50%. In these patients, during titration, the individual doses should be reduced. If higher doses are required, individual doses rather than dosing frequency should be increased. These patients should be monitored closely for the onset or increase in severity of the common adverse events (dry mouth, somnolence, asthenia, and dizziness) as indicators of potential overdose.

Use in Women Taking Oral Contraceptives: Tizanidine should be used with caution in women taking oral contraceptives, as clearance of tizanidine is reduced by approximately 50% in such patients. In these patients, during titration, the individual doses should be reduced.

INFORMATION FOR THE PATIENT

Patients should be advised of the limited clinical experience with tizanidine both in regard to duration of use and the higher doses required to reduce muscle tone (see WARNINGS).

Because of the possibility of tizanidine lowering blood pressure, patients should be warned about the risk of clinically significant orthostatic hypotension (see WARNINGS).

Because of the possibility of sedation, patients should be warned about performing activities requiring alertness, such as driving a vehicle or operating machinery (see WARNINGS). Patients should also be instructed that the sedation may be additive when tizanidine is taken in conjunction with drugs (baclofen, benzodiazepines) or substances (*e.g.,* alcohol) that act as CNS depressants.

CARCINOGENESIS, MUTAGENESIS, AND IMPAIRMENT OF FERTILITY

No evidence for carcinogenicity was seen in two dietary studies in rodents. Tizanidine was administered to mice for 78 weeks at doses up to 16 mg/kg, which is equivalent to 2 times the maximum recommended human dose on a mg/m^2 basis. Tizanidine was also administered to rats for 104 weeks at doses up to 9 mg/kg, which is equivalent to 2.5 times the maximum recommended human dose on a mg/m^2 basis. There was no statistically significant increase in tumors in either species.

Tizanidine was not mutagenic or clastogenic in the following *in vitro* assays: the bacterial Ames test and the mammalian gene mutation test and chromosomal aberration test in Chinese hamster cells. It was also negative in the following *in vivo* assays: the bone marrow micronucleus test in mice, the bone marrow micronucleus and cytogenecity test in Chinese hamsters, the dominant lethal mutagenicity test in mice, and the unscheduled DNA synthesis (UDS) test in mice.

Tizanidine did not affect fertility in male rats at doses of 10 mg/kg, approximately 2.7 times the maximum recommended human dose on a mg/m^2 basis, and in females at doses of 3 mg/kg, approximately equal to the maximum recommended human dose on a mg/m^2 basis; fertility was reduced in males receiving 30 mg/kg (8 times the maximum recommended human dose on a mg/m^2 basis) and in females receiving 10 mg/kg (2.7 times the maximum recommended human dose on a mg/m^2 basis). At these doses, maternal behavioral effects and clinical signs were observed including marked sedation, weight loss, and ataxia.

PREGNANCY CATEGORY C

Reproduction studies performed in rats at a dose of 3 mg/kg, equal to the maximum recommended human dose on a mg/m^2 basis, and in rabbits at 30 mg/kg, 16 times the recommended human dose on a mg/m^2 basis, did not show evidence of teratogenicity. Tizanidine at doses that are equal to and up to 8 times the maximum recommended human dose on a mg/m^2 basis increased gestation duration in rats. Prenatal and postnatal pup loss was increased and developmental retardation occurred. Postimplantation loss was increased in rabbits at doses of 1 mg/kg or greater, equal to or greater than 0.5 times the maximum recommended human dose on a mg/m^2 basis. Tizanidine has not been studied in pregnant women. Tizanidine should be given to pregnant women only if clearly needed.

LABOR AND DELIVERY

The effect of tizanidine on labor and delivery is unknown.

NURSING MOTHERS

It is not known whether tizanidine is excreted in human milk, although as a lipid soluble drug, it might be expected to pass into breast milk.

GERIATRIC USE

Tizanidine should be used with caution in elderly patients because clearance is decreased four-fold.

PEDIATRIC USE

There are no adequate and well-controlled studies to document the safety and efficacy of tizanidine in children.

DRUG INTERACTIONS:

In vitro studies of cytochrome P450 isoenzymes using human liver microsomes indicate that neither tizanidine nor the major metabolites are likely to affect the metabolism of other drugs metabolized by cytochrome P450 isoenzymes.

Acetaminophen: Tizanidine delayed the T_{max} of acetaminophen by 16 minutes. Acetaminophen did not affect the pharmacokinetics of tizanidine.

Alcohol: Alcohol increased the AUC of tizanidine by approximately 20% while also increasing its C_{max} by approximately 15%. This was associated with an increase in side effects of tizanidine. The CNS depressant effects of tizanidine and alcohol are additive.

Oral Contraceptives: No specific pharmacokinetic study was conducted to investigate interaction between oral contraceptives and tizanidine. Retrospective analysis of population pharmacokinetic data following single and multiple dose administration of 4 mg tizanidine, however, showed that women concurrently taking oral contraceptives had 50% lower clearance of tizanidine compared to women not on oral contraceptives (see PRECAUTIONS).

ADVERSE REACTIONS:

In multiple-dose, placebo controlled clinical studies, 264 patients were treated with tizanidine and 261 with placebo. Adverse events, including severe adverse events, were more frequently reported with tizanidine than with placebo.

Common Adverse Events Leading to Discontinuation: Forty-five of 264 (17%) patients receiving tizanidine and 13 of 261 (5%) patients receiving placebo in three multiple dose, placebo-controlled clinical studies discontinued treatment for adverse events. When patients withdrew from the study, they frequently had more than one reason for discontinuing. The adverse events most frequently leading to withdrawal of tizanidine treated patients in the controlled clinical studies were asthenia (3%), somnolence (3%), dry mouth (3%), increased spasm or tone (2%), and dizziness (2%).

Most Frequent Adverse Clinical Events Seen in Association With the Use of Tizanidine: In multiple dose, placebo-controlled clinical studies involving 264 patients with spasticity, the most frequent adverse events were dry mouth, somnolence/sedation, asthenia, and dizziness. Three-quarters of the patients rated the events as mild to moderate and one-quarter of the patients rated the events as being severe. These events appeared to be dose related.

Adverse Events Reported in Controlled Studies: The events cited reflect experience gained under closely monitored conditions of clinical studies in a highly selected patient population. In actual clinical practice or in other clinical studies, these frequency estimates may not apply, as the conditions of use, reporting behavior, and the kinds of patients treated may differ. TABLE 1 lists treatment emergent signs and symptoms that were reported in greater than 2% of patients in three multiple dose, placebo-controlled studies who received tizanidine where the frequency in the tizanidine group was at least as common as in the placebo group. These events are not necessarily related to tizanidine treatment. For comparison purposes, the corresponding frequency of the event (per 100 patients) among placebo treated patients is also provided.

TABLE 1 Multiple Dose, Placebo-Controlled Studies - Frequent (>2%) Adverse Events Reported for Which Tizanidine Incidence is Greater than Placebo

Event	Placebo (N=261) %	Tizanidine (N=264)%
Dry Mouth	10	49
Somnolence	10	48
Asthenia (tiredness)	16	41
Dizziness	4	16
UTI	7	10
Infection	5	6
Constipation	1	4
Liver function tests abnormal	<1	3
Vomiting	0	3
Speech disorder	0	3
Amblyopia (blurred vision)	<1	3
Urinary frequency	2	3
Flu syndrome	2	3
SGPT/ALT increased	<1	3
Dyskinesia	0	3
Nervousness	<1	3
Pharnygitis	1	3
Rhinitis	2	3

In the single dose, placebo-controlled study involving 142 patients with spasticity, the patients were specifically asked if they had experienced any of the four most common adverse events: dry mouth, somnolence (drowsiness), asthenia (tiredness), and dizziness. In addition, hypotension and bradycardia were observed. The occurrence of the adverse events are summarized in TABLE 2. Other events were, in general, reported at a rate of 2% or less.

TABLE 2 Single Dose, Placebo-Controlled Study - Common Adverse Events Reported

Event	Placebo (N=48)%	Tizanidine 8 mg (N=45) %	Tizanidine 16 mg (N=49) %
Somnolence	31	78	92
Dry mouth	35	76	88
Asthenia	40	67	78
Dizziness	4	22	45
Hypotension	0	16	33
Bradycardia	0	2	10

Other Adverse Events Observed During the Evaluation of Tizanidine: Tizanidine was administered to 1187 patients in additional clinical studies where adverse event information was available. The conditions and duration of exposure varied greatly, and included (in overlapping categories) double-blind and open-label studies, uncontrolled and controlled studies, inpatient and outpatient studies, and titration studies. Untoward events associated with the exposure were recorded by clinical investigators using terminology of their own choosing. Consequently, it is not possible to provide a meaningful estimate of the proportion of individuals experiencing adverse events without first grouping similar types of untoward events into a smaller number of standardized event categories.

In the tabulations that follow, reported adverse events were classified using a standard COSTART-based dictionary terminology. The frequencies presented, therefore, represent the proportion of the 1187 patients exposed to tizanidine who experienced an event of the type cited on at least one occasion while receiving tizanidine. All reported events are included except those already listed in TABLE 1. If the COSTART term for an event was so general as to be uninformative, it was replaced with a more informative term. It is important to emphasize that, although the events reported occurred during treatment with tizanidine, they were not necessarily caused by it.

Events are further categorized by body system and listed in order of decreasing frequency according to the following definitions: frequent adverse events are those occurring on one or more occasions in at least 1/100 patients (only those not already listed in the tabulated results from placebo-controlled studies appear in this listing); infrequent adverse events are those occurring in 1/100 to 1/1000 patients.

Body as a Whole: *Frequent:*fever; *Infrequent:*allergic reaction, monillasis, malaise, abscess, neck pain, sepsis, cellulitis, death, overdose; *Rare:*carcinoma, congenital anomaly, suicide attempt.

Cardiovascular System: *Infrequent:*vasodilation, postural hypotension, syncope, migraine, arrhythmia; *Rare:*angina pectoris, coronary artery disorder, heart failure, myocardial infarct, phlebitis, pulmonary embolus, ventricular extrasystoles, ventricular tachycardia.

Digestive System: *Frequent:*abdomen pain, diarrhea, dyspepsia; *Infrequent:*dysphagia, cholelithiasis, fecal impaction, flatulence, gastrointestinal hemorrhage, hepatitis, melena; *Rare:* gastroenteritis, hematemesis, hepatoma, intestinal obstruction, liver damage.

Hemic and Lymphatic System: *Infrequent:*ecchymosis, hypercholesteremia, anemia, hyperlipemia, leukopenia, leukocytosis, sepsis; *Rare:*petechia, purpura, thrombocythemia, thrombocytopenia.

Metabolic and Nutritional System: *Infrequent:*edema, hypothyroidism, weight loss; *Rare:* adrenal cortex insufficiency, hyperglycemia, hypokalemia, hyponatremia, hypoproteinemia, respiratory acidosis.

Musculoskeletal System: *Frequent:*myasthenia, back pain; *Infrequent:*pathological fracture, arthralgia, arthritis, bursitis.

Nervous System: *Frequent:*depression, anxiety, paresthesia; *Infrequent:*tremor, emotional lability, convulsion, paralysis, thinking abnormal, vertigo, abnormal dreams, agitation, depersonalization, euphoria, migraine, stupor, dysautonomia, neuralgia; *Rare:*dementia, hemoplagia, neuropathy.

Respiratory System: *Infrequent:*sinusitis, pneumonia, bronchitis; *Rare:*asthma.

Skin and Appendages: *Frequent:*rash, sweating, skin ulcer; *Infrequent:*pruritus, dry skin, acne, alopecia, urticaria; *Rare:*exfoliative dermatitis, herpes simplex, herpes zoster, skin carcinoma.

Special Senses: *Infrequent:*ear pain, tinnitus, deafness, glaucoma, conjunctivitis, eye pain, optic neuritis, otitis media, retinal hemorrhage, visual field defect; *Rare:*iritis, keratitis, optic atrophy

Urogenital System: *Infrequent:*urinary urgency, cystitis, menorrhagia, pyelonephritis, urinary retention, kidney calculus, uterine fibroids enlarged, vaginal moniliasis, vaginitis; *Rare:* albuminuria, glycosuria, hematuria, metrorrhagia.

DRUG ABUSE AND DEPENDENCE:

Abuse potential was not evaluated in human studies. Rats were able to distinguish tizanidine from saline in a standard discrimination paradigm, after training, but failed to generalize the effects of morphine, cocaine, diazepam or phenobarbital to tizanidine. Monkeys were shown to self-administer tizanidine in a dose-dependent manner, and abrupt cessation of tizanidine produced transient signs of withdrawal at doses >35 times the maximum recommended human dose on a mg/m^2 basis. These transient withdrawal signs (increased locomotion, body twitching, and aversive behavior toward the observer) were not reversed by naloxone administration.

OVERDOSAGE:

One significant overdosage of tizanidine has been reported. Attempted suicide by a 46 year-old male with multiple sclerosis resulted in coma very shortly after the ingestion of one-hundred 4 mg tizanidine tablets. Pupils were not dilated and nystagmus was not present. The patient had marked respiratory depression with Cheyne-Stokes respiration. Gastric lavage and forced diuresis with furosemide and mannitol were instituted. The patient recovered several hours later without sequelae. Laboratory findings were normal.

Should overdosage occur, basic steps to ensure the adequacy of an airway and the monitoring of cardiovascular and respiratory systems should be undertaken. For the most recent information concerning the management of overdose, contact a poison control center.

DOSAGE AND ADMINISTRATION:

A single oral dose of 8 mg of tizanidine reduces muscle tone in patients with spasticity for a period of several hours. The effect peaks at approximately 1 to 2 hours and dissipates between 3 to 6 hours. Effects are dose-related.

Although single doses of less than 8 mg have not been demonstrated to be effective in controlled clinical studies, the dose-related nature of tizanidine's common adverse events make it prudent to begin treatment with single oral doses of 4 mg. Increase the dose gradually (2 to 4 mg steps) to optimum effect (satisfactory reduction of muscle tone at a tolerated dose).

The dose can be repeated at 6 to 8 hour intervals, as needed, to a maximum of three doses in 24 hours. The total daily dose should not exceed 36 mg.

Experience with single doses exceeding 8 mg and daily doses exceeding 24 mg is limited. There is essentially no experience with repeated, single, daytime doses greater than 12 mg or total daily doses greater than 36 mg (see WARNINGS).

PATIENT INFORMATION:

Tizanidine is used for treatment of increased muscle tone associated with spasticity.

Inform your physician if you are pregnant or nursing.

Inform your physician if you have kidney disease or liver impairment.

May cause significant hypotension; Do not rapidly arise from a prone position.

Inform your physician if you are taking concurrent antihypertensive medication.

May cause sedation; use caution while driving or operating hazardous machinery.

Hallucinations have been reported; be aware of this possibility.

Inform your physician if you are taking any other medications, including over-the-counter drugs (*e.g.* acetaminophen).

Do not drink alcohol with tizanidine.

Oral contraceptives can prolong the effect of tizanidine.

May cause dry mouth, sleepiness, slowed heart rate, weakness, and dizziness.

May be taken with or without food.

HOW SUPPLIED:

Tizanidine HCl is available as 4 mg white tablets, embossed with the Athena logo and "594" on one side and cross-scored on the other.

Storage: Store at 15-30°C (59-86°F). Dispense in containers with child resistant closure.

TOBRAMYCIN *(002355)*

CATEGORIES: Aminoglycosides; Anti-Infectives; Antibacterials; Antibiotics; Antimicrobials; EENT Drugs; Eye, Ear, Nose, & Throat Preparations; Ocular Infections; Ophthalmics; Topical; Pregnancy Category B; Sales > $100 Million; FDA Approval Pre 1982

BRAND NAMES: *Oftalmotrisol-T*; **Tobrex**
(International brand names outside U.S. in italics)

FORMULARIES: Aetna; BC-BS; Medi-Cal; PCS

DESCRIPTION:

Tobramycin 0.3% is a sterile topical ophthalmic antibiotic formulation prepared specifically for topical therapy of external ophthalmic infections.

Each gram of tobramycin ophthalmic ointment contains: *Active:* Tobramycin 0.3% (3 mg). *Preservative:* Chlorobutanol 0.5%.*Inactives:* Mineral Oil, White Petrolatum.

Each ml of tobramycin solution contains: *Active:* tobramycin 0.3% (3 mg). *Preservative:* Benzalkonium Chloride 0.01% (0.1 mg).*Inactives:* Boric Acid, Sodium Sulfate, Sodium Chloride, Tyloxapol, Sodium Hydroxide and/or Sulfuric Acid (to adjust pH) and Purified Water.

Tobramycin is a water-soluble aminoglycoside antibiotic active against a wide variety of gram-negative and gram-positive ophthalmic pathogens.

Chemical name: O-(3-amino-3-deoxy-a-D-gluco- pyranosyl-(1→4))-O-(2,6-diamino-2,3,6-trideoxy-a-D-ribohexo-pyranosyl -(1→6))-2-deoxystreptamine.

CLINICAL PHARMACOLOGY:

In Vitro Data: *In vitro* studies have demonstrated tobramycin is active against susceptible strains of the following microorganisms: Staphylococci, including *S. aureus* and *S. epidermidis* (coagulase-positive and coagulase-negative), including penicillin-resistant strains.

Streptococci, including some of the Group A-beta-hemolytic species, some nonhemolytic species, and some *Streptococcus pneumoniae.*

Pseudomonas aeruginosa, Escherichia coli, Klebsiella pneumoniae, Enterobacter aerogenes, Proteus mirabilis, Morganella morganii, most*Proteus vulgaris* strains, *Haemophilus influenzae* and *H. aegyptius, Moraxella lacunata, Acinetobacter calcoaceticus* and some *Neisseria* species. Bacterial susceptibility studies demonstrate that in some cases, microorganisms resistant to gentamicin retain susceptibility to tobramycin.

INDICATIONS AND USAGE:

Tobramycin is a topical antibiotic indicated in the treatment of external infections of the eye and its adnexa caused by susceptible bacteria. Appropriate monitoring of bacterial response to topical antibiotic therapy should accompany the use of Tobrex. Clinical studies have shown tobramycin to be safe and effective for use in children.

CONTRAINDICATIONS:

Tobramycin Ophthalmic Ointment and Ophthalmic Solution are contraindicated in patients with known hypersensitivity to any of its components.

WARNINGS:

NOT FOR INJECTION INTO THE EYE. Sensitivity to topically applied aminoglycosides may occur in some patients. If a sensitivity reaction to tobramycin occurs, discontinue use. Remove contact lenses before applying ointment or solution.

PRECAUTIONS:

GENERAL

As with other antibiotic preparations, prolonged use may result in overgrowth of nonsusceptible organisms, including fungi. If superinfection occurs, appropriate therapy should be initiated. Ophthalmic ointments may retard corneal wound healing.

Cross-sensitivity to other aminoglycoside antibiotics may occur; if hypersensitivity develops with this product, discontinue use and institute appropriate therapy.

INFORMATION FOR THE PATIENT

Ophthalmic Ointment: Do not touch tube tip to any surface, as this may contaminate the ointment.

Ophthalmic Solution: Do not touch dropper tip to any surface, as this may contaminate the solution.

PREGNANCY CATEGORY B

Reproduction studies in three types of animals at doses up to thirty-three times the normal human systemic dose have revealed no evidence of impaired fertility or harm to the fetus due to tobramycin. There are, however, no adequate and well-controlled studies in pregnant women. Because animal studies are not always predictive of human response, this drug should be used during pregnancy only if clearly needed.

NURSING MOTHERS

Because of the potential for adverse reactions in nursing infants from Tobrex, a decision should be made whether to discontinue nursing the infant or discontinue the drug, taking into account the importance of the drug to the mother.

ADVERSE REACTIONS:

The most frequent adverse reactions to tobramycin ophthalmic ointment and ophthalmic solution are hypersensitivity and localized ocular toxicity, including lid itching and swelling, and conjunctival erythema. These reactions occur in less than three of 100 patients treated with tobramycin. Similar reactions may occur with the topical use of other aminoglycoside antibiotics. Other adverse reactions have not been reported from tobramycin therapy; however, if topical ocular tobramycin is administered concomitantly with systemic aminoglycoside antibiotics, care should be taken to monitor the total serum concentration.

In clinical trials, tobramycin ophthalmic ointment produced significantly fewer adverse reactions (3.7%) than did Garamycin Ophthalmic Ointment (10.6%).

OVERDOSAGE:

Clinically apparent signs and symptoms of an overdose of tobramycin ophthalmic ointment and ophthalmic solution (punctate keratitis, erythema, increased lacrimation, edema and lid itching) may be similar to adverse reaction effects seen in some patients.

DOSAGE AND ADMINISTRATION:

OPHTHALMIC OINTMENT

In mild to moderate disease, apply a half-inch ribbon into the affected eye(s) two or three times per day. In severe infections, instill a half-inch ribbon into the affected eye(s) every three to four hours until improvement, following which treatment should be reduced prior to discontinuation.

How to Apply tobramycin ointment

1. Tilt your head back.

2. Place a finger on your cheek just under your eye and gently pull down until a "V" pocket is formed between your eyeball and your lower lid.

3. Place a small amount (about 1/2 inch) of tobramycin in the "V" pocket. Do not let the tip of the tube touch your eye.

4. Look downward before closing your eye.

OPHTHALMIC SOLUTION

In mild to moderate disease, instill one or two drops into the affected eye(s) every four hours. In severe infections, instill two drops into the eye(s) hourly until improvement, following which treatment should be reduced prior to discontinuation.

HOW SUPPLIED:

OPHTHALMIC OINTMENT

3.5 g sterile ointment in opthalmic tube, containing tobramycin 0.3% (3 mg/g).

Storage: Store at 8°-27°C (46°- 80°F).

OPHTHALMIC SOLUTION

5 ml sterile solution in Drop-Tainer dispenser, containing tobramycin 0.3% (3 mg/ml).

Storage: Store at 8°-27°C (46°- 80°F).

HOW SUPPLIED - RATED THERAPEUTICALLY EQUIVALENT:

Solution - Ophthalmic - 0.3 %

5 ml	$14.18	Tobramycin, HL Moore Drug Exch	00839-7610-85
5 ml	$14.95	Tobramycin, Major Pharms	00904-2970-05

Solution/Drops - Ophthalmic - 0.3 %

5 ml	$4.03	Tobramycin, H.C.F.A. F F P	99999-2355-01

HOW SUPPLIED - NOT RATED EQUIVALENT:

Ointment - Ophthalmic; Top - 0.3 %

3.5 gm	**$19.69**	**TOBREX, Alcon**	**00065-0644-35**

TOBRAMYCIN SULFATE *(002356)*

CATEGORIES: Aminoglycosides; Anti-Infectives; Antibiotics; Antimicrobials; Bone Infections; EENT Drugs; Eye, Ear, Nose, & Throat Preparations; Infections; Intra-Abdominal Infections; Meningitis; Peritonitis; Respiratory Tract Infections; Septicemia; Skin Infections; Urinary Tract Infections; Pregnancy Category D; FDA Approval Pre 1982

BRAND NAMES: **Nebcin**; Tobramycin In Sodium Chloride

WARNING:
Patients treated with Tobramycin Sulfate Injection, USP, and other aminoglycosides should be under close clinical observation, because these drugs have an inherent potential for causing ototoxicity and nephrotoxicity.
Neurotoxicity, manifested as both auditory and vestibular ototoxicity, can occur. The auditory changes are irreversible, are usually bilateral, and may be partial or total. Eighth-nerve impairment and nephrotoxicity may develop, primarily in patients having preexisting renal damage and in those with normal renal function to whom aminoglycosides are administered for longer periods or in higher doses than those recommended. Other manifestations of neurotoxicity may include numbness, skin tingling, muscle twitching, and convulsions. The risk of aminoglycoside-induced hearing loss increases with the degree of exposure to either high peak or high trough serum concentrations. Patients who develop cochlear damage may not have symptoms during therapy to warn them of eighth-nerve toxicity, and partial or total irreversible bilateral deafness may continue to develop after the drug has been discontinued.
Rarely, nephrotoxicity may not become apparent until the first few days after cessation of therapy. Aminoglycoside-induced nephrotoxicity usually is reversible.
Renal and eighth-nerve function should be closely monitored in patients with known or suspected renal impairment and also in those whose renal function is initially normal but who develop signs of renal dysfunction during therapy. Peak and trough serum concentrations of aminoglycosides should be monitored periodically during therapy to assure adequate levels and to avoid potentially toxic levels. Prolonged serum concentrations above 12 mcg/ml should be avoided. Rising trough levels (above 2 mcg/ml) may indicate tissue accumulation. Such accumulation, excessive peak concentrations, advanced age, and cumulative dose may contribute to ototoxicity and nephrotoxicity (see PRECAUTIONS.) Urine should be examined for decreased specific gravity and increased excretion of protein, cells, and casts. Blood urea nitrogen, serum creatinine, and creatinine clearance should be measured periodically. When feasible, it is recommended that serial audiograms be obtained in patients old enough to be tested, particularly high-risk patients. Evidence of impairment of renal, vestibular, or auditory function requires discontinuation of the drug or dosage adjustment.
Tobramycin should be used with caution in premature and neonatal infants because of their renal immaturity and the resulting prolongation of serum half-life of the drug.
Concurrent and sequential use of other neurotoxic and/or nephrotoxic antibiotics, particularly other aminoglycosides (*e.g.,* amikacin, streptomycin, neomycin, kanamycin, gentamicin, and paromomycin), cephaloridine, viomycin, polymyxin B, colistin, cisplatin, and vancomycin, should be avoided. Other factors that may increase patient risk are advanced age and dehydration.
Aminoglycosides should not be given concurrently with potent diuretics, such as ethacrynic acid and furosemide. Some diuretics themselves cause ototoxicity, and intravenously administered diuretics enhance aminoglycoside toxicity by altering antibiotic concentrations in serum and tissue.
Aminoglycosides can cause fetal harm when administered to a pregnant woman (see PRECAUTIONS).

DESCRIPTION:

Tobramycin sulfate, a water-soluble antibiotic of the aminoglycoside group, is derived from the actinomycete *Streptomyces tenebrarius.*Tobramycin sulfate, Injection, is a clear and colorless sterile aqueous solution for parenteral administration.

Tobramycin sulfate is *O*-3-amino-3-deoxy-α-D -glucopyranosyl- (1→4)-*O*-[2,6-diamino-2,3,6 -trideoxy-α-D-*ribo*- hexopyranosyl-(1→6)] -2- deoxy-L-streptamine, sulfate (2:5)(salt) and has the chemical formula $(C_{18}H_{37}N_5O_9)_2 \cdot 5H_2SO_4$. The molecular weight is 1,425.39.

Each ml also contains phenol as a preservative (5 mg, multiple-dose vials; 1.25 mg ADD-Vantage vials), sodium bisulfite (3.2 mg, multiple-dose vials; 1.6 mg, ADD-Vantage vials), 0.1 mg edetate disodium, and water for injection, qs. Sulfuric acid and/or sodium hydroxide may have been added to adjust the pH.

CLINICAL PHARMACOLOGY:

Tobramycin is rapidly absorbed following intramuscular administration. Peak serum concentrations of tobramycin occur between 30 and 90 minutes after intramuscular administration. Following an intramuscular dose of 1 mg/kg of body weight, maximum serum concentrations reach about 4 mcg/ml, and measurable levels persist for as long as 8 hours. Therapeutic serum levels are generally considered to range from 4 to 6 mcg/ml. When tobramycin sulfate is administered by intravenous infusion over a 1-hour period, the serum concentrations are similar to those obtained by intramuscular administration. Tobramycin sulfate is poorly absorbed from the gastrointestinal tract.

In patients with normal renal function, except neonates, tobramycin sulfate administered every 8 hours does not accumulate in the serum. However, in those patients with reduced renal function and in neonates, the serum concentration of the antibiotic is usually higher and can be measured for longer periods of time than in normal adults. Dosage for such patients must, therefore, be adjusted accordingly (see DOSAGE AND ADMINISTRATION).

Following parenteral administration, little, if any, metabolic transformation occurs, and tobramycin is eliminated almost exclusively by glomerular filtration. Renal clearance is similar to that of endogenous creatinine. Ultrafiltration studies demonstrate that practically no serum protein binding occurs. In patients with normal renal function, up to 84% of the dose is recoverable from the urine in 8 hours and up to 93% in 24 hours.

CLINICAL PHARMACOLOGY: *(cont'd)*

Peak urine concentrations ranging from 75 to 100 mcg/ml have been observed following the intramuscular injection of a single dose of 1 mg/kg. After several days of treatment, the amount of tobramycin excreted in the urine approaches the daily dose administered. When renal function is impaired, excretion of tobramycin sulfate is slowed, and accumulation of the drug may cause toxic blood levels.

The serum half-life in normal individuals is 2 hours. An inverse relationship exists between serum half-life and creatinine clearance, and the dosage schedule should be adjusted according to the degree of renal impairment (see DOSAGE AND ADMINISTRATION). In patients undergoing dialysis, 25% to 70% of the administered dose may be removed, depending on the duration and type of dialysis.

Tobramycin can be detected in tissues and body fluids after parenteral administration. Concentrations in bile and stools ordinarily have been low, which suggests minimum biliary excretion. Tobramycin has appeared in low concentration in the cerebrospinal fluid following parenteral administration, and concentrations are dependent on dose, rate of penetration, and degree of meningeal inflammation. It has also been found in sputum, peritoneal fluid, synovial fluid, and abscess fluids, and it crosses the placental membranes. Concentrations in the renal cortex are several times higher than the usual serum levels.

Probenecid does not affect the renal tubular transport of tobramycin.

Tobramycin acts by inhibiting synthesis of protein in bacterial cells.*In vitro* tests demonstrate that tobramycin is bactericidal.

Tobramycin has been shown to be active against most strains of the following organisms both *in vitro* and in clinical infection (see INDICATIONS AND USAGE):

Gram-positive aerobes: *Staphylococcus aureus*

Gram-negative aerobes: *Citrobacter* species;*Enterobacter* species; *Escherichia coli; Klebsiella* species; *Morganella morganii; Pseudomonas aeruginosa; Proteus mirabilis; Proteus vulgaris; Providencia* species;*Serratia*species

Aminoglycosides have a low order of activity against most gram-positive organisms, including *Streptococcus pyogenes, Streptococcus pneumoniae,* and enterococci.

Although most strains of enterococci demonstrate *in vitro*resistance, some strains in this group are susceptible. *In vitro* studies have shown that an aminoglycoside combined with an antibiotic that interferes with cell-wall synthesis affects some enterococcal strains synergistically. The combination of penicillin G and tobramycin results in a synergistic bactericidal effect *in vitro* against certain strains of *Enterococcus faecalis.* However, this combination is not synergistic against other closely related organisms, e.g., *Enterococcus faecium.* Speciation of enterococci alone cannot be used to predict susceptibility. Susceptibility testing and tests for antibiotic synergism are emphasized.

Cross resistance between aminoglycosides may occur.

SUSCEPTIBILITY TESTS

Diffusion Techniques: Quantitative methods that require measurement of zone diameters give the most precise estimates of susceptibility of bacteria to antimicrobial agents. One such procedure is the National Committee for Clinical Laboratory Standards (NCCLS)-approved procedure.[1] This method has been recommended for use with disks to test susceptibility to tobramycin. Interpretation involves correlation of the diameters obtained in the disk test with minimum inhibitory concentrations (MIC) for tobramycin.

Reports from the laboratory giving results of the standard single-disk susceptibility test with a 10-mcg tobramycin disk should be interpreted according to the criteria in TABLE 1.

TABLE 1

Zone Diameter(mm)	Interpretation
≥15	(S) Susceptible
13-14	(I) Intermediate
≤12	(R) Resistant

A report of "Susceptible" indicates that the pathogen is likely to be inhibited by generally achievable blood levels. A report of "Intermediate" suggests that the organism would be susceptible if high dosage is used or if the infection is confined to tissues and fluids in which high antimicrobial levels are obtained. A report of "Resistant" indicates that achievable concentrations are unlikely to be inhibitory and other therapy should be selected.

Standardized procedures require the use of laboratory control organisms. The 10-mcg tobramycin disk should give the following zone diameters (TABLE 2):

TABLE 2

Organism	Zone Diameter (mm)
E. coli ATCC 25922	18-26
P. aeruginosa ATCC 27853	19-25
S. aureus ATCC 25923	19-29

Dilution Techniques: Broth and agar dilution methods, such as those recommended by the NCCLS,[2] may be used to determine MICs of tobramycin. MIC test results should be interpreted according to the following criteria (TABLE 3):

TABLE 3

MIC (mcg/ml)	Interpretation
≤4	(S) Susceptible
8	(I) Intermediate
≥16	(R) Resistant

As with standard diffusion methods, dilution procedures require the use of laboratory control organisms. Standard tobramycin powder should give the following MIC values (TABLE 4):

TABLE 4

Organism	MIC Range (mcg/ml)
E. faecalis ATCC 29212	8.0-32.0
E. coli ATCC 25922	0.25-1
P. aeruginosa ATCC 27853	0.12-2
S. aureus ATCC 29213	0.12-1

INDICATIONS AND USAGE:

Tobramycin sulfate is indicated for the treatment of serious bacterial infections caused by susceptible strains of the designated microorganisms in the diseases listed below:

Septicemia in the neonate, child, and adult caused by *P. aeruginosa, E. coli,* and *Klebsiella* sp

Lower respiratory tract infection s caused by *P. aeruginosa,Klebsiella* sp, *Enterobacter* sp, *Serratia* sp,*E. coli,* and *S. aureus* (penicillinase- and non-penicillinase-producing strains)

Serious central-nervous-system infections (meningitis) caused by susceptible organisms

INDICATIONS AND USAGE: *(cont'd)*

Intra-abdominal infections , including peritonitis, caused by *E. coli, Klebsiella* sp, and *Enterobacter* sp

Skin, bone, and skin structure infections caused by *P. aeruginosa, Proteus* sp, *E. coli, Klebsiella* sp, *Enterobacter* sp, and *S. aureus.*

Complicated and recurrent urinary tract infections caused by *P.aeruginosa, Proteus* sp (indole-positive and indole-negative),*E. coli, Klebsiella* sp, *Enterobacter* sp,*Serratia* sp, *S. aureus, Providencia* sp, and *Citrobacter* sp

Aminoglycosides, including tobramycin sulfate, are not indicated in uncomplicated initial episodes of urinary tract infections unless the causative organisms are not susceptible to antibiotics having less potential toxicity. Tobramycin sulfate may be considered in serious staphylococcal infections when penicillin or other potentially less toxic drugs are contraindicated and when bacterial susceptibility testing and clinical judgment indicate its use.

Bacterial cultures should be obtained prior to and during treatment to isolate and identify etiologic organisms and to test their susceptibility to tobramycin. If susceptibility tests show that the causative organisms are resistant to tobramycin, other appropriate therapy should be instituted. In patients in whom a serious life-threatening gram-negative infection is suspected, including those in whom concurrent therapy with a penicillin or cephalosporin and an aminoglycoside may be indicated, treatment with tobramycin sulfate may be initiated before the results of susceptibility studies are obtained. The decision to continue therapy with tobramycin sulfate should be based on the results of susceptibility studies, the severity of the infection, and the important additional concepts discussed in the BOXED WARNING above.

CONTRAINDICATIONS:

A hypersensitivity to any aminoglycoside is a contraindication to the use of tobramycin. A history of hypersensitivity or serious toxic reactions to aminoglycosides may also contraindicate the use of any other aminoglycoside because of the known cross-sensitivity of patients to drugs in this class.

WARNINGS:

See BOXED WARNING. Tobramycin sulfate contains sodium bisulfite, a sulfite that may cause allergic-type reactions, including anaphylactic symptoms and life-threatening or less severe asthmatic episodes, in certain susceptible people. The overall prevalence of sulfite sensitivity in the general population is unknown and probably low. Sulfite sensitivity is seen more frequently in asthmatic than in nonasthmatic people.

PRECAUTIONS:

Serum and urine specimens for examination should be collected during therapy, as recommended in the BOXED WARNING. Serum calcium, magnesium, and sodium should be monitored.

Peak and trough serum levels should be measured periodically during therapy. Prolonged concentrations above 12 mcg/ml should be avoided. Rising trough levels (above 2 mcg/ml) may indicate tissue accumulation. Such accumulation, advanced age, and cumulative dosage may contribute to ototoxicity and nephrotoxicity. It is particularly important to monitor serum levels closely in patients with known renal impairment.

A useful guideline would be to perform serum level assays after 2 or 3 doses, so that the dosage could be adjusted if necessary, and at 3- to 4-day intervals during therapy. In the event of changing renal function, more frequent serum levels should be obtained and the dosage or dosage interval adjusted according to the guidelines provided in the DOSAGE AND ADMINISTRATION section.

In order to measure the peak level, a serum sample should be drawn about 30 minutes following intravenous infusion or 1 hour after an intramuscular injection. Trough levels are measured by obtaining serum samples at 8 hours or just prior to the next dose of tobramycin sulfate. These suggested time intervals are intended only as guidelines and may vary according to institutional practices. It is important, however, that there be consistency within the individual patient program unless computerized pharmacokinetic dosing programs are available in the institution. These serum-level assays may be especially useful for monitoring the treatment of severely ill patients with changing renal function or of those infected with less susceptible organisms or those receiving maximum dosage.

Neuromuscular blockade and respiratory paralysis have been reported in cats receiving very high doses of tobramycin (40 mg/kg). The possibility of prolonged or secondary apnea should be considered if tobramycin is administered to anesthetized patients who are also receiving neuromuscular blocking agents, such as succinylcholine, tubocurarine, or decamethonium, or to patients receiving massive transfusions of citrated blood. If neuromuscular blockade occurs, it may be reversed by the administration of calcium salts.

Cross-allergenicity among aminoglycosides has been demonstrated.

In patients with extensive burns, altered pharmacokinetics may result in reduced serum concentrations of aminoglycosides. In such patients treated with tobramycin sulfate, measurement of serum concentration is especially important as a basis for determination of appropriate dosage.

Elderly patients may have reduced renal function that may not be evident in the results of routine screening tests, such as BUN or serum creatinine. A creatinine clearance determination may be more useful. Monitoring of renal function during treatment with aminoglycosides is particularly important in such patients.

An increased incidence of nephrotoxicity has been reported following concomitant administration of aminoglycoside antibiotics and cephalosporins.

Aminoglycosides should be used with caution in patients with muscular disorders, such as myasthenia gravis or parkinsonism, since these drugs may aggravate muscle weakness because of their potential curare-like effect on neuromuscular function.

Aminoglycosides may be absorbed in significant quantities from body surfaces after local irrigation or application and may cause neurotoxicity and nephrotoxicity.

Aminoglycosides have not been approved for intraocular and/or subconjunctival use. Physicians are advised that macular necrosis has been reported following administration of aminoglycosides, including tobramycin, by these routes.

See BOXED WARNING regarding concurrent use of potent diuretics and concurrent and sequential use of other neurotoxic or nephrotoxic drugs.

The inactivation of tobramycin and other aminoglycosides by β-lactam-type antibiotics (penicillins or cephalosporins) has been demonstrated *in vitro* and in patients with severe renal impairment. Such inactivation has not been found in patients with normal renal function who have been given the drugs by separate routes of administration.

Therapy with tobramycin may result in overgrowth of nonsusceptible organisms. If overgrowth of nonsusceptible organisms occurs, appropriate therapy should be initiated.

Pregnancy Category D: Aminoglycosides can cause fetal harm when administered to a pregnant woman. Aminoglycoside antibiotics cross the placenta, and there have been several reports of total irreversible bilateral congenital deafness in children whose mothers received streptomycin during pregnancy. Serious side effects to mother, fetus, or newborn have not

PRECAUTIONS: *(cont'd)*

been reported in the treatment of pregnant women with other aminoglycosides. If tobramycin is used during pregnancy or if the patient becomes pregnant while taking tobramycin, she should be apprised of the potential hazard to the fetus.

Usage in Children: See INDICATIONS AND USAGEand DOSAGE AND ADMINISTRATION.

ADVERSE REACTIONS:

Neurotoxicity: Adverse effects on both the vestibular and auditory branches of the eighth nerve have been noted, especially in patients receiving high doses or prolonged therapy, in those given previous courses of therapy with an ototoxin, and in cases of dehydration. Symptoms include dizziness, vertigo, tinnitus, roaring in the ears, and hearing loss. Hearing loss is usually irreversible and is manifested initially by diminution of high-tone acuity. Tobramycin and gentamicin sulfates closely parallel each other in regard to ototoxic potential.

Nephrotoxicity: Renal function changes, as shown by rising BUN, NPN, and serum creatinine and by oliguria, cylindruria, and increased proteinuria, have been reported, especially in patients with a history of renal impairment who are treated for longer periods or with higher doses than those recommended. Adverse renal effects can occur in patients with initially normal renal function.

Clinical studies and studies in experimental animals have been conducted to compare the nephrotoxic potential of tobramycin and gentamicin. In some of the clinical studies and in the animal studies, tobramycin caused nephrotoxicity significantly less frequently than gentamicin. In some other clinical studies, no significant difference in the incidence of nephrotoxicity between tobramycin and gentamicin was found.

Other reported adverse reactions possibly related to tobramycin sulfate include anemia, granulocytopenia, and thrombocytopenia; and fever, rash, exfoliative dermatitis, itching, urticaria, nausea, vomiting, diarrhea, headache, lethargy, pain at the injection site, mental confusion, and disorientation. Laboratory abnormalities possibly related to tobramycin sulfate include increased serum transaminases (AST [SGOT], ALT [SGPT]); increased serum LDH and bilirubin; decreased serum calcium, magnesium, sodium, and potassium; and leukopenia, leukocytosis, and eosinophilia.

OVERDOSAGE:

Signs and Symptoms: The severity of the signs and symptoms following a tobramycin overdose are dependent on the dose administered, the patient's renal function, state of hydration, and age and whether or not other medications with similar toxicities are being administered concurrently. Toxicity may occur in patients treated more than 10 days, in adults given more than 5 mg/kg/day, in children given more than 7.5 mg/kg/day, or in patients with reduced renal function where dose has not been appropriately adjusted.

Nephrotoxicity following the parenteral administration of an aminoglycoside is most closely related to the area under the curve of the serum concentration versus time graph. Nephrotoxicity is more likely if trough blood concentrations fail to fall below 2 mcg/ml and is also proportional to the average blood concentration. Patients who are elderly, have abnormal renal function, are receiving other nephrotoxic drugs, or are volume depleted are at greater risk for developing acute tubular necrosis. Auditory and vestibular toxicities have been associated with aminoglycoside overdose. These toxicities occur in patients treated longer than 10 days, in patients with abnormal renal function, in dehydrated patients, or in patients receiving medications with additive auditory toxicities. These patients may not have signs or symptoms or may experience dizziness, tinnitus, vertigo, and a loss of high-tone acuity as ototoxicity progresses. Ototoxicity signs and symptoms may not begin to occur until long after the drug has been discontinued.

Neuromuscular blockade or respiratory paralysis may occur following administration of aminoglycosides. Neuromuscular blockade, respiratory failure, and prolonged respiratory paralysis may occur more commonly in patients with myasthenia gravis or Parkinson's disease. Prolonged respiratory paralysis may also occur in patients receiving decamethonium, tubocurarine, or succinylcholine. If neuromuscular blockade occurs, it may be reversed by the administration of calcium salts but mechanical assistance may be necessary.

If tobramycin were ingested, toxicity would be less likely because aminoglycosides are poorly absorbed from an intact gastrointestinal tract.

Treatment: In all cases of suspected overdosage, call your Regional Poison Control Center to obtain the most up-to-date information about the treatment of overdose. This recommendation is made because, in general, information regarding the treatment of overdose may change more rapidly than the package insert. In managing overdosage, consider the possibility of multiple drug overdoses, interaction among drugs, and unusual drug kinetics in your patient.

The initial intervention in a tobramycin overdose is to establish an airway and ensure oxygenation and ventilation. Resuscitative measures should be initiated promptly if respiratory paralysis occurs.

Patients who have received an overdose of tobramycin and who have normal renal function should be adequately hydrated to maintain a urine output of 3 to 5 ml/kg/hr. Fluid balance, creatinine clearance, and tobramycin plasma levels should be carefully monitored until the serum tobramycin level falls below 2 mcg/ml.

Patients in whom the elimination half-life is greater than 2 hours or whose renal function is abnormal may require more aggressive therapy. In such patients, hemodialysis may be beneficial.

DOSAGE AND ADMINISTRATION:

Tobramycin sulfate may be given intramuscularly or intravenously. ADD-Vantage vials are not for intramuscular administration. Recommended dosages are the same for both routes. The patient's pretreatment body weight should be obtained for calculation of correct dosage. It is desirable to measure both peak and trough serum concentrations (see BOXED WARNING and PRECAUTIONS).

Administration for Patients With Normal Renal Function—Adults With Serious Infections: 3 mg/kg/day in 3 equal doses every 8 hours (see TABLE 5.)

Adults With Life-Threatening Infections: Up to 5 mg/kg/day may be administered in 3 or 4 equal doses (see TABLE 5.) The dosage should be reduced to 3 mg/kg/day as soon as clinically indicated. To prevent increased toxicity due to excessive blood levels, dosage should not exceed 5 mg/kg/day unless serum levels are monitored (see BOXED WARNING and PRECAUTIONS).

Children: 6 to 7.5 mg/kg/day in 3 or 4 equally divided doses (2 to 2.5 mg/kg every 8 hours or 1.5 to 1.89 mg/kg every 6 hours).

Premature or Full-Term Neonates 1 Week of Age or Less: Up to 4 mg/kg/day may be administered in 2 equal doses every 12 hours.

It is desirable to limit treatment to a short term. The usual duration of treatment is 7 to 10 days. A longer course of therapy may be necessary in difficult and complicated infections. In such cases, monitoring of renal, auditory, and vestibular functions is advised, because neurotoxicity is more likely to occur when treatment is extended longer than 10 days.

Administration for Patients With Impaired Renal Function: Whenever possible, serum tobramycin concentrations should be monitored during therapy.

DOSAGE AND ADMINISTRATION: *(cont'd)*

TABLE 5 Dosage Schedule Guide For Adults With Normal Renal Function (Dosage at 8-Hour Intervals)

For Patient Weighing		Usual Dose for Serious Infections		Maximum Dose for Life-Threatening Infections (Reduce as soon as possible)	
kg	lb	1 mg/kg q8h (Total, 3mg/kg/day)		1.66 mg/kg q8h (Total, 5mg/kg/day)	
		mg/dose q8h	ml/dose*	mg/dose q8h	ml/dose*
120	264	120 mg	3 ml	200 mg	5 ml
115	253	115 mg	2.9 ml	191 mg	4.75 ml
110	242	110 mg	2.75 ml	183 mg	4.5 ml
105	231	105 mg	2.6 ml	175 mg	4.4 ml
100	220	100 mg	2.5 ml	166 mg	4.2 ml
95	209	95 mg	2.4 ml	158 mg	4 ml
90	198	90 mg	2.25 ml	150 mg	3.75 ml
85	187	85 mg	2.1 ml	141 mg	3.5 ml
80	176	80 mg	2 ml	133 mg	3.3 ml
75	165	75 mg	1.9 ml	125 mg	3.1 ml
70	154	70 mg	1.75 ml	116 mg	2.9 ml
65	143	65 mg	1.6 ml	108 mg	2.7 ml
60	132	60 mg	1.5 ml	100 mg	2.5 ml
55	121	55 mg	1.4 ml	91 mg	2.25 ml
50	110	50 mg	1.25 ml	83 mg	2.1 ml
45	99	45 mg	1.1 ml	75 mg	1.9 ml
40	88	40 mg	1 ml	66 mg	1.6 ml

* Applicable to all product forms except Tobramycin Sulfate, Pediatric, Injection.

Following a loading dose of 1 mg/kg, subsequent dosage in these patients must be adjusted, either with reduced doses administered at 8-hour intervals or with normal doses given at prolonged intervals. Both of these methods are suggested as guides to be used when serum levels of tobramycin cannot be measured directly. They are based on either the creatinine clearance level or the serum creatinine level of the patient because these values correlate with the half-life of tobramycin. The dosage schedule derived from either method should be used in conjunction with careful clinical and laboratory observations of the patient and should be modified as necessary. Neither method should be used when dialysis is being performed.

Reduced Dosage At 8-Hour Intervals: When the creatinine clearance rate is 70 ml or less per minute or when the serum creatinine value is known, the amount of the reduced dose can be determined by multiplying the normal dose from TABLE 5 by the percent of normal dose from the accompanying nomogram (for this nomogram, please see original package insert).

An alternate rough guide for determining reduced dosage at 8-hour intervals (for patients whose steady-state serum creatinine values are known) is to divide the normally recommended dose by the patient's serum creatinine.

Normal Dosage At Prolonged Intervals: If the creatinine clearance rate is not available and the patient's condition is stable, a dosage frequency *in hours* for the dosage given in TABLE 5 can be determined by multiplying the patient's serum creatinine by 6.

Dosage in Obese Patients: The appropriate dose may be calculated by using the patient's estimated lean body weight plus 40% of the excess as the basic weight on which to figure mg/kg.

Intramuscular Administration: Tobramycin sulfate may be administered by withdrawing the appropriate dose directly from a vial or by using a prefilled Hyporet. ADD-Vantage vials are not for intramuscular administration.

Intravenous Administration: For intravenous administration, the usual volume of diluent (0.9% Sodium Chloride Injection or 5% Dextrose Injection) is 50 to 100 ml for adult doses. For children, the volume of diluent should be proportionately less than that for adults. The diluted solution usually should be infused over a period of 20 to 60 minutes. Infusion periods of less than 20 minutes are not recommended because peak serum levels may exceed 12 mcg/ml (see BOXED WARNING).

Use of ADD-Vantage Tobramycin Sulfate Vials: ADD-Vantage tobramycin sulfate vials are not intended for multiple use and should not be used with a syringe in the conventional way. These products are intended for use only with Abbott ADD-Vantage diluent containers and in those instances in which the physician's order specified 60-mg or 80-mg doses. Use within 24 hours after activation.

Tobramycin sulfate should not be physically premixed with other drugs but should be administered separately according to the recommended dose and route.

Prior to administration, parenteral drug products should be inspected visually for particulate matter and discoloration whenever solution and container permit.

Store at controlled room temperature 59° to 86°F (15° to 30°C).

REFERENCES:

1. National Committee for Clinical Laboratory Standards, Performance standards for antimicrobial disk susceptibility tests—4th ed. Approved Standard NCCLS Document M2-A4, Vol 10, No. 7, NCCLS, Villanova, PA, 1990.
2. National Committee for Clinical Laboratory Standards. Methods for dilution antimicrobial susceptibility tests for bacteria that grow aerobically—2nd ed. Approved Standard NCCLS Document M7-A2, Vol 10, No 8, NCCLS, Villanova, PA, 1990.

HOW SUPPLIED - RATED THERAPEUTICALLY EQUIVALENT:

Injection, Dry-Soln - Intravenous - 60 mg/vial

6 ml x 25	**$173.11**	**NEBCIN, Lilly**	**00002-7293-25**

Injection, Dry-Soln - Intravenous - 80 mg/vial

8 ml x 25	**$194.11**	**NEBCIN, Lilly**	**00002-7294-25**
25's	**$194.11**	**NEBCIN, Lilly**	**00002-7381-25**

Injection, Solution - Intramuscular; - 10 mg/ml

2 ml	**$3.65**	**NEBCIN, Lilly**	**00002-0501-01**
2 ml	$4.95	Tobramycin Sulfate, Abbott	00074-3577-01
2 ml x 25	$60.00	Tobramycin Sulfate, Raway	00686-8900-24
2 ml x 25	$76.99	Tobramycin Sulfate, Vial, Marsam	00209-8900-24
6 ml	$9.74	Tobramycin Sulfate, Abbott	00074-3254-03
8 ml	$10.92	Tobramycin Sulfate, Abbott	00074-3255-03

Injection, Solution - Intramuscular; - 40 mg/ml

1.5 ml	$9.50	Tobramycin Sulfate, Abbott	00074-3582-01
1.5 ml x 10	$65.63	Tobramycin Sulfate, Lederle Parenterals	00205-3027-45
1.5 ml x 24	**$169.06**	**NEBCIN, Lilly**	**00002-0509-24**
1.5 ml x 25	$164.90	Tobramycin Sulfate, Syringe, Marsam	00209-8920-34
1.5 ml x 25	$164.90	Tobramycin Sulfate, Geneva Pharms	00781-3776-73
2 ml	**$7.28**	**NEBCIN, Lilly**	**00002-1499-01**
2 ml	$9.83	Tobramycin Sulfate, Abbott	00074-3578-01
2 ml	$10.66	Tobramycin Sulfate, Abbott	00074-3583-01
2 ml x 10	$67.44	Tobramycin Sulfate, Lederle Parenterals	00205-3027-04
2 ml x 10	$73.69	Tobramycin Sulfate, Lederle Parenterals	00205-3027-46
2 ml x 24	**$189.22**	**NEBCIN, Lilly**	**00002-0503-24**
2 ml x 25	$98.00	Tobramycin Sulfate, Raway	00686-8950-24

HOW SUPPLIED - RATED THERAPEUTICALLY EQUIVALENT: *(cont'd)*

2 ml x 25	$135.94	Tobramycin Sulfate, Astra USA	00186-1783-04
2 ml x 25	$136.56	Tobramycin Sulfate, Bristol Myers Squibb	00003-2725-10
2 ml x 25	$153.48	Tobramycin Sulfate, Vial, Marsam	00209-8950-24
2 ml x 25	**$182.11**	**NEBCIN, Lilly**	**00002-1499-25**
2 ml x 25	$184.59	Tobramycin Sulfate, Syringe, Marsam	00209-8922-34
2 ml x 25	$184.59	Tobramycin Sulfate, Geneva Pharms	00781-3774-72
2 ml x 25	$184.69	Tobramycin Sulfate, Bristol Myers Squibb	00003-2725-25
2 ml x 25	$344.40	Tobramycin Sulfate, Gensia Labs	00703-9402-04
30 ml	$73.92	Tobramycin Sulfate, Bristol Myers Squibb	00003-2725-30
30 ml	$74.00	Tobramycin Sulfate, Raway	00686-8970-20
30 ml	$197.51	Tobramycin Sulfate, Gensia Labs	00703-9416-01
30 ml x 1	$89.94	Tobramycin Sulfate, Vial, Marsam	00209-8970-20
30 ml x 5	$369.06	Tobramycin Sulfate, Astra USA	00186-1784-01
30 ml x 6	**$655.59**	**NEBCIN, Lilly**	**00002-7090-16**
30 ml x 10	$1011.56	Tobramycin Sulfate, Lederle Parenterals	00205-3027-08
50 ml	$245.77	Tobramycin Sulfate, Abbott	00074-3590-02

Solution - Ophthalmic - 0.3 %

5 ml	$9.90	Tobrasol, Ocusoft	54799-0513-05
5 ml	$13.38	Tobramycin Sulfate, Aligen Independ	00405-6145-05
5 ml	$13.50	Tobramycin Sulfate, Steris Labs	00402-0914-05
5 ml	$13.50	Tobramycin Sulfate, Falcon Ophthalmics	61314-0643-05
5 ml	$14.25	Aktob, Akorn	17478-0290-10
5 ml	$14.82	Tobramycin Sulfate, United Res	00677-1535-20
5 ml	$14.96	Tobramycin Sulfate, Schein Pharm (US)	00364-3014-53
5 ml	$15.05	Tobramycin Sulfate, Fougera	00168-0254-03
5 ml	$15.50	Tobramycin Sulfate, Goldline Labs	00182-7044-62
5 ml	$19.69	TOBREX, Alcon	00065-0643-05

HOW SUPPLIED - NOT RATED EQUIVALENT:

Injection, Solution - Intramuscular; - 40 mg/ml

40 ml x 6	**$655.59**	**NEBCIN, Lilly**	**00002-7040-16**

Injection, Solution - Intravenous - 1.2 gm

6's	**$655.59**	**NEBCIN, Lilly**	**00002-7382-16**

Injection, Solution - Intravenous - 60 mg/50 ml

50 ml	$13.98	TOBRAMYCIN SULFATE IN NS, Abbott	00074-3469-13

Injection, Solution - Intravenous - 80 mg/50 ml

50 ml	$14.64	TOBRAMYCIN IN SODIUM CHLORIDE, Abbott	00074-1984-14

Injection, Solution - Intravenous - 80 mg/100 ml

100 ml	$14.64	TOBRAMYCIN SULFATE IN NS, Abbott	00074-3470-23

Solution - Ophthalmic - 0.3 %

5 ml	$13.44	Tobramycin Sulfate, Qualitest Pharms	00603-7345-37
5 ml	$17.19	Tobramycin Sulfate, Rugby	00536-2980-65

TOCAINIDE HYDROCHLORIDE *(002357)*

CATEGORIES: Antiarrhythmic Agents; Arrhythmia; Cardiovascular Drugs; Pregnancy Category C; FDA Approved 1984 Nov

BRAND NAMES: **Tonocard**

FORMULARIES: Aetna

COST OF THERAPY: $880.59 (Arrhythmia; Tablet; 400 mg; 3/day; 365 days)

WARNING:

BLOOD DYSCRASIAS: Agranulocytosis, bone marrow depression, leukopenia, neutropenia, aplastic/hypoplastic anemia, thrombocytopenia and sequelae such as septicemia and septic shock have been reported in patients receiving tocainide HCl. Most of these patients received tocainide HCl within the recommended dosage range. Fatalities have occurred (with approximately 25 percent mortality in reported agranulocytosis cases). Since most of these events have been noted during the first 12 weeks of therapy, it is recommended that complete blood counts, including white cell, differential and platelet counts be performed, optimally, at weekly intervals for the first three months of therapy; and frequently thereafter. Complete blood counts should be performed promptly if the patient develops any signs of infection (such as fever, chills, sore throat, or stomatitis), bruising, or bleeding. If any of these hematologic disorders is identified, tocainide HCl should be discontinued and appropriate treatment should be instituted if necessary. Blood counts usually return to normal within one month of discontinuation. Caution should be used in patients with pre-existing marrow failure or cytopenia of any type. (See ADVERSE REACTIONS.)

PULMONARY FIBROSIS: Pulmonary fibrosis, interstitial pneumonitis, fibrosing alveolitis, pulmonary edema, and pneumonia have been reported in patients receiving tocainide HCl. Many of these events occurred in patients who were seriously ill. Fatalities have been reported. The experiences are usually characterized by bilateral infiltrates on x-ray and are frequently associated with dyspnea and cough. Fever may or may not be present. Patients should be instructed to promptly report the development of any pulmonary symptoms such as exertional dyspnea, cough or wheezing. Chest x-rays are advisable at that time. If these pulmonary disorders develop, tocainide HCl should be discontinued. (See ADVERSE REACTIONS.)

DESCRIPTION:

Tocainide HCl is a primary amine analog of lidocaine with antiarrhythmic properties useful in the treatment of ventricular arrhythmias. The chemical name for tocainide hydrochloride is 2-amino-*N*-(2,6-dimethylphenyl) propanamide hydrochloride. Its empirical formula is $C_{11}H_{16}N_2O \cdot HCl$, with a molecular weight of 228.72.

Tocainide hydrochloride is a white crystalline powder with a bitter taste and is freely soluble in water. It is supplied as 400 mg and 600 mg tablets for oral administration. Each tablet contains the following inactive ingredients: hydroxypropyl methylcellulose, iron oxide, magnesium stearate, methylcellulose, polyethylene glycol, and titanium dioxide.

CLINICAL PHARMACOLOGY:

Action: Tocainide, like lidocaine, produces dose dependent decreases in sodium and potassium conductance, thereby decreasing the excitability of myocardial cells. In experimental animal models, the dose-related depression of sodium current is more pronounced in ischemic tissue than in normal tissue.

Electrophysiology: Tocainide is a Class I antiarrhythmic compound with electrophysiologic properties in man similar to those of lidocaine, but dissimilar from quinidine, procainamide, and disopyramide.

In studies of isolated dog Purkinje fibers, tocainide in concentrations of 1-50 mcg/ml had no significant effect on resting membrane potential, but reduced the amplitude and rate of depolarization (dv/dt) of the action potential. Tocainide decreased the effective refractory period (ERP) to a lesser extent than the action potential duration (APD) resulting in an increase in the ERP/APD ratio.

In patients with cardiac disease, tocainide HCl produced no clinically significant changes in sinus nodal function, effective refractory periods, or intracardiac conduction times when studied under electrophysiologic testing procedures.

Tocainide, like lidocaine, characteristically does not prolong ventricular depolarization (QRS duration) or repolarization (QT intervals) as measured by electrocardiography. Theoretically, therefore, tocainide HCl may be useful in the treatment of ventricular arrhythmias associated with a prolonged QT interval.

Patients who respond to lidocaine also respond to tocainide HCl in a majority of cases. Failure to respond to lidocaine usually predicts failure to respond to tocainide HCl, but there are exceptions to this.

In a controlled comparison with quinidine, 600 mg b.i.d. of tocainide HCl produced a mean reduction of 42 percent in PVC count, compared to a 54 percent reduction by quinidine 300 mg every 6 hours. Among all patients entered into the study, about one-fifth of tocainide recipients and one- third of quinidine recipients had 75 percent or greater reductions in PVC count or had elimination of ventricular tachycardia.

Pharmacokinetics: Following oral administration of tocainide, peak plasma concentrations occur within 0.5 to 2 hours. The average plasma half-life in patients is approximately 15 hours. Although the effective plasma concentration may vary from patient to patient, the usual therapeutic plasma range (as defined by 50-80 percent PVC suppression) is 4-10 mcg/ml (18-45 micromole/l), expressed as tocainide hydrochloride. Tocainide is approximately 10 percent bound to plasma protein.

In contrast to lidocaine, tocainide undergoes negligible first pass hepatic degradation. Following oral administration, the bioavailability of tocainide HCl approaches 100 percent. The extent of its bioavailability is unaffected by food. Tocainide has no cardioactive metabolites. Approximately 40 percent of the administered dose of tocainide is excreted unchanged in the urine. Acidification of the urine has not been shown to significantly alter tocainide excretion in the urine, but alkalinization of the urine results in a significant decrease in the percent of tocainide excreted unchanged in the urine. Animal data indicate that tocainide crosses the blood-brain barrier; however, it has less lipid solubility than lidocaine.

Hemodynamics: Cardiac catheterization studies in man utilizing intravenous tocainide infusions (0.5-0.75 mg/kg/min over 15 min) have shown that tocainide usually produces a small degree of depression of parameters of left ventricular function, such as left ventricular dP/dt, and left ventricular end diastolic pressure. There were usually no changes in cardiac output or clinical evidence of increasing congestive heart failure in the well-compensated patients studied. Small but statistically significant increases in aortic and pulmonary arterial pressures have been consistently observed and are probably related to small increases in vascular resistance. When used concomitantly with a beta-blocking drug, tocainide further reduced cardiac index and left ventricular dP/dt and further increased pulmonary wedge pressure.

No clinically significant changes in heart rate, blood pressure, or signs of myocardial depression were observed in a study of 72 post-myocardial infarction patients receiving long-term therapy with oral tocainide HCl at usual doses (400 mg q8h). When tocainide was administered orally at a dose of 120 mg/kg to anesthetized dogs (14 times the initial maximum dose recommended for humans), a negative inotropic effect was observed: the rate of change of left ventricular pressure decreased by up to 29 percent of control at 3 hours after administration. This effect was not observed at lower doses (60 mg/kg). Tocainide has been used safely in patients with acute myocardial infarction and various degrees of congestive heart failure. It has, however, a small negative inotropic effect and can increase peripheral resistance slightly. It therefore should be used cautiously in patients with known heart failure, particularly if a beta blocker is given as well. (See PRECAUTIONS.)

INDICATIONS AND USAGE:

Tocainide HCl is indicated for the treatment of documented ventricular arrhythmias, such as sustained tachycardia, that, in the judgment of the physician, are life-threatening. Because of the proarrhythmic effects of tocainide HCl, as well as its potential for other serious adverse effects,(see WARNINGS), its use to treat lesser arrhythmias is not recommended. Treatment of patients with asymptomatic ventricular premature contractions should be avoided.

Initiation of treatment with tocainide HCl, as with other antiarrhythmic agents used to treat life-threatening arrhythmias, should be carried out in the hospital. It is essential that each patient given tocainide HCl be evaluated electrocardiographically and clinically prior to, and during, therapy with tocainide HCl to determine whether the response to tocainide HCl supports continued treatment.

Antiarrhythmic drugs have not been shown to enhance survival in patients with ventricular arrhythmias.

CONTRAINDICATIONS:

Patients who are hypersensitive to this product or to local anesthetics of the amide type.

Patients with second or third degree atrioventricular block in the absence of an artificial ventricular pacemaker.

WARNINGS:

Mortality: In the National Heart, Lung and Blood Institute's Cardiac Arrhythmia Suppression Trial (CAST), a long-term, multi-centered, randomized, double-blind study in patients with asymptomatic non-life- threatening ventricular arrhythmias who had had myocardial infarctions more than six days but less than two years previously, an excessive mortality or non-fatal cardiac arrest rate was seen in patients treated with encainide or flecainide (56/730) compared with that seen in patients assigned to matched placebo-treated groups (22/725). The average duration of treatment with encainide or flecainide in this study was ten months.

The applicability of these results to other populations (*e.g.,* those without recent myocardial infarctions) or to other antiarrhythmic drugs is uncertain, but at present it is prudent to consider any antiarrhythmic agent to have a significant risk in patients with structural heart disease.

Acceleration of Ventricular Rate: Acceleration of ventricular rate occurs infrequently when antiarrhythmics are administered to patients with atrial flutter or fibrillation (see ADVERSE REACTIONS.)

PRECAUTIONS:

General: In patients with known heart failure or minimal cardiac reserve, tocainide HCl should be used with caution because of the potential for aggravating the degree of heart failure.

Caution should be used in the institution or continuation of antiarrhythmic therapy in the presence of signs of increasing depression of cardiac conductivity.

In patients with severe liver or kidney disease, the rate of drug elimination may be significantly decreased (see DOSAGE AND ADMINISTRATION.)

Since antiarrhythmic drugs may be ineffective in patients with hypokalemia, the possibility of a potassium deficit should be explored and, if present, the deficit should be corrected.

Like all other oral antiarrhythmics, tocainide HCl has been reported to increase arrhythmias in some patients (see ADVERSE REACTIONS.)

Information for the Patient: Patients should be instructed to promptly report the development of bruising or bleeding; any signs of infections such as fever, chills, sore throat, or soreness and ulcers in the mouth; any pulmonary symptoms, such as exertional dyspnea, cough, or wheezing; rash.

Laboratory Tests: As with other antiarrhythmics, abnormal liver function tests, particularly in the early stages of therapy, have been reported. Periodic monitoring of liver function should be considered. Hepatitis and jaundice have been reported in some patients.

Carcinogenesis, Mutagenesis, and Impairment of Fertility: The carcinogenic potential of tocainide was studied in mice using oral doses up to 300 mg/kg/day (about 6 times the maximum recommended human dose) for up to 94 weeks in males and 102 weeks in females and in rats at doses up to 200 mg/kg/day for 24 months. Tocainide did not affect the type or incidence of neoplasia in the two studies.

Tocainide did not show any mutagenic potential when evaluated *in vivo* in the micronucleus test using mice at oral doses up to 187.5 mg/kg/day (about 7 times the usual human dose). Also, no mutagenic activity was seen *in vitro* in the Ames microbial mutagen test or in the mouse lymphoma forward mutation assay.

Reproduction and fertility studies in rats showed no adverse effects on male or female fertility at oral doses up to 200 mg/kg/day (about 8 times the usual human dose).

Pregnancy, Teratogenic Effects, Pregnancy Category C: In a teratogenicity study in rabbits, tocainide was administered orally at doses of 25, 50, and 100 mg/kg/day (about 1 to 4 times the usual human dose). No evidence of a drug-related teratogenic effect was noted; however, these doses were maternotoxic and produced a dose-related increase in abortions and stillbirths. In a teratogenicity study in rats, an oral dose of 300 mg/kg/day (about 12 times the usual human dose) showed no evidence of treatment-related fetal malformations, but maternotoxicity and an increase in fetal resorptions were noted. An oral dose of 30 mg/kg/day (about twice the usual human dose) did not produce any adverse effects.

In reproduction studies in rats at maternotoxic oral doses of 200 and 300 mg/kg/day (about 8 and 12 times the usual human dose, respectively), dystocia, and delayed parturition occurred which was accompanied by an increase in stillbirths and decreased survival in offspring during the first week postpartum. Growth and viability of surviving offspring were not affected for the remainder of the lactation period.

There are no adequate and well-controlled studies in pregnant women. Tocainide HCl should be used during pregnancy only if the potential benefit justifies the potential risk to the fetus.

Nursing Mothers: It is not known whether tocainide is secreted in human milk. Because many drugs are secreted in human milk and because of the potential for serious adverse reactions in nursing infants from tocainide HCl, a decision should be made whether to discontinue nursing or to discontinue the drug, taking into account the importance of the drug to the mother.

Pediatric Use: Safety and effectiveness in children have not been established.

DRUG INTERACTIONS:

Tocainide and lidocaine are pharmacodynamically similar. The concomitant use of these two agents may cause an increased incidence of adverse reactions, including central nervous system adverse reactions such as seizure.

Specific interaction studies with cimetidine, digoxin, metoprolol and warfarin have been conducted, no clinically significant interaction was seen with cimetidine, digoxin or warfarin; but tocainide and metoprolol had additive effects on wedge pressure and cardiac index. Tocainide HCl has also been used in open studies with digitalis, beta-blocking agents, other antiarrhythmic agents, anticoagulants, and diuretics, without evidence of clinically significant interactions. Nevertheless, caution should be exercised in the use of multiple drug therapy.

Tocainide HCl is equally effective in digitalized and non-digitalized patients. In 17 patients with refractory ventricular arrhythmias on concomitant therapy, serum digoxin levels (1.1 ± 0.4 ng/ml) remained in the expected normal range (0.5-2.5 ng/ml) during tocainide administration.

ADVERSE REACTIONS:

Tocainide HCl commonly produces minor, transient, nervous system and gastrointestinal adverse reactions, but is otherwise generally well tolerated. Tocainide HCl has been evaluated in both short-term (n = 1,358) and long-term (n = 262) controlled studies as well as a compassionate use program. Dosages were lower in most of the controlled studies (1200 mg/day) and higher in the compassionate use program (1800 mg and more). In long-term (2-6 months) controlled studies, the most frequent adverse reactions were dizziness/vertigo (15.3 percent), nausea (14.5 percent), paresthesia (9.2 percent), and tremor (8.4 percent). These reactions were generally mild, transient, dose-related and reversible with a reduction in dosage, by taking the drug with food, or by therapy discontinuation. Tremor, when present, may be useful as a clinical indicator that the maximum dose is being approached. Adverse reactions leading to therapy discontinuation occurred in 21 percent of patients in long-term controlled trials and were usually related to the nervous system or digestive system.

Adverse reactions occurring in greater than one percent of patients from the short-term and long-term controlled studies appear in the following table (TABLE 1):

An additional group of about 2,000 patients has been treated in a program allowing for the use of tocainide HCl under compassionate use circumstances. These patients were seriously ill with the large majority on multiple drug therapy, and comparatively high doses of tocainide HCl were used. Fifty- four percent of the patients continued in the program for one year or longer, and 12 percent were treated for longer than three years, with the longest duration of therapy being nine years. Adverse reactions leading to therapy discontinuation occurred in 12 percent of patients (usually central nervous system effects or rash). A tabulation of adverse reactions occurring in one percent or more of patients follows (TABLE 2):

Adverse reactions occurring in less than one percent of patients in either the controlled studies or the compassionate use program or since the drug was marketed are as follows:

Body as a Whole: Septicemia; septic shock; syncope; vaso-vagal episodes; edema; fever; chills; cinchonism; asthenia; malaise.

Cardiovascular: Ventricular fibrillation; extension of acute myocardial infarction; cardiogenic shock; pulmonary embolism; angina; AV block; hypertension; claudication; increased QRS duration; pleurisy/pericarditis; prolonged QT interval; right bundle branch block; cardiomegaly; sinus arrest; vasculitis; orthostatic hypotension; cold extremities.

ADVERSE REACTIONS: *(cont'd)*

TABLE 1

	Percent of Patients Controlled Studies	
	Short-term (n = 1,358)	**Long-term (n = 262)**
Body As A Whole		
Tiredness/drowsiness/fatigue/lethargy/lassitude/sleepiness	1.6	0.8
Hot/cold feelings	0.5	1.5
Cardiovascular		
Hypotension	3.4	2.7
Bradycardia	1.8	0.4
Palpitations	1.8	0.4
Chest pain	1.6	0.4
Conduction disorders	1.5	0.0
Left ventricular failure	1.4	0.0
Digestive		
Nausea	15.2	14.5
Vomiting	8.3	4.6
Anorexia	1.2	1.9
Diarrhea/loose stools	0.0	3.8
Nervous System/Psychiatric		
Dizziness/vertigo	8.0	15.3
Paresthesia	3.5	9.2
Tremor	2.9	8.4
Confusion/disorientation/hallucinations	2.1	2.7
Headache	2.1	4.6
Nervousness	1.5	0.4
Altered mood/awareness	1.5	3.4
Incoordination/unsteadiness/walking disturbances	1.2	0.0
Anxiety	1.1	1.5
Ataxia	0.2	3.0
Skin		
Diaphoresis	5.1	2.3
Rash/skin lesion	0.4	8.4
Special Senses		
Blurred vision/visual disturbances	1.3	1.5
Tinnitus/hearing loss	0.4	1.5
Nystagmus	0.0	1.1

TABLE 2

	Percent of Patients Compassionate Use (n=1927)
Cardiovascular	
Increased ventricular arrhythmias/PVCs	10.9
CHF/progression of CHF	4.0
Tachycardia	3.2
Hypotension	1.8
Conduction disorders	1.3
Bradycardia	1.0
Digestive	
Nausea	24.6
Anorexia	11.3
Vomiting	9.0
Diarrhea/loose stools	6.8
Musculoskeletal	
Arthritis/arthralgia	4.7
Myalgia	1.7
Nervous System/Psychiatric	
Dizziness/vertigo	25.3
Tremor	21.6
Nervousness	11.5
Confusion/disorientation/hallucinations	11.2
Altered mood/awareness	11.0
Ataxia	10.8
Paresthesia	9.2
Skin	
Rash/skin lesion	12.2
Diaphoresis	8.3
Lupus	1.6
Special Senses	
Blurred vision/vision disturbances	10.0
Nystagmus	1.1

Digestive: Hepatitis, jaundice (see PRECAUTIONS), abnormal liver function tests; pancreatitis; abdominal pain/discomfort; constipation; dysphagia; gastrointestinal symptoms (including dyspepsia); stomatitis; dry mouth; thirst.

Hematologic: Agranulocytosis; bone marrow depression; aplastic/hypoplastic anemia; hemolytic anemia; anemia; leukopenia; neutropenia; thrombocytopenia; eosinophilia.

Metabolic and Immune: Hypersensitivity Reaction (including some of the following symptoms or signs: rash, fever, joint pains, abnormal liver function tests, eosinophilia); increased ANA.

Musculoskeletal: Muscle cramps; muscle twitching/spasm; neck pain; pain radiating from neck; pressure on shoulder.

Nervous System/Psychiatric: Coma; convulsions/seizures; myasthenia gravis; depression; psychosis; psychic disturbances; agitation; decreased mental acuity; dysarthria; impaired memory; increased stuttering/slurred speech; insomnia/sleeping disturbances; local anesthesia; dream abnormalities.

Respiratory: Respiratory arrest; pulmonary edema; pulmonary fibrosis; fibrosing alveolitis; pneumonia; interstitial pneumonitis; dyspnea; hiccough; yawning.

Skin: Stevens-Johnson syndrome; exfoliative dermatitis; erythema multiforme; urticaria; alopecia; pruritus; pallor/flushed face.

Special Senses: Diplopia; earache; taste perversion/smell perversion.

Urogenital: Urinary retention; polyuria/increased diuresis.

Agranulocytosis, bone marrow depression, leukopenia, neutropenia, aplastic/hypoplastic anemia, and thrombocytopenia have been reported (0.18 percent) in patients receiving tocainide HCl in controlled trials and the compassionate use program. Most of these events have been noted during the first 12 weeks of therapy. (See BOXED WARNING.)

Pulmonary fibrosis, interstitial pneumonitis, fibrosing alveolitis, pulmonary edema, and pneumonia, have been reported in patients receiving tocainide HCl. The incidence of pulmonary fibrosis (including interstitial pneumonitis and fibrosing alveolitis) was 0.11 percent in controlled trials and the compassionate use program. These events usually occurred in seriously ill patients. Symptoms of these pulmonary disorders and/or x-ray changes usually occurred following 3-18 weeks of therapy. Fatalities have been reported. (See BOXED WARNING.)

A number of disorders, in which a causal relationship with tocainide HCl has not been established, have been reported in seriously ill patients. These include: renal failure, renal dysfunction, myocardial infarction, cerebrovascular accidents and transient ischemic attacks. These disorders may be related to the patient's underlying condition.

DRUG ABUSE AND DEPENDENCE:

Drug withdrawal after chronic treatment has not shown any indication of psychological or physical dependence.

OVERDOSAGE:

The initial and most important signs and symptoms of overdosage would be expected to be related to the central nervous system. Other adverse reactions, such as gastrointestinal disturbances, may follow. (See ADVERSE REACTIONS.)

Should convulsions or cardiopulmonary depression or arrest develop, the patency of the airway and adequacy of ventilation must be assured immediately. Should convulsions persist despite ventilatory therapy with oxygen, small increments of anticonvulsive agents may be given intravenously. Examples of such agents include a benzodiazepine (*e.g.,* diazepam), an ultrashort-acting barbiturate (*e.g.,* thiopental or thiamylal), or a short-acting barbiturate (*e.g.,* pentobarbital or secobarbital).

The oral LD_{50} of tocainide was calculated to be about 800 mg/kg in mice, 1000 mg/kg in rats, and 230 mg/kg in guinea pigs; deaths were usually preceded by convulsions.

Studies in normal individuals to date indicate that tocainide has a hemodialysis clearance approximately equivalent to its renal clearance.

DOSAGE AND ADMINISTRATION:

The dosage of tocainide HCl must be individualized on the basis of antiarrhythmic response and tolerance, both of which are dose-related. Clinical and electrocardiographic evaluation (including Holter monitoring if necessary for evaluation) are needed to determine whether the desired antiarrhythmic response has been obtained and to guide titration and dose adjustment. Adverse effects appearing shortly after dosing, for example, suggest a need for dividing the dose further with a shorter dose-interval. Loss of arrhythmia control prior to the next dose suggests use of a shorter dose interval and/or a dose increase. Absence of a clear response suggests reconsideration of therapy.

The recommended initial dosage is 400 mg every 8 hours. The usual adult dosage is between 1200 and 1800 mg/day in a three dose daily divided regimen. Doses beyond 2400 mg per day have been administered infrequently. Patients who tolerate the t.i.d. regimen may be tried on a twice daily regimen with careful monitoring.

Some patients, particularly those with renal or hepatic impairment, may be adequately treated with less than 1200 mg/day.

HOW SUPPLIED:

No. 3409 -Tablets Tonocard, 400 mg, are oval, yellow, scored; film-coated tablets, coded 707 on one side and Tonocard on the other side.

No. 3410 -Tablets Tonocard, 600 mg, are oblong, yellow, scored, film-coated tablets, coded 709 on one side and Tonocard on the other side.

Storage: Store below 40°C (104°C), preferably between 15°C and 30°C (59°F and 86°F). Store in a well-closed container.

HOW SUPPLIED - EQUIVALENTS NOT AVAILABLE:

Tablet, Plain Coated - Oral - 400 mg

100's	$80.42	TONOCARD, Astra Merck	61113-0707-68
100's	$84.95	TONOCARD, Astra Merck	61113-0707-28

Tablet, Plain Coated - Oral - 600 mg

100's	$102.50	TONOCARD, Astra Merck	61113-0709-68
100's	$107.05	TONOCARD, Astra Merck	61113-0709-28

TOLAZAMIDE *(002358)*

CATEGORIES: Antidiabetic Agents; Blood Glucose Regulators; Diabetes; Diabetes Mellitus; Hormones; Hyperglycemia; Sulfonylureas; Vascular Disorders, Cerebral/Peripheral; Weight Loss; Pregnancy Category C; FDA Approval Pre 1982

BRAND NAMES: *Diabewas*; *Diadutos*; *Norglycin*; Tolamide; *Tolanase*; **Tolinase**; *Tolisan*
(International brand names outside U.S. in italics)

FORMULARIES: Aetna; BC-BS; FHP; Medi-Cal

DESCRIPTION:

These tablets contain tolazamide, an oral blood glucose lowering drug of the sulfonylurea class. Tolazamide is white or creamy-white powder with a melting point of 165° to 173° C. The solubility of tolazamide at pH 6.0 (mean urinary pH) is 27.8 mg per 100 ml.

The chemical names for tolazamide are (1) Benzenesulfonamide, *N*-((hexahydro-1*H*-azepin-1-yl) amino) carbonyl)-4-methyl-; (2) 1- (Hexahydro-1*H*-azepin-1-yl)-3-(*p*-tolylsulfonyl)urea and its molecular weight is 311.40.

Tolinase tablets for oral administration are available as scored, white tablets containing 100 mg, 250 mg tolazamide. Inactive ingredients: calcium sulfate, docusate sodium, magnesium stearate, methylcellulose, sodium alginate.

CLINICAL PHARMACOLOGY:

MECHANISM OF ACTION

Tolazamide appears to lower the blood glucose acutely by stimulating the release of insulin from the pancreas, an effect dependent upon functioning beta cells in the pancreatic islets. The mechanism by which tolazamide lowers blood glucose during long-term administration has not been clearly established. With chronic administration in Type II diabetic patients, the blood glucose lowering effect persists despite a gradual decline in the insulin secretory response to the drug. Extrapancreatic effects may be involved in the mechanism of action of oral sulfonylurea hypoglycemic drugs.

Some patients who are initially responsive to oral hypoglycemic drugs, including tolazamide tablets, may become unresponsive or poorly responsive over time. Alternatively, tolazamide tablets may be effective in some patients who have become unresponsive to one or more other sulfonylurea drugs.

In addition to its blood glucose lowering actions, tolazamide produces a mild diuresis by enhancement of renal free water clearance.

CLINICAL PHARMACOLOGY: *(cont'd)*

PHARMACOKINETICS

Tolazamide is rapidly and well absorbed from the gastrointestinal tract. Peak serum concentrations occur at three to four hours following a single oral dose of the drug. The average biological half-life of the drug is seven hours. The drug does not continue to accumulate in the blood after the first four to six doses are administered. A steady or equilibrium state is reached during which the peak and nadir values do not change from day to day after the fourth to sixth doses.

Tolazamide is metabolized to five major metabolites ranging in hypoglycemic activity from 0-70%. They are excreted principally in the urine. Following a single oral dose of tritiated tolazamide, 85% of the dose was excreted in the urine and 7% in the feces over a five-day period. Most of the urinary excretion of the drug occurred within the first 24 hours post administration.

When normal fasting nondiabetic subjects are given a single 500 mg dose of tolazamide orally, a hypoglycemic effect can be noted within 20 minutes after ingestion with a peak hypoglycemic effect occurring in two to four hours. Following a single oral dose of 500 mg tolazamide, a statistically significant hypoglycemic effect was demonstrated in fasted nondiabetic subjects 20 hours after administration. With fasting diabetic patients, the peak hypoglycemic effect occurs at four to six hours. The duration of maximal hypoglycemic effect in fed diabetic patients is about ten hours, with the onset occurring at four to six hours and with the blood glucose levels beginning to rise at 14 to 16 hours. Single dose potency of tolazamide in normal subjects has been shown to be 6.7 times that of tolbutamide on a milligram basis. Clinical experience in diabetic patients has demonstrated tolazamide to be approximately five times more potent than tolbutamide on a milligram basis, and approximately equivalent in milligram potency to chlorpropamide.

INDICATIONS AND USAGE:

Tolazamide tablets are indicated as an adjunct to diet to lower the blood glucose in patients with noninsulin dependent diabetes mellitus (Type II) whose hyperglycemia cannot be satisfactorily controlled by diet alone.

In initiating treatment for noninsulin-dependent diabetes, diet should be emphasized as the primary form of treatment. Caloric restriction and weight loss are essential in the obese diabetic patient. Proper dietary management alone may be effective in controlling the blood glucose and symptoms of hyperglycemia. The importance of regular physical activity should also be stressed and cardiovascular risk factors should be identified and corrective measures taken where possible.

If this treatment program fails to reduce symptoms and/or blood glucose, the use of an oral sulfonylurea or insulin should be considered. Use of tolazamide must be viewed by both the physician and patient as a treatment in addition to diet and not as a substitute for diet or as a convenient mechanism for avoiding dietary restraint. Furthermore, loss of blood glucose control on diet alone may be transient thus requiring only short-term administration of tolazamide.

During maintenance programs, tolazamide should be discontinued if satisfactory lowering of blood glucose is no longer achieved. Judgments should be based on regular clinical and laboratory evaluations.

In considering the use of tolazamide in asymptomatic patients, it should be recognized that controlling the blood glucose in noninsulin-dependent diabetes has not been definitely established to be effective in preventing the long-term cardiovascular or neural complications of diabetes.

CONTRAINDICATIONS:

Tolazamide tablets are contraindicated in patients with: 1) known hypersensitivity or allergy to tolazamide; 2) diabetic ketoacidosis, with or without coma. This condition should be treated with insulin; 3) Type I diabetes, as sole therapy.

SPECIAL WARNING ON INCREASED RISK OF CARDIOVASCULAR MORTALITY

The administration of oral hypoglycemic drugs has been reported to be associated with increased cardiovascular mortality as compared to treatment with diet alone or diet plus insulin. This warning is based on the study conducted by the University Group Diabetes Program (UGDP), a long-term prospective clinical trial designed to evaluate the effectiveness of glucose-lowering drugs in preventing or delaying vascular complications in patients with noninsulin-dependent diabetes. The study involved 823 patients who randomly assigned to one of four treatment groups (DIABETES, 19 (supp.2):747-830, 1970.)

UGDP reported that patients treated for five to eight years with diet plus a fixed dose of tolbutamide (1.5 grams per day) had a rate of cardiovascular mortality approximately 2.5 times that of patients with diet alone. A significant increase in total mortality was not observed, but the use of tolbutamide was discontinued based on the increase in cardiovascular mortality, thus limiting the opportunity for the study to show an increase in overall mortality. Despite controversy regarding the interpretation of these results, the findings of the UGDP study provide an adequate basis for this warning. The patient should be informed of the potential risks and advantages of tolazamide and of alternative modes of therapy.

Although only one drug in the sulfonylurea class (tolbutamide) was included in this study, it is prudent from a safety standpoint to consider that this warning may also apply to other oral hypoglycemic drugs in this class, in view of their close similarities in mode of action and chemical structure.

PRECAUTIONS:

GENERAL

Hypoglycemia: All sulfonylurea drugs are capable of producing severe hypoglycemia. Proper patient selection and dosage and instructions are important to avoid hypoglycemic episodes. Renal or hepatic insufficiency may cause elevated blood levels of tolazamide and the latter may also diminish gluconeogenic capacity, both of which increase the risk of serious hypoglycemic reactions. Elderly, debilitated, or malnourished patients and those with adrenal or pituitary insufficiency are particularly susceptible to the hypoglycemic action of glucose lowering drugs. Hypoglycemia may be difficult to recognize in the elderly and in people who are taking beta-adrenergic blocking drugs. Hypoglycemia is more likely to occur when caloric intake is deficient, after severe or prolonged exercise, when alcohol is ingested, or when more than one glucose-lowering drug is used.

Loss of Control of Blood Glucose: When a patient stabilized on any diabetic regimen is exposed to stress such as fever, trauma, infection, or surgery, loss of control of blood glucose may occur. At such times it may be necessary to discontinue tolazamide tablets and administer insulin.

The effectiveness of any hypoglycemic drug, including tolazamide, in lowering blood glucose to a desired level decreases in many patients over a period of time, which may be due to progression of the severity of the diabetes or to diminished responsiveness to the drug. This phenomenon is known as secondary failure to distinguish it from primary failure in which the drug is ineffective in an individual patient when first given. Adequate adjustment of dose and adherence to diet should be assessed before classifying a patient as a secondary failure.

PRECAUTIONS: *(cont'd)*

INFORMATION FOR THE PATIENT

Patients should be informed of the potential risks and advantages of tolazamide and of alternative modes of therapy. They should also be informed about the importance of adherence to dietary instructions, of a regular exercise program, and of regular testing of urine and/or blood glucose.

The risks of hypoglycemia, its symptoms and treatment, and conditions that predispose to its development should be explained to patients and responsible family members. Primary and secondary failure should also be explained.

LABORATORY TESTS

Blood and urine glucose should be monitored periodically. Measurement of glycosylated hemoglobin may be useful in some patients.

CARCINOGENICITY

In a bioassay for carcinogenicity, rats and mice of both sexes were treated with tolazamide for 103 weeks at low and high doses. No evidence of carcinogenicity was found.

PREGNANCY CATEGORY C

Teratogenic Effects: Tolazamide, administered to pregnant rats at ten times the human dose, decreased litter size but did not produce teratogenic effects in the offspring. In rats treated at a daily dose of 14 mg/kg no reproductive aberrations or drug related fetal anomalies were noted. At an elevated dose of 100 mg/kg per day there was a reduction in the number of pups born and an increased perinatal mortality. There are, however, no adequate and well-controlled studies in pregnant women. Because animal reproduction studies are not always predictive of human response, tolazamide is not recommended for the treatment of the pregnant diabetic patient. Serious consideration should also be given to the possible hazards of the use of tolazamide in women of child bearing age and in those who might become pregnant while using the drug.

Because recent information suggests that abnormal blood glucose levels during pregnancy are associated with a higher incidence of congenital abnormalities, many experts recommend that insulin be used during pregnancy to maintain blood glucose levels as close to normal as possible.

Nonteratogenic Effects: Prolonged severe hypoglycemia (four to ten days) has been reported in neonates born to mothers who were receiving a sulfonylurea drug at the time of delivery. This has been reported more frequently with the use of agents with prolonged half-lives. If tolazamide is used during pregnancy, it should be discontinued at least two weeks before the expected delivery date.

NURSING MOTHERS

Although it is not known whether tolazamide is excreted in human milk, some sulfonylurea drugs are known to be excreted in human milk. Because the potential for hypoglycemia in nursing infants may exist, a decision should be made whether to discontinue nursing or to discontinue the drug, taking into account the importance of the drug to the mother. If the drug is discontinued and if diet alone is inadequate for controlling blood glucose, insulin therapy should be considered.

PEDIATRIC USE

Safety and effectiveness in children have not been established.

DRUG INTERACTIONS:

The hypoglycemic action of sulfonylureas may be potentiated by certain drugs including nonsteroidal anti-inflammatory agents and other drugs that are highly protein bound, salicylates, sulfonamides, chloramphenicol, probenecid, coumarins, monoamine oxidase inhibitors, and beta-adrenergic blocking agents. When such drugs are administered to a patient receiving tolazamide, the patient should be closely observed for hypoglycemia. When such drugs are withdrawn from a patient receiving tolazamide, the patient should be observed closely for loss of control.

Certain drugs tend to produce hyperglycemia and may lead to loss of control. These drugs include the thiazides and other diuretics, corticosteroids, phenothiazines, thyroid products, estrogens, oral contraceptives, phenytoin, nicotinic acid, sympathomimetics, calcium channel blocking drugs, and isoniazid. When such drugs are administered to a patient receiving tolazamide, the patient should be closely observed for loss of control. When such drugs are withdrawn from a patient receiving tolazamide, the patient should be observed closely for hypoglycemia.

A potential interaction between oral miconazole and oral hypoglycemic agents leading to severe hypoglycemia has been reported. Whether this interaction also occurs with the intravenous, topical or vaginal preparations of miconazole is not known.

ADVERSE REACTIONS:

Tolazamide tablets have generally been well tolerated. In clinical studies in which more than 1,784 diabetic patients were specifically evaluated for incidence of side effects, only 2.1% were discontinued from therapy because of side effects.

Hypoglycemia: See PRECAUTIONS and OVERDOSAGE.

Gastrointestinal Reactions: Cholestatic jaundice may occur rarely; tolazamide tablets should be discontinued if this occurs. Gastrointestinal disturbances, e.g., nausea, epigastric fullness, and heartburn, are the most common reactions and occurred in 1% of patients treated during clinical trials. They tend to dose-related and may disappear when dosage is reduced.

Dermatologic Reactions: Allergic skin reactions, e.g., pruritus, erythema, urticaria, and morbilliform or maculopapular eruptions, occurred in 0.4% of patients treated during clinical trials. These may be transient and may disappear despite continued use of tolazamide; if skin reactions persist, the drug should be discontinued.

Porphyria cutanea tarda and photosensitivity reactions have not been reported with sulfonylureas.

Hematologic Reactions: Leukopenia, agranulocytosis, thrombocytopenia, hemolytic anemia, aplastic anemia, and pancytopenia have been reported with sulfonylureas.

Metabolic Reactions: Hepatic porphyria and disulfiram-like reactions have been reported with sulfonylureas; however, disulfiram-like reactions with tolazamide have been reported very rarely.

Cases of hyponatremia have been reported with tolazamide and all other sulfonylureas, most often in patients who are on other medications or have medical conditions known to cause hyponatremia or increase release of antidiuretic hormone. The syndrome of inappropriate antidiuretic hormone (SIADH) secretion has been reported with certain other sulfonylureas, and it has been suggested that these sulfonylureas may augment the peripheral (antidiuretic) action of ADH and/or increase release of ADH.

Miscellaneous: Weakness, fatigue, dizziness, vertigo, malaise and headache were reported infrequently in patients treated during clinical trials. The relationship to therapy with tolazamide is difficult to assess.

OVERDOSAGE:

Overdosage of sulfonylureas, including tolazamide tablets, can produce hypoglycemia.

Mild hypoglycemic symptoms without loss of consciousness or neurologic findings should be treated aggressively with oral glucose and adjustment in drug dosage and/or meal patterns. Close monitoring should continue until the physician is assured the patient is out of danger. Severe hypoglycemic reactions with coma, seizure, or other neurological impairment occur infrequently, but constitute medical emergencies requiring immediate hospitalization. If hypoglycemic coma is suspected or diagnosed, the patient should be given a rapid intravenous injection of concentrated (50%) glucose solution. This should be followed by a continuous infusion of a more dilute (10%) glucose solution at a rate which will maintain the blood glucose at a level above 100 mg/dl. Patients should be closely monitored for a minimum of 24 to 48 hours since hypoglycemia may recur after apparent clinical recovery.

DOSAGE AND ADMINISTRATION:

There is no fixed dosage regimen for the management of diabetes mellitus with tolazamide tablets or any other hypoglycemic agent. In addition to the usual monitoring of urinary glucose, the patient's blood glucose must also be monitored periodically to determine the minimum effective dose for the patient; to detect primary failure, i.e., inadequate lowering of blood glucose at the maximum recommended doses of medication; and to detect secondary failure, i.e., loss of adequate blood glucose response after an initial period of effectiveness. Glycosylated hemoglobin levels may also be of value in monitoring the patient's response to therapy.

Short-term administration of tolazamide may be sufficient during periods of transient loss of control in patients usually controlled well on diet.

USUAL STARTING DOSE

The usual starting dose of tolazamide tablets for the mild to moderately severe Type II diabetic patient is 100-250 mg daily administered with breakfast or the first main meal. Generally, if the fasting blood glucose is less than 200 mg/dl, the starting dose is 100 mg/day as a single daily dose. If the fasting blood glucose value is greater than 200 mg/dl, the starting dose is 250 mg/day as a single dose. If the patient is malnourished, underweight, elderly, or not eating properly, the initial therapy should be 100 mg once a day. Failure to follow an appropriate dosage regimen may precipitate hypoglycemia. Patients who do not adhere to their prescribed dietary regimen are more prone to exhibit unsatisfactory response to drug therapy.

TRANSFER FROM OTHER HYPOGLYCEMIC THERAPY

Patients Receiving Other Oral Antidiabetic Therapy: Transfer of patients from other oral antidiabetes regimens of tolazamide should be done conservatively. When transferring patients from oral hypoglycemic agents other than chlorpropamide to tolazamide, no transition period or initial or priming dose is necessary. When transferring from chlorpropamide, particular care should be exercised to avoid hypoglycemia.

Tolbutamide: If receiving less than 1 gm/day, begin at 100 mg of tolazamide per day. If receiving 1 gm or more per day, initiate at 250 mg of tolazamide per day as a single dose.

Chlorpropamide: 250 mg of chlorpropamide may be considered to provide approximately the same degree of blood glucose control 250 mg of tolazamide. The patient should be observed carefully for hypoglycemia during the transition period from chlorpropamide to tolazamide (one to two weeks) due to the prolonged retention of chlorpropamide in the body and the possibility of subsequent overlapping drug effects.

Acetohexamide: 100 mg of tolazamide may be considered to provide approximately the same degree of blood glucose control as 250 mg of acetohexamide.

Patients Receiving Insulin: Some Type II diabetic patients who have been treated only with insulin may respond satisfactorily to therapy with tolazamide. If the patient's previous insulin dosage has been less than 20 units, substitution of 100 mg of tolazamide per day as a single daily dose may be tried. If the previous insulin dosage was less than 40 units, but more than 20 units, the patient should be placed directly on 250 mg of tolazamide per day as a single dose. If the previous insulin dosage was greater than 40 units, the insulin dosage should be decreased by 50% and 250 mg of tolazamide per day started. The dosage of tolazamide should be adjusted weekly (or more often in the group previously requiring more than 40 units of insulin). During this conversion period when both insulin and tolazamide are being used, hypoglycemia may rarely occur. During insulin withdrawal, patients should test their urine for glucose and acetone at least three times daily and report results to their physician. The appearance of persistent acetonuria with glycosuria indicates that the patients is a Type I diabetic who requires insulin therapy.

MAXIMUM DOSE

Daily doses of greater than 1000 mg are not recommended. Patients will generally have no further response to doses larger than this.

USUAL MAINTENANCE DOSE

The usual maintenance dose is in the range of 100-1000 mg/day with the average maintenance dose being 250-500 mg/day. Following initiation of therapy, dosage adjustment is made in increments of 100 mg to 250 mg at weekly intervals based on the patients's blood glucose response.

DOSAGE INTERVAL

Once a day therapy is usually satisfactory. Doses up to 500 mg/day should be given as single dose in the morning. 500 mg once daily is as effective as 250 mg twice daily. When a dose of more than 500 mg/day is required, the dose may be divided and given twice daily.

In elderly patients, debilitated or malnourished patients, and patients with impaired renal or hepatic function, the initial and maintenance dosing should be conservative to avoid hypoglycemic reactions (see PRECAUTIONS.)

Store at controlled room temperature 15-30°C (59-86°F).

HOW SUPPLIED - RATED THERAPEUTICALLY EQUIVALENT:

Tablet, Uncoated - Oral - 100 mg

100's	$5.03	Tolazamide, United Res	00677-0953-01
100's	$5.03	Tolazamide, H.C.F.A. F F P	99999-2358-01
100's	$7.88	Tolazamide, US Trading	56126-0122-11
100's	$10.40	Tolazamide, Schein Pharm (US)	00364-0721-01
100's	$10.50	Tolazamide, Qualitest Pharms	00603-6096-21
100's	$10.60	Tolazamide, Mutual Pharm	53489-0151-01
100's	$10.65	Tolazamide, Zenith Labs	00172-2978-60
100's	$10.65	Tolazamide, Goldline Labs	00182-1677-01
100's	$10.80	Tolazamide 100, Major Pharms	00904-0234-60
100's	$11.00	Tolazamide, Rugby	00536-4738-01
100's	$11.20	Tolazamide, Martec Pharms	52555-0291-01
100's	$11.54	Tolazamide, Aligen Independ	00405-5024-01
100's	$12.49	Tolazamide, HL Moore Drug Exch	00839-7014-06
100's	$17.15	Tolazamide 100, Major Pharms	00904-0234-61
100's	$19.89	Tolazamide, Schein Pharm (US)	00364-0721-90
100's	**$28.12**	**TOLINASE, Pharmacia & Upjohn**	**00009-0070-02**
250's	$12.57	Tolazamide, H.C.F.A. F F P	99999-2358-02
500's	$25.15	Tolazamide, H.C.F.A. F F P	99999-2358-03
1000's	$50.30	Tolazamide, H.C.F.A. F F P	99999-2358-04

HOW SUPPLIED - RATED THERAPEUTICALLY EQUIVALENT: *(cont'd)*

Tablet, Uncoated - Oral - 250 mg

100's	$9.38	Tolazamide, United Res	00677-0954-01
100's	$9.38	Tolazamide, H.C.F.A. F F P	99999-2358-05
100's	$19.07	Tolazamide, US Trading	56126-0103-11
100's	$21.51	Tolazamide, Qualitest Pharms	00603-6097-21
100's	$21.75	Tolazamide, Mutual Pharm	53489-0152-01
100's	$21.80	Tolazamide, Zenith Labs	00172-2979-60
100's	$22.26	Tolazamide, HL Moore Drug Exch	00839-6755-06
100's	$22.50	Tolazamide, Rugby	00536-4739-01
100's	$22.58	Tolazamide, Schein Pharm (US)	00364-0720-01
100's	$22.90	Tolazamide, Martec Pharms	52555-0292-01
100's	$23.70	Tolazamide, Voluntary Hosp	53258-0173-01
100's	$25.15	Tolazamide, Aligen Independ	00405-5025-01
100's	$26.95	Tolazamide, Mylan	00378-0217-01
100's	$33.50	Tolazamide, Schein Pharm (US)	00364-0720-90
100's	$34.36	Tolazamide 250, Major Pharms	00904-0235-61
100's	$35.00	Tolazamide, Voluntary Hosp	53258-0173-13
100's	$46.60	Tolazamide, Goldline Labs	00182-1645-89
100's	**$59.37**	**TOLINASE, Pharmacia & Upjohn**	**00009-0114-05**
100's	**$63.40**	**TOLINASE, Pharmacia & Upjohn**	**00009-0114-06**
200's	$18.76	Tolazamide, United Res	00677-0954-04
200's	$18.76	Tolazamide, H.C.F.A. F F P	99999-2358-06
200's	$35.90	Tolazamide 250, Major Pharms	00904-0235-25
200's	$36.40	Tolazamide, Qualitest Pharms	00603-6097-23
200's	$39.90	Tolazamide, Mutual Pharm	53489-0152-04
200's	$42.00	Tolazamide, Zenith Labs	00172-2979-61
200's	$42.00	Tolazamide, Goldline Labs	00182-1645-04
200's	**$117.13**	**TOLINASE, Pharmacia & Upjohn**	**00009-0114-04**
250's	$23.45	Tolazamide, H.C.F.A. F F P	99999-2358-07
250's	$51.40	Tolazamide, Rugby	00536-4739-02
500's	$46.90	Tolazamide, H.C.F.A. F F P	99999-2358-08
500's	$66.30	Tolazamide 250, Major Pharms	00904-0235-40
500's	$94.50	Tolazamide, Zenith Labs	00172-2979-70
500's	$99.80	Tolazamide, Rugby	00536-4739-05
500's	$105.00	Tolazamide, Aligen Independ	00405-5025-02
1000's	$93.80	Tolazamide, United Res	00677-0954-10
1000's	$93.80	Tolazamide, H.C.F.A. F F P	99999-2358-09
1000's	$179.55	Tolazamide, Zenith Labs	00172-2979-80
1000's	$179.55	Tolazamide, Goldline Labs	00182-1645-10
1000's	$179.62	Tolzamide, HL Moore Drug Exch	00839-6755-16
1000's	$189.56	Tolazamide, Qualitest Pharms	00603-6097-32
1000's	$191.00	Tolazamide, Mutual Pharm	53489-0152-10
1000's	$201.05	Tolazamide, Aligen Independ	00405-5025-03
1000's	**$571.88**	**TOLINASE, Pharmacia & Upjohn**	**00009-0114-02**

Tablet, Uncoated - Oral - 500 mg

100's	$17.40	Tolazamide, United Res	00677-0955-01
100's	$17.40	Tolazamide, H.C.F.A. F F P	99999-2358-10
100's	$31.45	Tolazamide, Aligen Independ	00405-5026-01
100's	$40.43	Tolazamide, Qualitest Pharms	00603-6098-21
100's	$40.45	Tolazamide, Zenith Labs	00172-2980-60
100's	$40.45	Tolazamide, Goldline Labs	00182-1679-01
100's	$40.45	Tolazamide 500, Major Pharms	00904-0236-60
100's	$40.45	Tolazamide, Martec Pharms	52555-0293-01
100's	$42.40	Tolazamide, Rugby	00536-4744-01
100's	$43.25	Tolazamide, Schein Pharm (US)	00364-0722-01
100's	$43.34	Tolazamide, HL Moore Drug Exch	00839-7016-06
100's	$44.00	Tolazamide, Mutual Pharm	53489-0153-01
100's	$51.50	Tolazamide, Mylan	00378-0551-01
100's	$67.15	Tolazamide 500, Major Pharms	00904-0236-61
100's	$67.30	Tolazamide, Schein Pharm (US)	00364-0722-90
100's	**$113.92**	**TOLINASE, Pharmacia & Upjohn**	**00009-0477-06**
250's	$43.50	Tolazamide, H.C.F.A. F F P	99999-2358-11
500's	$87.00	Tolazamide, H.C.F.A. F F P	99999-2358-12
500's	$153.12	Tolazamide, Qualitest Pharms	00603-6098-28
500's	$190.00	Tolazamide, Mutual Pharm	53489-0153-05
1000'S	$87.00	Tolazamide, Zenith Labs	00172-2980-70
1000's	$111.65	Tolazamide 500, Major Pharms	00904-0236-40

TOLAZOLINE HYDROCHLORIDE *(002359)*

CATEGORIES: Alpha Receptor Blocking Agents; Cardiovascular Drugs; Hypertension; Vascular Disorders, Cerebral/Peripheral; Vasodilating Agents; Pregnancy Category C; FDA Approved 1985 Feb

BRAND NAMES: **Priscoline**

DESCRIPTION:

Tolazoline HCl, USP, is a peripheral vasodilator available in ampuls for intravenous administration. Each milliliter of sterile, aqueous solution contains tolazoline hydrochloride USP, 25 mg; tartaric acid ACS, 6.5 mg; and hydrous sodium citrate USP, 6.5 mg. Tolazoline hydrochloride is 4,5-dihydro-2-(phenylmethyl)-1*H*-imidazole monohydrochloride.

Tolazoline hydrochloride USP is a white to off-white crystalline powder. Its solutions are slightly acid to litmus. It is freely soluble in water and in alcohol. Its molecular weight is 196.68.

CLINICAL PHARMACOLOGY:

Tolazoline HCl is a direct peripheral vasodilator with moderate competitive alpha-adrenergic blocking activity. It decreases peripheral resistance and increases venous capacitance. It has the following additional actions: (1) sympathomimetic, including cardiac stimulation; (2) parasympathomimetic, including gastrointestinal tract stimulation that is blocked by atropine; and (3) histamine-like, including stimulation of gastric secretion and peripheral vasodilatation. Tolazoline HCl given intravenously produces vasodilatation, primarily due to a direct effect on vascular smooth muscle, and cardiac stimulation; the blood pressure response depends on the relative contributions of the two effects. Tolazoline HCl usually reduces pulmonary arterial pressure and vascular resistance.

In neonates the half-life of tolazoline HCl ranges from 3 to 10 hours.

INDICATIONS AND USAGE:

Tolazoline HCl is indicated for the treatment of persistent pulmonary hypertension of the newborn ("persistent fetal circulation") when systemic arterial oxygenation cannot be satisfactorily maintained by usual supportive care (supplemental oxygen and/or mechanical ventilation).

Tolazoline HCl should be used in a highly supervised setting, where vital signs, oxygenation, acid-base status, fluid, and electrolytes can be monitored and maintained.

CONTRAINDICATIONS:

Tolazoline HCl is contraindicated in patients with hypersensitivity to tolazoline.

WARNINGS:

Tolazoline HCl stimulates gastric secretion and may activate stress ulcers. Through this mechanism, it can produce significant hypochloremic alkalosis. Pretreatment of infants with antacids may prevent gastrointestinal bleeding.

Patients should be observed closely for signs of systemic hypotension, and supportive therapy should be instituted if needed.

In patients with mitral stenosis, parenterally administered tolazoline HCl may produce a rise or fall in pulmonary artery pressure and total pulmonary resistance; therefore it must be used with caution in patients with known or suspected mitral stenosis.

PRECAUTIONS:

General: The effects of tolazoline HCl on pulmonary vessels may be pH dependent. Acidosis may decrease the effect of tolazoline HCl.

Carcinogenesis, Mutagenesis, and Impairment of Fertility: Long-term carcinogenicity studies in animals have not been performed with tolazoline HCl.

Pregnancy Category C: Animal reproduction studies have not been conducted with tolazoline HCl. It is also not known whether tolazoline HCl can cause fetal harm when administered to a pregnant woman or can affect reproduction capacity. Tolazoline HCl should be given to a pregnant woman only if clearly needed.

Nursing Mothers: It is not known whether this drug is excreted in human milk. Because many drugs are excreted in human milk, caution should be exercised when tolazoline HCl is administered to a nursing woman.

ADVERSE REACTIONS:

The following adverse reactions have been observed, but there are insufficient data to support an estimate of their frequency:

Cardiovascular: Hypotension, tachycardia, cardiac arrhythmias, hypertension, pulmonary hemorrhage.

Digestive and Hepatic: Gastrointestinal hemorrhage, nausea, vomiting, diarrhea, hepatitis.

Skin: Flushing, increased pilomotor activity with tingling or chilliness, rash.

Hematologic: Thrombocytopenia, leukopenia.

Renal: Edema, oliguria, hematuria.

OVERDOSAGE:

Acute Toxicity: Oral LD_{50}'s (mg/kg): mice, 400; rats, 1200.

Signs and Symptoms: Signs and symptoms of overdosage may include increased pilomotor activity, peripheral vasodilatation, skin flushing, and, in rare instances, hypotension and shock.

Treatment: In treating hypotension, it is most important to place the patient's head low and administer intravenous fluids. Epinephrine should not be used, since large doses of tolazoline HCl may cause "epinephrine reversal" (further reduction in blood pressure, followed by an exaggerated rebound).

DOSAGE AND ADMINISTRATION:

An initial dose of 1 to 2 mg/kg, via scalp vein, followed by an infusion of 1 to 2 mg/kg per hour have usually resulted in significant increases in arterial oxygen. There is very little experience with infusions lasting beyond 36 to 48 hours. Response, if it occurs, can be expected within 30 minutes after the initial dose.

Note: Parenteral drug products should be inspected visually for particulate matter and discoloration prior to administration, whenever solution and container permit.

Store between 15 and 30°C (59-86°F). Protect from light.

HOW SUPPLIED - EQUIVALENTS NOT AVAILABLE:

Injection, Repository - Intramuscular; - 25 mg/ml

4 ml $47.89 PRISCOLINE, AMPULS 25, Novartis 00083-6733-04

TOLBUTAMIDE *(002360)*

CATEGORIES: Antidiabetic Agents; Blood Glucose Regulators; Central Nervous System Agents; Diabetes; Diagnostic Agents; Hormones; Hyperglycemia; Pancreatic Function; Sulfonylureas; Pregnancy Category C; FDA Approval Pre 1982

BRAND NAMES: *Abemin*; *Aglicem*; *Aglycid*; *Ansulin*; *Arcosal*; *Artosin*; *Diabecid-R*; *Diaben*; *Diatol*; *Dolipol*; *Fordex*; *Glucosulfa*; *Glyconon*; *Guabeta*; *Mobenol*; *Noglucor*; *Novobutamide*; *Orabet*; **Orinase**; Orinase Diagnostic; *Orsinon*; *Rastinon*; *Raston*; *Tolbusal*; *Tolbutamida Valdecases*; *Tolsiran*
(International brand names outside U.S. in italics)

FORMULARIES: Aetna; BC-BS; FHP; Medi-Cal; WHO

DESCRIPTION:

These tablets contain tolbutamide, an oral blood glucose lowering drug of the sulfonylurea category. Tolbutamide is a pure white crystalline compound practically insoluble in water but forming water-soluble salts with alkalies.

The chemical names for tolbutamide are: (1) Benzenesulfonamide,*N*-((butylamino)carbonyl)-4-methyl; (2) 1-Butyl-3-(*p*-tolylsulfonyl)urea and its molecular weight is 270.35.

Each Orinase tablet for oral administration contains 250 mg or 500 mg tolbutamide. Inactive ingredients: colloidal silicon dioxide, croscarmellose sodium, magnesium stearate, pregelatinized starch.

CLINICAL PHARMACOLOGY:

MECHANISM OF ACTION

Tolbutamide appears to lower blood glucose acutely by stimulating the release of insulin from the pancreas, an effect dependent upon functioning beta cells in the pancreatic islets. The mechanism by which tolbutamide lowers blood glucose during long-term administration has not been clearly established. With chronic administration in Type II diabetic patients, the blood glucose lowering effect persists despite a gradual decline in the insulin secretory response to the drug. Extrapancreatic effects may be involved in the mechanism of action of oral sulfonylurea hypoglycemic drugs.

Some patients who are initially responsive to oral hypoglycemic drugs, including tolbutamide tablets, may become unresponsive or poorly responsive over time. Alternatively, Tolbutamide may be effective in some patients who have become unresponsive to one or more other sulfonylurea drugs.

CLINICAL PHARMACOLOGY: *(cont'd)*

PHARMACOKINETICS

When administered orally, the tolbutamide in tolbutamide tablets is readily absorbed from the gastrointestinal tract. Absorption is not impaired and glucose lowering and insulin releasing effects are not altered if the drug is taken with food. Detectable levels are present in the plasma within twenty minutes after oral ingestion of a 500 mg Tolbutamide tablet, with peak levels occurring at three to four hours and only small amounts detectable at 24 hours. The half-life of tolbutamide is 4.5 to 6.5 hours. As tolbutamide has no p-amino group, it cannot be acetylated, which is one of the common modes of metabolic degradation for the antibacterial sulfonamides. However, the presence of the p-methyl group is oxidized to form a carboxyl group, converting tolbutamide into the totally inactive metabolite 1-butyl-3-p-carboxy-phenylsulfonylurea, which can be recovered in the urine within 24 hours in amounts accounting for up to 75% of the administered dose.

The major tolbutamide metabolite has been found to have no hypoglycemic or other action when administered orally and IV to both normal and diabetic subjects. This tolbutamide metabolite is highly soluble over the critical acid range of urinary pH values, and its solubility increases with increase in pH. Because of the marked solubility of the tolbutamide metabolite, crystalluria does not occur. A second metabolite, 1-butyl-3-(p-hydroxymethyl) phenyl sulfonylurea also occurs to a limited extent. It is an inactive metabolite.

The administration of 3 grams of tolbutamide to either nondiabetic or tolbutamide-responsive diabetic subjects will, in both instances, occasion a gradual lowering of blood glucose. Increasing the dose to 6 grams does not usually cause a response which is significantly different from that produced by the 3 g dose of Tolbutamide solution, nondiabetic fasting adults exhibit a 30% or greater reduction in blood glucose within one hour, following which the blood glucose gradually returns to the fasting level over six to twelve hours. Following the administration of a 3 g dose of Tolbutamide solution, tolbutamide responsive diabetic patients show a gradually progressive blood glucose lowering effect, the maximal response being reached between five to eight hours after ingestion of a single 3 g dose. The blood glucose then rises gradually and by the 24th hour has usually returned to pretest levels. The magnitude of the reduction, when expressed in terms of the percent of the pretest blood glucose, tends to be similar to the response seen in the nondiabetic subject.

INDICATIONS AND USAGE:

Tolbutamide tablets are indicated as an adjunct to diet to lower the blood glucose in patients with noninsulin-dependent diabetes whose hyperglycemia cannot be satisfactorily controlled by diet alone. In initiating treatment for noninsulin dependent diabetes, diet should be emphasized as the primary form of treatment. Caloric restriction and weight loss are essential in the obese diabetic patient. Proper dietary management alone may be effective in controlling the blood glucose and symptoms of hyperglycemia. The importance of regular physical activity should also be stressed and cardiovascular risk factors should be identified and corrective measures taken where possible.

If this treatment program fails to reduce symptoms and/or blood glucose, the use of an oral sulfonylurea or insulin should be considered. Use of Tolbutamide must be viewed by both the physician and patient as a treatment in addition to diet, and not as a substitute for diet or as a convenient mechanism for avoiding dietary restraint. Furthermore, loss of blood glucose control on diet alone may be transient, thus requiring only short-term administration of Tolbutamide.

During maintenance programs, Tolbutamide should be discontinued if satisfactory lowering of blood glucose is no longer achieved. Judgments should be based on regular clinical and laboratory evaluations.

In considering the use of Tolbutamide in asymptomatic patients, it should be recognized that controlling the blood glucose in noninsulin-dependent diabetes has not been definitely established to be effective in preventing the long-term cardiovascular or neural complications of diabetes.

CONTRAINDICATIONS:

Tolbutamide tablets are contraindicated in patients with: 1) known hypersensitivity or allergy to Tolbutamide; 2) diabetic ketoacidosis, with or without coma. This condition should be treated with insulin. 3) Type I diabetes, as sole therapy.

SPECIAL WARNING ON INCREASED RISK OF CARDIOVASCULAR MORTALITY

The administration of oral hypoglycemic drugs has been reported to be associated with increased cardiovascular mortality as compared to treatment with diet alone or diet plus insulin. This warning is based on the study conducted by the University Group Diabetes Program (UGDP), a long-term prospective clinical trial designed to evaluate the effectiveness of glucose-lowering drugs in preventing or delaying vascular complications in patients with noninsulin-dependent diabetes. The study involved 823 patients who were randomly assigned to one of four treatment groups (Diabetes, 19 (supp.2):747-830, 1970.)

UGDP reported that patients treated for five to eight years with diet plus a fixed dose of tolbutamide (1.5 grams per day) had a rate of cardiovascular mortality approximately 2 1/2 times that of patients with diet alone. A significant increase in total mortality was not observed, but the use of tolbutamide was discontinued based on the increase in cardiovascular mortality, thus limiting the opportunity for the study to show an increase in overall mortality. Despite controversy regarding the interpretation of these results, the findings of the UGDP study provide an adequate basis for this warning. The patient should be informed of the potential risks and advantages of tolbutamide tablets and of alternative modes of therapy.

Although only one drug in the sulfonylurea class (tolbutamide) was included in this study, it is prudent from a safety standpoint to consider that this warning may also apply to other oral hypoglycemic drugs in this class, in view of their close similarities in mode of action and chemical structure.

PRECAUTIONS:

GENERAL

Hypoglycemia: All sulfonylurea drugs are capable of producing severe hypoglycemia. Proper patient selection and dosage and instructions are important to avoid hypoglycemic episodes. Renal or hepatic insufficiency may cause elevated blood levels of tolbutamide and the latter may also diminish gluconeogenic capacity, both of which increase the risk of serious hypoglycemic reactions. Elderly, debilitated or malnourished patients and those with adrenal or pituitary insufficiency are particularly susceptible to the hypoglycemic action of glucose lowering drugs. Hypoglycemia may be difficult to recognize in the elderly and people who are taking beta-adrenergic blocking drugs. Hypoglycemia is more likely to occur when caloric intake is deficient, after severe or prolonged exercise, when alcohol is ingested, or when more than one glucose lowering drug is used.

Loss of Control of Blood Glucose: When a patient stabilized on any diabetic regimen is exposed to stress such as fever, trauma, infection, or surgery, loss of blood glucose control may occur. At such times it may be necessary to discontinue tolbutamide tablets and administer insulin.

The effectiveness of any hypoglycemic drug, including Tolbutamide, in lowering blood glucose to a desired level decreases in patients over a period of time, which may be due to progression of the severity of the diabetes or to diminished responsiveness to the drug. This phenomenon is known as secondary drug failure to distinguish it from primary failure in

PRECAUTIONS: *(cont'd)*

which the drug is ineffective in an individual patient when first given. Adequate adjustment of dose and adherence to diet should be assessed before classifying a patient as a secondary failure.

INFORMATION FOR THE PATIENT

Patients should be informed of the potential risks and advantages of Tolbutamide and of alternative modes of therapy. They should also be informed about the importance of adherence to dietary instructions, of a regular exercise program, and of regular testing of urine and/or blood glucose.

The risks of hypoglycemia, its symptoms and treatment, and conditions that predispose to its development should be explained to patients and responsible family members. Primary and secondary failure should also be explained.

LABORATORY TESTS

Blood and urine glucose should be monitored periodically. Measurement of glycosylated hemoglobin may be useful in some patients.

A metabolite of tolbutamide in urine may give a false positive reaction for albumin if measured by the acidification-after-boiling test, which causes the metabolite to precipitate. There is no interference with the sulfosalicylic acid test.

CARCINOGENESIS, AND MUTAGENICITY

Bioassay for carcinogenicity was performed in both sexes of rats and mice following ingestion of tolbutamide for 78 weeks. No evidence of carcinogenicity was found.

Tolbutamide has also been demonstrated to be nonmutagenic in the Ames salmonella/mammalian microsome mutagenicity test.

PREGNANCY CATEGORY C

Teratogenic Effects: Tolbutamide has been shown to be teratogenic in rats given doses 25 to 100 times the human dose. In some studies, pregnant rats given high doses of tolbutamide have shown increased mortality in offspring and ocular and bony abnormalities. Repeat studies in other species (rabbits) have not demonstrated a teratogenic effect. There are no adequate and well controlled studies in pregnant women. Tolbutamide is not recommended for the treatment of pregnant diabetic patients. Serious consideration should also be given to the possible hazards of the use of Tolbutamide in women of child-bearing age and in those who might become pregnant while using the drug.

Because recent information suggests that abnormal blood glucose levels during pregnancy are associated with a higher incidence of congenital abnormalities, many experts recommend that insulin be used during pregnancy to maintain blood glucose levels as close to normal as possible.

Nonteratogenic Effects: Prolonged severe hypoglycemia (four to ten days) has been reported in neonates born to mothers who were receiving a sulfonylurea drug at the time of delivery. This has been reported more frequently with the use of agents with prolonged half lives. If Tolbutamide is used during pregnancy, it should be discontinued at least two weeks before the expected delivery date.

NURSING MOTHERS

Although it is not known whether tolbutamide is excreted in human milk, some sulfonylurea drugs are known to be excreted in human milk. Because the potential for hypoglycemia in nursing infants may exist, a decision should be made whether to discontinue nursing or to discontinue the drug, taking into account the importance of the drug to the mother. If the drug is discontinued and if diet alone is inadequate for controlling blood glucose, insulin therapy should be considered.

PEDIATRIC USE

Safety and effectiveness in children have not been established.

DRUG INTERACTIONS:

The hypoglycemic action of sulfonylureas may be potentiated by certain drugs including nonsteroidal anti-inflammatory agents and other drugs that are highly protein bound, salicylates, sulfonamides, chloramphenicol, probenecid, coumarins, monoamine oxidase inhibitors, and beta adrenergic blocking agents. When such drugs are administered to a patient receiving Tolbutamide, the patient should be closely observed for hypoglycemia. When such drugs are withdrawn from a patient receiving Tolbutamide, the patient should be observed closely for loss of control.

Certain drugs tend to produce hyperglycemia and may lead to loss of control. These drugs include the thiazides and other diuretics, corticosteroids, phenothiazines, thyroid products, estrogens, oral contraceptives, phenytoin, nicotinic acid, sympathomimetics, calcium channel blocking drugs and isoniazid. When such drugs are administered to a patient receiving Tolbutamide, the patient should be closely observed for loss of control of blood glucose. When such drugs are withdrawn from a patient receiving Tolbutamide, the patient should be observed closely for hypoglycemia.

A potential interaction between oral miconazole and oral hypoglycemic agents leading to severe hypoglycemia has been reported. Whether this interaction also occurs with the intravenous, topical or vaginal preparations of miconazole is not known.

ADVERSE REACTIONS:

Hypoglycemia: See PRECAUTIONS and OVERDOSAGE.

Gastrointestinal Reactions: Cholestatic jaundice may occur rarely; tolbutamide tablets should be discontinued if this occurs. Gastrointestinal disturbances, e.g. nausea, epigastric fullness, and heartburn, are the most common reactions and occurred in 1.4% of patients treated during clinical trials. They tend to be dose-related and may disappear when dosage is reduced.

Dermatologic Reactions: Allergic skin reactions, e.g. pruritus, erythema, urticaria, and morbilliform or maculopapular eruptions, occurred in 1.1% of patients treated during clinical trials. These may be transient and may disappear despite continued use of Tolbutamide; if skin reactions persist, the drug should be discontinued.

Porphyria cutanea tarda and photosensitivity reactions have been reported with sulfonylureas.

Hematologic Reactions: Leukopenia, agranulocytosis, thrombocytopenia, hemolytic anemia, aplastic anemia, and pancytopenia have been reported with sulfonylureas.

Metabolic Reactions: Hepatic porphyria and disulfiram-like reactions have been reported with sulfonylureas.

Endocrine Reactions: Cases of hyponatremia and the syndrome of inappropriate antidiuretic hormone (SIADH) secretion have been reported with this and other sulfonylureas.

Miscellaneous Reactions: Headache and taste alterations have occasionally been reported with tolbutamide administration.

OVERDOSAGE:

Overdosage of sulfonylureas, including tolbutamide tablets, can produce symptoms of hypoglycemia.

Mild hypoglycemia symptoms without loss of consciousness or neurologic findings should be treated aggressively with oral glucose and adjustments in drug dosage and/or meal patterns. Close monitoring should continue until the physician is assured the patient is out of danger.

OVERDOSAGE: *(cont'd)*

Severe hypoglycemic reactions with coma, seizure, or other neurological impairment occur infrequently but constitute medical emergencies requiring immediate hospitalization. If hypoglycemic coma is suspected or diagnosed, the patient should be given a rapid intravenous injection of concentrated (50%) glucose solution. This should be followed by a continuous infusion of a more dilute (10%) glucose solution at a rate which will maintain the blood glucose level above 100 mg/dl. Patients should be closely monitored for a minimum of 24 to 48 hours, since hypoglycemia may recur after apparent clinical recovery.

DOSAGE AND ADMINISTRATION:

There is no fixed dosage regimen for the management of diabetes mellitus with tolbutamide tablets or any other hypoglycemic agent. In addition to the usual monitoring of urinary glucose, the patient's blood glucose must also be monitored periodically to determine the minimum effective dose for the patient; to detect primary failure, i.e. inadequate lowering of blood glucose at the maximum recommended dose of medication; and to detect secondary failure, i.e. loss of adequate blood glucose response after an initial period of effectiveness. Glycosylated hemoglobin levels may also be of value in monitoring the patient's response to therapy.

Short-term administration of Tolbutamide may be sufficient during periods of transient loss of control in patients usually controlled well on diet.

USUAL STARTING DOSE

The usual starting dose is 1 to 2 grams daily. This may be increased or decreased depending on individual patient response. Failure to follow an appropriate dosage regimen may precipitate hypoglycemia. Patients who do not adhere to their prescribed dietary regimens are more prone to exhibit unsatisfactory response to drug therapy.

Transfer From Other Hypoglycemic Therapy Patients Receiving Other Antidiabetic Therapy: Transfer of patients from other oral antidiabetes regimens to Tolbutamide should be done conservatively. When transferring patients from oral hypoglycemic agents other than chlorpropamide to Tolbutamide, no transition period and no initial or priming doses are necessary. When transferring patients from chlorpropamide, however, particular care should be exercised during the first two weeks because of the prolonged retention of chlorpropamide in the body and the possibility that subsequent overlapping drug effects might provoke hypoglycemia.

Patients Receiving Insulin: Patients requiring 20 units or less of insulin daily may be placed directly on Tolbutamide and insulin abruptly discontinued. Patients whose insulin requirement is between 20 and 40 units daily may be started on therapy with Tolbutamide with a concurrent 30 to 50% reduction in insulin dose, with further daily reduction of the insulin when response to tolbutamide is observed. In patients requiring more than 40 units of insulin daily, therapy with Tolbutamide may be initiated in conjunction with a 20% reduction in insulin dose the first day, with further careful reduction of insulin as response is observed. Occasionally, conversion to Tolbutamide in the hospital may be advisable in candidates who require more than 40 units of insulin daily. During this conversion period when both insulin and Tolbutamide are being used, hypoglycemia may rarely occur. During insulin withdrawal, patients should test their urine for glucose and acetone at least three times daily and report results to their physician. The appearance of persistent acetonuria with glycosuria indicates that the patient is a Type I diabetic patient who requires insulin therapy.

MAXIMUM DOSE

Daily doses of greater than 3 grams are not recommended.

USUAL MAINTENANCE DOSE

The maintenance dose is in the range of 0.25-3 grams daily. Maintenance doses above 2 grams are seldom required.

DOSAGE INTERVAL

The total daily dose may be taken either in the morning or in divided doses through the day. While either schedule is usually effective, the divided dose system is preferred by some clinicians from the standpoint of digestive tolerance.

In elderly, debilitated or malnourished patients and patients with impaired renal or hepatic function, the initial and maintenance dosing should be conservative to avoid hypoglycemic reactions (see PRECAUTIONS.)

Store at controlled room temperature 15-30° C (59-86° F).

HOW SUPPLIED - RATED THERAPEUTICALLY EQUIVALENT:

Tablet, Uncoated - Oral - 250 mg

100's	$12.00	Tolbutamide, UDL	51079-0560-20

Tablet, Uncoated - Oral - 500 mg

100's	$2.95	Tolbutamide, Raway	00686-2245-10
100's	$4.58	Tolbutamide, H.C.F.A. F F P	99999-2360-01
100's	$5.25	Tolbutamide, Harber Pharm	51432-0462-03
100's	$6.00	Tolbutamide, Eon Labs Mfg	00185-0535-01
100's	$6.30	Tolbutamide 500, Major Pharms	00904-0223-60
100's	$6.65	Tolbutamide, Zenith Labs	00172-2245-60
100's	$6.65	Tolbutamide, Goldline Labs	00182-1084-01
100's	$7.90	Tolbutamide, United Res	00677-0592-01
100's	$7.95	Tolbutamide, HL Moore Drug Exch	00839-6253-06
100's	$9.25	Tolbutamide, Raway	00686-4062-13
100's	$9.77	Tolbutamide 500, Major Pharms	00904-0223-61
100's	$10.00	Tolbutamide, Voluntary Hosp	53258-0162-01
100's	$10.98	Tolbutamide, Qualitest Pharms	00603-6121-21
100's	$11.06	Tolbutamide, Schein Pharm (US)	00364-0477-01
100's	$11.65	Tolbutamide, Vangard Labs	00615-1514-13
100's	$12.17	Tolbutamide, Aligen Independ	00405-5031-01
100's	$12.20	Tolbutamide, Goldline Labs	00182-1084-89
100's	$12.40	Tolbutamide, Mylan	00378-0215-01
100's	$12.40	Tolbutamide, Rugby	00536-4668-01
100's	$15.00	Tolbutamide, Voluntary Hosp	53258-0162-13
100's	**$27.20**	**ORINASE, Pharmacia & Upjohn**	**00009-0100-11**
200's	$9.16	Tolbutamide, H.C.F.A. F F P	99999-2360-03
200's	**$53.77**	**ORINASE, Pharmacia & Upjohn**	**00009-0100-02**
500's	$12.40	Tolbutamide, Raway	00686-2245-12
500's	$14.95	Tolbutamide, H & H Labs	46703-0087-05
500's	$22.67	Tolbutamide, HL Moore Drug Exch	00839-6253-12
500's	$22.90	Tolbutamide, H.C.F.A. F F P	99999-2360-04
500's	$25.90	Tolbutamide, United Res	00677-0592-05
500's	$26.50	Tolbutamide, Zenith Labs	00172-2245-70
500's	$26.50	Tolbutamide, Goldline Labs	00182-1084-05
500's	$33.75	Tolbutamide, Rugby	00536-4668-05
500's	$54.40	Tolbutamide, Mylan	00378-0215-05
1000's	$45.00	Tolbutamide, Eon Labs Mfg	00185-0535-10
1000's	$45.80	Tolbutamide, H.C.F.A. F F P	99999-2360-02
1000's	$51.90	Tolbutamide, Zenith Labs	00172-2245-80
1000's	$53.12	Tolbutamide, Qualitest Pharms	00603-6121-32
1000's	$55.95	Tolbutamide 500, Major Pharms	00904-0223-80
1000's	$60.00	Tolbutamide, Schein Pharm (US)	00364-0477-02
1000's	$65.47	Tolbutamide, HL Moore Drug Exch	00839-6253-16
1000's	$65.85	Tolbutamide, Rugby	00536-4668-10

HOW SUPPLIED - RATED THERAPEUTICALLY EQUIVALENT:
(cont'd)

1000's	$72.28	Tolbutamide, Amer Preferred	53445-1084-00
1000's	$81.96	Tolbutamide Tablets 500 Mg, Aligen Independ	00405-5031-03

HOW SUPPLIED - NOT RATED EQUIVALENT:
Injection, Lyphl-Soln - Intravenous - 1 gm/vial

20 ml	**$54.92**	**Orinase Diagnostic, Pharmacia & Upjohn**	**00009-0741-01**

TOLMETIN SODIUM *(002361)*

CATEGORIES: Analgesics; Anti-Inflammatory Agents; Antiarthritics; Antipyretics; Arthritis; Central Nervous System Agents; NSAIDS; Nonsteroidal Anti-Inflammatory; Osteoarthritis; Pain; Pregnancy Category C; FDA Approval Pre 1982; Patent Expiration 1990 Aug

BRAND NAMES: *Donison*; *Midocil*; *Reutol*; *Safitex*; **Tolectin**
(International brand names outside U.S. in italics)

FORMULARIES: Aetna; BC-BS; CIGNA; FHP; Foundation; Humana; Kaiser; Medco; Medi-Cal; PruCare; United

COST OF THERAPY: $287.43 (Arthritis; Capsule; 400 mg; 3/day; 365 days)

PRIMARY ICD9: 715.99 (Osteoarthritis, Unspecified, Multiple Sites)

DESCRIPTION:

Tolmetin Sodium 200 mg tablets for oral administration contain tolmetin sodium as the dihydrate in an amount equivalent to 200 mg of tolmetin (scored for 100 mg). Each tablet contains 18 mg (0.784 mEq) of sodium and the following inactive ingredients: cellulose, magnesium stearate, silicon dioxide, corn starch and talc.

Tolmetin Sodium capsules for oral administration contain tolmetin sodium as the dihydrate in an amount equivalent to 400 mg of tolmetin. Each capsule contains 36 mg (1.568 mEq) of sodium and the following inactive ingredients: gelatin, magnesium stearate, corn starch, talc, FD&C Red No. 3, FD&C Yellow No. 6 and titanium dioxide.

Tolmetin Sodium 600 mg tablets for oral administration contain tolmetin sodium as the dihydrate in an amount equivalent to 600 mg of tolmetin. Each tablet contains 54 mg (2.35 mEq) of sodium and the following inactive ingredients: cellulose, silicon dioxide, crospovidone, hydroxypropyl methyl cellulose, magnesium stearate, polyethylene glycol, corn starch, titanium dioxide, FD&C Yellow No. 6 and D&C Yellow No. 10.

The pKa of tolmetin is 3.5 and tolmetin sodium is freely soluble in water.

Tolmetin sodium is a nonsteroidal anti-inflammatory agent.

CLINICAL PHARMACOLOGY:

Studies in animals have shown tolmetin sodium to posses anti- inflammatory, analgesic, and antipyretic activity. In the rat, tolmetin sodium prevents the development of experimentally induced polyarthritis and also decreases established inflammation.

The mode of action of tolmetin sodium is not known. However, studies in laboratory animals and man have demonstrated that the anti-inflammatory action of tolmetin sodium is *not* due to pituitary-adrenal stimulation. Tolmetin Sodium inhibits prostaglandin synthetase *in vitro* and lowers the plasma level of prostaglandin E in man. This reduction in prostaglandin synthesis may be responsible for the anti- inflammatory action. Tolmetin Sodium does not appear to alter the course of the underlying disease in man.

In patients with rheumatoid arthritis and in normal volunteers, tolmetin sodium is rapidly and almost completely absorbed with peak plasma levels being reached within 30-60 minutes after an oral therapeutic dose. In controlled studies, the time to reach peak tolmetin plasma concentration is approximately 20 minutes longer following administration of a 600 mg tablet, compared to an equivalent dose given as 200 mg tablets. The clinical meaningfulness of this finding, if any, is unknown. Tolmetin displays a biphasic elimination from the plasma consisting of a rapid phase with a half-life of one to 2 hours followed by a slower phase with a half-life of about 5 hours. Peak plasma levels of approximately 40 mcg/ml are obtained with a 400 mg oral dose. Essentially all of the administered dose is recovered in the urine in 24 hours either as an inactive oxidative metabolite or as conjugates of tolmetin. An 18-day multiple dose study demonstrated no accumulation of tolmetin when compared with a single dose.

In two fecal blood loss studies of 4 to 6 days duration involving 15 subjects each, tolmetin sodium did not induce an increase in blood loss over that observed during a 4-day drug-free control period. In the same studies, aspirin produced a greater blood loss than occurred during the drug-free control period, and a greater blood loss than occurred during the tolmetin sodium treatment period. In one of the two studies, indomethacin produced a greater fecal blood loss than occurred during the drug-free control period; in the second study, indomethacin did not induce a significant increase in blood loss.

Tolmetin Sodium is effective in treating both the acute flares and in the long-term management of the symptoms of rheumatoid arthritis, osteoarthritis and juvenile rheumatoid arthritis.

In patients with either rheumatoid arthritis or osteoarthritis, tolmetin sodium is as effective as aspirin and indomethacin in controlling disease activity, but the frequency of the milder gastrointestinal adverse effects and tinnitus was less than in aspirin-treated patients, and the incidence of central nervous system adverse effects was less than in indomethacin-treated patients.

In patients with juvenile rheumatoid arthritis, tolmetin sodium is as effective as aspirin in controlling disease activity, with a similar incidence of adverse reactions. Mean SGOT values, initially elevated in patients on previous aspirin therapy, remained elevated in the aspirin group and decreased in the tolmetin sodium group.

Tolmetin Sodium has produced additional therapeutic benefit when added to a regimen of gold salts and, to a lesser extent, with corticosteroids. Tolmetin Sodium should not be used in conjunction with salicylates since greater benefit from the combination is not likely, but the potential for adverse reactions is increased.

INDICATIONS AND USAGE:

Tolmetin Sodium is indicated for the relief of signs and symptoms of rheumatoid arthritis and osteoarthritis. Tolmetin Sodium is indicated in the treatment of acute flares and the long-term management of the chronic disease.

Tolmetin Sodium is also indicated for treatment of juvenile rheumatoid arthritis. The safety and effectiveness of tolmetin sodium have not been established in children under 2 years of age see PRECAUTIONS, Pediatric Use and DOSAGE AND ADMINISTRATION.

CONTRAINDICATIONS:

Anaphylactoid reactions have been reported with tolmetin sodium as with other nonsteroidal anti-inflammatory drugs. Because of the possibility of cross-sensitivity to other nonsteroidal anti-inflammatory drugs, particularly zomepirac sodium, anaphylactoid reactions may be more likely to occur in patients who have exhibited allergic reactions to these compounds. For this reason, tolmetin sodium should not be given to patients in whom aspirin and other nonsteroidal anti-inflammatory drugs induce symptoms of asthma, rhinitis, urticaria or other symptoms of allergic or anaphylactoid reactions. Patients experiencing anaphylactoid reactions on tolmetin sodium should be treated with conventional therapy, such as epinephrine, antihistamines and/or steroids.

WARNINGS:

RISK OF GI ULCERATION, BLEEDING AND PERFORATION WITH NSAID THERAPY

Serious gastrointestinal toxicity such as bleeding, ulceration, and perforation, can occur at any time, with or without warning symptoms, in patients treated chronically with NSAID (Nonsteroidal Anti-Inflammatory Drug) therapy. Although minor upper gastrointestinal problems, such as dyspepsia, are common, usually developing early in therapy, physicians should remain alert for ulceration and bleeding in patients treated chronically with NSAID's even in the absence of previous GI tract symptoms. In patients observed in clinical trials of several months to two years duration, symptomatic upper GI ulcers, gross bleeding or perforation appear to occur in approximately 1% of patients treated for 3-6 months, and in about 2-4% of patients treated for one year. Physicians should inform patients about the signs and/or symptoms of serious GI toxicity and what steps to take if they occur.

Studies to date have not identified any subset of patients not at risk of developing peptic ulceration and bleeding. Except for a prior history of serious GI events and other risk factors known to be associated with peptic ulcer disease, such as alcoholism, smoking, etc., no risk factors (*e.g.*, age, sex) have been associated with increased risk. Elderly or debilitated patients seem to tolerate ulceration or bleeding less well than other individuals and most spontaneous reports of fatal GI events are in this population. Studies to date are inconclusive concerning the relative risk of various NSAID's in causing such reactions. High doses of any NSAID probably carry a greater risk of these reactions, although controlled clinical trials showing this do not exist in most cases. In considering the use of relatively large doses (within the recommended dosage range), sufficient benefit should be anticipated to offset the potential increased risk of GI toxicity.

PRECAUTIONS:

GENERAL

Because of ocular changes observed in animals and of reports of adverse eye findings with nonsteroidal anti-inflammatory agents, it is recommended that patients who develop visual disturbances during treatment with tolmetin sodium have ophthalmologic evaluations.

As with other nonsteroidal anti-inflammatory drugs, long-term administration of tolmetin to animals has resulted in renal papillary necrosis and other abnormal renal pathology. In humans, there have been reports of acute interstitial nephritis with hematuria, proteinuria, and occasionally nephrotic syndrome.

A second form of renal toxicity has been seen in patients with prerenal conditions leading to a reduction in renal blood flow or blood volume, where the renal prostaglandins have a supportive role in the maintenance of renal perfusion. In these patients administration of an NSAID may cause a dose dependent reduction in prostaglandin formation and may precipitate overt renal decompensation. Patients at greatest risk of this reaction are those with heart failure, liver dysfunction, those taking diuretics, and the elderly. Discontinuation of NSAID therapy is typically followed by recovery to the pretreatment state.

Since tolmetin sodium and its metabolites are eliminated primarily by the kidneys, patients with impaired renal function should be closely monitored, and it should be anticipated that they will require lower doses.

Tolmetin Sodium prolongs bleeding time. Patients who may be adversely affected by prolongation of bleeding time should be carefully observed when tolmetin sodium is administered.

In patients receiving concomitant tolmetin sodium-steroid therapy, any reduction in steroid dosage should be gradual to avoid the possible complications of sudden steroid withdrawal.

Peripheral edema has been reported in some patients receiving tolmetin sodium therapy. Therefore, as with other nonsteroidal anti-inflammatory drugs, tolmetin sodium should be used with caution in patients with compromised cardiac function, hypertension, or other conditions predisposing to fluid retention.

The antipyretic and anti-inflammatory activities of the drug may reduce fever and inflammation, thus diminishing their utility as diagnostic signs in detecting complications of presumed noninfectious, non- inflammatory painful conditions.

As with other nonsteroidal anti-inflammatory drugs, borderline elevations of one or more liver tests may occur in up to 15% of patients. These abnormalities may progress, may remain essentially unchanged, or may be transient with continued therapy. The SGPT (ALT) test is probably the most sensitive indicator of liver dysfunction. Meaningful (3 times the upper limit of normal) elevations of SGPT or SGOT (AST) occurred in controlled clinical trials in less than 1% of patients. A patient with symptoms and/or signs suggesting liver dysfunction, or in whom an abnormal liver test has occurred, should be evaluated for evidence of the development of more severe hepatic reaction while on therapy with tolmetin sodium. Severe hepatic reactions, including jaundice and fatal hepatitis, have been reported with tolmetin sodium as with other nonsteroidal anti-inflammatory drugs. Although such reactions are rare, if abnormal liver tests persist or worsen, if clinical signs and symptoms consistent with liver disease develop, or if systemic manifestations occur (*e.g.*, eosinophilia, rash, etc.), tolmetin sodium should be discontinued.

CARCINOGENESIS, MUTAGENESIS, AND IMPAIRMENT OF FERTILITY

Tolmetin sodium did not possess any carcinogenic liability in the following long- term studies: a 24-month study in rats at doses as high as 75 mg/kg/day, and an 18-month study in mice at doses as high as 50 mg/kg/day.

No mutagenic potential of tolmetin sodium was found in the Ames Salmonella-Microsomal Activation Test.

Reproductive studies revealed no impairment of fertility in animals. Effects on parturition have been shown, however, as with other prostaglandin inhibitors. This information is detailed in the Pregnancy section below.

PREGNANCY CATEGORY C

Reproduction studies in rats and rabbits at doses up to 50 mg/kg (1.5 times the maximum clinical dose based on a body weight of 60 kg) revealed no evidence of teratogenesis or impaired fertility due to tolmetin sodium. However, tolmetin sodium is an inhibitor of prostaglandin synthetase. Drugs in this class have known effects on the fetal cardiovascular system which may cause constriction of the ductus arteriosus *in utero* during the third trimester of pregnancy, which may result in persistent pulmonary hypertension of the newborn.

PRECAUTIONS: *(cont'd)*

There are no adequate and well-controlled studies in pregnant women. Tolmetin Sodium should be used during pregnancy only if the potential benefit justifies the potential risk to the fetus.

Non-Teratogenic Effects: Prostaglandin inhibitors have also been shown to increase the incidence of dystocia and delayed parturition in animals.

NURSING MOTHERS

Tolmetin Sodium has been shown to be secreted in human milk. Because of the possible adverse effects of prostaglandin inhibiting drugs on neonates, use in nursing mothers should be avoided.

PEDIATRIC USE

The safety and effectiveness of tolmetin sodium for children under 2 years of age have not been established.

LABORATORY TESTS

Because serious GI tract ulceration and bleeding can occur without warning symptoms, physicians should follow chronically treated patients for the signs and symptoms of ulceration and bleeding and should inform them of the importance of this follow-up see WARNINGS, Risk of GI Ulceration, Bleeding and Perforation with NSAID Therapy.

DRUG/LABORATORY TEST INTERACTION

The metabolites of tolmetin sodium in urine have been found to give positive tests for proteinuria using tests which rely on acid precipitation as their endpoint (*e.g.,* sulfosalicylic acid). No interference is seen in the tests for proteinuria using dye-impregnated commercially available reagent strips (*e.g.* Albustix, Uristix, etc.).

INFORMATION FOR THE PATIENT

Tolmetin Sodium, like other drugs of its class, is not free of side effects. The side effects of these drugs can cause discomfort and, rarely, there are more serious side effects, such as gastrointestinal bleeding, which may result in hospitalization and even fatal outcomes.

NSAID's (Nonsteroidal Anti-Inflammatory Drugs) are often essential agents in the management of arthritis, but they also may be commonly employed for conditions which are less serious. Physicians may wish to discuss with their patients the potential risks (see WARNINGS, PRECAUTIONS, and ADVERSE REACTIONS) and likely benefits of NSAID treatment, particularly when the drugs are used for less serious conditions where treatment without NSAID's may represent an acceptable alternative to both the patient and physician.

DRUG INTERACTIONS:

The *in vitro* binding of warfarin to human plasma proteins is unaffected by tolmetin, and tolmetin does not alter the prothrombin time of normal volunteers. However, increased prothrombin time and bleeding have been reported in patients on concomitant tolmetin sodium and warfarin therapy. Therefore, caution should be exercised when administering tolmetin sodium to patients on anticoagulants.

In adult diabetic patients under treatment with either sulfonylureas or insulin there is no change in the clinical effects of either tolmetin sodium or the hypoglycemic agents.

Caution should be used if tolmetin sodium is administered concomitantly with methotrexate. Tolmetin sodium and other nonsteroidal anti- inflammatory drugs have been reported to reduce the tubular secretion of methotrexate in an animal model, possibly enhancing the toxicity of methotrexate.

Drug - Food Interaction: In a controlled single dose study, administration of tolmetin sodium with milk had no effect on peak plasma tolmetin concentrations, but decreased total tolmetin bioavailability by 16%. When tolmetin sodium was taken immediately after a meal, peak plasma tolmetin concentrations were reduced by 50% while total bioavailability was again decreased by 16%.

ADVERSE REACTIONS:

The adverse reactions which have been observed in clinical trials encompass observations in about 4370 patients treated with tolmetin sodium, over 800 of whom have undergone at least one year of therapy. These adverse reactions, reported below by body system, are among those typical of nonsteroidal anti-inflammatory drugs and, as expected, gastrointestinal complaints were most frequent. In clinical trials with tolmetin sodium, about 10% of patients dropped out because of adverse reactions, mostly gastrointestinal in nature.

Incidence Greater Than 1%: The following adverse reactions which occurred more frequently than 1 in 100 were reported in controlled clinical trials.

Gastrointestinal: Nausea (11%), dyspepsia,* gastrointestinal distress,* abdominal pain,* diarrhea,* flatulence,* vomiting,* constipation, gastritis, and peptic ulcer. Forty percent of the ulcer patients had a prior history of peptic ulcer disease and/or were receiving concomitant anti-inflammatory drugs including corticosteroids, which are known to produce peptic ulceration.

Body as a Whole: Headache,* asthenia,* chest pain

Cardiovascular: Elevated blood pressure,* edema*

Central Nervous System: Dizziness,* drowsiness, depression

Metabolic/Nutritional: Weight gain,* weight loss*

Dermatologic: Skin irritation

Special Senses: Tinnitus, visual disturbance

Hematologic: Small and transient decreases in hemoglobin and hematocrit not associated with gastrointestinal bleeding have occurred. These are similar to changes reported with other nonsteroidal anti- inflammatory drugs.

Urogenital: Elevated BUN, urinary tract infection

*Reactions occurring in 3% to 9% of patients treated with tolmetin sodium. Reactions occurring in fewer than 3% of the patients are unmarked.

Incidence Less Than 1%: (Causal Relationship Probable) The following adverse reactions were reported less frequently than 1 in 100 in controlled clinical trials or were reported since marketing. The probability exists that there is a causal relationship between tolmetin sodium and these adverse reactions.

Gastrointestinal: Gastrointestinal bleeding with or without evidence of peptic ulcer, perforation, glossitis, stomatitis, hepatitis, liver function abnormalities

Body as a Whole: Anaphylactoid reactions, fever, lymphadenopathy, serum sickness

Hematologic: Hemolytic anemia, thrombocytopenia, granulocytopenia, agranulocytosis

Cardiovascular: Congestive heart failure in patients with marginal cardiac function

Dermatologic: Urticaria, purpura, erythema multiforme, toxic epidermal necrolysis

Urogenital: Hematuria, proteinuria, dysuria, renal failure

Incidence Less Than 1%: (Causal Relationship Unknown) Other adverse reactions were reported less frequently than 1 in 100 in controlled clinical trials or were reported since marketing, but a causal relationship between tolmetin sodium and the reaction could not be determined. These rarely reported reactions are being listed as alerting information for the physician since the possibility of a causal relationship cannot be excluded.

Body as a Whole: Epistaxis

ADVERSE REACTIONS: *(cont'd)*

Special Senses: Optic neuropathy, retinal and macular changes

OVERDOSAGE:

In the event of overdosage, the stomach should be emptied by inducing vomiting or by gastric lavage followed by the administration of activated charcoal.

DOSAGE AND ADMINISTRATION:

In adults with rheumatoid arthritis or osteoarthritis, the recommended starting dose is 400 mg three times daily (1200 mg daily), preferably including a dose on arising and a dose at bedtime. To achieve optimal therapeutic effect the dose should be adjusted according to the patient's response after one to two weeks. Control is usually achieved at doses of 600-1800 mg daily in divided doses (generally t.i.d.). Doses larger than 1800 mg/day have not been studied and are not recommended.

The recommended starting dose for children (2 years and older) is 20 mg/kg/day in divided doses (t.i.d. or q.i.d.). When control has been achieved, the usual dose ranges from 15 to 30 mg/kg/day. Doses higher than 30 mg/kg/day have not been studied and, therefore, are not recommended.

A therapeutic response to tolmetin sodium can be expected in a few days to a week. Progressive improvement can be anticipated during succeeding weeks of therapy. If gastrointestinal symptoms occur, tolmetin sodium can be administered with antacids other than sodium bicarbonate. Tolmetin Sodium bioavailability and pharmacokinetics are not significantly affected by acute or chronic administration of magnesium and aluminum hydroxides; however, bioavailability is affected by food or milk (see DRUG INTERACTIONS, Drug-Food Interactions.)

Store at controlled room temperature (15-30°C, 59-86°F). Protect from light.

HOW SUPPLIED - RATED THERAPEUTICALLY EQUIVALENT:

Capsule, Gelatin - Oral - 400 mg

30's	$7.87	Tolmetin Sodium, H.C.F.A. F F P	99999-2361-01
100's	$26.25	Tolmetin Sodium, United Res	00677-1424-01
100's	$26.25	Tolmetin Sodium, H.C.F.A. F F P	99999-2361-02
100's	$68.95	Tolmetin Sodium, H N Norton Co.	50732-0900-01
100's	$72.87	Tolmetin Sodium, Mutual Pharm	53489-0507-01
100's	$74.50	Tolmetin Sodium, Geneva Pharms	00781-2182-01
100's	$75.50	Tolmetin Sodium, Goldline Labs	00182-1931-01
100's	$77.61	Tolmetin Sodium, Purepac Pharm	00228-2520-10
100's	$78.45	Tolmetin Sodium, Major Pharms	00904-7653-60
100's	$78.95	Tolmetin Sodium, Harber Pharm	51432-0657-03
100's	$79.90	Tolmetin Sodium, Parmed Pharms	00349-8963-01
100's	$80.00	Tolmetin Sodium, Aligen Independ	00405-5035-01
100's	$80.00	Tolmetin Sodium, Qualitest Pharms	00603-6130-21
100's	$80.00	Tolmetin Sodium, Novopharm (US)	55953-0815-40
100's	$80.99	Tolmetin Sodium, HL Moore Drug Exch	00839-7671-06
100's	$81.30	Tolmetin Sodium, Teva	00093-0213-01
100's	$81.46	Tolmetin Sodium, Schein Pharm (US)	00364-2507-01
100's	$85.04	Tolmetin Sodium, Rugby	00536-5509-01
100's	$85.95	Tolmetin Sodium, Mylan	00378-5200-01
100's	$89.50	Tolmetin Sodium, Goldline Labs	00182-1931-89
100's	$92.19	Tolmetin Sodium, Vangard Labs	00615-0351-13
100's	**$101.63**	**TOLECTIN DS, McNeil Lab**	**00045-0414-60**
100's	**$106.21**	**TOLECTIN DS, McNeil Lab**	**00045-0414-10**
500's	$131.25	Tolmetin Sodium, United Res	00677-1424-05
500's	$131.25	Tolmetin Sodium, Mutual Pharm	53489-0507-05
500's	$131.25	Tolmetin Sodium, H.C.F.A. F F P	99999-2361-03
500's	$327.51	Tolmetin Sodium, H N Norton Co.	50732-0900-05
500's	$337.50	Tolmetin Sodium, Goldline Labs	00182-1931-05
500's	$373.58	Tolmetin Sodium, Purepac Pharm	00228-2520-50
500's	$380.00	Tolmetin Sodium, Aligen Independ	00405-5035-02
500's	$380.00	Tolmetin Sodium, Novopharm (US)	55953-0815-70
500's	$383.45	Tolmetin Sodium, Major Pharms	00904-7653-40
500's	$385.25	Tolmetin Sodium, Teva	00093-0213-05
500's	$388.13	Tolmetin Sodium, HL Moore Drug Exch	00839-7671-12
500's	**$491.05**	**TOLECTIN DS, McNeil Lab**	**00045-0414-70**
1000's	$262.50	Tolmetin Sodium, H.C.F.A. F F P	99999-2361-04
1000's	$722.00	Tolmetin Sodium, Novopharm (US)	55953-0815-80

Tablet - Oral - 200 mg

100's	$49.75	Tolmetin Sodium, Duramed Pharms	51285-0846-02

Tablet - Oral - 400 mg

100's	$75.50	Tolmetin Sodium, Duramed Pharms	51285-0847-02
500's	$358.65	Tolmetin Sodium, Duramed Pharms	51285-0847-04

Tablet - Oral - 600 mg

100's	$96.50	Tolmetin Sodium, Duramed Pharms	51285-0848-02

Tablet, Uncoated - Oral - 200 mg

100's	$46.09	Tolmetin Sodium, Mutual Pharm	53489-0506-01
100's	$51.00	Tolmetin Sodium, United Res	00677-1425-01
100's	$52.37	Tolmetin Sodium, Aligen Independ	00405-5033-01
100's	$60.74	Tolmetin Sodium, HL Moore Drug Exch	00839-7729-06
100's	**$64.06**	**TOLECTIN 200, McNeil Lab**	**00045-0412-60**

Tablet, Uncoated - Oral - 600 mg

100's	$85.92	Tolmetin Sodium, Aligen Independ	00405-5034-01
100's	$88.13	Tolmetin Sodium, United Res	00677-1447-01
100's	$88.13	Tolmetin Sodium, Geneva Pharms	00781-1428-01
100's	$88.13	Tolmetin Sodium, H.C.F.A. F F P	99999-2361-05
100's	$89.50	Tolemtin Sodium, Harber Pharm	51432-0794-03
100's	$94.30	Tolmetin Sodium, Purepac Pharm	00228-2480-10
100's	$95.00	Tolmetin Sodium, Goldline Labs	00182-1932-01
100's	$95.00	Tolmetin Sodium, Novopharm (US)	55953-0817-40
100's	$95.03	Tolmetin Sodium, HL Moore Drug Exch	00839-7690-06
100's	$95.06	Tolmetin Sodium, Qualitest Pharms	00603-6131-21
100's	$95.25	Tolmetin Sodium, Major Pharms	00904-7694-60
100's	$98.78	Tolmetim Sodium, Schein Pharm (US)	00364-2523-01
100's	$99.00	Tolmetin Sodium, Parmed Pharms	00349-8964-01
100's	$105.95	Tolmetin Sodium, Mylan	00378-0313-01
100's	$105.95	Tolmetin Sodium, Rugby	00536-4681-01
100's	$110.00	Tolmetin Sodium, Vangard Labs	00615-3564-13
100's	$120.00	Tolmetin Sodium, Goldline Labs	00182-1932-89
100's	**$123.32**	**TOLECTIN 600, McNeil Lab**	**00045-0416-60**
500's	$412.41	Tolmetin Sodium, Aligen Independ	00405-5034-02
500's	$440.65	Tolmetin Sodium, H.C.F.A. F F P	99999-2361-06
500's	$451.37	Tometin Sodium, HL Moore Drug Exch	00839-7690-12
500's	$497.51	Tolmetin Sodium, Purepac Pharm	00228-2480-50
500's	**$595.97**	**TOLECTIN 600, McNeil Lab**	**00045-0416-70**

TOPIRAMATE *(003312)*

CATEGORIES: Anticonvulsants; Antiepileptics; Carbonic Anhydrase Inhibitors; Central Nervous System Agents; Convulsions; Epilepsy; Epilepticus; FDA Approved 1996 Dec; Pregnancy Category C; Seizures; Tonic-Clonic Seizures

BRAND NAMES: **Topamax**

PRIMARY ICD9: 345.90 (Epilepsy, Unspecified, Without Mention of Intractable)

DESCRIPTION:

Topiramate is a sulfamate-substituted monosaccharide that is intended for use as an antiepileptic drug. Topamax is available as 25 mg, 100 mg, and 200 mg round tablets for oral administration.

Topiramate is a white crystalline powder with a bitter taste. Topiramate is most soluble in alkaline solutions containing sodium hydroxide or sodium phosphate and having a pH of 9 to 10. It is freely soluble in acetone, chloroform, dimethylsulfoxide, and ethanol. The solubility in water is 9.8 mg/ml. Its saturated solution has a pH of 6.3. Topiramate has the molecular formula $C_{12}H_{21}NO_8S$ and a molecular weight of 339.36. Topiramate is designated chemically as 2,3:4,5-bis-*O*-(1-methylethylidene)-β-D-fructopyranose sulfamate.

Topamax tablets contain the following inactive ingredients: lactose monohydrate, pregelatinized starch, microcrystalline cellulose, sodium starch glycolate, magnesium stearate, purified water, carnauba wax, hydroxypropyl methylcellulose, titanium dioxide, polyethylene glycol, synthetic iron oxide (100 and 200 mg tablets) and polysorbate 80.

CLINICAL PHARMACOLOGY:

MECHANISM OF ACTION

The precise mechanism by which topiramate exerts its antiseizure effect is unknown; however, electrophysiological and biochemical studies of the effects of topiramate on cultured neurons have revealed three properties that may contribute to topiramate's antiepileptic efficacy. First, action potentials elicited repetitively by a sustained depolarization of the neurons are blocked by topiramate in a time-dependent manner, suggestive of a state-dependent sodium channel blocking action. Second, topiramate increases the frequency at which γ-aminobutyrate (GABA) activates $GABA_A$receptors, and enhances the ability of GABA to induce a flux of chloride ions into neurons, suggesting that topiramate potentiates the activity of this inhibitory neurotransmitter. This effect was not blocked by flumazenil, a benzodiazepine antagonist, nor did topiramate increase the duration of the channel open time, differentiating topiramate from barbiturates that modulate $GABA_A$ receptors. Third, topiramate antagonizes the ability of kainate to activate the kainate/AMPA (α-amino-3-hydroxy-5-methylisoxazole-4-propionic acid; non-NMDA) subtype of excitatory amino acid (glutamate) receptor, but has no apparent effect on the activity of N-methyl-D-aspartate (NMDA) at the NMDA receptor subtype. These effects of topiramate are concentration-dependent within the range of 1 μM to 200 μM.

Topiramate also inhibits some isoenzymes of carbonic anhydrase (CA-II and CA-lV). This pharmacologic effect is generally weaker than that of acetazolamide, a known carbonic anhydrase inhibitor, and is not thought to be a major contributing factor to topiramate's antiepileptic activity.

PHARMACODYNAMICS

Topiramate has anticonvulsant activity in rat and mouse maximal electroshock seizure (MES) tests. Topiramate is only weakly effective in blocking clonic seizures induced by the $GABA_A$ receptor antagonist, pentylenetetrazole. Topiramate is also effective in rodent models of epilepsy, which include tonic and absence-like seizures in the spontaneous epileptic rat (SER) and tonic and clonic seizures induced in rats by kindling of the amygdala or by global ischemia.

PHARMACOKINETICS

Absorption of topiramate is rapid, with peak plasma concentrations occurring at approximately 2 hours following a 400 mg oral dose. The relative bioavailability of topiramate from the tablet formulation is about 80% compared to a solution. The bioavailability of topiramate is not affected by food.

The pharmacokinetics of topiramate are linear with dose proportional increases in plasma concentration over the dose range studied (200 to 800 mg/day). The mean plasma elimination half-life is 21 hours after single or multiple doses. Steady state is thus reached in about 4 days in patients with normal renal function. Topiramate is 13-17% bound to human plasma proteins over the concentration range of 1-250 mcg/ml.

METABOLISM AND EXCRETION

Topiramate is not extensively metabolized and is primarily eliminated unchanged in the urine (approximately 70% of an administered dose). Six metabolites have been identified in humans, none of which constitutes more than 5% of an administered dose. The metabolites are formed via hydroxylation, hydrolysis, and glucuronidation. There is evidence of renal tubular reabsorption of topiramate. In rats, given probenecid to inhibit tubular reabsorption, along with topiramate, a significant increase in renal clearance of topiramate was observed. This interaction has not been evaluated in humans. Overall, plasma clearance is approximately 20 to 30 ml/min in humans following oral administration.

PHARMACOKINETIC INTERACTIONS

(see also DRUG INTERACTIONS)

Antiepileptic Drugs: Potential interactions between topiramate and standard AEDs were assessed in controlled clinical pharmacokinetic studies in patients with epilepsy. The effect of these interactions on mean plasma AUCs are summarized in TABLE 3.

SPECIAL POPULATIONS

Renal Impairment: The clearance of topiramate was reduced by 42% in moderately renally impaired (creatinine clearance 30-69 ml/min/1.73m²) and by 54% in severely renally impaired subjects (creatinine clearance <30 ml/min/1.73m²) compared to normal renal function subjects (creatinine clearance >70 ml/min/1.73m²). Since topiramate is presumed to undergo significant tubular reabsorption, it is uncertain whether this experience can be generalized to all situations of renal impairment. It is conceivable that some forms of renal disease could differentially affect glomerular filtration rate and tubular reabsorption resulting in a clearance of topiramate not predicted by creatinine clearance. In general, however, use of one-half the usual dose is recommended in patients with moderate or severe renal impairment.

Hemodialysis: Topiramate is cleared by hemodialysis. Using a high efficiency, counterflow, single pass-dialysate hemodialysis procedure, topiramate dialysis clearance was 120 ml/min with blood flow through the dialyzer at 400 ml/min. This high clearance (compared to 20-30 ml/min total oral clearance in healthy adults) will remove a clinically significant amount of topiramate from the patient over the hemodialysis treatment period. Therefore, a dose adjustment may be required (see DOSAGE AND ADMINISTRATION).

Hepatic Impairment: In hepatically impaired subjects, the clearance of topiramate may be decreased; the mechanism underlying the decrease is not well understood.

Age, Gender, and Race: Clearance of topiramate was not affected by age (18-67 years), gender, or race.

CLINICAL PHARMACOLOGY: *(cont'd)*

Pediatric Pharmacokinetics: Pharmacokinetics of topiramate were evaluated in patients ages 4 to 17 years receiving one or two other antiepileptic drugs. Pharmacokinetic profiles were obtained after one week at doses of 1, 3, and 9 mg/kg/day. Clearance was independent of dose. Although the relationship between age and clearance among patients of pediatric age has not been systematically evaluated, it appears that the weight adjusted clearance of topiramate is higher in pediatric patients than in adults.

CLINICAL STUDIES:

The effectiveness of topiramate as an adjunctive treatment for partial onset seizures was established in five multicenter, randomized, double-blind, placebo-controlled trials, two comparing several dosages of topiramate and placebo and three comparing a single dosage with placebo, in patients with a history of partial onset seizures, with or without secondarily generalization.

Patients in these studies were permitted a maximum of two antiepileptic drugs (AEDs) in addition to topiramate or placebo. In each study, patients were stabilized on optimum dosages of their concomitant AEDs during an 8-12 week baseline phase. Patients who experienced at least 12 (or 8, for 8-week baseline studies) partial onset seizures, with or without secondarily generalization, during the baseline phase were randomly assigned to placebo or a specified dose of topiramate in addition to their other AEDs.

Following randomization, patients began the double-blind phase of treatment. Patients received active drug beginning at 100 mg per day; the dose was then increased by 100 mg or 200 mg/day increments weekly or every other week until the assigned dose was reached, unless intolerance prevented increases. After titration, patients entered an 8- or 12-week stabilization period. The numbers of patients randomized to each dose, and the actual mean, and median doses in the stabilization period are shown in TABLE 1.

TABLE 1 Topiramate Dose Summary During the Stabilization Periods of Each of Five Double-Blind, Placebo-Controlled, Add-On Trials

			Target Topiramate Dosage (mg/day)				
Protocol	Stabilization Dose	Placebo*	200	400	600	800	1000
YD	N	42	42	40	41	-	-
	Mean Dose	5.9	200	390	556	-	-
	Median Dose	6.0	200	400	600	-	-
YE	N	44	-	-	40	45	40
	Mean Dose	9.7	-	-	544	739	796
	Median Dose	10.0	-	-	600	800	1000
Y1	N	23	-	19	-	-	-
	Mean Dose	3.8	-	395	-	-	-
	Median Dose	4.0	-	400	-	-	-
Y2	N	30	-	-	28	-	-
	Mean Dose	5.7	-	-	522	-	-
	Median Dose	6.0	-	-	600	-	-
Y3	N	28	-	-	-	25	-
	Mean Dose	7.9	-	-	-	568	-
	Median Dose	8.0	-	-	-	600	-

* Placebo dosages are given as the number of tablets. Placebo target dosages were as follows: Protocol Y1, 4 tablets/day; Protocols YD and Y2, 6 tablets/day; Protocol Y3, 8 tablets/day; Protocols YE, 10 tablets/day.

In all add-on trials, the reduction in seizure rate from baseline during the entire double-blind phase was measured. Responder rate (fraction of patients with at least a 50% reduction) was also measured. The median percent reductions in seizure rates and the responder rates by treatment group for each study are shown in TABLE 2.

TABLE 2 Median Percent Seizure Rate Reduction and Percent Responders in Five Double-Blind, Placebo-Controlled, Add-On Trials

			Target Topiramate Dosage (mg/day)				
Protocol	Efficacy Results	Placebo*	200	400	600	800	1000
YD	N	45	45	45	46	-	-
	Median % Reduction	11.6	27.2 *	47.5 †	44.7 ‡	-	-
	% Responders	18	24	44 §	46 §	-	-
YE	N	47	-	-	48	48	47
	Median % Reduction	1.7	-	-	40.8 ‡	41.0 ‡	36.0 ‡
	% Responders	9	-	-	40 ‡	41 ‡	36 §
Y1	N	24	-	23	-	-	-
	Median % Reduction	1.1	-	40.7 ‖	-	-	-
	% Responders	8	-	35 §	-	-	-
Y2	N	30	-	-	30	-	-
	Median % Reduction	-12.2	-	-	46.4 ¶	-	-
	% Responders	10	-	-	47 ‡	-	-
Y3	N	28	-	-	-	28	-
	Median % Reduction	-20.6	-	-	-	24.3 ‡	-
	% Responders	0	-	-	-	43 ‡	-

Comparisons with placebo: * p=0.080; † p ≤0.010; ‡p ≤0.001; § p ≤0.050; ‖ p=0.065; ¶p ≤0.005

‡†Subset analyses of the antiepileptic efficacy of topiramate in these studies showed no differences as a function of gender, race, age, baseline seizure rate, or concomitant AED.

INDICATIONS AND USAGE:

Topiramate is indicated as adjunctive therapy for the treatment of adults with partial onset seizures.

CONTRAINDICATIONS:

Topiramate is contraindicated in patients with a history of hypersensitivity to any component of this product.

WARNINGS:

Withdrawal of AEDs: Antiepileptic drugs, including topiramate, should be withdrawn gradually to minimize the potential of increased seizure frequency.

Cognitive/Neuropsychiatric Adverse Events: Adverse events most often associated with the use of topiramate were central nervous system-related. The most significant of these can be classified into two general categories: 1) psychomotor slowing, difficulty with concentration, and speech or language problems, in particular, word-finding difficulties and 2) somnolence

WARNINGS: *(cont'd)*

or fatigue. Additional nonspecific CNS effects occasionally observed with topiramate as add-on therapy include dizziness or imbalance, confusion, memory problems, and exacerbation of mood disturbances (*e.g.*, irritability and depression).

Reports of psychomotor slowing, speech and language problems, and difficulty with concentration and attention were common. Although in some cases these events were mild to moderate, they at times led to withdrawal from treatment. The incidence of psychomotor slowing is only marginally dose-related, but both language problems and difficulty with concentration or attention clearly increased in frequency with increasing dosage in the five double-blind trials (see TABLE 5). Somnolence and fatigue were the most frequently reported adverse events during clinical trials with topiramate. These events were generally mild to moderate and occurred early in therapy. While the incidence of somnolence does not appear to be dose-related, that of fatigue increases at dosages above 400 mg/day.

PRECAUTIONS:

GENERAL

Kidney Stones: A total of 32/2086 (1.5%) of pabents exposed to topiramate during its development reported the occurrence of kidney stones, an incidence about 2-4 times that expected in a similar, untreated population. As in the general population, the incidence of stone formation among topiramate treated patients was higher in men.

An explanation for the association of topiramate and kidney stones may lie in the fact that topiramate is a weak carbonic anhydrase inhibitor. Carbonic anhydrase inhibitors (*e.g.*, acetazolamide or dichlorphenamide) promote stone formation by reducing urinary citrate excretion and by increasing urinary pH. The concomitant use of topiramate with other carbonic anhydrase inhibitors may create a physiological environment that increases the risk of kidney stone formation, and should therefore be avoided.

Increased fluid intake increases the urinary output, lowering the concentration of substances involved in stone formation. Hydration is recommended to reduce new stone formation.

Paresthesia: Paresthesia, an effect associated with the use of other carbonic anhydrase inhibitors, appears to be a common effect of topiramate.

Adjustment of Dose in Renal Failure: The major route of elimination of unchanged topiramate and its metabolites is via the kidney. Dosage adjustment may be required (see DOSAGE AND ADMINISTRATION).

Decreased Hepatic Function: In hepatically impaired patients, topiramate should be administered with caution as the clearance of topiramate may be decreased.

INFORMATION FOR THE PATIENT

Patients, particularly those with predisposing factors, should be instructed to maintain an adequate fluid intake in order to minimize the risk of renal stone formation (See PRECAUTIONS, General, for support regarding hydration as a preventative measure).

Patients should be warned about the potential for somnolence, dizziness, confusion, and difficulty concentrating and advised not to drive or operate machinery until they have gained sufficient experience on topiramate to gauge whether it adversely affects their mental and/or motor performance.

CARCINOGENESIS, MUTAGENESIS, AND IMPAIRMENT OF FERTILITY

An increase in urinary bladder tumors was observed in mice given topiramate (20, 75, and 300 mg/kg) in the diet for 21 months. The elevated bladder tumor incidence, which was statistically significant in males and females receiving 300 mg/kg, was primarily due to the increased occurrence of a smooth muscle tumor considered histomorphologically unique to mice. Plasma exposures in mice receiving 300 mg/kg were approximately 0.5 to 1 times steady state exposures measured in patients receiving topiramate monotherapy at the recommended human dose (RHD) of 400 mg, and 1.5 to 2 times steady state topiramate exposures in patients receiving 400 mg of topiramate plus phenytoin. The relevance of this finding to human carcinogenic risk is uncertain. No evidence of carcinogenicity was seen in rats following oral administration of topiramate for 2 years at doses up to 120 mg/kg (approximately 3 times the RHD on a mg/m^2 basis). Topiramate did not demonstrate genotoxic potential when tested in a battery of *in vitro* and *in vivo* assays. Topiramate was not mutagenic in the Ames test or the *in vitro* mouse lymphoma assay; it did not increase unscheduled DNA synthesis in rat hepatocytes *in vitro*; and it did not increase chromosomal aberrations in human lymphocytes *in vitro* or in rat bone marrow *in vivo*. No adverse effects on male or female fertility were observed in rats at doses up to 100 mg/kg (2.5 times the RHD on a mg/m^2 basis).

PREGNANCY CATEGORY C

Topiramate has demonstrated selective developmental toxicity, including teratogenicity, in experimental animal studies. When oral doses of 20, 100, or 500 mg/kg were administered to pregnant mice during the period of organogenesis, the incidence of fetal malformations (primarily craniofacial defects) was increased at all doses. The low dose is approximately 0.2 times the recommended human dose (RHD=400 mg/day) on a mg/m^2 basis. Fetal body weights and skeletal ossification were reduced at 500 mg kg in conjunction with decreased maternal body weight gain.

In rat studies (oral doses of 20, 100, and 500 mg/kg or 0.2, 2.5, 30 and 400mg/kg), the frequency of limb malformations (ectrodactyly, micromelia, and amelia) was increased among the offspring of dams treated with 400 mg/kg (10 times the RHD on a mg/m^2 basis) or greater during the organogenesis period of pregnancy. Embryotoxicity (reduced fetal body weights, increased incidence of structural variations) was observed at doses as low as 20 mg/kg (0.5 times the RHD on a mg/m^2basis). Clinical signs of maternal toxicity were seen at 400 mg/kg and above, and maternal body weight gain was reduced during treatment with 100 mg/kg or greater.

In rabbit studies (20, 60, and 180 mg/kg or 10, 35. and 120 mg/kg orally during organogenesis), embryo/fetal mortality was increased at 35 mg/kg (2 times the RHD on a mg/m^2 basis) or greater, and teratogenic effects (primarily rib and vertebral malformations) were observed at 120 mg/kg (6 times the RHD on a mg/m^2 basis). Evidence of maternal toxicity (decreased body weight gain, clinical signs, and/or mortality) was seen at 35 mg/kg and above.

When female rats were treated during the latter part of gestation and throughout lactation (0.2, 4, 20, and 100 mg/kg or 2, 20, and 200 mg/kg), offspring exhibited decreased viability and delayed physical development at 200 mg kg (5 times the RHD on a mg/m^2 basis) and reductions in pre- and/or postweaning body weight gain at 2 mg/kg (0.05 times the RHD on a mg/m^2 basis) and above. Maternal toxicity (decreased body weight gain, clinical signs) was evident at 100 mg/kg or greater.

In a rat embryo/fetal development study with a postnatal component (0.2, 2.5, 30 or 400 mg/kg during organogenesis; noted above), pups exhibited delayed physical development at 400 mg/kg (10 times the RHD on a mg/m^2 basis) and persistent reductions in body weight gain at 30 mg/kg (1 times the RHD on a mg/m^2 basis) and higher. There are no studies using topiramate in pregnant women. Topiramate should be used during pregnancy only if the potential benefit outweighs the potential risk to the fetus.

LABOR AND DELIVERY

In studies of rats where dams were allowed to deliver pups naturally, no drug related effects on gestation length or parturition were observed at dosage levels up to 200 mg/kg/day.

The effect of topiramate on labor and dellvery in humans is unknown.

PRECAUTIONS: *(cont'd)*

NURSING MOTHERS

Topiramate is excreted in the milk of lactating rats. It is not known if topiramate is excreted in human milk. Since many drugs are excreted in human milk, and because the potential for serious adverse reactions in nursing infants to topiramate is unknown, the potential benefit to the mother should be weighed against the potential risk to the infant when considering recommendations regarding nursing.

PEDIATRIC USE

Safety and effectiveness in children have not been established. The pharmacokinetic profile of topiramate was studied in patients between the ages of 4 and 17 years. (See CLINICAL PHARMACOLOGY, Pediatric Pharmacokinetics).

GERIATRIC USE

In clinical trials, 2% of patients were over 60. No age related difference in effectiveness or adverse effects were seen. There were no pharmacokinetic differences related to age alone, although the possibility of age-associated renal functional abnormalities should be considered.

RACE AND GENDER EFFECTS

Evaluation of efficacy and safety in clinical trials has shown no race or gender related effects.

DRUG INTERACTIONS:

Antiepileptic Drugs: Potential interactions between topiramate and standard AEDs were assessed in controlled clinical pharmacokinetic studies in patients with epilepsy. The effect of these interactions on mean plasma AUCs are summarized in TABLE 3.

In TABLE 3, the second column (AED concentration) describes what happens to the concentration of the AED listed in the first column when topiramate is added.

The third column (topiramate concentration) describes how the coadministration of a drug listed in the first column modifies the concentration of topiramate in experimental settings when topiramate was given alone.

TABLE 3 Summary of AED Interactions with Topiramate

AED Co-administered	AED Concentration	Topiramate Concentration
Phenytoin	NC or 25% increase *	48% decrease
Carbamazepine (CBZ)	NC	40% decrease
CBZ epoxide †	NC	NE
Valproic acid	11% decrease	14% decrease
Phenobarbital	NC	NE
Primidone	NC	NE

* Plasma concentration increased 25% in some patients, generally those on a b.i.d. dosing regimen of phenytoin.
† is not administered but is an active metabolite of carbamazepine.
NC less than 10% change in plasma concentration.
AED Antiepileptic drug.
NE Not Evaluated.

OTHER DRUG INTERACTIONS

Digoxin: In a single-dose study, serum digoxin AUC was decreased by 12% with concomitant topiramate administration. The clinical relevance of this observation has not been established.

CNS Depressants: Concomitant administration of topiramate and alcohol or other CNS depressant drugs has not been evaluated in clinical studies. Because of the potential of topiramate to cause CNS depression, as well as other cognitive and/or neuropsychiatric adverse events, topiramate should be used with extreme caution if used in combination with alcohol and other CNS depressants.

Oral Contraceptives: In an interaction study with oral contraceptives using a combination product containing norethindrone and ethinyl estradiol, topiramate did not significantly affect the clearance of norethindrone. The mean total exposure to the estrogenic component decreased by 18%, 21%, and 30% at daily doses of 200, 400, and 800 mg/day, respectively. Therefore, efficacy of oral contraceptives may be compromised by topiramate. Patients taking oral contraceptives should be asked to report any change in their bleeding patterns. The effect of oral contraceptives on the pharmacokinetics of topiramate is not known.

Others: Concomitant use of topiramate, a weak carbonic anhydrase inhibitor, with other carbonic anhydrase inhibitors (*e.g.*, acetazolamide or dichlor phenamide) may create a physiological environment that increases the risk of renal stone formation, and should therefore be avoided.

Laboratory Tests: There are no known interactions of topiramate with commonly used laboratory tests.

ADVERSE REACTIONS:

The most commonly observed adverse events associated with the use of topiramate at dosages of 200 to 400 mg/day in controlled trials, that were seen at greater frequency in topiramate-treated patients and did not appear to be dose-related were: somnolence, dizziness, ataxia, speech disorders and related speech problems, psychomotor slowing, nystagmus, and paresthesia (see TABLE 4). The most common dose-related adverse events at dosages of 200 to 1000 mg/day were: fatigue, nervousness, difficulty with concentration or attention, confusion, depression, anorexia, language problems, anxiety, mood problems, cognitive problems not otherwise specified, weight decreased, and tremor (see TABLE 5).

In controlled clinical trials, 11% of patients receiving topiramate 200 to 400 mg/day as adjunctive therapy discontinued due to adverse events. This rate appeared to increase at dosages above 400 mg/day. Adverse events associated with discontinuing therapy included somnolence, dizziness, anxiety, difficulty with concentration or attention, fatigue, and paresthesia and increased at dosages above 400 mg/day.

Approximately 28% of the 1715 individuals with epilepsy who received topiramate at dosages of 200 to 1600 mg/day in clinical studies discontinued treatment because of adverse events; an individual patient could have reported more than one adverse event. These adverse events were: psychomotor slowing (4.1%), difficulty with memory (3.3%), fatigue (3.3%), confusion (3.2%), somnolence (3.2%), difficulty with concentration/attention (2.9%), anorexia (2.9%), depression (2.6%), dizziness (2.6%), weight decrease (2.5%), nervousness (2.2%), ataxia (2.2%), paresthesia (2.0%), and language problems (2.0%).

Incidence in Controlled Clinical Trials - Add-On Therapy: TABLE 4 lists treatment-emergent adverse events that occurred in at least 1 % of patients treated with 200 to 400 mg/day topiramate in controlled trials that were numerically more common at this dose than in the patients treated with placebo. In general, most patients who experienced adverse events during the first eight weeks of these trials no longer experienced them by their last visit.

The prescriber should be aware that these data were obtained when topiramate was added to concurrent antiepileptic drug therapy and cannot be used to predict the frequency of adverse events in the course of usual medical practice where patient characteristics and other factors may differ from those prevailing during clinical studies. Similarly, the cited frequencies cannot be directly compared with data obtained from other clinical investigations involving

ADVERSE REACTIONS: *(cont'd)*

different treatments, uses, or investigators. Inspection of these frequencies, however, does provide the prescribing physician with a basis to estimate the relative contribution of drug and non-drug factors to the adverse event incidences in the population studied.

TABLE 4 Incidence (%) of Treatment-Emergent Adverse Events in Placebo-Controlled, Add-On Trials * †
Events that occurred in at least 1% of topiramate-treated patients and occurred more frequently in topiramate-treated than placebo-treated patients

Body System/Adverse Event ‡	Placebo (N=174)	Topiramate Dosage (mg/day) 200-400 (N=113)	600-1,000 (N=247)
Body as a Whole - General Disorders			
Asthenia	1.1	8.0	4.5
Back Pain	4.0	6.2	2.0
Chest Pain	2.3	4.4	2.0
Influenza-Like Symptoms	2.9	3.5	3.2
Leg Pain	2.3	3.5	2.4
Hot Flushes	1.7	2.7	0.8
Body Odor	0.0	1.8	0.0
Edema	1.1	1.8	1.2
Rigors	0.0	1.8	0.4
Central & Peripheral Nervous System Disorders			
Dizziness	14.4	28.3	32.4
Ataxia	6.9	21.2	17.0
Speech Disorders/Related Speech Problems	2.9	16.8	13.8
Nystagmus	11.5	15.0	15.0
Paresthesia	3.4	15.0	14.6
Tremor	6.3	10.6	13.8
Language Problems	0.6	6.2	11.7
Coordination Abnormal	1.7	5.3	3.6
Hypoaesthesia	1.1	2.7	0.8
Gastrointestinal System Disorders			
Nausea	6.3	11.5	13.8
Dyspepsia	5.2	8.0	5.7
Abdominal Pain	2.9	5.3	7.3
Constipation	0.6	5.3	3.2
Dry Mouth	1.1	2.7	3.2
Gingivitis	0.0	1.8	0.4
Hearing and Vestibular Disorders			
Hearing Decreased	1.1	1.8	1.6
Metabolic and Nutritional Disorders			
Weight Decrease	2.3	7.1	12.6
Musculoskeletal System Disorders			
Myalgia	1.1	1.8	1.6
Platelet, Bleeding and Clotting Disorders			
Epistaxis	1.1	1.8	0.8
Psychiatric Disorders			
Somnolence	10.3	30.1	25.9
Psychomotor Slowing	2.3	16.8	25.1
Nervousness	7.5	15.9	20.6
Difficulty with Memory	2.9	12.4	12.6
Confusion	5.2	9.7	15.0
Depression	6.3	8.0	13.4
Difficulty with Concentration/Attention	1.1	8.0	15.4
Anorexia	4.0	5.3	11.3
Agitation	1.7	4.4	4.0
Mood Problems	1.7	3.5	10.1
Aggressive Reaction	0.6	2.7	4.0
Apathy	0.0	1.8	4.5
Depersonalization	0.6	1.8	1.6
Emotional Liability	1.1	1.8	2.4
Reproductive Disorders, Female	(N=39)	(N=24)	(N=42)
Breast Pain, Female	0.0	8.3	0.0
Dysmenorrhea	2.6	8.3	0.0
Menstrual Disorder	0.0	4.2	0.0
Respiratory System Disorders			
Upper Respiratory Infection	11.5	12.4	12.1
Pharyngitis	2.9	7.1	2.8
Sinusitis	4.0	4.4	4.0
Dyspnea	1.1	1.8	3.2
Skin and Appendages Disorders			
Rash	4.0	4.4	3.2
Pruritus	1.1	1.8	3.2
Sweating Increased	0.0	1.8	0.4
Urinary System Disorders			
Hematuria	0.6	1.8	0.8
Vision Disorders			
Diplopia	6.3	14.2	14.6
Vision Abnormal	2.9	14.2	10.5
Eye pain	1.1	1.8	2.0
White Cell and Res Disorders			
Leukopenia	0.6	2.7	1.6

* Patients in these add-on trials were receiving 1 to 2 concomitant antiepileptic drugs in addition to topiramate or placebo.
† Values represent the percentage of patients reporting a given adverse event. Patients may have reported more than one adverse event during the study and can be included in more than one adverse event category.
‡ Adverse events reported by at least 1% of patients in the topiramate 200-400 mg/day group and more common than in the placebo group are listed in this table.

Other Adverse Events Observed: Other events that occurred in more than 1% of patients treated with 200 to 400 mg of topiramate in placebo-controlled trials but with equal or greater frequency in the placebo group were: fatigue, headache, injury, anxiety, rash, pain, convulsions aggravated, coughing, gastroenteritis, rhinitis, back pain, hot flushes, bronchitis, abnormal gait, involuntary muscle contractions, and epistaxis.

Other Adverse Events Observed During All Clinical Trials: Topiramate, initiated as adjunctive therapy, has been administered to 1715 patients with epilepsy during all clinical studies. During these studies, all adverse events were recorded by the clinical investigators using terminology of their own choosing. To provide a meaningful estimate of the proportion of individuals having adverse events, similar types of events were grouped into a smaller number of standardized categories using modified WHOART dictionary terminology. The frequencies presented represent the proportion of 1715 topiramate-treated patients who experienced an event of the type cited on at least one occasion while receiving topiramate. Reported events are included except those already listed in the previous table, those too general to be informative, and those not reasonably associated with the use of the drug.

ADVERSE REACTIONS: *(cont'd)*

TABLE 5 Incidence (%) of Dose-Related Adverse Events From Five Placebo-Controlled, Add-On Trials

Adverse Event (N=174)	Placebo (N=45)	Topiramate Dosage (mg/day) 200 (N=68)	400 (N=247)	600-1000
Fatigue	14.4	11.1	11.8	30.8
Nervousness	7.5	13.3	17.6	20.6
Difficulty with Concentration/Attention	1.1	6.7	8.8	15.4
Confusion	5.2	8.9	10.3	15.0
Depression	6.3	8.9	7.4	13.4
Anorexia	4.0	4.4	5.9	11.3
Language Problems	0.6	2.2	8.8	11.7
Anxiety	5.2	2.2	2.9	9.3
Mood problems	1.7	0.0	5.9	10.1
Cognitive problems NOS	0.6	0.0	0.0	4.0
Weight decrease	2.3	4.4	8.8	12.6
Tremor	6.3	13.3	8.8	13.8

Events are classified within body system categories and enumerated in order of decreasing frequency using the following definitions: *frequent* occurring in at least 1/100 patients; *infrequent* occurring in 1/100 to 1/1000 patients; *rare* occurring in fewer than 1/1000 patients.

Autonomic Nervous System Disorders: *Infrequent:* vasodilation

Body as a Whole: *Frequent:* fatigue, fever, malaise *Infrequent:* syncope, halitosis, abdomen enlarged *Rare:* alcohol intolerance, substernal chest pain, sudden death

Cardiovascular Disorders, General: *Infrequent:* hypertension, hypotension, postural hypotension

Central & Peripheral Nervous System Disorders: *Frequent:* hypokinesia, vertigo, stupor, convulsions grand mal, hyperkinesea, hypertonia *Infrequent:* leg cramps, hyporeflexia, neuropathy, migraine, apraxia, hyperaesthesia, dyskinesia, hyperreflexia, dysphonia, scotoma, ptosis, dystonia, visual field defect, coma, encephalopathy, fecal incontinence, upper motor neuron lesion *Rare:* cerebellar syndrome, EEG abnormal, tongue paralysis.

Endocrine Disorders: *Infrequent:* goiter *Rare:* thyroid disorder.

Gastrointestinal System Disorders: *Frequent:* diarrhea, vomiting, flatulence, gastroenteritis *Infrequent:* gum hyperplasia, hemorrhoids, tooth caries, stomabtis, dysphagia, melena, gastritis, saliva increased, hiccough, gastroesophageal reflux, tongue edema, esophagitis *Rare:* eructation

Hearing and Vestibular Disorders: *Frequent:* tinnitus *Rare:* earache, hyperacusis

Heart Rate and Rhythm Disorders: *Frequent:* palpitation *Infrequent:* AV block, bradycardia, bundle branch block *Rare:* arrhythmia, arrhythmia atrial, fibrillation atrial

Liver and Biliary System Disorders: *Infrequent:* SGPT increased, SGOT increased, gall bladder disorder *Rare:* gamma-GT increased

Metabolic and Nutritional Disorders: *Frequent:* weight increase *Infrequent:* thirst, hypokalemia, alkaline phosphatase increased, dehydrabon, hypocalcemia, hyperlipemia, acidosis, hyperglycemia, creatinine increased, hyperchloremia, xerophthalmia *Rare:* diabetes mellitus, hypernatremia, abnormal serum folate, hyponatremia, hypocholesterolemia, hypoglycemia, hypophosphatemia

Musculoskeletal System Disorders: *Frequent:* arthralgia, muscle weakness *Infrequent:* arthrosis, osteoporosis

Myo-, Endo-, Pericardial and Valve Disorders: *Infrequent:* angina pectoris

Neoplasms: *Infrequent:* basal cell carcinoma, thrombocythemia *Rare:* polycythemia

Platelet, Pleeding, and Clotting Disorders: *Infrequent:* gingival bleeding, purpura, thrombocytopenia, pulmonary embolism

Psychiatric Disorders: *Frequent:* insomnia, personality disorder, impotence. hallucination, euphoria, psychosis, libido decreased, suicide attempt *Infrequent:* paranoid reaction, appetite increased, delusion, paranoia, delirium, abnormal dreaming, neurosis *Rare:* libido increased, manic reaction

Red Blood Cell Disorders: *Frequent:* anemia *Rare:* marrow depression, pancytopenia

Reproductive Disorders, Female: *Frequent:* intermenstrual bleeding, leukorrhea, menorrhagia, vaginitis, amenorrhea

Reproductive Disorders, Male: *Infrequent:* ejaculation disorder, breast discharge

Respiratory System Disorders: *Frequent:* coughing, bronchitis *Infrequent:* asthma, bronchospasm *Rare:* laryngismus

Skin and Appendages Disorders: *Frequent:* acne, alopecia *Infrequent:* dermatitis, nail disorder, folliculitis, dry skin, urticaria, skin discoloration, eczema, photosensitivity reaction, erythematous rash, seborrhoea, sweating decreased, abnormal hair texture *Rare:* chloasma

Special Senses Other, Disorders: *Frequent:* taste perversion *Infrequent:* taste loss, parosmia

Urinary System Disorders:

Frequent: urinary tract infection, micturition frequency, urinary incontinence, dysuria, renal calculus.

Infrequent: urinary retention, face edema, renal pain, nocturia, albuminuria, polyuria, oliguria.

Vascular (Extracardiac) Disorders: *Infrequent:* flushing, deep vein thrombosis, phlebitis *Rare:* vasospasm

Vision Disorders: *Frequent:* conjunctivitis *Infrequent:* abnormal accommodation, photophobia, abnormal lacrimation, strabismus, color blindness, myopia, mydriasis *Rare:* cataract, corneal opacity, iritis

White Cell and Reticuloendothelial System Disorders: *Infrequent:* lymphadenopathy, eosinophilia, lymphopenia, granulocytopenia, lymphocytosis

DRUG ABUSE AND DEPENDENCE:

The abuse and dependence potential of topiramate has not been evaluated in human studies.

OVERDOSAGE:

In acute topiramate overdose, if the ingestion is recent, the stomach should be emptied immediately by lavage or by induction of emesis. Activated charcoal has not been shown to adsorb topiramate *in vitro*. Therefore, its use in overdosage is not recommended. Treatment should be appropriately supportive. Hemodialysis is an effective means of removing topiramate from the body. However, in the few cases of acute overdosage reported, hemodialysis has not been necessary.

DOSAGE AND ADMINISTRATION:

In the controlled add-on trials, no correlation has been demonstrated between trough plasma concentrations of topiramate and clinical efficacy. No evidence of tolerance has been demonstrated in humans. Doses above 400 mg/day (600, 800, and 1000 mg/day) have not been shown to improve responses.

The recommended total daily dose of topiramate as adjunctive therapy is 400 mg/day in two divided doses. A daily dose of 200 mg/day has inconsistent effects and is less effective than 400 mg/day. It is recommended that therapy be initiated at 50 mg/day followed by titration to an effective dose. Daily doses above 1600 mg have not been studied.

TABLE 5 The Recommended Daily Dose for Topiramate

	AM Dose	PM Dose
Week 1	none	50 mg
Week 2	50 mg	50 mg
Week 3	50 mg	100 mg
Week 4	100 mg	100 mg
Week 5	100 mg	150 mg
Week 6	150 mg	150 mg
Week 7	150 mg	200 mg
Week 8	200 mg	200 mg

It is not necessary to monitor topiramate plasma concentrations to optimize topiramate therapy. On occasion, the addition of topiramate to phenytoin may require an adjustment of the dose of phenytoin to achieve optimal clinical outcome. Addition or withdrawal of phenytoin and/or carbamazepine during adjunctive therapy with topiramate may require adjustment of the dose of topiramate. Because of the bitter taste, tablets should not be broken.

Topiramate can be taken without regard to meals.

Patients with Renal Impairment: In renally impaired subjects (creatinine clearance less than 70 ml/min/1.73m^2), one half of the usual adult dose is recommended. Such patients will require a longer time to reach steady-state at each dose.

Patients Undergoing Hemodialysis: Topiramate is cleared by hemodialysis at a rate that is 4 to 6 times greater than a normal individual. Accordingly, a prolonged period of dialysis may cause topiramate concentration to fall below that required to maintain an anti-seizure effect. To avoid rapid drops in topiramate plasma concentration during hemodialysis a supplemental dose of topiramate may be required. The actual adjustment should take into account 1) the duration of dialysis period, 2) the clearance rate of the dialysis system being used, and 3) the effective renal clearance of topiramate in the patient being dialyzed.

Patients with Hepatic Disease: In hepatically impaired patients topiramate plasma concentrations may be increased. The mechanism is not well understood.

PATIENT INFORMATION:

Topiramate is used for the treatment of adults with epilepsy.

Kidney stone formation has been reported. Patients should drink plenty of fluids.

Inform your physician if you are taking any other medicines.

Topiramate may cause oral contraceptive failure.

Inform your doctor if you are pregnant or nursing.

May cause sleepiness, dizziness, incoordination, speech disorders, slowing of motor skills, involuntary eye movement, and numbness/tingling of the extremeties.

Patients should use caution while driving or operating hazardous machinery.

May be taken with or without food. Do not break tablets in half. Take as recommended by physician.

HOW SUPPLIED:

Topomax is available as debossed, coated, round tablets in the following strengths and colors: 25 mg white (coded "TOP" on one side; "25" on the other); 100 mg yellow (coded "TOPOMAX" on one side; "100" on the other); 200 mg salmon (coded "TOPOMAX" on one side; "200" on the other).

Topomax tablets should be stored in tightly-closed containers at controlled room temperature, (59 to 86° F, 15 to 30° C). Protect from moisture.

HOW SUPPLIED - EQUIVALENTS NOT AVAILABLE:

Tablet - Oral - 25 mg

25 mg x 60 $64.80 TOPAMAX, McNeil Lab 00045-0639-65

Tablet - Oral - 100 mg

100 mg x 60 $147.60 TOPAMAX, McNeil Lab 00045-0641-65

Tablet - Oral - 200 mg

200 mg x 60 $172.80 TOPAMAX, McNeil Lab 00045-0642-65

TOPOTECAN HYDROCHLORIDE *(003288)*

CATEGORIES: Antineoplastics; Chemotherapy; Camptothecin Derivative; Oncologic Drugs; Ovarian Carcinoma; Pregnancy Category D; FDA Approved 1996 May

BRAND NAMES: **Hycamtin**

WARNING:
Topotecan hydrochloride for injection should be administered under the supervision of a physician experienced in the use of cancer chemotherapeutic agents. Appropriate management of complications is possible only when adequate diagnostic and treatment facilities are readily available. Therapy with topotecan hydrochloride should not be given to patients with baseline neutrophil counts of less than 1500 cells/mm^3. In order to monitor the occurrence of bone marrow suppression, primarily neutropenia, which may be severe and result in infection and death, frequent peripheral blood cell counts should be performed on all patients receiving topotecan hydrochloride.

DESCRIPTION:

Topotecan hydrochloride is a semi-synthetic derivative of camptothecin and is an anti-tumor drug with topoisomerase I-inhibitor activity.

Topotecan hydrochloride is supplied as a sterile lyophilized, buffered, light yellow to greenish powder available in single-dose vials. Each vial contains topotecan hydrochloride equivalent to 4 mg of topotecan as free base. The reconstituted solution ranges in color from yellow to yellow-green and is intended for administration by intravenous infusion.

Inactive ingredients are mannitol, 48 mg, and tartaric acid, 20 mg. Hydrochloric acid and sodium hydroxide may be used to adjust the pH. The solution pH ranges from 2.5 to 3.5. The chemical name for topotecan hydrochloride is (*S*)-10–[(dimethylamino) methyl]-4–ethyl-4,9–dihydroxy-1 *H*-pyrano[3',4': 6,7] indolizino [1,2–b]quinoline-3, 14–(4*H*, 12*H*)-dione monohydrochloride. It has the molecular formula $C_{23}H_{23}N_3O_5 \cdot HCl$ and a molecular weight of 457.9.

It is soluble in water and melts with decomposition at 213° to 218°C.

CLINICAL PHARMACOLOGY:

MECHANISM OF ACTION

Topoisomerase I relieves torsional strain in DNA by inducing reversible single strand breaks. Topotecan binds to the topoisomerase I-DNA complex and prevents religation of these single strand breaks. The cytotoxicity of topotecan is thought to be due to double strand DNA damage produced during DNA synthesis when replication enzymes interact with the ternary complex formed by topotecan, topoisomerase I and DNA. Mammalian cells cannot efficiently repair these double strand breaks.

PHARMACOKINETICS

The pharmacokinetics of topotecan have been evaluated in cancer patients following doses of 0.5 to 1.5 mg/m^2 administered as a 30–minute infusion. Topotecan exhibits multiexponential pharmacokinetics with a terminal half-life of 2 to 3 hours. Total exposure (AUC) is approximately dose-proportional. Binding of topotecan to plasma proteins is about 35%.

Metabolism and Elimination: Topotecan undergoes a reversible pH dependent hydrolysis of its lactone moiety; it is the lactone form that is pharmacologically active. At pH ≤4 the lactone is exclusively present whereas the the ring-opened hydroxy-acid form predominates at physiologic pH. *In vitro* studies in human liver microsomes indicate that metabolism of topotecan to an N-demethylated metabolite represents a minor metabolic pathway.

In humans, about 30% of the dose is excreted in the urine and renal clearance is an important determinant of topotecan elimination (see Special Populations).

SPECIAL POPULATIONS

Gender: The overall mean topotecan plasma clearance in male patients was approximately 24% higher than in female patients, largely reflecting difference in body size.

Geriatrics: Topotecan pharmacokinetics have not been specifically studied in an elderly population, but population pharmacokinetic analysis in female patients did not identify age as a significant factor. Decreased renal clearance, common in the elderly, is a more important determinant of topotecan clearance.

Race: The effect of race on topotecan pharmacokinetics has not been studied.

Renal Impairment: In patients with mild renal impairment (creatinine clearance of 40 to 60 mL/min.), topotecan plasma clearance was decreased to about 67% of the value in patients with normal renal function. In patients with moderate renal impairment (Cl_{cr} of 20 to 39 mL/min.), topotecan plasma clearance was reduced to about 34% of the value in control patients, with an increase in half-life. Mean half-life, estimated in three renally impaired patients, was about 5.0 hours. Dosage adjustment is recommended for these patients (see DOSAGE AND ADMINISTRATION).

Hepatic Impairment: Plasma clearance in patients with hepatic impairment (serum bilirubin levels between 1.7 and 15.0 mg/dl) was decreased to about 67% of the value in patients without hepatic impairment. Topotecan half-life increased slightly, from 2.0 hours to 2.5 hours, but these hepatically impaired patients tolerated the usual recommended topotecan dosage regimen (see DOSAGE AND ADMINISTRATION.)

Drug Interactions: Pharmacokinetic studies of the interaction of topotecan with concomitantly administered medications have not been formally investigated. *In vitro* inhibition studies using marker substrates known to be metabolized by human P450 CYP1A2, CYP2A6, CYP2C8/9, CYP2C19, CYP2D6, CYP2E, CYP3A or CYP4A or dihydropyrimidine dehydrogenase indicate that the activities of these enzymes were not altered by topotecan. Enzyme inhibition by topotecan has not been evaluated *in vivo*.

PHARMACODYNAMICS

The dose-limiting toxicity of topotecan is leukopenia. White blood cell count decreases with increasing topotecan dose or topotecan AUC. When topotecan is administered at a dose of 1.5 mg/m^2/day for 5 days, an 80 to 90% decrease in white blood cell count at nadir is typically observed after the first cycle of therapy.

CLINICAL STUDIES:

Topotecan hydrochloride was studied in four clinical trials of 452 patients with metastatic ovarian carcinoma. All patients had disease that had recurred on, or was unresponsive to, a platinum-containing regimen. Patients in these four studies received an initial dose of 1.5 mg/m^{2}given by intravenous infusion over 30 minutes for 5 consecutive days, starting on day one of a 21–day course.

Two of the studies, involving 223 patients given topotecan, are mature enough for evaluation (although survival results are incomplete). Topotecan was compared with paclitaxel in a randomized trial involving 112 patients treated with topotecan (1.5 mg/m^2/day x 5 days starting on day one of a 21–day course) and 114 patients treated with paclitaxel (175 mg/m^2 over 3 hours on day 1 of a 21–day course). All patients had recurrent ovarian cancer after a platinum-containing regimen or had not responded to at least one prior platinum-containing regimen. Patients who did not respond to the study therapy, or who progressed, could be given the alternative treatment.

Response rates, response duration and time to progression are shown in TABLE 1.

CLINICAL STUDIES: *(cont'd)*

TABLE 1 Efficacy of Topotecan vs. Paclitaxel in Ovarian Cancer

Parameter	Topotecan HCl		Paclitaxel
Complete Response Rate	5.4%		3.5%
Partial Response Rate	14.3%		8.8%
Overall Response Rate	19.6%		12.3%
95% Confidence Interval	12.8% to 28.2%		6.9 to 19.7%
(p-value)		(0.092)	
RESPONSE DURATION (WEEKS)			
Median	32.1		23.1
95% Confidence Interval	24.1† to ∞		23.1† to 24.4
hazard-ratio			
(Topotecan: paclitaxel)		0.424	
(p-value)		(0.224)	
TIME TO PROGRESSION (WEEKS)			
Median	23.1		14.0
95% Confidence Interval	17.1† to 29.6†		11.9† to 18.3†
hazard-ratio			
(Topotecan: paclitaxel)		0.578	
(p-value)		(0.002)	

The calculation for duration of response was based on the interval between first response and time to progression.
† Value corresponds to a censored event; i.e., patient had not yet progressed.

The time to response was longer with topotecan compared to paclitaxel with a mean of 10 weeks (range 3.1 to 24.1) vs 7 weeks (range 2.4 to 12.3). Consequently, the efficacy of topotecan may not be achieved if patients are withdrawn from treatment prematurely.

In the crossover phase, 5 of 53 (9.4%) patients who received topotecan after paclitaxel had a partial response and 1 of 37 (2.7%) patients who received paclitaxel after topotecan had a complete response.

Topotecan was active in patients who had developed resistance to platinum-containing therapy, defined as tumor progression while on, or tumor relapse within 6 months after completion of, a platinum-containing regimen. One complete and seven partial responses were seen in 60 patients, for a response rate of 13%. In the same study, there were no complete responders and four partial responders on the paclitaxel arm, for a response rate of 7%.

The adverse reaction profile for paclitaxel in this study was consistent with the product's approved labeling; the adverse reaction profile for topotecan in this study was consistent with that observed in all 452 patients from the four ovarian cancer clinical trials (see ADVERSE REACTIONS).

Topotecan was also studied in an open-label, non-comparative trial in 111 patients with recurrent ovarian cancer after treatment with a platinum-containing regimen, or who had not responded to one prior platinum-containing regimen. The response rate was 14% (95% CI=7.9% to 20.9%). The median duration of response was 18 weeks (range 5 to 42 weeks). The time to progression was 8.4 weeks (range: 0.7 to 72.1 weeks).

INDICATIONS AND USAGE:

Topotecan hydrochloride is indicated for the treatment of patients with metastatic carcinoma of the ovary after failure of initial or subsequent chemotherapy.

CONTRAINDICATIONS:

Topotecan hydrochloride is contraindicated in patients who have a history of hypersensitivity reactions to topotecan or to any of its ingredients. Topotecan should not be used in patients who are pregnant or breast-feeding, or those with severe bone marrow depression.

WARNINGS:

Bone marrow suppression (primarily neutropenia) is the dose-limiting toxicity of topotecan. Neutropenia is not cumulative over time.

Neutropenia: Severe (grade 4, <500 cells/mm^3) neutropenia was most common during course 1 of treatment (60% of patients) and occurred in 40% of all courses, with a median duration of 7 days. The nadir neutrophil count occurred at a median of 11 days. Prophylactic G-CSF was given in 27% of courses after the first cycle. Therapy-related sepsis or febrile neutropenia occurred in 26% of patients and sepsis was fatal in 0.7%.

Thrombocytopenia: Grade 4 thrombocytopenia (<25,000/mm^3) occurred in 26% of patients and in 9% of courses, with a median duration of 5 days and platelet nadir at a median of 15 days. There were no episodes of serious bleeding. Platelet transfusions were given to 13% of patients and in 4% of courses.

Anemia: Severe anemia (grade 3/4, <8 gm/dl) occurred in 40% of patients and in 16% of courses. Median nadir was at Day 15. Transfusions were needed in 56% of patients and in 23% of courses.

Monitoring of Bone Marrow Function: Topotecan should only be administered in patients with adequate bone marrow reserves, including baseline neutrophil counts of at least 1,500 cells/mm^{3}and platelet count at least 100,000/mm^3. Frequent monitoring of peripheral blood cell counts should be instituted during treatment with topotecan. Patients should not be treated with subsequent courses of topotecan until neutrophils recover to > 1,000 cells/mm^3, platelets recover to > 100,000 cells/mm3 and hemoglobin levels recover to 9.0 mg/dL, (with transfusion if necessary). Severe myelotoxicity has been reported when topotecan is used in combination with cisplatin (see DRUG INTERACTIONS).

Pregnancy: Topotecan may cause fetal harm when administered to a pregnant woman. The effects of topotecan on pregnant women have not been studied. If topotecan is used during a patient's pregnancy, or if a patient becomes pregnant while taking topotecan, she should be warned of the potential hazard to the fetus. Fecund women should be warned to avoid becoming pregnant. In rabbits, a dose of 0.10 mg/kg/day (about equal to the clinical dose on a mg/m^2 basis) given on days 6 through 20 of gestation caused maternal toxicity, embryolethality, and reduced fetal body weight. In the rat, a dose of 0.23 mg/kg/day (about equal to the clinical dose on a mg/m^2 basis) given for 14 days before mating through gestation day six caused fetal resorption, microphthalmia, pre-implant loss, and mild maternal toxicity. A dose of 0.10 mg/kg/day (about half the clinical dose on a mg/m^2 basis) given to rats on days six through 17 of gestation caused an increase in post-implantation mortality. This dose also caused an increase in total fetal malformations. The most frequent malformations were of the eye (microphthalmia, anophthalmia, rosette formation of the retina, coloboma of the retina, ectopic orbit), brain (dilated lateral and third ventricles), skull and vertebrae.

PRECAUTIONS:

General: Inadvertent extravasation with topotecan has been associated with only mild local reactions such as erythema and bruising.

Hematology: Monitoring of bone marrow function is essential (see WARNINGS and DOSAGE AND ADMINISTRATION).

Carcinogenesis, Mutagenesis, and Impairment of Fertility: Carcinogenicity testing of topotecan has not been performed. Topotecan, however, is known to be genotoxic to mammalian cells and is a probable carcinogen. Topotecan was mutagenic to L5178Y mouse lymphoma cells and clastogenic to cultured human lymphocytes with and without metabolic activation. It was also clastogenic to mouse bone marrow. Topotecan did not cause mutations in bacterial cells.

Pregnancy Category D: See WARNINGS.

Nursing Mothers: It is not known whether the drug is excreted in human milk. Breast-feeding should be discontinued when women are receiving topotecan (see CONTRAINDICATIONS).

Pediatric Use: Safety and effectiveness in pediatric patients have not bee established.

DRUG INTERACTIONS:

Concomitant administration of G-CSF can prolong the duration of neutropenia, so if G-CSF is to be used, it should not be initiated until day 6 of the course of therapy, 24 hours after completion of treatment with topotecan.[1]

Myelosuppression was more severe when topotecan was given in combination with cisplatin in Phase I studies. In a reported study on concomitant administration of cisplatin 50 mg/m^2 and topotecan at a dose of 1.25 mg/m^2/day x 5 days, one of three patients had neutropenia for 12 days and a second patient died with neutropenic sepsis. There are no adequate data to define a safe and effective regimen for topotecan and cisplatin in combination.

ADVERSE REACTIONS:

Data in the following section are based on the experience of 452 patients with metastatic ovarian carcinoma treated with topotecan. Table 2 lists the principal hematologic toxicities and Table 3 lists non-hematologic toxicities occurring in at least 19% of patients.

TABLE 2 Summary of Hematologic Adverse Events in Patients Receiving Topotecan Hydrochloride

	Patients n=452	Courses n=2375
Neutropenia		
<1,500 cells/mm^3	98	78
<500 cells/mm^3	81	40
Leukopenia		
<3,000 cells/mm^3	98	77
<1,000 cells/mm^3	32	11
Thrombocytopenia		
<75,000 cells/mm^3	63	39
<25,000 cells/mm^3	26	9
Anemia		
<10 g/dl	95	76
<8 g/dl	40	16
Sepsis or fever/infection with Grade 4 neutropenia	26	7
Platelet transfusions	13	4
RBC transfusions	56	23

TABLE 3A Summary of Non-hematologic Adverse Events in Patients Receiving Topotecan Hydrochloride

Non-hematologic Adverse Events	All Grades: % Incidence		Grade 3: % Incidence	
	n=452 Patients	n=2375 Courses	n=452 Patients	n=2375 Courses
Gastrointestinal				
Nausea	77	50	10	3
Vomiting	58	26	6	3
Diarrhea	42	19	4	1
Constipation	39	18	2	<1
Abdominal Pain	33	13	4	<1
Stomatitis	24	9	2	<1
Anorexia	19	8	2	<1
Body as a Whole				
Fatigue	37	25	6	2
Fever	34	13	1	<1
Asthenia	21	10	3	<1
Skin and Appendages				
Alopecia	59	62	NA	NA

Premedications were not routinely used in these clinical studies.

TABLE 3B Summary of Non-hematologic Adverse Events in Patients Receiving Topotecan Hydrochloride

Non-hematologic Adverse Events	Grade 4: % Incidence	
	n=452 Patients	n=2375 Courses
Gastrointestinal		
Nausea	<1	<1
Vomiting	3	<1
Diarrhea	<1	<1
Constipation	1	<1
Abdominal Pain	2	<1
Stomatitis	<1	<1
Anorexia	0	0
Body as a Whole		
Fatigue	0	0
Fever	<1	<1
Asthenia	1	<1
Skin and Appendages		
Alopecia	NA	NA

Premedications were not routinely used in these clinical studies.

ADVERSE REACTIONS: *(cont'd)*

Hematologic: (See WARNINGS.)

Gastrointestinal: The incidence of nausea was 77% (10% grade 3/4) and vomiting occurred in 58% (9% grade 3/4) of patients (see TABLE 3A and TABLE 3B). The prophylactic use of antiemetics was not routine in patients treated with topotecan. Forty-two percent of patients had diarrhea (5% grade 3/4), 39% constipation (3% grade 3/4) and 33% had abdominal pain (6% grade 3/4).

Skin/Appendages: Total alopecia (Grade 3) occurred in 42% of patients.

Central and Peripheral Nervous System: Headache (21%) was the most frequently reported neurologic toxicity. Parasthesia occurred in 9% of patients but was generally Grade 1.

Liver/Biliary: Grade 1 transient elevations in SGOT/AST and SGPT/ALT occurred in 5% of patients. Greater elevations, grade 3/4, occurred in <1%. Grade 3/4 eleveated bilirubin occurred in <3% of patients.

Respiratory: Dyspnea (20%); Grade 3/4 dyspnea (4%). TABLE 4 shows the grade 3/4 hematologic and major non-hematologic adverse events in the topotecan/paclitaxel comparator trial.

TABLE 4 Comparative Toxicity Profiles for Ovarian Cancer Patients Randomized to Receive Topotecan Hydrochloride or Paclitaxel

Adverse Event	Topotecan HCl		Paclitaxel	
	Pts n=112 %	Courses n=555 %	Pts n=114 %	Courses n=550 %
Hematologic Grade 3/4				
Grade 4 neutropenia (<500 cells/ml)	79.5	36.7	21.9	8.5
Grade 3/4 Anemia (Hgb < 8 g/dl)	40.5	16.0	6.3	2.0
Grade 4 Thrombocytopenia (<25,000 plts/ml)	25.3	9.6	1.8	0.4
Fever/Grade 4 neutropenia	23.2	5.4	2.6	0.5
Documented Sepsis	5.4	1.1	1.8	0.4
Death related to Sepsis	1.8	0.4	0.0	0.0
Non-Hemotologic Grade 3/4				
Gastrointestinal				
Abdominal pain	5.4	1.1	3.5	0.9
Constipation	5.4	1.1	0.0	0.0
Diarrhea	6.3	1.6	0.9	0.2
Intestinal Obstruction	4.5	1.1	4.4	0.9
Nausea	8.9	3.1	1.8	0.4
Stomatitis	0.9	0.2	0.9	0.2
Vomiting	9.8	2.0	2.6	0.5
Constitutional				
Anorexia	3.6	0.2	0.0	0.0
Dyspnea	6.3	1.8	5.3	1.3
Fatigue	8.0	2.2	5.3	2.0
Malaise	1.8	0.5	1.8	0.4
Neuromuscular				
Arthralgia	0.9	0.2	3.5	0.5
Asthenia	5.4	1.8	3.5	1.3
Headache	0.9	0.2	1.8	0.9
Myalgia	0.0	0.0	2.6	1.6
Pain	5.4	1.1	10.5	2.2

Premedications were not routinely used in patients randomized to topotecan hydrochloride, while patients receiving paclitaxel received routine pretreatment with corticosteroids, diphenhydramine, and histamine receptor type 2 blockers.

OVERDOSAGE:

There is no known antidote for overdosage with topotecan hydrochloride. The primary anticipated complication of overdosage would consist of bone marrow suppression.

The LD_{10} in mice receiving single intravenous infusions of topotecan hydrochloride was 75 mg/m^2(CI 95%: 47 to 97).

DOSAGE AND ADMINISTRATION:

Prior to administration of the first course of topotecan hydrochloride, patients must have a baseline neutrophil count of > 1500 cells/mm^3 and a platelet count of >100,000 cells/mm^3. The recommended dose of topotecan is 1.5 $mg/m^2$by intravenous infusion over 30 minutes daily for 5 consecutive days, starting on day one of a 210day course. A minimum of four courses is recommended because median time to response in three clinical trials was 9 to 12 weeks. In the event of severe neutropenia during any course, the dose should be reduced by 0.25 mg/m^2 for subsequent courses. Alternatively, in the event of severe neutropenia, G-CSF may be administered following the subsequent course (before resorting to dose reduction) starting from Day 6 of the course (24 hours after completion of topotecan administration).

ADJUSTMENT OF DOSE IN SPECIAL POPULATIONS

Hepatic Impairment: No dosage adjustment appears to be required for treating patients with impaired hepatic function (plasma bilirubin >1.5 to <10 mg/dl).

Renal Functional Impairment: No dosage adjustment appears to be required for treating patients with mild renal impairment (Cl_{cr} 40 to 60 ml/min). Dosage adjustment to 0.75 mg/m^2 is recommended for patients with moderate renal impairment (20 to 39 ml/min). Insufficient data are available in patients with severe renal impairment to provide a dosage recommendation.

Elderly Patients: No dosage adjustment appears to be needed in the elderly, other than adjustments related to renal function.

PREPARATION FOR ADMINISTRATION

Precautions: Topotecan hydrochloride is a cytotoxic anticancer drug. As with other potentially toxic compounds, topotecan should be prepared under a vertical laminar flow hood while wearing gloves and protective clothing. If topotecan solution contacts the skin, wash the skin immediately and thoroughly with soap and water. If topotecan contacts mucous membranes, flush thoroughly with water.

Preparation for Intravenous Administration: Each topotecan 4 mg vial is reconsitituted with 4 mL Sterile Water for Injection. Then the appropriate volume of the reconstituted solution is diluted in either 0.9% Sodium Chloride Intravenous Infusion or 5% Dextrose Intravenous Infusion prior to administration.

Because the lyophilized dosage form contains no antibacterial preservative, the reconstituted product should be used immediately.

DOSAGE AND ADMINISTRATION: *(cont'd)*

STABILITY

Unopened vials of topotecan hydrochloride are stable until the date indicated on the package when stored between 20° and 25°C (68° and 77°F) and protected from light in the original package. Because the vials contain no preservatives, contents should be used immediately after reconstitution.

Reconstituted vials of topotecan hydrochloride diluted for infusion are stable at approximately 20° to 25°C (68° to 77°F) and ambient lighting conditions for 24 hours.

REFERENCES:

1. Rowinsky, et al. Phase 1 and pharmacologic study of high doses of the topoisomerase I inhibitor topotecan with granulocyte colony-stimulating factor in patients with solid tumors. J Clin Oncol. 1996; 14: 1224–1235. **2.** Recommendations for the safe handling of parenteral antineoplastic drugs. NIH Publication No. 83–2621. For sale by the Superintendent of Documents, US Government Printing Office, Washington, DC 20402. **3.** AMA Council Report. Guidelines for handling parenteral antineoplastics. JAMA 1985;253(11): 1590–1592. **4.** National Study Commission on Cytotoxic Exposure-recommendations for handling cytotoxic agents. Available from Louis P. Jeffry, Chairman, National Study Commission on Cytotoxic Exposure. Massachusetts College of Pharmacy and Allied Health Sciences, 179 Longwood Avenue, Boston, Massachusetts, 02115. **5.** Clinical Oncological Society of Australia. Guidelines and recommendations for safe handling of antineoplastic agents. Med J Austr. 1983;1: 426–428. **6.** Jones RB, et al. Safe handling of chemotherapeutic agents: A report from the Mount Sinai Medical Center. CA-A Cancer Journal for Clinicians 1983; Sep./Oct.: 258–263. **7.** American Society of Hospital Pharmacists Technical Assistance Bulletin on Handling Cytotoxic and Hazardous Drugs. Am J Hos Pharm 1990;47: 1033–1049. **8.** OSHA Work-Practice guidelines for personnel dealing with cytotoxic (antineoplastic) drugs. Am J Hosp Pharm 1986;43: 1193–1204.

HOW SUPPLIED:

Topotecan hydrochloride for injection is supplied in 4 mg (free base) single-dose vials, in packages of 5 vials.

Storage: Store the vials protected from light in the original cartons at controlled room temperature between 20° and 25°C (68° and 77°F).

Handling and Disposal: Procedures for proper handling and disposal of anticancer drugs should be used. Several guidelines on this subject have been published.[2–8] There is no general agreement that all of the procedures recommended in the guidelines are necessary or appropriate.

HOW SUPPLIED - EQUIVALENTS NOT AVAILABLE:

Injection - Intravenous - 4 mg

4 mg vials x 5 $2,437.50 HYCAMTIN, SKB Pharms 00007-4201-05

TOREMIFENE CITRATE *(003273)*

CATEGORIES: Antineoplastics; Breast Carcinoma; Cancer; Chemotherapy; Oncologic Drugs; Tumors; FDA Unapproved

BRAND NAMES: **Fareston**

Prescribing information not available at time of publication.

TORSEMIDE *(003179)*

CATEGORIES: Antihypertensives; Cardiovascular Drugs; Cirrhosis; Congestive Heart Failure; Diuretics; Edema; Electrolytic, Caloric-Water Balance; Heart Failure; Hypertension; Loop Diuretics; FDA Class 1S ("Standard Review"); FDA Approved 1993 Aug

BRAND NAMES: **Demadex**; Presaril; *Unat*
(International brand names outside U.S. in italics)

COST OF THERAPY: $177.93 (Edema; Tablet; 10 mg; 1/day; 365 days) vs. Potential Cost of $5,887.41 (Edema)

DESCRIPTION:

Torsemide is a diuretic of the pyridine-sulfonylurea class. Its chemical name is 1-isopropyl-3-[(4-*m*-toluidino-3-pyridyl)sulfonyl]urea.

Its empirical formula is $C_{16}H_{20}N_4O_3S$, its pKa is 7.1, and its molecular weight is 348.43.

Demadex is a white to off-white crystalline powder. The tablets for oral administration also contain lactose NF, crospovidone NF, povidone USP, microcrystalline cellulose NF, and magnesium stearate NF. Torsemide ampuls for intravenous injection contain a sterile solution of torsemide (10 mg/ml), polyethylene glycol-400 NF, tromethamine USP, and sodium hydroxide NF (as needed to adjust pH) in water for injection USP.

CLINICAL PHARMACOLOGY:

Mechanism of Action: Micropuncture studies in animals have shown that torsemide acts from within the lumen of the thick ascending portion of the loop of Henle, where it inhibits the $Na^+/K^+/2Cl^-$ carrier system. Clinical pharmacology studies hav e confirmed this site of action in humans, and effects in other segments of the nephron have not been demonstrated. Diuretic activity thus correlates better with the rate of drug excretion in the urine than with the concentration in the blood.

Torsemide increases the urinary excretion of sodium, chloride, and water, but it does not significantly alter glomerular filtration rate, renal plasma flow, or acid-base balance.

Pharmacokinetics and Metabolism: The **bioavailability** of torsemide tablets is approximately 80%, with little intersubject variation; the 90% confidence interval is 75% to 89%. The drug is absorbed with little first-pass metabolism, and the serum concentration reaches its peak (C_{max}) within one hour after oral administration. C_{max} and area under the serum concentration-time curve (AUC) after oral administration are proportional to dose over the range of 2.5 to 200 mg. Simultaneous food intake delays the time to C_{max} by about 30 minutes, but overall bioavailability (AUC) and diuretic activity are unchanged. Absorption is essentially unaffected by renal or hepatic dysfunction.

The **volume of distribution** of torsemide is 12 to 15 liters in normal adults or in patients with mild to moderate renal failure or congestive heart failure. In patients with hepatic cirrhosis, the volume of distribution is approximately doubled.

In normal subjects the **elimination half-life** of torsemide is approximately 3.5 hours. Torsemide is cleared from the circulation by both hepatic metabolism (approximately 80% of total clearance) and excretion into the urine (approximately 20% of total clearance in patients with normal renal function). The major metabolite in humans is the carboxylic acid derivative, which is biologically inactive. Two of the lesser metabolites possess some diuretic activity, but for practical purposes metabolism terminates the action of the drug.

CLINICAL PHARMACOLOGY: *(cont'd)*

Because torsemide is extensively bound to plasma protein (>99%), very little enters tubular urine via glomerular filtration. Most renal clearance of torsemide occurs via active secretion of the drug by the proximal tubules into tubular urine.

In patients with decompensated congestive heart failure, hepatic and renal clearance are both reduced, probably because of hepatic congestion and decreased renal plasma flow, respectively. The total clearance of torsemide is approximately 50% of that seen in healthy volunteers, and the plasma half-life and AUC are correspondingly increased. Because of reduced renal clearance, a smaller fraction of any given dose is delivered to the intraluminal site of action, so at any given dose there is less natriuresis in patients with congestive heart failure than in normal subjects.

In patients with renal failure, renal clearance of torsemide is markedly decreased but total plasma clearance is not significantly altered. A smaller fraction of the administered dose is delivered to the intraluminal site of action, and the natriuretic action of any given dose of diuretic is reduced. A diuretic response in renal failure may still be achieved if patients are given higher doses. The total plasma clearance and elimination half-life of torsemide remain normal under the conditions of impaired renal function because metabolic elimination by the liver remains intact.

In patients with hepatic cirrhosis, the volume of distribution, plasma half-life, and renal clearance are all increased, but total clearance in unchanged.

The pharmacokinetic profile of torsemide in healthy elderly subjects is similar to that in young subjects except for a decrease in renal clearance related to the decline in renal function that commonly occurs with aging. However, total plasma clearance and elimination half- life remain unchanged.

Clinical Effects: The diuretic effects of torsemide begin within 10 minutes of intravenous dosing and peak within the first hour. With oral dosing, the onset of diuresis occurs within one hour and the peak effect occurs during the first or second hour. Independent of the route of administration, diuresis lasts about six to eight hours. In healthy subjects given doses, the dose-response relationship for sodium excretion is linear over the dose range of 2.5 to 20 mg. The increase in potassium excretion is negligible after a single dose of up to 10 mg and only slight (5 to 15 mEq) after a single dose of 20 mg.

Torsemide has been studied in controlled rials in patients with New York Heart Association Class II to Class IV **congestive heart failure**. Patients who received 10 to 20 mg of daily torsemide in these studies achieved significantly greater reductions in weight and edema than did patients who received placebo.

In single-dose studies in patients with **nonanuric renal failure**, high doses of torsemide (20 to 200 mg) caused marked increases in water and sodium excretion. In patients with nonanuric renal failure severe enough to require hemodialysis, chronic treatment with up to 200 mg of daily torsemide has not been shown to change steady-state fluid retention. Chronic use of any diuretic in renal disease has not been studied in adequate and well-controlled trials. When patients in a study of acute renal failure received total daily doses of 520 to 1200 mg of torsemide, 26% experienced seizures; seizures were also seen in similar patients who received comparatively high doses of furosemide, but not in similar patients who received placebo.

When given with aldosterone antagonists, torsemide also caused increases in sodium and fluid excretion in patients with edema or ascites due to **hepatic cirrhosis**. Urinary sodium excretion rate relative to the urinary excretion rate of torsemide is less in cirrhotic patients than in healthy subjects (possibly because of the hyperaldosteronism and resultant sodium retention that are characteristic of portal hypertension and ascites). However, because of the increased renal clearance of torsemide in patients with hepatic cirrhosis, these factors tens to balance each other, and the result is an overall natriuretic response that is similar to that seen in healthy subjects. Chronic use of any diuretic in hepatic disease has not been studied in adequate and well-controlled trials.

In patients with **essential hypertension**, torsemide has been shown in controlled studies to lower blood pressure when administered once a day at doses of 5 to 10 mg. The antihypertensive effect is near maximal after four to six weeks of treatment, but it may continue to increase for up to 12 weeks. Systolic and diastolic supine and standing blood pressures are reduced. There is no significant orthostatic effect, and there is only a minimal peak-trough difference in blood pressure reduction.

The antihypertensive effects of torsemide are, like those of other diuretics, on the average greater in black patients (a low-renin population) than in non-black patients.

When torsemide is first administered, daily urinary sodium excretion increases for at least a week. With chronic administration, however, daily sodium loss comes into balance with dietary sodium intake. If the administration of torsemide is suddenly stopped, blood pressure returns to pretreatment levels over several days, without overshoot.

Torsemide has been administered together with β-adrenergic blocking agents, ACE inhibitors, and calcium-channel blockers. Adverse drug interactions have not been observed, and special dosage adjustment has not been necessary.

INDICATIONS AND USAGE:

Torsemide is indicated for the treatment of edema associated with congestive heart failure, renal disease, or hepatic disease. Chronic use of any diuretic in renal or hepatic disease has not been studied in adequate and well-controlled trials.

Torsemide intravenous injection is indicated when a rapid onset of diuresis is desired or when oral administration is impractical.

Torsemide is indicated for the treatment of hypertension alone or in combination with other antihypertensive agents.

CONTRAINDICATIONS:

Torsemide is contraindicated in patients with known hypersensitivity to torsemide or to sulfonylureas.

Torsemide is contraindicated in patients who are anuric.

WARNINGS:

Hepatic Disease With Cirrhosis And Ascites: Torsemide should be used with caution in patients with hepatic disease with cirrhosis and ascites, since sudden alterations of fluid and electrolyte balance may precipitate hepatic coma. In these patients, diuresis with torsemide (or any other diuretic) is best initiated in the hospital. To prevent hypokalemia and metabolic alkalosis, an aldosterone antagonist or potassium-sparing drug should be used concomitantly with torsemide.

Ototoxicity: Tinnitus and hearing loss (usually reversible) have been observed after rapid intravenous injection of other loop diuretics and have also been observed after oral torsemide. It is not certain that these events were attributable to torsemide. Ototoxicity

WARNINGS: *(cont'd)*

has also been seen in animal studies when very high plasma levels of torsemide were induced. Administered intravenously, torsemide should be injected slowly over two minutes, and single doses should not exceed 200 mg.

Volume And Electrolyte Depletion: Patients receiving should be observed for clinical evidence of electrolyte imbalance, hypovolemia, or prenatal azotemia. Symptoms of these disturbances may include one or more of the following: dryness of the mouth, thirst, weakness, lethargy, drowsiness, restlessness, muscle pains or cramps, muscular fatigue, hypotension, oliguria, tachycardia, nausea, and vomiting. Excessive diuresis may cause dehydration, blood-volume reduction, and possible thrombosis and embolism, especially in elderly patients. In patients who develop fluid and electrolyte imbalances, hypovolemia, or prenatal azotemia, the observed laboratory changes may include hyper- or hyponatremia, hyper- or hypochloremia, hyper- or hypokalemia, acid-base abnormalities, and increased blood urea nitrogen. If any of these occur, torsemide should be discontinued until the situation is corrected; torsemide may be restarted at a lower dose.

In controlled studies in the United States, torsemide was administered to hypertensive patients at doses of 5 mg or 10 mg daily. After six weeks at these doses, the mean decrease in serum potassium was approximately 0.1 mEq/L. The percentage of patients who had a serum potassium level below 3.5 mEq/L at any time during the studies was essentially the same in patients who received torsemide (1.5%) as in those who received placebo (3%). In patients followed for one year, there was no further change in mean serum potassium levels. In patients with congestive heart failure, hepatic cirrhosis, or renal disease treated with torsemide at doses higher than those studied in U.S. antihypertensive trials, hypokalemia was observed with greater frequency, in a dose-related manner.

In patients with cardiovascular disease, especially those receiving digitalis glycosides, diuretic-induced hypokalemia may be a risk factor for the development of arrhythmias. The risk of hypokalemia is greatest in patients with cirrhosis of the liver, in patients experiencing a brisk diuresis, in patients who are receiving inadequate oral intake of electrolytes, and in patients receiving concomitant therapy with corticosteroids or ACTH.

Periodic monitoring of serum potassium and other electrolytes is advised in patients treated with torsemide.

PRECAUTIONS:

LABORATORY VALUES

Potassium: See statement in WARNINGS.

Calcium: Single doses of torsemide increased the urinary excretion of calcium by normal subjects, but serum calcium levels were slightly increased in four- to six-week hypertension trials. In a long-term study of patients with congestive heart failure, the average one-year change in serum calcium was a decrease of 0.10 mg/dL (0.02 mmol/L). Among 426 patients treated with torsemide for an average of 11 months, hypocalcemia was not reported as an adverse event.

Magnesium: Dingle doses of torsemide caused healthy volunteers to increase the urinary excretion of magnesium, but serum magnesium levels were slightly increased in four- to six-week hypertension trials. In long-term hypertension studies, the average one- year change in serum magnesium was an increase of 0.03 mg/dL (0.01 mmol/L). Among 426 patients treated with torsemide for an average of 11 months, one case of hypomagnesemia (1.3 mg/dL (0.53 mmol/L)) was reported as an adverse event.

In a long-term clinical study of torsemide in patients with congestive heart failure, the estimated annual change in serum magnesium was an increase of 0.2 mg/dL (0.08 mmol/L), but these data are confounded by the fact that many of these patients received magnesium supplements. In a four-week study in which magnesium supplementation was not given, the rate of occurrence of serum magnesium levels below 1.7 mg/dL (0.70 mmol/L was 6% and 9% in the groups receiving 5 mg and 10 mg of torsemide, respectively.

Blood Urea Nitrogen (Bun), Creatinine, And Uric Acid: Torsemide produces small dose-related increases in each of these laboratory values. In hypertensive patients who received 10 mg of torsemide daily for six weeks, the mean increase in blood urea nitrogen was 1.8 mg/dL (0.6 mmol.L), the mean in serum creatinine was 0.05 mg/dL (4 mcgmol/L), and the mean increase in serum uric acid was 1.2 mg/dL (70 mcmol/L). Little further change occurred with long-term treatment, and all changes reversed when treatment was discontinued.

Symptomatic gout has been reported in patients receiving torsemide, but its incidence has been similar to that in patients receiving placebo.

Glucose: Hypertensive patients who received 10 mg of daily torsemide experienced a mean increase in serum glucose concentration of 5.5 mg/dL (0.3 mmol/L) after six weeks of therapy, with a further increase of 1.8 mg/dL (0.1 mmol/L) during the subsequent year. In long-term studies in diabetics, mean fasting glucose values were not significantly changed from baseline. Cases of hyperglycemia have been reported but are uncommon.

Serum Lipids: In the controlled short-term hypertension studies in the United States, daily doses of 5,10, and 20 mg of torsemide were associated with increases in total plasma cholesterol of 4, 4, and 8 mg/dL (0.10 to 0.20 mmol/L), respectively. The changes subsided during chronic therapy.

In the same short-term hypertension studies, daily doses of 5, 10, and 20 mg of torsemide were associated with mean increases in plasma triglycerides of 16, 13, and 71 mg/dL (0.15 to 0.80 mmmol/L), respectively.

In long-term studies of 5 to 20 mg of torsemide daily, no clinically significant differences from baseline lipid values were observed after one year of therapy.

Other: In long-term studies in hypertensive patients, torsemide has been associated with small mean decreases in hemoglobin, hematocrit, and erythrocyte count and small mean increases in white blood cell count, platelet count, and serum alkaline phosphatase. Although statistically significant, all of these changes were medically inconsequential. No significant trends have been observed in any liver enzyme tests other than alkaline phosphatase.

CARCINOGENESIS, MUTAGENESIS, AND IMPAIRMENT OF FERTILITY

No overall increase in tumor incidence was found when torsemide was given to rats and mice throughout their lives at dose up to 9 mg/kg/day (rats) and 32 mg/kg/day (mice). On a body-weight basis, these doses are 27 to 96 times a human dose of 20 mg; on a body-surface-area basis, they are 5 to 8 times this dose. In the rat study, the high-dose female group demonstrated renal tubular injury, interstitial inflammation, and a statistically significant increase in renal adenomas and carcinomas. The tumor incidence in this group was, however, not much higher than the incidence sometimes seen in historical controls. Similar signs of chronic non-neoplastic renal injury have been reported in high- dose animal studies of other diuretics such as furosemide and hydrochlorothiazide.

PRECAUTIONS: *(cont'd)*

No mutagenic activity was detected in any of a variety of *in vivo* and *in vitro* tests of torsemide and its major human metabolite. The tests included the Ames test in bacteria (with and without metabolic activation), tests for chromosome aberrations and sister-chromatid exchanges in human lymphocytes, tests for various nuclear anomalies in cells found in hamster and murine bone marrow, tests for unscheduled DNA synthesis in mice and rats, and others.

In doses up to 25 mg/kg/day (75 times a human dose of 20 mg on a body-weight basis; 13 times this dose on a body-surface-area basis), torsemide had no adverse effect on the reproductive performance of male or female rats.

PREGNANCY CATEGORY B

There was no fetotoxicity or teratogenicity in rats treated with up to 5 mg/kg/day of torsemide (on a mg/kg basis, this is 15 times a human dose of 20 mg/day; on a mg/m^2 basis, 1.7 times this dose). Fetal and maternal toxicity (decrease in average body weight, increase in fetal resorption, and delayed fetal ossification) occurred in rabbits and rats given doses 4 (rabbits) and 5 (rats) times larger. Adequate and well-controlled studies have not been carried out in pregnant women.

Because animal reproduction studies are not always predictive of human response, this drug should be used during pregnancy only if clearly needed.

LABOR AND DELIVERY

The effect of torsemide on labor and delivery is unknown.

NURSING MOTHERS

It is not known whether torsemide is excreted in human milk. Because many drugs are excreted in human milk, caution should be exercised when torsemide is administered to a nursing woman.

GERIATRIC USE

Of the total number of patients who received torsemide in U.S. clinical studies, 24% were 65 or older while about 4% were 75 or older. No specific age-related differences in effectiveness or safety were observed between younger patients and elderly patients.

PEDIATRIC USE

Safety and effectiveness in children have not been established.

Administration of another loop diuretic to severely premature infants with edema due to patent ductus arteriosus and hyaline membrane disease has occasionally been associated with renal calcifications, sometimes barely visible on x-ray but sometimes in staghorn form, filling the renal pelves. Some of these calculi have been dissolved, and hypercalciuria has been reported to have decreased, when chlorothiazide has been coadministered along with the loop diuretic. In other premature neonates with hyaline membrane disease, another loop diuretic has been reported to increase the risk of persistent patent ductus arteriosus, possibly through a prostaglandin-E-mediated process. The use of torsemide in such patients has not been studied.

DRUG INTERACTIONS:

In patients with essential hypertension, torsemide has been administered together with β-blockers, ACE inhibitors, and calcium- channel blockers. In patients with congestive heart failure, torsemide has been administered together with digitalis glycosides, ACE inhibitors, and organic nitrates. None of these combined uses was associated with new or unexpected adverse events.

Torsemide does not affect the protein binding of **glyburide** or of **warfarin**, the anticoagulant effect of **phenprocoumon** (a related coumarin derivative), or the pharmacokinetics of **digoxin** or **carvedilol** (a vasodilator/β-blocker). In healthy subjects, coadministration of torsemide was associated with significant reduction in the renal clearance of **spironolactone**, with corresponding increases in the AUC. However, clinical experience indicates that dosage adjustment of either agent is not required.

Because torsemide and salicylates compete for secretion by renal tubules, patients receiving high doses of **salicylates** may experience salicylate toxicity when torsemide is concomitantly administered. Also, although possible interactions between torsemide and **nonsteroidal anti-inflammatory agents (including aspirin)** have not been studied, coadministration of these agents with another loop diuretic (furosemide) has occasionally been associated with renal dysfunction.

The natriuretic effect of torsemide (like that of many other diuretics) is partially inhibited by the concomitant administration of **indomethacin**. This effect has been demonstrated for torsemide under conditions of dietary sodium restriction (50 mEq/day) but not in the presence of normal sodium intake (150 mEq/day).

The pharmacokinetic profile and diuretic activity of torsemide are not altered by **cimetidine** or **spironolactone**. Coadministration of **digoxin** is reported to increase the area under the curve for torsemide by 50%, but dose adjustment of torsemide is not necessary.

Concomitant use of torsemide and cholestyramine has not been studied in humans but, in a study of animals, coadministration of cholestyramine decreased the absorption of orally administered torsemide. If torsemide and cholestyramine are used concomitantly, simultaneous administration is not recommended.

Coadministration of **probenecid** reduces secretion of torsemide into the proximal tubule and thereby decreases the diuretic activity of torsemide.

Other diuretics are known to reduce the renal clearance of **lithium**, inducing a high risk of lithium toxicity, so coadministration of lithium and diuretics should be undertaken with great caution, if at all. Coadministration of lithium and torsemide has not been studied.

Other diuretics have been reported to increase the ototoxic potential of**aminoglycoside antibiotics** and of **ethacrynic acid**, especially in the presence of impaired renal function. These potential interactions with torsemide have not been studied.

ADVERSE REACTIONS:

At the time of approval, torsemide had been evaluated for safety in approximately 4000 subjects: over 800 of these subjects received torsemide for at least six months, and over 380 were treated for more than one year. Among these subjects were 564 who received torsemide during U.S.-based trials in which 274 other subjects received placebo.

The reported side effects of torsemide were generally transient, and there was no relationship between side effects and age, sex, race, or duration of therapy. Discontinuation of therapy due to side effects occurred in 3.5% of U.S. patients treated with torsemide and in 4.4% of patients treated with placebo. In studies conducted in the United States and Europe, discontinuation rates due to side effects were 3.0% (38/1250) with torsemide and 3.4% (13/380) with furosemide in patients with congestive heart failure, 2.0% (8/409) with torsemide and 4.8% (11/230) with furosemide in patients with renal insufficiency, and 7.6% (13/170) with torsemide and 0% (0/33) with furosemide in

patients with cirrhosis.

The most common reasons for discontinuation of therapy with torsemide were (in descending order of frequency) dizziness, headache, nausea, weakness, vomiting, hyperglycemia, excessive urination, hyperuricemia, hypokalemia, excessive thirst, hypovolemia, impotence, esophageal hemorrhage, and dyspepsia. Dropout rates for these adverse events ranged from 0.1% to 0.5%.

ADVERSE REACTIONS: *(cont'd)*

The side effects considered possibly or probably related to study drug that occurred in U.S. placebo-controlled trials in more than 1% of patients treated with torsemide are shown in the table below.

TABLE 1 Torsemide, Adverse Reactions
Reactions Possibly or Probably Drug-Related U.S. Placebo-Controlled Studies Incidence (Percentages of Patients)

	Torsemide (N=564)	Placebo (N=274)
headache	7.3	9.1
excessive urination	6.7	2.2
dizziness	3.2	4.0
rhinitis	2.8	2.2
asthenia	2.0	1.5
diarrhea	2.0	1.1
ECG abnormality	2.0	0.4
cough increase	2.0	1.5
constipation	1.8	0.7
nausea	1.8	0.4
arthralgia	1.8	0.7
dyspepsia	1.6	0.7
sore throat	1.6	0.7
myalgia	1.6	0.7
chest pain	1.2	0.4
insomnia	1.2	1.5
edema	1.1	1.1
nervousness	1.1	0.4

The daily doses of torsemide used in these trials ranged from 1.25 to 20 mg, with most patients receiving 5 to 10 mg; the duration of treatment ranged from one to 52 days, with a median of 41 days. Of the side effects listed in the table, only "excessive urination" occurred significantly more frequently in patients treated with torsemide than in patients treated with placebo, 4% of those treated with 5 mg of daily torsemide, and 15% of those treated with 10 mg. The complaint of excessive urination was generally not reported as an adverse event among patients who received torsemide for cardiac, renal, or hepatic failure.

Serious adverse events reported in the clinical studies for which a drug relationship could not be excluded were atrial fibrillation, chest pain, diarrhea, digitalis intoxication, gastrointestinal hemorrhage, hyperglycemia, hyperuricemia, hypokalemia, hypotension, hypovolemia, shunt thrombosis, rash rectal bleeding, syncope, and ventricular tachycardia.

Angioedema has been reported in a patient exposed to torsemide who was later found to be allergic to sulfa drugs.

Of the adverse reactions during placebo-controlled trials listed without taking into account assessment of relatedness to drug therapy, arthritis and various other nonspecific musculoskeletal problems were more frequently reported in association with torsemide than with placebo, even though gout was somewhat more frequently associated with placebo. These reactions did not increase in frequency or severity with the dose of torsemide. One patient in the group treated with torsemide withdrew due to myalgia, and one in the placebo group withdrew due to gout.

Hypokalemia: See statement in WARNINGS.

OVERDOSAGE:

There is no human experience with overdoses of torsemide, but the signs and symptoms of overdosage can be anticipated to be those of excessive pharmacologic effect: dehydration, hypovolemia, hypotension, hyponatremia, hypokalemia, hypochloremic alkalosis, and hemoconcentration. Treatment of overdosage should consist of fluid and electrolyte replacement.

Laboratory determinations of serum levels of torsemide and its metabolites are not widely available.

No data are available to suggest physiological maneuvers (*e.g.*, maneuvers to change the pH of the urine) that might accelerate elimination of torsemide and its metabolites. Torsemide is not dialyzable, so hemodialysis will not accelerate elimination.

DOSAGE AND ADMINISTRATION:

General: Torsemide tablets may be given at any time in relation to a meal, as convenient. Special dosage adjustment in the elderly is not necessary.

Because of the high bioavailability of torsemide, oral and intravenous doses are therapeutically equivalent, so patients may be switched to and from the intravenous form with no change in dose. torsemide intravenous injection should be administered slowly over a period of two minutes.

Before administration, the solution of torsemide should be visually inspected for discoloration and particulate matter. If either is found, the ampul should not be used.

Congestive Heart Failure: The usual initial dose is 10 mg or 20 mg of once-daily oral or intravenous torsemide. If the diuretic response is inadequate, the dose should be titrated upward by approximately doubling until the desired diuretic response is obtained. Single doses higher than 200 mg have not been adequately studied.

Chronic Renal Failure: The usual initial dose of torsemide is 20 mg of once-daily oral or intravenous torsemide. If the diuretic response is inadequate, the dose should be titrated upward by approximately doubling until the desired diuretic response is obtained. Single doses higher than 200 mg have not been adequately studied.

Chronic use of any diuretic in renal disease has not been studied in adequate and well-controlled trials.

Hepatic Cirrhosis: The usual initial is 5 to 10 mg of once-daily oral or intravenous torsemide, administered together with an aldosterone antagonist or a potassium-sparing diuretic. If the diuretic response is inadequate, the dose should be titrated upward by approximately doubling until the desired diuretic response is obtained. Single doses higher than 40 mg have not been adequately studied.

Chronic use of any diuretic in hepatic disease has not been studied in adequate and well-controlled trials.

Hypertension: The usual initial dose is 5 mg once daily. If the 5 mg dose does not provide adequate reduction in blood pressure within four to six weeks, the dose may be increased to 10 mg once daily. If the response to 10 mg is insufficient, an additional antihypertensive agent should be added to the treatment regimen.

HOW SUPPLIED:

Torsemide for oral administration is available as white, scored tablets containing 5, 10, 20, or 100 mg of torsemide. The 5, 10 and 20 mg tablets are oval. The 100 mg tablet is capsule shaped.

Each tablet is debossed on the scored side with the Boehringer Mannheim logo and a portion (102, 103, 104, or 105) of the National Drug Code. On the opposite side, the tablet is debossed with 5, 10, 20, or 100 to indicate the dose.

HOW SUPPLIED: *(cont'd)*

Torsemide for intravenous injection is supplied in clear ampuls containing 2 ml (20 mg,) or 5 ml (50 mg) of a 10 mg/ml sterile solution.

Storage: Store all dosage forms at controlled room temperature, 15-30°C (59-86°F). Do not freeze.

(Boehringer Mannheim, 7/94, 626222)

HOW SUPPLIED - EQUIVALENTS NOT AVAILABLE:

Injection, Solution - Intravenous - 10 mg/ml

2 ml x 10	$35.75	DEMADEX, Boehringer Mannheim	53169-0108-80
5 ml x 10	$50.50	DEMADEX, Boehringer Mannheim	53169-0108-81

Tablet, Uncoated - Oral - 5 mg

100's	$43.75	DEMADEX, Boehringer Mannheim	53169-0102-01
100's	$45.00	DEMADEX, Boehringer Mannheim	53169-0102-60

Tablet, Uncoated - Oral - 10 mg

100's	$48.75	DEMADEX, Boehringer Mannheim	53169-0103-01
100's	$48.75	DEMADEX, Boehringer Mannheim	53169-0103-60

Tablet, Uncoated - Oral - 20 mg

100's	$52.50	DEMADEX, Boehringer Mannheim	53169-0104-60
100's	$56.25	DEMADEX, Boehringer Mannheim	53169-0104-01

Tablet, Uncoated - Oral - 100 mg

100's	$216.25	DEMADEX, Boehringer Mannheim	53169-0105-01
100's	$222.50	DEMADEX, Boehringer Mannheim	53169-0105-60

TRAMADOL HYDROCHLORIDE *(003255)*

CATEGORIES: Analgesics; Central Nervous System Agents; Opiate Agonists (Controlled); Pain; FDA Class 1S ("Standard Review"); FDA Approved 1995 Mar; Top 200 Drugs

BRAND NAMES: *Contramal*; *Exopen*; *Mabron*; *Tadol*; *Tradol* (Mexico); *Tramal* (Germany); *Tramed*; *Tramol*; *Tridol*; **Ultram**; *Zipan*
(International brand names outside U.S. in italics)

DESCRIPTION:

Ultram (tramadol hydrochloride) is a centrally acting analgesic. The chemical name for tramadol hydrochloride is (±)*cis*-2- [(dimethylamino)methyl]-1-(3-methoxyphenyl cyclohexanol hydrochloride. The molecular weight of tramadol hydrochloride is 299.8.

Tramadol hydrochloride is a white, bitter, crystalline and odorless powder. It is readily soluble in water and ethanol and has a pKa of 9.41. The water/n-octanol partition coefficient is 1.35 at pH 7. Ultram tablets contain 50 mg of tramadol hydrochloride and are white in color. Inactive ingredients in the tablet are corn starch, hydroxypropyl methylcellulose, lactose, magnesium stearate, microcrystalline cellulose, polyethylene glycol, polysorbate 80, sodium starch glycolate, titanium dioxide and wax.

CLINICAL PHARMACOLOGY:

PHARMACODYNAMICS

Tramadol is a centrally acting synthetic analgesic compound that is not derived from natural sources nor is it chemically related to opiates. Although its mode of action is not completely understood from animal tests, at least two complementary mechanisms appear applicable; binding to μ-opioid receptors and inhibition of reuptake of norepinephrine and serotonin. Tramadol opioid activity derives from low affinity binding of the parent compound to μ-opioid receptors and higher affinity binding of the M1 metabolite. In animal models, M1 is up to 6 times more potent than tramadol in producing analgesia and 200 times more potent in μ-opioid binding. The contribution to human analgesia of tramadol relative to M1 is unknown.

Tramadol-induced antinociception is only partially antagonized by the opiate antagonist naloxone in several animal tests. In addition, tramadol has been shown to inhibit reuptake of norepinephrine and serotonin *in vitro*, as have some other opioid analgesics. These latter mechanisms may contribute independently to the overall analgesic profile of tramadol. Onset of analgesia in humans is evident within one hour after administration and reaches a peak in approximately two to three hours. Peak plasma concentrations are reached about two hours after administration, which correlates closely with the time to peak pain relief.

Apart from analgesia, tramadol administration may produce a constellation of symptoms (including dizziness, somnolence, nausea, constipation, sweating and pruritus) similar to that of an opioid. However, tramadol causes significantly less respiratory depression than morphine. In contrast to morphine, tramadol has not been shown to cause histamine release. At therapeutic doses, tramadol has no effect on heart rate, left- ventricular function or cardiac index. Orthostatic changes in blood pressure have been observed.

PHARMACOKINETICS

Absorption: Racemic tramadol is rapidly and almost completely absorbed after oral administration. The mean absolute bioavailability of a 100 mg oral dose is approximately 75%. Oral administration of tramadol with food does not significantly affect its rate or extent of absorption. Therefore, tramadol can be administered without regard to food. The mean peak (± SD) plasma concentration of racemic tramadol is 308 ± 78 ng/ml and occurs at approximately two hours after a single 100 mg oral dose in healthy subjects. At this dose, the mean peak plasma concentration of the active mono-*O*-desmethyl metabolite, racemic M1 is 55 ± 20 ng/ml and occurs approximately three hours post-dose. The separate [+]- and [-]-enantiomers of tramadol generally follow a parallel time course in plasma after a single 100 mg oral dose of tramadol. Following 100 mg oral administration of tramadol the maximum plasma concentrations of the [-]-enantiomer of tramadol are somewhat lower than those of the [+]-enantiomer (148 ± 33 vs. 168 ± 36 ng/ml respectively). The [-]-M1 enantiomer is present at slightly higher plasma concentrations than the [+]-M1 enantiomer (35 ± 10 vs. 26 ± 13 ng/ml respectively). At steady state following a 100 mg q.i.d. regimen of tramadol, 3 out of 18 subjects formed relatively low amounts of [+]-M1, while their [-]-M1 formation remained similar to that of other subjects. This is believed not to be clinically significant.

Plasma concentrations of racemic tramadol are predictable over a 50 mg to 100 mg single-dose range. This is also true under multiple-dose conditions. Steady state is achieved after two days of dosing tramadol by a 100 mg q.i.d. regimen (maximum plasma concentration was 592 ± 177 ng/ml). The plasma half-life of tramadol following a single and multiple dosing was 6 and 7 hours, respectively. This increase in half-life upon multiple dosing is not considered to be clinically significant or to warrant dosage adjustment for chronic use.

Mean plasma racemic tramadol and racemic M1 concentration-versus-time profiles following a single 100 mg oral dose of tramadol and following twenty-nine 100 mg doses four times daily.

Distribution: The volume of distribution of tramadol was 2.6 and 2.9 liters/kg in male and female subjects, respectively following a 100 mg intravenous dose. The binding of tramadol to human plasma proteins is approximately 20% and binding also appears to be independent

CLINICAL PHARMACOLOGY: *(cont'd)*

of concentration up to 10 mcg/ml. Saturation of plasma protein binding occurs only at concentrations outside the clinically relevant range. Although not confirmed in humans, tramadol has been shown in rats to cross the blood-brain barrier.

Metabolism: Tramadol is extensively metabolized after oral administration. Approximately 30% of the dose is excreted in the urine as unchanged drug, whereas 60% of the dose is excreted as metabolites. The remainder is excreted either as unidentified or an unextractable metabolites. The major metabolic pathways appear to be *N*- and *O*-demethylation and glucuronidation or sulfation in the liver. Only the one metabolite (mono-*O*-desmethyl-tramadol denoted M1) is pharmacologically active. Production of M1 is dependent on the CYP2D6 isoenzyme of cytochrome P-450.

Elimination: The mean terminal plasma elimination half-lives of racemic tramadol and racemic M1 are 6.3 ± 1.4 and 7.4 ± 1.4 hours respectively. The plasma elimination half-life of racemic tramadol increased from approximately six hours to seven hours upon multiple dosing.

SPECIAL POPULATIONS

Renal: Impaired renal function results in a decreased rate and extent of excretion of tramadol and its active metabolite M1. In patients with creatinine clearances of less than 30/ml/min adjustment of the dosing regimen is recommended (see DOSAGE AND ADMINISTRATION). The total amount of tramadol and M1 removed during a dialysis period is less than 7% of the administered dose.

Hepatic: Metabolism of tramadol and M1 is reduced in patients with advanced cirrhosis of the liver resulting in a larger area under the serum-concentration-versus-time curve for tramadol and longer tramadol and M1 elimination half-lives (13 hrs. for tramadol and 19 hrs. for M1). In cirrhotic patients adjustment of the dosing regimen is recommended (see DOSAGE AND ADMINISTRATION).

Age: Healthy elderly subjects aged 65 to 75 years have plasma tramadol concentrations and elimination half-lives comparable to those observed in healthy subjects less than 65 years of age. In subjects over 75 years maximum serum concentrations are slightly elevated (208 vs. 162 ng/ml) and the elimination half-life is slightly prolonged (7 vs. 6 hours) compared to subjects 65 to 75 years of age. Adjustment of the daily dose is recommended for patients older than 75 years (see DOSAGE AND ADMINISTRATION).

Gender: The absolute bioavailability of tramadol was 73% in males and 79% in females. The plasma clearance was 6.4 ml/min/kg in males and 5.7 ml/min/kg in females following a 100 mg IV dose of tramadol. Following a single oral dose, and after adjusting for body weight, females had a 12% higher peak tramadol concentration and a 35% higher area under the concentration-time curve compared to males. This difference may not be of any clinical significance.

CLINICAL STUDIES:

Tramadol hydrochloride has been given in single oral doses of 50, 75, 100, 150 and 200 mg to patients with pain following surgical procedures (orthopedic, gynecological, cesarean section) and pain following oral surgery (extraction of impacted molars).

In single-dose models of pain following oral surgery, pain relief was demonstrated in some patients at doses of 50 mg and 75 mg. A dose of 100 mg tramadol tended to provide analgesia superior to codeine sulfate 60 mg, but it was not effective as the combination of aspirin 650 mg with codeine phosphate 60 mg. In single-dose models of pain following surgical procedures, 150 mg provided analgesia generally comparable to the combination of acetaminophen 650 mg with propoxyphene napsylate 100 mg, with a tendency toward later peak effect.

Tramadol hydrochloride has been studied in three long-term controlled trials involving a total of 820 patients, with 530 patients receiving tramadol. Patients with chronic conditions such as low back pain, cancer, neuropathic pain and orthopedic and joint conditions entered a double-blind phase of one to three months. Average daily doses of approximately 250 mg of tramadol in divided doses produced analgesia comparable with five doses of acetaminophen 300 mg with codeine phosphate 30 mg (Tylenol with Codeine #3) daily five doses of aspirin 325 mg with codeine phosphate 30 mg daily and with two to three doses of acetaminophen 500 mg with oxycodone hydrochloride 5 mg (Tylox) daily. Following the double-blind period, some patients took tramadol in an open period for up to two years.

INDICATIONS AND USAGE:

Tramadol is indicated for the management of moderate to moderately severe pain.

CONTRAINDICATIONS:

Tramadol should not be administered to patients who have previously demonstrated hypersensitivity to tramadol or in cases of acute intoxication with alcohol, hypnotics, centrally acting analgesics, opioids or psychotropic drugs.

WARNINGS:

Seizure Risk: Tramadol causes seizures in animal models, and a few seizures have been reported in humans receiving excessive single oral doses (700 mg) or large intravenous doses (300 mg). Administration of tramadol may enhance the seizure risk in patients taking MAO inhibitors, neuroleptics, other drugs that reduce the seizure threshold patients with epilepsy, or patients otherwise at increased risk for seizure. In animal studies, naloxone administration increased the risk of convulsions.

Use with CNS Depressants: Tramadol should be used with caution and in reduced dosages when administered to patients receiving CNS depressants such as alcohol, opioids, anesthetic agents, phenothiazines, tranquilizers or sedative hypnotics.

Use with MAO Inhibitors: Tramadol should be used with great caution in patients taking monoamine oxidase inhibitors, since tramadol inhibits the uptake of norepinephrine and serotonin.

PRECAUTIONS:

Respiratory Depression: When large doses of tramadol are administered with anesthetic medications or alcohol, respiratory depression may result. Cases of intraoperative respiratory depression, usually with large intravenous doses of tramadol and with concurrent administration of respiratory depressants, have been reported in foreign experience. Such cases should be treated as overdoses (see OVERDOSAGE.) Tramadol should be administered cautiously in patients at risk for respiratory depression.

Increased Intracranial Pressure or Head Trauma: Tramadol should be used with caution in patients with increased intracranial pressure or head injury. Pupillary changes (miosis) from tramadol may obscure the existence, extent or course of intracranial pathology. Clinicians should also maintain a high index of suspicion for adverse drug reaction when evaluating altered mental status in these patients if they are receiving tramadol.

Acute Abdominal Conditions: The administration of tramadol may complicate the clinical assessment of patients with acute abdominal conditions.

PRECAUTIONS: *(cont'd)*

Patients Physically Dependent on Opioids: Tramadol is not recommended for patients who are dependent on opioids. Patients who have recently taken substantial amounts of opioids may experience withdrawal symptoms. Because of the difficulty in assessing dependence in patients who have previously received substantial amounts of opioid medication, caution should be used in the administration of tramadol to such patients.

Use in Renal and Hepatic Disease: Impaired renal function results in a decreased rate and extent of excretion of tramadol and its active metabolite M1. In patients with creatinine clearances of less than 30 ml/min, dosing reduction is recommended (see DOSAGE AND ADMINISTRATION).

Metabolism of tramadol and M1 is reduced in patients with advanced cirrhosis of the liver. In cirrhotic patients, dosing reduction is recommended (see DOSAGE AND ADMINISTRATION).

With the prolonged half-life in these conditions, achievement of steady state is delayed, so that it may take several days for elevated plasma concentrations to develop.

Information for the Patient: Patients being treated with tramadol should receive the following information:

Tramadol may impair mental or physical abilities required for the performance of potentially hazardous tasks such as driving a car or operating machinery.

Carcinogenesis, Mutagenesis, and Impairment of Fertility: Tramadol was not mutagenic in the following assays: Ames *Salmonella* microsomal activation test, CHO/HPRT mammalian cell assay, mouse lymphoma assay (in the absence of metabolic activation), dominant lethal mutation tests in mice, chromosome aberration test in Chinese hamsters, and bone marrow micronucleus tests in mice and Chinese hamsters. Weakly mutagenic results occurred in the presence of metabolic activation in the mouse lymphoma assay and micronucleus test in rats. Overall, the weight of evidence from these tests indicates that tramadol does not pose a genotoxic risk to humans.

A slight, but statistically significant, increase in two common murine tumors, pulmonary and hepatic, was observed in a mouse carcinogenicity study, particularly in aged mice (dosing orally up to 30 mg/kg for approximately two years, although the study was not done with the Maximum Tolerated Dose). This finding is not believed to suggest risk in humans. No such finding occurred in a rat carcinogenicity study.

No effects on fertility were observed for tramadol at oral dose levels up to 50 mg/kg in male rats and 75 mg/kg in female rats.

Pregnancy, Teratogenic Effects, Pregnancy Category C: There are no adequate and well-controlled studies in pregnant women. Tramadol should be used during pregnancy only if the potential benefit justifies the potential risk to the fetus.

Tramadol has been shown to be embryotoxic and fetotoxic in mice, rats and rabbits at maternally toxic doses 3 to 15 times the maximum human dose or higher (120 mg/kg in mice, 25 mg/kg or higher in rats and 75 mg/kg or higher in rabbits), but was not teratogenic at these dose levels. No harm to the fetus due to tramadol was seen at doses that were not maternally toxic.

No drug-related teratogenic effects were observed in progeny of mice, rats or rabbits treated with tramadol by various routes (up to 140 mg/kg for mice, 80 mg/kg for rats or 300 mg/kg for rabbits). Embryo and fetal toxicity consisted primarily of decreased fetal weights, skeletal ossification and increased supernumerary ribs at maternally toxic dose levels. Transient delays in developmental or behavioral parameters were also seen in pups from rat dams allowed to deliver. Embryo and fetal lethality were reported only in one rabbit study at 300 mg/kg, a dose that would cause extreme maternal toxicity in the rabbit.

In peri- and post-natal studies in rats, progeny of dams receiving oral (gavage) dose levels of 50 mg/kg or greater had decreased weights, and pup survival was decreased early in lactation at 80 mg/kg (6 to 10 times the maximum human dose). No toxicity was observed for progeny of dams receiving 8, 10, 20, 25 or 40 mg/kg. Maternal toxicity was observed at all dose levels, but effects on progeny were evident only at higher dose levels where maternal toxicity was more severe.

Labor and Delivery: Tramadol should not be used in pregnant women prior to or during labor unless the potential benefits outweigh the risks, because safe use in pregnancy has not been established. Tramadol has been shown to cross the placenta. The mean ratio of serum tramadol in the umbilical veins compared to maternal veins was 0.83 for 40 women given tramadol during labor.

The effect of tramadol, if any, on the later growth, development, and functional maturation of the child is unknown.

Nursing Mothers: Tramadol is not recommended for obstetrical preoperative medication or for post-delivery analgesia in nursing mothers because its safety in infants and newborns has not been studied. Following a single IV 100 mg dose of tramadol, the cumulative excretion in breast milk within 16 hours postdose was 100 mcg of tramadol (0.1% of the maternal dose) and 27 mcg of M1.

Pediatric Use: The pediatric use of tramadol is not recommended because safety and efficacy in patients under 16 years of age have not been established.

Geriatric Use: In subjects over the age of 75 years, serum concentrations are slightly elevated and the elimination half-life is slightly elevated and the elimination half-life is slightly prolonged. The aged also can be expected to vary more widely in their ability to tolerate adverse drug effects. Daily doses in excess of 300 mg are not recommended in patients over 75 (see DOSAGE AND ADMINISTRATION).

DRUG INTERACTIONS:

Tramadol does not appear to induce its own metabolism in humans, since observed maximal plasma concentrations after multiple oral doses are higher than expected based on single-dose data. Tramadol is a mild inducer of selected drug metabolism pathways measured in animals.

Concomitant administration of tramadol hydrochloride with **carbamazepine** causes a significant increase in tramadol metabolism, presumably through metabolic induction by carbamazepine. Patients receiving chronic carbamazepine doses of up to 800 mg daily may require up to twice the recommended dose of tramadol.

Tramadol is metabolized to M1 by the CYP2D6 P-450 isoenzyme.**Quinidine** is a selective inhibitor of that isoenzyme; so that concomitant administration of quinidine and tramadol results in increased concentrations of tramadol and reduced concentrations of M1. The clinical consequences of this effect have not been fully investigated, and the effect on quinidine concentrations is unknown.

Concomitant administration of tramadol with **cimetidine** does not result in clinically significant changes in tramadol pharmacokinetics. Therefore, no alteration of the tramadol dosage regimen is recommended.

Interactions with **MAO Inhibitors** due to interference with detoxification mechanisms, have been reported for some centrally acting drugs (see WARNINGS).

ADVERSE REACTIONS:

Tramadol hydrochloride was administered to 550 patients during the double-blind or open-label extension periods in U.S. studies of chronic nonmalignant pain. Of these patients, 375 were 65 years old or older. TABLE 1 reports the cumulative incidence rate of adverse reactions by 7, 30 and 90 days for the most frequent reactions (5% or more by 7 days). The most frequently reported events were in the central nervous system and gastrointestinal system. Although the reactions listed in the table are felt to be probably related to tramadol administration, the reported rates also include some events that may have been due to underlying disease or concomitant medication. The overall incidence rates of adverse experiences in these trials were similar for tramadol and the active control groups, Tylenol with Codeine #3 (acetaminophen 300 mg with codeine phosphate 30 mg), and aspirin 325 mg with codeine phosphate 30 mg. (TABLE 1)

TABLE 1 Cumulative Incidence of Adverse Reactions for Tramadol HCl In Chronic Trials of Nonmalignant Pain

	Up to 7 Days	Up to 30 Days	Up to 90 Days
Dizziness/Vertigo	26%	31%	33%
Nausea	24%	34%	40%
Constipation	24%	38%	46%
Headache	18%	26%	32%
Somnolence	16%	23%	25%
Vomiting	9%	13%	17%
Pruritus	8%	10%	11%
"CNS Stimulation"	7%	11%	14%
Asthenia	6%	11%	12%
Sweating	6%	7%	9%
Dyspepsia	5%	9%	13%
Dry Mouth	5%	9%	10%
Diarrhea	5%	6%	10%

[1] "CNS Stimulation" is a composite of nervousness, anxiety, agitation, tremor, spasticity, euphoria, emotional lability and hallucinations.

Incidence Less Than 5% Possibly Casually Related: TABLE 2 lists adverse reactions that occurred with an incidence of less than 5% in clinical trials, and for which the possibility of a casual relationship with tramadol exists. Reactions are separated according to whether the incidence was greater than 1%. (TABLE 2)

TABLE 2 Possibly Tramadol HCl Related Adverse Reactions with an Incidence of Less Than 5%

	Incidence of Adverse Reaction	
Body System	**From 1% to <5%**	**Less Than 1%**
Body as a Whole	Malaise	Allergic reaction; Accidental injury; Weight loss
Cardiovascular	Vasodilation	Syncope; Orthostatic hypotension; Tachycardia
Central Nervous System	Anxiety; Confusion; Coordination disturbance; Euphoria; Nervousness; Sleep disorder	Seizure (seeWARNINGS); Paresthesia; Cognitive dysfunction; Hallucinations; Tremor; Amnesia; Difficulty in concentration; Abnormal gait
Gastrointestinal	Abdominal pain; Anorexia; Flatulence	
Musculoskeletal	Hypertonia	
Respiratory		Dyspnea
Skin	Rash	Urticaria, Vesicles
Special Senses	Visual disturbance	Dysgeusia
Urogenital	Urinary retention; Urinary frequency; Menopausal symptoms	Dysuria; Menstrual disorder

Other Adverse Experiences, Causal Relationship Undetermined: A variety of other adverse events were reported infrequently in patients taking tramadol during clinical trials. A causal relationship between tramadol and these events has not been determined. However, the most significant events are listed below as alerting information to the physician:

Body as a whole: Suicidal tendency.

Cardiovascular: Abnormal ECG, hypertension, myocardial ischemia, palpitations.

Central Nervous System: Migraine.

Gastrointestinal: Gastrointestinal bleeding, hepatitis, stomatitis.

Laboratory abnormalities: Creatinine increase, elevated liver enzymes, hemoglobin decrease, proteinuria.

Sensory: Cataracts, deafness, tinnitus.

DRUG ABUSE AND DEPENDENCE:

Although tramadol can produce drug dependence of the μ-opioid type (like codeine or dextropropoxyphene) and potentially may be abused, there has been little evidence of abuse in foreign clinical experience. In clinical trials, tramadol produced effects similar to an opioid, and at supratherapeutic doses was recognized as an opioid in subjective/behavioral studies. Tolerance development has been reported to be relatively mild and withdrawal, when present, is not considered to be as severe as that produced by other opioids. Part of tramadol's activity is believed derived from its active metabolite, which is responsible for some delay on onset of activity and some extension of the duration of μ-opioid activity. Delayed μ-opioid activity is believed to reduce a drug's abuse liability.

An assay for tramadol is not included in routine urine screens for drugs of abuse.

OVERDOSAGE:

Few cases of overdoses with tramadol have been reported. Estimates of ingested dose in foreign fatalities have been in the range of 3 to 5 g. A 3 g intentional overdose in a patient in the clinical studies produced emesis and no sequelae. The lowest dose reported to be associated with fatality was possibly between 500 and 1000 mg in a 40 kg woman, but details of the case are not completely known.

Serious potential consequences of overdosage are respiratory depression and seizure. Naloxone will reverse some, but not all, symptoms caused by overdosage with tramadol so that general supportive treatment is recommended. Primary attention should be given to the assurance of adequate respiratory exchange. Hemodialysis is not expected to be helpful because it removes only a small percentage of the administered dose. Convulsions occurring in mice following the administration of toxic doses of tramadol could be suppressed with barbiturates or benzodiazepines, but were increased with naloxone. Naloxone did not change the lethality of an overdose in mice.

DOSAGE AND ADMINISTRATION:

For the treatment of painful conditions tramadol 50 mg to 100 mg can be administered as needed for relief every four to six hours, not to exceed 400 mg per day. For moderate pain tramadol 50 mg may be adequate as the initial dose, and for more severe pain, tramadol 100 mg is usually more effective as the initial dose.

Individualization of Dose: Available data do not suggest that a dosage adjustment is necessary in elderly patients 65 to 75 years of age unless they also have renal or hepatic impairment. For elderly patients**over 75 years old,** not more than 300 mg/day in divided doses as above is recommended. In all patients with **creatine clearance less than 30 ml/min,** it is recommended that the dosing interval of tramadol be increased to 12 hours with a maximum daily dose of 200 mg. Since only 7% of an administered dose is removed by hemodialysis, **dialysis patients** can receive their regular dose on the day of dialysis. The recommended dose for patients with **cirrhosis** is 50 mg every 12 hours. Patients receiving chronic **carbamazepine** doses up to 800 mg daily may require up to twice the recommended dose of tramadol.

PATIENT INFORMATION:

Tramadol HCl is used to relieve moderate to severe pain. This drug should be used as directed and only for the period of time determined by the physician. This drug can cause dizziness or tiredness and in some cases nausea, constipation and headache. Avoid the use of alcohol or other depressants' such as sleeping pills or tranquilizers. Be especially careful when performing potentially hazardous tasks such as driving or operating machinery while taking this drug. Please tell your pharmacist or physician if you are pregnant or nursing.

HOW SUPPLIED:

Ultram (tramadol hydrochloride) 50 mg tablet (white, film-coated capsule-shaped tablet) engraved "McNeil" on one side and "659" on the other side.

Ultram (tramadol hydrochloride) 50 mg tablet, bottles of 100 tablets, and packages of 100 unit doses in blister packs (10 cards of 10 tablets each).

Dispense in a tight container. Store at controlled room temperature (15° to 30°C, 59° to 86°F).

HOW SUPPLIED - EQUIVALENTS NOT AVAILABLE:

Tablet, Uncoated - Oral - 50 mg

100's	$60.00	ULTRAM, McNeil Lab	00045-0659-60
100's	$66.00	ULTRAM, McNeil Lab	00045-0659-10

TRANDOLAPRIL *(003286)*

CATEGORIES: ACE Inhibitors; Angiotensin Converting Enzyme Inhibitors; Hypertension; Pregnancy Category C; Pregnancy Category D; FDA Approved 1996 Apr

BRAND NAMES: *Gopten* (Australia, England, France, Germany); **Mavik**; *Odrik* (Australia, England, France); *Udrik* (Germany)
(International brand names outside U.S. in italics)

PRIMARY ICD9: 401.1 (Essential Hypertension)

WARNING:
Use in Pregnancy: When used in pregnancy during the second and third trimesters, ACE inhibitors can cause injury and even death to the developing fetus. When pregnancy is detected, trandolapril should be discontinued as soon as possible. See **WARNINGS, Fetal/Neonatal Morbidity and Mortality.**

DESCRIPTION:

Trandolapril is the ethyl ester prodrug of a nonsulfhydryl angiotensin converting enzyme (ACE) inhibitor, trandolaprilat. Trandolapril is chemically described as (2S,3aR,7aS)-1-[(S)-N-[(S)-1-Carboxy-3-phenylpropyl]alanyl] hexahydro-2-indolinecarboxylic acid, 1-ethyl ester. Its empirical formula is $C_{24}H_{34}N_2O_5$.

Trandolapril is a colorless, crystalline substance that is soluble (>100 mg/ml) in chloroform, dichloromethane, and methanol. Mavik tablets contain 1 mg, 2 mg, or 4 mg of trandolapril for oral administration. Each tablet also contains corn starch, croscarmellose sodium, hydroxypropyl methylcellulose, iron oxide, lactose, povidone, sodium stearyl fumarate.

CLINICAL PHARMACOLOGY:

MECHANISM OF ACTION

Trandolapril is deesterified to the diacid metabolite, trandolaprilat, which is approximately eight times more active as an inhibitor of ACE activity. ACE is a peptidyl dipeptidase that catalyzes the conversion of angiotensin I to the vasoconstrictor, angiotensin II. Angiotensin II is a potent peripheral vasoconstrictor that also stimulates secretion of aldosterone by the adrenal cortex and provides negative feedback for renin secretion. The effect of trandolapril in hypertension appears to result primarily from the inhibition of circulating and tissue ACE activity thereby reducing angiotensin II formation, decreasing vasoconstriction, decreasing aldosterone secretion, and increasing plasma renin. Decreased aldosterone secretion leads to diuresis, natriuresis, and a small increase of serum potassium. In controlled clinical trials, treatment with trandolapril alone resulted in mean increases in potassium of 0.1 mEq/L. (See PRECAUTIONS.)

ACE is identical to kininase II, an enzyme that degrades bradykinin, a potent peptide vasodilator; whether increased levels of bradykinin play a role in the therapeutic effect of trandolapril remains to be elucidated.

While the principal mechanism of antihypertensive effect is thought to be through the renin-angiotensin-aldosterone system, trandolapril exerts antihypertensive actions even in patients with low-renin hypertension. Trandolapril was an effective antihypertensive in all races studied. Both black patients (usually a predominantly low-renin group) and non-black patients responded to 2 to 4 mg of trandolapril.

PHARMACOKINETICS AND METABOLISM

Pharmacokinetics: Trandolapril's ACE-inhibiting activity is primarily due to its diacid metabolite, trandolaprilat. Cleavage of the ester group of trandolapril, primarily in the liver, is responsible for conversion. Absolute bioavailability after oral administration of trandolapril is about 10% as trandolapril and 70% as trandolaprilat. After oral trandolapril under fasting conditions, peak trandolapril levels occur at about one hour and peak trandolaprilat levels occur between 4 and 10 hours. The elimination half lives of trandolapril and trandolaprilat are about 6 and 10 hours, respectively, but, like all ACE inhibitors, trandolaprilat also has a prolonged terminal elimination phase, involving a small fraction of administered drug, probably representing binding to plasma and tissue ACE. During multiple dosing of trandolapril, there is no significant accumulation of trandolaprilat. Food slows absorption of trandolapril, but does not effect AUC or C_{max} of trandolaprilat or C_{max} of trandolapril.

CLINICAL PHARMACOLOGY: *(cont'd)*

Metabolism and Excretion: After oral administration of trandolapril, about 33% of parent drug and metabolites are recovered in urine, mostly as trandolaprilat, with about 66% in feces. The extent of the absorbed dose which is biliary excreted has not been determined. Plasma concentrations (C_{max} and AUC of trandolapril and C_{max} of trandolaprilat) are dose proportional over the 1-4 mg range, but the AUC of trandolaprilat is somewhat less than dose proportional. In addition to trandolaprilat, at least 7 other metabolites have been found, principally glucuronides or deesterification products.

Serum protein binding of trandolapril is about 80%, and is independent of concentration. Binding of trandolaprilat is concentration-dependent, varying from 65% at 1000 ng/mL to 94% at 0.1 ng/mL, indicating saturation of binding with increasing concentration.

The volume of distribution of trandolapril is about 18 liters. Total plasma clearances of trandolapril and trandolaprilat after approximately 2 mg IV doses are about 52 liters/hour respectively. Renal clearance of trandolaprilat varies from 1-4 liters/hour, depending on dose.

SPECIAL POPULATIONS

Pediatric: Trandolapril pharmacokinetics have not been evaluated in patients <18 years of age.

Geriatric and Gender: Trandolapril pharmacokinetics have been investigated in the elderly (>65 years) and in both genders. The plasma concentration of trandolapril is increased in elderly and young hypertensive patients. The pharmacokinetics of trandolapril and trandolaprilat and inhibition of ACE activity are similar in male and female elderly hypertensive patients.

Race: Pharmacokinetic differences have not been evaluated in different races.

Renal Insufficiency: Compared to normal subjects, the plasma concentrations of trandolapril and trandolaprilat are approximately 2-fold greater and renal clearance is reduced by about 85% in patients with creatinine clearance below 30 ml/min and in patients on hemodialysis. Dosage adjustment is recommended in renally impaired patients. (See DOSAGE AND ADMINISTRATION.)

Hepatic Insufficiency: Following oral administration in patients with mild to moderate alcoholic cirrhosis, plasma concentrations of trandolapril and trandolaprilat were, respectively, 9-fold and 2-fold greater than in normal subjects, but inhibition of ACE activity was not affected. Lower doses should be considered in patients with hepatic insufficiency. (See DOSAGE AND ADMINISTRATION.)

Drug Interactions: Trandolapril did not affect the plasma concentration (pre-dose and 2 hours post-dose) of oral digoxin (0.25 mg). Coadministration of trandolapril and cimetidine led to an increase of about 44% in C_{max} for trandolapril, but no difference in the pharmacokinetics of trandolaprilat or in ACE inhibition. Coadministration of trandolapril and furosemide led to an increase of about 25% in the renal clearance of trandolaprilat, but no effect was seen on the pharmacokinetics of furosemide or trandolaprilat or on ACE inhibition.

PHARMACODYNAMICS AND CLINICAL EFFECTS

A single 2-mg dose of trandolapril produces 70 to 85% inhibition of plasma ACE activity at 4 hours with about 10% decline at 24 hours and about half the effect manifest at 8 days. Maximum ACE inhibition is achieved with a plasma trandolaprilat concentration of 2 ng/ml. ACE inhibition is a function of trandolaprilat concentration, not trandolapril concentration. The effect of trandolapril on exogenous angiotensin I was not measured.

Four placebo-controlled dose response studies were conducted using once-daily oral dosing of trandolapril in doses from 0.25 to 16 mg per day in 827 black and non-black patients with mild to moderate hypertension. The minimal effective once-daily dose was 1 mg in non-black patients and 2 mg in black patients. Further decreases in trough supine diastolic blood pressure were obtained in non-black patients with higher doses. There was a slightly greater effect on the reduction in blood pressure, but no difference on systolic pressure with b.i.d. dosing. During chronic therapy, the maximum reduction in blood pressure with any dose is achieved within one week. Following 6 weeks of monotherapy in placebo-controlled trials in patients with mild to moderate hypertension, once-daily doses of 2 to 4 mg lowered supine or standing systolic/diastolic blood pressure 24 hours after dosing by an average 7-10/4-5 mmHg below placebo responses in non-black patients. Once-daily doses of 2 to 4 mg lowered blood pressure 4-6/3-4 mmHg in black patients. Trough to peak ratios for effective doses ranged from 0.5 to 0.9. There were no differences in response between men and women, but responses were somewhat greater in patients under 60 than in patients over 60 years old. Abrupt withdrawal of trandolapril has not been associated with a rapid increase in blood pressure.

Administration of trandolapril to patients with mild to moderate hypertension results in a reduction of supine, sitting and standing blood pressure to about the same extent without compensatory tachycardia.

Symptomatic hypotension is infrequent, although it can occur in patients who are salt- and/or volume-depleted. (See WARNINGS.) Use of trandolapril in combination with thiazide diuretics gives a blood pressure lowering effect greater than that seen with either agent alone, and the additional effect of trandolapril is similar to the effect of monotherapy.

INDICATIONS AND USAGE:

Trandolapril is indicated for the treatment of hypertension. It may be used alone or in combination with other antihypertensive medication such as hydrochlorothiazide.

In considering the use of trandolapril, it should be noted that in controlled trials ACE inhibitors (for which adequate data are available) cause a higher rate of angiodema in black than in non-black patients. (See WARNINGS, Angiodema.)

CONTRAINDICATIONS:

Trandolapril is contraindicated in patients who are hypersensitive to this product and in patients with a history of angiodema related to previous treatment with an ACE inhibitor.

WARNINGS:

ANAPHYLACTOID AND POSSIBLY RELATED ACTIONS

Presumably because angiotensin converting enzyme inhibitors affect the metabolism of eicosanoids and polypeptides, including endogenous bradykinin, patients receiving ACE inhibitors, including trandolapril, may be subject to a variety of adverse reactions, some of them serious.

ANGIOEDEMA

Angioedema of the face, extremities, lips, tongue, glottis, and larynx has been reported in patients treated with ACE inhibitors including trandolapril. Symptoms suggestive of angioedema or facial edema occurred in 0.13% of trandolapril-treated patients. Two of the four cases were life-threatening and resolved without treatment or with medication (corticosteroids). Angioedema associated with laryngeal edema can be fatal. If laryngeal stridor or angioedema of the face, tongue or glottis occurs, treatment with trandolapril should be discontinued immediately, the patient treated in accordance with accepted medical care and carefully observed until the swelling disappears. In instances where swelling is confined to the face and lips, the condition generally resolves without treatment; antihistamines may be useful in relieving symptoms. **Where there is involvement of the tongue, glottis, or larynx,**

WARNINGS: *(cont'd)*

likely to cause airway obstruction, emergency therapy, including but not limited to subcutaneous epinephrine solution 1:1,000 (0.3 to 0.5 ml) should be promptly administered. (See Information for the Patient and ADVERSE REACTIONS)

Anaphylactoid Reactions During Desensitization: Two patients undergoing desensitizing treatment with hymenoptera venom while receiving ACE inhibitors sustained life-threatening anaphylactoid reactions. In the same patients, these reactions did not occur when ACE inhibitors were temporarily withheld, but they reappeared when the ACE inhibitors were inadvertently readministered.

Anaphylactoid Reactions During Membrane Exposure: Anaphylactoid reactions have been reported in patients dialyzed with high-flux membranes and treated concomitantly with an ACE inhibitor. Anaphylactoid reactions have also been reported in patients undergoing low-density lipoprotein apheresis with dextran sulfate absorption.

HYPOTENSION

Trandolapril can cause symptomatic hypotension. Like other ACE inhibitors, trandolapril has only rarely been associated with symptomatic hypotension in uncomplicated hypertensive patients. Symptomatic hypotension is most likely to occur in patients who have been salt- or volume-depleted as a result of prolonged treatment with diuretics, dietary salt restriction, dialysis, diarrhea, or vomiting. Volume and/or salt depletion should be corrected before initiating treatment with trandolapril. (See DRUG INTERACTIONS and ADVERSE REACTIONS.) In controlled and uncontrolled studies, hypotension was reported as an adverse event in 0.6 percent of patients and led to discontinuations in 0.1% of patients.

In patients with concomitant congestive heart failure, with or without associated renal insufficiency, ACE inhibitor therapy may cause excessive hypotension, which may be associated with oliguria or azotemia, and rarely, with acute renal failure and death. In such patients, trandolapril therapy should be started at the recommended dose under close medical supervision. These patients should be followed closely during the first 2 weeks of treatment and, thereafter, whenever the dosage of trandolapril or diuretic is increased. (See DOSAGE AND ADMINISTRATION.) Care in avoiding hypotension should also be taken in patients with ischemic heart disease, aortic stenosis, or cerebrovascular disease.

If symptomatic hypotension occurs, the patient should be placed in the supine position and, if necessary, normal saline may be administered intravenously. A transient hypotensive response is not a contraindication to further doses; however, lower doses of trandolapril or reduced concomitant therapy should be considered.

NEUTROPENIA/AGRANULOCYTOSIS

Another ACE inhibitor, captopril, has been shown to cause agranulocytosis and bone marrow depression rarely in patients with uncomplicated hypertension, but more frequently in patients with renal impairment, especially if they also have a collagen-vascular disease such as systemic lupus erythematosus or scleroderma. Available data from clinical trials of trandolapril are insufficient to show that trandolapril does not cause agranulocytosis at similar rates. As with other ACE inhibitors, periodic monitoring of white blood cell counts in patients with collagen-vascular disease and/or renal disease should be considered.

HEPATIC FAILURE

ACE inhibitors rarely have been associated with a syndrome of cholestatic jaundice, fulminant hepatic necrosis, and death. The mechanism of this syndrome is not understood. Patients receiving ACE inhibitors who develop jaundice should discontinue the ACE inhibitor and receive appropriate medical follow-up.

FETAL/NEONATAL MORBIDITY AND MORTALITY

ACE inhibitors can cause fetal and neonatal morbidity and death when administered to pregnant women. Several dozen cases have been reported in the world literature. When pregnancy is detected, ACE inhibitors should be discontinued as soon as possible.

The use of ACE inhibitors during the second and third trimesters of pregnancy has been associated with fetal and neonatal injury, including hypotension, neonatal skull hypoplasia, anuria, reversible or irreversible renal failure, and death. Oligohydramnios has also been reported, presumably resulting from decreased fetal renal function; oligohydramnios in this setting has been associated with fetal limb contractures, craniofacial deformation, and hypoplastic lung development. Prematurity, intrauterine growth retardation, and patent ductus arteriosus have also been reported, although it is not clear whether these occurrences were due to the ACE inhibitor exposure.

These adverse effects do not appear to have resulted from intrauterine ACE-inhibitor exposure that has been limited to the first trimester. Mothers whose embryos and fetuses are exposed to ACE inhibitors only during the first trimester should be so informed. Nonetheless, when patients become pregnant, physicians should make every effort to discontinue the use of trandolapril as soon as possible.

Rarely (probably less often than once in every thousand pregnancies), no alternative to ACE inhibitors will be found. In these rare cases, the mothers should be apprised of the potential hazards to their fetuses, and serial ultrasound examinations should be performed to assess the intra-amniotic environment.

If oligohydramnios is observed, trandolapril should be discontinued unless it is considered life-saving for the mother. Contraction stress testing (CST), a non-stress test (NST), or biophysical profiling (BPP) may be appropriate, depending upon the week of pregnancy.

Patients and physicians should be aware, however, that oligohydramnios may not appear until after the fetus has sustained irreversible injury.

Infants with histories of *in utero* exposure to ACE inhibitors should be closely observed for hypotension, oliguria, and hyperkalemia. If oliguria occurs, attention should be directed toward support of blood pressure and renal perfusion. Exchange transfusions or dialysis may be required as a means of reversing hypotension and/or substituting for disordered renal function.

Doses of 0.8 mg/kg/day (9.4 mg/m^2/day) in rabbits, 1000 mg/kg/day (7000 mg/m^2/day) in rats, and 25 mg/kg/day (295 mg/m^2/day) in cynomolgus monkeys did not produce teratogenic effects. These doses represent 10 and 3 times (rabbits), 1250 and 2564 times (rats), and 312 and 108 times (monkeys) the maximum projected human dose of 4 mg based on body-weight and body-surface-area, respectively assuming a 50 kg woman.

PRECAUTIONS:

GENERAL

Impaired Renal Function

As a consequence of inhibiting the renin-angiotensin system, changes in renal function may be anticipated in susceptible individuals. In patients with severe heart failure whose renal function may depend on the activity of the renin-angiotensin-aldosterone system, treatment with ACE inhibitors, including trandolapril, may be associated with oliguria and/or progressive azotemia and rarely with acute renal failure and/or death.

In hypertensive patients with unilateral or bilateral renal artery stenosis, increases in blood urea nitrogen and serum creatinine have been observed in some patients following ACE inhibitor therapy. These increases were almost always reversible upon discontinuation of the ACE inhibitor and/or diuretic therapy. In such patients, renal function should be monitored during the first few weeks of therapy.

PRECAUTIONS: *(cont'd)*

Some hypertensive patients with no apparent preexisting renal vascular disease have developed increases in blood urea and serum creatinine, usually minor and transient, especially when ACE inhibitors have been given concomitantly with a diuretic. This is more likely to occur in patients with preexisting renal impairment. Dosage reduction and/or discontinuation of any diuretic and/or the ACE inhibitor may be required.

Evaluation of hypertensive patients should always include assessment of renal function. (See DOSAGE AND ADMINISTRATION.)

Hyperkalemia and potassium-sparing diuretics

In clinical trials, hyperkalemia (serum potassium >6.00 mEq/L) occurred in approximately 0.4 percent of hypertensive patients receiving trandolapril. In most cases, elevated serum potassium levels were isolated values, which resolved despite continued therapy. None of these patients were discontinued from the trials because of hyperkalemia. Risk factors for the development of hyperkalemia include renal insufficiency, diabetes mellitus, and the concomitant use of potassium-sparing diuretics, potassium supplements, and/or potassium-containing salt substitutes, which should be used cautiously, if at all, with trandolapril. (See DRUG INTERACTIONS.)

Cough

Presumably due to the inhibition of the degradation of endogenous bradykinin, persistent nonproductive cough has been reported with all ACE inhibitors, always resolving after discontinuation of therapy. ACE inhibitor-induced cough should be considered in the differential diagnosis of cough. In controlled trials of trandolapril, cough was present in 2% of trandolapril patients and 0% of patients given placebo. There was no evidence of a relationship to dose.

Surgery/Anesthesia

In patients undergoing major surgery or during anesthesia with agents that produce hypotension, trandolapril will block angiotensin II formation secondary to compensatory renin release. If hypotension occurs and is considered to be due to this mechanism, it can be corrected by volume expansion.

INFORMATION FOR THE PATIENT

Angioedema

Angioedema, including laryngeal edema, may occur at any time during treatment with ACE inhibitors, including trandolapril. Patients should be advised and told to report immediately any signs or symptoms suggesting angioedema (swelling of face, extremities, eyes, lips, tongue, difficulty in swallowing or breathing) and to stop taking the drug until they have consulted with their physician. (See WARNINGS and ADVERSE REACTIONS.)

Symptomatic Hypotension

Patients should be cautioned that light-headedness can occur, especially during the first days of trandolapril therapy, and should be reported to a physician. If actual syncope occurs, patients should be told to stop taking the drug until they have consulted with their physician. (See WARNINGS.)

All patients should be cautioned that inadequate fluid intake, excessive perspiration, diarrhea, or vomiting, resulting in reduced fluid volume, may precipitate an excessive fall in blood pressure with the same consequences of light-headedness and possible syncope.

Patients planning to undergo any surgery and/or anesthesia should be told to inform their physician that they are taking an ACE inhibitor that has a long duration of action.

Hyperkalemia

Patients should be told not to use potassium supplements or salt substitutes containing potassium without consulting their physician. (See PRECAUTIONS.)

Neutropenia

Patients should be told to report promptly any indication of infection (*e.g.*, sore throat, fever) which could be a sign of neutropenia.

Pregnancy

Female patients of childbearing age should be told about the consequences of second- and third-trimester exposure to ACE inhibitors, and they should also be told that these consequences do not appear to have resulted from intrauterine ACE-inhibitor exposure that has been limited to the first trimester. These patients should be asked to report pregnancies to their physicians as soon as possible.

NOTE: As with many other drugs, certain advice to patients being treated with trandolapril is warranted. This information is intended to aid in the safe and effective use of this medication. It is not a disclosure of all possible adverse or intended effects.

CARCINOGENESIS, MUTAGENESIS, AND IMPAIRMENT OF FERTILITY

Long-term studies were conducted with oral trandolapril administered by gavage to mice (78 weeks) and rats (104 and 106 weeks). No evidence of carcinogenic potential was seen in mice dosed up to 25 mg/kg/day (85 mg/m^2/day) or rats dosed up to 8 mg/kg/day (60 mg/m^2/day). These doses are 313 and 32 times (mice), and 100 and 23 times (rats) the maximum recommended human daily dose (MRHDD) of 4 mg based on body-weight and body-surface-area, respectively assuming a 50 kg individual. The genotoxic potential of trandolapril was evaluated in the microbial mutagenicity (Ames) test, the point mutation and chromosome aberration assays in Chinese hamster V79 cells, and the micronucleus test in mice. There was no evidence of mutagenic or clastogenic potential in these *in vitro* and *in vivo* assays.

Reproduction studies in rats did not show any impairment of fertility at doses up to 100 mg/kg/day (710 mg/m^2/day) of trandolapril, or 1250 and 260 times the MRHDD on the basis of body-weight and body-surface-area, respectively.

PREGNANCY CATEGORY C(FIRST TRIMESTER) AND PREGNANCY CATEGORY D (SECOND AND THIRD TRIMESTERS)

See WARNINGS, Fetal/Neonatal Morbidity and mortality.

NURSING MOTHERS

Radiolabeled trandolapril or its metabolites are secreted in rat milk. Trandolapril should not be administered to nursing mothers.

GERIATRIC USE

In placebo-controlled studies of trandolapril, 31.1% of patients were 60 years and older, 20.1% were 65 years and older, and 2.3% were 75 years and older. No overall differences in effectiveness or safety were observed between these patients and younger patients. (Greater sensitivity of some older individual patients cannot be ruled out).

PEDIATRIC USE

The safety and effectiveness of trandolapril in pediatric patients have not been established.

DRUG INTERACTIONS:

CONCOMITANT DIURETIC THERAPY

As with other ACE inhibitors, patients on diuretics, especially those on recently instituted diuretic therapy, may experience an excessive reduction of blood pressure after initiation of therapy with trandolapril. The possibility of exacerbation of hypotensive effects with trandolapril may be minimized by either discontinuing the diuretic or cautiously increasing salt intake prior to initiation of treatment with trandolapril. If it is not possible to discontinue the diuretic, the starting dose of trandolapril should be reduced. (See DOSAGE AND ADMINISTRATION.)

DRUG INTERACTIONS: *(cont'd)*

AGENTS INCREASING SERUM POTASSIUM

Trandolapril can attentuate potassium loss caused by thiazide diuretics and increase serum potassium when used alone. Use of potassium-sparing diuretics (spironolactone, triamterene, or amiloride), potassium supplements, or potassium-containing salt substitutes concomitantly with ACE inhibitors can increase the risk of hyperkalemia. If concomitant use of such agents is indicated, they should be used with caution and with appropriate monitoring of serum potassium. (See PRECAUTIONS.)

LITHIUM

Increased serum lithium levels and symptoms of lithium toxicity have been reported in patients receiving concomitant lithium and ACE inhibitor therapy. These drugs should be coadministered with caution, and frequent monitoring of serum lithium levels is recommended. If a diuretic is also used, the risk of lithium toxicity may be increased.

OTHER

No clinically significant interaction has been found between trandolaprilat and food, cimetidine, digoxin, or furosemide. The anticoagulant effect of warfarin was not significantly changed by trandolapril.

ADVERSE REACTIONS:

The safety experience in U.S. placebo-controlled trials included 1067 hypertensive patients, of whom 831 received trandolapril. Nearly 200 hypertensive patients received trandolapril for over one year in open-label trials. In controlled trials, withdrawals for adverse events were 2.1% on placebo and 1.4% on trandolapril. Adverse events considered at least possibly related to treatment occurring in 1% of trandolapril-treated patients and more common on trandolapril than placebo, pooled for all doses, are shown below, together with the frequency of discontinuation of treatment because of these events.

TABLE 1 ADVERSE EVENTS IN PLACEBO-CONTROLLED TRIALS

	Trandolapril (N=832) % incidence (%Discontinuance)	Placebo (N=237) % incidence (%Discontinuance)
Cough	1.9 (0.1)	0.4 (0.4)
Dizziness	1.3 (0.2)	0.4 (0.4)
Diarrhea	1.0 (0.0)	0.4 (0.0)

Headache and fatigue were all seen in more than 1% of trandolapril-treated patients but were more frequently seen on placebo. Adverse events were not usually persistent or difficult to manage.

Clinical adverse experiences possibly or probably related or of uncertain relationship to therapy occurring in 0.3% to 1.0% (except as noted) of the patients treated with trandolapril (with or without concomitant calcium ion antagonist or diuretic) in controlled or uncontrolled trials (N=1134) and less frequent, clinically significant events seen in clinical trials or post-marketing experience (the rarer events are in italics) include (listed by body system):

General Body Function: chest pain

Cardiovascular: AV first degree block, bradycardia, edema, flushing, hypotension, palpitations.

Central Nervous System: drowsiness, insomnia, paresthesia, vertigo.

Dermatologic: pruritus, rash, pemphigus.

Eye, Ear, Nose, Throat: epistaxis, throat inflammation, upper respiratory tract infection.

Emotional, Mental, Sexual States: anxiety, impotence, decreased libido.

Gastrointestinal: abdominal distention, abdominal pain/cramps, constipation, dyspepsia, diarrhea, vomiting, *pancreatitis.*

Hemopoietic: *decreased leukocytes, decreased neutrophils.*

Metabolism and Endocrine: *increased creatinine, increased potassium,* increased SGPT (ALT).

Musculoskeletal System: extremity pain, muscle cramps, gout.

Pulmonary: dyspnea.

Angioedema: Angioedema has been reported in 4 (0.13%) patients receiving trandolapril in U.S. and foreign studies. Angioedema associated with laryngeal edema may be fatal. If angioedema of the face, extremities, lips, tongue, glottis, and/or larynx occurs, treatment with trandolapril should be discontinued and appropriate therapy instituted immediately. (See WARNINGS)

Hypotension: In hypertensive patients, symptomatic hypotension occurred in 0.6 percent and near syncope occurred in 0.2 percent. Hypotension or syncope was a cause for discontinuation of therapy in 0.1 percent of hypertensive patients.

Fetal/Neonatal Morbidity and Mortality: See WARNINGS, Fetal Neonatal Morbidity and Mortality.

Cough: See PRECAUTIONS, Cough.

Clinical Laboratory Test Findings

Hematology: (See WARNINGS.) Low white blood cells, low neutrophils, low lymphocytes, thrombocytopenia.

Serum Electrolytes: Hyperkalemia (See PRECAUTIONS.) hyponatremia.

Creatinine and Blood Urea Nitrogen: Increases in creatinine levels occurred in 1.1 percent of patients receiving trandolapril alone and 7.3 percent of patients treated with trandolapril, a calcium ion antagonist and a diuretic. None of these increases required discontinuation of treatment. Increases in these laboratory values are more likely to occur in patients with renal insufficiency or those pretreated with a diuretic and, based on experience with other ACE inhibitors, would be expected to be especially likely in patients with renal artery stenosis. (See PRECAUTIONS and WARNINGS.)

Liver function tests: Occasional elevation of transaminases at the rate of 3× upper normals occurred in 0.8% of patients and persistent increase in bilirubin occurred in 0.2% of patients. Discontinuation for elevated liver enzymes occurred in 0.2 percent of patients.

OVERDOSAGE:

No data are available with respect to overdosage in humans. The oral LD_{50} of trandolapril in mice was 4875 mg/Kg in males and 3990 mg/Kg in females. In rats, an oral dose of 5000 mg/Kg caused low mortality (1 male out of 5; 0 females). In dogs, an oral dose of 1000 mg/Kg did not cause mortality and abnormal clinical signs were not observed. In humans the most likely clinical manifestation would be symptoms attributable to severe hypotension.

Laboratory determinations of serum levels of trandolapril and its metabolites are not widely available, and such determinations have, in any event, no established role in the management of trandolapril overdose. No data are available to suggest that physiological maneuvers (*e.g.,* maneuvers to change the pH of the urine) might accelerate elimination of trandolapril and its metabolites. Trandolaprilat is removed by hemodialysis. Angiotensin II could presumably serve as a specific antagonist antidote in the setting of trandolapril overdose, but angiotensin II is essentially unavailable outside of scattered research facilities. Because the hypotensive effect of trandolapril is achieved through vasodilation and effective hypovolemia, it is reasonable to treat trandolapril overdose by infusion of normal saline solution.

DOSAGE AND ADMINISTRATION:

The recommended initial dosage of trandolapril for patients not receiving a diuretic is 1 mg once daily in non-black patients and 2 mg in black patients. Dosage should be adjusted according to the blood pressure response. Generally, dosage adjustments should be made at intervals of at least 1 week. Most patients have required dosages of 2 to 4 mg once daily. There is little clinical experience with doses above 8 mg.

Patients inadequately treated with once-daily dosing at 4 mg may be treated with twice-daily dosing. If blood pressure is not adequately controlled with trandolapril monotherapy, a diuretic may be added.

In patients who are currently being treated with a diuretic, symptomatic hypotension occasionally can occur following the initial dose of trandolapril. To reduce the likelihood of hypotension, the diuretic should, if possible, be discontinued two to three days prior to beginning therapy with trandolapril. (See WARNINGS.) Then, if blood pressure is not controlled with trandolapril alone, diuretic therapy should be resumed. If the diuretic cannot be discontinued, an initial dose of 0.5 mg trandolapril should be used with careful medical supervision for several hours until blood pressure has stabilized. The dosage should subsequently be titrated (as described above) to the optimal response. (See WARNINGS, PRECAUTIONS, and DRUG INTERACTIONS.)

Concomitant administration of trandolapril with potassium supplements, potassium salt substitutes, or potassium-sparing diuretics can lead to increases of serum potassium. (See PRECAUTIONS.)

DOSAGE ADJUSTMENT IN RENAL IMPAIRMENT OR HEPATIC CIRRHOSIS

For patients with creatinine clearance <30 ml/min or with hepatic cirrhosis, the recommended starting dose, based on clinical and pharmacokinetic data, is 0.5 mg daily. Patients should subsequently have their dosage titrated (as described above) to the optimal response.

PATIENT INFORMATION:

Trandolapril is used for the treatment of high blood pressure. Discontinue use and contact your doctor if you become pregnant. If swelling of the extremities, face, eyes, lips, tongue or difficulty in swallowing or breathing occur, stop taking the drug and immediately see your physician.

Inform your physician or pharmacist if you are taking any other medicines.

Inform your physician if you have kidney or liver disease.

May be taken with or without food.

May cause cough, dizziness or diarrhea; notify your physician or pharmacist if this continues.

HOW SUPPLIED:

Storage: Store at controlled room temperature: 20°-25°C (68°-77°F).

HOW SUPPLIED - EQUIVALENTS NOT AVAILABLE:

Tablet - Oral - 1 mg

1 mg x 100	$60.00	MAVIK, Knoll Pharms	00048-5805-01
1 mg x 100	$60.00	MAVIK, Knoll Pharms	00048-5805-41

Tablet - Oral - 2 mg

2 mg x 100	$60.00	MAVIK, Knoll Pharms	00048-5806-01
2 mg x 100	$60.00	MAVIK, Knoll Pharms	00048-5806-41

Tablet - Oral - 4 mg

4 mg x 100	$60.00	MAVIK, Knoll Pharms	00048-5807-01
4 mg x 100	$60.00	MAVIK, Knoll Pharms	00048-5807-41

TRANEXAMIC ACID *(002365)*

CATEGORIES: Blood Formation/Coagulation; Coagulants and Anticoagulants; Dental; Fibrinolytic & Proteolytic; Hemophilia; Hemorrhage; Hemostatics; Prostatectomy, Hemorrhage In*; Pregnancy Category B; FDA Approved 1986 Dec
* Indication not approved by the FDA

BRAND NAMES: *Amcacid; Amchafibrin; Amexan; Antivoff; Cyclokapron;* **Cyklokapron**; *Exacyl; Frenolyse; Hexakapron; Transamin*
(International brand names outside U.S. in italics)

DESCRIPTION:

Each tablet contains 50 mg of tranexamic acid. Each ml of the sterile solution for intravenous injection contains 100 mg tranexamic acid and Water for injection to 1 ml.

Chemical Name: trans-4-(aminomethyl)cyclohexanecarboxylic acid. *Empirical Formula:* C8H15NO2. *Molecular Weight:* 157.2

Tranexamic acid is a white crystalline powder. Inert ingredients in the tablets are microcrystalline cellulose, talc, magnesium stearate, silicon dioxide, and povidone. The aqueous solution for injection has a pH of 6.5-7.5.

CLINICAL PHARMACOLOGY:

Tranexamic acid is a competitive inhibitor of plasminogen activation, and at much higher concentrations, a noncompetitive inhibitor of plasmin, actions similar to aminocaproic acid. Tranexamic acid is about 10 times more potent *in vitro* than aminocaproic acid.

Tranexamic acid binds more strongly than aminocaproic acid to both the strong and weak receptor sites of the plasminogen molecule in a ratio corresponding to the difference in potency between the compounds.

Transexamic acid in a concentration of 1 mg per ml does not aggregate platelets *in vitro.* Transexamic acid in concentrations up to 10 mg per ml blood has no influence on the platelet count, the coagulation time or various coagulation factors in whole blood or citrated blood from normal subjects. On the other hand, tranexamic acid in concentrations of 10 mg and 1 mg per ml blood prolongs the thrombin time.

The plasma protein binding of tranexamic acid is about 3% at therapeutic plasma levels and seems to be fully accounted for by its binding to plasminogen. Tranexamic acid does not bind to serum albumin.

Absorption of tranexamic acid after oral administration in humans represents approximately 30-50% of the ingested dose and bioavailability is not affected by food intake.

After an intravenous dose of 1 g, the plasma concentration time curve shows a triexponential decay with a half-life of about 2 hours for the terminal elimination phase. The initial volume of distribution is about 9-12 liters. Urinary excretion is the main route of elimination via glomerular filtration. Overall renal clearance is equal to overall plasma clearance (110-116 ml/min) and more than 95% of the dose is excreted in the urine as the unchanged drug. Excretion of tranexamic acid is about 90% at 24 hours after intravenous administration of 10 mg per kg body weight. After oral administration of 10-15 mg per kg body weight, the cumulative urinary excretion at 24 hours is 39% and at 48 hours, 41% of the ingested dose or

CLINICAL PHARMACOLOGY: *(cont'd)*

78% and 82% of the absorbed material. Only a small fraction of the drug is metabolized. After oral administration, 1% of the dicarboxylic acid and 0.5% of the acetylated compound are excreted.

The plasma peak level after 1 g orally is 8 mg per L and after 2 g, 15 mg per L, both obtained three hours after dosing.

An antifibrinolytic concentration of tranexamic acid remains in different tissues for about 17 hours, and in the serum, up to seven or eight hours.

The concentration of tranexamic acid in a number of other tissues is lower than in blood. In breast milk the concentration is about one hundredth of the serum peak concentration obtained. Tranexamic acid concentration in cerebrospinal fluid is about one tenth of that of plasma. The drug passes into the aqueous humour, the concentration being about one tenth of the plasma concentration.

Tranexamic acid has been detected in semen where it inhibits fibrinolytic activity but does not influence sperm migration.

INDICATIONS AND USAGE:

Tranexamic acid is indicated in patients with hemophilia for short term use (two to eight days) to reduce or prevent hemorrhage and reduce the need for replacement therapy during and following tooth extraction.

CONTRAINDICATIONS:

Tranexamic Acid is contraindicated:

1. In patients with acquired defective color vision, since this prohibits measuring one endpoint that should be followed as a measure of toxicity (See WARNINGS).

2. In patients with subarachnoid hemorrhage. Anecdotal experience indicates that cerebral edema and cerebral infarction may be caused by Tranexamic Acid in such patients.

WARNINGS:

Focal areas of retinal degeneration have developed in cats, dogs and rats following oral or intravenous tranexamic acid at doses between 250 to 1600 mg/kg/day (6 to 40 times the recommended usual human dose) from 6 days to 1 year. The incidence of such lesions has varied from 25% to 100% of animals treated and was dose-related. At lower doses some lesions have appeared to be reversible.

Limited data in cats and rabbits showed retinal changes in some animals with doses as low as 126 mg/kg/day (only about 3 times the recommended human dose) administered for several days to two weeks.

No retinal changes have been reported or noted in eye examinations in patients treated with tranexamic acid for weeks to months in clinical trials.

However, visual abnormalities, often poorly characterized, represent the most frequently reported postmarketing adverse reaction in Sweden. For patients who are to be treated continually for longer than several days, an ophthalmological examination, including visual acuity, color vision, eye-ground and visual fields, is advised, before commencing and at regular intervals during the course of treatment. Transexamic acid should be discontinued if changes in examination results are found.

PRECAUTIONS:

General: The dose of Tranexamic Acid should be reduced in patients with renal insuficiency because of the risk of accumulation. (See DOSAGE AND ADMINISTRATION.)

Carcinogenesis, Mutagenesis, and Impairment of Fertility: As increased incidence of leukemia in male mice receiving tranexamic acid in food at a concentration of 4.8% (equivalent to doses as high as 5/g/kg/day) may have been related to treatment. Female mice were not included in this experiment.

Hyperplasia of the biliary tract and cholangioma and adenocarcinoma of the intrahepatic biliary system have been reported in one strain of rats after dietary administration of doses exceeding the maximum tolerated dose for 22 months. Hyperplastic, but not neoplastic, lesions were reported at lower doses. Subsequent long term dietary administration studies in a different strain of rat, each with an exposure level equal to the maximum level employed in the earlier experiment, have failed to show much hyperplastic/neoplastic changes in the liver. No mutagenic activity has been demonstrated in several *in vitro* and *in vivo* test systems.

Pregnancy Category B: Reproduction studies performed in mice, rats, and rabbits have not revealed any evidence of impaired fertility or adverse effects on the fetus due to tranexamic acid.

There are no adequate and well-controlled studies in pregnant women. However, tranexamic acid is known to pass the placenta and appears in cord blood at concentrations approximately equal to maternal concentration. Because animal reproduction studies are not always predictive of human response, this drug should be used during pregnancy only if clearly needed.

Nursing Mothers: Tranexamic acid is present in the mother's milk at a concentration of about a hundredth of the corresponding serum levels. Caution should be exercised when Tranexamic acid is administered to a nursing woman.

Pediatric Use: The drug has had limited use in children, principally in connection with tooth extraction. The limited data suggest that dosing instructions for adults can be used for children needing Tranexamic acid therapy.

ADVERSE REACTIONS:

Gastrointestinal disturbances (nausea, vomiting, diarrhea) may occur but disappear when the dosage is reduced. Giddiness and hypotension have been reported occasionally. Hypotension has been observed when intravenous injection is too rapid. To avoid this response, the solution should not be injected more rapidly than 1 ml per minute. This adverse reaction has not been reported with oral administration.

OVERDOSAGE:

There is no known case of overdosage of Tranexamic acid. Symptoms of overdosage may be nausea, vomiting orthostatic symptoms, and/or hypotension.

DOSAGE AND ADMINISTRATION:

For Dental Extraction In Patients With Hemophilia: Immediately before surgery, substitution therapy is given together with tranexamic acid, 10 mg per kg body weight I.V. After surgery, 25 mg per kg body weight are given orally three to four times daily for two to eight days.

Alternatively, tranexamic acid can be administered entirely orally, 25 mg per kg body weight 3 to 4 times a day beginning one day prior to surgery.

Parenteral therapy, 10 mg per kg body weight 3 to 4 times daily can be used for patients unable to take oral medication.

For intravenous infusion, Tranexamic Acid Injection may be mixed with most solutions for infusion such as electrolyte solutions, carbohydrate solutions, amino acid solutions and Dextran solutions. The mixture should be prepared the same day the solution is to be used.

DOSAGE AND ADMINISTRATION: *(cont'd)*

TABLE 1 NOTE: For patients with moderate to severe impaired renal function, the following dosages are recommended:

Serum Creatinine (micromol/L)	Tranexamic Acid Dosage I.V. Dose	Tablets
120-250(1.36-2.83 mg/dl)	10 mg/kg BID	15 mg/kg BID
250-500(2.83-5.66 mg/dl)	10 mg/kg daily	15 mg/kg daily
>500(>5.66 mg/dl)	10 mg/kg every 48 hours or 5 mg/kg every 24 hours	15 mg/kg every 48 hours or 7.5 mg/kg every 24 hours

Heparin may be added to Tranexamic Acid Injection. Tranexamic Acid Injection should NOT be mixed with blood. The drug is a synthetic amino acid, and should NOT be mixed with solutions containing penicillin.

HOW SUPPLIED:

Storage: Store Tranexamic Acid tablets and injections at room temperature (15°-30° C).

HOW SUPPLIED - EQUIVALENTS NOT AVAILABLE:

Injection, Solution - Intravenous - 100 mg/ml

10 ml x 10 $16.23 CYKLOKAPRON, Pharmacia & Upjohn 00016-1114-08

Tablet, Uncoated - Oral - 500 mg

100's $315.00 CYKLOKAPRON, Pharmacia & Upjohn 00016-0114-00

TRANYLCYPROMINE SULFATE *(002366)*

CATEGORIES: Antidepressants; Central Nervous System Agents; Depression; Neuroleptics; MAO Inhibitors; Monoamine Oxidase Inhibitors; Psychotherapeutic Agents; Seasonal Affective Disorder*; FDA Approved 1985 Aug

* Indication not approved by the FDA

BRAND NAMES: **Parnate**; *Sicoton*

(International brand names outside U.S. in italics)

FORMULARIES: Aetna; PCS

COST OF THERAPY: $123.66 (Depression; Tablet; 10 mg; 3/day; 90 days)

PRIMARY ICD9: 311 (Depressive Disorder, Not Elsewhere Classified)

DESCRIPTION:

BEFORE PRESCRIBING, THE PHYSICIAN SHOULD BE FAMILIAR WITH THE ENTIRE CONTENTS OF THIS PRESCRIBING INFORMATION.

Chemically, tranylcypromine sulfate is (±)-*trans*-2-phenylcyclopropylamine sulfate (2:1).

Each round, rose-red, film-coated tablet is imprinted with the product name Parnate and SKF and contains tranylcypromine sulfate equivalent to 10 mg of tranylcypromine. Inactive ingredients consist of gelatin, lactose, cellulose, citric acid, croscarmellose sodium, talc, magnesium stearate, iron oxide, D&C Red No. 7, FD&C Blue No. 2, FD&C Yellow No. 6, FD&C Red No. 40, titanium dioxide and trace amounts of other inactive ingredients.

NOTE: Parnate (tranylcypromine sulfate) tablets have been changed from rose-red sugar-coated tablets to rose-red film-coated tablets. The film-coated tablets differ in size from the sugar-coated tablets, but the drug content remains unchanged.

CLINICAL PHARMACOLOGY:

Tranylcypromine is a non-hydrazine monoamine oxidase inhibitor with a rapid onset of activity. It increases the concentration of epinephrine, norepinephrine and serotonin in storage sites throughout the nervous system and, in theory, this increased concentration of monoamines in the brain stem is the basis for its antidepressant activity. When tranylcypromine is withdrawn, monoamine oxidase activity is recovered in 3 to 5 days, although the drug is excreted in 24 hours.

INDICATIONS AND USAGE:

For the treatment of Major Depressive Episode Without Melancholia.

Tranylcypromine sulfate should be used in adult patients who can be closely supervised. It should rarely be the first antidepressant drug given. Rather, the drug is suited for patients who have failed to respond to the drugs more commonly administered for depression.

The effectiveness of tranylcypromine sulfate has been established in adult outpatients, most of whom had a depressive illness which would correspond to a diagnosis of Major Depressive Episode Without Melancholia. As described in the American Psychiatric Association's Diagnostic and Statistical Manual, third edition (DSM III). Major Depressive Episode implies a prominent and relatively persistent (nearly every day for at least 2 weeks) depressed or dysphoric mood that usually interferes with daily functioning and includes at least 4 of the following 8 symptoms: change in appetite, change in sleep, psychomotor agitation or retardation, loss of interest in usual activities or decrease in sexual drive, increased fatigability, feelings of guilt or worthlessness, slowed thinking or impaired concentration and suicidal ideation or attempts.

The effectiveness of tranylcypromine sulfate in patients who meet the criteria for Major Depressive Episode with Melancholia (endogenous features) has not been established.

Summary of Contraindications Tranylcypromine sulfate should not be administered in combination with any of the following: MAO inhibitors or dibenzazepine derivatives; sympathomimetics (including amphetamines); some central nervous system depressants (including narcotics and alcohol); antihypertensive, diuretic, antihistaminic, sedative or anesthetic drugs; bupropion HCl; buspirone HCl; dextromethorphan; cheese or other foods with a high tyramine content; or excessive quantities of caffeine.

Tranylcypromine sulfate should not be administered to any patient with a confirmed or suspected cerebrovascular defect or to any patient with cardiovascular disease, hypertension or history of headache.

(For complete discussion of CONTRAINDICATIONS and WARNINGS, see below.)

CONTRAINDICATIONS:

Tranylcypromine Sulfate Is Contraindicated:

1. In Patients With Cerebrovascular Defects Or Cardiovascular Disorders: Tranylcypromine sulfate should not be administered to any patient with a confirmed or suspected cerebrovascular defect or to any patient with cardiovascular disease or hypertension.

2. In The Presence Of Pheochromocytoma: Tranylcypromine sulfate should not be used in the presence of pheochromocytoma since such tumors secrete pressor substances.

CONTRAINDICATIONS: *(cont'd)*

3. In Combination With Mao Inhibitors Or With Dibenzazepine-Related Entities: Tranylcypromine sulfate should not be administered together or in rapid succession with other MAO inhibitors or with dibenzazepine- related entities. Hypertensive crises or severe convulsive seizures may occur in patients receiving such combinations.

In patients being transferred to tranylcypromine sulfate from another MAO inhibitor or from a dibenzazepine-related entity, allow a medication-free interval of at least a week, then initiate tranylcypromine sulfate using half the normal starting dosage for at least the first week of therapy. Similarly, at least a week should elapse between the discontinuance of tranylcypromine sulfate and the administration of another MAO inhibitor or a dibenzazepine-related entity, or the readministration of tranylcypromine sulfate.

The following list includes some other MAO inhibitors, dibenzazepine-related entities and tricyclic antidepressants.

Other Mao Inhibitors:

Furazolidone Furoxone (Roberts Laboratories)
Isocarboxazid Marplan (Roche Laboratories)
Pargyline HCl Eutonyl (Abbott Laboratories)
Pargyline HCl and Eutron
methyclothiazide (Abbott Laboratories)
Phenelzine sulfate Nardil (Parke-Davis)
Procarbazine HCl Matulane (Roche Laboratories)

Dibenzazepine-Related and Other Tricyclics:

Amitriptyline HCl Elavil (Merck Sharp & Dohme)
Endep (Roche Products)
Perphenazine and Etrafon amitriptyline HCl (Schering)
Triavil (Merck Sharp & Dohme)
Clomipramine Anafranil hydrochloride (Ciba-Geigy)
Desipramine HCl Norpramin (Marion Merrell Dow)
Pertofrane (Rhone-Poulenc Rorer Pharmaceuticals)
Imipramine HCl Janimine (Abbott Laboratories)
Tofranil (Geigy Pharmaceuticals)
Nortriptyline HCl Aventyl(Eli Lilly & Co.)
Pamelor (Sandoz)
Protriptyline HCl Vivactil (Merck Sharp & Dohme)
Doxepin HCl, Adapin (Fisons)
Sinequan (Roerig)
Carbamazepine,Tegretol (Geigy Pharmaceuticals)
Cyclobenzaprine HCl, Flexeril (Merck Sharp & Dohme)
Amoxapine, Asendin (Lederle)
Maprotiline HCl, Ludiomil (CIBA)
Trimipramine maleate, Surmontil (Wyeth-Ayerst Laboratories)

4. In Combination With Bupropion: The concurrent administration of a MAO inhibitor and bupropion hydrochloride (Wellbutrin, Burroughs Wellcome) is contraindicated. At least 14 days should elapse between discontinuation of a MAO inhibitor and initiation of treatment with bupropion hydrochloride.

5. In Combination With Selective Serotonin Reuptake Inhibitors (SSRI): As a general rule, tranylcypromine sulfate should not be administered in combination with any SSRI. There have been reports of serious, sometimes fatal, reactions (including hyperthermia, rigidity, myoclonus, autonomic instability with possible rapid fluctuations of vital signs, and mental status changes that include extreme agitation progressing to delirium and coma) in patients receiving fluoxetine (Prozac, Lilly) in combination with a monoamine oxidase inhibitor (MAOI), and in patients who have recently discontinued fluoxetine and are then started on a MAOI. Some cases presented with features resembling neuroleptic malignant syndrome. Therefore, fluoxetine and other SSRIs should not be used in combination with a MAOI, or within 14 days of discontinuing therapy with a MAOI. Since fluoxetine and its major metabolite have very long elimination half-lives, at least 5 weeks should be allowed after stopping fluoxetine before starting a MAOI.

At least 2 weeks should be allowed after stopping sertraline (Zoloft, Roerig) or paroxetine (Paxil, SmithKline Beecham Pharmaceuticals) before starting a MAOI.

6. In combination with buspirone: Tranylcypromine sulfate should not be used in combination with buspirone HCl (Buspar, Mead Johnson), since several cases of elevated blood pressure have been reported in patients taking MAO inhibitors who were then given buspirone HCl. At least 10 days should elapse between the discontinuation of tranylcypromine sulfate and the institution of buspirone HCl.

7. In combination with sympathomimetics: Tranylcypromine sulfate should not be administered in combination with sympathomimetics, including amphetamines, and over-the-counter drugs such as cold, hay fever or weight-reducing preparations that contain vasoconstrictors.

During tranylcypromine sulfate therapy, it appears that certain patients are particularly vulnerable to the effects of sympathomimetics when the activity of certain enzymes is inhibited. Use of sympathomimetics and compounds such as guanethidine, methyldopa, reserpine, dopamine, levodopa and tryptophan with tranylcypromine sulfate may precipitate hypertension, headache and related symptoms. In addition, use with tryptophan may precipitate disorientation, memory impairment and other neurologic and behavioral signs.

8. In combination with meperidine: Do not use meperidine concomitantly with MAO inhibitors or within 2 or 3 weeks following MAOI therapy. Serious reactions have been precipitated with concomitant use, including coma, severe hypertension or hypotension, severe respiratory depression, convulsions, malignant hyperpyrexia, excitation, peripheral vascular collapse and death. It is thought that these reactions may be mediated by accumulation of 5-HT (serotonin) consequent to MAO inhibition.

9. In combination with dextromethorphan: The combination of MAO inhibitors and dextromethorphan has been reported to cause brief episodes of psychosis or bizarre behavior.

10. In combination with cheese or other foods with a high tyramine content: Hypertensive crises have sometimes occurred during tranylcypromine sulfate therapy after ingestion of foods with a high tyramine content. In general, the patient should avoid protein foods in which aging or protein breakdown is used to increase flavor. In particular, patients should be instructed not to take foods such as cheese (particularly strong or aged varieties), sour cream, Chianti wine, sherry, beer (including nonalcoholic beer), liqueurs, pickled herring, anchovies, caviar, liver, canned figs, raisins, bananas or avocados (particularly if overripe), chocolate, soy sauce, sauerkraut, the pods of broad beans (fava beans), yeast extracts, yogurt, meat extracts or meat prepared with tenderizers.

CONTRAINDICATIONS: *(cont'd)*

11. In patients undergoing elective surgery: Patients taking tranylcypromine sulfate should not undergo elective surgery requiring general anesthesia. Also, they should not be given cocaine or local anesthesia containing sympathomimetic vasoconstrictors. The possible combined hypotensive effects of tranylcypromine sulfate and spinal anesthesia should be kept in mind. Tranylcypromine sulfate should be discontinued at least 10 days prior to elective surgery.

Additional Contraindications: In general, the physician should bear in mind the possibility of a lowered margin of safety when tranylcypromine sulfate (tranylcypromine sulfate) is administered in combination with potent drugs.

1. Tranylcypromine sulfate should not be used in combination with some central nervous system depressants such as narcotics and alcohol, or with hypotensive agents. A marked potentiating effect on these classes of drugs has been reported.

2. Anti-parkinsonism drugs should be used with caution in patients receiving tranylcypromine sulfate since severe reactions have been reported.

3. Tranylcypromine sulfate should not be used in patients with a history of liver disease or in those with abnormal liver function tests.

4. Excessive use of caffeine in any form should be avoided in patients receiving tranylcypromine sulfate.

WARNING TO PHYSICIANS: Tranylcypromine sulfate is a potent agent with the capability of producing serious side effects: Tranylcypromine sulfate is not recommended in those depressive reactions where other antidepressant drugs may be effective. **It should be reserved for patients who can be closely supervised and who have not responded satisfactorily to the drugs more commonly administered for depression.**

Before prescribing, the physician should be completely familiar with the full material on dosage, side effects and contraindications on these pages, with the principles of MAO inhibitor therapy and the side effects of this class of drugs. Also, the physician should be familiar with the symptomatology of mental depressions and alternate methods of treatment to aid in the careful selection of patients for tranylcypromine sulfate therapy. In depressed patients, the possibility of suicide should always be considered and adequate precautions taken.

Pregnancy Warning: Use of any drug in pregnancy, during lactation or in women of childbearing age requires that the potential benefits of the drug be weighed against its possible hazards to mother and child.

Animal reproductive studies show that tranylcypromine sulfate passes through the placental barrier into the fetus of the rat, and into the milk of the lactating dog. The absence of harmful action of tranylcypromine sulfate on fertility or on postnatal development by either prenatal treatment or from the milk of treated animals has not been demonstrated. Tranylcypromine is excreted in human milk.

Warning To The Patient: Patients should be instructed to report promptly the occurrence of headache or other unusual symptoms, *i.e.,* palpitation and/or tachycardia, a sense of constriction in the throat or chest, sweating, dizziness, neck stiffness, nausea or vomiting.

Patients should be warned against eating the foods listed in Section 9 under CONTRAINDICATIONS while on tranylcypromine sulfate therapy. Also, they should be told not to drink alcoholic beverages. The patient should also be warned about the possibility of hypotension and faintness, as well as drowsiness sufficient to impair performance of potentially hazardous tasks such as driving a car or operating machinery.

Patients should also be cautioned not to take concomitant medications, whether prescription or over-the-counter drugs such as cold, hay fever or weight-reducing preparations, without the advice of a physician. They should be advised not to consume excessive amounts of caffeine in any form. Likewise, they should inform other physicians, and their dentist, about their use of tranylcypromine sulfate.

WARNINGS:

Hypertensive Crises: The most important reaction associated with tranylcypromine sulfate is the occurrence of hypertensive crises which have sometimes been fatal.

These crises are characterized by some or all of the following symptoms: occipital headache which may radiate frontally, palpitation, neck stiffness or soreness, nausea or vomiting, sweating (sometimes with fever and sometimes with cold, clammy skin) and photophobia. Either tachycardia or bradycardia may be present, and associated constricting chest pain and dilated pupils may occur. **Intracranial bleeding, sometimes fatal in outcome, has been reported in association with the paradoxical increase in blood pressure.**

In all patients taking tranylcypromine sulfate blood pressure should be followed closely to detect evidence of any pressor response. It is emphasized that full reliance should not be placed on blood pressure readings, but that the patient should also be observed frequently.

Therapy should be discontinued immediately upon the occurrence of palpitation or frequent headaches during tranylcypromine sulfate therapy. These signs may be prodromal of a hypertensive crisis.

Important: Recommended Treatment In Hypertensive Crises: If a hypertensive crisis occurs, tranylcypromine sulfate should be discontinued and therapy to lower blood pressure should be instituted immediately. Headache tends to abate as blood pressure is lowered. On the basis of present evidence, phentolamine (available as Regitine*) is recommended. (The dosage reported for phentolamine is 5 mg IV) Care should be taken to administer this drug slowly in order to avoid producing an excessive hypotensive effect. Fever should be managed by means of external cooling. Other symptomatic and supportive measures may be desirable in particular cases. Do not use parenteral reserpine.

PRECAUTIONS:

Hypotension: Hypotension has been observed during tranylcypromine sulfate therapy. Symptoms of postural hypotension are seen most commonly but not exclusively in patients with pre-existent hypertension; blood pressure usually returns rapidly to pretreatment levels upon discontinuation of the drug. At doses above 30 mg daily, postural hypotension is a major side effect and may result in syncope. Dosage increases should be made more gradually in patients showing a tendency toward hypotension at the beginning of therapy. Postural hypotension may be relieved by having the patient lie down until blood pressure returns to normal.

Also, when tranylcypromine sulfate is combined with those phenothiazine derivatives or other compounds known to cause hypotension, the possibility of additive hypotensive effects should be considered.

Other Precautions There have been reports of drug dependency in patients using doses of tranylcypromine significantly in excess of the therapeutic range. Some of these patients had a history of previous substance abuse. The following withdrawal symptoms have been reported: restlessness, anxiety, depression, confusion, hallucinations, headache, weakness and diarrhea.

Drugs which lower the seizure threshold, including MAO inhibitors, should not be used with Amipaque†. As with other MAO inhibitors, tranylcypromine sulfate (tranylcypromine sulfate) should be discontinued at least 48 hours before myelography and should not be resumed for at least 24 hours postprocedure.

PRECAUTIONS: *(cont'd)*

In depressed patients, the possibility of suicide should always be considered and adequate precautions taken. Exclusive reliance on drug therapy to prevent suicidal attempts is unwarranted, as there may be a delay in the onset of therapeutic effect or an increase in anxiety and agitation. Also, some patients fail to respond to drug therapy or may respond only temporarily.

MAO inhibitors may have the capacity to suppress anginal pain that would otherwise serve as a warning of myocardial ischemia.

The usual precautions should be observed in patients with impaired renal function since there is a possibility of cumulative effects in such patients.

Older patients may suffer more morbidity than younger patients during and following an episode of hypertension or malignant hyperthermia.

Older patients have less compensatory reserve to cope with any serious adverse reaction. Therefore, tranylcypromine sulfate should be used with caution in the elderly population.

Although excretion of tranylcypromine sulfate is rapid, inhibition of MAO may persist up to 10 days following discontinuation.

Because the influence of tranylcypromine sulfate on the convulsive threshold is variable in animal experiments, suitable precautions should be taken if epileptic patients are treated.

Some MAO inhibitors have contributed to hypoglycemic episodes in diabetic patients receiving insulin or oral hypoglycemic agents. Therefore, tranylcypromine sulfate should be used with caution in diabetics using these drugs.

Tranylcypromine sulfate may aggravate coexisting symptoms in depression, such as anxiety and agitation.

Use tranylcypromine sulfate with caution in hyperthyroid patients because of their increased sensitivity to pressor amines.

Tranylcypromine sulfate should be administered with caution to patients receiving Antabuse‡. In a single study, rats given high intraperitoneal doses of *d* or *l* isomers of tranylcypromine sulfate plus disulfiram experienced severe toxicity including convulsions and death. Additional studies in rats given high oral doses of racemic tranylcypromine sulfate and disulfiram produced no adverse interaction.

ADVERSE REACTIONS:

Overstimulation which may include increased anxiety, agitation and manic symptoms is usually evidence of excessive therapeutic action. Dosage should be reduced, or a phenothiazine tranquilizer should be administered concomitantly.

Patients may experience restlessness or insomnia; may notice some weakness, drowsiness, episodes of dizziness or dry mouth; or may report nausea, diarrhea, abdominal pain or constipation. Most of these effects can be relieved by lowering the dosage or by giving suitable concomitant medication.

Tachycardia, significant anorexia, edema, palpitation, blurred vision, chills and impotence have each been reported.

Headaches without blood pressure elevation have occurred.

Rare instances of hepatitis and skin rash have been reported.

Impaired water excretion compatible with the syndrome of inappropriate secretion of antidiuretic hormone (SIADH) has been reported.

Tinnitus, muscle spasm, tremors, myoclonic jerks, numbness, paresthesia, urinary retention and retarded ejaculation have been reported.

Hematologic disorders including anemia, leukopenia, agranulocytosis and thrombocytopenia have been reported.

Post-Introduction Reports: The following are spontaneously reported adverse events temporally associated with tranylcypromine sulfate therapy. No clear relationship between tranylcypromine sulfate and these events has been established. Localized scleroderma, flare-up of cystic acne, ataxia, confusion, disorientation, memory loss, urinary frequency, urinary incontinence, urticaria, fissuring in corner of mouth, akinesia.

OVERDOSAGE:

Symptoms: The characteristic symptoms that may be caused by overdosage are usually those described above.

However, an intensification of these symptoms and sometimes severe additional manifestations may be seen, depending on the degree of overdosage and on individual susceptibility. Some patients exhibit insomnia, restlessness and anxiety, progressing in severe cases to agitation, mental confusion and incoherence. Hypotension, dizziness, weakness and drowsiness may occur, progressing in severe cases to extreme dizziness and shock. A few patients have displayed hypertension with severe headache and other symptoms. Rare instances have been reported in which hypertension was accompanied by twitching or myoclonic fibrillation of skeletal muscles with hyperpyrexia, sometimes progressing to generalized rigidity and coma.

Treatment: Gastric lavage is helpful if performed early. Treatment should normally consist of general supportive measures, close observation of vital signs and steps to counteract specific symptoms as they occur, since MAO inhibition may persist. The management of hypertensive crises is described under WARNINGS in the HYPERTENSIVE CRISES section.

External cooling is recommended if hyperpyrexia occurs. Barbiturates have been reported to help relieve myoclonic reactions, but frequency of administration should be controlled carefully because tranylcypromine sulfate may prolong barbiturate activity. When hypotension requires treatment, the standard measures for managing circulatory shock should be initiated. If pressor agents are used, the rate of infusion should be regulated by careful observation of the patient because an exaggerated pressor response sometimes occurs in the presence of MAO inhibition. Remember that the toxic effect of tranylcypromine sulfate may be delayed or prolonged following the last dose of the drug. Therefore, the patient should be closely observed for at least a week. It is not known if tranylcypromine is dialyzable.

DOSAGE AND ADMINISTRATION:

Dosage should be adjusted to the requirements of the individual patient. Improvement should be seen within 48 hours to 3 weeks after starting therapy.

The usual effective dosage is 30 mg per day, usually given in divided doses. If there are no signs of improvement after a reasonable period (up to 2 weeks), then the dosage may be increased in 10 mg per day increments at intervals of 1 to 3 weeks; the dosage range may be extended to a maximum of 60 mg per day from the usual 30 mg per day.

HOW SUPPLIED:

Parnate is supplied as round, rose-red, film-coated tablets imprinted with the product name PARNATE and SKF and contains tranylcypromine sulfate equivalent to 10 mg of tranylcypromine, in bottles of 100 with a desiccant.

Store between 15° and 30°C (59° and 86°F).

* phentolamine mesylate USP, Ciba.

† metrizamide, Sanofi Winthrop Pharmaceuticals.

HOW SUPPLIED: *(cont'd)*

‡ disulfiram, Wyeth-Ayerst Laboratories.

HOW SUPPLIED - EQUIVALENTS NOT AVAILABLE:

Tablet, Plain Coated - Oral - 10 mg

100's	$45.80	PARNATE, SKB Pharms	00007-4471-20

TRAZODONE HYDROCHLORIDE *(002367)*

CATEGORIES: Antianxiety Drugs; Antidepressants; Anxiety; Central Nervous System Agents; Depression; Psychotherapeutic Agents; Selective Serotonin Reuptake Inhibitors; Agoraphobia*; Panic Disorder*; Pregnancy Category C; FDA Approval Pre 1982

* Indication not approved by the FDA

BRAND NAMES: *Beneficat*; *Bimaran*; *Deprax*; *Desirel*; **Desyrel**; *Manegan*; *Molipaxin*; *Pragmarel*; *Sideril*; *Taxagon*; *Thombran*; *Trazalon*; *Trazolan*; Trazon-150; *Trazonil*; *Trittico*

(International brand names outside U.S. in italics)

FORMULARIES: Aetna; BC-BS; CIGNA; FHP; Foundation; Humana; Kaiser; Medco; Medi-Cal; PCS; PruCare; United

COST OF THERAPY: $13.58 (Depression; Tablet; 50 mg; 3/day; 90 days) vs. Potential Cost of $2,456.15 (Depression)

PRIMARY ICD9: 311 (Depressive Disorder, Not Elsewhere Classified)

DESCRIPTION:

Trazodone hydrochloride, (abbreviated here as trazodone HCl), is an antidepressant chemically unrelated to tricyclic, tetracyclic, or other known antidepressant agents. It is a triazolopyridine derivative designated as 2-(3-(4-(3-chlorophenyl)-1 - piperazinyl) propyl-1,2,4-triazolo(4,3-a)pyridi n-3 (2H)-one hydrochloride. Trazodone HCl is a white odorless crystalline powder which is freely soluble in water. Its molecular weight is 408.3. The empirical formula is $C_{19}H_{22}ClN_5O$°HCl.

Trazodone HCl is supplied for oral administration in 50 mg, 100 mg, 150 mg, and 300 mg tablets.

Trazodone HCl Tablets, 50 mg, contain the following inactive ingredients: dibasic calcium phosphate, castor oil, microcrystalline cellulose, ethylcellulose, FD&C Yellow No. 6 (aluminum lake), lactose, magnesium stearate, povidone, sodium starch glycolate, and starch (corn).

Trazodone HCl Tablets, 100 mg, contain the following inactive ingredients: dibasic calcium phosphate, castor oil, microcrystalline cellulose, ethylcellulose, lactose, magnesium stearate, povidone, sodium starch glycolate, and starch (corn).

Trazodone HCl Tablets, 150 mg, contain the following in active ingredients: microcrystalline cellulose, FD&C Yellow No. 6 (aluminum lake), magnesium stearate, pre-gelatinized starch, and stearic acid.

Trazodone HCl Tablets, 300 mg, contain the following inactive ingredients: microcrystalline cellulose, yellow ferric oxide, magnesium stearate, sodium starch glycolate, pregelatinized starch, and stearic acid.

CLINICAL PHARMACOLOGY:

The mechanism of trazodone HCl's antidepressant action in man is not fully understood. In animals, trazodone HCl selectively inhibits serotonin uptake by brain synaptosomes and potentiates the behavioral changes induced by the serotonin precursor, 5-hydroxytryptophan. Cardiac conduction effects of trazodone HCl in the anesthetized dog are qualitatively dissimilar and quantitatively less pronounced than those seen with tricyclic antidepressants. Trazodone HCl is not a monoamine oxidase inhibitor and, unlike amphetamine-type drugs, does not stimulate the central nervous system.

In man, trazodone HCl is well absorbed after oral administration without selective localization in any tissue. When trazodone HCl is taken shortly after ingestion of food, there may be an increase in the amount of drug absorbed, a decrease in maximum concentration and a lengthening in the time to maximum concentration. Peak plasma levels occur approximately one hour after dosing when trazodone HCl is taken on an empty stomach or two hours after dosing when taken with food. Elimination of trazodone HCl is biphasic, consisting of an initial phase (half-life 3-6 hours) followed by a slower phase (half-life 5-9 hours), and is unaffected by the presence or absence of food. Since the clearance of trazodone HCl from the body is sufficiently variable, is some patients trazodone HCl may accumulate in the plasma.

For those patients who responded to trazodone HCl, one-third of the inpatients and one-third of the outpatients had a significant therapeutic response by the end of the first week of treatment. Three-fourths of all responders demonstrated a significant therapeutic effect by the end of the second week. One-fourth of responders required 2-4 weeks for a significant therapeutic response.

INDICATIONS AND USAGE:

Trazodone HCl is indicated for the treatment of depression. The efficacy of trazodone HCl has been demonstrated in both inpatient and outpatient settings and for depressed patients with and without prominent anxiety. The depressive illness of patients studied corresponds to the Major Depressive Episode criteria of the American Psychiatric Association's Diagnostic and Statistical Manual, III.[a]

Major Depressive Episode implies a prominent and relatively persistent (nearly every day for at least two weeks) depressed or dysphoric mood that usually interferes with daily functioning, and includes at least four of the following eight symptoms: change in appetite, change in sleep, psychomotor agitation or retardation, loss of interest in usual activities or decrease in sexual drive, increased fatigability, feelings of guilt or worthlessness, slowed thinking or impaired concentration, and suicidal ideation or attempts.

CONTRAINDICATIONS:

Trazodone HCl is contraindicated in patients hypersensitive to trazodone HCl.

WARNINGS:

TRAZODONE HAS BEEN ASSOCIATED WITH THE OCCURRENCE OF PRIAPISM. IN APPROXIMATELY 1/3 OF THE CASES REPORTED, SURGICAL INTERVENTION WAS REQUIRED AND, IN A PORTION OF THESE CASES, PERMANENT IMPAIRMENT OF ERECTILE FUNCTION OR IMPOTENCE RESULTED. MALE PATIENTS WITH PROLONGED OR INAPPROPRIATE ERECTIONS SHOULD IMMEDIATELY DISCONTINUE THE DRUG AND CONSULT THEIR PHYSICIAN.

If an erection should persist, promptly contact Bristol-Myers USPG Medical Services Department (812/429-5591 or 812/429-5000).

WARNINGS: *(cont'd)*

The detumescence of priapism and drug-induced penile erections by the intracavernosal injection of alpha-adrenergic stimulants such as epinephrine and metaraminol has been reported.[b-g] For one case of priapism (of some 12-24 hours' duration) in a trazodone HCl-treated patient in whom the intracavernosal injection of epinephrine was accomplished, prompt detumescence occurred with return of normal erectile activity.

This procedure should be performed under the supervision of a urologist or a physician familiar with the procedure and should not be initiated without urologic consultation if the priapism has persisted for more than 24 hours.

Trazodone HCl is not recommended for use during the initial recovery phase of myocardial infarction.

Caution should be used when administering trazodone HCl to patients with cardiac disease, and such patients should be closely monitored, since antidepressant drugs (including trazodone HCl) have been associated with the occurrence of cardiac arrhythmias. Recent clinical studies in patients with pre-existing cardiac disease indicate that trazodone HCl may be arrhythmogenic in some patients in that population. Arrhythmias identified include isolated PVC's, ventricular couplets, and in two patients short episodes (3-4 beats) of ventricular tachycardia.

PRECAUTIONS:

GENERAL

The possibility of suicide in seriously depressed patients is inherent in the illness and may persist until significant remission occurs. Therefore, prescriptions should be written for the smallest number of tablets consistent with good patient management.

Hypotension, including orthostatic hypotension and syncope, has been reported to occur in patients receiving trazodone HCl. Concomitant administration of antihypertensive therapy with trazodone HCl may require a reduction in the dose of the antihypertensive drug.

Little is known about the interaction between trazodone HCl and general anesthetics; therefore, prior to elective surgery, trazodone HCl should be discontinued for as long as clinically feasible.

As with all antidepressants, the use of trazodone HCl should be based on the consideration of the physician that the expected benefits of therapy outweigh potential risk factors.

INFORMATION FOR THE PATIENT

Because priapism has been reported to occur in patients receiving trazodone HCl, patients with prolonged or inappropriate penile erection should immediately discontinue the drug and consult with the physician(see WARNINGS.)

Antidepressants may impair the mental and/or physical ability required for the performance of potentially hazardous tasks, such as operating an automobile or machinery; the patient should be cautioned accordingly.

Trazodone HCl may enhance the response to alcohol, barbiturates, and other CNS depressants.

Trazodone HCl should be given shortly after a meal or light snack. Within any individual patient, total drug absorption may be up to 20% higher when the drug is taken with food rather than on an empty stomach. The risk of dizziness/lightheadedness may increase under fasting conditions.

LABORATORY TESTS

Occasional low white blood cell and neutrophil counts have been noted in patients receiving trazodone HCl. These were not considered clinically significant and did not necessitate discontinuation of the drug; however, the drug should be discontinued in any patient whose white blood cell count or absolute neutrophil count falls below normal levels. White blood cell and differential counts are recommended for patients who develop fever and sore throat (or other signs of infection) during therapy.

THERAPEUTIC INTERACTIONS

Concurrent administration with electroshock therapy should be avoided because of the absence of experience in this area.

There have been reports of increased and decreased prothrombin time occurring in Coumadinized patients who take trazodone HCl.

CARCINOGENESIS, MUTAGENESIS, AND IMPAIRMENT OF FERTILITY

No drug-or dose-related occurrence of carcinogenesis was evident in rats receiving trazodone HCl in daily oral doses up to 300 mg/kg for 18 months.

PREGNANCY CATEGORY C

Trazodone HCl has been shown to cause increased fetal resorption and other adverse effects on the fetus in two studies using the rat when given at dose levels approximately 30-50 times the proposed maximum human dose. There was also an increase in congenital anomalies in one of three rabbit studies at approximately 15-50 times the maximum human dose. There are no adequate and well-controlled studies in pregnant women. Trazodone HCl should be used during pregnancy only if the potential benefit justifies the potential risk to the fetus.

NURSING MOTHERS

Trazodone HCl and/or its metabolites have been found in the milk of lactating rats, suggesting that the drug may be secreted in human milk. Caution should be exercised when trazodone HCl is administered to a nursing woman.

PEDIATRIC USE

Safety and effectiveness in children below the age of 18 have not been established.

DRUG INTERACTIONS:

Increased serum digoxin or phenytoin levels have been reported to occur in patients receiving trazodone HCl concurrently with either of those two drugs.

It is not known whether interactions will occur between monoamine oxidase (MAO) inhibitors and trazodone HCl. Due to the absence of clinical experience, if MAO inhibitors are discontinued shortly before or are to be given concomitantly with trazodone HCl, therapy should be initiated cautiously with gradual increase in dosage until optimum response is achieved.

ADVERSE REACTIONS:

Because the frequency of adverse drug effects is affected by diverse factors (*e.g.,* drug dose, methods of detection, physician judgment, disease under treatment, etc.) a single meaningful estimate of adverse event incidence is difficult to obtain. This problem is illustrated by the variation in adverse event incidence observed and reported from the inpatients and outpatients treated with trazodone HCl. It is impossible to determine precisely what accounts for the differences observed.

CLINICAL TRIAL REPORTS

The table below, (TABLE 1), is presented solely to indicate the relative frequency of adverse events reported in representative controlled clinical studies conducted to evaluate the safety and efficacy of trazodone HCl.

ADVERSE REACTIONS: *(cont'd)*

The figures cited cannot be used to predict precisely the incidence of untoward events in the course of usual medical practice where patient characteristics and other factors often differ from those which prevailed in the clinical trials. These incidence figures, also, cannot be compared with those obtained from other clinical studies involving related drug products and placebo as each group of drug trials is conducted under a different set of conditions.

TABLE 1

	Treatment-Emergent Symptom Incidence Inpts		Outpts	
	T	**P**	**T**	**P**
Number of Patients	142	95	157	158
% of Patients Reporting				
ALLERGIC				
Skin Condition/Edema	2.8	1.1	7.0	1.3
AUTONOMIC				
Blurred Vision	6.3	4.2	14.7	3.8
Constipation	7.0	4.2	7.6	5.7
Dry Mouth	14.8	8.4	33.8	20.3
CARDIOVASCULAR				
Hypertension	2.1	1.1	1.3	*
Hypotension	7.0	1.1	3.8	0.0
Shortness of Breath	*	1.1	1.3	0.0
Syncope	2.8	2.1	4.5	1.3
Tachycardia/Palpitations	0.0	0.0	7.0	7.0
CNS				
Anger/Hostility	3.5	6.3	1.3	2.5
Confusion	4.9	0.0	5.7	7.6
Decreased Concentration	2.8	2.1	1.3	0.0
Disorientation	2.1	0.0	*	0.0
Dizziness/Lightheadedness	19.6	5.3	28.0	15.2
Drowsiness	23.9	6.3	40.8	19.6
Excitement	1.4	1.1	5.1	5.7
Fatigue	11.3	4.2	5.7	2.5
Headache	9.9	5.3	19.8	15.8
Insomnia	9.9	10.5	6.4	12.0
Impaired Memory	1.4	0.0	*	*
Nervousness	14.8	10.5	6.4	8.2
GASTROINTESTINAL/ABDOMINAL/GASTRIC				
Disorder	3.5	4.2	5.7	4.4
Bad Taste in Mouth	1.4	0.0	0.0	0.0
Diarrhea	0.0	1.1	4.5	1.9
Nausea/Vomiting	9.9	1.1	12.7	9.5
MUSCOLOSKELETAL				
Musculoskeletal Aches/Pains	5.6	3.2	5.1	2.5
NEUROLOGICAL				
Incoordination	4.9	0.0	1.9	0.0
Paresthesia	1.4	0.0	0.0	*
Tremors	2.8	1.1	5.1	3.8
SEXUAL FUNCTION				
Decreased Libido	*	1.1	1.3	*
OTHER				
Decreased Appetite	3.5	5.3	0.0	*
Eyes Red/Tired/Itching	2.8	0.0	0.0	0.0
Head Full-Heavy	2.8	0.0	0.0	0.0
Malaise	2.8	0.0	0.0	0.0
Nasal/Sinal Congestion	2.8	0.0	5.7	3 2
Nightmares/Vivid Dreams	*	1.1	5.1	5.7
Sweating/Clamminess	1.4	1.1	*	*
Tinnitus	1.4	0.0	0.0	*
Weight Gain	1.4	0.0	4.5	1.9
Weight Loss	*	3.2	5.7	2.5

* Incidence less than 1%.
T = Trazodone HCl
P = Placebo

Occasional sinus bradycardia has occurred in long-term studies.

In addition to the relatively common (*i.e.,* greater than 1%) untoward events enumerated above, the following adverse events have been reported to occur in association with the use of trazodone HCl in the controlled clinical studies: akathisia, allergic reaction, anemia, chest pain, delayed urine flow, early menses, flatulence, hallucinations/delusions, hematuria, hypersalivation, hypomania, impaired speech, impotence, increased appetite, increased libido, increased urinary frequency, missed periods, muscle twitches, numbness, and retrograde ejaculation.

POSTINTRODUCTION REPORTS

Although the following adverse reactions have been reported in trazodone HCl users, the causal association has neither been confirmed nor refuted.

Voluntary reports received since market introduction include the following: agitation, alopecia, apnea, ataxia, breast enlargement, diplopia, edema, extrapyramidal symptoms, grand mal seizures, hallucinations, hemolytic anemia, hyperbilirubinemia, leukonychia, jaundice, lactation, liver enzyme alterations, methemoglobinemia, nausea/vomiting (most frequently), paresthesia, priapism (See WARNINGS and **PRECAUTIONS, Information for Patients**; some patients may require surgical intervention), pruritus, psychosis, rash, stupor, inappropriate ADH syndrome, tardive dyskinesia, unexplained death, urinary incontinence, urinary retention, urticaria, vasodilation, vertigo, and weakness.

Cardiovascular system effects which have been reported include the following: conduction block, orthostatic hypotension and syncope, palpitations, bradycardia, atrial fibrillation, myocardial infarction, cardiac arrest, arrhythmia, and ventricular ectopic activity, including ventricular tachycardia (see WARNINGS.)

OVERDOSAGE:

Animal Oral LD_{50}

The oral LD_{50} of the drug is 610 mg/kg in mice, 486 mg/kg in rats, and 560 mg/kg rabbits.

SIGNS AND SYMPTOMS

Death from overdose has occurred in patients ingesting trazodone HCl and other drugs concurrently (namely, alcohol; alcohol + chloral hydrate + diazepam; amobarbital; chlordiazepoxide; or meprobamate).

The most severe reactions reported to have occurred with overdose of trazodone HCl alone have been priapism, respiratory arrest, seizures, and EKG changes. The reactions reported most frequently have been drowsiness and vomiting. Overdosage may cause an increase in incidence or severity of any of the reported adverse reactions (see ADVERSE REACTIONS.)

OVERDOSAGE: *(cont'd)*

TREATMENT

There is no specific antidote for trazodone HCl. Treatment should be symptomatic and supportive in the case of hypotension or excessive sedation. Any patient suspected of having taken an overdose should have the stomach emptied by gastric lavage. Forced diuresis may be useful in facilitating elimination of the drug.

DOSAGE AND ADMINISTRATION:

The dosage should be initiated at a low level and increased gradually, noting the clinical response and any evidence of intolerance. Occurrence of drowsiness may require the administration of a major portion of the daily dose at bedtime or a reduction of dosage. Trazodone HCl should be taken shortly after a meal or light snack. Symptomatic relief may be seen during the first week, with optimal antidepressant effects typically evident within two weeks. Twenty-five percent of those who respond to trazodone HCl require more than two weeks (up to four weeks) of drug administration.

USUAL ADULT DOSAGE

An initial dose of 150 mg/day in divided doses is suggested. The dose may be increased by 50 mg/day every three to four days. The maximum dose for out patients usually should not exceed 400 mg/day in divided doses. Inpatients (*i.e.,* more severely depressed patients) may be given up to but not in excess of 600 mg/day in divided doses.

MAINTENANCE

Dosage during prolonged maintenance therapy should be kept at the lowest effective level. Once an adequate response has been achieved, dosage may be gradually reduced, with subsequent adjustment depending on therapeutic response.

Although there has been no systematic evaluation of the efficacy of trazodone HCl beyond six weeks, it is generally recommended that a course of antidepressant drug treatment should be continued for several months.

Store at room temperature. Protect from temperatures above 104°F (40°C).

Dispense in tight, light-resistant container (USP).

REFERENCES:

a. Williams JBW, Ed: Diagnostic and Statistical Manual of Mental Disorders-III, American Psychiatric Association, May, 1980. **b.**Brindley GS: New treatment for priapism. *Lancet*July 28, 1984, ii: 220. **c.** Goldstein I, et al: Pharmacologic detumescence: The alternative to surgical shunting. *J Urology*1986;135(4:PEII):308A. **d.** Brindley GS: Pilot experiments on the actions of drugs injected into the human corpus cavernosum penis. *Br J Pharmacol* 1986;87:495-500. **e.** Padma-Nathan H, et al: Treatment of prolonged or priapistic erections following intracavernosal papaverine therapy. *Semin Urol* 1986;4(4):236-238. **f.** Lue TF, et al: Priapism: A refined approach to diagnosis and treatment. *J Urology* 1986;136:104-110. **g.** Fabre LF, Feighner JP: Long-term therapy for depression with trazodone. *J Clin Psychiatry*1983;44(1):17-21.

HOW SUPPLIED - RATED THERAPEUTICALLY EQUIVALENT:

Tablet, Plain Coated - Oral - 50 mg

100's	$5.03	Trazodone, United Res	00677-1133-01
100's	$6.97	Trazodone HCl, H.C.F.A. F F P	99999-2367-01
100's	$11.72	Trazodone Hcl, US Trading	56126-0368-11
100's	$13.88	Trazodone Hcl, IDE-Interstate	00814-7980-14
100's	$14.00	Trazodone Hcl, Raway	00686-0427-20
100's	$23.28	Trazodone Hcl, Barr	00555-0489-02
100's	$24.07	Trazodone Hcl, Qualitest Pharms	00603-6144-21
100's	$25.20	Trazodone Hcl 50, Major Pharms	00904-3990-60
100's	$25.53	Trazodone HCl, Bristol Myers Squibb	00003-3296-31
100's	$26.00	Trazodone Hcl, Sidmak Labs	50111-0433-01
100's	$26.26	Trazodone Hcl, Lederle Pharm	00005-3787-23
100's	$26.80	Trazodone Hcl, Martec Pharms	52555-0260-01
100's	$28.41	Trazodone HCl, Teva	00093-0637-01
100's	$28.60	Trazodone Hcl Tablets 50 Mg, Aligen Independ	00405-5036-01
100's	$28.65	Trazodone Hcl, Goldline Labs	00182-1259-01
100's	$28.65	Trazodone Hcl, Mutual Pharm	53489-0510-01
100's	$28.72	Trazodone Hcl, Purepac Pharm	00228-2439-10
100's	$28.75	Trazodone HCl, Warner Chilcott	00047-0577-24
100's	$29.00	Trazodone Hcl, Dupont Pharma	00056-0261-70
100's	$30.71	Trazodone Hcl, HL Moore Drug Exch	00839-7251-06
100's	$35.56	Trazodone HCl, Geneva Pharms	00781-1807-01
100's	$36.70	Trazodone Hcl, Medirex	57480-0369-01
100's	$36.75	Trazodone HCl, Schein Pharm (US)	00364-2109-01
100's	$37.90	Trazodone HCl, Geneva Pharms	00781-1807-13
100's	$41.73	Trazodone Hcl, Parmed Pharms	00349-8906-01
100's	$41.73	Trazodone HCl, Rugby	00536-4715-01
100's	$43.00	Trazodone Hcl, Goldline Labs	00182-1259-89
100's	$43.51	Trazodone Hcl 50, Major Pharms	00904-3990-61
100's	$45.15	Trazodone Hcl, Vangard Labs	00615-2578-13
100's	**$130.49**	**DESYREL, Bristol Myers Squibb**	**00087-0775-41**
100's	**$139.06**	**DESYREL, Bristol Myers Squibb**	**00087-0775-42**
250's	$17.42	Trazodone HCl, H.C.F.A. F F P	99999-2367-02
250's	$40.25	Trazodone HCl, Rugby	00536-4715-02
500's	$25.15	Trazodone Hcl, United Res	00677-1133-05
500's	$34.85	Trazodone HCl, H.C.F.A. F F P	99999-2367-03
500's	$63.80	Trazodone Hcl 50, Major Pharms	00904-3990-40
500's	$65.05	Trazodone Hcl, Elkins Sinn	00641-4016-88
500's	$99.30	Trazodone Hcl, Qualitest Pharms	00603-6144-28
500's	$105.56	Trazodone Hcl, Barr	00555-0489-04
500's	$128.00	Trazodone Hcl, Goldline Labs	00182-1259-05
500's	$128.00	Trazodone Hcl, Sidmak Labs	50111-0433-02
500's	$131.85	Trazodone Hcl, Martec Pharms	52555-0260-05
500's	$142.15	Trazodone HCl, Rugby	00536-4715-05
500's	$143.35	Trazodone Hcl, Parmed Pharms	00349-8906-05
500's	$143.60	Trazodone Hcl, Purepac Pharm	00228-2439-50
500's	$150.00	Trazodone HCl, Geneva Pharms	00781-1807-05
500's	$150.00	Trazodone Hcl, Mutual Pharm	53489-0510-05
600's	$270.00	Trazodone Hcl, Medirex	57480-0369-06
1000's	$50.30	Trazodone Hcl, Sidmak Labs	50111-0433-03
1000's	$69.70	Trazodone HCl, H.C.F.A. F F P	99999-2367-04
1000's	$130.15	Trazodone Hcl, Elkins Sinn	00641-4016-89
1000's	$221.65	Trazodone Hcl, Goldline Labs	00182-1259-10
1000's	$226.00	Trazodone Hcl, Martec Pharms	52555-0260-10
1000's	$247.20	Trazodone HCl, Schein Pharm (US)	00364-2109-02
1000's	$260.00	Trazodone Hcl, Mutual Pharm	53489-0510-10
1000's	$269.90	Trazodone HCl, Teva	00093-0637-10
1000's	$274.81	Trazodone Hcl Tablets 50 Mg, Aligen Independ	00405-5036-03
1000's	$284.25	Trazodone HCl, Geneva Pharms	00781-1807-10
1000's	$284.30	Trazodone Hcl, HL Moore Drug Exch	00839-7251-16
1000's	**$1133.88**	**DESYREL, Bristol Myers Squibb**	**00087-0775-43**

Tablet, Plain Coated - Oral - 100 mg

100's	$11.70	Trazodone HCl, H.C.F.A. F F P	99999-2367-05
100's	$11.93	Trazodone, United Res	00677-1134-01
100's	$22.95	Trazodone Hcl, IDE-Interstate	00814-7982-14
100's	$23.90	Trazodone Hcl, US Trading	56126-0369-11
100's	$30.00	Trazadone Hcl, Raway	00686-0428-20
100's	$36.75	TRAZONDONE HCL, Barr	00555-0490-02

HOW SUPPLIED - RATED THERAPEUTICALLY EQUIVALENT: *(cont'd)*

100's	$39.75	Trazodone Hcl 100, Major Pharms	00904-3991-60
100's	$41.00	Trazodone Hcl, Qualitest Pharms	00603-6145-21
100's	$41.00	Trazodone Hcl, Sidmak Labs	50111-0434-01
100's	$41.78	Trazodone Hcl, HL Moore Drug Exch	00839-7252-06
100's	$42.45	Trazodone Hcl, Mutual Pharm	53489-0511-01
100's	$42.50	Trazodone Hcl, Goldline Labs	00182-1260-01
100's	$44.25	Trazodone Hcl, Martec Pharms	52555-0261-01
100's	$44.59	Trazodone HCl, Bristol Myers Squibb	00003-3227-41
100's	$45.11	Trazodone Hcl, Lederle Pharm	00005-3788-23
100's	$46.43	Trazodone HCl, Teva	00093-0638-01
100's	$47.62	Trazodone HCl, Schein Pharm (US)	00364-2110-01
100's	$48.00	Trazodone Hcl, Dupont Pharma	00056-0262-70
100's	$48.66	TRAZODONE HCL, Warner Chilcott	00047-0578-24
100's	$48.66	Trazodone Hcl, Purepac Pharm	00228-2441-10
100's	$48.82	Trazodone Hcl Tablets 100 Mg, Aligen Independ	00405-5037-01
100's	$59.45	Trazodone, Rugby	00536-4688-01
100's	$59.45	Trazodone Hcl, Geneva Pharms	00781-1808-01
100's	$64.00	Trazodone Hcl, Medirex	57480-0370-01
100's	$70.18	Trazodone Hcl, Parmed Pharms	00349-8907-01
100's	$74.40	Trazodone Hcl, Goldline Labs	00182-1260-89
100's	$76.94	Trazodone Hcl, Vangard Labs	00615-2579-13
100's	$76.94	Trazodone HCl, Geneva Pharms	00781-1808-13
100's	$78.43	Trazodone Hcl 100, Major Pharms	00904-3991-61
100's	**$228.04**	**DESYREL, Bristol Myers Squibb**	**00087-0776-41**
100's	**$242.81**	**DESYREL, Bristol Myers Squibb**	**00087-0776-42**
250's	$29.25	Trazodone HCl, H.C.F.A. F F P	99999-2367-06
500's	$58.50	Trazodone HCl, H.C.F.A. F F P	99999-2367-07
500's	$59.65	Trazodone Hcl, United Res	00677-1134-05
500's	$59.65	Trazodone Hcl, HL Moore Drug Exch	00839-7252-12
500's	$97.05	Trazodone Hcl 100, Major Pharms	00904-3991-40
500's	$165.12	Trazodone Hcl, Qualitest Pharms	00603-6145-28
500's	$173.65	Trazodone Hcl, Elkins Sinn	00641-4017-88
500's	$174.56	TRAZONDONE HCL, Barr	00555-0490-04
500's	$180.00	Trazodone Hydrochloride, Mutual Pharm	53489-0511-05
500's	$187.00	Trazodone Hcl, Goldline Labs	00182-1260-05
500's	$187.00	Trazodone Hcl, Sidmak Labs	50111-0434-02
500's	$192.50	Trazodone Hcl, Geneva Pharms	00781-1808-05
500's	$196.70	Trazodone Hcl, Martec Pharms	52555-0261-05
500's	$220.50	Trazodone, Rugby	00536-4688-05
600's	$454.00	Trazodone Hcl, Medirex	57480-0370-06
1000's	$117.00	Trazodone HCl, H.C.F.A. F F P	99999-2367-08
1000's	$119.30	Trazodone Hcl, Sidmak Labs	50111-0434-03
1000's	$210.00	Trazodone Hcl, Aligen Independ	00405-5037-03
1000's	$300.00	Trazodone Hcl, Mutual Pharm	53489-0511-10
1000's	$341.00	Trazodone Hcl, Goldline Labs	00182-1260-10
1000's	$375.00	Trazodone HCl, Schein Pharm (US)	00364-2110-02
1000's	$441.08	Trazodone HCl, Teva	00093-0638-10
1000's	**$1981.53**	**DESYREL, Bristol Myers Squibb**	**00087-0776-43**

Tablet, Plain Coated - Oral - 150 mg

100's	$58.43	Trazodone HCl, H.C.F.A. F F P	99999-2367-09
100's	$67.43	Trazodone Hcl, United Res	00677-1302-01
100's	$70.35	DOTAZONE, Major Pharms	00904-3992-60
100's	$77.20	Trazodone Hcl, Qualitest Pharms	00603-6146-21
100's	$78.75	Trazodone Hcl, Harber Pharm	51432-0456-03
100's	$79.06	Trazodone Hcl, Parmed Pharms	00349-8824-01
100's	$79.58	Trazodone Hcl, HL Moore Drug Exch	00839-7507-06
100's	$81.12	Trazodone Hcl, Aligen Independ	00405-5038-01
100's	$88.50	Trazodone Hcl, Goldline Labs	00182-1298-01
100's	$89.27	Trazodone HCl, Schein Pharm (US)	00364-2300-01
100's	$89.90	Trazodone Hcl, Martec Pharms	52555-0132-01
100's	$89.98	Trazodone, Geneva Pharms	00781-1826-01
100's	$94.45	Trazodone Hcl, Sidmak Labs	50111-0441-01
100's	$96.88	Trazodone HCl, Warner Chilcott	00047-0716-24
100's	$96.88	Trazodone HCl, Rugby	00536-4689-01
100's	**$196.46**	**DESYREL DIVIDOSE, Bristol Myers Squibb**	**00087-0778-43**
250's	$146.07	Trazodone HCl, H.C.F.A. F F P	99999-2367-10
250's	$184.90	Trazodone Hcl, Major Pharms	00904-3392-70
250's	$184.90	Trazodone Hcl, Major Pharms	00904-3992-70
250's	$189.95	Trazodone Hcl, Parmed Pharms	00349-8824-25
250's	$242.20	Trazodone HCl, Rugby	00536-4689-02
500's	$292.15	Trazodone HCl, H.C.F.A. F F P	99999-2367-11
500's	$340.20	Trazodone Hcl, Sidmak Labs	50111-0441-02
500's	$356.87	Trazodone Hcl, HL Moore Drug Exch	00839-7507-12
500's	**$923.35**	**DESYREL DIVIDOSE, Bristol Myers Squibb**	**00087-0778-44**

HOW SUPPLIED - NOT RATED EQUIVALENT:

Tablet, Plain Coated - Oral - 300 mg

100's	**$349.66**	**DESYREL, Bristol Myers Squibb**	**00087-0796-41**

TRETINOIN *(002368)*

CATEGORIES: Acne; Acne Vulgaris; Cell Stimulants/Proliferants; Dermatologicals; Orphan Drugs; Skin/Mucous Membrane Agents; Topical; Vitamin A; Cervical Carcinoma*; Photodamaged Skin*; Pregnancy Category C; Sales > $100 Million; FDA Approval Pre 1982; Top 200 Drugs

* Indication not approved by the FDA

BRAND NAMES: *Aberel* (France); *Aberela*; *A-Acido*; *Acid A Vit*; *Acnavit*; *Acta*; *Airol* (Mexico); *Alten*; *Avitcid*; *Avitoin*; *Cordes-Vas*; *Cordes VAS* (Germany); *Derm A*; *Dermairol*; *Dermojuventus*; *Effederm* (France); *Epi-Aberel* (Germany); *Eudyna* (Germany); *Locacid*; *Locion De Tretinoina*; *Relief*; Renova; *Retavit*; *Retiderma*; **Retin-A**; *Retin A* (France); Retinoic Acid; *Retiol*; *Retrieve Cream*; *SteiVAA*; *Stieva-A* (Mexico); *Stieva A* (Canada); *Vitamin A Acid* (Canada)

(International brand names outside U.S. in italics)

FORMULARIES: Aetna; BC-BS; FHP; PCS

DESCRIPTION:

Retin-A Gel, Cream and Liquid, containing tretinoin are used for the topical treatment of acne vulgaris. Retin-A Gel contains tretinoin (retinoic acid, vitamin A acid) in either of two strengths, 0.025% or 0.01% by weight in a gel vehicle of butylated hydroxytoluene, hydroxypropyl cellulose and alcohol (denatured with *tert*-butyl alcohol and brucine sulfate) 90% w/w. Retin-A (tretinoin) Cream contains tretinoin in either of three strengths, 0.1%, 0.5%, or 0.025% by weight, in a hydrophilic cream vehicle of stearic acid, isopropyl myristate, polyoxyl 40 stearate, stearyl alcohol, xanthan gum, sorbic acid, butylated hydroxytoluene, and purified water. Retin-A Liquid contains tretinoin 0.05% by weight, polyethylene glycol 400, butylated hydroxytoluene and alcohol (denatured with *tert*-butyl alcohol and brucine sulfate) 55%. Chemically, tretinoin is *all-trans*-retinoic acid.

CLINICAL PHARMACOLOGY:

Although the exact mode of action of tretinoin is unknown, current evidence suggests that topical tretinoin decreases cohesiveness of follicular epithelial cells with decreased micro-comedo formation. Additionally, tretinoin stimulates mitotic activity and increased turnover of follicular epithelial cells causing extrusion of the comedones.

INDICATIONS AND USAGE:

Tretinoin is indicated for topical application in the treatment of acne vulgaris. The safety and efficacy of the long-term use of this product in the treatment of other disorders have not been established.

CONTRAINDICATIONS:

Use of the product should be discontinued if hypersensitivity to any of the ingredients is noted.

PRECAUTIONS:

General: If a reaction suggesting sensitivity or chemical irritation occurs, use of the medication should be discontinued. Exposure to sunlight, including sunlamps, should be minimized during the use of tretinoin, and patients with sunburn should be advised not to use the product until fully recovered because of heightened susceptibility to sunlight as a result of the use of tretinoin. Patients who may be required to have considerable sun exposure due to occupation and those with inherent sensitivity to the sun should exercise particular caution. Use of sunscreen products and protective clothing over treated areas is recommended when exposure cannot be avoided. Weather extremes, such as wind or cold, also may be irritating to patients under treatment with tretinoin.

Tretinoin acne treatment should be kept away from the eyes, the mouth, angles of the nose, and mucous membranes. Topical use may induce severe local erythema and peeling at the site of application. If the degree of local irritation warrants patients should be directed to use the medication less frequently, discontinue use temporarily, or discontinue use altogether. Tretinoin has been reported to cause severe irritation on eczematous skin and should be used with utmost caution in patients with this condition.

Carcinogenesis: Long-term animal studies to determine the carcinogenic potential of tretinoin have not been performed. Studies in hairless albino mice suggest that tretinoin may accelerate the tumorigenic potential of weakly carcinogenic light from a solar simulator. In other studies, when lightly pigmented hairless mice treated with tretinoin were exposed to carcinogenic doses of UVB light, the incidence and rate of development of skin tumors was reduced. Due to significantly different experimental conditions, no strict comparison of these disparate data is possible. Although the significance of these studies to man is not clear, patients should avoid or minimize exposure to sun.

Pregnancy, Teratogenic Effects, Pregnancy Category C: Oral tretinoin has been shown to be teratogenic in rats when given in doses 1000 times the topical human dose. Oral tretinoin has been shown to be fetotoxic in rats when given in doses 500 times the topical human dose. Topical tretinoin has not been shown to be teratogenic in rats and rabbits when given in doses of 100 and 320 times the topical human dose, respectively (assuming a 50 kg adult applies 250 mg of 0.1% cream topically). However, at these topical doses, delayed ossification of a number of bones occurred in both species. These changes may be considered variants of normal development and are usually corrected after weaning. There are no adequate and well-controlled studies in pregnant women. Tretinoin should be used during pregnancy only if the potential benefit justifies the potential risk to the fetus.

Nursing Mothers: It is not known whether this drug is excreted in human milk. Because many drugs are excreted in human milk, caution should be exercised when tretinoin is administered to a nursing woman.

Gels Are Flammable. Note: Keep away from heat and flame. Keep tube tightly closed.

DRUG INTERACTIONS:

Concomitant topical medication, medicated or abrasive soaps and cleansers, soaps and cosmetics that have a strong drying effect, and products with high concentrations of alcohol, astringents, spices or lime should be used with caution because of possible interaction with tretinoin. Particular caution should be exercised in using preparations containing sulfur, resorcinol, or salicylic acid with tretinoin. It also is advisable to "rest" a patient's skin until the effects of such preparations subside before use of tretinoin is begun.

ADVERSE REACTIONS:

The skin of certain sensitive individuals may become excessively red, edematous, blistered, or crusted. If these effects occur, the medication should either be discontinued until the integrity of the skin is restored, or the medication should be adjusted to a level the patient can tolerate. True contact allergy to topical tretinoin is rarely encountered. Temporary hyper- or hypopigmentation has been reported with repeated application of tretinoin. Some individuals have been reported to have heightened susceptibility to sunlight while under treatment with tretinoin. To date, all adverse effects of tretinoin have been reversible upon discontinuance of therapy (see DOSAGE AND ADMINISTRATION.)

OVERDOSAGE:

If medication is applied excessively, no more rapid or better results will be obtained and marked redness, peeling, or discomfort may occur. Oral ingestion of the drug may lead to the same side effects as those associated with excessive oral intake of Vitamin A.

DOSAGE AND ADMINISTRATION:

Tretinoin Gel, Cream or Liquid should be applied once a day, before retiring, to the skin where acne lesions appear, using enough to cover the entire affected area lightly.

Liquid: The liquid may be applied using a fingertip, gauze pad, or cotton swab. If gauze or cotton is employed, care should be taken not to oversaturate it to the extent that the liquid would run into areas where treatment is not intended.

Gel: Excessive application results in "pilling" of the gel, which minimizes the likelihood of over application by the patient.

Application may cause a transitory feeling of warmth or slight stinging. In cases where it has been necessary to temporarily discontinue therapy or to reduce the frequency of application, therapy may be resumed or frequency of application increased when the patients become able to tolerate the treatment.

Alterations of vehicle, drug concentration, or dose frequency should be closely monitored by careful observation of the clinical therapeutic response and skin tolerance.

During the early weeks of therapy, an *apparent* exacerbation of inflammatory lesions may occur. This is due to the action of the medication on deep, previously unseen lesions and should not be considered a reason to discontinue therapy.

Therapeutic results should be noticed after two to three weeks but more than six weeks of therapy may be required before definite beneficial effects are seen.

Once the acne lesions have responded satisfactorily, it may be possible to maintain the improvement with less frequent applications, or other dosage forms.

DOSAGE AND ADMINISTRATION: *(cont'd)*

Patients treated with tretinoin acne treatment may use cosmetics, but the areas to be treated should be cleansed thoroughly before the medication is applied (See PRECAUTIONS.)

PATIENT INFORMATION:

Tretinoin is used to treat acne. It is available in a cream, gel or topical solutions. Tretinoin may cause your skin to be sensitive to the sun, wind and extreme cold. The most common side effects include skin that becomes excessively red, edematous, blistered, or crusted. If these effects occur, the medication should either be discontinued or the dosage lowered to something tolerated by your skin. Tretinoin should be applied lightly to the skin where the acne is prior to bedtime. Your skin may get a warm or tingling feeling after you apply the medication. You may notice acne worsening when therapy is started. This occurs when the medication begins to work on acne that is not visible from the surface. Treatment should not be discontinued.

HOW SUPPLIED:

Storage Conditions: Retin-A Liquid, 0.05% and Retin-A Gel, 0.025% and 0.01%: store below 86°F. Retin-A Cream, 0.1%, 0.05%, and 0.025%: store below 80°F.

HOW SUPPLIED - EQUIVALENTS NOT AVAILABLE:

Cream - Topical - 0.025 %

20 gm	**$26.10**	**RETIN-A, Ortho Pharm**	**00062-0165-01**
45 gm	**$49.44**	**RETIN-A, Ortho Pharm**	**00062-0165-02**

Cream - Topical - 0.05 %

20 gm	$27.06	RETIN - A, Ortho Pharm	00062-0175-12
45 gm	$50.82	RETIN - A, Ortho Pharm	00062-0175-13

Cream - Topical - 0.10 %

20 gm	**$31.56**	**RETIN-A, Ortho Pharm**	**00062-0275-23**
45 gm	**$59.28**	**RETIN-A, Ortho Pharm**	**00062-0275-01**

Gel - Topical - 0.010 %

15 gm	$21.00	RETIN - A, Ortho Pharm	00062-0575-44
45 gm	$49.74	RETIN - A, Ortho Pharm	00062-0575-46

Gel - Topical - 0.025 %

15 gm	$21.24	RETIN - A, Ortho Pharm	00062-0475-42
45 gm	$50.16	RETIN - A, Ortho Pharm	00062-0475-45

Liquid - Topical - 0.05 %

28 ml	**$41.58**	**RETIN-A, Ortho Pharm**	**00062-0075-07**

Powder

1 gm	$56.10	RETINOIC ACID, Paddock Labs	00574-0647-01

TRETINOIN, RETINOIC ACID *(003233)*

CATEGORIES: Acute Promyelocytic Leukemia; Leukemia; Orphan Drugs; Pharmaceutical Adjuvants; Vitamin A; FDA Approved 1995 Nov

BRAND NAMES: **Vesanoid**

WARNING:

1. Experienced Physician and Institution: Patients with acute promyelocytic leukemia (APL) are at high risk in general and can have severe adverse reactions to tretinoin. Tretinoin should therefore be administered under the supervision of a physician who is experienced in the management of patients with acute leukemia and in a facility with laboratory and supportive services sufficient to monitor drug tolerance and protect and maintain a patient compromised by drug toxicity, including respiratory compromise. Use of tretinoin requires that the physician concludes that the possible benefit to the patient outweighs the following known adverse effects of the therapy.

2. Retinoic Acid-APL Syndrome: About 25% of patients with APL treated with tretinoin have experienced a syndrome called the retinoic-acid-APL (RA-APL) syndrome characterized by fever, dyspnea, weight gain, radiographic pulmonary infiltrates and pleural or pericardial effusions. This syndrome has occasionally been accompanied by impaired myocardial contractility and episodic hypotension. It has been observed with or without concomitant leukocytosis. Endotracheal intubation and mechanical ventilation have been required in some cases due to progressive hypoxemia, and several patients have expired with multiorgan failure. The syndrome generally occurs during the first month of treatment, with some cases reported following the first dose of tretinoin. The management of the syndrome has not been defined rigorously, but high-dose steroids given at the first suspicion of the RA-APL syndrome appear to reduce morbidity and mortality. At the first signs suggestive of the syndrome (unexplained fever, dyspnea and/or weight gain, abnormal chest auscultatory findings or radiographic abnormalities), high-dose steroids (dexamethasone 10 mg intravenously administered every 12 hours for 3 days or until the resolution of symptoms) should be immediately initiated, irrespective of the leukocyte count. The majority of patients do not require termination of tretinoin therapy during treatment of the RA-APL syndrome.

3. Leukocytosis at Presentation and Rapidly Evolving Leukocytosis During Tretinoin Treatment: During tretinoin treatment about 40% of patients will develop rapidly evolving leukocytosis. Patients who present with high WBC at diagnosis (>5x10(9)/L) have an increased risk of a further rapid increase in WBC counts. Rapidly evolving leukocytosis is associated with a higher risk of life-threatening complications. If signs and symptoms of the RA-APL syndrome are present together with leukocytosis, treatment with high-dose steroids should be initiated immediately. Some investigators routinely add chemotherapy to tretinoin treatment in the case of patients presenting with a WBC count of >5x10(9)/L or in the case of a rapid increase in WBC count for patients leukopenic at start of treatment, and have reported a lower incidence of the RA-APL syndrome. Consideration could be given to adding full-dose chemotherapy (including an anthracycline if not contraindicated) to the tretinoin therapy on day 1 or 2 for patients presenting with a WBC count of >5x10(9)/L, or immediately, for patients presenting with a WBC count of <5x10(9)/L, if the WBC count reaches greater than or equal to 6x10(9)/L by day 5, or greater than or equal to 10x(9)/L by day 10, or greater than or equal to 15x10(9)/L by day 28.

4. Teratogenic Effects. Pregnancy Category D: See WARNINGS. There is a high risk that a severely deformed infant will result if tretinoin is administered during pregnancy. If, nonetheless, it is determined that tretinoin represents the best available treatment for a pregnant woman or a woman of childbearing potential, it must be assured that the patient has received full information and warnings of the risk to the fetus if she were to be pregnant and of the risk of possible contraception failure and has been instructed in the need to use two reliable forms of contraception simultaneously during therapy and for 1 month following discontinuation of therapy, and has acknowledged her understanding of the need for using dual contraception, unless abstinence is the chosen method. Within 1 week prior to the institution of tretinoin therapy, the patient should have blood or urine collected for a serum or urine pregnancy test with a sensitivity of at least 50 mIU/L. When possible tretinoin therapy should be delayed until a negative result from this test is obtained. When a delay is not possible the patient should be placed on two reliable forms of contraception. Pregnancy testing and contraception counseling should be repeated monthly throughout the period of tretinoin treatment.

DESCRIPTION:

Tretinoin is a retinoid that induces maturation of acute promyelocytic leukemia (APL) cells in culture. It is available in a 10 mg soft gelatin capsule for oral administration. Each capsule also contains beeswax, butylated hydroxyanisole, edetate disodium, hydrogenated soybean oil flakes, hydrogenated vegetable oils and soybean oil. The gelatin capsule shell contains glycerin, yellow iron oxide, red iron oxide, titanium dioxide, methylparaben and propylparaben. Chemically, tretinoin is all-trans retinoic acid and is related to retinol (Vitamin A). It is a yellow to light orange crystalline powder with a molecular weight of 300.44.

CLINICAL PHARMACOLOGY:

MECHANISM OF ACTION

Tretinoin is not a cytolytic agent but instead induces cytodifferentiation and decreased proliferation of APL cells in culture and *in vivo.* In APL patients, tretinoin treatment produces an initial maturation of the primitive promyelocytes derived from the leukemic clone, followed by a repopulation of the bone marrow and peripheral blood by normal, polyclonal hematopoietic cells in patients achieving complete remission (CR). The exact mechanism of action of tretinoin in APL is unknown.

PHARMACOKINETICS

Tretinoin activity is primarily due to the parent drug. In human pharmacokinetics studies, orally administered drug was well absorbed into the systemic circulation, with approximately two-thirds of the administered radiolabel recovered in the urine. The terminal elimination half-life of tretinoin following initial dosing is 0.5 to 2 hours in patients with APL. There is evidence that tretinoin induces its own metabolism. Plasma tretinoin concentrations decrease on average to one-third of their day 1 values during 1 week of continuous therapy. Mean $\pm$ SD peak tretinoin concentrations decreased from 394 $\pm$ 89 to 138 $\pm$ 139 ng/mL, while area under the curve (AUC) values decreased from 537 $\pm$ 191 ng h/mL to 249 $\pm$ 185 ng h/mL during 45 mg/m^2 daily dosing in 7 APL patients. Increasing the dose to "correct" for this change has not increased response.

Absorption: A single 45 mg/m^2 (~80 mg) oral dose to APL patients resulted in a mean $\pm$ SD peak tretinoin concentration of 347$\pm$ 266 ng/mL. Time to reach peak concentration was between 1 and 2 hours.

Distribution: The apparent volume of distribution of tretinoin has not been determined. Tretinoin is greater than 95% bound in plasma, predominately to albumin. Plasma protein binding remains constant over the concentration range of 10 to 500 ng/mL.

Metabolism: Tretinoin metabolites have been identified in plasma and urine. Cytochrome P450 (CYP) enzymes have been implicated in the oxidative metabolism of tretinoin. Metabolites include 13-*cis* retinoic acid, 4-oxo *trans* retinoic acid, 4-oxo *cis* retinoic acid, and 4-oxo *trans* retinoic acid glucuronide. In APL patients, daily administration of a 45 mg/m^2 dose of tretinoin resulted in an approximately tenfold increase in the urinary excretion of 4-oxo trans retinoic acid glucuronide after 2 to 6 weeks of continuous dosing, when compared to baseline values.

Excretion: Studies with radiolabeled drug have demonstrated that after the oral administration of 2.75 and 50 mg doses of tretinoin, greater than 90% of the radioactivity was recovered in the urine and feces. Based upon data from 3 subjects, approximately 63% of radioactivity was recovered in the urine within 72 hours and 31% appeared in the feces within 6 days.

Special Populations: The pharmacokinetics of tretinoin have not been separately evaluated in women, in members of different ethnic groups, or in individuals with renal or hepatic insufficiency.

CLINICAL STUDIES:

Tretinoin has been investigated in 114 previously treated APL patients and in 67 previously untreated ("de novo") patients in one open-label, uncontrolled, single investigator clinical study (Memorial Sloan-Kettering Cancer Center [MSKCC]) and in two cohorts of compassionate cases treated by multiple investigators under the auspices of the National Cancer Institute (NCI). All patients received 45 mg/m^2/day as a divided oral dose for up to 90 days or 30 days beyond the day that CR was reached. Results are shown in TABLE 1.

TABLE 1

	MSKCC		NCl Cohort 1		NCl Cohort 2	
	Relapsed n-20	**de Novo n=15**	**Relapsed* n=48**	**de Novo n=14**	**Relapsed n=46**	**de Novo n=38**
Complete Remission	16 (80%)	11 (73%)	24 (50%)	5 (35%)	24 (52%)	26 (68%)
Median Survival (Mo)	10.8	NR	5.8	0.5	8.8	NR
Median Follow-up (Mo)	9.9	42.9	5.6	1.2	8.0	13.1
RA-APL Syndrome	4 (20%)	5 (33%)	10 (21%)	8 (43%)	NA	NA

NR = Not Reached
NA = Not Available
* Including 9 chemorefractory patients
† Including 8 patients who received chemotherapy but failed to enter remission

CLINICAL STUDIES: *(cont'd)*

The median time to CR was between 40 and 50 days (range: 2 to 120 days. Most patients in these studies received cytotoxic chemotherapy during the remission phase. These results compare to the 30% to 50% CR rate and ≤6 month median survival reported for cytotoxic chemotherapy of APL in the treatment of relapse. Ten of 15 pediatric cases achieved CR (8 of 10 males and 2 of 5 females). There were insufficient patients of Black, Hispanic, or Asian derivation to estimate relative response rates in these groups, but responses were seen in each category. Responses were seen in 3 of 4 patients for whom cytogenetic analysis failed to detect the t(15;17) translocation typically seen in APL. The t(15;17) translocation results in the PML/RARα gene, which appears necessary for this disease. Molecular genetic studies were not conducted in these cases, but it is likely they represent cases with a masked translocation giving rise to PML/RARα. Responses to tretinoin have not been observed in cases in which PML/RARα fusion has been shown to be absent.

INDICATIONS AND USAGE:

Tretinoin capsules are indicated for the induction of remission in patients with acute promyelocytic leukemia (APL), French-American-British (FAB) classification M3 (including the M3 variant), characterized by the presence of the t(15;17) translocation and/or the presence of the PML/RARα gene who are refractory to, or who have relapsed from, anthracycline chemotherapy, or for whom anthracycline-based chemotherapy is contraindicated. Tretinoin is for the induction of remission only. The optimal consolidation or maintenance regimens have not been defined, but all patients should receive an accepted form of remission consolidation and/or maintenance therapy for APL after completion of induction therapy with tretinoin.

CONTRAINDICATIONS:

Tretinoin is contraindicated in patients with a known hypersensitivity to retinoids. Tretinoin should not be given to patients who are sensitive to parabens, which are used as preservatives in the gelatin capsule.

WARNINGS:

Pregnancy Category D: See BOXED WARNING. Tretinoin has teratogenic and embryotoxic effects in mice, rats, hamsters, rabbits and pigtail monkeys, and may be expected to cause fetal harm when administered to a pregnant woman. Tretinoin causes fetal resorptions and a decrease in live fetuses in all animals studied. Gross external, soft tissue and skeletal alterations occurred at doses higher than 0.7 mg/kg/day in mice, 2 mg/kg/day in rats, 7 mg/kg/day in hamsters, and at a dose of 10 mg/kg/day, the only dose tested, in pigtail monkeys (about 1/20, 1/4, and 1/2 and 4 times the human dose, respectively, on a mg/m^2 basis). There are no adequate and well controlled studies in pregnant women. Although experience with humans administered tretinoin is extremely limited, increased spontaneous abortions and major human fetal abnormalities related to the use of other retinoids have been documented in humans. Reported defects include abnormalities of the CNS, musculoskeletal system, external ear, eye, thymus and great vessels; and facial dysmorphia, cleft palate, and parathyroid hormone deficiency. Some of these abnormalities were fatal. Cases of IQ scores less than 85, with or without obvious CNS abnormalities, have also been reported. All fetuses exposed during pregnancy can be affected and at the present time there is no antepartum means of determining which fetuses are and are not affected. Effective contraception must be used by all females during tretinoin therapy and for 1 month following discontinuation of therapy. Contraception must be used even when there is a history of infertility or menopause, unless a hysterectomy has been performed. Whenever contraception is required, it is recommended that two reliable forms of contraception be used simultaneously, unless abstinence is the chosen method. If pregnancy does occur during treatment, the physician and patient should discuss the desirability of continuing or terminating the pregnancy.

Patients Without The t(15;17) Translocation: Initiation of therapy with tretinoin may be based on the morphological diagnosis of acute promyelocytic leukemia. Confirmation of the diagnosis of APL should be sought by detection of the t(15;17) genetic marker by cytogenetic studies. If these are negative, PML/RARα fusion should be sought using molecular diagnostic techniques. The response rate of other AML subtypes to tretinoin has not been demonstrated; therefore, patients who lack the genetic marker should be considered for alternative treatment.

Retinoic Acid-APL (RA-APL) Syndrome: In up to 25% of patients with APL treated with tretinoin, a syndrome occurs which can be fatal (see BOXED WARNING and ADVERSE REACTIONS).

Leukocytosis at Presentation and Rapidly Evolving Leukocytosis During Tretinoin Treatment: See BOXED WARNING.

Pseudotumor Cerebri: Retinoids, including tretinoin, have been associated with pseudotumor cerebri (benign intracranial hypertension), especially in pediatric patients. Early signs and symptoms of pseudotumor cerebri include papilledema, headache, nausea and vomiting and visual disturbances. Patients with these symptoms should be evaluated for pseudotumor cerebri, and, if present, appropriate care should be instituted in concert with neurological assessment. Lipids. Up to 60% of patients experienced hypercholesterolemia and/or hypertriglyceridemia, which were reversible upon completion of treatment. The clinical consequences of temporary elevation of triglycerides and cholesterol are unknown, but venous thrombosis and myocardial infarction have been reported in patients who ordinarily are at low risk for such complications.

Elevated Liver Function Test Results: Elevated liver function test results occur in 50% to 60% of patients during treatment. Liver function test results should be carefully monitored during treatment and consideration be given to a temporary withdrawal of tretinoin if test results reach greater than five times the upper limit of normal values. However, the majority of these abnormalities resolve without interruption of tretinoin or after completion of treatment.

PRECAUTIONS:

GENERAL

Tretinoin has potentially significant toxic side effects in APL patients. Patients undergoing therapy should be closely observed for signs of respiratory compromise and/or leukocytosis (see BOXED WARNING). Supportive care appropriate for APL patients; *e.g.,* prophylaxis for bleeding, prompt therapy for infection, should be maintained during therapy with tretinoin.

LABORATORY TESTS

The patient's hematologic profile, coagulation profile, liver function test results, and triglyceride and cholesterol levels should be monitored frequently.

EFFECT OF FOOD

No data on the effect of food on the absorption of tretinoin are available. The absorption of retinoids as a class has been shown to be enhanced when taken together with food.

CARCINOGENESIS, MUTAGENESIS, AND IMPAIRMENT OF FERTILITY

No long-term carcinogenicity studies with tretinoin have been conducted. In short-term carcinogenicity studies, tretinoin at a dose of 30 mg/kg/day (about 2 times the human dose on a mg/m^2 basis) was shown to increase the rate of diethylnitrosamine (DEN)-induced mouse liver adenomas and carcinomas. Tretinoin was negative when tested in the Ames and Chinese hamster V79 cell HGPRT assays for mutagenicity. A twofold increase in the sister

PRECAUTIONS: *(cont'd)*

chromatid exchange (SCE) has been demonstrated in human diploid fibroblasts, but other chromosome aberration assays, including an *in vitro* assay in human peripheral lymphocytes and an *in vivo* mouse micronucleus assay, did not show a clastogenic or aneuploidogenic effect. Adverse effects on fertility and reproductive performance were not observed in studies conducted in rats at doses up to 5 mg/kg/day (about 2/3 the human dose on a mg/m^2 basis). In a 6-week toxicology study in dogs, minimal to marked testicular degeneration, with increased numbers of immature spermatozoa, were observed at 10 mg/kg/day (about 4 times the equivalent human dose in mg/m^2).

NURSING MOTHERS

It is not known whether this drug is excreted in human milk. Because many drugs are excreted in human milk, and because of the potential for serious adverse reactions from tretinoin in nursing infants, mothers should discontinue nursing prior to taking this drug.

PEDIATRIC USE

There are limited clinical data on the pediatric use of tretinoin. Of 15 pediatric patients (age range: 1 to 16 years) treated with tretinoin, the incidence of complete remission was 67%. Safety and effectiveness in pediatric patients below the age of 1 year have not been established. Some pediatric patients experience severe headache and pseudotumor cerebri, requiring analgesic treatment and lumbar puncture for relief. Increased caution is recommended in the treatment of pediatric patients. Dose reduction may be considered for pediatric patients experiencing serious and/or intolerable toxicity; however; the efficacy and safety of tretinoin at doses lower than 45 mg/m^2/day have not been evaluated in the pediatric population.

DRUG INTERACTIONS:

Limited clinical data on potential drug interactions are available. As tretinoin is metabolized by the hepatic CYP system, there is a potential for alteration of pharmacokinetics parameters in patients administered concomitant medications that are also inducers or inhibitors of this system. Medications that generally induce hepatic CYP enzymes include rifampicin, glucocorticoids, phenobarbital and pentobarbital. Medications that generally inhibit hepatic CYP enzymes include ketoconazole, cimetidine, erythromycin, verapamil, diltiazem and cyclosporin. To date there are no data to suggest that co-use with these medications increases or decreases either efficacy or toxicity of tretinoin.

DRUG-DRUG INTERACTIONS

In 13 patients who had received daily doses of tretinoin for 4 consecutive weeks, administration of ketoconazole (400 to 1200 mg oral dose) 1 hour prior to the administration of the tretinoin dose on day 29 led to a 72% increase (218 ± 224 versus 375 ± 285 ng h/mL) in tretinoin mean plasma AUC. The precise CYP system involved in these interactions has not been specified; CYP, 3A4, 2C8 and 2E have been implicated in various preliminary reports.

ADVERSE REACTIONS:

Virtually all patients experience some drug related toxicity, especially headache, fever, weakness, and fatigue. These adverse effects are seldom permanent or irreversible nor do they usually require interruption of therapy. Some of the adverse events are common in patients with APL, including hemorrhage, infections, gastrointestinal hemorrhage, disseminated intravascular coagulation, pneumonia, septicemia, and cerebral hemorrhage.

The following describes the adverse events, regardless of drug relationship, that were observed in patients treated with tretinoin.

Typical Retinoid Toxicity: The most frequently reported adverse events were similar to those described in patients taking high doses of vitamin A and included headache (86% of patients), fever (83%), skin/mucous membrane dryness (77%), bone pain (77%), nausea/vomiting (57%), rash (54%), mucositis (26%), pruritus (20%), increased sweating (20%), visual disturbances (17%), ocular disorders (17%), alopecia (14%), skin changes (14%), changed visual acuity (6%), bone inflammation (3%), visual field defects (3%).

RA-APL Syndrome: APL patients treated with tretinoin have experienced a syndrome characterized by fever, dyspnea, weight gain, radiographic pulmonary infiltrates and pleural or pericardial effusions. This syndrome has occasionally been accompanied by impaired myocardial contractility and episodic hypotension and has been observed with or without concomitant leukocytosis. Some patients have expired due to progressive hypoxemia and multiorgan failure. The syndrome generally occurs during the first month of treatment, with some cases reported following the first dose of tretinoin. The management of the syndrome has not been defined rigorously, but high-dose steroids given at the first signs of the syndrome appear to reduce morbidity and mortality. Treatment with dexamethasone, 10 mg intravenously administered every 12 hours for 3 days or until resolution of symptoms, should be initiated without delay at the first suspicion of symptoms (one or more of the following: fever, dyspnea, weight gain, abnormal chest auscultatory findings or radiographic abnormalities). Sixty percent or more of patients treated with tretinoin may require high-dose steroids because of these symptoms. The majority of patients do not require termination of tretinoin therapy during treatment of the syndrome.

Body as a Whole: General disorders related to tretinoin administration and/or associated with APL included malaise (66%), shivering (63%), hemorrhage (60%), infections (58%), peripheral edema (52%), pain (37%), chest discomfort (32%), edema (29%), disseminated intravascular coagulation (26%), weight increase (23%), injection site reactions (17%), anorexia (17%), weight decrease (17%), myalgia (14%), flank pain (9%), cellulitis (8%), face edema (6%), fluid imbalance (6%), pallor (6%), lymph disorders (6%), acidosis (3%), hypothermia (3%), ascites (3%).

Respiratory System Disorders: Respiratory system disorders were commonly reported in APL patients administered tretinoin. The majority of these events are symptoms of the RA-APL syndrome (see BOXED WARNING). Respiratory system adverse events included upper respiratory tract disorders (63%), dyspnea (60%), respiratory insufficiency (26%), pleural effusion (20%), pneumonia (14%), rales (14%), expiratory wheezing (14%), lower respiratory tract disorders (9%), pulmonary infiltration (6%), bronchial asthma (3%), pulmonary edema (3%), larynx edema (3%), unspecified pulmonary disease (3%).

Ear Disorders: Ear disorders were consistently reported, with earache or feeling of fullness in the ears reported by 23% of the patients. Hearing loss and other unspecified auricular disorders were observed in 6% of patients, with infrequent (<1%) reports of irreversible hearing loss.

Gastrointestinal Disorders: GI disorders included GI hemorrhage (34%), abdominal pain (31%), other gastrointestinal disorders (26%), diarrhea (23%), constipation (17%), dyspepsia (14%), abdominal distention (11%), hepatosplenomegaly (9%), hepatitis (3%), ulcer (3%), unspecified liver disorder (3%).

Cardiovascular and Heart Rate and Rhythm Disorders: Arrhythmias (23%), flushing (23%), hypotension (14%), hypertension (11%), phlebitis (11%), cardiac failure (6%) and for 3% of patients: cardiac arrest, myocardial infarction, enlarged heart, heart murmur, ischemia, stroke, myocarditis, pericarditis, pulmonary hypertension, secondary cardiomyopathy.

Central and Peripheral Nervous System Disorders and Psychiatric: Dizziness (20%), paresthesias (17%), anxiety (17%), insomnia (14%), depression (14%), confusion (11%), cerebral hemorrhage (9%), intracranial hypertension (9%), agitation (9%), hallucination (6%) and for 3% of patients: abnormal gait, agnosia, aphasia, asterixis, cerebellar edema, cerebellar disorders, convulsions, coma, CNS depression, dysarthria, encephalopathy, facial paralysis, hemiplegia, hyporeflexia, hypotaxia, no light reflex, neurologic reaction, spinal cord disorder, tremor, leg weakness, unconsciousness, dementia, forgetfulness, somnolence, slow speech.

Urinary System Disorders: Renal insufficiency (11%), dysuria (9%), acute renal failure (3%), micturition frequency (3%), renal tubular necrosis (3%), enlarged prostate (3%).

Miscellaneous Adverse Events: Isolated cases of erythema nodosum, basophilia and hyperhistaminemia, Sweet's syndrome, organomegaly, hypercalcemia, pancreatitis and myositis have been reported.

OVERDOSAGE:

There has been no experience with acute overdosage in humans. The maximal tolerated dose in patients with myelodysplastic syndrome or solid tumors was 195 mg/m^2/day. The maximal tolerated dose in pediatric patients was lower at 60 mg/m^2/day. Overdosage with other retinoids has been associated with transient headache, facial flushing, cheilosis, abdominal pain, dizziness and ataxia. These symptoms have quickly resolved without apparent residual effects.

DOSAGE AND ADMINISTRATION:

The recommended dose is 45 mg/m^2/day administered as two evenly divided doses until complete remission is documented. Therapy should be discontinued 30 days after achievement of complete remission or after 90 days of treatment, whichever occurs first. If after initiation of treatment of tretinoin the presence of the [(15;17) translocation is not confirmed by cytogenetics and/or by polymerase chain reaction studies and the patient has not responded to tretinoin, alternative therapy appropriate for acute myelogenous leukemia should be considered. Tretinoin is for the induction of remission only. Optimal consolidation or maintenance regimens have not been determined. All patients should therefore receive a standard consolidation and/or maintenance chemotherapy regimen for APL after induction therapy with tretinoin, unless otherwise contraindicated.

PATIENT INFORMATION:

Tretinoin is used to induce remission in certain types of leukemia. Do not use if you are pregnant or nursing or if you are allergic to retinoids. Take two times daily as directed by your doctor. May cause headache, fever, weakness, fatigue, stomach or intestinal upset, skin and mucous membrane dryness, rash, bleeding, and infections. Inform your doctor or pharmacist if these effects occur.

HOW SUPPLIED:

Vesanoid is supplied as 10 mg capsules, two-tone (lengthwise), orange-yellow and reddish-brown and imprinted Vesanoid 10 Roche. Supplied in high density polyethylene, opaque Prescription Pak Bottles of 100 capsules with child-resistant closure. Store at 15°C to 30°C (59°F to 86°F). Protect from light.

HOW SUPPLIED - EQUIVALENTS NOT AVAILABLE:

Capsule - Oral - 10 mg

100's $1,260.00 VESANOID, Roche 00004-0250-01

TRIAMCINOLONE *(002370)*

CATEGORIES: Adrenal Corticosteroids; Adrenal Hyperplasia; Adrenal Insufficiency; Adrenocortical Insufficiency; Airway Obstruction; Anemia; Ankylosing Spondylitis; Antiarthritics; Arthritis; Aspiration Pneumonitis; Asthma; Atopic Dermatitis; Bursitis; Cancer; Carditis; Chemotherapy; Chorioretinitis; Choroiditis; Colitis; Conjunctivitis; Corneal Ulcer; Dermatitis; Dermatitis Herpetiformis; Dermatologicals; Diuresis; Drug Hypersensitivity; Enteritis; Epicondylitis; Erythema Multiforme; Erythroblastopenia; Gouty Arthritis; Herpes; Herpes Zoster; Hormones; Hypercalcemia; Inflammation; Iridocyclitis; Keratitis; Leukemia; Lupus Erythematosus; Lymphoma; Meningitis; Multiple Sclerosis; Mycosis Fungoides; Nephrotic Syndrome; Osteoarthritis; Pain; Pemphigus; Pneumoconiosis; Pneumonitis; Proteinuria; Psoriasis; Purpura; Retinochoroiditis; Rhinitis; Sarcoidosis; Serum Sickness; Spondylitis; Synovitis; Synovitis of Osteoarthritis; Tenosynovitis; Thrombocytopenia; Thrombocytopenic Purpura; Thyroiditis; Trichinosis; Tuberculosis; Ulcerative Colitis; Uveitis; FDA Approval Pre 1982

BRAND NAMES: *Adcortyl*; *Aristcort*; Aristo-Pak; **Aristocort**; *Delphicort*; *Extracort*; Kenacort; *Ledercort*; *Oricort*; *Triaminoral*
(International brand names outside U.S. in italics)

FORMULARIES: Aetna; BC-BS; CIGNA; FHP; Humana; Kaiser; Medco; Medi-Cal; PruCare; United; PCS

COST OF THERAPY: $24.63 (Asthma; Tablet; 4 mg; 1/day; 365 days)

PRIMARY ICD9: 493.90 (Asthma, Unspecified, Without Mention of Status Asthmaticus)

DESCRIPTION:

Triamcinolone is a synthetic adrenocorticosteroid. Aristocort tablets contain triamcinolone, 9-Fluoro-11β, 16α, 17,21-tetrahydroxypregna-1,4-diene-3,20-dione.

Aristocort Tablets contain 1, 2, 4, or 8 mg triamcinolone.

Inactive Ingredients: Corn Starch Dibasic Calcium Phosphate, Docusate Sodium, Lactose, Magnesium Stearate, Microcrystalline Cellulose, Red 30, Sodium Benzoate, Sodium Starch Glycolate and Yellow 10.

CLINICAL PHARMACOLOGY:

Triamcinolone is primarily glucocorticoid in action and has potent anti-inflammatory, hormonal and metabolic effects common to cortisone-like drugs. It is essentially devoid of mineralocorticoid activity when administered in therapeutic doses, causing little or no sodium retention, with potassium excretion minimal or absent. The body's immune responses to diverse stimuli are also modified by its action.

INDICATIONS AND USAGE:

Endocrine Disorders:

Primary or secondary adrenocortical insufficiency (hydrocortisone or cortisone is the first choice; synthetic analogs may be used in conjunction with mineralocorticoids where applicable; in infancy mineralocorticoid supplementation is of particular importance).

Congenital adrenal hyperplasia

Nonsuppurative thyroiditis

Hypercalcemia associated with cancer

INDICATIONS AND USAGE: *(cont'd)*

Rheumatic Disorders: As adjunctive therapy for short-term administration (to tide the patient over an acute episode or exacerbation) in:
Psoriatic arthritis
Rheumatoid arthritis, including juvenile rheumatoid arthritis (selected cases may require low-dose maintenance therapy)
Ankylosing spondylitis
Acute and subacute bursitis
Acute nonspecific tenosynovitis
Acute gouty arthritis
Posttraumatic osteoarthritis
Synovitis of osteoarthritis
Epicondylitis
Collagen Diseases: During an exacerbation or as maintenance therapy in selected cases of:
Systemic lupus erythematosus
Acute rheumatic carditis
Dermatologic Diseases:
Pemphigus
Bullous dermatitis herpetiformis
Severe erythema multiforme (Stevens-Johnson syndrome)
Exfoliative dermatitis
Mycosis fungoides
Severe psoriasis
Severe seborrheic dermatitis
Allergic States: Control of severe or incapacitating allergic conditions intractable to adequate trials of conventional treatment:
Seasonal or perennial allergic rhinitis
Bronchial asthma
Contact dermatitis
Atopic dermatitis
Serum sickness
Drug hypersensitivity reactions
Ophthalmic Diseases: Severe acute and chronic allergic and inflammatory processes involving the eye and its adnexa such as:
Allergic conjunctivitis
Keratitis
Allergic corneal marginal ulcers
Herpes zoster ophthalmicus
Iritis and iridocyclitis
Chorioretinitis
Anterior segment inflammation
Diffuse posterior uveitis and choroiditis
Optic neuritis
Sympathetic ophthalmia
Respiratory Disease:
Symptomatic sarcoidosis
Loeffler's syndrome not manageable by other means
Berylliosis
Fulminating or disseminated pulmonary tuberculosis when used concurrently with appropriate antituberculous chemotherapy
Aspiration pneumonitis
Hematologic Disorders:
Idiopathic thrombocytopenic purpura in adults
Secondary thrombocytopenia in adults
Acquired (autoimmune) hemolytic anemia
Erythroblastopenia (RBC anemia)
Congenital (erythroid) hypoplastic anemia
Neoplastic Diseases: For palliative management of:
Leukemias and lymphomas in adults
Acute leukemia of childhood
Edematous States:
To induce a diuresis or remission of proteinuria in the nephrotic syndrome, without uremia, of the idiopathic type or that due to lupus erythematosus
Gastrointestinal Diseases: To tide the patient over a critical period of the disease in:
Ulcerative colitis
Regional enteritis
Nervous System:
Acute exacerbations of multiple sclerosis
Miscellaneous:
Tuberculous meningitis with subarachnoid block or impending block when used concurrently with appropriate antituberculous chemotherapy
Trichinosis with neurologic or myocardial involvement

CONTRAINDICATIONS:

Systemic fungal infections.
Sensitivity to the drug or any of its components.

WARNINGS:

In patients on corticosteroid therapy subjected to unusual stress, increased dosage of rapidly acting corticosteroids before, during, and after the stressful situation is indicated.

Corticosteroids may mask some signs of infection, and new infections may appear during their use. There may be decreased resistance and inability to localize infection when corticosteroids are used.

Prolonged use of corticosteroids may produce posterior subcapsular cataracts, glaucoma with possible damage to the optic nerves, and may enhance the establishment of secondary ocular infections due to fungi or viruses.

WARNINGS: *(cont'd)*

Usage in Pregnancy: Since adequate human reproduction studies have not been done with corticosteroids the use of these drugs in pregnancy, nursing mothers or women of childbearing potential requires that the possible benefit of the drug be weighed against the potential hazards to the mother and embryo or fetus. Infants born of mothers who have received substantial doses of corticosteroids during pregnancy should be carefully observed for signs of hypoadrenalism.

Average and large doses of hydrocortisone or cortisone can cause elevation of blood pressure, salt and water retention, and increased excretion of potassium. These effects are less likely to occur with triamcinolone except when used in large doses. Dietary salt restriction and potassium supplementation may be necessary. All corticosteroids increase calcium excretion.

While on Corticosteroid Therapy, Patients Should NOT Be Vaccinated Against Smallpox. Other immunization procedures should not be undertaken in patients who are on corticosteroids, especially on high doses, because of possible hazards of neurological complications and lack of antibody response.

The use of triamcinolone in active tuberculosis should be restricted to those cases of fulminating or disseminated tuberculosis in which the corticosteroid is used for the management of the disease in conjunction with appropriate antituberculous regimen.

If corticosteroids are indicated in patients with latent tuberculosis or tuberculin reactivity, close observation is necessary as reactivation of the disease may occur. During prolonged corticosteroid therapy, these patients should receive chemoprophylaxis.

Children who are on immunosuppressant drugs are more susceptible to infections than healthy children. Chickenpox and measles, for example, can have a more serious or even fatal course in children on immunosuppressant corticosteroids. In such children, or in adults who have not had these diseases, particular care should be taken to avoid exposure. If exposed, therapy with varicella zoster immune globulin (VZIG) or pooled intravenous immunoglobulin (IVIG), as appropriate, may be indicated. If chickenpox develops, treatment with antiviral agents may be considered.

PRECAUTIONS:

Drug-induced secondary adrenocortical insufficiency may be minimized by gradual reduction of dosage. This type of relative insufficiency may persist for months after discontinuation of therapy; therefore, in any situation of stress occurring during that period, hormone therapy should be reinstituted. Since mineralocorticoid secretion may be impaired, salt and/or a mineralocorticoid should be administered concurrently.

There is an enhanced effect of corticosteroids on patients with hypothyroidism and in those with cirrhosis.

Corticosteroids should be used cautiously in patients with ocular herpes simplex because of possible corneal perforation.

The lowest possible dose of corticosteroids should be used to control the condition under treatment, and when reduction in dosage is possible, the reduction should be gradual.

Psychic derangements may appear when corticosteroids are used, ranging from euphoria, insomnia, mood swings, personality changes and severe depression to frank psychotic manifestations. Also, existing emotional instability or psychotic tendencies may be aggravated by corticosteroids.

Aspirin should be used cautiously in conjunction with corticosteroids in hypoprothrombinemia.

Steroids should be used with caution in nonspecific ulcerative colitis if there is a probability of impending perforation, abscess or other pyogenic infection, diverticulitis, fresh intestinal anastomoses, active or latent peptic ulcer, renal insufficiency, hypertension, osteoporosis, and myasthenia gravis.

Growth and development of infants and children on prolonged corticosteroid therapy should be carefully observed.

Although controlled clinical trials have shown corticosteroids to be effective in speeding the resolution of acute exacerbations of multiple sclerosis they do not show that they affect the ultimate outcome or natural history of the disease. The studies do show that relatively high doses of corticosteroids are necessary to demonstrate a significant effect. (See DOSAGE AND ADMINISTRATION.)

Since complications of treatment with glucocorticoid are dependent on the size of the dose and the duration of treatment a risk/benefit decision must be made in each individual case as to dose and duration of treatment and as to whether daily or intermittent therapy should be used.

Information for the Patient: Patients who are on immunosuppressant doses of corticosteroids should be warned to avoid exposure to chickenpox or measles and, if exposed, to obtain medical advice.

ADVERSE REACTIONS:

Fluid and electrolyte disturbances: Sodium retention, fluid retention, congestive heart failure in susceptible patients, potassium loss, hypokalemic alkalosis, hypertension.

Musculoskeletal: Muscle weakness, steroid myopathy, loss of muscle mass, osteoporosis, vertebral compression fractures, aseptic necrosis of femoral and humeral heads, pathologic fracture of long bones.

Gastrointestinal: Peptic ulcer with possible subsequent perforation and hemorrhage, pancreatitis, abdominal distention, ulcerative esophagitis.

Dermatologic: Impaired wound healing, thin fragile skin, petechiae and ecchymoses, facial erythema, increased sweating, may suppress reactions to skin tests.

Neurological: Convulsions, increased intracranial pressure with papilledema (pseudotumor cerebri) usually after treatment, vertigo, headache.

Endocrine: Menstrual irregularities, development of cushingoid state, suppression of growth in children, secondary adrenocortical and pituitary unresponsiveness, particularly in times of stress, as in trauma, surgery or illness, decreased carbohydrate tolerance, manifestations of latent diabetes mellitus, increased requirements for insulin or oral hypoglycemic agents in diabetics.

Ophthalmic: Posterior subcapsular cataracts, increased intraocular pressure, glaucoma, exophthalmos.

Metabolic: Negative nitrogen balance due to protein catabolism.

Hypersensitivity Reactions: Anaphylactoid reactions have been reported rarely with products of this class.

DOSAGE AND ADMINISTRATION:

GENERAL PRINCIPLES

1. The initial dosage of triamcinolone may vary from 4 to 48 mg per day depending on the specific disease entity being treated. In situations of less severity lower doses will generally suffice while in selected patients higher initial doses may be required. The initial dosage should be maintained or adjusted until a satisfactory response is noted. If after a reasonable period of time there is a lack of satisfactory clinical response, the drug should be discontinued and the patient transferred to other appropriate therapy. **IT SHOULD BE EM-**

DOSAGE AND ADMINISTRATION: *(cont'd)*

PHASIZED THAT DOSAGE REQUIREMENTS ARE VARIABLE AND MUST BE INDIVIDUALIZED ON THE BASIS OF THE DISEASE UNDER TREATMENT AND THE RESPONSE ON THE PATIENT. After a favorable response is noted, the proper maintenance dosage should be determined by decreasing the initial drug dosage in small increments at appropriate time intervals until the lowest dosage is reached which will maintain an adequate clinical response. It should be kept in mind that constant monitoring is needed in regard to drug dosage. Included in the situation which may make dosage adjustment necessary are changes in clinical status secondary to remissions or exacerbations in the disease process, the patient's individual drug responsiveness, and the effect of patient exposure to stressful situations not directly related to the disease entity under treatment; in this latter situation it may be necessary to increase the dosage of triamcinolone for a period of time consistent with the patient's condition. It after long-term therapy the drug is to be stopped, it is recommended that it be withdrawn gradually rather than abruptly.

2. Dosage should be individualized according to the severity of the disease and the response of the patient. For infants and children, the recommended dosage should be governed by the same considerations rather than by strict adherence to the ratio indicated by age or body weight.

3. Hormone therapy is an adjunct to, and not a replacement for, conventional therapy.

4. The severity, prognosis and expected duration of the disease and the reaction of the patient to medication are primary factors in determining dosage.

5. If a period of spontaneous remission occurs in a chronic condition, treatment should be discontinued.

6. Blood pressure, body weight, routine laboratory studies, including 2-hour postprandial blood glucose and serum potassium, and a chest X-ray should be obtained at regular intervals during prolonged therapy. Upper GI X-rays are desirable in patients with known or suspected peptic ulcer disease.

7. Suppression of autogenous pituitary function, a common effect of exogenous corticosteroids administration, may be reduced, modified or minimized by revision of dose schedules. The time of maximum corticoid effect is from midnight to 8 AM and minimal during the intervening hours. Use of a single daily dose at or about 8 AM will be effective in most conditions, will lower corticoid overload and will cause the least interference with the diurnal system of endogenous secretion and hypothalamopituitary-adrenal function; alternate-day dosage in some conditions in certain severe disorders requiring long-term and/or high dose maintenance levels have proven both clinically effective and less likely to produce adverse reactions.

8 Alternate-Day Therapy: After the conventional dose has been established, some patients may be maintained on alternate-day therapy. It has been shown that the activity of the adrenal cortex varies throughout the day, being greatest from about midnight to 8:00 AM. Exogenous corticoid suppresses this activity least when given at the time of maximum activity. A 48 hour interval appears to be necessary since shorter intervals are accompanied by adrenal suppression similar to that of conventional daily divided doses. Therefore, with the alternate-day dose plan, a total 48-hour requirement is given every other day at 8:00 AM. As with other regimens, the minimum effective dose level should be sought.

The maximum daily morning dose not associated with lasting adrenocorticoid suppression is 8 mg.

SPECIFIC DOSAGE RECOMMENDATIONS

Endocrine Disorders: Wide variation in dosage requirements for the endocrine disorders such as *congenital adrenal hyperplasia, non-suppurative thyroiditis,* and *hypercalcemia* associated with cancer precludes specific recommendation except for*adrenocortical insufficiency* where the dose is usually 4-12 mg daily in addition to mineralocorticoid therapy.

Rheumatic Disorders: Rheumatoid arthritis; acute gouty arthritis; ankylosing spondylitis; and *selected cases* of *psoriatic arthritis;* in *acute* and *subacute bursitis;* and in*acute nonspecific tenosynovitis.* The initial suppressive dose of triamcinolone in these conditions ranges from 8 to 16 mg per day, although the occasional patient may require higher doses.

Patients may show an early or a delayed effect, characterized by a reduction in the inflammatory reaction and in joint swelling, together with alleviation of pain and stiffness, resulting in an increased range of motion of the affected joints or tissues. Maintenance doses are adjusted to keep symptoms at a level tolerable to the patient. Rapid reduction of the steroid or its abrupt discontinuance may result in recurrence or even exacerbation of signs and symptoms. Short-term administration is desirable as a rule. Triamcinolone is ordinarily administered as a single morning dose, daily or on alternate days depending on the need of the patient. Occasional patients may secure more effective relief on divided daily doses, either 2 to 4 times daily.

Collagen Diseases: *Systemic Lupus Erythematosus:* The initial dose is usually 20 to 32 mg daily continued until the desired response is obtained, when reduced maintenance levels are sought. Patients with more severe symptoms may require higher initial doses, 48 mg or more daily, and higher maintenance doses. Although some patients with systemic lupus erythematosus appear to have spontaneous remissions or to tolerate the disorder in its milder forms for prolonged periods of time, adjustment of dosage scheduling to reduce adverse suppression of the pituitary-adrenal axis may be useful.

Acute Rheumatic Carditis: In severely ill patients with carditis, pericardial effusion and/or congestive heart failure, corticosteroid therapy is effective in the control of the acute and severe inflammatory changes and may be lifesaving. Initial dose of triamcinolone may be from 20 to 60 mg daily, and clinical response is usually rapid and the drug can then be reduced. Maintenance therapy should be continued for at least 6 to 8 weeks and is seldom required beyond a period of 3 months. Corticosteroid therapy does not preclude conventional treatment, including antibiotics and salicylization.

Dermatological Disorders: *Pemphigus; bullous dermatitis herpetiformis; severe erythema multiforme* (Stevens-Johnson syndrome);*exfoliative dermatitis;* and *mycosis fungoides.* The initial dose is 8 to 16 mg daily. In these conditions, as well as in certain allergic dermatoses, *alternate-day* administration has been found effective and apparently less likely to produce adverse side effects.

Severe psoriasis: Triamcinolone may produce reduction or remission of the disabling skin manifestations following initial doses of 8 to 16 mg daily. The period of maintenance is dependent on the clinical response. Corticosteroid reduction or discontinuation of therapy should be attempted with caution since relapse may occur and may appear in more aggravated form, the so-called "rebound phenomenon."

Allergic States: Triamcinolone is administered is doses of 8 to 12 mg daily in acute seasonal or perennial *allergic rhinitis.* Intractable cases may require high initial and maintenance doses. In*bronchial asthma,* 8 to 16 mg daily are usually effective. The usual therapeutic measures for control of bronchial asthma should be carried out in addition to triamcinolone therapy. In both allergic rhinitis and bronchial asthma, therapy is directed at alleviation of acute distress and chronic long-term use of corticosteroids is neither desirable nor often essential. Some patients may be maintained on alternate-day therapy. In such conditions as *contact dermatitis* and atopic dermatitis, topical therapy may be supplemented with short courses of triamcinolone by mouth in doses of 8 to 16 mg daily. In severely ill patients with *serum sickness,* epinephrine may be the drug of choice for immediate therapy, often supplemented by antihistamines.

DOSAGE AND ADMINISTRATION: *(cont'd)*

Triamcinolone is frequently useful as adjunctive treatment in such cases, with the dosage determined by the severity of the disorder, the speed with which therapeutic response is desired and the response of the patient to initial therapy.

Ophthalmological Diseases: Allergic conjunctivitis; keratitis; iridocyclitis; chorioretinitis; anterior segment inflammation; diffuse posterior uveitis and choroiditis, optic neuritis and sympathetic ophthalmia. Initial doses range from 12 to 40 mg daily depending on the severity of the condition, the nature and degree of involvement of ocular structure, but response is usually rapid and therapy of short-term duration.

Respiratory Diseases: Symptomatic sarcoidosis; Loeffler's syndrome' berylliosis; and in certain cases of fulminating or disseminated pulmonary tuberculosis when concurrently accompanied by appropriate antituberculous chemotherapy. Initial doses are usually in the range of 16 to 48 mg daily.

Hematologic Disorders: Idiopathic and secondary thrombocytopenia in adults, acquired (autoimmune) hemolytic anemia; erythroblastopenia (RBC anemia;) congenital (erythroid) hypoplastic anemia. Triamcinolone is used to produce a remission of symptoms and may, in some instances, produce an apparent regression of abnormal cellular blood elements to normal states, temporary or permanent. The recommended dose varies between 16 to 60 mg daily, with reduction after adequate clinical response.

Neoplastic Diseases: Acute leukemia in childhood. The usual dose of triamcinolone is 1 mg per kilogram of body weight daily, although as much as 2 mg per kilogram may be necessary. Initial response is usually seen within 6 to 21 days and therapy continued from 4 to 6 weeks.

Acute leukemia and lymphoma in adults: The usual dose of triamcinolone is 16 to 40 mg daily, although it may be necessary to give as much as 100 mg daily in leukemia. Triamcinolone therapy in these neoplasias is only palliative and not curative. Other therapeutic and supportive measures must be used when appropriate.

Edematous States: *Nephrotic Syndrome:* Triamcinolone may be used to induce a diuresis or remission of proteinuria in the nephrotic syndrome, without uremia, of the idiopathic type or that due to lupus erythematosus. The average dose is 16 to 20 mg (up to 48 mg) daily until diuresis occurs. The diuresis may be massive and usually occurs by the 14th day, but occasionally may be delayed. After diuresis begins it is advisable to continue treatment until maximal or complete chemical and clinical remission occurs, at which time the dosage should be reduced gradually and then discontinued. In less severe cases maintenance dosages of as little as 4 mg daily may be adequate. Alternatively and when maintenance therapy may be prolonged, triamcinolone may be administered on alternate-day dose schedules.

Miscellaneous: *Tuberculous Meningitis:* Triamcinolone may be useful when accompanied by appropriate antituberculous therapy when there is subarachnoid block or impending block. The average dosage is 32 to 48 mg daily in either single or divided doses (TABLE 1.

TABLE 1

	Anti-inflammatory Relative Potency		Frequently Used Tablet Strength (mg)		Tablet X Potency Equivalent Value
Hydrocortisone	1	X	20	=	20
Prednisolone	4	X	5	=	20
Triamcinolone	5	X	4	=	20
Dexamethasone	25	X	0.75	=	18.75

HOW SUPPLIED:

Store at Controlled Room Temperature 15-30°C (59-86°F).

HOW SUPPLIED - EQUIVALENTS NOT AVAILABLE:

Tablet, Uncoated - Oral - 2 mg

100's	**$72.52**	**ARISTOCORT, Fujisawa Pharm (US)**	**57317-0601-10**

Tablet, Uncoated - Oral - 4 mg

16's	$9.72	Triamcinolone, Qualitest Pharms	00603-6170-14
16's	$10.45	TRIAMCINOLONE 4, Major Pharms	00904-0884-44
16's	$13.50	Triamcinolone, Horizon Pharms	60904-0454-35
16's	$20.89	ARISTO-PAK, Fujisawa USA	00469-5123-16
30's	**$41.44**	**ARISTOCORT, Fujisawa Pharm (US)**	**57317-0600-30**
100's	$6.75	Triamcinolone, HL Moore Drug Exch	00839-5009-06
100's	$7.90	Triamcinolone 4, Major Pharms	00904-0884-60
100's	$7.95	Triamcinolone, Schein Pharm (US)	00364-0352-01
100's	$10.75	Triamcinolone, Consolidated Midland	00223-2110-01
100's	$14.25	Triamcinolone, IDE-Interstate	00814-8000-14
100's	$112.80	KENACORT, Bristol Myers Squibb	00003-0512-50
100's	**$131.23**	**ARISTOCORT, Fujisawa Pharm (US)**	**57317-0600-10**
1000's	$79.00	Triamcinolone, Consolidated Midland	00223-2110-02

Tablet, Uncoated - Oral - 8 mg

50's	$96.49	KENACORT, Bristol Myers Squibb	00003-0518-40
50's	**$112.05**	**ARISTOCORT, Fujisawa USA**	**00469-5125-50**

TRIAMCINOLONE ACETONIDE *(002371)*

CATEGORIES: Adrenal Corticosteroids; Adrenal Hyperplasia; Adrenal Insufficiency; Airway Obstruction; Allergies; Alopecia; Alopecia Areata; Anemia; Anti-Inflammatory Agents; Antiasthmatics/Bronchodilators; Antimicrobials; Arthritis; Aspiration Pneumonitis; Asthma; Bursitis; Carditis; Colitis; Conjunctivitis; Corneal Ulcer; Dental; Dermatitis; Dermatologicals; Dermatoses; Diuresis; EENT Drugs; Edema; Enteritis; Epicondylitis; Erythema Multiforme; Eye, Ear, Nose, & Throat Preparations; Glucocorticoids; Gouty Arthritis; Granuloma Annulare; Herpes; Herpes Zoster; Hormones; Hypercalcemia; Inflammation; Inflammatory Lesions; Keloids; Lesions; Leukemia; Lichen Simplex Chronicus; Lupus Erythematosus; Lymphoma; Meningitis; Multiple Sclerosis; Necrobiosis Lipoidica; Nephrotic Syndrome; Ocular Infections; Ophthalmics; Osteoarthritis; Pemphigus; Pneumoconiosis; Pneumonitis; Proteinuria; Pruritus; Psoriasis; Purpura; Respiratory & Allergy Medications; Retinochoroiditis; Rhinitis; Sarcoidosis; Skin/Mucous Membrane Agents; Spondylitis; Steroids; Sulfonamides; Synovitis; Synovitis of Osteoarthritis; Tenosynovitis; Thrombocytopenia; Thyroiditis; Trichinosis; Tuberculosis; Ulcerative Colitis; Uveitis; Pregnancy Category C; Sales > $100 Million; FDA Approval Pre 1982; Top 200 Drugs

BRAND NAMES: Acetocot; *Adcortyl* (England); *Adcortyl in Orabase* (England); *Albicort*; *Ahbina*; Aricin; *Aristocort*; *Aristocort* ; *Aristocort A*; *Aristocort C* (Canada); *Aristocort D* (Canada); *Aristocort R* (Canada); Aristocort Topical; Aristogel; Azmacort; Cenocort A-40; Cinalog; Cinolar; *Cinolone*; Cinonide 40; *Delphi Creme*; *Delphicort* (Germany); Delta-Tritex; *Denkacort Forte*; *Dermacort*; *Facort*; Flutex; *Ftorocort*; *Gemicort*; *Generlog*; Kena-Plex 40; Kenac; *Kenacort*; *Kenacort A*; *Kenacort*

A I.A.-I.D.; *Kenacort A I.M.*; *Kenacort A in Orabase*; *Kenacort-A* (Australia); *Kenacort-A IM*; *Kenacort-A in Orabase*; *Kenacort-A Intra-articular Intra-dermal*; *Kenacort-A IA ID*; *Kenacort A IA ID*; *Kenacort E*; *Kenacort IM* (Mexico); *Kenacort Retard* (France); *Kenacort T*; *Kenacort T Munnsalve*; Kenaject-40; **Kenalog**; *Kenalog-10*; *Kenalog-40* (Canada); *Kenalog Dental* (Mexico); *Kenalog in Orabase* (Australia, Canada); *Kenalone*; Kenonel; *Ledercort* (England); *Ledercort A*; Nasacort; *Nincort*; Oracort; *Oralog*; Oralone; *Oramedy*; *Rheudenolon*; *Shincort*; Sholog K; Tac; Tramacort 40; Tri-Kort; Triacet; Triacort; *Triaderm* (Canada); Triam-A; Triamcinair; *Triamcort*; Triamcot; Triamonide 40; Trianide; Triatex; *Tricort*; *Tricot*; Triderm; *Trigon*; Trilog; *Trinlog*; Trylone A; Trymex; *Unicilone*; *Unif*; *Volon A*; *Volon A Antibiotikafrei* (Germany); *Volon A 10* (Germany); *Volon A 40* (Germany); *Volon A Spray*
(International brand names outside U.S. in italics)

FORMULARIES: BC-BS; FHP; Foundation

COST OF THERAPY: $474.79 (Asthma; Aerosol; 100 mcg; 0.6/day; 365 days)

PRIMARY ICD9: 493.90 (Asthma, Unspecified, Without Mention of Status Asthmaticus)

DESCRIPTION:

Nasal and Oral Inhalers and AQ Nasal Spray: Triamcinolone acetonide, USP, Nasal Inhaler, is a glucocorticosteroid with a molecular weight of 434.51 and with the chemical designation 9-Fluoro-11β, 16α, 17,21-tetrahydroxypregna-1, 4-diene-3,20-dione cyclic 16,17-acetal with acetone. ($C_{24}H_{31}FO_6$).

Oral Inhaler: Triamcinolone acetonide Oral Inhaler is a metered-dose aerosol unit containing a microcrystalline suspension of triamcinolone acetonide in the propellant dichlorodifluoromethane and dehydrated alcohol USP 1% w/w. Each canister contains 60 mg triamcinolone acetonide. Each actuation releases approximately 200 mcg triamcinolone acetonide, of which approximately 100 mcg are delivered from the unit (*in vitro* testing). There are at least 240 actuations in one triamcinolone acetonide aerosol canister. After 240 actuations, the amount delivered per actuation may not be consistent and the unit should be discarded.

AQ Nasal Spray: Triamcinolone Acetonide AQ Nasal Spray is an unscented, thixotropic, water-based metered-dose pump spray formulation unit containing a microcrystalline suspension of triamconolone acetonide in an aqueous medium. Microcrystalline cellulose, carboxymethylcellulose sodium, polysorbate 80, dextrose, benzalkonium chloride, and edetate disodium are contained in this aqueous medium; hydrochloric acid or sodium hydroxide may be added to adjust the pH to a target of 5.0 within a range of 4.5 and 6.0.

Each bottle contains 9.075 mg triamcinolone acetonide. Each actuation delivers 55 mcg triamcinolone acetonide from the nasal actuator to the patient (estimated from *in vitro* testing) after an initial priming of 5 sprays. It will remain adequately primed for 2 weeks. If the product is not used for more than 2 weeks, then it can be adequately reprimed with one spray. There are at least 120 actuations in one triamcinolone acetonide AQ nasal spray bottle. **After 120 actuations, the amount of triamcinolone acetonide delivered per actuation may not be consistent and the unit should be discarded.** In the manufacturer's original package insert, patients are provided with a check-off form to track usage in the Information for Patients tear-off sheet.

Nasal Inhaler: Triamcinolone acetonide Nasal Inhaler is a metered-dose aerosol unit containing a microcrystalline suspension of triamcinolone acetonide in dichlorodifluoromethane and dehydrated alcohol USP 0.7% w/w. Each canister contains 15 mg triamcinolone acetonide. Each actuation releases approximately 55 mcg triamcinolone acetonide from the nasal actuator to the patient (estimated from *in vitro* testing). There are at least 100 actuations in one triamcinolone acetonide Nasal Inhaler canister. **After 100 actuations, the amount delivered per actuation may not be consistent and the unit should be discarded.** Patients are provided with a check-off card to track usage as part of the Information for Patients tear-off sheet.

Dental Paste: Each gram of triamcinolone acetonide in Orabase provides 1 mg (0.1%) triamcinolone acetonide in emollient dental paste containing gelatin, pectin, and carboxymethylcellulose sodium is a plastibase (plasticized Hydrocarbon Gel), a polyethylene and mineral oil gel base.

Injection-10: (For Intra-articular, Intrabursal or Intradermal Use)

Triamcinolone acetonide (sterile triamcinolone acetonide suspension, USP) provides triamcinolone acetonide, a synthetic corticosteroid with marked anti-inflammatory action, in a sterile aqueous suspension suitable for intradermal, intra-articular, and intrabursal injection into tendon sheaths. The preparation is NOT suitable for IV or IM use. Each ml of the sterile aqueous suspension provides 10 mg triamcinolone acetonide, with sodium chloride for isotonicity, 0.9% (w/v) benzyl alcohol as preservative, 0.75% carboxymethylcellulose sodium, and 0.04%, polysorbate 80; sodium hydroxide or hydrochloric may have been added to adjust pH between 5.0 and 7.5. At the time of manufacture, the air in the container is replaced by nitrogen. The chemical name is 9-fluoro- 11β,16α,17,21-tetrahyroxypregna-1,4-diene -3,20-dione cyclic 16,17- acetal with- acetone.

Injection-40: (Not for IV or Intradermal Use).

Triamcinolone acetonide (sterile triamcinolone acetonide suspension, USP) provides triamcinolone acetonide, a synthetic corticosteroid with marked anti-inflammatory action. Each ml of the sterile aqueous suspension provides 40 mg triamcinolone acetonide, with sodium chloride for isotonicity, 0.9% (w/v) benzyl alcohol as preservative, 0.75% carboxymethylcellulose sodium, and 0.04%, polysorbate 80. Sodium hydroxide or hydrochloric may have been added to adjust pH between 5.0 and 7.5. At the time of manufacture, the air in the container is replaced by nitrogen.

Aerosol Spray, Cream, and Ointment: (For Dermatologic Use Only)

The topical corticosteroids constitute a class of primarily synthetic steroids used as anti-inflammatory and antipruritic agents. The steroids in the class include triamcinolone acetonide. The chemical name is 9- Fluoro-11β,16β,17, 21- tetrahyroxypregna-1,4-diene-3,20-dione cyclic 16,17-acetal with acetone.

Aerosol Spray: A two-second application which covers an area approximately the size of the hand, delivers an amount of triamcinolone acetonide not exceeding 0.2. After spraying, the nonvolatile vehicle remaining on the skin contains approximately 0.2% triamcinolone acetonide. Each gram of spray provides 0.147 mg triamcinolone acetonide in a vehicle of isopropyl palmitate, dehydrated alcohol (10.3%) and isobutane propellant.

Cream: (All Strengths) Each gram of 0.025%, 0.1% and 0.5% triamcinolone acetonide cream provides 0.25% mg, 1 mg or 5 mg triamcinolone acetonide, respectively, in a vanishing cream base containing propylene glycol, cetearyl alcohol (and) ceteareth-20 white petrolatum, sorbitol solution, glyceryl monostearate, polyethylene glycol monostearate, simethicone, sorbic acid, and purified water.

Ointment: (All Strengths) Each gram of 0.025%, 0.1%, and 0.5% triamcinolone acetonide ointment provides 0.25 mg, 1 mg, or 5 mg triamcinolone acetonide, respectively in Plastibase (Plasticized Hydrocarbon Gel), a polyethylene and mineral oil gel base.

CLINICAL PHARMACOLOGY:

Oral Inhaler: The precise mechanism of the action of the inhaled drug is unknown. However, use of the inhaler makes it possible to provide effective local steroid activity with minimal systemic effect.

Triamcinolone acetonide is a more potent derivative of triamcinolone. Although triamcinolone itself is approximately one to two times as potent as prednisone in animal models of inflammation, triamcinolone acetonide is approximately 8 times more potent than prednisone.

Pharmacokinetic studies with radiolabeled triamcinolone acetonide have been carried out by the oral route and intravenous route in several species. The pharmacokinetic behavior of the triamcinolone acetonide was similar in all species within each route of administration. The major portion of the dose was eliminated in the feces irrespective of route of administration with only one species (rabbit) showing significant urinary excretion of radioactivity.

The results of studies in which triamcinolone acetonide was administered as an aerosol showed rapid disappearance of radioactivity from the lungs comparable to that observed following oral administration with peak blood levels occurring in one to two hours. Virtually no radioactivity was present in the lung and trachea 24 hours after dosing.

Based upon intravenous dosing of triamcinolone acetonide phosphate ester, the half-life of triamcinolone acetonide was reported to be 88 minutes. The volume of distribution (Vd) reported was 99.5 L (SD ± 27.5) and clearance was 45.2 L/hour (SD ± 9.1) for triamcinolone acetonide. The plasma half-life of corticoids does not correlate well with the biologic half-life.

Three metabolites of triamcinolone acetonide have been identified. They are 6β-hydroxytriamcinolone acetonide, 21-carboxytriamcinolone acetonide and 21-carboxy-6β-hydroxytriamcinolone acetonide. All three metabolites are expected to be substantially less active than the parent compound due to (a) the dependence of anti-inflammatory activity on the presence of anti-inflammatory activity on the presence of a 21-hydroxyl group, (b) the decreased activity observed upon 6-hydroxylation, and (c) the markedly increased water solubility favoring rapid elimination. There appeared to be some quantitative differences in the metabolites among species. No differences were detected in metabolic pattern as a function of route of administration.

Nasal Inhaler and AQ Nasal Spray: Triamcinolone acetonide is a more potent derivative of triamcinolone. Although triamcinolone itself is approximately one to two times as potent as prednisone in animal models of inflammation, triamcinolone acetonide is approximately 8 times more potent than prednisone.

Although the precise mechanism of corticosteroid antiallergic action is unknown, corticosteroids are very effective. However, they do not have an immediate effect on allergic signs and symptoms. When allergic symptoms are very severe, local treatment with recommended doses (microgram) of any available topical corticosteroids are not as effective as treatment with larger doses (milligram) of oral or parenteral formulations. When corticosteroids are prematurely discontinued symptoms may not recur for several days.

Based upon intravenous dosing of triamcinolone acetonide phosphate ester, the half-life of triamcinolone acetonide was reported to be 88 minutes. The volume of distribution (Vd) reported was 99.5 L (SD ± 27.5) and clearance was 45.2 L/hour (SD ± 9.1) for triamcinolone acetonide. The plasma half-life of corticosteroids does not correlate well with the biologic half-life.

Pharmacokinetic characterization of the triamcinolone acetonide AQ nasal spray formulation was determined in both normal subjects and in patients with allergic rhinitis. Single dose intranasal administration of 220 mcg of the AQ nasal spray in normal subjects and patients demonstrated minimal absorption of triamcinolone acetonide. The mean peak plasma concentration was approximately 0.5ng/mL (range: 0.1 to 1.0 ng/mL) and occurred at 1.5 hours post dose. THe mean plasma drug concentration was less than 0.06 ng/mL at 12 hours, and below the assay detection limit at 24 hours. The average terminal half-life was 3.1 hours. The range of mean $AUC_{0-\infty}$ values was 1.4 ng·hr/mL between doses of 110 mcg to 440 mcg in both patients and healthy volunteers. Dose proportionality was demonstrated in both normal subjects and in allergic rhinitis patients following single intranasal doses of 110 mcg or 220 mcg triamcinolone acetonide AQ nasal spray. The C_{max} and AUC of the 440 mcg dose increased less than proportionally when compared to 110 and 220 mcg doses.

When administered intranasally to humans at 440 mcg/day dose, the peak plasma concentration was <1 ng/ml and occurred on average at 3.4 hours (range 0.5 - 8.0 hours) post dosing. The apparent half-life was 4.0 hours (range 1.0 - 7.0 hours); however, this value probably reflects lingering absorption. Intranasal doses below 440 mcg/day gave sparse data and did not allow for the calibration of meaningful pharmacokinetic parameters.

In animal studies using rats and dogs, three metabolites of triamcinolone acetonide have been identified. They are 6β-hydroxytriamcinolone acetonide, 21-carboxytriamcinolone acetonide and 21-carboxy-6β-triamcinolone acetonide. All three metabolites are expected to be substantially less active than the parent compound due to (a) the dependence of anti-inflammatory activity on the presence of 21-hydroxyl group, (b) the decreased activity observed upon —hydroxylation, and (c) the markedly increased water solublity favoring rapid elimination. There appeared to be some quantitative differences in the metabolites among species. No differences were detected in metabolic pattern as a function of route of adminstration.

INDIVIDUALIZATION OF DOSAGE

Nasal Inhaler: Individual patients will experience a variable time to onset and degree of symptom relief when using triamcinolone acetonide. It is recommended that dosing be started at 220 mcg once a day and the effect be assessed in four to seven days.

Adults and Children 12 Years of Age and Older: Some relief can be expected in approximately two-thirds of patients within four to seven days. If greater effect is desired an increase of dose to 440 mcg once a day can be tried. If adequate relief has not been obtained by the third week of triamcinolone acetonide treatment, consideration to alternate forms of treatment should be considered.

A dose-response between 110 mcg/day (one spray/nostril/day) and 440 mcg/day (four sprays/nostril/day) is not clearly discernible. In general, in the clinical trials the highest dose tended to provide relief sooner. This suggests an alternative approach to starting therapy with triamcinolone acetonide (*e.g.,* starting treatment with 440 mcg (four sprays/nostril/day) and then, depending on the patient's response, decreasing the dose by one spray per day every four to seven days).

Although triamcinolone acetonide may be used at 220 mcg/day or 440 mcg/day divided into two or four times a day, the degree of relief does not seem to be significantly different compared to once-a-day dosing. As with other nasal corticosteroids, the vehicle used to deliver the corticosteroid may cause symptoms that are difficult to distinguish from the patient's rhinitis symptoms. Thus, depending upon the balance between these vehicle side effects and the benefits of treatment, in determining the optimal dose for the relief of symptoms, individual patients may need to have a trial of high and low doses.

Children 6 Through 11 Years of Age: In children 6 through 11 years of age, it is recommended that dosing be started at 220 mcg as two sprays (55 mcg/spray) in each nostril once a day. In clinical trials, significant relief of rhinitis symptoms in children was observed as early as the fourth day of treatment and generally, it took one to two weeks to achieve maximum benefit. If adequate relief has not been obtained by the third week of treatment, alternate forms of treatment should be considered.

CLINICAL PHARMACOLOGY: *(cont'd)*

In general, it is always desirable to titrate an individual patient to the minimum effective dose to reduce the possibility of side effects. In clinical trials, after symptoms have been brought under control at the recommended starting doses, reducing the daily dose to 110 mcg (one spray in each nostril oncer per day) has been shown to be effective in controlling symptoms in approximatley one-half of adult patients being treated long-term for allergic rhinitis. (See PRECAUTIONS, WARNINGS, PRECAUTIONSInformation for the Patient, and ADVERSE REACTIONS).

AQ Nasal Spray: It is recommended that dosing be started at 220 mcg as 2 sprays in each nostril once daily for adults and children 12 years and older.

An improvement in some patient symptoms may be seen within the first day of treatment, and generally, it takes one week of treatment to reach maximum benefit. Initial assessment for response should be made during this time frame and periodically until the patient's symptoms are stabilized. If adequate relief of symptoms has not been obtained after 3 weeks of treatment, triamcinolone acetonide AQ nasal spary should be discontinued.

It is always desirable to titrate an individual patient to the minimum effective dose to reduce the possibility of side effects. Therefore, when the maximum benefit has been achieved and symptoms have been controlled, reducing the dose to 110 mcg (one spray in each nostril once per day) has been shown to be effective in maintaining control of the allergic rhinitis symptoms in patients who were initially controlled at 220 mcg/day. (See PRECAUTIONS, WARNINGS, PRECAUTIONSInformation for the Patient, and ADVERSE REACTIONS.)

Aerosol Spray, Cream, and Ointment Topical corticosteroids share anti-inflammatory, antipruritic and vasoconstrictive actions.

The mechanism of anti-inflammatory activity of the topical corticosteroids is unclear. Various laboratory methods, including vasoconstrictor assays, are used to compare and predict potencies and/or clinical efficacies of the topical corticosteroids. There is some evidence to suggest that a recognizable correlation exists between vasoconstrictor potency and therapeutic efficacy in man.

PHARMACOKINETICS

The extent of percutaneous absorption of topical corticosteroids is determined by many factors including the vehicle, the integrity of the epidermal barrier, and the use of occlusive dressings.

Topical corticosteroids can be absorbed from normal intact skin. Inflammation and/or other disease processes in the skin increase percutaneous absorption. Occlusive dressings substantially increase the percutaneous absorption of topical corticosteroids. Thus, occlusive dressings may be a valuable therapeutic adjunct for treatment of resistant dermatoses (see DOSAGE AND ADMINISTRATION).

Once absorbed through the skin, topical corticosteroids are handled through pharmacokinetic pathways similar to systematically administered corticosteroids. Corticosteroids are bound to plasma proteins in varying degrees. Corticosteroids are metabolized primarily in the liver and are then excreted by the kidneys. Some of the topical corticosteroids and their metabolites are also excreted into the bile.

CLINICAL STUDIES:

Nasal Inhaler In double-blind, parallel, placebo-controlled clinical trials of seasonal and perennial allergic rhinitis, in adults and adolescentes in fixed total daily doses of 110, 220 and 440 mcg per day, the responses to aerosolized triamcinolone acetonide demonstrated a statistically significant improvement over placebo. In open label trials where the doses were sometimes adjusted according to patients' signs and symptoms, the daily doses and regimens varied. The most commonly used dose was 110 mcg per day.

The Nasal Inhaler, at a dose of 220 mcg once daily, has also been studied in two double blind placebo controlled trials of two and four weeks duration in children ages 6 through 11 years with seasonal and perennial allergic rhinitis. These trials included 162 males and 91 females. The nasal inhaler, administered at a fixed dose of 220 mcg once daily resulted in consistent and statistically significant reductions of allergic rhinitis symptoms over vehicle placebo.

In attempting to determine if systemic absorption played a role in the response to triamcinolone acetonide, a clinical study comparing intranasal and depot intramuscular triamcinolone acetonide was conducted. The doses used were based on bioavailability studies of each formulation. The final doses of triamcinolone acetonide 440 mcg once a day and Kenalog-40, 4 mg intramuscularly once a week, were chosen to deliver comparable total amounts of weekly triamcinolone acetonide. However, the weekly injection yielded sustained plasma levels throughout the dosing interval while the daily triamcinolone acetonide application resulted in daily peak and trough concentrations, the mean of which was 3.5 times below the Kenalog plasma levels. Both topical triamcinolone acetonide and intramuscular Kenalog-40 were clinically effective. In addition, in some studies there was evidence of improvement of eye symptoms. This suggests that triamcinolone acetonide, at least to some degree is acting by a systemic mechanism.

In order to evaluate the effects of systemic absorption on the Hypothalamic-Pituitary-Adrenal (HPA) axis, triamcinolone acetonide to adults in doses of 440 mcg once a day was compared to placebo and 42 days of a single morning dose of prednisone 10 mg. Adrenal response to a six-hour cosyntropin stimulation test suggests that intranasal triamcinolone acetonide 440 mcg/day for six weeks did not measurably affect adrenal activity. Conversely, oral prednisone at 10 mg/day significantly reduced the response to ACTH.

No evidence of adrenal axis suppression was observed in 26 pediatric patients exposed for 6 weeks to systemic levels of triamcinolone acetonide higher than the systemic levels observed following administration of the maximum recommended dose of triamcinolone acetonide nasal inhaler.

AQ Nasal Spray: The safety and efficacy of triamcinolone acetonide AQ nasal spray has been evaluated in 10 double-blind, placebo-controlled clinical trials of two to four weeks in duration in adults and children 12 years and older with seasonal or perennial allergic rhinitis. The number of patients treated with the AQ nasal spray in these studies was 1266; of these patients, 675 were male and 591 were female.

Overall, the results of these clinical trials showed that triamcinolone acetonide AQ nasal spray 220 mcg once daily (2 sprays in each nostril) when compared to placebo provides statistically significant relief of nasal symptoms including sneezing, stuffiness, discharge, and itching.

INDICATIONS AND USAGE:

Oral Inhaler: Triamcinolone acetonide Oral Inhaler is indicated only for patients who require chronic treatment with corticosteroids for the control of the symptoms of bronchial asthma. Such patients would include those already receiving systemic corticosteroids and selected patients who are inadequately controlled on a non-steroid regimen and in whom steroid therapy has been withheld because of concern over potential adverse effects.

Triamcinolone acetonide oal ihaler is *NOT* indicated:

1. For relief of asthma which can be controlled by bronchodilators and other non-steroid medications.
2. In patients who require systemic corticosteroid treatment infrequently.
3. In the treatment of non-asthmatic bronchitis.

INDICATIONS AND USAGE: *(cont'd)*

AQ Nasal Spray: Triamcinolone Acetonide AQ Nasal Spray is indicated for the treatment of seasonal and perennial allergic rhinitis symptoms.

Nasal Inhaler: Triamcinolone acetonide Nasal Inhaler is indicated for the nasal treatment of seasonal and perennial allergic rhinitis symptoms in adults and children 6 years of age and older.

Dental Paste: Triamcinolone acetonide dental paste is indicated for adjunctive treatment and for the temporary relief of symptoms associated with oral inflammatory lesions and ulcerative resulting from trauma.

INJECTION-10: *Intra-Articular:* Triamcinolone acetonide Injection-10 is indicated for intra-articular or intrabursal administration, and for injection into tendon sheaths, as adjunctive therapy for short-term administration (to tide the patient over an acute episode or exacerbation) in: synovitis of osteoarthritis, rheumatoid arthritis, acute and subacute bursitis, acute gouty arthritis, epicondylitis, acute nonspecific, tenospecific, and posttraumatic osteoarthritis.

Intradermal: Intralesional administration is indicated for the treatment of keloids, discoid lupus erythematosus, necrobiosis, lipoidica, diabeticorum, alopecia areata, and localized hypertrophic, infiltrated, inflammatory lesions of: licheplanus, psoriatic plaques, granuloma annulare, and lichen simplex chronicus (neurodermatitis). This drug may be useful in cystic tumors of an aponeurosis or tendon (ganglia).

INJECTION-40: *Intramuscular:* When oral therapy is not feasible or is temporarily undesirable in the judgement of the physician, triamcinolone acetonide Injection-40 is indicated for *IM* use as follows:

Endocrine disorders: Nonsuppurative thyroiditis

Rheumatic disorders: As adjunctive therapy for short-term administration (to side the patient over an acute episode or exacerbation) in: posttraumatic osteoarthritis; synovitis of osteoarthritis; rheumatoid arthritis; acute and subacute bursitis; epicondylitis; acute nonspecific tenosynovitis; acute gouty arthritis; psoriatic arthritis; ankylosing spondylitis; juvenile rheumatoid arthritis.

Collagen disease: During an exacerbation or as maintenance therapy in selected cases of: systemic lupus erythematosus; acute rheumatic carditis.

Dermatologic diseases: Pemphigus: severe erythema multiforme (Stevens-Johnson syndrome); exfoliative dermatitis; bullous dermatitis herpetiformis; severe seborrheic dermatitis; severe psoriasis.

Allergic states: Controls of severe or incapacitating allergic conditions intractable to adequate trials of conventional treatment in: bronchial asthma; contact dermatitis; atopic dermatitis; seasonal or perennial allergic rhinitis.

Ophthalmic diseases: Severe chronic allergic and inflammatory processes involving the eye, such as: herpes zoster ophthalmicus; iritis; iridocyclitis; chorioretinitis; diffuse posterior uveitis and choroiditis; optic neuritis; sympathetic ophthalmia; anterior segment inflammation.

Gastrointestinal diseases: To tide the patient over a critical period of disease in: ulcerative colitis (systemic therapy); regional enteritis (systemic therapy).

Respiratory diseases: Symptomatic sarcoidosis; berylliosis; aspiration pneumonitis.

Hematologic disorders: Acquired (autoimmune) hemolytic anemia.

Neoplastic diseases: For palliative management of: leukemias and lymphomas in adults; acute leukemia of childhood.

Edematous state: To induce diuresis or remission of proteinuria in the nephrotic syndrome without uremia, of the idiopathic type or that due to lupus erythematosus.

Intra-Articular: This drug is indicated for the intra-articular or intrabursal administration, and for injections into tendon sheaths as adjunctive therapy for short-term administration (to tide the patient over an acute episode or exacerbation) in: synovitis of osteoarthritis; rheumatoid arthritis; epicondylitis; acute nonspecific tenosynovitis; post traumatic osteoarthritis

Aerosol Spray: Triamcinolone acetonide aerosol spray is indicated for relief of the inflammatory and pruritic manifestations of corticosteroid-responsive dermatoses.

Cream: (All Strengths) Indicated for relief of the inflammatory and pruritic manifestations of corticosteroid-responsive dermatoses.

Ointment: (All Strengths) Indicated for relief of the inflammatory and pruritic manifestations of corticosteroid-responsive dermatoses.

CONTRAINDICATIONS:

Oral Inhaler: Triamcinolone acetonide Oral Inhaler is contraindicated in the primary treatment of status asthmaticus or other acute episodes of asthma where intensive measures are required.

Oral and Nasal Inhalers and AQ Nasal Spray: Hypersensitivity to any of the ingredients of this preparation contraindicates its use.

Aerosol Spray, Cream and Ointment: Topical corticosteroids are contraindicated in those patients with a history of hypersensitivity to any of the components of the preparations.

WARNINGS:

Oral Inhaler: Particular care is needed in patients who are transferred from systemically active corticosteroids to triamcinolone acetonide Oral Inhaler because deaths due to adrenal insufficiency have occurred in asthmatic patients during and after transfer from systemic corticosteroids to aerosolized steroids in recommended doses. After withdrawal from systemic corticosteroids, a number of months is usually required for recovery of hypothalamic-pituitary- adrenal (HPA) function. For some patients who have received large doses of oral steroids for long periods of time before therapy with triamcinolone acetonide Oral Inhaler is initiated, recovery may be delayed for one year or longer. During this period of HPA suppression, patients may exhibit signs and symptoms of adrenal insufficiency when exposed to trauma, surgery or infections, particularly gastroenteritis or other conditions with acute electrolyte loss. Although triamcinolone acetonide Oral Inhaler may provide control of asthmatic symptoms during these episodes, in recommended doses it supplies only normal physiological amounts of corticosteroid systemically and does NOT provide the increased systemic steroid which is necessary for coping with these emergencies.

During periods of stress or a severe asthmatic attack, patients who have been recently withdrawn from systemic corticosteroids should be instructed to resume systemic steroids (in large doses) immediately and to contact their physician for further instruction. These patients should also be instructed to carry a warning card indicating that they may need supplementary systemic steroids during periods of stress or a severe asthma attack.

WARNINGS: *(cont'd)*

Localized infections with *Candida albicans* have occurred infrequently in the mouth and pharynx. These areas should be examined by the treating physician at each patient visit. The percentage of positive mouth and throat cultures *Candida albicans*did not change during a year of continuous therapy. The incidence of clinically apparent infection is low (2.5%). These infections may disappear spontaneously or may require treatment with appropriate antifungal therapy or discontinuance of treatment with triamcinolone acetonide Oral Inhaler.

Triamcinolone acetonide Oral Inhaler is not to be regarded as a bronchodilator and is not indicated for rapid relief of bronchospasm.

Patients should be instructed to contact their physician immediately when episodes of asthma which are not responsive to bronchodilators occur during the course of treatment with triamcinolone acetonide Oral Inhaler. During such episodes, patients may require therapy with systemic corticosteroids.

There is no evidence that control of asthma can be achieved by the administration of triamcinolone acetonide Oral Inhaler in amounts greater than the recommended doses, which appear to be the therapeutic equivalent of approximately 10 mg/day of oral prednisone.

Transfer of patients from systemic steroid therapy to triamcinolone acetonide Oral Inhaler may unmask allergic conditions previously suppressed by the systemic steroid therapy, e.g., rhinitis, conjunctivitis, and eczema.

Nasal Inhaler: The replacement of a systemic corticosteroid with a topical corticoid can be accompanied by signs of adrenal insufficiency and, in addition, some patients may experience symptoms of withdrawal, *e.g.* joint and/or muscular pain, lassitude and depression. Patients previously treated for prolonged periods with systemic corticosteroids and transferred to topical corticoids should be carefully monitored for acute adrenal insufficiency in response to stress. In those patients who have asthma or other clinical conditions requiring long-term systemic corticosteroid treatment, too rapid a decrease in systemic corticosteroids may cause a severe exacerbation of their symptoms.

Children who are on immunosuppressant drugs are more susceptible to infections than healthy children. Chickenpox and measles, for example, can have a more serious or even fatal course in children on immunosuppressant doses of corticosteroids. In such chcildren, or in adults who have not had these diseases, particular care should be taken to avoid exposure. If exposed, therapy with varicella zoster immune globulin (VZIG) or pooled intravenous immunoglobulin (IVIG), as appropriate, may be indicated. If chickenpox develops, treatment with antiviral agents may be considered.

The use of triamcinolone acetonide nasal inhaler with alternate-day systemic prednisone could increase the likelihood of hypothalamic-pituitary-adrenal (HPA) suppression compared to a therapeutic dose of either one alone. Therefore, triamcinolone acetonide nasal inhaler should be used with caution in patients already receiving alternate-day prednisone treatment for any disease.

AQ Nasal Spray: The replacement of a systemic corticosteroid can be accompanied by signs of adrenal insufficiency and, in addition, some patients may experience symptoms of withdrawal; *e.g.,* joint and/or muscular pain, lassitude and depression. Patients previously treated for prolonged periods with systemic corticosteroids and transferred to topical corticosteroids should be carefully monitored for acute adrenal insufficiency in response to stress. In those patients who have asthma or other clinical conditions requiring long-term systemic corticosteroid treatment, too rapid a decrease in systemic corticosteroids may cause a severe exacerbation of their symptoms.

Children who are on immunosuppressant drugs are more susceptible to infections than healthy children. Chickenpox and measles, for example, can have a more serious or even fatal course in children on immunosuppressant doses of corticosteroids. In such children, or in adults who have not had these diseases, particular care should be taken to avoid exposure. If exposed, therapy with varicella-zoster immune globulin (VZIG) or pooled intravenous immunoglobulin (IVIG), as appropriate may be indicated. If chickenpox develops, treatment with antiviral agents may be considered.

The use of triamcinolone acetonide AQ nasal spray with alternate day systemic prednisone could increase the likelihood of hypothalamic-pituitary-adrenal (HPA) suppression compared to a therapeutic dose of either one alone. Therefore, triamcinolone acetonide nasal spray should be used with caution in patients already receiving alternate day prednisone treatment for any disease.

PRECAUTIONS:

GENERAL

In clinical studies with triamcinolone acetonide administered intranasally, the development of localized infections of the nose and pharynx with *Candida albicans* has rarely occurred. When such an infection develops it may require treatment with appropriate local therapy and discontinuance of treatment with triamcinolone acetonide nasal inhaler or AQ nasal spray.

Triamcinolone acetonide administered intranasally has been shown to be minimally absorbed into the systemic circulation in humans. Patients with active rhinitis showed absorption similar to that found in normal volunteers.

Nasal Inhaler: Triamcinolone acetonide at 440 mcg/day for 42 days did not measurably affect adrenal response to a six hour cosyntropin test. In the same study prednisone 10 mg/day significantly reduced adrenal response to ACTH over the same period (see CLINICAL STUDIES).

AQ Nasal Spray: Daily doses of 220 mcg or 440 mcg triamcinolone acetonide AQ nasal spray, 10 mg prednisone each was compared to placebo. Adrenal response to six-hour cosyntropin test showed that triamcinolone acetonide AQ nasal spray in doses of 220 or 440 mcg/day for six weeks had no statistically significant effect on adrenal activity. In the same study prednisolone 10 mg/day significantly reduced adrenal response to synthetic ACTH over the same period.

Either Triamcinolone Acetonide Nasal Inhaler or AQ Nasal Spray should be used with caution, if at all, in patients with active or quiescent tuberculous infections of the respiratory tract or in patients with untreated fungal, bacterial, or systemic viral infections or ocular herpes simplex.

Because of the inhibitory effect of corticosteroids on wound healing in patients who have experienced recent nasal septal ulcers, nasal surgery or trauma, a corticosteroid should be used with caution until healing has occurred. As with other nasally inhaled corticosteroids, nasal septal perforations have been reported in rare instances.

When used inexcessive doses, systemic corticosteroid effects such as hypercorticism and adrenal suppression may appear. If such changes occur, triamcinolone acetonide nasal inhaler should be discontinued slowly, consistent with accepted procedures for discontinuing oral steroid therapy.

Oral and Nasal Inhalers and AQ Nasal Spray: When used at excessive doses, systemic corticosteroid effects such as hypercorticism and adrenal suppression may appear. If such changes occur, triamcinolone acetonide Nasal Inhaler / AQ Nasal Spray should be discontinued slowly, consistent with accepted procedures for discontinuing oral steroid therapy.

Aerosol Spray, Cream and Ointment: Systemic absorption of topical corticosteroids has produced reversible hypothalamic-pituitary-adrenal (HPA) axis suppression, manifestations of Cushing's syndrome, hyperglycemia, and glucosuria in some patients.

PRECAUTIONS: *(cont'd)*

Conditions which augment systemic absorption include the application of the more potent steroids, use over large surface areas, prolonged use, and the addition of occlusive dressings.

Therefore, patients receiving a large dose of any potent topical steroid applied to a large surface area or under an occlusive dressing should be evaluated periodically for evidence of HPA axis suppression by using the urinary free cortisol and ACTH stimulation tests, and for the impairment of thermal homeostasis. If HPA axis suppression or elevation of the body temperature occurs, an attempt should be made to withdraw the drug, to reduce the frequency of application, substitute a less potent steroid, or use a sequential approach when utilizing the occlusive technique.

Recovery of HPA axis function and thermal homostasis are generally prompt and complete upon discontinuation of the drug. Infrequently, signs and symptoms of steroid withdrawal may occur, requiring supplemental systemic corticosteroids. Occasionally, a patient may develop a sensitivity reaction to a particular occlusive dressing material or adhesive and a substitute material may be necessary.

Children may absorb proportionally larger amounts of topical corticosteroids and thus be more susceptible to systemic toxicity (see Pediatric Use).

If irritation develops, topical corticosteroids should be discontinued and appropriate therapy instituted.

In the presence of dermatological infections, the use of an appropriate antifungal or antibacterial agent should be instituted. If a favorable response does not occur promptly, the corticosteroid should be discontinued until the infection has been adequately controlled.

Oral Inhaler: During withdrawal from oral steroids, some patients may experience symptoms of systemically active steroid withdrawal, e.g., joint and/or muscular pain, lassitude and depression, despite maintenance or even improvement of respiratory function (see DOSAGE AND ADMINISTRATIONfor details). Although steroid withdrawal effects are usually transient and not severe, severe and even fatal exacerbation of asthma can occur if the previous daily oral corticosteroid requirement had significantly exceeded 10 mg/day of prednisone or equivalent.

In responsive patients, inhaled corticosteroids will often permit control of asthmatic symptoms with less suppression of HPA function than therapeutically equivalent oral doses of prednisone. Since triamcinolone acetonide is absorbed into the circulation and can be systemically active, the beneficial effects of triamcinolone acetonide Oral Inhaler in minimizing or preventing HPA dysfunction may be expected only when recommended dosages are not exceeded.

Suppression of HPA function has been reported in volunteers who received 400 mcg daily of triamcinolone acetonide. In addition, suppression of HPA function has been reported in some patients who have received recommended doses for as little as 6 to 12 weeks. Since the response of HPA function to inhaled corticosteroids is highly individualized, the physician should consider this information when treating patients.

Because of the possibility of systemic absorption of inhaled corticosteroids, patients treated with these drugs should be observed carefully for any evidence of systemic corticosteroid effects including suppression of growth in children. Particular care should be taken in observing patients postoperatively or during periods of stress for evidence of a decrease in adrenal function.

The long-term effects of triamcinolone acetonide inhaler in human subjects are not completely known, although patients have received triamcinolone acetonide Oral Inhaler on a continuous basis for periods of two years or longer. While there has been no clinical evidence of adverse experiences, the local effects of the agent on developmental or immunologic processes in the mouth, pharynx, trachea and lung are also unknown.

Triamcinolone Acetonide Oral Inhaler should be used with caution, if at all, in patients with active or quiescent tuberculous infections of the respiratory tract or in patients with untreated fungal, bacterial, or systemic viral infections or ocular herpes simplex. The potential effects of long-term administration of triamcinolone acetonide Oral Inhaler on lung or other tissues are unknown. However, pulmonary infiltrates with eosinophilia have occurred in patients receiving other inhaled corticosteroids.

INFORMATION FOR THE PATIENT

Patients being treated with triamcinolone acetonide Nasal Inhaler or AQ Nasal Spray should receive the following information and instructions.

Patients who are on immunosuppressant doses of corticosteroids should be warned to avoid exposure to chickenpox or measles and, if exposed, to obtain medical advice.

Patients should use triamcinolone acetonide Nasal Inhaler / AQ Nasal Spray at regular intervals since its effectiveness depends on its regular use. A decrease in symptoms may occur as soon as 12 hours after starting steroid therapy and generally can be expected to occur within a few days of initiating therapy in allergic rhinitis. The patient should take the medication as directed and should not exceed the prescribed dosage. The patient should contact the physician if symptoms do not improve after three weeks, or if the condition worsens. Nasal irritation and/or burning or stinging after use of the spray occur only rarely with this product. The patient should contact the physician if they occur.

Nasal Inhaler: For the proper use of this unit and to attain maximum improvement, the patient should read and follow the accompanying patient instructions carefully. Spraying triamcinolone acetonide directly onto the nasal septum should be avoided. Because the amount dispensed per puff may not be consistent, it is important to shake the canister well. Also, the canister should be discarded after 100 actuations.

AQ Nasal Spray: For the proper use of this unit and to attain maximum improvement, the patient should read and follow the accompanying patient instructions carefully. It is important to shake the bottle well before each use. **Also, the bottle should be discarded after 120 actuations since the amount of triamcinolone acetonide delivered thereafter per actuation may be substantially less than 55 mcg of drug.** Do not transfer any remaining suspension to another bottle.

Oral and Nasal Inhalers and AQ Nasal Spray: Patients who are on immunosuppressant doses of corticosteroids should be warned to avoid exposure to chickenpox or measles and, if exposed, to obtain medical advice.

Aerosol Spray, Cream and Ointment: Patients using topical corticosteroids should receive the following information and instructions:

This medication is to be used as directed by the physician. It is for external use only; avoid contact with the eyes and inhalation of the spray.

Patients should be advised not to use this medication for any disorder other than for which it was prescribed.

The treated skin area should not be bandaged or otherwise covered or wrapped as to be occlusive unless directed by the physician.

Patients should report any signs of local adverse reactions especially under occlusive dressing.

Parents of pediatric patients should be advised not to use tight- fitting diapers or plastic pants on a child being treated in the diaper area, as these garments may constitute occlusive dressings.

PRECAUTIONS: *(cont'd)*

LABORATORY TESTS

Aerosol Spray, Cream and Ointment: A urinary free cortisol test and ACTH stimulation test may be helpful in evaluating HPA axis suppression.

CARCINOGENESIS, MUTAGENESIS, AND IMPAIRMENT OF FERTILITY

Oral and Nasal Inhalers: No evidence of treatment-related carcinogenicity was demonstrated after two years of once daily oral administration of triamcinolone acetonide at a maximum daily dose of 1.0 mcg/kg/day (6.1 mcg/m²/day) in male or female rats and 3.0 mcg/kg/day (12.9 mcg/m²/day in male or female mice.

Male and female rats which were administered oral triamcinolone acetonide at doses as high as 15 mcg/kg/day (110 mcg/m²/day, as calculated on a surface area basis) exhibited no evidence of impaired fertility. The maximum human dose, for comparison, is 6.3 mcg/kg/day (240 mcg/m²/day). However, a few female rats which received maternally toxic doses of 8 or 15 mcg/kg/day (60 mcg/m²/day or 110 mcg/m²/day, respectively, as calculated on a surface area basis) exhibited dystocia and prolonged delivery. Developmental toxicity, which included increases in fetal resorptions and stillbirths and decreases in pup body weight and survival, also occurred at the maternally toxic doses (2.5 - 15.0 mcg/kg/day or 20 - 110 mcg/m²/day, as calculated on a surface area basis). Reproductive performance of female rats and effects on fetuses and offspring were comparable between groups that received placebo and non-toxic or marginally toxic doses (0.5 and 1.0 mcg/kg/day or 3.8 mcg/m²/day and 7.0 mcg/m²/day).

AQ Nasal Spray: No evidence of treatment-related carcinogenicity was demonstrated after two years of once daily gavage of triamcinolone acetonide at doses of 0.05, 0.2, and 1.0 mcg/kg (approximately 0.2. 0.7, and 4.0% of the recommended clinical dose on a mcg/m²basis) in the mouse. Mutagenesis studies with triamcinolone acetonide have not been carried out.

No evidence of impaired fertility was manifested when oral doses of up to 15.0 mcg/kg (55.0% of the recommended clinical dose on a mcg/m²basis) were administered to female and male rats. However, triamconolone acetonide at oral doses of 8.0 mcg/kg (approximately 30.0% of the recommended clinical dose on a mcg/m²basis) caused dystocia and prolonged delivery and at oral doses of 5.0 mcg/kg (approximately 20.0 % of the recommended clinical dose on a mcg/m² basis) and above caused increases in fetal resorptions and stillbirths and decreases in pup body weight and survival. At a lower dose of 1.0 mcg/kg (approximately 4.0% of the recommended clinical dose on a mcg/m² basis), it did not induce the aforementioned effects.

Aerosol Spray, Cream and Ointment: Long-term animal studies have not been performed to evaluate the carcinogenic potential or the effect on fertility of topical corticosteroids.

Studies to determine mutagenicity with prednisolone and hydrocortisone showed negative results.

PREGNANCY CATEGORY C

Oral and Nasal Inhalers: Like other corticoids, triamcinolone acetonide has been shown to be teratogenic in rats and rabbits. Teratogenic effects, which occurred in both species at 0.02, 0.04 and 0.08 mg/kg/day (approximately 135, 270 and 540 mcg/m²/day in the rat and 320, 640 and 1280 mcg/m²/day in the rabbit, as calculated on a surface area basis), included a low incidence of cleft palate and/or internal hydrocephaly and axial skeletal defects. Teratogenic effects, including CNS and cranial malformations, have also been observed in non-human primates at 0.5 mg/kg/day (approximately 6.7 mg/m²/day). The doses of 0.02, 0.04, 0.08, and 0.5 mg/kg/day used in these toxicology studies are approximately 12.8, 25.5, 51, and 318.7 times the minimum recommended dose of 110 mcg of triamcinolone acetonide per day and 3.2, 6.4, 12.7, and 80 times the maximum recommended dose of 440 mcg of triamcinolone acetonide per day based on a patient body weight of 70 kg. Administration of aerosol by inhalation to pregnant rats and rabbits produced embryotoxic and fetotoxic effects which were comparable to those produced by administration by other routes. There are no adequate and well-controlled studies in pregnant women. Triamcinolone acetonide should be used during pregnancy only if the potential benefit justifies the potential risk to the fetus.

Experience with oral corticoids since their introduction in pharmacologic as opposed to physiologic doses suggests that rodents are more prone to teratogenic effects from corticoids than humans. In addition, because there is a natural increase in glucocorticoid production during pregnancy, most women will require a lower exogenous steroid dose and many will not need corticoid treatment during pregnancy.

AQ Nasal Spray: Pregnancy Category C. Triamcinolone acetonide has been shown to be teratogenic at inhalational doses of 20, 40, and 80 mcg/kg in rats (approximately 0.75, 1.5, and 3.0 times the recommended clinical dose on a mcg/m² basis, respectively), in rabbits at the same doses (approximately 1.5, 3.0, and 6.0 the recommended clinical dose on a mcg/m² basis, respectively) and in monkeys, at an inhalational dose of 500 mcg/kg (approximately 37.0 times the recommended clinical dose on a mcg/m²basis.) Dose-related teratogenic effects in rats and rabbits included cleft palate and/or internal hydrocephaly and axial skeltal defects whereas the effects observed in the monkey were CNS and/or cranial malformations. There are no adequate and well-contolled studies in pregnant women. Triamcinolone acetonide should be used in pregnancy only if the potential benefit justifies the potential risk to the fetus.

Experience with oral corticoids since their introduction in pharmacologic as opposed to physiologic doses suggests that rodents are more prone to teratogenic effects from corticoids than humans. In addition, because there is a natural increase in glucocorticoid production during pregnancy, most women will require a lower exogenous steroid dose and many will not need corticoid treatment during pregnancy.

Oral and Nasal Inhalers and AQ Nasal Spray: *Nonteratogenic Effects:* Hypoadrenalism may occur in infants born of mothers receiving corticosteroids during pregnancy. Such infants should be carefully observed.

Aerosol Spray, Cream and Ointment: Category C. *Teratogenic Effects:* Corticosteroids are generally teratogenic in laboratory animals when administered systemically at relatively low dosage levels. The more potent corticosteroids have been shown to be teratogenic after dermal application in laboratory animals. There are no adequate and well- controlled studies in pregnant women on teratogenic effects from topically applied corticosteroids. Therefore, topical corticosteroids should be used during pregnancy only if the potential benefit justifies the potential risk to the fetus. Drugs of this class should not be used extensively on pregnant patients, in large amounts, or for long periods of time.

NURSING MOTHERS

Nasal Inhaler/AQ Nasal Spray: It is not known whether triamcinolone acetonide is excreted in human milk. Because other corticosteroids are excreted in human milk, caution should be exercised when triamcinolone acetonide Nasal Inhaler / AQ Nasal Spray is administered to nursing women.

Aerosol Spray, Cream and Ointment: It is not known whether topical administration of corticosteroids could result in sufficient systemic absorption to produce detectable quantities in breast milk. Systemically administered corticosteroids are secreted into breast milk in quantities **not** likely to have a deleterious effect on the infant. Nevertheless, caution should be exercised when topical corticosteroids are administered to a nursing woman.

PRECAUTIONS: *(cont'd)*

PEDIATRIC USE

Safety and effectiveness have not been established in children below the age of 6. Oral corticosteroids have been shown to cause growth suppression in children and teenagers, particularly with higher doses over extended periods. If a child or teenager on any corticosteroid appears to have growth suppression, the possibility that they are particularly sensitive to this effect of steroids should be considered.

Aerosol Spray, Cream and Ointment: Pediatric patients may demonstrate greater susceptibility to topical corticosteroid-induced HPA axis suppression and Cushing's syndrome than mature patients because of a larger skin surface area to body weight ratio.

HPA axis suppression, Cushing's syndrome, and intracranial hypertension have been reported in children receiving topical corticosteroids. Manifestation of adrenal suppression in children include linear growth retardation, delayed weight gain, low plasma cortisol levels, and absence of response to ACTH stimulation. Manifestations of intracranial hypertension include bulging fontanelles, headaches, and bilateral papilledema.

Administration of topical corticosteroids to children should be limited to the least amount compatible with an effective therapeutic regimen. Chronic corticosteroid therapy may interfere with the growth and development of children.

Oral Inhaler: Safety and effectiveness have not been established in children below the age of 6. Oral corticoids have been shown to cause growth suppression in children and teenagers, particularly with higher doses over extended periods. If a child or teenager on any corticoid appears to have growth suppression, the possibility that they are particularly sensitive to this effect of steroids should be considered.

> **Note:** The following statement below is required by the Federal government's Clean Air Act for all products containing or manufactured with chlorofluorocarbons (CFC's):
> **WARNING:** This product contains CFC-12, a substance which harms public health and environment by destroying ozone in the upper atmosphere.

ADVERSE REACTIONS:

Oral Inhaler: A few cases of oral candidiasis have been reported (see WARNINGS). In addition, some patients receiving triamcinolone acetonide Oral Inhaler have experienced hoarseness, dry throat, irritated throat and dry mouth. Increased wheezing and cough have been reported infrequently as has facial edema. These adverse effects have generally been mild and transient.

Nasal Inhaler: *Adults and Children 12 Years of Age and Older:* In controlled and uncontrolled studies, 1257 patients received treatment with intranasal triamcinolone acetonide. Adverse reactions are based on the 567 patients who received a product similar to the marketed triamcinolone acetonide canister.

These patients were treated for an average of 48 days (range 1 to 117 days). The 145 patients enrolled in uncontrolled studies received treatment from 1 to 820 days (average 332 days). The most prevalent adverse experience was headache, being reported by approximately 18% of the patients who received triamcinolone acetonide nasal inhaler irritation was reported by 2.8% of the patients receiving triamcinolone acetonide. Other nasopharyngeal side effects were reported by fewer than 5% of the patients who received triamcinolone acetonide and included: dry mucous membranes, naso-sinus congestion, throat discomfort, sneezing, and epistaxis. The complaints do not usually interfere with treatment and in the controlled and uncontrolled studies approximately 1% of patients have discontinued because of these nasal adverse effects.

In the event of accidental overdose, an increased potential for these adverse experiences may be expected, but systemic adverse experiences are unlikely (see OVERDOSAGE).

Children Ages 6 Through 11 Years of Age: Adverse event data in children 6 through 11 years of age are derived from two controlled clinical trials of two and four weeks duration. In these trials, 127 patients received fixed doses of 220 mcg/day of triamcinolone for an average of 22 days (range 8 to 33 days). Adverse events occurring at an incidence of 3% or greater and more common among children reated with 220 mcg triamcinolone acetonide daily than vehicle placebo were:

TABLE 1 Adverse Events (3% Or Greater) In Children Ages 6 Through 11

Adverse Events	220 mcg of Triamcinolone Acetonide Daily (n=127)	Vehicle Placebo (n=322)
Epistaxis	11.0%	9.3%
Cough	9.4%	9.3%
Fever	7.9%	5.6%
Nausea	6.3%	3.1%
Throat Discomfort	5.5%	5.3%
Otitis	4.7%	3.7%
Dyspepsia	4.7%	2.2%

Adverse events occurring at a rate of 3% or greater that were more common in the placebo group were: upper respiratory tract infection, headache, and concurrent infection.

Only 1.6% of patients discontinued due to adverse experiences. No patient discontinued due to a serious adverse event related to triamcinolone acetonide nasal inhaler therapy.

Though not observed in controlled clinical trials of triamcinolone acetonide nasal inhaler in children, cases of nasal septum perforation among pediatric users have been reported in post marketing surveillance of this product.

AQ Nasal Spray: In placebo-controlled, double-blind and open-label clinical studies, 1483 patients received treatment with triamcinolone acetonide aqeous nasal spray. These patients were treated for an average duration of 50.7 days. In the controlled trials (2-5 weeks duration) from which the following adverse reaction data is derived, 1394 patients were treated with the Triamcinolone Acetonide AQ Nasal Spray for an average of 18.7 days. In the long-term, open-label study, the 172 patients received treatment for an average duration of 286 days.

TABLE 2 Adverse Events Occurring at an Incidence of 2% or Greater and More Common Among Patients Treated with 220 mcg Triamcinolone Acetonide Daily Than Placebo

Adverse Events	Triamcinolone Acetonide 220 mcg (N=857) %	Placebo (N=962)%
Increase in cough	2.1	1.5
Epistaxis	2.7	0.8
Pharyngitis	5.1	3.6

Also, these adverse events occurring at an incidence of 2% or greater and more common among patients treated with placebo than 220 mcg triamcinolone acetonide daily were: Headache and Rhinitis.

ADVERSE REACTIONS: *(cont'd)*

Nasal septum perforation was reported in one patient although relationship to Triamcinolone Acetonide AQ Nasal Spray has not been established.

In the event of accidental overdosage, an increased potential for these adverse experiences may be expected, but systemic adverse experiences are unlikely. (See OVERDOSAGE.)

Aerosol Spray, Cream and Ointment: The following local adverse reactions are reported infrequently with topical corticosteroids, but may occur more frequently with the use of occlusive dressing (reactions are listed in an approximate decreasing order of occurrence): burning, itching, irritation, dryness, folliculitis, hypertrichosis, acneiform eruptions, hypopigmentation, perioral dermatitis, allergic contact dermatitis, maceration of the skin, secondary infection, skin atrophy, striae, and miliaria.

OVERDOSAGE:

Nasal Inhaler: Acute overdosage with this dosage form is unlikely. The acute topical application of the entire 15 mg of the canister would most likely cause nasal irritation and headache. It would be unlikely to see acute systemic adverse effects if the nasal application of the 15 mg of triamcinolone acetonide was administered all at once.

AQ Nasal Spray: Like any other nasally administered corticosteroid acute overdosing is unlikely in view of the total amount of active ingredient present. In the event that the entire contents of the bottle were administered all at once, via either oral or nasal application, clinically significant systemic adverse events would most likely not result. The patient may experience some gastrointestinal upset.

Aerosol Spray, Cream and Ointment: Topically applied corticosteroids can be absorbed in sufficient amounts to produce systemic effects (see General).

DOSAGE AND ADMINISTRATION:

ORAL INHALER: All patients should be instructed that the triamcinolone acetonide Oral Inhaler must be used on a regular daily basis rather than *prn*. Reliable dosage delivery cannot be assured after 240 actuations and patients should be cautioned against longer use of individual canisters.

Good oral hygiene including rinsing of the mouth after inhalation is recommended.

Adults: The usual dosage is two inhalations (approximately 200 mcg) given three to four times a day. The maximum daily intake should not exceed 16 inhalations (1600 mcg) in adults. Higher initial doses (12 to 16 inhalations per day) may be advisable in patients with more severe asthma, the dosage then being adjusted downward according to the response of the patient. In some patients maintenance can be accomplished when the total daily dose is given on a twice a day schedule.

Children 6 to 12 years of age: The usual dosage is two inhalations (100 to 200 mcg) given three or four times a day according to the response of the patient. The maximal daily intake should not exceed 12 inhalations (1200 mcg) in children 6 to 12 years of age. Insufficient clinical data exist with respect to the administration of triamcinolone acetonide Oral Inhaler in children below the age of 6. The long-term effects of inhaled steroids on growth are still under evaluation.

Patients receiving bronchodilators by inhalation should be advised to use the bronchodilator before triamcinolone acetonide Oral Inhaler in order to enhance penetration of triamcinolone acetonide into the bronchial tree. After use of an aerosol bronchodilator, several minutes should elapse before use of the triamcinolone acetonide Oral Inhaler to reduce the potential toxicity from the inhaled fluorocarbon propellants in the two aerosols.

Different considerations must be given to the following groups of patients in order to obtain the full therapeutic benefit of triamcinolone acetonide Oral Inhaler:

Patients Not Receiving Systemic Steroids: The use of triamcinolone acetonide Oral Inhaler is straightforward in patients who are inadequately controlled with non-steroid medications but in whom systemic steroid therapy has been withheld because of concern over potential adverse reactions. In patients who respond to triamcinolone acetonide, an improvement in pulmonary function is usually apparent within one to two weeks after the start of triamcinolone acetonide Oral Inhaler.

Patients Receiving Systemic Steroids: In those patients dependent on systemic steroids, transfer to triamcinolone acetonide Oral Inhaler and subsequent management may be more difficult because recovery from impaired adrenal function is usually slow. Such suppression has been known to last up to 12 months or longer. Clinical studies, however, have demonstrated that triamcinolone acetonide Oral Inhaler may be effective in the management of these asthmatic patients and may permit replacement or significant reduction in the dosage of systemic corticosteroids.

The patient's asthma should be reasonably stable before treatment with triamcinolone acetonide Oral Inhaler is started. Initially, the inhaler should be used concurrently with the patient's usual maintenance dose of systemic steroid. After approximately one week, gradual withdrawal of the systemic steroid is started by reducing the dose. The next reduction is made after an interval of one or two weeks, depending on the response of the patient. Generally, these decrements should not exceed 2.5 mg of prednisone or its equivalent. A slow rate of withdrawal cannot be overemphasized. During withdrawal, some patients may experience symptoms of systemically active steroid withdrawal, e.g., joint and/or muscular pain, lassitude and depression, despite maintenance or even improvement of respiratory function. Such patients should be encouraged to continue with the inhaler but should be watched carefully for objective signs of adrenal insufficiency, such as hypotension and weight loss. If evidence of adrenal insufficiency occurs, the systemic steroid dose should be boosted temporarily and thereafter further withdrawal should continue more slowly. No clinical studies have been conducted evaluating triamcinolone acetonide with alternate day prednisone regimens. However, based on the results of such a study with another inhaled corticosteroid, inhaled corticosteroids generally are not recommended for chronic use with alternate day prednisone regimens (see WARNINGS).

During periods of stress or a severe asthma attack, transfer patients will require supplementary treatment with systemic steroids. Exacerbations of asthma which occur during the course of treatment with triamcinolone acetonide Oral Inhaler should be treated with a short course of systemic steroid which is gradually tapered as these symptoms subside. There is no evidence that control of asthma can be achieved by administration of triamcinolone acetonide Oral Inhaler in amounts greater than the recommended doses.

Contents under pressure. Do not puncture. Do not use or store near heat or an open flame. Exposure to temperatures above 120°F may cause bursting. Never throw container into fire or incinerator. Keep out of reach of children.

Store at room temperature.

Nasal Inhaler and AQ Nasal Spray: A decrease in symptoms may occur as soon as 12 hours after starting steroid therapy and generally can be expected to occur within a few days of initiating therapy in allergic rhinitis.

If improvement is not evident after 2-3 weeks, the patient should be re-evaluated or discontinue treatment. (See CLINICAL PHARMACOLOGY, Individualization Of Dosage).

Adults and Children 12 years of age and older: The recommended starting dose of triamcinolone acetonide Nasal Inhaler is 220 mcg per day given as two sprays (approximately 55 mcg/spray) in each nostril once a day. If needed, the dose may be increased to 440 mcg per day (approximately 55 mcg/spray) either as once a day dosage or divided up to four times a day (*i.e.,* twice a day [two sprays/nostril] or four times a day [one spray/nostril]). After the desired effect is obtained, some patients may be maintained on a dose of as little as one spray (approximately 55 mcg) in each nostril once a day (total daily dose 110 mcg per day).

Children 6 Through 11 Years of Age: The recommended starting dose of triamcinolone acetonide nasal ihaler is 220 mcg per day given as two sprays (55 mcg/spray) in each nostril once a day. Once the maximal effect has been achieved, it always desirable to titrate the patient to the minimum effective dose.

Triamcinolone Acetonide Nasal Inhaler is not recommended for children below 6 years of age since adequate numbers of patients have not been studied in this age group.

Directions for Use: Illustrated Patient's Instructions for use accompany each package of **Triamcinolone Acetonide** Nasal Inhaler.

CONTENTS UNDER PRESSURE. DO NOT PUNCTURE. AVOID SPRAYING IN EYES. DO NOT USE OR STORE NEAR HEAT OR OPEN FLAME. EXPOSURE TO TEMPERATURES ABOVE 120œ F MAY CAUSE BURSTING. NEVER THROW CONTAINER INTO FIRE OR INCINERATOR. KEEP OUT OF REACH OF CHILDREN.

NOTE: THE FOLLOWING STATEMENT IS REQUIRED BY THE FEDERAL GOVERNMENT'S CLEAN AIR ACT FOR ALL PRODUCTS CONTAINING OR MANUFACTURED WITH CHLOROFLUOROCARBONS (CFC'S):

WARNING: Contains CFC-12, a substance which harms public health and enviroment by destroying ozone in the upper atmosphere. A notice similar to the above WARNING has been placed in the Information for the Patient portion of this monograph pursuant to EPA regulations.

DENTAL PASTE

Press a small dab (about 1/4 inch) to the lesion until a thin film develops. A larger quantity may be required for coverage of some lesions. For optimal results use only enough to coat the lesion with a thin film. Do not rub in. Attempting to spread this preparation may result in a granular, gritty sensation, however, a smooth slippery film develops.

The preparation should be applied at bedtime to permit steroid contact with the lesion throughout the night. Depending on the severity of symptoms, it may be necessary to apply the preparation two or three times a day, preferably after meals. If significant repair or regeneration has not occurred in seven days, further investigation is advisable.

INJECTION-10

Dosage: The initial dose for intra-articular or intrabursal administration and for injection into tendon sheaths may vary from 2.5 to 5 mg for smaller joints and from 5 to 15 mg for larger joints depending on the specific disease entity being treated. Single injections into several joints for multiple locus involvement, up to 20 mg or more, have been given without incident. For intradermal administration, the initial dose of triamcinolone acetonide will vary depending upon the specific disease entity being treated but should be limited to 1.0 mg (0.1 ml) per injection site, since larger volumes are more likely to produce cutaneous atrophy. Multiple sites (separated by one centimeter or more) may be injected, keeping in mind that the greater the *total volume* employed the more corticosteroids become available for possible systemic absorption and subsequent corticosteroid effects. Such injections may be repeated, if necessary, at weekly or less frequent intervals.

The lower dosages in the initial dosage range of triamcinolone acetonide may produce the desired effect when the corticosteroid is administered to provide a localized concentration. The site of the injection and the volume of the injection should be carefully considered when triamcinolone acetonide is administered for this purpose. The initial dosage should be maintained for this purpose. The initial dosage should be maintained or adjusted until a satisfactory response is noted. If after a reasonable period of time there is a lack of satisfactory clinical response, this drug should be discontinued and the patient transferred to other appropriate therapy. IT SHOULD BE EMPHASIZED THAT DOSAGE REQUIREMENTS ARE VARIABLE AND MUST BE INDIVIDUALIZED ON THE BASIS OF THE DISEASE UNDER TREATMENT AND THE RESPONSE OF THE PATIENT. After a favorable response is noted, the proper maintenance dosage should be determined by decreasing the initial drug dosage in small increments at appropriate time intervals until the lowest dosage which will maintain an adequate clinical response is reached. It should be kept in mind that constant monitoring is needed in regard to drug dosage. Included in the situations which may make dosage adjustments necessary are changes in clinical status secondary to remissions or exacerbations in the disease process, the patient's individual drug responsiveness, and the effect of the patient's individual drug responsiveness,a nd the effect of the patient exposure to stressful situations not directly related to the disease entity under treatment; in this latter situation it may be necessary to increase the dosage of this drug for a period of time consistent with the patients's condition. If the drug is to be stopped after long-term therapy, it is recommended that it be withdrawn gradually rather than abruptly.

ADMINISTRATION

Shake the vial before use to insure a uniform suspension. Prior to withdraw, inspect suspension for clumping or granular appearance (agglomeration). An agglomerated product results from exposure to freezing temperatures and should not be used. After withdraw, inject without delay to prevent settling in the syringe. Careful technique should be employed to avoid the possibility of entering a blood vessel or introducing infection.

Routine laboratory studies, such as urinalysis, two-hour postprandial blood sugar, determination of blood pressure and body weight, and a chest x-ray should be made at regular intervals during prolonged therapy. Upper GI x-rays are desirable with an ulcer history or significant dyspepsia.

For treatment of joints, the usual intra-articular Injection technique as described in standard textbooks, should be followed. If excessive amount of synovial fluid is present in the joint, some but not all, should be aspirated to aid in the relief of pain and to prevent undue dilation of the steroid.

With intra-articular or intrabursal administration, and with injection of this drug into tendon sheaths, the use of a local anesthetic is used, its package insert should be read with care and all the precautions connected with its use should be observed. It should be injected into the surrounding soft tissues prior to the injection of the injection of the corticosteroid. A small amount of the anesthetic solution may be instilled into the joint.

In treating acute nonspecific tenosynovitis, care should be taken to insure that the injection of this drug is made into the tendon sheath rather than the tendon substance. Epicondylitis (tennis elbow) may be treated by infiltrating the preparation into the area of greatest tenderness.

For treatment of dermal lesions, inject this drug directly into the lesion, i.e, intradermally or sometimes subcutaneously. For accuracy of dosage measurement and ease of administration, it is preferable to employ a tuberculin syringe and a small-bore needle (23 to 25 gauge). Ethyl chloride spray may be used to alleviate the discomfort of the injection.

Injection-40: The initial dose may vary from 2.5 to 60 mg per day. Depending on the specific disease entity being treated. In situations of less severity, lower doses will generally suffice while in selected patients higher initial doses may be required. Usually the parenteral dosage

DOSAGE AND ADMINISTRATION: *(cont'd)*

ranges are about 1/3 to 1/2 of the oral dose given every 12 hours. However in certain overwhelming, acute, life-threatening situations, administrations of dosages exceeding the usual dosages may be justified and may be in multiples of the usual dosages.

The initial dosage should be maintained or adjusted until a satisfactory response is noted. If after a reasonable period of time there is a lack of satisfactory clinical response, this drug should be discontinued and the patient transferred to other appropriate therapy.

IT SHOULD BE EMPHASIZED THAT DOSAGE REQUIREMENTS ARE VARIABLE AND MUST BE INDIVIDUALIZED ON THE BASIS OF THE DISEASE UNDER TREATMENT AND THE RESPONSE OF THE PATIENT. After a favorable response is noted, the proper maintenance dosage should be determined by decreasing the initial drug dosage in small increments at appropriate time intervals until the lowest dosage which will maintain an adequate clinical response is reached. It should be kept in mind that constant monitoring is needed in regard to drug dosage. Included in the situations which may make dosage adjustments necessary are changes in clinical status secondary to remissions or exacerbations in the disease process, the patient's individual drug responsiveness, and the effect of the patient's individual drug responsiveness,a nd the effect of the patient exposure to stressful situations not directly related to the disease entity under treatment; in this latter situation it may be necessary to increase the dosage of this drug for a period of time consistent with the patients's condition. If the drug is to be stopped after long-term therapy, it is recommended that it be withdrawn gradually rather than abruptly.

DOSAGE

Systemic: Although this drug may be administered for most initial therapy, most physicians's prefer to adjust the dose orally until adequate control is attained. IM administration provides a sustained or depot action which can be used to supplement or reduce initial oral therapy. With IM therapy, greater supervision of the amount of steroid used is made possible in the patient who is inconsistent in following an oral dosage schedule. In maintenance therapy, the patient-to-patient response is not uniform and, therefore, the dose must be individualized for optimal control.

For Adults And Children Over 12 Years Of Age: The suggested initial dose is 60 mg, **injected deeply into the gluteal muscle.** Subcutaneous fat atrophy may occur if care is not taken to inject the preparation intramuscularly. Dosage is usually adjusted within the range of 40 to 80 mg depending upon the patient response and duration of relief. However, some patients may be well controlled on dosages as low as 20 mg or less patients with hay fever or pollen asthma who are not responding to pollen administration and other conventional therapy may obtain a remission of symptoms lasting throughout the pollen season after one injection of 40 to 100 mg.

For Children From 6 To 12 Tears Of Age: The suggested initial dose is 40 mg, although dosage depends more upon the severity of symptoms than on age or weight. There is insufficient clinical experience with this drug to recommend its use in children under six years of age.

LOCAL

For intra-articular or intra-bursal administration and for injection into tendon sheaths, the initial dose of this drug may vary from 2.5 to 5 mg for smaller joints and from 5 to 15 mg for larger joints depending on the specific disease entity being treated, (A more dilute form of sterile triamcinolone acetonide Suspension USP is available). For adults, doses of up to 10 mg for smaller areas and up to 40 mg for larger areas have usually been sufficient to alleviate symptoms. Single injections into several joints for multiple locus involvement, up to a total of 80 mg, have been given without undue reactions. A single local infection of triamcinolone acetonide is frequently sufficient, but several injections may be needed for adequate relief of symptoms. The lower dosages in the initial dosage range of triamcinolone acetonide may produce the desired effect when the corticosteroid is administered to provide a localized concentration. The site of injection and the volume of the injection should be carefully considered when triamcinolone acetonide is administered for this purpose.

ADMINISTRATION

General: Shake the vial before use to insure a uniform suspension. Prior to withdraw, inspect suspension for clumping or granular appearance (agglomeration). An agglomerated product results from exposure to freezing temperatures and should not be used. After withdraw, inject without delay to prevent settling in the syringe. Careful technique should be employed to avoid the possibility of entering a blood vessel or introducing infection.

Routine laboratory studies, such as urinalysis, two-hour postprandial blood sugar, determination of blood pressure and body weight, and a chest x-ray should be made at regular intervals during prolonged therapy. Upper GI x-rays are desirable with an ulcer history or significant dyspepsia.

Systemic: For systemic therapy, injection should be made **deeply into the gluteal muscles** to insure IM delivery. For adults, a minimum needle length of 1 1/2 inches is recommended. In obese patients, a longer needle may be required. Use alternate sites for subsequent injections.

Local: For treatment of joints, the usual intra-articular Injection technique as described in standard textbooks, should be followed. If excessive amount of synovial fluid is present in the joint, some but not all, should be aspirated to aid in the relief of pain and to prevent undue dilation of the corticosteroid.

With intra-articular or intrabursal administration, and with injection of this drug into tendon sheaths, the use of a local anesthetic is used, its package insert should be read with care and all the precautions connected with its use should be observed. It should be injected into the surrounding soft tissues prior to the injection of the injection of the corticosteroid. A small amount of the anesthetic solution may be instilled into the joint.

In treating acute nonspecific tenosynovitis, care should be taken to insure that the injection of this drug is made into the tendon sheath rather than the tendon substance. Epicondylitis (tennis elbow) may be treated by infiltrating the preparation into the area of greatest tenderness.

AEROSOL SPRAY

Directions for use of the spray can are provided on the label. The preparation may be applied to any surface area of the body, but when it is sprayed about the face, care should be taken to see that the eyes are covered, and that inhalation of the spray is avoided.

Three or four applications daily of triamcinolone acetonide aerosol spray are generally adequate.

Occlusive Dressing Technique

Occlusive dressings may be used for the management of psoriasis or other recalcitrant conditions. Spray a small amount of the preparation onto the lesion, cover a small amount of the preparation onto the lesion, cover with pliable nonporous film, and seal the edges. If needed, additional moisture may be provided by covering the lesion with a dampened clean cotton cloth before the nonporous film is applied or by briefly wetting the affected the area with water immediately prior to applying the medication. The frequency of changing dressings is best determined on an individual basis. It may be convenient to apply the spray under an occlusive dressing in the evening and to remove the dressing in the morning (*i.e.*, 12-hour occlusion). When utilizing the 12-hour occlusion regimen, additional spray should be applied, without occlusion, during the day. Reapplication is essential at each dressing change.

If an infection develops, the use of occlusive dressings should be discontinued and appropriate antimicrobial therapy instituted.

DOSAGE AND ADMINISTRATION: *(cont'd)*

Cream: (All Strengths) Apply triamcinolone acetonide cream, 0.025% to the affected area two to four times daily. Rub in gently.

Apply the 0.1% or the 0.5% strength as appropriate, to the affected area two or three times daily. Rub gently.

Occlusive Dressing Technique

Occlusive dressings may be used for the management of psoriasis or other recalcitrant conditions. Spray a small amount of the preparation onto the lesion, cover a small amount of the preparation onto the lesion, cover with pliable nonporous film, and seal the edges. If needed, additional moisture may be provided by covering the lesion with a dampened clean cotton cloth before the nonporous film is applied or by briefly wetting the affected the area with water immediately prior to applying the medication. The frequency of changing dressings is best determined on an individual basis. It may be convenient to apply the spray under an occlusive dressing in the evening and to remove the dressing in the morning (*i.e.*, 12-hour occlusion). When utilizing the 12-hour occlusion regimen, additional spray should be applied, without occlusion, during the day. Reapplication is essential at each dressing change.

If an infection develops, the use of occlusive dressings should be discontinued and appropriate antimicrobial therapy instituted.

Cream: (All Strengths) Apply triamcinolone acetonide cream, 0.025% to the affected area two to four times daily. Rub in gently.

Apply the 0.1% or the 0.5% strength as appropriate, to the affected area two or three times daily. Rub gently.

OCCLUSIVE DRESSING TECHNIQUE

Occlusive dressings may be used for the management of psoriasis or other recalcitrant conditions. Spray a small amount of the preparation onto the lesion, cover a small amount of the preparation onto the lesion, cover with pliable nonporous film, and seal the edges. If needed, additional moisture may be provided by covering the lesion with a dampened clean cotton cloth before the nonporous film is applied or by briefly wetting the affected the area with water immediately prior to applying the medication. The frequency of changing dressings is best determined on an individual basis. It may be convenient to apply the spray under an occlusive dressing in the evening and to remove the dressing in the morning (*i.e.*, 12-hour occlusion). When utilizing the 12-hour occlusion regimen, additional spray should be applied, without occlusion, during the day. Reapplication is essential at each dressing change.

If an infection develops, the use of occlusive dressings should be discontinued and appropriate antimicrobial therapy instituted.

Ointment: (All Strengths) Apply a thin film of triamcinolone acetonide 0.225% to the affected area two or four times daily.

Apply a thin film of the 0.1% or the 0.5% triamcinolone acetonide ointment as appropriate, to the affected areas tow or three times daily.

OCCLUSIVE DRESSING TECHNIQUE

Occlusive dressings may be used for the management of psoriasis or other recalcitrant conditions. Spray a small amount of the preparation onto the lesion, cover a small amount of the preparation onto the lesion, cover with pliable nonporous film, and seal the edges. If needed, additional moisture may be provided by covering the lesion with a dampened clean cotton cloth before the nonporous film is applied or by briefly wetting the affected the area with water immediately prior to applying the medication. The frequency of changing dressings is best determined on an individual basis. It may be convenient to apply the spray under an occlusive dressing in the evening and to remove the dressing in the morning (*i.e.*, 12-hour occlusion). When utilizing the 12-hour occlusion regimen, additional spray should be applied, without occlusion, during the day. Reapplication is essential at each dressing change.

If an infection develops, the use of occlusive dressings should be discontinued and appropriate antimicrobial therapy instituted.

Storage: Store at controlled room temperature, 15-30°C (59-86°F). Protect from light; freezing, and heat.

PATIENT INFORMATION:

Triamcinolone acetonide is a corticosteroid product used primarily for its ability to decrease inflammation and relieve irritation. It is available as a nasal inhaler or an oral inhaler to decrease inflammation in the lungs of those with asthma or allergies. Proper technique for using an oral inhaler or a nasal inhaler is important to getting maximum effectiveness from the drug. Your pharmacist or physician can evaluate your technique. Inhalers should be shaken prior to use. The plastic inhaler should be washed regularly and allowed to dry. You should rinse your mouth with water after taking puffs from your oral inhaler. A cream, lotion and ointment are used to relieve itching and inflammation on the skin. The skin should not be tightly bandaged where the medication is applied. This includes diapers on babies being treated for rash. This medication should not be stopped abruptly but should be slowly discontinued. If you notice any signs of infection, or lack of cuts healing please contact your physician immediately. This medication works slowly and should not be used to treat conditions requiring quick relief of symptoms. For example, the inhalers should not be used to treat immediate breathing difficulties. This medication should be taken exactly as prescribed by your physician.

HOW SUPPLIED:

AQ NASAL SPRAY

Nasacort (Triamcinolone Acetonide AQ Nasal Spray is a nonchlorofluorocarbon (CFC) containing metered-dose pump spray which will provide 120 actuations. Net weight of the bottle contents is 16.5 grams.

It is supplied in a high-density polyethylene container with a metered-dose pump unit, nasal adapter, and patient instructions

Storage: Store at controlled room temperature, 15-30°C (59-86°F).

HOW SUPPLIED - RATED THERAPEUTICALLY EQUIVALENT:

Cream - Topical - 0.025 %

2.3 kg	$20.61	Triamcinolone, HL Moore Drug Exch	00839-6127-48
2.3 kg	$25.29	Triamcinolone Acetonide, Thames Pharma	49158-0139-22
2.3 kg	$32.39	Triamcinolone Acetonide, Clay Park Labs	45802-0063-29
15 gm	$1.04	Triamcinolone Acetonide, Clay Park Labs	45802-0063-35
15 gm	$1.12	Triamcinolone Acetonide, United Res	00677-0743-40
15 gm	$1.12	Triamcinolone Acetonide, GW Labs	00713-0226-15
15 gm	$1.12	Triamcinolone Acetonide, H.C.F.A. F F P	99999-2371-18
15 gm	$1.20	Triamcinolone Acetonide, Thames Pharma	49158-0139-20
15 gm	$1.28	Triamcinolone, HL Moore Drug Exch	00839-6127-47
15 gm	$1.30	Triamcinolone Acetonide, Goldline Labs	00182-1216-51
15 gm	$1.30	Triamcinolone Acetonide, Harber Pharm	51432-0776-10
15 gm	$1.38	Triamcinolone Acetonide, NMC Labs	23317-0300-15
15 gm	$1.41	Triamcinolone Acetonide, Qualitest Pharms	00603-7850-74
15 gm	$1.45	Triamcinolone Acetonide, Major Pharms	00904-2738-36
15 gm	$1.65	Triamcinolone Acetonide, Rugby	00536-5245-20
15 gm	$1.65	ARICIN, IDE-Interstate	00814-0850-93
15 gm	$1.70	Triamcinolone Acetonide, Fougera	00168-0003-15

HOW SUPPLIED - RATED THERAPEUTICALLY EQUIVALENT:
(cont'd)

15 gm	$1.74	Triamcinolone Acetonide, Schein Pharm (US)	00364-7211-72
15 gm	$1.90	Triamcinolone Acetonide, Consolidated Midland	00223-4449-15
15 gm	$2.14	Triamcinolone Acetonide, Geneva Pharms	00781-7030-27
15 gm	**$7.39**	**KENALOG, Bristol Myers Squibb**	**00003-0172-22**
30 gm	$2.25	Triamcinolone Acetonide, H.C.F.A. F F P	99999-2371-19
30 gm	$5.25	FLUTEX, Syosset Labs	47854-0575-05
60 gm	$3.00	FLUTEX, Syosset Labs	47854-0575-07
60 gm	$4.50	Triamcinolone Acetonide, H.C.F.A. F F P	99999-2371-20
60 gm	$13.13	ARISTOCORT, Fujisawa Pharm (US)	57317-0082-60
80 gm	$2.62	Triamcinolone Acetonide, H.C.F.A. F F P	99999-2371-21
80 gm	$2.80	Triamcinolone Acetonide, Thames Pharma	49158-0139-21
80 gm	$2.81	Triamcinolone Acetonide, Clay Park Labs	45802-0063-36
80 gm	$3.27	Triamcinolone Acetonide, Qualitest Pharms	00603-7850-90
80 gm	$3.31	Triamcinolone Acetonide, HL Moore Drug Exch	00839-6127-46
80 gm	$3.45	Triamcinolone Acetonide, Rugby	00536-5245-30
80 gm	$3.50	Triamcinolone Acetonide, Goldline Labs	00182-1216-53
80 gm	$3.50	Triamcinolone Acetonide, Major Pharms	00904-2738-11
80 gm	$3.50	Triamcinolone Acetonide, NMC Labs	23317-0300-80
80 gm	$3.57	Triamcinolone Acetonide, Harber Pharm	51432-0776-13
80 gm	$3.60	ARICIN, IDE-Interstate	00814-0850-97
80 gm	$4.00	Triamcinolone Acetonide, Fougera	00168-0003-80
80 gm	$4.25	Triamcinolone Acetonide, Geneva Pharms	00781-7030-29
80 gm	$4.32	Triamcinolone Acetonide, Schein Pharm (US)	00364-7211-60
80 gm	$6.00	Triamcinolone Acetonide, United Res	00677-0743-46
80 gm	$6.00	Triamcinolone Acetonide, GW Labs	00713-0226-80
80 gm	**$21.97**	**KENALOG, Bristol Myers Squibb**	**00003-0172-68**
454 gm	$7.67	Triamcinolone Acetonide, Clay Park Labs	45802-0063-05
454 gm	$8.60	Triamcinolone Acetonide, Thames Pharma	49158-0139-16
454 gm	$8.95	Triamcinolone Acetonide, Harber Pharm	51432-0776-20
454 gm	$9.00	Triamcinolone Acetonide, Major Pharms	00904-2738-27
454 gm	$9.18	Triamcinolone Acetonide, NMC Labs	23317-0300-16
454 gm	$9.35	Triamcinolone Acetonide, Goldline Labs	00182-1216-45
454 gm	$9.44	Triamcinolone Acetonide, H.C.F.A. F F P	99999-2371-22
454 gm	$18.75	Triamcinolone Acetonide, Rugby	00536-5245-98
454 gm	$34.05	Triamcinolone Acetonide, United Res	00677-0743-44
480 gm	$9.35	Triamcinolone Acetonide, Geneva Pharms	00781-7030-16
2270 gm	$170.25	Triamcinolone Acetonide, H.C.F.A. F F P	99999-2371-16
2383.5 gm	$178.76	Triamcinolone Acetonide, H.C.F.A. F F P	99999-2371-17

Cream - Topical - 0.1 %

1 oz	$5.95	FLUTEX CREAM 0.1 %, Syosset Labs	47854-0576-05
2.268 kg	$92.24	Triamcinolone Acetonide, Rugby	00536-5225-27
2.3 kg	$60.18	Triamcinolone Acetonide, HL Moore Drug Exch	00839-6126-48
2.3 kg	$63.20	Triamcinolone Acetonide, Thames Pharma	49158-0140-22
2.3 kg	$75.59	Triamcinolone Acetonide, Clay Park Labs	45802-0064-29
2.3 kg	$77.49	Triamcinolone Acetonide 1, NMC Labs	23317-0301-05
2.3 kg	$79.38	Triamcinolone Acetate, Goldline Labs	00182-1217-46
2.3 kg	$167.98	Triamcinolone Acetonide, United Res	00677-0747-47
2.38 kg	**$139.63**	**KENALOG, Bristol Myers Squibb**	**00003-0506-89**
5 pound	$66.42	Triamcinolone Acetonide, Major Pharms	00904-2741-33
15 gm	$0.90	Triamcinolone Acetonide, Syosset Labs	47854-0576-16
15 gm	$1.11	Triamcinolone Acetonide, United Res	00677-0747-40
15 gm	$1.11	Triamcinolone Acetonide, GW Labs	00713-0225-15
15 gm	$1.11	Triamcinolone Acetonide, H.C.F.A. F F P	99999-2371-03
15 gm	$1.11	Triamcinolone Acetonide, H.C.F.A. F F P	99999-2371-04
15 gm	$1.30	Triamcinolone Acetonide, Clay Park Labs	45802-0064-35
15 gm	$1.30	Triamcinolone Acetonide, Thames Pharma	49158-0140-20
15 gm	$1.52	Triamcinolone Acetonide 1, NMC Labs	23317-0301-15
15 gm	$1.70	Triamcinolone Acetate, Goldline Labs	00182-1217-51
15 gm	$1.74	Triamcinolone Acetonide, HL Moore Drug Exch	00839-6126-47
15 gm	$1.96	Triamcinolone Acetonide, Fougera	00168-0004-15
15 gm	$2.01	TRIACET, Teva	00093-0937-15
15 gm	$2.01	Triamcinolone Acetonide, Qualitest Pharms	00603-7851-74
15 gm	$2.03	Triamcinolone Acetonide, Rugby	00536-5225-20
15 gm	$2.04	Triamcinolone Acetonide, Schein Pharm (US)	00364-7212-72
15 gm	$2.05	Triamcinolone, Geneva Pharms	00781-7036-27
15 gm	$2.05	Triamcinolone Acetonide, Major Pharms	00904-2741-36
15 gm	$2.25	Triamcinolone Acetonide, Consolidated Midland	00223-4448-15
15 gm	$8.84	ARISTOCORT R, Fujisawa USA	00469-5108-15
15 gm	$10.74	ARISTOCORT A, Fujisawa Pharm (US)	57317-0052-15
15 gm	**$10.97**	**KENALOG, Bristol Myers Squibb**	**00003-0506-20**
20 gm	$1.48	Triamcinolone Acetonide, H.C.F.A. F F P	99999-2371-05
20 gm	$4.75	KENONEL, Marnel Pharceut	00682-4300-20
	$21.95	Triamcinolone, Geneva Pharms	00781-7036-16
30 gm	$1.80	Triamcinolone Acetonide, Thames Pharma	49158-0140-08
30 gm	$2.22	Triamcinolone Acetonide, H.C.F.A. F F P	99999-2371-06
30 gm	$2.33	ARICIN, IDE-Interstate	00814-0851-72
30 gm	$2.50	Triamcinolone Acetonide, Schein Pharm (US)	00364-7212-56
30 gm	$5.25	TRIDERM, Del Ray Lab	00316-0170-01
60 gm	$4.44	Triamcinolone Acetonide, H.C.F.A. F F P	99999-2371-07
60 gm	$21.54	ARISTOCORT R, Fujisawa USA	00469-5108-60
60 gm	**$26.75**	**KENALOG, Bristol Myers Squibb**	**00003-0506-46**
60 gm	$27.48	ARISTOCORT A, Fujisawa Pharm (US)	57317-0052-60
80 gm	$3.28	Triamcinolone Acetonide, H.C.F.A. F F P	99999-2371-08
80 gm	$3.80	Triamcinolone Acetonide, Thames Pharma	49158-0140-21
80 gm	$4.10	Triamcinolone Acetonide, Clay Park Labs	45802-0064-36
80 gm	$4.64	Triamcinolone Acetonide, Qualitest Pharms	00603-7851-90
80 gm	$4.79	Triamcinolone Acetonide, HL Moore Drug Exch	00839-6126-46
80 gm	$4.80	Triamcinolone Acetonide, Schein Pharm (US)	00364-7212-60
80 gm	$4.88	ARICIN, IDE-Interstate	00814-0851-97
80 gm	$4.95	Triamcinolone Acetate, Goldline Labs	00182-1217-53
80 gm	$5.05	TRIACET, Teva	00093-0937-81
80 gm	$5.06	Triamcinolone Acetonide 1, NMC Labs	23317-0301-80
80 gm	$5.10	Triamcinolone Acetonide, Rugby	00536-5225-30
80 gm	$5.10	Triamcinolone Acetonide, Major Pharms	00904-2741-11
80 gm	$5.15	Triamcinolone Acetonide, Fougera	00168-0004-80
80 gm	$5.15	Triamcinolone, Geneva Pharms	00781-7036-29
80 gm	$5.92	Triamcinolone Acetonide, United Res	00677-0747-46
80 gm	$5.92	Triamcinolone Acetonide, GW Labs	00713-0225-80
80 gm	**$32.34**	**KENALOG, Bristol Myers Squibb**	**00003-0506-49**
90 gm	$8.13	TRIDERM, Del Ray Lab	00316-0170-03
240 gm	$17.76	Triamcinolone Acetonide, H.C.F.A. F F P	99999-2371-09
240 gm	$67.96	ARISTOCORT R, Fujisawa USA	00469-5108-24
240 gm	$109.51	ARISTOCORT A, Fujisawa USA	00469-5102-24
454 gm	$16.00	Triamcinolone Acetonide, Thames Pharma	49158-0140-16
454 gm	$17.71	Triamcinolone Acetonide, Clay Park Labs	45802-0064-05
454 gm	$17.79	Triamcinolone Acetonide, H.C.F.A. F F P	99999-2371-10
454 gm	$18.55	Triamcinolone Acetonide, Major Pharms	00904-2741-27
454 gm	$19.42	Triamcinolone Acetonide 1, NMC Labs	23317-0301-16
454 gm	$19.97	Triamcinolone Acetonide, Fougera	00168-0004-16
454 gm	$20.85	Triamcinolone Acetonide, Rugby	00536-5225-98
454 gm	$22.05	Triamcinolone Acetate, Goldline Labs	00182-1217-45
454 gm	$33.59	Triamcinolone Acetonide, United Res	00677-0747-44

HOW SUPPLIED - RATED THERAPEUTICALLY EQUIVALENT:
(cont'd)

480 gm	$20.00	Triamcinolone Acetonide, Schein Pharm (US)	00364-7212-16
2270 gm	$167.98	Triamcinolone Acetonide, H.C.F.A. F F P	99999-2371-01
2378.25 gm	$103.72	ARISTOCORT R, Fujisawa USA	00469-5108-05
2383.5 gm	$176.37	Triamcinolone Acetonide, H.C.F.A. F F P	99999-2371-02

Cream - Topical - 0.5 %

15 gm	$2.80	Triamcinolone Acetonide, Thames Pharma	49158-0141-20
15 gm	$2.96	Triamcinolone, HL Moore Drug Exch	00839-6128-47
15 gm	$2.98	Triamcinolone Acetonide, United Res	00677-0751-40
15 gm	$2.98	Triamcinolone Acetonide, H.C.F.A. F F P	99999-2371-11
15 gm	$3.13	Triamcinolone Acetonide, Clay Park Labs	45802-0065-35
15 gm	$3.35	Triamcinolone Acetonide, Goldline Labs	00182-1218-51
15 gm	$3.90	ARICIN, IDE-Interstate	00814-0852-93
15 gm	$3.95	Triamcinolone Acetonide, Qualitest Pharms	00603-7852-74
15 gm	$4.20	Triamcinolone Acetonide, Fougera	00168-0002-15
15 gm	$4.28	Triamcinolone Acetonide, Schein Pharm (US)	00364-7213-72
15 gm	$4.28	Triamcinolone Acetonide, Rugby	00536-5200-20
15 gm	$4.40	Triamcinolone Acetonide, Major Pharms	00904-2744-36
15 gm	$5.19	Triamcinolone Acetonide, Harber Pharm	51432-0778-10
15 gm	$8.28	CINALOG, Embrex Economed	38130-0047-15
15 gm	$24.00	ARISTOCORT, Fujisawa USA	00469-5110-15
20 gm	$3.98	Triamcinolone Acetonide, H.C.F.A. F F P	99999-2371-12
20 gm	$5.00	Triamcinolone Acetonide, Consolidated Midland	00223-4443-20
20 gm	**$36.54**	**KENALOG, Bristol Myers Squibb**	**00003-1483-20**
	$22.00	Flutex Cream 0.5 %, Syosset Labs	47854-0577-13
30 gm	$5.88	Triamcinolone Acetonide, H.C.F.A. F F P	99999-2371-13
240 gm	$26.20	FLUTEX, Syosset Labs	47854-0577-11
240 gm	$47.76	Triamcinolone Acetonide, H.C.F.A. F F P	99999-2371-14
240 gm	$236.51	ARISTOCORT HP, Fujisawa USA	00469-5110-24
454 gm	$88.98	Triamcinolone Acetonide, H.C.F.A. F F P	99999-2371-15

Lotion - Topical - 0.025 %

60 ml	$7.05	Triamcinolone Acetonide, Harber Pharm	51432-0811-17
60 ml	$7.70	Triamcinolone Acetonide, Rosemont	00832-8560-60
60 ml	$8.20	Triamcinolone Acetonide, Major Pharms	00904-2739-03
60 ml	$8.95	Triamcinolone Acetonide, Consolidated Midland	00223-6635-60
60 ml	**$30.75**	**KENALOG, Bristol Myers Squibb**	**00003-0173-60**

Lotion - Topical - 0.1 %

60 ml	$6.90	Triamcinolone Acetonide, United Res	00677-1572-31
60 ml	$6.90	Triamcinolone Acetonide, H.C.F.A. F F P	99999-2371-23
60 ml	$7.30	Triamcinolone Acetonide, Thames Pharma	49158-0211-32
60 ml	$8.28	Triamcinolone Acetonide, Qualitest Pharms	00603-7855-49
60 ml	$8.76	Triamcinolone Acetonide, HL Moore Drug Exch	00839-6726-50
60 ml	$8.78	Triamcinolone Acetonide, Schein Pharm (US)	00364-7346-58
60 ml	$8.80	Triamcinolone Acetonide, Goldline Labs	00182-1777-68
60 ml	$9.00	Triamcinolone Acetonide, Major Pharms	00904-2742-03
60 ml	$9.74	Triamcinolone Acetonide, Rugby	00536-2360-61
60 ml	$9.95	Triamcinolone Acetonide, Consolidated Midland	00223-6636-60
60 ml	$28.90	Triamcinolone Acetonide, Morton Grove	60432-0561-60
60 ml	**$34.52**	**KENALOG, Bristol Myers Squibb**	**00003-0502-70**

Ointment - Topical - 0.025 %

2.3 kg	$27.42	Triamcinolone Acetonide, Rugby	00536-5190-27
2.3 kg	$32.39	Triamcinolone Acetdnide, Clay Park Labs	45802-0054-29
15 gm	$1.04	Triamcinolone Acetdnide, Clay Park Labs	45802-0054-35
15 gm	$1.07	Triamcinolone Acetate, HL Moore Drug Exch	00839-6392-47
15 gm	$1.12	Triamcinolone Acetonide, GW Labs	00713-0229-15
15 gm	$1.12	Triamcinolone Acetonide, H.C.F.A. F F P	99999-2371-34
15 gm	$1.30	Triamcinolone Acetonide, Goldline Labs	00182-1394-51
15 gm	$1.30	Triamcinolone Acetonide, Harber Pharm	51432-0782-10
15 gm	$1.33	Triamcinolone Acetonide, Schein Pharm (US)	00364-7359-72
15 gm	$1.34	Triamcinolone Acetonide, Qualitest Pharms	00603-7858-74
15 gm	$1.35	Triamcinolone Acetonide, Rugby	00536-5190-20
15 gm	$1.85	Triamcinolone Acetonide, Consolidated Midland	00223-4447-15
80 gm	$2.55	Triamcinolone Acetate, HL Moore Drug Exch	00839-6392-46
80 gm	$2.81	Triamcinolone Acetdnide, Clay Park Labs	45802-0054-36
80 gm	$2.83	Triamcinolone Acetonide, H.C.F.A. F F P	99999-2371-35
80 gm	$3.45	Triamcinolone Acetonide, Rugby	00536-5190-30
80 gm	$3.50	Triamcinolone Acetonide, Goldline Labs	00182-1394-53
80 gm	$3.57	Triamcinolone Acetonide, Harber Pharm	51432-0782-13
80 gm	$4.20	Triamcinolone Acetonide, Fougera	00168-0005-80
80 gm	$6.00	Triamcinolone Acetonide, GW Labs	00713-0229-80
80 gm	**$18.37**	**KENALOG, Bristol Myers Squibb**	**00003-0495-60**
454 gm	$7.67	Triamcinolone Acetdnide, Clay Park Labs	45802-0054-05
454 gm	$9.35	Triamcinolone Acetonide, Goldline Labs	00182-1394-45
454 gm	$9.35	Triamcinolone Acetonide, H.C.F.A. F F P	99999-2371-36
454 gm	$10.35	Triamcinolone Acetonide, Rugby	00536-5190-98
2270 gm	$170.25	Triamcinolone Acetonide, H.C.F.A. F F P	99999-2371-33

Ointment - Topical - 0.1 %

2.268 kg	$92.23	Triamcinolone Acetonide, Rugby	00536-5180-27
2.3 kg	$77.75	Triamcinolone Acetonide, Clay Park Labs	45802-0055-29
15 gm	$1.12	Triamcinolone Acetonide, United Res	00677-0753-40
15 gm	$1.12	Triamcinolone Acetonide, GW Labs	00713-0228-15
15 gm	$1.12	Triamcinolone Acetonide, H.C.F.A. F F P	99999-2371-25
15 gm	$1.30	Triamcinolone Acetonide, Thames Pharma	49158-0160-20
15 gm	$1.36	Triamcinolone Acetonide, Clay Park Labs	45802-0055-35
15 gm	$1.52	Triamcinolone Acetonide, NMC Labs	23317-0306-15
15 gm	$1.55	Triamcinolone Acetate, HL Moore Drug Exch	00839-6391-47
15 gm	$1.70	Triamcinolone Acetonide, Goldline Labs	00182-1395-51
15 gm	$1.95	Triamcinolone Acetonide, Consolidated Midland	00223-4446-15
15 gm	$1.98	Triamcinolone Acetonide, Geneva Pharms	00781-7033-27
15 gm	$1.99	Triamcinolone Acetonide, Fougera	00168-0006-15
15 gm	$2.01	Triamcinolone Acetonide, Qualitest Pharms	00603-7859-74
15 gm	$2.03	Triamcinolone Acetonide, Rugby	00536-5180-20
15 gm	$2.05	Triamcinolone Acetonide, Schein Pharm (US)	00364-7360-72
15 gm	$2.05	Triamcinolone Acetonide, Major Pharms	00904-2743-36
15 gm	$8.84	ARISTOCORT R, Fujisawa USA	00469-5112-15
15 gm	**$10.96**	**KENALOG, Bristol Myers Squibb**	**00003-0508-20**
	$16.00	Triamcinolone Acetonide, Thames Pharma	49158-0160-16
30 gm	$1.80	Triamcinolone Acetonide, Thames Pharma	49158-0160-08
30 gm	$2.25	Triamcinolone Acetonide, H.C.F.A. F F P	99999-2371-26
30 gm	$5.25	TRIDERM, Del Ray Lab	00316-0175-01
60 gm	$4.50	Triamcinolone Acetonide, H.C.F.A. F F P	99999-2371-27
60 gm	$20.68	ARISTOCORT, Fujisawa Pharm (US)	57317-0112-60
60 gm	**$26.48**	**KENALOG, Bristol Myers Squibb**	**00003-0508-56**
60 gm	$28.62	ARISTOCORT A, Fujisawa USA	00469-5105-60
80 gm	$2.80	Triamcinolone Acetonide, Thames Pharma	49158-0160-21
80 gm	$4.20	Triamcinolone Acetonide, H.C.F.A. F F P	99999-2371-28
80 gm	$4.21	Triamcinolone Acetonide, Clay Park Labs	45802-0055-36
80 gm	$4.79	Triamcinolone Acetate, HL Moore Drug Exch	00839-6391-46
80 gm	$4.88	ARICIN, IDE-Interstate	00814-0854-97
80 gm	$4.95	Triamcinolone Acetonide, Goldline Labs	00182-1395-53

HOW SUPPLIED - RATED THERAPEUTICALLY EQUIVALENT: *(cont'd)*

80 gm	$5.06	Triamcinolone Acetonide, NMC Labs	23317-0306-80
80 gm	$5.10	Triamcinolone Acetonide, Rugby	00536-5180-30
80 gm	$5.10	Triamcinolone Acetonide, Geneva Pharms	00781-7033-29
80 gm	$5.10	Triamcinolone Acetonide, Major Pharms	00904-2743-11
80 gm	$5.15	Triamcinolone Acetonide, Fougera	00168-0006-80
80 gm	$5.43	Triamcinolone Acetonide, Harber Pharm	51432-0780-13
80 gm	$6.00	Triamcinolone Acetonide, GW Labs	00713-0228-80
80 gm	$8.13	TRIDERM, Del Ray Lab	00316-0175-03
240 gm	$18.00	Triamcinolone Acetonide, H.C.F.A. F F P	99999-2371-29
240 gm	$67.96	ARISTOCORT R, Fujisawa USA	00469-5112-24
240 gm	**$94.07**	**KENALOG, Bristol Myers Squibb**	**00003-0508-60**
454 gm	$18.90	Triamcinolone Acetonide, Clay Park Labs	45802-0055-05
454 gm	$19.38	Triamcinolone Acetonide, H.C.F.A. F F P	99999-2371-30
454 gm	$19.40	Triamcinolone Acetonide, Goldline Labs	00182-1395-45
454 gm	$20.50	Triamcinolone Acetonide, Major Pharms	00904-2743-27
454 gm	$20.85	Triamcinolone Acetonide, Rugby	00536-5180-98
454 gm	$34.05	Triamcinolone Acetonide, United Res	00677-0753-44
2270 gm	$111.05	ARISTOCORT R, Fujisawa USA	00469-5112-05
2270 gm	$170.25	Triamcinolone Acetonide, H.C.F.A. F F P	99999-2371-24

Ointment - Topical - 0.5 %

15 gm	$3.09	Triamcinolone Acetonide, Clay Park Labs	45802-0049-35
15 gm	$3.33	Triamcinolone Acetonide, H.C.F.A. F F P	99999-2371-31
15 gm	$3.35	Triamcinolone Acetonide, Goldline Labs	00182-5068-51
15 gm	$4.28	Triamcinolone Acetonide, Rugby	00536-5170-20
15 gm	$5.19	Triamcinolone Acetonide, Harber Pharm	51432-0783-10
20 gm	$5.00	Triamcinolone Acetonide, Consolidated Midland	00223-4444-20
240 gm	$55.92	Triamcinolone Acetonide, H.C.F.A. F F P	99999-2371-32
240 gm	$209.56	ARISTOCORT, Lederle Pharm	00005-5178-57

Paste - Dental - 0.1 %

5 gm	$3.82	Triamcinolone Acetonide, United Res	00677-1200-36
5 gm	$3.82	Triamcinolone, HL Moore Drug Exch	00839-7403-41
5 gm	$3.82	Triamcinolone Acetonide, H.C.F.A. F F P	99999-2371-37
5 gm	$4.65	Triamcinolone Acetonide, Qualitest Pharms	00603-7870-69
5 gm	$5.00	Triamcinolone, Thames Pharma	49158-0231-03
5 gm	$6.09	Triamcinolone, Rugby	00536-5210-93
5 gm	$6.10	ORADENT DENTAL PASTE 0.1%, Major Pharms	00904-3643-68
5 gm	$6.40	Triamcinolone Acetonide, Goldline Labs	00182-5047-49
5 gm	$6.62	Triamcinolone Acetonide, Aligen Independ	00405-1610-45
5 gm	$8.89	Triamcinolone Dental Paste, Schein Pharm (US)	00364-2218-53
5 gm	$9.86	Traimcinolone In Orabase, Taro Pharms (US)	51672-1267-05
5 gm	$9.98	Triamcinolone Acetonide, Geneva Pharms	00781-7039-39
5 gm	**$12.33**	**KENALOG IN ORABASE, Bristol Myers Squibb**	**00003-0496-20**

HOW SUPPLIED - NOT RATED EQUIVALENT:

Aerosol - Inhalation - 100 mcg

20 gm	$43.36	AZMACORT, Rhone-Poulenc Rorer	00075-0060-37

Aerosol - Nasal - 55 mcg

10 gm	$39.18	NASACORT, Rhone-Poulenc Rorer	00075-1505-43

Aerosol, Spray - Topical - 3.3 mg/50gm

63 gm	**$24.27**	**KENALOG, Bristol Myers Squibb**	**00003-0501-62**

Injection, Solution - Intravenous - 40 mg/ml

1 ml	$4.66	Triamcinolone Acetonide, HL Moore Drug Exch	00839-6287-82
1 ml x 25	$81.25	Triamcinolone Acetonide, Consolidated Midland	00223-8691-25
5 ml	$6.50	Triamcinolone Acetonide, Consolidated Midland	00223-8691-05
5 ml	$8.54	Triamcinolone Acetonide, Balan	00304-1336-55
5 ml	$19.20	Triamcinolone Acetonide, Rugby	00536-9810-65

Injection, Susp - Intra-Articular - 10 mg/ml

5 ml	**$6.95**	**KENALOG-10, Bristol Myers Squibb**	**00003-0494-20**

Injection, Susp - Intra-Articular - 40 mg/ml

1 ml	$4.70	Triamcinolone Acetonide, Steris Labs	00402-0204-01
1 ml	**$5.39**	**KENALOG-40, Bristol Myers Squibb**	**00003-0293-05**
1 ml	$6.70	Triamcinolone Acetonide, Goldline Labs	00182-1141-85
1 ml x 25	$167.50	Triamcinolone Acetonide, Schein Pharm (US)	00364-6728-46
5 ml	$4.92	Triamcinolone Acetonide, Lannett	00527-0103-65
5 ml	$8.95	KEN-JEC, AF Hauser	52637-0540-05
5 ml	$9.85	Triamcinolone Acetonide, Insource	58441-0116-05
5 ml	$10.00	TRAMACORT-40, Bolan Pharm	44437-0204-05
5 ml	$11.50	ACETOCOT, C O Truxton	00463-1100-05
5 ml	$14.10	TRIAM-A, Hyrex Pharms	00314-3400-75
5 ml	$14.93	Triamcinolone Acetonide, General Inj & Vac	52584-0204-05
5 ml	$15.00	TAC-40, Parnell Pharm	50930-0204-05
5 ml	$16.30	Triamcinolone Acetonide, United Res	00677-0600-20
5 ml	$17.50	TRIAMONIDE, Forest Pharms	00456-0781-05
5 ml	$17.60	Triamcinolone Acetonide, Major Pharms	00904-0886-05
5 ml	$17.96	Triamcinolone Acetonide, HL Moore Drug Exch	00839-6287-25
5 ml	$18.00	Triamcinolone Acetonide, Steris Labs	00402-0204-05
5 ml	$19.25	Triamcinolone Acetonide, Geneva Pharms	00781-3116-75
5 ml	$19.80	Triamcinolone Acetonide, IDE-Interstate	00814-8008-38
5 ml	$22.05	Triamcinolone Acetonide, Goldline Labs	00182-1141-62
5 ml	$22.25	Triamcinolone Acetonide, Schein Pharm (US)	00364-6728-53
5 ml	$30.45	KENAJECT-40-, Mayrand Pharms	00259-0355-05
10 ml	**$40.74**	**KENALOG-40, Bristol Myers Squibb**	**00003-0293-28**
10 ml x 25	**$1044.05**	**KENALOG-40, Bristol Myers Squibb**	**00003-0293-55**

Injection, Susp - Intradermal - 3 mg/ml

5 ml	$8.95	TAC-3, Allergan	00023-0218-05

Ointment - Topical - 0.05 %

454 gm	$24.45	Triamcinolone Acetonide, Carolina Med	46287-0010-16

Powder

5 gm	$48.80	Triamcinolone Acetonide, Paddock Labs	00574-0450-05
10 gm	$6.60	Triamcinolone Acetonide, Paddock Labs	00574-0450-10

TRIAMCINOLONE DIACETATE *(002372)*

CATEGORIES: Adrenal Corticosteroids; Adrenal Hyperplasia; Adrenal Insufficiency; Airway Obstruction; Alopecia; Anemia; Antiarthritics; Arthritis; Asthma; Bursitis; Colitis; Conjunctivitis; Corneal Ulcer; Dermatitis; Diuresis; Granuloma Annulare; Herpes; Hormones; Hypercalcemia; Laryngeal Edema; Leukemia; Lupus Erythematosus; Lymphoma; Meningitis; Multiple Sclerosis; Osteoarthritis; Pain; Pneumoconiosis; Proteinuria; Psoriasis; Purpura; Retinochoroiditis; Rhinitis; Sarcoidosis; Spondylitis; Tenosynovitis; Thrombocytopenia; Thyroiditis; Trichinosis; Tuberculosis; Urticaria; Uveitis; FDA Approval Pre 1982

BRAND NAMES: Amcort; **Aristocort Forte**; Aristocort Suspension; Articulose-L.A.; Cenocort Forte; Kenacort; *Ledercort*; Sholog A; Tramacort-D; Tri-Med; Triam-Forte; Triamcot; Triamolone 40; Trilone; Tristo-Plex; Tristoject; Trylone D; U-Tri-Lone

(International brand names outside U.S. in italics)

Prescribing information not available at time of publication.

HOW SUPPLIED - EQUIVALENTS NOT AVAILABLE:

Injection, Solution - Intramuscular; - 40 mg/ml

1 ml	**$6.29**	**ARISTOCORT FORTE, Fujisawa Pharm (US)**	**57317-0202-01**
5 ml	$3.70	Triamcinolone Diacetate, Americal Pharm	54945-0567-41
5 ml	$6.46	Triamcinolone Diacetate, Insource	58441-0113-05
5 ml	$7.75	TRIAMCOT, C O Truxton	00463-1091-05
5 ml	$8.00	Triamcinolone Diacetate, Consolidated Midland	00223-8690-05
5 ml	$8.00	TRAMACORT-D, Bolan Pharm	44437-0182-75
5 ml	$8.98	Triamcinolone Diacetate, General Inj & Vac	52584-0042-05
5 ml	$10.33	U-TRI-LONE, UAD Labs	00785-8047-05
5 ml	$10.38	Triamcinolone Diacetate, HL Moore Drug Exch	00839-5057-25
5 ml	$11.01	Triamcinolone Diacetate, Rugby	00536-9800-65
5 ml	$11.05	Triamcinolone Diacetate, Steris Labs	00402-0042-05
5 ml	$11.34	Triamcinolone Diacetate, United Res	00677-0981-20
5 ml	$11.40	TRIAM FORTE, Hyrex Pharms	00314-0775-75
5 ml	**$12.53**	**ARISTOCORT FORTE, Fujisawa Pharm (US)**	**57317-0202-05**
5 ml	$12.75	Triamcinolone Diacetate, Major Pharms	00904-0885-05
5 ml	$13.35	Triamcinolone Diacetate, IDE-Interstate	00814-8007-38
5 ml	$13.75	Triamcinolone Diacetate, Goldline Labs	00182-3064-62
5 ml	$18.85	TRISTOJECT, Mayrand Pharms	00259-0323-05

Injection, Solution - Intravenous - 25 mg/ml

5 ml	$20.30	ARISTOCORT, Fujisawa Pharm (US)	57317-0203-05

Injection, Susp - Intra-Articular - 40 mg/ml

5 ml	$12.50	TRIAMOLONE, Forest Pharms	00456-1060-05

Syrup - Oral - 2 mg/5ml

120 ml	$20.21	ARISTOCORT, Lederle Pharm	00005-4421-58

Syrup - Oral - 4 mg/5ml

120 ml	$33.25	KENACORT DIACETATE, Bristol Myers Squibb	00003-0465-41

TRIAMCINOLONE HEXACETONIDE *(002373)*

CATEGORIES: Adrenal Corticosteroids; Alopecia; Alopecia Areata; Arthritis; Bursitis; Epicondylitis; Gouty Arthritis; Granuloma Annulare; Hormones; Inflammatory Lesions; Keloids; Lesions; Lichen Planus; Lichen Simplex Chronicus; Lupus Erythematosus; Necrobiosis Lipoidica; Osteoarthritis; Synovitis; Synovitis of Osteoarthritis; Tenosynovitis; Tumors; FDA Approval Pre 1982

BRAND NAMES: **Aristospan Intralesional**; Aristospan Parenteral

DESCRIPTION:

5 mg/ml-Parenteral: for Intralesional Administration.

20 mg/ml-Parenteral: for Intra-articular Administration.

Not For Intravenous Use.

Intralesional: A sterile suspension containing 5 mg/mL of micronized triamcinolone hexacetonide in the following inactive ingredients:

Polysorbate 80 NF............. 0.20% w/v.

Sorbitol Solution USP......... 50.00% v/v.

Water for Injection qs ad.... 100.00% V.

Hydrochloric Acid and Sodium Hydroxide, if required, to adjust pH to 4.5-6.5.

Preservative:

Benzyl Alcohol................ 0.90% w/v.

Intra-Articular: A sterile suspension containing 20 mg/mL of micronized triamcinolone hexacetonide in the following inactive ingredients:

Polysorbate 80 NF.............. 0.40% w/v.

Sorbitol Solution USP.......... 50.00% v/v.

Water for Injection qs ad..... 100.00% V.

Hydrochloric Acid and Sodium Hydroxide, if required, to adjust pH to 4.5-6.5.

Preservative: Benzyl Alcohol................. 0.90% w/v.

The hexacetonide ester of the potent glucocorticoid triamcinolone is relatively insoluble (0.0002% at 25° C in water).

When injected intralesionally, sublesionally, or intra-articularly, it can be expected to be absorbed slowly from the injection site.

Chemically triamcinolone hexacetonide USP is 9-Fluoro-11beta, 16alpha, 17,21-tetrahydroxypregna- 1,4-diene-3,20-dione cyclic 16,17-acetal with acetone 21-(3,3-dimethylbutyrate).

Molecular weight is 532.65.

CLINICAL PHARMACOLOGY:

Naturally occurring glucocorticoids (hydrocortisone), which also have salt-retaining properties, are used as replacement therapy in adrenocortical deficiency states. Their synthetic analogs are primarily used for their potent anti-inflammatory effects in disorders of many organ systems.

Glucocorticoids cause profound and varied metabolic effects. In addition, they modify the body's immune responses to diverse stimuli.

INDICATIONS AND USAGE:

Intralesional: Intralesional or sublesional Triamcinolone Hexacetonide is indicated for the following:

Keloids

Localized hypertrophic, infiltrated, inflammatory lesions of: lichen planus, psoriatic plaques, granuloma annulare and lichen simplex chronicus (neurodermatitis)

Discoid lupus erythematosus

Necrobiosis lipoidica diabeticorum

Alopecia areata

They may also be useful in cystic tumors of an aponeurosis or tendon (ganglia).

Sterile Triamcinolone Hexacetonide Suspension is indicated as adjunctive therapy for short-term administration (to tide the patient over an acute episode or exacerbation) in:

Synovitis of osteoarthritis Acute and subacute bursitis Epicondylitis

INDICATIONS AND USAGE: *(cont'd)*

Posttraumatic osteoarthritis Rheumatoid arthritis Acute gouty arthritis Acute nonspecific tenosynovitis

CONTRAINDICATIONS:

Systemic fungal infections.

WARNINGS:

In patients on corticosteroid therapy subjected to any unusual stress, increased dosage of rapidly acting corticosteroids before, during, and after the stressful situation is indicated.

Corticosteroids may mask some signs of infection, and new infections may appear during their use. There may be decreased resistance and inability to localize infection when corticosteroids are used.

Prolonged use of corticosteroids may produce posterior subcapsular cataracts, glaucoma with possible damage to the optic nerves, and may enhance the establishment of secondary ocular infections due to fungi or viruses.

Use in Pregnancy: Since adequate human reproduction studies have not been done with corticosteroids, the use of these drugs in pregnancy, nursing mothers, or women of childbearing potential requires that the possible benefits of the drug be weighed against the potential hazards to the mother and embryo or fetus. Infants born of mothers who have received substantial doses of corticosteroids during pregnancy should be carefully observed for signs of hypoadrenalism.

Average and large doses of cortisone or hydrocortisone can cause elevation of blood pressure, salt and water retention, and increased excretion of potassium. These effects are less likely to occur with the synthetic derivatives except when used in large doses. Dietary salt restriction and potassium supplementation may be necessary. All corticosteroids increase calcium excretion.

While on corticosteroid therapy patients should not be vaccinated against smallpox.

Other immunization procedures should not be undertaken in patients who are on corticosteroids, especially in high doses, because of possible hazards of neurological complications and lack of antibody response.

The use of triamcinolone hexacetonide suspension in active tuberculosis should be restricted to those cases of fulminating or disseminated tuberculosis in which the corticosteroid is used for the management of the disease in conjunction with appropriate antituberculous regimen.

If corticosteroids are indicated in patients with latent tuberculosis or tuberculin reactivity, close observation is necessary as reactivation of the disease may occur. During prolonged corticosteroid therapy, these patients should receive chemoprophylaxis.

Because rare instances of anaphylactoid reactions have occurred in patients receiving parenteral corticosteroid therapy, appropriate precautionary measures should be taken prior to administration, especially when the patient has a history of allergy to any drug.

Intralesional or sublesional injection of excessive dosage whether by single or multiple injection into any given area may cause cutaneous or subcutaneous atrophy.

Postinjection flare (following intra-articular use) and charcot-like arthropathy have been associated with parenteral corticosteroid therapy.

PRECAUTIONS:

Drug-induced secondary adrenocortical insufficiency may be minimized by gradual reduction of dosage. This type of relative insufficiency may persist for months after discontinuation of therapy; therefore, in any situation of stress occurring during that period, hormone therapy should be reinstituted. Since mineralocorticoid secretion may be impaired, salt and/or a mineralocorticoid should be administered concurrently.

There is an enhanced effect of corticosteroids in patients with hypothyroidism and in those with cirrhosis.

Corticosteroids should be used cautiously in patients with ocular herpes simplex for fear of corneal perforation.

The lowest possible dose of corticosteroids should be used to control the condition under treatment, and when reduction in dosage is possible, the reduction must be gradual.

Psychic derangements may appear when corticosteroids are used, ranging from euphoria, insomnia, mood swings, personality changes, and severe depression to frank psychotic manifestations. Also, existing emotional instability or psychotic tendencies may be aggravated by corticosteroids.

Aspirin should be used cautiously in conjunction with corticosteroids in hypoprothrombinemia.

Steroids should be used with caution in nonspecific ulcerative colitis, if there is a probability of impending perforation, abscess or other pyogenic infection, also in diverticulitis, fresh intestinal anastomoses, active or latent peptic ulcer, renal insufficiency, hypertension, osteoporosis, and myasthenia gravis.

Growth and development of infants and children on prolonged corticosteroid therapy should be carefully followed.

The following additional precautions apply for parenteral corticosteroids.

Intra-articular injection of a corticosteroid may produce systemic as well as local effects.

Appropriate examination of any joint fluid present is necessary to exclude a septic process.

A marked increase in pain accompanied by local swelling, further restriction of joint motion, fever, and malaise are suggestive of septic arthritis. If this complication occurs and the diagnosis is confirmed, appropriate antimicrobial therapy should be instituted.

Local injection of a steroid into a previously infected joint is to be avoided.

Corticosteroids should not be injected into unstable joints.

The slower rate of absorption by intramuscular administration should be recognized.

Atrophy at the site of injection has been reported.

Routine laboratory studies, such as urinalysis, two-hour postprandial blood sugar, determination of blood pressure and body weight, and a chest X-ray should be made at regular intervals during prolonged therapy. Upper GI X-rays are desirable in patients with an ulcer history or significant dyspepsia.

ADVERSE REACTIONS:

Fluid and Electrolyte Disturbances: Sodium retention; fluid retention; congestive heart failure in susceptible patients; potassium loss; hypokalemic alkalosis; hypertension.

Musculoskeletal: Muscle weakness; steroid myopathy; loss of muscle mass; osteoporosis; vertebral compression fractures; aseptic necrosis of femoral and humeral heads; pathologic fracture of long bones.

Gastrointestinal Peptic ulcer with possible subsequent perforation and hemorrhage; pancreatitis; abdominal distention; ulcerative esophagitis.

Dermatologic: Impaired wound healing; thin fragile skin; petechiae and ecchymoses; facial erythema; increased sweating; may suppress reactions to skin tests.

ADVERSE REACTIONS: *(cont'd)*

Neurological: Convulsions; increased intracranial pressure with papilledema (pseudotumor cerebri) usually after treatment; vertigo; headache.

Endocrine: Menstrual irregularities; development of Cushingoid state; suppression of growth in children; secondary adrenocortical and pituitary unresponsiveness, particularly in times of stress, as in trauma, surgery, or illness; decreased carbohydrate tolerance; manifestations of latent diabetes mellitus; increased requirements for insulin or oral hypoglycemic agents in diabetics.

Ophthalmic: Posterior subcapsular cataracts; increased intraocular pressure; glaucoma; exophthalmos.

Metabolic: Negative nitrogen balance due to protein catabolism.

The following additional adverse reactions are related to parenteral and intralesional corticosteroid therapy:

Rare instances of blindness associated with intralesional therapy around the orbit or intranasally.

Hyperpigmentation or hypopigmentation.

Sterile abscess.

Subcutaneous and cutaneous atrophy.

Anaphylactoid reactions have been reported rarely with products of this class.

DOSAGE AND ADMINISTRATION:

GENERAL

The initial dosage of triamcinolone hexacetonide suspension may vary from 2 to 48 mg per day depending on the specific disease entity being treated. In situations of less severity, lower doses will generally suffice while in selected patients higher initial doses may be required.

Usually the parenteral dosage ranges are one-third to one-half the oral dose given every 12 hours. However, in certain overwhelming, acute, life-threatening situations, administration in dosages exceeding the usual dosages may be justified and may be in multiples of the oral dosages.

The initial dosage should be maintained or adjusted until a satisfactory response is noted. If after a reasonable period of time there is a lack of satisfactory clinical response, Triamcinolone hexacetonide should be discontinued and the patient transferred to other appropriate therapy. It should be emphasized that dosage requirements are variable and must be individualized on the basis of the disease under treatment and the response of the patient. After a favorable response is noted, the proper maintenance dosage should be determined by decreasing the initial drug dosage in small increments at appropriate time intervals until the lowest dosage which will maintain an adequate clinical response is reached. It should be kept in mind that constant monitoring is needed in regard to drug dosage. Included in the situations which may make dosage adjustments necessary are changes in clinical status secondary to remissions or exacerbations in the disease process, the patients individual drug responsiveness, and the effect of patient exposure to stressful situations not directly related to the disease entity under treatment; in this latter situation it may be necessary to increase the dosage of triamcinolone hexacetonide for a period of time consistent with the patients condition. If after long-term therapy the drug is to be stopped, it is recommended that it be withdrawn gradually rather than abruptly.

DIRECTIONS FOR USE

Strict aseptic administration technique is mandatory. Topical ethyl chloride spray may be used locally before injection. The syringe should be gently agitated to achieve uniform suspension before use. Since this product has been designed for ease of administration, a small bore needle (not smaller than 24 gauge) may be used.

DILUTION

Intralesional: Triamcinolone hexacetonide suspension may be diluted, if desired, with dextrose and sodium chloride injection USP, (5% and 10% dextrose), sodium chloride injection USP, or sterile water for injection USP.

The optimum dilution, ie, 1:1, 1:2, 1:4, should be determined by the nature of the lesion, its size, the depth of injection, the volume needed, and location of the lesion. In general, more superficial injections should be performed with greater dilution. Certain conditions, such as keloids, require a less dilute suspension such as 5 mg/mL, with variation in dose and dilution as dictated by the condition of the individual patient. Subsequent dosage, dilution, and frequency of injections are best judged by the clinical response.

The suspension may also be mixed with 1% or 2% lidocaine hydrochloride, using the formulations which do not contain parabens. Similar local anesthetics may also be used. Diluents containing methylparaben, propylparaben, phenol, etc. should be avoided since these compounds may cause flocculation of the steroid. These dilutions will retain full potency for one week, but care should be exercised to avoid contamination of the vials contents and the dilutions should be discarded after 7 days.

INTRALESIONAL OR SUBLESIONAL

Average Dose: up to 0.5 mg per square inch of affected skin injected intralesionally or sublesionally. The frequency of subsequent injections is best determined by the clinical response. If desired, the vial may be diluted as indicated under DIRECTIONS FOR USE.

A lesser initial dosage range of triamcinolone hexacetonide may produce the desired effect when the drug is administered to provide a localized concentration. The site of the injection and the volume of the injection should be carefully considered when triamcinolone hexacetonide is administered for this purpose.

DILUTION

Intra-articular: Triamcinolone hexacetonide suspension may be mixed with 1% or 2% lidocaine hydrochloride, using the formulations which do not contain parabens.

Similar local anesthetics may also be used. Diluents containing methylparaben, propylparaben, phenol, etc, should be avoided since these compounds may cause flocculation of the steroid. These dilutions will retain full potency for one week, but care should be exercised to avoid contamination.

INTRA-ARTICULAR

Average dose—2 to 20 mg (0.1 ml to 1.0 ml)

The dose depends on the size of the joint to be injected, the degree of inflammation, and the amount of fluid present. In general, large joints (such as knee, hip, shoulder) require 10 to 20 mg. For small joints (such as interphalangeal, metacarpophalangeal), 2 to 6 mg may be employed. When the amount of synovial fluid is increased, aspiration may be performed before administering triamcinolone hexacetonide.

Subsequent dosage and frequency of injections can best be judged by clinical response.

The usual frequency of injection into a single joint is every three or four weeks, and injection more frequently than that is generally not advisable. To avoid possible joint destruction from repeated use of intra-articular corticosteroids, injection should be as infrequent as possible, consistent with adequate patient care. Attention should be paid to avoiding deposition of drug along the needle path which might produce atrophy.

HOW SUPPLIED - EQUIVALENTS NOT AVAILABLE:

Injection, Solution - Intravenous - 5 mg/ml

5 ml	$11.94	ARISTOSPAN, Fujisawa Pharm (US)	57317-0206-05

Injection, Solution - Intravenous - 20 mg/ml

1 ml	$8.18	ARISTOSPAN, Fujisawa Pharm (US)	57317-0205-01
5 ml	$18.40	ARISTOSPAN, Fujisawa Pharm (US)	57317-0205-05

TRIAMTERENE *(002374)*

CATEGORIES: Antihypertensives; Cirrhosis; Congestive Heart Failure; Diuresis; Diuretics; Edema; Electrolytic, Caloric-Water Balance; Heart Failure; Hyperaldosteronism; Nephrotic Syndrome; Potassium Sparing Diuretics; Renal Drugs; Pregnancy Category B; FDA Approval Pre 1982

BRAND NAMES: *Amterene; Diarrol; Diuteren;* **Dyrenium**; *Dytac; Jatropur; Reviten; Suloton; Triamteril; Trian; Urocaudal*
(International brand names outside U.S. in italics)

FORMULARIES: Aetna; Medi-Cal

COST OF THERAPY: $289.08 (Edema; Capsule; 100 mg; 2/day; 365 days)

> **WARNING:**
> Abnormal elevation of serum potassium levels (greater than or equal to 5.5 mEq/liter) can occur with all potassium-sparing agents, including triamterene. Hyperkalemia is more likely to occur in patients with renal impairment, and diabetes (even without evidence of renal impairment), elderly or severely ill patients. Since uncorrected hyperkalemia may be fatal, serum potassium levels must be monitored at frequent intervals especially in patients receiving triamterene, when dosages are changed or with any illness that may influence renal function.

DESCRIPTION:

Dyrenium (triamterene) is a potassium-conserving diuretic.

Triamterene is 2,4,7-triamino-6-phenylpteridine. Its molecular weight is 253.27. At 50°C, triamterene is slightly soluble in water. It is soluble in dilute ammonia, dilute aqueous sodium hydroxide and dimethylformamide. It is sparingly soluble in methanol.

Each capsule for oral administration, with opaque red cap and body, contains triamterene, 50 or 100 mg, and is imprinted with the product name Dyrenium, and strength (50 or 100) and SKF. Inactive ingredients consist of benzyl alcohol, cetylpyridinium chloride, D&C Red No. 33, FD&C Yellow No. 6, gelatin, lactose, magnesium stearate, povidone, sodium lauryl sulfate, titanium dioxide and trace amounts of other inactive ingredients.

CLINICAL PHARMACOLOGY:

Triamterene has a unique mode of action; it inhibits the reabsorption of sodium ions in exchange for potassium and hydrogen ions at that segment of the distal tubule under the control of adrenal mineralocorticoids (especially aldosterone). This activity is not directly related to aldosterone secretion or antagonism; it is a result of a direct effect on the renal tubule.

The fraction of filtered sodium reaching this distal tubular exchange site is relatively small, and the amount which is exchanged depends on the level of mineralocorticoid activity. Thus, the degree of natriuresis and diuresis produced by inhibition of the exchange mechanism is necessarily limited. Increasing the amount of available sodium and the level of mineralocorticoid activity by the use of more proximally acting diuretics will increase the degree of diuresis and potassium conservation.

Triamterene occasionally causes increases in serum potassium which can result in hyperkalemia. It does not produce alkalosis because it does not cause excessive excretion of titratable acid and ammonium.

Triamterene has been shown to cross the placental barrier and appear in the cord blood of animals.

PHARMACOKINETICS

Onset of action is 2 to 4 hours after ingestion. In normal volunteers the mean peak serum levels were 30 ng/ml at three hours. The average percent of drug recovered in the urine (0-48 hours) was 21%. Triamterene is primarily metabolized to the sulfate conjugate of hydroxytriamterene. Both the plasma and urine levels of this metabolite greatly exceed triamterene levels. Triamterene is rapidly absorbed, with somewhat less than 50% of the oral dose reaching the urine. Most patients will respond to triamterene during the first day of treatment. Maximum therapeutic effect, however, may not be seen for several days. Duration of diuresis depends on several factors, especially renal function, but it generally tapers off 7 to 9 hours after administration.

INDICATIONS AND USAGE:

Triamterene is indicated in the treatment of edema associated with congestive heart failure, cirrhosis of the liver, and the nephrotic syndrome; also in steroid-induced edema, idiopathic edema, and edema due to secondary hyperaldosteronism.

Triamterene may be used alone or with other diuretics either for its added diuretic effect or its potassium-conserving potential. It also promotes increased diuresis when patients prove resistant or only partially responsive to thiazides or other diuretics because of secondary hyperaldosteronism.

Usage in Pregnancy: The routine use of diuretics in an otherwise healthy woman is inappropriate and exposes mother and fetus to unnecessary hazard. Diuretics do not prevent development of toxemia of pregnancy, and there is no satisfactory evidence that they are useful in the treatment of developed toxemia.

Edema during pregnancy may arise from pathological causes or from the physiologic and mechanical consequences of pregnancy. Diuretics are indicated in pregnancy when edema is due to pathologic causes, just as they are in the absence of pregnancy (see PRECAUTIONS). Dependent edema in pregnancy, resulting from restriction of venous return by the expanded uterus, is properly treated through elevation of the lower extremities and use of support hose; use of diuretics to lower intravascular volume in this case is illogical and unnecessary. There is hypervolemia during normal pregnancy which is harmful to neither the fetus nor the mother (in the absence of cardiovascular disease), but which is associated with edema, including generalized edema, in the majority of pregnant women. If this edema produces discomfort, increased recumbency will often provide relief. In rare instances, this edema may cause extreme discomfort which is not relieved by rest. In these cases, a short course of diuretics may provide relief and may be appropriate.

CONTRAINDICATIONS:

Anuria. Severe or progressive kidney disease or dysfunction with the possible exception of nephrosis. Severe hepatic disease. Hypersensitivity to the drug.

Triamterene should not be used in patients with preexisting elevated serum potassium, as is sometimes seen in patients with impaired renal function or azotemia, or in patients who develop hyperkalemia while on the drug. Patients should not be placed on dietary potassium supplements, potassium salts, or potassium-containing salt substitutes in conjunction with triamterene.

Triamterene should not be given to patients receiving other potassium-sparing agents such as spironolactone, amiloride hydrochloride, or other formulations containing triamterene. Two deaths have been reported in patients receiving concomitant spironolactone and triamterene or Dyazide. Although dosage recommendations were exceeded in one case and in the other serum electrolytes were not properly monitored, these two drugs should not be given concomitantly.

WARNINGS:

There have been isolated reports of hypersensitivity reactions; therefore, patients should be observed regularly for the possible occurrence of blood dyscrasias, liver damage, or other idiosyncratic reactions.

Periodic BUN and serum potassium determinations should be made to check kidney function, especially in patients with suspected or confirmed renal insufficiency. It is particularly important to make serum potassium determinations in elderly or diabetic patients receiving the drug; these patients should be observed carefully for possible serum potassium increases.

If hyperkalemia is present or suspected, an electrocardiogram should be obtained. If the ECG shows no widening of the QRS or arrhythmia in the presence of hyperkalemia, it is usually sufficient to discontinue triamterene and any potassium supplementation and substitute a thiazide alone. Sodium polystyrene sulfonate (Kayexalate, Winthrop) may be administered to enhance the excretion of excess potassium. **The presence of a widened QRS complex or arrhythmia in association with hyperkalemia requires prompt additional therapy.** For tachyarrhythmia, infuse 44 mEq of sodium bicarbonate or 10 ml of 10% calcium gluconate or calcium chloride over several minutes. For asystole, bradycardia, or A-V block transvenous pacing is also recommended.

The effect of calcium and sodium bicarbonate is transient and repeated administration may be required. When indicated by the clinical situation, excess K^+ may be removed by dialysis or oral or rectal administration of Kayexalate. Infusion of glucose and insulin has also been used to treat hyperkalemia.

PRECAUTIONS:

GENERAL

Triamterene tends to conserve potassium rather than to promote the excretion as do many diuretics and, occasionally, can cause increases in serum potassium which, in some instances, can result in hyperkalemia. In rare instances, hyperkalemia has been associated with cardiac irregularities.

Electrolyte imbalance often encountered in such diseases as congestive heart failure, renal disease, or cirrhosis may be aggravated or caused independently by any effective diuretic agent including triamterene. The use of full doses of a diuretic when salt intake is restricted can result in a low-salt syndrome.

Triamterene can cause mild nitrogen retention which is reversible upon withdrawal of the drug and is seldom observed with intermittent (every-other-day) therapy.

Triamterene may cause a decreasing alkali reserve with the possibility of metabolic acidosis.

By the very nature of their illness, cirrhotics with splenomegaly sometimes have marked variations in their blood pictures. Since triamterene is a weak folic acid antagonist, it may contribute to the appearance of megaloblastosis in cases where folic acid stores have been depleted. Therefore, periodic blood studies in these patients are recommended. They should also be observed for exacerbations of underlying liver disease.

Triamterene has elevated uric acid, especially in persons predisposed to gouty arthritis.

Triamterene has been reported in renal stones in association with other calculus components. Triamterene should be used with caution in patients with histories of renal stones.

INFORMATION FOR THE PATIENT

To help avoid stomach upset, it is recommended that the drug be taken after meals.

If a single daily dose is prescribed, it may be preferable to take it in the morning to minimize the effect of increased frequency of urination on nighttime sleep.

If a dose is missed, the patient should not take more than the prescribed dose at the next dosing interval.

LABORATORY TESTS

Hyperkalemia will rarely occur in patients with adequate urinary output, but it is a possibility if large doses are used for considerable periods of time. If hyperkalemia is observed, Triamterene should be withdrawn. The normal adult range of serum potassium is 3.5 to 5.0 mEq per liter with 4.5 mEq often being used for a reference point. Potassium levels persistently above 6 mEq per liter require careful observation and treatment. Normal potassium levels tend to be higher in neonates (7.7 mEq per liter) than in adults.

Serum potassium levels do not necessarily indicate true body potassium concentration. A rise in plasma pH may cause a decrease in plasma potassium concentration and an increase in the intracellular potassium concentration. Because triamterene conserves potassium, it has been theorized that in patients who have received intensive therapy or been given the drug for prolonged periods, a rebound kaliuresis could occur upon abrupt withdrawal. In such patients withdrawal of triamterene should be gradual.

DRUG/LABORATORY TEST INTERACTIONS

Triamterene and quinidine have similar fluorescence spectra; thus, triamterene will interfere with the fluorescent measurement of quinidine.

CARCINOGENESIS, MUTAGENESIS, AND IMPAIRMENT OF FERTILITY

Long-term studies to determine the carcinogenic potential of triamterene are not available. Studies to determine the mutagenic potential of triamterene are not available. Reproductive studies have been performed in rats at doses up to 30 times the human dose and have revealed no evidence of impaired fertility.

PREGNANCY, TERATOGENIC EFFECTS, PREGNANCY CATEGORY B

Reproduction studies have been performed in rats at doses up to 30 times the human dose and have revealed no evidence of impaired fertility or harm to the fetus due to triamterene. There are, however, no adequate and well-controlled studies in pregnant women. Because animal reproductive studies are not always predictive of human response, this drug should be used during pregnancy only if clearly needed.

Nonteratogenic Effects: Triamterene has been shown to cross the placental barrier and appear in the cord blood of animals; this may occur in humans. The use of triamterene in pregnant women requires that the anticipated benefit be weighed against possible hazards to the fetus. These possible hazards include adverse reactions which have occurred in the adult.

PRECAUTIONS: *(cont'd)*

Nursing Mothers: Triamterene appears in animal milk; this may occur in humans. If use of the drug is deemed essential, the patient should stop nursing.

Pediatric Use: Safety and effectiveness in children have not been established.

DRUG INTERACTIONS:

Caution should be used when lithium and diuretics are used concomitantly because diuretic-induced sodium loss may reduce the renal clearance of lithium and increase serum lithium levels with risk of lithium toxicity. Patients receiving such combined therapy should have serum lithium levels monitored closely and the lithium dosage adjusted if necessary.

A possible interaction resulting in acute renal failure has been reported in a few subjects when indomethacin, a nonsteroidal anti-inflammatory agent, was given with triamterene. Caution is advised in administering nonsteroidal anti-inflammatory agents with triamterene.

The effects of the following drugs may be potentiated when given together with triamterene: antihypertensive medication, other diuretics, preanesthetic and anesthetic agents, skeletal muscle relaxants (nondepolarizing).

Potassium-sparing agents should be used with caution in conjunction with angiotensin-converting enzyme (ACE) inhibitors due to an increased risk of hyperkalemia.

The following agents, given together with triamterene, may promote serum potassium accumulation and possibly result in hyperkalemia because of the potassium-sparing nature of triamterene, especially in patients with renal insufficiency: blood from blood bank (may contain up to 30 mEq of potassium per liter of plasma or up to 65 mEq per liter of whole blood when stored for more than 10 days); low-salt milk (may contain up to 60 mEq of potassium per liter); potassium-containing medications (such as parenteral penicillin G potassium); salt substitutes (most contain substantial amounts of potassium).

Triamterene may raise blood glucose levels; for adult-onset diabetes, dosage adjustments of hypoglycemic agents may be necessary during and after therapy; concurrent use with chlorpropamide may increase the risk of severe hyponatremia.

ADVERSE REACTIONS:

Adverse effects are listed in decreasing order of frequency; however, the most serious adverse effects are listed first regardless of frequency. All adverse effects occur rarely (that is, one in 1000, or less).

Hypersensitivity: anaphylaxis, rash, photosensitivity.

Metabolic: hyperkalemia, hypokalemia.

Renal: azotemia, elevated BUN and creatinine, renal stones, acute interstitial nephritis (rare), acute renal failure (one case of irreversible renal failure has been reported).

Gastrointestinal: jaundice and/or liver enzyme abnormalities, nausea and vomiting, diarrhea.

Hematologic: thrombocytopenia, megaloblastic anemia.

Central Nervous System: weakness, fatigue, dizziness, headache, dry mouth.

OVERDOSAGE:

In the event of overdosage it can be theorized that electrolyte imbalance would be the major concern, with particular attention to possible hyperkalemia. Other symptoms that might be seen would be nausea and vomiting, other G.I. disturbances, and weakness. It is conceivable that some hypotension could occur. As with an overdose of any drug, immediate evacuation of the stomach should be induced through emesis and gastric lavage. Careful evaluation of the electrolyte pattern and fluid balance should be made. There is no specific antidote.

Reversible acute renal failure following ingestion of 50 tablets of a product containing a combination of 50 mg triamterene and 25 mg hydrochlorothiazide has been reported.

The oral LD_{50} in mice is 380 mg/kg. The amount of drug in a single dose ordinarily associated with symptoms of overdose or likely to be life-threatening is not known.

Although triamterene is 67% protein-bound, there may be some benefit to dialysis in cases of overdosage.

DOSAGE AND ADMINISTRATION:

Adult Dosage

Dosage should be titrated to the needs of the individual patient. When used alone, the usual starting dose is 100 mg twice daily after meals. When combined with another diuretic or antihypertensive agent, the total daily dosage of each agent should usually be lowered initially and then adjusted to the patient's needs. The total daily dosage should not exceed 300 mg. Please refer to Precautions-General.

When triamterene is added to other diuretic therapy or when patients are switched to triamterene from other diuretics, all potassium supplementation should be discontinued.

HOW SUPPLIED:

Capsules: 50 mg in bottles of 100 and 100 mg in bottles of 100.

Storage: Store at controlled room temperature (59° to 86° F). Protect from light.

HOW SUPPLIED - EQUIVALENTS NOT AVAILABLE:

Capsule, Gelatin - Oral - 50 mg

100's	$34.15	DYRENIUM 50, SKB Pharms	00108-3806-20

Capsule, Gelatin - Oral - 100 mg

100's	$39.60	DYRENIUM, SKB Pharms	00108-3807-21
100's	$42.90	DYRENIUM, SKB Pharms	00108-3807-20

TRIAZOLAM *(002375)*

CATEGORIES: Anxiolytics, Sedatives, Hypnotic; Benzodiazepines; Central Nervous System Agents; Hypnotics; Insomnia; Sedatives/Hypnotics; Pregnancy Category X; DEA Class CIV; Sales > $100 Million; FDA Approved 1982 Nov; Patent Expiration 1993 Sep

BRAND NAMES: *Dumozolam*; **Halcion**; *Novidorm*; *Nuctane*; *Somese*; *Somniton*; *Songar*; *Tialam*; *Trialam*
(International brand names outside U.S. in italics)

FORMULARIES: Aetna; BC-BS; Medi-Cal

COST OF THERAPY: $3.70 (Insomnia; Tablet; 0.25 mg; 1/day; 7 days)

DESCRIPTION:

Halcion Tablets contain triazolam, a triazolobenzodiazepine hypnotic agent.

Triazolam is a white crystalline powder, soluble in alcohol and poorly soluble in water. It has a molecular weight of 343.21.

The chemical name for triazolam is 8-chloro-6-(o-chlorophenyl)-1-methyl -4H-s-triazolo-(4,3-α)(1,4) benzodiazepine.

DESCRIPTION: *(cont'd)*

Each Halcion tablet, for oral administration, contains 0.125 mg or 0.25 mg of triazolam.

Inactive Ingredients: *0.125 mg:* cellulose, corn starch, docusate sodium, lactose, magnesium stearate, silicon dioxide, sodium benzoate; *0.25 mg:* cellulose, corn starch, docusate sodium, FD&C Blue No. 2, lactose, magnesium stearate, silicon dioxide, sodium benzoate.

CLINICAL PHARMACOLOGY:

Triazolam is a hypnotic with a short mean plasma half-life reported to be in the range of 1.5 to 5.5 hours. In normal subjects treated for 7 days with four times the recommended dosage, there was no evidence of altered systemic bioavailability, rate of elimination, or accumulation. Peak plasma levels are reached within 2 hours following oral administration. Following recommended doses of Halcion, triazolam peak plasma levels in the range of 1 to 6 ng/ml are seen. The plasma levels achieved are proportional to the dose given.

Triazolam and its metabolites, principally as conjugated glucuronides, which are presumably inactive, are excreted primarily in the urine. Only small amounts of unmetabolized triazolam appear in the urine. The two primary metabolites accounted for 79.9% of urinary excretion. Urinary excretion appeared to be biphasic in its time course.

Triazolam tablets 0.5 mg, in two separate studies, did not affect the prothrombin times or plasma warfarin levels in male volunteers administered sodium warfarin orally.

Extremely high concentrations of triazolam do not displace bilirubin bound to human serum albumin *in vitro*.

Triazolam ^{14}C was administered orally to pregnant mice. Drug-related material appeared uniformly distributed in the fetus with ^{14}C concentrations approximately the same as in the brain of the mother.

In sleep laboratory studies, triazolam tablets significantly decreased sleep latency, increased the duration of sleep, and decreased the number of nocturnal awakenings. After 2 weeks of consecutive nightly administration, the drug's effect on total wake time is decreased, and the values recorded in the last third of the night approach baseline levels. On the first and/or second night after drug discontinuance (first or second post-drug night), total time asleep, percentage of time spent sleeping, and rapidity of falling asleep frequently were significantly less than on baseline (predrug) nights. This effect is often called "rebound" insomnia.

The type and duration of hypnotic effects and the profile of unwanted effects during administration of benzodiazepine drugs may be influenced by the biologic half-life of administered drug and any active metabolites formed. When half-lives are long, the drug or metabolites may accumulate during periods of nightly administration and be associated with impairments of cognitive and motor performance during waking hours; the possibility of interaction with other psychoactive drugs or alcohol will be enhanced. In contrast, if half-lives are short, the drug and metabolites will be cleared before the next dose is ingested, and carry-over effects related to excessive sedation or CNS depression should be minimal or absent. However, during nightly use for an extended period pharmacodynamic tolerance or adaptation to some effects of benzodiazepine hypnotics may develop. If the drug has a short half-life of elimination, it is possible that a relative deficiency of the drug or its active metabolites (*i.e.,* in relationship to the receptor site) may occur at some point in the interval between each night's use. This sequence of events may account for two clinical findings reported to occur after several weeks of nightly use of rapidly eliminated benzodiazepine hypnotics: 1) increased wakefulness during the last third of the night and 2) the appearance of increased daytime anxiety after 10 days of continuous treatment.

INDICATIONS AND USAGE:

Triazolam is indicated for the short-term treatment of insomnia (generally 7-10 days). Use for more than 2-3 weeks requires complete reevaluation of the patient (see WARNINGS).

Prescriptions for triazolam should be written for short-term use (7-10 days) and it should not be prescribed in quantities exceeding a 1-month supply.

CONTRAINDICATIONS:

Triazolam tablets are contraindicated in patients with known hypersensitivity to this drug or other benzodiazepines.

Benzodiazepines may cause fetal damage when administered during pregnancy. An increased risk of congenital malformations associated with the use of diazepam and chlordiazepoxide during the first trimester of pregnancy has been suggested in several studies. Transplacental distribution has resulted in neonatal CNS depression following the ingestion of therapeutic doses of a benzodiazepine hypnotic during the last weeks of pregnancy.

Triazolam is contraindicated in pregnant women. If there is a likelihood of the patient becoming pregnant while receiving triazolam, she should be warned of the potential risk to the fetus. Patients should be instructed to discontinue the drug prior to becoming pregnant. The possibility that a woman of childbearing potential may be pregnant at the time of institution of therapy should be considered.

WARNINGS:

Sleep disturbance may be the presenting manifestation of a physical and/or psychiatric disorder. Consequently, a decision to initiate symptomatic treatment of insomnia should only be made after the patient has been carefully evaluated.

The failure of insomnia to remit after 7-10 days of treatment may indicate the presence of a primary psychiatric and/or medical illness.

Worsening of insomnia or the emergence of new abnormalities of thinking or behavior may be the consequence of an unrecognized psychiatric or physical disorder. These have also been reported to occur in association with the use of triazolam.

Because some of the adverse effects of triazolam appear to be dose related (see PRECAUTIONS and DOSAGE AND ADMINISTRATION), it is important to use the smallest possible effective dose. Elderly patients are especially susceptible to dose related adverse effects.

An increase in daytime anxiety has been reported for triazolam after as few as 10 days of continuous use. In some patients this may be a manifestation of interdose withdrawal (see CLINICAL PHARMACOLOGY). If increased daytime anxiety is observed during treatment, discontinuation of treatment may be advisable.

A variety of abnormal thinking and behavior changes have been reported to occur in association with the use of benzodiazepine hypnotics including triazolam. Some of these changes may be characterized by decreased inhibition, e.g. aggressiveness and extroversion that seem excessive, similar to that seen with alcohol and other CNS depressants (*e.g.,* sedative/hypnotics). Other kinds of behavioral changes have also been reported, for example, bizarre behavior, agitation, hallucinations, depersonalization. In primarily depressed patients, the worsening of depression, including suicidal thinking, has been reported in association with the use of benzodiazepines.

It can rarely be determined with certainty whether a particular instance of the abnormal behaviors listed above is drug induced, spontaneous in origin, or a result of an underlying psychiatric or physical disorder. Nonetheless, the emergence of any new behavioral sign or symptom of concern requires careful and immediate evaluation.

WARNINGS: *(cont'd)*

Because of its depressant CNS effects, patients receiving triazolam should be cautioned against engaging in hazardous occupations requiring complete mental alertness such as operating machinery or driving a motor vehicle. For the same reason, patients should be cautioned about the concomitant ingestion of alcohol and other CNS depressant drugs during treatment with triazolam tablets.

As with some, but not all benzodiazepines, anterograde amnesia of varying severity and paradoxical reactions have been reported following therapeutic doses of triazolam. Data from several sources suggest that anterograde amnesia may occur at a higher rate with triazolam than with other benzodiazepine hypnotics.

PRECAUTIONS:

General: In elderly and/or debilitated patients it is recommended that treatment with triazolam tablets be initiated at 0.125 mg to decrease the possibility of development of oversedation, dizziness, or impaired coordination.

Some side effects reported in association with the use of triazolam appear to be dose related. These include drowsiness, dizziness, light-headedness, and amnesia.

The relationship between dose and what may be more serious behavioral phenomena is less certain. Specifically, some evidence, based on spontaneous marketing reports, suggests that confusion, bizarre or abnormal behavior, agitation, and hallucinations may also be dose related, but this evidence is inconclusive. In accordance with good medical practice it is recommended that therapy be initiated at the lowest effective dose (see DOSAGE AND ADMINISTRATION).

Cases of "traveler's amnesia" have been reported by individuals who have taken triazolam to induce sleep while traveling, such as during an airplane flight. In some of these cases, insufficient time was allowed for the sleep period prior to awakening and before beginning activity. Also, the concomitant use of alcohol may have been a factor in some cases.

Caution should be exercised if triazolam is prescribed to patients with signs or symptoms of depression that could be intensified by hypnotic drugs. Suicidal tendencies may be present in such patients and protective measures may be required. Intentional overdosage is more common in these patients, and the least amount of drug that is feasible should be available to the patient at any one time.

The usual precautions should be observed in patients with impaired renal or hepatic function, chronic pulmonary insufficiency, and sleep apnea. In patients with compromised respiratory function, respiratory depression and apnea have been reported infrequently.

Information for the Patient: The text of a patient package insert is printed at the end of this insert. To assure safe and effective use of triazolam, the information and instructions provided in this patient package insert should be discussed with patients.

Laboratory Tests: Laboratory tests are not ordinarily required in otherwise healthy patients.

Carcinogenesis, Mutagenesis, and Impairment of Fertility: No evidence of carcinogenic potential was observed in mice during a 24-month study with triazolam in doses up to 4,000 times the human dose.

Pregnancy, Teratogenic Effects, Pregnancy Category X: See CONTRAINDICATIONS.

Non-teratogenic effects: It is to be considered that the child born of a mother who is on benzodiazepines may be at some risk for withdrawal symptoms from the drug, during the postnatal period. Also, neonatal flaccidity has been reported in an infant born of a mother who had been receiving benzodiazepines.

Nursing Mothers: Human studies have not been performed; however, studies in rats have indicated that triazolam and its metabolites are secreted in milk. Therefore, administration of triazolam to nursing mothers is not recommended.

Pediatric Use: Safety and efficacy of triazolam in children below the age of 18 have not been established.

DRUG INTERACTIONS:

Both pharmacodynamic and pharmacokinetic interactions have been reported with benzodiazepines. In particular, triazolam produces additive CNS depressant effects when co-administered with other psychotropic medications, anticonvulsants, antihistamines, ethanol, and other drugs which themselves produce CNS depression.

Pharmacokinetic interactions can occur when triazolam is administered along with drugs that interfere with its metabolism. Specific examples, documented with evidence from controlled trials, show that the co-administration of either cimetidine or erythromycin with triazolam causes an approximate doubling of the elimination half-life and plasma levels of triazolam. Consequently, consideration of dose reduction may be appropriate in patients treated concomitantly with either cimetidine or erythromycin and triazolam.

ADVERSE REACTIONS:

During placebo-controlled clinical studies in which 1003 patients received triazolam Tablets, the most troublesome side effects were extensions of the pharmacologic activity of triazolam, e.g. drowsiness, dizziness, or light-headedness.

The figures cited below are estimates of untoward clinical event incidence among subjects who participated in the relatively short duration (*i.e.,* 1 to 42 days) placebo-controlled clinical trials of triazolam. The figures cannot be used to predict precisely the incidence of untoward events in the course of usual medical practice where patient characteristics and other factors often differ from those in clinical trials. These figures cannot be compared with those obtained from other clinical studies involving related drug products and placebo, as each group of drug trials is conducted under a different set of conditions.

Comparison of the cited figures, however, can provide the prescriber with some basis for estimating the relative contributions of drug and nondrug factors to the untoward event incidence rate in the population studied. Even this use must be approached cautiously, as a drug may relieve a symptom in one patient while inducing it in others. (For example, an anticholinergic, anxiolytic drug may relieve dry mouth (a sign of anxiety) in some subjects but induce it (an untoward event) in others. (TABLE 1)

TABLE 1

Number of Patients % Patients Reporting: Central Nervous System	Halcion 1003	Placebo 997
Drowsiness	14.0	6.4
Headache	9.7	8.4
Dizziness	7.8	3.1
Nervousness	5.2	4.5
Light-headedness	4.9	0.9
Coordination, disorders/ataxia	4.6	0.8
Gastrointestinal		
Nausea/vomiting	4.6	3.7

ADVERSE REACTIONS: *(cont'd)*

In addition to the relatively common (*i.e.,* 1% or greater) untoward events enumerated above, the following adverse events have been reported less frequently (*i.e.,* 0.9% to 0.5%): euphoria, tachycardia, tiredness, confusional states/memory impairment, cramps/pain, depression, visual disturbances.

Rare (*i.e.,* less than 0.5%) adverse reactions included constipation, taste alterations, diarrhea, dry mouth, dermatitis/allergy, dreaming/nightmares, insomnia, paresthesia, tinnitus, dysesthesia, weakness, congestion, death from hepatic failure in a patient also receiving diuretic drugs.

In addition to these untoward events for which estimates of incidence are available, the following adverse events have been reported in association with the use of triazolam and other benzodiazepines: amnestic symptoms (anterograde amnesia with appropriate or inappropriate behavior), confusional states (disorientation, derealization, depersonalization, and/or clouding of consciousness), dystonia, anorexia, fatigue, sedation, slurred speech, jaundice, pruritus, dysarthria, changes in libido, menstrual irregularities, incontinence, and urinary retention. Other factors may contribute to some of these reactions, e.g. concomitant intake of alcohol or other drugs, sleep deprivation, an abnormal premorbid state, etc.

Other events reported include: paradoxical reactions such as stimulation, mania, an agitational state (restlessness, irritability, and excitation), increased muscle spasticity, sleep disturbances, hallucinations, delusions, aggressiveness, falling, somnambulism, syncope, inappropriate behavior and other adverse behavioral effects. Should these occur, use of the drug should be discontinued.

The following events have also been reported: chest pain, burning tongue/glossitis/stomatitis.

Laboratory analyses were performed on all patients participating in the clinical program for triazolam. The following incidences of abnormalities were observed in patients receiving triazolam and the corresponding placebo group. None of these changes were considered to be of physiological significance (TABLE 2).

TABLE 2

Number of Patients - % of Patients Reporting:	Halcion 380		Placebo 361	
	Low	High	Low	High
HEMATOLOGY				
Hematocrit	*	*	*	*
Hemoglobin	*	*	*	*
Total WBC count	1.7	2.1	*	1.3
Neutrophil count	1.5	1.5	3.3	1.0
Lymphocyte count	2.3	4.0	3.1	3.8
Monocyte count	3.6	*	4.4	1.5
Eosinophil count	10.2	3.2	9.8	3.4
Basophil count	1.7	2.1	*	1.8
URINALYSIS				
Albumin	-	1.1	-	*
Sugar	-	*	-	*
RBC/HPF	-	2.9	-	2.9
WBC/HPF	-	11.7	-	7.9
BLOOD CHEMISTRY				
Creatinine	2.4	1.9	3.6	1.5
Bilirubin	*	1.5	1.0	*
SGOT	*	5.3	*	4.5
Alkaline phosphatase	*	2.2	*	2.6

* Less than 1%

When treatment with triazolam is protracted, periodic blood counts, urinalysis, and blood chemistry analyses are advisable. Minor changes in EEG patterns, usually low-voltage fast activity, have been observed in patients during therapy with triazolam and are of no known significance.

DRUG ABUSE AND DEPENDENCE:

Controlled Substance: Triazolam is a controlled substance under the Controlled Substance Act, and triazolam tablets have been assigned to Schedule IV.

Abuse, Dependence and Withdrawal: Withdrawal symptoms, similar in character to those noted with barbiturates and alcohol (convulsions, tremor, abdominal and muscle cramps, vomiting, sweating, dysphoria, perceptual disturbances and insomnia), have occurred following abrupt discontinuance of benzodiazepines, including triazolam. The more severe symptoms are usually associated with higher dosages and longer usage, although patients at therapeutic dosages given for as few as 1-2 weeks can also have withdrawal symptoms and in some patients there may be withdrawal symptoms (daytime anxiety, agitation) between nightly doses (see CLINICAL PHARMACOLOGY). Consequently, abrupt discontinuation should be avoided and a gradual dosage tapering schedule is recommended in any patient taking more than the lowest dose for more than a few weeks. The recommendation for tapering is particularly important in any patient with a history of seizure.

The risk of dependence is increased in patients with a history of alcoholism, drug abuse, or in patients with marked personality disorders. Such dependence-prone individuals should be under careful surveillance when receiving triazolam. As with all hypnotics, repeat prescriptions should be limited to those who are under medical supervision.

OVERDOSAGE:

Because of the potency of triazolam, some manifestations of overdosage may occur at 2 mg, four times the maximum recommended therapeutic dose (0.5 mg).

Manifestations of overdosage with triazolam tablets include somnolence, confusion, impaired coordination, slurred speech, and ultimately, coma. Respiratory depression and apnea have been reported with overdosages of triazolam. Seizures have occasionally been reported after overdosages.

Death has been reported in association with overdoses of triazolam by itself, as it has with other benzodiazepines. In addition, fatalities have been reported in patients who have overdosed with a combination of a single benzodiazepine, including triazolam, and alcohol; benzodiazepine and alcohol levels seen in some of these cases have been lower than those usually associated with reports of fatality with either substance alone.

As in all cases of drug overdosage, respiration, pulse, and blood pressure should be monitored and supported by general measures when necessary. Immediate gastric lavage should be performed. An adequate airway should be maintained. Intravenous fluids may be administered.

Flumazenil, a specific benzodiazepine receptor antagonist, is indicated for the complete or partial reversal of the sedative effects of benzodiazepines and may be used in situations when an overdose with a benzodiazepine is known or suspected. Prior to the administration of flumazenil, necessary measures should be instituted to secure airway, ventilation and intravenous access. Flumazenil is intended as an adjunct to, not as a substitute for, proper management of benzodiazepine overdose. Patients treated with flumazenil should be monitored for re- sedation, respiratory depression, and other residual benzodiazepine effects for an appropriate period after treatment. **The prescriber should be aware of a risk of seizure in**

OVERDOSAGE: *(cont'd)*

association with flumazenil treatment, particularly in long-term benzodiazepine users and in cyclic antidepressant overdose. The flumazenil package insert including CONTRAINDICATIONS, WARNINGS and PRECAUTIONS should be consulted to prior use.

Experiments in animals have indicated that cardiopulmonary collapse can occur with massive intravenous doses of triazolam. This could be reversed with positive mechanical respiration and the intravenous infusion of norepinephrine bitartrate or metaraminol bitartrate. Hemodialysis and forced diuresis are probably of little value. As with the management of intentional overdosage with any drug, the physician should bear in mind that multiple agents may have been ingested by the patient.

The oral LD_{50} in mice is greater than 1,000 mg/kg and in rats is greater than 5,000 mg/kg.

DOSAGE AND ADMINISTRATION:

It is important to individualize the dosage of triazolam tablets for maximum beneficial effect and to help avoid significant adverse effects.

The recommended dose for most adults is 0.25 mg before retiring. A dose of 0.125 mg may be found to be sufficient for some patients (*e.g.,* low body weight). A dose of 0.5 mg should be used only for exceptional patients who do not respond adequately to a trial of a lower dose since the risk of several adverse reactions increases with the size of the dose administered. A dose of 0.5 mg should not be exceeded.

In geriatric and/or debilitated patients the recommended dosage range is 0.125 mg to 0.25 mg. Therapy should be initiated at 0.125 mg in this group and the 0.25 mg dose should be used only for exceptional patients who do not respond to a trial of the lower dose. A dose of 0.25 mg should not be exceeded in these patients.

As with all medications, the lowest effective dose should be used.

Store at controlled room temperature 15°-30° C (59°-86° F).

PATIENT PACKAGE INSERT:

The text of the patient insert for triazolam is set forth below.

Introduction: Triazolam is intended to help you sleep. It is one of several benzodiazepine sleeping pills that have generally similar properties. Anyone who is considering using one of these medications should be aware of both their benefits and several important risks and limitations, including diminishing effectiveness with continued use and the possible development of dependence (addiction) and possibly mental changes particularly when the drugs are used for more than a few days to a week. This patient information statement is intended to provide you with knowledge about this class of medications in general and about triazolam in particular that will be useful to guide you in the safe use of this product, **But It Should Not Replace A Discussion Between You And Your Physician About The Risks And Benefits Of Triazolam.**

This leaflet will focus on the beneficial and adverse effects of all members of this class of medications, as well as some specific information about triazolam. There are some differences among these products, and your physician may wish to discuss any specific advantages and disadvantages of particular members of this drug class with you.

Effectiveness Of Benzodiazepine Sleeping Pills: Benzodiazepine sleeping pills are effective medications and are relatively free of serious problems when they are used for **short-term**management of sleep problems (insomnia). insomnia is not always the same. It may be reflected in difficulty in falling asleep, frequent awakening during the night, and/or early morning awakening. Insomnia is often transient in nature, responding to brief treatment with sleeping pills. Use for more than a short while requires discussion with your physician about the risks and benefits of prolonged use.

SIDE EFFECTS

Common Side Effects: The most common side effects of benzodiazepine sleeping pills are related to the ability of the medications to make you sleepy; drowsiness, dizziness, lightheadedness, and difficulty with coordination. Users must be cautious about engaging in hazardous activities requiring complete mental alertness, e.g. operating machinery or driving a motor vehicle. Do not take alcohol while using triazolam. Benzodiazepine sleeping pills should not be used with other medications or substances that may cause drowsiness, without discussing said use with your physician.

How sleepy you are the day after you use one of these sleep medications depends on your individual response and on how quickly the product is eliminated from your body. The larger the dose, the more likely an individual will experience next day residual effects such as drowsiness. For this reason, it is important to use the lowest effective dose for each individual patient. Benzodiazepines that are eliminated rapidly, (*e.g.,* triazolam) tend to cause less next day drowsiness but may cause more withdrawal problems the day after use (see PATIENT PACKAGE INSERT, Special Concerns).

SPECIAL CONCERNS

Memory Problems: All benzodiazepine sleeping pills can cause a special type of amnesia (memory loss) in which a person may not recall events occurring during some period of time, usually several hours, after taking a drug. This is ordinarily not a problem, because the person taking a sleeping pill intends to be asleep during this vulnerable period of time. It can be a problem when the drugs are taken to induce sleep while traveling, such as during an airplane flight, because the person may awake before the effect of the drug is gone. This has been called "traveler's amnesia". Triazolam is more likely than other members of the class to cause this problem.

Tolerance/Withdrawal Phenomena: Some loss of effectiveness or adaptation to the sleep inducing effects of these medications may develop after nightly use for more than a few weeks and there may be a degree of dependence that develops. For the benzodiazepine sleeping pills that are eliminated quickly from the body, a relative deficiency of the drug may occur at some point in the interval between each night's use. This can lead to (1) increased wakefulness during the last third of the night, and (2) the appearance of increased signs of daytime anxiety or nervousness. These two events have been reported in particular for triazolam.

There can be more severe 'withdrawal' effects when a benzodiazepine sleeping pill is stopped. Such effects can occur after discontinuing these drugs following use for only a week or two, but may be more common and more severe after longer periods of continuous use. One type of withdrawal phenomenon is the occurrence of what is known as 'rebound insomnia'. That is, on the first few nights after the drug is stopped, insomnia is actually worse than before the sleeping pill was given. Other withdrawal phenomena following abrupt stopping of benzodiazepine sleeping pills range from mild unpleasant feelings to a major withdrawal syndrome which may include abdominal and muscle cramps, vomiting, sweating, tremor, and rarely, convulsions. These more severe withdrawal phenomena are uncommon.

Dependence/Abuse Phenomena: All benzodiazepine sleeping pills can cause dependence (addiction), especially when used regularly for more than a few weeks or at higher doses. Some people develop a need to continue taking these drugs, either at the prescribed dose or at increasing doses, not so much for continued therapeutic effect, but rather, to avoid withdrawal phenomena and/or to achieve nontherapeutic effects. Individuals who have been dependent on alcohol or other drugs may be at particular risk of becoming dependent on drugs in this class, but all people appear to be at some risk. This possibility must be considered before extending the use of these drugs for more than a few weeks.

PATIENT PACKAGE INSERT: *(cont'd)*

Mental and Behavioral Changes: A variety of abnormal thinking and behavior changes have been reported to occur in association with the use of benzodiazepine sleeping pills. Some of these changes are like the release of inhibition seen in association with alcohol, e.g. aggressiveness and extroversion that seem out of character. Others, however, can be more unusual and more extreme, such as confusion, bizarre behavior, agitation, hallucinations, depersonalization, and worsening of depression, including suicidal thinking. It is rarely clear whether such events are induced by the drug being taken, are caused by some underlying illness or are simply spontaneous happenings. In fact, worsened insomnia may in some cases be associated with illnesses that were present before the medication was used. In any event, the most important fact is to understand that regardless of the cause, users of these medications should promptly report any mental or behavioral changes to their doctor.

Effects on Pregnancy: Certain benzodiazepines have been linked to birth defects when administered during the early months of pregnancy. In addition, the administration of benzodiazepines during the last weeks of pregnancy has been associated with sedation of the fetus. Consequently, the use of this drug should be avoided at any time during pregnancy.

Safe Use Of Benzodiazepine Sleeping Pills: To assure the safe and effective use of triazolam, you should adhere to the following cautions:

1. Triazolam is a prescription medication and, therefore, should be used only as directed by your doctor. Follow your doctor's advice about how to take it, when to take it, and how long to take it. As with other prescription medication, triazolam should be taken only by the individual for whom it is prescribed.

2. Do not extend your use of triazolam beyond 7-10 days without first consulting your physician.

3. If you develop any unusual and disturbing thoughts or behavior during treatment with triazolam, you should discuss such problems with your physician.

4. Inform your physician about any alcohol consumption and medicine you are taking now, including drugs you may buy without a prescription. Do not use alcohol while taking triazolam.

5. Do not take triazolam in circumstances where a full night's sleep and elimination of the drug from the body are not possible before you would again need to be active and functional, e.g. an overnight flight of less than 7-8 hours, because amnestic episodes have been reported in such situations.

6. Do not increase the prescribed dose except on the advice of your physician.

7. Until you experience how this medication affects you, do not drive a car or operate potentially dangerous machinery, etc.

8. Be aware that you may experience an increase in sleep difficulties (rebound insomnia) on the first night or two after discontinuing triazolam.

9. Inform your physician if you are planning to become pregnant, if you are pregnant, or if you become pregnant while you are taking this medicine. The use of triazolam should be avoided at any time during pregnancy.

HOW SUPPLIED - RATED THERAPEUTICALLY EQUIVALENT:

Tablet, Plain Coated - Oral - 0.125 mg

10's	$4.84	Triazolam, H.C.F.A. F F P	99999-2375-04
10's	**$6.78**	**HALCION, Pharmacia & Upjohn**	**00009-0010-06**
10's	$61.63	Triazolam, Par Pharm	49884-0453-62
100's	$48.42	Triazolam, H.C.F.A. F F P	99999-2375-05
100's	$58.14	Triazolam, Roxane	00054-4858-06
100's	$59.68	Triazolam, Greenstone	59762-3717-01
100's	$60.22	Triazolam, Schein Pharm (US)	00364-2598-33
100's	$60.80	Triazolam, Qualitest Pharms	00603-6186-10
100's	$61.00	Triazolam, Geneva Pharms	00781-1441-83
100's	$61.63	Triazolam, Goldline Labs	00182-0175-13
100's	$64.00	Triazolam, Roxane	00054-8858-25
100's	$64.87	Triazolam, Aligen Independ	00405-0192-10
100's	$65.25	Triazolam, Geneva Pharms	00781-1441-13
100's	**$67.80**	**HALCION, Pharmacia & Upjohn**	**00009-0010-38**
100's	**$67.83**	**Halcion, Pharmacia & Upjohn**	**00009-0010-32**
500's	$242.10	Triazolam, H.C.F.A. F F P	99999-2375-06
500's	$282.14	Triazolam, Greenstone	59762-3717-03
500's	$283.00	Triazolam, Roxane	00054-4858-29
500's	$289.41	Triazolam, Qualitest Pharms	00603-6186-28
500's	$291.56	Triazolam, Par Pharm	49884-0453-05
500's	$295.97	Triazolam, Geneva Pharms	00781-1441-05
500's	$306.90	Triazolam, Aligen Independ	00405-0192-02
500's	**$329.13**	**HALCION, Pharmacia & Upjohn**	**00009-0010-11**

Tablet, Plain Coated - Oral - 0.25 mg

10's	$5.28	Triazolam, H.C.F.A. F F P	99999-2375-01
10's	**$7.42**	**HALCION, Pharmacia & Upjohn**	**00009-0017-58**
10's	$67.17	Triazolam, Par Pharm	49884-0454-62
100's	$52.86	Triazolam, H.C.F.A. F F P	99999-2375-02
100's	$60.57	Triazolam, Rugby	00536-5648-21
100's	$63.05	Triazolam, Roxane	00054-4859-06
100's	$64.73	Triazolam, Schein Pharm (US)	00364-2599-33
100's	$65.24	Triazolam, Greenstone	59762-3718-01
100's	$66.68	Triazolam, Geneva Pharms	00781-1442-83
100's	$66.93	Triazolam, Qualitest Pharms	00603-6187-10
100's	$67.17	Triazolam, Goldline Labs	00182-0176-13
100's	$67.22	Triazolam, Geneva Pharms	00781-1442-13
100's	$69.00	Triazolam, Roxane	00054-8859-25
100's	$70.70	Triazolam, Aligen Independ	00405-0193-10
100's	**$74.15**	**HALCION, Pharmacia & Upjohn**	**00009-0017-55**
500's	$264.30	Triazolam, H.C.F.A. F F P	99999-2375-03
500's	$307.26	Triazolam, Greenstone	59762-3718-03
500's	$309.00	Triazolam, Roxane	00054-4859-29
500's	$315.43	Triazolam, Schein Pharm (US)	00364-2599-05
500's	$317.78	Triazolam, Qualitest Pharms	00603-6187-28
500's	$318.53	Triazolam, Goldline Labs	00182-0176-05
500's	$318.53	Triazolam, Par Pharm	49884-0454-05
500's	$323.36	Triazolam, Geneva Pharms	00781-1442-05
500's	$335.29	Triazolam, Aligen Independ	00405-0193-02
500's	**$359.57**	**HALCION, Pharmacia & Upjohn**	**00009-0017-02**

TRICHLORMETHIAZIDE *(002376)*

CATEGORIES: Antihypertensives; Cirrhosis; Congestive Heart Failure; Diuretics; Edema; Electrolytic, Caloric-Water Balance; Glomerulonephritis; Heart Failure; Hypertension; Nephrotic Syndrome; Renal Drugs; Renal Failure; Thiazides; Pregnancy Category C; FDA Approval Pre 1982

BRAND NAMES: *Achletin*; *Anatran*; Aquacot; Aquazide; Aquex; *Carvacron*; *Deltowin*; *Diu-Fortan*; Diurese; *Doqua*; *Esmarin*; *Fluitran*; *Flute*; *Futory*; *Iopran*; *Kuromegu*; Marazide II; **Metahydrin**; Naqua; *Trichlon*; Trichlorex; Trichlormas; *Tricozide*; *Wupin*; *Zoyran*
(International brand names outside U.S. in italics)

FORMULARIES: Medi-Cal

DESCRIPTION:

Trichlormethiazide tablets contain trichlormethiazide, USP for use as an antihypertensive and diuretic drug. They are to be taken orally.

Trichlormethiazide is a member of a class of antihypertensive and diuretic drugs known as benzothiadiazines. The empirical formula is $C_8H_8Cl_3N_3O_4S_2$ with a molecular weight of 380.65; the chemical name is 6-Chloro-3-(dichloromethyl)-3,4-dihydro-2*H*-1,2,4-benzothiadiazine -7-sulfonamide 1,1- dioxide

Trichlormethiazide is a white or practically white crystalline powder. It is very slightly soluble in water and sparingly soluble in alcohol.

Each tablet contains 2 mg or 4 mg of trichlormethiazide.

The inactive ingredients for trichlormethiazide 2 mg tablets include corn starch, FD&C Red No. 40, lactose, and magnesium stearate.

The inactive ingredients for trichlormethiazide 4 mg tablets include corn starch, D&C Yellow No. 10 Al Lake, FD&C Blue No.1 Al Lake, lactose, and magnesium stearate.

CLINICAL PHARMACOLOGY:

The thiazide (benzothiadiazine) diuretics are a class of drug products that have close structural similarity and many similar pharmacological, physiochemical, and pharmacokinetic properties. The thiazide diuretics, including trichlormethiazide, are used generally as adjunctive medication to control the edema associated with various diseases and in the management of hypertension. (See INDICATIONS AND USAGE).

Thiazide diuretics enhance the renal excretion of sodium chloride and water by interfering with the transport of sodium ions across the renal tubular epithelium, primarily in the cortical diluting segment of the nephron. The thiazides also evoke a significant augmentation of potassium excretion, possibly due to the increased amount of sodium reaching the distal tubular site of sodium-potassium exchange. Long-term thiazide therapy can cause mild metabolic alkalosis associated with hypokalemia and hypochloremia.

The glomerular filtration rate is decreased by thiazides. This is of little significance in affecting primary drug action, but may be of clinical importance in patients with diminished renal reserve, contributing to decreased diuretic efficacy. When the glomerular filtration rate falls below 20 ml per minute, the thiazides may not be effective.

Thiazides may decrease uric acid excretion in man, thus increasing the plasma uric acid concentration.

Thiazides may induce hyperglycemia, aggravate existing diabetes mellitus, or precipitate diabetes in prediabetic patients. The exact mechanism of action causing these effects is not certain.

The excretion of certain other ions is affected by the thiazide diuretics: magnesium excretion is enhanced, leading to hypomagnesemia, calcium excretion is decreased relative to that of sodium iodide and bromide excretion occurs by renal mechanisms similar to those for chloride, possibly leading to slight iodide depletion and allowing chloruretic agents to be useful in the management of bromide intoxication.

Thiazide diuretics have antihypertensive activity *per se* in hypertensive patients and also may augment the actions of other antihypertensive drugs. The full mechanism of antihypertensive action is not known. Therapy for hypertension is often initiated with a thiazide diuretic which induces diuresis, natriuresis, depletion of extracellular fluid, and reduction of cardiac output. Direct arteriolar dilatation may play a role.

Plasma renin activity is elevated during thiazide therapy. The aldosterone secretion rate is increased slightly but significantly this contributes to the hypokalemia caused by thiazides.

Paradoxically, thiazides decrease urine volume in patients with diabetes insipidus, and thirst and water consumption decrease.

At maximal therapeutic doses, all thiazides are approximately equal in their diuretic and antihypertensive activities. The comparative effective daily dose range for chlorothiazide is 250 to 2000 mg; for hydrochlorothiazide 20 to 150 mg; and for trichlormethiazide 2 to 8 mg.

Thiazides are absorbed rapidly from the gastrointestinal tract. Most show demonstrable diuresis within an hour, and peak effects occur 3 to 6 hours after oral administration. Distribution is essentially limited to the extracellular fluid space, with little, if any, accumulation in tissues other than the kidneys. The duration of diuretic action of thiazides is determined by the rate of excretion. Chlorothiazide and hydrochlorothiazide act for six to 12 hours; trichlormethiazide for 24 hours. In general, thiazides with relatively long durations of action show proportionately high degrees of plasma protein-binding. Most thiazides are excreted primarily as unchanged drug in the urine.

Thiazides pass readily through the placenta to the fetus, and also appear in the milk of nursing mothers.

INDICATIONS AND USAGE:

Trichlormethiazide tablets are indicated as adjunctive therapy in edema associated with congestive heart failure, hepatic cirrhosis, and corticosteroid and estrogen therapy.

Trichlormethiazide tablets are indicated for the treatment of edema due to various forms of renal dysfunction, such as nephrotic syndrome, acute glomerulonephritis, and chronic renal failure.

Trichlormethiazide tablets are indicated in the management of hypertension either as the sole therapeutic agent or to enhance the effectiveness of other antihypertensive drugs in the more severe forms of hypertension.

Trichlormethiazide tablets are indicated in pregnancy only when the edema is due to pathologic causes. (See PRECAUTIONS, Pregnancy, Teratogenic Effects, Pregnancy Category B, and PRECAUTIONS, Nonteratogenic Effects). The routine use of diuretics in an otherwise healthy woman is inappropriate and exposes the mother and fetus to unnecessary hazard. Diuretics do not prevent development of toxemia of pregnancy, and there is no satisfactory evidence that they are useful in the treatment of toxemia. Edema during pregnancy may arise from pathologic causes or from the physiologic and mechanical consequences of pregnancy. Dependent edema in pregnancy, resulting from restriction of venous return by the expanded uterus, is properly treated through elevation of the lower extremities and use of support hose; use of diuretics to lower intravascular volume in this case is illogical and unnecessary. During normal pregnancy there is hypervolemia which is harmful to neither the fetus nor the mother (in the absence of cardiovascular disease), but which is associated with edema, including generalized edema, in the majority of pregnant women. If this edema produces discomfort, increased recumbency will often provide relief. In rare instances, this edema may cause extreme discomfort which is not relieved by rest. In these cases, a short course of diuretics may be appropriate and provide relief.

CONTRAINDICATIONS:

Trichlormethiazide tablets are contraindicated in patients with anuria and in those who are allergic to this drug, to other thiazides or to other sulfonamide-derived drugs. The routine use of thiazides is contraindicated in otherwise healthy pregnant women with mild edema. (See INDICATIONS AND USAGE and PRECAUTIONS, Pregnancy Category C.)

WARNINGS:

Thiazides should be used with caution in severe renal disease. In patients with renal disease thiazides may precipitate azotemia. Cumulative effects of the drug may develop in patients with impaired renal function.

Thiazides should be used with caution in patients with impaired hepatic function or progressive liver disease, since minor alterations of fluid and electrolyte balance may precipitate hepatic coma.

Thiazides may add to or potentiate the action of other antihypertensive drugs. Potentiation occurs with ganglionic or peripheral adrenergic blocking drugs.

Hypersensitivity reactions may occur in patients with a history of allergy, including aspirin sensitivity or bronchial asthma.

The exacerbation or activation of systemic lupus erythematosus has been reported.

Lithium should generally not be given with diuretics because the latter reduce its renal clearance and increase the risk of lithium toxicity.

PRECAUTIONS:

GENERAL

Periodic determinations of serum electrolytes should be done at appropriate intervals. Serum and urine electrolyte determinations are particularly important when the patient is vomiting excessively, having diarrhea, or receiving parenteral fluids. Thiazides may cause hyponatremia, hypochloremic alkalosis, hypokalemia, hypomagnesemia, and changes in serum and urine calcium. All patients receiving thiazide therapy should be observed for the clinical warning signs of fluid or electrolyte imbalance, irrespective of cause, including dryness of mouth, thirst, weakness, lethargy, drowsiness, restlessness, muscular pains, fatigue, or cramps, hypotension, tachycardia, oliguria, and gastrointestinal disturbances such as nausea and vomiting.

Hypokalemia may develop with trichlormethiazide as with other potent diuretics, including other thiazides, especially when the diuresis is brisk or when severe cirrhosis is present, or during the concomitant use of corticosteroids or ACTH. Hypokalemia poses an increased risk in digitalized patients and patients with cirrhosis, since decreases in the serum potassium concentration can precipitate serious arrhythmias during digitalis therapy, and in cirrhotic patients low potassium levels may precipitate hepatic coma. Thiazides should be discontinued immediately if signs of impending hepatic coma appear.

Chloride deficit are usually mild and usually do not require treatment except under extraordinary circumstances, as in liver or renal disease. Hypochloremic alkalosis may occur with hypokalemia, especially if patients are losing additional potassium and chloride from vomiting, diarrhea, gastrointestinal disease, or potassium-losing renal diseases.

Dilutional hyponatremia may occur or be aggravated during thiazide therapy in edematous patients especially in hot weather. Appropriate therapy is water restriction; salt should not be administered unless the hyponatremia is life threatening. In actual body salt depletion, appropriate replacement is the therapy of choice, however.

Serum and urine electrolyte determinations are particularly important to diagnose and treat electrolyte disturbances.

Hyperuricemia may occur in patients receiving thiazides or related diuretics. While usually asymptomatic, frank gout may occur in patients with a history of gout, a familial predisposition to gout, or chronic renal failure.

Insulin or oral hypoglycemic drug requirements may be altered in patients with diabetes mellitus because thiazides and related diuretics can produce hyperglycemia and glycosuria. Latent diabetes mellitus may become manifest during thiazide administration. Reversible oculomotor paresis has occurred as a manifestation of thiazide-induced glucose intolerance.

The antihypertensive effects of thiazides may be enhanced in post-sympathectomy patients.

If progressive renal impairment becomes evident during thiazide therapy, careful reappraisal of therapy is necessary with consideration given to withholding or discontinuing diuretic dosing. Nonprotein nitrogen, blood urea nitrogen, or serum creatinine levels should be determined since these will be increased in renal impairment.

INFORMATION FOR THE PATIENT

Physicians should give the following information and instructions to patients receiving thiazide diuretics. This information is intended to aid in the safe and effective use of this medication. It is not a disclosure of possible adverse or intended effects.

1. This drug must be taken on a regular schedule to be effective. Take as prescribed. Do not skip doses. If a dose is missed, do not double the dose. Do not take extra doses.

2. Use of this drug with other medications should be done only with a physician's advice. If other drugs are required for control of edema or hypertension, the patients should understand the need for compliance with the total therapeutic program.

3. This drug should be used only by the patient for whom it is prescribed. Do not allow anyone else to take this medication.

4. Pregnancy or plans for pregnancy should be discussed with the physician.

5. Since thiazides appear in breast milk, it is recommended that the baby not be breast fed.

6. The patient should be alerted to the possibilities of various side effects which might occur during thiazide therapy, including particularly changes in the control or severity of concurrent illnesses such as liver or kidney disease, diabetes mellitus, systemic lupus erythematosus, and gout.

7. The patient should be alerted to the effects of diuresis, including excessive losses of sodium, chloride and especially potassium, and how to provide for replacement.

8. Dietary instructions should be provided.

9. As required, return for laboratory tests.

LABORATORY TESTS

Since thiazides affect many organ functions, the safe and effective use of these drugs may require pretreatment and periodic laboratory tests. They may be helpful in following the patient's initial response or status after prolonged therapy in avoiding or identifying possible adverse reactions, as in patients who are vomiting or who have serious diseases such as severe hepatic disease, renal disease, diabetes mellitus or gout, in patients who are receiving concomitant medications such as digitalis glycosides or corticosteroids. The following procedures (not necessarily inclusive) should be considered in patient monitoring:

serum electrolyte determinations, especially sodium potassium, chloride, and bicarbonate

serum uric acid and blood glucose

serum creatinine or blood urea nitrogen

liver function tests, including serum transaminases, alkaline phosphatase, and bilirubin levels

electrocardiograms, especially in patients on digitalis glycosides

PRECAUTIONS: *(cont'd)*

DRUG/LABORATORY TEST INTERACTIONS

Thiazides can affect the laboratory test values for electrolytes, such as sodium, potassium, chloride, calcium, magnesium, and iodide, and for glucose uric acid, blood urea nitrogen, and serum creatinine. Thiazides may also interfere with diagnostic testing as follows:

(a) due to pharmacologic or metabolic effects

thiazides may cause false-negative results with the phentolamine and the tyramine tests for pheochromocytoma by attenuating the hypertensive response to tyramine

thiazides may compete with phenolsulfonphthalein (PSP) for renal tubular secretion, resulting in decreased urinary excretion of PSP.

thiazides may cause sulfobromophthalein (BSP) retention, probably due to a reduction in plasma volume and a resultant decrease in hepatic blood flow

thiazides may decrease urinary cortisol excretion, possibly due to changes in cortisol secretion, renal handling or metabolism

thiazides may decrease serum protein-bound iodine, although usually not to subnormal levels, without signs of thyroid disturbance

thiazides may cause increases in serum amylase levels, some reported increases being up to two times pretreatment levels. However, the fact that acute pancreatitis has occurred in patients on thiazides should also be kept in mind

(b) due to interference with laboratory analysis procedures

thiazides, except for chlorothiazide, may interfere with assays of total urinary estrogens and of estriol

thiazides may interfere with urinary 17-hydroxycorticosteroids measurements

CARCINOGENESIS, MUTAGENESIS, AND IMPAIRMENT OF FERTILITY

Long-term dosing studies have not been done with trichlormethiazide to determine whether this drug has carcinogenic potential. No study has been done to determine whether trichlormethiazide is mutagenic.

PREGNANCY CATEGORY B

Teratogenic Effects: Reproduction studies have been performed with trichlormethiazide in rats at doses 250 to 1250 times the recommended human daily dose and have revealed no evidence of impaired fertility or harm to the fetus. There are, however, no adequate and well-controlled studies in pregnant women. Since thiazides cross the placental barrier, their use may expose the fetus to other possible hazards, such as fetal or neonatal jaundice or thrombocytopenia. Trichlormethiazide tablets should be used during pregnancy only if clearly needed and when the potential benefits to the mother justify the potential risks to the infant.

Nonteratogenic Effects: Thiazides cross the placenta and appear in cord blood. Infants born to mothers treated with diuretics have shown changes in body water and electrolytes, although not of apparent clinical significance. Fetal or neonatal jaundice and thrombocytopenia have been reported in newborn infants of women receiving thiazides. There is an unconfirmed report of neonatal hemolysis in two infants attributed to maternal thiazide therapy.

NURSING MOTHERS

Thiazides can decrease milk production. Additionally, thiazides appear in breast milk. Thrombocytopenia can occur in the nursing infant when the mother is taking a thiazide diuretic. Because of the potential for unwanted adverse effects in nursing infants from trichlormethiazide tablets, a decision should be made whether to discontinue nursing or to discontinue the drug, taking into account the importance of the drug to the mother.

PEDIATRIC USE

Thiazide diuretics have been shown to be effective and safe in children when used as recommended. (See INDICATIONS AND USAGEand DOSAGE AND ADMINISTRATION).

DRUG INTERACTIONS:

The following are generally recognized potential thiazide drug interactions (not necessarily inclusive):

Digitalis Glycosides: Thiazides may produce hypokalemia, hypomagnesemia, and hypercalcemia which may predispose the patient to digitalis toxicity. Periodic serum electrolyte determinations may be required, and correction of electrolyte abnormalities, particularly hypokalemia, should be undertaken, either prophylactically or therapeutically. Electrocardiographic monitoring of the patient may be required to evaluate the patient's cardiac status initially and to control treatment.

Corticosteroids (and ACTH): Concomitant use with thiazides may enhance potassium loss. Periodic serum electrolyte determinations may be required, and correction of electrolyte abnormalities, particularly hypokalemia, should be undertaken.

Insulin Preparations And Oral Sulfonylureas: Thiazides may antagonize the hypoglycemic effects of these agents. Dosage adjustment may be necessary.

Diazoxide: Concomitant use of thiazides and diazoxide may potentiate the hyperglycemic, hyperuricemic, and antihypertensive effects of both drugs.

Methyldopa, Reserpine, Guanethidine Sulfate, Prazosin Hydrochloride, And Beta-Adrenergic Receptor Blockers: Concomitant use of a thiazide with most other antihypertensive drugs produces a more pronounced and antihypertensive response than when either drug is used as the sole therapeutic agent. Severe postural hypotension may result if a thiazide is added to the regimen of a patient stabilized on certain hypotensive agents, such as methyldopa, guanethidine sulfate, or prazosin.

Cholestyramine: Cholestyramine may bind thiazides in the gut. Thiazides should be taken at least one hour before cholestyramine.

Lithium Carbonate: Lithium toxicity has been reported in patients receiving thiazides. Renal clearance of lithium is decreased in patients on long-term thiazide treatment, and lithium therapy has been reported in some cases to be associated with morphological changes in the kidneys. Serum lithium concentrations should be measured frequently in such patients also on thiazides.

Tubocurarine And Gallamine: Thiazides may cause prolonged neuromuscular blockade in patients receiving nondepolarizing neuromuscular blocking agents, such as tubocurarine chloride or gallamine.

Probenecid: Thiazide-induced uric acid retention is blocked by probenecid.

Fenfluramine: Fenfluramine has been reported to enhance the blood pressure lowering effect and plasma norepinephrine levels resulting from use with hydrochlorothiazide in obese patients.

Indomethacin: The concomitant administration of indomethacin to hypertensive patients being treated with thiazide diuretics has resulted in partial loss of control of the lowered blood pressure. A possible explanation is inhibition of prostacyclin biosynthesis by indomethacin.

Anticholinergics: Drugs with significant anticholinergic effects on the gastrointestinal tract may delay gastric emptying and enhance the resorption of thiazides.

Sympathomimetic Agents: A decrease in arterial responsiveness to vasopressors (norepinephrine, phenylephrine), of uncertain clinical significance, has been reported during thiazide therapy.

ADVERSE REACTIONS:

The following adverse reactions have been observed, but there is not enough systematic data collection to support an estimate of their frequency.

Gastrointestinal System: pancreatitis; jaundice (intrahepatic cholestatic jaundice), acute cholecystitis; vomiting; diarrhea; nausea; gastric irritation; anorexia; cramping; constipation.

Central Nervous System: vertigo; headache; xanthopsia; dizziness; paresthesias.

Hematologic: aplastic anemia; thrombocytopenia; agranulocytosis; leukopenia.

Dermatologic-Hypersensitivity: anaphylactoid reactions; necrotizing angiitis (vasculitis, cutaneous vasculitis); purpura; photosensitivity; urticaria; rash.

Cardiovascular: orthostatic hypotension may occur and be aggravated by alcohol, barbiturates, or narcotics.

Other: hyperuricemia; hyperglycemia; glycosuria; muscle spasm; weakness; restlessness.

Whenever adverse reactions are moderate or severe, the dosage should be reduced or therapy withdrawn.

OVERDOSAGE:

Accidental or suicidal poisoning with thiazide diuretics has been reported infrequently.

Signs and Symptoms: Diuresis is to be expected; lethargy of varying degrees may appear and may progress to coma within a few hours, with minimal depression of respiration and cardiovascular function and without significant serum electrolyte changes or dehydration. The mechanism of CNS depression with thiazide overdosage is unknown. GI irritation and hypermotility may occur, temporary elevation of BUN has been reported, and serum electrolyte change could occur especially in patients with impaired renal function.

Treatment: Evacuate gastric contents, taking care to prevent aspiration, especially in the stuporous or comatose patient. GI effects are usually of short duration but may require symptomatic treatment.

Monitor serum electrolyte levels and renal function; institute supportive measures as required individually to maintain hydration, electrolyte balance, respiration, and cardiovascular-renal functions.

DOSAGE AND ADMINISTRATION:

Therapy should be individualized according to patient response. Dosage should be titrated to gain maximal therapeutic response and to establish the minimal dose possible to maintain that response.

ADULTS

Edematous Conditions: The usual oral dosage of trichlormethiazide tablets for diuretic effect is 1 to 4 mg daily.

Hypertension: The usual oral dosage of trichlormethiazide tablets for antihypertensive effect is 2 or 4 mg tablet once daily.

CHILDREN

Edematous Conditions or Hypertension: The oral dosage of trichlormethiazide tablets for children over 6 months of age is determined as follows: 0.07 mg/kg 24 hr or 2 mg sqM 24 hr orally as a single dose or divided into two doses.

Dispense in tight containers.

HOW SUPPLIED - EQUIVALENTS NOT AVAILABLE:

Tablet, Uncoated - Oral - 2 mg

100's	$3.00	Trichlormethiazide, Harber Pharm	51432-0883-03
100's	$35.65	NAQUA, Schering	00085-0822-03
100's	**$43.38**	**METAHYDRIN, Hoechst Marion Roussel**	**00068-0062-01**

Tablet, Uncoated - Oral - 4 mg

100's	$3.34	Trichlormethiazide, Qualitest Pharms	00603-6193-21
100's	$3.40	NIAZIDE, Major Pharms	00904-0340-60
100's	$3.50	Trichlormethiazide, Harber Pharm	51432-0884-03
100's	$4.69	Trichlormethiazide, United Res	00677-0361-01
100's	$6.20	Trichlormethiazide, Goldline Labs	00182-0517-01
100's	$7.30	Trichlormethiazide, Rugby	00536-3770-01
100's	$9.74	Trichlormethiazide, Camall	00147-0143-10
100's	$29.38	DIURESE, Amer Urologicals	00539-0801-01
100's	$61.58	NAQUA, Schering	00085-0547-03
100's	**$71.94**	**METAHYDRIN, Hoechst Marion Roussel**	**00068-0063-01**
1000's	$9.00	Trichlormethiazide, Calvin Scott	17224-0509-10
1000's	$18.00	AQUACOT, C O Truxton	00463-6248-10
1000's	$19.53	Trichlormethiazide, United Res	00677-0361-10
1000's	$19.58	Trichlormethiazide, HL Moore Drug Exch	00839-5011-16
1000's	$20.95	NIAZIDE, Major Pharms	00904-0340-80
1000's	$55.82	Trichlormethiazide, Camall	00147-0143-20
1000's	$231.25	DIURESE, Amer Urologicals	00539-0801-10

TRICHLOROACETIC ACID *(002377)*

CATEGORIES: Keratolytic Agents; Mucous Membrane Agents; Pharmaceutical Adjuvants; Skin/Mucous Membrane Agents; FDA Pre 1938 Drugs

BRAND NAMES: *Averuk*; *Beruciaporri*; Tri-Chlor; Tri-Verzone; *Verrupor*
(International brand names outside U.S. in italics)

Prescribing information not available at time of publication.

HOW SUPPLIED - EQUIVALENTS NOT AVAILABLE:

Crystals

30 gm	$13.58	Trichloroacetic Acid, Mallinckrodt	00406-2924-34
120 gm	$11.70	Trichloroacetic Acid, Paddock Labs	00574-0677-04
125 gm	$13.94	Trichloroacetic Acid, Mallinckrodt	00406-2924-11
125 gm	$15.28	Trichloroacetic Acid, Mallinckrodt	00406-2928-01
454 gm	$36.33	Trichloroacetic Acid, Paddock Labs	00574-0677-16
480 gm	$45.83	Trichloroacetic Acid, Mallinckrodt	00406-2924-03
500 gm	$49.70	Trichloroacetic Acid, Mallinckrodt	00406-2928-03

Solution - Topical

15 ml	$5.95	TRI-VERZONE, Dynapedic	10360-1002-01

TRIDIHEXETHYL CHLORIDE *(002379)*

CATEGORIES: Anticholinergic Agents; Antimuscarinics/Antispasmodics; Autonomic Drugs; Gastrointestinal Drugs; Peptic Ulcer; Ulcer; Pregnancy Category C; FDA Approval Pre 1982

BRAND NAMES: **Pathilon**

FORMULARIES: Medi-Cal

DESCRIPTION:

Tridihexethyl chloride is a synthetic anticholinergic quaternary ammonium compound chemically described as (3-cyclohexyl-3-hydroxy-3-phenyl-propyl)triethylammonium chloride. It is soluble in H_2O, in methanol and chloroform.

Tridihexethyl Cl oral tablets contains 25 mg of tridihexethyl chloride and the following inactive ingredients: Corn Starch, D&C Red #7, Dibasic Calcium Phosphate, Ethylcellulose, Hydroxypropyl Methylcellulose, Magnesium Stearate, Sodium Starch Glycolate, Stearic Acid, Titanium Dioxide and other ingredients.

CLINICAL PHARMACOLOGY:

As no assay method is available for determination of tridihexethyl chloride in blood, information as to its absorption must be indirectly derived. Gastrointestinal absorption of Tridihexethyl Cl appears to be relatively rapid based on reduction of gastric secretion within 60 minutes following a single oral dose.

Tridihexethyl Cl has atropine-like anticholinergic activity. Maximal antisecretory activity occurs two hours after administration. Following ingestion of a single 25 mg dose, fasting or caffeine-induced gastric secretion is inhibited for 4-5 hours; a 50 or 100 mg dose acts for about 6-8 hours.

Oral dosing with 100 mg Tridihexethyl Cl causes, within 90 minutes, a definite inhibition of motility of the proximal small intestine with no marked gastric or duodenal atonicity. Gastrointestinal motility is reduced for about 4-6 hours after single 25 or 50 mg oral doses.

INDICATIONS AND USAGE:

Effective for use as adjunctive therapy in the treatment of peptic ulcer.

CONTRAINDICATIONS:

Glaucoma; obstructive uropathy (for example, bladder neck obstruction due to prostatic hypertrophy); obstructive disease of the gastrointestinal tract (as in achalasia, paralytic ileus, pyloroduodenal stenosis, etc); intestinal atony of the elderly or debilitated patient; unstable cardiovascular status; severe ulcerative colitis; toxic megacolon complicating ulcerative colitis; myasthenia gravis.

WARNINGS:

In the presence of a high environmental temperature, heat prostration can occur with drug use (fever & heat stroke due to decreased sweating).

Diarrhea may be an early symptom of incomplete intestinal obstruction, especially in patients with ileostomy or colostomy. In this instance, treatment with this drug would be inappropriate and possibly harmful.

PRECAUTIONS:

GENERAL

Use with caution in patients with:

Autonomic neuropathy

Hepatic or renal disease

Early evidence of ileus

Ulcerative colitis—large doses may suppress intestinal motility to the point of producing a paralytic ileus and the use of this drug may precipitate or aggravate the serious complication of toxic megacolon

Hyperthyroidism, coronary heart disease, congestive heart failure, cardiac arrhythmias, hypertension and non-obstructing prostatic hypertrophy

Hiatal hernia associated with reflux esophagitis since anticholinergic drugs may aggravate this condition

It should be noted that the use of anticholinergic drugs in the treatment of gastric ulcer may produce a delay in gastric emptying time (antral stasis) and may complicate such therapy.

Do not rely on the use of the drug in the presence of complication of biliary tract disease.

Investigate any tachycardia before giving anticholinergic (atropine- like) drugs since they may increase the heart rate.

INFORMATION FOR THE PATIENT

Tridihexethyl chloride may produce drowsiness or blurred vision. In this event, the patient should be warned not to engage in activities requiring mental alertness such as operating a motor vehicle or other machinery or perform hazardous work while taking this drug.

CARCINOGENESIS, MUTAGENESIS, AND IMPAIRMENT OF FERTILITY

Long term studies in animals to evaluate the carcinogenic potential of Tridihexethyl Cl or studies to evaluate the mutagenic potential of Tridihexethyl Cl have not been conducted. A reproduction study has been performed in rats with Tridihexethyl Cl at a dose 11 to 15 times the human dose and has revealed no evidence of impaired fertility.

PREGNANCY, TERATOGENIC EFFECTS, PREGNANCY CATEGORY C

Animal reproduction studies to determine the teratogenic potential have not been conducted with Tridihexethyl Cl. It is also not known whether Tridihexethyl Cl can cause fetal harm when administered to a pregnant woman or can affect reproduction capacity. Tridihexethyl Cl should be given to a pregnant woman only clearly needed.

NURSING MOTHERS

It is not known whether Tridihexethyl Cl is secreted in human milk. Pups reared by lactating rats treated with Tridihexethyl Cl had depressed growth rates. Because many drugs are excreted in human milk and because of the potential for serious adverse reactions in nursing infants from Tridihexethyl Cl, a decision should be made whether to discontinue nursing or to discontinue the drug taking into account the importance of the drug to the mother.

DRUG INTERACTIONS:

There are no known interactions of Tridihexethyl Cl with other drugs commonly used in the treatment of peptic ulcer.

ADVERSE REACTIONS:

Adverse reactions may include xerostomia; urinary hesitancy and retention; blurred vision; decreased sweating; tachycardia; palpitations; mydriasis; dilatation of the pupil; cycloplegia; increased ocular tension; loss of taste; headaches; nervousness; drowsiness; weakness; dizziness; insomnia; nausea; vomiting; impotence; suppression of lactation; constipation; bloated feeling; severe allergic reaction or drug idiosyncrasies including anaphylaxis; urticaria and other dermal manifestation; some degree of mental confusion and/or excitement, especially in elderly persons.

OVERDOSAGE:

Signs and Symptoms Acute overdosage of anticholinergic agents can produce dry mouth, difficulty swallowing, marked thirst; blurred vision, photophobia; flushed, hot, dry skin; rash; hyperthermia; palpitations, tachycardia with weak pulse, elevated blood pressure; urinary urgency with difficulty in micturition; abdominal distention; restlessness, confusion, delirium and other signs suggestive of an acute toxic psychosis.

OVERDOSAGE: *(cont'd)*

Treatment Treatment is symptomatic and consists of general supportive measures, along with immediate gastric emptying. Supportive management includes maintenance of an airway and attention to vital signs, and may include administration of activated charcoal to reduce absorption and facilitate drug elimination. Physostigmine, because of its own toxicities, is generally reserved for life-threatening complications in anticholinergic drug overdosage. There have been no reports of such serious reactions with Tridihexethyl Cl.

DOSAGE AND ADMINISTRATION:

For effective therapeutic results, in particular with anticholinergic drugs, it is absolutely necessary to titrate dosage against the patient's individual needs and response.

The average oral adult dose is 25 to 50 mg of Tridihexethyl chloride, 3 to 4 times per day. The usual bedtime dose has been 50 mg. A few patients are well controlled on as little as 10 mg 3 times per day, while some require as much as 75 mg 4 times per day. The suggested initial dose is 25 mg 3 times per day before meals and 50 mg at bedtime.

Store at Controlled Room Temperature 15°-30°C (59°-86°F).

HOW SUPPLIED - EQUIVALENTS NOT AVAILABLE:

Tablet, Coated - Oral - 25 mg

100's $66.32 PATHILON, Lederle Pharm 00005-5079-23

TRIENTINE HYDROCHLORIDE *(002380)*

CATEGORIES: Chelating Agents; Cirrhosis; Heavy Metal Antagonists; Orphan Drugs; Wilson's Disease; Pregnancy Category C; FDA Approved 1985 Nov

BRAND NAMES: Cuprid; **Syprine**

DESCRIPTION:

Trientine hydrochloride is *N,N'*-bis (2-aminoethyl) -1,2 ethanediamine dihydrochloride. It is a white to pale yellow crystalline hygroscopic powder. It is freely soluble in water, soluble in methanol, slightly soluble in ethanol, and insoluble in chloroform and ether.

The empirical formula is $C_6H_{18}N_4 \cdot 2HCl$ with a molecular weight of 219.2.

Trientine hydrochloride is a compound for removal of excess copper from the body. Syprine (Trientine Hydrochloride) is available as 250 mg capsules for oral administration. Capsules Syprine contain gelatin, iron oxides, stearic acid, and titanium dioxide as inactive ingredients.

CLINICAL PHARMACOLOGY:

INTRODUCTION

Wilson's disease (hepatolenticular degeneration) is an autosomal inherited metabolic defect resulting in an inability to maintain a near-zero balance of copper. Excess copper accumulates possibly because the liver lacks the mechanism to excrete free copper into the bile. Hepatocytes store excess copper but when their capacity is exceeded copper is released into the blood and is taken up into extrahepatic sites. This condition is treated with a low copper diet and the use of chelating agents that bind copper to facilitate its excretion from the body.

Clinical Summary: Forty-one patients (18 male and 23 female) between the ages of 6 and 54 with a diagnosis of Wilson's disease and who were intolerant of d-penicillamine were treated in two separate studies with trientine hydrochloride. The dosage varied from 450 to 2400 mg per day. The average dosage required to achieve an optimal clinical response varied between 1000 mg and 2000 mg per day. The mean duration of trientine hydrochloride therapy was 48.7 months (range 2-164 months). Thirty-four of the 41 patients improved, 4 had no change in clinical global response, 2 were lost to follow-up and one showed deterioration in clinical condition. One of the patients who improved while on therapy with trientine hydrochloride experienced a recurrence of the symptoms of systemic lupus erythematosus which had appeared originally during therapy with penicillamine. Therapy with trientine hydrochloride was discontinued. No other adverse reactions, except iron deficiency, were noted among any of these 41 patients.

One investigator treated 13 patients with trientine hydrochloride following their development of intolerance to d-penicillamine. Retrospectively, he compared these patients to an additional group of 12 patients with Wilson's disease who were both tolerant of and controlled with d-penicillamine therapy, but who failed to continue any copper chelation therapy. The mean age at onset of disease of the latter group was 12 years as compared to 21 years for the former group. The trientine hydrochloride group received d-penicillamine for an average of 4 years as compared to an average of 10 years for the non-treated group.

Various laboratory parameters showed changes in favor of the patients treated with trientine hydrochloride. Free and total serum copper, SGOT, and serum bilirubin all showed mean increases over baseline in the untreated group which were significantly larger than with the patients treated with trientine hydrochloride. In the 13 patients treated with trientine hydrochloride, previous symptoms and signs relating to d-penicillamine intolerance disappeared in 8 patients, improved in 4 patients, and remained unchanged in one patient. The neurological status in the trientine hydrochloride group was unchanged or improved over baseline, whereas in the untreated group, 6 patients remained unchanged and 6 worsened. Kayser-Fleischer rings improved significantly during trientine hydrochloride treatment.

The clinical outcome of the two groups also differed markedly. Of the 13 patients on therapy with trientine hydrochloride (mean duration of therapy 4.1 years; range 1 to 13 years), all were alive at the data cutoff date, and in the non-treated group (mean years with no therapy 2.7 years; range 3 months to 9 years), 9 of the 12 died of hepatic disease.

PHARMACOKINETICS

Data on the pharmacokinetics of trientine hydrochloride are not available. Dosage adjustment recommendations are based upon clinical use of the drug (see DOSAGE AND ADMINISTRATION.)

CLINICAL STUDIES:

PRECLINICAL STUDIES

Chelating Properties: Studies in animals have shown that trientine hydrochloride has cupriuretic activities in both normal and copper-loaded rats. In general, the effects of trientine hydrochloride on urinary copper excretion are similar to those of equimolar doses of penicillamine, although in one study they were significantly smaller.

HUMAN STUDIES

Renal clearance studies were carried out with penicillamine and trientine hydrochloride on separate occasions in selected patients treated with penicillamine for at least one year. Six-hour excretion rates of copper were determined off treatment and after a single dose of 500 mg of penicillamine or 1.2 g of trientine hydrochloride. The mean urinary excretion rates of copper found in TABLE 1.

In patients *not* previously treated with chelating agents, a similar comparison was made in TABLE 2.

CLINICAL STUDIES: *(cont'd)*

TABLE 1

No. of Patients	Single Dose Treatment	Basal Excretion Rate (mg Cu + +/6hr)	Test-dose Excretion Rate (mcg Cu + +/6hr)
6	Trientine, 1.2 g	19	234
4	Penicillamine, 500 mg	17	320

TABLE 2

No. of Patients	Single Dose Treatment	Basal Excretion Rate (mg Cu + +/6hr)	Test-dose Excretion Rate (mcg Cu + +/6hr)
8	Trientine, 1.2 g	71	1326
7	Penicillamin, 500 mg	68	1074

These results demonstrate that trientine is effective as a cupriuretic agent in patients with Wilson's disease although on a molar basis it appears to be less potent or less effective than penicillamine. Evidence from a radio-labelled copper study indicates that the different cupriuretic effect between these two drugs could be due to a difference in selectivity of the drugs for different copper pools within the body.

INDICATIONS AND USAGE:

Trientine is indicated in the treatment of patients with Wilson's disease who are intolerant of penicillamine. Clinical experience with trientine is limited and alternate dosing regimens have not been well-characterized; all endpoints in determining an individual patient's dose have not been well defined. Trientine and penicillamine cannot be considered interchangeable. Trientine should be used when continued treatment with penicillamine is no longer possible because of intolerable or life endangering side effects.

Unlike penicillamine, trientine is not recommended in cystinuria or rheumatoid arthritis. The absence of a sulfhydryl moiety renders it incapable of binding cystine and, therefore, it is of no use in cystinuria. In 15 patients with rheumatoid arthritis, trientine was reported not to be effective in improving any clinical or biochemical parameter after 12 weeks of treatment.

Trientine is not indicated for treatment of biliary cirrhosis.

CONTRAINDICATIONS:

Hypersensitivity to this product.

WARNINGS:

Patient experience with trientine hydrochloride is limited (see CLINICAL PHARMACOLOGY.) Patients receiving trientine should remain under regular medical supervision throughout the period of drug administration. Patients (especially women) should be closely monitored for evidence of iron deficiency anemia.

PRECAUTIONS:

GENERAL

There are no reports of hypersensitivity in patients who have been administered trientine hydrochloride for Wilson's disease. However, there have been reports of asthma, bronchitis and dermatitis occurring after prolonged environmental exposure in workers who use trientine hydrochloride as a hardener of epoxy resins. Patients should be observed closely for signs of possible hypersensitivity.

INFORMATION FOR THE PATIENT

Patients should be directed to take trientine on an empty stomach, at least one hour before meals or two hours after meals and at least one hour apart from any other drug, food, or milk. The capsules should be swallowed whole with water and should not be opened or chewed. Because of the potential for contact dermatitis, any site of exposure to the capsule contents should be washed with water promptly. For the first month of treatment, the patient should have his temperature taken nightly, and he should be asked to report any symptoms such as fever or skin eruption.

LABORATORY TESTS

The most reliable index for monitoring treatment is the determination of free copper in the serum, which equals the difference between quantitatively determined total copper and ceruloplasmin-copper. Adequately treated patients will usually have less than 10 mcg free copper/dl of serum.

Therapy may be monitored with a 24 hour urinary copper analysis periodically (*i.e.*, every 6-12 months). Urine must be collected in copper-free glassware. Since a low copper diet should keep copper absorption down to less than one milligram a day, the patient probably will be in the desired state of negative copper balance if 0.5 to 1.0 milligram of copper is present in a 24-hours collection of urine.

CARCINOGENESIS, MUTAGENESIS, AND IMPAIRMENT OF FERTILITY

Data on carcinogenesis, mutagenesis, and impairment of fertility are not available.

PREGNANCY

Pregnancy Category C: Trientine hydrochloride was teratogenic in rats at doses similar to the human dose. The frequencies of both resorptions and fetal abnormalities, including hemorrhage and edema, increased while fetal copper levels decreased when trientine hydrochloride was given in the material diets of rats. There are no adequate and well-controlled studies in pregnant women. trientine should be used during pregnancy only if the potential benefit justifies the potential risk to the fetus.

NURSING MOTHERS

It is not known whether this drug is excreted in human milk. Because many drugs are excreted in human milk, caution should be exercised when trientine is administered to a nursing mother.

PEDIATRIC USE

Controlled studies of the safety and effectiveness of trientine in children have not been conducted. It has been used clinically in children as young as 6 years with no reported adverse experiences.

DRUG INTERACTIONS:

In general, mineral supplements should not be given since they may block the absorption of trientine. However, iron deficiency may develop, especially in children and menstruating or pregnant women, or as a result of the low copper diet recommended for Wilson's disease. If necessary, iron may be given in short courses, but since iron and trientine each inhibit absorption of the other, two hours should elapse between administration of trientine and iron.

DRUG INTERACTIONS: *(cont'd)*

It is important that trientine be taken on an empty stomach, at least one hour before meals or two hours after meals and at least one hour apart from any other drug, food, or milk. This permits maximum absorption and reduces the likelihood of inactivation of the drug by metal binding in the gastrointestinal tract.

ADVERSE REACTIONS:

Clinical experience with trientine has been limited. The following adverse reactions have been reported in patients with Wilson's disease who were on therapy with trientine hydrochloride: iron deficiency, systemic lupus erythematosus (see CLINICAL PHARMACOLOGY.)

Trientine is not indicated for treatment of biliary cirrhosis, but in one study of 4 patients treated with trientine hydrochloride for primary biliary cirrhosis, the following adverse reactions were reported: heartburn; epigastric pain and tenderness; thickening, fissuring and flaking of the skin; hypochromic abdominal pain, melena; anorexia; malaise; cramps; muscle pain; weakness; rhabdomyolysis. A causal relationship of these reactions to drug therapy should not be rejected or established.

OVERDOSAGE:

There is a report of an adult woman who ingested 30 g of trientine hydrochloride without apparent ill effect. No other data on overdosage are available.

DOSAGE AND ADMINISTRATION:

Systemic evaluation of dose and/or interval between dose has not been done. However, on limited clinical experience, the recommended initial dose of trientine is 500 - 750 mg/day for children and 750 - 1250 mg/day for adults given in divided doses two, three or four times daily. This may be increased to a maximum of 2000 mg/day for adults or 1500 mg/day for children age 12 or under. The daily dose of trientine should be increased only when the clinical response is not adequate or the concentration of free serum copper is persistently above 20 mcg/dl. Optimal long-term maintenance dosage should be determined at 6 - 12 month intervals (see PRECAUTIONS, Laboratory Tests.)

It is important that trientine be given on an empty stomach, at least one hour before meals or two hours after meals and at least one hour apart from any other drug, food, or milk. The capsules should be swallowed whole with water and should not be opened or chewed.

Storage: Keep container tightly closed. Store at 2 - 8°C (36 - 46°F).

HOW SUPPLIED - EQUIVALENTS NOT AVAILABLE:

Capsule, Gelatin - Oral - 250 mg

100's $90.16 SYPRINE, Merck 00006-0661-68

TRIETHANOLAMINE POLYPEPTIDE OLEATE CONDENSATE *(002381)*

CATEGORIES: Cerumenolytics; EENT Drugs; Ear Wax; Eye, Ear, Nose, & Throat Preparations; Otic Preparations; Otologic; Pregnancy Category C; FDA Approval Pre 1982

BRAND NAMES: **Cerumenex**

FORMULARIES: BC-BS

DESCRIPTION:

Cerumenex Eardrops contain Triethanolamine Polypeptide Oleate-Condensate (10%). Inactive Ingredients: Chlorbutanol 0.5%, Propylene Glycol and Water. Triethanolamine Polypeptide Oleate is a hygroscopic-miscible solution with low surface tension and optimal viscosity of 50-90 cps. It also has a slightly acid pH range (5.6-6.0) to approximate the surface of a normal ear canal.

CLINICAL PHARMACOLOGY:

Cerumenex Eardrops emulsify and disperse excess or impacted earwax. The triethanolamine polypeptide oleate, a surfactant, in a hygroscopic vehicle lyses cerumen to facilitate removal by subsequent water irrigation.

INDICATIONS AND USAGE:

For removal of impacted cerumen prior to ear examination, otologic therapy and/or audiometry.

CONTRAINDICATIONS:

Perforated tympanic membrane or otitis media is considered a contraindication to the use of this medication in the external ear canal.

A history of hypersensitivity to Cerumenex Eardrops or to any of its components is also a contraindication to the use of this medication.

WARNINGS:

Discontinue promptly if sensitization or irritation occurs.

PRECAUTIONS:

GENERAL

It is recommended that the following precautions be observed in prescribing and administration of this agent:

Extreme caution is indicated in patients with demonstrable dermatologic idiosyncrasies or with history or allergic reactions is general.

Exposure of the ear canal to the Cerumenex Eardrops should be limited to 15-30 minutes.

When administering Cerumenex Eardrops, care must be taken to avoid undue exposure of the skin outside the ear during the instillation and the flushing out of the medication. If the medication comes in contact with the skin, the area should be washed with soap and water. Use of proper technique (see DOSAGE AND ADMINISTRATION) will help avoid such undue exposure.

Cerumenex Eardrops should be used only with caution in external otitis.

INFORMATION FOR THE PATIENT

Patients should be cautioned to avoid placing the applicator tip into the ear canal.

Patients should be cautioned to gently flush the ear with lukewarm water.

Patients should be warned to use Cerumenex Eardrops in ears only. Surrounding skin should be promptly rinsed of any excess drops.

Patients should be instructed not to leave Cerumenex Eardrops in the ear for longer than 30 minutes. A second application may be made, if needed, but more frequent use must be indicated by the physician.

PRECAUTIONS: *(cont'd)*

Patients must be instructed not be exceed the time of exposure, nor to use medication more frequently than directed by the physician.

Patients should be advised to discontinue the use of the medication in case of a possible reaction and to consult their physician promptly.

CARCINOGENESIS, MUTAGENESIS, AND IMPAIRMENT OF FERTILITY

Long-term animal studies have not been performed to evaluate the carcinogenic potential or the effect on fertility of Cerumenex Eardrops.

PREGNANCY, TERATOGENIC EFFECTS, PREGNANCY CATEGORY C

Animal reproduction studies have not yet been conducted with Cerumenex Eardrops. It is also not known whether Cerumenex Eardrops can cause fetal harm when administered to a pregnant woman or can affect reproduction capacity. Cerumenex Eardrops should be given to a pregnant woman only if clearly needed.

NURSING MOTHERS

It is not known whether this drug is excreted in human milk. Because many drugs are excreted in human milk, caution should be exercised when Cerumenex Eardrops are administered to a nursing mother.

PEDIATRIC USE

Safety and effectiveness in children have not been established.

ADVERSE REACTIONS:

CLINICAL REACTIONS OF POSSIBLE ALLERGIC ORIGIN

Localized dermatitis reactions were reported in about 1% of 2,700 patients treated, ranging from a very mild erythema and pruritus of the external canal to a severe eczematoid reaction involving the external ear and periauricular tissue, generally with duration of 2-10 days. Other reactions which have been reported in connection with the use of Cerumenex Eardrops include allergic contact dermatitis, skin ulcerations, burning and pain at the application site and skin rash.

DOSAGE AND ADMINISTRATION:

1. Fill ear canal with Cerumenex Eardrops with the patient's head tilted at a 45° angle.

2. Insert cotton plug and allow to remain 15-30 minutes.

3. Then gently flush with lukewarm water, using a soft rubber syringe (avoid excessive pressure). Exposure of skin outside the ear to the drug should be avoided. The procedure may be repeated if the first application fails to clear the impaction.

FOR EXTERNAL USE IN THE EAR ONLY

Store at Controlled Room Temperature 15°-30°C (59°-86°F)

HOW SUPPLIED - EQUIVALENTS NOT AVAILABLE:

Liquid - Otic - 10 %

6 ml	$16.15	CERUMENEX, Purdue Frederick	00034-5490-06
12 ml	$25.87	CERUMENEX, Purdue Frederick	00034-5490-12

TRIFLUOPERAZINE HYDROCHLORIDE *(002382)*

CATEGORIES: Antipsychotics/Antimanics; Anxiety; Central Nervous System Agents; Neuroleptics; Phenothiazine Tranquilizers; Psychotherapeutic Agents; Psychotic Disorders; Tranquilizers; Skeletal Muscle Hyperactivity*; Vertigo/Motion Sickness/Vomiting*; FDA Approval Pre 1982

* Indication not approved by the FDA

BRAND NAMES: *Calmazine*; *Domilium*; *Eskazine*; *Espazine*; *Flupazine*; *Fluzine*; *Jatroneural*; *Modalina*; *Nerolet*; *Novoflurazine*; *Psyrazine*; *Sedizine*; **Stelazine**; Suprazine; *Terfluzine*; Tfp

(International brand names outside U.S. in italics)

FORMULARIES: Aetna; BC-BS; Medi-Cal

COST OF THERAPY: $16.65 (Psychotic Disorders; Tablet; 2 mg; 2/day; 90 days) vs. Potential Cost of $3,628.44 (Psychoses)

INDICATIONS AND USAGE:

For the management of the manifestations of psychotic disorders.

Trifluoperazine HCl is effective for the short-term treatment of generalized non-psychotic anxiety. However, trifluoperazine HCl is not the first drug to be used in therapy for most patients with non-psychotic anxiety because certain risks associated with its use are not shared by common alternative treatments (*i.e.,* benzodiazepines).

When used in the treatment of non-psychotic anxiety, trifluoperazine HCl should not be administered at doses of more than 6 mg per day or for longer than 12 weeks because the use of trifluoperazine HCl at higher doses or for longer intervals may cause persistent tardive dyskinesia that may prove irreversible (see WARNINGS).

The effectiveness of trifluoperazine HCl as a treatment for non-psychotic anxiety was established in a 4-week clinical multicenter study of outpatients with generalized anxiety disorder (DSM-III). This evidence does not predict that trifluoperazine HCl will be useful in patients with other non-psychotic conditions in which anxiety, or signs that mimic anxiety, are found (*i.e.,* physical illness, organic mental conditions, agitated depression, character pathologies, etc.).

Trifluoperazine HCl has not been shown effective in the management of behavioral complications in patients with mental retardation.

CONTRAINDICATIONS:

A known hypersensitivity to phenothiazines, comatose or greatly depressed states due to central nervous system depressants, and, in cases of existing blood dyscrasias, bone marrow depression and pre-existing liver damage.

WARNINGS:

Tardive Dyskinesia: Tardive dyskinesia, a syndrome consisting of potentially irreversible, involuntary, dyskinetic movements, may develop in patients treated with neuroleptic (antipsychotic) drugs. Although the prevalence of the syndrome appears to be highest among the elderly, especially elderly women, it is impossible to rely upon prevalence estimates to predict, at the inception of neuroleptic treatment, which patients are likely to develop the syndrome. Whether neuroleptic drug products differ in their potential to cause tardive dyskinesia is unknown.

Both the risk of developing the syndrome and the likelihood that it will become irreversible are believed to increase as the duration of treatment and the total cumulative dose of neuroleptic drugs administered to the patient increase. However, the syndrome can develop, although much less commonly, after relatively brief treatment periods at low doses.

WARNINGS: *(cont'd)*

There is no known treatment for established cases of tardive dyskinesia, although the syndrome may remit, partially or completely, if neuroleptic treatment is withdrawn. Neuroleptic treatment itself, however, may suppress (or partially suppress) the signs and symptoms of the syndrome and thereby may possibly mask the underlying disease process. The effect that symptomatic suppression has upon the long-term course of the syndrome is unknown.

Given these considerations, neuroleptics should be prescribed in a manner that is most likely to minimize the occurrence of tardive dyskinesia. Chronic neuroleptic treatment should generally be reserved for patients who suffer from a chronic illness that 1) is known to respond to neuroleptic drugs, and, 2) for whom alternative, equally effective, but potentially less harmful treatments are *not* available or appropriate. In patients who do require chronic treatment, the smallest dose and the shortest duration of treatment producing a satisfactory clinical response should be sought. The need for continued treatment should be reassessed periodically.

If signs and symptoms of tardive dyskinesia appear in a patient on neuroleptics, drug discontinuation should be considered. However, some patients may require treatment despite the presence of the syndrome.

For further information about the description of tardive dyskinesia and its clinical detection, please refer to the sections on PRECAUTIONS and ADVERSE REACTIONS.

Neuroleptic Malignant Syndrome (NMS) A potentially fatal symptom complex sometimes referred to as Neuroleptic Malignant Syndrome (NMS) has been reported in association with antipsychotic drugs. Clinical manifestations of NMS are hyperpyrexia, muscle rigidity, altered mental status and evidence of autonomic instability (irregular pulse or blood pressure, tachycardia, diaphoresis, and cardiac dysrhythmias).

The diagnostic evaluation of patients with this syndrome is complicated. In arriving at a diagnosis, it is important to identify cases where the clinical presentation includes both serious medical illness (*e.g.,* pneumonia, systemic infection, etc.) and untreated or inadequately treated extrapyramidal signs and symptoms (EPS). Other important considerations in the differential diagnosis include central anticholinergic toxicity, heat stroke, drug fever and primary central nervous system (CNS) pathology.

The management of NMS should include 1) immediate discontinuation of antipsychotic drugs and other drugs not essential to concurrent therapy, 2) intensive symptomatic treatment and medical monitoring, and 3) treatment of any concomitant serious medical problems for which specific treatments are available. There is no general agreement about specific pharmacological treatment regimens for uncomplicated NMS.

If a patient requires antipsychotic drug treatment after recovery from NMS, the potential reintroduction of drug therapy should be carefully considered. The patient should be carefully monitored, since recurrences of NMS have been reported.

An encephalopathic syndrome (characterized by weakness, lethargy, fever, tremulousness and confusion, extrapyramidal symptoms, leukocytosis, elevated serum enzymes, BUN and FBS) has occurred in a few patients treated with lithium plus a neuroleptic. In some instances, the syndrome was followed by irreversible brain damage. Because of a possible causal relationship between these events and the concomitant administration of lithium and neuroleptics, patients receiving such combined therapy should be monitored closely for early evidence of neurologic toxicity and treatment discontinued promptly if such signs appear. This encephalopathic syndrome may be similar to or the same as neuroleptic malignant syndrome (NMS).

Patients who have demonstrated a hypersensitivity reaction (*e.g.,* blood dyscrasias, jaundice) with a phenothiazine should not be re-exposed to any phenothiazine, including trifluoperazine HCl, unless in the judgment of the physician the potential benefits of treatment outweigh the possible hazard.

Trifluoperazine HCl Concentrate contains sodium bisulfite, a sulfite that may cause allergic-type reactions including anaphylactic symptoms and life-threatening or less severe asthmatic episodes in certain susceptible people. The overall prevalence of sulfite sensitivity in the general population is unknown and probably low. Sulfite sensitivity is seen more frequently in asthmatic than in non-asthmatic people.

Trifluoperazine HCl may impair mental and/or physical abilities, especially during the first few days of therapy. Therefore, caution patients about activities requiring alertness (*e.g.,* operating vehicles or machinery).

If agents such as sedatives, narcotics, anesthetics, tranquilizers or alcohol are used either simultaneously or successively with the drug, the possibility of an undesirable additive depressant effect should be considered.

Usage in Pregnancy: Safety for the use of trifluoperazine HCl during pregnancy has not been established. Therefore, it is not recommended that the drug be given to pregnant patients except when, in the judgment of the physician, it is essential. The potential benefits should clearly outweigh possible hazards. There are reported instances of prolonged jaundice, extrapyramidal signs, hyperreflexia or hyporeflexia in newborn infants whose mothers received phenothiazines.

Reproductive studies in rats given over 600 times the human dose showed an increased incidence of malformations above controls and reduced litter size and weight linked to maternal toxicity. These effects were not observed at half this dosage. No adverse effect on fetal development was observed in rabbits given 700 times the human dose nor in monkeys given 25 times the human dose.

Nursing Mothers: There is evidence that phenothiazines are excreted in the breast milk of nursing mothers. Because of the potential for serious adverse reactions in nursing infants from trifluoperazine, a decision should be made whether to discontinue nursing or to discontinue the drug, taking into account the importance of the drug to the mother.

PRECAUTIONS:

General: Given the likelihood that some patients exposed chronically to neuroleptics will develop tardive dyskinesia, it is advised that all patients in whom chronic use is contemplated be given, if possible, full information about this risk. The decision to inform patients and/or their guardians must obviously take into account the clinical circumstances and the competency of the patient to understand the information provided.

Thrombocytopenia and anemia have been reported in patients receiving the drug. Agranulocytosis and pancytopenia have also been reported—warn patients to report the sudden appearance of sore throat or other signs of infection. If white blood cell and differential counts indicate cellular depression, stop treatment and start antibiotic and other suitable therapy.

Jaundice of the cholestatic type of hepatitis or liver damage has been reported. If fever with grippe-like symptoms occurs, appropriate liver studies should be conducted. If tests indicate an abnormality, stop treatment.

One result of therapy may be an increase in mental and physical activity. For example, a few patients with angina pectoris have complained of increased pain while taking the drug. Therefore, angina patients should be observed carefully and, if an unfavorable response is noted, the drug should be withdrawn.

Because hypotension has occurred, large doses and parenteral administration should be avoided in patients with impaired cardiovascular systems. To minimize the occurrence of hypotension after injection, keep patient lying down and observe for at least 1/2 hour. If hypotension occurs from parenteral or oral dosing, place patient in head-low position with

PRECAUTIONS: *(cont'd)*

legs raised. If a vasoconstrictor is required, Levophed* and Neo-Synephrine† are suitable. Other pressor agents, including epinephrine, should not be used as they may cause a paradoxical further lowering of blood pressure.

Since certain phenothiazines have been reported to produce retinopathy, the drug should be discontinued if ophthalmoscopic examination or visual field studies should demonstrate retinal changes.

An antiemetic action of trifluoperazine HCl may mask the signs and symptoms of toxicity or overdosage of other drugs and may obscure the diagnosis and treatment of other conditions such as intestinal obstruction, brain tumor and Reye's syndrome.

With prolonged administration at high dosages, the possibility of cumulative effects, with sudden onset of severe central nervous system or vasomotor symptoms, should be kept in mind.

Neuroleptic drugs elevate prolactin levels; the elevation persists during chronic administration. Tissue culture experiments indicate that approximately 1/3 of human breast cancers are prolactin-dependent *in vitro*, a factor of potential importance if the prescribing of these drugs is contemplated in a patient with a previously detected breast cancer. Although disturbances such as galactorrhea, amenorrhea, gynecomastia and impotence have been reported, the clinical significance of elevated serum prolactin levels is unknown for most patients. An increase in mammary neoplasms has been found in rodents after chronic administration of neuroleptic drugs. Neither clinical nor epidemiologic studies conducted to date, however, have shown an association between chronic administration of these drugs and mammary tumorigenesis; the available evidence is considered too limited to be conclusive at this time.

Chromosomal aberrations in spermatocytes and abnormal sperm have been demonstrated in rodents treated with certain neuroleptics.

Because phenothiazines may interfere with thermoregulatory mechanisms, use with caution in persons who will be exposed to extreme heat.

As with all drugs which exert an anticholinergic effect, and/or cause mydriasis, trifluoperazine should be used with caution in patients with glaucoma.

Phenothiazines may diminish the effect of oral anticoagulants.

Phenothiazines can produce alpha-adrenergic blockade.

Concomitant administration of propranolol with phenothiazines results in increased plasma levels of both drugs.

Antihypertensive effects of guanethidine and related compounds may be counteracted when phenothiazines are used concurrently.

Thiazide diuretics may accentuate the orthostatic hypotension that may occur with phenothiazines.

Phenothiazines may lower the convulsive threshold; dosage adjustments of anticonvulsants may be necessary. Potentiation of anticonvulsant effects does not occur. However, it has been reported that phenothiazines may interfere with the metabolism of Dilantin‡ and thus precipitate Dilantin toxicity.

Drugs which lower the seizure threshold, including phenothiazine derivatives, should not be used with AmipaqueS. As with other phenothiazine derivatives, trifluoperazine HCl should be discontinued at least 48 hours before myelography, should not be resumed for at least 24 hours postprocedure and should not be used for the control of nausea and vomiting occurring either prior to myelography or postprocedure with Amipaque.

The presence of phenothiazines may produce false-positive phenylketonuria (PKU) test results.

Long-Term Therapy: To lessen the likelihood of adverse reactions related to cumulative drug effect, patients with a history of long-term therapy with trifluoperazine HCl and/or other neuroleptics should be evaluated periodically to decide whether the maintenance dosage could be lowered or drug therapy discontinued.

ADVERSE REACTIONS:

Drowsiness, dizziness, skin reactions, rash, dry mouth, insomnia, amenorrhea, fatigue, muscular weakness, anorexia, lactation, blurred vision and neuromuscular (extrapyramidal) reactions.

Neuromuscular (Extrapyramidal) Reactions: These symptoms are seen in a significant number of hospitalized mental patients. They may be characterized by motor restlessness, be of the dystonic type, or they may resemble parkinsonism.

Depending on the severity of symptoms, dosage should be reduced or discontinued. If therapy is reinstituted, it should be at a lower dosage. Should these symptoms occur in children or pregnant patients, the drug should be stopped and not reinstituted. In most cases barbiturates by suitable route of administration will suffice. (Or, injectable BenadrylII may be useful). In more severe cases, the administration of an anti-parkinsonism agent, except levodopa, usually produces rapid reversal of symptoms. Suitable supportive measures such as maintaining a clear airway and adequate hydration should be employed.

Motor Restlessness: Symptoms may include agitation or jitteriness and sometimes insomnia. These symptoms often disappear spontaneously. At times these symptoms may be similar to the original neurotic or psychotic symptoms. Dosage should not be increased until these side effects have subsided.

If this phase becomes too troublesome, the symptoms can usually be controlled by a reduction of dosage or change of drug. Treatment with anti-parkinsonian agents, benzodiazepines or propranolol may be helpful.

Dystonias: Symptoms may include: spasm of the neck muscles, sometimes progressing to torticollis; extensor rigidity of back muscles, sometimes progressing to opisthotonos; carpopedal spasm, trismus, swallowing difficulty, oculogyric crisis and protrusion of the tongue.

These usually subside within a few hours, and almost always within 24 to 48 hours, after the drug has been discontinued.

In mild cases, reassurance or a barbiturate is often sufficient.*In moderate cases*, barbiturates will usually bring rapid relief.*In more severe adult cases*, the administration of an anti-parkinsonism agent, except levodopa, usually produces rapid reversal of symptoms. Also, intravenous caffeine with sodium benzoate seems to be effective. *In children*, reassurance and barbiturates will usually control symptoms. (Or, injectable Benadryl may be useful.) Note: See Benadryl prescribing information for appropriate children's dosage. If appropriate treatment with anti-parkinsonism agents or Benadryl fails to reverse the signs and symptoms, the diagnosis should be reevaluated.

Pseudo-parkinsonism: Symptoms may include: mask-like facies; drooling; tremors; pill-rolling motion; cogwheel rigidity; and shuffling gait. Reassurance and sedation are important. In most cases these symptoms are readily controlled when an anti-parkinsonism agent is administered concomitantly. Anti-parkinsonism agents should be used only when required. Generally, therapy of a few weeks to 2 to 3 months will suffice. After this time patients should be evaluated to determine their need for continued treatment. (Note: Levodopa has not been found effective in pseudo-parkinsonism.) Occasionally it is necessary to lower the dosage of trifluoperazine HCl or to discontinue the drug.

ADVERSE REACTIONS: *(cont'd)*

Tardive Dyskinesia: As with all antipsychotic agents, tardive dyskinesia may appear in some patients on long-term therapy or may appear after drug therapy has been discontinued. The syndrome can also develop, although much less frequently, after relatively brief treatment periods at low doses. This syndrome appears in all age groups. Although its prevalence appears to be highest among elderly patients, especially elderly women, it is impossible to rely upon prevalence estimates to predict at the inception of neuroleptic treatment which patients are likely to develop the syndrome. The symptoms are persistent and in some patients appear to be irreversible. The syndrome is characterized by rhythmical involuntary movements of the tongue, face, mouth or jaw (*e.g.*, protrusion of tongue, puffing of cheeks, puckering of mouth, chewing movements). Sometimes these may be accompanied by involuntary movements of extremities. In rare instances, these involuntary movements of the extremities are the only manifestations of tardive dyskinesia. A variant of tardive dyskinesia, tardive dystonia, has also been described.

There is no known effective treatment for tardive dyskinesia; anti-parkinsonism agents do not alleviate the symptoms of this syndrome. If clinically feasible, it is suggested that all antipsychotic agents be discontinued if these symptoms appear. Should it be necessary to reinstitute treatment, or increase the dosage of the agent, or switch to a different antipsychotic agent, the syndrome may be masked.

It has been reported that fine vermicular movements of the tongue may be an early sign of the syndrome and if the medication is stopped at that time the syndrome may not develop.

Adverse Reactions Reported with Trifluoperazine HCl or Other Phenothiazine Derivatives: Adverse effects with different phenothiazines vary in type, frequency, and mechanism of occurrence, i.e., some are dose-related, while others involve individual patient sensitivity. Some adverse effects may be more likely to occur, or occur with greater intensity, in patients with special medical problems, e.g., patients with mitral insufficiency or pheochromocytoma have experienced severe hypotension following recommended doses of certain phenothiazines.

Neuroleptic Malignant Syndrome (NMS) has been reported in association with antipsychotic drugs. (See WARNINGS).

Not all of the following adverse reactions have been observed with every phenothiazine derivative, but they have been reported with one or more and should be borne in mind when drugs of this class are administered: extrapyramidal symptoms (opisthotonos, oculogyric crisis, hyperreflexia, dystonia, akathisia, dyskinesia, parkinsonism) some of which have lasted months and even years—particularly in elderly patients with previous brain damage; grand mal and petit mal convulsions, particularly in patients with EEG abnormalities or history of such disorders; altered cerebrospinal fluid proteins; cerebral edema; intensification and prolongation of the action of central nervous system depressants (opiates, analgesics, antihistamines, barbiturates, alcohol), atropine, heat, organophosphorus insecticides; autonomic reactions (dryness of mouth, nasal congestion, headache, nausea, constipation, obstipation, adynamic ileus, ejaculatory disorders/impotence, priapism, atonic colon, urinary retention, miosis and mydriasis); reactivation of psychotic processes, catatonic-like states; hypotension (sometimes fatal); cardiac arrest; blood dyscrasias (pancytopenia, thrombocytopenic purpura, leukopenia, agranulocytosis, eosinophilia, hemolytic anemia, aplastic anemia); liver damage (jaundice, biliary stasis); endocrine disturbances (hyperglycemia, hypoglycemia, glycosuria, lactation, galactorrhea, gynecomastia, menstrual irregularities, false-positive pregnancy tests); skin disorders (photosensitivity, itching, erythema, urticaria, eczema up to exfoliative dermatitis); other allergic reactions (asthma, laryngeal edema, angioneurotic edema, anaphylactoid reactions); peripheral edema; reversed epinephrine effect; hyperpyrexia; mild fever after large IM doses; increased appetite; increased weight; a systemic lupus erythematosus-like syndrome; pigmentary retinopathy; with prolonged administration of substantial doses, skin pigmentation, epithelial keratopathy, and lenticular and corneal deposits.

EKG changes—particularly nonspecific, usually reversible Q and T wave distortions—have been observed in some patients receiving phenothiazine tranquilizers. Although phenothiazines cause neither psychic nor physical dependence, sudden discontinuance in long-term psychiatric patients may cause temporary symptoms, e.g., nausea and vomiting, dizziness, tremulousness.

Note: There have been occasional reports of sudden death in patients receiving phenothiazines. In some cases, the cause appeared to be cardiac arrest or asphyxia due to failure of the cough reflex.

OVERDOSAGE:

(See also ADVERSE REACTIONS).

SYMPTOMS—Primarily involvement of the extrapyramidal mechanism producing some of the dystonic reactions described above. Symptoms of central nervous system depression to the point of somnolence or coma. Agitation and restlessness may also occur. Other possible manifestations include convulsions, EKG changes and cardiac arrhythmias, fever and autonomic reactions such as hypotension, dry mouth and ileus.

TREATMENT—It is important to determine other medications taken by the patient since multiple dose therapy is common in overdosage situations. Treatment is essentially symptomatic and supportive. Early gastric lavage is helpful. Keep patient under observation and maintain an open airway, since involvement of the extrapyramidal mechanism may produce dysphagia and respiratory difficulty in severe overdosage. **Do not attempt to induce emesis because a dystonic reaction of the head or neck may develop that could result in aspiration of vomitus.**

Extrapyramidal symptoms may be treated with anti-parkinsonism drugs, barbiturates or Benadryl. See prescribing information for these products. Care should be taken to avoid increasing respiratory depression. If administration of a stimulant is desirable, amphetamine, dextroamphetamine or caffeine with sodium benzoate is recommended. Stimulants that may cause convulsions (*e.g.*, picrotoxin or pentylenetetrazol) should be avoided.

If hypotension occurs, the standard measures for managing circulatory shock should be initiated. If it is desirable to administer a vasoconstrictor, Levophed and Neo-Synephrine are most suitable. Other pressor agents, including epinephrine, are not recommended because phenothiazine derivatives may reverse the usual elevating action of these agents and cause a further lowering of blood pressure.

Limited experience indicates that phenothiazines are *not*dialyzable.

DOSAGE AND ADMINISTRATION:

Adults: Dosage should be adjusted to the needs of the individual. The lowest effective dosage should always be used. Dosage should be increased more gradually in debilitated or emaciated patients. When maximum response is achieved, dosage may be reduced gradually to a maintenance level. Because of the inherent long action of the drug, patients may be controlled on convenient b.i.d. administration; some patients may be maintained on once-a-day administration.

When trifluoperazine HCl is administered by intramuscular injection, equivalent oral dosage may be substituted once symptoms have been controlled.

Note: Although there is little likelihood of contact dermatitis due to the drug, persons with known sensitivity to phenothiazine drugs should avoid direct contact.

DOSAGE AND ADMINISTRATION: *(cont'd)*

Elderly Patients: In general, dosages in the lower range are sufficient for most elderly patients. Since they appear to be more susceptible to hypotension and neuromuscular reactions, such patients should be observed closely. Dosage should be tailored to the individual, response carefully monitored, and dosage adjusted accordingly. Dosage should be increased more gradually in elderly patients.

Non-psychotic Anxiety: Usual dosage is 1 or 2 mg twice daily. Do not administer at doses of more than 6 mg per day or for longer than 12 weeks.

Psychotic Disorders: *Oral:*Usual starting dosage is 2 mg to 5 mg b.i.d. (Small or emaciated patients should always be started on the lower dosage.)

Most patients will show optimum response on 15 mg or 20 mg daily, although a few may require 40 mg a day or more. Optimum therapeutic dosage levels should be reached within 2 or 3 weeks.

When the Concentrate dosage form is to be used, it should be added to 60 ml (2 fl oz) or more of diluent *just prior to administration* to insure palatability and stability. Vehicles suggested for dilution are: tomato or fruit juice, milk, simple syrup, orange syrup, carbonated beverages, coffee, tea or water. Semisolid foods (soup, puddings, etc.) may also be used.

Intramuscular (for prompt control of severe symptoms): Usual dosage is 1 mg to 2 mg (1/2 to 1 ml) by deep intramuscular injection q4 to 6h, p.r.n. More than 6 mg within 24 hours is rarely necessary.

Only in very exceptional cases should intramuscular dosage exceed 10 mg within 24 hours. Injections should not be given at intervals of less than 4 hours because of a possible cumulative effect.

Note: Trifluoperazine HCl Injection has been usually well tolerated and there is little, if any, pain and irritation at the site of injection.

This solution should be protected from light. This is a clear, colorless to pale yellow solution; a slight yellowish discoloration will not alter potency. If markedly discolored, solution should be discarded.

Psychotic Children: Dosage should be adjusted to the weight of the child and severity of the symptoms. These dosages are for children, ages 6 to 12, who are hospitalized or under close supervision.

Oral: The starting dosage is 1 mg administered once a day or b.i.d. Dosage may be increased gradually until symptoms are controlled or until side effects become troublesome.

While it is usually not necessary to exceed dosages of 15 mg daily, some older children with severe symptoms may require higher dosages.

Intramuscular: There has been little experience with the use of trifluoperazine HCl Injection in children. However, if it is necessary to achieve rapid control of severe symptoms, 1 mg (1/2 ml) of the drug may be administered intramuscularly once or twice a day.

* norepinephrine bitartrate, Sanofi Winthrop Pharmaceuticals.
† phenylephrine hydrochloride, Sanofi Winthrop Pharmaceuticals.
‡ phenytoin, Parke-Davis.
S metrizamide, Sanofi Winthrop Pharmaceuticals.
II diphenhydramine hydrochloride, Parke-Davis.

HOW SUPPLIED - RATED THERAPEUTICALLY EQUIVALENT:

Concentrate - Oral - 10 mg/ml

60 ml	**$108.00**	**STELAZINE 10, SKB Pharms**	**00108-4901-42**

Tablet, Plain Coated - Oral - 1 mg

100's	$8.40	Trifluoperazine Hcl, United Res	00677-0691-01
100's	$8.44	Trifluoperazine Hcl, HL Moore Drug Exch	00839-6560-06
100's	$10.46	Trifluoperazine Hcl, US Trading	56126-0313-11
100's	$54.40	Trifluoperazine HCl, Geneva Pharms	00781-1030-01
100's	$56.85	Trifluoperazine HCl, Geneva Pharms	00781-1030-13
100's	**$60.95**	**STELAZINE, SKB Pharms**	**00108-4903-20**

Tablet, Plain Coated - Oral - 2 mg

100's	$9.25	Trifluoperazine Hcl, HL Moore Drug Exch	00839-6416-06
100's	$10.10	Trifluoperazine Hcl, United Res	00677-0692-01
100's	$12.90	Trifluoperazine Hcl, US Trading	56126-0314-11
100's	$34.50	Trifluoperazine Hcl, Harber Pharm	51432-0489-03
100's	$40.30	Trifluoperazine Hcl 2, Major Pharms	00904-0561-60
100's	$44.81	Trifluoperazine HCl, H.C.F.A. F F P	99999-2382-01
100's	$80.24	Trifluoperazine HCl, Geneva Pharms	00781-1032-01
100's	$83.85	Trifluoperazine HCl, Geneva Pharms	00781-1032-13
100's	**$89.90**	**STELAZINE, SKB Pharms**	**00108-4904-20**
1000's	$275.95	Trifluoperazine Hcl, Harber Pharm	51432-0489-06
1000's	$448.10	Trifluoperazine HCl, H.C.F.A. F F P	99999-2382-02
1000's	$561.76	Trifluoperazine HCl, Geneva Pharms	00781-1032-10

Tablet, Plain Coated - Oral - 5 mg

100's	$10.60	Trifluoperazine Hcl, United Res	00677-0693-01
100's	$12.02	Trifluoperazine Hcl, HL Moore Drug Exch	00839-6417-06
100's	$14.33	Trifluoperazine Hcl, US Trading	56126-0315-11
100's	$34.50	Trifluoperazine Hcl, Harber Pharm	51432-0490-03
100's	$40.10	Trifluoperazine Hcl 5, Major Pharms	00904-0562-60
100's	$50.30	Trifluoperazine Hcl, H.C.F.A. F F P	99999-2382-03
100's	$100.98	Trifluoperazine HCl, Geneva Pharms	00781-1034-01
100's	$105.52	Trifluoperazine HCl, Geneva Pharms	00781-1034-13
100's	**$113.15**	**STELAZINE, SKB Pharms**	**00108-4906-20**
1000's	$345.00	Trifluoperazine Hcl, Harber Pharm	51432-0490-06
1000's	$503.00	Trifluoperazine Hcl, H.C.F.A. F F P	99999-2382-04
1000's	$706.82	Trifluoperazine HCl, Geneva Pharms	00781-1034-10

Tablet, Plain Coated - Oral - 10 mg

100's	$13.55	Trifluoperazine Hcl, United Res	00677-0694-01
100's	$14.85	Trifluoperazine Hcl, US Trading	56126-0316-11
100's	$15.53	Trifluoperazine Hcl, HL Moore Drug Exch	00839-6561-06
100's	$54.50	Trifluoperazine Hcl 10, Major Pharms	00904-0563-60
100's	$55.00	Trifluoperazine Hcl, Harber Pharm	51432-0491-03
100's	$57.45	Trifluoperazine Hcl, H.C.F.A. F F P	99999-2382-05
100's	$152.24	Trifluoperazine HCl, Geneva Pharms	00781-1036-01
100's	$159.09	Trifluoperazine HCl, Geneva Pharms	00781-1036-13
100's	**$170.55**	**STELAZINE, SKB Pharms**	**00108-4907-20**
1000's	$550.00	Trifluoperazine Hcl, Harber Pharm	51432-0491-06
1000's	$574.50	Trifluoperazine Hcl, H.C.F.A. F F P	99999-2382-06
1000's	$1065.62	Trifluoperazine HCl, Geneva Pharms	00781-1036-10

HOW SUPPLIED - NOT RATED EQUIVALENT:

Injection, Solution - Intramuscular - 2 mg/ml

10 ml x 1	**$49.55**	**STELAZINE, SKB Pharms**	**00108-4902-01**
10 ml x 20	**$741.75**	**STELAZINE, SKB Pharms**	**00108-4902-12**

TRIFLUPROMAZINE *(002383)*

CATEGORIES: Central Nervous System Agents; Nausea; Phenothiazine Tranquilizers; Psychotherapeutic Agents; Psychotic Disorders; Tranquilizers; Vertigo/Motion Sickness/Vomiting; Vomiting; FDA Approval Pre 1982

BRAND NAMES: **Vesprin**

DESCRIPTION:

Vesprin is a phenothiazine derivative. It is available for parenteral use in multiple dose vials providing 10 or 20 mg triflupromazine hydrochloride per ml, with 1.5% (w/v) benzyl alcohol as a preservative and sodium chloride for isotonicity. The pH has been adjusted to 3.5 to 5.2 with sodium hydroxide and/or hydrochloric acid. At the time of manufacture, the air in the vials is replaced by nitrogen.

CLINICAL PHARMACOLOGY:

Experimental and clinical studies suggest that the phenothiazine derivatives act on the hypothalamus. These drugs are believed to depress various components of the mesodiencephalic activating system, which is involved in the control of basal metabolism and body temperature, wakefulness, vasomotor tone, emesis, and hormonal balance. In addition, the drugs exert a peripheral autonomic effect in varying degrees. However, the site and mode of action of phenothiazine derivatives including triflupromazine have not been completely elucidated.

INDICATIONS AND USAGE:

Vesprin Injection is effective in the management of the manifestations of psychotic disorders (excluding psychotic depressive reactions) and for the control of severe nausea and vomiting.

Vesprin has not been shown effective in the management of behavioral complications in patients with mental retardation.

CONTRAINDICATIONS:

Phenothiazine are contraindicated in patients with suspected or established subcortical brain damage, with or without hypothalamic damage, since a hyperthermic reaction with temperatures in excess of 104°F may occur in such patients, sometimes not until 14 to 16 hours after drug administration. Total body ice-packing is recommended for such a reaction; antipyretics may also be useful.

Phenothiazine compounds should not be used in patients receiving large doses of hypnotics.

As with other phenothiazine compounds, triflupromazine is contraindicated in comatose or severely depressed states.

The presence of blood dyscrasia or liver damage precludes the use of triflupromazine.

WARNINGS:

The extrapyramidal symptoms which can occur secondary to administration of triflupromazine may be confused with the central nervous system signs of an undiagnosed primary disease responsible for the vomiting, e.g. Reye's Syndrome or other encephalopathy. The use of triflupromazine and other potential hepatotoxins should be avoided in children and adolescents whose signs and symptoms suggest Reye's Syndrome.

TARDIVE DYSKINESIA

Tardive dyskinesia, a syndrome consisting of potentially irreversible, involuntary, dyskinetic movements may develop in patients treated with neuroleptic (antipsychotic) drugs. Although the prevalence of the syndrome appears to be highest among the elderly, especially elderly women, it is impossible to rely upon prevalence estimates to predict, at the inception of neuroleptic treatment, which patients are likely to develop the syndrome. Whether neuroleptic drug products differ in their potential to cause tardive dyskinesia is unknown.

Both the risk of developing the syndrome and the likelihood that it will become irreversible are believed to increase as the duration of treatment and the total cumulative dose of neuroleptic drugs administered to the patient increase. However, the syndrome can develop, although much less commonly, after relatively brief treatment periods at low doses.

There is no known treatment for established cases of tardive dyskinesia, although the syndrome may remit, partially or completely, if neuroleptic treatment is withdrawn, Neuroleptic treatment, itself, however, may suppress (or partially suppress) the signs and symptoms of the syndrome and thereby may possibly mask the underlying disease process. The effect that symptomatic suppression has upon the long-term course of the syndrome is unknown.

Given these considerations, neuroleptics should be prescribed in a manner that is most likely to minimize the occurrence of tardive dyskinesia. Chronic neuroleptic treatment should generally be reserved for patients who suffer from a chronic illness that, 1) is known to respond to neuroleptic drugs, and, 2) for whom alternative, equally effective, but potentially less harmful treatments are *not* available or appropriate. In the patients who do require chronic treatment, the smallest dose and the shortest duration of treatment producing a satisfactory clinical response should be sought. The need for continued treatment should be reassessed periodically.

If signs and symptoms of tardive dyskinesia appear in a patient on neuroleptics, drug discontinuation should be considered. However, some patients may require treatment despite the presence of the syndrome.

(For further information about the description of tardive dyskinesia and its clinical detection, please refer to the sections on PRECAUTIONS, Information for the Patient and ADVERSE REACTIONS, Tardive Dyskinesia.)

The use of this drug may impair the mental and physical abilities required for driving a car or operating heavy machinery.

Potentiation of the effect of alcohol may occur with the use of this drug.

USAGE IN PREGNANCY

The safety for the use of this drug during pregnancy has not been established; therefore, the possible hazards should be weighed against the potential benefits when administering this drug to pregnant patients.

PRECAUTIONS:

GENERAL

Antiemetic Effect: The antiemetic action of triflupromazine may mask the signs and symptoms of overdosage of other drugs and may obscure the diagnosis and treatment of other conditions such as intestinal obstruction, brain tumor, and Reye's Syndrome (See WARNINGS.)

Because of the possibility of cross-sensitivity, this drug should be used cautiously in patients who have developed cholestatic jaundice, dermatoses, or other allergic reactions to phenothiazine derivatives.

PRECAUTIONS: *(cont'd)*

Psychotic patients on large doses of a phenothiazine drug who are undergoing surgery should be watched carefully for possible hypotensive phenomena. Moreover, it should be remembered that reduced amounts of anesthetics or central nervous system depressants may be necessary. It is generally not recommended that triflupromazine be used prior to spinal anesthesia.

Although this is not a general feature of triflupromazine, potentiation of central nervous system depressants (opiates, analgesics, antihistamines, barbiturates, alcohol) may occur. The effects of atropine may be potentiated in some patients receiving triflupromazine.

Phenothiazines should be used with caution in patients with a history of convulsive disorders, since grand mal convulsions have been known to occur.

Patients with special medical disorders such as mitral valve insufficiency or pheochromocytoma, and patients who have exhibited idiosyncrasy to other centrally acting drugs may experience severe reactions to phenothiazine compounds.

The parenteral administrations of triflupromazine may sometimes cause postural hypotension; to preclude its occurrence, patients should be kept under close clinical supervision, in a recumbent position, if necessary.

Facilities should be available fro periodic checking of hepatic function, renal function, and the blood picture. Renal function of patients on long-term therapy should be monitored; if BUN (blood urea nitrogen) becomes abnormal, treatment should be discontinued.

As with any phenothiazine, the physician should be alert to the possible development of "silent pneumonias" in patients under treatment with triflupromazine.

Neuroleptic drugs elevate prolactin levels; the elevation persists during chronic administration. Tissue culture experiments indicate that approximately one-third of human breast cancers are prolactin dependent*in vitro*, a factor of potential importance if the prescription of these drugs is contemplated in a patient with a previously detected breast cancer. Although disturbances such as galactorrhea, amenorrhea, gynecomastia, and impotence have been reported, the clinical significance of elevated serum prolactin levels is unknown for most patients. An increase in mammary neoplasms has been found in rodents after chronic administration of neuroleptic drugs. Neither clinical studies nor epidemiologic studies conducted to date, however, have shown an association between chronic administration of these drugs and mammary tumorigenesis; the available evidence is considered too limited to be conclusive at this time.

INFORMATION FOR THE PATIENT

Given the likelihood that some patients exposed chronically to neuroleptics will develop tardive dyskinesia, it is advised that all patients in whom chronic use is contemplated be given, if possible, full information about this risk. The decision to inform patients and/or their guardians must obviously take into account the clinical circumstances and the competency of the patient to understand the information provided.

ADVERSE REACTIONS:

Central Nervous System: The side effects most frequently reported with phenothiazine compounds are extrapyramidal symptoms including pseudoparkinsonism, dystonia, dyskinesia, akathisia, oculogyric crises, opisthotonos, and hyperreflexia. Most often, these extrapyramidal symptoms are reversible; however, they may be persistent (see ADVERSE REACTIONS). With any given phenothiazine derivative, the incidence and severity of such reactions depend more on individual patient sensitivity than on other factors, but dosage level and patient age are also determinants.

Extrapyramidal reactions may be alarming, and the patient should be forewarned and reassured. These reactions can usually be controlled by administration of antiparkinsonian drugs such as Benztropine Mesylate and by subsequent reduction in dosage.

Tardive Dyskinesia: See WARNINGS. The syndrome is characterized by involuntary choreoathetoid movements which variously involve the tongue, puffing of the cheeks, puckering of the mouth, chewing movements), trunk and extremities. The severity of the syndrome and the degree of impairment produced vary widely.

The syndrome may become clinically recognizable either during treatment, upon dosage reduction, or upon withdrawal if treatment. Early detection of tardive dyskinesia is important. To increase the likelihood of detecting the syndrome at the earliest possible time, the dosage of neuroleptic drugs should be reduced periodically (if clinically possible) and the patient observed for signs of the disorder. This maneuver is critical, since neuroleptic drugs may mask the signs of the syndrome.

Drowsiness or lethargy, if they occur, may necessitate a reduction in dosage; the induction of a catatonic-like state has been known to occur with dosages far in excess of the recommended amounts. As with other phenothiazine compounds, reactivation or aggravation of psychotic processes may be encountered.

Phenothiazine derivatives have been known to cause, in some patients, restlessness, excitement, or bizarre dreams.

Autonomic Nervous System: Hypertension and fluctuation in blood pressure have been reported with triflupromazine.

Patients with pheochromocytoma, cerebral vascular or renal insufficiency appear to be particularly prone to hypotensive reactions with phenothiazine compounds and should therefore be observed closely when the drug is administered. If severe hypotension should occur, supportive measures including the use of intravenous vasopressor drugs should be instituted immediately. Levarterenol Bitartrate Injection and Phenylephrine Hydrochloride Injection are suitable drugs for this purpose. *Epinephrine should not be used* since phenothiazine derivatives have been found to reverse its action, resulting in a further lowering of blood pressure.

Autonomic reactions including nausea and loss of appetite, salivation, polyuria, perspiration, dry mouth, headache and constipation may occur. Autonomic effects can usually be controlled by reducing or temporarily discontinuing dosage.

In some patients, phenothiazine derivatives have caused blurred vision, glaucoma, bladder paralysis, fecal impaction, paralytic ileus, tachycardia, or nasal congestion.

Metabolic and Endocrine: Weight change, peripheral edema, abnormal lactation, gynecomastia, menstrual irregularities, false results on pregnancy tests, impotency in men, and increased libido in women have all been known to occur in some patients on phenothiazine therapy.

Allergic Reactions: Skin disorders such as itching, erythema, urticaria, seborrhea, photosensitivity, eczema, and even exfoliative dermatitis have been reported with phenothiazine derivatives. The possibility of anaphylactoid reactions occurring in some patients should be borne in mind.

Hematologic: Routine blood counts are advisable during therapy since blood dyscrasias including leukopenia, agranulocytosis, thrombocytopenic or nonthrombocytopenic purpura, eosinophilia and pancytopenia have been observed with phenothiazine derivatives. Furthermore, if any soreness of the mouth, gums, or throat, or any symptoms of upper respiratory infection occur and confirmatory leukocyte count indicates cellular depression, therapy should be discontinued and other appropriate measures instituted immediately.

ADVERSE REACTIONS: *(cont'd)*

Hepatic: Liver damage as manifested by cholestatic jaundice or biliary stasis have been observed with phenothiazine derivatives, particularly during the first months of therapy; treatment should be discontinued if this occurs. An increase in cephalin flocculation, sometime accompanied by alterations in other liver function tests has been reported in patients receiving phenothiazine who have had no clinical evidence of liver damage.

Others: Sudden, unexpected, and unexplained deaths have been reported in hospitalized psychotic patients receiving phenothiazines. Previous brain damage or seizures may be predisposing factors; high doses should be avoided in known seizure patients. Several patients have shown sudden flare-ups of psychotic behavior patterns shortly before death. Autopsy findings have usually revealed acute fulminating pneumonia or pneumonitis, aspiration of gastric contents, or intramyocardial lesions.

The following adverse reactions have also occurred with phenothiazine derivatives: systemic lupus erythematosus-like syndrome, hypotension severe enough to cause fatal cardiac arrest, altered electrocardiographic and electroencephalographic tracings, altered cerebrospinal fluid proteins, cerebral edema, potentiation of heat and of phosphorus insecticides, asthma, laryngeal edema, angioneurotic edema, and pigmentary retinopathy; with long-term use, skin pigmentation and lenticular and corneal opacities.

DOSAGE AND ADMINISTRATION:

PSYCHOTIC DISORDERS

Institutionalized Adult Patients: Optimum dosage levels must be determined individually in each patient.

The recommended intramuscular dose is 60 mg up to a maximum total daily dose of 150 mg.

Noninstitutionalized Adult Patients: Use the same regimen as outlined for institutionalized patients.

Children: As in adult therapy, optimum dosage levels must be determined individually for each patients.

When intramuscular use is indicated in children, the recommended range is 0.2 to 0.25 mg/kg (1/10 to 1/8 mg/lb) up to a maximum total daily dose of 10 mg. The drug should not be administered to children under 2 1/2 years of age.

NAUSEA AND VOMITING

For adults, the recommended dosage range for prophylaxis as well as for treatment is 1 mg up to a maximum total daily dose of 3 mg intravenously or 5 to 15 mg as a single dose which may be repeated every four hours up to a maximum total daily dose of 60 mg intramuscularly.

For elderly or debilitated patients, the recommended intramuscular dosage is 2.5 mg up to a maximum total daily dose of 15 mg.

Triflupromazine should generally not be used in children under 2 1/2 years of age. It should not be used in conditions for which children's dosages have not been established. Dosage and frequency of administration should be adjusted according to the severity of the symptoms and response of the patient. The duration of activity following intramuscular administration may last up to 12 hours. Subsequent doses may be given by the same route if necessary.

For children, the recommended dosage is a range of 0.2 to 0.25 mg/kg (1/10 to 1/8 mg/lb) up to a maximum total daily dose of 10 mg intramuscularly. Intravenous administration is not recommended for children.

STORAGE

Store the injection at room temperature; protect from light. Injection: avoid freezing. Parenteral solutions may vary in color from essentially colorless to light amber. If a solution has become any darker than light amber or is discolored in any other way, it should not be used.

HOW SUPPLIED - EQUIVALENTS NOT AVAILABLE:

Injection, Solution - Intramuscular; - 10 mg/ml

10 ml	$47.53	VESPRIN, Bristol Myers Squibb	00003-0987-70

Injection, Solution - Intramuscular; - 20 mg/ml

1 ml x 1	$13.00	VESPRIN, Bristol Myers Squibb	00003-0920-20

TRIFLURIDINE *(002384)*

CATEGORIES: Anti-Infectives; Antivirals; Conjunctivitis; EENT Drugs; Eye, Ear, Nose, & Throat Preparations; Herpes; Herpes Simplex; Keratitis; Keratoconjunctivitis; Lesions; Ocular Infections; Ophthalmics; Topical; Uveitis; Viral Agents; Viral Agents, Ophthalmological; FDA Approval Pre 1982

BRAND NAMES: *Aflomin*; *TFT*; *Triherpin*; *Viromidin*; *Virophta*; **Viroptic**
(International brand names outside U.S. in italics)

FORMULARIES: Aetna; BC-BS; Medi-Cal; PCS

DESCRIPTION:

Viroptic is the brand name for trifluridine (also known as trifluorothymidine, F_3TdR_1,F_3T), an antiviral drug for topical treatment of epithelial keratitis caused by Herpes simplex virus. The chemical name of trifluridine is 2'-deoxy-5-(trifluoromethyl)uridine.

Viroptic sterile ophthalmic solution contains 1% trifluridine in an aqueous solution with acetic acid and sodium acetate (buffers), sodium chloride, and thimerosal 0.001% (added as a preservative).

CLINICAL PHARMACOLOGY:

Trifluridine is a fluorinated pyrimidine nucleoside with *in vitro* and *in vivo* activity against Herpes simplex virus, types 1 and 2 and vacciniavirus. Some strains of Adenovirus are also inhibited *in vitro*.

Trifluridine interferes with DNA synthesis in cultured mammalian cells. However, its antiviral mechanism of action is not completely known.

In vitro perfusion studies on excised rabbit corneas have shown that trifluridine penetrates the intact cornea as evidenced by recovery of parental drug and its major metabolite, 5-carboxy-2'-deoxyuridine, on the endothelial side of the cornea. Absence of the corneal epithelium enhances the penetration of trifluridine approximately two-fold.

Intraocular penetration of trifluridine occurs after topical instillation of trifluridine into human eyes. Decreased corneal integrity or stromal or uveal inflammation may enhance the penetration of trifluridine into the aqueous humor. Unlike the results of ocular penetration of trifluridine *in vitro*, 5-carboxy-2'-deoxyuridine was not found in detectable concentrations within the aqueous humor of the human eye.

Systemic absorption of trifluridine following therapeutic dosing with trifluridine appears to be negligible. No detectable concentrations of trifluridine or 5-carboxy-2'-deoxyuridine were found in the sera of adult healthy normal subjects who had trifluridine instilled into their eyes seven times daily for 14 consecutive days.

INDICATIONS AND USAGE:

Trifluridine ophthalmic solution, 1% is indicated for the treatment of primary keratoconjunctivitis and recurrent epithelial keratitis due to Herpes simplex virus, types 1 and 2. Trifluridine is also effective in the treatment of epithelial keratitis that has not responded clinically to the topical administration of idoxuridine or when ocular toxicity or hypersensitivity to idoxuridine has occurred. In a smaller number of patients found to be resistant to topical vidarabine, trifluridine was also effective.

The clinical efficacy of trifluridine in the treatment of stromal keratitis and uveitis due to Herpes simplex virus or ophthalmic infections caused by vacciniavirus and Adenovirus has not been established by well-controlled clinical trials. Trifluridine has not been shown to be effective in the prophylaxis of Herpes simplex virus keratoconjunctivitis and epithelial keratitis by well-controlled clinical trials. Trifluridine is not effective against bacterial, fungal or chlamydial infections of the cornea or nonviral trophic lesions.

During controlled multicenter clinical trials, 92 of 97 (95%) patients (78 of 81 with dendritic and 14 of 16 with geographic ulcers) responded to trifluridine therapy as evidenced by complete corneal re-epithelialization within the 14-day therapy period. In these controlled studies, 56 of 75 (75%) patients (49 of 58 with dendritic and 7 of 17 with geographic ulcers) responded to idoxuridine therapy. The mean time to corneal re-epithelialization for dendritic ulcers (6 days) and geographic ulcers (7 days) was similar for both therapies. In other clinical studies, trifluridine was evaluated in the treatment of Herpes simplex virus keratitis in patients who were unresponsive or intolerant to the topical administration of idoxuridine or vidarabine. Trifluridine was effective in 138 of 150 (92%) patients (109 of 114 with dendritic and 29 of 36 with geographic ulcers) as evidenced by corneal re-epithelialization. The mean time to corneal re-epithelialization was 6 days for patients with dendritic ulcers and 12 days for patients with geographic ulcers.

CONTRAINDICATIONS:

Trifluridine ophthalmic solution, 1%, is contraindicated for patients who develop hypersensitivity reactions or chemical intolerance to trifluridine.

WARNINGS:

The recommended dosage and frequency of administration should not be exceeded (see DOSAGE AND ADMINISTRATION.)

PRECAUTIONS:

General: Trifluridine ophthalmic solution, 1% should be prescribed only for patients who have a clinical diagnosis of herpetic keratitis.

Trifluridine may cause mild local irritation of the conjunctiva and cornea when instilled but these effects are usually transient.

Although documented *in vitro* viral resistance to trifluridine has not been reported following multiple exposure to trifluridine, the possibility exists of viral resistance development.

Carcinogenesis, Mutagenesis, and Impairment of Fertility: *Mutagenic Potential:* Trifluridine has been shown to exert mutagenic, DNA-damaging and cell-transforming activities in various standard *in vitro* test systems, and clastogenic activity in *Vicia faba* cells. It did not induce chromosome aberrations in bone marrow cells of male or female rats following a single subcutaneous dose of 100 mg/kg, but was weakly positive in female, but not in male, rats following daily subcutaneous administration at 700 mg/kg/day for 5 days.

Although the significance of these test results is not clear or fully understood, there exists the possibility that mutagenic agents may cause genetic damage in humans.

Oncogenic Potential: Lifetime carcinogenicity bioassays in rats and mice given daily subcutaneous doses of trifluridine have been performed. Rats tested at 1.5, 7.5 and 15 mg/kg/day had increased incidences of adenocarcinomas of the intestinal tract and mammary glands, hemangiosarcomas of the spleen and liver, carcinosarcomas of the prostate gland and granulosa-thecal cell tumors of the ovary. Mice were tested at 1,5 and 10 mg/kg/day; those given 10 mg/kg/day trifluridine had significantly increased incidences of adenocarcinomas of the intestinal tract and uterus. Those given 10 mg/kg/day also had a significantly increased incidence of testicular atrophy as compared to vehicle control mice.

Pregnancy, Teratogenic Effects, Pregnancy Category C: Trifluridine was not teratogenic at doses up to 5.0 mg/kg/day (23 times the estimated human exposure) when given subcutaneously to rats and rabbits. However, fetal toxicity consisting of delayed ossification of portions of the skeletal occurred at dose levels of 2.5 and 5.0 mg/kg/day produced fetal death and resorption in rabbits. In both rats and rabbits, 1.0 mg/kg/day (5 times the estimated human exposure) was a no-effect levels. There were no teratogenic or fetotoxic effects after topical application of trifluridine ophthalmic solution 1% (approximately 5 times the estimated human exposure() to the eyes of rabbits on the 6th through 18th days of pregnancy.[1] In a non-standard test, trifluridine solution has been shown to be teratogenic when injected directly into the yolk sac of chicken eggs.[2] There are no adequate and well-controlled studies in pregnant women. Trifluridine ophthalmic solution 1% should be used during pregnancy only if the potential benefit justifies the potential risk to the fetus.

Nursing Mothers: It is unlikely that trifluridine is excreted in human milk after ophthalmic instillation of trifluridine because of the relatively small dosage (≤5.0 mg/day), its dilution in body fluids and its extremely short half-life (approximately 12 minutes). The drug should not be prescribed for nursing mothers unless the potential benefits outweigh the potential risks.

DRUG INTERACTIONS:

The following drugs have been administered topically to the eye and concurrently with trifluridine in a limited number of patients without apparent evidence of adverse interaction: antibiotics—chloramphenicol, erythromycin, polymyxin B sulfate, bacitracin, gentamicin sulfate, tetracycline HCl, sodium sulfacetamide, neomycin sulfate; steroids—dexamethasone, dexamethasone sodium phosphate, prednisolone acetate, prednisolone sodium phosphate, hydrocortisone, fluorometholone; and other ophthalmic drugs—atropine sulfate, scopolamine hydrobromide, naphazoline hydrochloride, cyclopentolate hydrochloride, homatropine hydrobromide, pilocarpine, 1-epinephrine hydrochloride, sodium chloride.

ADVERSE REACTIONS:

The most frequent adverse reactions reported during controlled clinical trials were mild, transient burning or stinging upon instillation (4.6%) and palpebral edema (2.8%). Other adverse reactions in decreasing order of reported frequency were superficial punctate keratopathy, epithelial keratopathy, hypersensitivity reaction, stromal edema, irritation, keratitis sicca, hyperemia, and increased intraocular pressure.

OVERDOSAGE:

Overdosage by ocular instillation is unlikely because any excess solution should be quickly expelled from the conjunctival sac.

Acute overdosage by accidental oral ingestion of trifluridine has not occurred. However, should such ingestion occur, the 75 mg dosage of trifluridine in a 7.5 ml bottle of trifluridine is not likely to produce adverse effects. Single intravenous doses of 15-30 mg/kg/day in

OVERDOSAGE: *(cont'd)*

children and adults with neoplastic disease produce reversible bone marrow depression as the only potentially serious toxic effect and only after 3-5 courses of therapy.[3] The acute oral LD_{50} in the mouse and rat was 4379 mg/kg or higher.

DOSAGE AND ADMINISTRATION:

Instill one drop of trifluridine ophthalmic solution, 1% onto the cornea of the affected eye every two hours while awake for a maximum daily dosage of nine drops until the corneal ulcer has completely re-epithelialized. Following re-epithelialization, treatment for an additional seven days of one drop every four hours while awake for a minimum daily dosage of five drops is recommended.

If there are no signs of improvement after seven days of therapy or complete re-epithelialization has not occurred after 14 days of therapy, other forms of therapy should be considered. Continuous administration of trifluridine for periods exceeding 21 days should be avoided because of potential ocular toxicity.

Store under refrigeration 2 to 8°C (36 to 46°F).

ANIMAL PHARMACOLOGY:

Animal Toxicology: Corneal wound healing studies in rabbits showed that trifluridine did not significantly retard closure of epithelial wounds. However, mild toxic changes such as intracellular edema of the basal cell layer, mild thinning of the overlying epithelium and reduced strength of stromal wounds were observed.

Whereas instillation of trifluridine into rabbit eyes during a subchronic toxicity study produced some degree of corneal epithelial thinning, a 12-month chronic toxicity study in rabbits in which trifluridine was instilled into eyes in intermittent, multiple, full-therapy courses showed no drug-related changes in the cornea.

REFERENCES:

1. Itoi M, Getter JW, Kaneko N, et al: Teratogenicities of ophthalmic drugs. I. Antiviral ophthalmic drugs. *Arch Ophthalmol* 1975;93:46-51. **2.** Kury G, Crosby RJ: The teratogenic effect of 5-trifluoromethyl-2'-deoxyuridine in chicken embryos. *Toxicol Appl Pharmacol* 1967;11:72-80. **3.** Ansfield FJ, Ramirez G: Phase I and II studies of 2'-deoxy-5-(trifluoromethyl)-uridine (NSC-75520).*Cancer Chemother Rep* 1971;55(pt 1):205-208.

HOW SUPPLIED - RATED THERAPEUTICALLY EQUIVALENT:

Solution - Ophthalmic - 10 mg/ml

7.5 ml $53.14 VIROPTIC, Glaxo Wellcome 00173-0968-02

TRIHEXYPHENIDYL HYDROCHLORIDE

(002385)

CATEGORIES: Anticholinergic Agents; Antiparkinson Agents; Autonomic Drugs; Central Nervous System Agents; Extrapyramidal Movement Disorders; Neuromuscular; Parkinsonism; Phenothiazines; FDA Approval Pre 1982

BRAND NAMES: *Acamed*; *Anti-Spas*; *Aparkane*; *Apo-Trihex*; **Artane**; *Bentex*; *Hexinal*; *Hipokinon*; *Novohexidyl*; *Pacitane*; *Pargitan*; *Parkinane*; *Parkines*; *Parkisonal*; *Partane*; *Stobrun*; Tremin; *Tridyl*; Trihexane; Trihexidyl; *Trihexin*; Trihexy; *Triphen*; Tritane

(International brand names outside U.S. in italics)

FORMULARIES: Aetna; BC-BS; FHP; Medi-Cal; PCS

COST OF THERAPY: $71.83 (Parkinsonism; Tablet; 2 mg; 3/day; 365 days)

CLINICAL PHARMACOLOGY:

Trihexyphenidyl HCl is the substituted piperidine salt, 3-(1-piperidyl)-1-phenyl-cyclohexyl-1-propanol hydrochloride, which exerts a direct inhibitory effect upon the parasympathetic nervous system. It also has a relaxing effect on smooth musculature; exerted both directly upon the muscle tissue itself and indirectly through an inhibitory effect upon the parasympathetic nervous system. Its therapeutic properties are similar to those of atropine although undesirable side effects are ordinarily less frequent and severe than with the latter.

INDICATIONS AND USAGE:

The drug is indicated as an adjunct in the treatment of all forms of parkinsonism (postencephalitic, arteriosclerotic, and idiopathic). It is often useful as adjuvant therapy when treating these forms of parkinsonism with levodopa. Additionally, it is indicated for the control of extrapyramidal disorders caused by central nervous system drugs such as the dibenzoxazepines, phenothiazines, thioxanthenes, and butyrophenones.

Sequels: For maintenance therapy after patients have been stabilized on trihexyphenidyl hydrochloride in conventional dosage forms (tablets or elixir).

WARNINGS:

Patients to be treated with Trihexyphenidyl HCl should have a gonioscope evaluation and close monitoring of intraocular pressures at regular periodic intervals.

PRECAUTIONS:

Although Trihexyphenidyl HCl is not contraindicated for patients with cardiac, liver, or kidney disorders, or with hypertension, such patients should be maintained under close observation. Since the use of Trihexyphenidyl HCl may in some cases continue indefinitely and since it has atropine-like properties, patients should be subjected to constant and careful long-term observation to avoid allergic and other untoward reactions. Inasmuch as Trihexyphenidyl HCl possesses some parasympatholytic activity, it should be used with caution in patients with glaucoma, obstructive disease of the gastrointestinal or genitourinary tracts, and in elderly males with possible prostatic hypertrophy. Geriatric patients, particularly over the age of 60, frequently develop increased sensitivity to the actions of drugs of this type, and hence, require strict dosage regulation. Incipient glaucoma may be precipitated by parasympatholytic drugs such as trihexyphenidyl HCl.

Tardive dyskinesia may appear in some patients on long-term therapy with antipsychotic drugs or may occur after therapy with these drugs has been discontinued. Antiparkinsonism agents do not alleviate the symptoms of tardive dyskinesia, and in some instances may aggravate them. However, parkinsonism and tardive dyskinesia often coexist in patients receiving chronic neuroleptic treatment, and anticholinergic therapy with Trihexyphenidyl HCl may relieve some of these parkinsonism symptoms.

ADVERSE REACTIONS:

Minor side effects, such as dryness of the mouth, blurring of vision, dizziness; mild nausea or nervousness, will be experienced by 30 to 50 percent of all patients. These sensations, however, are much less troublesome with Trihexyphenidyl HCl than with belladonna alkaloids and are usually less disturbing than unalleviated parkinsonism. Such reactions tend to

ADVERSE REACTIONS: *(cont'd)*

become less pronounced, and even to disappear, as treatment continues. Even before these reactions have remitted spontaneously, they may often be controlled by careful adjustment of dosage form, amount of drug, or interval between doses.

Isolated instances of suppurative parotitis secondary to excessive dryness of the mouth, skin rashes, dilatation of the colon, paralytic ileus, and certain psychiatric manifestations such as delusions and hallucinations, plus one doubtful case of paranoia all of which may occur with any of the atropine-like drugs, have been reported rarely with Trihexyphenidyl HCl.

Patients with arteriosclerosis or with a history of idiosyncrasy to other drugs may exhibit reactions of mental confusion, agitation, disturbed behavior, or nausea and vomiting. Such patients should be allowed to develop a tolerance through the initial administration of a small dose and gradual increase in dose until an effective level is reached. If a severe reaction should occur, administration of the drug should be discontinued for a few days and then resumed at a lower dosage. Psychiatric disturbances can result from indiscriminate use (leading to overdosage) to sustain continued euphoria.

Potential side effects associated with the use of any atropine-like drugs include constipation, drowsiness, urinary hesitancy or retention, tachycardia, dilation of the pupil, increased intraocular tension, weakness, vomiting, and headache.

The occurrence of angle-closure glaucoma due to long-term treatment with trihexyphenidyl hydrochloride has been reported.

DOSAGE AND ADMINISTRATION:

Dosage should be individualized. The initial dose should be low and then increased gradually, especially in patients over 60 years of age. Whether Trihexyphenidyl HCl may best be given before or after meals should be determined by the way the patient reacts. Postencephalitic patients, who are usually more prone to excessive salivation, may prefer to take it after meals and may, in addition, require small amounts of atropine which, under such circumstances, is sometimes an effective adjuvant. If Trihexyphenidyl HCl tends to dry the mouth excessively, it may be better to take it before meals, unless it causes nausea. If taken after meals, the thirst sometimes induced can be allayed by mint candies, chewing gum or water.

Trihexyphenidyl HCl in Idiopathic Parkinsonism: As initial therapy for parkinsonism, 1 mg of Trihexyphenidyl HCl in tablet or elixir form may be administered the first day. The dose may then be increased by 2 mg increments at intervals of three to five days, until a total of 6 to 10 mg is given daily. The total daily dose will depend upon what is found to be the optimal level. Many patients derive maximum benefit from this daily total of 6 to 10 mg, but some patients, chiefly those in the postencephalitic group, may require a total daily dose of 12 to 15 mg.

Trihexyphenidyl HCl in Drug-Induced Parkinsonism: The size and frequency of dose of Trihexyphenidyl HCl needed to control extrapyramidal reactions to commonly employed tranquilizers, notably the phenothiazines, thioxanthenes, and butyrophenones, must be determined empirically. The total daily dosage usually ranges between 5 and 15 mg although, in some cases, these reactions have been satisfactorily controlled on as little as 1 mg daily. It may be advisable to commence therapy with a single 1 mg dose. If the extra pyramidal manifestations are not controlled in a few hours, the subsequent doses may be progressively increased until satisfactory control is achieved. Satisfactory control may sometimes be more rapidly achieved by temporarily reducing the dosage of the tranquilizer on instituting Trihexyphenidyl HCl therapy and then adjusting dosage of both drugs until the desired ataractic effect is retained without onset of extrapyramidal reactions.

It is sometimes possible to maintain the patient on a reduced Trihexyphenidyl HCl dosage after the reactions have remained under control for several days. Instances have been reported in which these reactions have remained in remission for long periods after Trihexyphenidyl HCl therapy was discontinued.

Concomitant Use of Trihexyphenidyl HCl with Levodopa: When Trihexyphenidyl HCl is used concomitantly with levodopa, the usual dose of each may need to be reduced. Careful adjustment is necessary, depending on side effects and degree of symptom control. Trihexyphenidyl HCl dosage of 3 to 6 mg daily, in divided doses, is usually adequate.

Concomitant Use of Trihexyphenidyl HCl with Other Parasympathetic Inhibitors: Trihexyphenidyl HCl may be substituted, in whole or in part, for other parasympathetic inhibitors. The usual technique is partial substitution initially, with progressive reduction in the other medication as the dose of trihexyphenidyl HCl is increased.

Trihexyphenidyl Hcl Tablets And Elixir: The total daily intake of Trihexyphenidyl HCl tablets or elixir is tolerated best if divided into 3 doses and taken at mealtimes. High doses (>10 mg daily) may be divided unto 4 parts, with 3 doses administered at mealtimes and the fourth at bedtime.

Trihexyphenidyl HCl Sequels: Because of the relatively high dosage in each controlled release capsule, this dosage form should not be used for initial therapy. After patients are stabilized on trihexyphenidyl HCl in conventional dosage forms (tablet or elixir), for convenience of administration they may be switched to the controlled release capsules on a milligram per milligram total daily dose basis, as a single dose after breakfast or in two divided doses 12 hours apart. Most patients will be adequately maintained on the controlled release form, but some may develop an exacerbation of parkinsonism and have to be returned to the conventional form.

Store at Controlled Room Temperature 15-30°C (59-86°F).

Elixir: Store at Controlled Room Temperature 15-30°C (59-86°F). DO NOT FREEZE.

Sequels Sustained Release Capsules: Store at Controlled Room Temperature 15°-30°C (59°-86°F).

HOW SUPPLIED - RATED THERAPEUTICALLY EQUIVALENT:

Elixir - Oral - 2 mg/5ml

480 ml	$20.00	Trihexyphenidyl Hcl, Liquipharm	54198-0107-16
480 ml	**$32.94**	**ARTANE, Lederle Pharm**	**00005-4440-65**

Tablet - Oral - 5 mg

100's	$32.54	Trihexyphenidyl Hydrochloride, H.C.F.A. F F P	99999-2385-01

Tablet, Uncoated - Oral - 2 mg

100's	$6.56	Trihexyphenidyl Hydrochloride, US Trading	56126-0317-11
100's	$12.36	Trihexyphenidyl Hydrochloride 2s, Aligen Independ	00405-5061-01
100's	$12.81	Trihexyphenidyl Hcl, HL Moore Drug Exch	00839-1699-06
100's	$13.50	Trihexyphenidyl Hcl, Harber Pharm	51432-0466-03
100's	$14.25	Trihexyphenidyl Hcl 2, Major Pharms	00904-2041-60
100's	$14.53	Trihexyphenidyl Hcl, Vangard Labs	00615-0675-13
100's	$14.60	TRI-HEXANE, Rugby	00536-4723-01
100's	$14.75	Trihexyphenidyl Hcl, Goldline Labs	00182-0627-01
100's	$15.00	Trihexyphenidyl Hcl, Consolidated Midland	00223-2126-01
100's	$15.39	Trihexyphenidyl, Schein Pharm (US)	00364-0408-01
100's	$15.95	Trihexyphenidyl Hcl 2, Major Pharms	00904-2041-61
100's	**$16.39**	**ARTANE, Lederle Pharm**	**00005-4434-23**
100's	$18.84	Trihexyphenidyl, Schein Pharm (US)	00364-0408-90
100's	$20.33	Trihexyphenidyl Hcl, Martec Pharms	52555-0335-01
100's	**$21.50**	**ARTANE, Lederle Pharm**	**00005-4434-60**
1000's	$34.99	Trihexyphenidyl Hcl, Amer Preferred	53445-0627-00

HOW SUPPLIED - RATED THERAPEUTICALLY EQUIVALENT: *(cont'd)*

1000's	$94.84	Trihexyphenidyl Hcl, HL Moore Drug Exch	00839-1699-16
1000's	$94.85	TRI-HEXANE, Rugby	00536-4723-10
1000's	$101.60	Trihexyphenidyl Hcl 2, Major Pharms	00904-2041-80
1000's	$101.85	Trihexyphenidyl Hydrohloride, United Res	00677-0362-10
1000's	$105.00	Trihexyphenidyl Hcl, Goldline Labs	00182-0627-10
1000's	$117.19	Trihexyphenidyl, Schein Pharm (US)	00364-0408-02
1000's	**$121.21**	**ARTANE, Lederle Pharm**	**00005-4434-34**
1000's	$135.00	Trihexyphenidyl Hcl, Consolidated Midland	00223-2126-02
1000's	$135.00	Trihexyphenidyl Hcl, Harber Pharm	51432-0466-06

Tablet, Uncoated - Oral - 5 mg

100's	$6.54	Trihexyphenidyl Hcl, US Trading	56126-0318-11
100's	$20.25	Trihexyphenidyl Hcl, Qualitest Pharms	00603-6241-21
100's	$22.50	Trihexyphenidyl Hcl, Harber Pharm	51432-0468-03
100's	$25.50	TRIHEXANE, Rugby	00536-4724-01
100's	$25.50	Trihexyphenidyl Hcl 5, Major Pharms	00904-2050-60
100's	$27.50	Trihexyphenidyl Hcl, Consolidated Midland	00223-2127-01
100's	$27.60	Trihexyphenidyl Hcl, Goldline Labs	00182-0628-01
100's	$27.87	Trihexyphenidyl Hcl 5, Major Pharms	00904-2050-61
100's	$29.28	Trihexyphenidyl Hcl, HL Moore Drug Exch	00839-1698-06
100's	$30.55	Trihexyphenidyl, Schein Pharm (US)	00364-0409-01
100's	$31.06	Trihexyphenidyl Hydrochloride 5s, Aligen Independ	00405-5062-01
100's	**$32.58**	**ARTANE, Lederle Pharm**	**00005-4436-23**
100's	$32.73	Trihexyphenidyl, Schein Pharm (US)	00364-0409-90
100's	**$37.59**	**ARTANE, Lederle Pharm**	**00005-4436-60**
100's	$40.78	TRIHEXIPHENIDYL HCL, Martec Pharms	52555-0337-01
1000's	$43.28	Trihexyphenidyl Hcl, Amer Preferred	53445-0628-00
1000's	$227.50	Trihexyphenidyl Hcl, Consolidated Midland	00223-2127-02
1000's	$230.50	Trihexyphenidyl Hcl 5, Major Pharms	00904-2050-80
1000's	$255.00	Trihexyphenidyl Hcl, Goldline Labs	00182-0628-10
1000's	$255.00	Trihexyphenidyl Hcl 5, Harber Pharm	51432-0468-06
1000's	$255.02	Trihexyphenidyl, Schein Pharm (US)	00364-0409-02

TRIMEPRAZINE TARTRATE *(002387)*

CATEGORIES: Allergies; Antihistamines; Dermatitis; Eczema; Pruritus; Respiratory & Allergy Medications; Urticaria; FDA Approval Pre 1982

BRAND NAMES: *Nedeltran*; *Panectyl*; **Temaril**; *Theralene*; *Vallergan*; *Variargil*
(International brand names outside U.S. in italics)

Prescribing information not available at time of publication.

HOW SUPPLIED - EQUIVALENTS NOT AVAILABLE:

Capsule, Gelatin, Sustained Action - Oral - 5 mg

100's	**$105.13**	**TEMARIL, Allergan**	**00023-4750-11**

Syrup - Oral - 2.5 mg/5ml

120 ml	**$20.40**	**TEMARIL, Allergan**	**00023-4754-04**

Tablet, Coated - Oral - 2.5 mg

100's	**$65.43**	**TEMARIL, Allergan**	**00023-4741-10**
1000's	**$494.50**	**TEMARIL, Allergan**	**00023-4741-90**

TRIMETHADIONE *(002388)*

CATEGORIES: Anticonvulsants; Central Nervous System Agents; Convulsions; Epilepsy; Neuromuscular; Oxazolidinedione Anticonvulsant; Seizures; FDA Approval Pre 1982

BRAND NAMES: *Mino Aleviatin*; **Tridione**
(International brand names outside U.S. in italics)

FORMULARIES: PCS

> WARNING:
> BECAUSE OF ITS POTENTIAL TO PRODUCE FETAL MALFORMATIONS AND SERIOUS SIDE EFFECTS, TRIMETHADIONE SHOULD ONLY BE UTILIZED WHEN OTHER LESS TOXIC DRUGS HAVE BEEN FOUND INEFFECTIVE IN CONTROLLING PETIT MAL SEIZURES.

DESCRIPTION:

Tridione (trimethadione) is an antiepileptic agent. An oxazolidinedione compound, it is chemically identified as 3,5,5-trimethyloxozolidine-2,4-dione.

Tridione is a synthetic, water-soluble, white, crystalline powder. It is supplied in capsular, tablet, and liquid forms for oral use only.

Inactive Ingredients: *300 mg Capsule:* Corn starch, FD&C Blue No. 1, FD&C Red No. 3, FD&C Yellow No. 6, gelatin, titanium dioxide and artificial flavor. *150 mg Dulcet Tablet:* Corn starch, lactose, magnesium stearate, magnesium trisilicate, sucrose and natural/synthetic flavor. *Solution:* FD&C Yellow No. 6, methylparaben, sucrose, water and natural/synthetic flavors.

CLINICAL PHARMACOLOGY:

Trimethadione has been shown to prevent pentylenetetrazol-induced and thujone-induced seizures in experimental animals; the drug has a less marked effect on seizures induced by picrotoxin, procaine, cocaine, or strychnine. Unlike the hydantoins and antiepileptic barbiturates, trimethadione does not modify the maximal seizure pattern in patients undergoing electroconvulsive therapy.

Trimethadione has a sedative effect that may increase to the point of ataxia when excessive doses are used. A toxic dose of the drug in animals (approximately 2 g/kg) produced sleep, unconsciousness, and respiratory depression.

Trimethadione is rapidly absorbed from the gastrointestinal tract. It is demethylated by liver microsomes to the active metabolite, dimethadione.

Approximately 3% of a daily dose of trimethadione is recovered in the urine as unchanged drug. The majority of trimethadione is excreted slowly by the kidney in the form of dimethadione.

INDICATIONS AND USAGE:

Trimethadione is indicated for the control of petit mal seizures that are refractory to treatment with other drugs.

CONTRAINDICATIONS:

Trimethadione is contraindicated in patients with a known hypersensitivity to the drug.

WARNINGS:

Trimethadione may cause serious side effects. Strict medical supervision of the patient is mandatory, especially during the initial year of therapy.

Trimethadione should be withdrawn promptly if skin rash appears, because of the grave possibility of the occurrence of exfoliative dermatitis or severe forms of erythema multiforme. Even a minor acneiform or morbilliform rash should be allowed to clear completely before treatment with trimethadione is resumed; reinstitute therapy cautiously.

A complete blood count should be done prior to initiating therapy with trimethadione, and at monthly intervals thereafter. A marked depression of the blood count is an indication for withdrawal of the drug. If no abnormality appears within 12 months, the interval between blood counts may be extended. A moderate degree of neutropenia with or without a corresponding drop in the leukocyte count is not uncommon. Therapy need not be withdrawn unless the neutrophil count is 2500 or less; more frequent blood examinations should be done when the count is less than 3,000. Other blood dyscrasias, including leukopenia, eosinophilia, thrombocytopenia, pancytopenia, agranulocytosis, hypoplastic anemia, and fatal aplastic anemia, have occurred. Patients should be advised to report immediately such signs and symptoms as sore throat, fever, malaise, easy bruising, petechiae, or epistaxis, or others that may be indicative of an infection or bleeding tendency. Trimethadione should ordinarily not be used in patients with severe blood dyscrasias.

Liver function tests should be done prior to initiating therapy with trimethadione, and at monthly intervals thereafter. Hepatitis has been reported rarely. Jaundice or other signs of liver dysfunction are an indication for withdrawal of the drug. Trimethadione should ordinarily not be used in patients with severe hepatic impairment.

A urinalysis should be done prior to initiating therapy with trimethadione and at monthly intervals thereafter. Fatal nephrosis has been reported. Persistent or increasing albuminuria, or the development of any other significant renal abnormality, is an indication for withdrawal of the drug. Trimethadione should ordinarily not be used in patients with severe renal dysfunction.

Hemeralopia has occurred; this appears to be an effect of trimethadione on the neural layers of the retina, and usually can be reversed by a reduction in dosage. Scotomata are an indication for withdrawal of the drug. Caution should be observed when treating patients who have diseases of the retina or optic nerve.

Manifestations of systemic lupus erythematosus have been associated with the use of trimethadione as they have with the use of certain other anticonvulsants. Lymphadenopathies simulating malignant lymphoma have occurred. Lupus-like manifestations or lymph node enlargement are indications for withdrawal of the drug. Signs and symptoms may disappear after discontinuation of therapy, and specific treatment may be unnecessary.

A myasthenia gravis-like syndrome has been associated with the chronic use of trimethadione. Symptoms suggestive of this condition are indications for withdrawal of the drug.

Drugs known to cause toxic effects similar to those of trimethadione should be avoided or used only with extreme caution during therapy with trimethadione.

USAGE DURING PREGNANCY AND LACTATION

There are multiple reports in the clinical literature which indicate that the use of anticonvulsant drugs during pregnancy results in an increased incidence of birth defects in the offspring. Data are more extensive with respect to trimethadione, paramethadione, phenytoin and phenobarbital than with other anticonvulsant drugs.

Therefore, anticonvulsant drugs such as trimethadione should be administered to women of childbearing potential only if they are clearly shown to be essential in the management of their seizures. Effective means of contraception should accompany the use of trimethadione in such patients. If a patient becomes pregnant while taking trimethadione, termination of the pregnancy should be considered. A patient who requires therapy with trimethadione and who wishes to become pregnant should be advised of the risks.

Reports have suggested that the maternal ingestion of anticonvulsant drugs, particularly barbiturates, is associated with a neonatal coagulation defect that may cause bleeding during the early (usually within 24 hours of birth) neonatal period. The possibility of the occurrence of this defect with the use of trimethadione should be kept in mind. The defect is characterized by decreased levels of vitamin K-dependent clotting factors, and prolongation of either the prothrombin time or the partial thromboplastin time, or both. It has been suggested that prophylactic Vitamin K be given to the mother one month prior to, and during delivery, and to the infant, intravenously, immediately after birth.

The safety of trimethadione for use during lactation has not been established.

PRECAUTIONS:

Abrupt discontinuation of trimethadione may precipitate petit mal status. Trimethadione should always be withdrawn gradually unless serious adverse effects dictate otherwise. In the latter case, another anticonvulsant may be substituted to protect the patient.

Usage during Pregnancy and Lactation: See WARNINGS.

ADVERSE REACTIONS:

The following side effects, some of them serious, have been associated with the use of trimethadione:

Gastrointestinal: nausea, vomiting, abdominal pain, gastric distress.

CNS/Neurologic: drowsiness, fatigue, malaise, insomnia, vertigo, headache, paresthesias, precipitation of grand mal seizures, increased irritability, personality changes. Drowsiness usually subsides with continued therapy. If it persists, a reduction in dosage is indicated.

Hematologic: bleeding gums, epistaxis, retinal and petechial hemorrhages, vaginal bleeding, neutropenia, leukopenia, eosinophilia, thrombocytopenia, pancytopenia, agranulocytosis, hypoplastic anemia, and fatal aplastic anemia.

Dermatologic: acneiform or morbilliform skin rash that may progress to exfoliative dermatitis or to severe forms of erythema multiforme.

Other: hiccups, anorexia, weight loss, hair loss, changes in blood pressure, albuminuria, hemeralopia, photophobia, diplopia.

Fatal nephrosis has occurred.

Hepatitis has been reported rarely.

Lupus erythematosus, and lymphadenopathies simulating malignant lymphoma, have been reported.

Pruritus associated with lymphadenopathy and hepatosplenomegaly has occurred in hypersensitive individuals.

A myasthenia gravis-like syndrome has been reported.

OVERDOSAGE:

Symptoms of acute trimethadione overdosage include drowsiness, nausea, dizziness, ataxia, visual disturbances. Coma may follow massive overdosage.

OVERDOSAGE: *(cont'd)*

Gastric evacuation, either by induced emesis, or by lavage, or both, should be done immediately. General supportive care, including frequent monitoring of the vital signs and close observations of the patient, are required.

Alkalinization of the urine has been reported to enhance the renal excretion of dimethadione, the active metabolite of trimethadione.

A blood count and a careful evaluation of hepatic and renal function should be done following recovery.

DOSAGE AND ADMINISTRATION:

Trimethadione is administered orally.

Usual Adult Dosage: 0.9-2.4 grams daily in 3 or 4 equally divided doses (*i.e.,* 300-600 mg 3 or 4 times daily).

Initially, give 0.9 gram daily; increase this dose by 300 mg at weekly intervals until therapeutic results are seen or until toxic symptoms appear.

Maintenance dosage should be the least amount of drug required to maintain control.

Children's Dosage: Usually 0.3-0.9 gram daily in 3 or 4 equally divided doses.

HOW SUPPLIED:

Tridione Capsules (trimethadione capsules, USP), 300 mg are white. *Recommended storage:* Store capsules below 77°F (25°C).

Tridione Dulcet Tablets (trimethadione tablets, USP), 150 mg are white chewable tablets. *Recommended storage:* Store Dulcet tablets in refrigerator (2° - 8°C) to minimize crystallization. However, some crystallization not harmful to product may occur. Keep tightly closed.

Tridione Solution (trimethadione oral solution, USP) is supplied as 1.2 g per fluid ounce (40 mg per ml). *Recommended storage:* Store solution below 86°F (30°C).

HOW SUPPLIED - EQUIVALENTS NOT AVAILABLE:

Capsule, Gelatin - Oral - 300 mg

100's $42.69 TRIDIONE, Abbott **00074-3709-01**

Tablet, Chewable - Oral - 150 mg

100's $37.66 TRIDIONE, DULCET, Abbott **00074-3753-01**

TRIMETHOBENZAMIDE HYDROCHLORIDE

(002390)

CATEGORIES: Antiemetics; Gastrointestinal Drugs; Nausea; Nausea and Vomiting; Vertigo/Motion Sickness/Vomiting; Vomiting; Anterior Pituitary/Hypothalmic Function*; FDA Approval Pre 1982

* Indication not approved by the FDA

BRAND NAMES: *Anaus*; Arrestin; Benzacot; Bio-Gan; *Elen*; *Ibikin*; Navogan; Stemetic; T-Gen; Tebamide; Tegamide; Ti-Plex; Ticon; **Tigan**; Tiject-20; Triban; Tribenzagan; Trimazide

(International brand names outside U.S. in italics)

FORMULARIES: Aetna; BC-BS; FHP

WARNING:

Caution should be exercised when administering trimethobenzamide hydrochloride to children for the treatment of vomiting. Antiemetics are not recommended for treatment of uncomplicated vomiting in children and their use should be limited to prolonged vomiting of known etiology. There are three principal reasons for caution:

1. There has been some suspicion that centrally acting antiemetics may contribute, in combination with viral illnesses (a possible cause of vomiting in children), to development of Reye's syndrome, a potentially fatal acute childhood encephalopathy with visceral fatty degeneration, especially involving the liver. Although there is no confirmation of this suspicion, caution is nevertheless recommended.

2. The extrapyramidal symptoms which can occur secondary to trimethobenzamide hydrochloride may be confused with the central nervous system signs of an undiagnosed primary disease responsible for the vomiting, e.g., Reye's syndrome or other encephalopathy.

3. It has been suspected that drugs with hepatotoxic potential, such as trimethobenzamide, may unfavorably alter the course of Reye's syndrome. Such drugs should therefore be avoided in children whose signs and symptoms (vomiting) could represent Reye's syndrome. It should also be noted that salicylates and acetaminophen are hepatotoxic at large doses. Although it is not known that at usual doses they would represent a hazard in patients with the underlying hepatic disorder of Reye's syndrome, these drugs, too, should be avoided in children whose signs and symptoms could represent Reye's syndrome, unless alternative methods of controlling fever are not successful.

DESCRIPTION:

Chemically, trimethobenzamide HCl is N-(p-(2-(dimethylamino) -ethoxy) benzyl)-3,4,5-trimethoxybenzamide hydrochloride. It has a molecular weight of 424.93.

CLINICAL PHARMACOLOGY:

The mechanism of action of trimethobenzamide hydrochloride as determined in animals is obscure, but may be the chemoreceptor trigger zone (CTZ), an area in the medulla oblongata through which emetic impulses are conveyed to the vomiting center; direct impulses to the vomiting center apparently are not similarly inhibited. In dogs pretreated with trimethobenzamide HCl, the emetic response to apomorphine is inhibited, while little or no protection is afforded against emesis induced by intragastric copper sulfate.

INDICATIONS AND USAGE:

Trimethobenzamide hydrochloride is indicated for the control of nausea and vomiting.

CONTRAINDICATIONS:

The injectable form of trimethobenzamide hydrochloride in children, the suppositories in premature or newborn infants, and use in patients with known hypersensitivity to trimethobenzamide are contraindicated. Since the suppositories contain benzocaine they should not be used in patients known to be sensitive to this or similar local anesthetics.

WARNINGS:

Trimethobenzamide hydrochloride may produce drowsiness. Patients should not operate motor vehicles or other dangerous machinery until their individual responses have been determined. Reye's syndrome has been associated with the use of Trimethobenzamide hydrochloride and other drugs, including antiemetics, although their contribution, if any, to the cause and course of the disease hasn't been established. This syndrome is characterized by an abrupt onset shortly following a non-specific febrile illness, with persistent, severe vomiting, lethargy, irrational behavior, progressive encephalopathy leading to coma, convulsions and death.

Usage in Pregnancy: Trimethobenzamide hydrochloride was studied in reproduction experiments in rats and rabbits and no teratogenicity was suggested. The only effects observed were an increased percentage of embryonic resorptions or stillborn pups in rats administered 20 mg and 100 mg/kg and increased resorptions in rabbits receiving 100 mg/kg. In each study these adverse effects were attributed to one or two dams. The relevance to humans is not known. Since there is no adequate experience in pregnant or lactating women who have received this drug, safety in pregnancy or in nursing mothers has not been established.

PRECAUTIONS:

During the course of acute febrile illness, encephalitides, gastroenteritis, dehydration and electrolyte imbalance, especially in children and the elderly or debilitated, CNS reactions such as opisthotonos, convulsions, coma and extrapyramidal symptoms have been reported with and without use of trimethobenzamide hydrochloride or other antiemetic agents. In such disorders caution should be exercised in administering trimethobenzamide hydrochloride, particularly to patients who have recently received other CNS-acting agents (phenothiazines, barbiturates, belladonna derivatives). It is recommended that severe emesis should not be treated with an antiemetic drug alone; where possible the cause of vomiting should be established. Primary emphasis should be directed toward the restoration of body fluids and electrolyte balance, the relief of fever and relief of the causative disease process. Overhydration should be avoided since it may result in cerebral edema.

The antiemetic effects of trimethobenzamide hydrochloride may render diagnosis more difficult in such conditions as appendicitis and obscure signs of toxicity due to overdosage of other drugs.

DRUG INTERACTIONS:

Usage with Alcohol: Concomitant use of alcohol with trimethobenzamide hydrochloride may result in an adverse drug interaction.

ADVERSE REACTIONS:

There have been reports of hypersensitivity reactions and Parkinson-like symptoms. There have been instances of hypotension reported following parenteral administration to surgical patients. There have been reports of blood dyscrasias, blurring of vision, coma, convulsions, depression of mood, diarrhea, disorientation, dizziness, drowsiness, headache, jaundice, muscle cramps and opisthotonos. If these occur, the administration of the drug should be discontinued. Allergic-type skin reactions have been observed; therefore, the drug should be discontinued at the first sign of sensitization. While these symptoms will usually disappear spontaneously, symptomatic treatment may be indicated in some cases.

DOSAGE AND ADMINISTRATION:

(See WARNINGS and PRECAUTIONS.)

Dosage should be adjusted according to the indication for therapy, severity of symptoms and the response of the patient.

CAPSULES, 250 MG AND 100 MG

Usual Adult Dosage: One 250 mg capsule t.i.d. or q.i.d.

Usual Children's Dosage: 30 to 90 lbs: One or two 100 mg capsules t.i.d. or q.i.d.

SUPPOSITORIES, 200 MG (NOT TO BE USED IN PREMATURE OR NEWBORN INFANTS)

Usual Adult Dosage: One suppository (200 mg) t.i.d. or q.i.d.

Usual Children's Dosage: *Under 30 lbs:* One-half suppository (100 mg) t.i.d. or q.i.d. *30 to 90 lbs:* One-half to one suppository (100 to 200 mg) t.i.d. or q.i.d.

SUPPOSITORIES, PEDIATRIC, 100 MG (NOT TO BE USED IN PREMATURE OR NEWBORN INFANTS)

Usual Children's Dosage: *Under 30 lbs:* One suppository (100 mg) t.i.d. or q.i.d. *30 to 90 lbs:* One to two suppositories (100 to 200 mg) t.i.d. or q.i.d.

INJECTABLE, 100 MG/ML (NOT RECOMMENDED FOR USE IN CHILDREN)

Usual Adult Dosage: 2 ml (200 mg) t.i.d. or q.i.d. intramuscularly. *NOTE:* The injectable for is intended for intramuscular administration only; it is not recommended for intravenous use.

Intramuscular administration may cause pain, stinging, burning, redness and swelling at the site of injection. Such effects may be minimized by deep injection into the upper outer quadrant of the gluteal region, and by avoiding the escape of solution along the route.

HOW SUPPLIED - RATED THERAPEUTICALLY EQUIVALENT:

Injection, Solution - Intramuscular - 100 mg/ml

2 ml	$54.69	Trimethobenzamide Hcl Inj, Solopak Labs	39769-0062-02
2 ml x 10	$25.53	Trimethobenzamide HCl, Sanofi Winthrop	00024-1955-03
2 ml x 10	**$33.79**	**TIGAN, Beecham**	**00029-4085-22**
2 ml x 25	$56.50	Trimethobenzamide Hcl, Steris Labs	00402-0690-82
2 ml x 25	$70.63	Trimethobenzamide HCl, Schein Pharm (US)	00364-6762-42
2 ml x 25	**$117.18**	**TIGAN, Beecham**	**00029-4087-22**
20 ml	$8.68	Trimethobenzamide Hcl, HL Moore Drug Exch	00839-6676-33
20 ml	$9.32	Trimethobenzamide Hcl, Steris Labs	00402-0164-20
20 ml	$10.00	Trimethobenzamide Hcl, Consolidated Midland	00223-8700-20
20 ml	$13.51	Trimethobenzamide HCl, Schein Pharm (US)	00364-6762-55
20 ml	$14.25	Trimethobenzamide Hcl, IDE-Interstate	00814-8064-44
20 ml	**$24.03**	**TIGAN, Beecham**	**00029-4086-22**

HOW SUPPLIED - NOT RATED EQUIVALENT:

Capsule, Gelatin - Oral - 100 mg

100's	**$39.15**	**TIGAN, Beecham**	**00029-4082-30**
100's	**$42.67**	**TIGAN, Roberts Labs**	**54092-0186-01**

Capsule, Gelatin - Oral - 250 mg

100's	$34.55	Trimethobenzamide Hcl, Qualitest Pharms	00603-6256-21
100's	$35.30	Trimethobenzamide Hcl, Goldline Labs	00182-1396-01
100's	$35.95	Trimethobenzamide Hcl, United Res	00677-1383-01
100's	$36.48	Trimethobenzamide HCl, Rugby	00536-4727-01
100's	$37.80	Trimethobenzamide Hcl, Aligen Independ	00405-5066-01
100's	$39.50	Trimethobenzamide Hcl, Pecos	59879-0115-01
100's	$39.75	Trimethobenzamide Hcl, Major Pharms	00904-3291-60
100's	**$51.45**	**TIGAN, Beecham**	**00029-4083-30**
500's	**$244.21**	**TIGAN, Beecham**	**00029-4083-32**

HOW SUPPLIED - NOT RATED EQUIVALENT: *(cont'd)*

Suppository - Rectal - 100 mg

10's	$3.70	TEBAMIDE PEDIATRIC, GW Labs	00713-0107-09
10's	$4.97	Trimethobenzamide Hcl, Clay Park Labs	45802-0723-90
10's	$5.00	Trimethobenzamide Hcl, Paddock Labs	00574-7220-10
10's	$5.35	Trimethobenzamide Hcl, Major Pharms	00904-2735-15
10's	$5.75	Trimethobenzamide HCl, Schein Pharm (US)	00364-7347-10
10's	$5.75	Trimethobenzamide Hcl, Qualitest Pharms	00603-8150-10
10's	$5.80	T-GEN, Goldline Labs	00182-1428-23
10's	$6.38	Trimethobenzamide HCl, Rugby	00536-0211-19
10's	$6.75	Trimethobenzamide Hcl, Bio Pharm	59741-0305-09
10's	$6.90	TI-PLEX 100, Medi-Plex Pharm	59010-0335-10
10's	$6.99	Trimethobenzamide HCl, Cypress Pharm	60258-0503-10
10's	$10.07	Navogan, Intl Ethical	11584-0421-01
10's	$10.75	Trimethobenzamide, Elge	58298-0140-10
10's	**$16.40**	**TIGAN PEDIATRIC, Beecham**	**00029-4088-38**
50's	$23.50	Trimethobenzamide Hcl, Clay Park Labs	45802-0723-32
50's	$29.35	Trimethobenzamide Hcl, Bio Pharm	59741-0305-50
100's	$12.25	Trimethobenzamide Hcl, Bio Pharm	59741-0305-49

Suppository - Rectal - 200 mg

10's	$4.08	TEBAMIDE ADULT, GW Labs	00713-0108-09
10's	$4.90	Trimethobenzamide Hcl, Clay Park Labs	45802-0724-90
10's	$6.05	Trimethobenzamide Hcl, Paddock Labs	00574-7222-10
10's	$6.14	Trimethobenzamide Hcl, Qualitest Pharms	00603-8151-10
10's	$6.50	T-GEN, Goldline Labs	00182-1427-23
10's	$6.50	Trimethobenzamide Hcl, Rose Laboratories	42037-0136-10
10's	$7.25	Trimethobenzamide Hcl, Consolidated Midland	00223-5905-10
10's	$7.29	Trimethobenzamide HCl, Cypress Pharm	60258-0502-10
10's	$7.43	Trimethobenzamide HCl, Schein Pharm (US)	00364-7348-10
10's	$8.05	Trimethobenzamide Hcl, Major Pharms	00904-2736-15
10's	$9.07	Trimethobenzamide HCl, Rugby	00536-0221-19
10's	$12.54	Trimethobenzamide, Elge	58298-0145-10
10's	$13.95	Trimethobenzamide Hcl, Bio Pharm	59741-0304-09
10's	**$19.46**	**TIGAN, Beecham**	**00029-4084-38**
50's	$15.75	Trimethobenzamide Hcl, Bio Pharm	59741-0304-49
50's	$16.50	Trimethobenzamide Hcl, Rose Laboratories	42037-0136-50
50's	$19.54	TEBAMIDE ADULT, GW Labs	00713-0108-50
50's	$21.85	Trimethobenzamide Hcl, Paddock Labs	00574-7222-50
50's	$29.30	T-GEN, Goldline Labs	00182-1427-19
50's	$34.50	Trimethobenzamide Hcl, Consolidated Midland	00223-5905-50
50's	$49.10	Trimethobenzamide, Elge	58298-0145-50
50's	**$88.07**	**TIGAN, Beecham**	**00029-4084-39**
100's	$48.45	Trimethobenzamide Hcl, Bio Pharm	59741-0304-50

TRIMETHOPRIM *(002391)*

CATEGORIES: Anti-Infectives; Antibacterials; Antimicrobials; Infections; Sulfonamides; Urinary Anti-Infectives; Urinary Antibacterial; Urinary Tract Infections; Pregnancy Category C; FDA Approval Pre 1982

BRAND NAMES: *Abaprim*; *Alprim*; *Bactin*; *Idotrim*; *Ipral*; *Lidaprim*; *Methoprim*; *Monotrim*; *Primosept*; Primsol; **Proloprim**; *Syraprim*; *TMP-Ratiopharm*; *Tiempe*; *Trimexazole*; *Trimopan*; Trimpex; *Triprim*; *Unitrim*; *Wellcoprim*
(International brand names outside U.S. in italics)

FORMULARIES: Aetna; BC-BS; WHO

DESCRIPTION:

Trimethoprim is 2,4-diamino-5-(3,4,5-trimethoxybenzyl) pyrimidine. It is a white to light yellow, odorless, bitter compound with a molecular weight of 290.3.

CLINICAL PHARMACOLOGY:

Trimethoprim is rapidly absorbed following oral administration. It exists in the blood as unbound, protein-bound and metabolized forms. Ten to twenty percent of trimethoprim is metabolized, primarily in the liver; the remainder is excreted unchanged in the urine. The principal metabolites of trimethoprim are the 1-and 3-oxides and the 3'- and 4'- hydroxy derivatives. The free form is considered to be the therapeutically active form. Approximately 44% of trimethoprim is bound to plasma proteins.

Mean peak plasma concentrations of approximately 1.0 mcg/ml occur 1 to 4 hours after oral administration of a single 100-mg dose. A single 200-mg dose will result in plasma concentrations approximately twice as high. The half-life of trimethoprim ranges from 8 to 10 hours. However, patients with severely impaired renal function exhibit an increase in the half-life of trimethoprim, which requires either dosage regimen adjustment or not using the drug in such patients (see DOSAGE AND ADMINISTRATION). During a 13-week study of trimethoprim administered at a dosage of 50 mg q.i.d., the mean minimum steady-state concentration of the drug was 1.1 mcg/ml. Steady-state concentrations were achieved within 2 to 3 days of chronic administration and were maintained throughout the experimental period.

Excretion of trimethoprim is primarily by the kidneys through glomerular filtration and tubular secretion. Urine concentrations of trimethoprim are considerably higher than are the concentrations in the blood. After a single oral dose of 100 mg, urine concentrations of trimethoprim ranged from 30 to 160 mcg/ml during the 0- to 4-hour period and declined to approximately 18 to 91 mcg/ml during the 8- to 24-hour period. A 200-mg single oral dose will result in trimethoprim urine concentrations approximately twice as high. After oral administration, 50% to 60% of trimethoprim is excreted in urine within 24 hours, approximately 80% of this being unmetabolized trimethoprim.

Since normal vaginal and fecal flora are the source of most pathogens causing urinary tract infections, it is relevant to consider the distribution of trimethoprim into these sites. Concentrations of trimethoprim in vaginal secretions are consistently greater than those found simultaneously in the serum, being typically 1.6 times the concentrations of simultaneously obtained serum samples. Sufficient trimethoprim is excreted in the feces to markedly reduce or eliminate trimethoprim-susceptible organisms from the fecal flora. The dominant non-*Enterobacteriaceae* fecal organisms, *Bacteroides* spp. and *Lactobacillus* spp., are not susceptible to trimethoprim concentrations obtained with the recommended dosage.

Trimethoprim also passes the placental barrier and is excreted in breast milk.

Microbiology: Trimethoprim blocks the production of tetrahydrofolic acid from dihydrofolic acid by binding to and reversibly inhibiting the required enzyme, dihydrofolate reductase. This binding is very much stronger for the bacterial enzyme than for the corresponding mammalian enzyme. Thus, trimethoprim selectively interferes with bacterial biosynthesis of nucleic acids and proteins.

In vitro serial dilution tests have shown that the spectrum of antibacterial activity of trimethoprim includes the common urinary tract pathogens with the exception of *Pseudomonas aeruginosa.* (TABLE 1)

The recommended quantitative disc susceptibility method[1,2] may be used for estimating the susceptibility of bacteria to trimethoprim. With this procedure, reports from the laboratory giving results using the 5-mcg trimethoprim disc should be interpreted according to the

CLINICAL PHARMACOLOGY: *(cont'd)*

TABLE 1

Representative Minimum Inhibitory Concentrations for Trimethoprim-Susceptible Organisms

Bacteria	Trimethoprim MIC - mcg/ml(Range)
Escherichia coli	0.05 - 1.5
Proteus mirabilis	0.5 - 1.5
Klebsiella pneumoniae	0.5 - 5.0
Enterobacter species	0.5 - 5.0
Staphylococcus species (coagulase-negative)	0.15 - 5.0

following criteria: Organisms producing zones of 16 mm or greater are classified as susceptible, whereas those producing zones of 11 to 15 mm are classified as having intermediate susceptibility. A report from the laboratory of "Susceptible to trimethoprim" or "Intermediate susceptibility to trimethoprim" indicates that the infection is likely to respond when, as in uncomplicated urinary tract infections, effective therapy is dependent upon the urine concentration of trimethoprim. Organisms producing zones of 10 mm or less are reported as resistant, indicating that other therapy should be selected.

Dilution methods for determining susceptibility are also used, and results are reported as the minimum drug concentration inhibiting microbial growth (MIC).[3] If the MIC is 8 mcg per ml or less, the microorganism is considered "susceptible". If the MIC is 16 mcg per ml or greater, the microorganism is considered "resistant."

INDICATIONS AND USAGE:

For the treatment of initial episodes of uncomplicated urinary tract infections due to susceptible strains of the following organisms:*Escherichia coli, Proteus mirabilis, Klebsiella pneumoniae, Enterobacter* species and coagulase-negative *Staphylococcus* species, including *S. saprophyticus.*

Cultures and susceptibility tests should be performed to determine the susceptibility of the bacteria to trimethoprim. Therapy may be initiated prior to obtaining the results of these tests.

CONTRAINDICATIONS:

Trimethoprim is contraindicated in individuals hypersensitive to trimethoprim and in those with documented megaloblastic anemia due to folate deficiency.

WARNINGS:

Serious hypersensitivity reactions have been reported rarely in patients on trimethoprim therapy. Trimethoprim has been reported rarely to interfere with hematopoiesis, especially when administered in large doses and/or for prolonged periods.

The presence of clinical signs such as sore throat, fever, pallor or purpura may be early indications of serious blood disorders.

PRECAUTIONS:

General: Trimethoprim should be given with caution to patients with possible folate deficiency. Folates may be administered concomitantly without interfering with the antibacterial action of trimethoprim. Trimethoprim should also be given with caution to patients with impaired renal or hepatic function. If any clinical signs of a blood disorder are noted in a patient receiving trimethoprim, a complete blood count should be obtained and the drug discontinued if a significant reduction in the count of any formed blood element is found.

Drug/Laboratory Test Interactions: Trimethoprim can interfere with a serum methotrexate assay as determined by the competitive binding protein technique (CBPA) when a bacterial dihydrofolate reductase is used as the binding protein. No interference occurs, however, if methotrexate is measured by a radioimmunoassay (RIA).

The presence of trimethoprim may also interfere with the Jaffe alkaline picrate reaction assay for creatinine resulting in overestimations of about 10% in the range of normal values.

CARCINOGENESIS, MUTAGENESIS, AND IMPAIRMENT OF FERTILITY

Carcinogenesis: Long-term studies in animals to evaluate carcinogenic potential have not been conducted with trimethoprim.

Mutagenesis: Trimethoprim was demonstrated to be nonmutagenic in the Ames assay. No chromosomal damage was observed in human leukocytes cultured *in vitro* with trimethoprim; the concentration used exceeded blood levels following therapy with trimethoprim.

Impairment of Fertility: No adverse effects on fertility or general reproductive performance were observed in rats given trimethoprim in oral dosages as high as 70 mg/kg/day for males and 14 mg/kg/day for females.

Pregnancy, Teratogenic Effects, Pregnancy Category C: Trimethoprim has been shown to be teratogenic in the rat when given in doses 40 times the human dose. In some rabbit studies, the overall increase in fetal loss (dead and resorbed and malformed conceptuses) was associated with doses 6 times the human therapeutic dose.

While there are no large well-controlled studies on the use of trimethoprim in pregnant women, Brumfitt and Pursell,[4] in a retrospective study, reported the outcome of 186 pregnancies during which the mother received either placebo or trimethoprim in combination with sulfamethoxazole. The incidence of congenital abnormalities was 4.5% (3 of 66) in those who received placebo and 3.3% (4 of 120) in those receiving trimethoprim plus sulfamethoxazole. There were no abnormalities in the 10 children whose mothers received the drug during the first trimester. In a separate survey, Brumfitt and Pursell also found no congenital abnormalities in 35 children whose mothers had received trimethoprim plus sulfamethoxazole at the time of conception or shortly thereafter.

Because trimethoprim may interfere with folic acid metabolism, trimethoprim should be used during pregnancy only if the potential benefit justifies the potential risk to the fetus.

Nonteratogenic Effects: The oral administration of trimethoprim to rats at a dose of 70 mg/kg/day commencing with the last third of gestation and continuing through parturition and lactation caused no deleterious effects on gestation or pup growth and survival.

Nursing Mothers: Trimethoprim is excreted in human milk. Because trimethoprim may interfere with folic acid metabolism, caution should be exercised when trimethoprim is administered to a nursing woman.

Pediatric Use: The safety of trimethoprim in infants under two months of age has not been demonstrated. The effectiveness of trimethoprim has not been established in children under 12 years of age.

DRUG INTERACTIONS:

Trimethoprim may inhibit the hepatic metabolism of phenytoin. Trimethoprim, given at a common clinical dosage, increased the phenytoin half-life by 51% and decreased the phenytoin metabolic clearance rate by 30%. When administering these drugs concurrently, one should be alert for possible excessive phenytoin effect.

ADVERSE REACTIONS:

The adverse effects encountered most often with trimethoprim were rash and pruritus. Other adverse effects reported involved the gastrointestinal and hematopoietic systems.

Dermatologic: Rash, pruritus and phototoxic skin eruptions. At the recommended dosage regimens of 100 mg bid or 200 mg qd, each for 10 days, the incidence of rash is 2.9% to 6.7%. In clinical studies which employed high doses of trimethoprim, an elevated incidence of rash was noted. These rashes were maculopapular, morbilliform, pruritic and generally mild to moderate, appearing 7 to 14 days after the initiation of therapy.

Hypersensitivity: There have been rare reports of exfoliative dermatitis, erythema multiforme, Stevens-Johnson syndrome, Lyell syndrome, anaphylaxis and aseptic meningitis.

Gastrointestinal: Epigastric distress, nausea, vomiting and glossitis. Elevation of serum transaminase and bilirubin.

Hematologic: Thrombocytopenia, leukopenia, neutropenia, megaloblastic anemia and methemoglobinemia.

Miscellaneous: Fever, increases in BUN and serum creatinine levels.

OVERDOSAGE:

Acute: Signs of acute overdosage with trimethoprim may appear following ingestion of 1 gram or more of the drug and include nausea, vomiting, dizziness, headaches, mental depression, confusion and bone marrow depression (see Chronic).

Treatment consists of gastric lavage and general supportive measures. Acidification of the urine will increase renal elimination of trimethoprim. Peritoneal dialysis is not effective and hemodialysis only moderately effective in eliminating the drug.

Chronic: Use of trimethoprim at high doses and/or for extended periods of time may cause bone marrow depression manifested as thrombocytopenia, leukopenia and/or megaloblastic anemia. If signs of bone marrow depression occur, trimethoprim should be discontinued and the patient should be given leucovorin, 3 to 6 mg intramuscularly daily for three days, or as required to restore normal hematopoiesis.

DOSAGE AND ADMINISTRATION:

The usual oral adult dosage is 100 mg (one tablet) every 12 hours or 200 mg (two tablets) every 24 hours, each for 10 days. The use of trimethoprim in patients with a creatinine clearance of less than 15 ml/min is not recommended. For patients with a creatinine clearance of 15 to 30 ml/min, the dose should be 50 mg every 12 hours.

The effectiveness of trimethoprim has not been established in children under 12 years of age.

REFERENCES:

1. Bauer AW, Kirby WMM, Sherris JC, Turck M: Antibiotic Susceptibility Testing by standardized Single Disk Method, *Am J Clin Pathol 45*:493-496, 1966. **2.** Approved Standard ASM-2 Performance Standards for Antimicrobial Disc Susceptibility Test; National Committee for Clinical Laboratory Standards, 771 East Lancaster Avenue, Villanova, Pennsylvania 19085. **3.** Ericsson HM, Sherris JC: Antibiotic Sensitivity Testing. Report of an International Collaborative Study. *Acta Pathol Microbiol Scand* (B) (Suppl 217): 1-90, 1971. **4.** Brumfitt W, Pursell R: Trimethoprim/Sulfamethoxazole in the Treatment of Bacteriuria in Women.*J Infect Dis 128* (Suppl): S657-S663, 1973.

HOW SUPPLIED - RATED THERAPEUTICALLY EQUIVALENT:

Tablet, Uncoated - Oral - 100 mg

100's	$16.43	Trimethoprim, H.C.F.A. F F P	99999-2391-01
100's	$18.74	Trimethoprim, Qualitest Pharms	00603-6264-21
100's	$19.29	Trimethoprim, Major Pharms	00904-1646-60
100's	$20.00	Trimethoprim, Teva	00332-2158-09
100's	$21.43	Trimethoprim, Major Pharms	00904-1646-61
100's	$22.71	Trimethoprim, US Trading	56126-0409-11
100's	$22.80	Trimethoprim, Schein Pharm (US)	00364-0649-01
100's	$24.00	Trimethoprim 100, Goldline Labs	00182-1536-01
100's	$25.23	Trimethoprim, Rugby	00536-4686-01
100's	$25.23	Trimethoprim, HL Moore Drug Exch	00839-7284-06
100's	$68.42	TRIMPEX, Roche	00004-0127-01
100's	**$82.78**	**PROLOPRIM, Glaxo Wellcome**	**00173-0820-55**

Tablet, Uncoated - Oral - 200 mg

100's	$24.38	Trimethoprim, H.C.F.A. F F P	99999-2391-02
100's	$32.00	Trimethoprim, Teva	00332-2159-09
100's	$32.18	Trimethoprim, Qualitest Pharms	00603-6265-21
100's	$32.52	Trimethoprim, HL Moore Drug Exch	00839-7433-06
100's	$42.70	Trimethoprim, Rugby	00536-4683-01
100's	$42.70	Trimethoprim, Major Pharms	00904-1647-60
100's	$42.70	Trimethoprim, Major Pharms	00904-1647-61
100's	**$165.56**	**PROLOPRIM, Glaxo Wellcome**	**00173-0825-55**

TRIMETREXATE GLUCURONATE *(003189)*

CATEGORIES: AIDS Related Complex; Anti-Infectives; Antibacterials; Antimicrobials; Antineoplastics; Antiprotozoals; Antivirals; Methotrexate Analog; Orphan Drugs; Pneumocystis Carinii Pneumonia; Pneumonia; Lung Cancer*; FDA Class 1P ("Priority Review"); FDA Approved 1993 Dec
* Indication not approved by the FDA

BRAND NAMES: **Neutrexin**

FORMULARIES: Medi-Cal

> **WARNING:**
> TRIMETREXATE GLUCURONATE FOR INJECTION MUST BE USED WITH CONCURRENT LEUCOVORIN (LEUCOVORIN PROTECTION) TO AVOID POTENTIALLY SERIOUS OR LIFE-THREATENING TOXICITIES (SEE PRECAUTIONS AND DOSAGE AND ADMINISTRATION).

DESCRIPTION:

Neutrexin is the brand name for trimetrexate glucuronate. Trimetrexate, a 2,4-diaminoquinazoline, non-classical folate antagonist, is a synthetic inhibitor of the enzyme dihydrofolate reductase (DHFR). Neutrexin is available as a sterile lyophilized powder in single-dose vials, each containing timetrexate glucuronate equivalent to 25 mg of trimetrexate without any preservatives or excipients. The powder is reconstituted prior to intravenous infusion (See DOSAGE AND ADMINISTRATION, Reconstitution And Dilution.) Trimetrexate glucuronate is chemically known as 2,4-diamino-5-methyl-6-((3,4,5-trimethoxyanilino)methyl) quinazoline mono-D-glucuronate and has the following structure.

The empirical formula for trimetrexate glucuronate is $C_{19}H_{23}N_5O_3{\cdot}C_6H_{10}O_7$ with a molecular weight of 563.56. The active ingredient, trimetrexate free base, has an empirical formula of $C_{19}H_{23}N_5O_3$ with a molecular weight of 369.42. Trimetrexate glucuronate for injection is a pale greenish-yellow powder or cake. Trimetrexate glucuronate is soluble in water (>50 mg/

DESCRIPTION: *(cont'd)*

ml), whereas trimetrexate free base is practically insoluble in water (<0.1 mg/ml). The pKa of trimetrexate free base in 50% methanol/water is 8.0. The logarithm$_{10}$ of the partition coefficient of trimetrexate free base between octanol and water is 1.63.

CLINICAL PHARMACOLOGY:

MECHANISM OF ACTION

In vitro studies have shown that trimetrexate is a competitive inhibitor of dihydrofolate reductase (DHFR) from bacterial, protozoan, and mammalian sources. DHFR catalyzes the reduction of intracellular dihydrofolate to the active coenzyme tetrahydrofolate. Inhibition of DHFR results in the depletion of this coenzyme, leading directly to interference with thymidylate biosynthesis, as well as inhibition of folate-dependent formyltransferase, and indirectly to inhibition of purine biosynthesis. The end result is disruption of DNA, RNA, and protein synthesis, with consequent cell death.

Leucovorin (folinic acid) is readily transported into mammalian cells by an active, carrier-mediated process and can be assimilated into cellular folate pools following its metabolism. *In vitro* studies have shown that leucovorin provides a source of reduced folates necessary for normal cellular biosynthetic processes. Because the *Pneumocystis carinii* organism lacks the reduced folate carrier-mediated transport system, leucovorin is prevented from entering the organism. Therefore, at concentrations achieved with therapeutic doses of trimetrexate plus leucovorin, the selective transport of trimetrexate, but not leucovorin, into the *Pneumocystis carinii* organism allows the concurrent administration of leucovorin to protect normal host cells from the cytotoxicity of trimetrexate without inhibiting the antifolate's inhibition of *Pneumocystis carinii*. It is not known if considerably higher doses of leucovorin would affect trimetrexate's effect on *Pneumocystis carinii*.

MICROBIOLOGY

Trimetrexate inhibits, in a dose-related manner, *in vitro* growth of the trophozoite stage of rat *Pneumocystis carinii* cultured on human embryonic lung fibroblast cells. Trimetrexate concentrations between 3 and 54.1 mcM were shown to inhibit the growth of trophozoites. Leucovorin alone at a concentration of 10 mcM did not alter either the growth of the trophozoites or the anti-pneumocystis activity of trimetrexate. Resistance to trimetrexate's antimicrobial activity against*Pneumocystis carinii* has not been studied.

PHARMACOKINETICS

Trimetrexate pharmacokinetics were assessed in six patients with acquired immunodeficiency syndrome (AIDS) who had *Pneumocystic carinii* pneumonia (4 patients) or toxoplasmosis (2 patients). Trimetrexate was administered intravenously as a bolus injection at a dose of 30 mg/m^2/day along with leucovorin 20 mg/m^{2}every 6 hours for 21 days. Trimetrexate clearance (mean ± SD) was 38 ± 15 ml/min/m^2 and volume of distribution at steady state (Vd$_{SS}$) was 20 ± 8 L/m^2. The plasma concentration time profile declined in a biphasic manner over 24 hours with a terminal half- life of 11 ± 4 hours.

The pharmacokinetics of trimetrexate without the concomitant administration of leucovorin have been evaluated in cancer patients with advanced solid tumors using various dosage regimens. The decline in plasma concentrations over time has been described by either biexponential or triexponential equations. Following the single-dose administration of 10 to 130 mg/m^{2}to 37 patients, plasma concentrations were obtained for 72 hours. Nine plasma concentration time profiles were described as biexponential. The alpha phase half-life was 57 ± 28 minutes, followed by a terminal phase with a half-life of 16 ± 3 hours. The plasma concentrations in the remaining patients exhibited a triphasic decline with half-lives of 8.6 ± 6.5 minutes, 2.4 ± 1.3 hours, and 17.8 ± 8.2 hours.

Trimetrexate clearance in cancer patients has been reported as 53 ± 41 ml/min (14 patients) and 32 ± 18 ml/min/m^2(23 patients) following single-dose administration. After a five-day infusion of trimetrexate to 16 patients, plasma clearance was 30 ± 8 ml/min/m^2.

Renal clearance of trimetrexate in cancer patients has varied from about 4 ± 2 ml/min/m^2 to 10 ± 6 ml/min/m^2. Ten to 30% of the administered dose is excreted unchanged in the urine. Considering the free fraction of trimetrexate, active tubular secretion may possibly contribute to the renal clearance of trimetrexate. Renal clearance has been associated with urine flow, suggesting the possibility of tubular reabsorption as well.

The Vd$_{SS}$ of trimetrexate in cancer patients after single-dose administration and for whom plasma concentrations were obtained for 72 hours was 36.9 ± 17.6 L/m^2 (n=23) and 0.62 ± 0.24 L/kg (n=14). Following a constant infusion of trimetrexate for five days, Vd$_{SS}$ was 32.8 ± 16.6 L/m^2. The volume of the central compartment has been estimated as 0.17 ± 0.08 L/kg and 4.0 ± 2.9 L/m^2.

There have been inconsistencies in the reporting of trimetrexate protein binding. The *in vitro* plasma protein binding of trimetrexate using ultrafiltration is approximately 95% over the concentration range of 18.75 to 1000 ng/ml. There is a suggestion of capacity limited binding (saturable binding) at concentrations greater than about 1000 ng/ml, with free fraction progressively increasing to about 9.3% as concentration is increased to 15 mcg/ml. Other reports have declared trimetrexate to be greater than 98% bound at concentrations of 0.1 to 10 mcg/ml; however, specific free fractions were not stated. The free fraction of trimetrexate also has been reported to be about 15 to 16% at a concentration of 60 mcg/ml, increasing to about 20% at a trimetrexate concentration of 6 mcg/ml.

Trimetrexate metabolism in man has not been characterized. Preclinical data strongly suggest that the major metabolic pathway is oxidative O- demethylation, followed by conjugation to either glucuronide or the sulfate. N-demethylation and oxidation is a related minor pathway. Preliminary findings in humans indicate the presence of a glucuronide conjugate with DHFR inhibition and a demethylated metabolite in urine.

The presence of metabolite(s) in human plasma following the administration of trimetrexate is suggested by the differences seen in trimetrexate plasma concentrations when measured by HPLC and a nonspecific DHFR inhibition assay. The profiles are similar initially, but diverge with time; concentrations determined by DHFR being higher than those determined by HPLC. This suggests the presence of one or more metabolites with DHFR inhibition activity. After intravenous administration of trimetrexate to humans, urinary recovery averaged about 40%, using a DHFR assay, in comparison to 10% urinary recovery as determined by HPLC, suggesting the presence of one or more metabolites that retain inhibitory activity against DHFR. Fecal recovery of trimetrexate over 48 hours after intravenous administration ranged from 0.09 to 7.6% of the dose as determined by DHFR inhibition and 0.02 to 5.2% of the dose as determined by HPLC.

The pharmacokinetics of trimetrexate have not been determined in patients with renal insufficiency or hepatic dysfunction.

INDICATIONS AND USAGE:

Trimetrexate glucuronate for injection with concurrent leucovorin administration (leucovorin protection) is indicated as an alternative therapy for the treatment of moderate-to-severe*Pneumocystis carinii* pneumonia (PCP) in immunocompromised patients, including patients with the acquired immunodeficiency syndrome (AIDS), who are intolerant of, or are refractory to, trimethoprim- sulfamethoxazole therapy or for whom trimethoprim-sulfamethoxazole is contraindicated.

INDICATIONS AND USAGE: *(cont'd)*

This indication is based on the results of a randomized, controlled double-blind trial comparing trimetrexate glucoronate with concurrent leucovorin protection (TMTX/LV) to trimethoprim-sulfamethoxazole (TMP/SMX) in patients with moderate-to-severe *Pneumocystis carinii* pneumonia, as well as results of a Treatment IND. These studies are summarized below:

Trimetrexate Glucoronate Comparative Study with TMP/SMX: This double-blind, randomized trial initiated by the AIDS Clinical Trials Group (ACTG) in 1988 was designed to compare the safety and efficacy of TMTX/LV to that of TMP/SMX for the treatment of histologically confirmed, moderate-to-severe PCP, defined as (A-a) baseline gradient >30 mmHG, in patients with AIDS.

Of the 220 patients with histologically confirmed PCP, 109 were randomized to receive TMTX/LV and 111 to TMP/SMX. Study patients were randomized to TMTX/LV treatment were to receive 45 mg/m^2 of TMTX daily for 21 days plus 20 mg/m^2 of LV every 6 hours for 24 days. Those randomized to TMP/SMX were to receive 5 mg/kg TMP plus 25 mg/kg SMX four times daily for 21 days.

Response to therapy, defined as alive and off ventilatory support at completion of therapy, with no change in anti-pneumocystis therapy, or addition of supraphysiologic doses of steroids, occurred in fifty percent of patients in each treatment group.

The observed mortality in the TMTX/LV treatment group was approximately twice that in the TMP/SMX treatment group (95% CII: 0.99 - 4.11). Thirty of 109 (27%) patients treated with TMTX/LV and 18 of 111 (16%) patients receiving TMP/SMX died during the 21-day treatment course or 4-week follow-up period. Twenty-seven of 30 deaths in the TMTX/LV arm were attributed to PCP; all 18 deaths in the TMP/SMX arm were attributed to PCP.

A significantly smaller proportion of patients who received TMTX/LV compared to TMP/SMX failed therapy due to toxicity (10% vs. 25%), and a significantly greater proportion of patients failed due to lack of efficacy (40% vs. 24%). Six patients (12%) who responded to TMLX/LV relapsed during the one-month follow-up period; no patient responding to TMP/SMX relapsed during this period. Information is not available as to whether these patients received prophylaxis therapy for PCP.

Treatment IND: The FDA granted a treatment IND for trimetrexate glucoronate with leucovorin protection in February 1988 to make trimetrexate glucoronate therapy available to HIV-infected patients with histologically confirmed PCP who had disease refractory to or who were intolerant of TMP/SMX and/or intravenous pentamidine.

Over 500 physicians in the United States participated in the Treatment IND. Of the first 753 patients had been enrolled of whom 577 were evaluable for efficacy. Of these 227 patients were intolerant of both TMP/SMX and pentamidine (IST - patients intolerant of both standard therapies), 146 were tolerant of one therapy and refractory to the other (RIST - patients refractory to one therapy and intolerant to the other) and 204 were refractory to both therapies (RST - refractory to both standard therapies). This was a very ill patient population; 38% required ventilatory support at entry (TABLE 1). These studies did not have concurrent control groups.

TABLE 1 TREATMENT IND - Baseline Characteristics

	IST (n=227)	RIST (n=146)	RST (n=204)	TOTAL (n=577)
Ventilatory Support Required	39	50	129	218
n (%)	(17)	(34)	(63)	(38)
Median Days on Standard Therapy	10	12	16	14
First Episode of PCP	104	103	190	397
n (%)	(46)	(71)	(93)	(69)

The overall survival rate one month after completion of TMTX/LV as salvage therapy was 48%. Patients who had not responded to treatment with both TMP/SMX and pentamidine, of whom 63% required mechanical ventilation at entry, achieved a survival rate of 25% following treatment with TMTX/LV. Survival was 67% in patients who were intolerant to both TMP/SMX and pentamidine (TABLE 2).

TABLE 2 TREATMENT IND
Survival Rate One Month After Completion of Trimetrexate Glucoronate Therapy

	IST	RIST	RST
All Patients	153/227 (67%)	73/146 (50%)	50/204 (25%)
Baseline Ventilatory Support	9/39 (23%)	15/50 (30%)	18/129 (14%)
No Baseline Ventilatory Support	144/188 (77%)	58/96 (60%)	32/75 (43%)

In the Treatment IND, 12% of the patients discontinued trimetrexate glucoronate therapy (with leucovorin protection) for toxicity.

CONTRAINDICATIONS:

Trimetrexate glucuronate for injection is contraindicated in patients with clinically significant sensitivity to trimetrexate, leucovorin, or methotrexate.

WARNINGS:

Trimetrexate glucuronate for injection must be used with concurrent leucovorin to avoid potentially serious or life-threatening complications including bone marrow suppression, oral and gastrointestinal mucosal ulceration, and renal and hepatic dysfunction. Leucovorin therapy must extend for 72 hours past the last dose of trimetrexate glucoronate. Patients should be informed that failure to take the recommended dose and duration of leucovorin can lead to fatal toxicity. Patients should be closely monitored for the development of serious hematologic adverse reactions (see PRECAUTIONS and DOSAGE AND ADMINISTRATION).

Trimetrexate glucoronate can cause fetal harm when administered to a pregnant woman. trimetrexate has been shown to be fetotoxic and teratogenic in rats and rabbits. Rats administered 1.5 and 2.5 mg/kg/day intravenously on gestational days 6-15 showed substantial postimplantation loss and severe inhibition of maternal weight gain. Trimetrexate administered intravenously to rats at 0.5 and 1.0 mg/kg/day on gestational days 6-15 retarded normal fetal development and was teratogenic. Rabbits administered trimetrexate intravenously at daily doses of 2.5 and 5.0 mg/kg/day on gestational days 6-18 resulted in significant maternal and fetal toxicity. In rabbits, trimetrexate at 0.1 mg/kg/day was teratogenic in the absence of significant maternal toxicity. These effects were observed using doses 1/20 to 1/2 the equivalent human therapeutic dose based on a mg/m^2 basis. Teratogenic effects included skeletal, visceral, ocular, and cardiovascular abnormalities. If trimetrexate glucoronate is used during pregnancy, or if the patient becomes pregnant while taking this drug, the patient should be apprised of the potential hazard to the fetus. Women of childbearing potential should be advised to avoid becoming pregnant.

PRECAUTIONS:

GENERAL

Patients receiving trimetrexate glucuronate for injection may experience severe hematologic, hepatic, renal, and gastrointestinal toxicities. Caution should be used in treating patients with impaired hematologic, renal, or hepatic function. Patients who require concomitant therapy with nephrotoxic, myelosuppressive, or hepatotoxic drugs should be treated with trimetrexate glucoronate at the discretion of the physician and monitored carefully. To allow for full therapeutic doses of trimetrexate glucoronate, treatment with zidovudine should be discontinued during trimetrexate glucoronate therapy.

Trimetrexate glucoronate-associated myelosuppression, stomatitis, and gastrointestinal toxicities generally can be ameliorated by adjusting the dose of leucovorin. Mild elevations in transaminases and alkaline phosphatase have been observed with trimetrexate glucoronate administration and are usually not cause for modification of trimetrexate glucoronate therapy (see DOSAGE AND ADMINISTRATION). Seizures have been reported rarely (<1%) in AIDS patients receiving trimetrexate glucoronate; however, a causal relationship has not been established. An anaphylactoid reaction has been reported in a cancer patient receiving trimetrexate glucoronate as a bolus injection.

Trimetrexate glucoronate has not been evaluated clinically for the treatment of concurrent pulmonary conditions such as bacterial, viral, or fungal pneumonia or mycobacterial diseases. *In vitro* activity has been observed against *Toxoplasma gondii, Mycobacterium avium* complex, gram positive cocci, and gram negative rods. If clinical deterioration is observed in patients, they should be carefully evaluated for other possible causes of pulmonary disease and treated with additional agents as appropriate.

LABORATORY TESTS

Patients receiving trimetrexate glucoronate with leucovorin protection should be seen frequently by a physician. Blood tests to assess the following parameters should be performed at least twice a week during therapy: hematology (absolute neutrophil counts (ANC), platelets), renal function (serum creatinine, BUN), and hepatic function (AST, ALT, alkaline phosphatase).

DRUG INTERACTIONS:

Since trimetrexate is metabolized by a P450 enzyme system, drugs that induce or inhibit this drug metabolizing enzyme system may elicit important drug-drug interactions that may alter trimetrexate plasma concentrations. Agents that might be coadministered with trimetrexate in AIDS patients for other indications that could elicit this activity include erythromycin, rifampin, rifabutin, ketoconazole, and fluconazole.*In vitro* perfusion of isolated rat liver has shown that cimetidine caused a significant reduction in trimetrexate metabolism and that acetaminophen altered the relative concentration of trimetrexate metabolites possibly by competing for sulfate metabolites. Based on an *in vitro* rat liver model, nitrogen substituted imidazole drugs (clotrimazole, ketoconazole, miconazole) were potent, non-competitive inhibitors of trimetrexate metabolism. Patients medicated with these drugs and trimetrexate should be carefully monitored.

CARCINOGENESIS, MUTAGENESIS, AND IMPAIRMENT OF FERTILITY

Long term studies in animals to evaluate the carcinogenic potential of trimetrexate have not been performed. Trimetrexate was not mutagenic when tested using the standard Ames *Salmonella* mutagenicity assay with and without metabolic activation. Trimetrexate did not induce mutations in Chinese hamster lung cells or sister-chromatid exchange in Chinese hamster ovary cells. Trimetrexate did induce an increase in the chromosomal aberration frequency of cultured Chinese hamster lung cells; however, trimetrexate showed no clastogenic activity in a mouse micronucleus assay.

No studies have been conducted to evaluate the potential of trimetrexate to impair fertility. However, during standard toxicity studies conducted in mice and rats, degeneration of the testes and spermatocytes including the arrest of spermatogenesis was observed.

PREGNANCY CATEGORY D

See WARNINGS.

NURSING MOTHERS

It is not known if trimetrexate is excreted in human milk. Because many drugs are excreted in human milk and because of the potential for serious adverse reactions in nursing infants from trimetrexate, it is recommended that breast feeding be discontinued if the mother is treated with trimetrexate glucoronate.

PEDIATRIC USE

The safety and effectiveness of trimetrexate glucoronate for the treatment of histologically confirmed PCP has not been established for patients under 18 years of age. Two children, ages 15 months and 9 months, were treated with trimetrexate and leucovorin using a dose of 45 mg/m²of trimetrexate per day for 21 days and 20 mg/m²of leucovorin per day for 24 days. There were no serious or unexpected adverse effects.

ADVERSE REACTIONS:

Because many patients who participated in clinical trials of trimetrexate glucoronate (trimetrexate glucoronate for injection) had complications of advanced HIV disease, it is difficult to distinguish adverse events caused by trimetrexate glucoronate from those resulting from underlying medical conditions. TABLE 3 lists the adverse events that occurred in ≥1% of the patients who participated in the Comparative Study of trimetrexate glucoronate plus leucovorin versus TMP/SMX.

Laboratory toxicities were generally manageable with dose modification of trimetrexate/leucovorin (see DOSAGE AND ADMINISTRATION).

TABLE 4 lists the adverse events resulting in discontinuation of study therapy in the trimetrexate glucoronate comparative study with TMP/SMX. Twenty-nine percent of the patients on the TMP/SMX arm discontinued therapy due to adverse events compared to 10% of the patients treated with TMTX/LV (p<0.001).

Hematologic toxicity was the principal dose-limiting side effect. An anaphylactoid reaction has been reported in a cancer patient receiving trimetrexate glucoronate as a bolus injection.

OVERDOSAGE:

Trimetrexate glucuronate for injection administered without concurrent leucovorin can cause lethal complications. There has been no extensive experience in humans receiving single intravenous doses of trimetrexate greater than 90 mg/m²/day with concurrent leucovorin. The toxicities seen at this dose were primarily hematologic. In the event of overdose, trimetrexate glucoronate should be stopped and leucovorin should be administered at a dose of 40 mg/m² every 6 hours for 3 days. The LD_{50} of intravenous trimetrexate in mice is 62 mg/kg (186 mg/m²).

DOSAGE AND ADMINISTRATION:

Caution: Trimetrexate glucuronate for injection must be administered with concurrent leucovorin (leucovorin protection) to avoid potentially serious or life-threatening toxicities. Leucovorin therapy must extend for 72 hours past the last dose of trimetrexate glucoronate.

DOSAGE AND ADMINISTRATION: *(cont'd)*

TABLE 3 Comparison of Adverse Events Reported for ≥1% of Patients

Adverse Events	Number and Percent (%) of Patients with Adverse Events TMTX/LV (n=109)	TMP/SMX (n=111)
Non-Laboratory Adverse Events:		
Fever	9 (8.3)	14 (12.6)
Rash/Pruritus	6 (5.5)	14 (12.6)
Nausea/Vomiting	5 (4.6)[a]	15 (13.5)[a]
Confusion	3 (2.8)	3 (2.7)
Fatigue	2 (1.8)	0 (0.0)
Hematologic Toxicity:		
Neutropenia (≤1000/mm³)	33 (30.3)	37 (33.3)
Thrombocytopenia (≤75,000/mm³)	11 (10.1)	17 (15.3)
Anemia (Hgb <8 g/dL)	8 (7.3)	10 (9.0)
Hepatotoxicity:		
Increased AST (>5 x ULN[b])	15 (13.8)	10 (9.0)
Increased ALT (>5 x ULN)	12 (11.0)	13 (11.7)
Increased Alkaline Phosphatase (>5 x ULN)	5 (4.6)	3 (2.7)
Increased Bilirubin (2.5 x ULN)	2 (1.8)	1 (0.9)
Renal:		
Increased Serum Creatinine (>3 x ULN)	1 (0.9)	2 (1.8)
Electrolyte Imbalance:		
Hyponatremia	5 (4.6)	10 (9.0)
Hypocalcemia	2 (1.8)	0 (0.0)
No. of Patients With at Least one Adverse Event[c]	58 (53.2)	60 (54.1)

[a]statistically significant difference between treatment groups (Chi-square: p=0.022)
[b]ULN = Upper limit of normal range
[c]Patients could have reported more than one adverse event; therefore the sum of adverse events exceeds the number of patients

TABLE 4 Adverse Events Resulting in Discontinuation of Therapy

Adverse Events	Number and Percent (%) of Patients Discontinued for Adverse Events[b]Adverse Events TMTX/LV (n=109)	TMP/SMX (n=111)
Non-Laboratory Adverse Events:		
Rash/Pruritus	3 (2.8)	5 (4.5)
Fever	2 (1.8)	4 (3.6)
Nausea/Vomiting	1 (0.9)	8 (7.2)
Neurologic Toxicity	1 (0.9)[c]	2 (1.8)
Hematologic Toxicity:		
Neutropenia (≤1000/mm³)	4 (3.7)	6 (5.4)
Thrombocytopenia (≤75,000/mm³)	0 (0.0)	4 (3.6)
Anemia (Hgb < 8 g/dl)	0 (0.0)	4 (3.6)
Hepatotoxicity:		
Increased AST (>5 x ULN[a])	3 (2.8)	9 (8.1)
Increased ALT (>5 x ULN)	1 (0.9)	4 (3.6)
Increased Alkaline Phosphatase (>5 x ULN)	0 (0.0)	1 (0.9)
Electrolyte Imbalance:		
Hyponatremia	0 (0.0)	3 (2.7)
No. of Patients Discontinuing Therapy Due to an Adverse Event[b]	11 (10.1)[d]	32 (28.8)d

[a]ULN = Upper limit of normal range
[b]Patients could discontinue therapy due to more than one toxicity; therefore the sum exceeds number of patients who discontinued due to toxicity
[c]Patient discontinued TMTX/LV due to seizure, though causal relationship could not be established
[d]Statistically significant difference between treatment groups (Chi-square: p<0.001)

Trimetrexate glucuronate for injection is administered at a dose of 45 mg/m² once daily by intravenous infusion over 60-90 minutes. Leucovorin must be administered daily during treatment with trimetrexate glucoronate and for 72 hours past the last dose of trimetrexate glucoronate. Leucovorin may be administered intravenously at a dose of 20 mg/m²over 5 to 10 minutes every 6 hours for a total daily dose of 80 mg/m², or orally as 4 doses of 20 mg/m²spaced equally throughout the day. The oral dose should be rounded up to the next higher 25 mg increment. The recommended course of therapy is 21 days of trimetrexate glucoronate and 24 days of leucovorin.

DOSAGE MODIFICATIONS

Hematologic toxicity: Trimetrexate glucuronate for injection and leucovorin doses should be modified based on the worst hematologic toxicity according to the following table. If leucovorin is given orally, doses should be rounded up to the next higher 25 mg increment.

TABLE 5A Dose Modifications For Hematologic Toxicity

Toxicity Grade	Neutrophils (Polys and Bands)	Platelets	Recommended Dosage of Neutrexin
1	>1000/mm³	>75,000/mm³	45 mg/m² once daily
2	750-1000/mm³	50,000-75,000/mm³	45 mg/m² once daily
3	500-749/mm³	25,000-49,999/mm³	22 mg/m² once daily
4	<500/mm³	>25,000/mm³	Day 1-9 Discontinue Day 10-21 Interrupt up to 96 hrs[a]

Hepatic toxicity: Transient elevations of transaminases and alkaline phosphatase have been observed in patients treated with trimetrexate glucoronate. Interruption of treatment is advisable if transaminase levels or alkaline phosphatase levels increase to >5 times the upper limit of normal range.

Renal toxicity: Interruption of trimetrexate glucoronate is advisable if serum creatinine levels increase to >2.5 mg/dl and the elevation is considered to be secondary to trimetrexate glucoronate.

Other toxicities: Interruption of treatment is advisable in patients who experience severe mucosal toxicity that interferes with oral intake. Treatment should be discontinued for fever (oral temperature ≥105°F/40.5°C) that cannot be controlled with antipyretics.

Leucovorin therapy must extend for 72 hours past the last dose of trimetrexate glucoronate.

RECONSTITUTION AND DILUTION

Trimetrexate glucuronate for injection should be reconstituted with 2 ml of 5% Dextrose Injection, USP or Sterile Water for Injection, USP, to yield a concentration of 12.5 mg of trimetrexate per ml (complete dissolution should occur within 30 seconds). The reconstituted product will appear as a pale greenish-yellow solution and must be inspected visually for

DOSAGE AND ADMINISTRATION: *(cont'd)*

TABLE 5B Dose Modifications For Hematologic Toxicity

Toxicity Grade	Neutrophils (Polys and Bands)	Platelets	Recommended Dosage of Leucovorin
1	>1000/mm^3	>75,000/mm^3	20 mg/m^2 every 6 hours
2	750-1000/mm^3	50,000-75,000/mm^3	40 mg/m^2 every 6 hours
3	500-749/mm^3	25,000-49,999/mm^3	40 mg/m^2 every 6 hours
4	<500/mm^3	>25,000/mm^3	40 mg/m^2 every 6 hours

[a]If Grade 4 hematologic toxicity occurs prior to Day 10, Neutrexin should be discontinued. Leucovorin (40 mg/m^2, q6h) should be administered for an additional 72 hours. If Grade 4 hematologic toxicity occurs at Day 10 or later, Neutrexin may be held up to 96 hours to allow counts to recover. If counts recover to Grade 3 within 96 hours, Neutrexin should be administered at a dose of 22 mg/m^2 and leucovorin maintained at 40 mg/m^2, q6h. When counts recover to Grade 2 toxicity, Neutrexin dose may be increased to 45 mg/m^2, but the leucovorin dose should be maintained at 40 mg/m^2 for the duration of treatment. If counts do not improve to ≤Grade 3 toxicity within 96 hours, Neutrexin should be discontinued. Leucovorin at a dose of 40 mg/m^2,q6h should be administered for 72 hours following the last dose of Neutrexin.

particulate matter prior to dilution.**Do not use if cloudiness or precipitate is observed, solution should be filtered (0.22 mcm) prior to dilution.** Trimetrexate glucoronate should not be reconstituted with solutions containing either chloride ion or leucovorin, since precipitation occurs instantly.

After reconstitution, the solution is stable under refrigeration or at room temperature for up to 24 hours. Do not freeze reconstituted solution. Discard any unused portions after 24 hours.

Reconstituted solution should be further diluted with 5% Dextrose Injection, USP, to yield a final concentration of 0.25 to 2 mg of trimetrexate per ml. The diluted solution should be administered by intravenous infusion over 60 minutes. Trimetrexate glucoronate should not be mixed with solutions containing either chloride ion or leucovorin, since precipitation occurs instantly. It is stable under refrigeration or at room temperature for up to 24 hours. Do not freeze. Discard any unused portion after 24 hours after initial reconstitution. The intravenous line must be flushed thoroughly with at least 10 ml of 5% Dextrose Injection, USP, before and after administering trimetrexate glucoronate.

Leucovorin protection may be administered prior to or following trimetrexate glucoronate. In either case the intravenous line must be flushed thoroughly with at least 10 ml of 5% Dextrose Injection, USP. Leucovorin calcium for injection should be diluted according to the instructions in the leucovorin package insert, and administered over 5 to 10 minutes every 6 hours.

Caution: Parenteral products should be inspected visually for particulate matter and discoloration prior to administration, whenever solution and container permit. Trimetrexate glucoronate forms a precipitate instantly upon contact with chloride ion or leucovorin, therefore it should not be added to solutions containing sodium chloride or other anions. Trimetrexate glucoronate and leucovorin solutions must be administered separately. Intravenous lines should be flushed with at least 10 ml of 5% Dextrose Injection, USP, between trimetrexate glucoronate and leucovorin infusions.

HANDLING AND DISPOSAL

If trimetrexate glucoronate for injection contacts the skin or mucosa, immediately wash thoroughly with soap and water. Procedures for proper disposal of cytotoxic drugs should be considered. Several guidelines on this subject have been published (1-5).

HOW SUPPLIED:

Trimetrexate glucuronate for injection is supplied as a sterile lyophilized powder in 5 ml, single-dose vials. Each 5 ml vial contains trimetrexate glucuronate equivalent to 25 mg of trimetrexate. The vials are packaged and available in four market presentations as listed below:

Bulk Pack: 4 trays of 25 vials per shrink-wrapped tray

10 pack: 10 vials in a white chip-board carton

25 pack: 25 vials per shrink-wrapped tray

50 pack: 2 trays of 25 vials per shrink-wrapped tray

Starter pack: 21vials per shrink-wrapped tray; presented in combination with 28 vials of Leucovorin Calcium for Injection in a shrink-wrapped tray, each vial contains 50 mg of leucovorin as the calcium salt.

Store at controlled room temperature 15 to 30°C (59 to 86°F). **Protect from exposure to light.**

REFERENCES:

1. AMA Council Report, Guidelines for Handling Parenteral Antineoplastics. *Journal of the American Medical Association*March 15, 1985. **2.** Clinical Oncological Society of Australia: Guidelines and Recommendations for Safe Handling of Antineoplastic Agents. *Medical Journal of Australia* 1: 426-428, 1983. **3.** Jones RB, et al. Safe Handling of Chemotherapeutic Agents: A report from the Mount Sinai Medical Center. *CA - A Cancer Journal for Clinicians* Sept/Oct, 258-263, 1983. **4.** American Society of Hospital Pharmacists Technical Assistance Bulletin on Handling Cytotoxic Drugs in Hospitals. *American Journal of Hospital Pharmacy* 42: 131-137, 1985. **5.** OSHA Work Practice Guidelines for Personnel Dealing with Cytotoxic (Antineoplastic) Drugs. *American Journal of Hospital Pharmacy* 43: 1193-1204, 1986.(US Bioscience, Inc. 94/05, LB3003PA)

HOW SUPPLIED - EQUIVALENTS NOT AVAILABLE:

Injection, Solution - Intravenous - 25 mg

10's $550.00 NEUTREXIN, US Bioscience 58178-0020-10

Injection, Solution - Intravenous - 40 mg/vial

1's $41.65 NEUTREXIN, US Bioscience 58178-0020-01

50's $2273.75 NEUTREXIN, US Bioscience 58178-0020-50

TRIMIPRAMINE MALEATE *(002392)*

CATEGORIES: Antidepressants; Central Nervous System Agents; Depression; Psychotherapeutic Agents; Tricyclics; Tricyclic Antidepressants; Pregnancy Category C; FDA Approval Pre 1982

BRAND NAMES: *Rhotrimine*; *Stangyl*; *Sumontil*; **Surmontil**
(International brand names outside U.S. in italics)

FORMULARIES: Aetna

COST OF THERAPY: $178.41 (Depression; Capsule; 25 mg; 3/day; 90 days)

PRIMARY ICD9: 311 (Depressive Disorder, Not Elsewhere Classified)

DESCRIPTION:

Trimipramine maleate is 5-(3-dimethylamino-2-methylpropyl)-10,11-dihydro-5H-dibenz (b,f) azepine acid maleate (racemic form).

Trimipramine maleate capsules contain trimipramine maleate equivalent to 25 mg, 50 mg, or 100 mg of trimipramine as the base. The inactive ingredients present are FD&C Blue 1, gelatin, lactose, magnesium stearate, and titanium dioxide. The 25 mg dosage strength also contains D&C Yellow 10 and FD&C Yellow 6; the 50 mg dosage strength also contains D&C Red 28, FD&C Red 40, and FD&C Yellow 6.

Trimipramine maleate is prepared as a racemic mixture which can be resolved into levorotatory and dextrorotatory isomers. The asymmetric center responsible for optical isomerism is marked in the formula by an asterisk. Trimipramine maleate is an almost odorless, white or slightly cream-colored, crystalline substance, melting at 140-144° C. It is very slightly soluble in ether and water, is slightly soluble in ethyl alcohol and acetone, and freely soluble in chloroform and methanol at 20° C.

CLINICAL PHARMACOLOGY:

Trimipramine maleate is an antidepressant with an anxiety-reducing sedative component to its action. The mode of action of Trimipramine maleate on the central nervous system is not known. However, unlike amphetamine-type compounds it does not act primarily by stimulation of the central nervous system. It does not act by inhibition of the monoamine oxidase system.

INDICATIONS AND USAGE:

Trimipramine maleate is indicated for the relief of symptoms of depression. Endogenous depression is more likely to be alleviated than other depressive states. In studies with neurotic outpatients, the drug appeared to be equivalent to amitriptyline in the less-depressed patients but somewhat less effective than amitriptyline in the more severely depressed patients. In hospitalized depressed patients, trimipramine and imipramine were equally effective in relieving depression.

CONTRAINDICATIONS:

Trimipramine maleate is contraindicated in cases of known hypersensitivity to the drug. The possibility of cross-sensitivity to other dibenzazepine compounds should be kept in mind. Trimipramine maleate should not be given in conjunction with drugs of the monoamine oxidase inhibitor class (*e.g.,* tranylcypromine, isocarboxazid or phenelzine sulfate). The concomitant use of monoamine oxidase inhibitors (MAOI) and tricyclic compounds similar to Trimipramine maleate has caused severe hyperpyretic reactions, convulsive crises, and death in some patients. At least two weeks should elapse after cessation of therapy with MAOI before instituting therapy with Trimipramine maleate. Initial dosage should be low and increased gradually with caution and careful observation of the patient. The drug is contraindicated during the acute recovery period after a myocardial infarction.

WARNINGS:

Usage in Children: This drug is not recommended for use in children, since safety and effectiveness in the pediatric age group have not been established.

General: Extreme caution should be used when this drug is given to patients with any evidence of cardiovascular disease because of the possibility of conduction defects, arrhythmias, myocardial infarction, strokes, and tachycardia.

Caution is advised in patients with increased intraocular pressure, history of urinary retention, or history of narrow-angle glaucoma because of the drug's anticholinergic properties; hyperthyroid patients or those on thyroid medication because of the possibility of cardiovascular toxicity; patients with a history of seizure disorder, because this drug has been shown to lower the seizure threshold; patients receiving guanethidine or similar agents, since Trimipramine maleate may block the pharmacologic effects of these drugs.

Since the drug may impair the mental and/or physical abilities required for the performance of potentially hazardous tasks, such as operating an automobile or machinery, the patient should be cautioned accordingly.

PRECAUTIONS:

The possibility of suicide is inherent in any severely depressed patient and persists until a significant remission occurs. When a patient with a serious suicidal potential is not hospitalized, the prescription should be for the smallest amount feasible.

In schizophrenic patients activation of the psychosis may occur and require reduction of dosage or the addition of a major tranquilizer to the therapeutic regime.

Manic or hypomanic episodes may occur in some patients, in particular those with cyclic-type disorders. In some cases therapy with Trimipramine maleate must be discontinued until the episode is relieved, after which therapy may be reinstituted at lower dosages if still required.

Concurrent administration of Trimipramine maleate and electroshock therapy may increase the hazards of therapy. Such treatment should be limited to those patients for whom it is essential. When possible, discontinue the drug for several days prior to elective surgery.

There is evidence that cimetidine inhibits the elimination of tricyclic antidepressants. Downward adjustment of Trimipramine maleate dosage may be required if cimetidine therapy is initiated; upward adjustment if cimetidine therapy is discontinued.

Patients should be warned that the concomitant use of alcoholic beverages may be associated with exaggerated effects.

It has been reported that tricyclic antidepressants can potentiate the effects of catecholamines. Similarly, atropinelike effects may be more pronounced in patients receiving anticholinergic therapy.

Therefore, particular care should be exercised when it is necessary to administer tricyclic antidepressants with sympathomimetic amines, local decongestants, local anesthetics containing epinephrine, atropine or drugs with an anticholinergic effect. In resistant cases of depression in adults, a dose of 2.5 mg/kg/day may have to be exceeded. If a higher dose is needed, ECG monitoring should be maintained during the initiation of therapy and at appropriate intervals during stabilization of dose.

Pregnancy Category C: Trimipramine maleate has shown evidence of embryo-toxicity and/or increased incidence of major anomalies in rats or rabbits at doses 20 times the human dose. There are no adequate and well-controlled studies in pregnant women. Trimipramine maleate should be used during pregnancy only if the potential benefit justifies the potential risk to the fetus.

Semen studies in man (four schizophrenics and nine normal volunteers) revealed no significant changes in sperm morphology. It is recognized that drugs having a parasympathetic effect, including tricyclic antidepressants, may alter the ejaculatory response.

Chronic animal studies showed occasional evidence of degeneration of seminiferous tubules at the highest dose of 60 mg/kg/day.

Trimipramine maleate should be used with caution in patients with impaired liver function.

Chronic animal studies showed occasional occurrence of hepatic congestion, fatty infiltration, or increased serum liver enzymes at the highest dose of 60 mg/kg/day.

PRECAUTIONS: *(cont'd)*

Both elevation and lowering of blood sugar have been reported with tricyclic antidepressants.

ADVERSE REACTIONS:

Note: The pharmacological similarities among the tricyclic antidepressants require that each of the reactions be considered when Trimipramine maleate is administered. Some of the adverse reactions included in this listing have not in fact been reported with Trimipramine maleate.

Cardiovascular: Hypotension, hypertension, tachycardia, palpitation, myocardial infarction, arrhythmias, heart block, stroke.

Psychiatric: Confusional states (especially the elderly) with hallucinations, disorientation, delusions; anxiety, restlessness, agitation; insomnia and nightmares; hypomania; exacerbation of psychosis.

Neurological: Numbness, tingling, paresthesias of extremities; incoordination, ataxia, tremors; peripheral neuropathy; extrapyramidal symptoms; seizures, alterations in EEG patterns; tinnitus; syndrome of inappropriate ADH (antidiuretic hormone) secretion.

Anticholinergic: Dry mouth and, rarely, associated sublingual adenitis; blurred vision, disturbances of accommodation, mydriasis, constipation, paralytic ileus; urinary retention, delayed micturition, dilation of the urinary tract.

Allergic: Skin rash, petechiae, urticaria, itching, photosensitization, edema of face and tongue.

Hematologic: Bone-marrow depression including agranulocytosis, eosinophilia; purpura; thrombocytopenia. Leukocyte and differential counts should be performed in any patient who develops fever and sore throat during therapy; the drug should be discontinued if there is evidence of pathological neutrophil depression.

Gastrointestinal: Nausea and vomiting, anorexia, epigastric distress, diarrhea, peculiar taste, stomatitis, abdominal cramps, black tongue.

Endocrine: Gynecomastia in the male; breast enlargement and galactorrhea in the female; increased or decreased libido, impotence; testicular swelling; elevation or depression of blood-sugar levels.

Other: Jaundice (simulating obstructive); altered liver function; weight gain or loss; perspiration; flushing; urinary frequency; drowsiness, dizziness, weakness, and fatigue; headache; parotid swelling; alopecia.

Withdrawal Symptoms: Though not indicative of addiction, abrupt cessation of treatment after prolonged therapy may produce nausea, headache, and malaise.

OVERDOSAGE:

SIGNS AND SYMPTOMS

The response of the patient to toxic overdosage of tricyclic antidepressants may vary in severity and is conditioned by factors such as age, amount ingested, amount absorbed, interval between ingestion and start of treatment. Trimipramine maleate is not recommended for infants or young children. Should accidental ingestion occur in any amount, it should be regarded as serious and potentially fatal.

CNS abnormalities may include drowsiness, stupor, coma, ataxia, restlessness, agitation, hyperactive reflexes, muscle rigidity, athetoid and choreiform movements, and convulsions. Cardiac abnormalities may include arrhythmia, tachycardia, ECG evidence of impaired conduction, and signs of congestive failure. Other symptoms may include respiratory depression, cyanosis, hypotension, shock, vomiting, hyperpyrexia, mydriasis, and diaphoresis.

Treatment is supportive and symptomatic as no specific antidote is known. Depending upon need the following measures can be considered:

1. Trimipramine maleate is not recommended for use in infants and children. Hospitalization with continuous cardiac monitoring for up to 4 days is recommended for children who have ingested Trimipramine maleate in any amount. This is based on the reported greater sensitivity of children to acute overdosage with tricyclic antidepressants.

2. Blood and urine levels may not reflect the severity of the poisoning and are mostly of diagnostic value.

3. CNS involvement, respiratory depression, or cardiac arrhythmia can occur suddenly; hospitalization and close observation are necessary, even when the amount ingested is thought to be small or initial toxicity appears slight. Patients with any alteration of ECG should have continuous cardiac monitoring for at least 72 hours and be observed until well after the cardiac status has returned to normal; relapses may occur after apparent recovery.

4. The slow intravenous administration of physostigmine salicylate has been reported to reverse most of the cardiovascular and CNS effects of overdosage with tricyclic antidepressants. In adults, 1 to 3 mg has been reported to be effective. In children, start with 0.5 mg and repeat at 5-minute intervals to determine the minimum effective dose; do not exceed 2.0 mg. Avoid rapid injection, to reduce the possibility of physostigmine-induced convulsions. Because of the short duration of action of physostigmine, it may be necessary to repeat doses at 30- to 60-minute intervals as necessary.

5. In the alert patient, empty the stomach rapidly by induced emesis, followed by lavage. In the obtunded patient, secure the airway with a cuffed endotracheal tube before beginning lavage (do not induce emesis). Instillation of activated-charcoal slurry may help reduce absorption of trimipramine.

6. Minimize external stimulation to reduce the tendency to convulsions. If anticonvulsants are necessary, diazepam, short-acting barbiturates, paraldehyde, or methocarbamol may be useful. Do not use barbiturates if MAO inhibitors have been taken recently.

7. Maintain adequate respiratory exchange. Do not use respiratory stimulants.

8. Shock should be treated with supportive measures, such as intravenous fluids, oxygen, and corticosteroids. Digitalis may increase conduction abnormalities and further irritate an already sensitized myocardium. If congestive heart failure necessitates rapid digitalization, particular care must be exercised.

9. Hyperpyrexia should be controlled by whatever external means available, including ice packs and cooling sponge baths if necessary.

10. Hemodialysis, peritoneal dialysis, exchange transfusions, and forced diuresis have been generally reported as ineffective in tricyclic poisoning.

DOSAGE AND ADMINISTRATION:

Dosage should be initiated at a low level and increased gradually, noting carefully the clinical response and any evidence of intolerance.

Lower dosages are recommended for elderly patients and adolescents. Lower dosages are also recommended for outpatients as compared to hospitalized patients who will be under close supervision. It is not possible to prescribe a single dosage schedule of Trimipramine maleate that will be therapeutically effective in all patients. The physical psychodynamic factors contributing to depressive symptomatology are very complex; spontaneous remissions or exacerbations of depressive symptoms may occur with or without drug therapy. Consequently, the recommended dosage regimens are furnished as a guide which may be modified by factors such as the age of the patient, chronicity and severity of the disease, medical condition of the patient, and degree of psychotherapeutic support.

DOSAGE AND ADMINISTRATION: *(cont'd)*

Most antidepressant drugs have a lag period of ten days to four weeks before a therapeutic response is noted. Increasing the dose will not shorten this period but rather increase the incidence of adverse reactions.

USUAL ADULT DOSE

Outpatients and Office Patients: Initially, 75 mg/day in divided doses, increased to 150 mg/day. Dosages over 200 mg/day are not recommended. Maintenance therapy is in the range of 50 to 150 mg/day. For convenient therapy and to facilitate patient compliance, the total dosage requirement may be given at bedtime.

Hospitalized Patients: Initially, 100 mg/day in divided doses. This may be increased gradually in a few days to 200 mg/day, depending upon individual response and tolerance. If improvement does not occur in 2 to 3 weeks, the dose may be increased to the maximum recommended dose of 250 to 300 mg/day.

Adolescent and Geriatric Patients: Initially, a dose of 50 mg/day is recommended, with gradual increments up to 100 mg/day, depending upon patient response and tolerance.

Maintenance: Following remission, maintenance medication may be required for a longer period of time, at the lowest dose that will maintain remission. Maintenance therapy is preferably administered as a single dose at bedtime. To minimize relapse, maintenance therapy should be continued for about three months.

Keep bottles tightly closed.

Dispense in a tight container.

Protect capsules packaged in blister strips from moisture.

HOW SUPPLIED - EQUIVALENTS NOT AVAILABLE:

Capsule, Gelatin - Oral - 25 mg

100's	$66.08	SURMONTIL, Wyeth Labs	00008-4132-01

Capsule, Gelatin - Oral - 50 mg

100's	$108.14	SURMONTIL, Wyeth Labs	00008-4133-01

Capsule, Gelatin - Oral - 100 mg

100's	$157.20	SURMONTIL, Wyeth Labs	00008-4158-01

TRIOXSALEN *(002393)*

CATEGORIES: Depigmenting/Pigmenting Agents; Dermatologicals; Hypopigmentation; Lesions; Photosensitizer; Pigmenting Agents; Skin/Mucous Membrane Agents; Vitiligo; FDA Approval Pre 1982

BRAND NAMES: *Neosoralen*; *Puvadin*; **Trisoralen**
(International brand names outside U.S. in italics)

DESCRIPTION:

To facilitate repigmentation in vitiligo, increase tolerance to solar exposure and enhance pigmentation.

Caution: This Is Potent Drug. Trisoralen (Trioxsalen) is the first synthetic psoralen compound made available to the medical profession. It possesses greater activity than Methoxsalen[1,2,3,4] yet the LD_{50} of (Trioxsalen) is six times that of Methoxsalen. The chemical name for this drug is (4,5', 8- Trimethylpsoralen).

CLINICAL PHARMACOLOGY:

Pigment Formation With Trioxsalen: The normal pigmentation of the skin is due to melanin which is produced in the cytoplasm of the melanocytes located in the basal layers of the epidermis at its junction with the dermis. Melanin is formed by the oxidation of tyrosine to DOPA (Dihydroxyphenylalanine) with tyrosinase as catalyst. This enzymatic reaction, however, must be activated by radiant energy in the form of ultraviolet light, preferably between 2900 and 3800 angstroms (black light)[10].

The exact mechanism of the action of psoralens in the process of melanogenesis is not known. One group of investigators feel that the psoralens have a specific effect on the epidermis or, more specifically, on the melanocytes. Another group feels that the primary response to the psoralens is an inflammatory one and that the process of melanogenesis is secondary.

INDICATIONS AND USAGE:

Trioxsalen, taken approximately two hours before measured periods of exposure to ultraviolet facilitates:

Repigmentation Of Idiopathic Vitiligo: [12,13,14]Repigmentation, not equally reversible in every patient, will vary in completeness, time of onset, and duration. The rate of completeness of pigmentation with respect to locations of lesions, occurs more rapidly on fleshy regions, such as the face, abdomen, and buttocks, and less rapidly over bony areas such as the dorsum of the hands and feet. Repigmentation may begin after a few weeks; however, significant results may take as long as six to nine months, and repigmentation, at the optimum level, may, in some cases, require maintenance dosage to retain the new pigment. If follicular repigmentation is not apparent after three months of daily treatment, treatment should be discontinued as a failure.

Increasing Tolerance To Sunlight: [14] In blond persons and those with fair complexions who suffer painful reactions when exposed to sunlight, Trioxsalen aids in increasing resistance to solar damage. Certain persons who are allergic to sunlight or exhibit sun sensitivity may be benefited by the protective action of Trioxsalen[5]. In albinism, Trioxsalen will increase the tolerance of the skin to sunlight, although no pigment is formed[6,7,8]. This protective action seems to be related to the thickening of the horny layer and retention of melanin which produced a thickened, melanized stratum corneum and formation of a stratum lucidum[9,10].

Enhancing Pigmentation: [3,4] The use of Trioxsalen accelerates pigmentation only when the administration of the drug is followed by exposure of the skin to sunlight or ultraviolet irradiation. The increase in pigmentation is not immediate but occurs gradually within a few days of repeated exposure and may become equivalent in a degree to that achieved by a full summer of sun exposure. Since sufficient pigmentation will have been formed within two weeks of continuous therapy, the use of trioxsalen should not be continued beyond this period. Pigmentation can be maintained by periodic exposure to sunlight.

CONTRAINDICATIONS:

In those diseases associated with photosensitivity, such as porphyria, acute lupus erythematosus, or leukoderma of infectious origin. To date, the safety of this drug in young persons (12 and under), has not been established and is, therefore contraindicated. No preparation with any photosensitizing capacity, internal or external should be used concomitantly with Trioxsalen therapy.

WARNINGS:

Trioxsalen Is A Potent Drug: Read entire brochure before prescribing or dispensing this medication. The dosage of this medication should not be increased. The dosage of trioxsalen and exposure time should not be increased. Overdosage and/or overexposure may result in serious burning and blistering. When used to increase tolerance to sunlight or accelerate tanning, trioxsalen total dosage should not exceed 28 tablets, taken in daily single doses of two tablets on a continuous or interrupted regimen. To prevent harmful effects, the physician should carefully instruct the patient to adhere to the prescribed dosage schedule and procedure.

PRECAUTIONS:

Accidental Overdosage: If an overdose of trioxsalen (Trioxsalen) or ultraviolet light has been taken, emesis should be encouraged. The individual should be kept in a darkened room for eight hours or until cutaneous reactions subside. The treatment for severe reactions resulting from overdosage or over-exposure should follow accepted procedures for treatment of severe burns. There have not been any clinical reports or tests to verify that more severe reactions may result from the concomitant ingestion of furocoumarin-containing food while on trioxsalen therapy; but the physician should warn the patient that taking limes, figs, parsley, parsnips, mustard, carrots, and celery, might be dangerous.

ADVERSE REACTIONS:

Severe burns can result from excessive sunlight or sun lamp ultraviolet exposure. Occasionally, there may occur gastric discomfort; to minimize the gastric effect, the tablets may be taken with milk or after a meal. Some patients who are unable to tolerate 10 mg will tolerate 5 mg. This dosage produces the same therapeutic effect but more slowly.

DOSAGE AND ADMINISTRATION:

(Adults and Children over 12 years of age)

Vitiligo: Two tablets daily, taken two to four hours before measured periods of ultraviolet exposure or fluorescent black light[10](See suggested sun exposure guide.) (TABLE 1).

To increase tolerance to sunlight and/or enhance pigmentation: Two tablets daily, taken two hours before measured periods of exposure to sun or ultraviolet irradiation. Not to be continued for longer than 14 days. The dosage should **NOT** be increased, as severe burning may occur. (See suggested sun exposure guide.) (TABLE 1).

The exposure time to sunlight should be limited according to the following plan:

TABLE 1 Suggested Sun Exposure Guide

	Basic Skin Color: Light	Medium
Initial Exposure	15 min.	20 min.
Second Exposure	20 min.	25 min.
Third Exposure	25 min.	30 min.
Fourth Exposure	30 min.	35 min.
Subsequent Exposure	Gradually increase exposure based on erythema and tenderness.	
Sunglasses should be worn during exposure and the lips protected with a light-screening lipstick[10].		
Sun-Lamp Exposure: Should be initiated according to directions of the sun-lamp manufacturer.		

REFERENCES:

1. Pathak, M.A., and Fitzpatrick, T.B.,: Bioassay of Natural and Synthetic furocoumarins (Psoralens). J. Invest. Dermat. 32, 509-518, 1959. **2.** Pathak, M.A.; Fellman, J.H.; and Kaufman, K.D.,: The Effect of Structural Alterations on the Erythemal Activity of Furocoumarins: Psoralens. J. Invest. Dermat. 35, 165-183, 1960. **3.** Lerner, R.M., and Lerner, A.B.,: Dermatologic Medications, Second Edition, Year book Publishers, Pages 98-99. **4.** Pathak, M.A., and Fitzpatrick, T.B.,: Relationship of Molecular Configuration to the Activity of Furocoumarins Which Increase the Cutaneous Responses Following Long Wave Ultraviolet Radiation. J. Invest. Dermat. 32, No. 2, 255-262, 1959. **5.** Becker, S.W., Jr.,: Prevention of Sunburn and Light Allergy with Methoxsalen. G.P. 19, 115-117, 1959. **6.** Hu, F.; Fosnaugh, R.P., and Lesney, P.F.,: Studies on Albinism, Arch. Dermat. 83, 723-729, 1961. **7.** Lerner, A.B.,; Denton, C.R.; and Fitzpatrick, T.B.,: Clinical and Experimental Studies on 8- Methoxypsoralen in Vitiligo. J. Invest. Dermat. 20, 878, 1958. **8.** Sulzberger, M.B., and Lerner, A.B.,: Suntanning-Potentiation with Oral Medication. J.A.M.A., 167, 2077-2079, 1958. **9.** Becker, S.W., Jr.,: Effects of 8-Methoxypsoralen and Ultraviolet Light on Human Skin. Science, 127, 878, 1958. **10.** Stegmaier, O.C.,: The Use of Methoxsalen in Suntanning. J. Invest. Dermat. 32, No. 2, 345-349, 1959. **11.** Fitzpatrick, T.B.,: Current Therapy, W.B. Saunders Co., Page 515, 1958. **12.** Fitzpatrick, T.B.; Arndt, K.A.; El Mofty, A.M. and Pathak, M.A.: Hydroquinone and Psoralens in Therapy of Hypermelanosis and Vitiligo, ARCH. DERM. 93, 589-600, 1966. **13.** Becker, S.W., Jr.,: Psoralen Phototherapeutic Agents, J.A.M.A., 202, 422-424, 1967. **14.** El Mofty, A.M.: Vitiligo and Psoralens, PERGAMON PRESS INC., Long Island City, New York, 1st Edition, 1968.

HOW SUPPLIED:

Storage: Store at controlled room temperature (15°-30° C) 59°-86° F.

HOW SUPPLIED - EQUIVALENTS NOT AVAILABLE:

Tablet, Uncoated - Oral - 5 mg

28's	$67.19	TRISORALEN, ICN Pharms	00187-0303-28
100's	$200.13	TRISORALEN, ICN Pharms	00187-0303-01

TRIPELENNAMINE HYDROCHLORIDE *(002394)*

CATEGORIES: Allergic Reactions; Allergies; Anaphylactic Reactions; Angioedema; Antihistamines; Conjunctivitis; Respiratory & Allergy Medications; Rhinitis; Urticaria; FDA Approval Pre 1982

BRAND NAMES: *Azaron*; **PBZ**; Pelamine; Pyribenzamine; Triplen
(International brand names outside U.S. in italics)

FORMULARIES: Aetna; Medi-Cal

DESCRIPTION:

Tripelennamine hydrochloride is an antihistamine for oral administration. Tripelennamine hydrochloride is 2-(Benzyl(2-(dimethylamino)ethyl)amino)pyridine monohydrochloride.

CLINICAL PHARMACOLOGY:

Antihistamines are competitive antagonists of histamine, which also produce central nervous system effects (both stimulant and depressant) and peripheral anticholinergic, atropine-like effects (*e.g.,* drying).

INDICATIONS AND USAGE:

Perennial and seasonal allergic rhinitis; vasomotor rhinitis; allergic conjunctivitis due to inhalant allergens and foods; mild, uncomplicated allergic skin manifestations of urticaria and angio-edema; amelioration of allergic reactions to blood or plasma; dermographism; anaphylactic reactions as adjunctive therapy to epinephrine and other standard measures after the acute manifestations have been controlled.

CONTRAINDICATIONS:

PBZ should not be used in premature infants, neonates, or nursing mothers; patients receiving MAO inhibitors; patients with narrow-angle glaucoma, stenosing peptic ulcer, symptomatic prostatic hypertrophy, bladder neck obstruction, pyloroduodenal obstruction, lower respiratory tract symptoms (including asthma), or hypersensitivity to tripelennamine or related compounds.

WARNINGS:

Antihistamines often produce drowsiness and may reduce mental alertness in children and adults. Patients should be warned about engaging in activities requiring mental alertness (*e.g.,* driving a car, operating machinery or hazardous appliances). In elderly patients, approximately 60 years or older, antihistamines are more likely to cause dizziness, sedation and hypotension.

Patients should be warned that the central nervous system effects of PBZ may be additive with those of alcohol and other CNS depressants (*e.g.,* hypnotics, sedatives, tranquilizers, antianxiety agents).

Antihistamines may produce excitation, particularly in children.

Usage in Pregnancy: Although no tripelennamine-related teratogenic potential or other adverse effects on the fetus have been observed in limited animal reproduction studies, the safe use of this drug in pregnancy or during lactation has not been established. Therefore, the drug should not be used during pregnancy or lactation unless, in the judgment of the physician, the expected benefits outweigh the potential hazards.

Usage in Children: In infants and children particularly, antihistamines in overdosage may produce hallucinations, convulsions and/or death.

PRECAUTIONS:

PBZ, like other antihistamines, has atropine-like, anticholinergic activity and should be used with caution in patients with increased intraocular pressure, hyperthyroidism, cardiovascular disease, hypertension, or history of bronchial asthma.

ADVERSE REACTIONS:

The most frequent adverse reactions to antihistamines are sedation or drowsiness; sleepiness; dryness of the mouth, nose, and throat; thickening of bronchial secretions; dizziness; disturbed coordination; epigastric distress.

Other adverse reactions which may occur are: fatigue; chills; confusion; restlessness; excitation; hysteria; nervousness; irritability; insomnia; euphoria; anorexia; nausea; vomiting; diarrhea; constipation; hypotension; tightness in the chest; wheezing; blurred vision; diplopia; vertigo; tinnitus; convulsions; headache; palpitations; tachycardia; extrasystoles; nasal stuffiness; urinary frequency; difficult urination; urinary retention; leukopenia; hemolytic anemia; thrombocytopenia; agranulocytosis; aplastic anemia; allergic or hypersensitivity reactions, including drug rash, urticaria, anaphylactic shock, and photosensitivity. Although the following may have been reported to occur in association with some antihistamines, they have not been known to result from the use of PBZ: excessive perspiration, tremor, paresthesias, acute labyrinthitis, neuritis and early menses.

OVERDOSAGE:

Signs and Symptoms: The greatest danger from acute overdosage with antihistamines is their central nervous system effects which produce depression and/or stimulation.

In children, stimulation predominates initially in a syndrome which may include excitement, hallucinations, ataxia, incoordination, athetosis, and convulsions followed by postictal depression. Dry mouth, fixed dilated pupils, flushing of the face, and fever are common and resemble the syndrome of atropine poisoning.

In adults, CNS depression (*i.e.,* drowsiness, coma) is more common. CNS stimulation is rare; fever and flushing are uncommon.

In both children and adults, there can be a terminal deepening of coma and cardiovascular collapse; death can occur, especially in infants and children. *Treatment:* There is no specific therapy for acute overdosage with antihistamines. General symptomatic and supportive measures should be instituted promptly and maintained for as long as necessary.

In the conscious patient, vomiting should be induced even though it may have occurred spontaneously. If vomiting cannot be induced, gastric lavage is indicated. Adequate precautions must be taken to protect against aspiration, especially in infants and children. Charcoal slurry or other suitable agent should be instilled into the stomach after vomiting or lavage. Saline cathartics or milk of magnesia may be of additional benefit.

In the unconscious patient, the airway should be secured with a cuffed endotracheal tube before attempting to evacuate the gastric contents. Intensive supportive and nursing care is indicated, as for any comatose patient.

If breathing is significantly impaired, maintenance of an adequate airway and mechanical support of respiration is the safest and most effective means of providing for adequate oxygenation of tissues to prevent hypoxia (especially brain hypoxia during convulsions).

Hypotension is an early sign of impending cardiovascular collapse and should be treated vigorously. Although general supportive measures are important, specific treatment with intravenous infusion of a vasopressor (*e.g.,* levarterenol bitartrate) titrated to maintain adequate blood pressure may be necessary.

Do *not* use CNS stimulants.

Convulsions should be controlled by careful titration of a short-acting barbiturate, repeated as necessary.

Ice packs and cooling sponge baths can aid in reducing the fever commonly seen in children.

DOSAGE AND ADMINISTRATION:

PBZ

Dosage should be individualized.

Usual Adult Dose: 25 to 50 mg every four to six hours. As little as 25 mg may control symptoms, but as much as 600 mg daily may be given in divided doses, if necessary.

Children and Infants: 5 mg/kg/24 hours or 150 mg/m^2/24 hours divided into four to six doses. Do not exceed maximum total dose of 300 mg/24 hours.

PBZ-SR

Dosage should be individualized according to the needs and response of the response.

Adults: One 100 mg PBZ-SR tablet in the morning and one in the evening is generally adequate. In difficult cases, one 100 mg PBZ-SR tablet every 8 hours may be required.

Children: PBZ-SR tablets are not intended for use in children.

Note: PBZ-SR extended-release tablets must be swallowed whole and never crushed or chewed.

Do not store above 86°F (30°C). Protect from light.

HOW SUPPLIED - RATED THERAPEUTICALLY EQUIVALENT:

Tablet, Uncoated - Oral - 50 mg

100's	$6.75	Tripelennamine, Consolidated Midland	00223-2097-01
100's	$6.85	Tripelennamine, Schein Pharm (US)	00364-0281-01
100's	$21.67	PBZ, Novartis	00028-0117-01
250's	$12.00	TRIPLEN-50, IDE-Interstate	00814-8080-22
1000's	$43.50	TRIPLEN-50, IDE-Interstate	00814-8080-30
1000's	$47.38	Tripelennamine, Schein Pharm (US)	00364-0281-02
1000's	$47.50	Tripelennamine, Consolidated Midland	00223-2097-02

HOW SUPPLIED - NOT RATED EQUIVALENT:

Tablet, Coated, Sustained Action - Oral - 100 mg

100's	$35.69	PBZ-SR, Novartis	00028-0048-01

Tablet, Uncoated - Oral - 25 mg

100's	$14.28	PBZ, Novartis	00028-0111-01

TRIPROLIDINE HYDROCHLORIDE *(002396)*

CATEGORIES: Allergies; Alkylamines; Antihistamines; Respiratory & Allergy Medications; FDA Approval Pre 1982

BRAND NAMES: *Actidilon*; Harber-Fed
(International brand names outside U.S. in italics)

Prescribing information not available at time of publication.

HOW SUPPLIED - EQUIVALENTS NOT AVAILABLE:

Syrup - Oral - 1.25 mg/5ml

480 ml	$4.80	Triprolidine Hcl, Consolidated Midland	00223-6332-01
3840 ml	$29.99	Triprolidine Hcl, Consolidated Midland	00223-6332-02

Tablet, Uncoated - Oral - 2.5 mg

100's	$2.63	Harber-Fed, Harber Pharm	51432-0472-03

TROGLITAZONE *(003319)*

CATEGORIES: Antidiabetic Agents; Blood Glucose Regulators; Diabetes; Hyperglycemia; Pregnancy Category B; Thiazdidinedione

BRAND NAMES: **Rezulin**

PRIMARY ICD9: 250.1 (Type I (insulin dependent) diabetes)

DESCRIPTION:

Troglitazone is an oral antihyperglycemic agent which acts primarily by decreasing insulin resistance. Troglitazone is used in the management of type II diabetes (noninsulin-dependent diabetes mellitus (NIDDM) also known as adult-onset diabetes). It improves sensitivity to insulin in muscle and adipose tissue and inhibits hepatic gluconeogenesis. Troglitazone (± 5-[[4-[3,4-dihydro-6-hydroxy-2,5,7,8-tetramethyl-2H-1-benzopyran-2-yl)methoxy]phenyl]methyl]-2,4-thiazolidinedione) is not chemically or functionally related to either the sulfonylreas, the biguanides, or the α-glucosidase inhibitors. The molecule contains 2 chiral centers, with each of the 4 stereoisomers having similar pharmacologic effects.

Troglitazone is a white to yellowish crystalline compound; it may have a faint, characteristic odor. Troglitazone has a molecular formula of $C_{24}H_{27}NO_5S$ and a molecular weight of 441.55 daltons. It is soluble in N,N-dimethylformamide or acetone; sparingly soluble in ethyl acetate; slightly soluble in acetonitrile, anhydrous ethanol, or ether; and practically insoluble in water.

Rezulin is available as 200 and 400 mg tablets for oral administration formulated with the following excipients: croscarmellose sodium, hydroxypropyl methylcellulose, magnesium stearate, microcrystalline cellulose, polyethylene glycol 400, polysorbate 80, povidone, purified water, silicon dioxide, titanium dioxide, and synthetic iron oxides.

CLINICAL PHARMACOLOGY:

MECHANISM OF ACTION

Troglitazone is a thiazolidinedione antidiabetic agent that lowers blood glucose by improving target cell response to insulin It has a unique mechanism of action that is dependent on the presence of insulin for activity. Troglitazone decreases hepatic glucose output and increases insulin-dependent glucose disposal in skeletal muscle. Its mechanism of action is thought to involve binding to nuclear receptors (PPAR) that regulate the transcription of a number of insulin responsive genes critical for the control of glucose and lipid metabolism. Unlike sulfonylureas, troglitazone is not an insulin secretagogue.

In animal models of diabetes, troglitazone reduces the hyperglycemia, hyperinsulinemia, and hypertriglyceridemia characteristic of insulin-resistant states such as type II diabetes. Plasma lactate and ketone body formation are also decreased. The metabolic changes produced by troglitazone result from the increased responsiveness of insulin-dependent tissues and are observed in numerous animal models of insulin resistance. Treatment with troglitazone did not affect pancreatic weight, islet number or glucagon content, but did increase regranulation of the pancreatic beta cells in rodent models of insulin resistance.

Since troglitazone enhances the effects of circulating insulin (by decreasing insulin resistance), it does not lower blood glucose in animal models that lack endogenous insulin.

PHARMACOKINETICS AND DRUG METABOLISM

Maximum plasma concentration (C_{max}) and the area under plasma concentration-time curve (AUC) of troglitazone increase proportionally with increasing doses over the dose range of 200 to 600 mg/day (TABLE 1). Following daily drug administration, steady-state plasma concentrations of troglitazone are reached within 3 to 5 days.

TABLE 1 Mean (± SD) Steady-State Pharmacokinetic of Troglitazone in 21 Normal Volunteers

Dose (mg/day)	C_{max} (mcg/ml)	AUC (mcg·hr/ml)	CL/F* (ml/min)
200	0.90 (0.36)	7.4 (2.4)	500 (187)
400	1.61 (0.69)	13.4 (5.5)	601 (324)
600	2.82 (1.03)	22.1 (6.8)	496 (166)

* CL/F = Apparent oral clearance.

Absorption: Troglitazone is absorbed rapidly following oral administration; the time for maximum plasma concentration (T_{max}) occurs within 2 to 3 hours. Food increases the extent of absorption by 30% to 85%; thus troglitazone should be taken with a meal to enhance systemic drug availability.

CLINICAL PHARMACOLOGY: *(cont'd)*

Distribution: Mean apparent volume of distribution (V/F) of troglitazone following multiple-dose administration ranges from 10.5 to 26.5 L/kg of body weight. Troglitazone is extensively bound (>99%) to serum albumm. [^{14}C]troglitazone partitions into red blood cells (-5% of whole blood radioactivity).

Metabolism: In 6 healthy male volunteers given a single 400 mg dose of [^{14}C]troglitazone after 14 days of treatment with 400 mg troglitazone tablets, the major metabolites found in the plasma were the sulfate conjugate (Metabolite 1), followed by the quinone metabolite (Metabolite 3). Only 3.1% of the dose was detected in the urine; this was primarily in the form of the glucuronide conjugate (Metabolite 2), which is present in negligible amounts in the plasma. In both normal volunteers and patients with type II diabetes, steady-state levels of Metabolite 1 are 6 to 7 times that of troglitazone and Metabolite 3.

Troglilazone incubated with expressed human P450 1A1, 1A2, 2A6, 2B6, 2D6, 2E1, and 3A4 in the presence and absence of known inhibitors of these enzymes showed no Metabolite 3 formation above levels in control samples. Incubation of Metabolite 3 with human liver microsomes suggests that it is not subject to further metabolism.

The inhibitory profile of troglitazone against the 7 major P450 isozymes was characterized using human liver microsomes. Troglitazone was bound to inhibit 3A4, 2C9, and 2C19 by 40% to 67% at a concentration of 11 mcg/ml. Since the highest peak concentrations expected to be achieved on 600 mg once daily is in the range of 1 to 3 mcg/ml, inhibition may not be clinically important. The results of *in vivo* drug interaction studies tend to support this observation (see DRUG INTERACTIONS); caution should be observed when troglitazone is used in combination with drugs known to be metabolized by one of these enzymes. The inhibitory characteristics of Metabolite 3 have not been investigated directly.

Excretion: Following oral administration of [^{14}C]troglitazone, approximately 88% of the radioactivity is recovered in feces (85%) and urine (3%). Unchanged troglitazone zone is not recovered in urine following oral administration. Mean plasma elimination half-life of troglitazone ranges from 16 to 34 hours.

SPECIAL POPULATIONS

Renal Insufficiency: In patients with various degrees of renal function, the apparent clearance of total and unbound troglitazone and the plasma elimination half-life of troglitazone, Metabolite 1, and Metabolite 3 do not correlate with creatinine clearance. Thus, dose adjustment in patients with renal dysfunction is not necessary (see DOSAGE AND ADMINISTRATION).

Hepatic Insufficiency: Troglitazone, Metabolite 1, and Metabolite 3 plasma concentrations in patients with chronic liver disease (Childs-Pugh Grade B or C) were increased by approximately 30%, 400% and 100%, respectively, compared to those in healthy subjects without hepatic dysfunction. There was no changes in plasma protein binding. No adverse events were noted in any group that were attributed to drug. Nevertheless, troglitazone should be used with caution in patients with hepatic disease.

Geriatrics: Steady-state pharmacokinetics of troglitazone, Metabolite 1, and Metabolite 3 in healthy elderly subjects are comparable to those seen in young adults.

Pediatrics: Pharmacokinetic data in the pediatric population are not available.

Gender: Plasma concentrations of troglitazone and its metabolites are similar in men and women.

Ethnicity: Pharmacokinetics of troglitazone and its metabolites are similar among various ethnic groups.

PHARMACODYNAMICS AND CLINICAL EFFECTS

Clinical studies demonstrate that troglitazone improves insulin sensitivity in insulin-resistant patients. Troglitazone increases insulin-dependent glucose disposal, reduces hepatic gluconeogenesis, and enhances cellular responsiveness to insulin and thus, improves dysfunctional glucose homeostasis. In patients with type II diabetes, the decreased insulin resistance produced by troglitazone causes decreases in serum glucose, plasma insulin, and hemoglobin A_{1C}. These effects are independent of weight loss and persist with troglitazone treatment.

Following troglitazone treatment, LDL, HDL, and total cholesterol (total-C) increase, although total-C/HDL and LDL/HDL ratios do not change. The increase in total cholesterol is due to the increase in HDL and LDL cholesterol. Despite the observed increase in total and LDL cholesterol, ApoB fraction levels are not increased. Patients treated with troglitazone and concomitant insulin exhibit an initial reduction in triglyceride levels. With the reduction in insulin doses that may occur following troglitazone therapy, some attenuation of the triglyceride reduction may occur.

Phamacokinetic estimators of systemic troglitazone exposure do not improve the prediction of pharmacodynamic response beyond that obtained based upon knowledge of the administered dose.

Troglitazone has only been shown to exert its antihyperglycemic effect in the presence of insulin. Because troglitazone does not stimulate insulin secretion, hypoglycemia in patients treated with troglitazone alone is not to be expected. Because of this insulin-dependent mechanism of action, troglitazone should not be used in patients with type I diabetes.

CLINICAL STUDIES:

Two clinical studies were conducted to evaluate the effects of troglitazone on glycemic control and insulin dose in patients with type II diabetes who were being treated with insulin.

In one 6-month, double-blind, placebo-controlled study in insulin-treated type II diabetic patients receiving a mean of 73 (range 27-143) units/day of insulin with a mean baseline HbA_{1C} of 9.42 (range 7.04-12.48), troglitazone (200 or 600 mg/day) or placebo was added to the insulin therapy. Investigators were instructed to reduce insulin doses only if two consecutive FSGs were ≤100 mg/dl. Troglitazone-treated patients showed a significant ($p<0.0001$) reduction in HbA_{1C}compared with patients who received placebo (see TABLE 2).

Thirty percent of patients treated with 200 mg troglitazone and 57% of patients treated with 600 mg troglitazone had an HbA_{1C} value below 8% at the end of the study compared with 11% of placebo-treated patients. Accompanying this improvement in glycemic control was a significant ($p<0.0001$) decrease in exogenous insulin dosage of 15% in the 200 mg troglitazone treatment group and 42% in the 600 mg troglitazone treatment group compared with 1% in the placebo group.

A second 6-month, double-blind, placebo-controlled study in insulin-treated type II diabetics who previously were poorly controlled on oral agents receiving 30 to 150 units insulin/day assessed the use of troglitazone in reducing exogenous insulin dosage while improving glycemic control as measured by capillary blood glucose.

Patients treated with 200 mg (N=75) and 400 mg (N=76) troglitazone had their insulin doses decreased by 41% and 58%, respectively, compared to a reduction of insulin dose in the placebo group (N=71) of 14% while maintaining or improving glycemic control. Forty-one percent of the patients in the 400 mg group decreased their insulin injection frequency an average from 3 to 1 injections per day, 19% of patients receiving placebo decreased their injection frequency an average from 3 to 2 injections per day. Insulin therapy was discontinued in 15% of patients in the 400 mg troglitazone group compared to 7% in the 200 mg group and 1.5% in the placebo group.

A greater than 50% reduction in insulin dose was achieved by 51% of patients on 200 mg and 70% on 400 mg once daily as compared to 17% on placebo.

CLINICAL STUDIES: *(cont'd)*

TABLE 2 Mean Change From Baseline at 6 Months

Parameter	Placebo	Troglitazone 200 mg	Troglitazone 600 mg
N	**118**	**116**	**116**
HbA_{1C}%			
Mean Baseline	9.43 (0.10)	9.51 (0.10)	9.32 (0.11)
Mean change from baseline (SE)*	-0.12 (0.10)	-0.84 (0.10)	-1.41 (0.10)
Adjusted mean difference from placebo (SE)	—	-0.72 (0.14)†	-1.29 (0.14)†
Percent mean change from baseline	-1.3	-8.8	-15.1
Insulin daily dosage, units			
Mean baseline (SE)	75 (3.3)	73 (3.4)	71 (2.9)
Mean change from baseline	1 (2.1)	-11 (2.1)	-29 (2.2)
Adjusted mean difference from placebo (SE)	—	-12 (3.0)†	-30 (3.0)†
Percent mean change from baseline	1	-15	-42

* p<0.0001

An extended open-label study of troglitazone (N=17), has followed insulin-treated type II diabetic patients for up to 9 months. Following 9 months of treatment with 400 mg of troglitazone, mean HbA_{1C} levels were decreased by 0.8% compared with baseline values of 11.8% ± 2.0% (mean ± SD). The mean insulin daily dose decreased by 71% (42 units/day) in these seventeen patients.

INDICATIONS AND USAGE:

Troglitazone is indicated for use in patients with type II diabetes currently on insulin therapy whose hyperglycemia is inadequately controlled (HbA_{1C}>8.5%) despite insulin therapy of over 30 units per day given as multiple injections.

Management of type II diabetes should include diet control. Caloric restriction, weight loss, and exercise are essential for the proper treatment of the diabetic patient. This is important not only in the primary treatment of type II diabetes, but in maintaining the efficacy of drug therapy. Prior to initiation of troglitazone therapy, secondary causes of poor glycemic control (*e.g.*, infection or poor injection technique) should be investigated and treated.

CONTRAINDICATIONS:

Troglitazone is contraindicated in patients with known hypersensitivity or allergy to troglitazone or any of its components.

PRECAUTIONS:

GENERAL

Because of its mechanism of action, troglitazone is active only in the presence of insulin. Therefore, troglitazone should not be used in type I diabetes or for the treatment of diabetic keto-acidosis.

Hepatic: During all clinical studies in North America (N=2510 patients), a total of 20 troglitazone-treated patients were withdrawn from treatment because of liver function test abnormalities. Two of the 20 patients developed reversible jaundice. Both had liver biopsies which were consistent with an idiosyncratic drug reaction (see ADVERSE REACTIONS, Laboratory Abnormalities).

Hypoglycemia: Patients receiving troglitazone in combination with insulin may be at risk for hypoglycemia and a reduction in the dose of insulin may be necessary. Hypoglycemia has not been observed during the administration of troglitazone as monotherapy and would not be expected based on the mechanism of action.

Ovulation: In premenopausal anovulatory patients with insulin resistance, troglitazone treatment may result in resumption of ovulation. **These patients may be at risk for pregnancy.**

Hematologic: Across all clinical studies, hemoglobin declined by 3 to 4% in troglitazone-treated patients compared with 1 to 2% in those treated with placebo. White blood cell counts also declined slightly in troglitazone-treated patients compared to those treated with placebo. These changes occurred within the first four to eight weeks of therapy. Levels stabilized and remained unchanged for up to two years of continuing therapy. These changes may be due to the dilutional effects of increased plasma volume and have not been associated with any significant hematologic clinical effects (See ADVERSE REACTIONS, Laboratory Abnormalities).

INFORMATION FOR THE PATIENT

Troglitazone should be taken with meals. If the dose is missed at the usual meal, it may be taken at the next meal. If the dose is missed on one day, the dose should not be doubled the following day.

It is important to adhere to dietary instructions and to regularly have blood glucose and glycosylated hemoglobin tested. During periods of stress such as fever, trauma, infection, or surgery, insulin requirements may change and patients should seek the advice of their physician.

When using combination therapy with insulin, the risks of hypoglycemia, its symptoms and treatment, and conditions that predispose to its development should be explained to patients and their family members.

CARCINOGENESIS, MUTAGENESIS, AND IMPAIRMENT OF FERTILITY

Troglltazone was administered daily for 104 weeks to male rats at 100, 400, or 800 mg/kg and to female rats at 25, 50, or 200 mg/kg. Maximum plasma troglitazone AUC values based on parent compound represent exposures 12- and 47-fold higher for male and female rats, respectively, than human exposure of 400 mg daily. Troglitazone was not carcinogenic in male rats at any dose tested. In female rats, there was a statistically significant increase in sarcomatous tumors at the high dose (47-fold greater than estimated human exposure of parent compound). However, these findings are of unknown clinical relevance as this dose was associated with excessive mortality and is considered to have surpassed the maximum tolerated dose. No tumors of any type were increased in female rats at 25 and 50 mg/kg at exposures of 5- to 14-fold higher than in humans based on AUC of parent compound. In a 104-week study in mice given 50, 400, or 800 mg/kg, incidence of hemangiosarcoma was increased in females at 400 mg/kg and in both sexes at 800 mg/kg; incidence of hepatocellular carcinoma was increased in females at 800 mg/kg. The lowest dose with increased tumor incidence (400 mg/kg) was associated with AUC values of parent compound that were at least 16-fold higher than the human exposure. No tumors of any type were increased in mice at 50 mg/kg at exposures 2- to 4-fold higher than in humans based on AUC of parent compound.

Troglitazone has neither mutagenic in bacteria nor clastogenic in bone marrow of mice. Equivocal increases in chromosome aberrations were observed in an *in vitro* Chinese hamster lung cell assay. In mouse lymphoma cell gene mutations assays, results were equivocal when conducted with a microtiter technique and negative with an agar plate technique. A liver unscheduled DNA synthesis assay in rats was negative.

PRECAUTIONS: *(cont'd)*

No adverse effects on fertility or reproduction were observed in male or female rats given 40, 200, or 1000 mg/kg daily prior to and throughout mating and gestation. AUC at these doses was estimated to be 2- to 8-fold higher than the human exposure.

PREGNANCY CATEGORY B

Troglitazone was not teratogenic in rats given up to 2000 mg/kg or rabbits given up to 1000 mg/kg during organogenesis. Compared to human exposure of 400 mg daily, estimated exposures based on AUC at these doses were up to 8-fold higher in rats and up to 6-fold higher in rabbits. Body weights of fetuses and offspring of rats given 2000 mg/kg during gestation were decreased. Delayed postnatal development, attributed to decreased body weight, was observed in offspring of rats given 40, 200, or 1000 mg/kg during late gestation and lactation periods; no effects were observed in offspring of rats given 10 or 20 mg/kg.

There are no adequate and well-controlled studies in pregnant women. Troglitazone should not be used during pregnancy unless the potential benefit justifies the potential risk to the fetus.

Because current information strongly suggests that abnormal blood glucose levels during pregnancy are associated with a higher incidence of congenital abnormalities as well as increased neonatal morbidity and mortality, most experts recommend that insulin be used during pregnancy to maintain blood glucose levels as close to normal as possible.

NURSING MOTHERS

It is not known whether troglitazone is secreted in human milk. Troglitazone is secreted in the milk of lactating rats. Because many drugs are excreted in human milk, troglitazone should not be administered to a breast-feeding woman.

PEDIATRIC USE

Safety and effectiveness in pediatric patients have not been established.

GERIATRIC USE

Twenty-two percent of patients in clinical trials of troglitazone were 65 and over. No differences in effectiveness and safety were observed between these patients and younger patients.

USE IN PATIENTS WITH HEART FAILURE

Heart enlargement without microscopic changes has been observed in rodents at exposures exceeding 14 times the AUC of the 400 mg human dose. Serial echocardiographic evaluations in monkeys treated chronically at maximum achieveable exposures (3-5 times the human exposure at the 400 mg dose) did not reveal changes in heart size or function. In a 2-year echocardiographic clinical study using 600 to 800 mg/day of troglitazone in patients with type II diabetes, no increase in left ventricular mass or decrease in cardiac output was observed. The methodology employed was able to detect a change of about 10% or more in left ventricular mass.

In animal studies, troglitazone treatment was associated with increases of 6% to 15% in plasma volume. In a study of 24 normal volunteers, an increase in plasma volume of 6% to 8% compared to placebo was observed following 6 weeks of troglitazone treatment.

No increased incidence of adverse events potentially related to volume expansion (*e.g.*, congestive heart failure) have been observed during controlled clinical trials. However, patients with New York Heart Association (NYHA) Class III and IV cardiac status were not studied during clinical trials. Therefore, caution is advised during the administration of troglitazone to patients with NYHA Class III or IV cardiac status.

DRUG INTERACTIONS:

Cholestyramine: Concomitant administration of cholestyramine with troglitazone reduces the absorption of troglitazone by approximately 70%; thus coadministration of cholestyramine and troglitazone is not recommended.

Acetaminophen: Coadministration of acetaminophen and troglitazone does not alter the phamacokinetics of either drug.

Warfarin: Troglitazone has no clinically significant effect on prothrombin time when administered to patients receiving chronic warfarin therapy.

Sulfonylureas: Coadministration of troglitazone with glyburide does not appear to alter troglitazone or glyburide pharmacokinetics, but may further decrease fasting plasma glucose. There are insufficient data on the use of troglitazone with sulonylureas to establish the efficacy of this combination.

Metformin: No information is available on the use of troglitazone with metformin.

Ethanol: A single administration of a moderate amount of alcohol did not increase the risk of acute hypoglycemia in troglitazone-treated patients with type II diabetes mellitus.

Terfenadine: Coadministration of troglitazone with terfenadine decreases plasma concentrations of terfenadine and its active metabolite by 50 to 70% and may reduce the effectiveness of terfenadine.

Oral Contraceptives: Administration of troglitazone with an oral contraceptive containing ethinyl estradiol and norethindrone reduced the plasma concentrations of both by approximately 30%. These changes could result in loss of contraception.

The above interactions with terfenadine and oral contraceptives suggest that troglitazone may induce drug metabolism by CYP3A4. These findings should be considered when prescribing other CYP3A4 substrates such as cyclosporine, tacrolimus and some HMG-CoA reductase inhibitors.

ADVERSE REACTIONS:

In general, troglitazone is well-tolerated. Two patients in the clinical studies developed reversible jaundice with findings on liver biopsy consistent with idiosyncratic drug reaction (see PRECAUTIONS, General).

The overall incidence and types of adverse reactions reported in placebo-controlled clinical trials for troglitazone-treated patients and placebo-treated patients are shown in TABLE 3. In patients treated with troglitazone in glyburide-controlled studies (N=550) or uncontrolled studies (N=510), the safety profile of troglitazone appeared similar to that displayed in TABLE 3. The incidence of withdrawls during clinical trials was similar for patients treated with placebo or troglitazone (4%).

Types of adverse event seen when troglitazone was used concomitantly with insulin (N=542) were similar to those during troglitazone monotherapy (N=1731), although hypoglycemia occurred on insulin combination therapy. (See PRECAUTIONS).

LABORATORY ABNORMALITIES

Hematologic: Small decreases in hemoglobin, hematocrit, and neutrophil counts (within the normal range) were more common in troglitazone-treated than placebo-treated patients and may be related to increased plasma volume observed with troglitazone treatment. Hemoglobin decreases to below the normal range occurred in 5% of troglitazone-treated and 4% of placebo-treated patients.

Lipids: Small changes in serum lipids have been observed (see CLINICAL PHARMACOLOGY, Pharmacodynamics and Clinical Effects).

Serum Transaminase Levels: During controlled clinical trials, 2.2% of troglitazone treated patients had reversible elevations in AST or ALT greater than 3 times the upper limit of normal, compared with 0.6% of patients receiving placebo. Hyperbilirubinemia (>1.25 upper

ADVERSE REACTIONS: *(cont'd)*

TABLE 3 North American Placebo-Controlled Clinical Studies: Adverse Events Reported at a Frequency ≥5% of Troglitazone-Treated Patients

	% of Patients	
	Placebo (N=492)	Troglitazone (N=1450)
Infection	22	18
Headache	11	11
Pain	14	10
Accidental injury	6	8
Asthenia	5	6
Dizziness	5	6
Back pain	4	6
Nausea	4	6
Rhinitis	7	5
Diarrhea	6	5
Urinary tract infection	6	5
Peripheral edema	5	5
Pharyngitis	4	5

limit of normal) was found in 0.7% of troglitazone treated patients compared with 1.7% of patients receiving placebo. In the population of patients treated with troglitazone, mean and median values for bilirubin, AST, ALT, alkaline phosphatase, and GGT were decreased at the final visit compared with baseline, while values for LDH were increased slightly (see PRECAUTIONS, General, Hepatic.

DOSAGE AND ADMINISTRATION:

The current insulin dose should be combined upon initiation of troglitazone therapy. Troglitazone therapy should be initiated at 200 mg once daily in patients on insulin therapy. For patients not responding adequately, the dose of troglitazone should be increased after approximately 2 to 4 weeks.The usual dose of troglitazone is 400 mg once daily. The maximum recommended daily dose is 600 mg. It is recommended that the insulin dose be decreased by 10% to to 25% when fasting plasma glucose concentrations decrease to less than 120 mg/dl in patients receiving concomitant insulin and troglitazone. Further adjustments should be individualized based on glucose-lowering response. Troglitazone should be taken with a meal.

Patients with Renal Insufficiency: Dose adjustment in patients with renal insufficiency is not required (see CLINICAL PHARMACOLOGY, Pharmacokinetics and Drug Metabolism).

Patients with Hepatic Impairment: Troglitazone should be used with caution in patients with hepatic disease (see CLINICAL PHARMACOLOGY, Pharmacokinetics and Drug Metabolism).

PATIENT INFORMATION:

Troglitazone is used along with insulin for the treatment of type II diabetes.

Consult your physician if you are taking cholestyramine, other oral antidiabetes drugs, terfenadine or oral contraceptives.

Do not use if you are pregnant or breast feeding.

Consult your physician if you have liver disease.

May cause infection, headache, pain, accidental injury, weakness, dizziness, back pain, nausea, or runny nose.

Take with meals. If a dose is missed, take it at the next meal. If a dose is missed on one day, do not double the dose the following day.

Follow good dietary instruction and have regular blood tests performed.

When using combined therapy with insulin, hypoglycemia may result. Patients and relatives should be aware of the symptoms and treatment.

HOW SUPPLIED:

Rezulin is available in 200 and 400 mg tablets:*200 mg tablets:* yellow, oval, non-scored, film-coated tablet with "PD 352" debossed on one side, and "200" on the other. *400 mg tablets:* tan, oval, non-scored, film-coated tablet with "PD 353" debossed on one side, and "400" on the other.

Storage: Store at controlled room temperature 20°C-25°C (68°F-77°F). Protect from moisture and humidity.

HOW SUPPLIED - EQUIVALENTS NOT AVAILABLE:

Tablet, Film-Coated - Oral - 200 mg

30's	$104.40	REZULIN, Parke-Davis	00071-0352-15
90's	$313.20	REZULIN, Parke-Davis	00071-0352-23

Tablet, Film-Coated - Oral - 400 mg

30's	$160.20	REZULIN, Parke-Davis	00071-0353-15
90's	$480.60	REZULIN, Parke-Davis	00071-0353-23

TROLEANDOMYCIN *(002398)*

CATEGORIES: Anti-Infectives; Antibiotics; Antimicrobials; Infections; Lincosamides/Macrolides; Pharyngitis; Pneumonia; Respiratory Tract Infections; Streptococcal Infection; Rheumatic Fever*; FDA Approval Pre 1982

* Indication not approved by the FDA

BRAND NAMES: **Tao**

DESCRIPTION:

Tao (troleandomycin) is a synthetically derived acetylated ester of oleandomycin, an antibiotic elaborated by a species of *Streptomyces antibioticus.* It is a white crystalline compound, insoluble in water, but readily soluble and stable in the presence of gastric juice. The compound has a molecular weight of 814 and corresponds to the empirical formula $C_{41}H_{67}NO_{15}$.

CLINICAL PHARMACOLOGY:

Tao is an antibiotic shown to be active *in vitro* against the following gram-positive organisms:

Streptococcus pyogenes

Diplococcus pneumoniae

Susceptibility plate testing: If the Kirby-Bauer method of disc sensitivity is used, a 15 mcg oleandomycin disc should give a zone of over 18 mm when tested against a troleandomycin sensitive bacterial strain.

INDICATIONS AND USAGE:

Diplococcus Pneumoniae: Pneumococcal pneumonia due to susceptible strains.

Streptococcus Pyogenes: Group A beta-hemolytic streptococcal infections of the upper respiratory tract.

Injectable benzathine penicillin G is considered by the American Heart Association to be the drug of choice in the treatment and prevention of streptococcal pharyngitis and in long term prophylaxis of rheumatic fever.

Troleandomycin is generally effective in the eradication of streptococci from the nasopharynx. However, substantial data establishing the efficacy of Tao in the subsequent prevention of rheumatic fever are not available at present.

CONTRAINDICATIONS:

Troleandomycin is contraindicated in patients with known hypersensitivity to this antibiotic.

WARNINGS:

Use in Pregnancy: Safety for use in pregnancy has not been established.

The administration of troleandomycin has been associated with an allergic type of cholestatic hepatitis. Some patients receiving troleandomycin for more than two weeks or in repeated courses have shown jaundice accompanied by right upper quadrant pain, fever, nausea, vomiting, eosinophilia, and leukocytosis. These changes have been reversible on discontinuance of the drug. Liver function tests should be monitored in patients on such dosage, and the drug discontinued if abnormalities develop. Reports in the literature have suggested that the concurrent use of ergotamine-containing drugs and troleandomycin may induce ischemic reactions. Therefore, the concurrent use of ergotamine-containing drugs and troleandomycin should be avoided. Troleandomycin should be administered with caution to patients concurrently receiving estrogen containing oral contraceptives.

Studies in chronic asthmatic patients have suggested that the concurrent use of theophylline and troleandomycin may result in elevated serum concentrations of theophylline. Therefore, it is recommended that patients receiving such concurrent therapy be observed for signs of theophylline toxicity, and that therapy be appropriately modified if such signs develop.

PRECAUTIONS:

Troleandomycin is principally excreted by the liver.

Caution should be exercised in administering the antibiotic to patients with impaired hepatic function.

ADVERSE REACTIONS:

The most frequent side effects of troleandomycin preparations are gastrointestinal, such as abdominal cramping and discomfort, and are dose related. Nausea, vomiting, and diarrhea occur infrequently with usual oral doses.

During prolonged or repeated therapy, there is a possibility of overgrowth of nonsusceptible bacteria or fungi. If such infections occur, the drug should be discontinued and appropriate therapy instituted.

Mild allergic reactions such as urticaria and other skin rashes have occurred. Serious allergic reactions, including anaphylaxis, have been reported.

DOSAGE AND ADMINISTRATION:

Clinical judgment based on the type of infection and its severity should determine dosage within the below listed ranges.

Adults: 250 to 500 mg 4 times a day

Children: 125 to 250 mg (3-5 mg/lb or 6.6 to 11 mg/kg) every 6 hours

When used in streptococcal infection, therapy should be continued for ten days.

HOW SUPPLIED:

TAO Capsules 250 mg: Each capsule contains troleandomycin equivalent to 250 mg of oleandomycin: bottles of 100.

HOW SUPPLIED - EQUIVALENTS NOT AVAILABLE:

Capsule, Gelatin - Oral - 250 mg

100's	$93.74	TAO, Roerig	00049-1590-66

TROMETHAMINE *(002399)*

CATEGORIES: Acidosis; Alkalinizing Agents; Cardiac Arrest; Electrolyte Solutions; Electrolytic, Caloric-Water Balance; Homeostatic & Nutrient; Metabolic Acidosis; Urinary Alkalinizers; Pregnancy Category C; FDA Approval Pre 1982

BRAND NAMES: **Tham**; *Thamacetat* (France); *Thamesol*
(International brand names outside U.S. in italics)

DESCRIPTION:

For the prevention and correction of severe metabolic acidosis.

Tromethamine solution is a sterile, nonpyrogenic 0.3 M solution of tromethamine, adjusted to a pH of approximately 8.6 with glacial acetic acid. It is administered by intravenous injection, by addition to ACD blood for priming cardiac bypass equipment and by injection into the ventricular cavity during cardiac arrest.

Each 100 ml contains tromethamine 3.6 g (30 mEq) in water for injection. The solution is hypertonic (380 mOsm/liter, calc.) in relation to the extracellular fluid (280 mOsm/liter).

The solution contains no bacteriostat, antimicrobial agent or added buffer (except acetic acid for pH adjustment) and is intended only for use as a single-dose injection. When smaller doses are required the unused portion should be discarded.

Tromethamine solution is a parenteral systemic alkalizer and fluid replenisher.

Tromethamine, USP (sometimes called "tris" or "tris buffer") is chemically designated 2-amino-2-(hydroxymethyl)-1, 3-propanediol, a solid readily soluble in water, also classified as an organic amine buffer. Water for Injection, USP is chemically designated H_2O.

CLINICAL PHARMACOLOGY:

When administered intravenously as a 0.3 M solution, tromethamine acts as a proton acceptor and prevents or corrects acidosis by actively binding hydrogen ions (H+). It binds not only cations of fixed or metabolic acids, but also hydrogen ions of carbonic acid, thus increasing bicarbonate anion (HCO3-). Tromethamine also acts as an osmotic diuretic, increasing urine flow, urinary pH, and excretion of fixed acids, carbon dioxide and electrolytes. A significant fraction of tromethamine (30% at pH 7.40) is not ionized and therefore is capable of reaching equilibrium in total body water. This portion may penetrate cells and may neutralize acidic ions of the intracellular fluid.

The drug is rapidly eliminated by the kidney; 75% or more appears in the urine after eight hours. Urinary excretion continues over a period of three days.

CLINICAL PHARMACOLOGY: *(cont'd)*

Water is an essential constituent of all body tissues and accounts for approximately 70% of total body weight. Average normal adult daily requirement ranges from two to three liters (1.0 to 1.5 liters each for insensible water loss by perspiration and urine production).

Water balance is maintained by various regulatory mechanisms.

Water distribution depends primarily on the concentration of electrolytes in the body compartments and sodium (Na+) plays a major role in maintaining physiologic equilibrium.

INDICATIONS AND USAGE:

Tromethamine solution is indicated for the prevention and correction of metabolic acidosis. In the following conditions it may help to sustain vital functions and thus provide time for treatment of the primary disease:

Metabolic Acidosis Associated With Cardiac Bypass Surgery: Tromethamine solution has been found to be primarily beneficial incorrecting metabolic acidosis which may occur during or immediately following cardiac bypass surgical procedures.

Correction Of Acidity Of Acd Blood In Cardiac Bypass Surgery: It is well known that ACD blood is acidic and becomes more acidic on storage. Tromethamine effectively corrects this acidity. Tromethamine solution may be added directly to the blood used to prime the pump-oxygenator. When ACD blood is brought to a normal pH range the patient is spared an initial acid load. Additional tromethamine may be indicated during cardiac bypass surgery should metabolic acidosis appear.

Metabolic Acidosis Associated With Cardiac Arrest: Acidosis is nearly always one of the consequences of cardiac arrest and, in some instances, may even be a causative factor in arrest. It is important therefore, that the correction of acidosis should be started promptly with other resuscitative efforts. By correcting acidosis, tromethamine solution has caused the arrested hear to respond to resuscitative efforts after standard methods alone had failed. In these cases, tromethamine was given intraventricularly. It is to be noted, however, that such precariously ill patients often have died subsequently of causes unrelated to the administration of tromethamine. With administration by the peripheral venous route, metabolic acidosis has been corrected in a majority of patients. The success in reinstitution of cardiac rhythm by this means probably has not been of the same order of magnitude as with the intraventricular route.

CONTRAINDICATIONS:

Tromethamine solution is contraindicated in anuria and uremia.

WARNINGS:

Large doses of tromethamine solution may depress ventilation, as a result of increased blood pH and reduced CO_2 concentration. Thus, dosage should be adjusted so that blood pH is not allowed to increase above normal. In situations in which respiratory acidosis may be present concomitantly with metabolic acidosis, the drug may be used with mechanical assistance to ventilation.

Care must be exercised to prevent perivascular infiltration since this can cause inflammation, necrosis and sloughing of tissue. Venospasm and intravenous thrombosis, which may occur during infusion, can be minimized by insuring that the injection needle is well within the largest available vein and that solutions are slowly infused. Intravenous catheters are recommended. If perivascular infiltration occurs, institute appropriate countermeasures. (See ADVERSE REACTIONS.)

Tromethamine solution should be administered slowly and in amounts sufficient only to correct the existing acidosis, and to avoid overdosage and alkalosis. Overdosage in terms of total drug and/or too rapid administration, may cause hypoglycemia of a prolonged duration (several hours). Therefore, frequent blood glucose determinations should be made during and after therapy.

Extreme care should be exercised in patients with renal disease or reduced urinary output because of potential hyperkalemia and the possibility of a decreased excretion of tromethamine. In such patients, the drug should be used cautiously with electrocardiographic monitoring and frequent serum potassium determinations.

Because clinical experience has been limited generally to short-term use, the drug should not be administered for more than a period of one day except in a life-threatening situation.

The intravenous administrations of tromethamine solution can cause fluid and/or solute overloading resulting in dilution of serum electrolyte concentrations, overhydration, congested states or pulmonary edema.

Additives may be incompatible. Consult with pharmacist, if available. When introducing additives, use aseptic technique, mix thoroughly and do not store.

PRECAUTIONS:

Blood pH, PCO_2 bicarbonate, glucose and electrolyte determinations should be performed before, during and after administration of tromethamine solution.

While it has not been shown that the drug increases coagulation time in humans, this possibility should be kept in mind since this has been noted experimentally in dogs.

Do not administer unless solution is clear and seal is intact. Discard unused portion.

Pregnancy Category C: Animal reproduction studies have not been conducted with tromethamine. It is also not known whether tromethamine can cause fetal harm when administered to a pregnant woman or can affect reproduction capacity. Tromethamine should be given to a pregnant woman only if clearly needed.

Carcinogenesis, Mutagenesis, and Impairment of Fertility: Studies of tromethamine in animals to evaluate the effect of fertility have not been conducted.

Pediatric Use: hypoglycemia may occur when this product is used in premature and even full-term neonates. See WARNINGS and ADVERSE REACTIONS.

ADVERSE REACTIONS:

Generally, side effects have been infrequent.

Respiratory: Although the incidence of ventilatory depression is low, it is important to keep in mind that such depression may occur. Respiratory depression may be more likely to occur in patients who have chronic hypoventilation or those who have been treated with drugs which depress respiration. In patients associated with respiratory acidosis, tromethamine should be administered with mechanical assistance to ventilation.

Vascular: Extreme care should be taken to avoid perivascular infiltration. Local tissue damage and subsequent sloughing may occur if extravasation occurs. Chemical phlebitis and venospasm also have been reported.

Hematologic: Transient depression of blood glucose may occur. Reactions which may occur because of the solution or the technique of administration include febrile response, infection at the site of injection, venous thrombosis or phlebitis extending from the site of injection extravasation and hypervolemia.

If an adverse reaction does occur, discontinue the infusion, evaluate the patient, institute appropriate therapeutic countermeasures and save the remainder of the fluid for examination if deemed necessary.

OVERDOSAGE:

Too rapid administration and/or excessive amounts of tromethamine may cause alkalosis, hypoglycemia, overhydration or solute overload. In the event of overdosage, discontinue the infusion, evaluate the patient and institute appropriate countermeasures. (See WARNINGS, PRECAUTIONS, and ADVERSE REACTIONS.)

The LD_{50} values for the acute intravenous toxicity of tromethamine are influenced by the rate of infusion of the dose administered.

Intravenous LD_{50}Mice: 3500 mg/kg

Intravenous LD_{50}Rats: 2300 mg/kg

DOSAGE AND ADMINISTRATION:

Tromethamine solution is administered by slow intravenous infusion, by addition to pump-oxygenator ACD blood or other priming fluid or by injection into the ventricular cavity during cardiac arrest. For infusion by peripheral vein, a large needle should be used in the largest antecubital vein or an indwelling catheter placed in a large vein of an elevated limb to minimize chemical irritation of the alkaline solution during infusion. Catheters are recommended.

Dosage and rate of administration should be carefully supervised to avoid overtreatment (alkalosis). Pretreatment and subsequent determinations of blood values (*e.g.*, pH, PCO_2, PO_2, glucose and electrolytes) and urinary output should be made as necessary to monitor dosage and progress of treatment. In general, dosage should be limited to an amount sufficient to increase blood pH to normal limits (7.35 to 7.45) and to correct acid-base derangements.

The total quality to be administered during the period of illness will depend upon the severity and progression of the acidosis. The possibility of some retention of tromethamine, especially in patients with impaired renal function, should be kept in mind.

The intravenous dosage of tromethamine solution may be estimated from the buffer base deficit of the extracellular fluid in mEq/liter determined by means of the Siggaard-Andersen nomogram. The formula found in TABLE 1 is intended as a general guide.

TABLE 1
Tromethamine Solution (ml of 0.3 M) Required = Body Weight (kg) × Base Deficit (mEq/liter) × 1.1*
* Factor of 1.1. accounts for an approximate reduction of 10% in buffering capacity due to the presence of sufficient acetic acid to lower pH of the 0.3 M solution to approximately 8.6.

Thus, a 70 kg patient with a buffer base deficit ("negative base excess") of 5 mEq/liter would require 70 x 5 x 1.1 = 385 ml of tromethamine solution containing 13.9 g (115 mEq) of tromethamine. The need for administration of additional tromethamine solution is determined by serial determinations of the existing base deficit.

Correction of Metabolic Acidosis Associated With Cardiac Bypass Surgery: An average dose of approximately 9.0 ml/kg (324 mg/kg) has been used in clinical studies with tromethamine solution. This is equivalent to a total dose of 630 ml (189 mEq) for a 70 kg patient.

A total single dose of 500 ml (150 mEq) is considered adequate for most adults. Larger single doses (up to 1000 ml) may be required in unusually severe cases.

It is recommended that individual doses should not exceed 500 mg/kg (227 mg/lb) over a period of not less than one hour. Thus, for a 70 kg (154 pound) patient the dose should not exceed a maximum of 35 g per hour (1078 ml of a 0.3 M solution). Repeated determinations of pH and other clinical observations should be used as a guide to the need for repeat doses.

Correction of Acidity of Acd Blood in Cardiac Bypass Surgery: The pH of stored blood ranges from 6.80 to 6.22 depending upon the duration of storage. The amount of tromethamine solution used to correct this acidity ranges from 0.5 to 2.5 g (15 to 77 ml of a 0.3 M solution) added to each 500 ml of ACD blood used for priming the pump-oxygenator. Clinical experience indicates that 2 g (62 ml of a 0.3 M solution) added to 500 ml of ACD blood is usually adequate.

Correction of Metabolic Acidosis Associated With Cardiac Arrest: In the treatment of cardiac arrest, tromethamine solution should be given at the same time that other standard resuscitative measures, including manual systole, are being applied. If the chest is open, tromethamine solution is injected directly into the ventricular cavity.

From 2 to 6 g (62 to 185 ml of a 0.3 M solution) should be injected immediately. **Do Not Inject Into The Cardiac Muscle.**

If the chest is not open, from 3.6 to 10.8 g (111 to 333 ml of a 0.3 M solution) should be injected immediately into a larger peripheral vein. Additional amounts may be required to control acidosis persisting after cardiac arrest is reversed.

Parenteral drug products should be inspected visually for particulate matter and discoloration prior to administration, whenever solution and container permit. (See CONTRAINDICATIONS.)

(Abbott)

HOW SUPPLIED - EQUIVALENTS NOT AVAILABLE:

Injection, Solution - Intravenous - 36 mg/ml

500 ml $140.41 THAM, Abbott 00074-1593-04

TROPICAMIDE *(002400)*

CATEGORIES: Anticholinergic Agents; Antitussives/Expectorants/Mucolytics; Cycloplegics/Mydriatics; Diagnostic Agents; EENT Drugs; Eye, Ear, Nose, & Throat Preparations; Mydriasis; Mydriatics; Mydriatics & Cycloplegics; Ophthalmics; FDA Approval Pre 1982

BRAND NAMES: *Alcon-Mydril*; I-Picamide; Infi-Cyle; Mydral; *Mydramide*; **Mydriacyl**; Mydriafair; *Mydriaticum*; *Mydrin-M*; Ocu-Tropic; *Optacyl*; *Sandol*; Spectro-Cyl; Tropicacyl; *Tropimil*; Tropistorz; *Visumidriatic*
(International brand names outside U.S. in italics)

FORMULARIES: Aetna; FHP; Medi-Cal; WHO

DESCRIPTION:

Tropicamide is an anticholinergic prepared as a sterile topical ophthalmic solution in two strengths.

Chemical Name: Benzeneacetamide, N-ethyl-alpha- (hydroxymethyl)-N-(4-pyridinylmethyl)-.

Active Ingredients Per ml: Tropicamide 0.5% or 1.0%. *Preservative:* Benzalkonium Chloride 0.01%. *Inactive:* Sodium Chloride, Edetate Disodium, Hydrochloric Acid and/or Sodium Hydroxide (to adjust pH), Purified Water.

CLINICAL PHARMACOLOGY:

This anticholinergic preparation blocks the responses of the sphincter muscle of the iris and the ciliary muscle to cholinergic stimulation, dilating the pupil (mydriasis). The stronger preparation (1.0%) also paralyzes accommodation.

This preparation acts rapidly and the duration of activity is relatively short. The weaker strength may be useful in producing mydriasis with only slight cycloplegia.

INDICATIONS AND USAGE:

For mydriasis and cycloplegia for diagnostic procedures.

CONTRAINDICATIONS:

Contraindicated in persons with primary glaucoma or a tendency toward glaucoma (*e.g.,* narrow anterior chamber angle), and in persons showing hypersensitivity to any component of this preparation.

WARNINGS:

For topical use only—not for injection.

Reproductive studies have not been performed in animals. There is not adequate information on whether this drug may affect fertility in human males or females or have a teratogenic potential or other adverse effect on the fetus. This preparation may cause CNS disturbances which may be dangerous in infants and children. Possibility of occurrence of psychotic reaction and behavioral disturbance due to hypersensitivity to anticholinergic drugs should be borne in mind.

PRECAUTIONS:

In the elderly and others where increased intraocular pressure may be encountered, mydriatics and cycloplegics should be used cautiously. To avoid inducing angle closure glaucoma, an estimation of the depth of the angle of the anterior chamber should be made. The lacrimal sac should be compressed by digital pressure for two to three minutes after instillation to avoid excessive systemic absorption.

Patient Warning: Do not touch dropper tip to any surface, as this may contaminate the solution.

Patient should be advised not to drive or engage in other hazardous activities while pupils are dilated. Patient may experience sensitivity to light and should protect eyes in bright illumination during dilation. Parents should be warned not to get this preparation in their child's mouth and to wash their own hands and the child's hands following administration.

ADVERSE REACTIONS:

Increased intraocular pressure. Psychotic reactions, behavioral disturbances, and cardiorespiratory collapse in children and some adults with this class of drugs have been reported. Transient stinging, dryness of the mouth, blurred vision, photophobia with or without corneal staining, tachycardia, headache, parasympathetic stimulation, or allergic reaction may occur.

DOSAGE AND ADMINISTRATION:

For refraction, one or two drops of 1.0% solution in the eye(s), repeated in five minutes. If patient is not seen within 20 to 30 minutes, an additional drop may be instilled to prolong mydriatic effect. For examination of fundus, one or two drops of 0.5% solution 15 or 20 minutes prior to examination. Individuals with heavily pigmented irides may require larger doses.

HOW SUPPLIED - RATED THERAPEUTICALLY EQUIVALENT:

Solution - Ophthalmic - 0.5 %

2 ml	$4.27	OPTICYL, Optopics	52238-0850-02
15 ml	$4.18	Tropicamide, H.C.F.A. F F P	99999-2400-02
15 ml	$5.04	OPTICYL, Optopics	52238-0850-15
15 ml	$6.95	SPECTRO CYL, Spectrum Scitfc	53268-0590-12
15 ml	$7.50	Tropicamide, Martec Pharms	52555-0089-10
15 ml	$9.05	Mydral, Ocusoft	54799-0529-15
15 ml	$9.38	Tropicacyl, Akorn	17478-0101-12
15 ml	**$21.56**	**MYDRIACYL 1/2 % OPTHALMIC, Alcon-PR**	**00998-0354-15**

Solution - Ophthalmic - 1 %

2 ml	$4.27	Tropicamide, H.C.F.A. F F P	99999-2400-03
2 ml	$5.63	OPTICYL, Optopics	52238-0851-02
2 ml	$6.20	Mydral, Ocusoft	54799-0528-02
2 ml	$7.56	TROPICACYL, Akorn	17478-0102-20
3 ml	**$6.87**	**MYDRIACYL, Alcon**	**00065-0355-03**
15 ml	$6.30	Tropicamide, IDE-Interstate	00814-8116-42
15 ml	$6.31	OPTICYL, Optopics	52238-0851-15
15 ml	$7.95	SPECTRO CYL, Spectrum Scitfc	53268-0585-12
15 ml	$9.20	Tropicamide, Martec Pharms	52555-0090-10
15 ml	$9.38	TROPICACYL, Akorn	17478-0102-12
15 ml	$9.50	Tropicamide, Steris Labs	00402-0780-15
15 ml	$9.95	MYDRAL OPHTHALMIC, Ocusoft	54799-0528-12
15 ml	$10.42	Tropicamide, Aligen Independ	00405-6150-15
15 ml	**$22.81**	**MYDRIACYL 1% OPHTHALMIC, Alcon-PR**	**00998-0355-15**

HOW SUPPLIED - NOT RATED EQUIVALENT:

Solution - Ophthalmic - 0.5 %

2 ml	$4.27	Tropicamide, Apotex	60505-7506-01
15 ml	$5.04	Tropicamide, Apotex	60505-7506-05

Solution - Ophthalmic - 1 %

2 ml	$4.75	Spectro-Cyl, Spectrum Scitfc	53268-0585-59
2 ml	$5.19	Infi-Cyle, Infinity Pharm	58154-0585-59
2 ml	$5.63	Tropicamide, Apotex	60505-7505-01
15 ml	$6.31	Tropicamide, Apotex	60505-7505-05
15 ml	$7.33	INFI-CYLE, Infinity Pharm	58154-0585-64

TUBOCURARINE CHLORIDE *(002403)*

CATEGORIES: Analeptics; Anesthesia; Autonomic Drugs; Curare Derivatives; Diagnostic Agents; Myasthenia Gravis; Neuromuscular Blocking Agents; Non-Depolarizing Muscle Relaxants; Skeletal Muscle Relaxants; FDA Approval Pre 1982

> **WARNING:**
> This drug should only be administered by adequately trained individuals who are familiar with its actions, characteristics, and hazards (see WARNINGS).

DESCRIPTION:

Tubocurarine is the active ingredient of the curare-producing plant, *Chondodendron tomentosum.* Turbocurarine chloride injection is a nondepolarizing neuromuscular blocking agent for intravenous injection. Each ml of sterile, clear, aqueous, isotonic solution provides 3 mg crystalline tubocurarine chloride (equivalent to 20 units of curare activity), not more than 1 mg sodium bisulfite, 9 mg benzyl alcohol as a preservative, and sodium chloride for isotonicity; pH is adjusted between 2.5 and 5.0 with hydrochloric acid and sodium bicarbonate. At the time of manufacture, the air in the vial is replaced with nitrogen.

Tubocurarine chloride is a quaternary ammonium compound designated chemically as (+)-tubocurarine chloride hydrochloride pentahydrate.

$C_{37}H_{41}ClN_2O_6 \cdot HCl \cdot 5H_2O$/MW 771.73/CAS-6989-98-6

CLINICAL PHARMACOLOGY:

Following intravenous administration, tubocurarine chloride is rapidly distributed to the neuromuscular junction and interrupts the transmission of nerve impulses to skeletal muscles at the myoneural junction. The drug produces a competitive (nondepolarizing block of cholinergic receptors of the motor endplate without change in the resting potential of the postjunctional membrane to produce a flaccid paralysis of skeletal muscles.

Generally, maximum relaxation occurs within a mean time of approximately six minutes from the start of an adequate intravenous dose (onset of muscular relaxation is usually unpredictable following intramuscular administration) of tubocurarine chloride. Duration of action varies according to dosage, administration procedure, general anesthetic employed, and measurement employed. For rough comparison only, a paralyzing dose of 0.6 mg/kg of tubocurarine chloride is followed by recovery of twitch tension to 25 percent of control within approximately 80 minutes (supramaximal ulnar nerve stimulation, monitored by quantitation of force-of-thumb adduction).

Nondepolarizing muscle relaxants are longer acting than depolarizing muscle relaxants.

The paralysis following intravenous injection of an effective dose of tubocurarine chloride is selective initially and usually appears in the following muscles consecutively: levator muscles of eyelids, muscles of mastification, limb muscles, abdominal muscles, muscles of the glottis and finally the intercostal muscles and the diaphragm. Recovery generally occurs in the reverse order. Tubocurarine chloride has no direct effect on the uterus or other smooth muscles.

Repeated doses of tubocurarine chloride produce a cumulative effect. The duration of action, and possibly the magnitude of neuromuscular blockade may be altered by dehydration, hypothermia, hypocalcemia, hypokalemia, excess magnesium, acid-base imbalance, or by some carcinomas.

Histamine release may be triggered following administration of tubocurarine chloride (see General).

PHARMACOKINETICS

Plasma concentrations of tubocurarine chloride between 5 a nd 50 mcg/ml are approximately 40 to 45 percent bound to plasma proteins, mainly globulins. Redistribution into the tissues occurs following a single dose consistent with a three-compartment open model; the terminal half-life is approximately 3.9 hours. Following a large single dose or when repeated doses are administered, the tissues become saturated and factors of degradation and excretion by the liver and kidneys directly influence the intensity and duration of action. When tissue compartments are saturated, the drug may persist up to 24 hours and prolonged neuromuscular blockade can result if additional doses are administered within this period.

Tubocurarine is recovered unchanged mainly in the urine; doses of 0.2 or 0.5 mg/kg were followed by excretion of approximately 33 to 43 percent of dose 6 to 24 hours following administration. Tubocurarine is also excreted to a lesser extent by the biliary tract through a specific organic cation secretion mechanism with up to 11 percent of a dose being recovered in the bile in 24 hours. Approximately one percent of a dose undergoes hepatic metabolism (N-demethylation); the metabolite is excreted in the bile.

Prolonged neuromuscular blockade may occur in patients with impaired renal function (see General.)

Tubocurarine chloride has been identified in the cerebrospinal fluid in amounts unlikely to produce any pharmacological effects; minute quantities have also been detected in saliva.

In spite of low lipid solubility and complete ionization at physiologic pH range, the placental transfer and fetal distribution of tubocurarine has been reported (see Pregnancy.) When the drug is administered during delivery, blood levels in the newborn are directly related to the maternal dose and the time interval between injection and delivery. Although most infants do not grossly manifest drug effect following delivery, myoneural block has been reported in the newborn following the administration of repeated doses of tubocurarine chloride to the mother (245 mg total) for prolonged management of eclampsia.

INDICATIONS AND USAGE:

Tubocurarine chloride is indicated as an adjunct to anesthesia to induce skeletal-muscle relaxation. It may be employed to reduce the intensity of muscle contractions in pharmacologically or electrically induced convulsions; and to facilitate the management of patients undergoing mechanical ventilation.

Tubocurarine chloride also may be used as a diagnostic agent for myasthenia gravis when the results of tests with neostigmine or edrophonium are inconclusive.

CONTRAINDICATIONS:

Neuromuscular blocking agents are contraindicated in patients with known hypersensitivity to any of the components of the preparations.

WARNINGS:

NEUROMUSCULAR BLOCKING AGENTS SHOULD BE ADMINISTERED IN CAREFULLY INDIVIDUALIZED DOSES BY OR UNDER THE SUPERVISION OF EXPERIENCED CLINICIANS WHO ARE FAMILIAR WITH THE POTENTIAL COMPLICATIONS THAT MIGHT OCCUR FOLLOWING ADMINISTRATION OF THESE DRUGS. THESE DRUGS SHOULD NOT BE ADMINISTERED UNLESS FACILITIES FOR INTUBATION OF THE TRACHEA, ARTIFICIAL RESPIRATION, OXYGEN THERAPY, AND ANTAGONISTIC AGENTS FOR REVERSING A NONDEPOLARIZING BLOCK ARE IMMEDIATELY AVAILABLE. THE CLINICIAN MUST BE PREPARED TO ASSIST OR CONTROL RESPIRATION.

Tubocurarine chloride must be used with extreme caution during prolonged administration or as a diagnostic test in patients with myasthenia gravis, since prolonged respiratory paralysis may occur (see DOSAGE AND ADMINISTRATION). In such patients, a peripheral nerve stimulator may be valuable in monitoring response to the drug.

Particular care should be taken when tubocurarine chloride is used in patients with respiratory deficiencies or pulmonary disorders, since severe respiratory difficulty may occur.

Turbocurarine chloride injection, USP, contains sodium bisulfite, a sulfite that may cause allergic-type reactions, including anaphylactic symptoms and life-threatening or less severe asthmatic episodes, in certain susceptible people. The overall prevalence of sulfite sensitivity is seen more frequently in asthmatic than in nonasthmatic people.

PRECAUTIONS:

GENERAL

During the time the drug is exerting its effect and until the patients fully regains consciousness, *it is important that he be carefully watched for signs of respiratory embarrassment.*

Neuromuscular blocking agents should be used with caution in patients with poor renal perfusion or renal disease, hepatic or cardiovascular disease, or impaired endocrine function.

Neuromuscular blocking agents should be used with caution in patients in whom a sudden increase of histamine release is a definite hazard.

Hypotension, secondary to histamine release or ganglionic blockade, may occur following rapid injection or large doses of tubocurarine chloride.

Muscle relaxants have little to no effect on consciousness, pain threshold or cerebration. Therefore, they should always be used with adequate anesthesia.

DRUG/LABORATORY TEST INTERACTIONS

It has been reported that in patients with tetanus, continuous administration of tubocurarine in large doses results in production of a factor that interferes with the detection of catecholamines in urine when assayed fluorometrically.

CARCINOGENESIS, MUTAGENESIS, AND IMPAIRMENT OF FERTILITY

Long-term studies in animals have not been performed with neuromuscular blocking agents to evaluate carcinogenic or mutagenic potential, or possible impairment of fertility in males or females.

PREGNANCY CATEGORY C

Teratogenic Effects: Tubocurarine chloride has produced intrauterine growth retardation and limb deformities resembling clubfoot when administered intramuscularly to rat fetuses between 16 and 19 days gestation, and when injected into chick embryos between 5 and 15 days incubation. The incidence of growth retardation and limb deformity in the rat fetuses ranged from 21 to 23 percent and 7 to 8 percent, respectively.

There are no adequate and well-controlled studies in pregnant women. Neuromuscular blocking agents should be used during pregnancy only if the potential benefit justifies the potential risk to the fetus.

Nonteratogenic Effects: Prolonged administration of large doses of tubocurarine chloride, such as were used in the management of tetanus in a patient during early pregnancy, may be associated with fetal contractures. Following a total dose of approximately 1.3 g of tubocurarine chloride injected intravenously and intramuscularly over a period of ten days to a 10 to 12 week pregnant woman suffering from severe generalized tetanus, the infant was born at term with joint contractures. The condition was attributed to immobilization of the fetus at the time of joint formation.

LABOR AND DELIVERY

Neuromuscular blocking agents are usually well tolerated by the neonate if used during delivery, especially cesarean section delivery, provided that the interval between drug administration and delivery is reasonably short (1 to 10 minutes). Longer time intervals between drug use and delivery may impair the newborn's ability to breathe due to skeletal muscle weakness (see CLINICAL PHARMACOLOGY, Pharmacokinetics.)

NURSING MOTHERS

It is not known whether neuromuscular blocking agents are excreted in human milk. Because many drugs are excreted in human milk. Because many drugs are excreted in human milk, caution should be exercised when any neuromuscular blocking agent is administered to a nursing woman.

PEDIATRIC USE

Tubocurarine chloride has been successfully used to induce muscle relaxation in pediatric patients. However, premature infants and neonates may be more sensitive to nondepolarizing agents; infants and children exhibit the same widely variable responses as do adults.

It has been reported that doses based on body weight appear to be suitable for children (as for adults) whereas doses based on body surface area are more accurate for premature infants and neonates. Incremental doses of 0.20 mg may constitute a useful practical titration to obtain satisfactory conditions in infants and neonates.

DRUG INTERACTIONS:

When administered concurrently, the following drugs may interact with tubocurarine chloride:

Certain Antibiotics: Parenteral administration of high doses of certain antibiotics may intensify or resemble the neuromuscular blocking action of muscle relaxants. The following antibiotics have been associated with various degrees of paralysis: aminoglycosides (*i.e.,* neomycin, streptomycin, kanamycin, gentamicin, dihydrostreptomycin), bacitracin, polymyxin B, colistin, sodium colistimethate and tetracyclines. Synergism between intravenously injected tobramycin and curare has also been reported. Prolonged apnea, in the presence of low pseudocholinesterase levels and abnormal liver function tests, has been associated with intravenously injected clindamycin therapy. If muscle relaxants and antibiotics which may block neuromuscular transmission must be administered simultaneously, the patient should be observed closely for unexpected prolongation of respiratory depression.

Inhalation Anesthetics: The administration of neuromuscular blocking agents to patients anesthetized with volatile liquid anesthetic agents (*i.e.,* cyclopropane, diethyl ether, enflurane, fluroxene, halothane, isoflurane, methoxyflurane, and penthrane) will usually result in a dose related enhancement of neuromuscular blockade and an increase in duration of action. During anesthesia with halothane, ketamine hydrochloride may enhance the neuromuscular blockade produced by tubocurarine chloride. Nitrous oxide in oxygen, intravenous narcotics, and most other intravenous anesthetic adjuvants do not greatly affect the degree and duration of neuromuscular blockade.

Other Muscle Relaxants: Synergism has been demonstrated when nondepolarizing muscle relaxants (*i.e.,* gallamine triethiodide and tubocurarine chloride) are injected concurrently.

Synergistic or antagonistic effects may result when depolarizing and nondepolarizing muscle relaxants (*i.e.,* succinylcholine and tubocurarine chloride) are administered consecutively. The extent and type of interaction is greatly dependent upon the doses, and the sequence and timing of the injections. Under normal circumstances, when depolarizing and nondepolarizing muscle relaxants are to be administered consecutively, the effect of one should be allowed to dissipate prior to the administration of the other.

Magnesium Sulfate: Potentiation of the neuromuscular blocking effects of tubocurarine chloride were observed in patients with preeclamptic toxemia treated with intramuscular injections of magnesium sulfate prior to cesarean section.

Opiate Analgesics: Additive respiratory depressant effects may occur.

Potassium-Depleting Agents: (*i.e.,* amphotericin B, thiazide dieretics, furosemide, ethacrynic acid,chlorthalidone, carbonic anhydrase inhibitors, corticosteroids, corticotropin)—May cause an increased sensitivity to neuromuscular blocking agents. Adequate potassium serum levels should be assured prior to elective surgery.

Quinidine: Clinical cases strongly suggest that quinidine injected shortly after recovery causes recurrent paralysis in patients who received injections of either depolarizing or nondepolarizing muscle relaxants during surgery.

DRUG INTERACTIONS: *(cont'd)*

Calcium salts, Diazepam, Lithium carbonate, MAO inhibitors, Propranolol, Quinine salts, excessively high IV doses of Lidocaine, and Trimethaphan: Intensification and/or prolongation of the effect of curare-containing preparations may result.

ADVERSE REACTIONS:

The most frequently noted adverse reaction to neuromuscular blocking agents is an extended duration of the drugs' pharmacologic actions. prolonged neuromuscular effects may vary from skeletal muscle weakness to profound skeletal muscle relaxation resulting in respiratory insufficiency or apnea.

Potential adverse effects following administration of curare-containing preparations are listed below by body system.

Body as a Whole: Sudden histamine release may be evidenced by one or more of the following: erythema, edema, skin rash, flushing, tachycardia, arterial hypotension, bronchospasm and circulatory collapse. Isolated cases of allergic or anaphylactoid type reactions have been reported.

Cardiovascular System: Cases of cardiac arrhythmias, cardiac arrest, bradycardia, and hypotension are documented for all muscle relaxants. Due to their marked sensitivity to nondepolarizing agents, premature children and neonates may experience a higher frequency of these reactions.

Respiratory System: Prolonged apnea and respiratory depression have occurred following administration of muscle relaxants. Many physiological factors, drug interactions and individual sensitivities may contribute to the prolongation of respiratory paralysis (see CLINICAL PHARMACOLOGY and PRECAUTIONS).

OVERDOSAGE:

Prolonged effects of a nondepolarizing neuromuscular blocking agent may be manifested by extended skeletal muscle weakness, decreased respiratory reserve, low tidal volume or apnea. A peripheral nerve stimulator may be used to assess the degree of residual neuromuscular blockade. In general, recovery of the patient does not require measures beyond effective manual or mechanical ventilation and maintenance of an open airway until complete recovery of normal respiration is assured.

When prolonged effects of neuromuscular blockade are manifest, cholinesterase antagonists (*e.g.,* neostigmine methylsulfate, pyridostigmine bromide, or edrophonium chloride) may be administered adjunctively to inhibit the enzymatic hydrolysis of acetylcholine, permitting acetylcholine to accumulate and displace the nondepolarizing muscle relaxant at the cholinergic receptors of the postjunctional membrane. Sufficiently excessive doses of nondepolarizing muscle relaxants have no antidote. Intravenous injections of neostigmine or pyridostigmine should be accompanied or preceded by an intravenous injection of atropine sulfate or its equivalent to minimize muscarinic cholinergic side effects, notably excessive secretions and bradycardia. (Consult package inserts for complete prescribing information prior to administering antagonistic agents.) Care should be taken to avoid underventilation when antagonistic agents are administered.

Satisfactory reversal can be judged by return of skeletal muscle tone and respiration; a peripheral nerve stimulator may also be used to monitor restoration of twitch height. Because the duration of action of a nondepolarizing neuromuscular blocking agent may exceed that of the antagonist, careful observation for evidence of recurrent neuromuscular blockade is essential.

If hypotension develops following administration of tubocurarine chloride, the etiology should be determined and treatment, if indicated, should be directed at the etiology. When it is due to ganglionic blockade, hypotension may be treated with fluid load and vasopressors which act at the adrenergic receptors, as required.

The intravenous LD_{50} of tubocurarine chloride in mice and rabbits is 0.18 and 0.187 mg/kg, respectively.

DOSAGE AND ADMINISTRATION:

Dosage of tubocurarine chloride should always be individualized after assessment of clinical factors that might alter the action of the drug. If enhanced sensitivity is suggested (see CLINICAL PHARMACOLOGY, WARNINGS, and PRECAUTIONS), fractional dosage is advised initially to avoid overdosage.

The following intravenous dosages are for 70 kg adult patients having no suggested alteration of sensitivity and are intended to serve as guidelines only.

AS AN ADJUNCT TO ANESTHESIA TO INDUCE SKELETAL MUSCLE RELAXATION

Because of its marked variability of patient response to tubocurarine chloride it is advisable to administer the drug in incremental dose until the desired level of relaxation is achieved. If inhalation anesthetics or other drugs known to enhance curarization are employed, the initial dose of the muscle relaxant should be reduced and the response used as a guide to incremental doses (see DRUG INTERACTIONS).

Generally, effective doses for the average adult patient (70 kg) will be approximately 0.1 to 0.2 mg/kg for paresis of limb musculature, 0.4 to 0.5 mg/kg for abdominal relaxation, and 0.5 to 0.6 mg/kg for endotracheal intubation. During prolonged procedures, incremental doses may be repeated in 40 to 60 minutes as required.

TO REDUCE THE INTENSITY OF MUSCLE CONTRACTION IN PHARMACOLOGICALLY OR ELECTRICALLY INDUCED CONVULSIONS

Equipment, antagonists, oxygen and personnel capable of managing airway obstruction, underventilation and apnea should be readily available during the use of tubocurarine chloride for electroshock therapy. Patients should be observed closely until consciousness is regained in the event respiratory failure develops.

Tubocurarine chloride may be administered as a slow intravenous injection (1 to 1 1/2 minutes) until head drop occurs. Individualized dosage may be calculated on the basis of 0.1 to 0.2 mg/kg (amount anticipated to produce limb paresis).

IN THE DIAGNOSIS OF MYASTHENIA GRAVIS

Tubocurarine chloride has been useful as a diagnostic agent in patients suspected of having myasthenia gravis, since small doses of the drug produce a profound exaggeration of the syndrome. The test should be performed by personnel familiar with the hazards involved; advance preparation should be made for treating any untoward side effects.

The usual dose is 6 to 20 percent of the adult dose anticipated to produce limb paresis. The test should be terminated within two or three minutes by intravenous injection of 2 mg neostigmine methylsulfate; otherwise the marked exaggeration of myasthenia symptoms may be dangerous.

DRUG INCOMPATIBILITIES

Neuromuscular blocking agents are unstable in alkaline solutions. Because of the high pH of barbiturate solutions, a precipitate may form if they are combined with turbocurarine chloride injection. Separate injections are recommended. A single needle and intravenous tube attached to a threeway stopcock apparatus can readily be adapted to this method if it is desirable to utilize as few of the patient's veins as possible.

DOSAGE AND ADMINISTRATION: *(cont'd)*

A solution of trimethaphan camsylate in tubocurarine chloride at a concentration of 1 g and 60 mg, respectively, per liter of 5 percent dextrose in water, develops a haze in three hours.

GENERAL

Parenteral drug products should be inspected visually for particulate matter and discoloration, whenever solution and container permit. Turbocurarine chloride injection should be clear and colorless; solutions which have developed more than a faint color should not be used.

Storage: Store at room temperature; avoid excessive heat.

HOW SUPPLIED - RATED THERAPEUTICALLY EQUIVALENT:

Injection, Solution - Intramuscular; - 3 mg/ml

5 ml	$12.97	Tubocurarine Chloride, Abbott	00074-8066-15
10 ml	$11.32	Tubocurarine Chloride, Lilly	00002-1685-01
10 ml x 10	$85.63	Tubocurarine Chloride, Bristol Myers Squibb	00003-0950-15
20 ml	$18.43	Tubocurarine Chloride Inj., Abbott	00074-3386-04
20 ml x 10	$158.50	Tubocurarine Chloride, Bristol Myers Squibb	00003-0950-35

TYPHOID VACCINE *(002405)*

CATEGORIES: Biologicals; Fever; Immunologic; Serums, Toxoids and Vaccines; Typhoid Fever; Vaccines; FDA Pre 1938 Drugs

BRAND NAMES: Typhim Vi; *Typhoral*; *Typhovax*; *Typh-Vax*; *Typh-Vax Oral*; *Tyrix Vi*; *Vivotif* (Germany); Vivotif Berna; *Vivotif Berna Capsule*; *Vivotif Oralt Vaccin*; *Zerotyph*
(International brand names outside U.S. in italics)

FORMULARIES: WHO

DESCRIPTION:

VIVOTIF BERNA (TYPHOID VACCINE LIVE ORAL TY 21A)

Vivotif Berna (Typhoid Vaccine Live Oral Ty 21a) is a live attenuated vaccine for oral administration. The vaccine contains the attenuated strain *Salmonella typhi* 21a.

Vivotif Berna Vaccine is manufactured by the Swiss Serum and Vaccine Institute. The vaccine strain is grown under controlled conditions in medium containing a digest of bovine tissues, an acid digest of casein, dextrose and galactose. The bacteria are collected by centrifugation, mixed with stabilizer containing lactose and amino acids, and lyophilized. The lyophilized bacteria are filled into gelatin capsules which are coated with organic solution to render them resistant to dissolution in stomach acid. The enteric-coated capsules are then packaged in 4-capsule blisters for distribution. The contents of each enteric-coated capsule are shown in TABLE 1.

TABLE 1 Contents of one enteric-coated capsule of Vivotif Berna Vaccine

Viable*S. typhi* Ty 21a	2-6 x 10^9 colony-forming units
Non-viable*S. typhi* Ty 21a	5-50 x 10^9 bacterial cells
Sucrose	26-130 mg
Ascorbic acid	1-5 mg
Amino acid mixture	1.4-7 mg
Lactose	100-180 mg
Magnesium stearate	3.6-4.4 mg

TYPHOID VACCINE

Typhoid Vaccine, USP is a saline suspension containing not more than 1000 million Salmonella typhosa (Ty-2 strain) organisms per ml. After growing on veal infusion agar (containing 0.5 percent sodium chloride, 2 percent peptone, and 5 percent agar), the bacteria are washed off the medium, suspended in buffered sodium chloride injection, and killed by a combination of phenol and heat. Phenol (0.5 percent) is added to the final vaccine as preservative. Typhoid Vaccine, USP is tested for safety, potency, and purity and standardized according to F.D.A. Additional Standards for Bacterial Vaccines, 21 C.F.R. 620. 10-620.15.

CLINICAL PHARMACOLOGY:

VIVOTIF BERNA (TYPHOID VACCINE LIVE ORAL TY 21A)

Salmonella typhi is the etiological agent of typhoid fever, an acute, febrile enteric disease. This vaccine will not afford protection against species of *Salmonella* other than *Salmonella typhi*or other bacteria that cause enteric disease.

There are approximately 500 cases of typhoid fever per year diagnosed in the United States (1). In 62% of these patients (statistics from 1977-1979) the disease was acquired outside of the United States while in 38% of the patients the disease was acquired within the United States (2). Of the diseases acquired during foreign travel 50% of the cases were contracted in Mexico, 20% in Asian countries and 15% in India. The majority of the remaining cases were acquired in the Caribbean basin, South and Central America, North Africa, and Southern Europe (2). Typhoid fever is considered to be endemic in most areas of Central and South Africa, North and Central Africa, Southeast Asia and the Indian Subcontinent (3).

Of the disease acquired in the United States 23% of the cases were associated with typhoid carriers, 24% were due to food outbreaks, 23% were associated with the ingestion of contaminated food or water, 6% due to household contact with an infected person and 4% following exposure to*S. typhi* in a laboratory setting.

The majority of typhoid cases respond favorably to antibiotic therapy. However, the emergence of chloramphenicol or ampicillin-resistant strains has greatly complicated therapy. Even with appropriate antibiotic therapy there were 7 deaths among 901 acute typhoid cases reported in the United States from 1977-1979 (2). Approximately 3-5% of acute typhoid cases result in the development of chronic carrier state (4). These non- symptomatic carriers are the natural reservoir for *S.typhi* and can serve to maintain the disease in its endemic state or to directly infect individuals (2). Eradication of the carrier state by antibiotic therapy has been unsuccessful (5).

Virulent strains of *S. typhi* upon ingestion are able to pass through the stomach acid barrier, colonize the intestinal tract, penetrate the lumen and enter the lymphatic system and blood stream, thereby causing disease. One possible mechanism by which disease may be prevented is by evoking a local immune response in the intestinal tract. Such local immunity may be induced by oral ingestion of a live attenuated strain of *S. typhi* undergoing an aborted infection.

The ability of *S. typhi* to cause disease and to induce a protective immune response is dependent upon the bacteria processing a complete lipopolysaccharide (6, 7). The *S. typhi* Ty 21a vaccine strain, by virtue of a reduction in enzymes essential for lipopolysaccharide biosynthesis, is restricted in its ability to produce complete lipopolysaccharide (8, 9). However, a sufficient quantity of complete lipopolysaccharide is synthesized to evoke a protective immune response. Despite low levels of lipopolysaccharide synthesis, the cells lyse before regaining a virulent phenotype due to the intracellular build-up of intermediates during lipopolysaccharide synthesis (5, 8, 9).

CLINICAL PHARMACOLOGY: *(cont'd)*

The efficacy of the *S. typhi* Ty 21a strain has been evaluated in a series of double-blind field trials. The first trial was performed in Alexandria, Egypt with a study population of 32,388 children aged 6 to 7 years. Three doses of vaccine, in the form of a freshly reconstituted suspension administered after ingestion of 1 g of bicarbonate, were given on alternate days. Immunization resulted in a 95% decrease in the incidence of typhoid fever over a 3-year period of surveillance (5, 10).

A series of field trials were subsequently performed in Santiago, Chile to evaluate efficacy when the vaccine strain was administered in the form of an acid-resistant enteric-coated capsule. The initial trial involved 91,954 school-aged children, and compared 1 or 2 doses of vaccine given one week apart. After 33 months of surveillance vaccine efficacy was 21% for the single dose schedule and 54% for the 2-dose schedule (11). A further field trial was performed in Santiago, Chile involving 109,594 school-aged children (12). Three doses of enteric-coated capsules were administered either on alternate days (short immunization schedule) or 21 days apart (long immunization schedule). Following 36 months of surveillance vaccination resulted in a 67% decrease in the incidence of typhoid fever in the short immunization schedule group and a 49% reduction in the long immunization schedule group. After 48 months of surveillance the short immunization schedule resulted in a 68% decrease in typhoid fever (13). An undiminished level of protection was observed during the fifth year of surveillance. A field trial was next conducted in Santiago, Chile to determine the relative efficacy of 2, 3 and 4 doses of enteric-coated vaccine administered on alternate days to school-aged children. Relative vaccine efficacy as determined by comparison of disease incidence within the three vaccinated groups was highest for the four dose regimen. An additional field trial to determine vaccine efficacy was conducted in Plaju, Indonesia involving 22,001 individuals approximately 3 to 50 years of age. Due to logistical considerations three doses of enteric-coated capsules were administered at weekly intervals, a schedule known to provide suboptimal protection (12). After two years of surveillance vaccine efficacy for all age groups was 41%. It should be noted that vaccine efficacy was 36% for subjects 3 to 14 years of age and 60% for those 15 to 44 years of age.

At present, the precise mechanism(s) by which Vivotif Berna Vaccine confers protection against typhoid fever is unknown. However, it is known that immunization of adult subjects can elicit a humoral anti-*S.typhi* LPS antibody response. Taking advantage of this fact, the seroconversion rate was compared between adults living in an endemic area (Chile) and non-endemic areas (United States and Switzerland) after the ingestion of 3 doses of vaccine. Comparable seroconversion rates were seen between these groups. Other studies in North American volunteers have shown that the Ty 21a strain is capable of providing significant protection to an experimental challenge of *S. typhi*.

Because of the very low incidence of typhoid fever in United States citizens, efficacy studies are not currently feasible in this population. However, the above observations support the expectation that Vivotif Berna Vaccine will provide protection to recipients from non-typhoid endemic areas such as the United States.

INDICATIONS AND USAGE:

VIVOTIF BERNA (TYPHOID VACCINE LIVE ORAL TY 21A)

Vivotif Berna Vaccine is indicated for immunization of adults and children greater than 6 years of age against disease caused by *Salmonella typhi*. Results from clinical studies indicate that adults and children greater than 6 years of age may be protected against typhoid fever following the oral ingestion of 4 doses of Vivotif Berna Vaccine. Immunization (ingestion of all 4 doses of Vivotif Berna Vaccine) should be completed at least 1 week prior to potential exposure to *S. typhi*.

Routine immunization against typhoid fever is not recommended in the United States of America. Selective immunization against typhoid fever is recommended under the following circumstances: 1) expected intimate exposure to a house-hold contact with typhoid fever, 2) travelers to areas of the world with a risk of exposure to typhoid fever, and 3) workers in microbiology laboratories with expected frequent contact with *S. typhi* (14).

Not all recipients of Vivotif Berna Vaccine will be fully protected against typhoid fever. Travelers should take all necessary precautions to avoid contact or ingestion of potentially contaminated food or water sources. There is no evidence to support the use of typhoid vaccine to control common source outbreaks, disease following natural disasters or in persons attending rural summer camps.

Vivotif Berna Vaccine will not afford protection against enteric microorganisms other than *S. typhi*. An optimal booster dose has not yet been established. However, it is recommended that a booster dose consisting of 4 vaccine capsules taken on alternate days be given every 5 years under conditions of repeated or continued exposure to typhoid fever (seeDOSAGE AND ADMINISTRATION).

Typhoid fever continues to be an important disease in many parts of the world. Travelers entering such areas are at risk to contracting typhoid fever following the ingestion of contaminated food or water. Parenterally administered typhoid vaccine has been shown to be effective at reducing the incidence of disease in such endemic areas. However, immunization with such vaccines is frequently accompanied by adverse reactions such pain and/or swelling at the injection site, fever, malaise and headache.

TYPHOID VACCINE

Typhoid Vaccine, USP is indicated for active immunization against typhoid fever. Based on data obtained from field studies, it has been estimated that typhoid vaccine is 70% or more effective in preventing typhoid fever, depending in part on the degree of exposure.

Routine immunization against typhoid is no longer recommended for persons residing in the United States. Selective immunization is indicated in the following situations:

1. Intimate exposure to a known typhoid carrier, as would occur with continued household contact.

2. Foreign travel to areas where typhoid fever is endemic.

Although at one time typhoid immunization was suggested for persons attending summer camps or for residents of areas where flooding has occurred, there are no data to support continuation of such practices.[1,2]

CONTRAINDICATIONS:

VIVOTIF BERNA (TYPHOID VACCINE LIVE ORAL TY 21A)

Hypersensitivity to any component of the vaccine or the enteric-coated capsule.

Safety of the vaccine has not been demonstrated in persons deficient in their ability to mount a humoral or cell-mediated immune response, due to either a congenital or acquired immunodeficient state including treatment with immunosuppressive or antimitotic drugs. The vaccine should not be administered to these persons regardless of benefits.

TYPHOID VACCINE

Administration should be postponed in the presence of acute respiratory or other active infection.

A severe systemic or allergic reaction following a prior dose is a contraindication to further use.[3]

WARNINGS:

VIVOTIF BERNA (TYPHOID VACCINE LIVE ORAL TY 21A)

Vivotif Berna (Typhoid Vaccine Live Oral Ty 21a) is not to be taken during an acute febrile illness or in the face of acute gastrointestinal illness. Postpone taking the vaccine if persistent diarrhea or vomiting is occurring (see PRECAUTIONS.)

PRECAUTIONS:

VIVOTIF BERNA (TYPHOID VACCINE LIVE ORAL TY 21A)

General: The vaccine should not be administered to persons during an acute febrile illness or acute gastrointestinal illness. The vaccine should not be administered to individuals receiving sulfonamides and antibiotics since these agents may be active against the vaccine strain and prevent a sufficient degree of multiplication to occur in order to induce a protective immune response. The vaccine should not be administered to persons with a known hypersensitivity to any vaccine component or medium component (see DESCRIPTION.)

Information for the Patient: It is essential that all 4 doses of vaccine be taken at the prescribed alternate day interval to obtain a maximal protective immune response. Vaccine potency is dependent upon storage under refrigeration [between 2°C and 8°C (35.6°F-46.4°F)]. The vaccine should be stored under refrigeration at all times. It is essential to replace unused vaccine in the refrigerator between doses. The vaccine capsule should be swallowed approximately 1 hour before a meal with a cold or luke-warm (temperature not to exceed body temperature (*e.g.,* 37°C (98.6°F)) drink. Care should be taken not to chew the vaccine capsule. The vaccine capsule should be swallowed as soon as after placing in the mouth as possible.

Carcinogenesis, Mutagenesis, and Impairment of Fertility: Long-term studies in animals with Vivotif Berna Vaccine have not been performed to evaluate carcinogenic potential, mutagenic potential or impairment of fertility.

Pregnancy Category C: Animal reproduction studies have not been conducted with Vivotif Berna Vaccine. It is not known whether Vivotif Berna Vaccine can cause fetal harm when administered to pregnant woman or can affect reproduction capacity. Vivotif Berna Vaccine should be given to a pregnant woman only if clearly needed.

Nursing Mothers: There is no data to warrant the use of this product in nursing mothers. It is not known if Vivotif Berna Vaccine is excreted in human milk.

Pediatric Use: The safety and efficacy of Vivotif Berna Vaccine has not been established in children under 6 years of age. This product is therefore not recommended for use in children under 6 years of age.

TYPHOID VACCINE

A sterile syringe and needle should be used for each patient to prevent transmission of hepatitis B virus and other infectious agents from one person to another.

Specific information concerning use of typhoid vaccine during pregnancy is not available. However, as with other inactivated bacterial vaccines, its use is not contraindicated during pregnancy unless the intended recipient has manifested significant systemic or allergic reactions following administration of prior doses. Use of typhoid vaccine during pregnancy should be individualized to reflect actual need.

Before the injection of any biological, the physician should take all precautions known for prevention of allergic or any other side reactions. This should include: A review of the patient's history regarding possible sensitivity; the ready availability of epinephrine 1:1000 and other appropriate agents used for control of immediate allergic reactions; and a knowledge of the recent literature pertaining to use of the biological concerned.

ADVERSE REACTIONS:

VIVOTIF BERNA (TYPHOID VACCINE LIVE ORAL TY 21A)

Several lots of Vivotif Berna Vaccine have been evaluated in several field trials both in adults and in school-aged children. Objectively monitored side-effects, e.g., abdominal pain, diarrhea, vomiting, fever, headache and skin rash, did not occur at a statistically higher frequency in the vaccinated group as compared to a placebo group (11). Post- marketing surveillance outside of the United States has found that side- effects are infrequent, transient, and resolve of their own accord. Reported adverse reactions include nausea, abdominal cramps, vomiting, skin rash or urticaria in the trunk and/or extremities.

TYPHOID VACCINE

Most recipients of typhoid vaccine experience some degree of local and systemic response, usually beginning within 24 hours of administration and persisting for one or two days.

Local reactions are usually manifested by erythema, induration, and tenderness and should be expected in all those injected intracutaneously.

Systemic manifestations may include malaise, headache, myalgia, and elevated temperature.

OVERDOSAGE:

VIVOTIF BERNA (TYPHOID VACCINE LIVE ORAL TY 21A)

Five to 8 doses of Vivotif Berna Vaccine containing between 3-10 x 10^{10} viable vaccine organisms were administered to 155 healthy adult males. The dosage was, at a minimum, 5-fold higher than the currently recommended dose. No significant reactions, (*e.g.,* vomiting, acute abdominal distress or fever) were observed. At the recommended dosage the *S. typhi* Ty 21a vaccine strain is not excreted in the feces. However, clinical studies in volunteers have shown that overdosing can increase the possibility of shedding the *S. typhi* Ty 21a vaccine in the feces (15).

DOSAGE AND ADMINISTRATION:

VIVOTIF BERNA (TYPHOID VACCINE LIVE ORAL TY 21A)

The blister containing the vaccine capsules should be inspected to ensure that the foil seal and capsules are intact.

One capsule is to be swallowed approximately 1 hour before a meal with a cold or luke-warm [temperature not to exceed body temperature (*e.g.,* 37°C (98.6°F))]. drink on alternate days, e.g., days 1, 3, 5 and 7. The vaccine capsule should not be chewed and should be swallowed as soon after placing in the mouth as possible. A complete immunization schedule is the ingestion of 4 vaccine capsules as described above. Unless a complete immunization schedule is followed, an optimum immune response may not be achieved. Not all recipients of Vivotif Berna Vaccine will be fully protected against typhoid fever. Travelers should take all necessary precautions to avoid contact or ingestion of potentially contaminated food or water.

Booster Use: The optimum booster schedule for Vivotif Berna has not been determined. Efficacy has been shown to persist for at least 5 years. Further, there is no experience with Vivotif Berna Vaccine as a booster in persons previously immunized with parenteral typhoid vaccine. Despite these limitations it is recommended that a booster dose consisting of four vaccine capsules taken on alternate days be given every 5 years under conditions of repeated or continued exposure to typhoid fever.

Storage: Vivotif Berna Vaccine is not stable when exposed to ambient temperatures. Vivotif Berna Vaccine should therefore be shipped and stored between 2°C and 8°C (35.6-46.4°F). Each package of vaccine shows an expiration date. This expiration date is valid only if the product has been maintained at 2°C-8°C (35.6-46.4°F).

DOSAGE AND ADMINISTRATION: *(cont'd)*

TYPHOID VACCINE

Primary Immunization

1. Adults and children over 10 years of age: Two doses of 0.5 ml each, administered subcutaneously, at an interval of four or more weeks.

2. Children less than 10 years of age: Two doses of 0.25 ml each, administered subcutaneously, at an interval of four or more weeks. In instances where there is insufficient time for two doses administered at the specified intervals, three doses of the appropriate volume may be given at weekly intervals.

Booster Doses

1. Adults and children over 10 years of age: 0.5 ml, administered subcutaneously, or 0.1 ml, injected intracutaneously (intradermally).

2. Children 6 months to 10 years of age: 0.25 ml, administered subcutaneously, or 0.1 ml, intracutaneously (intradermally).

Under conditions of continued or repeated exposure, a booster dose should be given at least every three years. In instances where an interval of more than three years has elapsed since primary immunization or the last booster dose, a single booster dose is considered sufficient; it is not necessary to repeat the primary immunizing series.

Shake vial vigorously before withdrawing each dose.

Before injection, the rubber diaphragm of the vial and the skin over the site to be injected should be cleansed and prepared with a suitable germicide.

After insertion of the needle, aspirate to help avoid inadvertent injection into a blood vessel.

REFERENCES:

Vivotif Berna (Typhoid Vaccine Live Oral Ty 21a) 1. Centers for Disease Control. Annual summary 1980: reported morbidity and mortality in the United States. MMWR. *29:*12-17, 1981. **2.** Taylor, D.N., R.A. Pollard, P.A. Blake. Typhoid in the United States and the Risk to the International Traveler. J. Infect. Dis.*148:* 599-602, 1983. **3.** Levine, M.M., R.E. Black, C. Lanata, and the Chilean Typhoid Committee. Precise estimation of the numbers of chronic carriers of *Salmonella typhi* in Santiago, Chile, an endemic area. J. Infect. Dis. *146:* 724-726, 1982. **4.** Ames, W.R., M. Robbins. Age and sex as factors in the development of the typhoid carrier state, and a model for estimating carrier prevalence. Am. J. Public Health *33:* 221-230, 1943. **5.** Germanier, R. Typhoid Fever. In, Bacterial Vaccines. R. Germanier (ed.) p. 137-165, 1984. **6.** Germanier, R. Immunity in experimental salmonellosis. I. Protection induced by rough mutants of*Salmonella typhimurium.* Infect. Immun. *2:* 309-315, 1970. **7.** Germanier, R., E. Furer. Immunity in experimental salmonellosis II. Basis for the avirulence and protective capacity of Gal E mutants of *Salmonella typhimurium.* Infec. Immun. *4:*663-673, 1971. **8.** Germanier, R., E. Furer. Isolation and characterization of Gal E mutant Ty 21a of *Salmonella typhi:* a candidate strain for a live, oral typhoid vaccine. J. Infect. Dis.*131:* 553-558, 1975. **9.** Germanier, R., E. Furer. Characteristics of the attenuated oral vaccine strain *S. typhi* Ty 21a. Develop. Biol. Standard, *53:* 3-7, 1983. **10.** Wahdan, M.H., C. Serie, Y. Cerisier, S. Sallam, R. Germanier. A controlled field trial of live *Salmonella typhi* strain Ty 21a oral vaccine against typhoid: three-year results. J. Infect. Dis. *145:* 292-296, 1982. **11.** Levine, M.M., R.E. Black, C. Ferreccio, M.L. Clements, C. Lanata, J. Rooney, R. Germanier, A. Schuster, H. Rodriguez, J.M. Borgono, H. Lobos, I. Prenzel, C. Ristorio, M.E. Pinto. The efficacy of attenuated *S. typhi* oral vaccine strain Ty 21a evaluated in controlled field trials. In, Development of Vaccines and Drugs against Diarrhea. 11th Noble Conference, Stockholm, 1985, p. 90-101. J. Holmgren, A. Lindberg and R. Mollby (eds.). Studentlitteratur, Lund, Sweden, 1986. **12.** Levine, M.M., C. Ferreccio, R.E. Black, R. Germanier, Chilean Typhoid Committee. Large-Scale Field Trial of Ty 21a Live Oral Typhoid Vaccine in Enteric-Coated Capsule Formulation. Lancet *1:*1049-1052, 1987. **13.** Cryz, S.J., Jr., E. Furer, M.M. Levine. Zur Wirksamkeit des oralen, attenuierten *Salmonella Typhi* Ty 21a Lebendimpfstoffes in kontrollierten Feldversuchen, Schweiz. Med. Wschr. *118:* 467-470, 1988. **14.** Reports of the Committee on Infectious Diseases. Twenty-first edition, p 373-374, American Academy of Pediatrics, 141 Northwest Point Blvd., P.O. Box 927, Elk Grove Village, IL 60009-0827, 1988. **15.** Gilman, R.H., R.B. Hornick, W.E. Woodward, H.L. DuPont, M.J. Snyder, M.M. Levine, J.P. Libonati. Evaluation of a UDP-Glucose-4- epimeraseless mutant of *Salmonella typhi* as a live oral vaccine. J. Infect. Dis. *136:* 717-723, 1988. **Typhoid Vaccine 1.** Recommendation of the Public Health Service Advisory Committee on Immunization Practices—Typhoid Vaccine. Morbidity and Mortality Weekly Report 27 (No. 27): 231, 1978. **2.** Report of the Committee on Infectious Diseases, American Academy of Pediatrics, 1982 (Red Book). **3.** Recommendations of the Public Health Service Advisory Committee on Immunization Practices—General Recommendations on Immunization. Morbidity and Mortality Weekly Report 29 (No.7): 76, 1980.

HOW SUPPLIED - EQUIVALENTS NOT AVAILABLE:

Capsule, Gelatin, Sustained Action - Oral

4's	$32.45	VIVOTIF BERNA, Berna Prod	58337-0003-01

Injection, Susp - Subcutaneous - 8 unit/ml

0.5 ml	$32.44	TYPHIM VI, Connaught Labs	49281-0790-01
5 ml	$11.76	Typhoid Vaccine, Wyeth Labs	00008-0343-01
10 ml	$19.38	Typhoid Vaccine, Wyeth Labs	00008-0343-02
10 ml	$573.75	TYPHIM VI, Connaught Labs	49281-0790-20

UNDECYLENIC ACID *(002408)*

CATEGORIES: Anti-Infectives; Antifungals; Pharmaceutical Adjuvants; Skin/Mucous Membrane Agents; FDA Pre 1938 Drugs

BRAND NAMES: Fungoid

DESCRIPTION:

Undecylenic Acid is chemically 10-hendecenoic acid having an empirical formula $C_{11}H_{20}O_2$ and the chemical bond structure $CH_2 = CH(CH_2)_8CO_2H$. Undecylenic Acid is a colorless to pale yellow liquid which is soluble in water, alcohol, chloroform and ether. It is a fungistatic agent employed in the treatment of tinea pedis, tinea capitis, ringworm and dermatophytosis.

Active Ingredients: Undecylenic Acid 25%

Inactive Ingredients: PEG 8, Benzalkonium Chloride, Chloroxylenol.

INDICATIONS AND USAGE:

For the effective treatment of tinea pedis (athlete's foot). Relieves itching, scaling, cracking, burning, soreness, irritation and discomfort.

WARNINGS:

DO NOT USE ON CHILDREN UNDER TWO YEARS OF AGE UNLESS DIRECTED BY A PODIATRIST, DERMATOLOGIST or PHYSICIAN. FOR EXTERNAL USE ONLY. KEEP OUT OF THE REACH FOR CHILDREN. Avoid contact with eyes. if irritation occurs or if there is no improvement within 4 weeks, discontinue use and consult a PODIATRIST, DERMATOLOGIST or PHYSICIAN. Do not use for diaper rash. Do not use on patients sensitive to any of the ingredients in this product. Not effective on scalp or nail surfaces.

DOSAGE AND ADMINISTRATION:

Clean the affected area and dry thoroughly. Apply a thin layer of the product over the affected area twice daily (morning and night) or as directed by a PODIATRIST, DERMATOLOGIST OR PHYSICIAN. Supervise children in the use of this product. Pay special attention to spaces between the toes, wear well-fitting, ventilated shoes and change shoes and socks at least once a daily. Use daily for 4 weeks. If condition persists longer, consult your PODIATRIST, DERMATOLOGIST OR PHYSICIAN.

HOW SUPPLIED:

Available in a 1 oz. (29.57 ml) plastic bottle with controlled dropper.

Store at controlled room temperature 15°-30°C (59°-86°F).

See lot number and expiration date printed on bottle.

HOW SUPPLIED - EQUIVALENTS NOT AVAILABLE:

Solution - Topical - 25 %

30 ml $9.25 FUNGOID, Pedinol Pharma 00884-3194-01

UREA *(002411)*

CATEGORIES: Cell Stimulants/Proliferants; Dermatologicals; Diuretics; Electrolytic, Caloric-Water Balance; Glaucoma; Hormones; Intracranial Pressure; Intraocular Pressure; Keratolytic Agents; Ophthalmics; Pharmaceutical Adjuvants; Pressure, Intracranial; Pressure, Intraocular; Relaxants/Stimulants, Uterine; Skin/Mucous Membrane Agents; Pregnancy Category C; FDA Approval Pre 1982

BRAND NAMES: *Alphadrate*; *Anti-Dessechement*; *Aquadrate*; *Basodexan*; Carmol-20; *Fenuril*; Gord-Urea; Harber-Mol; Polygeline; **Ureaphil**
(International brand names outside U.S. in italics)

FORMULARIES: WHO

DESCRIPTION:

This drug will be abbreviated here as: "Urea (synth.)"

Urea (synth.) is a synthetic urea prepared as a white, sterile, nonpyrogenic lyophilized powder for reconstitution with 5 or 10% Dextrose Injection, USP or 10% invert sugar injection to provide a clear, colorless, hypertonic solution for intravenous infusion.

Each 150 ml bottle of Urea (synth.) contains urea 40 g with citric acid, 1 mg added as buffering agent.

May contain sodium hydroxide for pH adjustment. 666 mOsm/liter calculated on the basis of contents of bottle reconstituted to one liter with water for injection.

As determined by depression of freezing point, a theoretically isotonic solution of urea in water has a concentration of 1.63%.

Sterile urea contains no bacteriostat or antimicrobial agent and is intended for use only after reconstitution as a single-dose injection. When smaller doses are required the unused portion should be discarded.

Urea (synth.) when reconstituted as a 30% solution of urea is a hypertonic osmotic dehydrating agent.

Urea, USP, is the diamide of carbonic acid, chemically designated carbamide (CH4N2O), solid crystals, soluble in water.

CLINICAL PHARMACOLOGY:

The reduction of intracranial edema and abnormally elevated cerebrospinal fluid pressure which occurs following intravenous administration of hypertonic urea solution, depends upon osmotic pressure gradients between the blood, extracellular and intracellular fluid compartments. Thus, the primary mechanism of action appears to be physical. Hypertonic urea rapidly increases blood tonicity thus effecting a greater urea concentration gradient in the blood that in the extravascular fluid. This results in transudation of fluid from the tissues, including the brain and cerebrospinal fluid into the blood.

As the concentration of urea in the glomerular filtrate increases, reabsorption of a proportional amount of water is prevented. Such retardation of proximal tubular reabsorption increases the rate and volume of urine flow.

INDICATIONS AND USAGE:

When administered as a 30% solution, this preparation is indicated for the reduction of intracranial pressure (in the control of cerebral edema) and of intraocular pressure.

CONTRAINDICATIONS:

Urea (synth.) should not be used in patients with severely impaired renal function, active intracranial bleeding or marked dehydration. Frank liver failure is also a contraindication for use.

Urea (synth.) should not be infused in veins of the lower extremities of elderly patients because phlebitis and thrombosis of superficial and deep veins may occur.

WARNINGS:

Discard solution if not used within 24 hours after reconstitution.

Urea (synth.) may cause depletion of electrolytes which can result in hyponatremia and hypokalemia. Early signs of such depletion may indicate the need for supplementation before serum levels are reduced.

Extreme care is essential to prevent accidental extravasation of the solution at the site of injection since this may cause local reactions ranging from mild irritation to tissue necrosis.

If used in patients with some liver impairment, urea should be administered with great caution since there may be a significant rise in blood ammonia levels.

PRECAUTIONS:

An indwelling urethral catheter should be used in comatose patients receiving urea for injection to insure bladder emptying.

Rapid intravenous administration of hypertonic solutions of urea may be associated with hemolysis as well as a direct effect on the cerebral vasomotor centers which may result in increased capillary bleeding. These effects usually can be avoided by not exceeding an infusion rate of 4 ml per minute. Solutions of urea should not be administered through the same administration set through which blood is being infused.

Although arterial oozing has been reported as a nuisance when intracranial surgery is performed on patients following treatment with urea, it has not been a significant problem. However, sterile urea should not be used in the presence of active intracranial bleeding unless such use is preliminary to prompt surgical intervention to control hemorrhage. It should be kept in mind that reduction of brain edema induced by urea may result in reactivation of intracranial bleeding.

In the presence of kidney disease, urea should be administered with caution. Mild elevation of blood urea nitrogen does not preclude its use or continued use, but frequent laboratory studies should be made to determine if kidney function is adequate to eliminate the infused urea as well as that produced endogenously.

Patients exhibiting a temporary reduction in urine volume are generally able to maintain a satisfactory elimination of urea. However, if diuresis does not follow the injection of urea to such patients within 6 to 12 hours, the drug should be withdrawn pending further evaluation of renal function.

As with other infused solutions, Urea (synth.) (Sterile Urea, USP) may temporarily maintain circulatory volume and blood pressure in spite of considerable blood loss. Consequently, when excessive blood loss occurs within a short period of time, blood replacement should be adequate and simultaneous with the infusion of urea.

PRECAUTIONS: *(cont'd)*

Hypothermia when used with urea infusion may increase the risk of venous thrombosis and hemoglobinuria.

Pregnancy Category C: Animal reproduction studies have not been conducted with Sterile Urea, USP. It is also not known whether sterile urea can cause fetal harm when given to a pregnant woman or can affect reproduction capacity. Sterile Urea, USP should be given to a pregnant woman only if clearly needed.

Nursing Mothers: It is not known whether this drug is excreted in human milk. Because many drugs are excreted in human milk, caution should be exercised when sterile urea is administered to a nursing mother.

Do not administer unless seal of urea container is intact and reconstituted solution is clear. Discard unused portion.

ADVERSE REACTIONS:

Headaches (reported to be similar to those which occur in some patients following lumbar puncture), nausea and vomiting, occasionally syncope and disorientation have been known to occur following intravenous administration. Less often reported is a transient agitated confusional state. No serious reactions have been noted when solutions have been infused slowly provided renal function is not seriously impaired or there is no evidence of active intracranial bleeding. Chemical phlebitis and thrombosis near the site of injection have been reported infrequently.

Reactions which may occur because of the solution (reconstituted) or the technique of administration include febrile response, infection at the site of injection, venous thrombosis or phlebitis extending from the site of injection, extravasation and hypervolemia.

If an adverse reaction does occur, discontinue the infusion, evaluate the patient, institute appropriate therapeutic countermeasures and save the remainder of the fluid for examination if deemed necessary.

OVERDOSAGE:

In the event of overdosage as reflected by unusually elevated blood urea nitrogen (BUN) levels, discontinue the drug, evaluate the patient and institute corrective measures as indicated. See PRECAUTIONS and DOSAGE AND ADMINISTRATION.

DOSAGE AND ADMINISTRATION:

Urea (synth.) (Sterile Urea, USP) is administered as a 30% solution by slow intravenous infusion. The rate of injection should not exceed 4 ml per minute.

Sterile urea is prepared by adding an appropriate volume of 5 or 10% Dextrose Injection, USP or 10% invert sugar injection. The desired diluent can be added directly to the urea container.

To prepare 135 ml of a 30% solution of sterile urea, the contents of one 40 g container are mixed with 105 ml of the diluent, or two such containers are mixed with 210 ml of diluent to prepare 270 ml of a 30% solution. Each milliliter of a 30% solution provides 300 mg of urea.

Urea (synth.) should be freshly prepared in each case. Discard any unused portion.

The amount to be administered is generally estimated on the basis of grams of urea per kilogram of body weight. Dosage must also take into account the clinical condition of the patient, especially the state of hydration, electrolyte balance and integrity of renal function. The total daily dose should not exceed 120 g of urea.

For the reduction of increased intracranial or intraocular pressure the adult dose ranges from 1 to 1.5 g (3.3 to 5 ml) per kilogram of body weight; or 0.45 to 0.68 g (1.5 to 2.3 ml) per pound of body weight.

In children the dosage ranges from 0.5 to 1.5 g/kg of body weight. In young children up to 2 years of age as little as 0.1 g/kg may be adequate.

Parenteral drug products (reconstituted) should be inspected visually for particulate matter and discoloration prior to administration, whenever solution and container permit. See PRECAUTIONS.

Protect from freezing and extreme heat.

HOW SUPPLIED - EQUIVALENTS NOT AVAILABLE:

Cream - Topical - 20 %

454 gm $16.34 CARMOL-20, Syntex Labs 00033-2651-20

Injection, Dry-Soln - Intravenous - 40 gm

40 gm $70.25 UREAPHIL 40 G, Abbott 00074-1592-02

UROFOLLITROPIN *(002416)*

CATEGORIES: Anterior Pituitary/Hypothalmic Function; Fertility Agents; Gonadotropins; Hormones; In Vitro Fertilization; Infertility; Ovarian Disease, Polycystic; Ovulation, Induction of; Polycystic Ovarian Syndrome; Pregnancy Category X

BRAND NAMES: **Metrodin**

FORMULARIES: Aetna; BC-BS

DESCRIPTION:

Metrodin (urofollitropin for injection) is a preparation of gonadotropin extracted from the urine of postmenopausal women. Each ampule of Metrodin contains 75 IU of follicle-stimulating hormone (FSH) activity in not more than 0.83 mg of extract, plus 10 mg lactose in a sterile, lyophilized form. Urofollitropin is administered by intramuscular injection.

Metrodin contains an acidic, water soluble glycoprotein biologically standardized for FSH gonadotropin activity in terms of the Second International Reference Preparation for Human Menopausal Gonadotropins, established in September, 1964 by the Expert Committee on Biological Standards of the World Health Organization. Negligible amounts (less than 1 IU per 75 IU FSH) of luteinizing hormone (LH) activity are contained in Metrodin.

CLINICAL PHARMACOLOGY:

Urofollitropin stimulates ovarian follicular growth in women who do not have primary ovarian failure. Treatment with urofollitropin in most instances results only in follicular growth and maturation. In order to effect ovulation in the absence of an endogenous LH surge, human chorionic gonadotropin (hCG) must be given following the administration of urofollitropin when clinical and laboratory assessment of the patient indicates that sufficient follicular maturation has occurred.

CLINICAL STUDIES:

The results of the clinical experience and effectiveness of the administration of urofollitropin to 80 PCO patients in 189 courses of therapy are summarized below. All patients had received extensive prior therapy with clomiphene citrate, without success, and many had failed to conceive or hyperstimulated following treatment with Pergonal (menotropins for Injection, USP) (TABLE 1).

TABLE 1

	%
Patients ovulating	88
Patients pregnant	30
Patients aborting	25*
Multiple pregnancies	17*
Hyperstimulation syndrome (% patients)	6

* Based on total pregnancies.

INDICATIONS AND USAGE:

Urofollitropin and hCG given in a sequential manner are indicated for the induction of ovulation in patients with polycystic ovarian syndrome (PCO) who have an elevated LH/FSH ratio and who have failed to respond to adequate clomiphene citrate therapy.

Urofollitropin and hCG may also be used to stimulate the development of multiple oocytes in ovulatory patients participating in an *in vitro* fertilization program.

SELECTION OF PATIENTS

1. Before treatment with urofollitropin is instituted, a through gynecologic and endocrinologic evaluation must be performed. This should include a hysterosalpingogram (to rule out uterine and tubal pathology) and documentation of anovulation by means of basal body temperature, serial vaginal smears, examination of cervical mucus, determination of serum (or urinary) progesterone, urinary pregnanediol, and endometrial biopsy. Patients with tubal pathology should receive urofollitropin only if enrolled in an *in vitro* fertilization program.

2. Primary ovarian failure should be excluded by the determination of gonadotropin levels.

3. Careful examination should be made to rule out the presence of early pregnancy.

4. Patients in late reproductive life have a greater predilection to endometrial carcinoma as well as a higher incidence of anovulatory disorders. Cervical dilation and curettage should always be done for diagnosis before starting urofollitropin therapy in such patients who demonstrate abnormal uterine bleeding or other signs of endometrial abnormalities.

5. Evaluation of the husband's fertility potential should be included in the workup.

CONTRAINDICATIONS:

Urofollitropin is contraindicated in women who exhibit:

1. High levels of FSH indicating primary ovarian failure.

2. Uncontrolled thyroid or adrenal dysfunction.

3. An organic intracranial lesion such as a pituitary tumor.

4. The presence of any cause of infertility other than anovulation, as stated in the "Indications" unless they are candidates for Assisted Reproductive Technologies.

5. Abnormal bleeding of undetermined origin (see Selection of Patients.)

6. Ovarian cysts or enlargement not due to polycystic ovarian syndrome.

7. Prior hypersensitivity to urofollitropin.

8. Urofollitropin is contraindicated in women who are pregnant and may cause fetal harm when administered to a pregnant woman. There are limited human data on the effects of urofollitropin when administered during pregnancy.

WARNINGS:

Urofollitropin is a drug that should only be used by physicians who are thoroughly familiar with infertility problems. It is a potent gonadotropic substance capable of causing mild to severe adverse reactions. Gonadotropin therapy requires a certain time commitment by physicians and supportive health professionals, and its use requires the availability of appropriate monitoring facilities (see PRECAUTIONS, Laboratory Tests). It must be used with a great deal of care.

Overstimulation of the Ovary During Urofollitropin Therapy: Ovarian Enlargement: Mild to moderate uncomplicated ovarian enlargement, which may be accompanied by abdominal distension and/or abdominal pain, occurs in approximately 20% of those treated with urofollitropin and hCG, and generally regresses without treatment within two or three weeks.

In order to minimize the hazard associated with the occasional abnormal ovarian enlargement which may occur with urofollitropin-hCG therapy, the lowest dose consistent with expectation of goods results should be used. Careful monitoring of ovarian response can further minimize the risk of overstimulation.

If the ovaries are abnormally enlarged on the last day of urofollitropin therapy, hCG should not be administered in this course of therapy. This will reduce the chances of development of the Ovarian Hyperstimulation Syndrome.

The Ovarian Hyperstimulation Syndrome (OHSS): OHSS is a medical event distinct from uncomplicated ovarian enlargement. OHSS may progress rapidly (within 24 hours to several days) to become a serious medical event. It is characterized by an apparent dramatic increase in vascular permeability which can result in a rapid accumulation of fluid in the peritoneal cavity, thorax, and potentially, the pericardium. The early warning signs of development of OHSS are severe pelvic pain, nausea, vomiting, and weight gain. The following symptomatology has been seen with cases of OHSS: abdominal pain, abdominal distension, gastrointestinal symptoms including nausea, vomiting and diarrhea, severe ovarian enlargement, weight gain, dyspnea, and oliguria. Clinical evaluation may reveal hypovolemia, hemoconcentration, electrolyte imbalances, ascites, hemoperitoneum, pleural effusions, hydrothorax, acute pulmonary distress, and thromboembolic events (see Pulmonary and Vascular Complications.) Transient liver function test abnormalities suggestive of hepatic dysfunction, which may be accompanied by morphologic changes on liver biopsy, have been reported in association with the Ovarian Hyperstimulation Syndrome (OHSS).

OHSS occurred in approximately 6.0% of patients treated with urofollitropin therapy in the initial clinical trials, in patients treated for anovulation due to polycystic ovarian syndrome. During studies for *in vitro* fertilization, four cases of OHSS were reported followed 1,586 treatment cycles (0.25%). Cases of OHSS are more common, more severe, and more protracted if pregnancy occurs. OHSS develops rapidly; therefore, patients should be followed for at least two weeks after hCG administration. Most often, OHSS occurs after treatment has been discontinued and reaches its maximum at about seven to ten days following treatment. Usually, OHSS resolves spontaneously with the onset of menses. If there is evidence that OHSS may be developing prior to hCG administration (see PRECAUTIONS, Laboratory Tests), the hCG should be withheld.

If OHSS occurs, treatment should be stopped and the patient should be hospitalized. Treatment is primarily symptomatic and should consist of bed rest, fluid and electrolyte management, and analgesics if needed. The phenomenon of hemoconcentration associated with fluid loss into the peritoneal cavity, pleural cavity, and the pericardial cavity has been seen to occur and should be thoroughly assessed in the following manner: 1) fluid intake and output, 2) weight, 3) hematocrit, 4) serum and urinary electrolytes, 5) urine specific gravity, 6) BUN and creatinine, and 7) abdominal girth. These determinations are to be performed daily or more often if the need arises.

With OHSS there is an increased risk of injury to the ovary. The ascitic, pleural, and pericardial fluids should not be removed unless absolutely necessary to relieve symptoms such as pulmonary distress or cardiac tamponade. Pelvic examination may cause rupture of an ovarian cyst, which may result in hemoperitoneum, and should therefore be avoided. If this does occur, and if bleeding becomes such that surgery is required, the surgical treatment should be designed to control bleeding and to retain as much ovarian tissue as possible. Intercourse should be prohibited in those patients in whom significant ovarian enlargement occurs after ovulation because of the danger of hemoperitoneum resulting from ruptured ovarian cysts.

The management of OHSS may be divided into three phases: the acute, the chronic, and the resolution phases. Because the use of diuretics can accentuate the diminished intravascular volume, diuretics should be avoided except in the late phase of resolution as described below.

Acute Phase: Management during the acute phase should be designed to prevent hemoconcentration due to loss of intravascular volume to the third space and to minimize the risk of thromboembolic phenomena and kidney damage. Treatment is designed to normalize electrolytes while maintaining an acceptable but somewhat reduced intravascular volume. Full correction of the intravascular volume deficit may lead to an unacceptable increase in the amount of third space fluid accumulation. Management includes administration of limited intravenous fluids, electrolytes, and human serum albumin. Monitoring for the development of hyperkalemia is recommended.

Chronic Phase: After stabilizing the patient during the acute phase, excessive fluid accumulation in the third space should be limited by instituting severe potassium, sodium, and fluid restriction.

Resolution Phase: A fall in hematocrit and an increasing urinary output without an increased intake are observed due to the return of third space fluid to the intravascular compartment. Peripheral and/or pulmonary edema may result if the kidneys are unable to excrete third space fluid as rapidly as it is mobilized. Diuretics may be indicated during the resolution phase if necessary to combat pulmonary edema.

Pulmonary and Vascular Complications: The following paragraph describes serious medical events reported following gonadotropin therapy.

Serious pulmonary conditions (*e.g.,* atelectasis, acute respiratory distress syndrome) have been reported. In addition, thromboembolic events both in association with, and separate from the Ovarian Hyperstimulation Syndrome have been reported. Intravascular thrombosis and embolism, which may originate in venous or arterial vessels, can result in reduced blood flow to critical organs or the extremities. Sequelae of such events have included venous thrombophlebitis, pulmonary embolism, pulmonary infarction, cerebral vascular occlusion (stroke), and arterial occlusion resulting in loss of limb. In rare cases, pulmonary complications and/or thromboembolic events have resulted in death.

Multiple Births: Reports of multiple births have been associated with urofollitropin-hCG treatment, including triplet and quintuplet gestations. In clinical studies with urofollitropin, 83% of the pregnancies following therapy resulted in single births and 17% in multiple births. The patient and her husband should be advised of the potential risk of multiple births before starting treatment.

PRECAUTIONS:

General: Careful attention should be given to diagnosis in candidates for urofollitropin therapy (see INDICATIONS AND USAGE, Selection of Patients.)

Information for the Patient: Prior to the therapy with urofollitropin, patients should be informed of the duration of treatment and monitoring of their condition that will be required. Possible adverse reactions (see ADVERSE REACTIONS) and the risk of multiple births should also be discussed.

Laboratory Tests: In most instances, treatment with urofollitropin results only in follicular growth and maturation. In order to effect ovulation, hCG must be given following the administration of urofollitropin when clinical assessment of the patient indicates that sufficient follicular maturation has occurred. This may be estimated by measuring serum (or urinary) estrogen levels and sonographic visualization of the ovaries. The combination of both estradiol levels and ultrasonography is useful for monitoring the growth and development of follicles, timing hCG administration, as well as detecting ovarian enlargement and minimizing the risk of the Ovarian Hyperstimulation Syndrome and multiple gestation.

Urinary and/or plasma estrogen determinations provide an indirect index of follicular maturity since as the follicles grow and develop, they secrete estrogens in increasing amounts. However, plasma and/or urinary estrogen levels represent the sum of ovarian activity. It is recommended that the number of growing follicles be confirmed using ultrasonography because plasma and/or urinary estrogens do not give an indication of the number of follicles.

Other clinical parameters which may have potential use for monitoring urofollitropin therapy include:

1. Changes in the vaginal cytology,

2. Appearance and volume of the cervical mucus,

3. Spinnbarkeit, and

4. Ferning of the cervical mucus.

The above clinical indices provide an indirect estimate of the estrogenic effect upon the target organs and, therefore, should only be used adjunctively with more direct estimates of follicular development, i.e. serum estradiol and ultrasonography.

The clinical confirmation of ovulation, with the exception of pregnancy, is obtained by direct and indirect indices of progesterone production. The indices most generally used are as follows:

1. A rise in basal body temperature,

2. Increase in serum progesterone, and

3. Menstruation following the shift in basal body temperature.

When used in conjunction with indices of progesterone production, sonographic visualization of the ovaries will assist in determining if ovulation has occurred. Sonographic evidence of ovulation may include the following:

1. Fluid in the cul-de-sac,

2. Ovarian stigmata, and

3. Collapsed follicle.

Because of the subjectivity of the various tests for the determination of follicular maturation and ovulation, it cannot be overemphasized that the physician should choose tests with which he/she is thoroughly familiar.

Carcinogenesis and Mutagenesis: Carcinogenicity and mutagenicity studies have not been performed.

Pregnancy Category X: See "Contraindications."

PRECAUTIONS: *(cont'd)*

Nursing Mothers: It is not known whether this drug is excreted in human milk. Because many drugs are excreted in human milk, caution should be exercised if urofollitropin is administered to a nursing woman.

DRUG INTERACTIONS:

No clinically significant drug/drug or drug/food interactions have been reported during urofollitropin therapy.

ADVERSE REACTIONS:

The following adverse reactions reported during urofollitropin therapy are listed in decreasing order of potential severity:

1. Pulmonary and vascular complications (see WARNINGS),
2. Ovarian Hyperstimulation Syndrome (see WARNINGS),
3. Adnexal torsion (as a complication of ovarian enlargement),
4. Mild to moderate ovarian enlargement,
5. Abdominal pain,
6. Sensitivity to urofollitropin, (Febrile reactions which may be accompanied by chills, musculoskeletal aches, joint pains, malaise, headache, and fatigue have occurred after the administration of urofollitropin. It is not clear whether or not these were pyrogenic responses or possible allergic reactions.)
7. Ovarian cysts,
8. Gastrointestinal symptoms (nausea, vomiting, diarrhea, abdominal cramps, bloating),
9. Pain, rash, swelling, and/or irritation at the site of injection,
10. Breast tenderness,
11. Headache,
12. Dermatological symptoms (dry skin, body rash, hair loss, hives),
13. Hemoperitoneum has been reported during menotropins therapy and, therefore, may also occur during urofollitropin therapy.

The following medical events have been reported subsequent to pregnancies resulting from urofollitropin therapy:

1. Ectopic pregnancy
2. Congenital abnormalities

(Three incidents of chromosomal abnormalities and four birth defects have been reported followed urofollitropin-hCG or urofollitropin, Pergonal (menotropins for injection, USP)-hCG therapy in clinical trials for stimulation prior to *in vitro* fertilization. The aborted pregnancies included one Trisomy 13, one Trisomy 18, and one fetus with multiple congenital anomalies (hydrocephaly, omphalocele, and meningocele). One meningocele, one external ear defect, one dislocated hip and ankle, and one dilated cardiomyopathy in presence of maternal Systemic Lupus Erythematosus were reported. None of these events was thought to be drug-related. The incidence dose not exceed that found in the general population.)

There have been infrequent reports of ovarian neoplasms, both benign and malignant, in woman who have undergone multiple drug regimens for ovulation induction; however, a casual relationship has been established.

DRUG ABUSE AND DEPENDENCE:

There have been no reports of abuse or dependence with urofollitropin.

OVERDOSAGE:

Aside from possible ovarian hyperstimulation and multiple gestations (see WARNINGS), little is known concerning the consequences of acute overdosage with urofollitropin.

DOSAGE AND ADMINISTRATION:

Dosage: The dose of urofollitropin to produce maturation of the follicle must be individualized for each patient. It is recommended that the initial dose to any patient should be 75 IU of urofollitropin per day, **ADMINISTERED INTRAMUSCULARLY**, for seven to twelve days followed by hCG, 5,000 U to 10,000 U, one day after the last dose of urofollitropin. Administration of urofollitropin may exceed twelve days if inadequate follicle development is indicated by estrogen and/or ultrasound measurement. The patient should be treated until indices of estrogenic activity, as indicated under "Precautions," are equivalent to or greater than those of the normal individual. If serum or urinary estradiol determinations or ultrasonographic visualizations are available, they may be useful as a guide to therapy. If the ovaries are abnormally enlarged on the last day of urofollitropin therapy, hCG should not be administered in this course of therapy; this will reduce the chances of development of the Ovarian Hyperstimulation Syndrome. If there is evidence of ovulation but no pregnancy, repeat this dosage regimen for at least two more courses before increasing the dose of urofollitropin to 150 IU of FSH per day for seven to twelve days. As before, this dose should be followed by 5,000 U to 10,000 U of hCG one day after the last dose of urofollitropin. If evidence of ovulation is present, but pregnancy dose not ensue, repeat the same dose for two more course. Doses larger than this are not routinely recommended.

During treatment with both urofollitropin and hCG and during a two week post-treatment period, patients should be examined at least every other day for signs of excessive ovarian stimulation. It is recommended that urofollitropin administration be stopped if the ovaries become abnormally enlarged or abdominal pain occurs. Most instances of OHSS occur after treatment has been discontinued and reach their maximum at about seven to ten days post-ovulation. Patients should be followed for at least two weeks after hCG administration.

The couple should be encouraged to have intercourse daily, beginning on the day prior to the administration of hCG until ovulation becomes apparent from the indices employed for the determination of progestational activity. Care should be taken to ensure insemination. In the light of the foregoing indices and parameters mentioned, it should become obvious that, unless a physician is willing to devote considerable time to these patients and be familiar with and conduct the necessary laboratory studies, he/she should not use urofollitropin.

Assisted Reproductive Technologies; For Assisted Reproductive Technologies, therapy with urofollitropin should be initiated in the early follicular phase (cycle day 2 or 3) at a dose of 150 IU per day, until sufficient follicular development is attained. In most cases, therapy should not exceed ten days.

Administration: Dissolve the contents of one ampule of urofollitropin in one to two ml of sterile saline and **ADMINISTER INTRAMUSCULARLY** immediately. Any unused reconstituted material should be discarded. Parenteral drug products should be inspected visually, for particulate matter and discoloration prior to administration, whenever solution and container permit.

HOW SUPPLIED:

Metrodin is supplied in a sterile, lyophilized form as a white to off-white powder or pellet in ampules containing 75 IU FSH activity.

Lyophilized powder may be stored refrigerated or at room temperature (3°-25°C/37°-77°F). Protect from light. Use immediately after reconstitution. Discard unused material.

HOW SUPPLIED - EQUIVALENTS NOT AVAILABLE:

Injection, Solution - Intramuscular - 75 unit

1's	$59.67	METRODIN, Serono Labs	44087-6075-01
10's	$558.14	METRODIN, Serono Labs	44087-6075-03
100's	$5413.27	METRODIN, Serono Labs	44087-6075-04

Injection, Solution - Intramuscular - 150 unit

1's	$114.55	METRODIN, Serono Labs	44087-6150-01

UROKINASE *(002417)*

CATEGORIES: Angiography; Anticoagulants/Thrombolytics; Blood Formation/Coagulation; Catheter; Embolism; Myocardial Infarction; Pulmonary Embolism; Thrombolytic Agents; Thrombolytic Enzymes; Thrombosis; Pregnancy Category B; FDA Pre 1938 Drugs

BRAND NAMES: **Abbokinase**

COST OF THERAPY: $6,363.68 (Pulmonary Embolism; Injection; 250,000 unit/vial; 16/day; 1 days)

DESCRIPTION:

Injection and Open-Cath: Urokinase is an enzyme (protein) produced by the kidney, and found in the urine. There are two forms of urokinase differing in molecular weight but having similar clinical effects. Abbokinase (urokinase for injection) is a thrombolytic agent obtained from human kidney cells by tissue culture techniques and is primarily the low molecular weight form. It is supplied as a sterile lyophilized white powder containing mannitol (25 mg/vial), Albumin (Human) (250 mg/vial), and sodium chloride (50 mg/vial).

Injection: Abbokinase (urokinase for injection) should be used in hospitals where the recommended diagnostic and monitoring techniques are available. Thrombolytic therapy should be considered in all situations where the benefits to be achieved outweigh the risk of potentially serious hemorrhage. When internal bleeding does occur, it may be more difficult to manage than that which occurs with conventional anticoagulant therapy.

Urokinase treatment should be instituted as soon as possible after onset of pulmonary embolism, preferably no later than seven days after onset. Any delay in instituting lytic therapy to evaluate the effect of heparin decreases the potential for optimal efficacy.[1]

When urokinase is used for treatment of coronary artery thrombosis associated with evolving transmural myocardial infarction, therapy should be instituted within six hours of symptom onset.

Thin translucent filaments may occasionally occur in reconstituted Abbokinase vials, but do not indicate any decrease in potency of this product. No clinical problems have been associated with these filaments. See DOSAGE AND ADMINISTRATION section.

Following reconstitution with 5 ml of Sterile Water for Injection, USP, it is a clear, slightly straw-colored solution; each ml contains 50,000 IU of urokinase activity, 0.5% mannitol, 5% Albumin (Human), and 1% sodium chloride. The pH is adjusted with sodium hydroxide and/or hydrochloric acid prior to lyophilization.

Abbokinase is for intravenous and intracoronary infusion only.

IV Catheter Clearance: Each ml of reconstituted Abbokinase Open-Cath solution contains 5000 IU of urokinase activity, 5 mg gelatin, 15 mg mannitol, 1.7 mg sodium chloride and 4.6 mg monobasic sodium phosphate anhydrous. The pH is adjusted with sodium hydroxide and/or hydrochloric acid prior to lyophilization.

CLINICAL PHARMACOLOGY:

Urokinase acts on the endogenous fibrinolytic system. It is converts plasminogen to the enzyme plasmin. Plasmin degrades fibrin clots as well as fibrinogen and other plasma proteins.

Intravenous infusion of urokinase in doses recommended for lysis of pulmonary embolism is followed by increased fibrinolytic activity. This effect disappears within a few hours after discontinuation, but a decrease in plasma levels of fibrinogen and plasminogen and an increase in the amount of circulating fibrin (ogen) degradation products may persist for 12-24 hours.[2,3] There is a lack of correlation between embolus resolution and changes in coagulation and fibrinolytic assay results.

Information is incomplete about the pharmacokinetic properties in man. Urokinase administered by intravenous infusion is cleared rapidly by the liver. The serum half-life in man is 20 minutes or less. Patients with impaired liver function (*e.g.,* cirrhosis) would be expected to show a prolongation in half-life. Small fractions of an administered dose are excreted in bile and urine.

IV Catheter Clearance: When used as directed for IV catheter clearance, only small amounts of urokinase may reach the circulation; therefore, therapeutic serum levels are not expected to be achieved. Nevertheless, one should be aware of the clinical pharmacology of urokinase.

INDICATIONS AND USAGE:

Pulmonary Embolism: Abbokinase (urokinase for injection) is indicated in adults:

For the lysis of acute massive pulmonary emboli, defined as obstruction of blood flow to a lobe or multiple segments.

For the lysis of pulmonary emboli accompanied by unstable hemodynamics, i.e. failure to maintain blood pressure without supportive measures.

The diagnosis should be confirmed by objective means, such as pulmonary angiography via an upper extremity vein, or non-invasive procedures such as lung scanning.

Angiographic and hemodynamic measurements demonstrate a more rapid improvement with lytic therapy than with heparin therapy.[4-8]

Coronary Artery Thrombosis: Abbokinase has been reported to lyse acute thrombi obstructing coronary arteries, associated with evolving transmural myocardial infarction.[9] The majority of patients who received Abbokinase by intracoronary infusion within six hours following onset of symptoms showed recanalization of the involved vessel.

IT HAS BEEN ESTABLISHED THAT INTRACORONARY ADMINISTRATION OF ABBOKINASE DURING EVOLVING TRANSMURAL MYOCARDIAL INFARCTION RESULTS IN SALVAGE OF MYOCARDIAL TISSUE, NOR THAT IT REDUCES MORTALITY. THE PATIENTS WHO MIGHT BENEFIT FROM THIS THERAPY CANNOT BE DEFINED.

IV Catheter Clearance: Abbokinase is indicated for the restoration of patency to intravenous catheters, including central venous catheters, obstructed by clotted blood or fibrin.[10,11]

CONTRAINDICATIONS:

Injection and IV Catheter Clearance: Because thrombolytic therapy increases the risk of bleeding, urokinase is contraindicated in the following situations: (See WARNINGS.)

Active internal bleeding

History of cerebrovascular accident

CONTRAINDICATIONS: *(cont'd)*

Recent (within two months) intracranial or intraspinal surgery

Recent trauma including cardiopulmonary resuscitation

Intracranial neoplasm, arteriovenous malformation, or aneurysm

Known bleeding diathesis

Severe uncontrolled arterial hypertension

IV Catheter Clearance: There have been no reports, however, which would suggest a contraindication for the use of urokinase for IV catheter clearance.

WARNINGS:

INJECTION

Bleeding: The aim of urokinase is the production of sufficient amounts of plasmin for lysis of intravascular deposits of fibrin; however, fibrin deposits which provide hemostasis, for example, at sites of needle puncture, will also lyse, and bleeding from such sites may occur.

Intramuscular injections and nonessential handling of the patient must be avoided during treatment with urokinase. Venipunctures should be performed carefully and as infrequently as possible.

Should an arterial puncture be necessary (except for intracoronary administration), upper extremity vessels are preferable. Pressure should be applied for at least 30 minutes, a pressure dressing applied, and the puncture site checked frequently for evidence of bleeding.

In the following conditions, the risks of therapy may be increased and should be weighed against the anticipated benefits:

Recent (within 10 days) major surgery, obstetrical delivery, organ biopsy, previous puncture of non-compressible vessels

Recent (within 10 days) serious gastrointestinal bleeding

High likelihood of a left heart thrombus, e.g. mitral stenosis with atrial fibrillation

Subacute bacterial endocarditis

Hemostatic defects including those secondary to severe hepatic or renal disease

Pregnancy

Cerebrovascular disease

Diabetic hemorrhagic retinopathy

Any other condition in which bleeding might constitute a significant hazard or be particularly difficult to manage because of its location

Should serious spontaneous bleeding (not controlled by local pressure) occur, the infusion of urokinase should be terminated immediately, and treatment instituted as described under ADVERSE REACTIONS.

USE OF ANTICOAGULANTS

Concurrent use of anticoagulants with intravenous administration of Abbokinase is not recommended. However, concurrent use of heparin may be required during intracoronary administration of Abbokinase. A clinical study[9] with concurrent use of heparin and Abbokinase during intracoronary administration has demonstrated no tendency toward increased bleeding that would not be attributable to the procedure or Abbokinase alone. Nevertheless, careful monitoring for excessive bleeding is advised.

ARRHYTHMIAS

Rapid lysis of coronary thrombi has been reported occasionally to cause atrial or ventricular dysrhythmias as a result of reperfusion requiring immediate treatment. Careful monitoring for arrhythmias should be maintained during and immediately following intracoronary administration of Abbokinase.

IV CATHETER CLEARANCE

Excessive pressure should be avoided when Abbokinase solution is injected into the catheter. Such force could cause rupture of the catheter or expulsion of the clot into the circulation. During attempts to determine catheter occlusion, vigorous suction should not be applied due to possible damage to the vascular wall or collapse of soft-wall catheters.

Catheters may be occluded by substances other than fibrin clots such as drug precipitates. Abbokinase solution is not effective in such cases and there is the possibility that the substances may be forced into the vascular system.

PRECAUTIONS:

LABORATORY TESTS

Injection: Before commencing thrombolytic therapy, obtain a hematocrit, platelet count, and a thrombin time (TT), activated partial thromboplastin time (APTT), or prothrombin time (PT). If heparin has been given, it should be discontinued unless it is to be used in conjunction with Abbokinase for intracoronary administration. TT or APTT should be less than twice the normal control value before thrombolytic therapy is started.

During the infusion, coagulation tests and/or measures of fibrinolytic activity may be performed if desired. Results do not, however, reliably predict either efficacy or a risk of bleeding. The clinical response should be observed frequently, and vital signs, i.e. pulse, temperature, respiratory rate and blood pressure, should be checked at least every four hours. The blood pressure should not be taken in the lower extremities to avoid dislodgment of possible deep vein thrombi.

Following the intravenous infusion *before (re) instituting heparin,* the TT or APTT should be less than twice the upper limits of normal. Following intracoronary infusion of Abbokinase, blood coagulation parameters should be determined and heparin therapy continued as appropriate.

CARCINOGENICITY

Injection and IV Catheter Clearance: Adequate data are not available on the long-term potential for carcinogenicity in animals or humans.

PREGNANCY CATEGORY B

Reproduction studies have been performed in mice and rats at doses up to 1,000 times the human dose and have revealed no evidence of impaired fertility or harm to the fetus due to urokinase. There are, however, no adequate and well-controlled studies in pregnant women. Because animal reproduction studies are not always predictive of human response, this drug should be used during pregnancy only if clearly needed.

NURSING MOTHERS

It is known whether this drug is excreted in human milk. Because many drugs are excreted in human milk, caution should be exercised when urokinase is administered to a nursing woman.

PEDIATRIC USE

Safety and effectiveness in children have not been established.

DRUG INTERACTIONS:

INJECTION

The interaction of urokinase with other drugs has not been studied. Drugs that alter platelet function should not be used. Common examples are: aspirin, indomethacin and phenylbutazone.

DRUG INTERACTIONS: *(cont'd)*

Although a bolus dose of heparin is recommended prior to intracoronary use of urokinase, oral anticoagulants or heparin should not be given concurrently with large doses of urokinase such as those used for pulmonary embolism. Concomitant use of intravenous urokinase and oral anticoagulants or heparin may increase the risk of hemorrhage. (See WARNINGS.)

ADVERSE REACTIONS:

THE FOLLOWING ADVERSE REACTIONS HAVE BEEN ASSOCIATED WITH INTRAVENOUS THERAPY BUT MAY ALSO OCCUR WITH INTRACORONARY ARTERY INFUSION.

Bleeding

Injection And IV Catheter Clearance: The type of bleeding associated with thrombolytic therapy can be placed into two broad categories:

Superficial or surface bleeding, observed mainly at invaded or disturbed sites (*e.g.,* venous cutdowns, arterial punctures, sites of recent surgical intervention, etc.).

Internal bleeding, involving, e.g., the gastrointestinal tract, genitourinary tract, vagina, or intramuscular, retroperitoneal, or intracranial sites.

Several fatalities due to intracranial or retroperitoneal hemorrhage have occurred during thrombolytic therapy.

Should serious bleeding occur, urokinase infusion should be discontinued and, if necessary, blood loss and reversal of the bleeding tendency can be effectively managed with whole blood (fresh blood preferable), packed red blood cells and cryoprecipitate or fresh frozen plasma. Dextran should not be used. Although the use of aminocaproic acid (ACA, AMICAR) in humans as an antidote for urokinase has not been documented, it may be considered in an emergency situation.

Allergic Reactions

In vitro tests with urokinase, as well as intradermal tests in humans, gave no evidence of induced antibody formation. Relatively mild allergic type reactions, e.g., bronchospasm and skin rash, have been reported. When such reactions occur, they usually respond to conventional therapy. In addition, rare cases of anaphylaxis have been reported.

Miscellaneous

Fever and chills, including shaking chills (rigors), nausea and/or vomiting, transient hypotension or hypertension, dyspnea, tachycardia, cyanosis, back pain, hypoxemia, and acidosis have been reported together and separately. Rare cases of myocardial infarction have also been reported. A cause and effect relationship has not been established.

Aspirin is not recommended for treatment of fever.

DOSAGE AND ADMINISTRATION:

ABBOKINASE IS INTENDED FOR INTRAVENOUS AND INTRACORONARY INFUSION ONLY.

PULMONARY EMBOLISM: PREPARATION

Injection: Reconstitute Abbokinase (urokinase for injection) by aseptically adding 5 ml of Sterile Water for Injection, USP, to the vial. (It is important that Abbokinase be reconstituted *only* with Sterile Water for Injection, USP, *without* preservatives. Bacteriostatic Water for Injection should *not* be used.) Each vial should be visually inspected for discoloration (slightly straw-colored solution) and for the presence of particulate material. Highly colored solutions should not be used. Because Abbokinase contains no preservatives, it should not be reconstituted until immediately before using. Any unused portion of the reconstituted material should be discarded.

To minimize formation of filaments, avoid shaking the vial during reconstitution. Roll and tilt the vial to enhance reconstitution. The solution may be terminally filtered, e.g. through a 0.45 micron or smaller cellulose membrane filter. No other medication should be added to this solution.

Reconstituted Abbokinase is diluted with 0.9% Sodium Chloride Injection, USP or 5% Dextrose Injection, USP, prior to intravenous infusion. See TABLE 1, Dose Preparation, Pulmonary Embolism.

Administration

Administer Abbokinase (urokinase for injection) by means of a constant infusion pump that is capable of delivering a total volume of 195 ml. The following table may be used as an aid in the preparation of Abbokinase (urokinase for injection) for administration.

TABLE 1 Dose Preparation-Pulmonary Embolism

Weight (pounds)	Total Dose* Urokinase (IU)	Number Vials Abbokinase (urokinase for injection)	Volume of Abbokinase After Reconstitution (ml)** +	Volume of Diluent (ml) =	Final Volume (ml)
81-90	2,250,000	9	45	150	195
91-100	2,500,000	10	50	145	195
101-110	2,750,000	11	55	140	195
111-120	3,000,000	12	60	135	195
121-130	3,250,000	13	65	130	195
131-140	3,500,000	14	70	125	195
141-150	3,750,000	15	75	120	195
151-160	4,000,000	16	80	115	195
161-170	4,250,000	17	85	110	195
171-180	4,500,000	18	90	105	195
181-190	4,750,000	19	95	100	195
191-200	5,000,000	20	100	95	195
201-210	5,250,000	21	105	90	195
211-220	5,500,000	22	110	85	195
221-230	5,750,000	23	115	80	195
231-240	6,000,000	24	120	75	195
241-250	6,250,000	25	125	70	195
Infusion Rate:	Priming Dose 15 ml/10 min***		Dose for 12-Hour Period 15 ml/hr for 12 hrs		

* Priming dose + dose administered during 12-hour period.
** After addition of 5 ml of Sterile Water for Injection, USP, per vial. (See Preparation.)
*** Pump rate = 90 ml/hr

A priming dose of 2,000 IU/Ib (4,400 IU/kg) of Abbokinase is given as the Abbokinase-0.9% Sodium Chloride Injection or 5% Dextrose Injection admixture at a rate of 90 ml/hour over a period of 10 minutes. This is followed by a continuous infusion of 2,000 IU/Ib/hr (4,400 IU/kg/hr) of Abbokinase at a rate of 15 ml/hour for 12 hours. Since some Abbokinase admixture will remain in the tubing at the end of an infusion pump delivery cycle, the following flush procedure should be performed to insure that the total dose of Abbokinase is administered. A solution of 0.9% Sodium Chloride Injection or 5% Dextrose Injection approximately equal in

DOSAGE AND ADMINISTRATION: *(cont'd)*

amount to the volume of the tubing in the infusion set should be administered via the pump to flush the Abbokinase admixture from the entire length of the infusion set. The pump should be set to administer the flush solution at the continuous infusion rate of 15 ml/hour.

Anticoagulation After Terminating

Urokinase Treatment: At the end of urokinase therapy, treatment with heparin by continuous intravenous infusion is recommended to prevent recurrent thrombosis. Heparin treatment without a loading dose, should not begin until the thrombin time has decreased to *less than twice* the normal control value (approximately 3 to 4 hours after completion of the infusion). See manufacturer's prescribing information for proper use of heparin. This should then be followed by oral anticoagulants in the conventional manner.

LYSIS OF CORONARY ARTERY THROMBI[9]

Preparation

Reconstitute three (3) 250,000 IU vials of Abbokinase by aseptically adding 5 ml of Sterile Water for Injection, USP, to each vial. (It is important that Abbokinase be reconstituted *only* with Sterile Water for Injection, USP, *without*preservatives. Bacteriostatic Water for Injection should *not* be used.) Each vial should be visually inspected for discoloration (Slightly straw-colored solution) and for the presence of particulate material. Highly colored solutions should not be used. Because Abbokinase contains no preservatives, it should not be reconstituted until immediately before using. Any unused portion of the reconstituted material should be discarded.

To minimize formation of filaments, avoid shaking the vial during reconstitution. Roll and tilt the vial to enhance reconstitution. The solution may be terminally filtered, e.g. through a 0.45 micron or smaller cellulose membrane filter.

Add the contents of the three (3) reconstituted Abbokinase vials to 500 ml of 5% Dextrose Injection, USP. The following solution admixture will have a concentration of approximately 1500 IU per ml. No other medication should be added to the solution.

The admixture should be administered immediately as described under Administration. Any solution remaining after administration should be discarded.

NOTE: Adsorption of drug from dilute protein solution to various materials has been reported in the literature. Therefore, the directions for Preparation and Administration must be followed to assure that significant drug loss does not occur.

Administration

Prior to the infusion of Abbokinase, a bolus dose of heparin ranging from 2500 to 10,000 units should be administered intravenously. Prior heparin administration should be considered when calculating the heparin dose for this procedure. Following the bolus dose of heparin, the prepared Abbokinase solution should be infused into the occluded artery at a rate of 4 ml per minute (6000 IU per minute) for periods up to 2 hours. In a clinical study the average total dose of Abbokinase utilized for lysis of coronary artery thrombi was 500,000 IU.[9]

To determine response to Abbokinase therapy, periodic angiography during the infusion is recommended. It is suggested that the angiography be repeated at approximately 15 minute intervals. Abbokinase therapy should be continued until the artery is maximally opened, usually 15 to 30 minutes after the initial opening. Following the infusion, coagulation parameters should be determined. It is advisable to continue heparin therapy after the artery is opened by Abbokinase.

When Abbokinase was administered selectively into thrombosed coronary arteries via coronary catheter within 6 hours following onset of symptoms of acute transmural myocardial infarction, 60% of the occlusions were opened.[9]

IV CATHETER CLEARANCE

BECAUSE ABBOKINASE OPEN-CATH POWDER CONTAINS NO PRESERVATIVE, RECONSTITUTED SOLUTION SHOULD BE USED IMMEDIATELY AFTER RECONSTITUTION. DISCARD ANY UNUSED PORTION.

Preparation of Solution

Univial:

1. Remove protective cap. Turn plunger-stopper a quarter turn and press to force diluent into lower chamber.

2. Roll and tilt to effect solution. Use only a clear, essentially colorless solution.

3. Sterilize top of stopper with a suitable germicide.

4. Insert needle through the center of stopper until tip is barely visible. Withdraw dose.

It is recommended that vigorous shaking be avoided during reconstitution; roll and tilt to enhance reconstitution.

Parenteral drug products should be inspected visually for particulate matter and discoloration prior to administration, whenever solution and container permit.

Administration

When the following procedure is used to clear a central venous catheter, the patient should be instructed to exhale and hold his breath any time the catheter is not connected to IV tubing or a syringe. This is to prevent air from entering the open catheter.

Aseptically disconnect the IV tubing connection at the catheter hub and attach a 10 ml syringe. Determine occlusion of the catheter by *gently* attempting to aspirate blood from the catheter with the 10 ml syringe. If aspiration is not possible, remove the 10 ml syringe and attach a 1 ml tuberculin syringe filled with prepared Abbokinase to the catheter. Slowly and gently inject an amount of Abbokinase equal to the volume of the catheter. Aseptically remove the tuberculin syringe and connect a 5 ml syringe to the catheter. Wait at least 5 minutes before attempting to aspirate the drug and residual clot with the 5 ml syringe. Repeat aspiration attempts every 5 minutes. If the catheter is not open within 30 minutes, the catheter may be capped allowing Abbokinase to remain in the catheter for 30 to 60 minutes before again attempting to aspirate. A second injection of Abbokinase may be necessary in resistant cases.

When patency is restored, aspirate 4 to 5 ml of blood to assure removal of all drug and clot residual. Remove the blood-filled syringe and replace it with a 10 ml syringe filled with 0.9% Sodium Chloride Injection, USP. The catheter should then be gently irrigated with this solution to assure patency of the catheter. After the catheter has been irrigated, remove the 10 ml syringe and aseptically reconnect sterile IV tubing to the catheter hub.

REFERENCES:

1. Sherry S, et al. Thrombolytic therapy in thrombosis: A National Institutes of Health consensus development conference. *Ann Intern Med.* 1980;93:141-144. **2.** Bang NU. Physiology and biochemistry of fibrinolysis. In: Bang NU, Beller FK, Deutsch E, Mammen EF, eds. *Thrombosis and Bleeding Disorders.* New York, NY: Academic Press; 1971:292-327. **3.** McNicol GP. The fibrinolytic enzyme system. *Postgrad Med J.* August 1973;49 (suppl 5): 10-12. **4.** Sasahara AA, Hyers TM, Cole CM, et al. The urokinase pulmonary embolism trial. *Circulation.* 1973;47 (suppl 2):1-108. **5.** Urokinase pulmonary embolism trial study group: Urokinase-streptokinase embolism trial. *JAMA.* 1974;229:1606-1613. **6.** Sasahara AA, Bell WR, Simon TL, et al. The Phase II urokinase-streptokinase pulmonary embolism trial, *Thrombos Diathes Haemorrh* (Stuttg). 1975;33:464-476. **7.** Bell WR. Thrombolytic therapy: A comparison between urokinase and streptokinase, *Sem Thromb Hemost.* 1975;2:1-13. **8.** Fratantoni JC, Ness P, Simon TL. Thrombolytic therapy: Current status.*N Eng J Med.* 1975;293:1073-1078. **9.** Tennant SN, Campbell WB, et al. Intracoronary thrombolysis in acute myocardial infarction: Comparison of the efficacy of urokinase to streptokinase.*Circulation.* 1984;69:756-760. **10.** Lawson M, et al. The use of urokinase to restore the patency of occluded central venous catheters. *Am J Intravenous Therapy and Clinical Nutrition.*

REFERENCES: *(cont'd)*

1982;9:29-32. **11.** Glynn MFX, et al. Therapy for thrombotic occlusion of long-term intravenous alimentation catheters.*Journal of Parenteral and Enteral Nutrition.* 1980;4:387-390.(Injection: Abbott, 5/93, 06-8868-R10)(IV Catheter Clearance: Abbott, 9/93, 06-8909-R7)

HOW SUPPLIED:

Injection: Abbokinase (urokinase for injection) is supplied as a sterile lyophilized preparation (NDC 0074-6109-05). Each vial contains 250,000 IU urokinase activity, 25 mg mannitol, 250 mg Albumin (Human), and 50 mg sodium chloride. Store Abbokinase powder at 2° to 8°C.

IV Catheter Clearance: Abbokinase Open-Cath (urokinase for catheter clearance) is supplied as a sterile lyophilized preparation in single dose Univial packages of 1 ml and 1.8 ml.

Storage: Store powder below 77°F (25°C). Avoid freezing.

HOW SUPPLIED - EQUIVALENTS NOT AVAILABLE:

Injection, Lyphl-Soln - Intravenous - 5,000 unit/ml

1 ml	$49.04	ABBOKINASE, OPEN-CATH, Abbott	00074-6111-01

Injection, Lyphl-Soln - Intravenous - 9,000 unit/vial

1's	$85.52	ABBOKINASE, OPEN-CATH, Abbott	00074-6145-02

Injection, Lyphl-Soln - Intravenous - 250,000 unit/vi

1's	$397.73	ABBOKINASE, Abbott	00074-6109-05

URSODIOL *(002418)*

CATEGORIES: Cholelitholytic Agents; Gall Stone Dissolution Agents; Gastrointestinal Drugs; Pregnancy Category B; FDA Approved 1987 Dec

BRAND NAMES: **Actigall**; *Arsacol*; *Cholit-Ursan*; *Destolit*; *Deursil*; *Litanin*; *Ursochol*; *Ursolvan*; *Ursotan*
(International brand names outside U.S. in italics)

FORMULARIES: BC-BS; Medi-Cal; PCS

DESCRIPTION:

SPECIAL NOTE: Gallbladder stone dissolution with ursodiol treatment requires months of therapy. Complete dissolution does not occur in all patients and recurrence of stones within 5 years has been observed in up to 50% of patients who do dissolve their stones on bile acid therapy. Patients should be carefully selected for therapy with ursodiol, and alternative therapies should be considered.

Ursodiol is an agent intended for dissolution of radiolucent gallstones. It is available as 300-mg capsules suitable for oral administration.

Actigall is ursodiol (ursodeoxycholic acid), a naturally occurring bile acid found in small quantities in normal human bile and in large quantities in the biles of certain species of bears. It is a bitter-tasting, white powder freely soluble in ethanol, and in glacial acetic acid, slightly soluble in chloroform, sparingly soluble in ether, and practically insoluble in water. The chemical name for ursodiol is 3α,7β-dihydroxy-5β-cholan-24-oic acid ($C_{24}H_{40}O_4$). Ursodiol has a molecular weight of 392.56.

Actigall Inactive Ingredients: Gelatin; iron oxide; magnesium stearate; colloidal silicon dioxide; starch; and titanium dioxide.

CLINICAL PHARMACOLOGY:

About 90% of a therapeutic dose of ursodiol is absorbed in the small bowel after oral administration. After absorption, ursodiol enters the portal vein and undergoes efficient extraction from portal blood by the liver (*i.e.*, there is a large "first pass" effect) where it is conjugated with either glycine or taurine and is then secreted into the hepatic bile ducts. Ursodiol in bile is concentrated in the gallbladder and expelled into the duodenum in gallbladder bile via the cystic and common ducts by gallbladder contractions provoked by physiologic response to eating. Only small quantities of ursodiol appear in the systemic circulation and very small amounts are excreted into urine. The sites of the drug's therapeutic actions are in the liver, bile and gut lumen.

Beyond conjugation, ursodiol is not altered or catabolized appreciably by the liver or intestinal mucosa. A small proportion of orally administered drug undergoes bacterial degradation with each cycle of enterohepatic circulation. Ursodiol can be both oxidized and reduced at the 7-carbon, yielding either 7-keto-lithocholic acid or lithocholic acid, respectively. Further, there is some bacterially catalyzed deconjugation of glyco- and tauro-ursodeoxycholic acid in the small bowel. Free ursodiol, 7-keto-lithocholic acid and lithocholic acid are relatively insoluble in aqueous media and larger proportions of these compounds are lost from the distal gut into the feces. Reabsorbed free ursodiol is reconjugated by the liver. Eighty percent of lithocholic acid formed in the small bowel is excreted in the feces, but the 20% that is absorbed is sulfated at the 3-hydroxyl group in the liver to relatively insoluble lithocholyl conjugates which are excreted into bile and lost in feces. Absorbed 7-keto-lithocholic acid is stereospecifically reduced in the liver to chenodiol.

Lithocholic acid causes cholestatic liver injury and can cause death from liver failure in certain species unable to form sulfate conjugates. Lithocholic acid is formed by 7-dehydroxylation of the dihydroxy bile acids (ursodiol and chenodiol) in the gut lumen. The 7-dehydroxylation reaction appears to be alpha-specific, i.e., chenodiol is more efficiently 7-dehydroxylated than ursodiol and for equimolar doses of ursodiol and chenodiol, levels of lithocholic acid appearing in bile are lower with the former. Man has the capacity to sulfate lithocholic acid. Although liver injury has not been associated with ursodiol therapy, a reduced capacity to sulfate may exist in some individuals, but such a deficiency has not yet been clearly demonstrated.

PHARMACODYNAMICS

Ursodiol suppresses hepatic synthesis and secretion of cholesterol, and also inhibits intestinal absorption of cholesterol. It appears to have little inhibitory effect on synthesis and secretion into bile of endogenous bile acids, and does not appear to effect secretion of phospholipids into bile.

With repeated dosing, bile ursodeoxycholic acid concentrations reach a steady state in about 3 weeks. Although insoluble in aqueous media, cholesterol can be solubilized in at least two different ways in the presence of dihydroxy bile acids. In addition to solubilizing cholesterol in micelles, ursodiol acts by an apparently unique mechanism to cause dispersion of cholesterol as liquid crystals in aqueous media. Thus, even though administration of high doses (*e.g.*, 15-18 mg/kg/day) does not result in a concentration of ursodiol higher than 60% of the total bile acid pool, ursodiol-rich bile effectively solubilizes cholesterol. The overall effect of ursodiol is to increase the concentration level at which saturation of cholesterol occurs.

The various actions of ursodiol combine to change the bile of patients with gallstones from cholesterol-precipitating to cholesterol-solubilizing, thus resulting in bile conducive to cholesterol stones dissolution.

After ursodiol dosing is stopped, the concentration of the bile acid in bile falls exponentially, declining to about 5-10% of its steady-state level in about 1 week.

CLINICAL STUDIES:

On the basis of clinical trial results in a total of 868 patients with radiolucent gallstones treated in 8 studies (three in the U.S. involving 282 patients, one in the U.K. involving 130 patients and four in Italy involving 456 patients) for periods ranging from 6-78 months with ursodiol doses ranging from about 5 to 20 mg/kg/day, an ursodiol dose of about 8-10 mg/kg/day appeared to be the best dose. With an ursodiol dose of about 10 mg/kg/day complete stone dissolution can be anticipated in about 30% of unselected patients with uncalcified gallstones <20 mm in maximal diameter treated for up to two years. Patients with calcified gallstones prior to treatment, or patients who develop stone calcification or gallbladder nonvisualization on treatment, and patients with stones larger than 20 mm in maximal diameter rarely dissolve their stones. The chance of gallstone dissolution is increased up to 50% in patients with floating or floatable stones (*i.e.,* those with high cholesterol content), and is inversely related to stone size for those less than 20 mm in maximal diameter. Complete dissolution was observed in 81% of patients with stones up to 5 mm in diameter. Age, sex, weight, degree of obesity and serum cholesterol level are not related to the chance of stone dissolution with ursodiol.

A nonvisualizing gallbladder by oral cholecystogram prior to the initiation of therapy is not a contraindication to ursodiol therapy (the group of patients with nonvisualizing gallbladders in the ursodiol studies had complete stone dissolution rates similar to the group of patients with visualizing gallbladders). However, gallbladder nonvisualization developing during ursodiol treatment predicts failure of complete stone dissolution and in such cases therapy should be discontinued.

Partial stone dissolution occurring within 6 months of beginning therapy with ursodiol appears to be associated with a >70% chance of eventual complete stone dissolution with further treatment; partial dissolution observed within one year of starting therapy indicates 40% probability of complete dissolution.

Stone recurrence after dissolution with ursodiol therapy was seen within 2 years in 8/27 (30%) of patients in the U.K. studies,. Of 16 patients in the U.K. study whose stones had previously dissolved on chenodiol but later recurred, 11 had complete dissolution on ursodiol. Stone recurrence has been observed in up to 50% of patients within 5 years of complete stone dissolution on ursodiol therapy. Serial ultrasonographic examinations should be obtained to monitor for recurrence of stones, bearing in mind that radiolucency of the stones should be established before another course of ursodiol is instituted. A prophylactic dose of ursodiol has not been established.

ALTERNATIVE THERAPIES

Watchful Waiting: Watchful waiting has the advantage that no therapy may ever be required. For patients with silent or minimally symptomatic stones, the rate of development of moderate to severe symptoms or gallstone complications is estimated to be between 2% and 6% per year, leading to a cumulative rate of 7% to 27% in five years. Presumably the rate is higher for patients already having symptoms.

CHOLECYSTECTOMY

Surgery offers the advantage of immediate and permanent stone removal, but carries a high risk in some patients. About 5% of cholecystectomized patients have residual symptoms or retained common duct stones. The spectrum of surgical risk varies as a function of age and the presence of disease other than cholelithiasis (TABLE 1):

TABLE 1 Mortality Rates for Cholecystectomy in the U.S. (National Halothane Study, JAMA 1966; 197:775-8) 27,600 Cholecystectomies (Smoothed Rates) Deaths/1000 Operations***

	Age (Yrs)	Cholecystectomy	Cholecystectomy + Common Duct Exploration
Low Risk Patients*			
Women	0-49	.54	2.13
	50-69	2.80	10.10
Men	0-49	1.04	4.12
	50-69	5.41	19.23
High Risk Patients**			
Women	0-49	12.66	47.62
	50-69	17.24	58.82
Men	0-49	24.39	90.91
	50-69	33.33	111.11

* In good health or with moderate systemic disease.
** With severe or extreme systemic disease.
*** Includes both elective and emergency surgery.

Women in good health or who have only moderate systemic disease, and are under 49 years of age the lowest surgical mortality rate (0.054); men in all categories have a surgical mortality rate twice that of women. Common duct exploration quadruples the rates in all categories. The rates rise with each decade of life and increase tenfold or more in all categories with severe or extreme systemic disease.

INDICATIONS AND USAGE:

Ursodiol is indicated for patients with radiolucent, noncalcified gallbladder stones <20 mm in greatest diameter in whom elective cholecystectomy would be undertaken except for the presence of increased surgical risk due to systemic disease, advanced age, idiosyncratic reaction to general anesthesia, or for those patients who refuse surgery. Safety of use of ursodiol beyond 24 months is not established.

CONTRAINDICATIONS:

1. Ursodiol will not dissolve calcified cholesterol stones, radiopaque stones or radiolucent bile pigment stones. Hence, patients with such stones are not candidates for ursodiol therapy.

2. Patients with compelling reasons for cholecystectomy including unremitting acute cholecystitis, cholangitis, biliary obstruction, gallstone pancreatitis or biliary-gastrointestinal fistula are not candidates for ursodiol therapy.

3. Allergy to bile acids.

PRECAUTIONS:

Liver Tests: Ursodiol therapy has not been associated with liver damage.

Lithocholic acid, a naturally occurring bile acid, is known to be a liver-toxic metabolite. This bile acid is formed in the gut from ursodiol less efficiently and in smaller amounts than that seen from chenodiol. Lithocholic acid is detoxified in the liver by sulfation and although man appears to be an efficient sulfater, it is possible that some patients may have a congenital or acquired deficiency in sulfation, thereby predisposing them to lithocholate-induced liver damage.

Abnormalities in liver enzymes have not been associated with ursodiol therapy and in fact ursodiol has been shown to decrease liver enzyme levels in liver disease. However, patients given ursodiol should have SGOT (AST) and SGPT (ALT) measured at the initiation of therapy and thereafter as indicated by the particular clinical circumstances.

PRECAUTIONS: *(cont'd)*

Carcinogenesis, Mutagenesis, and Impairment of Fertility: Ursodeoxycholic acid was tested in two-year oral carcinogenicity studies in CD-1 mice and Sprague-Dawley rats at daily doses of 50, 250, and 1000 mg/kg/day. It was not tumorigenic in mice. In the rat study, it produced statistically significant dose-related increased incidences of pheochromocytomas of adrenal medulla in males (p=0.014, Peto trend test) and females (p=0.004, Peto trend test.) A 78-week rat study employing intrarectal instillation of lithocholic acid and tauro-deoxycholic acid, metabolites of ursodiol and chenodiol, has been conducted. These bile acids alone did not produce any tumors. A tumor-promoting effect of both metabolites was observed when they were co-administered with a carcinogenic agent. Results of epidemiologic studies suggest that bile acids might be involved in the pathogenesis of human colon cancer in patients who had undergone a cholecystectomy, but direct evidence is lacking. Ursodiol is not mutagenic in the Ames test. Dietary administration of lithocholic acid to chickens is reported to cause hepatic adenomatous hyperplasia.

Pregnancy Category B: Reproduction studies have been performed in rats and rabbits with ursodiol doses up to 200-fold the therapeutic dose and have revealed no evidence of impaired fertility or harm to the fetus at doses of 20 to 100-fold the human dose in rats and at 5-fold the human dose (highest dose tested) in rabbits. Studies employing 100 to 200-fold the human dose in rats have shown some reduction in fertility rate and litter size. There have been no adequate and well-controlled studies of the use of ursodiol in pregnant women, but inadvertent exposure of 4 women to therapeutic doses of the drug in the first trimester of pregnancy during the ursodiol trials led to no evidence of effects on the fetus or newborn baby. Although it seems unlikely, the possibility that ursodiol can cause fetal harm cannot be ruled out; hence, the drug is not recommended for use during pregnancy.

Nursing Mothers: It is not known whether ursodiol is excreted in human milk. Because many drugs are excreted in human milk, caution should be exercised when ursodiol is administered to a nursing mother.

Pediatric Use: The safety and effectiveness of ursodiol in children have not been established.

DRUG INTERACTIONS:

Bile acid sequestering agents such as cholestyramine and colestipol may interfere with the action of ursodiol by reducing its absorption. Aluminum-based antacids have been shown to absorb bile acids in vitro and may be expected to interfere with ursodiol in the same manner as the bile acid sequestering agents. Estrogens, oral contraceptives and clofibrate (and perhaps other liquid-lowering drugs) increase hepatic cholesterol secretion, and encourage cholesterol gallstone formation and hence may counteract the effectiveness of ursodiol.

ADVERSE REACTIONS:

Gastrointestinal: Ursodiol given in doses of 8-10 mg/kg/day rarely causes diarrhea (<1%). One study in which a placebo control was not used was associated with a 6% incidence of mild, transient diarrhea not requiring termination of therapy or lowering of ursodiol dose. One patient with ulcerative colitis in the ursodiol studies developed diarrhea on therapy. In the National Cooperative Gallstone Study, the incidence of diarrhea was 27.1% in the placebo group.

Dermatologic: One patient in the ursodiol studies with preexisting psoriasis apparently developed exacerbation of itching on ursodiol, which remitted on withdrawal of the drug.

Other: In two ongoing double-blind, placebo-controlled ursodiol studies in the U.S., for which the treatment codes have not yet been broken the following minor events have been reported:

Pruritus, rash, urticaria, dry skin, sweating, hair thinning, nausea, vomiting, dyspepsia, metallic taste, abdominal pain, biliary pain, cholecystitis, diarrhea, constipation, stomatitis, flatulence, headache, fatigue, anxiety, depression, sleep disorder, arthralgia, myalgia, back pain, cough, rhinitis.

Since these studies are ongoing and blinded, incidence rates in the ursodiol and placebo groups cannot be calculated, nor has it been established whether the reactions listed are associated with ursodiol.

OVERDOSAGE:

Neither accidental nor intentional overdosing with ursodiol has been reported. Doses of ursodiol in the range of 16-20 mg/kg/day have been tolerated for 6-37 months without symptoms by 7 patients. The LD_{50} for ursodiol in rats is over 5000 mg/kg given over 7-10 days and over 7500 mg/kg for mice. The most likely manifestation of severe overdose with ursodiol would probably be diarrhea, which should be treated symptomatically.

DOSAGE AND ADMINISTRATION:

The recommended dose for ursodiol treatment of radiolucent gallbladder stones is 8-10 mg/kg/day given in 2 or 3 divided doses.

Ultrasound images of the gallbladder should be obtained at 6-month intervals for the first year of ursodiol therapy to monitor gallstone response. If gallstones appear to have dissolved, ursodiol therapy should be continued and dissolution confirmed on a repeat ultrasound examination within 1 to 3 months. Most patients who eventually achieve complete stone dissolution will show partial or complete dissolution at the first on-treatment reevaluation. If partial stone dissolution is not seen by 12 months of ursodiol therapy, the likelihood of success is greatly reduced.

Storage: Do not store above 86° F (30° C).

HOW SUPPLIED - EQUIVALENTS NOT AVAILABLE:

Capsule, Gelatin - Oral - 300 mg

100's	**$207.57**	**ACTIGALL, Novartis**	**57267-0153-30**

VALACYCLOVIR HYDROCHLORIDE *(003265)*

CATEGORIES: Anti-Infectives; Antimicrobials; Antivirals; Fever Blisters; Herpes Genitalis; Herpes Zoster; Infections; Lesions; Varicella; Varicella Zoster; Viral Agents; FDA Class 1S ("Standard Review"); FDA Approved 1995 Jun

BRAND NAMES: **Valtrex**

DESCRIPTION:

Valacyclovir hydrochloride is the hydrochloride salt of L-valyl ester of the antiviral drug acyclovir.

Valtrex caplets are for oral administration. Each caplet contains valacyclovir hydrochloride equivalent to 500 mg valacyclovir and the inactive ingredients carnauba wax, colloidal silicon dioxide, crospovidone, FD&C Blue No. 2 Lake, hydroxypropyl methylcellulose, magnesium stearate, microcrystalline cellulose, polyethylene glycol, polysorbate 80, povidone, and titanium dioxide. The blue, film-coated caplets are printed with edible white ink.

The chemical name of valacyclovir hydrochloride is *L*-valine, 2- [(2-amino-1,6-dihydro-6-oxo-9*H*-purin-9-yl)methoxy]ethyl ester, monohydrochloride.

DESCRIPTION: *(cont'd)*

Valacyclovir hydrochloride is a white to off-white powder with a molecular formula $C_{13}H_{20}N_6O_4$•HCl and a molecular weight of 360.80. The maximum solubility in water at 25°C is 174 mg/ml. The pk_a's for valacyclovir hydrochloride are 1.90, 7.47, and 9.43.

CLINICAL PHARMACOLOGY:

MICROBIOLOGY

Valacyclovir hydrochloride is rapidly converted to acyclovir which has demonstrated antiviral activity against herpes simplex virus types 1 (HSV-1) and 2 (HSV-2) and varicella-zoster virus (VZV) both *in vitro* and *in vivo*. In cell culture, acyclovir's highest antiviral activity is against HSV-1, followed in decreasing order of potency against HSV-2 and VZV.

The inhibitory activity of acyclovir is highly selective due to its affinity for the enzyme thymidine kinase (TK) encoded by HSV, VZV, and EBV. This viral enzyme converts acyclovir into acyclovir monophosphate, a nucleotide analogue. The monophosphate is further converted into diphosphate by cellular guanylate kinase and into triphosphate by a number of cellular enzymes. *In vitro*, acyclovir triphosphate stops replication of herpes viral DNA. This is accomplished in three ways: 1) competitive inhibition of viral DNA polymerase, 2) incorporation and termination of the growing DNA chain, and 3) inactivation of the viral DNA polymerase. The greater antiviral activity of acyclovir against HSV compared to VZV is due to its more efficient phosphorylation by the viral TK.

Antiviral Activities: The quantitative relationship between the *in vitro* susceptibility of herpes viruses to antivirals and the clinical response to therapy has not been established in humans, and virus sensitivity testing has not been standardized. Sensitivity testing results, expressed as the concentration of drug required to inhibit by 50% the growth of virus in cell culture (IC_{50}), vary greatly depending upon a number of factors. Using a plaque-reduction assay, the IC_{50} against herpes simplex virus isolates from 0.02 to 13.5 mcg/ml for HSV-1 and from 0.01 to 9.9 g/ml for HSV-2. The IC_{50} for acyclovir against most laboratory strains and clinical isolates of VZV ranges from 0.12 to 10.8 mcg/ml. Acyclovir also demonstrates activity against the Oka vaccine strain of VZV with a mean IC_{50} of 1.35 mcg/ml.

Drug Resistance: Resistance to VZV to antiviral nucleoside analogues can result from qualitative or quantitative changes in the viral TK or DNA polymerase. Clinical isolates of VZV with reduced susceptibility to acyclovir have been recovered from patients with AIDS. In these cases, TK-deficient mutants of VZV have been recovered.

Resistance of HSV to antiviral necleoside analogues occurs by the same mechanism as resistance to VZV. While most of the acyclovir-resistant mutants isolates thus far from immunocomprimised patients have been found to be TK-deficient mutants, other mutants involving the viral TK gene (TK partial and TK altered) and DNA polymerase have also been isolated. TK-negative mutants may cause severe disease in immunocompromised patients. The possibility of viral resistance to valacyclovir (and therefore acyclovir) should be considered in patients who show poor clinical response during therapy.

After oral administration, valacyclovir hydrochloride is rapidly absorbed from the gastrointestinal tract and nearly completely converted to acyclovir and *L*-valine by first-pass intestinal and/or hepatic metabolism.

PHARMACOKINETICS

The pharmacokinetics of valacyclovir and acyclovir after oral administration of valacyclovir have been investigated in 12 volunteer studies involving 253 adults.

Absorption and Bioavailability: The absolute bioavailability of acyclovir after administration of valacyclovir is 54.5% ± 9.1% as determined following a 1 g oral dose of valacyclovir and a 350 mg intravenous acyclovir dose to 12 healthy volunteers. Acyclovir bioavailability from the administration of valacyclovir is not altered by administration with food (30 minutes after an 873 Kcal breakfast, which included 51 grams of fat).

There was a lack of dose proportionality in acyclovir maximum concentration (C_{max}) and area under the acyclovir concentration-time curve (AUC) after single-dose administration of 100 mg, 250 mg, 500 mg, 750 mg, and 1 g of valacyclovir to eight healthy volunteers. The mean C_{max} (± S.D.) was 0.83 (± 0.14), 2.15 (± 0.50), 3.28 (± 0.83), 4.17 (± 1.14), and 5.65 (± 2.37) mcg/ml, respectively; and the mean AUC (± S.D.) was 2.28 (± 0.40), 5.76 (± 0.60), 11.59 (± 1.79), 14.11 (± 3.54), and 19.52 (± 6.04) hr•mcg/ml, respectively.

There was also a lack of dose proportionality in acyclovir C_{max} and AUC after the multiple-dose administration of 250 mg, 500 mg, and 1 g of valacyclovir administered four times daily for 11 days in parallel groups of eight healthy volunteers. The mean C_{max} (± S.D.) was 2.11 (± 0.33), 3.69 (± 0.87), and 4.96 (± 0.64) mcg/ml, respectively, and the mean AUC (± S.D.) was 5.66 (± 1.09), 9.88 (± 2.01), and 15.70 (± 2.27) hr•mcg/ml, respectively.

There is no accumulation of acyclovir after the administration of valacyclovir at the recommended dosage regimen in healthy volunteers with normal renal function.

Distribution: The binding of valacyclovir to human plasma proteins ranged from 13.5% to 17.9%.

Metabolism: After oral administration, valacyclovir hydrochloride is rapidly absorbed from the gastrointestinal tract. Valacyclovir is rapidly and nearly completely converted to acyclovir and *L*-valine by first-pass intestinal and/or hepatic metabolism. Acyclovir is converted to a small extent to inactive metabolites by aldehyde oxidase and by alcohol and aldehyde dehydrogenase. Neither valacyclovir nor acyclovir metabolism is associated with liver microsomal enzymes. Plasma concentrations of unconverted valacyclovir are low and transient, generally becoming non-quantifiable by 3 hours after administration. Peak plasma valacyclovir concentrations are generally less than 0.5 mcg/ml at all doses. After single-dose administration of 1 g of valacyclovir HCl, average plasma valacyclovir concentrations observed were 0.5, 0.4, and 0.8 mcg/ml in patients with hepatic dysfunction, renal insufficiency, and in healthy volunteers who received concomitant cimetidine and probenecid, respectively.

Elimination: The pharmacokinetic disposition of acyclovir delivered by valacyclovir is consistent with previous experience from intravenous and oral acyclovir. Following the oral administration of a single 1 g dose of radiolabeled valacyclovir to four healthy subjects, 45.60% and 47.12% of administered radioactivity was recovered in urine and feces over 96 hours, respectively. Acyclovir accounted for 88.60% of the radioactivity excreted in the urine. Renal clearance of acyclovir following the administration of a single 1 g dose of valacyclovir HCl to 12 healthy volunteers was approximately 255 ± 86 ml/min which represents 41.9% of total acyclovir apparent plasma clearance.

The plasma elimination half-life of acyclovir typically averaged 2.5 to 3.3 hours in all studies of valacyclovir HCl in volunteers with normal renal function.

End-Stage Renal Disease (ESRD): Following administration of valacyclovir HCl to volunteers with ESRD, the average acyclovir half-life is approximately 14 hours. During hemodialysis, the acyclovir half-life is approximately 4 hours. Approximately one-third of acyclovir in the body is removed by dialysis during a 4-hour hemodialysis session. Apparent plasma clearance of acyclovir in dialysis patients was 86.3 ± 21.3 ml/min/1.73 m^2, compared to 679.16 ± 162.76 ml/min/1.73 m^2 in healthy volunteers.

Reduction in dosage is recommended in patients with renal impairment (see DOSAGE AND ADMINISTRATION.)

CLINICAL PHARMACOLOGY: *(cont'd)*

Geriatrics: After single-dose administration of 1 g of valacyclovir HCl in healthy geriatric volunteers (n=9, mean age ± S.D. = 74.0 ± 5.4 years), the half-life of acyclovir was 3.11 ± 0.51 hours, compared to 2.91 ± 0.63 hours in healthy volunteers (n=33, mean age ± S.D. = 41.2 ± 10.1 years). Dosage modification may be necessary in geriatric patients with reduced renal function (see DOSAGE AND ADMINISTRATION.)

Pediatrics: Valacyclovir pharmacokinetics have not been evaluated in pediatric patients.

Liver Disease: Administration of valacyclovir HCl to patients with moderate (biopsy-proven cirrhosis) or severe (with and without ascites and biopsy-proven cirrhosis) liver disease indicated that the rate but not the extent of conversion of valacyclovir to acyclovir is reduced, and the acyclovir half-life is not affected. Dosage modification is not recommended for patients with cirrhosis.

HIV Disease: In nine patients with advanced HIV disease (CD4 cell counts <150 cells/mm^3) who received valacyclovir HCl at a dosage of 1 g four times daily for 30 days, the pharmacokinetics of valacyclovir and acyclovir were not different from that observed in healthy volunteers (see WARNINGS.)

CLINICAL STUDIES:

Herpes Zoster Infections: Two randomized double-blind clinical trials in immunocompetent patients with localized herpes zoster were conducted. Valacyclovir HCl was compared to placebo in patients less than 50 years of age, and to acyclovir in patients greater than 50 years of age. All patients were treated within 72 hours of appearance of zoster rash. In patients less than 50 years of age, the median time to cessation of new lesion formation was two days for those treated with valacyclovir HCl compared to three days for those treated with placebo. In patients greater than 50 years of age, the median time to cessation of new lesions was three days in patients treated with either valacyclovir HCl or acyclovir. In patients less than 50 years of age, no difference was found with respect to the duration of pain after rash healing (post-herpetic neuralgia) between the recipients of valacyclovir HCl and placebo. In patients greater than 50 years of age who reported pain after rash healing (post-herpetic neuralgia), there was a nonsignificant trend toward a shorter median duration of pain after healing in patients treated with valacyclovir HCl for 7 or 14 days (40 or 43 days) compared to patients treated with acyclovir for 7 days (59 days).

Initial Genital Herpes: In a randomized, double-blind trial, immunocompetent adults with first episode genital herpes who presented within 72 hours of symptom onset were randomized to receive for 10 days valacyclovir hydrochloride 1000 twice daily (n=323) or acyclovir 200 mg 5 times a day (n=320). For both treatment groups; the median time to lesion healing was 9 days, the median time to cessation of pain was 5 days, the median time to cessation of viral shedding was 3 days.

Recurrent Genital Herpes: Two double-blind placebo-controlled trials in immunocompetent patients with recurrent genital herpes were conducted. Patients self-initiated therapy within 24 hours of the first sign or symptom of a recurrent genital herpes episode.

In one study, patients were randomized to receive 5 days of treatment with either valacyclovir hydrochloride 500 mg twice daily (n=360) or placebo (n=259). The median time to lesion healing was 4 days in the group receiving valacyclovir hydrochloride versus 6 days in the placebo group, and the median time to cessation of viral shedding in patients with at least one positive culture (42% of the overall study population) was 2 days in the group receiving valacyclovir hydrochloride 500 mg versus 4 days in the placebo group. The median item to cessation of the pain was 3 days in the group receiving valacyclovir hydrochloride 500 mg versus 4 days in the placebo group. Results supporting efficacy were replicated in a second trial.

INDICATIONS AND USAGE:

Herpes Zoster: Valacyclovir HCl is indicated for the treatment of herpes zoster (shingles).

Genital Herpes: Valacyclovir hydrochloride is indicated for treatment of the initial episode and for the episodic treatment of recurrent genital herpes.

CONTRAINDICATIONS:

Valacyclovir HCl is contraindicated in patients with a known hypersensitivity or intolerance to valacyclovir, acyclovir, or any component of the formulation.

WARNINGS:

Thrombotic thrombocytopenic purpura/hemolytic uremic syndrome (TTP/HUS), in some cases resulting in death, has occurred in patients with advanced HIV disease and also in allogenic bone marrow transplant and renal transplant recipients participating in clinical trials of valacyclovir HCl at doses of 8 grams per day.

PRECAUTIONS:

Efficacy of valacyclovir HCl has not been established for the treatment of disseminated herpes zoster, or suppression of recurrent genital herpes, or in immunocompromised patients.

Dosage adjustment is recommended when administering valacyclovir HCl to patients with renal impairment (see DOSAGE AND ADMINISTRATION.) Caution should also be exercised when administering valacyclovir HCl to patients receiving potentially nephrotoxic agents since this may increase the risk of renal dysfunction and/or the risk of reversible central nervous system symptoms such as those that have been reported in patients treated with intravenous acyclovir.

INFORMATION FOR THE PATIENT

Herpes Zoster: There are no data on treatment initiated more than 72 hours after onset of the zoster rash. Patients should be advised to initiate treatment with valacyclovir HCl as soon as possible after a diagnosis of herpes zoster.

Genital Herpes: Patients should be informed that valacyclovir HCl is not a cure for genital herpes. There are no data evaluating whether valacyclovir HCl will prevent transmission of infection to others. Because genital herpes is a sexually transmitted disease, patients should avoid contact with lesions or intercourse when lesions are present to avoid infecting partners. Genital herpes can also be transmitted in the absence of symptoms through asymptomatic viral shedding. If medical management of a genital herpes recurrence is indicates, patients should be advised to initiate therapy at the first sign or symptom of an episode.

There are no data on the effectiveness of treatment initiated more than 72 hours after the onset of signs and symptoms of a first episode of genital herpes or more than 24 hours of the onset of signs and symptoms of a recurrent episode.

CARCINOGENESIS, MUTAGENESIS, AND IMPAIRMENT OF FERTILITY

The data presented below include references to the peak steady-state acyclovir AUC observed in humans treated with 1 g valacyclovir given orally three times a day to treat herpes zoster. Plasma drug concentrations in animal studies are expressed as multiples of human exposure to acyclovir (see CLINICAL PHARMACOLOGY, Pharmacokinetics.)

Valacyclovir was noncarcinogenic in lifetime carcinogenicity bioassays at single daily doses (gavage) of up to 120 mg/kg/day for mice and 100 mg/kg/day for rats. There was no significant difference in the incidence of tumors between treated and control animals, nor did

PRECAUTIONS: *(cont'd)*

valacyclovir shorten the latency of tumors. Plasma concentrations of acyclovir were equivalent to human levels in the mouse bioassay and 1.4 to 2.3 times human levels in the rat bioassay.

Valacyclovir was tested in five genetic toxicity assays. An Ames assay was negative in the absence or presence of metabolic activation. Also negative were an *in vitro* cytogenetic study with human lymphocytes and a rat cytogenetic study at a single oral dose of 3000 mg/kg (8 to 9 times human plasma levels).

In the mouse lymphoma assay, valacyclovir was negative in the absence of metabolic activation. In the presence of metabolic activation (76% to 88% conversion to acyclovir), valacyclovir was weakly mutagenic.

A mouse micronucleus assay was negative at 250 mg/kg but weakly positive at 500 mg/kg (acyclovir concentrations 26 to 51 times human plasma levels).

Valacyclovir did not impair fertility or reproduction in rats at 200 mg/kg/day (6 times human plasma levels).

PREGNANCY, TERATOGENIC EFFECTS, PREGNANCY CATEGORY B

Valacyclovir was not teratogenic in rats or rabbits given 400 mg/kg (which results in exposures of 10 and 7 times human plasma levels, respectively) during the period of major organogenesis. There are no adequate and well-controlled studies of valacyclovir or acyclovir in pregnant women. A prospective epidemiologic registry of acyclovir use during pregnancy has been ongoing since 1984. As of December 1994, outcomes of live births have been documented in 380 women exposed to systemic acyclovir during the first trimester of pregnancy. The occurrence rate of birth defects approximates that found in the general population. However, the small size of the registry is insufficient to evaluate the risk for less common defects or to permit reliable and definitive conclusions regarding the safety of acyclovir in pregnant women and their developing fetuses. Valacyclovir should be used during pregnancy only if the potential benefit justifies the potential risk to the fetus.

Pregnancy Exposure Registry: To monitor maternal-fetal outcomes of pregnant women exposed to valacyclovir. Glaxo Wellcome maintains a Valacyclovir in Pregnancy Registry. Physicians are encouraged to register their patients by calling (800) 722-9292, ext. 39437.

NURSING MOTHERS

There is no experience with valacyclovir. However, acyclovir concentrations have been documented in breast milk in two women following oral administration of acyclovir and ranged from 0.6 to 4.1 times corresponding plasma levels. These concentrations would potentially expose the nursing infant to a dose of acyclovir as high as 0.3 mg/kg/day. Valacyclovir should be administered to a nursing mother with caution and only when indicated.

PEDIATRIC USE

Safety and effectiveness of valacyclovir in pediatric patients have not been established.

GERIATRIC USE

Of the total number of patients included in clinical studies of valacyclovir, 810 were age 65 or older, and 339 were age 75 or older. A total of 34 volunteers age 65 or older completed a pharmacokinetic trial of valacyclovir. The pharmacokinetics of acyclovir following single- and multiple-dose oral administration of valacyclovir in geriatric volunteers varied with renal function. Dosage reduction may be required in geriatric patients, depending on the underlying renal status of the patient (see CLINICAL PHARMACOLOGY) and DOSAGE AND ADMINISTRATION.

DRUG INTERACTIONS:

The administration of cimetidine and probenecid, separately or together, reduced the rate but not the extent of conversion of valacyclovir to acyclovir. Acyclovir C_{max} was increased 8.4% ± 27.8%, 22.5% ± 25.3%, and 29.6% ± 27.5% by cimetidine, probenecid, and combination treatment (concomitant cimetidine and probenecid administration), respectively. Acyclovir AUC (0 to 24) was increased 31.9% ± 22.9%, 49.0% ± 27.9%, and 77.9% ± 38.6% by cimetidine, probenecid, and combination treatment, respectively. The renal clearance of acyclovir was reduced by approximately 23.5% ± 9.6%, 33.0% ± 10.4%, and 46% ± 11.2% with cimetidine, probenecid, and combination treatment, respectively, resulting in higher plasma acyclovir concentrations. Thiazide diuretics did not affect acyclovir pharmacokinetics after administration of valacyclovir in a geriatric population.

An additive increase in acyclovir AUC and C_{max} was observed when valacyclovir was administered to healthy volunteers who were taking cimetidine, probenecid, or a combination of both cimetidine and probenecid (see CLINICAL PHARMACOLOGY, Pharmacokinetics.)

ADVERSE REACTIONS:

Adverse events reported by greater than 2% of a given treatment group in clinical trials of valacyclovir are listed in TABLES 1A and 1B.

TABLE 1A Incidence (%) of Adverse Events in Herpes Zoster Study Populations

Adverse Event	Valacyclovir HCl 1 g 3 × daily (n = 967)	Acyclovir 800 mg 5 × daily (n = 376)	Placebo (n = 195)
Nausea	15	19	8
Headache	14	13	12
Vomiting	6	8	3
Diarrhea	5	7	6
Constipation	4	5	3
Asthenia	4	5	4
Dizziness	3	6	2
Abdominal Pain	3	3	2
Anorexia	2	3	2

TABLE 1B Incidence (%) of Adverse Events in Genital Herpes Study Populations

Adverse Event	Valacyclovir HCl 1 g 3 × daily (n = 1194)	Valacyclovir HCl 500 mg 2 × daily (n=359)	Acyclovir 800 mg 5 × daily (n = 822)	Placebo (n = 439)
Nausea	6	6	7	8
Headache	16	17	12	14
Vomiting	1	1	2	<1
Diarrhea	4	5	3	6
Constipation	<1	1	1	1
Asthenia	2	1	2	4
Dizziness	3	2	2	3
Abdominal Pain	2	3	2	3
Anorexia	<1	<1	<1	<1

OVERDOSAGE:

There have been no reports of overdosage from the administration of valacyclovir HCl. However, it is known that precipitation of acyclovir in renal tubules may occur when the solubility (2.5 mg/ml) is exceeded in the intratubular fluid. In the event of acute renal failure and anuria, the patient may benefit from hemodialysis until renal function is restored (see DOSAGE AND ADMINISTRATION.)

DOSAGE AND ADMINISTRATION:

Valacyclovir HCl caplets may be given without regard to meals.

HERPES ZOSTER

The recommended dosage of valacyclovir HCl for the treatment of herpes zoster is 1 g (two 500 mg caplets) orally three times daily for 7 days. Therapy should be initiated at the earliest sign or symptom of herpes zoster and is most effective when started within 48 hours of the onset of zoster rash. No data are available on efficacy of treatment started greater than 72 hours after rash onset.

GENITAL HERPES

Initial Episodes: The recommended dosage of valacyclovir for treatment of initial genital herpes is 1 gram twice daily for 10 days.

There are no data on the effectiveness of treatment with valacyclovir when initiated more than 72 hours after the onset of signs and symptoms. Therapy was most effective when administered within 48 hours of the onset of signs and symptoms.

Recurrent Episodes: The recommended dosages of valacyclovir HCl for the treatment of recurrent genital herpes is 500 mg twice daily for 5 days. If medical management of a genital herpes recurrence is indicated, patients should be advised to initiate therapy at the first sign or symptom of an episode. There are no data on the effectiveness of treatment with valacyclovir HCl when initiated more than 24 hours after the onset of signs or symptoms.

Patients with Acute or Chronic Renal Impairment: In patients with reduced renal function, dosage reduction is recommended.

TABLE 2 Dosage Adjustments for Renal Impairment

Creatinine Clearance (ml/min)	Dosage for Herpes Zoster	Dosage for Genital Herpes: Initial Treatment	Recurrent Episodes
≥50	1 g every 8 hours	1 g every 12 hours	500 mg every 12 hours
30 - 49	1 g every 12 hours	1 g every 12 hours	500 mg every 12 hours
10 - 29	1 g every 24 hours	1 g every 24 hours	500 mg every 24 hours
<10	500 mg every 24 hours	500 mg every 24 hours	500 mg every 24 hours

Hemodialysis: During hemodialysis, the half-life of acyclovir after administration of valacyclovir HCl is approximately 4 hours. About one-third of acyclovir in the body is removed by dialysis during a 4-hour hemodialysis session. Patients requiring hemodialysis should receive the recommended dose of valacyclovir HCl after hemodialysis.

Peritoneal Dialysis: There is no information specific to administration of valacyclovir in patients receiving peritoneal dialysis. The effect of chronic ambulatory peritoneal dialysis (CAPD) and continuous arteriovenous hemofiltration/dialysis (CAVHD) on acyclovir pharmacokinetics has been studied. The removal of acyclovir after CAPD and CAVHD is less pronounced than with hemodialysis, and the pharmacokinetic parameters closely resemble those observed in patients with ESRD not receiving hemodialysis. Therefore, supplemental doses of valacyclovir should not be required following CAPD or CAVHD.

HOW SUPPLIED:

Valtrex caplets (blue, film-coated, capsule-shaped tablets) containing valacyclovir hydrochloride equivalent to 500 mg valacyclovir and printed with "Valtrex 500 mg".

Store at 15° to 25°C (59° to 77°F).

HOW SUPPLIED - EQUIVALENTS NOT AVAILABLE:

Tablet, Uncoated - Oral - 500 mg

42's	$115.92	VALTREX, Glaxo Wellcome	00173-0933-03
100's	$282.00	VALTREX, Glaxo Wellcome	00173-0933-56

VALPROATE SODIUM *(003326)*

CATEGORIES: Anticonvulsants; Antiepileptics; Bipolar Disorder; Central Nervous System Agents; Convulsions; Epilepsy; FDA Approved 1997 Jan; Pregnancy Category D; Seizures; Valproic Acid Derivatives

BRAND NAMES: **Depacon**; *Depakene* (Japan); *Depakin*; *Depakine* (France); *Depakine Chrono*; *Depakine Druppels*; *Depalept*; *Encorate*; *Epilim* (Australia); *Epilim Chrono*; *Leptilan*; *Orfil*; *Orfiril*; *Petilin*; *Valcote*; *Valeptol*; *Valoin*; *Valpakine*; *Valparin*; *Valporal*; *Valpro* (Australia); *Valprolan*; *Valproline ECT*
(International brand names outside U.S. in italics)

WARNING:
HEPATIC FAILURE RESULTING IN FATALITIES HAS OCCURRED IN PATIENTS RECEIVING VALPROIC ACID AND ITS DERIVATIVES. EXPERIENCE HAS INDICATED THAT CHILDREN UNDER THE AGE OF TWO YEARS ARE AT A CONSIDERABLY INCREASED RISK OF DEVELOPING FATAL HEPATOTOXICITY, ESPECIALLY THOSE ON MULTIPLE ANTICONVULSANTS, THOSE WITH CONGENITAL METABOLIC DISORDERS, THOSE WITH SEVERE SEIZURE DISORDERS ACCOMPANIED BY MENTAL RETARDATION, AND THOSE WITH ORGANIC BRAIN DISEASE. WHEN VALPROATE SODIUM FOR INJECTION IS USED IN THIS PATIENT GROUP, IT SHOULD BE USED WITH EXTREME CAUTION AND AS A SOLE AGENT. THE BENEFITS OF THERAPY SHOULD BE WEIGHED AGAINST THE RISKS. ABOVE THIS AGE GROUP, EXPERIENCE IN EPILEPSY HAS INDICATED THAT THE INCIDENCE OF FATAL HEPATOTOXICITY DECREASES CONSIDERABLY IN PROGRESSIVELY OLDER PATIENT GROUPS.
THESE INCIDENTS USUALLY HAVE OCCURRED DURING THE FIRST SIX MONTHS OF TREATMENT. SERIOUS OR FATAL HEPATOTOXICITY MAY BE PRECEDED BY NON-SPECIFIC SYMPTOMS SUCH AS MALAISE, WEAKNESS, LETHARGY, FACIAL EDEMA, ANOREXIA, AND VOMITING. IN PATIENTS WITH EPILEPSY, A

LOSS OF SEIZURE CONTROL MAY ALSO OCCUR. PATIENTS SHOULD BE MONITORED CLOSELY FOR APPEARANCE OF THESE SYMPTOMS. LIVER FUNCTION TESTS SHOULD BE PERFORMED PRIOR TO THERAPY AND AT FREQUENT INTERVALS THEREAFTER, ESPECIALLY DURING THE FIRST SIX MONTHS.

Teratogenicity: VALPROATE CAN PRODUCE TERATOGENIC EFFECTS SUCH AS NEURAL TUBE DEFECTS (*e.g.,* SPINA BIFIDA). ACCORDINGLY, THE USE OF VALPROATE PRODUCTS IN WOMEN OF CHILDBEARING POTENTIAL REQUIRES THAT THE BENEFITS OF ITS USE BE WEIGHED AGAINST THE RISK OF INJURY TO THE FETUS.

DESCRIPTION:

Valproate sodium is the sodium salt of valproic acid designated as sodium 2-propylpentanoate. Valproate sodium has a molecular weight of 166.2. It occurs as an essentially white and odorless, crystalline, deliquescent powder.

Depacon solution is available in 5 ml single-dose vials for intravenous injection. Each ml contains valproate sodium equivalent to 100 mg valproic acid, edetate disodium 0.40 mg, and water for injection to volume. The pH is adjusted to 7.6 with sodium hydroxide and/or hydrochloric acid. The solution is clear and colorless.

CLINICAL PHARMACOLOGY:

Valproate sodium exists as the valproate ion in the blood. The mechanisms by which valproate exerts its therapeutic effects have not been established. It has been suggested that its activity in epilepsy is related to increased brain concentrations of gamma-aminobutyric acid (GABA).

PHARMACOKINETICS

Bioavailability

Equivalent doses of intravenous (IV) valproate and oral valproate products are expected to result in equivalent C_{max}, C_{min}, and total systemic exposure to the valproate ion. However, the rate of valproate ion absorption may vary with the formulation used. These differences should be of minor clinical importance under the steady state conditions achieved in chronic use in the treatment of epilepsy.

Administration of divalproex sodium tablets and IV valproate (given as a one hour infusion), 250 mg every 6 hours for 4 days to 18 healthy male volunteers resulted in equivalent AUC, C_{max}, C_{min} as steady state, as well as after the first dose. The T_{max} after IV valproate sodium occurs at the end of the one hour infusion, while the T_{max} after oral dosing with divalproex sodium occurs at approximately 4 hours. Because the kinetics of unbound valproate are linear, bioequivalence between valproate sodium and divalproex sodium up to the maximum recommended dose of 60 mg/kg/day can be assumed. The AUC and C_{max} resulting from administration of IV valproate 500 mg as a single one hour infusion and a single 500 mg dose of valproic acid syrup to 17 healthy male volunteers were also equivalent.

Patients maintained on valproic acid doses of 750 mg to 4250 mg daily (given in divided doses every 6 hours) as oral divalproex sodium alone (n=24) or with another stabilized antiepileptic drug [carbamazepine (n=15), phenytoin (n=11), or phenobarbital (n=1)], showed comparable plasma levels for valproic acid when switching from oral divalproex sodium to IV valproate (1-hour infusion).

Distribution

Protein Binding: The plasma protein binding of valproate is concentration dependent and the free fraction increases from approximately 10% at 40 mcg/ml to 18.5% at 130 mcg/ml. Protein binding of valproate is reduced in the elderly, in patients with chronic hepatic diseases, in patients with renal impairment, and in the presence of other drugs (*e.g.,* aspirin). Conversely, valproate may displace certain protein-bound drugs (*e.g.,* phenytoin, carbamazepine, warfarin, and tolbutamide). (See DRUG INTERACTIONS for more detailed information on the pharmacokinetic interactions of valproate with other drugs.)

CNS Distribution: Valproate concentration in cerebrospinal fluid (CSF) approximate unbound concentrations in plasma (about 10% of total concentration).

Metabolism

Valproate is metabolized almost entirely by the liver. In adult patients on monotherapy, 30-50% of an administered dose appears in urine as a glucuronide conjugate. Mitochondrial β-oxidation is the other major metabolic pathway, typically accounting for over 40% of the dose. Usually, less than 15-20% of the dose is eliminated by other oxidative mechanisms. Less than 3% of an administered dose is excreted unchanged in urine.

The relationship between dose and total valproate concentration is nonlinear; concentration does not increase proportionally with the dose, but rather, increases to a lesser extent due to saturable plasma protein binding. The kinetics of unbound drug are linear.

Elimination

Mean plasma clearance and volume of distribution for total valproate are 0.56 L/hr/1.73 m^2 and 11 L/1.73 m^2, respectively. Mean terminal half-life for valproate monotherapy after a 60 minute intravenous infusion of 1000 mg was 16 ± 3.0 hours.

The estimates cited apply primarily to patients who are not taking drugs that affect hepatic metabolizing enzyme systems. For example, patients taking enzyme-inducing antepileptic drugs (carbamazepine, phenytoin, and phenobarbital) will clear valproate more rapidly. Because of these changes in valproate clearance, monitoring of antiepileptic concentrations should be intensified whenever concomitant antiepileptics are introduced or withdrawn.

Special Populations

Neonates: Children within the first two months of life have a markedly decreased ability to eliminate valproate compared to older children and adults. This is a result of reduced clearance (perhaps due to delay in development of glucuronosyl transferase and other enzyme systems involved in valproate elimination) as well as increased volume of distribution (in part due to decreased plasma protein binding). For example, in one study, the half-life in children under 10 days ranged from 10 to 67 hours compared to a range of 7 to 13 hours in children greater than 2 months.

Children: Pediatric patients (*i.e.,* between 3 months and 10 years) have 50% higher clearances expressed on weight (*i.e.,* ml/min/kg) than do adults. Over the age of 10 years, children have pharmacokinetic parameters that approximate those of adults.

Elderly: The capacity of elderly patients (age range: 68 to 89 years) to eliminate valproate has been shown to be reduced compared to younger adults (age range: 22 to 26). Intrinsic clearance is reduced by 39%; the free fraction is increased by 44%. Accordingly, the initial dosage should be reduced in the elderly. (See DOSAGE AND ADMINISTRATION.)

Gender: There are no differences in the body surface area adjusted unbound clearance between males and females (4.8 ± 0.17 and 4.7 ± 0.07 L/hr/1.73 m^2, respectively).

Race: The effects of race on the kinetics of valproate have not been studied.

Liver Disease: (See BOXED WARNING, CONTRAINDICATIONS, WARNINGS.) Liver disease impairs the capacity to eliminate valproate. In one study, the clearance of free valproate was decreased by 50% in 7 patients with cirrhosis and by 16% in 4 patients with acute hepatitis, compared with 6 healthy subjects. In that study, the half-life of valproate was increased from 12 to 18 hours. Liver disease is also associated with decreased albumin concentrations and larger unbound fractions (2 to 2.6 fold increase) of valproate. Accordingly, monitoring of total concentrations may be misleading since free concentrations may be substantially elevated in patients with hepatic disease whereas total concentrations may appear to be normal.

Renal Disease: A slight reduction (27%) in the unbound clearance of valproate has been reported in patients with renal failure (creatinine clearance <10 ml/minute); however, hemodialysis typically reduces valproate concentrations by about 20%. Therefore, no dosage adjustment appears to be necessary in patients with renal failure. Protein binding in these patients is substantially reduced; thus, monitoring total concentrations may be misleading.

PLASMA LEVELS AND CLINICAL EFFECT

The relationship between plasma concentration and clinical response is not well documented. One contributing factor is the nonlinear, concentration dependent protein binding of valproate which affects the clearance of the drug. Thus, monitoring of total serum valproate cannot provide a reliable index of the bioactive valproate species.

For example, because the plasma protein binding of valproate is concentration dependent, the free fraction increases from approximately 10% at 40 mcg/ml to 18.5% at 130 mcg/ml. Higher than expected free fractions occur in the elderly, in hyperlipidemic patients, and in patients with hepatic and renal diseases.

Epilepsy: The therapeutic range in epilepsy is commonly considered to be 50 to 100 mcg/ml of total valproate, although some patients may be controlled with lower or higher plasma concentrations.

Equivalent doses of valproate sodium and divalproex sodium yield equivalent plasma levels of the valproate ion (see Pharmacokinetics).

CLINICAL STUDIES:

The studies described in the following section were conducted with oral divalproex sodium products.

EPILEPSY

The efficacy of divalproex sodium in reducing the incidence of complex partial seizures (CPS) that occur in isolation or in association with other seizure types was established in two controlled trials.

In one, multiclinic, placebo controlled study employing an add-on design (adjunctive therapy), 144 patients who continued to suffer eight or more CPS per 8 weeks during an 8 week period of monotherapy withdoses of either carbamazepine or phenytoin sufficient to assure plasma concentrations within the "therapeutic range" were randomized to receive, in addition to their original antiepilepsy drug (AED), either divalproex sodium or placebo. Randomized patients were to be followed for a total of 16 weeks. TABLE 1 presents the findings.

TABLE 1 Adjunctive Therapy Study Median Median Incidence of CPS per 8 Weeks

Add-on Treatment	Number of Patients	Baseline Incidence	Experimental Incidence
Divalproex Sodium	75	16.0	8.9*
Placebo	69	14.5	11.5

* Reduction from baseline statistically significantly greater for divalproex sodium than placebo at p ≤0.05 level.

This study shows that the proportion of patients achieving any particular level of improvement was consistently higher for divalproex sodium than for placebo. For example, 45% of patients treated with divalproex sodium had a ≥50% reduction in complex partial seizure rate compared to 23% of patients treated with placebo.

The second study assessed the capacity of divalproex sodium to reduce the incidence of CPS when administered as the sole AED. The study compared the incidence of CPS among patients randomized to either a high or low dose treatment arm. Patients qualified for entry into the randomized comparison phase of this study only if 1) they continued to experience 2 or more CPS per 4 weeks during an 8 to 12 week long period of monotherapy with adequate doses of AED (*i.e.,* phenytoin, carbamazepine, phenobarbital, or primidone) and 2) they made a successful transition over a two week interval to divalproex sodium. Patients entering the randomized phase were then brought to their assigned target dose, gradually tapered off their concomitant AED and followed for an interval as long as 22 weeks. Less than 50% of the patients randomized, however, completed the study. In patients converted to divalproex sodium monotherapy, the mean total valproate concentrations during monotherapy were 71 and 123 mcg/ml in the low dose and high dose groups, respectively.

TABLE 2 presents the findings for all patients randomized who had at least one post-randomization assessment.

TABLE 2 Monotherapy Study Median Incidence of CPS Per 8 Weeks

Treatment	Number of Patients	Baseline Incidence	Randomized Phase Incidence
High dose divalproex sodium	131	13.2	10.7*
Low dose divalproex sodium	134	14.2	13.8

* Reduction from baseline statistically greater for high dose than low dose at p ≤0.05 level.

This study shows that the proportion of patients achieving any particular level of reduction was consistently higher for high dose divalproex sodium than for low dose divalproex sodium. For example, when switching from carbamazepine, phenytoin, phenobarbital, or primidone monotherapy to high dose divalproex sodium monotherapy, 63% of patients experienced no change or a reduction in complex partial seizure rates compared to 54% of patients receiving low dose divalproex sodium.

INDICATIONS AND USAGE:

Valproate sodium injection is indicated as an intravenous alternative in patients for whom oral administration of valproate products is temporarily not feasible in the following conditions:

Valproate sodium is indicated as monotherapy and adjunctive therapy in the treatment of patients with complex partial seizures that occur either in isolation or in association with other types of seizures.

Valproate sodium is also indicated for use as sole and adjunctive therapy in the treatment of patients with simple and complex absence seizures, and adjunctively in patients with multiple seizure types that include absence seizures.

Simple absence is defined as very brief clouding of the sensorium or loss of consciousness accompanied by certain generalized epileptic discharges without detectable clinical signs. Complex absence is the term used when other signs are also present. (SEE WARNINGS FOR STATEMENT REGARDING FATAL HEPATIC DYSFUNCTION.)

CONTRAINDICATIONS:

VALPROATE SODIUM INJECTION SHOULD NOT BE ADMINISTERED TO PATIENTS WITH HEPATIC DISEASE OR SIGNIFICANT HEPATIC DYSFUNCTION.

Valproate sodium injection is contraindicated in patients with known hypersensitivity to the drug.

WARNINGS:

Hepatic failure resulting in fatalities has occurred in patients receiving valproic acid. These incidents usually have occurred during the first six months of treatment. Serious or fatal hepatotoxicity may be preceded by non-specific symptoms such as malaise, weakness, lethargy, facial edema, anorexia, and vomiting. In patients with epilepsy, a loss of seizure control may also occur. Patients should be monitored closely for appearance of these symptoms. Liver function tests should be performed prior to thereapy and at frequent intervals thereafter, especially during the first six months of valproate therapy. However, physicans should not rely totally on serum biochemistry since these tests may not be abnormal in all instances, but should also consider the result of careful interim medical history and physical examination.

Caution should be observed when administering valproate products to patients with a prior history of hepatic disease. Patients on multiple anticonvulsants, children, those with congenital metabolic disorders, those with severe seizure disorders accompanied by mental retardation, and those with organic brain disease may be at particular risk. Experience has indicated that children under the age of two years are at a considerably increased risk of developing fatal hepatotoxicity, especially those with the aforementioned conditions. When valproate sodium is used in this patient group, it should be used with extreme caution and as a sole agent. The benefits of therapy should be weighed against the risks. Use of valproate sodium has not been studied in children below the age of 2 years. Above this age group, experience with valproate products in epilepsy has indicated that the incidence of fatal hepatotoxicity decreases considerably in progressively older patient groups.

The drug should be discontinued immediately in the presence of significant hepatic dysfunction, suspected or apparent. In some cases, hepatic dysfunction has progressed in spite of discontinuation of drug.

The frequency of adverse effects (particularly elevated liver enzymes and thrombocytopenia [see PRECAUTIONS]) may be dose-related. In a clinical trial of divalproex sodium as monotherapy in patients with epilepsy, 34/126 patients (27%) receiving approximately 50 mg/kg/day on average, had at least one value of platelets $\leq 75 \times 10^9$/L. Approximately half of these patients had treatment discontinued, with return of platelet counts to normal. In the remaining patients, platelet counts normalized with continued treatment. In this study, the probability of thrombocytopenia appeared to increase significantly at total valproate concentrations of ≥110 mcg/ml (females) or ≥135 mcg/ml (males). The therapeutic benefit which may accompany the higher doses should therefore be weighed against the possibility of a greater incidence of adverse effects.

A study was conducted to evaluate the effect of IV valproate in the prevention of post-traumatic seizures in patients with acute head injuries. Patients were randomly assigned to receive either IV valproate given for one week (followed by oral valproate products for either one or six months per random treatment assignment) or IV phenytoin given for one week (followed by placebo). In this study, the incidence of death was found to be higher in the two groups assigned to valproate treatment compared to the rate in those assigned to the IV phenytoin treatment group (13% vs 8.5%, respectively). Many of these patients were critically ill with multiple and/or severe injuries, and evaluation of the causes of death did not suggest any specific drug-related causation. Further, in the absence of a concurrent placebo control during the initial week of intravenous therapy, it is impossible to determine if the mortality rate in the patients treated with valproate with greater or less than that expected in a similar group not treated with valproate, or whether the rate seen the IV phenytoin treated patients was lower than would be expected. Nonetheless, until further information is available, it seems prudent not to use valproate sodium in patients with acute head trauma for the prophylaxis of post-traumatic seizures.

USAGE IN PREGNANCY

ACCORDING TO PUBLISHED AND UNPUBLISHED REPORTS, VALPROIC ACID MAY PRODUCE TERATOGENIC EFFECTS IN THE OFFSPRING OF HUMAN FEMALES RECEIVING THE DRUG DURING PREGNANCY.

THERE ARE MULTIPLE REPORTS IN THE CLINICAL LITERATURE WHICH INDICATE THAT THE USE OF ANTIEPILEPSY DRUGS DURING PREGNANCY RESULT IN AN INCREASED INCIDENCE OF BIRTH DEFECTS IN THE OFFSPRING. ALTHOUGH DATA ARE MORE EXTENSIVE WITH RESPECT TO TRIMETHADIONE, PARAMETHADIONE, PHENYTOIN, AND PHENOBARBITAL, REPORTS INDICATE A POSSIBLE SIMILAR ASSOCIATION WITH THE USE OF OTHER ANTIEPILEPSY DRUGS. THEREFORE, ANTIEPILEPSY DRUGS SHOULD BE ADMINISTERED TO WOMEN OF CHILDBEARING POTENTIAL ONLY IF THEY ARE CLEARLY SHOWN TO BE ESSENTIAL IN THE MANAGEMENT OF THEIR SEIZURES.

THE INCIDENCE OF NEURAL TUBE DEFECTS IN THE FETUS MAY BE INCREASED IN MOTHERS RECEIVING VALPROATE DURING THE FIRST TRIMESTER OF PREGNANCY. THE CENTERS FOR DISEASE CONTROL (CDC) HAS ESTIMATED THE RISK OF VALPROIC ACID EXPOSED WOMEN HAVING CHILDREN WITH SPINA BIFIDA TO BE APPROXIMATELY 1 TO 2%.

OTHER CONGENITAL ANOMALIES (*e.g.*, CRANIOFACIAL DEFECTS, CARDIOVASCULAR MALFORMATIONS, AND ANOMALIES INVOLVING VARIOUS BODY SYSTEMS), COMPATIBLE AND INCOMPATIBLE WITH LIFE, HAVE BEEN REPORTED. SUFFICIENT DATA TO DETERMINE THE INCIDENCE OF THESE CONGENITAL ANOMALIES IS NOT AVAILABLE.

THE HIGHER INCIDENCE OF CONGENITAL ANOMALIES IN ANTIEPILEPSY DRUG-TREATED WOMEN WITH SEIZURE DISORDERS CANNOT BE REGARDED AS A CAUSE AND EFFECT RELATIONSHIP. THERE ARE INTRINSIC METHODOLOGIC PROBLEMS IN OBTAINING ADEQUATE DATA ON DRUG TERATOGENICITY IN HUMANS; GENETIC FACTORS OR THE EPILEPTIC CONDITION ITSELF, MAY BE MORE IMPORTANT THAN DRUG THERAPY IN CONTRIBUTING TO CONGENITAL ANOMALIES.

PATIENTS TAKING VALPROATE MAY DEVELOP CLOTTING ABNORMALITIES. A PATIENT WHO HAD LOW FIBRINOGEN WHEN TAKING MULTIPLE ANTICONVULSANTS INCLUDING VALPROATE GAVE BIRTH TO AN INFANT WITH AFIBRINOGENEMIA WHO SUBSEQUENTLY DIED OF HEMORRHAGE. IF VALPROATE IS USED IN PREGNANCY THE CLOTTING PARAMETERS SHOULD BE MONITORED CAREFULLY.

HEPATIC FAILURE RESULTING IN THE DEATH OF A NEWBORN AND OF AN INFANT, HAVE BEEN REPORTED FOLLOWING THE USE OF VALPROATE DURING PREGNANCY.

Animal studies have demonstrated valproate-induced teratogenicity. Increased frequencies of malformations as well as intrauterine growth retardation and death, have been observed in mice, rats, rabbits, and monkeys following prenatal exposure to valproate. Malformations of the skeletal system are the most common structural abnormalities produced in experimental animals, but neural tube closure defects have been seen in mice exposed to maternal plasma valproate concentrations exceeding 230 mcg/ml (2.3 times the upper limit of the human therapeutic range) during susceptible periods of embryonic development. Administration of an oral dose of 200 mg/kg/day or greater (50% of the maximum human daily dose or greater on a mg/m^2 basis) to pregnant rats during organogenesis produced malformations (skeletal, cardiac, and urogenital) and growth retardation in the offspring. These doses resulted the peak maternal plasma valproate levels of approximately 340 mcg/ml or greater (3.4 times the upper limit of the human therapeutic range or greater). Behavioral deficits have been reported in the offspring of rats given a dose of 200 mg/kg/day throughout most of pregnancy. An oral dose of 350 mg/kg/day (2 times the maximum human daily dose on a mg/m^2 basis) produced skeletal and visceral malformations in rabbits exposed during organogenesis. Skeletal malformations, growth retardation, and death were observed in rhesus monkeys following administration of an oral dose of 200 mg/kg/day (equal to the maximum human daily dose on a mg/m^2 basis) during organogenesis. This dose resulted in peak maternal plasma valproate levels of approximately 280 mcg/ml (2.8 times the upper limit of the human therapeutic range).

The prescribing physician will wish to weigh the benefits of therapy against the risks in treating or counseling women of childbearing potential. If this drug is used during pregnancy, or if the patient becomes pregnant while taking this drug, the patient should be apprised of the potential hazard to the fetus.

Antiepilepsy drugs should not be discontinued abruptly in patients in whom the drug is administered to prevent major seizures because of the strong possibility of precipitating status epilepticus with attendant hypoxia and threat to life. In individual cases where the severity and frequency of the seizure disorder are such that the removal of medication does not pose a serious threat to the patient, discontinuation of the drug may be considered prior to and during pregnancy, although it cannot be said with any confidence that even minor seizures do not pose some hazard to the developing embryo or fetus.

Tests to detect neural tube and other defects using current accepted procedures should be considered a part of routine prenatal care in childbearing women receiving valproate.

PRECAUTIONS:

HEPATIC DYSFUNCTION

See BOXED WARNING, CONTRAINDICATIONS, WARNINGS.

GENERAL

Because of reports of thrombocytopenia (see WARNINGS), inhibition of the secondary phase of platelet aggregation, and abnormal coagulation parameters, (*e.g.*, low fibrinogen), platelet counts and coagulation tests are recommended before initiating therapy and at periodic intervals. It is recommended that patients receiving valproate sodium be monitored for platelet count and coagulation parameters prior to planned surgery. In a clinical trial of divalproex sodium as monotherapy in patients with epilepsy, 34/126 patients (27%) receiving approximately 50 mg/kg/day on average, had at least one value of platelets $\leq 75 \times 10^9$/L. Approximately half of these patients had treatment discontinued, with return of platelet counts to normal. In the remainng patients, platlet counts normalized with continued treatment. In this study, the probability of thrombocytopenia appeared to increase significantly at total valproate concentrations of ≥110 mcg/ml (females) or ≥135 mcg/ml (males). Evidence of hemorrhage, bruising, or a disorder of hemostasis/coagulation is an indication for reduction of the dosage or withdrawal of therapy.

Hyperammonemia with or without lethargy or coma has been reported and may be present in the absence of abnormal liver function tests. Asymptomatic elevations of ammonia are more common and when present require more frequent monitoring. If clinically significant symptoms occur, valproate sodium therapy should be modified or discontinued.

Since valproate sodium may interact with concurrently administered drugs which are capable of enzyme induction, periodic plasma concentration determinations of valproate and concomitant drugs are recommended during the early course of therapy. (See DRUG INTERACTIONS.)

Valproate is partially eliminated in the urine as a keto-metabolite which may lead to false interpretation of the urine ketone test.

There have been reports of altered thyroid function tests associated with valproate. The clinical significance of these is unknown.

INFORMATION FOR THE PATIENT

Since valproate sodium may produce CNS depression, especially when combined with another CNS depressant (*e.g.*, alcohol) patients should be advised not to engage in hazardous activities, such as driving an automobile or operating machinery, until it is known that they do not become drowsy from the drug.

CARCINOGENESIS, MUTAGENESIS, AND IMPAIRMENT OF FERTILITY

Carcinogenesis: Valproic acid was administered orally to Sprague Dawley rats and ICR (HA/ICR) mice at doses of 80 and 170 mg/kg/day (approximately 10 to 50% of the maximum human daily dose on a mg/m^2 basis) for two years. A variety of neoplasms were observed in both species. The chief findings were a statistically significant increase in the incidence of subcutaneous fibrosarcomas in high dose male rats receiving valpoic acid and a statically significant dose-related trend for benign pulmonary adenomas in male mice receiving valproic acid. The significance of these findings for humans is unknown.

Mutagenesis: Valproate was not mutagenic in an *in vivo* bacterial assay (Ames test), did not produce dominant lethal effects in mice, and did not increase chromosome aberration frequency in an *in vivo* cytogenic study in rats. Increased frequencies of sister chromatid exchange (SCE) have been reported in a study of epileptic children taking valproate, but this association was not observed in another study conducted in adults. There is some evidence that increase SCE frequencies may be associated with epilepsy. The biological significance of an increase in SCE frequency is not known.

Fertility: Chronic toxicity studies in juvenile and adult rats and dogs demonstrated reduced spermatogenesis and testicular atrophy at oral doses of 400 mg/kg/day or greater in rats (approximately equivalent to or greater than the maximum human daily dose on a mg/m^2 basis) and 150 mg/kg/day or greater in dogs (approximately 1.4 times the maximum human daily dose or greater on a mg/m^2 basis). Segment I fertility studies in rats have shown oral doses up to 350 mg/kg/day (approximately equal to the maximum human daily dose on a mg/m^2 basis) for 60 days to have no effect on fertility. THE EFFECT OF VALPROATE ON TESTICULAR DEVELOPMENT AND ON SPERM PRODUCTION AND FERTILITY IN HUMANS IS UNKNOWN.

PREGNANCY CATEGORY D

See WARNINGS.

NURSING MOTHERS

Valproate is excreted in breast milk. Concentratons in breast milk have been reported to be 1-10% of serum concentrations. It is not known what effect this would have on a nursing infant. Consideration should be given to discontinuing nursing when valproate is administered to a nursing woman.

PEDIATRIC USE

Experience with oral valproate has indicated that children under the age of two years are at a considerably increased risk of developing fatal hepatotoxicity, especially those with the aforementioned conditions (see BOXED WARNING). The safety of valproate sodium has not been studied in individual below the age of 2 years. If a decision is made to use valproate

PRECAUTIONS: *(cont'd)*

sodium in this age group, it should be used with extreme caution and as a sole agent. The benefits of therapy should be weighed against the risks. Above the age of 2 years, experience in epilepsy has indicated that the incidence of fatal hepatotoxicity decreases considerably in progressively older patient groups.

Younger children, especially those receiving enzyme-inducing drugs, will require larger maintenance doses to attain targeted total and unbound valproic acid concentrations.

The variability in free fraction limits the clinical usefulness of monitoring total serum valproic acid concentrations. Interpretation of valproic acid concentrations in children should include consideration of factors that affect hepatic metabolism and protein binding.

No unique safety concerns were identified in the 24 patients age 2 to 17 years who received valproate acid in clinical trials.

The basic toxicology and pathologic manifestations of valproate sodium in neonatal (4-day old) and juvenile (14-day old) rats are similar to those seen in young adult rats. However, additional findings, including renal alterations in juvenile rats and renal alterations and retinal dyspalsia in neonatal rats, have been reported. These findings occurred at 240 mg/kg/day, a dosage approximately equivalent to the human maximum recommended daily dose on a mg/m^2 basis. They were not seen at 90 mg/kg, or 40% of the maximum human daily dose on a mg/m^2 basis.

GERIATRIC USE

No unique safety concerns were identified in the 19 patients >65 years of age receiving valproate sodium in clinical trials.

DRUG INTERACTIONS:

EFFECTS OF CO-ADMINISTERED DRUGS ON VALPROATE CLEARANCE

Drugs that affect the level of expression of hepatic enzymes, particularly those that elevate levels of glucuronosyl transferases, may increase the clearance of valproate. For example, phenytoin, carbamazepine, and phenobarbital (or primidone) can double the clearance of valproate. Thus, patients on monotherapy will generally have longer half-lives and higher concentrations than patients receiving polytherapy with antiepilepsy drugs.

In contrast, drugs that are inhibitors of cytochrome P450 isozymes, (*e.g.,* antidepressants), may be expected to have little effect on valproate clearance because cytochrome P450 microsomal mediated oxidation is a relatively minor secondary metabolic pathway compared to glucuronidation and beta-oxidation.

Because of these changes in valproate clearance, monitoring of valproate and concomitant drug concentrations should be increased whenever enzyme inducing drugs are introduced or withdrawn.

The following list provides information about the potential for an influence of several commonly prescribed medications on valproate pharmacokinetics. The list is not exhaustive nor could it be, since new interactions are continuously being reported.

DRUGS FOR WHICH A POTENTIALLY IMPORTANT INTERACTION HAS BEEN OBSERVED

Aspirin: A study involving the co-administration of aspirin at antipyretic doses (11 to 16 mg/kg) with valproate to pediatric patients (n=6) revealed a decrease in protein binding and an inhibition of metabolism of valproate. Valproate free fraction was increased 4-fold in the presence of aspirin compared to valproate alone. The β-oxidation pathway consisting of 2-E-valproic acid, 3-OH-valproic acid, and 3-keto valproic acid was decreased from 25% of total metabolites excreted on valproate alone to 8.3% in the presence of aspirin. Caution should be observed if valproate and aspirin are to be co-administered.

Felbamate: A study involving the co-administration of 1200 mg/day of felbamate with valproate to patients with epilepsy (n=10) revealed an increase in mean valproate peak concentration by 35% (from 86 to 115 mcg/ml) compared to valproate alone. Increasing the felbamate dose to 2400 mg/day increased the mean valproate peak concentration to 133 mcg/ml (another 16% increase). A decrease in valproate dosage may be necessary when felbamate therapy is initiated.

Rifampin: A study involving the administration of a single dose of valproate (7 mg/kg) 36 hours after 5 nights of daily dosing with rifampin (600 mg) revealed a 40% increase in the oral clearance of valproate. Valproate dosage adjustment may be necessary when it is co-administered with rifampin.

DRUGS FOR WHICH EITHER NO INTERACTION OR A LIKELY CLINICALLY UNIMPORTANT INTERACTION HAS BEEN OBSERVED

Antacids: A study involving the co-administration of valproate 500 mg with commonly administered antacids (Maalox, Trisogel, and Titralac - 160 mEq doses) did not reveal any effect on the extent of absorption of valproate.

Chlorpromazine: A study involving the administration of 100 to 300 mg/day of chlorpromazine to schizophrenic patients already receiving valproate (200 mg twice a day) revealed a 15% increase in trough plasma levels of valproate.

Haloperidol: A study involving the administration of 6 to 10 mg/day of haloperidol to schizophrenic patients already receiving valproate (200 mg twice a day) revealed no significant changes in valproate trough plasma levels.

Cimetidine and Ranitidine: Cimetidine and ranitidine do not affect the clearance of valproate.

EFFECTS OF VALPROATE ON OTHER DRUGS

Valproate has been found to be a weak inhibitor of some P450 isozymes, epoxide hydrase, and glucuronyl transferases.

The following list provides information about the potential for an influence of valproate co-administration on the pharmacokinetics or pharmacodynamics of several commonly prescribed medications. The list is not exhaustive, since new interactions are continuously being reported.

DRUGS FOR WHICH A POTENTIALLY IMPORTANT VALPROATE INTERACTION HAS BEEN OBSERVED

Carbamazepine/Carbamazepine-10, 11-Epoxide: Serum levels of carbamazepine (CBZ) decreased 17% while that of carbamazepine-10, 11-epoxide (CBZ-E) increased by 45% upon co-administration of valproate and CBZ to epileptic patients.

Clonazepam: The concomitant use of valproic acid and clonazepam may induce absence status in patients with a history of absence type seizures.

Diazepam: Valproate displaces diazepam from its plasma albumin binding sites and inhibits its metabolism. Co-administration of valproate (1500 mg daily) increased the free fraction of diazepam (10 mg) by 90% in healthy volunteers (n=6). Plasma clearance and volume of distribution for free diazepam were reduced by 25% and 20%, respectively, in the presence of valproate. The elimination half-life of diazepam remained unchanged upon addition of valproate.

Ethosuximide: Valproate inhibits the metabolism of ethosuximide. Administration of a single ethosuximide dose of 500 mg with valproate (800 to 1600 mg/day) to healthy volunteers (n=6) was accompanied by a 25% increase in elimination half-life of ethosuximide and a 15% decrease in its total clearance as compared to ethosuximide alone. Patients receiving valproate and ethosuximide, especially along with other anticonvulsants, should be monitored for alterations in serum concentrations of both drugs.

DRUG INTERACTIONS: *(cont'd)*

Lamotrigine: In steady-state study involving 10 healthy volunteers, the elimination half-life of lamotrigine increased from 26 to 70 hours with valproate co-administration (a 165% increase). The dose of lamotrigine should be reduced when co-administered with valproate.

Phenobarbital: Valproate was found to inhibit the metabolism of phenobarbital. Co-administration of valproate (250 mg twice a day for 14 days) with phenobarbital to normal subjects (n=6) resulted in a 50% increase in half-life and a 30% decrease in plasma clearance of phenobarbital (60 mg single-dose). The fraction of phenobarbital dose excreted unchanged increased by 50% in presence of valproate.

There is evidence for sever CNS depression, with or without significant elevations of barbiturate or valproate serum concentrations. All patients receiving concomitant barbiturate therapy should be closely monitored for neurological toxicity. Serum barbiturate concentrations should be obtained, if possible, and the barbiturate dosage decreased, if appropriate.

Primidone: Which is metabolized to a barbiturate, may be involved in a similar interaction with valproate.

Phenytoin: Valproate displaces phenytoin from its plasma albumin binding sites and inhibits its hepatic metabolism. Co-administration of valproate (400 mg three times a day) with phenytoin (250 mg) in normal volunteers (n=7) was associated with a 60% increase in the free fraction of phenytoin. Total plasma clearance and apparent volume of distribution of phenytoin increased 30% in the presence of valproate. Both the clearance and appparent volume of distribution of free phenytoin were reduced by 25%.

In patients with epilepsy, there have been reports of breakthrough seizures occurring with the combination of valproate and phenytoin. The dosage of phenytoin should be adjusted as required by the clinical situation.

Tolbutamide: From *in vitro* experiments, the unbound fraction of tolbutamide was increased from 20% to 50% when added to plasma sample taken from patients treated with valproate. The clinical relevance of this displacement is unknown.

Warfarin: In an *in vitro* study, valproate increased the unbound fraction of warfarin by up to 32.6%. The therapeutic relevance of this is unknown; however, coagulation tests should be monitored if valproate therapy is instituted in patients taking anticoagulants.

Zidovudine: In six patients who were seropositive for HIV, the clearance of zidovudine (100 mg every 8 hours) was decreased by 38% after administration of valproate (250 or 500 mg every 8 hours); the half-life of zidovudine was unaffected.

DRUGS FOR WHICH EITHER NO INTERACTION OR A LIKELY CLINICALLY UNIMPORTANT INTERACTION HAS BEEN OBSERVED

Acetaminophen: Valproate had no effect on any of the pharmacokinetic parameters of acetaminophen when it was concurrently administered to three epileptic patients.

Amitriptyline/Nortriptyline: Administration of a single oral 50 mg dose of amitriptyline to 15 normal volunteers (10 males and 5 females) who received valproate (500 mg twice a day) resulted in a 21% decrease in plasma clearance of amitriptyline and a 34% decrease in the net clearance of nortriptyline.

Clozapine: In psychotic patients (n=11), no interaction was observed when valproate was co-administered with clozapine.

Lithium: Co-administration of valproate (500 mg twice a day) and lithium carbonate (300 mg three times a day) to normal volunteers (n=16) had no effect on the steady-state kinetics of lithium.

Lorazepam: Concomitant administration of valproate (500 mg twice a day) and lorazepam (1 mg twice a day) in normal volunteers (n=9) was accompanied by a 17% decrease in the plasma clearance of lorazepam.

Oral Contraceptive Steroids: Administration of a single-dose of ethinyloestradiol (50 mcg)/levonorgestrel (250 mcg) to 6 women on valproate (200 mg twice a day) therapy for 2 months did not reveal any pharmacokinetic interaction.

ADVERSE REACTIONS:

The adverse events that can result from valproate sodium use include all of those associated with oral forms or valproate. The following describes experience specifically with valproate sodium. Valproate sodium has been generally well tolerated in clinical trials involving 111 healthy adult male volunteers and 352 patients with epilepsy, given at doses of 125 to 6000 mg (total daily dose). A total of 2% of patients discontinued treatment with valproate sodium due to adverse events. The most common adverse events leading to discontinuation were 2 cases each of nausea/vomiting and elevated amylase. Other adverse events leading to discontinuation were hallucinations, pneumonia, headache, injection site reaction, and abnormal gait. Dizziness and injection site pain were observed more frequently at a 100 mg/ml infusion rate than at rates up to 33 mg/min. At a 200 mg/min rate, dizziness and taste perversion occurred more frequently than at a 100 mg/min rate. The maximum rate of infusion studied was 200 mg/min.

Adverse events reported by at least 0.5% of all subjects/patients in clinical trials of valproate sodium are summarized in TABLE 3.

TABLE 3 Adverse Events Reported During Studies of Valproate Sodium

Body System/Event	N=463
Body as a Whole	
Chest Pain	1.7%
Headache	4.3%
Injection Site Inflammation	0.6%
Injection Site Pain	2.6%
Injection Site Reaction	2.4%
Pain (unspecified)	1.3%
Cardiovascular	
Vasodilation	0.9%
Dermatologic	
Sweating	0.9%
Digestive System	
Abdominal Pain	1.1%
Diarrhea	0.9%
Nausea	3.2%
Vomiting	1.3%
Nervous System	
Dizziness	5.2%
Euphoria	0.9%
Hypesthesia	0.6%
Nervousness	0.9%
Paresthesia	0.9%
Somnolence	1.7%
Tremor	0.6%
Respiratory	
Pharyngitis	0.6%
Special Senses	
Taste Perversion	1.9%

ADVERSE REACTIONS: *(cont'd)*

EPILEPSY

Based on placebo-controlled trial of adjunctive therapy for treatment of complex partial seizures, divalproex sodium was generally well tolerated with most adverse events rated as mild to moderate in severity. Intolerance was the primary reason for discontinuation in the divalproex sodium-treated patients (6%), compared to 1% of placebo-treated patients.

TABLE 4 lists treatment-emergent adverse events which were reported by ≥5% of divalproex sodium-treated patients and for which the incidence was greater than in the placebo group, in the placebo-controlled trial of adjunctive therapy for treatment of complex partial seizures. Since patients were also treated with other antiepilepsy drugs, it is not possible, in most cases, to determine whether the adverse events can be ascribed to divalproex sodium alone, or the combination of divalproex sodium and other antiepilepsy drugs.

TABLE 4 Adverse Events Reported by ≥5% of Patients Treated with Divalproex Sodium During Placebo-Controlled Trial of Adjunctive Therapy for Complex Partial Seizures

Body System/Event	Divalproex Sodium % (n=77)	Placebo % (n=70)
Body as a Whole		
Headache	31	21
Asthenia	27	7
Fever	6	4
Gastrointestinal System		
Nausea	48	14
Vomiting	27	7
Abdominal Pain	23	6
Diarrhea	13	6
Anorexia	12	0
Dyspepsia	8	4
Constipation	5	1
Nervous System		
Somnolence	27	11
Tremor	25	6
Dizziness	25	13
Diplopia	16	9
Amblyopia/Blurred Vision	12	9
Ataxia	8	1
Nystagmus	8	1
Emotional Lability	6	4
Thinking Abnormal	6	0
Amnesia	5	1
Respiratory System		
Flu Syndrome	12	9
Infection	12	6
Bronchitis	5	1
Rhinitis	5	4
Other		
Alopecia	6	1
Weight Loss	6	0

TABLE 5 lists treatment-emergent adverse events which were reported by ≥5% of patients in the high dose divalproex sodium group, and for which the incidence was greater than in the low dose group, in a controlled trial of divalproex sodium monotherapy treatment of complex partial seizures. Since patients were being titrated off another antiepilepsy drug during the first portion of the trial, it is not possible, in many cases, to determine whether the following adverse events can be ascribed to divalproex sodium alone, or the combination of divalproex sodium and other antiepilepsy drugs.

TABLE 5 Adverse Events Reported by ≥5% of Patients in the High Dose Group in the Controlled Trial of Divalproex Sodium Monotherapy for Complex Partial Seizures

Body System/Event	High Dose % (n=131)	Low Dose % (n=134)
Body as a Whole		
Asthenia	21	10
Digestive System		
Nausea	34	26
Diarrhea	23	19
Vomiting	23	15
Abdominal Pain	12	9
Anorexia	11	4
Dyspepsia	11	10
Hemic/Lymphatic System		
Thrombocytopenia	24	1
Ecchymosis	5	4
Metabolic /Nutritional		
Weight Gain	9	4
Peripheral Edema	8	3
Nervous System		
Tremor	57	19
Somnolence	30	18
Dizziness	18	13
Insomnia	15	9
Nervousness	11	7
Amnesia	7	4
Nystagmus	7	1
Depression	5	4
Respiratory System		
Infection	20	13
Pharyngitis	8	2
Dyspnea	5	1
Skin Appendages		
Alopecia	24	13
Special Senses		
Amblyopia/Blurred Vision	8	4
Tinnitus	7	1

* Headache was the only adverse event that occurred in ≥5% of patients in the high dose group and at an equal or greater incidence in the low dose group.

The following additional adverse events were reported by greater than 1% but less than 5% of the 358 patients treated with divalproex sodium in the controlled trials of complex partial seizures:

Body as a Whole: Back pain, chest pain, malaise.

Cardiovascular System: Tachycardia, hypertension, palpitation.

Digestive System: Increased appetite, flatulence, hematemesis, eructation, pancreatis, periodontal abscess.

Hemic and Lymphatic System: Petechia.

Metabolic and Nutritional Disorders: SGOT increased, SGPT increased.

ADVERSE REACTIONS: *(cont'd)*

Musculoskeletal System: Myalgia, twitching, arthralgia, leg cramps, myasthenia.

Nervous System: Anxiety, confusion, abnormal gait, paresthesia, hypertonia, incoordination, abnormal dreams, personality disorder.

Respiratory System: Sinusitis, cough increased, pneumonia, epistaxis.

Skin and Appendages: Rash, pruritus, dry skin.

Special Senses: Taste perversion, abnormal vision, deafness, otitis media.

Urogenital System: Urinary incontinence, vaginitis, dysmenorrhea, amenorrhea, urinary frequency.

OTHER PATIENT POPULATIONS

Adverse events that have been reported with all dosage forms of valproate from epilepsy trials, spontaneous reports, and other sources are listed below by body system.

Gastrointestinal: The most commonly reported side effects at the initiation of therapy are nausea, vomiting, and indigestion. These effects are usually transient and rarely require discontinuation of therapy. Diarrhea, abdominal cramps, and constipation have been reported. Both anorexia with some weight loss and increased appetite with weight gain have also been reported. The administration of delayed-release divalproex sodium may result in reduction of gastrointestinal side effects in some patients using oral therapy.

CNS Effect: Sedative effects have occurred in patients receiving valproate alone but occur most often in patients receiving combination therapy. Sedation usually abates upon reduction of the other antiepileptic medication. Tremor (may be dose-related), hallucinations, ataxia, headache, nystagmus, diplopia, asterixis, "spots before eyes", dysarthria, dizziness, confusion, hypesthesia, vertigo, and incoordination. Rare cases of coma, have occurred in patients receiving valproate alone or in conjunction with phenobarbital. In rare instances encephalophathy, with fever has developed shortly after the introduction of valproate monotherapy without evidence of hepatic dysfunction or inappropriate plasma levels; all patients recovered after the drug was withdrawn. Several reports have noted reversible cerebral atrophy and dementia in association with valproate therapy.

Dermatologic: Transient hair loss, skin rash, photosensitivity, generalized pruritus, erythema multiforme, and Stevens-Johnson syndrome. Rare cases of toxic epidermal necrolysis have been reported including a fatal case in a 6 month old infant taking valproate and several other concomitant medications. An additional case of toxic epidermal necrosis resulting in death was reported in a 35 year old patient with AIDS taking several concomitant medications and with a history of multiple cutaneous drug reactions.

Psychiatric: Emotional upset, depression, psychosis, aggression, hyperactivity, hostility, and behavioral deterioration.

Musculoskeletal: Weakness.

Hematologic: Thrombocytopenia and inhibition of the secondary phase of platelet aggretion may be reflected in altered bleeding time, petechiae, bruising, hematoma formation, epistaxis, and frank hemorrhage (see PRECAUTIONS, General and DRUG INTERACTIONS). Relative lymphocytosis, macrocytosis, hypofibrinogenemia, leukopenia, eosinophilia, anemia including macrocytic with or without folate deficiency, bone marrow suppression, pancytopenia, aplastic anemia, and acute intermittent porphyria.

Hepatic: Minor elevations of transaminases (*e.g.,* SGOT and SGPT) and LDH are frequent and appear to be dose-related. Occasionally, laboratory test results include increases in serum bilrubin and abnormal changes in other liver function tests. These results may reflect potentially serious hepatotoxicity (see WARNINGS).

Endocrine: Irregular menses, secondary amenorrhea, breast enlargement, galactorrhea, and parotid gland swelling. Abnormal thyroid function tests (see PRECAUTIONS).

Pancreatic: Acute pancreatitis including fatalitites.

Metabolic: Hyperammonemia, (see PRECAUTIONS), hyponatremia, and inappropriate ADH secretion. There have been rare reports of Fanconi's syndrome occurring chiefly in children. Decreased carnitine concentrations have been reported although the clinical relevance is undetermined. Hyperglycemia has occurred and was associated with a fatal outcome in a patient with preexistent nonketotic hyperglycinemia.

Genitourinary: Enuresis and urinary tract infection.

Special Senses: Hearing loss, either, reversible or irreversible, has been reported; however, a cause and effect relationship has not been established. Ear pain has also been reported.

Other: Edema of the extremities, lupus erythematosus, bone pain, cough increased, pneumonia, otitis media, bradycardia, cutaneous vasculitis, and fever.

MANIA

Although valproate sodium has not been evaluated for safety and efficacy in the treatment of manic episodes associated with bipolar disorder, the following adverse events not listed above were reported by 1% or more of patients from two placebo-controlled clinical trials of divalproex sodium tablets.

Body as a Whole: Chills, neck pain, neck rigidity.

Cardiovascular System: Hypotension, postural hypotension.

Digestive System: Fecal incontinence, gastroenteritis, glossitis.

Musculoskeletal System: Arthrosis.

Nervous System: Agitation, catatonic reaction, hypokinesia, reflexes increased, tardive dyskinesia, vertigo.

Skin and Appendages: Furunculosis, maculopapular rash, seborrhea.

Special Senses: Conjunctivitis, dry eyes, eye pain.

Urogenital System: Dysuria.

MIGRAINE

Although valproate sodium has not been evaluated for safety and efficacy in the treatment of migraine headaches, the following adverse events not listed above were reported by 1% or more of patients from two placebo-controlled clinical trials of divalproex sodium tablets.

Body as a Whole: Face edema.

Digestive System: Dry mouth, stomatitis.

Urogenital System: Cystitis, metrorrhagia, and vaginal hemorrhage.

OVERDOSAGE:

Overdosage with valproate may result in somnolence, heart block, and deep coma. Fatalities have been reported; however patients have recovered from valproate serum concentrations as high as 2120 mcg/ml.

In overdose situations, the fraction of drug not bound to protein is high and hemodialysis or tandem hemodialysis plus hemoperfusion may result in significant removal of drug. General supportive measures should be applied with particular attention to the maintenance of adequate urinary output.

Naloxone has been reported to reverse the CNS depressant effects of valproate overdosage. Because naloxone could theoretically also reverse the antiepilepsy effects of valproate, it should be used with caution in patients with epilepsy.

DOSAGE AND ADMINISTRATION:

VALPROATE SODIUM FOR INTRAVENOUS USE ONLY.

Use of valproate sodium for periods of more than 14 days has not been studied. Patients should be switched to oral valproate products as soon as it is clinically feasible.

Valproate sodium should be administered as a 60 minute infusion (but not more than 20 mg/min) with the same frequency as the oral products, although plasma concentration monitoring and dosage adjustments may be necessary.

INITIAL EXPOSURE TO VALPROATE

The following dosage recommendations were obtained from studies utilizing oral divalproex sodium products.

Complex Partial Seizures: For adults and children 10 years of age or older.

Monotherapy (Initial Therapy): Valproate sodium has not been systematically studied as initial therapy. Patients should initiate therapy at 10 to 15 mg/kg/day. The dosage should be increased by 5 to 10 mg/kg/week to achieve optimal clinical response. Ordinarily, optimal clinical response is acieved at a daily doses below 60 mg/kg/day. If satisfactory clinical response has not been achieved, plasma levels should be measured to determine whether or not they are in the usually accepted therapeutic range (50 to 100 mcg/ml). No recommendation regarding the safety of valproate for use at doses above 60 mg/kg/day can be made.

The probability of thrombocytopenia increases significantly at total trough valproate plasma concentrations above 110 mcg/ml in females and 135 mcg/ml in males. The benefit of improved seizure control with higher doses should be weighed against the possibility of a greater incidence of adverse reactions.

Conversion to Monotherapy: Patients should initiate therapy at 10 to 15 mg/kg/day. The dosage should be increased by 5 to 10 mg/kg/week to achieve optimal clinical response. Ordinarily, optimal clinical response is achieved at daily doses below 60 mg/kg/day. If satisfactory clinical response has not been achieved, plasma levels should be measured to determine whether or not they are in the usually accepted therapeutic range (50 -100 mcg/ml). No recommendation regarding the safety of valproate for use at doses above 60 mg/kg/day can be made. Concomitant antiepilepsy drug (AED) dosage can ordinarily be reduced by approximately 25% every 2 weeks. This reduction may be started at initiation of vaproate sodium therapy, or delayed by 1 to 2 weeks if there is a concern that seizures are likely to occur with a reduction. The speed and duration of withdrawal of the concomitant AED can be highly variable, and patients should be monitored closely during this period for increased seizure frequency.

Adjunctive Therapy: Valproate sodium may be added to the patient's regimen at a dosage of 10 to 15 mg/kg/day. The dosage may be increased by 5 to 10 mg/kg/week to achieve optimal clinical response. Ordinarily, optimal clinical response is acheived at daily doses below 60 mg/kg/day. If satisfactory clinical response has not been achieved, plasma levels should be measured to determine whether or not they are in the usually accepted therapeutic range (50 - 100 mcg/ml). No recommendation regarding the safety of valproate for use at doses above 60 mg/kg/day can be made. If the total daily dose exceeds 250 mg, it should be given in divided doses.

In a study of adjunctive therapy for complex partial seizures in which patients were receiving either carbamazepine or phenytoin in addition to divalproex sodium, no adjustment of carbamazepine or phenytoin dosage was needed (see CLINICAL STUDIES). However, since valproate may interact with these or other concurrently administered AEDs as well as other drugs (see DRUG INTERACTIONS), periodic plasma concentration determinations of concomitant AEDs are recommended during the early course of therapy (see DRUG INTERACTIONS).

Simple and Complex Absence Seizures: The recommended intial dose is 15 mg/kg/day, increasing at one week intervals by 5 to 10 mg/kg/day until seizures are controlled or side effects preclude further increases. The maximum recommended dosage is 60 mg/kg/day. If the total daily dose exceeds 250 mg, it should be given in divided doses.

A good correlation has not been established between daily dose, serum concentrations, and therapeutic effect. However, therapeutic valproate serum concentrations for most patients with absence seizures is considered to range from 50 to 100 mcg/ml. Some patients may be controlled with lower or higher serum concentrations (see CLINICAL PHARMACOLOGY).

As the valproate sodium dosage is titrated upward, blood concentrations of phenobarbital and/or phenytoin may be affected (see PRECAUTIONS).

Antiepilepsy drugs should not be abruptly discontinued in patients in whom the drug is administered to prevent major seizures because of the strong possibility of precipitating status epilepticus with attendant hypoxia and threat to life.

REPLACEMENT THERAPY

When switching from oral valproate products, the total daily dose of valproate sodium should be equivalent to the total daily dose of the oral valproate product (see CLINICAL PHARMACOLOGY), and should be administered as a 60 minute infusion (but not more that 20 mg/min) with the same frequency as the oral products, although plasma concentration monitoring and dosage adjustments may be necessary. Patients receiving doses near the maximum recommended daily dose of 60 mg/kg/day, particularly those not receiving enzyme-inducing drugs, should be monitored more closely. If the total daily dose exceeds 250 mg, it should be given in a divided regimen. However, the equivalence shown between valproate sodium and oral valproate products (divalproex sodium) at steady state was only evaluated in an every 6 hour regimen. Whether, when valproate sodium is given less frequently (*i.e.,* twice or three times a day), trough levels fall below those that result from an oral dosage form given via the same regimen. For this reason, when valproate sodium is given twice or three times a day, close monitoring of trough plasma levels may be needed.

GENERAL DOSING ADVICE

Dosing in Elderly Patients: Due to a decrease in unbound clearance of valproate, the starting dose should be reduced; the ultimate therapeutic dose should be achieved on the basis of clinical response.

Dose-Related Adverse Events: The frequency of adverse effects (particularly elevated liver enzymes and thrombocytopenia) may be dose-related. The probability of thrombocytopenia appears to increase significantly at total valproate concentrations of ≥110 mcg/ml (females) or ≥135 mcg/ml (males) (see PRECAUTIONS). The benefit of improved therapeutic effect with higher doses should be weighed against the possibility of a greater incidence of adverse reactions.

ADMINISTRATION

Rapid infusion of valproate sodium has been associated with an increase in adverse events. Infusion times of less than 60 minutes or rates of infusion >20 mg/min have not been studied in patients with epilepsy (see ADVERSE REACTIONS).

Valproate sodium should be administered intravenously as a 60 minute infusion, as noted above. It should be diluted with at least 50 ml of a compatible diluent. Any unused portion of the vial contents should be discarded.

Parenteral drug products should be inspected visually for particulate matter and discoloration prior to administration whenever solution and container permit.

DOSAGE AND ADMINISTRATION: *(cont'd)*

COMPATIBILITY AND STABILITY

Valproate was found to be physically compatible and chemically stable in the following parenteral solutions for at least 24 hours when stored in glass or polyvinyl chloride (PVC) bags at controlled room temperature 15-30°C (59-86°F).

dextrose (5%) injection, USP

sodium chloride (0.9%) injection, USP

lactated ringer's injection, USP

HOW SUPPLIED:

Depacon (valproate sodium injection), equivalent to 100 mg of valproic acid per ml, is a clear, colorless solution in 5 ml single-dose vials, available in trays of 10 vials.

Recommended Storage: Store vials at controlled room temperature 15-30°C (59-86°F). No preservatives have been added. Unused portion of container should be discarded.

VALPROIC ACID *(002419)*

CATEGORIES: Anticonvulsants; Antiepileptics; Central Nervous System Agents; Convulsions; Epilepsy; Neuromuscular; Seizures; Bipolar Disorder*; Mania*; Pregnancy Category D; FDA Approval Pre 1982

* Indication not approved by the FDA

BRAND NAMES: *Convulex; Cryoval* (Mexico); **Depakene**; *Depakin*; *Depakine*; *Epilim*; *Leptilan*; Myproic Acid; *Orfiril* (Germany); *Valporal*; *Valprosid* (Mexico)
(International brand names outside U.S. in italics)

FORMULARIES: Aetna; BC-BS; FHP; Medi-Cal; PCS; WHO

COST OF THERAPY: $189.50 (Epilepsy; Capsule; 250 mg; 4/day; 365 days)

WARNING:
HEPATIC FAILURE RESULTING IN FATALITIES HAS OCCURRED IN PATIENTS RECEIVING VALPROIC ACID. EXPERIENCE HAS INDICATED THAT CHILDREN UNDER THE AGE OF TWO YEARS ARE AT A CONSIDERABLY INCREASED RISK OF DEVELOPING FATAL HEPATOTOXICITY, ESPECIALLY THOSE ON MULTIPLE ANTICONVULSANTS, THOSE WITH CONGENITAL METABOLIC DISORDERS, THOSE SEVERE SEIZURE DISORDERS ACCOMPANIED BY MENTAL RETARDATION, AND THOSE WITH ORGANIC BRAIN DISEASE. WHEN VALPROIC ACID PRODUCTS ARE USED IN THIS PATIENT GROUP, IT SHOULD BE USED WITH EXTREME CAUTION AND AS A SOLE AGENT. THE BENEFITS OF SEIZURE CONTROL SHOULD BE WEIGHED AGAINST THE RISKS. ABOVE THIS AGE GROUP, EXPERIENCE HAS INDICATED THAT THE INCIDENCE OF FATAL HEPATOTOXICITY DECREASES CONSIDERABLY IN PROGRESSIVELY OLDER PATIENT GROUPS.
THESE INCIDENTS USUALLY HAVE OCCURRED DURING THE FIRST SIX MONTHS OF TREATMENT. SERIOUS OR FATAL HEPATOTOXICITY MAY BE PRECEDED BY NON-SPECIFIC SYMPTOMS SUCH AS LOSS OF SEIZURE CONTROL, MALAISE, WEAKNESS, LETHARGY, FACIAL EDEMA, ANOREXIA AND VOMITING. PATIENTS SHOULD BE MONITORED CLOSELY FOR APPEARANCE OF THESE SYMPTOMS. LIVER FUNCTION TESTS SHOULD BE PERFORMED PRIOR TO THERAPY AND AT FREQUENT INTERVALS THEREAFTER, ESPECIALLY DURING THE FIRST SIX MONTHS.

DESCRIPTION:

Valproic acid is a carboxylic acid designated as 2-propylpentanoic acid. It is also known as dipropylacetic acid.

Valproic acid (pKa 4.8) has a molecular weight of 144 and occurs as a colorless liquid with a characteristic odor. It is slightly soluble in water (1.3 mg/ml) and very soluble in organic solvents.

Valproic acid capsules and syrup are antiepileptics for oral administration. Each soft elastic capsule contains 250 mg valproic acid. The syrup contains the equivalent of 250 mg valproic acid per 5 ml as the sodium salt.

CLINICAL PHARMACOLOGY:

Valproic acid ia an antiepileptic agent which dissociates to the valproate ion in the gastrointestinal tract. The mechanism by which valproate exerts its antiepileptic effects has not yet been established. It has been suggested that its activity is related to increased brain levels of gamma-aminobutyric acid (GABA).

Valproic acid is rapidly absorbed after oral administration. Peak plasma concentrations of valproate ion are observed one to four hours after a single dose of valproic acid. A slight delay in absorption occurs when the drug is administered with meals but this does not affect the total absorption.

Accordingly, administration of oral valproate products with food, and substitution among the various valproic acid and divalproex sodium products should be without consequence. Nonetheless, any changes in dosage administration or the addition or discontinuance of concomitant drugs, should ordinarily be accompanied by close monitoring of clinical status and valproate plasma concentrations.

The plasma half-life of valproate is typically in the range of six to sixteen hours. Half-lives in the lower part of the range are usually found in patients taking other antiepileptic drugs capable of enzyme induction.

Valproate is primarily metabolized in the liver. The major metabolic routes are glucuronidation, mitochondrial beta oxidation, and microsomal oxidation. The major metabolites formed are the glucuronide conjugate, 2- propyl-3-keto-pentanoic acid, and 2-propyl-hydroxypentanoic acids. Other unsaturated metabolites have been reported. The major route of elimination of these metabolites is in the urine.

Patients on monotherapy will generally have longer half-lives and higher concentrations of valproate at a given dosage than patients receiving polytherapy. This is primarily due to enzyme induction caused by other antiepileptics, which results in enhanced clearance of valproate by glucuronidation and microsomal oxidation. Because of these changes in valproate clearance, monitoring of antiepileptic concentrations should be intensified whenever concomitant antiepileptics are introduced or withdrawn.

CLINICAL PHARMACOLOGY: *(cont'd)*

The therapeutic range is commonly considered to be 50 to 100 mcg/ml of total valproate, although some patients may be controlled with lower or higher plasma concentrations.[4] Valproate is highly bound (90%) to plasma proteins in the therapeutic rang; however, protein binding is concentration-dependent and decreases at high valproate concentrations. The binding is variable among patients, and may be affected by fatty acids or by highly bound drugs such as salicylate. Some clinicians favor monitoring free valproate concentrations, which may more accurately reflect CNS penetration of valproate. As yet, a consensus on the therapeutic range of free concentrations has not been established; however; monitoring total and free valproate may be informative when there are changes in clinical status, concomitant medication or valproate dosage.

INDICATIONS AND USAGE:

Valproic acid is indicated for use as sole and adjunctive therapy in the treatment of simple and complex absence seizures, and adjunctively in patients with multiple seizure types which include absence seizures.

Simple absence is defined as very brief clouding of the sensorium or loss of consciousness, accompanied by certain generalized epileptic discharges without other detractable clinical signs. Complex absence is the term used when other signs are also present.

SEE WARNINGS FOR STATEMENT REGARDING FATAL HEPATIC DYSFUNCTION.

CONTRAINDICATIONS:

VALPROIC ACID SHOULD NOT BE ADMINISTERED TO PATIENTS WITH HEPATIC DISEASE OR SIGNIFICANT DYSFUNCTION.

Valproic acid is contraindicated in patients with known hypersensitivity to the drug.

WARNINGS:

Hepatic failure resulting in fatalities has occurred in patients receiving valproic acid. These incidents usually have occurred during the first six months of treatment. Serious or fatal hepatotoxicity may be preceded by non-specific symptoms such as loss of seizure control, malaise, weakness, lethargy, facial edema, anorexia and vomiting. Liver function tests should be performed prior to therapy and at frequent intervals thereafter, especially during the first six months. However, physicians should not rely totally on serum biochemistry since these tests may not be abnormal in all instances, but should also consider the results of careful interim medical history and physical examination. Caution should be observed when administering valproic acid to patients with a prior history of hepatic disease. Patients on multiple anticonvulsants, children, those with congenital metabolic disorders, those with severe seizure disorders accompanied by mental retardation, and those with organic brain disease may be at particular risk. Experience has indicated that children under the age of two years are at a considerably increased risk of developing fatal hepatotoxicity, especially those with the aforementioned conditions. When valproic acid products are used in this patient group, it should be with extreme caution and as a sole agent. The benefits of seizure control should be weighed against the risks. Above this age group, experience has indicated that the incidence of fatal hepatotoxicity decreases considerably in progressively older patient groups.

The drug should be discontinued immediately in the presence of significant hepatic dysfunction, suspected or apparent. In some cases, hepatic dysfunction has progressed in spite of discontinuation of drug.

The frequency of adverse effects (particularly elevated liver enzymes) may be dose-related. The benefit of improved seizure control which may be accompanied at higher doses should therefore be weighed against the possibility of a greater incidence of adverse effects.

Usage in Pregnancy: ACCORDING TO PUBLISHED AND UNPUBLISHED REPORTS, VALPROIC ACID MAY PRODUCE TERATOGENIC EFFECTS IN THE OFFSPRING OF HUMAN FEMALES RECEIVING THE DRUG DURING PREGNANCY.

THERE ARE MULTIPLE REPORTS IN THE CLINICAL LITERATURE WHICH MAY INDICATE THAT THE USE OF ANTIEPILEPTIC DRUGS DURING PREGNANCY RESULTS IN AN INCREASED INCIDENCE OF BIRTH DEFECTS IN THE OFFSPRING. ALTHOUGH DATA ARE MORE EXTENSIVE WITH RESPECT TO TRIMETHADIONE, PARAMETHADIONE, PHENYTOIN, AND PHENOBARBITAL, REPORTS INDICATE A POSSIBLE SIMILAR ASSOCIATION WITH THE USE OF OTHER ANTIEPILEPTIC DRUGS. THEREFORE, ANTIEPILEPTIC DRUGS SHOULD BE ADMINISTERED TO WOMEN OF CHILDBEARING POTENTIAL ONLY IF THEY ARE CLEARLY SHOWN TO BE ESSENTIAL IN THE MANAGEMENT OF SEIZURES.

THE INCIDENCE OF NEURAL TUBE DEFECTS IN THE FETUS MAY BE INCREASED IN MOTHERS RECEIVING VALPROATE DURING THE FIRST TRIMESTER OF PREGNANCY. THE CENTERS FOR DISEASE CONTROL (CDC) HAS ESTIMATED THE RISK OF VALPROIC ACID EXPOSED TO WOMEN HAVING CHILDREN WITH SPINA BIFIDA TO BE APPROXIMATELY 1 TO 2%[1].

OTHER CONGENITAL ANOMALIES (EG, CRANIOFACIAL DEFECTS, CARDIOVASCULAR MALFORMATIONS AND ANOMALIES INVOLVING VARIOUS BODY SYSTEMS), COMPATIBLE AND INCOMPATIBLE WITH LIFE, HAVE BEEN REPORTED. SUFFICIENT DATA TO DETERMINE THIS INCIDENCE OF THESE CONGENITAL ANOMALIES IS NOT AVAILABLE.

THE HIGHER INCIDENCE OF CONGENITAL ANOMALIES IN ANTIEPILEPTIC DRUG-TREATED WOMEN WITH SEIZURE DISORDERS CANNOT BE REGARDED AS A CAUSE AND EFFECT RELATIONSHIP. THERE ARE INTRINSIC METHODOLOGIC PROBLEMS IN ATTAINING ADEQUATE DATA ON DRUG TERATOGENICITY IN HUMANS; GENETIC FACTORS OR THE EPILEPTIC CONDITION ITSELF, MAY BE MORE IMPORTANT THAN DRUG THERAPY IN CONTRIBUTING TO CONGENITAL ANOMALIES.

PATIENTS TAKING VALPROATE MAY DEVELOP CLOTTING ABNORMALITIES. A PATIENT WHO HAD LOW FIBROGEN WHEN TAKING MULTIPLE ANTICONVULSANTS INCLUDING VALPROATE GAVE BIRTH TO AN INFANT WHO SUBSEQUENTLY DIED OF HEMORRHAGE. IF VALPROATE IS USED IN PREGNANCY, THE CLOTTING PARAMETERS SHOULD BE MONITORED CAREFULLY.

HEPATIC FAILURE RESULTING IN THE DEATH OF A NEWBORN AND OF AN INFANT, HAVE BEEN REPORTED FOLLOWING THE USE OF VALPROATE DURING PREGNANCY.

ANIMAL STUDIES HAVE ALSO DEMONSTRATED VALPROATE INDUCED TERATOGENICITY. Studies in rats and human females demonstrated placental transfer of the drug. Doses greater than 65 mg/kg/day given to pregnant rats and mice produced skeletal abnormalities in the offspring, primarily involving ribs and vertebrae; doses greater than 150 mg/kg/day given to pregnant rabbits produced fetal resorptions and (primarily) soft-tissue abnormalities in the offspring. In rats a dose-related delay in the onset of parturition was noted. Potential growth and survival of the progeny were adversely affected, particularly when the drug administration spanned the entire gestation and early lactation period.

Antiepileptic drugs should not be discontinued in patients in whom the drug is administered to prevent seizures because of the strong possibility of precipitating status epilepticus with attendant hypoxia and threat to life. In individual cases where the severity and frequency of the seizure disorder are such that the removal of medication does not pose a serious threat to

WARNINGS: *(cont'd)*

the patient, discontinuation of the drug may be considered prior to and during pregnancy, although it cannot be said with any confidence that even minor seizures do not pose some hazard to the developing embryo or fetus.

The prescribing physicians will wish to weigh these considerations in treating or counseling epileptic women of childbearing potential.

Tested to detect neural tube and other defects using current accepted procedures should be considered a part of routine prenatal care in childbearing women receiving valproate.

PRECAUTIONS:

Hepatic Dysfunction: see BOXED WARNING, CONTRAINDICATIONS, AND WARNINGS.

General: Because of reports of thrombocytopenia, inhibition of the secondary phase of platelet aggregation, and abnormal coagulation parameters, (*e.g.,* low fibrinogen), platelet counts and coagulation tests are recommended before initiating therapy and at periodic intervals. It is recommended that patients receiving valproic acid be monitored for platelet count and coagulation parameters prior to planned surgery. Evidence of hemorrhage, bruising or a disorder of hemostasis/coagulation is an indication for reduction of the dosage or withdrawal of therapy.

Hyperammonemia with or without lethargy or coma has been reported and may be present in the absence of abnormal liver function tests. Asymptomatic elevations of ammonia are more common and when present require more frequent monitoring. If clinically significant symptoms occur, valproic acid therapy should be modified or discontinued.

Since valproate may interact with concurrently administered antiepileptic drugs, periodic plasma concentrations of concomitant antiepileptic drugs are recommended during the early course of therapy (see DRUG INTERACTIONS.)

Valproate is partially eliminated in the urine as a keto-metabolite which may lead to a false interpretation of the urine ketone test.

There have also been reports of altered thyroid function tests associated with valproate. The clinical significance of these is unknown.

Information for the Patient: Since valproic acid products may produce CNS depression, especially when combined with another CNS depressant (*e.g.,* alcohol), patients should be advised an automobile or operating dangerous machinery, until it is known that they do not become drowsy from the drug.

Carcinogenesis: Valproic acid was administered to Sprague Dawley rats and ICR (HA/ICR) mice at doses of 0, 80. and 170 mg/kg/day for two years. A variety of neoplasms were observed in both species. The chief findings were a statistically significant increase in the incidence of subcutaneous fibrosarcomas in high dose male rats receiving valproic acid and a statistically significant dose-related trend for benign pulmonary adenomas in male mice receiving valproic acid. The significance of these findings for man is unknown.

Mutagenesis: Studies on valproate have been performed using bacterial and mammalian systems. These studies have provided no evidence of a mutagenic potential for valproate.

Fertility: Chronic toxicity studies in juvenile and adult rats and dogs demonstrated that 200 mg/kg/day in rats and greater than 90 mg/kg/day in dogs. Segment I fertility studies in rats have shown doses up to 350 mg/kg/day for 60 days to have no effect on fertility. THE EFFECT OF VALPROATE ON TESTICULAR DEVELOPMENT AND ON SPERM PRODUCTION AND FERTILITY IN HUMANS IS UNKNOWN.

Pregnancy Category D: See WARNINGS

Nursing Mothers: Valproate is excreted in breast milk. Concentrations in breast milk have been reported to be 1-10% of serum concentrations. It is not known what effect this would have on a nursing infant. Caution should be exercised when valproic acid is administered to a nursing woman.

DRUG INTERACTIONS:

Valproate may potentiate the CNS depressants (*i.e.,* alcohol., benzodiazepines, etc.)

The concomitant administration of valproate with drugs that exhibit extensive protein binding (*e.g.,* aspirin, carbamazepine, dicumarol. and phenytoin) may result in alteration of serum drug concentrations.

There is evidence that valproate can cause an increase in serum phenobarbital concentrations by impairment of non-renal clearance. This phenomenon can result in severe cns depression. The combination of valproate and phenobarbital has also been reported to produce cns depression without significant elevations of barbiturate or valproate serum concentrations. All patients receiving concomitant barbiturate therapy should be closely monitored for neurological toxicity. Serum barbiturate concentrations should be obtained, if possible and the barbiturate dosage decreased, if appropriate.

Primidone is metabolized into a barbiturate and, therefore, may also be involved in a similar or identical interaction.

There have also been reports of breakthrough seizures occurring with the combination of valproate and phenytoin. Most reports have noted a decrease in total plasma phenytoin concentration. However, increases in total phenytoin serum concentrations have been reported. An initial fall with subsequent increase in total phenytoin concentrations has also been reported. In addition, a decrease in total serum phenytoin with an increase in the free vs. Protein bound phenytoin concentrations has been reported. The dosage of phenytoin should be adjusted as required by the clinical situation.

The concomitant use of valproic acid and clonazepam may produce absence status in patients with a history of absence type seizures.

There is inconclusive evidence regarding the effects of valproate on serum ethosuximide concentrations. Patients receiving valproate and ethosuximide, especially along with other anticonvulsants, should be monitored for alterations in serum concentrations of both drugs.

Caution is recommended when valproate is used with drugs affecting coagulation (*e.g* aspirin, warfarin). See ADVERSE REACTIONS.

Evidence suggests that there is an association between the use of certain antiepileptics and failure of oral contraceptives. One explanation for this interaction is that enzyme-inducing antiepileptics effectively lower plasma concentrations of the relevant steroid hormones, resulting in unimpaired ovulation. However, other mechanisms, not related to enzyme induction may contribute to the failure of oral contraceptives. While valproate is not a significant enzyme inducer, and, therefore, would not be expected to decrease concentrations of steroid hormones, clinical data about the interaction of valproate with oral contraceptives is minimal.[2]

ADVERSE REACTIONS:

Since valproic acid has usually been used with other antiepileptic drugs, it is not possible, in most cases, to determine whether the following adverse reactions can be ascribed to valproic acid alone, or the combination of drugs.

ADVERSE REACTIONS: *(cont'd)*

Gastrointestinal: The most commonly reported side effects at the initiation of therapy are nausea, vomiting, and indigestion. These effects are usually transient and rarely require discontinuation of therapy. Diarrhea, abdominal cramps and constipation have been reported. Some patients experiencing gastrointestinal side effects may benefit by converting therapy from valproic acid to divalproex sodium.[3].

CNS Effects: Sedative effects have occurred in patients receiving valproate alone but occur most often in patients receiving combination therapy. Sedation usually abates upon reduction of other antiepileptic medication. Tremor (may be dose-related), hallucinations, ataxia, headache, nystagmus, diplopia, asterixis, "spots before eyes", dysarthria, dizziness, and incoordination. Rare cases of coma have been noted in patients receiving valproic acid alone or in conjunction with phenobarbital. In rare instances encephalopathy with fever has developed shortly after the introduction of valproate monotherapy without evidence of hepatic dysfunction or inappropriate plasma levels; all patients recovered after the drug was withdrawn.

Dermatologic: Transient hair loss, skin rash, photosensitivity, generalized pruritus, erythema multiforme, and Stevens-Johnson syndrome. A case of fatal epidermal necrolysis has been reported in a 6 month old infant taking valproate and several other concomitant medications.

Psychiatric: Emotional upset, depression, psychosis, aggression, hyperactivity and behavioral deterioration.

Musculoskeletal: Weakness.

Hematologic: Thrombocytopenia and inhibition of the secondary phase of platelet aggregation may be reflected in altered bleeding time, petechiae, bruising, hematoma formation and frank hemorrhage DRUG INTERACTIONS. Relative lymphocytosis, macrocytosis, hypofibrinogenemia, leukopenia, eosinophilia, anemia, bone marrow suppression, and acute intermittent porphyria.

Hepatic: Minor elevations of transaminases (*e.g.*SGOT and SGPT) and LDH are frequent and appear to be dose related. Occasionally, laboratory test results include increases in serum bilirubin and abnormal changes in other liver function tests. These results may reflect potentially serious hepatotoxicity. (see WARNINGS.)

Endocrine: Irregular menses, secondary amenorrhea, breast enlargement, galactorrhea, and parotid gland swelling. Abnormal thyroid function tests (see PRECAUTIONS.)

Pancreatic: Acute pancreatitis, including fatalities.

Metabolic: Hyperammonemia (see PRECAUTIONS), hyponatremia, and inappropriate ADH secretion.

There have been rare reports of Fanconi's syndrome occurring chiefly in children.

Decreased carnitine concentrations have been reported although the clinical relevance is undetermined.

Hyperglycinemia has occurred and was associated with a fatal outcome in a patient with preexisting nonketotic hyperglycinemia.

Other: Edema of the extremities.

OVERDOSAGE:

Overdosage with valproate may result in deep coma.

Since valproic acid is absorbed very rapidly, the benefit of gastric lavage or emesis will vary with time since ingestion. General supportive measures should be applied with particular attention to the maintenance of adequate urinary output.

Naloxone has been reported to reverse the CNS depressant effects of valproate overdosage. Because naloxone could theoretically also reverse the antiepileptic effects of valproate, it should be used with caution.

DOSAGE AND ADMINISTRATION:

Valproic acid is administered orally. The recommended initial dose is 15 mg/kg/day, increasing at one week intervals by 5 to 10 mg/kg/day, until seizures are controlled or side effects preclude further increases. The maximum recommended dosage is 60 mg/kg/day. If the total daily dose exceeds 250 mg, it should be given in a divided regimen.

TABLE 1 is a guide for the initial daily dose of valproic acid (15 mg/kg/day).

TABLE 1

Weight (kg)	(lb)	Total Daily Dose (mg)	Number of Capsules or Teaspoonfuls of Syrup: Dose 1	Dose 2	Dose 3
10-24.9	22-54.9	250	0	0	1
25-39.9	55-87.9	500	1	0	1
40-59.9	88-131.9	750	1	1	1
60-74.9	132-164.9	1,000	1	1	2
75-89.9	165-197.9	1,250	2	1	2

The frequency of adverse effects (particularly elevated liver enzymes) may be dose related. The benefits of improved seizure control with higher doses should be weighed against the possibility of a greater incidence of adverse reactions.

A good correlation has not been established between daily dose, serum concentration and therapeutic effect. However, therapeutic valproate serum concentrations for most patients will range from 50 to 100 mcg/ml. Some patients may be controlled with lower or higher serum concentrations(see CLINICAL PHARMACOLOGY.)

As the valproic acid dosage is titrated upward, blood concentrations of phenobarbital and/or phenytoin may be affected. (see PRECAUTIONS.)

Patients who experience G.I. irritation may benefit from administration of the drug with food or by slowly building up the dose from an initial low level.

THE CAPSULES SHOULD BE SWALLOWED WITHOUT CHEWING TO AVOID LOCAL IRRITATION OF THE MOUTH AND THROAT.

REFERENCES:

1. Centers for Disease Control, Valproate: A New cause of Birth Defects-report from Italy and Follow-up from France, *Morbidity and Mortality Weekly Report* 32(33): 438-439, August 26, 1983. **2.** Mattson, RH et al. Use of Oral Contraceptives by Women with Epilepsy,*JAMA* 256(2): 238-240, July 11, 1986. **3.** Wilder, BJ et al, Gastrointestinal Tolerance of Divalproex Sodium, *Neurology* 33: 808-811, June, 1983. **4.** Hurst DL. Expanded therapeutic range of valproate. *Pediatr Neurol.* 1987; 3: 342-344.

HOW SUPPLIED:

Storage: Store capsules at 59-77°F (15-25°C). Store syrup below 86°F (30°C).

HOW SUPPLIED - RATED THERAPEUTICALLY EQUIVALENT:

Capsule, Elastic - Oral - 250 mg

100's	$12.98	Valproic Acid, H.C.F.A. F F P	99999-2419-01
100's	$13.73	Valproic Acid, United Res	00677-1079-01
100's	$16.40	Valproic Acid, US Trading	56126-0106-11
100's	$25.05	Valproic Acid, Rugby	00536-4779-01
100's	$27.50	Valproic Acid, Solvay Pharms	00032-4120-06
100's	$28.00	Valproic Acid, Harber Pharm	51432-0469-03

HOW SUPPLIED - RATED THERAPEUTICALLY EQUIVALENT: *(cont'd)*

100's	$28.75	Valproic Acid, Qualitest Pharms	00603-6334-21
100's	$32.20	Valproic Acid, Rosemont	00832-1007-00
100's	$33.59	Valproic Acid, Purepac Pharm	00228-2455-10
100's	$34.44	Valproic Acid, Martec Pharms	52555-0325-01
100's	$36.10	Valproic Acid, Aligen Independ	00405-5094-01
100's	$36.10	Valproic Acid, Geneva Pharms	00781-2203-01
100's	$36.25	Valproic Acid, Sidmak Labs	50111-0852-01
100's	$37.50	Valproic Acid, Parmed Pharms	00349-8735-01
100's	$37.50	Valproic Acid, Intl Labs	00665-4120-06
100's	$40.49	Valproic Acid, HL Moore Drug Exch	00839-7840-06
100's	$41.05	Valproic Acid, Schein Pharm (US)	00364-0822-01
100's	$42.51	Valproic Acid, HL Moore Drug Exch	00839-7180-06
100's	$44.90	Valporic Acid, Goldline Labs	00182-1754-01
100's	$47.10	Valproic Acid, Rugby	00536-4477-01
100's	$47.10	Valproic Acid 250, Major Pharms	00904-2101-60
100's	$47.10	Valproic Acid, Major Pharms	00904-7765-60
100's	**$113.75**	**DEPAKENE, Abbott**	**00074-5681-11**
100's	**$116.34**	**DEPAKENE, Abbott**	**00074-5681-13**
500's	$99.13	Valproic Acid, Rugby	00536-4779-05

Syrup - Oral - 250 mg/5ml

5 ml	$75.80	Valproic Acid, Xactdose	50962-0226-05
480 ml	$28.51	Valproic Acid, H.C.F.A. F F P	99999-2419-02
480 ml	$34.41	Valproic Acid, United Res	00677-1155-33
480 ml	$37.95	Valproic Acid, Harber Pharm	51432-0670-20
480 ml	$45.00	Valproic Acid, Major Pharms	00904-2103-16
480 ml	$46.75	Valproic Acid, Qualitest Pharms	00603-1840-58
480 ml	$46.77	Valproic Acid Syrup, Schein Pharm (US)	00364-2139-16
480 ml	$46.80	Syrup Oral, Aligen Independ	00405-3890-16
480 ml	$46.80	Valproic Acid, Copley Pharm	38245-0633-07
480 ml	$49.01	Valproic Acid, HL Moore Drug Exch	00839-7195-69
480 ml	$50.00	Valproic Acid, Hi Tech Pharma	50383-0792-16
480 ml	$56.00	Valproic Acid, Morton Grove	60432-0621-16
480 ml	$68.25	Valproic Acid, Goldline Labs	00182-6115-40
480 ml	$69.17	Valproic Acid, Rugby	00536-2390-85
480 ml	$69.17	Valproic Acid Syrup, Geneva Pharms	00781-6701-16
480 ml	**$118.90**	**DEPAKENE, Abbott**	**00074-5682-16**

VALSARTAN *(003320)*

CATEGORIES: Angiotensin II Inhibitors; Antihypertensives; Cardiovascular Drugs; FDA Approved 1996 Feb; Hypertension; Pregnancy Category C, 1st Trimester; Pregnancy Category D, 2nd & 3rd Trimesters

BRAND NAMES: **Diovan**

> WARNING:
> **Use In Pregnancy: When used in pregnancy during the second and third trimesters, drugs that act directly on the renin-angiotensin system can cause injury and even death to the developing fetus. When pregnancy is detected, valsartan should be discontinued as soon as possible. See WARNINGS, Fetal/Neonatal Morbidity and Mortality.**

DESCRIPTION:

Diovan is a nonpeptide, orally active, and specific angiotensin II antagonist acting on the AT_1 receptor subtype.

Valsartan is chemically described as *N*-(1-oxopentyl)-N-[[2'-(1*H*-tetrazol-5-yl)[1,1'-biphenyl]-4-yl]methyl]-L-valine. Its empirical formula is $C_{24}H_{29}N_5O_3$, and its molecular weight is 435.5.

Valsartan is a white to practically white fine powder. It is soluble in ethanol and methanol and slightly soluble in water.

Diovan is available as capsules for oral administration, containing either 80 mg or 160 mg of valsartan. The inactive insredients of the capsules are cellulose compounds, crospovidone, gelatin, iron oxides, magnesium stearate, povidone, sodium lauryl sulfate, and titanium dioxide.

CLINICAL PHARMACOLOGY:

MECHANISM OF ACTION

Angiotensin II is formed from angiotensin I in a reaction catalyzed by angiotensin-converting enzyme (ACE, kininase II). Angiotensin II is the principal pressor agent of the renin-angiotensin system, with effects that include vasoconstriction, stimulation of synthesis and release of aldosterone, cardiac stimulation, and renal reabsorption of sodium. Valsartan blocks the vasoconstrictor and aldosterone-secreting effects of angiotensin II by selectively blocking the binding of angiotensin II to the AT_1 receptor in many tissues, such as vascular smooth muscle and the adrenal gland. Its action is therefore independent of the pathways for angiotensin II synthesis.

There is also an AT_2 receptor found in many tissues, but AT_2 is not known to be associated with cardiovascular homeostasis. Valsartan has much greater affinity (about 20,000-fold) for the AT_1 receptor than for the AT_2receptor. The primary metabolite of valsartan is essentially inactive with an affinity for the AT_1 receptor about one 200th that of valsartan itself.

Blockade of the renin-angiotensin system with ACE inhibitors, which inhibit the biosynthesis of angiotensin II from angiotensin I, is widely used in the treatment of hypertension. ACE inhibitors also inhibit the degradation of bradykinin, a reaction also catalyzed by ACE. Because valsartan does not inhibit ACE (kininase II), it does not affect the response to bradykinin. Whether this difference has clinical relevance is not yet known. Valsartan does not bind to or block other hormone receptors or ion channels known to be important in cardiovascular regulation.

Blockade of the angiotensin II receptor inhibits the negative regulatory feedback of angiotensin II on renin secretion, but the resulting increased plasma renin activity and angiotensin II circulating levels do not overcome the effect of valsartan on blood pressure.

PHARMACOKINETICS

Valsartan peak plasma concentration is reached 2 to 4 hours after dosing. Valsartan shows bi-exponential decay kinetics following intravenous administration, with an average elimination half-life of about 6 hours. Absolute bioavailability for the capsule formulation is about 25% (range 10%-35%). Food decreases the exposure (as measured by AUC) to valsartan by about 40% and peak plasma concentration (C_{max}) by about 50%. AUC and C_{max} values of valsartan increase approximately linearly with increasing dose over the clinical dosing range. Valsartan does not accumulate appreciably in plasma following repeated administration.

CLINICAL PHARMACOLOGY: *(cont'd)*

METABOLISM AND ELIMINATION

Valsartan, when administered as an oral solution, is primarily recovered in feces (about 83% of dose) and urine (about 13% of dose). The recovery is mainly as unchanged drug, with only about 20% of dose recovered as metabolites. The primary metabolite, accounting for about 9% of dose, is valeryl 4-hydroxy valsartan. The enzyme(s) responsible for valsartan metabolism have not been identified but do not seem to be CYP 450 isozymes.

Following intravenous administration, plasma clearance of valsartan is about 2 L/h and its renal clearance is 0.62 L/h (about 30% of total clearance).

DISTRIBUTION

The steady state volume of distribution of valsartan after intravenous administration is small (17 L), indicating that valsartan does not distribute into tissues extensively. Valsartan is highly bound to serum proteins (95%), mainly serum albumin.

SPECIAL POPULATIONS

Pediatric: The pharmacokinetics of valsartan have not been investigated in patients <18 years of age.

Geriatric: Exposure (measured by AUC) to valsartan is higher by 70% and the half-life is longer by 35% in the elderly than in the young. No dosage adjustment is necessary (see DOSAGE AND ADMINISTRATION).

Gender: Pharmacokinetics of valsartan does not differ significantly between males and females.

Renal Insufficiency: There is no apparent correlation between renal function (measured by creatinine clearance) and exposure (measured by AUC) to valsartan in patients with different degrees of renal impairment. Consequently, dose adjustment is not required in patients with mild-to-moderate renal dys function. No studies have been performed in patients with severe impairment of renal function (creatinine clearance < 10 ml/min) or patients undergoing dialysis, and it is not known whether valsartan is removed by hemodialysis. In the case of severe renal disease, exercise care with dosing of valsartan (see DOSAGE AND ADMINISTRATION).

Hepatic Insufficiency: On average, patients with mild-to-moderate chronic liver disease have twice the exposure (measured by AUC values) to valsartan of healthy volunteers (matched by age, sex and weight). In general, no dosage adjustment is needed in patients with mild-to-moderate liver disease. Care should be exercised in patients with liver disease (see DOSAGE AND ADMINISTRATION).

PHARMACODYNAMICS AND CLINICAL EFFECTS

Valsartan inhibits the pressor effect of angiotensin II infusions. An oral dose of 80 mg inhibits the pressor effect by about 80% at peak with approximately 30% inhibition persisting for 24 hours. No information on the effect of larger doses is available.

Removal of the negative feedback of angiotensin II causes a 2- to 3-fold rise in plasma renin and consequent rise in angiotensin II plasma concentration in hypertensive patients. Minimal decreases in plasma aldosterone were observed after administration of valsartan; very little effect on serum potassium was observed.

In multiple-dose studies in hypertensive patients with stable renal insufficiency and patients with renovascular hypertension, valsartan had no clinically significant effects on glomerular filtration rate, filtration fraction, creatinine clearance, or renal plasma flow.

In multiple-dose studies in hypertensive patients, valsartan had no notable effects on total cholesterol, fasting triglycerides, fasting serum glucose, or uric acid.

The antihypertensive effects of valsartan were demonstrated principally in 7 placebo-controlled, 4- to 12-week trials (one in patients over 65) of dosages from 10 to 320 mg/day in patients with baseline diastolic blood pressures of 95-115. The studies allowed comparison of once-daily and twice-daily regimens of 160 mg/day; comparison of peak and trough effects; comparison (in pooled data) of response by gender, age, and race; and evaluation of incremental ef fects of hydrochlorothiazide.

Administration of valsartan to patients with essential hypertension results in a significant reduction of sitting, supine, and standing systolic and diastolic blood pressure, usually with little or no orthostatic change.

In most patients, after administration of a single oral dose, onset of antihypertensive activity occurs at approximately 2 hours, and maximum reduction of blood pressure is achieved within 6 hours. The antihypertensive effect persists for 24 hours after dosing, but there is a decrease from peak effect at lower doses (40 mg) presumably reflecting loss of inhibition of angiotensin II. At higher doses, however (160 mg), there is little difference in peak and trough effect. During repeated dosing, the reduction in blood pressure with any dose is substantially present within 2 weeks, and maximal reduction is generally attained after 4 weeks. In long-term follow-up studies (without placebo control), the effect of valsartan appeared to be maintained for up to two years. The antihypertensive effect is independent of age, gender or race. The latter finding regarding race is based on pooled data and should be viewed with caution, because antihypertensive drugs that affect the renin-angiotensin system (that is, ACE inhibitors and angiotensin-II blockers) have generally been found to be less effective in low-renin hypertensives (frequently blacks) than in high-renin hypertensives (frequently whites). In pooled, randomized, controlled trials of valsartan that included a total of 140 blacks and 830 whites, valsartan and an ACE-inhibitor control were generally at least as effective in blacks as whites. The explanation for this difference from previous findings is unclear.

Abrupt withdrawal of valsartan has not been associated with a rapid increase in blood pressure.

The blood pressure lowering effect of valsartan and thiazide-type diuretics are approximately additive.

The 7 studies of valsartan monotherapy included over 2000 patients randomized to various doses of valsartan and about 800 patients randomized to placebo. Doses below 80 mg were not consistently distinguished from those of placebo at trough, but doses of 80, 160 and 320 mg produced dose-related decreases in systolic and diastolic blood pressure, with the difference from placebo of approximately 6-9/3-5 mmHg at 80-160 mg and 9/6 mmHg at 320 mg. In a controlled trial the addition of HCTZ to valsartan 80 mg resulted in additional lowering of systolic and diastolic blood pressure by approximately 6/3 and 12/5 mmHg for 12.5 and 25 mg of HCTZ, respectively, compared to valsartan 80 mg alone.

Patients with an inadequate response to 80 mg once daily were titrated to either 160 mg once daily or 80 mg twice daily, which resulted in a comparable response in both groups.

In controlled trials, the antihypertensive effect of once-daily valsartan 80 mg was similar to that of once-daily enalapril 20 mg or once-daily lisinopril 10 mg.

There was essentially no change in heart rate in valsartan-treated patients in controlled trials.

INDICATIONS AND USAGE:

Valsartan is indicated for the treatment of hypertension. It may be used alone or in combination with other antihypertensive agents.

CONTRAINDICATIONS:

Valsartan is contraindicated in patients who are hypersensitive to any component of this product.

WARNINGS:

FETAL/NEONATAL MORBIDITY AND MORTALITY

Drugs that act directly on the renin-angiotensin system can cause fetal and neonatal morbidity and death when administered to pregnant women. Several dozen cases have been reported in the world literature in patients who were taking angiotensin-converting enzyme inhibitors. When pregnancy is detected, valsartan should be discontinued as soon as possible.

The use of drugs that act directly on the renin-angiotensin system during the second and third trimesters of pregnancy has been associated with fetal and neonatal injury, including hypotension, neonatal skull hypoplasia, anuria, reversible or irreversible renal failure, and death. Oligohydramnios has also been reported, presumably resulting from decreased fetal renal function; oligohydramnios in this setting has been associated with fetal limb contractures, craniofacial deformation, and hypoplastic lung development. Prematurity, intrauterine growth retardation, and patent ductus arteriosus have also been re ported, although it is not clear whether these occurrences were due to exposure to the drug.

These adverse effects do not appear to have resulted from intrauterine drug exposure that has been limited to the first trimester. Mothers whose embryos and fetuses are exposed to an angiotensin II receptor antagonist only during the first trimester should be so informed. Nonetheless, when patients become pregnant, physicians should advise the patient to discontinue the use of valsartan as soon as possible.

Rarely (probably less often than once in every thousand pregnancies), no alternative to a drug acting on the renin-angiotensin system will be found. In these rare cases, the mothers should be apprised of the potential hazards to their fetuses, and serial ultrasound examinations should be performed to assess the intra-amniotic environment.

If oligohydramnios is observed, valsartan should be discontinued unless it is considered life-saving for the mother. Contraction stress testing (CST), a nonstress test (NST), or biophysical profiling (BPP) may be appropriate, depending upon the week of pregnancy. Patients and physicians should be aware, however, that oligohydramnios may not appear until after the fetus has sustained irreversible injury.

Infants with histories of *in utero* exposure to an angiotensin II receptor antagonist should be closely observed for hypotension, oliguria, and hyperkalemia. If oliguria occurs, attention should be directed toward support of blood pressure and renal perfusion. Exchange transfusion or dialysis may be required as means of reversing hypotension and/or substituting for disordered renal function.

No teratogenic effects were observed when valsartan was administered to pregnant mice and rats at oral doses up to 600 mg/kg/day and to pregnant rabbits at oral doses up to 10 mg/kg/day. However, significant decreases in fetal weight, pup birth weight, pup survival rate, and slight delays in developmental milestones were observed in studies in which parental rats were treated with valsartan at oral, maternally toxic (reduction in body weight gain and food consumption) doses of 600 mg/kg/day during organogenesis or late gestation and lactation. In rabbits, fetotoxicity (*i.e.*, resorptions, litter loss, abortions, and low body weight) associated with maternal toxicity (mortality) was observed at doses of 5 and 10 mg/kg/day. The no observed adverse effect doses of 600, 200 and 2 mg/kg/day in mice, rats and rabbits represent 9, 6, and 0.1 times, respectively, the maximum recommended human dose on a mg/m^2 basis. (Calculations assume an oral dose of 320 mg/day and a 60-kg patient.)

HYPOTENSION IN VOLUME- AND/OR SALT-DEPLETED PATIENTS

Excessive reduction of blood pressure was rarely seen (0.1%) in patients with uncomplicated hypertension. In patients with an activated renin-angiotensin system, such as volume- and/or salt-depleted patients receiving high doses of diuretics, symptomatic hypotension may occur. This condition should be corrected prior to administration of valsartan, or the treatment should start under close medical supervision.

If hypotension occurs, the patient should be placed in the supine position and, if necessary, given an intravenous infusion of normal saline. A transient hypotensive response is not a contraindication to further treatment, which usually can be continued without difficulty once the blood pressure has stabilized.

PRECAUTIONS:

GENERAL

Impaired Hepatic Function: As the majority of valsartan is eliminated in the bile, patients with mild-to-moderate hepatic impairment, including patients with biliary obstructive disorders, showed lower valsartan clearance (higher AUCs). Care should be exercised in administering valsartan to these patients.

Impaired Renal Function: As a consequence of inhibiting the renin-angiotensin-aldosterone system, changes in renal function may be anticipated in susceptible individuals. In patients whose renal function may depend on the activity of the renin-angiotensin-aldosterone system (*e.g.*, patients with severe congestive heart failure), treatment with angiotensin-converting enzyme inhibitors and angiotensin receptor antagonists have been associated with oliguria and/ or progressive azotemia and (rarely) with acute renal failure and/or death. Valsartan would be expected to behave similarly.

In studies of ACE inhibitors in patients with unilateral or bilateral renal artery stenosis, increases in serum creatinine or blood urea nitrogen have been reported. In a 4-day trial of valsartan in 12 patients with unilateral renal artery stenosis, no significant increases in serum creatinine or blood urea nitrogen were observed. There has been no long-term use of valsartan in patients with unilateral or bilateral renal artery stenosis, but an effect similar to that seen with ACE inhibitors should be anticipated.

INFORMATION FOR THE PATIENT

Pregnancy: Female patients of childbearing age should be told about the consequences of second- and third-trimester exposure to drugs that act on the renin-angiotensin system, and they should also be told that these consequences do not appear to have resulted from intrauterine drug exposure that has been limited to the first trimester. These patients should be asked to report pregnancies to their physicians as soon as possible.

CARCINOGENESIS, MUTAGENESIS, AND IMPAIRMENT OF FERTILITY

There was no evidence of carcinogenicity when valsartan was administered in the diet to mice and rats for up to 2 years at doses up to 160 and 200 mg/kgl day, respectively. These doses in mice and rats are about 2.6 and 6 times, respectively, the maximum recommended human dose on a mg/m^2 basis. (Calculations assume an oral dose of 320 mg/day and a 60-kg patient).

Mutagenicity assays did not reveal any valsartan-related effects at either the gene or chromosome level. These assays included bacterial mutagenicity tests with *Salmonella* (Ames) and *E coli*; a gene mutation test with Chinese hamster V79 cells; a cytogenetic test with Chinese hamster ovary cells; and a rat micronucleus test.

Valsartan had no adverse effects on the reproductive performance of male or female rats at oral doses up to 200 mglkg/day. This dose is 6 times the maximum recommended human dose on a mg/m^2 basis. (Calculations assume an oral dose of 320 mg/day and a 60-kg patient).

PREGNANCY CATEGORIES C (FIRST TRIMESTER) AND D (SECOND AND THIRD TRIMESTERS)

See WARNINGS, Fetal/Neonatal Morbidity and Mortality.

PRECAUTIONS: *(cont'd)*

NURSING MOTHERS

It is not known whether valsartan is excreted in human milk, but valsartan was excreted in the milk of lactating rats. Because of the potential for adverse effects on the nursing infant, a decision should be made whether to discontinue nursing or discontinue the drug, taking into account the importance of the drug to the mother.

PEDIATRIC USE

Safety and effectiveness in pediatric patients have not been established.

GERIATRIC USE

In the controlled clinical trials of valsartan, 1214 (36.2%) of patients treated with valsartan were 65 years and 265 (7.9%) were >75 years. No overall difference in the efficacy or safety of valsartan was observed in this patient population, but greater sensitivity of some older individuals cannot be ruled out.

DRUG INTERACTIONS:

No clinically significant pharmacokinetic interactions were observed when valsartan was coadministered with amlodipine, atenolol, cimetidine, digoxin, furosemide, glibenclamide, hydrochlorothiazide, or indomethacin. The valsartan-atenolol combination was more antihypertensive than either component, but it did not lower the heart rate more than atenolol alone.

Coadministration of valsartan and warfarin did not change the pharmacokinetics of valsartan or the time-course of the anticoagulant properties of warfarin.

CYP 450 Interactions: The enzyme(s) responsible for valsartan metabolism have not been identified but do not seem to be CYP 450 isozymes. The inhibitory or induction potential of valsartan on CYP 450 is also unknown.

ADVERSE REACTIONS:

Valsartan has been evaluated for safety in more than 4000 patients, including over 400 treated for over 6 months, and more than 160 for over 1 year. Adverse experiences have generally been mild and transient in nature and have only infrequently required discontinuation of therapy. The overall incidence of adverse experiences with valsartan was similar to placebo.

The overall frequency of adverse experiences was neither dose-related nor related to gender, age, race, or regimen. Discontinuation of therapy due to side effects was required in 2.3% of valsartan patients and 2.0% of placebo patients. The most common reasons for discontinuation of therapy with valsartan were headache and dizziness.

The adverse experiences that occurred in placebo-controlled clinical trials in at least 1 % of patients treated with valsartan and at a higher incidence in valsartan (n=2316) than placebo (n=888) patients included viral infection (3% vs. 2%), fatigue (2% vs.1%), and abdominal pain (2% vs.1%).

Headache, dizziness, upper respiratory infection, cough, diarrhea, rhinitis, sinusitis, nausea, pharyngitis, edema, and arthralgia occurred at a more than 1% rate but at about the same incidence in placebo and valsartan patients.

In trials in which valsartan was compared to an ACE inhibitor with or without placebo, the incidence of dry cough was significantly greater in the ACE-inhibitor group (7.9%) than in the groups who received valsartan (2.6%) or placebo (1.5%). In a 129-patient trial limited to patients who had had dry cough when they had previously received ACE inhibitors, the incidences of cough in patients who received valsartan, HCTZ, or lisinopril were 20%, 19%, and 69% respectively (p<0.001).

Dose-related orthostatic effects were seen in less than 1% of patients. An increase in the incidence of dizziness was observed in patients treated with valsartan 320 mg (8%) compared to 10 to 160 mg (2% to 4%).

Valsartan has been used concomitantly with hydrochlorothiazide without evidence of clinically important adverse interactions.

Other adverse experiences that occurred in controlled clinical trials of patients treated with valsartan (>0.2% of valsartan patients) are listed below. It cannot be determined whether these events were causally related to valsartan.

Body as a Whole: Allergic reaction and asthenia

Cardiovascular: Palpitations

Dermatologic: Pruritus and rash

Digestive: Constipation, dry mouth, dyspepsia, and flatulence

Musculoskeletal: Back pain, muscle cramps, and myalgia

Neurologic and Psychiatric: Anxiety, insomnia, paresthesia, and somnolence

Respiratory: Dyspnea

Special Senses: Vertigo

Urogenital: Impotence

Other reported events seen less frequently in clinical trials included chest pain, syncope, anorexia, vomiting, and angioedema.

CLINICAL LABORATORY TEST FINDINGS

In controlled clinical trials, clinically important changes in standard laboratory parameters were rarely associated with administration of valsartan.

Creatinine: Minor elevations in creatinine occurred in 0.8% of patients taking valsartan and 0.6% given placebo in controlled clinical trials.

Hemoglobin and Hematocrit: Greater than 20% decreases in hemoglobin and hematocrit were observed in 0.4% and 0.8%, respectively, of valsartan patients, compared with 0.1% and 0.1% in placebo-treated patients. One valsartan patient discontinued treatment for microcytic anemia.

Liver function tests: Occasional elevations (greater than 150%) of liver chemistries occurred in valsartan-treated patients. Three patients (< 0.1%) treated with valsartan discontinued treatment for elevated liver chemistries.

Neutropenia: Neutropenia was observed in 1.9% of patients treated with valsartan and 0.8% of patients treated with placebo.

Serum Potassium: Greater than 20% increases in serum potassium were observed in 4.4% of valsartan-treated patients compared to 2.9% of placebo-treated patients. No patient treated with valsartan discontinued therapy for hyperkalemia.

OVERDOSAGE:

Limited data are available related to overdosage in humans. The most likely manifestations of overdosage would be hypotension and tachycardia; bradycardia could occur from parasympathetic (vagal) stimulation. If symptomatic hypotension should occur, supportive treatment should be instituted.

It is not known whether valsartan or its active metabolite can be removed by hemodialysis.

OVERDOSAGE: *(cont'd)*

Valsartan was without grossly observable adverse effects at single oral doses up to 2000 mg/kg in rats and up to 1000 mg/kg in marmosets, except for salivation and diarrhea in the rat and vomiting in the marmoset at the highest dose (60 and 37 times, respectively, the maximum recommended human dose on a mg/m^2 basis). (Calculations assume an oral dose of 320 mg/day and a 60-kg patient).

DOSAGE AND ADMINISTRATION:

The recommended starting dose of valsartan is 80 mg once daily when used as monotherapy in patients who are not volume-depleted. Valsartan may be used over a dose range of 80 mg to 320 mg daily, administered once-a-day.

The antihypertensive effect is substantially present within 2 weeks and maximal reduction is generally attained after 4 weeks. If additional antihypertensive effect is required, the dosage may be increased to 160 mg or 320 mg or a diuretic may be added. Addition of a diuretic has a greater effect than dose increases beyond 80 mg.

No initial dosage adjustment is required for elderly patients, for patients with mild or moderate renal impairment, or for patients with mild or moderate liver insufficiency. Care should be exercised with dosing of valsartan in patients with hepatic or severe renal impairment.

Valsartan may be administered with other antihypertensive agents.

Valsartan may be administered with or without food.

PATIENT INFORMATION:

Valsartan is used for the treatment of hypertension.

Do not use during pregnancy or if nursing.

Inform physician if you have kidney or liver disease. May cause headache, dizziness, viral infection, fatigue, cough, or abdominal pain.

Take with or without food.

HOW SUPPLIED:

Diovan is available as capsules containing valsartan 80 mg or 160 mg. Capsules are imprinted as follows:

80 mg Capsule - Light grey/light pink opaque, imprinted CG FZF

160 mg Capsule - Dark grey/light pink opaque, imprinted CG GOG

Store below 30°C (86°F). Protect from moisture. Dispense in tight container (USP).

HOW SUPPLIED - EQUIVALENTS NOT AVAILABLE:

Capsule - Oral - 80 mg

80 mg x 100 $114.04 DIOVAN, Novartis 00083-4000-01

VANCOMYCIN HYDROCHLORIDE *(002420)*

CATEGORIES: Anesthesia; Anti-Infectives; Antibiotics; Antimicrobials; Bone Infections; Colitis; Dental; Endocarditis; Enterocolitis; Respiratory Tract Infections; Septicemia; Skin Infections; Pregnancy Category C; Sales > $100 Million; FDA Approval Pre 1982

BRAND NAMES: *Diatracin*; Lyphocin; **Vancocin**; Vancoled; Vancor
(International brand names outside U.S. in italics)

FORMULARIES: BC-BS; PCS; WHO

COST OF THERAPY: $14.00 (Infections; Injection; 1 gm/vial; 2/day; 7 days) vs. Potential Cost of $7,048.46 (DRG 79, Respiratory Infections)

PRIMARY ICD9: 136.9 (Unspecified Infections And Parasitic Diseases)

DESCRIPTION:

Injection: Vancocin HCl (vancomycin hydrochloride injection) in the Galaxy plastic container (PL 2040) contains vancomycin as vancomycin hydrochloride. It is a tricyclic glycopeptide antibiotic derived from*Amycolatopsis orientalis* formerly *Nocardia orientalis*). The molecular formula is $C_{66}H_{75}C_{12}H_9O_{24}$·HCl and the molecular weight is 1,4865.73. 500 mg of the base are equivalent to 0.34 mmol.

Oral: THIS PREPARATION FOR THE TREATMENT OF COLITIS IS FOR ORAL USE ONLY AND IS NOT SYSTEMICALLY ABSORBED. VANCOMYCIN HCL MUST BE GIVEN ORALLY FOR TREATMENT OF STAPHYLOCOCCAL ENTEROCOLITIS AND ANTIBIOTIC-ASSOCIATED PSEUDOMEMBRANOUS COLITIS PRODUCED BY Clostridium Difficile. ORALLY ADMINISTERED VANCOMYCIN HCL IS Not EFFECTIVE FOR OTHER TYPES OF INFECTION.

PARENTERAL ADMINISTRATION OF VANCOMYCIN HCL IS NOT EFFECTIVE FOR TREATMENT OF STAPHYLOCOCCAL ENTEROCOLITIS AND ANTIBIOTIC-ASSOCIATED PSEUDOMEMBRANOUS COLITIS PRODUCED BY Clostridium Difficile. IF PARENTERAL VANCOMYCIN THERAPY IS DESIRED, USE VANCOMYCIN HCL (STERILE VANCOMYCIN HYDROCHLORIDE, USP), INTRAVENOUS.

Vancomycin HCl for Oral Solution (Vancomycin Hydrochloride for Oral Solution, USP) and Pulvules Vancomycin HCl (Vancomycin Hydrochloride Capsules, USP), contain chromatographically purified vancomycin hydrochloride, a tricyclic glycopeptide antibiotic derived from Nocardia orientalis (formerly Streptomyces Orientalis).

Vancomycin HCl for Oral Solution contains vancomycin hydrochloride equivalent to 10 g or 1 g vancomycin.

CLINICAL PHARMACOLOGY:

Vancomycin is poorly absorbed after oral administration; it is given intravenously for therapy of systemic infections. Intramuscular injection is painful.

In subjects with normal kidney function, multiple intravenous dosing of 1 g of vancomycin (15 mg/kg)infused over 60 minutes produces mean plasma concentrations of approximately 63 mcg/mL immediately at the completion of infusion, mean plasma concentrations of approximately 23 mcg/mL 2 hours after infusion, and mean plasma concentrations of approximately 8 mcg/mL 11 hours after the end of the infusion. Multiple dosing of 500 mg infused over 30 minutes produces mean plasma concentrations of about 49 mcg/mL at the completion of infusion, mean plasma concentrations of about 19 mcg/mL 2 hours after infusion, and mean plasma concentrations of about 10 mcg/mL 6 hours after infusion. The plasma concentrations during multiple dosing are similar to those after a single dose.

The mean elimination half-life of vancomycin from plasma is 4 to 6 hours in subjects with normal renal function. In the first 24 hours, about 75% of an administered dose of vancomycin is excreted in urine by glomerular filtration. Mean plasma clearance is about 0.058 L/kg/h, and mean renal clearance is about 0.048 L/kg/h. Renal dysfunction slows excretion of vancomycin. In anephric patients, the average half-life of elimination is 7.5 days. The distribution coefficient is from 0.3 to 0.43 L/kg. There is no apparent metabolism of the

CLINICAL PHARMACOLOGY: *(cont'd)*

drug. About 60% of an intraperitoneal dose of vancomycin administered during peritoneal dialysis is absorbed systemically in 6 hours. Serum concentrations of about 10 mcg/mL are achieved by intraperitoneal injection of 30 mg/kg of vancomycin. Vancomycin is not effectively removed by either hemodialysis or peritoneal dialysis; there have been no reports of vancomycin clearance with hemoperfusion and hemofiltration.

Total systemic and renal clearance of vancomycin may be reduced in the elderly.

Vancomycin is approximately 55% serum protein bound as measured by ultrafiltration at vancomycin serum concentrations of 10 to 100 mcg/mL. After IV administration of vancomycin, inhibitory concentrations are present in pleural, pericardial, ascitic, and synovial fluids; in urine; in peritoneal dialysis fluid; and in atrial appendage tissue. Vancomycin HCl does not readily diffuse across normal meninges into the spinal fluid; but, when the meninges are inflamed, penetration into the spinal fluid occurs.

MICROBIOLOGY

The bactericidal action of vancomycin results primarily from inhibition of cell-wall biosynthesis. In addition, vancomycin alters bacterial-cell-membrane permeability and RNA synthesis. There is no cross-resistance between vancomycin and other antibiotics.

Vancomycin is active against staphylococci, including *Staphylococcus Aureus* and *Staphylococcus Epidermidis* (including heterogeneous methicillin-resistant strains); streptococci, including*Streptococcus Pyogenes, Streptococcus Pneumoniae* (including penicillin-resistant strains), *Streptococcus Agalactiae*, the viridans group, *Streptococcus Bovis*, and enterococci (eg,*Enterococcus Faecalis* [formerly *Streptococcus Faecalis*]); *Clostridium Difficile* (eg, toxigenic strains implicated in pseudomembranous enterocolitis); and diphtheroids. Other organisms that are susceptible to vancomycin *in vitro* include *Listeria Monocytogenes, Lactobacillus* species, *Actinomyces* species, *Clostridium* species, and *Bacillus* species.

Vancomycin is not active *in vitro* against gram-negative bacilli, mycobacteria, or fungi.

Synergy: The combination of vancomycin and an aminoglycoside acts synergistically *in vitro* against many strains of *S. aureus*, nonenterococcal group D streptococci, enterococci, and *Streptococcus* species (viridans group).

SUSCEPTIBILITY TESTING

Diffusion Techniques: Quantitative methods that require measurement of zone diameters provide reproducible estimates of the susceptibility of bacteria to antimicrobial compounds. One such standardized procedure[1,3] that has been recommended for use with disks to test the susceptibility of microorganisms to vancomycin uses the 30-mcg vancomycin disk. Interpretation involves correlation of the diameter obtained in the disk test with the MIC for vancomycin.

Reports from the laboratory providing results of the standard single-disk susceptibility test with a 30-mcg vancomycin disk should be interpreted according to the following criteria:

TABLE 1

Zone Diameter (mm)	Interpretation
≥12	Susceptible (S)
10-11	Intermediate (I)
≤9	Resistant (R)

A report of "Susceptible" indicates that the pathogen is likely to be inhibited by usually achievable concentrations of the antimicrobial compound in blood. A report of "Intermediate" indicates that the result should be considered equivocal, and, if the microorganism is not fully susceptible, to alternative clinically feasible drugs, the test should be repeated. This category implies possible clinical applicability in body sites where the drug is physiologically concentrated or in situations where high dosage of drug can be used. This category also provides a buffer zone that prevents small uncontrolled technical factors from causing major discrepancies in interpretation. A report of "Resistant" indicates that usually achievable concentrations of the antimicrobial compound in the blood are unlikely to be inhibitory and that other therapy should be selected.

Measurement of the MIC or MBC and achieved antimicrobial compound concentrations may be appropriate to guide therapy in some infections. (See Clinical Pharmacology section for further information on drug concentrations achieved in infected body sites and other pharmacokinetic properties of this antimicrobial drug product.)

Standardized susceptibility test procedures require the use of laboratory control organisms. The 30-mcg vancomycin disk should provide the following zone diameters in these laboratory test quality control strains:

TABLE 2

Microorganism	Zone Diameter (mm)
S. aureus ATCC 25923	15-19

Dilution Techniques: Quantitative methods that are used to determine minimum inhibitory concentrations provide reproducible estimates of the susceptibility of bacteria to antimicrobial compounds. One such standardized procedure uses a standardized dilution method[2,3](broth, agar, microdilution) or equivalent with vancomycin powder. The MIC values obtained should be interpreted according to the following criteria:

TABLE 3

MIC (mcg/mL)	Interpretation
≤4	Susceptible (S)
8	Intermediate (I)
≥16	Resistant (R)

Interpretation should be as stated above for results using diffusion techniques.

As with standard diffusion techniques, dilution methods require the use of laboratory control microorganisms. Standard vancomycin powder should provide the following MIC values:

TABLE 4

Microorganism	MIC (mcg/mL)
S. aureus ATCC 29213	0.5-2
S. faecalis ATCC 29212	1-4

INDICATIONS AND USAGE:

Injection: Vancomycin HCl (Sterile Vancomycin Hydrochloride,USP) is indicated for the treatment of serious or severe infections caused by susceptible strains of methicillin-resistant (beta-lactam-resistant) staphylococci. It is indicated for penicillin-allergic patients, for patients who cannot receive or who have failed to respond to other drugs, including the penicillins or cephalosporins, and for infections caused by vancomycin-susceptible organisms that are resistant to other antimicrobial drugs. Vancomycin HCl is indicated for initial therapy when methicillin-resistant staphylococci are suspected, but after susceptibility data are available, therapy should be adjusted accordingly.

Vancomycin HCl is effective in the treatment of staphylococcal endocarditis. Its effectiveness has been documented in other infections due to staphylococci, including septicemia, bone infections, lower respiratory tract infections, and skin and skin-structure infections. When staphylococcal infections are localized and purulent, antibiotics are used as adjuncts to appropriate surgical measures.

Vancomycin HCl has been reported to be effective alone or in combination with an aminoglycoside for endocarditis caused by *Streptococcus viridans* or *S. bovis*. For endocarditis caused by enterococci (eg, *E. faecalis*), Vancomycin HCl has been reported to be effective only in combination with an aminoglycoside.

Vancomycin HCl has been reported to be effective for the treatment of diphtheroid endocarditis. Vancomycin HCl has been used successfully in combination with either rifampin, an aminoglycoside, or both in early-onset prosthetic valve endocarditis caused by *S. epidermidis*or diphtheroids.

Specimens for bacteriologic cultures should be obtained in order to isolate and identify causative organisms and to determine their susceptibilities to Vancomycin HCl.

The parenteral form of Vancomycin HCl may be administered orally for treatment of antibiotic-associated pseudomembranous colitis caused by *C. difficile* and Staphylococcal Enterocolitis.

Parenteral administration of Vancomycin HCl alone is of unproven benefit for these indications.

Vancomycin HCl is not effective by the oral route for other types of infection.

Although no controlled clinical efficacy studies have been conducted, intravenous vancomycin has been suggested by the American Heart Association and the American Dental Association as prophylaxis against bacterial endocarditis in penicillin-allergic patients who have congenital heart disease or rheumatic or other acquired valvular heart disease when these patients undergo dental procedures or surgical procedures of the upper respiratory tract.

Note: When selecting antibiotics for the prevention of bacterial endocarditis, the physician or dentist should read the full joint statement of the American Heart Association and the American Dental Association.

ORAL

Vancomycin HCl (vancomycin hydrochloride) is administered orally for treatment of staphylococcal enterocolitis and antibiotic-associated pseudomembranous colitis produced by *C. Difficile*. Parenteral administration of Vancomycin HCl is not effective for the above indications; therefore, Vancomycin HCl must be given orally for these indications. Orally administered Vancomycin HCl is not effective for other types of infection.

CONTRAINDICATIONS:

Vancomycin HCl is contraindicated in patients with known hypersensitivity to this antibiotic.

WARNINGS:

Rapid bolus administration (eg, over several minutes) may be associated with exaggerated hypotension, including shock, and, rarely, cardiac arrest.

Vancomycin HCl injection should be administered over a period of not less than 60 minutes to avoid rapid-infusion-related reactions.

Stopping the infusion usually results in prompt cessation of these reactions.

Ototoxicity has occurred in patients receiving Vancomycin HCl. It may be transient or permanent.

It has been reported mostly in patients who have been given excessive doses, who have an underlying hearing loss, or who are receiving concomitant therapy with another ototoxic agent, such as an aminoglycoside. Vancomycin should be used with caution in patients with renal insufficiency because the risk of toxicity is appreciably increased by high, prolonged blood concentrations.

Dosage of Vancomycin HCl must be adjusted for patients with renal dysfunction (see PRECAUTIONS and DOSAGE AND ADMINISTRATION).

Pseudomembranous colitis has been reported with nearly all antibacterial agents, including vancomycin, and may range in severity from mild to life-threatening. Therefore, it is important to consider this diagnosis in patients who present with diarrhea subsequent to the administration of antibacterial agents.

Treatment with antibacterial agents alters the normal flora of the colon and may permit overgrowth of clostridia. Studies indicate that a toxin produced by *Clostridium difficile* is a primary cause of "antibiotic-associated colitis." After the diagnosis of pseudomembranous colitis has been established, therapeutic measures should be initiated. Mild cases of pseudomembranous colitis usually respond to drug discontinuation alone. In moderate to severe cases, consideration should be given to management with fluids and electrolytes, protein supplementation, and treatment with an antibacterial drug clinically effective against *C. difficile* colitis.

PRECAUTIONS:

General: Clinically significant serum concentrations have been reported in some patients who have taken multiple oral doses of vancomycin for active C Difficile-induced pseudomembranous colitis.

Prolonged use of Vancomycin HCl may result in the overgrowth of nonsusceptible organisms. Careful observation of the patient is essential. If superinfection occurs during therapy, appropriate measures should be taken.

In order to minimize the risk of nephrotoxicity when treating patients with underlying renal dysfunction or patients receiving concomitant therapy with an aminoglycoside, serial monitoring of renal function should be performed and particular care should be taken in following appropriate dosing schedules (see DOSAGE AND ADMINISTRATION.)

Serial tests of auditory function may be helpful in order to minimize the risk of ototoxicity.

Reversible neutropenia has been reported in patients receiving Vancomycin HCl (see ADVERSE REACTIONS.) Patients who will undergo prolonged therapy with Vancomycin HCl or those who are receiving concomitant drugs that may cause neutropenia should have periodic monitoring of the leukocyte count.

Vancomycin HCl is irritating to tissue and must be given by a secure intravenous route of administration. Pain, tenderness, and necrosis occur with intramuscular injection of Vancomycin HCl or with inadvertent extravasation. Thrombophlebitis may occur, the frequency and severity of which can be minimized by slow infusion of the drug and by rotation of venous access sites.

There have been reports that the frequency of infusion-related events (including hypotension, flushing, erythema, urticaria, and pruritus) increases with the concomitant administration of anesthetic agents. Infusion-related events may be minimized by the administration of Vancomycin HCl as a 60-minute infusion prior to anesthetic induction.

PRECAUTIONS: *(cont'd)*

The safety and efficacy of vancomycin administered by the intrathecal (intralumbar or intraventricular) route or by the intraperitoneal route have not been established by adequate and well-controlled trials.

Reports have revealed that administration of sterile vancomycin HCl by the intraperitoneal route during continuous ambulatory peritoneal dialysis (CAPD) has resulted in a syndrome of chemical peritonitis. To date, this syndrome has ranged from a cloudy dialysate alone to a cloudy dialysate accompanied by variable degrees of abdominal pain and fever. This syndrome appears to be short-lived after discontinuation of intraperitoneal vancomycin.

Pregnancy Category C: Animal reproduction studies have not been conducted with Vancomycin HCl. It is also not known whether Vancomycin HCl can affect reproduction capacity. In a controlled clinical study, the potential ototoxic and nephrotoxic effects of vancomycin on infants were evaluated when the drug was administered to pregnant women for serious staphylococcal infections complicating intravenous drug abuse. Vancomycin HCl was found in cord blood. No sensorineural hearing loss or nephrotoxicity attributable to Vancomycin HCl was noted. One infant whose mother received Vancomycin HCl in the third trimester experienced conductive hearing loss that was not attributed to the administration of Vancomycin HCl. Because the number of patients treated in this study was limited and Vancomycin HCl was administered only in the second and third trimesters, it is not known whether Vancomycin HCl causes fetal harm.

Vancomycin HCl should be given to a pregnant woman only if clearly needed.

Nursing Mothers: Vancomycin HCl is excreted in human milk. Caution should be exercised when Vancomycin HCl is administered to a nursing woman. Because of the potential for adverse events, a decision should be made whether to discontinue nursing or to discontinue the drug, taking into account the importance of the drug to the mother.

Pediatric Use: In premature neonates and young infants, it may be appropriate to confirm desired vancomycin serum concentrations.

Concomitant administration of vancomycin and anesthetic agents has been associated with erythema and histamine-like flushing in children (see ADVERSE REACTIONS.) The potential for toxic effects in children from chemicals that may leach from the plastic containers into the single- dose, premixed intravenous preparation has not been determined.

Geriatrics: The natural decrement of glomerual filtration with increasing age may lead to elevated vancomycin serum concentrations if dosage is not adjusted. Vancomycin dosage schedules should be adjusted in elderly patients (see DOSAGE AND ADMINISTRATION.)

DRUG INTERACTIONS:

Concomitant administration of vancomycin and unaesthetic agents has been associated with erythema and histamine-like flushing (see PRECAUTIONS, Pediatric Use) and anaphylactoid reactions (see ADVERSE REACTIONS.)

Concurrent and/or sequential systemic or topical use of other potentially neurotoxic and/or nephrotoxic drugs, such as amphotericin B, aminoglycosides, bacitracin, polymyxin B, colistin, viomycin, or cisplatin, when indicated, requires careful monitoring.

ADVERSE REACTIONS:

Infusion-Related Events: During or soon after rapid infusion of Vancomycin HCl, patients may develop anaphylactoid reactions, including hypotension (see ANIMAL PHARMACOLOGY), wheezing, dyspnea, urticaria, or pruritus. Rapid infusion may also cause flushing of the upper body ("red neck") or pain and muscle spasm of the chest and back. These reactions usually resolve within 20 minutes but may persist for several hours. Such events are infrequent if Vancomycin HCl is given by a slow infusion over 60 minutes. In studies of normal volunteers, infusion-related events did not occur when Vancomycin HCl was administered at a rate of 10 mg/min or less.

Nephrotoxicity: Rarely, renal failure, principally manifested by increased serum creatinine or BUN concentrations, especially in patients given large doses of Vancomycin HCl, has been reported.

Cases of interstitial nephritis have also been reported rarely. Most of these have occurred in patients who were given aminoglycosides concomitantly or who had preexisting kidney dysfunction. When Vancomycin HCl was discontinued, azotemia resolved in most patients.

Gastrointestinal: Onset of pseudomembranous colitis symptoms may occur during or after antibiotic treatment (See WARNINGS.)

Ototoxicity: A few dozen cases of hearing loss associated with Vancomycin HCl have been reported. Most of these patients had kidney dysfunction or a preexisting hearing loss or were receiving concomitant treatment with an ototoxic drug.

Vertigo, dizziness, and tinnitus have been reported rarely.

Hematopoietic: Reversible neutropenia, usually starting 1 week or more after onset of therapy with Vancomycin HCl or after a total dose of more than 25 g, has been reported for several dozen patients. Neutropenia appears to be promptly reversible when Vancomycin HCl is discontinued.

Thrombocytopenia has rarely been reported.

Although a causal relationship has not been established, reversible agranulocytosis (granulocytes $<500/mm^3$) has been reported rarely.

Phlebitis: Inflammation at the injection site has been reported.

Miscellaneous: Infrequently, patients have been reported to have had anaphylaxis, drug fever, nausea, chills, eosinophilia, rashes, including exfoliative dermatitis, Stevens-Johnson syndrome, and rare cases of vasculitis in association with administration of Vancomycin HCl.

Chemical peritonitis has been reported following intraperitoneal administration of vancomycin (see PRECAUTIONS.)

OVERDOSAGE:

Supportive care is advised, with maintenance of glomerular filtration, Vancomycin is poorly removed by dialysis. Hemofiltration and hemoperfusion with polysulfone resin have been reported to result in increased vancomycin clearance. The median lethal intravenous dose is 319 mg/kg in rats and 400 mg/kg in mice.

To obtain up-to-date information about the treatment of overdose, a good resource is your certified Regional Poison Control Center. Telephone numbers of certified poison control centers are listed in the Physicians $GenR_x$. In managing overdosage, consider the possibility of multiple drug overdoses, interaction among drugs, and unusual drug kinetics in your patient.

DOSAGE AND ADMINISTRATION:

INJECTION

Vancomycin HCl injection is intended for intravenous use only. A concentration of no more than 10 mg/mL is recommended. An infusion of 10 mg/min or less is associated with fewer infusion-related events (See ADVERSE REACTIONS.)

DOSAGE AND ADMINISTRATION: *(cont'd)*

Patients With Normal Renal Function

Adults: The usual daily intravenous dose is 2 g divided either as 500 mg every 6 hours or 1 g every 12 hours. Each dose should be administered over a period of at least 60 minutes. Other patient factors, such as age or obesity, may call for modification of the usual daily intravenous dose.

Children: The usual intravenous dosage of Vancocin HCl is 10 mg/kg per dose given every 6 hours. Each dose should be administered over a period of at least 60 minutes.

Neonates: In neonates and young infants, the total daily intravenous dosage maybe lower. In both neonates and infants, an initial dose of 15 mg/kg is suggested, followed by 10 mg/kg every 12 hours for neonates in the first week of life and every 8 hours thereafter up to the age of 1 month. Each dose should be administered over 60 minutes. Close monitoring of serum concentrations of vancomycin may be warranted in these patients.

Patients With Impaired Renal Function And Elderly Patients

Dosage adjustment must be made in patients with impaired renal function. In the elderly, dosage reductions greater than expected may be necessary because of decreased renal function. Measurement of vancomycin serum concentrations can be helpful in optimizing therapy, especially in seriously ill patients with changing renal function. Vancomycin serum concentrations can be determined by use of microbiologic assay, radioimmunoassay, fluorescence polarization immunoassay, fluorescence immunoassay, or high-pressure liquid chromatography.

If creatinine clearance can be measured or estimated accurately, the dosage for most patients with renal impairment can be calculated by using the following table. The dosage of Vancomycin HCl per day in mg is about 15 times the glomerular filtration rate in mL/min:

TABLE 5

Dosage Table For Vancomycin In Patients With Impaired Renal Function (Adapted from Moellering et al.)

Creatinine Clearance mL/min	Vancomycin Dose mg/24 h
100	1,545
90	1,390
80	1,235
70	1,080
60	925
50	770
40	620
30	465
20	310
10	155

The initial dose should be no less than 15 mg/kg, even in patients with mild to moderate renal insufficiency.

The table is not valid for functionally anephric patients. For such patients, an initial dose of 15 mg/kg of body weight should be given to achieve prompt therapeutic serum concentrations. The dose required to maintain stable concentrations is 1.9 mg/kg/24 h. In patients with marked renal impairment, it may be more convenient to give maintenance doses of 250 to 1,000 mg once every several days rather than administering the drug on a daily basis. In anuria, a dose of 1,000 mg every 7 to 10 days has been recommended.

When only the serum creatinine concentration is known, the following formula (based on sex, weight, and age of the patient) may be used to calculate creatinine clearance. Calculated creatinine clearances (mL/min) are only estimates. The creatinine clearance should be measured promptly.

TABLE 6

Men: [Weight (kg) × (140 - age in years)] ÷ [72 × serum creatinine concentration (mg/dL)]

Women: 0.85 × above value

The serum creatinine must represent a steady state of renal function. Otherwise, the estimated value for creatinine clearance is not valid. Such a calculated clearance is an overestimate of actual clearance in patients with conditions: (1)characterized by decreasing renal function, such as shock, severe heart failure, or oliguria; (2)in which a normal relationship between muscle mass and total body weight is not present, such as obese patients or those with liver disease, edema, or ascites; and (3) accompanied by debilitation, malnutrition, or inactivity.

The safety and efficacy of vancomycin administration by the intrathecal (intralumbar or intraventricular)routes have not been assessed.

Intermittent infusion is the recommended method of administration.

Directions For Use Of Vancocin HCl in Galaxy plastic container (PL 2040): Vancocin HCl in Galaxy plastic container (PL 2040) is for intravenous administration only.

Storage: Store in a freezer capable of maintaining a temperature at or below -20°C (-4°F).

Thawing of Plastic Containers

1. Thaw frozen containers at room temperature (25°C [77°F]) or under refrigeration (5°C [41°F]). DO NOT FORCE THAW BY IMMERSION IN WATER BATHS OR BY MICROWAVE IRRADIATION.

2. Check for minute leaks by squeezing the bag firmly. If leaks are detected, discard solution because sterility may be impaired.

3. DO NOT ADD SUPPLEMENTARY MEDICATION.

4. Visually inspect the container for particulate matter and discoloration. Components of the solution may precipitate in the frozen state and should dissolve with little or no agitation after the solution has reached room temperature. Potency is not affected. If after visual inspection, the solution is discolored or remains cloudy, an insoluble precipitate is noted, or any seals or outlet ports are not intact, the container should be discarded.

5. The thawed solution in Galaxy plastic container(PL 2040) remains chemically stable for 72 hours at room temperature (25°C [77°F]) or for 30 days when stored under refrigeration (5°C [41°F]).

6. Do not refreeze thawed antibiotics.

Preparation for Intravenous Administration

1. Suspend container from eyelet support

2. Remove protector from outlet port at bottom of container

3. Attach administration set. Refer to complete directions accompanying set.

4. Use sterile equipment.

Caution: Do not use plastic containers in series connections. Such use could result in an embolism due to residual air being drawn from the primary container before administration of the fluid from the secondary container is complete.

DOSAGE AND ADMINISTRATION: *(cont'd)*

ORAL

Adults: The usual daily dosage for Staphylococcus enterocolitis and antibiotic-associated pseudomembranous colitis produced by *C. difficile* is 500 mg to 2 g administered orally in 3 or 4 divided doses for 7 to 10 days.

Children: The usual daily dosage is 40 mg/kg in 3 or 4 divided doses for 7 to 10 days. The total daily dosage should not exceed 2 g.

Preparation And Stability: Vancomycin HCl (vancomycin Hydrochloride) For Oral Solution.

The contents of the 10-g vial may be mixed with distilled or deionized water (115 mL) for oral administration. When mixed with 115 mL of water, each 6 mL provide approximately 500 mg of vancomycin. The contents of the 1-g vial may be mixed with distilled or deionized water (20 mL).

When reconstituted with 20 mL, each 5 mL contains approximately 250 mg of vancomycin. Mix thoroughly to dissolve. These mixtures may be kept for 2 weeks in a refrigerator without significant loss of potency.

The appropriate oral solution dose may be diluted in 1 oz of water and given to the patient to drink. The diluted material may be administered via nasogastric tube. Common flavoring syrups maybe added to the solution to improve the taste for oral administration.

ANIMAL PHARMACOLOGY:

In animal studies, hypotension and bradycardia occurred in dogs receiving an intravenous infusion of vancomycin hydrochloride, 25 mg/kg, at a concentration of 25 mg/mL and an infusion rate of 13.3 mL/min.

REFERENCES:

1. National Committee for Clinical Laboratory Standards, Performance standards for antimicrobial disk susceptibility test—4th ed. Approved Standards NCCLS Document M2-A4, Vol 10, No 7, NCCLS, Villanova, PA, April 1990. **2.** National Committee for Clinical Laboratory Standards, Methods for dilution antimicrobial susceptibility tests for bacteria that grow aerobically—2nd ed. Approved Standard NCCLS Document M7-A2, Vol 10, No 8, NCCLS, Villanova, PA April 1990. **3.** National Committee for Clinical Laboratory Standards, Performance standards for antimicrobial susceptibility testing—4th Informational Supplement, NCCLS Document M100-S4 (ISBN 1-56238-172-5), Vol 12, No 20, NCCLS, Villanova, PA December 1992. **4.** Moellering RC, Krogstad DJ, Greenblatt DJ: Vancomycin therapy in patients with impaired renal function: A nomogram for dosage. *Ann Intern Med* 1981;94:343.(Eli Lilly, 11/04/93,PA 0481 AMP)

HOW SUPPLIED:

Vancocin HCl (vancomycin hydrochloride injection) is supplied as a frozen, iso-osmotic, premixed solution in a 100-mL single dose Galaxy plastic container (PL 2040) in the following vancomycin-equivalent dose: 500 mg/100-mL container (no 7467), Store at or below - 20°C (-4°F). See DIRECTIONS FOR USE OF VANCOCIN HCl (vancomycin hydrochloride injection) in Galaxy plastic container (PL 2040).

HOW SUPPLIED - RATED THERAPEUTICALLY EQUIVALENT:

Injection, Conc-Soln - Intravenous - 1 gm/vial

1 g x 10	$140.41	Vancomycin HCl, Schein Pharm (US)	00364-2473-91
1 gm	$20.35	LYPHOCIN, Fujisawa USA	00469-2840-40
1 gm	$22.62	VANCOMYCIN HCL, Abbott	00074-6535-01
1 gm	$22.62	Vancomycin HCl, Abbott	00074-6535-49
1 gm	$62.87	Sterile Vancomycin Hcl, Abbott	00074-6533-01
1 gm	$62.87	VANCOMYCIN HCL, Abbott	00074-6533-49
1 gm x 10	$115.15	VANCOLED, Lederle Parenterals	00205-3154-15
1 gm x 10	**$160.81**	**VANCOCIN HCL 1, Lilly**	**00002-7298-10**
1 gm x 10	$420.00	Vancomycin HCl, Voluntary Hosp	53258-8284-04
1 gm x 10	$516.00	VANCOMYCIN HCL, Voluntary Hosp	53258-2840-40
5 gm	$57.56	VANCOLED, Lederle Parenterals	00205-3154-05
500 mg x 10	$57.56	VANCOLED, Lederle Parenterals	00205-3154-88

Injection, Conc-Soln - Intravenous - 500 mg

1's	$8.56	STERILE VANCOMYCIN HCL, Elkins Sinn	00641-2777-41
1's	$11.32	VANCOMYCIN HCL, Abbott	00074-6534-01
1's	$11.32	VANCOMYCIN HCL, Abbott	00074-6534-49
1's	$31.45	VANCOMYCIN HCL, Abbott	00074-4332-49
10 ml	**$7.80**	**VANCOCIN HCL, Lilly**	**00002-1444-01**
10 ml	$218.75	LYPHOCIN 500, Fujisawa USA	00469-2210-30
10 ml x 10	$70.00	Vancomycin HCl, Schein Pharm (US)	00364-2472-33
10's	$149.50	Vancomycin Hcl, Harber Pharm	51432-0473-10
25's	$645.00	Vancomycin Hcl, Voluntary Hosp	53258-2210-03
500 mg	$31.45	STERILE VANCOMYCIN HCL, Abbott	00074-4332-01
500 mg x 10	**$82.80**	**VANCOCIN HCL 500, Lilly**	**00002-7297-10**

Injection, Dry-Soln - Intravenous - 10 gm

100 ml x 1	**$156.01**	**VANCOCIN HCL INJ 10, Lilly**	**00002-7355-01**

Injection, Solution - Intravenous - 5 gm

1's	$132.03	VANCOMYCIN HCL, Abbott	00074-6509-49
1's	$141.43	VANCOMYCIN HCL, Abbott	00074-6509-01
100 ml	$89.38	LYPHOCIN, Fujisawa USA	00469-2951-00

HOW SUPPLIED - NOT RATED EQUIVALENT:

Capsule, Gelatin - Oral - 125 mg

20's	**$94.50**	**VANCOCIN HCL, Lilly**	**00002-3125-42**

Capsule, Gelatin - Oral - 250 mg

20's	**$189.01**	**VANCOCIN HCL, Lilly**	**00002-3126-42**

Injection, Conc-Soln - Intravenous - 500 mg

100 ml x 12	**$132.05**	**VANCOCIN, Lilly**	**00002-7467-12**

Powder - Oral - 10 gm

10 gm	**$276.21**	**VANCOCIN HCL, Lilly**	**00002-2372-37**

Powder, Reconstitution - Oral - 1 gm/bottle

1 gm x 6	**$205.21**	**VANCOCIN HCL, Lilly**	**00002-5105-16**

VARICELLA VACCINE *(003195)*

CATEGORIES: Biologicals; Chickenpox; Immunologic; Serums, Toxoids and Vaccines; Vaccines; FDA Approved 1995 Mar

BRAND NAMES: **Varivax**; Varivax Vaccine

FORMULARIES: Aetna

DESCRIPTION:

Varivax (Varicella Vaccine) is a preparation of the Oka/Merck strain of live attenuated varicella virus. The virus was initially obtained from a child with natural varicella, then introduced into human embryonic lung cell cultures, adapted to and propagated in embryonic guinea pig cell cultures and finally propagated in human diploid cell cultures (WI-38). Further passage of the virus for varicella vaccine was performed at Merck Research Laboratories

DESCRIPTION: *(cont'd)*

(MRL) in human diploid cell cultures (MRC-5) that were free of adventitious agents. This live, attenuated varicella vaccine is a lyophilized preparation containing sucrose, phosphate, glutamate, and processed gelatin as stabilizers.

Varicella vaccine, when reconstituted as directed, is a sterile preparation for subcutaneous administration. Each 0.5 ml dose contains the following: a minimum of 1350 PFU (plaque forming units) of Oka/Merck varicella virus when reconstituted and stored at room temperature for 30 minutes, approximately 25 mg of sucrose, 12.5 mg hydrolyzed gelatin, 3.2 mg sodium chloride, 0.5 mg monosodium L-glutamate, 0.45 mg of sodium phosphate dibasic, 0.08 mg of potassium phosphate monobasic, 0.08 mg of potassium chloride; residual components of MRC-5 cells including DNA and protein; and trace quantities of sodium phosphate monobasic, EDTA, neomycin, and fetal bovine serum. The product contains no preservative.

To maintain potency, the lyophilized vaccine must be kept frozen at an average temperature of -15°C (+5°F) or colder and must be used before the expiration date (see HOW SUPPLIED, Stability and Storage.) Storage in a frost-free freezer with an average temperature of -15°C (+5°F) or colder is acceptable.

CLINICAL PHARMACOLOGY:

Varicella is a highly communicable disease in children, adolescents, and adults caused by the varicella-zoster virus. The disease usually consists of 300 to 500 maculopapular and/or vesicular lesions accompanied by a fever (oral temperature ≥100°F) in up to 70% of individuals.[1,2] Approximately 3.5 million cases of varicella occurred annually from 1980-1994 in the United States with the peak incidence occurring in children five to nine years of age.[3] The incidence rate of chickenpox is 8.3-9.1% per year in children 1-9 years of age.[4] The attack rate of natural varicella following household exposure among healthy susceptible children was shown to be 87%.[2]Although it is generally a benign, self-limiting disease, varicella may be associated with serious complications (*e.g.*, bacterial superinfection, pneumonia, encephalitis, Reye's Syndrome), and/or death.

Evaluation of Clinical Efficacy Afforded by Varicella Vaccine Clinical Data in Children: In combined clinical trials[5] of varicella vaccine at doses ranging from 1,000-17,000 PFU, the majority of subjects who received varicella vaccine and were exposed to wild-type virus were either completely protected from chickenpox or developed a milder form (for clinical description see below) of the disease. The protective efficacy of varicella vaccine was evaluated in three different ways: 1) by comparing chickenpox rates in vaccinees versus historical controls, 2) by assessment of protection from disease following household exposure, and 3) by a placebo- controlled, double-blind clinical trial.

In early clinical trials,[5] a total of 4142 children received 1000-1625 PFU of attenuated virus per dose of varicella vaccine and have been followed for up to six years post-single-dose vaccination. In this group there was considerable variation in chickenpox rates among studies and study sites, and much of the reported data were acquired by passive follow-up. It was observed that 2.1%-3.6% of vaccines per year reported chickenpox (called breakthrough cases). This represents an approximate 67% (57-77%) decrease from the total number of cases expected based on attack rates in children aged over 1-9 over this same period (8.3-9.1%).[4,6]In those who developed breakthrough chickenpox postvaccination, the majority experienced mild disease (median number of lesions <50). In one study, a total of 47% (27/58) of breakthrough cases had <50 lesions compared with 8% (7/92) in unvaccinated individuals, and 7% (4/58) of breakthrough cases had >300 lesions compared with 50% (46/92) in unvaccinated individuals.[7] In studies of vaccinated children who contracted chickenpox after a household exposure, 57% (31/54) of the cases reported <50 lesions, while 1.9% (1/54) reported >300 lesions with an oral temperature above 100°F.

In later clinical trials[5] with current vaccine, a total of 1164 children received 2900-9000 PFU of attenuated virus per dose of varicella vaccine and have been followed for up to three years post single-dose vaccination. It was observed that 0.2%-1.0% of vaccinees per year reported breakthrough chickenpox for up to three years post single-dose vaccination. This represents an approximate 93% decrease from the total number of cases expected based on attack rates in children aged 1-9 over this same period (8.3%-9.1%).[3,26] In those who developed breakthrough chickenpox postvaccination, the majority experienced mild disease.

Among a subset of vaccinees who were actively followed, 259 were exposed to an individual with chickenpox in a household setting. There were no reports of breakthrough chickenpox in 80% of exposed children; 20% reported a mild form of chickenpox.[5] This represents a 77% reduction in the expected number of cases when compared to the historical attack rate of varicella following household exposure to chickenpox of 87% in unvaccinated individuals.[2]

Although no placebo-controlled trial was carried out with varicella vaccine using the current vaccine, a placebo-controlled trial was conducted using a formulation containing 17,000 PFU per dose.[4,8]In this trial, a single dose of varicella vaccine protected 96-100% of children against chickenpox over a two-year period. The study enrolled healthy individuals 1 to 14 years of age (n=491 vaccine, n=465 placebo). In the first year, 8.5% of placebo recipients contracted chickenpox, while no vaccine recipient did, for a calculated protection rate of 100% during the first varicella season. In the second year, when only a subset of individuals agreed to remain in the blinded study (n=163 vaccine, n=161 placebo), 96% protective efficacy was calculated for the vaccine group compared to placebo.

There are insufficient data to assess the rate of protection against the complications of chickenpox (*e.g.*, encephalitis, hepatitis, pneumonia) in children.

Clinical Data in Adolescents and Adults: Although no placebo-controlled trial was carried out in adolescents and adults, efficacy was determined by evaluation of protection when vaccinees received 2 doses of varicella vaccine 4 to 8 weeks apart and were subsequently exposed to chickenpox in a household setting.[5] In up to two years of active follow-up, 17 of 64 (27%) vaccinees reported breakthrough chickenpox following household exposure; of the 17 cases, 12 (71%) reported <50 lesions, 5 reported 50-300 lesions, and none reported >300 lesions with an oral temperature above 100°F. In combined clinical studies of adolescents and adults (n=1019) who received two doses of varicella vaccine and later developed breakthrough chickenpox (42 of 1019), 25 of 42 (60%) reported <50 lesions, 16 of 42 (38%) reported 50-300 lesions, and 1 of 42 (2%) reported >300 lesions and an oral temperature above 100°F.[5]

The attack rate of unvaccinated adults exposed to a single contact in a household has not been previously studied. When compared to the previously reported attack rate of natural varicella of 87% following household exposure among unvaccinated children, this represents an approximate 70% reduction in the expected number of cases in the household setting.[2]

There are insufficient data to assess the rate protection of varicella vaccine against the serious complications of chickenpox in adults (*e.g.,* encephalitis, hepatitis, pneumonitis) and during pregnancy (congenital varicella syndrome).

Immunogenicity of Varicella Vaccine: Clinical trials with several formulations of the vaccine containing attenuated virus ranging from 1000 to 17,000 PFU per dose have demonstrated that varicella vaccine induces detectable immune responses in a high proportion of individuals and is generally well tolerated in healthy individuals ranging from 12 months to 55 years of age.[4,5,9-15]

Seroconversion as defined by the acquisition of any detectable varicella antibodies (gpELISA >0.3, a highly sensitive assay which is not commercially available) was observed in 97% of vaccinees at approximately 4-6 weeks postvaccination in 6889 susceptible children 12 months to 12 years of age. Rates of breakthrough disease were significantly lower among children with varicella antibody titers ≥5 compared to children with titers <5. Titers ≥5 were induced

CLINICAL PHARMACOLOGY: *(cont'd)*

in approximately 76% of children vaccinated with a single dose of vaccine at 1000-17,000 PFU per dose. In a multicenter study involving susceptible adolescents and adults 13 years of age and older, two doses of varicella vaccine administered four to eight weeks apart induced a seroconversion rate (gpELISA >0.3) of approximately 75% in 539 individuals four weeks after the first dose and of 99% in 479 individuals four weeks after the second dose. The average antibody response in vaccinees who received the second dose eight weeks after the first dose was higher than that in those, who received the second dose four weeks after the first dose. In another multicenter study involving adolescents and adults, two doses of varicella vaccine administered eight weeks apart induced a seroconversion rate (gpELISA >0.3) of 94% in 142 individuals six weeks after the first dose and 99% in 122 individuals six weeks after the second dose.[5]

Varicella vaccine also induces cell-mediated immune responses in vaccinees. The relative contributions of humoral immunity and cell-mediated immunity to protection from chickenpox are unknown.

Persistence of Immune Response: Studies in vaccinees examining chickenpox breakthrough rates over 5 years showed the lowest rates (0.2- 2.9%) in the first two years postvaccination, with somewhat higher but stable rates in the third through fifth year. The severity of reported breakthrough chickenpox, as measured by number of lesions and maximum temperature, appeared not to increase with time since vaccination.[5]

In clinical studies involving healthy children who received 1 dose of vaccine, detectable varicella antibodies (gpELISA >0.3) were present in 98.8% (3775/3822) at 1 year, 98.9% (1057/1069) at 2 years, 97.5% (548/562) at 3 years, and 99.5% (220/221) at 4 years postvaccination. Antibody levels were present at least one year in 97.2% (423/435) of healthy adolescents and adults who received two doses of live varicella vaccine separated by 4 to 8 weeks. A boost in antibody levels has been observed in vaccinees following exposure to natural varicella which could account for the apparent long-term persistence of antibody levels after vaccination in these studies. The duration of protection from varicella obtained using varicella vaccine in the absence of wild-type boosting in unknown. Varicella vaccine also induces cell-mediated immune responses in vaccinees. The relative contributions of humoral immunity and cell-mediated immunity to protection from chickenpox are unknown.

Transmission: In the placebo-controlled trial, transmission of vaccine virus was assessed in household settings (during the 8-week postvaccination period) in 416 susceptible placebo recipients who were household contacts of 445 vaccine recipients. Of the 416 placebo recipients, three developed chickenpox and seroconverted, nine reported a varicella-like rash and did not seroconvert, and six had no rash but seroconverted. If vaccine virus transmission occurred, it did so at a very low rate and possibly without recognizable clinical disease in contacts. These cases may represent either natural varicella from community contacts or a low incidence of transmission of vaccine virus from vaccinated contacts (see PRECAUTIONS.)[4,16]

Herpes Zoster: Overall, 9454 healthy children (12 months to 12 years of age) and 1648 adolescents and adults (13 years of age and older) have been vaccinated with Oka/Merck live attenuated varicella vaccine in clinical trials. Eight cases of herpes zoster have been reported in children during 44,994 person years of follow-up in clinical trials, resulting in a calculated incidence of at least 18 cases per 100,000 person years. The completeness of this reporting has not been determined. One case of herpes zoster has been reported in the adolescent and adult age group during 7826 person years of follow-up in clinical trials resulting in a calculated incidence of 12.8 cases per 100,000 person years.[5]

All nine cases were mild and without sequelae. Two cultures (one child and one adult) obtained from vesicles were positive for wild-type varicella zoster virus as confirmed by restriction endonuclease analysis.[5,17] The long-term effect of varicella vaccine on the incidence of herpes zoster, particularly in those vaccinees exposed to natural varicella, is unknown at present.

In children, the reported rate of zoster in vaccine recipients appears not to exceed that previously determined in a population-based study of healthy children who had experienced natural varicella.[5,18,19]The incidence of zoster in adults who have had natural varicella infection is higher than that in children.[20]

Reye's Syndrome: Reye's Syndrome has occurred in children and adolescents following natural varicella infection, the majority of whom had received salicylates.[21] In clinical studies in healthy children and adolescents in the United States, physicians advised varicella vaccine recipients not to use salicylates for six weeks after vaccination. There were no reports of Reye's Syndrome in varicella vaccine recipients during these studies.

Studies with Other Vaccines: In combined clinical studies involving 1080 children 12 to 36 months of age, 653 received varicella vaccine and M-M-R*II (Measles, Mumps, and Rubella Virus Vaccine Live) concomitantly at separate sites and 427 received the vaccines six weeks apart. Seroconversion rates and antibody levels were comparable between the two groups at approximately six weeks post-vaccination to each of the virus vaccine components. No differences were noted in adverse reactions reported in those who received varicella vaccine concomitantly with M-M-R II (Measles, Mumps, and Rubella Virus Vaccine Live) at separate sites and those who received varicella vaccine and M-M-R II (Measles, Mumps, and Rubella Virus Vaccine Live) at different times (see DRUG INTERACTIONS, Use with Other Vaccines.)[5]

In a clinical study involving 318 children 12 months to 42 months of age, 160 received an investigational vaccine (a formulation combining measles, mumps, rubella, and varicella in one syringe) concomitantly with booster doses of DTaP (diphtheria, tetanus, acellular pertussis) and OPV (oral poliovirus vaccine) while 144 received M-M-R II (Measles, Mumps, and Rubella Virus Vaccine Live) concomitantly with booster doses of DTaP and OPV followed by varicella vaccine 6 weeks later. At six weeks postvaccination, seroconversion rates for measles, mumps, rubella, and varicella and the percentage of vaccines whose titers were boosted for diphtheria, tetanus, pertussis, and polio were comparable between the two groups, but anti- varicella levels were decreased when the investigational vaccine containing varicella was administered concomitantly with DTaP. No clinically significant differences were noted in adverse reactions between the two groups.[5]

In another clinical study involving 307 children 12 to 18 months of age, 150 received an investigational vaccine (a formulation combining measles, mumps, rubella, and varicella in one syringe) concomitantly with a booster dose of PedvaxHIB* [Haemophilus b Conjugate Vaccine (Meningococcal Protein Conjugate)] while 130 received M-M-R-II (Measles, Mumps, and Rubella Virus Vaccine Live) concomitantly with a booster dose of PedvaxHIB followed by varicella vaccine 6 weeks later. At six weeks postvaccination, seroconversion rates for measles, mumps, rubella, and varicella, and geometric mean titers for PedvaxHIB were comparable between the two groups, but anti-varicella levels were decreased when the investigational vaccine containing varicella was administered concomitantly with PedvaxHIB. No clinically significant differences in adverse reactions were seen between the two groups.[5]

Varicella vaccine is recommended for subcutaneous administration. However, during clinical trials, some children received varicella vaccine intramuscularly resulting in seroconversion rates similar to those in children who received the vaccine by the subcutaneous route.[22] Persistance of antibody and efficacy in those receving intramuscular injections have not been defined.

INDICATIONS AND USAGE:

Varicella vaccine is indicated for vaccination against varicella in individuals 12 months of age and older.

Revaccination: The duration of protection of varicella vaccine is unknown at present and the need for booster doses is not defined. However, a boost in antibody levels has been observed in vaccinees following exposure to natural varicella as well as following a booster dose of varicella vaccine administered four to six years postvaccination.[5]

In a highly vaccinated population, immunity for some individuals may wane due to lack of exposure to natural varicella as a result of shifting epidemiology. Post-marketing surveillance studies are ongoing to evaluate the need and timing for booster vaccination.

Vaccination with varicella vaccine may not result in protection of all healthy, susceptible children, adolescents, and adults (see CLINICAL PHARMACOLOGY.)

CONTRAINDICATIONS:

A history of hypersensitivity to any component of the vaccine, including gelatin.

A history of anaphylactoid reaction to neomycin (each dose of reconstituted vaccine contains trace quantities of neomycin).

Individuals with blood dyscrasias, leukemia, lymphomas of any type, or other malignant neoplasms affecting the bone marrow or lymphatic systems.

Individuals receiving immunosuppressive therapy. Individuals who are on immunosuppressant drugs are more susceptible to infections than healthy individuals. Vaccination with live attenuated varicella vaccine can result in a more extensive vaccine-associated rash or disseminated disease in individuals on immunosuppressant doses of corticosteroids.

Individuals with primary and acquired immunodeficiency states, including those who are immunosuppressed in association with AIDS or other clinical manifestations of infection with human immunodeficiency virus;[23] cellular immune deficiencies; and hypogammaglobulinemic and dysgammaglobulinemic states.

A family history of congenital or hereditary immunodeficiency, unless the immune competence of the potential vaccine recipient is demonstrated.

Active untreated tuberculosis.

Any febrile respiratory illness or other active febrile infection.

Pregnancy; the possible effects of the vaccine on fetal development are unknown at this time. However, natural varicella is known to sometimes cause fetal harm. If vaccination of postpubertal females is undertaken, pregnancy should be avoided for three months following vaccination. (see PRECAUTIONS, Pregnancy)

WARNINGS:

Children and adolescents with acute lymphoblastic leukemia (ALL) in remission can receive the vaccine under an investigational protocol. More information is available by contacting the varicella vaccine coordinating center, Bio-Pharm Clinical Services, Inc., 4 Valley Square, Blue Bell, PA 19422 (215) 283-0897.

PRECAUTIONS:

General: Adequate treatment provisions, including epinephrine injection (1:1000), should be available for immediate use should an anaphylactoid reaction occur.

The duration of protection from varicella infection after vaccination with varicella vaccine is unknown.

It is not known whether varicella vaccine given immediately after exposure to natural varicella virus will prevent illness.

Vaccination should be deferred for at least 5 months following blood or plasma transfusions, or administration of immune globulin or varicella immune globulin or varicella zoster immune globulin (VZIG).[24]

Following administration of varicella vaccine, any immune globulin including VZIG should not be given for 2 months thereafter unless its use outweighs the benefits of vaccination.[24]

Vaccine recipients should avoid use of salicylates for 6 weeks after vaccination with varicella vaccine as Reye's Syndrome has been reported following the use of salicylates during natural varicella infection (see CLINICAL PHARMACOLOGY, Reye's Syndrome.)

Individuals vaccinated with varicella vaccine may potentially be capable of transmitting the vaccine virus to close contacts (see CLINICAL PHARMACOLOGY, Transmission.)

Therefore, vaccine recipients should avoid close association with susceptible high risk of individuals (*e.g.*, newborns, pregnant women, immunocompromised persons).

The potential risk of transmission of vaccine virus should be weighed against the risk of transmission of natural varicella virus in such circumstances.

the safety and efficacy of varicella vaccine have not been established in children and young adults who are known to be infected with human immunodeficiency viruses with an without evidence of immunosuppression (see also CONTRAINDICATIONS).

Care is to be taken by the health care provider for safe and effective use of varicella vaccine.

The health care provider should question the patient, parent, or guardian about reactions to a previous dose of varicella vaccine or a similar product.

the health care provider should obtain the previous immunization history of the vaccinee.

Varicella vaccine should not be injected into a blood vessel.

Vaccination should be deferred in patients with a family history of congenital or hereditary immunodeficiency until the patient's own immune system has been evaluated.

A separate sterile needle and syringe should be used for administration of each dose of varicella vaccine to prevent transfer of infectious diseases.

Needles should be disposed of properly and not be recapped.

Information for the Patient: The health care provider should inform the patient, parent or guardian of the benefits and risks of varicella vaccine.

Patients, parents, or guardians should be instructed to report any adverse reactions to their health care provider.

The U.S. Health Department of Health and Human Services has established a Vaccine Adverse Event Reporting System (VAERS) to accept all reports of suspected adverse events after the administration of any vaccine, including but not limited to the reporting of events required by the National Childhood Vaccine Injury Act of 1986.[25]. The VAERS toll-free number for VAERS forms and information is 1-800-822-7967.

Pregnancy should be avoided for three months following vaccination.

Carcinogenesis, Mutagenesis, and Impairment of Fertility: Varicella vaccine has not been evaluated for its carcinogenic or mutagenic potential, or its potential to impair fertility.

Pregnancy Category C: Animal reproduction studies have not been conducted with varicella vaccine. It is also not known whether varicella vaccine can cause fetal harm when administered to a pregnant woman or can affect reproduction capacity. Therefore, varicella vaccine should not be administered to pregnant females; furthermore, pregnancy should be avoided for three months following vaccination (see CONTRAINDICATIONS.)

PRECAUTIONS: *(cont'd)*

Nursing Mothers: It is not known whether varicella vaccine virus is secreted in human milk. Therefore, because some viruses are secreted in human milk, caution should be exercised if varicella vaccine is administered to a nursing woman.

Pediatric Use: No clinical data are available on safety or efficacy of varicella vaccine in children less than one year of age and administration to infants under twelve months of age is not recommended.

DRUG INTERACTIONS:

See PRECAUTIONS, General, regarding the administration of immune globulins, salicylates, and transfusions.

Use with Other Vaccines: Results from clinical studies indicate that varicella vaccine can be administered concomitantly with M-M- R II (Measles, Mumps, and Rubella Virus Vaccine Live).

Limited data from an experimental product containing varicella vaccine suggest that varicella vaccine can be administered concomitantly with a DTaP (diphtheria, tetanus, acellular pertussis) and PedvaxHIB using separate sites and syringes (see CLINICAL PHARMACOLOGY, Studies with other Vaccines.)[5] However, there are no data relating to simultaneous administration of varicella vaccine with DTO or OPV.

ADVERSE REACTIONS:

In clinical trials,[4,5,9-15] Varicella vaccine was administered to 11,102 healthy children, adolescents, and adults. Varicella vaccine was generally well tolerated.

In a double-blind placebo controlled study among 914 healthy children and adolescents who were serologically confirmed to be susceptible to varicella, the only adverse reactions that occurred at a significantly ($p<0.05$) greater rate in vaccine recipients than in placebo recipients were pain and redness at the injection site.[4]

Children 1 to 12 Years of Age: In clinical trials involving healthy children monitored for up to 42 days after a single dose of varicella vaccine, the frequency of fever, injection-site complaints, or rashes were reported as follows: (TABLE 1)

TABLE 1 Fever, Local Reactions, or Rashes (%) In Children 0 to 42 Days Postvaccination

Reaction	N	Post dose 1	Peak Occurrence In Postvaccination Days
Fever ≥102°F (39°C) Oral	8827	14.7%	0-42
Injection-site complaints (pain/soreness, swelling) and/or erythema, rash, pruritus, hematoma, induration, stiffness)	8916	19.3%	0-2
Varicella-like rash (injection site)	8916	3.4%	8-19
Median number of lesions		2	
Varicella-like rash (generalized)	8916	3.8%	5-26
Median number of lesions		5	

In addition, the most frequently (≥1%) reported adverse experiences, without regard to causality, are listed in decreasing order of frequency: upper respiratory illness, cough, irritability/nervousness fatigue, disturbed sleep, diarrhea, loss of appetite, vomiting, otitis, diaper rash/contact rash, headache, teething, malaise, abdominal pain, other rash, nausea, eye complaints, chills, lymphadenopathy, myalgia, lower respiratory illness, allergic reactions (including allergic rash, hives) stiff neck, heat rash/prickly heat, arthralgia, eczema/dry skin/dermatitis, constipation, itching.

Pneumonitis has been reported rarely (<1%) in children vaccinated with varicella vaccine; a casual relationship has not been established.

Febrile seizures have occurred rarely (<0.1%) in children vaccinated with varicella vaccine; a casual relationship has not been established.

Adolescents and Adults 13 Years of Age and Older: In clinical trials involving healthy adolescents and adults, the majority of whom received two doses of varicella vaccine and were monitored for up to 42 days after any dose, the frequency of fever, injection-site complaints, or rashes were reported as follows: (TABLES 2A and 2B)

TABLE 2A Fever, Local Reactions, or Rashes (%) in Adolescents and Adults 0-42 Days Postvaccination

Reaction	N	Post Dose 1	Peak Occurrence in Postvaccination Days
Fever ≥100°F (37.7°C) Oral	1584	10.2%	
Injection-site complaints (soreness, erythema, swelling, rash, pruritus, pyrexia, hematoma, induration numbness)	1606	24.4%	0-2
Varicella-like rash (injection site)	1606	3%	6-20
Median number of lesions		2	
Varicella-like rash (generalized)	1606	5.5%	7-21
Median number of lesions		5	

TABLE 2B Fever, Local Reactions, or Rashes (%) in Adolescents and Adults 0-42 Days Postvaccination

Reaction	N	Post Dose 2	Peak Occurrence in Postvaccination Days
Fever ≥100°F (37.7°C) Oral	956	9.5%	0-42
Injection-site complaints (soreness, erythema, swelling, rash, pruritus, pyrexia, hematoma, induration numbness)	955	32.5%	0-2
Varicella-like rash (injection site)	955	1%	0-6
Median number of lesions		2	
Varicella-like rash (generalized)	955	0.9%	0-23
Median number of lesions		5.5	

In addition, the most frequently (≥1%) reported adverse experiences, without regard to causality, are listed in decreasing order of frequency: upper respiratory illness, headache, fatigue, cough, myalgia, disturbed sleep, nausea, malaise, diarrhea, stiff neck, irritability/nervousness, lymphadenopathy, chills, eye complaints, abdominal pain, loss of appetite, arthralgia, otitis, itching, vomiting, other rashes, constipation, lower respiratory illness, allergic reactions (including allergic rash, hives), contact rash, cold/canker sore.

As with any vaccine, there is the possibility that broad use of the vaccine could reveal adverse reactions not observed in clinical trials.

DOSAGE AND ADMINISTRATION:

FOR SUBCUTANEOUS ADMINISTRATION Do not inject intravenously

Children 12 months to 12 years of age should receive a single 0.5 ml dose administered subcutaneously.

Adolescents and adults 13 years of age and older should receive a 0.5 ml dose administered subcutaneously at elected date and a second 0.5 ml dose 4 to 8 weeks later.

Varicella vaccine is for subcutaneous administration. The outer aspect of the upper arm (deltoid) is the preferred site of injection.

Varicella vaccine **MUST BE STORED FROZEN** at an average temperature of - 15°C (+5°F) or colder is acceptable. The diluent should be stored separately at room temperature or in the refrigerator. To reconstitute the vaccine, first withdraw 0.7 ml of diluent into the syringe to be used for reconstitution. Inject all the diluent in the syringe into the vial of lyophilized vaccine and gently agitate to mix thoroughly. Withdraw the entire contents into a syringe, change the needle, and inject the total volume (about 0.5 ml) of reconstituted vaccine subcutaneously, preferably into the outer aspect of the upper arm (deltoid) or the anterolateral thigh.**IT IS RECOMMENDED THAT THE VACCINE BE ADMINISTERED IMMEDIATELY AFTER RECONSTITUTION, TO MINIMIZE LOSS OF POTENCY. DISCARD IF RECONSTITUTED VACCINE IS NOT USED WITHIN 30 MINUTES.**

Caution: A sterile syringe free of preservatives, antiseptics, and detergents should be used for each injection and/or reconstitution of varicella vaccine because these substances may inactivate the vaccine virus.

It is important to use a separate sterile syringe and needle for each patient to prevent transmission of infectious agents from one individual to another.

To reconstitute the vaccine, use only the diluent supplied, since it is free of preservatives or other anti-viral substances which might inactivate the vaccine virus.

Do not freeze reconstituted vaccine.

Do not give immune globulin including Varicella Zoster Immune Globulin concurrently with varicella vaccine (see also PRECAUTIONS).

Parenteral drug products should be inspected visually for particulate matter and discoloration prior to administration, whenever solution and container permit. Varicella vaccine when reconstituted is a clear, colorless to pale yellow liquid.

REFERENCES:

1. Balfour, H.H.; et al.: Acyclovir treatment of varicella in otherwise healthy children, Pediatr., *116:*633-639, 1990. **2.** Ross, A.H.: Modification of chickenpox in family contacts by administration of gamma globulin, N. Engl. J. Med. *267:*369-376, 1962. **3.** Preblud, S.R.: Varicella: Complications and Costs, Pediatrics, *78* (4 Pt 2): 728-735, 1986. **4.** Weibel, R.E.; et al.: Live Attenuated Varicella Virus Vaccine, N. Engl. J. Med.*310* (22):1409-1415, 1984. **5.** Unpublished data; files of Merck Research Laboratories. **6.** Wharton, M.; et al.: Health Impact of Varicella in the 1980's. Thirtieth Interscience Conference on Antimicrobial Agents and Chemotherapy, (Abstract #1138), 1990. **7.** Bernstein, H.H.; et al.; Clinical Survey of Natural Varicella COmpared with Breakthrough Varicella After Immunization with Live Attenuated Oka/Merck Varicella Vaccine. Pediatrics *92*:833-837, 1993. **8.** Kuter, B.J.; et al.: Oka/Merck Varicella Vaccine in Healthy Children: Final Report of a 2-Year Efficacy Study and 7-Year Follow-up Studies, Vaccine, *9*:643-647, 1991. **9.** Arbeter, A.M.; et al.: Varicella Vaccine Trials in Healthy Children, A Summary of Comparative and Follow-up Studies, AJDC *138:*434-438, 1984. **10.** Weibel, R.E.; et al.: Live Oka/Merck Varicella Vaccine in Healthy Children, JAMA *254* (17):2435-2439, 1985. **11.** Chartrand, D.M.; et al.: New Varicella Vaccine Production Lots in Healthy Children and Adolescents, Abstracts of the 1988 Interscience Conference Antimicrobial Agents and Chemotherapy: *237* (Abstract #731). **12.** Johnson, C.E.; et al.: Live Attenuated Vaccine in Healthy 12 to 24 month old Children, Pediatrics *81:*512-518, 1988. **13.** Gershon, A.A.; et al.: Immunization of Healthy Adults with Live Attenuated Varicella Vaccine, Journal of Infectious Diseases,*158* (1): 132-137, 1988. **14.** Gershon, A.A.; et al.: Live Attenuated Varicella Vaccine: Protection in Healthy Adults Compared with Leukemic Children, Journal of Infectious Diseases, *161*:661-666, 1990. **15.** White, C.J.; et al.; Varicella Vaccine (Varivax) in Healthy Children and Adolescents: Results From Clinical Trials, 1987 to 1989, Pediatrics, *875* (5):604-610, 1991. **16.** Asano, Y.; et al.: Contact Infection from Live Varicella Vaccine Recipients, Lancet*1* (7966):965, 1976. **17.** Hammerschlag, M.R.; et al.: Herpes Zoster in an Adult Recipient of Live Attenuated Varicella Vaccine, J Infect Dis *160* (3);535-537, 1989. **18.** White, C.J.: Letters to the Editor, Pediatrics *318*:354, 1992. **19.** Guess H.A.; et al.: Epidemiology of Herpes Zoster in Children and Adolescents: A Population Based Study, Pediatrics *76* (4):512-517, 1985. **20.** Ragozzino, M.; et al.: Population-Based Study of Herpes Zoster and Its Sequelae, Medicine *61* (5):310-316, 1982. **21.** Morbidity and Mortality Weekly Report *34* (1): 13-16, Jan. 11, 1985. **22.** Dennehy, P.H.; et al.: Immunogenicity of Subcutaneous Versus Intramuscular Oka/Merck Varicella Vaccination in Healthy Children, Pediatrics *88* (3):604-607, 1991. **23.** Center for Disease Control: Immunization of Children Infected with Human T-Lymphotropic Virus Type III/ Lymohadenopathy - Associated Virus, Annals of Internal Medicine, *106*:75-78, 1987. **24.** Recommendations of the Advisory Committee on Immunization Practices (ACIP); General Recommendations on Immunization, MMWR*43* (No.RR- 1):15-18, January 28, 1994. **25.** Vaccine Adverse Event Reporting System - United States, MMWR *39* (41):730-733, 1990.

HOW SUPPLIED:

Varivax is supplied as follows: (1) a single-dose vial of lyophilized vaccine, (package A); and (2) a box of 10 vials of diluent (package B).

Varivax is supplied as follows: (1) a box of 10 single-dose vials of lyophilized vaccine (package A), and (2) a box of 10 vials of diluent (package B).

Stability and Storage: Varivax retains a potency level of 1500 PFU or higher per dose for at least 18 months in a frost-free freezer with an average temperature of -15°C (+5°F) or colder.

Varivax has a minimum potency level approximately 1350 PFU 30 minutes after reconstitution at room temperature (20-25°C, 68- 77°F).

For information regarding stability at temperatures other than those recommended for storage call 1-800-9-Varivax.

During shipment, to ensure that there is no loss of potency, the vaccine must be maintained at a temperature of -20°C (-4°F) or colder.

Before reconstitution, store the lyophilized vaccine in a freezer at an average temperature of -15°C (+5°F) or colder. Storage in a frost-free freezer with an average temperature of -15°C (+5°F) or colder is acceptable.

Before reconstitution, protect from light.

The diluent should be stores separately at room temperature, or in the refrigerator.

HOW SUPPLIED - EQUIVALENTS NOT AVAILABLE:

Injection, Solution - Intravenous

1's	**$49.93**	**VARIVAX VACCINE, Merck**	**00006-4826-00**
10's	**$493.00**	**VARIVAX VACCINE, Merck**	**00006-4827-00**

VARICELLA-ZOSTER IMMUNE GLOBULIN (HUMAN) *(003337)*

CATEGORIES: Blood Derivatives; Chickenpox; Immune Globulin; Immunologic; Immunomodulators; Plasma Fractions, Human; Varicella; Varicella Zoster

BRAND NAMES: VZIG; **Varicella Zoster Immune Globulin**

DESCRIPTION:

Varicella-Zoster Immune Globulin (Human) (VZIG) is a sterile 10.0 to 18.0% solution of the globulin fraction of human plasma, primarily immunoglobulin G (IgG) in 0.3M glycine.[1] VZIG contains no preservative. VZIG is derived from adult human plasma selected for high titers of varicella-zoster antibodies.[2] Plasma pools are fractionated by ethanol precipitation of the proteins according to Methods 6 and 9 of Cohn. A widely utilized solvent-detergent viral

DESCRIPTION: *(cont'd)*

inactivation process is also used.[3] Each milliliter contains 100 to 180 mg of protein, principally IgG, and trace amounts of IgA and IgM. The product is to be administered by intramuscular injection. The recommended dose is based on body weight.

CLINICAL PHARMACOLOGY:

This product contains IgG class varicella-zoster antibodies representative of the contributions of the large number of normal persons who donated plasma to the pool from which the product was derived. Upon absorption into the circulation, the antibodies persist for one month or longer. The precise concentration of varicella-zoster antibodies that must be achieved or maintained in order to attenuate Varicella is not known. In the clinical studies demonstrating its efficacy, VZIG was given within 96 hours of chickenpox exposure.[4,5]

When administered as described below, the product has been shown to significantly reduce mortality and morbidity from varicella among immunodeficient children. Lack of treatment of such patients has been associated with a mortality of 7%, a pneumonia rate of 25%, an encephalitis rate of 5%, and widespread pox (more than 100 pox):in 87%.[6,7] Clinical studies have shown that VZIG was able to significantly modify the expected severity of chickenpox, and that the observed frequencies of death (1%), pneumonia (6%), encephalitis (0%), and widespread pox (27%) were less than one quarter of those observed in the past when hyperimmune globulin was not given.[4] Although controlled clinical studies of VZIG efficacy in susceptible neonates, infants and healthy adults have not been done to date, it is expected that VZIG will also attenuate VZV infection in these groups.[8]

INDICATIONS AND USAGE:

VZIG is intended for the passive immunization of exposed, susceptible individuals who are at greater risk of complications from varicella than healthy children. High-risk groups include immunocompromised children, newborns of mothers with varicella shortly before or after delivery, premature infants, immunocompromised adults and normal susceptible adults[8] and may also include susceptible high risk infants less than a year of age.

Immunocompromised Children: VZIG is recommended for passive immunization of susceptible, immunocompromised children after significant exposure to chickenpox or zoster. These children include those with primary cellular immune deficiency disorders or neoplastlc diseases and those currently receiving immunosuppressive treatments. Although VZIG administration has been shown to reduce the severity of disease and decrease the rate of complications, severe varicella and death may still occur in exposed immunocompromised children despite VZIG administration. Antiviral chemotherapy should be considered if significant clinical varicella develops after VZIG administration.

Newborns of Mothers with Varicella Shortly before or After Delivery: VZIG is indicated for newborns of mothers who develop chickenpox within 5 days before or within 48 hours after delivery.[9-11] Despite VZIG administration some of these neonates may still develop varicella[10-15] which can be severe or fatal.[8] Antiviral chemotherapy should be considered in neonates who develop clinical varicella following VZIG administration.

Premature Infants: Although the risk of post-natally acquired varicella in the premature infant is unknown, it has been judged prudent to administer VZIG to exposed premature infants of 28 weeks gestation or more if their mothers have a negative or uncertain history of varicella.[8] Premature infants of less than 28 weeks gestation or birth weight of less than 1000 g should be considered for VZIG regardless of maternal history since they may not yet have acquired transplacental maternal antibody.

Full Term Infants Less than 1 Year of Age: Mortality from varicella in the first year of life is 4 times higher than that in older children, but lower than mortality in immunocompromised children or normal adults.[16,17] The decision to administer VZIG to infants less than one year of age should be evaluated on an individual basis. After careful evaluation of the type of exposure, susceptibility to varicella including maternal history of varicella and zoster, and presence of underlying disease, VZIG may be administered to selected infants.

Immunocompromised Adults: The complication rate for immunocompromised adults who contract varicella is likely to be substantially greater than for normal adults. Approximately 90% of immunocompromised adults with negative or unknown histories of prior varicella are likely to be immune. After a careful evaluation, which might include the measurement of antibody to Varicella-Zoster virus by a reliable and sensitive assay such as Fluorescent Antibody to Membrane Antigen (FAMA), adults who are believed susceptible should receive VZIG.

Healthy Adults: Chickenpox can be severe in normal adults. The decision to administer VZIG to an adult should be evaluated on an individual basis. Approximately 90% of adults with negative or uncertain histories of varicella will be immune. The objective is to modify rather than prevent illness in hopes of inducing lifelong immunity. The clinician should consider the patient's health status, type of exposure, and likelihood of previous unrecognized varicella infection in deciding whether to administer VZIG. Adults who are older siblings of large families and adults whose children have had varicella are more likely to be immune. If reliable and sensitive tests for varicella antibody are available, they might be used to determine susceptibility, if time permits. If, after careful evaluation, a normal adult with significant exposure to varicella is believed susceptible, VZIG may be administered.

Pregnant Women: Pregnant women may be at higher risk of complications of chickenpox than healthy adults.[18] They should be evaluated the same way as other adults. There is no evidence that administration of VZIG to a susceptible, pregnant woman will prevent viremia, fetal infection or congenital varicella syndrome. Therefore the primary indication for VZIG in pregnant women is to prevent complications of varicella in a susceptible adult patient rather than to prevent intrauterine infection. Pregnant women should be evaluated for type of exposure and history of previous infection as described for healthy adults.

Timing of VZIG After Varicella or Zoster Exposure: Greatest effectiveness of treatment is to be expected when it is begun within 96 hours after exposure; treatment after 96 hours is of uncertain value. There is no evidence that established infections with Varicella-Zoster virus can be modified by VZIG. There is no indication for the prophylactic use of VZIG in immunodeficient children or adults when there is a past history of varicella, unless the patient has undergone bone marrow transplantation.

Multiple Exposures: The duration of protection from a single dose of VZIG is not known. Therefore a second dose of VZIG should be considered when high risk patients have second exposures to Varicella-Zoster.

CONTRAINDICATIONS:

A history of prior severe reaction associated with the administration of human immune globulin, or severe thrombocytopenia.

WARNINGS:

The parenteral administration of any biologic should be surrounded by every precaution for the prevention and arrest of allergic and other untoward reactions.

Persons with immunoglobulin A deficiency have the potential for developing antibodies to immunoglobulin A and could have anaphylactic reactions to subsequent administration of blood products that contain immunoglobulin A. Therefore VZIG should be given to such persons only if the expected benefits outweigh the potential risks.

PRECAUTIONS:

Prepare the skin with 70% alcohol. Inject VZIG intramuscularly. NEVER ADMINISTER THIS MATERIAL INTRAVENOUSLY. Draw back on the plunger of the syringe to be certain that the needle is not in a blood vessel. A separate sterile disposable syringe and needle should be used for each individual patient to prevent the transmission of hepatitis viruses or other infectious agents from one person to another.

This product is made from human plasma and like other plasma products carries the possibility for transmission of blood-borne viral agents. The risk for transmission of recognized blood-borne viruses (*i.e.,* HIV-1, HIV-2, Hepatitis-B Virus, and Hepatitis C Virus) is considered to be extremely low because of the viral inactivation and removal properties inherent in the Cohn cold-ethanol precipitation procedure used for purification of immune globulin products.[19-21] Until 1993, cold ethanol manufactured immune globulins licensed in the U.S. had not been documented to transmit any viral agent. However, during a brief period in late 1993 to early 1994, an intravenous immune globulin made by one U.S. manufacturer was associated with transmission of Hepatitis C virus.[22] This was determined to be an isolated incident only related to one product not specifically treated by a viral inactivation process.[23] To further reduce the risk of enveloped viruses like Hepatitis C Virus, VZIG is also treated with a widely utilized solvent-detergent viral inactivation process.[3] Because new blood-borne viruses may yet emerge, VZIG like other blood products should be given only if a benefit is expected.

Although systemic allergic reactions are rare (see ADVERSE REACTIONS) epinephrine should be available for treatment of acute symptoms.

Antibodies present in immune globulin preparations may interfere with the immune response to live virus vaccines such as measles, mumps, and rubella. Therefore vaccination with live virus vaccines should be deferred until approximately five months after administration of Varicella Zoster Immune Globulin (Human). Persons who received VZIG within 14 days of live virus vaccination should be revaccinated with the live virus vaccine 5 months later.[24]

Administration of VZIG will result in false-positive tests for immunity to VZV for approximately two months after receiving VZIG. Therefore serodiagnostic tests to determine immunity to VZV should not be performed within 2 months of VZIG administration.

Pregnancy Category C: Animal reproduction studies have not been conducted with Varicella Zoster Immune Globulin (Human). It is also not known whether VZIG can cause fetal harm when administered to a pregnant woman or can affect reproduction capacity. VZIG should be given to a pregnant woman only if clearly needed. [21CFR 201.57 (f)][8]

Although pregnant women have not received the product in controlled studies, clinical use of other immunoglobulin preparations such as Rh immune globulin administered during pregnancy suggests that there are no known adverse effects on the fetus from the immune globulin itself.

ADVERSE REACTIONS:

The most frequent adverse reaction to VZIG is local discomfort at injection site. Pain, redness, or swelling occur at the injection site in about one in 100 patients. Less frequent adverse reactions are gastrointestinal symptoms, malaise, headache, rash and respiratory symptoms, which occur in approximately 1 in 500 patients. Severe reactions such as angioneurotic edema and anaphylactic shock are rare (less than 1 in 1000 patients). VZIG is prepared in the same manner as Immune Globulin (Human) and other immune globulins, and may be expected to resemble these globulins in ability to stimulate allotypic or other antiglobulin antibodies, and to react with such antibodies generated in response to prior injection of human globulin, or in response to transfusion of blood.[25]

OVERDOSAGE:

Although no data are available, clinical experience with other immunoglobulin preparations suggests that the only manifestations would be pain and tenderness at the injection site.

DOSAGE AND ADMINISTRATION:

Administer the product by deep intramuscular injection in the gluteal muscle, or in a physician-directed site if there are contraindications to the gluteal site. NEVER ADMINISTER THIS MATERIAL INTRAVENOUSLY. The recommended dose of VZIG is based on body weight according to the schedule in TABLE 1.

TABLE 1 Dosing Schedule for VZIG

Weight of Patients: Kilograms	Weight of Patients: Pounds	Units	Dose: Number of Vials
0-10	0-22	125	1 @ 125 units
10.1-20	22.1-44	250	2 @ 125 units
20.1-30	44.1-66	375	3 @ 125 units
30.1-40	66.1-88	500	4 @ 125 units
Over 40	Over 88	625	1 @ 625 units or 5 @ 125 units

Since VZIG does not contain a preservative administer the entire contents of each vial. Each 125 unit vial contains 125 units of antibody to varicella-zoster virus in a volume of approximately 1.25 ml and each 625 unit vial contains 625 units of antibody in a volume of approximately 6.25 ml. For patients weighing 10 kilograms or less, 125 units (1.25 ml) may be given in a single injection site. For patients weighing more than 10 kilograms, we recommend that no more than 2.5 ml be given in a single injection site, however some clinicians elect to give larger or smaller volumes.

The number of units required to prevent pneumonia and death and to reduce the number of pox is unknown. The proposed dosage regimen was found to be effective in significantly modifying the expected severity of chickenpox and reducing the observed frequency of death, pneumonia and encephalitis to less than 25% of the expected rate without treatment.

Parenteral drug products should be inspected visually for particulate matter and discoloration prior to administration whenever solution and container permit.

To prevent the transmission of hepatitis viruses or other infectious agents from one person to another, a separate sterile disposable syringe and needle should be used for each individual patient.

REFERENCES:

1. Janeway CA, and Rosen FS. The gamma globulins. *New England Journal of Medicine* 275:826-831, 1966. **2.** Zaia JA, Levin MJ, Wright GG, Grady GF. A practical method for the preparation of varicella zoster immune globulin. *J. Infect. Dis.* 137:601-604, 1978. **3.** Horowitz B, Wiebe ME, Lippin A, et al. Inactivation of viruses in labile blood derivatives. *Transfusion* 25:516-522, 1985. **4.** Zaia JA, Levin MJ, Preblud SR, Leszczynski J, et al. Evaluation of varicella-zoster immune globulin: protection of immunosuppressed children after household exposure to varicella. *J. Infect. Dis.*147:737-743, 1983. **5.** Levin MJ, Nelson WL, Preblud SR, Zaia JA. Clinical trials with varicella-zoster virus immunoglobulins, in Movell A, Nydegger (eds) Clinical use of intravenous immunoglobulins. London, *Academic Press*, 1986. **6.** Ross AH. Modification of chickenpox in family contact by administration of gamma globulin. *New England Journal of Medicine* 267:369-376,1962. **7.** Feldman S, Hughes WT, Daniel CB. Varicella in children with cancer, seventy-seven cases. *Pediatrics* 56:388-397,1975. **8.** Recommendations of the Immunization Practices Advisory Committee. Varicella-Zoster Immune Globulin for the prevention of chickenpox. *MMWR* vol. 33 (7):84-100, Feb. 1984. **9.** Meyers JD. Congenital varicella in term infants: risk reconsidered. *J. lnfect. Dis.* 129:215 217, 1974. **10.** Hanngren K, Grandien M, Granstrom G. Effect of zoster immunoglobulin for varicella prophylaxis in the newborn. Scand. *J. lnfect. Dis.* 17:343-347, 1985. **11.** Preblud SR, Nelson WL, Levin MJ, Zaia JA. Modification of congenital varicella with VZIG. Abstract No. 317 of the 26th Interscience Conference on Antimicrobial Agents and Chemotherapy, 1986. **12.** Gustafson TL, Shehab Z, Brunell PA. Outbreak of varicella in a newborn intensive care nursery. *Am. J. Dis. Child.* 138: 548-

REFERENCES: *(cont'd)*

550,1984. **13.** Bakshi SS, Miller TC, Kaplan M, et al. Failure of Varicella-Zoster immunoglobulin in modification of severe congenital varicella. *Pediatr. Infect. Dis.* 5:699-702, 1986. **14.** King SM, Gorensek M, Ford-Jones EL, Read SE. Fatal varicella-zoster infection in a newborn treated with varicella-zoster immunoglobulin. *Pediatr. Infect. Dis.* 5:588-589, 1986. **15.** Holland P, Issacs D, Moxon ER. Fatal neonatal varicella infection. *Lancet* 2: 1156, 1986. **16.** Preblud SR. Age-specific risks of varicella complications. *Pediatrics* 69:14-17, 1981. **17.** Preblud SR, Bergman DJ, Vernon LL. Deaths from varicella in infants. *Pediatr. Infect. Dis.* 4:503-507, 1985. **18.** Paryani SG, Arvin AM. Intrauterine infection with varicella-zoster virus after maternal varicella. *New England J. of Medicine* 314: 1542-46,1986. **19.** Bossell, et al. Safety of therapeutic immune globulin preparations with respect to transmission of human T-lymphotropic virus type III/lymphodenopathy-associated virus infection. *MMWR* vol. 35 (14): 231-233, April 11,1986. **20.** Wells MA, Wittek AE, Epstein JS, et al. Inactivation and partition of human T-cell lymphotropic virus, type III, during ethanol fractionation of plasma. *Transfusion* 26: 210-213,1986. **21.** McIver J, Grady G. Immunoglobulin preparations. In: Churchill WH and Kurtz SR, (ed): *Translusion Medicine.* Boston: Blackwell, 1988. **22.** Schneider L, Geha R. Outbreak of Hepatitis C associated with intravenous immunoglobulin administration - United States, October 1993 - June 1994. *MMWR* vol. 43 (28):505-509, July 22, 1 994. **23.** Yu MW, Mason 8L, Guo ZP, Tankersley DL et al. Hepatitis C transmission associated with intravenous immunoglobulins. *The Lancet*, May 6,1995, 345: 1173-1174. **24.** General Recommendations on Immunization: recommendations of the Advisory Committee on Immunization Practices. *MMWR* vol. 43 (No. RR-1): 17, Jan. 1994. **25.** Stiehm ER. Standard and special human immune serum globulins as therapeutic agents. *Pediatrics* 63:301-319, 1979.

HOW SUPPLIED:

The product is supplied in glass vials in two single use dosage forms.

Storage: The product should be stored between 2°C and 8°C (35.6°F to 46.4°F). DO NOT FREEZE.

HOW SUPPLIED - EQUIVALENTS NOT AVAILABLE:

Injection - Intramuscular - 125 u

1.250 ml	$99.60	VARICELLA ZOSTER IMMUNE GLOBULIN, Am Red Cross	52769-0118-02

Injection - Intramuscular - 625 u

6.250 ml	$448.20	VARICELLA ZOSTER IMMUNE GLOBULIN, Am Red Cross	52769-0118-10

VASOPRESSIN *(002422)*

CATEGORIES: Abdominal Distention; Antidiuretics; Diabetes; Diabetes Insipidus; Hormones; Pituitary; Roentgenography; Pregnancy Category C; FDA Pre 1938 Drugs

BRAND NAMES: **Pitressin**

DESCRIPTION:

Vasopressin Injection, USP Synthetic is a sterile, aqueous solution of synthetic vasopressin (8-Arginine vasopressin) of the posterior pituitary gland.

It is substantially free from the oxytocic principle and is standardized to contain 20 pressor units/ml. The solution contains 0.5% Chloretone (chlorobutanol) (chloroform derivative) as a preservative. The acidity of the solution is adjusted with acetic acid.

CLINICAL PHARMACOLOGY:

The antidiuretic action of vasopressin is ascribed to increasing reabsorption of water by the renal tubules.

Vasopressin can cause contraction of smooth muscle of the gastrointestinal tract and of all parts of the vascular bed, especially the capillaries, small arterioles and venules with less effect on the smooth musculature of the large veins. The direct effect on the contractile elements is neither antagonized by adrenergic blocking agents nor prevented by vascular denervation.

Following subcutaneous or intramuscular administration of vasopressin injection, the duration of antidiuretic activity is variable but effects are usually maintained for 2-8 hours.

The majority of a dose of vasopressin is metabolized and rapidly destroyed in the liver and kidneys. Vasopressin has a plasma half-life of about 10 to 20 minutes. Approximately 5% of a subcutaneous dose of vasopressin is excreted in urine unchanged after four hours.

CONTRAINDICATIONS:

Anaphylaxis or hypersensitivity to the drug or its components.

INDICATIONS AND USAGE:

Vasopressin Injection, USP is indicated for prevention and treatment of postoperative abdominal distention, in abdominal roentgenography to dispel interfering gas shadows, and in diabetes insipidus.

WARNINGS:

This drug should not be used in patients with vascular disease, especially disease of the coronary arteries, except with extreme caution. In such patients, even small doses may precipitate anginal pain, and with larger doses, the possibility of myocardial infarction should be considered.

Vasopressin may produce water intoxication. The early signs of drowsiness, listlessness, and headaches should be recognized to prevent terminal coma and convulsions.

PRECAUTIONS:

General: Vasopressin should be used cautiously in the presence of epilepsy, migraine, asthma, heart failure or any state in which a rapid addition to extracellular water may produce hazard for an already overburdened system.

Chronic nephritis with nitrogen retention contraindicates the use of vasopressin until reasonable nitrogen blood levels have been attained.

Information for the Patient: Side effects such as blanching of skin, abdominal cramps, and nausea may be reduced by taking 1 or 2 glasses of water at the time of vasopressin administration. These side effects are usually not serious and probably will disappear within a few minutes.

Laboratory Tests: Electrocardiograms (ECG) and fluid and electrolyte status determinations are recommended at periodic intervals during therapy.

Pregnancy Category C: Animal reproduction studies have not been conducted with Vasopressin Injection, USP. It is also not known whether Vasopressin Injection, USP can cause fetal harm when administered to a pregnant woman or can affect reproduction capacity. Vasopressin Injection, USP should be given to a pregnant woman only if clearly needed.

Labor and Delivery: Doses of vasopressin sufficient for an antidiuretic effect are not likely to produce tonic uterine contractions that could be deleterious to the fetus or threaten the continuation of the pregnancy.

Nursing Mothers: Caution should be exercised when Vasopressin Injection, USP is administered to a nursing woman.

DRUG INTERACTIONS:

1) The following drugs may potentiate the antidiuretic effect of vasopressin when used concurrently: carbamazepine; chlorpropamide; clofibrate; urea; fludrocortisone; tricyclic antidepressants. 2) The following drugs may decrease the antidiuretic effect of vasopressin when used concurrently: demeclocycline; norepinephrine; lithium; heparin; alcohol. 3) Ganglionic blocking agents may produce a marked increase in sensitivity to the pressor effects of vasopressin.

ADVERSE REACTIONS:

Local or systemic allergic reactions may occur in hypersensitive individuals. The following side effects have been reported following the administration of vasopressin.

Body as a Whole: anaphylaxis (cardiac arrest and/or shock) has been observed shortly after injection of vasopressin.

Cardiovascular: cardiac arrest, circumoral pallor, arrhythmias, decreased cardiac output, angina, myocardial ischemia, peripheral vasoconstriction and gangrene.

Gastrointestinal: abdominal cramps, nausea, vomiting, passage of gas.

Nervous System: tremor, vertigo, "pounding" in head.

Respiratory: bronchial constriction.

Skin and Appendages: sweating, urticaria, cutaneous gangrene.

OVERDOSAGE:

Water intoxication may be treated with water restriction and temporary withdrawal of vasopressin until polyuria occurs. Severe water intoxication may require osmotic diuresis with mannitol, hypertonic dextrose, or urea alone or with furosemide.

DOSAGE AND ADMINISTRATION:

Vasopressin Injection, USP may be administered subcutaneously or intramuscularly.

Ten units of Vasopressin Injection, USP (0.5 ml) will usually elicit full physiologic response in adult patients; 5 units will be adequate in many cases. Vasopressin Injection, USP should be given intramuscularly at three- or four-hour intervals as needed. The dosage should be proportionately reduced for children. (For an additional discussion of dosage, consult the sections below.)

When determining the dose of Vasopressin Injection, USP for a given case, the following should be kept in mind.

It is particularly desirable to give a dose not much larger than is just sufficient to elicit the desired physiologic response. Excessive doses may cause undesirable side effects—blanching of the skin, abdominal cramps, nausea—which, though not serious, may be alarming to the patient. Spontaneous recovery from such side effects occurs in a few minutes. It has been found that one or two glasses of water given at the time Vasopressin Injection, USP is administered reduce such symptoms.

Abdominal Distention: In the average postoperative adult patient, give 5 units (0.25 ml) initially, increase to 10 units (0.5 ml) at subsequent injections if necessary. It is recommended that Vasopressin Injection, USP be given intramuscularly and that injections be repeated at three-or four-hour intervals as required. Dosage to be reduced proportionately for children.

Vasopressin Injection, USP used in this manner will frequently prevent or relieve postoperative distension. These recommendations apply also to distention complicating pneumonia or other acute toxemias.

Abdominal Roentgenography: For the average case, two injections of 10 units each (0.5 ml) are suggested. These should be given two hours and one-half hour, respectively, before films are exposed. Many roentgenologists advise giving an enema prior to the first dose of Vasopressin Injection, USP.

Diabetes Insipidus: Vasopressin Injection, USP may be given by injection or administered intranasally on cotton pledgets, by nasal spray, or by dropper. The dose by injection is 5 to 10 units (0.25 to 0.5 ml) repeated two or three times daily as needed. When Vasopressin Injection, USP is administered intranasally by spray or on pledgets, the dosage and interval between treatments must be determined for each patient.

Storage: Store between 15 and 25°C (59 and 77°F).

HOW SUPPLIED - EQUIVALENTS NOT AVAILABLE:

Injection, Solution - Intramuscular; - 20 unit/ml

0.5 ml x 25	$75.00	Vasopressin, Am Regent	00517-0510-25
0.5 ml x 25	$84.75	Vasopressin, Voluntary Hosp	53258-2990-00
1 ml	**$80.63**	**PITRESSIN, Parke-Davis**	**00071-4200-03**
1 ml x 25	$135.00	Vasopressin, Am Regent	00517-1020-25
1 ml x 25	$150.00	Vasopressin, Voluntary Hosp	53258-3020-00
1 ml x 25	$181.25	Vasopressin, Fujisawa USA	00469-3020-00
1 x 25	**$107.88**	**PITRESSIN, Parke-Davis**	**00071-4200-45**
1 x 25	**$201.48**	**PITRESSIN, Parke-Davis**	**00071-4200-46**
10 ml	$69.02	Vasopressin, Fujisawa USA	00469-3020-30

VECURONIUM BROMIDE *(002424)*

CATEGORIES: Analeptics; Anesthesia; Autonomic Drugs; Endotracheal Intubation; Intubation; Muscle Relaxants; Muscles; Neuromuscular Blocking Agents; Non-Depolarizing Muscle Relaxants; Skeletal Muscle Relaxants; Pregnancy Category C; FDA Approved 1984 Apr

BRAND NAMES: **Norcuron**

FORMULARIES: WHO

> WARNING:
> This drug should be administered by adequately trained individuals familiar with its actions, characteristics, and hazards

DESCRIPTION:

Vecuronium bromide for injection is a nondepolarizing neuromuscular blocking agent of intermediate duration, chemically designated as piperidinium, 1-((2β, 3α, 5α, 16β, 17β)-3, 17-bis (acetyloxy-2-(1-piperidinyl) androstan-16-yl) -1-methyl -, bromide.

Its chemical formula is $C_{34}H_{57}BrN_2O_4$ with molecular weight 637.74.

Norcuron is supplied as a sterile nonpyrogenic freeze-dried buffered cake of very fine microscopic crystalline particles for intravenous injection only. Each 10 ml vial contains 10 mg vecuronium bromide, 20.75 mg citric acid anhydrous, 16.25 mg sodium phosphate dibasic anhydrous, 97 mg mannitol (to adjust tonicity), sodium hydroxide and/or phosphoric acid to buffer and adjust to a pH of 4. Each 20 ml vial contains 20 mg of vecuronium bromide, 41.5 mg citric acid anhydrous, 32.5 mg sodium phosphate dibasic anhydrous, 194

DESCRIPTION: *(cont'd)*

mg mannitol (to adjust tonicity), sodium hydroxide and/or phosphoric acid to buffer and adjust to a pH of 4. Bacteriostatic water for injection, USP when supplied contains 0.9% w/v BENZYL ALCOHOL, WHICH IS NOT FOR USE IN NEWBORNS.

CLINICAL PHARMACOLOGY:

Vecuronium bromide for injection is a nondepolarizing neuromuscular blocking agent possessing all of the characteristic pharmacological actions of this class of drugs (curariform). It acts by competing for cholinergic receptors at the motor end-plate. The antagonism to acetylcholine is inhibited and neuromuscular block is reversed by acetylcholinesterase inhibitors such as neostigmine. edrophonium, and pyridostigmine. Vecuronium bromide is about 1/3 more potent than pancuronium; the duration of neuromuscular blockade produced by vecuronium bromide is shorter than that of pancuronium at initially equipotent doses. The time to onset of paralysis decreases and the duration of maximum effect increases with increasing vecuronium bromide doses. The use of a peripheral nerve stimulator is recommended in assessing the degree of muscular relaxation with all neuromuscular blocking drugs. The ED_{90} (dose required to produce 90% suppression of the muscle twitch response with balanced anesthesia) has averaged 0.057 mg/kg (0.049 to 0.062 mg/kg in various studies). An initial vecuronium bromide dose of 0.08 to 0.10 mg/kg generally produces first depression of twitch in approximately 1 minute, good or excellent intubation conditions within 2.5 to 3 minutes, and maximum neuromuscular blockade within 3 to 5 minutes of injection in most patients.

Under balanced anesthesia, the time to recovery to 25% of control (clinical duration) is approximately 25 to 40 minutes after injection and recovery is usually 95% complete approximately 45-65 minutes after injection of intubating dose. The neuromuscular blocking action of vecuronium bromide is slightly enhanced in the presence of potent inhalation anesthetics. If vecuronium bromide is first administered more than 5 minutes after the start of the inhalation of enflurane, isoflurane, or halothane, or when steady state has been achieved, the intubating dose of vecuronium bromide may be decreased by approximately 15% (see DOSAGE AND ADMINISTRATION.) Prior administration of succinylcholine may enhance the neuromuscular blocking effect of vecuronium bromide and its duration of action. With succinylcholine as the intubating agent, initial doses of 0.04-0.06 mg/kg of vecuronium bromide will produce complete neuromuscular block with clinical duration of action of 25-30 minutes. If succinylcholine is used prior to vecuronium bromide, the administration of vecuronium bromide should be delayed until the patient starts recovering from succinylcholine-induced neuromuscular blockade. The effect of prior use of other nondepolarizing neuromuscular blocking agents on the activity of vecuronium bromide has not been studied (see DRUG INTERACTIONS.)

Repeated administration of maintenance doses of vecuronium bromide has little or no cumulative effect on the duration of neuromuscular blockade. Therefore, repeat doses can be administered at relatively regular intervals with predictable results. After an initial dose of 0.08 to 0.10 mg/kg under balanced anesthesia, the first maintenance dose (suggested maintenance dose is 0.010 to 0.015 mg/kg) is generally required within 25 to 40 minutes; subsequent maintenance doses, if required, may be administered at approximately 12 to 15 minute intervals. Halothane anesthesia increases the clinical duration of the maintenance dose only slightly. Under enflurane a maintenance dose of 0.010 mg/kg is approximately equal to 0.015 mg/kg dose under balanced anesthesia.

The recovery index (time from 25% to 75% recovery) is approximately 15-25 minutes under balanced or halothane anesthesia. When recovery from vecuronium bromide neuromuscular blocking effect begins, it proceeds more rapidly than recovery from pancuronium. Once spontaneous recovery has started, the neuromuscular block produced by vecuronium bromide is readily reversed with various anticholinesterase agents, e.g., pyridostigmine, neostigmine, or edrophonium in conjunction with an anticholinergic agent such as atropine or glycopyrrolate. Rapid recovery is a finding consistent with vecuronium bromide short elimination half-life, although there have been occasional reports of prolonged neuromuscular blockade in patients in the intensive care unit (See PRECAUTIONS.)

The administration of clinical doses of vecuronium bromide is not characterized by laboratory or clinical signs of chemically mediated histamine release. This does not preclude the possibility of rare hypersensitivity reactions (see ADVERSE REACTIONS.)

Pharmacokinetics: At clinical doses of 0.04-0.10 mg/kg, 60-80% of vecuronium bromide is usually bound to plasma protein. The distribution half-life following a single intravenous dose (range 0.025-0.280 mg/kg) is approximately 4 minutes. Elimination half-life over this sample dosage range is approximately 65-75 minutes in healthy surgical patients and in renal failure patients undergoing transplant surgery.

In late pregnancy, elimination half-life may be shortened to approximately 35-40 minutes. The volume of distribution at steady state is approximately 300-400 ml/kg; systemic rate of clearance is approximately 3-4.5 ml/minute/kg. In man, urine recovery of vecuronium bromide varies from 3-35% within 24 hours. Data derived from patients requiring insertion of a T-tube in the common bile duct suggests that 25-50% of a total intravenous dose of vecuronium may be excreted in bile within 42 hours. Only unchanged vecuronium has been detected in human plasma following use during surgery. In addition, its 3-desacetylmetabolite has been rarely detected in human plasma following prolonged clinical use in the ICU. (See PRECAUTIONS, Long Term Use in ICU.) One metabolite, 3-desacetyl vecuronium, has been recovered in the urine of some patients in quantities that account for up to 10% of injected dose; 3-desacetyl vecuronium has also been recovered by T-tube in some patients accounting for up to 25% of the injected dose.

This metabolite has been judged by animal screening (dogs and cats) to have 50% or more of the potency of vecuronium bromide; equipotent doses are of approximately the same duration as vecuronium bromide in dogs and cats. Biliary excretion accounts for about half the dose of vecuronium bromide within 7 hours in the anesthetized rats. Circulatory bypass of the liver (cat preparation) prolongs recovery from vecuronium bromide. Limited data derived from patients with cirrhosis or cholestasis suggests that some measurements of recovery may be doubled in such patients. In patients with renal failure, measurements of recovery do not differ significantly from similar measurements in healthy patients.

Studies involving routine hemodynamic monitoring in good risk surgical patients reveal that the administration of vecuronium bromide in doses up to three times that needed to produce clinical relaxation (0.15 mg/kg did not produce clinically significant changes in systolic, diastolic or mean arterial pressure. The heart rate, under similar monitoring, remained unchanged in some studies and was lowered by a mean of up to 8% in other studies. A large dose of 0.28 mg/kg administered during a period of no stimulation, while patients were being prepared for coronary artery bypass grafting was not associated with alterations in rate-pressure- product or pulmonary capillary wedge pressure. Systemic vascular resistance was lowered slightly and cardiac output was increased insignificantly. (The drug has not been studied in patients with hemodynamic dysfunction secondary to cardiac valvular disease). Limited clinical experience with use of vecuronium bromide during surgery for pheochromocytoma has shown that administration of this drug is not associated with changes in blood pressure or heart rate.

Unlike other nondepolarizing skeletal muscle relaxants, vecuronium bromide has no clinically significant effects on hemodynamic parameters. Vecuronium bromide will not counteract those hemodynamic changes or known side effects produced by or associated with anesthetic agents, other drugs or various other factors known to alter hemodynamics.

INDICATIONS AND USAGE:

Vecuronium bromide is indicated as an adjunct to general anesthesia, to facilitate endotracheal intubation and to provide skeletal muscle relaxation during surgery or mechanical ventilation.

CONTRAINDICATIONS:

Vecuronium bromide is contraindicated in patients known to have a hypersensitivity to it.

WARNINGS:

VECURONIUM BROMIDE SHOULD BE ADMINISTERED IN CAREFULLY ADJUSTED DOSAGE BY OR UNDER THE SUPERVISION OF EXPERIENCED CLINICIANS WHO ARE FAMILIAR WITH ITS ACTIONS AND THE POSSIBLE COMPLICATIONS THAT MIGHT OCCUR FOLLOWING ITS USE. THE DRUG SHOULD NOT BE ADMINISTERED UNLESS FACILITIES FOR INTUBATION, ARTIFICIAL RESPIRATION, OXYGEN THERAPY, AND REVERSAL AGENTS ARE IMMEDIATELY AVAILABLE. THE CLINICIAN MUST BE PREPARED TO ASSIST OR CONTROL RESPIRATION. TO REDUCE THE POSSIBILITY OF PROLONGED NEUROMUSCULAR BLOCKADE AND OTHER POSSIBLE COMPLICATIONS THAT MIGHT OCCUR FOLLOWING LONG-TERM USE IN THE ICU. VECURONIUM BROMIDE OR ANY OTHER NEUROMUSCULAR BLOCKING AGENT SHOULD BE ADMINISTERED IN CAREFULLY ADJUSTED DOSES BY OR UNDER THE SUPERVISION OF EXPERIENCED CLINICIANS WHO ARE FAMILIAR WITH ITS ACTIONS AND WHO ARE FAMILIAR WITH APPROPRIATE PERIPHERAL NERVE STIMULATOR MUSCLE MONITORING TECHNIQUES (See PRECAUTIONS.) In patients who are known to have myasthenia gravis or the myasthenic (Eaton-Lambert) syndrome, small doses of vecuronium bromide may have profound effects. In such patients, a peripheral nerve stimulator and use of a small test dose may be of value in monitoring the response to administration of muscle relaxants.

PRECAUTIONS:

GENERAL

Renal Failure: Vecuronium bromide is well tolerated without clinically significant prolongation of neuromuscular blocking effect in patients with renal failure who have been optimally prepared for surgery by dialysis. Under emergency conditions in anephric patients some prolongation of neuromuscular blockade may occur; therefore, if anephric patients cannot be prepared for non-elective surgery, a lower initial dose of vecuronium bromide should be considered.

Altered Circulation Time: Conditions associated with slower circulation time in cardiovascular disease, old age, edematous states resulting in increased volume of distribution may contribute to delay in onset time, therefore dosage should not be increased.

Hepatic Disease: Experience in patients with cirrhosis or cholestasis has revealed prolonged recovery time in keeping with the role the liver plays in vecuronium bromide metabolism and excretion (see CLINICAL PHARMACOLOGY, Pharmacokinetics.) Data currently available do not permit dosage recommendations in patients with impaired liver function.

Long-term Use in ICU: In the intensive care unit, long-term use of neuromuscular blocking drugs to facilitate mechanical ventilation may be associated with prolonged paralysis and/or skeletal muscle weakness, that may be first noted during attempts to wean such patients from the ventilator. Typically, such patients receive other drugs such as broad spectrum antibiotics, narcotics and/or steroids and may have electrolyte imbalance and diseases which lead to electrolyte imbalance, hypoxic episodes of varying duration, acid-base imbalance and extreme debilitation, any of which may enhance the actions of a neuromuscular blocking agent. Additionally, patients immobilized for extended periods frequently develop symptoms consistent with disuse muscle atrophy. The recovery picture may vary from regaining movement and strength in all muscles to initial recovery of movement of the facial and small muscles of the extremities then to the remaining muscles. In rare cases recovery may be over an extended period of time and may even, on occasion, involve rehabilitation. Therefore, when there is a need for long-term mechanical ventilation, the benefits-to-risk ratio of neuromuscular blockade must be considered.

Continuous infusion or intermittent bolus dosing to support mechanical ventilation, has not been studied sufficiently to support dosage recommendations. IN THE INTENSIVE CARE UNIT, APPROPRIATE MONITORING. WITH THE USE OF A PERIPHERAL NERVE STIMULATOR TO ASSESS THE DEGREE OF NEUROMUSCULAR BLOCKADE IS RECOMMENDED TO HELP PRECLUDE POSSIBLE PROLONGATION OF THE BLOCKADE. WHENEVER THE USE OF VECURONIUM BROMIDE OR ANY NEUROMUSCULAR BLOCKING AGENT IS CONTEMPLATED IN THE ICU, IT IS RECOMMENDED THAT NEUROMUSCULAR TRANSMISSION BE MONITORED CONTINUOUSLY DURING ADMINISTRATION AND RECOVERY WITH THE HELP OF A NERVE STIMULATOR. ADDITIONAL DOSES OF VECURONIUM BROMIDE OR ANY OTHER NEUROMUSCULAR BLOCKING AGENT SHOULD NOT BE GIVEN BEFORE THERE IS A DEFINITE RESPONSE TO T_1OR TO THE FIRST TWITCH. IF NO RESPONSE IS ELICITED, INFUSION ADMINISTRATION SHOULD BE DISCONTINUED UNTIL A RESPONSE RETURNS.

Severe Obesity or Neuromuscular Disease: Patients with severe obesity or neuromuscular disease may pose airway and/or ventilatory problems requiring special care before, during and after the use of neuromuscular blocking agents such as vecuronium bromide.

Malignant Hyperthermia: Many drugs used in anesthetic practice are suspected of being capable of triggering a potentially fatal hypermetabolism of skeletal muscle known as malignant hyperthermia. There are insufficient data derived from screening in susceptible animals (swine) to establish whether or not vecuronium bromide is capable of triggering malignant hyperthermia.

C.N.S.: Vecuronium bromide has no known effect on consciousness, the pain threshold or cerebration. Administration must be accompanied by adequate anesthesia or sedation.

Inhalational Anesthetics: Use of volatile inhalational anesthetics such as enflurane, isoflurane, and halothane with vecuronium bromide will enhance neuromuscular blockade. Potentiation is most prominent with use of enflurane and isoflurane. With the above agents the initial dose of vecuronium bromide may be the same as with balanced anesthesia unless the inhalational anesthetic has been administered for a sufficient time at a sufficient dose to have reached clinical equilibrium (see CLINICAL PHARMACOLOGY.)

Antibiotics: Parenteral/intraperitoneal administration of high doses of certain antibiotics may intensify or produce neuromuscular block on their own. The following antibiotics have been associated with various degrees of paralysis: aminoglycosides (such as neomycin, streptomycin, kanamycin, gentamicin, and dihydrostreptomycin); tetracyclines, bacitracin, polymyxin B; colistin; and sodium colistimethate. If these or other newly introduced antibiotics are used in conjunction with vecuronium bromide, unexpected prolongation of neuromuscular block should be considered a possibility.

Other: Experience concerning injection of quinidine during recovery from use of other muscle relaxants suggests that recurrent paralysis may occur. This possibility must also be considered for vecuronium bromide. Vecuronium bromide induced neuromuscular blockade has been counteracted by alkalosis and enhanced by acidosis in experimental animals (cat). Electrolyte imbalance and diseases which lead to electrolyte imbalance, such as adrenal cortical insuffi-

PRECAUTIONS: *(cont'd)*

ciency, have been shown to alter neuromuscular blockade. Depending on the nature of the imbalance, either enhancement or inhibition may be expected. Magnesium salts, administered for the management of toxemia of pregnancy may enhance the neuromuscular blockade.

DRUG/LABORATORY TEST INTERACTIONS

None known.

CARCINOGENESIS, MUTAGENESIS, AND IMPAIRMENT OF FERTILITY

Long-term studies in animals have not been performed to evaluate carcinogenic or mutagenic potential or impairment of fertility.

PREGNANCY CATEGORY C

Animal reproduction studies have not been conducted with vecuronium bromide. It is also not known whether vecuronium bromide can cause fetal harm when administered to a pregnant woman or can affect reproduction capacity. Vecuronium bromide should be given to a pregnant woman only if clearly needed.

PEDIATRIC USE

Infants under 1 year of age but older than 7 weeks also tested under halothane anesthesia, are moderately more sensitive to vecuronium bromide on a mg/kg basis than adults and take about 1 1/2 times as long to recover information presently available does not permit recommendations for usage in neonates.

DRUG INTERACTIONS:

Prior administration of succinylcholine may enhance the neuromuscular blocking effect of vecuronium bromide for injection and its duration of action. If succinylcholine is used before vecuronium bromide the administration of vecuronium bromide should be delayed until the succinylcholine effect shows signs of wearing off. With succinylcholine as the intubating agent, initial doses of 0.04-0.06 mg/kg of vecuronium bromide may be administered to produce complete neuromuscular block with clinical duration of action of 25-30 minutes (see CLINICAL PHARMACOLOGY.)

The use of vecuronium bromide before succinylcholine, in order to attenuate some of the side effects of succinylcholine, has not been sufficiently studied.

Other nondepolarizing neuromuscular blocking agents (pancuronium, d-tubocurarine, metocurine, and gallamine) act in the same fashion as does vecuronium bromide, therefore these drugs and vecuronium bromide may manifest an additive effect when used together. There are insufficient data to support concomitant use of vecuronium bromide and other competitive muscle relaxants in the same patient.

ADVERSE REACTIONS:

The most frequent adverse reaction to nondepolarizing blocking agents as a class consists of an extension of the drug's pharmacological action beyond the time period needed. This may vary from skeletal muscle weakness to profound and prolonged skeletal muscle paralysis resulting in respiration insufficiency or apnea.

Inadequate reversal of the neuromuscular blockade is possible with vecuronium bromide as with all curariform drugs. These adverse reactions are managed by manual or mechanical ventilation until recovery is judged adequate. Little or no increase in intensity of blockade or duration of action with vecuronium bromide is noted from the use of thiobarbiturates, narcotic analgesics, nitrous oxide, or droperidol. (See OVERDOSAGE for discussion of other drugs used in anesthetic practice which also cause respiratory depression.)

Prolonged to profound extensions of paralysis and/or muscle weakness as well as muscle atrophy have been reported after long-term use to support mechanical ventilation in the intensive care unit (see PRECAUTIONS).The administration of vecuronium bromide has been associated with rare instances of hypersensitivity reactions (bronchospasm, hypotension and/or tachycardia, sometimes associated with acute urticaria or erythema); (see also CLINICAL PHARMACOLOGY).

OVERDOSAGE:

The possibility of iatrogenic overdosage can be minimized by carefully monitoring muscle twitch response to peripheral nerve stimulation.

Excessive doses of vecuronium bromide produces enhanced pharmacological effects. Residual neuromuscular blockage beyond the time period needed may occur with vecuronium bromide as with other neuromuscular blockers. This may be manifested by skeletal muscle weakness, decreased respiratory reserve, low tidal volume, or apnea. A peripheral nerve stimulator may be used to assess the degree of residual neuromuscular blockade from other causes of decreased respiratory reserve.

Respiratory depression may be due either wholly or in part to other drugs used during the conduct of general anesthesia such as narcotics, thiobarbiturates and other central nervous system depressants.

Under such circumstances the primary treatment is maintenance of a patient airway and manual or mechanical ventilation until complete recovery of normal respiration is assured. Regonol (pyridostigmine bromide) injection, neostigmine, or edrophonium, in conjunction with atropine or glycopyrrolate will usually antagonize the skeletal muscle relaxant action of vecuronium bromide. Satisfactory reversal can be judged by adequacy of skeletal muscle tone and by adequacy of respiration. A peripheral nerve stimulator may also be used to monitor restoration of twitch height. Failure of prompt reversal (within 30 minutes) may occur in the presence of extreme debilitation, carcinomatosis, and with concomitant use of certain broad spectrum antibiotics, or anesthetic agents and other drugs which enhance neuromuscular blockade or cause respiratory depression of their own. Under such circumstances the management is the same as that of prolonged neuromuscular blockade. Ventilation must be supported by artificial means until the patient has resumed control of his respiration. Prior to the use of reversal agents, reference should be made to the specific package insert of the reversal agent.

DOSAGE AND ADMINISTRATION:

Vecuronium bromide for injections is for intravenous use only.

This drug should be administered by or under the supervision of experienced clinicians familiar with the use of neuromuscular blocking agents. Dosage must be individualized in each case. The dosage information which follows is derived from studies based upon units of drug per unit of body weight and is intended to serve as a guide only, especially regarding enhancement of neuromuscular blockade of vecuronium bromide by volatile anesthetics and by prior use of succinylcholine (see DRUG INTERACTIONS). Parenteral drug products should be inspected visually for particulate matter and discoloration prior to administration whenever solution and container permit.

To obtain maximum clinical benefits of vecuronium bromide and to minimize the possibility of overdosage, the monitoring of muscle twitch response to peripheral nerve stimulation is advised.

The recommended initial dose of vecuronium bromide is 0.08 to 0.10 mg/kg (1.4 to 1.75 times the ED_{90}) given as an intravenous bolus injection. This dose can be expected to produce good or excellent non-emergency intubation conditions in 2.5 to 3 minutes after injection. Under balanced anesthesia, clinically required neuromuscular blockade lasts approximately 25-30 minutes, with recovery to 25% of control achieved approximately 25 to 40

DOSAGE AND ADMINISTRATION: *(cont'd)*

minutes after injection and recovery to 95% of control achieved approximately 45-65 minutes after injection. In the presence of potent inhalation anesthetics, the neuromuscular blocking effect of vecuronium bromide is enhanced. If vecuronium bromide is first administered more than 5 minutes after the start of inhalation agent or when steady state has been achieved, the initial vecuronium bromide dose may be reduced by approximately 15%, i.e., 0.060 to 0.085 mg/kg.

Prior administration of succinylcholine may enhance the neuromuscular blocking effect and duration of action of vecuronium bromide. If intubation is performed using succinylcholine, a reduction of initial dose of vecuronium bromide to 0.04-0.06 mg/kg with inhalation anesthesia and 0.05-0.06 mg/kg with balanced anesthesia may be required.

During prolonged surgical procedures, maintenance doses of 0.010 to 0.015 mg/kg of vecuronium bromide are recommended; after the initial vecuronium bromide injection, the first maintenance dose will generally be required within 25 to 40 minutes. However, clinical criteria should be used to determine the need for maintenance doses.

Since vecuronium bromide lacks clinically important cumulative effects, subsequent maintenance doses, if required, may be administered at relatively regular intervals for each patient, ranging approximately from 12 to 15 minutes under balanced anesthesia, slightly longer under inhalation agents (If less frequent administration is desired, higher maintenance doses may be administered).

Should there be reason for the selection of larger doses in individual patients, initial doses ranging from 0.15 mg/kg up to 0.28 mg/kg have been administered during surgery under halothane anesthesia without ill effects to the cardiovascular system being noted as long as ventilation is properly maintained (see CLINICAL PHARMACOLOGY.)

Use by Continuous Infusion: After an intubating dose of 80-100 mcg/kg, a continuous infusion of 1 mcg/kg/min can be initiated approximately 20-40 min later. Infusion of vecuronium bromide should be initiated only after early evidence of spontaneous recovery from the bolus dose. Long-term intravenous infusion to support mechanical ventilation in the intensive care unit has not been studied sufficiently to support dosage recommendations (see PRECAUTIONS.)

The infusion of vecuronium bromide should be individualized for each patient. The rate of administration should be adjusted according to the patient's twitch response as determined by peripheral nerve stimulation. An initial rate of 1 mcg/kg/min is recommended, with the rate of the infusion adjusted thereafter to maintain a 90% suppression of twitch response. Average infusion rates may range from 0.8 to 1.2 mcg/kg/min.

Inhalation anesthetics, particularly enflurane and isoflurane may enhance the neuromuscular blocking action of nondepolarizing muscle relaxants. In the presence of steady-state concentrations of enflurane or isoflurane, it may be necessary to reduce the rate of infusion 25-60 percent, 45-60 min after the intubating dose. Under halothane anesthesia it may not be necessary to reduce the rate of infusion.

Spontaneous recovery and reversal of neuromuscular blockade following discontinuation of vecuronium bromide infusion may be expected to proceed at rates comparable to that following a single bolus dose (see CLINICAL PHARMACOLOGY.)

Infusion solutions of vecuronium bromide can be prepared by mixing vecuronium bromide with an appropriate infusion solution such as 5% glucose in water, 0.9% NaCl, 5% glucose in saline, or Lactated Ringers.

Unused portions of infusion solutions should be discarded.

Infusion rates of vecuronium bromide can be individualized for each patient using the following table (TABLE 1):

TABLE 1

Drug Delivery Rate (mcg/kg/min)	Infusion Delivery Rate (ml/kg/min) 0.1 mg/ml*	0.2 mg/ml†
0.7	0.007	0.0035
0.8	0.008	0.0040
0.9	0.009	0.0045
1.0	0.010	0.0050
1.1	0.011	0.0055
1.2	0.012	0.0060
1.3	0.013	0.0065

* 10 mg of Norcuron in 100 ml solution
† 20 mg of Norcuron in 100 ml solution

TABLE 2 is guideline for ml/min delivery for a solution of 0.1 mg.ml (10 mg in 100 ml) with an infusion pump.

TABLE 2 Norcuron Infusion Rate - ml/min

Amount of Drug mcg/kg/min	Patient Weight - kg 40	50	60	70	80	90	100
0.7	0.28	0.35	0.42	0.49	0.56	0.63	0.70
0.8	0.32	0.40	0.48	0.56	0.64	0.72	0.80
0.9	0.36	0.45	0.54	0.63	0.72	0.81	0.90
1.0	0.40	0.50	0.60	0.70	0.80	0.90	1.00
1.1	0.44	0.55	0.66	0.77	0.88	0.99	1.10
1.2	0.48	0.60	0.72	0.84	0.96	1.08	1.20
1.3	0.52	0.65	0.78	0.91	1.04	1.17	1.30

NOTE: If a concentration of 0.2 mg/ml is used (20 mg in 100 ml), the rate should be decreased by one-half.

Dosage in Children: Older children (10 to 17 years of age) have approximately the same dosage requirements (mg/kg) as adults and may be managed the same way. Younger children (1 to 10 years of age), may require a slightly higher initial dose and may also require supplementation slightly more often than adults.

Infants under one year of age but older than 7 weeks are moderately more sensitive to vecuronium bromide on a mg/kg basis than adults and take about 1 1/2 times as long to recover. (See also PRECAUTIONS, Pediatric Use.) Information presently available does not permit recommendation on usage in neonates (see PRECAUTIONS.) There are insufficient data concerning continuous infusion of vecuronium in children, therefore no dosing recommendations can be made.

Compatibility: Vecuronium bromide is compatible in solution with:

0.9% NaCl solution	5% glucose in saline
5% glucose in water	Lactated Ringers
Sterile water for injection	

Use within 24 hours of mixing with the above solutions.

Parenteral drug products should be inspected visually for particulate matter and discoloration prior to administration whenever solution and container permit.

HOW SUPPLIED:

Norcuron 10 ml vials (10 mg vecuronium bromide) and 10 ml prefilled syringes of diluent (bacteriostatic water for injection, USP) 22 g 1/4" needle. 10 ml vials (10 mg vecuronium bromide) and 10 ml vials of diluent (bacteriostatic water for injection, USP). 10 ml vials (10 mg vecuronium bromide) only; DILUENT NOT SUPPLIED. 20 ml vials (20 mg vecuronium bromide) only; DILUENT NOT SUPPLIED.

Storage : 15-30°C (59-86°F). Protect from light.

AFTER RECONSTITUTION

When reconstituted with supplied bacteriostatic water for injection: CONTAINS BENZYL ALCOHOL, WHICH IS NOT INTENDED FOR USE IN NEWBORNS. Use within 5 days. May be stored at room temperature or refrigerated.

When reconstituted with sterile water for injection or other compatible IV solutions; Refrigerate vial. Use within 24 hours. Single use only. Discard unused portion.

HOW SUPPLIED - RATED THERAPEUTICALLY EQUIVALENT:

Injection, Lyphl-Soln - Intravenous - 10 mg/10ml

10 ml	$259.58	NORCURON, Organon	00052-0441-60
10 ml with dilu	$239.31	NORCURON, Organon	00052-0441-17
10 ml without d	$230.26	NORCURON, Organon	00052-0441-15

Injection, Solution - Intravenous - 20 mg

10's	$440.47	NORCURON, Organon	00052-0442-46

VELNACRINE *(003152)*

CATEGORIES: Acetylcholine Protector; Alzheimer's Disease; Anticholinergic Agents; Central Nervous System Agents; Dementia; Neuromuscular; FDA Unapproved

BRAND NAMES: **Mentane**

Prescribing information not available at time of publication.

VENLAFAXINE HYDROCHLORIDE *(003166)*

CATEGORIES: Antidepressants; Central Nervous System Agents; Depression; Psychotherapeutic Agents; Selective Serotonin Reuptake Inhibitors; FDA Class 1S ("Standard Review"); FDA Approved 1993 Dec; Top 200 Drugs

BRAND NAMES: **Effexor**

FORMULARIES: Medi-Cal; PCS

DESCRIPTION:

Venlafaxine HCl is a structurally novel antidepressant for oral administration. It is chemically unrelated to tricyclic, tetracyclic, or other available antidepressant agents. It is designated (R/S)-1-[2-(dimethylamino)-1-(4-methoxyphenyl)ethyl] cyclohexanol hydrochloride or (±)-1-[α-[(dimethylamino)methyl]-p-methoxybenzyl] cyclohexanol hydrochloride and has the empirical formula of $C_{17}H_{27}NO_2HCl$. Its molecular weight is 313.87.

Venlafaxine hydrochloride is a white to off-white crystalline solid with a solubility of 572 mg/ml in water (adjusted to ionic strength of 0.2 M with sodium chloride). Its octanol:water (0.2 M sodium chloride) partition coefficient is 0.43.

Compressed tablets contain venlafaxine hydrochloride equivalent to 25 mg, 37.5 mg, 50 mg, 75 mg, or 100 mg venlafaxine. Inactive ingredients consist of cellulose, iron oxides, lactose, magnesium stearate, and sodium starch glycolate.

CLINICAL PHARMACOLOGY:

Pharmacodynamics: The mechanism of the antidepressant action of venlafaxine in humans is believed to be associated with its potentiation of neurotransmitter activity in the CNS. Preclinical studies have shown that venlafaxine and its active metabolite, O-desmethylvenlafaxine (ODV), are potent inhibitors of neuronal serotonin and norepinephrine reuptake and weak inhibitors of dopamine reuptake. Venlafaxine and ODV have no significant affinity for muscarinic, histaminergic, or α-1 adrenergic receptors *in vitro*. Pharmacologic activity at these receptors is hypothesized to be associated with the various anticholinergic, sedative, and cardiovascular effects seen with other psychotropic drugs. Venlafaxine and ODV do not possess monoamine oxidase (MAO) inhibitory activity.

Pharmacokinetics: Venlafaxine is well absorbed and extensively metabolized in the liver. O-desmethylvenlafaxine (ODV) is the only major active metabolite. On the basis of mass balance studies, at least 92% of a single dose of venlafaxine is absorbed. Approximately 87% of a venlafaxine dose is recovered in the urine within 48 hours as either unchanged venlafaxine (5%), unconjugated ODV (29%), conjugated ODV (26%), or other minor inactive metabolites (27%). Renal elimination of venlafaxine and its metabolites is the primary route of excretion. The relative bioavailability of venlafaxine from a tablet was 100% when compared to an oral solution. Food has no significant effect on the absorption of venlafaxine or on the formation of ODV.

The degree of binding of venlafaxine to human plasma is 27% ± 2% at concentrations ranging from 2.5 to 2215 ng/ml. The degree of ODV binding to human plasma is 30% ± 12% at concentrations ranging from 100 to 500 ng/ml. Protein-binding-induced drug interactions with venlafaxine are not expected.

Steady-state concentrations of both venlafaxine and ODV in plasma were attained within 3 days of multiple-dose therapy. Venlafaxine and ODV exhibited linear kinetics over the dose range of 75 to 450 mg total dose per day (administered on a q8h schedule). Plasma clearance, elimination half-life and steady-state volume of distribution were unaltered for both venlafaxine and ODV after multiple-dosing. Mean ± SD steady-state plasma clearance of venlafaxine and ODV is 1.3 ± 0.6 and 0.4 ± 0.2 l/h/kg, respectively; elimination half-life is 5 ± 2 and 11 ± 2 hours, respectively; and steady-state volume of distribution is 7.5 ± 3.7 l/kg and 5.7 ± 1.8 l/kg, respectively. When equal daily doses of venlafaxine were administered as either b.i.d. or t.i.d. regimens, the drug exposure (AUC) and fluctuation in plasma levels of venlafaxine and ODV were comparable following both regimens.

Age and Gender: A pharmacokinetic analysis of 404 venlafaxine-treated patients from two studies involving b.i.d. and t.i.d. regimens showed that dose-normalized trough plasma levels of either venlafaxine or ODV were unaltered due to age or gender differences. Dosage adjustment based upon the age or gender of a patient is generally not necessary (see DOSAGE AND ADMINISTRATION.)

Liver Disease: In 9 patients with hepatic cirrhosis, the pharmacokinetic disposition of both venlafaxine and ODV was significantly altered after oral administration of venlafaxine. Venlafaxine elimination half-life was prolonged by about 30%, and clearance decreased by about 50% in cirrhotic patients compared to normal subjects. ODV elimination half-life was prolonged by about 60% and clearance decreased by about 30% in cirrhotic patients compared to normal subjects. A large degree of intersubject variability was noted. Three patients with more severe cirrhosis had a more substantial decrease in venlafaxine clearance (about 90%) compared to normal subjects.

Dosage adjustment is necessary in these patients (see DOSAGE AND ADMINISTRATION.)

Renal Disease: In a renal impairment study, venlafaxine elimination half-life after oral administration was prolonged by about 50% and clearance was reduced by about 24% in renally impaired patients (GFR=10-70 ml/min), compared to normal subjects. In dialysis patients, venlafaxine elimination half-life was prolonged by about 180% and clearance was reduced by about 57% compared to normal subjects. Similarly, ODV elimination half-life was prolonged by about 40% although clearance was unchanged in patients with renal impairment (GFR=10-70 ml/min) compared to normal subjects. In dialysis patients, ODV elimination half-life was prolonged by about 142% and clearance was reduced by about 56%, compared to normal subjects. A large degree of intersubject variability was noted.

Dosage adjustment is necessary in these patients (see DOSAGE AND ADMINISTRATION.)

CLINICAL STUDIES:

The efficacy of venlafaxine HCl as a treatment for depression was established in 5 placebo-controlled, short-term trials. Four of these were 6-week trials in outpatients meeting DSM-III or DSM-III-R criteria for major depression: two involving dose titration with venlafaxine HCl in a range of 75 to 225 mg/day (t.i.d. schedule), the third involving fixed venlafaxine HCl doses of 75, 225, and 375 mg/day (t.i.d. schedule), and the fourth involving doses of 25, 75, and 200 mg/day (b.i.d. schedule). The fifth was a 4-week study of inpatients meeting DSM-III-R criteria for major depression with melancholia whose venlafaxine HCl doses were titrated in a range of 150 to 375 mg/day (t.i.d. schedule). In these 5 studies, venlafaxine HCl was shown to be significantly superior to placebo on at least 2 of the following 3 measures: Hamilton Depression Rating Scale (total score), Hamilton depressed mood item, and Clinical Global Impression—Severity of Illness rating. Doses from 75 to 225 mg/day were superior to placebo in outpatient studies and a mean dose of about 350 mg/day was effective in inpatients. Data from the 2 fixed-dose outpatient studies were suggestive of a dose-response relationship in the range of 75 to 225 mg/day. There was no suggestion of increased response with doses greater than 225 mg/day.

While there were no efficacy studies focusing specifically on an elderly population, elderly patients were included among the patients studied. Overall, approximately 2/3 of all patients in these trials were women. Exploratory analyses for age and gender effects on outcome did not suggest any differential responsiveness on the basis of age or sex.

INDICATIONS AND USAGE:

Venlafaxine HCl is indicated for the treatment of depression.

The efficacy of venlafaxine HCl in the treatment of depression was established in 6-week controlled trials of outpatients whose diagnoses corresponded most closely to the DSM-III or DSM-III-R category of major depressive disorder and in a 4-week controlled trial of inpatients meeting diagnostic criteria for major depressive disorder with melancholia (see CLINICAL PHARMACOLOGY.)

A major depressive episode implies a prominent and relatively persistent depressed or dysphoric mood that usually interferes with daily functioning (nearly every day for at least 2 weeks); it should include at least 4 of the following 8 symptoms: change in appetite, change in sleep, psychomotor agitation or retardation, loss of interest in usual activities or decrease in sexual drive, increased fatigue, feelings of guilt or worthlessness, slowed thinking or impaired concentration, and a suicide attempt or suicidal ideation.

The effectiveness of venlafaxine HCl in long-term use, that is, for more than 4 to 6 weeks, has not been systematically evaluated in controlled trials. Therefore, the physician who elects to use venlafaxine HCl for extended periods should periodically re-evaluate the long-term usefulness of the drug for the individual patient.

CONTRAINDICATIONS:

Venlafaxine HCl is contraindicated in patients known to be hypersensitive to it.

Concomitant use in patients taking monoamine oxidase inhibitors (MAOIs) is contraindicated (see WARNINGS.)

WARNINGS:

POTENTIAL FOR INTERACTION WITH MONOAMINE OXIDASE INHIBITORS

Adverse reactions, some of which were serious, have been reported in patients who have recently been discontinued from a monoamine oxidase inhibitor (MAOI) and stated on venlafaxine HCl, or who have recently had venlafaxine HCl therapy discontinued prior to initiation of an MAOI. These reactions have included tremor, myoclonus, diaphoresis, nausea, vomiting, flushing, dizziness, hyperthermia with features resembling neuroleptic malignant syndrome, seizures, and death. In patients receiving antidepressants with pharmacological properties similar to venlafaxine in combination with a monoamine oxidase inhibitor, there have also been reports of serious, sometimes fatal, reactions. For a selective serotonin reuptake inhibitor, these reactions have included hyperthermia, rigidity, myoclonus, autonomic instability with possible rapid fluctuations of vital signs, and mental status changes that include extreme agitation progressing to delirium and coma. Some cases presented with featured resembling neuroleptic malignant syndrome. Severe hyperthermia and seizures, sometimes fatal, have been reported in association with the combined use of tricyclic antidepressants and MAOIs. These reactions have also been reported in patients who have recently discontinued these drugs and have been started on an MAOI. Therefore, it is recommended that venlafaxine HCl not be used in combination with an MAOI, or within at least 14 days of discontinuing treatment with an MAOI. Based on the half-life of venlafaxine HCl, at least 7 days should be allowed after stopping venlafaxine HCl before starting an MAOI.

Sustained Hypertension: Venlafaxine treatment is associated with sustained increases in blood pressure. (1) In a premarketing study comparing three fixed doses of venlafaxine (75, 225, and 375 mg/day) and placebo, a mean increase in supine diastolic blood pressure (SDBP) of 7.2 mm Hg was seen in the 375 mg/day group at week 6 compared to essentially no changes in the 75 and 225 mg/day groups and a mean decrease in SDBP of 2.2 mm Hg in the placebo group. (2) An analysis for patients meeting criteria for sustained hypertension (defined as treatment-emergent SDBP ≥ 90 mm Hg *and* ≥ 10 mm Hg above baseline for 3 consecutive visits) revealed a dose-dependent increase in the incidence of sustained hypertension for venlafaxine (TABLE 1):

An analysis of the patients with sustained hypertension and the 19 venlafaxine patients who were discontinued from treatment because of hypertension (<1% of total venlafaxine-treated group) revealed that most of the blood pressure increases were in a modest range (10-15 mm Hg, SDBP). Nevertheless, sustained increases of this magnitude could have adverse consequences. Therefore, it is recommended that patients receiving venlafaxine have regular monitoring of blood pressure. For patients who experience a sustained increase in blood pressure while receiving venlafaxine, either dose reduction or discontinuation should be considered.

TABLE 1

Probability of Sustained Elevation in SDBP (Pool of Premarketing Venlafaxine Studies)

Treatment Group	Incidence of Sustained Elevation in SDBP
Venlafaxine	
< 100 mg/day	3%
101-200 mg/day	5%
201-300 mg/day	7%
300 mg/day	13%
Placebo	2%

PRECAUTIONS:

GENERAL

Anxiety and Insomnia: Treatment—emergent anxiety, nervousness, and insomnia were more commonly reported for venlafaxine-treated patients compared to placebo-treated patients in a pooled analysis of short-term, double-blind, placebo-controlled depression studies (TABLE 2):

TABLE 2

Symptom	Venlafaxine n = 1033	Placebo n = 609
Anxiety	6%	3%
Nervousness	13%	6%
Insomnia	18%	10%

Anxiety, nervousness, and insomnia led to drug discontinuation in 2%, 2%, and 3%, respectively, of the patients treated with venlafaxine in the phase 2-3 depression studies.

Changes in Appetite and Weight: Treatment-emergent anorexia was more commonly reported for venlafaxine-treated (11%) than placebo-treated patients (2%) in the pool of short-term, double-blind, placebo-controlled depression studies. A dose-dependent weight loss was often noted in patients treated with venlafaxine for several weeks. Significant weight loss, especially in underweight depressed patients, may be an undesirable result of venlafaxine treatment. A loss of 5% or more of body weight occurred in 6% of patients treated with venlafaxine compared with 1% of patients treated with placebo and 3% of patients treated with another antidepressant. However, discontinuation for weight loss associated with venlafaxine was uncommon (0.1% of venlafaxine-treated patients in the phase 2-3 depression trials).

Activation of Mania/Hypomania: During phase 2-3 trials, hypomania or mania occurred in 0.5% of patients treated with venlafaxine. Activation of mania/hypomania has also been reported in a small proportion of patients with major affective disorder who were treated with other marketed antidepressants. As with all antidepressants, venlafaxine HCl should be used cautiously in patients with a history of mania.

Seizures: During premarketing testing, seizures were reported in 0.26% (8/3082) of venlafaxine-treated patients. Most seizures (5 of 8) occurred in patients receiving doses of 150 mg/day or less. Venlafaxine HCl should be used cautiously in patients with a history of seizures. It should be discontinued in any patient who develops seizures.

Suicide: The possibility of a suicide attempt is inherent in depression and may persist until significant remission occurs. Close supervision of high-risk patients should accompany initial drug therapy. Prescriptions for venlafaxine HCl should be written for the smallest quantity of tablets consistent with good patient management in order to reduce the risk of overdose.

Use in Patients With Concomitant Illness: Clinical experience with venlafaxine HCl in patients with concomitant systemic illness is limited. Caution is advised in administering venlafaxine HCl to patients with diseases or conditions that could affect hemodynamic responses or metabolism. Venlafaxine HCl has not been evaluated or used to any appreciable extent in patients with a recent history of myocardial infarction or unstable heart disease. Patients with these diagnoses were systematically excluded from many clinical studies during the product's premarketing testing. Evaluation of the electrocardiograms for 769 patients who received venlafaxine HCl in 4- to 6- week double-blind placebo-controlled trials, however, showed that the incidence of trial-emergent conduction abnormalities did not differ from that with placebo. The mean heart rate in venlafaxine HCl-treated patients was increased relative to baseline by about 4 beats per minute.

In patients with renal impairment (GFR = 10-70 ml/min) or cirrhosis of the liver, the clearances of venlafaxine and its active metabolite were decreased, thus prolonging the elimination half-lives of these substances. A lower dose may be necessary (see DOSAGE AND ADMINISTRATION.) Venlafaxine HCl, like all antidepressants, should be used with caution in such patients.

INFORMATION FOR THE PATIENT

Physicians are advised to discuss the following issues with patients for whom they prescribe venlafaxine HCl:

Interference with Cognitive and Motor Performance: Clinical studies were performed to examine the effects of venlafaxine on behavioral performance of healthy individuals. The results revealed no clinically significant impairment of psychomotor, cognitive, or complex behavior performance. However, since any psychoactive drug may impair judgment, thinking, or motor skills, patients should be cautioned about operating hazardous machinery, including automobiles, until they are reasonably certain that venlafaxine HCl therapy does not adversely affect their ability to engage in such activities.

Pregnancy: Patients should be advised to notify their physician if they become pregnant or intend to become pregnant during therapy.

Nursing: Patients should be advised to notify their physician if they are breast-feeding an infant.

Concomitant Medication: Patients should be advised to inform their physicians if they are taking, or plan to take, any prescription or over- the-counter drugs, since there is a potential for interactions.

Alcohol: Although venlafaxine HCl has not been shown to increase the impairment of mental and motor skills caused by alcohol, patients should be advised to avoid alcohol while taking venlafaxine HCl.

Allergic Reactions: Patients should be advised to notify their physician if they develop a rash, hives, or a related allergic phenomenon.

Laboratory Tests There are no specific laboratory tests recommended.

CARCINOGENESIS, MUTAGENESIS, AND IMPAIRMENT OF FERTILITY

Carcinogenesis: Venlafaxine was given by oral gavage to mice for 18 months at doses up to 120 mg/kg/per day, which was 16 times, on a mg/kg basis, and 1.7 times on a mg/m^{2}basis, the maximum recommended human dose. Venlafaxine was also given to rats by oral gavage for 24 months at doses up to 120 mg/kg per day. In rats receiving the 120 mg/kg dose, plasma levels of venlafaxine were 1 times (male rats) and 6 times (female rats) the plasma levels of patients receiving the maximum recommended human dose. Plasma levels of the O-desmethyl metabolite were lower in rats than in patients receiving the maximum recommended dose. Tumors were not increased by venlafaxine treatment in mice or rats.

PRECAUTIONS: *(cont'd)*

Mutagenicity: Venlafaxine and the major human metabolite, O- desmethylvenlafaxine (ODV), were not mutagenic in the Ames reverse mutation assay in Salmonella bacteria or the CHO/HGPRT mammalian cell forward gene mutation assay. Venlafaxine was also not mutagenic in the *in vitro* BALB/c-3T3 mouse cell transformation assay, the sister chromatid exchange assay in cultured CHO cells, or the *in vivo* chromosomal aberration assay in rat bone marrow. ODV was not mutagenic in the *in vitro* CHO cell chromosomal aberration assay. There was a clastogenic response in the *in vivo* chromosomal aberration assay in rat bone marrow in male rats receiving 200 times, on a mg/kg basis, or 50 times, on a mg/m^2 basis, the maximum human daily dose. The no effect dose was 67 times (mg/kg) or 17 times (mg/m^2) the human dose.

Impairment of Fertility: Reproduction and fertility studies in rats showed no effects on male or female fertility at oral doses of up to 8 times the maximum recommended human daily dose on a mg/kg basis, or up to 2 times on a mg/m^2 basis.

PREGNANCY, TERATOGENIC EFFECTS, PREGNANCY CATEGORY C

Venlafaxine did not cause malformations in offspring of rats or rabbits given doses up to 11 times (rat) or 12 times (rabbit) the maximum recommended human daily dose on a mg/kg basis, or 2.5 times (rat) and 4 times (rabbit) the human daily dose on a mg/m^2 basis. However, in rats, there was a decrease in pup weight, an increase in stillborn pups, and an increase in pup deaths during the first 5 days of lactation, when dosing began during pregnancy and continued until weaning. The cause of these deaths is not known. These effects occurred at 10 times (mg/kg) or 2.5 times (mg/m^2) the maximum human daily dose. The no effect dose for rat pup mortality was 1.4 times the human dose on a mg/kg basis or 0.25 times the human dose on a mg/m^{2}basis. There are no adequate and well-controlled studies in pregnant women. Because animal reproduction studies are not always predictive of human response, this drug should be used during pregnancy only if clearly needed.

LABOR AND DELIVERY

The effect of venlafaxine HCl on labor and delivery in humans is unknown.

NURSING MOTHERS

It is not known whether venlafaxine hydrochloride or its metabolites are excreted in human milk. Because many drugs are excreted in human milk, caution should be exercised when venlafaxine HCl is administered to a nursing woman.

PEDIATRIC USE

Safety and effectiveness in individuals below 18 years of age have not been established.

GERIATRIC USE

Of the 2,897 patients in phase 2-3 depression studies with venlafaxine HCl, 12% (357) were 65 years of age or over. No overall differences in effectiveness or safety were observed between these patients and younger patients, and other reported clinical experience has not identified differences in response between the elderly and younger patients. However, greater sensitivity of some older individuals cannot be ruled out.

DRUG INTERACTIONS:

As with all drugs, the potential for interaction by a variety of mechanisms is a possibility.

Drugs Highly Bound to Plasma Protein: Venlafaxine is not highly bound to plasma proteins; therefore, administration of venlafaxine HCl to a patient taking another drug that is highly protein bound should not cause increased free concentrations of the other drug.

Lithium: The steady-state pharmacokinetics of venlafaxine administered as 50 mg every 8 hours were not affected when a single 600 mg oral dose of lithium was administered to 12 healthy male subjects. O- desmethylvenlafaxine (ODV) was also unaffected. Venlafaxine had no effect on the pharmacokinetics of lithium.

Diazepam: Under steady-state conditions for venlafaxine administered as 50 mg every 8 hours, a single 10 mg dose of diazepam did not appear to affect the pharmacokinetics of either venlafaxine or ODV in 18 healthy male subjects. Venlafaxine also did not have any affect on the pharmacokinetics of diazepam or its active metabolite, desmethyldiazepam.

Administration of venlafaxine HCl did not affect the psychomotor and psychometric effects induced by diazepam.

Cimetidine: Concomitant administration of cimetidine and venlafaxine HCl in a steady-state study for both drugs resulted in inhibition of first- pass metabolism of venlafaxine in 18 healthy subjects. The oral clearance of venlafaxine was reduced by about 43%, and the exposure (AUC) and maximum concentration (C_{max}) of the drug were increased by about 60%. However, co-administration of cimetidine had no apparent effect on the pharmacokinetics of ODV, which is present in much greater quantity in the circulation than is venlafaxine. Consequently, the overall pharmacological activity of venlafaxine plus ODV is expected to increase only slightly, and no dosage adjustment should be necessary for most normal adults. However, for patients with pre-existing hypertension, and for elderly patients or patients with hepatic dysfunction, the interaction associated with the concomitant use of venlafaxine HCl and cimetidine is not known and potentially could be more pronounced. Therefore, caution is advised with such patients.

Alcohol: A single dose of ethanol (0.5 g/kg) had no effect on the pharmacokinetics of venlafaxine or ODV when venlafaxine was administered as a 50 mg dose every 8 hours in 15 healthy male subjects. The administration of venlafaxine HCl in a stable regimen did not exaggerate the psychomotor and psychometric effects induced by ethanol in these same subjects when they were not receiving venlafaxine HCl.

Drugs that Inhibit Cytochrome $P_{450}IID_6$Metabolism: *In vitro* studies indicate that venlafaxine is metabolized to its active metabolite, ODV, by cytochrome $P_{450}IID_6$, the isoenzyme that is responsible for the genetic polymorphism seen in the metabolism of many antidepressants. Therefore, the potential exists for a drug interaction between venlafaxine HCl and drugs that inhibit cytochrome $P_{450}IID_6$ metabolism. Drug interactions that reduce the metabolism of venlafaxine to ODV could potentially increase the plasma concentrations of venlafaxine and lower the concentrations of the active metabolite.

Drugs Metabolized by Cytochrome $P_{450}IID_6$: *In vitro* studies indicate that venlafaxine is a relatively weak inhibitor of cytochrome $P_{450}IID_6$. However, the clinical significance of this finding is unknown.

Monoamine Oxidase Inhibitors: See CONTRAINDICATIONS and WARNINGS.

CNS-Active Drugs: The risk of using venlafaxine in combination with other CNS-active drugs has not been systematically evaluated (except in the case of lithium and diazepam, as noted above). Consequently, caution is advised if the concomitant administration of venlafaxine and such drugs is required.

Electroconvulsive Therapy: There are no clinical data establishing the benefit of electroconvulsive therapy combined with venlafaxine HCl treatment.

ADVERSE REACTIONS:

Associated With Discontinuation of Treatment: Nineteen percent (537/2897) of venlafaxine patients in phase 2-3 depression studies discontinued treatment due to an adverse event. The more common events (≥1%) associated with discontinuation and considered to be drug-related (*i.e.,* those events associated with dropout at a rate approximately twice or greater for venlafaxine compared to placebo) included (TABLE 3):

ADVERSE REACTIONS: *(cont'd)*

TABLE 3

CNS	**Venlafaxine**	**Placebo**
Somnolence	3%	1%
Insomnia	3%	1%
Dizziness	3%	—
Nervousness	2%	—
Dry mouth	2%	—
Anxiety	2%	1%
Gastrointestinal		
Nausea	6%	1%
Urogenital		
Abnormal ejaculation*	3%	—
Other		
Headache	3%	1%
Asthenia	2%	—
Sweating	2%	—

* Percentages based on the number of males.
—Less than 1%

INCIDENCE IN CONTROLLED TRIALS

Commonly Observed Adverse Events in Controlled Clinical Trials: The most commonly observed adverse events associated with the use of venlafaxine HCl (incidence of 5% or greater) and not seen at an equivalent incidence among placebo-treated patients (*i.e.,* incidence for venlafaxine HCl at least twice that for placebo), derived from the 1% incidence (TABLE 4) below, were asthenia, sweating, nausea, constipation, anorexia, vomiting, somnolence, dry mouth, dizziness, nervousness, anxiety, tremor, and blurred vision as well as abnormal ejaculation/orgasm and impotence in men.

Adverse Events Occurring at an Incidence of 1% or More Among Venlafaxine HCl- Treated Patients: The (TABLE 4) that follows enumerates adverse events that occurred at an incidence of 1% or more, and were more frequent than in the placebo group, among venlafaxine HCl-treated patients who participated in short-term (4- to 8-week) placebo-controlled trials in which patients were administered doses in a range of 75 to 375 mg/day. This (TABLE 4) shows the percentage of patients in each group who had at least one episode of an event at some time during their treatment. Reported adverse events were classified using a standard COSTART-based Dictionary terminology.

The prescriber should be aware that these figures cannot be used to predict the incidence of side effects in the course of usual medical practice where patient characteristics and other factors differ from those which prevailed in the clinical trials. Similarly, the cited frequencies cannot be compared with figures obtained from other clinical investigations involving different treatments, uses and investigators. The cited figures, however, do provide the prescribing physician with some basis for estimating the relative contribution of drug and nondrug factors to the side effect incidence rate in the population studied.

Dose Dependency of Adverse Events: A comparison of adverse event rates in a fixed-dose study comparing venlafaxine HCl 75, 225, and 375 mg/day with placebo revealed a dose dependency for some of the more common adverse events associated with venlafaxine HCl use, as shown in the (TABLE 5) that follows. The rule for including events was to enumerate those that occurred at an incidence of 5% or more for at least one of the venlafaxine groups and for which the incidence was at least twice the placebo incidence for at least one venlafaxine HCl group. Tests for potential dose relationships for these events (Cochran-Armitage Test, with a criterion of exact 2-sided p-value ≤ 0.05) suggested a dose- dependency for several adverse events in this list, including chills, hypertension, anorexia, nausea, agitation, dizziness, somnolence, tremor, yawning, sweating, and abnormal ejaculation.

Adaptation to Certain Adverse Events: Over a 6-week period, there was evidence of adaptation to some adverse events with continued therapy (*e.g.,* dizziness and nausea), but less to other effects (*e.g.,* abnormal ejaculation and dry mouth).

Vital Sign Changes: Venlafaxine HCl treatment (averaged over all dose groups) in clinical trials was associated with a mean increase in pulse rate of approximately 3 beats per minute, compared to no change for placebo. It was associated with mean increases in diastolic blood pressure ranging from 0.7 to 2.5 mm Hg averaged over all dose groups, compared to mean decreases ranging from 0.9 to 3.8 mm Hg for placebo. However, there is a dose dependency for blood pressure increase(see WARNINGS.)

Laboratory Changes: Of the serum chemistry and hematology parameters monitored during clinical trials with venlafaxine HCl, a statistically significant difference with placebo was seen only for serum cholesterol, i.e., patients treated with venlafaxine HCl had mean increases from baseline of 3 mg/dl, a change of unknown clinical significance.

ECG Changes: In an analysis of ECGs obtained in 769 patients treated with venlafaxine HCl and 450 patients treated with placebo in controlled clinical trials, the only statistically significant difference observed was for heart rate, i.e., a mean increase from baseline of 4 beats per minute for venlafaxine HCl.

Other Events Observed During The Premarketing Evaluation Of Venlafaxine: During its premarketing assessment, multiple doses of venlafaxine HCl were administered to 2181 patients in phase 2 and 3 studies. The conditions and duration of exposure to venlafaxine HCl varied greatly, and included (in overlapping categories) open and double-blind studies, uncontrolled and controlled studies, inpatient and outpatient studies, fixed-dose and titration studies. Untoward events associated with this exposure were recorded by clinical investigators using terminology of their own choosing. Consequently, it is not possible to provide a meaningful estimate of the proportion of individuals experiencing adverse events without first grouping similar types of untoward events into a smaller number of standardized event categories.

In the tabulations that follow, reported adverse events were classified using a standard COSTART-based Dictionary terminology. The frequencies presented, therefore, represent the proportion of the 2181 patients exposed to multiple doses of venlafaxine HCl who experienced an event of the type cited on at least one occasion while receiving venlafaxine HCl. All reported events are included except those already listed in (TABLE 4) and those events for which a drug cause was remote. If the COSTART term for an event was so general as to be uninformative, it was replaced with a more informative term. It is important to emphasize that, although the events reported occurred during treatment with venlafaxine HCl, they were not necessarily caused by it.

Events are further categorized by body system and listed in order of decreasing frequency according to the following definition: frequent adverse events are those occurring on one or more occasions in at least 1/100 patients (only those not already listed in the tabulated results from placebo-controlled trials appear in this listing); infrequent adverse events are those occurring in 1/100 to 1/1000 patients; rare events are those occurring in fewer than 1/1000 patients.

Body As A Whole: *Frequent:* accidental injury, malaise, neck pain; *Infrequent:* abdomen enlarged, allergic reaction, cyst, face edema, generalized edema, hangover effect, hernia, intentional injury, moniliasis, neck rigidity, overdose, chest pain substernal, pelvic pain, photosensitivity reaction, suicide attempt; *Rare:* appendicitis, body odor, carcinoma, cellulitis, halitosis, ulcer, withdrawal syndrome.

ADVERSE REACTIONS: *(cont'd)*

TABLE 4 Treatment-Emergent Adverse Experience Incidence in 4- to 8-Week Placebo-Controlled Clinical Trials [1]

Body System	Preferred Term	Effexor (n=1033)	Placebo (n=609)
Body as a Whole	Headache	25%	24%
	Asthenia	12%	6%
	Infection	6%	5%
	Chills	3%	—
	Chest Pain	2%	1%
	Trauma	2%	1%
Cardiovascular	Vasodilation	4%	3%
	Increased blood pressure/hypertension	2%	—
	Tachycardia	2%	—
	Postural hypotension	1%	—
Dermatological	Sweating	12%	3%
	Rash	3%	2%
	Pruritus	1%	—
Gastrointestinal	Nausea	37%	11%
	Constipation	15%	7%
	Anorexia	11%	2%
	Diarrhea	8%	7%
	Vomiting	6%	2%
	Dyspepsia	5%	4%
	Flatulence	3%	2%
Metabolic	Weight loss	1%	—
Nervous System	Somnolence	23%	9%
	Dry mouth	22%	11%
	Dizziness	19%	7%
	Insomnia	18%	10%
	Nervousness	13%	6%
	Anxiety	6%	3%
	Tremor	5%	1%
	Abnormal dreams	4%	3%
	Hypertonia	3%	2%
	Paresthesia	3%	2%
	Libido decreased	2%	—
	Agitation	2%	—
	Confusion	2%	1%
	Thinking abnormal	2%	1%
	Depersonalization	1%	—
	Depression	1%	—
	Urinary retention	1%	—
	Twitching	1%	—
Respiration	Yawn	3%	—
Special Senses	Blurred vision	6%	2%
	Taste perversion	2%	—
	Tinnitus	2%	—
	Mydriasis	2%	—
Urogenital System	Abnormal ejaculation/orgasm	12%[2]	—[2]
	Impotence	6%[2]	—[2]
	Urinary frequency	3%	2%
	Urination impaired	2%	—
	Orgasm disturbance	2%[3]	—[3]
	Menstrual disorder	1%[3]	—[3]

[1] Events reported by at least 1% of patients treated with Effexor (venlafaxine hydrochloride) are included, and are rounded to the nearest %. Events for which the Effexor incidence was equal to or less than placebo are not listed in the (TABLE 4), but included the following: abdominal pain, pain, back pain, flu syndrome, fever, palpitation, increased appetite, myalgia, arthralgia, amnesia, hypesthesia, rhinitis, pharyngitis, sinusitis, cough increased, urinary tract infection, and dysmenorrhea[3].
— Incidence less than 1%.
[2] Incidence based on number of male patients.
[3] Incidence based on number of female patients.

TABLE 5 Treatment-Emergent Adverse Experience Incidence in a Dose Comparison Trial

Body System/Preferred Term	Placebo (n=92)	Effexor (mg/day) 75 (n=89)	225 (n=89)	375 (n=88)
Body as a Whole				
Abdominal pain	3.3%	3.4%	2.2%	8.0%
Asthenia	3.3%	16.9%	14.6%	14.8%
Chills	1.1%	2.2%	5.6%	6.8%
Infection	2.2%	2.2%	5.6%	2.3%
Cardiovascular System				
Hypertension	1.1%	1.1%	2.2%	4.5%
Vasodilation	0.0%	4.5%	5.6%	2.3%
Digestive System				
Anorexia	2.2%	14.6%	13.5%	17.0%
Dyspepsia	2.2%	6.7%	6.7%	4.5%
Nausea	14.1%	32.6%	38.2%	58.0%
Vomiting	1.1%	7.9%	3.4%	6.8%
Nervous System				
Agitation	0.0%	1.1%	2.2%	4.5%
Anxiety	4.3%	11.2%	4.5%	2.3%
Dizziness	4.3%	19.1%	22.5%	23.9%
Insomnia	9.8%	22.5%	20.2%	13.6%
Libido decreased	1.1%	2.2%	1.1%	5.7%
Nervousness	4.3%	21.3%	13.5%	12.5%
Somnolence	4.3%	16.9%	18.0%	26.1%
Tremor	0.0%	1.1%	2.2%	10.2%
Respiratory System				
Yawn	0.0%	4.5%	5.6%	8.0%
Skin and Appendages				
Sweating	5.4%	6.7%	12.4%	19.3%
Special Senses				
Abnormality of accommodation	0.0%	9.1%	7.9%	5.6%
Urogenital System				
Abnormal ejaculation/orgasm	0.0%	4.5%	2.2%	12.5%
Impotence	0.0%	5.8%	2.1%	3.6%
(Number of men)	(n=63)	(n=52)	(n=48)	(n=56)

Cardiovascular System: *Frequent:* migraine;*Infrequent:* angina pectoris, extrasystoles, hypotension, peripheral vascular disorder (mainly cold feet and/or cold hands), syncope, thrombophlebitis; *Rare:* arrhythmia, first-degree atrioventricular block, bradycardia, bundle branch block, mitral valve disorder, mucocutaneous hemorrhage, sinus bradycardia, varicose vein.

ADVERSE REACTIONS: *(cont'd)*

Digestive System: *Frequent:* dysphagia, eructation;*Infrequent:* colitis, tongue edema, esophagitis, gastritis, gastroenteritis, gingivitis, glossitis, rectal hemorrhage, hemorrhoids, melena, stomatitis, stomach ulcer, mouth ulceration; *Rare:* cheilitis, cholecystitis, cholelithiasis, hematemesis, gum hemorrhage, hepatitis, ileitis, jaundice, oral moniliasis, intestinal obstruction, proctitis, increased salivation, soft stools, tongue discoloration, esophageal ulcer, peptic ulcer syndrome.

Endocrine System: *Rare:* goiter, hyperthyroidism, hypothyroidism.

Hemic And Lymphatic System: *Frequent:* ecchymosis;*Infrequent:* anemia, leukocytosis, leukopenia, lymphadenopathy, lymphocytosis, thrombocythemia, thrombocytopenia, WBC abnormal;*Rare:* basophilia, cyanosis, eosinophilia, erythrocytes abnormal.

Metabolic And Nutritional: *Frequent:* peripheral edema, weight gain; *Infrequent:* alkaline phosphatase increased, creatinine increased, diabetes mellitus, edema, glycosuria, hypercholesteremia, hyperglycemia, hyperlipemia, hyperuricemia, hypoglycemia, hypokalemia, SGOT increased, thirst; *Rare:* alcohol intolerance, bilirubinemia, BUN increased, gout, hemochromatosis, hyperkalemia, hyperphosphatemia, hypoglycemic reaction, hyponatremia, hypophosphatemia, hypoproteinemia, SGPT increased, uremia.

Musculoskeletal System: *Infrequent:* arthritis, arthrosis, bone pain, bone spurs, bursitis, joint disorder, myasthenia, tenosynovitis; *Rare:* osteoporosis.

Nervous System: *Frequent:* emotional lability, trismus, vertigo; *Infrequent:* apathy, ataxia, circumoral paresthesia, CNS stimulation, euphoria, hallucinations, hostility, hyperesthesia, hyperkinesia, hypertonia, hypotonia, incoordination, libido increased, myoclonus, neuralgia, neuropathy, paranoid reaction, psychosis, psychotic depression, sleep disturbance, abnormal speech, stupor, torticollis;*Rare:* akathisia, akinesia, alcohol abuse, aphasia, bradykinesia, cerebrovascular accident, loss of consciousness, delusions, dementia, dystonia, hypokinesia, neuritis, nystagmus, reflexes increased.

Respiratory System: *Frequent:* bronchitis, dyspnea;*Infrequent:* asthma, chest congestion, epistaxis, hyperventilation, laryngismus, laryngitis, pneumonia, voice alteration;*Rare:* atelectasis, hemoptysis, hypoxia, pleurisy, pulmonary embolus, sleep apnea, sputum increased.

Skin And Appendages: *Infrequent:* acne, alopecia, brittle nails, contact dermatitis, dry skin, herpes simplex, herpes zoster, maculopapular rash, urticaria; *Rare:* skin atrophy, exfoliative dermatitis, fungal dermatitis, lichenoid dermatitis, hair discoloration, eczema, furunculosis, hirsutism, skin hypertrophy, leukoderma, psoriasis, pustular rash, vesiculobullous rash.

Special Senses: *Frequent:* abnormal vision, ear pain;*Infrequent:* cataract, conjunctivitis, corneal lesion, diplopia, dry eyes, exophthalmos, eye pain, otitis media, parosmia, photophobia, subconjunctival hemorrhage, taste loss, visual field defect;*Rare:* blepharitis, chromatopsia, conjunctival edema, deafness, glaucoma, hyperacusis, keratitis, labyrinthitis, miosis, papilledema, decreased pupillary reflex, scleritis.

Urogenital System: *Frequent:* anorgasmia, dysuria, hematuria, metrorrhagia*, urination impaired, vaginitis*;*Infrequent:* albuminuria, amenorrhea*, kidney calculus, cystitis, leukorrhea, menorrhagia*, metrorrhagia*, nocturia, bladder pain, breast pain, kidney pain, polyuria, prostatitis*, pyelonephritis, pyuria, urinary incontinence, urinary urgency, uterine fibroids enlarged*, uterine hemorrhage*, vaginal hemorrhage*, vaginal moniliasis*;*Rare:* abortion*, breast engorgement, breast enlargement, calcium crystalluria, female lactation*, hypomenorrhea*, menopause*, prolonged erection*, uterine spasm*.

*Based on the number of male or female patients as appropriate.

DRUG ABUSE AND DEPENDENCE:

Controlled Substance Class: Venlafaxine HCl is not a controlled substance.

Physical And Psychological Dependence: *In vitro* studies revealed that venlafaxine has virtually no affinity for opiate, benzodiazepine, phencyclidine (PCP), or N-methyl-D-aspartic acid (NMDA) receptors.

Venlafaxine was not found to have any significant CNS stimulant activity in rodents. In primate drug discrimination studies, venlafaxine showed no significant stimulant or depressant abuse liability.

While the discontinuation effects of venlafaxine HCl have not been systematically evaluated in controlled clinical trials, a retrospective survey of new events occurring during taper or following discontinuation revealed the following six events that occurred at an incidence of at least 5% and for which the incidence for venlafaxine HCl was at least twice the placebo incidence: asthenia, dizziness, headache, insomnia, nausea, and nervousness. Therefore, it is recommended that the dosage be tapered gradually and the patient monitored (see DOSAGE AND ADMINISTRATION.)

While venlafaxine HCl has not been systematically studied in clinical trials for its potential for abuse, there was no indication of drug-seeking behavior in the clinical trials. However, it is not possible to predict on the basis of premarketing experience the extent to which a CNS active drug will be misused, diverted, and/or abused once marketed. Consequently, physicians should carefully evaluate patients for history of drug abuse and follow such patients closely, observing them for signs of misuse or abuse of venlafaxine HCl (*e.g.,* development of tolerance, incrementation of dose, drug-seeking behavior).

OVERDOSAGE:

Human Experience: There were 14 reports of acute overdose with venlafaxine HCl, either alone or in combination with other drugs and/or alcohol, among the patients included in the premarketing evaluation. The majority of the reports involved ingestions in which the total dose of venlafaxine HCl taken was estimated to be no more than several-fold higher than the usual therapeutic dose. The 3 patients who took the highest doses were estimated to have ingested approximately 6.75 g, 2.75 g, and 2.5 g. The resultant peak plasma levels of venlafaxine for the latter 2 patients were 6.24 and 2.35 mcg ml, respectively, and the peak plasma levels of O-desmethylvenlafaxine were 3.37 and 1.30 mcg ml, respectively. Plasma venlafaxine levels were not obtained for the patient who ingested 6.75 g of venlafaxine. All 14 patients recovered without sequelae. Most patients reported no symptoms. Among the remaining patients, somnolence was the most commonly reported symptom. The patient who ingested 2.75 g of venlafaxine was observed to have 2 generalized convulsions and a prolongation of QTc to 500 msec, compared with 450 msec at baseline. Mild sinus tachycardia was reported in 2 of the other patients.

Management: Treatment should consist of those general measures employed in the management of overdosage with any antidepressant. Ensure an adequate airway, oxygenation, and ventilation. Monitoring of cardiac rhythm and vital signs is recommended. General supportive and symptomatic measures are also recommended. Use of activated charcoal, induction of emesis, or gastric lavage should be considered. Due to the large volume of distribution of venlafaxine hydrochloride, forced diuresis, dialysis, hemoperfusion and exchange transfusion are unlikely to be of benefit. No specific antidotes for venlafaxine HCl are known.

In managing overdosage, consider the possibility of multiple drug involvement. The physician should consider contacting a poison control center on the treatment of any overdose.

DOSAGE AND ADMINISTRATION:

Initial Treatment: The recommended starting dose for venlafaxine HCl is 75 mg/day, administered in two or three divided doses, taken with food. Depending on tolerability and the need for further clinical effect, the dose may be increased to 150 mg/day. If needed, the dose should be further increased up to 225 mg/day. When increasing the dose, increments of up to 75 mg/day should be made at intervals of no less than 4 days. In outpatient settings there was no evidence of usefulness of doses greater than 225 mg/day for moderately depressed patients, but more severely depressed inpatients responded to a mean dose of 350 mg/day. Certain patients, including more severely depressed patients, may therefore respond more to higher doses, up to a maximum of 375 mg/day, generally in three divided doses.

Dosage For Patients With Hepatic Impairment: Given the decrease in clearance and increase in elimination half-life for both venlafaxine and ODV that is observed in patients with hepatic cirrhosis compared to normal subjects (see CLINICAL PHARMACOLOGY), it is recommended that the total daily dose be reduced by 50% in patients with moderate hepatic impairment. Since there was much individual variability in clearance between patients with cirrhosis, it may be necessary to reduce the dose even more than 50%, and individualization of dosing may be desirable in some patients.

Dosage For Patients With Renal Impairment: Given the decrease in clearance for venlafaxine and the increase in elimination half-life for both venlafaxine and ODV that is observed in patients with renal impairment (GFR = 10-70 ml/min) compared to normals (see CLINICAL PHARMACOLOGY), it is recommended that the total daily dose be reduced by 25% in patients with mild to moderate renal impairment. It is recommended that the total daily dose be reduced by 50% and the dose be withheld until the dialysis treatment is completed (4 hrs) in patients undergoing hemodialysis. Since there was much individual variability in clearance between patients with renal impairment, individualization of dosing may be desirable in some patients.

Dosage For Elderly Patients: No dose adjustment is recommended for elderly patients on the basis of age. As with any antidepressant, however, caution should be exercised in treating the elderly. When individualizing the dosage, extra care should be taken when increasing the dose.

Maintenance/Continuation/Extended Treatment: There is no body of evidence available to answer the question of how long a patient should continue to be treated with venlafaxine HCl. It is generally agreed that acute episodes of major depression require several months or longer of sustained pharmacologic therapy. Whether the dose of antidepressant needed to induce remission is identical to the dose needed to maintain and/or sustain euthymia is unknown.

Discontinuing Venlafaxine HCl: When discontinuing venlafaxine HCl after more than 1 week of therapy, it is generally recommended that the dose be tapered to minimize the risk of discontinuation symptoms. Patients who have received venlafaxine HCl for 6 weeks or more should have their dose tapered gradually over a 2-week period.

Switching Patients To Or From A Monoamine Oxidase Inhibitor: At least 14 days should elapse between discontinuation of an MAOI and initiation of therapy with venlafaxine HCl. In addition, at least 7 days should be allowed after stopping venlafaxine HCl before starting an MAOI (see CONTRAINDICATIONS and WARNINGS).

PATIENT INFORMATION:

Venlafaxine HCl is used in the treatment of depression. Any medication that works on the central nervous system has the potential to cause drowsiness. Those taking venlafaxine should use caution while driving or operating machinery. Avoid alcohol consumption as well. This medication has been reported to interact with a class of drugs called the monoamine oxidase inhibitors. Please consult your physician if you have taken one of these medications or have been prescribed one by another physician. This medication should be taken with food and taken as prescribed. This medication should not be discontinued abruptly but should be tapered over time.

HOW SUPPLIED:

Effexor (venlafaxine HCl tablets) is available in the following dosage strengths (expressed in equivalent amounts of venlafaxine): *25 mg:* peach, shield-shaped tablet with "25" and a "W" on one side and "701" on scored reverse side. *37.5 mg:* peach, shield-shaped tablet with "37.5" and a "W" on one side and "781" on scored reverse side. *50 mg:* peach, shield-shaped tablet with "50" and a "W" on one side and "703" on scored reverse side. *75 mg:* peach, shield-shaped tablet with "75" and a"W" on one side and "704" on scored reverse side. 100 mg, peach, shield-shaped tablet with "100" and a"W" on one side and "705" on scored reverse side.

The appearance of these tablets is a trademark of Wyeth-Ayerst Laboratories.

Store at controlled room temperature, 20°C to 25°C (68°F to 77°F), in a dry place.

Dispense in a well-closed container as defined in the USP.

HOW SUPPLIED - EQUIVALENTS NOT AVAILABLE:

Tablet, Uncoated - Oral - 25 mg

100's	$95.45	EFFEXOR, Wyeth Labs	00008-0701-01
100's	$95.45	EFFEXOR, Wyeth Labs	00008-0701-02

Tablet, Uncoated - Oral - 37.5 mg

100's	$98.31	EFFEXOR, Wyeth Labs	00008-0781-01
100's	$98.31	EFFEXOR, Wyeth Labs	00008-0781-02

Tablet, Uncoated - Oral - 50 mg

100's	$101.25	EFFEXOR, Wyeth Labs	00008-0703-01
100's	$101.25	EFFEXOR, Wyeth Labs	00008-0703-02

Tablet, Uncoated - Oral - 75 mg

100's	$107.34	EFFEXOR, Wyeth Labs	00008-0704-01
100's	$107.34	EFFEXOR, Wyeth Labs	00008-0704-02

Tablet, Uncoated - Oral - 100 mg

100's	$113.78	EFFEXOR, Wyeth Labs	00008-0705-01
100's	$113.78	EFFEXOR, Wyeth Labs	00008-0705-02

VERAPAMIL HYDROCHLORIDE *(002425)*

CATEGORIES: Angina; Antianginals; Antiarrhythmic Agents; Antihypertensives; Arrhythmia; Atrial Fibrillation; Calcium Channel Blockers; Cardiovascular Drugs; Fibrillation; Heart Flutter; Hypertension; Tachycardia; Migraine*; Pregnancy Category C; Sales > $500 Million; FDA Approval Pre 1982; Patent Expiration 1992 Dec; Top 200 Drugs

* Indication not approved by the FDA

BRAND NAMES: *Akilen*; *Anpec*; *Apo-Verap* (Canada); *Arpamyl LP* (France); *Azupamil* (Germany); *Berkatens* (England); **Calan**; Calan SR; *Calaptin*; *Calaptin 240 SR*; *Cardiabeltin*; *Cardiagutt* (Germany); *Caveril*; *Civicor*; *Civicor Retard*; *Coraver*; *Cordilox* (England); *Cordilox SR*; *Corpamil*; *Dignover* (Germany); *Dilacoran* (Mexico); *Dilacoran HTA* (Mexico); *Flamon*; *Geangin* (England); *Harteze*; *Hexasoptin*; *Hexasoptin Retard*; *Hormitol* (Japan); *Ikacor*; *Ikapress*; *Inselon*; Isoptin; *Isoptin Retard* (Germany); Isoptin SR; *Isoptine* (France); *Isoptino*; *Magotiron* (Japan); *Manidon*; *Manidon Retard*; *Novo-Veramil* (Canada); *Praecicor* (Germany); *Quasar*;

Rapam; *Robatelan* (Japan); *Securon* (England); *Univer*; *Vasolan* (Japan); *Vasomil*; *Vasopten*; *Veracaps SR*; *Veracor*; *Verahexal* (Germany); *Veraloc*; *Veramex* (Germany); *Veramil*; *Verapin*; *Verapress 240 SR*; *Verdilac* (Mexico); Verelan; *Verelan SR*; *Verpal*; *Verpamil*; *Vetrimil*
(International brand names outside U.S. in italics)

FORMULARIES: Aetna; BC-BS; CIGNA; FHP; Foundation; Humana; Kaiser; Medco; Medi-Cal; PCS; PruCare; United; WHO

COST OF THERAPY: $56.72 (Angina; Tablet; 80 mg; 3/day; 365 days)

DESCRIPTION:

Tablets: Verapamil (verapamil HCl) is a calcium ion influx inhibitor (slow-channel blocker or calcium ion antagonist) available for oral administration in film-coated tablets containing 40 mg, 80 mg, or 120 mg of verapamil hydrochloride.

Verapamil HCl is an almost white, crystalline powder, practically free of odor, with a bitter taste. It is soluble in water, chloroform, and methanol. Verapamil HCl is not chemically related to other cardioactive drugs.

Sustained-Release/Extended-Release Tablets: Verapamil HCl Sustained Release is a calcium ion influx inhibitor (slow-channel blocker or calcium ion antagonist).

The tablets/caplets are designed for sustained release of the drug in the gastrointestinal tract; sustained- release characteristics are not altered when the caplet is divided in half.

Verapamil HCl is an almost white, crystalline powder, practically free of odor, with a bitter taste. It is soluble in water, chloroform, and methanol. Verapamil HCl is not chemically related to other cardioactive drugs.

The chemical formula (for both forms) is Benzeneacetonitrile, α-(3-((2-(3,4- dimethoxyphenyl) ethyl)methylamino)propyl)-3-4,-dimethoxy-α-(1-methylethyl) -,monohydrochloride.

Capsules: Verapamil hydrochloride is a calcium influx inhibitor (slow channel blocker or calcium ion antagonist). Verapamil hydrochloride is available for oral administration as a 240 mg hard gelatin capsule (dark blue cap/yellow body), a 180 mg hard gelatin capsule (light gray cap/yellow body), and a 120 mg hard gelatin capsule (yellow cap/yellow body). These pellet filled capsules provide a sustained-release of the drug in the gastrointestinal tract.

Chemical name: Benzenacetonitrile, α-(3-((2-(3,4-dimethoxyphenyl)-ethyl) methylamino)propyl)-3,4-dimethoxy-α-(1- methylethyl)monohydrochloride.

Verapamil HCl is an almost white, crystalline powder, practically free of odor, with a bitter taste. It is soluble in water, chloroform and methanol. Verapamil HCl is not structurally related to other cardioactive drugs.

CLINICAL PHARMACOLOGY:

Verapamil HCl is a calcium ion influx, inhibitor (slow-channel blocker or calcium ion antagonist) that exerts its pharmacologic effects by modulating the influx of ionic calcium across the cell membrane of the arterial smooth muscle as well as in conductile and contractile myocardial cells.

MECHANISM OF ACTION

Angina: The precise mechanism of action of verapamil HCl as an antianginal agent remains to be fully determined, but includes the following two mechanisms:

1. Relaxation and Prevention of Coronary Artery Spasm: Verapamil HCl dilates the main coronary arteries and coronary arterioles, both in normal and ischemic regions, and is a potent inhibitor of coronary artery spasm, whether spontaneous or ergonovine-induced. This property increases myocardial oxygen delivery in patients with coronary artery spasm and is responsible for the effectiveness of verapamil HCl in vasospastic (Prinzmetal's or variant) as well as unstable angina at rest. Whether this effect plays any role in classical effort angina is not clear, but studies of exercise tolerance have not shown an increase in the maximum exercise rate-pressure product, a widely accepted measure of oxygen utilization. This suggests that, in general, relief of spasm or dilation of coronary arteries is not an important factor in classical angina.

2. Reduction of Oxygen Utilization: Verapamil HCl regularly reduces the total peripheral resistance (afterload) against which the heart works both at rest and at a given level of exercise by dilating peripheral arterioles. This unloading of the heart reduces myocardial energy consumption and oxygen requirements and probably accounts for the effectiveness of verapamil HCl in chronic stable effort angina.

Arrhythmia: Electrical activity through the AV node depends, to a significant degree, upon calcium influx through the slow channel. By decreasing the influx of calcium verapamil HCl prolongs the effective refractory period within the AV node and slows AV conduction in a rate-related manner. This property accounts for the ability of verapamil HCl to slow the ventricular rate in patients with chronic atrial flutter or atrial fibrillation.

Normal sinus rhythm is usually not affected, but in patients with sick sinus syndrome, verapamil HCl may interfere with sinus-node impulse generation and may induce sinus arrest or sinoatrial block. Atrioventricular block can occur in patients without preexisting conduction defects (see WARNINGS.) Verapamil HCl decreases the frequency of episodes of paroxysmal supraventricular tachycardia.

Verapamil HCl does not alter the normal atrial action potential or intraventricular conduction time, but in depressed atrial fibers it decreases amplitude, velocity of depolarization, and conduction velocity. Verapamil HCl may shorten the antegrade effective refractory period of the accessory bypass tract. Acceleration of ventricular rate and/or ventricular fibrillation has been reported in patients with atrial flutter or atrial fibrillation and a coexisting accessory AV pathway following administration of verapamil HCl (see WARNINGS.)

Verapamil HCl has a local anesthetic action that is 1.6 times that of procaine on an equimolar basis. It is not known whether this action is important at the doses used in man.

Essential Hypertension: Verapamil HCl exerts antihypertensive effects by decreasing systemic vascular resistance, usually without orthostatic decreases in blood pressure or reflex tachycardia; bradycardia (rate less than 50 beats/min) is uncommon (1.4%). During isometric or dynamic exercise verapamil HCl does not alter systolic cardiac function in patients with normal ventricular function.

Verapamil HCl does not alter total serum calcium levels. However, one report suggested that calcium levels above the normal range may alter the therapeutic effect of verapamil HCl.

PHARMACOKINETICS AND METABOLISM

More than 90% of the orally administered dose of verapamil is absorbed. Because of rapid biotransformation of verapamil during its first pass through the portal circulation, bioavailability ranges from 20% to 35%. Peak plasma concentrations are reached between 1 and 2 hours after oral administration. Chronic oral administration of 120 mg of verapamil every 6 hours resulted in plasma levels of verapamil ranging from 125 to 400 ng/ml, with higher values reported occasionally. A nonlinear correlation between the verapamil dose administered and verapamil plasma levels does exist. In early dose titration with verapamil a relationship exists between verapamil plasma concentration and prolongation of the PR interval. However, during chronic administration this relationship may disappear. The mean elimination half-life in single-doses studies ranged from 2.8 to 7.4 hours. In these same studies, after repetitive dosing, the half-life increased to a range from 4.5 to 12.0 hours (after less than 10 consecutive doses given 6 hours apart). Half-life of verapamil may increase

CLINICAL PHARMACOLOGY: *(cont'd)*

during titration. Aging may affect the pharmacokinetics of verapamil. Elimination half-life may be prolonged in the elderly. In healthy men, orally administered verapamil undergoes extensive metabolism in the liver. Twelve metabolites have been identified in plasma; all except norverapamil are present in trace amounts only. Norverapamil can reach steady-state plasma concentrations approximately equal to those of verapamil itself. The cardiovascular activity of norverapamil appears to be approximately 20% that of verapamil. Approximately 70% of an administered dose is excreted as metabolites in the urine and 16% or more in the feces within 5 days. About 3% to 4% is excreted in the urine as unchanged drug. Approximately 90% is bound to plasma proteins. In patients with hepatic insufficiency, metabolism is delayed and elimination half-life prolonged up to 14 to 16 hours (see PRECAUTIONS); the volume of distribution is increased and plasma clearance reduced to about 30% of normal. Verapamil clearance values suggest that patients with liver dysfunction may attain therapeutic verapamil plasma concentrations with one third of the oral daily dose required for patients with normal liver function.

In randomized, single dose, crossover studies using healthy volunteers, administration of verapamil extended-release tablets with food produced lower peak concentrations, delayed time to peak, and lesser total absorption (AUC), than when the product was administered to fasting subjects. Similar results were demonstrated for plasma norverapamil. Food thus produces decreased bioavailability (AUC) but a narrower peak to trough ratio. Good correlation of dose and response is not available, but controlled studies of extended-release verapamil have shown effectiveness of doses similar to the effective doses of immediate-release verapamil.

After four weeks of oral dosing (120 mg q.i.d.), verapamil and norverapamil levels noted in the cerebrospinal fluid with estimated partition coefficient of 0.06 for verapamil HCl and 0.04 for norverapamil.

No relationship has been established between the plasma concentration of verapamil and a reduction in blood pressure

In multiple dose studies under fasting conditions, the bioavailability, measured by AUC, of extended-release verapamil was similar to immediate release verapamil; rates of absorption were, of course, different.

HEMODYNAMICS AND MYOCARDIAL METABOLISM

Verapamil HCl reduces afterload and myocardial contractility. Improved left ventricular diastolic function in patients with HCM and those with coronary heart disease has also been observed with verapamil HCl therapy. In most patients, including those with organic cardiac disease, the negative inotropic action of verapamil HCl is countered by reduction of afterload, and cardiac index is usually not reduced. However in patients with severe left ventricular dysfunction (*e.g.*, pulmonary wedge pressure above 20 mm Hg or ejection fraction less than 30%), or in patients taking beta-adrenergic blocking agents or other cardiodepressant drugs, deterioration of ventricular function may occur (see DRUG INTERACTIONS.)

PULMONARY FUNCTION

Verapamil HCl does not induce bronchoconstriction and, hence, does not impair ventilatory function.

INDICATIONS AND USAGE:

Verapamil HCl tablets are indicated for the treatment of the following:

Angina

1. Angina at rest including Vasospastic (Prinzmetal's variant) angina; Unstable (crescendo, pre-infarction) angina

2. Chronic stable angina (classic effort-associated angina)

Arrhythmias

1. In association with digitalis for the control of ventricular rate at rest and during stress in patients with chronic atrial flutter and/or atrial fibrillation ([Ss]ee WARNINGS).

2. Prophylaxis of repetitive paroxysmal supraventricular tachycardia

Essential Hypertension

CONTRAINDICATIONS:

Verapamil HCl tablets are contraindicated in:

1. Severe left ventricular dysfunction ([Ss]ee WARNINGS)

2. Hypotension (systolic pressure less than 90 mm Hg) or cardiogenic shock

3. Sick sinus syndrome (except in patients with a functioning artificial ventricular pacemaker)

4. Second- or third-degree AV block (except in patients with a functioning artificial ventricular pacemaker)

5. Patients with atrial flutter or atrial fibrillation and an accessory bypass tract (*e.g.*, Wolff-Parkinson-White, Lown-Ganong-Levine syndromes). See WARNINGS.

6. Patients with known hypersensitivity to verapamil hydrochloride.

WARNINGS:

Heart Failure: Verapamil HCl has a negative inotropic effect, which in most patients is compensated by its afterload reduction (decreased systemic vascular resistance) properties without a net impairment of ventricular performance. In clinical experience with 4,954 patients, 87 (1.8%) developed congestive heart failure or pulmonary edema. Verapamil HCl should be avoided in patients with severe left ventricular dysfunction (*e.g.*, ejection fraction less than 30%) or moderate to severe symptoms of cardiac failure and in patients with any degree of ventricular dysfunction if they are receiving a beta-adrenergic blocker (See DRUG INTERACTIONS.) Patients with milder ventricular dysfunction should, if possible, be controlled with optimum doses of digitalis and/or diuretics before verapamil HCl treatment. **(Note interactions with digoxin under PRECAUTIONS.)**

Hypotension: Occasionally, the pharmacologic action of verapamil HCl may produce a decrease in blood pressure below normal levels, which may result in dizziness or symptomatic hypotension. The incidence of hypotension observed in 4,954 patients enrolled in clinical trials was 2.5%. In hypertensive patients, decreases in blood pressure below normal are unusual. Tilt-table testing (60 degrees) was not able to induce orthostatic hypotension.

Elevated Liver Enzymes: Elevations of transaminases with and without concomitant elevations in alkaline phosphatase and bilirubin have been reported. Such elevations have sometimes been transient and may disappear even with continued verapamil HCl treatment. Several cases of hepatocellular injury related to verapamil HCl have been proven by rechallenge; half of these had clinical symptoms (malaise, fever, and/or right upper quadrant pain), in addition to elevation of SGOT, SGPT, and alkaline phosphatase. Periodic monitoring of liver function in patients receiving verapamil HCl is therefore prudent.

Accessory Bypass Tract (Wolff-Parkinson-White or Lown-Ganong-Levine): Some patients with paroxysmal and/or chronic atrial fibrillation or atrial flutter and a coexisting accessory AV pathway have developed increased antegrade conduction across the accessory pathway bypassing the AV node, producing a very rapid ventricular response or ventricular fibrillation after receiving intravenous verapamil HCl (or digitalis). Although a risk of this occurring with oral verapamil HCl has not been established, such patients receiving oral verapamil HCl may

WARNINGS: *(cont'd)*

be at risk and its use in these patients is contraindicated (see CONTRAINDICATIONS.) Treatment is usually DC-cardioversion. Cardioversion has been used safety and effectively after oral verapamil HCl.

Atrioventricular Block: The effect of verapamil HCl on AV conduction and the SA node may cause asymptomatic first-degree AV block and transient bradycardia, sometimes accompanied by nodal escape rhythms. PR-interval prolongation is correlated with verapamil HCl plasma concentrations especially during the early titration phase of therapy. Higher degrees of AV block, however, were infrequently (0.8%) observed. Marked first-degree block or progressive development to second- or third-degree AV block requires a reduction in dosage or, in rare instances, discontinuation of verapamil HCl and institution of appropriate therapy, depending on the clinical situation.

Patients with Hypertrophic Cardiomyopathy (IHSS): In 120 patients with hypertrophic cardiomyopathy (most of them refractory or intolerant to propranolol) who received therapy with verapamil HCl at doses up to 720 mg/day, a variety of serious adverse effects were seen. Three patients died in pulmonary edema; all had severe left ventricular outflow obstruction and a past history of left ventricular dysfunction. Eight other patients had pulmonary edema and/or severe hypotension; abnormally high (greater than 20 mm Hg) pulmonary wedge pressure and a marked left ventricular outflow obstruction were present in most of these patients. Concomitant administration of quinidine (see DRUG INTERACTIONS) preceded the severe hypotension in 3 of the 8 patients (2 of whom developed pulmonary edema). Sinus bradycardia occurred in 11% of the patients, second-degree AV block in 4%, and sinus arrest in 2%. It must be appreciated that this group of patients had a serious disease with a high mortality rate. Most adverse effects responded well to dose reduction, and only rarely did verapamil HCl use have to be discontinued.

PRECAUTIONS:

GENERAL

Use in Patients with Impaired Hepatic Function: Since verapamil HCl is highly metabolized by the liver, it should be administered cautiously to patients with impaired hepatic function. Severe liver dysfunction prolongs the elimination half-life of verapamil HCl to about 14 to 16 hours; hence, approximately 30% of the dose given to patients with normal liver function should be administered to these patients. Careful monitoring for abnormal prolongation of the PR interval or other signs of excessive pharmacologic effects (see OVERDOSAGE) should be carried out.

Use in Patients with Attenuated (Decreased) Neuromuscular Transmission: It has been reported that verapamil HCl decreases neuromuscular transmission in patients with Duchenne's muscular dystrophy, and that verapamil HCl prolongs recovery from the neuromuscular blocking agent vecuronium. It may be necessary to decrease the dosage of verapamil HCl when it is administered to patients with attenuated neuromuscular transmission.

Use in Patients With Impaired Renal Function: About 70% of an administered dose of verapamil HCl is excreted as metabolites in the urine. Verapamil HCl is excreted by hemodialysis. Until further data are available, verapamil HCl should be administered cautiously to patients with impaired renal function. These patients should be carefully monitored for abnormal prolongation of the PR interval or other signs of overdosage (see OVERDOSAGE.)

CARCINOGENESIS, MUTAGENESIS, AND IMPAIRMENT OF FERTILITY

An 18-month toxicity study in rats, at a low multiple (6-fold) of the maximum recommended human dose, and not the maximum tolerated dose, did not suggest a tumorigenic potential. There was no evidence of a carcinogenic potential of verapamil HCl administered in the diet of rats for two years at doses of 10, 35, and 120 mg/kg/day or approximately 1, 3.5, and 12 times, respectively, the maximum recommended human daily dose (480 mg/day or 9.6 mg/kg/day).

Verapamil HCl was not mutagenic in the Ames test in 5 test strains at 3 mg per plate with or without metabolic activation.

Studies in female rats at daily dietary doses up to 5.5 times (55 mg/kg/day) the maximum recommended human dose did not show impaired fertility. Effects on male fertility have not been determined.

PREGNANCY CATEGORY C

Reproduction studies have been performed in rabbits and rats at oral doses up to 1.5 (15 mg/kg/day) and 6 (60 mg/kg/day) times the human oral daily dose, respectively, and have revealed no evidence of teratogenicity. In the rat, however, this multiple of the human dose was embryocidal and retarded fetal growth and development, probably because of adverse maternal effects reflected in reduced weight gains of the dams. This oral dose has also been shown to cause hypotension in rats. There are no adequate and well-controlled studies in pregnant women. Because animal reproduction studies are not always predictive of human response, this drug should be used during pregnancy only if clearly needed. Verapamil HCl crosses the placental barrier and can be detected in umbilical blood at delivery.

LABOR AND DELIVERY

It is not known whether the use of verapamil HCl during labor or delivery has immediate or delayed adverse effects on the fetus, or whether it prolongs the duration of labor or increases the need for forceps delivery or other obstetric intervention. Such adverse experiences have not been reported in the literature, despite a long history of use of verapamil HCl in Europe in the treatment of cardiac side effects of beta-adrenergic agonist agents used to treat premature labor.

NURSING MOTHERS

Verapamil HCl is excreted in human milk. Because of the potential for adverse reactions in nursing infants from verapamil HCl, nursing should be discontinued while verapamil HCl is administered.

PEDIATRIC USE

Safety and efficacy of verapamil HCl in children below the age of 18 years have not been established.

Animal Pharmacology and/or Animal Toxicology: In chronic animal toxicology studies verapamil HCl caused lenticular and/or suture line changes at 30 mg/kg/day or greater and frank cataracts at 62.5 mg/kg/day or greater in the beagle dog but not in the rat. Development of cataracts due to verapamil HCl has not been reported in man.

DRUG INTERACTIONS:

Beta-Blockers: Controlled studies in small numbers of patients suggest that the concomitant use of verapamil HCl and oral beta-adrenergic blocking agents may be beneficial in certain patients with chronic stable angina or hypertension, but available information is not sufficient to predict with confidence the effects of concurrent treatment in patients with left ventricular dysfunction or cardiac conduction abnormalities. Concomitant therapy with beta-adrenergic blockers and verapamil HCl may result in additive negative effects on heart rate, atrioventricular conduction and/or cardiac contractility.

In one study involving 15 patients treated with high doses of propranolol (median dose, 480 mg/day; range 160 to 1,280 mg/day) for severe angina, with preserved left ventricular function (ejection fraction greater than 35%), the hemodynamic effects of additional therapy with verapamil HCl were assessed using invasive methods. The addition of verapamil HCl to

DRUG INTERACTIONS: *(cont'd)*

high-dose beta-blockers induced modest negative inotropic and chronotropic effects that were not severe enough to limit short-term (48 hours) combination therapy in this study. These modest cardiodepressant effects persisted for greater than 6 but less than 30 hours after abrupt withdrawal of beta-blockers and were closely related to plasma levels of propranolol. The primary verapamil/beta-blocker interaction in this study appeared to be hemodynamic rather than electrophysiologic.

In other studies verapamil HCl did not generally induce significant negative inotropic, chronotropic, or dromotropic effects in patients with preserved left ventricular function receiving low or moderate doses of propranolol (less than or equal to 320 mg/day); in some patients, however, combined therapy did produce such effects. Therefore, if combined therapy is used, close surveillance of clinical status should be carried out. Combined therapy should usually be avoided in patients with atrio-ventricular conduction abnormalities and those with depressed left ventricular function.

Asymptomatic bradycardia (36 beats-min) with a wandering atrial pacemaker has been observed in a patient receiving concomitant timolol (a beta-adrenergic blocker) eyedrops and oral verapamil HCl.

A decrease in metoprolol and propranolol clearance has been observed when either drug is administered concomitantly with verapamil HCl. A variable effect has been seen when verapamil HCl and atenolol were given together.

Digitalis: Clinical use of verapamil HCl in digitalized patients has shown the combination to be well tolerated if digoxin doses are properly adjusted. However, chronic verapamil HCl treatment can increase serum digoxin levels by 50% to 75% during the first week of therapy, and this can result in digitalis toxicity. In patients with hepatic cirrhosis the influence of erapamil HCl on digoxin kinetics is magnified. Verapamil HCl may reduce total body clearance and extrarenal clearance of digitoxin by 27% and 29%, respectively. Maintenance and digitalization doses should be reduced when verapamil HCl is administered, and the patient should be reassessed to avoid over- or underdigitalization. Whenever overdigitalization is suspected, the daily dose of digitalis should be reduced or temporarily discontinued. On discontinuation of verapamil HCl use, the patient should be reassessed to avoid underdigitalization.

Antihypertensive Agents: Verapamil HCl administered concomitantly with oral antihypertensive agents (*e.g.,* vasodilators, angiotensin-converting enzyme inhibitors, diuretics, beta-blockers) will usually have an additive effect on lowering blood pressure. Patients receiving these combinations should be appropriately monitored. Concomitant use of agents that attenuate alpha-adrenergic function with verapamil HCl may result in a reduction in blood pressure that is excessive in some patients. Such an effect was observed in one study following the concomitant administration of verapamil HCl and prazosin.

ANTIARRHYTHMIC AGENTS

Disopyramide: Until data on possible interactions between verapamil HCl and disopyramide are obtained, disopyramide should not be administered within 48 hours before or 24 hours after verapamil HCl administration.

Flecainide: A study in healthy volunteers showed that the concomitant administration of flecainide and verapamil HCl may have additive effects on myocardial contractility, AV conduction, and repolarization. Concomitant therapy with flecainide and verapamil HCl may result in additive negative inotropic effect and prolongation of atrioventricular conduction.

Quinidine: In a small number of patients with hypertrophic cardiomyopathy (HCM), concomitant use of verapamil HCl and quinidine resulted in significant hypotension. Until further data are obtained, combined therapy of verapamil HCl and quinidine in patients with hypertrophic cardiomyopathy should probably be avoided.

The electrophysiologic effects of quinidine and verapamil HCl on AV conduction were studied in 8 patients. Verapamil HCl significantly counteracted the effects of quinidine on AV conduction. There has been a report of increased quinidine levels during verapamil HCl therapy.

OTHER

Nitrates: Verapamil HCl has been given concomitantly with short- and long-acting nitrates without any undesirable drug interactions. The pharmacologic profile of both drugs and the clinical experience suggest beneficial interactions.

Cimetidine: The interaction between cimetidine and chronically administered verapamil HCl has not been studied. Variable results on clearance have been obtained in acute studies of healthy volunteers; clearance of verapamil HCl was either reduced or unchanged.

Lithium: Pharmacokinetic and pharmacodynamic interactions between oral verapamil HCl and lithium have been reported. The former may result in a lowering of serum lithium levels in patients receiving chronic stable oral lithium therapy. The latter may result in an increased sensitivity to the effects of lithium. Patients receiving both drugs must be monitored carefully.

Carbamazepine: Verapamil therapy may increase carbamazepine concentrations during combined therapy. This may produce carbamazepine side effects such as diplopia, headache, ataxia, or dizziness.

Rifampin: Therapy with rifampin may markedly reduce oral verapamil HCl bioavailability.

Phenobarbital: Phenobarbital therapy may increase verapamil HCl clearance.

Cyclosporin: Verapamil HCl therapy may increase serum levels of cyclosporin.

Theophylline: Verapamil HCl may inhibit the clearance and increase the plasma levels of theophylline.

Inhalation Anesthetics: Animal experiments have shown that inhalation anesthetics depress cardiovascular activity by decreasing the inward movement of calcium ions. When used concomitantly, inhalation anesthetics and calcium antagonists, such as verapamil HCl, should each be titrated carefully to avoid excessive cardiovascular depression.

Neuromuscular Blocking Agents: Clinical data and animal studies suggest that verapamil HCl may potentiate the activity of neuromuscular blocking agents (curare-like and depolarizing). It may be necessary to decrease the dose of verapamil HCl and/or the dose of the neuromuscular blocking agent when the drugs are used concomitantly.

ADVERSE REACTIONS:

Serious adverse reactions are uncommon when verapamil HCl therapy is initiated with upward dose titration within the recommended single and total daily dose. See WARNINGS for discussion of heart failure, hypotension, elevated liver enzymes, AV block, and rapid ventricular response. Reversible (upon discontinuation of verapamil HCL) non-obstructive, paralytic ileus has been infrequently reported in association with the use of verapamil HCl. The following reactions, (TABLE 1), to orally administered verapamil HCl occurred at rates greater than 1.0% or occurred at lower rates but appeared clearly drug-related in clinical trials in 4,954 patients:

Elevated liver enzymes: (see WARNINGS.)

In clinical trials related to the control of ventricular response in digitalized patients who had atrial fibrillation or flutter, ventricular rates below 50 at rest occurred in 15% of patients and asymptomatic hypotension occurred in 5% of patients.

ADVERSE REACTIONS: *(cont'd)*

TABLE 1

Constipation	7.3%
Dizziness	3.3%
Nausea	2.7%
Hypotension	2.5%
Headache	2.2%
Edema	1.9%
CHF, Pulmonary edema	1.8%
Fatigue	1.7%
Dyspnea	1.4%
Bradycardia (HR <50/min)	1.4%
AV block total (1°,2°,3°)	1.2%
2° and 3°	0.8%
Rash	1.2%
Flushing	0.6%

The following reactions, reported in 1.0% or less of patients, occurred under conditions (open trials, marketing experience) where a causal relationship is uncertain; they are listed to alert the physician to a possible relationship.

Cardiovascular: Angina pectoris, atrioventricular dissociation, chest pain, claudication, myocardial infarction, palpitations, purpura (vasculitis), syncope.

Digestive System: Diarrhea, dry mouth, gastrointestinal distress, gingival hyperplasia.

Hemic and Lymphatic: Ecchymosis or bruising.

Nervous System: Cerebrovascular accident, confusion, equilibrium disorders, insomnia, muscle cramps, paresthesia, psychotic symptoms, shakiness, somnolence.

Skin: Arthralgia and rash, exanthema, hair loss, hyperkeratosis, macules, sweating urticaria, Stevens-Johnson syndrome, erythema multiforme.

Special Senses: Blurred vision.

Urogenital: Gynecomastia, galactorrhea/hyperprolactinemia, increased urination, spotty menstruation, impotence.

Treatment of Acute Cardiovascular Adverse Reactions: The frequency of cardiovascular adverse reactions that require therapy is rare; hence, experience with their treatment is limited. Whenever severe hypotension or complete AV block occurs following oral administration of verapamil HCl, the appropriate emergency measure should be applied immediately; e.g., intravenously administered norepinephrine bitartrate, atropine sulfate, isoproterenol HCl (all in the usual dose), or calcium gluconate (10% solution). In patients with hypertrophic cardiomyopathy (IHSS), alpha-adrenergic agents (phenylephrine HCl, metaraminol bitartrate, or methoxamine HCL) should be used to maintain blood pressure, and isoproterenol and norepinephrine should be avoided. If further support is necessary, dopamine HCl or dobutamine HCl may be administered. Actual treatment and dosage should depend on the severity of the clinical situation and the judgment and experience of the treating physician.

OVERDOSAGE:

Treat all verapamil HCl overdoses as serious and maintain observation for at least 48 hours (especially verapamil SR) and preferably under continuous hospital care. Delayed pharmacodynamic consequences may occur with the sustained-release formulation. Verapamil HCl is known to decrease gastrointestinal transit time. Treatment of overdosage should be supportive. Beta-adrenergic stimulation or parenteral administration of calcium solutions may increase calcium ion flux across the slow channel, and have been used effectively in treatment of deliberate overdosage with verapamil HCl. Verapamil HCl cannot be removed by hemodialysis. Clinically significant hypotensive reactions or fixed high-degree AV block should be treated with vasopressor agents or cardiac pacing, respectively. Asystole should be handled by the usual measures, including cardiopulmonary resuscitation.

DOSAGE AND ADMINISTRATION:

TABLETS

The dose of verapamil Hcl must be individualized by titration. The usefulness and safety of dosages exceeding 480 mg/day have not been established; therefore, this daily dosage should not be exceeded. Since the half-life of verapamil HCl increases during chronic dosing, maximum response may be delayed.

Angina: Clinical trials show that the usual dose is 80 mg to 120 mg three times a day. However, 40 mg three times a day may be warranted in patients who may have an increased response to verapamil HCl (*e.g.,* decreased hepatic function, elderly, etc). Upward titration should be based on therapeutic efficacy and safety evaluated approximately eight hours after dosing. Dosage may be increased at daily (*e.g.,* patients with unstable angina) or weekly intervals until optimum clinical response is obtained.

Arrhythmias: The dosage in digitalized patients with chronic atrial fibrillation (see PRECAUTIONS) ranges from 240 to 320 mg/day in divided (t.i.d. or q.i.d.) doses. The dosage for prophylaxis of PSVT (non-digitalized patients) ranges from 240 to 480 mg/day in divided (t.i.d. or q.i.d.) doses. In general, maximum effects for any given dosage will be apparent during the first 48 hours of therapy.

Essential Hypertension: Dose should be individualized by titration. The usual initial monotherapy dose in clinical trials was 80 mg three times a day (240 mg/day). Daily dosages of 360 and 480 mg have been used but there is no evidence that dosages beyond 360 mg provided added effect. Consideration should be given to beginning titration at 40 mg three times per day in patients who might respond to lower doses, such as the elderly or people of small stature. The antihypertensive effects of verapamil HCl are evident within the first week of therapy. Upward titration should be based on therapeutic efficacy, assessed at the end of the dosing interval.

SUSTAINED RELEASE TABLETS

Essential Hypertension: The dose of this form should be individualized by titration and should be administered with food. Initiate therapy with 180 mg of sustained-release verapamil HCl given in the morning. Lower initial doses of 120 mg a day may be warranted in patients who may have an increased response to verapamil HCl (*e.g.,* the elderly or small people). Upward titration should be based on therapeutic efficacy and safety evaluated weekly and approximately 24 hours after the previous dose. The antihypertensive effects of verapamil HCl Sustained release are evident within the first week of therapy.

If adequate response is not obtained with 180 mg of verapamil HCl Sustained release, the dose may be titrated upward in the following manner:

(a) 240 mg each morning

(b) 180 mg each morning plus 180 mg each evening; or 240 mg each morning plus 120 mg each evening,

(c) 240 mg every 12 hours

When switching from immediate-release to sustained-release verapamil the total daily dose in mg may remain the same.

Store at 59 to 86°F (15 to 30°C) and protect from light. Dispense in tight, light-resistant containers.

DOSAGE AND ADMINISTRATION: *(cont'd)*

CAPSULES-ESSENTIAL HYPERTENSION

The dose of verapamil HCl should be individualized by titration. The usual daily dose of sustained-release verapamil, in clinical trials has been 240 mg given by mouth once daily in the morning. However, initial doses of 120 mg a day may be warranted in patients who may have an increased response to verapamil (*e.g.,* elderly, small people, etc.). Upward titration should be based on therapeutic efficacy and safety evaluated approximately 24 hours after dosing. The antihypertensive effects of verapamil HCl are evident within the first week of therapy.

If adequate response is not obtained with 120 of verapamil HCl, the dose may be titrated upward in the following manner:

(a) 180 mg in the morning.

(b) 240 mg in the morning.

(c) 360 mg in the morning.

(d) 480 mg in the morning.

Verapamil HCl sustained-release capsules are for once-a-day administration. When switching from immediate-release verapamil to verapamil HCl capsules, the same total daily dose of verapamil HCl can be used.

As with immediate-release verapamil, dosages of verapamil HCl capsules should be individualized and titration may be needed in some patients.

Store at controlled room temperature 15-30°C (59-86°F), protected from moisture.

Dispense in a tight, light-resistant container as defined in USP.

PATIENT INFORMATION:

Verapamil HCl is known as a calcium channel blocker. It is taken to treat high blood pressure, to relieve some chest pains in patients with angina, or to treat some problems with heart rhythms. Verapamil has several drug interactions, make sure your physician and pharmacist known all the medicines you are taking so they may properly advise you. Verapamil HCl is excreted in breast milk. It may be necessary to change therapy or provide an alternate to breast milk. The most common side effect is constipation. This may be relieved with dietary modification (more fiber) or laxatives. Sustained release tablets should be taken with food. They should not be broken or crushed. Doses may need some adjustment, make sure to have your condition monitored regularly.

HOW SUPPLIED - RATED THERAPEUTICALLY EQUIVALENT:

Injection, Solution - Intravenous - 2.5 mg/ml

2 ml	$2.35	Verapamil Hcl 2.5, Abbott	00074-4011-01
2 ml	$3.47	Verapamil Hcl 2.5, Abbott	00074-1144-01
2 ml	$4.86	Verapamil Hcl 2.5, Abbott	00074-4000-01
2 ml	$6.75	Verapamil Hcl, Intl Medication	00548-1470-00
2 ml	$12.99	ISOPTIN, Knoll Labs	00044-1816-21
2 ml	$30.63	Verapamil Hcl Hcl, Solopak Labs	39769-0100-02
2 ml x 5	$9.38	Verapamil Hcl, Am Regent	00517-0501-72
2 ml x 5	$12.19	Verapamil Hcl, Am Regent	00517-5402-05
2 ml x 10	$26.84	Verapamil HCl, Sanofi Winthrop	00024-2110-03
2 ml x 10	$29.53	Verapamil HCl, Sanofi Winthrop	00024-2110-41
2 ml x 10	$121.14	Verapamil Hcl, Fujisawa USA	00469-5000-10
2 ml x 10	$122.47	ISOPTIN, Knoll Labs	00044-1815-07
4 ml	$2.42	Verapamil Hcl 2.5, Abbott	00074-4011-02
4 ml	$3.92	Verapamil Hcl 2.5, Abbott	00074-1144-02
4 ml	$5.23	Verapamil Hcl, Abbott	00074-1143-15
4 ml	$12.20	Verapamil Hcl, Intl Medication	00548-1471-00
4 ml	$36.88	Verapamil Hcl Hcl, Solopak Labs	39769-0100-05
4 ml x 5	$13.44	Verapamil Hcl, Am Regent	00517-5404-05
4 ml x 10	$18.00	Verapamil Hcl, Voluntary Hosp	53258-5000-02
4 ml x 10	$218.72	Verapamil Hcl, Fujisawa USA	00469-5000-20

Tablet - Oral - 240 mg

100's	$120.85	Verapamil Hcl ER, Mylan	00378-0411-01
1000's	$598.22	Verapamil Hcl ER, Mylan	00378-0411-10

Tablet, Coated, Sustained Action - Oral - 180 mg

100's	$38.25	Verapamil HCl, H.C.F.A. F F P	99999-2425-01
100's	$52.43	Verapamil Hcl, United Res	00677-1518-01
100's	$52.43	Verapamil Hcl, Geneva Pharms	00781-1239-01
100's	$97.75	Verapamil HCl, Qualitest Pharms	00603-6359-21
100's	$97.80	Verapamil Hcl, Rugby	00536-5675-01
100's	$97.80	Verapamil Hcl, Major Pharms	00904-7871-60
100's	$97.80	Verapamil Hcl, Major Pharms	00904-7931-60
100's	$97.80	Verapamil Hcl, H N Norton Co.	50732-0915-01
100's	$98.00	Verapamil Hcl, Martec Pharms	52555-0536-01
100's	$99.27	Verapamil Hcl, Caremark	00339-5811-12
100's	$101.57	Verapamil Hcl, Zenith Labs	00172-4286-60
100's	$101.57	Verapamil Hcl, Goldline Labs	00182-1969-01
100's	$102.95	Verapamil Hcl, Aligen Independ	00405-5101-01
100's	$105.50	Verapamil HCl, Rugby	00536-5630-01
100's	$105.62	Verapamil NCl, Schein Pharm (US)	00364-2590-01
100's	$107.20	Verapamil, HL Moore Drug Exch	00839-7878-06
100's	$111.00	Verapamil HCl, Warner Chilcott	00047-0472-24
100's	**$112.86**	**CALAN SR, Searle**	**00025-1911-31**
100's	$112.86	ISOPTIN SR, Knoll Labs	00044-1825-02
100's	**$118.50**	**CALAN SR, Searle**	**00025-1911-34**
100's	$118.50	ISOPTIN SR, Knoll Labs	00044-1825-12
500's	$191.25	Verapamil HCl, H.C.F.A. F F P	99999-2425-02
500's	$464.65	Verapamil Hcl, H N Norton Co.	50732-0915-05
500's	$482.45	Verapamil Hcl, Zenith Labs	00172-4286-70
500's	$482.45	Verapamil Hcl, Goldline Labs	00182-1969-05

Tablet, Coated, Sustained Action - Oral - 240 mg

100's	$38.25	Verapamil HCl, H.C.F.A. F F P	99999-2425-03
100's	$53.93	Verapamil Hcl, United Res	00677-1453-01
100's	$53.93	Verapamil Hcl, Geneva Pharms	00781-1018-01
100's	$103.00	Verapamil Hcl, H N Norton Co.	50732-0901-01
100's	$107.45	Verapamil HCl, Qualitest Pharms	00603-6360-21
100's	$110.00	Verapamil Hcl, Harber Pharm	51432-0529-03
100's	$111.20	Verapamil Hcl, Aligen Independ	00405-5102-01
100's	$111.95	Verapamil Hcl, Martec Pharms	52555-0537-01
100's	$112.79	Verapamil Hcl, Caremark	00339-5809-12
100's	$113.00	Verapamil HCl, Rugby	00536-5674-01
100's	$113.19	Verapamil SR, HL Moore Drug Exch	00839-7670-06
100's	$113.70	Verapamil ER, Schein Pharm (US)	00364-2567-01
100's	$116.20	Verapamil Hcl, Zenith Labs	00172-4280-60
100's	$116.20	Verapamil Hcl, Goldline Labs	00182-1970-01
100's	$119.26	Verapamil HCl ER, Rugby	00536-4823-01
100's	$120.85	Verapamil HCl, Warner Chilcott	00047-0474-24
100's	$126.80	Verapamil SR, Major Pharms	00904-7723-60
100's	**$129.12**	**CALAN SR, Searle**	**00025-1891-31**
100's	$129.12	ISOPTIN SR, Knoll Labs	00044-1826-02
100's	**$135.57**	**CALAN SR, Searle**	**00025-1891-34**

HOW SUPPLIED - RATED THERAPEUTICALLY EQUIVALENT: *(cont'd)*

100's	$135.57	ISOPTIN SR, Knoll Labs	00044-1826-10
300's	$114.75	Verapamil HCl, H.C.F.A. F F P	99999-2425-04
300's	**$407.87**	**CALAN SR, Searle**	**00025-1891-45**
500's	$191.25	Verapamil HCl, H.C.F.A. F F P	99999-2425-05
500's	$269.65	Verapamil Hcl, United Res	00677-1453-05
500's	$495.00	Verapamil Hcl, Rugby	00536-5674-05
500's	$499.23	Verapamil HCl, HL Moore Drug Exch	00839-7670-12
500's	$536.67	Verapamil Hcl, Rugby	00536-4823-05
500's	$553.90	Verapamil Hcl, Martec Pharms	52555-0537-05
500's	$553.92	Verapamil HCl, Schein Pharm (US)	00364-2567-05
500's	$553.92	Verapamil Hcl, H N Norton Co.	50732-0901-05
500's	$575.24	Verapamil Hcl, Zenith Labs	00172-4280-70
500's	$575.24	Verapamil Hcl, Goldline Labs	00182-1970-05
500's	$598.25	Verapamil HCl, Warner Chilcott	00047-0474-30
500's	$629.95	Verapamil Hcl, Major Pharms	00904-7723-40
500's	**$639.16**	**CALAN SR, Searle**	**00025-1891-51**
500's	$639.16	ISOPTIN SR, Knoll Labs	00044-1826-03

Tablet, Plain Coated - Oral - 40 mg

100's	$21.45	Verapamil HCl, H.C.F.A. F F P	99999-2425-06
100's	$26.15	Verapamil Hcl, Qualitest Pharms	00603-6356-21
100's	$26.29	Verapamil Hcl, Watson Labs	52544-0404-01
100's	$26.75	Verapamil HCl, Geneva Pharms	50752-0305-05
100's	$27.25	Verapamil Hcl, Major Pharms	00904-7799-60
100's	$27.31	Verapamil Hcl, Caremark	00339-5857-12
100's	$27.47	Verapamil Hcl, HL Moore Drug Exch	00839-7921-06
100's	$27.66	Verapamil Hcl, Rugby	00536-5624-01
100's	$27.66	Verapamil HCl, Geneva Pharms	00781-1014-01
100's	$29.70	Verapamil Hcl, Goldline Labs	00182-1601-01
100's	$30.74	ISOPTIN, Knoll Labs	00044-1821-02
100's	$32.27	ISOPTIN, Knoll Labs	00044-1821-10
100's	**$33.17**	**CALAN, Searle**	**00025-1771-31**

Tablet, Plain Coated - Oral - 80 mg

50's	$2.59	Verapamil HCl, H.C.F.A. F F P	99999-2425-07
50's	$14.95	Verapamil Hcl, Mutual Pharm	53489-0154-02
100's	$5.18	Verapamil Hcl, United Res	00677-1130-01
100's	$5.18	Verapamil HCl, H.C.F.A. F F P	99999-2425-08
100's	$8.93	Verapamil Hcl, IDE-Interstate	00814-8280-14
100's	$10.71	Verapamil Hcl, US Trading	56126-0360-11
100's	$14.25	Verapamil Hcl, Martec Pharms	52555-0179-01
100's	$21.18	Verapamil Hcl, HL Moore Drug Exch	00839-7253-06
100's	$21.18	Verapamil Hcl, HL Moore Drug Exch	00839-7267-06
100's	$21.32	Verapamil HCl, Lederle Pharm	00005-3446-43
100's	$21.50	Verapamil Hcl, Qualitest Pharms	00603-6357-21
100's	$21.65	Verapamil Hcl, Goldline Labs	00182-1300-01
100's	$22.05	Verapamil Hcl, Major Pharms	00904-2920-60
100's	$22.43	Verapamil Hcl, Watson Labs	52544-0343-01
100's	$22.43	Verapamil Hcl, Watson Labs	52544-0344-01
100's	$22.50	Verapamil Hcl, Harber Pharm	51432-0403-03
100's	$23.50	Verapamil Hcl, Mutual Pharm	53489-0154-01
100's	$23.55	Verapamil Hcl, Caremark	00339-5621-12
100's	$23.56	Verapamil HCl, Rugby	00536-4931-01
100's	$23.84	Verapamil Hcl, Purepac Pharm	00228-2473-10
100's	$23.90	Verapamil HCl, Geneva Pharms	50752-0306-05
100's	$25.92	Verapamil Hcl, Aligen Independ	00405-5099-01
100's	$26.86	Verapamil Hcl, Parmed Pharms	00349-8624-01
100's	$27.60	Verapamil HCl, Schein Pharm (US)	00364-2111-01
100's	$27.65	Verapamil, Geneva Pharms	00781-1016-01
100's	$27.70	Verapamil HCl, Warner Chilcott	00047-0328-24
100's	$27.70	Verapamil Hcl, Mylan	00378-0512-01
100's	$32.70	Verapamil Hcl, Medirex	57480-0374-01
100's	$34.25	Verapamil HCl, Schein Pharm (US)	00364-2111-90
100's	$35.65	Verapamil Hcl, Major Pharms	00904-2920-61
100's	$42.09	Verapamil Hcl, Goldline Labs	00182-1300-89
100's	$42.09	Verapamil, Geneva Pharms	00781-1016-13
100's	$44.19	Verapamil Hcl, Vangard Labs	00615-2518-13
100's	$44.22	ISOPTIN, Knoll Labs	00044-1822-02
100's	$46.77	ISOPTIN, Knoll Labs	00044-1822-10
100's	**$47.72**	**CALAN, Searle**	**00025-1851-31**
250's	$12.95	Verapamil HCl, H.C.F.A. F F P	99999-2425-09
500's	$25.85	Verapamil Hcl, Sidmak Labs	50111-0486-01
500's	$25.90	Verapamil Hcl, United Res	00677-1130-05
500's	$25.90	Verapamil HCl, H.C.F.A. F F P	99999-2425-10
500's	$53.15	Verapamil Hcl, Major Pharms	00904-2920-40
500's	$83.95	Verapamil Hcl, Watson Labs	52544-0343-05
500's	$83.95	Verapamil Hcl, Watson Labs	52544-0344-05
500's	$98.48	Verapamil Hcl, HL Moore Drug Exch	00839-7253-12
500's	$98.75	Verapamil HCl, Rugby	00536-4931-05
500's	$98.80	Verapamil Hcl, Goldline Labs	00182-1300-05
500's	$99.40	Verapamil HCl, Geneva Pharms	50752-0306-08
500's	$106.71	Verapamil Hcl Tablets 80 Mg, Aligen Independ	00405-5099-02
500's	$107.00	Verapamil Hcl, Mutual Pharm	53489-0154-05
500's	$112.50	Verapamil Hcl, Harber Pharm	51432-0403-05
500's	$119.20	Verapamil Hcl, Purepac Pharm	00228-2473-50
500's	$119.68	Verapamil Hcl, Parmed Pharms	00349-8624-05
500's	$120.50	Verapamil HCl, Warner Chilcott	00047-0328-30
500's	$120.50	Verapamil HCl, Schein Pharm (US)	00364-2111-05
500's	$120.75	Verapamil, Geneva Pharms	00781-1016-05
500's	$212.16	ISOPTIN, Knoll Labs	00044-1822-05
500's	**$228.93**	**CALAN, Searle**	**00025-1851-51**
600's	$203.00	Verapamil Hcl, Medirex	57480-0374-06
750's	$299.89	Verapamil Hcl, Glasgow Pharm	60809-0120-55
750's	$299.89	Verapamil Hcl, Glasgow Pharm	60809-0120-72
1000's	$51.80	Verapamil HCl, H.C.F.A. F F P	99999-2425-11
1000's	$93.50	Verapamil Hcl, Sidmak Labs	50111-0486-02
1000's	$116.35	Verapamil Hcl, Qualitest Pharms	00603-6357-32
1000's	$130.45	Verapamil Hcl, Major Pharms	00904-2920-80
1000's	$150.00	Verapamil Hcl, Goldline Labs	00182-1300-10
1000's	$160.45	Verapamil Hcl, Watson Labs	52544-0343-10
1000's	$160.45	Verapamil Hcl, Watson Labs	52544-0344-10
1000's	$167.00	Verapamil HCl, Rugby	00536-4931-10
1000's	$181.50	Verapamil Hcl, Sidmak Labs	50111-0486-03
1000's	$188.93	Verapamil Hcl, HL Moore Drug Exch	00839-7267-16
1000's	$190.15	Verapamil Hcl, Parmed Pharms	00349-8624-10
1000's	$190.15	Verapamil Hcl, Parmed Pharms	00349-8628-10
1000's	$191.20	Verapamil HCl, Geneva Pharms	50752-0306-09
1000's	$192.03	Verapamil Hcl, Purepac Pharm	00228-2473-96
1000's	$205.00	Verapamil Hcl, Mutual Pharm	53489-0154-10
1000's	$207.40	Verapamil HCl, Schein Pharm (US)	00364-2111-02
1000's	$247.45	Verapamil, Geneva Pharms	00781-1016-10
1000's	$247.50	Verapamil Hcl, Mylan	00378-0512-10

HOW SUPPLIED - RATED THERAPEUTICALLY EQUIVALENT: *(cont'd)*

1000's	$406.69	ISOPTIN, Knoll Labs	00044-1822-04
1000's	**$438.82**	**CALAN, Searle**	**00025-1851-52**

Tablet, Plain Coated - Oral - 120 mg

100's	$8.25	Verapamil Hcl, United Res	00677-1131-01
100's	$8.25	Verapamil HCl, H.C.F.A. F F P	99999-2425-12
100's	$9.66	Verapamil Hcl, US Trading	56126-0361-11
100's	$13.43	Verapamil Hcl, IDE-Interstate	00814-8281-14
100's	$27.90	Verapamil Hcl, Qualitest Pharms	00603-6358-21
100's	$28.27	Verapamil Hcl, HL Moore Drug Exch	00839-7254-06
100's	$28.27	Verapamil Hcl, HL Moore Drug Exch	00839-7268-06
100's	$28.55	Verapamil Hcl, Goldline Labs	00182-1301-01
100's	$29.20	Verapamil Hcl, Major Pharms	00904-2924-60
100's	$29.75	Verapamil HCl, Geneva Pharms	50752-0307-05
100's	$29.93	Verapamil Hcl, Watson Labs	52544-0345-01
100's	$29.93	Verapamil Hcl, Watson Labs	52544-0346-01
100's	$30.25	Verapamil Hcl, Mutual Pharm	53489-0155-01
100's	$30.83	Verapamil, Caremark	00339-5622-12
100's	$30.85	Verapamil Hcl, Martec Pharms	52555-0180-01
100's	$30.86	Verapamil Hcl, Purepac Pharm	00228-2475-10
100's	$32.50	Verapamil HCl, Rugby	00536-4932-01
100's	$34.65	Verapamil Hcl Tablets 120 Mg, Aligen Independ	00405-5100-01
100's	$34.65	Verapamil Hcl, Sidmak Labs	50111-0487-01
100's	$34.94	Verapamil Hcl, Parmed Pharms	00349-8625-01
100's	$34.94	Verapamil Hcl, Parmed Pharms	00349-8629-01
100's	$35.30	Verapamil HCl, Schein Pharm (US)	00364-2112-01
100's	$35.40	Verapamil HCl, Geneva Pharms	00781-1017-01
100's	$35.45	Verapamil HCl, Warner Chilcott	00047-0329-24
100's	$35.45	Verapamil Hcl, Mylan	00378-0772-01
100's	$43.45	Verapamil Hcl, Medirex	57480-0375-01
100's	$47.54	Verapamil Hcl, Major Pharms	00904-2924-61
100's	$56.11	Verapamil HCl, Schein Pharm (US)	00364-2112-90
100's	$56.16	Verapamil Hcl, Goldline Labs	00182-1301-89
100's	$56.16	Verapamil HCl, Geneva Pharms	00781-1017-13
100's	$57.85	Verapamil Hcl, Vangard Labs	00615-2532-13
100's	$59.80	ISOPTIN, Knoll Labs	00044-1823-02
100's	$62.40	ISOPTIN, Knoll Labs	00044-1823-10
100's	**$64.52**	**CALAN, Searle**	**00025-1861-31**
250's	$20.62	Verapamil HCl, H.C.F.A. F F P	99999-2425-13
500's	$41.25	Verapamil HCl, H.C.F.A. F F P	99999-2425-14
500's	$63.18	Verapamil Hcl, Balan	00304-1704-05
500's	$74.75	Verapamil Hcl, Major Pharms	00904-2924-40
500's	$91.85	Verapamil Hcl, Qualitest Pharms	00603-6358-28
500's	$99.00	Verapamil Hcl, Goldline Labs	00182-1301-05
500's	$112.64	Verapamil HCl, Rugby	00536-4932-05
500's	$115.45	Verapamil Hcl, Watson Labs	52544-0345-05
500's	$115.45	Verapamil Hcl, Watson Labs	52544-0346-05
500's	$129.75	Verapamil HCl, Geneva Pharms	50752-0307-08
500's	$129.80	Verapamil Hcl, Aligen Independ	00405-5100-02
500's	$129.80	Verapamil Hcl, Sidmak Labs	50111-0487-02
500's	$142.00	Verapamil Hcl, Mutual Pharm	53489-0155-05
500's	$154.30	Verapamil Hcl, Purepac Pharm	00228-2475-50
500's	$155.10	Verapamil HCl, Warner Chilcott	00047-0329-30
500's	$155.10	Verapamil HCl, Schein Pharm (US)	00364-2112-05
500's	$155.25	Verapamil HCl, Geneva Pharms	00781-1017-05
500's	$160.20	Verapamil Hcl, Parmed Pharms	00349-8625-05
500's	$160.20	Verapamil Hcl, Parmed Pharms	00349-8629-05
500's	$167.40	Verapamil Hcl, Mylan	00378-0772-05
500's	$287.05	ISOPTIN, Knoll Labs	00044-1823-05
600's	$270.80	Verapamil Hcl, Medirex	57480-0375-06
1000's	$82.50	Verapamil Hcl, Watson Labs	52544-0345-10
1000's	$82.50	Verapamil Hcl, Watson Labs	52544-0346-10
1000's	$82.50	Verapamil Hcl, Mutual Pharm	53489-0155-10
1000's	$82.50	Verapamil HCl, H.C.F.A. F F P	99999-2425-15
1000's	$233.55	Verapamil HCl, Geneva Pharms	50752-0307-09
1000's	$255.08	Verapamil Hcl, HL Moore Drug Exch	00839-7268-16
1000's	$295.19	Verapamil Hcl, Purepac Pharm	00228-2475-96
1000's	$320.40	Verapamil Hcl, Parmed Pharms	00349-8625-10
1000's	$550.19	ISOPTIN, Knoll Labs	00044-1823-04
1000's	**$593.65**	**CALAN, Searle**	**00025-1861-52**

HOW SUPPLIED - NOT RATED EQUIVALENT:

Capsule, Gelatin, Sustained Action - Oral - 120 mg

100's	$107.66	VERELAN 120, Lederle Pharm	00005-2490-23

Capsule, Gelatin, Sustained Action - Oral - 180 mg

100's	$112.76	VERELAN, Lederle Pharm	00005-2489-23

Capsule, Gelatin, Sustained Action - Oral - 240 mg

100's	$127.28	VERELAN 240, Lederle Pharm	00005-2491-23

Tablet, Coated, Sustained Action - Oral - 120 mg

100's	**$89.05**	**CALAN SR 120, Searle**	**00025-1901-31**
100's	$89.05	ISOPTIN SR, Knoll Labs	00044-1827-02
100's	**$93.50**	**CALAN SR 120, Searle**	**00025-1901-34**
100's	$93.50	ISOPTIN SR, Knoll Labs	00044-1827-12

Tablet, Coated, Sustained Action - Oral - 180 mg

100's	$98.50	Verapamil HCl, West Point Pharma	59591-0286-68
100's	$111.00	Verapamil HCl, Sidmak Labs	50111-0879-01

Tablet, Coated, Sustained Action - Oral - 240 mg

100's	$103.75	Verapamil HCl, West Point Pharma	59591-0280-68
100's	$118.00	Verapamil HCl, Sidmak Labs	50111-0880-01
500's	$580.00	Verapamil HCl, Sidmak Labs	50111-0880-02

Tablet, Plain Coated - Oral - 40 mg

100's	$9.75	Verapamil HCl, Harber Pharm	51432-0881-03

VIDARABINE *(002426)*

CATEGORIES: Anti-Infectives; Antimicrobials; Antivirals; Conjunctivitis; EENT Drugs; Eye, Ear, Nose, & Throat Preparations; Encephalitis; Herpes; Herpes Simplex; Herpes Simplex Encephalitis; Keratitis; Keratoconjunctivitis; Lesions; Topical; Viral Agents; Viral Agents, Ophthalmological; Pregnancy Category C; FDA Approval Pre 1982

BRAND NAMES: *Arasena*; **Vira-A**
(International brand names outside U.S. in italics)

FORMULARIES: Aetna; BC-BS

DESCRIPTION:

Vira-A is the trade name for vidarabine (also known as adenine arabinoside and Ara-A), an antiviral drug. Vira-A is a purine nucleoside obtained from fermentation cultures of *Streptomyces antibioticus*.

INFUSION

Each milliliter of sterile suspension contains 200 milligrams of vidarabine monohydrate equivalent to 187.4 milligrams of vidarabine. Each milliliter contains 0.1 milligram Phemerol (benzethonium chloride) as a preservative; sodium phosphate, USP, 1.8 milligrams, and sodium biphosphate, USP, 4.8 milligrams as buffering agents. Hydrochloric acid may have been added to adjust pH. Vira-A is a white, crystalline solid with this empirical formula: $C_{10}H_{13}N_5O_4 \cdot H_2O$. The molecular weight is 285.2; the solubility is 0.45 mg/ml at 25°C; and the melting point ranges from 260° to 270°C. The chemical name is 9-β-D-arabinofuranosyladenine monohydrate.

OPHTHALMIC OINTMENT

Each gram of the ophthalmic ointment contains 30 mg of vidarabine monohydrate equivalent to 28.11 mg of vidarabine in a sterile, inert, petrolatum base.

CLINICAL PHARMACOLOGY:

INFUSION

Following intravenous administration, Vira-A is rapidly deaminated into arabinosylhypoxanthine (Ara-Hx), the principal metabolite, which is promptly distributed into the tissues. Peak Ara-Hx and Ara-A plasma levels ranging from 3 to 6 mcg/ml and 0.2 to 0.4 mcg/ml, respectively, are attained after slow intravenous infusion of Vira-A doses of 10 mg/kg of body weight. These levels reflect the rate of infusion and show no accumulation across time. The mean half-life of Ara-Hx is 3.3 hours. Ara-Hx penetrates into the cerebrospinal fluid (CSF) to give a CSF/plasma ratio of approximately 1:3.

Excretion of Vira-A is principally via the kidneys. Urinary excretion is constant over 24 hours. Forty-one to 53% of the daily dose is recovered in the urine as Ara-Hx with 1 to 3% appearing as the parent compound. There is no evidence of fecal excretion of drug or metabolites. In patients with impaired renal function Ara-Hx may accumulate in the plasma and reach levels several-fold higher than those described above.

Vira-A possesses *in vitro* and *in vivo* antiviral activity against *Herpes virus* simplex (Herpes simplex virus) types 1 and 2.

The antiviral mechanism of action has not yet been established. The drug is converted into nucleotides which appear to be involved with the inhibition of viral replication. In KB cells infected with Herpes simplex virus type 1, Vira-A inhibits viral DNA synthesis. Vira-A is rapidly deaminated to Ara-Hx, the principal metabolite, in cell cultures, laboratory animals, and humans.

Ara-Hx also possesses *in vitro* antiviral activity but this activity is significantly less than the activity of Vira-A.

OPHTHALMIC OINTMENT

Vira-A is a purine nucleoside obtained from fermentation cultures of*Streptomyces antibioticus*. Vira-A possesses *in vitro* and *in vivo* antiviral activity against herpes simplex types 1 and 2, Varicella-Zoster, and Vaccinia viruses. Except for Rhabdovirus and Oncornavirus, Vira-A does not display *in vitro* antiviral activity against other RNA or DNA viruses, including Adenovirus.

The antiviral mechanism of action has not been established. Vira-A appears to interfere with the early steps of viral DNA synthesis. Vira-A is rapidly deaminated to arabinosylhypoxanthine (Ara-Hx), the principle metabolite. Ara-Hx also possesses *in vitro* antiviral activity but this activity is less than that of Vira-A. Because of the low solubility of Vira-A, trace amounts of both Vira-A and Ara-Hx can be detected in the aqueous humor only if there is an epithelial defect in the cornea. If the cornea is normal, only trace amount of Ara-Hx can be recovered from the aqueous humor.

Systemic absorption of Vira-A should not be expected to occur following ocular administration and swallowing lacrimal secretions. In laboratory animals, Vira-A is rapidly deaminated in the gastrointestinal tract to Ara-Hx.

In contrast to topical idoxuridine, Vira-A demonstrated less cellular toxicity in the regenerating corneal epithelium of the rabbit.

INDICATIONS AND USAGE:

INFUSION

Vira-A is indicated in the treatment of Herpes simplex virus encephalitis. Controlled studies indicated that Vira-A therapy will reduce the mortality caused by Herpes simplex virus encephalitis from 70 to 28% 30 days following onset. In a larger uncontrolled study of 75 patients with biopsy-proven herpes simplex encephalitis, the mortality 6 months from onset was 39%, similar to 44% in the initial controlled study at 6 months.

Morbidity from both studies one year after onset was: normal 53%, moderately debilitated 29%, and severely damaged 18%. Vira-A does not appear to alter morbidity and resulting serious neurological sequelae in the comatose patient. Therefore early diagnosis and treatment are essential.

Herpes simplex virus encephalitis should be suspected in patients with a history of an acute febrile encephalopathy associated with disordered mentation, altered level of consciousness and focal cerebral signs.

Studies which may support the suspected diagnosis include examination of cerebrospinal fluid and localization of an intra-cerebral lesion by brain scan, electroencephalography or computerized axial tomography (CAT).

Brain biopsy is required in order to confirm the etiological diagnosis by means of viral isolation in cell cultures.

Detection of Herpes simplex virus in the biopsied brain tissue can also be reliably done by specific fluorescent antibody techniques. Detection of Herpes virus-like particles by electron microscopy or detection of intranuclear inclusions by histopathologic techniques only provides a presumptive diagnosis.

OPHTHALMIC OINTMENT

Vira-A ophthalmic ointment, 3%, is indicated for the treatment of acute keratoconjunctivitis and recurrent epithelial keratitis due to herpes simplex virus types 1 and 2. It is also effective in superficial keratitis caused by Herpes simplex virus which has not responded to topical idoxuridine or when toxic or hypersensitivity reactions to idoxuridine have occurred. The effectiveness of Vira-A ophthalmic ointment, 3%, against stromal keratitis and uveitis due to Herpes simplex virus has not been established.

The clinical diagnosis of keratitis caused by herpes simplex virus is usually established by the presence of typical dendritic or geographic lesions on slit-lamp examination.

In controlled and uncontrolled clinical trials, an average of seven and nine days of continuous Vira-A ophthalmic ointment, 3%, therapy was required to achieve corneal re-epithelialization. In the controlled trials, 70 of 81 subjects (86%) re-epithelialized at the end of three weeks of therapy. In the uncontrolled trials, 101 of 142 subjects (71%) re-epithelialized at the end of three weeks. Seventy-five percent of the subjects in these uncontrolled trials had either not healed previously or had developed hypersensitivity to topical idoxuridine therapy.

INDICATIONS AND USAGE: *(cont'd)*

The following topical antibiotics: gentamicin,erythromycin, chloramphenicol; or topical steroids: prednisolone or dexamethasone have been administered concurrently with Vira-A ophthalmic ointment, 3%, without an increase in adverse reactions.

CONTRAINDICATIONS:

Vira-A is contraindicated in patients who develop hypersensitivity reactions to it.

WARNINGS:

INFUSION

Vira-A should not be administered by the intramuscular or subcutaneous route because of its low solubility and poor absorption.

There are no reports available to indicate that Vira-A for infusion is effective in the management of encephalitis due to varicella-zoster or vaccinia viruses. Vira-A is not effective against infections caused by adenovirus or RNA viruses. It is also not effective against bacterial or fungal infections. There are no data to support efficacy of Vira-A against cytomegalovirus, vaccinia virus, or smallpox virus.

OPHTHALMIC OINTMENT

Normally, corticosteroids alone are contraindicated in Herpes simplex virus infections of the eye. If Vira-A ophthalmic ointment, 3%,is administered concurrently with topical corticosteroid therapy, corticosteroid-induced glaucoma or cataract formation and progression of a bacterial or viral infection.

Vira-A is not effective against RNA virus or adenoviral ocular infections. It is also not effective against bacterial, fungal, or chlamydial infections of the cornea or non-viral trophic ulcers.

Although viral resistance to Vira-A has not been observed, this possibility may exist.

PRECAUTIONS:

GENERAL

Infusion: Treatment should be discontinued in the patient with a brain biopsy negative for Herpes simplex virus in cell culture.

Special care should be exercised when administering Vira-A to patients susceptible to fluid overloading or cerebral edema. Examples are patients with CNS infections and impaired renal function.

Patients with impaired renal function, such as post-operative renal transplant recipients, may have a slower rate of renal excretion of Ara-Hx. Therefore, the dose of Vira-A may need to be adjusted according to the severity of impairment. These patients should be carefully monitored.

Patients with impaired liver function should also be observed for possible adverse effects.

Although clear evidence of adverse experience in humans from simultaneous Vira-A and allopurinol administration has not been reported, laboratory studies indicate that allopurinol may interfere with Vira-A metabolism. Therefore, caution is recommended when administering Vira-A to patients receiving allopurinol.

Ophthalmic Ointment: The diagnosis of keratoconjunctivitis due to herpes simplex virus should be established clinically prior to prescribing Vira-A ophthalmic ointment, 3%.

Patients should be forewarned that Vira-A ophthalmic ointment, 3%, like any ophthalmic ointment, may produce a temporary visual haze.

LABORATORY TESTS

Infusion: Appropriate hematologic tests are recommended during Vira-A administration since hemoglobin, hematocrit, white blood cells, and platelets may be depressed during therapy.

Some degree of immunocompetence must be present in order for Vira-A to achieve clinical response.

CARCINOGENESIS, MUTAGENESIS, AND IMPAIRMENT OF FERTILITY

Carcinogenesis: Chronic parenteral (IM) studies of vidarabine have been conducted in mice and rats.

In the mouse study, there was a statistically significant increase in liver tumor incidence among the vidarabine-treated females. In the same study, some vidarabine-treated male mice developed kidney neoplasia. No renal tumors were found in the vehicle-treated control mice or the vidarabine-treated female mice.

In the rat study, intestinal, testicular, and thyroid neoplasia occurred with greater frequency among the vidarabine-treated animals than in the vehicle-treated controls. The increases in thyroid adenoma incidence in the high-dose (50 mg/kg) males and the low-dose (30 mg/kg) females were statistically significant.

Hepatic megalocytosis, associated with vidarabine treatment, has been found in short-and long-term rodent (rat and mouse) studies. It is not clear whether or not this represents a preneoplastic change.

Mutagenesis: Results of *in vitro* experiments indicate that vidarabine can be incorporated into mammalian DNA and can induce mutation in mammalian cells (mouse L5178Y cell line). Thus far, *in vivo* studies have not been as conclusive, but there is some evidence (dominant lethal assay in mice) that vidarabine may be capable of producing mutagenic effects in male germ cells.

It has also been reported that vidarabine causes chromosome breaks and gaps when added to human leukocytes *in vitro*. While the significance of these effects in terms of mutagenicity is not fully understood, there is a well-known correlation between the ability of various agents to produce such effects and their ability to produce heritable genetic damage.

PREGNANCY CATEGORY C

Infusion: Vira-A given parenterally is teratogenic in rats and rabbits. Doses of 5 mg/kg or higher given intramuscularly to pregnant rabbits during organogenesis induced fetal abnormalities. Doses of 3 mg/kg or less did not induce teratogenic changes in pregnant rabbits. Vira-A doses ranging from 30 to 250 mg/kg were given intramuscularly to pregnant rats during organogenesis; signs of maternal toxicity were induced at doses of 100 mg/kg or higher and frank fetal anomalies were found at doses of 150 to 250 mg/kg.

A safe dose for the human embryo or fetus has not been established.

There are no adequate and well controlled studies in pregnant women, Vira-A should be used during pregnancy only if the potential benefit justifies the potential risk to the fetus.

Ophthalmic Ointment: Ten percent Vira-A ointment applied to 10% of the body surface during organogenesis induced fetal abnormalities in rabbits. When 10% Vira-A ointment was applied to 2% to 3% of the body surface of rabbits, no fetal abnormalities were found. This dose greatly exceeds the total recommended ophthalmic dose in humans. The possibility of embryonic or fetal damage in pregnant women receiving Vira-A ophthalmic ointment, 3%, is remote. The topical ophthalmic dose is small, and the drug relatively insoluble. Its ocular penetration is very low. However, a safe dose for a human embryo or fetus has not been established. There are no adequate and well controlled studies in pregnant women. Vira-A should be used during pregnancy only of the potential benefit justifies the potential risk to the fetus.

PRECAUTIONS: *(cont'd)*

NURSING MOTHERS

It is not known whether Vira-A is excreted in human milk. Because many drugs are excreted in human milk and because of the potential tumorigenicity shown for Vira-A in animal studies, a decision should be made whether to discontinue nursing or to discontinue the drug, taking into account the importance of the drug to the mother.

Ophthalmic Ointment Only: However, breast milk excretion is unlikely because Vira-A is rapidly deaminated in the gastrointestinal tract.

ADVERSE REACTIONS:

INFUSION

The principal adverse reactions involve the gastrointestinal tract and are anorexia, nausea, vomiting, and diarrhea. These reactions are mild to moderate, and seldom require termination of Vira-A therapy.

CNS disturbances have been reported at therapeutic doses. These are tremor, dizziness, hallucinations, confusion, psychosis, and ataxia.

Hematologic clinical laboratory changes noted in controlled and uncontrolled studies were a decrease in hemoglobin or hematocrit, white blood cell count, and platelet count. SGOT elevations were also observed. Other changes occasionally observed were decreases in reticulocyte count and elevated total bilirubin.

Other symptoms which have been reported are weight loss, malaise, pruritus, rash, hematemesis, and pain at the injection site.

OPHTHALMIC OINTMENT

Lacrimation, foreign body sensation, conjunctival injection, burning, irritation, superficial punctae keratitis, pain, photophobia, punctal occlusion, and sensitivity have been reported with Vira-A ophthalmic ointment, 3%. The following have also been reported but appear disease- related: uveitis, stromal edema, secondary glaucoma, trophic defects, corneal vascularization, and hyphema.

OVERDOSAGE:

INFUSION

Acute massive overdose of the intravenous form has been reported without any serious evidence of adverse effect. Because of the low solubility of Vira-A, acute water overloading would pose a greater threat to the patient than Vira-A. Doses of Vira-A over 20 mg/kg/day can produce bone marrow depression with concomitant thrombocytopenia and leukopenia. If a massive overdose of the intravenous form occurs, hematologic, liver, and renal functions should be carefully monitored.

OPHTHALMIC OINTMENT

Acute massive overdosage by oral ingestion of the ophthalmic ointment has not occurred. However, the rapid deamination to arabinosylhypoxanthine should preclude any difficulty. The oral LD_{50} for vidarabine is greater than 5020 mg/kg in mice and rats. No untoward effects should results from ingestion of the entire contents of a tube.

Overdosage by ocular instillation is unlikely because any excess should be expelled from the conjunctival sac. Too frequent administration should be avoided.

DOSAGE AND ADMINISTRATION:

INFUSION

CAUTION - THE CONTENTS OF THE VIAL MUST BE DILUTED IN AN APPROPRIATE INTRAVENOUS SOLUTION PRIOR TO ADMINISTRATION. RAPID OR BOLUS INJECTION MUST BE AVOIDED.

Dosage : Herpes simplex virus encephalitis - 15 mg/kg/day for 10 days.

Method of Preparation: Each 5-ml vial contains 1 gram of Vira-A (200 mg per ml of suspension). The solubility of Vira-A in intravenous infusion fluids is limited. Each one mg of Vira-A requires 2.22 ml of intravenous infusion fluid for complete solubilization. Therefore, each one liter of intravenous infusion fluid will solubilize a maximum of 450 mg of Vira-A.

Any appropriate intravenous solution is suitable for use as a diluent*EXCEPT* biologic or colloidal fluids (*e.g.,* blood products, protein solutions, etc.).

Shake the Vira-A vial well to obtain a homogeneous suspension before measuring and transferring.

Prepare the Vira-A solution for intravenous administration by aseptically transferring the proper dose of Vira-A into an appropriate intravenous infusion fluid. The intravenous infusion fluid used to prepare the Vira-A solution should be prewarmed to 35 to 40°C (95 to 100°F) to facilitate solution of the drug following its transference. Depending on the dose to be given, more than one liter of intravenous infusion fluid may be required. Thoroughly agitate the prepared admixture until*completely* clear. Complete solubilization of the drug, as indicated by a completely clear solution, is ascertained by careful visual inspection. Final filtration with an in-line membrane filter (0.45 μ pore size or smaller) is necessary.

Dilution should be made just prior to administration and used at least within 48 hours. Subsequent agitation, shaking, or Inversion of the bottle is unnecessary once the drug is completely in solution. DO NOT REFRIGERATE THE DILUTION.

Administration: Using aseptic technique, slowly infuse the total daily dose by intravenous infusion (prepared as discussed above) at a constant rate over a 12- to 24-hour period.

OPHTHALMIC OINTMENT

Administer approximately one half inch of Vira-A ophthalmic ointment, 3%, into the lower conjunctival sac five times daily at three hour internals.

If there are no signs of improvement after 7 days, or complete re- epithelialization has not occurred by 21 days, other forms of therapy should be considered. Some severe cases may require longer treatment.

After re-epithelialization has occurred, treatment for an additional seven days at a reduced dosage (such as twice daily) is recommended in order to prevent recurrence.

ANIMAL PHARMACOLOGY:

Acute Toxicity: The Intraperitoneal LD_{50} for Vira-A ranged from 3,890 to 4,500 mg/kg in mice, and from 2,239 to 2,512 mg/kg in rats, suggesting a low order of toxicity to a single parenteral dose. Hepatic megalocytosis was observed in rats after single, intraperitoneal injections at doses near and exceeding the LD_{50} value. The hepatic megalocytosis appeared to regress completely over several months. Acute intravenous LD_{50} values could not be obtained because of the limited solubility of Vira-A.

Subacute Toxicity: Rats, dogs, and monkeys have been given daily intramuscular injections of Vira-A as a 20% suspension for 28 days. These animal species showed dose related decreases in hemoglobin, hematocrit, and lymphocytes. Bone marrow depression was also observed in monkeys. Except for localized, injection-site injury and weight gain inhibition or loss, rats tolerated daily doses up to 150 mg/kg, and dogs tolerated daily doses up to 50 mg/kg. Megalocytosis was not seen in the rats dosed by the intramuscular route for 28 days. Rhesus monkeys were particularly sensitive to Vira-A. Daily intramuscular doses of 15 mg/kg were

ANIMAL PHARMACOLOGY: *(cont'd)*

tolerable, but doses of 25 mg/kg or higher induced progressively severe clinical signs of CNS toxicity. Three monkeys given slow intravenous infusions of Vira-A in solution at a dose of 15 mg/kg daily for 28 days had no significant adverse reactions.

HOW SUPPLIED - EQUIVALENTS NOT AVAILABLE:

Ointment - Ophthalmic - 3 %

3.5 gm	$20.77	VIRA-A, Parke-Davis	00071-3677-07

VINBLASTINE SULFATE *(002427)*

CATEGORIES: Antineoplastics; Breast Carcinoma; Cancer; Chemotherapy; Choriocarcinoma; Hodgkin's Disease; Kaposi's Sarcoma; Letterer-Siwe Disease; Lymphoma; Mycosis Fungoides; Oncologic Drugs; Sarcoma; Testicular Carcinoma; Lung Cancer*; Pregnancy Category D; FDA Approval Pre 1982

* Indication not approved by the FDA

BRAND NAMES: **Velban**; Velsar

FORMULARIES: BC-BS; Medi-Cal; WHO

WARNING:
Caution - This preparation should be administered by individuals experienced in the administration of vinblastine sulfate. It is extremely important that needle be properly positioned in the vein before this product is injected. If leakage into surrounding tissue should occur during intravenous administration of vinblastine sulfate, it may cause considerable irritation. The injection should be discontinued immediately, and any remaining portion of the dose should then be introduced into another vein. Local injection of hyaluronidase and the application of moderate heat to the area of leakage help disperse the drug and are thought to minimize discomfort and the possibility of cellulitis.
FATAL IF GIVEN INTRATHECALLY. FOR INTRAVENOUS USE ONLY.
See WARNINGS section for the treatment of patients given intrathecal vinblastine sulfate.

DESCRIPTION:

Vinblastine sulfate is the salt of an alkaloid extracted from *Vinca rosea* Linn, a common flowering herb known as the periwinkle (more properly known as *Catharanthus roseus* G. Don). Previously, the generic name was vincaleukoblastine, abbreviated VLB, It is a stathmokinetic oncolytic agent. When treated in vitro with this preparation, growing cells are arrested in metaphase.

Chemical and physical evidence indicate that vinblastine sulfate has the empirical formula $C_{46}H_{58}N_4O_9{\cdot}H_2SO_4$ and that it is a dimeric alkaloid containing both indole and dihydroindole moieties.

Vials of vinblastine sulfate contain 10 mg (0.011 mmol) of vinblastine sulfate, in the form of a lyophilized plug, without excipients. When sodium chloride solution is added prior to injection, the pH of the resulting solution lies in the range of 3.5 to 5.

CLINICAL PHARMACOLOGY:

Experimental data indicate that the action of vinblastine sulfate is different from that of other recognized antineoplastic agents. Tissue-culture studies suggest an interference with metabolic pathways of amino acids leading from glutamic acid to the citric acid cycle and to urea. In vivo experiments tend to confirm the in vitro results. A number of studies in vitro and vivo have demonstrated that vinblastine sulfate produces a stathmokinetic effect and various atypical mitotic figures. The therapeutic responses, however, are not fully explained by the cytologic changes, since these changes are sometimes observed clinically and experimentally in the absence of any oncolytic effects.

Reversal of the antitumor effect of vinblastine sulfate by glutamic acid or tryptophan has been observed. In addition, glutamic acid and aspartic acid have protected more from lethal doses of vinblastine sulfate. Aspartic acid was relatively ineffective in reversing the antitumor effect.

Other studies indicate that vinblastine sulfate has an effect on cell-energy production required for mitosis and interferes with nucleic acid synthesis. The mechanism of action of vinblastine sulfate has been related to the inhibition of microtubule formation in the mitotic spindle, resulting in an arrest of dividing cells at the metaphase stage.

Pharmacokinetic studies in patients with cancer have shown a triphasic serum decay pattern following rapid intravenous injection. The initial, middle, and terminal half-lives are 3.7 minutes, 1.6 hours, and 24.8 hours respectively. The volume of the central compartment is 70% of body weight, probably reflecting very rapid tissue binding to formed elements of the blood. Extensive reversible tissue binding occurs. Low body stores are present at 48 and 72 hours after injection. Since the major route of excretion may be through the biliary system, toxicity from this drug may be increased when there is hepatic excretory insufficiency. Following injection of tritiated vinblastine in the human cancer patient, 10% of the radioactivity was found in feces and 14% in the urine; the remaining activity was not accounted for. Similar studies in dogs demonstrated that, over 9 days, 30% to 36% of radioactivity was found in the bile and 12% to 17% in the urine. A similar study in the rat demonstrated that the highest concentrations of radioactivity were found in the lung, liver, spleen, and kidney 2 hours after injection.

HEMATOLOGIC EFFECTS

Clinically, leukopenia is an expected effect of vinblastine sulfate, and the level of the leukocyte count is an important guide to therapy with this drug. In general, the larger the dose employed, the more profound and longer lasting the leukopenia will be. The fact that the white-blood-cell count returns to normal levels after drug-induced leukopenia is an indication that the white-cell-producing mechanism is not permanently depressed. Usually, the white count has completely returned to normal after the virtual disappearance of white cell from the peripheral blood.

Following therapy with vinblastine sulfate, the nadir in white-blood-cell count may be expected to occur 5 to 10 days after the last day of drug administration. Recovery of the white blood count is fairly rapid thereafter and is usually complete within another 7 to 14 days. With the smaller doses employed for maintenance therapy, leukopenia may not be a problem.

Although the thrombocyte count ordinarily is not significantly lowered by therapy with vinblastine sulfate, patients whose bone marrow has been recently impaired by prior therapy with radiation or with other oncolytic drugs may show thrombocytopenia (less than 200,000 platelets/mm^3). When other chemotherapy or radiation has not been employed previously,

CLINICAL PHARMACOLOGY: *(cont'd)*

thrombocyte reduction below the level of 200,000/mm^3 is rarely encountered, even when vinblastine sulfate may be causing significant leukopenia. Rapid recovery from thrombocytopenia within a few days is the rule.

The effect of vinblastine sulfate upon the red-cell count and hemoglobin is usually insignificant when other therapy does not complicate the picture. It should be remembered, however, that patients with malignant disease may exhibit anemia even in the absence of any therapy.

INDICATIONS AND USAGE:

Vinblastine sulfate is indicated in the palliative treatment of the following:

I. Frequently Responsive Malignancies

Generalized Hodgkin's disease (Stages III and IV, Ann Arbor modification of Rye staging system)

Lymphocytic lymphoma (nodular and diffuse, poorly and well differentiated)

Histiocytic lymphoma

Mycosis fungoides (advanced stages)

Advanced carcinoma of the testis

Kaposi's sarcoma

Letterer-Siwe disease (histiocytosis X)

II. Less Frequently Responsive Malignancies

Choriocarcinoma resistant to other chemotherapeutic agents.

Carcinoma of the breast, unresponsive to appropriate endocrine surgery and hormonal therapy

Current principles of chemotherapy for many types of cancer include the concurrent administration of several antineoplastic agents. For enhanced therapeutic effect without additive toxicity, agents with different dose-limiting clinical toxicities and different mechanisms of action are generally selected. Therefore, although vinblastine sulfate is effective as a single agent in the aforementioned indications, it is usually administered in combination with other antineoplastic drugs. Such combination therapy produces a greater percentage of response than does a single agent regimen. These principles have been applied, for example, in the chemotherapy of Hodgkin's disease.

Hodgkin's Disease: Vinblastine sulfate has been shown to be one of the most effective single agents for the treatment of Hodgkin's disease. Advanced Hodgkin's disease has also been successfully treated with several multiple drug regimens that included vinblastine sulfate. Patients who had relapses after treatment with the MOPP program—mechlorethamine hydrochloride (nitrogen mustard), vincristine sulfate (Oncovin (Vincristine Sulfate Injection, Lilly)), prednisone, and procarbazine - have likewise responded to combination-drug therapy that included vinblastine sulfate. A protocol using cyclophosphamide in place of nitrogen mustard and vinblastine sulfate instead of Oncovin is an alternative therapy for previously untreated patients with advanced Hodgkin's disease.

Advanced testicular germinal-cell cancers (embryonal carcinoma, teratocarcinoma, and choriocarcinoma) are sensitive to vinblastine sulfate alone, but better clinical results are achieved when vinblastine sulfate is administered concomitantly with other antineoplastic agents. The effect of bleomycin is significantly enhanced if vinblastine sulfate is administered 6 to 8 hours, prior to the administration of bleomycin; this schedule permits more cells to be arrested during metaphase, the stage of the cell cycle in which bleomycin is active.

CONTRAINDICATIONS:

Vinblastine sulfate is contraindicated in patients who have significant granulocytopenia unless this is a result of the disease being treated. It should not be used in the presence of bacterial infections. Such infections must be brought under control prior to the initiation of therapy with vinblastine sulfate.

WARNINGS:

This product is for intravenous use only. It should be administered by individuals experienced in the administration of vinblastine sulfate. The intrathecal administration of vinblastine sulfate has resulted in death. Syringes containing this product should be labeled "WARNING - FOR INTRAVENOUS USE ONLY."

The following treatment successfully arrested progressive paralysis in a single patient mistakenly given the related vinca alkaloid, vincristine sulfate, intrathecally. If vinblastine sulfate is mistakenly administered intrathecally, this treatment is recommended and should be initiated immediately after the intrathecal injection.

1. Remove as much spinal fluid as can be safely done through the lumbar access.

2. Insert a catheter in a lateral cerebral ventricle for the purpose of flushing the subarachnoid space from above with removal through a lumbar access.

3. Initiate flushing through the cerebral catheter with lactated Ringer's solution infused at the rate of 150 ml/h.

4. As soon as fresh frozen plasma becomes available, infuse fresh frozen plasma, 25 ml, diluted in 1 L of Lactated Ringer's solution through the cerebral ventricular catheter at the rate of 75 ml/h with removal through the lumbar access. The rate of infusion should be adjusted to maintain a protein level in the spinal fluid of 150 mg/dl.

5. Administer 10 g of glutamic acid intravenously over 24 hours followed by 500 mg 3 times daily by mouth for 1 month or until neurological dysfunction stabilizes. The role of glutamic acid in this treatment is not certain and may not be essential.

The use of this treatment has not been reported following intrathecal vinblastine sulfate.

USAGE IN PREGNANCY

Caution is necessary with the administration of all oncolytic drugs during pregnancy. Information on the use of vinblastine sulfate during human pregnancy is very limited. Animal studies with vinblastine sulfate suggest that teratogenic effects may occur. Vinblastine sulfate can cause fetal harm when administered to a pregnant woman. Laboratory animals given this drug early in pregnancy suffer resorption of the conceptus; surviving fetuses demonstrate gross deformities. There, are no adequate and well-controlled studies in pregnant women. If this drug is used during pregnancy, or if the patient becomes pregnant while receiving this drug, she should be apprised of the potential hazard to the fetus. Women of childbearing potential should be advised to avoid becoming pregnant.

Aspermia has been reported in man. Animal studies show metaphase arrest and degenerative changes in germ cells.

WARNINGS: *(cont'd)*

Leukopenia (granulocytopenia) may reach dangerously low levels following administration of the higher recommended doses. It is therefore important to follow the dosage technique recommended under the DOSAGE AND ADMINISTRATION. Stomatitis and neurologic toxicity, although not common or permanent, can be disabling.

PRECAUTIONS:

GENERAL

Toxicity may be enhanced in the presence of hepatic insufficiency.

If leukopenia with less than 2,000 white blood cells/mm^3 occurs following a dose of vinblastine sulfate, the patient should be watched carefully for evidence of infection until the white-blood-cell count has returned to a safe level.

When cachexia or ulcerated areas of the skin surface are present, there may be a more profound leukopenic response to the drug; therefore, its use should be avoided in older persons suffering from either of these conditions.

In patients with malignant-cell infiltration of the bone marrow, the leukocyte and platelet counts have sometimes fallen precipitously after moderate doses of vinblastine sulfate. Further use of the drug in such patients is inadvisable.

Acute shortness of breath and severe bronchospasm have been reported following the administration of vinca alkaloids. These reactions have been encountered most frequently when the vinca alkaloid was used in combination with mitomycin-C and may require aggressive treatment, particularly when there is pre-existing pulmonary dysfunction. The onset may be within minutes or several hours after the vinca is injected and may occur up to 2 weeks following a dose of mitomycin.

The use of small amounts of vinblastine sulfate daily for long periods is not advised, even though the resulting total weekly dosage may be similar to that recommended. Little or no added therapeutic effect has been demonstrated when such regimens have been used. *Strict adherence to the recommended dosage schedule is very important.* When amounts equal to several times the recommended weekly dosage were given in 7 daily installments for long periods, convulsions, severe and permanent central-nervous-system damage and even death occurred.

Care must be taken to avoid contamination of the eye with concentrations of vinblastine sulfate used clinically. If accidental contamination occurs, severe irritation (or, if the drug was delivered under pressure, even corneal ulceration) may result. The eye should be washed with water immediately and thoroughly.

It is not necessary to use preservative-containing solvents if unused portions of the remaining solutions are discarded immediately. Unused preservative-containing solutions should be refrigerated for future use.

INFORMATION FOR THE PATIENT

The patient should be warned to report immediately the appearance of sore throat, fever, chills, or sore mouth. Advice should be given to avoid constipation, and the patient should be made aware that alopecia may occur and that jaw pain and pain in the organs containing tumor tissue may occur. The latter is thought possibly to result from swelling of tumor tissue during its response to treatment. Scalp hair will regrow to its pretreatment extent even with continued treatment with vinblastine sulfate. Nausea and vomiting, although not common, may occur. Any other serious medical event should be reported to the physician.

LABORATORY TESTS

Since dose-limiting clinical toxicity is the result of depression of the white-blood-cell count, it is imperative that this count be obtained just before the planned dose of vinblastine sulfate. Following administration of vinblastine sulfate, a fall in the white-blood-cell count may occur. The nadir of this fall is observed from 5 to 10 days following a dose. Recovery to pretreatment levels is usually observed from 7 to 14 days after treatment. These effects will be exaggerated when preexisting bone marrow damage is present and also with the higher recommended doses (see DOSAGE AND ADMINISTRATION). The presence of this drug or its metabolites in blood or body tissues is not known to interfere with clinical laboratory tests.

CARCINOGENESIS, MUTAGENESIS, AND IMPAIRMENT OF FERTILITY

Aspermia has been reported in man. Animal studies suggest that teratogenic effects may occur. See WARNINGS regarding impaired fertility. Animal studies have shown metaphase arrest and degenerative changes in germ cells. Amenorrhea has occurred in some patients treated with the combination consisting of an alkylating agent, procarbazine, prednisone, and vinblastine sulfate. Its occurrence was related to the total dose of these 4 agents used. Recovery of menses was frequent. The same combination of drugs given to male patients produced azoospermia; if spermatogenesis did return, it was not likely to do so with less than 2 years of unmaintained remission.

Mutagenicity: Tests in *Salmonella typhimurium* and with the dominant lethal assay in mice failed to demonstrate mutagenicity. Sperm abnormalities have been noted in mice. Vinblastine sulfate has produced an increase in micronuclei formation in bone marrow cells of mice; however, since vinblastine sulfate inhibits mitotic spindle formation, it cannot be concluded that this is evidence of mutagenicity. Additional studies in mice demonstrated no reduction in fertility of males. Chromosomal translocations did occur in male mice. First-generation male offspring of these mice were not heterozygous translocation carriers.

In vitro tests using hamster lung cells in culture have produced chromosomal changes, including chromatid breaks and exchanges, whereas tests using another type of hamster cell failed to demonstrate mutation. Breaks and aberrations were not observed on chromosome analysis of marrow cells patients being treated with this drug.

It is not clear from the literature how this drug affects synthesis of DNA and RNA. Some believe that there is no interference. Others believe that vinblastine interferes with nucleic acid metabolism but may not do so by direct effect but possibly as the result of biochemical disturbance in some other part of the molecular organization of the cell. No inhibition of RNA synthesis occurred in rat hepatoma cells exposed in culture to noncytotoxic levels of vinblastine. Conflicting results have been noted by others regarding interference with DNA synthesis.

Carcinogenesis: There is no currently available evidence to indicate that vinblastine sulfate itself has been carcinogenic in humans since the inception of its clinical use in the late 1950's. Patients treated for Hodgkin's disease have developed leukemia following radiation therapy and administration of vinblastine sulfate in combination with other chemotherapy including agents known to intercalate with DNA. It is not known to what extent vinblastine sulfate may have contributed to the appearance of leukemia. Available data in rats and mice have failed to demonstrate clearly evidence of carcinogenesis when the animals were treated with the maximum tolerated dose and with one half that dose for 6 months. This testing system demonstrated that other agents were clearly carcinogenic, whereas vinblastine sulfate was in the group of drugs causing slightly increased or the same tumor incidence as controls in one study and 1.5 to twofold increase in tumor incidence over controls in another study.

PREGNANCY CATEGORY D

(See WARNINGS.)

Vinblastine sulfate should be given to a pregnant woman only if clearly needed. Animal studies suggest that teratogenic effects may occur.

PRECAUTIONS: *(cont'd)*

PEDIATRIC USAGE

The dosage schedule for children is indicated under DOSAGE AND ADMINISTRATION.

NURSING MOTHERS

It is not known whether this drug is excreted in human milk. Because many drugs are excreted in human milk and because of the potential for serious adverse reactions from vinblastine sulfate in nursing infants, a decision should be make whether to discontinue nursing or the drug, taking into account the importance of the drug to the mother.

DRUG INTERACTIONS:

Vinblastine sulfate should not be diluted with solvents that raise or lower the pH of the resulting solution from between 3.5 and 5. Solutions should be made with normal saline (with or without preservative) and should not be combined in the same container with any other chemical. Unused portions of the remaining solutions that do not contain preservative should be discarded immediately.

The simultaneous oral or intravenous administration of phenytoin and antineoplastic chemotherapy combinations that included vinblastine sulfate has been reported to have reduced blood levels of the anticonvulsant and to have increased seizure activity. Dosage adjustment should be based on serial blood level monitoring. The contribution of vinblastine sulfate to this interaction is not certain. The interaction may result from either reduced absorption of phenytoin or an increase in the rate of its metabolism and elimination.

ADVERSE REACTIONS:

Prior to the use of the drug, patients should be advised of the possibility of untoward symptoms.

In general the incidence of adverse reactions attending the use of vinblastine sulfate appears to be related to the size of the dose employed. With the exception of epilation, leukopenia, and neurologic side effects, adverse reactions generally have not persisted for longer than 24 hours. Neurologic side effects are not common; but when they do occur, they often last for more than 24 hours. Leukopenia, the most common adverse reaction, is usually the dose-limiting factor.

The following are manifestations that have been reported as adverse reactions, in decreasing order of frequency. The most common adverse reactions are underlined:

Hematologic: Leukopenia (granulocytopenia), anemia, thrombocytopenia (myelosuppression).

Dermatologic: Alopecia is common. A single case of light sensitivity associated with this product has been reported.

Gastrointestinal: Constipation, anorexia, nausea, vomiting, abdominal pain, ileus, vesiculation of the mouth, pharyngitis, diarrhea, hemorrhagic enterocolitis, bleeding from an old peptic ulcer, rectal bleeding.

Neurologic: Numbness of digits (paresthesias), loss of deep tendon reflexes, peripheral neuritis, mental depression, headache, convulsions.

Cardiovascular: Hypertension. Cases of unexpected myocardial infarction and cerebrovascular accidents have occurred in patients undergoing combination chemotherapy with vinblastine, bleomycin, and cisplatin. Raynaud's phenomenon has also been reported with this combination.

Pulmonary: See PRECAUTIONS.

Miscellaneous: Malaise, bone pain, weakness, pain in tumor-containing tissue, dizziness, jaw pain, skin vesiculation, hypertension, Raynaud's phenomenon when patients are being treated with vinblastine sulfate in combination with bleomycin and cis-platinum for testicular cancer. The syndrome of inappropriate secretion of antidiuretic hormone has occurred with higher than recommended doses.

Nausea and vomiting usually may be controlled with ease by antiemetic agents. When epilation develops, it frequently is not total; and, in some cases, hair regrows while maintenance therapy continues.

Extravasation during intravenous injection may lead to cellulitis and phlebitis. If the amount of extravasation is great, sloughing may occur.

OVERDOSAGE:

Signs and Symptoms: Side effects following the use of vinblastine sulfate are dose related. Therefore, following administration of more than the recommended dose, patients can be expected to experience these effects in an exaggerated fashion. (See CLINICAL PHARMACOLOGY, CONTRAINDICATIONS, WARNINGS, PRECAUTIONS, and ADVERSE REACTIONS.) There is no specific antidote. In addition, neurotoxicity similar to that with Oncovin may be observed. Since the major route of excretion may be through the biliary system, toxicity from this drug may be increased when there is hepatic insufficiency.

Treatment: To obtain up-to-date information about the treatment of overdose, a good resource is your certified Regional Poison Control Center. In managing overdosage consider the possibility of multiple drug overdoses, interaction among drugs, and unusual drug kinetics in your patient. Overdoses of vinblastine sulfate have been reported rarely. The following is provided to serve as a guide should such an overdose be encountered.

Supportive care should include the following: (1) prevention of side effects that result from the syndrome of inappropriate secretion of antidiuretic hormone (this would include restriction of the volume of daily fluid intake to that of the urine output plus insensible loss and perhaps the administration of a diuretic affecting the function of the loop of Henle and the distal tubule; (2) administration of an anticonvulsant; (3) prevention of ileus; (4) monitoring the cardiovascular system; and (5) determining daily blood counts for guidance in transfusion requirements and assessing the risk of infection. The major effect of excessive doses of vinblastine sulfate will be myelosuppression, which may be life threatening. There is no information regarding the effectiveness of dialysis nor of cholestyramine for the treatment of overdosage.

Vinblastine sulfate in the dry state is irregularly and unpredictably absorbed from the gastrointestinal tract following oral administration. Absorption of the solution has not been studied. If vinblastine is swallowed, activated charcoal in a water slurry may be given by mouth along with a cathartic. The use of cholestyramine in this situation has not been reported.

Symptoms of overdose will appear when greater-than-recommended doses are given. Any dose of vinblastine sulfate that results in elimination of platelets and neutrophils from blood and marrow and their precursors from marrow should be considered life threatening. The exact dose that will do this in all patients is unknown. Overdoses occurring during prolongs, consecutive-day infusions may be more toxic than the same total dose given by rapid intravenous injection. The intravenous median lethal dose in mice is 10 mg/kg body weight; in rats, it is 2.9 mg/kg. The oral median lethal dose in rats is 7 mg/kg.

Protect the patient's airway and support ventilation and perfusion. Meticulously monitor and maintain, within acceptable limits, the patient's vital signs, blood gases, serum electrolytes, etc. Absorption of drugs from the gastrointestinal tract may be decreased by giving activated charcoal, which, in many cases, is more effective than emesis or lavage; consider charcoal instead of or in addition to gastric emptying if the drug has been swallowed. Repeated doses of charcoal over time may hasten elimination of some drugs that have been absorbed. Safeguard the patient's airway when employing gastric emptying or charcoal.

DOSAGE AND ADMINISTRATION:

Caution: It is extremely important that the needle be properly positioned in the vein before this product is injected.

If leakage into surrounding tissue should occur during intravenous administration of vinblastine sulfate, it may cause considerable irritation. The injection should be discontinued immediately, and any remaining portion of the dose should then be introduced into another vein. Local injection of hyaluronidase and the application of moderate heat to the area of leakage help disperse the drug and are thought to minimize discomfort and the possibility of cellulitis.

There are variations in the depth of the leukopenic response that follows therapy with vinblastine sulfate. For this reason,it is recommended that the drug be given no more frequently than *once every 7 days.* It is wise to initiate therapy for adults by administering a single intravenous dose of 3.7 mg/m^2 of body surface area (bsa); the initial dose for children should be 2.5 mg/m^2. Thereafter, white-blood-cell counts should be made to determine the patient's sensitivity to vinblastine sulfate. A reduction of 50% in the dose of vinblastine sulfate is recommended for patients having a direct serum bilirubin value above 3 mg/100 ml. Since metabolism and excretion are primarily hepatic, no modification is recommended for patients with impaired renal function.

A simplified and conservative incremental approach to dosage at*weekly intervals* may be outlined in TABLE 1.

TABLE 1

	Adults	Children
First dose	3.7 mg/m^2 bsa	2.5 mg/m^2 bsa
Second dose	5.5 mg/m^2 bsa	3.75 mg/m^2 bsa
Third dose	7.4 mg/m^2 bsa	5.0 mg/m^2 bsa
Fourth dose	9.25 mg/m^2 bsa	6.25 mg/m^2 bsa
Fifth dose	11.1 mg/m^2 bsa	7.5 mg/m^2 bsa

The above-mentioned increases may be used until a maximum dose (not exceeding 1.8 mg/m^2 bsa for adults and 12.5 mg/m^2 bsa for children) is reached. The dose should not be increased after that dose which reduces the white-cell count to approximately 3,000 cells/mm^3. In some adults, 3.7 mg/m^2 bsa may produce this leukopenia; other adults may require more than 11.1 mg/m^2 bsa; and, very rarely, as much as 18.5 mg/m^2 bsa may be necessary. For most adult patients, however, the weekly dosage will prove to be 5.5 to 7.4 mg/m^2 bsa.

When the dose of vinblastine sulfate which will produce the above degree of leukopenia has been established, a dose of *1 increment smaller* than this should be administered at weekly intervals for maintenance. Thus, the patient is receiving the maximum dose that does not cause leukopenia. *It should be emphasized that, even though 7 days have elapsed, the next dose of vinblastine sulfate should not be given until the white-cell count has returned to at least 4,000/mm^3.* In some cases, oncolytic activity may be encountered before leukopenic effect. When this occurs, there is no need to increase the size of subsequent doses (see PRECAUTIONS).

The duration of maintenance therapy varies according to the disease being treated and the combination of antineoplastic agents being used. There are differences of opinion regarding the duration of maintenance therapy with the same protocol for a particular disease; for example, various durations have been used with the MOPP program in treating Hodgkin's disease. Prolonged chemotherapy for maintaining remissions involves several risks, among which are life-threatening infectious diseases, sterility, and possibly the appearance of other cancers through suppression of immune surveillance.

In some disorders, survival following complete remission may not be as prolonged as that achieved with shorter periods of maintenance therapy. On the other hand, failure to provide maintenance therapy in some patients may lead to unnecessary relapse; complete remissions in patients with testicular cancer, unless maintained for at least 2 years, often result in early relapse.

To prepare a solution containing 1 mg of vinblastine sulfate/ml, add 10 ml of Sodium Chloride Injection (preserved with phenol or benzyl alcohol) to the 10 mg of vinblastine sulfate in the sterile vial. Other solutions are not recommended. The drug dissolves instantly to give a clear solution. After a solution has been made in this way and a portion of it has been removed from a vial, the remainder of the vial's contents may be stored in a refrigerator for future use for 30 days without significant loss of potency.

The dose of vinblastine sulfate (calculated to provide the desired amount) may be injected either into the tubing of a running intravenous infusion or directly into a vein. The latter procedure is readily adaptable to outpatient therapy. In either case the injection may be completed in about 1 minute. If care is taken to insure that the needle is securely within the vein and that no solution containing vinblastine sulfate is spilled extravascularly, cellulitis and/or phlebitis will not occur. To minimize further the possibility of extravascular spillage, it is suggested that the syringe and needle be rinsed with venous blood before withdrawal of the needle. The dose should not be diluted in large volumes of diluent (*i.e.,* 100 to 250 ml) or given intravenously for prolonged periods (ranging from 30 to 60 minutes or more), since this frequently results in irritation of the vein and increases the chance of extravasation.

Because of the enhanced possibility of thrombosis, it is considered inadvisable to inject a solution of vinblastine sulfate into an extremity in which the circulation is impaired or potentially impaired by such conditions as compressing or invading neoplasm, phlebitis, or varicosity.

Parenteral drug products should be inspected visually for particulate matter and discoloration prior to administration, whenever solution and container permit.

It is not necessary to use preservative-containing solvents if unused portions of the remaining solution are discarded immediately. Unused preservative-containing solutions should be refrigerated for future use.

Procedures for proper handling and disposal of anticancer drugs should be considered. Several guidelines on this subject have been published. There is no general agreement that all of the procedures recommended in the guidelines are necessary or appropriate.

Special Dispensing Information: When dispensing vinblastine sulfate in other than the original container, (*e.g.,* a syringe containing a specific dose), it is imperative that it be packaged in an overwrap bearing the statement "DO NOT REMOVE COVERING UNTIL MOMENT OF INJECTION. FATAL IF GIVEN INTRATHECALLY. FOR INTRAVENOUS USE ONLY" (see WARNINGS).

The vials should be stored in a refrigerator (2 to 8°C, or 36 to 46°F) to assure extended stability.

HOW SUPPLIED - RATED THERAPEUTICALLY EQUIVALENT:

Injection, Lyphl-Soln - Intravenous - 10 mg

10 ml $37.50 Vinblastine Sulfate, Schein Pharm (US) 00364-2447-54

Injection, Solution - Intravenous - 1 mg/ml

10 ml $38.92 VELBAN, Lilly 00002-1452-01

HOW SUPPLIED - NOT RATED EQUIVALENT:

Injection, Solution - Intravenous - 1 mg/ml

10 ml	$21.25	Vinblastine Sulfate, Harber Pharm	51432-0419-10
10 ml	$32.50	Vinblastine Sulfate, Voluntary Hosp	53258-2780-03
10 ml	$33.13	Vinblastine Sulfate, Fujisawa USA	00469-2780-30
10 ml	$34.50	Vinblastine Sulfate, Voluntary Hosp	53258-1620-03
25 ml	$53.00	Vinblastine Sulfate, Harber Pharm	51432-0478-10

VINCRISTINE SULFATE *(002428)*

CATEGORIES: Antineoplastics; Cancer; Chemotherapy; Hodgkin's Disease; Leukemia; Lymphoma; Neuroblastoma; Oncologic Drugs; Rhabdomyosarcoma; Wilms' Tumor; Pregnancy Category D; FDA Approved 1984 Mar

BRAND NAMES: **Oncovin**; Vincasar Pfs; Vincrex

FORMULARIES: BC-BS; Medi-Cal; WHO

WARNING:
Caution - This preparation should be administered by individuals experienced in the administration of Oncovin. It is extremely important that the intravenous needle or catheter be properly positioned before any vincristine is injected. Leakage into surrounding tissue during intravenous administration of Oncovin may cause considerable irritation. If extravasation occurs, the injection should be discontinued immediately, and any remaining portion of the dose should then be introduced into another vein. Local injection of hyaluronidase and the application of moderate heat to the area of leakage help disperse the drug and are thought to minimize discomfort and the possibility of cellulitis.
FATAL IF GIVEN INTRATHECALLY. FOR INTRAVENOUS USE ONLY.
See WARNINGS for the treatment of patients given intrathecal Oncovin.

DESCRIPTION:

Oncovin (Vincristine Sulfate, USP, Lilly) is the salt of an alkaloid obtained from a common flowering herb, the periwinkle plant (*Vinca rosea Linn).* Originally known as leurocristine, it has also been referred to as LCR and VCR. The empirical formula for vincristine sulfate is:

$C_{46}H_{56}N_4O_{10} \cdot H_2SO_4$.

It has a molecular weight of 923.04.

Vincristine sulfate is a white to off-white powder. It is soluble in methanol, freely soluble in water, but only slightly soluble in 95% ethanol. In 98% ethanol, vincristine sulfate has an ultraviolet spectrum with maxima at 221 nm (8 + 47,100).

Each ml contains vincristine sulfate, 1 mg (1.08 μmol); mannitol, 100 mg; methylparaben, 1.3 mg; propylparaben, 0.2 mg; and water for injection, qs. Acetic acid and sodium acetate have been added for pH control. The pH of Oncovin Solution ranges from 3.5 to 5.5. This product is a sterile solution for cancer/oncolytic use.

CLINICAL PHARMACOLOGY:

The mechanisms of action of Oncovin remain under investigation.[1] The mechanism of action of Oncovin has been related to the inhibition of microtubule formation in the mitotic spindle, resulting in an arrest of dividing cells at the metaphase stage.

Central-nervous-system leukemia has been reported in patients undergoing otherwise successful therapy with Oncovin. This suggests that Oncovin does not penetrate well into the cerebrospinal fluid.

Pharmacokinetic studies in patients with cancer have shown a triphasic serum decay pattern following rapid intravenous injection. The initial, middle, and terminal half-lives are 5 minutes, 2.3 hours, and 85 hours respectively; however, the range of the terminal half-life in humans is from 19 to 155 hours. The liver is the major excretory organ in humans and animals; about 80% of an injected dose of Oncovin appears in the feces and 10% to 20% can be found in the urine. Within 15 to 30 minutes after injection, over 90% of the drug is distributed from the blood into tissue, where it remains tightly, but not irreversibly, bound.[2]

Current principles of cancer chemotherapy involve the simultaneous use of several agents. Generally, each agent used has a unique toxicity and mechanism of action so that therapeutic enhancement occurs without additive toxicity. It is rarely possible to achieve equally good results with single-agent methods of treatment. Thus, Oncovin is often chosen as part of polychemotherapy because of lack of significant bone-marrow suppression (at recommended doses) and of unique clinical toxicity (neuropathy). See DOSAGE AND ADMINISTRATIONfor possible increased toxicity when used in combination therapy.

INDICATIONS AND USAGE:

Oncovin is indicated in acute leukemia.

Oncovin has also been shown to be useful in combination with other oncolytic agents in Hodgkin's disease,[3] non-Hodgkin's malignant lymphomas[4-6] (lymphocytic, mixed-cell, histiocytic, undifferentiated, nodular, and diffuse types), rhabdomyosarcoma,[7] neuroblastoma,[8] and Wilms' tumor.[9]

CONTRAINDICATIONS:

Patients with the demyelinating form of Charcot-Marie-Tooth syndrome should not be given Oncovin. Careful attention should be given to those conditions listed under Warnings and Precautions.

WARNINGS:

This preparation is for intravenous use only. It should be administered by individuals experienced in the administration of Oncovin. The intrathecal administration of Oncovin usually results in death. Syringes containing this product should be labeled "WARNING—FOR IV USE ONLY."

Extemporaneously prepared syringes containing this product must be packaged in an overwrap which is labeled "DO NOT REMOVE COVERING UNTIL MOMENT OF INJECTION. FATAL IF GIVEN INTRATHECALLY. FOR INTRAVENOUS USE ONLY."

Treatment of patients following intrathecal administration of Oncovin has included immediate removal of spinal fluid and flushing with Lactated Ringer's, as well as other solutions and has not prevented ascending paralysis and death. In one case, progressive paralysis in an adult was arrested by the following treatment initiated immediately after the intrathecal injection:

WARNINGS: *(cont'd)*

1. As much spinal fluid was removed as could be safely done through lumbar access.
2. The subarachnoid space was flushed with Lactated Ringer's solution infused continuously through a catheter in a cerebral lateral ventricle at the rate of 150 ml/h. The fluid was removed through a lumbar access.
3. As soon as fresh frozen plasma became available, the fresh frozen plasma, 25 ml, diluted in 1 L of Lactated Ringer's solution was infused through the cerebral ventricular catheter at the rate 75 ml/h with removal through the lumbar access. The rate of infusion was adjusted to maintain a protein level in the spinal fluid of 150 mg/dl.
4. Glutamic acid, 10 g, was given intravenously over 24 hours followed by 500 mg 3 times daily by mouth for 1 month or until neurological dysfunction stabilized. The role of glutamic acid in this treatment is not certain and may not be essential.

Pregnancy Category D: Oncovin can cause fetal harm when administered to a pregnant woman. When pregnant mice and hamsters were given doses of Oncovin that caused the resorption of 23% to 85% of fetuses, fetal malformations were produced in those that survived. Five monkeys were given since doses of Oncovin between days 27 and 34 of their pregnancies; 3 of the fetuses were normal at term, and 2 viable fetuses had grossly evident malformations at term.[10] In several animal species, Oncovin can induce teratogenesis as well as embryo death at doses that are nontoxic to the pregnant animal. There are no adequate and well-controlled studies in pregnant women. If this drug is used during pregnancy or if the patient becomes pregnant while receiving this drug, she should be apprised of the potential hazard to the fetus. Women of childbearing potential should be advised to avoid becoming pregnant.

PRECAUTIONS:

General: Acute uric acid nephropathy, which may occur after the administration of oncolytic agents, has also been reported with Oncovin. In the presence of leukopenia or a complicating infection, administration of the next dose of Oncovin warrants careful consideration.

If central-nervous-system leukemia is diagnosed, additional agents may be required because Oncovin does not appear to cross the blood-brain barrier in adequate amounts.

Particular attention should be given to dosage and neurologic side effects if Oncovin is administered to patients with preexisting neuromuscular disease and when other drugs with neurotoxic potential are also being used.

Acute shortness of breath and severe bronchospasm have been reported following the administration of vinca alkaloids. These reactions have been encountered most frequently when the vinca alkaloid was used in combination with mitomycin-C and may require aggressive treatment, particularly when there is preexisting pulmonary, dysfunction. The onset of these reactions may occur minutes to several hours after the vinca alkaloid is injected and may occur up to 2 weeks following the dose of mitomycin. Progressive dyspnea requiring chronic therapy may occur. Oncovin should not be read ministered.

Care must be taken to avoid contamination of the eye with concentrations of Oncovin used clinically. If accidental contamination occurs, severe irritation (or, if the drug was delivered under pressure, even corneal ulceration) may result. The eye should be washed immediately and thoroughly.

Laboratory Tests: Because dose-limiting clinical toxicity is manifested as neurotoxicity, clinical evaluation (*e.g.,* history, physical examination) is necessary to detect the need for dosage modification. Following administration of Oncovin, some individuals may have a fall in the white-blood-cell count or platelet count, particularly when previous therapy or the disease itself has reduced bone-marrow function. Therefore, a complete blood count should be done before administration of each dose. Acute elevation of serum uric acid may also occur during induction of remission in acute leukemia; thus, such levels should be determined frequently during the first 3 to 4 weeks of treatment or appropriate measures taken to prevent uric acid nephropathy. The laboratory performing these tests should be consulted for its range of normal values.

Carcinogenesis, Mutagenesis, and Impairment of Fertility: Neither in vivo nor in vitro laboratory tests have conclusively demonstrated the mutagenicity of this product.[10] Fertility following treatment with Oncovin alone for malignant disease has not been studied in humans. Clinical reports of both male and female patients who received multiple-agent chemotherapy that included Oncovin indicate that azoospermia and amenorrhea can occur in postpubertal patients. Recovery occurred many months after completion of chemotherapy in some but not all patients. When the same treatment is administered to prepubertal patients, permanent azoospermia and amenorrhea are much less likely.[12-18]

Patients who received chemotherapy with Oncovin in combination with anticancer drugs known to be carcinogenic have developed second malignancies. The contributing role of Oncovin in this development has not been determined. No evidence of carcinogenicity was found following intraperitoneal administration of Oncovin in rats and mice, although this study was limited.[10]

Pregnancy Category D: See WARNINGS.

Nursing Mothers: It is not known whether this drug is excreted in human milk. Because many drugs are excreted in human milk and because of the potential for serious adverse reactions due to Oncovin in nursing infants a decision should be made either to discontinue nursing or the drug, taking into account the importance of the drug to the mother.

DRUG INTERACTIONS:

The simultaneous oral or intravenous administration of phenytoin and antineoplastic chemotherapy combinations that included vincristine sulfate has been reported to reduce blood levels of the anticonvulsant and to increase seizure activity.[11] Dosage adjustment should be based on serial blood level monitoring. The contribution of vincristine sulfate to this interaction is not certain. The interaction may result from reduced absorption of phenytoin and an increase in the rate of its metabolism and elimination.

Oncovin should not be diluted in solutions that raise or lower the pH outside the range of 3.5 to 5.5. It should not be mixed with anything other than normal saline or glucose in water.

Whenever solution and container permit, parenteral drug products should be inspected visually for particulate matter and discoloration prior to administration.

Procedures for proper handling and disposal of anticancer drugs should be considered. Several guidelines on this subject have been published.[20-25] There is no general agreement that all of the procedures recommended in the guidelines are necessary or appropriate.

ADVERSE REACTIONS:

PRIOR TO THE USE OF THIS DRUG, PATIENTS AND/OR THEIR PARENTS/ GUARDIAN SHOULD BE ADVISED OF THE POSSIBILITY OF UNTOWARD SYMPTOMS.

ADVERSE REACTIONS: *(cont'd)*

IN GENERAL, ADVERSE REACTIONS ARE REVERSIBLE AND ARE RELATED TO DOSAGE. THE MOST COMMON ADVERSE REACTION IS HAIR LOSS; THE MOST TROUBLESOME ADVERSE REACTIONS ARE NEUROMUSCULAR IN ORIGIN.

WHEN SINGLE, WEEKLY DOSES OF THE DRUG ARE EMPLOYED, THE ADVERSE REACTIONS OF LEUKOPENIA, NEURITIC PAIN, AND CONSTIPATION OCCUR BUT ARE USUALLY OF SHORT DURATION (*I.E.,* LESS THAN 7 DAYS). WHEN THE DOSAGE IS REDUCED, THESE REACTIONS MAY LESSEN OR DISAPPEAR. THE SEVERITY OF SUCH REACTIONS SEEMS TO INCREASE WHEN THE CALCULATED AMOUNT OF DRUG IS GIVEN IN DIVIDED DOSES. OTHER ADVERSE REACTIONS, SUCH AS HAIR LOSS, SENSORY LOSS, PARESTHESIA, DIFFICULTY IN WALKING, SLAPPING GAIT, LOSS OF DEEP-TENDON REFLEXES, AND MUSCLE WASTING, MAY PERSIST FOR AT LEAST AS LONG AS THERAPY IS CONTINUED. GENERALIZED SENSORIMOTOR DYSFUNCTION MAY BECOME PROGRESSIVELY MORE SEVERE WITH CONTINUED TREATMENT, SOME NEUROMUSCULAR DIFFICULTIES MAY PERSIST FOR PROLONGED PERIODS IN SOME PATIENTS. REGROWTH OF HAIR MAY OCCUR WHILE MAINTENANCE THERAPY CONTINUES.

THE FOLLOWING ADVERSE REACTIONS HAVE BEEN REPORTED:

Hypersensitivity: Rare cases of allergic-type reactions, such as anaphylaxis, rash, and edema, that are temporally related to vincristine therapy have been reported in patients receiving vincristine as a part of multidrug chemotherapy regimens.

Gastrointestinal: Constipation, abdominal cramps, weight loss, nausea, vomiting, oral ulceration, diarrhea, paralytic ileus, intestinal necrosis and/or perforation, and anorexia have occurred. Constipation may take the form of upper-colon impaction, and, on physical examination, the rectum may be empty. Colicky abdominal pain coupled with an empty rectum may mislead the physician. A flat film of the abdomen is useful in demonstrating this condition. All cases have responded to high enemas and laxatives. A routine prophylactic regimen against constipation is recommended for all patients receiving Oncovin. Paralytic ileus (which mimics the "surgical abdomen") may occur, particularly in young children. The ileus will reverse itself with temporary discontinuance of Oncovin and with symptomatic care.

Genitourinary: Polyuria, dysuria, and urinary retention due to bladder atony have occurred. Other drugs known to cause urinary retention (particularly in the elderly) should, if possible, be discontinued for the first few days following administration of Oncovin.

Cardiovascular: Hypertension and hypotension have occurred. Chemotherapy combinations that have included vincristine sulfate, when given to patients previously treated with mediastinal radiation, have been associated with coronary artery disease and myocardial infarction. Causality has not been established.

Neurologic: Frequently, there is a sequence to the development of neuromuscular side effects. Initially, only sensory impairment and paresthesia may be encountered. With continued treatment, neuritic pain and, later, motor difficulties may occur. There have been no reports of any agent that can reverse the neuromuscular manifestations that may accompany therapy with Oncovin. Loss of deep-tendon reflexes, foot drop, ataxia, and paralysis have been reported with continued administration. Cranial nerve manifestations, including isolated paresis and/or paralysis of muscles controlled by cranial motor nerves, may occur in the absence of motor impairment elsewhere; extraocular and laryngeal muscles are those most commonly involved. aw pain, pharyngeal pain, parotid gland pain, bone pain, back pain, limb pain, and myalgias have been reported; pain in these areas may be severe. Convulsions, frequently with hypertension, have been reported in a few patients receiving Oncovin. Several instances of convulsions followed by coma have been reported in children. Transient cortical blindness and optic atrophy with blindness have been reported.

Pulmonary: See PRECAUTIONS.

Endocrine: Rare occurrences of a syndrome attributable to inappropriate antidiuretic hormone secretion have been observed in patients treated with Oncovin. This syndrome is characterized by high urinary sodium excretion in the presence of hyponatremia; renal or adrenal disease, hypotension, dehydration, azotemia, and clinical edema are absent. With fluid deprivation, improvement occurs in the hyponatremia and in the renal loss of sodium.

Hematologic: Oncovin does not appear to have any constant or significant effect on platelets or red blood cells. Serious bone-marrow depression is usually not a major dose-limiting event. However, anemia, leukopenia, and thrombocytopenia have been reported. Thrombocytopenia, if present when therapy with Oncovin is begun, may actually improve before the appearance of marrow remission.

Skin: Alopecia and rash have been reported.

Other: Fever and headache have occurred.

OVERDOSAGE:

Side effects following the use of Oncovin are dose related. In children under 13 years of age, death has occurred following doses of Oncovin that were 10 times those recommended for therapy. Severe symptoms may occur in this patient group following dosages of 3 to 4 mg/m^2. Adults can be expected to experience severe symptoms after single doses of 3 mg/m^2 or more (see ADVERSE REACTIONS). Therefore, following administration of doses higher than those recommended, patients can be expected to experience exaggerated side effects. Supportive care should include the following: (1) prevention of side effects resulting from the syndrome of inappropriate antidiuretic hormone secretion (preventive treatment would include restriction of fluid intake and perhaps the administration of a diuretic affecting the function of Henle's loop and the distal tubule); (2) administration of anticonvulsants; (3) use of enemas or cathartics to prevent ileus (in some instances, decompression of the gastrointestinal tract may be necessary); (4) monitoring the cardiovascular system; and (5) determining daily blood counts for guidance in transfusion requirements.

Folinic acid has been observed to have a protective effect in normal mice that were administered lethal doses of Oncovin (*Cancer Res*1963;23:1390). Isolated case reports suggest that folinic acid may be helpful in treating humans who have received an overdose of Oncovin. It is suggested that 100 mg of folinic acid be administered intravenously every 3 hours for 24 hours and then every 6 hours for at least 48 hours. Theoretically (based on pharmacokinetic data), tissue levels of Oncovin can be expected to remain significantly elevated for at least 72 hours. Treatment with folinic acid does not eliminate the need for the above-mentioned supportive measures.

Most of an intravenous dose of Oncovin is excreted into the bile after rapid tissue binding (see CLINICAL PHARMACOLOGY). Because only very small amounts of the drug appear in dialysate, hemodialysis is not likely to be helpful in cases of overdosage. An increase in the severity of side effects may be experienced by patients with liver disease that is severe enough to decrease biliary excretion.

Enhanced fecal excretion of parenterally administered vincristine has been demonstrated in dogs pretreated with cholestyramine. There are no published clinical data on the use of cholestyramine as an antidote in humans.

There are no published clinical data on the consequences of oral ingestion of vincristine. Should oral ingestion occur, the stomach should be evacuated. Evacuation should be followed by oral administration of activated charcoal and a cathartic.

DOSAGE AND ADMINISTRATION:

This preparation is for intravenous use only (see WARNINGS).

Neurotoxicity appears to be dose related. Extreme care must be used in calculating and administering the dose of Oncovin since overdosage may have a very serious or fatal outcome.

The concentration of vincristine contained in all vials and Hyporets of Oncovin is 1 mg/ml. Do not add extra fluid to the vial prior to removal of the dose. Withdraw the solution of Oncovin into an accurate dry syringe, measuring the dose carefully. Do not add extra fluid to the vial in an attempt to empty it completely.

Caution — It is extremely important that the intravenous needle or catheter be properly positioned before any vincristine is injected. Leakage into surrounding tissue during intravenous administration of Oncovin may cause considerable irritation. If extravasation occurs, the injection should be discontinued immediately and any remaining portion of the dose should then be introduced into another vein. Local injection of hyaluronidase and the application of moderate heat to the area of leakage will help disperse the drug and may minimize discomfort and the possibility of cellulitis.

Oncovin must be administered via an intact, free-flowing intravenous needle or catheter. Care should be taken that there is no leakage or swelling occurring during administration (see BOXED WARNING).

The solution may be injected either directly into a vein or into the tubing of a running intravenous infusion (see DRUG INTERACTIONSbelow). Injection of Oncovin should be accomplished within 1 minute.

The drug is administered intravenously *at weekly intervals.*

The usual dose of Oncovin for children is 2 mg/m^2. For children weighing 10 kg or less, the starting dose should be 0.05 mg/kg, administered once a week. The usual dose of Oncovin for adults is 1.4 mg/m^2. A 50% reduction in the dose of Oncovin is recommended for patients having a direct serum bilirubin value above 3 mg/100 ml.[19]

Oncovin should not be given to patients while they are receiving radiation therapy through ports that include the liver. When Oncovin is used in combination with L-asparaginase, Oncovin should be given 12 to 24 hours before administration of the enzyme in order to minimize toxicity; administering L-asparaginase before Oncovin may reduce hepatic clearance of Oncovin.

Special Dispensing Information: When dispensing Oncovin in other than the original container, (*e.g.,* a syringe containing a specific dose), it is imperative that it be packaged in an overwrap bearing the statement: "DO NOT REMOVE COVERING UNTIL MOMENT OF INJECTION. FATAL IF GIVEN INTRATHECALLY. FOR INTRAVENOUS USE ONLY" (see WARNINGS).

Storage: This product should be refrigerated.

REFERENCES:

1. Watanabe K, West WL: Calmodulin, activated cyclic nucleotide phosphodiesterase, microtubules, and vinca alkaloids. *Fed Proc*1982; 41:2292. **2.** Nelson RL: The comparative clinical pharmacology and pharmacokinetics of vindesine, vincristine, and vinblastine in human patients with cancer.*Med Pediatr Oncol* 1982;10:115. **3.** DeVita VT Jr, Serpick AA, Carbone PP: Combination chemotherapy in the treatment of advanced Hodgkin's disease. *Ann Intern Med*1970;73:881. **4.** Bagley CM Jr, DeVita VT Jr, Berard CW, et al: Advanced lymphosarcoma: Intensive cyclical chemotherapy with cyclophosphamide, vincristine, and prednisone. *Ann Intern Med* 1972;73: 227. **5.** Lowenbraun S, DeVita VT, Serpick AA: Combination chemotherapy with nitrogen mustard, vincristine, procarbazine, and prednisone in lymphosarcoma and reticulum cell sarcoma. *Cancer* 1970;25:1018. **6.** Luce JK, Gamble JF, Wilson HE, et al: Combined cyclophosphamide, vincristine, and prednisone therapy of malignant lymphoma. *Cancer*1971;28:306. **7.** Wilbur JR, Sutow WW, Sullivan MP, et al: Successful treatment of rhabdomyosarcoma with combination chemotherapy and radiotherapy. *Am Soc Clin Oncology* April 7, 1971. **8.** Sullivan MP, Nora AH, Kulapongs P, et al: Evaluation of vincristine sulfate and cyclophosphamide chemotherapy for metastatic neuroblastoma.*Pediatrics* 1969;44:685. **9.** Vietti TJ, Sullivan MP, Haggard ME, et al: Vincristine sulfate and radiation therapy in metastatic Wilms tumor. *Cancer* 1970;25:12. **10.** International Agency for Research on Cancer, Monograph on the evaluation of the carcinogenic risk of chemicals to humans, suppl 4, October 1982. **11.** Grossman SA, Sheidler VR, Gilbert MR: Decreased phenytoin levels in patients receiving chemotherapy. *Am J Med*1989;87:505. **12.** Roeser HP, Stocks AE, Smith AJ: Testicular damage due to cytotoxic drugs and recovery after cessation of therapy. *Aust NZ J Med*1978;8:250. **13.** Chapman R, Sutcliffe SB, Malpas JS: Male gonadal dysfunction in Hodgkin's disease. *JAMA* 1981;245:1323. **14.** Sherins RJ, DeVita VT: Effect of drug treatment for lymphoma on male reproductive capacity. *Ann Intern Med*1981;79:216. **15.** DeVita VT: The consequences of the chemotherapy of Hodgkin's disease.*Cancer* 1981;47:1. **16.** Horning SJ, Hoppe RT, Kaplan HS, et al: Female reproductive potential after treatment for Hodgkin's disease. *N Engl J Med*1981;304: 1377. **17.** Blatt J, Poplack DG, Sherins RJ: Testicular function in boys after chemotherapy for acute lymphoblastic leukemia. *N Engl J Med*1981;304:1121. **18.** Siris ES, Leventhal BG, Vaitukaitis JL: Effect of childhood leukemia and chemotherapy on puberty and reproductive function in girls. *N Engl J Med* 1976;294:1143. **19.** DeVita VT Jr, Hellman S, Rosenberg SA (eds): *Cancer, principles and Practice of Oncology,* ed 2. Philadelphia, J.B. Lippincott Co, 1985. **20.** Recommendations for the safe handling of parenteral antineoplastic drugs. NIH Publication No. 83-2621, US Government Printing Office, Washington DC 20402. **21.** Council on Scientific Affairs: Guidelines for handling parenteral antineoplastics. *JAMA* 1985;253:1590. **22.** National Study Commission on Cytotoxic Exposure—Recommendations for handling cytotoxic agents. Available from Louis P. Jeffrey, ScD, Director of Pharmacy Services, Rhode Island Hospital, 593 Eddy Street, Providence, Rhode Island 02902. **23.** Clinical Oncological Society of Australia: Guidelines and recommendations for safe handling of antineoplastic agents. *Med J Aust* 1983;1:426. **24.** Jones RB, et al: Safe handling of chemotherapeutic agents: A report from the Mount Sinai Medical Center. *CA* (Sept/Oct) 1983;33:258. **25.** American Society of Hospital Pharmacists: Technical assistance bulletin on handling cytotoxic drugs in hospitals. *Am J Hosp Pharm* 1985;42:131.*Hyporet (disposable syringe, Lilly)

HOW SUPPLIED - RATED THERAPEUTICALLY EQUIVALENT:

Injection, Solution - Intravenous - 1 mg/ml

1 ml	$15.00	Vincristine Sulfate, Harber Pharm	51432-0476-01
1 ml	**$34.62**	**ONCOVIN, Lilly**	**00002-7194-01**
1 ml hyporets x	**$107.28**	**ONCOVIN, Lilly**	**00002-7198-09**
1 ml x 10	$37.08	VINCASAR PFS, Pharmacia & Upjohn	00013-7456-86
2 ml	$38.25	Vincristine Sulfate, Schein Pharm (US)	00364-2448-52
2 ml	$40.00	Vincristine, Voluntary Hosp	53258-0352-01
2 ml	**$69.22**	**ONCOVIN, Lilly**	**00002-7195-01**
2 ml x 3	**$211.08**	**ONCOVIN, Lilly**	**00002-7199-09**
5 ml	$150.00	Vincristine, Voluntary Hosp	53258-0352-02
5 ml	**$156.21**	**ONCOVIN, Lilly**	**00002-7196-01**

Injection, Solution - Intravenous - 2 mg/vial

2 ml x 10	$74.15	VINCASAR PFS 2, Pharmacia & Upjohn	00013-7466-86

HOW SUPPLIED - NOT RATED EQUIVALENT:

Injection, Solution - Intravenous - 1 mg/ml

1 ml	$20.00	Vincristine, Voluntary Hosp	53258-0352-00
1 ml	$30.16	Vincristine Sulfate, Steris Labs	00402-1028-01
2 ml	$30.00	Vincristine Sulfate, Harber Pharm	51432-0477-02
2 ml	$38.25	Vincristine Sulfate, Steris Labs	00402-1028-02
5 ml	$56.99	Vincristine Sulfate, Balan	00304-2201-55
5 ml	$73.13	Vincristine Sulfate, Harber Pharm	51432-0475-05

VINORELBINE TARTRATE *(003190)*

CATEGORIES: Antineoplastics; Cancer; Chemotherapy; Cytotoxic Agents; Lung Cancer; Oncologic Drugs; Tumors; Breast Carcinoma*; FDA Class 1P ("Priority Review"); FDA Approved 1994 Dec; Patent Expiration 1998 Dec
* Indication not approved by the FDA

BRAND NAMES: **Navelbine**

FORMULARIES: Medi-Cal

COST OF THERAPY: $1,272.33 (Lung Cancer; Injection; 10 mg/ml; 0.75/day; 30 days)

PRIMARY ICD9: 162.9 (Malignant Neoplasm of Bronchus and Lung, Unspecified)

WARNING:
Navelbine (vinorelbine tartrate) injection should be administered under the supervision of a physician experienced in the use of cancer chemotherapeutic agents. This product is for intravenous use only. Intrathecal administration of other vinca alkaloids has resulted in death. Syringes containing this product should be labeled "WARNING - NAVELBINE FOR INTRAVENOUS USE ONLY."

Severe granulocytopenia resulting in increased susceptibility to infection may occur. Granulocyte counts should be >/-1000 cells mm3 prior to the administration of Navelbine. The dosage should be adjusted according to complete blood counts with differentials obtained on the day of treatment.

Caution - It is extremely important that the intravenous needle or catheter be properly positioned before Navelbine is injected. Improper administration of Navelbine may result in extravasation causing local necrosis and/or thrombophlebitis (see DOSAGE AND ADMINISTRATION, Administration Precautions.)

DESCRIPTION:

Navelbine (vinorelbine tartrate) Injection is for intravenous administration. Each vial contains vinorelbine tartrate equivalent to 10 mg (1 ml vial) or 50 mg (5 ml vial) vinorelbine in Water for Injection. No preservatives or other additives are present. The aqueous solution is sterile and nonpyrogenic.

Vinorelbine tartrate is a semi-synthetic vinca alkaloid with antitumor activity. The chemical name is 3',4'-didehydro-4'-deoxy-*C*'- norvincaleukoblastine [*R*-(*R**,*R**)-2,3- dihydroxybutanedioate (1:2)(salt)].

Vinorelbine is a white to yellow or light brown amorphous powder with the molecular formula $C_{45}H_{54}N_4O_8 \cdot 2C_4H_6O_6$ and molecular weight of 1079.12. The aqueous solubility is >1000 mg/ml in distilled water. The pH of Navelbine Injection is approximately 3.5.

CLINICAL PHARMACOLOGY:

Vinorelbine is a vinca alkaloid that interferes with microtubule assembly. The vinca alkaloids are structurally similar compounds comprised of two multiringed units, vindoline and catharanthine. unlike other vinca alkaloids, the catharanthine unit is the site of structural modification for vinorelbine. The antitumor activity of vinorelbine is thought to be due primarily to inhibition of mitosis at metaphase through its interaction with tubulin. Like other vinca alkaloids, vinorelbine may also interfere with: 1) amino acid, cyclic AMP, and glutathione metabolism, 2) calmodulin-dependent Ca^{++}-transport ATPase activity, 3) cellular respiration, and 4) nucleic acid and lipid biosynthesis. In intact tectal plates from mouse embryos, vinorelbine, vincristine, and vinblastine inhibited mitotic microtubule formation at the same concentration (2 μM), inducing a blockade of cells at metaphase. Vincristine produced depolymerization of axonal microtubules at 5 μM, but vinblastine and vinorelbine did not have this effect until concentrations of 30 μM and 40 μM, respectively. These data suggest relative selectivity of vinorelbine for mitotic microtubules.

Pharmacokinetics: The pharmacokinetics of vinorelbine were studied in 49 patients who received doses of 30 mg/m²in four clinical trials. Doses were administered by 15- to 20-minute constant rate infusions. Following intravenous administration, vinorelbine concentration in plasma decays in a triphasic manner. The initial rapid decline primarily represents distribution of drug to peripheral compartments followed by metabolism and excretion of the drug during subsequent phases. The prolonged terminal phase is due to relatively slow efflux of vinorelbine from peripheral compartments. The terminal phase half-life averages 27.7 to 43.6 hours and the mean plasma clearance ranges from 0.97 to 1.26 L/hr/kg. Steady state volume of distribution (V_{ss}) values range from 25.4 to 40.1 L/kg.

Vinorelbine demonstrated high binding to platelets and lymphocytes. The free fraction was approximately 0.11 in pooled human plasma over a concentration range of 234 to 1169 ng/ml. The binding to plasma constituents in cancer patients ranged from 79.6% to 91.2%. Vinorelbine binding was not altered in the presence of cisplatin, 5-fluorouracil, or doxorubicin.

Vinorelbine undergoes substantial hepatic elimination in humans, with large amounts recovered in feces after intravenous administration to humans. One metabolite, deacetylvinorelbine, has been shown to possess antitumor activity. This metabolite has been detected but not quantified in human plasma. The effects of renal or hepatic dysfunction on the disposition of vinorelbine have not been assessed, but based on experience with other anticancer vinca alkaloids, dose adjustments are recommended for patients with impaired hepatic function (see DOSAGE AND ADMINISTRATION.)

The disposition of radiolabeled vinorelbine given intravenously was studied in a limited number of patients. Approximately 18% of the administered dose was recovered in the urine and 46% in the feces. Incomplete recovery in humans is consistent with results in animals where recovery is incomplete, even after prolonged sampling times. As separate study of the urinary excretion of vinorelbine using specific chromatographic analytical methodology showed that 10.9% ± 0.7% of a 30 mg/m² intravenous dose was excreted unchanged in the urine.

The pharmacokinetics of vinorelbine are not influenced by the concurrent administration of cisplatin with Navelbine (see DRUG INTERACTIONS.)

CLINICAL STUDIES:

Data from two controlled clinical studies (823 patients), as well as additional data from more than 100 patients enrolled in two uncontrolled clinical trials, support the use of Navelbine in patients with advanced non-small cell lung cancer (NSCLC). In a large European clinical trial, 612 patients with Stage III or IV NSCLC, no prior chemotherapy, and WHO Performance Status of 0, 1, or 2 were randomized to treatment with single-agent Navelbine (30 mg/m²/week), Navelbine (30 mg/m²/week) plus cisplatin (120 mg/m²days 1 and 29, then every 6 weeks), and vindesine (3 mg/m²/week for 7 weeks, then every other week) plus cisplatin (120 mg/m² days 1 and 29, than every 6 weeks). Navelbine plus cisplatin produced longer survival times than vindesine plus cisplatin (median survival 40 weeks vs. 32 weeks, P=0.03). The median survival time for patients receiving single-agent Navelbine was similar to that observed with vindesine plus cisplatin (31 weeks vs. 32 weeks). The 1-year survival rates were 35% for Navelbine plus cisplatin, 27% for vindesine plus cisplatin, and 30% for single-agent Navelbine. The overall objective response rate (all partial responses) was significantly higher in the patients treated with Navelbine plus cisplatin (28%) than in those treated with vindesine plus cisplatin (19%, P=0.03) and in those treated with single-agent Navelbine (14%, P<0.001). The response rates reported for vindesine plus cisplatin and single-agent Navelbine were not significantly different. Significantly less nausea, vomiting, alopecia, and neurotoxicity were observed in patients receiving single- agent Navelbine compared to those receiving the combination of vindesine and cisplatin.

Single-agent Navelbine was studied in a North American, randomized clinical trial in which patients with Stage IV NSCLC, no prior chemotherapy, and Karnofsky Performance Status ≥70 were treated with Navelbine (30 mg/m²) weekly or 5-fluorouracil (5-FU) (425 mg/m²IV bolus) plus leucovorin (LV) (20 mg/m² IV bolus) daily for 5 days every 4 weeks. A total of 211 patients were randomized at a 2:1 ratio to Navelbine (143) or 5-FU/LV (68). Navelbine showed improved survival time compared to 5-FU/LV. In an intent-to-treat analysis, the median survival time for patients receiving Navelbine was 30 weeks and for those receiving 5-FU/LV was 22 weeks (P=0.06). The 1-year survival rates were 24 % (±4% S.E.) for Navelbine and 16% (±5% S.E.) for the 5-FU/Lv group, using the Kaplan-Meier product-limit estimates. The median survival time with 5-FU/LV was similar to, or slightly better than, that usually observed in untreated patients with advanced NSCLC, suggesting that the difference was not related to some unknown detrimental effect of 5-FU/LV therapy. The response rates (all partial responses) for Navelbine and 5 FU/LV were 12% and 3%, respectively. Quality-of-life (QOL) was also an endpoint in this study. Patients completed a modified Southwest Oncology Group QOL questionnaire which assessed the domains of role functioning, physical functioning, symptom distress, and global QOL. Quality-of-life was not adversely affected by Navelbine when compared to control.

A dose-ranging study of Navelbine (20, 25, or 30 mg/m²/week) plus cisplatin (120 mg/m²days 1 and 29, then every 6 weeks) in 32 patients with NSCLC demonstrated a median survival of 44 weeks. There were no responses at the lowest dose level; the response rate was 33% in the 21 patients treated at the two highest dose levels.

INDICATIONS AND USAGE:

Navelbine is indicated as a single agent or in combination with cisplatin for the first-line treatment of ambulatory patients with unresectable, advanced non-small cell lung cancer (NSCLC). In patients with Stage IV NSCLC, Navelbine is indicated as a single agent or in combination with cisplatin. In Stage III NSCLC, Navelbine is indicated in combination with cisplatin.

CONTRAINDICATIONS:

Administration of Navelbine is contraindicated in patients with pretreatment granulocyte counts <1000 cells/mm³ (see WARNINGS.)

WARNINGS:

Navelbine should be administered in carefully adjusted doses by or under the supervision of a physician experienced in the use of cancer chemotherapeutic agents.

Patients treated with Navelbine should be frequently monitored for myelosuppression both during and after therapy. Granulocytopenia is dose- limiting. Granulocyte nadirs occur between 7 and 10 days after dosing with granulocyte count recovery usually within the following 7 to 14 days. Complete blood counts with differentials should be performed and results reviewed prior to administering each dose of Navelbine. Navelbine should not be administered to patients with granulocyte counts <1000 cells/mm³. Patients developing severe granulocytopenia should be monitored carefully for evidence of infection and/or fever. See DOSAGE AND ADMINISTRATION for recommended dose adjustments for granulocytopenia.

Pregnancy Category D: Navelbine may cause fetal harm if administered to a pregnant woman. A single dose of vinorelbine has been shown to be embryo- and/or fetotoxic in mice and rabbits at doses of 9 mg/m² and 5.5 mg/m², respectively (one-third and one- sixth the human dose). At nonmaternotoxic doses, fetal weight was reduced and ossification was delayed. There are no studies in pregnant women. If Navelbine is used during pregnancy, or if the patient becomes pregnant while receiving this drug, the patient should be apprised of the potential hazard to the fetus. Women of childbearing potential should be advised to avoid becoming pregnant during therapy with Navelbine.

PRECAUTIONS:

GENERAL

Most drug-related adverse events of Navelbine are reversible. If severe adverse events occur, Navelbine should be reduced in dosage or discontinued and appropriate corrective measures taken. reinstitution of therapy with Navelbine should be carried out with caution and alertness as to possible recurrence of toxicity.

Navelbine should be used with extreme caution in patients whose bone marrow reserve may have been compromised by prior irradiation or chemotherapy, or whose marrow function is recovering from the effects of previous chemotherapy (see DOSAGE AND ADMINISTRATION.)

Acute shortness of breath and severe bronchospasm have been reported infrequently following the administration of Navelbine and other vinca alkaloids, most commonly when the vinca alkaloid was used in combination with mitomycin. These adverse events may require treatment with supplemental oxygen, bronchodilators, and/or corticosteroids, particularly when there is pre-existing pulmonary dysfunction.

Care must be taken to avoid contamination of the eye with concentrations of Navelbine used clinically. Severe irritation of the eye has been reported has been reported with accidental exposure to another vinca alkaloid. If exposure occurs, the eye should immediately be thoroughly flushed with water.

INFORMATION FOR THE PATIENT

Patients should be informed that the major acute toxicities of Navelbine are related to bone marrow toxicity, specifically granulocytopenia with increased susceptibility to infection. They should be advised to report fever or chills immediately. Women of childbearing potential should be advised to avoid becoming pregnant during treatment.

LABORATORY TESTS

Since dose-limiting clinical toxicity is the result of depression of the white blood cell count, it is imperative that complete blood counts with differentials be obtained and reviewed on the day of treatment prior to each dose of Navelbine (see ADVERSE REACTIONS, Hematologic.)

Hepatic: There is no evidence that the toxicity of Navelbine is enhanced in patients with elevated liver enzymes. No data are available for patients with severe baseline cholestasis, but the liver plays an important role in the metabolism of Navelbine. Because clinical experience in patients with severe liver disease is limited, caution should be exercised when administering Navelbine to patients with severe hepatic injury or impairment (see DOSAGE AND ADMINISTRATION.)

CARCINOGENESIS, MUTAGENESIS, AND IMPAIRMENT OF FERTILITY

The carcinogenic potential of Navelbine has not been studied. Vinorelbine has been shown to affect chromosome number and possibly structure *in vivo* (polyploidy in bone marrow cells from Chinese hamsters and positive micronucleus test in mice). It was not mutagenic in the Ames test and gave inconclusive results in the mouse lymphoma TK Locus assay. The significance of these or other short term test results for human risk is unknown. Vinorelbine

PRECAUTIONS: *(cont'd)*

did not affect fertility to a statistically significant extent when administered to rats on either a once weekly (9 mg/m^2, approximately one-third the human dose) or alternate day schedule (4.2 mg/m^2, approximately one-seventh the human dose) prior to and during mating. However, biweekly administration for 13 or 26 weeks in the rat at 2.1 and 7.2 mg/m^2 (approximately one- fifteenth and one-fourth the human dose) resulted in decreased spermatogenesis and prostate/seminal vesicle secretion.

PREGNANCY CATEGORY D

See WARNINGS.

NURSING MOTHERS

It is not known whether the drug is excreted in human milk. Because many drugs are excreted in human milk and because of the potential for serious adverse reactions in nursing infants from Navelbine, it is recommended that nursing be discontinued in women who are receiving therapy with Navelbine.

PEDIATRIC USE

Safety and effectiveness have not been established.

GERIATRIC USE

Of the total number of patients in North American clinical studies of IV Navelbine, approximately one-third were 65 years of age or greater. No overall differences in effectiveness or safety were observed between these patients and younger patients. Other reported clinical experience has not identified differences in responses between the elderly and younger patients, but greater sensitivity of some older individuals cannot be ruled out.

DRUG INTERACTIONS:

Acute pulmonary reactions have been reported with Navelbine and other anticancer vinca alkaloids used in conjunction with mitomycin. Although the pharmacokinetics of vinorelbine are not influenced by the concurrent administration of cisplatin, the incidence of granulocytopenia with Navelbine used in combination with cisplatin is significantly higher than with single-agent Navelbine.

ADVERSE REACTIONS:

Granulocytopenia is the major dose-limiting toxicity with Navelbine. Dose adjustments are required for hematologic toxicity and hepatic insufficiency (see DOSAGE AND ADMINISTRATION.)

Data in the following table are based on the experience of 365 patients (143 patients with NSCLC; 222 patients with advanced breast cancer) treated with IV Navelbine as a single agent in three clinical studies. The dosing schedule in each study was 30 mg/m^2 Navelbine on a weekly basis.

TABLE 1 Summary of Adverse Events in 365 Patients Receiving Single-Agent Navelbine*†

Adverse Event		All Patients (n=365) (% Incidence)	NSCLC (n=143) (% Incidence)
Bone Marrow			
Granulocytopenia	<2,000 cells/mm^3	90	80
	<500 cells/mm^3	36	
29			
Leukopenia	<4,000 cells/mm^3	92	81
	<1,000 cells/mm^3	15	
12			
Thrombocytopenia	<100,000 cells/mm^3	5	4
	<50,000 cells/mm^3	1	1
Anemia	<11 g/dL	83	77
	<8 g/dL		9
Hospitalizations due to granulocytopenic complications		9	8

* None of the reported toxicities were influenced by age. Grade based on modified criteria from the National Cancer Institute.

† Patients with NSCLC had not yet received prior chemotherapy. The majority of the remaining patients had received prior chemotherapy.

TABLE 2

Adverse Event	All Grades (%Incidence) All Patients	All Grades NSCLC	Grade 3 (%Incidence) All Patients	Grade 3 NSCLC	Grade 4 (%Incidence) All Patients	Grade 4 NSCLC
Clinical Chemistry Elevations						
Total Bilirubin (n=351)	13	9	4	3	3	2
SGOT (n=346)	67	54	5	2	1	1
General						
Asthenia	36	27	7	5	0	0
Injection Site Reactions	28	38	2	5	0	0
Injection Site Pain	16	13	2	5	0	0
Phlebitis	7	10	<1	1	0	0
Digestive						
Nausea	44	34	2	1	0	0
Vomiting	20	15	2	1	0	0
Constipation	35	29	3	2	0	0
Diarrhea	17	13	1	1	0	0
Peripheral Neuropathy‡	25	20	1	1	<1	0
Dyspnea	7	3	2	2	1	0
Alopecia	12	12	≤1	1	0	0

‡ Incidence of paresthesia plus hypesthesia.

Hematologic: Granulocytopenia was the major dose-limiting toxicity with Navelbine; it was generally reversible and not cumulative over time. Granulocyte nadirs occurred 7 to 10 days after the dose, with granulocyte recovery usually within the following 7 to 14 days. Granulocytopenia resulted in hospitalizations for fever and/or sepsis in 8% of patients. Septic deaths occurred in approximately 1% of patients. Prophylactic hematologic growth factors have not been routinely used with Navelbine. If medically necessary, growth factors may be administered at recommended doses no earlier than 24 hours after the administration of cytotoxic chemotherapy. Growth factors should not be administered in the period 24 hours before the administration of chemotherapy.

Grade 3 or 4 anemia occurred in 1% of patients, although blood products were administered to 18% of patients who received Navelbine. Grade 3 or 4 thrombocytopenia was reported in 1% of patients.

Neurologic: Mild to moderate peripheral neuropathy manifested by paresthesia and hypesthesia were the most frequently reported neurologic toxicities. Loss of deep tendon reflexes occurred in less than 5% of patients. The development of severe peripheral neuropathy was infrequent (1%) and generally reversible.

ADVERSE REACTIONS: *(cont'd)*

Skin: Alopecia was reported in 12% of patients and was usually mild.

Like other anticancer vinca alkaloids, Navelbine is a moderate vesicant. Injection site reactions, including erythema, pain at injection site, and vein discoloration occurred in approximately one-third of patients; 5% were severe. Chemical phlebitis along the vein proximal to the site of injection was reported in 10% of patients.

Gastrointestinal: Mild or moderate nausea occurred in 34% of patients treated with Navelbine; severe nausea was infrequent (<2%). Prophylactic administration of antiemetics was not routine in patients treated with single-agent Navelbine. Due to the low incidence of severe nausea and vomiting with single-agent Navelbine, the use of serotonin antagonists is generally not required. Constipation occurred in 29% of patients, with paralytic ileus occurring in 1%. Vomiting, diarrhea, anorexia, and stomatitis were usually mild or moderate and each occurred in less than 20% of patients.

Hepatic: Transient elevations of liver enzymes were reported without clinical symptoms.

Cardiovascular: Chest pain was reported in 5% of patients. Most reports of chest pain were in patients who had either a history of cardiovascular disease or tumor within the chest. There have been rare reports of myocardial infarction.

Pulmonary: Shortness of breath was reported in 3% of patients; it was severe in 2% (see PRECAUTIONS, General.) Interstitial pulmonary changes were documented in a few patients.

Other: Fatigue occurred in 27% of patients. It was usually mild or moderate but tended to increase with cumulative dosing.

Other toxicities that have been reported in less than 5% of patients include jaw pain, myalgia, arthralgia, and rash. Hemorrhagic cystitis and the syndrome of inappropriate ADH secretion were each reported in <1% of patients.

Combination Use: In a randomized study, 206 patients received treatment with Navelbine plus cisplatin and 206 patients received single-dose Navelbine. The toxicity profile of cisplatin is known (see full prescribing information for cisplatin.) The incidence of severe nausea and vomiting was 30% for Navelbine/cisplatin compared to <2% for single- agent Navelbine. Cisplatin did not appear to increase the incidence of neurotoxicity observed with single-agent Navelbine. However, myelosuppression, specifically Grade 3 and 4 granulocytopenia, was greater with the combination of Navelbine/cisplatin (79%) than with single-agent Navelbine (53%). The incidence of fever and infection may be increased with the combination.

OVERDOSAGE:

There is no known antidote for overdoses of Navelbine. The primary anticipated complications of overdosage would consist of bone marrow suppression and peripheral neurotoxicity. If overdosage occurs, general supportive measures together with appropriate blood transfusions and antibiotics should be instituted as deemed necessary by the physician.

DOSAGE AND ADMINISTRATION:

The usual initial dose of Navelbine is 30 mg/m^2 administered weekly. The recommended method of administration is an intravenous injection over 6 to 10 minutes. In controlled trials, single-agent Navelbine was given weekly until progression or dose-limiting toxicity. Navelbine was used at the same dose in combination with 120 mg/m^2 of cisplatin, given on days 1 and 29, then every 6 weeks.

No dose adjustments are required for renal insufficiency. If moderate or severe neurotoxicity develops, Navelbine should be discontinued. The dosage should be adjusted according to hematologic toxicity or hepatic insufficiency, whichever results in the lower dose.

Dose Modifications for Hematologic Toxicity: Granulocyte counts should be ≥1000 cells/mm^3 prior to the administration of Navelbine. Adjustments in the dosage of Navelbine should be based on granulocyte counts obtained on the day of treatment according to TABLE 3.

TABLE 3 Dose Adjustments Based on Granulocyte Counts

Granulocytes (cells/mm^3) on Days of Treatment	Dose of Navelbine (mg/m^2)
≥1500	30
1000 to 1499	15
<1000	Do not administer. Repeat granulocyte count in 1 week. If 3 consecutive weekly doses are held because granulocyte count is <1000 cells/mm^3, discontinue Navelbine.

Note: For patients who, during treatment with Navelbine, have experienced fever and/or sepsis while granulocytopenic or had 2 consecutive weekly doses held due to granulocytopenia, subsequent doses of Navelbine should be:
22.5 mg/m^2 for granulocytes ≥1500 cells/mm^3
11.25 mg/m^2 for granulocytes 1000 to 1499 cells/mm^3

Dose Modification for Hepatic Insufficiency: Navelbine should be administered with caution to patients with hepatic insufficiency. In patients who develop hyperbilirubinemia during treatment with Navelbine, the dose should be adjusted for total bilirubin according to TABLE 4.

TABLE 4 Dose Modification Based on Total Bilirubin

Total Bilirubin (mg/dL)	Dose of Navelbine (mg/m^2)
≤2.0	30
2.1 to 3.0	15
>3.0	7.5

Dose Modification for Concurrent Hematologic Toxicity and Hepatic Insufficiency: In patients with both hematologic toxicity and hepatic insufficiency, the lower of the doses determined from Table 3 and Table 4 should be administered.

Administration Precautions: Caution - Navelbine must be administered intravenously. It is extremely important that the intravenous needle or catheter be properly positioned before any Navelbine is injected. Leakage into surrounding tissue during intravenous administration of Navelbine may cause considerable irritation, local tissue, necrosis, and/or thrombophlebitis. If extravasation occurs, the injection should be discontinued immediately, and any remaining portion of the dose should then be introduced into another vein. Since there are no established guidelines for treatment of extravasation injuries with Navelbine, institutional guidelines may be used. The *ONS Chemotherapy Guidelines* provide additional recommendations for the prevention of extravasation injuries.[1]

As with other toxic compounds, caution should be exercised in handling and preparing the solution of Navelbine. Skin reactions may occur with accidental exposure. The use of gloves is recommended. If the solution of Navelbine contacts the skin or mucosa, immediately wash the skin or mucosa thoroughly with soap and water. Severe irritation of the eye has been reported with accidental contamination of the eye with another vinca alkaloid. If this happens with Navelbine, the eye should be flushed with water immediately and thoroughly.

DOSAGE AND ADMINISTRATION: *(cont'd)*

Procedures for proper handling and disposal of anticancer drugs should be used. Several guidelines on this subject have been published.[2-8]there is no general agreement that all of the procedures recommended in the guidelines are necessary or appropriate.

Navelbine Injection is a clear, colorless to pale yellow solution. Parenteral drug products should be visually inspected for particulate matter and discoloration prior to administration whenever solution and container permit. If particulate matter is seen, Navelbine should not be administered.

Preparation for Administration: Navelbine Injection must be diluted in either a syringe or IV bag using one of the recommended solutions. The diluted Navelbine should be administered over 6 to 10 minutes into the side port of a free-flowing IV **closest to the IV bag** followed by flushing with at least 75 to 125 ml of one of the solutions. Diluted Navelbine may be used for up to 24 hours under normal room light when stored in polypropylene syringes or polyvinyl chloride bags at 5° to 30°C (41° to 86°F).

Syringe: The calculated dose of Navelbine should be diluted to a concentration between 1.5 and 3.0 mg/ml. The following solutions may be used for dilution:

5% Dextrose Injection, USP

0.9 Sodium Chloride Injection, USP

IV Bag: The calculated dose of Navelbine should be diluted to a concentration between 0.5 and 2 mg/ml. The following solutions may be used for dilution:

5% Dextrose Injection, USP

0.9% Sodium Chloride Injection, USP

0.45% Sodium Chloride Injection, USP

5% Dextrose and 0.45% Sodium Chloride Injection, USP

Ringer's Injection, USP

Lactated Ringer's Solution, USP

Stability: Unopened vials of Navelbine are stable until the date indicated on the package when stored under refrigeration at 2° to 8° (36° to 46°F) and protected from light in the carton. Unopened vials of Navelbine are stable at temperatures up to 25°C (77°F) for up to 72 hours. This product should not be frozen.

HOW SUPPLIED:

Navelbine Injection is a clear to colorless to pale yellow solution in Water for Injection, containing 10 mg vinorelbine per ml. Navelbine Injection is available in single-use, clear glass vials with black elastomeric stoppers and royal blue caps, individually packaged in a carton.

Store the vials under refrigeration at 2° to 8°C (36° to 46°F) in the carton. Protect from light. DO NOT FREEZE.

REFERENCES:

1. ONS Clinical Practice Committee. Cancer Chemotherapy Guidelines: Recommendations for the management of vesicant extravasation, hypersensitivity, and anaphylaxis. Pittsburgh, Pa: Oncology Nursing Society; 1992:1-4. **2.** Recommendations for the safe handling of parenteral antineoplastic drugs. Washington, DC: Division of Safety, National Institutes of Health; 1983. US Dept of Health and Human Services, Public Health Service publication NIH 83-2621. **3.** AMA Council on Scientific Affairs. Guidelines for handling parenteral antineoplastics. *JAMA.* 1985;253:1590-1591. **4.** National Study Commission on Cytotoxic Exposure. Recommendations for handling cytotoxic agents. 1987. Available from Louis P. Jeffrey, Chairman, National Study Commission on Cytotoxic Exposure. Massachusetts College of Pharmacy and Allied Health Sciences, 179 Longwood Avenue, Boston, MA, 02115. **5.** Clinical Oncological Society of Australia. Guidelines and recommendations for safe handling of antineoplastic agents. *Med J Australia.* 1983;1:426-428. **6.** Jones RB, Frank R, Mass T. Safe handling of chemotherapeutic agents: a report from the Mount Sinai Medical Center. *CA-A Cancer J for Clin.* 1983;33:258-263. **7.** American Society of Hospital Pharmacists. ASHP technical assistance bulletin on handling cytotoxic and hazardous drugs. *Am J Hosp Pharm.* 1990;47:1033-1049. **8.** Yodaiken RE, Benet D. OSHA work-practice guidelines for personnel dealing with cytotoxic (antineoplastic) drugs. *Am J Hosp Pharm.* 1986;43:1193-1204.

HOW SUPPLIED - EQUIVALENTS NOT AVAILABLE:

Injection, Solution - Intravenous - 10 mg/ml

1 ml	$56.55	NAVELBINE, Glaxo Wellcome	00173-0656-01
5 ml	$282.74	NAVELBINE, Glaxo Wellcome	00173-0656-44

VITAMIN A *(002429)*

CATEGORIES: Homeostatic & Nutrient; Vitamin A; Vitamins; FDA Approval Pre 1982

BRAND NAMES: *A313*; *Acaren*; *Acon*; *Afaxin*; Alphalin; Aquasol A; *Ariovit*; *Arovit*; *Atunol*; *Avibon*; *Avimin*; *Avipur*; *Avitin*; *Axerol*; *Bagovit*; *Biovit A*; *Dagravit*; Del-Vi-A; *Dolce*; *Euvitol*; *Ido A 50*; *Idrurto A*; *Oculotect*; *Ro-A-Vit*; Solaneed; Vi-Dom-A; *Vogan (International brand names outside U.S. in italics)*

FORMULARIES: Aetna; WHO

DESCRIPTION:

Water-miscible vitamin A Palmitate 50,000 USP Units (15 mg retinol)/ml with 0.5% chlorobutanol as preservative; 12% polysorbate 80, 0.1% citric acid, 0.03% butylated hydroxyanisole, 0.03% butylated hydroxytoluene; and sodium hydroxide to adjust pH.

THIS IS A STERILE PRODUCT FOR INTRAMUSCULAR INJECTION

Aquasol A Parenteral (water-miscible vitamin A) provides 50,000 USP Units of vitamin A per ml a retinol ($C_{20}H_{30}O$) in the form of vitamin A palmitate, a light yellow to amber oil.

Ordinarily oil-soluble, the vitamin A in this product has been water solubilized by special processing* and is available in a water solution for intramuscular injection.

One USP Unit is equivalent to one international unit (IU) and to 0.3 mcg of retinol or 0.6 mcg of beta-carotene.

CLINICAL PHARMACOLOGY:

Beta-carotene, retinol, and retinal have effective and reliable vitamin A activity. Retinal and retinol are in chemical equilibrium in the body and have equivalent antixerophthalmic activity. Retinal combines with the rod pigment, opsin, in the retina to form rhodopsin, necessary for visual dark adaptation. Vitamin A prevents retardation of growth and preserves the epithelial cells integrity. Normal adult liver storage is sufficient to satisfy two years' requirements of Vitamin A.

Vitamin A is readily absorbed from the gastrointestinal tract, where the biosynthesis of vitamin A from beta-carotene takes place. Vitamin A absorption requires bile salts, pancreatic lipase, and dietary fat. It is transported in the blood to the liver by the chylomicron fraction of the lymph. Vitamin A is stored in Kupffer cells of the liver mainly as the palmitate. Normal serum vitamin A is 80-300 Units per 100 ml (plasma range is 30-70 mcg per dl) and for carotenoids 270-753 Units per 100 ml. The normal adults liver contains approximately 100 to 300 micrograms per gram, mostly as retinol palmitate.

* Oil-soluble vitamin A water solubilized with polysorbate 80.

INDICATIONS AND USAGE:

Vitamin A injection is effective for the treatment of vitamin A deficiency.

The parenteral administration is indicated when the oral administration is not feasible as in anorexia, nausea, vomiting, pre- and post- operative conditions, or it is not available as in the "Malabsorption syndrome" with accompanying steatorrhea.

CONTRAINDICATIONS:

The intravenous administration. Hypervitaminosis A. Sensitivity to any of the ingredients in this preparation.

Use in Pregnancy: Safety of amounts exceeding 6,000 Units of vitamin A daily during pregnancy has not been established at this time. The use of vitamin A in excess of the recommended dietary allowance may cause fetal harm when administered to a pregnant woman. Animal reproduction studies have shown fetal abnormalities associated with overdose in several species. Malformations of the central nervous system, the eye, the palate, and the urogenital tract are recorded. Vitamin A in excess of the recommended dietary allowance is contraindicated in women who are or may become pregnant. If vitamin A is used during pregnancy, or if the patient becomes pregnant while taking vitamin A, the patient should be apprised of the potential hazard to the fetus.

WARNINGS:

Avoid overdosage. Keep out of the reach of children.

PRECAUTIONS:

General: Protect from light. Prolonged daily dose administration over 25,000 Units vitamin A should be under close supervision. Blood level assays are not a direct measure of liver storage. Liver storage should be adequate before discontinuing therapy. Single vitamin A deficiency is rare. Multiple vitamin deficiency is expected in any dietary deficiency.

Carcinogenesis: There are no studies that show that administration of vitamin A will cause or prevent cancer.

Pregnancy Category X: See CONTRAINDICATIONSsection.

Nursing Mothers: The U.S. Recommended Daily Allowance (RDA) of vitamin A (5,000 Units) is recommended for nursing mothers.

DRUG INTERACTIONS:

Women on oral contraceptives have shown a significant increase in plasma vitamin A levels.

ADVERSE REACTIONS:

See OVERDOSAGE. Anaphylactic shock and death have been reported using the intravenous route. Allergic reactions have been reported rarely with administration of Aquasol A Parenteral including one case of an anaphylactoid type reaction.

OVERDOSAGE:

The following amounts have been found to be toxic orally. Toxicity manifestations depend on the age, dosage, size, and duration of administration.

ACUTE TOXICITY

single dose (25,000 Units/kg body weight)

Infant: 350,000 Units

Adult: Over 2 million Units

CHRONIC TOXICITY

(4,000 Units/kg body weight for 6 to 15 months)

Infants 3 to 6 months old: 18,500 Units (water dispersed)/day for one to three months.

Adult: 1 million Units daily for three days; 50,000 Units daily for longer than 18 months; 500,000 Units daily for two months.

Hypervitaminosis A Syndrome

1. General manifestations: Fatigue, malaise, lethargy, abdominal discomfort, anorexia, and vomiting.

2. Specific manifestations:

a. Skeletal: Slow growth, hard tender cortical thickening over the radius and tibia, migratory arthralgia and premature closure of the epiphysis.

b. Central Nervous System: Irritability, headache, and increased intracranial pressure as manifested by bulging fontanels, papilledema, and exophthalmos.

c. Dermatologic: Fissures of the lips, drying and cracking of the skin, alopecia, scaling, massive desquamation, and increased pigmentation.

d. Systemic: Hypomenorrhea, hepatosplenomegaly, jaundice, leukopenia, vitamin A plasma level over 1,200 Units/100 ml.

THE TREATMENT OF HYPERVITAMINOSIS A CONSISTS OF IMMEDIATE WITHDRAWAL OF THE VITAMIN ALONG WITH SYMPTOMATIC AND SUPPORTIVE TREATMENT.

DOSAGE AND ADMINISTRATION:

For intramuscular use.

I. Adults: 100,000 Units daily for three days followed by 50,000 daily for two weeks.

II. Children 1 to 8 years old: 17,500 to 35,000 Units daily for 10 days.

III. Infants: 7,500 to 15,000 Units daily for 10 days.

Follow-up therapy with an oral therapeutic multi-vitamin preparation, containing 10,000 to 20,000 Units vitamin A for persons over 8 years old and 5,000 to 10,000 Units for infants and children, is recommended daily for two months. In malabsorption, the parenteral route must be used for an equivalent preparation.

Poor dietary habits should be corrected and an abundant and well-balanced dietary intake should be prescribed.

HOW SUPPLIED - RATED THERAPEUTICALLY EQUIVALENT:

Capsule, Elastic - Oral - 50,000 unit

100's	$2.50	Vitamin A, Apotheca	12634-0344-01
100's	$4.12	Vitamin A, Rugby	00536-4784-01
100's	$4.22	Vitamin A, H.C.F.A. F F P	99999-2429-01
100's	$5.50	Vitamin A Solubilized, Consolidated Midland	00223-1790-01
100's	$11.23	DEL VI A, Del Ray Lab	00316-0135-01
100's	$72.36	AQUASOL A, Astra USA	00186-4301-00
1000's	$18.75	Vitamin A, Apotheca	12634-0344-10
1000's	$32.50	Vitamin A Solubilized, Consolidated Midland	00223-1790-02
1000's	$42.20	Vitamin A, H.C.F.A. F F P	99999-2429-02

HOW SUPPLIED - NOT RATED EQUIVALENT:

Capsule, Elastic - Oral - 25,000 unit

100's	$2.25	Vitamin A, Rexall	00122-3124-34
100's	$3.75	Vitamin A, Consolidated Midland	00223-1750-01
100's	$4.50	Vitamin A, Consolidated Midland	00223-1751-01
100's	$41.61	AQUASOL A, Astra USA	00186-4291-00
1000's	$16.75	Vitamin A, Consolidated Midland	00223-1740-02
1000's	$27.50	Vitamin A, Consolidated Midland	00223-1751-02
1000's	$29.50	Vitamin A, Consolidated Midland	00223-1750-02

Injection, Solution - Intramuscular - 50,000 unit/ml

2 ml x 10	$197.34	AQUASOL A, Astra USA	00186-4239-62

VITAMIN B COMPLEX *(002434)*

CATEGORIES: Homeostatic & Nutrient; Multivitamins; Vitamin B Complex; Vitamins; FDA Pre 1938 Drugs

BRAND NAMES: B-Complex-100; B-Ject; B-Plex; Becomject-100; Bee-Comp W/C; Key-Plex; Lanoplex; Lysiplex; Mechol; Morplex; Pluri-B; Proticuleen; Rubavance; Vitabix

Prescribing information not available at time of publication.

HOW SUPPLIED - RATED THERAPEUTICALLY EQUIVALENT:

Injection, Solution - Intramuscular;

10 ml	$9.44	B Complex With C & B-12, HL Moore Drug Exch	00839-6363-30

HOW SUPPLIED - NOT RATED EQUIVALENT:

Capsule, Gelatin - Oral

100's	$2.99	Vitamin B Complex, Balan	00304-0479-01
1000's	$35.18	Vitamin B Complex, Balan	00304-0479-00

Injection, Solution - Intramuscular;

10 ml	$7.95	BEE-COMP W/C, AF Hauser	52637-0110-10
10 ml	$9.12	KEY-PLEX UNIVIAL, Hyrex Pharms	00314-0912-70
30 ml	$1.80	LANOPLEX, Lannett	00527-0108-58
30 ml	$3.63	Liver, Iron,B-Complex W/B-12, Rugby	00536-1233-75
30 ml	$3.65	LIVER, IRON,B-COMPLEX W/B-12, Americal Pharm	54945-0569-53
30 ml	$4.29	Vitamin B Complex 100, McGuff	49072-0057-30
30 ml	$5.75	Vitamin B Complex 100, Steris Labs	00402-0010-30
30 ml	$8.00	B Complex H.P., C O Truxton	00463-1007-30
30 ml	$11.30	B-JECT, Hyrex Pharms	00314-0010-30
30 ml	$15.00	Vitamin B Complex 100, Pasadena	00418-6222-30

Tablet, Uncoated - Oral

100's	$14.05	B-PLEX, Raway	00686-3514-13

VITAMIN B COMPLEX; VITAMIN C *(002435)*

CATEGORIES: Blood Formation/Coagulation; Caloric Agents; Deficiency Anemias; Electrolytic, Caloric-Water Balance; Geriatric Vitamins; Homeostatic & Nutrient; Multivitamins; Vitamin B Complex; Vitamins; FDA Pre 1938 Drugs

BRAND NAMES: B-Plex; Becomject-100; Berocca; Berovite; Berplex; Berroplex; Beta-C-Plex; Cota-B-Plex; Dialyvite; Formula B Plus; Harberplex; **Larobec**; Lipo-Nicin; Megaton; Nervidox 6; Neurin Bc; Neurobion; Neurodep; Neuroforte-Six; Nutriject; Orabex-Tf; Parplex; Rubroben-1000; Scorbex/12; Therobec; Vitaplex

DESCRIPTION:

Active ingredients are as follows (TABLE 1):

TABLE 1

Each Larobec tablet contains:	Quantity	U.S. RDA—Adults and children 4 or more years of age
Water-Soluble Vitamins		
Vitamin C (ascorbic acid)	500 mg	60 mg
Vitamin B1 (as thiamine mononitrate)	15 mg	1.5 mg
Vitamin B2 (riboflavin)	15 mg	1.7 mg
Niacin (as niacinamide)	100 mg	20 mg
Pantothenic acid (as calcium d-pantothenate)	18 mg	10 mg
Folic acid	0.5 mg	0.4 mg
Vitamin B12 (cyanocobalamin)	5 mcg	6 mcg

Each tablet also contains acacia, calcium sulfate, carnauba wax, hydrogenated vegetable oil, magnesium oxide, magnesium stearate, povidone, shellac, sodium benzoate, sugar and talc with the following dyes: FD&C Yellow No. 6, D&C Yellow No. 10 and titanium dioxide.

Larobec is a prescription-only oral multivitamin tablet specially formulated for patients who require prophylactic or therapeutic nutritional supplementation of water-soluble vitamins and are receiving levodopa therapy for Parkinson's disease and syndrome. Larobec provides Therapeutic levels of ascorbic acid, vitamins B1, B2, niacin, pantothenic acid and folic acid and a Supplemental level of vitamin B12 Without pyridoxine (vitamin B6), which has been reported to reduce the clinical benefits of levodopa therapy.

CLINICAL PHARMACOLOGY:

Vitamins are essential for maintenance of normal metabolic functions including hematopoiesis. The water-soluble vitamins play vital roles in the conversion of carbohydrate, protein and fat into tissue and energy. Thiamine (B1) acts as a coenzyme in carbohydrate metabolism. Riboflavin (B2) functions as a coenzyme in the electron transport system associated with conversion of tissue oxidations into usable energy. Niacin serves as a coenzyme in oxidation-reduction reactions in tissue respiration. Pantothenic Acid functions as a coenzyme in various metabolic acetylation reactions. Folic Acid and Cyanocobalamin (B12)are metabolically interrelated. They are essential to nucleic acid synthesis and normal maturation of red blood cells. Ascorbic Acid (C) performs a vital function in the process of cellular respiration, and is involved in both carbohydrate and amino acid metabolism. It is essential for collagen formation and tissue repair.

The water-soluble vitamins (B-complex and C) are not significantly stored by the body; excess quantities are excreted in the urine. They must be replenished regularly through diet or other means to maintain essential tissue levels. Thus these vitamins are rapidly depleted in conditions interfering with their intake or absorption.

INDICATIONS AND USAGE:

Larobec is indicated for supportive nutritional supplementation when a water-soluble vitamin formulation (without pyridoxine) is required prophylactically or therapeutically in patients who are undergoing treatment with levodopa.

CONTRAINDICATIONS:

Larobec is contraindicated in patients known to be hypersensitive to any of its components.

WARNINGS:

Administration of vitamin B6 may be required if signs of pyridoxine deficiency develop. Folic acid in doses above 0.1 mg daily may obscure pernicious anemia. Larobec is not intended for treatment of pernicious anemia or other megaloblastic anemias where vitamin B12 is deficient. Neurologic involvement may develop or progress, despite temporary remission of anemia, in patients with vitamin B12 deficiency who receive supplemental folic acid and who are inadequately treated with B12.

PRECAUTIONS:

General: Certain patients may require additional nutritional supplementation with fat-soluble vitamins and minerals according to the dietary habits of the individual. Larobec is not intended for treatment of severe specific vitamin deficiencies.

Information for the Patient: Because toxic reactions have been reported with injudicious use of certain vitamins, urge patients to follow your specific instructions regarding dosage regimen.

As with any medication, advise patients to keep Larobec out of reach of children.

ADVERSE REACTIONS:

Adverse reactions have been reported with specific vitamins, but generally at levels substantially higher than those in Larobec.

However, allergic and idiosyncratic reactions are possible at lower levels.

DOSAGE AND ADMINISTRATION:

Usual adult dosage: one tablet daily.

HOW SUPPLIED - EQUIVALENTS NOT AVAILABLE:

Elixir - Oral - 10 mg/1 mg/40 m

480 ml	$9.68	MEGATON, Hyrex Pharms	00314-0080-16

Injection, Lyphl-Soln - Intramuscular;

1's	$22.50	NERVIDOX 6, Teral Labs	51234-0120-10
10 ml	$7.00	Vitamin B-Complex W/B-12 And C, Consolidated Midland	00223-7216-10
10 ml	$7.50	Vitamin B Complex C W/B-12, Consolidated Midland	00223-7243-10
10 ml	$9.53	B Complex With C & B12 Inj, Schein Pharm (US)	00364-2262-54
10 ml	$9.53	B Complex With C & B-12, Steris Labs	00402-0123-11
10 ml	$9.95	NEUROBION 1000, OTC Pharm	55959-0131-01
10 ml	$10.07	B COMPLEX WITH C & B-12, United Res	00677-1349-21
10 ml	$10.91	Pluri-B with C, Lyophilized Covial, Pasadena	00418-6781-10
10 ml	$11.75	Neurin-Bc Injection, Sorter	53879-0303-10
10 ml	$12.38	Vitamin B-Complex W/C & B-12, Rugby	00536-2081-70
10 ml	$13.43	Vitamin B-Complex, IDE-Interstate	00814-8456-40
10 ml	$13.60	B Complex With C & B-12 Inj, Goldline Labs	00182-3005-63
10 ml	$15.00	Nutriject, Llorens Pharm	54859-0401-10
10 ml	$17.70	NEUROFORTE-SIX, Intl Ethical	11584-1018-06
10 ml	$22.50	NEURO B12 FORTE, AJ Bart	49326-0154-10
10's	$8.95	B-PLEX 100 LYO WITH C & B-12, Merit Pharms	30727-0301-70
30 ml	$7.65	Vitamin B Complex 100, Major Pharms	00904-0890-30
30 ml	$22.45	BECOMJECT-100, Mayrand Pharms	00259-0294-30
1000 ml	$9.06	DEXTROSE WITH VITAMINS, McGaw	00264-1970-00
1000 ml x 6	$33.18	DEXTROSE WITH VITAMINS, McGaw	00264-1972-00

Tablet, Uncoated - Oral

100's	$6.75	Formula-B, Major Pharms	00904-2630-60
100's	$7.34	B-C W/Folic Acid, Geneva Pharms	00781-1101-01
100's	$7.70	B-Complex Vitamins, Copley Pharm	38245-0151-10
100's	$8.31	Therapeutic Vitamin, Rugby	00536-5536-01
100's	$9.63	PARPLEX, Parmed Pharms	00349-8076-01
100's	$10.20	B-Plex, Goldline Labs	00182-4063-01
100's	$10.40	Vitamin Complex, Aligen Independ	00405-5103-01
100's	$12.38	Therobec, Qualitest Pharms	00603-5969-21
100's	$13.49	MOR-PLEX, HL Moore Drug Exch	00839-6769-06
100's	$18.22	B-C W/Folic Acid Plus, Geneva Pharms	00781-1102-01
100's	$24.15	Nephplex Rx, Nephro-Tech	59528-0317-01
100's	$28.95	Neo Vite, Pharmacist Choice	54979-0166-01
100's	$29.50	B-PLEX, Goldline Labs	00182-4062-01
250's	$18.75	Formula B, Major Pharms	00904-2630-70

VITAMIN E *(002438)*

CATEGORIES: Emollients; Skin/Mucous Membrane Agents; Amyotrophic Lateral Sclerosis*; Antiparkinson Agents*; Cancer*; Parkinsonism*; FDA Pre 1938 Drugs
* Indication not approved by the FDA

BRAND NAMES: *Bio E*; *Davitamon E*; *Detulin*; *E Perle*; *Ephynal*; Lactinol-E; *Optovit-E*; Tocopherol; *Vita-E*
(International brand names outside U.S. in italics)

Prescribing information not available at time of publication.

HOW SUPPLIED - EQUIVALENTS NOT AVAILABLE:

Cream - Topical - 10 %/3500 unit

60 gm	$5.00	LACTINOL-E CREME, Pedinol Pharma	00884-4990-02

WARFARIN SODIUM *(002444)*

CATEGORIES: Anticoagulants; Anticoagulants/Thrombolytics; Atrial Fibrillation; Blood Formation/Coagulation; Coagulants and Anticoagulants; Coronary Occlusion; Embolism; Fibrillation; Myocardial Infarction; Pulmonary Embolism; Thrombosis; Stroke*; Pregnancy Category X; Sales > $100 Million; FDA Approval Pre 1982; Top 200 Drugs
* Indication not approved by the FDA

BRAND NAMES: *Aldocumar*; *Athrombin*; *Coumadan Sodico*; **Coumadin**; *Coumadine* (France); *Marevam*; *Marevan* (Australia, England); *Orfarin*; Panwarfin; Sofarin; *UniWarfin*; *Waran*; *Warfilone* (Canada)
(International brand names outside U.S. in italics)

FORMULARIES: Aetna; BC-BS; CIGNA; DoD; FHP; Humana; Kaiser; Medco; Medi-Cal; PCS; PruCare; United; WHO

COST OF THERAPY: $112.78 (Thrombosis; Tablet; 5 mg; 1/day; 365 days)

DESCRIPTION:

Crystalline warfarin sodium, is an anticoagulant which acts by inhibiting vitamin K-dependent coagulation factors. Chemically, it is 3- (α-acetonylbenzyl) -4 -hydroxycoumarin and is a racemic mixture of the R and S enantiomers. Crystalline warfarin sodium is an isopropanol clathrate. The crystallization of warfarin sodium virtually eliminates trace impurities present in amorphous warfarin sodium. Its empirical formula is $C_{19}H_{15}NaO_4$.

Crystalline warfarin sodium occurs as a white, odorless, crystalline powder, is discolored by light and is very soluble in water; freely soluble in alcohol; very slightly soluble in chloroform and in ether.

COUMADIN TABLETS

Coumadin Tablets for oral use also contain: *All strengths:* Lactose, starch and magnesium stearate; *1 mg:* D&C Red 6; *2 mg:* FD&C Blue 2 and FD&C Red 40; *2-1/2 mg:* FD&C Blue 1 and D&C Yellow 10; *4 mg:* FD&C Blue 1 Lake; *5 mg:* FD&C Yellow 6; *7-1/2 mg:* D&C Yellow 10 and FD&C Yellow 6; *10 mg:* Dye Free.

COUMADIN FOR INJECTION

Coumadin for Injection is supplied as a sterile, lyophilized powder, which, after reconstitution with 2.7 ml sterile Water for Injection, contains: Warfarin sodium: 2 mg/ml; Sodium Phosphate, Dibasic, Heptahydrate: 4.98 mg/ml; Sodium Phosphate, Monobasic, Monohydrate: 0.194 mg/ml Sodium Chloride: 0.1 mg/ml; Mannitol: 38.0 mg/ml; Sodium Hydroxide, as needed for pH adjustment to: 8.1 to 8.3.

CLINICAL PHARMACOLOGY:

Warfarin sodium and other coumarin anticoagulants act by inhibiting the synthesis of vitamin K dependent clotting factors, which include Factors II, VII, IX and X, and the anticoagulant proteins C and S. Half-lives of these clotting factors are as follows: Factor II - 60 hours, VII - 4-6 hours, IX - 24 hours, and X - 48-72 hours. The half-lives of proteins C and S are approximately 8 hours and 30 hours, respectively. The resultant *in vivo* effect is a sequential depression of Factors VII, IX, X and II activities. Vitamin K is an essential cofactor for the post ribosomal synthesis of the vitamin K dependent clotting factors. The vitamin promotes the biosynthesis of γ-carboxyglutamic acid residues in the proteins which are essential for biological activity. warfarin sodium is thought to interfere with clotting factor synthesis by inhibition of the regeneration of vitamin K_1 epoxide. The degree of depression is dependent upon the dosage administered. Therapeutic doses of warfarin sodium decrease the total amount of the active form of each vitamin K dependent clotting factor made by the liver by approximately 30% to 50%.

An anticoagulation effect generally occurs within 24 hours after drug administration. However, peak anticoagulant effect may be delayed 72 to 96 hours. The duration of action of a single dose of racemic warfarin sodium is 2 to 5 days. The effects of warfarin sodium may become more pronounced as effects of daily maintenance doses overlap. Anticoagulants have no direct effect on an established thrombus, nor do they reverse ischemic tissue damage. However, once a thrombus has occurred, the goal of anticoagulant treatment is to prevent further extension of the formed clot and prevent secondary thromboembolic complications which may result in serious and possibly fatal sequelae.

PHARMACOKINETICS

Warfarin sodium is a racemic mixture of the R- and S- enantiomers. The S-enantiomer exhibits 2-5 times more anticoagulant activity than the R-enantiomer in humans, but generally has a more rapid clearance.

Absorption: Warfarin sodium is essentially completely absorbed after oral administration with peak concentration generally attained within the first 4 hours.

Distribution: There are no differences in the apparent volumes of distribution after intravenous and oral administration of single doses of warfarin sodium solution. warfarin sodium distributes into a relatively small apparent volume of distribution of about 0.14 liter/kg. A distribution phase lasting 6 to 12 hours is distinguishable after rapid intravenous or oral administration of an aqueous solution. Using a one compartment model, and assuming complete bioavailability, estimates of the volumes of distribution of R- and S-warfarin sodium are similar to each other and to that of the racemate. Concentrations in fetal plasma approach the maternal values, but warfarin sodium has not been found in human milk (see WARNINGS, Lactation.) Approximately 99% of the drug is bound to plasma proteins.

Metabolism: The elimination of warfarin sodium is almost entirely by metabolism. Warfarin sodium is stereoselectively metabolized by hepatic microsomal enzymes (cytochrome P-450) to inactive hydroxylated metabolites (predominant route) and by reductases to reduced metabolites (warfarin sodium alcohols). The warfarin sodium alcohols have minimal anticoagulant activity. The metabolites are principally excreted into the urine; and to a lesser extent into the bile. The metabolites of warfarin sodium that have been identified include dehydrowarfarin sodium, two diastereoisomer alcohols, 4'-, 6-, 7-, 8- and 10-hydroxywarfarin sodium. The Cytochrome P-450 isozymes involved in the metabolism of warfarin sodium include 2C9, 2C19, 2C8, 2C18, 1A2, and 3A4. 2C9 is likely to be the principal form of human liver P-450 which modulates the *in vivo* anticoagulant activity of warfarin sodium.

Excretion: The terminal half-life of warfarin sodium after a single dose is approximately one week; however, the effective half-life ranges from 20 to 60 hours, with a mean of about 40 hours. The clearance of R- warfarin sodium is generally half that of S-warfarin sodium, thus as the volumes of distribution are similar, the half-life of R-warfarin sodium is longer than that of S-warfarin sodium. The half-life of R-warfarin sodium ranges from 37 to 89 hours, while that of S-warfarin sodium ranges from 21 to 43 hours. Studies with radiolabeled drug have demonstrated that up to 92% of the orally administered dose is recovered in urine. Very little warfarin sodium is excreted unchanged in urine. Urinary excretion is in the form of metabolites.

Elderly: There are no significant age-related differences in the pharmacokinetics of racemic warfarin sodium. Limited information suggests that there is no difference in the clearance of S-warfarin sodium in elderly versus young subjects. However, there may be a slight decrease in the clearance of R-warfarin sodium in the elderly compared to the young. Older patients (60 years or older) appear to exhibit greater than expected PT/INR response to the anticoagulant effects of warfarin sodium. As patient age increases, less warfarin sodium is required to produce a therapeutic level of anticoagulation. The cause of the increased responsiveness to warfarin sodium is not known.

Renal Dysfunction: Renal clearance is considered to be a minor determinant of anticoagulant response to warfarin sodium. No dosage adjustment is necessary for patients with renal failure.

Hepatic Dysfunction: Hepatic dysfunction can potentiate the response to warfarin sodium through impaired synthesis of clotting factors and decreased metabolism of warfarin sodium.

CLINICAL PHARMACOLOGY: *(cont'd)*

The administration of warfarin sodium via the intravenous (IV) route should provide the patient with the same concentration of an equal oral dose, but maximum plasma concentration will be reached earlier. However, the full anticoagulant effect of a dose of warfarin sodium may not be achieved until 72-96 hours after dosing, indicating that the administration of IV warfarin sodium should not provide any increased biological effect or earlier onset of action.

MECHANICAL AND BIOPROSTHETIC HEART VALVES

In a prospective, randomized, open label, positive-controlled study (Mok, et al, 1985) in 254 patients, the thromboembolic-free interval was found to be significantly greater in patients with mechanical prosthetic heart valves treated with warfarin sodium alone compared with dipyridimole-aspirin (p<0.005) and pentoxifylline-aspirin (p<0.05) treated patients. Rates of thromboembolic events in these groups were 2.2, 8.6, and 7.9/100 patient years, respectively. Major bleeding rates were 2.5, 0.0, and 0.9/100 patient years, respectively.

In a prospective, open label, clinical trial (Saour, et al, 1990) comparing moderate (INR 2.65) vs. high intensity (INR 9.0) warfarin sodium therapies in 258 patients with mechanical prosthetic heart valves, thromboembolism occurred with similar frequency in the two groups (4.0 and 3.7 events/100 patient years, respectively). Major bleeding was more common in the high intensity group (2.1 events/100 patient years) vs. 0.95 events/100 patient years in the moderate intensity group.

In a randomized trial (Turpie, et al, 1988) in 210 patients comparing two intensities of warfarin sodium therapy (INR 2.0-2.25 vs. INR 2.5-4.0) for a three month period following tissue heart valve replacement, thromboembolism occurred with similar frequency in the two groups (major embolic events 2.0% vs 1.9%, respectively and minor embolic events 10.8% vs. 10.2%, respectively). Major bleeding complications were more frequent with the higher intensity (major hemorrhages 4.6%) vs. none in the lower intensity group.

CLINICAL STUDIES:

Atrial Fibrillation (AF): In five prospective randomized controlled clinical trials involving 3711 patients with nonrheumatic AF, warfarin sodium significantly reduced the risk of systemic thromboembolism including stroke (See TABLE 1) The risk reduction ranged from 60 % to 86% in all except one trial (CAFA: 45%) which stopped early due to published positive results from two of these trials. The incidence of major bleeding in these trials ranged from 0.6 to 2.7% (See TABLE 1) Meta-analysis findings of these studies revealed that the effects of warfarin sodium in reducing thromboembolic events including stroke were similar at either moderately high INR (2.0-4.5) or low INR (1.4-3.0). There was a significant reduction in minor bleeds at the low INR. Similar data from clinical studies in valvular atrial fibrillation patients are not available.

TABLE 1A Clinical Studies Of Warfarin Sodium In Non-Rheumatic AF Patients

Study	N: Warfarin Treated Patients	N: Control Patient	PT Ratio	INR
AFASAK	335	336	1.5-2.0	2.8-4.2
SPAF	210	211	1.3-1.8	2.0-4.5
BAATAF	212	208	1.2-1.5	1.5-2.7
CAFA	187	191	1.3-1.6	2.0-3.0
SPINAF	260	265	1.2-1.5	1.4-2.8

* All study results of warfarin sodium vs. control are based on intention-to-treat analysis and include ischemic stroke and systemic thromboembolism, excluding hemorrhage and transient ischemic attacks.

TABLE 1B Clinical Studies Of Warfarin Sodium In Non-Rheumatic AF Patients cont'd

Study	Thromboembolism % Risk Reduction	Thromboembolism pValue	% Major Bleeding Warfarin Treated Patients	% Major Bleeding Control Patient
AFASAK	60	0.027	0.6	0.0
SPAF	67	0.01	1.9	1.9
BAATAF	86	<0.05	0.9	0.5
CAFA	45	0.25	2.7	0.5
SPINAF	79	0.001	2.3	1.5

Myocardial Infarction: WARIS (The Warfarin Sodium Re-Infarction Study) was a double-blind, randomized study of 1214 patients 2 to 4 weeks post- infarction treated with warfarin sodium to a target INR of 2.8 to 4.8. (But note that a lower INR was achieved and increased bleeding was associated with INR's above 4.0; see DOSAGE AND ADMINISTRATION.) The primary endpoint was a combination of total mortality and recurrent infarction. A secondary endpoint of cerebrovascular events was assessed. Mean follow-up of the patients was 37 months. The results for each endpoint separately, including an analysis of vascular death, are provided in the following table:

TABLE 2

Event	Warfarin (n=607)	Placebo (n=607)	RR (95%CI)	% Risk Reduction (p-Value)
Total Patient Years of Follow-Up	2018	1944		
Total Mortality	94 (4.7/100 py)	123 (6.3/100 py)	0.76 (0.60, 0.97)	24 (p=0.030)
Vascular Death	82 (4.1/100 py)	105 (5.4/100 py)	0.78 (0.60, 1.02)	22 (p=0.068)
Recurrent MI	82 (4.1/100 py)	124 (6.4/100 py)	0.66 (0.51, 0.85)	34 (p=0.001)
Cardiovascular Event	20 (1.0/100 py)	44 (2.3/100 py)	0.46 (0.28, 0.75)	54 (p=0.002)

RR = Relative Risk
Risk Reduction = (I-RR)
CI = Confidence Interval
MI = Myocardial Infarction
py = patient years

INDICATIONS AND USAGE:

Warfarin sodium is indicated for the prophylaxis and/or treatment of venous thrombosis and its extension, and pulmonary embolism.

Warfarin sodium is indicated for the prophylaxis and/or treatment of the thromboembolic complications associated with atrial fibrillation and/or cardiac valve replacement.

INDICATIONS AND USAGE: *(cont'd)*

Warfarin sodium is indicated to reduce the risk of death, recurrent myocardial infarction, and thromboembolic events such as stroke or systemic embolization after myocardial infarction.

CONTRAINDICATIONS

Anticoagulation is contraindicated in any localized or general physical condition or personal circumstance in which the hazard of hemorrhage might be greater than the potential clinical benefits of anticoagulation, such as:

Pregnancy: Warfarin sodium is contraindicated in women who are or may become pregnant because the drug passes through the placental barrier and may cause fatal hemorrhage to the fetus *in utero.* Furthermore, there have been reports of birth malformations in children born to mothers who have been treated with warfarin sodium during pregnancy.

Embryopathy characterized by nasal hypoplasia with or without stippled epiphyses (chondrodysplasia punctata) has been reported in pregnant women exposed to warfarin sodium during the first trimester. Central nervous system abnormalities also have been reported, including dorsal midline dysplasia characterized by agenesis of the corpus callosum, Dandy-Walker malformation, and midline cerebellar atrophy. Ventral midline dysplasia, characterized by optic atrophy, and eye abnormalities have been observed. Mental retardation, blindness, and other central nervous system abnormalities have been reported in association with second and third trimester exposure. Although rare, teratogenic reports following *in utero* exposure to warfarin sodium include urinary tract anomalies such as single kidney, asplenia, anencephaly, spina bifida, cranial nerve palsy, hydrocephalus, cardiac defects and congenital heart disease, polydactyly, deformities of toes, diaphragmatic hernia, and corneal leukoma, cleft palate, cleft lip, schizencephaly, and microcephaly.

Spontaneous abortion and still birth are known to occur and a higher risk of fetal mortality is associated with the use of warfarin sodium. Low birth weight and growth retardation have also been reported.

Women of childbearing potential who are candidates for anticoagulant therapy should be carefully evaluated and the indications critically reviewed with the patient. If the patient becomes pregnant while taking this drug, she should be apprised of the potential risks to the fetus, and the possibility of termination of the pregnancy should be discussed in light of those risks.

Hemorrhagic tendencies or blood dyscrasias.

Recent or contemplated surgery of:

(1) central nervous system;

(2) eye;

(3) traumatic surgery resulting in large open surfaces.

Bleeding tendencies associated with active ulceration or overt bleeding of:

(1) gastrointestinal, genitourinary or respiratory tracts;

(2) cerebrovascular hemorrhage;

(3) aneurysms-cerebral, dissecting aorta;

(4) pericarditis and pericardial effusions;

(5) bacterial endocarditis.

Threatened abortion ,eclampsia, and preeclampsia

Inadequate laboratory facilities

Unsupervised patients with senility , alcoholism, psychosis, or lack of patient cooperation

Spinal puncture and other diagnostic or therapeutic procedures with potential for uncontrollable bleeding.

Miscellaneous: major regional, lumbar block anesthesia, and malignant hypertension.

WARNINGS:

The most serious risks associated with anticoagulant therapy with sodium warfarin sodium are hemorrhage in any tissue or organ and, less frequently(0.1%), necrosis and/or gangrene of skin and other tissues. The risk of hemorrhage is related to the level of intensity and the duration of anticoagulant therapy. Hemorrhage and necrosis have in some cases been reported to result in death or permanent disability. Necrosis appears to be associated with local thrombosis and usually appears within a few days of the start of anticoagulant therapy. In severe cases of necrosis, treatment through debridement or amputation of the affected tissue, limb, breast or penis has been reported. Careful diagnosis is required to determine whether necrosis is caused by an underlying disease. warfarin sodium therapy should be discontinued when warfarin sodium is suspected to be the cause of developing necrosis and heparin therapy may be considered for anticoagulation. Although various treatments have been attempted, no treatment for necrosis has been considered uniformly effective. See below for information on predisposing conditions. These and other risks associated with anticoagulant therapy must be weighed against the risk of thrombosis or embolization in untreated cases.

It cannot be emphasized too strongly that treatment of each patient is a highly individualized matter. Warfarin sodium, a narrow therapeutic range (index) drug, may be affected by factors such as other drugs and dietary Vitamin K. Dosage should be controlled by periodic determinations of prothrombin time (PT) /International Normalized Ratio (INR) or other suitable coagulation tests. Determinations of whole blood clotting and bleeding times are not effective measures for control of therapy. Heparin prolongs the one-stage PT. When heparin and warfarin sodium are administered concomitantly, refer below to CONVERSION FROM HEPARIN THERAPY for recommendations.

Caution should be observed when warfarin sodium is administered in any situation or in the presence of any predisposing condition where added risk of hemorrhage or necrosis is present.

Anticoagulation therapy with warfarin sodium may enhance the release of atheromatous plaque emboli, thereby increasing the risk of complications from systemic cholesterol microembolization, including the "purple toes syndrome." Discontinuation of warfarin sodium therapy is recommended when such phenomena are observed.

Systemic atheroemboli and cholesterol microemboli can present with a variety of signs and symptoms including purple toes syndrome, livedo reticularis, rash, gangrene, abrupt and intense pain in the leg, foot, or toes, foot ulcers, myalgia, penile gangrene, abdominal pain, flank or back pain, hematuria, renal insufficiency, hypertension, cerebral ischemia, spinal cord infarction, pancreatitis, symptoms stimulating polyarteritis, or any other sequelae of vascular compromise due to embolic occlusion. The most commonly involved visceral organs are the kidneys followed by the pancreas, spleen, and liver. Some cases have progressed to necrosis or death.

Purple toes syndrome is a complication of oral anticoagulation characterized by a dark, purplish or mottled color of the toes, usually occurring between 3-10 weeks, or later, after the initiation of therapy with warfarin sodium or related compounds. Major features of this syndrome include purple color of plantar surfaces and sides of the toes that blanches on moderate pressure and fades with elevation of the legs; pain and tenderness of the toes;

WARNINGS: *(cont'd)*

waxing and waning of the color over time. While the purple toes syndrome is reported to be reversible, some cases progress to gangrene or necrosis which may require debridement of the affected area, or may lead to amputation.

A severe elevation (> 50 seconds) in activated partial thromboplastin time (aPTT) with a PT/INR in the desired range has been identified as an indication of increased risk of postoperative hemorrhage.

The decision to administer anticoagulants in the following conditions must be based upon clinical judgment in which the risks of anticoagulant therapy are weighed against the benefits:

Lactation: Warfarin sodium appears in the milk of nursing mothers in an inactive form. Infants nursed by warfarin sodium treated mothers had no change in prothrombin times (PTs). Effects in premature infants have not been evaluated.

Severe to moderate hepatic or renal insufficiency.

Infectious diseases or disturbances of intestinal flora: sprue, antibiotic therapy.

Trauma which may result in internal bleeding.

Surgery or trauma: resulting in large exposed raw surfaces.

Indwelling catheters.

Severe to moderate hypertension.

Known or suspected deficiency in protein C mediated anticoagulant response: Hereditary or acquired deficiencies of protein C or its cofactor, protein S, have been associated with tissue necrosis following warfarin sodium administration. (Tissue necrosis may occur in the absence of protein C deficiency). Not all patients with these conditions develop necrosis, and tissue necrosis occurs in patients without these deficiencies. Inherited resistance to activated protein C has been described in many patients with venous thromboembolic disorders but has not yet been evaluated as a risk factor for tissue necrosis. The risk associated with these conditions, both for recurrent thrombosis and for adverse reaction, is difficult to evaluate since it does not appear to be the same for everyone. Decisions about testing and therapy must be made on an individual basis. It has been reported that concurrent anticoagulation therapy with heparin for 5 to 7 days during initiation of therapy with warfarin sodium may minimize the incidence of tissue necrosis. Warfarin sodium therapy should be discontinued when warfarin sodium is suspected to be the cause of developing necrosis and heparin therapy may be considered for anticoagulation.

Miscellaneous: polycythemia vera, vasculitis, severe diabetes

Minor and severe allergic/hypersensitivity reactions and anaphylactic reactions have been reported.

In patients with acquired or inherited warfarin sodium resistance, decreased therapeutic responses to warfarin sodium have been reported. Exaggerated therapeutic responses have been reported in other patients.

Patients with congestive heart failure may exhibit greater than expected PT/INR response to warfarin sodium, thereby requiring more frequent laboratory monitoring, and reduced doses of warfarin sodium.

Concurrent use of anticoagulants with streptokinase or urokinase is not recommended and may be hazardous. (Please note recommendations accompanying these preparations.)

PRECAUTIONS:

GENERAL

Periodic determination of PT/INR or other suitable coagulation test is essential.

Numerous factors, alone or in combination, including travel, changes in diet, environment, physical state and medication may influence response of the patient to anticoagulants. It is generally good practice to monitor the patient's response with additional PT determinations in the period immediately after discharge from the hospital, and whenever other medications are initiated, discontinued or taken irregularly. The following factors are listed for reference; however, other factors may also affect the anticoagulant response.

Drugs may interact with warfarin sodium through pharmacodynamic or pharmacokinetic mechanisms. Pharmacodynamic mechanisms for drug interactions with warfarin sodium are synergism (impaired hemostasis, reduced clotting factor synthesis), competitive antagonism (Vitamin K), and altered physiological control loop for vitamin K metabolism (hereditary resistance). Pharmacokinetic mechanisms for drug interactions with warfarin sodium are mainly enzyme induction, enzyme inhibition, and reduced plasma protein binding. It is important to note that some drugs may interact by more than one mechanism.

The following factors, alone or in combination, may be responsible for INCREASED PT/INR response:

Endogenous Factors:

Blood Dyscrasias: See CONTRAINDICATIONS	Infectious Hepatitis
Cancer	Jaundice
Collagen Vascular Disease	Hyperthyroidism
Congestive Heart Failure	Poor Nutritional State
Diarrhea	Steatorrhea
Elevated Temperature	Vitamin K Deficiency
Hepatic Disorders	

Exogenous Factors: Potential drug interactions with warfarin sodium are listed below by drug class and by specific drugs.

Classes of Drugs

Adrenergic Stimulants, Central	Diuretics‡
Alcohol Abuse Reduction Preparations	Fungal medications, Systemic‡
Analgesics	Gastric Acidity and Peptic Ulcer Agents ‡
Anesthetics, Inhalation	Gastrointestinal, Ulcerative ColitisAgents
Antiarrhythmics	Gout Treatment Agents
Antibiotics:	Hemorrheologic Agents
Aminoglycosides (oral)	Hepatotoxic Drugs
Cephalosporins, paternal	Hyperglycemic Agents
Macrolides	Hypertensive Emergency Agents
Miscellaneous	Hypnotics‡
Penicillins, intravenous, high dose	Monoamine Oxidase Inhibitors
Sulfonamides, long acting	Narcotics, prolonged
Tetracyclines	Non-steroidal Anti-inflammatory Agents
Anticoagulants	Pyschostimulants
Anticonvulsants‡	Pyrazolones
Antidepressants‡	Salicylates
Antimalarial Agents	Steroids, Adrenocortical ‡
Antineoplastics‡	Steroids, Anabolic (17-Alkyl Testosterone Derivatives)
Antiparasitic/Antimicrobials	Thrombolytics
Antiplatelet Drugs/Effects	Thyroid Drugs
Antithyroid Drugs	Tuberculosis Agents‡
Beta-Adrenergic Blockers	Uricsuric Agents
Bromelains	Vaccines
Cholelitholytic Agents	Vitamins‡
Diabetes Agents, Oral	

Specific Drugs Reported

Acetaminophen	Mefenamic
Alcohol‡	Methimazole‡

PRECAUTIONS: *(cont'd)*

Allopurinol
Aminosalicylic Acid
Aminodarone HCl
Aspirin
Cefamandole
Cefazolin
Cefoperazone
Cefotetan
Cefoxitin
Ceftriaxone
Chenodiol
Chloramphenicol
Chloral Hydrate‡
Chlorpropamide
Cholestyramine‡
Cimetidine
Ciprofloxacin
Clarithromycin
Clofibrate
Coumadin Overdose
Cyclophosphamide‡
Danazol
Dextran
Dextrothyroxine
Diazoxide
Diclofenac
Dicumarol
Diflunsial
Disulfiram
Doxycycline
Erthromycin
Ethacrynic Acid
Fenoprofen
Fluconazole
Fluorouracil
Glucagon
Halothane
Heparin
Ibuprofen
Ifosamide
Indomethacin
Influenza Virus Vaccine
Itraconazole
Ketoprofen
Ketorolac
Levamisole
Levothyroxine
Liothyronine
Lovastatin
Methyldopa
Methylphenidate
Methylsalicylate Ointment (Topical)
Miconazole
Moricizine HCl‡
Nalidixic Acid
Naproxen
Neomycin
Norfloxacin
Ofloxacin
Olsalazine
Omeprazole
Oxaprozin
Oxymetholone
Paroxetine
Penicillin G, intravenous
Pentoxifylline
Phenylbutazone
Phenytoin‡
Piperacillin
Piroxicam
Prednisone‡
Propafenone
Propoxyphene
Propranolol
Propylthiouracil‡
Quinidine
Quinine
Ranitidine‡
Sertaline
Simvastatin
Stanozolol
Streptokinase
Sulfamethizole
Sulfamethoxazole
Sulfinpyrazone
Sulfisoxazole
Sulindac
Tamoxifen
Tetracycline
Thyroid
Ticacillin
Ticlopidine
Tissue Plasminogen Activator (t-PA)
Tolbutamide
Trimethoprim/Sulfamethoxazole
Urokinase
Valproate
Vitamin E

‡ Increased and decreased PT/INR responses have been reported.

Other factors affecting blood elements which may modify hemostasis:dietary deficiencies; prolonged hot weather; unreliable PT/INR determinations

The following factors, alone or in combination, may be responsible for DECREASED PT response :

Endogenous Factors:

Edema
Hereditary Warfarin Resistance
Hyperlipemia
Hypothyroidism
Nephrotic Syndrome

Exogenous Factors: Potential drug interactions with warfarin sodium are listed below by drug class and by specific drugs.

Classes of Drugs

Adrenal Cortical Steroid Inhibitors
Antacids
Antianxiety Agents
Antiarrhythmics‡
Antibiotics‡
Anticonvulsants‡
Antidepressants‡
Antineoplastics‡
Antipsychotic Medications
Antithyroid Drugs‡
Barbiturates
Diuretics‡
Enteral Nutritional Supplments
Fungal Medications, Systemic
Gastric Acidity and Peptic Ulcer Agents‡
Hypnotics‡
Hypolipidemics‡
Immunosuppressives
Oral Contraceptives, Estrogen Containing
Steroids, Adrenocortical‡
Tuberculosis Agents‡
Vitamins‡

Specific Drugs Reported

Alcohol‡
Aminoglutethimide
Amobarbital
Azathioprine
Butabarbital
Butalbital
Carbamazepine
Chloral Hydrate
Chlordiazepoxide
Chlorthalidone
Cholestyramine‡
Corticotropin
Cortisone
Coumadin Underdosage
Cyclophosphamide‡
Dicloxaxillin
Ethchlorvynol
Glutethimide
Griseofulvin
Haloperidol
Meprobamate
Methimazole‡
Moricizine HCl‡
Nafcillin
Paraldehyde
Pentobarbital
Phenobarbital
Phenytoin‡
Phenytoin‡
Phenytoin‡
Prednisone‡
Primidone
Propylthiouracil‡
Ranitidine‡
Rifampin
Secobarbital
Spironolactone
Sucralfate
Trazodone
Vitamin C (High Dose)
Vitamin K

Also:

Diet high in in vitamin K

Unreliable PT/INR determinations

‡ Increased and decreased PT/INR responses have been reported.

Because a patient may be exposed to a combination of the above factors, the net effect of warfarin sodium PT/INR response may be unpredictable. More frequent PT/INR monitoring is therefore advisable. Medications of unknown interaction with coumarins are best regarded with caution. When these medications are started or stopped, more frequent PT monitoring is advisable.

It has been reported that concomitant administration of warfarin sodium and ticlopidine may be associated with cholestatic hepatitis.

PRECAUTIONS: *(cont'd)*

Effect on Other Drugs: Coumarins may also affect the action of other drugs. Hypoglycemic agents (chlorpropamide and tolbutamide) and anticonvulsants (phenytoin and phenobarbital) may accumulate in the body as a result of interference with either their metabolism or excretion.

Special Risk Patients: Warfarin sodium is a narrow therapeutic range (index) drug, and caution should be observed when warfarin sodium is administered to certain patients such as the elderly or debilitated or when administered in any situation or physical condition where added risk of hemorrhage is present.

Intramuscular (IM) injections of concomitant medications should be confined to the upper extremities which permits easy access for manual compression, inspections for bleeding and use of pressure bandages.

Caution should be observed when warfarin sodium is administered concomitantly with nonsteroidal anti-inflammatory drugs (NSAIDs), including aspirin, to be certain that no change in anticoagulation dosage is required. In addition to specific drug interactions that might affect PT, NSAIDS, including aspirin, can inhibit platelet aggregation, and can cause gastrointestinal bleeding, peptic ulceration and/or perforation.

Acquired or inherited warfarin sodium resistance should be suspected if large daily doses of warfarin sodium are required to maintain a patient's PT/INR within a normal therapeutic range.

INFORMATION FOR THE PATIENT

The objective of anticoagulant therapy is to decrease the clotting ability of the blood so that thrombosis is prevented, while avoiding spontaneous bleeding. Effective therapeutic levels with minimal complications are in part dependent upon cooperative and well-instructed patients who communicate effectively with their physician. Patients should be advised: Strict adherence to prescribed dosage schedule is necessary. Do not take or discontinue any other medication, except on advice of physician. Avoid alcohol consumption. Do not take warfarin sodium during pregnancy and do not become pregnant while taking it (See CONTRAINDICATIONS.) Avoid any activity or sport that may result in traumatic injury. Prothrombin time tests and regular visits to the physician or clinic are needed to monitor therapy. If the prescribed dose of warfarin sodium therapy is forgotten, notify the physician immediately. Take the dose as soon as possible on the same day but do not take a double dose of warfarin sodium the next day in order to make up for the missed doses. The amount of Vitamin K in food may affect therapy with warfarin sodium. Eat a normal, balanced diet maintaining a consistent amount of Vitamin K. Avoid drastic changes in dietary habits, such as eating large amounts of green leafy vegetables. Contact the physician if any illness, such as diarrhea, infection or fever develops. Notify physician immediately if any unusual bleeding or symptoms occur. Signs and symptoms of bleeding include pain, swelling or discomfort, prolonged bleeding from cuts, increased menstrual flow or vaginal bleeding, nosebleeds or bleeding of gums from brushing, unusual bleeding, bruising, red or dark brown urine, red or tar black stools, headache, dizziness, or weakness. If therapy with warfarin sodium is discontinued, patients should be cautioned that the anticoagulant effects of warfarin sodium may persist for about 2 to 5 days.

CARCINOGENESIS, MUTAGENESIS, AND IMPAIRMENT OF FERTILITY

Carcinogenicity and mutagenicity studies have not been performed with warfarin sodium. The reproductive effects of warfarin sodium have not been evaluated.

PREGNANCY CATEGORY X

See CONTRAINDICATIONS.

PEDIATRIC USE

Safety and effectiveness in pediatric patients below the age of 18 have not been established in randomized, controlled clinical trials. However, the use of warfarin sodium in pediatric patients is well-documented for the prevention and treatment of thromboembolic events. Difficulty achieving and maintaining therapeutic PT/INR ranges in the pediatric patient has been reported. More frequent PT/INR determinations are recommended because of possible changing warfarin sodium requirements.

ADVERSE REACTIONS:

POTENTIAL ADVERSE REACTIONS TO WARFARIN SODIUM MAY INCLUDE

Fatal or nonfatal hemorrhage from any tissue or organ: This is a consequence of the anticoagulant effect. The signs, symptoms, and severity will vary according to the location and degree or extent of the bleeding. Hemorrhagic complications may present as paralysis; paresthesia; headache, chest, abdomen, joint, muscule, or other pain; dizziness, shortness of breath, difficult breathing or swallowing; unexplained swelling; weakness; hypotension; or unexplained shock. Therefore, the possibility of hemorrhage should be considered in evaluating the condition of any anticoagulated patient with complaints which do not indicate an obvious diagnosis. Bleeding during anticoagulant therapy does not always correlate with PT/INR. (See OVERDOSAGE, Treatment.)

Bleeding: which occurs when the PT/INR is within the therapeutic range warrants diagnostic investigation since it may unmask a previously unsuspected lesion, e.g., tumor, ulcer, etc.

Necrosis of skin and other tissues. (See WARNINGS.)

Adverse reactions reported infrequently include: Hypersensitivity reactions, systemic cholesterol microembolization, purple toes syndrome, vasculitis, hepatitis, cholestatic hepatic injury, jaundice, elevated liver enzymes, fever, dermatitis, including bullous eroptions, urticaria, abdominal pain including cramping, asthenia, nausea, vomiting, diarrhea, headache, pruritis, alopecia, and paresthesia.

Rare events of tracheal or tracheobronchial calcification have been reported in association with long-term warfarin sodium therapy. The clinical significance of this event is unknown.

Priapism has been associated with anticoagulant administration, however, a causal relationship has not been established.

OVERDOSAGE:

Signs and Symptoms: Suspected or overt abnormal bleeding (*e.g.,* appearance of blood in stools or urine, hematuria, excessive menstrual bleeding, melena, petechiae, excessive bruising or persistent oozing from superficial injuries) are early manifestations of anticoagulation beyond a safe and satisfactory level.

Treatment: Excessive anticoagulation, with or without bleeding, may be controlled by discontinuing warfarin sodium therapy and if necessary, by administration of oral or parenteral vitamin K_1. (Please see recommendations accompanying vitamin K_1preparations prior to use.)

Such use of vitamin K_1 reduces response to subsequent warfarin sodium therapy. Patients may return to a pretreatment thrombotic status following the rapid reversal of a prolonged PT/INR. Resumption of warfarin sodium administration reverses the effect of vitamin K, and a therapeutic PT/INR can again be obtained by careful dosage adjustment. If rapid anticoagulation is indicated, heparin may be preferable for initial therapy.

If minor bleeding progresses to major bleeding, give 5 to 25 mg (rarely up to 50 mg) parenteral vitamin K_1. In emergency situations of severe hemorrhage, clotting factors can be returned to normal by administering 200 to 500 ml of fresh whole blood or fresh frozen plasma, or by giving commercial Factor IX complex.

OVERDOSAGE: *(cont'd)*

A risk of hepatitis and other viral diseases is associated with the use of these blood products; Factor IX complex is also associated with an increased risk of thrombosis. Therefore, these preparations should be used only in exceptional or life-threatening bleeding episodes secondary to warfarin sodium overdosage.

Purified Factor IX preparations should not be used because they cannot increase the levels of prothrombin, Factor VII and Factor X which are also depressed along with the levels of Factor IX as a result of warfarin sodium treatment. Packed red blood cells may also be given if significant blood loss has occurred. Infusions of blood or plasma should be monitored carefully to avoid precipitating pulmonary edema in elderly patients or patients with heart disease.

DOSAGE AND ADMINISTRATION:

The dosage and administration of warfarin sodium must be individualized for each patient according to the particular patient's PT/INR response to the drug. The dosage should be adjusted based upon the patient's PT/INR. (See Laboratory Control below for full discussion on INR.)

Venous Thromboembolism (including pulmonary embolism): Available clinical evidence indicates that an INR or 2.0-3.0 is sufficient for prophylaxis and treatment of venous thromboembolism and minimizes the risk of hemorrhage associated with higher INRs.

Atrial Fibrillation: Five recent clinical trials evaluated the effects of warfarin sodium in patients with nonvalvular atrial fibrillation (AF). Meta-analysis findings of these studies revealed that the effects of warfarin sodium in reducing thromboembolic events including stroke were similar at either moderately high INR (2.0-4.5) or low INR (1.4-3.0). There was a significant reduction in minor bleeds at the low INR. Similar data from clinical studies in valvular atrial fibrillation patients are not available. The trials in non-valvular atrial fibrillation support the American College of Chest Physicians' (ACCP) recommendation that an INR of 2.0-3.0 be used for long term warfarin sodium therapy in appropriate AF patients.

Post-Myocardial Infarction: In post-myocardial infarction patients, warfarin sodium therapy should be initiated early (2-4 weeks post-infarction) and dosage should be adjusted to maintain an INR of 2.5-3.5 long-term. The recommendation is based on the results of the WARIS study in which treatment was initiated 2 to 4 weeks after infarction. In patients thought to be at an increased risk of bleeding complications or on aspirin therapy, maintenance of warfarin sodium therapy at the lower end of the INR range is recommended.

Mechanical and Bioprosthetic Heart Valves: In patients with mechanical heart valves, long term prophylaxis with warfarin sodium to an INR of 2.5-3.5 is recommended. In patients with bioprosthetic heart valves, based on limited data, the American College of Chest Physicians recommends warfarin sodium therapy to an INR of 2.0-3.0 for 12 weeks after valve insertion. In patients with additional risk factors such as atrial fibrillation or prior thromboembolism, consideration should be given for longer term therapy.

Recurrent Systemic Embolism: In cases where the risk of thromboembolism is great, such as in patients with recurrent systemic embolism, a higher INR may be required.

An INR of greater than 4.0 appears to provide no additional therapeutic benefit in most patients and is associated with a higher risk of bleeding.

Initial Dosage: The dosing of warfarin sodium must be individualized according to patient's sensitivity to the drug as indicated by the PT/INR. Use of a large loading dose may increase the incidence of hemorrhagic and other complications, does not offer more rapid protection against thrombi formation, and is not recommended. Low initiation doses are recommended for elderly and/or debilitated patients and patients with potential to exhibit greater than expected PT/INR response to warfarin sodium (See PRECAUTIONS). It is recommended that warfarin sodium therapy be initiated with a dose of 2 to 5 mg per day with dosage adjustments based on the results of PT/INR determinations.

Maintenance: Most patients are satisfactorily maintained at a dose of 2 to 10 mg daily. Flexibility of dosage is provided by breaking scored tablets in half. The individual dose and interval be gauged by the patient's prothrombin response.

Duration of Therapy: The duration of therapy in each patient should be individualized. In general, anticoagulant therapy should be continued until the danger of thrombosis and embolism has passed.

Missed Dose: The anticoagulant effect of warfarin sodium persists beyond 24 hours. If the patient forgets to take the prescribed dose of warfarin sodium at the scheduled time, the dose should be taken as soon as possible on the same day. The patient should not take the missed dose by doubling the daily dose to make up for missed doses, but should refer back to his or her physician.

Intravenous Route of Administration: Warfarin sodium for injection provides an alternate administration route for patients who cannot receive oral drugs. The I.V. dosages would be the same as those that would be used orally if the patient could take the drug by the oral route. Warfarin sodium for injection should be administered as a slow bolus injection over 1 to 2 minutes into a peripheral vein. It is not recommended for intramuscular administration. The vial should be reconstituted with 2.7 mL of sterile Water for Injection and inspected for particulate matter and/or discoloration immediately prior to use. Do not use if either particulate matter and/or discoloration is noted. After reconstitution, warfarin sodium for injection is chemically and physically stable for 4 hours at room temperature. It does not contain any antimicrobial preservative and, thus, care must be taken to assure the sterility of the prepared solution. The vial is not recommended for multiple use and unused solution should be discarded.

LABORATORY CONTROL

The PT reflects the depression of Vitamin K dependent Factors VII, X, and II. There are several modifications of the one-stage PT and the physician should become familiar with the specific method used in his laboratory. The degree of anticoagulation indicated by any range of PTs may be altered by the type of thromboplastin used; the appropriate therapeutic range must be base don the experience of each laboratory. The PT should be determined daily after the administration of the initial dose until PT/INR results stabilize in the therapeutic range. Intervals between subsequent PT/INR determinations should be based upon the physician's judgement of the patient's reliability and response to warfarin sodium in order to maintain the individual within the therapeutic range. Acceptable intervals for PT/INR determinations are normally within the range of one to four weeks after a stable dosage has been determined. To ensure adequate control, it is recommended that additional PT test are done when other warfarin sodium products are interchanged with warfarin sodium and also if other medications are coadministered with warfarin sodium (See PRECAUTIONS).

Different thromboplastin reagents vary substantially in their sensitivity to warfarin sodium-induced effects on PT. To define the appropriate therapeutic regimen it is important to be familiar with the sensitivity of the thromboplastin reagent used in the laboratory and its relationship to the International Reference Preparation (IRP), a sensitive thromboplastin reagent prepared from human brain.

A system of standardizing the PT in oral anticoagulant control was introduced by the World Health Organization in 1983. It is based upon the determination of an International Normalized Ratio (INR) which provides a common basis for communication of PT results and interpretations of therapeutic ranges. The INR system of reporting is based on a logarithmic relationship between the PT ratios of the test and reference preparation. The INR

DOSAGE AND ADMINISTRATION: *(cont'd)*

is the PT ratio that would be obtained if the International Reference Preparation (IRP), which has an ISI of 1.0 were used to perform the test. Early clinical studies of oral anticoagulants, which formed the basis for recommended therapeutic ranges of 1.5 to 2.5 times control mean normal PT, used sensitive human brain thromboplastin. When using the less sensitive rabbit brain thromboplastins commonly employed in PT assays today, adjustments must be made to the targeted PT range that reflect this decrease in sensitivity.

The INR can be calculated as:

$$\text{INR} = (\text{observed PT ratio})^{\text{ISI}}$$

where the ISI (International Sensitivity Index) is the correction factor in the equation that relates the PT ratio of the local reagent to the reference preparation and is a measure of the sensitivity of a given thromboplastin to reduction of Vitamin K —dependent coagulation factors; the lower the ISI, the more sensitive the reagent and the closer the derived INR will be to the observed PT ratio [1]

The proceedings and recommendations of the 1992 National Conference on Antithrombotic Therapy [2-4] review and evaluate issues related to oral anticoagulant therapy and the sensitivity of thromboplastin reagents and provide additional guidelines for defining the appropriate therapeutic regimen.

The conversion of the INR to PT ratios for the less intense (INR 2.0-3.0) and more intense (INR 2.5-3.5) therapeutic range recommended by the ACCP for thromboplastins over a range of ISI values shown in TABLE 3.[5]

TABLE 3 Relationship Between INR and PT Ratios For Thromboplastins With Different ISI Values

		PT RATIOS			
	ISI	ISI	ISI	ISI	ISI
	1.0	1.4	1.8	2.3	2.8
INR=2.0-3.0	2.0-3.0	1.6-2.2	1.5-1.8	1.4-1.6	1.3-1.5
INR=2.5-3.5	2.5-3.5	1.9-2.4	1.7-2.0	1.5-1.7	1.4-1.6

TREATMENT DURING DENTISTRY AND SURGERY

The management of patients who undergo dental and surgical procedures requires close liaison between attending physicians, surgeons and dentists. PT/INR determination is recommended just prior to any dental or surgical procedure. In patients undergoing minimal invasive procedures who must be anticoagulated prior to, during, or immediately following these procedures, adjusting the dosage of warfarin sodium to maintain the PT at the low end of the therapeutic range may safely allow for continued anticoagulation. The operative site should be sufficiently limited and accessible to permit the effective use of local procedures for hemostasis. Under these conditions, dental and surgical procedures may be performed without undue risk of hemorrhage. Some dental or surgical procedures may necessitate the interruption of warfarin sodium therapy. When discontinuing warfarin sodium even for a short period of time, the benefits and risks should be strongly considered.

CONVERSION FROM HEPARIN THERAPY

Since the anticoagulant effect of warfarin sodium is delayed, heparin is preferred initially for rapid anticoagulation. Conversion to warfarin sodium may begin concomitantly with heparin therapy or may be delayed 3 to 6 days. To ensure continuous anticoagulation, it is advisable to continue full dose heparin therapy and the warfarin sodium therapy be overlapped with heparin for 4 to 5 days, until warfarin sodium has produced the desired therapeutic response as determined by PT/INR. When warfarin sodium has produced the desired PT/INR, heparin may be discontinued.

Warfarin sodium may increase the aPTT test. During initial therapy with warfarin sodium, the interference with heparin anticoagulation is of minimal clinical significance. As heparin may affect the PT/INR, patients receiving both heparin and warfarin sodium should have blood for PT ratio/INR determination drawn at least:

5 hours after the last IV bolus dose of heparin, or

4 hours after cessation of a continuous IV infusion of heparin, or

24 hours after the last subcutaneous heparin injection.

REFERENCES:

1. Poller, L. : Laboratory Control of Anticoagulant Therapy. Seminars in Thrombosis and Hemostasis, Vol. 12, No.1, pp. 13-19, 1986. **2.** Hirsh, J.: Is the Dose of Warfarin Sodium Prescribed by American Physicians Unnecessarily High?*Arch Int Med,*Vol. 147, pp. 769- 771, 1987. **3.** Cook, D.J., Guyatt, H.G., Laupacis, A., Sackett, D.L.: Rules of Evidence and CLinical Recommendations on the Use of Antithrombotic Agents. Chest ACCP Consensus Conference on Antithrombotic Therapy. *Chest*, Vol. 12, (Suppl), pp.305S-311S, 1992 **4.** Hirsh, J., Dalen, J., Deykin, D., Poller, L.: Oral Anticoagulants Mechanism of Action. Clinical Effectiveness, and Optimal Therapeutic Range. Chest ACCP Consensus Conference on Antithrombotic Therapy. *Chest*, Vol.102 (Suppl), pp.312S-326S, 1992 **5.** Hirsh, J., M.D., F.C.C.P.: Hamilton Civic Hospitals Research Center, Hamilton, Ontario, Personal Communication.

PATIENT INFORMATION:

Warfarin sodium is used to decrease the clotting ability of the blood to prevent thrombosis. Do not use if you are pregnant or have bleeding tendencies. Inform your doctor of any other medications you are taking, including over the counter drugs. Take as directed by your doctor. Avoid alcohol or activities that could result in injury or bleeding. Carry identification stating you are taking warfarin. May cause bleeding, bruising, diarrhea, infection or fever. Inform your doctor or pharmacist if these effects occur.

HOW SUPPLIED:

Tablets: For oral use, single scored, imprinted numerically and packaged in bottles of 30, 100, 1000 and Hospital Blister Packs of 100.

Coumadin oral tablets are available in 1, 2, 2-1/2, 4, 5, 7-1/2, and 10 mg of crystalline warfarin sodium with one face inscribed with the word COUMADIN, single scored and imprinted numerically with the 1, 2, 2-1/2, 4, 5, 7-1/2, or 10 superimposed, and on the other face inscribed with the word "DuPont."

Protect from Light. Store in carton until contents have been used. Store at controlled room temperature (59°-86°F, 15°-30° C). Dispense in a tight, light resistant container as defined in the USP.

Injection: Available for intravenous use only. Not recommended for intramuscular administration. Reconstitute with 2.7 mL of sterile Water for Injection to yield 2 mg/mL. Net contents 5.4 mg lyophilized powder. Maximum yield 2.5 mL.

Protect from light. Keep vial in box until used. Store at controlled room temperature (59°-86°F, 15°-30° C)

After reconstitution, store at controlled room temperature (59°-86°F, 15°-30° C) and use within 4 hours. Do not refrigerate. Discard any unused solution.

HOW SUPPLIED - EQUIVALENTS NOT AVAILABLE:

Injection, Solution - Intravenous - 5 mg

1's $18.75 COUMADIN, Du Pont Merck 00590-0324-35

HOW SUPPLIED - EQUIVALENTS NOT AVAILABLE: *(cont'd)*

Tablet, Uncoated - Oral - 1 mg

100's	**$45.35**	**COUMADIN, Dupont Pharma**	**00056-0169-70**
100's	**$45.35**	**COUMADIN, Dupont Pharma**	**00056-0169-75**
1000's	**$453.75**	**COUMADIN, Dupont Pharma**	**00056-0169-90**

Tablet, Uncoated - Oral - 2 mg

30's	**$14.20**	**COUMADIN, Dupont Pharma**	**00056-0170-30**
100's	**$47.35**	**COUMADIN, Dupont Pharma**	**00056-0170-70**
100's	**$47.35**	**COUMADIN, Dupont Pharma**	**00056-0170-75**
1000's	**$473.50**	**COUMADIN, Dupont Pharma**	**00056-0170-90**

Tablet, Uncoated - Oral - 2.5 mg

30's	**$14.65**	**COUMADIN, Dupont Pharma**	**00056-0176-30**
100's	**$48.80**	**COUMADIN, Dupont Pharma**	**00056-0176-70**
100's	**$48.80**	**COUMADIN, Dupont Pharma**	**00056-0176-75**
1000's	**$488.00**	**COUMADIN, Dupont Pharma**	**00056-0176-90**

Tablet, Uncoated - Oral - 4 mg

100's	**$49.15**	**COUMADIN, Dupont Pharma**	**00056-0168-70**
100's	**$49.15**	**COUMADIN, Dupont Pharma**	**00056-0168-75**
1000's	**$491.50**	**COUMADIN, Dupont Pharma**	**00056-0168-90**

Tablet, Uncoated - Oral - 5 mg

30's	**$14.85**	**COUMADIN, Dupont Pharma**	**00056-0172-30**
100's	$30.90	Warfarin Sodium, United Res	00677-0794-01
100's	**$49.50**	**COUMADIN, Dupont Pharma**	**00056-0172-70**
100's	**$49.50**	**COUMADIN, Dupont Pharma**	**00056-0172-75**
1000's	**$494.95**	**COUMADIN, Dupont Pharma**	**00056-0172-90**

Tablet, Uncoated - Oral - 7.5 mg

100's	**$72.60**	**COUMADIN, Dupont Pharma**	**00056-0173-70**
100's	**$72.60**	**COUMADIN, Dupont Pharma**	**00056-0173-75**

Tablet, Uncoated - Oral - 10 mg

100's	**$75.30**	**COUMADIN, Dupont Pharma**	**00056-0174-70**
100's	**$75.30**	**COUMADIN, Dupont Pharma**	**00056-0174-75**

WATER FOR INJECTION, STERILE *(002445)*

CATEGORIES: Electrolytic, Caloric-Water Balance; Irrigating Solutions; Otic Preparations; Otologic; Pharmaceutical Aids; Vertigo/Motion Sickness/Vomiting; FDA Approval Pre 1982

BRAND NAMES: Bacteriostatic Water; Sterile Water; Water

FORMULARIES: Medi-Cal; WHO

Prescribing information not available at time of publication.

HOW SUPPLIED - RATED THERAPEUTICALLY EQUIVALENT:

Injection, Solution - Intravenous

10 ml	$1.40	Sterile Water, Abbott	00074-4887-10
10 ml	$1.40	Water, Abbott	00074-4887-25
10 ml x 25	$9.82	Water, Fujisawa USA	00469-0185-25
10 ml x 25	$23.13	Sterile Water, Fujisawa USA	00469-0185-15
20 ml	$1.76	Sterile Water, Abbott	00074-4887-20
20 ml x 25	$34.38	WATER, Fujisawa USA	00469-0185-20
30 ml	$1.88	BACTERIOSTATIC WATER, Abbott	00074-3977-03
30 ml	$2.08	BACTERIOSTATIC WATER, Hyrex Pharms	00314-0794-30
50 ml	$2.53	Sterile Water, Abbott	00074-4887-50
50 ml x 25	$39.69	Water, Fujisawa USA	00469-0185-50
100 ml	$3.49	Sterile Water, Abbott	00074-4887-99
250 ml	$9.11	Sterile Water, McGaw	00264-7850-20
500 ml x 10	$5.78	Sterile Water, McGaw	00264-1850-10
500 ml x 24	$9.11	Sterile Water For Injection, McGaw	00264-7850-10
1000 ml	$9.97	Sterile Water, Baxter Hlthcare	00338-0013-04
1000 ml	$10.47	Sterile Water, Abbott	00074-7990-09
1000 ml x 12	$10.04	Sterile Water, McGaw	00264-7850-00
2000 ml	$9.10	Sterile Water, Baxter Hlthcare	00338-0013-06
2000 ml	$17.94	Water, Abbott	00074-7118-07

Liquid - Irrigation - 100 %

1000 ml	$5.45	Sterile Water, Baxter Hlthcare	00338-0003-44
2000 ml	$8.38	Sterile Water, Baxter Hlthcare	00338-0003-46
3000 ml	$15.00	Sterile Water, Baxter Hlthcare	00338-0003-47
5000 ml	$20.70	Sterile Water, Baxter Hlthcare	00338-0003-49

Solution - Irrigation - 100 %

250 ml	$11.18	Sterile Water, Baxter Hlthcare	00338-0004-02
250 ml	$11.74	Sterile Water, Abbott	00074-6139-02
500 ml	$11.18	Sterile Water, Baxter Hlthcare	00338-0004-03
500 ml	$11.74	Sterile Water, Abbott	00074-6139-03
500 ml x 12	$12.29	Sterile Water, McGaw	00264-2101-10
1000 ml	$6.18	Water, Baxter Hlthcare	00338-0002-04
1000 ml	$7.49	Sterile Water, Abbott	00074-7973-05
1000 ml	$10.86	Sterile Water, Abbott	00074-6139-09
1000 ml	$11.53	Sterile Water, Baxter Hlthcare	00338-0004-04
1000 ml	$14.39	Sterile Water, Abbott	00074-7139-09
1000 ml x 12	$12.06	Sterile Water, McGaw	00264-2101-00
1500 ml	$14.82	Sterile Water, Abbott	00074-6139-06
1500 ml	$15.74	Sterile Water, Baxter Hlthcare	00338-0004-05
1500 ml	$19.58	WATER, Abbott	00074-7139-06
2000 ml	$11.54	Sterile Water, Abbott	00074-7973-07
2000 ml x 6	$19.38	Sterile Water, McGaw	00264-2101-50
3000 ml	$17.25	Sterile Water, Abbott	00074-7973-08
4000 ml x 4	$22.20	Sterile Water, McGaw	00264-2101-70

HOW SUPPLIED - NOT RATED EQUIVALENT:

Inhalant - Inhalation

3 ml x 100	$24.20	WATER FOR INHALATION, Dey Labs	49502-0810-03
5 ml x 100	$24.20	WATER FOR INHALATION, Dey Labs	49502-0810-05
2000 ml	$12.10	Water, Abbott	00074-7907-07

Injection, Solution - Intravenous

5 ml	$1.64	Sterile Water, Abbott	00074-4027-02
5 ml x 25	$14.10	Sterile Water, Gensia Labs	00703-7503-04
5 ml x 25	$14.69	Sterile Water, Am Regent	00517-3005-25
5 ml x 25	$19.06	WATER, Fujisawa USA	00469-5185-25
5 ml x 25	$20.00	Water, Consolidated Midland	00223-8979-05
5 ml x 100	$36.88	Sterile Water, Am Regent	00517-0990-75
10 ml	$1.80	Water, Steris Labs	00402-1057-10
10 ml	$1.80	DILUENT, Major Pharms	00904-0895-10
10 ml	$2.17	Sterile Water, Abbott	00074-4044-02
10 ml	$10.35	Water, Rugby	00536-3615-04

HOW SUPPLIED - NOT RATED EQUIVALENT: *(cont'd)*

10 ml x 25	$18.25	Water for Injection, P.F., Pasadena	00418-2441-10
10 ml x 25	$19.69	Sterile Water, Am Regent	00517-3010-25
10 ml x 25	$21.00	Sterile Water, Gensia Labs	00703-7514-04
10 ml x 25	$21.25	BACTERIOSTATIC WATER, Fujisawa USA	00469-0249-25
10 ml x 25	$22.50	Water, Consolidated Midland	00223-8980-10
10 ml x 25	$23.50	Water for Injection, B.A., Pasadena	00418-2461-10
10 ml x 25	$43.75	Water, Consolidated Midland	00223-8884-10
20 ml	$2.83	Sterile Water, Abbott	00074-4029-03
20 ml x 25	$22.19	Sterile Water, Am Regent	00517-3020-25
20 ml x 25	$23.50	Water for Injection, P.F., Pasadena	00418-2441-20
20 ml x 25	$26.10	Water, Gensia Labs	00703-7515-04
25 x 30 ml	$48.25	Water for Injection, Parabens, Pasadena	00418-2471-66
30 ml	$0.72	Water Injectable, Lannett	00527-0118-58
30 ml	$0.92	Water, Insource	58441-0102-30
30 ml	$1.83	Bacteriostatic Water, Geneva Pharms	00781-3130-90
30 ml	$1.99	BACTERIOSTATIC H2O, HL Moore Drug Exch	00839-5180-36
30 ml	$2.25	Water, Steris Labs	00402-1057-30
30 ml	$2.45	Water, Goldline Labs	00182-0741-66
30 ml	$2.45	Water, Goldline Labs	00182-3116-66
30 ml	$2.45	Bacteriostatic Water, United Res	00677-0329-23
30 ml	$2.50	Water Bacteriostatic, C O Truxton	00463-1084-30
30 ml	$2.50	DILUENT, Major Pharms	00904-0895-30
30 ml	$3.75	Water, Rugby	00536-2610-75
30 ml	$35.93	BACTERIOSTATIC WATER, Am Regent	00517-0662-25
30 ml x 25	$12.19	BACTERIOSTATIC WATER, Elkins Sinn	00641-2800-45
30 ml x 25	$24.30	BACTERIOSTATIC WATER, Gensia Labs	00703-7556-04
30 ml x 25	$28.25	Water, Fujisawa USA	00469-2250-25
30 ml x 25	$29.68	BACTERIOSTATIC WATER, Fujisawa USA	00469-2249-25
30 ml x 25	$36.50	Water for Injection, B.A., Pasadena	00418-2461-66
30 ml x 25	$43.75	Water, Consolidated Midland	00223-8883-30
30 ml x 100	$67.98	Water Injectable, Lannett	00527-0118-57
50 ml x 10	$11.76	Water, Gensia Labs	00703-7597-03
50 ml x 25	$30.94	Sterile Water, Am Regent	00517-3050-25
100 ml	$4.10	Sterile Water, Abbott	00074-1490-01
100 ml x 10	$17.28	Water, Gensia Labs	00703-7518-03
100 ml x 25	$54.00	Water, Consolidated Midland	00223-8982-70
100 ml x 25	$68.75	Sterile Water, Fujisawa USA	00469-2185-25
250 ml	$9.73	Sterile Water, Abbott	00074-1590-02
250 ml x 12	$5.35	Sterile Water, McGaw	00264-1920-20
500 ml	$6.37	Water, Abbott	00074-1590-03
500 ml fill/100	$9.37	Sterile Water, McGaw	00264-1920-01
500 ml x 12	$10.20	Sterile Water, McGaw	00264-1920-10
650 ml fill/100	$6.36	Sterile Water, McGaw	00264-1920-03
1000 ml	$11.56	Sterile Water, Abbott	00074-1590-05
1000 ml x 6	$11.01	Sterile Water, McGaw	00264-1920-00
2000 ml x 6	$22.40	Sterile Water, McGaw	00264-1920-50

Solution - Irrigation - 100 %

500 ml	$3.33	Sterile Water For Irrigation, HL Moore Drug Exch	00839-6675-83

YELLOW FEVER VACCINE *(001292)*

CATEGORIES: Immunologic; Serums, Toxoids and Vaccines; Vaccines; Yellow Fever Vaccine; FDA Pre 1938 Drugs

BRAND NAMES: Yf-Vax

FORMULARIES: WHO

Prescribing information not available at time of publication.

HOW SUPPLIED - EQUIVALENTS NOT AVAILABLE:

Injection, Lyphl-Susp - Subcutaneous - 2000 unit

1's	$236.63	YF-VAX, Connaught Labs	49281-0915-01
5's	$189.38	YF-VAX, Connaught Labs	49281-0915-05

YOHIMBINE HYDROCHLORIDE *(002450)*

CATEGORIES: Alpha Receptor Blocking Agents; Antihypertensives; Autonomic Drugs; Cardiovascular Drugs; Impotence; Mydriatics; Parasympatholytics; Sympatholytic Agents; Hypertension*; FDA Pre 1938 Drugs
* Indication not approved by the FDA

BRAND NAMES: **Actibine**; Aphrodyne; Dayto-Himbin; Erex; Thybine; Yocon; Yohimbine Hcl; Yohimex; Yomax

DESCRIPTION:

Yohimbine is a 3α-15α-20β-17α-hydroxy Yohimbine-16α-carboxylic acid methyl ester. The alkaloid is found in Rubaceae and related trees. Also in Rauwolfia Serpentina (L) Benth.

Yohimbine is an indolalkylamine alkaloid with chemical similarity to reserpine. It is a crystalline powder, odorless. Each compressed tablet contains 5.4 mg of Yohimbine Hydrochloride. Also contains: colloidal silicon dioxide, lactose, magnesium stearate, microcrystalline cellulose, pregelatinized starch and stearic acid.

CLINICAL PHARMACOLOGY:

Yohimbine blocks presynaptic alpha-2-adrenergic receptors. Its action or peripheral blood vessels resembles that of reserpine, though it is weaker and of short duration. Yohimbine's peripheral autonomic nervous system effect is to increase parasympathetic (cholinergic) and decrease sympathetic (adrenergic) activity. It is to be noted that in male sexual performance, erection is linked to cholinergic activity and to alpha-2 adrenergic blockade which may theoretically result in increased penile inflow, decreased penile blood outflow or both. Yohimbine exerts a stimulating action on the mood and may increase anxiety. Such actions have not been adequately studied or related to dosage although they appear to require high doses of the drug. Yohimbine has a mild anti- diuretic action, probably via stimulation of hypothalamic centers and release of posterior pituitary hormone.

Reportedly, Yohimbine exerts no significant influence on cardiac stimulation and other effects mediated by β-adrenergic receptors, its effect on blood pressure, if any would be to lower it; however, no adequate studies are at hand to quantitate this effect in terms of yohimbine dosage.

INDICATIONS AND USAGE:

Yohimbine hydrochloride is indicated as a sympathicolytic and mydriatic. It may have activity as an aphrodisiac.

CONTRAINDICATIONS:

Renal diseases, and patient's sensitive to the drug. In view of the limited and inadequate information at hand, no precise tabulation can be offered of additional contraindications.

WARNINGS:

Generally, this drug is not proposed for use in females and certainly must not be used during pregnancy. Neither is this drug proposed for use in pediatric, geriatric or cardio-renal patients with gastric or duodenal ulcer history. Nor should it be used in conjunction with mood-modifying drugs such as antidepressants, or in psychiatric patients in general.

ADVERSE REACTIONS:

Yohimbine readily penetrates the (CNS) and produces a complex pattern of responses in lower doses than those required to produce peripheral α-adrenergic blockade. These include, anti-diuresis, a general picture of central excitation including elevation of blood pressure and heart rate, increased motor activity, nervousness, irritability and tremor. Sweating, nausea and vomiting are common after parenteral administration of the drug.[1,2] Also, dizziness, headache skin flushing reported when used orally.[1,3]

DOSAGE AND ADMINISTRATION:

Experimental dosage reported in treatment of erectile impotence:[1,3,4] one tablet (5.4 mg) 3 times a day, to adult males taken orally. Occasional side effects reported with this dosage is to be reduced to 1/2 tablet 3 times a day followed by gradual increases to 1 tablet 3 times a day. Reported therapy not more than 10 weeks.[3]

REFERENCES:

1. A. Morales et al., New England Journal of Medicine: 1221. November 12, 1981. **2.** Goodman, Gilman - The Pharmacological basis of Therapeutics 6th ed., p. 176-188,McMillan. **3.** Weekly Urological Clinical letter, 27:2, July 4, 1983. **4.** A. Morales et al., The Journal of Urology 128:45-47, 1982.

HOW SUPPLIED - RATED THERAPEUTICALLY EQUIVALENT:

Tablet - Oral - 5.4 mg

100's	$20.00	Yohimbine Hcl, Duramed Pharms	51285-0877-02
1000's	$195.00	Yohimbine Hcl, Duramed Pharms	51285-0877-05

HOW SUPPLIED - NOT RATED EQUIVALENT:

Tablet, Uncoated - Oral - 5.4 mg

30's	$18.78	YOCON, Palisades Pharms	53159-0001-30
100's	$10.95	Yohimbine Hcl, Eon Labs Mfg	00185-0998-01
100's	$12.15	Yohimbine Hcl, Concord Labs	20254-0017-01
100's	$13.88	Yohimbine Hcl, IDE-Interstate	00814-8600-14
100's	$15.23	Yohimbine Hcl, H N Norton Co.	50732-0820-01
100's	$17.19	Yohimbine HCl, Rugby	00536-4989-01
100's	$17.20	Yohimbine Hydrochloride, United Res	00677-1417-01
100's	$17.55	Yohimbine Hcl, Major Pharms	00904-3255-60
100's	$17.85	Yohimbine Hcl, Mikart	46672-0111-10
100's	$17.95	Yohimbine Hcl, Jerome Stevens	50564-0509-01
100's	$18.00	Yohimbine Hcl, Goldline Labs	00182-1625-01
100's	$18.44	Yohimbine Hcl, Aligen Independ	00405-5200-01
100's	$18.63	Yohimbine Hcl, HL Moore Drug Exch	00839-7538-06
100's	$18.63	Yohimbine Hcl, HL Moore Drug Exch	00839-7822-06
100's	$18.70	YOHIMEX, Kramer Labs	55505-0100-15
100's	$18.75	Yohimbine Hcl, Royce	51875-0361-01
100's	$18.95	Yohimbine Hcl, Martec Pharms	52555-0538-01
100's	$19.50	Yohimbine Hcl, Pharmacist Choice	54979-0159-01
100's	$19.50	Yohimbine Hcl, Econolab	55053-0730-01
100's	$19.71	Yohimbine Hcl, Vintage Pharms	00254-6377-28
100's	$19.71	Yohimbine Hcl, Qualitest Pharms	00603-6430-21
100's	$19.87	APHRODYNE, Star Pharms FL	00076-0401-03
100's	$20.55	Yohimbine, Caraco Pharm	57664-0199-08
100's	$20.76	Yovital, Bradley Pharms	00482-0017-10
100's	$24.95	MEDEREK, Med Tek Pharms	52349-0280-10
100's	**$27.50**	**ACTIBINE, Consolidated Midland**	**00223-2391-01**
100's	$27.50	Yohimbine Hcl, Consolidated Midland	00223-2392-01
100's	$29.00	Erex, Ion	11808-0400-01
100's	$35.00	VIRITAB, AJ Bart	49326-0208-90
100's	$39.00	YOCON, Palisades Pharms	53159-0001-01
250's	$36.34	Yohimbine Hydrochloride Tablets 5.4 Mg, Mikart	46672-0111-25
500's	$44.00	Yohimbine Hcl, United Res	00677-1417-05
500's	$81.65	Yohimbine HCl, Rugby	00536-4989-05
500's	$85.75	Yohimbine Hcl, Aligen Independ	00405-5200-02
1000's	$89.95	Yohimbine Hcl, Eon Labs Mfg	00185-0998-10
1000's	$93.45	Yohimbine Hydrochloride Tablets 5.4 Mg, Mikart	46672-0111-11
1000's	$115.40	Yohimbine Hcl, Concord Labs	20254-0017-04
1000's	$131.25	Yohimbine Hcl, Major Pharms	00904-3255-80
1000's	$140.00	Yohimbine Hcl, H N Norton Co.	50732-0820-10
1000's	$167.67	Yohimbine Hcl, HL Moore Drug Exch	00839-7538-16
1000's	$175.00	Yohimbine Hcl, Royce	51875-0361-04
1000's	$178.85	APHRODYNE, Star Pharms FL	00076-0401-04
1000's	$179.36	Yohimbine Hcl, Vintage Pharms	00254-6377-38
1000's	$179.36	Yohimbine Hcl, Qualitest Pharms	00603-6430-32
1000's	$199.90	Yohimbine, Caraco Pharm	57664-0199-18
1000's	**$250.00**	**ACTIBINE, Consolidated Midland**	**00223-2391-02**
1000's	$250.00	Yohimbine Hcl, Consolidated Midland	00223-2392-02
1000's	$331.48	YOCON, Palisades Pharms	53159-0001-10

ZAFIRLUKAST *(003303)*

CATEGORIES: Airway Obstruction; Asthma; Leukotriene Receptor Antagonist; Respiratory & Allergy Medications; Respiratory Muscle Relaxant; Smooth Muscle Relaxants; Pregnancy Category B; FDA Approved 1996 Aug

BRAND NAMES: Accolate

PRIMARY ICD9: 493.9 (Asthma, Unspecified, Without Mention of Status Asthmaticus)

DESCRIPTION:

Zafirlukast is a synthetic, selective peptide leukotriene receptor antagonist (LTRA), with the chemical name 4-(5-cyclopentyloxy-carbonylamino-1-methyl-indol-3-ylmethyl) -3-methoxy-N-o-tolylsulfonylbenzamide. The molecular weight of zafirlukast is 575.7.

The empirical formula is $C_{31}H_{33}N_3O_6S$.

Zafirlukast, a fine white to pale yellow amorphous powder, is practically insoluble in water. It is slightly soluble in methanol and freely soluble in tetrahydrofuran, dimethylsulfoxide, and acetone.

Accolate is supplied as a 20 mg tablet for oral administration. *Inactive Ingredients:* Film-coated tablets containing croscarmellose sodium, lactose, magnesium stearate, microcrystalline cellulose, povidone, hydroxypropylmethylcellulose and titanium dioxide.

CLINICAL PHARMACOLOGY:

GENERAL

Zafirlukast is a selective and competitive receptor antagonist of leukotriene D_4 and E_4(LTD_4 and LTE_4), components of slow-reacting substance of anaphylaxis (SRSA). Cysteinyl leukotriene production and receptor occupation have been correlated with the pathophysiology of asthma, including airway edema, smooth muscle constriction, and altered cellular activity associated with the inflammatory process, which contribute to the signs and symptoms of asthma. Patients with asthma were found in one study to be 25–100 times more sensitive to the bronchoconstricting activity of inhaled LTD_4 than nonasthmatic subjects.

In vitro studies demonstrated that zafirlukast antagonized the contractile activity of three leukotrienes (LTC_4, LTD_4 and LTE_4) in conducting airway smooth muscle from laboratory animals and humans. Zafirlukast prevented intradermal LTD_4–induced increases in cutaneous vascular permeability and inhibited inhaled LTD_4–induced influx of eosinophils into animal lungs. Inhalation challenge studies in sensitized sheep showed that zafirlukast suppressed the airway responses to antigen; this included both the early- and late-phase response and the nonspecific hyperresponsiveness.

In humans, zafirlukast inhibited bronchoconstriction caused by several kinds of inhalational challenges. Pretreatment with single oral doses of zafirlukast inhibited the bronchoconstriction caused by sulfur dioxide and cold air in patients with asthma. Pretreatment with single doses of zafirlukast attenuated the early- and late-phase reaction caused by inhalation of various antigens such as grass, cat dander, ragweed, and mixed antigens in patients with asthma. Zafirlukast also attenuated the increase in bronchial hyperresponsiveness to inhaled histamine that followed inhaled allergen challenge.

CLINICAL PHARMACOKINETICS AND BIOAVAILABILITY

Zafirlukast is rapidly absorbed following oral administration. The absolute bioavailability of zafirlukast is unknown. Peak plasma concentrations are achieved 3 hours after dosing.

The mean terminal half-life of zafirlukast is approximately 10 hours in both normal subjects and patients with asthma. Steady-state plasma concentrations of zafirlukast are proportional to the dose and predictable from single-dose pharmacokinetic data.

Zafirlukast is extensively metabolized. Following oral administration of a radiolabeled dose, urinary excretion accounts for approximately 10% of the dose and the remainder is excreted in feces. Unmetabolized zafirlukast is not detected in urine. *In vitro* studies using human liver microsomes showed that the hydroxylated metabolites of zafirlukast are formed through the cytochrome P450 2C9 (CYP2C9) enzyme pathway. Additional *in vitro* studies utilizing human liver microsomes show that zafirlukast inhibits the cytochrome P450 CYP3A4 and CYP2C9 isoenzymes at concentrations close to the clinically achieved plasma concentrations. The metabolites of zafirlukast found in plasma are at least 90 times less potent as LTD_4 receptor antagonists than zafirlukast in a standard *in vitro* test of activity.

Cross-study comparisons in patients ranging from 7 years to greater than 65 years of age show that mean dose (mg/kg) normalized AUC and C_{max} increase and plasma clearance (CL) decreases with increasing age. In patients above 65 years of age, there is an approximately 2–3 fold greater C_{max} and AUC compared to young adult patients.

In a study of patients with hepatic impairment (biopsy-proven cirrhosis), there was a 50–60% greater C_{max} and AUC compared to normal subjects.

Based on a cross-study comparison, there are no apparent differences in the pharmacokinetics of zafirlukast between renally impaired patients and normal subjects.

In two separate studies, one using a high fat and the other a high protein meal, administration of zafirlukast with food reduced the mean bioavailability by approximately 40%.

In the concentration range of 0.25–10 mcg/ml, zafirlukast is >99% bound to plasma proteins, predominantly albumin.

CLINICAL STUDIES:

Three U.S. double-blind, randomized, placebo-controlled, 13–week clinical trials in 1,380 patients with mild-to-moderate asthma demonstrated that zafirlukast improved daytime asthma symptoms, nighttime awakenings, mornings with asthma symptoms, rescue beta$_2$–agonist use, FEV_1, and morning peak expiratory flow rate. In these studies, the patients had a mean baseline FEV_1 of approximately 75% of predicted normal and a mean baseline beta-agonist requirement of approximately 4–5 puffs of albuterol per day. The results of the largest of the trials are shown in TABLE 1.

TABLE 1 Mean Change from Baseline at Study Endpoint

	Zafirlukast 20 mg twice daily N=514	Placebo N=248
Daytime Asthma symptom score (0-3 scale)	-0.44*	-0.25
Nighttime Awakenings (number per week)	-1.27*	-0.43
Mornings with Asthma Symptoms (days per week)	-1.32*	-0.75
Rescue β_2-agonist use (puffs per day)	-1.15*	-0.24
FEV_1 (L)	+0.15*	+0.05
Morning PEFR (L/min)	+22.06*	+7.63
Evening PEFR (L/min)	+13.12	+10.14

* p<0.05, compared to placebo

In a second and smaller study, the effect of zafirlukast on most efficacy parameters was comparable to the active control (inhaled cromolyn sodium 1600 mcg four times per day) and superior to placebo at endpoint for decreasing rescue beta-agonist use.

In these trials, improvement in asthma symptoms occurred within one week of initiating treatment with zafirlukast. The role of zafirlukast in the management of patients with more severe asthma, patients receiving antiasthma therapy other than as-needed, inhaled beta$_2$–agonists, or as an oral or inhaled corticosteroid-sparing agent remains to be fully characterized.

INDICATIONS AND USAGE:

Zafirlukast is indicated for the prophylaxis and chronic treatment of asthma in adults and children 12 years of age and older.

CONTRAINDICATIONS:

Zafirlukast is contraindicated in patients who are hypersensitive to zafirlukast or any of its inactive ingredients.

WARNINGS:

Zafirlukast is not indicated for use in the reversal of bronchospasm in acute asthma attacks, including status asthmaticus. Therapy with zafirlukast can be continued during acute exacerbations of asthma.

Coadministration of zafirlukast with warfarin results in a clinically significant increase in prothrombin time (PT). Patients on oral warfarin anticoagulant therapy and zafirlukast should have their prothrombin times monitored closely and anticoagulant dose adjusted accordingly. (See DRUG INTERACTIONS.)

PRECAUTIONS:

Information for the Patient: Zafirlukast is indicated for the chronic treatment of asthma and should be taken regularly as prescribed, even during symptom-free periods. Zafirlukast is not a bronchodilator and should not be used to treat acute episodes of asthma. Patients receiving zafirlukast should be instructed not to decrease the dose or stop taking any other antiasthma medications unless instructed by a physician. Women who are breast-feeding should be instructed not to take zafirlukast (See PRECAUTIONS, Nursing Mothers.) Alternative antiasthma medication should be considered in such patients.

The bioavailability of zafirlukast may be decreased when taken with food. Patients should be instructed to take zafirlukast at least 1 hour before or 2 hours after meals.

Carcinogenesis, Mutagenesis, and Impairment of Fertility: In two-year carcinogenicity studies, zafirlukast was administered at oral daily doses of 10, 100, and 300 mg/kg to mice and 40, 400, and 2000 mg/kg to rats. Male mice given 300 mg/kg/day of zafirlukast had a greater incidence of hepatocellular adenomas as compared to concurrent controls; female mice at this dose showed a greater incidence of whole body histocytic sarcomas. Male and female rats given 2000 mg/kg/day of zafirlukast had a greater incidence of urinary bladder transitional cell papillomas as compared to concurrent controls. Pharmacokinetic data show that the plasma concentrations in mice at non-tumorigenic (100 mg/kg) and tumorigenic (300 mg/kg) doses of zafirlukast were approximately 70 times and 220 times, respectively, the plasma concentrations at the maximum recommended human daily oral dose. For rats, plasma concentrations at the non-tumorigenic (400 mg/kg) and tumorigenic (2000 mg/kg) doses of zafirlukast were approximately 170 times and 200 times, respectively, the plasma concentrations in humans at the maximum recommended human daily oral dose. The clinical significance of these findings for the long-term use of zafirlukast is unknown.

In mutagenicity studies, there was no evidence of mutagenic potential in reverse (*S. typhimurium* and *E. coli*) or forward point mutation (CHO-HGPRT and mouse lymphoma) assays or in two assays for chromosomal aberrations (human peripheral blood lymphocyte clastogenic assay and the rat bone marrow micronucleus assay).

Reproduction and fertility studies in rats showed no effect on fertility due to zafirlukast at doses up to 2000 mg/kg (approximately 400 times in the maximum recommended daily oral dose on mg/m^2 basis). In the one-year toxicity studies in dogs, zafirlukast produced an increase in absolute and relative uterine and ovarian weights at an oral dose of 150 mg/kg, resulting in approximately 85 times the systemic exposure (AUC_{0-12h}) in humans at the maximum recommended human oral daily dose.

Pregnancy Category B: No teratogenicity was observed at oral doses up to 1600 mg/kg/day in mice (approximately 160 times the maximum recommended human daily oral dose on a mg/m^2 basis), 2000 mg/kg/day in rats (approximately 400 times the maximum recommended human daily oral dose on a mg/m^2 basis) and 2000 mg/kg/day in cynomolgus monkeys (approximately 800 times the maximum recommended human daily oral dose on a mg/m^2 basis). At 2000 mg/kg/day in rats, maternal toxicity and deaths were seen with increased incidence of early fetal resorption. Spontaneous abortions occurred in cynomolgus monkeys at a maternally toxic dose of 2000 mg/kg/day orally. There are no adequate and well-controlled trials in prenant women. Because animal reproduction studies are not always predictive of human response, zafirlukast should be used during pregnancy only if clearly needed.

Nursing Mothers: Zafirlukast is excreted in breast milk. Following repeated 40–mg twice-a-day dosing in healthy women, average steady-state concentrations of zafirlukast in breast milk were 50 ng/ml compared to 255 ng/ml in plasma. Because of the potential for tumorigenicity shown for zafirlukast in mouse and rat studies and the enhanced sensitivity of neonatal rats and dogs to the adverse effects of zafirlukast, zafirlukast should not be administered to mothers who are breast-feeding.

Pediatric Use: The safety and effectiveness of zafirlukast in pediatric patients below the age of 12 years have not been established.

DRUG INTERACTIONS:

In a drug interaction study in 16 healthy male volunteers, coadministration of multiple doses of zafirlukast (160 mg/day) to steady state with a single 25–mg dose of warfarin resulted in a significant increase in the mean AUC (+63%) and half-life (+36%) of S-warfarin. The mean prothrombin time (PT) increased by approximately 35%. This interaction is probably due to an inhibition by zafirlukast of the cytochrome P450 2C9 isoenzyme system. Patients on oral warfarin anticoagulant therapy and zafirlukast should have their prothrombin times monitored closely and anticoagulant dose adjusted accordingly (see WARNINGS.) No formal drug-drug interaction studies with zafirlukast and other drugs known to be metabolized by the cytochrome P450 2C9 isoenzyme (*e.g.*, tolbutamide, phenytoin, carbamazepine) have been conducted; however, care should be exercised when zafirlukast is co-administered with these drugs.

In a drug interaction study in 16 healthy male volunteers, co-administration of zafirlukast (320 mg/day), with terfenadine (60 mg twice daily) to steady state resulted in a decrease in the C_{max} (-66%) and AUC (-54%) of zafirlukast. No effect of zafirlukast on terfenadine plasma concentrations or ECG parameters (*i.e.*, QTc interval) was seen. No formal drug-drug interaction studies between zafirlukast and other drugs known to be metabolized by the P450 3A4 (CYP 3A4) isoenzyme (*e.g.*, dihydropyridine calcium-channel blockers, cyclosporin, cisapride, astemizole) have been conducted. As zafirlukast is known to be an inhibitor of CYP 3A4 *in vitro*, it is reasonable to employ appropriate clinical monitoring when these drugs are coadministered with zafirlukast.

In a drug interaction study in 11 asthmatic patients, co-administration of a single dose of zafirlukast (40 mg) with erythromycin (500 mg three times daily for 5 days) to steady state resulted in decreased mean plasma levels of zafirlukast by approximately 40% due to a decrease in zafirlukast bioavailability.

Co-administration of zafirlukast (80 mg/day) at steady state with a single dose of a liquid theophylline preparation (6 mg/kg) in 13 asthmatic patients resulted in decreased mean plasma levels of zafirlukast by approximately 30%, but no effect on plasma theophylline levels was observed.

Co-administration of zafirlukast (40 mg/day) with aspirin (650 mg four times daily) resulted in mean increased plasma levels of zafirlukast by approximately 45%.

In a single-blind, parallel-group, 3–week study in 39 healthy female subjects taking oral contraceptives, 40 mg twice daily of zafirlukast had no significant effect on ethinyl estradiol plasma concentrations or contraceptive efficacy.

ADVERSE REACTIONS:

The safety database for zafirlukast consists of more than 4,000 healthy volunteers and patients who received zafirlukast, of which 1723 were asthmatics enrolled in trials of 13 weeks duration or longer. A total of 671 patients received zafirlukast for 1 year or longer. The majority of the patients were 18 years of age or older; however 222 patients between the age of 12 and 18 years received zafilukast.

A comparison of adverse events reported by ≥1% of zafirlukast-treated patients, and at rates numerically greater than in placebo-treated patients, is shown for all trials in TABLE 2.

ADVERSE REACTIONS: *(cont'd)*

TABLE 2

Adverse Event	Zafirlukast (N=4058)	Placebo (N=2032)
Headache	12.9%	11.7%
Infection	3.5%	3.4%
Nausea	3.1%	2.0%
Diarrhea	2.8%	2.1%
Pain (generalized)	1.9%	1.7%
Asthenia	1.8%	1.6%
Abdominal Pain	1.8%	1.1%
Accidental Injury	1.6%	1.5%
Dizziness	1.6%	1.5%
Myalgia	1.6%	1.5%
Fever	1.6%	1.1%
Back Pain	1.5%	1.2%
Vomiting	1.5%	1.1%
SGPT Elevation	1.5%	1.1%
Dyspepsia	1.3%	1.2%

The frequency of less common adverse events was comparable between zafirlukast and placebo.

Although the frequency of hepatic transaminase elevations was comparable between zafirlukast and placebo-treated patients, a single case of symptomatic hepatitis and hyperbilirubinemia, without other attributable cause, occurred in a patient who had received 40 mg/day of zafirlukast for 100 days. In this patient, the liver enzymes returned to normal within 3 months of stopping zafirlukast.

In clinical trials, an increased proportion of zafirlukast patients over the age of 55 years reported infections as compared to placebo-treated patients. A similar finding was not observed in other age groups studied. These infections were mostly mild or moderate in intensity and predominantly affected the respiratory tract. Infections occurred equally in both sexes, were dose-proportional to total milligrams of zafirlukast exposure, and were associated with coadministration of inhaled corticosteroids. The clinical significance of this finding is unknown.

OVERDOSAGE:

No deaths occurred at oral zafirlukast doses of 2000 mg/kg in mice (approximately 200 times the maximum recommended human daily oral dose on a mg/m^2 basis), 2000 mg/kg in rats (approximately 400 times the maximum recommended daily oral dose on a mg/m^2 basis), and 500 mg/kg in dogs (approximately 330 times the maximum recommended human daily oral dose on a mg/m^2 basis).

There is no experience to date with zafirlukast in overdose in humans. It is reasonable to employ the usual supportive measures in the event of an overdose (*e.g.*, remove unabsorbed material from the gastrointestinal tract, employ clinical monitoring, and institute supportive therapy, if required).

DOSAGE AND ADMINISTRATION:

The recommended dose of zafirlukast is 20 mg twice daily in adults and children 12 years and older. Since food reduces the bioavailability of zafirlukast, zafirlukast should be taken at least 1 hour before or 2 hours after meals.

Elderly Patients: Based on cross-study comparisons, the clearance of zafirlukast is reduced in elderly patients (65 years of age and older), such that C_{max} and AUC are approximately twice those of younger adults. In clinical trials, a dose of 20 mg twice daily was not associated with an increase in the overall incidence of adverse events or withdrawals because of adverse events in elderly patients.

Patients with Hepatic Impairment: The clearance of zafirlukast is reduced in patients with stable alcoholic cirrhosis such that the C_{max} and AUC are approximately 50–60% greater than those of normal adults. Zafirlukast has not been evaluated in patients with hepatitis or in long-term studies of patients with cirrhosis.

Patients with Renal Impairment: Dosage adjustment is not required for patients with renal impairment.

Pediatric Patients: The safety and effectiveness of zafirlukast in pediatric patients below the age of 12 years have not been established.

PATIENT INFORMATION:

Zafirlukast is for the prevention and chronic treatment of asthma; it is not for acute asthma attacks.

Do not take this drug if you are nursing.

Inform your doctor if you are pregnant or if you are taking aspirin, antibiotics, blood thinning medications or any other asthma medicine.

Take this medicine 1 hour before or 2 hours after meals.

May cause headache, infection, nausea, diarrhea or generalized pain. Inform your physician or pharmacist if this occurs.

HOW SUPPLIED:

Accolate 20 mg Tablets are white, round, biconvex, coated tablets identified with "ZENECA" debossed on one side and "ACCOLATE 20" debossed on the other side.

Store at controlled room temperature, (20°-25°) (68°-77° F). Protect from light and moisture. Dispense in the original air-tight container.

HOW SUPPLIED - EQUIVALENTS NOT AVAILABLE:

Tablet - Oral - 20 mg

20 mg tablets x	$87.50	ACCOLATE, Zeneca Pharms	00310-0402-39
20 mg x 60	$52.50	ACCOLATE, Zeneca Pharms	00310-0402-00

ZALCITABINE *(003076)*

CATEGORIES: AIDS Related Complex; Anti-Infectives; Antivirals; HIV Infection; Nucleoside Analogue Drugs; Orphan Drugs; Viral Agents; Pregnancy Category C; FDA Class 1P ("Priority Review"); FDA Approved 1992 Jun

BRAND NAMES: D.D.C.; ddC; Dideoxycytidine; **HIVID**

FORMULARIES: Medi-Cal; PCS

COST OF THERAPY: $2,517.62 (AIDS; Tablet; 0.750 mg; 3/day; 365 days)

WARNING:
THE USE OF ZALCITABINE HAS BEEN ASSOCIATED WITH SIGNIFICANT CLINICAL ADVERSE REACTIONS, SOME OF WHICH ARE POTENTIALLY FATAL. ZALCITABINE CAN CAUSE SEVERE PERIPHERAL NEUROPATHY AND BECAUSE OF THIS SHOULD BE USED WITH EXTREME CAUTION IN PATIENTS WITH PRE-EXISTING NEUROPATHY. ZALCITABINE MAY ALSO RARELY CAUSE PANCREATITIS AND PATIENTS WHO DEVELOP ANY SYMPTOMS SUGGESTIVE OF PANCREATITIS WHILE USING ZALCITABINE SHOULD HAVE THERAPY SUSPENDED IMMEDIATELY UNTIL THIS DIAGNOSIS IS EXCLUDED.
RARE OCCURRENCES OF LACTIC ACIDOSIS IN THE ABSENCE OF HYPOXEMIA AND SEVERE HEPATOMEGALY WITH STEATOSIS HAVE BEEN REPORTED WITH THE USE OF NUCLEOSIDE ANALOGUES, INCLUDING ZIDOVUDINE AND ZALCITABINE, AND ARE POTENTIALLY FATAL. IN ADDITION, RARE CASES OF HEPATIC FAILURE AND DEATH CONSIDERED POSSIBLY RELATED TO UNDERLYING HEPATITIS B AND ZALCITABINE MONOTHERAPY HAVE BEEN REPORTED (SEE WARNINGS and PRECAUTIONS).
BECAUSE OF CLINICAL UNCERTAINTY REGARDING THE MOST APPROPRIATE USE OF NUCLEOSIDE ANALOGUES, IT IS RECOMMENDED THAT THE DECISIONS REGARDING THE USE OF ZALCITABINE THERAPY BE MADE IN CONSULTATION WITH A PHYSICIAN EXPERIENCED IN THE TREATMENT OF HIV-INFECTED PERSONS (SEE INDICATIONS AND USAGE and CLINICAL STUDIES).

DESCRIPTION:

Hivid is the Hoffmann-La Roche brand of zalcitabine [formerly called 2'3'-dideoxycytidine (ddC)], a synthetic pyrimidine nucleoside analogue active against the human immunodeficiency virus (HIV). Hivid is available as film-coated tablets for oral administration in strengths of 0.375 mg and 0.750 mg. Each tablet also contains the inactive ingredients lactose, microcrystalline cellulose, croscarmellose sodium, magnesium stearate, hydroxypropyl methylcellulose, polyethylene glycol and polysorbate 80 along with the following colorant system: 0.375 mg tablet — synthetic brown, black, red and yellow iron oxides, and titanium dioxide; 0.750 mg tablet — synthetic black iron oxide and titanium dioxide. The chemical name for zalcitabine is 4-amino-1-beta-D-2',3'-dideoxyribofuranosyl-2-(1H)-pyrimidone or 2',3'-dideoxycytidine with the molecular formula $C_9H_{13}N_3O_3$ and a molecular weight of 211.22.

Zalcitabine is a white to off-white crystalline powder with an aqueous solubility of 76.4 mg/ml at 25°C.

CLINICAL PHARMACOLOGY:

Mechanism of Action: Zalcitabine is a synthetic nucleoside analogue of the naturally occurring nucleoside 2'- deoxycytidine in which the 3'-hydroxyl group is replaced by hydrogen. Within cells, zalcitabine is converted to the active metabolite, dideoxycytidine 5'-triphosphate (ddCTP), by cellular enzymes. ddCTP serves as an alternative substrate to deoxycytidine triphosphate (dCTP) for HIV-reverse transcriptase and inhibits the *in vitro* replication of HIV-1 by inhibition of viral DNA synthesis. This inhibition has been demonstrated *in vitro* in human primary cell cultures and in established cell lines. In DNA biosynthesis, DNA chain extension occurs through the formation of a phosphodiester bridge between the 3'-hydroxyl group of the growing end of a DNA chain and the 5'- phosphate group of the incoming deoxynucleotide. Because ddCTP lacks the 3'-hydroxyl group required for chain elongation, its incorporation into a growing DNA chain leads to premature chain termination. ddCTP serves as a competitive inhibitor of the natural substrate, dCTP, for the active site of DNA polymerase and thus further inhibits viral as well as cellular DNA synthesis.

The active metabolite, ddCTP, also has a high affinity for cellular DNA polymerase beta and mitochondrial DNA polymerase gamma and has been reported to be incorporated into the DNA of cells in culture. Furthermore, the cellular DNA polymerase beta is able to utilize ddCTP causing chain termination.

The half-life of ddCTP in established cell lines and in human peripheral blood mononuclear cells in culture has been determined to be in the range of 2.6 to 10 hours.

Microbiology: The anti-HIV activity of zalcitabine was determined in a variety of human T-cell lines infected with different strains of HIV. The *in vitro* anti-HIV activity of zalcitabine varied greatly depending upon the time between virus infection and zalcitabine treatment of cell cultures, the ratio of the number of infectious virus particles to the number of cells, the kind of assay and the cell type used. When established cell lines were infected with a large excess of virus per cell and drug added soon after infection, the concentration of zalcitabine required to inhibit HIV-1 replication by 50% (ID_{50}) was generally in the range of 30 nM to 500 nM (1 nM = 0.21 ng/ml). In these cell lines, >95% inhibition of viral replication was achieved with 100 nM to 1000 nM zalcitabine. Zalcitabine blocked virus- induced cytopathic effects in cell lines in culture at a concentration of 30 nM to 300 nM. In assays measuring the inhibition of p24 viral antigen, the ID_{50} of zalcitabine was in the range of 1 nM to 500 nM, and the 90% inhibitory concentration (ID_{90}) was in the range of 500 Nm to 1000 Nm. In peripheral blood mononuclear cell cultures infected with HIV-1 (LAV strain) at a low ratio of virus to cells and assayed for HIV-reverse transcriptase, ID_{50} and ID_{90} values for zalcitabine were determined to be 11 Nm and 100 Nm, respectively. In monocyte/macrophage cultures infected with HIV (Ba-L strain) and treated with zalcitabine, the ID_{90} value was <10 nM when assayed for viral p24 antigen. However, viral replication in monocyte/macrophage cultures infected with a lymphotropic isolate of HIV (LAV-1 strain) was not inhibited at 100,000 nM. Comparative studies of the antiviral activity of zalcitabine against HIV-1 and HIV-2 *in vitro* revealed no significant difference in sensitivity between the two viruses when activity was determined by measuring viral cytopathic effect.

The results of cytotoxicity studies in various cell lines demonstrated that the concentration of the drug necessary to inhibit the cell growth by 50% (EC_{50}) was in the range of 5000 nM to >100,000 nM. *In vitro* combination studies have demonstrated that zalcitabine and zidovudine have an additive or synergistic antiviral effect, depending on the cell line used, without increased cytotoxicity over that observed for either agent alone.

Resistance to Zalcitabine: The emergence of HIV variants with reduced susceptibility (resistance) to zalcitabine has been demonstrated in a small number of patients who have received more than 1 year of zalcitabine monotherapy. Reduced sensitivity has been associated with point mutations at codons 65 (Lys to Arg or Asn), 74 (Leu to Val), 69 (Thr to Asp), 75 (Val to Thr), 184 (Met to Val) and 215 (Tyr to Cys) in the pol gene that encodes the viral enzyme, reverse transcriptase. These mutations are interactive with other reverse-transcriptase inhibitors. The Tyr to Cys mutation at position 215 may arise in virus that has already undergone the principal mutation (Thr to Tyr) to zidovudine resistance at this position. Resistance to zidovudine caused by the position 215 mutation (Thr to Tyr) is suppressed by the change in zalcitabine sensitivity at position 74 (Leu to Val), restoring zidovudine sensitivity. Combination therapy with zalcitabine and zidovudine does not appear to prevent the emergence of zidovudine-resistant isolates. Additionally, the point mutations at positions 74, 75 and 184 are associated with resistance to didanosine (ddI), that at position 75 with resistance to stavudine (D4T), and those at positions 65 (Lys to Arg) and 184 (Met to Val) with resistance to lamivudine (3TC).

Pharmacokinetics: The pharmacokinetics of zalcitabine has been evaluated in studies in HIV-infected patients following 0.01 mg/kg, 0.03 mg/kg and 1.5 mg oral doses, and a 1.5 mg intravenous dose administered as a 1-hour infusion.

Absorption and Bioavailability in Adults: Following oral administration to HIV-infected patients, the mean absolute bioavailability of zalcitabine was >80% (30% CV, range 23% to 124%, n=19). The absorption rate of a 1.5 mg oral dose of zalcitabine (n=20) was reduced when administered with food. This resulted in a 39% decrease in mean maximum plasma concentrations (C_{max}) from 25.2 ng/ml (35% CV, range 11.6 to 37.5 ng/ml) to 15.5 ng/ml (24% CV, range 9.1 to 23.7 ng/ml), and a twofold increase in time to achieve maximum plasma concentrations from a mean of 0.8 hours under fasting conditions to 1.6 hours when the drug was given with food. The extent of absorption (as reflected by AUC) was decreased by 14%, from 72 ng°hr/ml (28% CV, range 43 to 119 ng°hr/ml) to 62 ng°hr/ml (23% CV, range 42 to 91 ng°hr/ml). The clinical relevance of these decreases is unknown. Absorption of zalcitabine does not appear to be reduced in patients with diarrhea not caused by an identified pathogen.

Distribution in Adults: The steady-state volume of distribution following IV administration of a 1.5 mg dose of zalcitabine averaged 0.534 (± 0.127) l/kg (24% CV, range 0.304 to 0.734 l/kg, n=20). Cerebrospinal fluid obtained from 9 patients at 2 to 3.5 hours following 0.06 mg/kg or 0.09 mg/kg IV infusion showed measurable concentrations of zalcitabine. The CSF: plasma concentration ratio ranged from 9% to 37% (mean 20%), demonstrating penetration of the drug through the blood-brain barrier. The clinical relevance of these ratios has not been evaluated.

Metabolism and Elimination in Adults: Zalcitabine is phosphorylated intracellularly to zalcitabine triphosphate, the active substrate for HIV-reverse transcriptase. Concentrations of zalcitabine triphosphate are too low for quantitation following administration of therapeutic doses to humans.

Zalcitabine does not undergo a significant degree of metabolism by the liver. The primary metabolite of zalcitabine that has been identified is dideoxyuridine (ddU), which accounts for less than 15% of an oral dose in both urine and feces (n=4). Approximately 10% of an orally administered radiolabeled dose of zalcitabine appears in the feces (n=10), comprised primarily of unchanged drug and ddU. Renal excretion of unchanged drug appears to be the primary route of elimination, accounting for approximately 80% of an intravenous dose and 60% of an orally administered dose within 24 hours after dosing (n=19). The mean elimination half-life is 2 hours and generally ranges from 1 to 3 hours in individual patients. Total clearance following an intravenous dose averaged 285 ml/min (29% CV, range 165 to 447 ml/min, n=20). Renal clearance averaged approximately 235 ml/min or about 80% of total clearance (30% CV, range 129 to 348 ml/min, n=20). Renal clearance exceeds glomerular filtration rate suggesting renal tubular secretion contributes to the elimination of zalcitabine by the kidneys.

In patients with impaired kidney function, prolonged elimination of zalcitabine may be expected. Preliminary results from 7 patients with renal impairment (estimated CrCl <55 ml/min) indicate that the half-life was prolonged (up to 8.5 hours) in these patients compared to those with normal renal function. Maximum plasma concentrations were higher in some patients after a single dose (see PRECAUTIONS.)

In patients with normal renal function, the pharmacokinetics of zalcitabine was not altered during 3 times daily multiple dosing (n=9). Accumulation of drug in plasma during this regimen was negligible. The drug was <4% bound to plasma proteins, indicating that drug interactions involving binding-site displacement are unlikely (see DRUG INTERACTIONS).

Pharmacokinetics in Children: Limited pharmacokinetic data have been reported for 5 HIV-positive children using doses of 0.03 and 0.04 mg/kg zalcitabine administered orally every 6 hours.[1] The mean bioavailability of zalcitabine in these children was 54% and mean apparent systemic clearance was 150 ml/min/m^2. Due to the small number of subjects and different analytical techniques, it is difficult to make comparisons between pediatric and adult data.

CLINICAL STUDIES:

ZALCITABINE MONOTHERAPY

The indication for zalcitabine use as monotherapy is based on the results of CPCRA 002, a Phase 2/3 randomized, multicenter, open-label study in which zalcitabine was compared to didanosine as treatment for patients with advanced HIV infection (median CD4 cell count = 37 cells/mm^3) who were clinically intolerant to zidovudine, or who had met criteria for having disease progression while receiving zidovudine.[2] Patients in this study had a mean of 17.5 months of prior zidovudine use. The results demonstrate that zalcitabine was at least as efficacious as didanosine in terms of time to an AIDS-defining event or death, while for survival alone the results favored zalcitabine. However, most of the patients (66%) in either group had disease progression over the median 16 months of follow-up. Overall rates of study drug tolerance, discontinuation and adverse events were similar for the two groups, although the types of events were different.

The effect of therapy with zalcitabine or didanosine on either disease progression or survival in patients with demographic characteristics similar to those studied in CPCRA 002 has not been studied in placebo- controlled clinical trials. A clinical study (N3300/ACTG 114) has demonstrated zidovudine to be superior to zalcitabine as monotherapy for advanced HIV disease (CD4 cell count ≤200 cells/mm^3) in zidovudine-naive patients.[3,4] The final analysis of this study indicated that 134 patients (42%) in the zalcitabine group with a median follow-up of 85 weeks and 120 patients (38%) in the zidovudine group with a median follow-up of 96 weeks died with a relative risk for mortality of zidovudine to zalcitabine of 0.54.

COMBINATION THERAPY

Zidovudine-Naive Patients: The use of zalcitabine in combination with zidovudine in zidovudine-naive patients is based on two small clinical studies (N3447/ACTG 106 and BW 34,225-02) showing a greater rise in CD4 cell counts, which was maintained longer with combination therapy when compared to zidovudine monotherapy.[5,6]

There have been no results from controlled studies of combination therapy with primary clinical endpoints of disease progression or death in patients who were naive to antiretroviral therapy when combination therapy was initiated.

Zidovudine-Exposed Patients: The use of zalcitabine in combination with zidovudine in patients who have previously received zidovudine is based on the results from a subgroup analysis of a Phase 3, randomized, double- blind clinical trial (ACTG 155). ACTG 155 was a comparative study (n=1001) of zalcitabine alone or in combination with zidovudine versus zidovudine alone in patients with an entry CD4 cell count ≤300 cells/mm^3 who had previously received zidovudine for 6 months or more.

Overall, there were no significant treatment differences in disease progression or death for the three study groups. However, for those patients on combination zalcitabine and zidovudine with baseline CD4 cell counts between 150 to 300 cells/mm^3 at entry, there were fewer study endpoints of disease progression when compared to the zidovudine monotherapy group but

CLINICAL STUDIES: *(cont'd)*

not the zalcitabine monotherapy group. There were too few deaths in the ≥150 cells/mm³ subgroup for an effect on survival alone to be assessed. All treatment arms eventually showed decline in CD4 cell count despite treatment although for the combination arm there was an initial increase for patients with CD4 cell counts ≥150 cells/mm³. Further studies are ongoing to confirm clinical benefit from combination therapy.

INDICATIONS AND USAGE:

Zalcitabine Monotherapy: Zalcitabine is indicated for the treatment of HIV infection in adults with advanced HIV disease who either are intolerant to zidovudine or who have disease progression while receiving zidovudine.

Combination Therapy of Zalcitabine and Zidovudine: Zalcitabine in combination with zidovudine is indicated for the treatment of selected patients with advanced HIV disease (CD4 cell count ≤300 cells/mm³). In zidovudine-naive patients this indication is based on greater increases in CD4 cell counts that were maintained longer for patients treated with combination therapy as compared to zidovudine monotherapy. There have been no studies showing clinical benefit from combination therapy in zidovudine-naive patients. For patients with prior zidovudine exposure, this indication is based on a subgroup analysis of clinical data that showed a clinical benefit only for those patients with a CD4 count ≥150 cells/mm³at the time of the initiation of therapy. No benefit from combination therapy has been observed from studies of zidovudine-exposed patients with CD4 cell counts <150 cells/mm³, and combination therapy is therefore not currently recommended for these patients (see CLINICAL STUDIES).

CONTRAINDICATIONS:

Zalcitabine is contraindicated in patients with clinically significant hypersensitivity to zalcitabine or to any of the excipients contained in the tablets.

WARNINGS:

SIGNIFICANT CLINICAL ADVERSE REACTIONS, SOME OF WHICH ARE POTENTIALLY FATAL, HAVE BEEN REPORTED WITH ZALCITABINE MONOTHERAPY AND WITH ZALCITABINE IN COMBINATION WITH ZIDOVUDINE. THE COMPLETE PRESCRIBING INFORMATION FOR ZIDOVUDINE SHOULD BE CONSULTED BEFORE COMBINATION THERAPY WITH ZALCITABINE IS INITIATED. PATIENTS WITH DECREASED CD4 CELL COUNTS APPEAR TO HAVE AN INCREASED INCIDENCE OF ADVERSE EVENTS. IF PATIENTS DEVELOP UNEXPECTED SERIOUS ADVERSE REACTIONSWHILE ON THERAPY WITH EITHER OF THESE AGENTS, DISCONTINUE THERAPY IMMEDIATELY AND REPORT THE EVENT TO THE MANUFACTURER OR FDA.

Peripheral Neuropathy: THE MAJOR CLINICAL TOXICITY OF ZALCITABINE IS PERIPHERAL NEUROPATHY, WHICH OCCURRED IN 22% TO 35% OF SUBJECTS TREATED IN PHASE 2/3 MONOTHERAPY STUDIES DEPENDING ON SEVERITY AND PRESUMED RELATIONSHIP TO DRUG. By comparison, neuropathy occurred in 0% to 14% of zidovudine-treated patients. In ACTG 155, rates of peripheral neuropathy were similar among patients treated with zalcitabine monotherapy and zalcitabine in combination with zidovudine.

Zalcitabine-related peripheral neuropathy is a sensorimotor neuropathy characterized initially by numbness and burning dysesthesia involving the distal extremities. These symptoms may be followed by sharp shooting pains or severe continuous burning pain if the drug is not withdrawn. The neuropathy may progress to severe pain requiring narcotic analgesics and is potentially irreversible. In some patients, symptoms of neuropathy may initially progress despite discontinuation of zalcitabine. With prompt discontinuation of zalcitabine, the neuropathy is usually slowly reversible.

There are no data regarding the use of zalcitabine in patients with preexisting peripheral neuropathy since these patients were excluded from clinical trials; therefore, zalcitabine should be used with extreme caution in these patients. Individuals with moderate or severe peripheral neuropathy, as evidenced by symptoms accompanied by objective findings, are advised to avoid zalcitabine.

Zalcitabine should be stopped promptly when moderate discomfort from numbness, tingling, burning or pain of the extremities progresses, or any related symptoms occur that are accompanied by an objective finding.

Pancreatitis: PANCREATITIS, WHICH HAS BEEN FATAL IN SOME CASES, HAS BEEN OBSERVED WITH THE ADMINISTRATION OF ZALCITABINE ALONE OR THE COMBINATION OF ZALCITABINE WITH ZIDOVUDINE. Pancreatitis is an uncommon complication of zalcitabine monotherapy or in combination with zidovudine, occurring in 1.1% of patients. The occurrence of asymptomatic elevated serum amylase of any etiology while on zalcitabine monotherapy was 1.6%.

Patients with a history of pancreatitis or known risk factors for the development of pancreatitis should be followed more closely while on zalcitabine therapy. Of 528 zalcitabine-treated patients enrolled in an expanded- access safety study (N3544), who had a history of prior pancreatitis or increased amylase, 28 (5.3%) developed pancreatitis and an additional 23 (4.4%) developed asymptomatic elevated serum amylase. There are no apparent difference in the occurrence of pancreatitis between the two doses of zalcitabine in the expanded-access trial (N3544).

Treatment with zalcitabine monotherapy or zalcitabine in combination with zidovudine should be stopped immediately if clinical signs or symptoms (nausea, vomiting, abdominal pain) or if abnormalities in laboratory values (hyperamylasemia associated with dysglycemia, rising triglyceride level, decreasing serum calcium) suggestive of pancreatitis should occur. If clinical pancreatitis develops during zalcitabine administration, it is recommended that zalcitabine be permanently discontinued. Treatment with zalcitabine should also be interrupted if treatment with another drug known to cause pancreatitis (*e.g.,* intravenous pentamidine) ir required (see DRUG INTERACTIONS.)

Hepatic Toxicity: RARE OCCURRENCES OF LACTIC ACIDOSIS IN THE ABSENCE OF HYPOXEMIA AND SEVERE HEPATOMEGALY WITH STEATOSIS HAVE BEEN REPORTED WITH THE USE OF NUCLEOSIDE ANALOGUES, INCLUDING ZIDOVUDINE AND ZALCITABINE, AND ARE POTENTIALLY FATAL.[7,8]IN ADDITION, RARE CASES OF HEPATIC FAILURE (ONE WHICH COINCIDED WITH RENAL FAILURE) AND DEATH CONSIDERED POSSIBLY RELATED TO UNDERLYING HEPATITIS B AND ZALCITABINE MONOTHERAPY HAVE BEEN REPORTED. Treatment with zalcitabine in patients with preexisting liver disease, liver enzyme abnormalities, a history of ethanol abuse or hepatitis should be approached with caution. Zalcitabine should be interrupted or discontinued in the setting of deterioration of liver function tests, hepatic steatosis, progressive hepatomegaly or unexplained lactic acidosis. In clinical trials, drug interruption was recommended if liver function tests exceeded >5 times the upper limit of normal.

Other Serious Toxicities

a) Oral Ulcers: Severe oral ulcers occurred in approximately 3% of patients receiving zalcitabine in CPCRA 002 and ACTG 155; less severe oral ulcerations have occurred at higher frequencies in other clinical trials.

WARNINGS: *(cont'd)*

b) Esophageal Ulcers: Infrequent cases of esophageal ulcers have also been attributed to zalcitabine therapy. Interruption of zalcitabine should be considered in patients who develop esophageal ulcers that do not respond to specific treatment for opportunistic pathogens in order to assess a possible relationship to zalcitabine.

c) Cardiomyopathy/Congestive Heart Failure: Cardiomyopathy and congestive heart failure in patients with AIDS have been associated with the use of nucleoside analogues. Infrequent cases have been reported in patients receiving zalcitabine. Treatment with zalcitabine in patients with baseline cardiomyopathy or history of congestive heart failure should be approached with caution.

d) Anaphylactoid Reaction: An anaphylactoid reaction was reported in a patient receiving both zalcitabine and zidovudine. In addition, there have been several reports of urticaria without other signs of anaphylaxis.

BECAUSE SEVERE ADVERSE EFFECTS MAY BE ATTRIBUTABLE TO EITHER THE ZALCITABINE OR THE ZIDOVUDINE COMPONENTS OF COMBINATION THERAPY, THE COMPLETE PRODUCT INFORMATION FOR ZIDOVUDINE SHOULD BE CONSULTED BEFORE INITIATION OF COMBINATION THERAPY OR REINSTITUTION OF MONOTHERAPY WITH ZIDOVUDINE FOLLOWING AN ADVERSE REACTION.

PRECAUTIONS:

GENERAL

The safety profile of zalcitabine in children younger than 13 years of age has not been established.

1. Renal Impairment: Patients with renal impairment (estimated creatinine clearance <55 ml/min) may be at a greater risk of toxicity from zalcitabine due to decreased drug clearance. Dosage adjustment is recommended in these patients (see DOSAGE AND ADMINISTRATION.)

2. Lymphoma: High doses of zalcitabine, administered for 3 months to $B_6C_3F_1$ mice (resulting in plasma concentrations over 1000 times those seen in patients taking the recommended doses of zalcitabine) induced an increased incidence of thymic lymphoma. Although the pathogenesis of the effect is uncertain, a predisposition to chemically induced thymic lymphoma and high rates of spontaneous lymphoreticular neoplasms have previously been noted in this strain of mice.

The incidence of lymphomas was reviewed in 13 comparative studies conducted by Roche, the NIAID and the NCI, as well as 7 Roche expanded-access studies that included zalcitabine. In 1 study, ACTG 155, a statistically significant increased rate of lymphomas was seen in patients receiving zalcitabine or combination zalcitabine and zidovudine compared to zidovudine alone (rates of 0, 1.3 and 2.3 per 100 person years for zidovudine, zalcitabine, and combination zalcitabine and zidovudine, respectively; log rank p-value=0.01, pooling zalcitabine and combination zalcitabine and zidovudine vs. zidovudine, p-value=0.003). Based on review of the literature, the incidence of lymphomas in HIV-infected patients with advanced disease on zidovudine monotherapy would be expected to be approximately 1 to 2 per 100 person years of follow-up.

None of the other comparative studies evaluated showed a statistically significant difference in rates of lymphomas in patients receiving either zalcitabine monotherapy or combination zalcitabine and zidovudine. Additional information about ongoing studies will further address this issue. A high incidence of non-Hodgkin's B cell lymphomas (NHL) has been described in a wide variety of immune deficiency states including inherited immunodeficiency states, patients receiving cancer chemotherapy for treatment of prior unrelated malignancies, organ transplant patients and patients with AIDS.

INFORMATION FOR PATIENTS

Patients should be informed that zalcitabine is not a cure for HIV infection and that they may continue to develop illnesses associated with advanced HIV infection including opportunistic infections. Since it is frequently difficult to determine whether symptoms are a result of drug effect or underlying disease manifestation, patients should be encouraged to report all changes in their condition to their physician. Patients should be informed that the use of zalcitabine or other antiretroviral drugs does not preclude the ongoing need to maintain practices designed to prevent transmission of HIV. Women of childbearing age should use effective contraception while using zalcitabine.

Patients should be instructed that the major toxicity of zalcitabine is peripheral neuropathy. Pancreatitis and hepatic toxicity are other serious and potentially life-threatening toxicities that have been reported in patients treated with zalcitabine monotherapy or in combination with zidovudine. Patients should be advised of the early symptoms of these conditions and instructed to promptly report them to their physician. Since the development of peripheral neuropathy appears to be dose-related to zalcitabine, patients should be advised to follow their physicians' instructions regarding the prescribed dose.

LABORATORY TESTS

Complete blood counts and clinical chemistry tests should be performed prior to initiating zalcitabine monotherapy or combination therapy with zalcitabine and zidovudine and at appropriate intervals thereafter. Baseline testing of serum amylase and triglyceride levels should be performed in individuals with a prior history of pancreatitis, increased amylase, those on parenteral nutrition or with a history of ethanol abuse.

CARCINOGENESIS, MUTAGENESIS, AND IMPAIRMENT OF FERTILITY

Carcinogenesis: Carcinogenicity studies in animals have not yet been completed.

Mutagenesis: Ames tests using 7 different tester strains, with and without metabolic activation, were performed with no evidence of mutagenicity. Chinese hamster lung cell tests, with and without metabolic activation, and mouse lymphoma cell tests were performed and there was no evidence of mutagenicity. An unscheduled DNA synthesis assay was performed in rat hepatocytes with no increases in DNA repair. An *in vitro* mammalian cell transformation assay was positive at doses of 500 mcg/ml and higher. Human peripheral blood lymphocytes were exposed to zalcitabine, with and without metabolic activation; at 1.5 mcg/ml and higher, dose-related increases in chromosomal aberration were seen. Oral doses of zalcitabine at 2500 and 4500 mg/kg were clastogenic in the mouse micronucleus assay.

Impairment of Fertility: Fertility and reproductive performance were assessed in rats at plasma concentrations up to 2142 times those achieved with the maximum recommended human dose (MRHD) based on AUC measurements. No adverse effects on rate of conception or general reproductive performance were observed. The highest dose was associated with embryolethality and evidence of teratogenicity. The next lower dose studied (plasma concentrations equivalent to 485 times the MRHD) was associated with a lower frequency of embryotoxicity but no teratogenicity. The fertility of F1 males was significantly reduced at a calculated dose of 2142 (but not 485) times the MRHD (based on AUC measurements) in a teratology study in which rat mothers were dosed on gestation days 7 to 15. No adverse effects were observed on the fertility of parents or F1 generation in the study of fertility and general reproductive performance or in the perinatal and postnatal reproduction study.

PRECAUTIONS: *(cont'd)*

PREGNANCY CATEGORY C

Teratogenic Effects: Zalcitabine has been shown to be teratogenic in mice at calculated exposure levels of 1365 and 2730 times that of the MRHD (based on AUC measurements). In rats, zalcitabine was teratogenic at a calculated exposure level of 2142 times the MRHD but not at an exposure level of 485 times the MRHD. In a perinatal and postnatal study in the rat, a high incidence of hydrocephalus was observed in the F1 offspring derived from liters of dams treated with 1071 (but not 485) times the MRHD (based on AUC measurements). There are no adequate and well-controlled studies of zalcitabine in pregnant women. Zalcitabine should be used during pregnancy only if the potential benefit justifies the potential risk to the fetus. Fertile women should not receive zalcitabine unless they are using effective contraception during therapy. If pregnancy occurs, physicians are encouraged to report such cases by calling (800) 526-6367.

Nonteratogenic Effects: Increased embryolethality was observed in pregnant mice at doses 2730 times the MRHD and in pregnant rats above 485 (but not 98) times the MRHD (based on AUC measurements). Average fetal body weight was significantly decreased in mice at doses of 1365 times the MRHD and in rats at 2142 times the MRHD (based on AUC measurements). In a perinatal and postnatal study, the learning and memory of a significant number of Fl offspring were impaired, and they tended to stay hyperactive for a longer period of time. These effects, observed at a calculated exposure level of 1071 (but not 485) times the MRHD (based on AUC measurements), were considered to result from extensive damage to or gross underdevelopment of the brain of these F1 offspring consistent with the finding of hydrocephalus.

NURSING MOTHERS

It is not known whether zalcitabine is excreted in human milk. Because many drugs are excreted in human milk and the potential exists for serious adverse reactions from zalcitabine in nursing infants, a decision should be made whether to discontinue nursing or to discontinue the drug, taking into account the importance of the drug to the mother. It is currently recommended practice in the United States that HIV-infected women do not breastfeed infants regardless of the use of antiretroviral agents.

PEDIATRIC USE

Safety and effectiveness of zalcitabine in combination with zidovudine or as monotherapy in HIV-infected children younger than 13 years of age has not been established.

DRUG INTERACTIONS:

There was no significant pharmacokinetic interaction between zidovudine and zalcitabine when single doses of zalcitabine (1.5 mg) and zidovudine (200 mg) were coadministered to 12 HIV-positive patients.

Following administration of a single oral 1.5 mg dose of zalcitabine alone during probenecid treatment (500 mg at 8 and 2 hours before and 4 hours after zalcitabine dosing) to 12 HIV-positive patients, mean renal clearance decreased from 310 ml/min (28% CV) to 180 ml/min (22% CV) and AUC increased from 59 ng°hr/ml (27% CV) to 91 ng°hr/ml (22% CV), indicating an increase in exposure of approximately 50% to zalcitabine. Mean $T_{1/2}$of zalcitabine increased from 1.7 to 2.5 hours (see PRECAUTIONS.)

Administration of a single dose of 1.5 mg zalcitabine with a single dose of 800 mg cimetidine to 12 HIV-positive patients resulted in a decrease in renal clearance from 224 ml/min (27% CV) to 171 ml/min (39% CV) and an increase in AUC from 75 ng°hr/ml (29% CV) to 102 ng°hr/ml (35% CV)(see PRECAUTIONS) indicating an increase in exposure of approximately 36% to zalcitabine.

Concomitant administration of Maalox TC (30 ml) with a single dose of 1.5 mg zalcitabine to 12 HIV-positive patients resulted in a decrease in mean C_{max} from 25.2 ng/ml (28% CV) to 18.4 ng/ml (34% CV) and AUC from 75 ng°hr/ml (29% CV, n=10) to 58 ng°hr/ml (36% CV, n=10) indicating a decrease in bioavailability of approximately 25% to zalcitabine (see PRECAUTIONS.)

Administration of a single dose of 1.5 mg zalcitabine with 20 mg metoclopramide (10 mg 1 hour before and 10 mg 4 hours after zalcitabine dose) to 12 HIV-positive patients resulted in a decrease in AUC from 69 ng·hr/ml (16% CV) to 62 ng·hr/ml (21% CV) indicating a decrease in bioavailability of approximately 10% (see PRECAUTIONS.)

Administration of a single dose of 1.5 mg to zalcitabine during loperamide treatment (4 mg 16 hours before zalcitabine, 2 mg at 10 and 4 hours before zalcitabine and 2 mg 2 hours after the zalcitabine dose) to 12 HIV-positive patients with diarrhea resulted in no significant pharmacokinetic interaction between zalcitabine and loperamide.

The concomitant use of zalcitabine with drugs that have the potential to cause peripheral neuropathy should be avoided where possible. Drugs that have been associated with peripheral neuropathy include chloramphenicol, cisplatin, dapsone, disulfiram, ethionamide, glutethimide, gold, hydralazine, iodoquinol, isoniazid, metronidazole, nitrofurantoin, phenytoin, ribavirin and vincristine. Concomitant use of zalcitabine with didanosine is not recommended.

Treatment with zalcitabine should be interrupted when the use of a drug that has the potential to cause pancreatitis is required. Death due to fulminant pancreatitis possibly related to intravenous pentamidine and zalcitabine has been reported. If intravenous pentamidine is required to treat *Pneumocystis carinii* pneumonia, treatment with zalcitabine should be interrupted (see WARNINGS.)

Drugs such as amphotericin, foscarnet and aminoglycosides may increase the risk of developing peripheral neuropathy or other zalcitabine-associated toxicities by interfering with the renal clearance of zalcitabine (thereby raising systemic exposure). Patients who require the use of one of these drugs with zalcitabine should have frequent clinical and laboratory monitoring with dosage adjustment for any significant change in renal function. Concomitant administration of probenecid or cimetidine decreases the elimination of zalcitabine, most likely by inhibition of renal tubular secretion of zalcitabine. Patients receiving these drugs in combination with zalcitabine should be monitored for signs of toxicity and the dose of zalcitabine reduced if warranted.

Absorption of zalcitabine is moderately reduced (approximately 25%) when coadministered with magnesium/aluminum containing antacid products. The clinical significance of this reduction is not known, hence zalcitabine is not recommended to be ingested simultaneously with magnesium/aluminum containing antacids. Bioavailability is mildly reduced (approximately 10%) when zalcitabine and metoclopramide are coadministered (see CLINICAL PHARMACOLOGY.)

ADVERSE REACTIONS:

(See WARNINGS.) TABLES 1 and 2A and B summarize the clinical adverse events that occurred in ≥1% of patients in the comparative monotherapy trial (ACTG 155) of zidovudine and zalcitabine monotherapies vs. zalcitabine and zidovudine combination therapy, respectively.

ADVERSE REACTIONS: *(cont'd)*

TABLE 1 Percentage of Patients with Clinical Adverse Experiences Considered Unassessable or at Least Possibly Related to Study Drug and ≥ Grade III [a] Occurring in ≥1% of Patients in CPCRA 002

	CPCRA 002[b] ZDV Intolerant or Failure n=437	
Body System/Adverse Event	**Zalcitabine 0.750 mg q8h[c] n=237**	**ddl 250 mg q12h[c] n=230**
Systemic		
Fatigue	3.8	2.6
Abdominal Pain	3.0	7.0
Headache	2.1	1.3
Fever	1.7	0.4
Gastrointestinal		
Oral Lesions/Stomatitis	3.0	0
Vomiting/Nausea	3.4	7.0
Diarrhea	2.5	17.0
Hepatic		
Abnormal Hepatic Function	8.9	7.0
Neurological		
Convulsions	1.3	2.2
Peripheral Neuropathy	28.3	13.0
Skin		
Rash/Pruritus/Urticaria	3.4	3.9
Metabolic and Nutrition		
Elevated Amylase	3.4	5.2
Pancreatitis	0	1.7

[a]Grade II Adverse Events possibly or probably related to treatment or unassessable were included if study drug dosage was changed or interrupted.
[b]Median duration of treatment was 34 weeks for both zalcitabine and didanosine groups.
[c]Zalcitabine and ddl dosed by body weight. Only 1 zalcitabine patient and 3 ddl patients received 0.375 mg q8h and 167 mg q12h, respectively.

TABLE 2A Percentage of Patients with Clinical Adverse Experiences Considered Unassessable [a] or at Least Possibly Related to Study Drug in ≥1% of Patients in ACTG 155[b]

	Zalcitabine		ZDV		Zalcitabine + ZDV	
	Mod/Sev LT/Death	**Sev/LT Death**	**Mod/Sev LT/Death**	**Sev/LT Death**	**Mod/Sev LT/Death**	**Sev/LT Death**
Activity/Sleep						
Insomnia	0.7	0.0	2.8	0.4	4.2	0.2
Liver/Gall Bladder						
LDH, ABN, Lab Results	0.7	0.7	1.4	0.4	0.7	0.0
GGT Abnormal	2.8	2.8	3.5	3.2	0.9	0.7
Lower G.I.						
Constipation	0.4	0.0	1.1	0.4	1.4	0.2
Melena	1.1	0.0	0.4	0.0	0.2	0.0
Flatulence, Gas	0.7	0.0	1.4	0.0	0.7	0.0
Diarrhea	9.5	0.4	10.6	1.4	10.6	1.2
Lymph System, Platelets, SPL						
Lymphadenopathy	1.4	0.4	1.1	0.0	0.5	0.0
Metabolic/Nutrition						
Hypoglycemia	6.3	1.8	6.3	1.1	7.8	1.4
Triglyceride Abnormal, NEC	0.7	0.7	1.4	0.7	0.2	0.0
Hypophosphatemia	2.1	0.7	1.8	0.4	1.2	0.5
Hypernatremia	0.4	0.0	1.1	1.1	1.4	0.5
Hyponatremia	3.5	0.0	1.4	0.4	1.2	0.0
Bilirubin, Inc.	4.9	2.1	5.3	2.8	5.4	2.6
Appetite, Loss of	3.9	0.0	6.7	0.0	7.3	0.9
Abnormal Weight Loss, Nos	4.9	0.7	6.3	1.1	9.4	0.5
Hypomagnesemia	1.1	0.4	0.7	0.0	0.5	0.2
Hypocalcium	2.1	1.1	1.8	0.7	2.1	0.7
Creatinine	1.1	0.4	0.4	0.0	1.4	0.7
Amylase, Inc.	8.1	4.9	2.8	1.4	4.2	2.1
Hyperglycemia	5.6	1.1	3.9	2.1	4.5	1.6
Musculoskeletal						
Joint Pain	1.1	0.0	0.4	0.0	1.9	0.0
Weakness Leg Muscle	2.1	0.0	1.8	0.0	4.2	0.0
Myalgia Muscle Pain	6.0	0.4	10.2	1.8	8.0	0.5
Muscle Weakness, Upper	0.7	0.0	2.1	0.0	1.4	0.0
CPR Elevated	0.7	0.4	1.4	1.1	1.2	1.2
Weakness, Gen. Muscle, Nos	0.4	0.4	1.4	0.0	1.9	0.5
Neurological						
Dizziness	1.1	0.0	1.4	0.0	1.4	0.0
Confusion	1.8	0.4	0.7	0.0	0.5	0.0
Loss of Memory	1.8	0.0	0.0	0.0	0.5	0.2
Concentration, DEC	1.1	0.0	0.7	0.0	0.5	0.0

[a]Adverse events listed in this category were considered unassessible or the relationship was not specified by the investigator.
[b]A total of 1001 patients (428 on zalcitabine and ZDV; 286 on ZDV; 287 on zalcitabine) were randomized. Ten patients were excluded from the ACTG analyses: 7 never received study medication; 3 were lost to follow-up within the first 2 weeks of treatment. Those 3 patients (2 on combination zalcitabine and ZDV; 1 on ZDV) are included in this safety table.

TABLES 3 and 4 summarize severe or life-threatening laboratory abnormalities occurring in zalcitabine monotherapy Protocol CPCRA 002 and zalcitabine monotherapy and combination therapy with zidovudine in ACTG 155, respectively.

Monotherapy and Combination Trials: Clinical adverse experiences of all intensities (except ACTG 155 whose events are at least moderate in severity) and at least possibly related to zalcitabine that occurred in <1% of the patients in N3544 (expanded access), CPCRA 002 (comparative monotherapy trial), and ACTG 155 (zalcitabine monotherapy or combination zalcitabine with zidovudine) and in <3% of the patients in N3300/ACTG 114 (comparative monotherapy trial) are listed below by body system. Several of these events occurred in slightly higher rates in other studies:

ADVERSE REACTIONS: *(cont'd)*

TABLE 2B Percentage of Patients with Clinical Adverse Experiences Considered Unassessable [a] or at Least Possibly Related to Study Drug in ≥1% of Patients in ACTG 155[b]

	Zalcitabine Mod/Sev LT/Death	Zalcitabine Sev/LT Death	ZDV Mod/Sev LT/Death	ZDV Sev/LT Death	Zalcitabine + ZDV Mod/Sev LT/Death	Zalcitabine + ZDV Sev/LT Death
Psychological						
Anxiety State Unspecified	0.7	0.0	1.4	0.4	1.2	0.0
Depression	2.1	0.4	3.9	0.4	4.0	0.7
Renal						
Dysuria	0.7	0.0	1.1	0.0	1.2	0.0
Urination (Frequency)	0.4	0.0	1.8	0.4	1.2	0.0
Reproduction						
Vaginal Discharge	0.0	0.0	1.1	0.0	0.0	0.0
Respiratory						
Nasal Discharge	3.5	0.0	6.0	0.0	6.4	0.2
Cough	6.3	0.0	7.7	0.0	8.2	0.2
Rales/Rhonchi	1.1	0.0	0.7	0.0	0.0	0.0
Dyspnea/Respiratory Distress	2.8	0.7	5.6	0.0	2.8	0.0
Skin						
Pruritic Disorder	4.9	1.1	4.2	0.4	4.0	0.5
Rash	11.2	2.1	8.8	1.4	9.4	0.7
Night Sweats	2.8	0.7	2.5	0.0	3.8	0.5
Chills Night Sweats	1.1	0.0	0.7	0.0	0.7	0.0
Lip Blister, Lesions	1.1	0.4	0.0	0.0	0.2	0.0
Special Senses						
Ear Problem, Pain	0.0	0.0	1.1	0.0	0.5	0.0
Smell Dysfunction	1.1	0.4	0.0	0.0	0.0	0.0
Systemic, General Body						
Fever/Febrile	16.8	4.9	17.6	9.2	16.2	3.8
Malaise Fatigue	13.3	1.8	17.3	2.8	18.1	3.5
Headache	12.3	1.4	16.2	1.8	15.3	2.6
Chest Pain, Unspec.	1.4	0.4	3.9	0.4	2.8	0.2
General Debilitation	1.1	0.0	1.8	0.4	0.2	0.0
Chills	1.4	0.7	1.1	0.0	2.1	0.5
Upper G.I.						
Acute Pharyngitis	1.8	0.0	1.1	0.0	2.4	0.0
Oral Ulcers[c]	7.0	3.2	2.8	0.0	5.6	0.9
Nausea	3.5	0.7	7.0	1.1	8.2	0.5
Dysphagia	4.2	0.4	1.1	0.0	3.5	0.7
Vomiting	3.5	1.1	4.6	1.4	6.6	0.7
Swallowing, Painful	2.1	0.4	1.1	0.0	2.1	0.5
Mouth Lesion	3.2	1.1	1.4	0.7	2.6	0.2
Abdominal Pain	8.1	1.4	7.7	1.4	7.1	1.9

[a]Adverse events listed in this category were considered unassessible or the relationship was not specified by the investigator.
[b]A total of 1001 patients (428 on zalcitabine and ZDV; 286 on ZDV; 287 on zalcitabine) were randomized. Ten patients were excluded from the ACTG analyses: 7 never received study medication; 3 were lost to follow-up within the first 2 weeks of treatment. Those 3 patients (2 on combination zalcitabine and ZDV; 1 on ZDV) are included in this safety table.
[c]Adverse events combined to form this category.
Note: Certain laboratory abnormalities were also recorded as clinical events and are included in this table.

TABLE 3 Percentage of Patients with Protocol Grade 3-4 Laboratory Abnormalities

CPCRA 002[a] ZDV Intolerant or Failure n=437

Laboratory Abnormality	Zalcitabine 0.750 mg q8h[b] n=237	ddI 250 mg q12h[b] n=230
Anemia (<7.5 gm/dl)	8.4	7.4
Leukopenia (<1500 cells/mm^3)	13.1	9.6
Eosinophilia (>1000 cells/mm^3 or 25%)	2.5	1.7
Neutropenia (<750 cells/mm^3)	16.9	11.7
Thrombocytopenia (<50,000 cells/mm^3)	1.3	4.8
SGOT (>5 x ULN)	7.6	5.7

[a]Median duration of treatment was 34 weeks for both the zalcitabine and ddI groups.
[b]Zalcitabine and ddI dosed by body weight. Only 1 zalcitabine patient and 3 ddI patients received 0.375 mg q8h and 167 mg q12h, respectively.
Note: Elevated amylase is listed with clinical adverse experiences in TABLE 1.

TABLE 4 Percentage of Patients with Grade 3/4 Laboratory Abnormalities [a] in ACTG 155

Laboratory Abnormality	Zalcitabine n=285	ZDV n=283	Zalcitabine + ZDV n=423
Anemia (<7.5 gm/dl)	6	4.2	5.7
Leukopenia (<1500 cells/mm^3)	9.1	12.7	13.9
Neutropenia (<750 cells/mm^3)	15.1	18.7	22.7
Eosinophilia (>1000 or 25%)	6.3	4.6	5.0
Thrombocytopenia (<50,000 cells/mm^3)	2.8	2.1	3.1
SGPT (>250 U/l)	3.2	3.9	3.1
SGOT (>250 U/l)	3.2	4.2	3.5
Alkaline Phosphatase (>625 U/l)	1.4	1.1	1.2

[a]Several other laboratory abnormalities were recorded as clinical adverse experiences included in TABLE 2.

Body as a Whole: asthenia, cachexia, chest tightness or pain, chills, cutaneous/allergic reaction, debilitation, difficulty moving, dry eyes/mouth, edema, facial pain or swelling, fatigue, fever, flank pain, flushing, increased sweating, lymphadenopathy, malaise, night sweats, pain, pelvic/groin pain, rigors, weight decrease.

Cardiovascular: abnormal cardiac movement, arrhythmia, atrial fibrillation, cardiac failure, cardiac dysrhythmias, cardiomyopathy, heart racing, hypertension, palpitation, subarachnoid hemorrhage, syncope, tachycardia, ventricular ectopy.

ADVERSE REACTIONS: *(cont'd)*

Endocrine/Metabolic: abnormal triglycerides, abnormal lipase, altered serum glucose, diabetes mellitus, glycosuria, gout, hot flushes, hyperglycemia, hyperkalemia, hyperlipemia, hypernatremia, hyperuricemia, hypocalcemia, hypokalemia, hypomagnesemia, increased nonprotein nitrogen, polydipsia.

Gastrointestinal: abdominal bloating or cramps, acute pancreatitis, anal/rectal pain, anorexia, bleeding gums, colitis, constipation, dental abscess, dry mouth, dyspepsia, dysphagia, enlarged abdomen, epigastric pain, eructation, esophageal pain, esophageal ulcers, esophagitis, flatulence, gagging with pills, gastritis, gastrointestinal hemorrhage, gingivitis, glossitis, gum disorder, heartburn, hemorrhagic pancreatitis, hemorrhoids, increased saliva, left quadrant pain, melena, nausea & vomiting, odynophagia, painful sore gums, pancreatitis, rectal hemorrhage, rectal mass, rectal ulcers, salivary gland enlargement, sore tongue, sore throat, tongue disorder, tongue ulcer, toothache, unformed/loose stools, vomiting.

Hematologic: absolute neutrophil count alteration, anemia, epistaxis, decreased hematocrit, granulocytosis, hemoglobinemia, leukopenia, neutrophilia, platelet alteration, purpura, thrombocytopenia, thrombus, unspecified hematologic toxicity, white blood cell alteration.

Hepatic: abnormal gamma-glutamyl transferase, abnormal lactate dehydrogenase, bilirubinemia, cholecystitis, decreased alkaline phosphatase, hepatitis, hepatocellular damage, hepatomegaly, increased alkaline phosphatase, increased SGOT, increased SGPT.

Musculoskeletal: arthralgia, arthritis, arthropathy, arthrosis, back pain, backache, bone pains/aches, bursitis, cold extremities, extremity pain, increased creatine phosphokinase, joint pain, joint inflammation, joint swelling, leg cramps, muscle weakness, muscle disorder, muscle stiffness, muscle cramps, myalgia, myopathy, myositis, neck pain, rib pain, stiff neck.

Neurological: abnormal coordination, aphasia, ataxia, Bell's palsy, confusion, convulsion, decreased concentration, decreased neurological function, disequilibrium, dizziness, dysphonia, facial nerve palsy, focal motor seizures, grand mal seizure, hyperkinesia, hypertonia, hypokinesia, memory loss, migraine, neuralgia, neuritis, paralysis, seizures, speech disorder, status epilepticus, stupor, tremor, twitch, vertigo.

Psychological: acute psychotic disorder, acute stress reaction, agitation, amnesia, anxiety, confusion, decreased motivation, decreased sexual desire, depersonalization, depression, emotional lability, euphoria, hallucination, impaired concentration, insomnia, manic reaction, mood swings, nervousness, paranoid state, somnolence, suicide attempt.

Respiratory: acute nasopharyngitis, chest congestion, coughing, cyanosis, dry nasal mucosa, dyspnea, flu-like symptoms, hemoptysis, pharyngitis, sinus congestion, sinus pain, sinusitis, wheezing.

Skin: acne, alopecia, bullous eruptions, carbuncle/furuncle, cellulitis, cold sore, dermatitis, dry skin, dry rash desquamation, erythematous rash, exfoliative dermatitis, finger inflammation, follicular rash, impetigo, infection, itchy rash, lip blisters/lesions, macular/papular rash, maculopapular rash, moniliasis, mucocutaneous/skin disorder, nail disorder, photosensitivity reaction, pruritus, skin disorder, skin lesions, skin fissure, skin ulcer, urticaria.

Special Senses: abnormal vision, blurred vision, burning eyes, decreased taste, decreased vision, ear pain/problem, ear blockage, eye abnormality, eye inflammation, eye itching, eye pain, eye irritation, eye redness, eye hemorrhage, fluid in ears, hearing loss, increased tears, loss of taste, mucopurulent conjunctivitis, parosmia, photophobia, taste perversion, tinnitus, unequal-sized pupils, xerophthalmia, yellow sclera.

Urogenital: abnormal renal function, acute renal failure, albuminuria, bladder pain, dysuria, genital lesion/ulcer, increased blood urea nitrogen, micturition frequency, nocturia, painful penis sore, penile edema, polyuria, renal cyst, renal calculus, testicular swelling, toxic nephropathy, urinary retention, vaginal itch, vaginal ulcer, vaginal pain, vaginal/cervix disorder.

OVERDOSAGE:

Acute Overdosage: Inadvertent pediatric overdoses have occurred with doses up to 1.5 mg/kg zalcitabine. The children had prompt gastric lavage and treatment with activated charcoal and had no sequelae. Mixed overdoses including zalcitabine and other drugs have led to drowsiness and vomiting (with zalcitabine or placebo, zidovudine and cotrimoxazole), or increased ggt (with 18.75 mg zalcitabine with zidovudine and lormetazam) or increased creatinine phosphokinase (with zalcitabine or placebo, zidovudine, fluconazole, dapsone and wine). There is no experience with acute zalcitabine overdosage at higher doses and sequelae are unknown. There is no known antidote for zalcitabine overdosage. It is not known whether zalcitabine is dialyzable by peritoneal dialysis or hemodialysis.

Chronic Overdosage: In an initial dose-finding study in which zalcitabine was administered at doses 25 times (0.25 mg/kg q8h) the currently recommended dose, 1 patient discontinued zalcitabine after 1 1/2 weeks of treatment subsequent to the development of a rash and fever.

In the early Phase 1 studies, all patients receiving zalcitabine at approximately 6 times the current total daily recommended dose experienced peripheral neuropathy by week 10. Eighty percent of patients who received approximately 2 times the current total daily recommended dose experienced peripheral neuropathy by week 12.

DOSAGE AND ADMINISTRATION:

The recommended monotherapy regimen is one 0.750 mg tablet of zalcitabine orally every 8 hours (2.25 mg zalcitabine total daily dose). The recommended combination regimen is one 0.750 mg tablet of zalcitabine orally, administered concomitantly with 200 mg of zidovudine every 8 hours (2.25 mg zalcitabine total daily dose and 600 mg zidovudine total daily dose). Based on preliminary data, the recommended zalcitabine dosage reduction for patients with impaired renal function is: creatinine clearance 10 to 40 ml/min: 0.750 mg of zalcitabine q12h; creatinine clearance <10 ml/min: 0.750 mg of zalcitabine q24h.

Monitoring of Patients: Periodic complete blood counts and clinical chemistry tests should be performed. Serum amylase levels should be monitored in those individuals who have a history of elevated amylase, pancreatitis, ethanol abuse, who are on parenteral nutrition or who are otherwise at high risk of pancreatitis. Careful monitoring for signs or symptoms suggestive of peripheral neuropathy is recommended, particularly in individuals with a low CD4 cell count or who are at a greater risk of developing peripheral neuropathy while on therapy (see WARNINGS.)

Dose Adjustment for Monotherapy with Zalcitabine and in Combination Therapy with Zalcitabine and Zidovudine: For toxicities in patients receiving monotherapy that are likely to be associated with zalcitabine (*e.g.,* peripheral neuropathy, severe oral ulcers, pancreatitis, elevated liver function tests especially in patients with chronic Hepatitis B) zalcitabine should be interrupted or dose reduced. FOR SEVERE TOXICITIES OR THOSE PERSISTING AFTER DOSE REDUCTION, ZALCITABINE SHOULD BE INTERRUPTED. For recipients of combination therapy with zalcitabine and zidovudine, dose adjustments for either drug should be based on the known toxicity profile of the individual drugs. For toxicities that have been associated with either zalcitabine or zidovudine (*e.g.,* hepatic toxicity), both drugs should be interrupted or dose reduced. For any interruption of zalcitabine, and especially if zalcitabine is permanently discontinued, the zidovudine dosage schedule should be adjusted from 200 mg q8h to 100 mg q4h as recommended in the complete product information for zidovudine. FOR SEVERE TOXICITIES OR TOXICITIES IN WHICH THE CAUSATIVE DRUG IS UNCLEAR OR THOSE PERSISTING AFTER DOSE INTERRUPTION OR REDUCTION OF ONE DRUG, THE OTHER DRUG SHOULD ALSO BE INTER-

DOSAGE AND ADMINISTRATION: *(cont'd)*

RUPTED OR DOSE-REDUCED. PHYSICIANS SHOULD REFER TO THE COMPLETE PRODUCT INFORMATION FOR ZIDOVUDINE FOR A DESCRIPTIONOF KNOWN ZIDOVUDINE-ASSOCIATED ADVERSE REACTIONS.

Patients developing moderate discomfort with signs or symptoms of peripheral neuropathy should stop zalcitabine. Zalcitabine-associated peripheral neuropathy may continue to worsen despite interruption of zalcitabine. Zalcitabine should be reintroduced at 50% dose — 0.375 mg q8h only if all findings related to peripheral neuropathy have improved to mild symptoms. Zalcitabine may be permanently discontinued if patients experience severe discomfort related to peripheral neuropathy or moderate discomfort that progresses. If other moderate to severe clinical adverse reactions or laboratory abnormalities (such as increased liver function tests) occur, then zalcitabine in those patients receiving monotherapy or both zalcitabine and zidovudine for those on combination treatment, should be interrupted until the adverse reaction abates. Zalcitabine or zidovudine monotherapy or zalcitabine and zidovudine combination therapy should then be carefully reintroduced at lower doses if appropriate. If adverse reactions recur at the reduced dose, therapy should be discontinued. The minimum effective dose of zalcitabine in combination with zidovudine for the treatment of adult patients with advanced HIV infection has not been established.

In patients with poor bone marrow reserve, particularly those patients with advanced symptomatic HIV disease, frequent monitoring of hematologic indices is recommended to detect serious anemia or granulocytopenia (see WARNINGS.) Significant toxicities, such as anemia (hemoglobin of <7.5 gm/dl or reduction of >25% of baseline) and/or granulocytopenia (granulocyte count of <750 cells/mm³ or reduction of >50% from baseline), may require a treatment interruption of zalcitabine and zidovudine until evidence of marrow recovery is observed (see WARNINGS.) For less severe anemia or granulocytopenia, a reduction in daily dose of zidovudine in those patients receiving combination therapy may be adequate. In patients who experience hematologic toxicity, reduction in hemoglobin may occur as early as 2 to 4 weeks after initiation of therapy, and granulocytopenia usually occurs after 6 to 8 weeks of therapy. In patients who develop significant anemia, dose modification does not necessarily eliminate the need for transfusion. If marrow recovery occurs following dose modification, gradual increases in dose may be appropriate depending on hematologic indices and patient tolerance. For more details, refer to the complete product information for zidovudine.

REFERENCES:

1. Pizzo PA, Butler K, Balis F, et al. Dideoxycytidine alone and in an alternating schedule with zidovudine in children with symptomatic human immunodeficiency virus infection. *J Pediatr.*1990; 117(5):799-808. **2.** Abrams DI, Goldman AI, Launer C, et al. A comparative trial of didanosine or zalcitabine after treatment with zidovudine in patients with human immunodeficiency virus infection. *N Engl J Med.* 1994; 330(10)657-662. **3.** Follansbee S, Drew L, Olson R, el al. The efficacy of zalcitabine (ddC, zalcitabine) versus zidovudine (ZDV) as monotherapy in ZDV-naive patients with advanced HIV disease; a randomized, double-blind, comparative trial (ACTG 114; N3300). IXth International Conference on AIDS/IV STD World Congress, Berlin, Germany, June 7-11, 1993. Poster PO-B26-2113. **4.** Remick S, Follansbee S, Olson R, et al. Safety and tolerance of zalcitabine (ddc, zalcitabine) in a double-blind comparative trial (ACTG 114; N3300). IXth International Conference on AIDS/IV STD World Congress, Berlin, Germany, June 7-11, 1993. Poster PO-B26-2115. **5.** Meng T-C, Fischl MA, Boota AM, et al. Combination therapy with zidovudine and dideoxycytidine in patients with advanced human immunodeficiency virus infection. *Ann Intern Med.* 1992; 116(1):13-20. **6.** Schooley R and the Wellcome Resistance Study Collaborative Group. Trial of ZDV/ddl vs ZDV/ddC vs ZDV in HIV-infected patients with CD4 cell counts less than 300: Preliminary Results. Fourth European Conference on Clinical Aspects and Treatment of HIV Infection, Milan, Italy, March 16-18, 1994, 052. **7.** "Dear Doctor" letter, Burroughs Wellcome Co., June 1, 1993. **8.** Food and Drug Administration Antiviral Drugs Advisory Committee Meeting, "Mitochondrial Damage Associated with Nucleoside Analogues," Rockville, MD, Sept. 21, 1993.

HOW SUPPLIED:

Hivid 0.375 mg tablets are oval, beige, film-coated tablets with "Hivid 0.375" imprinted on one side and "Roche" on the other side. Hivid 0.750 mg tablets are oval, gray, film- coated tablets with "Hivid 0.750" imprinted on one side and "Roche" on the other side.

The tablets should be stored in tightly closed bottles at 59° to 86°F (15° to 30°C).

HOW SUPPLIED - EQUIVALENTS NOT AVAILABLE:

Tablet, Uncoated - Oral - 0.375 mg

100's $183.42 HIVID, Roche **00004-0220-01**

Tablet, Uncoated - Oral - 0.750 mg

100's $229.92 HIVID, Roche **00004-0221-01**

ZIDOVUDINE *(002451)*

CATEGORIES: AIDS Related Complex; Anti-Infectives; Antimicrobials; Antivirals; HIV Infection; Immunomodulators; Infections; Nucleoside Analogue Drugs; Orphan Drugs; Viral Agents; Pregnancy Category C; Sales > $100 Million; FDA Approved 1987 Mar; Patent Expiration 1994 Feb

BRAND NAMES: AZT; **Retrovir**; *Retrovis*
(International brand names outside U.S. in italics)

FORMULARIES: Aetna; BC-BS; Medi-Cal; PCS

COST OF THERAPY: $3,488.45 (AIDS; Capsule; 100 mg; 6/day; 365 days)

> **WARNING:**
> ZIDOVUDINE MAY BE ASSOCIATED WITH HEMATOLOGIC TOXICITY INCLUDING GRANULOCYTOPENIA AND SEVERE ANEMIA PARTICULARLY IN PATIENTS WITH ADVANCED HIV DISEASE (SEE WARNINGS.) PROLONGED USE OF ZIDOVUDINE HAS BEEN ASSOCIATED WITH SYMPTOMATIC MYOPATHY SIMILAR TO THAT PRODUCED BY HUMAN IMMUNODEFICIENCY VIRUS. RARE OCCURRENCES OF POTENTIALLY FATAL LACTIC ACIDOSIS IN THE ABSENCE OF HYPOXEMIA, AND SEVERE HEPATOMEGALY WITH STEATOSIS HAVE BEEN REPORTED WITH THE USE OF CERTAIN ANTIRETROVIRAL NUCLEOSIDE ANALOGUES..

DESCRIPTION:

Zidovudine [formerly called azidothymidine (AZT)], is a pyrimidine nucleoside analogue active against human immunodeficiency virus (HIV).

The chemical name of zidovudine is 3'-azido-3'-deoxythymidine.

Zidovudine is a white to beige, odorless, crystalline solid with a molecular weight of 267.24 and a solubility of 20.1 mg/ml in water at 25°C. The molecular formula is $C_{10}H_{13}N_5O_4$.

Tablets: Retrovir tablets are for oral administration. Each film-coated tablet contains 300 mg of zidovudine and the inactive ingredients hydroxypropyl methylcellulose, magnesium stearate, microcrystalline cellulose, polyethylene glycol, sodium starch glycolate, and titanium dioxide.

DESCRIPTION: *(cont'd)*

Capsules: Retrovir capsules are for oral administration. Each capsule contains 100 mg of zidovudine and the inactive ingredients corn starch, magnesium stearate, microcrystalline cellulose, and sodium starch glycolate. The 100 mg empty hard gelatin capsule, printed with edible black ink, consists of black iron oxide, dimethylpolysiloxane, gelatin, pharmaceutical shellac, soya lecithin, and titanium dioxide. The blue band around the capsule consists of gelatin and FD&C Blue No. 2.

Syrup: Retrovir syrup is for oral administration. Each teaspoonful (5 ml) of Retrovir syrup contains 50 mg of zidovudine and the inactive ingredients sodium benzoate 0.2% (added as a preservative), citric acid, flavors, glycerin, and liquid sucrose. Sodium hydroxide may be added to adjust pH.

Intravenous Infusion: Retrovir IV infusion is a sterile solution for intravenous infusion only. Each ml contains 10 mg zidovudine in Water for Injection. Hydrochloric acid and/or sodium hydroxide may have been added to adjust the pH to approximately 5.5. Retrovir IV infusion contains no preservatives.

CLINICAL PHARMACOLOGY:

MICROBIOLOGY

Mechanism of Action: Zidovudine is a synthetic nucleoside analogue of the naturally occurring nucleoside, thymidine, in which the 3'-hydroxy (-OH) group is replaced by an azido ($-N_3$) group. Within cells, zidovudine is converted to the active metabolite, zidovudine 5'-triphosphate (AztTP), by the sequential action of the cellular enzymes. Zidovudine 5'-triphosphate inhibits the activity of the HIV reverse transcriptase both by competing for utilization with the natural substrate, deoxythymidine 5'-triphosphate (dTTP), and by its incorporation into viral DNA. The lack of a 3'-OH group in the incorporated nucleoside analogue prevents the formation of the 5' to 3' phosphodiester linkage essential for DNA chain elongation and, therefore, the viral DNA growth is terminated. The active metabolite AztTP is also a weak inhibitor of the cellular DNA polymerase-alpha and mitochondrial polymerase-gamma and has been reported to be incorporated into the DNA of cells in culture.

In Vitro HIV Susceptibility: The *in vitro* anti-HIV activity of zidovudine was assessed by infecting cell lines of lymphoblastic and monocytic origin and peripheral blood lymphocytes with laboratory and clinical isolates of HIV. The IC_{50} and IC_{90} values (50% and 90% inhibitory concentrations) were 0.003 to 0.013 and 0.03 to 0.13 mcg/ml), respectively (1nM=0.27 ng/ml). The IC_{50} and IC_{90} values of HIV isolates recovered from 18 untreated AIDS/ARC patients were in the range of 0.003 to 0.013 mcg/ml and 0.03 to 0.3 mcg/ml, respectively. Zidovudine showed antiviral activity in all acutely infected cell lines; however, activity was substantially less in chronically infected cell lines. In drug combination studies with zalcitabine, didanosine, lamivudine, saquinavir, indinavir, ritonavir, nevirapine, delavirdine, or interferon-alpha, zidovudine showed additive to synergistic activity in cell culture. The relationship between the *in vitro* susceptibility of HIV to reverse transcriptase inhibitors and the inhibition of HIV replication in humans has not been established.

Drug Resistance: HIV isolates with reduced sensitivity to zidovudine have been selected *in vitro* and were also recovered from patients treated with zidovudine. Genetic analysis of the isolates showed mutations which results in five amino acid substitutions (Met41→Leu, A67→Asn, Lys70→Arg, Thr215→Tyr or Phe, and Lys219→Gln) in the viral reverse transcriptase. In general, higher levels of resistance were associated with greater number of mutations with 215 mutation being the most significant.

Cross Resistance: The potential for cross-resistance between HIV reverse transcriptase inhibitors and protease inhibitors is low because the different enzyme targets involved. Combination therapy with zidovudine plus zalcitabine or didanosine does not appear to prevent the emergence of zidovudine-resistant isolates. Combination therapy with zidovudine plus lamivudine delayed the emergence of mutations conferring resistance to zidovudine. In some patients harboring zidovudine-resistant virus, combination with zidovudine plus lamivudine restored phenotypic sensitivity to zidovudine by 12 weeks of treatment. HIV isolates with multi-drug resistance to zidovudine, didanosine, zalcitabine, stavudine, and lamivudine were recovered from a small number of patients treated for ≥1 year with the combination of zidovudine and didanosine or zalcitabine. The pattern of resistant mutations in the combination therapy was different (Ala62→Val, Val75→Ile, Phe77→116Tyr, and Gln→151Met) from monotherapy, with mutation 151 being most significant for multidrug resistance. Site-directed mutagenesis studies showed that these mutations could also result in resistance to zalcitabine, lamivudine, and stavudine.

PHARMACOKINETICS

Adults: The pharmacokinetics of zidovudine has been evaluated in 22 adult HIV-infected patients in a Phase 1 dose-escalation study.

After oral dosing (capsules), zidovudine was rapidly absorbed from the gastrointestinal tract with peak serum concentrations occurring within 0.5 to 1.5 hours. Dose-independent kinetics was observed over the range of 2 mg/kg every 8 hours to 10 mg/kg every 4 hours. The mean zidovudine half-life was approximately 1 hour and ranged from 0.78 to 1.93 hours following oral dosing.

Following intravenous dosing, dose-dependent kinetics was observed over the range of 1 to 5 mg/kg with a mean zidovudine half-life of 1.1 hours (range 0.48 to 2.86 hours). Total body clearance averaged 1900 ml/min/70 kg, and the apparent volume of distribution was 1.6 L/kg. At a dose of 7.5 mg/kg every 4 hours, total body clearance was calculated to be about 1200 ml/min/70 kg, with no change in half-life. Renal clearance is estimated to be 400 ml/min/70 kg, indicating glomerular filtration and active tubular secretion by the kidneys. Zidovudine plasma protein binding is 34% to 38%, indicating that drug interactions involving binding site displacement are not anticipated. The mean steady-state peak and trough concentrations of zidovudine at 2.5 mg/kg every 4 hours were 1.06 and 0.12 mcg/ml, respectively.

Zidovudine is rapidly metabolized to 3'-azido-3'-deoxy-5'-*O*-β-*D*-glucopyranuronosylthymidine (GZDV) which has an apparent elimination half-life of 1 hour (range 0.61 to 1.73 hours). Following oral administration, urinary recovery of zidovudine and GZDV accounted for 14% and 74% of the dose, respectively, and the total urinary recovery averaged 90% (range 63% to 95%), indicating a high degree of absorption. Following intravenous administration, urinary recoveries of zidovudine and GZDV accounted for 18% and 60% of the dose, respectively, and the total urinary recovery averaged 77% (range 64% to 98%). However, as a result of first-pass metabolism, the average oral capsule bioavailability of zidovudine is 65% (range 52% to 75%). A second metabolite, 3'-amino-3'-deoxythymidine (AMT), has been identified in the plasma following single dose intravenous administration of zidovudine. AMT area-under-the-curve (AUC) was one-fifth of the AUC of zidovudine and had a half-life of 2.7 ± 0.7 hours. In comparison, GZDV AUC was about 3-fold greater than the AUC of zidovudine.

Additional pharmacokinetic data following intravenous dosing indicated dose-independent kinetics over the range of 1 to 5 mg/kg with a mean zidovudine half-life of 1.1 hours (range 0.48 to 2.86 hours). Total body clearance averaged 1900 ml/min/70 kg and the apparent volume of distribution was 1.6 L/kg. Renal clearance is estimated to be 400 ml/min/70 kg, indicating glomerular filtration and active tubular secretion by the kidneys. Zidovudine plasma protein binding is 34% to 38%, indicating that drug interactions involving binding site displacement are not anticipated.

CLINICAL PHARMACOLOGY: *(cont'd)*

The zidovudine cerebrospinal fluid (CSF)/plasma concentration ratio was determined in 39 patients receiving chronic therapy with zidovudine. The median ratio measured in 50 paired samples drawn 1 to 8 hours after the last dose of zidovudine was 0.6.

Adults with Impaired Renal Function: The pharmacokinetics of zidovudine has been evaluated in patients with impaired renal function following a single 200 mg oral dose. In 14 patients (mean creatinine clearance 18 ± 2 ml/min), the half-life of zidovudine was 1.4 hours compared to 1.0 hour for control subjects with normal renal function; AUC values were approximately twice those of controls. Additionally, GZDV half-life in these patients was 8.0 hours (vs 0.9 hours for control) and AUC was 17 times higher than for control subjects. The pharmacokinetics and tolerance were evaluated in a multiple-dose study in patients undergoing hemodialysis (n=5) or peritoneal dialysis (n=6). Patients received escalating doses of zidovudine up to 200 mg five times daily for 8 weeks. Daily doses of 500 mg or less were well tolerated despite significantly elevated plasma levels of GZDV. Apparent oral clearance of zidovudine was approximately 50% of that reported in patients with normal renal function. The plasma concentrations of AMT are not known in patients with renal insufficiency. Daily oral doses of 300 to 400 mg should be appropriate in HIV-infected patients with severe renal dysfunction (see DOSAGE AND ADMINISTRATION, Dose Adjustment. Hemodialysis and peritoneal dialysis appear to have a negligible effect on the removal of zidovudine, whereas GZDV elimination is enhanced.

Pediatrics: The pharmacokinetics and bioavailability of zidovudine have been evaluated in 21 HIV-infected children, aged 6 months through 12 years, following intravenous doses administered over the range of 80 to 160 mg/m^2 every 6 hours, and following oral doses of the intravenous solution administered over the range of 90 to 240 mg/m^2 every 6 hours. After discontinuation of the IV infusion, zidovudine plasma concentrations decayed biexponentially, consistent with two-compartment pharmacokinetics. Proportional increases in AUC and in zidovudine concentrations were observed with increasing dose, consistent with dose-independent kinetics over the dose range studied. The mean terminal half-life and total body clearance across all dose levels administered were 1.5 hours and 30.9 ml/min/kg, respectively. These values compare to mean half-life and total body clearance in adults of 1.1 hours and 27.1 ml/min/kg.

The mean oral bioavailability of 65% was independent of dose. This value is the same as the bioavailability in adults. Doses of 180 mg/m^2 four times daily in pediatric patients produced similar systemic exposure (24 hour AUC 10.7 hr·mcg/ml) as doses of 200 mg six times daily in adult patients (10.9 hr·mcg/ml).

The pharmacokinetics of zidovudine has been studied in neonates from birth to 3 months of life. In one study of the pharmacokinetics of zidovudine in women during the last trimester of pregnancy, zidovudine elimination was determined immediately after birth in 8 neonates who were exposed to zidovudine *in utero.* The half-life was 13.0 ± 5.8 hours. In another study, the pharmacokinetics of zidovudine was evaluated in pediatric patients (ranging in age of 1 day to 3 months) of normal birth weight for gestational age and with normal renal and hepatic function. In neonates less than or equal to 14 days old, mean ± SD total body clearance was 10.9 ± 4.8 ml/min/kg (n=18) and half-life was 3.1 ± 1.2 hours (n=21). In neonates and infants greater than 14 days, total body clearance was 19.0 ± 4.0 ml/min/kg (n=16) and half-life was 1.9 ± 0.7 hours (n=18). Bioavailability was 89% ± 19% (n=15) in the younger age group and decreased to 61% ± 19% (n=17) in infants older than 14 days.

Concentrations of zidovudine in cerebrospinal fluid were measured after both intermittent oral and IV drug administration in 21 pediatric patients during Phase 1 and Phase 2 studies. The mean zidovudine CSF/plasma concentration ratio measured at an average time of 2.2 hours postdose at oral doses of 120 to 240 mg/m^2 was 0.52 ± 0.44 (n=28); after an IV infusion of doses of 80 to 160 mg/m^2 over 1 hour, the mean CSF/plasma concentration ratio was 0.87 ± 0.66 (n=23) at 3.2 hours after the start of the infusion. During continuous IV infusion, mean steady-state CSF/plasma ratio was 0.26 ± 0.17 (n=28).

As in adult patients, the major route of elimination in pediatric patients was by metabolism to GZDV. After IV dosing, about 29% of the dose was excreted in the urine unchanged and about 45% of the dose was excreted as GZDV. Overall, the pharmacokinetics of zidovudine in pediatric patients greater than 3 months of age is similar to that of zidovudine in adult patients.

Pregnancy: The pharmacokinetics of zidovudine has been studied in a Phase 1 study of eight women during the last trimester of pregnancy. As pregnancy progressed, there was no evidence of drug accumulation. The pharmacokinetics of zidovudine was similar to that of nonpregnant adults. Consistent with passive transmission of the drug across the placenta, zidovudine concentrations in infant plasma at birth were essentially equal to those in maternal plasma at delivery. Although data are limited, methadone maintenance therapy in five pregnant women did not appear to alter zidovudine pharmacokinetics. However, in another patient population, a potential for interaction has been identified (see PRECAUTIONS.)

Nursing Mothers: The U.S. Public Health Service Centers for Disease Control and Prevention advises HIV-infected women not to breast feed to avoid postnatal transmission of HIV to a child who may not be infected. After administration of a single dose of 200 mg zidovudine to 13 HIV-infected women, the mean concentration of zidovudine was similar in human milk and serum (see PRECAUTIONS, Nursing Mothers).

Effect of Food on Absorption: *Capsules:* Administration of zidovudine capsules with food decreased peak plasma concentrations by greater than 50%, however bioavailability as determined by AUC may not be affected. *Tablets:* In a single-dose study of 23 healthy volunteers, the mean ± SD relative bioavailability of the zidovudine 300–mg tablet relative to three 100–mg zidovudine capsules was 110 ± 18%. After administration of the 300–mg zidovudine tablet or three 100–mg zidovudine capsules, the mean ± SD C_{max} values were 1.81 ± 0.52 and 1.50 ± 0.46 mcg/ml, respectively. The effect of food on the absorption of zidovudine from the tablet formulation is not known. *Syrup:* In a multiple dose bioavailability study conducted in 12 HIV-infected adults receiving doses of 100 or 200 mg every 4 hours, zidovudine syrup was demonstrated to be bioequivalent to zidovudine capsules with respect to area under the zidovudine plasma concentration-time curve (AUC). The rate of absorption of zidovudine syrup was greater than that of zidovudine capsules, as indicated by mean times to peak concentration of 0.5 and 0.8 hours, respectively. Mean values for steady-state peak concentration (dose-normalized to 200 mg) were 1.5 and 1.2 mcg/ml for syrup and capsules, respectively.

CLINICAL STUDIES:

Description of Clinical Studies: Therapy with zidovudine has been shown to prolong survival and decrease the incidence of opportunistic infections in patients with advanced HIV disease at the initiation of therapy and to delay disease progression in asymptomatic HIV-infected patients.

Other randomized studies suggest that the duration of the clinical benefit of monotherapy with zidovudine is time-limited.

Combination Therapy-Adults: ACTG175 was a randomized, double-blind, controlled trial that compared zidovudine 200 three times daily; didanosine 200 mg twice daily; zidovudine plus didanosine; and zidovudine plus zalcitabine 0.75 mg three times daily. A total of 2467 HIV-infected adults with baseline CD4 counts of 200 to 500 cells/mm^3(mean=352) and no prior AIDS-defining event enrolled with the following demographics: male (82%), Caucasian (70%), mean age of 35 years, asymptomatic HIV infection (81%), and prior antiretroviral use (57%, mean duration=89.5 weeks). The overall median duration of study treatment was 118 weeks. The incidence of AIDS-defining events or death is shown in TABLE 1.

TABLE 1 First AIDS-Defining Event or Death and Death Only by Study Arm and Antiviral Experience

Antiretroviral Experience	Event	Treatment: Zidovudine	Didanosine	Zidovudine plus Didanosine	Zidovudine plus Zalcitabine
Overall	No. of patients	619	620	613	615
	AIDS/ Death	96 (16%)	71 (11%)	66 (11%)	76 (12%)
	Death only	54 (9%)	29 (5%)	31 (5%)	40 (7%)
Naive	No. of patients	269	268	263	267
	AIDS/ Death	32 (12%)	23 (9%)	20 (8%)	16 (6%)
	Death only	18 (7%)	11 (4%)	11(4%)	9 (3%)
Experienced	No. of patients	350	352	350	348
	AIDS/ Death	64 (18%)	48 (14%)	45 (13%)	60 (17%)
	Death only	36 (10%)	18 (5%)	20 (6%)	31 (9%)

Zidovudine in combination with certain antiretroviral agents has been shown to be superior to monotherapy in one or more of the following: delaying death, delaying development of AIDS, increasing CD4 cell counts, and decreasing plasma HIV RNA. Use of zidovudine in come combinations is based on surrogate marker data. The complete prescribing information for each drug should be consulted before combination therapy which included zidovudine is initiated.

Pregnant Women and Their Neonates: The utility of zidovudine for the prevention of maternal-fetal HIV transmission was demonstrated in a randomized, double-blind, placebo-controlled trial (ACTG 076) conducted in HIV-infected pregnant women with CD4 cell counts of 200 to 1818 cells/mm^3 (median in the treated group: 560 cells/mm^3) who had little or no previous exposure to zidovudine. Oral zidovudine was initiated between 14 and 34 weeks of gestation (median 11 weeks of therapy) followed by intravenous administration of zidovudine during labor and delivery. After birth, infants received oral zidovudine syrup for 6 weeks. The study showed a statistically significant difference in the incidence of HIV infection in the neonates (based on viral culture from peripheral blood) between the group receiving zidovudine and the group receiving placebo. Of 363 neonates evaluated in the study, the estimated risk of HIV infection was 7.8% in the group receiving zidovudine and 24.9% in the placebo group, a relative reduction in transmission risk of 68.7%. Zidovudine was well tolerated by mothers and infants. There was no difference in pregnancy-related adverse events between the treatment groups.

Dose Frequency Study: A randomized, double-blind, dose-frequency study of zidovudine in 320 patients with AIDS or advanced ARC was conducted to assess the safety and tolerability of 600 mg zidovudine per day given as either 100 mg every 4 hours or as 300 mg every 12 hours for 48 weeks. No significant difference was detected between the two dose frequencies with regard to adverse experiences or hematologic abnormalities. Although this study was not designed to determine efficacy, no differences in the frequency of or in time to opportunistic infections, neoplasms, or death were noted between treatment groups. Changes in CD4 cell counts and β_2–microglobulin levels were similar between treatment groups.

INDICATIONS AND USAGE:

Zidovudine is indicated for the treatment of HIV-infection when antiretroviral therapy is waranted (see CLINICAL STUDIES.)

The duration of clinical benefit from antiretroviral therapy may be limited. Alterations in antiviral therapy should be considered if disease progression occurs during treatment.

Maternal-Fetal HIV Transmission: Zidovudine is also indicated for the prevention of maternal-fetal HIV transmission as part of a regimen that includes oral zidovudine beginning between 14 and 34 weeks of gestation, intravenous zidovudine during labor, and administration of zidovudine syrup to the newborn after birth. The efficacy of this regimen for preventing HIV transmission in women who have received zidovudine for a prolonged period before pregnancy has not been evaluated. The safety of zidovudine for the mother or fetus during the first trimester of pregnancy has not been assessed (see CLINICAL STUDIES.)

CONTRAINDICATIONS:

Zidovudine tablets, capsules, syrup, and IV infusion are contraindicated for patients who have potentially life-threatening allergic reactions to any of the components of the formulations.

WARNINGS:

Before combination therapy with zidovudine is initiated, consult the complete prescribing information for each drug. The safety profile of zidovudine plus other antiretroviral agents reflects the individual safety profiles of each component.

The incidence of adverse reactions appears to increase with disease progression, and patients should be monitored carefully, especially as disease progression occurs.

Bone Marrow Suppression: Zidovudine should be used with extreme caution in patients who have bone marrow compromise evidenced by granulocyte count <1000 cells/mm^3 or hemoglobin <9.5 g/dl. In patients with advanced symptomatic HIV disease, anemia and neutropenia were the most significant adverse events observed (see ADVERSE REACTIONS.) There have been reports of pancytopenia associated with the use of zidovudine, which was reversible in most instances after discontinuance of the drug.

However, significant anemia in many cases required dose adjustment, discontinuation of zidovudine, and/or blood transfusions has occurred during treatment with zidovudine alone or in combination with other antiretrovirals. Frequent blood counts are strongly recommended in patients with advanced HIV disease who are treated with zidovudine. For HIV-infected individuals and patients with asymptomatic or early HIV disease, periodic blood counts are recommended. If anemia or neutropenia develops, dosage adjustments may be necessary (see DOSAGE AND ADMINISTRATION.)

Myopathy: Myopathy and myositis with pathological changes, similar to that produced by HIV disease, have been associated with prolonged use of zidovudine.

Lactic Acidosis/Severe Hepatomegaly with Steatosis: Rare occurrences of potentially fatal lactic acidosis in the absence of hypoxemia, and severe hepatomegaly with steatosis have been reported with the use of antiretroviral nucleoside analogues. Lactic acidosis should be considered whenever a patient receiving therapy with zidovudine develops unexplained tachypnea, dyspnea, or fall in serum bicarbonate level. Under these circumstances, therapy with zidovudine should be suspended until the diagnosis of lactic acidosis has been excluded.

WARNINGS: *(cont'd)*

Caution should be exercised when administering zidovudine to any patient, particularly obese women, with hepatomegaly, hepatitis, or other known risk factor for liver disease. These patients should be followed closely while on therapy with zidovudine. The significance of elevated aminotransferase levels suggesting hepatic injury in HIV-infected patients prior to starting zidovudine or while on zidovudine is unclear. Treatment with zidovudine should be suspended in the setting of rapidly elevating aminotransferase levels, progressive hepatomegaly, or metabolic/lactic acidosis of unknown etiology.

Other Serious Adverse Reactions: Several serious adverse events have been reported with use of zidovudine in clinical practice. Reports of pancreatitis, sensitization reactions (including anaphylaxis in one patient), vasculitis, and seizures have been rare. These adverse events, except for sensitization, have also been associated with HIV disease. Changes in skin and nail pigmentation have been associated with the use of zidovudine.

PRECAUTIONS:

General: Zidovudine is eliminated from the body primarily by renal excretion following metabolism in the liver (glucuronidation). In patients with severely impaired renal function, dosage reduction is recommended (see CLINICAL PHARMACOLOGY, Pharmacokinetics and DOSAGE AND ADMINISTRATION. Although very little data are available, patients with severely impaired hepatic function may be at greater risk of toxicity.

Information for Patients: Zidovudine is not a cure for HIV infection, and patients may continue to acquire illnesses associated with HIV infection, including opportunistic infections. Therefore, patients should be advised to seek medical care for any significant change in their health status.

The safety and efficacy of zidovudine in treating women, intravenous drug users, and racial minorities[7-9] is not significantly different than that observed in white males.

Patients should be informed that the major toxicities of zidovudine are neutropenia and/or anemia. The frequency and severity of these toxicities are greater in patients with more advanced disease and in those who initiate therapy later in the course of their infection. They should be told that if toxicity develops, they may require transfusions or dose modifications including possible discontinuation. They should be told of the extreme importance of having their blood counts followed closely while on therapy, especially for patients with advanced symptomatic HIV disease. They should be cautioned about the use of other medications, including ganciclovir and interferon-alpha, that may exacerbate the toxicity of zidovudine (see DRUG INTERACTIONS.) Patients should be informed that other adverse effects of zidovudine include nausea and vomiting. Patients should also be encouraged to contact their physician if they experience muscle weakness, shortness of breath, symptoms of hepatitis or pancreatitis, or any other unexpected adverse events while being treated with zidovudine.

Zidovudine tablets, capsules and syrup are for oral ingestion only. Patients should be told of the importance of taking zidovudine exactly as prescribed. They should be told not to share medication and not to exceed the recommended dose. Patients should be told that the long-term effects of zidovudine are unknown at this time.

Pregnant women considering the use of zidovudine during pregnancy for prevention of HIV-transmission to their infants should be advised that transmission may still occur in some cases despite therapy. The long-term consequences of *in utero* and infant exposure to zidovudine are unknown.

HIV-infected pregnant women should be advised not to breast-feed to avoid postnatal transmission of HIV to a child who may not yet be infected.

Patients should be advised that therapy with zidovudine has not been shown to reduce the risk of transmission of HIV to others through sexual contact or blood contamination.

Carcinogenesis, Mutagenesis, Impairment of Fertility: Zidovudine was administered orally at three dosage levels to separate groups of mice and rats (60 females and 60 males in each group). Initial single daily doses were 30, 60, and 120 mg/kg/day in mice and 80, 220, and 600 mg/kg/day in rats. The doses in mice were reduced to 20, 30, and 40 mg/kg/day after day 90 because of treatment-related anemia, whereas in rats only the high dose was reduced to 450 mg/kg/day on day 91 and then to 300 mg/kg/day on day 279.

In mice, seven late-appearing (after 19 months) vaginal neoplasms (five nonmetastasizing squamous cell carcinomas, one squamous cell papilloma, and one squamous polyp) occurred in animals given the highest dose. One late-appearing squamous cell papilloma occurred in the vagina of a middle dose animal. No vaginal tumors were found at the lowest dose.

In rats, two late-appearing (after 20 months), non-metastasizing vaginal squamous cell carcinomas occurred in animals given the highest dose. No vaginal tumors occurred at the low or middle dose in rats. No other drug-related tumors were observed in either sex of either species.

It is not known how predictive the results of rodent carcinogenicity studies may be for humans. At doses that produced tumors in mice and rats, the estimated drug exposure (as measured by AUC) was approximately 3 times (mouse) and 24 times (rat) the estimated human exposure at the recommended therapeutic dose of 100 mg every 4 hours.

No evidence of mutagenicity (with or without metabolic activation) was observed in the Ames *Salmonella* mutagenicity assay at concentrations up to 10 mcg per plate, which was the maximum concentration that could be tested because of the antimicrobial activity of zidovudine against the *Salmonella* species. In a mutagenicity assay conducted in L5178Y/TK$^{+/-}$ mouse lymphoma cells, zidovudine was weakly mutagenic in the absence of metabolic activation only at the highest concentrations tested (4000 and 5000 mcg/ml). In the presence of metabolic activation, the drug was weakly mutagenic at concentrations of 1000 mcg/ml and higher. In an *in vitro*mammalian cell transformation assay, zidovudine was positive at concentrations of 0.5 mcg/ml and higher. In an *in vitro* cytogenetic study performed in cultured human lymphocytes, zidovudine induced dose-related structural chromosomal abnormalities at concentrations of 3 mcg/ml and higher. No such effects were noted at the two lowest concentrations tested, 0.3 and 1 mcg/ml. In an *in vivo* cytogenetic study in rats given a single intravenous injection of zidovudine at doses of 37.5 to 300 mg/kg, there were no treatment-related structural or numerical chromosomal alterations in spite of plasma levels that were as high as 453 mcg/ml 5 minutes after dosing.

In two *in vivo* micronucleus studies (designed to measure chromosome breakage or mitotic spindle apparatus damage) in male mice, oral doses of zidovudine 100 to 1000 mg/kg/day administered once daily for approximately 4 weeks induced dose-related increases in micronucleated erythrocytes. Similar results were also seen after 4 or 7 days of dosing at 500 mg/kg/day in rats and mice.

In a study involving 11 AIDS patients, it was reported that the seven patients who were receiving zidovudine (1200 mg/day) as their only medication for 4 weeks to 7 months showed a chromosome breakage frequency of 8.29 ± 2.65 breaks per 100 peripheral lymphocytes. This was significantly ($P < 0.05$) higher than the incidence of 0.5 ± 0.29 breaks per 100 cells that was observed in the four AIDS patients who had not received zidovudine.

No effect on male or female fertility (judged by conception rates) was seen in rats given zidovudine orally at doses up to 450 mg/kg/day.

Pregnancy Category C: Oral teratology studies in the rat and in the rabbit at doses up to 500 mg/kg/day revealed no evidence of teratogenicity with zidovudine. Zidovudine treatment resulted in embryo/fetal toxicity as evidenced by an increase in the incidence of fetal resorptions in rats given 150 or 450 mg/kg/day and rabbits given 500 mg/kg/day. The doses used in the teratology studies resulted in peak zidovudine plasma concentrations (after one-half of the daily dose) in rats 66 to 226 times, and in rabbits 12 to 87 times, mean steady-state peak human plasma concentrations (after one-sixth of the daily dose) achieved with the recommended daily dose (100 mg every 4 hours). In an *in vitro* experiment with fertilized mouse oocytes, zidovudine exposure resulted in a dose-dependent reduction in blastocyst formation. In an additional teratology study in rats, a dose of 3000 mg/kg/day (very near the oral median lethal dose in rats of 3683 mg/kg) caused marked maternal toxicity and an increase in the incidence of fetal malformations. This dose resulted in peak zidovudine plasma concentrations 350 times peak human plasma concentrations. (Estimated area-under-the-curve [AUC] in rats at this dose level was 300 times the daily AUC in humans given 600 mg per day.) No evidence of teratogenicity was seen in this experiment at doses of 600 mg/kg/day or less.

A randomized, double-blind, placebo-controlled trial was conducted in HIV-infected pregnant women to determine the utility of zidovudine for the prevention of maternal-fetal HIV-transmission (see CLINICAL STUDIES.) Congenital abnormalities occurred with similar frequency between neonates born to mothers who received zidovudine and neonates born to mothers who received placebo. Abnormalities were either problems in embryogenesis (prior to 14 weeks) or were recognized on ultrasound before or immediately after initiation of study drug.

Antiretroviral Pregnancy Registry: To monitor maternal-fetal outcomes of pregnant women exposed to zidovudine, an Antiretroviral Pregnancy Registry has been established. Physicians are encouraged to register patients by calling (800) 722-9292, ext. 39437.

Nursing Mothers: The U.S. Public Health Service Centers for Disease Control and Prevention advises HIV-infected women not to breast-feed to avoid postnatal transmission of HIV to a child who may not yet be infected. Zidovudine is excreted in human milk (see CLINICAL PHARMACOLOGY, Pharmacokinetics).

Pediatric Use: Zidovudine has been studied in HIV-infected pediatric patients over 3 months of age who have HIV-related symptoms or who are asymptomatic with abnormal laboratory values indicating significant HIV-related immunosuppression.(See CLINICAL STUDIES), ADVERSE REACTIONS, and DOSAGE AND ADMINISTRATION.

DRUG INTERACTIONS:

Ganciclovir: Use of zidovudine in combination with ganciclovir increases the risk of hematologic toxicities in some patients with advanced HIV disease. Should the use of this combination become necessary in the treatment of patients with HIV disease, dose reduction or interruption of one or both agents may be necessary to minimize hematologic toxicity. Hematologic parameters, including hemoglobin, hematocrit, and white blood cell count with differential, should be monitored frequently in all patients receiving this combination.

Interferon-alpha: Hematologic toxicities have also been seen when zidovudine is used concomitantly with interferon-alpha. As with the concomitant use of zidovudine and ganciclovir, dose reduction or interruption of one or both agents may be necessary, and hematologic parameters should be monitored frequently.

Bone Marrow Suppressive Agents/Cytotoxic Agents: Coadministration of zidovudine with drugs that are cytotoxic or which interfere with RBC/WBC number or function (*e.g.*, dapsone, flucytosine, vincristine, vinblastine, or adriamycin) may increase the risk of hematologic toxicity.

Probenecid: Limited data suggest that probenecid may increase zidovudine levels by inhibiting glucuronidation and/or by reducing renal excretion of zidovudine. Some patients who have used zidovudine concomitantly with probenecid have developed flu-like symptoms consisting of myalgia, malaise, and/or fever and maculopapular rash.

Phenytoin: Phenytoin plasma levels have been reported to be low in some patients receiving zidovudine, while in one case a high level was documented. However, in a pharmacokinetic interaction study in which 12 HIV-positive volunteers received a single 300 mg phenytoin dose alone and during steady-state zidovudine conditions (200 mg every 4 hours), no change in phenytoin kinetics was observed. Although not designed to optimally assess the effect of phenytoin on zidovudine kinetics, a 30% decrease in oral zidovudine clearance was observed with phenytoin.

Methadone: In a pharmacokinetic study of nine HIV-positive patients receiving methadone-maintenance (30 to 90 mg daily) concurrent with 200 mg of zidovudine every 4 hours, no changes were observed in the pharmacokinetics of methadone upon initiation of therapy with zidovudine and after 14 days of treatment with zidovudine. No adjustments in methadone-maintenance requirements were reported. For four patients, the mean zidovudine AUC was elevated two-fold, while for five patients, the value was equal to that of control patients. The exact mechanism and clinical significance of these data are unknown.

Fluconazole: The coadministration of fluconazole with zidovudine has been reported to interfere with the oral clearance and metabolism of zidovudine. In a pharmacokinetic interaction study in which 12 HIV-positive men received zidovudine 200 mg every 8 hours alone and in combination with fluconazole 400 mg daily, fluconazole increased the zidovudine AUC (74%; range 28% to 173%) and the zidovudine half-life (128%; range -4% to 189%) at steady-state. The clinical significance of this interaction is unknown.

Atovaquone: Data from 14 HIV-infected volunteers who were given atovaquone tablets 750 mg every 12 hours with zidovudine 200 mg every 8 hours showed a 24% ± 12% decrease in zidovudine oral clearance, leading to a 35% ± 23% increase in plasma zidovudine AUC. The glucuronide metabolite:parent ratio decreases from a mean of 4.5 when zidovudine was administered alone to 3.1 when zidovudine was administered with atovaquone tablets. Zidovudine had no effect on atovaquone pharmacokinetics.

Valproic Acid: The concomitant administration of valproic acid 250 mg (n=5) or 500 mg (n=1) every 8 hours and zidovudine 100 mg orally every 8 hours for 4 days to six HIV-infected, asymptomatic male volunteers, resulted in a 79% ± 61% (mean ± SD) increase in the plasma zidovudine AUC and a 22% ± 10% decrease in the plasma GZDV AUC as compared to the administration of zidovudine in the absence of valproic acid. The GDZV/zidovudine urinary excretion ratio decreased 58% ± 12%. Because no change in the zidovudine plasma half-life occurred, these results suggest that valproic acid may increase the oral bioavailability of zidovudine through inhibition of first-pass metabolism. Although clinical significance of this interaction is unknown, patients should be monitored more closely for a possible increase in zidovudine-related adverse effects. The effect of zidovudine on the pharmacokinetics of valproic acid was not evaluated.

Lamivudine: Zidovudine and lamivudine were coadministered to 13 asymptomatic HIV-positive patients in a single-center, open-label, randomized, crossover study. No significant differences were observed in AUC∞ or total clearance for lamivudine or zidovudine when the two drugs were administered together. Coadministration of zidovudine with lamivudine resulted in an increase of 39% ± 62% (mean ± SD) in C_{max} of zidovudine.

Other Agents: Preliminary data from a drug interaction study (n=10) suggest that coadministration of 200 mg zidovudine and 600 mg rifampin decreases the area under the plasma concentration curve by an average of 48% ± 34%. However, the effect of the once daily

DRUG INTERACTIONS: *(cont'd)*

dosing of rifampin on multiple daily doses of ID is unknown. Some nucleoside analogues affecting DNA replication, such as ribavirin, antagonize the *in vitro* antiviral activity of zidovudine against HIV; concomitant use of such drugs should be avoided.

ADVERSE REACTIONS:

The adverse events reported during intravenous administration of zidovudine IV infusion are similar to those reported with oral administration; granulocytopenia and anemia were reported most frequently. Long-term intravenous administration beyond 2 to 4 weeks has not been studied in adults and may enhance hematologic adverse events. Local reaction, pain, and slight irritation during intravenous administration occur infrequently.

Monotherapy: *Adults:* The frequency and severity of adverse events associated with the use of oral zidovudine in adults are greater in patients with more advanced infection at the time of initiation of therapy. TABLE 2 summarizes the relative incidence of hematologic adverse events observed in clinical studies by severity of HIV disease present at the start of treatment with oral zidovudine (TABLE 2).

TABLE 2

Stage of Disease	Zidovudine Daily Dose* (mg)	Granulocytopenia (<750 cells/mm^3)	Anemia (Hgb< 8.0 g/dl)
Asymptomatic			
ACTG 019[3]	500	1.8%†	1.1%†
Early HIV Disease (CD4 >200 cells/mm^3)			
ACTG 016[4]	1200	4%	4%
Advanced HIV Disease (CD4 >200 cells/mm^3)			
BW 02[1]	1500	10%†	3%†‡
(CD4 ≤200 cells/mm^3)			
ACTG 002[10]	600	37%	29%
BW 02[1]	1500	47%	29%‡

* The currently recommended dose is 500 to 600 mg daily.
† Not statistically significant compared to placebo.
‡ Anemia = Hgb <7.5 g/dl.

The anemia reported in patients with advanced HIV disease receiving zidovudine appeared to be the result of impaired erythrocyte maturation as evidenced by macrocytosis while on drug. Although mean platelet counts in patients receiving zidovudine were significantly increased compared to mean baseline values, thrombocytopenia did occur in some of these patients with advanced disease. Twelve percent of patients receiving zidovudine compared to 5% of patients receiving placebo had >50% decreases from baseline platelet count. Mild drug-associated elevations in total bilirubin levels have been reported as an uncommon occurrence in patients treated for asymptomatic HIV infection.

The HIV-infected adults participating in these clinical trials often had baseline symptoms and signs of HIV disease and/or experienced adverse events at some time during study. It was often difficult to distinguish adverse events possibly associated with administration of zidovudine from underlying signs of HIV disease or intercurrent illnesses. TABLE 3 summarizes clinical adverse events or symptoms which occurred in at least 5% of all patients with advanced HIV disease treated with 1500 mg/day of zidovudine in the original placebo-controlled study. Of the items listed in the table, only severe headache, nausea, insomnia, and myalgia were reported at a significantly greater rate in patients receiving zidovudine (TABLE 3).

TABLE 3 Percentage (%) of Patients with Clinical Events in Advanced HIV Disease (BW 02)

Adverse Event	Zidovudine 1500 mg/day* (n=144) %	Placebo (n=137) %
Body as a Whole		
Asthenia	19	18
Diaphoresis	5	4
Fever	16	12
Headache	42	37
Malaise	8	7
Gastrointestinal		
Anorexia	11	8
Diarrhea	12	18
Dyspepsia	5	4
GI Pain	20	19
Nausea	46	18
Vomiting	6	3
Musculoskeletal		
Myalgia	8	2
Nervous		
Dizziness	6	4
Insomnia	5	1
Paresthesia	6	3
Somnolence	8	9
Respiratory		
Dyspnea	5	3
Skin		
Rash	17	15
Special Senses		
Taste Perversion	5	8

* The currently recommended oral dose is 500 to 600 mg/daily.

All events of a severe or life-threatening nature were monitored for adults in the placebo-controlled studies in early HIV disease and asymptomatic HIV infection. Data concerning the occurrence of additional signs or symptoms were also collected. No distinction was made in reporting events between those possibly associated with the administration of the study medication and those due to the underlying disease. TABLES 4 and 5 summarize all those events reported at a statistically significant greater incidence for patients receiving zidovudine in these studies:

Several serious adverse events have been reported with the use of zidovudine in clinical practice. Myopathy and myositis with pathological changes, similar to that produced by HIV disease, have been associated with prolonged use of zidovudine. Reports of hepatomegaly with steatosis, hepatitis, pancreatitis, lactic acidosis, sensitization reactions (including anaphylaxis in one patient), hyperbilirubinemia, vasculitis, and seizures have been rare. These adverse events, except for sensitization, have also been associated with HIV disease. A single case of macular edema has been reported with the use of zidovudine.

ADVERSE REACTIONS: *(cont'd)*

TABLE 4 Percentage (%) of Patients with Adverse Events in Early HIV Disease (ACTG 016)

Adverse Event	Zidovudine 1200 mg/day* (n=361) %	Placebo (n=352) %
Body as a Whole		
Asthenia	69	62
Gastrointestinal		
Dyspepsia	6	1
Nausea	61	41
Vomiting	25	13

* The currently recommended oral dose is 500 to 600 mg/daily.

TABLE 5 Percentage (%) of Patients with Adverse Events* in Asymptomatic HIV Infection (ACTG 019)

Adverse Event	Zidovudine 500 mg/day (n=453) %	Placebo (n=428)%
Body as a Whole		
Asthenia	8.6†	5.8
Headache	62.5	52.6
Malaise	53.2	44.9
Gastrointestinal		
Anorexia	20.1	10.5
Constipation	6.4†	3.5
Nausea	51.4	29.9
Vomiting	17.2	9.8
Nervous		
Dizziness	17.9†	15.2

* Reported ≥5% of study population.
† Not statistically significant versus placebo.

Additional adverse events reported in clinical trials at a rate not significantly different from placebo are listed below. Selected events from post-marketing clinical experience with zidovudine are also included. Many of these events may also occur as part of HIV disease. The clinical significance of the association between treatment with zidovudine and these events is unknown.

Body as a Whole: abdominal pain, back pain, body odor, chest pain, chills, edema of the lip, fever, flu syndrome, hyperalgesia.

Cardiovascular: syncope, vasodilation.

Gastrointestinal: bleeding gums, constipation, diarrhea, dysphagia, edema of the tongue, eructation, flatulence, mouth ulcer, rectal hemorrhage.

Hemic and Lymphatic: lymphadenopathy.

Musculoskeletal: arthralgia, muscle spasm, tremor, twitch.

Nervous: anxiety, confusion, depression, dizziness, emotional lability, loss of mental acuity, nervousness, paresthesia, somnolence, vertigo.

Respiratory: cough, dyspnea, epistaxis, hoarseness, pharyngitis, rhinitis, sinusitis.

Skin: acne, changes in skin and nail pigmentation, pruritus, rash, sweat, urticaria.

Special senses: amblyopia, hearing loss, photophobia, taste perversion.

Urogenital: dysuria, polyuria, urinary frequency, urinary hesitancy.

Pediatrics: Anemia and granulocytopenia among children with advanced HIV disease receiving zidovudine occurred with similar incidence to that reported for adults with AIDS or advanced ARC (See ADVERSE REACTIONS. Management of neutropenia and anemia included, in some cases, dose modification and/or blood product transfusions. In the open-label studies, 17% had their dose modified (generally a reduction in dose by 30%) due to anemia and 25% had their dose modified (temporary discontinuation or dose reduction by 30%) for neutropenia. Four pediatric patients had zidovudine permanently discontinued for neutropenia. TABLE 6 summarizes the occurrence of anemia (Hgb <7.5 g/dl) and granulocytopenia (<750 cells/mm^3) among 124 children receiving zidovudine for a mean of 267 days (range 3 to 855 days).

TABLE 6

Advanced Pediatric HIV Disease	Granulocytopenia (<750 cells/mm^3) n	%	Anemia (Hgb <7.5 g/dl) n	%
(n=124)	48	39	28*	23

* Twenty-two children received one or more transfusions due to a decline in hemoglobin to <7.5 g/dl; an additional 15 children were transfused for hemoglobin levels >7.5 g/dl. Fifty-nine percent of the patients transfused had a pre-study history of anemia or transfusion requirement.

Macrocytosis was observed among the majority of pediatric patients enrolled in the studies.

In the open-label studies involving 124 children, 16 clinical adverse events were reported by 24 children. No event was reported by more than 5.6% of the study populations. Due to the open-label design of the studies, it was difficult to determine possible events related to the use of zidovudine versus disease-related events. Therefore, all clinical events reported as associated with therapy with zidovudine or of unknown relationship to therapy with zidovudine are presented in TABLE 7.

The clinical adverse events reported among adult recipients of zidovudine may also occur in pediatric patients.

Use for the Prevention of Maternal-Fetal Transmission of HIV: In a randomized, double-blind, placebo-controlled trial in HIV-infected women and their neonates conducted to determine the utility of zidovudine for the prevention of maternal-fetal HIV transmission, zidovudine syrup at 2 mg/kg was administered every 6 hours for 6 weeks to neonates beginning within 12 hours after birth. The most commonly reported adverse experiences were anemia (hemoglobin <9.0 g/dl) and neutropenia (<1000 cells/mm^3). Anemia occurred in 22% of the neonates who received zidovudine and in 12% of the neonates who received placebo. The mean difference in hemoglobin values was less than 1.0 g/dl for neonates receiving zidovudine compared to neonates receiving placebo. No neonates with anemia required transfusion and all hemoglobin values spontaneously returned to normal within 6 weeks after completion of therapy with zidovudine. Neutropenia was reported with similar frequency in the group that received zidovudine (21%) and in the group that received placebo (27%). The long-term consequences of *in utero* and infant exposure to zidovudine are unknown.

TABLE 7 Percentage (%) of Pediatric Patients with Clinical Events in Open Label Studies

Adverse Event	n	%
Body as a Whole		
Fever	4	3.2
Phlebitis*/Bacteremia	2	1.6
Headache	2	1.6
Gastroinstestinal		
Nausea	1	0.8
Vomiting	6	4.8
Abdominal Pain	4	3.2
Diarrhea	1	0.8
Weight Loss	1	0.8
Nervous		
Insomnia	3	2.4
Nervousness/Irritability	2	1.6
Decreased Reflexes	7	5.6
Seizure	1	0.8
Cardiovascular		
Left Ventricular Dilation	1	0.8
Cardiomyopathy	1	0.8
S_3 Gallop	1	0.8
Congestive Heart Failure	1	0.8
Generalized Edema	1	0.8
ECG Abnormality	3	2.4
Urogenital		
Hematuria/Viral Cystitis	1	0.8

* Peripheral vein IV catheter site.

OVERDOSAGE:

Cases of acute overdoses in both pediatric patients and adults have been reported with doses up to 50 grams. None were fatal. The only consistent finding in these cases of overdose was spontaneous or induced nausea and vomiting. Hematologic changes were transient and not severe. Some patients experienced nonspecific CNS symptoms such as headache, dizziness, drowsiness, lethargy, and confusion. One report of a grand mal seizure possibly attributable to zidovudine occurred in a 35-year-old male 3 hours after ingesting 36 grams of zidovudine. No other cause could be identified. All patients recovered without permanent sequelae. Hemodialysis and peritoneal dialysis appear to have a negligible effect on the removal of zidovudine while elimination of its primary metabolite, GZDV, is enhanced.

DOSAGE AND ADMINISTRATION:

ORAL FORMS

Adults: The recommended total oral daily dose of zidovudine is 600 mg per day in divided doses in combination with other antiretroviral agents and 500 mg (100 mg every 4 hours while awake) or 600 mg per day in divided doses for monotherapy. The effectiveness of this dose compared to higher dosing regimens in improving the neurologic dysfunction associated with HIV disease is unknown. A small randomized study found a greater effect of higher doses of zidovudine on improvement of neurological symptoms in patients with pre-existing neurological disease.

Pediatrics: The recommended oral dose in pediatric patients 3 months to 12 years of age is 180 mg/m^2 every 6 hours (720 mg/m^2 per day), not to exceed 200 mg every 6 hours.

Maternal-Fetal HIV Transmission: The recommended oral dosing regimen for administration to pregnant women (>14 weeks of pregnancy) and their newborn neonates is:

Maternal Dosing: 100 mg orally 5 times per day until the start of labor. (See CLINICAL STUDIES) During labor and delivery, intravenous zidovudine should be administered at 2 mg/kg (total body weight) over 1 hour followed by a continuous intravenous infusion of 1 mg/kg/h (total body weight) until clamping of the umbilical cord.

Neonatal Dosing: 2 mg/kg orally every 6 hours starting within 12 hours after birth and continuing through 6 weeks of age. Neonates unable to receive oral dosing may be administered zidovudine intravenously at 1.5 mg/kg, infused over 30 minutes, every 6 hours. (See PRECAUTIONS) if hepatic disease or renal insufficiency is present.

Monitoring of Patients: Hematologic toxicities appear to be related to pretreatment bone marrow reserve and to dose and duration of therapy. In patients with poor bone marrow reserve, particularly in patients with advanced symptomatic HIV disease, frequent monitoring of hematologic indices is recommended to detect serious anemia or granulocytopenia (see WARNINGS.) In patients who experience hematologic toxicity, reduction in hemoglobin may occur as early as 2 to 4 weeks, and granulocytopenia usually occurs after 6 to 8 weeks.

Dose Adjustment: Significant anemia (hemoglobin of <7.5 g/dl or reduction of >25% of baseline) and/or significant granulocytopenia (granulocyte count of <750 cells/mm^3 or reduction of >50% from baseline) may require a dose interruption until evidence of marrow recovery is observed (see WARNINGS.) For less severe anemia or granulocytopenia, a reduction in daily dose may be adequate. In patients who develop significant anemia, dose modification does not necessarily eliminate the need for transfusion. If marrow recovery occurs following dose modification, gradual increases in dose may be appropriate depending on hematologic indices and patient tolerance.

In end-stage renal disease patients maintained on hemodialysis or peritoneal dialysis, recommended oral dosing is 100 mg every 6 to 8 hours (see CLINICAL PHARMACOLOGY, Pharmacokinetics.

There are insufficient data to recommend dose adjustment of zidovudine in patients with impaired hepatic function.

INTRAVENOUS INFUSION

For adults with symptomatic HIV infection, including AIDS, the recommended intravenous dose is 1 mg/kg infused over 1 hour. This dose should be administered every 4 hours around the clock (6 mg/kg/daily). The effectiveness of this dose compared to higher dosing regimens in improving the neurologic dysfunction associated with HIV disease is unknown (see INDICATIONS AND USAGE.) A small randomized study found a greater effect of higher doses of zidovudine on improvement of neurological symptoms in patients with pre-existing neurological disease.

For asymptomatic HIV infection, the recommended intravenous dose for adults is 1 mg/kg every 4 hours while awake (5 mg/kg daily).

Patients should receive zidovudine IV infusion only until oral therapy can be administered. The intravenous dosing regimen equivalent to the oral administration of 100 mg every 4 hours is approximately 1 mg/kg intravenously every 4 hours.

In end-stage renal disease patients maintained on hemodialysis or peritoneal dialysis, recommended dosing is 1 mg/kg every 6 to 8 hours (see CLINICAL PHARMACOLOGY, Pharmacokinetics.

There are insufficient data to recommend dose adjustment of zidovudine in patients with impaired hepatic function.

DOSAGE AND ADMINISTRATION: *(cont'd)*

Method of Preparation: Zidovudine IV infusion must be diluted prior to administration. The calculated dose should be removed from the 20 ml vial and added to 5% Dextrose Injection solution to achieve a concentration no greater than 4 mg/ml. Admixture in biologic or colloidal fluids (*e.g.*, blood products, protein solutions, etc.) is not recommended.

After dilution, the solution is physically and chemically stable for 24 hours at room temperature and 48 hours if refrigerated at 2° to 8°C (36° to 46°F). Care should be taken during admixture to prevent inadvertent contamination. As an additional precaution, the diluted solution should be administered within 8 hours if stored at 25°C (77°F) or 24 hours if refrigerated at 2° to 8°C to minimize potential administration of a microbially contaminated solution.

Parenteral drug products should be inspected visually for particulate matter and discoloration prior to administration whenever solution and container permit. Should either be observed, the solution should be discarded and fresh solution prepared.

Administration: Zidovudine IV infusion is administered intravenously at a constant rate over one hour. Rapid infusion or bolus injection should be avoided. Zidovudine IV infusion should not be given intramuscularly.

REFERENCES:

1. Fischl MA, Richman DD, Grieco MH, et al. The efficacy of azidothymidine (AZT) in the treatment of patients with AIDS and AIDS-related complex. A double-blind, placebo-controlled trial. *N Engl J Med.* 1987;317: 185-191. 2. Richman DD, Fischl MA, Grieco MH, et al. The toxicity of azidothymidine (AZT) in the treatment of patients with AIDS and AIDS-related complex. A double-blind, placebo-controlled trial. *N Engl J Med.* 1987;317:192-197. 3. Volberding PA, Lagakos SW, Koch MA, et al. Zidovudine in asymptomatic human immunodeficiency virus infection. A controlled trial in persons with fewer than 500 CD4-positive cells per cubic millimeter.*N Engl J Med.* 1990;322:941-949. 4. Fischl MA, Richman DD, Hansen N, et al. The safety and efficacy of zidovudine in the treatment of patients with mildly symptomatic HIV infection. A double-blind, placebo-controlled trial. *Annals Internal Med.* 1990;112:727-737. 5. Meng T-C, Fischl MA, Boota AM, et al. Combination therapy with zidovudine and dideoxycytidine in patients with advanced human immunodeficiency virus infection. *Ann Intern Med.* 1992;116:13-20. 6. Schooley R and the Wellcome Resistance Study Collaborative Group. Trial of ZDV/ddI vs ZDV/ddC vs ZDV in HIV-infected patients with CD4 cell counts less than 300: Preliminary Results. Fourth European Conference on Clinical Aspects and Treatment of HIV infection, Milan, Italy, March 16-18, 1994, 052. 7. Creagh-Kirk T, Doi P, Andrews E, et al. Survival experience among patients with AIDS receiving zidovudine. Follow-up of patients in a compassionate plea program.*JAMA.* 1988;260:3009-3015. 8. Lagakos S, Fischl MA, Stein DS, Lim L, Volberding P. Effects of zidovudine therapy in minority and other subpopulations with early HIV infection. *JAMA.* 1991;266:2709-2712. 9. Easterbrook PJ, Keruly JC, Creagh-Kirk T, et al. Racial and ethnic differences in outcome in zidovudine-treated patients with advanced HIV disease. *JAMA.* 1991;266:2713-2718. 10. Fischl M, Parker C, Pettinelli C, Wulfsohn M, Hirsch M, Collier A, et al. A randomized controlled trial of a reduced daily dose of zidovudine in patients with the acquired immunodeficiency syndrome. *N Engl J Med.* 1990;323:1009-1014.

HOW SUPPLIED:

Tablets: Retrovir tablets 300 mg (biconvex, white, round, film-coated) containing 300 mg zidovudine, one side engraved "GXCW3" and "300" on the other side.

Capsules: Retrovir capsules 100 mg (white, opaque cap and body with a dark blue band) containing 100 mg zidovudine and printed with "Wellcome" and unicorn logo on cap and "Y9C" and "100" on body. Protect from moisture.

Syrup: Retrovir syrup (colorless to pale yellow, strawberry-flavored) containing 50 mg zidovudine in each teaspoonful (5 ml).

Intravenous Infusion: Retrovir IV infusion, 10 mg zidovudine in each ml.

Storage: Store all products at 15° to 25°C (59° to 77°F) and protect from light.

HOW SUPPLIED - EQUIVALENTS NOT AVAILABLE:

Capsule, Gelatin - Oral - 100 mg

100's $159.29 RETROVIR, Glaxo Wellcome 00173-0108-55

Injection, Conc, w/Buf - Intravenous - 10 mg/ml

20 ml x 10 $172.30 RETROVIR, Glaxo Wellcome 00173-0107-93

Syrup - Oral - 50 mg/5ml

240 ml $38.23 RETROVIR, Glaxo Wellcome 00173-0113-18

Tablet - Oral - 300 mg

60's $286.72 RETROVIR, Glaxo Wellcome 00173-0501-00

ZILEUTON *(003257)*

CATEGORIES: Allergies; Antiasthmatics/Bronchodilators; Asthma; EENT Drugs; Eye, Ear, Nose, & Throat Preparations; Lipoxygenase Inhibitors; Respiratory & Allergy Medications; FDA Approved 1996 Dec

BRAND NAMES: **Zyflo**

DESCRIPTION:

Zileuton is an orally active inhibitor of 5-lipoxygenase, the enzyme that catalyzes the formation of leukotrienes from arachidonic acid. Zileuton has the chemical name (±)-l-(l-Benzo[b] thien-2- ylethyl)-l -hydroxyurea. Zileuton has the molecular formula $C_{11}H_{12}N_2O_2S$ and molecular weight of 236.29. It is a racemic mixture (50:50) of R(+) and S(-) enantiomers. Zileuton is a practically odorless, white, crystalline powder that is soluble in methanol and ethanol, slightly soluble in acetonitrile and practically insoluble in water and hexane. The melting point ranges from 144.2°C to 145.2°C. Zyflo tablets for oral administration is supplied in one dosage strength containing 600 mg of zileuton.

Zyflo Inactive Ingredients: crospovidone, hydroxypropyl cellulose, hydroxypropyl methylcellulose, magnesium stearate, microcrystalline cellulose, pregelatinized starch, propylene glycol, sodium starch glycolate, talc, and titanium dioxide.

CLINICAL PHARMACOLOGY:

MECHANISM OF ACTION

Zileuton is a specific inhibitor of 5-lipoxygenase and thus inhibits leukotriene (LTB_4, LTC_4, LTD_4 and LTE_4) formation. Both the R(+) and S(-) enantiomers are pharmacologically active as 5-lipoxygenase inhibitors in *in vitro* systems. Leukotrienes are substances that induce numerous biological effects including augmentation of neutrophil and eosinophil migration, neutrophil and monocyte aggregation, leukocyte adhesion, increased capillary permeability, and smooth muscle contraction. These effects contribute to inflammation, edema, mucous secretion, and bronchoconstriction in the airways of asthmatic patients. Sulfido-peptide leukotrienes (LTC_4, LTD_4, LTE_4, also known as the slow-releasing substances of anaphylaxis) and LTB_4, a chemoattractant for neutrophils and eosinophils, can be measured in a number of biological fluids including bronchoalveolar lavage fluid (BALF) from asthmatic patients.

CLINICAL PHARMACOLOGY: *(cont'd)*

Zileuton is an orally active inhibitor of *ex vivo* LTB_4 formation in several species, including dogs, monkeys, rats, sheep, and rabbits. Zileuton inhibits arachidonic acid-induced ear edema in mice, neutrophil migration in mice in response to polyacrylamide gel, and eosinophil migration into the lungs of antigen-challenged sheep.

Zileuton inhibits leukotriene-dependent smooth muscle contractions *in vitro* in guinea pig and human airways. The compound inhibits leukotriene-dependent bronchospasm in antigen and arachidonic acid-challenged guinea pigs. In antigen-challenged sheep, zileuton inhibits late-phase bronchoconstriction and airway hyperactivity. In humans, pretreatment with zileuton attenuated bronchoconstriction caused by cold air challenge in patients with asthma.

PHARMACOKINETICS

Zileuton is rapidly absorbed upon oral administration with a mean time to peak plasma concentration (T_{max}) of 1.7 hours and a mean peak level (C_{max}) of 4.98 mcg/ml. The absolute bioavailability of zileuton is unknown. Systemic exposure (mean AUC) following 600 mg zileuton administration is 19.2 mcg/hr/ml. Plasma concentrations of zileuton are proportional to dose, and steady-state levels are predictable from single-dose pharmacokinetic data. Administration of zileuton with food resulted in a small but statistically significant increase (27%) in zileuton C_{max} without significant changes in the extent of absorption (AUC) or T_{max}. Therefore, zileuton can be administered with or without food (see DOSAGE AND ADMINISTRATION).

The apparent volume of distribution (V/F) of zileuton is approximately 1.2 L/kg. Zileuton is 93% bound to plasma proteins, primarily to albumin, with minor binding to αl-acid glycoprotein.

Elimination of zileuton is predominantly via metabolism with a mean terminal half-life of 2.5 hours. Apparent oral clearance of zileuton is 7.0 ml/min/kg. Zileuton activity is primarily due to the parent drug. Studies with radiolabeled drug demonstrated that orally administered zileuton is well absorbed into the systemic circulation with 94.5% and 2.2% of the radiolabeled dose recovered in urine and feces, respectively. Several zileuton metabolites have been identified in human plasma and urine. These include two diastereomeric O-glucuronide conjugates (major metabolites) and an N-dehydroxylated metabolite of zileuton. The urinary excretion of the inactivated N-dehydroxylated metabolite and unchanged zileuton each accounted for less than 0.5% of the dose. *In vitro* studies utilizing human liver microsomes have shown that zileuton and its N-dehydroxylated metabolite can be oxidatively metabolized by the cytochrome P450 isoenzymes 1A2, 2C9 and 3A4 (CYP1A2, CYP2C9 and CYP3A4).

SPECIAL POPULATIONS

Effect of Age: Zileuton pharmacokinetics were similar in healthy elderly subjects (>65 years) compared to healthy younger adults (18 to 40 years).

Effect of Gender: Across several studies, no significant gender effects were observed on the pharmacokinetics of zileuton.

Renal insufficiency: The pharmacokinetics of zileuton were similar in healthy subjects and in subjects with mild, moderate, and severe renal insufficiency. In subjects with renal failure requiring hemodialysis, zileuton pharmacokinetics were not altered by hemodialysis and a very small percentage of the administered zileuton dose (<0.5%) was removed by hemodialysis. Hence, dosing adjustment in patients with renal dysfunction or undergoing hemodialysis is not necessary.

Hepatic Insufficiency: Zileuton is contraindicated in patients with active liver disease (see CONTRAINDICATIONS and PRECAUTIONSHepatic Effects).

CLINICAL STUDIES:

Two double-blind, parallel, placebo-controlled, multicenter studies have established the efficacy of zileuton in the treatment of asthma. Three hundred seventy-three (373) patients were enrolled in the 6-month, double blind phase of Study 1, and 401 patients were enrolled in the 3-month double-blind phase of Study 2. In these studies, the patients were mild-to-moderate asthmatics who had a mean baseline FEV_1 of approximately 2.3 liters and who used inhaled beta-agonists as needed, the mean being approximately 6 puffs of albuterol per day from a metered-dose inhaler. In each study, patients were randomized to receive either zileuton 400 mg four times daily, zileuton 600 mg four times daily, or placebo. Only the zileuton 600 mg four times daily dosage regimen was shown to be efficacious by demonstrating statistically significant improvement across several parameters.

Efficacy endpoints measured in Study 1 are shown in TABLE 1 as mean change from baseline to the end of the study (six months). Statistically significant differences from placebo at the p<0.05 level are indicated by an asterisk(*). Similar results were observed after three months in Study 2.

TABLE 1 Mean Change From Baseline To End Of Study (Six Month Study)

Efficacy Endpoint	Zileton 600 mg 4x Daily	Placebo
Trough FEV_1 (L)	0.27	0.14
AM PEFR (L/min)	30.60*	5.04
PM PEFR (L/min)	24.59*	7.98
β-Agonist Use (puffs/day)	-1.77*	-0.22
Daily Symptom Score (0-3 Scale)	-0.49*	-0.28
Nocturnal Symptom Score (0-3 Scale)	-0.29*	-0.04

Of all the patients in Study 1 and Study 2, 7.0% of those administered zileuton 600 mg four times daily required systemic corticosteroid therapy for exacerbation of asthma, whereas 18.7% of the placebo group required corticosteroid treatment. This difference was statistically significant.

In these trials there was a statistically significant improvement from baseline in FEV_1, which occurred 2 hours after initial administration of zileuton. This mean increase was approximately 0.10 L greater than that in placebo-treated patients.

These studies evaluated patients receiving as-needed inhaled beta-agonist as their only asthma therapy. In this patient population, post-hoc analyses suggested that individuals with lower FEV_1 values at baseline showed a greater improvement.

The role of zileuton in the management of patients with more severe asthma, patients receiving anti-asthma therapy other than as-needed, inhaled beta-agonists, or patients receiving it as an oral or inhaled corticosteroid sparing agent remains to be fully characterized.

INDICATIONS AND USAGE:

Zileuton is indicated for the prophylaxis and chronic treatment of asthma in adults and children 12 years of age and older.

CONTRAINDICATIONS:

'leuton tablets are contraindicated in patients with:

'e liver disease or transaminase elevations greater than or equal to three times the upper 'f normal (≥3 × ULN) (see PRECAUTIONSHepatic Effects).

CONTRAINDICATIONS: *(cont'd)*

Hypersensitivity to zileuton or any of its inactive ingredients.

WARNINGS:

Zileuton is not indicated for use in the reversal of bronchospasm in acute asthma attacks, including status astmaticus. Therapy with zileuton can be continued during acute exacerbations of asthma.

PRECAUTIONS:

Hepatic: Elevations of one or more liver function tests may occur during zileuton therapy. These laboratory abnormalities may progress, remain unchanged, or resolve with continued therapy. In a few cases, initial transaminase elevations were first noted after discontinuing treatment, usually within 2 weeks. The ALT (SGPT) test is considered the most sensitive indicator of liver injury. In placebo-controlled clinical trials, the frequency of ALT elevations greater than or equal to three times the upper limits of normal (3 x ULN) was 1.9% for zileuton treated patients, compared with 0.2% for placebo-treated patients.

In a long-term safety surveillance study, 2458 patients received zileuton in addition to their usual asthma care and 489 received their usual asthma care. In patients treated for up to 12 months with zileuton in addition to their usual asthma care, 4.6% developed an ALT of at least 3×ULN, compared with 1.1% of patients receiving only their usual asthma care. Sixty-one percent of these elevations occurred during the first two months of zileuton therapy. After two months of treatment, the rate of new ALT elevations ≥3×ULN stabilized at a mean of 0.30% per month for patients receiving zileuton-plus usual-asthma care compared with 0.11% per month for patients receiving usual asthma care alone. Of the 61 zileuton plus usual asthma care patients with ALT elevations between 3 to 5×ULN, 32 patients (52%) had ALT values decrease to below 2×ULN while continuing zileuton therapy. Twenty-one of the 61 patients (34%) had further increases in ALT levels to ≥5×ULN and were withdrawn from the study in accordance with the study protocol. In patients who discontinued zileuton, elevated ALT levels returned to <2×ULN in an average of 32 days (range 1-111 days).

In controlled and uncontrolled clinical trials involving more than 5000 patients treated with zileuton, the overall rate of ALT elevation ≥3×ULN was 3.2%. In these trials, one patient developed symptomatic hepatitis with jaundice, which resolved upon discontinuation of therapy. An additional 3 patients with transaminase elevations developed mild hyperbilirubinemia that was less than three times the upper limit of normal. There was no evidence of hypersensitivity or other alternative etiologies for these findings. In subsequent analyses, females over the age of 65 appeared to be at an increased risk for ALT elevations. Patients with pre-existing transaminase elevations may also be at an increased risk for ALT elevations (see CONTRAINDICATIONS).

It is recommended that hepatic transaminases be evaluated at initiation of, and during therapy with, zileuton. Serum ALT should be monitored before treatment begins, once-a-month for the first 3 months, every two to three months for the remainder of the first year, and periodically thereafter for patients receiving long-term zileuton therapy. If clinical signs and/or symptoms of liver dysfunction (*e.g,* right upper quadrant pain, nausea, fatigue, lethargy, pruritus, jaundice, or "flu-like" symptoms) develop or transaminase elevations greater than 5 times the ULN occur, zileuton should be discontinued and transaminase levels followed until normal.

Since treatment with zileuton may result in increased hepatic transaminases, zileuton should be used with caution in patients who consume substantial quantities of alcohol and/or have a past history of liver disease.

Information for the Patient: Patients should be told that:

Zileuton is indicated for the chronic treatment of asthma and should be taken regularly as prescribed, even during symptom-free periods.

Zileuton is not a bronchodilator and should not be used to treat acute episodes of asthma.

When taking zileuton, they should not decrease the dose or stop taking any other antiasthma medications unless instructed by a physician.

While using zileuton, medical attention should be sought if short-acting bronchodilators are needed more often than usual, or if more than the maximum number of inhalations of short-acting bronchodilator treatment prescribed for a 24-hour period are needed.

The most serious side effect of zileuton is elevation of liver enzyme tests and that, while taking zileuton, they must return for liver enzyme test monitoring on a regular basis.

If they experience signs and/or symptoms of liver dysfunction (*e.g.,* right upper quadrant pain, nausea, fatigue, lethargy, pruritus, jaundice, or "flu-like" symptoms), they should contact their physician immediately.

Zileuton can interact with other drugs and that, while taking zileuton, they should consult their doctor before starting or stopping any prescription or non-prescription medicines.

Carcinogenesis, Mutagenesis, and Impairment of Fertility: In 2-year carcinogenicity studies, increases in the incidence of liver, kidney, and vascular tumors in female mice and a trend towards an increase in the incidence of liver tumors in male mice were observed at 450 mg/kg/day (providing approximately 4 times [females] or 7 times [males] the systemic exposure [AUC] achieved at the maximum recommended human daily oral dose). No increase in the incidence of tumors was observed at 150 mg/kg/day (providing approximately 2 times the systemic exposure [AUC] achieved at the maximum recommended human daily oral dose). In rats, an increase in the incidence of kidney tumors was observed in both sexes at 170 mg/kg/day (providing approximately 6 times [males] or 14 times [females] the systemic exposure [AUC] achieved at the maximum recommended human daily oral dose). No increased incidence of kidney tumors was seen at 80 mg/kg/day (providing approximately 4 times [males] or 6 times [females] the systemic exposure [AUC] achieved at the maximum recommended human daily oral dose). Although a dose-related increased incidence of benign Leydig cell tumors was observed, Leydig cell tumorogenesis was prevented by supplementing male rats with testosterone.

Zileuton was negative in genotoxicity studies including bacterial reverse mutation (Ames) using *S. typhimurium* and *E. coli,* chromosome aberration in human lymphocytes, *in vitro* unscheduled DNA synthesis (UDS), in rat hepatocytes with or without zileuton pretreatment and in mouse and rat kidney cells with zileuton pretreatment, and mouse micronucleus assays. However, a dose-related increase in DNA adduct formation was reported in kidneys and livers of female mice treated with zileuton. Although some evidence of DNA damage was observed in a UDS assay in hepatocytes isolated from Aroclor-1254 treated rats, no such finding was noticed in hepatocytes isolated from monkeys, where the metabolic profile of zileuton is more similar to that of humans.

In reproductive performance/fertility studies, zileuton produced no effects on fertility in rats at oral doses up to 300 mg/kg/day (providing approximately 8 times [male rats] and 18 times [female rats] the systemic exposure [AUC] achieved at the maximum recommended human daily oral dose). Comparative systemic exposure (AUC) is based on measurements in male rats or nonpregnant female rats at similar dosages. However, reduction in fetal implants was observed at oral doses of 150 mg/kg/day and higher (providing approximately 9 times the systemic exposure [AUC] achieved at the maximum recommended human daily oral dose). Increases in gestation length, prolongation of estrous cycle, and increases in stillbirths were observed at oral doses of 70 mg/kg/day and higher (providing approximately 4 times the systemic exposure (AUC) achieved at the maximum recommended human daily oral dose).

PRECAUTIONS: *(cont'd)*

In a perinatal/postnatal study in rats, reduced pup survival and growth were noted at an oral dose of 300 mg/kg/day (providing approximately 18 times the systemic exposure [AUC] achieved at the maximum recommended human daily oral dose).

Pregnancy, Teratogenic Effects, Pregnancy Category C: Developmental studies indicated adverse effects (reduced body weight and increased skeletal variations) in rats at an oral dose of 300 mg/kg/day (providing approximately 18 times the systemic exposure [AUC] achieved at the maximum recommended human daily oral dose). Comparative systemic exposure [AUC] is based on measurements in nonpregnant female rats at a similar dosage. Zileuton and/or its metabolites cross the placental barrier of rats. Three of 118 (2.5%) rabbit fetuses had cleft palates at an oral dose of 150 mg/kg/day (equivalent to the maximum recommended human daily oral dose on a mg/m^2 basis). There are no adequate and well-controlled studies in pregnant women. Zileuton should be used during pregnancy only if the potential benefit justifies the potential risk to the fetus.

Nursing Mothers: Zileuton and/or its metabolites are excreted in rat milk. It is not known if zileuton is excreted in human milk. Because many drugs are excreted in human milk, and because of the potential for tumorogenicity shown for zileuton in animal studies, a decision should be made whether to discontinue nursing or to discontinue the drug, taking into account the importance of the drug to the mother.

Pediatric Use: The safely and effectiveness of zileuton in pediatric patients under 12 years of age have not been established.

DRUG INTERACTIONS:

In a drug-interaction study in 16 healthy volunteers, co-administration of multiple doses of zileuton (800 mg every 12 hours) and theophylline (200 mg every 6 hours) for 5 days resulted in a significant decrease (approximately 50%) in steady-state clearance of theophylline, an approximate doubling of theophylline AUC, and an increase in theophylline C_{max} by 73%). The elimination half-life of theophylline was increased by 24%. Also, during co-administration, theophylline-related adverse events were observed more frequently than after theophylline alone. Upon initiation of zileuton in patients receiving theophylline, the theophylline dosage should be reduced by approximately one half and plasma theophylline concentrations monitored. Similarly, when initiating therapy with theophylline in a patient receiving zileuton, the maintenance dose and/or dosing interval of theophylline should be adjusted accordingly and guided by serum theophylline determinations (see WARNINGS).

Concomitant administration of multiple doses of zileuton (600 mg every 6 hours) and warfarin (fixed daily dose obtained by titration in each subject) to 30 healthy male volunteers resulted in a 15% decrease in R-warfarin clearance and an increase in AUC of 22%. The pharmacokinetics of S-warfarin were not affected. These pharmacokinetic changes were accompanied by a clinically significant increase in prothrombin times. Monitoring of prothrombin time, or other suitable coagulation tests, with the appropriate dose titration of warfarin is recommended in patients receiving concomitant zileuton and warfarin therapy (see WARNINGS).

Co-administration of zileuton and propranolol results in a significant increase in propranolol concentrations. Administration of a single 80 mg dose of propranolol in 16 healthy male volunteers who received zileuton 600 mg every 6 hours for 5 days resulted in a 42% decrease in propranolol clearance. This resulted in an increase in propranolol C_{max}, AUC, and elimination half-life by 52%, 104%, and 25%, respectively. There was an increase in β-blockade and decrease in heart rate associated with the co-administration of these drugs. Patients on zileuton and propranolol should be closely monitored and the dose of propranolol reduced as necessary (see WARNINGS). No formal drug-drug interaction studies between zileuton and other beta-adrenergic blocking agents (*i.e.,* β-blockers) have been conducted. It is reasonable to employ appropriate clinical monitoring when these drugs are co-administered with zileuton.

In a drug interaction study in 16 healthy volunteers, co-administration of multiple doses of terfenadine (600 mg every 12 hours) and zileuton (600 mg every 6 hours) for 7 days resulted in a decrease in clearance of terfenadine by 22% leading to a statistically significant increase in mean AUC and C_{max} of terfenadine of approximately 35%. This increase in terfenadine plasma concentration in the presence of zileuton was not associated with a significant prolongation of the QTc interval. Although there was no cardiac effect in this small number of healthy volunteers, given the high inter-individual pharmacokinetic variability of terfenadine, co-administration of zileuton and terfenadine is not recommended.

Drug-drug interaction studies conducted in healthy volunteers between zileuton and prednisone and ethinyl estradiol (oral contraceptive), drugs known to be metabolized by the P450 3A4 (CYP3A4) isoenzyme, have shown no significant interaction. However, no formal drug-drug interaction studies between zileuton and dihydropyridine, calcium channel blockers, cyclosporine, cisapride, and astemizole, also metabolized by CYP3A4 have been conducted. It is reasonable to employ appropriate clinical monitoring when these drugs are co-administered with zileuton.

Drug-drug interaction studies in healthy volunteers have been conducted with zileuton and digoxin, phenytoin, sulfasalazine, and naproxen. There was no significant interaction between zileuton and any of these drugs.

Co-administration of zileuton and theophylline results in, on average, an approximate doubling of serum theophylline concentrations. Theophylline dosage in these patients should be reduced and serum theophylline concentrations monitored closely (see DRUG INTERACTIONS).

ADVERSE REACTIONS:

In clinical studies a total of 5542 patients have been exposed to zileuton in clinical trials, 2252 of them for greater than 6 months and 742 for greater than 1 year.

Adverse events most frequently occurring (frequency ≥3%) in zileuton-treated patients and at a frequency greater than placebo-treated patients are summarized in TABLE 2.

TABLE 2 Proportion of Patients Experiencing Adverse Events in Placebo-Controlled Studies in Asthma

Body System/Event	Zileuton 600 mg 4 x Daily % Occurrence (N=475)	Placebo % Occurrence (N=491)
Body As A Whole		
Headache	24.6	24.0
Pain (unspecified)	7.8	5.3
Abdominal Pain	4.6	2.4
Asthenia	3.8	2.4
Accidental Injury	3.4	2.0
Digestive System		
Dyspepsia	8.2*	2.9
Nausea	5.5	3.7
Musculoskeletal		
Myalgia	3.2	2.9

* p≤0.05 vs placebo

ADVERSE REACTIONS: *(cont'd)*

Less common adverse events occurring at a frequency of greater than 1% and more commonly in zileuton-treated patients included: arthralgia, chest pain, conjunctivitis constipation, dizziness, fever, flatulence, hypertonia, insomnia, lymphadenopathy, malaise, neck pain/rigidity, nervousness, pruritus, somnolence, urinary tract infection, vaginitis, and vomiting.

The frequency of discontinuation from the asthma clinical studies due to any adverse event was comparable between zileuton (9.7%) and placebo-treated (8. 4%) groups.

In placebo-controlled clinical trials, the frequency of ALT elevations ≥3×ULN was 1.9% for zileuton-treated patients, compared with 0.2% for placebo-treated patients. In controlled and uncontrolled trials, one patient developed symptomatic hepatitis with jaundice, which resolved upon discontinuation of therapy. An additional 3 patients with transaminase elevations developed mild hyperbilirubinemia that was less than three times the upper limit of normal. There was no evidence of hypersensitivity or other alternative etiologies for these findings. Zileuton is contraindicated in patients with active liver disease or transaminase elevations greater than or equal to 3×ULN (see CONTRAINDICATIONS). It is recommended that hepatic transaminases be evaluated at initiation of and during therapy with zileuton (see PRECAUTIONS, Hepatic Effects).

Occurrences of low white blood cell count ≤2.8×10^9/L) were observed in 1.0% of 1673 patients taking zileuton and 0.6% of 1056 patients taking placebo in placebo-controlled studies. These findings were transient and the majority of cases returned toward normal or baseline with continued zileuton dosing. All remaining cases returned toward normal or baseline after discontinuation of zileuton. Similar findings were also noted in a long-term safety surveillance study of 2458 patients treated with zileuton plus usual asthma care versus 489 patients treated only with usual asthma care for up to one year. The clinical significance of these observations is not known.

In the long-term safety surveillance trial of zileuton plus usual asthma care versus usual asthma care alone, a similar adverse event profile was seen as in other clinical trials.

OVERDOSAGE:

Human experience of acute overdose with zileuton is limited. A patient in a clinical trial took between 6.6 and 9.0 grams of zileuton in a single dose. Vomiting was induced and the patient recovered without sequelae. Zileuton is not removed by dialysis. Should an overdose occur, the patient should be treated symptomatically and supportive measures instituted as required. If indicated elimination of unabsorbed drug should be achieved by emesis or gastric lavage; usual precautions should be observed to maintain the airway. A Certified Poison Control Center should be consulted for up-to-date information on management of overdose with zileuton.

The oral minimum lethal doses in mice and rats were 500-4000 and 300-1000 mg/kg in various preparations, respectively (providing greater than 3 and 9 times the systemic exposure [AUC] achieved at the maximum recommended human daily oral dose, respectively). No deaths occurred but nephritis was reported in dogs at an oral dose of 1000 mg/kg (providing in excess of 12 times the systemic exposure [AUC] achieved at the maximum recommended human daily oral dose).

DOSAGE AND ADMINISTRATION:

The recommended dosage of zileuton for the symptomatic treatment of patients with asthma is one 600 mg tablet four times a day for a total daily dose of 2400 mg. For ease of administration, zileuton may be taken with meals and at bedtime. Hepatic transaminases should be evaluated prior to initiation of zileuton and periodically during treatment (see PRECAUTIONS, Hepatic Effects).

PATIENT INFORMATION:

Zileuton is used for the chronic treatment of asthma in adults and children age 12 years and older.

Zileuton should be taken regularly as prescribed, even during symptom-free periods.

Zileuton is not a bronchodilator and should not be used to treat acute episodes of asthma.

Do not decrease the dose, or stop taking any other antiasthma medications unless instructed by your physician.

Contact your physician immediately if short-acting bronchodilators are needed more often than usual, or if the maximum number of inhalations of short-acting bronchodilator treatment prescribed for a 24-hour period are needed.

Return to see your physician for liver enzyme test monitoring on a regular basis.

Contact your physician immediately if you experience right upper quadrant pain, nausea, fatigue, lethargy, yellowing of the skin or eyes, flu-like symptoms, or if you experience uncomfortable sensations leading to scratching.

Zileuton may be taken with or without food.

Inform your physician if you are pregnant, intend to become pregnant, or if you are nursing an infant.

HOW SUPPLIED:

ZYFLO Filmtab Tablets are available as 1 dosage strength: 600 mg white ovaloid tablets with single bisect, debossed on bisect side with Abbott logo and ZL (Abbo-Code), and 600 on the opposite side.

Recommended storage: Store tablets at controlled room temperature between 20°-25°C, (68°-77°F). See USP. Protect from light.

HOW SUPPLIED - EQUIVALENTS NOT AVAILABLE:

Tablet - Oral - 600 mg

120's	$75.00	ZYFLO, Abbott	00074-8036-22

ZINC *(002452)*

CATEGORIES: Electrolytic, Caloric-Water Balance; Homeostatic & Nutrient; Mineral Supplements; Replacement Solutions; Vitamins; FDA Pre 1938 Drugs

Prescribing information not available at time of publication.

HOW SUPPLIED - EQUIVALENTS NOT AVAILABLE:

Injection, Solution - Intravenous - 1 mg/ml

10 ml	$52.50	Zinc Sulfate, Fujisawa USA	00469-6300-30
30 ml	$91.25	Zinc Sulfate, Fujisawa USA	00469-6310-50

ZINC ACETATE *(003264)*

CATEGORIES: Chelating Agents; Heavy Metal Antagonists; Orphan Drugs; Wilson's Disease; FDA Unapproved

Prescribing information not available at time of publication.

ZINC CHLORIDE *(002454)*

CATEGORIES: Electrolytic, Caloric-Water Balance; Homeostatic & Nutrient; Mineral Supplements; Replacement Solutions; Vitamins; FDA Approved 1986 Jun

BRAND NAMES: Zinc Trace Element

Prescribing information not available at time of publication.

HOW SUPPLIED - EQUIVALENTS NOT AVAILABLE:

Injection, Conc-Soln - Intravenous - 1 mg/ml

10 ml	$3.72	Zinc 1, Abbott	00074-4090-01
50 ml	$16.72	Zinc 1, Abbott	00074-4526-05

ZINC OXIDE *(002456)*

CATEGORIES: Antipruritics/Local Anesthetics; Skin/Mucous Membrane Agents

BRAND NAMES: *Biogena Baby*; Ken Tox; *OZ*; *Zinkolie*
(International brand names outside U.S. in italics)

FORMULARIES: WHO

Prescribing information not available at time of publication.

HOW SUPPLIED - EQUIVALENTS NOT AVAILABLE:

Cream - Topical

30 gm	$2.50	KEN TOX, Kenyon Drug	12535-0229-16

Ointment - Topical

30 gm	$1.26	Zinc Oxide, Qualitest Drugs	52446-0969-78

ZINC SULFATE *(002459)*

CATEGORIES: Electrolytic, Caloric-Water Balance; Homeostatic & Nutrient; Mineral Supplements; Pharmaceutical Adjuvants; Replacement Solutions; Vitamins; Zinc Salts; FDA Approved 1987 May

BRAND NAMES: *Z Span*; Zinc-220; Zinca-Pak; Zincate; *Zincomed*
(International brand names outside U.S. in italics)

Prescribing information not available at time of publication.

HOW SUPPLIED - EQUIVALENTS NOT AVAILABLE:

Capsule, Gelatin - Oral - 220 mg

100's	$8.60	ZINCATE, Paddock Labs	00574-9167-01
100's	$13.31	Zinc Sulfate, Upsher Smith	00245-0080-11
1000's	$62.15	ZINCATE, Paddock Labs	00574-9167-10

Injection, Solution - Intravenous - 1 mg/ml

10 ml	$44.38	ZINCA-PAK, Solopak Labs	39769-0043-10
10 ml x 25	$62.19	Zinc Sulfate, Am Regent	00517-6110-25

Injection, Solution - Intravenous - 5 mg/ml

5 ml	$61.25	ZINCA-PAK, Solopak Labs	39769-0045-05
5 ml x 25	$124.69	Zinc Sulfate, Am Regent	00517-8105-25

ZOLPIDEM TARTRATE *(003145)*

CATEGORIES: Anxiolytics, Sedatives, Hypnotic; Central Nervous System Agents; Hypnotics; Imidazopyridines; Insomnia; Sedatives/Hypnotics; DEA Class CIV; FDA Class 1S ("Standard Review"); Sales > $100 Million; FDA Approved 1992 Dec; Patent Expiration 2006 Oct; Top 200 Drugs

BRAND NAMES: **Ambien**; *Niotal*; *Stilnoct*; *Stilnox* (France, Germany)
(International brand names outside U.S. in italics)

FORMULARIES: PCS

COST OF THERAPY: $11.24 (Insomnia; Tablet; 10 mg; 1/day; 7 days)

DESCRIPTION:

Zolpidem tartrate, is a non-benzodiazepine hypnotic of the imidazopyridine class and is available in 5 mg and 10 mg strength tablets for oral administration.

Chemically, zolpidem is N,N,6-trimethyl-2-p-toyl-imidazo(1,2,-a)pyridine-3-acetamide L-(+)-tartrate (2:1).

Zolpidem tartrate is a white to off-white crystalline powder that is sparingly soluble in water, alcohol, and propylene glycol. It has a molecular weight of 764.88.

Each Ambien tablet includes the following inactive ingredients: hydroxypropyl methylcellulose, lactose, magnesium stearate, microcrystalline cellulose, polyethylene glycol, sodium starch glycolate, titanium dioxide; the 5 mg tablet also contains FD&C Red No. 40, iron oxide colorant, and polysorbate 80.

CLINICAL PHARMACOLOGY:

PHARMACODYNAMICS

Subunit modulation of the $GABA_a$ receptor chloride channel macromolecular complex is hypothesized to be responsible for sedative, anticonvulsant, anxiolytic, and myorelaxant drug properties. The major modulatory site of the $GABA_a$ receptor complex is located on its alpha (α) subunit and is referred to as the benzodiazepine (BZ) or Ω receptor. At least three subtypes of the Ω receptor have been identified.

While zolpidem is a hypnotic agent with a chemical structure unrelated to benzodiazepines, barbiturates, or other drugs with known hypnotic properties, it interacts with a GABA-BZ receptor complex and shares some of the pharmacological properties of the benzodiazepines. In contrast to the benzodiazepines, which non-selectively bind to and activate all three omega receptor subtypes, zolpidem *in vitro* binds the (ω_1) receptor preferentially. The (Ω_1) receptor is found primarily on the Lamina IV of the sensorimotor cortical regions, substantia nigra (pars reticulata), cerebellum molecular layer, olfactory bulb, ventral thalamic complex, pons, inferior colliculus, and globus pallidus. This selective binding of zolpidem on the (Ω_1) receptor is not absolute, but it may explain the relative absence of myorelaxant and anticonvulsant effects in animal studies as well as the preservation of deep sleep (stages 3 and 4) in human studies of zolpidem at hypnotic doses.

CLINICAL PHARMACOLOGY: *(cont'd)*

PHARMACOKINETICS

The pharmacokinetic profile of zolpidem tartrate is characterized by rapid absorption from the GI tract and a short elimination half-life ($T_{1/2}$) in healthy subjects. In a single- dose crossover study in 45 healthy subjects administered 5 and 10 mg zolpidem tartrate tablets, the mean peak concentrations (C_{max}) were 59 (range: 29 to 113) and 121 (range: 58 to 272) ng/ml, respectively, occurring at a mean time (T_{max}) of 1.6 hours for both. The mean zolpidem tartrate elimination half-life was 2.6 (range: 1.4 to 4.5) and 2.5 (range: 1.4 to 3.8) hours, for the 5 and 10 mg tablets, respectively. Zolpidem tartrate is converted to inactive metabolites that are eliminated primarily by renal excretion. Zolpidem tartrate demonstrated linear kinetics in the dose range of 5 to 20 mg. Total protein binding was found to be 92.5 ± 0.1% and remained constant, independent of concentration between 40 and 790 ng/ml. Zolpidem did not accumulate in young adults following nightly dosing with 20 mg zolpidem tartrate tablets for 2 weeks.

A food-effect study in 30 healthy male volunteers compared the pharmacokinetics of zolpidem tartrate 10 mg when administered while fasting or 20 minutes after a meal. Results demonstrated that with food, mean AUC and C_{max}were decreased by 15% and 25% respectively, while mean $T_{max}$was prolonged by 60% (from 1.4 to 2.2 hr). The half-life remained unchanged. These results suggest that, for faster sleep onset, zolpidem tartrate should not be administered with or immediately after a meal.

In the elderly, the dose for zolpidem tartrate should be 5 mg (see PRECAUTIONSand DOSAGE AND ADMINISTRATION). This recommendation is based on several studies in which the mean C_{max}, $T_{1/2}$, and AUC were significantly increased when compared to results in young adults. In one study of eight elderly subjects (> 70 years), the means for C_{max}, $T_{1/2}$, and AUC significantly increased by 50% (255 vs 284 ng/ml), 32% (2.2 vs 2.9 hr), and 64% (955 vs 1,562 ng · hr/ml), respectively, as compared to younger adults (20 to 40 years) following a single 20 mg oral zolpidem dose. Zolpidem tartrate did not accumulate in elderly subjects following nightly oral dosing of 10 mg for 1 week.

The pharmacokinetics of zolpidem tartrate in eight patients with chronic hepatic insufficiency were compared to results in healthy subjects. Following a single 20 mg oral zolpidem dose, mean C_{max} and AUC were found to be two times (250 vs 499 ng/ml) and five times (788 vs 4,203 ng · hr/ml) higher, respectively, in hepatically compromised patients. T_{max} did not change. The mean half-life in cirrhotic patients of 9.9 hr (range: 4.1 to 25.8 hr) was greater than that observed in normals of 2.2 hr (range: 1.6 to 2.4 hr). Dosing should be modified accordingly in patients with hepatic insufficiency (see PRECAUTIONS and DOSAGE AND ADMINISTRATION).

The pharmacokinetics of zolpidem tartrate were studied in 11 patients with end-stage renal failure (mean Cl_{cr}= 6.5 ± 1.5 ml/min) undergoing hemodialysis three times a week, who were dosed with zolpidem 10 mg orally each day for 14 to 21 days. No statistically significant differences were observed for C_{max}, T_{max}, half-life, and AUC between the first and last days of drug administration when baseline concentration adjustments were made. On day 1, C_{max} was 172 ± 29 ng/ml (range: 46 to 344 ng/ml). After repeated dosing for 14 or 21 days, C_{max} was 203 ± 32 ng/ml (range 28 to 316 ng/ml). On day 1, $T_{max}$was 1.7 ± 0.3 hr (range 0.5 to 3.0 hr); after repeated dosing T_{max} 0.8 ± 0.2 hr (range 0.5 to 2.0 hr). This variation is accounted for by noting that last-day serum sampling began 10 hours after the previous dose, rather than after 24 hours. This resulted in residual drug concentration and a shorter period to reach maximal serum concentration. On day 1, $T_{1/2}$ was 2.4 ± 0.4 hr (range 0.4 to 5.1 hr). After repeated dosing, $T_{1/2}$ was 2.5 ± 0.4 hr (range: 0.7 to 4.2 hr). AUC was 796 ± 159 ng · hr/ml after the first dose and 818 ± 170 ng · hr/ml after repeated dosing. Zolpidem was not hemodialyzable. No accumulation of unchanged drug appeared after 14 or 21 days. Zolpidem tartrate pharmacokinetics were not significantly different in renally impaired patients. No dosage adjustment is necessary in patients with compromised renal function. As a general precaution, these patients should be closely monitored.

POSTULATED RELATIONSHIP BETWEEN ELIMINATION RATE OF HYPNOTICS AND THEIR PROFILE OF COMMON UNTOWARD EFFECTS

The type and duration of hypnotic effects and the profile of unwanted effects during administration of hypnotic drugs may be influenced by the biologic half- life of administered drug and any active metabolites formed. When half-lives are long, drug or metabolites may accumulate during periods of nightly administration and may be associated with impairment of cognitive and/or motor performance during waking hours; the possibility of interaction with other psychoactive drugs or alcohol will be enhanced. In contrast, if half-lives, including half-lives of active metabolites, are short, drug and metabolites will be cleared before the next dose is ingested, and carryover effects related to excessive sedation or CNS depression should be minimal or absent. Zolpidem tartrate has a short half-life and no active metabolites. During nightly use for an extended period, pharmacodynamic tolerance or adaptation to some effects of hypnotics may develop. If the drug has a short elimination half-life, it is possible that a relative deficiency of the drug or its active metabolites (*i.e.,* in relationship to the receptor site) may occur at some point in the interval between each night's use. This sequence of events may account for two clinical findings reported to occur after several weeks of nightly use of other rapidly eliminated hypnotics, namely, increased wakefulness during the last third of the night, and the appearance of increased signs of daytime anxiety. Increased wakefulness during the last third of the night as measured by polysomnography has not been observed in clinical trials with zolpidem tartrate.

CONTROLLED TRIALS SUPPORTING SAFETY AND EFFICACY

Transient Insomnia: Normal adults experiencing transient insomnia (n=462) during the first night in a sleep laboratory were evaluated in a double blind, parallel group, single-night trial comparing two doses of zolpidem (7.5 and 10 mg) and placebo. Both zolpidem doses were superior to placebo on objective (polysomnographic) measures of sleep latency, sleep duration, and number of awakenings.

Chronic insomnia: Adult outpatients, with chronic insomnia (n=75) were evaluated in a double-blind, parallel group, 5-week trial comparing two doses of zolpidem tartrate (10 and 15 mg) and placebo. On objective (polysomnographic) measures of sleep latency and sleep efficiency, zolpidem 15 mg was superior to placebo for all 5 weeks; zolpidem 10 mg was superior to placebo on sleep latency for the first 4 weeks and on sleep efficiency for weeks 2 and 4. Zolpidem was comparable to placebo on number of awakenings at both doses studied.

Adult outpatients (n=141) with chronic insomnia were evaluated in a double-blind, parallel group, 4-week trial comparing two doses of zolpidem (10 and 15 mg) and placebo. Zolpidem 10 mg was superior to placebo on a subjective measure of sleep latency for all 4 weeks, and on subjective measures of total sleep time, number of awakenings, and sleep quality for the first treatment week. Zolpidem 15 mg was superior to placebo on a subjective measure of sleep latency for the first 3 weeks, on a subjective measure of total sleep time for the first week, and on number of awakenings and sleep quality for the first 2 weeks.

Next-day residual effects: There was no evidence of residual next-day effects seen with zolpidem tartrate in several studies utilizing the Multiple Sleep latency Test (MSLT), the Digit Symbol Substitution Test (DSST), and patient ratings of alertness. In one study involving elderly patients, there was a small but statistically significant decrease in one measure of performance, the DSST, but no impairment was seen in the MSLT study.

Rebound effects: There was no objective (polysomnographic) evidence of rebound insomnia at recommended doses seen in studies evaluating sleep on the nights following discontinuation of zolpidem tartrate. There was subjective evidence of impaired sleep in the elderly on the first posttreatment night at doses above the recommended elderly dose of 5 mg.

CLINICAL PHARMACOLOGY: *(cont'd)*

Memory impairment: Two small studies (n=6 and n=9) utilizing objective measures of memory yielded little evidence for memory impairment following the administration of zolpidem tartrate. There was subjective evidence from adverse event data for anterograde amnesia occurring in association with the administration zolpidem tartrate, predominantly at doses above 10 mg.

Effects on sleep stages: In studies that measured the percentage of sleep time spent in each sleep stage, zolpidem tartrate has generally been shown to preserve sleep stages. Sleep time spent in stages 3 and 4 (deep sleep) was found comparable to placebo with only inconsistent, minor changes in REM (paradoxical) sleep at the recommended dose.

INDICATIONS AND USAGE:

Zolpidem tartrate is indicated for the short-term treatment of insomnia. Hypnotics should generally be limited to 7 to 10 days of use; and reevaluation of the patient is recommended if they are to be taken for more than 2 to 3 weeks.

Zolpidem tartrate should not be prescribed in quantities exceeding a 1-month supply (see WARNINGS).

Zolpidem tartrate has been shown to decrease sleep latency and increase the duration of sleep for up to 5 weeks in controlled clinical studies (see CLINICAL PHARMACOLOGY).

CONTRAINDICATIONS:

None known.

WARNINGS:

Since sleep disturbances may be the presenting manifestation of a physical and/or psychiatric disorder, symptomatic treatment of the insomnia should be initiated only after a careful evaluation of the patient. The failure of insomnia to remit after 7 to 10 days of treatment may indicate the presence of a primary psychiatric and/or medical illness which should be evaluated. Worsening of insomnia or the emergence of new thinking or behavior abnormalities may be the consequence of an unrecognized psychiatric or physical disorder. Such findings have emerged during the course of treatment with sedative/hypnotic drugs, including zolpidem tartrate. Because some of the important adverse effects of zolpidem tartrate appear to be dose related (see PRECAUTIONS and DOSAGE AND ADMINISTRATION), it is important to use the smallest possible effective dose, especially in the elderly.

A variety of abnormal thinking and behavior changes have been reported to occur in association with the use of sedative/hypnotics. Some of these changes may be characterized by decreased inhibition (*e.g.,* aggressiveness and extroversion that seemed out of character), similar to effects produced by alcohol and other CNS depressants. Other reported behavioral changes have included bizarre behavior, agitation, hallucinations, and depersonalization. Amnesia and other neuropsychiatric symptoms may occur unpredictably. In primarily depressed patients, worsening of depression, including suicidal thinking, has been reported in association with the use of sedative/hypnotics.

It can rarely be determined with certainty whether a particular instance of the abnormal behaviors listed above are drug induced, spontaneous in origin, or a result of an underlying psychiatric or physical disorder. Nonetheless, the emergence of any new behavioral sign or symptom of concern requires careful and immediate evaluation.

Following the rapid dose decrease or abrupt discontinuation of sedative/hypnotics, there have been reports of signs and symptoms similar to those associated with withdrawal from other CNS-depressant drugs (see DRUG ABUSE AND DEPENDENCE).

Zolpidem tartrate, like other sedative/hypnotic drugs, has CNS-depressant effects. Due to the rapid onset of action, zolpidem tartrate should only be ingested immediately prior to going to bed. Patients should be cautioned against engaging in hazardous occupations requiring complete mental alertness or motor coordination such as operating machinery or driving a motor vehicle after ingesting the drug, including potential impairment of the performance of such activities that may occur the day following ingestion of zolpidem tartrate. Zolpidem tartrate showed additive effects when combined with alcohol and should not be taken with alcohol. Patients should also be cautioned about possible combined effects with other CNS-depressant drugs. Dosage adjustments may be necessary when zolpidem tartrate is administered with such agents because of the potentially additive effects.

PRECAUTIONS:

GENERAL

Use In The Elderly And/Or Debilitated Patients: Impaired motor and/or cognitive performance after repeated exposure or unusual sensitivity to sedative/hypnotic drugs is a concern in the treatment of elderly and/or debilitated patients. Therefore, the recommended zolpidem tartrate dosage is 5 mg in such patients (see DOSAGE AND ADMINISTRATION) to decrease the possibility of side effects. These patients should be closely monitored.

Use In Patients With Concomitant Illness: Clinical experience with zolpidem tartrate in patients with concomitant systemic illness is limited. Caution is advisable in using zolpidem tartrate in patients with diseases or conditions that could affect metabolism or hemodynamic responses. Although preliminary studies did not reveal respiratory depressant effects at hypnotic doses of zolpidem tartrate in normals, precautions should be observed if zolpidem tartrate is prescribed to patients with compromised respiratory function, since sedative/hypnotics have the capacity to depress respiratory drive. Post-marketing reports or respiratory insufficiency, most of which involved patients with pre-existing respiratory impairment, have been received. Data in end-stage renal failure patients repeatedly treated with zolpidem tartrate did not demonstrate drug accumulation or alterations in pharmacokinetic parameters. No dosage adjustment in renally impaired patients is required; however, these patients should be closely monitored (see Pharmacokinetics). A study in subjects with hepatic impairment did reveal prolonged elimination in this group; therefore, treatment should be initiated with 5 mg in patients with hepatic compromise, and they should be closely monitored.

Use In Depression: As with other sedative/hypnotic drugs, zolpidem tartrate should be administered with caution to patients exhibiting signs or symptoms of depression. Suicidal tendencies may be present in such patients and protective measures may be required. Intentional overdosage is more common in this group of patients; therefore, the least amount of drug that is feasible should be prescribed for the patient at any one time.

INFORMATION FOR THE PATIENT

Patient information is provided at the end of this monograph. To assure safe and effective use of zolpidem tartrate, this information and instructions provided in the patient information section should be discussed with patients (see PATIENT PACKAGE INSERT).

LABORATORY TESTS

There are no specific laboratory tests recommended.

DRUG/LABORATORY TEST INTERACTIONS

Zolpidem is not known to interfere with commonly employed clinical laboratory tests.

CARCINOGENESIS, MUTAGENESIS, AND IMPAIRMENT OF FERTILITY

Carcinogenesis: Zolpidem was administered to rats and mice for 2 years at dietary dosages of 4, 18, and 80 mg/kg/day. In mice, these doses are 26 to 520 times or 2 to 35 times the maximum 10 mg human dose on a mg/kg or mg/m^2 basis, respectively. In rats these doses are 43 to 876 times or 6 to 115 times the maximum 10 mg human dose on a mg/kg or mg/m^2 basis, respectively. No evidence of carcinogenic potential was observed in mice. Renal lipocarcinomas were seen in 4/100 rats (3 males, 1 female) receiving 80 mg/kg/day and a renal lipoma was observed in one male rat at the 18 mg/kg/day dose. Incidence rates of lipoma and liposarcoma for zolpidem were comparable to those seen in historical controls and the tumor findings are thought be a spontaneous occurrence.

Mutagenesis: Zolpidem did not have mutagenic activity in several tests including the Ames test, genotoxicity in mouse lymphoma cells *in vitro,* chromosomal aberration in cultured human lymphocytes, unscheduled DNA synthesis in rat hepatocytes *in vitro,* and the micronucleus test in mice.

Impairment of Fertility: In a rat reproduction study, the high dose (100 mg/base/kg) of zolpidem resulted in irregular estrus cycles and prolonged precoital intervals, but there was no effect on male or female fertility after daily oral doses of 4 to 100 mg base/mg or 5 to 130 times the recommended human dose in mg/m^2. No effects on any other fertility parameters were noted.

PREGNANCY CATEGORY B

Teratogenic Effects: Studies to assess the effects of zolpidem on human reproduction and development have not been conducted.

Teratology studies were conducted in rats and rabbits.

In rats, adverse maternal and fetal effects occurred at 20 and 100 mg base/kg and included dose-related maternal lethargy and ataxia and a dose-related trend to incomplete ossification of fetal skull bones. Under-ossification of various fetal bone indicated a delay in maturation and is often seen in rats treated with sedative/hypnotic drugs. There were no teratogenic effects after zolpidem administration. The no-effect dose for maternal or fetal toxicity was 4 mg base/kg or 5 times the maximum human dose on a mg/m^2 basis.

In rabbits, dose-related maternal sedation and decreased weight gain occurred at all doses tested. At the high dose, 16 mg base/kg, there was an increase in postimplantation fetal loss and underossification of sternebrae in viable fetuses. These fetal findings in rabbits are often secondary to reductions in maternal weight gain. There were no frank teratogenic effects. The no-effect dose for fetal toxicity was 4 mg base/kg or 7 times the maximum human dose on a mg/m^2 basis.

Because animal reproduction studies are not always predictive of human response, this drug should be used during pregnancy only if clearly needed.

Nonteratogenic Effects: Studies to assess the effects on children whose mother took zolpidem during pregnancy have not been conducted. However, children born of mothers taking sedative/hypnotic drugs may be at some risk for withdrawal symptoms from the drug during the postnatal period. In addition, neonatal flaccidity has been reported in infants born of mothers who received sedative/hypnotic drugs during pregnancy.

LABOR AND DELIVERY

Zolpidem tartrate has no established use in labor and delivery.

NURSING MOTHERS

Studies in lactating mothers indicate that the half-life of zolpidem is similar to that in young normal volunteers (2.6 ± 0.3 hr). Between 0.004 and 0.019% of the total administered dose is excreted into milk, but the effect of zolpidem on the infant is unknown.

In addition, in a rat study, zolpidem inhibited the secretion of milk. The no-effect dose was 4 mg base/kg or 6 times the recommended human dose in mg/m^2.

The use of zolpidem tartrate in nursing mothers is not recommended.

PEDIATRIC USE

Safety and effectiveness in children below the age of 18 have not been established.

DRUG INTERACTIONS:

CNS-ACTIVE DRUGS

Zolpidem tartrate was evaluated in healthy volunteers in single-dose interaction studies for several CNS drugs. A study involving haloperidol and zolpidem revealed no effect of haloperidol on the pharmacokinetics or pharmacodynamics of zolpidem. Imipramine in combination with zolpidem produced no pharmacokinetic interaction other a 20% decrease in peak levels of imipramine, but there was an additive effect of decreased alertness. Similarly, chlorpromazine in combination with zolpidem produced no pharmacokinetic interaction, but there was an additive effect of decreased alertness and psychomotor performance. The lack of a drug interaction following single-dose administration does not predict a lack following chronic administration.

An additive effect on psychomotor performance between alcohol and zolpidem was demonstrated.

Since the systemic evaluation of zolpidem tartrate in combination with other CNS-active drugs have been limited, careful consideration should be given to the pharmacology of any CNS-active drug to be used with zolpidem. Any drug with CNS-depressant effects could potentially enhance the CNS- depressant effects of zolpidem.

OTHER DRUGS

A study involving cimetidine/zolpidem and ranitidine/zolpidem combinations revealed no effect of either drug on the pharmacokinetics or pharmacodynamics of zolpidem. Zolpidem had no effect on digoxin kinetics and did not effect prothrombin time when given with warfarin in normal subjects. Zolpidem's sedative/hypnotic effect was reversed by flumazenil; however, no significant alterations in zolpidem pharmacokinetics were found.

ADVERSE REACTIONS:

ASSOCIATED WITH DISCONTINUATION OF TREATMENT

Approximately 4% of 1,701 patients who received zolpidem at all doses (1.25 to 90 mg) in U.S. pre-marketing clinical trial discontinued treatment because of an adverse clinical event. Events most commonly associated with discontinuation from U.S. trials were daytime drowsiness (0.5%), dizziness (0.4%), headache (0.5%), nausea (0.6%), and vomiting (0.5%).

Approximately 6% of 1,320 patients who received zolpidem at all doses (5 to 50 mg) in similar foreign trials discontinued treatment because of an adverse event. Events most commonly associated with discontinuation from these trials were daytime drowsiness (1.6%), amnesia (0.6%), dizziness (0.6%), headache (0.6%), nausea (0.6%).

INCIDENCE IN CONTROLLED CLINICAL TRIALS

Most Commonly Observed Adverse Events In Controlled Trials: During short-term treatment (up to 10 nights) with zolpidem tartrate at doses up to 10 mg, the most commonly observed adverse events associated with the use of zolpidem and seen at statistically significant differences from placebo-treated patients were drowsiness (reported by 2% of zolpidem patients), dizziness (1%), and diarrhea(1%). During longer- term treatment (28 to 35 nights) with zolpidem at doses up to 10 mg, the most commonly observed adverse events associated with the use of zolpidem and seen at statistically significant differences from placebo-treated patients were dizziness (5%) and drugged feelings (3%).

Adverse Events Observed At An Incidence Of ≥ 1% In Controlled Trials: TABLE 1 and TABLE 2 enumerate treatment-emergent adverse event frequencies that were observed at an incidence equal to 1% or greater among patients with insomnia who received zolpidem tartrate in U.S. placebo-controlled trials. Events reported by investigators were classified

SUPPLIER PROFILES

1st Texas *see* Scherer

3M Pharms *NDC Code:* **00089**
3M Phamaceuticals Inc. **612-733-1110**
Bldg. 275-3W-01 3M Center **800-423-5146**
St. Paul, MN 55144-1000
Medical Product Sales Volume: $250,000,000
Total Employees: 1,000
Ownership: 3M *FAX:* 612-733-3451
Distribution: Manufacturer of Branded Pharmaceuticals
CEO: L.D. DeSimone/Chairman & CEO
W. George Meredith/Group VP
Harry Hammerly/EVP
Marketing: John Sampson/Marketing Director
Gary Cann/National Sales Manager
Mike Downing/Business Development
Production: James Vaughan/Plant Administration
Research: Joan K Backhaus/Advance Regulatory Officer
Bert Slade/Clinical Research Director
Bob Nelson/Global Technical Director
Florence Wong/Regulatory Affairs Manager
Ray Steffen/Medical Services Spclst
Federal Procurement Eligibility: Medicaid Rebate

999 Pharm *NDC Code:* **A00211**
999 Pharmaceutical Co.
Beijing, CHINA
Medical Product Sales Volume: $300,000,000
Total Employees: 6,000
Ownership: Public
Distribution: Manufacturer of Pharmaceuticals
CEO: Zhao Xinxian/Chairman

Abana Pharms *NDC Code:* **12463**
Abana Pharmaceuticals. Inc. **205-988-4588**
P.O. Box 360388 **800-828-1969**
Birmingham, AL 35236
Total Employees: 50
Ownership: PRIVATE *FAX:* 205-988-3294
Distribution: Distributor of Branded Pharmaceuticals
CEO: Dale E. Eads/President
Perry N. Cole/VP - Executive VP
Marketing: John W. Fuqua/VP Sales and Marketing
Federal Procurement Eligibility: Medicaid Rebate

Abbott *NDC Code:* **00074**
Abbott Laboratories **847-937-6100**
100 Abbott Park Road **800-633-9110**
Abbott Park, IL 60064-3500
Medical Product Sales Volume: $11,013,500,000
Total Employees: 52,817
Ownership: Public *FAX:* 847-937-1511
Distribution: Manufacturer of Branded Pharmaceuticals
CEO: Duane L. Burnham/Chairman & CEO
Gary P. Coughlan/CFO
Thomas R. Hodgson/President & COO
Paul N. Clark/Pres Pharmaceutical Div.
John C. Kane/SVP Ross Products
David A. Thompson/SVP Diagnostics
John G. Kringel/SVP Hospital Products
J. Duncan McIntyre/SVP International Operations
Robert L. Parkinson, Jr./VP European Operations
Ellen M. Walvoord/Human Resources
Marketing: Deryk David/Dir Prof. Communications
Susan Sherwood/Creative Services
Mark Trudeau/Product Mgr BIAXIN
Ron Lloyd/Product Mgr HYTRIN
Production: Joseph S. Jenckes/VP Washington, D.C.
Don G. Wright/VP Corp. Quality & Reg. Affairs
Research: Andre Pernet/Dir Worldwide Pharm Devel
Donald C Buell/Director Healthcare
Rose Feder/Mgr Medical Information Sys Dvlpmnt
James C Lierman/Dir Market Development
John D Opem/Mgr Abbott Information Services
Michael S Perlman/Sr Information Manager
Gregory G Pugh/Mgr Data Management
Joaquin M Valdes/Assoc Medical Director
Federal Procurement Eligibility: Medicaid Rebate

Able Labs *NDC Code:* **53265**
Able Labs **908-754-2253**
6 Hollywood Court
South Plainfield, NJ 07080
Medical Product Sales Volume: $17,000,000
Total Employees: 170
Ownership: AL Labs
Distribution: Manufacturer of Generic Suppositories
CEO: Robert A. Pudlak/SVP Finance & Administration
Production: Mark M. Fenton/VP Regulatory and Technical Affairs
Robert S. Mills/VPOperations
Federal Procurement Eligibility: Medicaid Rebate

Acme United *NDC Code:* **00924**
Acme United Corp
75 Kings Highway Cutoff
Fairfield, CT 06430
Ownership: PRIVATE

Adria *see* Pharmacia & Upjohn

Adv Remedies *NDC Code:* **57685**
Advanced Remedies, Inc. **201-386-5566**
72-6 Veronica Ave. **800-922-0547**
Sommerset, NJ 08873
Ownership: Sidmak Labs *FAX:* 201-386-9280
Distribution: Manufacturer of Ophthalmic Generics

Advance Bio *NDC Code:* **00518**
Advance Biofactures Corp
35 Wilbur Street
Lynbrook, NY 11563
Ownership: PRIVATE

Advanced Nutritional *NDC Code:* **10888**
Advanced Nutritional Technology, Inc.
6988 Sierra Court **800-624-6543**
Dublin, CA 94568
Ownership: PRIVATE
Distribution: Manufacturer of OTC's

AF Hauser *NDC Code:* **52637**
A.F. Hauser Co., Inc. **219-464-2309**
4401 East U.S. Hwy #30
Valparaiso, IN 46383
Total Employees: 10
Ownership: PRIVATE *FAX:* 219-464-8035
Distribution: Distributor of Branded, Generic, and Topical Pharmaceuticals
CEO: Allen F. Hauser/President and CEO
Leora Hauser/VP, Secretary & Treasurer
Janet Hauser/VP
Marketing: Dave Hauser/VP, Director of Sales and Purchasing

Affymax *see* Glaxo Wellcome

Agouron Pharm *NDC Code:* **63010**
Agouron Pharmaceuticals, Inc. **619-622-3000**
10350 North Torrey Pines Rd. **800-585-6050**
La Jolla, CA 92037-1020
Total Employees: 358
Ownership: Public *FAX:* 800-585-6052
Distribution: Pharmaceutical company specializing in drug design
CEO: Peter Johnson/President & CEO
Steven S. Cowell/VP of Finance & CFO
R. Kent Snyder/VP of Business Development
Gary E. Friedman/VP & General Counsel
Donna Nichols/Dir, Corporate Communications
Marketing: Geoff Altman/Dir Mktg & Sales
Bill Denby/Dir Mktg Managed Care
Research: Barry D. Quart, Pharm.D./VP, Regulatory Affairs
Robert C. Jackson, PhD/VP of Research & Development
Neil J. Clendeninn MD, PhD./VP Clinical Affairs

AH Robins *see* Elkins Sinn

AH Robins *NDC Code:* **00031**
A.H. Robins Company, Inc. **610-688-4400**
555 E. Lancaster Avenue
Saint Davids, PA 19087
Total Employees: 1,322
Ownership: Wyeth Ayerst
Distribution: Manufacturer of Branded Pharmaceuticals
Research: Emily Morley/Director Regulatory Affrs
Federal Procurement Eligibility: Medicaid Rebate
Medical Product Subsidiaries (Listed Separately):
Elkins-Sinn

AJ Bart *NDC Code:* **49326**
A. J. Bart Inc.
Box 813
Gurabo, PR 00778
Ownership: PRIVATE
Medical Product Subsidiaries (Listed Separately):
Laboratorios PR

Akorn *NDC Code:* **17478**
Akorn, Inc. **847-236-3800**
150 South Wyckles Road **800-535-7155**
Decatur, IL 62522
Medical Product Sales Volume: $35,000,000
Total Employees: 300
Ownership: Public *FAX:* 847-236-3823
Distribution: Manufacturer of Generic Ophthalmics
CEO: John N. Kapoor/Chairman
Joseph A. Yazbeck/Founder
Barry D. LeBlanc/President
Harold Koch/Senior Vice President
Marketing: Craig V. Smith/Vice President, Sales
Federal Procurement Eligibility: Medicaid Rebate

Alba Pharma *NDC Code:* **10023**
Alba Pharmacal Corporation
P.O. Box 813
Gurabo, PR 00778
Ownership: PRIVATE

Alcon *NDC Code:* **00065**
Alcon Laboratories, Inc. **817-293-0450**
6201 South Freeway
Fort Worth, TX 76134
Medical Product Sales Volume: $200,000,000
Total Employees: 2,500
Ownership: Nestle *FAX:* 817-551-4630
Distribution: Manufacturer of Branded Ophthalmologicals
CEO: Edgar H. Schollmaier/President & C.E.O.
T.R.G. Sear/Executive VP
Richard H. Sisson/Executive VP
Marketing: Blaise McGoey/VP, General Manager Marketing
Production: Walter J. Klein/Director Manufacturing Operations
Bruce C. Rudy/VP Corp. Mfg. & Engineering
Research: Dr. Dilip Raval/SVP Research & Development
Robert W Brobst/Dir Data Administration
Edwin Dorsey/Director Analy R&D
Robert B Hackett/Director Toxicology
Kay M Harris/Mgr Regulatory Affairs
William H Hubregs/VP Corporate Reg Affairs
Sharon L Mcallister/Science Librarian
T.O. Mcdonald/Sr Dir Worldwide Clinical
Larry J Oliver/Mgr Quality Information Systems
Mary B Pencis/Assoc Dir Intl Reg Affair
Robert E Roehrs/Sr Dir Regulatory Affairs
Ronald J Trancik/Director Dermatology
Bill York/VP Research
Federal Procurement Eligibility: Medicaid Rebate
Medical Product Subsidiaries (Listed Separately):
Alcon-PR
Alcon Surgical

Alcon Surgical — *NDC Code:* **08065**
Alcon Surgical — **817-293-0450**
6201 South Freeway
Fort Worth, TX 76134
Total Employees: 91
Ownership: Alcon Labs — *FAX:* 817-551-4615
Distribution: Manufacturer of Branded Ophthalmologicals

Alcon-PR — *NDC Code:* **00998**
Alcon Puerto Rico, Inc. — **817-293-0450**
6201 South Freeway
Fort Worth, TX 76134
Total Employees: 250
Ownership: Alcon Labs
Distribution: Manufacturer of Branded Pharmaceuticals
Federal Procurement Eligibility: Medicaid Rebate

Aligen Independ — *NDC Code:* **00405**
Aligen Independent Laboratories, Inc. — **307-733-0570**
3510 North Lake Creek Dr.
Jackson, WY 83001
Total Employees: 15
Ownership: PRIVATE — *FAX:* 307-733-0572
Distribution: Distributor of Generics
CEO: Michael Simon/President
Marketing: Fred Morgan/Director of Marketing
Federal Procurement Eligibility: Medicaid Rebate

ALK — *NDC Code:* **53298**
ALK Laboratories Inc. — **203-877-4782**
27 Village Lane — **800-325-7354**
Wallingford, CT 06492-2426
Total Employees: 400
Ownership: PRIVATE
Distribution: Manufacturer of Allergen Products
Marketing: Judith Broggi/Proj Mgr
Production: Jack Shumway/Dir Reg Affairs
Medical Product Subsidiaries (Listed Separately):
Berkeley Biolog

Allen & Hanburys *see* Glaxo Wellcome

Allergan — *NDC Code:* **00023**
Allergan Inc. — **714-752-4500**
2525 DuPont Drive — **800-347-4500**
Irvine, CA 92623-9534
Medical Product Sales Volume: $884,000,000
Total Employees: 5,160
Ownership: Public — *FAX:* 714-246-4217
Distribution: Manufacturer of Branded Ophthalmologicals
CEO: Gavin S. Herbert/Chairman
Willaim C. Shepard/President & CEO
Richard M. Haugen/EVP and COO
Vicente Anido, Jr.,PhD/Pres, Americas Region & Corp VP
Warren B. Brainard/SVP, Pan-Asia Region
Michael J. Donohoe/Corp. VP & Pres, Europe
Jeffrey B. D'Eliscu/Corp. VP, Corp. Communicat.
Bert Moyer/Corp VP & CFO
Marketing: Mike Ball/SVP, US Mktg
Production: Jackie J. Schiavo/SVP Worldwide Operations
Research: Lester J. Kaplan, PhD/Corp. VP Pharm. R&D
Richard C Courtney/Dir Clinical Research
Judith M Leon/Manager Clinical Research
Margaret Murray/Director Project Mgmt
Robin L Nelson/Dir, Research Compliance
Federal Procurement Eligibility: Medicaid Rebate
Medical Product Subsidiaries (Listed Separately):
Allergan Med
Pacific Pharma

Allergan-Amer — *NDC Code:* **11980**
Allergan America — **714-951-0455**
2525 DuPont Drive
Irvine, CA 92623
Ownership: Allergan — *FAX:* 714-380-4056
Distribution: Manufacturer of Branded Ophthalmics
CEO: W. Richard Ulmer/President
Marketing: Jim Largent/Director of Marketing
Russ Trenary/Director In-Line Market Planning
Kay Ford/Group Marketing Manager
Steve Guida/VP Worldwide Marketing
Lloyd Malchow/Director of National Sales
Production: John Hendrick/VP Manufacturing
Federal Procurement Eligibility: Medicaid Rebate

Alliance Pharm — *NDC Code:* **59449**
Alliance Pharmaceutical Inc. — **619-558-4300**
P.O. Box 429
Richmond, TX 74406-0429
Total Employees: 200
Ownership: Public
Distribution: Manufacturer of Imaging Agents

Allscrips Pharm — *NDC Code:* **54569**
Allscrips Pharmaceuticals Inc. — **847-680-3515**
1033 Butterfield Road — **800-654-0889**
Vernon Hills, IL 60061-1360
Total Employees: 170
Ownership: PRIVATE
Distribution: Distributor for In-Office Physician Dispensing
CEO: Michael E. Cahr
Marketing: Cindy Green/Dir, Marketing
Production: Brian Ward/VP of Pharmacy Services

Alpha Therapeutic — *NDC Code:* **49669**
Alpha Therapeutic Corp. — **213-225-2221**
5555 Valley Boulevard — **800-421-0008**
Los Angeles, CA 90032
Medical Product Sales Volume: $400,000,000
Total Employees: 2,600
Ownership: Green Cross — *FAX:* 213-227-9053
Distribution: Manufacturer of Blood Products

Alpha Therapeutic *(cont'd)*
CEO: H. Edward Matveld/President & Chairman
Marketing: Pete DeHart/Senior VP Sales & Marketing
Carolyn Siegal/VP Business Development
Dennis Flanaghan/Director of Sales
Production: Willi Zuniga/SVP, Manufacturing Operations
Research: William Craig, PhD/VP, Research and Development
Jonathan Goldsmith, MD/VP, Clinical Affairs, Medical Director
Federal Procurement Eligibility: Medicaid Rebate

Alphagen Labs — *NDC Code:* **59743**
Alphagen Laboratories Inc. — **770-475-8973**
11525 N. Fulton Industrial Blvd.
Alpharetta, GA 30201
Total Employees: 6
Ownership: PRIVATE — *FAX:* 770-751-1792
Distribution: Specialty Distributor
CEO: Daniel C. Hauck/Pres
Federal Procurement Eligibility: Medicaid Rebate

Alpharma — *NDC Code:* **00472**
Alpharma U.S. Pharmaceuticals Division — **410-298-1000**
333 Cassell Dr., Ste 3500 — **800-638-9096**
Baltimore, MD 21244
Total Employees: 850
Ownership: PRIVATE — *FAX:* 410-298-6343
Distribution: Manufacturer of Liquid Generics
CEO: Thomas L. Anderson/President
James J. Pappas/VP Finance
Marketing: Ben Maizel/VP Sales & Marketing
Jeannie Dunk/Contract Manager
Production: Arnold O. Lawing/VP Operations
William C. Clements/V.P Quality Affairs
Research: Stanley A. Kaplan, PhD/SVP R&D, Reg. Affairs
Federal Procurement Eligibility: Medicaid Rebate

Alra Labs — *NDC Code:* **51641**
Alra Laboratories, Inc. — **708-244-9440**
3850 Clearview Count — **800-248-2572**
Gurnee, IL 60031
Total Employees: 75
Ownership: PRIVATE — *FAX:* 708-244-9464
Distribution: Manufacturer of Generics
CEO: Dr. Raj Bhutani/President
Marketing: Jane Manarik/P.R.
Production: George Mocogni/Controller
Federal Procurement Eligibility: Medicaid Rebate

Altaire Pharm — *NDC Code:* **59390**
Altaire Pharmaceuticals Inc.
Ownership: PRIVATE
Federal Procurement Eligibility: Medicaid Rebate

Altana — *NDC Code:* **25463**
Altana, Inc.
60 Baylis Road
Melville, NY 11747
Medical Product Sales Volume: $200,000,000
Total Employees: 9,214
Ownership: Public
Distribution: Manufacturer of Pharmaceuticals
Medical Product Subsidiaries (Listed Separately):
Fougera
Pharmaderm
Savage Labs

Altana Inc *see* Fougera

Alza — *NDC Code:* **17314**
Alza Corporation — **415-494-5000**
950 Page Mill Road, P.O. Box 10950 — **800-233-5222**
Palo Alto, CA 94303-0802
Medical Product Sales Volume: $34,000,000
Total Employees: 1,071
Ownership: Public/Ciba Geigy AG — *FAX:* 415-494-5121
Distribution: Manufacturer of Controlled-Release Products
CEO: Dr. Alejandro Zaffaroni/Co-Chairman
Ernest Mario/Co-Chairman & CEO
Harold Fethe/VP, Human Resources
David R. Hoffman/VP, Treasurer
Peter Staple/VP, General Counsel
Marketing: Jim Butler/VP, Sales & Marketing
John Satler/Manager, Sales Services
Production: Dr. Gary V. Fulscher/SVP, Operations
Michael Paulik/VP, Operations
Research: Samuel Saks, MD/SVP, Medical Affairs
Dr. Felix Theeuwes/President, Alza Research & Development / Chief Scientist
Marilou S. Cramer/Dir, Clinical Sciences
Mary E. Prevo/VP, Environmental Product Safety
Janne Wissel/VP, Regulatory Affairs / Quality Management
Federal Procurement Eligibility: Medicaid Rebate
Medical Product Subsidiaries (Listed Separately):
Therapeutic Discovery

Am Generics — *NDC Code:* **58634**
American Generics Inc. — **518-725-1800**
34 West Fulton St.
Gloversville, NY 12078
Medical Product Sales Volume: $2,500,000
Total Employees: 7
Ownership: PRIVATE — *FAX:* 518-725-1869
Distribution: Distributor of Generics/Brand drugs
CEO: Dr. V. Ravi Chandran/President & CEO
Marketing: Ali Novin
Production: Mohammed Nuralam
Research: Steven Kinne

Am Pharms — *NDC Code:* **58605**
America Pharmaceuticals, Inc. — **205-942-6415**
120 Summit Parkway/Suite 101
Birmingham, AL 35209
Ownership: PRIVATE
Distribution: Distributor of Pharmaceuticals
Marketing: Mary Ann Ortegas

Am Red Cross — *NDC Code:* **52769**
American Red Cross Blood Services — **202-737-8300**
1616 North Fort Myer Dr.
Rosslyn, VA 22209
Ownership: PRIVATE
CEO: Fred Katz/Sr. Medical Director
Federal Procurement Eligibility: Medicaid Rebate

Am Regent — *NDC Code:* **00517**
American Regent Inc. — **516-924-4000**
1 Luitpold Drive
Shirley, NY 11967
Total Employees: 300
Ownership: Luitpold Pharm — *FAX:* 516-924-1731
Distribution: Manufacturer of Generics
CEO: Raif Lange
Marketing: Mary Jane Helenek
Production: Fred Pratt
Research: Dr. Chin Wu
Federal Procurement Eligibility: Medicaid Rebate

Amend Drug Chem — *NDC Code:* **17317**
Amend Drug & Chemical Company — **201-926-0333**
83 Cordier St.
Irvington, NJ 07111
Total Employees: 11
Ownership: PRIVATE
Distribution: Distributor of Powder Forms of Generics

Amer Preferred — *NDC Code:* **53445**
American Preferred Pharmaceutical, Inc. — **501-661-5557**
P.O. Box 23007
Little Rock, AR 72221
Ownership: PRIVATE
Federal Procurement Eligibility: Medicaid Rebate

Amer Urologicals — *NDC Code:* **00539**
American Urologicals, Inc. — **305-962-2900**
7881 Hollywood Blvd., Suite 4
Pembroke Pines, FL 33024
Total Employees: 2
Ownership: PRIVATE
Distribution: Specialty Distributor
CEO: Marvin Lund/President
Federal Procurement Eligibility: Medicaid Rebate

Americal Pharm — *NDC Code:* **54945**
Americal Pharmaceuticals, Inc. — **714-579-7545**
1340 N. Jefferson St.
Anaheim, CA 92807
Total Employees: 50
Ownership: Akorn
Distribution: Specialty Manufacturer

American Cyanamid — *NDC Code:* **P00005**
American Cyanamid Company — **201-831-2000**
One Cyanamid Plaza
Wayne, NJ 07470
Medical Product Sales Volume: $2,870,000,000
Total Employees: 26,550 — *Telex:* 219136-ACYIN UR
Ownership: American Home Products — *FAX:* 201-831-3151
CEO: Albert J. Costello/Chairman
Frank W. Atlee/President
David Bethune/Group VP Medical
Jeff Hoyak/Dir Public Affairs
Marketing: George J. Vuturo, PhD/VP Industry Affairs, Lederle
Ken Pitzer/Product Mgr VERElan
John Gargiulo/Product Mgr SUPRAX
Kevin Poulos/Product Mgr ZOSYN
Michael J. Paradiso/Product Mgr TETRAMUNE
Richard Johnson/Product Mgr ZIAC
Research: Charles Homey, MD/President, Medical Research Div.
Joseph L Dabronzo/Assist Dir Intl Drug Srv
Loretta L Dente/Drug Surveillance Coord
Kristen Palmer/Medical Information Assoc
Beverly A Wallo/Sr Data Coordinator
Medical Product Subsidiaries (Listed Separately):
Immunex
Lederle Labs
Lederle Parenterals
Lederle Piperacillin
Lederle-Praxis
Storz

American Home Prod — *NDC Code:* **P00008**
American Home Products Corporation — **201-660-5000**
Five Giralda Farm
Madison, NJ 07940
Medical Product Sales Volume: $14,088,300,000
Total Employees: 59,747
Ownership: Public — *FAX:* 201-660-5771
Distribution: Manufacturer of Drugs and Specialty Foods
CEO: John R. Stafford/Chariman & CEO
Bernard Canavan, MD/President
Robert G. Blount/CFO
Stanley F. Barshay/SVP
Joseph R. Bock/SVP
Louis L. Hoynes,Jr./SVP & General Counsel
John L. Skule/VP Corporate Affairs
Fred Hassan/Group VP Pharmaceuticals
Rene R. Lewin/Human Resources
Medical Product Subsidiaries (Listed Separately):
American Cyanamid

American Home Prod *(cont'd)*
Ayerst Labs
Elkins-Sinn
Genetics Institute
AH Robins
Whitehall
Wyeth-Ayerst

Amgen *NDC Code:* **55513**
Amgen
1840 Dehavilland Drive
Thousand Oaks, CA 91320-1789
805-447-1000
800-772-6436
Medical Product Sales Volume: $2,198,100,000
Total Employees: 4,646
Ownership: Public *FAX:* 805-447-1985
Distribution: Biotechnology Manufacturer
CEO: Gordon Binder/Chairman & CEO
Kevin W. Sharer/President
Robert S. Attiyeh/CFO
George Vandeman/SVP Sec. & Gen'l Counsel
Daryl Hill/SVP Asia-Pacific
Steven M. Odre/VP Intellectual Property
Robert Attiyeh/SVP Finance & Devel.
Edward F. Garnett/Human Resources
Marketing: Stan Benson/SVP Sales & Marketing
David Boyden/Manager, Neupogen Marketing
Craig L. Brooks/VP, Marketing
Michael Savin/Director, Mktg
Production: N. Kirby Alton/SVP, Therapeutic Product Development
Dennis Fenton/SVP, Operations
Linda Wudl/VP, Quality Assurance
Research: Daniel Vapnek/SVP Research
Bruce W. Altrock/VP Biology and Biochemistry
George Morstyn/VP ,Clinical Devel.
Lawrence M. Souza/VP ,Exploratory Research
Art Cohen, PhD/Director of Pharmacology
J Marion Anderson/Mgr, CRA Development
Peter Armerding/Manager, Information Technology
Diane M Ascoli/Manager, Clinical Data
Moraye B Bear/Manager, Biostatics
Sandy Garofolo/Manager, Professional Serv
Michael R Downing/Sr Dir, Product Development
Ronald P Evens/Dir, Professional Services
Alan B Forsythe/Dir, Corporate Biomedical Information
Sarah Swanson/Regulatory Affairs Associate Dir
Rachel A. Wagner/Publishing Manager
Federal Procurement Eligibility: Medicaid Rebate
Medical Product Subsidiaries (Listed Separately):
Kirin-Amgen
Synergen

Amid *NDC Code:* **00493**
Amid Laboratories, Inc.
P.O. Box 1024
Oxford, MS 38655
Ownership: PRIVATE

Amide Pharm *NDC Code:* **52152**
Amide Pharmaceuticals, Inc.
101 East Main Street
Little Falls, NJ 07424
201-890-1440
Total Employees: 25
Ownership: PRIVATE
Federal Procurement Eligibility: Medicaid Rebate

Ampharco *NDC Code:* **59015**
AmPharco Inc.
9549a Bolsa Ave.
Westminster, CA 92683
714-531-3560
Total Employees: 9
Ownership: PRIVATE
Distribution: Importer

Anabolic *NDC Code:* **00722**
Anabolic Inc.
17802 Gillette
Irvine, CA 92614
Ownership: PRIVATE
Distribution: Distributor/Manufacturer of Generics

Anaquest *see* Ohmeda Pharm

Anesta *see* BTG Pharms

Apex *see* Gensia Labs

Apotex *NDC Code:* **60505**
Apotex Inc.
150 Signet Dr.
Weston, ON M9L 1T9, CANADA
416-749-9300
800-268-0599
Medical Product Sales Volume: $185,000,000
Total Employees: 500
Ownership: PRIVATE *FAX:* 416-749-9578
Distribution: Distributor/Manufacturer of Generics
CEO: Bernard Sherman/Chairman
Medical Product Subsidiaries (Listed Separately):
Yorpharm

Apotheca *NDC Code:* **12634**
Apotheca Inc.
1622 North 16th Street
Phoenix, AZ 85006
Ownership: PRIVATE

Apothecon *NDC Code:* **00003, 59772, 62269**
Apothecon Inc. Div. Bristol-Myers Squibb
777 Scudders Mill Road
Plainsburo, NJ 08536
609-243-6000
800-321-1335
Medical Product Sales Volume: $500,000,000

Apothecon *(cont'd)*
Total Employees: 4,000
Ownership: Bristol-Myers Squibb *FAX:* 609-243-6973
Distribution: Manufacturer of Generics
Federal Procurement Eligibility: Medicaid Rebate

Arco Pharms *NDC Code:* **00275**
Arco Pharmaceuticals, Inc.
105 Orville Drive
Bohemia, NY 11716
516-567-9500
Ownership: Nature's Bounty *FAX:* 516-563-1623
CEO: Arthur Rudolph/Chairman of the Board
Harvey Kamil/Executive VP
Marketing: Barry Drucker/Senior VP of Sales
Production: James Taylor/VP Production
Abe Kleinman/VP Manufacturing

Arcola *NDC Code:* **00070**
Arcola Laboratories
P.O. Box 5092
Collegeville, PA 19426-0107
215-454-8000
800-727-6737
Ownership: Rhone-Poulenc Rorer *FAX:* 609-395-1147

Areo All-Gas,TH *NDC Code:* **10014**
Aero All Gas Co.
3150 Main St.
Hartford, CT 06120
Ownership: PRIVATE

Ares-Serono *NDC Code:* **P44087**
Ares-Serono Group
15B Chemin des Mines
Geneva CH-1211, SWITZERLAND
022-764431
Medical Product Sales Volume: $855,000,000
Total Employees: 3,658
Ownership: Public
Distribution: Manufacturer of Branded Pharmaceuticals
CEO: Fabio Bertarelli/CEO
Ernesto Bertarelli/Deputy CEO
Research: Kamel Besseghir/Mgr Drug Surveillance
Jean-Yves Le Cotonnec/Corp Dir-Clin Pharm/Safe
Gerard Farmer
Andrew Galazka/Corporate Clinical Dir Resch
Madeleine Rouiller/Regulatory Affairs Mgr
Medical Product Subsidiaries (Listed Separately):
Interpharm Labs
Serono Labs

Armstrong Pharm *NDC Code:* **A00050**
Armstrong Pharmaceuticals, Inc.
76 Elm Street
New Canaan, CT 06840
203-966-4170
Medical Product Sales Volume: $13,908,000
Total Employees: 140
Ownership: Medeva plc *FAX:* 203-966-4763
Distribution: OEM Supplier of Inhalers
CEO: H.R. Shepherd/Chairman & CEO
Harvey Mintzer/President
Augustine Lawlor/VP, CFO & SEC
Benjamin Shepard/E.V.P

Arzol Chem *NDC Code:* **12870**
Arzol Chemical
208 Benton Road, P.O. Box 91
North Haverhill, NH 03774
603
Medical Product Sales Volume: $282,000
Total Employees: 5
Ownership: PRIVATE *FAX:* 603-787-6889
Distribution: Wholesale
CEO: Stanley C. Hartell
Marketing: Donna Hartell/Assistant Manager

Ascher *NDC Code:* **00225**
B.F. Ascher & Company, Inc.
15501 West 109th Street
Lenexa, KS 66219
913-888-1880
Total Employees: 85
Ownership: PRIVATE *FAX:* 913-888-2250
Distribution: Specialty Manufacturer
CEO: James J. Ascher/President
C. Steven Bennett/Controller
Marketing: James J. Ascher, Jr./Dir of Mktg
Research: Charles H. Borchers/Dir Scientific & Legal Aff.
Federal Procurement Eligibility: Medicaid Rebate

Astra Merck *NDC Code:* **61113**
Astra/Merck Group of Merck & Company
725 Chesterbrook Blvd.
Wayne, PA 19087-5677
Medical Product Sales Volume: $1,000,000,000
Total Employees: 900
Ownership: Merck/Astra
Distribution: Manufacturer of Branded Pharmaceuticals

Astra USA *NDC Code:* **00186**
Astra USA, Inc.
50 Otis Street
Westborough, MA 01581-4500
508-366-1100
800-225-6333
Medical Product Sales Volume: $350,000,000
Total Employees: 1,200 *Telex:* 6810105
Ownership: Astra AB *FAX:* 508-366-7406
Distribution: Manufacturer of Branded Pharmaceuticals
CEO: Mats Nilsson/Chairman
Jan Larson/President
Marketing: Andrew Heath/Vice President
Bill Albrect/Product Mgr TOPROL
David Segar/Dir Sales Adm.
Production: William Harnett/Vice President, Operations
Research: Gerard Boyce/Vice President, Research
Leslie Williams, D.V.M./Assoc Dir, Product Safety
William Gray, Jr., MD/Sr. Dir, Medical Services
David J. Pizzi/Mgr, Drug Regulatory Affairs

Astra USA *(cont'd)*
Mary E. Rice/Mgr, Medical Information
Federal Procurement Eligibility: Medicaid Rebate

Athena *NDC Code:* **59075**
Athena Neurosciences Inc.
800 Gateway Blvd.
S. San Francisco, CA 94080
415-877-0900
Medical Product Sales Volume: $28,000,000
Total Employees: 330
Ownership: Public *FAX:* 415-877-8370
Distribution: Branded Pharmaceuticals and Biotech Development Company
CEO: John Groom/President & CEO
Morgan L. Beatty, PhD/Vice President, Technical Operations
Lisabeth F. Murphy/Vice President, Legal Affairs, General Counsel, and Secretary
Jan D. Wallace, MD/Vice President, Clinical and Regulatory Affairs
Kevin R. Davidge/Vice President, Finance
Marketing: Micheal D. Coffee/Vice President, Sales & Marketing
Research: Paulette E. Setler, PhD/Senior Vice President, Corporate Development and Chief Scientific Officer
Ivan M. Lieberburg, PhD/VP of Alzheimer's Research

Atley Pharms *NDC Code:* **59702**
Atley Pharmaceuticals
Rt. 2 Box 217B
Beaver Dam, VA 23015
804-550-1979
Total Employees: 17
Ownership: PRIVATE *FAX:* 804-550-1979
Distribution: Specialty Distributor
CEO: John Henry Attkisson/President
Blake Kelley/EVP
Elizabeth Attkisson/Secretary/Treasurer
Federal Procurement Eligibility: Medicaid Rebate

Ayerst *NDC Code:* **00046**
Ayerst Laboratories, Inc.
170 Rador Chester Rd.
Saint Davids, PA 19087
215-688-4400
800-950-5099
Ownership: Wyeth-Ayerst *FAX:* 215-688-2762
Distribution: Manufacturer of Branded Pharmaceuticals
CEO: Bernard Canavan, MD/Chairman
Fred Hassan/President
Marketing: Robert Essner/SVP Sales & Marketing
Jay Rachelli/Director Wyeth Marketing
Joseph Mahady/Director Ayerst Marketing
Frank Corcoran/Dir Marketing Plng. & New Products
Research: William N. Warden/Exec Dir Marketing Research & Plng.
Federal Procurement Eligibility: Medicaid Rebate

B F Ascher *see* Ascher

B-D *see* BD Microbiology

Bajamar Chem *NDC Code:* **44184**
Bajamar Chemical Co., Inc.
P.O. Box 12411
St. Louis, MO 63132
314-997-3414
Total Employees: 23
Ownership: PRIVATE *FAX:* 314-997-2948
Distribution: Specialty Manufacturer
CEO: Harvey Mizes/President
Marketing: Barry Mizes/VP Marketing
Federal Procurement Eligibility: Medicaid Rebate

Baker Cummins *see* Baker Norton Pharms

Baker Cummins Derm *NDC Code:* **58174**
Baker Cummins Dermatologicals, Inc.
8800 N.W. 36th Street
Miami, FL 33178
800-842-6704
Medical Product Sales Volume: $778,790
Total Employees: 55
Ownership: Baker Cummins *FAX:* 305-770-5035
Distribution: Manufacturer of Dermatologicals
CEO: Charles Hsiao, PhD/President
Marketing: Gary Draper/SVP Mktg & Sales
Production: Randy Glover/VP Miami Operations
Jane Hsiao, PhD/Chief Regulatory Officer
Research: John Whisnant, MD/SVP Research & Development

Baker Norton Pharms *NDC Code:* **00575**
Baker Norton Pharmaceuticals, Inc.
DBA Baker Cummins Dermatolo
4400 Biscayne Blvd.
Miami, FL 33137
305-590-2200
800-347-4774
Medical Product Sales Volume: $56,724,056
Total Employees: 500
Ownership: Ivax *FAX:* 305-590-2252
Distribution: Manufacturer of Branded Pharmaceuticals
CEO: Philip Frost, MD/Chairman
Barry Strumwasser/President
Marketing: Gary Draper/SVP Marketing & Sales
Production: Randy Glover/VP Miami Ops
Research: John Whisnant, MD/SVP Research & Development
Federal Procurement Eligibility: Medicaid Rebate
Medical Product Subsidiaries (Listed Separately):
Baker Cummins Derm

Balan *NDC Code:* **00304**
J. J. Balan Inc.
5725 Forster Ave.
Brooklyn, NY 11234
718-251-8663
Total Employees: 5
Ownership: PRIVATE
Distribution: Distributor of Generics
Federal Procurement Eligibility: Medicaid Rebate
Medical Product Subsidiaries (Listed Separately):
Balan JJ

Barnes-Hind *see* Vision Pharms

Barr *NDC Code:* **00555**
Barr Laboratories, Inc. **914-362-1100**
2 Quaker Road **800-222-0190**
Pomona, NY 10970
Medical Product Sales Volume: $58,000,000
Total Employees: 270
Ownership: Public *FAX:* 914-353-3843
Distribution: Manufacturer & Distributor of Generics
CEO: Bruce Downey/Chairman of the Board, CEO & Pres
Gerald F. Price/EVP
Paul M. Bisaro/Chief Financial Officer & Gen'l Counsel
Charles Mayr/Dir of Corporate Communications
Catherine F. Higgins/VP Human Resources
Bruce Hooey/Chief Information Officer
Marketing: Timothy Catlett/VP Sales & Marketing
Charles Mayr/Dir of Corp. Communications
Production: Ezzeldin A. Hamza/SVP R&D
Mary Petit/VP Quality Control
Federal Procurement Eligibility: Medicaid Rebate

Barre *see* Alpharma

Barre-National *see* Alpharma

Barre-NMC *see* Alpharma

Bartor Pharcal *NDC Code:* **10116**
Bartor Pharmacal Co.
70 High St.
Rye, NY 10580
Ownership: PRIVATE
Distribution: Specialty Manufacturer

Basel *see* Novartis

BASF *NDC Code:* **A00129**
BASF Group **49-6 21 600**
Basf Aktiengesellschaft, 38 Carl-Boch-Strasse
Ludwigshafen D-6700, GERMANY
Medical Product Sales Volume: $1,310,000,000
Total Employees: 128,105
Ownership: Public *FAX:* 49-6 21 604 2525
Distribution: Manufacturer of Chemicals
CEO: Dr. Hans Albers/Chairman
Jurgen Strube/Group Chairman
J. Dieter Stein/Chairman North America
Medical Product Subsidiaries (Listed Separately):
Boots Pharm
Knoll Pharm

Baucom Labs *NDC Code:* **54696**
Baucom Labs
Ownership: PRIVATE

Bausch and Lomb *NDC Code:* **24208**
Bausch and Lomb Pharmaceuticals, Inc. **813-975-7775**
8500 Hidden River Pky. **800-227-1427**
Tampa, FL 33637-1014
Total Employees: 350
Ownership: Public *FAX:* 813-975-7757
Distribution: Manufacturer of Generic Ophthalmics
CEO: Daniel E. Gill/Chairman of the Board
Alan P. Dozier/President, Bausch & Lomb Pharm Div.
Marketing: Dave Jarosz/VP Mktg
Production: Tony Caracciolo/VP of Production
Federal Procurement Eligibility: Medicaid Rebate

Baxter Hlthcare *see* Fenwal Labs

Baxter Hlthcare *NDC Code:* **00338, 57234**
Baxter Healthcare Corp. **847-546-6311**
Rt 12 Rt 120 and Wilson Rd
Round Lake, IL 60073
Medical Product Sales Volume: $8,100,000,000
Total Employees: 61,300
Ownership: Public *FAX:* 847-270-4668
Distribution: Manufacturer/Distributor of Hospital Supplies
CEO: William B. Graham/Senior Chairman
Vernon R. Loucks Jr./Chairman & CEO
Arthur F. Staubitz/President
Harry M. Jansen Kraemer, Jr./SVP
Research: John Wesley/VP Medical Affairs
Sandra Coleman/Product Information
Steven Hoff/Reg Affairs, Mgr Renal Division
Richard Kandler/Assoc Dir Clinical Studies Fenwall Div
Marcia Marconi/VP, Regulatory Affairs
Harold E Sargent/Corporate Research and Technical Services
David Behrens/Mgr Computer Graphics and Information Management
Federal Procurement Eligibility: Medicaid Rebate
Medical Product Subsidiaries (Listed Separately):
Baxter Edwards
Baxter Hlthcare
Baxter Hyland
Baxter Pharm

Baxter Hyland *NDC Code:* **00944**
Hyland Therapeutics **818-956-3200**
550 N. Brand Avenue
Glendale, CA 91203
Ownership: Baxter Healthcare
Distribution: Manufacturer of Branded Pharmaceuticals
CEO: Carl Brooks/President
Anita Bessler/EVP Therapeutics
Marketing: Dr. Rene deVreker/Director New Product Planning
Norm Miller/Business Manager U.S. Sales
Production: John Bacich/VP Manufacturing Operations
Research: Henry S. Kingdon, MD/VP R&D, Med'l Dir
Teresa Habern/Intl Reg Affairs Assoc
Pamela Koo/Mgr, Reimbrsmnt Policy/Prog

Baxter Hyland *(cont'd)*
Susan Liu-Maruya/Clinical Project Manager
Federal Procurement Eligibility: Medicaid Rebate

Bayer *NDC Code:* **00026**
Bayer Corp Pharmaceutical Div **203-937-2000**
400 Morgan Lane
West Haven, CT 06516
Medical Product Sales Volume: $2,700,000,000
Total Employees: 1,600
Ownership: Bayer AG *FAX:* 203-934-8553
Distribution: Manufacturer of Branded Pharmaceuticals
CEO: Helge Wehmeier/CEO
Horst K. Wallrabe/President
Ralph M. Galustian/EVP
Marketing: Gerald B. Rosenberg/SVP, Marketing and Sales
R. James Lamb/VP, Sales
David Kelemen/Product Mgr ADALAT
Mark Hansen/Product Mgr CIPRO
Mary S. Marinaccio/Product Mgr TRASYLOL
Vincent Heidenreich/Mgr Advertising & Sales Promo.
Hank Osipa/Mgr Sales Training
Research: Lawrence E. Posner,MD/SVP, Medical Research
Arthur D. Edwards/Asst. Dir, Regulatory Affairs
Carl E Calcagni/Dir Regulatory Affairs
David Goldman/Dir Product Development
Allen H Heller/Dir Clinical Pharmacology
Kevin Higgins/Dir Professional Services
Marissa Seligman/Mgr Scientific Pblctns
Paula A Sonnino/Manager Information Services
Leslie Wilson/Mgr Socio-Econom Studies
Federal Procurement Eligibility: Medicaid Rebate
Medical Product Subsidiaries (Listed Separately):
Miles Allergy
Miles Cutter
Schein

Bayer AG *NDC Code:* **P00026**
Bayer AG **49-214-301**
Bayerwerk
51368 Leverkusen, GERMANY
Medical Product Sales Volume: $31,532,900,000
Total Employees: 142,200
Ownership: Public *FAX:* 49-214-308-11 46
Distribution: Manufacturer of Chemicals
CEO: Dr. Manfred Schneider/Chairman
Dr. H. Wunderlich/Dep. Chairman
Research: Gerd Aichinger/Regulatory Affairs Mgr
Jan Dycka/Head Statistical Dept
Wolfgang Ebsen/Regulatory Affairs
Margitta Feldsieper/Clin Qual Assur Officer
Reiner Frey/Clin Project Leader
Wolfram Hoffmann/Study Director Toxicology
Dietlind Kammacher/Regulatory Affairs
Uwe Keup/Hea Regulatory Affairs
Udo Klein/Head Regulatory Affairs
Reinhard Kobelt/Project Leader Clinical Rsch
Ursula Streicher-Saied/Head Reg Compliance Int'L
Kurt Troll/Head Of Marketing Service
Thomas R Weighrauch/Dir Head Intl Clinical R&D
Knut Zellerhoff/Head Proj Coordination
Medical Product Subsidiaries (Listed Separately):
Bayer Pharm
Miles

Bayer Pharm *NDC Code:* **00192**
Bayer Pharmaceuticals **203-937-2000**
400 West Morgan Lane
West Haven, CT 06516
Ownership: Bayer AG *FAX:* 203-934-8553
Distribution: Manufacturer of Branded Pharmaceuticals
Federal Procurement Eligibility: Medicaid Rebate

BD Microbiology *NDC Code:* **00011**
Becton Dickinson Microbiology Systems **410-771-0100**
250 Schilling Circle
Cockeysville, MD 21030
Medical Product Sales Volume: $10,000,000
Total Employees: 100
Ownership: Becton-Dickinson *FAX:* 410-584-7121
Distribution: Manufacturer of Branded Pharmaceuticals
CEO: Anthony Pasquarelli/President
Marketing: Joy Sussman/Manager Marketing Communications
Greg Wills/Director of Marketing
Ronald Spivey/Marketing Logistics Manager

Beach Pharms *NDC Code:* **00486**
Beach Pharmaceuticals, Division of Beach Products, Inc. **864-277-7282**
201 Delaware Street **800-845-8210**
Greenville, SC 29605
Ownership: PRIVATE *FAX:* 864-277-8045
CEO: Richard B. Jenkins/CEO
Richard Stephan Jenkins/VP
Marketing: Clete Harmon/Director of Q.A.
Federal Procurement Eligibility: Medicaid Rebate
Medical Product Subsidiaries (Listed Separately):
Pharm Associates

Becton Dickinson *NDC Code:* **08290**
Becton Dickinson & Company Inc.
9450 South State Street **800-526-4650**
Sandy, UT 84070
Medical Product Sales Volume: $2,260,000,000
Total Employees: 18,500
Ownership: Public
Distribution: Manufacturer of Laboratory & Medical Products
CEO: Wesley J. Howe/Chairman
Clateo Castellini/Sector President - Medical
Walter M. Miller/Sector President - Diagnostic
Alfred J. Battaglia/Group President
E. Ralph Biggadike/Group President

Becton Dickinson *(cont'd)*
Production: James W. Hulse/VP Quality & Regulatory Affairs
Thomas A. Reichert, MD/VP Medical Affairs
Research: Donald S. Hetzel/VP R&D
Medical Product Subsidiaries (Listed Separately):
Becton Dickinson

Bedford *NDC Code:* **10130**
Bedford Laboratories Div. Ben Venue Laboratories, Inc.
Ownership: PRIVATE

Bedford Labs *NDC Code:* **55390**
Bedford Laboratories **216-232-3320**
300 Northfield Road
Bedford, OH 44146
Total Employees: 10
Ownership: Benvenue Laboratories *FAX:* 216-232-2772
Distribution: Distributor of Generic Injectables

Beecham *NDC Code:* **00029**
Beecham Division Smithkline Beecham **615-764-5141**
1250 South Collegeville Rd.
Collegeville, PA 19426
Ownership: Smithkline Beecham
Distribution: Manufacturer of Branded Pharmaceuticals
Federal Procurement Eligibility: Medicaid Rebate

Bergen Brunswig *NDC Code:* **24385**
Bergen Brunswig Corp. **714-385-4000**
4000 Metropolitan Drive
Orange, CA 92668
Medical Product Sales Volume: $5,000,000,000
Total Employees: 3,700
Ownership: Public *FAX:* 714-385-1442
Distribution: Pharmaceutical Distributor
CEO: R.E. Martini/Chairman
Donald Roden/President & CEO
Neil Dimick/EVP & CFO
Philip Engle/President, Drug Operations
Marketing: Michael Quinn/EVP Sales & Marketing
Chris Fribourg/VP Merchandising & Promotion

Berlex Labs *NDC Code:* **50419**
Berlex Laboratories **201-694-4100**
300 Fairfield Road
Wayne, NJ 07470
Medical Product Sales Volume: $238,000,000
Total Employees: 800
Ownership: Schering AG *FAX:* 201-942-1610
Distribution: Manufacturer of Branded Pharmaceuticals & Imaging Agents
CEO: Jorge Raul Engel/President & CEO
Robert S. Cohen/EVP & COO
Dr. Alan D. Rudzik/EVP Research & Development
Marketing: Fred Scheel/Director Marketing Communications
Elise Klein/Dir Marketing Pharm. & Imaging
Robert E. Liptrot/Executive Director Sales
John Trombetta/Director, Market Research
Marilyn Bonito/Promotional Administrator
George Fortier/Product Mgr BETAPACE
Production: Dr. C.R. Willis, Jr./VP Operations
Research: Lorene Connolly/Mgr Library Services
James T Crowe/Head Drug Devel Systems
Michael Flashner/Director Pharm Proj Dev
Lawrence M Gifford/Dir Medical Affairs
Peter Hinderling/Dir Clinical Pharmacology
Federal Procurement Eligibility: Medicaid Rebate

Berna Prod *NDC Code:* **58337**
Berna Products Corp. **305-443-2900**
4216 Ponce De Leon Blvd. **800-533-5899**
Coral Gables, FL 33146
Total Employees: 9
Ownership: PRIVATE
Distribution: Distributor of Vaccines
CEO: Andres Murai Jr./President
Marketing: Mike O'Neal/Regional Sales Mgr
Wallis Quayle/Regional Sales Mgr
Production: Dr. S.J. Cryz, Jr./Director of
Research: Dr. S.J. Cryz, Jr./Director of

Best Generics *see* Goldline Labs

Beta Derma *NDC Code:* **53062**
Beta Dermaceuticals, Inc. **210-349-9326**
P.O. Box 691106
San Antonio, TX 78269-1106
Medical Product Sales Volume: $466,263
Total Employees: 8
Ownership: PRIVATE *FAX:* 210-349-9363
Distribution: Manufacturer of Dermatologics
CEO: Henry Rangel/President
Production: W. Dewitt Moore
Federal Procurement Eligibility: Medicaid Rebate

Bio Pharm *NDC Code:* **59741**
Bio Pharm, Inc. **215-949-3711**
10 H Runway Rd.
Levitown, PA 19057
Total Employees: 5
Ownership: PRIVATE
Distribution: Specialty Distributor
Federal Procurement Eligibility: Medicaid Rebate

Bio Tech Gen *see* BTG Pharms

Bio-Pharm *NDC Code:* **A00196**
Bio-Pharm Clinical Services, Inc. **215-283-0770**
4 Valley Square, 512 Township Line Rd.
Blue Bell, PA 19422
Total Employees: 470
Ownership: PRIVATE *FAX:* 215-283-0733
Distribution: Contract Research
CEO: John Cullen, J.D./COO
Stuart J. Hamill, PhD/President
Gerri Henwood, PhD/President & CEO
Marketing: Charlene Richter
Production: Kathleen Krakauer, PhD/Dir Clinical Writing
Barbara Schryver, PhD/Director Clinical Writing
Laura Webb/Director, Clinical Writing
Lilliam Kingsbury, PhD/VP Biostatistics
Charles Gombar, MD/VP Clinical Monitoring
Gerri Henwood/President & CEO
Spencer Hudson/Senior Biostatistician
Barbara T Nagle/VP Training
Dorothy McGill/VP Medical Affairs
Lori Ferris/VP Clinical Data Coordination
Steve Boccardo/VP Information Systems
Steve Preiss/VP Programming
John Santoro/VP Data Management
Ted M Smith/VP Pharmacoeconomics
Research: Joe Tempio

Bio-Tech Pharm *NDC Code:* **53191**
Bio-Tech Pharmacal, Inc. **501-443-9148**
P.O. Box 1992 **800-345-1199**
Fayetteville, AR 72702
Ownership: PRIVATE *FAX:* 501-443-5643

Biocraft *see* Teva

Biogen *NDC Code:* **59627**
Biogen Inc. **617-252-9200**
14 Cambridge Center
Cambridge, MA 02142
Medical Product Sales Volume: $149,300,000
Total Employees: 900
Ownership: Public *FAX:* 617-864-8900
Distribution: Biotech Development Company (License Intron A & Hepatitis B Vac.)
CEO: James L. Vincent/Chairman & CEO
James R. Tobin/President
Micheal J. Astrue/VP, General Counsel
Marketing: Kenneth M. Bake/VP Mktg & Sales
Production: Dr. Irwin D. Smith/VP Development Operations
James C. Mullen/VP, Operations
Michael R. Slater/VP Regulatory Affairs
Research: Dr. Irving H. Fox/VP, Medical Affairs
Joseph M. Davie/VP Research

Bioline Labs *see* Goldline Labs

Blansett Pharma *NDC Code:* **51674**
Blansett Pharmacal Co. Inc. **501-758-8635**
3304 Pike Avenue
North Little Rock, AR 72118
Medical Product Sales Volume: $500,000
Total Employees: 6
Ownership: PRIVATE
Federal Procurement Eligibility: Medicaid Rebate

Block Drug *NDC Code:* **10158**
Block Drug Company, Inc. **201-434-3000**
257 Cornelison Ave. **800-356-6500**
Jersey City, NJ 07302
Medical Product Sales Volume: $624,000,000
Total Employees: 3,301
Ownership: Public *FAX:* 201-332-2362
Distribution: Manufacturer of RX/OTC Pharmaceuticals
CEO: Leonard Block/Sr. Chairman
James A. Block/Chairman
Thomas R. Block/President
Marketing: Donald H. LeSeiur/ExecVP U.S. Marketing
Production: Gilbert Seymann/VP Operations
Research: Thomas Ritchey, PhD/VP Regulatory Affairs
Frederick A. Curro, DMD. PhD/VP Deputy Dir, R&D
Phil Hozeny/Assoc Dir Admin & Info

Bluco *NDC Code:* **10160**
Bluco Inc. **313-513-4500**
28350 Schoolcraft
Livonia, MI 48180
Medical Product Sales Volume: $800,000
Total Employees: 8
Ownership: PRIVATE *FAX:* 313-513-4507
Distribution: Surgical and Medical Supply
CEO: Sandye R. Booy/President
Marketing: S.H. Blustein
Production: John Booy

Blue Cross *see* Halsey Drug

Blue Ridge Labs *see* Hoechst Marion Roussel

Boc Group *NDC Code:* **A00133**
BOC Group plc **0276-77222**
Chertsy Rd., Windlesham
Surrey GU20, UNITED KINGDOM
Medical Product Sales Volume: $1,085,000,000
Total Employees: 40,088
Ownership: Public *FAX:* 0276-7133
Distribution: Manufacturer of Gases
CEO: R. V. Giordano/Chairman
P. Bosonnet/Dep. Chairman
P. J. Rich/President
Medical Product Subsidiaries (Listed Separately):
Anaquest

Bock Pharma *NDC Code:* **00563**
Bock Pharmacal Company **314-579-0770**
P.O. Box 419056 **800-727-2625**
St. Louis, MO 63141-9056
Medical Product Sales Volume: $90,000,000
Total Employees: 400
Ownership: PRIVATE *FAX:* 314-579-0348
Distribution: Specialty Distribution, Branded Pharmaceuticals
CEO: Lawrence B. Moskoff/CEO
William B. Moskoff/President
Marketing: John McCall/VP, Sales and Marketing
William D. Ballantyne/Dir, Marketing
Research: Dave Byron/VP, Scientific Affairs
Federal Procurement Eligibility: Medicaid Rebate

Boehringer Mannheim *NDC Code:* **53169**
Boehringer Mannheim Corporation, Therapeutics Division **301-216-3900**
101 Orchard Ridge Dr. **800-628-2672**
Gaithersburg, MD 20878
Medical Product Sales Volume: $1,600,000,000
Total Employees: 403
Ownership: Roche AG
Distribution: Manufacturer of Branded Pharmaceuticals
CEO: John Melville/VP, Therapeutics US
J. Barry Buzogany, Esq./VP Legal
Rich Voss/Executive Director Business Development
Greg Fulton/Director, Marketing
Alan L. Lichtenstein/Director, Human Resources
Marketing: Jeanne Riley/Director, Market Research
Tony Yost/Executive Director, Sales
Research: Patricia Young, PhD/VP Regulatory Affairs

Boehringer Pharms *NDC Code:* **00597**
Boehringer Ingelheim Pharmaceuticals Inc. **203-798-9988**
900 Ridgebury Road
Ridgefield, CT 06877-0368
Ownership: Boehringer Ingelheim GMBH *FAX:* 203-791-6234
Distribution: Manufacturer of Branded Pharmaceuticals
CEO: Louis Fernandez/Chairman
Werner Gerstenberg/CEO & President
Marketing: Ian R. Mills/SVP, Marketing and Sales
Douglas Wilson, PhD/Pulmonary Group Dir
Steve Schmidt/Dir Marketing Communications
Susan Badders/Product Mgr ATROVENT
Gary Nichols/Dir Sales Training & Devel.
Production: Dr. W. Polonius/VP Production
Martin Kaplan/Dir, Drug Regulatory Affairs
Research: Chester Wood, MD/Sen Assoc Dir Clinical Res
Margaret Wecker, PhD/Assoc Dir Clinical Res
Ersen Arseven/Grp Dir Intl Data Mgt
Reiner Becker/VP Corp Planning
Penelope A Bowers/Associate Medical Dir
David R Brill/Assoc Dir Drug Reg Affair
Cynthia S Dommisse/Mgr Regulatory Affairs
Holly D Dursema/Manager Drug Reg Affairs
John J Elliott/Mgr Medical Information Services
Tricia Gregory/Mgr Medical Data Management
Lisa D Hanin/Mgr Drug Reg Affairs
Loretta M Kearney/Mgr Medical Services
Linda J M Macgregor/Mgr Medical Information Services
Patricia A Morrow/Mgr Prod Public Relations
Margaret Norman/Manager Information Services
Gerhard S Sharon/Mgr Medical Communication
Charlie Willmer/Manager Medical Systems
Federal Procurement Eligibility: Medicaid Rebate
Medical Product Subsidiaries (Listed Separately):
Isis Pharm
Lee Labs
Roxane

Bolan Pharm *NDC Code:* **44437**
Bolan Pharmaceutical, Inc. **817-268-6110**
828 Mountain Terrace
Hurst, TX 76053
Medical Product Sales Volume: $200,000
Total Employees: 4
Ownership: PRIVATE *FAX:* 817-268-6147
Distribution: Specialty Distributor
CEO: Sidney L. Boyd
Federal Procurement Eligibility: Medicaid Rebate

Bolar *see* Circa Pharm

Boots Pharm *NDC Code:* **00524**
Boots Pharmaceuticals, Inc. **708-405-7400**
300 Tri-State International Cent Ste.200 **800-323-1817**
Lincolnshire, IL 60069
Medical Product Sales Volume: $270,000,000
Total Employees: 1,500
Ownership: BASF
Distribution: Manufacturer of Branded Pharmaceuticals
CEO: Gordon Solway/Chairman
Carter Eckert/President & CEO
Charles Defesche/EVP
Marketing: John Fowler/VP Sales & Marketing
Thomas Thurman/VP New Product Marketing
Research: Hans A De Haan/Med Dir Cardiovascular
Ian K Lee/Sr Medical Director
Rona B Mcgreevy/Manager Medical Info
Anthony M Orlando/Director/Stat & Clinical Info
David H Warnock/Mgr Regulatory Affairs
Federal Procurement Eligibility: Medicaid Rebate
Medical Product Subsidiaries (Listed Separately):
Boots Pharms

Boots Pharms *see* Knoll Pharms

Boyle Pharm *NDC Code:* **00222**
Boyle & Company Pharmaceuticals **818-441-0284**
1613 Chelsea Road, Suite 313
San Marino, CA 91108
Total Employees: 9
Ownership: PRIVATE
CEO: Susan Boyle/President

Bracco DXS *NDC Code:* **00270**
Bracco Diagnostics, Inc. **609-897-2000**
107 College Road East **800-631-5245**
Princeton, NJ 08540
Total Employees: 400
Ownership: Bracco Spa
Distribution: Manufacturer of Imaging Agents
CEO: Michael Tweedle,Phd/President
John Cornille/Dir

Bradley Pharms *NDC Code:* **00482**
Bradley Pharmaceuticals, Inc. **201-882-1505**
383 Route 46 West **800-929-9300**
Fairfield, NJ 07006-2402
Medical Product Sales Volume: $12,800,000
Total Employees: 100
Ownership: Public *FAX:* 201-575-5366
Distribution: Manufacturer of Branded Pharmaceuticals
CEO: Daniel Glassman/President
Alan V. Gallantar/Controller
Marketing: Gene Goldberg/Vice President
John DeMartino/Director, Trade Relations
Production: Albert Fleischner, PhD/VP, Mfg., R&D
Research: Bob Corbo/VP, Quality Assurance and Quality Control
Federal Procurement Eligibility: Medicaid Rebate
Medical Product Subsidiaries (Listed Separately):
Kenwood Laboratories
Doak Dermatologies

Braintree *NDC Code:* **52268**
Braintree Laboratories Inc. **617-843-2202**
60 Columbian Street
Braintree, MA 02185-0929
Ownership: PRIVATE *FAX:* 617-843-7932
Distribution: Specialty Manufacturer
CEO: Harry Keegan/President
Jack DiPalma/MD/Medical Director
Marketing: Peter C. Kenney/VP Marketing
Research: Mark B. Cleveland, PhD/VP New Product Development
Federal Procurement Eligibility: Medicaid Rebate

Breckenridge *NDC Code:* **51991**
Breckenridge Inc.
P.O. Box 206 **800-367-3395**
Boca Raton, FL 33429
Ownership: PRIVATE
Federal Procurement Eligibility: Medicaid Rebate

Bristol Labs *see* Mead Johnson

Bristol-Myers Squibb *NDC Code:* **00087, 00153**
Bristol-Myers Squibb Co. **212-546-4000**
345 Park Avenue **800-631-5244**
New York, NJ 10154-0037
Medical Product Sales Volume: $15,065,000,000
Total Employees: 51,200
Ownership: Public *FAX:* 212-546-4020
Distribution: Manufacturer of Branded Pharmaceuticals
CEO: Charles A. Heimbold, Jr./President, Chairman & CEO
Kenneth E. Weg/EVP and President, Pharmaceutical Group
Michael E. Autera/EVP
John L. McGoldrick/SVP & General Counsel
Michael F. Mee/SVP & CFO
Charles G. Tharp, PhD/SVP, Human Resources
Samuel L. Barker, PhD/President, U.S. Pharmaceuticals, Pharmaceutical Group
Peter R. Dolan/President, Mead Johnson Nutritional Group
John L. Skule/VP, Public Affairs
Richard L. Thompson/VP, Government Affairs
Federal Procurement Eligibility: Medicaid Rebate
Medical Product Subsidiaries (Listed Separately):
Bristol Labs
Bristol Myers
Bristol-Myers Squibb
Squibb-Mark
Mead Johnson
Westwood

Brown Pharm *see* ICN Pharms

BTG Pharms *NDC Code:* **54396**
BTG Pharmaceuticals Corp. **708-913-1144**
70 Wood Avenue South
Iselin, NJ 08830
Medical Product Sales Volume: $1,020,212
Total Employees: 24
Ownership: Public *FAX:* 708-913-9919
Distribution: Distributor/Manufacturer of Branded Pharmaceuticals
CEO: Marvin P. Loeb/Chairman
Stephen M. Simes/President & CEO
Stephen A. Bourne, CPA/Treasurer, Controller
Bruce N. Barron/VP, CFO
Research: Samuel A. Pasquale, MD/Consulting Clin. Research Dir

Burroughs Wellcome *see* Glaxo Wellcome

BYK-Gulden *see* Altana

C & M Pharm *NDC Code:* **00398**
C & M Pharmacal, Inc. **810-548-7846**
1721 Maple Lane **800-423-5173**
Hazel Park, MI 48030
Medical Product Sales Volume: $1,000,000
Total Employees: 35
Ownership: PRIVATE *FAX:* 810-548-0913
CEO: Elliott Milstein/President
Donald St. Pierre/Gen'l Mgr & VP
Jodi Anstandig/Controller
Marketing: Claudia Sinta/Marketing Manager

C M C *see* Consolidated Midland

C O Truxton *NDC Code:* **00463**
C.O. Truxton, Inc. **609-365-4118**
136 Harding Avenue
Bellmawr, NJ 08103
Total Employees: 25
Ownership: PRIVATE
Distribution: Distributor of Brands & Generics
Marketing: Gerg Devine/Manager
Federal Procurement Eligibility: Medicaid Rebate

Calvin Scott *NDC Code:* **17224**
Calvin-Scott & Company, INC. **505-294-8825**
209 Eubank NE
Albuquerque, NM 87123
Medical Product Sales Volume: $5,000,000
Total Employees: 23
Ownership: PRIVATE
Distribution: Specialty Manufacturer of Bariatric Pharmaceuticals
Marketing: H. A. Lattimer
Production: Marsha M. Goachee

Camall *NDC Code:* **00147**
Camall Company, Inc. **810-752-9683**
P.O. Box 307 **800-521-6720**
Romeo, MI 48065-0307
Total Employees: 24
Ownership: PRIVATE *FAX:* 810-752-6226
Distribution: Manufacturer of Generics
CEO: Eugene M. Schmall, I/Chairman & President
Eugene M. Schmall, II/Dir New Prod. Development
Marketing: Sidney R. Schmall/VP Marketing & Sales
Production: Leslie W. Smith/VP of Operations
Federal Procurement Eligibility: Medicaid Rebate

Caraco Pharm *NDC Code:* **57664**
Caraco Pharmaceutical Laboratories, Ltd. **313-871-8400**
1150 Elijah McCoy Drive
Detroit, MI 48202
Medical Product Sales Volume: $3,000,000
Total Employees: 40
Ownership: PRIVATE *FAX:* 313-871-8314
Distribution: Manufacturer of Generics
CEO: C. Arnold Curry, MD
Marketing: Sherman N. Ginn/VP Sales & Mktg
Jean Heider/Mgr Sales Administrator
Production: William R. Hurd/COO, Pres
Research: James Chao/VP R&D
Federal Procurement Eligibility: Medicaid Rebate

Caremark *NDC Code:* **00339**
Caremark Inc. **312-967-1910**
2215 Sanders Rd NB5N **800-933-0303**
Northbrook, IL 60062
Ownership: Baxter Hlthcare
Distribution: Distributor of Generics

Carnrick *NDC Code:* **00086**
Carnrick Laboratories, Inc. Division GWCarnick Co. **201-267-2670**
65 Horse Hill Road
Cedar Knolls, NJ 07927
Total Employees: 175
Ownership: PRIVATE *FAX:* 201-267-2289
Distribution: Manufacturer of Branded Pharmaceuticals
CEO: Edmond J. Bergeron/President & CEO
Research: Wayne E. Sokoly/Director of Technical Services
Dolores M. Fortunes/Mgr Reg Affairs
Federal Procurement Eligibility: Medicaid Rebate

Carolina Med *NDC Code:* **46287**
Carolina Medical Products **919-753-7111**
P.O. Box 147
Farmville, NC 27828
Medical Product Sales Volume: $2,000,000
Total Employees: 20
Ownership: PRIVATE *FAX:* 919-753-3882
Distribution: Specialty Manufacturer
CEO: James Olsen/Pres
Henry Smith/VP

Centeon *NDC Code:* **00053**
Centeon LLC **215-454-8000**
1020 First Avenue
King of Prussia, PA 19406
Medical Product Sales Volume: $232,000,000
Total Employees: 2,000
Ownership: Rhone-Poulenc Rorer *FAX:* 215-540-8160
Distribution: Manufacturer of Branded Plasma Products
CEO: John A. Sedor/SVP & General Manager
Marketing: Lyn Wiesinger/VP Marketing Worldwide
Research: Garrett Bergman, MD/Dir, Medical & Scientific Affairs
Stewart Mueller/Dir Reg Affairs
Judith A Polowczuk/Mgr Regulatory Affairs
Federal Procurement Eligibility: Medicaid Rebate

Center Laboratories *see* Ctr Labs Hermal

Century Pharms *NDC Code:* **00436**
Century Pharmaceuticals **317-849-4210**
10377 Hague Road
Indianapolis, IN 46256
Total Employees: 15
Ownership: PRIVATE *FAX:* 317-849-4263
Distribution: Distributor/Manufacturer of Generics
CEO: Ross A. Deardorff, R.Ph./President

Cerenex Pharm *see* Glaxo Wellcome

Cetus *see* Chiron Thera

Cetylite Inds *NDC Code:* **10223**
Cetylite Industries, Inc. **609-665-6111**
9051 River Road **800-257-7740**
Pennsauken, NJ 08110
Medical Product Sales Volume: $4,000,000
Total Employees: 27
Ownership: PRIVATE *FAX:* 609-665-5408
CEO: Stanley L. Wachman/President
Burton I. Katzman/VP Sales

CFH Labs LP *NDC Code:* **00136**
CFH Laboratories LP
114 American Rd.
Morris Plains, NJ 07950
Ownership: PRIVATE

Challenge Prod *NDC Code:* **50467**
Challenge Products Incorporated **314-348-2227**
Lake Road 54-22 **800-322-9800**
Osage Beach, MO 65065
Medical Product Sales Volume: $1,200,000
Total Employees: 12
Ownership: Public *FAX:* 314-348-2228
Distribution: Distributor to Dental Office or Pharmacy
Production: Laura Melvin/Quality Assurance

Charter Labs *NDC Code:* **50550**
Charter Laboratories, Inc.
1200 Paco Way
Lakewood, NJ 08701
Ownership: PRIVATE

Chase *NDC Code:* **54429**
Chase Laboratories **201-589-8181**
280 Chestnut Street
Newark, NJ 07105
Medical Product Sales Volume: $60,000,000
Total Employees: 500
Ownership: Sobel NV
Distribution: Manufacturer of Generics
CEO: Richard Remaly/President
Federal Procurement Eligibility: Medicaid Rebate
Medical Product Subsidiaries (Listed Separately):
Banner Gelatin

Chelsea Labs *NDC Code:* **46193**
Chelsea Labs, Inc.
2021 East Roosevelt Blvd.
Monroe, NC 28110
Ownership: Rugby Labs
Distribution: Manufacturer of Generics

Chemrich Labs *NDC Code:* **10235**
Chemrich Laboratories
5211 Telegraph Rd.
Los Angeles, CA 90022
Ownership: PRIVATE
Federal Procurement Eligibility: Medicaid Rebate

Chiron Thera *NDC Code:* **53905**
Chiron Therapeutics **510-601-3440**
4560 Horton Street **800-244-7668**
Emeryville, CA 94608-2997
Total Employees: 200 *Telex:* 4992659
Ownership: Chiron *FAX:* 510-601-3435
Distribution: Manufacturer of Branded Pharmaceuticals
CEO: Ed Penhoet/President
Marketing: Edward Kenney/VP, Sales & Marketing
Tom Dezao/Marketing Group Director
Herbert Lee/Director, Professional Services
Production: Renato Fuchs, PhD/SVP Mfg & Devel Ops
Research: Pablo Valenzuela, PhD/SVP Biologicals R&D
Federal Procurement Eligibility: Medicaid Rebate
Medical Product Subsidiaries (Listed Separately):
Central Pharm

Ciba *see* Novartis

Ciba Vision *NDC Code:* **58768, 00058**
Ciba Vision Ophthalmics **770-418-4000**
11460 Johns Creek Parkway **800-845-6585**
Duluth, GA 30155
Medical Product Sales Volume: $200,000,000
Total Employees: 208
Ownership: Ciba Vision Corp
Distribution: Manufacturer of Branded Ophthalmics & Generics
CEO: Steve Martin/President
Marketing: Dan Myers/VP Sales and Marketing
Harry Diamond/Dir Trade & Managed Care
Production: Tom Elder/Executive Director, Logistics
Research: Howard Shlevin/VP Research, Product & Business Development
T. Al Reaves, PhD/Dir Clinical Research
Lawrence D Mandt/Director Regulatory Affairs & Quality Assurance
Federal Procurement Eligibility: Medicaid Rebate

Circa Pharm *NDC Code:* **00725**
Circa Pharmaceuticals Inc. **516-842-8383**
33 Ralph Avenue **800-872-0159**
Copiague, NY 11726-0030
Medical Product Sales Volume: $15,600,000
Total Employees: 490
Ownership: Watson Pharm *FAX:* 516-842-8630
Distribution: Manufacturer of Generics
CEO: Melvin Sharoky, MD/Chairman
Thomas P. Rice/COO & CFO
Marketing: Patricia Anderson/National Sales Mgr
Federal Procurement Eligibility: Medicaid Rebate
Medical Product Subsidiaries (Listed Separately):
Circa
Somerset
Hercon Labs
Hi-Tech

Circle Pharms *NDC Code:* **00659**
Circle Pharmaceuticals, Inc. **317-842-5463**
6320 Rucker Rd. **800-444-9296**
Indianapolis, IN 46220
Ownership: Century Pharm
CEO: William J. Mooney/President
Marketing: Kathleen Mooney/Director, Marketing

CIS *NDC Code:* **45567**
CIS-US, Inc.
10 Deanglo Drive
Bedford, MA 01730
Ownership: Atomic Energy Sa
Distribution: Manufacturer of Diagnostic Agents

Clay Park Labs *NDC Code:* **45802**
Clay Park Laboratories, Inc. **212-901-2800**
1700 Bathgate Avenue
Bronx, NY 10457
Medical Product Sales Volume: $52,000,000
Total Employees: 525
Ownership: Agis-Careline Group *FAX:* 212-294-8324
Distribution: Distributor/Manufacturer of Generic Topicals
CEO: Morton H. Katz/Vice President
Bernard Ettinger/President & CEO
Giora Carni/EVP
Jeremy Block/Chief Tech Off
Marketing: Samuel Sirkin/Director of
Production: Shabbir Barrot/Director of
Federal Procurement Eligibility: Medicaid Rebate

Clincl Formula *NDC Code:* **51822**
Clinical Formula LLC DBA AHC Pharmacal Inc. **714-631-0149**
888 West 16th St
Newport Beach, CA 92663
Total Employees: 35
Ownership: PRIVATE *FAX:* 714-631-0745
Distribution: Manufacturer of Pharmaceuticals
Production: Ken Kutanakit/Plant Mgr

Colgate Oral *NDC Code:* **00126**
Colgate Oral Pharmaceuticals **214-233-2800**
14335 Gillis Road
Dallas, TX 75244
Ownership: Colgate-Palmolive Co. *FAX:* 214-239-6854
Distribution: Manufacturer of Dental Products
CEO: Nick Vinke/President & General Mgr
Marketing: Robert Rubbinaccio/Marketing Manager, U.S.
Production: Tom Collins
John Trentacosti/Quality
Research: Dave Saar
Federal Procurement Eligibility: Medicaid Rebate

Colgate-Hoyt Labs *see* Colgate Oral

Colmed *see* Rosemont

Compumed *NDC Code:* **00403**
Compumed Inc.
1517 Edward Ave.
Harahan, LA 70123
Ownership: PRIVATE

Connaught Merieux *NDC Code:* **11793, 49281**
Connaught Laboratories, Inc. **717-839-7187**
Route 611, P.O. Box 187
Swiftwater, PA 18370
Ownership: Connaught *FAX:* 717-839-7235
Distribution: Manufacturer of Vaccines
CEO: David Williams/President
Gary Ebert/VP Operations
Marketing: Doug Reynolds/VP Marketing
James Brown/VP Sales
Laurie Michel/Dir Govt. Affair and Public Policy
Research: Linda L Buzzar/Clinical Research Assoc
Gordon Campbell/Mgr Emerging Technology
Cynthia Dukes/Clin Research Manager
Kenneth P Guito/Clincal Research Mgr
Michael J Hensley/Dir Reg Affairs Intl
Sanford Kaufman/Director Public Affairs
Sandra Konnecke/Mgr Scientific Systems
Donald H Marks/Dir Of Clinical Research
Carol Negron/Sr Clinical Data Coord
Federal Procurement Eligibility: Medicaid Rebate

Consolidated Midland *NDC Code:* **00223**
Consolidated Midland Corp. **914-279-6108**
16-20 Main St.
Brewster, NY 10509
Medical Product Sales Volume: $1,000,000
Total Employees: 14
Ownership: PRIVATE
Distribution: Distributor/Manufacturer of Generics

Consolidated Midland *(cont'd)*
CEO: Frank Debora/President

Contract Pharma *NDC Code:* **10267**
Contract Pharmacal Corp.
160 Commerce Dr.
Hauppauge, NY 11788
Ownership: PRIVATE

Convatec *NDC Code:* **00519**
Convatec Div. Bristol-Myers Squibb
P.O. Box 5254 **800-582-6514**
Princeton, NJ 08543-5254
Ownership: Bristol-Myers Squibb

Cook-Waite Labs *NDC Code:* **00961**
Cook-Waite Laboratories **212-907-2712**
90 Park Avenue
New York, NY 10016
Ownership: Sanofi Winthrop
Distribution: Manufacturer of Dental Anesthetics

Cooper Cos *NDC Code:* **P00058**
Cooper Companies, Inc. **212-557-2690**
1 Bridge Plaza N. 6th Flr.
Fort Lee, NJ 07024-7502
Medical Product Sales Volume: $45,000,000
Total Employees: 700
Ownership: Public
CEO: Gary A. Singer/Co-Chairman
Bruce D. Sturman/Co-Chairman
Steven G. Singer/EVP & C. Admin. Ofcr. & Sec.
Robert S. Weiss/VP & Treasurer & CFO
Medical Product Subsidiaries (Listed Separately):
Cooper Vision Pharm

Cooper Laboratories *see* Cooper Cos

Cooper Vision Pharm *NDC Code:* **59426**
Cooper Vision Pharmaceuticals, Inc. **714-366-8692**
930-A Calle Negocio
San Clemente, CA 92673
Ownership: Cooper Cos
Distribution: Manufacturer of Optical Products
Federal Procurement Eligibility: Medicaid Rebate

Coopervision *see* Cooper Cos

Copley Pharm *NDC Code:* **38245**
Copley Pharmaceutical, Inc. **617-821-6111**
25 John Road **800-325-6111**
Canton, MA 02021
Medical Product Sales Volume: $142,158,000
Total Employees: 500
Ownership: Public *FAX:* 617-821-4068
Distribution: Manufacturer of Generics
CEO: Gabriel R. Cipau, PhD/President & CEO
Kenneth Larsen/Chairman
Jane C.I. Hirsh/President International
Marketing: Julie Trendowicz/VP Sales & Marketing
Donald V. Kowalski/Dir of Trade Relations
Production: Madhu Balachandron/EVP Operations
Research: Jerome Skelly, PhD/VP Scientific Affairs
Whe-Yong W Lolo/Research & Development
Federal Procurement Eligibility: Medicaid Rebate

Cord Labs *see* Geneva Pharms

Crandall Assoc *NDC Code:* **00392**
Crandall Associate, Inc. **313-939-2310**
32529 Mound Road
Warren, MI 48093
Medical Product Sales Volume: $100,000
Total Employees: 2
Ownership: PRIVATE
Federal Procurement Eligibility: Medicaid Rebate

Creighton Prod *see* Geneva Pharms

Ctr Labs *NDC Code:* **00268**
Center Laboratories **516-767-1800**
35 Channel Drive
Port Washington, NY 11050
Ownership: E M INDUSTRIES (E Merck AG) *FAX:* 516-767-4229
CEO: Alan Pernick/President
Marketing: Rick Aloi/National Sales Manager
Production: Brian Woods/Product Manager
Federal Procurement Eligibility: Medicaid Rebate

Ctr Labs Hermal *NDC Code:* **48017**
Center Labs Hermal Dermatology
Group **518-475-0175**
163 Delaware Ave **800-437-6251**
Delmar, NY 12054-1313
Total Employees: 50
Ownership: PRIVATE *FAX:* 518-475-0180
Distribution: Distributor of Branded Generic Topicals
CEO: James R. Tombros/General Manager
Research: Jeanette Borger/Marketing Services Manager

Curatek Pharms *NDC Code:* **55326**
Curatek Pharmaceuticals Limited Partnership
3773 Howard Hughes Pky, Ste 350N **800-332-7680**
Las Vegas, NV 89109
Total Employees: 7
Ownership: Limited Partnership
Distribution: Specialty Manufacturer
CEO: Robert J. Borgman/President
John E. Presutti/Vice President
Research: Robert J. Borgman/President
Federal Procurement Eligibility: Medicaid Rebate

Cutter *see* Miles

Cygnus Therapeutics *NDC Code:* **A00065**
Cygnus Therapeutics Systems **415-369-4300**
400 Penobscot Drive
Redwood City, CA 94063
Medical Product Sales Volume: $5,057,000
Total Employees: 278
Ownership: Public *FAX:* 415-369-5318
Distribution: Developer of Transdermal Systems
CEO: G.W. Cleary, PhD/Chairman
Gregory Lawless, PhD/Pres & CEO
L. Clayton/VP &CFO
C.G. Arnold/VP
G.R. Hooper/VP
Thomas Spencer/VP

Cypress Pharm *NDC Code:* **60258**
Cypress Pharmaceutical, Inc. **601-856-4393**
135 Industrail Blvd.
Madison, MS 39110
Ownership: PRIVATE *FAX:* 601-853-1567
Distribution: Specialty Distributor
Federal Procurement Eligibility: Medicaid Rebate

Cytogen *NDC Code:* **A00014**
Cytogen Corp. **609-987-8200**
600 College Road East
Princeton, NJ 08540-5380
Medical Product Sales Volume: $10,851,000
Total Employees: 260
Ownership: Public
Distribution: Biotech Development Company
CEO: George W. Ebright/Chairman & CEO
Martin D. Cleary/Group VP & CFO
Dr. Thomas J. McKearn/President
William J. Ryan/VP, Gen. Counsel & Secretary
Marketing: James H. Geddes/Group VP, Marketing & Sales
Research: John D. Rodwell, PhD/VP Research & Development

D-M Pharm *see* Teva

Danbury Pharm *NDC Code:* **00591**
Danbury Pharmacal **203-744-7200**
P.O. Box 296 **800-553-4044**
Danbury, CT 06813
Total Employees: 277
Ownership: Schein Pharm *FAX:* 914-225-1763
Distribution: Manufacturer of Generics
Production: J. Cayado/VP, Operations
Research: E. Cohen/VP Scientific Operations
Federal Procurement Eligibility: Medicaid Rebate

Daniels Pharms *see* Jones Medical

Dartmouth Pharms *NDC Code:* **58869**
Dartmouth Pharmaceuticals, Inc. **508-748-3209**
37 Pine Hill Lane
Marion, MA 02738-1149
Total Employees: 12
Ownership: PRIVATE *FAX:* 508-748-3132
Distribution: Distributor of Branded Pharmaceuticals
CEO: Micheal J. Greco
Federal Procurement Eligibility: Medicaid Rebate

Dayton Labs *NDC Code:* **52041**
Dayton Laboratories Inc. **305-594-0988**
3307 NW 74th Avenue **800-446-0255**
Miami, FL 33172
Total Employees: 11
Ownership: PRIVATE
Distribution: Specialty Manufacturer
Marketing: Renaldo Farinis

Del Ray Lab *NDC Code:* **00316**
Del Ray Laboratories, Inc. **205-853-8247**
22 20th Avenue Northwest
Birmingham, AL 35215
Medical Product Sales Volume: $1,000,000
Total Employees: 10
Ownership: PRIVATE *FAX:* 205-853-8257
Distribution: Manufacturer of Corticosteroids
CEO: Raymond Delaney/President

Deliz *NDC Code:* **58238**
Deliz Pharmaceutical Corp
Box 29765
San Juan, PR 92907-0765
Ownership: PRIVATE

Delmont Labs *NDC Code:* **48532**
Delmont Laboratories, Inc. **610-543-2747**
P.O. Box 269 **800-562-5541**
Swarthmore, PA 19081
Total Employees: 9
Ownership: PRIVATE *FAX:* 610-543-6298
Distribution: Manufacturer of Branded Biologicals
CEO: David J. Ganfield, PhD/President & Owner
Federal Procurement Eligibility: Small Business

Delta Drug *NDC Code:* **00827**
Delta Drug Co. **904-733-3193**
9282 San Jose Blvd., #2804
Jacksonville, FL 32257
Ownership: PRIVATE

Delta Pharma *NDC Code:* **53706**
Delta Pharmaceuticals **805-772-1592**
800 Lockner Road
Columbia, SC 29210
Ownership: PRIVATE
Federal Procurement Eligibility: Medicaid Rebate

Denison Pharms *NDC Code:* **00295**
Denison Pharmaceuticals, Inc. **401-723-5500**
P.O. Box 1305
Pawtucket, RI 02862
Medical Product Sales Volume: $3,000,000
Total Employees: 40
Ownership: PRIVATE

Derm Prod of TX *see* Galderma

Dermik Labs *NDC Code:* **00066**
Dermik Laboratories, Inc. **610-454-3050**
500 Arcola Road **800-727-6737**
Collegeville, PA 19426
Medical Product Sales Volume: $100,000,000
Total Employees: 600
Ownership: Rhone-Poulenc Rorer
Distribution: Manufacturer of Branded Dermatologicals
CEO: Robert Bitterman/VP RPR Dermatologicals
Marketing: Keith Greathouse/Exec Dir WW Marketing
Robert Moccia/Dir of Sales
Production: Raymond Tobey/VP & Technical Dir
Research: Dr. Todd Plott/Director Medical Affairs
Federal Procurement Eligibility: Medicaid Rebate

Dermol Pharm *NDC Code:* **50744**
Dermol Pharmaceuticals, Inc. **404-977-7779**
3807 Roswell Road **800-334-7779**
Marietta, GA 30062
Ownership: PRIVATE

Dey Labs *NDC Code:* **49502**
Dey Laboratories, Inc. **707-224-3200**
2751 Napa Valley Corporate Drive **800-755-5560**
Napa, CA 94558
Medical Product Sales Volume: $150,000,000
Total Employees: 500
Ownership: Lipha S A/E Merck *FAX:* 707-224-3235
Distribution: Manufacturer of Generic Inhalants
CEO: Charles Rice/CEO
Marketing: Robert Mozak/VP Sales & Marketing
Todd Galles/Product Mgr
Production: Gary Michard/VP Operations
Federal Procurement Eligibility: Medicaid Rebate

Dista *NDC Code:* **00777**
Dista Products Co. **317-276-4000**
2542 Lilly Corp Center
Indianapolis, IN 46285
Ownership: Lilly
Distribution: Manufacturer of Branded Pharmaceuticals
CEO: W. Seymour Holt/VP General Mgr
Federal Procurement Eligibility: Medicaid Rebate

Dixon Shane *NDC Code:* **17236**
Dixon Shane Inc. **215-673-7770**
256 Geiger Road **800-262-7770**
Philadelphia, PA 19115
Total Employees: 20
Ownership: PRIVATE *FAX:* 215-673-3445
Distribution: Distributor of Generics
Marketing: Jeffrey Kamal/Vice President
Federal Procurement Eligibility: Medicaid Rebate

Doak Dermatologics *NDC Code:* **10337**
Doak Dermatologics Div. **516-333-7222**
67 Sylvester Street **800-645-3191**
Westbury Long Island, NY 11590
Medical Product Sales Volume: $2,000,000
Total Employees: 28
Ownership: PRIVATE *FAX:* 516-334-5135

Dorasol Labs *NDC Code:* **00471**
Dorasol Laboratories
P.O. Box 363906
San Juan, PR 00936-3906
Ownership: PRIVATE

Dow Hickam *NDC Code:* **00514**
Dow Hickam Pharmaceuticals **713-240-1000**
P.O. Box 2006
Sugarland, TX 77478
Medical Product Sales Volume: $18,000,000
Total Employees: 150
Ownership: Mylan *FAX:* 713-240-0003
Distribution: Specialty Manufacturer
CEO: Dow B. Hickam/President
Marketing: William W. Richardson/VP Sales
Production: Dewayne Dickey/Director Operations
Research: Robin F. Scamuffa/Director Technical Affairs
Robin F Scamuffa/Dir Technical Affairs
Barbara T Smith/Research Associate
Federal Procurement Eligibility: Medicaid Rebate

Drug Industries *NDC Code:* **00261**
Drug Industries **313-869-5500**
13700 Woodward Ave.
Detroit, MI 48203
Total Employees: 9
Ownership: PRIVATE
Distribution: Specialty Manufacturer

Du Pont *see* DuPont Radiopharms

Du Pont Critical *see* Dupont Pharma

Du Pont Merck *NDC Code:* **00590**
DuPont Merck Pharma **302-992-4240**
DuPont Merck Plaza, Centre Rd. **800-441-9861**
Wilmington, DE 19805
Ownership: Du Pont Merck
Distribution: Manufacturer of Branded Pharmaceuticals
Research: Paul Friedman, MD/President, Research
Federal Procurement Eligibility: Medicaid Rebate

Dunhall Pharms *NDC Code:* **00217**
Dunhill Pharmaceuticals, Inc. **501-787-5232**
P.O. Box 100
Gravette, AR 72736
Ownership: PRIVATE
Distribution: Distributor/Manufacturer of Generics
Federal Procurement Eligibility: Medicaid Rebate

Dupont Pharma *NDC Code:* **00056**
DuPont Pharma **302-992-5000**
DuPont Merck Plaza, Centre Road **800-441-9861**
Wilmington, DE 19805
Medical Product Sales Volume: $1,100,000,000
Total Employees: 4,460
Ownership: Du Pont/Merck *FAX:* 302-995-0671
Distribution: Manufacturer of Branded Pharmaceuticals
CEO: Paul Howes/President & CEO
Michael Miller/SVP & CFO
Maida Milone/SVP Legal, Gvt. Affairs
Production: Richard Davis/SVP Quality Assurance & Regulatory Compliance
Research: Paul Friedman, MD/Pres Research
Teresa P Dowling/Director Profess Srvcs
Federal Procurement Eligibility: Medicaid Rebate
Medical Product Subsidiaries (Listed Separately):
Du Pont Pharma
Endo Labs

DuPont Radiopharms *NDC Code:* **11994**
DuPont Radiopharmaceutical Division
331 Treble Cove Road
North Billerica, MA 01862
Total Employees: 700
Ownership: Du Pont Merck
Distribution: Radiopharmaceuticals

Dura *NDC Code:* **51479**
Dura Pharmaceuticals, Inc. **619-457-2553**
5880 Pacific Center Blvd.
San Diego, CA 92121-4204
Medical Product Sales Volume: $23,500,000
Total Employees: 150
Ownership: Public
Distribution: Specialty Brand Manufacturer
Research: Maryann Christopher/Mgr Clinical Research
Kathleen Heffernan/Mgr Regulatory Affairs
Charles W Prettyman/VP Development Reg Affair
Federal Procurement Eligibility: Medicaid Rebate

Duramed Pharms *NDC Code:* **51285**
Duramed Pharmaceuticals, Inc. **513-731-9900**
5040 Duramed Road **800-543-8338**
Cincinnati, OH 45213
Medical Product Sales Volume: $43,900,000
Total Employees: 303
Ownership: Public *FAX:* 513-731-5270
Distribution: Manufacturer of Generics
CEO: E. Thomas Arington/CEO & President
Timothy J. Holt/CFO
Judy Hattendorf/Human Resources
Marketing: Jeffrey T. Arington/SVP Mktg, Sales & Science
Production: Allen Marko/VP Manufacturing
Phil Rose/VP Marketing & Managed Care
Federal Procurement Eligibility: Medicaid Rebate

Dynapedic *NDC Code:* **10360**
Dynapedic
Ownership: PRIVATE

Dynapharm *NDC Code:* **55516**
Dynapharm, Inc. **619-453-5818**
P.O. Box 2141
Del Mar, CA 92014
Ownership: PRIVATE

E Z Em *NDC Code:* **10361**
E Z Em Co, Inc. **516-333-8230**
717 Main Street **800-544-4624**
Westbury, NY 11590
Medical Product Sales Volume: $93,417,000
Total Employees: 1,000
Ownership: PRIVATE *FAX:* 516-333-8278
Distribution: Manufacturer of Contrast Agents
CEO: Howard S. Stern/Chairman & CEO
Daniel R. Martin/President & COO
Marketing: Kay N. Hatch/VP, Marketing
Production: Craig Burk/VP, Production
Research: Joseph A. Riina/SVP Technical Affairs
Gloria Riina/Director of Clinical Affairs

East TX O2 *NDC Code:* **10363**
East Texas Oxygen Co.
4608 Highway 271
Tyler
Ownership: PRIVATE

Eastman Kodak *NDC Code:* **58472**
Eastman Kodak Company **716-724-4000**
343 State Street
Rochester, NY 14650

Eastman Kodak *(cont'd)*
Medical Product Sales Volume: $4,917,000,000
Total Employees: 132,600
Ownership: Public
Distribution: Manufacturer of Chemicals & Photography Equipment
CEO: Kay Whitmore/President

Econolab *NDC Code:* **55053**
Econolab **313-427-0821**
P.O. Box 85543
Westland, MI
Ownership: PRIVATE
Federal Procurement Eligibility: Medicaid Rebate

ECR Pharms *NDC Code:* **00095**
ECR Pharmaceuticals **800-527-1955**
P.O. Box 71600
Richmond, VA 23233
Medical Product Sales Volume: $2,200,000
Total Employees: 40
Ownership: E Claiborn Robins Co *FAX:* 804-527-1959
Distribution: Distributor of Branded Pharmaceuticals
CEO: E.C. Robins, Jr./President
D.S. Caskey/Vice President of Pharmaceutical Operations
Marketing: Charles W. Wesley/Sales and Marketing
William Selberis
Research: Robert S. Murphey/Senior VP
Federal Procurement Eligibility: Medicaid Rebate

Edwards Pharms *NDC Code:* **00485**
Edwards Pharmaceuticals, Inc. **601-837-8182**
111 Mulberry Street **800-543-9560**
Ripley, MS 38663
Medical Product Sales Volume: $500,000
Total Employees: 5
Ownership: PRIVATE *FAX:* 601-837-1473
Distribution: Distributer of Branded Generics
CEO: Linda White Freeman/President
Federal Procurement Eligibility: Medicaid Rebate Woman Owned Minority Owned

Effcon Labs *NDC Code:* **55806**
Effcon Laboratories Inc. **404-428-7011**
P.O. Box 7499
Marietta, GA 30065
Total Employees: 5
Ownership: PRIVATE *FAX:* 404-428-6811
Distribution: Specialty Manufacturer
CEO: Ed R. Burklow/President
Marketing: Kent Burklow

Elder Pharm *see* ICN Pharms

Elge *NDC Code:* **58298**
Elge, Inc.
P.O. Box 944
Richmond, TX 77406
Ownership: PRIVATE

Eli Lilly *see* Lilly

Elkins Sinn *NDC Code:* **00641**
Elkins Sinn Div. AH Robins Co, Inc. **609-424-3700**
170 Radnor Chester Rd. 2nd Floor **800-257-8349**
Saint Davids, PA 19087
Total Employees: 556
Ownership: AH Robins *FAX:* 609-424-8747
Distribution: Manufacturer of Generics
CEO: Joseph J. Beschel/VP & General Manager
Research: Thelma C Hilibrand/Dir Reg Affairs
Federal Procurement Eligibility: Medicaid Rebate

Embrex Economed *NDC Code:* **38130**
Embrex/Economed Pharmaceuticals, Inc. **919-226-1091**
P.O. Box 3303
Burlington, NC 27215
Total Employees: 5
Ownership: PRIVATE *FAX:* 919-229-5475
CEO: Cary D. Allred/President
Marketing: Kevin Pack/Director of Marketing
Federal Procurement Eligibility: Medicaid Rebate

Emerson Labs *NDC Code:* **00802**
Emerson Laboratories **214-792-5848**
1008 Whitaker
Texarkana, TX 75501
Ownership: PRIVATE

Endo Labs *NDC Code:* **60951**
Endo Laboratories, L.L.C. **302-663-6887**
4301 Lancaster Pike
Wilmington, DE 19880
Ownership: Dupont Merck
Distribution: Manufacturer of Generics

Enzon *NDC Code:* **57665**
Enzon, Inc. **908-980-4500**
20 Kingsbridge Road
Piscataway, NJ 08854-3998
Medical Product Sales Volume: $11,000,000
Total Employees: 85
Ownership: Public *FAX:* 908-980-5911
Distribution: Biotechnology Manufacturer
CEO: Peter Tombros/President & CEO
John A. Caruso/VP Business Development & General Counsel
Kenneth J. Zuerblis/VP Finance & CFO
Marketing: Kimberly Cooper/Corporate Communications Specialist

Enzon *(cont'd)*
Production: Anna T. Viau/Senior Director; Regulatory & Medical Affairs
Research: Dr. Jeffrey McGuire/VP Research & Chief Scientific Officer
Dr. Robert G.L. Shorr/VP Science & Technology
Kwok L. Shum/Senior Director, Pharmacology & Toxicology
Federal Procurement Eligibility: Medicaid Rebate
Medical Product Subsidiaries (Listed Separately):
Enzon Labs, Inc.

Eon Labs Mfg *NDC Code:* **00185**
Eon Labs Manufacturing, Inc. **718-276-8600**
227-15 North Conduit Avenue **800-526-0225**
Laurelton, NY 11413
Total Employees: 200
Ownership: Eon Labs, Inc. *FAX:* 718-949-3120
Distribution: Manufacturer of Generics
CEO: Dr. Bernhard Hampl/President & CEO
David Gransee/Assistant Secretary
Marketing: Sherrie M. Bradley/SVP, Sales, Mktg
Production: Sadie Ciganek/VP, Regulatory Affairs
Dr. Pranab Bhattacharyya/VP, Quality Management
Federal Procurement Eligibility: Medicaid Rebate

Equipharm *NDC Code:* **57779**
Equipharm Corp. **914-354-8787**
P.O. Box D3700
Pomona, NY 10970
Total Employees: 10
Ownership: PRIVATE *FAX:* 914-354-8703
Distribution: Specialty Distributor
CEO: A.P. Bedrosian

Erbamont *see* Pharmacia & Upjohn

Erie Medical *NDC Code:* **20371**
Erie Medical, Division of GCENCO Inc.
10225 82nd Avenue
Kenosha, WI 53142
Ownership: PRIVATE

ESI Lederle *NDC Code:* **59911**
ESI Lederle, Inc. **215-989-5900**
555 East Lancaster **800-950-5099**
Radnor, PA 19087
Ownership: Wyeth-Ayerst *FAX:* 215-688-2762
Distribution: Distributor of Generics
CEO: Michael Dey, PhD/VP & General Manager
Federal Procurement Eligibility: Medicaid Rebate

Ethex *NDC Code:* **58177**
Ethex Corporation **314-567-3307**
10888 Metro Court
St. Louis, MO 63043
Medical Product Sales Volume: $17,000,000
Total Employees: 50
Ownership: KV Pharmaceutical Company *FAX:* 314-567-0701
Distribution: Distributor of Specialty Generics
CEO: Michael S. Anderson/President, CEO
Marketing: Robert Shanks/VP Mktg
Marco Polizzi/Product Mgr
Christopher Keith/Product Mgr
Tricia Wetzel/Mktg Svcs Mgr
Ann McBride/Customer Service Supervisor
Federal Procurement Eligibility: Medicaid Rebate

Ethitek Pharms *NDC Code:* **54686**
Ethitek Pharmaceuticals Company **847-675-6611**
7701 N. Austin Ave.
Skokie, IL 60077
Medical Product Sales Volume: $100,000
Total Employees: 2
Ownership: PRIVATE *FAX:* 847-675-0252
Distribution: Specialty Manufacturer
CEO: Irving C. Udell/Managing Director
Production: Dennis Emig/Operations Manager

Eveready Drugs *NDC Code:* **57548**
Eveready Drugs Ltd. **212-249-1050**
1229 Third Avenue
New York, NY 10021
Total Employees: 11
Ownership: PRIVATE
Distribution: Specialty Distributor
CEO: Alan Rosenblum/President

Everett Labs *NDC Code:* **00642**
Everett Laboratories, Inc. **201-674-8455**
71 Glenwood Place
East Orange, NJ 07017
Total Employees: 24
Ownership: PRIVATE *FAX:* 201-674-0933
Distribution: Manufacturer of Branded Pharmaceuticals
CEO: Everett G. Felper/CEO & President
Hariett Felper/Secretary & Treasurer
Marketing: John Giordano/EVP, Director of Marketing
Federal Procurement Eligibility: Medicaid Rebate

F A Mitchell *NDC Code:* **10770**
F.A. Mitchell Co., Inc. **617-244-1523**
15 Churchill Terrace
Newtonville, MA 02160
Ownership: PRIVATE
Federal Procurement Eligibility: Medicaid Rebate

Falcon Ophthalmics *NDC Code:* **61314**
Falcon Ophthalmics, Inc.
6201 South Freeway
Fort Worth, TX 76134-2099
Ownership: PRIVATE

Family Pharm *NDC Code:* **52735**
Family Pharmacy
P.O. Box 1027 **800-333-7347**
Southeastern, PA 19398-1027
Total Employees: 4
Ownership: PRIVATE *FAX:* 614-261-7360
Distribution: Distributor of Generics
Federal Procurement Eligibility: Medicaid Rebate

Faulding *see* Purepac Pharm

Faulding Pharm (US) *NDC Code:* **61703**
Faulding, Inc. **908-527-9100**
200 Elmora Ave.
Elizabeth, NJ 07207
Medical Product Sales Volume: $61,000,000
Total Employees: 340
Ownership: Public *FAX:* 908-527-0649
Distribution: OEM Supplier
CEO: Richard F. Moldin/Chairman, Pres & CEO
Lee H. Cracker/CFO, Secy. & Tres.
Garth Boehm, MD/EVP

Fenwal Labs *NDC Code:* **00942**
Fewal Div. Baxter Health Care
Rt 120 and Wilson Rd.
Round Lake, IL 60073
Ownership: Baxter Hlthcare

Ferndale Labs *NDC Code:* **00496**
Ferndale Laboratories, Inc. **313-548-0900**
780 West Eight Mile Road
Ferndale, MI 48220
Medical Product Sales Volume: $18,000,000
Total Employees: 185
Ownership: PRIVATE *FAX:* 313-548-0279
Distribution: Specialty Manufacturer
CEO: James T. McMillan/Chairman & CEO
David Beens/President & COO
Marketing: Gary Tessoff/Sales and Marketing Director
Production: Hank Rosen/VP, Operations
Pravin Patel/VP Business Development
Stephen Goldner/VP Reg. Affairs
Research: Randall Wagner/Dir
Federal Procurement Eligibility: Medicaid Rebate

Ferring Labs *NDC Code:* **55566**
Ferring Pharmaceuticals **914-333-8900**
120 White Plains Road, Suite 400
Tarrytown, NY 10591
Total Employees: 18
Ownership: Ferring Bv *FAX:* 914-631-1992
Distribution: Specialty Manufacturer
CEO: Frederik Paulson/CEO
Joseph T. Curti, MD/President
Marketing: Wayne C. Anderson/VP, Sales and Marketing
Production: Dr. I Nudleman/Dir, Regulatory Affairs
Research: Ronald Nardi, PhD/VP, Scientific Affairs

Fielding *NDC Code:* **00421**
Fielding Company **314-567-5462**
112 Weldon Parkway
Maryland Heights, MO 63043
Total Employees: 10
Ownership: Distributor of Vitamins
CEO: William E. Georges
Marketing: Melissa E. Georges/Marketing Executive
Federal Procurement Eligibility: Medicaid Rebate

Fisons *NDC Code:* **00585**
Fisons Corp. **716-475-9000**
755 Jefferson Rd. **800-234-2475**
Rochester, NY 14623
Medical Product Sales Volume: $200,000,000
Total Employees: 325 *Telex:* 4441031 AREX RUI
Ownership: Fisons plc *FAX:* 716-272-3958
Distribution: Manufacturer of Branded Pharmaceuticals
CEO: Dr. Brian W. Tempest
Stuart Wallis/CEO
Marketing: Elizabeth Likly/VP Marketing
Thomas C. Parker/VP Sales
Kim M. Baily/Mktg Svcs Mgr
Kay Cook/Corp. Comm. Mgr
Joyce L. Miller/Mgr Labeling & Prom Adv
Production: Russell D. Gilbert/VP, Manufacturing
Dr. Robert B. Parker/Sr. Dir Regulatory Affairs
Research: Barry W. Steiger/SVP R&D
Peter Johnson, PhD/Dir R&D Worldwide
Michael J. Tidd/VP Medical Affairs
Federal Procurement Eligibility: Medicaid Rebate
Medical Product Subsidiaries (Listed Separately):
Lotus

Fisons plc *NDC Code:* **P00585**
Fisons plc **47-323-2525**
Fisons House, Princess Street
Ipswich Suffolk IP1 1QH, UNITED KINGDOM
Medical Product Sales Volume: $1,862,000,000
Total Employees: 14,336
Ownership: Rhone-Poulenc Rorer *FAX:* 47-323-1540
Distribution: Manufacturer of Branded Pharmaceuticals
CEO: Patrick V. M. Egan/Chairman
Stuart Wallis/President
Medical Product Subsidiaries (Listed Separately):
Fisons
Medeva plc

Fleming *NDC Code:* **00256**
Fleming and Co. **314-343-8200**
1600 Fenpark Drive
Fenton, MO 63026
Total Employees: 110
Ownership: PRIVATE *FAX:* 314-343-8203
Distribution: Manufacturer of Branded Pharmaceuticals
CEO: Tom Fleming/President
Ted Feller/EVP
Marketing: M. T. Fleming/Marketing Director
Research: Ted Feller
Federal Procurement Eligibility: Medicaid Rebate

Flemington Pharm *see* Fleming

Flemming Pharms *NDC Code:* **60976**
Flemming Pharmaceuticals Inc.
11 Greenway Plaza, Ste 1115
Houston, TX 77046
Ownership: PRIVATE

Flint Labs *see* Knoll Pharms

Fluoritab *NDC Code:* **00288**
Fluoritab Corp. **313-847-3623**
Box 507
Temperance, MI 48182
Total Employees: 1
Ownership: PRIVATE *FAX:* 313-847-3985
Distribution: Distributor of Fluoride Products
CEO: Lanice Andress/President

Forest Labs *NDC Code:* **10418**
Forest Laboratories, Inc. **212-421-7850**
300 Prospect Street
Inwood, NY 11696
Medical Product Sales Volume: $446,900,000
Total Employees: 1,612
Ownership: Public *FAX:* 212-750-9152
Distribution: Manufacturer of Branded Pharmaceuticals
CEO: Howard Solomon/President
Kenneth E. Goodman/VP Finance
Raymond Stafford/VP
William J. Candee III/Secretary
Bernard McGovern/Human Resources
Marketing: Phillip M. Satow/EVP Marketing
Tom Nee/Product Mgr AEROBID
Marjorie Nichols/Product Mgr FLUMADINE
Production: Ronald F. Albano/VP Licensing
Mary Prehn/Dir, New Products Development & Market Research
Research: Lawrence S. Olanoff, MD, PhD/VP Scientific Affairs
Kim M Antonacci/Clin Information Officer
Donald H Waters/Dir Biochemistry/Pharmaco
Medical Product Subsidiaries (Listed Separately):
Forest Pharm
Gilbert Labs
Inwood Labs
UAD Labs
Pharmax Ltd

Forest Pharms *NDC Code:* **00456**
Forest Pharmaceuticals, Inc. **314-344-8870**
13622 Lakefront Drive
St. Louis, MO 63045
Total Employees: 180
Ownership: Forest Labs *FAX:* 314-344-4435
Distribution: Manufacturer of Generics & Brands
CEO: Michael F. Baker/EVP Sales
William B. Sparks/EVP Finance
Research: Laura LeKemeyer/Supervisor, Scientific Affairs
Federal Procurement Eligibility: Medicaid Rebate

Fougera *NDC Code:* **00168**
E. Fougera Div Altana Inc. **516-454-6996**
60 Baylis Road **800-645-9833**
Melville, NY 11747
Total Employees: 200
Ownership: Altana Inc *FAX:* 516-756-7017
Distribution: Manufacturer of Generic Topicals
CEO: George Cole/CEO
Kevin Sheil/Senior VP
Art Dulik/Senior VP, Finance
Marketing: Nancy Zappala/Sales Coordinator
Federal Procurement Eligibility: Medicaid Rebate

Foxmeyer *NDC Code:* **52297**
FoxMeyer Corporation **214-446-4800**
1220 Senlac Drive
Carrollton, TX 75006
Total Employees: 10,000
Ownership: Public *FAX:* 214-446-4499
Distribution: Distributor of Pharmaceuticals
CEO: Tom Anderson/President
Marketing: Michael Webster/SVP Sales & Mktg
William Jones/SVP National Accounts

Fresenius *NDC Code:* **49230**
Fresenius USA, Inc.
2637 Shadelands Dr.
Walnut Creek, CA 949598
Ownership: PRIVATE

Fujisawa Pharm (US) *NDC Code:* **57317**
Fujisawa Pharmaceutical Co. **708-317-8800**
3 Parkway North, 3rd Floor **800-888-7704**
Deerfield, IL 60015-2548
Ownership: Fujisawa
Distribution: Manufacturer of Branded & Generic Pharmaceuticals
CEO: Hatsuo Aoki/Chairman & CEO
Production: S. Trippi/VP Operations

Fujisawa Pharm (US) *(cont'd)*
Research: James K. Shook/VP R&D Operations
Josh Vijya/Sr. Associate, Safety Information Ctr
Federal Procurement Eligibility: Medicaid Rebate
Medical Product Subsidiaries (Listed Separately):
Fujisawa Lyphomed

Fujisawa USA *NDC Code:* **00469**
Fujisawa USA, Inc.
800-888-7704
Deerfield, IL 60015
Ownership: Fujisawa
Distribution: Manufacturer of Generic Injectables
Federal Procurement Eligibility: Medicaid Rebate

Galderma *NDC Code:* **00299**
Galderma Laboratories, Inc. **817-263-2600**
P.O. Box 331329
Fort Worth, TX 76163
Total Employees: 150
Ownership: Nestle/L'oreal *FAX:* 817-263-2639
Distribution: Manufacturer of Topicals
CEO: Steve Clark/President
Marketing: Harold W. Barnett/Dir of Marketing
Federal Procurement Eligibility: Medicaid Rebate

Gallipot *NDC Code:* **51552**
Gallipot, Inc. **612-681-9517**
2020 Silver Bell Rd. #11-12
St. Paul, MN 55122-1050
Medical Product Sales Volume: $2,500,000
Total Employees: 9
Ownership: PRIVATE *FAX:* 612-681-9001
Distribution: Manufacturer of Chemicals
CEO: Michael J. Jones

Gate Pharms *NDC Code:* **57844**
Gate Pharmaceuticals **215-256-8400**
650 Cathill Road **800-292-4283**
Sellersville, PA 18960
Ownership: Teva *FAX:* 215-256-7855
Distribution: Distributor of Branded Pharmaceuticals
CEO: Barry R. Edwards/Executive Director
Marketing: Dale Benner/Product Manager
Federal Procurement Eligibility: Medicaid Rebate

Gebauer Chem *NDC Code:* **00386**
Gebauer Company **216-271-5252**
9410 St. Catherine Avenue **800-321-9348**
Cleveland, OH 44104
Total Employees: 25
Ownership: PRIVATE *FAX:* 216-271-5335
CEO: E.W. Rose, Jr./Chairman
John A. Giltinan/President
Marketing: Margie Kruse
Production: Ron Coleman
Research: Kiera Black
Federal Procurement Eligibility: Medicaid Rebate

Geigy *see* Novartis

Genderm *NDC Code:* **52761**
Genderm Corporation **708-634-7373**
600 Knightsbridge Parkway
Lincolnshire, IL 60069
Medical Product Sales Volume: $35,000,000
Total Employees: 140
Ownership: PRIVATE *FAX:* 708-634-2008
Distribution: Manufacturer of Dermatologicals
CEO: Joel E. Bernstein, MD/Chairman
Frank R. Pollard/President & CEO
Frank I. Brisben/EVP
Marketing: Jean Rumsfield/Dir, Marketing
Research: Brian J Coe/Assoc Dir, Drug Discovery
Jessie Coe/Director Mis
Patrice L Flynn/Assoc Dir Clinical Research
Gary Knappenberger/Dir Regulatory Affairs
Joan Para/Manager Medical Information
Federal Procurement Eligibility: Medicaid Rebate
Medical Product Subsidiaries (Listed Separately):
Genderm

Genentech *NDC Code:* **50242**
Genentech, Inc. **415-266-1000**
460 Point San Bruno Blvd.
South San Francisco, CA 94080
Medical Product Sales Volume: $795,000,000
Total Employees: 2,331
Ownership: Public/Roche Holding Ltd *FAX:* 415-583-2163
Distribution: Biotechnology Manufacturer
CEO: Arthur D. Levinson/President & CEO
Robert A. Swanson/Chairman
William D. Young/SVP
David W. Beier/VP Government Affairs
Marketing: Richard B. Brewer/VP Sales & Marketing
Edmon R. Jennings/VP Sales
Bonnie Matlock/Assoc Dir Immun. & Endocrin. Prods.
Russ Belden/Product Mgr ACTIVASE
John Foster/Product Mgr PULMOZYME
Production: Paul F. Hohenschuh/VP Manufacturing
M. David McFarlane, PhD/VP Regulatory Affairs
Richard D. Ring/VP Quality & Product Development
Barry M. Sherman, MD/VP Medical Affairs
Henry Fuchs, MD/Associate Dir, Medical Affairs
Research: Arthur D. Levinson, PhD/SVP Research & Development
Hugh Nial, MD/VP Research Discovery
William F. Bennett, PhD/Cardiovascular Research
Phillip W. Berman, PhD/Immunology
Stuart E. Biolder, PhD/Process Sciences
Tim Gregory, PhD/Process Sciences
William S. Hancock, PhD/Analytical Chemistry
Dennis J. Henner, PhD/Cell Genetics
Robert D. Hershberg, PhD/Process Sciences

Genentech *(cont'd)*
Paula Jardieu, PhD/Immunology
Andrew J.S. Jones, D. Phil./Process Sciences
Anthony A. Kossiakoff, PhD/Protein Engineering
Laurence A. Lasky, PhD/Immunology
Ted Love, MD/Research Physician
Jennie P. Mather, PhD/Process Sciences
Ernst Rinderknecht, PhD/Process Sciences
Gordon A. Vehar, PhD/Cardiovascular Research
James A. Wells, PhD/Protein Engineering
Kathryn A Burg/Manager Quality Affairs
Janice Castillo/Director
Sandra J Hecker/Head Of Medical Writing
Irene Loeffler/Mgr Biomedical Records
Daniel P Maher/Mgr Product Development
Barbara H Mcclellan/Mgr Phase Iv Clinical Trials
Polly Moore/Dir Information Resource
Stuart E Nixon/Mgr Clinical Data Services
Charlene M Pagel/Clinical Research Assist
Carol Riccomini/Data Base Administrator
James D Richards/Mgr Information Technology
Federal Procurement Eligibility: Medicaid Rebate
Medical Product Subsidiaries (Listed Separately):
Scios Nova

General Generics *NDC Code:* **50272**
General Generics Incorporated **601-234-0130**
P.O. Box 510 **800-647-6196**
Oxford, MS 38655
Ownership: PRIVATE *FAX:* 601-234-9335
Distribution: Distributor of Generics

General Inj & Vac *NDC Code:* **52584**
General Injectables & Vaccines, Inc. **703-688-4121**
U.S. Highway 52, P.O. Box 9
Bastian, VA 24314-0009
Total Employees: 350
Ownership: PRIVATE
Distribution: Specialty Distributor

Generix Drug *see* Goldline Labs

Genetco *NDC Code:* **00302**
Genetco, Inc. **516-585-1000**
711 Union Parkway
Ronkonkama, NY 11779
Ownership: PRIVATE
Distribution: Distributor of Generics
Federal Procurement Eligibility: Medicaid Rebate

Geneva Pharms *NDC Code:* **00781, 50752**
Geneva Pharmaceuticals Inc. **303-466-2400**
2555 W. Midway Boulevard **800-525-8747**
Broomfield, CO 80038-0446
Medical Product Sales Volume: $210,000,000
Total Employees: 1,200
Ownership: Novartis *FAX:* 303-438-4600
Distribution: Distributor of Generics
CEO: Charles Lay/President
Terry P. Ruth/EVP, Finance & Administration
Mary Beth Wallingford/VP, Controller
Marketing: Joe Papa/SVP, Sales & Marketing
Russ Secter/Marketing Dir
Production: George Seaback/SVP Operations
Research: Paul Jarosz/SVP Development
Ron Hartmann, RPh, MBA/Manager, Government Affairs
Federal Procurement Eligibility: Medicaid Rebate

Gensia Labs *NDC Code:* **00703**
Gensia Laboratories Inc. **619-546-8300**
19 Huges
Irvine, CA 92618
Medical Product Sales Volume: $70,000,000
Total Employees: 400
Ownership: Public *FAX:* 619-453-0095
Distribution: Manufacturer of Injectables
CEO: David F. Hale/Chairman, President & CEO
Patrick Walsh/EVP COO Gensia Labs
Carl F. Boboski/EVP
David D. Burgess/VP Finance, CFO & Treasurer
Thomas P. Donahoe/VP, General Counsel
Paul K. Laikind, PhD/VP Corporate Development
Marketing: Stephen C. Eisold/VP & Gen Mgr Gensia Pharm
Jeffrey M. Yordon/VP Sales-Marketing Multisource
Nicholas Yeo/Director of Marketing, Europe
Production: Chester Damecki/VP, G.M. Multisource + Operations
Jack W. Reich, PhD/VP Regulatory Affairs
Research: Dr. Harry E. Gruber/VP Research
David A. Shapiro, MD/VP Clinical Research
Dr. Ronald R. Tuttle/VP New Drug Discovery
Walter Singleton, MD/VP Medical & Pharm. Development
Ruth Wikberg-Leonardi/Mgr Regulatory Affairs
Federal Procurement Eligibility: Medicaid Rebate

Genzyme *NDC Code:* **58468**
Genzyme Corporation **617-252-7500**
One Kendall Square **800-745-4447**
Cambridge, MA 02139-1562
Medical Product Sales Volume: $310,000,000
Total Employees: 1,100
Ownership: Public *FAX:* 617-252-7600
Distribution: Biotechnology Manufacturer
CEO: Henri A. Termeer/Chairman, President & CEO
Geoffrey F. Cox, PhD/SVP Operations
David D. Fleming/SVP, Pres Diagnostics
Elliott D. Hillback Jr/SVP & CEO
Mark A. Hofer/VP & General Counsel
Evan M. Lebson/VP & Treasurer
David J. McLachlan/SVP, Finance, CFO
Gregory D. Phelps/SVP, Corporate Development
James A. Warren/Corporate Controller
Erik Tambuyzer, PhD/VP Diagnostic Bus. Devel.

Genzyme *(cont'd)*
Marketing: Paul Hastings/VP Global Marketing Ther Div
Mike Raab/Product Manager
Production: Lisa Raines/VP Government Rel
David Foster/Dir Government Rel
Research: James R. Rasmussen, PhD/SVP Research
Alan E. Smith, PhD/SVP Research
Richard Moscicki, MD/VP Clinical Medical & Reg Affairs
Federal Procurement Eligibility: Medicaid Rebate

Geriatric Pharm *NDC Code:* **00249**
Geriatric Pharm. Corporation **414-272-2552**
P.O. Box 99
Butler, WI 53007
Total Employees: 20
Ownership: Hauck
Federal Procurement Eligibility: Medicaid Rebate

Gilbert Labs *NDC Code:* **00535**
Gilbert Laboratories
13622 Lakefront Dr.
Saint Louis, MO 63045
Medical Product Sales Volume: $1,000,000
Total Employees: 9
Ownership: PRIVATE
Distribution: Specialty Manufacturer

Gilead Sciences *NDC Code:* **61958**
Gilead Sciences, Inc.
353 Lakeside Drive **800-939-9009**
Foster City, CA 94404
Ownership: PRIVATE *FAX:* 800-693-9099

GIV *see* General Inj & Vac

Glades Pharms *NDC Code:* **59366**
Glades Pharmaceuticals **305-567-1319**
255 Alhambra Circle, Ste 1000 **800-452-3371**
Coral Gables, FL 33134
Total Employees: 30
Ownership: Stiefel Labs *FAX:* 305-443-3467
Distribution: Manufacturer of Generic Topicals
CEO: Brendan Murphy/President
Marketing: Alina Castaneda/Executive Assistant
Federal Procurement Eligibility: Medicaid Rebate

Glasgow Pharm *NDC Code:* **60809**
Glasgow Pharmaceuticals
890 North L Rogers Wells Blvd.
Glasgow, KY 42142-1209
Ownership: PRIVATE

Glaxo Dermatology *see* Glaxo Wellcome

Glaxo Wellcome *NDC Code:* **00173**
Glaxo Wellcome Inc. **919-483-2100**
1011 North Arendell Avenue
Zebulon, NC 27597
Medical Product Sales Volume: $3,680,000,000
Total Employees: 4,000
Ownership: Glaxo Wellcome plc *FAX:* 919-248-2381
Distribution: Manufacturer of Branded Pharmaceuticals
CEO: Robert Ingram/President & CEO
Federal Procurement Eligibility: Medicaid Rebate
Medical Product Subsidiaries (Listed Separately):
Allen & Hanburys
Glaxo Dermatology
Cerenex Pharm
Affymax

Glaxo Wellcome plc *NDC Code:* **P00173**
Glaxo Wellcome plc **44-171-493-4060**
Landsdowne House, Berkley Square
London W1X 6BQ, United Kingdom
Medical Product Sales Volume: $14,284,000,000
Total Employees: 65,702
Ownership: Public *FAX:* 44-171-408-0228
Distribution: Manufacturer of Branded Pharmaceuticals
CEO: Sir Richard Sykes/Deputy Chairman and CEO
Sean Lance/Dir Europe; Chief Operating Officer
John D. Coombe/CFO

Glenbrook Labs *see* Sanofi Winthrop

Glenwood *NDC Code:* **00516**
Glenwood, Inc. **201-569-0050**
83 North Summit Street **800-542-0772**
Tenafly, NJ 07670
Medical Product Sales Volume: $2,000,000
Total Employees: 35
Ownership: PRIVATE *FAX:* 201-567-4443
Distribution: Specialty Manufacturer
CEO: Michael Fuhrmann/CEO
Christopher Fuhrmann/President
David Fuhrmann/VP, Operations
Douglas A. Sears/Medical Director
Marketing: Brian Fuhrmann/VP Sales & Marketing

Global Pharm *see* Global Pharm

Global Pharm *NDC Code:* **00115**
Global Pharmaceutical Corporation **215-289-2220**
Castor and Kensington Avenues
Philadelphia, PA 19124
Total Employees: 40
Ownership: Global Pharm
Distribution: Manufacturer of Generic Pharmaceuticals
CEO: Max L. Mendelsohn/President & CEO
Cornel C. Spiegler/CFO
Joseph Storella/COO
Marketing: Gary R. Dubin/Dir Business Development and Sales

Global Pharm *(cont'd)*
Research: Pieter Groenewoud/VP Research and Development
Federal Procurement Eligibility: Medicaid Rebate

Global Source *NDC Code:* **59618**
Global Source Mgt. & Consulting Inc. **305-921-0006**
3001 North 29th Street
Hollywood, FL 33020
Ownership: PRIVATE
Distribution: Importer
Federal Procurement Eligibility: Medicaid Rebate

GM Pharms *NDC Code:* **58809**
GM Pharmaceuticals Inc. **817-784-8661**
P.O. Box 150312
Arlington, TX 76015
Total Employees: 9
Ownership: PRIVATE
Distribution: Specialty Manufacturer
CEO: Odes W. Mitchell/President

Goldline Labs *NDC Code:* **00182**
Goldline Laboratories, Inc. **305-491-4002**
1900 West Commercial Boulevard **800-327-4114**
Fort Lauderdale, FL 33309
Medical Product Sales Volume: $400,000,000
Total Employees: 450
Ownership: Ivax *FAX:* 305-492-7399
Distribution: Distributor of Generics
CEO: William F. Schreck/President
Marketing: William Mescall/VP, Sales & Mktg
Production: William L. Wasserman/Dir Packaging
Arnold Schacter/Dir Quality - Regulatory Affairs
Federal Procurement Eligibility: Medicaid Rebate

Good Sense *NDC Code:* **70030**
Good Sense **616-673-8451**
117 Water Street
Allegan, MI 49010
Ownership: Perrigo
Distribution: Manufacturer of Generics

Gordon Labs *NDC Code:* **10481**
Gordon Laboratories **215-789-3055**
6801 Ludlow Street
Upper Darby, PA 19082
Ownership: PRIVATE

Great S Labs *NDC Code:* **51301**
Great Southern Laboratories **713-530-3077**
10863 Rockley Road
Houston, TX 77099
Ownership: PRIVATE
Federal Procurement Eligibility: Medicaid Rebate

Greenstone *NDC Code:* **59762**
Greenstone Company **616-323-4000**
7171 Portage Road 7025-298-103 **800-253-8600**
Kalamazoo, MI 49001
Medical Product Sales Volume: $100,000,000
Total Employees: 100
Ownership: Upjohn *FAX:* 616-232-5251
Distribution: Distributor of Generics
Federal Procurement Eligibility: Medicaid Rebate

Grupak Labs *NDC Code:* **57801**
215-791-3010
2222 South 12th Street **800-666-6166**
Allentown, PA 18103
Ownership: PRIVATE *FAX:* 215-791-3632
Federal Procurement Eligibility: Medicaid Rebate

Guardian Labs *NDC Code:* **00327**
Guardian Laboratories Div. United Guardian, Inc. **516-273-0900**
P.O. Box 18050
Hauppauge, NY 11788
Medical Product Sales Volume: $3,000,000
Total Employees: 50
Ownership: PRIVATE *FAX:* 516-273-0858
Distribution: Specialty Manufacturer
CEO: Alfred R. Globus/Chairman, CEO
Kenneth H. Globus/President
Robert S. Rubinger/EVP, Secretary
Federal Procurement Eligibility: Medicaid Rebate

GW Labs *NDC Code:* **00713**
G & W Labs. **908-753-2000**
111 Coolidge Street
South Plainfield, NJ 07080
Medical Product Sales Volume: $6,000,000
Total Employees: 100
Ownership: PRIVATE *FAX:* 908-752-9264
Distribution: Distributor/Manufacturer of Generics
CEO: Burton Greenblatt/President
Marketing: Joel Zaklin/VP Sales & Marketing
Production: Robert Devine/Director of Production
Research: Dr. Kripanath Borah/Dir of Research
Federal Procurement Eligibility: Medicaid Rebate

Gynex *see* BTG Pharms

Gynomed Pharm *see* Gynopharma

Gynopharma *NDC Code:* **54765**
Gynopharma, Inc. **908-725-3100**
50 Division Street **800-322-4966**
Somerville, NJ 08876
Total Employees: 100
Ownership: PRIVATE *FAX:* 908-725-5838
Distribution: Specialty Manufacturer
CEO: Roderick L. Mackenzie/Chairman
Robert S. Cohen/President, CEO
Marketing: Sherry Bump/Dir Mktg
Doug McNamee/VP Sales
Research: Robin Foldesy,PhD/Research & Development
Tracy Romano/Clinical Research Associate

H & H Labs *NDC Code:* **46703**
H. & H. Laboratories
Ownership: PRIVATE

H N Norton Co. *NDC Code:* **50732**
H N Norton Co. **318-688-4800**
8910 Linwood Avenue **800-346-2207**
Shreveport, LA 71106
Medical Product Sales Volume: $14,600,000
Total Employees: 190
Ownership: Ivax *FAX:* 318-688-2125
Distribution: Distributor & Manufacturer of Generics
CEO: George Lukacs/President
Production: Russ McMahen/Production VP
Federal Procurement Eligibility: Medicaid Rebate

H R Cenci Labs *see* HR Cenci

H.C.F.A. F F P *NDC Code:* **99999**
HCFA Federal Financial Participation
Upper Limits Price (for Medicare)
Maximum Allowable Cost
Ownership: PRIVATE

Halsey Drug *NDC Code:* **00879**
Halsey Drug Company **718-467-7500**
1827 Pacific Street
Brooklyn, NY 11233
Medical Product Sales Volume: $20,225,000
Total Employees: 160
Ownership: Public *FAX:* 718-493-1575
Distribution: Manufacturer of Generics
CEO: Rosendo Ferran/President & CEO
Federal Procurement Eligibility: Medicaid Rebate
Medical Product Subsidiaries (Listed Separately):
Cenci Labs
Houba, Inc.

Hamilton Pharma *NDC Code:* **60322**
Hamilton Pharma, Inc. **415-855-5050**
340 Kingland Street **800-773-3678**
Nutley, NJ 07110
Ownership: Syntex Labs *FAX:* 415-852-1569
Distribution: Manufacturer of Generics
Federal Procurement Eligibility: Medicaid Rebate

Harber Pharm *NDC Code:* **51432**
Harber Pharmaceutical **201-348-3700**
350 Meadowlands Parkway
Secaucus, NJ 07094
Ownership: PRIVATE
Distribution: Distributor of Generics
Federal Procurement Eligibility: Medicaid Rebate

Hassle *see* Astra USA

Hauser *see* AF Hauser

Hauser Pharmaceuticals *see* AF Hauser

Henry Schein *NDC Code:* **00404**
Henry Schein **516-843-5500**
135 Duryea Road **800-772-4346**
Melville, NY 11747
Medical Product Sales Volume: $830,000
Total Employees: 3,200
Ownership: Schein Pharm *FAX:* 516-843-5658
CEO: Stanley M. Bergman/CEO
Steven Paladino/CFO
Leonard A. David/Human Resources

Heran Pharm *NDC Code:* **50434**
Heran Pharmaceutical Inc. **512-680-2969**
130 Longridge
San Antonio, TX 78228
Total Employees: 7
Ownership: PRIVATE
Distribution: Specialty Manufacturer

Herbert Labs *see* Allergan

Hercon Labs *NDC Code:* **49730**
Hercon Laboratories Corp.
York, PA
Ownership: Circa Pharm
Research: Joseph J Sobecki/Dir Regulatory Affairs
Federal Procurement Eligibility: Medicaid Rebate

Hermal Pharmaceutical Laborato *see* Ctr Labs Hermal

Hi Tech Pharma *NDC Code:* **50383**
Hi Technology Pharmacal Co., Inc. **516-789-8228**
369 Bayview Avenue
Amityville, NY 11701

Hi Tech Pharma *(cont'd)*
Medical Product Sales Volume: $16,000,000
Total Employees: 130
Ownership: Circa Pharm
Distribution: Manufacturer of Liquid Generics
CEO: Bernard Seltzer/CEO
Federal Procurement Eligibility: Medicaid Rebate

Highland Pkging *NDC Code:* **55782**
Highland Packaging Co.
6244 Lemay Ferry Road
St. Louis, MO 63129
Ownership: PRIVATE

Hill Dermac *NDC Code:* **28105**
Hill Dermaceuticals, Inc. **407-896-8280**
598 A Herndon Avenue
Orlando, FL 32814
Total Employees: 35
Ownership: PRIVATE *FAX:* 407-896-8280
Distribution: Manufacturer of Dermatologicals
CEO: Jerry S. Roth
Marketing: Jerry S. Roth
Production: Elaine Cox
Research: Rosario G. Ramirez, MD/Dir Med/Reg Affairs
Federal Procurement Eligibility: Medicaid Rebate

Hirsch Ind *NDC Code:* **50673**
Hirsch Industries, Inc. **804-355-4500**
4912 West Broad St.
Richmond, VA 23230
Total Employees: 2
Ownership: PRIVATE *FAX:* 804-741-4198
Distribution: Speciality Manufacturer
CEO: Jerry I. Hirsch/President

HL Moore *see* HL Moore Drug Exch

HL Moore Drug Exch *NDC Code:* **00839**
HL Moore Drug Exchange Div
Parkway Distributors **203-225-4621**
389 John Downey Drive
New Britain, CT 06050
Medical Product Sales Volume: $275,000,000
Total Employees: 500
Ownership: Public *FAX:* 203-223-2382
Distribution: Distributor of Generics
CEO: Mark Karp/President
Marketing: Gary Savage/Director of Marketing
John Dillaway/VP National Accounts
Production: Anthony J. Malafronte, RPh/Manager, Regulatory Affairs
Federal Procurement Eligibility: Medicaid Rebate

Hoechst Marion Roussel *NDC Code:* **00088, 00039, 00068**
Hoechst Marion Roussel, Inc. **816-966-4000**
P.O. Box 9627 **800-633-1610**
Kansas City, MO 64134-0627
Medical Product Sales Volume: $2,600,000,000
Total Employees: 6,600
Ownership: Hoechst AG *FAX:* 816-966-3270
Distribution: Manufacturer of Branded Pharmaceuticals
CEO: Peter C. Ladell/Pres Hoechst Marion Roussel N.A.
Edward Connolly/VP Community Affairs
Gary D. Street/VP, General Patent Counsel
Marketing: Kim Carroll/Product Mgr CARDIZEM
Production: Jerry B. Hedrick, Jr./VP Government Affairs
Al S. Baker
Research: Frank L. Douglas, PhD/Head, Global Research
Judith Hemberger/SVP, Global Drug Regulatory Affairs
John M. Orwin, MD/Managing Dir, Clinical Research
Michele R Flicker
Kirk H Hoffman/Mgr Medical Information
John Y Kimbrell/Sr Dir Scientific Info
Stanley C Mcdermott/Clin Trials Manager
Kristi S Wyatt/Dir Copy Approval
Federal Procurement Eligibility: Medicaid Rebate
Medical Product Subsidiaries (Listed Separately):
Blue Ridge Labs
Rugby Labs
Merrell
Hoechst Roussel

Hoffman La Roche *see* Roche

Hollister-Stier *see* Miles Spokane

Holloway Pharm *see* Abana Pharms

Hope Pharms *NDC Code:* **60267**
Hope Pharmaceuticals Inc.
2961 West MacArthur Blvd., Ste 130
Santa Ana, CA 92704
Ownership: PRIVATE

Hoprich *NDC Code:* **60155**
Hoprich Co. Inc. **812-474-0440**
2300 North Burkhardt
Evansville, IN 47715
Ownership: PRIVATE *FAX:* 812-474-0445

Horizon Pharm *NDC Code:* **59630**
Horizon Pharmaceutical Corp. **404-442-9707**
1125 Northmeadow Pky, Ste 130
Roswell, GA 30076
Medical Product Sales Volume: $1,500,000
Total Employees: 20
Ownership: PRIVATE *FAX:* 404-442-9594
Distribution: Specialty Distributor
CEO: Brent Dixon/President

Horizon Pharm *(cont'd)*
Marketing: Greg Hauck/VP Sales & Mktg
Federal Procurement Eligibility: Medicaid Rebate

Horizon Pharms *NDC Code:* **60904**
Horizon Pharmaceuticals, Inc.
1833 West Plantside Dr.
Louisville, KY 40299
Ownership: PRIVATE

Horizon Prod Co *NDC Code:* **54580**
Horizon Products Company **303-688-9694**
2339 Mount Royal DR.
Castle Rock, CO 80104
Total Employees: 11
Ownership: PRIVATE
Distribution: Specialty Manufacturer
Federal Procurement Eligibility: Medicaid Rebate

Horus *see* Boehringer Pharms

Horus Therapeutics *NDC Code:* **59229**
Horus Therapeutics, Inc. **716-292-4820**
2320 Brighton-Henrietta Line
Rochester, NY 14623
Medical Product Sales Volume: $1,000,000
Total Employees: 20
Ownership: PRIVATE *FAX:* 716-292-4836
Distribution: Specialty Manufacturer
CEO: Bernard C. Ouellette/President
Production: Dr. James Cappola/SVP Medical Affairs
Federal Procurement Eligibility: Medicaid Rebate

Hoyt Labs *see* Colgate Oral

HR Cenci *NDC Code:* **00556**
HR Cenci Labs., Inc. **209-268-4401**
P.O. Box 12524
Fresno, CA 93778
Medical Product Sales Volume: $5,000,000
Total Employees: 35
Ownership: Halsey Drug *FAX:* 209-237-5957
Distribution: Manufacturer of Generic Powders & Liquids
CEO: Herman F. Cenci/President
Production: Norma Banks/Director, Regulatory Affairs
Federal Procurement Eligibility: Medicaid Rebate

HR Cenci Labs *see* HR Cenci

Hsn Redi-Med In *NDC Code:* **53506**
Redi-Med, Inc. **404-929-0961**
801-N North Blacklawn Road
Conyers, GA 30207
Total Employees: 34
Ownership: PRIVATE

Huckaby Pharma *NDC Code:* **58407**
Huckaby Pharmacal, Inc. **502-222-4700**
6316 Old Lagrange Road
Crestwood, KY 40014
Total Employees: 12
Ownership: PRIVATE
Federal Procurement Eligibility: Medicaid Rebate

Hudson *NDC Code:* **25077**
The Hudson Corporation **516-567-9500**
90 Orville Drive
Bohemia, NY 11716
Ownership: Nature's Bounty
Distribution: Manufacturer of Generics

Humco Holding Grp *NDC Code:* **00395**
Humco Holding Group Inc. **214-793-3174**
1008 Whitaker Street
Texarkana, TX 75501
Medical Product Sales Volume: $7,000,000
Total Employees: 70
Ownership: PRIVATE

Humphrey *see* Allergan

Hynson, Wescott, & Dunning *see* BD Microbiology

Hyrex Pharms *NDC Code:* **00314**
Hyrex Pharmaceuticals **901-794-9050**
3494 Democrat Road
Memphis, TN 38118
Medical Product Sales Volume: $2,200,000
Total Employees: 39
Ownership: PRIVATE *FAX:* 901-794-9051
Distribution: Specialty Manufacturer
CEO: Malcolm H. Baker/Chairman
James E. Baker/President
Frank Polk Baker/EVP
Marketing: James Segerson/Director, Sales
Federal Procurement Eligibility: Medicaid Rebate

ICI Americas *see* Zeneca

ICI Pharm *see* Zeneca Pharms

ICI Pharma *see* Zeneca Pharms

ICI Pharma PR *see* IPR

ICN Pharms *NDC Code:* **00187**
I.C.N. Pharmaceuticals, Inc. **714-545-0113**
3300 Hyland Avenue **800-548-5100**
Costa Mesa, CA 92626

ICN Pharms *(cont'd)*
Medical Product Sales Volume: $414,027,000
Total Employees: 5,858
Ownership: Public *FAX:* 714-641-7275
Distribution: Specialty Manufacturer
CEO: Milan Panic/Chairman
Adam Jerney/COO, Exectutive Vice President
David Watt/General Counsel
Marketing: J. Julian/SVP Worldwide Marketing
Production: Dr. Robert Little
Research: Devron Averett, PhD/SVP Research & Development
Humberto Fernandez, MD/VP Worldwide Clinical Regulatory Affairs
Cheri Jones/Dir Corporate Regulatory Affairs
Anil K. Hiteshi/Manager, Regulatory Affairs
Federal Procurement Eligibility: Medicaid Rebate
Medical Product Subsidiaries (Listed Separately):
ICN Galenika

IDE-Interstate *NDC Code:* **00814**
IDE Interstate **516-957-8300**
1500 New Horizons Blvd. **800-666-8100**
Amityville, NY 11701-1130
Medical Product Sales Volume: $60,000,000
Total Employees: 114
Ownership: PRIVATE *FAX:* 516-957-1678
Distribution: Distributor of Generics

Immunex *NDC Code:* **58406**
Immunex Corp. **206-587-0430**
51 University Street **800-466-8639**
Seattle, WA 98101
Medical Product Sales Volume: $156,600,000
Total Employees: 750
Ownership: Public *FAX:* 800-441-6303
Distribution: Biopharmaceutical Manufacturer
CEO: Edward V. Fritzky/Chairman & CEO
Leonard R. Stevens/SVP, Marketing
Scott G. Hallquist/SVP, General Counsel, & Secy.
Douglas G. Southern/SVP, Treasurer & CFO
Peggy V. Phillips/SVP, Pharmaceutical Development
Douglas E. Williams, PhD/SVP, Discovery Research
Production: Susan K. Erb/VP, Facilities & Materials
Research: F. Ann Hayes, MD/VP, Clinical Development
Federal Procurement Eligibility: Medicaid Rebate

Immuno-US *NDC Code:* **54129**
Immuno-U.S., Inc. **313-652-7872**
1200 Parkdale Rd.
Rochester, MI 48307-1744
Total Employees: 19
Ownership: PRIVATE
Distribution: Specialty Manufacturer
Federal Procurement Eligibility: Medicaid Rebate

Infinity Pharm *NDC Code:* **58154**
Infinity Pharmaceuticals
P.O. Box 939
Abita Spring, AL 70420
Ownership: PRIVATE

Insource *NDC Code:* **58441**
InSource, Inc. **703-688-4178**
Rt 2, P.O. Box 39 **800-366-3829**
Bland, VA 24315-0039
Medical Product Sales Volume: $20,000,000
Total Employees: 50
Ownership: PRIVATE *FAX:* 703-688-4962
Distribution: Specialty Distributor

Institute Merieux *NDC Code:* **P50361**
Institute Merieux
17 rue Bourgelat
Lyon 69002, FRANCE
Medical Product Sales Volume: $978,000,000
Total Employees: 6,760
Ownership: Rhone-Poulenc SA
Distribution: Manufacturer of Vaccines
CEO: Alain Merieux/President
Research: Caraux
Jean Caraux/Med Dir Immunoprotein
Nadine Roiron/Pharmacist Quality Assur
Medical Product Subsidiaries (Listed Separately):
Connaught

Interpharm *NDC Code:* **53746**
Interpharm Inc. **516-349-1731**
3 Fairchild Avenue
Plainview, NY 11803
Medical Product Sales Volume: $8,000,000
Total Employees: 52
Ownership: PRIVATE *FAX:* 516-349-0989
Distribution: Manufacturer of Generic Drugs
CEO: Bhupat Sutaria
Marketing: Robert Sutaria
Research: Dr. M. Sutaria
Federal Procurement Eligibility: Medicaid Rebate

Intl Ethical *NDC Code:* **11584**
International Ethical Laboratories Inc. **809-765-3510**
1021 Americo Miranda Ave Reparto
San Juan, PR 00921
Medical Product Sales Volume: $950,000
Total Employees: 11
Ownership: PRIVATE *FAX:* 809-767-1110
Distribution: Manufacturer of Respiratory Drugs
CEO: Sammy Diaz/President
Roberto Landron/Vice President, Treasurer

Intl Labs *NDC Code:* **00665**
International Laboratories Div. Solvay **404-578-2007**
901 Sawyer Road **800-241-1643**
Marietta, GA 30062

Intl Labs *(cont'd)*
Total Employees: 120
Ownership: Solvay Pharm
Distribution: Manufacturer of Generics
Federal Procurement Eligibility: Medicaid Rebate

Intl Medication *NDC Code:* **00548**
International Medication Systems Ltd. **818-442-6757**
1886 Santa Anita Avenue
South El Monte, CA 91733
Medical Product Sales Volume: $39,000,000
Total Employees: 675
Ownership: Medeva
Distribution: Manufacturer of Injectables
CEO: Randall Wall/President
Federal Procurement Eligibility: Medicaid Rebate

Intl Pharm Prod *see* Americal Pharm

Invamed *NDC Code:* **52189**
Invamed, Inc. **201-575-3303**
2400 Rt 130 North
Dayton, NJ 08810
Medical Product Sales Volume: $2,000,000
Total Employees: 25
Ownership: PRIVATE
Federal Procurement Eligibility: Medicaid Rebate

Inverness *see* Somerset

Inwood Labs *NDC Code:* **00258**
Inwood Laboratories **212-471-8000**
300 Prospect Street
Inwood, NY 11096
Total Employees: 65
Ownership: Forest Labs
Distribution: Distributor of Generics
Production: Robert Glickstein/VP Manufacturing
Richard S. Overton/VP Operations & Facilities
Federal Procurement Eligibility: Medicaid Rebate

Iolab *see* Ciba Vision

Ion *NDC Code:* **11808**
Ion Laboratories Inc. **817-589-7257**
7431 Pebble Dr. **800-666-0045**
Fort Worth, TX 76118-6945
Total Employees: 18
Ownership: PRIVATE *FAX:* 817-284-0531
Federal Procurement Eligibility: Medicaid Rebate

IPR *NDC Code:* **54921**
IPR Pharmaceuticals, Inc. **809-750-5353**
South Main Street
Carolina, PR 98419-1967
Medical Product Sales Volume: $4,000,000
Total Employees: 363
Ownership: Zeneca *FAX:* 809-750-5332
Distribution: Manufacturer of Generics
CEO: Ruben Freyre/President & Gen. Mgr
Marketing: Antonio Del Rosario/Commercial Dir
Production: Nelson Perez/Pharmaceutical Operations Director
Research: Shirley Suarez/Drug Regulatory Affairs
Federal Procurement Eligibility: Medicaid Rebate

Iso-Tex Dxs *NDC Code:* **50914**
Iso Tex Diagnostics, Inc. **713-482-1231**
P.O. Box 909 **800-477-4839**
Friendswood, TX 77546
Total Employees: 7
Ownership: PRIVATE *FAX:* 713-482-1070
CEO: Thomas J. Maloney/President

J and J Medcl *NDC Code:* **56091**
Johnson and Johnson Medical, Inc.
2500 Arbrook Blvd.
Arlington, TX 76004-3130
Ownership: PRIVATE

J J Balan *see* Balan

Jacobus Pharm *NDC Code:* **49938**
Jacobus Pharmaceutical Co. **609-921-7447**
37 Cleveland Lane
Princeton, NJ 08540
Total Employees: 12
Ownership: PRIVATE
Distribution: Specialty Manufacturer
Federal Procurement Eligibility: Medicaid Rebate

James Alexander *NDC Code:* **46414**
James Alexander Corporation **908-362-9266**
845 Rt 94
Blairstown, NJ 07825
Ownership: PRIVATE *FAX:* 908-362-5019

Janssen Phar *NDC Code:* **50458**
Janssen Pharmaceutica, Inc. **609-730-2000**
P.O. Box 200
Titusville, NJ 08560-0200
Medical Product Sales Volume: $1,050,000,000
Total Employees: 11,000
Ownership: Johnson & Johnson *FAX:* 908-524-9118
Distribution: Manufacturer of Branded Pharmaceuticals
CEO: Paul Janssen, MD,PhD/Chairman
Ronald Gelbman/Chairman
Paulo Costa/CEO
Larry G. Pickering/President
David R. Sheffield/VP, Finance
Marketing: David Roche/EVP Sales & Marketing
William Weldon/VP, Marketing

Janssen Phar *(cont'd)*
Karen McCormick/Group Product Dir, Office Prods.
Terence Downer/VP, Corporate Development
Mitch Walker/Consumer Marketing Director
Mark Perlotto/Product Mgr PROPULSID
Ellen McDonald/Product Mgr SPORANOX
Tom Anderson/Product Mgr RISPERDAL
David Mallegol/Dir Marketing Comm
John Reardon/Mgr Training & Devel.
Production: Diane Parks/VP Operations
Claudia Wolbach/Regulatory Affairs
Roy Cosan/Exec Dir, New Product Development
Henry Avallone/Exec Dir Reg Compliance
Research: Charles P Barranco/Mgr Clinical Research
Eva Chin Carey/Dir R&D Project Planning
Douglas N Dobak/Executive Dir Reg Affairs
Alice T M Hsuan/Vice President
Mark A Klausner/Dir Medical Affairs
Kenneth B Leahy/Exec Director Fin & Admin
Dorothy A Lowenhaupt/Mgr Clinical Operations
Tom Manion/Mgr Research Information Service
Carolyn E Maranca/Mgr Regulatory Affairs
Linda Roemer/Dir Science Information
Carol Slusser/Mgr Medical Writing
Ruth Wasserman/Director Reg Affairs
Federal Procurement Eligibility: Medicaid Rebate

JB Roerig *see* Roerig

Jerome Stevens *NDC Code:* **50564**
Jerome Stevens Pharmaceuticals, Inc **516-567-1113**
60 Da Vinci Drive
Bohemia, NY 11716
Ownership: PRIVATE
Distribution: Distributor/Manufacturer of Generics
Federal Procurement Eligibility: Medicaid Rebate

JJ Balan *see* Balan

Jmed *see* Jones Medical

JMI *see* Jones Medical

Johnson & Johnson *NDC Code:* **P00137**
Johnson & Johnson **908-524-0400**
One Johnson & Johnson Plaza
New Brunswick, NJ 08933
Medical Product Sales Volume: $21,620,000,000
Total Employees: 89,300
Ownership: Public *FAX:* 908-524-3300
Distribution: Manufacturer of Healthcare Products
CEO: Ralph S. Larsen/Chairman & CEO
Robert J. Darnetta/CFO
Roger S. Fine/Human Resources
Robert Wilson/Vice Chairman
Ronald Gelbman/Dir Pharm & Diagnostics
James Lenehan/Dir Consumer Pharm & Professional Group
Christian Koffman/Worldwide Chairman, Consumer & Personal Care Group
Robert Z. Gussin, PhD/VP Science & Technology
Roger S. Fine/VP Administration
Willard D. Nielsen/VP, Public Affairs
Medical Product Subsidiaries (Listed Separately):
Janssen Pharmaceutica
Lifescan
Neutrogena
Ortho Diagnostic Systems
Ortho/Mcneil Pharmaceutical

Jones Medical *NDC Code:* **52604, 00689**
Jones Medical Industries, Inc. **314-576-6100**
P.O. Box 46903
St Louis, MO 63146
Medical Product Sales Volume: $10,200,000
Total Employees: 508
Ownership: Public *FAX:* 314-469-5749
Distribution: Specialty Manufacturer
CEO: Dennis M. Jones/CEO
Judith A. Jones/CFO
Marketing: Michael T. Bramblett/Executive Vice President
Bruce Ashman/VP Sales & Marketing — Endocrine Products
Gerald Garner/VP Sales & Marketing — Hospital Products

Jordan Pharms *NDC Code:* **58196**
Jordan Pharmaceuticals, Inc.
20612 Canada Rd,
Lake Forest, CA 92630
Ownership: PRIVATE

K-V Pharm *see* KV Pharms

Kabi Pharmacia *see* Pharmacia & Upjohn

Kabi Vitrum *NDC Code:* **00601**
Kabi Vitrum, Inc. **919-553-3831**
P.O. Box 597
Clayton, NC 27520
Total Employees: 110
Ownership: Kabi Pharmacia AB
Distribution: Manufacturer of Branded Pharmaceuticals
Federal Procurement Eligibility: Medicaid Rebate
Medical Product Subsidiaries (Listed Separately):
Kabi Pharmacia

Kanetta *see* Sanofi Winthrop

Keene Pharms *NDC Code:* **00588**
Keene Pharmaceuticals, Inc. **817-645-8083**
303 South Mockingbird
Keene, TX 76059
Medical Product Sales Volume: $500,000
Total Employees: 5
Ownership: PRIVATE

Kendall Mcgaw *see* McGaw

Kenneth A Manne *NDC Code:* **10706**
Kenneth A. Manne Co.
P.O. Box 825
Johns Island, SC 29457-0825
Ownership: PRIVATE

Kenwood Labs *see* Bradley Pharms

Kenyon Drug *NDC Code:* **12535**
Kenyon Drug Inc. **319-363-9426**
P.O. Box 1546
Cedar Rapids, IA 52406
Ownership: PRIVATE

Key *see* Schering

King Pharm *see* General Inj & Vac

King Pharms *NDC Code:* **60793**
King Pharmaceuticals Inc. **615-989-8000**
501 Fifth Street **800-336-7783**
Bristol, TN 37620
Total Employees: 269
Ownership: Insource Williams *FAX:* 423-989-6232
Distribution: Manufacturer and distributor of generic and brand name drugs

Kingswood Labs *see* Century Pharms

Kirkman *NDC Code:* **00098**
Kirkman Laboratories, Inc. **503-245-4551**
5321 SW 33rd Dr.
Portland, OR 97201-1120
Medical Product Sales Volume: $500,000
Total Employees: 10
Ownership: PRIVATE *FAX:* 503-243-6815
CEO: Stanley N. Bachman/Chairman & President
Russell B. Swartz/VP
Marketing: Dr. Kenneth W. Gores/Director, New Products

Kirkman Sales *NDC Code:* **58223**
Kirkman Sales Company **503-694-1600**
P.O. Box 1009 **888-547-5626**
Wilsonville, OR 97070
Medical Product Sales Volume: $500,000
Total Employees: 8
Ownership: PRIVATE *FAX:* 503-682-0838
Distribution: Distributor of Fluoride
CEO: Ken Humphrey/CEO
James G. Hall/Vice President
Marketing: H. B. Humphrey
Production: Karleen Day
Federal Procurement Eligibility: Medicaid Rebate

Knoll Labs *NDC Code:* **00044**
Knoll Pharmaceutical Co. **800-526-1072**
199 Cherry Hill Road
Parsippany, NJ 07054
Medical Product Sales Volume: $190,000,000
Total Employees: 880
Ownership: BASF
Distribution: Manufacturer of Branded Pharmaceuticals
CEO: Gerald E. Bendele/President
Marketing: John L. Parsons, Jr./VP, Marketing and Sales
John Kalimtzis/Product Mgr ISOPTIN
Production: Robert W. Ashworth, PhD/Dir, Regulatory Affairs
Carl Zolna/Mgr Product Information
Research: Keiko Aogaichi/Director Cvim Research
Candis J Banks/Mgr Clinicla Research
Diana L Gowe/Info Specialist
Leonard G Marcoci Jr/Director M.I.S.
Andrea C Kay/Assist Dir Medical Onc & Imm
Theodore Kramer/Assoc Dir Internal Med
Joanne Lustig/Mgr Medical & Scientific Info
Beverly A Novrit/Assoc Dir Clinical Rsch
Mark D Pepper/Assoc Dir Medical Affairs
Steve G Svokos/VP Reg And Tech Affairs
Federal Procurement Eligibility: Medicaid Rebate

Knoll Pharms *NDC Code:* **00048**
Knoll Pharmaceutical Co. Div of BASF
199 Cherry Hill Road **800-526-1072**
Parsippany, NJ 07054
Ownership: BASF
Distribution: Manufacturer of Branded Pharmaceuticals
Federal Procurement Eligibility: Medicaid Rebate

Kodak *see* Eastman Kodak

Kraft Pharm *NDC Code:* **00796**
Kraft Pharmaceutical Company, Inc.
1442 Klosterman Avenue
Oreland, PA 19075
Ownership: PRIVATE

Kramer Labs *NDC Code:* **55505**
Kramer Laboratories, Inc. **305-223-1287**
8778 Southwest 8Th Street **800-824-4894**
Miami, FL 33174

Kramer Labs *(cont'd)*
Medical Product Sales Volume: $8,000,000
Total Employees: 5
Ownership: PRIVATE *FAX:* 305-223-5510
Distribution: Specialty Distributor
CEO: Guido Mendoza
Marketing: Gloria Rodriguez/Vice President

Kramer P I *NDC Code:* **52083**
Kramer Pharmacal, Inc. **305-594-0988**
3307 N.W. 74Th Avenue
Miami, FL 33122
Medical Product Sales Volume: $500,000
Total Employees: 5
Ownership: PRIVATE

Krasity Med *NDC Code:* **00736**
Krasity's Medical and Surgical Supply, Inc.
1825 Bailey St.
Dearborn, MI 48124
Ownership: PRIVATE

KV Pharms *NDC Code:* **10609**
KV Pharmaceutical Co. **314-645-6600**
2503 S. Hanley Road
St. Louis, MO 63144
Medical Product Sales Volume: $43,500,000
Total Employees: 400
Ownership: Public *FAX:* 314-645-6732
Distribution: Specialty Manufacturer
CEO: Victor Hermelin/Chairman
Marc S. Hermelin/V. Chairman
Ted Wood/President & CEO
M.I. Kirschner/VP
Gerald Mitchell/VP, Finance
Alan Johnson/Secy.
Raymond F. Chiostri/VP
Research: Hal Herring/Dir Quality Assurance

Labs Atral *NDC Code:* **53862**
Laboratorios Atral Sarl **203-637-8957**
36 Twin Lakes Lane
Riverside, CT 06878
Ownership: PRIVATE
Distribution: Specialty Manufacturer

Lafayette Pharms *NDC Code:* **59081**
Lafayette Pharmaceuticals Inc. **317-447-3129**
P.O. Box 4499 **800-428-7843**
Lafayette, IN 47903-4499
Total Employees: 60
Ownership: PRIVATE *FAX:* 317-447-6913
Distribution: Specialty Manufacturer
CEO: Herbert A. Hoebel/President & CEO
Marketing: Lynne Hamilton Lang/Vice President, Sales & Marketing
Robert A. Sharp/Vice President, Regulatory Affairs
Production: James E. Kudla/Plant Manager

Landry *NDC Code:* **00538**
713-528-0808
2405-A Smith Street
Houston, TX 77006
Total Employees: 6
Ownership: PRIVATE

Lannett *NDC Code:* **00527**
The Lannett Co., Inc. **215-333-9000**
9000 State Road
Philadelphia, PA 19136
Medical Product Sales Volume: $1,000,000
Total Employees: 40
Ownership: Public *FAX:* 215-333-9004
Distribution: Manufacturer of Generics
CEO: Barry Weisberg/President & CEO
William Farber/Chairman & President
Audrey Farber/Secretary & Treasurer
Federal Procurement Eligibility: Medicaid Rebate

Laser *NDC Code:* **00277**
Laser, Inc. **219-663-1165**
2200 West 97th Pl.
Crown Point, IN 46307
Total Employees: 13
Ownership: PRIVATE
CEO: Donald A. Laser/Chairman nad President
J.N. Allegretti, RPh/General Manager
Federal Procurement Eligibility: Medicaid Rebate

Lederle Parenterals *NDC Code:* **00205**
Lederle Parenterals, Inc. **914-733-5000**
Middletown Road **800-533-3753**
Pearl River, NY 10965
Ownership: Lederle Labs
Distribution: Manufacturer of Branded Pharmaceuticals
Federal Procurement Eligibility: Medicaid Rebate

Lederle Pharm *NDC Code:* **00005**
Lederle Pharmaceutical Div. American Cyanamid **914-732-5000**
170 Randor Chester Road; 2nd Floor **800-533-3753**
Saint Davids, PA 19087
Medical Product Sales Volume: $1,760,000,000
Total Employees: 25,000
Ownership: American Cyanamid
Distribution: Manufacturer of Branded Pharmaceuticals
CEO: Lawrence Tilton/President
Michael J. Marquard/VP & Gen. Mgr Lederle Labs
Frank C. Condella, Jr., RPh/VP Gen. Mgr Lederle Standard
Marketing: Armondo Anido/VP Anti-Infectives
Tim Catlatt/VP Cardiovascular

Lederle Pharm *(cont'd)*
Lisa Egbuonu-Davis/VP Public & Gov't. Affairs
George J. Vuturo PhD/VP Industry Affairs
Jeff Hoyak/Dir Public Affairs
Production: Harriet Kiltie, MD/VP Regulatory Affairs
Jerry Johnson, MD/Dir Scientific & Medical Services
Linda Marcy/Regulatory Affairs
Research: Peter A Ascione/Manager Drug Reg Affairs
Lawrence G Bassin/Dir Prod Surv/Epidemiolog
Andrea M Brillaud/Mgr Medical Services
Robert E Desjardins/VP Clinical Research
Claude P George/Dir Clinical Research
Eric R Jacoby/Planning Information Mgr
David H Mason Jr/VP Scientific Affairs/Med Dir
Harriet Laine/Mgr Medical Writing Services
Martin P Lefkowitz/Dir Clinical Development
Cindy M Mason/Dept Head Clinical Info
Vern G De Vries/Sr Dir Us Reg Affairs
Earl F Walker/Assist Dir For Labeling
Rona S Wasserman/Assoc Dir Medical Editorial
David H Wu/Dir Prof Medical Services
Federal Procurement Eligibility: Medicaid Rebate
Medical Product Subsidiaries (Listed Separately):
Lederle
Lederle Parenterals
Lederle Piperacillin
Lederle Standard
Praxis
Storz

Lederle Piperacillin *NDC Code:* **00206**
Lederle Piperacillin, Inc. **914-733-5000**
170 Radnor Chester Road **800-533-3753**
Saint Davids, PA 19087
Ownership: Lederle Labs
Distribution: Manufacturer of Branded Pharmaceuticals
Federal Procurement Eligibility: Medicaid Rebate

Lederle Standard *see* Lederle Pharm

Lederle-Praxis *NDC Code:* **53124**
Lederle-Praxis Biologicals Division **716-272-7000**
211 Bailey Road
West Henrietta, NY 14586-9728
Medical Product Sales Volume: $325,000,000
Total Employees: 170
Ownership: Lederle
Federal Procurement Eligibility: Medicaid Rebate

Lee Pharma *NDC Code:* **23558**
Lee Pharmaceuticals, Inc. **818-442-3141**
1444 Santa Anita Avenue
South El Monte, CA 91733
Medical Product Sales Volume: $13,380,000
Total Employees: 117
Ownership: Public *FAX:* 818-443-1561
Distribution: OEM Supplier
CEO: Dr. Henry Lee/Chairman
Ronald G. Lee/President
Michael Agresti/VP, Treasurer & Secretary

Lemax *NDC Code:* **23594**
Lemax Pharm. Corp. **305-598-2333**
6915 S. W. 92 Court
Miami, FL 33173
Medical Product Sales Volume: $100,000
Total Employees: 3
Ownership: PRIVATE

Lemmon *see* Teva

Leo Pharm *see* Lilly

Lilly *NDC Code:* **00002**
Eli Lilly and Co. **317-276-2000**
Lilly Corporate Center Drop Code 2542 **800-545-5979**
Indianapolis, IN 46285
Medical Product Sales Volume: $7,346,600,000
Total Employees: 29,200
Ownership: Public *FAX:* 317-276-6331
Distribution: Manufacturer of Branded Pharmaceuticals
CEO: Randall Tobias/President & CEO
Charles E. Golden/CFO
Richard D. Wood/Chairman
Earl B. Herr, Jr., PhD/EVP
Gene L. Step/EVP & Pres, Pharmaceutical Div.
Sidney Taurel/Lilly Pharm. Pres
Mitch Daniels/Pres N.A. Pharm.
Michael Hanson/Dir Internal Medical Unit
James Harper/Dir Endocrine Unit
Robert Postlethwait/Dir CNS Unit
William Ringo/Dir Anti-Infectives & Generic Drugs
Gino Santini/VP Corp Strategy & Bus Devel
Pedro P. Granadillo/Human Resources
Marketing: Eurelio M. Cavalier/Group VP Sales
Alan Clark/VP US Sales & Mktg
Gary Clark/VP Marketing Planning & Development
Robert A. Luginbill/GM Integrated Disease Mgt
Joe Burkett/Manager of Marketing Services
Mike Swearingen/Mgr Marketing Svcs
Jim Lancaster/Product Mgr PROZAC
Jack Tupman/Product Mgr LORABID
Lynn Dines/Product Mgr AXID
Jim Cusick/Product Mgr HUMULIN
Production: Joseph C. Cook, Jr./VP, Production Operations
Robert H. Williams, PhD/VP Quality & Environ.
Thomas Trainer/VP Information Technology
Research: Mel Perelman, PhD/EVP & President, Research
Thomas L. Emmick, PhD/VP Research
W. Leigh Thompson, PhD, MD/EVP Research
Jean A Allan/Clin Rsch Administrator
Carol M Andrejasich/Sr Clinical Resrch Admin
John A Bartley/Manager

Lilly *(cont'd)*
Sandra K Bower/Dept Head Creative Srvs
Douglas L Cocks/Mgr Corp Affairs Research
Carol J Fouts-Johnson/Dept Head Medical Plns & Chemo
S Michael Harrill/Manager Medical Plans
Donald G Hoffman/Head Toxicology Info
Martin D Hynes/Dir Quality Assur-R&D
Nancy L Langwith/Dir Medical Information Systems
John E Mccullough/Mgr Pharm Projects
Steven R Merten/Department Head
David J Miner/Head Pharm Regulatory Aff
Max W Talbott/Dir Medical Reg Affairs
W Leigh Thompson/Exec Vice President
Steven B Whittaker/Department Head
Federal Procurement Eligibility: Medicaid Rebate
Medical Product Subsidiaries (Listed Separately):
Dista
PCS Health Systems
Ranbaxy Pharm
STC Pharm

Liposome *NDC Code:* **61799**
The Liposome Company
1 Research Way
Princeton, NJ 08540
Ownership: PRIVATE

Liquipharm *NDC Code:* **54198**
Liquipharm, Inc. **310-558-3344**
10716 Mc Cune Ave.
Los Angeles, CA 90034
Total Employees: 18
Ownership: PRIVATE *FAX:* 310-558-8367
Distribution: Manufacturer of Generic Liquid Pharmaceuticals
CEO: Barry Sugarman/B.S. Engr/President
A.P. Bedrosian/Executive VP
Marketing: Sam Masters
Production: Jos'e Beristein
Federal Procurement Eligibility: Medicaid Rebate

Loch Pharm *see* Bedford Labs

Logen Pharm *NDC Code:* **00820**
Logen Pharmaceutical, Inc. **305-493-6487**
60 Pierces Road **800-252-8889**
Newburgh, NY 12550
Ownership: PRIVATE *FAX:* 305-493-6427
Federal Procurement Eligibility: Medicaid Rebate

Lorvic *NDC Code:* **00273**
Lorvic Corporation **314-524-7444**
8810 Frost Avenue
St Louis, MO 63134
Medical Product Sales Volume: $3,000,000
Total Employees: 92
Ownership: PRIVATE

Lotus *see* Fisons

Lotus Biochem *NDC Code:* **59417**
Lotus Biochemical Corporation
P.O. Box 3586 **800-355-6556**
Radford, VA 24143
Total Employees: 40
Ownership: PRIVATE *FAX:* 800-688-6625
Distribution: Specialty Manufacturer
Marketing: J. J. Link/VP Marketing

Lu Chem Pharmaceuticals, Inc. *see* H N Norton Co.

Luitpold *see* Am Regent

Lunsco *NDC Code:* **48534, 10892**
Lunsco, Inc. **703-980-4358**
Route 2 Box 62 **800-624-8614**
Pulaski, VA 24301
Ownership: Lunsco *FAX:* 703-980-4484

Lyne Labs *NDC Code:* **00374**
Lyne Laboratories **508-583-8700**
10 Burke Drive
Brockton, MA 02401
Total Employees: 50
Ownership: PRIVATE *FAX:* 508-583-9120
Distribution: Distributor/Manufacturer of Generics

Lyphomed *see* Fujisawa USA

Macnary *NDC Code:* **55982**
Macnary Ltd.
25000 Pitkin, Ste 130
Spring, TX 77386
Ownership: PRIVATE

Major Pharms *NDC Code:* **00904**
Major Pharmaceuticals Inc.
31778 Enterprise Dr.
Livonia, MI 48150
Medical Product Sales Volume: $110,000,000
Total Employees: 700
Ownership: Great Lakes
Distribution: Distributor of Generics
Marketing: Rita M. Clay/Marketing Adm.
Federal Procurement Eligibility: Medicaid Rebate
Medical Product Subsidiaries (Listed Separately):
Murray Drug
TX Drug Reps

Mallinckrodt *NDC Code:* **00406**
Mallinckrodt Inc. **314-530-2000**
16305 Swingley Ridge Drive **800-325-8888**
Chesterfield, MO 63017
Total Employees: 2,000
Ownership: PRIVATE
Distribution: Manufacturer of Branded and Generic Pharmaceuticals
CEO: C. Ray Holman/Chairman & CEO
Mack G. Nichols/COO
Michael J. Collins/President, Pharmaceutical Specialties Division
Daniel E. Wood/President, Industrial Specialties Division
Mike Milosovisch/President, Pharmaceutical Chemicals Division
Marketing: Tricia Wetzel/Pharmaceutical Specialties Div., National Account Manager
Production: Richard Hoyt/General Mngr., Manufacturing, Specialty Products
Research: Carl O. Quicksall/VP, Science & Technology
Medical Product Subsidiaries (Listed Separately):
Baker

Mallinckrodt Medcl *NDC Code:* **00019**
Mallinckrodt Medical, Inc. **314-895-2000**
675 McDonnell Boulevard **800-822-2075**
St. Louis, MO 63134
Medical Product Sales Volume: $1,010,000,000
Total Employees: 4,790
Ownership: Imcera *FAX:* 314-895-7225
Distribution: Manufacturer of Diagnostic/Imaging Agents
CEO: C.R. (Ray) Holman/President & CEO
William J. Mercer/SVP and Group Executive
Robert G. Moussa/SVP and Group Executive
J. Eugene Fox/SVP, Science & Technology
Thomas R. Trotter/VP, GM, Mallin. Sensor Systems
Charles R. Clark/VP, GM, Anesthesiology
David Morra/Vice President, GM, Cardiology
Peter Vermeeren/VP, General Manager-Nuclear Medical
James C. Carlile/VP, General Manager-Radiology
Marketing: Richard Martin/Director, Marketing-Nuclear Medical
John Q. Hesemann/Director Marketing-Radiology
Patrick W. Coleman/Director, Marketing-Anesthesia
Production: Robert F. Ingham/Manager, Product Registrations
Research: R.A. Virage/Director, Research and Development
Donald Lankin/Assoc Dir Intl Clinical Rsch

Manufac Chems *NDC Code:* **00148**
Manufacturing Chemists **317-823-6878**
5767 Thunderbird Road
Indianapolis, IN 46236
Ownership: PRIVATE
Distribution: Manufacturers of Pharmaceuticals

Marion Labs *see* Hoechst Marion Roussel

Marion Merrell Dow *see* Hoechst Marion Roussel

Marlop Pharms *NDC Code:* **12939**
Marlop Pharmaceuticals, Inc. **212-796-1570**
P.O. Box 536
Bronx, NY 10471
Total Employees: 3
Ownership: PRIVATE
Federal Procurement Eligibility: Medicaid Rebate

Marnel Pharceut *NDC Code:* **00682**
Marnel Pharmaceuticals, Inc. **318-232-1396**
206 Luke Drive
Lafayette, LA 70506
Total Employees: 5
Ownership: PRIVATE *FAX:* 318-232-1491
Distribution: Specialty Brand Distributor
Marketing: Juliet McKay
Federal Procurement Eligibility: Medicaid Rebate

Marsam *NDC Code:* **00209**
Marsam Pharmaceuticals Inc. **609-424-5600**
P.O. Box 1022
Cherry Hill, NJ 08003
Medical Product Sales Volume: $30,000,000
Total Employees: 108
Ownership: Schein *FAX:* 609-751-8784
Distribution: OEM Manufacturer of Generic Injectables
CEO: Marvin Samson/President
Judith U. Arnoff, RPh/VP
Robert A. St. Pierre/CPA, Controller
Marketing: E. T. Lillard/VP Sales
Edward J. Moylan, RPh/Dir Business Devel.
Production: Howard C. Zell, PhD/Dir Regulatory Affairs
Andrew B. Samson/Purchasing Director
Dennis M. Barnoski/Dir Manufacturing
William H. Miele, PhD/Mgr Quality Assurance
Research: Fakral Sayeed, PhD/VP Scientific Affairs

Martec Pharms *NDC Code:* **52555**
Martec Pharmaceuticals, Inc. **816-241-4144**
1800 North Topping Ave. **800-822-6782**
Kansas City, MO 64120
Total Employees: 25
Ownership: Ratiopharm Gmbh/Mepha AG *FAX:* 816-483-5432
Distribution: Distributer/Manufacturer of Generic Pharmaceuticals
CEO: Richard G. Spears/President
Klaus Lichtenberger/Executive VP
Dave McMillin/Dir of Operations
Marketing: Sara J. Miller/VP, Marketing
Production: Paul T. Sudhaker/Scientific Affairs
Federal Procurement Eligibility: Medicaid Rebate

Mason Distbtrs *NDC Code:* **11845**
Mason Distributors, Inc. **305-624-5557**
5105 Northwest 159th Street **800-327-6005**
Hialeah, FL 33014

Mason Distbtrs *(cont'd)*
Medical Product Sales Volume: $35,000,000
Total Employees: 200
Ownership: PRIVATE *FAX:* 800-328-3944
Distribution: Distributor of Generics
CEO: Carlos Rodriguez/President
Marketing: Sonia Rodriguez
Production: Cary Gonzalez
Federal Procurement Eligibility: Medicaid Rebate

Mason Pharms *NDC Code:* **12758**
Mason Pharmaceuticals, Inc.
6578 Willowbrae Way
Sacremento, CA 95831
Total Employees: 15
Ownership: Mason Dist
CEO: M.C. Horning, Jr./President
Marketing: Angela Horning/Director of Marketing

Mass Biol Labs *NDC Code:* **14362**
Mass. Public Health Bio. Lab. **617-983-6400**
305 South Street
Jamaica Plain, MA 02130
Ownership: PRIVATE
Research: Ann Dodds-Frerichs/Regulatory Affair Manager
Federal Procurement Eligibility: Medicaid Rebate

Mayrand Pharms *NDC Code:* **00259**
Mayrand Pharmaceuticals **910-761-5075**
4 Dundas Circle **800-334-0514**
Greenburo, NC 27407
Medical Product Sales Volume: $5,000,000
Total Employees: 65
Ownership: Goody's Manufacturing *FAX:* 910-723-1897
Distribution: Specialty Manufacturer
CEO: Robert G. Boulton/Chairman and President
Marketing: James Rose/Director, Marketing
Production: Ed Pyatte/Director, Production
Larry Diesbach/Dir Quality Compliance
Research: Robert P. Halliday,PhD/EVP, Research
Federal Procurement Eligibility: Medicaid Rebate

McGaw *see* Gensia Labs

McGaw *NDC Code:* **00264**
McGaw, Inc. **714-660-2000**
P.O. Box 19791
Irvine, CA 92714-9791
Medical Product Sales Volume: $309,400,000
Total Employees: 2,000
Ownership: Ivax
Distribution: Manufacturer of IV Solutions
CEO: James Sweeney/Chairman
Norwick Godspeed/President
Marketing: Edward Quilty/VP Sales & Marketing
Production: Diane Gerst/Manager, Regulatory Affairs

McGregor *NDC Code:* **11089**
Mc Gregor Pharmaceuticals **813-530-4361**
8420 Ulmerton Road, Suite 408
Largo, FL 34641
Medical Product Sales Volume: $75,000
Total Employees: 3
Ownership: PRIVATE *FAX:* 813-530-5569

McGuff *NDC Code:* **49072**
Mc Guff Company, Inc. **714-545-2491**
3629 West Mac Arthur 202
Santa Ana, CA 92704
Medical Product Sales Volume: $3,000,000
Total Employees: 13
Ownership: PRIVATE *FAX:* 714-540-5614
Distribution: Distributer of Generics
CEO: Ronald M. McGuff/President
Marketing: R. Scott Nixon/Sales Manager

McKesson Medalist *NDC Code:* **37937**
McKesson Medalist **415-983-8300**
One Post Street
San Francisco, CA 94104
Ownership: McKesson
Distribution: Distributor of Generics

McKesson Valu-Rite *NDC Code:* **49348**
McKesson Valu-Rite **415-983-8300**
One Post Street
San Francisco, CA 94104
Ownership: McKesson
Distribution: Distributor of Generics

McNeil Lab *NDC Code:* **00045**
McNeilab Inc.
Rt. 202 South
Raritan, NJ 08869
Medical Product Sales Volume: $900,000,000
Total Employees: 8,000
Ownership: Johnson & Johnson
Distribution: Manufacturer of Branded Pharmaceuticals
CEO: Thomas E. Nystrom/VP, Finance
Marketing: Thomas L. Bishop/Exec Dir, Product Management
Production: William F. O'Brien/VP Operations
Research: Melvin R. Toews, MD/VP, Scientific Affairs
Edward G Brann/Mgr Regulatory Affairs
Allyne Z Cheifet/Mgr Regulatory Affairs
Vivian A Chester/Exec Dir Reg Affairs
Jose F Gonzalez/Exec Dir Medical Services
Helen J Hohman/Manager Information Services
Gary P Horowitz/Sr Dir Regulatory Affairs
Barbara H Korberly/Director Medical Affairs
Sherry L Montgomery/Dir Scientific Information Resources
J Ellen Scheel/Mgr Medical Communication

McNeil Lab *(cont'd)*
Diane C Shaffer/Mgr Library & Information Svs
Patricia E Stewart/VP Research & Development
Anthony R Temple/Exec Dir Medical Affairs
Federal Procurement Eligibility: Medicaid Rebate

MCR/American Pharma *see* Am Pharms

MD Pharm *NDC Code:* **43567**
M D Pharmaceutical Inc. **714-556-3941**
3501 West Garry Avenue
Santa Ana, CA 92704
Medical Product Sales Volume: $130,000,000
Total Employees: 65
Ownership: Medeva plc *FAX:* 714-556-0315
Distribution: Manufacturer of Generics
CEO: Edward Griffith
Marketing: Mark S. Bursack/Sales & Mktg Director
Federal Procurement Eligibility: Medicaid Rebate

ME Pharm *NDC Code:* **58607**
ME Pharmaceuticals Inc. **317-962-4410**
P.O. Box 565
Richmond, IN 47375
Total Employees: 19
Ownership: Vesco
Distribution: Manufacturer of Vitamins

Mead Johnson *see* Bristol-Myers Squibb

Mead Johnson *NDC Code:* **00015**
Mead Johnson and Co.
P.O. Box 4000
Princeton, NJ 08543-4000
Medical Product Sales Volume: $1,000,000,000
Total Employees: 10,000
Ownership: Bristol-Myers Squibb
Distribution: Manufacturer of Chemotherapy Products
Federal Procurement Eligibility: Medicaid Rebate

Med Derm Pharms *NDC Code:* **45565**
Med Derm Pharmaceuticals Inc. **615-477-3991**
P.O. Box 5193
Kingsport, TN 37663
Ownership: PRIVATE
Federal Procurement Eligibility: Medicaid Rebate

Med Tech System *NDC Code:* **57424**
Medical Technology Systems, Inc. **813-576-6311**
12920 N. Automobile Blvd.
Clearwater, FL 34622
Total Employees: 5
Ownership: PRIVATE

Med Tek Pharms *NDC Code:* **52349**
Med Tek Pharmaceuticals **901-853-5333**
721 Chaney Cove
Collierville, TN 38017
Medical Product Sales Volume: $500,000
Total Employees: 9
Ownership: Cord *FAX:* 901-853-5339
Distribution: Specialty Manufacturer
CEO: Dan H. DeLoach
Federal Procurement Eligibility: Medicaid Rebate

Medcl Prods Labs *NDC Code:* **10733**
Medical Products Laboratories, Inc. **215-677-2700**
9990 Global Road **800-523-0191**
Philadelphia, PA 19115
Medical Product Sales Volume: $5,000,000
Total Employees: 150
Ownership: PRIVATE *FAX:* 215-677-7736
Distribution: Manufacturer of Dental Pharmaceutical
CEO: Dr. H.G. Stone/Secretary
Production: Arun Patel/Q.A. Manager

Medcl Prods Panamerc *NDC Code:* **00576**
Medical Products Panamerica, Inc. **305-545-6524**
647 West Flagler Street
Miami, FL 33130
Ownership: PRIVATE

Medco Lab *NDC Code:* **11940**
Medco Lab., Inc. **712-255-8770**
716 West 7Th Street
Sioux City, IA 51102-0864
Ownership: PRIVATE *FAX:* 712-255-4064
Distribution: Distributor of Topical Pharmaceuticals
CEO: William Winckler/President

Medco Supply *NDC Code:* **00764**
Medco Supply Co., Inc. **317-282-6112**
705 South Nichols Avenue
Muncie, IN 47303
Medical Product Sales Volume: $2,000,000
Total Employees: 8
Ownership: PRIVATE

Medeva Pharms *NDC Code:* **53014**
Medeva Pharmaceuticals, Inc. **817-545-7791**
4550 Buckingham Road
Fort Worth, TX 76155
Total Employees: 375
Ownership: Medeva plc *FAX:* 817-354-7820
Distribution: Specialty Manufacturer
CEO: Bruce W. Simpson/President & CEO
Marketing: Tom Parker/VP, Sales and Marketing
Production: Ray Iankowski/Dir, Regulatory Affairs
Federal Procurement Eligibility: Medicaid Rebate

Medi Physics *NDC Code:* **17156**
Medi Physics, Inc. DBA Amersham Healthcare **708-593-6300**
2636 S. Clearbrook Dr. **800-323-0668**
Arlington Heights, IL 60005
Medical Product Sales Volume: $20,000,000
Total Employees: 100
Ownership: Amersham *FAX:* 708-593-8236
Distribution: Manufacturer of Radiopharmaceuticals
CEO: Alan F. Herbert/President
Marketing: John McCarthy/VP Sales & Mktg
Production: Thomas Springer/Dir Ops
Research: Dr. Peter Knox/Dir R&D

Medi-Plex Pharm *NDC Code:* **59010**
Medi-Plex Pharmaceuticals, Inc. **804-527-1950**
3981 Deep Rock Rd
Richmond, VA 23233
Medical Product Sales Volume: $500,000
Total Employees: 19
Ownership: ECR Pharm *FAX:* 804-527-1959
Distribution: Distributor of Branded Generics
CEO: E. C. Robins, Jr.
Davis Caskey/Pharm Ops

Medi-Rx Pharm *NDC Code:* **00645**
Medi Rx Pharmaceutical, Inc.
45 North Palmer
Houston, TX 77003
Ownership: PRIVATE

Medicis *NDC Code:* **99207**
Medicis Pharmaceutical Corp. **602-808-8800**
4343 E. Camelback Rd., Suite 250 **800-845-1313**
Phoenix, AZ 85018
Medical Product Sales Volume: $25,300,000
Total Employees: 157
Ownership: Public *FAX:* 602-808-0822
Distribution: Developer and Marketer of Dermatologicals
CEO: Jonah Shacknai/Chairman & CEO
Mark A. Prygocki, Sr./CFO & Secretary
Adriane Carlino/Human Resources
Marketing: Pamela J. Doyle/VP
Ralph Bohrer/VP Sales
Production: Joseph Cooper/VP
Research: Eugene H. Gans, PhD/Chair, Central Research Com.
Federal Procurement Eligibility: Medicaid Rebate

Medimmune *NDC Code:* **60574**
MedImmune Inc. **301-417-0770**
35 West Watkins Mill Road
Gaithersburg, MD 20878
Medical Product Sales Volume: $16,200,000
Total Employees: 254
Ownership: Public *FAX:* 301-527-4200
Distribution: Biotech Development Company
CEO: Wayne T. Hockmeyer, PhD/Chairman & CEO
David M. Mott/President & COO
Franklin H. Top, Jr/EVP & Medical Director
Marketing: David P. Wright/EVP, Sales and Marketing
Research: James F. Young, PhD/SVP, Research & Development
Bogdan Dziurzynski/SVP Reg Affairs & Quality Assur

Medirex *NDC Code:* **57480**
Medirex, Inc. **201-227-4774**
20 Chapin Road Unit H, P.O. Box 731
Pine Brook, NJ 07058
Medical Product Sales Volume: $1,000,000
Total Employees: 19
Ownership: Sidmak Labs *FAX:* 201-227-0779
Distribution: Distributor of Generics
CEO: Eric Sorensen/President
Marketing: Gary Mauldin/Sales Manager
Production: Robert Cushman/VP, Operations
Federal Procurement Eligibility: Medicaid Rebate

Medtronic *NDC Code:* **58281**
Medtronic Inc. **612-572-5000**
800 53rd Ave. N.E.
Minneapolis, MN 55421
Medical Product Sales Volume: $600,000,000
Total Employees: 8,314
Ownership: Public
Distribution: Manufacturer of Pacemakers
CEO: W. R. Wallin/Chairman
W. W. George/President & CEO

Melville *NDC Code:* **13143**
Melville Biologics **516-752-8754**
155 Duryea Road
Melville, NY 11741
Medical Product Sales Volume: $31,000,000
Total Employees: 150
Ownership: Medimmune
Distribution: Manufacturer of Blood Products
Federal Procurement Eligibility: Medicaid Rebate

Mepha AG *see* Martec Pharms

Merck *NDC Code:* **00006**
Merck and Company, Inc.
1 Merck Drive **800-672-6372**
Whitehouse Station, NJ 08889-0100
Medical Product Sales Volume: $6,550,500,000
Total Employees: 34,400
Ownership: Merck & Co
Distribution: Manufacturer of Branded Pharmaceuticals
CEO: David Anstice/Pres US Human Health
Keith Yothers/Bus. Mgr U.S. Human Health

Merck *(cont'd)*
Marketing: Michael Thomas/VP U.S. Human Health
Jerome C. Keller/VP Sales
J. Martin Carroll/VP Sales Human Health
Richard J. Glaser/VP Marketing, Vaccine Div.
Mary McKinney/Sr. Dir Innovation & Ops.
Jeffrey Holladay, MD/Health Education & Alliance Devel.
Matt Bennett/Dir Marketing Comm.
M. Skoien/Product Mgr VASOTEC
Jay Galeota/Product Mgr ZOCOR
S. Vignau/Product Mgr MEVACOR
Gail Ryan/Mgr Editorial Services
Production: James P. Hoffman, MD/VP Medical Services
Robert H. Hunter,R.Ph.,PhD/Dir Pharmacy Affairs
Roy W. Walker/Mgr Scientific Information
Research: Eve Slater, MD/SVP Clinical & Regulatory Devel.
Ivan L. Rubin/Exec Dir Bus. Strategy & Research
William B Abrams/Exec Dir Scientific Dev
Frances B Alvarez/Sr Labeling Documen Coord
Susan Schramm Apple/Sr Promotion Mgr
Douglas Archer/Assoc Dir/Promotion Mgmt
Elliott T Berger/Sr Dir Regulatory Affairs
Roger G Berlin/Executive Director
David W Blois/Exec Dir Reg Affairs
Scott A Bolenbaugh/Dir Health Economics
Bram Greenberg, MD/Exec Dir Medical Services
Dennis M Gross/Dir Strategic Planning
Charles C Leighton/Sr VP Admin/Scientific Pol
James T Molt/Dir Regulatory Affairs
Gail A Ryan/Mgr Editorial Services
Federal Procurement Eligibility: GSA Contract Medicaid Rebate

Merck Sharp & Dohme *see* Merck

Merieux *see* Institute Merieux

Merit Pharms *NDC Code:* **30727**
Merit Pharmaceuticals **213-227-4831**
2611 San Fernando Road **800-421-9657**
Los Angeles, CA 90065
Ownership: PRIVATE *FAX:* 213-227-4833

MGI Pharma *see* MGI Pharma

MGI Pharma *NDC Code:* **58063**
MGI Pharma, Inc. **612-935-7335**
9900 Bren Rd. East, Suite 300E Opus Center
Minnetonka, MN 55343
Medical Product Sales Volume: $4,300,000
Total Employees: 63
Ownership: Public *FAX:* 612-935-0468
Distribution: Specialty Manufacturer
CEO: Charles N. Blitzer/Chairman
Charles C. Muscoplat/EVP
James V. Adam/C.F.O.
Lori-jean Gille/Gen'l Counsel & Secretary
Jon C. Lee/VP, Sales & Mktg
Research: Susan Gallagher/Dir Clinical Development
Robin Dawe/Dir Product Development
John R. MacDonald/Dir Preclinical Pharm/Toxicology
Federal Procurement Eligibility: Medicaid Rebate

MGP *see* Morton Grove

Mikart *NDC Code:* **46672**
Mikart, Inc. **404-351-4510**
1750 Chattahoochee Avenue NW
Atlanta, GA 30318
Medical Product Sales Volume: $22,000,000
Total Employees: 165
Ownership: PRIVATE *FAX:* 404-350-0432
Distribution: Manufacturer of Generics
CEO: Miguel Arteche/President
Marketing: Cerie McDonald/EVP
Federal Procurement Eligibility: Medicaid Rebate

Miles *NDC Code:* **00161**
Miles Inc. **203-937-2000**
400 Morgan Lane
West Haven, CT 06516
Ownership: Public
Distribution: Manufacturer of Branded Pharmaceuticals
Federal Procurement Eligibility: Medicaid Rebate

Miles Allergy *see* Miles Spokane

Miles Pharmaceuticals *see* Bayer

Miles Spokane *NDC Code:* **00118**
Miles Inc. **509-489-5656**
400 Morgan Lane
West Haven, CT 06516
Ownership: Miles
CEO: Anthony Bonanzino/Director Operations
Federal Procurement Eligibility: Medicaid Rebate

Miles/Schein *see* Schein Pharm (US)

Milex Prod *NDC Code:* **00396**
Milex Products, Inc. **773-631-6484**
5915-21 Northwest Highway
Chicago, IL 60631
Total Employees: 245
Ownership: PRIVATE *FAX:* 773-631-8156
Distribution: Specialty Manufacturer - International Distribution
CEO: H.T. Milgrom/President
Marketing: Robert Shaw/VP, Sales Manager
Research: William Jeffries/Director, Research and Development

Millgood *NDC Code:* **53118**
Millgood Laboratories, Inc. **404-377-6538**
250 D Arizona Avenue, P.O. Box 170159
Atlanta, GA 30317
Total Employees: 4
Ownership: PRIVATE

Minette Pharm *NDC Code:* **10760**
Minette Pharmaceutical Corporation **716-834-1353**
2930 Genesse Street, P.O. Box 142
Buffalo, NY 14225
Ownership: PRIVATE
CEO: Charles McGuire/President

Misemer *NDC Code:* **00276**
417-881-0660
4553 South Campbell
Springfield, MO 65807
Total Employees: 11
Ownership: PRIVATE
Distribution: Speciality Manufacturer
CEO: Bill Hawkins/President

Mission Pharma *NDC Code:* **00178**
Mission Pharmacal Company **210-696-8400**
P.O. Box 786099 **800-531-3333**
San Antonio, TX 78278-6099
Ownership: PRIVATE *FAX:* 210-696-6010
Distribution: Branded Pharmaceuticals, Topicals, Vitamins & Nutritional Supplements
Marketing: Mike Schwartz/OTC National Sales Manager
Dan Kibbe/Pharmaceutical National Sales Manager
Michael Hausig/International Sales

MMS *NDC Code:* **52891**
Medical Market Specialties **201-239-3915**
P.O.Box 307
Cedar Grove, NJ 07009
Ownership: PRIVATE
Federal Procurement Eligibility: Medicaid Rebate

Modulus-III *NDC Code:* **53127**
Modulus I I I Inc. **203-938-3916**
10 Sunny View Drive
Redding, CT 06896
Ownership: PRIVATE

Moleculon *see* Faulding Pharm (US)

Monarch *NDC Code:* **61570**
Monarch Pharmaceuticals **800-776-3637**
355 Beecham Street
Bristol, TN 37620
Ownership: PRIVATE

Monsanto *NDC Code:* **P00014**
Monsanto Company **314-694-1000**
800 North Lindberg Blvd.
St. Louis, MO 63167
Medical Product Sales Volume: $1,531,000,000
Total Employees: 33,797
Ownership: Public
Distribution: Chemical Manufacturer
CEO: Robert B. Shapiro/President
Research: Denis Forster
Medical Product Subsidiaries (Listed Separately):
Searle

Morton Grove *NDC Code:* **60432**
Morton Grove Pharmaceuticals, Inc.
6451 West Main Street **800-346-6854**
Morton Grove, IL 60053
Total Employees: 130
Ownership: PRIVATE *FAX:* 847-967-5607
Distribution: Distributor of Liquid Generics
CEO: Brian Tambi/President, CEO, Chairman
Marketing: Carol J. Englen/Director, Sales & Marketing
Production: Louis E. Windecker/EVP
Research: William Henderscott, PhD/SVP, Scientific Affairs

Mova Pharms *NDC Code:* **55370**
Mova Pharmaceutical Corporation
P.O. Box 8639
Caguas, PR 00726
Ownership: PRIVATE

MS&D *see* Merck

MSD *see* Merck

Muro Pharm *NDC Code:* **00451**
Muro Pharmaceutical, Inc. **508-851-5981**
890 East Street
Tewksbury, MA 01876
Medical Product Sales Volume: $70,000,000
Total Employees: 300
Ownership: PRIVATE *FAX:* 508-851-7346
Distribution: Manufacturer of Branded Respiratory Products
CEO: George D. Behrakis/President, CEO
Erene Koukias/CFO
Brant Sayre/Director, Operations
Marketing: Peter R. Allen/Dir, Sales and Marketing
Dennis Mc Enaney/Advertising & Sales promotion
David Benn
Ellie Sullivan Eckhoff/Exhibit Manager
Kenneth Morse/Sales Director
Research: Joseph A Celona/Dir Regulatory Affairs
Federal Procurement Eligibility: Medicaid Rebate

Murray Drug *NDC Code:* **00150**
Murray Drug Corp. **502-753-6654**
415 South 4Th St.
Murray, KY 42071
Ownership: Major Pharm

Mutual Pharm *NDC Code:* **53489**
Mutual Pharmaceutical Company, Inc. **215-288-6500**
1100 Orthodox Street **800-523-3684**
Philadelphia, PA 19124-3131
Total Employees: 240
Ownership: United Res Labs *FAX:* 215-288-6559
Distribution: Manufacturer of Generics
CEO: Richard H. Roberts, MD, PhD/President
Robert Love/SVP Finance and Administration
Production: Donald Evans/SVP Operations
Robert Dettery/VP, Regulatory Affairs
Research: John Poole/SVP of Quality
Federal Procurement Eligibility: Medicaid Rebate

MY-K Labs *see* Rosemont

Mylan *NDC Code:* **00378**
Mylan Pharmaceuticals **304-599-2595**
P.O. Box 4310 **800-826-9526**
Morgantown, WV 26504
Medical Product Sales Volume: $392,860,000
Total Employees: 2,000
Ownership: Public *FAX:* 412-232-0123
Distribution: Manufacturer of Generics
CEO: Milan Puskar/Chairman & CEO - Mylan Labs
C.B. Todd/Pres Mylan Pharm.
Louis J. DeBone/EVP
John P. O'Donnell, PhD/EVP
Marketing: Robert Sanzen/VP Marketing Sales
Production: Charles H. Crunkleton/VP Manufacturing
Byron Witt/VP Quality Control
Richard Stupar/VP Purchasing
Research: Cheryl D. Blume, PhD/VP Scientific Affairs
Federal Procurement Eligibility: Medicaid Rebate
Medical Product Subsidiaries (Listed Separately):
Somerset
Dow Hickam
UDL Labs
Bertek

N Am Biologicals *NDC Code:* **59730**
NABI (North American Biologicals, Inc. **305-625-5303**
16500 N.W. 15th Avenue **800-458-4244**
Miami, FL 33169
Medical Product Sales Volume: $200,000,000
Total Employees: 2,000
Ownership: PRIVATE *FAX:* 305-625-0925
Distribution: Manufacturer of Blood Plasma Components
CEO: David Gury/President
Medical Product Subsidiaries (Listed Separately):
Univax

Nastech Pharm *NDC Code:* **A00094**
Nastech Pharmaceutical Company, Inc. **516-273-0101**
129 Oser Avenue
Hauppauge, NY 11788
Medical Product Sales Volume: $765,000
Total Employees: 10
Ownership: Public *FAX:* 516-273-0252
Distribution: Developer of Nasal Delivery Technology
CEO: Dr. Vincent Romeo/President & CEO
Research: William E. Gannon, Jr., MD/Dir of Medical Affairs

Nelson Pharm *NDC Code:* **55437**
612-542-3232
3101 Louisiana Ave. North
Minneapolis, MN 55424
Ownership: Paddock Labs

Nephro-Tech *NDC Code:* **59528**
Nephro-Tech, Inc.
Ownership: PRIVATE

Nephron *NDC Code:* **00487**
Nephron Pharmaceuticals Corporation **407-246-1389**
4121 34th Street
Orlando, FL 32811-6458
Medical Product Sales Volume: $1,000,000
Total Employees: 12
Ownership: PRIVATE *FAX:* 407-872-0001
Distribution: Manufacturer of Generic Inhalants
CEO: Steven F. Simmons/President
Production: Raul Lugo Jr./Manager

Neutrogena *NDC Code:* **10812**
Neutrogena Corp. **213-642-1150**
55760 West 96th Street **800-421-6857**
Los Angeles, CA 90045
Medical Product Sales Volume: $280,000,000
Total Employees: 840
Ownership: PRIVATE *FAX:* 213-337-5564
Distribution: Manufacturer of Toiletries
CEO: Lloyd Costen/Chairman & CEO
Dr. Mitchell Wortzman/Pres Dermatology Division
Marketing: Lori H. Bush/VP Mktg

Newton Indust *NDC Code:* **17113**
Newton Industries INC. **201-383-2332**
1 Hicks Avenue
Newton, NJ 07860
Total Employees: 50
Ownership: PRIVATE *FAX:* 201-383-3268

Newton Indust *(cont'd)*
Marketing: Luis M. Fernandez

Nexagen *see* Nexstar

Nexstar *NDC Code:* **56146**
NeXstar Pharmaceuticals, Inc. **303-546-7793**
2860 Wilderness Place
Boulder, CO 80301
Medical Product Sales Volume: $62,426,000
Total Employees: 543
Ownership: Public *FAX:* 303-444-0672
Distribution: OEM Supplier
CEO: Patric Mahaffy/President & CEO
Larry Gold, PhD/Chief Scientific Officer
M.E. Hart/VP & CFO
Paul G. Schmidt/VP, Drug Delivery Research
Ray Bendele/VP, Life Sciences
Mike Burke/VP, Business Development
Adam Cochran/VP & General Counsel
Bruce Eaton/VP, Research Chemistry (Medicinal)
Barbara Kazmier/VP, Human Resources
Barry Polisky/VP, Drug Discovery (Research operations)
Crispin Eley/VP, Pharmaceutical Operations
Dave Flamberg/VP, Compliance
Marketing: John F. Hannon/Director of Marketing
Barry Herron/VP, Sales & Marketing
Research: Nicole Myers/VP, Clinical Development
Stephen Campbell/Dir Reg Affairs/Adverse Effects
Linda Chaplin/Mgr Clinical Data Monitor
Deloris Secor/Mgr Documentation Control
Linda Schindler/Clinical Trials Liason
Phil Rutledge/Clinical Trials Liason
Regina Olsen-Raine/Clinical Trials Liason

NMC Laboratories *see* Alpharma

NMC Labs *NDC Code:* **23317**
N.M.C. Laboratories **718-326-1500**
70-36 83rd Street
Glendale, NY 11385
Total Employees: 150
Ownership: AL Labs *FAX:* 718-894-3218
Distribution: Manufacturer of Topicals
CEO: George S. Barrett/President & COO
Marketing: Frank C. Condella, Jr./VP Sales
Production: John B. de Brun, Jr./VP Operations
Ernesto Pulga/Regulatory Affairs Associate
Federal Procurement Eligibility: Medicaid Rebate

Nomax *NDC Code:* **51801**
Nomax, Inc. **314-961-2500**
40 North Rock Hill Road
St. Louis, MO 63119
Total Employees: 50
Ownership: PRIVATE *FAX:* 314-961-8923
Distribution: Specialty Manufacturer
CEO: C.L. Voellinger/Chairman & President
Marketing: Robert E. Hess/Director of Marketing
Production: Larry Jeske/Director of Production
Research: John Rogers, MD/Director of Research

Nordisk USA *see* Novo Nordisk Pharm

Northampton Medical *see* UCB Pharma Pharma Pharma

Norton *see* Baker Norton Pharms

Norwich Eaton *see* Procter Gamble Pharm

Novartis *NDC Code:* **00083, 58887, 00028, 57267, 17088, 00043, 00078**
Novartis Pharmaceutical Corp. **908-277-5000**
556 Morris Avenue **800-845-6585**
Summit, NJ 07901
Medical Product Sales Volume: $27,009,300,000
Total Employees: 116,178
Ownership: Novartis AG
Distribution: Pharmaceuticals, Generics, Consumer Health, Ophthalmics

Novartis AG *NDC Code:* **P00078**
Novartis **+41-61-324 8000**
Lichtstrasse 35
CH-4002 Basel, Switzerland
Medical Product Sales Volume: $27,009,300,000
Total Employees: 116,178
Ownership: Public *FAX:* +41-61-321-0985
Distribution: Pharmaceuticals, Generics, Consumer Health, Ophthalmics
CEO: Dr. Alex Krauer/Chairman
Dr. Daniel Vasella/President & CEO
Jan-J¨org Rudloff/Vice Chairman
Prof. Dr. Helmut Sihler/Vice Chairman
Dr. Raymund Breu/CFO
Alexandre F. Jetzer/Head of International Coordination, Human Resources, Legal and Taxes
Dr. Hans Kindler/Head of Novartis Services
Pierre Douaze/Head of Novartis Healthcare
Dr. Wolfgang Samo/Head of Novartis Agribusiness
David Pyott/Head of Novartis Nutrition
Marketing: Walter P von Wartburg/Communications
Production: Pierre Douaze/Pharmaceuticals
Wayne Yetter/CEO, US Pharmaceuticals
Roland Jeannet/Consumer Health
Dr. Oswla Sellemond/Generics
Dr. Glen Bradley/Ciba Vision
Dr. Wolfgang Samo/Crop Protection
Heinz Imhof/Seeds
Hans-Beat G¨urtler/Animal Health
David Pyott/Nutrition
Research: Daniel Wagni'ere/Group Technology

Novo Nordisk Pharm *NDC Code:* **00169**
Novo Nordisk Pharmaceutical Industries, Inc. **609-987-5800**
3612 Powhatan Road
Clayton, NC 27520
Medical Product Sales Volume: $400,000,000
Total Employees: 200
Ownership: Novo Nordisk A/S
Distribution: Importer of Insulin
CEO: Ken Capuano/President
Research: Daniel D Cugini/Mgr Product Safety
Deborah K Donnelly/Assoc Dir/Clinical Oper
Helle M Gawrylewski/Assoc Dir Scientific Info
Rex S Clements Jr/VP Medical Affairs
Robert J Moss/Dir Professional Services
Stephanie D Rais/Dir Regulatory Affairs
John A Scarlett/Sr VP Medical & Scien Affairs
Diane Wood/Mgr Regulatory Affairs

Novopharm (US) *NDC Code:* **55953**
Novopharm USA Inc. **708-882-4200**
165 East Commerce Drive, Suite 200 **800-635-5067**
Schaumburg, IL 60173-5326
Total Employees: 45
Ownership: Novopharm Canada *FAX:* 708-882-4232
Distribution: Manufacturer of Generic Pharmaceuticals
CEO: Robert Gunter/President & C.O.O.
Jim Moore/Dir of Finance
Marketing: Sidney Baron/VP, Sales and Mktg
Darla Day/Manager Key Accounts, Central Division
Jim Fletcher/Director, Operations
Sara Gunter/Director, Customer Affairs
Andy Gunter/Director, Managed Health Care
Arthur Maher/Director Field Sales
Larry Moyer/Dir Key Accounts, South Atlantic Region
Susan Eckdahl/Director, Marketing
Laura Welter/Mktg Mgr
Tom Kronovich/Mgr Key Accounts N. Eastern Div.
Pete Kamp/Mgr Key Accounts, South West Div.
Production: Real Duteau/VP Scientific Affairs
Federal Procurement Eligibility: Medicaid Rebate
Medical Product Subsidiaries (Listed Separately):
Granutec

Nutraceutical Labs *NDC Code:* **58916**
Nutraceutical Laboratories Inc. **414-886-6466**
P.O. Box 171 **800-593-1236**
Wheeling, IL 60090
Medical Product Sales Volume: $25,000
Total Employees: 1
Ownership: PRIVATE *FAX:* 414-886-6822
CEO: Will J. Lepeska/President
Federal Procurement Eligibility: Medicaid Rebate

Nutripharm Labs *NDC Code:* **51081**
Nutripharm Laboratories, Inc. **201-569-8502**
64 North Summit Street
Tenafly, NJ 07670
Ownership: Palisades Pharm *FAX:* 201-569-7416
Distribution: Specialty Manufacturer
Marketing: Leslie Seidler/EVP
Production: Cynthia Romanoff/General Manager

Nycomed *NDC Code:* **00407**
Nycomed, Inc. **47-296-3400**
101 Carnegie Center
Princeton, NJ 08540-9988
Medical Product Sales Volume: $1,240,000,000
Total Employees: 4,959
Ownership: Ivax Nycomed *FAX:* 47-296-3600
Distribution: Manufacturer of Pharmaceuticals
CEO: Terje Mikalsen/Chairman
Svein Asser/President
Marketing: Stein H. Annexstad/Dep. CEO, Marketing
Research: Per Erik Lillevold/Mgr Clinical R & D
Siv Winge/Engineer
Medical Product Subsidiaries (Listed Separately):
Sterling Winthrop Imaging

Oclassen Pharms *NDC Code:* **55515**
Oclassen Pharmaceuticals, Inc. **415-258-4500**
100 Pelican Way **800-288-4508**
San Rafael, CA 94901
Total Employees: 80
Ownership: PRIVATE *FAX:* 415-258-4550
Distribution: Distributor of Branded Pharmaceuticals
CEO: Glenn A. Oclassen/Chairman
Terry L. Johnson/President & CEO
Marketing: Anthony A DiTonno/VP, Marketing and Sales
Carolyn Logan/Director of Sales
Ross Dileo/Director, Regulatory Affairs
Research: Frank Killey, PhD/VP Research & Development
Federal Procurement Eligibility: Medicaid Rebate

Ocumed *NDC Code:* **51944**
Ocumed, Inc. **201-226-2330**
109 Kinderkamack Road
Montvale, NJ 07645
Total Employees: 50
Ownership: PRIVATE

Ocusoft *NDC Code:* **54799**
Ocusoft Inc. **281-342-3350**
P.O. Box 429 **800-233-5469**
Richmond, TX 77469
Medical Product Sales Volume: $5,000,000
Total Employees: 20
Ownership: PRIVATE *FAX:* 281-232-6015
CEO: Cynthia L. Barratt/President
Marketing: Rosemary Martinez/VP Sales & Mktg
Federal Procurement Eligibility: Medicaid Rebate

OHM *NDC Code:* **51660**
Ohm Laboratories, Inc. **908-297-3030**
P.O. Box 7397 **800-527-6481**
North Bruns, NJ 08902
Total Employees: 30
Ownership: PRIVATE *FAX:* 908-247-0268
Federal Procurement Eligibility: Medicaid Rebate

Ohmeda Pharm *NDC Code:* **10019**
Ohmeda Pharmaceutical Products Div. **908-647-9200**
110 Allen Road **800-262-3784**
Liberty Corner, NJ 07938
Medical Product Sales Volume: $250,000,000
Total Employees: 400
Ownership: Boc Group *FAX:* 908-604-7652
Distribution: Manufacturer of Anesthetics
CEO: Paul Thomas/President
Ron Martin/VP Finance
Marketing: Theresa Heggie/Dir Mktg
Production: Calvin Jobe/VP Operations
Ronald Quadrel/VP Division Quality
Research: Robert Capetola/VP R&D

OK State Dept Hlth *NDC Code:* **55385**
Oklahoma State Depatment of Health
1000 Northeast 10th St. Pharmacy Rm B14
Oklahoma City, OK 73117
Ownership: PRIVATE

Optopics *NDC Code:* **52238**
Optopics Laboratories Corp. **609-451-9350**
40 Main St. **800-223-0865**
Fairton, NJ 08200-0210
Medical Product Sales Volume: $2,000,000
Total Employees: 35
Ownership: PRIVATE *FAX:* 609-451-2177
Distribution: Specialty Manufacturer
CEO: Frank C. Nicholas/Chairman & CEO
Scott H. Nicholas/VP, Tech. Affairs Director
Marketing: Peter K. Nicholas/VP, Marketing
Federal Procurement Eligibility: Medicaid Rebate

Oral B Labs *NDC Code:* **00041**
Oral-B Laboratories, Inc. **415-961-8130**
600 Clipper Dr.
Belmont, CA 94002
Total Employees: 1,570
Ownership: Gillette
CEO: Glenn Archibald/President
Bill Hanigan/VP, Finance
Marketing: Robert Perry/Director, Marketing
Dwight Laursen/VP, Sales
Research: Gary Pitts/VP, Research and Development

Organon *NDC Code:* **00052**
Organon Inc. **201-325-4500**
375 Mount Pleasant Avenue
West Orange, NJ 07052
Medical Product Sales Volume: $259,000,000
Total Employees: 500 *Telex:* 138201
Ownership: Akzo *FAX:* 201-325-4589
Distribution: Manufacturer of Branded Pharmaceuticals
CEO: Brian Haigh/President
Craig Rothenberg/Manager of Public Relations
Marketing: David W. Dingwell/VP Marketing & Sales
Mike Nevinski/Director of Marketing
Joseph Serratelli/Director, Marketing
Jerry Sweeney/Director, Sales Training
Research: Ana M Arango Bossard/Sr Clinical Study Manager
Kirsten H Deutsche/Assist Dir Reg Affairs
Roy W Dodsworth/Dir Of Reg Affairs
Maureen Heu/Mgr Product Information
Harry J Housman/Vice President
Thomas Lang/Asst Dir Reg Affairs
Robert J Piraino/Dir Information Services
David L Wilson/Mgr Clinical Data Systems
William Yuan/Director Of Biometrics
Federal Procurement Eligibility: Medicaid Rebate

Organon Teknika *NDC Code:* **48642**
Organon Teknika Corporation **919-620-2000**
100 Akzo Avenue **800-682-2666**
Durham, NC 27712
Total Employees: 1,500
Ownership: Akzo *FAX:* 919-620-2107
CEO: Robert Timmins/President & CEO
Lloyd Moores/SVP Finance & Operations, CFO
Marketing: Micheal Cavanaugh/Dir Marketing-Diagnostic Prod.
Barry Warren/Dir Marketing-Immunodiagnostics
Harry Schricky/VP, Sales and Marketing
Research: R. Driscoll/VP, Research and Development

Ortega Pharm *NDC Code:* **00191**
Ortega Pharm. Co., Inc. **904-389-5558**
2923 Corinthian Avenue
Jacksonville, FL 32210
Medical Product Sales Volume: $500,000
Total Employees: 8
Ownership: PRIVATE

Ortho Biotech *NDC Code:* **59676**
Ortho Biotech **908-218-6000**
Route 202, P.O. Box 300
Raritan, NJ 08869
Ownership: Ortho Pharm *FAX:* 908-218-1416
Distribution: Biotech Manufacturer
Marketing: Lori Lonczak/Product Mgr PROCRIT
Federal Procurement Eligibility: Medicaid Rebate

Ortho Dx Systems *NDC Code:* **00562**
Ortho Diagnostic Systems, Inc.
US Hwy 1001 Rt. 202
Raritan, NJ 08869
Ownership: PRIVATE

Ortho Pharm *NDC Code:* **00062, 00107**
Ortho-McNeil Pharmaceutical Corp. **908-218-6000**
Route 202, P.O. Box 300 **800-542-5365**
Raritan, NJ 08869
Medical Product Sales Volume: $1,000,000,000
Total Employees: 10,000
Ownership: JOHNSON & JOHNSON *FAX:* 908-218-1416
Distribution: Manufacturer of Branded Pharmaceuticals
CEO: Eric P. Milledge/President
Carol Webb/President, Biotech Division
T. E. Nystrom/VP, Finance
Marketing: William Curnow/VP Marketing & Sales, Ortho
A. Wojatsek/VP Marketing & Sales, McNeil
W. Cordivari/VP Marketing & Sales, Derm.
Production: Joseph T. Anstatt/VP Operations
David E. Williams/VP Operations, Biotech
Research: W. Duncan, PhD/Chairman RW Johnson Res Institute
R. Cohn, PhD/SVP Preclinical Development
L. Itri, MD/SVP Medical Affairs
P. Peterson, MD, PhD/SVP Drug Discovery
Federal Procurement Eligibility: Medicaid Rebate
Medical Product Subsidiaries (Listed Separately):
Ortho Biotech

OTC Pharm *NDC Code:* **55959**
OTC Phamaceuticals **203-698-0297**
P.O. Box 677
Old Greenwich, CT 07870
Ownership: PRIVATE

Otsuka America Pharm *NDC Code:* **59148**
Otsuka America Pharmaceutical, Inc. **301-990-0300**
2440 Research Blvd.
Rockvile, MD 20850
Medical Product Sales Volume: $5,100,000
Total Employees: 286
Ownership: Otsuka *FAX:* 301-990-0036
Distribution: Distributor of Ophthalmics
CEO: T. Sato/President
Lloyd A. Tepper/Controller
Marketing: Charles Vaughn/Director of Marketing
Karen A. Kessnick/Associate Product Manager
Research: Lawrence L. Nussbaum/Dir, Medical Affairs

Owen/Galderma Labs *see* Galderma

Pacific Pharma *see* Allergan

Paco Pharm *NDC Code:* **52967**
Paco Pharmaceutical Services, Inc. **201-367-9000**
1200 Paco Way
Lakewood, NJ 08701
Medical Product Sales Volume: $64,000,000
Total Employees: 1,000
Ownership: West
Distribution: Contact Packaging
CEO: William G. Little/CEO

Paddock Labs *NDC Code:* **00574**
Paddock Laboratories, Inc. **612-546-4676**
3940 Quebec Avenue North **800-328-5113**
Minneapolis, MN 55427
Medical Product Sales Volume: $16,000,000
Total Employees: 135
Ownership: PRIVATE *FAX:* 612-546-4842
Distribution: Manufacturer of Generics
CEO: Bruce G. Paddock, R.Ph./Chairman & President
Jerry Menth/Director, Purchasing
Ed Maloney/Director, Operations
Marketing: Allan Slizewski/Director Sales & Marketing
Production: Martin A. Erickson, III, R.Ph./Professional Affairs
Research: Mary Beth Erstad/New Products
Federal Procurement Eligibility: Medicaid Rebate

Palisades Pharms *NDC Code:* **53159**
Palisades Pharmaceuticals, Inc. **201-569-8502**
P.O. Box 579
Tenafly, NJ 07670
Ownership: PRIVATE *FAX:* 201-569-7416
Distribution: Specialty Manufacturer
Marketing: Leslie Seidler/Exec VP
Production: Cynthia Romanoff/Gen'l Mgr
Federal Procurement Eligibility: Medicaid Rebate

Pam Am Labs *NDC Code:* **00525**
Pan American Labs, Inc. **504-89304097**
P.O. Box 8950
Mandeville, LA 70470-8950
Total Employees: 5
Ownership: PRIVATE
Distribution: Specialty Manufacturer
Federal Procurement Eligibility: Medicaid Rebate

Par Pharm *NDC Code:* **49884**
PAR Pharmaceutical, Inc. **914-425-7100**
One Ram Ridge Road **800-423-1032**
Spring Valley, NY 10977
Medical Product Sales Volume: $78,600,000
Total Employees: 400
Ownership: Public/Clal Pharm Ltd *FAX:* 914-425-7907
Distribution: Manufacturer of Generics
CEO: Kenneth I. Sawyer/President & CEO
Dennis O'Connor/CFO, VP
Marketing: Daniel O. Hayden/VP, Sales
Cori Bussetti/Marketing Specialist

Par Pharm *(cont'd)*
Production: Michelle Bonomi/Manager of Regulatory Affairs
Federal Procurement Eligibility: Medicaid Rebate
Medical Product Subsidiaries (Listed Separately):
Par Pharm

Parke-Davis *NDC Code:* **00071**
Parke Davis Div of Warner Lambert Co. **201-540-2000**
2800 Plymouth Rd. **800-223-0432**
Ann Arbor, MI 48106-1047
Medical Product Sales Volume: $1,750,000,000
Total Employees: 12,000
Ownership: Warner-Lambert *FAX:* 201-540-4624
Distribution: Manufacturer of Branded Pharmaceuticals
CEO: Anthony Wild, PhD/N.A. President
Harold F. Oberkfell/Latin Am. President
Michael Hoffman/VP Health Care Systems
Marketing: Robert W. Doyle/Dir Advertising Operations
Lynn Ebben/Product Mgr LOPID
Production: Felix Garcia/VP Manufacturing
Harry F. Tappen/Director, Market Research
David F. Rhodes/Drug Information Services
Research: Ron Cresswell/Chairman Parke-Davis Research
Dr. Wendell Wierenga/SVP, Pharmaceutical Research
D A Beechuk/Dir Clinical Pharmacy
Mary E Black/Assoc Dir Clinical Communicat
David Canter/VP Cardiovascular
Graham J Frank/VP Worldwide Clinical Research
Irwin G Martin/Sr Dir Worldwide Reg Affs
Richard N Spivey/Dir Ww Reg Affairs
Marie E Ulrey/Mgr Clinical Communications
Andrew Uprichard/Dir Pharm Research Div
William M Wardell/Sr VP Drug Development
Federal Procurement Eligibility: Medicaid Rebate

Parmed Pharms *NDC Code:* **00349**
Parmed Pharmaceuticals, Inc. **716-284-5666**
4220 Hyde Park Boulevard
Niagara Falls, NY 14305
Total Employees: 110
Ownership: AL Labs *FAX:* 716-284-8031
Distribution: Distributor of Generics
CEO: Dominick V. Palmo/VP & General Manager
Marketing: James W. Hillman/VP Direct Marketing
Bridget C. Borzecki/Mgr Mktg & Key Accounts
Production: Diane M. Linza/QC Reg. Surp.
Federal Procurement Eligibility: Medicaid Rebate

Parnell Pharm *NDC Code:* **50930**
Parnell Pharmaceuticals, Inc. **415-256-1800**
P.O. Box 5130
Larkspur, CA 94977
Total Employees: 10
Ownership: PRIVATE *FAX:* 415-256-8099
Distribution: Specialty Manufacturer
CEO: Francis W. Parnell MD/Chairman, President & CEO
Marketing: John F. Parnell/VP
Research: Paul W. Lofholm, Pharm. D/Dir, Scientific Affairs

Pasadena *NDC Code:* **00418**
Pasadena Research Labs **714-492-4030**
Suite 150, 942 Calle Negocio **800-223-9851**
San Clemente, CA 92673
Total Employees: 12
Ownership: PRIVATE *FAX:* 714-498-3613
Distribution: Distributor of Injectables
CEO: Tom Yankoff/Chairman & President
David Gencarella/EVP & General Manager
Marketing: Sally Razak/Director of Purchasing

Pasteur Merieux *see* Institute Merieux

PBH *see* Vision Pharms

PBI *see* Rosemont

Pecos *NDC Code:* **59879**
Pecos Pharmaceutical
25301 Cabot Rd 212-213
Laguna Hills, CA 92653
Ownership: PRIVATE
Federal Procurement Eligibility: Medicaid Rebate

Pedinol Pharma *NDC Code:* **00884**
Pedinol Pharmacal, Inc. **516-293-9500**
30 Banfi Plaza North **800-733-4665**
Farmingdale, NY 11735
Medical Product Sales Volume: $5,700,000
Total Employees: 40
Ownership: PRIVATE *FAX:* 516-293-7359
Distribution: Manufacturer of Topicals
CEO: Richard Strauss RPh/President
Federal Procurement Eligibility: Medicaid Rebate

Pegasus Med Svs *NDC Code:* **10974**
Pegasus Medical, Inc. **714-753-9055**
1 Technology Dr., Build 1C, Suite 525
Irvine, CA 92718
Ownership: PRIVATE

Penn Labs *NDC Code:* **58437**
Penn Laboratories, Inc.
1250 South Collegeville Rd.
Collegeville, PA 19426
Ownership: PRIVATE
Distribution: Distributor of Generics
Federal Procurement Eligibility: Medicaid Rebate

Pennex *NDC Code:* **00426**
Pennex Pharmaceuticals, Inc. **708-976-5617**
Pennex Drive **800-245-6110**
Verona, PA 15147
Total Employees: 300
Ownership: Good Health *FAX:* 412-826-4720
Distribution: Manufacturer of Generic Liquids & OTC's
CEO: Jack van Hulst/President
Marketing: Daryl Johnson/VP Sales & Marketing
Suzanne Gupta/Marketing Coordinator
Production: Louis E. Windecker/VP Manufacturing
Chris Nascone/Plant Manager

Pennex Pharm *see* Morton Grove

Perrigo *NDC Code:* **00113, 58948**
Perrigo Company **616-673-8451**
117 Water Street
Allegan, MI 49010
Medical Product Sales Volume: $571,000,000
Total Employees: 4,000
Ownership: Public *FAX:* 616-673-7535
Distribution: Manufacturer of Generic Pharmaceuticals
CEO: Michael J. Jandernoa/Chairman & CEO
Dick Hansen/President
Marketing: Paul Nicholson/VP Sales & Marketing
Medical Product Subsidiaries (Listed Separately):
Good Sense
Perrigo

Perry Med Prod *NDC Code:* **11763**
Perry Medical Products, Inc. **503-235-6417**
3580 Northeast Broadway
Portland, OR 97232
Ownership: PRIVATE

Person and Covey *NDC Code:* **00096**
Person and Covey, Inc. **818-240-1030**
616 Allen Ave., Box 25018
Glendale, CA 91221-5018
Medical Product Sales Volume: $7,500,000
Total Employees: 50
Ownership: PRIVATE *FAX:* 818-547-9821
Distribution: Specialty Manufacturer of Skin & Hair Care Products
CEO: Lorne V. Person/President
Cecil Stewart/Executive Vice President
Marketing: William Person/Director of Marketing
Production: Harald Eyzendooren/Director of Production

Pfeiffer Pharms *NDC Code:* **00927**
Pfeiffer Pharmaceuticals, Inc.
P.O. Box 4447
Atlanta, GA 30302
Ownership: PRIVATE
CEO: Charles M. Bentley/President & CEO
John C. Coyle/Director of Regulatory Affairs

Pfizer Labs *NDC Code:* **00069**
Pfizer Laboratories Div Pfizer Inc. **212-573-2323**
235 East 42nd Street; 5th Floor
New York, NY 10017-5755
Medical Product Sales Volume: $11,306,000,000
Total Employees: 46,500
Ownership: Public *FAX:* 212-573-7851
Distribution: Manufacturer of Branded Pharmaceuticals
CEO: William C. Steere, Jr./Chairman of the Board & CEO
Edward C. Bessey/Vice Chairman; Pres-US Pharm Group
David L. Shedlarz/CFO
Henry A. McKinnell, PhD/EVP & Chief Finacial Officer; Pres-Hosp. Products Group
Robert Neimeth/EVP; Pres-Int'l Pharm. Group
C.L. Clemente/SVP-Corp. Affairs; Secretary & Corp. Counsel
Paul S. Miller/SVP; General Counsel
Brian W. Barrett/VP; Pres, Northern Asia, Australasia, & Canada-Int'l Pharm Group
M. Kenneth Bowler/VP-Federal Govt. Regulations
Bruce R. Ellig/VP-Personnel
Donald F. Farley/VP; Pres-Food Science Group
David M. Fitzgerald/VP; Exec VP-Hosp Products Group & Pres, Howmedica Div.
George A. Forcier, PhD/VP-Quality Control
P. Nigel Gray/VP; Exec VP-Hosp Products Group & Pres, Medical Devices Div.
Gary N. Jortner/VP; Group VP, Disease Management-US Pharm Group
Karen Katen/VP; Exec VP-US Pharm Group
Alan G. Levin/Treasurer
Brower A. Merriam/VP; President Animal Hlth Group
John C. Mesloh/VP-Corp Purchasing
Victor Micati/VP, Pres Europe-International Pharm Group
William J. Robison/VP, Human Resources
Herbert V. Ryan/Controller
Craig Sexton, MD/VP; EVP-Central Research
Gerald H. Schulze/VP-Pharmaceutical Planning
Robert L. Shafer/VP-Public Affairs
David L. Shedlarz/VP-Finance
Frederick W. Telling, PhD/VP-Corp. Strategic Planning & Policy
Marketing: Gary Jortner/Group VP
George Flouty, MD/Medical Director
Steve Leder/Controller
Pat Kelly/Group VP
Howard Steinberg, MD/Medical Dir
Helen Lang/Dir of Finance
Research: John F. Niblack, PhD/EVP Research & Development
George M. Milne, Jr., PhD/VP; Pres-Central Research
Craig Saxton, MD/VP, EVP Central Research
Federal Procurement Eligibility: Medicaid Rebate
Medical Product Subsidiaries (Listed Separately):
Pfizer Pharm
Pfizer Roerig
Pfizer Roerig
Value Health

Pfizer Pharm *NDC Code:* **00663**
Pfizer Pharmaceuticals, Inc. **212-573-2323**
235 East 42nd Street
New York, NY 10017-5755
Medical Product Sales Volume: $1,800,000,000
Total Employees: 250
Ownership: Pfizer
Distribution: Manufacturer of Branded Pharmaceuticals
Federal Procurement Eligibility: Medicaid Rebate

Pharm America *NDC Code:* **51655**
Pharmaceutical Corp. Of America **317-573-8000**
12348 Hancock St.
Carmel, IN 46032
Ownership: PRIVATE
Distribution: Specialty Manufacturer

Pharm Assoc *NDC Code:* **00121**
Pharmaceutical Associates, Inc.
Subsidiary of Beach Products, Inc. **864-277-7282**
201 Delaware **800-845-8210**
Greenville, SC 29605
Ownership: Beach Products *FAX:* 864-277-8045
CEO: Richard B. Jenkins/CEO & President
Paul S. May/President, Pharmaceutical Associates, Inc.
Marketing: David Winchell/VP Sales and Marketing
Clete Harmon/Director of Q.A.
Federal Procurement Eligibility: Medicaid Rebate

Pharm Basics *see* Rosemont

Pharm Pkging Ctr *NDC Code:* **54383**
Pharmaceutical Packaging Center
3530 Pomona Blvd.
Pomona, CA 91768
Ownership: PRIVATE

Pharm Resources *see* Par Pharm

Pharm Tech Pkg *NDC Code:* **52803**
Pharm-Tech Packaging Corp. **201-887-8828**
58 Pearl Street **800-524-2732**
Hobart, NY 13788
Ownership: PRIVATE

Pharma Tek *NDC Code:* **39822**
Pharma Tek, Inc. **516-757-5522**
4 York Court
Northport, NY 11768
Medical Product Sales Volume: $7,000,000
Total Employees: 15
Ownership: PRIVATE
CEO: Dan J. Badia/President/CEO
Shirely Harmbuing/Vice President
Marketing: J. Granger
Production: J. Robin Liles
Research: Susan E. Badia

Pharmacaps *see* Advanced Nutritional

Pharmaceutical Basics *see* Pennex

Pharmacia *see* Pharmacia & Upjohn

Pharmacia & Upjohn *NDC Code:* **00009, 00013, 00016**
Pharmacia and Upjohn Copmany
7000 Portage Road **800-253-8600**
Kalamazoo, MI 49001
Medical Product Sales Volume: $7,286,000,000
Total Employees: 31,700
Ownership: Public
Distribution: Manufacturer of Branded Pharmaceuticals
CEO: Jan Ekberg/CEO
Robert C. Salisbury/CFO
Federal Procurement Eligibility: Medicaid Rebate

Pharmacist Choice *NDC Code:* **54979**
Pharmacist Choice, Inc. **541-747-5223**
2444 Ranch Drive
Springfield, OR 97477
Ownership: PRIVATE
Distribution: Specialty Manufacturer
Federal Procurement Eligibility: Medicaid Rebate

Pharmafair *see* Bausch and Lomb

Pharmics *NDC Code:* **00813**
Pharmics, Inc. **801-972-4138**
P.O. Box 27554 **800-456-4138**
Salt Lake City, UT 84127-0554
Total Employees: 6
Ownership: Public *FAX:* 801-972-4139
Distribution: Manufacturer of Branded Pharmaceuticals
CEO: Walter J. Plumb III/President
Marketing: Paul H. Bagley/General Manager
Research: Lester Partlow/Director of Research
Federal Procurement Eligibility: Medicaid Rebate

Phys Dispensing Rx *NDC Code:* **55289**
Physicians Dispensing Rx, Inc.
6000 NW 2nd St., Ste 800
Oklahoma City, OK 73127
Ownership: PRIVATE

Physicians Form *NDC Code:* **53261**
Physicians Formulary Services, Inc.
1101 East Colonial Drive **800-445-3689**
Orlando, FL 32803
Ownership: PRIVATE

Pilk Barnes Hind *see* Vision Pharms

Poly Pharms *NDC Code:* **50991**
Poly Pharmaceuticals, Inc. **601-776-3497**
200 North Archusa Ave
Quitman, MS 39355
Medical Product Sales Volume: $1,000,000
Total Employees: 25
Ownership: PRIVATE *FAX:* 601-776-3497
Distribution: Distributor of Branded Pharmaceuticals
CEO: James Brownlee, R.Ph./President
Federal Procurement Eligibility: Medicaid Rebate

Polymedica *see* Alcon-PR

Porton Prod *see* Speywood Pharm

Poythress *see* ECR Pharms

Pratt *see* Pfizer Labs

Praxis Bio *see* Lederle-Praxis

Primedics *NDC Code:* **00684**
Primedics Laboratories **213-770-3005**
15524 South Broadway Street **800-533-0173**
Gardenia, CA 90248
Total Employees: 9
Ownership: Irenda
Distribution: Manufacturer of Branded Pharmaceuticals
Marketing: Gregory A. Bambos/Vice President

Primus *NDC Code:* **55762**
Primus Pharmaceutical Inc. **912-923-4829**
RR 1, Box 2730
Juliette, GA 31046-9546
Total Employees: 7
Ownership: PRIVATE
Distribution: Specialty Manufacturer
Federal Procurement Eligibility: Medicaid Rebate

PRL Enterpr *NDC Code:* **53633**
P R L Enterprises Inc.
3380 Forest View Road
Rockford, IL 61109
Medical Product Sales Volume: $3,000,000
Total Employees: 24
Ownership: PRIVATE

Pro Prods Co *NDC Code:* **48015**
ProWay Inc., dba Professional Products Company
P.O. Box 1628
San Diego, CA 92112
Ownership: PRIVATE

Procordia AB *NDC Code:* **P00153**
Procordia AB **46-8-138000**
Lindhagensgatan 133
Stockholm S-11287, SWEDEN
Medical Product Sales Volume: $3,600,000,000
Total Employees: 100,000
Ownership: Public *FAX:* 46-8-6188607
Distribution: Conglomerate
CEO: Jan Ekberg/President
Medical Product Subsidiaries (Listed Separately):
Erbamont SP.A.
Kabi Pharmacia AB

Procter Gamble Mfg *NDC Code:* **37000**
Procter and Gamble Manufacturing Co. **513-983-1100**
8700 Mason Montgomery Road **800-448-4878**
Mason, OH 45040
Medical Product Sales Volume: $35,284,000,000
Total Employees: 103,000
Ownership: Public *FAX:* 513-983-9369
Distribution: Manufacturer of Household Products
CEO: John E. Pepper/Chairman
Erik G. Nelson/CFO
Benjamin L. Bethell/Human Resources
Durk I. Jager/President
Gerald V. Dirvin/EVP
Malcom Jozoff/SVP Health Care
Thomas A. Moore/Health Care, U.S.
Marketing: Robert J. Herbold/SVP Information, Advertising & Marketing Services
Lawrence D. Milligan/SVP Sales
Robert L. Wehling/VP Marketing Services
Research: Gordon F. Brunner/SVP Research & Development
Geoffrey Place/VP R&D, Health Care & Environment
Nancy H Allen/Mgr Regulatory Services
June E Austin/Regulatory Manager
Mark B Gelbert/Regulatory Affairs Mgr
Candice L Slough/Medical Affairs Manager
Michael D Young/Corporate Director
Medical Product Subsidiaries (Listed Separately):
P&G Pharmaceuticals

Procter Gamble Pharm *NDC Code:* **00149**
Procter & Gamble Pharmaceuticals **607-335-2111**
11450 Grooms Rd. **800-448-4878**
Cincinnati, OH 45242
Medical Product Sales Volume: $400,000,000
Total Employees: 3,023
Ownership: Procter & Gamble *FAX:* 607-335-2798
Distribution: Manufacturer of Branded Pharmaceuticals
CEO: G. Gilbert Cloyd/Division Manager, Norwich Div.
Donald R. Lee/Professional Affairs
Frederick H.Kruse/Manager, International
F.H. Kruse/Global Planning & Coordination
I.B. Simon/General Manager, Pharmaceuticals
Marketing: Jeffrey E. Hass/G.M. Europe
Robert J. Lazor/Manager, Sales Operations

Procter Gamble Pharm *(cont'd)*
T.M. Finn/Marketing
R.J. Lazor/Sales
E.A. Minton/Product Supply
G.E. Wentler/Product Developement
Production: Thomas L. Long/Manager, Manufacturing
David J. Manzo/Manager, Quality Assurance
E. Samuel Smith/Regulatory & Medical Affairs
Research: James L. Russell/Research & Product Development
J Curtis Gwilliam/Dir Mngmt Systms Dept
John D Mestler/Group Mgr Scientific Sys
Daniel J Michel/Coord Medical Communications
Elizabeth A Nies/Section Head
Robert P Peraza/Section Head, Information Svc
Terri Power/Assoc Medical Commun
Brandt Rowles/Mgr Academic Relations
Marilyn M Sherman/Group Leader
E Samuel Smith/Dir Reg & Medical Affairs
W. Hedgin/Research & Developement, Europe
Dr. M.D. Young/Regulatory and Clinical Developement
Federal Procurement Eligibility: Medicaid Rebate

Procyte *NDC Code:* **A00059**
Procyte Corp. **206-820-4548**
12040 115th Avenue Northeast
Kirkland, WA 98034-6900
Medical Product Sales Volume: $621,000
Total Employees: 36
Ownership: Public *FAX:* 206-820-4111
Distribution: OEM Supplier
CEO: Joseph Ashley/Chairman, CEO & President
Karen L. Hedine/VP
G.W. Duncan/VP
G.B. Jones/Secy.
Production: D.H.Fulle/Controller

Prosperous IMP *see* Deliz

Purdue Frederick *NDC Code:* **00034**
Purdue Frederick Co. **203-853-0123**
100 Connecticut Ave. **800-733-1333**
Norwalk, CT 06850-3590
Medical Product Sales Volume: $100,000,000
Total Employees: 450
Ownership: PRIVATE *FAX:* 203-838-1576
Distribution: Manufacturer of Branded Pharmaceuticals
CEO: Dr. Mortimer Sackler/Chairman & CEO
Dr. Raymond Sackler/President
Edward Albright/EVP & General Mgr
Marketing: Michael Friedman/Group VP Marketing & Sales
James H. Shriver/VP Sales
Research: Mark Chasin, PhD/VP Research & Development
Federal Procurement Eligibility: Medicaid Rebate

Purepac Pharm *see* Faulding Pharm (US)

Purepac Pharm *NDC Code:* **00228**
Purepac Pharmaceutical Co. Div. Faulding **908-527-9100**
200 Elmora Avenue **800-526-6978**
Elizabeth, NJ 07207
Medical Product Sales Volume: $70,000,000
Total Employees: 350
Ownership: Public/Kalipharm/Faulding *FAX:* 908-527-0649
Distribution: Manufacturer of Generics
CEO: Robert H. Bur/President
Marketing: Kenneth L. Hertzel/VP Sales & Marketing
Alison A. Marini/Sales Promotion Manager
Production: John Hoofnagle/VP Manufacturing
Federal Procurement Eligibility: Medicaid Rebate

Quad Pharm *see* Par Pharm

Qualitest Drugs *NDC Code:* **52446**
Qualitest Drugs, Inc. **205-859-4011**
1236 Jordan Street
Huntsville, AL 35811
Ownership: Qualitest Products *FAX:* 205-859-4021
Distribution: Distributor of Generics
Federal Procurement Eligibility: Medicaid Rebate

Qualitest Pharms *NDC Code:* **00603**
Qualitest Pharmaceuticals, Inc. **205-859-4011**
1236 Jordan Street **800-444-4011**
Huntsville, AL 35811
Total Employees: 100
Ownership: PRIVATE *FAX:* 205-859-4021
Distribution: Distributor of Generics
Marketing: Charles (Trey) Propst/Contracts Manager
Federal Procurement Eligibility: Medicaid Rebate
Medical Product Subsidiaries (Listed Separately):
Qualitest Drugs

Quality Res Pharms *NDC Code:* **52765**
Quality Research Pharmaceuticals Inc. **513-681-3260**
1117 Third Ave Southwest
Carmel, IN 46032
Ownership: PRIVATE

Quantum Pharm *see* American Home Prod

R and D Labs *NDC Code:* **54391**
R & D Laboratories, Inc.
4640 Admirality Way, Suite 710 **800-338-9066**
Marine Del Rey, CA 90292
Ownership: PRIVATE
CEO: Rhonda Makoff, PhD/President & CEO
Robert Weitzman/CFO
Marketing: Silvio M. Coccia/VP, Sales & Marketing

R/P Rorer Generics *see* Arcola

RA McNeil *NDC Code:* **12830**
R.A. McNeil Co. **615-265-8240**
1210 East Dallas Road **800-755-3033**
Chattanooga, TN 37405
Medical Product Sales Volume: $500,000
Total Employees: 3
Ownership: PRIVATE *FAX:* 615-265-7373
Distribution: Specialty Distributor
CEO: Ronald A. McNeil/President
Federal Procurement Eligibility: Medicaid Rebate

Rachelle Labs *NDC Code:* **00196**
Rachelle Laboratories, Inc. **219-842-3305**
16265 State Road 17
Culver, ID 46511
Total Employees: 64
Ownership: Halsey Drug *FAX:* 219-842-2519
Distribution: Manufacturer
CEO: George Krsek/President
Research: Roger Hulme

Raway *NDC Code:* **00686**
Raway Pharmacal Inc. **914-626-8133**
15 Granit Road
Accord, NY 12404
Medical Product Sales Volume: $500,000
Total Employees: 4
Ownership: PRIVATE
Distribution: Distributor of Topical Generics
CEO: Jack Burman/CEO

Reckitt & Colman *NDC Code:* **12496**
Reckitt & Colman Pharm., Inc.
1901 Hugenot Road- 110 **800-444-7599**
Richmond, VA 23235
Ownership: Reckitt & Colman plc *FAX:* 804-379-1215
Distribution: Consumer Package Goods Manufacturer

Recsei Labs *NDC Code:* **10952**
Recsei Laboratories **805-964-2912**
330 South Kellogg, Bldg. M
Goleta, CA 93117-3875
Medical Product Sales Volume: $230,000
Total Employees: 6
Ownership: PRIVATE
Distribution: Manufacturer of OTC Pharmaceuticals
CEO: Paul Recsei/CEO

Reed & Carnrick *NDC Code:* **00021**
Reed & Carnrick **201-434-3000**
257 Cornelison Avenue **800-526-6040**
Jersey City, NJ 07302
Medical Product Sales Volume: $50,600,000
Total Employees: 800
Ownership: Schwarz Pharma *FAX:* 201-981-1391
Distribution: Manufacturer of Branded Pharmaceuticals
CEO: John Spitznagel/President
Marketing: Peter Volk/VP Marketing
Joseph N. Noonberg/VP Sales
Production: Peter Casey/VP Operations
Research: Richard K. Bourne, PhD/VP Regulatory Affairs
Frederick A. Curro, DMD, PhD/VP Pharm. Development
Louis J Scotti/Dir New Business Develop
Federal Procurement Eligibility: Medicaid Rebate

Reese Chemical *NDC Code:* **10956**
Reese Chemical Co. **216-231-6441**
10617 Frank Ave.
Cleveland, OH 44106
Ownership: PRIVATE
Distribution: Manufacturer of Generics

Reg Svc *NDC Code:* **48433**
Regional Service Center, Inc.
17A Everberg Rd.
Woburn, MA 18011-1019
Ownership: PRIVATE

Reid-Provident *NDC Code:* **00063**
Reid-Provident
3991 Deep Rock Road
Richmond, VA 23233
Ownership: Solvay Pharm

Reid-Rowell *see* Solvay Pharms

Renal Division *NDC Code:* **00941**
Baxter Healthcare Corp Renal Division
1620 Waukegan Rd. Bldg. R
McGaw Park, IL 60085
Ownership: PRIVATE

Res Inds *NDC Code:* **00433**
Research Industries Corp. **801-562-0200**
6864 South, 300 West **800-453-8432**
Midvale, UT 84047-1001
Medical Product Sales Volume: $12,000,000
Total Employees: 225
Ownership: PRIVATE *FAX:* 801-565-6209
Distribution: Specialty Pharmaceutical Manufacturer
CEO: Gary L. Crocker/CEO
Marketing: Clyde H. Baker/Sr. Marketing VP
Ted Floyd/Pharmaceutical Customer Services
Debbie A. Orr/Customer Service Manager
Production: Micheal Kelly/Production VP
Research: Russ Hibbert/Dir, Research - Pharmaceuticals
Joe Todd/Dir, Research -Medical Devices

Respa Pharms *NDC Code:* **60575**
Respa Pharmaceuticals, Inc.
213 South Milwaukee Ave.
Lake Villa, IL 60046
Ownership: PRIVATE

Revlon *see* Rhone-Poulenc Rorer

Rexall *NDC Code:* **00122**
Rexall Drug Co. **305-561-2187**
851 Broken Sound Pky NW
Boca Raton, FL 33487-3693
Ownership: PRIVATE
Distribution: Distributor/Manufacturer of Generics

Rexall Rexall *NDC Code:* **60814**
Rexall Rexall Managed Care **305-561-2187**
851 Broken Sound Pky North West
Boca Raton, FL 33487
Ownership: Rexall
Distribution: Distributor of Generics

Rexar *NDC Code:* **00478**
Rexar Pharmacal **516-561-7662**
396 Rockaway Ave.
Valley Stream, NY 11581
Total Employees: 15
Ownership: Richwood
Distribution: Specialty Manufacturer
CEO: Philip Zotos/President
Marketing: Thad D. Demos/VP, Marketing
Production: Tom Gerontzos/VP, Operations
Medical Product Subsidiaries (Listed Separately):
Obetrol

Rhone-Poulenc Rorer *NDC Code:* **00075, 12516, 00195**
Rhone-Poulenc Rorer Pharmaceuticals, Inc.
500 Arcola Road **610-454-8000**
Collegeville, PA 19426-0996 **800-727-6737**
Medical Product Sales Volume: $5,420,600,000
Total Employees: 26,000
Ownership: Public/Rhone-Poulenc *FAX:* 610-454-3573
Distribution: Manufacturer of Branded Pharmaceuticals
CEO: Michel de Rosen/CEO
Mafred E. Karobath/CFO
Stuart Samuels/SVP & General Manager
Glenn Mattes/VP Div. Mgr Rorer
Marketing: Stephen Downs/VP
Research: Clarissa C Bencan/Mgr Drg Information Centr
Linda M Boyle/Mgr Medical Information Systems
Arthur W Fetter/Senior VP Drug Safety
Genevieve E Gadsden/Mgr Fda Communications
Gary T Shearman/VP Ww Regulatory Affairs
Cheryl A Shepard/Dir Ww Clinical & Reg Data Mt
Cheryl S Weinrich/Med Information Admin
Federal Procurement Eligibility: Medicaid Rebate
Medical Product Subsidiaries (Listed Separately):
Armour Pharm
Dermik Labs

Rhone-Poulenc SA *NDC Code:* **P00195**
Rhone-Poulenc SA **1-47681234**
25 quai Paul Donner
Courbevoie Cedex F-92408, FRANCE
Medical Product Sales Volume: $3,824,000,000
Total Employees: 89,051
Ownership: Public *FAX:* 1-681922
Distribution: Manufacturer of Chemicals
CEO: Jean-Rene Fourtou/Chairman
J. M. Bruel/Managing Dir
Igor Landau/Dir Health Care
Research: Martine Bayssas/Dir Clinical Research
David C P Brown/Deputy Director
Graham Copping/Director Toxicology Dept
Richard P Gural/Dir Worldwide Reg Affairs
Christine Lise Julow/Director Reg Affrs Europe
Celine Melcion/Deputy Dir Toxicology
Barbara Moigne/Sr Data Manager
Roland Poels/VP Medical Affairs-Europe
Edmond Roland/Head Cardiovascular Dept
Allan Rosetzsky/Sr Dir Medical Affairs
Philippe Zeisser/Dirmedical Development
Medical Product Subsidiaries (Listed Separately):
Fisons plc
Institut Merieux
Rhone-Poulenc Rorer

RIC *see* Res Inds

Richwood Pharm *NDC Code:* **58521**
Richwood Pharmaceutical Company, Inc. **606-282-2100**
7900 Tanner's Gate Lane, Suite 200 **800-536-7878**
Florence, KY 41042
Total Employees: 100
Ownership: PRIVATE *FAX:* 606-282-2103
Distribution: Distributor/Manufacturer of Branded Generic Pharmaceuticals
CEO: Roger D. Griggs/President
William Nuerge/COO
Marketing: Stefan Antonsson/VP of Marketing
Victor Vaughn/VP Sales
Production: Richard Costic/Dir of Manufacturing
Harry R. Painter/Product Director
Research: Ronald G. Browne, PhD
Medical Product Subsidiaries (Listed Separately):
Rexar Pharmacal
MANUFACTURING CHEMIST, INC. (MCI)

Rico Pharm *see* Teral Labs

RID *NDC Code:* **54807**
R.I.D. Inc. **213-268-0635**
609 North Mednik Avenue **800-834-7489**
Los Angeles, CA 90022
Medical Product Sales Volume: $1,200,000
Total Employees: 7
Ownership: PRIVATE *FAX:* 213-268-1336
Distribution: Distributer of Generics
CEO: Isras Chatkeon/Vice President
Federal Procurement Eligibility: Medicaid Rebate

Riker Labs *see* 3M Pharms

Robar *NDC Code:* **54171**
Robar Inc.
Ownership: PRIVATE

Roberts Labs *NDC Code:* **54092**
Roberts Laboratories Inc. **908-389-1182**
4 Industrial Way West **800-992-9306**
Eatontown, NJ 07724-2274
Medical Product Sales Volume: $113,380,000
Total Employees: 486 *Telex:* 9102501110RSCHGRP
Ownership: Public *FAX:* 908-389-1014
Distribution: Owner/Distributor of Branded and Generic Pharmaceuticals
CEO: Robert A. Vukovich, PhD/Chairman, Pres & CEO
Robert W. Loy/Executive VP, Operations and New Business Development
Peter M. Rogalin, CPA/VP, Treasurer, CFO
Marketing: John T. Spitznagel/Executive VP, Worldwide Sales & Marketing
Production: Moises Saporta/VP, Manufacturing Operations
Research: Philip Lang, PhD/Dir, Chemical Process Development
Andrew W. Karlan/VP, Worldwide Regulatory Affairs
Michael Petrone, MD/Dir, Medical Affairs

Robins *see* AH Robins

Roche *NDC Code:* **00004**
Hoffman LaRoche, Inc. **201-235-5000**
340 Kingsland Street
Nutley, NJ 07110
Medical Product Sales Volume: $1,100,000,000
Total Employees: 22,000
Ownership: Roche Holding Ltd *FAX:* 201-235-2036
Distribution: Manufacturer of Branded Pharmaceuticals
CEO: Irwin Lerner/President Hoffman-LaRoche Inc.
Patrick Zenner/President Roche Labs
Stephen G. Sudovar/SVP Pharm. Div.
Marketing: Carolyn Glynn/VP Public Policy & Comm.
Mike McGuire/Product Mgr ROCEPHIN
Laura Hill/Product Mgr TORADOL
Barbara Braun/Product Mgr BUMEX
Dan Kim/Product Mgr ROMAZICON
Research: Robert B Armstrong/Director Medical Affairs
Kennedy P Berkowitz/VP & Dir Public Affairs
Zofia E Dziewanowska/VP - Therapeutic Research
Samuel J Franco/Mgr Clinical Field Serv.
Edward W Mazure/Mgr Info/Communication
Richard I Raibman/Director Business Dev
Federal Procurement Eligibility: Medicaid Rebate
Medical Product Subsidiaries (Listed Separately):
Roche Prod

Roche Holding Ltd *NDC Code:* **P00004**
Roche Holding Ltd. **41-61-688-8888**
Grenzacherstrasse 1 24
CH-4002 Basel, SWITZERLAND
Medical Product Sales Volume: $12,754,100,000
Total Employees: 50,497
Ownership: Public *FAX:* 41-61-691-0014
Distribution: Manufacturer of Branded Pharmaceuticals
CEO: Fritz Gerber/Chairman
Henri B. Meier/CFO
Dr. A. F. Leuenberger/Dep. Chairman
Dr. L. Hoffmann/Dep. Chairman
Armin Kessler/CEO Pharmaceuticals Div
Franz Humer/COO Pharmaceuticals Div
Dr. F. Amrein/Sec.
Production: Peter Simon/Dir Pharm Operations
Research: Garry-Claude Berneker/Head Of Drug Safety 74/106
Wolf Blasi/Head Intl Clinical Research
Douglas E Busch/Head Research Information Serv
Ulrich Goetz/Information Manager
Gertrud M Huber/Drug Reg Affairs Mgr
Mathias Hukkelhoven/Mgr Regulatory Affairs
Medical Product Subsidiaries (Listed Separately):
Genentech
Roche Labs
Syntex

Roche Prod *NDC Code:* **00140**
Roche Products Inc. **201-235-5000**
P.O. Box 452
Manati, PR 00701
Ownership: Roche Labs
Distribution: Manufacturer of Branded Pharmaceuticals

Roerig *NDC Code:* **00049**
Roerig **212-573-2323**
235 East 42nd Street; 5th Floor DRAD
New York, NY 10017-5755
Ownership: Pfizer *FAX:* 212-808-8862
Distribution: Manufacturer of Branded Pharmaceuticals
Federal Procurement Eligibility: Medicaid Rebate

Roerig Pfizer *NDC Code:* **00662**
Roerig Pfizer **212-573-2323**
235 East 42nd Street; 5th Floor DRAD
New York, NY 10017-5755
Ownership: Pfizer
Federal Procurement Eligibility: Medicaid Rebate

Ronda Pharm *NDC Code:* **00675**
2622 Humboldt Street
Los Angeles, CA 90031
Ownership: PRIVATE

Rorer Pharm *see* Rhone-Poulenc Rorer

Rosemont *NDC Code:* **00832**
Rosemont Pharmaceutical Corporation **303-733-7207**
301 South Cherokee Street **800-445-8091**
Denver, CO 80223
Total Employees: 100
Ownership: Akzo Nobel BV *FAX:* 303-698-1005
Distribution: Manufacturer of Generic Pharmaceuticals
CEO: Wim B.J. Mens, PhD/President
Marketing: Raymond S. Wolski/Director, Sales & Marketing
Carla James/Marketing Assistant
Federal Procurement Eligibility: Medicaid Rebate

Ross Labs *see* Abbott

Roxane *NDC Code:* **00054**
Roxane Laboratories, Inc. **614-276-4000**
P.O. Box 16532
Columbus, OH 43216
Total Employees: 850
Ownership: Boehringer Ingleheim *FAX:* 614-274-0974
Distribution: Manufacturer of Brand & Generic Tablets, Capsules, and Liquids
CEO: Gerald C. Wojta/President
Production: Tom Eggleton/VP, Production
Sue A. Touse, R.Ph, J.D./Manager, Regulatory Affairs
Sean Alan/Director, Regulatory Affairs
Research: Michael Schoblelock/Manager, Clinical Research
Dr. Kirk Shepard/VP, Medical Affairs
Dr. Edward Brewton/VP, Scientific Affairs
Federal Procurement Eligibility: Medicaid Rebate

Royce *NDC Code:* **51875**
Royce Laboratories, Inc. **305-624-1500**
16600 N.W. 54 Avenue
Miami, FL 33014
Medical Product Sales Volume: $10,500,000
Total Employees: 135
Ownership: Public *FAX:* 305-621-8416
Distribution: Manufacturer of Generics
CEO: Patrick J. McEnany/Chairman and CEO
Robert Band/CPA, VP Finance/CFO
Marketing: Jack Bleau/EVP Sales & Marketing
Production: Mohammad Rahman/VP, Plant Operations
Dr. Loren Gelber/VP Regulatory Compliance
Research: Dr. Steven Miller/VP, R&D
Federal Procurement Eligibility: Medicaid Rebate

RSR Labs *see* General Inj & Vac

Ruckstuhl *see* Superior

Rugby *NDC Code:* **00536**
Rugby Laboratories., Inc. **516-536-8565**
898 Orlando Ave. **800-645-2158**
West Hempstead, NY 11552
Medical Product Sales Volume: $296,000,000
Total Employees: 770
Ownership: Hoechst Marion Roussel *FAX:* 516-536-4458
Distribution: Distributor/Manufacturer of Generics
CEO: Edward Mehrer/Chairman
Richard Frankovic/President & COO
Martin Zeiger/EVP
Marketing: Allan Egeth/VP Marketing
Research: Valerie M. Cameron/Dir Regulatory Affairs
Federal Procurement Eligibility: Medicaid Rebate
Medical Product Subsidiaries (Listed Separately):
Chelsea Labs

Rugby-Darby *see* Rugby

Russ Pharm *see* UCB Pharma

Rystan *NDC Code:* **00263**
Rystan Company, Inc. **973-256-3737**
P.O. Box 214
Little Falls, NJ 07424-0214
Total Employees: 16
Ownership: G.W.C. HEALTH, INC. *FAX:* 973-256-4083
Distribution: Specialty Manufacturer
CEO: Edmond J. Bergeron/President
Herbert Wagner/General Manager
Marketing: Donald H. Leaman,Jr./Director of Marketing
Production: Anil Patel, PhD/Quality Assurance
Federal Procurement Eligibility: Medicaid Rebate

S K Beecham *see* SKB Biols

Sandoz *see* Novartis

Sandoz Consumer *see* Novartis

Sandoz Pharm *see* Novartis

Sanofi Winthrop *NDC Code:* **00024**
Sanofi Winthrop Pharmaceuticals **212-907-2000**
90 Park Avenue
New York, NY 10016
Medical Product Sales Volume: $1,200,000,000
Total Employees: 1,550
Ownership: Sanofi
Distribution: Manufacturer of Branded Pharmaceuticals, Imaging Agents

Sanofi Winthrop *(cont'd)*
CEO: George Doherty/President
Robert DeLuccia/Pres Pharm Div
Daniel Welch/Pres Canada
James J. Boisvert/President International Div.
Dan Peters/President Sanofi Winthrop
Daniel Genter/VP Kanetta Generic Div.
Production: Jane Melville/Corp. VP Manufacturing
Research: Jack Dean/Pres Res Div
Chris J Bouvier/Dir Research Systems
Maryann Brennan/Site Mgr Information Service
Nancy L Durst/VP Strategic Issues
Teresa A Eagan/Training Manager
Romana R Farrington/Dir Regulatory Affairs
Charmaine R Fedick/Sr Clinical Research Manager
Keith Lasher/Clin Research Manager
Linda Nardone/VP Drug Reg Affairs
Federal Procurement Eligibility: Medicaid Rebate
Medical Product Subsidiaries (Listed Separately):
Cook-Waite Labs
Kanetta

Saron *NDC Code:* **00834**
Saron Pharmacal Corp. **813-898-8525**
7100 30th Avenue N.
St. Petersburg, FL 33710
Total Employees: 14
Ownership: PRIVATE

Savage Labs *NDC Code:* **00281**
Savage Laboratories **516-454-9071**
60 Baylis Road **800-231-0206**
Melville, NY 11747
Medical Product Sales Volume: $30,000,000
Total Employees: 125
Ownership: Altana *FAX:* 516-454-0732
Distribution: Specialty Manufacturer
CEO: George Cole/President
Marketing: Nancy McCutcheon/National Sales Manager
Janique Saunders/Sales Service Mgr
Production: Michael LaRocco/Director of Production
Research: Dave Pearce/Director of Research
Federal Procurement Eligibility: Medicaid Rebate

Scandipharm *NDC Code:* **58914**
Scandipharm, Inc. **205-991-8085**
22 Inverness Center Parkway
Birmingham, AL 35242
Total Employees: 60
Ownership: PRIVATE
Distribution: Specialty Manufacturer

Schein Pharm (US) *NDC Code:* **00364**
Schein Pharmaceutical, Inc. **973-593-5500**
100 Campus Drive
Florham Park, NJ 07932
Medical Product Sales Volume: $385,000,000
Total Employees: 1,700
Ownership: Miles *FAX:* 973-593-5640
Distribution: Brand & Multisource Pharmaceutical Manufacture and Distribution
CEO: Martin Sperber/Chairman & CEO
Michael Casey/EVP
James McGee/EVP & COO
Paul Feurfman/General Counsel
Darisn Ashraft/EVP & CFO
Marvin Samson/EVP
Marketing: Steven A. Basile/VP Marketing
Kenneth J. Chester/SVP Sales & Marketing
Production: Thomas T. Culkin, Pharm D./Dir Prof. & Form. Affairs
Federal Procurement Eligibility: Medicaid Rebate
Medical Product Subsidiaries (Listed Separately):
Danbury Pharm
Marsam
Steris Labs
Schein Bayer Pharm Serv
Eastern Distribution Center
Western Distribution Center

Scherer *NDC Code:* **11014, 00274**
R. P. Scherer North America **813-572-4000**
2725 Scherer Drive **800-237-0958**
St. Petersburg, FL 33716
Medical Product Sales Volume: $400,000,000
Total Employees: 4,000
Ownership: Public *FAX:* 813-573-1607
Distribution: Specialty Manufacturer of Capsules
CEO: Herbert Hugill/President
Marketing: William J. Jones/Marketing Mgr
Medical Product Subsidiaries (Listed Separately):
Scherer Labs TX

Schering *NDC Code:* **00085**
Schering-Plough Corporation **908-298-4000**
Galloping Hill Road **800-822-7000**
Kenilworth, NJ 07033
Medical Product Sales Volume: $3,640,000,000
Total Employees: 21,100
Ownership: Public *FAX:* 908-298-5354
Distribution: Manufacturer of Branded Pharmaceuticals
CEO: Robert P. Luciano/Chairman & CEO
Jack L. Wyszomierski/CFO
Richard J. Kogan/President & COO
Raul E. Cesan/EVP & Pres Pharm. Unit
David Stout/Pres Schering Labs
Donald R. Conklin/EVP & Pres Health Care Products
Rodolfo C. Bryce/President Schering International
Allan S. Kushen/SVP Public Affairs
Hugh A. D'Andrade/EVP Administration
Gordon C. O'Brien/Human Resources
Marketing: Tom Feitel/Dir, New Product Development
Leonard Camarda/VP Disease Mgt. & Managed Care
Steve Andrzejewski/Senior Dir., Marketing Allergy
Paul Huff/Product Mgr Claritin
Jason O'Neill/Product Mgr VANCENASE

Schering *(cont'd)*
Production: Maurice Greene, PhD/VP Quality Control
Robert Fidanza/Director Corporate Quality Assur.
Brian Morgan/Dir Pharmaceuticals Compliance
Research: Jonathan R. Spicehandler/President Research Div.
Alexander Z. Lane, MD, PhD/Pres, S.-P. Research
Donald R. Conklin/EVP, Pharm.
Dr. Peder K. Jensen/Sr. Dir, Clinical Research
John M Clayton/Sr VP Scientific & Reg Affairs
Wayne Coen/Mgr Worldwide Research Qa
Arthur Gertel/Dir Medical Communications
Elin R Krhoun/Mgr Regulatory Affairs
Barbara A Matlosz/Dir Regulatory Affairs
Kathleen M O'Brien/V P Research Services
Loretta A Simek/Mgr Regulatory Affairs
Gay Steinbrick/Director Drug Information
Diane J Zezza/Mgr Regulatory Affairs
Federal Procurement Eligibility: Medicaid Rebate
Medical Product Subsidiaries (Listed Separately):
Key
Warrick Pharm

Schiaperelli *see* SCS Pharm

Scholl *see* Schering

Schwarz Pharma (US) *NDC Code:* **00091, 00131**
Schwarz Pharma, Inc. **414-238-9994**
P.O. Box 2038 **800-319-8400**
Milwaukee, WI 53201
Medical Product Sales Volume: $113,000,000
Total Employees: 700
Ownership: Schwarz Pharma AG *FAX:* 414-238-0961
Distribution: Manufacturer of Branded Pharmaceuticals
CEO: Klaus Julicher/President
Marketing: Donald Lucas/VP, Sales and Marketing
Production: John Lee/VP, Pharmaceutical Operations
Research: H. Ron Stratton, PhD./VP, Drug Product Development
S. Pollock, R.Ph./Director, Regulatory Affairs
Federal Procurement Eligibility: Medicaid Rebate
Medical Product Subsidiaries (Listed Separately):
Central Pharm

Sclavo *NDC Code:* **42021**
Sclavo, Inc. **201-696-8300**
5 Mansard Court **800-526-5260**
Wayne, NJ 07470
Total Employees: 80
Ownership: PRIVATE *FAX:* 201-831-1208
CEO: G. Marucci/President
T. Vanni/EVP
Marketing: Martin King PhD/VP New Product Development

Scot Tussin *NDC Code:* **00372**
Scot Tussin Pharmacal Inc. **401-942-8555**
P.O. Box 8217 **800-638-7268**
Cranston, RI 02920-0217
Medical Product Sales Volume: $2,000,000
Total Employees: 20
Ownership: PRIVATE *FAX:* 401-942-5690
Distribution: Specialty Manufacturer of Antitussives for Prescription and Over The Counter Pharmaceuticals
CEO: Salvatore G. Scotti PhD/President
Michelle M. Scotti/VP
Production: K.M. Scotti/VP
Research: Dr. A. Di Pippo
Dr. D. Woodford
Federal Procurement Eligibility: GSA Contract

Scruggs *NDC Code:* **00329**
Scruggs Pharmacal Company, Inc.
P.O. Box 1024
Oxford, MS 38655
Ownership: PRIVATE

SCS Pharm *NDC Code:* **00905**
SCS Pharmaceuticals **708-982-7000**
P.O. Box 5110 **800-942-2566**
Chicago, IL 60680
Ownership: Searle *FAX:* 708-470-3851
Distribution: Manufacturer of Branded Pharmaceuticals
CEO: Al Heller/General Manager
Marketing: Donna Cassini/Product Manager
Research: Subhash Desai/Assoc Dir Clinical Affairs
Arnold Yeadon/Director Medical Affairs
Federal Procurement Eligibility: Medicaid Rebate

Searle *NDC Code:* **00025, 00014**
GD Searle and Co.
4901 Searle Okwy **800-323-1603**
Skokie, IL 60077
Ownership: Public
Distribution: Manufacturer of Branded Pharmaceuticals
Federal Procurement Eligibility: Medicaid Rebate

Seatrace *NDC Code:* **00551**
Seatrace Pharmaceuticals, Inc. **205-442-5023**
P.O. Box 363
Gadsden, AL 35902
Medical Product Sales Volume: $1,000,000
Total Employees: 8
Ownership: PRIVATE *FAX:* 205-442-5079
Distribution: Specialty Manufacturer
CEO: Hugh Campbell
Marketing: Ken Winsen
Research: Dr. T. Sam Roe

Seneca Pharms *NDC Code:* **47028**
Seneca Pharmaceuticals **919-783-6936**
P.O. Box 25021
Raleigh, NC 27611

Seneca Pharms *(cont'd)*
Medical Product Sales Volume: $1,000,000
Total Employees: 4
Ownership: PRIVATE *FAX:* 919-782-8234
Distribution: Manufacturer with Southeast Distribution
CEO: Nelson Hinton/President
Marketing: Tracey Nycek
Federal Procurement Eligibility: Medicaid Rebate

Serono Labs *NDC Code:* **44087**
Serono Laboratories, Inc. **617-982-9000**
100 Longwater Circle **800-283-8088**
Norwell, MA 02061
Medical Product Sales Volume: $173,000,000
Total Employees: 878
Ownership: Ares-Serono *FAX:* 617-871-6754
Distribution: Manufacturer of Fertility Products
CEO: Hisham Samra, MD/President
James L. McEvoy/VP Human Resources
Marketing: Ellen Frank, PhD/VP Marketing
Jim Worth/Director of Infertility Marketing
Production: Peter Grassam/VP Operations
Research: Jack Singer PhD/VP Research & Development
Jodi Klein Holmans/Sr Clinical Data Analyst
Sally M Kennedy/Med Research Specialist
Robert J Matis/Dir Post Marketing Rsch
David R Palan/Drug Information & Surv Assoc
Rosann J Reinhart/Dir Plng & Logistics
Deborah J Yerdon/Sr Reg Aff Associate

Sherwood-Davis & Geck *NDC Code:* **08880**
Sherwood-Davis & Geck **314-621-7788**
1915 Olive Street **800-325-7472**
St. Louis, MO 63103
Medical Product Sales Volume: $1,000,000,000
Total Employees: 8,600
Ownership: American Home Products *FAX:* 314-241-1673
Distribution: Specialty Manufacturer
CEO: David A. Low/President
Robert Egan/VP, U.S. Sales and Marketing
Trevor M. Pritchard/EVP International Sales and Marketing
J. Terry Broers/VP Finance and Administration
Susan C. Pfeffer/VP Human Resources
D. Graeme Thomas/VP Global Strategic Planning and R&D
Edwin Weichselbaum/VP Global Manufacturing & Engineering
Thomas Gonzalez/VP Global Quality Management
Frank J. Facile/VP Regulatory Affairs
Stanley N. Garber/Corporate Counsel
Federal Procurement Eligibility: Medicaid Rebate

Shionogi USA *NDC Code:* **45809**
Shionogi USA **310-540-1161**
3848 Carson Street #206
Torrence, CA 90503
Medical Product Sales Volume: $3,943,520
Total Employees: 3
Ownership: Shionogi *FAX:* 310-316-2549
Distribution: Importer
CEO: Mike Horikawa/VP
Marketing: Connie Thane/Marketing Manager
Production: Mike Horikawa/VP
Federal Procurement Eligibility: Medicaid Rebate

Shoals Pharm *NDC Code:* **47649**
404-475-4758
P.O. Box 1065
Alpharetta, GA 30239-1065
Total Employees: 4
Ownership: Hauck
Distribution: Specialty Manufacturer

Sidmak Labs *NDC Code:* **50111**
Sidmak Laboratories, Inc. **201-386-5566**
17 West Street, P.O. Box 371 **800-922-0547**
East Hanover, NJ 07936
Medical Product Sales Volume: $80,000,000
Total Employees: 600 *Telex:* 820811
Ownership: PRIVATE *FAX:* 201-386-9280
Distribution: Manufacturer of Generics
CEO: Satish Patel, PhD/President
Vinayak Bhalani/EVP
Louis Guerci/VP, Finance & Administration
Marketing: Mr. Loken Patel/Dir Of Sales
Production: Mr. P. Ajbani/Director of Production
Paul Rulon PhD/Director of Quality Control
Eileen Taylo/Regulatory Assistant
Research: Mr. D. Kumbhani/Director of Research
Federal Procurement Eligibility: Medicaid Rebate
Medical Product Subsidiaries (Listed Separately):
Advanced Remedies
Medirex
Medisol Labs

Sigma Tau Pharms *NDC Code:* **54482**
Sigma Tau Pharmaceuticals, Inc. **301-948-1041**
800 S. Frederick Avenue **800-447-0169**
Gaithersburg, MD 20877
Total Employees: 25
Ownership: Sigma-Tau Spa *FAX:* 301-948-8627
Distribution: Specialty Manufacturer
CEO: Claudio Cavazza PhD/Chairman & President
C. Kenneth Mehrling/Gen'l Mgr
Marketing: Barbara Bacon/VP Mktg & Sales
Federal Procurement Eligibility: Medicaid Rebate

Silarx Pharms *NDC Code:* **54838**
Silarx Pharmaceuticals, Inc. **914-352-4020**
19 West Street
Spring Valley, NY 10977
Total Employees: 30
Ownership: PRIVATE *FAX:* 914-352-4037
Distribution: Specialty Manufacturer
CEO: R. Desai/President

Silarx Pharms *(cont'd)*
Production: V. Patel
Research: C. Patel
Federal Procurement Eligibility: Medicaid Rebate

SKB Biols *NDC Code:* **58160**
SmithKline Beecham Biologicals
89 Rue De L'Institute
Rixensart Belgium
Ownership: Smithkline Beecham
Distribution: Manufacturer of Vaccines
Marketing: Eduardo Beruff/Director of Vaccines

SKB Pharms *NDC Code:* **00007, 00108**
SmithKline Beecham Pharmaceuticals **215-751-4000**
1250 South Collegeville Road **800-366-8900**
Collegeville, PA 19426
Medical Product Sales Volume: $8,867,000,000
Total Employees: 54,000
Ownership: Public *FAX:* 215-751-3400
Distribution: Manufacturer of Branded Pharmaceuticals
CEO: Jerry Karabelas/President N.A. Pharm.
J.P. Garnier/Chairman Pharm
Jan Leschly/CEO
Hugh R. Collum/Finance Dir
John C. Parker, Jr./SVP & Dir Information Resources
Tamar Howson/VP Dir, Worldwide Pharm. Bus. Development
Marketing: Howard Pien/VP Marketing
Research: Dr. George Post/Chairman of R&D
W Ford Calhoun/SVP, Dir Sci/Clinical Systems
Thomas Honohan/VP Worldwide Compliance
Robert L Powell/VP & Dir Ra & Pps
Federal Procurement Eligibility: Medicaid Rebate
Medical Product Subsidiaries (Listed Separately):
Beecham Labs
Fujisawa Smithkline
S K & F Labs
S K Beecham
Smithkline Consumer

SKCP *see* Beecham

Smith Kline & French *see* SKB Pharms

Smithkline Beecham *see* SKB Pharms

Smithkline Beecham plc *NDC Code:* **P00007**
SmithKline Beecham Plc **44-081-975-2000**
One New Horizons Court
Brentford, Middlesex TW8 9EP, UNITED KINGDOM
Medical Product Sales Volume: $10,874,100,000
Total Employees: 52,400
Ownership: Public *FAX:* 44-081-560-8399
Distribution: Manufacturer of Branded Pharmaceuticals
CEO: Henry Wendt/Chairman
Jan Leschly/Chief Executive
Hugh R. Collum/Finance Director & CFO
Harry C. Groome/Chairman, SKBeecham Consumer Brands
Dr. Jean-Pierre Garnier/Pres, World-Wide Pharmaceuticals
Dr. Jerry Karabelas/Pres, N.A. Pharmaceuticals
Dan Phelan/Human Resources
Research: Dr. George H. Poste/Chair., Pharmaceutical R&D
Alan Blick/Dir Information Sciences
Emily C Donnelly/Dir Transnatl Reg Affairs
Howard Fisher/Head Clinical Supplies
Tom Gallacher/Head Clinical Policies
Gerard J Marsat/Dir Ww Reg Compliance Gcp
Angie Mckenzie/Mgr Medical Systems Uk
David Moran/Dir & VP Clinical Operations
Sylvia Thompson/Clinical Research Manager
Alan W Tremper/Director Syntehtic Chem
Paul Wirdnam/Uk Database Manager
Medical Product Subsidiaries (Listed Separately):
Diversified Pharm Svcs
Smithkline Beecham

Soc Eze Sed Drs *NDC Code:* **10287**
Soc Eze Sedative Dressing Co.
P.O. Box 28
Gardendale, AL 35071
Ownership: PRIVATE

Sola/Barnes-Hind *see* Vision Pharms

Solopak Labs *NDC Code:* **39769**
Solopak Laboratories, Inc. **561-997-9999**
1845 Tonne Rd. **800-225-7656**
Elk Grove, IL 60007
Medical Product Sales Volume: $57,656,000
Total Employees: 543
Ownership: PRIVATE *FAX:* 561-998-3036
Distribution: Manufacturer of Generic Injectables
CEO: Patrick Welsh/Chairman
Otto Nonnenmann/CEO
Marketing: Don Franklin/Vice President
Elizabeth M. Carbon/Manager, Bids & Contracts
Production: Bob Polster/VP Manufacturing
Research: Dr. Allen Kay/Vice President
Federal Procurement Eligibility: Medicaid Rebate
Medical Product Subsidiaries (Listed Separately):
Solopak Med Prod

Solopak Mdcl *NDC Code:* **59747**
SoloPak Medical Products, Inc. **708-806-0080**
1845 Tonne Road
Elk Grove Village, IL 60007-5125
Medical Product Sales Volume: $17,761,702
Total Employees: 193
Ownership: Solpak Pharmaceuticals Inc. *FAX:* 708-806-0087
Distribution: Manufacturer of Pre-filled Syringes
CEO: Otto Nonnenmann
Production: Robert Polster
Research: Allen Kay

Solvay & CIE *NDC Code:* **P00032**
Solvay & CIE **32-2-509-6111**
33 Rue de Prince Albert, Ixelles
Brussels B-1050, BELGIUM
Medical Product Sales Volume: $1,100,000,000
Total Employees: 45,585
Ownership: Public *FAX:* 32-2-509-6617
Distribution: Manufacturer of Chemicals & Pharmaceuticals
CEO: Baron Daniel Janssen/Chairman
Medical Product Subsidiaries (Listed Separately):
Kali-Chemie AG
Solvay

Solvay Pharm *see* Intl Labs

Solvay Pharms *NDC Code:* **00032**
Solvay Pharmaceuticals, Inc. **770-578-9000**
901 Sawyer Road
Marietta, GA 30062
Medical Product Sales Volume: $100,000,000
Total Employees: 1,000
Ownership: Solvay & CIE
Distribution: Manufacturer of Branded Pharmaceuticals
CEO: David Dodd/President
Marketing: Lawrence Downey, MD/SVP Sales & Mktg
Research: Virginia O Ackerman/Director Reg Liason
Theresa Cheung/Regulatory Affairs
Evan M. Demestihas, MD/Sr. Director Medical & Professional Services
Andrew L Finn/VP Clinical Operations
Bradley Jeffries/Dir Clinical Research
Federal Procurement Eligibility: Medicaid Rebate
Medical Product Subsidiaries (Listed Separately):
Intl Labs
Reid-Provident

Somerset *NDC Code:* **39506**
Somerset Pharmaceuticals, Inc. **813-288-0040**
5215 West Laurel Street
Tampa, FL 33607-1729
Ownership: Mylan/Watson *FAX:* 813-282-0085
Distribution: Manufacturer of Branded Pharmaceuticals
CEO: Dana G. Barnett
Marketing: Tara Arcomano, R.Ph.
Research: Cheryl D. Blume, PhD/Director, Production and Research
Federal Procurement Eligibility: Medicaid Rebate

Sorter *NDC Code:* **53879**
Sorter Inc.
Ownership: PRIVATE

Speywood Pharm *NDC Code:* **55688**
Speywood Pharmaceuticals, Inc. **508-478-8900**
27 Maple Street
Milford, MA 01757
Total Employees: 19
Ownership: Porton Intl plc *FAX:* 508-478-1883
Distribution: Specialty Manufacturer
CEO: Peter J. Vichi/Director North America
Walter P. Rahn/Controller
Marketing: Frederick H. Garber/Marketing Manager
Federal Procurement Eligibility: Medicaid Rebate

Squibb Diagnostics *see* Bracco DXS

Squibb Westwood *see* Westwood Squibb

Squibb-Mark *NDC Code:* **57783**
Squibb-Mark, Generic **609-987-6812**
P.O. Box 4000
Princeton, NJ 08543
Ownership: Bristol-Myers Squibb
CEO: Thomas Ludlan/President
Marketing: Lee Burg/VP Sales
Nanci Bachman/Director, Marketing
Federal Procurement Eligibility: Medicaid Rebate

Stafford Miller *NDC Code:* **55372**
Stafford Miller Internationl Co.
257 Cornelison St
Jersy City, NJ 07302
Ownership: PRIVATE
Federal Procurement Eligibility: Medicaid Rebate

Star Pharms FL *NDC Code:* **00076**
Star Pharmaceuticals, Inc. **9545-971-9704**
1990 Northwest 44th St. **800-845-7827**
Pompano Beach, FL 33064
Medical Product Sales Volume: $1,000,000
Total Employees: 8
Ownership: PRIVATE *FAX:* 954-971-7718
Distribution: Manufacturer of Branded Pharmaceuticals
CEO: Scott L. Davidson/Chairman & President
Marketing: Stu Werner
Nalini Narain
Federal Procurement Eligibility: Medicaid Rebate

STC Pharm *see* Lilly

Steris Labs *NDC Code:* **00402**
Steris Labs **602-269-5120**
P.O. Box 23160 **800-692-9995**
Phoenix, AZ 85063-3160
Total Employees: 600
Ownership: Schein Pharm *FAX:* 602-269-7468
Distribution: Manufacturer of Generic Injectables, Ophthalmic and Otic Products
CEO: Gary Sielski/VP & Gen Mgr
Ron Crowe/VP Human Resources
Marketing: Michael Jay Blank/VP Marketing
Production: George Sheaffer/VP Engineering/Tech Services

Steris Labs *(cont'd)*
Research: Wanda Williams/Dir
Federal Procurement Eligibility: Medicaid Rebate

Sterling Drug *see* Sanofi Winthrop

Sterling Winthrop *see* Sanofi Winthrop

Sterling Winthrop Imaging *see* Nycomed

Stewart-Jackson *NDC Code:* **45985**
Stewart Jackson Pharmacal, Inc. **901-396-8285**
4200 Lamar Ave. #103
Memphis, TN 38118-6978
Ownership: PRIVATE
Federal Procurement Eligibility: Medicaid Rebate

Stiefel Labs *NDC Code:* **00145, 56083**
Stiefel Laboratories Inc. **305-443-3800**
255 Alhambra Circle, Suite 1000
Coral Gables, FL 33134
Ownership: PRIVATE *FAX:* 305-443-3467
Distribution: Manufacturer of Topicals
CEO: Werner K. Stiefel/Chairman, CEO
Charles W. Stiefel/President
Richard I. Fried/VP Finance
Marketing: Jon Jungquist/VP and Gen'l Manager
Production: J. Jay Pittman, Jr./President Manufacturing Division
Research: Daniel W. Nicolai/President, Stiefel Research Inc.
Federal Procurement Eligibility: Medicaid Rebate
Medical Product Subsidiaries (Listed Separately):
Durham Pharm
Glades Pharm

Storz Ophthalm *NDC Code:* **57706**
Storz Ophthalmics Inc. Div. American Cyanamid **914-733-5000**
401 North Middletown Road **800-533-3753**
Pearl River, NY 10965
Ownership: American Cyanamid

Stratus Pharms *NDC Code:* **58980**
Stratus Pharmaceuticals Inc.
P.O. Box 4632
Miami, FL 33265
Ownership: PRIVATE *FAX:* 305-254-6875
Distribution: Specialty Manufacturer
CEO: John Billoch/VP Operations
Federal Procurement Eligibility: Medicaid Rebate

Stuart Pharm *NDC Code:* **00038**
Stuart Pharmaceuticals **302-886-3000**
Concord Pike & New Murphy Road
Wilmington, DE 19897
Medical Product Sales Volume: $1,360,000,000
Total Employees: 2,800
Ownership: Zeneca *FAX:* 302-886-1667
Distribution: Manufacturer of Branded Pharmaceuticals
CEO: Robert C. Black/President
Jack Duncan/Dir
Marketing: Michael J. Rance/VP Business Development
Donald E. Frank/National Sales Manager
Production: Robert G. Milkovics
Research: Barbara Stepanek/Research Information
Federal Procurement Eligibility: Medicaid Rebate

Summit *see* Novartis

Superior *NDC Code:* **00144**
Superior Pharmaceutical Company **314-776-6160**
1385 Kemper Meadow Dr.
Cincinnati, OH 45240
Ownership: PRIVATE

Superpharm Labs *see* Goldline Labs

Syntex FP *NDC Code:* **42987**
Syntex FP, Inc. **415-855-5050**
340 Kingsland St.
Nutley, NJ 07110
Total Employees: 1,800
Ownership: Syntex
Distribution: Manufacturer of Branded Pharmaceuticals
Federal Procurement Eligibility: Medicaid Rebate

Syntex Labs *NDC Code:* **00033**
Syntex Laboratories, Inc. **415-855-5050**
3401 Hillview Avenue
Palo Alto, CA 94304
Medical Product Sales Volume: $2,123,000,000
Total Employees: 9,500
Ownership: Roche Holding Ltd *FAX:* 415-852-1569
Distribution: Manufacturer of Branded Pharmaceuticals
CEO: Paul E. Freiman/Chairman
Thomas W. Hoffmeister/Pres Syntex Laboratories
Hans A. Wolf/Vice Chairman, Chief Admin. Officer
John P. Munson/President, Syntex Intl.
Kenneth Taylor, MD, PhD/President
Marketing: Virgil Thompson/EVP Marketing
Henry Kirsch/SVP Marketing
Dr. Debbie Jo Blank/VP Pharmaceutical Marketing
Roberto Rosenkranz/Dir, New Product Development
Mary O'Hara/Marketing
Peter Smith/Product Mgr NAPROSYN
Amy Stephenson/Product Mgr ANAPROX
Jay Shepard/Product Mgr TORADOL
Production: Dr. Boyd Poulsen/SVP Pharmaceutical Development
Anthony Bourdakis/VP Reg. Affairs
Dr. Robert Sparks/VP Product Saftey & Compliance
John Lampson/Director, Legislative Compliance
Art Mandell/Director, Market Planning
Barbara Simkin/Manager, New Product Market

Syntex Labs *(cont'd)*
Research
David M. Hoffmeister/Attorney
Research: Dr. John H. Fried/Vice Chair, Pres Syntex Research
Dr. Robert A. Lewis/EVP & Dir Basic Research
Karl Agre/Dir Cv Clinical Research
Nancy R Baltis/Mgr Information Resource
Anthony Bourdakis/VP Reg Affrs & Corp Compl
Irwin A Heyman/VP & Director Its
Ruth Kasle/Mgr Corp Regulatory Info
Samuel Ladabaum/Dir Resrces & Intellignc
Pat K Lavette/Mgr Technical Information
Penny Lewis/Manager Of Training
Sarah L Peralo/Mgr Information Section
Robert L Roe/Ex Vp/Dir Medical Research
Keith Schmidt/Dir Sales Strategy
Kathy Trimble/Mgr Product Information Mgmnt
Carol Whiteley/New Product Develop Mgr
Rickey Wilson/VP Human Pharm Reg Affrs
Federal Procurement Eligibility: Medicaid Rebate
Medical Product Subsidiaries (Listed Separately):
Hamilton Pharm
Syntex FP
Syntex PR

Syntex PR *NDC Code:* **18393**
Syntex Laboratories (P R) **415-855-5050**
3401 Hillview Avenue
Palo Alto, CA 94304
Ownership: Syntex
Distribution: Manufacturer of Branded Pharmaceuticals
Federal Procurement Eligibility: Medicaid Rebate

Syosset Labs *NDC Code:* **47854**
Syosset Laboratories, Inc. **516-921-6306**
150 Eileen Way
Syosset, NY 11791
Medical Product Sales Volume: $3,500,000
Total Employees: 25
Ownership: Medicis Derm *FAX:* 516-921-7971
Distribution: Manufacturer of Dermatologicals
CEO: Mark Newman/President
Steven Victor/CEO
Marketing: Lou Barricelli/National Sales Manager
Production: Paul Gabel/Director of Production
Federal Procurement Eligibility: Medicaid Rebate

Takeda-Abbott Pharm *see* TAP Pharm

Talbert Phcy *NDC Code:* **44514**
Talbert Pharmacy warehouse
6603 Darin Way
Cypress, CA 90630
Ownership: PRIVATE

TAP Pharm *NDC Code:* **00300**
TAP Pharmaceuticals, Inc. **847-317-5700**
D387 AP6C 1 **800-622-2011**
Abbott Park, IL 60064-3500
Total Employees: 524
Ownership: Takeda-Abbott Pharm *FAX:* 847-317-5795
Distribution: Manufacturer of Branded Pharmaceuticals
CEO: Hank Pietraszek/CEO
Marketing: Donald V. Patton/VP Marketing
Research: John Seely, PhD./VP Research
Dean P. Sundberg/Director of Regulatory Affairs
S. Albert Edwards/Assoc Dir Regulatory Affairs
Janet M Eppers/Medical Services Spclst
Judy Decker Wargel/Reg Products Manager
Federal Procurement Eligibility: Medicaid Rebate

Taro Pharms (US) *NDC Code:* **51672**
Taro Pharmaceuticals U.S.A. Inc. **914-345-9001**
5 Skyline Drive **800-544-1449**
Hawthorne, NY 10532-9998
Medical Product Sales Volume: $25,000,000
Total Employees: 63
Ownership: Taro Pharm *FAX:* 914-345-8728
Distribution: Manufacturer of Generic Topicals
CEO: Barrie Levitt, MD/CEO
Peter Giallorenzo/SVP, and COO
Marketing: Rebecca Pike/VP, Sales and Marketing
Arlene Adoff/Director of Marketing
Research: Avi Yacobi, PhD
Federal Procurement Eligibility: Medicaid Rebate

TE Wm Pharm *NDC Code:* **51189**
T.E. Williams Pharm. **719-687-3092**
P.O. Box 312
Divide, CO 80814-0312
Total Employees: 4
Ownership: PRIVATE
Distribution: Specialty Manufacturer
Federal Procurement Eligibility: Medicaid Rebate

Teral Labs *NDC Code:* **51234**
Teral Laboratories
Box 813
Gurabo, PR 00778
Ownership: PRIVATE

Teregen Labs *NDC Code:* **52384**
Teregen Labs Pharmaceuticals **216-975-3134**
35104 Euclid #214, P.O. Box 5025 **800-848-0055**
Willowick, OH 44095
Total Employees: 9
Ownership: Gentere *FAX:* 216-975-9808
Distribution: Manufacturer of Generics
CEO: Dennis Sharpe

Teva *NDC Code:* **00093, 00332**
Teva Pharmaceuticals USA, Inc. **215-256-8400**
P.O. Box 904 **800-545-8800**
Sellersville, PA 18960
Medical Product Sales Volume: $220,000,000
Total Employees: 508
Ownership: Teva Pharm *FAX:* 215-256-7855
Distribution: Manufacturer of Generics
CEO: William A. Fletcher/President & CEO
Marketing: Eugene Cioschi/Manager, Pharmacy Promotions
Charles Krippendorf/VP, Sales
Nick Varano/Manager, Gov. Bids & Contracts
Production: Dr. Ronald Nedich/S.V.P, Operations
Research: Deborah Jaskot/Director, Regulatory Affairs
Marc Goshko/Dir, Scientific Affairs
Alison Thomas, R.Ph./Regulatory Affairs Assoc
Federal Procurement Eligibility: Medicaid Rebate
Medical Product Subsidiaries (Listed Separately):
Gate Pharm

Teva Pharm *NDC Code:* **17372**
Teva Pharmaceutical Industries Ltd. **003-926-7267**
5 Basel St. P.O. Box 3190
Petach Tikva 49131, ISRAEL
Medical Product Sales Volume: $587,000,000
Total Employees: 2,700 *Telex:* 381111 TEVPTA IL
Ownership: Public *FAX:* 003-923-4050
Distribution: Manufacturer of Branded and Generic Pharmaceuticals
CEO: Moshe Shamir/Chairman
Eli Hurvitz/President & CEO
Dr. Aaron Schwartz/Managing Director - Pharm. Div.
Dr. Yair Gibor/Medical Director
Research: Dr. Ben-Zion Weiner/VP R & D
Medical Product Subsidiaries (Listed Separately):
Lemmon

Thames Pharma *NDC Code:* **49158**
Thames Pharmacal Co., Inc. **516-737-1155**
2100 Fifth Ave. **800-225-1003**
Ronkonkoma, NY 11779
Medical Product Sales Volume: $10,000,000
Total Employees: 135
Ownership: PRIVATE *FAX:* 516-737-3185
Distribution: Distributor/Manufacturer of Generics
CEO: Harry Schlakman/CEO
Marketing: Paula Fierro/Sales Manager
Production: Eric Stern/EVP Operations
Federal Procurement Eligibility: Medicaid Rebate

TIE Pharm *NDC Code:* **55496**
TIE Pharmaceuticals
425 Madison Ave., Suite 605
New York, NY 10017
Ownership: PRIVATE

Time-Caps Labs *NDC Code:* **49483**
Time-Caps Labs **516-753-1110**
7 Micheal Ave.
Farmingdale, NY 11735
Total Employees: 37
Ownership: PRIVATE *FAX:* 516-753-2220
Research: Walter Epler/VP Regulatory Affairs

Tmk Pharm *NDC Code:* **59582**
TMK Pharmaceuticals
1505 West Reyolds St. **800-554-8399**
Plantcity, FL 33567
Total Employees: 11
Ownership: PRIVATE
Distribution: Specialty Manufacturer
Federal Procurement Eligibility: Medicaid Rebate

Topi-Cana *NDC Code:* **59197**
Topi-Cana Specialties **305-970-4539**
P.O. Box 636408 **800-829-6610**
Margate, FL 33063
Medical Product Sales Volume: $250,000
Total Employees: 2
Ownership: PRIVATE *FAX:* 305-977-0255
Distribution: Specialty Distributor
CEO: Jay Barrett/President

Torrance *NDC Code:* **00389**
Torrance Co. **616-327-0722**
800 Lenox Avenue **800-327-0722**
Portage, MI 49002
Medical Product Sales Volume: $500,000
Total Employees: 4
Ownership: PRIVATE *FAX:* 616-327-0763
Distribution: Distributor of Generics

Tpn Of New England *see* Immuno-US

Trinity Technologies *NDC Code:* **61355**
Trinity Technologies Corp. **810-778-5630**
28510 Hayes
Roseville, MI 48066
Medical Product Sales Volume: $2,000,000
Total Employees: 25
Ownership: Therapharm Holdings
Distribution: Manufacturer of Generics
Marketing: John Panlsen/Dir, Sales & Marketing
Federal Procurement Eligibility: Medicaid Rebate

TX Drug Reps *NDC Code:* **47202**
Texas Drug Reps Inc. **512-349-2695**
11722 Warfield
San Antonio, TX 78216
Ownership: Major Pharm
Distribution: Distributor of Generics

UAD Labs *NDC Code:* **00785**
UAD Laboratories, Inc. **314-344-8870**
13622 Lakefront Drive
St. Louis, MO 63045
Total Employees: 208
Ownership: Forest Labs *FAX:* 314-344-4435
Distribution: Specialty Manufacturer
CEO: James E. Smith/VP Operations
Research: Laura Lakemeyer/Supervisor, Scientific Affairs
Federal Procurement Eligibility: Medicaid Rebate

UCB Pharma Pharma Pharma *NDC Code:* **50474**
UCB Pharma Pharma Pharma, Inc. **770-437-5500**
1950 Lake Park Drive **800-477-7877**
Smyrna, GA 30080
Total Employees: 500
Ownership: UCB Pharma Pharma SA *FAX:* 770-437-5510
Distribution: Branded, Branded Generic, OTC Products, Research and Development
CEO: Tony Tebbott/President
Marketing: Veronique Cardon/Director, Marketing
Ralph Steinlight/Director,, Sales Administration
Production: Luc Vermeesch/Director, Operations
Research: Ernst Wulfert/Director
Federal Procurement Eligibility: Medicaid Rebate
Medical Product Subsidiaries (Listed Separately):
Northampton

UDL *NDC Code:* **51079**
UDL Laboratories, Inc. **815-282-1201**
P.O. Box 10319
Rockford, IL 61131-3019
Total Employees: 320
Ownership: Roderick Corporation (formerly known as T.C. Manufacturing Company, Inc.) A wholly owned subsidiary of Mylan Laboratories, Inc. *FAX:* 815-282-9391
Distribution: Distributer of Generic Pharmaceuticals in Oral Solid and Liquid Forms
CEO: Michael Reicher/President
Marketing: John Ford/Senior Vice President of Sales & Marketing
Production: Sherri MacDonald/Sr VP of Operations
Research: Anita Runyan, PhD,/R&D Director
Federal Procurement Eligibility: Medicaid Rebate

Unimed *NDC Code:* **A00100**
Unimed, Inc. **708-541-2525**
2150 E. Lake Cook Road - Suite 210
Buffalo Grove, IL 60089
Medical Product Sales Volume: $3,697,201
Total Employees: 33
Ownership: Public *FAX:* 708-541-2569
Distribution: Marketer of Pharmaceuticals
CEO: Dr. John Kapoor/Chairman
Stephen Simes/President & CEO
David Riggs/VP Finance & Administration, CFO
Russell W. Abraham/VP Operations
Marketing: Subh Sethi/VP Sales & Marketing

Unit Dose Laboratories *see* UDL

United Res *NDC Code:* **00677**
United Research Labs. **215-638-2626**
3600 Marshall Lane **800-523-3684**
Bensalem, PA 19020
Medical Product Sales Volume: $50,000,000
Total Employees: 120
Ownership: PRIVATE *FAX:* 215-638-6101
Distribution: Distributor of Generics
CEO: Richard H. Roberts MD, PhD/CEO
Marketing: Maurice Maleh/SVP Sales and Marketing
Lawrence Felzer/Group Mgr, Pricing & Contracts
Federal Procurement Eligibility: Medicaid Rebate
Medical Product Subsidiaries (Listed Separately):
Fort David Labs
Mutual Pharm

Univax *see* N Am Biologicals

Universal Labs *NDC Code:* **52906**
Universal Labs Inc.
1021 Americo Miranda Ave. Repto Metro
San Juan, PR 00921
Ownership: PRIVATE

Upjohn *see* Pharmacia & Upjohn

Upsher Smith *NDC Code:* **00245**
Upsher-Smith Laboratories, Inc. **612-473-4412**
14905-23rd Ave. North **800-328-3344**
Minneapolis, MN 55447
Total Employees: 200
Ownership: PRIVATE *FAX:* 612-476-4026
Distribution: Manufacturer of Specialty Brands
CEO: Kenneth L. Evenstad/Chairman, President & CEO
Larry Shelton/EVP
Marketing: Kade Kadrie/SVP Sales & Marketing
Production: George Tomaich/VP, Manufacturing
Research: Harvey M. Arbit/VP, Regulatory Affairs
Federal Procurement Eligibility: Medicaid Rebate

URL *see* United Res

US Bioscience *NDC Code:* **58178**
U. S. Bioscience, Inc. **610-832-0570**
One Tower Bridge,Ste 400 100 Front Street **800-447-3969**
West Conshohocken, PA 19428
Medical Product Sales Volume: $2,400,000
Total Employees: 150
Ownership: Public *FAX:* 610-832-4500
Distribution: Manufacturer of Branded Pharmaceuticals
CEO: Philip S. Schein/Chairman & CEO
Russell McLauchlan/President & COO

US Bioscience *(cont'd)*
Marketing: Alison Ayers/VP, Sales
R. Alan Birtchet/VP, Marketing
Barbara Deptula/Bus Unit Dir
Ellen Evans/Dir Bus Devel
Gary Mickey/Bus Unit Dir
Production: Donald O. Brown/SVP Pharm Operations
J. Paul Davignon/VP Product Devel
Martin Stogniew, PhD/Dir Anal. Chemistry
Barbara Scheffler/SVP, Clinical Oper. & Reg. Affairs
Wolfgang Oster, MD/VP, International CR, Medical & Reg Affairs
Charles Katzer/Dir, Pharm. Manuf. & Distrib.
Christine Smith/Dir, Reg. Affairs
Research: Robert Capizzi, MD/EVP Worldwide R&D
Robert Myers/VP Information Science
Paul Kennedy, PhD/Dir, Pharm. Technology
Ralph Reynolds, MD/Sr. Dir, Clinical Rsearch
Edith Mitchell, MD/Sr Dir, Clinical Research/Med Affairs
Mary Rose Keller/Dir,Clinical Research Support
John Conlon, PhD/DirBiostatistics
Federal Procurement Eligibility: Medicaid Rebate

US Pharm *NDC Code:* **52747**
U.S. Pharmaceutical Corp. **404-987-4745**
2401 C Mellon Court
Decatur, GA 30035
Total Employees: 43
Ownership: PRIVATE *FAX:* 404-987-4806
Distribution: Specialty Manufacturer
CEO: Rose M. Krebs/President
Marketing: Raymond F. Meyer/Dir of Mktg
Federal Procurement Eligibility: Medicaid Rebate

US Trading *NDC Code:* **56126**
United States Trading Corp. **310-558-4666**
10718 McCune Ave.
Los Angeles, CA 90034
Total Employees: 10
Ownership: PRIVATE
Distribution: Distributor of Generics
Federal Procurement Eligibility: Medicaid Rebate

USV *see* Rhone-Poulenc Rorer

Valmed *NDC Code:* **54627**
Valmed Inc. **508-393-1599**
203 South West Cutoff **800-477-0487**
Northboro, MA 01532
Total Employees: 20
Ownership: PRIVATE *FAX:* 508-393-6860
Distribution: Specialty Manufacturer
CEO: Allyn Taylor/President
Federal Procurement Eligibility: Small Business Woman Owned

Vangard Labs *NDC Code:* **00615**
Vangard Laboratories **502-651-6188**
P.O. Box 1268
Glasgow, KY 42142-1268
Total Employees: 20
Ownership: Midway Med
Distribution: Manufacturer of Generics
Federal Procurement Eligibility: Medicaid Rebate

Venture Pharm *NDC Code:* **59785**
Venture Pharmaceuticals Inc.
Florence, AL 35630
Ownership: PRIVATE

Veratex *NDC Code:* **17022**
Veratex Corporation **313-588-2970**
1304 East Maple Road
Troy, MI 48084
Medical Product Sales Volume: $30,000,000
Total Employees: 190
Ownership: Chemed
Distribution: Physician Distributor
CEO: James Daulin/Group Executive
Marketing: Nancy Gurdiner/SVP, Sales & Marketing

Vestar *see* Nexstar

Vintage Pharms *NDC Code:* **00254**
Vintage Pharmaceuticals Inc.
3241 Woodpark Blvd.
Charlotte, NC 28206
Ownership: PRIVATE

Viratek *NDC Code:* **53095**
Viratek Incorporated **714-545-0100**
3300 Hyland Avenue **800-548-5100**
Costa Mesa, CA 92626
Medical Product Sales Volume: $11,000,000
Total Employees: 68
Ownership: ICN Pharm/Public *FAX:* 714-556-0131
Distribution: Manufacturer of Branded Pharmaceuticals
CEO: Milan Panic/Chairman & CEO
Nils O. Johannesson/President
D.C. Watt/Secretary

Vision Pharms *NDC Code:* **00077**
Vision Pharmaceuticals LP **408-736-5462**
2525 DuPont Dr. **800-538-1680**
Irvine, CA 92715
Ownership: Pilkington *FAX:* 408-773-5282
Distribution: Manufacturer of Branded Pharmaceuticals
CEO: Gary Mulloy/President & CEO
Research: David Marcus/VP Regulatory Affairs

Vita-Rx *NDC Code:* **49727**
Vita-Rx Corporation **706-568-1881**
4625 Warm Springs Road **800-241-8276**
Columbus, GA 31908
Total Employees: 17
Ownership: PRIVATE *FAX:* 706-568-1886
Distribution: Distributor of Branded and Generic Injectibles, and Generic Pharmaceuticals
CEO: Charles R. Allen/President
Marketing: Wally Doolittle
Federal Procurement Eligibility: Medicaid Rebate

Vitaline *NDC Code:* **54022**
Vitaline Corporation **503-482-9231**
385 Williamson Way
Ashland, OR 97520
Total Employees: 44
Ownership: PRIVATE *FAX:* 503-482-9112
Distribution: Specialty Manufacturer
CEO: Celia Meese/President
Marketing: Jed D. Meese/Exec VP, Technical Director
Federal Procurement Eligibility: Medicaid Rebate

Vitarine Pharm *see* Eon Labs Mfg

Voluntary Hosp *NDC Code:* **53258, 00702**
Voluntary Hospitals America, Inc. **214-594-0722**
P.O. Box 160909
Irving, TX 75016
Medical Product Sales Volume: $35,000,000
Total Employees: 1,960
Ownership: PRIVATE
Distribution: Distributor of Generics

Vortech Pharms *NDC Code:* **00298**
Vortech Pharmaceuticals, Ltd. **313-584-4088**
P.O. Box 189
Dearborn, MI 48121
Total Employees: 17
Ownership: PRIVATE
Distribution: Manufacturer of Veterinary Pharmaceuticals
CEO: John A. Mac Neil/President

Wakefield Pharms *NDC Code:* **59310**
Wakefield Pharmaceuticals Inc. **770-664-1661**
1050 Cambridge Sq., Ste. C
Alpharetta, GA 30201
Total Employees: 30
Ownership: PRIVATE *FAX:* 770-664-1126
Distribution: Specialty Distributor of Branded Rx
CEO: Frank Byington/Pres & Chairman
Federal Procurement Eligibility: Medicaid Rebate

Wallace Labs *NDC Code:* **00037**
Wallace Laboratories Div. Carter-Wallace, Inc. **609-655-6000**
Half Acre Road
Cranbury, NJ 08512
Medical Product Sales Volume: $663,000,000
Total Employees: 4,020
Ownership: Public
Distribution: Manufacturer of Pharmaceuticals/Contraceptives
CEO: Henry Hoyt, Jr./Chairman
Charles O. Hoyt/Chairman of Executive Committee
Daniel J. Black/President
Herbert Sosman/VP Pharm,U.S.
Marketing: Thomas G. Gerstmeyer/VP Marketing
Stanley Kleiner/VP Sales
Research: Frank A Beebe/Manager Marketing Service
Judith S Burgess/Dir Data Management
William Diamantis/Dir Of Pharmacology
Anita Durso/Mgr Clinical Research
D Gevail Evans/Mgr Regulatory Affairs
Harry P Flanagan/VP Medical Affairs
Ana M Fontana/Exec Dir Reg Affairs
Caroline D Galbreath/Mgr Regulatory Affairs
Mark M Goldstein/Director Mis
Monroe I Klein/VP Regulatory Affairs
Elisabeth Neumann/Director Medical Services
James L Perhach/VP Clinical Pharmacology
Alberto Rosenberg/VP Clinical Research
Joseph P Soyka/Dir Medical Affairs
Federal Procurement Eligibility: Medicaid Rebate

Walnut Pharm *see* Akorn

Warner Chilcott *NDC Code:* **00047**
Warner Chilcott Inc. **201-540-2000**
100 Enterprise Drive, Ste 280 **800-521-8813**
Rockaway, NJ 07866
Medical Product Sales Volume: $90,000,000
Total Employees: 400
Ownership: Warner-Lambert *FAX:* 201-540-3283
Distribution: Manufacturer of Generics
CEO: Roger Boissonneauit/General Manager
Marketing: A. Dominick Musacchio/Dir Marketing
Gary Borchard/Manager, Sales & Marketing
Research: Charles Baton/Dir Hlth Care Econ/Policy
Harvey L Dickstein/VP Reg Affairs Admin
Lesley Fierro/Supervisor Drug Informatn
Eleonora C Gabriel/Director Drug Safety
David F Rhodes/Mgr Product/Form Info
Diane M Telliho/Mgr Drug Safety & Surv
Donald M Thall/Mgr Drug Safety/Epidem
Jan Worster/Dir Professional Services
Federal Procurement Eligibility: Medicaid Rebate

Warner-Lambert *NDC Code:* **P00071**
Warner-Lambert Company **201-540-2000**
170 Tabor Road
Morris Plains, NJ 07950

Warner-Lambert *(cont'd)*
Medical Product Sales Volume: $5,050,000,000
Total Employees: 34,000
Ownership: Public
Distribution: Manufacturer of Branded & Generic Pharmaceuticals
CEO: Melvin R. Goodes/Chairman & CEO
Lodewijk J.R. de Vink/President & COO
Joseph E. Smith/EVP, President Pharm. Sector
Fred Hassan/Group VP Pharmaceuticals
John F. Walsh/EVP, Pres, Consumer Prod. Sector
Ronald E. Zier/VP Public Affairs
Donald E. O'Neill/EVP
Earnest J. Larini/VP & CFO
Marketing: Michael Hall/National Account Sales Manager
Production: Philip M. Gross/VP, Pres Novon Products Group
Research: Ronald M. Cresswell, PhD/VP Chair, Pharm. Research
Pedro M. Cuatrecasas MD/VP, Parke-Davis Research
D J Bauer/Group Dir Pharm Mktg Sup
Elliot B Beck/Dir Intl Registration
Joseph D Clark/VP Reg & Scientific Affrs
Mary C Grasso/Assoc Dir Medical Affairs
Lawrence F Haverkost/Director New Products Pla
Louise S Kaufman/Senior Director
Robert J Monaghan/Dir Reg Affairs Intl
Susan J Sebastian/Med Communications Spec
Floyd Seidman/Mgr Pharm Labeling
Jerome Wilson/Dir Biostat & Data Mgmt
Medical Product Subsidiaries (Listed Separately):
Jouveinal SA
Parke-Davis
Warner Chilcott

Warrick Pharms *NDC Code:* **59930**
Warrick Pharmaceuticals Corp. **908-298-4000**
2000 Galloping Hill Road **800-822-7000**
Kenilworth, NJ 07033
Ownership: Schering *FAX:* 908-298-5354
Distribution: Manufacturer of Generic Pharmaceuticals
Federal Procurement Eligibility: Medicaid Rebate

Watson Labs *NDC Code:* **52544**
Watson Laboratories, Inc. **909-270-1400**
132A Business Center Drive
Corona, CA 91720
Medical Product Sales Volume: $94,900,000
Total Employees: 500
Ownership: Public
Distribution: Manufacturer of Generics
CEO: Dr. Allen Chao/President
Research: Neil E Sherman/Vice President Qa
Federal Procurement Eligibility: Medicaid Rebate
Medical Product Subsidiaries (Listed Separately):
Cicra Pharm

WC *see* Warner Chilcott

WE Pharm *NDC Code:* **59196**
WE Pharmaceuticals Inc. **619-788-9155**
P.O. Box 1142
Ramona, CA 92065
Total Employees: 24
Ownership: PRIVATE *FAX:* 619-788-9445
Distribution: Specialty Manufacturer of Respiratory Products
CEO: Craig Wheeler/President
Marketing: Tom Evangelisti
Production: Joe Salmon
Research: Scott Garner

Webcon *see* Alcon-PR

Webcon Pharm *see* Alcon

Weleda *NDC Code:* **00155**
Weleda Inc.
P.O. Box 769
Spring Valley, NY 10977
Ownership: PRIVATE

Wesley Pharma *NDC Code:* **00917**
Wesley Pharmacal Co. **215-698-2900**
114 Railroad Drive
Ivyland, PA 18974
Total Employees: 21
Ownership: PRIVATE

West Point Pharma *NDC Code:* **59591**
West Point Pharma **215-661-5000**
800-647-7770
West Point, PA 19486
Ownership: Merck
Distribution: Manufacturer of Generics
Federal Procurement Eligibility: Medicaid Rebate

West Ward Pharm *NDC Code:* **00143**
West-Ward Pharmaceutical Corp. **800-631-2174**
465 Industrial Way West
Eatontown, NJ 07724
Medical Product Sales Volume: $6,000,000
Total Employees: 91
Ownership: Hikma Pharm, Jordan *FAX:* 908-542-6150
Distribution: Manufacturer/Distributor of Generics
CEO: Nabil Rizk/General Manager and Pres
Marketing: Hal Zenenberg/Director of Marketing
Production: Martin Sheer/Director of Production
Research: Suresh Chokhavatia/Mgr Research & Development
Federal Procurement Eligibility: Medicaid Rebate

Westwood Squibb *NDC Code:* **00072**
Westwood-Squibb Pharmaceuticals, Inc. **716-887-3400**
100 Forest Avenue **800-333-0950**
Buffalo, NY 14213

Westwood Squibb *(cont'd)*
Medical Product Sales Volume: $100,000,000
Total Employees: 800
Ownership: Bristol-Myers Squibb
Distribution: Manufacturer of Branded Pharmaceuticals
CEO: Jeffrey B. Marsh/President
Marketing: Gary Duszynski/Sen Mgr, Managed Care Mktg
Tom Klein/Product Strategy Mgr
Jeffrey Dunbar/Customer Marketing Manager
Baetana Schucckler/Customer Marketing Manager
Production: Kathy B. Schrode, PhD/Dir Drug Regulatory Affairs
Federal Procurement Eligibility: Medicaid Rebate

WH Rorer *see* Rhone-Poulenc Rorer

Wharton *see* Rhone-Poulenc Rorer

Whitby *see* UCB Pharma

Whitby Pharm *see* Searle

Whitehall *NDC Code:* **00573**
Whitehall Labs
685 Third Avenue **212-986-1000**
New York, NY 10017
Total Employees: 744
Ownership: American Home Prod *FAX:* 212-878-5771
Marketing: Andrew Davis/SVP Marketing
Lyn Ciocca/VP Marketing
Holly Crosbie-Foote/VP Marketing
John Schmitt/VP Marketing
Research: Stephen Cristo/Mgr Regulatory Affairs
Psyzard J Cuprys/Assoc Dir Reg Affairs
Barry H Dash/Sr VP Scientific Affairs
Mary H Davis/Assoc Dir Reg Affairs
Sandy A Furey/Director Medical Affairs
David J George/Dir Tech Affairs
Jamie J Greene/Assoc Dir Of Clinical Resrch
Julie P Minn/Mgr Drug Information
Devra C Mintz/Asst Dir Medical Affairs
Iris H Shelton/Asst Dir Reg Affairs
Steven J Stravinski/VP Medical & Scientific Affairs
William R Thoden/Mgr Clinical Research
Joel A Waksman/Director Of Statistics
Federal Procurement Eligibility: Medicaid Rebate

Wilcole Pharm *NDC Code:* **58918**
Wilcole Pharmaceuticals, Inc.
Ownership: PRIVATE

Willen Drug *see* Baker Norton Pharms

William Labs *NDC Code:* **51101**
William Labs Inc. **908-340-1717**
727 Raritan Road
Clark, NJ 07066
Medical Product Sales Volume: $500,000
Total Employees: 5
Ownership: PRIVATE *FAX:* 908-340-1919
Distribution: Distributor of Branded Pharmaceuticals
CEO: Blanche Lichtenstein/President
Marketing: Ronni L. Faust/Vice President

Winsor Pharm *NDC Code:* **59004**
Winsor Pharmaceuticals, Inc. **804-254-4400**
1211 Sherwood Ave.
Richmond, VA 23261
Total Employees: 45
Ownership: Witby Pharm
Distribution: Distributor of Generics

Winthrop *see* Sanofi Winthrop

Wyeth Labs *NDC Code:* **00008**
Wyeth Laboratories, Inc. **610-688-4400**
170 Radnor Chester Road **800-950-5099**
Saint Davids, PA 19087
Medical Product Sales Volume: $3,859,144,000
Total Employees: 4,000
Ownership: American Home Prod *FAX:* 215-688-2762
Distribution: Manufacturer of Branded Pharmaceuticals
CEO: Bernard Canavan, MD/Chairman
Robert Essner/President
Joseph Mahady/Pres US Pharm Div
Marketing: Carrie Smith Cox/VP Women's Health
David Ridenour/VP Therapeutics
Marily Rhudy/VP Public Affairs
Jay Rachelli/Director, Wyeth Marketing
M. Dean/Product Mgr VERELEN
R. Repella/Product Mgr LODINE
K. Cancelliere/Product Mgr ISMO
J. Buchalter/Product Mgr PREMARIN
N. Marmontello/Product Mgr EFFEXOR
Ron Hayen/Dir Managed Healthcare Marketing
William Flanagan/Assoc Dir Marketing Comm.
Research: Robert Levy, MD/Pres Wyeth-Ayerst Research
William N. Warden/Exec Dir Marketing Research & Plng.
Patricia M Acri/Assoc Dir Drug Info
Joseph N Bathish/VP Regulatory Affairs
Marc W Deitch/Vice President Medical Affair
Eleanor M Delorme/Mgr Drg Regulatory Affrs
Steven R Eby/Drug Information Manager
Larry E Hare/Sr Dir Clinical Communication
Albert K Kellenbenz/Sr Dir R&D Computer Svc
Joan L Kennedy/Dir Clinical Data Mgm
Earl T Lewis/Sr Dir Medical Affairs
M Alex Michaels/VP Medical Affairs
Joseph L Morrison/Dir Regulatory Affairs
Gary L Neil/Executive Vice President
Emanuel J Russo/Director Pharm Affairs
Federal Procurement Eligibility: Medicaid Rebate
Medical Product Subsidiaries (Listed Separately):
Ayerst Labs
ESI-Pharma

Xactdose *NDC Code:* **50962**
Xactdose, Inc. **815-624-8523**
722 Progressive Lane
South-Beloit, IL 61080
Medical Product Sales Volume: $15,000,000
Total Employees: 40
Ownership: PRIVATE *FAX:* 815-624-8245
Distribution: Unit-Dose Packager
CEO: Warren Swanson
Production: Dian Campbell/Quality Assurance Manager

Yorpharm *NDC Code:* **61147**
Yorpharm Inc.
1641 Barclay Blvd.
Buffalo Grove, IL 60089
Total Employees: 200
Ownership: Apotex
Distribution: Manufacturer of Generic Injectables
CEO: Jeff Yordon/President

Zeneca *NDC Code:* **11511**
Zeneca Inc. **302-886-3000**
Concord Pike & New Murphy Road
Wilmington, DE 19897
Medical Product Sales Volume: $3,060,000,000
Total Employees: 7,900
Ownership: Imperial Chemical plc/Zeneca Ltd
Distribution: Manufacturer of Branded Pharmaceuticals
CEO: Robert C. Black/President
Tom McKillop, PhD/President Pharmaceuticals

Zeneca *(cont'd)*
Production: Robert G. Milkovies/VP Production
Research: Frank S Kondrad/Mgr Intl Strategic Planning
Frieda S Mecray/Librarian
Medical Product Subsidiaries (Listed Separately):
IPR Pharma
Stuart Pharm
Zeneca Pharm

Zeneca Group *NDC Code:* **P00310**
Zeneca Group plc **071-834-4444**
Millbank
London SW1P 3JF, UNITED KINGDOM
Medical Product Sales Volume: $9,184,100,000
Total Employees: 70,000
Ownership: Public *FAX:* 071-834-2042
Distribution: Manufacturer of Branded Pharmaceuticals
CEO: Sir Sydney Lipworth/Chairman
David Barnes/CEO
D. Friend/CEO, Pharmaceuticals
Medical Product Subsidiaries (Listed Separately):
Zeneca

Zeneca Pharms *NDC Code:* **00310**
Zeneca Pharmaceuticals Div. Zeneca Inc. **302-886-3000**
1800 Concord Pike **800-456-3669**
Wilmington, DE 19850-5437
Medical Product Sales Volume: $1,360,000,000
Total Employees: 3,000
Ownership: Zeneca *FAX:* 302-886-3119
Distribution: Manufacturer of Branded Pharmaceuticals
CEO: Robert C. Black/President
John C. Barber/VP, Business Development
W. James O'Shea/VP, Sales & Marketing
Marketing: Gene H. Zaiser/VP Sales
Christopher J. Iacono/VP Mktg
Howard A. Rosenberg/VP Commercial Planning
Alan J. Milbauer/VP External Affairs
William J. Simpson/National Business Director
Production: Robert G. Milkovics/VP Technical Operations
Research: David C. U'Prichard/EVP, Director
Ronald L. Krall/SVP Clinical Development
Frank M. Armstrong/VP Clinical/Medical Affairs
Jeffrey S. Rudolf/VP Pharmaceutical Development
A. Keith Willard/VP Biomedical Research
Federal Procurement Eligibility: Medicaid Rebate
Medical Product Subsidiaries (Listed Separately):
IPR Pharma

Zenith Labs *NDC Code:* **00172**
Zenith Laboratories, Inc. **201-767-1700**
140 Legrand Avenue **800-631-1583**
Northvale, NJ 07647
Medical Product Sales Volume: $96,000,000
Total Employees: 401
Ownership: Ivax *FAX:* 201-767-6873
Distribution: Manufacturer of Generics
CEO: Phillip Frost, MD
John H. Klein/President No. American Pharm
Bill Schreck/EVP Opeartions
Richard Friedman/VP Finance & CFO
Marketing: Lenora C. Gavalas/EVP Sales and Marketing
Production: Nicholas Maselli/VP Northvale Operations
Research: Subramanian Veerappan
Robert Monaghan/Director of Regulatory Affairs
Vincent Warren/Director of Analytical Research
Federal Procurement Eligibility: Medicaid Rebate

DIRECTORY OF AIDS DRUG ASSISTANCE PROGRAMS IN THE U.S., GUAM, AND VIRGIN ISLANDS

Listed by State or Territory

ALABAMA
Catherine Jackson
Direct And Service Branch
HIV/AIDS Divison
Alabama Department of Health
434 Monroe Street
Montgomery, AL 36130
(334) 613-5357, Fax: (334) 288-5021

ALASKA
Wendy Craytor
Division of Public Health
Alaska Department of Health and Social Services
P.O. Box 240249
Anchorage, AK 99524
(907) 269-8058, Fax: (907) 561-4239
wendyc@health.state.ak.us

ARIZONA
Steve Stephens/Judy Norton
Office of HIV/AIDS Services
Arizona Department of Health Services
3815 North Black Canyon Highway
Phoenix, AZ 85015
(602) 230-5838, Fax: (602) 230-5973

ARKANSAS
Claude Nesbit
Division of AIDS/STD
Arkansas Department of Health
4815 W. Markham St., Slot 33
Little Rock, AR 72205
(501) 661-2292, Fax: (501) 661-2082

CALIFORNIA
Michael Montgomery
Office of HIV/AIDS
California Department of Health Services
P.O. Box 942732
Sacramento, CA 94234
(916) 323-7357, Fax: (916) 327-3177

COLORADO
Karen Ringen
Govenor's AIDS Council
Colorado Department of Health
4300 Cherry Creek Drive, South
Denver, CO 80222
(303) 692-2719, Fax: (303) 782-5393

CONNECTICUT
Carol Ross
Department of Social Services
25 Sigourney St
Hartford, CT 06106
(860) 424-5144, Fax: (860) 951-9544

DELAWARE
Jim Welch
Division of Public Health
P.O. Box 637, Federal and Water St.
Dover, DE 19903
(302) 739-3032, Fax: (302) 739-6617

DISTRICT OF COLUMBIA
Anthony Marshall
Agency for HIV/AIDS
717 14th Street, NW, Suite 600
Washington, DC 20005
(202) 727-2500, Fax: (202) 727-8471

FLORIDA
Joseph May
HIV/ AIDS Program
Florida Department of Health
Building 6, Room 403,
1317 Winewood Blvd.
Tallahassee, FL 32399
(904) 413-0735, Fax: (904) 414-6719
mayj@hrs.state.fl.us

GEORGIA
Libby Brown
Ryan White Projects
Epidemiology and Prevention Branch
Georgia Department of Human Services
10th Floor, Room 400
2 Peachtree St., NW
Atlanta, GA 30303
(404) 657-3127, Fax: (404) 657-3133

GUAM
Charles Crisostomo, MPH
Bureau of Communicable Disease Control
Department of Public Health and Social Services
P.O. Box 2816
Agana, GU 96910
(671) 735-7142, Fax: (671) 734-1475

HAWAII
Suzanne Richmond - Crum
STD/AIDS Prevention Branch
State of Hawaii Department of Health
3627 Kilauea, Suite 306
Honolulu, HI 96816
(808) 732-0026, Fax: (808) 735-8529

IDAHO
Jean Stark
Bureau of Communicable Disease Prevention
STD/Aids Program
Idaho Department of Health and Welfare
450 West State St., 4th Floor
Boise, ID 83720
(208) 334-6526, Fax: (208) 332-7346

ILINOIS
Nancy Abraham
AIDS Activities Section
Illinois Department of Public Health
525 W. Jefferson, 1st Floor
Springfield, IL 62761
(217) 524-5983, Fax: (217) 524-6090

INDIANA
Jodie Patsiner
Indiana Community AIDS Action Network
3951 N. Meridian
Indianapolis, IN 46208
(317) 920-3190, Fax: (317) 383-6663

IOWA
Patricia Young
STD/ HIV Program
Iowa Department of Public Health
Lucas State Office Bldg., 1st Floor
321 E. 12th St.
Des Moines, IA 50319
(515) 242-5838, Fax: (515) 281-4529

KANSAS
Sally Finney Brazier, M. ED.
Bureau of Disease Control
Kansas Department of Health
Mills Building, Suite 605
109 South West 9th
Topeka, KS 66612
(913) 296-6036, Fax: (913) 296-4197

KENTUCKY
Anna Mayne
HIV/AIDS Program
Department for Public Health
275 East Main St.
Frankfort, KY 40621
(502) 564-6539, Fax: (502) 564-9865
amayne@mail.state.ky.us.

LOUISIANA
Beth Scalco/ Kira Radtke
HIV Program Office
Louisiana Department of Health and Hospitals
1600 Canal St., Ste. 900
New Orleans, LA 70112
(504) 568-7474, Fax: (504) 568-7044

MAINE
Jeanette Talbot
Department of Human Services
11 State House Station
221 State St.
Augusta, ME 04333
(207) 287-5060, Fax: (207) 287-5065

MARYLAND
Patricia Wilson, LCSWC
AIDS Administration
Maryland Department of Health and Mental Hygiene
500 N. Calvert St., 5th Flr.
Baltimore, MD 21202
(410) 474-5087, Fax: (410) 333-6333

MASSACHUSETTS
Thera Meehan/ Andy Epstein
HIV/ AIDS Bureau
Massachusetts Department of Public Health
3rd Floor, 250 Washington St.
Boston, MA 02108
(617) 624-5331, Fax: (617) 624-5399
tmeehan@madph.org/aepstein@madph.org

MICHIGAN
Shirley Ayers
HIV/AIDS Prevention and Intervention
Department of Public Health
P.O. Box 30035, 3500 Martin Luther King Blvd.
Lansing, MI 48909
(517)335-9333, Fax: (517) 335-8121

MISSISSIPPI
Robert Lowery
Ryan White Programs
Mississippi Department of Health
P.O. Box 1700, 2423 North State St.
Jackson, MS 39215
(601) 960-7723, Fax: (601) 960-7909

MISSOURI
John Hubbs
Office of HIV/AIDS Care
Missouri Department of Health
P.O. Box 570, 1730 East Elm St.
Jefferson City, MO 65102
(573) 751-4752, Fax: (573) 751-6447

MONTANA
Joe Merrifield
Department of Public Health and Human Services
P.O. Box 202951, 1400 Broadway
Helena, MT 59620
(406) 444-4744, Fax: (406) 444-2920
Jmerrifield@mt.gov

NEBRASKA
Lesa Rastede
Division of Disease Control
Nebraska Department of Health
P.O. Box 95007
301 Centennial Mall, South
Lincoln, NE 68509
(402) 471-0362, Fax: (402) 471-6426

NEVADA
Jane Fox/Terri Ignacio
HIV/ AIDS Program Office
State Health Division
505 E. King St., Room 304
Carson City, NV 89710
(702) 687-4800, Fax: (702) 687-4988

NEW HAMPSHIRE
Niel Twitchell
STD/HIV Program
Division of Public Health Services
6 Hazen Dr.
Health and Welfare Bldg.
Concord, NH 03301
(603) 271-4480, Fax: (603) 271-3745

NEW JERSEY
Carmine Grasso
Intervention and Care Services Unit
Division of AIDS Prevention and Control
New Jersey Department of Health
363 W. State St., CN 363
Trenton, NJ 08625
(609) 984-6125, Fax: (609) 292-4244

NEW MEXICO
Brenda Kenyon
HIV/AIDS/STD Bureau
Suite 1 (Marquez Place)
525 Camino De Los Marquez
Santa Fe, NM 87501
(505) 476-8465, Fax: (505) 476-8527

NEW YORK
Lanny Cross
AIDS Institute
New York Department of Health
P.O. Box 2052, Empire Station
Albany, NY 12220
(518) 459-1641, Fax: (518) 459-2749
LTC02@ health.state.ny.us

NORTH CAROLINA
Arthur Okrent
Division of Adult Health Promotion
NC Department of Environment, Health and Natural Resources
P.O. Box 27687
Raleigh, NC 27605
(919) 715-3118, Fax: (919) 715-3144
aokrent@mail.ehnr.state.nc.us

NORTH DAKOTA
Pam Vukelic
Division of Disease Control
North Dakota Department of Health
600 East Blvd.
Bismark, ND 58505
(701) 328-2378, Fax: (701)328-1412

OHIO
Sheila Egan
Ohio Department of Health
P.O. Box 118, 246 North High Street
Columbus, OH 43266
(614) 466-6669, Fax: (614) 728-4622

OKLAHOMA
Cindy Boerger, MSW
HIV/STD Service
Oklahoma Department of Health
1000 NE 10th & Stonewall
Oklahoma City, OK 73117
(405) 271-4636, Fax: (405) 271-5149

OREGON
Lisa McAuliffe
HIV Program
Oregon Health Division
800 NE Oregon St., Ste. 745
Portland, OR 97232
(503) 731-4438, Fax: (503) 731-4082

PENNSYLVANIA
John Folby
DPW
SPBP
P.O. Box 8021
Harrisburg, PA 17105-8021
(717) 772-6057, Fax: (717) 772-4309

PUERTO RICO
Maria Diaz
Pharmacy Section
Puerto Rico Department of Health
P.O. Box 70184
San Juan, PR 00936
(809) 274-5534, Fax: (809) 274-5523

RHODE ISLAND
Mary Marinelli, M. A. T.
Office of AIDS/STD
Rhode Island Department of Health
3 Capitol Hill, Room 105
Providence, RI 02908
(401) 277-0232, Fax: (401)272-3771

SOUTH CAROLINA
Earl Turner
Department of Health and Environmental Control
Box 101106, Mills-Jarret Complex
Columbia, SC 29211
(803) 737-4099, Fax: (803)737-3979

SOUTH DAKOTA
Dave Morgan
Communicable Disease Prevention and Control
South Dakota Department of Health
445 East Capitol
Pierre, SD 57501
(605) 773-3737, Fax: (605) 773-5509

TENNESSEE

Sharon Benton
Tennessee Department of Health
Cordell Hull Building, 4th Floor
426 5th Avenue, North
Nashville, TN 37247
(615) 741-0237, Fax: (615) 741-3857

TEXAS

Sheryl Skinner
HIV/STD Health Resources Division
Texas Department of Health
1100 West 49th Street
Austin, TX 78756
(512) 490-2510, Fax: (512) 490-2503

UTAH

Jodi Quintana - Pond
HIV/ AIDS Treatment & Care Program
Utah Department of Health
288 North, 1460 West
Salt Lake City, UT 84116
(801) 538-6225, Fax: (801) 538-6036
hlchs.jquintan@state.ut.us

U.S. VIRGIN ISLANDS

Stan Phillips
St. Thomas Hospital
48 Sugar Estate
St. Thomas, VI 00802
(809) 776-5466, Fax: (809) 777-4001

VERMONT

Mary Pierce
Vermont Department of Health
P.O. Box 70
Burlington, VT 05402
(802) 863-7245, Fax: (802) 863-7314

VIRGINIA

Anne Elam
Bureau of STD/ AIDS
Virginia Department of Health
Room 112, P.O. Box 2448
Richmond, VA 23218
(804) 225-4844, Fax: (804) 225-3517

WASHINGTON

Raleigh Watts/Tawney Harper
Office of Client Services
Washington State Department of Health
Mail Stop 7841, Airdustrial Park, Building #9
Olympia, WA 98504
(360) 664-2216, Fax: (360) 664-2216

WEST VIRGINIA

Robert Johnson, Sr.
Division of Surveillance & Disease Control
WV Department of Health
1442 Washington Street, East
Charleston, WV 25301
(304) 558-5358, Fax: (304) 558-6335

WISCONSIN

Richard Albertoni
Client Service Coordinator
Division of Health, Room 167
Wisconsin Department of Health and Social Services
1414 East Washington Avenue
Madison, WI 53703
(608) 267-6875, Fax: (608) 266-2906

WYOMING

Terrance Foley
Manager, HIV/AIDS Prevention Program
Wyoming Department of Health
Hathaway Building, 4th Floor
Cheyenne, WY 82002
(307) 777-5932, Fax: (307)777-5402

HEMATOLOGIC NORMAL VALUES

DIFFERENTIAL CELL COUNT OF BONE MARROW

Myeloid cells		
Neutrophilic series		
Myeloblasts	0.3%-5.0%	
Promyelocytes	1%-8%	
Myelocytes	5%-19%	
Metamyelocytes	9%-24%	
Bands	9%-15%	
Segmented cells	7%-30%	
Eosinophil precursors	0.5%-3.0%	
Eosinophils	0.5%-4.0%	
Basophilic series	0.2%-0.7%	
Erythroid cells		
Pronormoblasts	1%-8%	
Basophilic normoblasts		
Polychromatophilic normoblasts	7%-32%	
Orthochromatic normoblasts		
Megakaryocytes	0.1%	
Lymphoreticular cells		
Lymphocytes	3%-17%	
Plasma cells	0%-2%	
Reticulum cells	0.1%-2.0%	
Monocytes	0.5%-5.0%	
Myeloid/erythroid ratio	0.6-2.7	
Acid hemolysis test (Ham)	No hemolysis	
Carboxyhemoglobin		
Nonsmoker	<1%	
Smoker	2.1%-4.2%	
Cold hemolysis test (Donath-Landsteiner)	No hemolysis	
Complete blood count (see Table 3)		
Erythrocyte life span		
Normal	120 days	
^{51}Cr-labeled half-life	28 days	
Erythropoietin by radioimmunassay	9-33 mU/dl	
Ferritin, serum		
Male	15-200 µg/L	
Female	12-150 µg/L	
Folate, RBC	120-670 ng/ml	
Fragility, osmotic		
Hemolysis begins 0.45%-0.38% NaCl		
Hemolysis completed 0.33%-0.30% NaCl		
Haptoglobin, serum	100-300 mg/dl	
Hemoglobin		
Hemoglobin A_{1C}	0%-5% of total	
Hemoglobin A_2 by column	2%-3% of total	
Hemoglobin, fetal	<1% of total	
Hemoglobin, plasma	0%-5% of total	
Hemoglobin, serum	2-3 mg/ml	
Iron, serum		
Male	75-175 µg/dl	
Female	65-165 µg/dl	
Iron-binding capacity, total serum (TIBC)	250-450 µg/dl	
Iron turnover rate (plasma)	20-42 mg/24 hr	
Leukocyte alkaline phosphatase (LAP) score	30-150	
Methemoglobin	<1.8%	
Reticulocytes (see Table 3)		
Schilling test (urinary excretion of radiolabeled vitamin B_{12} after "flushing" intramuscular injection of B_{12})	6%-30% of oral dose within 24 hr	
Sedimentation rate	*Male*	*Female*
Wintrobe	0-5 mm/hr	0-15 mm/hr
Westergren	0-15 mm/hr	0-20 mm/hr
Transferrin saturation, serum	20%-50%	
Volume	*Male*	*Female*
Blood	52-83 ml/kg	50-75 ml/kg
Plasma	25-43 ml/kg	28-45 ml/kg
Red cell	20-36 ml/kg	19-31 ml/kg

COMPLETE BLOOD COUNT

Parameter	*Male*	*Female*
Hematocrit (%)	40-52	38-48
Hemoglobin (g/dl)	13.5-18.0	12-16
Erythrocyte count ($\times 10^{12}$ cells/L)	4.6-6.2	4.2-5.4
Reticulocyte count (%)	0.6-2.6	0.4-2.4
MCV (fL)	82-98	82-98
MCH (pg)	27-32	27-32
MCHC (g/dl)	32-36	32-36
WBC ($\times 10^9$ cells/L)	4.5-11.0	4.5-11.0
Segmented neutrophils	1.8-7.7	1.8-7.7
Average (%)	40-60	40-60
Bands (cells)	0-0.3	0-0.3
Average (%)	0-3	0-3
Eosinophils (cells $\times 10^9$/L)	0-0.5	0-0.5
Average (%)	0-5	0-5
Basophils (cells $\times 10^9$/L)	0-0.2	0-0.2
Average (%)	0-1	0-1
Lymphocytes (cells $\times 10^9$/L)	1.0-4.8	1.0-4.8
Average (%)	20-45	20-45
Monocytes (cells $\times 10^9$/L)	0-0.8	0-0.8
Average (%)	2-6	2-6
Platelet count (cells\x\10^9/L)	150-350	150-350

COAGULATION NORMAL VALUES

Template bleeding time	3.5-7.5 min
Clot retraction, qualitative	Apparent in 30-60 min; complete in 24 hr, usually in 6 hr
Coagulation time (Lee-White)	
Glass tubes	5-15 min
Siliconized tubes	20-60 min
Euglobulin lysis time	120-240 min
Factors II, V, VII, VIII, IX, X, XI, or XII	100% or 1.0 unit/ml
Fibrin degradation products	<10 µg/ml or titer ≤ 1.4
Fibrinogen	200-400 mg/ml
Partial thromboplastin time, activated	20-40 sec
Prothrombin time (PT)	11-14 sec
Thrombin time	10-15 sec
Whole blood clot lysis time	>24 hr

RENAL FUNCTION TESTS

ANION GAP

$Na^{+} - HCO^{+}{}^{-}_{3}$ 1 Cl^{-} = 12 ± 2 mEq/L

OSMOLALITY

$$\text{Osmolality (serum)} = 2\ \text{Na (mEq/L)} + \frac{\text{BUN (mg/dl)}}{2.8} + \frac{\text{glucose (mg/dl)}}{18}$$

BICARBONATE DEFICIT

HCO^{-}_{3} deficit = body weight (kg) × 0.4 (desired HCO^{-}_{3} − observed HCO^{-}_{3})

Glomerural filtration rate

$$GFR = \frac{Ucr \times V}{Pcr}$$

= 130 ± 20 ml/min in males

= 120 ± 15 ml/min in females

$$= \frac{\sim Ucr}{Pcr} \times 70$$

where

Ucr = urine creatinine (mg/dl)

Pcr = plasma creatinine (mg/dl)

V = urine volume/24 hr (ml/min)

RENAL PLASMA FLOW

$$RPF = \frac{Upah \times V}{Ppah}$$

= 700 ± 130 ml/min in males

= 600 ± 100 ml/min in females

where

Upah = urine para-aminohippuric acid (mg/dl)

V = urine volume/24 hr (ml/min)

Ppah = plasma para-aminohippuric acid (mg/dl)

SEMEN NORMAL VALUES

Liquefaction	Complete in 15 min
Morphology	>50% normal forms
Motility	>75% motile forms
pH	7.2-8.0
Spermatocrit	10%
Spermatocyte count	>50 million/ml
Volume	2.0-6.6 ml

SERUM NORMAL VALUES

Acetoacetate	0.3-2.0 mg/dl
Acid phosphatase	0-0.8 U/ml
Acid phosphatase, prostatic	2.5-12.0 IU/L
Albumin	3.0-5.5 g/dl
Aldolase	1-6 IU/L
Alkaline phosphatase	
15-20 years	40-200 IU/L
20-101 years	35-125 IU/L
Alpha-1 antitrypsin	200-500 mg/dl
ALT	0-40 IU/L
Ammonia	11-35 µmol/L
Amylase, serum	2-20 U/L
Anion gap	8-12 mEq/L (mmol/L)
Ascorbic acid	0.4-1.5 mg/dl
AST	5-40 IU/L
Bilirubin	
Total	0.2-1.2 mg/dl
Direct	0-0.4 mg/dl
Calcium, serum	8.7-10.6 mg/dl
Carbon dioxide, total	18-30 mEq/L (mmol/L)
Carcinoembryonic antigen, serum	<2.5 µg/L
Carotene (carotenoids)	50-300 µg/dl
C3 complement	55-120 mg/dl
C4 complement	14-51 mg/dl
Ceruloplasmin	15-60 mg/dl
Chloride, serum	95-105 mEq/L (mmol/L)
Cholesterol, total	
12-19 years	120-230 mg/dl
20-29 years	120-240 mg/dl
30-39 years	140-270 mg/dl
40-49 years	150-310 mg/dl
50-59 years	160-330 mg/dl
Copper	100-200 µg/dl
Creatine kinase, total	20-200 IU/L
Creatine kinase, isoenzymes	
MM fraction	94%-95%
MB fraction	0%-5%
BB fraction	0%-2%
Normal values in	
Heart	80% MM, 20% MB
Brain	100% BB
Skeletal, muscle	95% MM, 2% MB
Creatinine, serum	
Female adult	0.5-1.3 mg/dl
Male adult	0.7-1.5 mg/dl
Delta-aminolevulinic acid (ALA)	<200 µg/dl
α-Fetoprotein, serum	<40 µg/L
Folate, serum	1.9-14.0 ng/ml
Gamma glutamyl transpeptidase	
Male	12-38 IU/l
Female	9-31 IU/L
Gastrin	150 pg/ml
Glucose, serum (fasting)	70-115 mg/dl
Glucose-6-phosphate dehydrogenase	5-10 IU/g Hb
G6PD screen, qualitative	Negative
Haptoglobin	100-300 mg/dl
Hemoglobin A_2	0%-4% of total Hb
Hemoglobin F	0%-2% of total Hb
Immunoglobulin, quantitation	
IgG	700-1500 mg/dl
IaA	70-400 mg/dl
IgM	
Male	30-250 mg/dl
Female	30-300 mg/dl
IgD	0-40 mg/dl
Insulin, fasting	6-20 µU/ml
Iron-binding capacity	250-400 µg/dl
Iron, total, serum	40-150 µg/dl
Lactic acid	0.6-1.8 mEq/L
LDH, serum	20-220 IU/L
LDH isoenzymes	
LDH^1	20%-34%
LDH^2	28%-41%
LDH^3	15%-25%
LDH^4	3%-12%
LDH^5	6%-15%
Leucine aminopeptidase (LAP)	30-55 IU/L
Lipase	4-24 IU/dl
Magnesium, serum	1.5-2.5 mEq/L
5'-Nucleotidase	0.3-3.2 Bodansky units
Osmolality, serum	278-305 mOsm/kg serum water
Phenylalanine	3 mg/dl
Phosphorus, inorganic, serum	2.0-4.3 mg/dl
Potassium, plasma	3.1-4.3 mEq/L
Potassium, serum	3.5-5.2 mEq/L
Protein, total, serum	
2-55 years	5.0-8.0 g/dl
55-101 years	6.0-8.3 g/dl
Protein electrophoresis, serum	
Albumin	3.2-5.2 g/dl
Alpha-1	0.6-1.0 g/dl
Alpha-2	0.6-1.0 g/dl
Beta	0.6-1.2 g/dl
Gamma	0.7-1.5 g/dl
Sodium, serum	135-145 mEq/L
Sulfate	0.5-1.5 mg/dl
T_3 uptake	25%-45%
T_4	4-11 µg/dl
Triglycerides	
2-29 years	10-140 mg/dl
30-39 years	20-150 mg/dl
40-49 years	20-160 mg/dl
50-59 years	20-190 mg/dl
60-101 years	20-200 mg/dl
Urea nitrogen, serum	
2-65 years	5-22 mg/dl
Male	10-38 mg/dl
Female	8-26 mg/dl
Uric acid	